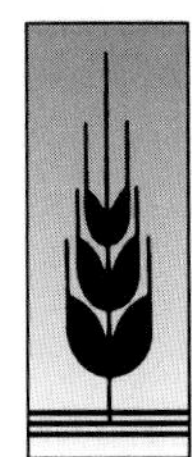

Modern Nutrition in Health and Disease

NINTH EDITION

EDITORS

MAURICE E. SHILS, M.D., Sc.D.

Professor Emeritus of Medicine
Cornell University Medical College
Consultant Emeritus (Nutrition)
Memorial Sloan-Kettering Cancer Center
New York City, New York
Adjunct Professor (Nutrition), Retired
Department of Public Health Sciences
Wake Forest University School of Medicine
Winston-Salem, North Carolina

JAMES A. OLSON, Ph.D.

Distinguished Professor of Liberal Arts & Sciences
Department of Biochemistry & Biophysics
Iowa State University
Ames, Iowa

MOSHE SHIKE, M.D.

Director of Clinical Nutrition
Memorial Sloan-Kettering Cancer Center
Professor of Medicine
Cornell University Medical College
New York City, New York

A. CATHARINE ROSS, Ph.D.

Professor and Head
Department of Veterinary Science
Professor
Nutrition Department
College of Health and Human Development
The Pennsylvania State University
University Park, Pennsylvania

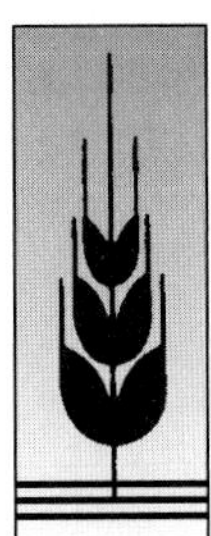

Modern Nutrition in Health and Disease

NINTH EDITION

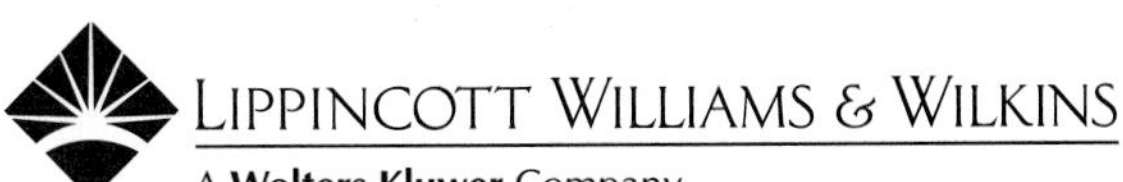

Philadelphia • Baltimore • New York • London
Buenos Aires • Hong Kong • Sydney • Tokyo

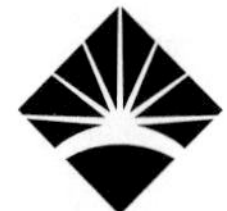

Editor: Donna Balado
Managing Editor: Jennifer Schmidt
Marketing Manager: Tara Williams
Production Editor: Jennifer D. Weir

351 West Camden Street
Baltimore, Maryland 21201-2436 USA

530 Walnut St.
Philadelphia, Pennsylvania 19106-3621 USA

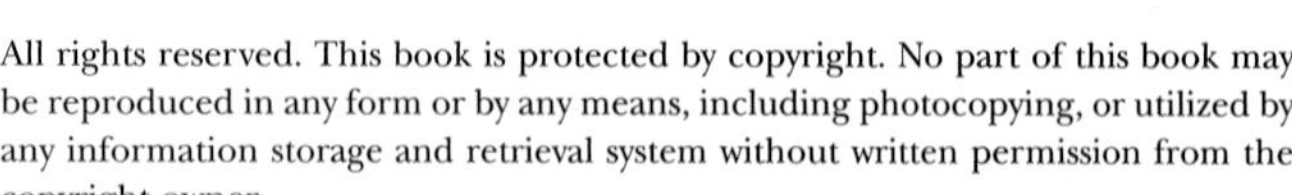

Printed in the United States of America

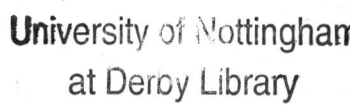

First Edition, 1955
Second Edition, 1960
Third Edition, 1964
Fourth Edition, 1968
Fifth Edition, 1973
Sixth Edition, 1980
Seventh Edition, 1988
Eighth Edition, 1994

Modern nutrition in health and disease/editors, Maurice E. Shils . . . .
[et al.].—9th ed.
p. cm.
Includes bibliographical references and index.
ISBN 0-683-30769-X
1. Nutrition. 2. Diet therapy. I. Shils, Maurice E. (Maurice Edward), 1914– .
QP141.M64 1998
613.2—dc21 98-38505
CIP

The publishers have made every effort to trace the copyright holders for borrowed material. If they have inadvertently overlooked any, they will be pleased to make the necessary arrangements at the first opportunity.

To purchase additional copies of this book, call our customer service department at **(800) 638-3030** or fax orders to **(301) 824-7390.** For other book services, including chapter reprints and large quantity sales, ask for the Special Sales Department. International customers should call **(301) 714-2324.**

Visit Lippincott Williams & Wilkins on the Internet: **http://www.lww.com.** Lippincott Williams & Wilkins customer service representatives are available from 8:30 am to 6:00 pm, EST.

02 03
3 4 5 6 7 8 9 10

Preface

The immediate predecessor of *Modern Nutrition in Health and Disease* was *Dietotherapy,* published in 1945 and edited by Drs. Michael Wohl and Robert Goodhart. With the same editors, its successor, the first edition of *Modern Nutrition in Health and Disease,* appeared in 1955. Its original objective has remained in succeeding editions: to serve as a comprehensive authoritative text and reference source reviewing the history, scientific base, and practice of nutrition for students, practitioners, and educators. The broad scope of nutritional sciences has relevance to all basic and applied biologic sciences, medicine, dentistry, dietetics, nursing, pharmacy, public health, and public policy.

This edition has 115 chapters and multiple sections of an Appendix, updated by 169 authors in 10 countries and from many scientific disciplines. To these authors we express our deep appreciation.

Thirty-five chapters review specific dietary components in depth; 18 others are concerned with the role of nutrition in integrated biologic systems; 5 review aspects of nutrition assessment; 41 cover a variety of clinical disorders; and 13 discuss public health and policy issues.

Thirty-six new chapters have been introduced designed to provide better understanding of the role of nutrition in integrated biologic systems and in other areas. These include general and specific aspects of molecular biology and genetics, ion channels, transmembrane signaling, and other topics—all in tutorial form. The matter of essential and conditionally essential nutrients is reviewed historically in the opening chapter and considered in separate chapters on individual essential nutrients and in those on taurine, homocysteine, glutamine, arginine, choline, and carnitine.

There are added chapters on nutritional issues in pediatrics, cardiovascular disorders, gastroenterology, cancer, hematology, and rheumatology. In the field of public health, new chapters address vegetarian diets, anthropology, "alternative" nutritional therapies, nutritional priorities in less industrialized countries, and risk assessment of nutrition-related environmental chemicals.

An extensive Appendix includes dietary reference recommendations from various national (including the new 1997 and 1998 U.S. Dietary Reference Intakes) and international agencies, multiple anthropometric tables, nutrient and nonnutrient contents of foods and beverages, numerous therapeutic diets and exchange lists, and other sources of nutritional information.

Relevant quantitative data have been expressed both in conventional and in international system (SI) units. The widespread use of the SI units in major publications in the United States and especially in other countries makes dual unitage useful to our readers.

We have endeavored to provide the breadth of coverage and quality of content required by this ever-changing discipline in its basic and clinical dimensions. We invite the comments and suggestions of our readers.

MAURICE EDWARD SHILS
Winston-Salem, NC
JAMES ALLEN OLSON
Ames, IA
MOSHE SHIKE
New York City, NY
A. CATHARINE ROSS
University Park, PA

Acknowledgments

The preparation, editing, and production of this extensive work has succeeded because of the expertise, effort, and dedication of many individuals in addition to the authors. The editors have worked with some personally, while others have been involved "behind the scenes" at the editorial, publication, and distribution stages.

At Williams and Wilkins, our interactions were primarily with Donna Balado, acquisitions editor; Victoria Vaughn, formerly senior managing editor; Jennifer Schmidt, managing editor; Jennifer Weir, production editor; and Anne K. Schwartz, copy editor. We express our appreciation to them for their guidance, knowledge, and cooperation in solving the numerous issues arising at various stages of planning, executing, and producing this work.

We are particularly indebted to Betty Shils, Beverly Satchell, Maggie Wheelock, and Denise Kowalski for enabling us to manage the enormous number of communications, records, manuscripts, and page proofs involved in the editing process.

To our respective spouses, Betty, Giovanna, Sherry, and Alex, we extend appreciation and thanks for their understanding and support of the increased demands on our time.

Contributors

STEVE F. ABCOUWER, Ph.D.
Assistant Biochemist, Department of Surgical Oncology
Massachusetts General Hospital
Instructor, Department of Surgery
Harvard Medical School
Boston, Massachusetts

PHYLLIS B. ACOSTA, Dr.P.H.
Director, Metabolic Diseases
Department of Pediatric Nutrition Research and Development
Ross Products Division, Abbott Laboratories
Columbus, Ohio

NANCY W. ALCOCK, Ph.D.
Professor, Department of Preventive Medicine and Community Health
University of Texas Medical Branch
Galveston, Texas

DAVID H. ALPERS, M.D.
Professor and Chief, Division of Gastroenterology
Washington University School of Medicine
St. Louis, Missouri

JAMES ANDERSON, M.D.
Professor, Medicine and Clinical Nutrition
Department of Internal Medicine
University of Kentucky
Chief, Endocrine
Metabolic Section
VA Medical Center
Lexington, Kentucky

AFTAB A. ANSARI, Ph.D.
Department of Pathology
Emory University School of Medicine
Atlanta, Georgia

LYNNE M. AUSMAN, D.Sc.
Scientist, Jean Mayer USDA Human Nutrition Research Center on Aging
Tufts University
Boston, Massachusetts
Professor, School of Nutrition Science and Policy
Tufts University
Medford, Massachusetts

STEPHEN BARRETT, M.D.
Consumer Advocate
Member, Board of Directors
National Council Against Health Fraud, Inc.
Allentown, Pennsylvania

RICHARD BAUMGARTNER, Ph.D.
Associate Professor, Division of Epidemiology
Department of Medicine
University of New Mexico
Albuquerque, New Mexico

GEORGE H. BEATON, Ph.D.
Professor Emeritus, Department of Nutritional Sciences
University of Toronto
Toronto, Ontario, Canada

ELIOT L. BERSON, M.D.
William F. Chatlos Professor of Ophthalmology
Harvard Medical School
Director, Berman-Gund Laboratory for the Study of Retinal Degenerations
Massachusetts Eye and Ear Infirmary
Boston, Massachusetts

WAYNE R. BIDLACK, Ph.D.
Dean, College of Agriculture
California State Polytechnic University, Pomona
Pomona, California

DIANE F. BIRT, Ph.D.
Professor, Eppley Institute for Research in Cancer and Department of Biochemistry and Molecular Biology
College of Medicine
University of Nebraska Medical Center
Omaha, Nebraska
Current address:
Department of Food Science and Human Nutrition
Iowa State University
Ames, Iowa

ABBY S. BLOCH, Ph.D., R.D.
Coordinator of Clinical Nutrition Research, Gastroenterology/Nutrition Service
Department of Medicine
Memorial Sloan-Kettering Cancer Center
New York City, New York

IRWIN G. BRODSKY, M.D., M.P.H.
Assistant Professor of Medicine and Nutrition
Department of Medicine
Endocrinology and Metabolism Section
University of Illinois at Chicago
Chicago, Illinois

REX O. BROWN, Pharm.D., BCNSP, FACN
Professor, Department of Clinical Pharmacy
University of Tennessee
Nutrition Support Pharmacist
Department of Pharmacy
Regional Medical Center at Memphis
University of Tennessee Medical Center
Memphis, Tennessee

RAYMOND F. BURK, M.D.
Professor of Medicine
Director, Division of Gastroenterology
Department of Medicine
Vanderbilt University
Nashville, Tennessee

DANIEL CERVANTES-LAUREAN, M.D.
Pulmonary-Critical Care Medicine Branch
National Heart, Lung, and Blood Institute
National Institutes of Health
Bethesda, Maryland

ISRAEL CHANARIN, M.D., F.R.C.Path.
Formerly, Chief, Division of Hematology
Medical Research Council
Northwick Park Hospital Centre
Harrow, Middlesex, United Kingdom

FRANCISCO CHEW, M.D.
Head, Maternal and Child Health Unit
Instituto de Nutricion de Centro America y Panama (INCAP)
Guatemala City, Guatemala

ROBERT CHIN, Jr., M.D.
Associate Professor of Medicine
Section on Pulmonary and Critical Care Medicine
Wake Forest University School of Medicine
Winston-Salem, North Carolina

GRAEME A. CLUGSTON, M.B., D.C.H., Ph.D.
Chief, Nutrition Section
World Health Organization
Geneva, Switzerland

STEVEN COHN, M.D.
Assistant Professor of Medicine, Division of Gastroenterology
Washington University School of Medicine
St. Louis, Missouri

J. JOSEPH CONNON, M.D., F.R.C.P. (Lond), F.R.C.P.C.
Professor of Medicine, Department of Medicine
University of Toronto
Toronto, Ontario, Canada

ARTHUR COOPER, M.D., M.S.
Associate Professor
Chief, Pediatric Surgical Critical Care
College of Physicians and Surgeons of Columbia University
Harlem Hospital Center
New York City, New York

ROBERT J. COUSINS, Ph.D.
Boston Family Professor of Nutrition
Food Science and Human Nutrition Department and Center for Nutritional Sciences
University of Florida
Gainesville, Florida

EARL B. DAWSON, Ph.D.
Associate Professor, Department of Obstetrics and Gynecology
University of Texas Medical Branch
Galveston, Texas

BESS DAWSON-HUGHES, M.D.
Chief, Calcium and Bone Metabolism Laboratory
Jean Mayer USDA Human Nutrition Research Center on Aging
Associate Professor of Medicine
Tufts University
Boston, Massachusetts

DOMINICK P. DEPAOLA, D.D.S., Ph.D.
President and Dean, College of Dentistry
Texas A&M University
Dallas, Texas
Current address:
President and Chief Executive Officer, Forsyth Dental Center
Boston, Massachusetts

WILLIAM H. DIETZ, M.D., Ph.D.
Director of Clinical Nutrition, New England Medical Center
Boston, Massachusetts
Current address:
Director, Division of Nutrition and Physical Activity
Centers for Disease Control and Prevention
Atlanta, Georgia

EUGENE P. DIMAGNO, M.D.
Professor of Medicine, Department of Internal Medicine
Director, Department of Gastroenterology Research Unit
Mayo Clinic
Rochester, Minnesota

JOHANNA DWYER, D.Sc., R.D.
Professor of Medicine and Community Health
Tufts University Schools of Medicine and Nutrition
Senior Scientist
Jean Mayer USDA Human Nutrition Research Center on Aging at Tufts University
Director, Frances Stern Nutrition Center
New England Medical Center
Boston, Massachusetts

LOUIS JACOB ELSAS II, M.D.
Professor and Director, Division of Medical Genetics
Pediatrics/Medicine/Biochemistry
School of Medicine
Emory University
Atlanta, Georgia

JOHN W. ERDMAN, Jr., M.D.
Professor, Department of Food Science and Human Nutrition
Director of Nutritional Sciences
University of Illinois
Urbana, Illinois

DAVID ERLIJ, M.D., Ph.D.
Professor of Physiology
State University of New York Health Science Center at Brooklyn
Brooklyn, New York

MARY P. FAINE, M.S., R.D.
Associate Professor and Director of Nutrition Education
Department of Prosthodontics
School of Dentistry
University of Washington
Seattle, Washington

VIRGIL F. FAIRBANKS, M.D.
Consultant, Mayo Clinic
Professor of Medicine and Laboratory Medicine
Mayo Clinic and Mayo Foundation
Rochester, Minnesota

ANNA M. FAN, Ph.D.
Chief, Pesticide and Environmental Toxicology Section
Office of Environmental Health Hazard Assessment
California Environmental Protection Agency
Berkeley, California

LAWRENCE FEINMAN, M.D.
Associate Professor, Department of Medicine
Mount Sinai School of Medicine (CUNY)
New York City, New York
Chief, Section of Gastroenterology
Veterans Affairs Medical Center
Bronx, New York

C. RICHARD FLEMING, M.D.[†]
David Murdoch Professor of Nutrition Science
Mayo Medical School
Chair, Division of Gastroenterology
Mayo Clinic
Jacksonville, Florida

JEFFREY S. FLIER, M.D.
Professor of Medicine, Harvard Medical School
Chief, Division of Endocrinology and Metabolism
Beth Israel Deaconess Medical Center
Boston, Massachusetts

ALLAN L. FORBES, M.D.
Medical Consultant (Foods and Nutrition)
Formerly, Director, Office of Nutrition and Food Sciences
Food and Drug Administration
Old Farm
Rockville, Maryland

GILBERT B. FORBES, M.D.
Professor of Pediatrics and Biophysics, Emeritus
School of Medicine and Dentistry
University of Rochester
Rochester, New York

ELLEN B. FUNG, Ph.D.
Postdoctoral Fellow
Division of Gastroenterology and Nutrition
Children's Hospital of Philadelphia
Philadelphia, Pennsylvania

ROBERT A. GABBAY, M.D., Ph.D.
Instructor, Harvard Medical School
Endocrine Division
Beth Israel Deaconess Medical Center
Boston, Massachusetts

CLAUDIO GALPERIN, M.D.
Postdoctoral Scholar
Division of Rheumatology/Allergy and Clinical Immunology
University of California at Davis
Davis, California
Current address:
Rua Albuquerque Lins
São Paulo, Brazil

J. BRUCE GERMAN, Ph.D.
The John Kinsella Endowed Chair of Food Science
University of California at Davis
Davis, California

M. ERIC GERSHWIN, M.D.
The Jack and Donald Chia Professor of Medicine
Chief, Division of Rheumatology/Allergy and Clinical Immunology
University of California at Davis
Davis, California

ELIZABETH J. GONG, M.Ph., M.S, R.D.
Nutrition Research Associate, Department of Nutrition
University of California at Davis
Davis, California

ANNE M. GRIFFITHS, M.D., F.R.C.P.C.
Associate Professor of Pediatrics, Faculty of Medicine
University of Toronto
Director, Inflammatory Bowel Diseases Program
Division of Gastroenterology and Clinical Nutrition
The Hospital for Sick Children
Toronto, Ontario, Canada

[†]Deceased.

SCOTT M. GRUNDY, M.D., Ph.D.
Chairman, Department of Clinical Nutrition
Professor of Internal Medicine
Director, Center for Human Nutrition
University of Texas Southwestern Medical Center at Dallas
Dallas, Texas

CHARLES H. HALSTED, M.D.
Professor, Department of Internal Medicine and Nutrition
University of California at Davis
Davis, California

EDWARD F. HAPONIK, M.D.
Professor of Internal Medicine
Chief, Section of Pulmonary and Critical Care Medicine
Wake Forest University School of Medicine
Winston-Salem, North Carolina

ALFRED E. HARPER, Ph.D.
Professor Emeritus, Department of Nutritional Sciences; Biochemistry
University of Wisconsin
Madison, Wisconsin

ROGER C. HARRIS, Ph.D.
Senior Research Fellow, Royal Veterinary College
University of London
London, England

JOHN N. HATHCOCK, Ph.D.
Director, Nutritional and Regulatory Science
Council for Responsible Nutrition
Washington, DC

FELIX P. HEALD, M.D.
Professor Emeritus of Pediatrics
University of Maryland School of Medicine
Baltimore, Maryland

ROBERT P. HEANEY, M.D.
John A. Creighton University Professor
Creighton University
Omaha, Nebraska

WILLIAM C. HEIRD, M.D.
Professor, Children's Nutrition Research Center
Department of Pediatrics
Baylor College of Medicine
Houston, Texas

VICTOR D. HERBERT, M.D., J.D.
Professor of Medicine, Mount Sinai School of Medicine
Chief of Hematology and The Nutrition Laboratory
Bronx Veteran Affairs Medical Center
New York City, New York

BASIL S. HETZEL, M.D.
Chairman, International Council for Control of Iodine Deficiency Disorders
Woman's and Children's Hospital
North Adelaide, Australia

STEVEN B. HEYMSFIELD, M.D.
Professor of Medicine, College of Physicians and Surgeons
Columbia University
Deputy Director, Obesity Research Center
Saint Lukes-Roosevelt Hospital
New York City, New York

L. JOHN HOFFER, M.D., C.M., Ph.D.
Associate Professor, Department of Medicine and Dietetics and Human Nutrition
McGill University
Senior Physician, Division of Endocrinology
Department of General Internal Medicine
Sir Mortimer B. Davis-Jewish General Hospital
Montreal, Quebec, Canada

MICHAEL F. HOLICK, M.D., Ph.D.
Professor of Medicine, Dermatology, and Physiology
Section of Endocrinology, Diabetes, and Metabolism in the Department of Medicine
Boston University School of Medicine
Boston, Massachusetts

EDWARD S. HORTON, M.D.
Professor, Department of Medicine
Harvard Medical School
Medical Director, Joslin Diabetes Center
Boston, Massachusetts

CHARLES HUGHES, M.D.
Professor of Medicine, Medical College of Wisconsin
Department of Cardiology
Department of Veteran Affairs
Clement J. Zablocki Medical Center
Milwaukee, Wisconsin

ERIC HULTMAN, M.D., Ph.D.
Professor Emeritus, Department of Medical Laboratory Sciences and Technology
Karolinska Institute, Division of Clinical Chemistry
Huddinge Hospital
Huddinge, Sweden

DIANE M. HUSE, R.D., M.S.
Assistant Professor of Nutrition, Mayo Medical School
Clinical Dietitian, Mayo Clinic
Rochester, Minnesota

ROBERT A. JACOB, Ph.D.
Research Chemist, USDA Western Research Center
Western Human Nutrition Research Center
Presidio of San Francisco, California

DOUGLAS R. JEFFERY, M.D., Ph.D.
Assistant Professor of Neurology, Department of Neurology
Wake Forest University School of Medicine
Winston-Salem, North Carolina

ALEXANDRA L. JENKINS
Research Associate, Department of Nutrition Sciences
University of Toronto
Toronto, Ontario, Canada

DAVID J. A. JENKINS, M.D., Ph.D.
Professor
Department of Nutrition Sciences
University of Toronto
Toronto, Ontario, Canada

MARGARET M. JOHNSON, M.D.
Senior Associate Consultant
Mayo Clinic at Jacksonville
Jacksonville, Florida

PATRICIA K. JOHNSTON, M.S., R.D., Dr.P.H.
Professor
Department of Nutrition
School of Public Health, Loma Linda University
Associate Dean
Loma Linda University
Loma Linda, California

PETER J. H. JONES, Ph.D.
Associate Professor of Human Nutrition
Director, School of Dietetics and Human Nutrition
McGill University
Montreal, Quebec

ROBERT KARP, M.D.
Medical Director
Pediatric Resource Center of Kings County Hospital Center
Professor of Pediatrics
State University of New York Health Science Center at Brooklyn
Brooklyn, New York

CARL L. KEEN, Ph.D.
Professor and Chair
Department of Nutrition
University of California at Davis
Davis, California

DARLENE G. KELLY, M.D., Ph.D.
Assistant Professor, Mayo Medical School
Consultant in Gastroenterology
Department of Internal Medicine
Mayo Foundation
Rochester, Minnesota

GERALD T. KEUSCH, M.D.
Professor of Medicine, Tufts University School of Medicine
New England Medical Center
Boston, Massachusetts

JANET C. KING, Ph.D.
Professor, Department of Nutritional Sciences
University of California at Berkeley
Berkeley, California
Director, Western Human Nutrition Research Center
USDA, ARS
San Francisco, California

SAMUEL KLEIN, M.D.
Professor of Medicine
Director, Center for Human Nutrition
Washington University School of Medicine
St. Louis, Missouri

JAMES P. KNOCHEL, M.D.
Chairman, Department of Internal Medicine
Presbyterian Hospital
Clinical Professor, Department of Internal Medicine
University of Texas Southwestern Medical School
Dallas, Texas

JOEL D. KOPPLE, M.D.
Professor of Medicine and Public Health
Schools of Medicine and Public Health
University of California at Los Angeles
Los Angeles, California
Chief, Division of Nephrology and Hypertension
Harbor-UCLA Medical Center
Torrance, California

PATRICIA KOSTKA, M.S., R.D.
Clinical Specialist Dietitian
Cardiopulmonary Rehabilitation Center
Department of Veteran Affairs
Clement J. Zablocki Medical Center
Milwaukee, Wisconsin

JANE M. KOTCHEN, M.D., M.P.H.
Professor, Department of Epidemiology/Medicine
Medical College of Wisconsin
Milwaukee, Wisconsin

THEODORE A. KOTCHEN, M.D.
Professor and Chairman, Department of Medicine
Medical College of Wisconsin
Milwaukee, Wisconsin

ELIZABETH A. KRALL, Ph.D.
Assistant Professor, School of Nutrition
Scientist II
Jean Mayer USDA Human Nutrition Research Center on Aging
Tufts University
Boston, Massachusetts

STANLEY KUBOW, Ph.D.
Associate Professor, School of Dietetics and Human Nutrition
McGill University
Montreal, Quebec

MARIE FANELLI KUCZMARSKI, Ph.D., R.D., L.D.
Associate Professor, Department of Nutrition and Dietetics
University of Delaware
Newark, Delaware

ROBERT J. KUCZMARSKI, Dr.P.H., R.D., L.D.
Nutrition Analyst, National Center for Health Statistics
Centers for Disease Control and Prevention
United States Public Health Service
Hyattsvile, Maryland

HELEN W. LANE, R.D., Ph.D.
Chief, Biomedical Operations Research Branch
NASA Chief Nutritionist
Johnson Space Center, NASA
Houston, Texas

JAMES E. LEKLEM, Ph.D.
Professor, Department of Nutrition and Food Management
Oregon State University
Corvallis, Oregon

ORVILLE A. LEVANDER, Ph.D.
Nutrient Requirements and Functions Laboratory
Human Nutrition Research Center
Agricultural Research Services
United States Department of Agriculture
Beltsville, Maryland

ROY J. LEVIN
Reader in Physiology, Department of Biomedical Science
University of Sheffield
Sheffield, England

CHARLES S. LIEBER, M.D.
Professor of Medicine and Pathology, Mount Sinai School of Medicine (CUNY)
New York City, New York
Chief, Section of Liver Disease and Nutrition
Director, Alcohol Research and Treatment Center and GI-Liver-Nutrition Training Program
Veterans Affairs Medical Center
Bronx, New York

STEPHEN F. LOWRY, M.D., F.A.C.S.
Professor of Surgery, Cornell University Medical College
New York City, New York
Current address:
Professor and Chairman, Department of Surgery
University of Medicine and Dentistry of New Jersey
New Brunswick, New Jersey

ALEXANDER R. LUCAS, M.D.
Professor of Psychiatry, Mayo Medical School
Division of Child and Adolescent Psychiatry
Mayo Clinic
Rochester, Minnesota

RICHARD D. MATTES, R.D., M.P.H., Ph.D.
Professor, Department of Foods and Nutrition
Purdue University
Lafayette, Indiana
Adjunct Associate Professor of Medicine, Division of Endocrinology and Metabolism
Indiana University School of Medicine
Indianapolis, Indiana

DWIGHT E. MATTHEWS, Ph.D.
Professor of Medicine and Chemistry
University of Vermont
Burlington, Vermont

DONALD B. McCORMICK, Ph.D.
Fuller E. Callaway Professor, Department of Biochemistry
Emory University
Atlanta, Georgia

N. GERALD McELVANEY, M.D.
Professor of Medicine, Clinical Investigation Unit
Beaumont Hospital
Dublin, Ireland

WILLIAM J. McGANITY, M.D., F.R.C.S. (Canada)
Ashbel Smith Professor Emeritus of Obstetrics and Gynecology
Department of Obstetrics and Gynecology
University of Texas Medical Branch
Galveston, Texas

DONALD S. McLAREN, M.D., Ph.D., D.T.M. and H., F.R.C.P.E.
Honorary Head, Nutritional Blindness Prevention Programme
Department of Preventive Ophthalmology
Institute of Ophthalmology
London, United Kingdom

STEPHEN H. McNAMARA, Esq.
Senior Partner
Hyman, Phelps, and McNamara, P.C.
Washington, DC

DONALD M. MOCK, M.D., Ph.D.
Professor and Director
Division of Digestive, Endocrine, Genetic, and Nutritional Disorders
University of Arkansas for Medical Sciences
Director, Department of Clinical Nutrition
Arkansas Children's Hospital
Little Rock, Arkansas

JOEL MOSS, M.D., Ph.D.
Chief, Pulmonary-Critical Care Medicine Branch
National Heart, Lung, and Blood Institute
National Institutes of Health
Bethesda, Maryland

JEANETTE M. NEWTON, M.D.
Fellow in Clinical Nutrition
University of California at Davis
Davis, California

FORREST H. NIELSEN, Ph.D.
Director and Research Nutritionist
Grand Forks Human Nutrition Research Center
United States Department of Agriculture
Grand Forks, North Dakota

MAN S. OH, M.D.
Professor of Medicine
Health Sciences Center at Brooklyn
State University of New York
Brooklyn, New York

JAMES A. OLSON, Ph.D.
Distinguished Professor of Liberal Arts and Sciences
Department of Biochemistry and Biophysics
Iowa State University
Ames, Iowa

ROBERT E. OLSON, M.D., Ph.D.
Professor Emeritus of Medicine
State University of New York at Stony Brook
Professor of Pediatrics
University of South Florida
Tampa, Florida

CAROLE A. PALMER, Ed.D., R.D.
Professor and Co-head, Division of Nutrition and Preventive Dentistry
Department of General Dentistry
School of Dental Medicine
Professor, School of Nutrition
Tufts University
Boston, Massachusetts

SHEAU-FANG PAN, M.A.
Obesity Research Center
St. Luke's Roosevelt Hospital Center
New York City, New York

F. XAVIER PI-SUNYER, M.D.
Professor of Medicine, College of Physicians and Surgeons
Columbia University
Director, Division of Endocrinology, Diabetes, and Nutrition
Director of Obesity Research Center
St. Luke's-Roosevelt Hospital Center
New York City, New York

NORA PLESOFSKY-VIG, Ph.D.
Research Scientist
Department of Genetics and Cell Biology and Plant Biology
University of Minnesota
St. Paul, Minnesota

ERIC T. POEHLMAN, Ph.D.
Professor of Medicine, Division of Pharmacology and Metabolic Research
University of Vermont
Burlington, Vermont

SARA A. QUANDT, Ph.D.
Associate Professor, Department of Public Health Sciences
Wake Forest University School of Medicine
Adjunct Associate Professor, Department of Anthropology
Wake Forest University
Winston-Salem, North Carolina

JEANNE I. RADER, Ph.D.
Director, Division of Science and Applied Technology
Department of Food Labeling
Center for Food Safety and Applied Nutrition
United States Food and Drug Administration
Washington, DC

MASSIMO RAIMONDO, M.D.
Resident, Division of Gastroenterology
Department of Internal Medicine
Mayo Clinic
Rochester, Minnesota

CHARLES J. REBOUCHE, Ph.D.
Associate Professor, Department of Pediatrics
University of Iowa
Iowa City, Iowa

A. CATHARINE ROSS, Ph.D.
Professor and Head, Department of Veterinary Science
Professor, Nutrition Department
College of Health and Human Development
The Pennsylvania State University
University Park, Pennsylvania

ROBERT M. RUSSELL, M.D.
Chief Scientist, Jean Mayer USDA Human Nutrition Research Center on Aging
Tufts University
Boston, Massachusetts
Professor, School of Nutrition Science and Policy
Tufts University
Medford, Massachusetts

HUGH A. SAMPSON, M.D.
Professor of Pediatrics; Director, Pediatric Clinical Research Center
Department of Pediatrics
Johns Hopkins University School of Medicine
Baltimore, Maryland
Current address:
Professor of Pediatrics
Mount Sinai School of Medicine
New York City, New York

PAUL D. SAVAGE, M.D.
Assistant Professor of Medicine
Wake Forest University School of Medicine
Winston-Salem, North Carolina

JAMES S. SCOLAPIO, M.D.
Fellow, Division of Gastroenterology
Mayo Clinic
Rochester, Minnesota

JOHN M. SCOTT, D.Sc.
Professor of Experimental Nutrition, Department of Biochemistry
Trinity College
Dublin, Ireland

CLAY F. SEMENKOVICH, M.D.
Associate Professor, Departments of Medicine and Cell Biology and Physiology
Washington University School of Medicine
St. Louis, Missouri

MOSHE SHIKE, M.D.
Director of Clinical Nutrition
Memorial Sloan-Kettering Cancer Center
Professor of Medicine
Cornell University Medical College
New York City, New York

MAURICE E. SHILS, M.D., Sc.D.
Professor Emeritus of Medicine
Cornell University Medical College
Consultant Emeritus (Nutrition)
Memorial Sloan-Kettering Cancer Center
New York City, New York
Adjunct Professor (Nutrition), Retired
Department of Public Health Sciences
Wake Forest University School of Medicine
Winston-Salem, North Carolina

JAMES D. SHULL, Ph.D.
Associate Professor, Eppley Institute for Research in Cancer
Department of Biochemistry and Molecular Biology
College of Medicine
University of Nebraska Medical Center
Omaha, Nebraska

GERARD P. SMITH, M.D.
Professor of Psychiatry (Behavioral Neuroscience)
Department of Psychiatry
Cornell University Medical College
New York City, New York

MICHELLE K. SMITH, M.D.
Clinical Research Fellow, Department of Surgery
Cornell University Medical College
New York City, New York

SCOTT M. SMITH, Ph.D.
Research Nutritionist, Biomedical Operations and Research
Johnson Space Center, NASA
Houston, Texas

NOEL W. SOLOMONS, M.D.
Senior Scientist and Coordinator
Center for Studies of Sensory Impairment, Aging and Metabolism
CESSIAM Hospital de Ojos-Oides
Guatemala City, Guatemala

WILEY W. SOUBA, M.D., Sc.D.
Chief, Surgical Oncology
Massachusetts General Hospital
Professor of Surgery
Harvard Medical School
Boston, Massachusetts

VIRGINIA A. STALLINGS, M.D.
Chief, Nutrition Section
Division of Gastroenterology and Nutrition
Department of Pediatrics
Childrens Hospital of Philadelphia
University of Pennsylvania School of Medicine
Philadelphia, Pennsylvania

WILLIAM F. STENSON, M.D.
Professor of Medicine, Department of Medicine
Washington University School of Medicine
St. Louis, Missouri

MARTHA H. STIPANUK, Ph.D.
Professor, Division of Nutritional Sciences
Cornell University
Ithaca, New York

BARBARA J. STOECKER, Ph.D.
Professor and Head, Department of Nutritional Sciences
Oklahoma State University
Stillwater, Oklahoma

TAKASHI SUGIMURA, M.D.
President Emeritus
National Cancer Center
Tokyo, Japan

VICHAI TANPHAICHITR, M.D., Ph.D.
Professor of Medicine
Director, Research Center
Faculty of Medicine, Ramathibodi Hospital, Mahidol University
Bangkok, Thailand

JAMES A. THOMAS
Professor, Department of Biochemistry and Biophysics
Iowa State University
Ames, Iowa

RAJPAL S. TOMAR, Ph.D.
Staff Toxicologist, Office of Environmental Health Hazard Assessment
California Environmental Protection Agency
Berkeley, California

BENJAMÍN TORÚN, M.D., Ph.D.
Senior Scientist
Head, Department of Nutrition and Health Unit
Instituto de Nutricion de Centro America y Panama (INCAP)
Professor of Basic and Human Nutrition
University of San Carlos de Guatemala
Guatemala City, Guatemala

MARET G. TRABER, Ph.D.
Research Associate Biochemist
Department of Molecular and Cell Biology
University of California Berkeley
Berkeley, California

A. STEWART TRUSWELL, M.D., F.R.C.P., F.R.A.C.P., F.F.P.H.M.
Professor of Human Nutrition, Department of Biochemistry
University of Sydney
Sydney, Australia

JUDITH R. TURNLUND, Ph.D.
Research Leader, Western Human Nutrition Research Center
United States Department of Agriculture
San Francisco, California

PENNY S. TURTEL, M.D.
Associate Attending, Department of Medicine
Monmouth Medical Center
Monmouth, New Jersey

JAIME URIBARRI, M.D.
Associate Professor of Medicine
Mount Sinai Medical School
New York City, New York

VIRGINIA UTERMOHLEN, M.D.
Associate Professor, Division of Nutritional Sciences
Cornell University
Ithaca, New York

JAMES W. VAN HOOK, M.D.
Assistant Professor of Obstetrics and Gynecology
Department of Obstetrics and Gynecology
University of Texas Medical Branch
Galveston, Texas

JERRY VOCKLEY, M.D., Ph.D.
Consultant and Associate Professor in Medical Genetics
Department of Medical Genetics
Mayo Clinic
Rochester, Minnesota

KEIJI WAKABAYASHI, Ph.D.
Chief, Cancer Prevention Division
National Cancer Center Research Institute
Tokyo, Japan

WEI WANG, Ph.D.
Instructor, College of Agriculture
California State Polytechnic University
Pomona, California

CONNIE M. WEAVER, Ph.D.
Professor and Head, Department of Foods and Nutrition
Purdue University
West Lafayette, Indiana

DONALD G. WEIR, M.D., F.R.C.P.I., F.R.C.P., F.A.C.P.
Professor, Department of Clinical Medicine
Trinity College
Dublin, Ireland

WALTER C. WILLET, M.D., Dr.P.H.
Professor of Epidemiology and Nutrition
Departments of Epidemiology and Nutrition
Harvard School of Public Health
Boston, Massachusetts

ALEXA W. WILLIAMS
Research Assistant, Department of Food Science and Human Nutrition
University of Illinois
Urbana, Illinois

DOUGLAS W. WILMORE, M.D.
Frank Sawyer Professor of Surgery
Harvard Medical School
Department of Surgery
Brigham and Women's Hospital
Boston, Massachusetts

THOMAS M. S. WOLEVER, M.D., Ph.D.
Associate Professor, Department of Nutrition Sciences
University of Toronto
Toronto, Ontario, Canada

LUCAS WOLF, M.D.
Fellow in Geographic Medicine and Infectious Diseases
Tufts University School of Medicine
New England Medical Center
Boston, Massachusetts

ANN M. YAKTINE, M.S.
Graduate Assistant, Eppley Institute for Research in Cancer
Department of Biochemistry and Molecular Biology
College of Medicine
University of Nebraska Medical Center
Omaha, Nebraska

STEVEN YOSHIDA, Ph.D.
Postdoctoral Scholar
Division of Rheumatology, Allergy and Clinical Immunology
University of California at Davis
Davis, California

STEVEN H. ZEISEL, M.D., Ph.D.
Professor and Chairman, Department of Nutrition
School of Public Health
Professor, Department of Medicine
School of Medicine
University of North Carolina at Chapel Hill
Chapel Hill, North Carolina

Contents

†Deceased.

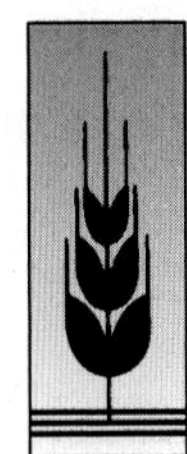

PART I.

Specific Dietary Components

1. Defining the Essentiality of Nutrients

ALFRED E. HARPER

THE CONCEPT OF NUTRITIONAL ESSENTIALITY

The concept of nutritional essentiality was firmly established less than 100 years ago. It arose from observations that certain diseases observed in human populations consuming poor diets could be prevented by including other foods in the diet and that failure of animals fed on diets composed of purified components or restricted to one or a few foodstuffs to grow and survive could similarly be corrected by including another food or an extract of the food in the diet. The food constituents that were found to prevent these problems were classified as indispensable (or essential) nutrients. Nutrients that could be deleted from the diet without causing growth failure or specific signs of disease were classified as dispensable (or nonessential).

This classification of nutrients served well through the 1950s as the basis of recommendations for treating dietary deficiency diseases, offering dietary advice to the public, and establishing food regulations and policy. As information about nutrients accrued, however, some essential nutrients were found to be synthesized from precursors, interactions among some nutrients in the diet were found to influence the need for others, and later, in some conditions, such as prematurity, certain pathologic states, and genetic defects, the ability of the body to synthesize several nutrients not ordinarily required was found to be so impaired that a dietary source was needed. As a result, the system of classifying nutrients simply as indispensable or dispensable has been modified to include a category of conditional essentiality (1).

Recently, associations observed between the risk of developing certain chronic and degenerative diseases and the consumption of some dispensable nutrients and nonnutrient components of foods, as well as the beneficial effects sometimes observed with high intakes of some essential nutrients, have raised questions about the adequacy of the present system of nutritional classification of food constituents (2–6). In this chapter evolution of the concept of nutritional essentiality is outlined and problems encountered in classifying food constituents on the basis of their effects on health and disease are identified.

Evolution of the Concept

Differences in the physical properties of foods and in their content of medicinal and toxic substances were considered to be important in the prevention and treatment of diseases in ancient times, but knowledge that foods contain many substances essential for life has been acquired only during the past two centuries (7–11). Although the Hippocratic physicians in Greece practiced a form of dietetic medicine some 2400 years ago, they had no understanding of the chemical nature of foods and believed that foods contained only a single nutritional principle—aliment (9). This belief persisted until the 19th century, but a few earlier observations presaged the concept of nutritional essentiality (11). During the 1670s, Sydenham, a British physician, observed that a tonic of iron filings in wine improved the condition of chlorotic (anemic) patients, and in the 1740s, Lind, a British naval surgeon, found that consumption of citrus fruits, but not typical shipboard foods and medicines, cured scurvy in sailors. McCollum (9) cites Sydenham's report as the first evidence of essentiality of a specific nutrient, but it was not recognized as such at the time.

Between 1770 and 1794, through experiments on the nature of respiration in guinea pigs and human subjects, Lavoisier and Laplace discovered that oxidation of carbon compounds in tissues was the source of energy for bodily functions (7). For the first time, a specific function of foods had been identified in chemical terms. Lavoisier and his colleagues also established the basic concepts of organic chemistry, thus opening the way for understanding the chemical nature of foods.

Scientists interested in animal production then began to examine food components as nutrients. The first evidence of nutritional essentiality of an organic food component—protein—was the observation of Magendie in 1816 that dogs fed only carbohydrate or fat lost considerable body protein and died within a few weeks, whereas dogs fed on foods containing protein remained healthy. A few years later, in 1827, Prout, a physician and scientist in London, proposed that the nutrition of higher animals could be explained by their need for the three major constituents of foods—proteins, carbohydrates, and fats—and the changes these undergo in the body. This explanation, which was widely accepted, sounded the death knell of the single aliment hypothesis of the Hippocratic physicians.

During the next two decades, knowledge of the needs

of animals for several mineral elements advanced. Chossat found that a calcium supplement prevented the mineral loss observed in birds fed a diet of wheat; Boussingalt, using the balance technique, showed that pigs required calcium and phosphorus for skeletal development and also noted that cattle deteriorated when deprived of salt for a prolonged period. Liebig, a leading German chemist with a major interest in agricultural problems, found that sodium was the major cation of blood and potassium of tissues. Thus, by 1850, at least six mineral elements (Ca, P, Na, K, Cl, and Fe) had been established as essential for higher animals (11).

During this time also, Liebig postulated that energy-yielding substances (carbohydrates, fats) and proteins together with a few minerals were the principles of a nutritionally adequate diet. Liebig's hypothesis, however, was questioned by Pereira (1847), who noted that diets restricted to a small number of foods were associated with development of diseases such as scurvy, and by Dumas, who observed that feeding children artificial milk containing the known dietary constituents had failed to prevent deterioration of their health during the siege of Paris (1870–71). Still, owing to his great prestige, Leibig's concept continued to dominate thinking throughout the 19th century (9).

In 1881, Lunin in Dorpat, and 10 years later, Socin in Basel, found that mice fed on diets composed of purified proteins, fats, carbohydrates, and a mineral mixture survived less than 32 days. Mice that received milk or egg yolk in addition remained healthy throughout the 60-day experiments. Lunin and Socin concluded that these foods must contain small amounts of unknown substances essential for life. Their observations, nonetheless, did not stimulate a vigorous search for essential nutrients in foods, probably because of the skepticism of prominent scientists. Von Bunge, in whose laboratories Lunin and Socin worked, attributed inadequacies of purified diets to mineral imbalances or failure to supply minerals as organic complexes. Voit, a colleague of Liebig, assumed that purified diets would be adequate if they could be made palatable.

During the early 1880s, Takaki, director general of the Japanese Navy, noted that about 30% of Japanese sailors developed beriberi, although this disease was not prevalent among British sailors, whose rations were higher in protein. When evaporated milk and meat were included in the rations of the Japanese Navy, the incidence of beriberi declined remarkably. He concluded correctly that beriberi was a dietary deficiency disease, but incorrectly that it was caused by an inadequate intake of protein. In the 1890s, Eijkman, an army physician in the Dutch East Indies who was concerned with the high incidence of beriberi in the prisons in Java (Indonesia), where polished rice was a staple, discovered that chickens fed on a military hospital diet consisting mainly of polished rice developed a neurologic disease resembling beriberi, whereas those fed rice with the pericarp intact remained healthy. He proposed that accumulation of starch in the intestine favored formation of a substance that acted as a nerve poison and that rice hulls contained an antidote.

Grijns extended Eijkman's investigations and showed through feeding trials with chickens that the protective substance in rice hulls could be extracted with water. In 1901, he concluded that beriberi was caused by the absence from polished rice of an essential nutrient present mainly in the hulls. He provided, for the first time, a clear concept of a dietary deficiency disease, but the broad implications of his discovery were not appreciated. The authors of a British report (8) noted that facts brought to light by research done between 1880 and 1901 had "little or no effect on orthodox views and teaching concerning human nutrition." Another 15 years of research was required before the concept that foods contained a variety of unidentified essential nutrients gained widespread acceptance.

Establishing the Concept

The first evidence of essentiality of a specific organic molecule was the discovery by Willcock and Hopkins (12) in 1906 that a supplement of the amino acid tryptophan prolonged the survival of mice fed on a diet in which the protein source was the tryptophan-deficient protein zein. The following year, Holst and Frölich in Norway reported that guinea pigs fed on dry diets with no fresh vegetables developed a disease resembling scurvy, which was prevented by feeding them fresh vegetables or citrus juices. This was further evidence that foods contained unidentified substances that protected against specific diseases (9, 10).

Also, in 1907, Hart and associates at Wisconsin initiated a direct test of the validity of Liebig's hypothesis that the nutritive value of foods and feeds could be predicted from measurements of their gross composition by chemical analysis. They fed heifers on different rations designed to contain essentially the same amounts of major nutrients and minerals, each composed of a single plant source—wheat, oats, or corn—using all parts of the plant. The study lasted 3 years and included two reproductive periods. Animals that ate the wheat plant ration failed to thrive and did not produce viable calves; those fed the corn plant ration grew well and reproduced successfully. The results of this study, published in 1911, demonstrated that Liebig's hypothesis was untenable and stimulated intensive investigation in the United States of nutritional defects in diets (13).

In experiments undertaken between 1909 and 1913 to compare the nutritional value of proteins, Osborne and Mendel at Yale had initially been unable to obtain satisfactory rates of growth of rats fed on purified diets. They solved this problem by including a protein-free milk preparation in the diets. They then demonstrated that proteins from different sources differed in nutritive value and discovered that lysine, sulfur-containing amino acids, and histidine were essential for the rat (14).

During this time, Hopkins also observed that including small amounts of protein-free extracts of milk in nutritionally inadequate, purified diets converted them into diets that supported growth (10). In 1912 he commented: "It is possible that what is absent from artificial diets . . . is of the nature of an organic complex . . . which the animal body cannot synthesize." In 1912 also, in a review of the literature on beriberi, scurvy, and pellagra, Funk in London, who had been trying to purify the antiberiberi principle from rice polishings, proposed that these diseases were caused by a lack in the diet of "special substances which are in the nature of organic bases, which we will call vitamines" (9).

In studies of the nutritional inadequacies of purified diets McCollum and Davis, at Wisconsin, noted that when part of the carbohydrate was supplied as unpurified lactose, growth of rats was satisfactory if the fat was supplied as butterfat. When butterfat was replaced by lard or olive oil, growth failure occurred. In 1913 they concluded that butterfat contained an unidentified substance essential for growth. Meanwhile, Osborne and Mendel observed that if they purified the protein-free milk included in their diets, growth failure of rats again occurred, but if they substituted milk fat for the lard in their diets, growth was restored. They also concluded in 1913 that milk fat contained an unidentified substance essential for life.

McCollum and Davis extracted the active substance from butterfat and transferred it to olive oil, which then promoted growth. They called this substance "fat-soluble A." They then tested their active extracts in a polished rice diet of the type used by Eijkman and Grijns and found that even though the diet contained fat-soluble A, it failed to support growth. The problem was remedied when they added water extracts of wheat germ or boiled eggs. They concluded that animals consuming purified diets required two unidentified factors—fat-soluble A and water-soluble B (presumably Grijns' antiberiberi factor) (9, 10). Thus, by 1915, six minerals, four amino acids, and three vitamins—A, B, and the antiscorbutic factor—had been identified as essential nutrients.

The concept that foods contained several organic substances that were essential for growth, health, and survival was by then generally accepted. By 1918, the importance of consuming a wide variety of foods to ensure that diets provided adequate quantities of these substances was being emphasized in health programs for the public in Great Britain and the United States, and by the League of Nations.

NUTRITIONAL CLASSIFICATION OF FOOD CONSTITUENTS

As discoveries of other unidentified nutrients in foods or feeds continued to be reported after the 1920s, sometimes on the basis of limited evidence, criteria were needed, both on scientific grounds and for regulatory purposes, for establishing the validity of such claims.

Criteria of Essentiality

Criteria for establishing whether or not a dietary constituent is an essential nutrient were implicit in the types of investigations that had provided the basis for the concept of nutritional essentiality. Later they were elaborated in more detail as follows:

1. The substance is required in the diet for growth, health, and survival
2. Its absence from the diet or inadequate intake results in characteristic signs of a deficiency disease and, ultimately, death
3. Growth failure and characteristic signs of deficiency are prevented only by the nutrient or a specific precursor of it, not by other substances
4. Below some critical level of intake of the nutrient, growth response and severity of signs of deficiency are proportional to the amount consumed
5. The substance is not synthesized in the body and is, therefore, required for some critical function throughout life

By 1950 some 35 nutrients had been shown to meet these criteria. Nutrients presently accepted as essential for humans and for which there are recommended dietary intakes (RDIs) or allowances (RDAs) are listed in Table 1.1.

Classification According to Essentiality

As knowledge of nutritional needs expanded, nutrients were classified according to their essentiality. This type of classification was applied initially to amino acids. In the early 1920s, Mendel used the term *indispensable* for amino acids that are not synthesized in the body. The term *nonessential* was used widely for those that are not required in the diet. This term was not considered satisfactory because these amino acids, although not required in the

Table 1.1
Nutrients Essential for Humans

Water	Energy sources
Amino acids	Fatty acids
Histidine	Linoleic
Isoleucine	α-Linolenic
Leucine	Minerals
Lysine	Calcium
Methionine	Phosphorus
Phenylalanine	Magnesium
Threonine	Iron
Tryptophan	Trace minerals
Valine	Zinc
Vitamins	Copper
Ascorbic acid	Manganese
Vitamins A, D, E, K	Iodine
Thiamin	Selenium
Riboflavin	Molybdenum
Niacin	Chromium
Vitamin B_6 (pyridoxine)	Electrolytes
Pantothenic acid	Sodium
Folic acid	Potassium
Biotin	Chloride
Vitamin B_{12} (cobalamin)	Ultratrace elements[a]

[a] *See Chapter 16.*

diet, are physiologically essential. Block and Bolling used the term *indispensable* for organic nutrients with carbon skeletons that are not synthesized in the body, and *dispensable,* which does not carry the broad implication of the term *nonessential,* for those with carbon skeletons that can be synthesized (15, 16).

Nutritional essentiality is characteristic of the species, not the nutrient. Arginine is required by cats and birds but not by humans. Also, it is not synthesized by the young of most species in amounts sufficient for rapid growth. It may, therefore, be either dispensable or indispensable depending on the species and stage of growth. Ascorbic acid (vitamin C), which is required by humans and guinea pigs, is not required by most species.

The Concept of Conditional Essentiality

Snyderman (17) found that premature infants, in whom many enzymes of amino acid metabolism develop late during gestation, required cystine and tyrosine (which are dispensable for most full-term infants) to ensure nitrogen retention and maintain their normal plasma levels. Cystine and tyrosine were thus essential for premature infants. Rudman and associates (18, 19) subsequently proposed the term *conditionally essential* for nutrients not ordinarily required in the diet but which must be supplied exogenously to specific populations that do not synthesize them in adequate amounts. They applied the term initially to dispensable nutrients needed by seriously ill patients maintained on total parenteral nutrition (TPN). The term now is used for similar needs that result from developmental immaturity, pathologic states, or genetic defects.

Developmental Immaturity. Cystine and tyrosine, as mentioned above, are conditionally essential for premature infants (17). McCormick (3) has suggested that because preterm infants lack the enzymes for elongation and desaturation of linoleic and α-linolenic acids, elongated derivatives of these fatty acids, which are precursors of eicosanoids and membrane phospholipids, should be considered conditionally essential for them.

Damage to the cones of the eye and decline in weight gain of infant monkeys fed a taurine-free diet were prevented by supplements of taurine. In premature infants maintained on TPN without taurine, plasma taurine concentration declined, and the b-wave of the electroretinogram was attenuated. Gaull (20) suggests that taurine becomes conditionally essential for children maintained on TPN because they cannot synthesize enough to meet the body's need.

Plasma and tissue carnitine concentrations are lower in newborn infants than in adults, but this condition has not been associated with any physiologic defect. In infants maintained on TPN without carnitine, however, plasma and tissue carnitine levels are low, and in one study, this was associated with impaired fat metabolism and reduced nitrogen retention, both corrected by carnitine supplementation. Hoppel (21) concluded from a comprehensive review of the evidence that carnitine may be conditionally essential for premature infants maintained on TPN but is not conditionally essential for adults.

Pathologic States. Some patients with cirrhosis of the liver require supplements of cysteine and tyrosine to maintain nitrogen balance and normal plasma levels of these amino acids. Plasma taurine concentration also declines in adults with low plasma cystine levels. Insufficient synthesis of these nutrients in cirrhotic patients has been attributed to impairment of the synthetic pathway in the diseased liver. In some cancer patients, plasma choline concentrations declined by 50% when they were maintained on TPN. This was attributed to precursors of choline bypassing the liver during feeding by TPN (18).

In human subjects suffering severe illness, trauma, or infections, muscle and plasma glutamine concentrations decrease, generally in proportion to the severity of the illness or injury. In animals, decreased glutamine concentrations are associated with negative nitrogen balance, decreased tissue protein synthesis, and increased protein degradation. In clinical trials, nitrogen balance and clinical responses of surgical patients were improved by provision of glutamine in parenteral fluids following surgery. These findings support the conclusion that glutamine utilization exceeds its synthesis in patients in hypercatabolic states, and thus glutamine becomes conditionally essential for them (22).

Genetic Defects. Conditional essentiality of nutrients is also observed in individuals with genetic defects in pathways for synthesis of biologically essential but nutritionally dispensable substances. Genetic defects of carnitine synthesis result in myopathies that can be corrected by carnitine supplements (3). Genetic defects in the synthesis of tetrahydrobiopterin, the cofactor for aromatic amino acid hydroxylases, result in phenylketonuria and impaired synthesis of some of the neurotransmitters for which aromatic amino acids are precursors (3). Tetrahydrobiopterin is thus conditionally essential for such individuals.

Criteria for Conditional Essentiality

Rudman and Feller (18) proposed three criteria for establishing conditional essentiality of nutrients: *(a)* decline in the plasma level of the nutrient into the subnormal range; *(b)* appearance of chemical, structural, or functional abnormalities; and *(c)* correction of both of these by a dietary supplement of the nutrient. All these criteria must be met to establish unequivocally that a nutrient is conditionally essential.

Conditional essentiality represents a qualitative change in requirements, i.e., the need for a nutrient that is ordinarily dispensable. Alterations in the need for an essential nutrient, from whatever cause, and health benefits from consumption of nonnutrients, dispensable nutrients, or essential nutrients in excess of amounts needed for normal physiologic function do not fit this category. Such situations should be dealt with separately.

MODIFICATION OF ESSENTIAL NUTRIENT NEEDS

Needs for essential nutrients may be influenced by *(a)* the presence in the diet of substances for which the nutrient is a precursor, that are precursors of the nutrient, or that interfere with the absorption or utilization of the nutrient; *(b)* imbalances and disproportions of other related nutrients; *(c)* some genetic defects; and *(d)* use of drugs that impair utilization of nutrients. These conditions do not alter basic requirements; they just increase or decrease the amounts that must be consumed to meet requirements. A few examples below illustrate the general characteristics of such effects.

Nutrient Interactions

Precursor-Product Relationships. Many substances that are physiologically, but not nutritionally, essential are synthesized from specific essential nutrients. If the products of the synthetic reactions are present in the diet, they may exert sparing effects that reduce the need for the precursor nutrients. Less phenylalanine and methionine are required, particularly by adults, when the diet includes tyrosine and cystine, for which they are, respectively, specific precursors. Birds, which do not synthesize arginine, have a high requirement for this amino acid. Inclusion in the diet of creatine, for which arginine is a precursor, reduces the need for arginine. Effects of this type, however, have not been explored extensively (23).

Precursors of Essential Nutrients. Tryptophan is a precursor of niacin. The need for niacin is therefore reduced by dietary tryptophan, but the efficiency of conversion differs for different species. The cat has an absolute requirement for niacin, but the rat converts tryptophan to niacin very efficiently. Human requirements for niacin are expressed as niacin-equivalents: 60 mg of dietary tryptophan equals 1 mg of niacin. ß-Carotene, and to a lesser extent other carotenoids, are precursors of retinol (vitamin A). Human requirements for vitamin A are expressed as retinol-equivalents: 1 μg retinol-equivalent equals 1 μg of retinol or 6 μg of ß-carotene. These are examples of interactions that alter the dietary need for essential nutrients (24). They are not examples of conditional essentiality.

Imbalances and Disproportions of Nutrients. High proportions of some nutrients in the diet can influence the need for others. This phenomenon was first recognized when additions of amino acids that stimulated growth of young rats fed on diets low in tryptophan and niacin were found to precipitate niacin deficiency—an example of a vitamin deficiency induced by an amino acid imbalance. With diets that contain adequate niacin but are low in tryptophan, amino acid disproportions increased the need for tryptophan and depressed growth (25). Many examples of this type of imbalance, involving a variety of amino acids, have been observed in young animals. The growth-depressing effects result from depressed food intake mediated through alterations in brain neurotransmitter concentrations (26).

Dietary imbalances can also increase needs for some mineral elements (23, 27). Disproportionate amounts of molybdenum and sulfate in the diet increase the dietary need for copper and precipitate copper deficiency in animals consuming an otherwise adequate amount of copper. Extra manganese in the diets of sheep or pigs increases the need for iron to prevent anemia, and excess iron reduces the absorption of manganese. The presence in the diet of phytic acid, which binds zinc as well as other multivalent cations, impairs zinc absorption and increases the need for zinc. Thus, phytic acid can precipitate zinc deficiency in both humans and animals.

Dietary needs for some essential nutrients are influenced by the proportions of macronutrients in the diet. The need for vitamin E in the diet increases as the amount of fat rich in polyunsaturated fatty acids is increased (28). Thiamin functions mainly as part of the cofactor for decarboxylation of the α-ketoacids arising from metabolism of carbohydrates and branched-chain amino acids; hence, the need for thiamin depends upon the relative proportions of fat, carbohydrate, and protein in the diet. Fat has long been known to exert a "thiamin-sparing" effect (29).

Genetic Defects

Individuals with genetic defects that limit conversion of a vitamin to its coenzyme form develop severe deficiency diseases. Defects in the utilization of biotin, cobalamin, folate, niacin, pyridoxine, and thiamin are known. Effects of some of these diseases are relieved by large doses of the vitamin, but the degree of response varies with the disease and among patients with the same defect (30). Intakes required to relieve or correct these conditions are well above the RDA. In the genetic disease acrodermatitis enteropathica, which impairs zinc absorption, the need for zinc is three to four times the RDI level (see Chapter 11).

Drug-Nutrient Interactions

Many types of drug-nutrient interactions increase the need for a nutrient. The drug may cause malabsorption, act as a vitamin antagonist, or impair mineral absorption (see Chapter 99). These and other conditions that alter the amounts of essential nutrients needed because of either interactions among dietary constituents or impairment of a metabolic function are not examples of conditional essentiality.

HEALTH BENEFITS NOT RELATED TO NUTRITIONAL ESSENTIALITY

For several decades after the concept of nutritional essentiality was established in the early 1900s, foods were primarily considered to be sources of essential nutrients required for critical physiologic functions that, if impaired by dietary deficiencies, caused specific diseases. Except for the debilitating effects of malnutrition, little consideration was given during this time to the idea that the type of diet consumed might influence development of diseases other than those caused by inadequate intakes of essential nutrients. By the 1950s, dietary deficiency diseases were virtually eliminated in industrialized nations. Improvements in nutrition, sanitation, and control of infectious diseases had resulted in immense improvements in health; life expectancy had lengthened, and chronic and degenerative diseases had become the major causes of death. This aroused interest in the possibility that susceptibility to such diseases might be influenced by the type of diet consumed.

Associations observed subsequently between diet composition, intakes of various individual diet components, and the incidence of heart disease and cancer have implicated food constituents such as fatty acids, fiber, carotenoids, various nonnutrient substances in plants, and high intakes of some essential nutrients (especially vitamins E and C, which can function as antioxidants) as factors influencing the risk of developing these diseases (6) (see Chapters 76, 80, and 81). This has led to proposals for modifying the criteria for essentiality or conditional essentiality to include dietary constituents reported to reduce the risk of chronic and degenerative diseases or to improve immune function, and for considering such effects of high intakes of essential nutrients as part of the basis for establishing RDIs (2–6).

The definitions for *essential* and *conditionally essential* nutrients are clear from the criteria used to establish them. If the definitions were broadened to include substances that provide some desirable effect on health but do not fit these criteria, the specificity of the current definitions would be lost. Providing a health benefit, as for example is the case with fiber, is obviously not an adequate criterion for classifying a food constituent as essential or conditionally essential. Altering the criteria for establishing RDIs on the basis of effects of intakes of essential nutrients that greatly exceed physiologic needs or amounts obtainable from usual diets would have similar consequences—the specificity of the term *RDI* would be lost.

Food Constituents Desirable for Health. A straightforward way of avoiding these problems is to treat food constituents that exert desirable or beneficial effects on health, but do not fit the criteria established for essentiality or conditional essentiality, as a separate category of food constituents termed *desirable (or beneficial) for health* (1). Another more general term for such substances, which embraces both beneficial and adverse effects, is *physiological modulators* (31). A dietary guideline for including plenty of fresh vegetables and fruits in diets as sources of both known and unidentified substances that may have desirable effects on health or in preventing disease has been readily accepted. Individual food constituents that may confer health benefits different from those of physiologically required quantities of essential nutrients, whether they are nonnutrients, dispensable nutrients, or essential nutrients in quantities exceeding those obtainable from diets, are more appropriately included in guidelines for health than in the RDI. Some nutrients and other food constituents that have prophylactic actions are presently dealt with in essentially this manner. Fiber and fluoride are discussed in dietary guideline publications, and this has been suggested as the most appropriate way of dealing with the potential beneficial effects of high intakes of antioxidant nutrients (32).

Fluoride, in appropriate dose, reduces susceptibility to dental caries without exerting a toxic effect. Whether fluoride meets criteria for essentiality, whether it is essential for tooth and bone development, or even if it should be considered a nutrient is controversial. Nonetheless, in low doses it acts as a prophylactic agent in protecting teeth against the action of bacteria. It is discussed in RDI and dietary guidelines publications on this basis, and it is certainly classified appropriately as a dietary constituent that provides a desirable health benefit.

Fiber has been long recognized to be beneficial for gastrointestinal function, to prevent constipation, and to relieve signs of diverticulosis. There is no basis for classifying fiber as an essential nutrient, but some forms of fiber that are transformed in the gastrointestinal tract into products that can be oxidized to yield energy fit the definition of nutrients. Without question it is a food constituent that provides a desirable health benefit when ingested in moderate amounts (33). Fiber is discussed with carbohydrates in RDI publications and with plant foods in dietary guidelines. A recommendation for inclusion of fiber in diets is appropriate, but recommended intakes should not be considered as RDIs, which are reference values for intakes of essential nutrients.

To develop a separate category of food constituents of this type (substances with desirable effects on health that are different from effects attributable to the physiologic functions of essential nutrients), specific criteria must be established to identify those to be included. Establishing appropriate criteria for assessing the validity of health claims for a category of food constituents that will include a variety of unrelated substances with different types of effects, many of which apply to only segments of the population, will be more complex than establishing criteria for assessing the validity of claims for essentiality of food constituents. The latter criteria apply uniformly to all substances proposed for inclusion and can be measured objectively. Assessing the effects of food constituents on health or in preventing disease involves a greater element of judgment and is more subjective than evaluating the essentiality of nutrients. Thus, claims for such effects must be evaluated especially critically.

In establishing criteria for assessing claims for desirable health benefits, consideration must be given to the need for subcategories of substances having different effects. Susceptibility to chronic and degenerative diseases is highly variable and may be influenced by many factors, including genetic differences among individuals or between populations, lifestyle, and diet-genetic interactions that can influence expression of genetic traits. Among questions that require answers are, Does the effect result from alteration of a basic mechanism that prevents a disease from developing or is it due to modulation of the disease process? Does the benefit apply to the entire population or only to individuals at risk? This has been a source of controversy in relation to dietary recommendations for reducing the risk of developing heart disease (34). The effects of dietary constituents on immunocompetence should be analyzed in a similar manner: Are they of general significance or of consequence only if the immune system is impaired? When is stimulation of the immune system beneficial and when might it have adverse effects?

An immense number of plant constituents with anticarcinogenic actions are currently under investigation. These constituents differ in both their effects on cells and the stage of tumor development at which they act, and some have both adverse and beneficial effects (35). A number of subcategories would seem to be needed for which specific criteria will be required.

Pharmacologic Effects of Nutrients. Nutrients that function in large doses as drugs fall logically into a separate category of pharmacologic agents (36). Nicotinic acid in large doses is used to lower serum cholesterol. This represents use of a nutrient as a drug (see Chapter 23). The effect is unrelated to its function as a vitamin required for oxidation of energy-yielding nutrients and can be achieved only by quantities that far exceed nutritional requirements or usual dietary amounts. Use of tryptophan as a sleep inducer (37) and of continuous intravenous infusions of magnesium in the treatment of preeclampsia or myocardial infarction fall into this category (38). Essential nutrients that fit this pattern are functioning as pharmacologic agents not as nutritional supplements, as are substances, such as aspirin or quinine, originally isolated from plants, that are used as medicines.

With the current state of knowledge, it is undoubtedly premature to try to resolve definitively the problems encountered in classifying food constituents that have desirable effects on health or have been implicated in disease prevention. Such actions are not related to the physiologic functions of essential nutrients. Nonetheless, even though solutions proposed at this stage must be considered tentative, an orderly resolution of questions relating to health effects of food constituents that do not fit current nutritional concepts must be started. The confusion that would be created by accommodating them through modifying the criteria for essentiality or conditional essentiality is to be avoided at all costs. They should be considered within the context of dietary guidelines for health, not as part of the scientifically based RDIs.

REFERENCES

1. Roche AF, ed. Nutritional essentiality: a changing paradigm. Report of the 12th Ross Conference on Medical Research. Columbus, OH: Ross Products Division, Abbott Laboratories, 1993.
2. Sauberlich HE, Machlin LJ, eds. Ann NY Acad Sci 1992; 669:1–404.
3. McCormick DB. The meaning of nutritional essentiality in today's context of health and disease. In: Roche AF, ed. Nutritional essentiality: a changing paradigm. Report of the 12th Ross Conference on Medical Research. Columbus, OH: Ross Products Division, Abbott Laboratories, 1993;11–15.
4. Institute of Medicine. How should recommended dietary allowances be revised? Washington, DC: National Academy Press, 1994;1–36.
5. Lachance P. Nutr Rev 1994;52:266–70.
6. Combs GF Jr. J Nutr 1996;126:2373S–6S.
7. Lusk G. Endocr Metab 1922;3:3–78.
8. Medical Research Council. Vitamins: a survey of present knowledge. London: H. M. Stationery Office, 1932;1–332.
9. McCollum EV. A history of nutrition. Boston: Houghton Mifflin, 1957.
10. Guggenheim KY. Nutrition and nutritional diseases. The evolution of concepts. Lexington, MA: DC Heath, 1981;1–378.
11. Harper AE. Nutritional essentiality: historical perspective. In: Roche AF, ed. Nutritional essentiality: a changing paradigm. Report of the 12th Ross Conference on Medical Research. Columbus, OH: Ross Products Division, Abbott Laboratories, 1993;3–11.
12. Willcock EG, Hopkins FG. J Physiol (Lond) 1906;35:88–102.
13. Maynard LA. Nutr Abstr Rev 1962;32:345–55.
14. Block RJ, Mitchell HH. Nutr Abstr Rev 1946;16:249–78.
15. Hawk PB, Oser BL, Summerson WH. Practical physiological chemistry. 13th ed. Philadelphia: Blackiston, 1954;1014–17.
16. Harper AE. J Nutr 1974;104:965–7.
17. Snyderman SE. Human amino acid metabolism. In: Velázquez A, Bourges H, eds. Genetic factors in nutrition. New York: Academic Press, 1984;269–78.
18. Rudman D, Feller A. J Am Coll Nutr 1986;5:101–6.
19. Chipponi JX, Bleier JC, Santi MT, et al. Am J Clin Nutr 1982;35;1112–16.
20. Gaull GE. J Am Coll Nutr 1986;5:121–5.
21. Hoppel C. Carnitine: conditionally essential? In: Roche AF, ed. Nutritional essentiality: a changing paradigm. Report of the 12th Ross Conference on Medical Research. Columbus, OH: Ross Products Division, Abbott Laboratories, 1993;52–7.
22. Smith RJ. Glutamine: conditionally essential? In: Roche AF, ed. Nutritional essentiality: a changing paradigm. Report of the 12th Ross Conference on Medical Research. Columbus, OH: Ross Products Division, Abbott Laboratories, 1993;46–51.
23. Scott ML. Nutrition of humans and selected animal species. New York: John Wiley & Sons, 1986;1–537.
24. National Research Council. Recommended dietary allowances. 10th ed. Washington, DC: National Academy Press, 1989.
25. Pant KC, Rogers QR, Harper AE. J Nutr 1972;102:117–30.
26. Gietzen DW. J Nutr 1993;123:610–25.
27. Hill CH. Mineral interrelationships. In: Prasad AS, ed. Trace elements in human health and disease. New York: Academic Press, 1976;281–300.
28. DuPont J, Holub BJ, Knapp HR, et al. Am J Clin Nutr 1996;63:991S–3S.
29. Gubler CJ. Thiamin. In: Machlin LJ, ed. Handbook of vitamins. New York: Marcel Dekker, 1984;245–98.
30. Mudd SH. Adv Nutr Res 1982;4:1–34.
31. Olson JA. J Nutr 1996;126:1208S–12S.
32. Jacob RA, Burri BJ. Am J Clin Nutr 1996;63:985S–90S.
33. Marlett JA. Dietary fiber: a candidate nutrient. In: Roche AF, ed. Nutritional essentiality: a changing paradigm. Report of the 12th Ross Conference on Medical Research. Columbus, OH: Ross Products Division, Abbott Laboratories, 1993;23–8.
34. Olson RE. Circulation 1994;90:2569–70.

35. Johnson IT, Williamson G, Musk SRR. Nutr Res Rev 1994;7:175–203.
36. Draper HH. J Nutr 1988;118:1420–1.
37. Hartmann EL. Effect of L-tryptophan and other amino acids on sleep. In: Diet and behavior: A multidisciplinary evaluation. Nutr Rev 1986;44(Suppl):70–3.
38. Shils ME, Rude RK. J Nutr 1996;126:2398S–403S.

SELECTED READINGS

Herbert V, ed. Symposium: prooxidant effects of antioxidant vitamins. J Nutr 1996;126(Suppl):1197S–227S.

Institute of Medicine. How should recommended dietary allowances be revised? Washington, DC: National Academy Press, 1994;1–36.

Nielsen FH, Johnson WT, Milne DB, eds. Workshop on new approaches, endpoints and paradigms for RDAs of mineral elements. J Nutr 1996;126(Suppl):2299S–495S.

Roche AF, ed. Nutritional essentiality: a changing paradigm. Report of the 12th Ross Conference on Medical Research. Columbus, OH: Ross Products Division, Abbott Laboratories, 1993.

Sauberlich HE, Machlin LJ, eds. Beyond deficiency. New views on the function and health effects of nutrients. Ann NY Acad Sci 1992;669:1–404.

2. Proteins and Amino Acids

DWIGHT E. MATTHEWS

Proteins are associated with all forms of life, and much of the effort to determine how life began has centered on how proteins were first produced. Amino acids joined together in long strings by peptide bonds form proteins, which twist and fold in three-dimensional space, producing centers to facilitate the biochemical reactions of life that either would run out of control or not run at all without them. Life could not have begun without enzymes, of which there are thousands of different types in the body. Proteins are prepared and secreted to act as cell-cell signals in the form of hormones and cytokines. Plasma proteins produced and secreted by the liver stabilize the blood by forming a solution of the appropriate viscosity and osmolarity. These secreted proteins also transport a variety of compounds through the blood.

The largest source of protein in higher animals is muscle. Through complex interactions, entire sheets of proteins slide back and forth to form the basis of muscle contraction and all aspects of our mobility. Muscle contraction provides for pumping oxygen and nutrients throughout the body, inhalation and exhalation in our lungs, and movement. Many of the underlying causes of noninfectious diseases are due to derangements in proteins. Molecular biology has provided much information about DNA and RNA, not so much to understand DNA per se, but to understand the purpose and function of the proteins that are translated from the genetic code.

Three major classes of substrates are used for energy: carbohydrate, fat, and protein. The amino acids in protein differ from the other two primary sources of dietary energy by inclusion of nitrogen (N) in their structures. Amino acids contain at least one N in the form of an amino group, and when amino acids are oxidized to CO_2 and water to produce energy, waste N is produced that must be eliminated. Conversely, when the body synthesizes amino acids, N must be available. The synthetic pathways of other N-containing compounds in the body usually require donation of N from amino acids or incorporation of amino acids per se into the compound being synthesized. Amino acids provide the N for DNA and RNA synthesis. Therefore, when we think of amino acid metabolism, we must think of N metabolism.

Protein and amino acids are also important to the energy metabolism of the body. As Cahill pointed out (1), protein is the second largest store of energy in the body after adipose tissue fat stores (Table 2.1). Carbohydrate is stored as glycogen, and while important for short-term energy needs, has very limited capacity for meeting energy needs beyond a few hours. Amino acids from protein are converted to glucose by the process called gluconeogenesis, to provide a continuing supply of glucose after the glycogen is consumed during fasting. Yet, protein stores must be conserved for numerous critical roles in the body. Loss of more than about 30% of body protein results in such reduced muscle strength for breathing, reduced immune function, and reduced organ function that death

Abbreviations: **ADP**—adenosine diphosphate; **AMP**—adenosine monophosphate; **ATP**—adenosine triphosphate; **A-V**—arteriovenous; **BCAA**—branched-chain amino acid; **GMP**—guanosine monophosphate; **IMP**—inosine monophosphate; **KIC**—α-ketoisocaproate; **mRNA**—messenger RNA; **N**—nitrogen; **PER**—protein efficiency ratio; **PRPP**—phosphoribosylpyrophosphate; **RDA**—recommended dietary allowance; **TCA**—cycle, tricarboxylic acid cycle; **TML**—trimethyllysine; **tRNA**—transfer RNA; **WHO/FAO/UNU**—World Health Organization/Food and Agriculture Organization/ United Nations University.

Table 2.1
Body Composition of a Normal Man in Terms of Energy Components

Component	Mass (kg)	Energy (kcal)	Availability[a] (days)
Body water and minerals	49	0	0
Protein	6	24,000	13
Glycogen	0.2	800	0.4
Fat	15	140,000	78
Total:	70	164,800	91.4

Data adapted from Cahill GF. N Engl J Med 1970;282:668–75.

[a]Availability is the duration for which the energy supply would last based upon an 1800 kcal/day resting energy consumption.

results. Hence, the body must adapt to fasting by conserving protein, as is seen by a dramatic decrease in N excretion within the first week of starvation.

Body protein is made up of 20 amino acids, each with different metabolic fates in the body, different activities in different metabolic pathways in different organs, and differing compositions in different proteins. When amino acids are released after absorption of dietary protein, the body makes a complex series of decisions concerning the fate of those amino acids: to oxidize them for energy, to incorporate them into proteins, or to use them in the formation of a number of other N-containing compounds. This chapter elucidates the complex pathways and roles amino acids play in the body, with a focus on nutrition. Since the inception of this book, this chapter has been authored by the late Hamish Munro, an excellent teacher who spent much of his life refining complex biochemical concepts into understandable terms. Professor Munro brought order into the apparently chaotic world of amino acid and protein metabolism through his classic four-volume series (2–5). Readers familiar with former versions of this chapter will find many of his views carried forward into the present chapter.

AMINO ACIDS

Basic Definitions

The amino acids that we are familiar with and all of those incorporated into mammalian protein are "alpha"-amino acids. By definition, they have a carboxyl-carbon group and an amino nitrogen group attached to a central α-carbon (Fig. 2.1). Amino acids differ in structure by substitution of one of the two hydrogens on the α-carbon with another functional group. Amino acids can be characterized by their functional groups, which are often classified at neutral pH as *(a)* nonpolar, *(b)* uncharged but polar, *(c)* acidic (negatively charged), and *(d)* basic (positively charged) groups.

Within any class there are considerable differences in shape and physical properties. Thus, amino acids are often arranged in other functional subgroups. For example, amino acids with an aromatic group—phenylalanine, tyrosine, tryptophan, and histidine—are often grouped, although tyrosine is clearly polar and histidine is also basic. Other common groupings are the aliphatic or neutral amino acids (glycine, alanine, isoleucine, leucine, valine, serine, threonine and proline). Proline differs in that its functional group is also attached to the amino group, forming a five-member ring. Serine and threonine contain hydroxy groups. The branched-chain amino acids (BCAAs: isoleucine, leucine, and valine) share common enzymes for the first two steps of their degradation. The acidic amino acids, aspartic acid and glutamic acid, are often referred to as their ionized, salt forms: *aspartate* and *glutamate.* These amino acids become *asparagine* and *glutamine* when an amino group is added in the form of an amide group to their carboxyl tails.

The sulfur-containing amino acids are methionine and cysteine. Cysteine is often found in the body as an amino acid dimer, *cystine,* in which the thiol groups (the two sulfur atoms) are connected to form a disulfide bond. Note the distinction between *cysteine* and *cystine*; the former is a single amino acid, and the latter is a dimer with different properties. Other amino acids that contain sulfur, such as homocysteine, are not incorporated into protein.

All amino acids are charged in solution: in water, the carboxyl group rapidly loses a hydrogen to form a carboxyl anion (negatively charged), while the amino group gains a hydrogen to become positively charged. An amino acid, therefore, becomes "bipolar" (often called a *zwitterion*) in solution, but without a net charge (the positive and negative charges cancel). However, the functional group may distort that balance. Acidic amino acids lose the hydrogen on the second carboxyl group in solution. In contrast, basic amino acids accept a hydrogen on the second N and form a molecule with a net positive charge. Although the other amino acids do not specifically accept or donate additional hydrogens in neutral solution, their functional groups do influence the relative polarity and acid-base nature of their bipolar portion, giving each amino acid different properties in solution.

The functional groups of amino acids also vary in size. The molecular weights of the amino acids are given in Table 2.2. Amino acids range from the smallest, glycine, to large and bulky molecules (e.g., tryptophan). Most amino acids crystallize as uncharged molecules when purified and dried. The molecular weights given in Table 2.2 reflect their molecular weights as crystalline amino acids. However, basic and acidic amino acids tend to form much more stable crystals as salts, rather than as free amino acids. Glutamic acid can be obtained as the free amino acid with a molecular weight of 147 and as its sodium salt, monosodium glutamate (MSG), which has a crystalline weight of 169. Lysine is typically found as a hydrogen chloride–containing salt. Therefore, when amino acids are represented by weight, it is important to know whether the weight is based on the free amino acid or on its salt.

Another important property of amino acids is optical activity. Except for glycine, which has a single hydrogen as its functional group, all amino acids have at least one chiral center: the α-carbon. The term *chiral* comes from

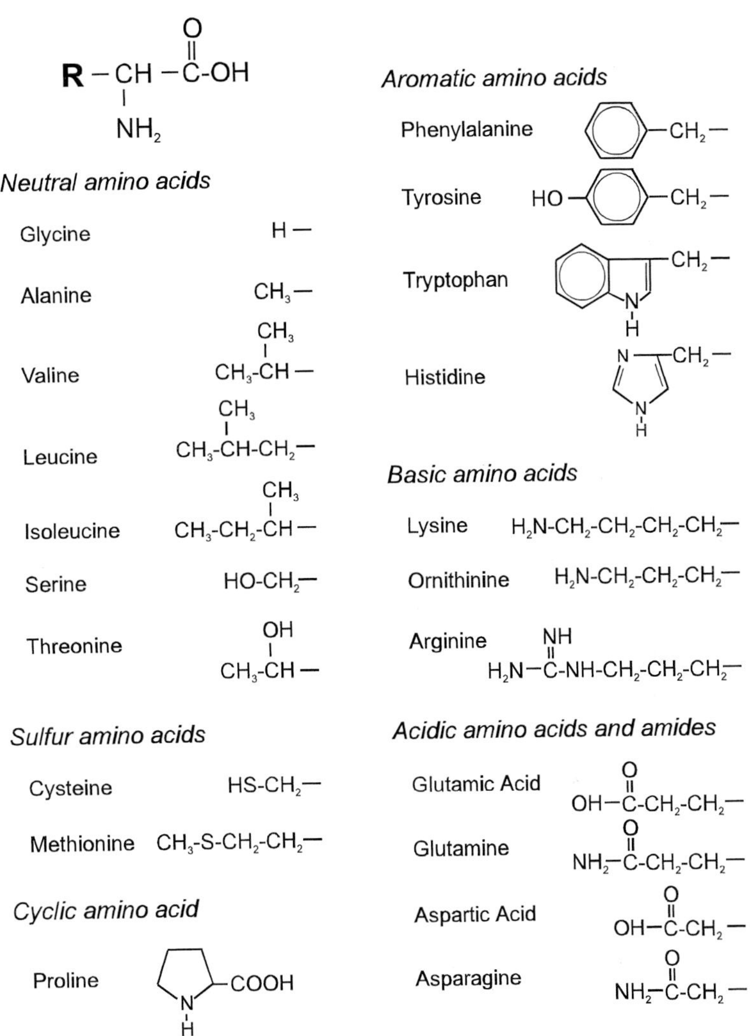

Figure 2.1. Structural formulas of the 21 common α-amino acids. The α-amino acids all have *(a)* a carboxyl group, *(b)* an amino group, and *(c)* a differentiating functional group attached to the α-carbon. The generic structure of amino acids is shown in the upper left corner with the differentiating functional marked *R*. The functional group for each amino acid is shown below. Amino acids have been grouped by functional class. Proline is the only amino acid whose entire structure is shown because of its "cyclic" nature.

Greek for *hand* in that these molecules have a left (*levo* or L) and right (*dextro* or D) handedness around the α-carbon atom. The tetrahedral structure of the carbon bonds allows two possible arrangements of a carbon center with the same four different groups bonded to it, which are not superimposable; the two configurations, called *stereoisomers*, are mirror images of each other. The body recognizes only the L form of amino acids for most reactions in the body, although some enzymatic reactions will operate with lower efficiency when given the D form. Because we do encounter some D amino acids in the foods we eat, the body has mechanisms for clearing these amino acids (e.g., renal filtration).

Any number of molecules could be designed that meet the basic definition of an amino acid: a molecule with a central carbon to which are attached an amino group, a carboxyl group, and a functional group. However, a relatively limited variety appear in nature, of which only 20 are incorporated directly into mammalian protein. Amino acids are selected for protein synthesis by binding with transfer RNA (tRNA). To synthesize protein, strands of DNA are transcribed into messenger RNA (mRNA). Different tRNA molecules bind to specific triplets of bases in mRNA. Different combinations of the 3 bases found in mRNA code for different tRNA molecules. However, the 3-base combinations of mRNA are recognized by only 20 different tRNA molecules, and 20 different amino acids are incorporated into protein during protein synthesis.

Of the 20 amino acids in proteins, some are synthesized de novo in the body from either other amino acids or simpler precursors. These amino acids may be deleted from our diet without impairing health or blocking growth; they are *nonessential* and *dispensable* from the diet. However, several amino acids have no synthetic pathways in humans; hence these amino acids are *essential* or *indispensable* to the diet. Table 2.2 lists the amino acids as essential or nonessential for humans. Both the standard 3-letter abbreviation and the 1-letter abbreviation used in representing amino acid sequences in proteins are also presented in Table 2.2 for each amino acid. Some nonessential amino

Table 2.2
Common Amino Acids in the Body

	Standard Abbreviation		
Molecular	3-Letter	1-Letter	Weight[a]
Essential amino acids			
Isoleucine	Ile	I	131
Leucine	Leu	L	131
Lysine	Lys	K	146
Methionine	Met	M	149
Phenylalanine	Phe	F	165
Threonine	Thr	T	119
Tryptophan	Trp	W	204
Valine	Val	V	117
Histidine[b]	His	H	155
Nonessential amino acids			
Alanine	Ala	A	89
Arginine	Arg	R	174
Aspartic acid	Asp	D	133
Asparagine	Asn	N	132
Glutamic acid	Glu	E	147
Glutamine	Gln	Q	146
Glycine	Gly	G	75
Proline	Pro	P	115
Serine	Ser	S	105
Conditionally essential amino acids			
Cysteine	Cys	C	121
Tyrosine	Tyr	Y	181
Some special amino acids			
Alloisoleucine	*a*Ile		131
Citrulline			175
Homocysteine			135
Hydroxylysine	Hyl		162
Hydroxyproline	Hyp		131
3-Methylhistidine			169
Ornithine	Orn		132

[a]Molecular weight is rounded to the nearest whole number and represents the number of grams per mole of amino acid. Because glutamine is degraded to glutamate when proteins are hydrolyzed, the sum of the glutamine and glutamate together is often abbreviated *Glx*. The same is true also for the sum of asparagine and aspartate: *Asx*. The 1-letter abbreviations are often used to indicate protein sequences.

[b]The essentiality for histidine has only been shown for infants, but probably small amounts are needed for adults as well (8).

acids may become *conditionally essential* under conditions when synthesis becomes limited or when adequate amounts of precursors are unavailable to meet the needs of the body (6–8). The history and rationale of the classification of amino acids in Table 2.2 is discussed in greater detail below.

Beside the 20 amino acids that are recognized by, and bind to, tRNA for incorporation into protein, other amino acids appear commonly in the body. These amino acids have important metabolic functions. For example, ornithine and citrulline are linked to arginine through the urea cycle. Other amino acids appear as modifications after incorporation into proteins; for example, hydroxyproline, produced when proline residues in collagen protein are hydroxylated, and 3-methylhistidine, produced by posttranslational methylation of select histidine residues of actin and myosin. Because no tRNA codes for these amino acids, they cannot be reused when a protein containing them is broken down (hydrolyzed) to its individual amino acids.

Amino Acid Pools and Distribution

The distribution of amino acids is complex. Not only are there 20 different amino acids incorporated into a variety of different proteins in a variety of different organs in the body, but amino acids are consumed in the diet from a variety of protein sources. In addition, each amino acid is maintained in part as a free amino acid in solution in blood and inside cells. Overall, a wide range of concentrations of amino acids exists across the various protein and free pools. Dietary protein is enzymatically hydrolyzed in the alimentary tract, releasing free individual amino acids that are then absorbed by the gut lumen and transported into the portal blood. Amino acids then pass into the systemic circulation and are extracted by different tissues. Although the concentrations of individual amino acids vary among different free pools such as plasma and intracellular muscle, the abundance of individual amino acids is relatively constant in a variety of proteins throughout the body and nature. Table 2.3 shows the amino acid composition of egg protein and muscle and liver proteins (9). The data are expressed as *moles* of amino acid. The historical expression of amino acids is on a weight basis (e.g., *grams* of amino acid). Comparing amino acids by weight skews the comparison toward the heaviest amino acids, making them appear more abundant than they are. For example, tryptophan (molecular weight, 204) appears almost three times as abundant as glycine (molecular weight, 75) when quoted in terms of weight.

An even distribution of all 20 amino acids would be 5% per amino acid, and the median distribution of individual amino acids centers around this figure for the proteins shown in Table 2.3. Tryptophan is the least common

Table 2.3
Amino Acid Concentrations in Muscle and Liver Protein and in High-Quality Egg Protein

	Composition (μmol/g protein)		
		Mammalian	
Amino Acid	Hen Egg	Muscle	Liver
Alanine	810	730	750
Arginine	360	380	328
Aspartate + asparagine	530	600	600
Cysteine	190	120	140
Glutamate + glutamine	810	990	800
Glycine	450	670	610
Histidine	150	180	170
Isoleucine	490	360	380
Leucine	650	610	690
Lysine	425	580	510
Methionine	200	170	170
Phenylalanine	340	270	310
Proline	350	430	430
Serine	770	480	510
Threonine	410	390	390
Tryptophan	80	55	80
Tyrosine	220	170	200
Valine	600	470	520

Data taken from Tables V and VII (pp. 343–4) of Block RJ, Weiss KW. Amino acid handbook: methods and results of analysis. Springfield, IL: Charles C Thomas, 1956.

amino acid in many proteins, but considering the effect of its large size on protein configuration, this is not surprising. Amino acids of modest size and limited polarity such as alanine, leucine, serine, and valine are relatively abundant in protein (8–10% each). While the abundance of the essential amino acids is similar across the protein sources in Table 2.3, a variety of vegetable proteins are deficient or low in some essential amino acids. In the body, a variety of proteins are particularly rich in specific amino acids that confer specific attributes to the protein. For example, collagen is a fibrous protein abundant in connective tissues and tendons, bone, and muscle. Collagen fibrils are arranged differently depending on the functional type of collagen. Glycine makes up about one-third of collagen, and there is also considerable proline and hydroxyproline (proline converted after it has been incorporated into collagen). The glycine and proline residues allow the collagen protein chain to turn tightly and intertwine, and the hydroxyproline residues provide for hydrogen-bond cross-linking. Generally, the alterations in amino acid concentrations do not vary so dramatically among proteins as they do in collagen, but such examples demonstrate the diversity and functionality of the different amino acids in proteins.

The abundance of different amino acids varies over a far wider range in the free pools of extracellular and intracellular compartments. Typical values for free amino acid concentrations in plasma and intracellular muscle are given in Table 2.4, which shows that amino acid concentrations vary widely in a given tissue and that free amino acids are generally inside cells. Although there is a significant correlation between free amino acid levels in plasma and muscle, the relationship is not linear (10). Amino acid concentrations range from a low of ≈20 μM for aspartic acid and methionine to a high of ≈500 μM for glutamine. The median level for plasma amino acids is 100 μM. There is no defined relationship between the nature of amino acids (essential vs. nonessential) and amino acid concentrations or type of amino acids (e.g., plasma concentrations of the three BCAAs range from 50 to 250 μM). Notably, the concentration of the acidic amino acids, aspartate and glutamate, is very low outside cells in plasma. In contrast, the concentration of glutamate is among the highest inside cells, such as muscle (Table 2.4).

It is important to bear in mind the differences in the relative amounts of N contained in extracellular and intracellular amino acid pools and in protein itself. A normal person has about 55 mg amino acid N/L outside cells in extracellular space and about 800 mg amino acid N/L inside cells, which means that free amino acids are about 15 times more abundant inside cells than outside (10). Furthermore, the total pool of free amino acid N is small compared with protein-bound amino acids. Multiplying the free pools by estimates of extracellular water (0.2 L/kg) and intracellular water (0.4 L/kg) provides a measure of the total amount of N present in free amino acids: 0.33 g N/kg body weight. In contrast, body composition studies show that the N content of the body is 24 g N/kg body weight (11, 12). Thus, free amino acids make up only about 1% of the total amino N pool, with 99% of the amino N being protein bound.

Table 2.4
Typical Concentrations of Free Amino Acids in the Body

Amino acid[a]		Concentration (mM) Plasma	Intracellular Muscle	Gradient Intracellular/Plasma
Aspartic acid	NE	0.02		
Phenylalanine	E	0.05	0.07	1.4
Tyrosine	CE	0.05	0.10	2.0
Methionine	E	0.02	0.11	5.5
Isoleucine	E	0.06	0.11	1.8
Leucine	E	0.12	0.15	1.3
Cysteine	CE	0.11	0.18	1.6
Valine	E	0.22	0.26	1.2
Ornithine		0.06	0.30	5.0
Histidine	E	0.08	0.37	4.6
Asparagine	NE	0.05	0.47	9.4
Arginine	NE	0.08	0.51	6.4
Proline	NE	0.17	0.83	4.9
Serine	NE	0.12	0.98	8.2
Threonine	E	0.15	1.03	6.9
Lysine	E	0.18	1.15	6.4
Glycine	NE	0.21	1.33	6.3
Alanine	NE	0.33	2.34	7.1
Glutamic acid	NE	0.06	4.38	73.0
Glutamine	NE	0.57	19.45	34.1
Taurine[b]		0.07	15.44	221.0

Data from Bergström J, Fürst P, Noree LO, et al. J Appl Physiol 1974;36:693–7.
[a]E, essential; NE, nonessential; CE, conditionally essential.
[b]Taurine is not an amino acid per se but is highly concentrated in free form in muscle.

Amino Acid Transport

The gradient of amino acids within and outside cells is maintained by active transport. Simple inspection of Table 2.4 shows that different transport mechanisms must exist for different amino acids to produce the range of concentration gradients observed. A variety of different transporters exist for different types and groups of amino acids (13–16). Amino acid transport is probably one of the more difficult areas of amino acid metabolism to quantify and characterize. The affinities of the transporters and their mechanisms of transport determine the intracellular levels of the amino acids. Generally, the essential amino acids have lower intracellular/extracellular gradients than do the nonessential amino acids (Table 2.4), and they are transported by different carriers. Amino acid transporters are membrane-bound proteins that recognize different amino acid shapes and chemical properties (e.g., neutral, basic, or anionic). Transport occurs both into and out of cells. Transport may be thought of as a process that sets the intracellular/extracellular gradient, or the transporters may be thought of as processes that set the rates of amino acid cellular influx and efflux, which then define the intracellular/extracellular gradients (13). Perhaps the more dynamic concept of transport defining flows of amino acids is more appropriate, but the gradient (e.g., intracellular muscle amino acid levels) is measurable, not the rates.

The transporters fall into two classes: sodium-independent and sodium-dependent carriers. The sodium-dependent carriers cotransport a sodium atom into the cell with the amino acid. The high extracellular/intracellular sodium gradient (140 mEq outside and 10 mEq inside) facilitates inward transport of amino acids by the sodium-dependent carriers. These transporters generally produce larger gradients and accumulations of amino acids inside cells than outside. The sodium entering the cell may be transported out via the sodium-potassium pump, which transports a potassium ion in for the removal of a sodium ion.

Few transporter proteins have been identified; most information concerning transport results from kinetic studies of membranes using amino acids and competitive inhibitors or amino acid analogues to define and characterize individual systems. Table 2.5 lists the amino acid transporters characterized to date and the amino acids they transport. The neutral and bulky amino acids (the BCAAs, phenylalanine, methionine, and histidine) are transported by system *L*. System *L* is sodium independent, operates with a high rate of exchange, and produces small gradients. Other important transporters are systems *ASC* and *A*, which use the energy available from the sodium ion gradient as a driving force to maintain a steep gradient for the various amino acids transported (e.g., glycine, alanine, threonine, serine, and proline) (13, 14). The anionic transporter (X_{AG-}) also produces a steep gradient for the dicarboxylic amino acids, glutamate and aspartate. Other important carriers are systems *N* and N^m for glutamine, asparagine, and histidine. System y^+ handles much of the transport of the basic amino acids. Some overall generalizations can be made in terms of the type of amino acid transported by a given carrier, but the system is not readily simplified because individual carrier systems transport several different amino acids, and individual amino acids are often transported by several different carriers with different efficiencies. Thus, amino acid gradients are formed and amino acids are transported into and out of cells via a complex system of overlapping carriers.

Table 2.5
Amino Acid Transporters

System	Amino Acid Transported	Tissue Location	pH Dependence
Sodium dependent			
A	Most neutrals (Ala, Ser)	Ubiquitous	Yes
ASC	Most neutrals	Ubiquitous	No
B	Most neutrals	Intestinal brush border	Yes
N	Gln, Asn, His	Hepatocytes	Yes
N^m	Gln, Asn	Muscle	No
Gly	Gly, sarcosine	Ubiquitous	
X_{AG-}	Glu, Asp	Ubiquitous	
Sodium independent			
L	Leu, Ile, Val, Met, Phe, Tyr, Trp, His	Ubiquitous	Yes
T	Trp, Phe, Tyr	Red blood cells, hepatocytes	No
y^+	Arg, Lys, Orn	Ubiquitous	No
asc	Ala, Ser, Cys, Thr	Ubiquitous	Yes

Data taken from compilations in refs. 13–15.

PATHWAYS OF AMINO ACID SYNTHESIS AND DEGRADATION

Several amino acids have their metabolic pathways linked to the metabolism of other amino acids. These codependencies become important when nutrient intake is limited or when metabolic requirements are increased. Two aspects of metabolism are reviewed here: the synthesis only of nonessential amino acids and the degradation of all amino acids. Degradation serves two useful purposes: *(a)* production of energy from the oxidation of individual amino acids (≈4 kcal/g protein, almost the same energy production as for carbohydrate) and *(b)* conversion of amino acids into other products. The latter is also related to amino acid synthesis; the degradation pathway of one amino acid may be the synthetic pathway of another amino acid. Amino acid degradation also produces other non–amino acid, N-containing compounds in the body. The need for synthesis of these compounds may also drain the pools of their amino acid precursors, increasing the need for these amino acids in the diet. When amino acids are degraded for energy rather than converted to other compounds, the ultimate products are CO_2, water, and urea. The CO_2 and water are produced through classical pathways of intermediary metabolism involving the tricarboxylic acid cycle (TCA cycle). Urea is produced because other forms of waste N, such as ammonia, are toxic if their levels rise in the blood and inside cells. For mammals, urea production is a means of removing waste N from the oxidation of amino acids in the form of a nontoxic, water-soluble compound.

This section discusses the pathways of amino acid metabolism. In all cases, much better and more detailed descriptions of the pathways can be found in standard textbooks of biochemistry. One caveat to the reader consulting such texts for reference information: mammals are not the only form of life. Several texts cover subject matter beyond mammalian systems and present material for pathways that are of little importance to human biochemistry. When consulting reference material, the reader needs to be aware of what organism contains the metabolic pathways and enzymes being discussed. The discussion below concerns human biochemistry. First, the routes of degradation of each amino acid when the pathway is directed toward oxidation of the amino acid for energy are discussed, then pathways of amino acid synthesis, and finally use of amino acids for other important compounds in the body.

Amino Acid Degradation Pathways

Complete amino acid degradation produces nitrogen, which is removed by incorporation into urea. Carbon skeletons are eventually oxidized to CO_2 via the TCA cycle. The TCA cycle (also known as the Krebs cycle or the citric acid cycle) oxidizes carbon for energy, producing CO_2 and water. The inputs to the cycle are acetyl-CoA and oxaloacetate forming citrate, which is degraded to α-ketoglutarate and then to oxaloacetate. Carbon skeletons from amino acids may enter the Krebs cycle via acetate as acetyl-CoA or via oxaloacetate/α-ketoglutarate, direct metabolites of the amino acids aspartate and glutamate, respectively. An alternative to complete oxidation of the carbon skeletons to CO_2 is the use of these carbon skeletons for formation of fat and carbohydrate. Fat is formed from elongation of acetyl units, and so amino acids whose carbon skeletons degrade to acetyl-CoA and ketones may alternatively be used for synthesis of fatty acids. Glucose is split in glycolysis to pyruvate, the immediate product of alanine. Pyruvate may be converted back to glucose by elongation to oxaloacetate. Amino acids whose degradation pathways go toward formation of pyruvate, oxaloacetate, or α-ketoglutarate may be used for glucose synthesis. Thus, the degradation pathways of many amino acids can be partitioned into two groups with respect to the disposal of their carbon: amino acids whose carbon skeleton may be used for synthesis of glucose (gluconeogenic amino acids) and those whose carbon skeletons degrade for potential use for fatty acid synthesis.

The amino acids that degrade directly to the primary gluconeogenic and TCA cycle precursors, pyruvate, oxaloacetate, and α-ketoglutarate, do so by rapid and reversible transamination reactions:

L-glutamate + oxaloacetate ↔ α-ketoglutarate + L-aspartate

(catalyzed by the enzyme aspartate aminotransferase) which of course is also

L-aspartate + α-ketoglutarate ↔ oxaloacetate + L-glutamate

and

L-alanine + α-ketoglutarate ↔ pyruvate + L-glutamate

is catalyzed by the enzyme alanine aminotransferase. Clearly, the amino N of these three amino acids can be rapidly exchanged, and each amino acid can be rapidly converted to/from a primary compound of gluconeogenesis and the TCA cycle. As shown below, compartmentation among different organ pools is the only limiting factor for complete and rapid exchange of the N of these amino acids.

The essential amino acids leucine, isoleucine, and valine are grouped together as the BCAAs because the first two steps in their degradation are common to all three amino acids:

$$\left.\begin{array}{r}\text{Leucine}\\ \text{Isoleucine}\\ \text{Valine}\end{array}\right\} \begin{array}{c}+\ \alpha\text{-ketoglutarate}\\ \leftrightarrow \text{glutamate} +\end{array} \left\{\begin{array}{l}\alpha\text{-ketoisocaproate}\\ \alpha\text{-keto-}\beta\text{-methylvalerate}\\ \alpha\text{-ketoisovalerate}\end{array}\right.$$

The reversible transamination to keto acids is followed by irreversible decarboxylation of the carboxyl group to liberate CO_2. The BCAAs are the only essential amino acids that undergo transamination and thus are unique among essential amino acids.

Together, the BCAAs, alanine, aspartate, and glutamate make up the pool of amino N that can move among amino acids via reversible transamination. As shown in Figure 2.2, glutamic acid is central to the transamination process. In addition, N can leave the transaminating pool via removal of the glutamate N by glutamate dehydrogenase or enter by the reverse process. The amino acid glutamine is intimately tied to glutamate as well; all glutamine is made from amidation of glutamate, and glutamine is degraded by removal of the amide N to form ammonia and glutamate. A similar process links asparagine and aspartate. Figure 2.2 shows that the center of N flow in the body is through glutamate. This role becomes even clearer when we look at how urea is synthesized in the liver. CO_2, ATP, and NH_3 enter the urea cycle to form carbamoyl phosphate, which condenses with ornithine to form citrulline (Fig. 2.3). The second N enters via aspartate to form arginosuccinate, which is then cleaved into arginine and fumarate. The arginine is hydrolyzed by arginase to ornithine, liberating urea. The resulting ornithine can reenter the urea cycle. As is mentioned briefly below, some amino acids may release ammonia directly (e.g., glutamine, asparagine, and glycine), but most transfer through glutamate first, which is then degraded to α-ketoglutarate and ammonia. The pool of aspartate in the body is small, and aspartate cannot be the primary transporter of the second N into urea synthesis. Rather, aspartate must act as arginine and ornithine do, as a vehicle for the introduction of the second N. If so, the second N is delivered by transamination via glutamate, which places glutamate at another integral point in the degradative disposal of amino acid N.

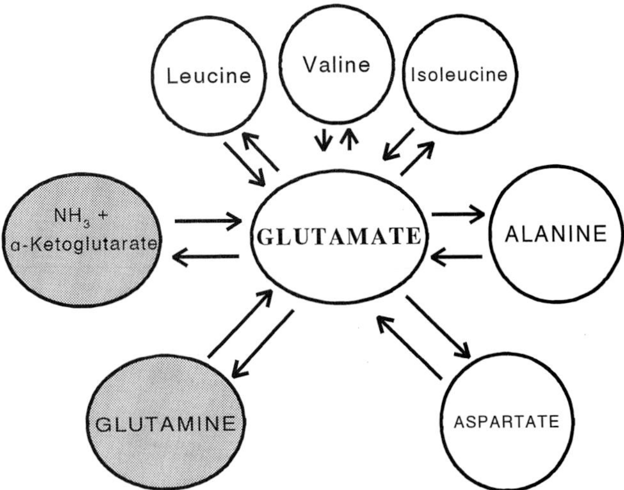

Figure 2.2. Movement of amino N around glutamic acid. Glutamate undergoes reversible transamination with several amino acids. Nitrogen is also removed from glutamate by glutamate dehydrogenase, producing α-ketoglutarate and ammonia. In contrast, the enzyme glutamine synthetase adds ammonia to glutamate to produce glutamine. Glutamine is degraded to glutamate by liberation of the amide N to release ammonia by a different enzymatic pathway (glutaminase).

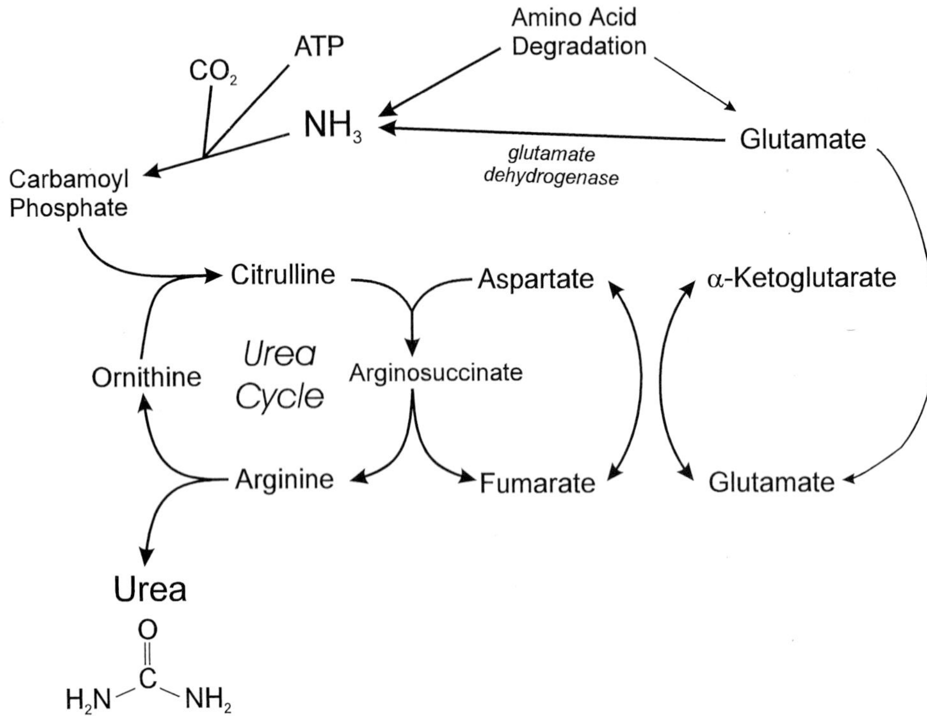

Figure 2.3. Urea cycle disposal of amino acid N. Urea synthesis incorporates one N from ammonia and another from aspartate. Ornithine, citrulline, and arginine sit in the middle of the cycle. Glutamate is the primary source for the aspartate N; glutamate is also an important source of the ammonia in the cycle.

An outline of the degradative pathways of the various amino acids is presented in Table 2.6. Rather than show individual reaction steps, the major pathways for degradation, including the primary endproducts, are presented. The individual steps may be found in textbooks of biochemistry or in reviews of the subject such as the very good chapter by Krebs (17). Because of the importance of transamination, most of the N from amino acid degradation appears via N transfer to α-ketoglutarate to form glutamate. In some cases, the aminotransferase catalyzes the transamination reaction with glutamate bidirectionally, as indicated in Figure 2.2, and these enzymes are distributed in many tissues. In other cases, the transamination reactions are liver specific and compartmentalized and specifically degrade, rather than reversibly exchange, nitrogen. For example, when leucine labeled with the stable isotopic tracer ^{15}N was infused into dogs for 9 hours, considerable amounts of ^{15}N were found in circulating glutamine, glutamate, alanine, the other two BCAAs, but not tyrosine (18, 19), indicating that the transamination of tyrosine was minimal.

Another reason why the entries in Table 2.6 do not show individual steps is that the specific metabolic pathways of all the amino acids are not clearly defined. For example, two pathways for cysteine are shown. Both are active, but how much cysteine is metabolized by which pathway is not as clear. Methionine is metabolized by conversion to homocysteine. The homocysteine is not directly converted to cysteine; rather, homocysteine condenses with a serine to form cystathionine, which is then split into

Table 2.6
Pathways of Amino Acid Degradation

Metabolic Pathway	*Important Enzymes*	Nitrogen End-Products	Carbon End-Products
Amino acids converted to other amino acids			
Asparagine	*Asparaginase*	Aspartate	$+NH_3$
Glutamine	*Glutaminase*	Glutamate	$+NH_3$
Arginine	*Arginase*	Ornithine	+Urea
Phenylalanine	*Phenylalanine hydroxylase*	Tyrosine	
Proline		Glutamate	
Cysteine		Taurine	
Transamination to form glutamate			
Alanine		Glutamate	Pyruvate
Aspartate		Glutamate	Oxaloacetate
Leucine		Glutamate	Ketones
Isoleucine		Glutamate	Succinate
Valine		Glutamate	Succinate
Ornithine		2 Glutamates	α-Ketoglutarate
Tyrosine		Glutamate	Ketone + fumarate
Cysteine		Glutamate	Pyruvate + SO_4^{-2}
Other pathways			
Serine	*Serine dehydratase*	NH_3	Pyruvate
Threonine	*Serine dehydratase*	NH_3	Ketobutyrate
Histidine	*Histidase*	NH_3	Urocanate
Tryptophan		NH_3	Kynurenine
Glycine		NH_3	CO_2
Methionine		NH_3	Ketobutyrate
Lysine		2 Glutamates	Acetate

cysteine, ammonia, and ketobutyrate. However, the original methionine molecule appears as ammonia and ketobutyrate; the cysteine carbon skeleton comes from the serine. So the entry in Table 2.6 shows methionine degraded to ammonia, yet this degradation pathway is the major synthetic pathway for cysteine. Because of the importance of the sulfur-containing amino acids (20), a more extensive discussion of the metabolic pathways of these amino acids may be found in Chapters 27 and 34.

Glycine is degraded by more than one possible pathway, depending upon the text you consult. However, the primary pathway appears to be the glycine cleavage enzyme system that breaks glycine into CO_2 and ammonia and transfers a methylene group to tetrahydrofolate (21). This is the predominant pathway in rat liver and in other vertebrate species (22). Although this reaction degrades glycine, its importance is the production of a methylene group that can be used in other metabolic reactions.

Synthesis of Nonessential Amino Acids

The essential amino acids are those that cannot be synthesized in sufficient amounts in the body and so must be supplied in the diet in sufficient amounts to meet the body's needs. Therefore, discussion of amino acid synthesis applies only to the nonessential amino acids. Nonessential amino acids fall into two groups on the basis of their synthesis: *(a)* amino acids that are synthesized by transferring a nitrogen to a carbon skeleton precursor that has come from the TCA cycle or from glycolysis of glucose and *(b)* amino acids synthesized specifically from other amino acids. Because this latter group of amino acids depends upon the availability of other specific amino acids, they are particularly vulnerable to becoming essential if the dietary supply of a precursor amino acid becomes limiting. In contrast, the former group is rarely rate limited in synthesis because of the ample precursor availability of carbon skeletons from the TCA cycle and from the labile amino-N pool of transaminating amino acids.

The pathways of nonessential amino acid synthesis are shown in Figure 2.4. As with amino acid degradation, glutamate is central to the synthesis of several amino acids by providing the N. Glutamate, alanine, and aspartate may share amino-N transaminating back and forth among them (Fig. 2.2). As Figure 2.4 is drawn, glutamate derives its N from ammonia with α-ketoglutarate, and that glutamate goes on to promote the synthesis of other amino acids. Under most circumstances, the transaminating amino acids shown in Figure 2.2 supply more than adequate amino N to glutamate. The transaminating amino acids provide a buffer pool of N that can absorb an increase in N from increased degradation or supply N when there is a drain. From this pool, glutamate provides material to maintain synthesis of ornithine and proline, the latter particularly important in synthesis of collagen and related proteins.

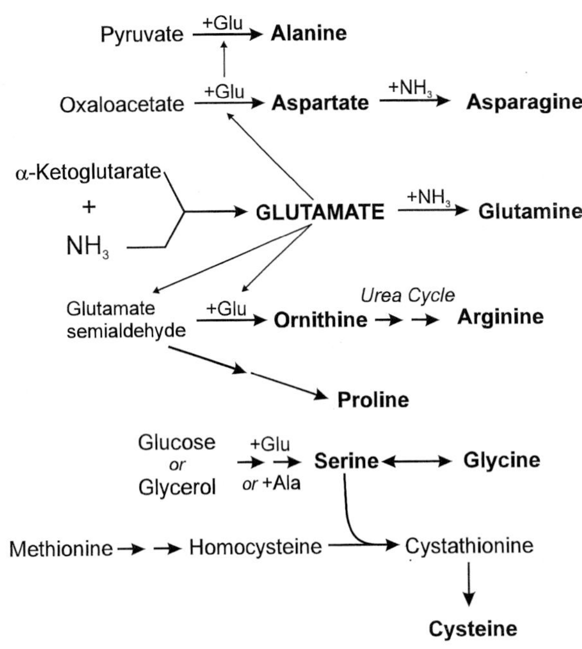

Figure 2.4. Pathways of synthesis of nonessential amino acids. Glutamate is produced from ammonia and α-ketoglutarate. That glutamate becomes the N source added to carbon precursors (pyruvate, oxaloacetate, glycolysis products of glucose, and glycerol) to form most of the other nonessential amino acids. Cysteine and tyrosine are different in that they require essential amino acid input for their production.

Serine may be produced from hydroxypyruvate derived either from glycolysis of glucose or from glycerol. Serine may then be used to produce glycine through a process that transfers a methylene group to tetrahydrofolate. This pathway could (and probably should) have been listed in Table 2.6 as a degradative pathway for serine. However, it is not usually considered an important means of degrading serine but as a source of glycine and one-carbon-unit generation (21, 22). On the other hand, the pathway backward from glycine to serine is also quite active in humans. When [^{15}N]glycine is given orally, the primary transfer of ^{15}N is to serine (23). Therefore, there is significant reverse synthesis of serine from glycine. The other major place where ^{15}N appeared was in glutamate and glutamine, indicating that the ammonia released by glycine oxidation is immediately picked up and incorporated into glutamate and the transaminating-N pool.

All of the amino acids shown in Figure 2.4 have *active* routes of synthesis in the body (17), in contrast to the essential amino acids for which no routes of synthesis exist in humans. This statement should be a simple definition of "essential" versus "nonessential." However, in nutrition, we define a "nonessential" amino acid as an amino acid that is *dispensable* from the diet (7). This definition is different from defining the presence or absence of enzymatic pathways for an amino acid's synthesis. For example, two of the nonessential amino acids depend upon degradation of essential amino acids for their production: cysteine and tyrosine. Although serine provides the carbon skeleton and amino group of cysteine, methionine provides the sulfur through condensation of homocysteine and serine to form cystathionine (20). The above discussion explains why neither the carbon skeleton nor amino group of serine are likely to be in short supply, but provision of sulfur from methionine may become limiting. Therefore, cysteine synthesis depends heavily upon the availability of the essential amino acid methionine. The same is true for tyrosine. Tyrosine is produced by hydroxylation of phenylalanine, which is also *the* degradative pathway of phenylalanine. The availability of tyrosine is strictly dependent upon the availability of phenylalanine and the liver's ability to perform the hydroxylation.

Incorporation of Amino Acids into Other Compounds

Table 2.7 lists some of the important products made from amino acids, directly or in part. The list is not inclusive and is meant to highlight important compounds in the body that depend upon amino acids for their synthesis. Amino acids are also used for the synthesis of taurine (20, 24, 25), the "amino acid–like" 2-aminoethanesulfonate found in far higher concentrations inside skeletal muscle than any amino acid (10). Glutathione, another important sulfur-containing compound (26, 27), is composed of glycine, cysteine, and glutamate.

Carnitine (28, 29) is important in the transport of long-chain fatty acids across the mitochondrial membrane before fatty acids can be oxidized. Carnitine is synthesized from ϵ-*N,N,N*-trimethyllysine (TML) (30). TML synthesis from free lysine has not been demonstrated in mammalian systems; rather TML appears to arise from methylation of peptide-linked lysine. The TML is released when proteins containing the TML are broken down (30). TML can also arise from hydrolysis of ingested meats. In contrast to 3-methylhistidine, TML can be found in proteins of both muscle and other organs such as liver (31). In rat muscle, TML is about one-eighth as abundant as 3-methylhistidine. Using comparisons of 3-methylhistidine to TML concentration in muscle protein and rates of 3-methylhistidine release in the rat (32), Rebouche estimated that protein breakdown in a rat would release about 2 μmol/day of TML, which could be used for the estimated 3 μmol/day of carnitine synthesized (30). These calculations suggest that carnitine requirements can be met from synthesis from TML from protein plus the carnitine from dietary intake.

Amino acids are the precursors for a variety of neurotransmitters that contain N. Glutamate may be an exception in that it is both a precursor for neurotransmitter production and is a primary neurotransmitter itself (33). Glutamate appears important in a variety of neurologic disorders from amyotrophic lateral sclerosis to Alzheimer's disease (34). Tyrosine is the precursor for catecholamine synthesis. Tryptophan is the precursor for serotonin synthesis. A variety of studies have reported the importance of plasma concentrations of these and other amino acids upon the synthesis of their neurotransmitter products; most commonly cited relationship is the increase in brain serotonin levels with administration of tryptophan.

Table 2.7
Important Products Synthesized from Amino Acids

Amino Acid	Incorporated Into
Arginine	Creatine
Aspartate	Purines and pyrimidines
Cysteine	Glutathione
	Taurine
Glutamate	Neurotransmitters
Glutamine	Purines and pyrimidines
Glycine	Creatine
	Porphryins (hemoglobin and cytochromes)
	Purines
Histidine	Histamine
Lysine	Carnitine
Methionine	One-carbon methylation/transfer reactions
	Creatine
	Choline
Serine	One-carbon methylation/transfer reactions
	Ethanolamine and choline
Tyrosine	Neurotransmitters
Tryptophan	Neurotransmitters

Creatine and Creatinine

Most of the creatine in the body is found in muscle, where it exists primarily as creatine phosphate. When muscular work is performed, creatine phosphate provides the energy through hydrolysis of its "high-energy" phosphate bond, forming creatine with transferal of the phosphate to form an ATP. The reaction is reversible and catalyzed by the enzyme ATP-creatine transphosphorylase (also known as creatine phosphokinase).

The original pathways of creatine synthesis from amino acid precursors were defined by Bloch and Schoenheimer in an elegant series of experiments using ^{15}N-labeled compounds (35). Creatine is synthesized outside muscle in a two-step process (Fig. 2.5). The first step occurs in the kidney and involves transfer of the guanidino group of arginine onto the amino group of glycine to form ornithine and guanidinoacetate. Methylation of the guanidinoacetate occurs in the liver via *S*-adenosylmethionine to create creatine. Although glycine donates a nitrogen and carbon backbone to creatine, arginine must be available to provide the guanidino group, as well as methionine to donate the methyl group. Creatine is then transferred to muscle where it is phosphorylated. When creatine phosphate is hydrolyzed to creatine in muscle, most of the creatine is rephosphorylated when ATP requirements are reduced, to restore the creatine phosphate supply. However, some of the muscle creatine pool is continually dehydrated by a nonenzymatic process forming creatinine. Creatinine is

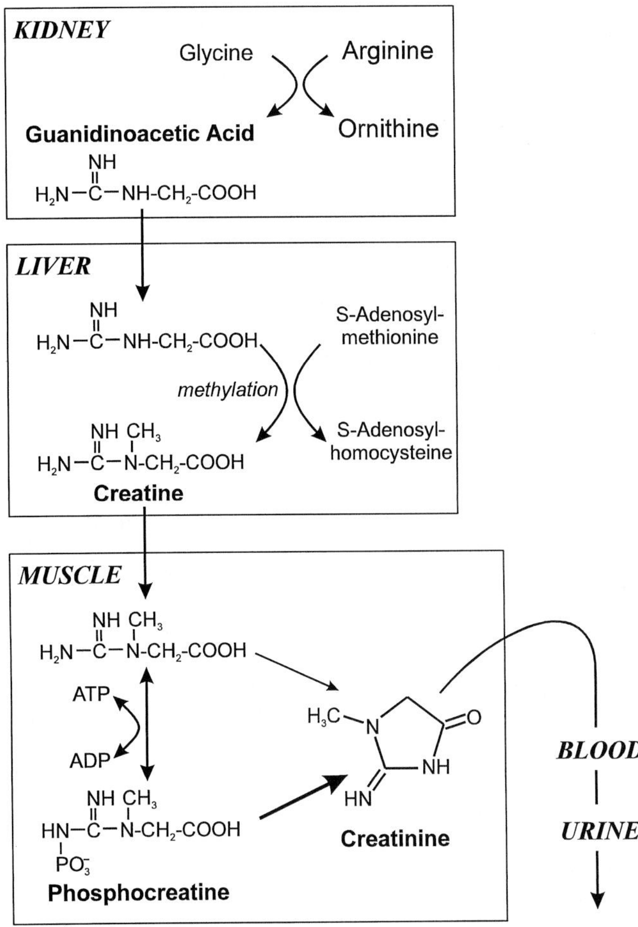

Figure 2.5. Synthesis of creatine and creatinine. Creatine is synthesized in the liver from guanidinoacetic acid synthesized in the kidney. Creatine taken up by muscle is primarily converted to phosphocreatine. Although there is some, limited direct dehydration of creatine directly to creatinine, most creatinine comes from dehydration of phosphocreatine. Creatinine is rapidly filtered by the kidney into urine.

not retained by muscle but is released into body water, removed by the kidney from blood, and excreted into urine (36).

The daily rate of creatinine formation is remarkably constant ($\approx$1.7% of the total creatine pool per day) and dependent upon the size of the creatine/creatine-phosphate pool, which is proportional to muscle mass (37). Thus, daily urinary output of creatinine has been used as a measure of total muscle mass in the body. Urinary creatinine excretion increases within a few days after a dietary creatine load, and several more days are required after removal of creatine from the diet before urinary creatinine excretion returns to baseline, indicating that creatine in the diet per se affects creatinine production (38). Therefore, consumption of creatine and creatinine in meat-containing foods increases urinary creatinine measurements. Although urinary creatinine measurements have been used primarily to estimate the adequacy of 24-hour urine collections, with adequate control of food composition and intake, creatinine excretion measurements are useful and accurate indices of body muscle mass (39, 40), especially when the alternatives are much more difficult and expensive radiometric approaches.

Purine and Pyrimidine Biosynthesis

The purines (adenine and guanine) and the pyrimidines (uracil and cytosine) are involved in many intracellular reactions when high-energy di- and triphosphates have been added. These compounds also form the building blocks of DNA and RNA. Purines are heterocyclic double-ring compounds synthesized with phosphoribosylpyrophosphate (PRPP) sugar as a base to which the amide N of glutamine is added, followed by attachment of a glycine molecule, a methylene group from tetrahydrofolate, and an amide N from another glutamine to form the imidazole ring. Then CO_2 is added, followed by the amino N of aspartic acid and another carbon to form the final ring to produce inosine monophosphate (IMP)—a purine attached to a ribose phosphate sugar. The other purines, adenine and guanine, are formed from inosine monophosphate by addition of a glutamine amide N or aspartate amino N to make guanosine monophosphate (GMP) or adenosine monophosphate (AMP), respectively. These compounds can be phosphorylated to high–energy di- and triphosphate forms: ADP, ATP, GDP, and GTP.

In contrast to purines, pyrimidines are not synthesized after attachment to a ribose sugar. The amide N of glutamine is condensed with CO_2 to form carbamoyl phosphate, which is further condensed with aspartic acid to make orotic acid—the pyrimidine's heterocyclic 6-member ring. The enzyme forming carbamoyl phosphate is present in many tissues for pyrimidine synthesis but is not the hepatic enzyme that makes urea (Fig. 2.3). However, a block in the urea cycle causing a lack of adequate amounts of arginine to prime the urea synthesis cycle in the liver will result in diversion of unused carbamoyl phosphate to orotic acid and pyrimidine synthesis (41). Uracil is synthesized as uridine monophosphate by forming orotidine monophosphate from orotic acid followed by decarboxylation. Cytosine is formed by adding the amide group of glutamine to uridine triphosphate to form cytidine triphosphate.

TURNOVER OF PROTEINS IN THE BODY

As indicated above, proteins in the body are not static. Just as every protein is synthesized, it is also degraded. Schoenheimer and Rittenberg first applied isotopically labeled tracers to the study of amino acid metabolism and protein turnover in the 1930s and first suggested that proteins are continually made and degraded in the body at different rates. We now know that the rate of turnover of proteins varies widely and that the rate of turnover of individual proteins tends to follow their function in the body, i.e., proteins whose concentrations must be regulated (e.g., enzymes) or that act as signals (e.g., peptide hormones) have relatively high rates of synthesis and degradation as a means of regulating concentrations. On the other hand, structural proteins such as collagen and myofibrillar proteins or secreted plasma proteins have relatively long lifetimes. However, there must be an overall balance between synthesis and breakdown of proteins. Balance in healthy adults who are neither gaining nor losing weight means that the amount of N consumed as protein in the diet will match the amount of N lost in urine, feces, and other routes. However, considerably more protein is mobilized in the body every day than is consumed (Fig. 2.6).

Although there is no definable entity such as "whole-body protein," the term is useful for understanding the amount of energy and resources spent in producing and breaking down protein in the body. Several methods using isotopically labeled tracers have been developed to quantitate the whole-body turnover of proteins. The concept and definition of whole-body protein turnover and these methods have been the subject of entire books (e.g., [42]). An important point of Figure 2.6 is that the overall turnover of protein in the body is several fold greater than the input of new dietary amino acids (43). A normal adult may consume 90 g of protein that is hydrolyzed and absorbed as free amino acids. Those amino acids mix with amino acids entering from protein breakdown from a variety of proteins. Approximately a third of the amino acids appear from the large, but slowly turning over, pool of muscle protein. In contrast, considerably more amino acids appear and disappear from proteins in the visceral and internal organs. These proteins make up a much smaller proportion of the total mass of protein in the body but have rapid synthesis and degradation rates. The overall result is that approximately 340 g of amino acids enter the free pool daily, of which only 90 g come from dietary amino acids. The question is how to assess the turnover of protein in the human body? As noted from Figure 2.6, the issue quickly becomes complex. Much effort has been spent in devising methods to quantify various aspects of protein metabolism in humans in meaningful terms. The methods that have been developed and applied with success to date are listed in Table 2.8. These methods, which range from simple and noninvasive to expensive and complicated, are described below.

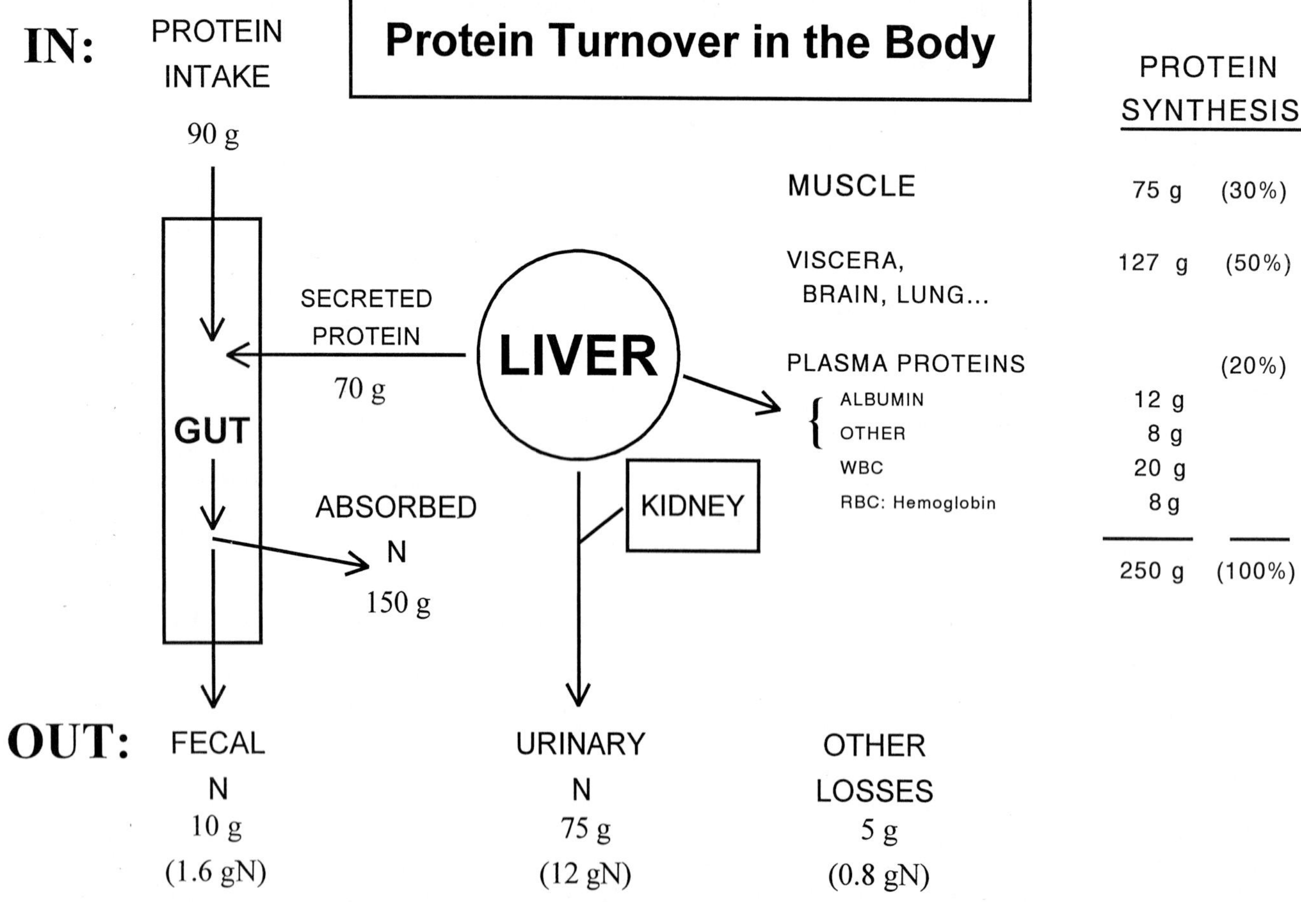

Figure 2.6. Relative rates of protein turnover and intake in a healthy 70-kg human. Under normal circumstances, dietary intake (IN = 90 g) matches N losses (OUT = 90 g). Protein breakdown then matches synthesis. Protein intake is only 90/(90 + 250) ≈ 25% of total turnover of N in the body per day. (Redrawn from Hellerstein MK, Munro HN. Interaction of liver and muscle in the regulation of metabolism in response to nutritional and other factors. In: Arias IM, Jakoby WB, Popper H, et al., eds. The liver: biology and pathobiology. 2nd ed. New York: Raven Press, 1988;965–83.)

Table 2.8
Methods of Measuring Protein Metabolism in Humans

- Nitrogen balance
- Arteriovenous measurement of amino acids and/or tracer across a tissue bed
- End-product method
- Turnover of individual components:
  - Essential amino acids (index of protein breakdown)
  - Nonessential amino acids (de novo synthesis and gluconeogenesis)
  - Urea (amino acid oxidation)
- Tracer *into* a specific protein to measure protein synthesis
- Tracer *out to* a specific protein to measure protein degradation

METHODS OF MEASURING PROTEIN TURNOVER AND AMINO ACID KINETICS

Nitrogen Balance

The oldest (and most widely used) method of following changes in body N is the N balance method. Because of its simplicity, the N balance technique is the standard of reference for defining minimum levels of dietary protein and essential amino acid intakes in humans of all ages (44, 45). Subjects are placed for several days on a specific level of amino acid and/or protein intake and their urine and feces are collected over a 24-h period to measure their N excretion. A week or more may be required before collection reflects adaptation to a dietary change. A dramatic example of adaption involves placing healthy subjects on a diet containing a minimal amount of protein. As shown in Figure 2.7, urinary N excretion drops dramatically in response to the protein-deficient diet over the first 3 days and stabilizes at a new lower level of N excretion by day 8 (46).

The N end-products excreted in the urine are not only end products of amino acid oxidation (urea and ammonia) but also other species such as uric acid from nucleotide degradation and creatinine (Table 2.9). Fortunately, most of the nonurea, nonammonia N is relatively constant over a variety of situations and is a relatively small proportion of the total N in the urine. Most of the N is excreted as urea, but ammonia N excretion increases significantly when subjects become acidotic, as is apparent in Table 2.9 when subjects have fasted for 2 days (47). Table 2.9 also illustrates how urea production is related to N intake and how the body adapts its oxidation of amino acids to follow amino acid supply (i.e., with ample supply, excess amino acids are oxidized and urea production is high, but with insufficient dietary amino acids, amino acids are conserved and urea production is greatly decreased).

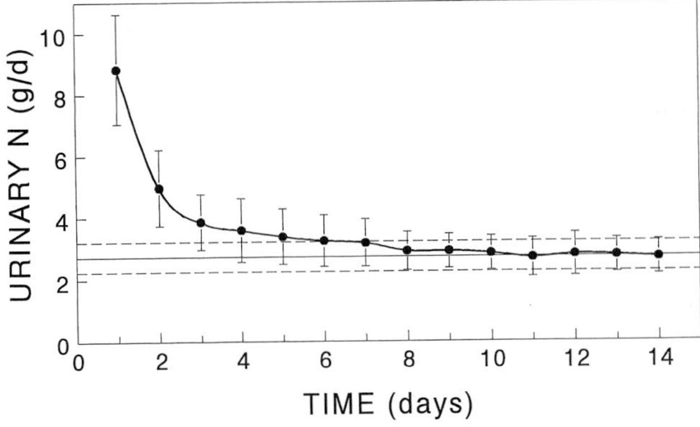

Figure 2.7. Time required for urinary N excretion to stabilize after changing from an adequate to a deficient protein intake in young men. *Horizontal solid and broken lines* are mean ± 1 standard deviation for N excretion at the end of the measurement period. (Data from NS Scrimshaw, Hussein MA, Murray E, et al., J Nutr 1972;102:1595–604.)

Nitrogen appears in the feces because the gut does not completely absorb all dietary protein and reabsorb all N secreted into the gastrointestinal tract (Fig. 2.6). In addition, N is lost from skin via sweat as well as via shedding of dead skin cells. There are also additional losses through hair, menstrual fluid, nasal secretions, and so forth. As N excretion in the urine decreases in the case of subjects on a minimal-protein diet (Fig. 2.7), it becomes increasingly important to account for N losses through nonurinary, nonfecal routes (48). The loss of N by these various routes is shown in Table 2.10. Most of the losses that are not readily measurable are minimal (<10% of total N loss under conditions of a protein-free diet when adaptation has greatly reduced urinary N excretion) and can be discounted by use of a simple offset factor for nonurinary, nonfecal N losses. The assessment of losses comes into play in the finer definition of zero balance as a function of dietary protein intake for the purpose of determining amino acid and protein requirements. As we shall see below, small changes in N balance corrections make significant changes in the assessment of protein requirements using N balance.

Although the N balance technique is very useful and easy to apply, it provides no information about the inner workings of the system. An interesting analogy for the N balance technique is illustrated in Figure 2.8 where the simple model of N balance is represented by a gumball machine. Balance is taken between "coins in" and "gumballs out." However, we should not conclude that the machine turns coins into gum, although that conclusion is easy to reach with the N balance method. What the N bal-

Table 2.9
Composition of the Major Nitrogen-Containing Species in Urine

N Species	High-Protein Diet	Low-Protein Diet (g N/day)	Fasting (day 2)
Urea	14.7 (87%)	2.2 (61%)	6.6 (75%)
Ammonia	0.5 (3%)	0.4 (11%)	1.0 (12%)
Uric acid	0.2 (1%)	0.1 (3%)	0.2 (2%)
Creatinine	0.6 (4%)	0.6 (17%)	0.4 (5%)
Undetermined	0.8 (5%)	0.3 (8%)	0.5 (6%)
Total	16.8 (100%)	3.6 (100%)	8.7 (100%)

Data compiled from reports by Folin (1905) and Cathcart (1907) cited in ref. 47.

Table 2.10
Obligatory Nitrogen Losses by Adult Men on a Protein-Free Diet

	Daily Nitrogen Loss	
	As Nitrogen (mg N/kg/day)	As Protein Equivalent (g protein/kg/day)
Urine	37	0.23
Feces	12	0.08
Cutaneous	3	0.02
Other	2	0.01
Total:	54	0.34
Upper limit (+2 standard deviations)	70	0.44

Data from Munro HN. Amino acid requirements and metabolism and their relevance to parenteral nutrition. In: Wilkinson AW, ed. Parenteral nutrition. London: Churchill-Livingstone, 1972;34–67.

ance technique fails to provide is information about what occurs *within* the system (i.e., inside the gumball machine). Inside the system is where the changes in whole-body protein synthesis and breakdown actually occur (shown as the smaller arrows into and out of the *Body N Pool* in Fig. 2.8). A further illustration of this point is made at the bottom of Figure 2.8 where a positive increase in N balance has been observed going from zero (case *0*) to positive balance (cases *A–D*). A positive N balance could be obtained with identical increases in N balance by any of four different alterations in protein synthesis and breakdown: a simple increase in protein synthesis (case *A*), a decrease in protein breakdown (case *C*), an increase in both protein synthesis and breakdown (case *B*), or a decrease in both (case *D*). The effect is the same positive N balance for all four cases, but the energy implications are considerably different. Because protein synthesis costs energy, cases *A* and *B* are more expensive,

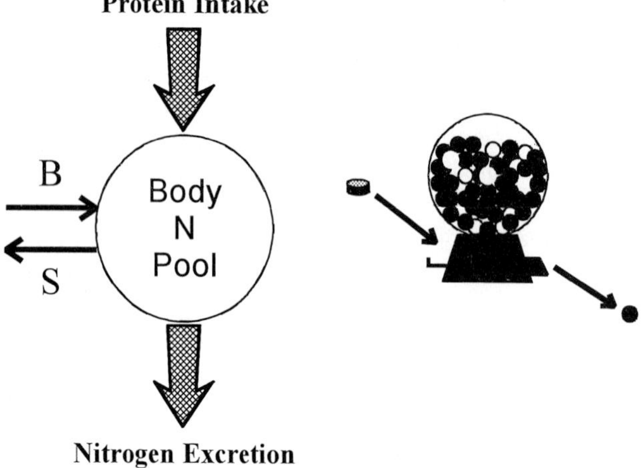

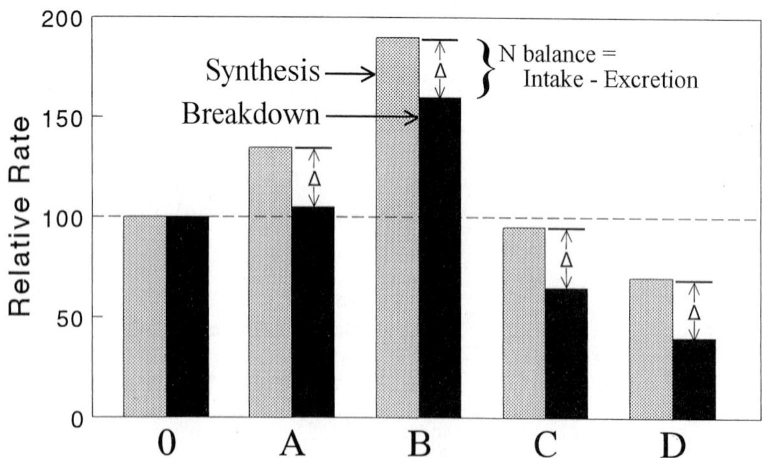

Figure 2.8. Illustration of the N balance technique. Nitrogen balance is simply the difference between input and output, which is similar to the introduction of a coin into a gumball machine resulting in a gumball being released. The perception of only the "in" and "out" observations is that the machine changed the coin directly into a gumball or that the dietary intake becomes directly the N excreted without consideration of amino acid entry from protein breakdown *(B)* or uptake for protein synthesis *(S)*. This point is further illustrated with four different hypothetical responses to a change from a zero N balance (case *0*) to a positive N balance (cases *A–D*). A positive N balance can be obtained by increasing protein synthesis *(A)*, by increasing synthesis more than breakdown *(B)*, by decreasing breakdown *(C)*, or by decreasing breakdown more than synthesis *(D)*. The N balance method does not distinguish among the four possibilities.

while cases *C* and *D* require less energy than the starting case, *0*. To resolve these four cases, we have to look directly at rates of protein turnover (breakdown and synthesis) using a labeled tracer.

Using Arteriovenous Differences to Define Organ Balances

Just as the N balance technique can be applied across the whole body, so can the balance technique be applied across a whole organ or tissue bed. These measurements are made from the blood delivered to the tissue and from the blood emerging from the tissue via catheters placed in an artery to define arterial blood levels and the vein draining the tissue to measure venous blood levels. The latter catheter makes the procedure particularly invasive when applied to organs such as gut, liver, kidney, or brain (49–52). Less invasive are measures of muscle metabolism inferred from measurement of arteriovenous (A-V) differences across the leg or arm (51). Measurements have even been made across fat depots (53). However, the A-V difference provides no information about the mechanism in the tissue that causes the uptake or release that is observed. More information is gleaned from measurement of amino acids that are not metabolized within the tissue, such as the release of essential amino acids tyrosine or lysine, which are not metabolized by muscle. Their A-V differences across muscle should reflect the difference between net amino acid uptake for muscle protein synthesis and release from muscle protein breakdown. 3-Methylhistidine, an amino acid produced by posttranslational methylation of selected histidine residues in myofibrillar protein, which cannot be reused for protein synthesis when it is released from myofibrillar protein breakdown, is quantitatively released from muscle tissue when myofibrillar protein is degraded (32, 54). Its A-V difference can be used as a specific marker of myofibrillar protein breakdown (55–57).

The limited data set of simple balance values across an organ bed is greatly enhanced when a tracer is administered and its balance is also measured across an organ bed. This approach allows a complete solution of the various pathways operating in the tissue for each amino acid tracer used. In some cases the measurement of tracer can become very complicated, requiring measurement of multiple metabolites to provide a true metabolite balance across the organ bed (58). Another approach using a tracer of a nonmetabolized essential amino acid has been described by Barrett et al. (59). This method requires a limited set of measurements with simplified equations to define specifically rates of protein synthesis and breakdown in muscle tissue. The conceptual simplicity of this approach with a limited set of measurements required makes it extremely useful for defining muscle-specific changes in response to a variety of perturbations (e.g., local infusion of insulin into the same muscle bed [60]). This approach has been expanded by others (61–63).

Tracer Methods Defining Amino Acid Kinetics

Isotopically labeled tracers are used to follow flows of *endogenous* metabolites in the body. The labeled tracers are identical to the endogenous metabolites in terms of chemical structure with substitution of one or more atoms with isotopes different from those usually present. The isotopes are substituted to make the tracers distinguishable (measurable) from the normal metabolites. We usually think first of the radioactive isotopes (e.g., ^{3}H for hydrogen and ^{14}C for carbon) as tracers that can be measured by the particles they emit when they decay, but there are also nonradioactive, stable isotopes that can be used. Because isotopes of the same atom only differ in the number of neutrons that are contained, they can be distinguished in a compound by mass spectrometry, which determines the abundance of compounds by mass. Most of the lighter elements have one *abundant* stable isotope and one or two isotopes of higher mass of *minor abundance*. The major and minor isotopes are ^{1}H and ^{2}H for hydrogen, ^{14}N and ^{15}N for nitrogen, ^{12}C and ^{13}C for carbon, and ^{16}O, ^{17}O, and ^{18}O for oxygen. Except for some isotope effects, which can be significant for both the radioactive (^{3}H) and nonradioactive (^{2}H) hydrogen isotopes, a compound that is isotopically labeled is essentially indistinguishable from the corresponding unlabeled endogenous compound in the body. Because they do not exist in nature and so little of the radioactive material is administered, radioisotopes are considered "weightless" tracers that do not add material to the system. Radioactive tracer data are expressed as counts or disintegrations per minute per unit compound. Because the stable isotopes are naturally occurring (e.g., $\approx$1% of all carbon in the body is ^{13}C), the stable isotope tracers are administered and measured as the "excess above the naturally occurring abundance" of the isotope in the body as either the *mole ratio* of the amount of tracer isotope divided by the amount of unlabeled material or the *mole fraction* (usually expressed as a percentage: *mole % excess* or *atom % excess*, the latter being an older, less appropriate term in the literature) (64).

The basis of most tracer measurements to determine amino acid kinetics is the simple concept of tracer dilution. This concept is illustrated in Figure 2.9 for the determination of the flow of water in a stream. If you infuse a dye of known concentration (enrichment) into the stream, go downstream after the dye has mixed well with the stream water, and take a sample of the dye, then you can calculate from the measured dilution of the dye the rate at which water must be flowing in the stream to make that dilution. The necessary information required is infusion rate of dye (tracer infusion rate) and measured concentration of the dye (enrichment or specific activity of the tracer). The calculated value is the flow of water through the stream (flux of unlabeled metabolite) causing the dilution. This simple dye-dilution analogy is the basis for almost all kinetic calculations in a wide range of for-

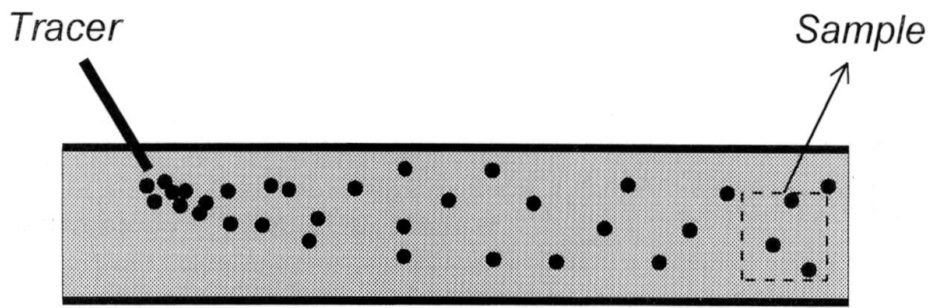

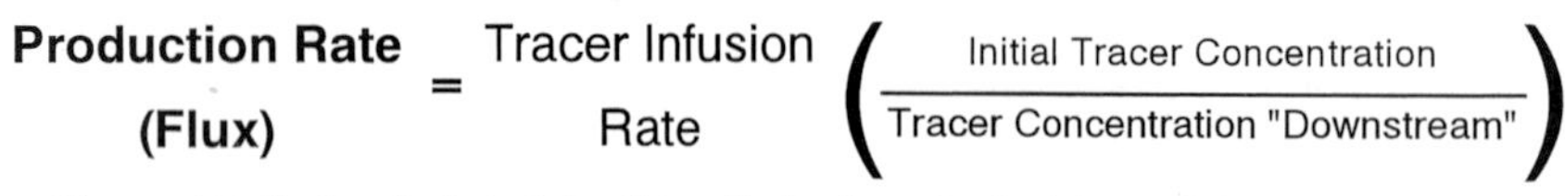

Production Rate (Flux) = Tracer Infusion Rate (Initial Tracer Concentration / Tracer Concentration "Downstream")

Figure 2.9. Basic principal of the "dye-dilution" method of determining tracer kinetics.

mats for a wide range of applications. A few of the more important approaches are discussed below.

Models for Whole-Body Amino Acid and Protein Metabolism

The limitations to using tracers to define amino acid and protein metabolism are largely driven by how the tracer is administered and where it is sampled. The simplest method of tracer administration is orally, but intravenous administration is preferred to deliver the tracer *systemically* (to the whole body) into the free pool of amino acids. The simplest site of sampling of the tracer dilution is also from the free pool of amino acids via blood. Therefore, most approaches to measuring amino acid and protein kinetics in the whole body using amino acid tracers assume a single, free pool of amino N, as shown in Figure 2.10. Amino acids enter the free pool from dietary amino acid intake (enteral or parenteral) and by amino acids released from protein breakdown. Amino acids leave the free pool by amino acid oxidation to end products (CO_2, urea, and ammonia) and from amino acid uptake for protein synthesis. The free amino acid pool can be viewed from the standpoint of all of the amino acids together (as discussed for the end-product method) or from the viewpoint of a single amino acid and its metabolism per se. The model in Figure 2.10 is called a "single-pool model" because protein is not viewed as a pool per se, but rather as a source of entry of unlabeled amino acids into the free pool, on the one hand, and a route of amino acid removal for protein synthesis on the other. Only a small portion of the proteins in the body are assumed to turn over during the time course of the experiment. Obviously, these assumptions are not true: many proteins in the body are turning over rapidly (e.g, most enzymes). Proteins that do turn over during the time course of the experiment will become labeled and appear as part of the free amino acid pool. However, these proteins make up only a fraction of the total protein; the remainder turn over slowly (e.g., muscle protein). Most amino acids entering via protein breakdown and leaving for new protein synthesis are coming from slowly turning over proteins. These flows are the *B* and *S* arrows of the traditional single-pool model of whole-body protein metabolism shown in Figure 2.10.

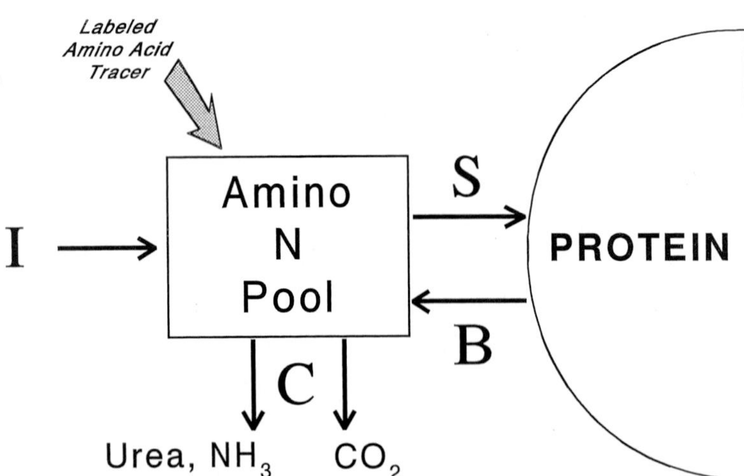

Figure 2.10. Single-pool model of whole-body protein metabolism measured with a labeled amino acid tracer. Amino acid enters the free pool from dietary intake *(I)* and amino acid released from protein breakdown *(B)* and leaves the free pool via amino acid oxidation *(C)* to urea, ammonia, and CO_2 and uptake for protein synthesis *(S)*.

End-Product Approach

The earliest model of whole-body protein metabolism in humans was applied by San Pietro and Rittenberg in 1953 using [^{15}N]glycine (65). Glycine was used as the first tracer because glycine is the only amino acid without an optically active α-carbon center and therefore is easy to synthesize with a ^{15}N label. At that time, measurement of the tracer in plasma glycine was very difficult. Thus, San Pietro and Rittenberg proposed a model based upon something that could be readily measured, urinary urea and ammonia. The assumption was that the urinary N end-products reflected the average enrichment in ^{15}N of all of the free amino acids being oxidized. Although glycine ^{15}N was the tracer, the tracee was assumed to be *all* free amino acids (assumed to be a single pool). However, it quickly became obvious that the system was more complicated and that a more complicated model and solution were required.

In essence, the method languished until 1969, when Picou and Taylor-Roberts (66) proposed a simpler method that also followed the glycine ^{15}N tracer into urinary N. Their method dealt only with the effect of the dilution of the ^{15}N tracer in the free amino acid pool as a whole, rather than invoking solution of tracer-specific equations of a specific model. Their assumptions were similar to those of the earlier Rittenberg approach in that they assumed that the ^{15}N tracer mixes (scatters) among the free amino acids in some distribution that is not required to be known but that represents amino acid metabolism per se. This distribution of ^{15}N tracer could be measured in the end products of amino acid metabolism, urea and ammonia. These assumptions allow the model to become "fuzzy" as shown in Figure 2.11, in that an explicit definition of the inner workings is not required. The [^{15}N]glycine tracer is administered (usually orally), and urine samples are obtained to measure the ^{15}N dilution in the free amino acid pool (67). The ^{15}N in the free amino acid pool is diluted with unlabeled amino acid entering from protein breakdown and from dietary intake. The turnover of the free pool (Q, typically expressed as mg N/kg/day) is calculated from the measured dilution of ^{15}N in the end products via the same approach illustrated in Figure 2.9:

$$Q = i/E_{UN}$$

where i is the rate of [^{15}N]glycine infusion (mg ^{15}N/kg/day), and E_{UN} is the ^{15}N enrichment in atom % excess ^{15}N in urinary N (urea and/or ammonia). The free pool is assumed to be in steady state (neither increasing or decreasing over time), and therefore, the turnover of amino acid will be equal to the rate of amino acids entering via whole-body protein breakdown *(B)* and dietary intake *(I)* and also equal to the rate of amino acids leaving via uptake for protein synthesis *(S)* and via amino acid oxidation to the end products urea and ammonia *(C)*:

$$Q = I + B = C + S$$

Because dietary intake should be known and urinary N excretion is measured, the rate of whole-body protein breakdown can be determined: $B = Q - I$, as well as the rate of whole-body synthesis: $S = Q - C$. In these calculations, the standard value of 6.25 g protein = 1 g N is used to interconvert protein and urinary N. Attention to the units (g of protein vs. g of N) is important, as both units are often used concurrently in the same report.

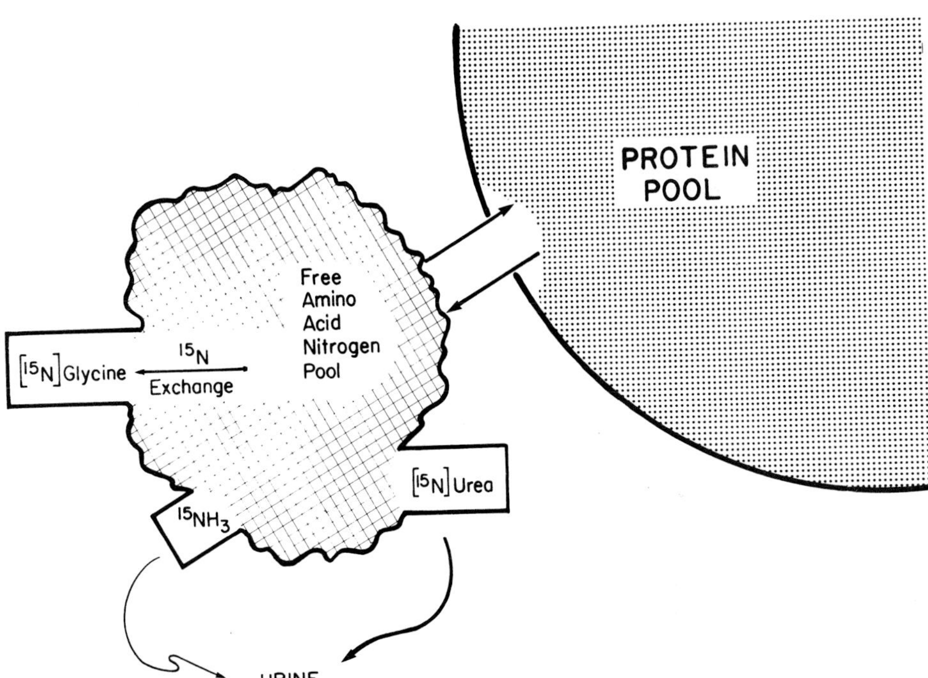

Figure 2.11. Model for measurement of protein turnover using [^{15}N]glycine as the tracer and measurement of the dilution of the ^{15}N tracer in urinary endproducts, urea and ammonia. (From Bier DM, Matthews DE. Fed Proc 1982;41:2679–85, with permission.)

Occasionally in the literature a term called "net protein balance" or "net protein gain" appears in papers. Net protein balance is defined as the difference between the measured protein synthesis and breakdown rates $(S - B)$, which can be determined from whole-body protein breakdown and synthesis measured as shown above. However, as can seen by rearranging the balance equation for Q above: $S - B = I - C$, which is simply the difference between intake and excretion, i.e., nitrogen balance. The $S - B$ term is a misnomer, in that it is based solely upon the N balance measurement, not upon the administration of the ^{15}N tracer.

There is no question that the end-product method of Picou and Taylor-Roberts is a cornerstone method for protein metabolic research in humans and is especially well suited for studies of infants and children because it is non-invasive, requiring only oral administration of tracer and collection only of urine. However, the end-product method is not without its problems; the most serious of which are mentioned below.

When the [^{15}N]glycine tracer is given orally at short intervals (e.g., every 3 h) the time required to reach a plateau in urinary urea ^{15}N is about 60 h regardless of whether adults (23, 68), children, or infants (69, 70) are studied. The delay in attaining a plateau is due to the time required for the ^{15}N tracer to equilibrate within the free glycine, serine, and urea pools (23, 67). An additional problem is plateau definition. Often the urinary urea ^{15}N time course does not show by either visual inspection or curve-fitting regression the anticipated single exponential rise to plateau. To avoid this problem, Waterlow et al. (71) suggested measuring the ^{15}N in ammonia after a *single dose* of [^{15}N]glycine. The advantage is that the ^{15}N tracer passes through the body ammonia pool within 24 hours. Tracer administration and urine collection are greatly simplified, and the modification does not depend on defining a plateau in urinary urea ^{15}N. The caveat here is the dependence of the single-dose end-product method upon *ammonia* metabolism. Urinary ammonia ^{15}N enrichment usually differs from urinary urea ^{15}N enrichment (72) because the amino-^{15}N precursor for ammonia synthesis is of renal origin, while the amino-^{15}N precursor for urea synthesis is of hepatic origin. Which enrichment should be used? Probably the urea ^{15}N, but it is difficult to prove either way (42).

The primary difficulty with the end-product method is highlighted from a report in which several different ^{15}N-labeled amino acid tracers, including ^{15}N-glycine and some ^{15}N-labeled proteins, were compared as tracers for the end-product method. Widely divergent results were determined for protein turnover (from 2.6 to 17.8 g/kg/day), depending upon the ^{15}N label administered (73). The differences reflect differences in the metabolism and distribution of the ^{15}N label when placed into different amino acids and illustrate how dependent the end-product approach is on the metabolism of the amino acid tracer. Therefore, it is difficult to determine whether a change in end-product ^{15}N enrichment may be attributable either to a change in protein turnover *or* to a change in the distribution of ^{15}N due to changes in tracer metabolism *that may be independent* of changes in protein metabolism. To make these distinctions, the kinetics of the amino acid tracer in the body must be measured as well.

Measurement of the Kinetics of Individual Amino Acids

As an alternative to measuring the turnover of the whole amino-N pool per se, the kinetics of an individual amino acid can be followed from the dilution of an infused tracer of that amino acid. The simplest models consider only essential amino acids that have no de novo synthesis. The kinetics of essential amino acids mimic the kinetics of protein turnover as shown in Figure 2.10. The same type of model can be constructed but cast specifically in terms of a single essential amino acid, and the same steady-state balance equation can be defined:

$$Q_{aa} = I_{aa} + B_{aa} = C_{aa} + S_{aa}$$

where Q_{aa} is the turnover rate (or flux) of the essential amino acid, I_{aa} is the rate at which the amino acid is entering the free pool from dietary intake, B_{aa} is the rate of amino acid entry from protein breakdown, C_{aa} is the rate of amino acid oxidation, and S_{aa} is the rate of amino acid uptake for protein synthesis. The most common method for defining amino acid kinetics has been a primed infusion of an amino acid tracer until isotopic steady state (constant dilution) is reached in blood. The flux for the amino acid is measured from the dilution of the tracer in the free pool. Knowing the tracer enrichment and infusion rate and measuring the tracer dilution in blood samples taken at plateau, the rate of unlabeled metabolite appearance is determined (64, 74, 75):

$$Q_{aa} = i_{aa} \cdot (E_i/E_p - 1)$$

where i_{aa} is the infusion rate of tracer with enrichment E_i (mole % excess) and E_p is the blood amino acid enrichment.

For a carbon-labeled tracer, the amino acid oxidation rate can be measured from the rate of $^{13}CO_2$ or $^{14}CO_2$ excretion (42, 64, 74). The choice of a carbon label that is quantitatively oxidized is critical. For example, the ^{13}C of an L-[1-^{13}C]leucine tracer is quantitatively released at the first irreversible step of leucine catabolism. In contrast, a ^{13}C-label in the leucine tail will end up in acetoacetate or acetyl-CoA, which may or may not be quantitatively oxidized. Other amino acids, such as lysine, have even more nebulous oxidation pathways.

Before the oxidized carbon-label is recovered in exhaled air, it must pass through the body bicarbonate pool. Therefore, information about body bicarbonate kinetics is required (76). To complete the oxidation rate calculation based upon the measured recovery of the administered carbon-label as CO_2, we must know what fraction of bicarbonate pool turnover is the release of CO_2 into exhaled air versus retention for alternative fates in the body. In general only about 80% of the bicarbonate produced is released immediately as expired CO_2, as determined from infusion of labeled bicarbonate and measurement of the fraction infused that is recovered in exhaled CO_2 (77). The other approximately 20% is retained in bone and metabolic pathways that "fix" carbon. The amount of bicarbonate retained is somewhat variable (ranging from 0 to 40% of its production) and needs to be determined when different metabolic situations are investigated. In cases in which the retention of bicarbonate in the body may change with metabolic perturbation, parallel studies measuring the recovery of an administered dose of ^{13}C- or ^{14}C-labeled bicarbonate are essential to interpretation of the oxidation results (78, 79).

The rate of amino acid release from protein breakdown and uptake for protein synthesis is calculated by subtracting dietary intake and oxidation from the flux of an essential amino acid—just as is done with the end-product method. The primary distinction is that the measurements are specific to a single amino acid's kinetics (μmol of amino acid per unit time) rather than in terms of N per se. Flux components can be extrapolated to whole-body protein kinetics by dividing the amino acid rates by the assumed concentration of the amino acid in body protein (as shown in Table 2.3).

The principal advantages to measuring the kinetics of an individual metabolite are that *(a)* the results are specific to *that* metabolite, improving the confidence of the measurement, and *(b)* the measurements can be performed quickly because turnover time of the free pool is usually rapid (a tracer infusion study can be completed in less than 4 hours using a priming dose to reduce the time required to come to isotopic steady state). Drawbacks to measuring the kinetics of an individual amino acid are that *(a)* an appropriately labeled tracer may not be available to follow the pathways of the amino acid being studied, especially with regard to amino acid oxidation, and *(b)* metabolism of amino acids occurs within cells, but the tracers are typically administered into and sampled from the blood outside cells. Amino acids do not freely pass through cells; they are transported. For the neutral amino acids (leucine, isoleucine, valine, phenylalanine, and tyrosine), transport in and out of cells may be rapid, and only a small concentration gradient between plasma and intracellular milieus exists (Table 2.4). However, even that small gradient limits exchange of intracellular and extracellular amino acids. For leucine, this phenomenon can be defined using α-ketoisocaproate (KIC), which is formed from leucine inside cells by transamination. Some of the KIC formed is then decarboxylated, but most of it is either reaminated to reform leucine (80) or released from cells into plasma. Thus, plasma KIC enrichment can be used as a marker of intracellular leucine enrichment from which it came (81).

Previous workers have shown that generally, plasma KIC enrichment is about 25% lower than plasma leucine enrichment (75, 81, 82). If plasma KIC enrichment is substituted for the plasma leucine tracer enrichment in the calculation of leucine kinetics, then the measured leucine flux and oxidation and, likewise, estimates of protein breakdown and synthesis are increased by about 25%. However, when protein metabolism is studied under two different conditions and the resulting leucine kinetics are compared, the same relative response is obtained regardless of whether leucine or KIC enrichment is used for the calculation of kinetics (81). The prudent approach is to measure both species and to note occasions when the KIC/leucine enrichment ratio has changed, to signal a possible change in the partitioning of amino acids between intracellular and extracellular spaces (83).

Use of KIC to represent intracellular leucine is an application of a *concept* that adds definition to the model shown in Figure 2.12 but does not require a more rigorous *model* to describe leucine kinetics. Because of confusion over a suitable model to describe leucine kinetics, a series of experiments were performed to develop a true multicompartmental model for the leucine-KIC system (84). Four leucine and three KIC pools were required to account for leucine kinetics. Clearly the kinetics of individual metabolites are far more complex than one- or two-compartment models. However, the conventional model using KIC as the precursor enrichment for calculating leucine kinetics as shown in Figure 2.12 agreed well with the multicompartmental model, which means that under many metabolic circumstances, the simpler approaches should accurately follow directional changes without requiring introduction of complicated compartmental models. These and intermediate models have been reviewed (75, 85), and the various assumptions, limitations, strengths, and weaknesses have been discussed. The leucine/KIC tracer system remains the single most applied measure of whole-body amino acid kinetics used to reflect changes in protein metabolism (83).

Most amino acids do not have a convenient metabolite that can be readily measured in plasma to define aspects of their intracellular metabolism, but an intracellular marker for leucine does not necessarily authenticate leucine as the tracer for defining whole-body protein metabolism. A variety of investigators have measured the turnover rate of many of the amino acids, both essential and nonessential, in humans, to define aspects of the metabolism of these amino acids. The general trend of these amino acid kinetic data has been reviewed by Bier (75). The fluxes of essential amino acids should represent their release rates from whole-body protein breakdown for postabsorptive humans in whom there is no dietary intake. Therefore, if the Waterlow model of Figure 2.10 is a reasonable representation of whole-body protein turnover, the individual rates of essential amino acid turnover should be proportional to each amino acid's content in body protein, and a linear relationship of amino acid flux and amino acid abundance in body protein should exist.

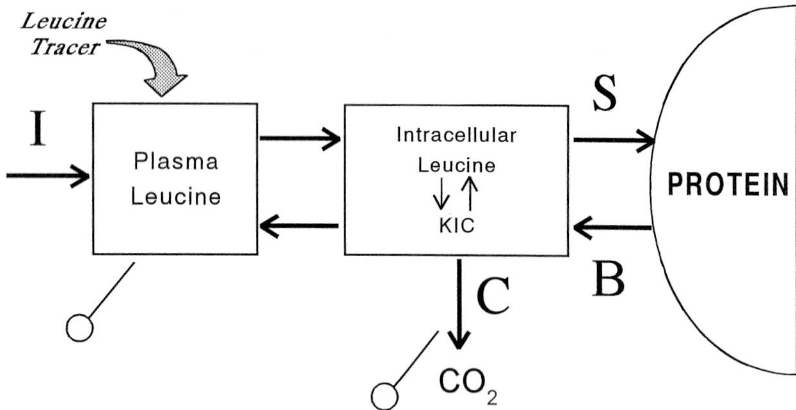

Figure 2.12. Two-pool model of leucine kinetics. The leucine tracer is administered to the plasma pool *(large arrow)* and sampled from plasma and/or from exhaled CO_2 *(circles with sticks)*. Plasma leucine exchanges with intracellular leucine where metabolism occurs: uptake for protein synthesis *(S)* or conversion to α-ketoisocaproate *(KIC)*. Oxidation *(C)* occurs from KIC. Unlabeled leucine enters into the free pool via dietary intake *(I)* or protein breakdown *(B)* into intracellular pools.

That relationship is shown in Figure 2.13 for data gleaned from a variety of studies in humans measured in the postabsorptive state (without dietary intake during the infusion studies) previously consuming diets of adequate N and energy intake. Amino acid flux is correlated with amino acid composition in protein across a variety of amino acid tracers and studies. This correlation suggests that even if there are problems in defining intracellular/extracellular concentration gradients of tracers to assess true intracellular events, changes in fluxes measured for the various essential amino acids reflect changes in breakdown in general.

Because nonessential amino acids are synthesized in the body, their fluxes are expected to exceed their expected flux based upon the regression line in Figure 2.13 by the amount of de novo synthesis that occurs. Because de novo synthesis and disposal of the nonessential amino acids would be expected to be based upon the metabolic pathways of individual amino acids, the degree to which individual nonessential amino acids lie above the line should also vary. For example, tyrosine is a nonessential amino acid because it is made by hydroxylation of phenylalanine, which is also the pathway of phenylalanine disposal. The rate of tyrosine de novo synthesis *is* the rate

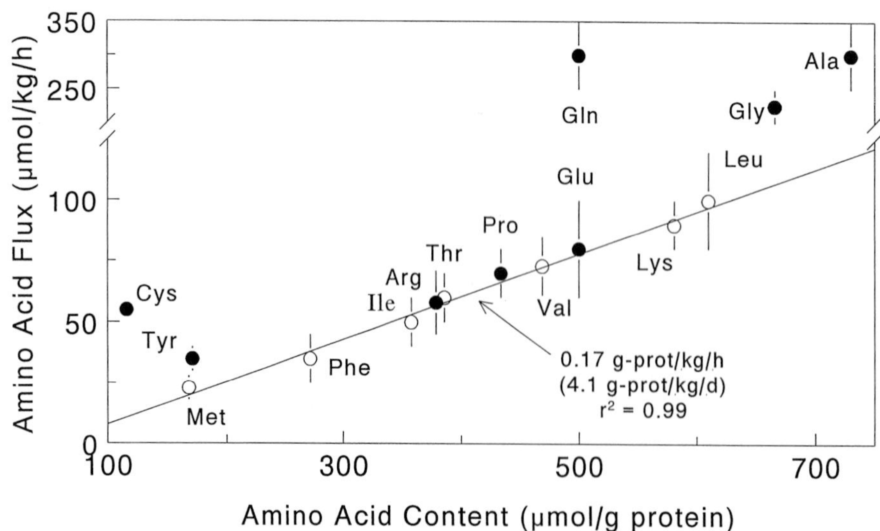

Figure 2.13. Fluxes of individual amino acids measured in postabsorptive humans are plotted against amino acid concentration in protein. *Closed circles* represent nonessential amino acids, and *open circles* represent essential amino acids. The *regression line* is for the flux of the essential amino acids versus their content in protein. *Error bars* represent the range of reported values that were taken from various reports in the literature of studies of amino acid kinetics in healthy humans eating adequate diets of N and energy intake studied in the postabsorptive state. The amino acid content of protein data are taken for muscle values from Table 2.3. The regression line slope of 4.1 g protein/kg/day is similar to other estimates of whole body protein turnover. (Redrawn from Bier DM. Diabetes Metab Rev 1989;5:111–32, with additional data added.)

of phenylalanine disposal. In the postabsorptive state, 10 to 20% of an essential amino acid's turnover goes to oxidative disposal. For phenylalanine, with a flux of about 40 μmol/kg/h, phenylalanine disposal produces about 6 μmol/kg/h of tyrosine. We would predict from the tyrosine content of body protein that tyrosine release from protein breakdown would be 21 μmol/kg/h and that the flux of tyrosine (tyrosine release from protein breakdown plus tyrosine production from phenylalanine) would be 21 + 6 = 27 μmol/kg/h. The measured tyrosine flux approximates this prediction (Fig. 2.13) (86).

Compared with tyrosine, which has a de novo synthesis component limited by phenylalanine oxidation, most nonessential amino acids have very large de novo synthesis components because of the metabolic pathways they are involved in. For example, arginine is at the center of the urea cycle (Fig. 2.3). Normal synthesis for urea is 8–12 g of N per day. That amount of urea production translates into an arginine de novo synthesis of approximately 250 μmol/kg/h, which is four times the expected 60 μmol/kg/h of arginine released from protein breakdown. As can be seen in Figure 2.13, however, the *measured* arginine flux approximates the arginine release from protein breakdown (87). The large de novo synthesis component does not exist in the measured flux. The explanation for this low flux is that the arginine involved in urea synthesis is very highly compartmentalized in the liver, and this arginine does not exchange with the tracer arginine infused intravenously.

Similar disparities are seen between the measured fluxes of glutamine and glutamate determined with intravenously infused tracers and their anticipated fluxes from their expected de novo synthesis components. The predicted flux for glutamate should include transamination with the BCAAs, alanine, and aspartate, as well as glutamate's contribution to the production and degradation of glutamine. However, the glutamate flux measured in postabsorptive adult subjects infused with [^{15}N]glutamate is 80 μmol/kg/h, barely above the anticipated rate of glutamate release from protein breakdown (Fig. 2.13). The size of the free glutamate pool was also determined in this study from the tracer dilution. The tracer-determined pool of glutamate was very small and approximated only the pool size predicted for extracellular water. The much larger intracellular pool that exists in muscle (Table 2.4) was not seen with the intravenously administered tracer. The flux measured for glutamine is considerably larger (350 μmol/kg/h), reflecting a large de novo synthesis component (Fig. 2.13). However, the pool size determined with the [^{15}N]glutamine tracer also was small—not much larger than glutamine in extracellular water. The large intracellular-muscle free pool of glutamine was not found (88). The results of this study showed that glutamine and glutamate tracers administered intravenously define pools of glutamine and glutamate that reflect primarily extracellular free glutamine and glutamate. The large intracellular pools (especially those in muscle) are tightly compartmentalized and do not readily mix with extracellular glutamine and glutamate. Intracellular events such as glutamate transamination are not detected by the glutamate tracer. The same is true of the glutamine tracer. However, the prominent role of glutamine in the body is *interorgan transport,* i.e., production by muscle and release for use by other tissues (89, 90), and that event is measured by the glutamine tracer (as is obvious from Fig. 2.13 in which the tracer-determined glutamine flux shows the highest measured flux of any amino acid).

The model in Figure 2.10 does not consider the potential first-pass effect that the splanchnic bed (gut and liver) has on regulating the delivery of nutrients from the oral route. Under normal circumstances, the amino acid tracer is infused intravenously to measure whole-body systemic kinetics. However, enterally delivered amino acids pass through the gut and liver before entering the systemic circulation. Any metabolism of these amino acids by gut or liver on the first pass during absorption will not be "seen" by an intravenously infused tracer in terms of systemic kinetics. Therefore, another pool with a second arrow showing the first-pass removal by gut and liver should precede the input arrow for I (Fig. 2.14) to indicate the role of the splanchnic bed. A fraction f of the dietary intake $(I \cdot f)$ is sequestered on the first-pass, and only $I \cdot (1 - f)$ enters the systemic circulation.

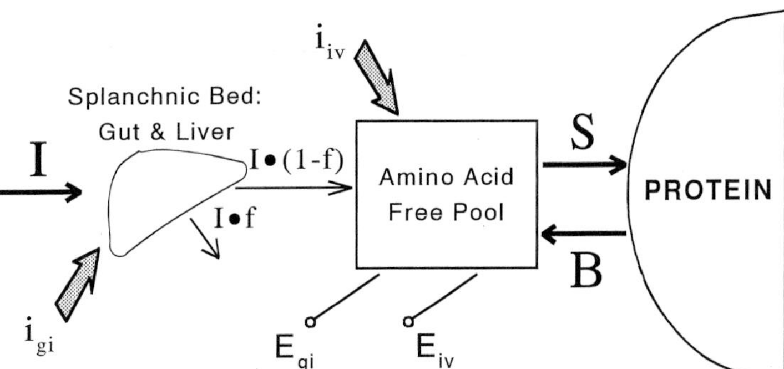

Figure 2.14. Model of whole-body protein metabolism for the fed state when first-pass uptake of dietary intake is considered. A labeled amino acid tracer is administered by the gastrointestinal route (i_{gi}) to follow dietary amino acid intake (I). The fraction of dietary amino acid sequestered on first pass by the splanchnic bed (f) can be determined by administering the tracer by both the gastrointestinal and the intravenous routes (i_{iv}) and comparing the enrichments in blood for the two tracers (E_{gi} and E_{iv}, respectively).

There are two ways to address this problem. The first does not evaluate the fraction sequestered explicitly but builds the tracer administration scheme into the first-pass losses. One simply adds the amino acid tracer to the dietary intake so that the tracer administration *is* the oral route (I_{gi}) and enrichments in blood (E_{gi}) come after any first-pass metabolism by the splanchnic bed (91, 92). This approach is especially useful for studying the effect of varying levels of amino acid intake, but it does not evaluate per se the amount of material sequestered by the splanchnic bed.

The second approach applies the tracer by both the intravenous route and the enteral route. The intravenous tracer infusion (I_{iv}) and plasma enrichment (E_{iv}) are used to determine systemic kinetics, and the enteral tracer infusion and its plasma enrichment determine systemic kinetics plus the effect of the first pass. By difference, the fraction, f, is readily calculated (93). This approach can be applied even in the postabsorptive state to determine basal uptake of amino acid tracers by the splanchnic bed. As shown in Table 2.11, a number of amino acids have been studied, and first-pass fractional uptake values for these different amino acids have been determined (93–101). In general, the splanchnic bed removes less of the essential amino acids but more than half of the nonessential amino acids on the first-pass—especially glutamate, which is almost entirely removed.

Synthesis of Specific Proteins

The above methods deal with measurements at the whole-body level but do not address specific proteins and their rates of synthesis and degradation. To do so requires obtaining samples of the proteins for purification. Some proteins are readily sampled (e.g., proteins in blood such as the lipoproteins, albumin, fibrinogen, and other secreted proteins). Other proteins require tissue sampling (e.g., muscle biopsy). If a protein (or group of proteins) can be sampled and purified, then its (their) synthetic rate can be determined directly from the rate of tracer incorporation. Proteins that turn over slowly (e.g., muscle protein or albumin) incorporate only a small amount of tracer during a tracer infusion. Because the incorporation rate of tracer is approximately linear during this time, protein synthesis can be measured by obtaining only two samples. This technique has been especially useful for evaluating protein synthesis of myofibrillar protein with a limited number of muscle biopsies (102, 103). For proteins that turn over at a faster rate, the tracer concentration rises exponentially in the protein toward a plateau value of enrichment that matches that of the precursor amino acids used for its synthesis (i.e., the intracellular amino acid enrichment). The types of protein that have been measured under these conditions have been the lipoproteins, especially apolipoprotein-B (apo-B) in very low density lipoprotein (VLDL) (104–106).

Table 2.11
First-Pass Sequestration of Enteral Amino and Keto Acid Tracers by the Gut and Liver in Humans

Amino Acid	Fraction Sequestered (f, %)	Reference
Leucine	17–21	(93, 94)
Phenylalanine	29–78	(93–95)
Alanine	70	(96)
Arginine	31–49	(97)
Glutamate	88–96	(98,99)
Glutamine	54–74	(98,100)
α-Ketoisocaproate	25–32	(101)

Determination of the protein fractional synthetic rate is a "precursor-product" method that requires knowledge of both the rate of tracer incorporation into the protein being synthesized and the enrichment of the amino acid precursor used for synthesis. For muscle, L-[1-^{13}C]leucine is often used as the tracer, and plasma KIC ^{13}C enrichment is used to approximate the intracellular muscle leucine enrichment (102). Various other schemes have been used to estimate intracellular liver amino acid tracer enrichment. Hippuric acid is excreted in urine after formation in the liver by conjugation of benzoic acid and glycine. Therefore, urinary hippuric acid can be used as an index of hepatic intracellular glycine ^{15}N enrichment (107, 108). Although the evidence is not specific, suggestions have been made that the hippuric acid does not accurately reflect the glycine precursor pool from which the export proteins are synthesized. However, in the absence of better approach, using the hippuric acid ^{15}N enrichment is clearly better than using another tracer where the hepatic intracellular enrichment is completely unknown. For proteins such as VLDL apo-B that turn over quickly (typically 4–8 hours), tracer incorporation into the protein will approach a plateau within the period of tracer infusion. If the tracer enrichment in the protein does not reach a plateau during the time course of the tracer infusion, curve fitting can usually predict the plateau. When the standard precursor-product relationship holds (i.e., the product is made only from the precursor), the protein plateau amino acid enrichment will reflect the precursor enrichment, simplifying the kinetic calculation (106). Cryer et al. (104) were able to use the plateau in VLDL apo-B to measure the precursor enrichment in normal subjects but still had to use urinary hippurate in hyperlipemic subjects who had large, slow-turnover VLDL pools that did not approach plateau during the course of the 8-h infusion.

Degradation of Specific Proteins

Measurement of protein degradation is much more limited in terms of the methods available. To measure protein degradation, the protein must be prelabeled. Three methods have been used: *(a)* removal of the protein from the body, followed by iodination with radioactive iodine, and reinjection into the body to follow the disappearance of the labeled protein; *(b)* administration of a labeled amino acid to label proteins via incorporation of the tracer during protein synthesis, followed by measurement of labeled amino acid release from degradation of the protein; and *(c)* use of posttranslational amino acids such as 3-methylhistidine.

The use of iodination limits this methodology to readily removable and reinjectable proteins (i.e., proteins in plasma). Therefore, the applications of this method are limited but it has found use in lipoprotein metabolism (109–111). The method is not without problems: proteins that are iodinated do not have the same structure after removal and iodination as they had before removal from the body, and the iodination process may cause untoward effects. However, properly applied, the method can be very specific for measuring the kinetics of select proteins.

Alternatively, proteins may be labeled by long infusions of amino acid tracer. After the tracer infusion is stopped, the tracer enrichment disappears quickly from plasma. At that point, serial sampling of the protein and measuring the decrease in tracer enrichment with time will give its degradation rate. However, another problem occurs: 80% or more of the amino acids released from protein breakdown are reused for synthesis of new proteins. Therefore the amino acid tracer from protein degradation is recycled into new proteins. Because there is generally not a large starting enrichment in the proteins being measured, recycling of low enrichments of tracer greatly complicates interpretation of the labeled protein data obtained by this method.

3-Methylhistidine and Other Posttranslational Amino Acids. In the body, a number of enzymes can modify the structure of proteins after they have been synthesized. The changes are generally modest, occur to specific amino acids, and are either the addition of a hydroxyl group (e.g., conversion of proline to hydroxyproline in collagen [112]) or methylation of N moieties of amino acid residues such as histidine or lysine. Because t-RNAs do not code for these hydroxylated or methylated amino acids, they are not reused for protein synthesis once the protein containing them is degraded. Of posttranslationally modified amino acids, 3-methylhistidine has found the most extensive application: the measurement of muscle myofibrillar protein breakdown (32, 113).

Because of the quantitative importance of muscle to whole-body protein metabolism, measurement of the release of 3-methylhistidine is an important tool for following breakdown of myosin and actin, which are both primary proteins in skeletal muscle and the primary proteins containing 3-methylhistidine (Fig. 2.15). Analyses of rat carcasses demonstrated that muscle accounts for three-quarters of the 3-methylhistidine pool in body proteins (32), and administered ^{14}C-3-methylhistidine has been shown to be quantitatively recovered in the urine of rats (114) and humans (115). There are caveats, however, to the use of 3-methylhistidine excretion for measurement of myofibrillar protein breakdown. Dietary meat will distort urinary 3-methylhistidine collection (116). As much as 5% of the 3-methylhistidine released in the urine may be acetylated in the liver first (a pathway that is much more predominant in the rat), and urinary samples may have to be hydrolyzed before measurement of 3-methylhistidine. Conversion of 3-methylhistidine to balenine (the dipeptide 3-methylhistidine-β-alanine) is of less importance in humans than in other species (117).

Myofibrillar protein and 3-methylhistidine are not specific to skeletal muscle, which means that urinary 3-methylhistidine measurement may not be specific to skeletal muscle protein breakdown (118, 119). The primary argument has been that even though skin and gut may have a small pool of myofibrillar protein compared to the large mass of protein found in skeletal muscle, skin and gut protein turn over rapidly by comparison and, therefore, continually contribute a significant amount of 3-methylhistidine to the urine. More-recent work suggests that skin and gut contributions, while noticeable, can be accommodated in the calculation of human skeletal muscle turnover from urinary 3-methylhistidine excretion (113, 117, 120).

A more specific approach to 3-methylhistidine measurement of skeletal muscle myofibrillar protein breakdown measures release of 3-methylhistidine from skeletal muscle via A-V blood measurements across a muscle bed, such as leg or arm (121). This measurement of protein breakdown from the 3-methylhistidine A-V difference can be combined with the A-V difference measurement of an essential amino acid that is not metabolized in muscle, such as tyrosine. In contrast to 3-methylhistidine, tyrosine released by protein breakdown is reused for protein synthesis. The A-V difference of tyrosine across an arm or leg defines net protein balance (i.e., the difference between protein breakdown and synthesis). Protein synthesis is, therefore, the difference of the 3-methylhistidine and tyrosine A-V difference measurements (56, 122). The results by this technique should be similar to those obtained by the tracer method of Barrett et al. (59).

CONTRIBUTION OF SPECIFIC ORGANS TO PROTEIN METABOLISM

Whole-Body Metabolism of Protein and Contributions of Individual Organs

From the above discussion of tracers of amino acid and protein metabolism, it is clear that the body is not static and that all compounds are being made and degraded over time. A general balance of the processes occurring is shown in Figure 2.6 for an average adult. In diabetics treated with insulin, Nair et al. measured leucine and phenylalanine kinetics in the whole body as well as leucine and phenylalanine tracer balances across a leg and across the splanchnic bed (123). This work measured directly in humans what has been assumed from a composite of the measurements shown in Figure 2.6. They found that

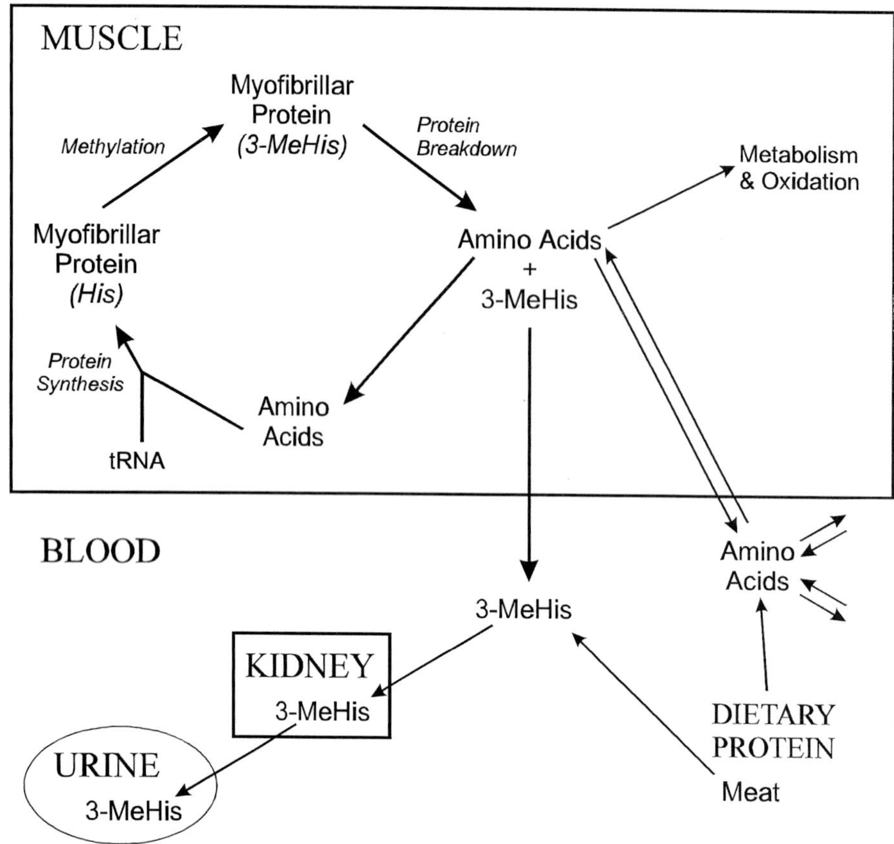

Figure 2.15. Schematic depiction of the formation and disposal of 3-methylhistidine in myofibrillar protein in humans. Because 3-methylhistidine is not reused for protein synthesis or oxidized/metabolized, its release into blood represents degradation of myofibrillar protein from tissues containing myosin and actin (muscle, smooth muscle such as gut, skin). In man, 3-methylhistidine is quantitatively excreted into urine; in rat, 3-methylhistidine is also acetylated in the liver before excretion in urine. Dietary intake of meat adds another source of 3-methylhistidine. (Figure drawn from previous descriptions of the metabolism of 3-methylhistidine (32).)

approximately 250 g of protein turns over in a day on the basis of the leucine and phenylalanine fluxes. Muscle protein turnover accounted for 65 g/day, and splanchnic protein turnover accounted for 62 g/day. If secreted proteins are synthesized at a rate of 48 g/day, then nonsplanchnic, nonmuscle organs account for another 75 g/day. The proportion of skeletal muscle mass in the body is consistent with skeletal muscle's contribution to whole-body protein turnover: skeletal muscle comprises about one-third of the protein in the body (11) and accounts for about one-quarter of the turnover.

If amino acids could be completely conserved (i.e., if none were oxidized for energy or synthesized into other compounds), then all amino acids released from proteolysis could be completely reincorporated into new protein synthesis. Obviously, that is not the case, and when there is no dietary intake, whole-body protein breakdown must exceed protein synthesis by an amount equal to net disposal of amino acids by oxidative and other routes. Therefore, we need to consume enough amino acids during the day to make up for the losses that occur both during this period and during the nonfed period. This concept becomes the basis for methods defining amino acid and protein requirements discussed below.

As shown in Figure 2.6*A*, if about 90 g of protein are eaten in a day, of which 10 g are lost in feces, the net absorption will be 80 g. In the process, considerably more protein is made and broken down. The total turnover of protein in the body, including both dietary intake and endogenous metabolism, is 90 + 250 = 340 g/day, of which oxidation of dietary protein accounts for (75 + 5)/340 = 24% of the turnover of protein in the body per day. When dietary protein intake is restricted, adaptation occurs whereby the body reduces N losses (Fig. 2.7), and protein intake/oxidation becomes a much smaller proportion of total protein turnover.

The preceding discussion defines turnover of protein in various parts of the body but does not integrate flows of material per se or highlight the relationship of amino acids to metabolites that are used for energy, such as glucose and fatty acids. Clearly, there must be interorgan cooperation to maintain protein homeostasis, simply because some tissues such as muscle have large amino acid reservoirs, yet all tissues have amino acid needs. A regular feeding schedule means that part of the day is a fasting period in which endogenous protein is used for energy and gluconeogenesis. The fed period then supplies amino acids from dietary protein to replenish these losses and

Table 2.12
Contribution of Different Organs and Tissues to Energy Expenditure

	Weight		Metabolic Rate	
Organ or Tissue	kg	(% of total)	kcal/kg/day	(% of total)
Kidneys	0.3	(0.5)	440	(8)
Brain	1.4	(2.0)	240	(20)
Liver	1.8	(2.6)	200	(21)
Heart	0.3	(0.5)	440	(9)
Muscle	28.0	(40.0)	13	(22)
Adipose tissue	15.0	(21.4)	4	(4)
Other (skin, gut, bone, etc.)	23.2	(33.0)	12	(16)
Total:	70.0	(100)		(100)

Data taken from Elia M. Organ and tissue contribution to metabolic rate. In: Kinney JM, Tucker HN, eds. Energy metabolism: determinants and cellular corollaries. New York: Raven Press, 1992:61–79.

provide additional amino acids that can be used for energy during the feeding portion as well. Such a normal diurnal feeding and fasting pattern causes movement of amino acids among organs, which takes on particular importance in situations of trauma and stress in which adaptation, or rather lack of adaptation, of amino acid metabolism to physiologic insults or pathophysiologic states occurs.

As Cahill and Aoki has emphasized (124), the first consideration of the body is to maintain and distribute energy supplies (oxygen and oxidative substrates). The caloric needs of different tissues in the body are shown in Table 2.12. As can be seen from the table, the brain makes up only about 2% of body weight yet has 20% of the energy needs (125). The brain also lacks the ability to store energy (e.g., glycogen depots), so it depends continually on delivery of energy substrates via the blood from other organs (Fig. 2.16). In the postabsorptive state, the primary energy substrate for the brain is glucose. In infancy and early childhood, when the brain makes up a significantly greater proportion of body mass, glucose production and use rates are proportionately higher (126). The pioneering studies of Cahill, Felig, and Wahren have provided us with a wealth of data concerning flows of amino acids and glucose from organ balance studies in humans studied over a range of nutritional states (50, 51, 127–129). Some basic concepts may be derived from these studies.

As shown in Figure 2.16*A*, in the postabsorptive state,

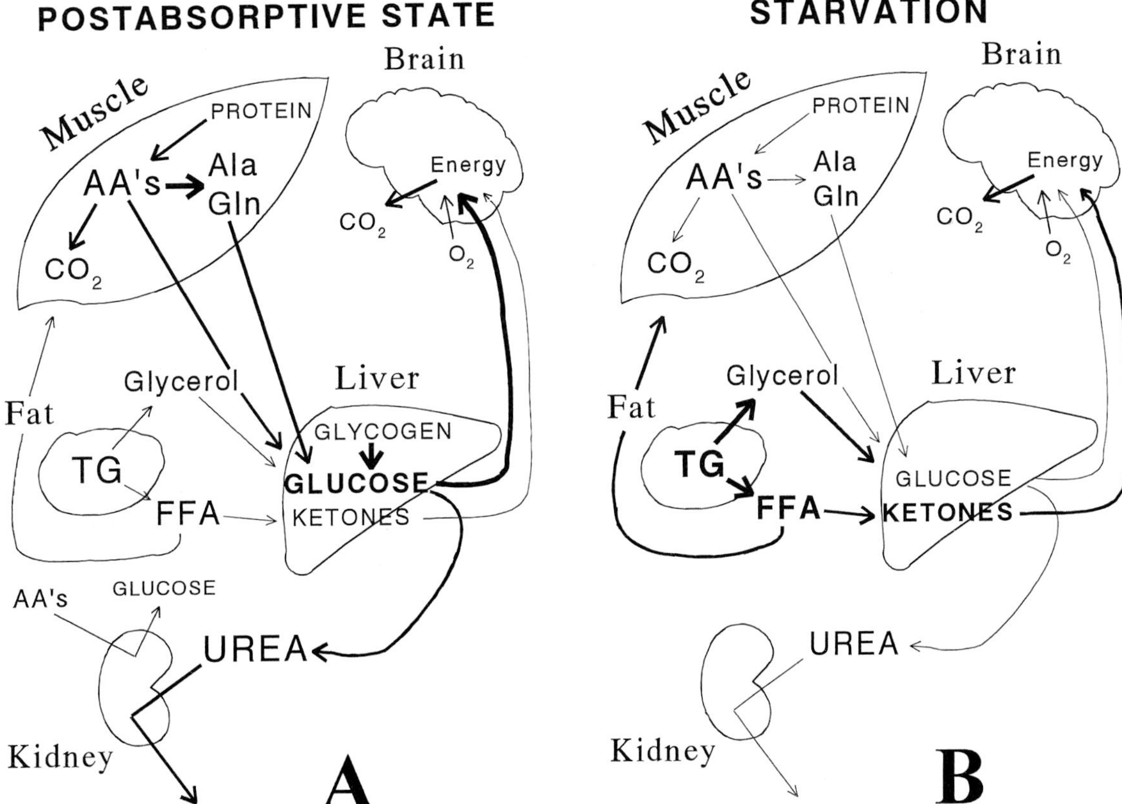

Figure 2.16. Interorgan flow of substrates in the body to maintain energy balance in the postabsorptive state (panel *A*) and after adaptation to starvation (panel *B*). The schematic diagrams are patterned after the work of Cahill. In all states, energy needs of the brain must be satisfied. In the postabsorptive state, glucose from liver glycogenolysis provides most of the glucose needed by the brain. After liver glycogen stores have been depleted (fasting state), gluconeogenesis from amino acids from muscle stores predominates as the glucose source. Eventually the body adapts to starvation by production and use of ketone bodies instead of glucose, thus sparing amino acid loss for gluconeogenesis. *AAs,* amino acids; *Ala,* alanine; *Gln,* glutamine; *TG,* triglycerides; *FFA,* free fatty acids. respectively. (Redrawn from Cahill GF Jr, Aoki TT. Partial and total starvation. In: Kinney JM, ed. Assessment of energy metabolism in health and disease, report of the first Ross conference on medical research. Columbus, Ohio: Ross Laboratories, 1980;129–34.)

the body provides energy for the brain in the form of glucose primarily from hepatic glycogenolysis and secondarily from glucose synthesis (gluconeogenesis) from amino acids. Other substrates (e.g., glycerol released from triglyceride lipolysis) may also be used for gluconeogenesis, but amino acids provide the bulk of the gluconeogenic substrate. The pathways of conversion are discussed above for those amino acids whose carbon skeletons can be easily rearranged to form gluconeogenic precursors. The remaining amino acids released from protein breakdown and not used for gluconeogenesis may be oxidized. The amino acid N released by this process is removed from the body by incorporation into urea via synthesis in the liver and excretion into urine via the kidney. Gluconeogenesis also occurs in the kidney, but the effect and magnitude are masked from A-V measurements because the kidney is also a glucose consumer. With respect to amino acids, the net effect of the kidney is the uptake and use of amino acids for gluconeogenesis (130, 131).

Role of Skeletal Muscle in Whole-Body Amino Acid Metabolism

Early A-V difference studies across the human leg or arm revealed that more than 50% of the amino acids released from skeletal muscle are in the form of alanine and glutamine (132), yet alanine and glutamine comprise less than 20% of amino acids in protein (Table 2.3). The specific purpose of the alanine and glutamine release is still not well defined. Several possible reasons exist. First, skeletal muscle will oxidize nonessential amino acids and the BCAAs in situ for energy. Because amino acid oxidation produces waste N and because ammonia is neurotoxic, release of waste N as ammonia must be avoided. Because both alanine and glutamine are readily synthesized from intermediates derived from glucose (alanine from transamination of pyruvate from glycolysis, and glutamine from α-ketoglutarate), they are excellent vehicles to remove waste N from muscle while avoiding ammonia release. Alanine removes one and glutamine removes two Ns per amino acid. These observations have led to the proposal of a glucose-alanine cycle in which glucose made by the liver is taken up by muscle, where glycolysis liberates pyruvate. The pyruvate is then transaminated to alanine and released from muscle. That alanine is extracted by the liver and transaminated to pyruvate that is then used for glucose synthesis (132). This scheme has been expanded to explain the use of BCAAs by muscle for energy and the disposal through alanine of their amino-N groups. Such a scheme resolves a problem related to the BCAAs. In contrast to the other essential amino acids, which are metabolized only in liver, the BCAAs are readily oxidized in other tissues, especially muscle. Thus, if the BCAAs, which comprise about 20% of amino acids in muscle protein, are oxidized for energy by the muscle, then the glucose-alanine cycle could provide a means of removal of the N that is generated in the process.

Whole-Body Adaptation to Fasting and Starvation

As indicated in Figure 2.16*A*, lipolysis (breakdown of adipose triglyceride to free fatty acids and glycerol) plays a lesser role in postabsorptive energy supply, especially to the brain. However, glycogen stores are limited and become depleted in less than 24 hours. That point in time when liver glycogen stores are exhausted is, by definition, the beginning of the *fasting* state. Now the glucose needs of the brain must be met completely by gluconeogenesis, which means sacrificing amino acids from protein. Because protein is critical to body function, from enzyme activity to muscle function related to breathing and circulation, unrestrained use of amino acids for glucose production would rapidly deplete protein, causing death in a matter of days. Clearly, this does not occur, because people may survive without food and obese subjects may be fasted for weeks without protein intake (1). Adaptation occurs in starvation by the brain's switching from a glucose-based to a ketone-based fuel supply. Free fatty acids released from lipolysis are converted in the liver into ketone bodies that can then be used by the brain and other tissues for energy. That conversion begins in the fasting state and is complete during long-term fasting periods (Fig. 2.16*B*). In starvation, tissues such as muscle may use free fatty acids directly for energy, and the brain uses ketone bodies. The body's dependence upon glucose as a fuel has been greatly reduced, thereby conserving protein. This adaptation process is complete within a week of onset of starvation (124).

The Fed State

Although the body can accommodate to starvation, it is not a normal occurrence. The adaptations seen in everyday life evolve around the postabsorptive period and the fed period. Basically, we go through our nights after completing absorption of the last meal using nutrient stores of glycogen and protein as depicted in Figure 2.16*A*. During the fed portion of the day the dietary intake of amino acids and glucose is used to replete protein and glycogen that were lost during the postabsorptive period; intake that exceeds amounts needed to replete nighttime losses are either oxidized or stored to increase protein, glycogen, or fat for growth or storage of excess calories. Although muscle contains the bulk of body protein, all organs are expected to lose protein during the postabsorptive period and, therefore, need repletion during the fed period. What is poorly understood is how the individual amino acids that enter through the diet are distributed among the various tissues in the amounts needed for each tissue. Just as each amino acid has its own separate metabolic pathways, the rates and fates of absorption and use are expected to differ among amino acids. Thus, dietary protein requirements cannot be discussed without also considering the requirements for individual amino acids.

Digestion and Absorption of Protein

Two organs have particular, potentially important, regulatory roles during feeding: the gut and liver. All dietary intake passes first through the gut and then through the liver via portal blood flow. Digestion of protein begins with pepsin secretion in gastric juice and with proteolytic enzymes secreted from the pancreas and the mucosa of the small intestine (133). These enzymes are secreted in their "pro" (or zymogen) form and become activated by cleavage of a small peptide portion. Pancreatic proenzymes become activated by intestinal enterokinase secreted into the intestinal juice to cleave trypsinogen to trypsin. The presence of dietary protein in the gut appears to signal secretion of the enzymes. As trypsin becomes activated, it binds to proteins to initiate hydrolysis. An excess of trypsin occurs when either more trypsin is secreted than there is protein present or when most of the dietary protein has been hydrolyzed. At this point the presence of unbound trypsin appears to signal a feedback regulation system to the pancreatic acinar cells to inhibit synthesis and secretion of trypsinogen. Some plants, such as soybeans, contain protein inhibitors of proteolytic enzymes such as trypsin. These proteins may often be denatured by heating (i.e., by cooking). Feeding unheated soybeans to rats results in hypertrophy of the pancreas, presumably caused by hypersecretion of pancreatic juices. The presumed mechanism is that the trypsin inhibitor in soy binds trypsin, which, in the free state, serves as a feedback inhibitor of pancreatic secretion (134).

The events of protein digestion and absorption as shown in Figure 2.17 are well established (133, 135–138). Proteins are successively broken down into smaller peptides on the basis of the amino acid residues targeted by the proteolytic enzymes. For example, pepsin has a relatively low specificity for neutral amino acids such as leucine or phenylalanine, whereas trypsin shows specificity for a basic target (lysine or arginine). In addition, exopeptidases attack the free ends of the peptide chains: pancreatic carboxypeptidases at the carboxyl terminus, and aminopeptidases secreted in intestinal juice at the amino terminus.

The free amino acids are absorbed by active transport into the mucosa by transporters specific to different types of amino acids (136, 137). At the same time, peptides, in particular di- and tripeptides, are assimilated on the luminal side intact. Peptide hydrolases present in the brush border and cytosol of the mucosal cells complete the hydrolysis of these peptides prior to their release into the portal blood system. There are specific transport systems for peptide uptake into mucosal cells, separate from the transporters for amino acids. It is thought that a quarter of dietary protein is absorbed as di- and tripeptides (139). For example, patients with the rare genetic Hartnup disease with a defect in renal and gut transport of selected amino acids cannot transport free tryptophan into

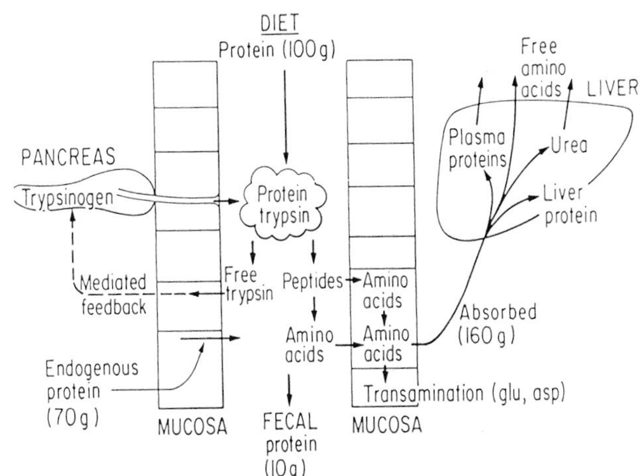

Figure 2.17. Digestion and absorption of dietary protein in the intestine. The secretion and feedback system of the pancreatic trypsinogen/trypsin is shown. In addition to the assumed dietary protein load of 100 g, an additional protein load of about 70 g occurs from secretion of protein and sloughing of mucosal cells. Under normal conditions, almost all of the protein is recovered by hydrolysis and absorption. Amino acids are absorbed by active transport through the mucosal cells into the portal blood system. Some amino acids are immediately metabolized by gut and liver during absorption. (From Crim MC, Munro HN. Protein and amino acid requirements and metabolism in relation to defined formula diets. In: Shils ME, ed. Defined formula diets for medical purposes. Chicago: American Medical Association, 1977;5–15, with permission.)

mucosal cells but do indeed absorb tryptophan when it is administered as a dipeptide (140, 141).

Figure 2.17 shows that in addition to dietary protein, protein is added directly to the lumen in the form of secreted proteins and sloughed cells. Because the small intestine is continually being remodeled with cells formed in the crypts migrating toward the villus tips, epithelial and other cells are continuously being sloughed off the tips of the villi. Although the exact amounts of protein secreted and cells sloughed are unknown, a reasonable estimate is that of the 70 g of protein added to the lumen, 20 g may come from secreted proteins and 50 g may come from sloughed cells (135). As indicated in Figure 2.17, most of this protein is efficiently reabsorbed.

To a limited but important extent, some proteins and large peptides enter intact directly from the gut into the basolateral blood. Absorption of intact proteins or large portions of proteins is a tenable physiologic explanation for numerous diseases involving food allergies and idiosyncrasies. The gut is generally viewed as an impermeable barrier that nutrients cross by active transport or where a break in the barrier occurs through cell injury. Small amounts of some proteins may pass this barrier by several possible mechanisms, such as through "leaks" between epithelial cell junctions or possibly by transport through uptake into vesicles from the lumen to the submucosal side of the epithelial cells (142). Again, the amount of protein entering intact is small, but it may be important in situations of immune response to the proteins or in delivery of some peptide drugs.

Gut and Liver as Metabolic Organs

The gut and liver facilitate absorption and delivery of dietary amino acids to the systemic blood and other tissues in the body. During this process, the gut and liver see all nutrients being absorbed and may sequester on the first pass during absorption any fraction of the dietary amino acids before these amino acid ever enter the systemic circulation. The liver has a natural role in this process as it is the organ that inactivates/modifies toxic substances in the blood. Therefore, the liver would be expected to regulate the flow of dietary amino acids into the systemic circulation following a meal. In addition, the liver is the only site in the body for metabolizing essential amino acids, except the BCAAs (which are metabolized by several tissues, most notably muscle). As mentioned above and discussed below, in terms of determining amino acid requirements, amino acids consumed during feeding in excess of the body's current needs would be expected to be oxidized. Therefore, a potential role for the liver is removal of excess amino acids, especially essential amino acids that cannot be oxidized in other tissues, on the first pass during amino acid absorption. The role of the gut and liver as active metabolic organs that metabolize dietary amino acids was shown in catheterized dogs by Elwyn et al. in 1968 (143). They demonstrated the active metabolism of the key nonessential amino acids, alanine, glutamine, and glutamate, and described how the BCAAs passed intact through the splanchnic bed. Several groups have shown similar results with respect to passage of amino acids following meal feeding in humans, using splanchnic bed and/or leg/arm A-V catheterization (51, 144–146). These studies have made several consistent observations.

As discussed above, the first observation was that most of the BCAAs in a meal pass through the splanchnic bed to be extracted and used by peripheral tissues. Later studies using labeled amino acid tracers administered enterally and intravenously (Fig. 2.14) showed that the BCAA leucine has the lowest fractional extraction by the gut and liver on the first pass when delivered enterally (Table 2.11). The amount of leucine oxidized by liver in the postabsorptive state is minimal (<2%) (93). Under conditions of feeding, the amount of enteral leucine extracted by the gut and liver on the first pass rose only slightly (94). However, the liver was shown to be a significant producer of KIC, indicating that the first step in BCAA metabolism is active, i.e., transamination. This step does not irreversibly remove leucine, rather it only forms a ketoacid that can be reconverted into leucine in a peripheral tissue such as muscle. Alternatively, the KIC produced by liver and released can be oxidized.

Of particular interest is the observation that the gut extracts glutamate and glutamine and releases alanine and ammonia (143). Early experiments with enteral glutamate infusion in dogs suggested that the glutamate sequestered is converted directly to alanine on the basis of glutamate uptake with resulting alanine release (147). Unfortunately, any interpretation of such an observation without proof from isotopic tracer studies would fall under the "gumball machine" analogy of Figure 2.8. Nonetheless, the observation is intriguing, especially in light of the consistent observation of a large A-V gradient for glutamine across the gut, indicating uptake (148–151).

PROTEIN AND AMINO ACID REQUIREMENTS

The most fundamental question in nutrition concerning protein and amino acids is simply, what amount of protein is required in the diets of humans to maintain health? This question has several parts. First, we must evaluate the intake of both protein and the amounts of the individual amino acids in that protein. Second, this question must be answered in humans *(a)* over the complete range of life and development, *(b)* in sickness and in health, and *(c)* under different conditions of work and environment. These questions and the methods used to answer them are discussed below in terms of their individual components.

When we discuss the amino acid composition of a specific protein source, we generally focus upon the amount of essential acids contained in it because these are the amino acids that are *indispensable* to our diet. Which amino acids are dispensable and which are indispensable was originally determined by testing whether a diet deficient in a particular amino acid would support growth in a rat. However, there are important species differences between rats and humans that limit the comparison of rat to man. Furthermore, the growth retardation model, which is effective with the rat, is not applicable to humans. An alternative for studying amino acid requirements in humans is the N balance technique. A diet that is adequate in total N but deficient in an essential (indispensable) amino acid cannot produce a positive N balance because protein can be synthesized only if each amino acid is present in adequate amounts. The nonessential amino acids can be synthesized if protein intake is adequate, but limited intake of an essential amino acid limits the amount of protein that can be synthesized. The body is then faced with a dietary excess of the other *nonlimiting* essential and nonessential amino acids that it cannot put into protein. Therefore, these amino acids must be oxidized to urea, and a negative N balance results.

The classic studies of Rose and colleagues measured N balance in humans fed diets deficient in individual amino acids. They determined that eight amino acids produced a negative N balance when they were deficient in the diet of adult humans (152–154). Although the enzymatic pathways are missing for synthesis of these essential amino acids, several of these amino acids (such as the BCAAs) have a catabolic pathway whose first step is reversible (i.e., transamination to form branched-chain keto acids). The rat growth model was used to show that growth can be supported by supplying the keto acids of these essential amino acids. Various formulations have been proposed for supplying the carbon skeleton of several essential amino acids (e.g., the BCAAs) without adding N, which is detrimental in disease states such as renal disease (155).

Another related question is whether dispensable, nonessential amino acids ever become indispensable. If a nonessential amino acid is used in the body faster than it is made, it becomes essential for that *condition* (6). Tyrosine and cysteine are made from phenylalanine and methionine, respectively, but if insufficient phenylalanine or methionine is consumed, tyrosine and cysteine also become deficient and *essential*. This question must be answered across the range of life from infancy to the elderly as well as in sickness and health. For example, enzymes for amino acid metabolism mature at different rates in the growing fetus and newborn infant. Histidine is essential in infants but not necessarily in healthy children or adults. Therefore, the classification of "essential" or "nonessential" depends upon species, maturation (i.e., infant, growing child, or adult), diet, nutritional status, and pathophysiologic condition. Also to be considered is whether a particular amino acid *given in excess of requirement* has properties that may ameliorate or improve a clinical condition. These considerations must somehow be evaluated for each population group in which they are important.

Protein Requirements

Determination of the protein requirement must consider both the amount of amino acid N and its quality (i.e., its ability to be digested and absorbed and its essential amino acid content). The simplest approach to measuring the nutritional quality of a protein is to measure the ability of that protein to promote growth in young growing animals, such as rats. Their growth depends on synthesis of new protein, which depends on essential amino acid intake. Because alterations in rat growth can be measured in several days, the growing rat is often used to compare differences in quality (composition) of protein/amino acid diets. Because this approach cannot ethically be applied to humans, other approaches for assessing *human* requirements have been applied: the *factorial method* and the *balance method*.

Factorial Method

When a person is placed on a protein-free diet, rates of amino acid oxidation and urea production decrease over several days as the body tries to conserve its resources, but amino acid oxidation and urea production do not drop to zero (Fig. 2.7). There is always some *obligatory* oxidation of amino acids and urea formation and miscellaneous losses of N (Table 2.10). The factorial method assesses all routes of loss possible for adult humans on an N-free diet. The minimum daily requirement of protein is assumed to be the amount that matches the sum of the various obligatory N losses.

Whereas nonurinary nonfecal N losses are often ignored in N balance studies of adequate protein intake, they are of critical importance in the assessment of protein requirements by the factorial method. A variety of studies have been performed to assess these losses, and the results are tabulated in a World Health Organization/Food and Agriculture Organization/ United Nations University (WHO/FAO/UNU) panel publication (156) and summarized again in a U.S. National Research Council report (157). The obligatory N losses include *(a)* urinary N, estimated to be 38 mg/kg/day of N; *(b)* fecal loss of enzymes and desquamated intestinal cells that cannot be fully reabsorbed, estimated to be 12 mg/kg/day; and *(c)* loss of N through sweat, hair, skin, and nail turnover and growth, menstrual flow, seminal fluid, ammonia in breath, nasal secretions, etc., estimated to be 2 to 3 mg/kg/day on a protein-free diet and 5 to 8 mg/kg/day with a normal protein intake (48). Summation of these directly measurable losses gives a total obligatory minimum daily loss of N of 54 mg/kg/day (range, 41–69 mg/kg/day), corresponding to a protein intake of 0.34 g/kg/day (where 1 g N = 6.25 g protein) (157).

This value of 54 mg/kg/day of N is an "average value," which must be raised if it is to indicate a requirement that will apply to most adults in the population. The 1973 WHO/FAO report (158) suggested a coefficient of variability among individuals of 15%. Adding twice this amount (+2 standard deviations) gives a protein requirement that includes 97.5% of the adult population; thus, the 0.34 g/kg/day protein becomes 0.44 g/kg/day after rounding off (45). For adults, the *dietary protein requirement* is considered to be this amount *plus* an adjustment for the inefficiency of use of dietary protein and for the quality (amino acid composition and digestibility) of the protein source consumed. For children and pregnant or lactating women, an additional (theoretically determined) amount of protein is added to this recommendation to account for growth and milk formation (157). Clearly this approach is based upon extrapolation of N losses from protein-starvation conditions and may reflect an adaptation to N deprivation, which may not reflect normal metabolism and N requirements of healthy humans near the actual requirement level. Hence, another method is needed to produce an alternative assessment of protein requirements.

Balance Method

In the balance method, subjects are fed varying amounts of protein or amino acids and the *balance* of a particular parameter—usually *N balance*—is measured. An adequate amount of dietary protein is that level of intake that will maintain a neutral or slightly positive N balance. The balance method can be used to titrate N intake in infants, children, and women during pregnancy, when the end point is a balance positive enough to allow appropriate accretion of new tissue. The balance method is also useful for testing the validity of the factorial method estimates. In general, N balance studies in which dietary protein intake is titrated give higher protein requirements than predicted by the factorial method.

There are several reasons for this result. The N balance method has important errors associated with it that are not minor (48, 158). Urine collections tend to underestimate N losses, and intake tends to be overestimated. Miscellaneous cutaneous and hair losses, which are "best guesses," may have small but substantial errors. However, these factors affect both methods. In the balance method, which "titrates" dietary intake to determine zero balance, the response to increasing protein intake is nonlinear. As protein intake is increased from a grossly deficient status toward an adequate status, the improvement in N balance is at first proportional to the amount of protein added to the diet. As the balance point is approached, however, the slope of the N balance–protein intake curve progressively decreases, i.e., more protein is required to achieve a zero N balance than is predicted by linear extrapolation (158). This refractoriness in reaching N equilibrium has been estimated to add 30% to the intake needed to equal output. As a result, the factorial method estimate of 0.44 g/kg/day is increased to a recommended intake of 0.57 g/kg/day (45).

Most studies of N balance have been performed at presumably adequate levels of energy intake. However, N balance is affected by energy intake. Energy intake below requirements causes the N balance measurement to become negative when protein intake is near the requirement. Most recommendations are based, nonetheless, on the assumption that energy intake is adequate (159). Another factor affecting N balance indirectly is the quality and digestibility of the protein being consumed. Generally it is assumed that protein of lesser quality and digestibility than egg white will be consumed. A correction factor that increases protein requirements by 25 to 30% is added to compensate for consumption of lesser-quality protein (156).

Table 2.13
Recommended Intakes of High-Quality Reference Protein for Normal Humans

Age (years)	Weight (kg)		Recommended Dietary Allowance of Protein (g/kg/day)	
0–0.5	6		2.2	
0.5–1	9		1.6	
1–3	13		1.2	
4–6	20		1.1	
7–10	28		1.0	
	Males	Females	Males	Females
11–14	45	46	1.0	1.0
15–18	66	55	0.9	0.8
19+	72–79	58–65	0.8	0.8

	(g/day)
Pregnancy add	+10
Lactation, 1st 6 months add	+15
Lactation, 2nd 6 months add	+12

Data from Food and Nutrition Board, National Research Council. Recommended dietary allowances. 10th ed. Washington, DC: National Academy Press, 1989.

Recommended Dietary Allowances for Protein

In 1989, the Food and Nutrition Board subcommittee of the U.S. National Research Council updated their recommended dietary allowances (RDAs) for protein and amino acids (157). The RDAs are largely based upon the 1985 FAO/WHO/UNU committee report (156). The RDA values for protein shown in Table 2.13 were based largely upon N balance data (rather than factorial method data) from studies using a high-quality, highly digestible source of protein. The protein intake values that produced zero N balance were then increased by two standard deviations to encompass 97.5% of the population to get the RDA for the reference protein. For example, from studies of young adult men, the value of 0.6 g/kg/day was increased to 0.75 g/kg/day.

The types of protein consumed in the United States were reviewed to determine both essential amino acid composition (see below) and digestibility. The RDA for the reference protein was then adjusted for imbalances in essential acids and protein digestibility where deemed important to produce the values shown in Table 2.13. (The reader is referred to ref. 157 for details.)

Special cases are cited in Table 2.13 in which growth and accretion of tissue must be accounted for in the RDAs: during pregnancy, during lactation, and in infants and children. In pregnancy, total protein deposited was estimated to be 925 g on the basis of maternal weight gain and an average birth weight at term. The rates of protein accretion were then divided by trimesters, with adjustments for variation in birth weight (+15%) and an assumed efficiency of conversion of dietary protein to fetal, placental, and maternal tissues (+70%) to produce increments in reference protein intake of +1.3, +6.1, and +10.7 g protein/day for the 1st, 2nd, and 3rd trimesters, respectively. These values were rounded to 10 g/day of additional protein for all trimesters to compensate for uncertainties about rates of tissue deposition and maintenance of those increases (Table 2.13) (157).

A factor to account for the additional protein intake required by women who are lactating was also added to values in Table 2.13. This addition was based upon the composition of human milk, the volume of milk produced, an adjustment for the estimated 70% conversion efficiency of dietary protein into newly synthesized milk protein, and a 25% increase to account for a two standard deviation variance among women. This value was also adjusted for duration of lactation.

Protein requirements for newborn infants include additional intake to account for the approximate 3.3 g protein/day accretion of growth of infants fed human milk (which includes a 25% increase to account for a two standard deviation variance). The RDA for older infants and children is based upon the 1985 WHO report (156), which used a modified factorial method. Rates of protein accretion due to growth were calculated by age group, increased by 50% to account for variability among children, and adjusted by a 70% conversion efficiency factor of dietary protein to body protein synthesis. This estimate was then increased by 25% (to account for a two standard deviation variance) to give the RDA.

Amino Acid Requirements

Recommendations for the intake of individual amino acids are largely based upon the pioneering work of W. C. Rose and his colleagues in the 1950s (152, 153). Irwin and Hegsted have reviewed these and other studies of amino acid requirement levels published before 1971 (160). Rose's studies are all N balance studies in which young male subjects were placed upon diets whose N intake consisted of a mixture of crystalline amino acids. The intake of a single amino acid could be altered, and the N balance measured. Because of the expense of the amino acid diets and the great difficulty in performing serial N balance studies at different intakes, Rose and colleagues were only able to study a very limited number of subjects per amino acid. Problems with interpreting the N balance data for a limited number of subjects cloud the extrapolation of these data to populations (161–163); yet these N-balance data remain the basis for the present amino acid recommendations in adults (Table 2.14). Rose's data have been confirmed in the more recent study of Inoue et al., also using the N balance technique (164), but the data set for requirements for individual amino acids is extremely slim.

An alternative approach has been taken by Young and colleagues (162, 165, 166), based upon the method of Harper and others to assess amino acid requirements in growing animals by using amino acid oxidation as an index of dietary sufficiency. Animals fed an insufficient amount of a specific individual amino acid reduce their oxidation of the deficient amino acid to obligatory levels. Oxidation of the dietary-deficient amino acid will remain at obligatory oxidation levels until the requirement level is met. Then, as dietary amino acid intake rises above requirement, the excess amino acid is oxidized. Therefore, a two-line curve should appear when amino acid oxidation is plotted against amino acid intake: a flat line below requirement (indicating obligatory oxidation) and a rising curve above the requirement (indicating oxidation of excess amino acid intake). The requirement level for the amino acid should be the intersection of the two curves, i.e., where oxidation of excess amino acid begins (167).

The amino acid oxidation curve has been assessed in growing animals placed on diets in which the intake of one amino acid is manipulated. A ^{14}C-labeled amino acid tracer of the manipulated amino acid is added to a test meal to measure oxidation as a function of dietary amino acid intake (168). This approach has been applied by Young and coworkers to assessing human amino acid requirements using *nonradioactive*, stable, isotopically labeled amino acid tracers. From the results of these studies, Young proposed that the present recommended essential amino acid requirements for isoleucine, leucine, lysine, phenylalanine/tyrosine, and valine be increased in healthy adults (165, 166). These estimates, which are 2 to 3 times the RDAs for adults (Table 2.14), have been challenged on methodologic and theoretical grounds by Millward et al. (169). Both Young (165, 166, 170) and Millward (171) have provided experimental data from stable isotope tracer studies in humans to support their arguments for and against increasing the recommended intakes of essential amino acids.

Zello et al. (172) have taken a different approach to the measurement of amino acid requirements using the oxidation of an amino acid tracer as an index. Rather than administer and measure the oxidation of an amino acid tracer of the amino acid that is being reduced in the diet, they use another essential amino acid tracer as the *indicator* of N balance. Nitrogen balance becomes negative when a single amino acid is deficient in the diet because the excess amino acids that cannot be incorporated into protein when one amino acid is deficient are oxidized, which increases urea production. As discussed above, measurement of the increase in urea production is fraught with problems, which is why direct oxidation of the indicator amino acid is measured using an amino acid tracer. When

Table 2.14
Estimates of Dietary Amino Acid Requirements (mg/kg/day) by Age Group

Amino Acid	Infants 3–4 months	Children 2–5 years	Children 10–12 years	Adults	Proposed by Young Adults[a]
Histidine	28	?	?	8–12[b]	
Isoleucine	70	31	28	10	23
Leucine	161	73	42	14	39
Lysine	103	64	44	12	30
Methionine + cysteine	58	27	22	13	15
Phenylalanine + tyrosine	125	69	22	14	39
Threonine	87	37	28	7	15
Tryptophan	17	12	3	4	6
Valine	93	38	25	10	20

Data in the first 4 columns were taken from ref. 157. Data for adults are based upon amounts of amino acids consumed to maintain N balance or to provide optimal growth in young children. Data for infants are based upon human or cow's milk consumption need for good growth.

[a]Data from Young and El-Koury (166) are based upon obligatory amino acid losses determined in part from amino acid tracer studies.

[b]Although no requirement for histidine has been quantified beyond infancy, 8–12 mg/kg/day has been recommended for adults.

dietary intake of the test amino acid is below requirement levels, oxidation of the indicator amino acid increases as excess amino acids are wasted. The key to this method is the availability of an indicator amino acid tracer whose oxidation can be accurately and precisely measured, which differs from the test amino acid being manipulated in the diet. Using this approach and [1-^{13}C]phenylalanine as the indicator amino acid, Zello et al. determined a requirement level for dietary lysine of 37 mg/kg/day (173), which supports Young's higher estimate of lysine requirements (Table 2.14).

Histidine, which is essential to the diet of the rat, has been hard to define as essential to the diet of adult humans (160). In the 1973 FAO/WHO report, no requirement for histidine was given for adults (158), but the 1985 WHO/FAO/UNU report (156) listed a requirement for histidine of 8–12 mg/kg/day (Table 2.14). This requirement in adults is based upon extrapolation of data from infants (157). The limited studies of adults indicate that the requirement for histidine may be less than 2 mg/kg/day (174). However, this requirement has not been clearly documented in normal subjects (154). Proving that histidine is essential in adults has largely been restricted to studies of renal failure (8). Why is it so difficult to determine whether histidine is essential in adults, using conventional dietary techniques, when there is little evidence that a metabolic pathway for histidine synthesis exists in humans (17)? The difficulties occur because the requirement for histidine is small and the stores of histidine in the body are large (8, 154). Histidine is particularly abundant in hemoglobin and carnosine (the dipeptide β-alanylhistidine, which is present in large quantities in muscle). Furthermore, gut flora synthesize an unknown amount of histidine, which may be absorbed and used. Histidine must be removed from the diet for more than a month to observe effects, and those effects are indirect measures of histidine insufficiency (a fall in hemoglobin and rise in serum iron) rather than alterations in conventional indices (N balance). Thus, even though little direct evidence for histidine synthesis in humans exists, our estimates for the necessity of dietary histidine intake in adults are still largely inferential.

In contrast to histidine, arginine is synthesized in large amounts in the body for the production of urea. However, like that of cysteine and tyrosine, synthesis of arginine depends upon the availability of precursors, ornithine and citrulline. Although adequate amounts of arginine, ornithine, and citrulline are normally present in the liver to operate the urea cycle, the synthesis of ornithine, from which arginine and citrulline are produced, may be limited (17). Because arginine is synthesized in the body from ornithine, it is *not* an essential amino acid, but it is *indispensable* for optimal growth in several species of young mammals (154).

Rose et al. observed an adequate N balance in adult subjects fed an arginine-free diet, and Snyderman et al. found no health problems or lack of weight gain in infants fed an arginine-free diet (8). Carey et al. (175) placed adult subjects on a diet devoid of arginine for 5 days. They measured indices of urea cycle activity: plasma ammonia concentration, daily urinary excretion of orotic acid, and urinary N excretion. They found no alterations due to the arginine-free diet. These results would lead to the conclusion that arginine is nonessential to the diet of humans; yet, there is little evidence that the body synthesizes ornithine from glutamate in substantial amounts (Fig. 2.4).

Castillo et al. simultaneously measured arginine, ornithine, and citrulline kinetics in healthy adults, using stable isotopically labeled tracers (87). Their studies show that the fluxes of all three amino acids are very low in blood and do not reflect the active urea cycle component, which appears to be highly compartmentalized in the liver. Ornithine and citrulline fluxes were comparable, but were only one-third the rate of arginine turnover, and a relatively small fraction of the ornithine tracer appeared in plasma arginine or citrulline. The low flux of ornithine suggests that very little synthesis occurs, but direct measurements of ornithine synthesis are lacking. Inferential measurements do suggest ornithine synthesis. For example, ^{15}N tracer is transferred from glycine into glutamate and into the metabolic products of glutamate, including ornithine and proline (23).

Assessment of Protein Quality

The quality of a protein is defined by its ability to support growth in animals. Higher-quality protein produces a faster growth rate. Such growth rate measurements evaluate the actual factors important in a protein: *(a)* pattern and abundance of essential amino acids, *(b)* relative amounts of nonessential and essential amino acids in the mixture, *(c)* digestibility when eaten, and *(d)* presence of toxic materials such as trypsin inhibitors or allergenic stimuli. Methods of determining the quality of a formula or protein source have generally fallen into two categories: empiric biologic assays and scoring systems.

Biologic Assays

It is assumed that the "highest quality protein" is protein that supports maximal growth of a young animal. Because rats grow quickly and have limited protein stores and a high metabolic rate, deficiencies and imbalances in amino acid patterns in young growing rats can be easily detected in a short period of time. The *protein efficiency ratio (PER)* is defined as the weight gained (in grams) divided by the amount of test protein consumed (in grams) by a young growing rat over several days. Obviously, duration of diet, age, starting body weight, and species of rat used are important variables. Typically, 21-day-old male rats fed 9 to 10% protein (by weight) for 10 days to 4 weeks are used. In one series of tests, casein produced a PER of 2.8; soy protein, 2.4; and wheat gluten, 0.4. Clearly, a casein diet produced much better growth (2.8 g of carcass weight increase for every gram of casein consumed) than gluten (0.4 g of carcass weight increase for every gram of gluten consumed). Such an approach has been useful in defining the relative efficacies of clinical formulas used in enteral and parenteral nutrition (176). The formula that provides the optimal mixture of essential and nonessential amino acids should induce the most rapid growth. Results from this method will be skewed in application to humans, depending upon the extent that human requirements for individual amino acids differ from those of the rat. However, the method has been very useful in comparing a new protein source against reference proteins, such as egg protein, and does evaluate other factors such as relative digestibility.

Scoring Systems

Rather than using growth in an animal species to indicate protein quality, a variety of methods have been developed to assign a quantitative value to the pattern of amino acids in a nutritional formula or to a particular dietary protein source. Thus, assignment is based on the amounts and importance of the individual amino acids in a formula. These "scoring" methods can be used to define protein quality in terms of amino acid content for any species. Block and Mitchell pointed out in 1946 that all amino acids have to be provided simultaneously at the sites of protein synthesis in the body in the same proportions that go into the protein (177). Assuming that any nonessential amino acid would not be limiting, they proposed that the value of a protein could be determined from the essential amino acid most limiting in abundance relative to the optimum amount needed. From this idea of "most limiting amino acid" came the concept of chemical scoring, which has been incorporated into the important reports assessing dietary needs of humans (157, 158, 178). The key to the method is that the test protein is defined "against" a reference protein, deemed to be of the "highest quality" in terms of amino acid composition. Historically, proteins that support maximal growth in animals were considered the proteins of "highest" quality. Those proteins from the most available sources for human consumption—eggs and cow milk—were consequently used as reference proteins. In 1973, the FAO/WHO adopted the amino acid requirement pattern recommended for various age groups (Table 2.14) as the basis for calculating chemical scores (158, 179). Some of the scoring patterns that have been used are shown in Table 2.15. Typically, data for the 2- to 5-year-old child are taken as most representative.

The scoring system is easy to apply because no animal studies or clinical studies are required to compare different nutritional formulations. The *chemical score* of a protein is calculated in two steps. First a score is calculated for each essential amino acid (EAA) in the protein against the reference protein:

$$\text{EAA score} = \frac{(\text{content of the EAA in the } \textit{test} \text{ protein/mixture})}{(\text{content of the EAA in } \textit{reference} \text{ protein/mixture})} \cdot 100$$

Next the lowest score is selected; the amino acid with the lowest score is defined as the *limiting amino acid*. The chemical score of the limiting amino acid is the protein's score. Typically, the limiting amino acids in dietary proteins are lysine, the sulfur-containing amino acids, threonine, and/or tryptophan. The BCAAs and phenylalanine/tyrosine are not usually limiting. The scoring method points out the obvious: proteins not balanced among the essential amino acids are not as good as those that are.

Ratio of Essential to Nonessential Amino Acids in Protein

Protein requirements diminish from infancy on (Table 2.13) because rates of accretion of new protein diminish with maturity. However, when the changes in requirements for essential amino acids in Table 2.14 are compared with the total protein requirements in Table 2.13 with age, a greater drop with age is seen in essential amino acid requirements than in protein requirements. Essential amino acids make up more than 30% of protein requirements in infancy and early childhood and drop to 20% in later childhood and 11% in adulthood. As essential amino

Table 2.15
Scoring Patterns of Amino Acid Requirements in Humans and of Egg and Body Proteins

Amino Acid	Infants 1 year	Children 2–5 years	Children 10–12 years	Adults	Hen Egg Protein	Body Protein
	(mg amino acid/g protein)					
Histidine	16	19	19	11	22	
Isoleucine	40	28	28	13	54	38
Leucine	93	66	44	19	86	65
Lysine	60	58	44	16	70	50
Methionine + cysteine	33	25	22	17	57	25
Phenylalanine + tyrosine	72	63	22	19	93	65
Threonine	50	34	28	9	47	25
Tryptophan	10	11	9	5	17	10
Valine	54	35	25	13	66	35

Data for humans and egg protein taken from ref. 157; data for body protein taken from ref. 166.

acids become a decreasingly important part of the amino acid requirements with age, nonessential amino acid intake could increase and become an increasingly greater proportion of our intake. However, such substitution does not necessarily happen. Except for possibly changing the type of protein eaten (e.g., decreased intake of milk proteins), we continue to eat protein presumably at or above the RDA. If that protein is of high quality, such as egg protein, it provides almost half of its amino acids as essential amino acids. Therefore, consumption of high-quality protein by adults at levels that meet the RDA for protein provide a severalfold excess of individual essential amino acids beyond requirements. In general, it is not hard for adults to meet the minimum for essential amino acid intake, as recommended or as proposed by Young (165), when protein is consumed at or above requirement.

Amino Acid Availability from Dietary Protein Sources

The above methods provide schemes for determining protein quality based upon either animal growth or amino acid composition using scoring. A particular drawback with the scoring system is that it does not consider other factors inherent in the test protein or the effect of how the protein is prepared for consumption. How food is prepared may significantly affect the bioavailibility of individual amino acids. As discussed above, some plants contain protein inhibitors of proteolytic digestive enzymes. Although soy protein is limiting in terms of its methionine content (180), rats fed soy protein grow poorly because of trypsin inhibition (134). Heat processing of the soy protein inactivates these inhibitors and improves growth (180).

However, heat processing itself may damage amino acids. For example, heat treatment of protein in the presence of reducing sugars can promote reactions altering the lysine amino groups in the protein. This reaction, called the Maillard, or "browning," reaction, can be seen in milk processing in which lactose reacts with lysine at high temperatures. Oxidative or alkaline processing conditions may alter other essential and nonessential amino acids, inducing loss of methionine or formation of amino acid products that have toxic properties. Likewise, storage conditions may affect the nutritional quality of the protein. Thus, processing or "cooking" the protein source as well as storage conditions and other factors must be considered in evaluating the quality of the protein.

Protein and Amino Acid Needs in Disease

Most of the discussion to this point has centered around amino acid and protein metabolism in normal individuals. Although the effect of disease on amino acid and protein requirements is beyond the limits of this introductory chapter, a few important general points need to be made. The first is that energy and protein needs are tied together, as illustrated in Figure 2.16. When metabolic rate rises, body protein is mobilized for use as a fuel (amino acid oxidation) and for supply of carbon for gluconeogenesis. Several disease states increase metabolic rate. The first is infection, in which the onset of fever is a hallmark of increased metabolic rate. The second is injury, be it trauma, burn injury, or surgery per se. Along with onset of a hypermetabolic state comes a characteristic increase in the loss of protein measured by increased urea production. Sir David Cuthbertson observed over 60 years ago that a simple bone fracture causes significant loss of N in the urine (181). Since then, numerous studies of the hypermetabolic state of injury and infection have been performed. For most people, the injuries suffered are minimal and self-limiting, i.e., the fever goes away in a couple of days or the injury heals. In normal, healthy people the impact of the injury on overall protein metabolism is as minimal as a bout of fasting. However, in chronic, long-term illness or in patients otherwise weakened by age or other factors, onset of a hypermetabolic state may produce a significant and dangerous loss of body N.

The second point is that while the diagnosis of a metabolic condition that needs correcting may be straightforward (e.g., finding an increased loss of N and wasting of body protein), correcting the problem by administration of nutritional support is not as simple. The underlying illness usually resists or complicates simple nutritional replacement of amino acids. Trauma and infection are classic problems in which prevention of N loss is very difficult. Supplying additional nutrients either enterally (by mouth or feeding tube) or parenterally (by intravenous administration) may blunt, but will not reverse, the N loss seen in injury (182, 183).

Simple tools have been used to identify the hypermetabolic state: indirect calorimetry to measure energy expenditure, and N balance to follow protein loss. These measurements have shown that blunting the N loss in such patients is not as simple as supplying more calories, more amino acids, or different formulations of amino acids. What becomes clear is that although a nutritional problem exists, nutritional replacement will not correct the problem; instead, the metabolic factors that cause the condition must be identified and corrected. Wilmore has categorized the factors that produce the hypermetabolic state into three groups: stress hormones (cortisol, catecholamines, glucagon), cytokines (tumor necrosis factor, interleukins, etc.), and lipid mediators (prostaglandins, thromboxanes, etc.) (182). Strategies have been developed to address these various components. For example, insulin and growth hormone have been administered to provide anabolic hormonal stimuli to improve N balance. Alternatively, studies have been conducted in healthy individuals in which one or more of the potential mediators are administered to determine its effect on amino acid and protein metabolism (183, 184). For example, studies of the infusion of individual hormones while isotopically labeled amino acid tracers are also infused have given us some insight into the mechanisms of hormone action upon the regulation of amino acid oxidation and protein breakdown and synthesis in humans (184).

There are areas in which administration of a specific amino acid may produce a pharmacologic effect in ameliorating the disease state; for example, administration of glutamine and arginine or limiting sulfur amino acid intake. Glutamine is the most highly concentrated amino acid in muscle cells and plasma (89). Glutamine is an important nutrient to many cells, especially the gut and white cells, where it may be used both as a source of energy and for such critical processes as the synthesis of nucleotides (185). Glutamine is an essential nutrient for cell culture media. Because a hallmark of injury is a drop in the intracellular level of muscle glutamine, presumably because of increased use by other tissues, glutamine has been proposed as a nutrient that becomes conditionally essential in trauma and infection (182).

Arginine is another nonessential amino acid with important properties for promoting immune system function. Arginine is the precursor for nitric oxide synthesis (186) and has been proposed as a nutrient for altering immune function and improving wound healing (187, 188). We believe that adequate ornithine is synthesized to maintain arginine supplies under normal conditions, but we do not know whether additional demands for arginine can be met endogenously or whether arginine becomes a conditionally indispensable nutrient. For example, Yu et al. (189) used stable isotope tracers to measure arginine kinetics in pediatric burn patients and determined little net de novo arginine synthesis, suggesting that under conditions of burn injury, insufficient arginine is made to meet the body's presumed increased need when the immune system is under challenge.

Elevated plasma homocysteine is an independent risk factor for vascular disease (190). Homocysteine is produced by hydrolysis of *S*-adenosylhomocysteine, which is derived from *S*-adenosylmethionine, a major methyl group donor (e.g., in creatine synthesis in Fig. 2.5). Homocysteine may be "remethylated" to methionine or degraded via condensation with serine to form cystathionine, which then goes on to form cysteine (Fig. 2.4). High concentrations of homocysteine occur when either or both of the disposal pathways of homocysteine are impaired. Because these reactions of homocysteine metabolism depend upon vitamin B_6 (pyridoxal 5′-phosphate) and folate, supplementation of the diet with vitamin B_6 and folate often is effective in lowering plasma homocysteine levels (190). Alternatively, the dietary intake of sulfur amino acids may be reduced by ingesting relatively more of a sulfur amino acid–poor dietary protein, such as soy protein.

While supplementation of specific amino acids or cofactors may produce beneficial responses, there may be occasions when supplementation produces undesirable effects on the disease state. Supplementing glutamine in the diets of cancer patients may be counterproductive because the glutamine (which is essential for fast-growing cell lines in culture) may promote accelerated tumor growth (191). Similarly, arginine supplementation may stimulate nitric oxide synthesis because of the increased availability of the precursor for its formation. However, nitric oxide production produces both helpful and detrimental effects (186). In these and other applications of specific nutrients, the use of isotopically labeled tracers is particularly helpful because the metabolic fate of the administered nutrient may be followed (labeled nitrate production from nitric oxide synthesis from ^{15}N-labeled arginine) as well as measurement of the promotion or suppression of protein synthesis and proteolysis in specific tissues. Amino acid and protein requirements in various diseases are quite difficult to assess and require a multifactorial approach. These are the real challenges facing us in nutrition today and in the days ahead.

REFERENCES

1. Cahill GF. N Engl J Med 1970;282:668–75.
2. Munro HN, Allison JB, eds. Mammalian protein metabolism, vol 1. New York: Academic Press, 1964.
3. Munro HN, Allison JB, eds. Mammalian protein metabolism, vol 2. New York: Academic Press, 1964.
4. Munro HN, ed. Mammalian protein metabolism, vol 3. New York: Academic Press, 1969.
5. Munro HN, ed. Mammalian protein metabolism, vol 4. New York: Academic Press, 1970.
6. Chipponi JX, Bleier JC, Santi MT, et al. Am J Clin Nutr 1982;35:1112–6.
7. Harper AE. Dispensable and indispensable amino acid interrelationships. In: Blackburn GL, Grant JP, Young VR, eds. Amino acids: metabolism and medical applications. Boston: John Wright, 1983;105–21.
8. Laidlaw SA, Kopple JD. Am J Clin Nutr 1987;46:593–605.
9. Block RJ, Weiss KW. Amino acid handbook: methods and results of analysis. Springfield, IL: Charles C Thomas, 1956.
10. Bergström J, Fürst P, Noree LO, et al. J Appl Physiol 1974;36:693–7.
11. Cohn SH, Vartsky D, Yasumura S, et al. Am J Physiol 1980;239:E524–30.
12. Heymsfield SB, Waki M, Kehayias J, et al. Am J Physiol 1991;261:E190–8.
13. Christensen HN. Physiol Rev 1990;70:43–77.
14. Souba WW, Pacitti AJ. J Parent Ent Nutr 1992;16:569–78.
15. Rennie MJ, Tadros L, Khogali S, et al. J Nutr 1994; 124(Suppl):1503S–8S.
16. Ellory JC. Amino acid transport systems in mamalian red cells. In: Yudilevich DL, Boyd CA, eds. Amino acid transport in animal cells. Manchester: Manchester University Press, 1987;106–19.
17. Krebs HA. The metabolic fate of amino acids. In: Munro HN, Allison JB, eds. Mammalian protein metabolism, vol I. New York: Academic Press, 1964;125–76.
18. Matthews DE, Ben Galim E, Bier DM. Anal Chem 1979;51:80–4.
19. Ben Galim E, Hruska K, Bier DM, et al. J Clin Invest 1980;66:1295–304.
20. Stipanuk MH. Annu Rev Nutr 1986;6:179–209.
21. Yoshida T, Kikuchi G. Arch Biochem Biophys 1970;139: 380–92.
22. Yoshida T, Kikuchi G. J Biochem (Tokyo) 1972;72:1503–16.
23. Matthews DE, Conway JM, Young VR, et al. Metabolism 1981;30:886–93.
24. Jacobsen JG, Smith LH Jr. Physiol Rev 1968;48:424–511.

25. Hayes KC. Nutr Rev 1985;43:65–70.
26. Meister A. Glutathione. In: Arias IM, Jakoby WB, Popper H, et al., eds. The liver: biology and pathobiology. 2nd ed. New York: Raven Press, 1988;401–17.
27. Beutler E. Annu Rev Nutr 1989;9:287–302.
28. Rebouche CJ, Paulson DJ. Annu Rev Nutr 1986;6:41–66.
29. Borum PR. Annu Rev Nutr 1983;3:233–59.
30. Rebouche CJ. Fed Proc 1982;41:2848–52.
31. Watkins CA, Morgan HE. J Biol Chem 1979;254:693–701.
32. Young VR, Munro HN. Fed Proc 1978;37:2291–300.
33. Shank RP, Aprison MH. Glutamate as a neurotransmitter. In: Kvamme E, ed. Glutamine and glutamate in mammals, vol 2. Boca Raton, FL: CRC Press, 1988;3–19.
34. Rothstein JD, Martin LJ, Kuncl RW. N Engl J Med 1992;326:1464–8.
35. Bloch K, Schoenheimer R. J Biol Chem 1941;138:167–94.
36. Heymsfield SB, Arteaga C, McManus C, et al. Am J Clin Nutr 1983;37:478–94.
37. Walser M. JPEN J Parenter Enteral Nutr 1987;11:73S–8S.
38. Crim MC, Calloway DH, Margen S. J Nutr 1975;105: 428–38.
39. Welle S, Thornton C, Totterman S, et al. Am J Clin Nutr 1996;63:151–6.
40. Wang Z-M, Gallagher D, Nelson M, et al. Am J Clin Nutr 1996;63:863–9.
41. Milner JA, Visek WJ. Nature 1973;245:211–2.
42. Waterlow JC, Garlick PJ, Millward DJ. Protein turnover in mammalian tissues and in the whole body. Amsterdam: North-Holland, 1978.
43. Hellerstein MK, Munro HN. Interaction of liver and muscle in the regulation of metabolism in response to nutritional and other factors. In: Arias IM, Jakoby WB, Popper H, et al., eds. The liver: biology and pathobiology. 2nd ed. New York: Raven Press, 1988;965–83.
44. Harper AE. Am J Clin Nutr 1985;41:140–8.
45. Munro HN. Historical perspective on protein requirements: objectives for the future. In: Blaxter K, Waterlow JC, eds. Nutritional adaptation in man. London: John Libbey, 1985;155–68.
46. Scrimshaw NS, Hussein MA, Murray E, et al. J Nutr 1972;102:1595–604.
47. Allison JB, Bird JWC. Elimination of nitrogen from the body. In: Munro HN, Allison JB, eds. Mammalian protein metabolism, vol 1. New York: Academic Press, 1964;483–512.
48. Munro HN. Amino acid requirements and metabolism and their relevance to parenteral nutrition. In: Wilkinson AW, ed. Parenteral nutrition. London: Churchill-Livingstone, 1972; 34–67.
49. Owen OE, Reichle FA, Mozzoli MA, et al. J Clin Invest 1981;68:240–52.
50. Owen OE, Morgan AP, Kemp HG, et al. J Clin Invest 1967;46:1589–95.
51. Wahren J, Felig P, Hagenfeldt L. J Clin Invest 1976;57:987–99.
52. Brundin T, Wahren J. Am J Physiol 1994;267:E648–55.
53. Frayn KN, Khan K, Coppack SW, et al. Clin Sci 1991;80:471–4.
54. Young VR, Haverberg LN, Bilmazes C, et al. Metabolism 1973;23:1429–36.
55. Pisters PWT, Pearlstone DB. Crit Rev Clin Lab Sci 1993;30:223–72.
56. Möller-Loswick A-C, Zachrisson H, Hyltander A, et al. Am J Physiol 1994;266:E645–52.
57. Louard RJ, Bhushan R, Gelfand RA, et al. J Clin Endocrinol Metab 1994;79:278–84.
58. Cheng KN, Dworzak F, Ford GC, et al. Eur J Clin Invest 1985;15:349–54.
59. Barrett EJ, Revkin JH, Young LH, et al. Biochem J 1987;245:223–8.
60. Gelfand RA, Barrett EJ. J Clin Invest 1987;80:1–6.
61. Biolo G, Chinkes D, Zhang X-J, et al. JPEN J Parenter Enteral Nutr 1992;16:305–15.
62. Biolo G, Fleming RYD, Maggi SP, et al. Am J Physiol 1995;268:E75–84.
63. Tessari P, Inchiostro S, Zanetti M, et al. Am J Physiol 1995;269:E127–36.
64. Wolfe RR. Radioactive and stable isotope tracers in biomedicine: principles and practice of kinetic analysis. New York: Wiley Liss, 1992.
65. San Pietro A, Rittenberg D. J Biol Chem 1953;201:457–73.
66. Picou D, Taylor-Roberts T. Clin Sci 1969;36:283–96.
67. Bier DM, Matthews DE. Fed Proc 1982;41:2679–85.
68. Steffee WP, Goldsmith RS, Pencharz PB, et al. Metabolism 1976;25:281–97.
69. Duffy B, Gunn T, Collinge J, et al. Pediatr Res 1981;15:1040–4.
70. Yudkoff M, Nissim I, McNellis W, et al. Pediatr Res 1987;21:49–53.
71. Waterlow JC, Golden MHN, Garlick PJ. Am J Physiol 1978;235:E165–74.
72. Fern EB, Garlick PJ, McNurlan MA, et al. Clin Sci 1981;61:217–8.
73. Fern EB, Garlick PJ, Waterlow JC. Clin Sci 1985;68:271–82.
74. Matthews DE, Motil KJ, Rohrbaugh DK, et al. Am J Physiol 1980;238:E473–9.
75. Bier DM. Diabetes Metab Rev 1989;5:111–32.
76. Saccomani MP, Bonadonna RC, Caveggion E, et al. Am J Physiol 1995;269:E183–92.
77. Allsop JR, Wolfe RR, Burke JF. J Appl Physiol 1978;45:137–9.
78. El-Khoury AE, Sánchez M, Fukagawa NK, et al. J Nutr 1994;124:1615–27.
79. Leese GP, Nicoll AE, Varnier M, et al. Eur J Clin Invest 1994;24:818–23.
80. Matthews DE, Bier DM, Rennie MJ, et al. Science 1981;214: 1129–31.
81. Matthews DE, Schwarz HP, Yang RD, et al. Metabolism 1982;31:1105–12.
82. Schwenk WF, Beaufrère B, Haymond MW. Am J Physiol 1985;249:E646–50.
83 Matthews DE. Ital J Gastroenterol 1993;25:72–8.
84. Cobelli C, Saccomani MP, Tessari P, et al. Am J Physiol 1991;261:E539–50.
85. Cobelli C, Saccomani MP. JPEN J Parenter Enteral Nutr 1991;15:45S–50S.
86. Tessari P, Barazzoni R, Zanetti M, et al. Am J Physiol 1996;271:E733–41.
87. Castillo L, Sánchez M, Vogt J, et al. Am J Physiol 1995;268: E360–7.
88. Darmaun D, Matthews DE, Bier DM. Am J Physiol 1986;251:E117–26.
89. Souba WW, Herskowitz K, Austgen TR, et al. JPEN J Parenter Enteral Nutr 1990;14:237S–43S.
90. Souba WW. Annu Rev Nutr 1991;11:285–308.
91. Cortiella J, Matthews DE, Hoerr RA, et al. Am J Clin Nutr 1988;48:988–1009.
92. Tessari P, Pehling G, Nissen SL, et al. Diabetes 1988;37:512–9.
93. Matthews DE, Marano MA, Campbell RG. Am J Physiol 1993;264:E109–18.
94. Hoerr RA, Matthews DE, Bier DM, et al. Am J Physiol 1991;260:E111–7.
95. Krempf M, Hoerr RA, Marks L, et al. Metabolism 1990;39:560–2.
96. Battezzati A, Brillon DJ, Matthews DE. J Investig Med 1995;43:401A.

97. Castillo L, Chapman TE, Yu YM, et al. Am J Physiol 1993;265:E532–9.
98. Matthews DE, Marano MA, Campbell RG. Am J Physiol 1993;264:E848–54.
99. Battezzati A, Brillon DJ, Matthews DE. Am J Physiol 1995;269:E269–76.
100. Hankard RG, Darmaun D, Sager BK, et al. Am J Physiol 1995;269:E663–70.
101. Harkin R, Battezzati A, Brillon DJ, et al. Am J Clin Nutr 1995;61:907.
102. Nair KS, Halliday D, Griggs RC. Am J Physiol 1988;254: E208–13.
103. Welle S, Thornton C, Statt M, et al. Am J Physiol 1994;267:E599–604.
104. Cryer DR, Matsushima T, Marsh JB, et al. J Lipid Res 1986;27:508–16.
105. Lichtenstein AH, Hachey DL, Millar JS, et al. J Lipid Res 1992;33:907–14.
106. Reeds PJ, Hachey DL, Patterson BW, et al. J Nutr 1992;122: 457–66.
107. Schauder P, Arends J, Schäfer G, et al. Klin Wochenschr 1989;67:280–5.
108. Arends J, Schäfer G, Schauder P, et al. Metabolism 1995;44:1253–8.
109. Pussell BA, Peake PW, Brown MA, et al. J Clin Invest 1985;76:143–8.
110. Brinton EA, Eisenberg S, Breslow JL. Arterioscler Thromb 1994;14:707–20.
111. Ikewaki K, Rader DJ, Schaefer JR, et al. J Lipid Res 1993;34:2207–15.
112. Laurent GJ. Am J Physiol 1987;252:C1–9.
113. Long CL, Dillard DR, Bodzin JH, et al. Metabolism 1988;37:844–9.
114. Young VR, Alexis SD, Baliga BS, et al. J Biol Chem 1972;247:3592–600.
115. Long CL, Haverberg LN, Young VR, et al. Metabolism 1975;24:929–35.
116. Elia M, Carter A, Bacon S, et al. Clin Sci 1980;59:509–11.
117. Rathmacher JA, Flakoll PJ, Nissen SL. Am J Physiol 1995;269:E193–8.
118. Millward DJ, Bates PC, Grimble GK, et al. Biochem J 1980;190:225–8.
119. Rennie MJ, Millward DJ. Clin Sci 1983;65:217–25.
120. Sjölin J, Stjernström H, Henneberg S, et al. Metabolism 1989;38:23–9.
121. Lundholm K, Bennegård K, Eden E, et al. Cancer Res 1982;42:4807–11.
122. Morrison WL, Gibson JNA, Rennie MJ. Eur J Clin Invest 1988;18:648–54.
123. Nair KS, Ford GC, Ekberg K, et al. J Clin Invest 1995;95:2926–37.
124. Cahill GF Jr, Aoki TT. Partial and total starvation. In: Kinney JM, ed. Assessment of energy metabolism in health and disease, report of the first Ross conference on medical research. Columbus, Ohio: Ross Laboratories, 1980;129–34.
125. Elia M. Organ and tissue contribution to metabolic rate. In: Kinney JM, Tucker HN, eds. Energy metabolism: determinants and cellular corollaries. New York: Raven Press, 1992;61–79.
126. Bier DM, Leake RD, Haymond MW, et al. Diabetes 1977;26:1016–23.
127. Owen OE, Felig P, Morgan AP, et al. J Clin Invest 1969;48:574–83.
128. Pozefsky T, Felig P, Tobin JD, et al. J Clin Invest 1969;48:2273–82.
129. Felig P, Owen OE, Wahren J, et al. J Clin Invest 1969;48:584–94.
130. Stumvoll M, Chintalapudi U, Perriello G, et al. J Clin Invest 1995;96:2528–33.
131. Cersosimo E, Judd RL, Miles JM. J Clin Invest 1994;93:2584–9.
132. Felig P. Annu Rev Biochem 1975;44:933–55.
133. Alpers DH. Digestion and absorption of carbohydrates and proteins. In: Johnson LR, Alpers DH, Christensen J, et al., eds. Physiology of the gastrointestinal tract. 3rd ed. New York: Raven Press, 1994;1723–49.
134. Green GM, Olds BA, Matthews G, et al. Proc Soc Exp Biol Med 1973;142:1162–7.
135. Crim MC, Munro HN. Protein and amino acid requirements and metabolism in relation to defined formula diets. In: Shils ME, ed. Defined formula diets for medical purposes. Chicago: American Medical Association, 1977;5–15.
136. Matthews DM. Protein absorption: development and present state of the subject. New York: Wiley-Liss, 1991.
137. Ganapathy V, Brandsch M, Leibach FH. Intestinal transport of amino acids and peptides. In: Johnson LR, Alpers DH, Christensen J, et al., eds. Physiology of the gastrointestinal tract. 3rd ed. New York: Raven Press, 1994;1773–94.
138. Freeman HJ, Kim YS. Annu Rev Med 1978;29:99–116.
139. Alpers DH. Fed Proc 1986;45:2261–7.
140. Asatoor AM, Cheng B, Edwards KDG, et al. Gut 1970;11: 380–7.
141. Jepsen JB. Hartnup disease. In: Stanbury JB, Wyngaarden JB, Fredrickson DS, eds. The metabolic basis of inherited disease. 4th ed. New York: McGraw-Hill, 1978;1563–77.
142. Gardner ML. Absorption of intact proteins and peptides. In: Johnson LR, Alpers DH, Christensen J, et al., eds. Physiology of the gastrointestinal tract. 3rd ed. New York: Raven Press, 1994;1795–820.
143. Elwyn DH, Parikh HC, Shoemaker WC. Am J Physiol 1968;215:1260–75.
144. Aoki TT, Brennan MF, Muller WA, et al. Am J Clin Nutr 1976;29:340–50.
145. DeFronzo RA, Felig P. Am J Clin Nutr 1980;33:1378–86.
146. Elia M, Livesey G. Clin Sci 1983;64:517–26.
147. Neame KD, Wiseman G. J Physiol 1957;135:442–50.
148. Windmueller HG. Adv Enzymol 1982;53:201–37.
149. Windmueller HG. Metabolism of vascular and luminal glutamine by intestinal mucosa in vivo. In: Häussinger D, Sies H, eds. Glutamine metabolism in mammalian tissues. Berlin: Springer-Verlag, 1984;61–77.
150. Cersosimo E, Williams PE, Radosevich PM, et al. Am J Physiol 1986;250:E622–8.
151. Abumrad NN, Williams P, Frexes-Steed M, et al. Diabetes Metab Rev 1989;5:213–26.
152. Rose WC, Wixom RL, Lockhart HB, et al. J Biol Chem 1955;217:987–95.
153. Rose WC. Nutr Abstr Rev 1957;27:631–47.
154. Visek WJ. Annu Rev Nutr 1984;4:137–55.
155. Walser M. Clin Sci 1984;66:1–15.
156. FAO/WHO/UNU. Energy and protein requirements. Geneva: World Health Organization technical series no. 724, 1985.
157. Food and Nutrition Board, National Research Council. Recommended dietary allowances. 10th ed. Washington, DC: National Academy Press, 1989.
158. FAO/WHO. Energy and protein requirements. Geneva: World Health Organization technical report series no. 522, 1973.
159. Young VR, Yu YM, Fukagawa NK. Acta Paediatr Scand 1991;80(Suppl)373:5–24.

160. Irwin MI, Hegsted DM. J Nutr 1971;101:539–66.
161. Millward DJ, Price GM, Pacy PJH, et al. Proc Nutr Soc 1990;49:473–87.
162. Young VR, Bier DM, Pellett PL. Am J Clin Nutr 1989;50: 80–92.
163. Young VR. Am J Clin Nutr 1987;46:709–25.
164. Inoue G, Komatsu T, Kishi K, et al. Amino acid requirements of Japanese young men. In: Blackburn GL, Grant JP, Young VR, eds. Amino acids: metabolism and medical applications. Boston: John Wright, 1983;55–62.
165. Young VR. J Nutr 1994;124(Suppl):1517S–23S.
166. Young VR, El-Khoury AE. Proc Natl Acad Sci USA 1995;92:300–4.
167. Young VR, Moldawer LL, Hoerr R, et al. Mechanisms of adaptation to protein malnutrition. In: Blaxter K, Waterlow JC, eds. Nutritional adaptation in man. London: John Libbey, 1985;189–217.
168. Kang-Lee YA, Harper AE. J Nutr 1977;107:1427–43.
169. Millward DJ, Rivers JPW. Eur J Clin Nutr 1988;42:367–93.
170. Marchini JS, Cortiella J, Hiramatsu T, et al. Am J Clin Nutr 1993;58:670–83.
171. Millward J. J Nutr 1994;124 Suppl:1509S–16S.
172. Zello GA, Wykes LJ, Ball RO, et al. J Nutr 1995;125:2907–15.
173. Zello GA, Pencharz PB, Ball RO. Am J Physiol 1993;264: E677–85.
174. Kopple JD, Swendseid ME. J Nutr 1981;111:931–42.
175. Carey GP, Kime Z, Rogers QR, et al. J Nutr 1987;117:1734–9.
176. Bjelton L, Sandberg G, Wennberg A, et al. Assessment of biological quality of amino acid solutions for intravenous nutrition. In: Kinney JM, Borum PR, eds. Perspectives in clinical nutrition. Baltimore: Urban & Schwarzenberg, 1989;31–41.
177. Block RJ, Mitchell HH. Nutr Abstr Rev 1946;16:249–78.
178. Reeds PJ. Proc Nutr Soc 1990;49:489–97.
179. Pellett PL. Am J Clin Nutr 1990;51:723–37.
180. Young VR, Scrimshaw NS, Torun B, et al. J Am Oil Chem Soc 1979;56:110–20.
181. Cuthbertson DP. Injury 1980;11:175–89.
182. Wilmore DW. N Engl J Med 1991;325:695–702.
183. Lowry SF. Proc Nutr Soc 1992;51:267–77.
184. Matthews DE, Battezzati A. Substrate kinetics and catabolic hormones. In: Kinney JM, Tucker HN, eds. Organ metabolism and nutrition: ideas for future critical care. New York: Raven Press, 1994;1–22.
185. Souba WW, Klimberg VS, Plumley DA, et al. J Surg Res 1990;48:383–91.
186. Griffith OW, Stuehr DJ. Annu Rev Physiol 1995;57:707–36.
187. Brittenden J, Heys SD, Ross J, et al. Clin Sci 1994;86:123–32.
188. Ziegler TR, Gatzen C, Wilmore DW. Annu Rev Med 1994;45:459–80.
189. Yu YM, Sheridan RL, Burke JF, et al. Am J Clin Nutr 1996;64:60–6.
190. Verhoef P, Stampfer MJ, Buring JE, et al. Am J Epidemiol 1996;143:845–59.
191. Souba WW. Ann Surg 1993;218:715–28.

SELECTED READINGS

Food and Nutrition Board, National Research Council. Recommended dietary allowances. 10th ed. Washington, DC: National Academy Press, 1989.

Munro HN, Allison JB. Mammalian protein metabolism, vol 1. New York: Academic Press, 1964.

Nissen S. Modern methods in protein nutrition and metabolism. San Diego: Academic Press, 1992.

Wolfe RR. Radioactive and stable isotope tracers in biomedicine: principles and practice of kinetic analysis. New York: Wiley Liss, 1992.

3. Carbohydrates

ROY J. LEVIN

HISTORICAL HIGHLIGHTS

The initial history of carbohydrates is the story of sugar cane and the human passion for sweetness. Although there is some dissension, sugar cane's origin is thought to be Papua New Guinea. It was probably cultivated from wild plants (still in existence) about 10,000 years ago at the time of the global Neolithic agricultural revolution. The slow diffusion of migrants carried it to India, Southeast Asia, and China. Sugar was mentioned by an Indian author in 325 BC. After the Arabs defeated the Romans, they brought the sugar cane from Persia to Europe and the Mediterranean where it failed to thrive, apart from the Moroccan coast. The returning Crusaders brought sugar to the European courts where it became an important and desirable luxury dietary constituent. Sugar cane was introduced to the Caribbean by Christopher Columbus on his second voyage, in 1493. The plants came from his father-in-law's plantation established in Madeira in 1492 (Canary Islands). They thrived and were dispersed to Central and South America and throughout the Caribbean. By the early 17th century, raw sugar was being handled by refineries in England and France. Beets (unlike sugar cane, which needed a tropical or semitropical climate) could be grown in temperate climates and were first recognized as a source of sugar by Marggraf in 1747. Napoleon used beets to bypass the British sugar blockade of the French Caribbean Islands; by 1813, approximately 35,000,000 kg (35,000 tonnes) were being produced. Sugar from beets now represents 40% of the world sugar market. Kirchoff, a Russian chemist, reported in 1812 that starch, the plant storage form of carbohydrate, when boiled with dilute acid gave rise to a sugar identical with that of grapes (glucose). Schmidt, in 1844, designated carbohydrates as compounds that contained C, H, and O and showed that sugar was found in the blood. Liver glycogen, the animal storage form of carbohydrate, was discovered by the outstanding French physiologist Claude Bernard in 1856. Sugar is now cultivated in practically every country in the world and is consumed as a basic or staple food.

DEFINITION

What are carbohydrates? The formal definition is a class of substances having the formula $C_n(H_2O)_n$, i.e., the molar ratio of C:H:O is 1:2:1. This definition, however, fails for oligosaccharides, polysaccharides, and sugar alcohols (viz., sorbitol, maltitol, mannitol, galactitol, and lactitol). Of the complex carbohydrate macromolecules known, the main member is plant starch (and the animal polymer glycogen), but the group includes pectins, cellulose, and gums. Simple carbohydrates include the hexose monosaccharides (glucose, galactose, and fructose) and the disaccharides maltose (glucose-glucose), sucrose (glucose-fructose), and lactose (glucose-galactose). Other carbohydrates include trioses (glycerose, $C_3H_6O_3$), tetroses (erythrose, $C_4H_8O_4$), and pentoses (ribose, $C_5H_{10}O_5$). The latter are important constituents of nucleic acids. In general, oligosaccharides yield two to ten monosaccharides on hydrolysis, while polysaccharides yield more than ten. The polysaccharides serve storage and structural functions. Starch is the storage carbohydrate of plants; glycogen is that of animals (liver contains up to 6% and muscle about 1%) and is often called animal starch. There are many different types of starch, depending on the plant source. Inulin, for example, is a starch found in the tubers and roots of dahlias, artichokes, and dandelions and when hydrolyzed yields only fructose; hence it is a fructosan. The oligosaccharide cellulose consists of glucose units linked by β(1-4) bonds to form long straight chains strengthened by hydrogen bonding. It is the chief structural framework of plants and cannot be easily digested by humans because they do not secrete an intestinal carbohydrase that attacks the β(1-4) linkage. It is often thought of as a dietary fiber that gives bulk to food. Bacterial enzymes, however, can break down cellulose. A small amount is probably hydrolyzed by this process in the colons of humans, but it has little nutritive value.

Dietary Carbohydrates

Carbohydrates (Fig. 3.1) thus exist as a vast family of naturally occurring compounds and derivatives of these compounds. Fortunately, only a small number of them are commercially significant and used in the food industry, while a similar number are of metabolic importance.

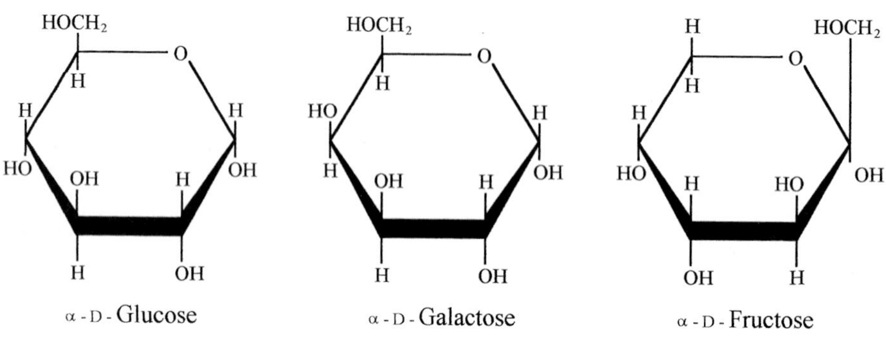

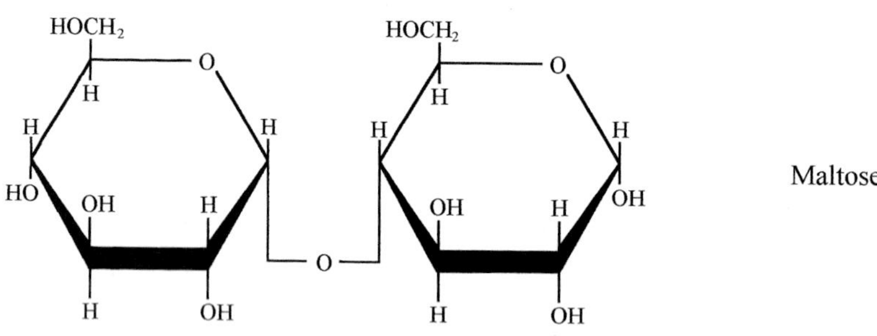

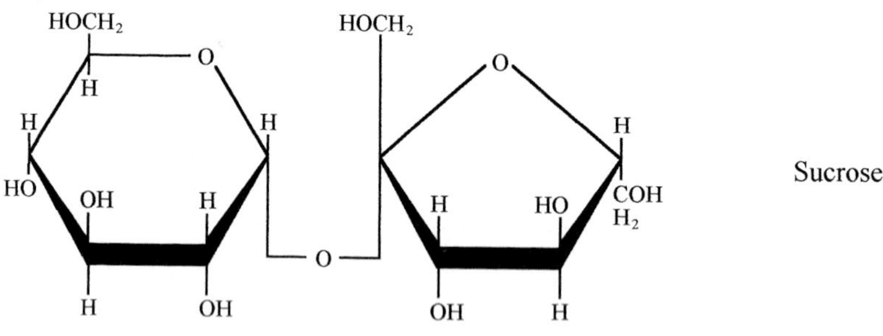

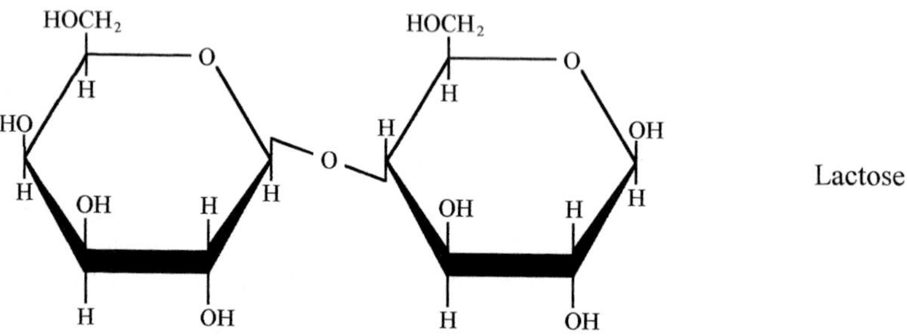

Figure 3.1. Structures of the common dietary monosaccharides and disaccharides in perspective, Haworth representation.

Table 3.1
Principal Dietary Carbohydrates

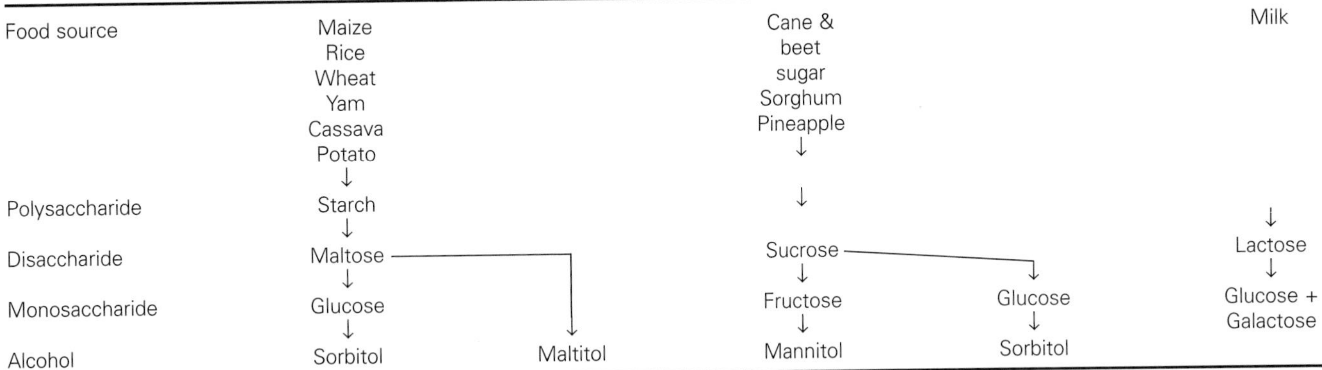

Food source	Maize Rice Wheat Yam Cassava Potato ↓		Cane & beet sugar Sorghum Pineapple ↓		Milk
Polysaccharide	Starch ↓		↓		↓
Disaccharide	Maltose ↓		Sucrose ↓		Lactose ↓
Monosaccharide	Glucose ↓	↓	Fructose ↓	Glucose ↓	Glucose + Galactose
Alcohol	Sorbitol	Maltitol	Mannitol	Sorbitol	

Dietary carbohydrate is a major nutrient for both man and omnivorous animals. Human adults in the Western world obtain approximately half their daily caloric requirements from dietary carbohydrates; in the developing countries, it is the major source. Of this ingested carbohydrate, some 60% is in the form of polysaccharides, mainly starch and glycogen, but the disaccharides sucrose and lactose represent 30% and 10%, respectively (Table 3.1). More recently, in a few Western countries, a significant intake of monosaccharide sugars (glucose and fructose) can be obtained from manufactured foods and drinks. Some oligosaccharides, such as raffinose and stachyose, are found in small amounts in various legumes. They cannot be broken down by the enzymes of the pancreas and small intestine, but they are digested by bacterial enzymes, especially in the colon.

The important dietary polysaccharides, starch and glycogen, have to be broken down into their constituent monosaccharides before they can be used for metabolic purposes. This breakdown is initially carried out by the carbohydrase α-amylase secreted by the salivary glands and the pancreas and completed by the barrier of disaccharidases in the brush border membrane of the mature enterocytes covering the villi of the small intestine (see Table 3.2 for the major intestinal glycosidases) (1).

Table 3.2
Major Glycosidases of the Mammalian Enterocyte Brush Border

Glycosidase	Enzyme Complex	Enzyme Activity
Maltase-sucrase	Sucrase-isomaltase	80% of maltase; some α-limit dextrinase; all of sucrase; most of isomaltase
Maltase-isomaltase		
Maltase-glucoamylase (2)	Glucoamylase	All glucoamylase; most of α-limit dextrinase; 20% maltase: small % isomaltase
Trehalase		All trehalase
Lactase	β-glycosidase	All neutral lactase and cellobiose
Glycosyl-ceramidase (phlorizin hydrolase)		Most of aryl-β-glycosidase

Adapted from Dahlqvist A, Semenza G. J Pediatr Gastroenterol 1988;4:857–67.

Starch

Starch, by far the most important dietary polysaccharide, consists only of glucose units and is thus a homopolysaccharide and is designated a glucosan or glucan. It is actually composed of two such homopolymers (Fig. 3.2): amylose, which has linear (1-4) linked α-D-glucose, and amylopectin, a highly branched form containing both (1-4) and (1-6) linkages at the branch points. Plants have both forms as insoluble, semicrystalline granules and differing ratios of amylopectin and amylose, depending on the plant source (Table 3.3). The salivary and pancreatic amylases act on the interior (1-4) linkages but cannot break the outer glucose-glucose links. Thus, the final breakdown products formed by the amylases are α(1-4)-linked disaccharides (maltose) and trisaccharides (maltotriose).

Starch Breakdown

The breakdown of starch begins in the mouth, with salivary amylase. It is often assumed that as this is swallowed into an acid stomach the enzymic carbohydrate breakdown is then stopped (although acid hydrolysis may still occur) because salivary amylase is inhibited by a pH below 4. However, starch and its end products and the proteins

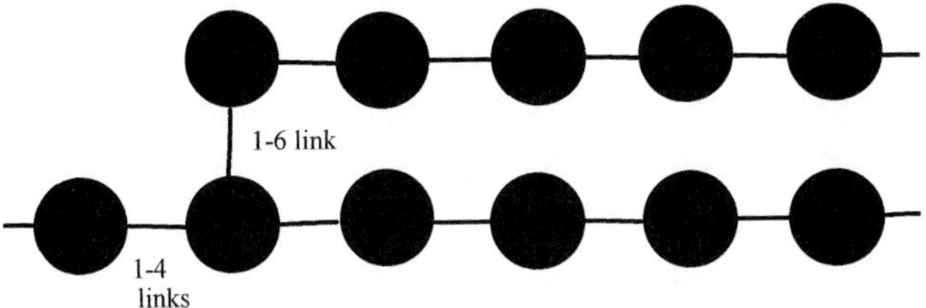

Figure 3.2. Starch is composed of amylose (15–20%) and amylopectin (80–85%). Amylose is a nonbranching helical chain structure of glucose residues, while amylopectin (a portion shown above) has branched chains of 24–30 glucose residues *(solid black)* joined by (1→4) glucosidic linkages with (1-6) linkages creating the branching points.

Table 3.3
Amylose and Amylopectin Content of Various Plant Starches

	Amylose (%)	Amylopectin (%)
Maize (standard)	24	76
Potato	20	80
Rice	18.5	81.5
Tapioca	16.7	83.3
Wheat	25	75

and amino acids present in a mixed meal all buffer the acid of the stomach, allowing hydrolysis to continue. The quantitative involvement of salivary amylase in the breakdown of starch is thus probably underestimated. Pancreatic α-amylase added to the emptying gastric contents (chyle) in the duodenum cannot hydrolyze the (1-6) branching links and has little specificity for the (1-4) links adjacent to the branching points. Amylase action thus produces large oligosaccharides (α-limit dextrins) containing on average about eight glucose units with one or more (1-6) links. These α-limit dextrins are split by the enzymic action of glucoamylase (α-limit dextrinase), which sequentially removes a single glucose unit from the nonreducing end of a linear α(1-4)-glucosyl oligosaccharide. Maltose and maltotriose are then broken down by secreted and brush border disaccharidases, especially sucrase-isomaltase, into free glucose, which is then transported into and across the enterocytes by hexose transporters (Table 3.4).

The initial breakdown of starch into α-limit dextrins, the intraluminal or cavital digestion phase, occurs mainly in the bulk fluid phase of the intestinal contents. In man, there appears to be little of the so-called contact or membrane digestion in which adsorption of amylase onto the brush border surface of enterocytes facilitates its enzymatic activity (2).

Normally α-amylase is not a limiting factor in the assimilation of starches in humans, but newborn babies and especially premature ones cannot assimilate starch because the pancreas secretes insufficient α-amylase to digest it. However, after a month, the secretion of α-amylase is satisfactory for full digestion (3).

Resistant Starch

Starch is usually eaten cooked. The heat of cooking gelatinizes the starch granules, increasing their susceptibility to enzymic (α-amylase) breakdown. However, a proportion of the starch, called resistant starch (RS), is undigestible even after prolonged incubation with the enzyme. In cereals, RS represents 0.4 to 2% of the dry matter; in potatoes, 1 to 3.5%; and in legumes, 3.5 to 5.7%. RS has been categorized as the sum of the starch and degradation products not absorbed in the small intestine of a healthy person (3a). There are three main categories: RS1, physically enclosed starch (partially milled grains and seeds); RS2, ungelatinized crystallite granules of the B-type x-ray pattern (as found in bananas and potatoes); and RS3, retrograded amylose (formed during the cooling of starch gelatinized by moist heating). Resistant starch escapes digestion in the small intestine, but it then enters the colon, where it can be fermented by the local resident bacteria (of which there are over 400 different types). In this respect, RS is somewhat similar to dietary fiber. Estimates of the RS and unabsorbed starch represent about 2 to 5% of the total starch ingested in the average Western diet. This approximates to less than 10 g carbohydrate/day (4). The end products of the fermentation of the RS in the colon are short-chain fatty acids (e.g., acetic, butyric, propionic), carbon dioxide, hydrogen, and methane (expelled as flatus).

Refractory starches stimulate bacterial growth in the colon. While the short-chain fatty acids stimulate crypt cell mitosis in animals, it is not known whether they do the same in the human colon (5). However, if the human colon is removed from the mainstream of foodstuffs flowing down the lumen of the gastrointestinal tract, then the colonocytes become defunctionalized and ionic absorption is reduced. Luminal short-chain fatty acids from bacterial fermentation are used by colonocytes as metabolic substrates and appear essential for normal colonic function (6).

Dietary Fiber

Dietary fiber was originally defined as "the remnants of plant cell walls not hydrolyzed by the alimentary enzymes

Table 3.4
Human Facilitated-Diffusion Glucose Transporter Family, GLUT 1–5

Type	Amino Acids (N)	Chromosome Location	K_m (mmol/L) for Hexose Uptake[a]	Major Expression Sites
GLUT 1 (red cell)	492	1	1–2 (red cells)	Placenta, brain, kidney, colon
GLUT 2 (liver)	524	3	15–20 (hepatocytes)	Liver, β-cell,kidney, small intestine
GLUT 3 (brain)	496	12	10 (Xenopus oocytes)	Brain, testis
GLUT 4 (muscle/fat)	509	17	5 (adipocytes)	Skeletal & heart muscle, brown & white fat
GLUT 5 (small intestine)	501	1	6–11* *(fructose) (*Xenopus* oocytes)	Small intestine, sperm

[a]The approximate K_m values refer to the uptake of glucose (fructose in the case of GLUT 5) in the designated tissue or cells in parentheses and are shown to give an approximate index of the affinity of the transporter for glucose.

of man" but the definition was subsequently modified to include "all plant polysaccharides and lignin which are resistant to hydrolysis by the digestive enzymes of man" (7). The fiber, both soluble and insoluble, is fermented by the luminal bacteria of the colon. High-fiber diets maintained for the long term reduce the incidence of colon cancer, but the mechanisms(s) involved rest on speculation, viz., its bulking action speeding colonic transit and reducing the absorption of luminal chemicals or the fiber absorbing the carcinogenic agents (5). (See also Chapter 43.)

Sugar Functions and Properties

Sugars, unlike starch, have an obvious impact on human taste—they are sweet. The classic view of taste recognizes four: sweet, sour, salty, and bitter, with all other taste sensations considered mixtures of these. A more modern concept is that sweetness is not a unitary quality, and individuals "taste" different sweetness qualities for different sweeteners. Human neonates recognize and like sweetness, which is not surprising since the lactose in their major food, human milk, gives it a sweet taste. Estimates of relative sweetness of various carbohydrates by humans are usually made against the standard, sucrose (100%). On this scale, glucose (sweet with a bitter side taste) is 61 to 70, fructose (sweet, fruity) 130 to 180, maltose (sweet, syrupy) 43 to 50, and lactose 15 to 40. It is speculated that during mankind's evolution, the quest for food, hence, energy, made primitive man recognize that sweetness indicated safety and energy. Hence, sweetness became a desirable quality.

Today, sugar (especially sucrose) is used extensively in foods to give sweetness, energy, texture, and bulk and also for appearance, preservation (by raising the osmotic pressure), and fermentation (in bread, alcoholic beverages). The palatability, appearance, and shelf life of a huge variety of foods and drinks are enhanced by adding sucrose, e.g., breads, cakes, and biscuits; preserves and jellies; confectionery; dairy products; cured, dried, and preserved meats; breakfast cereals; and frozen and canned vegetables. This "hidden sugar" makes the assessment of dietary sucrose intakes difficult.

GETTING GLUCOSE INTO CELLS—THE TRANSPORTERS

A major source of metabolic energy for most, if not all, mammalian cells is the oxidation of D-glucose. The lipid-rich membranes of such cells, however, are relatively impermeable to hydrophilic polar molecules such as glucose. Special transport processes have been developed to allow the cellular entry and exit of glucose. Carrier proteins located in the plasma membranes of cells can bind glucose and allow it to traverse the lipid membrane barrier, releasing the hexose into the cellular cytoplasm or body fluids.

Two distinct classes have been described: *(a)* a family of facilitative glucose transporters (Table 3.4) and *(b)* Na^+-glucose cotransporters (symporters). The former class are membrane integral proteins found on the surface of all cells. They transport D-glucose down its concentration gradient (from high to low), a process described as *facilitative diffusion.* The energy for the transfer comes from dissipation of the concentration difference of the glucose. Such glucose transporters allow glucose to enter cells readily, but they can also allow it to exit from cells according to the prevailing concentration difference. In contrast, the Na^+-glucose cotransporters participate in the uphill movement of D-glucose against its concentration difference, that is, they perform *active transport.* They are especially expressed in the specialized brush borders of the enterocytes of the small intestine and the epithelial cells of the kidney (proximal) tubule. They occur at lower levels in the epithelial cells lining the lung and in the liver (8). Cooperation between the two classes of glucose transporters, together with the hormones involved in carbohydrate metabolism, allows a fine control of glucose concentration in the plasma, maintaining a continuous supply of the body's main source of cellular energy.

The Human Facilitative-Diffusion Glucose Transporter Family

Five major hexose transporters have been identified and cloned since the characterization of the first, GLUT 1, by molecular cloning (9). They are numbered GLUT 1 to 5 in the order of their discovery and are all proteins with similar molecular structures containing between 492 and 524 amino acid residues. Mueckler et al. (9), using hydropathic and secondary structure predictions, proposed a two-dimensional orientation model of GLUT 1 in the plasma membrane (Fig. 3.3). The molecule has three major domains: *(a)* 12 α-helices spanning the membrane

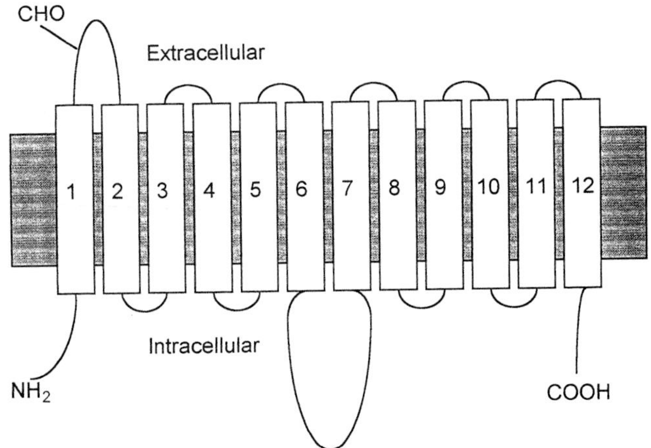

Figure 3.3. Highly schematic diagram illustrating the predicted secondary structure model of the glucose transporter molecule (GLUT 1) in the cell membrane *(shaded).* The putative membrane-spanning α-helices are shown as rectangles numbered 1–12 connected by chains *(lines)* of linked amino acids. (Adapted from Mueckler M, Caruso C, Baldwin SA, et al. Science 1985;229:941–5.)

with the N and C termini of the protein on the cytoplasmic side of the cell membrane, *(b)* an intracellular domain of 65 hydrophilic amino acids (between M6 and M7), and *(c)* an extracellular 33-amino-acid segment (between M1 and M2) containing the site for an asparagine-linked oligosaccharide at asparagine 45.

The prediction was that the polypeptide backbone of the molecule traverses or spans the plasma membrane 12 times. Both the amino- and carboxy-terminal ends of the molecule are on the cytoplasmic side of the membrane, while an N-glycosylation site is present on the first extracytoplasmic loop (M1 and M2). These basic topologic features have been confirmed by studies using proteolytic digestion and sequence-specific antibodies. GLUT 1, purified from human red cells and reconstituted in liposomes, appears to be predominantly in the α-helical form, and the transmembrane segments form α-helixes at right angles to the plane of the lipid membrane (10). The molecular structure of GLUT 1, shown in Figure 3.3, is, of course, a two-dimensional model. At present, the three-dimensional structure of the carrier in the membrane is not known. Studies using radiation inactivation of the carrier in intact red cells have indicated that GLUT 1 probably exists as homotetramer (11).

The structures, properties, expression sites, and roles of each of the five facilitative glucose transporter isoforms are briefly described below and summarized in Table 3.4. Because of the recognized importance of these transporters in health and disease, there have been numerous reviews (12–16), which should be consulted for greater detail.

GLUT 1 (Erythroid-Brain Carrier)

GLUT 1 is the glucose transporter in the human red cell. The first to be characterized by molecular cloning (9), it consists of 492 amino acid residues (Table 3.4). The gene for its expression is located on chromosome 1. GLUT 1 is widely distributed in many tissues including heart, kidney, adipose cells, fibroblasts, placenta, retina, and brain, but little is expressed in muscle or liver. Since there is particularly high expression in the endothelial cells of the microvessels of the brain, it forms part of the blood-brain barrier (17). The transport process for D-glucose in the red cell is asymmetrical, as the affinity (K_m) for D-glucose uptake is approximately 1 to 2 mmol/L while the K_m for the exit of glucose is 20 to 30 mmol/L. This asymmetry appears to be allosterically regulated by the binding of intracellular metabolites and inhibited by adenosine triphosphate (ATP) (18). The asymmetry allows the transporter to be effective when the extracellular glucose is low and the intracellular demand high.

GLUT 2 (Liver Glucose Transporter)

Many biochemical studies indicated that the glucose transporter in liver cells was distinct from that of the red cells. Moreover, adult liver cells had only very low levels of GLUT 1 mRNA. Cloning of the second glucose carrier, GLUT 2, was accomplished by screening rat and human cDNA libraries with a cDNA probe for GLUT 1. GLUT 2 has 55% identity in amino acid sequence with GLUT 1, and it displays the same topologic organization in the cell membrane as predicted for GLUT 1. Human GLUT 2 contains 524 amino acids (Table 3.4), compared with rat GLUT 1 of 522 residues, and they show 82% identity in amino acid sequences, an excellent example of conservation of structure between species. GLUT 2 is preferentially expressed in liver (sinusoidal membranes), kidney (tubule cells), small intestine (enterocytes), and the insulin-secreting β cells of the pancreas.

In the liver cell, GLUT 2 has a low affinity for glucose (K_m = 17 mmol/L) and shows symmetric transport, i.e., a similar K_m for influx and efflux. This high-capacity, low-affinity transporter is useful for rapid glucose efflux following gluconeogenesis. GLUT 2 can also transport galactose, mannose, and fructose (19). The ability to transport fructose is only seen with GLUT 2 and GLUT 5 (see below).

GLUT 3 (Brain Glucose Transporter)

GLUT 3 was originally cloned from a human fetal muscle cDNA library (20). It contains 496 amino acid residues (Table 3.4) and shows 64% identity with GLUT 1 and 52% identity with GLUT 2. Its amino acid sequence again suggests that its membrane topology is similar to that of GLUT 1 (Fig. 3.3). GLUT 3 mRNA appears to be present in all tissues, but its highest expression is in adult brain, kidney, and placenta. Adult muscle, however, shows only very low levels. In the brain, it is mainly expressed in neurons. A GLUT 3 mRNA is found in fibroblasts and in smooth muscle. Since both of these cell types are found in practically all tissues, the ubiquitous expression of GLUT 3 is understandable. Its affinity for glucose transport is relatively low ($K_m \approx$ 10 mmol/L) but significantly higher than that of GLUT 1 (17 mmol/L). A GLUT 3 is also found in spermatozoa. Such cells undertake glycolysis in the male genital tract, taking up glucose from epididymal fluid.

GLUT 4 (Insulin-Responsive Glucose Transporter)

Glucose is transported across the cell membranes of adipocytes (fat cells), and its rate of transport can be speeded up 20- to 30-fold within 2 or 3 minutes by addition of insulin, without evidence of protein synthesis. Studies showed that this stimulation of glucose transport was due in part to translocation of GLUT 1 from an intracellular pool into the membrane. Careful quantitative measurements showed, however, that this could account for only a 12- to 15-fold increase in glucose transport. It became obvious that another transporter would have to be involved to account for the much larger insulin-stimulated transport. This new transporter, GLUT 4, was first identified in rat adipocytes by use of a monoclonal antibody. Subsequently, it has been cloned from rat, mouse, and human DNA (19). It is a protein with 509 amino acid residues (Table 3.4), with 65% identity with GLUT 1, 54% identity with GLUT 2, and 58% identity with GLUT 3. Rat and mouse GLUT 4s have 95 and 96% identity, respectively, with human GLUT 4. As with the previous GLUT transporters, the two-dimensional orientation of the structure in the cell membrane is similar to that proposed for GLUT 1 (Fig. 3.3).

GLUT 4 is the major glucose transporter of the insulin-sensitive tissues, brown and white fat, and skeletal and cardiac muscle. It occurs primarily in intracellular vesicles in the cells of these tissues. Insulin stimulation causes a rapid increase in the number of glucose transporters on the membranes of these cells because the vesicles are translocated toward the membrane and then fuse with it, releasing the molecule. This process ensures a high density of glucose transporters, enhancing the ability to move glucose from the surrounding cellular fluid into the interior of the cell, i.e., increased V_{max} for glucose uptake. Because of this mechanism, the position of GLUT 4 and its regulation are important components of glucose homeostasis and its role in diabetes has been much studied.

Glut 5 (The Fructose Transporter?)

GLUT 5 was isolated from human (21), rat, and rabbit enterocyte cDNA libraries. It consists of 501 amino acid residues (Table 3.4), and has only 42%, 40%, 39%, and 42% identity with GLUTs 1, 2, 3, and 4, respectively. It is said to be primarily expressed in the jejunum (both in the brush border and basolateral membrane), but its mRNA has been detected, albeit at low levels, in human kidney, skeletal muscle, and adipocytes, microglial cells, and the blood-brain barrier. GLUT 5 appears to transport glucose poorly and is really the transporter for fructose. It is found in high concentrations in mature human spermatozoa (22), which are known to use fructose as an energy source (human seminal fluid contains high concentrations of fructose, which is manufactured by the seminal vesicles). In oocytes injected with GLUT 5 mRNA to effect GLUT 5 expression, the K_m for fructose uptake was 6 to 11 mmol/L.

Other Transporters

The major glucose transporters in cells have been the identified and cloned GLUTs 1–5. There are reports, however, of a possible GLUT 6 and GLUT 7.

GLUT 6 (Pseudogene-like Sequence)

A cDNA clone isolated from a human jejunum cDNA library hybridized to an approximately 11-kb transcript expressed at variable levels in all normal and tumor cells examined (22). The sequence of a partial-length GLUT 6 cDNA revealed approximately 80% identity with the human brain GLUT 3 transporter. However, because of multiple stop codons and frame shifts, the sequence could not encode a functional glucose transporter protein. The GLUT 6 gene was located on the long arm of human chromosome 5.

GLUT 7 (Hepatic Microsomal Glucose Transporter)

The existence of GLUT 7 has been reported. Unlike the others, it is an internal or intracellular transporter, possibly involved in the glucose-6-phosphatase complex found in the endoplasmic reticulum of hepatocytes. Glucose is produced in the liver by glycogenolysis and gluconeogenesis. The last stage of each of these processes is the removal of a phosphate group from glucose by the multicomponent enzyme glucose-6-phosphatase; the resultant free glucose is liberated into the lumen of the endoplasmic reticulum. To export the glucose into the bloodstream it must be transferred across the endoplasmic reticulum membrane. The transporter that does this job is called GLUT 7 (23). It has 65% identity of amino acids with GLUT 2. There is a unique sequence of 6 amino acids at the C terminus of GLUT 7 that appears to be involved in keeping the transporter in the endoplasmic reticulum membrane (19).

Study of Glucose Transporters by Use of Transgenic and Knock-Out Mice

Although a host of metabolic inhibitors are available for use in examining metabolic pathways, their specificities are often questionable. With molecular biologic techniques, however, metabolic pathways can be changed in quite specific ways, even in the intact animal. A protein (e.g., enzyme/carrier) can be overexpressed, expressed in a tissue that normally does not contain it, or eliminated in any particular cell type. Site-directed mutations allow a molecule to be dissected and particular component groups removed or altered so that their role in the molecule's functioning can be studied. Application of these techniques to the investigation of metabolic pathways and their regulation is just beginning (24). Recent examples involve the study of GLUT 1 and GLUT 4, which are responsible for transporting the bulk of the glucose from the blood, and investigating the role of GLUT 2 in glucose sensing in the insulin-secreting β cells of the pancreas. GLUTs 1 and 4 were altered in skeletal muscle and adipose tissue, respectively, (24) and the gene for GLUT 4 inactivated (25). In the case of GLUT 2, mice were created that did not express this transporter in the insulin-secreting cells of the pancreas (26). Brief comments about these studies show the new approaches fostered by molecular biologic techniques.

Transgenic mice were established that expressed high levels of human GLUT 1, and it was properly located in the muscle sarcolemma. The increase in the transporter created a 3- to 4-fold increase in glucose transport into specific tested muscles, confirming that GLUT 1 plays a major role in controlling glucose entry into resting muscle. Strangely, insulin did not increase the entry of glucose into the transgenic mice muscles despite the fact that GLUT 4 levels in these mice were the same as those of control mice. Possibly, the GLUT 1 levels are so high in the transgenic set that glucose is not limited any longer by transporter activity. Muscle glucose was 4- to 5-fold and glycogen 10-fold higher in the transgenic mice, even though they showed an 18 (fed) to 30% (fasted) decrease in plasma glucose concentration. Oral glucose loads did not increase plasma levels as much as in normal mice and glucose was more rapidly disposed of. Thus, changing the level of GLUT 1 transporters affected not only muscle metabolism but also whole animal responses.

Because increases in the insulin-responsive transporter GLUT 4 occur in human and rodent adipocytes and are associated with obesity, the question arises as to whether increasing the GLUT 4 levels in adipocytes plays a role in obesity. Transgenic mice were made that expressed human GLUT 4 in their adipocytes. Basal-level glucose transport into their adipocytes increased approximately 20-fold compared with controls, but insulin only stimulated glucose uptake by a factor of 2.5, rather than the 15-fold increase of controls. Again, the possible explanation is that glucose transport is so high in the transgenic adipocytes that the number of transporters activated by insulin makes little difference to the overall transport. While the fat cell size was unchanged in the transgenic mice, their number more than doubled, and body lipid nearly tripled, matching the increase in cell number. The results suggest that a specific increase in GLUT 4 in adipocytes plays a role in generating obesity.

Remarkably, mice created with an absence of GLUT 4 have nearly normal glucose homeostasis (25). Clearly, while GLUT 4 is critical to the handling of glucose in insulin-sensitive tissues, it does not appear to be essential for survival. Presumably, other mechanisms can substitute for the absence of GLUT 4.

The β cells of the pancreas first sense, then respond to, elevated blood glucose levels by secreting insulin. The glucose transporter in their cell membranes is GLUT 2; circumstantial evidence suggests that it may be involved in the glucose-sensing mechanism. However, studies in transgenic mice created to express a transforming ras protein in the β cells showed that these animals respond normally to a glucose load, even though their β cells do not express GLUT 2 (26). It is thus difficult to consider GLUT 2 part of the sensing apparatus.

One major difficulty in using transgenic and "knockout" mice is that the induced changes occur early on in the developing animal. Thus, the changes observed can be due to the presence or absence of the trans-gene at the time of the laboratory measurements or the genetic change could have initiated a plethora of events that caused the observed phenotype. Techniques are being developed, however, to overcome this serious problem.

BLOOD GLUCOSE—METABOLIC AND HORMONAL REGULATION

Metabolic

The concentration of glucose in the blood, set within the normal adult range of 3.9 to 5.8 mmol/L (70–105 mg/100 mL), is probably the most regulated of all substances. When a carbohydrate meal is ingested, the level may temporarily rise to 6.5 to 7.2 mmol/L, and during fasting it can fall to 3.3 to 3.9 mmol/L. One of the major reasons for closely regulating blood glucose levels is that the brain normally depends on a continuous supply, although it can adapt to lower levels or even use ketone bodies from fat breakdown (27) if adaptation occurs slowly. This becomes essential during starvation, since the adult human brain uses about 140 g/day of glucose (28), and only about 130 g/day of glucose can be obtained from noncarbohydrate sources. Injection of a hormone, such as insulin, that rapidly lowers the blood glucose level can lead to convulsions and even death if left uncorrected.

Glucose enters the blood pool (about 16 g) from a number of sources. In normal postabsorptive man, the plasma appearance rate is 8 to 10 g/h, the blood pool being replaced every 2 hours. At normal blood glucose levels, the liver is a net producer of glucose.

When the dietary carbohydrates in a meal are finally hydrolyzed to glucose, galactose, and fructose, after absorption these are transported by the portal blood flow into the liver and kidney. The rising level of glucose to the liver decreases the liver output of glucose. In the rat, uptake and output are equal at about 8.3 mmol/L. The glucose entering the blood during a meal is handled by the liver and peripheral tissues, the first step being phosphorylation. In the tissues, phosphorylation is by hexokinase, an enzyme subject to feedback inhibition by the product, glucose-6-phosphate. The liver enzyme, glucokinase, is not so affected, has a lower affinity for glucose, and can increase its activity over the normal range of glucose found in the portal blood. It thus appears to be ideal for handling the high levels of glucose that enter the portal blood during a carbohydrate meal. Both galactose and fructose can be converted into glucose by the hepatic cells, so little of either hexose is found in the peripheral circulation, and more than 95% of all circulating hexoses is glucose.

Cori Cycle

Glucose can be formed in the liver and kidney from two other groups of compounds that undergo gluconeogenesis. Those in the first group, such as some amino acids (especially alanine during starvation) and propionate, are converted into glucose without being recycled; those in the second group are formed from glucose during its partial metabolism in various tissues. Both muscle and red blood cells oxidize glucose to form lactate, which on entering the liver is resynthesized into glucose. This newly formed glucose is then available for recirculation back to the tissue, a process known as the Cori, or lactic acid, cycle. The Cori cycle may account for approximately 40% of the normal plasma glucose turnover.

In the case of adipose tissue, the cells hydrolyze fats (acylglycerols) and form glycerol that cannot be metabolized by the adipocytes. The glycerol diffuses from the cells, enters the blood, and is transported to the liver and kidneys where it is converted back into glucose. Finally, glucose is also released into the blood by glycogenolysis of the large store of glycogen in the liver.

Hormonal

The level of glucose in the blood is regulated by both hormonal and metabolic mechanisms. The major hormones controlling the glucose level are *(a)* insulin, *(b)* glucagon, and *(c)* epinephrine (adrenaline), but others such as *(d)* thyroid hormone, *(e)* glucocorticoids, and *(f)* growth hormone also play a role.

Insulin

Diabetes Mellitus—IDDM (Type I) and NIDDM (Type II). Insulin has a central role in regulating blood glucose. It is secreted by the β cells in the islets of Langerhans in the human pancreas; the daily output is some 40 to 50 units, which is about 15 to 20% of the amount stored in the gland. The glucose level in the blood controls insulin release; high blood glucose levels (hyperglycemia) cause secretion of insulin, low levels (hypoglycemia) inhibit. When the pancreas is unable to secrete insulin or secretes too little, the medical condition is known as diabetes mellitus. This disease, the third most prevalent in the Western world, is normally classified as type I, or insulin-dependent (IDDM), or type II, non-insulin-dependent (NIDDM). NIDDM accounts for approximately 90% of all diabetic patients. IDDM patients have an autoimmune disease of the β cells—they cannot make insulin and need daily injections of the hormone. IDDM affects children and younger adults predominantly and becomes manifest when about 80% of the β cells are destroyed. Those with NIDDM are mature adults. They have reduced secretion of the hormone and reduced metabolic response to it (peripheral insulin resistance). The cause(s) of this insulin resistance is still to be identified. There are conflicting findings about the role of GLUT 4 in the insensitivity. One group of workers has reported that there are no changes in GLUT 4 mRNA or protein (29), but others have found a small (18%) decrease (30). The insulin resistance may be due to a defect in translocation of GLUT 4 to the muscle membrane (19).

Mechanism of Insulin Secretion. The mechanism of the regulation of insulin secretion by the external glucose level has been studied using patch clamp techniques to control the ionic channels (see Chapter 38) in the β-cell membrane. The resting membrane potential of the β cells is maintained by the Na^+-K^+ ATPase and ATP-sensitive K^+ channels (K_{ATP} channels). Normally these are open, but they close following glucose metabolism, when there is a concomitant increase in the ATP:ADP ratio (31). This depolarizes the cell membrane and opens voltage-gated Ca^{2+} channels. The resulting increase in the intracellular free Ca^{2+} concentration activates secretion of insulin through exocytosis—the fusion of insulin-containing granules with the plasma membrane and the release of their contents (32). A number of drugs (sulfonylureas), such as tolbutamide and glibenclamide, cause insulin secretion by inhibiting the K_{ATP} channels of the β cells and are used medically to treat NIDDM. K_{ATP} channels are a heteromultimeric complex of the inward rectifier K^+ channel (K_{IR} 6.2) and a receptor for sulfonylureas, SUR1, a member of the ABC or traffic family of plasma membrane proteins (33).

Apart from a high level of glucose in the blood, a variety of compounds increase insulin secretion, including amino acids, free fatty acids, ketone bodies, and the hormones glucagon and secretin. In human pregnancy, the hormones placental lactogen, estrogens, and progestin all increase insulin secretion. Hence, insulin levels are higher in the pregnant than in the nonpregnant. Other hormones, such as epinephrine and norepinephrine (noradrenaline), inhibit its release. Inhibitory mechanisms are important as they protect individual β cells from overresponding and exhausting themselves (e.g., effects of chronic administration of growth hormone). Local controls by a host of autocrine, paracrine, and neurocrine substances (34) are thought to be involved in the inhibition of insulin secretion; these include the peptide pancreastatin, neuropeptide Y (NPY), somatostatin, calcitonin gene-related peptide (CGRP), galanin, and amylin (islet amyloid polypeptide or IAPP).

Insulin acts to lower blood glucose levels by facilitating its entrance into insulin-sensitive tissues and the liver. It does this by increasing the level of transporters in tissues such as muscle. In the liver, however, insulin stimulates storage of glucose as glycogen or enhances its metabolism via the glycolytic pathway. Surprisingly, glucose entry into liver cells is not mediated by changes in glucose transporter function, despite the fact that hepatocytes have these transporters present in their sinusoidal membranes (35). There is a functional specialization in the liver in regard to the disposition of GLUTs 1 and 2. GLUT 2 has higher expression in the periportal hepatocytes than in the perivenous hepatocytes. In the perivenous region, however, GLUT 1 is also present in the sinusoidal membranes of the hepatocytes, which form rows around the terminal hepatic venules. Periportal hepatocytes are more gluconeogenic than the more glycolytic perivenous cells (36). Why hepatocytes have GLUT 2 in their membranes is an enigma, as it is certainly not necessary for the ingress or egress of glucose. It has been suggested that GLUT 2 may be transporting fructose, since GLUT 5, the fructose transporter, is not expressed in the liver. However, GLUT 1 expression correlates well with the glycolytic activity of cells; in general, the higher the activity, the greater the concentration of GLUT 1. Thus, the presence of GLUT 1 in the perivenous liver cells may aid the efficient functioning of their glycolytic pathway.

While insulin has a primary influence on glucose homeostasis, it also influences many other cellular functions (Table 3.5). Glucose has a profound effect on the secretion of insulin, and insulin strongly affects the normal storage of ingested fuels and cellular growth and differentiation (as exemplified in Table 3.5). Thus, indirectly, glucose also influences these cellular events, which underscores the crucial role of glucose in influencing metabolism and catabolism, both directly and indirectly.

Glucagon

Glucagon is secreted by the α cells of the islets of Langerhans in the pancreas. A major stimulus for its secretion is hypoglycemia (low blood glucose levels). Glucagon acts on the hepatic cells of the liver to cause glycogenolysis, the breakdown of glycogen, by activating the enzyme phosphorylase. It also enhances gluconeogenesis (formation of glucose) from amino acids and lactate. Thus, the major actions of glucagon oppose those of insulin. The α and β cells in the islets have a close functional relationship with one another; there is intraislet regulation of glucagon by insulin and of insulin by glucagon (37). Because of this, it is claimed that it is difficult to separate the direct effects of changes in plasma glucose levels on glucagon secretion from the α cells from control of glucagon secretion by insulin. When plasma glucose levels increase about twofold, glucagon secretion is inhibited by concurrent changes in β cell activity rather than by the direct effects of glucose or insulin on the α cells (38).

Glucagon must attach to its specific receptor in the plasma membrane to activate cellular responses. This specific glucagon receptor is a member of a superfamily of guanine nucleotide–binding protein-coupled receptors, and it is also a member of a smaller subfamily of homologous receptors for peptides structurally related to glucagon GLP-1 (glucagon-like peptide-1), GIP (gastric inhibitory peptide), VIP (vasoactive intestinal peptide), secretin, GRF (growth hormone–releasing factor), and PACAP (pituitary adenylate cyclase–activating polypeptide). Using specific glucagon receptor mRNA expression in rat tissues, glucagon receptor mRNA was observed to be relatively abundant in liver, adipose tissue, and pancreatic islets, as expected, but also in heart, kidney, spleen, thymus, and stomach. Low levels were found in adrenal glands, small intestine, thyroid, and skeletal muscle. No expression was observed in testes, lung, large intestine, or brain (39).

Table 3.5
Influence of Glucose via Insulin

Positive Effects	Negative Effects
Glucose uptake	Pyruvate → glucose
Amino acid uptake	Apoptosis
Acetyl-CoA → fatty acid	Gene expression
Glucose → glycogen	
Protein synthesis	
DNA-synthesis	
Na^+ K^+ pump	
Gene expression	

Epinephrine

Epinephrine is secreted by the chromaffin cells of the adrenal medulla. It is often called the "fight or flight" hormone because stresses, such as fear, excitement, hypoglycemia, and blood loss, cause increased epinephrine output. It acts on liver and muscle to bring about glycogenolysis by stimulating phosphorylase, thus releasing glucose for muscle metabolism.

Thyroid

In humans, fasting blood glucose levels are elevated in hyperthyroid patients and lowered in hypothyroid patients. Thyroid hormones enhance the action of epinephrine in increasing glycolysis and gluconeogenesis and can potentiate the actions of insulin on glycogen synthesis and glucose utilization. They have a biphasic action in animals; at low doses they enhance glycogen synthesis in the presence of insulin, but at large doses they increase glycogenolysis.

Glucocorticoids

Glucocorticoids (11-oxysteroids) are secreted by the adrenal cortex. They increase gluconeogenesis and inhibit the utilization of glucose in the extrahepatic tissues; they are thus antagonistic to insulin's actions. The increased gluconeogenesis activated by the glucocorticoids involves increased protein catabolism in the tissues, enhanced uptake of amino acids by the liver, and increased activity of transaminases and other enzymes involved with hepatic gluconeogenesis.

Growth Hormone

Growth hormone is secreted by the anterior pituitary. Its secretion is enhanced by hypoglycemia. It has direct and indirect effects on decreasing glucose uptake in specific tissues such as muscle. Part of this effect may be due to the liberation of fatty acids from adipose tissue, which then inhibit glucose metabolism. If growth hormone is chronically administered, it causes persistent hyperglycemia, which stimulates the insulin secretion. The β

cells, however, finally become exhausted, and diabetes ensues.

TRANSEPITHELIAL HEXOSE TRANSPORT—INTESTINE AND KIDNEY

Na⁺-Glucose Cotransporters (SGLTs)

The intestine and the kidney are two major organs that have epithelia with the specific function of vectorially transferring hexoses across their cells into the bloodstream. In the intestine, the transporters of the mature enterocytes capture the hexoses from the lumen after breakdown of dietary polysaccharides into simple hexoses, D-glucose, D-galactose, and D-fructose. In the kidney, the cells of the proximal tubule capture the glucose from the glomerular filtrate to return it to the blood. These glucose transporters, localized in the brush border membranes of the epithelial cells, differ from the GLUT 1–5 type and share no sequence homology. They are thus members of quite a different protein family.

Moreover, they transport glucose across the cell membrane by having both hexose and Na^+ binding sites; thus the name Na^+-glucose cotransporters. They couple cellular glucose transfer to the inwardly directed electrochemical gradient of Na^+. The low intracellular concentration of Na^+ ions, maintained by Na^+-K^+ ATPase or the Na^+ pump at the basolateral borders of the cells, powers the uphill transfer of glucose through the agency of the cotransporter. The affinity of the sugar molecule for its cotransporter binding site is greater when the Na^+ ions are attached to the transporter than when they are removed. Thus the external binding of Na^+ and its subsequent intracellular debinding (because of the lower intracellular Na^+ ion concentration) causes the binding, then release, of glucose, allowing it to be transported uphill against its concentration gradient. It is then transported across the basolateral membranes of the cells of the small intestine and kidney, usually by GLUT 2, but in the S3 segments of straight kidney tubules GLUT 1 is found. In this part of the kidney, GLUT 1 is probably involved both in the transepithelial transfer of glucose and in its uptake from the blood to provide energy from cellular glycolysis.

The low concentration of the cotransporters in cell membranes (0.05–0.7%), their hydrophobic nature, and their sensitivity to proteolysis and denaturation made them nearly impossible to prepare by normal biochemical extraction and purification techniques. The first to be cloned and sequenced, by the technique known as functional expression cloning, was SGLT-1, the form found in the rabbit small intestine (40). Amphibian eggs of the toad *Xenopus laevis* can express almost any RNA that is injected into them and make the corresponding protein. Poly(A)*mRNA isolated from the rabbit small intestinal mucosa and microinjected into *Xenopus* oocytes stimulated Na^+-dependent uptake of the hexose analogue α-methyl glucoside that could be blocked by the plant glycoside phlorizin, a high-affinity competitor for the sugar site of the transporter (15). Phlorizin has no effect on the GLUT 1–5 transporters; they are inhibited by the mold metabolite phloretin, which is the aglycone of phlorizin. Phloretin has no effect on the Na^+-glucose transporter but blocks the GLUT 1–5 transporters. The predicted topologic organization of SGLT-1 in the cell membranes was surmised from its amino acids and, like the glucose transporter family, it is a large polypeptide with 12 putative membrane-spanning α-helices (Fig. 3.4). The polypeptide is glycosylated at one site, but this has little effect on its function (41). Radiation inactivation analysis of SGLT-1 suggests that the functional form in the membrane is a tetramer. Human SGLT-1 cDNA encodes a transporter with 84% amino acid sequence identity to the rabbit SGLT-1. It is composed of 664 amino acids. The gene for human SGLT-1 is located on chromosome 22 at q11.2→qter.

More recently, it has been shown that there are three different isoforms of the SGLT cotransporters, designated SGLT-1, SGLT-2 (672 amino acids), and SGLT-3 (16). The cotransporters SGLT-1 and -2 have different glucose-Na^+ coupling ratios, the former high-affinity cotransporter ($K_m \approx 0.8$ mmol/L), primarily expressed in the small intestine, transports each glucose molecule with two Na^+ ions, while the latter, lower-affinity ($K_m \approx 1.6$ mmol/L) cotransporter, expressed in the kidney tubules, transports glucose with one Na^+. SGLT-3, isolated from pig intestine, is a low-affinity cotransporter. It has approximately 60% homology in amino acid sequence to SGLT-2 (42).

Glucose-Galactose Malabsorption

The importance of human SGLT-1 for intestinal glucose absorption is exemplified in glucose-galactose malabsorption, a rare inborn error of glucose transport. This condition gives rise to a severe watery diarrhea in

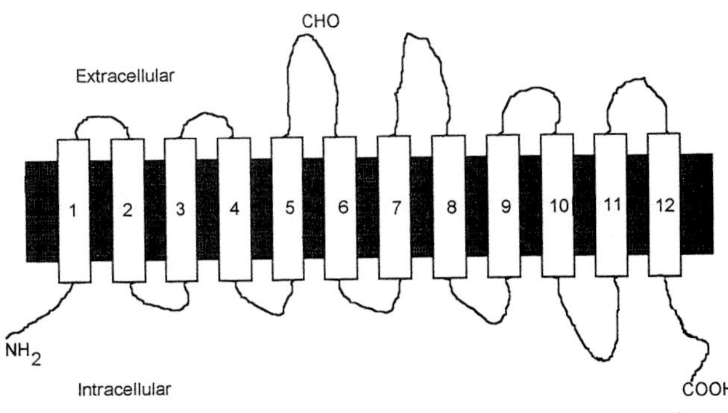

Figure 3.4. Highly schematic diagram illustrating the predicted secondary structure model of the Na^+-glucose-cotransporter (SGLT-1) molecule in the cell membrane *(solid)*. The putative membrane-spanning α-helices are shown as rectangles numbered 1–12 connected by linked amino-acid chains *(lines)*. An outer glycosylation site is shown *(CHO)*. It has little effect on carrier function. (Adapted from Wright EM, Turk E, Zabel B, et al. J Clin Invest 1991;88:1435–40.)

neonates, which is lethal unless glucose- and galactose-containing foods are removed from the diet. The diarrhea occurs because the unabsorbed hexoses enter the colon and are fermented into diarrheogenic compounds. The lack of hexose absorption in two sisters with the condition appears to be due to a single base change at nucleotide position 92, where a guanine is replaced by adenine. The mutation changed amino acid 28 of their SGLT-1 from aspartate to asparagine, making the SGLT-1 cotransporter defective and inactive. A single amino-acid alteration in the 664 that make up the molecule makes it unable to function as a cotransporter (43). Thus in humans who lack a functional SGLT-1, it appears that absorption of glucose and galactose cannot proceed normally. Experimental studies measuring the absorption of glucose in human jejunum in vivo showed that more than 95% of glucose absorption occurred by a carrier-mediated process, which agrees with the described pathophysiology of glucose-galactose malabsorption (44, 45).

Electrogenic Glucose-Linked Na^+ Transfer

Because SGLT cotransporters carry both glucose and Na^+ ions across the cell membrane without counterions, movement of the charged Na^+ ions creates an electrical potential difference across the cell membrane and subsequently across the epithelium. The transfer of glucose (or galactose) across the intestine or kidney tubule is called electrogenic (potential generating) or rheogenic (current generating). This electrical activity has been of inestimable value in the assessment of the kinetics of active hexose transport in native tissues and injected *Xenopus* eggs. This linking of the electrogenic Na^+ ion transfer with the hexose also enhances the net absorption of fluid across the small intestine. It is so effective that it overcomes the terrible excessive fluid secretory consequences of cholera toxin action in the small bowel and is a highly effective and cheap treatment to keep patients hydrated and alive. A simple solution of NaCl and glucose (or even rice water) has probably saved more lives than any drug!

Galactose

Metabolism and Transport. Galactose is a hexose monosaccharide whose dietary intake is usually in the form of the disaccharide lactose (milk sugar). Lactose is split by the digestive enzyme lactase into its hexose moities, glucose and galactose. Galactose shares the same transport mechanisms as glucose in the enterocytes, namely apical SGLT cotransporters and the basolateral GLUT 2. It enters the portal blood and is practically cleared in its passage through the liver, so that little or no galactose is seen in the systemic blood above 1 mmol/L, even after ingesting as much as 100 g of lactose. Ingestion of galactose without glucose, however, induces higher plasma concentrations. Alcohol is said to depress galactose uptake and metabolism by the liver, leading to an increased level in the blood (galactosemia). In the liver cells, it is converted by the enzyme galactokinase into galactose-1-phosphate. This, in turn, is converted by a two-stage enzymic transformation into glucose-1-phosphate, which is converted into glycogen. Although in theory glucose-1-phosphate can enter the glycolytic pathway, it does not normally do so to any great extent. Most tissues have enzymes that can metabolize galactose. However, even in the complete absence of dietary galactose, glucose can be converted into galactose and supply cellular needs for galactose if required. Many structural elements of cells and tissues (viz., glycoproteins and mucopolysaccharides) contain galactose.

Cataracts and Inborn Errors. Galactose levels in peripheral blood normally do not go above 1 mmol/L. If they do (galactosemia), then various tissues can remove it from the blood and convert it into galactitol (dulcitol) by the enzyme aldehyde reductase. As it is nonmetabolized, it builds up in the tissues and causes pathologic changes because of the high osmotic pressure created. In the lens of the eye, such a scenario causes cataracts (46). Cataracts can also occur in two inborn errors of galactose metabolism caused by deficiencies of the enzymes galactose-1-phosphate uridyltransferase and galactokinase. The former enzyme deficiency creates classical galactosemia. Unless it is treated promptly in the neonate by withdrawing galactose from the diet (taken in from the lactose content of normal milk), either death or severe mental retardation can occur. Cataracts can also occur as a complication of diabetes mellitus, in which blood glucose is raised to high levels.

Fructose

Metabolism and Transport. Fructose, a monosaccharide ketohexose, is present either as the free hexose (honey, soft drinks, sweets, biscuits, apples, pears) or is produced from hydrolysis of the dietary disaccharide sucrose (yielding glucose and fructose). In humans, it is absorbed largely intact into the portal blood and is almost totally cleared in a single passage through the liver. Thus, there is essentially no appreciable fructose in the blood. After a large oral dose of 1 g free fructose/kg body weight, the blood level will increase to 0.5 mmol/L in 30 minutes and then slowly decrease during the next 90 minutes. In the liver, fructose is phosphorylated by the abundant enzyme fructokinase into fructose-1-phosphate, which is cleaved by hepatic aldolase into glyceraldehyde and dihydroxyacetone phosphate (DHA phosphate). DHA phosphate is an intermediary metabolite in both the glycolytic and gluconeogenic pathways. Glyceraldehyde, while not intermediary in either pathway, can be converted by various liver enzymes into glycolytic intermediary metabolites available to be metabolized ultimately to produce glycogen. This glycogen can then be broken down into glucose by glycogenolysis.

Absorption. Although fructose is absorbed across the enterocytes of the small intestine, it is not a substrate for the SGLT cotransporters. The evidence for this is threefold: *(a)* fructose absorption is normal in those with glucose-galactose malabsorption, who have defective SGLT-1 cotransporters; *(b)* fructose absorption is not reduced by phlorizin, the classic inhibitor of SGLT-1 cotransporters; and *(c)* fructose absorption is neither Na^+-sensitive nor electrogenic like that of glucose or galactose. Recent studies on the expression of human GLUT 5 transporter in *Xenopus* oocytes showed that the transporter exhibited selectivity for high-affinity fructose transport that was not blocked by cytochalasin B, a potent inhibitor of facilitative glucose transport by glucose transporters (22). As GLUT 5 is also expressed in high levels in the brush border of enterocytes in the small intestine (47), the isoform is likely to be the fructose transporter of the small intestine. Indirect evidence for the likelihood of fructose transporting by GLUT 5 is the fact that it is expressed in high concentration in human spermatids and spermatozoa (47), cells known to metabolize fructose. GLUT 2, localized to the basolateral membrane of enterocytes, although having a much lower affinity for fructose transport than GLUT 5, probably mediates the exit of the absorbed fructose from the enterocytes into the blood. Recently, however, it has been reported that GLUT 5 is also localized on the basolateral membrane in the human jejunum (48), so fructose could also exit from the enterocytes by this transporter.

In humans, absorption of fructose from sucrose ingestion is more rapid than that from equimolar amounts of fructose ingestion. The numerous explanations for this phenomenon include differences in gastric emptying, enhanced fluid absorption initiated by the glucose entraining fructose, and cotransport of fructose and glucose by a disaccharidase-related transport system (49, 50).

Inborn Errors. Six genetically determined abnormalities in the metabolism of fructose have been described in humans (51). These are caused by deficiencies in fructokinase, aldolase A and B, fructose-1,6-diphosphatase, and glycerate kinase, and by fructose malabsorption. Limiting dietary fructose is favorable in each of these conditions except aldolase A deficiency. Fructokinase deficiency, manifest in the liver, causes fructosemia (high levels in blood) and fructosuria (excretion in urine). In contrast to the low levels of fructose observed in the blood of normal humans after ingestion of 1 g of free fructose/kg, the concentration in the fructokinase-deficient person approaches 3 mmol/L and is sustained for many hours. Despite the sustained high levels of fructose in the blood, cataracts do not develop, in sharp contrast to the cases of galactokinase deficiency and diabetes mellitus (see specific sections).

The three aldolases, A, B, and C, catalyze the reversible conversion of fructose-1-diphosphate into glyceraldehyde-3-phosphate and dihydroxyacetone phosphate. Each is coded for by a different gene: A is on chromosome 16, B on 9, and C on 17. Expression of the enzymes is regulated during development so that A is produced in embryonic tissues and adult muscle, B in adult liver, kidney, and intestine, and C in adult nervous tissue. Deficiency of A produces a syndrome of mental retardation, short stature, hemolytic anemia, and abnormal facies. The deficiency is probably detrimental because aldolase A is normally involved in fetal glycolysis. There is no treatment for the condition. Deficiency of aldolase B (hereditary fructose intolerance), the most frequent of the three deficiencies, was first observed in 1956 (52). When fructose is ingested, vomiting, failure to thrive, and liver dysfunction occur.

Deficiency of fructose-1-6-diphosphatase was described in 1970. Patients exhibit hypoglycemia, acidosis, ketonuria, and hyperventilation. Urinalysis shows many changes in organic acids, but excretion of glycerol is diagnostic. Treatment is to avoid dietary fructose.

D-Glyceric aciduria is rare and is caused by D-glycerate kinase deficiency. The presentation of the disease is highly variable, from no clinical symptoms to severe metabolic acidosis and psychomotor retardation, which suggests that perhaps among the 10 described cases, there are other, different enzyme deficiencies.

In fructose malabsorption, ingestion of the ketohexose in quantity creates abdominal bloating, flatulence, and diarrhea. Persons with this condition appear to have a defect in fructose absorption. No assessments of intestinal GLUT 5 or its controlling gene have yet been made in any of these patients. If either glucose or galactose is ingested with fructose, fructose absorption is enhanced, and often no symptoms of malabsorption occur (50, 51).

GLUCOSE STORAGE

Glycogen

Glucose is stored in the liver and muscles of animals and humans as the branched polymer glycogen; the equivalent polymer in plants is starch. Glycogen is more branched than amylopectin and has 10 to 18 long chains of α-D-glucopyranose residues (in $\alpha(1 \rightarrow 4)$ glucoside links) with branching by $\alpha(1 \rightarrow 6)$ glucoside bonds (Fig. 3.5). Although it occurs in concentrations of up to 6% of liver mass but only 1% of muscle, muscle mass is so much greater that it represents 3 to 4 times as much glycogen as in the liver. Muscle glycogen is mainly used by the muscle, but liver glycogen is for storage, export, and the maintenance of blood glucose. The liver has glycogen stores for only 12 to 18 hours of fasting; it then becomes glycogen depleted.

Formation and Breakdown of Glycogen

Glucose is first enzymically phosphorylated, then reacted with uridine triphosphate to give uridine diphosphate glucose (UDP-glucose). The enzyme glycogen synthetase fits this onto a preexisting glycogen chain (primer and/or protein backbone), splitting off the UDP. The glucose residue added by 1→4 linkages is attached at the

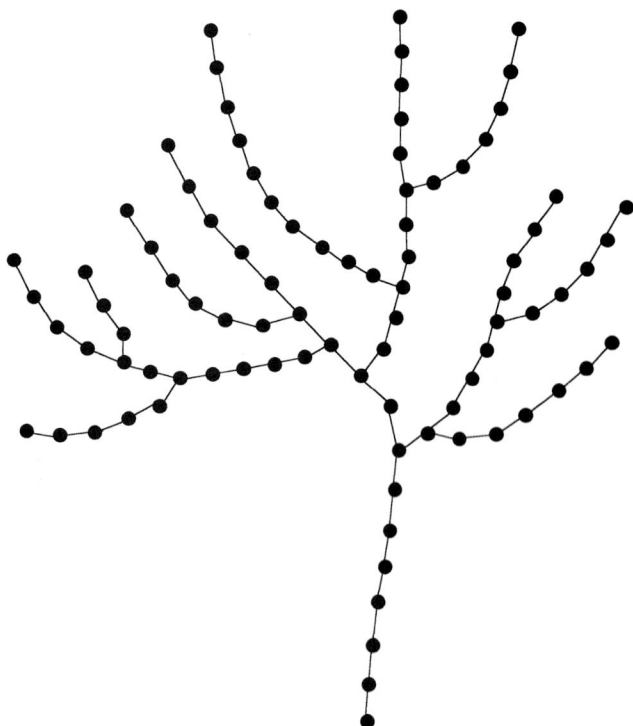

Figure 3.5. A highly schematic diagram of a portion of a glycogen molecule. Each *solid black circle* represents a glucose moiety joined by 1→4 and 1→6 links. The branching of the structure, caused by the 1→6 links, is more random than is shown.

outer end of the molecule so that the branches of the glycogen tree become elongated. After 11 glucose residues, another enzyme called the "branching enzyme" (amylol (1→4) → (1→6) transglucosidase) transfers part of the 1→4 chain of glucose residues (>6) to a neighboring chain to form a 1→6 link and create a branch point. Glycogen grows by further 1→4 and 1→6 additions. As the number increases the total number of reactive sites in the molecule also increases, which hastens both glycogenesis and glycogenolysis. Breakdown of glycogen is mediated by three enzymes: *(a)* phosphorylase acting at the 1→4 linkages; *(b)* α(1→4) → α(1→4) glucan transferase, which transfers a trisaccharide unit from one branch to another, exposing 1→6 branch points; and *(c)* the "debranching enzyme" (amylo(1→6)-glucosidase), which splits the linkage. Removal of the branch allows further action by the phosphorylase. In the liver and kidney (but not in muscle), a specific enzyme, glucose-6-phosphatase, dephosphorylates the glucose so that it can diffuse from the cells into the bloodstream. The enzymes controlling glycogen metabolism are regulated by a complex series of phosphorylations and dephosphorylations and by allosteric mechanisms under hormonal influence (see insulin and glucagon).

Glycogen Storage Diseases

Glycogen storage diseases include more than 10 genetic differences involving either enzymes or transporters. They are characterized as storing glycogen in abnormal quantity, location, or structure. Five types of glycogen storage disease have been described (53): type I (glucose-6-phosphatase deficiency), type II (acid α-glucoside deficiency), type III (amylo-1,6-glycosidase deficiency), type IV (branching enzyme deficiency), and type V (muscle phosphorylase deficiency), which was later expanded to at least seven types (type VI, liver phosphorylase or phosphorylase B kinase deficiency; type VII, muscle fructokinase deficiency). For details, consult the review by Hers (54). In types I, III, and VI, the liver cannot convert glycogen into glucose, causing hepatomegaly (enlarged liver), hypoglycemia, hypoinsulinism, hyperglucagonemia, hyperlipidemia, and growth retardation. In types V and VII (but also in type II and a subgroup of type VI), the muscle is affected and cannot provide glycolytic fuel for contraction. Symptoms are often mild, however, and become apparent only when young adulthood is reached and strenuous exercise is taken.

In a number of the glycogen storage diseases liver transplantation is the only "curative" treatment.

Carbohydrates and Athletic Performance

Carbohydrate present in muscle (300 g), liver (90 g), and body fluids (30 g) is the major fuel for physical performance. The ATP stored in muscle cells can only give high-power output for a few seconds. It can be resynthesized anaerobically for a further few seconds (5–8) by using the phosphate from creatinine phosphate. These short, intense bursts of muscular activity are found in sprints (100 meters), track and field events, and sports such as tennis, hockey, football, gymnastics, and weightlifting. If the maximum effort lasts for 30 seconds, then breakdown of muscle glycogen can supply the energy, with buildup of muscle lactic acid. Most physical activity, however, requires an energy source that can power muscles for longer periods. The duration and intensity of exercise determines the mix of fuel used. In resting or light activity, about 60% is from free fatty acids (FFAs) and triglycerides in muscles. At moderate levels of activity (approximately 50% of the maximum O_2 uptake), fat and carbohydrate contribute about equal amounts as energy sources. Carbohydrate, a prime energy source, becomes more and more important as the intensity of the exercise increases. The change to using carbohydrate is not a linear response but accelerates with the intensity of the work. Endurance athletes use more fat and so conserve the carbohydrate in muscle and liver, but it is that level that ultimately limits continued performance. Fatigue arises when the store becomes depleted. The store of carbohydrate usually suffices for just 2 to 3 hours of physical exertion.

Dietary Manipulation of Glycogen Stores—Carbohydrate Loading

Dietary manipulation can be used to increase the stores of glycogen in muscle and liver. Glycogen increases when more carbohydrate is eaten. The practice is called carbohydrate loading. The athlete has 3 days of exhausting physical exercise on a low-carbohydrate diet followed by 3 days of rest on a high-carbohydrate diet. In general, athletes dislike both phases; in the first, they feel exhausted both mentally and physically, and in the second, they feel bloated because the glycogen retains extra water. However, other feeding programs exist that do not use the carbohydrate depletion phase. For athletes in general, it makes sense to eat plenty of carbohydrate to maximize glycogen storage, as the usual training periods of several hours per day deplete it. There is little doubt that a high-carbohydrate diet improves glycogen storage and athletic performance (see also Chapter 47). What to advise athletes to ingest just before an event is difficult. Solid food is not advisable before strenuous exercise. A popular solution for athletes is drinking glucose/sweetened fruit juices. Fructose ingestion is said to cause less increase in blood glucose and insulin levels and thus a slower loss of muscle glycogen (see review 55).

Carbohydrate Intolerance

There is a range of clinical disorders in which sugar digestion or absorption is disturbed and gives rise to sugar intolerance, creating symptoms by the undigested or unabsorbed sugar and causing water to enter the intestine, which activates peristalsis and induces passage of frequent fluid stools. The undigested carbohydrate can also enter the colon and become fermented into diarrheic agents. The disorders are usually classified as *(a)* congenital or *(b)* secondary to some other disease, to impaired digestion of disaccharides, or to impaired absorption of the monosaccharides. The congenital deficiencies, although relatively rare, are life threatening; examples are sucrase-maltase deficiency (watery diarrhea after ingesting sucrose-containing foods), alactasia (absence of lactase, diarrhea from ingestion of milk), glucose-galactose malabsorption (diarrhea from ingestion of glucose, galactose, or lactose), and the very rare trehalase deficiency (intolerance to trehalose in mushrooms). Sugar intolerance secondary to underlying gastrointestinal disease is the commonest type, especially in pediatrics. Infections of the gastrointestinal tract, for example, often induce a temporary intolerance to lactose.

Lactose Intolerance. Adult mammals and most human groups after weaning keep only a fraction of the intestinal lactase activity of neonates (who need it to digest the lactose of breast milk). The persistence of lactase activity in Europeans has been regarded as the exception to the rule, since most human groups are hypolactasic and lactose malabsorbers (56). However, small amounts of dietary lactose, up to 250 mL of milk, can be tolerated by most adult lactose maldigesters. The decrease in lactase in adults is a programed event, and feeding high-lactose diets does not prevent the decrease. The mechanisms of the decline in activity have been studied in rats. As the animal matures, more and more mRNA message for lactase is needed to maintain the decreasing lactase activity in the enterocytes, suggesting that translational events may be of great importance in lactase gene expression (57).

Diagnosis of Carbohydrate Intolerance

Sugar Tolerance Tests. Clinical quantitative assessment of the efficiency of the digestion and absorption of carbohydrates in humans rests mainly on relatively simple tests in which carbohydrate loads (at least 50 g) are ingested and blood samples are taken to estimate the sugar levels attained at various time intervals after ingestion. The levels are then compared with those obtained in normal subjects. The most commonly used test is the oral glucose tolerance test (OGGT). Typically, nonpregnant adults take 75 g of glucose over 5 minutes and the glucose is estimated in serum at 0, 30, 60, 90, and 120 minutes. A pregnant woman takes 100 g of glucose and has another estimate at 180 minutes. A child takes 1.75 g/kg up to the maximum of 75 g (58). Values above normal indicate some form of inadequate handling of the ingested glucose. This test is often used to assess for diabetes mellitus. The reproducibility of the OGTT has been claimed to be poor, even when repeated in the same individual (59). An oral tolerance test also exists for galactose. As the liver is a major site of galactose metabolism, the test has been used to assess liver function. Similar oral tolerance tests exist for fructose and the disaccharides lactose (lactase deficiency) and sucrose (sucrase deficiency).

Breath Hydrogen Tests. Carbohydrates that have not been digested or absorbed reach the colon and become fermented by the resident bacteria. Hydrogen gas is produced and is excreted in the breath. Measuring breath hydrogen thus provides an estimate of whether malabsorption of a sugar or carbohydrate occurs (see also Chapter 57). It was first used to detect lactose intolerance and has since been used in numerous studies on carbohydrate intolerance (60). It has a number of weaknesses; for example, it gives no indication of the amount of carbohydrate absorbed before the sugar reached the colon, and the hydrogen in the breath is only a fraction of that formed.

Oral Tolerance Tests and the Glycemic Index. Nutritionists use a form of oral tolerance test to assess the so-called glycemic potential of different foods. A carbohydrate load is ingested and the level of blood sugar is measured over a period of time. The increments in blood glucose are then compared with equivalent increments from different foods by normalizing these values to a baseline obtained with glucose, usually by using the area under the 2-h glucose curve after feeding a 50-g carbohydrate portion, and expressing it as a percentage of the mean obtained after 50 g of glucose. This normalized figure, designated the *glycemic index* of the food (61), enjoyed considerable popularity in the dietetic management of diabetes and hypoglycemia. However, there is a large scatter in glycemic index for each group of foodstuffs, attributed to many factors such as its form when eaten, the way it is processed, how it is chewed, how it is emptied from the stomach, and the physiologic and metabolic responses of individuals. The glycemic index has been criticized as a crude index of questionable value (62), but it still has its adherents (63). What it does illustrate is that carbohydrate foods differ widely in their effects on blood glucose and hormonal responses after a meal. Diets with a low glycemic index, designated *lente,* have been claimed to be useful in diabetes, hyperlipidemia, and even healthy subjects. They appear to prolong satiety and hence lead to a better control of food intake (63).

Caries and Sugar

Dental caries is a disease created by bacterial plaque on the enamel of teeth. Gradual and progressive demineralization of the enamel, dentine, and cementum occurs. Many studies have suggested that carbohydrates, especially sugars and in particular sucrose, are important carie-promoting components of food. However, despite a huge amount of laboratory and clinical research, the relationship between sugar and caries is still poorly characterized. A major reason for this is the complexity of the problem, for the formation of caries involves multifactorial interactions such as nutrients and food components of diet, plaque bacteria, salivary flow and composition, minerals and fluoride status, genetics, age, and even the race of the individual (see also Chapter 66). The most common organism in dental plaque associated with caries is *Streptococcus mutans,* but other bacteria contribute. Most studies have focused on the acids (lactic and acetic) generated from sugars (sucrose) by the bacteria, but the complex formation and accumulation of plaque from the insoluble dextran made from sucrose is an important feature (64, 65).

Carbohydrates and Health

The mean annual consumption of sucrose plus fructose in developed countries is about 25% of the caloric intake. Fructose is more lipogenic than glucose. This high intake of sucrose (approximately 50 kg/year/person) has been contentiously implicated in influencing the health of humans, apart from caries, because a high consumption of sucrose/fructose in experimental animals (often rats) creates, among other things, hyperlipidemia, insulin resistance, hypertension, and diabetic-like tissue lesions (66). However, while a hyperlipidemic effect of sucrose and fructose has been demonstrated in a number of human studies, firm conclusions cannot be made because of great variations in the type of subjects, duration of intake, background diet, and study conditions (66). The general conclusion of an FDA-sponsored survey published in 1986 was that the present voluntary intake of sucrose and fructose is not harmful to humans (67). A more recent review, while accepting that the intake of sucrose was not a problem in normal individuals, suggested care when dealing with individuals with hypertriglyceridemia (68).

Glucose and Cerebral Functions

There is now good evidence that increases in plasma glucose can enhance learning in rodents and humans (69). Many drugs that impair learning and memory (e.g., opiates, γ-aminobutyric agonists, cholinergic antagonists) can have their actions reduced by glucose (70). Injecting glucose into the medial septum and into the amygdala of the brain in rats attenuates the inhibitory action of morphine in a trained avoidance task (69). It is suggested that glucose metabolites, such as pyruvate, may contribute to the mechanism by which glucose regulates brain cell function. Glucose has also been shown to enhance the memory of aged rodents and humans. In healthy humans 60 to 80 years old, glucose (50 g) was more effective than saccharin (27 mg) in improving narrative memory test performance (69), but it had no effect on performance of nonmemory tasks, i.e., attention, motor speed, or overall IQ. These actions of glucose showed an inverted U-shaped dose-response curve, the optimal glucose dose producing blood levels of 8.9 mmol/L (160 mg/dL). The effects of glucose on memory outlast the increased level of glucose in the plasma, indicating a stable improvement in function. Remarkably, glucose can also enhance memory and other cognitive functions in patients with Alzheimer's disease and young adults with Down's syndrome (69). These promising findings suggest that glucose or its metabolites may be harnessed to ameliorate the normal loss of mental function with age and the cruel degeneration of mental ability with Alzheimer's disease.

REFERENCES

1. Dahlqvist A, Semenza G. J Pediatr Gastroenterol 1988;4:857–67.
2. Ugolev AM, Delaey P. Biochim Biophys Acta 1973;300:102–28.
3. Gray GM. J Nutr 1992;122:172–7.

3a. Asp N-G, ed. Am J Clin Nutr 1994;59(Suppl 3):679S–794S.

4. Wursch P. World Rev Nutr Diet 1989;60:199–256.
5. Wursch P. Dietary fibre and unabsorbed carbohydrates. In: Gracey M, Kretchmer N, Rossi E, eds. Sugars in nutrition. Nestlé Nutrition Workshop series. New York: Raven Press, 1991;25:153–68.
6. Roediger EEW. Dis Colon Rectum 1990;33:858–62.
7. Trowell H, Southgate DT, Wolever TMS, et al. Lancet 1976;1:967.
8. Lee W-S, Kanai Y, Wells RG, et al. J Biol Chem 1994;269:12032–9.
9. Mueckler M, Caruso C, Baldwin SA, et al. Science 1985;229:941–5.
10. Alvarez J, Lee DC, Baldwin SA, et al. J Biol Chem 1987;262:3502–9.
11. Cuppoletti J, Jung CY, Green FA. J Biol Chem 1981;256:1305–6.
12. Bell GI, Kayano T, Buse JB, et al. Diabetes Care 1990;13:198–208.
13. Silverman M. Annu Rev Biochem 1991;60:757–94.
14. Thorens B. Annu Rev Physiol 1993;55:591–608.

15. Hediger MA, Rhoads DB. Physiol Rev 1994;74:993–1026.
16. Hediger MA, Kanai Y, You G. J Physiol 1995;482:7S–17S.
17. Maher F, Vanucci SJ, Simpson LA. FASEB J 1994;8:1003–11.
18. Diamond DL, Carruthers A. J Biol Chem 1993 284:6437–44.
19. Gould GW, Holman GD. Biochem J 1993;295:329–41.
20. Kayano T, Kukumoto H, Eddy RL, et al. J Biol Chem 1988;263:15245–8.
21. Kayano T, Burant CF, Fukumoto H, et al. J Biol Chem 1990;265:13726–82.
22. Burant CF, Takeda J, Brot-Laroche E. J Biol Chem 1992;267:14523–26.
23. Waddell ID, Zomerschoe G, Voice MW, et al. Biochem J 1992;286:173–7.
24. Koretsky AP. Physiol Rev 1995;75:667–88.
25. Katz EB, Stenbit AE, Hatton K. Nature 1995;377:151–6.
26. Tal M, Wu YJ, Leiser M, et al. Proc Natl Acad Sci USA 1992;89:5744–8.
27. Owen E, Morgan AP, Kemp HG, et al. J Clin Invest 1967;46:1589–95.
28. Cahill GF, Owen OE, Felig P. Physiologist 1968;11:97–102.
29. Pedersen O, Bak JF, Andersen P, et al. Diabetes 1990;39:865–70.
30. Dohm GL, Elton GW, Friedman E, et al. Am J Physiol 1991;260:E459–63.
31. Ashcroft FM, Harrison DE, Ashcroft SJH. Nature 1984;312:446–8.
32. Dunne MJ, Petersen OH. Biochim Biophys Acta (Rev Biomembranes) 1991;1071:67–82.
33. Inagaki N, Gonoi T, Clement IV, et al. Science 1995;270:1166–70.
34. Smith DM, Bloom SR. Biochem J 1995;23:336–40.
35. Thorens B, Cheng Z-Q, Brown D, et al. Am J Physiol 1990;259:C279–85.
36. Jungermann K, Katz N. Physiol Rev 1989;69:708–64.
37. Pipeleers D. Diabetologia 1987;30:277–91.
38. Asplin CM, Hollander P, Palmer JP. Diabetologia 1984;26:203–7.
39. Hansen LH, Abrahamsen N, Nishimura E. Peptides 1995;16:1163–6.
40. Hediger MA, Coady MJ, Ikeda T, et al. Nature 1987;330:379–81.
41. Wright EM, Turk E, Zabel B, et al. J Clin Invest 1991;88:1435–40.
42. Mackenzie B, Panayotova-Heiermann M, Loo DDF, et al. J Biol Chem 1994;269:22488–91.
43. Turk E, Zabel B, Mundlos S, et al. Nature 1991;350:354–6.
44. Fine KD, Santa Ana CA, Porter JL, et al. Gastroenterol 1993;105:1117–25.
45. Levin RJ. Digestion and absorption of carbohydrates—from molecules and membranes to humans. In: Asp N-G, ed. Carbohydrates in human nutrition. Am J Clin Nutr Suppl 3(Suppl) 1994;59:690S–98S.
46. Van Heyningen R. Nature 1959;184:194–5.
47. Davidson NO, Hausman AML, Ifkovits CA. Am J Physiol 1992;262:C795–C800.
48. Blakemore SJ, Aledo JC, James J, et al. Biochem J 1995;309:7–112.
49. Fujisawa T, Riby J, Kretchmer N. Gastroenterology 1991;101:360–7.
50. Riby JE, Fujisawa T, Kretchmer N. Am J Clin Nutr 1993;58(Suppl):748S–3S.
51. Hommes FA. Am J Clin Nutr 1993;58(Suppl):788S–95S.
52. Chambers RA, Pratt RTC. Lancet 1956;2:340–1.
53. Cori GT. Harvey Lect 1954;48:145–71.
54. Hers H-G. Glycogen storage diseases. In: Gracey M, Kretchmer N, Rossi E, eds. Sugars in nutrition, Nestlé Nutrition Workshop series. New York: Raven Press, 1991;249–65.
55. Stanton R. Sugars in the diet of athletes. In: Gracey M, Kretchmer N, Rossi E, eds. Sugars in nutrition, Nestlé Nutrition Workshop series. New York: Raven Press, 1991;267–78.
56. Kretchmer N. Gastroenterology 1971;61:805–13.
57. Nudell DM, Santiago NA, Zhu J-S. Am J Physiol 1993;265:G1108–15.
58. Potparic O, Gibson J, eds. A dictionary of clinical tests. Lancashire: Parthenon Publishing, 1993.
59. McDonald GW, Fisher GF, Burnham C. Diabetes 1965;14:473–80.
60. Levitt MD, Donaldsen RM. J Lab Clin Med 1970;75:937–45.
61. Jenkins DJA, Wolever TMS, Taylor RH, et al. Am J Clin Nutr 1981;34:362–66.
62. Marks V. Glycemic responses to sugar and starches. In: Dobbing J, ed. Dietary starches and sugars in man: a comparison. London: Springer-Verlag, 1989;151–67.
63. Bjorck I, Granfeldt Y, Liljeberg H, et al. Am J Clin Nutr 1994;59(Suppl):699S–705S.
64. Bowen W. Simple carbohydrates as microbiological substrates. In: Conning D, ed. Biological functions of carbohydrates. International symposium. 1993;64–7.
65. Navia JM. Carbohydrates and dental health. In: Asp N-G, ed. Carbohydrates in human nutrition. Am J Clin Nutr 1994;59(Suppl 3):719S–27S.
66. Shafrir E. Metabolism of disaccharides and monosaccharides with emphasis on sucrose and fructose and their lipogenic potential. In: Gracey M, Kretchmer N, Rossi E, eds. Sugars in nutrition. Nestlé Nutrition Workshop series. New York: Raven Press, 1991;131–52.
67. Glinsmann WH, Irausquin H, Park YK. Report of Sugars Task Force. Washington, DC: Food and Drug Adminstration, 1986.
68. Truswell AS. Food carbohydrates and plasma lipids—an update. In: Asp N-G, ed. Carbohydrates in human nutrition. Am J Clin Nutr 1994;59(Suppl 3):710S–8S.
69. Gold P. Am J Clin Nutr 1995;61(Suppl):987S–95S.
70. Gold P. Modulation of memory processing: enhancement of memory in rodents and humans. In: Butters N, Squire LR, eds. Neuropyschology of memory. New York: Guilford Press, 1992:402–14.

SELECTED READINGS

Asp N-G, ed. Carbohydrates in human nutrition. Am J Clin Nutr 1994;59(Suppl 3):679S–794S.

Bray TM, Stephen AM, eds. Starch in human nutrition. Can J Physiol Pharmacol 1991;69(Suppl):54–136.

Dobbing J, ed. Dietary starches and sugars in man: a comparison. London: Springer-Verlag, 1989.

Gould GW, Holman GD. The glucose transporter family: structure, function and tissue specific expression. Biochem J 1993;295:329–41.

Gracey M, Kretchmer N, Rossi E, eds. Sugars in nutrition. Nestlé Nutrition Workshop series. New York: Raven Press, 1991.

Greenberg RE, ed. New dimensions in carbohydrates. Am J Clin Nutr 1995;61(Suppl):915S–1011S.

Levin RJ. Dietary carbohydrate and the kinetics of intestinal functions in relation to hexose absorption. In: Dobbing J, ed. Dietary starches and sugars in man: a comparison. London: Springer-Verlag, 1989;89–117.

Thorens B. Glucose transporters in the regulation of intestinal, renal and liver glucose fluxes. Am J Physiol 1996;270:G541–53.

Vettorazzi G, Macdonald I, eds. Sucrose: nutritional and safety aspects. London: Springer-Verlag, 1988.

4. Lipids, Sterols, and Their Metabolites

PETER J. H. JONES and STANLEY KUBOW

HISTORICAL INTRODUCTION

In 1918, Aron first proposed that fat may be essential for normal growth and development of animals. Butter, apart from its caloric value, was deemed to have an important nutritional value because of the presence of certain lipid molecules. Evans and Burr (1927) subsequently demonstrated that a deficiency of fat severely affected both growth and reproduction of experimental animals, despite addition of the fat-soluble vitamins A, D, and E to the diet. These authors suggested that fat contained a new essential substance termed *vitamin F.* The work of Burr and Burr in 1929 first showed the nutritional importance of specific lipids in fat. Weanling rats fed a fat-free diet showed impaired growth, scaly skin, tail necrosis, and increased mortality, conditions that were reversed by feeding linoleic acid (C18:2n-6). In further work, the same authors described impaired fertility and augmented water consumption as additional symptoms of a deficiency of either C18:2n-6 or α-linolenic acid (C18:3n-3). The term *essential fatty acids* (EFA) was coined by Burr and Burr for those fatty acids (FA) not synthesized in mammals and for which deficiencies could be reversed by dietary addition.

Arachidonic acid (C20:4n-6) was determined to be an EFA in 1938. It was found to be approximately three times as effective as C18:2n-6 in relieving essential fatty acid deficiency (EFAD) symptoms. C18:2n-6 was subsequently found to undergo biotransformation to C20:4n-6; thus, C18:2n-6 was judged to be the primary unsaturated FA required in the diet by animals. Although various researchers were able to generate EFAD in different species by feeding EFA-deficient diets, EFAD was first described in the human in 1958. Infants fed a milk-based formula diet lacking EFA showed severe skin symptoms that were alleviated by addition of C18:2n-6.

In human adults, EFAD was subsequently described as a consequence of parenteral nutrition in which fat-free solutions containing only glucose, amino acids, electrolytes, and micronutrients were continuously infused. The resulting rashes and low plasma concentrations of polyunsaturated fatty acids (PUFA) were reversed by infusion of intravenous emulsions containing C18:2n-6. Holman et al. (1982) reported the first example of deficiency symptoms attributed to C18:3n-3 deficiency in a 6-year-old girl maintained parenterally for 5 months on a safflower-oil–based emulsion rich in C18:2n-6. Deficiency symptoms, including neuropathy and low serum concentrations of C18:3n-3, were corrected by changing the parenteral nutrition recipe to include soybean oil emulsion rich in n-3 FA (1). Neuringer et al. (2) in 1984 demonstrated C18:3n-3 deficiency in the offspring of rhesus monkeys showing a loss in visual activity. C18:3n-3 defi-

Abbreviations: **BS**—bile salt; **CH**—cholesterol; **CE**—cholesterol ester; **DG**—diglyceride; **EFA**—essential fatty acid; **EFAD**—essential fatty acid deficiency; **FA**—fatty acid; **HDL**—high-density lipoprotein; **IDL**—intermediate density lipoprotein; **LCFA**—long-chain fatty acid; **LDL**—low-density lipoprotein; **MCFA**—medium-chain fatty acid; **MCT**—medium-chain triglyceride; **MG**—monoglyceride; **MUFA**—monounsaturated fatty acid; **PAF**—platelet-activating factor; **PL**—phospholipids; **PUFA**—polyunsaturated fatty acid; **PG**—prostaglandin; **PGHS**—prostaglandin synthase; **SAFA**—saturated fatty acid; **SCFA**—short-chain fatty acid; **TG**—triglyceride; **VLCFA**—very long-chain fatty acid; **VLDL**—very low-density lipoprotein.

ciency was also described in nine patients who had received 0.02 to 0.09% of calories as n-3 FA via gastric tube feeding over a period of 2.5 to 12 years (3). The scaly dermatitis and depressed concentrations of n-3 FA in plasma and erythrocytes of the patients were reversed by supplementation with C18:3n-3.

CHEMISTRY AND STRUCTURE

Fats and lipids are defined as a class of compounds soluble in organic solvents, including acetone, ether, and chloroform. These compounds vary considerably in size and polarity, ranging from hydrophobic triglycerides (TGs) and sterol esters to more water-soluble phospholipids (PL) and cardiolipins. Dietary lipids also include cholesterol (CH) and phytosterols. Unlike other macronutrients, the non-water miscibility of lipids necessitates that these compounds receive specialized processing during digestion, absorption, transport, storage, and utilization. This specialization in metabolic handling distinguishes dietary lipids and their metabolites from other macronutrients.

Triglycerides and Fatty Acids

Triglycerides (TG), or triacylglycerols, make up by far the largest proportion of dietary lipids consumed by humans. A TG is composed of three FAs esterified to a glycerol molecule in one of three stereochemically distinct bonding positions: sn-1, sn-2, and sn-3. Variation in the type of FA and their bonding pattern to glycerol further increases the heterogeneity of TG composition. For most dietary oils, approximately 90% of the TG mass consists of FA. These FA are generally unbranched hydrocarbon chains with an even number of carbons, ranging from 4 to 26 carbon atoms. Smaller quantities of longer-chain FA have also been identified in mammalian tissues and thus may exist in human diets (4). Very long-chain fatty acids (VLCFA) predominate in the brain and specialized tissues, such as retina and spermatozoa (5). Adipose tissue contains FA of varying lengths.

In addition to differences in chain length, FA vary in the number and arrangement of double bonds along the hydrocarbon chain. Major FA are given in Figure 4.1. Systems for identifying the position of double bonds along the hydrocarbon chain entail carbon-counting from either

COMMON NAME	GENEVA NOMENCLATURE	CODE	FORMULA
butyric acid	butanoic acid	C4:0	$CH_3(CH_2)_2COOH$
caproic acid	hexanoic acid	C6:0	$CH_3(CH_2)_4COOH$
caprylic acid	octanoic acid	C8:0	$CH_3(CH_2)_6COOH$
capric acid	decanoic acid	C10:0	$CH_3(CH_2)_8COOH$
lauric acid	dodecanoic acid	C12:0	$CH_3(CH_2)_{10}COOH$
myristic acid	tetradecanoic acid	C14:0	$CH_3(CH_2)_{12}COOH$
palmitic acid	hexadecanoic acid	C16:0	$CH_3(CH_2)_{14}COOH$
stearic acid	octadecanoic acid	C18:0	$CH_3(CH_2)_{16}COOH$
palmitoleic acid	9-hexadecaenoic acid	C16:1, n-7 *cis*	$CH_3(CH_2)_5CH{=}CH(CH_2)_7COOH$
oleic acid	9-octadecaenoic acid	C18:1, n-9 *cis*	$CH_3(CH_2)_7CH{=}CH(CH_2)_7COOH$
elaidic acid	9-octadecaenoic acid	C18:1, n-9 *trans*	$CH_3(CH_2)_7CH{=}CH(CH_2)_7COOH$
linoleic acid	9,12-octadecadienoic acid	C18:2, n-6,9 all *cis*	$CH_3(CH_2)_4CH{=}CHCH_2CH{=}CH(CH_2)_7COOH$
α-linolenic acid	9,12,15-octadecatrienoic acid	C18:3, n-3,6,9 all *cis*	$CH_3CH_2CH{=}CHCH_2CH{=}CHCH_2CH{=}CH(CH_2)_7COOH$
γ-linolenic acid	6,9,12-octadecatrienoic acid	C18:3, n-6,9,12 all *cis*	$CH_3(CH_2)_4CH{=}CHCH_2CH{=}HCH_2CH{=}CH(CH_2)_4COOH$
columbinic acid	5,9,12-octatrienoic acid	C18: n-6 *cis*, 9 *cis*, 13 *trans*	$CH_3(CH_2)_4CH{=}CHCH_2CH{=}HCH_2CH{=}CHCH_2CH_2CH{=}CH(CH_2)_3COOH$
arachidic acid	eicosanoic acid	C20:0	$CH_3(CH_2)_{18}COOH$
behenic acid	docosanoic acid	C22:0	$CH_3(CH_2)_{20}COOH$
eicosenoic acid	11-eicosenoic acid	C20:1, n-9 *cis*	$CH_3(CH_2)_7CH{=}CH(CH_2)_9COOH$
erucic acid	13-docosaenoic acid	C22:1, n-9 *cis*	$CH_3(CH_2)_7CH{=}CH(CH_2)_{11}COOH$
brassidic acid	13-docosaenoic acid	C22:1, n-9 *trans*	$CH_3(CH_2)_7CH{=}CH(CH_2)_{11}COOH$
nervonic acid	15-tetracosaenoic acid	C24:1, n-9 *cis*	$CH_3(CH_2)_7CH{=}CH(CH_2)_{13}COOH$
"Mead" acid	5,8,11-eicosatrienoic acid	C20:3, n-9,12,15 all *cis*	$CH_3(CH_2)_7CH{=}CHCH_2CH{=}CHCH_2CH{=}CH(CH_2)_3COOH$
dihomo-γ-linolenic acid	8,11,14-eicosatetraenoic acid	C20:3, n-6,9,12 all *cis*	$CH_3(CH_2)_4CH{=}CHCH_2CH{=}HCH_2CH{=}CH(CH_2)_6COOH$
arachidonic acid	5,8,11,14-eicosatetraenoic acid	C20:4, n-6,9,12,15 all *cis*	$CH_3(CH_2)_4CH{=}CHCH_2CH{=}HCH_2CH{=}CHCH_2CH{=}CH(CH_2)_3COOH$
timnodonic acid	5,8,11,14,17-eicosapentaenoic acid	C20:5, n-3,6,9,12,15 all *cis*	$CH_3(CH_2CH{=}CH)_5(CH_2)_3COOH$
clupanodonic acid	7,10,13,16,19-docosapentaenoic acid	C22:n-3,6,9,12,15 all *cis*	$CH_3(CH_2CH{=}CH)_5(CH_2)_5COOH$
docosahexenoic acid	4,7,10,13,16,19-docosahexaenoic acid	C22:6, n-3,6,9,12,15,18 all *cis*	$CH_3(CH_2CH{=}CH)_6(CH_2)_2COOH$

Figure 4.1. Names, codes, and formulas of fatty acids mentioned in this chapter.

end of the molecule. The less common "delta" system of identification of double bonds counts from the carboxyl end of the fatty acyl chain. More commonly used is identification of the position of the first carbon of a double bond relative to the methyl terminus of the FA. Double bonds identified relative to the methyl end use the terms "n" or "ω" to indicate distance of the first bond along the carbon chain. For example, any FA described as n-6, or ω-6, has the initial double bond situated between the 6th and 7th carbon atoms from the methyl end. To contain a single double bond, a FA must be at least 12 carbon atoms in length. These monounsaturated fatty acids (MUFA) typically possess a double bond at the n-9 or n-7 position. Addition of further double bonds produces a PUFA. Each subsequent double bond invariably occurs three carbon atoms further along the carbon chain from the bond preceding it. Therefore, the number of double bonds within a FA is restricted by its chain length. FA with 18 carbon atoms or more that possess more than a single double bond will contain the first bond of their series only at the n-9, n-6, or n-3 position. For a 16-carbon atom FA, the first double bond may be located at the n-7 position. A maximum of 6 double bonds occurs in dietary FA.

The essentiality of a FA depends on the distance of the first double bond from the methyl terminus. During de novo FA formation, human biosynthetic enzymes can insert double bonds at the n-9 position or higher; however, these enzymes cannot insert double bonds at any position closer to the methyl end. For this reason, FA with double bonds at the n-6 and n-3 positions are, as individual classes, considered essential. These EFA must therefore be obtained from plants or other organisms that possess the enzymatic pathways for their construction. Mammalian tissues contain four families of PUFA (n-3, n-6, n-7, n-9) designated according to the number of carbon atoms from the terminal methyl group to the first carbon of the first double bond. Among all FA, only those of n-6 and n-3 classes are essential to the diet. All other FA can be synthesized by humans from an excess of dietary energy.

Double bonds in foods we consume most commonly occur in the *cis* configuration. *Trans* bonds, also present, are a result of hydrogenation, the process used to increase the viscosity of oils, and the microbial metabolism in ruminants. *Trans* bonds reduce internal rotational mobility of the fatty acyl chain and are less reactive to electrophilic additions such as halogenation, hydration, and hydrogenation (6, 7). Most dietary *trans* FA are monoenes, 18 carbons in length. The major *trans* FA, elaidic acid (C18:1n-9 *trans*) has a melting point of 44°C, versus 13°C for oleic acid (C18:1n-9).

Phospholipids

A limited amount of dietary lipid occurs as PL. PL are distinct from TG in that they contain polar head groups that confer amphipathic properties to the molecule. PL are insoluble amphophiles with a hydrophilic, often zwitterionic, head group, and hydrophobic tails composed of two longer-chain FA. These head groups are attached to the primary glycerol moiety via phosphate linkages. Polar head groups can vary in size and charge and include inositol, choline, serine, ethanolamine, and glycerol.

Sterols

CH, an amphipathic molecule, has a steroid nucleus and branched-hydrocarbon tail. CH is found in the diet both in the free form and esterified to FA, particularly C18:2n-6. CH is found only in foods of animal origin; plant oils are cholesterol free. Although free of CH, plant materials do contain phytosterols, compounds chemically related to CH. Common dietary phytosterols are listed in Figure 4.2. Phytosterols differ in their chemical side-chain configuration and steroid-ring–bonding pattern. The most common dietary phytosterols are β-sitosterol, campesterol, and stigmasterol. 5-α-Hydrogenation of phytosterols forms saturated phytosterols, including campestanol and sitostanol. Increasing evidence suggests that saturated phytosterols, such as sitostanol, inhibit CH absorption better than more hydrophilic plant sterols, such as β-sitosterol. These saturated phytosterols are found in very small amounts in normal diets but can be commercially produced.

DIETARY CONSIDERATIONS

Fat intake of the average North American diet represents 38% of total calories consumed (8, 9). Over 95% of the total fat intake is composed of TG; the remainder is in the form of PL, free FA, CH, and plant sterols. Total dietary TG in the North American diet is about 100 to 150 g per day. In addition to dietary intake, lipids enter the gastrointestinal tract by release from mucosal cells, biliary expulsion into the lumen, and bacterial action.

In almost no other instance can food choice influence nutrient composition as much as in the case of fats. As dietary TG vary widely in their FA composition, so does FA consumption (Table 4.1, see also more detailed tables of marine and nonmarine sources [Appendix Tables IV-A-19-A and B]). Large differences exist in the FA composition of oils from both plant and animal sources. Short-chain fatty acids (SCFA) (4 carbons) and medium-chain fatty acids (MCFA) (6 to 12 carbons) are found in vegetable oils and dairy fat, whereas fish oils and certain plants contain FA of the n-3 family. Long-chain n-3 FA can be found in a few terrestrial plants and range-fed nonruminant game animals. MUFA are found in plant oils, although meat fats also contain moderate amounts. As a rule, n-6 PUFA are found in vegetable fats and not in meat products, except in the case of C20:4n-6. Plant-derived oils vary widely in composition, largely because of genetic and environmental factors. In the case of animal fats, the composition of the feed also affects the final FA composition.

Intake of *trans* FA in the North American diet has not been firmly established, but it appears to range from 2 to

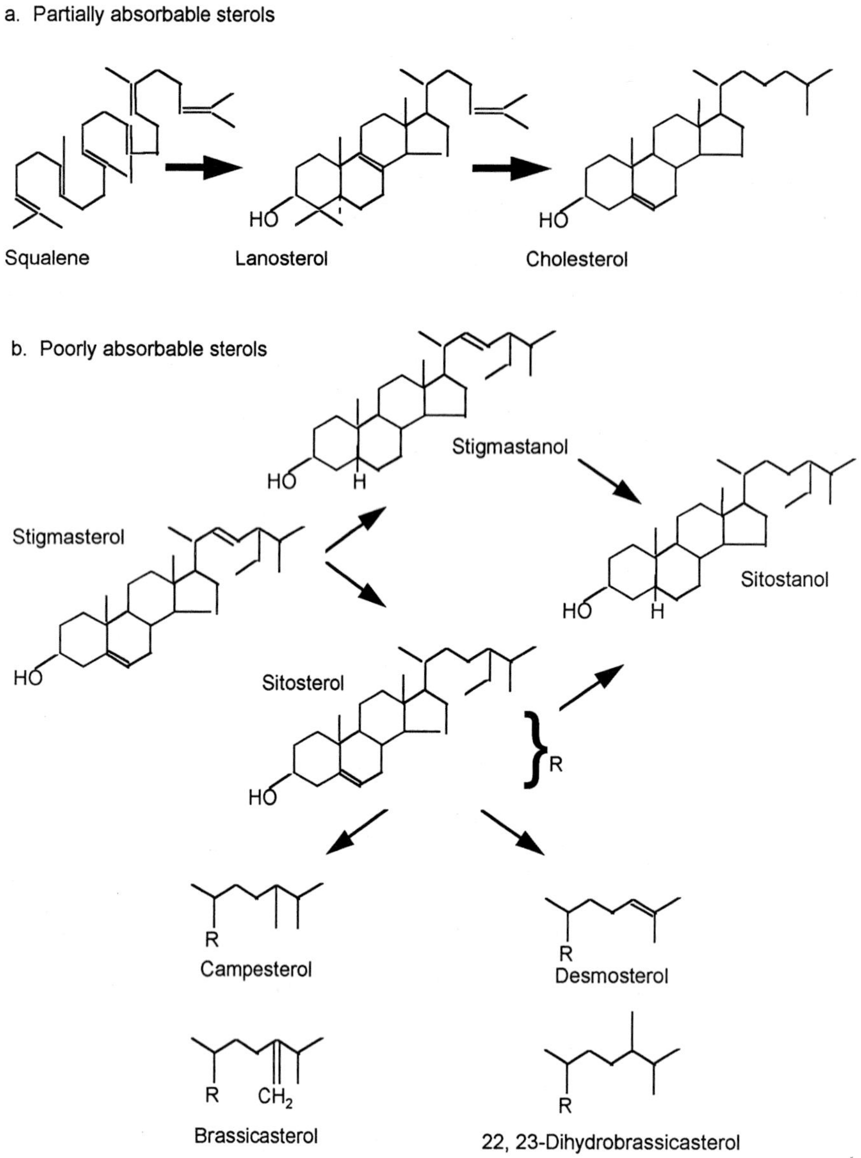

Figure 4.2. Molecular structure of the more important sterols in food (side chains only are shown for the bottom four structures).

7% of the total energy intake (7, 10). Amounts of *trans* FA in the diet have remained relatively constant over past decades, partly because the rise in vegetable fat consumption has been counterbalanced by a decline in the *trans* FA content of many foods made with vegetable fat (6). Methodological limitations in measuring the various isomeric forms of dietary *trans* FA contribute to the imprecision in our knowledge of consumption levels.

The dietary contribution of CH varies significantly across foods. Typically, 250 to 700 mg of CH is consumed each day in the North American diet, with the larger proportion esterified to FA. Reduction of dietary CH levels can be readily achieved by excluding animal fats from the diet.

North American diets typically contain about 250 mg/day of plant sterols, with vegetarian diets containing much larger amounts (11). Most plant sterols are found as β-sitosterol, campesterol, and stigmasterol.

DIGESTION AND ABSORPTION

Digestion in Mouth and Esophagus

Digestion of dietary lipids and their metabolites evokes a series of specific processes that enable absorption through the water-soluble environment of the gut (Table 4.2). Digestion begins in the oral cavity with salivation and mastication. Lingual lipase, released from the serous glands of the tongue with saliva, starts the hydrolysis of free FA from TG. Mechanical dispersion by chewing enlarges the surface area upon which lingual lipase can act. Lingual lipase cleaves at the sn-3 position, preferentially hydrolyzing shorter-chain FA found in foods, such as milk. Hydrolysis continues in the stomach, where gastric lipase promotes further lipid digestion, preferring TG containing SCFA. Fat entering the upper duodenum is 70% TG, with the remainder being a mixture of partially digested hydrolysis products.

Table 4.1
Average Triglyceride Fatty Acid Composition of Important Edible Fats[a]

		Average Fatty Acid Composition						
		Saturated			Mono- and Polyunsaturated			
Food	Average Fat%	Total[b]	16:0	18:0	18:1	18:2	18:3	20:4
Milk (cow)	3.5	65[b]	25	11	26	1–3	2	tr
Butter	80				26			
Pork	100	42	28	13	46	6–8	2	2
Beef	100	53	29	20	42	2	tr	—
Chicken	15	30	25	4	42	21	—	—
Egg	11				42			
Groundnut oil	100	19[c]	11	3	40–55[c]	20–43[c]		
Sesame oil	100	15	9	5	39	40	1	—
Soybean oil	100	15	11	4	23	51	7	—
Corn oil	100	13	11	2	25	55	tr	—
Sunflower seed oil	100	12	6	4	24	60–70	tr	—
Olive oil	100	17	14	3	71	10	tr	—
Cottonseed oil	100	30	25	3	18	51	tr	
Safflower seed oil	100	10	7	3	15[d]	75[d]	tr	
Palm oil	100	52	45	5	38	10	—	
Coconut oil	100	88[b]	8	3	6	2	—	
Palm kernel oil	100	80[b]	7	2	14	1	—	
Rapeseed oil	100	7	5	2	53	22	10[e]	
Cashew nut	68	24	14	10	30	35	tr	
Walnut	63	10	7	2	15	60	10	
Herring (menhaden)	16–25	30	19	4	13	1	1+[f]	
Mackerel[g]	25	25	17	5	18	1	#	

[a]*The figures given are approximations, as climate, species, fodder composition, etc. cause great variations. See also Appendices Tables IV A21a,b for additional information.*
[b]*The balance of saturated fatty acids is formed by fatty acids with chain lengths <12 (butter 14%) and 12 and 14 (butter 16%, coconut and palm kernel 65–70%).*
[c]*Circa 4% of C20:0 and C22:0, groundnuts from Argentina have relatively low C18:1 and high C18:2 concentrations.*
[d]*Also safflower seed oil with the reverse C18:1/18:2 composition is available.*
[e]*Contrary to new rapeseed varietes, such as Canbra and LEAR, old varieties of rapeseed oil and also mustard seed oil have 10% C20:In-9 and 30–50% C22:In-9.*
[f]*Menhaden herring oil has 11% C20:5n-3, 9% C22:6n-3, but Norwegian herring oil has 13% C20:In-9, 21% C22:In-11, 7% C20:5n-3, and 7% C22:6n-3.*
[g]*Depending on fishing grounds, mackerel oil is similar to menhaden or to Norwegian/North Sea herring.*

Intestinal Digestion

Intestinal digestion requires bile salts (BS) and pancreatic lipase. BS, PL, and sterols are the three principal lipid components of bile, the emulsifying fluid produced by the liver. BS consist of a steroid nucleus and an aliphatic side chain conjugated in an amide bond with taurine or glycine. The number and orientation of hydroxyl groups on the nucleus vary. The hydroxyl and ionized sulfonate or carboxylate groups of the conjugate make BS water soluble. Primary BS, defined as those synthesized directly from hepatic CH, include the tri- and dihydroxy bile salts, cholate and chenodeoxycholate, respectively. Secondary BS, including deoxycholate and lithocholate, are produced from primary BS via bacterial action on cholate and chenodeoxycholate in the gut, respectively. Further modification of secondary BS by hepatocytes or bacteria produces sulfate esters of lithocholate and ursodeoxycholate. Biliary phosphatidylcholine (PC), the main PL in bile, typically contains palmitic acid (C16:0) in the sn-1 position and an unsaturated 18- or 20-carbon FA in the sn-2 position.

Pancreatic lipase, the principal enzyme of TG digestion, hydrolyzes ester bonds at the sn-1 and sn-3 positions of the glycerol moiety (Fig. 4.3). BS inhibit lipase activity through displacement of the enzyme from its substrate at the surface of the lipid droplet. Colipase, also a pancreatic protein, reverses BS inhibition of pancreatic lipase by binding lipase, ensuring its adhesion to the droplet. Then, through its affinity to BS, PL, and CH, colipase facilitates

Table 4.2
Factors Involved in the Digestion of Fats

Source	Factor	Location of Action	Function
Food (breast milk)	Bile salt–stimulated lipase	Duodenum	Converts monoglycerides and free fatty acids to glycerol and free fatty acids
Oral cavity	Lingual lipase	Mouth; esophagus; stomach	Cleave triglycerdes at sn-3 position
Stomach	Gastric lipase	Stomach; duodenum	Cleave triglycerides at sn-3 position
Pancreas	Pancreatic lipase	Duodenum	Splitting of sn-1 and sn-3 positions
Liver	Bile salts	Duodenum	Emulsification of fats and reabsorption in small intestine and colon

shuttling of hydrolysis product monoglycerides (MG) and free FA from the lipid droplet into the BS-containing micelle. FA linked at the sn-2 position of MG, PL, and cholesterol esters (CE) are resistant to hydrolysis by lipase. Lipolysis by pancreatic lipase is extremely rapid, so MG and free FA production is faster than their subsequent incorporation into micelles (12). Synthesis of both lipase and colipase is stimulated by the hormone secretin and the presence of dietary TG in the small intestine. Release of BS and pancreatic lipase is also regulated humorally. The presence of amino acids and fat digestion products in the digesta evokes release of cholecystokinin (CCK) and secretin into the circulation. CCK then stimulates the production of exocrine pancreatic enzymes, while secretin enhances output of pancreatic electrolytes. CCK also induces synthesis of hepatic bile and its release through contraction of the gall bladder.

In breast-fed infants, TG are digested by the concerted action of gastric lipase, colipase-dependent pancreatic lipase, and a bile salt-stimulated lipase (BSSL) present in breast milk. Gastric lipase initiates digestion of the milk fat globule, and BSSL nonselectively converts the resulting MG and free FA to glycerol and free FA. This process increases absorptive efficiency.

Micellar solubilization of fat hydrolysis products occurs through the amphipathic actions of BS and PL, which are secreted at a ratio of approximately 1:3. CH is present in bile only in the unesterified form, which is the major sterol form (13). The polar termini of BS orient toward the aqueous milieu of the chyme, while the nonpolar termini containing hydrocarbon groups face the center of the micelle. BS and PL naturally aggregate so that nonpolar termini form a hydrophobic core. For micelles to form, a threshold concentration of BS must be reached, termed *the critical micellar concentration* (CMC). The typical biliary CMC of BS is 2 mM. BS concentrations within the proximal duodenum generally remain well in excess of this threshold.

Incorporation of MG hydrolyzed from TG into micelles increases the ability of the particle to solubilize free FA and CH. BS micelles generally possess the highest affinity for MG and unsaturated long-chain free fatty acids (LCFA) (14). Both diglycerides (DG) and TG have limited incorporation into micelles. Upon formation, mixed micelles containing FA, MG, CH, PL, and BS migrate to the unstirred water layer adjacent to the brush border surface.

Fat digestion has been the focus of clinical attention in light of the increasing global prevalence of obesity. Creation of fat substitutes that have properties similar to those of a naturally occurring fat, but which are resistant to the action of pancreatic lipase, has been actively pursued. Olestra, formed by chemical combination of sucrose with FA, possesses "mouthfeel" and texture similar to those of TG. However, Olestra passes through the intestine undigested and unabsorbed (15). The product is heat stable and has been approved for use in certain foods. The efficacy of Olestra in long-term weight control remains to be confirmed (16). Consumption of Olestra is not without risk of side effects, including anal leakage and reduced absorption of fat-soluble vitamins.

Absorption

Lipid absorption appears to occur in large part through passive diffusion. Micelles containing fat digestion products exist in dynamic equilibrium with each other; the peristaltic, churning action of the intestine maintains high intermicellar contact. This contact results in partitioning of constituents from more- to less-populated micelles, which equalizes the overall micellar concentration of digestion products. Thus, during digestion of a bolus of fat, micelles pick up evenly and rapidly the 2-MG and free FA that are released by the action of pancreatic lipase until the micelles are saturated with them.

Penetration of micelles across the unstirred water layer bordering the intestinal mucosal cells represents the first stage of absorption. Micelles, but not lipid droplets, approach and enter this water layer for two reasons. First, micelles are much smaller (30 to 100 Å) than emulsified droplets of fat (25,000 ± 20,000 Å). Second, the hydrophobic nature of the larger lipid droplet results in reduced solubilization at the site of the unstirred water layer.

Transport of micellar products across the unstirred water layer into the enterocyte is described in Figure 4.3. Micelles closest to the plasma membrane of the brush border partition their digestion products across the water envelope in a concentration-dependent fashion. Digestion products continue to be shuttled between micelles across the unstirred water layer, creating a chain-reaction effect. This action hinges on the lower cellular concentration of digestion products at the enterocyte. Intestinal fatty acid–binding proteins (FABP) assist in transmucosal shunting of digestion product FA and possibly MG and BS. Elevated FABP activity in the distal bowel is associated with higher FA absorption (17).

The overall efficiency of fat absorption in human adults is about 95%, more or less independent of the amount of fat consumed. However, the qualitative nature of the dietary fat influences overall efficiency. In general, efficiency increases with the degree of FA unsaturation (18). There is also evidence that as FA chain length increases, absorption efficiency decreases. Likewise, the positional distribution of FA on dietary TG is an important determinant of the eventual efficiency of absorption. Studies with structured lipids have shown that when octanoate, palmitate, or linoleate was substituted at different sn positions on a TG molecule, the positional distribution altered digestion, absorption, and lymphatic transport of these two FA (19, 20). The natural tendency of C16:0 to locate at the sn-2 position in breast milk may therefore explain the high digestibility of this milk fat. FA with chain lengths less than 12 carbon atoms are also absorbed passively by the gastric mucosa and taken up by the portal vein (21).

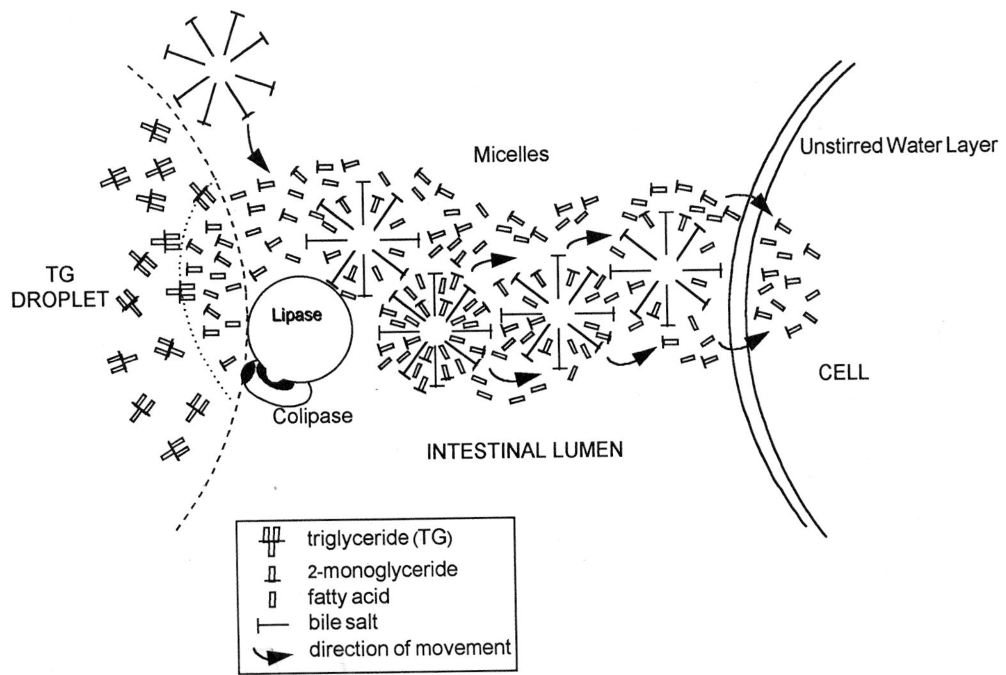

Figure 4.3. Transport hypothesis of fatty acids and 2-monoglycerides through lipase-mediated hydrolysis, micellar transfer, and cellular uptake stages.

Micellar BS are not absorbed with fat digestion products but are reabsorbed further along the gastrointestinal tract. Passive intestinal absorption of unconjugated BS occurs throughout the small intestine and colon. Active transport components predominate in the ileum and include the brush border membrane receptor, cytosolic bile acid–binding proteins and basolateral anion-exchange proteins. The enterohepatic recirculation of BS is approximately 97 to 98% efficient (22). Although bile acid production and secretion is normally not rate limiting in lipid absorption, it has been proposed that bile acid synthesis may be subnormal in infants. Dietary taurine supplementation results in higher bile acid excretion and FA absorption in preterm and small-for-gestational-age infants (23).

Digestion and Absorption of Phospholipids

Dietary PL constitute only a small portion of ingested lipid; however, PL are secreted in large quantities in bile. PL assist in emulsification of TG droplets as well as micellar solubilization of CH and other lipid-soluble components of the diet. PL, in particular PC, are also essential for stabilization of the micelle within the unstirred water layer. PL of both dietary and biliary origin are digested through cleavage by phospholipase A_2, a pancreatic enzyme secreted in bile. In contrast to pancreatic lipase, phospholipase A_2 cleaves FA at the sn-2 position of PL, yielding lysophosphoglycerides and free FA. These products undergo absorption through a process similar to that described above.

Digestion and Absorption of Sterols

CH within the intestine originates from both diet and bile. The amount of CH in the diet varies markedly depending on the degree of inclusion of foods from nonplant sources; biliary CH secretion is more consistent. Dietary and biliary CH differ in several ways. Dietary CH is up to 65% esterified, while biliary CH exists in free form, which probably explains the different absorption efficiencies of dietary (34%) and biliary (46%) CH (24). Biliary CH is also absorbed at a site more proximal within the small intestine.

CH, being hydrophobic, requires a specialized system so that digestion and absorption can occur within a water-soluble environment. The absorption efficiency for CH is much lower than that of TG. The major rate-limiting factor associated with the lower absorption of CH is its poor micellar solubility. Using various techniques, it has been demonstrated that 40 to 65% of CH is absorbed over the physiologic range of CH intakes in humans (23).

Digestion of dietary CE involves release of the esterified FA by a BS-dependent CE hydrolase secreted by the pancreas. Removal of esterified FA does not appear to be rate limiting; mixtures of free and esterified CH were absorbed with equal efficiency in rats (25). Free sterol then is solubilized within mixed micelles in the upper small intestine. Water-soluble lipid-exchange proteins of low molecular weight, located on the luminal side of the brush border membrane, may be involved in the transmembrane movement of CH and PL (26). The concentration of sphingomyelin within the apical membrane of the intestinal cell may also regulate the rate of CH uptake from micelles.

The amount of CH in the circulatory lipoproteins appears to be marginally responsive to the amount of dietary CH, within the normal physiologic range. Likely, compensatory changes in CH absorption (27) and biosynthesis (28) serve to maintain circulatory CH levels in the face of changes in dietary intake.

In contrast to CH, plant sterol absorption is very limited and differs across dietary phytosterols. For the major plant sterol, β-sitosterol, the typical absorption efficiency is 4 to 5%, about 1/10th that of CH (29). Absorption efficiency is higher for campesterol, about 10% (29), and almost nonexistent for sitostanol (30). This structure-specific discrimination depends on both the number of carbon atoms at the C24 position of the sterol side chain and the degree of hydrogenation of the sterol nucleus double bond. Differences in absorption across phytosterols are reflected in their circulating concentrations. Plasma campesterol levels are usually higher than those of sitosterol, while circulating levels of highly saturated sitostanol are almost nonquantifiable (11).

Phytosterol absorption is markedly reduced for two reasons. First, solubilization of phytosterols within micelles may be considerably lower than that of CH. Second, inadequate esterification of phytosterols may occur within the enterocyte membranes. Acylcoenzyme A:cholesterol acyltransferase (ACAT)-dependent esterification of CH is at least 60 times that of β-sitosterol (31).

Dietary phytosterols appear to compete with each other and with CH for absorption. Sitosterol consumption reduces absorption of CH, which in turn lowers circulating CH levels. Moreover, addition of sitostanol to diets lowers circulating levels of CH more than addition of nonsaturated plant sterols does (11), apparently through more effective reduction in absorption of CH and unsaturated FA (30). Saturated plant sterol esters, such as sitostanol esters, may be useful in lowering total and low-density-lipoprotein (LDL) CH levels in serum (32).

TRANSPORT AND METABOLISM

Solubility of Lipids

Transport of largely hydrophobic lipids through the circulation is achieved in large part by use of aggregates of lipids and protein, called *lipoproteins.* Principal lipid components of lipoproteins are TG, CH, CE, and PL. Protein constituents, termed *apolipoproteins* or *apoproteins,* increase both particle solubility and recognition by enzymes and receptors located at the outer surface of lipoproteins. The major lipoprotein classes are listed in Table 4.3 (32a). Lipoproteins differ in composition; however, all types feature hydrophilic apoproteins, PL polar head groups, and CH hydroxyl groups facing outward at the water interface, with PL acyl tails and CH steroid nuclei oriented toward the interior of the aggregate. CE and TG molecules form the core of the lipoprotein particle. In this manner, hydrophobic lipids can be internally solubilized and transported within a water medium. Lipoproteins represent a continuous spectrum of particles varying in size, density, composition, and function. Internal transport of lipids can be divided into exogenous and endogenous systems, reflecting lipids of dietary and internal origin, respectively.

Exogenous Transport System

The exogenous transport system transfers lipids of intestinal origin to peripheral and hepatic tissues (Fig. 4.4). Such lipids may originate from diet or secretions in the intestine. The exogenous system starts with reorganization in the enterocyte of absorbed FA, 2-MG, lysophospholipids, PL, smaller amounts of glycerol, CH, and phytosterols into molecules more readily packaged within the primary secretory unit, the chylomicron. Chylomicrons are assembled in the enterocyte endoplasmic reticulum membrane in conjunction with the Golgi apparatus. Chylomicron TG are reassembled predominantly via the monoacyl-glycerol pathway. Absorbed FA are activated by microsomal FA-CoA synthase to yield acyl-CoA, then combined sequentially with 2-MG through the action of mono- and diglyceride-acyltransferases. In addition, about 20% of TG resynthesis occurs by the α-glycerophosphate pathway. α-Glycerophosphate, synthesized de novo within the enterocyte from absorbed free glycerol or triose phosphates, combines with two fatty acyl-CoA units to form phosphatidic acid. After dephosphorylation, the 1,2-diglyceride is converted to TG by addition of a further fatty acyl-CoA. Phosphatidic acid is also converted to PL with addition of

Table 4.3
Physical-Chemical Characteristics of the Major Lipoprotein Classes

Lipoprotein	Density (g/dL)	Molecular Mass (daltons)	Diameter (nm)	Lipid (%)[a]		
				Triglyceride	Cholesterol	Phospholipid
Chylomicrons	0.95	1400×10^6	75–1200	80–95	2–7	3–9
VLDL	0.95–1.006	$10–80 \times 10^6$	30–80	55–80	5–15	10–20
IDL	1.006–1.019	$5–10 \times 10^6$	25–35	20–50	20–40	15–25
LDL	1.019–1.063	2.3×10^6	18–25	5–15	40–50	20–25
HDL	1.063–1.21	$1.7–3.6 \times 10^5$	5–12	5–10	15–25	20–30

From Ginsberg HN. Med Clin North Am 1994;78:1–20, with permission from WB Saunders.

[a] Percentage composition of lipids; apolipoproteins make up the rest. VLDL, very low-density lipoprotein; IDL, intermediate-density lipoprotein; LDL, low-density lipoprotein; HDL, high-density lipoprotein.

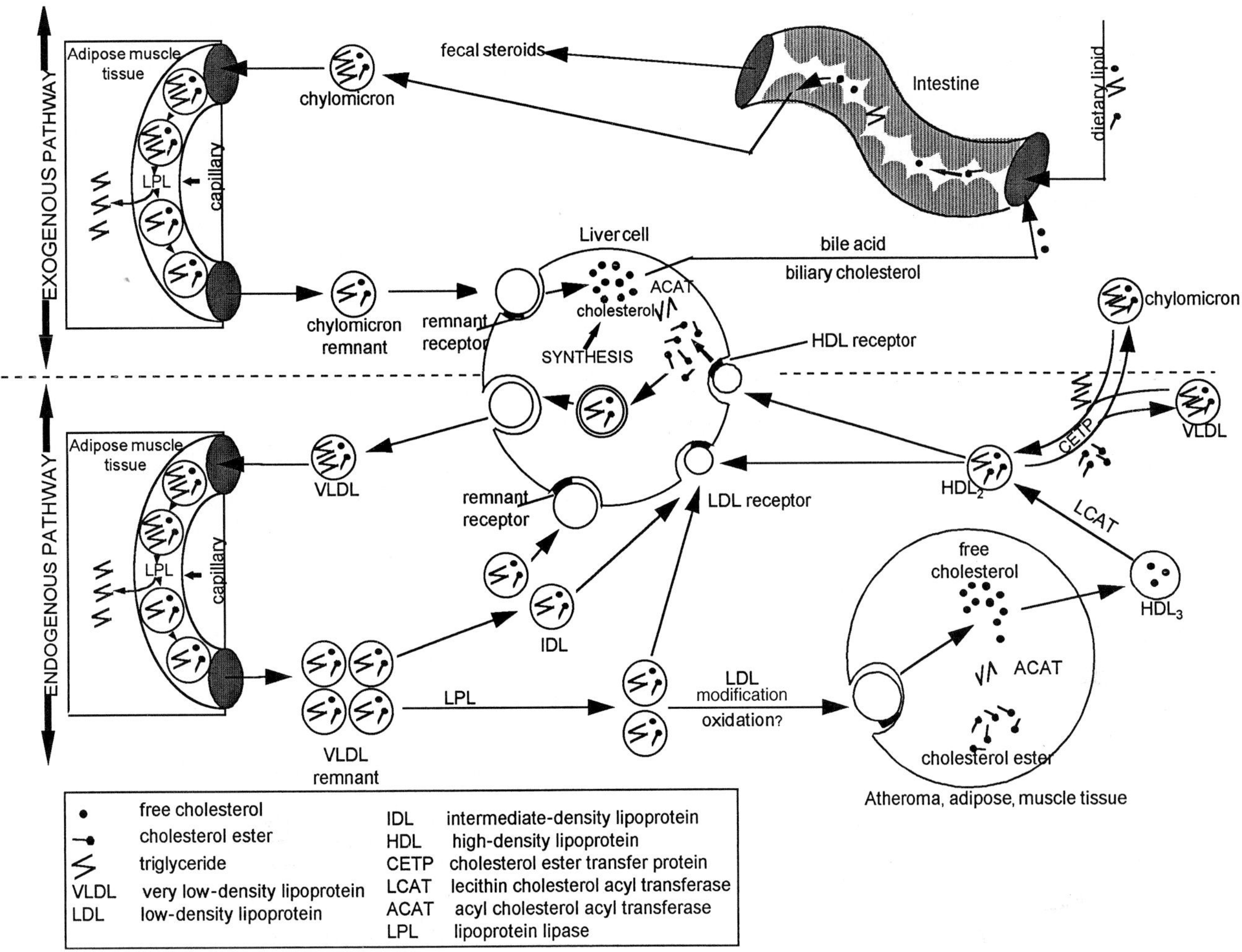

Figure 4.4. Exogenous and endogenous pathways of lipid transport.

FA, as is most lysophospholipid entering the enterocyte. The extent to which the phosphatidic acid pathway contributes to TG synthesis is influenced by the PL requirement of the enterocyte for chylomicron structure and assembly. Absorbed free CH is in large part reesterified using fatty acyl-CoA by acyl-CoA cholesterol acyltransferase (ACAT) located in microsomes (33).

Synthesis of new lipid appears to be a driving force in assembly and secretion of lipoproteins. Uptake of dietary long-chain fatty acids (LCFA), incorporation into TG by the glycerol-3-phosphate pathway, and assembly of lipoproteins all require fatty acid–binding protein (FABP) (34).

Not all FA require chylomicron incorporation and transport. FA less than 14 carbons in length and those containing several double bonds undergo, to a variable degree, direct internal transport via the portal circulation. Fats undergo direct portal transfer either as lipoprotein-bound TG or albumin-bound free (unesterified) FA. Portal transfer delivers FA to the liver faster than chylomicron transit. The FA structure-dependent specificity in these studies has raised questions about whether all FA can be considered equivalent in the context of energy and lipid metabolism. An accumulating body of evidence suggests that consumption of fats containing SCFA associated with portal transit results in higher rates of fat oxidation.

Chylomicrons released from mucosal cells circulate through the lymphatic system and reach the superior vena cava via the thoracic duct. Release into the circulation is followed by TG hydrolysis at the capillary surface of tissues by lipoprotein lipase. Hydrolysis of TG within the core of the chylomicron results in movement of FA into tissues and the subsequent production of TG-depleted chylomicron remnant particles. Chylomicron remnants then pick up CE from high-density lipoproteins (HDL) and are rapidly taken up by the liver.

Endogenous Transport System

The endogenous shuttle for lipids and their metabolites consists of three interrelated components. The first, involving very low-density lipoproteins (VLDL), intermediate-density lipoproteins (IDL), and LDL, coordinates movement of lipids from liver to peripheral tissues. The second, involving HDL, encompasses a series of events that returns lipids from peripheral tissues to liver. The third component of the system, not involving lipoproteins, effects the free FA–mediated transfer of lipids from storage reservoirs to metabolizing organs.

Components of the endogenous lipoprotein system are illustrated in Figure 4.4. The system begins with assembly of VLDL particles, mostly in the liver. Assembly of nascent VLDL starts in the endoplasmic reticulum and depends on the presence of adequate core lipids, CE, and TG. It has been estimated using stable isotope tracers that most TG FA within VLDL is preformed (35, 36). Some VLDL particles may also originate from intestinal tissue. Addition of surface lipids, mainly PL and free CH, occurs in the Golgi apparatus before the particle is secreted.

Following secretion of the VLDL particle into the circulation, a number of interchanges with tissues and lipoproteins occur. A major event is deposition of lipids into peripheral tissues. Hydrolysis of VLDL TG occurs through the action of lipoprotein lipase, an enzyme located on the endothelial side of vessel tissue, which mediates hydrolysis of chylomicron TG. Lipase-generated free FA can be used as energy sources or structural components for lipids, including PL, leukotrienes (LT), and thromboxanes (TXA), or converted back to TG and stored. TG and PL from both chylomicron remnants and LDL are also hydrolyzed by hepatic lipase. When hepatic lipase is absent, large LDL particles and TG-rich lipoproteins accumulate. Through TG depletion, the VLDL particle is converted to a denser, smaller, and cholesterol-rich, triglyceride-rich lipoprotein (TRL) remnant. High circulatory levels of TRL remnants are associated with progression of coronary artery disease. TRL remnants themselves can be cleared from plasma through hepatic lipoprotein receptors or be converted to smaller LDL. LDL is the major cholesterol-carrying lipoprotein. Although LDL levels are associated with heart disease risk in general, recent evidence suggests that a predominance of smaller, denser LDL particles in the circulation confers an elevated risk of coronary heart disease (37). An LDL receptor allows the liver to catabolize LDL. Modified or oxidized LDL can also be taken up by a scavenger receptor on macrophages in various tissues, including the arterial wall.

The second component of the endogenous transport system, perhaps nebulously termed *reverse CH transport,* involves movement of CH from peripheral tissues to the liver. Since 1975, when Miller and Miller (38) described the protective effect of HDL on atherosclerosis, much work has been undertaken to better understand the structure and function of HDL. HDL particles are highly heterogeneous, with subcomponents originating from both the intestinal tract and liver. It has been proposed that HDL particles participate in reverse CH transport by acquiring CH from tissues and other lipoproteins and transporting it to the liver for excretion. Circumstantial evidence suggests that elevated HDL levels are associated with reduced coronary risk in humans; the link between subnormal HDL levels and higher risk has been established (39).

The third component of the endogenous lipid transport system involves non-lipoprotein-associated movement of free FA through the circulation. These FA, largely products of cellular TG hydrolysis, are secreted by adipose tissue into plasma, where they bind with albumin. Recent evidence suggests that saturated fatty acids (SAFA) and C18:1n-9 are more slowly mobilized than PUFA, at a rate that is independent of their relative proportion in adipose tissue (40, 41). Albumin-bound FA are removed in a concentration gradient–dependent manner by metabolically active tissues and used largely as energy sources.

Apoproteins, Lipid Transfer Proteins, and Lipoprotein Metabolism

Interorgan movement of exogenous and endogenous lipids within lipoproteins is not incidental, but coordinated by a series of apoproteins. Apoproteins confer greater water solubility, coordinate the movement and activities of lipoproteins by modulating enzyme activity, and mediate particle removal from the circulation by specific receptors. Indeed, rates of synthesis and catabolism of the major lipoproteins are regulated to a large extent by apoproteins residing on a particular surface that is recognized by specific cellular receptors. Much has been learned about the role of apoproteins through the study of genetic defects and their effects on modification of apoprotein structure and thus lipoprotein function (42).

Lipoproteins vary in apoprotein content. Apolipoprotein B (Apo-B) is the major protein contained in chylomicrons, VLDL, IDL, and LDL particles. A larger Apo-B-100 is associated with VLDL and LDL of hepatic origin, while a lower-molecular-weight Apo-B-48 species is found in chylomicrons and intestinally derived VLDL. Apo-B-48 is thought to be generated from the same messenger RNA as Apo-B-100. During apoprotein assembly, hydrophobic Apo-B associates with PL in the endoplasmic reticulum immediately after translation and then requires the presence of adequate core lipid CE and TG. This process of assembly of Apo-B-containing lipoproteins may be influenced by FA composition.

Apoprotein E is synthesized in the liver and is present on all forms of lipoproteins. Apo-E binds both heparin-like molecules (which are present on all cells) and the LDL receptor. Apo-E displays genetic polymorphism; at least three alleles of the Apo-E gene produce six or more possible genotypes, which differ in their ability to bind the LDL receptor. Interactions between Apo-E genotype and CH absorption and synthesis have been suggested.

Most HDL particles contain apoproteins A-I, A-II, A-IV, and C. Apo-A-I and Apo-A-IV are believed to be activators of lecithin:cholesterol acyltransferase (LCAT), an enzyme that esterifies CH in plasma. Apo-A-I also appears to be the crucial structural protein for HDL. Three C apoproteins exist: Apo-C-I, Apo-C-II, and Apo-C-III; each possesses distinct functions and all are synthesized in the liver. Apo-C-II, present in chylomicrons, VLDL, IDL, and HDL, is important in activation of the enzyme lipoprotein lipase, along with Apo-E. Apo-C-III, present on chylomicrons, IDL, and HDL, may inhibit PL action.

Apoproteins play a role in interorgan lipid movement and distribution at several levels. For instance, VLDL are modified by lipoprotein lipase in peripheral tissues to form LDL particles. Apo-C-II, activating lipoprotein lipase, hydrolyzes VLDL and chylomicron TG. It is believed that HDL exchanges Apo-E and Apo-C for Apo-A-I and Apo-A-IV on chylomicrons in the circulation. Apo-E is important in the hepatic clearance of TG-depleted chylomicron remnants.

Apoproteins are critical in the removal of particles from the circulation. LDL is taken up into tissues by two processes, mostly in liver cells but also in adipocytes, smooth muscle cells, and fibroblasts. The first process is receptor dependent and involves the interaction of Apo-B-100 and LDL with specific LDL receptors on cell surfaces. Quantitatively, most LDL receptors exist in the liver (Fig. 4.4). Postcontact events involve clustering of these receptors in coated pits and LDL internalization. The second process is receptor independent. In contrast to receptor-dependent LDL uptake, receptor-independent transport is nonsaturable and does not appear to be regulated. The rate of receptor-independent transfer is low but increases as a direct function of plasma LDL levels; thus uptake by this pathway can be substantial at high plasma LDL levels.

The LDL receptor is sensitive to both the total amount and unesterified fraction of CH within the cell. Receptor integrity, particularly for LDL, is implicated in the progression of atherosclerosis. Individuals with genetically inherited abnormalities in their LDL receptors have greatly elevated LDL levels because of faulty receptor-apoprotein interactions (42). Likewise, genetic problems with apoprotein structure can result in similar elevations of LDL. CH in LDL particles can undergo chemical modification by oxidation and can then be taken up by macrophage LDL scavenger receptors in an unregulated fashion, potentially resulting in foam cell production and atherogenesis. Higher concentrations of CH also favor formation of β-VLDL, particles that float at a density of less than 1.006 but have β-electrophoretic mobility. β-VLDL can arise from chylomicron remnants or be formed by hepatocytes. These particles interact with LDL receptors on macrophages, depositing large amounts of CE into the macrophage. Substantial increases in CE content convert macrophages to foam cells. LDL receptors on macrophages do not appear to be suppressed as CE concentration increases, unlike those on fibroblasts or smooth muscle.

Formation of HDL also critically depends on apoproteins. Coalescence of PL-apoprotein complexes results in aggregation of Apo-A-I, Apo-A-II, Apo-A-IV, and possibly Apo-E to form nascent HDL particles. These CH-poor, smaller Apo-A-I-containing forms of HDL are heterogeneous in size and can be classified overall as pre-β or discoidal HDL. Subsequently, discoidal HDL changes in size and composition in plasma and extracellular spaces as a result of acquiring free CH from cell membranes of peripheral tissues. HDL-binding proteins have been identified on plasma membranes of cells, including macrophages, fibroblasts, hepatocytes, and adipocytes. Free CH taken up by HDL is esterified by LCAT and moves to the core of the HDL particle. LCAT transfers an sn2-acyl group of PC or phosphatidylethanolamine (PE) to the free hydroxyl residue of CH. Esterification prevents reentry of CH into peripheral cells. Phospholipid transfer protein (PLTP), which provides PC to HDL, also contributes to the compositional shifts in HDL. As HDL becomes enriched with CE, proteins Apo-C-II, and C-III are picked up from other lipoproteins to form three spherical categories of HDL. In order of increasing size and lipid content, these include HDL_3, HDL_{2a}, and HDL_{2b}. Spherical HDL likely go through repeated cycles of size increase and decrease over their circulatory life span of 2 to 3 days.

Spherical HDL can be removed from the circulation and metabolized via two routes. First, HDL_2 can transfer CE to either Apo-B-containing lipoproteins or directly to cells. CH moves from HDL_2 via cholesterol ester transfer protein (CETP), which mediates the transfer of CE from HDL_2 to VLDL and chylomicrons in exchange for TG. Apo-B-containing particles in turn transport CE to liver. CETP is produced in liver and associates with HDL. As a result of CETP, HDL_2 reconverts to the HDL_3 form. Other apoproteins on HDL that play a role in reverse CH transport and can activate LCAT include Apo-A-IV, Apo-C-I, and Apo-E. Secondly, entire particles of HDL_2 can be taken up by LDL receptors and possibly by a separate Apo-E receptor present on hepatocytes.

Actions of HDL other than reverse CH transport may include protection of lipoproteins from oxidative modification, direct removal of CH from atherosclerotic lesions, and a role in the metabolism of eicosanoids (39). HDL can inhibit oxidative modification of LDL in vitro and may contribute to HDL antiatherogenic potential in vivo (43).

Plasma albumin may also be important in reverse CH transport. Through passive diffusion, albumin picks up CH from peripheral cells and passes it to lipoproteins, including HDL and LDL. A large proportion of CH efflux persists in the absence of Apo-A-I, suggesting mainly albumin-dependent shuttling (44).

Dietary Factors That Influence Plasma Lipoproteins

Dietary factors profoundly influence lipoprotein levels and metabolism, which in turn alter an individual's susceptibility to atherosclerosis. Dietary fat, CH, fiber, protein, alcohol consumption, and energy balance all have major impact. Classic studies originally revealed that consumption of saturated fats elevated circulating total and LDL CH levels in humans (45). Plasma cholesterol-raising effects of SAFA, particularly myristic (C14:0) and C16:0 acids, are well established. Newer technologies that reduce saturated fat content in dairy products result in lower plasma CH levels when these products are consumed by humans (46). The CH-raising effect is believed to occur because the regulatory pool of liver CH is shifted from CE to free CH when hepatocytes become enriched with C14:0 and C16:0 acids. Higher levels of free CH in the liver suppress LDL receptor activity, driving up circulatory levels. Postmeal accumulation of VLDL is more prolonged in individuals consuming diets rich in SAFA than in those consuming diets containing n-6 PUFA (47).

Conversely, metabolic studies show that consumption of n-6 PUFA lowers circulatory CH values; however, epidemiologic data fail to demonstrate any direct protective effect of dietary PUFA on coronary heart disease risk. Consumption of n-3 PUFA is more strongly inversely correlated with the incidence of heart disease. Whether this action is due to lipid lowering or changing eicosanoid-related thrombosis susceptibility has not been firmly established. n-3 PUFA that lower circulating TG levels have only a minor impact on lipoprotein CH levels in humans (48).

Consumption of monounsaturated fats also results in lower CH levels, but to no greater extent than n-6 PUFA consumption. Consumption of *trans* FA raises LDL and lowers HDL levels in a dose-dependent fashion. It has been suggested recently that dietary *trans* fat consumption may increase CETP activity, explaining the higher circulatory LDL levels associated with *trans* fat consumption (49). The role of dietary CH in hyperlipidemia has engendered considerable debate. Within the range of normal CH intakes, changing dietary CH content seems to produce little alteration in circulating CH levels or subsequent metabolism (50). Certain individuals demonstrate a hypersensitivity to dietary CH, which may result in a misleading perception of the response to dietary CH within a population overall.

Dietary fiber also influences CH levels. In general, insoluble fibers, such as cellulose, hemicellulose, and lignin from grain and vegetables (see Chapter 3), have limited effects on CH levels, whereas more soluble forms, such as gums and pectins found in legumes and fruit, possess greater CH-lowering properties. Fiber exhibits CH-lowering action by at least three mechanisms other than simple replacement of hypercholesterolemic dietary ingredients. First, fiber may act as a bile acid–sequestering agent. Second, fiber likely reduces the rate of insulin rise by slowing carbohydrate absorption, thus slowing CH synthesis. Third, fiber may produce SCFA, which are absorbed by the portal circulation and inhibit CH synthesis.

Qualitative protein intake may also influence circulating CH levels, since consumption of animal protein leads to higher circulating CH levels than consumption of plant protein. Alcohol intake is somewhat arguably associated with heart disease risk. The relationship between alcohol consumption and CH levels is "J" shaped. At lower levels of intake, wine and spirits (but not beer) produce a more favorable lipid profile: lowering LDL and raising HDL CH values. Further, consumption of excess calories resulting in obesity is associated with higher circulating CH levels. Both CH and TG levels fall during weight loss (51). The distribution of excess weight appears to have a stronger association with circulating lipid level than the amount of weight (52). In summary, these dietary factors suggest that replacing energy-dense and saturated fat-rich, animal-based foods with those obtained from plant sources is warranted to maintain a desirable profile of circulating lipids.

OXIDATION AND CONVERSION OF LIPIDS TO OTHER METABOLITES

Fatty Acid Oxidation

In an individual of stable weight, the amount of fat consumed equals the quantity partitioned to meet energy needs. FA are a more efficient energy source than other macronutrients because of their high content in bonds between carbon and hydrogen. Such bonds are stronger and therefore contain more oxidizable energy than bonds between carbon and other atoms, as found in carbohydrates, protein, and alcohol. FA used for energy proceed through stages, including transport to oxidative tissues, transcellular uptake, mitochondrial transfer, and subsequent β-oxidation.

FA partitioned for oxidation are activated to fatty acyl-CoA, which are then transported into mitochondria to be oxidized. However, LCFA and their CoA derivatives cannot cross the mitochondrial membrane without carnitine, synthesized in humans from lysine and methionine. Transferase enzymes bind activated FA covalently to carnitine. After intramitochondrial transmission, FA are reactivated with CoA while carnitine recycles to the cytoplasmic surface.

Mitochondrial β-oxidation of FA entails the consecutive release of two-carbon acetyl-CoA units from the carboxyl terminus of the acyl chain. Prior to release of each unit, the β-carbon atoms of the acyl chain undergo cyclical degradation in four stages: dehydrogenation (removal of hydrogen), hydration (addition of water), dehydrogenation, and cleavage. Completion of these four reactions represents one cycle of β-oxidation. For unsaturated bonds within FA, the initial dehydrogenation reaction is omitted. The entire cycle is repeated until the fatty acyl chain is completely degraded. Absence of chain-shortened n-6 or n-3 FA in cellular or subcellular compartments indicates that once an FA begins cyclic degradation by β-oxidation, the process continues until the acyl chain is completely broken down.

Peroxisomal FA β-oxidation is similar to mitochondrial oxidation; yet there are several differences between these two organelles. First, very long acyl-CoA synthetase, the enzyme responsible for the activation of VLCFA, is present in peroxisomes and endoplasmic reticulum but not mitochondria, likely explaining why VLCFA are oxidized predominantly in peroxisomes. Second, the initial reaction in peroxisomal β-oxidation (desaturation of acyl-CoA) is catalyzed by an FAD-containing fatty acyl-CoA oxidase that is presumed to be the rate-limiting enzyme, whereas an acyl-CoA dehydrogenase is the first enzyme in the mitochondrial pathway. Third, peroxisomal β-oxidation is not directly coupled to the electron transfer chain that conserves energy via oxidative phosphorylation. In peroxisomes, electrons generated in the first oxidation step are transferred directly to molecular oxygen, yielding hydrogen peroxide that is disposed of by catalase, while energy produced in the second oxidation step (NAD^+ reduction) is conserved in the form of high-energy electrons of nicotinamide adenine dinucleotide (NADH). Fourth, the second (hydration) and third (NAD^+-dependent dehydrogenation) steps are catalyzed by a multifunctional protein that also displays δ^3,δ^2-enoyl-CoA isomerase activity required for oxidation of unsaturated FA.

Dietary Modulation of Fatty Acid Oxidation

Recently, considerable interest has surrounded structure-dependent induction of FA oxidation. Thus, food selection may influence the partitioning of dietary fat for oxidation or retention for storage and structural use in humans. This issue is of health interest for at least two reasons. First, consumption of fats associated with greater retention may result in an increased tendency toward obesity. Second, the greater accumulation of less preferentially oxidized FA in cells may confer structural/functional changes because of shifts in membrane PL FA patterns or in prostaglandin (PG):thromboxane (TXA) ratios. The influence of tissue FA composition on functional ability, such as insulin sensitivity, is well recognized (53).

Discriminative oxidation of certain FA is well defined; for others it has been suggested. Short- and medium-chain triglyceride (MCT) consumption is associated with increased energy production in humans, perhaps because of direct portal transfer of SCFA and MCFA from gut to liver. The lack of requirement for carnitine in mitochondrial membrane transit by SCFA may also be responsible for their more rapid oxidation. For LCFA, increasing evidence suggests that n-6 and n-3 PUFA are more rapidly oxidized for energy than are SAFA. In animals, labeled PUFA are more readily converted to carbon dioxide than are SAFA (54), while PUFA consumption exhibits greater thermogenic effect (55), oxygen consumption (56), and sympathetic nervous system stimulation (57). Whole-body FA balance data also support the concept that C18:2n-6 is more readily used for energy than are SAFA (58). Although these findings have yet to be confirmed in humans, consumption of fats containing PUFA appears to enhance the contribution of dietary fat to total energy production in healthy individuals (59) and influences the use of other FA for energy (60); however, mechanisms remain to be defined. Portal venous transfer rates, release rates of FA from adipose tissue, hepatic FA oxidation enzyme activities, and mitochondrial entry rates of FA generally increase with the degree of acyl chain unsaturation.

Peroxidative Modification of Lipids

Lipids are oxidized by reactive oxygen species produced as byproducts of normal metabolism. Reactive oxygen species include superoxide ($^{\cdot}O_2^-$), hydroxyl radical ($^{\cdot}OH$), hydrogen peroxide, singlet oxygen ($^1O_2$), and hypochlorous acid ($HOCl^-$). In healthy individuals, generation of reactive oxygen species should be in balance with antioxidant defenses. Circumstances that enhance oxidant exposure, such as increased formation of reactive oxygen species caused by chemicals and drugs, or that compromise antioxidant capability, such as decreased antioxidant vitamin levels because of malnutrition, are referred to as *oxidative stress*. Possible free radical effects on cells include oxidative damage to proteins, carbohydrates, and DNA. Oxidative stress has also long been known to be capable of inducing lipid oxidation and, in the presence of oxygen, lipid peroxidation of cell membranes.

It is generally accepted that lipid oxidation proceeds via a free radical mechanism called autoxidation, which includes initiation, propagation, and termination stages and predominantly occurs with PUFA. Polyunsaturated acyl chains of membrane PL are particularly sensitive to lipid peroxidation. Lipid oxidation, both nonenzymatic and enzymatic, is self-propagating in cellular membranes. Peroxidation of PUFA is classically depicted as a series of three or four basic reactions; however, the process becomes more complex as both the degree of unsaturation and severity of peroxidative conditions increases. The following initiation, propagation, and termination reactions characterize the general scheme of autoxidation:

1. Initiation:	$X^{\bullet} + LH^{\bullet} \rightarrow L^{\bullet} + XH$	
2. Propagation:	$L^{\bullet} + O_2 \rightarrow LOO^{\bullet}$	
3.	$LOO^{\bullet} + LH \rightarrow L^{\bullet} + LOOH$	
4. Termination:	$LO^{\bullet} + LO^{\bullet} \rightarrow$	nonradical polymers
5.	$LOO^{\bullet} + LOO^{\bullet} \rightarrow$	nonradical polymers
6.	$L^{\bullet} + L^{\bullet} \rightarrow$	nonradical polymers
7.	$LOO^{\bullet} + L^{\bullet} \rightarrow$	nonradical polymers

A peroxidation sequence in a membrane or PUFA is initiated by the attack of any free radical with sufficient reactivity to abstract a hydrogen atom from an allelic methylene group of an unsaturated FA; this includes the $HO^{\cdot}$ and $HO_2^{\cdot}$ radicals. The initiating free radical ($X^{\cdot}$) abstracts a hydrogen atom from the carbon chain, generating a lipid carbon-centered radical ($L^{\cdot}$, reaction 1). This carbon-centered lipid radical tends to be stabilized by a molecular rearrangement that produces a conjugated diene, which then readily reacts with molecular oxygen to yield a hydroperoxyl radical ($LOO^{\cdot}$, reaction 2). The peroxyl radical can propagate the oxidizing chain reaction by abstracting electrons from other susceptible PUFA, forming another lipid free radical and a molecule of lipid hydroperoxide (*LOOH*) (reaction 3). The overall chain reaction has a pyramidal effect through which a relatively few initiating radicals break down PUFA. These reactions continue until the chain is terminated, either by the combination of two radicals to form a nonradical product (reactions 4–7) or by termination of the propagation reaction in the presence of a hydrogen or an electron donor. Termination may also result from hydrogen abstraction from vitamin E (α-tocopherol) or another lipid antioxidant to form hydroperoxides. Vitamin E is termed a *chain-breaking antioxidant* because it donates a hydrogen atom to lipid radicals, thereby terminating the propagative process and lipid peroxidation. Lipid peroxidation can also be inhibited by reduction of lipid hydroperoxides by selenoperoxidases, such as glutathione (GSH)-peroxidase, to their corresponding alcohols.

Lipid peroxides are rapidly decomposed in vivo by metal ions and their complexes. The alkoxyl or peroxyl radical byproducts of lipid hydroperoxide breakdown can propagate the chain reaction of lipid peroxidation (61). Although lipid peroxides are highly toxic, they are poorly absorbed in vivo. The toxicity of peroxides has in part been attributed to their ability to oxidize the thiol groups of proteins, glutathione, and other sulfhydryl compounds and form insoluble deposits called *lipofuscin* in the artery wall or neural tissue (61).

The end products of lipid peroxidation include aldehydes and hydrocarbon gases. Short-chain aldehydes can attack amino groups on protein molecules to form cross-links between different protein molecules. The most commonly measured product is malondialdehyde (MDA), known to react with proteins and amino acids (Fig. 4.5). Several studies have shown a positive relationship between in vivo lipid peroxidation and urinary excretion of MDA. MDA adduct formation with proteins, PL, and nucleic acids may be a cause of pathology as MDA adducts with serine, lysine, ethanolamine, and guanidine have been detected in urine (62).

Lipid peroxidation has been implicated in the pathogenesis of diseases, including cancer and atherosclerosis. Although products of lipid peroxidation are readily measurable in blood, the significance and occurrence of lipid peroxidation is controversial. A major criticism has been that lipid peroxidation may not be initially involved in causing the underlying disease pathology, as excess production of lipid peroxidation byproducts could result from the primary disease process. Also, many analytic methods produce some disruption of cell structure. Such disruption could produce misleading findings, as lipid peroxidation may accompany tissue damage, although some recent studies have dissociated lipid peroxidation from in vitro cell death (63).

The PL components of cellular membranes are highly vulnerable to oxidative damage because of the susceptibility of their PUFA side chains to peroxidation. Membrane lipid peroxidation results in loss of PUFA, decreased membrane fluidity, and increased permeability of the membrane to substances such as Ca^{2+} ions. Lipid peroxidation can lead to loss of enzyme and receptor activity and have deleterious effects on membrane secretory functions. Continued lipid peroxidation can lead to complete loss of membrane integrity, as can be observed from the hemolysis associated with lipid peroxidation of erythrocyte membranes.

A wide range of dietary components has been reported to influence membrane susceptibility to oxidative damage. Cellular lipid peroxidation depends strongly on PUFA intake as well as intake of vitamin E and other lipid antioxidants. In isolated erythrocytes from human subjects, the production of lipid peroxidation products following hydrogen peroxide–induced oxidative stress has been measured as thiobarbituric acid–reactive substances (TBARS). Multivariate analysis showed that the unsaturation index was the best predictor of erythrocyte TBARS variability (64). A relatively stable C18:2n-6:vitamin E ratio in vegetable oils provides protection from risk of excessive lipid peroxidation and vitamin E deficiency at high PUFA intakes. Fish oils are an exception to the observation of a natural association between PUFA and vitamin E in edible fats and oils and the stability of PUFA to oxidation in the diet and body. The highly unsaturated n-3 pentanoic and hexanoic FA, found in abundance in fish and marine oils with relatively low vitamin E content, markedly increase the in vivo susceptibility of these oils to peroxidation (65). TBARS increased with higher concentrations of total n-3 PUFA in isolated human erythrocytes, whereas TBARS decreased with higher concentrations of total MUFA (64).

The effects of oxygen free radicals on membrane CH may be as important as the effects observed on membrane PL, since oxidized CH derivatives, the oxysterols or CH oxides, have been suggested to play a key role in development of atherosclerosis (66). This concept has been fostered by increasing evidence of the role of oxidatively modified lipoproteins in atherogenesis. CH readily undergoes oxidation (67), and the metabolites derived display a wide variety of actions on cellular metabolism, including

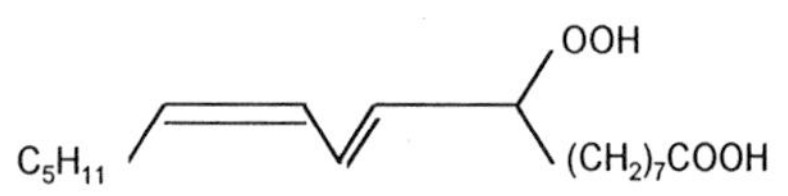

OOH
C_5H_{11} $(CH_2)_7COOH$

9-HYDROPEROXY-10-TRANS, 12-CIS-OCTADECADIENOIC ACID (LINOLEIC ACID-9-HYDROPEROXIDE)

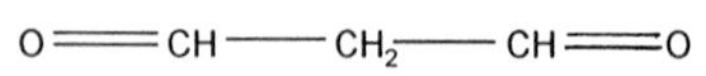

O═CH—CH_2—CH═O

MALONDIALDEHYDE

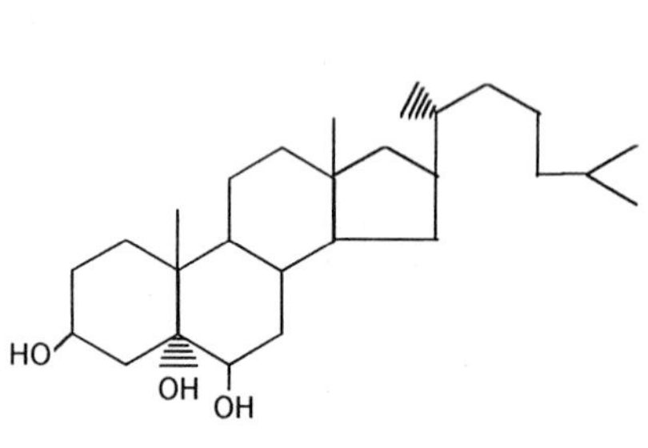

HO OH OH

CHOLESTANE-3β, 5α,6β-TRIOL (CHOLESTANETRIOL)

Figure 4.5. Three oxidation products associated with toxicity.

angiotoxic, mutagenic, and carcinogenic effects (66). Common CH oxidation products include cholesterol-5α,6α-epoxide, cholesterol-5β,6β-epoxide, and cholestane-3β,5α,6β triol (Fig. 4.5). CH oxides disturb endothelial integrity by perturbing vascular permeability, whereas purified CH has no effect. CH oxidation products have been detected in human serum lipoproteins and human atheromatous plaques (68). Substantial amounts of oxidized CH are detected in a variety of foods of animal origin exposed to oxidizing conditions (67). These highly atherogenic oxysterols may also be ingested and absorbed from processed foods or generated by free radical oxidation of lipoproteins. To date, however, it is unclear whether CH oxides merely serve as markers for oxidatively modified lipoproteins or if they contribute to the toxicity of oxidized lipoproteins. In addition, analysis of oxysterols is beset by such difficulties as artifact generation and decomposition of oxysterols during sample manipulation (67).

LDL oxidation has been implicated as a causal factor in development of human atherosclerosis (69). Unsaturated lipids in LDL are subject to peroxidative degradation, and the susceptibility of LDL to oxidation has been correlated with the degree of coronary atherosclerosis (70). Autoantibodies exist in human serum, and oxidized LDL is present in atherosclerotic plaque, indicating that oxidized LDL exists in vivo (71). Possible sources of oxidation include endothelial cells, smooth muscle cells, monocytes, macrophages, and other inflammatory cells. In the presence of the promoter copper, peroxidation of LDL results in formation of hydroxyalkenals and MDA, which modify Apo-B by reacting with its lysine amino groups. This modification of Apo-B could, in turn, impair its uptake by the LDL receptor. Oxidatively modified LDL may exert atherogenic effects via their cytotoxic and chemotactic properties and the promotion of LDL uptake by the scavenger receptors on macrophages leading to the formation of lipid-enriched foam cells.

Nutritional and biochemical studies suggest that diet can modulate the susceptibility of plasma LDL to oxidative degradation by altering the concentration of PUFA and antioxidants in the lipoprotein particle. The first targets of peroxidation in the oxidation of LDL are PUFA of PL on the LDL surface. In studies of LDL isolated from healthy humans and animals, a diet rich in C18:2n-6 increased the susceptibility of plasma LDL to copper-induced oxidation and to in vitro macrophage uptake, compared with a diet high in C18:1n-9 (72). C18:1n-9 and other MUFA do not contain the easily oxidized conjugated double bonds found in PUFA. Also, C18:1n-9 has a high affinity for transition metals, making them unavailable for LDL peroxidation. Depending on the dose used, subjects treated with n-3 PUFA showed either an increase or no change in LDL oxidation (73). Other studies have shown that increasing the amount of vitamin E in the LDL particle via oral supplementation decreased LDL susceptibility to in vitro oxidative damage (74). A difficulty with in vitro assays of plasma lipoprotein oxidation is that these assays are subject to influences by a variety of plasma substrates and conditions, making their relevance to physiologic situations uncertain. However, recent clinical evidence of protection against cardiovascular disease by vitamin E supplementation and the inhibition of atherosclerotic lesions in animals by antioxidants supports the oxidative hypothesis of atherosclerosis and the likely effectiveness of dietary antioxidants (75, 76). The lower incidence of cardiovascular disease in populations consuming more olive oil may be partly due to an inhibition of LDL oxidation by the antioxidant action of olive oil as well as by those antioxidants found in fruits and vegetables associated with the Mediterranean diet.

INTRACELLULAR MOVEMENT AND BIOSYNTHESIS OF LIPIDS

Fatty Acids

SAFA are biosynthesized in the extramitochondrial compartment by a group of enzymes known as FA synthetases. Compared with many animal species, human FA synthesis occurs predominantly in the liver and is much less active in adipose tissue. The FA biosynthetic pathway is almost identical in all organisms examined to date. The starting point is acetyl-CoA. Acetyl-CoA and oxaloacetate are cleaved from citrate, which is transported from the mitochondria. The first reaction in the FA biosynthetic pathway proper is the conversion of acetyl-CoA to malonyl-CoA by acetyl-CoA carboxylase, which is rate limiting for FA synthesis. Acetyl-CoA then combines sequentially with a series of malonyl-CoA molecules as follows:

$$\text{Acetyl-CoA} + 7\ \text{malonyl-CoA} + 14\ \text{NADPH} + 14\text{H}^+ \rightarrow \text{C16:0 (palmitic acid)} + 7\ CO_2 + 8\ \text{CoASH} + 14\ \text{NADP}^+ + 6\ H_2O$$

In mammals, complete de novo synthesis results in C16:0. Other FA can be formed from C16:0 by chain elongation via microsomal malonyl-CoA-dependent elongase. Mammals possess a series of desaturases and elongases to generate long-chain PUFA from the metabolism of C16:0, C18:0, C18:2n-6, and C18:3n-3 (Fig. 4.6). These reactions occur predominantly in the endoplasmic reticulum membranes. Desaturase reactions are catalyzed by membrane-bound desaturases with broad chain-length specificity, including Δ^9, Δ^6, Δ^5, and Δ^4 fatty acyl-CoA desaturases. These are involved in the desaturation of the C16:1n-7, C18:1n-9, C18:2n-6, and C18:3n-3 families. The Δ^4 desaturation required for formation of C22:6n-3 from C22:5n-3, and C22:5n-6 from C22:4n-6, respectively, involves three steps. These steps require an elongation reaction followed by membrane (microsomal) desaturation and shortening in peroxisomes. The desaturase enzymes are highly specific for the position of the double bond. The FA desaturase system involves three integral components: the desaturase, NADH-cytochrome b_5 reductase, and cytochrome b_5, which are constituents of microsomal membranes. Desaturases require electrons supplied mostly by

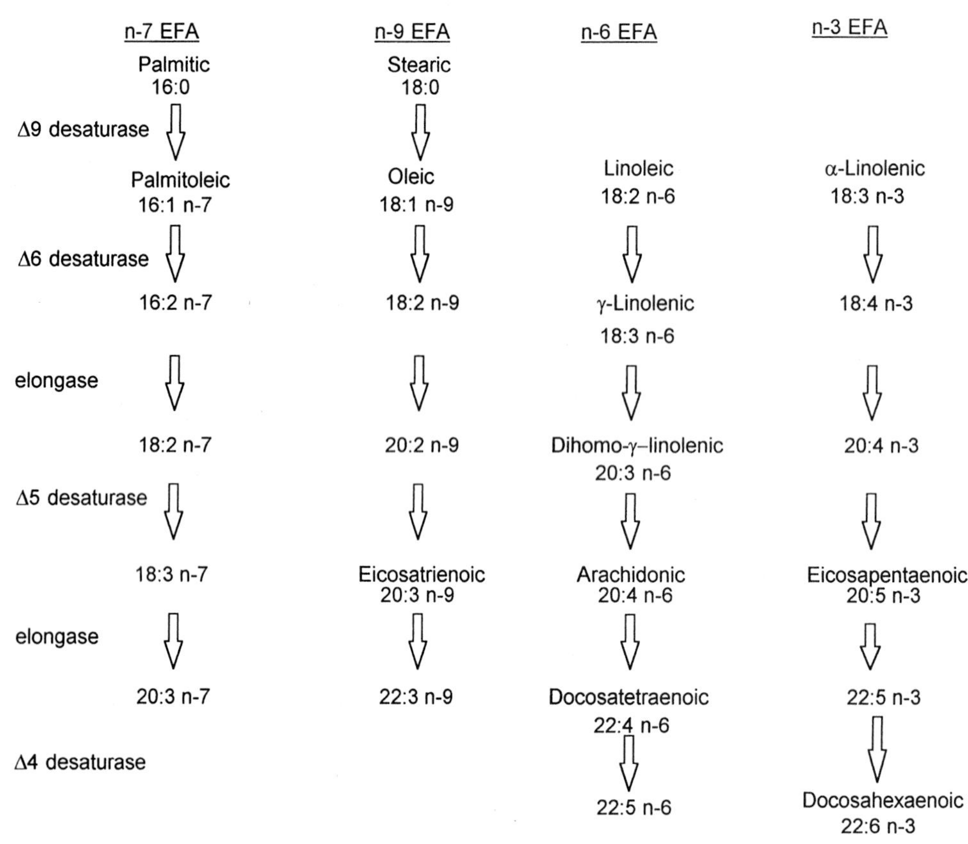

Figure 4.6. Effects of desaturase and elongase on essential fatty acids.

NADH-cytochrome b_5 reductase in addition to the activated substrate in the form of acyl-CoA.

Precursors for the n-7 and n-9 families of PUFA are MUFA that are synthesized via microsomal Δ^9 oxidative desaturation of C16:0 and C18:0 to form C16:1n-7 and C18:1n-9, respectively (Fig. 4.6). Additional double bonds can be introduced into existing MUFA C16:1n-7 and C18:1n-9 and also into C18:2n-6 via Δ^6 desaturase (Fig. 4.6). Until recently, humans and other mammals were thought incapable of synthesizing long-chain n-3 (C18: 3n-3) and n-6 (C18:2n-6) EFA. Recent studies, however, suggest that C18:2n-6 and C18:3n-3 can be synthesized in humans and other mammals via elongation of the dietary precursors C16:2n-6 and C16:3n-3, respectively (78). Edible green plants can contain up to 14% C16:2n-6 and C16:3n-3 (78). In a practical sense, a dietary supply of EFA is still important, since humans likely do not obtain enough 16-carbon precursors.

In mammals, FA from the n-3 and n-6 FA cannot be interconverted because of a lack of Δ^{12} or Δ^{15} desaturase enzymes, although such interconversions can take place in plants. Δ^6 Desaturase is the regulatory enzyme in these reactions and requires an n-9 *cis* double bond. Hence, *trans* FA, such as C18:1n-9 *trans,* formed either by rumen bacteria or by chemical hydrogenation of FA with *cis* double bonds, cannot be desaturated by this enzyme. The n-3, n-6, and n-9 FA families compete with each other, especially at the rate-limiting Δ^6 desaturase step. In general, desaturase enzymes display highest affinity for the most highly unsaturated substrate. The order of preference is α-linolenic family (n-3) > linoleic family (n-6) > oleic acid family (n-9) > palmitoleic acid family (n-7) > elaidic acid family (n-9, *trans*). Competition also exists among the families of PUFA for the elongase enzymes and for the acyl transferases involved in formation of PL.

Because of the competitive nature of FA desaturation and elongation, each class of EFA can interfere with the metabolism of the other. This competition has nutritional implications. An excess of n-6 EFA will reduce the metabolism of C18:3n-3, possibly leading to a deficit of its metabolites, including eicosapentanoic acid (C20:5n-3). This is a matter of concern in relation to infant formulas, which may contain an excess of C18:2n-6 with no balancing of n-3 EFA. Conversely, as long-chain n-3 EFA markedly decrease Δ^6 desaturation of C18:2n-6, excessive intake of fish oils could lead to impairment of C18:2n-6 metabolism and a deficit of n-6 EFA derivatives. High doses of fish oil in humans can cause a large reduction in the levels of C20:3n-6 in plasma PL, with a smaller effect on C20:4n-6 content (79). Although C18:1n-9 can inhibit Δ^6 desaturase activity, high dietary intakes are necessary. In the presence of C18:2n-6 or C18:3n-3, little desaturation of C18:1n-9 occurs. During EFAD, C20:3n-9 is synthesized from C18:1n-9 because of the nearly complete absence of competitive effects of n-3 and n-6 EFA. The presence of C20: 3n-9 in tissues instead of C20:4n-6, C20:5n-3, and C22:6n-3 indicates EFAD, which reverses on EFA feeding (80). In the catalytic hydrogenation of vegetable oils and fish oils for the production of some margarines and shortenings, a variety of geometric and positional isomers of unsaturated FA are formed in varying amounts. After absorption, these isomers may compete with the EFA and endogenously synthesized FA for desaturation and chain elongation.

In a phenomenon called *retroversion*, very long-chain C22 PUFA present in marine oils may be shortened by two carbons with concomitant saturation of a double bond. For example, C22:6n-3 is converted to C22:5n-3 and to C20:5n-3 (81). This peroxisomal pathway is also active in converting C22:5n-6 into C20:4n-6 (82). As a result of competition among various PUFA families for desaturases, elongases, and acyl transferases, and because of retroversion, a characteristic pattern of end products accumulates in tissue lipids for each family. Hence, the major PUFA product for the palmitoleate n-7 family is C20:3n-7; for the oleate n-9, C20:3n-9; and for linoleate, C20:4n-6 and some C20:3n-6. The most common products for the n-3 fatty acid family are C20:5n-3 and C22:6n-3.

The efficiency of the multistage synthesis of PUFA is unclear in the human. It has been suggested that activities of the various required desaturase and elongase enzymes differ with developmental stage or pathologic state. Regulation of desaturase activity could be of biologic importance, since the higher homologues of EFA are physiologically important regulatory metabolites.

Dietary factors and hormonal status can influence desaturase activities. Fat-free diets result in increased Δ^5 and Δ^6 desaturation, which may reflect a homeostatic response to maintain membrane fluidity (83). Protein and EFAD increase Δ^6 desaturase activity; conversely, low-protein diets and alcohol consumption decrease Δ^6 activity. Although glucose refeeding after a fast induces Δ^6 desaturase activity, a glucose-rich diet actually decreases enzymatic activity. Insulin stimulates Δ^6 desaturase activity; activity is depressed by glucagon, epinephrine, glucocorticoids, and thyroxines. Diabetes also depresses Δ^6, Δ^5, and Δ^4 desaturase activities, which are restored by insulin injection (84). Zinc may also play a role in the regulation of Δ^6 desaturase activity, as the dermal and growth effects of EFA and zinc deficiency are similar (85). This concept is supported by observations that administration of C18:3n-6, which bypasses the Δ^6 desaturase step, corrects most of the symptoms of zinc deficiency, whereas administration of C18:2n-6 has no effect. As the typical Western diet contains sufficient C20:4n-6, obtained from meat and dairy products, those with decreased desaturase activity could suffer from a deficiency of C20:3n-6, the precursor of the PG "1" series. Some authors have suggested that certain individuals may have increased need for EFA derivatives because of a disease condition, aging, or a metabolic block in desaturase activity. Evening primrose, borage, and black current seed oils contain C18:3n-6 that bypasses the step requiring Δ^6 desaturase and have been used therapeutically for a variety of clinical conditions, including psoriasis (86).

Cholesterol

Current evidence indicates that three distinct pathways modulate the intracellular transmission of CH. Separate translocational systems exist for endogenously synthesized and LDL-derived exogenous CH. A third transport system also exists for CH destined for steroid synthesis.

CH biosynthesis represents a major vector in the total body CH supply in humans, with up to about 75% being synthesized during consumption of the typical North American diet. Animal studies demonstrate that even though all organs incorporate acetate into sterol, the liver is the primary biosynthetic organ (87). Conversely, in humans, it has been estimated that the net contribution of liver biosynthesis does not exceed 10% of total CH biosynthesis. The role of extrahepatic organs in human cholesterogenesis remains undefined.

Acetate can be converted into mevalonic acid by a sequence of reactions starting with acetate + CoA + ATP → 1A acetyl-CoA + PP + AMP. However, most of the acetyl-CoA used for sterol synthesis is not derived from this reaction but rather is generated within the mitochondria by β-oxidation of FA or oxidative decarboxylation of pyruvate. Pyruvate is converted into citrate, which diffuses into the cytosol and is hydrolyzed to acetyl-CoA and oxaloacetate by citrate-ATP lyase:

$$\text{Citrate} + \text{ATP} + \text{CoA} \rightarrow \text{1A acetyl-CoA} + \text{oxaloacetate} + \text{ADP} + H_2O$$

Citrate participating in this reaction acts as a carrier to transport acetyl carbon across the mitochondrial membranes, which are impermeable to acetyl-CoA. Subsequently, in the cytosol, acetyl-CoA is converted into mevalonate:

$$2\ \text{acetyl-CoA} \rightarrow \text{acetoacetyl-CoA} + \text{CoA}$$
$$\text{Acetoacetyl-CoA} + \text{acetyl-CoA} + H_2 \rightarrow \text{HMG-CoA} + \text{CoA}$$
$$\text{HMG-CoA} + 2\ \text{NADPH} + 2\ H^+ \xrightarrow{\textit{HMG-CoA reductase}} \text{mevalonate} + 2\ \text{NADP}^+ + \text{CoA}$$

Mevalonic acid is phosphorylated, isomerized, and converted to geranyl- and farnesyl-pyrophosphate, which in turn form squalene. Squalene is then oxidized and cyclized to a steroid ring, lanosterol. In the last steps, lanosterol is converted into CH by the loss of three methyl groups, saturation of the side chain, and a shift of the double bond from Δ^8 to Δ^5. During the later stages of CH biosynthesis, intermediates are bound to a sterol carrier protein.

CH biosynthesis in humans is sensitive to a number of dietary factors. Adding CH to the diet at physiologic levels results in modest increases in circulating CH levels, with a mild reciprocal inhibition of synthesis (28, 50). Dietary fat selection exhibits a more pronounced influence on human cholesterogenesis, as consumption of polyunsaturated fats is associated with higher biosynthesis than other plant or animal fats. Differences in FA composition and levels of plant sterol levels may both be contributing factors (35). Higher meal frequency reduces biosynthesis rates in humans, which may explain the lower circulating CH synthesis rates seen in individuals consuming more numerous smaller meals (88). Insulin, which is associated with hepatic CH synthesis in animals, may be released in greater amounts when less frequent but larger meals are consumed. Circadian periodicity, with a maximum at night, is tied to the timing of meal consumption. Of dietary factors capable of modifying CH synthesis, energy restriction exhibits the greatest effect. Humans fasted for 24 hours exhibit complete cessation of CH biosynthesis (18). How synthesis responds to more minor energy imbalance has not been examined.

There is an emerging view that CH synthesis acts both passively and actively in relation to circulatory CH levels, depending on dietary perturbation. Passively, the liver responds to high CH levels through LDL receptor–mediated suppression of synthesis (42). The modest suppression in the face of increasing dietary and circulating levels reflects the limited hepatic contribution to total body production of CH (28). Substitution of PUFA for other fats results in a decreased ratio of hepatic intracellular free CH to esterified CH, which in turn upregulates both LDL receptor number and cholesterogenesis. In both of these ways, CH synthesis responds passively to external stimuli. In contrast, nonhepatic synthesis is less sensitive to dietary CH level and fat type, while together with hepatic synthesis, nonhepatic synthesis is more responsive to synthesis pathway substrate availability (89). In this manner, several dietary factors actively modify CH synthesis and levels. Such differential sensitivity may explain the more pronounced decrement in CH synthesis and levels occurring after energy deficit in humans.

CH serves as a required precursor for other important steroid compounds, including sex hormones, adrenocorticoid hormones, and vitamin D. Steroidal sex hormones, including estrogen, androgen, and progesterone, involve removal of the CH side chain at C-17 and rearrangement of the double bonds in the steroid nucleus. Corticosteroid hormone production involves similar rearrangements of the CH molecule. 7-Dehydrocholesterol is the precursor of cholecalciferol (vitamin D) formed at the skin surface through the action of ultraviolet irradiation. Steroid hormone metabolites are excreted principally through the urine. It is estimated that humans convert about 50 mg/day of CH to steroid hormones.

Vertebrates cannot convert plant sterols to CH. However, insects and prawns can transform phytosterols into steroid hormones or bile acids through a CH intermediate.

FUNCTIONS OF ESSENTIAL FATTY ACIDS

After ingestion, EFA (C18:2n-6 and C18:3n-3) are distributed between adipose TG, other tissue stores, and tissue structural lipids. A proportion of C18:2n-6 and C18:3n-3 provides energy, and these PUFA are oxidized more rapidly than are SAFA or MUFA. In contrast, long-chain PUFA derived from EFA (i.e., C20:3n-6, C20:4n-6, C20:5n-3, and C22:6n-3) are less readily oxidized. These acids, when present preformed in the diet, are incorporated into structural lipids about 20 times more efficiently than after synthesis from dietary C18:2n-6 and C18:3n-3. The liver is the site of most of the PUFA metabolism that transforms dietary 18-carbon EFA into long-chain PUFA with 20 or 22 carbons. Long-chain PUFA are transported to extrahepatic tissues for incorporation into cell lipids, even though there is differential uptake and acylation of PUFA among different tissues. The final tissue composition of long-chain PUFA is the result of the above complex processes along with the influence of dietary factors. The major elements in the diet that determine the final distribution of long-chain PUFA in cell PL include the relative proportions of n-3, n-6, and n-9 FA families, and the preformed long-chain PUFA versus their shorter-chain precursors (90).

Membrane structural PL contain high concentrations of PUFA and the 20- and 22-carbon PUFA that predominate from the two families of EFA. C20:4n-6 is the most important and abundant long-chain PUFA found in membrane PL and is the primary precursor of eicosanoids. The concentration of free C20:4n-6 is strictly regulated via phospholipases and acyltransferases. Most nonacylated C20:4n-6 is bound to cytosolic protein. In terms of EFA from the n-3 PUFA series, C20:5n-3 and C22:6n-3 are most prevalent in membrane PL. The long-chain PUFA derived from EFA are incorporated primarily in the 2-acyl position in bilayer PL of mammalian plasma, mitochondrial, and nuclear membranes. The 20-carbon FA, when released from their PL, can be transformed into intracellular metabolites (inositol triphosphate [IP_3] and diacylglycerol [DAG]) and extracellular metabolites (platelet-activating factor [PAF] and eicosanoids), which participate in many important cell-signaling responses. The relative proportions in tissue PL of C20:4n-6 and other long-chain PUFA (C18:3n-6, C20:4n-6, and C20:5n-3) are important, as these PUFA can compete for or inhibit enzymes involved in generation of intracellular and extracellular biologically active products. Also, dietary C18:1n-9, C18:2n-6, C18:2n-6 *trans*, C18:3n-6, C18:3n-3, and long-chain n-3 PUFA C20:5n-3 and C22:6n-3 can compete with C20:4n-6 for the acyltransferases for esterification into PL pools and thereby inhibit C20:4n-6-mediated membrane functions.

Membrane Functions and Integrity

As fragile membranes in erythrocytes and mitochondria are typical of EFAD, an early function attributed to EFA was their role as integral components of PL required for plasma and intracellular membrane integrity. EFAD results in a progressive decrease in C20:4n-6 in membrane PL, with a concomitant increase in C18:1n-9 and its product, C20:3n-9. The fluidity and other physical properties of membrane PL are largely determined by the chain length and degree of unsaturation of their component FA. These physical properties, in turn, affect the ability of PL to perform structural functions, such as the maintenance of normal activities of membrane-bound enzymes. Dietary SAFA, MUFA, and PUFA, major determinants of the composition of stored and structural lipids, alter the activity and affinity of receptors, membrane permeability, and transport properties (91).

The heterogeneity and selectivity of PUFA with respect to their tissue membrane distribution among different organs may be related to their structural and functional roles (91). For example, long-chain derivatives of n-3 PUFA are concentrated in biologic structures involved in fast movement, such as that required in transport mechanisms in the brain and its synaptic junction and in the retina (92). Approximately 50% of the PL in the disk membrane of the retinal rod outer segment in which rhodopsin resides contains C22:6n-3 (93). The C22:6n-3 is concentrated in the major PL classes, i.e., PC, PE, and phosphotidylserine (PS) in the disk membrane, whereas C20:4n-6 is found in the minor PL components, such as phosphatidylinositol (PI). This observation has led to speculation that C22:6n-3 plays a structural role in these membranes while C20:4n-6 may play a more functional role (94).

In addition to their structural role and their movement across membranes, structural lipids can also modulate cell function by acting as either intracellular mediators of signal transduction or modulators of cell-cell interactions. These actions are initiated by phospholipases. Phospholipase A_2 cleaves FA, usually PUFA, present at the 2 position of PL. PUFA released under action of phospholipase A_2 produce metabolites released extracellularly to act on other cells. These metabolites include PAF (a choline-containing PL with an acetate residue in the 2-position) and eicosanoids. Phospholipase C acts on phosphoinositides to break the bond between glycerol and phosphoric acid, releasing intracellularly diacylglycerols (DAG) and inositol phosphates (IP), which are involved in signal transduction. After receptor stimulation, DAG and IP act intracellularly as second messengers to activate protein kinase C and release intracellular stores of calcium, respectively (5). Activated protein kinase C mediates transduction of a wide variety of extracellular stimuli, such as hormones and growth factors, leading to regulation of such cellular processes as cell proliferation and differentiation. PL can act as a cofactor for some isoforms of protein kinase C by enhancing binding to DAG (95). In addition, unesterified PUFA can activate protein kinase C with differing potencies (96). As dietary PUFA can greatly modulate PUFA composition of structural lipids, generation of intra- and extracellular products can be greatly affected by dietary lipids. For example, thrombin-stimulated platelets from rabbits fed fish oil form less IP than platelets from those fed either corn or olive oil (97).

BIOSYNTHESIS AND FUNCTION OF EICOSANOIDS

Some of the most potent effects of PUFA are related to their enzymatic conversion into a series of oxygenated metabolites called *eicosanoids,* so-named because their precursors are PUFA with chain lengths of 20 carbon units. Eicosanoids include PG, thromboxane (TXA), leukotrienes (LT), hydroxy fatty acids, and lipoxins. PG and TXA are generated via cyclooxygenase (CO) enzymes, whereas LT, hydroxy acids, and lipoxins are produced from lipoxygenase (LO) metabolism. Under stimulation, rapid and transient synthesis of active eicosanoids activates specific receptors locally in the tissues in which they are formed. Eicosanoids modulate cardiovascular, pulmonary, immune, reproductive, and secretory functions in many cells. They are rapidly converted to their inactive forms by selective catabolic enzymes.

Humans depend on the dietary presence of the n-3 and n-6 structural families of PUFA for adequate biosynthesis of eicosanoids. There are three direct precursor FA from which eicosanoids are formed by the action of membrane-bound CO or specific LO enzyme systems: C20:3n-6, C20:4n-6, and C20:5n-3. A series of prostanoids and LT with different biologic properties are generated from each of these FA (Fig. 4.7). The first irreversible, committed step in the synthesis of PG and LT is a hydroperoxide-activated FA oxygenase action exerted by either prostaglandin H synthase (PGHS) or LO enzymes on the nonesterified precursor PUFA (Fig. 4.8).

Stimulation of normal cells via specific physiologic or pathologic stimuli, such as thrombin, adenosine diphosphate (ADP), or collagen, initiates a calcium-mediated cas-

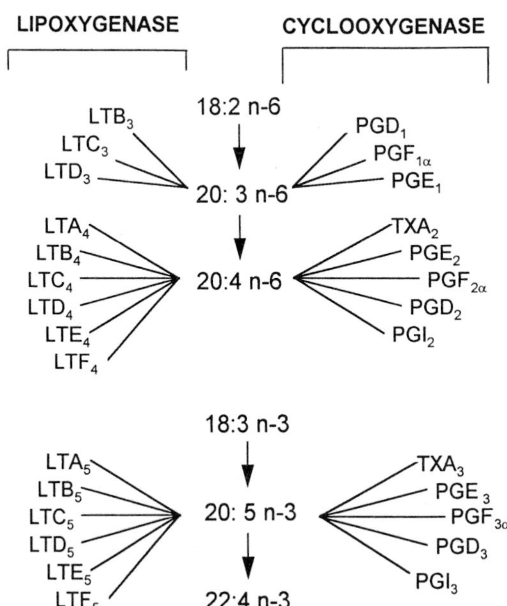

Figure 4.7. Formation of PG, TXA, and LT from DHGA (C20:3n-6), arachidonic acid (C20:4n-6), and EPA (C20:5n-3) via cyclooxygenase and lipoxygenase pathways. LT, leukotriene; PG, prostaglandin; TXA, thromboxane.

cade. This cascade involves phospholipase A_2 activation, which releases PUFA on position 2 of cell membrane. The greatest proportion of PUFA available to phospholipase A_2 action contains C20:4n-6. Hydrolytic release from PL esters appears to occur indiscriminantly with n-3 and n-6 types of PUFA and to involve all major classes of PL, such as PC, phosphatidyl ethanolamine (PE), and phosphatidyl inositol (PI). These FA serve as direct precursors for generation of eicosanoid products via CO and LO enzymatic action (Fig. 4.8). Enzymatic biotransformation of the PUFA precursors to PG is catalyzed via two PG synthase isozymes designated PGH synthase-1 (PGHS-1) and PGH synthase-2 (PGHS-2) (98). PGHS-1 is located in the ER and PGHS-2 is located in the nuclear envelope. Both forms are bifunctional enzymes that catalyze the oxygenation of C20:4n-6 to PGG_2 via CO reaction and the reduction of PGG_2 to form a transient hydroxyendoperoxide (PGH_2) via the peroxidase reaction (Fig. 4.8). The PGH_2 intermediate is rapidly converted to PGI_2 by vascular endothelial cells, to TXA_2 by an isomerase in platelets, or to other prostanoids, depending on the tissues involved. The PGHS-2 generates prostanoids associated with mitogenesis and inflammation and is inhibited by glucocorticoids. On the other hand, PGHS-1 is expressed only after cell activation and is inhibited by nonsteroidal antiinflammatory drugs such as aspirin but not by glucocorticoids.

C20:4n-6 can be oxygenated via the 5-, 12-, and 15-LO pathways (Fig. 4.7). From C20:4n-6, the 5-LO pathway generates mainly LTB_4, LTC_4, and LTD_4, which are implicated as important mediators in a variety of proliferative and synthetic immune responses. LTB_4 in particular has been indicated a key proinflammatory mediator in inflammatory and proliferative disorders (98). From C20:4n-6, the 12-LO pathway generates 12-L-hydroxyeicosatetranoic acid (12-HETE) and 12-hydroperoxyeicosatetranoic acid (12-HPETE). A proinflammatory response can be generated by 12-HETE in a variety of cell types. Products generated from C20:4n-6 metabolism by the 15-LO reaction include 15-hydroxyeicosatetranoic acid (15-HETE), which has antiinflammatory action and may inhibit 5- and 12-LO activities (99).

Since the major eicosanoids are synthesized from C20:4n-6, the availability of C20:4n-6 in PL pools of tissue may be a primary factor in regulating the quantities of eicosanoids synthesized by tissues in vivo. Also, the intensity of the n-6 eicosanoid signal from the released PUFA will be greater as C20:4n-6 becomes a greater proportion of the PUFA. The levels of C20:4n-6 in tissue PL pools are affected by the elongation and desaturation of dietary C18:2n-6 and by intake of C20:4n-6 (170–220 mg/day in the Western diet) (100). Although dietary concentrations of C18:2n-6 up to 2 to 3% of calories increase tissue C20:4n-6 concentrations, intake of C18:2n-6 above 3% of calories is poorly correlated with tissue C20:4n-6 content (101). Since C18:2n-6 constitutes approximately 6 to 8% of the North American diet, moderate dietary changes in C18:2n-6 would not be expected to modulate tissue C20:4n-6 levels. Intakes of C18:2n-6 above 12%, however, may actually decrease tissue C20:4n-6 because of inhibition of Δ_6 desaturase. In contrast, dietary C20:4n-6 is much more effective in enriching C20:4n-6 in tissue PL (101) and, compared with C18:2n-6, relatively low dietary levels

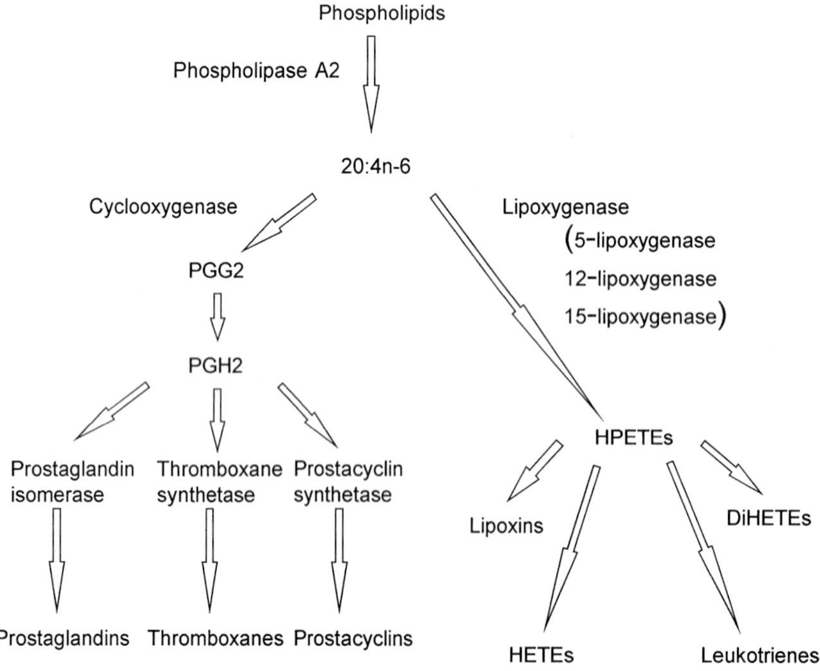

Figure 4.8. Major pathways of synthesis of eicosanoids from arachidonic acid. PG, prostaglandin; HPETE, hydroperoxyeicosatrienoic acid; HETE, hydroxy fatty acid; diHETE, dihydroxyeicosatetranoic acid. (From Innis SM. Essential dietary lipids. In: Ziegler EE, Filer LJ, eds. Present knowledge in nutrition. 7th ed. Washington, DC: ILSI Press, 1996;58–66, with permission.)

of C20:4n-6 may be physiologically significant in enhancing eicosanoid metabolism (100).

Feeding diets high in n-3 FA results in substitution of C20:4n-6 by n-3 PUFA in membrane PL. This can suppress the response of C20:4n-6-derived eicosanoids by decreasing availability of the C20:4n-6 precursor and by competitive inhibition of C20:5n-3 for eicosanoid biosynthesis (102). Although less pronounced than the effect observed with C20:5n-3 and C22:6n-3 dietary supplementation, C18:3n-3-enriched diets suppress PGE_2 production by peripheral blood mononuclear cells in monkeys (102). C18:3n-3 could competitively inhibit desaturation and elongation of C18:2n-6 for conversion into C20:4n-6. The eicosanoids derived from n-3 are homologues of those derived from C20:4n-6 with which they compete (Fig. 4.9), and they are associated with less active responses than n-6 eicosanoids when bound to the specific receptors.

Diets rich in competing and moderating FA (n-3 PUFA, C18:3n-6) may produce changes in the production of eicosanoids which are more favorable with respect to inflammatory reactions. For instance, the PGE_3 formed from C20:5n-3 has less inflammatory effect than PGE_2 derived from C20:4n-6. The LTB_5 derived from C20:5n-3 is substantially less active in proinflammatory functions than the LTB_4 formed from C20:4n-6, including the aggregation and chemotaxis of neutrophils. Two 15-LO products, 15-HEPE and 17-hydroxydocosahexanoic acid (17-HoDHE), are derived from C20:5n-3 and C22:6n-3, respectively (99). Both metabolites are potent inhibitors of LTB_4 formation.

Overproduction of C20:4n-6-derived eicosanoids has been implicated in many inflammatory and autoimmune disorders such as thrombosis, immune-inflammatory disease (e.g., arthritis, lupus nephritis), cancer, and psoriatic

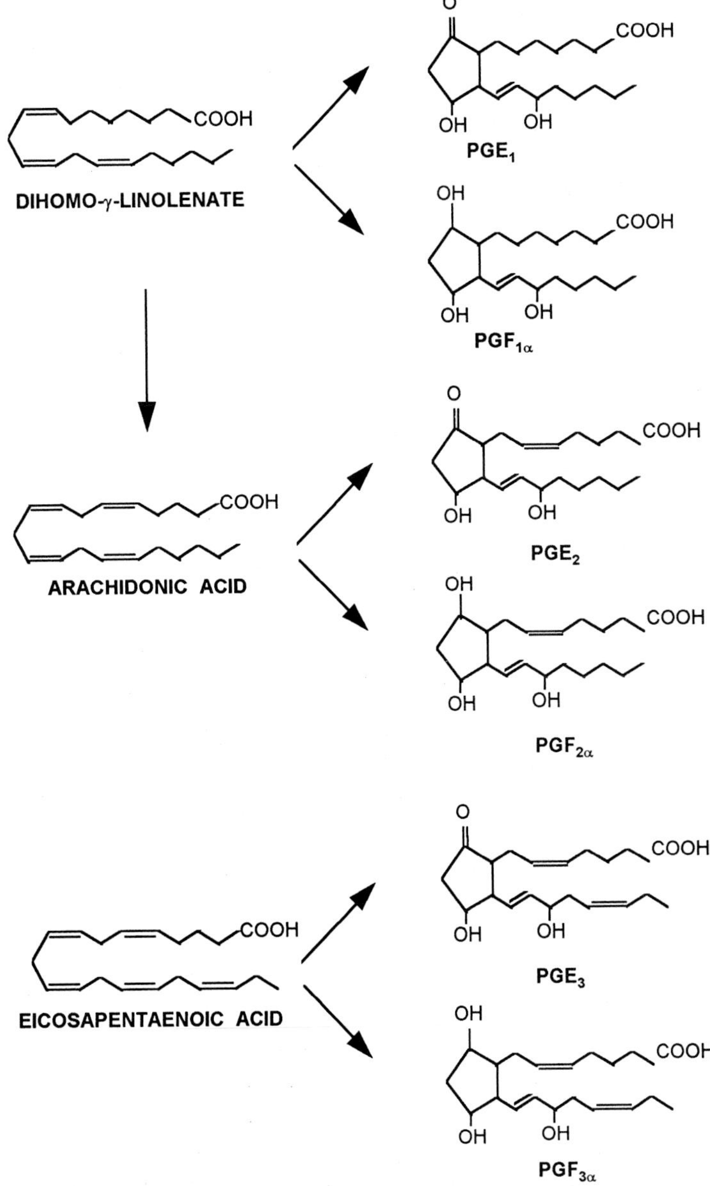

Figure 4.9. Prostaglandin formation.

skin lesions, among others. Because the typical American appears to maintain n-6 PUFA in PL near the maximal capacity, some have suggested that the n-6-rich diet in the United States may contribute to the incidence and severity of eicosanoid-mediated diseases such as thrombosis and arthritis (103). Because platelet aggregation and activation are indicated to play a critical role in progression toward vascular occlusion and myocardial infarction, the counterbalancing roles of TXA_2 and PGI_2 in cardiovascular functions have been emphasized. C20:4n-6 is required for platelet function as a precursor of the proaggregatory TXA_2. Biosynthesis of TXA_2 is the rate-limiting step in the aggregation of platelets, a key event in thrombosis. The effects of TXA_2 are counteracted by PGI_2, a potent antiaggregatory agent that prevents adherence of platelets to blood vessel walls. Due to displacement of C20:4n-6 from membrane PL by C18:2n-6, C18:3n-6, and C20:3n-6, stepwise increases in dietary C18:2n-6 from 3 to 40% of calories actually decreased platelet aggregation, indicating inhibition of eicosanoid synthesis by these n-6 PUFA. However, the antithrombotic influence of C18:2n-6 is substantially less than that observed after high intake of n-3 PUFA-rich fish oils (104). This has been related to the observations that PGI_3 generated from C20:5n-3 has antiaggregatory potency. Conversely, TXA_3 derived from C20:5n-3 has a very weak proaggregatory effect while TXA_2 synthesis is reduced (105). Chronic ingestion of aspirin (106) and n-3 PUFA reduces the intensity of TXA_2 biosynthesis, which could decrease rates of cardiovascular mortality. However, epidemiologic studies on the effects of dietary n-3 FA on cardiovascular disease have been inconsistent. A recent prospective study demonstrated no protective effect of fish consumption on cardiovascular disease mortality and morbidity (107), whereas another showed protective effects in elderly persons who ate only small amounts of fish (108). Results of several studies suggest that C18:3n-6 and n-3 EFA are involved in the regulation of cell-mediated immunity and that administration of these FA may be beneficial in suppressing pathologic immune responses. For example, subjects with rheumatoid arthritis fed fish oils high in n-3 PUFA have consistently obtained symptomatic benefit in doubly blinded, randomized, controlled trials (109). Although it appears that inhibition of the proinflammatory eicosanoids LTB_4 and PGE_2 can account for many of the protective effects of n-3 PUFA, decreased production of the cytokines interleukin-1β and tumor necrosis factor are also likely involved (110).

ESSENTIAL FATTY ACID REQUIREMENTS

n-6 Fatty Acid Requirements

In studies on EFA, C18:2n-6 and C20:4n-6 have been emphasized because mammals have an absolute requirement for the n-6 family of FA. EFA are required for stimulation of growth, maintenance of skin and hair growth, regulation of CH metabolism, lipotropic activity, and maintenance of reproductive performance, among other physiologic effects. On a molecular level, EFA are components of specific lipids and maintain the integrity and optimal levels of unsaturation of tissue membranes. Because EFA are necessary for normal function of all tissues, the list of symptoms of EFAD is long (111). Detailed studies on the symptoms of EFAD have been done in young rats, in which EFAD was found to be avoided by providing 1 to 2% of calories as C18:2n-6 (112). In these rat studies, classic signs of EFAD included reduced growth rates, scaly dermatitis with increased loss of water by a change of skin permeability, male and female infertility, and depressed inflammatory responses. Also observed during EFAD are kidney abnormalities, abnormal liver mitochondria, decreased capillary resistance, increased fragility of erythrocytes, and reduced contraction of myocardial tissue (113).

C18:2n-6 is specifically required in the skin to maintain the integrity of the epidermal water barrier. In this regard, C18:2n-6 seems to be required as an integral component of acylglucoceramides. Animals with EFAD lose considerable amounts of water through the skin, which limits growth rates. Repletion of C18:2n-6 at 1% of calories corrects excessive transepidermal water loss, and growth is restored (114). Although transdermal water loss during EFAD symptoms may reflect the role of C18:2n-6 as a key component of skin acylglucoceramides, the major metabolic effects of C18:2n-6 derive from its further metabolism to C20:4n-6 and thence to eicosanoids. In EFAD, platelet adherence and aggregation are impaired because of limited thromboxane synthesis secondary to limiting supplies of C20:4n-6 and possible inhibition by accumulated eicosatrienoic acid C20:3n-9. The action of eicosanoids in modulating the release of hypothalamic and pituitary hormones has been indicated to be a major factor in the role of the n-3 and n-6 EFA in supporting growth and development (103). The skin is subject to rapid infection, and surgical wounds heal very slowly in humans who have EFAD. This probably reflects the lack of C20:4n-6, which is required for eicosanoid-mediated protective inflammatory and immune cell functions and for tissue proliferation (103). Monocyte and macrophage function is defective in EFAD because eicosanoid production is impaired. The scaliness of the skin of an EFA-deficient patient has been ascribed to insufficient synthesis of PG, and the efficacy of various EFA of the n-6 type against the scaly dermatitis has been demonstrated at low dose levels.

Columbinic acid (C18:3n-6, 9, 13 *cis, cis, trans*), found in the seed oil of the columbine, *Aquilegia vulgaris,* and dihomocolumbinic acid (C20:3n-6, 9, 13 *cis, cis, trans*) have been used to differentiate the roles of EFA as structural components in biomembranes versus their roles as eicosanoid precursors (115). Neither columbinic acid nor dihomocolumbinic acid can be converted to PG; however, columbinic acid can be incorporated into membrane PL in contrast to dihomocolumbinic acid. As EFAD results in decreased tissue concentrations of C20:4n-6, EFAD symptoms are worsened further by dietary addition of dihomocolumbinic acid. Columbinic acid given to EFA-deficient rats, either orally or by topical skin application, efficiently restores their growth rate and normal skin function (114). When EFA-deficient rats treated with columbinic acid became pregnant, however, they died of inadequate labor during parturition, since uterine labor depends on normal PG biosynthesis (116).

One of the most often used and sensitive diagnostic indicators of EFAD in all species tested, including humans, is the triene (n-9):tetraene (n-6) ratio (111); C20:3n-9 (triene) is the major product derived from nonessential FAs. C20:4n-6 with four double bonds (tetraene) is the major metabolite of C18:2n-6. The triene:tetraene ratio in plasma remains below 0.4 when dietary EFA are adequate and increases to above 0.4 with EFAD. Dietary intake of adequate amounts of EFA decreases formation of triene as a consequence of competitive inhibition among families of PUFA for desaturases and acyl transferases. If EFA are not available, the biosynthesis of PUFA with three double bonds derived from C18:1n-9 and C16:n-7 continues, leading to the accumulation of n-9 FA, specifically C20:3n-9, resulting in turn in an increased plasma triene:tetraene ratio. Feeding diets with 0.1 to 0.5% of C18:2n-6 normalizes an abnormally high triene/tetraene ratio in a few days (117). The optimum dietary C18:2n-6 intake required for a ratio less than 0.4 and prevention of EFAD symptoms is 1 to 2% of total calories. The triene:tetraene ratio, however, does not resolve if the EFAD is caused by a lack of either n-3 or n-6 EFA, since adequate intake of either C18:2n-6 or C18:3n-3 prevents synthesis of C20:3n-9 (118).

The exact requirement for EFA in humans is not clearly defined but is apparently very low. The first study of EFAD, in human adults maintained for 6 months on a diet extremely low in fat, did not produce dramatic symptoms (119). It has been suggested that because adults contain approximately a kilogram of C18:2n-6 in body stores, depletion of EFA stores to produce deficiency symptoms would require maintaining an EFAD diet for more than 6 months. Most diets contain enough EFA or their metabolic products to meet daily EFA requirements; thus EFAD is relatively rare in humans. When it does occur in humans, some of the symptoms characteristic in animals, such as abnormal skin conditions, increased susceptibility to infection, and an increase in triene:tetraene ratio, are observed.

An important role for C20:4n-6 in optimal fetal development has been suggested because C20:4n-6 exerts growth-promoting effects (120). Crawford et al. (121) demonstrated that mothers of low-birth-weight infants had lower intakes of C18:2n-6 than mothers of normal-birth-weight infants. However, lower C20:4n-6 concentrations in plasma and in plasma PC have been associated with depressed intrauterine and extrauterine growth, despite adequate dietary C18:2n-6 levels (122). In a doubly blinded, randomized, controlled trial, depressed plasma PC C20:4n-6 concentrations induced by supplementation of formulas with C20:5n-3-rich marine oils were associated with slower growth rates in preterm infants (123). Supplementation of formula with a low C20:5n-3-concentration marine oil caused relatively minor decreases in plasma PC C20:4n-6 concentration and in weight-to-length ratio in preterm infants (124).

Long-chain EFA of 20- and 22-carbon chain length are incorporated about 10 times more efficiently into the developing brain than are the parent EFA. However, whether term or preterm infants have sufficient enzymatic activity to synthesize their own long-chain PUFA from EFA to meet their requirement for brain growth and development is controversial. Despite knowledge that the developing and mature brain can desaturate and elongate C18:2n-6 and C18:3n-3 to their respective long-chain PUFA products and that brain and retina can incorporate C20:4n-6 and C22:6n-3 from plasma, the quantitative importance of these two pathways is uncertain. Lower levels of C20:4n-6 in the red blood cell PL of formula-fed infants than in PL from breast milk–fed infants has led to debate about whether C20:4n-6 is essential for optimal central nervous system development in infants (125). The lower erythrocyte C20:4n-6 levels of formula-fed babies (vs. breast-fed babies) can be normalized by inclusion of C20:4n-6 in formula. Stable isotope studies have indicated in vivo C20:4n-6 synthesis in term infants, but the rate of this synthesis is low and only about 6% of total plasma C20:4n-6 is renewed in this manner (126). However, postmortem studies of brain FA composition showed that brain C20:4n-6 is maintained in formula-fed infants (127).

The concept has emerged that an optimal ratio of n-3 and n-6 FA is required in the diet because n-3 and n-6 families compete for eicosanoid production. Various authorities have recommended that at least 3% of daily calories be provided as linoleate, to prevent EFAD; however, equal amounts of C18:2n-6 and various SAFA have been recommended to reduce serum CH for the prevention of atherosclerosis (117). Advocacy for increased intake of vegetable oils rich in C18:2n-6 has resulted in C18:2n-6 consumption of approximately 6 to 7% of calories in the United States, leading to a ratio of n-6:n-3 PUFA consumption above 10 (117). Although this amount of C18:2n-6 may be beneficial for reduction of elevated plasma CH in those on a high-fat diet, it has been argued that an n-6:n-3 PUFA ratio exceeding 10 is imbalanced compared with n-6:n-3 ratios of 2 to 4 found in food lipids of hunter/gatherer societies (103, 117). There is concern that a high intake of C18:2n-6 relative to n-3 PUFA may lead to excessive or imbalanced eicosanoid production conducive to various pathophysiologies. The optimal n-6:n-3 ratio in the diet is not yet clear and may vary with developmental stage, the presence of long-chain EFA, and other factors. Some authorities have suggested that the n-6:n-3 EFA ratio should be in the range of 4:1 to 10:1 (128); others believe optimal n-6:n-3 ratios to be 4:1 or lower (129, 130).

n-3 Fatty Acid Requirements

Requirements for n-3 FA have been less definitive because it has been difficult to demonstrate their essentiality in animal studies; n-3 FA levels in mammalian tissues are generally much lower than n-6 FA levels. Biochemical studies have indicated differences in the metabolism and tissue distribution of the two series of EFA. C20:4n-6 and C20:3n-6 tend to predominate in liver and platelets, while the main biologic activity of long-chain n-3 EFA appears to reside in retina, testes, and the central nervous system. C18:3n-3 is similar to C18:2n-6 with regard to growth rate, capillary resistance, erythrocyte fragility, and mitochondrial function. Dietary C18:3n-3 and C20:5n-3 are inferior to C18:2n-6 and the other n-6 PUFA in resolving skin lesions and preventing transepidermal water loss. Because of the inability of C18:3n-3 to normalize all physiologic functions during EFAD and because EFA activities attributed to C18:3n-3 were also expressed equally or more potently by C18:2n-6, n-3 FA were until recently designated nonessential or partially essential.

In the past 15 years, studies have suggested that n-3 FA may be essential in development of neural tissue and visual function, beyond the requirement for n-6 FA, for which they can partially substitute. Across mammalian species, levels of C22:6 n-3 in brain and retinal PL are extremely stable despite wide variations in diet (131). The strong affinity of brain lipids for C22:6n-3 suggest a requirement for n-3 EFA, but this requirement is difficult to study because n-3 EFAD develops only under extreme dietary conditions (125, 131). In particular, C22:6n-3 is selectively retained by the brain, and depletion of C22:6n-3 is difficult after weaning. Multigenerational studies in rats have been needed to produce drastic reductions in brain C22:6n-3 levels. For example, feeding rats fat-free diets from weaning reduced retinal C22:6n-3 concentrations in adults by only 10 to 20%. In the first generation, feeding diets containing 2.5% C18:2n-6 and free of n-3 PUFA decreased C22:6n-3 concentrations by 60% and in the second generation by more than 87% (132).

An essential role for C22:6n-3 in brain and retinal PL was described by Neuringer and Connor, who demonstrated C18:3n-3 deficiency in rhesus monkeys fed during gestation diets with safflower oil (n-6:n-3 ratio of 255:1) as the sole source of fat (133). Their offspring reared on the same diet developed abnormal electroretinograms compared with those of the control group of offspring fed soybean oil (n-6:n-3 ratio of 7). Decreased concentrations of C18:3n-3 and long-chain n-3 PUFA in plasma PL were observed in offspring who showed loss of visual activity. Learning capacity, as tested in a spatial-reversal learning task, was not affected, possibly because of the observed compensatory increase of n-6 PUFA, particularly C22:5n-6, in PL. Retinal n-3 PUFA deficiency was reversed at the ages of 10 and 24 months by feeding a fish oil diet rich in C20:5n-3 and C22:6n-3 (133). Although such extremely high n-6:n-3 ratios rarely occur in human nutrition because of the wide availability of n-3 PUFA in foods, these ratios have been induced by total parenteral nutrition. A 6-year-old child developed peripheral neuropathy and periods of blurred vision after receiving total parenteral nutrition whose sole source of lipid was a safflower oil emulsion (1). After 5 months, she experienced episodes of numbness, weakness, inability to walk, leg pain, and blurred vision. Very low serum concentrations of C18:3n-3 and other n-3 PUFA were detected. Replacement of the lipid source by a soybean oil emulsion containing C18:3n-3 caused all symptoms of deficiency to disappear, and serum concentrations of n-3 PUFA returned to normal (1). Recent reports on neurologic symptoms in an infant, associated with a parentally fed C18:3n-3-poor formula, and deficiency symptoms in adults that were corrected by C18:3n-3 support the essentiality of this FA in the diet (1, 134). In the above cases, however, the C18:3n-3 deficiency symptoms could arguably be attributed to low levels of vitamin E or total EFAD (127).

As human brain gray matter and retinal membranes contain significant amounts of C22:6n-3, the requirement for n-3 EFA may be more critical during the last trimester of gestation and first months of life, when rapid accretion of these FA occurs in the central nervous system (125, 131). Brain PL acquires only long-chain derivatives of EFA, not their 18-carbon precursors, and C22:6n-3 is the predominant PUFA in PL in synaptosomal membranes and photoreceptors (131). C22:6n-3 also accounts for approximately 50 to 60% of FA in the PL of the photoreceptor disks that contain rhodopsin and the G-protein. Much of the C22:6n-3 acquired by the brain is accrued during the suckling period, when the brain undergoes rapid development. A number of animal studies have demonstrated an impairment in the visual process, altered learning behavior, and low brain C22:6n-3 content because of a deficiency in C18:3n-3 and its metabolites C20:5n-3 and C22:6n-3 (125, 131). Permanent learning defects and alterations in synaptic function in the brain, observed in EFAD during pregnancy, can be prevented by feeding n-3 EFA (133, 135). In addition, a correlation has been noted between diet-induced changes in C22:6n-3 in the retina and a modification of electrical potentials induced in rod outer segments by light stimulation (136).

Although adequate dietary intake of n-3 EFA appears to be critical for central nervous system development, the optimum requirements for n-3 EFA for infants are not known. Human milk provides both C18:3n-3 and C22:6n-3 that are often absent from most infant formulas on the market. Formula-fed infants thus depend on endogenous synthesis of long-chain PUFA. Infant formulas provide nutrition that results in growth rates equal or superior to those of breast milk-fed infants. There is a suggestion, however, that long-chain n-3 PUFA may not be synthesized from their parent EFA at optimal rates for brain development during the first few weeks after birth, particularly in preterm infants. Clandinin et al. (137) have indicated that the infant's requirement for neural accumulation of long-chain PUFA can be met by intake of long-chain PUFA alone, without endogenous synthesis. Using the FA composition of red blood cell PL as an index of cerebral membrane composition, infants fed human milk had a significantly better C22:6n-3 status than formula-fed infants (138). The extent to which diet-induced changes in red blood cell membranes reflect changes in brain PL is not clear. However, recent postmortem studies indicate a lower C22:6n-3 brain content in formula-fed infants than in infants receiving breast milk (139). In a randomized trial of n-3 PUFA supplementation of formulas fed to term infants, C22:6n-3-treated infants had better visual acuities than infants fed standard formula (140). Other work, however, has shown no effect of long-chain PUFA formula supplementation on visual, psychomotor, or mental development (141).

Preterm infants may be especially susceptible to n-3 EFAD because of their relatively immature desaturase and elongase enzyme systems and their low fat stores. In two randomized clinical trials, intake of formula containing marine oil by preterm infants normalized blood levels of C22:6n-3 and improved certain aspects of visual function relative to breast-fed infants (142). In one of the randomized studies, however, marine oil supplementation was associated with decreases in linear growth, some measures of cognitive development, and blood C20:4n-6 content. These results are of concern in view of the important role of C20:4n-6 in growth and development (123). However, a more physiologic formulation containing pure C22:6n-3 resulted in better cognitive and visual performance and a less detrimental effect on growth than the mixture of C20:5n-3 and C22:6n-3 given over a shorter interval (124, 143).

Pregnancy

Rapidly developing fetal organs, such as the liver and brain, incorporate large amounts of long-chain n-3 and n-6 EFA into membrane PL (144). The accumulation of EFA during human pregnancy has been approximated to be 620 g, which includes the demand for fetal, placental, mammary gland, and uterine growth and the increased maternal blood volume. On the basis of this estimate of expected EFA acquisition by maternal tissues and the conceptus, it is advised that maternal EFA consumption during pregnancy be increased from 3 to 4.5% of calories (145). In circumstances of relatively low dietary intake of n-6 EFA (i.e., 2 to 4% of calories), EFAD may be more likely to develop during periods of rapid cell division and growth.

Lactation

In well-nourished mothers, approximately 4 to 5% of total calories in human milk is present as C18:2n-6 and C18:3n-3, and a further 1% as long-chain PUFA derived from these FA, amounting to about 6% of total energy as EFA and its metabolites. The efficiency of conversion of dietary EFA into milk FA is not clear; however, an additional 1 to 2% of calories in the form of EFA is recommended during the first 3 months of lactation. Another 2 to 4% of calories above the basic requirement is recommended thereafter (145).

Infancy and Childhood

The optimum requirements for EFA of the n-6 and n-3 families for infants are still not known, although normal growth of infants depends on an adequate supply of EFA. Growing individuals apparently require a minimum of 1 to 4.5% of total calories as C18:2n-6 to ensure an adequate supply of EFA for tissue proliferation, membrane integrity, and eicosanoid formation (128, 146). The need for n-3 EFA has been indicated to be higher during growth and development. Estimates based upon FA compositional data from autopsy tissue and breast milk n-3 EFA concentrations have ranged from 0.5 to 1.2% of calories (146). The Canadian Nutrition Recommendations suggest infant dietary intakes of C18:3n-3 of 1% of energy in the absence of intake of long-chain n-3 PUFA, compared with C18:3n-3 of 0.5% of energy when a supply of long-chain n-3 EFA is available in the diet (128). However, the bioequivalency of C18:3n-3 and its long-chain products, C20:5n-3 and C22:6n-3, has not yet been determined, although long-chain PUFA clearly contribute to the C20:5n-3 and C22:6n-3 content of plasma and erythrocyte PL (131). Another question that needs to be addressed is whether long-chain PUFA, especially C22:6n-3, are conditionally essential for optimal visual and neural development of preterm and term infants.

Adults

For adults, appropriate minimum amounts of n-6 EFA are in the range of 1 to 4% of energy to prevent signs of EFAD (131). The C18:3n-3 requirements for adults are suggested to range from 0.2 to 0.3% of energy to 1% of energy, although more studies are needed to define the minimal requirements in humans (3, 147).

Nutrient Interrelationships

Several dietary components are known to affect EFA requirements because of their interactions with EFA use or metabolism. Dietary SAFA slightly increase EFA requirements, as evaluated by growth and dermal symptoms of deficiency and the triene:tetraene ratio in plasma (148). This effect has been related to the action of SAFA in raising plasma levels of CH that forms esters with PUFA, thereby depleting the availability of the EFA pool for PL. In addition, in several animal species, induction of serum CH via a high-CH diet can aggravate EFAD. *cis*-MUFA (mainly C18:1n-9 and its product C20:3n-9) can replace EFA in the lipids of EFAD animals and humans. High dietary levels of C18:1n-9 suppressed desaturation of EFA such that if dietary concentrations of C18:1n-9 were 10 times higher than that of C18:2n-6, triene:tetraene ratios indicating EFAD were observed (149). Partial hydrogenation of vegetable oils in the production of margarines and shortenings forms SAFA and a variety of *trans* and positional isomers. The estimated average daily *trans* FA intake is 8 to 10 g, or 6 to 8% of the total dietary FA. *Trans*-MUFA increase the EFA requirement in animals when fed at moderate levels and can influence the desaturase reactions critical to the metabolism of PUFA (150). *Trans*-FA can also raise plasma levels of LDL and total CH, which could further increase EFA use.

High-Risk Clinical Situations

Although development of human EFAD has traditionally been regarded as rare, use of the sensitive triene:tetraene ratio as a diagnostic index has recently indicated the existence of EFAD in a number of high-risk clinical conditions. EFAD appears to be exacerbated by increased metabolic demands associated with either growth or the hypermetabolism seen following stress, injury, or sepsis (151).

The supply of C18:2n-6 is of concern in premature infants because of their borderline stores of EFA and high caloric expenditure (151). Unless C18:2n-6 is supplied to premature infants in parenteral or enteral diets, early onset of EFAD may occur. Biochemical changes in the plasma and clinical signs indicating EFAD can develop rapidly within 5 to 10 days of life in premature infants (151, 152).

In patients receiving long-term parenteral nutrition without lipid, continuous glucose infusion results in high circulating levels of insulin that inhibit lipolysis and depress release of EFA from adipose fat stores (131). Development of EFAD in infants, children, and adults maintained on continuous fat-free or minimal-fat parenteral nutrition has been reversed by oral or intravenous administration of C18:2n-6 (151). Parenteral nutrition containing only amino acids and completely free of glucose does not produce evidence of EFAD (153). Clinical signs of EFAD include alopecia, scaly dermatitis, increased capillary fragility, poor wound healing, increased platelet aggregation, increased susceptibility to infection, fatty liver, and growth retardation in infants and children (153).

EFAD development has been described in several human diseases, including cystic fibrosis (154), acrodermatitis enteropathica (149), peripheral vascular disease (PVD) (155), and multiple sclerosis (156). Enteral supplementation of vegetable oils high in C18:2n-6 has been demonstrated to improve EFAD in patients with cystic fibrosis (154). Children with cystic fibrosis may require 7 to 10% of energy as C18:2n-6 to prevent reduced weight gain and growth, and infants with cystic fibrosis may require formula with a C18:2n-6 content above 12% of total calories (154, 157). Subjects with anorexia nervosa may have EFAD exhibited by plasma PL profiles showing lowered n-6 and n-3 PUFA concentrations (158). Low total plasma PUFA concentrations, particularly those of 20- and 22-carbon n-3 PUFA, have been noted in patients with acquired immune deficiency syndrome (AIDS) (159). Development of EFAD as measured by the triene:tetraene ratio has been demonstrated in elderly patients with PVD (160), in subjects with fat malabsorption after major intestinal resection, during low-fat, high-protein dietary supplementation for treatment of kwashiorkor (161), and after serious accidents and burns. Oral or intravenous feeding of C18:2n-6-containing TG corrects the biochemical and clinical abnormalities in these conditions.

ACKNOWLEDGMENTS

The authors extend special thanks to Catherine Vanstone for her invaluable contribution to researching and writing this chapter. The graphic art work of Helen Rimmer is also gratefully acknowledged. Finally, appreciation is extended to Fady Ntanios and Andrea Papamandjaris, who offered suggestions on improving the quality and composition of the chapter.

REFERENCES

1. Holman RT, Johnson SB, Hatch TF. Am J Clin Nutr 1982;35:617–23.
2. Neuringer M, Connor WE, Van Petten C, Barstad L. J Clin Invest 1984;73:272–6.
3. Bjerve KS. J Intern Med 1989;225(Suppl):171S–5S.
4. Poulos A, Beckman K, Johnson DW, et al. Adv Exp Med Biol 1992;318:331–40.
5. Poulos A. Lipids 1995;30:1–14.
6. Kris-Etherton PM, Yu S. Am J Clin Nutr 1997;65:1628S–44S.
7. ASCN Task Force on Trans Fatty Acids. Am J Clin Nutr 1996; 63:663–70.
8. Posner BM, Cupples LA, Franz MM, et al. Int J Epidemiol 1993;22:1014–25.
9. Anonymous. MMWR 1994;43;116–7, 123–5.
10. Chen ZY, Ratnayake WM, Fortier L, et al. Can J Physiol Pharmacol 1995;73:718–23.
11. Ling WH, Jones PJH. Life Sci 1995;57:195–206.
12. Vandermeers A, Vandermeers-Piret MC, Rathe J, et al. Biochim Biophys Acta 1974;370:257–68.
13. Hay DW, Carey MC. Hepatology 1990;12(Suppl):6S–14S.
14. Hofmann AF, Mekhijian HS. Bile acids and the intestinal absorption of fat and electrolytes in health and disease. In: Nair PP, Kritchevsky D, eds. The bile acids, vol 2. New York: Plenum Press, 1973.
15. Bergholz CM. Crit Rev Food Sci Nutr 1992;32:141–6.
16. Rolls BJ, Pirraglia PA, Jones MB, et al. Am J Clin Nutr 1992;56:84–92.
17. Reinhart GA, Mahan DC, Lepine AJ, et al. J Anim Sci 1993;71:2693–9.
18. Jones PJ, Scanu AM, Schoeller DA. J Lab Clin Med 1988;111:627–33.
19. Tso P, Karlstad MD, Bistrian BR, et al. Am J Physiol 1995;268:G568–77.
20. de Fouw NJ, Kivits GA, Quinlan PT, et al. Lipids 1994;29:765–70.
21. Bracco U. Am J Clin Nutr 1994;60(Suppl):1002S–9S.
22. Grundy SM, Metzger AL, Adler RD. J Clin Invest 1972;51:3026–43.

23. Wasserhess P, Becker M, Staab D. Am J Clin Nutr 1993;58:349–53.
24. Samuel P, McNamara DJ. J Lipid Res 1983;24:265–76.
25. Mattson FH, Jandacek RJ, Webb MR. J Nutr 1976;106:747–52.
26. Lipka G, Schulthess G, Thurnhofer H, et al. J Biol Chem 1995;270:5917–25.
27. Quintao EC, Sperotto G. Adv Lipid Res 1987;22:173–88.
28. Jones PJH, Pappu AS, Hatcher L, et al. Atheroscler Thromb 1996;16:1222–8.
29. Miettinen TA, Tilvis RS, Kesaniemi YA. Am J Epidemiol 1990;131:20–31.
30. Vanhanen HT, Miettinen TA. Clin Chim Acta 1992;205:97–107.
31. Child P, Kuksis A. Biochem Cell Biol 1986;64:847–53.
32. Miettinen TA, Puska P, Gylling H, et al. N Engl J Med 1995;333:1308–12.
32a. Ginsberg HN. Med Clin North Am 1994;78:1–20.
33. Sugiyama Y, Ishikawa E, Odaka H, et al. Atherosclerosis 1995;113:71–8.
34. Levy E, Mehran M, Seidman E. FASEB J 1995;9:626–35.
35. Leitch CA, Jones PJ. J Lipid Res 1993;34:157–63.
36. Hellerstein MK, Christiansen M, Kaempfer S, et al. J Clin Invest 1991;87:1841–52.
37. Austin MA, Hokanson JE, Brunzell JD. Curr Opin Lipidol 1994;5:395–403.
38. Miller GJ, Miller NE. Lancet 1975;1:16–9.
39. Barter PJ, Rye KA. Atherosclerosis 1996;121:1–12.
40. Raclot T, Groscolas R. J Lipid Res 1995;36:2164–73.
41. Connor WE, Lin DS, Colvis C. J Lipid Res 1996;37:290–8.
42. Brown MS, Goldstein JL. J Clin Invest 1983;72:743–7.
43. Mackness MI, Durrington PN. Atherosclerosis 1995;115:243–53.
44. Goldberg IJ. J Lipid Res 1996:37;693–707
45. Hegsted DM, McGandy RB, Myers ML, et al. Am J Clin Nutr 1965;17:281–295.
46. Noakes M, Nestel PJ, Clifton PM. Am J Clin Nutr 1996;63:42–6.
47. Bergeron N, Havel RJ. Arterioscler Thromb Vasc Biol 1996;16:497.
48. Harris WS. Lipids 1996;31:243–52.
49. van Tol A, Zock PL, van Gent T, et al. Atherosclerosis 1995;115:129–34.
50. Grundy SM, Barrett-Connor E, Rudel LL, et al. Arteriosclerosis 1988;8:95–101.
51. Andersen RE, Wadden TA, Bartlett SJ, et al. Am J Clin Nutr 1995;62:350–7.
52. Lemieux S, Prud'homme D, Moorjani S, et al. Atherosclerosis 1995;118:155–64.
53. Clandinin MT, Cheema S, Field CJ, et al. Ann NY Acad Sci 1993;683:151–63.
54. Leyton J, Drury PJ, Crawford MA. Br J Nutr 1987;57:383–93.
55. Takeuchi H, Matsuo T, Tokuyama K, et al. J Nutr 1995;125:920–5.
56. Shimomura Y, Tamura T, Suzuki M. J Nutr 1990;120:1291–6.
57. Matsuo T, Shimomura Y, Saitoh S, et al. Metab Clin Exp 1995;44:934–9.
58. Chen ZY, Menard CR, Cunnane SC. Am J Physiol 1995;268:R498–505.
59. Jones PJ, Schoeller DA. Metab Clin Exp 1988;37:145–51.
60. Clandinin MT, Wang LC, Rajotte RV, et al. Am J Clin Nutr 1995;61:1052–7.
61. Kubow S. Free Radic Biol Med 1992;12:63–81.
62. Draper HH, Hadley M. Xenobiotica 1990;20:901–7.
63. Welsch CW, Welsch MA, Huelskamp LJ, et al. Int J Oncol 1995;6:55–64.
64. Girelli D, Olivieri O, Stanzial AM, et al. Clin Chim Acta 1994;227:45–57.
65. Draper HH. Nutritional modulation of oxygen radical pathology. In: Draper HH, ed. Advances in nutritional research, vol 8. New York: Plenum Press, 1990;119–45.
66. Addis PB, Warner GJ. In: Aruoma OI, Halliwell B, eds. Free radicals and food additives. London: Taylor and Francis, 1991;77–119.
67. Smith LL. Lipids 1996;31:453–87.
68. Peng SK, Philips GA, Xia GZ, et al. Atherosclerosis 1987;64:1–6.
69. Holvoet P, Collen D. FASEB J 1994;8:1279–84.
70. Regnstrom J, Nilsson J, Tornvall P, et al. Lancet 1992;339:1183–6.
71. Palinski W, Rosenfeld ME, Yla-Herttuala S, et al. Proc Natl Acad Sci USA 1989;86:1372–6.
72. Louheranta AM, Porkkalasarataho EK, Nyyssönen MK, et al. Am J Clin Nutr 1996;63:698–703.
73. Bonanome A, Biasia F, Deluca M, et al. Am J Clin Nutr 1996;63:261–6.
74. Jialal I, Fuller CJ, Huet BA. Arterioscler Thromb Vasc Biol 1995;15:190–8.
75. Stephens NG, Parsons A, Schofield PM, et al. Lancet 1996;347:781–6.
76. Parker RA, Sabrah T, Cap M, et al. Arterioscler Thromb Vasc Biol 1995;15:349–58.
77. Geiger M, Mohammed BS, Sankarappa S, et al. Biochim Biophys Acta 1993;1170:137–42.
78. Cunnane SC, Ryan MA, Craig KS, et al. Lipids 1995;30:781–3.
79. Kinsella JE, Broughton KS, Whelan J. J Nutr Biochem 1990;1:123–41.
80. Holman RT. Biological activities of and requirement for polyunsaturated acids. In: Holman RT, ed. Progress in the chemistry of fats and other lipids, vol 9. New York: Pergamon Press, 1970;611–82.
81. Schlenk H, Sand DM, Gellerman JL. Biochim Biophys Acta 1969;187:201–7.
82. Hagve TA, Christophersen BO. Biochim Biophys Acta 1986;875:165–73.
83. Blond JP, Bezard J. Biochim Biophys Acta 1991;1084:255–60.
84. Mimouni V, Narce M, Huang YS, et al. Prostaglandin Leukotrienes Essent Fatty Acid 1994;50:43–7.
85. Cunnane SC. Prog Food Nutr Sci 1988;12:151–88.
86. Horrobin DF. Am J Clin Nutr 1993;57(Suppl):732S–6S.
87. Dietschy JM. Klin Wochenschr 1984;62:338–45.
88. Jenkins DJ, Khan A, Jenkins AL, et al. Metab Clin Exp 1995;44:549–55.
89. Wu-Pong S, Elias PM, Feingold KR. J Invest Dermatol 1994;102:799–802.
90. Galli C, Marangoni F, Galella G. Prostaglandin Leukotrienes Essent Fatty Acid 1993;48:51–5.
91. Murphy MG. J Nutr Biochem 1990;1:68–79.
92. Tinoco J. Prog Lipid Res 1982;21:1–45.
93. Stinson AM, Wiegand RD, Anderson RE. Exp Eye Res 1991;52:213–8.
94. Litman BJ, Mitchell DC. Lipids 1996;31(Suppl):193S–7S.
95. Huang KP. Trends Neurosci 1989;12:425–32.
96. Nishizuka Y. Science 1992;258:607–14.
97. Medini L, Colli S, Mosconi C, et al. Biochem Pharmacol 1990;39:129–33.
98. Goetzl EJ, An S, Smith WL. FASEB J 1995;9:1051–8.
99. Ziboh VA. Proc Soc Exp Biol Med 1994;205:1–11.
100. Li B, Birdwell C, Whelan J. J Lipid Res 1994;35:1869–77.
101. Whelan J, Surette ME, Hardardottir I, et al. J Nutr 1993;123:2174–85.
102. Wu D, Meydani SN, Meydani M, et al. Am J Clin Nutr 1996;63:273–80.
103. Lands WE. FASEB J 1992;6:2530–6.

104. Emken EA. Am J Clin Nutr 1992;56(Suppl):798S.
105. von Schacky C, Fischer S, Weber PC. J Clin Invest 1985;76:1626–31.
106. Anonymous. Lancet 1988;2:349–60.
107. Morris MC, Manson JE, Rosner B, et al. Am J Epidemiol 1995;142:166–75.
108. Kromhout D, Feskens EJ, Bowles CH. Int J Epidemiol 1995;24:340–5.
109. Kremer JM. Lipids 1996;31(Suppl):243S–7S.
110. Caughey GE, Mantzioris E, Gibson RA, et al. Am J Clin Nutr 1996;63:116–22.
111. Holman RT. Essential fatty acid deficiency. In: Holman RT, ed. Progress in the chemistry of fats and other lipids, vol 9, pt 2. New York: Pergamon Press, 1971;275–348.
112. Kinsella JE. α-Linolenic acid: functions and effects on linoleic acid metabolism and eicosanoid-mediated reactions. In: Kinsella JE, ed. Advances in food and nutrition research. San Diego: Academic Press, 1991;1–184.
113. Vergroesen AJ. Bibl Nutr Dieta 1976;23:19–26.
114. Hansen HS. Trends Biochem Sci 1986;11:263–5.
115. Houtsmuller UM. Prog Lipid Res 1981;20:889–96.
116. Paulsrud JR, Pensler L, Whitten CF, et al. Am J Clin Nutr 1972;25:897–904.
117. Kinsella JE, Lokesh B, Stone RA. Am J Clin Nutr 1990;52:1–28.
118. Mohrhauer H, Holman RT. J Lipid Res 1963;4:151–9.
119. Brown WR, Hansen AE, Burr GO, et al. J Nutr 1938;16:511–24.
120. Carlson SE. J Nutr 1996;126:1092–8.
121. Crawford MA, Costeloe K, Doyle W, et al. Essential fatty acids in early development. In: Bracco U, Deckelbaum RJ, eds. Polyunsaturated fatty acids in human nutrition. New York: Raven Press, 1992;93–110.
122. Koletzko B, Braun M. Ann Nutr Metab 1991;35:128–31.
123. Carlson SE, Cooke RJ, Werkman SH, et al. Lipids 1992;27:901–7.
124. Carlson SE, Werkman SH, Tolley EA. Am J Clin Nutr 1996;63:687–97.
125. Innis SM. Can J Physiol Pharmacol 1994;72:1483–92.
126. Koletzko B, Decsi T, Demmelmair H. Lipids 1996;31:79–83.
127. Makrides M, Neumann MA, Gibson RA. Lipids 1996;31:115–9.
128. Canada Health and Welfare, Health Protection Branch, Bureau of Nutritional Sciences. 1990 Nutrition Recommendations. Ottawa, 1990.
129. Bezard J, Blond JP, Bernard A, et al. Reprod Nutr Dev 1994; 34:539–68.
130. Gibson RA, Makrides M, Neumann MA, et al. J Pediatr 1994;125(Suppl):48S–55S.
131. Innis SM. Prog Lipid Res 1991;30:39–103.
132. Anderson GJ. J Lipid Res 1994;35:105–111.
133. Neuringer M, Connor WE. Nutr Rev 1986;44:285–94.
134. Bjerve KS, Fischer S, Wammer F, et al. Am J Clin Nutr 1989;49:290–300.
135. Galli C, Spagnuoli C, Boricio E, et al. Dietary essential fatty acids and prostaglandins. In: Cocceani F, Olley PM, eds. Advances in prostaglandins and thromboxane research. New York: Raven Press, 1978;181–9.
136. Wheeler TG, Benolken RM, Anderson RE. Science 1975;188:1312–4.
137. Clandinin MT, Chappell JE, Heim T. Prog Lipid Res 1981;20:901–4.
138. Carlson SE, Rhodes PG, Ferguson MG. Am J Clin Nutr 1986;44:798–804.
139. Farquharson J, Jamieson EC, Abbasi KA, et al. Arch Dis Child 1995;72:198–203.
140. Makrides M, Neumann MA, Simmer K, et al. Lancet 1995;345:1463–8.
141. Auestad N, Montalto MB, Wheeler RE, et al. Pediatr Res 1995;37:302A.
142. Carlson SE, Werkman SH, Rhodes PG, et al. Am J Clin Nutr 1993;58:35–42.
143. Werkman SH, Carlson SE. Lipids 1996;31:91–7.
144. Clandinin MT, Jumpsen J, Suh M. J Pediatr 1994;125(Suppl):25S–32S.
145. FAO/WHO Expert Consultation. The role of fats and oils in human nutrition. FAO food and nutrition paper 3. Rome, Italy: Food and Agriculture Organization, 1978.
146. European Society of Paediatric Gastroenterology and Nutrition. Acta Paediatr Scand 1987;336:1–14.
147. Bjerve KS, Fischer S, Alme K. Am J Clin Nutr 1987;46:570–6.
148. Alfin-Slater RB, Morris RS, Hansen H, et al. J Nutr 1965;87:168–72.
149. Holman RT. Adv Exp Med Biol 1977;83:515–34.
150. Lands WE, Blank ML, Nutter LJ, et al. Lipids 1966;1:224–9.
151. Sardesai VM. J Nutr Biochem 1992;3:154–67.
152. Farrell PM, Gutcher GR, Palta M, et al. Am J Clin Nutr 1988;48:220–9.
153. Stegink LD, Freeman JB, Wispe J, et al. Am J Clin Nutr 1977;30:388–93.
154. Mischler EH, Parrell SW, Farrell PM, et al. Pediatr Res 1986;20:36–41.
155. Kingsbury KJ, Brett C, Stovold R, et al. Postgrad Med J 1974;50:425–40.
156. Dworkin RH, Bates D, Millar JH, et al. Neurology 1984;34:1441–5.
157. van Egmond AW, Kosorok MR, Kosick R, et al. Am J Clin Nutr 1996;63:746–52.
158. Holman RT, Adams CE, Nelson RA, et al. J Nutr 1995;125:901–7.
159. Begin ME, Manku MS, Horrobin DF. Prostaglandins Leukotrienes Essent Fatty Acids 1989;37:135–7.
160. Friedman Z, Frolich JC. Pediatr Res 1979;13:932–6.
161. Naismith DJ. Br J Nutr 1973;30:567–76.
162. Innis SM. Essential dietary lipids. In: Ziegler EE, Filer LJ, eds. Present knowledge in nutrition. 7th ed. Washington, DC: ILSI Press, 1996;58–66.

SELECTED READINGS

Crawford MA, Costeloe K, Doyle W, et al. Essential fatty acids in early development. In: Bracco U, Deckelbaum RJ, eds. Polyunsaturated fatty acids in human nutrition. New York: Raven Press, 1992;93–110.

Groff JL, Gropper SS, Hunt SM. Advanced nutrition and human metabolism. 2nd ed. Minneapolis: West Publishing, 1995.

Grundy SM. Dietary fat. In: Ziegler EE, Filer LJ, eds. Present knowledge in nutrition. 7th ed. Washington, DC: ILSI Press, 1996;44–57.

Innis SM. Essential dietary lipids. In: Ziegler EE, Filer LJ, eds. Present knowledge in nutrition. 7th ed. Washington, DC: ILSI Press, 1996;58–66.

5. Energy Needs: Assessment and Requirements in Humans

ERIC T. POEHLMAN and EDWARD S. HORTON

HISTORICAL PERSPECTIVE

The understanding and assessment of energy requirements in humans have been enhanced by the advent of indirect calorimetry. In indirect calorimetry, the type and rate of substrate oxidation and energy are measured in vivo from gas exchange measurements. This method in combination with other measurement techniques permits investigation of numerous aspects of metabolism, heat production, energy requirements of physical activity, and altered energy metabolism in injury and disease. The development and interpretation of indirect calorimetry have represented a fundamental milestone for chemistry, biology, and medicine.

The high level of interest in indirect calorimetry over the past decades as a method of determining energy needs has resulted from several factors. Media and "lay" attention to food, exercise, and the prevention of obesity as important ways to improve lifestyle has been associated with greater awareness of indirect calorimetry. Moreover, commercial availability of improved and convenient equipment for measuring gaseous exchange in healthy humans and hospitalized patients has made indirect calorimetry readily available to both clinicians and scientists. At the same time, measurements of energy expenditure have assumed new importance in investigating and managing obesity.

Historical developments from 1650 to 1950 were primarily directed toward measuring basal metabolic rates. Discussions of gas exchange often start with the references to Lavoisier and his contemporaries, who were the first to demonstrate animal respiration (1). Lavoisier was studying the combustion and oxidation of metals. He gave the name *oxygene* to the material absorbed by the metal when heated in air. Moreover, he introduced the term *calorique* to describe heat. In collaboration with the physicist, Laplace, he conducted studies of the heat released in combustion, which laid the foundation for thermal chemistry. Later, Lavosier carried out elegant experiments to relate the uptake of oxygen by an animal to the output of CO_2 and heat. Heat production was measured by an ice calorimeter and helped to establish the science of calorimetry.

During the first half of the 1800s, techniques for chemical measurement of foods and other biologic materials were being developed and the scientific concepts of Lavoisier were still considered quite controversial. The second half of the 1800s saw a growth in organic and biochemistry. The gas exchange of nutrients upon oxidation was related to heat production in a bomb calorimeter. Such studies were extended to animals and then to men by the use of direct and indirect calorimetry. Voit established a center for investigators in Germany, and studies there led the way in establishing the relationship between gas exchange and calorimetry of the whole body (2). Such studies had widespread influence on calorimetry in Europe as well as in the United States, where Atwater (3), Benedict (4), Lusk (5), and DuBois (6) were particularly influential in advancing the field.

The measurement of gas concentration before World War II was largely gravimetric for chamber or room calorimeters and volumetric when measuring basal metabolic rates of individuals. The classic portable basal metabolic rate apparatus of Benedict (4) depended on a closed system, in which a container of oxygen would decrease in volume in proportion to the uptake of oxygen by the subject, while the CO_2 was absorbed but not measured. Oxygen consumption was then translated into calories per hour by assuming an amount of expired CO_2, which would yield a nonprotein respiratory quotient (RQ) of 0.82 and hence a caloric equivalent for oxygen of 4.825 kcal (20.19 kJ) liter^{-1}. The wartime events of the early 1940s provided a stimulus to develop more rapid and accurate methods of gas analysis, particularly for the new demands of combat aviation at higher altitudes. Following World War II, phys-

Abbreviations: **RMR**—resting metabolic rate; **TEF**—thermic effect of feeding.

ical methods of gas analysis began to dominate the field of gas exchange. Mass spectrometry was introduced for measuring both O_2 and CO_2, as well as paramagnetic analyzers for O_2 and infrared analyzers for CO_2.

A significant advancement in the 1980s was the use of doubly labeled water to measure energy expenditure in free-living individuals, the first noninvasive technique to do so accurately in free-living humans. The technique was first introduced by Lifson et al. in the 1950s (7) as an isotopic technique for measuring the CO_2 production rate in small animals. Unfortunately, it was not possible to apply the technique to humans because the dose required was cost prohibitive given the relatively poor sensitivity of isotope-ratio mass spectrometry at that time. Not for another 20 years did Lifson et al. describe the feasibility of applying the technique to measuring free-living energy expenditure in humans (8), an application later recognized by Schoeller et al. (9), who administered both ^{18}O- and ^{2}H-labeled water and followed the decay rates of each isotope in body water over 1 to 2 weeks. The difference in the decay rates then allowed calculation of the CO_2 production over that time period. For the first time, an accurate calculation of daily energy expenditure in free-living individuals was possible.

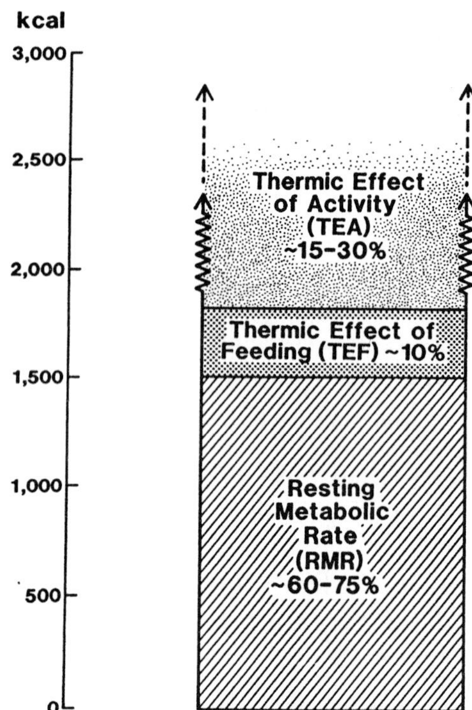

Figure 5.1. The components of daily energy expenditure.

KEY ASPECTS OF ENERGY EXPENDITURE

Changes in body energy content occur through changes in the balance between daily intake and energy expenditure. Energy intake is episodic, derived primarily from the carbohydrates, proteins, and fats in foods consumed. Total daily energy expenditure for theoretical and analytic purposes can be divided into several components (Fig. 5.1).

Resting Metabolic Rate

The *resting metabolic rate* (RMR) represents the largest portion of daily energy expenditure (60 to 75%) and is a measurement of the energy expended for maintenance of normal body functions and homeostasis. These processes include resting cardiovascular and pulmonary functions, the energy consumed by the central nervous system, cellular homeostasis, and other biochemical reactions involved in the maintenance of resting metabolism.

Another term to describe basal levels of energy expenditure is *basal metabolic rate* (BMR). While at the Mayo Clinic, Dr Boothby defined and popularized use of the BMR for the diagnosis of thyroid disorders. He defined this function as the energy expended by an individual bodily and mentally at rest in a thermoneutral environment 12 to 18 hours after a meal. Much to the inconvenience of the patient, measurements were done during the early morning hours when, in addition, the circadian rhythm of oxygen consumption was known to be low. Because of the increase in metabolism caused by the muscular and mental unrest introduced by this procedure, it is unlikely that the true basal metabolism was often measured. Therefore, for practical and conceptual reasons, the BMR is now rarely measured. In its place, we now measure what is referred to as the resting metabolic rate (or resting energy expenditure), which may be (but is not always) higher than the BMR.

The RMR is primarily related to the fat-free mass of the body and is also influenced by age, gender, body composition, and genetic factors. For example, the RMR decreases with advancing age (2 to 3%/decade), which is primarily attributed to the loss of fat-free mass. Males tend to have a higher RMR than females because of their greater body size. The dependency of the RMR on body composition must be considered when individuals of different age, sex, and physical activity status are compared. Other processes, such as sympathetic nervous system activity, thyroid hormone activity, and sodium-potassium pump activity, contribute to the variation in the RMR among individuals. (See WHO equations for predicting basal metabolic rates from body weights and heights for different age groups and both sexes and their derived data in Appendix Tables III-10-B to E).

Thermic Effect of Feeding

The thermic effect of feeding (TEF) is the increase in energy expenditure associated with food ingestion. The TEF represents approximately 10% of the daily energy expenditure and includes the energy costs of food absorption, metabolism, and storage. The magnitude of the TEF depends on several factors, including the caloric content and composition of the meal as well as the antecedent diet of the individual. Following meal ingestion, energy expenditure increases for 4 to 8 hours, its magnitude and duration depending on the quantity and type of macronutrient (i.e., protein, fat, or carbohydrate).

The TEF has been divided into subcomponents: obligatory and facultative thermogenesis. The obligatory component of the TEF is the energy cost associated with absorption and transport of nutrients and the synthesis and storage of protein, fat, and carbohydrate. The "excess" energy expended above the obligatory thermogenesis is the facultative thermogenesis and is thought to be partially mediated by sympathetic nervous system activity.

The TEF also decreases with advancing age and may be associated with development of insulin resistance (10). It is presently unclear how exercise training influences the TEF, although there is clearly some interaction between physical exercise and TEF. There is presently no evidence that gender influences postprandial thermogenesis.

Thermic Effect of Physical Activity

The most variable component of the daily energy expenditure is the thermic effect of physical activity (11). The component includes the energy expended above the RMR and the TEF and includes the energy expended through voluntary exercise and the energy devoted to involuntary activity such as shivering, fidgeting, and postural control. In sedentary individuals, the thermic effect of activity may be as low as 100 kcal/day; in highly active individuals it may approach 3000 kcal/day (see Chapter 47). Thus, physical activity represents a significant factor in the daily energy expenditure in humans because it is extremely variable and subject to voluntary control. Physical activity tends to decrease with advancing age; this decrease in physical activity may be associated with a loss of fat-free mass and an increase in adiposity. Males in general tend to have a greater caloric expenditure associated with physical activity than females, partially because of the greater energy cost of moving a larger body mass. Average values of the energy cost of different grades of physical activity for men and women are given in Appendix Tables III-A-11-D and E.

The RMR, TEF, and physical activity often overlap during the course of a normal day. Although daily variations in energy balance put individuals in a slight energy deficit or surplus, maintenance of a stable body weight depends on tight coupling of energy intake and energy expenditure over long periods of time. It is presently unclear which psychologic and/or physiologic factors influence the coupling of energy intake with energy expenditure to maintain energy balance.

METHODS OF MEASUREMENT

Many methods of measuring energy expenditure have become available over the years, and they vary in complexity, cost, and accuracy (12). It is important to gain an appreciation of the differences in the methods and of their applications in laboratory and other settings. The techniques used to measure total daily energy expenditure and its components are briefly described below. A more detailed explanation of the laboratory methods of measuring energy expenditure has been published (13).

The most widely used methods for measuring the energy expenditure involve indirect calorimetry. Direct calorimetry (measurement of heat loss from a subject) has been used to measure energy expenditure, but the high cost and complicated engineering of this method have discouraged investigators from using this approach.

Indirect Calorimetry

The term *indirect* refers to the estimation of energy production by measuring O_2 consumption and CO_2 production rather than by directly measuring heat transfer. This method requires a steady state of CO_2 production and respiratory exchange and subjects with a normal acid-base balance. To determine the RMR, measurements are usually taken with the subject in a supine or semireclined position after a 10- to 12-hour fast. Depending on the equipment, the subject typically breathes through a mouthpiece, face mask, or ventilated hood or is placed in a room calorimeter in which expired gases are collected. Typical RMR values range from 0.7 to 1.6 kcal/min, depending on the subject's body size, body composition, level of physical training, and gender. The room in which the measurements are made is usually darkened and quiet, and the volunteer remains undisturbed during the measurement process. Measurement of RMR typically lasts 30 minutes to 1 hour, whereas postprandial measurements frequently take 3 to 8 hours. These measurements are generally easily reproducible (with a coefficient of variation below 5%).

Several methods have been used to measure O_2 consumption and CO_2 production at rest. Generally, an "open circuit" method is used in which both ends of the system are open to atmospheric pressure and the subject's inspired and expired air are kept separate by means of a three-way respiratory valve or nonrebreathing mask. The expired gases are usually collected in a Douglas bag or Tissot respirometer for measurement of O_2 and CO_2 content. Hyperventilation may occur in subjects who are not well adapted to a mouthpiece and may result in inappropriately high levels of O_2 consumption and CO_2 production. When a mask is used, it is frequently difficult to obtain an airtight seal around the subject's nose and mouth.

To circumvent some of these problems, ventilated hoods have been developed in which the subject is fitted with a transparent hood equipped with a snugly fitting collar. Fresh air is drawn into the hood via an intake port, and expired air is drawn out of the hood by a motorized fan. The flow rate is measured by a pneumotachograph, and aliquots of the outflowing air are analyzed for O_2 consumption and CO_2 production after temperature and water vapor content have been adjusted. O_2 consumption and CO_2 production are calculated from the differences in their concentrations in the inflowing and outflowing air and the flow rate. Ventilated hoods are excellent for both short- and long-term measurements but are less useful in measuring the energy expenditure of physical activity; in the latter case the subject may find the hood uncomfortable, and there is a problem with dissipation of perspiration and water vapor.

Measurement of the energy expenditure of physical activity has traditionally presented several methodological challenges. Indirect calorimetry using a mouthpiece or face mask has been used to assess O_2 consumption and CO_2 production. This method generally yields reliable and accurate measurements of the energy cost of physical activity in a laboratory setting but provides no information about the energy cost of physical activity under free-living conditions because of the stationary nature of the equipment. Portable respirometers use a face mask with valves that direct expired air through collection tubes to a respirometer carried on the subject's back. The respirometer contains a flowmeter and a sampling device that collects an aliquot of expired gases for analysis at a later time. There are drawbacks to this method: first, there is an inherent delay in obtaining results, and second, the rate of energy expended during work performance is integrated over the entire period of gas collection.

In an attempt to avoid some of the problems associated with measurement of free-living physical activity, several less complicated (and less accurate) methods have been devised. These methods use physiologic measurements, observation, and records of physical activity, as well as activity diaries or recall. Heart-rate recording, used to measure energy expenditure, is based on the correlation between heart rate and oxygen consumption during moderate to heavy exercise (13, 14). The correlation, however, is much poorer at lower levels of physical activity, and a subject's heart rate may be altered by such events as anxiety or change in posture without significant changes in oxygen consumption.

It is possible to estimate energy expenditure over relatively long periods of time by measuring energy intake and changes in body composition. However, there are errors inherent in attempting an accurate determination of energy intake over several days, weeks, or months, as well as in the methods available for determination of body composition.

Time-motion studies have also been used to estimate the energy expenditure of physical activity in real-life situations. In time-motion studies, detailed records of physical activity are kept by an observer, and energy expenditure is estimated from the duration and intensity of the work performed. The major problem with this method is the marked individual variations in the energy costs of doing a particular task.

Physical activity diaries and physical activity recall instruments have been used to quantify the energy costs of different activities over a representative period of time. Record keeping is often inaccurate and may interfere with the subject's normal activities. Furthermore, the subject's recall of physical activity depends on his or her memory, which may not always be reliable. Measuring motion by devices such as a pedometer or an accelerometer may provide an index of physical activity (i.e., counts) but does not quantitate energy expenditure. In summary, measurement of free-living physical activity continues to be the most significant challenge in the field of energy metabolism.

In recent years, large respiration chambers have been built in laboratories. Such a chamber operates on the same principle as the ventilated hood system: it is essentially a large, airtight room in which temperature and humidity are controlled. Fresh air is drawn into the chamber and allowed to mix. Simultaneously, air is drawn from the chamber, and the flow rate is measured and analyzed continuously for O_2 and CO_2 content. The size of the room affords the subject sufficient mobility to sleep, eat, exercise, and perform normal daily routines, making detailed measurements of energy expenditure possible over a period of several hours or days. Room calorimeters are probably the best method currently available for conducting short-term studies (several days) of energy expenditure in humans when the object is to measure RMR, TEF, and the energy expenditure of physical activity. Physical activity level is quantified by a radar system that is activated by the subject's movement within the chamber. As with other movement devices, the radar system does not quantitate the intensity of activity. It is also likely, however, that free-living physical activity is blunted in the room calorimeter because of its confining nature. Thus room calorimeters do not offer the best model for examining adaptations in free-living physical activity. Although room calorimeters are moderately expensive to construct, they provide reliable information on daily energy expenditure and substrate oxidation.

Substrate Oxidation

The assessment of nutrient use is frequently used in combination with the assessment of energy expenditure. This area has been previously reviewed (14) and is briefly summarized in this chapter. When the measurement of $\dot{V}O_2$ is available (in liters of O_2 STPD [standard temperature (0°C), pressure (760 mm Hg), and dry] per minute), metabolic rate ($\dot{M}$), which corresponds to energy expenditure, can be calculated (in kJ/min) as follows:

$$\dot{M} = 20.3 \times \dot{V}O_2 \qquad (5.1)$$

where 20.3 is the mean value (in kJ/L) of the energy equivalent for the consumption of 1 L (STPD) of O_2. To take into account the heat generated by the oxidation of the three macronutrients (carbohydrates, fats, and proteins), three measurements must be performed: oxygen consumption ($\dot{V}O_2$), carbon dioxide production ($\dot{V}CO_2$), and urinary excretion (N). Simple equations for computing metabolic rate (or energy expenditure) from these three determinations are written in the following form:

$$\dot{M} = aVO_2 + bVCO_2 \ cN \quad (5.2)$$

The factors *a, b,* and *c* depend on the respective constants for the amount of O_2 used and the amount of CO_2 produced during oxidation of the three classes of nutrients (Table 5.1). An example of such a formula is given below:

$$\dot{M} = 16.18\ \dot{V}O_2 + 5.02\ \dot{V}CO_2 - 5.99\ N \quad (5.3)$$

where M is in kilojoules per unit of time, VO_2 and VCO_2 are in liters STPD per unit of time and N is in grams per unit of time. For example, if $\dot{V}O_2 = 600$ L/day, $\dot{V}CO_2 = 500$ L/day (respiratory quotient, or RQ = 0.83) and $N = 25$ g/day, then $M = 12{,}068$ kJ/day. The simpler equation (5.1) gives a value of 12,180 kJ per day.

Indirect calorimetry also allows computation of the nutrient oxidation rates in the whole body. An index of protein oxidation is obtained from the total amount of nitrogen excreted in the urine during the test period. One approach to calculating the nutrient oxidation rate is based on the O_2 consumption and CO_2 production due to the oxidation rates of the three nutrients, carbohydrate, fat, and protein, respectively. In a subject oxidizing c g/min of carbohydrate (as glucose) and f g/min of fat, and excreting n g/min of urinary nitrogen, the following equations, based on Table 5.1, can be used:

$$\dot{V}O_2 = 0.746c + 2.02f + 6.31n \quad (5.4)$$

and

$$\dot{V}CO_2 = 0.746c + 1.43f + 5.27n \quad (5.5)$$

We can solve equations 5.4 and 5.5 for the unknown c and f this way:

$$c = 4.59\ VCO_2 - 3.25\ VO_2 - 3.68n \quad (5.6)$$

$$f = 1.69\ VO_2 - 1.69\ VCO_2 - 1.72n \quad (5.7)$$

Because 1 g of urinary nitrogen arises from approximately 6.25 g protein, the protein oxidation rate p (in g/min) is given by the equation

$$p = 6.25n \quad (5.8)$$

Thus, indirect calorimetry allows calculation of net rates of nutrient oxidation. It is important to appreciate that indirect calorimetry measures the net appearance by oxidation of a substrate. Moreover, it is important to understand that there is a slight difference in the heat produced per liter of O_2 consumed when one compares carbohydrate, lipid, and protein oxidation. An examination of substrate oxidation has broadened our knowledge of the effects of environment (i.e., diet, exercise), disease, and nutrient requirements in humans.

Doubly Labeled Water

The doubly labeled water technique offers promise as a method of determining energy requirements in free-living populations and in subjects in whom traditional measures of energy expenditure, using indirect calorimetry, have proven impractical and difficult (e.g., infants and critically ill patients). The basis of this technique is that after a bolus dose of two stable isotopes of water (^2H_2O and $H_2{}^{18}O$), ^2H_2O is lost from the body in water alone, whereas $H_2{}^{18}O$ is lost not only in water but also as $C^{18}O_2$ via the carbonic anhydrase system (9). The difference in the two turnover rates is therefore related to the CO_2 production rate, and with a knowledge of the fuel mixture oxidized (from the composition of the diet), energy expenditure can be calculated.

The main advantages of the doubly labeled water technique are *(a)* it measures total daily energy expenditure, which includes an integrated measure of RMR, TEF, and the energy expenditure of physical activity; *(b)* it permits an unbiased measurement of free-living energy expenditure; and *(c)* measurements are conducted over extended periods of time (1 to 3 weeks). Thus, energy values derived from the doubly labeled water method are representative of the typical daily energy expenditure and therefore the daily energy needs of free-living adults. Furthermore, this technique provides an accurate estimate of free-living

Table 5.1
Energy Equivalent from Oxidation of Substrates

				Energy Equivalent (per gram)					
				Heat Released per Gram		VO_2		VCO_2	
Substrates	O_2 Consumed[a]	CO_2 Produced[a]	RQ[b]	kJ	kcal	kJ	kcal	kJ	kcal
Starch	0.829	0.829	1.00	17.6	4.20	21.2	5.06	21.2	5.06
Saccharose	0.786	0.786	1.00	16.6	3.96	21.1	5.04	21.1	5.04
Glucose	0.746	0.746	1.00	15.6	3.74	21.0	5.01	21.0	5.01
Lipid	2.019	1.427	0.71	39.6	9.46	19.6	4.69	27.7	6.63
Protein	1.010	0.844	0.83	19.7	4.70	19.0	4.66	23.3	5.58
Lactic acid	0.746	0.746	1.00	15.1	3.62	20.3	4.85	20.3	4.85

Data from Livesey G, Marinos E. Am J Clin Nutr 1988;47:608–627.
[a]In liters per gram of substrate oxidized.
[b]RQ, respiratory quotient.

Table 5.2
Advantages and Disadvantages of the Doubly Labeled Water Technique

Advantages	Disadvantages
Noninvasive and unobtrusive	Availability and expense of oxygen-18
Measurements are performed under free-living conditions	Reliance on isotope ratio mass spectrometry for analysis of samples
Measurements are performed over extended time periods (7–14 days)	A direct measurement of CO_2 production and O_2 consumption; the method does not measure substrate oxidation
Measurements can be used to estimate physical activity energy expenditure when combined with measurement of resting metabolic rate	The method is not suitable for epidemiological studies

physical activity. Daily free-living physical activity is calculated from the difference between the total daily energy expenditure and the combined energy expenditures of the RMR and TEF. Thus the doubly labeled water technique provides the most realistic estimate in free-living subjects of the average daily energy expenditure associated with physical activity.

Disadvantages of the doubly labeled water method are its expense and limited availability (Table 5.2). Consequently, the technique does not lend itself to epidemiologic studies or studies of large groups of subjects. However, this technique is now being used to examine energy requirements of persons in a variety of healthy and diseased states. With use of the doubly labeled water method, measurement of daily energy expenditure becomes a proxy measure of daily energy requirements.

Labeled Bicarbonate

The labeled bicarbonate (^{13}C or ^{14}C) method has recently won favor as a technique for measuring energy expenditure over shorter periods of time (several days) than those covered by the doubly labeled water method (15). When labeled bicarbonate is infused at a constant rate, it reaches a rapid equilibrium with the body's CO_2 pool. The extent of isotopic dilution depends on the rate of CO_2 production, provided there is not isotopic exchange or fixation. Thus variations in the dilution of isotope reflect variations in CO_2 production and hence energy expenditure. Because the method assesses CO_2 production rather than O_2 consumption, it requires assumptions about the respiratory quotient similar to those required by the doubly labeled water method.

In the final analysis, cost and the specific research questions generated should direct the selection of methods of measuring energy expenditure. Questions of substrate oxidation and its impact on the regulation of energy balance, for example, are most applicable to the techniques of indirect calorimetry using room calorimeters and ventilated hood systems. On the other hand, more reliable information on the adaptations of free-living subjects to environmental perturbations (exercise, dietary interventions, etc.) over long periods of time is provided by the use of the doubly labeled water method combined with indirect calorimetry systems.

CAN ENERGY INTAKE BE ACCURATELY MEASURED IN HUMANS?

Self-recorded food intake has been the traditional method of estimating energy requirements. However, available methods for estimating food intake are fraught with limitations and methodological problems. While there is a clear need to provide well-founded recommendations for dietary energy, there have been major technical, physiologic and conceptual problems in doing so. The establishment of individual energy requirements has been problematic because of reliance on *(a)* measurement of energy intake from self-recorded diaries and/or dietary interviews, *(b)* the use of a multiple of BMR (or RMR) to predict energy needs, and *(c)* the failure of current recommended daily energy requirements to take into account the diversity of the population with respect to body composition and physical activity. The shortcomings of each of these approaches are briefly discussed below.

Self-recording of energy intake depends on the cooperation of the volunteer, and the very act of recording energy intake may actually alter ingestive behavior, even in compliant volunteers who wish to "please" the investigator. Thus, recording food intake becomes an unreliable tool on which to base guidelines for determining energy needs. Several recent studies suggest consistent underreporting of actual energy intake when validated against measures of total daily energy expenditure from doubly labeled water (16–18). Data from our laboratory suggest a significant underreporting of energy intake by as much as 30% in older individuals, compared with measurement of daily energy expenditure (16). Underreporting was more pronounced in women (30%) than in men (15%). Thus, it is apparent that using measures of energy intake to estimate energy requirements lacks scientific credibility because of the uncertainty and unreliability of subject reporting.

An alternative method of estimating energy needs uses multiples of RMR (19). In this approach, estimates of daily energy expenditure are not derived directly but by a factorial approach in which RMR and the estimated energy expenditure from various physical activities are summed (20). This method suffers from a number of methodological problems. First, it does not consider the components of daily energy expenditure that contribute to individual variation in daily energy expenditure. These "neglected" components include *(a)* the TEF, which contributes approximately 10 to 15% of daily energy expenditure (21), and *(b)* the thermic effect of physical activity. Data from our laboratory showed that under free-living conditions, physical activity is highly variable in normal persons and can range from as low as 187 kcal/day to 1235 kcal/day (11, 16).

Furthermore, knowledge of RMR alone provides insufficient information for explaining variation in daily energy expenditure, as variation in RMR explains less than half of individual variation in daily energy expenditure (16).

Another "general method" of assessing energy needs is based on recommended daily allowances (22) (see Appendix Table II-A-2-a-1). The current RDAs divide the adult population into two age groups—those who are 19 to 50 years old and those 51 years old and older. The frequent use of the category of "51 and older" is recognized as inappropriate, because normal and diseased aging produces increased heterogeneity in almost all physiologic measurements. The physiologic status and energy requirements of individuals who are 50 to 60 years old are very different from those of persons who are 80 to 90 years old. Furthermore, the RDAs do not take into account energy recommendations for individuals who vary in physical activity or disease state. It is evident, however, that the use of a single energy value is far too crude an approach and should be abandoned for medical, nutritional, and planning purposes. These methods were necessitated, until recently, by the lack of a direct method to measure daily energy expenditure under free-living conditions.

The World Health Organization Consultative Panel has stated that future guidelines should be based on measurements of energy expenditure "if and when these became available" (19). As noted above, the doubly labeled water technique ($^{2}H_{2}{}^{18}O$) provides a measure of free-living energy expenditure. In the adult individual, daily energy expenditure defines the level of energy intake to maintain energy balance (23). Measurement of total daily energy expenditure with the doubly labeled water technique therefore acts as a proxy indicator of the amount of energy intake that is required to maintain energy balance and body energy stores.

ENERGY NEEDS OF SPECIFIC POPULATIONS

Below, we examine recent applications of doubly labeled water methodology in healthy and diseased older individuals to understand better daily energy requirements and the regulation of energy balance. We consider several diseases that are associated with negative energy balance and generalized wasting.

Heart Failure

Heart failure is an increasing important and frequent clinical problem, with the highest prevalence observed in the elderly (24). The incidence of heart failure increases 50-fold between the ages of 40 and 60 years. The unexplained loss of body weight and muscle mass are hallmark clinical features of end-stage congestive heart failure (25). It is unclear whether reduction in caloric intake or elevated caloric expenditure accounts for the negative energy balance and subsequent weight loss in advanced heart failure. Furthermore, daily energy requirements in heart failure are unknown.

Several studies have examined energy expenditure in heart failure. RMR, body composition, and dietary intake were examined in 20 heart failure patients with documented systolic dysfunction and compared with an age-matched cohort of 40 healthy elderly volunteers (26). RMR was measured by indirect calorimetric techniques and fat mass and fat-free mass were measured by dual-energy x-ray absorptiometry. Fat-free mass (lean body mass minus skeleton) was approximately 4 kg lower in heart failure patients, despite similar amounts of fat mass. Although lower fat-free mass was noted, the RMR was 18% higher in heart failure patients than in healthy controls (Fig. 5.2). These results suggest that heart failure patients have a higher RMR (for their metabolic size), which may contribute to their propensity for unexplained weight loss and musculoskeletal wasting.

Measurement of the RMR, however, only provides partial information on whether energy needs are indeed higher in congestive heart failure patients. Ultimately, the balance between daily energy expenditure and food intake regulates body composition in humans. Although recent work (26–28) provided evidence that resting energy requirements are higher in heart failure and that the magnitude of the increase in resting energy needs increases with symptom severity (27), it was unclear whether daily energy needs are higher in heart failure patients in their free-living environment. Accordingly, daily energy expenditure and physical activity were measured in free-living cachectic (12) and noncachectic (13) patients with heart failure and 50 healthy control volunteers, by doubly labeled water and indirect calorimetry methodology (29) (Table 5.3). As expected, fat mass and fat-free mass were lower in cachectic patients than in noncachectic patients and controls. Daily energy expenditure was lower ($P < .05$) in cachectic patients (1870 ± 347

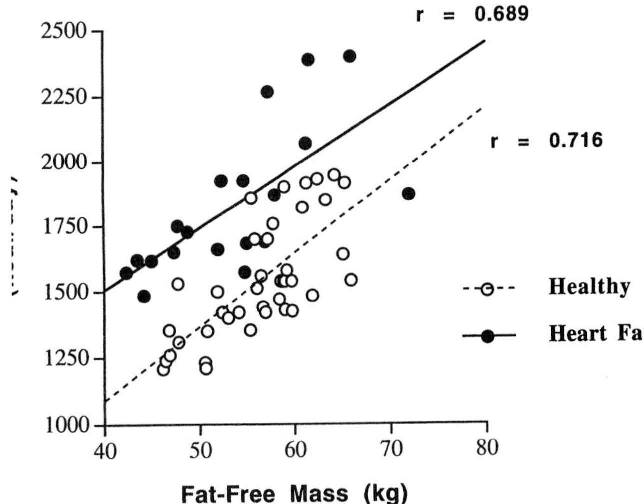

Figure 5.2. The relationship between resting metabolic rate and fat-free mass in healthy individuals and patients with heart failure. This figure shows that resting metabolic rate (per kg of fat-free mass) is higher in heart failure patients. (Adapted from Poehlman ET, Scheffers J, Gottlieb SS, et al. Ann Intern Med 1994;121:860–2).

Table 5.3
Daily Energy Expenditure,[a] Its Components and Energy Intake in Cachectic and Noncachectic Heart Failure Patients and Healthy Controls

Variable	Cachectic Patients	Noncachectic Patients	Healthy Controls
Daily energy expenditure (kcal/day)	1870 ± 347*	2349 ± 545	2543 ± 449
Resting metabolic rate (kcal/day)	1414 ± 210*	1698 ± 252	1561 ± 223
Physical activity energy expenditure	269 ± 307	416 ± 361	728 ± 223**

Adapted from Toth MJ, Gottlieb SS, Goran MI, et al. Am J Physiol 1997;272:E469–75.
[a]Values are mean ± SD.
* $P < .05$ less than noncachectic and healthy controls.
** $P < .05$ greater than noncachectic and cachectic.

kcal/day) than in noncachectic patients (2349 ± 545 kcal/day) and healthy controls (2543 ± 449 kcal/day) (Table 5.3). Differences in daily energy expenditure were due to lower ($P < .05$) free-living physical activity energy expenditure in cachectic (269 ± 307 kcal/day) and noncachectic patients (416 ± 361 kcal/day) compared with healthy controls (728 ± 374 kcal/day). Thus, the hypothesis that daily energy requirements are higher in heart failure patients is not supported by these initial studies using doubly labeled water methodology. Moreover, these findings underscore the need to measure daily energy expenditure in free-living patients accurately before drawing conclusions about the presence or absence of elevated daily energy expenditure and its relationship to weight loss. Because no evidence for an elevated daily energy expenditure in cachectic heart failure patients was found, the suggestion is that inadequate energy intake is a likely determinant of weight loss. Several factors including abdominal pain and distention, gastrointestinal hypomotility, and delayed gastric emptying have been suggested to contribute to anorexia in heart failure patients (25). The fact that daily energy expenditure was not elevated in noncachectic patients, however, argues against an elevated daily energy expenditure preceding weight loss.

Alzheimer's Disease

Alzheimer-type dementia, a growing health problem, is one of the leading causes of death among elderly people (30). The overall estimate is that more than 10% of persons over 65 suffer from senile dementia of the Alzheimer's type (31). Annual medical costs for Alzheimer's disease are estimated to be more than 40 billion dollars (32).

Unexplained weight loss is a frequent clinical finding in patients with Alzheimer's disease. The National Institute of Neurological and Communicative Disorders and Strokes Task Force on Alzheimer's Disease has included weight loss as a "clinical feature consistent with the diagnosis of Alzheimer's disease" (33). Moreover, it has been postulated that Alzheimer's disease may be characterized by dysfunction in body weight regulation (34).

Weight loss is due to a mismatch of energy intake with energy expenditure, which leads to low body weight, atrophy of muscle mass, and accelerated loss of functional independence in persons with Alzheimer's disease. Weight loss also increases the risks of decubitus ulcers, systemic infection, mortality, and greater consumption of health care resources (35, 36). Although it may not yet be possible to prevent, treat, or permanently alter the course of the underlying disease, identification and amelioration of nutritional problems may prove an ideal strategy for lessening the burden of the disease.

Is the energy imbalance associated with Alzheimer's disease caused by reduced energy intake, an elevated rate of energy expenditure, or a combination of both? Studies examining the caloric adequacy of diets of Alzheimer's patients as a potential contributor to weight loss (37–39) have yielded inconclusive results. This is not surprising, since the recording of food intake is an unreliable method that provides little useful information on an individual's actual habitual energy intake. Therefore, investigators have focused on the possibility that elevated energy expenditure contributes to unexplained weight loss in Alzheimer's patients. Several investigators found an elevated RMR in Alzheimer's patients, which might itself result in weight loss, (40–42), although these results remain controversial (43–46). A more important question, however, is whether free-living Alzheimer's patients have a higher daily energy expenditure than normal elderly persons.

Doubly labeled water methodology was used to examine the hypothesis that Alzheimer's patients are characterized by high levels of daily energy expenditure (47). Thirty Alzheimer's patients (73 ± 8 years of age; Mini-Mental score: 16 ± 8) and 103 healthy elderly persons (69 ± 7 years of age) were studied. Daily energy expenditure and its components (RMR and free-living physical activity) from doubly labeled water and indirect calorimetry were measured over a 10-day period. Fat-free mass tended to be lower in Alzheimer's patients (45 ± 9 kg) than in the healthy controls (49 ± 10 kg; $P = .07$), whereas no differences were noted in fat mass between groups. Daily energy expenditure was 14% lower in Alzheimer's patients (1901 ± 517 kcal/day) than in the controls (2213 ± 513 kcal/day; $P \leq .001$) because of a lower RMR (1287 ± 227 vs. 1418 ± 246 kcal/day; $P < .01$) and physical activity–related energy expenditure (425 ± 317 vs. 574 ± 342 kcal/day; $P < .05$) (Table 5.4). There were no differences between groups when energy expenditure was normalized for differences in fat-free mass. Thus, the lower energy expenditure in Alzheimer's patients is primarily due to their lower fat-free mass.

Daily energy expenditure was also examined in a subgroup ($N = 11$) of Alzheimer's patients who had lost significant body weight (5.6 ± 2.3 kg) within the previous year. A lower daily energy expenditure was found in

Table 5.4
Daily Energy Expenditure[a] and Its Components in Alzheimer's Patients and Healthy Elderly Persons

Variable	Alzheimer's Volunteers (N = 30)	Healthy Elderly (N = 103)
Daily energy expenditure (kcal/day)	1901 ± 517	2213 ± 513**
Resting metabolic rate (kcal/day)	1287 ± 227	1418 ± 246*
Physical activity energy expenditure (kcal/day)	425 ± 317	574 ± 342*

Adapted from Poehlman ET, Toth MJ, Goran MI, et al. Neurology 1997;997–1002.
[a]Values are listed as means ± SD.
*$P < .05$.
**$P < .01$.

cachectic Alzheimer's patients (1799 ± 474 kcal/day) than in noncachectic Alzheimer's patients (1960 ± 544 kcal/day) and healthy elderly controls (2213 ± 513 kcal/day; $P < .01$). Thus, daily energy expenditure is not higher, but lower in Alzheimer's patients, because of lower levels of resting and physical-activity–related energy expenditure and fat-free mass.

Collectively, the hypothesis that an increased daily energy expenditure contributes to weight loss in heart failure or Alzheimer's diseases is not supported by these findings. These findings, again, underscore the importance of assessing daily energy expenditure in free-living individuals before drawing conclusions regarding the presence or absence of a "hypermetabolic state."

Parkinson's Disease

Approximately 50% of patients afflicted with Parkinson's disease experience significant weight loss during the course of the disease. The suggestion has been made that inappropriately high levels of energy expenditure contribute to their unexplained weight loss. Several studies have compared differences in RMR between Parkinson's disease patients and an age-matched control population in an attempt to address this question. Several investigators (48–50) found an elevated RMR in Parkinson's disease patients, compared with healthy controls. The elevated RMR was at least partially attributed to tremor, rigidity, and a general dyskinesia in these patients.

More recently, total daily energy expenditure was assessed in Parkinson's patients to examine the hypothesis that free-living daily energy expenditure and its components (RMR and physical activity energy expenditure) are elevated (51). In contrast to the proposed hypothesis, daily energy expenditure was 15% lower in Parkinson's disease patients (2214 ± 460 kcal/day) than in healthy elderly controls (2590 ± 497 kcal/day). This was primarily due to lower physical activity energy expenditure (339 ± 366) in Parkinson's disease patients compared with that of the controls (769 ± 412 kcal/day). Thus, although excessive muscular activity in the form of rigidity and tremor may contribute to an elevated RMR (48–50), the overall effect of Parkinson's disease is to lower daily energy expenditure by reducing the energy expenditure associated with purposeful physical activity. Impairment of gain and movement associated with the signs and symptoms of Parkinson's disease probably promotes a reduction in physical activity.

The absence of an elevated daily energy expenditure suggests that an abnormally elevated daily energy expenditure is not a likely predisposing factor to weight loss. Thus, it is likely that a lower caloric intake is implicated in the weight loss of these patients. Swallowing disorders, impaired hand-to-mouth coordination, nausea, excessive saliva production, and delayed gastric emptying time may contribute to reduced energy intake in Parkinson's disease patients (52).

ACKNOWLEDGMENTS

Supported in part by a grant from the National Institute of Aging to ETP (RO1AG-07857), a Research Career and Development Award from the National Institute of Aging (KO4-AG00564) to ETP, Alzheimer's Association/Red Apple Companies Pilot Research Grants to ETP, GCRC RR-109 at the University of Vermont, and the American Association of Retired Persons Andrus Foundation to ETP.

REFERENCES

1. Holmes FL. Lavoisier and the chemistry of life. Madison: University of Wisconsin Press, 1985;3.
2. Voit E. Z Biol 1901;23:113–54.
3. Atwater W, Benedict F. 1905: Washington, DC: Carnegie Institute, publ no. 42, 1–193.
4. Benedict FG. Boston Med Surg J 1918;178:667–78.
5. Lusk G. The elements of the science of nutrition. 4th ed. Philadelphia: WB Saunders, 1928.
6. DuBois EF. Basal metabolism in health and disease. Philadelphia: Lea & Febiger, 1924.
7. Lifson N, Gordon GB, McClintock R. J Appl Physiol 1955;7: 704–10.
8. Lifson N, Little WS, Levitt DG, Henderson RM. J Appl Physiol 1975;39:657–64.
9. Schoeller DA, Ravussin E, Schutz Y, et al. Am J Physiol 1986: 250:R823–30.
10. Golay A, Schutz Y, Broquet C, et al. J Am Geriatr Soc 1983: 31:144–48.
11. Dauncey MJ. Can J Physiol Pharmacol 1990;68:17–27.
12. Horton ES. Energy intake and activity. In: Pollitt E, Amante P, eds. Current topics in nutrition and disease. New York: Alan R Liss, 1984;115–29.
13. Murgatroyd PR, Shetty PS, Prentice AM. Int J Obesity 1993;17: 549–68.
14. Schutz Y, Jequier E. Energy needs: assessment and requirements. In: Shils ME, ed. Modern nutrition in health and disease. 8th ed. Philadelphia: Lea & Febiger, 1994;101–11.
15. Elia M, Fuller N, Murgatroyd P. Proc Nutr Soc 1988;47:247–58.
16. Goran MI, Poehlman ET. Metabolism 1992;41:744–53.
17. Mertz W, Tsui JC, Judd JT, et al. Am J Clin Nutr 1991;54: 291–95.
18. Schoeller DA. Nutr Rev 1990;48:373–79.
19. World Health Organization, Food and Agriculture Organi-

zation, United Nations University. Energy and protein requirements. Geneva: World Health Organization, (Technical reports series, 724), 1985.
20. James WPT, Ferro-Luzzi A. Energy needs of the elderly: a new approach. In: Munro HN, Danford DE, eds. Human nutrition. A comprehensive treatise, vol 6: Nutrition, aging and the elderly. New York: Plenum Press, 1989;129–51.
21. Poehlman ET, Melby CL, Badylak SF. J Gerontol 1991;46: B54–8.
22. National Research Council. Recommended dietary allowances. 10th ed. Washington, DC: National Academy Press, 1989.
23. Schoeller DA. J Nutr 1988;118:1278–89.
24. Minotti J, Masie B. Circulation 1992;85:2323–5.
25. Pittman JG, Cohen P. N Engl J Med 1964:271:403–9.
26. Poehlman ET, Scheffers J, Gottlieb SS, et al. Ann Intern Med 1994;121:860–2.
27. Obisesan TO, Toth MJ, Donaldson K, et al. Am J Cardiol 1996;77:1250–3.
28. Riley M, Elborn JS, McKane WR, et al. Clin Sci 1991;80:633–9.
29. Toth MJ, Gottlieb SS, Goran MI, et al. Am J Physiol 1997;272:E469–75.
30. Council on Scientific Affairs: Dementia. JAMA 1985;256: 2234–8.
31. Evans DA, Funkenstein HH, Albert MS, et al. JAMA 1989; 262:2251–6.
32. Butler R. Bull NY Acad Med 1982;58:362–71.
33. McKhann G, Drachman D, Folstein M, et al. Neurology 1984;34:939–43.
34. White H, Pieper C, Schmader K, et al. J Am Geriatr Soc 1996;44:265–72.
35. Sandman PO, Adolfsson R, Nygren C, et al. J Am Geriatr Soc 1987;35:31–8.
36. Pinchcofsy-Devin GD, Kaminski JR. J Am Geriatr Soc 1986;34: 435–9.
37. Parvizi S, Nymon M. J Nutr Elderly 1982;2:15–9.
38. Bucht G, Sandman PO. Age Ageing 1990;19:S32–6.
39. Renvall MJ, Spindler AA, Ramsdell JW, et al. Am J Med Sci 1989;298:20–6.
40. Singh S, Mulley GP, Losowsky MS. Age Ageing 1988;17:21–8.
41. Adolfsson R, Bucht G, Lithner F, et al. Acta Med Scand 1989;208:387–8.
42. Wolf-Klein GP, Silverstone FA, Lansey SC, et al. Nutrition 1995;11:264–8.
43. Niskanen L, Piirainen M, Koljonen M. Age Ageing 1993;22: 132–7.
44. Prentice AM, Leavesley K, Murgatroyd PR, et al. Age Ageing 1989;18:158–67.
45. Donaldson KE, Carpenter WH, Toth MJ, et al. J Am Geriatr Soc 1996:44:1232–4.
46. Litchford MD, Wakefield LM. J Am Diet Assoc 1987;87:211–3.
47. Poehlman ET, Toth MJ, Goran MI, et al. Neurology 1997;48:997–1002.
48. Levi SL, Cox M, Lugon M, et al. Br Med J 1990;301:1256–7.
49. Brousselle E, Borson F, de Gonzalez JM, et al. Rev Neurol (Paris) 1991;147:46–51.
50. Markus H, Cox M, Tomkins A. Clin Sci 1992;83:199–204.
51. Toth MJ, Fishman PS, Poehlman ET. Neurology 1997;48:88–91.
52. Abbott RA, Cox M, Markus H, et al. Eur J Clin Nutr 1992;55:701–7.

SELECTED READINGS

Poehlman ET. Energy intake and energy expenditure in the elderly. Am J Hum Biol 1996;8:199–296.

Schwartz MW, Dallman MF, Woods SC. Hypothalamic response to starvation: implications for the study of wasting disorders. Am J Physiol 1995;269:R949–57.

6. Electrolytes, Water, and Acid-Base Balance

MAN S. OH and JAIME URIBARRI

REGULATION OF INTRA- AND EXTRACELLULAR VOLUME AND OSMOLALITY

The body fluid, an aqueous solution containing many electrolytes, consists of intracellular and extracellular compartments. The intracellular fluid is not a single large compartment; each cell has its own separate environment, communicating with other cells only via interstitial fluid and plasma. Consequently, cells in various tissues differ considerably in their solute content and concentrations.

Regardless of the nature of the solute and its electrical charge, however, osmotic equilibrium is maintained so that each particle of solute throughout the body is surrounded by the same number of water molecules. Since cell membranes are very permeable to water, osmolality is the same throughout the body fluids. Operation of normal metabolic functions of the body requires maintaining an optimal ionic strength in its environment, primarily the intracellular fluid, where most metabolic activities occur. The homeostatic mechanisms of the body are therefore constantly at work to provide such an environment.

Because the extracellular fluid (ECF) is not the site of major metabolic activity, substantial alteration in its ionic strength may occur without adverse effects on the body function. The main function of the ECF is to serve as a conduit between cells and between organs. The plasma is a route of rapid transit, and the interstitial fluid serves as a slow supply zone, which by flowing around the cell permits the entire cell surface to be used as an area of exchange. The ability of the ECF to function efficiently as a conduit requires maintenance of optimal extracellular volume, particularly of plasma volume, the vehicle of rapid transportation through the circulation.

An additional important function of the ECF is regulation of the intracellular volume and its ionic strength. Because of the requirement for osmotic equilibrium between the cells and the ECF, any alteration in extracellular osmolality is followed by an identical change in intracellular osmolality, which is usually accompanied by a reciprocal change in cell volume.

Although cells and organs can be supplied with substrate and relieved of metabolic products with a much slower circulation, normal circulation is required to supply sufficient oxygen for the body's metabolic needs. Normal plasma volume is a prerequisite for maintenance of normal circulation. Because plasma is in equilibrium with the interstitial fluid, the maintenance of normal plasma volume requires normal extracellular volume. A low extracellular volume can result in impaired organ perfusion, and an excessive extracellular volume may lead to vascular congestion and pulmonary edema.

Volumes of Body Fluid

Total body water can be determined by dilution of various substances including deuterium, tritium, and antipyrine. Total body water measured with antipyrine in hospitalized adults without fluid and electrolyte disorders is about 54% of the body weight. The fractional water content is higher in infants and children and decreases progressively with aging. The water content also depends on the body content of fat; women and obese persons, because of their higher fat content, tend to have less water for a given weight.

A useful short cut for calculation of total body water, using the fact that 54% of body weight in kg is body water, and 1 kg is 2.2 lb, is:

$$\text{Total body water (L)} = \text{Body weight (lb)}/4$$

For an obese subject, subtract 10% from the calculated body water, and for a lean person add 10%. For a very obese person, subtract 20%. Women have about 10% less body water than men for the same body weight.

Extracellular volume is measured directly, and the intracellular volume is estimated as the difference between total body water and extracellular volume. Measurement of total body water by dilution techniques is reproducible and reliable, but measurement of extracellular volume is not, because different markers have different volumes of distribution. Markers such as sodium, chloride, and bromide penetrate the cells to some extent, whereas markers such as mannitol, inulin, and sucrose do not penetrate certain parts of the ECF. Thus, depending on the type of marker used, ECF volume could vary from 27 to 53% of total body water (Table 6.1).

Extracellular volume measured with chloride and expressed as percentage of total body water varies from 42 to 53%, greater in older subjects and women. Extracellular volumes measured with inulin and sulfate are smaller, about 30 to 33% of total body water. For clinical application, a value of 40% of total body water will be considered to represent extracellular volume. Extracellular volume is further divided into three fractions: interstitial volume (28% of total body water), plasma volume (8%), and transcellular water volume (4%). Transcellular water includes luminal fluid of the gastrointestinal tract, the fluids of the central nervous system, fluid in the eye as well as the lubricating fluids at serous surfaces (Table 6.1).

Composition of Body Fluid

Extracellular Composition

The concentrations of electrolytes in plasma are easily measured and their values are well known. These concentrations increase by about 7% when expressed in plasma water, because about 7% of plasma is solids. Thus, plasma sodium is 140 meq/L but the concentration in plasma water is 151 meq/L. The concentrations of electrolytes in interstitial fluid differ from those in plasma because of differences in protein concentrations between plasma and interstitial fluid. The actual differences in electrolyte concentrations can be predicted by the Donnan equilibrium. With normal plasma protein concentrations, the concentrations of diffusible cations are higher in plasma water than in interstitial water by about 4%, while the concentrations of diffusible anions are lower in the plasma than in the interstitium by the same percentage. The concentrations of calcium and magnesium in the interstitial fluid are lower than the values predicted by the Donnan equilibrium, because these ions are substantially protein bound.

Interstitial fluid consists of two phases, the free phase and the gel phase. The latter is invested with a fibrous meshwork that is largely made up of collagen fibers that hold the cells together. A ground substance consists of glycosaminoglycans, which also limit the mobility of water, holding some of the bound water in an icelike lattice. That part of the interstitial fluid in the free form is what we usually regard as the free "interstitial fluid," which is a route for water and solutes from capillaries to lymphatics.

Intracellular Composition

While sodium, chloride, and bicarbonate are the main solutes in the ECF, potassium, magnesium, phosphate, and proteins are the dominant solutes in the cell. The intracellular concentrations of sodium and chloride cannot be measured accurately because of technical difficulties and are estimated by subtracting the extracellular amount from the total tissue value. Since concentrations of electrolytes in the ECF are high, a small error in extracellular water volume measurement causes a large error in the measurement of intracellular concentration of these ions. The concentration of bicarbonate is calculated from cell pH, and the bicarbonate concentration shown in Table 6.2 is based on the assumption that average cell pH is 7.0.

The electrolyte composition of intracellular fluid is not identical throughout the tissues. For example, the concentration of chloride in muscle is very low, about 3 meq/L, but it is 75 to 80 meq/L in erythrocytes. The concentration of potassium in the muscle cell is about 140 meq/L, but in the platelets only about 118 meq/L. The concentration of sodium in muscle and red blood cells is about 13 meq/L, but in leukocytes, about 34 meq/L. Because muscle represents the bulk of the body cell mass, it is customary to use the electrolyte concentration of the muscle cells as representative of the intracellular electrolyte concentration.

Because a substantial part of the anions inside the cell consists of polyvalent ions such as phosphate and protein, a total ionic concentration in the cell in meq/L is higher than that of the ECF, but osmolal concentrations of the extracellular and intracellular fluid are the same.

Table 6.1
Volumes of Body Fluid Compartments[a]

Intracellular volume	24 L (60%)
Extracellular volume	16.0 L (40%)
Interstitial volume	11.2 L (28%)
Plasma volume	3.2 L (8%)
Transcellular volume	1.6 L (4%)

[a]A normal man weighing 73 kg (160 lb) with 40 L of total body water is used as a model.

Osmolar Relations and Regulation

Measurement of Plasma Osmolality

The plasma osmolality can be measured with an osmometer or estimated as the sum of the concentration of all the solutes in the plasma. Because an osmometer does not distinguish between effective osmols and ineffective osmols, effective osmolality can only be estimated. Urea is the only ineffective osmol that has substantial con-

Table 6.2
Electrolyte Concentrations in Extracellular and Intracellular Fluids

	Plasma		Interstitial Fluid		Plasma Water		Cell Water in Muscle	
	(meq/L)	(mmol/L)	(meq/L)	(mmol/L)	(meq/L)	(mmol/L)	(meq/L)	(mmol/L)
Na^+	140	140	145.3	145.3	149.8	149.8	13	13
K^+	4.5	4.5	4.7	4.7	4.8	4.8	140	140
Ca^{2+}	5.0	2.5	2.8	2.8	5.3	5.3	1×10^{-7}	0.5×10^{-7}
Mg^{2+}	1.7	0.85	1.0	0.5	1.8	0.9	7.0	3.5
Cl^-	104	104	114.7	114.7	111.4	111.4	3	3
HCO_3^-	24	24	26.5	26.5	25.7	25.7	10	10
SO_4^{2-}	1	0.5	1.2	0.6	1.1	0.55	—	—
Phosphate	2	1.1[a]	2.3	1.3[a]	2.2	1.2[a]	107	57[b]
Protein	15	1	8	0.5	16	1	40	2.5[c]
Organic anions	5	5[d]	5.6	5.6[d]	5.3	5.3[d]	—	

[a]The calculation is based on the assumption that the pH of the extracellular fluid is 7.4 and the pK of H_2PO_4 is 6.8.
[b]The intracellular molal concentration of phosphate is calculated with the assumption that the pKs of organic phosphates are 6.1 and the intracellular pH 7.0.
[c]The calculation is based on the assumption that each mmol of intracellular protein has on average 15 meq, but the nature of cell proteins is not clearly known.
[d]The assumption is that all the organic anions are all univalent.

centration in the plasma. Still, its normal concentration is only 5 mosm/L. In the normal plasma, therefore, total osmolality is nearly equal to effective osmolality. Plasma osmolality is estimated as follows:

$$\text{Plasma osmolality} = \text{Plasma Na (meq/L)} \times 2 + \text{glucose (mg/dL)}/18 + \text{urea (mg/dL)}/2.8.$$

Many of the solutes that may accumulate abnormally in the body are anions of an acid (e.g., salicylate, glycolate, formate, lactate, β-hydroxybutyrate). These substances should not be added in estimating plasma osmolality, since they are largely balanced by sodium and therefore already included in the value when plasma sodium is multiplied by 2.

Nonelectrolyte solutes that accumulate abnormally in the serum, e.g., ethanol, isopropyl alcohol, ethylene glycol, methanol, and mannitol, will cause the measured osmolality to exceed the calculated osmolality, producing an osmolal gap. This osmolal gap is frequently a useful clinical clue to the presence of the toxic substances listed above. Accumulation of neutral and cationic amino acids can also cause a serum osmolal gap.

Control of Intracellular Volume: Concept of Effective Osmolality

When the osmolal concentration of the ECF increases by accumulation of solutes that are restricted to the ECF (e.g., glucose, mannitol, and sodium), osmotic equilibrium is reestablished as water shifts from the cell to the ECF, increasing intracellular osmolality to the same level as the extracellular osmolality. When the extracellular osmolality increases by accumulation of solutes that can enter the cell freely (e.g., urea and alcohol), the osmotic equilibrium is achieved by entry of those solutes into the cell. Such solutes are ineffective osmols. Since most of the solutes normally present in the ECF are effective osmols, loss of extracellular water will increase effective osmolality and hence cause water to shift from the cells. Reduction in extracellular osmolality either by loss of normal extracellular solutes or by retention of water reduces effective osmolality for the same reasons and hence causes water to shift into the cells.

Effect of Hyperglycemia on Serum Sodium. The permeability of a membrane for a given solute varies with the cell type. For example, glucose does not accumulate in the muscle. It does not enter the muscle cell freely, and when it enters the cell with the help of insulin, it is quickly metabolized. Thus, glucose is an effective osmol for the muscle cell (i.e., hyperglycemia will cause water to shift from the muscle cell). On the other hand, glucose is an ineffective osmol for red blood cells and liver and kidney cells, because it enters these cells freely. Glucose is generally categorized as an effective osmol because the muscle cells represent the largest body cell mass. Glucose enters some of the brain cells.

Accumulation of glucose or mannitol in the ECF is a well-known cause of hyponatremia. The relationship between change in serum sodium level and change in glucose concentration in a normal adult is about 1.5 meq/L of Na for 100 mg/dL of glucose. This figure is valid, however, only when the volume of distribution of glucose is somewhere between 40 and 50% of total body water. As the volume of distribution of glucose increases, the effect of glucose on serum sodium decreases progressively. Decreased volume of distribution of glucose has an opposite effect. The change in serum Na caused by hyperglycemia can be estimated with the following formula:

$$\Delta\text{Na (meq/L)} = (5.6 - 5.6a)/2,$$

where ΔNa is a reduction in serum Na in meq/L for each 100-mg increase in glucose, and a is the fraction of the volume of glucose distribution over total body water.

With marked expansion of extracellular volume (e.g., congestive heart failure and other edema-forming states), the volume of distribution of glucose represents a much greater fraction of total body water, and hence a fall in serum sodium caused by hyperglycemia would be much less than usual. For example, when the volume of distribution of glucose is 80% of total body water (0.8), the decrease in serum Na for 100 mg/dL rise in glucose would be only about 0.55 meq/L; $(5.5 - 5.5 \times 0.8)/2 = 0.55$. When the glucose volume is 20% of total body water, ΔNa would be 2.2 meq/L for 100 mg/dL increase in glucose.

Concept of Tonicity

In the strict sense, the tonicity of a solution is expressed only in reference to a physiologic system: a hypertonic solution is one that shrinks the cells, while a hypotonic solution causes them to swell. Tonicity may also be used to compare a given physiologic state with the normal state. The body fluid is called hypertonic if effective osmolality is increased, causing dehydration of the cells. When the term *tonicity* is applied to a fluid in vitro, it is used almost interchangeably with total osmolality. Thus, a solution that contains a high concentration of urea is called hypertonic. Similarly, urine is said to be hypertonic if its osmolality is high, regardless of the nature of its solute.

Osmolality and Specific Gravity

Whereas osmolality of fluid depends on osmolal concentration of its solute, specific gravity is determined by the weight of the solute relative to the volume it occupies in solution. Plasma protein contributes little to osmolality because of its low molal concentration, but it is the major factor determining specific gravity of plasma. Urinary specific gravity and osmolality usually change in parallel, but discrepancy between the two occurs with heavy proteinuria and severe glycosuria.

Signs and Symptoms of Abnormal Cell Volume and Electrolyte Concentrations

A variety of signs and symptoms appear with an increase or decrease in effective osmolality, which is accompanied by a reciprocal change in intracellular volume. Whether these manifestations are caused by abnormal cell volume or abnormal tonicity is not clearly known. Some clinical manifestations are probably caused by cell swelling and shrinkage.

In contrast, some cerebral manifestations of hyper- and hypoosmolality may persist even after the brain cell volume has been restored to normal. Since restoration of normal brain cell volume may not normalize electrolyte concentration, the persisting signs and symptoms may be attributed to abnormal electrolyte concentration in the brain cells rather than to the abnormal brain cell volume. The fact that some of the most serious cerebral manifestations of altered osmolality are related to brain cell volume and that brain cells have the capacity to regulate their volume with time may help explain why the rapidity as well as the extent of alteration in osmolality are important determinants of severity of symptoms.

Signs and Symptoms of Hypoosmolality. For obvious reasons, hypoosmolality without hyponatremia is physiologically impossible. There is no evidence that a reduced concentration of sodium ion in the extracellular fluid, without low effective osmolality, causes any adverse effect, except in the presence of severe hyperkalemia. Thus, when hyponatremia is caused by hyperglycemia or mannitol administration, the signs and symptoms are those of hyperosmolality and cell dehydration. When moderate hyponatremia is caused by salt depletion, some of the symptoms such as easy fatigability and muscle cramps and spasms attributed to hyponatremia, may be due at least in part to reduced effective vascular volume.

Most of the signs and symptoms of hyponatremia, which include nausea, vomiting, headache, papilledema, and mental confusion, originate in the central nervous system and are clearly due to brain swelling and increased intracranial pressure. Lethargy, weakness, hyper- and hyporeflexia, delirium, coma, psychosis, focal weakness, ataxia, aphasia, generalized rigidity, and seizure are probably caused by increased cell volume and reduced electrolyte concentration of the brain cells.

Gastrointestinal manifestations include abdominal cramps, temporary loss of sense of taste and flavor, decreased appetite, nausea, vomiting, salivation, and paralytic ileus. Cardiovascular effects of hypoosmolality are usually manifested as hypotension and other signs of low effective vascular volume. Hyponatremia can also be accompanied by muscle cramps, twitching, and rigidity, but these muscular manifestations may still result from hypoosmolality.

Signs and Symptoms of Hyperosmolality. Increased effective osmolality need not be accompanied by hypernatremia. Accumulation of effective solutes other than sodium salts in the extracellular fluid can cause hyperosmolality and cell dehydration but may be accompanied by normal or low serum sodium concentration. However, hypernatremia is always accompanied by hyperosmolality and cell dehydration. Since alteration of the concentration of sodium ion does not produce profound physiologic effects, any clinical signs and symptoms of hypernatremia are likely to be those of hyperosmolality and cell dehydration. Hence, if hyperosmolality is caused by glucose, mannitol, or glycerol, clinical manifestations will mimic those of hypernatremia despite the low serum sodium concentration.

As in the hypoosmolal states, the symptoms and signs of hyperosmolality depend on the rapidity of its development as well as the severity of hyperosmolality. A patient may be comatose when the serum sodium reaches 160 meq/L rapidly, whereas the patient may remain conscious with a serum sodium concentration of 190 meq/L if hypernatremia occurs gradually.

Most of the symptoms and signs of hyperosmolality are those that originate in the central nervous system. Acute hyperosmolality due to hypernatremia both in human subjects and in animals can lead to subdural, cortical, and subarachnoid hemorrhages because of sudden shrinkage of the brain cells. Depression of mental state ranges from lethargy to coma. Generalized seizure is also observed, although somewhat less commonly than in hypoosmolality. Muscular symptoms of hyperosmolality include muscular rigidity, tremor, myoclonus, hyperreflexia, spasticity, and rhabdomyolysis. In children, spasticity, chronic seizure disorder, and retardation of mental development may occur with chronic hyperosmolality.

Regulation of Intracellular Volume

When cells swell in response to extracellular hypoosmolality, the regulatory mechanism that works to reduce cellular solute content and thereby reduce their volume is referred to as volume regulatory decrease (VRD). In shrunken cells, the volume regulatory mechanisms work to increase the solute content of the cells and thereby increase their volume; this process is termed volume regulatory increase (VRI). Most cells are capable of volume regulation with both VRD and VRI. In contrast, the muscle cells do not have volume regulatory mechanisms.

Red blood cells of all species studied so far have shown a capacity to regulate the cell volume, but different species seem to use different mechanisms for volume regulation. In general, VRD in blood cells is achieved by loss of electrolytes, namely NaCl and KCl. The initial defense against brain swelling in hyponatremia also seems to include osmotic inactivation as well as osmotic disequilibrium; the brain osmolality is significantly higher than that of serum in animals made acutely hyponatremic in 2 hours.

As in the case of VRD, different species use different mechanisms to achieve VRI. VRI is accounted for by increases in Na, K, and Cl but also by other osmols, which have been collectively termed *idiogenic osmols*. However, since the nature of most of these osmols is now well known, such terminology is inappropriate.

The total contribution of electrolytes to the changes in tissue osmolality in the presence of hyperosmolality is estimated to be about 50 to 60%, and the remainder is accounted for by organic solutes. There are three major classes of organic substances that participate in VRI: polyols (sorbitol and myoinositol), methylamines (betaine and glycerophosphotidylcholine), and amino acids (taurine, glutamine, glutamic acid, aspartic acid). Among the organic solutes, amino acids are most important for VRI.

Unlike the muscle cells whose volumes remain chronically altered as long as effective osmolality is abnormal, brain cells can restore the volume to normal when effective osmolality remains chronically altered (Figs. 6.1 and 6.2). In acute hyponatremia, the brain cell volume is initially increased. If the hypoosmolal state persists, the brain cell volume is normalized over a few days, as the cellular solute content decreases. Sudden normalization of osmolality from a chronic hypoosmolal state then causes extracellular shift of water and hence shrinkage of the brain to a subnormal level. Similarly, in a chronic hyperosmolal state, brain volume is normalized by increasing total solute content of the brain, and a sudden reduction in osmolality from a chronic hyperosmolal state can therefore cause brain swelling.

Regulation of Extracellular Volume

Because the extracellular sodium concentration is maintained within a fairly narrow range through regulation of antidiuretic hormone (ADH) release, the extracellular volume depends primarily on its sodium content. In most clinical situations, the extracellular volume correlates well with vascular volume, which in turn correlates positively with the effective vascular volume, an imaginary volume that correlates with the cardiac output in relation to the tissue's demand for oxygen.

Hence, the main efferent mechanisms for regulation of extracellular volume are designed to sense the changes in effective vascular volume rather than the extracellular volume or vascular volume. This situation sometimes leads to a pathologic retention of salt. For example, salt is retained in congestive heart failure despite markedly expanded extracellular volume and vascular volume, because *effective* vascular volume is reduced.

Theoretically, there are two ways to alter the salt content of the body: to alter the intake of salt and to alter

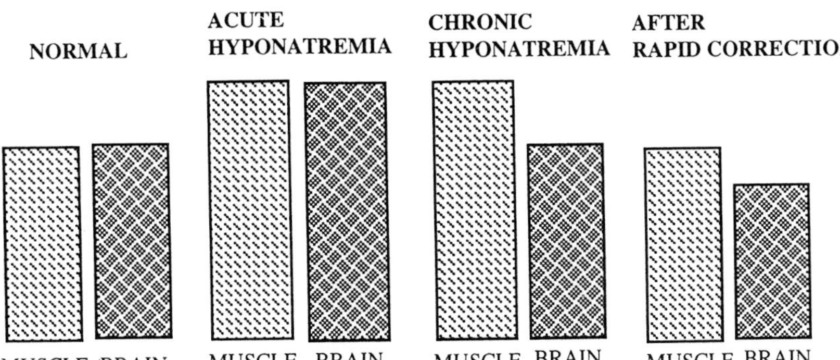

Figure 6.1. Cell volume regulation in hyponatremia. Note that both brain and muscle cell volume are increased in acute hyponatremia; in chronic hyponatremia, brain cell volume returns to normal, while muscle cell volume remains increased. With rapid correction of hyponatremia, muscle cell volume returns to normal, and brain becomes dehydrated.

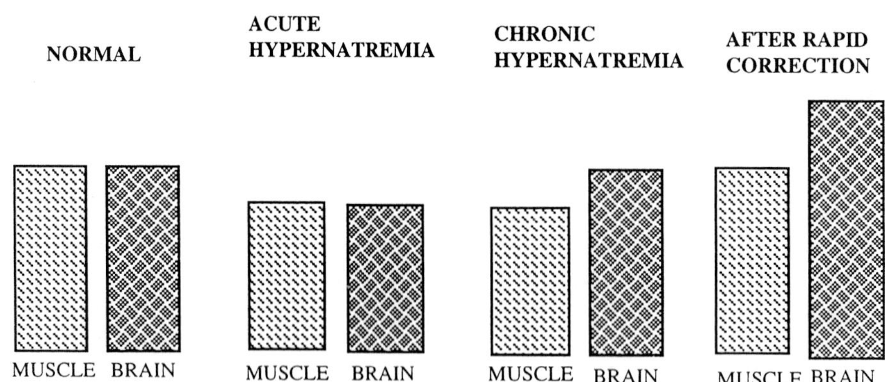

Figure 6.2. Cell volume regulation in hypernatremia. In acute hypernatremia, both muscle and brain cell volumes are reduced; in chronic hypernatremia, brain volume returns to normal. Rapid correction of hypernatremia normalizes muscle cell volume but causes brain edema.

renal salt output. There is no well-developed mechanism to change the behavior of salt intake in response to changes in effective vascular volume. Thus, the salt content of the body is altered primarily through changes in renal salt output, which can be achieved through physical and humoral factors. The physical factors for renal salt regulation work through changes in glomerular filtration rate (GFR) or changes in peritubular capillary oncotic and hydrostatic pressures. Humoral factors work primarily through their effects on renal tubular salt reabsorption, either by increasing or decreasing it, but they can also work via effects on physical factors. Figure 6.3 shows the nomenclature of the nephron sites, and Figure 6.4 summarizes various salt reabsorption mechanisms at different nephron sites.

A number of humoral factors are proven or suggested to participate in regulating renal salt output. Among these, those that have well-proven physiologic effects are aldosterone, catecholamines, angiotensin II, and perhaps ADH and prostaglandins. The proof for the physiologic relevance of some other hormones such as atrial natriuretic peptide, urodilatin, guanylin, uroguanylin, kallekreins and kinins, insulin, and glucagon is not very convincing at the moment. Figure 6.5 summarizes the regulation of effective vascular volume by various humoral and physical factors that affect renal output of salt.

Nonrenal Control of Water and Electrolyte Balance

Water is lost from the skin primarily as a means of eliminating heat. Water loss from the skin without sweat is called insensible perspiration. Sweat contains about 50 meq/L of sodium and 5 meq/L of potassium. Because the main purpose of water loss from the skin is elimination of

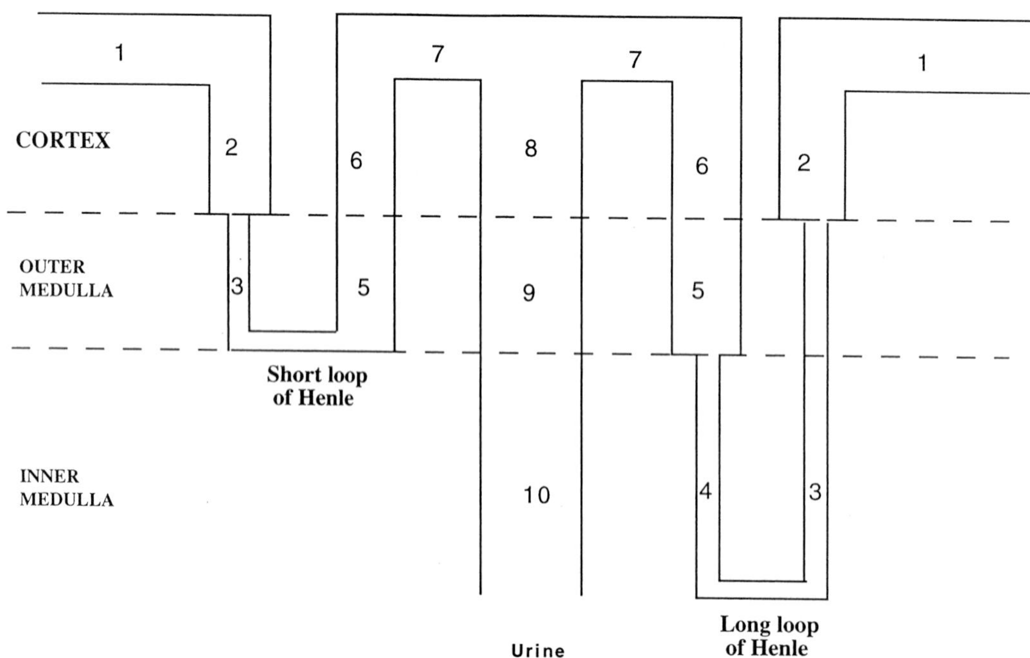

Figure 6.3. Anatomy of nephron. *1,* proximal convoluted tubule; *2,* proximal straight tubule; *3,* thin descending limb of Henle; *4,* thin ascending limb of Henle; *5,* medullary thick ascending limb of Henle; *6,* cortical thick ascending limb of Henle; *7,* distal convoluted tubule; *8,* cortical collecting duct; *9,* outer medullary collecting duct; *10,* inner medullary collecting duct.

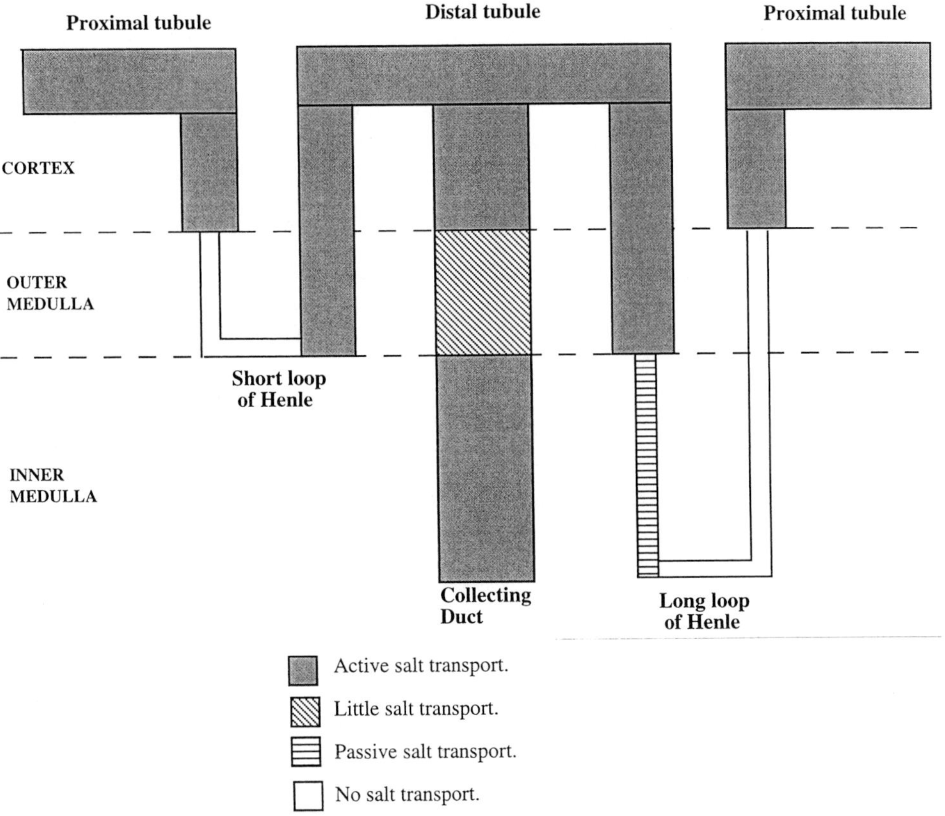

Figure 6.4. Salt transport in various nephron sites. *Solid,* active salt transport; *diagonal lines,* little salt transport; *horizontal lines,* passive salt transport; *clear areas,* no salt transport.

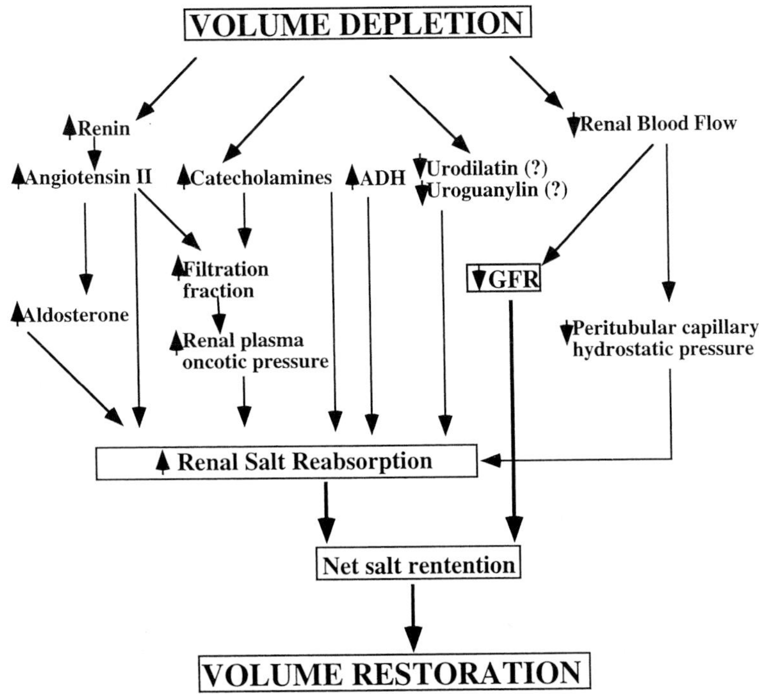

Figure 6.5. Regulation of effective vascular volume. Volume depletion leads to net renal salt retention, which in turn leads to restoration of volume. Net renal salt retention is achieved by increased renal salt transport and reduction of GFR. Increased renal salt transport is achieved by activation of humoral agents and physical factors. Among the humoral agents with well-proven physiologic effects are *aldosterone, angiotensin II, catecholamines,* and *ADH.* Physiologic impact of reduced production or *urodilatin* and *uroguanylin* is unclear. Physical factors that contribute to renal salt retention include decreased *peritubular hydrostatic pressure* and increased *plasma oncotic pressure.* Reduced renal plasma flow results in reduced GFR.

heat, water loss from the skin depends mainly on the amount of heat generated:

Water loss from the skin = 30 mL per 100 calories.

The water content of inspired air is less than that of expired air; hence, water is lost with respiration. Because the ventilatory volume is determined by the amount of CO_2 production, which is in turn determined by the caloric expenditure, the ventilatory water loss in normal environmental conditions also depends on caloric expenditure:

Respiratory water loss
= 13 mL per 100 calories at normal pCO_2.

By coincidence, the quantity of water lost during normal respiration is about equal to the metabolic water production. Hence, in calculating water balance, respiratory water loss may be ignored in the measurement of insensible water loss, provided that metabolic water gain is also ignored. Respiratory water loss increases with hyperventilation or fever, disproportionately to metabolic water production.

The net activity of the gastrointestinal (GI) tract to the level of the jejunum is secretion of water and electrolytes. The net activity from jejunum to colon is reabsorption. Most of the fluid entering the small intestine is absorbed there, and the remainder by the colon, leaving only about 100 mL of water to be excreted daily in the feces. The contents of the GI tract are isotonic with plasma, and any fluid that enters the GI tract becomes isotonic via secretion and reabsorption. Thus, if water is ingested and vomited, solute is lost from the body.

Routes of Fluid and Electrolyte Loss

Fluid and electrolytes may be lost from the GI tract for a variety of reasons such as diarrhea, vomiting or gastric drainage, and drainage or fistula from the bile ducts, pancreas, and intestine. Although diarrheal fluid is usually isotonic in terms of cations (Na and K), diarrhea caused by nonabsorbable solutes (e.g., lactulose, mannitol, sorbitol, or disaccharides, as in a patient with disaccharide malabsorption) causes greater water loss than electrolyte loss. Diarrheal fluid usually contains substantial amounts of bicarbonate and potassium; hence diarrhea tends to cause metabolic acidosis and hypokalemia. Because vomitus contains HCl, vomiting tends to produce metabolic alkalosis. The amount of HCl depends on the rate of acid secretion; when acid secretion is maximally stimulated, the concentration of HCl is about 100 meq/L. Because gastric fluid contains little Na in relation to water, vomiting without fluid intake tends to cause hypernatremia.

Obstruction of the bowel may cause transfer of fluid from the extracellular space into the intestinal lumen. Since the composition of the sequestered fluid is similar to that of the extracellular fluid, effective arterial volume will be reduced without much alteration in composition. The patient may give evidence of extracellular volume depletion without weight loss.

The loss through skin increases with fever, increased metabolism, sweating, and burns. The fluid lost through the skin is markedly hypotonic.

Water is lost through the lung with ventilation, and the amount depends on the ventilatory volume. Fever and hyperventilation increase water loss through the lung.

The kidney may lose sodium excessively in a number of situations, including diuretic therapy, aldosterone deficiency or unresponsiveness, and relief of urinary tract obstruction.

Miscellaneous losses include drainage from the pleural and peritoneal cavity, seepage from burns and transected lymphatics, and fluid loss during hemo- and peritoneal dialysis.

Types of Dehydration

Depending on the quantity of salt loss in relation to water loss, several types of dehydration are encountered. The net alteration in body composition is determined by the sum of the losses and gains. The net change in dehydration may be *(a)* isotonic dehydration, in which net salt and water loss are equal; *(b)* hypertonic dehydration, with loss of water alone or water in excess of salt; or *(c)* hypotonic dehydration, in which salt loss exceeds water loss (Fig. 6.6).

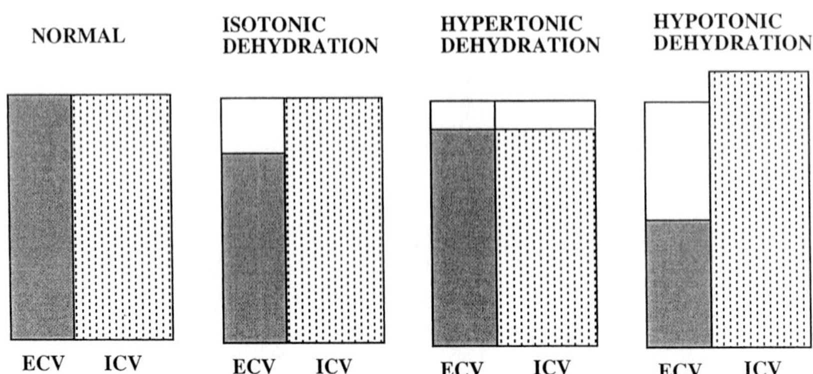

Figure 6.6. Changes in extracellular volume *(ECV)* and intracellular volume *(ICV)* in different types of dehydration. Note that for the same amount of total body water loss, ECV is lowest in hypotonic dehydration.

Isotonic Dehydration. Salt may be lost isotonically through the GI tract or directly from the ECF by aspiration of pleural effusion, ascites, etc. With GI fluid loss, salt is lost with an equal or larger water loss, and the osmolality of the body fluids is subsequently adjusted to isotonicity by oral intake of salt or urinary excretion of water. Isotonic fluid loss is borne completely by the extracellular fluid space. Treatment calls for isotonic salt solution.

Hypertonic Dehydration. The primary aberration in hypertonic dehydration is water deficit. Two major mechanisms account for abnormal water deficit: inadequacy of water intake and excessive water loss. Dehydration due to excessive water loss usually develops more rapidly than that due to reduced water intake. Inadequacy of water intake is always caused by either *(a)* defective thirst due to a defective thirst center or impaired consciousness or *(b)* lack of water or an inability to drink water.

Water loss may occur through the kidney (e.g., osmotic diuresis and diabetes insipidus) or through the nonrenal routes (e.g., sweating, osmotic diarrhea, vomiting of HCl). Loss of HCl with water is almost equivalent to the loss of pure water for the Na balance, since it leaves sodium bicarbonate behind replacing sodium chloride in the ECF.

Even when excessive water loss is the cause of hypertonic dehydration, one of the conditions that limit water intake must be present to maintain hypertonicity. Otherwise, stimulation of thirst by increased osmolality will lead to increased water drinking and correction of the hypernatremia.

Salt content of the body in hypertonic dehydration may be normal, increased, or decreased, and the extent of extracellular volume depletion depends on the degree of salt retention. On the other hand, intracellular volume depletion depends solely on the magnitude of hypertonicity. Salt administered or ingested in a state of water deficit is retained, resulting in increased salt content in the body.

The water required to lower the serum sodium concentration to a desired level can be determined with the following formula:

$$\text{Water requirement} = (\text{actual Na}/\text{goal Na} - 1) \times \text{TBW} = \Delta\text{Na}/\text{goal Na} \times \text{TBW}$$

where ΔNa is the difference between the actual and goal sodium concentration.

Water requirement calculated using this formula is based on the assumption that water is lost without gain or loss of salt. If salt retention is part of the reason for the hypernatremia, administering the total amount calculated by the above formula will overexpand volume. However, if the kidney is functioning normally, the excess salt and water will be excreted.

Rapid correction of hypernatremia to normal levels offers no advantage and is potentially harmful, as it may cause brain edema. It is advisable to reduce serum sodium at a rate no greater than 0.7 meq/L/h, or 10% of actual serum Na per day; in acute hypernatremia, the speed of correction can be faster.

Hypotonic Dehydration. Fluids lost from the body, especially GI tract loss, are almost always either hypotonic or isotonic in relation to serum sodium concentration, and loss of such fluid cannot cause hypotonicity of body fluid. Hypotonic dehydration usually occurs because the patient loses a salt solution and replaces it with water or with a solution containing less sodium and potassium than the fluid that has been lost.

In the presence of normal renal function, net loss of salt alone is difficult to achieve because the resultant hyponatremia would suppress ADH, resulting in water loss. Decreased effective vascular volume then causes the release of ADH to prevent further depletion of the extracellular volume, and hyponatremia develops.

Hypoosmolality of the ECF causes a shift of water into the cells to achieve osmotic equilibrium. Hence cell volume is increased despite extracellular volume contraction. Patients with hypotonic dehydration may thus show more evidence of compromised circulation for a given degree of body water loss than do patients with isotonic or hypertonic dehydration (Fig. 6.6). In addition, acute hyponatremia per se may also diminish vascular tone and cardiac output.

Hypotonic dehydration may be treated by estimating the amount of salt needed to restore the osmolality of the body fluids to normal, administering this amount of salt in the form of hypertonic saline, and adding normal saline to restore the extracellular volume. The sodium requirement to increase serum sodium concentration is calculated with the following equation:

$$\text{Na requirement} = \Delta\text{Na} \times \text{TBW (in L)},$$

where ΔNa is desired serum Na − actual serum Na.

Even though the administered sodium would be distributed mainly in the ECF, total body water is used for this calculation because an increase in serum Na is accompanied by an exactly proportionate increase in serum osmolality (Na × 2 = osmolality). Estimation of the amount of solutes required to increase serum osmolality must always be based on total body water, because extracellular osmolality cannot be increased without increasing intracellular osmolality to the same extent.

As an alternative therapeutic approach, one can raise serum Na levels with isotonic or hypotonic saline; as ECF volume increases, ADH is suppressed; as free water is excreted, serum sodium levels return to normal. This approach is recommended in patients who suffer more from hypovolemia than from hypotonicity. In patients with chronic hyponatremia, rapid correction of hyponatremia may be particularly dangerous because of the possible occurrence of central pontine myelinolysis, a demyelinating disease primarily of the central pons, which causes severe motor nerve dysfunction, e.g., quadriplegia. This complication is more likely to occur with rapid treatment of chronic hyponatremia than with acute hyponatremia. The complication may be avoided by increasing serum sodium more slowly (no faster than 8 meq/24 h; about 0.35 meq/h). Although hypertonic saline is the main culprit, administration of isotonic saline may also cause rapid correction of hyponatremia and central pontine myelinolysis.

Principles of Fluid Therapy

Goals of Salt and Water Replacement. The goal of therapy is to restore the patient to a state of normal hemodynamics and normal body fluid osmolality. There are several components in the program of water and electrolyte therapy: *(a)* existing deficits must be identified and made up; *(b)* daily basal requirements for sodium, potassium, and water must be supplied; and *(c)* ongoing losses must be quantified and provided for. Short-term parenteral therapy does not require inclusion of calcium, phosphate, and magnesium.

Basal Requirements. The basal requirement for water depends on sensible (urinary) and insensible losses of water. Fever increases respiratory water loss by increasing the vapor pressure of the expired air and increases loss of water from the skin by increasing the vapor pressure on the skin surface and the basal metabolic rate. Urinary loss of water depends on the total amount of solute excreted and urine osmolality. Solute excretion depends mainly on salt ingestion and protein intake, but sometimes the water requirement may be increased by severe glycosuria.

Daily Water Requirements. In the absence of fever and sweating, water loss through the skin is relatively fixed, but urinary water excretion varies greatly and depends on the total amount of solute to be excreted and urine osmolality. For example, if the total solute excretion is 600 mosm/day, the urine volume will be 500 mL if urine is concentrated to 1200 mosm/L and 15 L if urine osmolality is 40 mosm/L. For such a person, the minimum water requirement would be 1100 mL (500 mL for urinary water loss plus 600 mL for skin water loss at 2000 cal/day). On the other hand, the maximal allowable water intake would be 15.6 L. If the concentration mechanism is impaired and the kidney can increase urine osmolality to only 600 mosm/L, the minimum water requirement would be 1.6 L. Similarly, impaired urine dilution reduces the maximum allowable water intake. If urine can be diluted to only 300 mosm/L, the maximal allowable water intake decreases to 2.6 L (600/300 + 0.6).

Clearly, in the absence of abnormal urine concentration and dilution, a large range of water intake causes neither dehydration nor overhydration. However, for a variety of reasons, underestimating water requirement is safer than overestimating. First, the excessive amount of water gained with impaired urine dilution tends to be greater than the water deficit resulting from impaired urine concentration. Second, clinically, impaired urine dilution (e.g., syndrome of inappropriate ADH secretion [SIADH]) is more common than impaired urine concentration. Finally, if the patient is conscious, hypernatremia has thirst as an effective defense mechanism, whereas patients with severe hyponatremia often lapse into coma without warning.

Clinical problems and answers for this section are presented before the selected readings.

DISORDERS OF POTASSIUM METABOLISM

Total body K^+ in hospitalized adults is about 43 meq/kg body weight, and only about 2% of this is found in the ECF. The gradient of K concentration across the cell membrane determines the membrane potential (Em) according to the Nernst equation:

$$Em = -60 \log \text{intracellular } K^+/\text{extracellular } K^+$$

Intracellular K^+/extracellular K^+ is normally about 30, and therefore the normal Em is −90 mv.

The membrane potential tends to increase with hypokalemia and to decrease with hyperkalemia. In hypokalemia, both intra- and extracellular K^+ tend to decrease, but the extracellular concentration tends to decrease proportionately more than the intracellular concentration. Hence, intracellular K^+/extracellular K^+ tends to increase. In hyperkalemia, this ratio tends to decrease for the same reason.

Potassium Flux and Excretion

Control of Transcellular Flux of Potassium

Transmembrane electrical gradients cause diffusion of cellular K^+ out of cells and Na^+ into cells. Since the Na^+-K^+ ATPase pump, which reverses this process, is stimulated by insulin and β-catechols (through β_2-adrenergic receptors), alterations in levels of these hormones can affect K^+ transport and its serum levels. Efflux of K^+ can also be stimulated by acidosis and a rise in effective osmolality (Fig. 6.7). The effect of acidosis and alkalosis on transcellular K^+ flux depends not only on the pH but also on the type

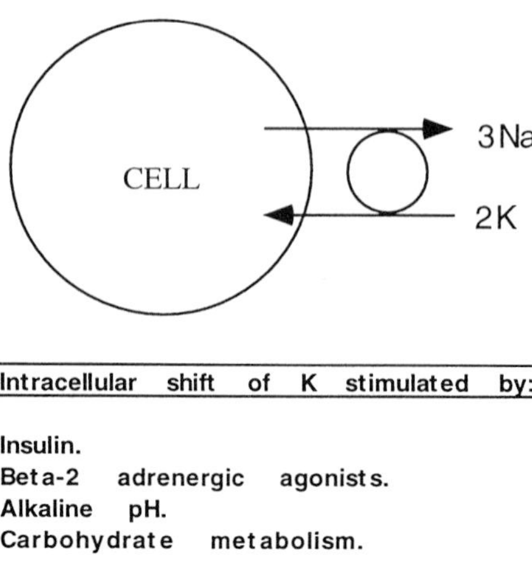

Figure 6.7. Transcellular shift of potassium.

of anion that accumulates. In general, metabolic acidosis causes greater K^+ efflux than respiratory acidosis. Metabolic acidosis due to inorganic acids (e.g., sulfuric acid and hydrochloric acid) causes greater K^+ efflux than that due to organic acids (e.g., lactic acid and keto acids). Acidosis causes efflux of K^+ from the cell because of a shift of H^+ into the cell in exchange for K^+. A modifying factor appears to be the anion accumulation in the cells. In organic acidosis, much H^+ entering the cell is balanced by organic anions, lactate and ketone anions, and therefore efflux of K^+ is prevented. In respiratory acidosis, bicarbonate accumulates in the cell to balance the incoming H^+. Alkalosis tends to lower serum K^+ levels. As with acidosis, K^+ influx varies with the type of alkalosis. In respiratory alkalosis, probably because of a drop in cellular bicarbonate concentration, K^+ influx is lower than in metabolic alkalosis. When pH is kept normal with increased concentration of bicarbonate and pCO_2, K^+ tends to move into the cells; accumulation of bicarbonate in the cell must be accompanied by Na^+ and K^+. Similarly, when pH is kept normal with low bicarbonate and low pCO_2, K^+ tends to move out of the cells.

Control of Renal Excretion of Potassium

About 90% of the daily K^+ intake (60–100 meq) is excreted in the urine, and 10% in the stools. Potassium filtered at the glomerulus is largely (70–80%) reabsorbed by active and passive mechanisms in the proximal tubule. In the ascending limb of Henle's loop, K^+ is further reabsorbed together with Na^+ and Cl, so that a very small amount is delivered into the distal nephron. The K^+ appearing in the urine is largely what has been secreted into the cortical collecting duct by mechanisms shown in Figure 6.8.

Na^+-K^+ ATPase located on the basolateral side of the cortical collecting duct pumps K into the cell while it pumps Na^+ out of the cell. Luminal Na enters the cell through Na channels, providing a continuous supply of Na. Because Na that has entered the cell and is then pumped out to the peritubular space is not followed one to one by Cl^-, an excess negative charge develops in the lumen, and K^+ is passively secreted through specialized K^+ channels to balance this charge. Aldosterone increases K^+ secretion by increasing passive entry of Na^+ from the lumen to the cell, thereby stimulating Na^+-K^+ ATPase activity. Aldosterone also stimulates Na^+-K^+ ATPase activity directly and increases passive K^+ secretion by enhancing the activity of the K^+ channel. The peritubular K^+ concentration and pH also influence K^+ secretion through their effects on Na^+-K^+ ATPase activity. High serum K^+ concentration and alkaline pH stimulate the enzyme activity, and low serum K^+ and acidic pH inhibit the activity.

Anions that accompany Na^+ and that penetrate the tubular membrane less readily than Cl^- allow greater luminal negativity and hence greater K^+ secretion. Examples of such anions include sulfate, bicarbonate, and anionic antibiotics such as penicillin and carbenicillin. Bicarbonate in the tubular fluid has an additional effect of enhancing potassium secretion apart from being a poorly reabsorbable anion. The luminal bicarbonate concentration is the main determinant of the luminal pH in the cortical collecting duct, and a high luminal bicarbonate concentration, through its effect on pH, increases K^+ secretion by the enhanced luminal K^+ channel activity. A marked increase in renal K^+ excretion in patients who vomit may be explained by this mechanism. ADH also appears to increase luminal K^+ channel activity. If tubular K^+ is washed away by rapid urine flow, more K^+ is secreted to satisfy the electrical gradient. Renal K^+ wasting during osmotic diuresis could be explained by this mechanism. The more Na^+ is presented to the distal nephron, the more can be absorbed and more K^+ secreted "in exchange." Increased Na^+ delivery to the collecting duct also increases renal K^+ excretion by its effect on urine flow. Figure 6.8 summarizes factors that influence K^+ secretion in the collecting duct.

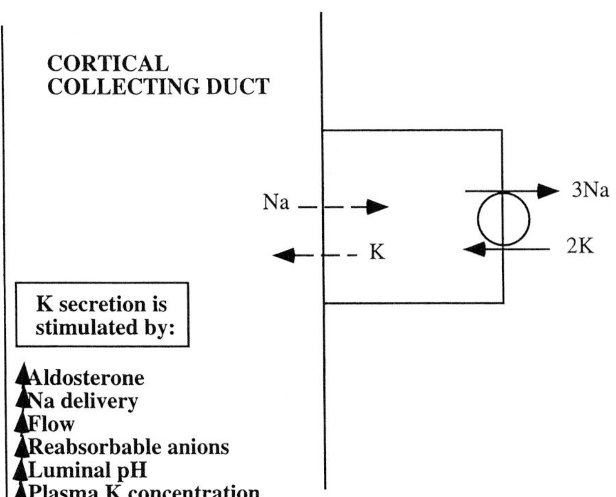

Figure 6.8. Factors that regulate K secretion in the collecting duct include high concentrations of plasma aldosterone, increased delivery of Na to the nephron site, increased urine flow, hyperkalemia, and increased concentrations of poorly reabsorbable anions such as sulfate and bicarbonate. Alkaline luminal pH also stimulates K secretion.

Plasma Renin Activity (PRA), Plasma Aldosterone Concentration (PA), and Abnormalities in K^+ Metabolism

Because abnormalities in PRA and PA are frequently either responsible for, or caused by, abnormalities in K^+ metabolism, it is important to understand their relationships. In general

1. Expansion of effective arterial volume caused by primary increase in aldosterone (primary aldosteronism) or by other mineralocorticoids suppresses PRA; when mineralocorticoids other than aldosterone are present in excess, they retain salt and water, and the resulting volume expansion suppresses both PRA and PA
2. Increased PRA always increases PA (secondary aldosteronism), unless the rise in PRA is caused by a primary defect in aldosterone secretion; PRA may be high because of

a. volume depletion secondary to renal or extrarenal salt loss
b. abnormality in renin secretion (e.g., reninoma [hemangiopericytoma of afferent arteriole], malignant hypertension, renal artery stenosis)
c. increased renin substrate production (e.g., oral contraceptives)

3. When renin is deficient primarily, aldosterone is always low (e.g., hyporeninemic hypoaldosteronism)
4. Elevated serum K^+ levels can directly stimulate the adrenal cortex to release aldosterone

Hypokalemia

Causes and Pathogenesis

Because the intracellular K^+ concentration greatly exceeds the extracellular concentration, K^+ shift into the cell can cause severe hypokalemia with little change in its intracellular concentration (Table 6.3). Alkalosis, insulin, and β_2-agonists can cause hypokalemia by stimulating Na^+-K^+ ATPase activity. The mechanism of cellular K^+ accumulation in periodic paralysis is not clearly understood. In barium poisoning, K^+ accumulates in the cell, and hypokalemia develops because inhibition of the K^+ channel by barium prevents K^+ efflux from the cell in the face of continuous cellular uptake of K^+ through the action of Na^+-K^+ ATPase. K^+ accumulates in the cell along with anions as the cell mass increases during nutritional recovery, because K^+ is the main intracellular cation. Poor intake of K^+ by itself rarely causes hypokalemia, because poor intake of K^+ is usually accompanied by poor caloric intake, which causes catabolism and release of K^+ from the tissues.

Vomiting and diarrhea are common causes of hypokalemia. Diarrhea causes direct K^+ loss in the stool, but in vomiting, hypokalemia results mainly from K^+ loss in the urine rather than in the vomitus. Vomiting causes metabolic alkalosis, and the subsequent renal excretion of bicarbonate leads to renal K^+ wasting.

Table 6.3
Causes of Hypokalemia

Intracellular shift (e.g., alkalosis, periodic paralysis, β_2-agonists, barium poisoning, insulin, nutritional recovery state)
Poor intake
Gastrointestinal loss (e.g., vomiting, diarrhea, drainage, laxative abuse)
Excessive renal loss
- 1° Aldosteronism (adrenal adenoma or hyperplasia); PRA is suppressed
- 2° Aldosteronism (the rise in aldosterone is secondary to rise in renin)
  - Malignant hypertension, renal artery stenosis, reninoma
  - Diuretics
  - Bartter's syndrome, Gitelman's syndrome
- Excess mineralocorticoids other than aldosterone (e.g., Cushing's syndrome, ACTH-producing tumor, licorice
- Chronic metabolic acidosis (e.g., type I and type II RTA).
- Delivery of poorly reabsorbed anions to the distal tubule (e.g., bicarbonate, ketone anions, carbenecillin
- Miscellaneous causes: magnesium deficiency, acute leukemia, Liddle's syndrome

Renal loss of K^+ is the most common cause of hypokalemia. Renal K^+ wasting occurs when increased aldosterone concentration is accompanied by adequate distal delivery of Na^+. In primary aldosteronism, distal delivery of Na^+ increases because increased NaCl reabsorption in the cortical collecting duct by the action of aldosterone inhibits salt reabsorption in the proximal tubule and Henle's loop. In secondary aldosteronism, hypokalemia occurs only in conditions that are accompanied by increased distal Na^+ delivery. Examples include renal artery stenosis, diuretic therapy, and malignant hypertension. Heart failure does not lead to hypokalemia despite secondary aldosteronism unless distal delivery of Na^+ is increased by diuretic therapy.

Bartter's syndrome is caused by defective NaCl reabsorption in the thick ascending limb of Henle, whereas in Gitelman's syndrome, the defect in NaCl reabsorption is in the distal convoluted tubule. Defective Na reabsorption proximal to the aldosterone-effective site results in increased delivery of Na to the cortical collecting duct and hence in hypokalemia. In chronic metabolic acidosis, hypokalemia probably develops because reduced proximal reabsorption of NaCl allows increased delivery of NaCl to the distal nephron. In licorice, renal K^+ wasting results from the sustained mineralocorticoid activity of cortisol as licorice inhibits the enzyme 11-β-hydroxy steroid dehydrogenase, which normally rapidly metabolizes cortisol in the kidney. Liddle's syndrome is caused by increased Na^+ channel activity in the collecting duct; accumulation of Na^+ in the cell leads to stimulation of Na^+-K^+ ATPase activity, resulting in increased K^+ secretion. Figure 6.9 shows a schematic approach to the differential diagnosis of hypokalemia (Table 6.3).

Clinical Manifestations

Low serum K^+ levels lead to characteristic electrocardiographic changes, alterations in cardiac rate, rhythm, and conduction, and to muscle weakness. Depletion of cellular K^+ leads to a number of structural and functional alterations in a variety of organs. These include skeletal muscle cell necrosis and acute rhabdomyolysis, nephrogenic diabetes insipidus (possibly due to inhibition of ADH by excess prostaglandin), and cardiac cell necrosis. K^+ depletion is often associated with metabolic alkalosis, in part because K^+ deficiency leads to increased renal production and retention of bicarbonate. Reduced insulin secretion and reduced intestinal motility are other common disorders of hypokalemia.

Hypokalemia produces abnormalities of rhythm and of rate of electrical conduction in the heart through alteration in several physiologic states. Alteration in ventricular repolarization leads to depression of the S-T segment, flattening and inversion of T waves, and appearance of U waves, the most common ECG abnormalities of hypokalemia. Combinations of altered states of polarization and conduction can produce arrhythmias, most com-

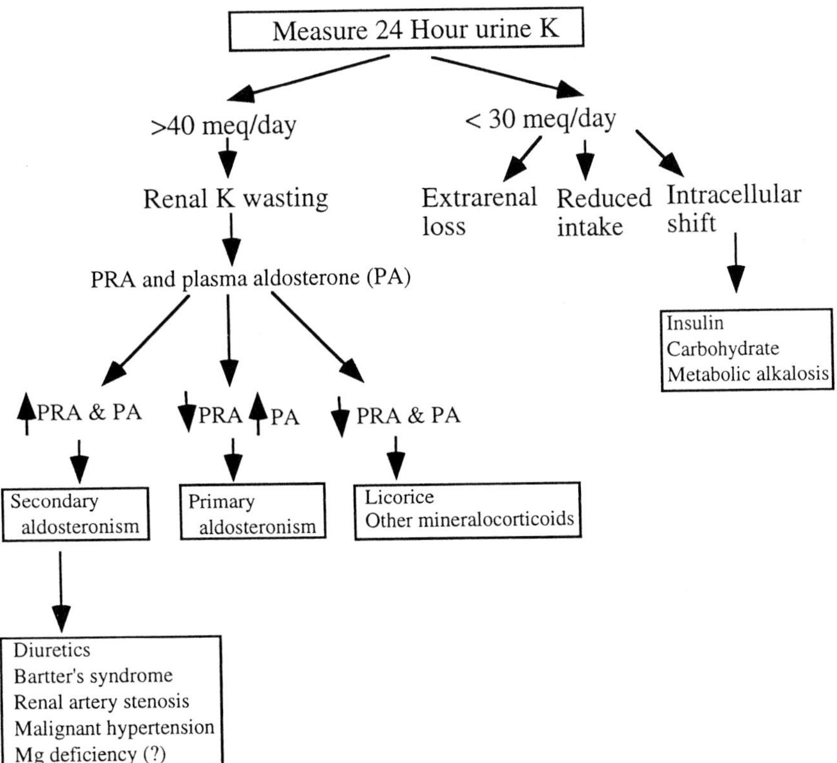

Figure 6.9. Differential diagnosis of hypokalemia. The first step is measuring 24-h urine K excretion. If the amount is more than 40 meq/day, it signifies renal wasting of K; less than 20 meq/L suggests an extrarenal cause. Once renal K wasting is suspected, measurement of PRA and plasma aldosterone will help differentiate among different causes of renal K wasting.

monly supraventricular and ventricular ectopic beats and tachycardia, A-V conduction disturbances, and ventricular fibrillation. Rapidly developing hypokalemia is more likely to produce abnormal cardiac function than more slowly developing hypokalemia. Potassium depletion intensifies digitalis toxicity through an unknown mechanism.

Treatment

Hypokalemia is usually treated either by potassium administration or by prevention of renal loss of potassium. Renal loss of potassium is prevented either by treating its cause (e.g., removal of aldosterone-producing adenoma or discontinuation of diuretics) or by administering potassium-sparing diuretics. The potassium-sparing diuretics in current use are aldosterone antagonists (e.g., spironolactone), triamterene, and amiloride. Aldosterone antagonists are effective in preventing renal potassium loss only if an increased mineralocorticoid concentration is responsible for hypokalemia. In Liddle's syndrome, spironolactone is ineffective because plasma aldosterone is reduced; triamterene and amiloride are effective regardless of the plasma aldosterone concentration. The daily dose of spironolactone ranges from 25 to 400 mg. The usual doses of triamterene range from 50 to 150 mg twice daily. Amiloride is administered at 5 mg/day and can be slowly increased up to 20 mg/day; it should be administered with food to avoid gastric irritation. Because reduced delivery of sodium to the distal nephron reduces potassium secretion, a low-salt diet helps reduce renal potassium loss from any cause, independent of the plasma aldosterone concentration.

In a nonemergency setting, potassium should be given orally as potassium chloride, potassium phosphate, or the salt of an organic acid. In the critical care setting, potassium is usually given intravenously and primarily as potassium chloride. The first goal in treating severe hypokalemia is elimination of cardiac arrhythmias. A decline in serum [K^+] of 1 meq/L generally indicates a loss of 150 to 200 meq of potassium and a decline of 2 meq/L, a loss in excess of 500 meq, but the relationship is not rigidly fixed. For example, in acidotic states, serum potassium may be high in the face of potassium depletion.

To initiate rapid intravenous administration of potassium, it may be useful to estimate the number of liters of ECF as body weight in kg $\times$ 0.2. This figure times the desired increment in serum potassium per liter represents the amount of potassium that can be safely given in 20 to 30 minutes without danger of hyperkalemia.

Although it is usually unnecessary to give potassium at a rate greater than 10 to 20 meq/h, a rate in excess of 100 meq/h may be needed in certain life-threatening situations (e.g., a patient with ketoacidosis, severe hypokalemia, and an ECG showing a dangerous arrhythmia). Glucose-containing solution should not be used as a vehicle for KCl when serum K^+ is to be increased rapidly; glucose stimulates insulin release, which, in turn, drives K^+ into cells.

Potassium at concentrations above 40 meq/L may produce pain at the infusion site and may lead to sclerosis of smaller vessels. When a concentration above 100 meq/L is used, a femoral line is preferable. It is advisable to avoid central venous infusion of potassium at high concentrations; depolarization of the conduction tissues may lead to cardiac arrest.

Hyperkalemia

Causes and Pathogenesis

Hyperkalemia may be caused by one of three mechanisms: *(a)* shift of potassium from the cells to the ECF, *(b)* increased potassium intake, and *(c)* reduced renal potassium excretion (Table 6.4). Hyperkalemic familial periodic paralysis, administration of succinylcholine in paralyzed patients, administration of cationic amino acids such as ε-aminocaproic acid, arginine, or lysine; rhabdomyolysis or hemolysis; and acute acidosis all cause hyperkalemia by extracellular potassium shift. Rhabdomyolysis and hemolysis cause hyperkalemia only when they are accompanied by renal failure.

Although hyperkalemia is not as predictable with organic acidosis as with inorganic acidosis in experimental situations, hyperkalemia is common in diabetic ketoacidosis and phenformin-induced lactic acidosis. The more frequent occurrence of hyperkalemia in clinical organic acidosis may be explained by the longer duration of acidosis and the presence of other factors such as dehydration and renal failure and insulin deficiency in diabetic ketoacidosis. Hyperkalemia can also occur in severe digitalis intoxication by extracellular shift of potassium, as digitalis inhibits the Na^+-K^+ ATPase pump.

The kidney's ability to excrete potassium is so great that hyperkalemia rarely occurs solely on the basis of increased intake of potassium. Thus, hyperkalemia is almost always due to impaired renal excretion. There are three major mechanisms of diminished renal potassium excretion: reduced aldosterone or aldosterone responsiveness, renal failure, and reduced distal delivery of sodium.

Table 6.4
Causes of Hyperkalemia

Pseudohyperkalemia
- Thrombocytosis, massive leukocytosis, use of tourniquet with fist exercise, in vitro hemolysis

True hyperkalemia
- Due to extracellular shift: acute acidosis (especially inorganic acidosis), catabolic states, periodic paralysis, succinylcholine, cationic amino acids, exercise while using a β-blocker, digitalis intoxication
- Due to excessive ingestion: rare if renal excretion of K is normal
- Decreased renal excretion
  - Hypoaldosteronism: Addison's disease; selective hypoaldosteronism (hyporeninemic hypoaldosteronism, heparin, congenital adrenal enzyme deficiencies, angiotensin-converting enzyme inhibitors)
  - Tubular unresponsiveness to aldosterone (pseudohypoaldosteronism type I and II): congenital, salt-losing nephropathy
  - Potassium-sparing diuretics
  - Severe dehydration

Aldosterone deficiency may be part of a generalized deficiency of adrenal hormones (e.g., Addison's disease) or it may represent a selective process (e.g., hyporeninemic hypoaldosteronism). Hyporeninemic hypoaldosteronism is the most common cause of all aldosterone deficiency states and by far the commonest cause of chronic hyperkalemia among nondialysis patients. Selective hypoaldosteronism can also occur with heparin therapy, which inhibits steroid production in the zona glomerulosa. In patients with reduced aldosterone secretion, any agent that limits the supply of renin or angiotensin II may provoke hyperkalemia; for example, ACE inhibitors, nonsteroidal antiinflammatory agents, and β-blockers. The latter may compound the tendency to hyperkalemia by interfering with potassium transport into cells. Renal tubular unresponsiveness to aldosterone (pseudohypoaldosteronism) may be congenital, but it is more often an acquired defect. This defect may involve only potassium secretion (pseudohypoaldosteronism type II) or sodium reabsorption as well as potassium secretion (pseudohypoaldosteronism type I). Most cases of so-called salt-losing nephritis appear to represent the latter defect. Severe volume depletion may cause hyperkalemia despite secondary hyperaldosteronism, because volume depletion causes a marked reduction in delivery of sodium to the cortical collecting duct.

Pseudohyperkalemia, defined as increased potassium concentration only in the local blood vessel or in vitro, has no physiologic consequences. Prolonged use of a tourniquet with fist exercises can increase the serum potassium level by as much as 1 meq/L. Thrombocytosis and severe leukocytosis cause pseudohyperkalemia through potassium release from the platelets and white blood cells, respectively, during blood clotting.

Clinical Manifestations

In severe hyperkalemia, paralysis of the skeletal muscle occurs. Rapidly ascending neuromuscular weakness or paralysis has been observed in very severe hyperkalemia. Hyperkalemia can also cause mental confusion and paresthesia. The main dangers of hyperkalemia are abnormalities of cardiac rhythm and of its rate of conduction.

Increased velocity of repolarization results in tall, peaked T waves with shortened QT intervals. This is the earliest sign of hyperkalemia, and it begins to appear when potassium concentration in serum rises above 5.5 meq/L. However, as was the case with hypokalemia, the rate of development of hyperkalemia is important in the development of cardiac rhythm abnormalities. Reduction in the resting potential of the cardiac conduction system and muscle by high extracellular potassium concentration is associated with slowing of conduction. As hyperkalemia worsens, P-waves flatten and QRS-complexes widen progressively, then the P-waves disappear entirely and the

QRS merge with the T waves simulating a sine wave. Other ECG findings include fascicular block and complete heart block (especially in digitalized subjects), ventricular tachycardia, flutter and fibrillation, and cardiac arrest.

Treatment

Hyperkalemia may be treated by removing potassium from the body, by shifting extracellular potassium into the cells, and by antagonizing potassium action on the membrane of the cardiac conduction system (Table 6.5). Potassium may be removed by several routes: through the GI tract with a potassium exchange resin given orally or by enema; through the kidney by diuretics, mineralocorticoids, and increased salt intake; and by hemodialysis or peritoneal dialysis. A potassium exchange resin, sodium polystyrene sulfonate (Kayexalate), is more effective when it is given with agents such as sorbitol or mannitol that cause osmotic diarrhea. One tablespoon of Kayexalate mixed with 100 mL of 10% sorbitol or mannitol can be given by mouth two to four times a day. When it is given as an enema, a larger quantity is given more frequently.

Hemodialysis can rapidly remove potassium from the body, but it takes time to set up the dialysis machine. Potassium can be shifted into cells with glucose and insulin or by increasing the blood pH with sodium bicarbonate. Bicarbonate was not very effective against hyperkalemia in patients with renal failure, but when given with insulin, bicarbonate appears to have a synergistic effect. Specific β_2-agonists such as salbutamol and albuterol drive K^+ into cells by stimulating the Na^+-K^+ ATPase. Antagonizing the action of potassium on the heart with intravenous calcium salts or hypertonic sodium solution has the fastest effect against hyperkalemia and is used in life-threatening hyperkalemia.

Prolonged administration of diuretics and a high-salt diet is an effective treatment for hyporeninemic hypoaldosteronism. This regimen ensures delivery of an adequate amount of sodium to the cortical collecting duct without causing further volume expansion. Mineralocorticoid may be required as an adjunct therapy for hyporeninemic hypoaldosteronism, and the agent most commonly used is a synthetic mineralocorticoid, fludrocortisone (Florinef). However, since renal salt retention may be important in the pathogenesis of hyporeninemic hypoaldosteronism, mineralocorticoid replacement may lead to salt retention and worsening of hypertension. Reduced potassium intake may be added to any of the methods recommended above in the long-term management of hyperkalemia.

Clinical problems and answers for this section are presented before the selected readings.

Table 6.5
Treatment of Hyperkalemia

- Reduction in body potassium content
  - Reduction in intake
  - Increased fecal excretion: potassium-exchange resin and sorbitol
  - Increased renal excretion: mineralocorticoids, increased salt intake, diuretics
  - Peritoneal or hemodialysis
- Intracellular shift of potassium
  - Glucose and insulin
  - Administration of alkali
  - β-Agonists: Salbutamol, albuterol
- Antagonizing the membrane effect of hyperkalemia
  - Calcium salts
  - Hypertonic sodium salts

PATHOPHYSIOLOGY OF WATER AND ANTIDIURETIC HORMONE METABOLISM

Regulation of Thirst and Antidiuretic Hormone Release

A rise in effective osmolality shrinks the hypothalamic osmoreceptor cells, which then signal the cerebral cortex (thirst center) and the ADH-releasing mechanism in the supraoptic and paraventricular nuclei. ADH is released from the posterior pituitary and carried by the circulation to the kidney, where it increases the permeability of the collecting ducts to water and enhances salt reabsorption in the outer medullary thick ascending limb of Henle's loop.

Decline in plasma osmolality of only 2 to 3% produces maximum suppression of ADH, so even mild clinical hyponatremia should produce maximally dilute urine (<100 mosm/L). ADH has two classes of receptors: V1 receptors cause increased vasomotor tone and certain metabolic effects, and V2 receptors are associated with antidiuresis. Vasopressinase, which normally breaks down ADH rapidly, may rise in pregnancy and occasionally causes polyuria. DDAVP, a synthetic analogue of arginine vasopressin, which resists vasopressinase and therefore has a prolonged effect, is useful in polyuria of pregnancy.

Because solute excretion is normal in water diuresis, osmolality of urine is very low. About 180 L of water is filtered daily; 160 L is reabsorbed in the proximal tubule and in the descending limb, and 20 L of dilute urine is delivered to the distal nephron. In the proximal tubule, water reabsorption passively follows salt reabsorption, whereas in the descending thin limb, water reabsorption is unaccompanied by salt reabsorption and in response to salt reabsorption in the ascending limbs. Both thin and thick ascending limbs of Henle and distal convoluted tubules are water impermeable, in the presence or absence of ADH. Reabsorption of water in the collecting duct is regulated by ADH (Fig. 6.10). With deficiency of ADH or tubular unresponsiveness to ADH, little water is reabsorbed in the collecting duct, and a large volume of dilute urine is excreted. In the presence of maximal ADH, urine can be concentrated up to 1200 mosm/L as water is reabsorbed in the cortical and medullary collecting duct. Osmotic concentration of the urine with the countercurrent mechanism results in medullary hypertonicity, sufficient ADH, and tubular membrane responsive to ADH.

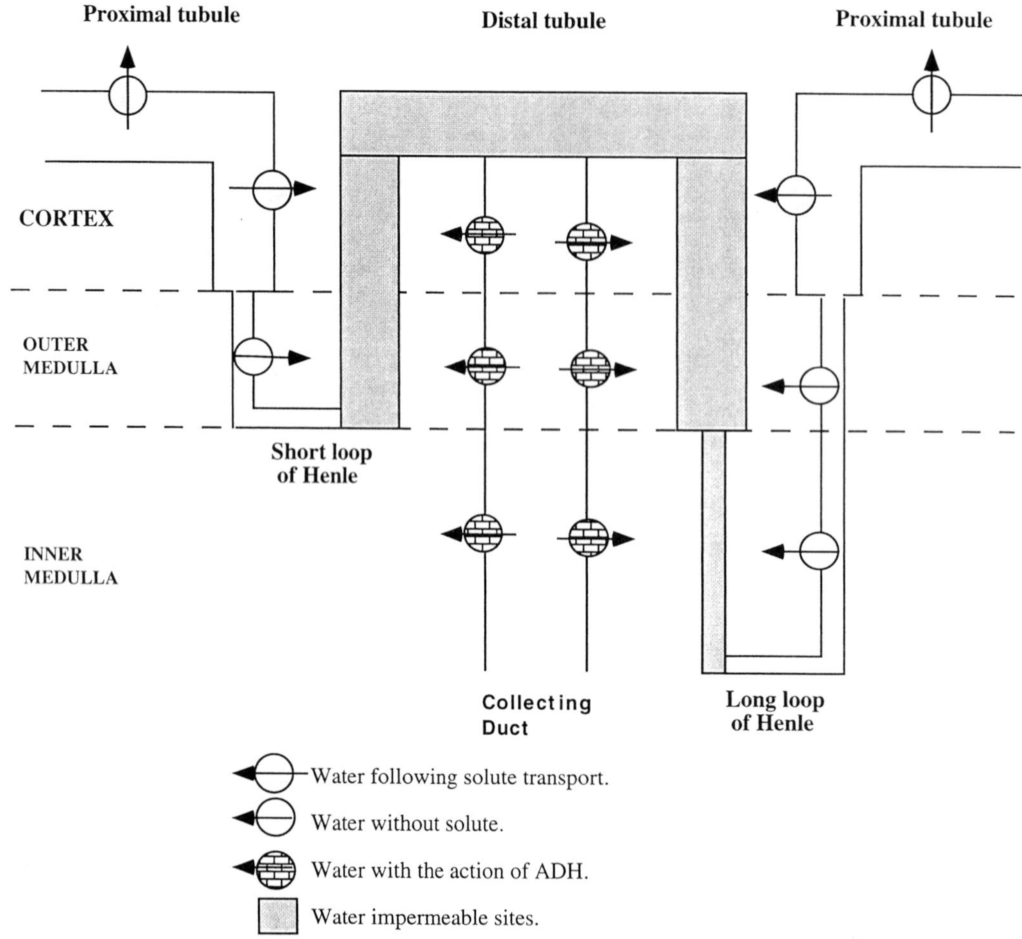

Figure 6.10. Transport of water at various nephron sites.

ADH release is also regulated by nonosmotic factors. Low effective arterial volume provokes thirst and ADH output, and high volume has the reverse effects. The effects are mediated through atrial stretch receptors and baroreceptors. α-Catechols suppress, and β-catechols enhance, ADH output. Prostaglandins inhibit the effect of ADH on the kidney. Angiotensin II stimulates thirst and ADH. Lack of glucocorticoid enhances ADH action on the kidney and may increase plasma ADH.

Physical and emotional stress (e.g., major surgery) enhance ADH output, possibly in part through emetic stimuli. Many drugs affect ADH release or action; for example, ethanol inhibits output of ADH. Lithium and demeclocycline inhibit the effect of ADH on the kidney. Chlorpropamide increases the action of ADH on the kidney. Some drugs may operate through emetic stimulus, one of the most potent physiologic stimuli to ADH release.

The urine may become osmotically concentrated in the absence of ADH if effective vascular volume is very low. The combination of reduced GFR and enhanced proximal reabsorption of filtrate reduces the volume of dilute urine formed in Henle's loop. This small volume moves so slowly down the collecting duct that even the limited permeability of the membrane permits withdrawal of a significant fraction of the water from the filtrate. Water retention by this mechanism may contribute to hyponatremia.

Polyuria

Polyuria is arbitrarily defined as urine volume in excess of 2.5 L/day (Table 6.6). There are two types of polyuria: osmotic diuresis and water diuresis.

Osmotic Diuresis. Osmotic diuresis is characterized by an excessive rate of solute excretion, in excess of 60 mosm/h, or 1440 mosm/day, in the adult. Urine osmolality is characteristically greater than that of plasma, but it need not be when it coexists with water diuresis. Only the

Table 6.6
Causes of Polyuria

Lack of ADH
Central diabetes insipidus
Suppression by excessive water intake: psychogenic, organic brain disease, iatrogenic
Excess vasopressinase: pregnancy
Failure of the kidney to respond to ADH
Congenital nephrogenic diabetes insipidus
Chronic renal failure
Acquired nephrogenic diabetes insipidus: certain drugs, structural and functional renal disorders

excessive solute excretion is the hallmark of osmotic diuresis. Solutes commonly responsible for osmotic diuresis include glucose, urea, mannitol, radiopaque media, and NaCl.

Water Diuresis. Water diuresis is characterized by excretion of a large volume of dilute urine. The cause of polyuria in water diuresis is reduced reabsorption of water in the collecting duct. Water is not reabsorbed in the collecting duct either because of the lack of ADH or unresponsiveness to ADH (nephrogenic diabetes insipidus). The lack of ADH is due to either primary deficiency (central diabetes insipidus) or physiologic suppression by low serum osmolality (primary polydipsia).

The deficiency of ADH is usually partial and, therefore, can be mild, moderate, or severe. In a rare instance, ADH can be made but cannot be released in response to a rise in osmolality of the ECF because of a defect involving the osmoreceptor cells (e.g., hypothalamic lesions). In such instances, ADH may be released in response to hypovolemia or to drugs.

Lack of ADH may have many causes, including idiopathic cell degeneration, tumors and granulomas, surgery involving the pituitary or nearby structures, trauma, infarction, and infection. When the diagnosis of central diabetes insipidus is made, the patient is usually treated with replacement of ADH as DDAVP via the nasal mucosa. Less commonly, low levels of ADH may have their effects boosted by drugs such as chlorpropamide. Since ADH deficiency is not an all-or-none phenomenon, urine osmolality may be very low with severe deficiency or fairly close to normal with mild deficiency.

Congenital nephrogenic diabetes insipidus is a rare disorder with severe polyuria, expressed only in males, and invariably evident in the neonate. It is treated with salt restriction and thiazide diuretics to produce a state of volume depletion; with reduced effective arterial volume, reabsorption of filtrate in the proximal tubule is increased, and less fluid is presented to the ascending limb where dilute urine is made. Acquired nephrogenic diabetes insipidus, which can be treated in the same manner, is caused by a number of disorders including amyloidosis, light-chain nephropathy, and hypercalcemia. Patients with chronic renal failure may also have varying degrees of unresponsiveness to ADH.

Primary polydipsia is defined as increased water drinking that is not caused by physiologically stimulated thirst (i.e., in the absence of hyperosmolality or volume depletion). In contrast, polydipsia in patients with diabetes insipidus or diabetic patients with marked glycosuria could be termed *secondary polydipsia,* since in these conditions polydipsia is secondary to thirst stimulation due to hyperosmolality. In primary polydipsia, ADH secretion is suppressed physiologically, and urine output is therefore increased markedly. When polydipsia is modest, serum Na remains within normal limits, but at the low range of normal, in contrast to high normal serum Na levels seen in patients with diabetes insipidus. Primary polydipsia is usually of psychogenic origin, hence the term *psychogenic polydipsia.*

Differential Diagnosis of Polyuria. The first step in the differential diagnosis should be measurement of urine osmolality. Osmotic diuresis is ruled out or diagnosed solely on the basis of the rate of osmolal excretion. Osmotic diuresis is defined as the excretion of osmols at a rate greater than 60 mosm/h, or 1440 mosm/day. For example, a urine output of 5 L/day at an osmolality of 400 mosm/L equals the osmolal excretion rate of 2000 mosm/day and therefore is an osmotic diuresis. On the other hand, excretion of 10 L of urine at 100 mosm/L gives only 1000 mosm/day and therefore is water diuresis.

For the differential diagnosis of water diuresis, the first step is determining the serum Na concentration. In diabetes insipidus, serum Na tends to be high normal, and in primary polydipsia, it tends to be low normal. However because of much overlap, a water-deprivation test is needed to confirm the diagnosis. Water is restricted overnight or until loss of 5% of the body weight. In primary polydipsia, maximum urine osmolality (>700 mosm/L) can usually be achieved by water restriction. A submaximal response that improves significantly upon administration of ADH indicates central diabetes insipidus; a submaximal response that fails to respond to ADH points to nephrogenic diabetes insipidus (Fig. 6.11).

Treatment. If the cause of polyuria is osmotic diuresis, the cause of the increased solute excretion must be removed. If the patient has glycosuria, diabetes should be controlled. If the patient is ingesting a high-protein diet, curtailing protein intake would reduce urea excretion.

If the cause is diabetes insipidus, the distinction should be made between nephrogenic and central (pituitary) diabetes insipidus. Administering ADH or stimulating ADH secretion is helpful only for pituitary diabetes insipidus. Exogenous ADH is available in three forms. Pitressin tannate in oil is administered intramuscularly. Desmopressin (dDAVP), a synthetic analogue of ADH, is administered intranasally, subcutaneously, or intravenously. A synthetic lysine vasopressin (lypressin, Diapid) is administered as a nasal spray. The usual dose of intranasal dDAVP is 0.1 or 0.2 mL twice daily by tube or by nasal spray, and the usual dose for Diapid is one to two sprays in each nostril four times a day.

Some patients may prefer oral agents, and the two that have been used extensively are chlorpropamide and thiazide diuretics. Chlorpropamide (100–250 mg/day) stimulates secretion of endogenous ADH and may also enhance the effect of ADH. Its use has been markedly curtailed since the advent of dDAVP. Thiazide diuretics produce vascular volume depletion and enhance reabsorption of fluid in the proximal tubule. Thus, they increase urine concentration by reducing delivery of fluid to the distal diluting segment of the nephron. Addition of a thiazide diuretic to chlorpropamide may prevent the hypo-

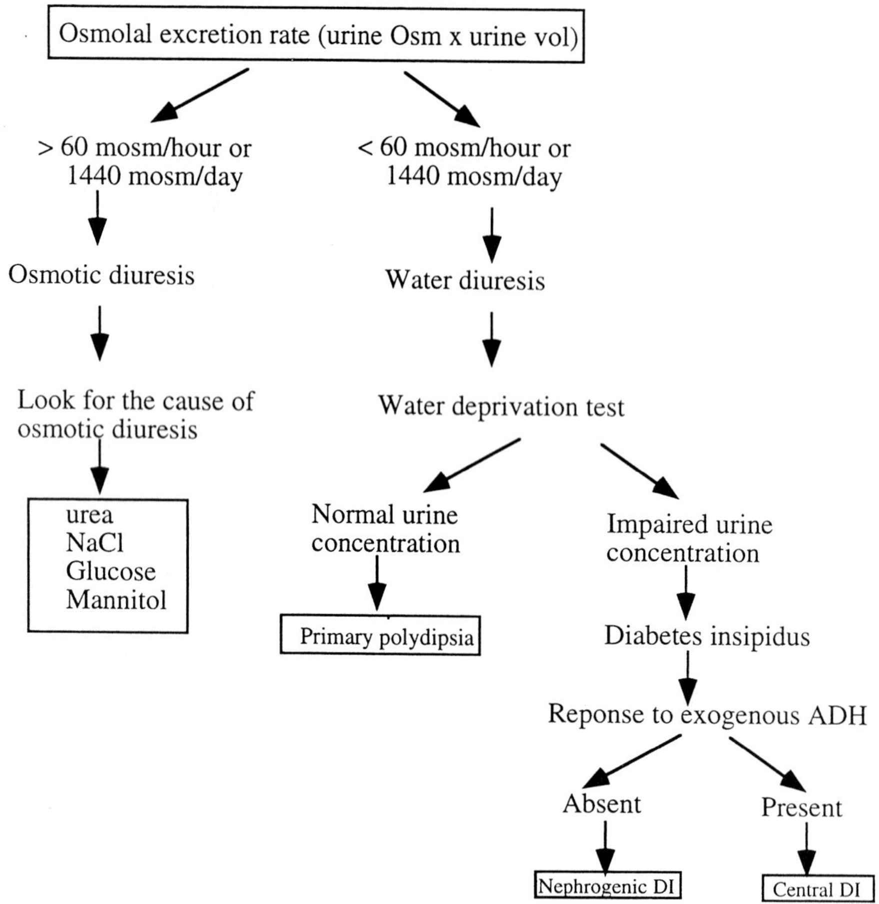

Figure 6.11. Differential diagnosis of polyuria.

glycemia that may occur if the latter is used alone. Two other drugs used for the treatment of central diabetes insipidus are clofibrate and carbamazepine. Since both drugs are less effective than chlorpropamide and have more serious side effects, they should be the last resources. Nephrogenic diabetes insipidus cannot be treated with ADH preparations or an agent that stimulates ADH release, but measures to reduce the distal delivery of salt and water (i.e., low-salt diet and thiazide diuretics) are effective.

Hyponatremia

Hyponatremia, the most common electrolyte disorder, is defined as a reduced plasma sodium concentration (<135 meq/L). Generally, clinical concern arises when the concentration is less than 130 meq/L.

The term *pseudohyponatremia* is applied to a spurious reduction in serum sodium concentration caused by a systematic error in the measurement. The common causes include hyperlipidemia, hyperproteinemia, or increased viscosity of the plasma. The error in measurement in pseudohyponatremia results from dilution of the sample. Measurements of serum sodium with a flame photometer can result in this type of error because the sample is always diluted in such measurements. The same error also occurs even with an ion-specific electrode method, if the sample is diluted (indirect method). In pseudohyponatremia, plasma osmolality, which is customarily measured without dilution, is normal.

However, a low plasma sodium concentration with a normal plasma osmolality need not indicate the presence of pseudohyponatremia; true hyponatremia may be accompanied by a normal plasma osmolality because of hyperglycemia, azotemia, or the presence of mannitol or alcohol. In hypergammaglobulinemic states such as multiple myeloma, serum sodium is falsely low because of displacement of serum water by γ-globulins, but, on the other hand, the sodium concentration is also truly low because cationic charges on γ-globulins displace sodium to maintain electrical neutrality.

A mechanism of pseudohyponatremia not widely appreciated is in vitro hemolysis, a well-known cause of pseudohyperkalemia. Since cell lysis does not change osmolality of the plasma, any rise in serum potassium must be met by a reciprocal decrease in serum sodium. However, the reduction in serum Na from hemolysis is somewhat greater than the increase in serum K, by a factor of 1.3, because hemoglobin released from the red cells causes additional reduction in serum Na as in hyperproteinemia. In pseudohyponatremia, effective osmolality is normal. Although in true hyponatremia, serum osmolality is usually low, it may also be normal; by coincidence, true

Table 6.7
Types of Hyponatremia According to Effective Osmolality

1. Normal effective osmolality: pseudohyponatremia (e.g., hyperlipidemia, hyperproteinemia, and in vitro hemolysis), accumulation of abnormal cations (e.g., lithium, γ-globulins)
2. Increased effective osmolality: hyperglycemia, mannitol infusion
3. Low effective osmolality: usual hyponatremia

reduction in serum sodium could be accompanied by accumulation of some solutes to give a normal serum osmolality (Table 6.7).

Causes and Pathogenesis

The immediate mechanisms responsible for a reduction in extracellular sodium concentration are *(a)* shift of water from the cell caused by accumulation of extracellular solutes other than sodium salts; *(b)* retention of excess water in the body; *(c)* loss of sodium; and *(d)* shift of sodium into the cells (Fig. 6.12). The appropriate physiologic response to hypotonicity is suppression of ADH release, which leads to rapid excretion of excess water and correction of hyponatremia. Persistence of hyponatremia indicates failure of this compensatory mechanism. In most instances, hyponatremia is maintained because the kidney fails to produce water diuresis, but sometimes ingestion of water in excess of the limits of normal renal compensation is responsible.

The reasons for the inability of the kidney to excrete water include *(a)* renal failure, *(b)* reduced delivery of glomerular filtrate to the distal nephron, and *(c)* the presence of ADH. The mechanism for impaired water excretion in renal failure is obvious and needs no further explanation. Reduced distal delivery of filtrate results from a low glomerular filtration rate and enhanced proximal tubular reabsorption of salt and water, and these states are most commonly caused by volume depletion.

Abnormal retention of water is the main reason for development of hyponatremia in most instances, and water retention is usually caused by ingestion or administration of hypotonic fluid. However, in certain clinical settings, water retention can occur despite administration of isotonic fluid. The latter phenomenon occurs when urine is excreted containing sodium and potassium at concentrations that exceed the sum of serum concentrations of the two ions. Excretion of hypertonic urine requires an increased amount of ADH in the presence of marked sodium diuresis. Clinical examples include a patient who receives a large amount of isotonic fluid in the immediate postoperative period, a patient with SIADH who is treated with isotonic fluid, and a patient who receives a thiazide diuretic.

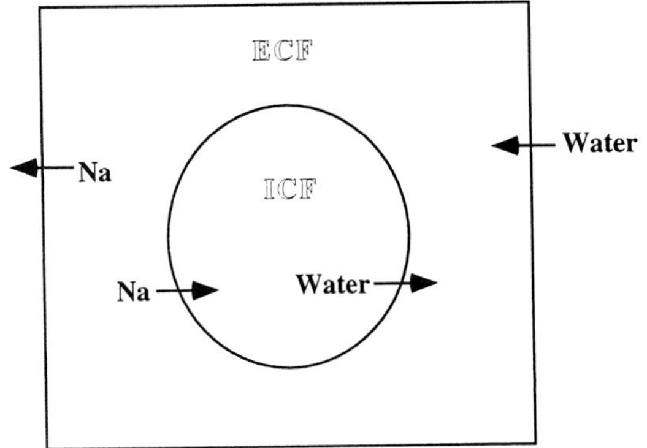

Figure 6.12. Pathogenetic mechanisms of hyponatremia. Hyponatremia is caused by one of four mechanisms: loss of Na from the body fluid, shift of Na into cells, gain of water from the outside, and shift of water from cells.

Normal dilution of urine requires delivery of adequate amounts of fluid to the diluting segment and reabsorption of solute without water at that segment. Increased body fluid tonicity causes release of ADH, which allows reabsorption of water in the collecting duct, helping to restore the body fluid tonicity. Thus, the response is considered appropriate when ADH is released in response to hypertonicity of the body fluid. However, release of ADH in the presence of hyponatremia is also not inappropriate if the effective arterial volume is reduced. ADH secretion is considered inappropriate when it occurs despite hyponatremia and despite a normal or increased effective arterial volume. The causes of SIADH include tumors, pulmonary diseases such as tuberculosis and pneumonia, central nervous system diseases, and drugs.

Hyponatremia in clinical states associated with reduced effective arterial volume such as congestive heart failure and cirrhosis of the liver is caused by a combination of reduced delivery of fluid to the distal nephron and increased secretion of ADH. Salt restriction and diuretics increase the severity of hyponatremia. ADH secretion may be present despite hyponatremia in myxedema and glucocorticoid deficiency states. It is not clear, however, whether ADH secretion in these conditions is truly inappropriate or appropriate.

Finally, mild hyponatremia may be caused by "resetting of the osmostat" at an osmolality lower than the usual level. In such cases, urine dilution occurs normally when the plasma osmolality is brought down below the reset level. Resetting of the osmostat is a form of SIADH, since ADH secretion occurs inappropriately at hyponatremic levels without evidence of reduced effective arterial volume. Patients with chronic debilitating diseases such as pulmonary tuberculosis often manifest this phenomenon (Table 6.8).

Diagnosis

The presence of a low plasma sodium level and normal osmolality suggests pseudohyponatremia but does not confirm it. By coincidence, true hyponatremia may be accompanied by a high concentration of urea or alcohol, resulting in normal osmolality. A more direct proof is demonstration of a normal sodium concentration using a sodium-specific electrode or demonstration of reduced water content of plasma. Pseudohyponatremia due to

Table 6.8
Causes of Hyponatremia According to Mechanisms of Maintenance

Increased water intake, e.g., primary polydipsia
Reduced renal water excretion
- Reduced delivery of fluid to the distal nephron because of low effective arterial volume (ADH release is usually stimulated as well)
  - Edema-forming states: heart failure, nephrotic syndrome, cirrhosis of the liver
  - Nonrenal sodium loss: gastrointestinal sodium loss, sweating
  - Renal sodium loss: thiazide diuretics, aldosterone deficiency
- Advanced renal failure
- Inappropriate secretion of ADH (SIADH)
  - Tumors
  - Pulmonary diseases
  - Central nervous system disorders
  - Drugs, e.g., chlorpropamide, barbiturate, morphine, indomethacin
  - Physical and emotional stress
  - Idiopathic
  - Reset osmostat
- Unknown mechanisms
  - Glucocorticoid deficiency
  - Myxedema

hyperlipidemia is caused by accumulation of chylomicrons, which consist mostly of triglyceride, and is obvious from the milky appearance of serum or plasma. Substantial hyponatremia due to hyperlipidemia requires accumulation of more than 5 to 6 g/dL of lipids, and this degree of hyperlipidemia does not occur with hypercholesterolemia alone. Each gram per deciliter of lipid falsely reduces serum sodium by 1.7 meq/L and each gram per deciliter of protein by 1.0 meq/L. Pseudohyponatremia due to hyperproteinemia can be confirmed by measurement of plasma proteins. Hyponatremia caused by mannitol or glucose is suspected from the history or by simultaneous measurements of plasma sodium, osmolality, and glucose.

In evaluating hyponatremia associated with hypoosmolality, the main concern is distinguishing between SIADH and hyponatremia from other causes, mainly volume-depletion states and edematous states. The major distinction between SIADH and other causes of hyponatremia lies in the status of effective arterial volume (EAV). EAV is normal or increased in the former and reduced in the latter. However, no single diagnostic test measures EAV with certainty. Physical examination is notoriously inaccurate in determining mild-to-moderate volume depletion. A more reliable method for estimating EAV uses measurements of urinary Na, serum urea nitrogen (SUN), serum creatinine, and serum uric acid. Urinary Na excretion above 20 meq/L, SUN below 10 mg/dL, serum creatinine below 1 mg/dL, and serum urate below 4.0 mg/dL all suggest normal or increased EAV. In contrast, measurement of urine osmolality has virtually no diagnostic value and often misleads physicians. Contrary to the common belief, urine osmolality in SIADH need not be greater than plasma osmolality. Furthermore, a high urine osmolality does not necessarily support the diagnosis of SIADH, because most other causes of hyponatremia are also accompanied by urine osmolality higher than plasma osmolality.

The only situation in which urine osmolality may be appropriately low in the presence of hyponatremia is the hyponatremia caused by primary polydipsia, and this is usually apparent when a careful history reveals polyuria and polydipsia (Fig. 6.13). In all other causes of hyponatremia, urine osmolality is inappropriately increased (i.e., greater than 100 mosm/L).

Treatment

Hyponatremia is treated either by addition of sodium or by removal of water. Salt is given to patients with hyponatremia due to salt depletion. Water is removed in hyponatremic states with normal or increased body sodium content. *The speed of correction of hyponatremia should depend on the speed of development and on the patient's symptoms.* Clearly, severe symptomatic hyponatremia is a life-threatening condition, but there are dangers associated with treatment of hyponatremia. In the past, volume overload was thought to be the main danger associated with administration of a large quantity of salt-containing solution. Now, central pontine myelinolysis is considered a major danger associated with rapid correction of hyponatremia. This demyelinating disease of the central pons and the other areas of the brain is characterized by motor nerve dysfunction including quadriplegia. This complication tends to occur more often with chronic hyponatremia than with acute hyponatremia and is more frequently observed in malnourished and debilitated patients. To minimize this complication, hyponatremia should be corrected at a rate less than 0.35 meq/L/h or less than 8 meq/24 h. Since the danger of central pontine myelinolysis is limited mainly to those with asymptomatic chronic hyponatremia, rapid correction (at a rate of 1–2 meq/L/h) should be restricted to those with acute symptomatic hyponatremia. Even then, there is no advantage in rapidly increasing serum sodium to a level above 125 meq/L.

For patients admitted with hypotonic dehydration and chronic asymptomatic hyponatremia, the traditional recommendation has been administration of isotonic saline. As the volume expansion suppresses ADH release induced by the low EAV, a rise in serum sodium concentration follows rapid water excretion, provided that renal function is adequate. Sometimes, rapid excretion of water following isotonic saline administration in these patients may lead to development of central pontine myelinolysis. Alternating 0.45% and 0.9% sodium chloride solutions may therefore be safer. If potassium depletion coexists, appropriate treatment is with 0.45% NaCl containing 40 meq/L potassium.

Acute Treatment. For hyponatremia with sodium depletion and symptomatic hypoosmolality, intravenous administration of sodium as hypertonic saline will correct hypoosmolality effectively. The amount of sodium neces-

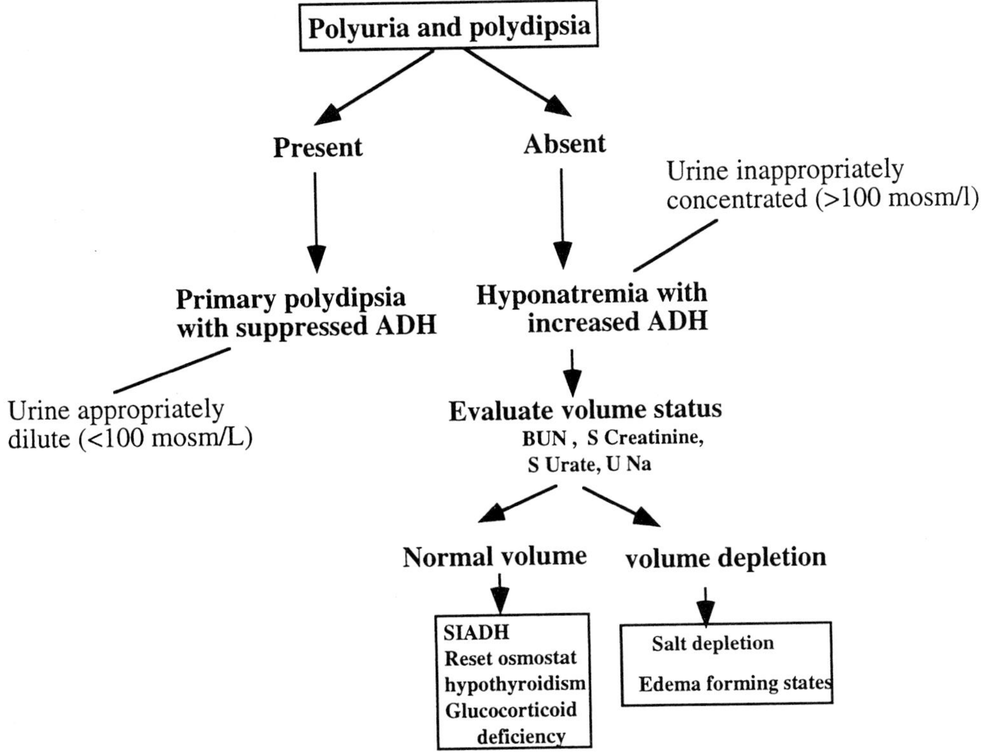

Figure 6.13. Differential diagnosis of hyponatremia.

sary to increase the sodium to a desired level is calculated as follows:

$$\text{Sodium requirement (meq)} = \text{TBW} \times \Delta\text{Na}$$

where ΔNa is the desired serum sodium level minus the actual serum sodium.

Sodium may be administered as a 3 or 5% NaCl solution. When accumulation of excess water is primarily responsible for hyponatremia, as in SIADH, water may be rapidly removed by intravenous administration of osmotic diuretics such as mannitol or urea. More readily available is a loop diuretic (e.g., furosemide) to be given simultaneously with hypertonic saline. Furosemide causes loss of water and sodium, but hypertonic saline replaces the lost sodium; the net result is removal of water. The response to furosemide cannot be predicted with precision, and frequent follow-up measurements of serum sodium levels must be made. There is no theoretical advantage to replacing exactly the amount of sodium lost in urine with hypertonic saline. Administration of hypertonic saline alone usually causes a salt and water diuresis, but addition of a loop diuretic makes correction of hyponatremia easier by preventing excretion of concentrated urine. Another advantage of a diuretic is prevention of fluid overload.

Chronic Treatment. Chronic hyponatremia may be treated by a reduction in water intake or by an increase in renal water excretion. Reduction of water intake is preferable but not always feasible. If water restriction is difficult or unsuccessful, the latter approach may be used. Increased renal water excretion can be achieved by the use of pharmacologic agents that interfere with urine concentration. Lithium and demeclocycline increase urine output by reducing production of cyclic adenosine monophosphate (AMP) and also interfering with its action. Demeclocycline is more effective and has fewer side effects, but it may cause nephrotoxicity in patients with liver disease.

Administration of a loop diuretic such as furosemide in conjunction with increased salt and potassium intake is safer for treating chronic hyponatremia than the above methods. The diuretic prevents high medullary interstitial osmolality by limiting reabsorption of salt in Henle's loop and hence prevents urine concentration. Increased salt and potassium intake increases water output by increasing delivery of solutes. There is evidence that ethacrynic acid may impair ADH-stimulated water movement across the collecting duct, and furosemide may have the same effect. Finally, vasopressin antagonists, not yet commercially available, may become an important addition to both chronic and acute treatment of hyponatremia in the future. Daily ingestion of urea has been used successfully, but again, it is not as practical as a loop diuretic.

Hypernatremia

Hypernatremia is defined as an increased sodium concentration in plasma water. Whereas hyponatremia may not be accompanied by hypoosmolality, hypernatremia is always associated with an increased effective plasma osmolality and hence with reduced cell volume. However, the extracellular volume in hypernatremia may be normal, decreased, or increased.

Causes and Pathogenesis

Hypernatremia is caused by loss of water, gain of sodium, or both (Table 6.9). Loss of water could be due to increased loss or reduced intake, and gain of sodium is due either to increased intake or to reduced renal excretion. Increased loss of water can occur through the kidney (e.g., in diabetes insipidus or osmotic diuresis), the GI tract (e.g., gastric suction or osmotic diarrhea), or the skin. Reduced water intake occurs most commonly in comatose patients or in those with a defective thirst mechanism. Less frequent causes of reduced water intake include continuous vomiting, lack of access to water, and mechanical obstruction such as esophageal tumor. The excess gain of sodium leading to hypernatremia is usually iatrogenic, e.g., from hypertonic saline infusion, accidental entry into maternal circulation during abortion with hypertonic saline, or administration of hypertonic sodium bicarbonate during cardiopulmonary resuscitation or treatment of lactic acidosis. Reduced renal sodium excretion leading to sodium gain and hypernatremia is usually in response to dehydration caused by primary water deficit.

Water depletion due to diabetes insipidus, osmotic diuresis, or insufficient water intake leads to secondary sodium retention in those who continue to ingest or are given sodium. Consequently, in chronic hypernatremia, sodium retention is more important than water loss. Whether hypernatremia is due to sodium retention or water loss can be determined by examination of the patient's volume status. For example, if a patient with a serum sodium level of 170 meq/L does not have obvious evidence of dehydration, hypernatremia is not caused entirely by water loss. To increase the serum sodium to 170 meq/L by water deficit alone, one would have to lose more than 20% of total body water.

Whereas the physiologic defense against hyponatremia is increased renal water excretion, the physiologic defense against hypernatremia is increased water drinking in response to thirst. Because thirst is such an effective and sensitive defense mechanism against hypernatremia, it is virtually impossible to increase serum sodium by more than a few milliequivalents per liter if the water drinking mechanism is intact. Therefore, in a patient with hypernatremia, there will always be a reason for reduced water intake (Table 6.9).

Table 6.9
Causes of Hypernatremia

Reduced water content of the body
Reduced water intake
Defective thirst due to altered mental state or thirst center defect
Inability to drink water
Lack of access to water
Increased water loss
Gastrointestinal loss: vomiting, osmotic diarrhea
Cutaneous loss: sweating and fever
Respiratory loss: hyperventilation and fever
Renal loss: diabetes insipidus, osmotic diuresis
Increased sodium content of the body
Increased intake
Hypertonic saline or sodium bicarbonate infusion
Ingestion of sea water
Renal salt retention: usually in response to primary water deficit

Treatment

Acute Treatment. Hypernatremia is treated by either addition of water or removal of sodium. The choice depends on the body sodium and water content. If water depletion is the cause of hypernatremia, water is added. If sodium excess is the cause, sodium must be removed. When the water deficit is severe, isotonic (0.9%) NaCl or 0.45% NaCl may be given initially to stabilize circulatory dynamics, followed by administration of hypotonic solutions to normalize the tonicity. Administration of 5% dextrose solution would also correct the extracellular volume depletion, but a larger volume is needed to expand the extracellular volume, and the ensuing rapid reduction of the plasma osmolality might result in cerebral edema. In acute symptomatic hypernatremia, serum sodium may be reduced by 6 to 8 meq/L in the first 3 to 4 h, but thereafter, the rate of decline should not exceed 1 meq/L/h. As with hyponatremia, chronic hypernatremia usually does not cause central nervous system symptoms and thus does not require rapid correction. A safe rate of correction is 0.7 meq/L/h, or about 10% of the serum sodium concentration over 24 h. The amount of water needed to correct hypernatremia can be estimated with the following equation:

$$\text{Water deficit (in liters)} = \text{TBW}\,(\text{Na}_2/\text{Na}_1 - 1) = \text{TBW} \times \Delta\,\text{Na}/\text{Na}_1$$

where Na_1 is the desired serum sodium level, Na_2 the observed serum sodium, TBW total body water, and ΔNa the difference between the desired and observed serum sodium levels.

In hypernatremia with excess sodium, reducing serum sodium with fluids usually initiates natriuresis, but if natriuresis does not occur promptly, sodium may be removed with diuretics. Furosemide plus 5% dextrose solution might be an appropriate regimen to treat hypernatremia associated with excess sodium. If a hypernatremic patient with sodium excess has renal failure, salt should be removed by dialysis.

Chronic Treatment. Hypernatremic disorders that require chronic preventive therapy include diabetes insipidus and primary hypodipsia. Although diabetes insipidus is often listed as a cause of hypernatremia, it does not cause hypernatremia in the absence of thirst defect. Treatment is therefore directed toward curtailment of polydipsia and polyuria. Subjects with primary hypodipsia should be educated to drink on schedule. In some instances, stimulation of the thirst center with chlorpropamide has been effective.

Clinical problems and answers for this section are presented before the selected readings.

ACID-BASE DISORDERS

Bicarbonate and CO_2 Buffer System

All body buffers are in equilibrium with protons (H^+) and therefore with pH as shown in the following equation:

$$pH = pK + \log A^-/HA$$

where A^- is a conjugate base of an acid HA.

Because HCO_3 and CO_2 are the major buffers of the body, pH is typically expressed as a function of their ratio, as in the Henderson-Hasselbalch equation:

$$pH = 6.1 + \log HCO_3^-/pCO_2 \times 0.03,$$

where 6.1 is the pK of the HCO_3^- and CO_2 buffer system, and 0.03 is the solubility coefficient of CO_2. The equation can be further simplified by combining the two constants, pK and solubility coefficient of CO_2:

$$\begin{aligned} pH &= 6.1 + \log HCO_3^-/pCO_2 \times 0.03 \\ &= 6.1 + \log 1/0.03 + \log HCO_3^-/pCO_2 \\ &= 7.62 + \log HCO_3^-/pCO_2 \\ &= 7.62 - \log pCO_2/HCO_3^- \\ &= 7.62 + \log HCO_3^- - \log CO_2. \end{aligned}$$

When H^+ is expressed in nanomoles instead of pH (a negative log value), pCO_2 can be related to HCO_3 in an equation:

$$H\ (nM) = 24 \times pCO_2\ (mm\ Hg)/HCO_3^-\ (mM)$$

The Henderson-Hasselbalch equation indicates that pH depends on HCO_3^-/pCO_2. pH increases when this ratio increases (alkalosis), and pH decreases when it decreases (acidosis). The ratio may be increased by increasing HCO_3^- (metabolic alkalosis) or by decreasing pCO_2 (respiratory alkalosis). The ratio may be decreased by decreasing HCO_3^- (metabolic acidosis) or increasing pCO_2 (respiratory acidosis).

Whole-Body Acid-Base Balance

Net Acid Production

On a typical American diet, the daily production of nonvolatile acid is about 90 meq/day. The main acids are sulfuric acid (about 40 meq/day), which originates from metabolism of sulfur-containing amino acids such as methionine and cystine, and incompletely metabolized organic acids (about 50 meq/day). The total amount of organic acid produced normally is much more than 50 meq/day, but the bulk of organic acid produced in the body is metabolized, and only a small amount is lost in the urine as organic anions, by escaping metabolism (e.g., citrate) or as a metabolic end product (e.g., urate). On typical American diets, the amount of alkali absorbed from the GI tract is about 30 meq/day. Thus, the net amount of acid produced daily can be estimated as the sum of sulfate and organic anions in the urine minus the net alkali absorbed from the GI tract.

Determination of the net alkali (or acid) content of diet is based on the metabolic fates of dietary chemicals after absorption into the body rather than their in vitro states. For example, dietary citric acid is considered neutral because it is metabolized to CO_2 and water in the body, whereas K^+ citrate is an alkali because it would be converted to K^+ bicarbonate after metabolism. Similarly, arginine Cl^- is an acid, because metabolism of arginine in the body results in formation of HCl. Thus, the net alkali value of diet is best determined by the total number of noncombustible cations (Na^+, K^+, Ca^{2+}, and Mg^{2+}) relative to the total number of noncombustible anions (Cl and P):

$$\text{Net alkali content} = (Na^+ + K^+ + Ca^{2+} + Mg^{2+}) - (Cl^- + 1.8\ P).$$

All units are expressed as meq/day except P, which is expressed as mmol/day. Only the above six ions are considered in the equation because other noncombustible ions are present in negligible amounts in normal food. Sulfate is not included here because the ion is formed in the body only after metabolism of sulfur-containing amino acids.

The amount of alkali absorbed from food does not equal the amount present in food, because absorption of divalent noncombustible ions, Ca^{2+}, Mg^{2+}, and P, is incomplete. Hence, traditionally, measurement of net GI alkali absorption required analysis of both food and stool, which necessitated prolonged collection of stool. Thus, net GI alkali absorption is expressed as net alkali of food minus net alkali of stool.

Analysis of food for measurement of net alkali content is cumbersome, and analysis of stool is even more cumbersome. Such analyses typically require admitting patients to a special metabolic unit. Recently, a new method was developed to measure net GI alkali absorption. In this new method, urine electrolytes, instead of diet and stool electrolytes, are measured. The method is based on the assumption that noncombustible ions absorbed from the GI tract are eventually excreted in the urine, and thus, individual amounts of these electrolytes excreted in the urine would equal those absorbed from the GI tract. Hence

$$\text{Net GI alkali absorption} = \text{urine } (Na^+ + K^+ + Ca^{2+} + Mg^{2+}) - \text{urine } (Cl^- + 1.8\ P)$$

and 24-h urine can be collected in outpatient settings, while the subjects are eating their usual diets. The amount of net alkali absorbed on typical American diet stated earlier, 30 meq/day, was measured by analysis of urine electrolytes using the above formula.

Net Acid Excretion

The most important function of the kidney in acid-base homeostasis is excretion of acid, which is tantamount to generation of alkali. Acid is excreted in the form of NH_4^+ and titratable acid. Another important function of the kidney is excretion of HCO_3. Although the main function of renal excretion of HCO_3^- is prevention of metabolic alkalosis, a small amount of bicarbonate is normally excreted in the urine (about 10 meq/day). Thus, net acid excretion, which is tantamount to net renal production of alkali, can be determined by subtracting HCO_3^- excretion from acid excretion.

$$\text{Net acid excretion} = \text{acid excretion} - HCO_3^- \text{ excretion}$$
$$= NH_4^+ + \text{titratable acid} - HCO_3^-$$

Normally about two-thirds of acid excretion occurs in the form of NH_4^+, but in acidosis, NH_4^+ excretion may increase as much as 10-fold. Excretion of titratable acid is usually modest because of the limited amount of buffer that produces titratable acid (i.e., phosphate, creatinine, and urate) but may be increased markedly in disease states (e.g., β-hydroxybutyrate in diabetic ketoacidosis). Maintenance of acid-base balance requires that net acid production equals net acid excretion (Fig. 6.14). Metabolic acidosis develops when net acid production exceeds net acid excretion, and metabolic alkalosis develops when net acid excretion exceeds net acid production.

Terminology

The terms *acidosis* and *alkalosis* refer to a pathologic process leading to acidic or alkaline pH, whereas acidemia and alkalemia refer to acidic and alkaline pH. Patients could have acidosis but actually have alkaline pH. For example, we may say that a patient has combined respiratory acidosis and metabolic alkalosis. Obviously, the patient cannot have acidic and alkaline pH at the same time, and therefore those terms must refer to pathologic processes. However, clinicians often use the terms interchangeably. For example, if someone says, "the patient has an acidotic pH," she means a low pH, not a pathologic process leading to a low pH.

Metabolic Acidosis

Classification by Net Acid Excretion

All metabolic acidoses result from reduction in bicarbonate content of the body with two minor and clinically unimportant exceptions: acidosis resulting from dilution of the body fluid by administration of a large amount of saline solution (dilution acidosis) and acidosis that results from shift of H^+ from the cell. Reduction in bicarbonate content may be due to a primary increase in acid production (extrarenal acidosis) or due to a primary reduction in net acid excretion (renal acidosis) (Table 6.10). In extrarenal acidosis, net acid excretion is markedly increased as the kidney compensates to overcome acidosis. On the other hand, net acid excretion may be restored to normal in chronic renal acidosis as acidosis stimulates renal H^+ excretion. Normal net acid excretion in the presence of acidemic pH suggests a defect in renal acid excretion, and therefore renal acidosis. If the renal acid excretion capacity is normal, net acid excretion should be supernormal in the presence of acidemic pH (Fig. 6.15).

Renal Acidosis. Renal acidosis is further classified into two types: uremic acidosis and renal tubular acidosis (RTA). In uremic acidosis, reduced net acid excretion results from reduced nephron mass (i.e., renal failure); in renal tubular acidosis, reduction in net acid excretion results from a specific tubular dysfunction. Because development of renal acidosis depends on the rate of net acid excretion as well as the rate of net acid production, which

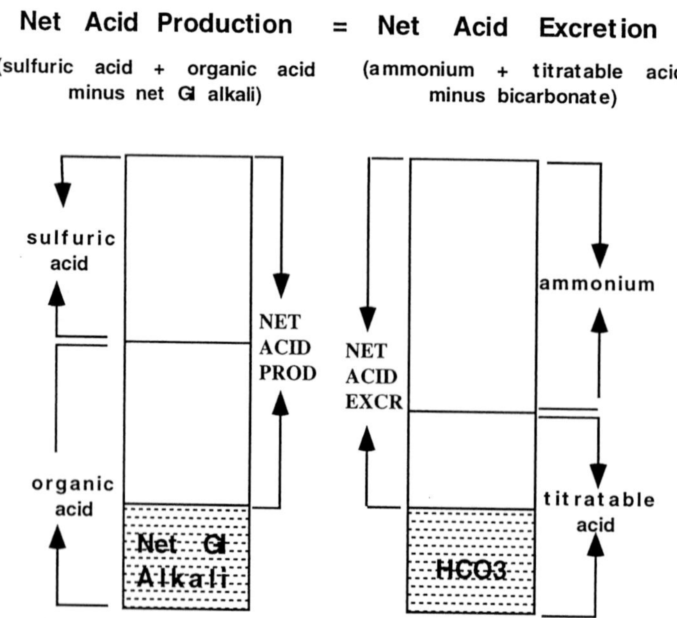

Figure 6.14. Balance between net acid excretion and net acid production. Net acid production is measured as the sum of sulfuric acid and organic acid minus net GI alkali. Net GI alkali represents a net amount of alkali absorbed from the GI tract from the food. Net acid excretion is measured as the sum of urine ammonium and titratable acid minus urine bicarbonate. In acid-base equilibrium, net acid production equals net acid excretion.

Table 6.10
Causes of Metabolic Acidosis According to Net Acid Excretion

Renal acidosis: absolute or relative reduction in net acid excretion
Uremic acidosis
Renal tubular acidosis
Distal renal tubular acidosis (type I)
Proximal renal tubular acidosis (type II)
Aldosterone deficiency or unresponsiveness (type IV)
Extrarenal acidosis: increase in net acid excretion
Gastrointestinal loss of bicarbonate
Ingestion of acids or acid precursors: ammonium chloride, sulfur, toluene
Acid precursors or toxins: salicylate, ethylene glycol, methanol, paraldehyde
Organic acidosis
L-Lactic acidosis
D-Lactic acidosis
Ketoacidosis

varies greatly according to the diet, the level of renal failure at which uremic acidosis develops varies greatly. On a usual diet, uremic acidosis can develop when the GFR falls below 20% of normal.

There are three types of RTA. Type I RTA, also called classical RTA or distal RTA, is characterized by an inability to reduce urine pH below 5.5. Since acidification of urine to a very low urine pH occurs at the collecting duct, the likely site of defect in type I RTA is the collecting duct, which is a part of the distal nephron, hence the term *distal RTA*. Because H^+ secretion in the collecting duct is somewhat impaired also in type IV RTA, some authors consider both type I and type IV RTA a form of distal RTA. Still, most authorities use type I RTA and distal RTA synonymously. In type I RTA, net acid excretion usually remains persistently below daily net acid production, and thus patients develop progressively more severe metabolic acidosis. Type I RTA can develop as a primary disorder or secondary to drug toxicity, tubulointerstitial renal diseases, or other renal diseases.

Type II RTA, also called proximal RTA, has defective proximal bicarbonate reabsorption characterized by a reduced renal bicarbonate threshold. Urine can be made free of bicarbonate and acidified normally when serum bicarbonate decreases to a low level. Most patients with proximal RTA have evidence of generalized proximal tubular dysfunction (i.e., Fanconi's syndrome), which is manifested by bicarbonaturia, aminoaciduria, glycosuria, phosphaturia, and uricosuria. Of these, renal glycosuria (glycosuria in the presence of normal blood glucose levels) is most useful in diagnosing Fanconi's syndrome. Type II RTA may be a primary disorder or secondary to genetic or acquired renal dysfunction. Hypokalemia is a characteristic finding of both type I and type II RTA but tends to be more severe in type I than in type II. A hybrid of types I and II RTA is called type III RTA.

Type IV RTA is caused by aldosterone deficiency or tubular unresponsiveness to aldosterone, resulting in impaired renal tubular potassium secretion and hence hyperkalemia. Although reduced H^+ secretion in the collecting duct plays a role, the major mechanism of acidosis in type IV RTA is hyperkalemia-induced impairment in ammonia production in the proximal tubule. Type IV RTA is far more common than either type I or type II RTA, and the most common cause of type IV RTA is hyporeninemic hypoaldosteronism (Table 6.10).

Organic Acidosis. Extrarenal acidosis may result from administration or ingestion of acid, overproduction of endogenous acid, or loss of bicarbonate. Among these, overproduction of endogenous acid, especially of lactic acid and keto acids, is the most important mechanism. Only marked overproduction leads to acidosis, because of the enormous capacity to metabolize organic acids. For example, about 1300 meq of lactic acid are produced daily in a normal person without resulting in acidosis.

Organic acids are titrated immediately by the body's

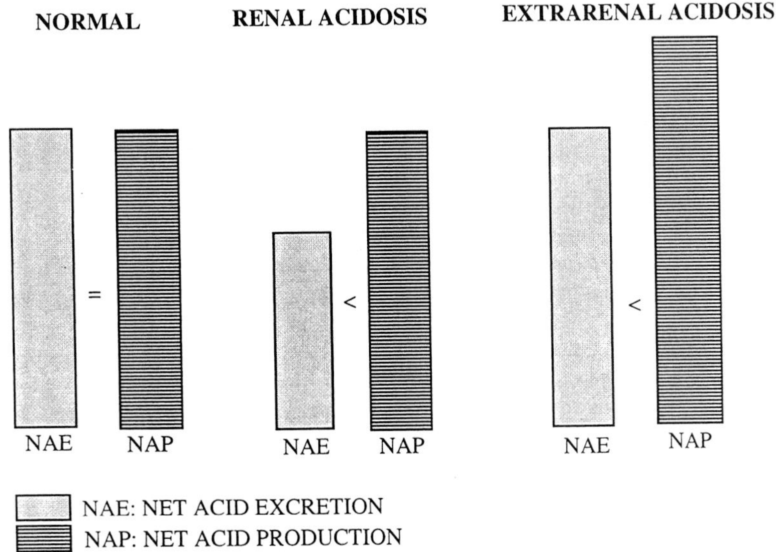

Figure 6.15. Relationship between net acid excretion and net acid production in renal and extrarenal acidosis.

alkaline buffers. When they react with bicarbonate, organic anions and CO_2 are formed. When the anions are retained in body fluid, the result is metabolic acidosis with increased anion gap. When the anions are excreted in the urine, the anion gap returns to normal, and acidosis becomes hyperchloremic. *Retention of these anions per se is not responsible for acidosis.* Their presence merely provides a clue to the mechanism of reduced bicarbonate concentration. Their removal from the body fluid, by dialysis or renal excretion, would not improve the pH. The retained organic anions are potential bicarbonate; when they are metabolized, bicarbonate is regenerated. Thus, loss of organic anions in the urine is tantamount to loss of bicarbonate. If an organic anion is entirely retained, subsequent metabolism results in the complete recovery of the lost alkali. Characteristically, organic acidosis is rapid in onset and in recovery.

Lactic Acidosis. Lactic acid is produced from pyruvic acid by the action of the enzyme lactic acid dehydrogenase (LDH) and the cofactor NADH. Metabolism of lactic acid requires its conversion back to pyruvic acid, using the same enzyme and NAD as a cofactor. For this reason, production and metabolism of lactic acid are reciprocally influenced by the same factors; increased concentration of pyruvic acid and an increased NADH:NAD ratio increase lactic acid production while reducing its metabolism. Consequently, in most cases of lactic acidosis, lactic acid production is increased, and at the same time, its metabolism is reduced.

By far the most common cause of lactic acidosis is tissue hypoxia, which results from circulatory shock, severe anemia, severe heart failure, acute pulmonary edema, cardiac arrest, carbon monoxide poisoning, seizures, vigorous muscular exercise, etc. Normally, lactic acid is produced by extrahepatic tissues and metabolized by the liver, but every organ in the body, except red blood cells, can produce and use lactic acid; red cells can only produce lactic acid. Lactic acidosis in acute alcoholism and severe liver disease is caused by impaired lactic acid metabolism (Table 6.11).

Lactic acidosis, unless specified, refers to the acidosis caused by L-lactic acid, the isomer normally produced in the human body. The enzyme, LDH, responsible for production of lactic acid in the human body is an L-isomer, and therefore only L-lactic acid is formed from human metabolism. D-Lactic acidosis, which is due to the accumulation of D-lactic acid, has been reported in humans.

Table 6.11
Causes of Lactic Acidosis

Tissue hypoxia, e.g., circulatory shock, hypoxemia, heart failure, anemia
Acute alcoholism
Drugs and toxins, e.g., phenformin, isoniazid
Diabetes mellitus
Leukemia
Idiopathic
Short bowel syndrome (D-lactic acidosis)

D-Lactic acidosis is characterized by severe acidosis and neurologic manifestations. The affected patients behave as if they are alcohol intoxicated despite normal blood ethanol levels. The mechanism of D-lactic acidosis is the colonic overproduction of D-lactic acid by bacteria. Necessary requirements for overproduction of D-lactic acid in the colon are delivery of a large amount of substrate to the colon (i.e., malabsorption syndrome) and proliferation of D-LDH-forming bacteria in the colon. Treatment of D-lactic acidosis is oral administration of antibiotics.

Ketoacidosis. Keto acids, acetoacetic acid and β-hydroxybutyric acid, are produced in the liver from free fatty acids (FFAs) and metabolized by the extrahepatic tissues. Unlike lactic acidosis, increased production of keto acids alone, not impaired use, is the mechanism for keto acid accumulation. Increased production requires a high concentration of FFAs and their conversion to keto acids in the liver. Insulin deficiency is responsible for increased mobilization of FFAs from the adipose tissue, and glucagon excess and insulin deficiency stimulate conversion of FFAs to keto acids in the liver.

Two major keto acids in the body are acetoacetic acid and β-hydroxybutyric acid. β-hydroxybutyric acid (BB) is produced from acetoacetic acid (AA) with the enzyme BB dehydrogenase and the cofactor NADH. The same enzyme and NAD are required to convert BB to AA. Consequently, the NADH:NAD ratio is the sole determinant of the BB:AA ratio. Clinical diagnosis of ketoacidosis is usually made with Acetest, which detects AA but not BB. Although BB is the predominant acid in typical ketoacidosis (the usual ratio of BB to AA is about 2.5 to 3.0), the reaction to Acetest represents a fair estimate of the total concentration of keto acids as long as the ratio remains normal. When the ratio of BB to AA is greatly increased, Acetest may be negative or only slightly positive despite retention of a large amount of total ketones in the form of BB. This condition, called β-hydroxybutyric acidosis, is commonly seen in alcoholic ketoacidosis.

Serum Anion Gap

The serum anion gap (AG) is estimated as

$$Na^+ - (Cl^- + HCO_3^-) \text{ or } (Na^+ + K^+) - (Cl^- + HCO_3^-).$$

Since the normal serum potassium concentration is quantitatively a minor component of serum electrolytes, the fluctuation in its concentration affects the overall result little, and hence the first of the two equations is more commonly used to estimate the anion gap, with a normal value of about 12 meq/L (8–16 meq/L). Some authors subtract the normal anion gap from the observed anion gap as we have defined it; calculated this way, the normal anion gap should be zero.

The term *anion gap* implies that there is a gap between cation and anion concentration, but there is no gap; the concentration of total cations in the serum must be exactly equal to the concentration of total anions. Although the total concentration of unmeasured anions (i.e., all anions other than chloride and bicarbonate) is about 23 meq/L, the anion gap, $Na^+ - (Cl^- + HCO_3^-)$, is only 12 meq/L because there are about 11 meq/L of unmeasured cations (i.e., all cations other than sodium). Let us assume that total serum cations = Na^+ + unmeasured cations (UC), and that total serum anions = $Cl^- + HCO_3^-$ + unmeasured anions (UA). Since total serum cations = total serum anions, $Na^+ + UC = (Cl^- + HCO_3^-) + UA$. Hence, $Na^+ - (Cl^- + HCO_3^-) = UA - UC$. Since $AG = Na^+ - (Cl + HCO_3^-)$, the anion gap (AG) = UA − UC (Fig. 6.16). The anion gap is estimated from concentrations of Na^+, Cl^-, and HCO_3^-, but alterations in anion gap can be predicted more readily from changes in unmeasured anions or unmeasured cations than from changes in Na, Cl, or HCO_3. Figure 6.16 shows this relationship graphically.

Clearly, a change in the anion gap must involve changes in UAs or UCs or a laboratory error involving the measurement of Na^+, Cl^-, or HCO_3^-. The anion gap can be increased by increased UA or decreased UC or by a laboratory error resulting in a false increase in serum Na^+ or a false decrease in serum Cl^- or HCO_3^-. AG can be decreased by decreased UA or increased UC or by laboratory errors resulting in a false decrease in serum Na^+ or a false increase in serum Cl^- or HCO_3^-. The equation also predicts that a change in UA may not change AG if UC is changed to the same extent in the same direction. For example, hypermagnesemia due to $MgSO_4$ intoxication does not reduce the AG although a high serum magnesium level increases UC, because the sulfate accumulation also causes an increase in UA. Decreased AG is most commonly due to reduction in serum albumin concentration, while increased AG is most often due to accumulation of anions of acids, such as sulfate, lactate, ketone anions. Since bromide is an unmeasured anion, bromide intoxication should lead to increased AG. However, bromide intoxication is accompanied by a low serum AG, because bromide causes a false increase in serum Cl^-.

A change in serum Na^+ usually does not cause a change in AG, because serum Cl^- usually changes in the same direction. For the same reason, HCO_3^- concentrations cannot be used to predict a change in AG. For example, when the serum HCO_3^- concentration increases in metabolic alkalosis, Cl^- concentration almost invariably decreases reciprocally to maintain electrical neutrality, so AG is unchanged. When HCO_3^- concentration decreases, Cl^- concentration may remain unchanged or increase. If bicarbonate is replaced by another anion, Cl^- concentration remains unchanged, hence normochloremic acidosis with increased AG (e.g., organic acidosis and uremic acidosis). When bicarbonate concentration decreases without another anion replacing it, electrical neutrality is maintained by a higher Cl^- concentration; hence, hyperchloremic acidosis with normal AG.

Proper interpretation of serum AG requires the knowledge of existence of conditions that influence AG even though they may have no effect on metabolic acidosis. For example, if a person with hypoalbuminemia develops lactic acidosis, the AG could be normal because the low albumin and the lactate accumulation have opposite effects on it.

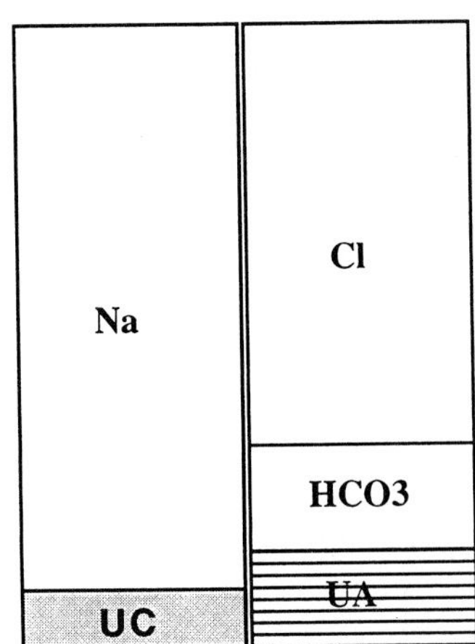

Figure 6.16. Anatomy of anion gap *(AG)*.

Diagnosis

One approach to the differential diagnosis of metabolic acidosis is to measure the serum AG. If the AG is increased, the likely conditions include organic acidosis, uremic acidosis, and acidosis due to certain toxins (Table 6.12). If the AG is normal, the likely conditions include renal tubular acidosis and acidosis due to diarrheal loss of bicarbonate. Contrary to the common misconception, most cases of uremic acidosis are accompanied by normal AG; only in advanced chronic renal failure and acute renal failure is AG increased. Furthermore, the vast majority of patients with ketoacidosis pass through a phase of hyperchloremic acidosis (normal AG) during the recovery phase.

Another approach to the differential diagnosis of meta-

Table 6.12
Classification of Metabolic Acidosis by Anion Gap

Metabolic acidosis with increased anion gap (normochloremic acidosis)
Ketoacidosis
Lactic acidosis, D-lactic acidosis
β-Hydroxybutyric acidosis
Uremic acidosis
Ingestion of toxins: salicylate, methanol, ethylene glycol
Metabolic acidosis with normal anion gap (hyperchloremic acidosis)
Renal tubular acidosis
Uremic acidosis (early)
Acidosis following respiratory alkalosis
Intestinal loss of bicarbonate
Administration of chloride-containing acid: HCl, NH_4Cl
Ketoacidosis during recovery phase

bolic acidosis is to classify it into renal and extrarenal acidosis. Two major causes of extrarenal acidosis are organic acidosis and diarrheal loss of bicarbonate. Organic acidosis is usually obvious from clinical findings (e.g., evidence of tissue hypoxia in lactic acidosis, or hyperglycemia and ketonemia in ketoacidosis). Diarrhea as the cause of metabolic acidosis is first suspected from the history, but history is often misleading, because the severity of diarrhea cannot easily be determined. The measurement of urine AG is useful in determining the severity of diarrhea. Urine AG, which is measured as urine ($Na^+ + K^+$) − urine Cl^-, is reduced or negative when diarrhea is severe. Diarrheal loss of bicarbonate leads to metabolic acidosis, which in turn causes increased urinary excretion of ammonium as a part of the renal compensatory mechanism. Vomiting causes metabolic alkalosis and hence urinary excretion of bicarbonate, leading to increased urine AG.

Once extrarenal acidosis is excluded, renal acidosis is the only alternative diagnosis. Of the two types of renal acidosis, uremic acidosis can be readily diagnosed by measuring serum creatinine and BUN. If renal acidosis is confirmed but uremic acidosis is ruled out, the diagnosis must be renal tubular acidosis (RTA). Among the three types of RTA, type IV RTA will be suspected by the presence of hyperkalemia. Hypokalemia suggests either type I or type II RTA. If spontaneous urine pH is below 5.5, type I RTA is ruled out. If urine pH is higher than 5.5, urine pH should be measured after administration of 40 mg of furosemide by mouth. If the urine pH remains above 5.5, the likely diagnosis is type I RTA.

Treatment

Restoration of normal blood pH and bicarbonate concentration is the ultimate aim of therapy for metabolic acidosis. Rapid restoration of normal pH is usually unnecessary and may be undesirable for several reasons. When the pH is increased acutely, restoration of a normal concentration of the red blood cell 2,3-DPG (diphosphoglycerate) lags behind. In addition, a sudden increase in extracellular pH can cause a paradoxical cerebrospinal fluid (CSF) acidosis. Rapid restoration of a normal serum bicarbonate level in metabolic acidosis would also be undesirable, because persistent hyperventilation would produce a very high blood pH.

The initial aim in the treatment of severe metabolic acidosis should be to increase the blood pH to a level at which adverse cardiovascular effects of severe acidemia can be avoided. Although the risk of acidosis varies with age and cardiovascular status, it is considered prudent, at least in older patients, to keep blood pH above 7.1 to 7.2. The blood pH may be increased by administration of alkali or by allowing alkali to be produced by metabolism of retained organic anions (OA^-) in the case of organic acidosis:

$$\begin{array}{c} OA^- + \underset{\substack{\uparrow \\ CO_2 + H_2O}}{H_2CO_3} \rightarrow OAH + HCO_3^- \end{array}$$

Successful treatment of the cause of organic acidosis increases the serum bicarbonate concentration by this mechanism. When ketoacidosis is treated with insulin and fluid, the outcome is usually predictable: a substantial increase in the plasma bicarbonate concentration. Thus, exogenous alkali is seldom necessary in ketoacidosis. In contrast, response to treatment in lactic acidosis is usually poor. In type A lactic acidosis (due to hypoxia), the prognosis depends on the cause of hypoxia. In most cases of circulatory shock, the prognosis is extremely poor. The prognosis of lactic acidosis due to acute alcohol intoxication is fairly good. With seizure-induced lactic acidosis, recovery is usually complete within hours after the control of the seizure.

Type B lactic acidosis can be treated with administration of alkali in the hope of spontaneous recovery, but administration of bicarbonate tends to be self-defeating because it increases lactic acid production. Rising cell pH increases glycolysis and therefore increases lactic acid production. Discouraged by the poor results of bicarbonate therapy and offering theoretical arguments against alkali therapy, some authors have recommended against using bicarbonate in the treatment of all types of lactic acidosis, but judicious use of bicarbonate is beneficial in severe acidosis.

Three types of alkali can be used for the treatment of metabolic acidosis: bicarbonate, salts of organic acids, and THAM (tromethamine). Organic salts used as a bicarbonate substitute include lactate, acetate, and citrate. Each milliequivalent of the organic salts produces 1 meq of bicarbonate. However, because they require metabolism, an increase in bicarbonate concentration is delayed. Furthermore, when metabolism is impaired (e.g., in lactic acidosis) organic salts may have no effect. The amount and speed of administration of bicarbonate and organic salts vary widely depending on the severity of acidosis.

THAM increases pH by producing HCO_3 in a reaction with H_2CO_3:

$$\begin{array}{c} THAM + \underset{\substack{\uparrow \\ CO_2 + H_2O}}{H_2CO_3} \rightarrow THAM\text{-}H^+ + HCO_3^- \end{array}$$

Because bicarbonate formation by THAM occurs at the expense of carbonic acid, rapid infusion of THAM results in a marked reduction in pCO_2; the rate should not exceed 2 mmol/min. Administration of THAM probably has no advantage in treatment of metabolic acidosis in most situations, but it should be more advantageous than bicarbonate in treating metabolic acidosis complicated by respiratory acidosis.

For a given quantity of administered bicarbonate, the serum bicarbonate level rises less in severe, than in mild, metabolic acidosis (i.e., the apparent volume of distribution of bicarbonate is greater in severe than mild metabolic acidosis). However, the absolute increase in pH for a given dose of bicarbonate administered is greater in more severe metabolic acidosis than in mild acidosis, because the increase in serum bicarbonate is proportionately greater, though less in absolute magnitude, with severe acidosis than with mild acidosis. In practice, however, there is no need to estimate bicarbonate requirements accurately to achieve a certain specific level. Since changes in pCO_2 following acute increase in serum bicarbonate cannot be accurately predicted, it is difficult to predict the pH for a given increase in bicarbonate. The best approach is to administer two to three ampules of sodium bicarbonate (44.5 or 50 meq per ampule) by intravenous injection and then repeat a blood gas measurement 20 to 30 min after bicarbonate injection to determine the need for further therapy.

For treatment of chronic acidosis, citrate (available as Shohl's solution) is more palatable than bicarbonate. For treatment of uremic acidosis in dialysis patients, sodium bicarbonate is the most commonly used alkali in hemodialysis fluids, and sodium lactate in peritoneal dialysis fluids.

Metabolic Alkalosis

At normal serum bicarbonate concentration, bicarbonate filtered at the glomerulus is virtually completely reabsorbed. As serum bicarbonate concentration rises above the normal level, bicarbonate reabsorption is incomplete, and bicarbonaturia begins. A slight increase in serum bicarbonate above 24 meq/L causes marked bicarbonaturia. Hence, when renal tubular bicarbonate handling and GFR are normal, it is very difficult to maintain a high plasma bicarbonate unless an enormous amount of bicarbonate is given.

Maintenance of metabolic alkalosis requires two conditions: a mechanism to increase plasma bicarbonate and a mechanism to maintain the increased concentration. Bicarbonate concentration may be increased by administration of alkali, gastric loss of HCl through vomiting or nasogastric suction, or renal generation of bicarbonate. Plasma bicarbonate concentration can be maintained at a high level if bicarbonate is not filtered at the glomerulus because of advanced renal failure or if filtered bicarbonate is absorbed avidly because of an increased renal threshold for bicarbonate. The two most common causes for increased renal bicarbonate threshold are volume depletion and K^+ depletion (Table 6.13).

The renal threshold for bicarbonate is increased in K^+ depletion because of enhanced tubular reabsorption of bicarbonate and a decrease in glomerular filtration rate, which could reduce the filtered load of bicarbonate. When metabolic alkalosis is caused by volume depletion of nonrenal causes, urinary excretion of Cl^- is reduced. Urinary Na^+ is an unreliable index of volume depletion in metabolic alkalosis, because excretion of bicarbonate may cause obligatory loss of Na despite volume depletion. Metabolic alkalosis accompanied by low urinary chloride can be corrected by administration of chloride-containing fluid (e.g., NaCl or KCl solution), hence the term *chloride-responsive metabolic alkalosis,* e.g., vomiting-induced alkalosis. Patients with chloride-responsive metabolic alkalosis are volume depleted. However, when volume depletion is caused by primary renal sodium loss, urinary loss of Cl^- is not reduced despite volume depletion. Metabolic alkalosis accompanied by normal excretion of chloride in urine is called chloride-resistant metabolic alkalosis (e.g., hypokalemia-induced alkalosis); administration of Cl^- does not correct alkalosis. In edema-forming conditions, administration of Cl^- may not improve metabolic alkalosis even though the pattern of urinary excretion of Cl^- would suggest chloride-responsive metabolic alkalosis, because fluid administration usually does not restore the effective vascular volume to normal. Common clinical conditions that increase serum bicarbonate levels are shown in Table 6.14.

Treatment

When the increased renal bicarbonate threshold in metabolic alkalosis is caused by reduced EAV and hypokalemia, correction of these abnormalities leads to rapid restoration of bicarbonate concentration in most patients. Correction of low EAV is accomplished by administration of normal saline or half-normal saline. Sometimes discontinuation of an offending agent (e.g., a diuretic) and restoration of normal salt intake suffices. If volume depletion is to be corrected, chloride must be given to replace the excreted bicarbonate, either as sodium chloride or as potassium chloride. In certain clinical situations such as edema-forming states, treatment of reduced EAV with salt solution is not effective. In such sit-

Table 6.13
Mechanisms and Causes of Maintaining High Extracellular Bicarbonate

Reduced effective arterial volume, e.g., diuretic therapy, vomiting, edema formation
Potassium deficiency
Chloride deficiency accompanied by volume depletion, e.g., vomiting
High pCO_2
Secondary hypoparathyroidism, e.g., milk-alkali syndrome, hypercalcemia of malignancy due to an osteolytic mechanism
Advanced renal failure

Table 6.14
Mechanisms and Causes of Increasing Extracellular Bicarbonate

Loss of HCl from the stomach, e.g., gastric suction, vomiting
Administration of bicarbonate or bicarbonate precursors, e.g., sodium lactate, sodium acetate, sodium citrate
Shift of H^+ into the cell, e.g., K^+ depletion
Rapid contraction of extracellular volume without loss of bicarbonate, e.g., contraction alkalosis by the use of loop diuretics
Increased renal excretion of acid, e.g., diuretic therapy, high aldosterone state, potassium depletion, high pCO_2, secondary hypoparathyroidism

uations, acetazolamide (Diamox), a carbonic anhydrase inhibitor, will treat metabolic alkalosis as well as edema. Acetazolamide administration usually reduces the renal bicarbonate threshold to a subnormal level, but bicarbonate threshold may remain supernormal despite the drug in severe volume depletion.

Correction of metabolic alkalosis by renal excretion of bicarbonate requires adequate renal function. In renal failure, metabolic alkalosis can be treated by administration of dilute HCl, by acidifying salts, or by dialysis. Acidifying salts include ammonium chloride, arginine chloride, and lysine chloride. Metabolism of these salts results in release of HCl, which then titrates bicarbonate. If continuous acid loss from the stomach is the cause of metabolic alkalosis, an inhibitor of acid secretion such as cimetidine, ranitidine, nizatidine, or famotidine is useful.

Respiratory Alkalosis

With the exception of respirator-induced alkalosis and voluntary hyperventilation, respiratory alkalosis always results from stimulation of the respiratory center. The two most common causes of respiratory alkalosis are hypoxic stimulation of the respiratory center and stimulation through the pulmonary receptors, caused by various lung lesions such as pneumonia, pulmonary congestion, and pulmonary embolism. Certain drugs, e.g., salicylate and progesterone, stimulate the respiratory center directly. Respiratory alkalosis is common in gram-negative sepsis; the mechanism is unclear. Blood pH tends to be extremely high when respiratory alkalosis is caused by psychogenic stimulation of the respiratory center, because the condition is usually superacute, and therefore there is no time for compensation (Table 6.15).

Table 6.15
Causes of Respiratory Alkalosis

Diseases of the lung: any intrapulmonary pathology such as pneumonia, pulmonary fibrosis, pulmonary congestion, pulmonary embolism
Hypoxemia
CNS lesions
Gram-negative sepsis
Drugs: salicylate, progesterone

Treatment

In chronic respiratory alkalosis, treatment is usually not needed because the excellent compensation restores the blood pH to normal or nearly normal values. In acute respiratory alkalosis due to psychogenic hyperventilation, the patient should be sedated to depress the respiratory center. pCO_2 can also be increased by the use of a rebreathing bag.

Respiratory Acidosis

The causes of respiratory acidosis are usually quite apparent. They include diseases of the lung (most common), respiratory muscle, respiratory nerve, thoracic cage, and airways, and suppression of the respiratory center by stroke, drugs such as phenobarbital, or severe hypothyroidism (Table 6.16).

Table 6.16
Causes of Respiratory Acidosis

Lung diseases: chronic obstructive lung disease, advanced interstitial lung disease, acute asthma
Thoracic deformity or airway obstruction
Diseases of respiratory muscle and nerve: myasthenia gravis, hypokalemic paralysis, botulism, amyotrophic lateral sclerosis, Guillain-Barré syndrome
Depression of the respiratory center: barbiturate intoxication, stroke

Treatment

Treatment should be directed toward removing the cause. If the cause cannot be removed quickly and the patient is in acute respiratory distress, mechanical ventilation with endotracheal intubation is indicated. However, the decision to intubate is more often based on hypoxemia than on respiratory acidosis.

Mixed Acid-Base Disorders

The term *mixed acid-base disorder* refers to a clinical condition in which two or more primary acid-base disorders coexist. They generally present with one obvious disturbance and what appears to be an inappropriate (excessive or inadequate) compensation. The "inappropriateness" of the compensatory process is the result of a separate primary disorder. The appropriate degrees of compensation for primary acid-base disorders have been determined by analysis of data from a large number of patients and are expressed as equations in Table 6.17. When the two disorders influence the blood pH in opposite directions, the blood pH is determined by the dominant disorder. If the disorders cancel out each other's effects, blood pH can be normal.

When there is any compensation for acid-base disorders, pCO_2 and HCO_3^- change in the same direction (i.e., both are high or both low). If pCO_2 and HCO_3^- are changed in opposite directions (e.g., pCO_2 is high and HCO_3^- is low, or pCO_2 is low and HCO_3^- is high), a mixed acid-base disorder is certain.

Appropriateness of compensation can be determined by consulting Table 6.17. Compensation can be excessive,

Table 6.17
Formulas for Predicting Normal Acid-Base Compensation[a]

Metabolic acidosis	$\Delta pCO_2 = \Delta HCO_3 \times 1.2 \pm 2$
Metabolic alkalosis[b]	$\Delta pCO_2 = \Delta HCO_3 \times 0.7 \pm 5$
Acute respiratory acidosis	$\Delta HCO_3 = \Delta pCO_2 \times 0.07 \pm 1.5$
Chronic respiratory acidosis	$\Delta HCO_3 = \Delta pCO_2 \times 0.4 \pm 3$
Acute respiratory alkalosis	$\Delta HCO_3 = \Delta pCO_2 \times 0.2 \pm 2.5$
Chronic respiratory alkalosis	$\Delta HCO_3 = \Delta pCO_2 \times 0.5 \pm 2.5$

[a] ΔHCO_3 and ΔpCO_2 represent the difference between normal and actual values.
[b] No matter how high the serum HCO_3 rises, pCO_2 rarely rises above 60 mm Hg in metabolic alkalosis.

insufficient, or appropriate. One can get an idea of the appropriateness of compensation from the degree of pH deviation without consulting the formula for normal compensation. In general, compensation is most effective in respiratory alkalosis (pH is often normalized), the next best is respiratory acidosis (pH may become normal), and the third best is metabolic acidosis. Compensation is least effective in metabolic alkalosis, partly because hypoxemia, an inevitable consequence of hypoventilation, stimulates ventilation. If a patient has low pCO_2 and low HCO_3^- with normal pH, the likely diagnosis is compensated respiratory alkalosis rather than compensated metabolic acidosis.

CLINICAL PROBLEMS AND ANSWERS

Regulation of Intra- and Extracellular Volume and Osmolality

Problems

1. A 45-year-old chronic alcoholic was brought in coma to the emergency room. The patient had the following laboratory values: serum Na, 115 meq/L; serum osmolality, 400 mosm/L; serum glucose, 1000 mg/dL; BUN, 42 mg/dL; and total serum osmolality, 400 mosm/L.
   a. Is the patient's intracellular volume (ICV) increased, decreased, or normal?
   b. When serum glucose is normalized by metabolism, will serum sodium increase, decrease, or remain the same?
   c. When glucose is normalized by metabolism, will extracellular osmolality increase, decrease, or remain the same?
2. Which of the following patients has an increased ICV?
   a. A diabetic patient with serum sodium of 110 meq/L and serum glucose of 2000 mg/dL?
   b. An alcoholic with serum sodium of 125 meq/L and serum alcohol of 500 mg/dL?
   c. A uremic patient with serum sodium of 150 meq/L and serum urea nitrogen of 140 mg/dL?
   d. A patient with serum sodium of 150 meq/L with anasarca?
   e. A patient who developed hyponatremia after receiving 200 g mannitol?
3. A patient weighing 120 lb has serum sodium level of 110 meq/L. How much sodium is needed to increase serum sodium to 120 meq/L? Assume that total body water volume is kept constant.
4. A patient has total body water of 40 L and serum Na concentration of 180 meq/L. What amount of water is required to reduce serum Na to 163 meq/L?
5. Match lettered conditions with numbered laboratory data.
   a) vomiting, b) diarrhea, c) diuretic therapy
   i) Low serum K, low serum bicarbonate, urine Cl more than the sum of urine Na and K
   ii) Low serum K, high serum bicarbonate, normal urine Cl
   iii) Low serum K, high serum bicarbonate, low urine Cl
6. Three patients with identical size, weight, and body composition are admitted to the hospital after acute weight loss of 5 lb overnight, but with different serum Na concentrations. Patient A has serum Na^+ of 120 meq/L; patient B, 140 meq/L; and patient C, 160 meq/L. Which patient do you think has the smallest extracellular volume?

Answers

1. a. The ICV is normal because effective serum osmolality is normal, even though total serum osmolality is increased; alcohol is not an effective osmol. The effective osmolality in this patient is $(115 \times 2) + (1000/18) = 285$ mosm/L.
   b. Metabolism of glucose will cause loss of osmols from the ECF, and hence a shift of water into the cells. Serum sodium therefore will increase.
   c. Extracellular osmolality decreases as glucose enters the cell and is metabolized.
2. b. Only this patient has reduced effective osmolality. The laboratory data do not show an actual value of sodium in Case e, but since mannitol causes hyponatremia by a shift of water from the intracellular fluid to the ECF, the intracellular volume must be decreased.
3. Sodium requirement = Δ serum $Na^+ \times$ TBW = $10 \times 30 = 300$ meq, where Δ serum Na^+ is actual serum Na^+ minus the goal serum Na^+, and total body water (TBW) is calculated as body weight (lb)/4. Although the administered Na^+ is going to remain mostly in the ECF, TBW is used to calculate the sodium requirement, because an increase in serum Na^+ causes an increase in serum osmolality that is exactly twice the value of the increase in serum Na^+. Of course, to calculate the amount of solute required to increase the serum osmolality, one must use TBW rather than ECV. An increase in extracellular osmolality is impossible without increasing intracellular osmolality to the same extent; otherwise, water will keep coming out of the cell.
4. The formula to calculate the amount of water removal to reduce serum Na^+ is (Δ serum Na^+/goal serum Na^+) $\times$ TBW; thus $(17/163) \times 40 = 4.17$ L.
5. a-iii, b-i, c-ii. Diarrhea causes loss of bicarbonate and K^+ in the stool, and thus hypokalemia and metabolic acidosis. Because the loss of bicarbonate in diarrhea is accompanied by loss of K^+ and Na^+, urinary excretion of Na^+ and K^+ tends to be less than that of Cl^-. The higher concentration of Cl^- in urine is accompanied by increased excretion of ammonium, which occurs in response to metabolic acidosis. Both vomiting and diuretic therapy cause hypokalemia and metabolic alkalosis, but the former is accompanied by low urine Cl^- as Cl^- is lost in the vomitus.
6. Patient A has the smallest ECV. Since they all started with the same TBW and lost the same amount of water

(5 lb), the current TBW must be the same for all three patients. Remember that acute weight loss is considered to be entirely water loss. Patient A has the smallest ECV, because A has the largest ICV. Patient A has the largest ICV, because ICV is inversely proportional to the effective osmolality, which is smallest in A.

Disorders of Potassium Metabolism

Problems

1. A 64-year-old man is admitted to the hospital with severe pneumonia, fever, and bacteremia. White blood cell count is 28,500 and platelet count, 700,000. As part of his general evaluation, a blood sample is sent for serum electrolyte concentrations. Serum potassium is reported to be 5.7 meq/L. Rapid evaluation of the electrocardiogram shows no abnormalities. The patient is not acidotic and renal function is nearly normal. What is the likely cause of this patient's hyperkalemia?
2. A 60-year-old woman with diabetes mellitus since age 48 is admitted to the hospital because of shortness of breath. Blood pressure is 160/107. She has slight edema. Serum Na^+, 140; Cl^-, 114; bicarbonate, 15; K^+, 6.5 meq/L. Blood glucose concentration is 170 mg/dL. She is treated with diuretics and with Kayexalate and sorbitol. Serum K^+ the next day is 4.0 meq/L. What is the likely cause of this patient's hyperkalemia?
3. A well-known actress in musical comedy complains of severe weakness and is afraid of falling off the stage during dance routines. The only remarkable physical findings are a transient drop in blood pressure upon standing up, sluggish tendon reflexes, and muscle weakness. ECG shows S-T depression and sagging T waves. An additional complaint is moderate polyuria. Urinary K^+ excretion is 9 meq in 24 h. Blood pH is normal. What is the likely cause of this patient's hypokalemia?

Answers

1. The likely cause is pseudohyperkalemia due to thrombocytosis. Leukocytosis can also cause pseudohyperkalemia, but only when white cell counts are extremely high. However,the absence of ECG abnormality should not be taken as evidence for pseudohyperkalemia, since chronic hyperkalemia, even when quite severe, is often accompanied by a normal ECG.
2. The most likely cause is hyporeninemic hypoaldosteronism, mainly because it is the commonest cause of chronic hyperkalemia. Furthermore, diabetic nephropathy is the most common pathology that causes hyporeninemic hypoaldosteronism. The presence of hypertension further suggests hyporeninemic hypoaldosteronism rather than Addison's disease. Lacking both glucocorticoids and mineralocorticoids, Addison's disease is expected to cause hypotension. Hypotension might also be expected in patients with hyporeninemic hypoaldosteronism, since they are lacking in both renin and aldosterone. However, they are usually hypertensive, suggesting that the effective volume is increased in these patients. In fact, the likely pathogenetic mechanism of the hyporeninemia in this condition is the primary volume expansion resulting from renal salt retention. Low serum bicarbonate is probably the result of type IV RTA, a common complication of hyporeninemic hypoaldosteronism.
3. Nonrenal loss of potassium, such as laxative abuse or diarrhea, is the likely cause of her hypokalemia. The clue is the low excretion of urine K^+. A diuretic therapy or primary hyperaldosteronism would be accompanied by a normal rate of K^+ excretion. Vomiting is also a common cause of hypokalemia, but the main route of K^+ loss in vomiting is the kidney rather than the stomach, as the increased urine bicarbonate causes renal K^+ wasting.

Water and ADH Metabolism

Problems

1. A 63-year-old man with alcoholic cirrhosis of the liver, weighing 120 lbs, was admitted to the hospital complaining of progressive weakness and vomiting for several days, but without neurologic abnormality. On examination, he had poor skin turgor and no subcutaneous fat. Serum Na^+ was 108 meq/L; Cl^-, 78 meq/L; K^+, 2.3 meq/L; HCO_3^-, 29 meq/L. Urine osmolality was 650 mosm/L; BUN, 15 mg/dL; serum creatinine, 1.1 mg/dL; uric acid, 5.5 mg/dL; urine Na, 45 meq/L; and urine pH, 7.5. The patient was treated with 1 L normal saline (154 meq/L of Na^+), with addition of 40 meq/L of K^+ every 6 h for the first 24 h. In 16 hours the serum Na^+ had risen to 121 meq/L, and in 24 hours to 128 meq/L. Three days later, the patient was unable to speak or swallow. CT scan and MRI of the brain showed a hypodense area in the central pons.
   a. Why was hyponatremia corrected so fast with normal saline? Did K^+ administration play a role?
   b. How do you explain the neurologic abnormality?
   c. Does urine osmolality on admission suggest SIADH? If the value had been 200 mosm/L, would you have ruled out SIADH?
   d. Does urine Na^+ on admission suggest SIADH or a volume depletion state?
2. A 65-year-old woman, weighing 150 lbs, was admitted to the hospital because her family felt she was weak and "not quite herself." She had no specific complaints and was able to answer questions. Physical examination suggested moderate dehydration, and the resident estimated her fluid loss at about 4 L. She had a 10-cm curved scar over the area of the frontal lobe of the brain, BUN was 45 mg/dL; creatinine, 1.3. Serum Na^+ was 182 meq/L; urine osmolality, 550 mosm/L; urinary Na^+, 75 meq/L. After pitressin was administered, the urine osmolality rose to 750 mosm/L.

True or False?

a. The patient's hypernatremia is entirely due to water loss.

b. CT scan of the head would show marked brain shrinkage consistent with severe hyperosmolality.

c. The patient has central diabetes insipidus.

d. The patient has a thirst defect as well as a defect in water conservation.

e. The patient should immediately receive an infusion of pitressin and water sufficient to lower her serum Na to 140 meq/L within the next 12–16 hours.

f. From the information given, can you prove that the patient does not have osmotic diuresis?

3. A 72-year-old healthy man ingests a diet that allows him to excrete a total of 800 mosm/day solute and 2 L water.

a. What will be his average urine osmolality on the diet indicated?

b. What would be his average urine osmolality if he increased salt intake and excreted 1000 mosm of solute and drank less water to decrease urine output to 1 L/day?

c. What would be his average urine osmolality if he reduced his food intake and excreted only 320 mosm of solute and drank enough water to increase urine output to 4 L/day?

d. What would his fluid balance be if he developed lung cancer and had a high blood level of ADH that prevented urine osmolality from falling below 400 mosm/L while ingesting the original diet and drinking the 4 L/day of water?

Answers

1. a. As volume depletion was corrected, water diuresis occurred. Administration of K^+ has almost the same effect as that of sodium for the following reasons. Potassium is retained mostly in the cell, and therefore it requires a shift of K^+ into the cells in exchange for extracellular shift of Na. Potassium in this case thus has the same effect on extracellular sodium concentration as sodium. Alternatively, if the administered K^+ is excreted in the urine, it will be accompanied by water. The loss of water causes a rise in serum Na^+.

b. A rapid increase in serum Na^+ in a patient with chronic hyponatremia can cause central pontine myelinolysis (CPM), and the patient has characteristic clinical findings of CPM.

c. Urine osmolality is rarely useful in differential diagnosis of hyponatremia, because virtually every patient with hyponatremia has inappropriately concentrated urine, i.e., urine osmolality in excess of 100 mosm/L in the presence of hyponatremia. The only exception is hyponatremia due to primary polydipsia, in which urine osmolality is expected to be less than 100 mosm/L. However, the polyuria and polydipsia of primary polydipsia make the diagnosis obvious. Urine osmolalities of 650 mosm/L and 200 mosm/L are both consistent with SIADH, but they are also consistent with most other causes of hyponatremia.

d. Urine Na^+ concentration on admission argues against dehydration. On the other hand, a high urine pH (7.5) indicates increased excretion of bicarbonate, which can cause Na^+ diuresis despite dehydration. When urine pH is high, urine Cl^- concentration is a more reliable indicator of the volume status.

2. a. False. If water deficit were the sole cause of hypernatremia, serum Na^+ concentration of 182 meq/L would require a loss of 9.2 L water for a person with total body water of 40 L. The amount of water deficit needed to raise serum Na^+ to 182 meq/L is calculated as (ΔNa $\times$ TBW)/goal Na^+ = (42 $\times$ 40)182 = 9.2 L. The patient was judged to be only moderately dehydrated by the resident, who estimated the loss of water at 4 L. Obviously, a big part of hypernatremia was caused by the retention of Na^+.

b. False. Because the hypernatremia was chronic as shown by the lack of severe neurologic abnormalities, the brain volume would be nearly normal.

c. True. Urine osmolality of 550 mosm/L is inappropriately low for the patient's severe hypernatremia, and therefore the patient has diabetes insipidus (DI). The subsequent response to exogenous ADH indicates that it was central DI.

d. True. The patient has deficiency of ADH and a thirst defect. In fact, if ADH deficiency were the only defect the patient had, the patient would have been polydipsic and polyuric but not hypernatremic.

e. False. Since the patient has chronic hypernatremia with a near normal brain volume, rapid correction of hyponatremia can cause brain edema and therefore should be avoided.

f. To rule out osmotic diuresis one must know the rate of solute excretion, which requires urine osmolality and urine volume. Since only urine osmolality is known, osmotic diuresis cannot be ruled out in this case.

3. a. 800 mosm/2 L = 400 mosm/L

b. 1000 mosm/1 L = 1000 mosm/L

c. 320 mosm/4 L = 80 mosm/L

d. The patient will retain water and develop hyponatremia.

Acid-Base Disorders

Problems

1. A 46-year-old alcoholic man with type I diabetes mellitus is brought to the hospital after he was discovered unconscious. In the ambulance, his vital signs were BP, 80/40 mm Hg; pulse, 120/min; respiration rate, 40/min. The chest and abdomen were normal, except for a surgical scar in the middle line of the upper abdomen. The ER physician subsequently learned that a day before the patient became ill, he drank whiskey and skipped his usual insulin dose. He gave no history of malabsorption syndrome. The laboratory tests on

admission to the ER showed the following. Urinalysis: 4+ glucose, 4+ ketones, 1+ protein, no RBC. Serum Na^+, 144 meq/L; Cl^-, 109 meq/L; K^+, 5.5 meq/L; CO_2, 14 mmol/L; glucose, 920 mg/dL; creatinine, 2.1 mg/dL; BUN, 90 mg/dL; serum ketone, 2+; serum lactate, 2.5 meq/L; measured serum osmolality, 360 mosm/L. Arterial blood gases: pH 7.32, pCO_2 28 mm Hg, pO_2 105 mm Hg on room air.
   a. Does the patient have ketoacidosis?
   b. Is the respiratory compensation appropriate?
   c. If net acid excretion had been 70 meq/day (usual normal value 40–100) in this patient at the time of admission, would this have ruled out renal acidosis?
2. The serum anion gap can be best predicted from the formula AG = unmeasured anion − unmeasured cation, where unmeasured anions are defined as any anions other than Cl and bicarbonate, and unmeasured cations any cations other than Na.
   a. Bromide is an unmeasured anion according to the above definition. However, bromide intoxication lowers anion gap. Why?
   b. Why is serum anion gap usually normal in hypermagnesemia due to $MgSO_4$?
   c. What is the effect of high serum Na^+ or Cl^- on serum anion gap?
3. HCO_3/pCO_2 determines pH. Normal blood pH is 7.4 with normal HCO_3^- of 24 mmol/L and normal pCO_2 of 40 mm Hg; the normal ratio is 24/40. If pCO_2 is 20 mm Hg and HCO_3^- 14 mM, will pH be higher or lower than 7.4?
4. Data: Serum Na^+, 138; K^+, 4.2 meq/L; Cl^-, 114, bicarbonate, 12 meq/L. Within seconds you know the diagnosis, hyperchloremic metabolic acidosis, and suspect two conditions: diarrhea and renal tubular acidosis (RTA).
   a. What serum electrolyte value argues against RTA in this patient?
   b. What is the commonest cause of type IV RTA?
   c. What test would you need to diagnose diarrhea as the cause?
   d. Do you think your diagnosis, hyperchloremic acidosis, is premature? What test is essential before such a conclusion ?
   e. If blood pH were 7.4, what would pCO_2 be? What would your diagnosis be? If a drug was responsible for this type of acid-base disorder, what would it be?
5. Why are there two phases of compensation (acute and chronic) for respiratory acidosis and respiratory alkalosis, but only one phase of compensation for metabolic acidosis and metabolic alkalosis?
6. Indicate whether the serum anion gap is increased (I), decreased (D), or unchanged (U) with the following.
   a. Low serum Na^+
   b. Low serum Cl^-
   c. Lithium intoxication
   d. Hypoalbuminemia
   e. Lactic acidosis
   f. Bromide intoxication
   g. Diarrhea-induced metabolic acidosis
   h. Hypermagnesemia due to $MgSO_4$ overdose

Answers

1. a. The increased serum anion gap suggests organic acidosis or advanced uremic acidosis. The serum creatinine of 2.1 mg/dL rules out advanced uremic acidosis. Among the organic acidoses, lactic acidosis is ruled out by the serum lactate level of only 2.5 meq/L (the value must be at least 6 meq/L). Usual ketoacidosis requires a stronger Acetest reaction. However, β-hydroxybutyric acidosis (a type of ketoacidosis) can occur with a modest elevation in acetoacetate, which Acetest primarily reacts with. D-Lactic acidosis does not occur in the absence of malabsorption syndrome.
   b. Yes. Using the formula for normal compensation in Table 6.17 shows that a pCO_2 of 28 mm Hg is an appropriate compensation for 14 meq/L bicarbonate.
   c. If net acid excretion were only 70 meq/day, you would have to suspect renal acidosis. In extrarenal acidosis, net acid excretion is not normal but markedly increased.
2. a. Bromide is measured as chloride in most hospital laboratories at higher than its actual concentration. This results in pseudohyperchloremia and hence a low serum anion gap.
   b. Because both unmeasured anion (sulfate) and unmeasured cation (Mg) are increased.
   c. The effects of high serum Na^+ or Cl^- on serum anion gap cannot be predicted without knowing how other ions are altered.
3. The pH would be higher than 7.4, because pCO_2 is exactly a half of the normal value, but bicarbonate is slightly higher than the normal value. Thus, bicarbonate/pCO_2 is slightly increased.
4. a. In types I and II RTA, serum K^+ is low, and in type IV RTA, serum K^+ is high. Therefore, a normal serum potassium concentration in this patient argues against RTA.
   b. Hyporeninemic hypoaldosteronism.
   c. Urine anion gap, which is expected to be reduced or negative. The low urine anion gap in diarrhea is due to increased renal excretion of ammonium.
   d. Chronic respiratory alkalosis can also be accompanied by low serum bicarbonate and high serum chloride concentrations. The blood pH will allow one to decide between chronic respiratory alkalosis and hyperchloremic metabolic acidosis. In the former, the blood pH would be slightly high or high normal, and in the latter, the blood pH would be low.
   e. The normal blood pH suggests chronic respiratory alkalosis more than chronic metabolic acidosis; the former is better compensated than the latter. Salicylate and progesterone are two drugs that can produce chronic respiratory alkalosis.
5. In respiratory acid-base disorders there are two distinct

stages of compensation. The first stage, which is completed within seconds, is due to tissue buffering. The second stage is due to renal compensation, which requires several days. Thus, no matter how acute respiratory acid-base disorder may be, the acute phase of compensation is always completed. In contrast, in metabolic acid-base disorders, there is only one stage of compensation, the ventilatory adjustment, which requires 12 to 24 hours to complete.

6. a, U; b, U; c, D; d, D; e, I; f, D; g, U; h, U.

TOPICAL READING LISTS

Regulation of Body Volumes and Osmolality

Briggs JP, Singh I, Sawaya BE, Schnerman J. Disorders of salt balance. In: Kokko JP, Tannen RL, eds. Fluid and electrolytes. 3rd ed. Philadelphia: WB Saunders, 1996.

Gullans SR, Verbalis JG. Control of brain volume during hyperosmolar and hypoosmolar conditions. Annu Rev Med 1993;44: 289–301.

Jensen MD, Kanaley JA, Roust LR, O'Brien PC, et al. Assessment of body composition with the use of dual-energy x-ray absorptiometry: evaluation and comparison with other methods. Mayo Clin Proc 1993;69:867–73.

Levin A, Klassen J, Halperin ML. Osmotic diuresis: the importance of counting the number of osmoles excreted. Clin Invest Med 1995;18:401–5.

McManus ML, Churchill KB, Strange K. Regulation of cell volume in health and disease. N Engl J Med 1995;333:1260–6.

Oh MS, Carroll HJ. Regulation of intracellular and extracellular volume. In: Arieff AI, DePronzo RA, eds. Fluid and electrolyte, and acid-base disorders. 2nd ed. Edinburgh: Churchill-Livingstone, 1995.

Videen JS, Micaelis T, Pinto P, Ross BD. Human cerebral osmolytes during chronic hyponatremia. A proton magnetic resonance spectroscopy study. J Clin Invest 1995;95:788–93.

Zardetto-Smith AM, Thunhorst RL, Cicha ML, Johnson AK. Afferent signaling and forebrain mechanisms in the behavioral control of extracellular volume. Ann NY Acad Sci 1993:689: 161–76.

Disorders of Potassium Metabolism

Allon M. Hyperkalemia in end-stage renal disease: mechanisms and management. J Am Soc Nephrol 1995;16:1134–8.

Gadallah MI, Abreo K, Work J. Liddle's syndrome, an under recognized entity: a report of four cases, including the first report in black individuals. Am J Kidney Dis 1995;25:829–35.

Gladziwa U, Schwarz R, Gittera H, et al. Chronic hypokalemia of adults: Gitelman's syndrome is frequent but classical Bartter's syndrome is rare. Nephrol Dial Transplant 1995;10:1607–13.

Greenberg S, Reiser IW, Chou SY, Porush J. Trimethoprim-sulfamethoxazole induces reversible hyperkalemia. Ann Intern Med 1993;119:291–5.

Howes LG. Which drugs affect potassium? Drug Safety 1995;12: 240–4.

Kamel KS, Ethier JH, Quaggin S, et al. Studies to determine the basis for hyperkalemia in recipients of a renal transplant who are treated with cyclosporine. J Am Soc Nephrol 1992;2: 1279–84.

Kamel KS, Quaggin S, Scheich A, Halperin ML. Disorders of potassium metabolism: an approach based on pathophysiology. Am J Kidney Dis 1994;24:597–613.

Kim HJ. Combined effect of bicarbonate and insulin with glucose in acute therapy of hyperkalemia in end-stage renal disease. Nephron 1996;72:476–82.

Kruse JA, Clark VL, Carlson RW, Geheb MA. Concentrated potassium chloride infusions in critically ill patients with hypokalemia. J Clin Pharmacol 1994;34:1077–82.

Pathophysiology of Water and ADH Metabolism

Ellis SJ. Severe hyponatremia: complications and treatment. Q J Med 1995;88:905–9.

Musch W, Thimpont J, Vandervelde D, et al. Combined fractional excretion of sodium and urea better predicts response to saline in hyponatremia than do usual clinical and biochemical parameters. Am J Med 1995;99:348–55.

Nora NA, Hedger R, Batlle DC. Severe acute peripartum hypernatremia. Am J Kidney Dis 1992;19:385–8.

Oh MS, Carroll HJ. Disorders of sodium metabolism: hypernatremia and hyponatrenia. Crit Care Med 1992;20:94–103.

Oh MS, Carroll HJ. Essential hypernatremia: is there such a thing? Nephron 1994;67:144–5.

Oh MS, Kim HJ, Carroll HJ. Recommendations for treatment of symptomatic hyponatremia. Nephron 1995;70:143–50.

Palevsky PM, Bhagrath R, Greenberg A. Hypernatremia in hospitalized patients. Ann Intern Med 1996;124:197–203.

Sterns RH, Cappuccio JD, Silver SM, Cohen ED. Neurologic sequelae after treatment of hyponatremia: a multicenter perspective, J Am Soc Nephrol 1994;4:1522–30.

Zarinetchi F, Berl T. Evaluation and management of severe hyponatremia. Adv Intern Med 1996;41:251–83.

Acid-Base Disorders

Battle D, Flores G. Underlying defects in distal renal tubular acidosis: new understandings. Am J Kidney Dis 1996;27:896–915.

Elisaf M, Merkouropoulos M, Tsianos EV, Siamopoulos KC. Acid-base and electrolyte abnormalities in alcoholic patients. Miner Electrolyte Metab 1994;20:274–81.

Halperin ML, Kamel KS. D-Lactic acidosis: turning sugars into acids in the gastrointestinal tract. Kidney Int 1996;49: 1–8.

Kitabchi AE, Wall BM. Diabetic ketoacidosis. Med Clin North Am 1995;79:9–37.

Laski ME, Kurtzman NA. Acid-base disorders in medicine. Dis Month 1996;42:511–25.

Oh MS. A new method for estimating G-I absorption of alkali. Kidney Int 1989;36:915–7.

Oh MS, Carroll HJ. The anion gap. N Engl J Med 1977;297:814–7.

Oh MS, Carroll HJ. Contributions to nephrology. Whole body acid-base balance. In: Berlyne GM, ed. The kidney today. Basel: Karger, 1992;100:89–104.

Sabatini S. The cellular basis of metabolic alkalosis. Kidney Int 1996;49:906–17.

Sulders YM, Frissen PH, Slaats EH, Siberbusch J. Renal tubular acidosis. Pathophysiology and diagnosis. Arch Intern Med 1996;156:1629–36.

Uribarri J, Douyon H, Oh MS. A reevaluation of the urinary parameters of acid production and excretion in patients with chronic renal acidosis. Kidney Int 1995;47:624–7.

7. Calcium

CONNIE M. WEAVER and ROBERT P. HEANEY

BIOLOGIC ROLES OF CALCIUM

In higher mammals, the most obvious role of calcium is structural or mechanical and is expressed in the mass, hardness, and strength of the bones and teeth. But calcium has another fundamental function: shaping key biologic proteins to activate their catalytic and mechanical properties. A significant portion of the regulatory apparatus calcium metabolism of the body is concerned with protection of this second function (e.g., all activities and roles of parathyroid hormone (PTH), calcitonin, and vitamin D). The structural role is discussed in greater detail in Chapter 83, while the cell metabolic, regulatory, and nutritional aspects of this critical element are discussed in this chapter.

Abbreviations: **Ca**—calcium; **ECF**—extracellular fluid; **PTH**—parathyroid hormone.

Calcium and the Cell

The calcium ion (Ca^{2+}) has an ionic radius of 0.99 Å and is able to form coordination bonds with up to 12 oxygen atoms (1). The combination of these two features makes calcium nearly unique among all cations in its ability to fit neatly into the folds of the peptide chain. By binding with the oxygen atoms of glutamic and aspartic acid residues projecting from the peptide backbone, calcium stiffens the protein molecule and fixes its tertiary structure. Magnesium and strontium, which are chemically similar to calcium in the test tube, have different ionic radii and do not bond so well with protein. Lead and cadmium ions, by contrast, substitute quite well for calcium, and in fact, lead binds to various calcium-binding proteins with greater avidity than does calcium itself. (Fortunately, neither element is present in significant quantity in the milieu in which living organisms thrive. Nevertheless, the ability of lead to bind to the calcium-binding proteins is a part of the basis for lead toxicity.)

Binding of calcium to a large number of cell proteins (see Table 7.1 for some examples) results in the activation of their unique functions (2). These proteins range from those involved with cell movement and muscle contraction to nerve transmission, glandular secretion, and even cell division. In most of these situations, calcium acts as both a signal transmitter from the outside of the cell to the inside and an activator of the functional proteins involved. In fact, ionized calcium is the most common signal transmitter in all of biology. It operates from bacterial cells all the way up to cells of highly specialized tissues in higher mammals.

When a cell is activated (e.g., a muscle fiber receives a nerve stimulus to contract), the first thing that happens is that calcium channels in the plasma membrane open to admit a few calcium ions into the cytosol. These bind immediately to a wide array of intracellular activator proteins, which in turn release a flood of calcium from the intracellular storage vesicles (the sarcoplasmic reticulum, in the case of muscle). This second step quickly raises cytosol calcium concentration and leads to activation of the contraction complex. Two of the many calcium-binding proteins are of particular interest here: *(a)* troponin c, after it has bound calcium, initiates a series of steps that lead to the actual muscle contraction; and *(b)* calmodulin, a second and widely distributed calcium-binding protein, activates the enzymes that break down glycogen to release energy for contraction. In this way, calcium ions both trigger the contraction and fuel the process. When the cell has completed its assigned task, the various pumps quickly lower the cytosol calcium concentration, and the cell

Table 7.1
Examples of Cell Proteins Binding or Activated by Calcium

Protein	Function
Calmodulin	Modulator/regulator of several protein kinases
Troponin C	Modulator of muscle contraction
Calretinin, retinin	Activator of guanyl cyclase
Calneurin B	Phosphatase
Protein kinase C	Widely distributed protein kinase
Phospholipase A_2	Synthesis of arachidonic acid
Caldesmon	Regulator of muscle contraction
Parvalbumin	Calcium storage
Calbindin	Calcium storage
Calsequestrin	Calcium storage

returns to a resting state. These processes are described in more detail below.

If all of the functional proteins of a cell were fully activated by calcium at the same time, the cell would rapidly self-destruct. For that reason, cells must keep free calcium ion concentrations in the cytosol at extremely low levels, typically on the order of 0.1 μmol. This is 10,000-fold lower than the concentration of calcium ion ($[Ca^{2+}]$) in the extracellular water outside the cell. Cells maintain this concentration gradient by a combination of mechanisms: *(a)* a cell membrane with limited calcium permeability; *(b)* ion pumps that move calcium rapidly out of the cytosol, either to the outside of the cell or into storage vesicles within the cell; and *(c)* a series of specialized proteins in the storage vesicles that have no catalytic function in their own right, but which serve only to bind (and hence sequester) large quantities of calcium. Low cytosolic $[Ca^{2+}]$ ensures that the various functional proteins remain dormant until the cell activates certain of them, which it does simply by letting $[Ca^{2+}]$ rise in critical cytosolic compartments.

OCCURRENCE AND DISTRIBUTION IN NATURE

Calcium is the fifth most abundant element in the biosphere (after iron, aluminum, silicon, and oxygen). It is the stuff of limestone and marble, coral and pearls, sea shells and egg shells, antlers and bones. Because calcium salts exhibit intermediate solubility, calcium is found both in solid form (rocks) and in solution. It was probably present in abundance in the watery environment in which life first appeared. Today, seawater contains approximately 10 mmol calcium per liter (approximately eight times higher than the calcium concentration in the extracellular water of higher vertebrates), and even fresh waters, if they support an abundant biota, typically contain calcium at concentrations of 1 to 2 mmol. In most soils, calcium exists as an exchangeable cation in the soil colloids. It is taken up by plants, whose parts typically contain from 0.1 to as much as 8% calcium. Generally, calcium concentrations are highest in the leaves, lower in the stems and roots, and lowest in the seeds.

In land-living mammals, calcium accounts for 2 to 4% of gross body weight. A 60-kg adult human female typically contains about 1000 to 1200 g (25–30 mol) of calcium in her body. More than 99% of that total is in the bones and teeth. About 1 g is in the plasma and extracellular fluid (ECF) bathing the cells, and 6 to 8 g in the tissues themselves (mostly sequestered in calcium storage vesicles inside cells, see above).

In the circulating blood, calcium concentration is typically 2.25 to 2.5 mmol. About 40 to 45% of this quantity is bound to plasma proteins, about 8 to 10% is complexed with ions such as citrate, and 45 to 50% is dissociated as free ions. In the ECF outside of the blood vessels, total calcium concentration is on the order of 1.25 mmol, which differs from the concentration in plasma because of the absence of most plasma proteins from the ECF. It is the calcium concentration in the ECF which the cells see, and which is tightly regulated by the parathyroid, calcitonin, and vitamin D hormonal control systems.

With advancing age, humans commonly accumulate calcium deposits in various damaged tissues, such as atherosclerotic plaques in arteries, healed granulomas, and other scars left by disease or injury, and often in the rib cartilages as well. These deposits are called dystrophic calcification and rarely amount to more than a few grams of calcium. These deposits are not caused by dietary calcium but by local injury, coupled with the widespread tendency of proteins to bind calcium. Calcification in tissues other than bones and teeth is generally a sign of tissue damage and cell death.

METABOLISM

Homeostatic Regulation

Plasma calcium, which is in exchange with ECF calcium, is tightly regulated at approximately 2.5 mM (9–10 mg/dL). If serum calcium concentration lies more than 10% away from the population mean, there is reason to suspect disease. The homeostatic regulation of serum calcium requires a system of controlling factors and feedback mechanisms (Fig. 7.1).

When plasma calcium concentration falls, the parathyroid gland is stimulated to release PTH. PTH promptly increases renal phosphate clearance, increases renal tubular reabsorption of calcium, activates bone resorption loci and augments osteoclast work at existing resorption loci, and activates vitamin D to enhance intestinal calcium absorption. Activation of vitamin D occurs in two steps. An initial hydroxylation by vitamin D 25-hydroxylase in a microsomal cytochrome enzyme system similar to the P450 system that occurs in the liver. The second hydroxylation by 25-OH-D-1α-hydroxylase in the proximal convoluted tubule cells of the kidney converts the vitamin to its active potent form, 1,25-dihydroxyvitamin D (1,25$(OH)_2$D), or calcitriol (see Chapter 18 for additional details.) This step is stimulated by PTH through a fall in serum phosphate. PTH and 1,25$(OH)_2$D act synergistically to enhance renal tubular reabsorption of calcium and to

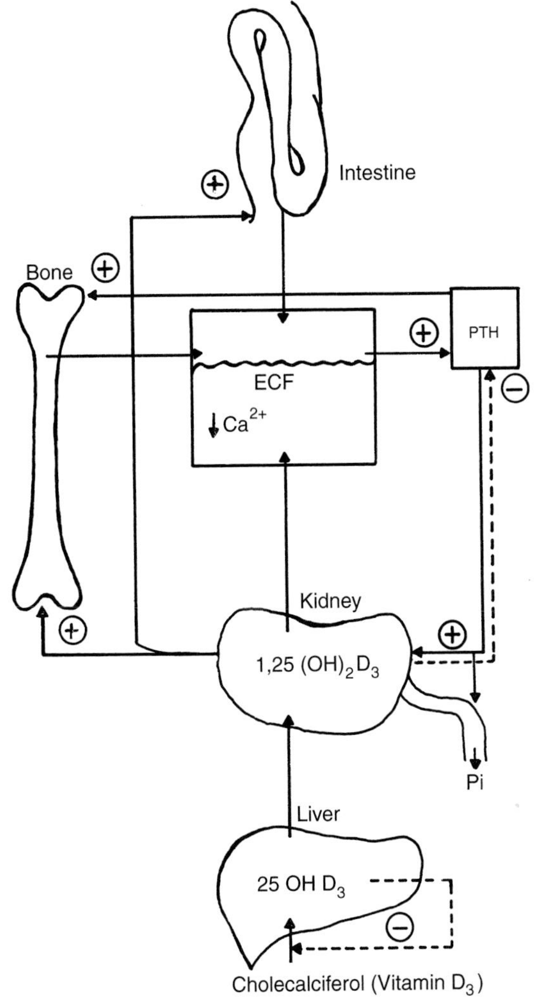

Figure 7.1. Homeostatic regulation of serum calcium depicting the positive and negative controls in effect when plasma calcium falls below 2.5 mM.

mobilize calcium stores from bone. PTH acts in a classical negative feedback loop to raise the ECF [Ca^{2+}], thereby closing the loop and reducing PTH release. Although this sophisticated regulatory mechanism allows a rapid response to correct transient hypocalcemia, in situations of a chronically deficient calcium diet it does so only with serious consequences to the skeleton.

When plasma calcium concentration rises in response to increased calcium absorption, increased tubular reabsorption, and bone resorption, the renal excretory threshold changes, and extra calcium is excreted in the urine.

In infants and children, a principal defense against hypercalcemia is release of calcitonin by the C cells of the thyroid gland. Calcitonin is a peptide hormone with binding sites in the kidney, bone, and central nervous system. Absorption of calcium from an 8-oz feeding in a 6-month-old infant dumps 150 to 220 mg calcium into the ECF. This is enough, given the small size of the ECF compartment at that age (1.5–2 L), to produce fatal hypercalcemia if other adjustments are not made. What happens is that calcitonin (CT) is released, in part in response to the rise in serum calcium concentration, but even before that, in response to gut hormones signaling coming absorption. This burst of CT slows or halts osteoclastic resorption, thus stopping bony release of calcium. Later, when absorption stops, CT levels fall also, and osteoclastic resorption resumes. By contrast, CT has little significance in adults because absorption is lower to begin with, and the ECF is vastly larger. As a result, absorptive calcemia from a high-calcium diet raises the ECF [Ca^{2+}] by only a few percentage points.

Absorption

Calcium usually is freed from complexes in the diet during digestion and is released in a soluble and probably ionized form for absorption. However, low-molecular-weight complexes, such as calcium oxalate and calcium carbonate, can be absorbed intact (3).

Fractional calcium absorption (absorptive efficiency) generally varies approximately inversely with intake, but the absolute quantity of calcium absorbed increases with intake (4, 5). However, only 20% of the variation in calcium absorption can be accounted for by the usual calcium intake that is thought to reflect calcium status (6). Rather, individuals seem to have preset absorptive efficiencies; approximately 60% of the variance in calcium absorption between individuals can be accounted for by their individual fractional calcium absorption (7).

An exception to the inverse relationship between fractional calcium absorption and load occurs in the presence of wheat bran given as extruded cereal. The enormous calcium-binding capacity of this fiber-rich food bound half of the calcium across the spectrum of usual dietary intakes (8).

Mechanisms of Absorption

Calcium absorption occurs by two pathways:

1. Transcellular: saturable (active) transfer that involves a calcium-binding protein, calbindin
2. Paracellular: a nonsaturable (diffusional) transfer that is a linear function of the calcium content of the chyme

The relationship between calcium intake and absorbed calcium is shown in Figure 7.2. At lower calcium intakes, the active component contributes to absorbed calcium. As calcium intakes increase and the active component becomes saturated, an increasing proportion of calcium is absorbed by passive diffusion. The figure illustrates that the adaptive component (i.e., the change in active transport produced by intakes that differ from the group mean) is rather small. This demonstrates our inefficiency in compensating for a fall in calcium intake.

Active absorption is more efficient in the duodenum and proximal jejunum where the pH is more acid (pH ≈ 6.0) and where calbindin is present. However, absorption is greater in the ileum where the residence time is greatest. Absorption from the colon accounts for about 5% of

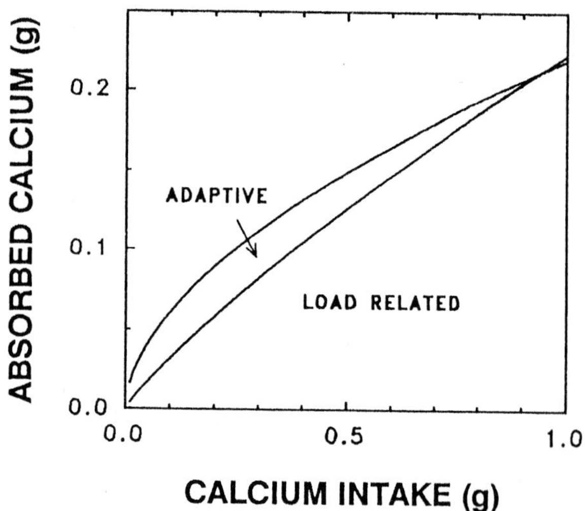

Figure 7.2. Relationship between calcium intake and absorbed calcium in women tested on their usual calcium intakes (adaptive) and in women tested with no prior exposure to the test load (load-related, a physiochemical effect).

the total absorption in normal individuals but may be important in patients with small bowel resections and where colonic bacteria break down dietary complexes.

Transcellular Calcium Transport. Calcium (and phosphorus) movement into the epithelial cells probably occurs through calcium channels or a transporter (9) down a steep gradient and does not require energy. The main regulator of transport across the epithelial cell against the energy gradient is $1,25(OH)_2D$. As illustrated in Figure 7.3, $1,25(OH)_2D$, which is responsive to serum calcium levels, regulates the synthesis of calbindin by DNA transcription upon binding of the vitamin with receptors in the nucleus. This affects the stability (i.e., translation) of the calbindin mRNA. Intestinal calbindin, a 9-kDa protein in mammals and a 28-kDa protein in birds, is capable of binding two Ca^{2+} per molecule. Calbindin operates by binding Ca^{2+} on the surface of the cell, then internalizing the ions via endocytic vesicles that probably fuse with lysosomes. After release of the bound calcium in the acidic lysosomal interior, the calbindin returns to the cell surface, and the Ca^{2+} ions exit the cell via the basolateral membrane (10). Calbindin serves both as a Ca^{2+} translocator and a cytosolic Ca^{2+} buffer (11). Using ion microscopic imaging of injected $^{44}Ca^{2+}$, calcium entry into the villus was observed in vitamin D–deficient chicks, but the rapid transfer of Ca^{2+} through the cytoplasm to the basolateral pole did not occur in the absence of the ability to synthesize calbindin (12).

Vitamin D–induced calcium transport also seems to involve activation of calcium-dependent ATP pumps to effect extrusion of calcium against an electrochemical gradient into the plasma. Relative Ca^{2+} binding capacities across the enterocyte are brush border = 1, calbindin = 4, and the ATP-dependent Ca^{2+} pump = 10, which ensures unidirectional transfer of Ca^{2+} (13).

Paracellular Calcium Transport. In the paracellular pathway, calcium transfer occurs between cells. Theoretically, this can be in both directions, but normally the predominant direction is from lumen into blood. Rate of transfer depends on calcium load and tightness of the junctions. Water probably carries calcium through the junctions by solvent drag (14). Citrate appears to enhance paracellular calcium transport (15).

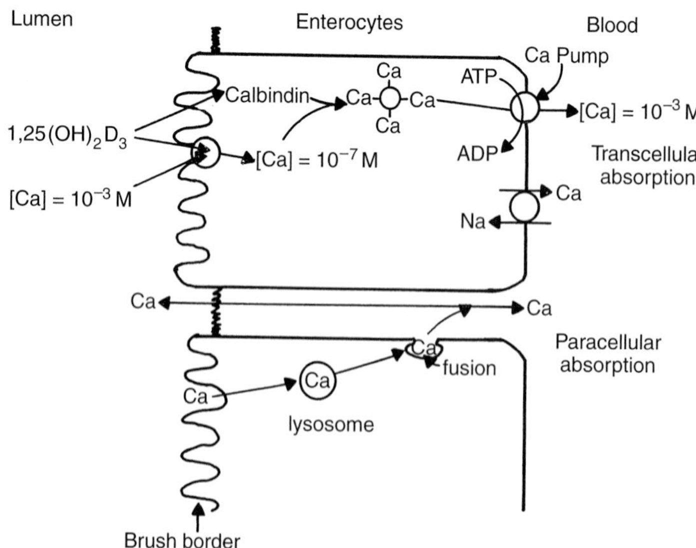

Figure 7.3. Calcium absorption showing active, transcellular absorption and passive, paracellular absorption. Paracellular absorption is bidirectional; transcellular absorption is unidirectional. Calcium enters the cytosol down a concentration gradient. Calcium is transported across the enterocyte against an uphill gradient with the aid of vitamin D-induced calbindin, probably at least partially via endosomes and lysosomes. Finally, it is extruded at the basolateral membrane, primarily via the ATP-dependent Ca^{2+} pump and secondarily via the Na^+/Ca^+ exchanger or by exocytosis.

Physiologic Factors Affecting Absorption

Various host factors affect fractional calcium absorption (Table 7.2). Vitamin D status, intestinal transit time, and mucosal mass are the best established (16). Phosphorus deficiency, as may occur through prolonged use of aluminum-containing antacids, can cause hypophosphatemia, increased circulating levels of $1,25(OH)_2D$ and elevated calcium absorption, hypercalciuria, bone pain, and increased bone resorption.

Stage of life cycle also influences calcium absorption. In infancy, absorption is dominated by diffusion. Therefore, the vitamin D status of the mother does not affect fractional calcium absorption of breast-fed infants. Both active and passive calcium transport are increased during pregnancy and lactation. Calbindin and plasma $1,25(OH)_2D$ and PTH levels increase during pregnancy. From midlife on, absorption efficiency declines by about 0.2 absorption percentage points per year, with an additional 2% decrease at menopause (17).

Decreased stomach acid, as occurs in achlorhydria, reduces the solubility of insoluble calcium salts (e.g., carbonate, phosphate), thereby reducing absorption of calcium unless fed with a meal (18). Absorption of calcium supplements improves when they are taken with food, perhaps by slowing gastric emptying and thereby extending the time in which the calcium-containing chyme is in contact with the absorptive surface.

Table 7.2
Physiologic Factors Affecting Calcium Absorption

Increased Absorption	Decreased Absorption
Vitamin D adequacy	Vitamin D deficiency
Increased mucosal mass	Decreased mucosal mass
Calcium deficiency	Menopause
Phosphorus deficiency	Old age
Pregnancy	Decreased stomach acid (without a meal)
Lactation	Rapid intestinal transit time
Mucosal permeability	

Excretion

Calcium is lost from the body in urine, feces, and sweat. Differences in losses between adult women and adolescent girls on equal and adequate calcium intakes are given in Figure 7.4. This figure demonstrates conservation of calcium at the kidney, for building bone during the rapid skeletal growth during puberty.

Turnover of the miscible calcium pool in healthy adults is about 16%/day and that of the rapidly exchanging component (of which the ECF is a part) about 40%/day. The filterable load of the kidney is determined by the glomerular filtration rate and the plasma concentration of ultrafilterable calcium (ionized plus that bound to low-molecular-weight anions). In adults, this is about 175 to 250 mmol per day (7–10 g per day). More than 98% of this calcium is reabsorbed by the renal tubule as the filtrate passes through the nephron, but 2.5 to 5 mmol (100–200 mg) is excreted in urine daily. Endogenous fecal excretory loss is similar to the amount excreted in urine. Loss in sweat is typically 0.4 to 0.6 mmol (16–24 mg) per day (19), and additional diurnal losses from shed skin, hair, and nails bring the total to as much as 1.5 mmol (60 mg) per day.

Endogenous Fecal Calcium

Fecal calcium includes calcium that is unabsorbed from the diet plus calcium that enters the gut from endogenous sources, including shed mucosal cells, saliva, gastric juices, pancreatic juice, and bile. Endogenous fecal calcium losses are approximately 2.5 to 3.0 mmol (100–120 mg) per day. These losses are inversely proportional to absorption efficiency and directly related to gut mass (and hence

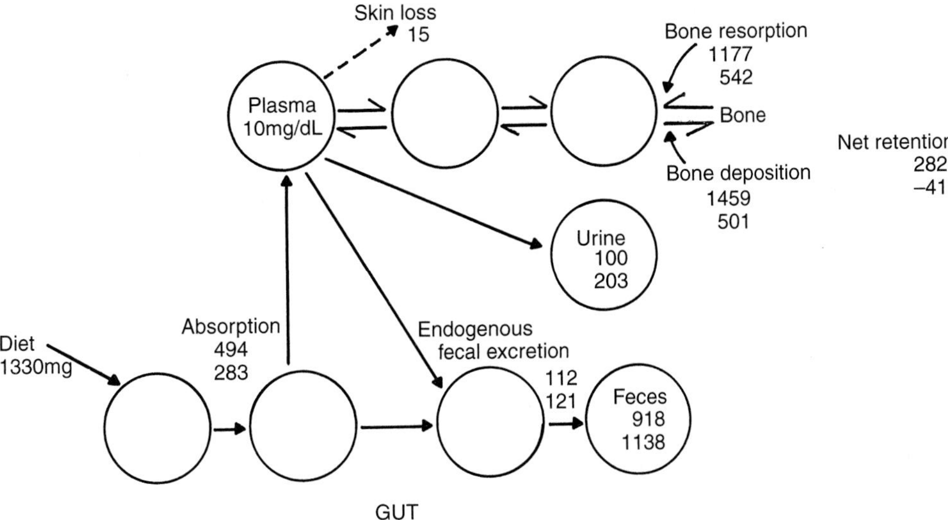

Figure 7.4. Calcium metabolism. Daily mass transfer in adult women *(lower values)* and adolescent girls *(upper values)*. Data were taken from reference 20, except skin loss in adults, taken from 19. *Circles* represent compartments determined from kinetic modeling and do not necessarily represent discrete physiologic entities.

to food intake). Urinary calcium increases during childhood up to adolescence. Endogenous fecal calcium values of adolescent girls and adult women (shown in Fig. 7.4) are not significantly different.

Urinary Excretion

Calcium losses in the urine are load dependent except during adolescence. During this period of rapid growth, absorbed calcium is diverted to bone growth at calcium intakes typically ingested, except for obligatory losses in urine, skin, and endogenous secretions (21).

Machinery for calcium transport described above for the intestinal epithelial cells is also present in the nephrons of the kidney, but it is not known if it is functional. Both processes are calcium-load dependent, stimulated by PTH and $1,25(OH)_2D$, and have a microvillar myosin I–calmodulin complex that could serve as a calcium transporter (22). Active transport occurs in the distal convoluted tubule against a concentration gradient. In the mammalian kidney, vitamin D regulation works through calbindin-D_{28}k, which binds four Ca^{2+} per molecule and shares no sequence homology with calbindin-D_9k of the intestine. This calcium-binding protein has been cloned and is regulated by both transcriptional and posttranscriptional mechanisms. Administration of $1,25(OH)_2D$ to rats induces calbindin-D_{28}k mRNA and vitamin D–receptor mRNA in vitamin D–sufficient animals (23). However, in the absence of vitamin D, hypercalciuria is not observed as would be predicted if mechanisms were similar to those in the gut. A fall in filtered load is associated with slight reductions in urine calcium. Even so, renal calcium clearance is reduced in vitamin D deficiency and increased in PTH deficiency, indicating that the major effect on conservation of calcium is exerted by PTH.

Paracellular transport dominates in the proximal tubule as reabsorption occurs across a concentration gradient, and it also occurs in the thick ascending limb of the loop of Henle, the distal nephron, and the collecting ducts. Tubular reabsorption decreases in postmenopausal women. Calcium resorption is determined by Na^+. For every 100 mmol of sodium excreted, approximately 0.5 to 1.5 mmol of calcium is pulled out with it in the urine.

DIETARY CONSIDERATIONS

Dietary sources and calcium intakes have altered considerably during human evolution. Early man derived calcium from roots, tubers, nuts, and beans in quantities believed to exceed 37.5 mmol (1500 g) per day (24) and perhaps up to twice this when consuming food to meet the caloric demands of a hunter-gatherer of contemporary body size. After domestication of grains, calcium intakes decreased substantially because the staple foods became grains (fruits), the plant parts that accumulate the least calcium. Consequently, the modern human consumes on average insufficient calcium to optimize bone density. The food group that supplies the bulk of the calcium in the Western diet is now the dairy food group.

Food Sources and Bioavailability

For adults, dairy products supply 72% of the calcium in the U.S. diet, grain products about 11%, and vegetables and fruits about 6% (25). Although corn tortillas processed with lime and dried beans provide the bulk of dietary calcium for some ethnic groups, it is difficult for most individuals to ingest enough calcium from foods available in a cereal-based economy without liberal consumption of dairy products. Thus, food manufacturers have developed calcium-fortified products, which have had limited market success. Many individuals have turned to dietary supplements to meet their calcium needs. However, it is prudent to remember that calcium is not the only nutrient important to health supplied by dairy products (Table 7.3). Users of milk in the U.S., compared to nonusers, get 35% more vitamin A, 38% more folate, 56% more riboflavin, 22% more magnesium, and 24% more potassium, in addition to 80% more calcium (26).

Aside from gross calcium content, potential calcium sources should be evaluated for bioavailability. Although calcium absorption efficiency varies inversely with load, fractional calcium absorption from various dairy products is similar, at approximately 30% (27). The calcium from most supplements is absorbed as well as that from milk, since solubility of the salts at neutral pH has little impact on calcium absorption (28). Absorption of one very soluble salt, calcium-citrate-malate (CCM), is better than that of other salts (29). Several plant constituents form indigestible salts with calcium, thereby decreasing absorption of calcium.

The most potent inhibitor of calcium absorption is oxalic acid, found in high concentration in spinach and rhubarb and to a lesser extent in sweet potatoes and dried beans (30). Calcium absorption from spinach is only 5%, compared with 27% from milk ingested at a similar load (31). When these two foods of dissimilar bioavailability are coingested during the same meal, calcium fractional

Table 7.3
Contribution of Foods Represented by the Milk Group to Nutrients Available in the U.S. Food Supply

Nutrient	%
Calcium	76.8
Phosphorus	35.7
Riboflavin	34.7
Potassium	21.1
Protein	20.6
Magnesium	19.8
Vitamin B_{12}	17.8
Fat	11.8
Vitamin B_6	16.7
Energy	9.9
Vitamin A	9.6

From the 1987–88 Nationwide Food Consumption Survey.

absorption from milk is depressed 30% of the difference between milk and spinach (fed alone) by the presence of spinach, and calcium fractional absorption from spinach is enhanced 37% of the difference between milk and spinach by the presence of milk (32). The absence of complete exchange and the failure to find equal absorption from the two foods intermediate between the values for the foods fed singly suggest that calcium does not completely form a common dietary pool as has been reported for iron and zinc.

Phytic acid, the storage form of phosphorus in seeds, is a modest inhibitor of calcium absorption. The phytic acid content of seeds, which depends on the phosphorus content of the soil in which the plants are grown, influences calcium absorption (33). Fermentation, as occurs during bread making, reduces phytic acid because of the phytase present in yeast, resulting in increased calcium absorption (34). Since the early balance studies of McCance and Widdowson, who reported negative calcium balance while consuming whole wheat products (35), it has been assumed that fiber negatively affects calcium balance through either physical entrapment or cationic binding with uronic acid residues (36). However, it is more likely that the phytic acid associated with fiber-rich foods is the component that affected balance, since purified fibers do not negatively affect calcium absorption (37). Only concentrated sources of phytate such as wheat bran ingested as extruded cereal (34) or dried beans (38) substantially reduce calcium absorption. For other plants rich in calcium (primarily the *Brassica* genus, which includes broccoli, kale, bok choy, cabbage, and mustard and turnip greens), calcium bioavailability is as good as that from milk (39). The *Brassica* are an anomaly in the plant kingdom in that they do not accumulate oxalate to detoxify excess calcium to protect against cell death.

Several foods and the number of servings required to equal the amount of calcium in one glass of milk are listed in Table 7.4.

True enhancers of calcium absorption have not been well characterized. Lactose appears to enhance calcium absorption in infants. However, in adults, calcium absorption from various dairy products is equivalent, regardless of the lactose content, chemical form of calcium, or presence of flavorings (29, 41).

Nutrient-Nutrient Interactions

Several nutrients and food constituents affect aspects of calcium homeostasis other than through a simple effect on digestibility and absorbability as described above. Several dietary components influence urinary calcium excretion. A major determinant of urinary calcium is urinary sodium, which reflects dietary sodium (42, 43). Sodium and calcium share some of the same transport systems in the proximal tubule, so that each 100-mmol (2.3 g) increment of sodium excreted by the kidney pulls out approximately 0.6 to 1.0 mmol (24–40) of accompanying calcium (44). Because urinary calcium losses account for 50% of the variability in calcium retention, dietary sodium has a tremendous potential influence on bone loss. In adult women, each extra gram of sodium per day is projected to produce an additional rate of bone loss of 1% per year if the calcium loss in the urine comes from the skeleton (45). A longitudinal study of postmenopausal women showed a negative correlation between urinary sodium excretion and bone density of the hip (42). The authors concluded, from the range of values available to them, that bone loss could have been prevented either by a daily dietary calcium increase of 891 mg calcium or by halving the daily sodium excretion.

Another dietary component that influences urinary calcium excretion is protein. Each gram of protein metabolized increases urinary calcium levels by about 1.75 mg; thus, doubling the amount of purified dietary proteins or amino acids in the diet increases urinary calcium by about 50% (46). The acid load of the sulfate produced in the metabolism of sulfur-containing amino acids is mainly responsible for increasing urinary calcium. However, protein-rich foods typically also contain phosphorus, which has a hypocalciuric effect, thereby offsetting the hypercalciuric effect of the protein. Although urinary calcium loss

Table 7.4
Food Sources of Bioavailable Calcium

Food	Serving Size (g)	Calcium Content[a] (mg)	Fractional Absorption[b] (%)	Estimated[3] Absorbable Ca/serving (mg)	Servings Needed to Equal 1 Glass of Milk
Milk (or 1 glass yogurt or 1½ oz. cheddar cheese)	240	300	32.1	96.3	1.0
Beans, dried	177	50	15.6	7.8	12.3
Broccoli	71	35	61.3	21.5	4.5
Cabbage	85	79	52.7	41.6	2.3
Kale	65	47	58.8	27.6	3.5
Spinach	90	122	5.1	6.2	15.5
Tofu, calcium set	126	258	31.0	80.0	1.2

Adapted from references 38–40.

[a]Adjusted for load; for milk, this is fractional absorption (Fx abs) = 0.889 − 0.0964 ln load; for low-oxalate vegetables, after adjusting by the ratio of fractional absorption determined for kale relative to milk at the same load, the equation becomes Fx abs = 0.959 − 0.0964 ln load.

[b]Calcium content (mg) × Fx abs.

is unchanged by inclusion of protein and phosphorus-rich foods such as meat, cereal, beans, and dairy products, the phosphorus increases the calcium content of the digestive secretions and therefore increases endogenous calcium losses in the feces. Thus, increasing consumption of protein-rich foods results in net calcium loss, which can exacerbate risks of a low calcium diet. The dietary calcium:protein ratio was more closely related to the rate of bone gain in young women than either dietary calcium or protein alone (47). At the other extreme, inadequate protein intakes compromise bone health and may contribute to osteoporosis in the elderly.

Although widely varying intakes of dietary phosphorus and calcium have produced no changes in calcium balance (48) (presumably because of the offset of increased endogenous secretion of calcium by decreased urinary calcium), some investigators have been concerned about the popular trend toward high phosphate consumption in soft drinks. Elevated PTH levels, if sustained, could lead to bone resorption, but this effect has been reported in diets that have both elevated phosphorus and low calcium levels (49). Other investigators (50) reported the same elevated PTH levels with lower calcium intakes without elevated phosphorus intakes. Thus, low calcium level alone accounts for the observed elevation in PTH.

Although caffeine in large amounts acutely increases urinary calcium (51), 24-h urinary calcium was not altered in a double-blind, placebo-controlled trial (52). Daily consumption of caffeine equivalent to 2 to 3 cups of coffee accelerated bone loss from the spine and total body in postmenopausal women who consumed less than 744 mg calcium per day (53). The relationship between caffeine intake and bone loss in this observational study may be due to a small decrease in calcium absorption (54) or to a confounding factor such as a probable inverse association between milk intake and caffeine intake.

Fat intake has a negative impact on calcium balance only during steatorrhea. In this condition, calcium forms insoluble soaps with fatty acids in the gut.

Increased use of calcium supplements and fortified foods have raised concern about high calcium intakes producing relative deficiencies of several minerals. High calcium intakes have produced relative magnesium deficiencies in rats (55); however, calcium intake does not affect magnesium retention in humans (56). Similarly, except for a single report in postmenopausal women (57), decreased zinc retention has not been associated with high calcium intakes. The nature of this interaction is controversial and requires further study. Iron absorption from nonheme sources is decreased by half from radiolabeled test meals in the presence of calcium intakes up to 300 mg calcium a day, after which there is no further reduction. Thus, practically speaking, it is prudent to set iron requirements assuming that individuals are going to ingest the amount of calcium in at least one glass of milk with each meal (58). The inhibition of iron absorption by calcium does not appear to be a gut effect and may involve competition with the transport of iron in the intestinal mucosa (59), possibly at the level of mobilferrin (see Chapter 10). Up to 12 weeks of calcium supplementation does not change iron status (60), probably because of compensating upregulation of iron absorption. Single-meal iron-absorption studies quite possibly exaggerate inhibitory effects that disappear in the context of the whole diet.

FUNCTIONS

Intracellular Messenger

Ionized calcium is the most common signal transduction element in cells because of its ability to reversibly bind to proteins. To effect a regulatory change, an internal or external stimulus (physical, electrical, or chemical) causes a change in [Ca^{2+}] at a specific site in the cell by releasing a store of Ca^{2+} from within or by causing Ca^{2+} to enter the cell from the outside (Fig. 7.4). [Ca^{2+}] is maintained at about 0.1 μM in the cytosol via many binding and specialized-extrusion proteins. This is necessary because Ca^{2+} is not metabolized like other second-messenger molecules. A released Ca^{2+} ion probably migrates less than 0.1 to 0.5 μm, existing as a free ion only about 50 μsec before encountering a binding protein. The endoplasmic reticulum (sarcoplasmic reticulum in muscles) with its Ca^{2+}-ATP pumps is the major intracellular calcium sink housing Ca^{2+}-binding proteins. Accumulation of Ca^{2+} in the cytosol would lead to cell death because it would precipitate phosphate (vital in energy transfer).

The plasma membrane is important in maintaining calcium homeostasis because the resting membrane is only slightly permeable to entering Ca^{2+}, and a Ca^{2+}-Mg^{2+}-ATPase pump pumps Ca^{2+} out of the cell cytosol back to the ECF space. The pump is activated by calmodulin, an intracellular Ca^{2+} receptor protein that lowers the K_m (Ca^{2+}) from 0.4 to 0.8 μM to 0.2 μM and increases the total capacity of the pump. Thus, a momentary increase in cytosolic [Ca^{2+}] caused by an influx of Ca^{2+} is quickly returned to preexcitation levels. Other less important pathways of Ca^{2+} flux across the plasma membrane include influx pathways, potential-operated (voltage-dependent) channels, receptor-operated channels, and Na^+ channels, and the efflux pathway, a Na^+-Ca^{2+}-exchange pathway maintained by the Na^+ pump. Calcium messenger systems include trigger proteins in excitable cells and sustained responses in nonexcitable and excitable cells (1).

Sustained Responses

When an external or internal stimulus such as a hormone or neurotransmitter binds to a receptor in the plasma membrane, a series of responses occur as depicted in Figure 7.5. Receptors can be G protein–coupled receptors as shown in the figure or receptor tyrosine kinases. The phospholipase C is activated, which breaks down phosphatidylinositol-4,5-bisphosphate (PIP_2) in the cell membrane into inositol-1,4,5-triphosphate ($InsP_3$) and di-

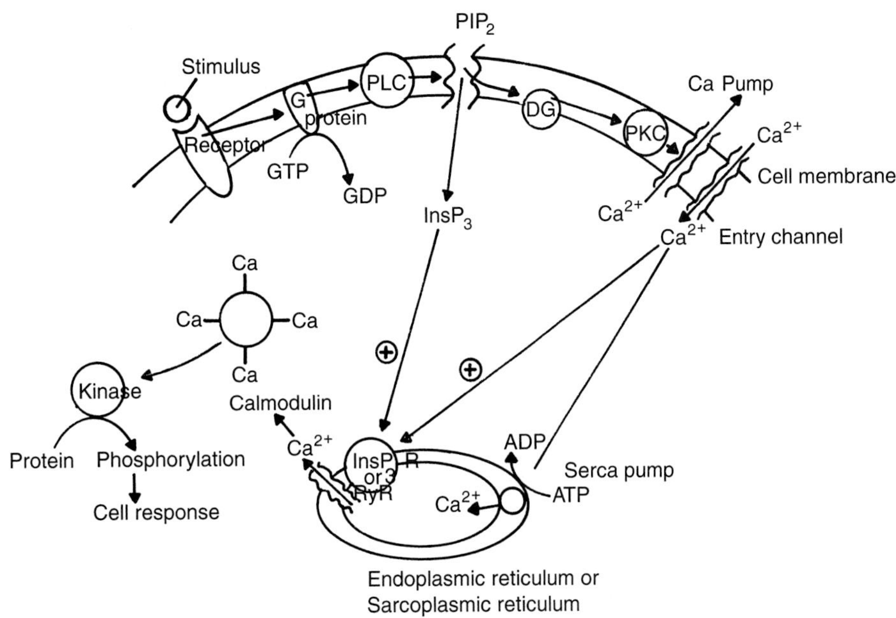

Figure 7.5. Intracellular Ca^{2+} signaling. Abbreviations: PLC, phospholipase C; $InsP_3$, inositol-1,4,5-triphosphate; GTP, guanosine triphosphate; GDP, guanosine diphosphate; PIP_2, phosphatidylinositol-4,5-bisphosphate; DG, diacylglycerol; PKC, protein kinase C; $InsP_{3R}$, $InsP_{3R}$ receptor; RYR, ryanodine receptor; Ca pump, plasma membrane Ca^{2+}-ATPase pump; SERCA, smooth endoplasmic reticulum Ca^{2+}-ATPase pump. (Adapted from Clapham DE. Cell 1995;80:259–68.)

acylglycerol (DG). Released into the cytosol, $InsP_3$ binds to receptors in the endoplasmic reticular (or sarcoplasmic reticular in muscles) membrane, which induces liberation of Ca^{2+} from internal stores. Ca^{2+} can also enter the cytosol via plasma membrane Ca^{2+}-selective voltage-independent channels. Cystolic Ca^{2+} concentrations can change from 0.1 μM to 10 μM. The increased cytosolic Ca^{2+} binds to calmodulin, which in turn activates kinases to phosphorylate specific proteins. This system accounts for the secretion of aldosterone from adrenal cells in response to angiotensin II, insulin secretion from β cells, and contraction of smooth muscles.

Meanwhile the lipid portion of PIP_2, DG, remains in the membrane and activates another membrane-attached enzyme, protein kinase C, which stimulates activity of the calcium pump. Thus, waves of Ca^{2+} are initiated by extra Ca^{2+} cycling in and out of cells (61). As Ca^{2+} concentration returns to resting levels following action of Ca^{2+} pumps, recovery occurs in about 1 second, setting the stage for another Ca^{2+} spike.

Trigger Proteins

Calcium receptor protein pathways are almost universal and are present in excitable and nonexcitable cells. They are important for fast switch processes in which Ca^{2+} acts as an on-off switch. Examples of excitable cells are skeletal muscle and neurons. Excitable cells contain voltage-dependent Ca^{2+} channels in the plasma membrane in addition to the system described above for nonexcitable cells, which allow dramatic increases in intracellular Ca^{2+}. Entering Ca^{2+} activates ryanodine receptors (RyR) to release Ca^{2+} from internal stores.

We have much to learn about how one diffusible ion can regulate such diverse cellular processes as proliferation, differentiation, neuronal adaptation, and movement.

Cofactor for Extracellular Enzymes and Proteins

Calcium is necessary to stabilize or allow maximal activity for a number of proteases and blood clotting enzymes. These functions are not significantly affected by changes in extracellular Ca^{2+} concentration. Those that do not seem to be calmodulin activated by the system described above include glyceraldehyde phosphate dehydrogenase, pyruvate dehydrogenase, and α-ketoglutarate dehydrogenase.

Bones and Teeth

The role of calcium in bones and teeth is described more fully in Chapter 83. Calcium exists primarily as the insoluble hydroxyapatite with the general formula $Ca_{10}(PO_4)_6\ (OH)_2$. Calcium comprises 39.9% of the weight of bone mineral.

Aside from the obvious structural role, the skeleton is an important reservoir of calcium to maintain plasma calcium concentrations. Mobilization of calcium from bone may involve as yet unidentified calcium-binding sites (62).

The bone calcium pool turns over every 10 to 12 years on average, but turnover does not occur in the teeth. Remodeling of bone continues throughout life. Bone-resorbing osteoclasts begin this process by extruding packets of citric and lactic acids to dissolve bone and proteolytic enzymes to digest organic matrix. Bone-forming osteoblasts then synthesize new bone to replace resorbed bone. Usually, these processes are coupled. Bone formation exceeds resorption during growth. Bone resorption exceeds formation during development of osteoporosis. Osteoblasts have receptors for PTH, $1,25(OH)_2D$, estrogen, and prostaglandin E_2. Osteoclasts have receptors for calcitonin. Bone resorption is enhanced by PTH and inhibited by calcitonin.

ASSESSMENT OF CALCIUM STATUS

Assessment of calcium nutrient status presents challenges unique among the nutrients. The skeleton, as noted in Chapter 83, functions as a very large calcium reserve both for maintenance of ECF calcium concentrations and for the critical cellular functions of calcium. This reserve is so large that calcium deficiency at a cell or tissue level is essentially never encountered, at least for nutritional reasons. However, since the mechanical function of the skeleton is directly proportional to skeletal mass, i.e., to the size of the calcium reserve, it follows that any reduction whatsoever in the reserve will result in a decrease in bone strength. In this sense, calcium is the only nutrient for which the reserve has a distinct function in its own right. The size of that reserve can be assessed by total-body bone mineral estimation using dual-energy x-ray absorptiometry (DEXA) (see Chapter 83). A problem arises in the interpretation of the results: the reserve can be low not only for nutritional causes but for other reasons as well, such as lack of adequate physical inactivity, weight loss, gonadal hormone deficiency, and various medical diseases and their treatments.

In a research setting, calcium balance (intake minus excretion) can be used to determine whether losses of calcium from the body are being met by the intake of the controlled diet. If an individual is in negative balance, calcium is being lost from bone. However, the calcium status of a free-living population on self-selected calcium intakes cannot be readily assessed.

The other aspect of calcium metabolism, the concentration of $[Ca^{2+}]$ in the blood and ECF, can, however, readily be measured. Low serum $[Ca^{2+}]$ usually mean some abnormality of parathyroid function; serum $[Ca^{2+}]$ is rarely ever low because of dietary calcium deficiency. This is basically because (as noted above) the skeleton serves as a very large calcium reserve and protects the ECF $[Ca^{2+}]$ essentially without limit. As described elsewhere in this chapter, it is the function of the parathyroid glands to draw down calcium from these reserves for the maintenance of ECF $[Ca^{2+}]$.

DEFICIENCY

Overt, uncomplicated calcium metabolic deficiencies are almost nonexistent given the large skeletal reserves as discussed above. One possible exception is the report in children aged 7 to 12 years on daily calcium intakes of 3.1 mol (125 mg) (61). Abnormal biochemistry values were observed including hypocalcemia, hypercalciuria, and elevated alkaline phosphatase levels.

Chronic inadequacy of calcium in the diet is one factor in the etiology of several disorders (64). Adequate calcium intakes have been definitely established as protective against osteoporosis and have been associated with reducing the risk of hypertension, colon cancer, lead poisoning, and kidney stones in patients with the short bowel syndrome.

The primary strategies for reducing the risk of osteoporosis are to maximize development of peak bone mass during growth and to reduce bone loss later in life. Achieving optimal calcium intakes is a goal for both of these aims. Further details on the role of calcium in preventing this debilitating disease may be found in Chapter 85. The role of calcium in ameliorating hypertension is less well documented than for osteoporosis but has been extensively studied in the last decade. The evidence is reviewed in an LSRO report (65). A recent metaanalysis (66) of randomized, controlled intervention trials showed that calcium supplementation has a small lowering effect on systolic blood pressure (−1.27 mm Hg) but not on diastolic blood pressure. However, a metaanalysis specifically confined to calcium supplementation trials with pregnant women showed a much more dramatic effect of calcium (67). Both systolic and diastolic blood pressures were significantly lowered (−5.40 mm Hg and −3.44 mm Hg, respectively). The odds ratio with calcium supplementation was 0.30 for pregnancy-induced hypertension, 0.38 for preeclampsia, and 0.69 for premature infants. In contrast, no effect of calcium supplementation was observed in women already consuming 24.5 mmol (980 mg) daily in the randomized, controlled trial of Calcium for Preeclampsia Prevention (CPEP) (68). Other groups that may be vulnerable to calcium deficiency–related hypertension include African Americans and the elderly.

The effect of dietary calcium in reducing the risk for colonic tumors has been suggested in a number of studies. Dietary calcium may protect against abnormal epithelial growth. One proposed mechanism is that Ca^{2+} precipitates bile acids and fatty acids that can otherwise stimulate colon cell proliferation. Intakes of 1800 mg/day for men and 1500 mg/day for women have been recommended to reduce the incidence of colon cancer (69). However, two prospective studies showed that the occurrence of colorectal adenoma was related neither to calcium intake nor to milk consumption (70). The role of calcium in colon cancer of humans requires further study.

High calcium intakes decrease the risk of kidney stones (see toxicity section below) (71). Unabsorbed calcium in the gut forms a highly insoluble oxalate salt in the colon, thereby reducing absorption of oxalate from the diet. Large calcium supplements are the accepted therapy for the kidney stone problem of intestinal hyperoxalosis.

REQUIREMENTS AND RECOMMENDED INTAKES

The calcium requirement is the amount of dietary calcium required to replace losses in the urine, feces, and sweat, plus the calcium needed for bone accretion during periods of skeletal growth. Calcium is a plateau nutrient; above a certain intake, little further increase in calcium retention can occur because the excess is excreted. Plateau intakes for achieving maximal calcium retention were used with other data to set the 1997 dietary reference intakes for calcium. Recommendations across the life span for adequate intakes of calcium by the National Academy of Science Food and Nutrition Board are given in Table 7.5. Calcium requirements throughout life are not uniform because of changes in skeletal growth and age-related changes in absorption and excretion.

Infancy

A term human infant contains approximately 0.65 to 0.75 mol (26–30 g) of calcium. During the first year of life, the rate of calcium deposition in relation to body size is higher than at any other period during life.

Childhood and Adolescence

Calcium accretion continues throughout childhood. Rate of growth slows between the ages of 2 and 8 years. Maximal accretion occurs during the pubertal growth spurt, which occurs for most girls between the ages of 12 and 14 years and for boys, 14 and 16 years. The intake required for mean maximal calcium retention in adolescent girls is 1300 mg/day (72). Between the ages of 9 and 17 years, approximately 45% of the adult skeleton is acquired. This represents a gain in bone mass of about 7 to 8%/year.

Several calcium or dairy supplementation trials have been conducted in children. They all demonstrate that calcium intake can positively influence bone accumulation (73–76). However, the differential gain in bone mass wanes after cessation of calcium supplementation (77).

Table 7.5
Adequate Calcium Intakes during the Life Span

Group	Adequate Intake (mg/day)
Infant	
Birth–6 months	210
6 months–1 year	270
Children	
1–5 years	500
4–8 years	800
Adolescents 9–18 years	1300
Adults	
19–50 years	1000
Over 50 years	1200
Pregnant and lactating	
14–18	1300
>19	1000

From Food and Nutrition Board, National Academy Press. Dietary reference intakes calcium, phosphorus, magnesium, vitamin D, and fluoride. Washington, DC: National Academy Press, 1997.

Peak Bone Mass

After adult height is achieved, calcium accretion continues during the phase of bone consolidation. At the end of consolidation, when the maximum amount of bone has been accumulated, the adult is said to have achieved his or her peak bone mass. In females, 90% of total body bone mineral content is achieved by age 16.9 years, 95% by 19.8 years, and 99% by age 22.1 years (78). However, the timing of peak bone mass varies with the skeletal site. The hip achieves peak bone mass first at approximately age 16.7 years for the trochanter, 17.2 years for the femoral neck, and 18.5 years for Ward's triangle, whereas the spine can add mass throughout most of the 2nd decade of life in females (79). The skull accumulates bone throughout life, as does the femur shaft (80).

Although 60 to 80% of peak bone mass is genetically predetermined, a number of environmental factors affect bone mass. The main determinant of bone density in adolescent girls is calcium intake (81). During this period, urinary calcium is relatively unaffected by calcium intake (72). Aside from calcium intake, other lifestyle choices that affect peak bone mass include physical activity, intake of other nutrients that affect calcium balance (covered elsewhere in this chapter), anorexia, and substance abuse. Beyond the timing of peak bone mass, lifestyle choices can affect rate of bone loss, but the window of opportunity to build bone has passed.

Adults

The mature female has 23 to 25 mol (920–1000 g) body calcium, and the mature male has approximately 30 mol (1200 g) body calcium. The population coefficient of variation around these means is about 15%. Total body bone mass remains relatively constant over the reproductive years, as decreases in the proximal femur and other sites after age 18 are offset by continued growth of the forearm, total spine, and head. Then age-related bone loss occurs, which varies with the individual, but occurs most rapidly during the first 3 years after menopause in women. The average adult loses bone at a rate of ~1%/year. Age-related decreases in calcium absorption and increases in urinary calcium contribute to this loss. These physiologic changes are more abrupt at the menopause in women. The explanation for bone loss during aging includes a variety of causes such as declining calcium intakes (discussed below), declining physical activity, decreased levels of gonadal hormones, decreased circulating levels of $1,25(OH)_2D$, and intestinal resistance to $1,25(OH)_2D$. The calcium intake required by older adults to achieve mean maximal retention or minimal loss was determined to be 1200 mg/day by the Panel on Calcium and Related

Nutrients (Table 7.5) using the balance data of Spencer et al (82).

Calcium intakes required to prevent bone loss also suffice to protect against risk of hypertension. The calcium intake threshold for reducing risk of high blood pressure is likely to be 12.5 to 15 mmol/day (500–600 mg/day). Optimal calcium intakes to reduce risk of other diseases are not known.

Pregnancy

Fetal skeletal calcium accretion is not great until the third trimester. During the third trimester, approximately 5 mmol/day (200 mg/day) of calcium is required for fetal growth. The mother's calcium absorption increases beginning by the second trimester to meet fetal demands and to store calcium for the subsequent lactational drain (83). At low calcium intakes, the mother's skeleton is compromised to meet calcium demands of the fetus, and the fetal skeleton is protected except at exceptionally low calcium intakes. In one study, calcium supplementation increased bone density of neonates of malnourished women in India (84). There is no evidence to date that multiple births are harmful to women, even on low calcium intakes.

During pregnancy, biologically active PTH falls, calcitonin increases during early pregnancy, and prolactin increases 10- to 20-fold.

Lactation

Calcium transfer to breast milk varies mainly with changes in volume; calcium concentration is relatively constant at 7 ± 0.65 mmol/L (280 ± 26 mg/L). Daily calcium transfer from maternal serum to breast milk increases from 4.2 mmol/day (168 mg/day) at 3 months following parturition to 7 mmol/day (280 mg/day) at 6 months following parturition. To meet this need, the maternal skeleton is depleted at a rate of about 1% per month; this loss is not prevented by calcium and vitamin D supplementation (85). A postlactation anabolic phase allows recovery of bone density to prelactation levels. Whether this recovery is complete in all individuals, such as older lactating women, is not known.

ADEQUACY OF CALCIUM INTAKE

The median calcium intakes by age, for males and females in the United States, collected by the USDA 1994 Continuing Survey of Food Intakes by Individuals (CSFII) and adjusted for day-to-day variation are shown in Figure 7.6, compared with the 1997 dietary reference intakes (DRIs) for calcium. It is obvious that the typical man consumes more calcium at all stages of life than do women. Calcium intakes are highest in boys during their adolescent growth spurt. In contrast, just as girls enter their period of most rapid skeletal growth, intakes decline. Calcium intakes of females were below the DRI for calcium above the age of 9 years. Low calcium intakes are also associated with low intakes of other nutrients, including vitamins B_6, B_{12}, thiamin, riboflavin, and magnesium (87).

Assessment of calcium intakes of populations is important for determining nutritional status and drawing conclusions about the relationship between diet and health

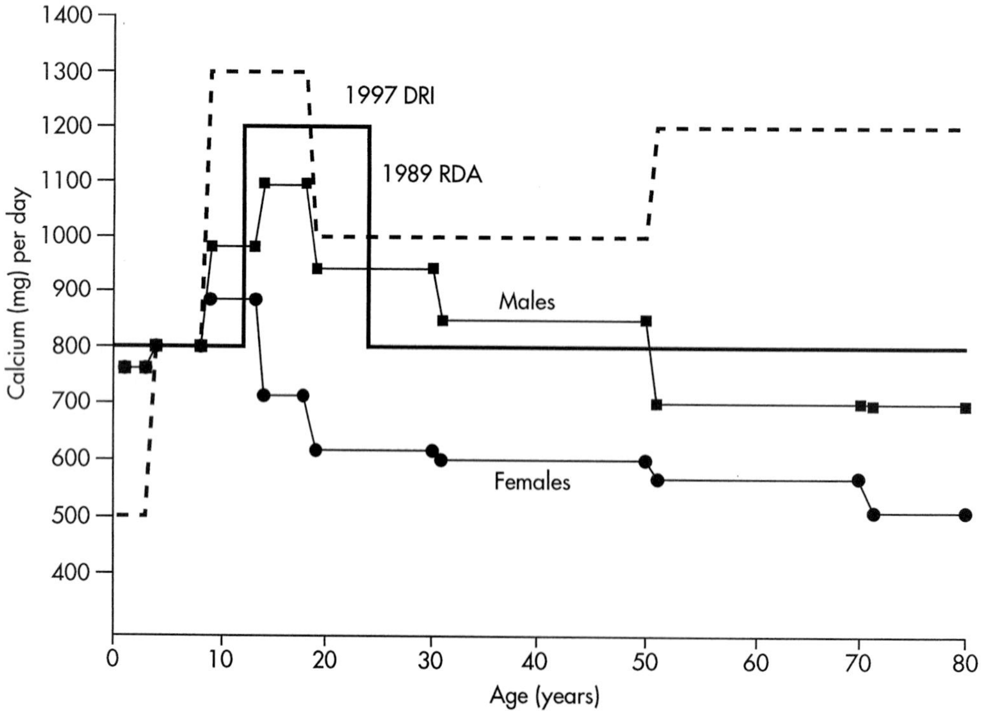

Figure 7.6. Mean calcium intakes by age for U.S. males and females assessed by 24-h dietary recall adjusted for day-to-day variation (86) compared with 1997 dietary reference intakes for calcium adequate intakes and the 1989 RDA. 40 mg Ca = 1 mmol.

and disease. However, assessing the usual calcium intake of an individual is fraught with errors. Calcium intake can be assessed with food-frequency questionnaires, diet recalls, or diet records or by duplicate plate analysis. The latter eliminates many of the errors associated with other methods but is not practical for assessing large groups of individuals. Food-frequency questionnaires assess calcium better than some nutrients because dairy foods are the major source of calcium, and individuals recall dairy product consumption reasonably well. However, hidden calcium taken in as food additives (anticaking agents, etc.), water, fortified foods, and components of pharmaceuticals can be easily overlooked. Diet recall and diet records suffer from errors in estimating portion size, from variability in food composition, and from inadequacies of existing food composition tables. Multiple diet records can improve the estimate of an individual's average calcium intake. However, the generally large variability in calcium intake from day to day precludes confidence in estimates of usual calcium intake of an individual (88, 89).

TOXICITY

Nutritional toxicity of calcium means an elevation of blood calcium levels (hypercalcemia) because of overconsumption of calcium, or an elevation of urine calcium excretion to the point that either the kidneys calcify or renal stones develop. Hypercalcemia, particularly if severe, results in lax muscle tone, constipation, large urine volumes, nausea, and ultimately confusion, coma, and death. It essentially never occurs from ingestion of natural food sources. A good illustration of the safety of food calcium sources is provided by nomadic, pastoral people, such as the Masai (90). Because their diets consist mostly of the milk of their herds and flocks, they have calcium intakes above 5000 mg/day (and often higher), roughly 5 to 10 times what people of industrialized nations ingest. Such pastoral people are not known to have an unusual incidence of hypercalcemia or kidney stones.

Hypercalcemia is reported only with ingestion of large quantities of calcium in the form of supplements, usually taken with absorbable alkali (which raises the pH of the urine and predisposes to calcium deposits in the kidneys). In the past, this outcome sometimes occurred in the treatment of peptic ulcer with large quantities of milk, calcium carbonate, and sodium bicarbonate and was termed the *milk alkali syndrome.* Even so, this complication was unusual, and most individuals can consume large quantities of calcium supplements for years without difficulty.

Kidney stones are not usually caused by dietary calcium. More often, individuals with kidney stones have high urine calcium levels because they have a renal leak of calcium. Accordingly, they often have some reduction of their skeletal calcium reserves. Lowering calcium intake in such individuals rarely affects their kidney stone problem but always leads to further reduction in bone mass. While high calcium intakes may contribute to kidney stone formation in certain susceptible individuals, in most individuals, the stone problem is actually helped by *increasing* calcium intakes (70). This is because urinary oxalate excretion is a more important risk factor for stones than is urinary calcium excretion. A high calcium diet binds oxalate of dietary origin in the gut and prevents its absorption, thereby reducing urinary oxalate load.

CLINICAL DISORDERS INVOLVING CALCIUM

As noted above, low calcium intakes, coupled with high obligatory calcium losses from the body, deplete skeletal calcium reserves. In other words, low intakes cause subnormal bone mass (and strength). This is one of the contributing causes of osteoporosis (covered in Chapter 85). Medical science recognizes no clear disorder of intracellular calcium regulation. However, cell injury, damage, or serious dysfunction is always associated with a rise in cytosolic calcium concentration, probably reflecting impaired ability of the cell to maintain the normal 10,000-fold gradient. Moreover, it is likely that the rise in cytosolic calcium worsens the cell damage and hastens cell death (91).

The most common disorders of calcium metabolism (other than osteoporosis, which is multifactorial in etiology), involve regulation of ECF [Ca^{2+}]. Usually these are due to disorders of parathyroid gland function and are not nutritional. As noted elsewhere in this chapter, the skeletal calcium reserves are so vast, relative to the size of the ECF [Ca^{2+}] compartment, that simple dietary deficiency of calcium essentially never compromises ECF [Ca^{2+}] regulation. There are, however, a few rare exceptions that are worth noting because they illustrate how the system operates.

During growth, when the demands of skeletal mineralization are highest, extremely low calcium diets may lead to hypocalcemia, despite maximal secretory output of the parathyroid glands. One consequence of hypersecretion of PTH is a lowering of serum phosphate levels. The combination of low calcium and low phosphorus levels in the ECF results both in undermineralization of newly deposited bone matrix and in osteoblast dysfunction. The result is rickets. Usually rickets is produced by vitamin D deficiency, by hypophosphatemia from other causes, or by osteoblast toxicity (see Chapter 83). However, as this example shows, it can sometimes be caused by calcium deficiency alone (89).

Another example of nutritional hypocalcemia occurs as a result of magnesium deficiency, most often noted in severe alcoholism or as a result of intestinal fistulas or malabsorption that causes excessive magnesium loss from the body. Magnesium, of course, is an essential cation for many cell metabolic processes (see Chapter 9), and with severe magnesium depletion, many organs and systems function abnormally. The system regulating ECF [Ca^{2+}] is an example. Both PTH release from the parathyroid glands and bony response to PTH depend on magnesium, and both are defective in magnesium deficiency (90). Evidence that both steps are impaired is provided by the fact that PTH levels in Mg-deficient patients fail to rise adequately in response to hypocalcemia, and exogenous PTH fails to elevate their bone remodeling as it should. Magnesium repletion corrects both problems.

ACKNOWLEDGMENTS

This work was supported in part by PHS grants AR40553, RR00750, and AR39221.

REFERENCES

1. Clapham DE. Cell 1995;80:259–68.
2. Carafoli E, Penniston JT. Sci Am 1985;253(5):70–8.
3. Hanes D, Weaver CM, Wastney ME. FASEB J 1995;9: A283(#1642).
4. Heaney RP, Saville PD, Recker RR. J Lab Clin Med 1975;85:881–90.
5. Heaney RP, Weaver CM, Fitzsimmons ML. J Bone Miner Metab 1990;5:1135–8.
6. Heaney RP. Am J Clin Nutr 1991;54:242S–57S.
7. Heaney RP, Weaver CM, Fitzsimmons ML, et al. J Bone Miner Res 1990;5:1139–42.
8. Weaver CM, Heaney RP, Teegarden D, et al. J Nutr 1996;126:303–7.
9. Wassermann RH, Fullmer CS. J Nutr 1995;125:1971S–79S.
10. Nemere I, Leathers V, Norman AW. J Biol Chem 1986;261: 16106–14.
11. Nemer I. J Nutr 1992;122:657–61.
12. Fullmer CS. J Nutr 1992;122:644–50.
13. Wassermann RH, Chandler JS, Meyer SA, et al. J Nutr 1992;122:662–71.
14. Korback U. J Nutr 1992;122:672–7.
15. Louie D, Zhong Z, Glover W. Gastroenterology 1993;104:A633.
16. Barger-Lux MJ, Heaney RP, Lanspa SJ, et al. J Clin Endocrinol Metab 1995;80:406–11.
17. Heaney RP, Recker RR, Steagman MR, et al. J Bone Miner Res 1989;4:469–75.
18. Recker RR. N Engl J Med 1985;43:133–7.
19. Charles P, Jenson FT, Mosekilde L, et al. Clin Sci 1983;65: 415–22.
20. Wastney ME, Ng J, Smith D, et al. Am J Physiol 1996;271: R208–16.
21. Matkovic V, Heaney RP. Am J Clin Nutr 1992;55:992–6.
22. Coluccio LM. Eur J Cell Biol 1991;56:286–94.
23. Christakos S, Gill R, Lee S, et al. J Nutr 1992;122:678–82.
24. Eaton SB, Konner M. N Engl J Med 1985;312:283–9.
25. US Department of Agriculture, Nationwide Food Consumption Survey 1987–1988, PB-92–500016. Washington, DC; US Government Printing Office, 1989.
26. Fleming KH, Heimback JT. J Nutr 1994;124:1426S–30S.
27. Nickel KP, Martin BR, Smith DL, et al. J Nutr 1996;126:1406–11.
28. Heaney RP, Recker RR, Weaver CM. Calcif Tissue Int 1990;46:300–4.
29. Andon MB, Peacock M, Kanerva RL, et al. J Am Coll Nutr 1996;15:313–16.
30. Heaney RP, Weaver CM. Am J Clin Nutr 1989;50:830–2.
31. Heaney RP, Weaver CM, Recker RR. Am J Clin Nutr 1988;47:707–9.
32. Weaver CM, Heaney RP. Calcif Tissue Int 1991;56:436–42.
33. Heaney RP, Weaver CM, Fitzsimmons ML. Am J Clin Nutr 1991;53:745–7.
34. Weaver CM, Heaney RP, Martin BR, et al. J Nutr 1991;121:1769–75.
35. McCance RA, Widdowson EM. J Physiol 1942;101:44–85.
36. James WPT, Branch WJ, Southgate DAT. Lancet 1978;1:638–9.
37. Heaney RP, Weaver CM. J Am Geriatr Soc 1995;43:1–3.
38. Weaver CM, Heaney RP, Proulx WR, et al. J Food Sci 1993;58(6):1401–3.
39. Heaney RP, Weaver CM, Hinders SM, et al. J Food Sci 1993;58:1378–80.
40. Weaver CM, Plawecki KL. Am J Clin Nutr 1994;59:1238S–41S.
41. Recker RR, Bammi A, Barger-Lux MG, Heaney RP. Am J Clin Nutr 1988;47:93–5.
42. Devine A, Criddle RA, Dick IM, et al. Am J Clin Nutr 1995;62:740–5.
43. Matkovic V, Ilich JZ, Andon WB, et al. Am J Clin Nutr 1995;62:417–25.
44. Itoh R, Suyama Y. Am J Clin Nutr 1996;63:735–40.
45. Shortt C, Madden A, Flynn A, et al. Eur J Clin Nutr 1988;42:595–603.
46. Heaney RP. J Am Diet Assoc 1993;93:1259–60.
47. Recker RR, Davis KM, Hinders SM, et al. JAMA 1992;268:2403–8.
48. Spencer H, Kramer L, Osis D, et al. J Nutr 1978;108:447–57.
49. Calvo MS, Kumar R, Heath H. J Clin Endocrinol Metab 1990;70:1334–40.
50. Barger-Lux MJ, Heaney RP. J Clin Endocrinol Metab 1993;76:103–7.
51. Hasling C, Sondergraad K, Charles P, et al. J Nutr 1992;122:1119–26.
52. Barger-Lux MJ, Heaney RP, Stegman MR. Am J Clin Nutr 1990;52:722–5.
53. Harris SS, Dawson-Hughes B. Am J Clin Nutr 1994;60:573–8.
54. Barger-Lux MJ, Heaney RP. Osteoporosis Int 1995;5:97–102.
55. Evans GE, Weaver CM, Harrington DD, et al. J Hypertens 1990;8:327–37.
56. Andon MB, Ilich JZ, Tzagournio MA, et al. Am J Clin Nutr 1996;63:950–3.
57. Wood RJ, Zheng JJ. Am J Clin Nutr 1997;65:1803–9.
58. Gleerup A, Rossander-Hulten L, Gramatkovski E, et al. Am J Clin Nutr 1995;61:97–104.
59. Halberg L, Rossander-Hulten L, Brune M, et al. Eur J Clin Nutr 1992;46:317–27.
60. Whiting SJ. Nutr Rev 1995;53:77–80.
61. Berridge MJ. Nature 1993;361:315–25.
62. Bronner F, Stein WD. J Nutr 1995;125:1987S–95S.
63. Pettifore JM. Am J Clin Nutr 1979;32:2477–83.
64. Barger-Lux MJ, Heaney RP. J Nutr 1994;124:1406S–11S.
65. Hamet P. J Nutr 1995;125:311S–400S.
66. Bucher HC, Guyatt GH, Cook RJ, et al. JAMA 1996;275:1113–7.
67. Bucher HC, Guyatt GH, Cook RJ, et al. JAMA 1996;275:1128–9.
68. Levine RJ, Hauth JC, Curet LB, et al. N Engl J Med 1997;337:69–76.
69. Garland CF, Garland FC, Gorham ED. Am J Clin Nutr 1991;54:193S–201S.
70. Kampman E, Giovannucci E, vant Veer P, et al. Am J Epidemiol 1994;139:16–29.
71. Curhan GC, Willett WC, Renion EB, et al. N Engl J Med 1993;328:833–8.
72. Jackman LA, Millane SS, Martin BR, et al. Am J Clin Nutr 1997;66:327–33.
73. Johnston CC Jr, Miller JZ, Slemenda CW, et al. N Engl J Med 1992;327:82–7.
74. Lloyd T, Andon MB, Rollings N, et al. JAMA 1993;270:841–4.

75. Lee WTK, Leung SS, Leung DMY, et al. Br J Nutr 1995;74:125–39.
76. Chan GM, Hoffman K, McMurry MM. J Pediatr 1995;126:551–6.
77. Lee WTK, Leung SSF, Leung DMY, et al. Am J Clin Nutr 1996;64;71–7.
78. Teegarden D, Proulx WR, Martin BR, et al. J Bone Miner Res 1995;10:711–5.
79. Matkovic V, Jelic T, Wardlaw GM, et al. J Clin Invest 1994;93:799–808.
80. Heaney RP, Barger-Lux MJ, Davies KM, et al. Osteoporosis Int 1997;7:426–30.
81. Matkovic V, Fortana D, Tominac C, et al. Am J Clin Nutr 1990;52:878–88.
82. Spencer K, Kramer L, Lesniak M, et al. Clin Orthop 1984;184:270–80.
83. Heaney RP, Skillman TG. J Clin Endocrinol Metab 1971;331:661–70.
84. Wargovich MJ. J Am Coll Nutr 1988;7:295–300.
85. Kalkwarf HJ, Specker BC, Bianchi DC, et al. N Engl J Med 1997;337:523–8.
86. Nusser SM, Carriquiry AL, Dodd KW, Fuller WA. J Am Stat Assoc 1996;1440–9.
87. Barger-Lux MJ, Heaney RP, Packard PT, et al. Clin Appl Nutr 1992;2:39–44.
88. Weaver CM, Martin BR, Peacock M. In: Burckhardt P, Heaney RP, eds. Nutritional aspects of osteoporosis. New York: Raven Press, 1995;7:123–8.
89. Barger-Lux MJ, Heaney RP. In: Burckhardt P, Heaney RP, eds. Nutritional aspects of osteoporosis. New York: Raven Press 1995;7:243–51.
90. Jackson RT, Latham MC. Am J Clin Nutr 1979;32:779–82.
91. Rasmussen H, Palmieri GMA. Altered cell calcium metabolism and human diseases. In: Rubin RP, Weiss GB, Putnsy JW Jr, eds. Calcium in biological systems. New York: Plenum Publishing, 1985;551–60.
92. Pettifor JM, Ross P, Moodley G, et al. Am J Clin Nutr 1979; 32:2477–83.
93. Anast CS, Gardner DW. Magnesium metabolism. In: Bronner F, Coburn JW, eds. Disorders of mineral metabolism, vol III. New York: Academic Press, 1981;423–506.

SELECTED READINGS

Anderson JJB, Garner SC, eds. Calcium and phosphorus in health and disease. Boca Raton, FL: CRC Press, 1996;1–395.

Barger-Lux MJ, Heaney RP. The role of calcium intake in preventing bone fragility, hypertention, and certain cancers. J Nutr 1994;124:1406S–1411S.

Bronner F, ed. Intracellular calcium regulation. New York: John Wiley & Sons, 1990;1–480.

Clapham DE. Calcium signaling. Cell 1995;80:259–68.

Nordin BEC, ed. Calcium in human biology. London: Springer-Verlag, 1988;1–481.

8. Phosphorus

JAMES P. KNOCHEL

Hypophosphatemia and phosphorus deficiency are exceptionally common among seriously ill, hospitalized patients. Although both conditions have many causes, they are most commonly seen during treatment of diabetic ketoacidosis (DKA) and alcoholic withdrawal and while administering nutrients to a starved or wasted patient (Table 8.1).

Refeeding a starved person or administering nutrients to an undernourished sick patient may result in a predictable derangement of blood composition, a variety of specific organ dysfunctions, and sudden death secondary to arrhythmias. This condition has been termed the *refeeding syndrome.* Old historical records describe epidemics of death when starving persons gained access to food, engorged themselves, then became sick and died. One report describes deaths of Jews in the first century who had been entrapped and starved by the Romans. Some escaped, stuffed themselves with food, and died. Flavius Josephus pointed out clearly that death occurred in those who overindulged themselves but not in those who were skillful enough to restrain their appetites (1). Similar descriptions of death during refeeding were related by physicians observing liberated prisoners during WWII. Although the appearance of anasarca suggested beriberi precipitated by feeding carbohydrates, incorporation of brewers' yeast did not prevent the disease. As foretold from biblical descriptions (1), it was finally realized that refeeding with small amounts of food or milk would prevent this disaster. Since laboratory measurements were not available then, it was never clearly appreciated that overly aggressive refeeding could cause serious derangements of plasma. However, more recent studies on patients with anorexia nervosa treated with parenteral nutrition or overzealously with a normal diet have shown that hypophosphatemia and phosphorus deficiency play major roles in their metabolic complications.

CHEMISTRY AND PROPERTIES OF PHOSPHORUS

At normal blood pH, phosphate ions exist as 4 parts of HPO_4^{-2} and 1 part of $H_2PO_4^{-1}$. Thus $(4 \times 2^-) + (1 \times 1^-) \div (4 + 1) = 1.8$, which is the average valence of PO_4 in arterial plasma. In most laboratories, phosphorus is reported as inorganic P, and its normal range is 3.0 to 4.5 mg/dL or since the molecular weight of P is 30, 1.0 to 1.5 mM. About 5 to 10% of phosphorus is bound to protein, so most of the element is freely filtered by the glomerulus.

Children have higher plasma phosphorus concentrations, which may result from growth hormone and insulin-like growth factor activities (2). Plasma phosphorus concentration regulates erythrocyte synthesis and stores of 2,3-diphosphoglycerate (2,3-DPG), which is bound to hemoglobin (3). This substance plays an important role in hemoglobin affinity for oxygen. When 2,3-DPG is elevated, as it is in children, hemoglobin releases its oxygen more easily, and blood hemoglobin concentration and hematocrits are set at lower values. Nevertheless, oxygen delivery to tissues is normal. This phenomenon is also seen in patients with end-stage renal disease. If phosphate-binding antacids are administered to cause hypophosphatemia, 2,3-DPG in erythrocytes falls, and blood hemoglobin levels rise to complement the reduction of oxygen delivery that would occur otherwise (2).

Metabolism of Phosphorus

Recommended Phosphorus Intake

The current recommendations for daily dietary intake (known as dietary reference intake) of phosphorus by the Food and Nutrition Board of the Institute of Medicine (3a) are as follows: *(a)* 0 to 6 months, 100 mg (provided by human milk); 6 to 12 months, 275 mg (provided by milk plus food); *(b)* 1 through 8 years, 460 to 500 mg; *(c)* age 9 to 18, 1250 mg; *(d)* age 19 to 70, 700 mg; and during pregnancy or lactation, 1250 mg.

Dietary Sources of Phosphorus

Protein-rich foods and cereal grains are rich sources of phosphorus. In the United States about one-half of dietary

Table 8.1
Causes of Hypophosphatemia

- Hypophosphatemia without phosphorus deficiency
  - Pseudohypophosphatemia
    - Mannitol
    - Bilirubin
    - Acute leukemia
  - Decreased dietary intake
  - Decreased intestinal absorption
    - Vitamin D deficiency
    - Malabsorption
    - Steatorrhea
    - Secretory diarrhea
    - Vomiting
    - PO_4^{-3}-binding antacids
  - Shift from serum into cells
    - Respiratory alkalosis
      - Sepsis
      - Heat stroke
      - Neuroleptic malignant syndrome
      - Hepatic coma
      - Salicylate poisoning
      - Gout
      - Panic attacks
      - Psychiatric depression
    - Hormonal effects
      - Insulin
      - Glucagon
      - Epinephrine
      - Androgens
      - Cortisol
      - Anovulatory hormones
    - Nutrient effects
      - Glucose
      - Fructose
      - Glycerol
      - Lactate
      - Amino acids
      - Xylitol
    - Cellular uptake syndromes
      - Recovery from hypothermia
      - Burkitt lymphoma
      - Histiocytic lymphoma
      - Acute myelomonocytic leukemia
      - Acute myelogenous leukemia
      - Chronic myelogenous leukemia in blast crisis
      - Treatment of pernicious anemia
      - Erythropoietin therapy
      - Erythrodermic psoriasis
      - Hungry bone syndrome
        - After parathyroidectomy
        - Acute leukemia
- Hypophosphatemia with phosphorus deficiency
  - Decreased dietary intake
  - Decreased intestinal absorption
    - Vitamin D deficiency
    - Malabsorption
    - Steatorrhea
    - Secretory diarrhea
    - Vomiting
    - PO_4^{-3}-binding antacids
  - Increased excretion into the urine
    - Hyperparathyroidism
    - Renal tubule defects
    - Fanconi syndrome
    - X-linked hypophosphatemic rickets
    - Hereditary hypophosphatemic rickets with hypercalciuria
    - Polyostotic fibrous dysplasia
    - Panostotic fibrous dysplasia
    - Neurofibromatosis
    - Kidney transplantation
    - Oncogenic osteomalacia
    - Aldosteronism
    - Licorice ingestion
    - Volume expansion
    - Inappropriate secretion of antidiuretic hormone
    - Mineralocorticoid administration
    - Corticosteroid therapy
    - Diuretics
    - Aminophylline therapy

phosphorus comes from milk, meat, poultry, and fish. Cereals provide 12%. Processed meats and cheese contain more phosphorus than natural products.

Absorption of Phosphorus

Phosphorus from soluble products such as meat is more available than that from other sources. Milk casein contains a phosphopeptide resistant to enzymatic hydrolysis; human milk, being lower in casein, may have more phosphorus available for absorption than cow's milk. Phytic acid in cereal grains reduces bioavailability. A low phytase content of corn and oats reduces phosphorus bioavailability, and accordingly, these grains may be rachitogenic (4).

Absorption of phosphorus occurs throughout the length of the small intestine and is under the control of vitamin D and specific phosphate transporters. Absorption is reduced by a number of phosphate-binding antacids.

Total Body Content of Phosphorus

A normal 70-kg man contains about 700 g (23 mol) of phosphorus. Eighty percent is contained in bone and 9% in skeletal muscle. Most intracellular phosphorus exists as organic compounds, such as creatine phosphate and adenosine monophosphate (AMP) and triphosphate (ATP). As potassium is the most concentrated cation in the cell, phosphate is the most abundant anion. Total tissue phosphorus and nitrogen contents exist in a molar ratio of 0.03 in health.

Renal Handling of Phosphorus

In health, the kidneys retain about 80% of phosphorus filtered by the glomerulus. The major regulators of phosphate balance by the kidney are glomerular filtration and parathyroid hormone. Phosphorus is reabsorbed mainly in the proximal tubule by active transport. Parathyroid hormone reduces phosphorus reabsorption by the proximal tubular cells. The fractional clearance rises with hyperphosphatemia and falls with hypophosphatemia. Expansion of extracellular volume independently raises phosphate clearance (2). Vitamin D plays a small role in renal phosphate balance. Nevertheless, serum phosphorus levels play a major role in renal conversion of 25-hydroxyvitamin D_3 to 1,25-dihydroxyvitamin D_3.

Functions of Phosphorus

Phosphorus is a critically important element in every cell of the body. It is a major component of bone where it exists as hydroxyapatite. Plasma membranes require phosphorus as a component of phospholipids. All energy production and storage in the body depend upon adequate sources of phosphorus, including adenosine triphosphate, creatine phosphate, and other phosphorylated compounds. Phosphorus is a critical component of virtually all enzymes, cellular messengers such as the G-proteins, and carbohydrate fuels. A number of hormones depend upon phosphorylation for their activation. Phosphorus is of vital importance for acid-base regulation, not only serving as one of the most important buffers at the bone surface but also in renal regulation of proton balance.

HYPOPHOSPHATEMIA

Hypophosphatemia without Phosphorus Deficiency

Hypophosphatemia, i.e., a plasma concentration below 2.5 mg/dL (0.83 mM), is especially common in hospitalized patients who are seriously ill. It commonly occurs in the absence of a total body phosphorus deficit. For example, hyperventilation and respiratory alkalosis can reduce plasma phosphorus to values as low as 0.3 mg/dL (0.1 mM) in normal persons. By reducing plasma pCO_2, cytosolic pCO_2 falls, intracellular pH rises, and phosphofructokinase activity increases, resulting in phosphorylation of glucose. As a result, cytosolic phosphate falls, plasma phosphate enters the cell, and hypophosphatemia follows. Hyperventilation, respiratory alkalosis, and hypophosphatemia in the absence of phosphorus deficiency can occur in hepatic coma, endotoxic sepsis and shock, severe pain, recovery from exercise, and hyperthermia due to either heat stroke or the neuroleptic malignant syndrome. Administration of glucose or amino acids stimulates release of insulin, or administration of insulin causes cellular uptake of phosphorus and hypophosphatemia (2).

Intravenous fructose is dangerous because it can cause severe liver injury and induce modest hypophosphatemia as a result of "phosphate trapping" (2, 5). In this process, fructose is converted in the liver to fructose-1-phosphate without feedback inhibition of continued fructose uptake. For example, when glucose is transported into a hepatocyte, the glucose-6-phosphate formed inhibits glucokinase, thereby downregulating the process of glucose uptake. In the case of fructose, fructose-1-phosphate does not inhibit fructokinase, and accordingly, the unregulated uptake of fructose goes on, resulting in hypophosphatemia. The cytosolic phosphate trapping causes a sharp elevation in the phosphorylation potential ($ATP \div (ADP \times P^i)$), which results in decreased mitochondrial respiration and decreased ATP production. Cytosolic hypophosphatemia activates AMP deaminase, which reduces the nucleotide pool. The resulting inosine monophosphate is irreversibly converted to uric acid. Injury resulting from intravenous (not oral) fructose is seen only in tissues capable of metabolizing fructose, including the liver, proximal tubules of the kidney, and probably the small intestinal epithelium.

Hypophosphatemia with Phosphorus Deficiency

Hypophosphatemia in association with phosphorus deficiency is most commonly seen in chronic alcoholics during withdrawal and in patients recovering from DKA. Chronic ingestion of ethanol in large quantities causes depletion of body phosphorus stores in both humans and experimental animals (2). Indeed, phosphorus deficiency in this setting may play an important role in alcoholic myopathy and acute rhabdomyolysis (Table 8.1).

Hypophosphatemia occurs in as many as 50% of hospitalized alcoholics (2). Most chronic alcoholics who are not acutely ill show either a normal or slightly depressed serum phosphorus concentration (6). Hospitalized alcoholic patients are commonly unable to eat for a period of days before admission to the hospital, because of alcoholic ketoacidosis or, alternatively, alcohol withdrawal. Two important factors generally explain hypophosphatemia in such patients. First, administration of intravenous fluids containing nutrients without phosphorus is commonly responsible. Second, the usual hyperventilation and respiratory alkalosis that prevails in withdrawing alcoholics may result in hypophosphatemia that may be severe. On the first day of hospitalization of alcoholic patients, before the decline of serum phosphorus, urinary phosphorus excretion rates may equal 1 g or more (7). This is a high phosphorus excretion for a person who has virtually no phosphorus intake. Phosphaturia in such instances has been ascribed to the associated ketoacidosis (8), lactic acidosis, or proximal tubular injury (7). Nevertheless, consequent to administration of nutrients, correction of volume depletion, reversal of ketoacidosis, and development of respiratory alkalosis, phosphorus virtually disappears from the urine. Thus, the development of hypophosphatemia is caused by a shift of phosphorus out of extracellular fluid into the intracellular compartment. Hypokalemia and hypomagnesemia occur less commonly in these patients.

Measurement of muscle composition in severe chronic alcoholics discloses a complex derangement in which total phosphorus and magnesium are abnormally low, and sodium, chloride, and calcium contents are abnormally high (6, 9, 10). In some patients, potassium content of skeletal muscle is also low. While the average value for total phosphorus content in alcoholic patients is 20.4 mmol/dg of dried fat-free muscle, some patients demonstrate values as low as 12 mmol/dg. If one assumes that all muscle tissue is uniformly affected and that skeletal muscle occupies 40% of the body mass, the total deficiency of phosphorus in skeletal muscle alone extrapolates to 1800 mmol in patients with the lower values.

The causes of phosphorus deficiency in chronic alcoholics are multifactorial. Chronic administration of intoxicating quantities of ethanol to dogs for 2 months causes equally severe phosphorus deficiency in skeletal muscle despite a generous intake of all essential nutrients, including phosphorus (9, 10). Our observations suggest that alcohol exerts toxicity on the muscle cell and is responsible for disorganization of muscle composition, despite a nutritious diet (11). The precise mechanism of these effects is unknown. Since ethanol interferes with sodium transport in a variety of tissues, including skeletal muscle (10, 11), and since phosphate transport in nearly all tissues examined depends upon normal sodium transport, perhaps deranged sodium transport is somehow responsible for loss of phosphate from muscle. It has been proposed that cytosolic production of the anion acetaldehyde during metabolism of ethanol may electrically dislocate phosphate from the cell (12).

Alcohol may also damage the proximal tubule epithelium of the kidney. It has been reported that urinary γ-glutamyltranspeptidase (GGT), a tubular brush border membrane enzyme and the fractional clearance of lysozyme, a marker of proximal tubular function, are elevated in 61% of chronic alcoholics (13). Reduced capacity for phosphate reabsorption is seen in 82% of hypophosphatemic alcoholics but in none who were normophosphatemic. Others have described a renal phosphorus leak causing hypophosphatemia that resolves on abstinence (7). Parathyroid hormone is inhibited by acute alcoholic intoxication and therefore is unlikely to be responsible for these abnormalities (15). Poor phosphorus intake, use of phosphate-binding antacids, impaired vitamin D metabolism, magnesium deficiency, vomiting, or diarrhea might also cause such a deficit of phosphorus.

Simple dietary deficiency as a cause of phosphorus deficiency and hypophosphatemia is very rare because phosphorus is abundant in all foods and is avidly retained by the kidney. However, if the diet is deprived of phosphorus while a person ingests a phosphate-binding drug (e.g., aluminum hydroxide gel) severe and potentially fatal phosphorus deficiency may occur. In fact, refeeding a diet containing inadequate phosphorus to a starving person may allow tissue to be resynthesized without adequate phosphorus. This refeeding or nutritional recovery syndrome is heralded by hypophosphatemia with or without hypokalemia, progressively severe weakness, and a multitude of tissue and organ dysfunctions described below in more detail.

Hyperparathyroidism causes only mild hypophosphatemia in most instances. Malabsorption of fat causes modest hypophosphatemia, mainly from urinary loss. Thus, steatorrhea causes reduced absorption of vitamin D, vitamin D deficiency, malabsorption of calcium, hypocalcemia, increased production of parathyroid hormone, phosphaturia, and hypophosphatemia.

Primary impairment of phosphorus absorption by the renal tubule is seen in several conditions, including X-linked hypophosphatemia and Fanconi syndrome. Dietary vitamin D deficiency and interference with vitamin D production in oncogenic osteomalacia are acquired causes. Extracellular volume-expanded states, including the syndrome of inappropriate secretion of antidiuretic hormone, and primary aldosteronism also reduce phosphorus absorption (2). Acute infusion of sodium chloride solutions causes phosphaturia and hypophosphatemia by two mechanisms. First, the resulting volume expansion per se appears to reduce tubular reabsorption of phosphorus, and in addition, acute reduction of serum calcium causes release of parathyroid hormone and phosphaturia.

Two important conditions causing excessive loss of phosphorus into the urine are chronic respiratory acidosis and DKA. A reduction in intracellular pH causes degradation of organic phosphates, which allows phosphorus to enter plasma. Both conditions, untreated, are usually associated with a normal or even elevated serum phosphorus concentration. Because of this, phosphorus is lost into the urine and depletion occurs. The associated osmotic diuresis in DKA abets phosphorus losses. Effective treatment of either condition unveils the phosphorus deficiency. Thus, relief from hypercarbia allows cell pH to rise, glucose phosphorylation increases, and phosphorus in serum falls to potentially very low levels. Treatment of DKA with insulin, fluids, and electrolytes results in rapid hypophosphatemia as phosphorus is taken up by cells.

Effect of Phosphorus Deficiency and Hypophosphatemia

Phosphorus deficiency impairs growth. This is seen especially in the various forms of vitamin D deficiency in humans, such as celiac sprue, and in diseases causing renal tubular loss of phosphorus. Numerous experimental studies have documented the role of phosphorus in growth. Early phosphorus deficiency is often associated with losses of potassium, magnesium, and nitrogen. Reductions in major cell components are almost invariably associated with abnormalities of cellular ion transport, eventually resulting in accumulation of sodium, chloride, calcium, and water.

Osteomalacia, defined as a defect in bone mineralization, often occurs in longstanding phosphorus deficiency. Experimental phosphorus deprivation in conjunction with phosphate-binding antacid ingestion in human volunteers (16) resulted in profound muscle weakness and bone pain. In clinical settings, vitamin D deficiency resulting from steatorrhea or in patients with tumors that produce a substance interfering with renal production of $1,25(OH)_2D_3$ eventually causes osteomalacia (17).

Distinct from osteomalacia, dietary phosphorus deprivation acutely results in skeletal demineralization, even before serum phosphorus levels fall (2). Although the substance responsible for this phenomenon is unknown, it appears to be either a hormone or a cytokine, but not parathyroid hormone. In normal adults, phosphorus deprivation causes release of calcium from the skeleton and hypercalcuria; however, hypercalemia does not occur. In contrast, in growing children or in adults with various diseases affecting bone, such as Paget's disease, hyperparathyroidism, or metastatic malignancy involving bone, the skeletal response to phosphorus deprivation is more brisk, and hypercalcemia may occur. In experimental animals, dissolution of hydroxyapatite from the skeleton with phosphorus deprivation is prevented by colchicine (18).

Myopathy and Rhabdomyolysis

Chronic phosphorus deficiency in man causes a proximal myopathy (19). Proximal muscle atrophy and weakness may be striking. Osteomalacia usually accompanies this disorder. Laboratory findings characteristically show normal creatine phosphokinase (CPK) and aldolase activities; phosphorus levels in serum are modestly depressed, calcium levels may be low or normal, and alkaline phosphatase activity is usually sharply elevated.

Selective phosphorus deficiency causes reversible injury to muscle cells of the dog (20). These changes include depressed resting muscle transmembrane electrical potential, increased cellular content of Na, Cl, and water, and decreased phosphorus content. Serum CPK activity is normal. Chronic phosphorus deficiency apparently does not cause acute rhabdomyolysis. However, acute hypophosphatemia may precipitate rhabdomyolysis if superimposed upon chronic phosphorus depletion (21, 22). Most cases have occurred either during acute alcohol withdrawal or in severe chronic alcoholism treated with nutrients devoid of phosphorus. In alcoholics, rhabdomyolysis usually appears within the first few days in the hospital and is marked by a sudden elevation of CPK activity. The clinical manifestations include severe muscle pain, profound weakness, muscle tenderness, stiffness, swelling, and rarely muscular paralysis and diaphragm failure. Some patients are relatively asymptomatic and show very few abnormal muscle findings despite severely elevated serum creatine kinase or aldolase activities. In either situation, muscle creatine kinase activity in serum is consistently elevated, sometimes exceeding 100,000 IU/L. Other classical laboratory findings may be seen, i.e., myoglobinuria, hyperkalemia, hypocalcemia, hyperuricemia, and hypoalbuminemia (23). Hypophosphatemia and phosphorus deficiency may be obscured by release of residual phosphate from necrotic skeletal muscle and correction of the hypophosphatemia (22).

Rhabdomyolysis during total parenteral nutrition (TPN) is very rare and has not been observed if important intracellular element deficiencies are prevented. Apparently, rhabdomyolysis does not occur with acute hypophosphatemia in the absence of preexisting damage to muscle cells (24). If chronically phosphorus-depleted dogs with hypophosphatemic myopathy are hyperalimented without phosphorus, their serum phosphorus levels rapidly decline to values below 1.0 mg/dL and they become very ill, displaying marked weakness, inability to swallow their secretions, muscle fasciculations, and, in some, convulsions. They also show a pronounced elevation of CPK activity in serum. Histologic examination of skeletal muscle shows frank rhabdomyolysis. However, if phosphorus-deficient dogs are hyperalimented with phosphorus, serum phosphorus does not fall, CPK activity does not increase, and muscle histology remains normal (21).

The apparent prerequisite that muscle injury must exist before hypophosphatemia can cause acute florid rhabdomyolysis expresses itself both positively and negatively in several clinical settings. Patients with chronic alcoholic myopathy develop frank rhabdomyolysis if they become acutely hypophosphatemic, and patients with the neuroleptic malignant syndrome (25) develop florid rhabdomyolysis that appears to correlate inversely with the degree of hypophosphatemia. Negative expressions of this relationship are exemplified by the rarity of rhabdomyolysis in the patient who becomes hypophosphatemic during treatment of DKA or in the patient with simple starvation who becomes hypophosphatemic during TPN therapy (26). Usually neither of the latter instances show evidence of preexisting skeletal muscle damage.

Normal dogs deprived of calories but otherwise fed a diet replete with all other nutrients develop acute hypophosphatemia when hyperalimented. They show no evidence of rhabdomyolysis (24). Organs were sampled to determine their total phosphorus, sodium, potassium, chloride, magnesium, and calcium content. Although hypophosphatemia appeared quickly and usually attained levels below 1 mg/dL by the 2nd or 3rd day of hyperalimentation, CPK levels did not become abnormally high. Total phosphorus content fell substantially in skeletal muscle, liver, and bone. In contrast, total phosphorus content of cerebral cortex, left ventricle, adrenal gland, pancreas, renal cortex, renal medulla, thyroid, and spleen remained within normal limits. Despite sharp reduction in total muscle phosphorus and inorganic phosphorus concentrations in serum, ATP, ADP, and inorganic content of muscle tissue remained normal in dogs with acute hypophosphatemia that were not already phosphorus deficient. Thus, the phosphorylation potential (855 mmol/L in control animals) remained essentially unchanged (863 mmol/L in the hypophosphatemic animals) (24).

In contrast to the acute hypophosphatemic model, chronic phosphorus deficiency caused a pronounced change in muscle content of high energy components. ATP, ADP, and inorganic phosphate each fell by approximately 50%, thus seriously reducing the total adenine nucleotide pool. In addition, the increased value for the phosphorylation potential indicates a reduced rate of mitochondrial respiration, hence a reduced rate of ATP synthesis (24).

Our studies also suggest that not only bone but also skeletal muscle is apparently an endogenous reservoir for phosphorus. Thus, in the event of acute phosphorus depletion causing hypophosphatemia, muscle phosphorus is rapidly mobilized to provide phosphorus for vital organs. A low value for ATP, such as that observed in dogs with chronic phosphorus deficiency, implies that such a cell is in jeopardy. Thus, in the event of a superimposed insult, such as more pronounced hypophosphatemia or perhaps anorexia from a variety of influences in the phosphorus-deficient state, ATP levels must necessarily fall further. Much evidence suggests that when ATP levels decline to critically low values, cellular death may supervene. Additional evidence indicates that if sodium transport is so impaired that sodium ions accumulate in muscle cytoplasm, sodium-calcium exchange is decreased (27), so that sufficient calcium may accumulate in the cell to activate lysosomal enzymes and lead to destruction of the cell.

An important species difference appears to exist between rats, dogs, and humans in terms of the effect of phosphorus depletion and hypophosphatemia on skeletal muscle (28). Humans and dogs respond to phosphorus depletion in a virtually identical manner. In contrast, rats fed a phosphorus-deficient diet without added phosphate-binding antacids showed no changes in sodium, adenine nucleotides, resting transmembrane potential difference, potassium, or water contents of skeletal muscle although serum phosphorus levels declined from 8.3 to 2.8 mg/dL (29). Similarly, there was only a very slight change in phosphate content of muscle and no change in calcium content or transport. It appears that in experimental phosphate depletion, dogs are the ideal model if one wishes to replicate human disease.

Hypophosphatemic Cardiomyopathy and Arrhythmias

Calculated cardiac stroke work increases after phosphorus administration in seriously ill patients with hypophosphatemia. These improvements occur independently of Starling effects and probably represent an improvement in myocardial contractility (2, 30, 31).

In phosphorus-deficient dogs (32), left ventricular end-diastolic pressure increased and stroke work decreased. Myocardial stroke work fell independently of the Frank-Starling effect. Left ventricular ejection velocity and ventricular contractility are both reduced by phosphorus deficiency (33). Isoproterenol, which usually increases stroke work of the left ventricle, fails to do so in the presence of phosphorus deficiency. The phosphorylation potential of left ventricular muscle became substantially elevated in dogs with chronic phosphorus deficiency. This occurred because of 30% reduction of cytosolic inorganic phosphate concentration. The resulting alteration of the phosphorylation potential implies that the capacity for mitochondrial energy production is reduced. All abnormalities return to normal with phosphorus repletion.

Phosphorus-depleted rats show reductions in myocardial inorganic phosphorus, glycogen, glucose-6-phosphate, cytidine triphosphate, phosphatidylcholine, phosphatidylethanolamine, and total phospholipid phosphorus (34) and impaired fatty acid oxidation. Such abnormalities of lipid metabolism suggest defective phospholipid biosynthesis and might explain cellular membrane injury. Others have shown that feeding growing pigs aluminum hydroxide gel to induce phosphorus deficiency causes low levels of ATP and glucose-6-phosphate in the myocardium (35).

Approximately 20% of hypophosphatemic patients show cardiac arrhythmias, even without underlying heart disease, hypokalemia, hypomagnesemia, hyperlactatemia, or hypoxia (36). After repletion of the anion, the severity of arrhythmias improves. Arrhythmias have been described in patients with anorexia nervosa who become hypophosphatemic (37). Hypophosphatemia in patients with acute myocardial infarction increases the risk for ventricular tachycardia (38).

In vivo metabolism of inorganic phosphorus and its compounds can be studied using ^{31}P nuclear magnetic resonance spectroscopy. Using this technique the concentrations of phosphocreatine and ATP in the normal human heart have been estimated to be 11.0 ± 2.7 (SD) and 6.9 ± 1.6 mmol/g wet weight, respectively (39). This technique should be useful for studying disorders of the heart associated with phosphorus deficiency and hypophosphatemia.

Respiratory Insufficiency

Several clinical reports have described patients treated with TPN who developed respiratory failure (2, 40). These patients became seriously ill because of respiratory acidosis and hypoxia. Most were in intensive care unit settings and were desperately ill, receiving glucose or amino acids intravenously. Some demonstrated abnormalities of central nervous system function or peripheral neuropathy. Although profound weakness or muscle paralysis in some of the patients suggested the Guillain-Barré syndrome, usually the cerebrospinal fluid was normal. Some could not be weaned off ventilators at the anticipated time.

Most patients who developed acute respiratory failure due to hypophosphatemia induced by TPN had serious preexisting conditions. These include chronic intestinal fistulas, malabsorption syndrome, Crohn's disease, ulcerative colitis, small bowel resection, exocrine pancreatic insufficiency, chronic alcoholism associated with malnutrition, and gastrointestinal cancer. Others have suffered from chronic respiratory acidosis or cor pulmonale. Serum phosphorus concentrations have been below 1.0 mg/dL when respiratory failure occurred. In some cases, the patients were also hypokalemic. However, respiratory failure persisted despite correction of hypokalemia, responding to subsequent administration of phosphate salts and correction of hypophosphatemia (41). Phosphorus-deficient dogs also show diminished diaphragm function as a result of muscular weakness (42).

One important study was conducted on eight such patients with a mean serum phosphorus level of 1.65 ± 0.54 mg/dL, to characterize contractility of the diaphragm during electrical phrenic nerve stimulation (43). Correction of hypophosphatemia resulted in a twofold increase in transdiaphragmatic pressure generated by phrenic nerve stimulation.

Oddly enough, frank clinically evident rhabdomyolysis almost never occurs in patients who have developed respiratory failure. As pointed out in the section dealing with rhabdomyolysis, the latter apparently does not appear to occur as a consequence of acute hypophosphatemia per se unless significant muscle cell injury preexists. Thus, almost all cases of hypophosphatemic rhabdomyolysis occur in alcoholics, who probably all have preexisting muscle cell damage. This relationship may also explain the observation that the respiratory insufficiency and hypophosphatemic neurologic syndromes are hardly ever seen in alcoholics after admission to the hospital, because rhabdomyolysis usually corrects their hypophosphatemia spontaneously. Chronic alcoholism apparently protects against hypophosphatemic respiratory failure. Most patients who develop hypophosphatemic respiratory insufficiency have slowly become hypophosphatemic during administration of nutrients following correction of respiratory acidosis. In these patients, muscle cells have presumably not been damaged sufficiently for hypophosphatemic rhabdomyolysis to occur.

Erythrocyte Dysfunction

Phosphorus deficiency impairs oxygen release from hemoglobin (44) and rarely causes hemolysis (45, 46). The red cell is the only tissue in the body that produces 2,3-diphosphoglycerate (44). 2,3-DPG is bound to hemoglobin and serves to enhance dissociation of oxygen from the hemoglobin molecule. The interaction of 2,3-DPG with oxyhemoglobin has been well characterized. Deficiency of erythrocyte 2,3-DPG impairs release of oxygen from oxyhemoglobin, thus causing hypoxia (44). Coexistent acidosis reverses this effect by the Bohr effect (47). Reduced 2,3-DPG in erythrocytes may play an important role in neurologic disturbances that occur in hypophosphatemia (44).

As pointed out above, the vast majority of patients with DKA become hypophosphatemic during treatment. However, in most, there has not been adequate time for development of severe phosphorus deficiency. Because they usually recover rapidly with appropriate treatment, serum phosphorus levels recover spontaneously upon resumption of food intake and 2,3-DPG levels ordinarily do not fall (2). On the other hand, newly discovered diabetics who have been out of control for prolonged periods have more opportunity to develop serious phosphorus depletion (2).

Hemolysis in hypophosphatemia is rare. Superimposed events, such as alcoholic ketoacidosis or coincidental aspirin poisoning requiring hemodialysis, have also been present (2). Serum phosphorus concentration was less than 0.5 mg/dL. Severe acidosis, quite independently of hypophosphatemia, may inhibit phosphofructokinase and in turn inhibit synthesis of 2,3-DPG and ATP (47). If ATP levels fall below 15% of normal, hemolysis may supervene (48). That the bulk of patients with DKA are not severely phosphorus deficient probably explains why frank hemolysis has never been reported in such patients. Simple improvement of acidosis in most patients with DKA leads to correction of the metabolic abnormalities despite hypophosphatemia.

Leukocyte Dysfunction

Hypophosphatemia and phosphorus deficiency cause a 50% reduction in chemotactic, phagocytic, and bactericidal activity of granulocytes. Leukocyte ATP levels fall (49). All abnormalities are corrected by phosphate repletion or in vitro by incubation of the leukocytes with adenosine and phosphate. These effects are seen only when hypophosphatemia is severe.

The mechanism by which hypophosphatemia impairs granulocytic function is probably related to impaired ATP synthesis. Microtubule contractions regulate the mechanical properties of leukocytes, thus pseudopod and vacuole formation. Microfilaments require ATP as their source of energy (2, 50). Actin and myosin are found in the cytoplasm of granulocytes. Phosphorus deficiency is also associated with a rise in intracellular calcium, which may independently impair phagocytosis (51). Hypophosphatemia not only limits mechanical functions of the granulocyte but also may impair the requirement for increased rate of synthesis of phosphoinositides and other organic phosphate compounds that are necessary for bactericidal activity during phagocytosis (52).

Platelet Disorders

Malnourished dogs treated with parenteral hyperalimentation without adequate phosphate become hypophosphatemic and show seven abnormalities of platelet function and structure (53): *(a)* thrombocytopenia; *(b)* increased platelet diameter suggesting shortened platelet survival; *(c)* megakaryocytosis of the marrow; *(d)* 5- to 10-fold acceleration of the rate of labeled platelet disappearance from blood; *(e)* impaired clot retraction; *(f)* a 50% reduction in platelet ATP content; and *(g)* hemorrhage into the gut and skin. Of note, none of these abnormalities is seen if phosphorus supplements are provided. Despite these abnormalities, there appears to be little evidence that hypophosphatemia is a primary cause of hemorrhage in man.

Metabolic Acidosis

Three mechanisms permit urinary excretion of hydrogen ions. First, disodium hydrogen phosphate (Na_2HPO_4) is converted to monosodium dihydrogen phosphate (NaH_2PO_4) by exchange of luminal Na^+ for cellular H^+, and the hydrogen ions thus excreted are measurable as titratable acidity. Second, ammonia produced in the tubular cell diffuses into the tubular lumen and combines with H^+ to become NH_4^+. Third, a small quantity of hydrogen is excreted as free hydrogen ion, thus accounting for the acid pH. The acid pH facilitates formation of NH_4^+ in the tubular lumen. Since the ammonium ion is essentially not reabsorbable, ammonium excretion is enhanced in proportion to urinary acidification.

Severe metabolic acidosis may occur in the presence of phosphate deficiency and severe hypophosphatemia (54). Removal of phosphorus from the diet and simultaneous administration of phosphate-binding antacids leads to prompt mobilization of bone mineral and hypercalciuria (55). As hypophosphatemia becomes more severe, phosphate ions virtually disappear from the urine, thereby eliminating the capacity to excrete hydrogen ions as titratable acid.

Ordinarily, metabolic acidosis would be expected to augment renal production of ammonia. However, in phosphate deficiency, NH_3 formation decreases, presumably as a result of higher intracellular pH (56), and reduces urinary acidification by formation of NH_4^+ (57). Thereby, the decrease in ammonia production and unavailability of buffer phosphate in the urine substantially reduce excretion of metabolic acids.

One would predict that metabolic acidosis would regularly develop when excretion of titratable acid or ammonium into the urine is severely limited. However, metabolic acidosis in phosphorus deficiency is rare. The explanation lies in the fact that during mobilization of bone mineral, there also occurs mobilization of carbonate, which is an important component of bone apatite. During osteolysis associated with phosphorus deprivation, sufficient carbonate is mobilized from bone to titrate all metabolic acid retained in the body. However, should something prevent mobilization of bone mineral, then severe metabolic acidosis may occur. This has been described in experimental vitamin D deficiency and in children with severe lactase deficiency and protein-calorie malnutrition during refeeding without adequate phosphate in the diet (54). Addition of phosphate to their diet increased excretion of titratable acid into the urine and corrected metabolic acidosis. In experimental phosphorus deficiency, administration of diphosphonate or colchicine to impede calcium mobilization from bone causes metabolic acidosis (18).

Nervous System Dysfunction

Nervous system dysfunction is a well-recognized complication of severe hypophosphatemia. Hyperalimented malnourished dogs become hypophosphatemic and develop ataxia, convulsions, and death (21, 58). Experimental human phosphorus deficiency caused weakness, apathy, and intention tremors (16) and made patients bedridden.

A wide spectrum of clinical manifestations have been reported involving almost all levels of the nervous system from higher cortical function, brainstem, to peripheral nerves and muscle. The most florid examples of hypophosphatemia-induced nervous system dysfunction have been reported during the course of nutritional recovery syndrome. In such patients, hypophosphatemia usually occurs after approximately 1 week or more of hyperalimentation with solutions of glucose and/or amino acids not containing enough phosphorus to prevent hypophosphatemia. The sequence of abnormalities consists of irritability, apprehension, muscular weakness, numbness, paresthesias, dysarthria, confusion, obtundation, convulsive seizures, coma, and death (59, 60). Such a clinical state could be confused with that of delirium tremens in the alcoholic, because even lucid visual and auditory hallucinations may occur (61, 62). One report (44) described paresthesias about the mouth and limbs, mental obtundation, and hyperventilation in three of eight patients who became hypophosphatemic during hyperalimentation. At the same time, these patients displayed a sharp drop in red cell 2,3-DPG content that correlated with slowing of the electroencephalogram. Both abnormalities disappeared and the patients recovered symptomatically when hypophosphatemia was corrected. Most notably, such symptoms do not occur when adequate phosphorus is provided to prevent hypophosphatemia during hyperalimentation. Emphasis has been placed upon the importance of central nervous system complications in patients who slowly develop severe hypophosphatemia during the course of TPN (2, 44, 58–60).

Symptoms of brainstem dysfunction, such as ptosis, dysphagia, dysphonia, impaired ability to swallow secretions, respiratory weakness, and hypercarbia in a setting of profound muscle weakness, have been reported. Distortions in color perception and even amblyopia may occur. Some patients with slowly developing hypophosphatemia develop all clinical features of the Guillain-Barré syndrome with ascending paralysis, areflexia and respiratory muscle paralysis (2). Other cases closely resemble Wernicke's encephalopathy, in which dramatic improvement has been observed following correction of hypophosphatemia. However, when hypophosphatemia is prolonged, recovery after correction may be delayed. Asterixis has also been described. Peripheral neuropathy documented by nerve conduction studies has also been reported. Psychiatric manifestations may include paranoid delusions, extreme anxiety, and visual and auditory hallucinations. A syndrome resembling encephalitis has been described in children with malnutrition who became ill after 1 week of refeeding. Although phosphorus levels were not measured, the possibility of hypophosphatemia seems likely. These children developed coarse tremors resembling parkinsonism, mainly involving the upper extremities but also the legs, neck, and tongue. They remained alert. Hypotonia has also been described in infants undergoing treatment for protein-calorie malnutrition (63). There appeared to be a positive correlation between the reduction in serum phosphate and the occurrence of death during treatment. Obviously, all levels of nervous system dysfunction may be seen. As one might suspect, smooth muscle function is also apparently affected by severe hypophosphatemia as evinced by ileus.

In patients who develop syndromes of central or peripheral nervous system dysfunction and also in those who develop respiratory failure as a result of hypophosphatemia, rhabdomyolysis is virtually nonexistent. Presumably, the apparent requirement for preexistent skeletal muscle injury is missing. Failure to develop rhabdomyolysis results in inexorable and progressive hypophosphatemia and thus permits full expression of nervous system failure.

Treatment of Hypophosphatemia

Milk is an excellent source of phosphorus, containing 33 mmol/L (100 mg/dL). Phosphate salts are also available for oral use. They are less likely to cause diarrhea in phosphorus-deficient patients than in normal persons. Phosphorus salts cannot be given by intramuscular or subcutaneous injection, but sodium phosphate and potassium phosphate are available for intravenous use. The potassium salt should be given when hypokalemia and hypophosphatemia coexist. Two recent prospective studies on hypophosphatemic patients in acute intensive care unit situations show that a 15-mmol dose of either sodium or potassium phosphate may be given in 100 mL of 0.9% sodium chloride intravenously over a period of 2 hours (64). A second study shows that depending on the severity of hypophosphatemia, doses ranging from 0.16 to 0.64 mmol/kg may be given over a period of 1 or 2 hours as a single dose on a daily basis (65). Serum phosphorus should be measured within several hours after the infusion and at least daily under such conditions. Oral administration of phosphate salts or milk should be resumed as quickly as possible (2). A safe dosage regimen for treatment of alcoholics who are hypophosphatemic, phosphorus deficient, hypokalemic, and hypomagnesemic is the infusion each 8 to 12 h of 1 L of 0.5 normal sodium chloride in 5% glucose containing 9 mmol of potassium phosphate and 4.2 mmol of magnesium sulfate (2.0 mL of 50% $MgSO_4$ solution).

Hyperphosphatemia should be avoided because it can cause severe hypocalcemia and crystal deposition in important structures including blood vessels, the eye, lung, heart, and kidney. Fatal alveolar diffusion block has occurred, especially if the patient is alkalotic. Patients treated with parenteral nutrition should receive adequate amounts of phosphate to prevent hypophosphatemia (see Chapter 101).

HYPERPHOSPHATEMIA

Hyperphosphatemia in adults is defined as an elevation of serum phosphorus above 5 mg/dL (1.67 mmol/L) and is a common finding with many causes. Spurious hyperphosphatemia may occur in patients with thrombocytosis when blood is allowed to clot to obtain serum. Undelayed collection of plasma from heparinized samples will show lower values. Certain autoanalyzers cause spurious hyperphosphatemia because of chemical interference. Abnormal positively charged serum proteins, as in plasma cell dyscrasias, may bind phosphorus and cause marked elevations exceeding 13 mg/dL (4.3 mM).

Decreased renal excretion of phosphorus is the most common cause of hyperphosphatemia. Since parathyroid hormone (PTH) is phosphaturic, hyperphosphatemia is a cardinal feature of hypoparathyroidism, either as a primary disorder or in patients whose renal cAMP response to PTH is abnormal (pseudohypoparathyroidism type I) or those whose phosphaturic response to PTH is suppressed (pseudohypoparathyroidism type II) (2).

Severe hypomagnesemia causes marked suppression of PTH in plasma despite hypocalcemia but does not usually cause hyperphosphatemia (66, 67). Hyperphosphatemia occurs in tumoral calcinosis, pseudoxanthoma elasticum, infantile hypophosphatasia, and hyperostosis because of decreased renal excretion. Untreated severe hyperthyroidism apparently increases cellular catabolism sufficiently to elevate serum phosphorus in some patients despite increased phosphorus loss in the urine. Acromegaly or administration of growth hormone causes hyperphosphatemia. Presumably, the higher phosphorus levels in children partly reflect growth hormone activity (68) or insulin-like growth factor I activity (69). Hyperphosphatemia occurs in untreated adrenal insufficiency because of volume-contraction metabolic acidosis and possibly reduced glomerular permeability. Mild hyperphosphatemia may occur with biphosphonate therapy because of increased tubular reabsorption of phosphorus.

Hyperphosphatemia, sometimes with levels up to 46 mg/dL, has occurred secondary to increased absorption from the gut following administration of excess phosphate salts by mouth or from the colon as a result of enemas that contain phosphorus. Overmedication with vitamin D and production of vitamin D by granulomatous tissue as in sarcoidosis and tuberculosis can cause hyperphosphatemia (2). Both acute metabolic and acute respiratory acidosis may decompose cellular organic phosphates, reduce phosphorylation, and result in diffusion of phosphorus from the cell and hyperphosphatemia. Lactic acidosis is especially important as a cause of hyperphosphatemia. Reduced insulin levels secondary to clonidine administration also can cause hyperphosphatemia. Cellular release of phosphorus may cause hyperphosphatemia, particularly in rhabdomyolysis, infarction of other tissues, or hemolysis. The tumor lysis syndrome, usually seen in patients whose tumor responds briskly to chemotherapy, consists of hyperphosphatemia, hypocalcemia, hyperkalemia, metabolic acidosis, hyperuricemia, and, in many cases, acute renal failure. Severe hyperphosphatemia after intravenous infusion of phosphate salts is a particular danger in patients who are acidotic or oliguric. Finally, infusion of compounds containing phospholipids for parenteral nutrition has caused hyperphosphatemia.

Treatment of Hyperphosphatemia

Hyperphosphatemia is potentially serious because of potential metastatic calcification. Before initiating treatment for hyperphosphatemia, its cause should be identified and corrected whenever possible. Although only an approximate guide, a calcium-phosphorus product (serum Ca in mg/dL × serum P in mg/dL) above 70 indicates a potential threat of calcification. Calcification is more likely to occur in the presence of an elevated blood pH or elevated level of parathyroid hormone.

In the absence of renal insufficiency, hydration or volume expansion by infusing hypotonic saline will increase fractional clearance of phosphorus by the kidney. Aluminum-based antacids will bind phosphorus in the gut and prevent absorption. Although long-term use of these compounds may result in aluminum toxicity, their use for a short time in acute hyperphosphatemia is safe and may be very helpful. Hyperphosphatemia in the presence of renal insufficiency often requires either peritoneal dialysis or hemodialysis.

REFERENCES

1. Complete works of Flavius Josephus, book V, chapter XIII, paragraph 4, p 569. Grand Rapids, MI: Kreger Publications, 1981.
2. Knochel JP, Agarwal R. Hypophosphatemia and hyperphosphatemia. In: Brenner B, ed. The kidney. 5th ed. Philadelphia: WB Saunders, 1996;1086–133.
3. Guest GM, Rapoport S. Am J Dis Child 1939;58:1072–89.
4. Simons AW, Versteegh HAJ, Jongbloed AW, et al. J Nutr 1990;64:525–40.
5. Bode JC, Zelder O, Rumpelt HJ, Wittkamp W. Eur J Clin Invest 1973;3:436–41.
6. Anderson R, Cohen M, Haller R, et al. Miner Electrolyte Metab 1980;4:106–12.
7. DeMarchi S, Cecchin E, Basile A, et al. N Engl J Med 1993;329:1927–34.
8. Elisaf M, Merkouropoulos M, Tsianos EV, Siamopoulos KC. Miner Electrolyte Metab 1994;20:274–81.
9. Blachley JD, Ferguson ER, Carter NW, Knochel JP. Trans Assoc Am Physicians 1980;93:110–22.
10. Ferguson ER, Blachley JD, Carter NW, Knochel JP. Am J Physiol 246(Renal Fluid Electrolyte Physiol) 1984;15:F700–9.
11. Blachley JD, Johnson JH, Knochel JP. Am J Med Sci 1985;289:22–6.
12. Veech RL, Gates DN, Crutchfield C, et al. Alcohol Clin Exp Res 1994;18:1040–56.
13. Angeli P, Gatta A, Caregaro L, et al. Gastroenterology 1991;100:502–12.
14. Deleted.
15. Peng T, Cooper CW, Munson PL. Endocrinology 1972; 91:586–93.
16. Lotz M, Zisman E, Bartter FC. N Engl J Med 1968;278:409–15.
17. Cai Q, Hodgson SF, Kao PC, et al. N Engl J Med 1994;330:1679–81.
18. Emmett M, Goldfarb S, Agus ZS, et al. J Clin Invest 1977;59:291–8.
19. Ravid M, Robson M. JAMA 1976;236:1380.
20. Fuller TJ, Carter NC, Barcenas C, Knochel JP. J Clin Invest 1976;57:1019–24.
21. Knochel JP, Barcenas C, Cotton JR, et al. J Clin Invest 1978;62:1240–6.
22. Knochel JP, Bilbrey GL, Fuller TJ, Carter NW. Ann NY Acad Sci 1975;252:274–86.
23. Knochel JP. Am J Med 1992;72:521–35.
24. Knochel JP, Haller R, Ferguson E. Phosphate and minerals in health and disease. In: Massry SG, Ritz E, Jahn H, eds. Advances in experimental medicine and biology, vol 128. New York: Plenum Press, 1980;323–34.
25. Harsch H. J Clin Psychiatry 1987;48:328–33.
26. Wada S, Nagase T, Koike Y, et al. Intern Med 1992;31:478–82.
27. Welsh DG, Lindinger MI. J Appl Physiol 1996;80:1263–9.
28. Knochel JP. Adv Exp Biol Med 1982;151:191–8.
29. Kretz J, Sommer G, Boland R, et al. Klin Wochenschr 1980;58:833–7.
30. Zazzo JF, Troche G, Ruel P, Maintenant J. Intensive Care Med 1995;21:826–31.
31. Bollaert PE, Levy B, Nace L, et al. Chest 1995;107:1698–701.
32. Fuller TJ, Nichols WW, Brenner BJ, et al. J Clin Invest 1978;62:1194.
33. Fuller TJ, Nichols WW, Brenner BJ, Peterson JC. Adv Exp Biol Med 1977;103:395–400.
34. Brautbar N, Baczynski R, Carpenter C, et al. Am J Physiol 1982;242:F699–F704.
35. Haglin L, Essen-Gustavsson B, Lindholm A. Acta Vet Scand 1994;35:263–71.
36. Venditti FJ, Marotta C, Panezai FR, et al. Miner Electrolyte Metab 1987;13:19–25.
37. Beumont PJ, Large M. Med J Aust 1991;155:519–522.
38. Ognibene A, Ciniglio R, Greifenstein A, et al. South Med J 1994;87:65–9.
39. Bottomley PA, Hardy CJ, Roemer PB. Magn Reson Med 1990;14:425–34.
40. Fiaccadori E, Coffsini E, Fracchia C, et al. Chest 1994;105:1392–8.
41. Newman JH, Neff TA, Ziporin P. N Engl J Med 1977;296:1101–3.
42. Planas RF, McBrayer RH, Koen PA. Adv Exp Med Biol 1982;151:283–90.
43. Aubier M, Murciano D, Lecogguic Y, et al. N Engl J Med 1985;313:420–4.
44. Travis SF, Sugerman HJ, Ruberg RL, et al. N Engl J Med 1971;285:763–8.
45. Lichtman MA, Miller DR, Cohen J, Waterhouse C. Ann Intern Med 1971;74:562–8.
46. Jacob HS, Amsden P. N Engl J Med 1971;285:1446.
47. Astrup P. Adv Exp Med Biol 1970;6:67.
48. Nakoa K, Wada T, Kamiyana T. Nature 1962;194:877–8.
49. Craddock PR, Yawata Y, Van Santen L, et al. N Engl J Med 1974;290:1403.
50. Stossel TP. N Engl J Med 1974;290:717–23.
51. Kiersztejn M, Chervu I, Smogorzewski M, et al. J Am Soc Nephrol 1992;2:1484–9.
52. Lichtman MA. N Engl J Med 1974;290:1432–3.
53. Yawata Y, Hebbel RP, Silvis S, et al. J Lab Clin Med 1974;84:643–53.
54. Kohaut EC, Klish WJ, Beachler CW, Hill LL. Am J Clin Nutr 1977;30:861.
55. Pronove P, Bell NH, Bartter FC. Metabolism 1961;10:364–71.
56. Gold LW, Massry SG, Arieff AI, Coburn JW. J Clin Invest 1973;52:2556–62.
57. Arruda JAL, Julka NK, Rubinstein H, et al. Metabolism 1980;29:826–36.
58. Yawata Y, Craddock P, Hebbel R, et al. Clin Res 1973;31:729.

59. Silvis SE, DiBartolomeo AG, Aaker HM. Am J Gastroenterol 1980;73:215–22.
60. Silvis SE, Paragas PD. J Lab Clin Med 1972;62:513–20.
61. Treloar A, Crook M, Parker L, Doig R. Lancet 1991;338:1467–8.
62. Zurkirchen MA, Misteli M, Conen D. Schweiz Med Wochenschr 1994;124:1807–12.
63. Freiman I, Pettifor JM, Moodley GM. J Pediatr Gastroenterol Nutr 1982;1:547–50.
64. Rosen GH, Boullata JI, O'Rangas EA, et al. Crit Care Med 1995;23:1204–10.
65. Clark CL, Sacks GS, Dickerson RN, et al. Crit Care Med 1995;23:1504–11.
66. Shils ME. Medicine (Baltimore) 1969;48:61–85.
67. Shils ME. Magnesium. In: Shils ME, Young VR, eds. Modern nutrition in health and disease. 8th ed. Philadelphia: Lea & Febiger, 1994;164–84.
68. Haramati A, Mulroney SE, Lumpkin MD. Pediatr Nephrol 1990;4:387–91.
69. Suzuki K, Nonaka K, Ichihara K, et al. Bone Miner 1986;1:51–8.

9. Magnesium

MAURICE E. SHILS

Magnesium plays an essential role in a wide range of fundamental biologic reactions. Hence, it is not surprising that deficiency in the organism may lead to serious biochemical and symptomatic changes. Kruse and associates made the first systematic observations of magnesium deficiency in rats and dogs in the early 1930s (1). The first description of clinical depletion in man, published in 1934, involved a small number of patients with various underlying diseases (2). In the early 1950s, Flink initiated studies documenting depletion of this ion in alcoholics and in patients on magnesium-free intravenous solutions (3). Although the diets ordinarily consumed by healthy Americans do not appear to lead to clinically significant depletion, an increasing number of clinical disorders have been associated with depletion.

BIOCHEMISTRY AND PHYSIOLOGY

Magnesium is involved in more than 300 essential metabolic reactions, and the number increases with new discoveries in molecular biology. Magnesium ion (Mg^{2+}) forms complexes with a variety of organic molecules having biologic activities. The relatively high—in comparison with other electrolytes—extracellular and intracellular concentrations of Mg^{2+} tend to favor binding to such molecules. The binding of functional groups is, in descending order: phosphates > carboxylates > hydroxyls, in terms of both relative importance and binding affinities (4). Mg^{2+} is essential for many enzymatic reactions and has two general interactions: *(a)* Mg^{2+} binds to the substrate, thereby forming a complex with which the enzyme interacts, as in the reaction of kinases with MgATP, and *(b)* Mg^{2+} binds directly to the enzyme and alters its structure and/or serves a catalytic role (e.g., exonuclease, topoisomerase, and RNA- and DNA polymerases) (5, 6). Other divalent metal ions (especially Mn^{2+}) activate many of the same enzymes but usually have less specificity and/or are present in much smaller quantities. Because of the weak binding of Mg^{2+} to proteins, activated enzymes are not necessarily isolated in the metal-bound form. Consequently, Mg^{2+} must be added for in vitro reactions, whereas in vivo, the background Mg^{2+} concentration usually suffices to stimulate the enzyme.

Adenosine triphosphate (ATP) has a strategic position in "free-energy" currency for virtually all cellular processes by providing high-energy phosphate. It exists in all cells primarily as magnesium ATP^{2-} (MgATP).

Enzyme Interactions

Some examples of the numerous enzymes in both classes mentioned above will emphasize the important role of magnesium (7–9). They include hexokinase, which phosphorylates glucose by way of MgATP and other enzymes necessary for the glycolytic cycle. Magnesium is required in steps of the citric acid cycle; three of the four key enzymes in the gluconeogenesis pathway from non-carbohydrate sources require magnesium. It is required in lipid metabolism; amino acid activation via RNA and DNA polymerases; the transketolase reaction involving thiamin; and the transfer of CO^2 to biotin in carboxylation reactions. Glutathione, a key intracellular antioxidant, has a Mg^{2+} requirement for its synthesis. The ubiquitin-proteosome pathway of protein degradation (see Chapter 2) also requires Mg^{2+} and ATP. Protein kinases, enzymes that catalyze the transfer of the α-phosphate from MgATP (e.g., in intracellular signaling), now number more than 100 (10).

The second messenger, cyclic adenosine monophosphate (cAMP), formed from MgATP and the enzyme adenylate cyclase, is activated by Mg^{2+} through its two binding sites (11). cAMP is involved in many reactions, including secretion of parathyroid hormone (PTH) by its gland (12); in addition, PTH exerts at least some of its physiologic effects through the formation and actions of cAMP (13).

Structural Modifications

The negatively charged ribose phosphate structure of nucleic acids has an affinity for Mg^{2+}; the resulting stabilization of numerous ribonucleotides and deoxyribonucleotides induces important physicochemical changes—all having biologic effects (4, 14, 15); hence "RNA science eventually became magnesium science" (14). In addition, the binding of hydrated Mg^{2+} by transfer RNA (tRNA) and modified tRNA and its DNA analogues results in structures that cannot be duplicated by the binding of other metals (4, 6, 14). Magnesium, calcium, and some other cations react with hydrophilic polyanionic carboxylates and phosphates of the various membrane components to stabilize the membrane and thereby affect fluidity and permeability.

Extracellular and Intracellular Magnesium Interrelations

In the early 1970s, it was noted that the magnesium ion modulated muscle tension (16) and that its intracellular concentration increased with epinephrine stimulation of lipolysis in adipocytes (17). The availability of ^{28}Mg enabled transport studies in cardiac cells and revealed that the free intracellular (cytosolic) magnesium concentration $[Mg^{2+}]_i$ was 1 mmol or lower (18), appreciably less than had been postulated. More-sensitive methods of measuring intracellular concentrations have advanced our understanding of magnesium transport, cellular homeostasis, and its regulatory role (19, 20). Of the approximately 500 mmol of total intracellular magnesium in the adult human, about 90 to 95% of that in the cytosol is bound to ligands such as ATP, ADP, citrate, proteins, and nucleic acids. The small remainder is free Mg^{2+}. What processes maintain or modify the relationships between total and ionized internal and external magnesium?

Transport across Plasma Membranes. $[Mg^{2+}]_i$ is maintained far from electrochemical equilibrium with external $[Mg^{2+}]$ ($[Mg^{2+}]_e$), indicating that the plasma membrane must contain transport mechanisms to extrude this ion; otherwise, magnesium would gradually accumulate intracellularly (21). Studies from a variety of tissues and species indicate that a Na^+-dependent Mg^{2+} efflux is a common mechanism for maintaining the intracellular homeostasis. There are some exceptions and other evidence for a Na^+-independent transport system (22, 23) as well as transporters that depend on hormones and others inhibited by calcium channel blockers, which suggests a role for Ca^{2+} in Mg^{2+} efflux (24). Because of the difficulties in studying the molecular aspects of Mg^{2+} transporters in eukaryocytes, investigations have been made in certain bacteria, in which four distinct regulating systems have been found (22, 25).

Ion Exchange across the Plasma Membrane. Cytosolic Mg^{2+} exchanges readily with extracellular magnesium; however, the level of the cytosolic free ion is highly regulated. For example, intact isolated cells from various rat tissues placed in a normal magnesium medium maintain their usual $[Mg^{2+}]_i$ despite a many-fold increase in external $[Mg^{2+}]$ (22, 26–27). Similarly, cells depleted of Mg^{2+} and then bathed in a medium of supernormal Mg^{2+} concentration gradually accumulate Mg^{2+} until the normal concentration is reached and then maintain that level (27).

Stimulated Intracellular Magnesium Exchanges. Perfused rat livers and hearts and isolated hepatocytes and myocytes release Mg^{2+} into the medium upon stimulation with certain adrenergic agonists or cAMP (28). Reverse movement of Mg^{2+} occurred with carbachol stimulation of the muscarinic receptor, causing a decrease in cytosolic cAMP levels (28) (Fig. 9.1). The observed fluxes were rapid, the quantities released or taken up within a few minutes were equal and accounted for approximately 5 to 10% of total cellular ionized magnesium. Such data suggest that the flux mechanisms are activated by appropriate hormones and are associated with redistribution of ionized magnesium from or into various intracellular compartments.

Mg^{2+} plays a role in ion channels (see Chapter 38). For example, in myocardial cells, Mg^{2+} produces inward rectification in at least four different potassium channels by plugging the open channel as outward current begins to flow. It also modulates the outwardly directed potassium current and the inwardly directed low-threshold calcium current (29). Stimulation of the K_{ATP} channel by MgATP activates this channel in intact pancreatic β cells; hence MgATP is an intracellular regulator of insulin secretion (30).

Cell Surface Receptors. Finding that ATP, ADP, and adenosine act directly on surface receptors led to the discovery of classes of such receptors, designated as purinoceptors (31, 32). These widely distributed receptors with many actions have been subdivided into P1 (adenosine-stimulated) purinoceptors and various subtypes of P2 purinoceptors, which are activated by ATP and ADP.

Cell Migration. Levels of extracellular Mg^{2+} and Ca^{2+} can affect the adhesive and migratory activities of many cell types. For example, in the early stages of cutaneous wound

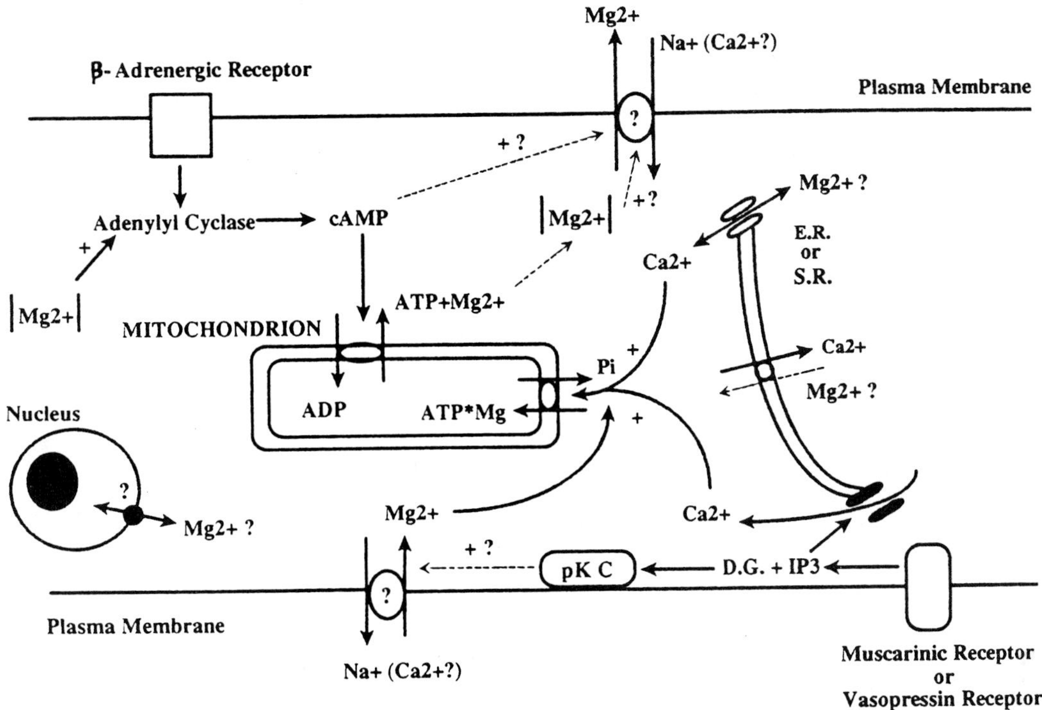

Figure 9.1. Schema of regulation of cellular Mg^{2+} homeostasis in the mammalian cell. The pathways are indicated for cellular Mg^{2+} release *(upper section)* and for its uptake *(lower section)*. Stimulated by β-adrenergic agonists, cAMP is increased in the cytosol, which modulates mitochondrial adenine nucleotide translocase and increases the efflux of Mg^{2+} from the mitochondrion by means of an exchange of one Mg-ATP for ADP. Activation of muscarinic receptors (in cardiac cells) or vasopressin receptors (in the liver) may stimulate a Mg^{2+} influx mechanism either by decreasing cAMP or by enhancing protein kinase C activity by diacylglycerol *(D.G.)*. Vasopressin receptor activation is coupled with production of inositol triphosphate *(IP3)* from phosphatidylinositol bisphosphate, which induces release of Ca^{2+} from the endoplasmic reticulum *(E.R.)* or the sarcoplasmic reticulum *(S.R.)*. Calcium ion release may be associated with either Mg^{2+} influx or Mg redistribution in the nucleus or endoplasmic reticulum. (From Romani A, Marfella C, Scarpa A. Miner Electrolyte Metab 1993;19:282–289, with permission.)

repair, in which cell migration into the wound is initiated, $[Mg^{2+}]$ increased and $[Ca^{2+}]$ decreased in the wound fluid. The data suggest that such ionic changes affect integrins and E-cadherins in activating the phenotypes of cells involved in wound healing (33).

ANALYTIC PROCEDURES

A variety of methods have been developed to measure magnesium in foods, excreta, blood, cells, and cell compartments.

Total Magnesium. Atomic absorption spectrometry (AAS) has been widely used to determine total magnesium in many sources and still remains the reference method (34). Clinical laboratories now almost exclusively use one of the various chromophores in automated instruments, with varying precision compared with AAS; however, with experience and proper calibration, these methods are acceptable (35). Inductively coupled plasma emission spectroscopy is useful for determination of a number of minerals including magnesium in serum, urine and, after wet ashing, stool or foods (36).

Ionized Magnesium and Ion-Selective Electrodes (ISEs). Electrodes have been developed with increasingly specific resins, which can measure ionized magnesium in serum, plasma, whole blood, and cells (21, 37). Calcium ion and lipophilic cations (e.g., acetylcholine and cation substitutes) may interfere. The current clinical chemistry literature indicates that ISEs from various manufacturers differ in accuracy from each other and from AAS and may give misleading results in sera with low magnesium concentrations (38, 39). Huijgen et al. have reviewed the combination of methods that allows measurement of all known serum magnesium parameters (37).

Magnetic Resonance Spectroscopy (MRS). A number of metabolites exist in equilibrium between uncomplexed and complexed Mg^{2+}. Because the resonances of such molecules may shift upon Mg^{2+} complexation, MR spectra can provide information on $[Mg^{2+}]_i$. ATP is the most useful endogenous indicator because of the ^{31}P nuclei and its high concentration and broad distribution in cells. The observed shift difference between α and β phosphate resonances is the parameter of choice. This method is used to measure $[Mg^{2+}]_i$ noninvasively in many tissues and cells. Technical issues in methodology have been discussed (40–42). Exogenous MRS indicators have been developed to measure cytosolic Mg^{2+}; such indicators gain sensitivity and selectivity, for example, by using fluoridated compounds, because essentially no fluoride background resonance normally exists in cells. Biologic and technical issues with these indicators have been reviewed (40).

Fluorescent Indicators. Several indicators (e.g., FURAPTRA) undergo a change in fluorescence on binding to Mg^{2+}. The measurable shift in the excitation spectrum allows determination by a ratio method of the ion concentration in cell suspensions and in individual cells. Calibration and a number of metabolic issues must be considered in using this method (21, 40).

[Σ Citrate]:[Σ Isocitrate] Ratio

Free $[Mg^{2+}]$ in cytoplasm can be measured from the variation in the [Σ citrate]:[Σ isocitrate] ratio in the aconitase reaction because this varies with $[Mg^{2+}]_i$ (43).

Magnesium Isotopes. Isotopes have been used as biologic tracers to follow the absorption, distribution, and excretion of the magnesium ion. The radioisotope ^{28}Mg has been used in human studies (44). Its value is limited by its radioactivity, its short half-life of 21.3 h, and its short supply. The percentage of distribution of stable magnesium in nature is 78.99% ^{24}Mg, 10.0% ^{25}Mg, and 11.01 ^{26}Mg. The latter has been used for tracer studies (47), including absorption studies in man (45). The ^{25}Mg:^{26}Mg ratio has been used to measure intestinal absorption (46).

Energy-Dispersive X-ray Analysis. Energy-dispersive x-ray analysis has been used to measure intracellular $[Mg^{2+}]$ in sublingual epithelial cells and atrial biopsy specimens in various conditions (47).

BODY COMPOSITION

The distribution of magnesium in various body compartments of apparently healthy adult individuals is summarized in Table 9.1. Somewhat more than half of the total is in bone, with almost all of the rest in soft tissue. Magnesium is the most abundant divalent mineral cation in cells and is second only in electrolyte quantity to monovalent potassium. Reference values for magnesium in serum, in blood cells, and in infants and children are given in references 48 and 48a. While bone has the largest amounts, much of this is either within the hydration shell or on the crystal surface (49). The amount of magnesium lost in sweat is very small in comparison to other cations. For example, in a 10-km run in 40.5 minutes with an average body weight (fluid) loss of 1.45 kg, the actual ion losses per kg of weight loss were Na, 800 mg; K, 200 mg; Ca, 20 mg; and Mg, 5 mg (50).

Most intracellular magnesium exists in bound form. Measured by ^{31}P MRS, frog muscle cells contained 5.8 mmol/L magnesium bound to ATP, 1.7 mmol/L to phosphocreatine, and 0.3 mmol/L to myosin; the free $[Mg^{2+}]_i$ was 0.6 mmol/L (51).

HOMEOSTASIS

Homeostasis of the individual with respect to a mineral depends on the amounts ingested, the efficiency of intestinal and renal absorption and excretion, and all other factors affecting them. A schema for magnesium balance is given in Figure 9.2.

Table 9.1
Distribution and Concentrations of Magnesium (Mg) in a Healthy Adult (Total body: 833–1170 mmol[a], or 20–28 g)

Site	Percentage of Total Body Mg	Concentration or Content
Bone	53	0.5% of bone ash
Muscle	27	9 mmol/kg wet weight
Soft tissue	19	9 mmol/kg wet weight
Adipose tissue	0.012	0.8 mmol/kg wet weight[b]
Erythrocytes	0.5	1.65–2.73 mmol/L[c]
Serum	0.3	0.88 ± 0.06 mm/L[d]
% total		
free	65	0.56 ± 0.05 mmol/L[e]
complexed	8	
bound	27	
Mononuclear blood cells[f]		2.91 ± 0.6 fmol/cell[g] 2.79 ± 0.6 fmol/cell[h] 3.00 ± 0.4 fmol/cell[i]
Platelets		2.26 ± 0.29 mmol/L[j]
$[Mg^{2+}]_i$[k]		0.5–1.0 mmol/L
Cerebrospinal fluid		1.25 mmol/L
free 55%		
complexed 45%		
Secretions		
Saliva, gastric, bile		0.3–0.7 mmol/L
Sweat		0.3 mmol/L (38°C)[l] 0.09 mmol/h[m]

[a]1 mmol = 2 mEq = 24.3 mg.
[b]From Snyder et al. Report of the Task Group on Reference Man. Elmsford, NY: Pergamon Press, 1975;306.
[c]Magnesium falls slowly with aging.
[d]Similar at various ages.
[e]From Huijgen HJ, Van Ingen HE, Kok WT, et al. Clin Biochem 1996;29:261–6.
[f]Monocytes and lymphocytes in venous blood.
[g]From Elin, Hossini. Clin Chem 1985;31:377–80. 1 fmol = 24.3 fg.
[h]From Reinhart et al. Clin Clim Acta 1987;167:187–95.
[i]From Yang et al. J Am Coll Nutr 1990;9:328.
[j]From Niemala et al. Clin Chem 1996;42:S280.
[k]Intracellular free magnesium concentration.
[l]From Consolazio et al. J Nutr 1963;79:407.
[m]From Wenk C, Kohut M, Kunz G, et al. Z Ernahrungswiss 1993;32:301–7.

Dietary Intake

Magnesium is widely distributed in plant and animal sources but in differing concentrations (see Appendix Table IV-A-22). The major food sources of the element beyond childhood to ages 60 to 65 in the United States as percentages of the daily intake have been listed (52). Vegetables, fruits, grains, and animal products accounted for approximately 16% each; dairy product contributions fell from about 20% in adolescents to about 10% for those beyond the third decade; beverages of various types yielded percentages of about 4% among adolescents, increasing to 15% in older age groups.

Daily per capita availability in the U.S. food supply increased by 9.4% from 1981 to 1990, at which date it was 350 mg (14.5 mmol) ([53] and Table 58 therein). This figure, based on disappearance data, differs markedly from actual intake data. For example, the mean daily *analyzed*

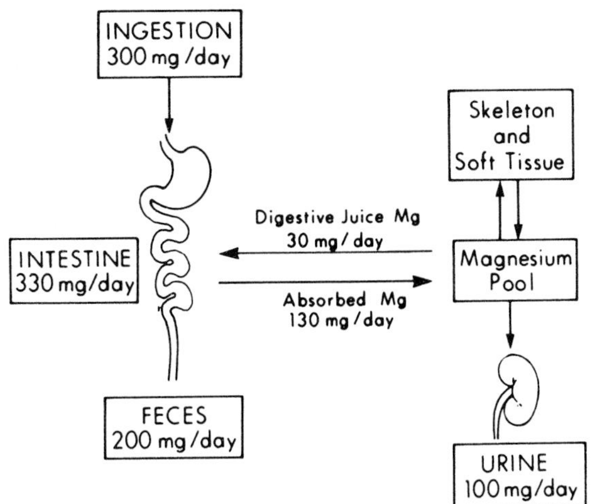

Figure 9.2. Magnesium homeostasis in man. A schematic representation of its metabolic economy indicating *(a)* its relatively poor absorption from the alimentary tract, *(b)* its distribution into a number of tissue pools with major distribution into bone, and *(c)* its dependence on the kidney for excretion. Homeostasis depends upon the integrity of intestinal and renal absorptive processes. (From Slatapolsky E. In: Klahr S, ed. Pathophysiology of calcium, magnesium and phosphorus metabolism in the kidney and body fluids. New York: Plenum Publishing, 1984, with permission.)

intakes in the Total Diet Study for females ages 14 to 16 years, 25 to 30, and 60 to 65 were 194 mg (8.08 mmol), 189 mg (7.88 mmol), and 187 mg (7.79 mmol), respectively. For males in the same age groups, the intakes were 297 mg (12.38 mmol), 294 mg (12.25 mmol), and 250 mg (10.42 mmol), respectively (54).

When calculating individual intake from food composition tables, caution is advised because "there is less than 75% analytical data for important sources of this food component" (55). An example is the analyzed versus calculated values (using the USDA database) for the 234 foods in the U.S. FDA Total Dietary Study for eight age-sex groups, representing the core items of the U.S. food supply. The analyzed figures were 115 to 124% greater than the calculated values (unadjusted for missing values in the database) among the age groups reported (52, 54). Inadequate or few data exist for this ion in a number of products ([53] and Table 58 therein).

Intestinal Absorption

The fractional absorption of ingested magnesium by healthy humans is influenced by its dietary concentration and the presence of inhibiting or promoting dietary components. Based upon the time of appearance of ^{28}Mg in the blood following its oral ingestion, absorption began within 1 hour, stabilized at the rate of 4 to 6%/h from the 2nd to 8th hour, then decreased rapidly, and ceased at the 10th hour (56). When small amounts of magnesium were fed in the form of a standard meal supplemented by varying amounts of magnesium (57) or when Mg was given as ^{28}Mg (58), fractional absorption fell progressively from approximately 65 to 70% with intake of 7 to 36 mg (0.3–1.5 mmol) down to 11 to 14% with intake of 960 to 1000 mg (40 mmol). Absorption of magnesium as a function of intake is curvilinear (Fig. 9.3) and reflects a saturable process with passive diffusion. Estimates of the fractions absorbed by each process were 10 and 7%, respectively (57). Similar absorptive processes appear to occur in children (59).

Data on absorption fractions from balance studies using differing diets have been quite variable, ranging from 35 to 70% (60). When free-living adults eating self-selected diets were evaluated periodically over the course of a year, the mean absorptive fraction averaged 21% with average intake of 323 mg (13.4 mmol) by men and 27% with average intake of 234 mg (9.75 mmol) by women (61).

Sites of Absorption. Absorption studies in the rat by various techniques, including intact intestinal absorption, everted sacs, in vivo perfusion (summarized in [62, 63]), and stripped mucosa (64) show that magnesium is absorbed along the entire intestine, small and large; in some reports, colonic uptake is the greater. Evidence suggests that in the human, colonic absorption of magnesium is probable (63).

Influence of Other Ions. Long-term balance studies in healthy individuals, for the most part, indicate that increasing oral calcium intake does not significantly affect magnesium absorption or retention (65–67). Some reports indicate decreased magnesium absorption at high levels of phosphate, whereas others found no consistent effect (62, 68).

A major increase in zinc intake (from 12 to 142 mg/day) decreased magnesium absorption and balance

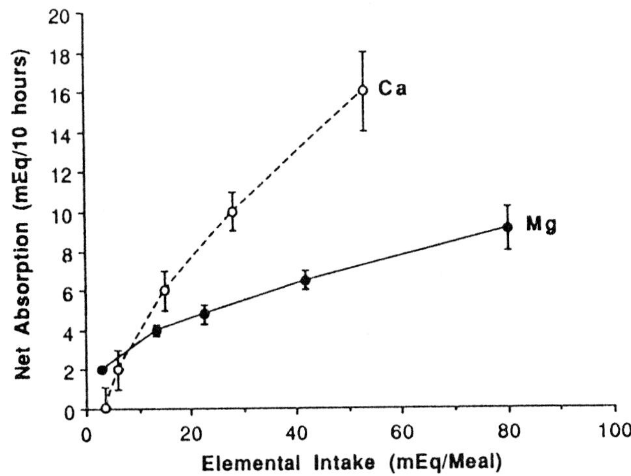

Figure 9.3. Net magnesium and calcium absorption in healthy humans. The data were obtained under conditions described in reference 57 and in the text. Mean values S.E. are indicated by *vertical bars.* The absorption data for magnesium represent a curved function compatible with a saturable process (at about 10 mEq/meal in this study) and a linear function reflecting passive diffusion at higher intakes. (From Fine KD, Santa Ana CA, Porter JL, et al. J Clin Invest 1991;88:396–402, with permission.)

very significantly (69). Vitamin B_6 depletion induced in young women was associated with negative magnesium balance because of increased urinary excretion (70). Hypochlorhydria following short-term administration of the gastric proton-pump inhibitor, omeprazole, did not change the intestinal absorption of magnesium, calcium, phosphorus, or zinc (71).

Increased amounts of magnesium in the diet have been associated with either decreased calcium absorption (65) or no effect (57, 72). Increased amounts of absorbable oral magnesium have been noted to decrease phosphate absorption, perhaps secondary to formation of insoluble magnesium phosphate (57). Although increased magnesium intake may not affect calcium absorption, renal tubular mechanisms may increase calcium excretion (57); conversely, decreased absorption of magnesium associated with high phosphate intake did not change magnesium balance because of associated decreased urinary excretion of magnesium (57).

Increased intakes of dietary fiber have been reported to decrease magnesium utilization in humans, presumably by decreasing absorption. However, the introduction of uncontrolled variables—including multiple differences between dietary components in addition to fiber contents—complicates interpretation of the data (72a, 72b). When isolated fiber has been added to a basal diet, the effects of fiber per se have been negative for dephytinized barley fiber (72c) and positive for cellulose (72d).

Absorbability of Magnesium Salts in Humans. The fractional absorption of a salt depends on its solubility in intestinal fluids and the amounts ingested, e.g., 5 mmol (120 mg) of the acetate in gelatin capsules has been found to be an optimal dose in terms of net absorption. Absorption of enteric-coated magnesium chloride is 67% less than that of the acetate in gelatin capsules (57). Magnesium citrate has high solubility, even in water, whereas magnesium oxide is poorly soluble even in acid solution. Magnesium oxide and various salts in large doses act as an osmotic laxative, with resultant diarrhea; the physician faced with a diarrhea of uncertain etiology should consider measuring fecal magnesium levels (72).

Magnesium Absorption: Any Relation to Calcitriol? While there is some uncertainty in the literature, there are data indicating that magnesium absorption in many individuals is not truly calcitriol dependent, as are calcium and phosphate. When patients with impaired calcium absorption were given vitamin D or its active form, those with both osteomalacia and osteoporosis had equivocal improvement in magnesium absorption (73), whereas those with osteomalacia or hypo- or hyperparathyroidism had only small increases, compared with calcium (74). Magnesium was absorbed by individuals with no detectable plasma calcitriol and, in contrast to calcium absorption, there was no significant correlation between plasma calcitriol and magnesium absorption (75). Individuals with absorptive hypercalciuria resulting from increased intestinal calcium absorption have normal magnesium absorption (76, 77).

Calcitriol did not increase net magnesium absorption in the stripped mucosa of the rat duodenum (78), ileum, or colon (64), but it markedly increased calcium absorption in the duodenum (78). The influence of magnesium depletion in rats on expression of the vitamin D–dependent protein in the proximal intestine that facilitates calcium absorption (calbindin D_{9k}) has been reported as negative (79) or positive(80). Other contradictory data from studies on this issue in the rat are reviewed in reference 62.

The effects of various gastrointestinal disorders on absorption are discussed below in the section on disease-related depletion.

Renal Regulation

Filtration and Tubular Absorption

The kidney plays a critical role in excreting the absorbed magnesium that is not retained for tissue growth or turnover replacement (26, 81). About 10% (roughly 100 mmol or 2400 mg) of the total body magnesium is normally filtered daily through the glomeruli in the healthy adult; of this only about 5% is excreted in the urine. Approximately 75% of the serum magnesium is ultrafilterable at the glomeruli. The fractional absorption of the filtered load in the various segments of the nephron is summarized in Figure 9.4.

Hormonal and Other Regulator Influences on Absorption

Micropuncture studies in rodents showed that in the absence of hormonal influences, magnesium transport is a passive process occurring in the paracellular space and driven by transcellular transport of NaCl and the potential difference. Arginine, vasopressin, glucagon, calcitonin, PTH, and (to a lesser degree) an adrenergic agonist and insulin, when added individually to the bath of mouse segments of the cortical thick ascending limb of loop of Henle, significantly increased magnesium absorption (82). Proof that magnesium balance is normally regulated hormonally would require that certain changes in serum magnesium levels liberate one or more of these hormones into the blood and act on the tubule (82).

Although the regulatory mechanisms are unclear, a number of conditions affect absorption, principally in the ascending thick limb. Inhibition occurs with hypermagnesemia and hypercalcemia (26, 81). Decreased magnesium intake in experimental animals and humans rapidly decreases magnesium excretion, even before serum/plasma magnesium levels fall below the normal range (26, 83).

The close relationship between magnesium and potassium is clearly demonstrated in renal function. In the rat and man, magnesium depletion results in K^+ loss. In the deficient rat, K^+ entry into the tubule lumen occurs at a

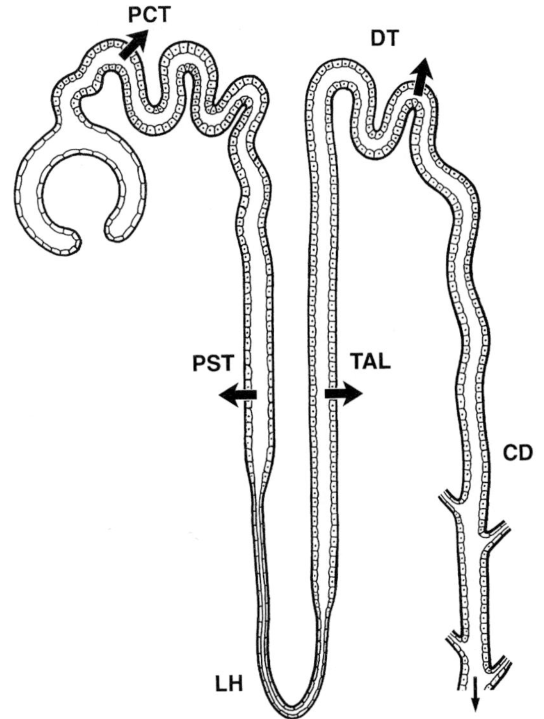

Figure 9.4. Fractional segmental reabsorption of filtered magnesium in the nephron. The percentage absorption of filtered Mg^{2+} has been determined by micropuncture techniques in various laboratory animals as the magnesium proceeds through the nephron. In the rat, approximately 10 to 20% of the Mg^{2+} is reabsorbed in the proximal convoluted tubule *(PCT)*; this is only 25 to 30% that of Na^+ and Ca^{2+} in this segment. Magnesium reabsorption in the superficial and juxtamedullary proximal straight tubule *(PST)* is small, varying up to 5% depending on its luminal concentration. The major site for Mg^{2+} reabsorption is the thick ascending limb *(TAL)* of the loop of Henle *(LH)*, primarily in its cortical portion. Here, 50 to 60% of magnesium leaves the lumen. The descending limb reabsorbs about 20% of the filtered load as a substantial amount of water is removed. In the distal convoluted tubule *(DT)* a little more than one-half of the magnesium remaining is absorbed, for a net fractional reabsorption of about 5%. Even less is reabsorbed in the collecting ducts *(CD)*. There may be a balance in the ducts between absorption and secretion.

distal site and is associated with a rise in plasma aldosterone levels (84).

Tissue Sources

Extracellular and intracellular magnesium and that in bone compartments enter into the homeostatic mechanism. Human iliac crest changes indicate a broad range of loss during depletion with a weighted average of 18%, or 1.2 mmol/kg body weight (85). In young magnesium-deficient rats, the major body loss is from bone (approximately 15% of that in bone) with much less from muscle; however, age and duration of study affect the amounts lost (85). During starvation in a human obesity study, significant amounts of magnesium were lost, partly from loss of lean body mass, with an additional amount lost from bone as well as muscle, which was associated with acidosis (86). In an experimental human study of about 3-weeks' duration with resulting asymptomatic hypomagnesemia, there was no significant decrease in muscle magnesium; presumably bone and soft tissues were the sources of loss (87).

ASSESSING MAGNESIUM NUTRITURE

For public health as well as for individual need, procedures for assessing magnesium status are desirable. The available evaluation methods fall into five general classes.

Dietary Assessment

A dietitian or physician can do a rough but rapid evaluation of the probable level of intake of individuals from information on the usual frequency of intakes of the food groups making major contributions to magnesium intake. However, other evaluation methods are necessary because inadequate dietary intake per se is usually not the primary cause of depletion in clinical situations.

Clinical Evaluation

Clinical evaluation includes a history and physical examination taken by a health practitioner sensitive to the causes, signs, and symptoms associated with magnesium depletion. This usually provides enough information to decide whether the individual is at no risk, is already at risk, or is symptomatically depleted. Risk factors are listed in Table 9.2. Symptoms and signs of deficiency are given in Table 9.3. Hypermagnesemia may also be a clinical problem (see last section). Laboratory tests are often key in establishing the correct diagnosis.

Laboratory Analyses: Serum/Plasma, Urine, and Blood Cells

Total, Bound, and Ionized Serum Magnesium. In otherwise healthy laboratory animals and humans, instituting a magnesium-restricted diet results in a fairly early and progressive decline in total serum magnesium. In contrast, there are a number of reports of normal serum/plasma levels associated with a variety of illnesses but with low values in various blood cells and other organs (see below). Consequently, total serum/plasma magnesium values in such situations may be considered unreliable indicators of depletion. This has stimulated the search for more reliable laboratory markers for magnesium status.

Magnesium bound to protein and other serum/plasma ligands varies with changes in the concentrations of such ligands and in acid-base conditions; acidosis decreases bonding, and alkalosis increases it. The level of ionized magnesium may be more relevant under certain circumstances than that of total magnesium (37, 88). Improved ISEs for determining ionized magnesium in whole blood, serum, and plasma greatly simplify this determination; they are available commercially but require calibration (38, 39).

Erythrocytes. In experimental human magnesium deficiency, the magnesium content of red cells measured following hemolysis decreases more slowly and to a lesser

Table 9.2
Risk Factors for Magnesium Depletion

Gastrointestinal disorders
- Partial bowel obstruction; motility disorders[a]
- Inflammatory bowel diseases
- Gluten enteropathy (celiac disease); sprue syndromes
- Intestinal fistulas, bypass, or resection
- Pancreatitis
- Immune diseases with villous atrophy
- Radiation enteritis
- Fatty acid malabsorption
  - Lymphangiectasia;
  - Bile insufficiency
- Ileal dysfunction
- Primary idiopathic hypomagnesemia
- Gastrointestinal infections (viral, bacterial, protozoan)
  - Malabsorption
  - Vomiting/diarrhea

Renal dysfunction with excessive urine losses (see Table 9.4)
- Tubular disorders
- Metabolic or hormonal disorders
- Nephrotoxic and diuretic drugs

Endocrine disorders (see Table 9.4)
- Hyperaldosteronism
- Hyperparathyroidism with hypercalcemia
- Postparathyroidectomy ("hungry bone" syndrome)
- Hyperthyroidism
- Diabetes mellitus

Pediatric genetic, congenital, and infectious disorders
- Primary idiopathic hypomagnesemia
- Renal wasting syndromes (see Table 9.4)
  - Bartter's syndrome (see Table 9.4)
  - Gitleman's syndrome
- Infants born of diabetic mothers
- Transient neonatal hypomagnesemic hypocalcemia
- Poor intake; vomiting/diarrhea
  - Protein-energy malnutrition

Inadequate intake, provision, and/or retention or dilution of magnesium
- Alcoholism
- Chronic infusion or ingestion of solutions or diets insufficient in magnesium
- Hypercatabolic states (burns, trauma), usually associated with above entry
- Postcardiac and transplantation surgery
- Hyperthermia

[a]Secondary to poor intake and/or loss of small bowel contents; malabsorption is the key factor in other conditions in this category.

extent than does total serum magnesium (89). Magnesium ion concentrations measured by ^{31}P MRS in erythrocytes of healthy volunteers on a magnesium-deficient diet for 3 weeks and in erythrocytes of other hypomagnesemic patients were significantly lower than those in the baseline period of normal magnesemic groups; in all subjects, $[Mg^{2+}]_i$ correlated with serum levels (90). Recent MRS data on erythrocytes of end-stage renal patients on dialysis did not support older data claiming that such patients have intracellular magnesium depletion (91).

Blood Mononuclear Cells. Reports indicate that magnesium concentrations in human mononuclear cells are a better guide to magnesium nutriture than is the serum level (92, 93), but there are contradictory reports (94–96).

Urine Levels As Indicators. In an individual with normal renal function, 24-h magnesium excretion that is more than 10 to 15% of the amount ingested from an adequate diet suggests good nutriture. When there is a major reduction in the amounts ingested and/or absorbed, there is a fairly rapid and progressive reduction in urinary excretion of this ion by the normal kidney; in early stages of such depletion, total serum magnesium may still be within normal limits, but urine levels may be significantly reduced (24, 97). In situations in which renal magnesium wasting occurs (Table 9.4), the resulting hypomagnesemia (e.g., [0.7 mmol/L) is associated with urinary magnesium excretion of more than 1 mmol/day (98, 101) (Fig. 9.5). Such a relationship suggests renal tubular dysfunction if the cause of the hypomagnesemia is otherwise uncertain.

Magnesium Load/Retention Test

The intravenous load or retention test provides an estimate of the proportion of infused magnesium that is retained over a given period (99, 100). Persons retaining more than the percentage retained by magnesium-replete individuals (e.g., 20–25%) are considered to have some body depletion. The test was initially validated in weanling rats and then in mature rats given differing amounts of magnesium, while magnesium was measured in plasma, urine, and bone (99). A suggested clinical protocol that

Table 9.3
Symptoms and Signs of Magnesium Depletion

Neuromuscular
- Paresthesias (facial, hands, feet)[a,b]
- Positive Trousseau's sign[a,c]
- Positive Chvostek's sign[a,d]
- Normal or depressed deep tendon reflexes despite hypocalcemia[a]
- Spontaneous carpopedal spasm (tetany)[a]
- Generalized muscle spasticity[a]
- Tremor, muscle fasciculations, myoclonic jerks
- Athetoid and choreiform movements
- Focal and generalized seizures[e]
- Personality changes—mild to severe[a]

Gastrointestinal
- Anorexia[a,f]
- Nausea and vomiting[a,f]

Cardiovascular
- ECG changes—compatible with hypokalemia and/or hypocalcemia[a]
- Arrhythmias—usually drug and disease related

Clinical laboratory findings
- Hypomagnesemia[a] (usually, but not always in clinical states)
- Hypokalemia[a,g]
- Hypocalcemia[a,g] and hypocalciuria[a]
- Urine magnesium low, but level depends on etiology (see text)
- Electromyographic changes[h]

Hypocitraturia

[a]Noted in study of severe experimental Mg depletion (89).
[b]Numbness/tingling are among the earliest symptoms.
[c]Carpal spasm when sphygmomanometer pressure is raised above the systolic.
[d]Facial muscle twitching when the area of the facial nerve is tapped.
[e]With or without coma—more common in children.
[f]Heralding an exacerbation of neuromuscular symptoms.
[g]The presence of both hypokalemia and hypocalcemia without other obvious cause suggests magnesium depletion.
[h]Rapid, high-pitched firing potentials noted in study of severe experimental Mg depletion (89).

Table 9.4
Metabolic, Hormonal, and Drug Influences on Renal Magnesium Excretion

Increased excretion
Acidosis—e.g., fasting, ketoacidosis
Alcoholism
Diuresis
Diuretics—e.g., thiazides, high dose, loop diuretics
Osmotic—e.g., glucose, mannitol
Hypermagnesemia[a]
Hypercalcemia/hypercalciuria
Hyperaldosteronism
Hyperparathyroidism[b]
Hyperthyroidism
Increased extracellular fluid volume
Mineralocorticoids
Phosphate depletion
Potassium depletion
Renal tubular dysfunction
Familial renal wasting syndromes
Primary magnesuric hypomagnesemia; Bartter's and related syndromes
Postrenal obstruction
Postrenal transplantation
Acute tubulointerstitial nephritis
Tubular acidosis
Nephrotoxic drugs—e.g., amphotericin; cisplatin, pentamidine, aminoglycosides; cyclosporine
Decreased excretion
Alkalosis
Antidiuretic hormone
Calcitonin
Contracted extracellular fluid volume
Familial hypocalcuric hypercalcemia
Glucagon
Hypocalcemia
Hypomagnesemia
Hypothyroidism
Lithium
K^+ and Mg^{2+} sparing diuretics
Renal failure, advanced

[a]When associated with excessive magnesium infusion/injection.
[b]Secondary to hypercalcemia.

has been tested in a relatively large number of hypomagnesemic patients, chronic alcoholics, and animal controls has been published (100). It is an invasive, time-consuming, nonstandardized, and expensive test, requiring hospitalization or other close supervision for the partial or full 24 hours after infusion, with careful urine collection for laboratory analysis. This type of test again raises the important question of how much depletion must occur in various body pools before magnesium deficiency becomes biochemically and clinically significant.

Combined Laboratory Testing

An algorithm combining serum magnesium level with renal excretion and the load test is presented in Figure 9.5. While blood and urine levels together with history usually suffice to make the diagnosis, the load test may be included when semiqualitative data on the severity of pool depletion is desired or when the urinary data are equivocal (101).

Enzymatic Reactions

Despite the numerous enzymatic reactions for which Mg^{2+} is essential, there is no clinically useful diagnostic enzymatic reaction for detecting deficiency.

Classic Balance Studies

The long-term and expensive metabolic studies used to estimate normal human requirements are not applicable to the study of sick patients. They are discussed in the next section.

NEEDS FOR HEALTH?

Intake Standards. For healthy older children, adolescents, and adults, the primary approach has been the balance study. For infants and young children, the figures are based primarily on estimates of magnesium intakes of milk and other foods that allow good development. Such data have been transmuted into the dietary reference intakes (RDIs) in the United States (101a) and similar standards in other countries. (See Appendix Tables II-A-2 to A-8.) The new U.S. reference intakes for magnesium are given in Table 9.5 (see also Appendix Table II-A-2-b-3) with comparison to the 1989 RDA figures (101b). Both are based on estimates of intake that meet the needs of 97 to 98% of healthy individuals. The chief difference is in higher levels in the DRI for all ages beyond 8 years.

Are Americans at Risk for Deficiency? Estimates of magnesium intakes in NHANES III (1988–91) indicated that children 2 to 11 years grouped by gender, age, and race/ethnicity had median intakes well above their RDA. Those ages 1 to 5 years in the lower fifth percentile took in about 90% of the RDA, which includes a safety factor (53–55). On the other hand, males and females from 12 to

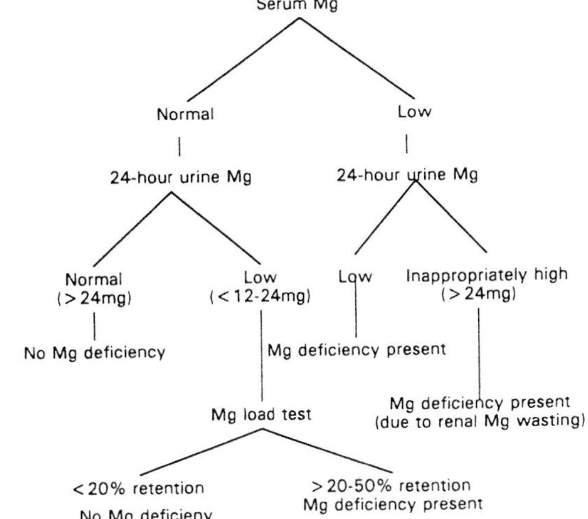

Figure 9.5. Algorithm of a diagnostic approach to suspected magnesium deficiency, in which urine magnesium levels are emphasized to distinguish the key factors leading to magnesium depletion. (From Al Ghamdi SMG, Cameron EC, Sutton RAL. Am J Kidney Dis 1994;24: 737–752, with permission.)

Table 9.5
Comparison of 1989 and 1997 Recommendations for Daily Intakes of Magnesium (mg)

	1989[a]			1997[b]	
Age (years)	Male	Female	Age (years)	Male	Female
0–0.5	40	40	0–0.5	30[c]	30[c]
0.5–1.0	60	60	0.5–1.0	75[d]	75[d]
1–3	80	80	1–3	80	80
4–6	120	120	4–8	130	130
7–10	170	170	9–13	240	240
11–14	270	280	14–18	410	360
15–18	400	300	19–30	400	310
19–24	350	280	31–50	420	320
25–50	350	280	51–70	420	320
51+	350	280	>70	420	320
Pregnant		320	Pregnancy		
Lactating				≤18	400
1st 6 months		355		19–30	350
2nd 6 months		355		31–50	360
			Lactating		
				≤18	360
				19–30	310
				31–50	320

[a]Food and Nutrition Board, National Research Council. Recommended dietary allowances. 10th ed. Washington, DC: National Academy Press, 1989, end table (101b).

[b]Food and Nutrition Board, Institute of Medicine. Dietary reference intakes for calcium, phosphorus, magnesium, vitamin D, and fluoride. Washington, DC: National Academy Press, 1997 (101a).

[c]Intake from human milk by healthy breast-fed infants.

[d]Human milk plus solid food.

more than 60 years, grouped by race and ethnicity, with the exception of non-Hispanic white males, had low median intakes in terms of the RDA (53).

The basis for the claims that many adolescents and adults in the United States are at risk of magnesium depletion rests on the accuracy of two indices: the dietary intake data summarized in NHANES and the RDA. If either or both of these are seriously inaccurate, the extent of potential depletion will be either higher or lower. The *Third Report on Nutrition Monitoring in the United States* (1995) analyzed intake in relation to the RDA for age and gender; it concluded that magnesium presents a potential public health issue requiring further study (53). One reason given was that in 1988–91, the medium intakes of magnesium from food were lower than the RDAs in various population groups. The report accepts the dietary intakes as "low" without questioning the reliability of the RDAs. Interestingly, the 1989 nutrition monitoring report did not consider magnesium a current health issue (55). On the basis of the 1997 DRI (Table 9.5), a higher percentage of adolescents and adults will be deemed at risk by these criteria. The new tables for this nutrient and a brief explanation of the various reference intakes are given in Appendix Table II-A-2-b, b3, and b4.

The median magnesium intake of many Americans also appears inadequate to those who argue that the *median* magnesium intake should be approximately 600 mg/day. As was recently stated, "extensive metabolic balance studies done by the USDA Research Service showed that the ratio of dietary calcium to magnesium that best maintained equilibrium (i.e., output equaling intake) was 2:1" (102). The reference is to Hathaway, who reviewed publications on various aspects of magnesium and presented many tables, brief summaries, and detailed data (without any statistical analysis) from a large number of balance studies performed in the 1930s to 1950s (many with USDA support) in various institutions around the world (103). Review of this report fails to reveal any statements claiming a preferred ratio of dietary calcium:magnesium of 2:1 or recommending a median daily magnesium intake of about 600 mg. In her brief summary and conclusions, Hathaway stated specifically that "Studies with adults indicate that young women require abut 300 mg of magnesium a day and young men between 300 and 400 mg and protein intakes about 70 and 80 gms, respectively" (103). Her only summary statement relating magnesium and calcium was a general one: "Its [magnesium's] relation to calcium and phosphorus intakes and metabolism seems to be more complicated [compared with protein] as the requirements seem to be interrelated" (103). Later research supports Hathaway's opinion; magnesium and calcium are now known to be interrelated in a number of mimic/antagonist relations. However, chemical or metabolic evidence for a 2:1 dietary interrelationship does not exist.

Criteria for Evaluating Magnesium Nutriture in Health

Adequacy of Dietary Intake Data. The section on dietary intake noted that laboratory analysis of foods revealed a magnesium content 115 to 124% greater than those calculated by tables of food composition (52–54) and that a number of foods have not yet been thoroughly analyzed. Dietary intake data must be considered only semiquantitative; they probably should have confidence limits applied on the basis of the variability of such data.

Lack of Evidence for Significant Depletion. Serum magnesium was determined by AAS in 15,820 individuals in the NHANES I (1971–74) survey; 95% of adults ages 18 to 74 years had serum levels in the range of 0.75 to 0.96 mmol/L (1.50–1.92 mEq/L) with a mean of 0.85 mmol/L. The levels of the fifth percentile were at or above the lower levels of normal (i.e., 0.70–0.73 mmol/L (104).

Adequacy of the Current RDAs. A recent critique of previous—including the 10th—RDAs for magnesium noted that most of the published human balance data referenced in its various editions often did not meet the criteria for acceptable methodology (105). The balance studies (usually short term) were done mostly in adolescents and younger adults, and balance data presented for pregnant women were less than adequate (105). Published data about the elderly were meager (106). The need was pointed out for improved definition of acceptable standards, evaluation of the optimum base (i.e., weight, fat-free mass, or lean body mass), documentation of the accepted data, and more awareness of the ways in which homeostatic mechanisms conserve body magnesium. While the database of the 1997 reference values (Table 9.5) has eliminated the poorer studies, a question remains as to the accuracy of many balance studies in terms of adherence to acceptable methodology.

EXPERIMENTAL MAGNESIUM DEFICIENCY

A large number of different laboratory and domestic animals, some subhuman primates, and human subjects have been studied in the course of magnesium deficiency induced by diets low in this element (107).

Laboratory Animals

Hypomagnesemia is the hallmark of experimental magnesium depletion in all species, but other manifestations often vary. Although most studied, the rat is strikingly different from other species in certain of its acute deficiency signs, including hyperemia of ears and feet induced by histamine release from basophils, hyperirritability associated with characteristic and usually fatal tonic-clonic convulsions, high levels of serum calcium with low inorganic phosphate, and decreased circulating PTH in response to the hypercalcemia. Mice on the same diet did not have hyperemia, became hypocalcemic in association with hypomagnesemia, and often died with a single abrupt and massive convulsion (108). Deficient dogs and monkeys—also on diets of the same composition—developed spasticity, weakness, tremors, and occasionally nonfatal convulsions with hypocalcemia; increasing calcium intake did not increase serum calcium or prevent the neuromuscular changes (109).

Other changes in deficient young rats include reduced growth rate, alopecia, and skin lesions. Chronic deficiency in the rat leads to edema, hypertrophic gums, leukocytosis, and splenomegaly. Various thymic abnormalities have also been noted (110). Crystalluria in the kidney with calcification and degenerative changes in various organs, especially the kidney, muscle, heart, and aorta, are prominent in deficient rats (111–112), guinea pigs (113), dogs (114), and certain other species maintained on low-magnesium diets, particularly when the calcium content is high compared with that of human diets (109, 113).

Humans

Symptomatic human deficiency has been induced experimentally by dietary restriction. Deficiency also occurs in a number of predisposing and complicating disease states (Tables 9.2 and 9.4). In the single depletion study in which signs and symptoms occurred, plasma magnesium fell progressively in six subjects to levels that were only 10 to 30% those of control periods, while erythrocyte magnesium declined more slowly and to a lesser degree (89). Urine (Fig. 9.6) and fecal magnesium decreased to

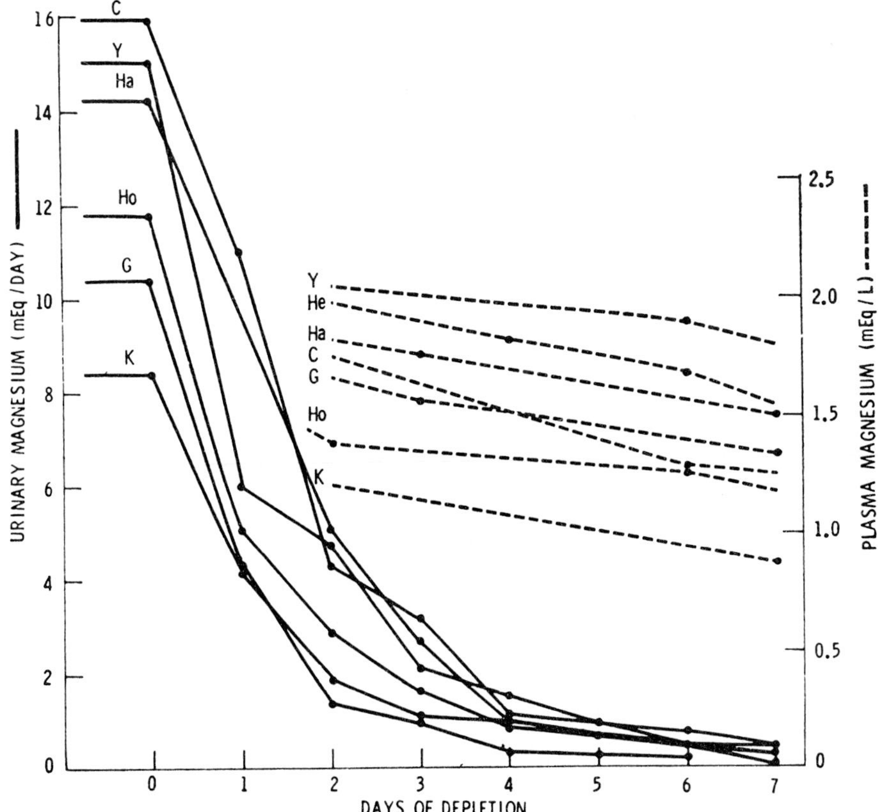

Figure 9.6. Plasma and urinary magnesium in the week following omission of magnesium from the diet in human experimental deficiency. Rapid decrease in urinary excretion occurred in six subjects. By the 10th day, all plasma values except that of subject Y were more than two standard deviations below the normal mean. (From Shils ME. Medicine (Baltimore) 1969;48:61–85.)

extremely low levels within 7 days. In one subject (Fig. 9.7) and the other four consistently symptomatic patients, hypomagnesemia, hypocalcemia, and hypokalemia were present. Good intestinal absorption of calcium and low urinary output resulted in positive calcium balance. Serum phosphate was variable. Negative potassium balance resulted from increased urinary loss. Serum sodium remained normal, and the subjects were in positive sodium balance. Abnormal neuromuscular function (Table 9.3) occurred in five of the seven subjects after deficiency periods ranging from 25 to 110 days. All symptoms and signs (including personality changes and gastrointestinal symptoms) reverted to normal with reinstitution of magnesium.

In other detailed investigations of experimental magnesium depletion in human subjects in 1958, 1960, and 1966 (reviewed in [89]), marked decreases in fecal and urinary output occurred, but symptoms and signs of deficiency did not. More recently, hypomagnesemia has been induced by formula feeding for 3-week periods for physiologic studies (100, 115).

The signs and symptoms noted above in experimental deficiency and still others have been described individually or in various combinations in clinical cases of hypomagnesemia (Table 9.3). The closest disease-related condition to uncomplicated experimental human magnesium deficiency is congenital primary (idiopathic) hypomagnesemia related to a specific defect in intestinal absorption of this ion (59, 116). Hypomagnesemia, hypomagnesuria, hypocalcemia, and hypokalemia with tetany (often with convulsions), occurred in infants and were corrected or prevented with magnesium supplements. Calcium and vitamin D supplements without magnesium were ineffective in maintaining normocalcemia (116).

Metabolic Correlates

Sequence of Changes in Human Deficiency

Observations made during experimental studies and during clinical deficiency are the bases for this schema of changes during deficiency and repletion. The initiating factor appears to be failure of the normal heterionic exchange of bone calcium for magnesium at the labile bone mineral surface (117). Impaired receptor responsiveness to PTH of the osteoclasts follows, with reduced active bone resorption (118). Hypocalcemia progresses despite the increasing levels of circulating PTH that may occur at this stage (109, 119).

As depletion progresses, PTH secretion diminishes to very low levels despite adequate intraparathyroid gland hormonal reserves (119, 120). Signs of severe magnesium depletion are now present: hypomagnesemia with very low circulating PTH, hypocalcemia and hypocalciuria with positive calcium balance, hypokalemia with loss of body potassium, sodium retention, and neuromuscular and other clinical signs and symptoms (89).

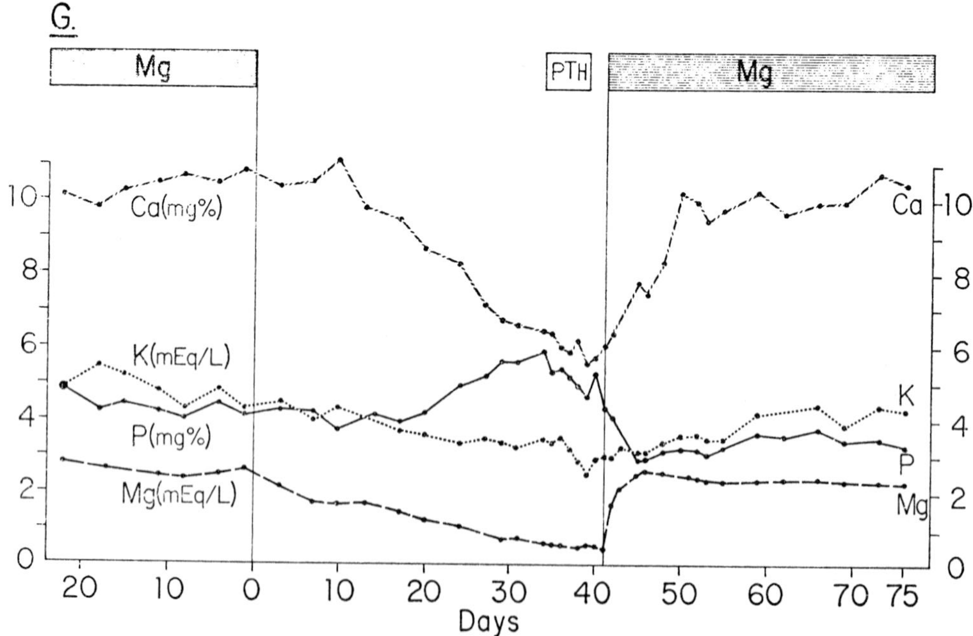

Figure 9.7. The course of blood chemistries in a subject subsisting before, during, and after a period on a diet very restricted in magnesium *(Mg)*. Mg was omitted after the patient was on the control diet for 1 month. The rise in serum inorganic phosphate *(P)* with Mg depletion in this patient was unique among the depleted subjects. On depletion day 25, Trousseau's and Chvostek's signs first occurred, and the former became progressively stronger as plasma calcium *(Ca)*, Mg, and potassium *(K)* continued to decline. These electrolyte changes were noted in all symptomatic subjects. On depletion day 35, PTH *(PTH)* was given i.m. at 50 units t.i.d. for 5 days; this had no effect on plasma Ca but appeared to decrease P. On day 41, anorexia, nausea, paresthesias, and generalized muscle spasticity developed; 17 mEq of Mg was then given i.v. with rapid improvement. This was followed by similar amounts of Mg i.m. 12 and 15 hours later. Dietary Mg (40 mEq/day) was resumed on the third repletion day. Note the characteristic delay in the return to normal of serum Ca and K. (From Shils ME. Medicine (Baltimore) 1969;48:61–85.)

Following administration of adequate magnesium, serum magnesium levels rise rapidly, presumably with increased heterionic calcium exchange but with little or no detectable change in circulating calcium in this early phase. Despite an increase in circulating PTH, the serum calcium response is delayed, presumably until osteoclast receptors to PTH regain responsiveness (118). When calcium levels increase, plasma PTH levels decline appropriately. The delayed rise in serum potassium is presumably secondary to the period required to restore the normal activity of the cellular membrane Na-K ATPase, Na-K-Cl cotransporter, or K channels (121). Clinical signs and symptoms tend to disappear in a matter of hours to a few days, although serum calcium and potassium usually have not reached normal levels.

Additional Effects of Deficiency

Magnesium, Calcium, and PTH Interactions. Extracellular Mg^{2+} plays various roles, including regulation of PTH secretion. It is essential in the formation of cAMP through its binding at two sites in adenylate cyclase, which in turn stimulates PTH secretion (10). When Mg^{2+} is absent or present at very low levels in culture medium for explants of bovine parathyroid glands or rat parathyroid tissue, there is little PTH secretion despite a low [Ca^{2+}], which suggests that Mg^{2+} is essential for hormone synthesis. However, when the minimum [Mg^{2+}] necessary for such synthesis is present, increasing [Mg^{2+}] and/or [Ca^{2+}] progressively suppresses secretion (reviewed in [122, 123]). Extracellular Ca^{2+} and Mg^{2+} do not act directly but rather modulate a cell-surface, extracellular, Ca^{2+}-sensing receptor; the resulting inward current mobilizes intracellular Ca^{2+} stores, presumably by activating phosphoinositide-specific phospholipase C on a pathway to inhibition of PTH secretion (124). These results support the in vitro and in vivo findings that extracellular [Mg^{2+}] has an appreciably smaller effect than [Ca^{2+}] in suppressing PTH secretion (122).

PTH Levels in Deficient Human Subjects. Development of the immunologic method for measuring the circulating PTH level (the iPTH assay) was a major advance in understanding the magnesium–parathyroid gland relationship. The earliest reported use of this method on a deficient individual with idiopathic malabsorptive defect suggested a failure of synthesis or secretion (or both) of PTH (125). As more iPTH assays were performed on deficiency patients, a more complex situation became apparent: magnesium deficiency resulted in high, low, or normal PTH levels (119, 122), depending in part on the severity of the deficiency and the reaction of osteoclast receptors to PTH (118) (see below).

Patients with marked hypomagnesemia and hypocalcemia respond to a rapid intravenous injection of a magnesium bolus with a major rise in serum iPTH levels within 1 minute, from an undetectable baseline; very rapid elevation of serum magnesium levels is not associated with any detectable rise in serum calcium levels over the next 0.5 to 6 hours. It was concluded that the magnesium-depleted parathyroid gland could synthesize PTH but needed magnesium to induce secretion (119, 120). Eumagnesemic normal subjects given the same magnesium infusion had the expected rise in serum magnesium levels, but their iPTH level declined significantly (119).

PTH Response in Depleted Rats. Circulating PTH in rats, in contrast to humans and other species, responded appropriately to the rising calcium levels induced by magnesium deficiency (126, 127). Severely magnesium-depleted rats could secrete large amounts of iPTH when hypocalcemia was induced by depletion of either calcium or vitamin D (127).

Bone Changes and Resistance to PTH. Resistance to PTH was predicted from the normal or elevated iPTH levels found in some hypomagnesemic and hypocalcemic patients and also by the relative refractoriness of deficient laboratory species and humans after administration of parathyroid extract (reviewed in [122]). Such resistance has been confirmed in dogs with chronic magnesium depletion, which show markedly reduced uptake of synthetic bovine PTH perfused into isolated tibias (118). This correlated with a significant depression in cAMP production by the deficient dogs, whose bones had a histologic picture of skeletal inactivity with virtually no osteoid.

Wallach reviewed the multiple effects of magnesium deficiency on skeletal morphology and composition. Depressed bone growth, abnormal bone formation, and osteopenia occur, with some species variability (49). In vitro rat bone studies conducted years ago suggested that magnesium somehow stimulated the normal process of bone resorption (128). Studies with cultured rat osteoclasts demonstrated that Mg^{2+} is essential for their adhesion to bone (an early critical step in bone resorption) and that Ca^{2+} diminishes such adhesion (129).

Vitamin D Resistance. The usual calcemic effect of vitamin D and its active metabolites calcidiol and calcitriol is blunted—even with high doses—in the presence of magnesium deficiency induced under a variety of conditions in humans, including rickets (130), intestinal malabsorption (131), and idiopathic (132) or surgically induced hypoparathyroidism (133). Hypomagnesemic hypercalcemic rats were also resistant (133). Although serum calcitriol levels were low in most depleted humans, serum magnesium, PTH, and calcium levels rose in response to magnesium administration (114, 134–136). Low calcitriol levels were frequent in magnesium-deficient patients and persisted for 5 to 13 days after magnesium therapy, despite normal magnesium, PTH, and calcium responses (135). It has been suggested that magnesium depletion may partially impair the stimulatory effect of PTH on hydroxylation of calcidiol to calcitriol (115). Others found that administering magnesium together with calcidiol resulted in a rise in serum calcitriol levels to normal, but magnesium administration without the calcidiol elicited little or no rise in this hormone (137). Further study is necessary to determine the cause and significance of the depressed calcidiol and calcitriol concentrations in magnesium-depleted patients. Nonetheless, normal calcitriol levels are clearly not essential for correction of hypomagnesemic hypocalcemia.

Magnesium depletion in rats did not affect normal conversion of calcidiol to calcitriol in vivo nor did it modify the in vitro activity of the 1α-hydroxylase in renal mitochondria (133). It was concluded that vitamin D resistance induced by magnesium depletion is the consequence of impaired skeletal response to calcitriol.

Renal Citrate Reabsorption. Magnesium-deficient patients have markedly lower urinary citrate content secondary to increased renal tubular citrate reabsorption (138). The low urinary citrate is an additional risk factor for renal stone formation in hyperoxaluric hypomagnesemic patients.

Lipids, Lipoproteins, and Prostanoids. Magnesium deficiency in rats has been associated with increased serum/plasma phospholipid (139, 140) and triglyceride (140) levels, variable total cholesterol (139, 140) levels, low free cholesterol (140) levels, increased levels of oleic and linoleic acids, decreased stearic and arachidonic acid levels, and modifications of lipoprotein concentrations (140) Plasma prostanoid (PGE_2, $PGF_{2\alpha}$, 6-keto-$PGF_{1\alpha}$, and TBX^2) levels were significantly higher in both plasma and tissues of deficient rats than in controls (141). In contrast to pair-fed controls, the hyperlipidemia in magnesium-depleted young rats was associated with increased oxidation of very low density (VLDLs) and low-density lipoproteins (LDLs). Increased lipid oxidation occurred in liver, heart, and muscle of the deficient rats (142). Magnesium depletion, by inhibiting adenylate cyclase activity and thereby lowering cAMP levels, may permit increased cyclooxygenase activity and stimulation of prostanoid synthesis (140).

Because certain biochemical and pathologic changes differ in the magnesium-deficient rat and in other species, experimental comparison with other species is necessary before generalizing the lipid and prostanoid changes noted above. Lipid alterations have been reported in hypomagnesemic human subjects; however, they are often complicated by factors related to underlying lipoprotein abnormalities occurring in diabetes, coronary artery disease, myocardial infarction, and other diseases.

DISEASE-RELATED (CONDITIONED) DEPLETION

Experimental versus Clinical Depletion

Unlike experimental magnesium depletion in humans and various species of laboratory animals, the clinical literature dealing with magnesium deficiency reports large variations in the concentrations of magnesium found in serum, various blood cells, and biopsy specimens of muscle and bone (reviewed in [143]). These marked and inconsistent variations emphasize the difficulty in ascribing cause and effect to a specific nutrient deficiency in uncontrolled situations in sick individuals. Normal cellular metabolism and homeostasis depend critically on an adequate supply of energy and essential nutrients. A deficiency of any one nutrient (e.g., magnesium, sodium, potassium, phosphate, or nitrogen) has a negative impact on retention of others (144). Magnesium deficiency depletes potassium (89), and potassium depletion reduces cellular magnesium (145). The adverse effects of major loss of lean body mass and acidosis on magnesium status have been noted (86). The clinical situation may be further complicated by a hypercatabolic state, hormonal imbalance, and various medications.

Prevalence

The many risk factors for magnesium depletion (Tables 9.2 and 9.4) suggest that this condition is not a rare occurrence in acutely or chronically ill patients. Of 2300 patients surveyed in a Veterans Administration hospital, 6.9% were hypomagnesemic; 11% of patients having routine magnesium determinations were hypomagnesemic. When patients were hypokalemic, hypomagnesemia occurred in 42%; 29% of those with hypophosphatemia were hypomagnesemic, 27% of those with hyponatremia, and 22% of those with hypocalcemia (146). The true prevalence of magnesium depletion is not known, because this ion is not included in routine electrolyte testing in many clinics or hospitals (147). Similar high rates of depletion have been reported in studies of ICU patients (148–150).

Gastrointestinal Disorders

Gastrointestinal disorders (Table 9.2) may lead to magnesium depletion in various ways. Persistent nausea, cramping, or abdominal pain may seriously impair intake. Vomiting of upper tract (stomach) contents is not associated with significant losses of magnesium, but persistent loss of large volumes from the small intestine for any reason will cause serious loss of magnesium (5–10 mmol/L). Crohn's and Whipple's diseases, gluten-induced enteropathy (celiac disease), lymphangiectasia, enteral fistulas, radiation enteritis, and surgically induced bowel resection, as well as other malabsorption syndromes impair magnesium absorption. These conditions are among the more common disease-related causes of depletion, in part, because of their chronic nature. Any condition that significantly increases the amount of unabsorbed fatty acids in the lumen will significantly reduce magnesium (and calcium) absorption by precipitating them as fatty soaps (i.e., bile insufficiency secondary to biliary obstruction or to damage or resection of the terminal ileum). Additional resection or disease of the colonic epithelium probably contributes to magnesium loss, because evidence suggests that the colon is a site of magnesium absorption. A large number of infections by bacteria, protozoa, and other parasites and viruses induce loss of magnesium by all of these mechanisms. Gastrointestinal damage (gastritis, cirrhosis, pancreatitis) induced by chronic alcoholic intake also affects magnesium status adversely in other ways.

Renal Disorders

Magnesium Wasting

Clinical depletion is induced by metabolic disorders that lead to renal magnesium wasting, including the hypercalcemia of hyperparathyroidism and malignancy, genetic disease, alcoholism, and diabetes mellitus. Thiazide diuretics in medium-strength dosages generally cause relatively little magnesium loss but may do so if ingested in large amounts over long periods; potassium loss may be more significant. Loop diuretics (e.g., furosemide) acting on the main site of tubular absorption are more likely to induce magnesium losses with chronic use (98, 121). Cisplatin nephrotoxicity has caused magnesium and potassium losses, which may occur rapidly and may persist for months or even years after discontinuation of the drug (98, 151). Provision of the drug with extensive hydration provides some protection.

Not all hypercalcemic conditions are associated with magnesium wasting. Familial hypocalciuric hypercalcemia (152) and lithium carbonate (153) used in the treatment of manic depression are associated with hypercalcemia, hypermagnesemia, and decreased excretion of calcium and magnesium.

Following release of a unilateral or bilateral ureteral obstruction, absolute and fractional urinary magnesium excretion increases from the obstructed kidney(s). This parallels the increase in sodium and calcium during the postobstructive diureses; however, the magnesuria persists well beyond the sodium and water diuresis (154). Magnesium wasting may also occur with various nephritides and following kidney transplant.

Primary hypomagnesemia (59) and congenital renal wasting syndromes (98) reflect deficiencies secondary to malabsorption in the intestine and kidney tubule, respectively. They are differentiated clinically by a very low urinary output in the former and a relatively high output in the latter.

Hypomagnesemia may occur in Bartter's syndrome (presenting below the age of 6 years with urinary potassium wasting, hypokalemia, alkalosis, normal or increased urinary calcium, and hyperaldosteremia, hyperreninemia, and increased urinary PGE_2), but usually in a minority of 20 to 36% (96, 98). A similar syndrome has been described with normal juxtaglomerular apparatus and severe hypokalemia that responded to large amounts of magnesium (155). The milder Gitelman's (or Welt's) syndrome frequently presents in adult life; it also has renal potassium wasting with resultant hypokalemia and alkalosis but with hypocalciuria and with most having hypomagnesemia with magnesium wasting (98). These and other related conditions have been summarized (98).

Chronic Renal Failure

While filtration through the glomeruli is progressively reduced, magnesium excretion continues to balance intake until the filtration rate falls below approximately 30% of normal; consequently, serum magnesium levels are within the normal range up to this time. Renal balancing factors include an increasing osmotic load, increased sodium excretion, increased calcium concentration in the tubule, and acidosis, all of which increase fractional magnesium excretion (156). If there is also tubular damage, magnesium wasting may occur; hypomagnesemia may result despite concomitant azotemia.

Magnesium in Dialysis Patients. Hemo- and peritoneal dialysis decrease magnesium together with other substances accumulated in blood because of severely impaired filtration. When the fluxes of plasma magnesium were determined using high-efficiency hemodialysis, a magnesium-free dialysate reduced the plasma magnesium from a high level (mean, 1.35 mmol/L [3.3 mg/dL]) to low normal (mean, 0.66 mmol/L [1.6 mg/dL]) in 2.5 h. A magnesium level of 0.6 mg/dL in the dialysate was well tolerated (157). It was suggested that approximately 0.5 g/day of magnesium carbonate be given orally with this dialysate level to minimize hypercalcemia and allow a doubling of intravenous calcitriol (157a).

Alcohol and Alcoholism

Magnesium depletion has been noted with high frequency in chronic alcoholics. The many causes include poor intake (as alcohol calories replace nutritious foods by choice or necessity) exacerbated by gastrointestinal problems such as nausea, vomiting, gastritis, and diarrhea, and increased urinary loss as the result of the direct action of alcohol, ketosis, and the frequent use of diuretics (158, 159).

It has been suggested that magnesium depletion in chronic alcoholics may play a role in cardiovascular disease by increasing the platelet aggregation that occurs with deficiency (159); in addition, osteoporosis, which is common in alcoholics, may be partly due to alcohol-induced transient cycles of hypoparathyroidism followed by rebound hyperparathyroidism (160). With age and relative weight, alcoholism is among the three most common associations for hypertension in men and women (161, 162).

Diabetes Mellitus

Diabetes mellitus is probably the most common disorder associated with magnesium depletion (100, 163). More than 30% of ambulatory diabetic patients without renal insufficiency were hypomagnesemic on a multifactorial basis (163). A significant negative correlation was noted between serum/plasma magnesium and blood glycohemoglobin levels in insulin-dependent pregnant women, with significant relationships to the rates of spontaneous abortion and malformation (164). About one-third of infants born to diabetic mothers were hypomagnesemic during the first 3 days of life. Similar negative correlations were noted between plasma and muscle magnesium and glycohemoglobin levels in adult insulin-dependent diabetes mellitus (IDDM) (165). In one group of children with IDDM, serum magnesium, calcium, PTH, calcitriol, and osteocalcin levels were lower than in age- and sex-matched controls (166); in another series, magnesium and potassium were low in skeletal muscle (167). Following oral magnesium supplementation, these values increased significantly. Supplementation also decreased the insulin requirement (168). When very elderly patients with normal serum magnesium and glucose levels but subnormal erythrocyte magnesium concentrations were given oral daily magnesium supplements, their erythrocyte magnesium levels rose, accompanied by net increases in insulin secretion and action (169).

Magnesium depletion in diabetic ketoacidosis occurs in part because of acidosis-induced cellular loss. Many such patients have normal or elevated serum magnesium (because of decreased glomerular filtration with volume contraction), but administration of fluid and insulin (particularly with intermittent relatively large amounts of the latter) without supplementary magnesium soon induces low serum levels indicating low tissue levels (170).

Intracellular magnesium concentration is reduced in muscle and in various blood cells of type II diabetics (100, 171). One cause of depletion appears to be increased urinary losses accompanying glycosuria-induced osmotic diuresis. Because insulin normally increases intracellular magnesium concentration, the insulin lack or resistance of the two types of diabetics has been suggested as a cause of reduced intracellular magnesium. Magnesium-deficient type II diabetics with decreased red cell magnesium had increased sensitivity to platelet aggregation, which was reduced by magnesium supplements (159).

Hypertension

The possible relationship of hypertension to magnesium nutriture has been examined by a number of approaches. In epidemiologic studies in which hypertension was correlated with dietary food records, magnesium intake was not associated with blood pressure in black girls 9 and 10 years old. In white girls of the same age, higher magnesium intake was associated with decreased diastolic pressure; however, this effect disappeared after adjustment for dietary fiber intake (172). In a 4-year follow-up of 1248 male health professionals, the same relationship was noted; namely, hypertension was inversely related to the intakes of magnesium and dietary fiber. Only dietary fiber, however, had an independent inverse association (161). With adult females in a similar type of study, dietary magnesium (and calcium) was independently inversely related to hypertension (162). Reports relating serum magnesium levels in hypertensives to those in nonhypertensives are inconsistent; magnesium levels were lower in both sexes with hypertension (173), were lower in men but not in women (174), or did not differ in either gender from controls (175, 176).

The results of intervention studies are much more relevant. In uncontrolled studies, hypertensive patients on thiazide diuretics given magnesium supplements exhibited subsequent drop in blood pressure (177, 178), whereas in a controlled study, magnesium supplements had no significant effect after 6 months (179). When a magnesium supplement was compared with placebo in patients not on diuretics who had either mild-to-moderate (180) or mild hypertension (181), there was no decline in blood pressure at 1 or 3 months, respectively; in contrast, the same magnesium salt in another study produced a small but significant decrease only in the diastolic pressure of women with mild-to-moderate hypertension (182). An 8-month controlled study in subjects with mild hypertension compared placebo with either magnesium or potassium salts alone or together; potassium alone or given with magnesium caused a significant reduction in pressure, but magnesium had no added effect (183). In yet other controlled clinical trials, supplemental magnesium had no effect on the blood pressure of individuals with high-normal or mild hypertension (184, 186). In this study, when some of the subjects with low pretreatment urinary magnesium levels were given magnesium, their blood pressure fell significantly; however, this change was observed mainly in association with increased urinary excretion of sodium (186).

Erythrocytes of patients with essential hypertension had elevated levels of intracellular calcium and sodium, but the magnesium level and pH were low; these differences were exacerbated by salt loading salt-sensitive individuals and blunted by a calcium channel blocker (187). Hypertensive patients with left ventricular hypertrophy (LVH)—a prognostic factor for congestive heart failure and a risk factor for myocardial infarction and sudden death—had lower erythrocyte magnesium levels than hypertensive patients without LVH. The LVH patients had evidence of insulin resistance; insulin infusion increased their intracellular magnesium levels significantly over those of patients without LVH (188). Lack of insulin rather than hypertension appeared to cause the low red cell magnesium concentration.

The *Third Report on Nutrition Monitoring in the United States* (53) classified magnesium as a potential public health issue. This claim was made in part "because epidemiological and clinical studies have suggested that certain of these minerals are associated with hypertension (potassium and possibly magnesium)" (53). The stated support for this "possible" relationship is: "Limited evidence suggests that low serum levels of magnesium may be associated with an increased risk of hypertension" (53), and only two papers were cited (161, 162). These references were cited inaccurately in the third report; they did not report serum magnesium levels, nor did the authors of reference 161 find an association between dietary magnesium intake and hypertension in males when dietary fiber was factored into the data.

Protein-Energy Malnutrition

Magnesium depletion has occurred in children with inadequate food intakes in association with malabsorption, persistent vomiting and/or diarrhea, and infection. Serum or plasma magnesium was noted to be low in a significant proportion of such children in various studies in Africa (189), whereas in a study in Central America, 50% of serum magnesium values were below 0.65 mmol/L on admission (190).

Postparathyroidectomy Hypomagnesemia

Symptomatic hypomagnesemia may follow parathyroidectomy for primary hyperparathyroidism in association with the expected hypocalcemia, presumably as part of the "hungry bone" syndrome that results from rapid uptake of calcium and magnesium by bone. Muscle weakness, tremor, and mental changes can be reversed by magnesium supplementation despite continuing low calcium levels (191).

Cardiovascular Disease

Various statements above have indicated the importance of magnesium in cardiovascular function. This section evaluates the literature on the possible relationship of this nutrient to various aspects of heart disease, particularly coronary artery disease (CAD). For many years, researchers have tried to assess the relationship between CAD prevalence and ingestion of "hard" water (i.e., water relatively high in calcium but also containing, in various proportions, magnesium, fluoride, phosphates, and other ions). An inverse relationship between the magnesium content of water and CAD has been claimed (192, 193), denied (194, 195), or stated to be uncertain (196). Serious difficulties exist in collecting accurate data about water composition and consumption over long periods, changes in water sources and treatment methods, population shifts, intakes of other sources of magnesium, and a large number of other variables, such as diet, and in proper execution of case-controlled or randomized studies (196).

Depressed magnesium status has been implicated as a causative factor for both dysrhythmias and myocardial infarction. Older literature cited low serum/plasma magnesium levels in individuals complaining of chest pain or with proven myocardial infarction upon, or soon after, admission; most of these reports were either uncontrolled or otherwise inadequate. More-recent studies suggest that other significant events contributed to the reported low serum values (reviewed in [143]): *(a)* the time blood is drawn following onset of chest pain is important, since magnesium leaves the infarcted myocytes; *(b)* the prior and often chronic use of diuretics and cardiac glycosides by patients with heart disease may induce depletion of magnesium as well as potassium and contribute to arrhythmias; *(c)* postinfarction lipolysis (also induced by ethanol withdrawal, epinephrine, and surgery) releases serum fatty acids that lower serum magnesium levels; and *(d)* the degree of pain per se affects magnesium levels. Similarly, the decreased magnesium content of ischemic hearts at postmortem examination is attributable to many factors, including previous medications, extent of previous myocardial damage, and sampling sites.

Dietary magnesium intakes (comparing those of highest and lowest quartiles) were not a significant predictor of the occurrence of ischemic heart disease in a 16-year observation period of 2512 males, ages 45 to 59, when age, smoking, and energy and alcohol intakes were considered (196a).

Magnesium Infusion in Myocardial Infarction

A number of controlled studies supported the conclusion that intravenous magnesium given early after suspected myocardial infarction reduced the frequency of serious arrhythmias and mortality (197–200). These observations were supported by several metaanalyses (201, 202). In addition, the report of a major, randomized, double-blinded, placebo-controlled study, the Leicester Intravenous Magnesium Intervention Trial (LIMIT-2), indicated some benefit with magnesium (203). Mortality from all causes was 7.8% in the magnesium-treated group of 1019 patients and 10.3% in the placebo group of 1002 patients ($P = .04$). Left ventricular failure was reduced by an average of 25% ($P = .009$) in the magnesium group, as followed in the coronary care unit. The authors also concluded that magnesium was acting pharmacologically rather than correcting an existing deficit, that it did not affect progression to acute infarction in those with unstable CAD, and that it did not have antiarrhythmic action. A follow-up report on those who survived this study for 1.0 to 5.5 years indicated that the magnesium-treated group had 21% lower mortality from ischemic heart disease and 16% lower all-cause mortality than the controls (204).

The Fourth International Study of Infarct Survival (ISIS-4) was a much larger randomized trial than LIMIT-2 of patients having suspected myocardial infarction. This study compared the benefits of three different treatments with each other and with placebo-treated or "open" control groups (205). In comparing intravenous magnesium sulfate (2216 patients) with open controls (2103 patients), no significant reduction was found in 5-week mortality, either overall (magnesium, 7.64%; controls, 7.24%) or in any subgroup examined (i.e., treated early or late, presence or absence of fibrinolytic or antiplatelet therapies, or high risk of death). There was a significant *excess* of mortality with magnesium treatment in heart-failure patients or in those suffering from cardiogenic shock. Intravenous magnesium was concluded to be ineffective. The differences among the metaanalyses, LIMIT-2, and the ISIS 4 megatrial have led to continuing and divergent opinion on this subject (206–208).

Rasmussen and colleagues, who had been proponents of magnesium infusion at the time of suspected infarction (200), found that daily oral administration of magnesium hydroxide (15 mmol, or 360 mg, over a 1-year period) to survivors of an acute myocardial infarction resulted in no differences in the incidences of reinfarction, sudden death, or coronary artery bypass grafting, compared with placebo (209).

Magnesium in Cardiac Surgery or Organ Transplantation

Cardiopulmonary bypass (CPB), used in cardiac and organ transplant procedures greatly expands the extracellular fluid volume (ECF) because of infusion of blood and/or blood derivatives (e.g., up to 2500 mL/m^2 increases the ECF volume between 20 and 30%). Associated with this procedure are lactic acidosis, metabolic alkalosis, hemodilution, extracellular ion shifts, binding of Ca^{2+} and Mg^{2+} to stored blood products, and decreased serum [K^+], [Na^+], [Ca^{2+}], and [Mg^{2+}] (210). A significant number of candidates for cardiac surgery (211) or liver transplantation (212) are hypomagnesemic preoperatively, primarily because of poor intake and medications. Magnesium levels decrease further with ECF expansion and increased excretion stimulated by loop diuretics. Magnesium administration given once intraoperatively after the termination of CPB elevated the depressed serum magnesium transiently; this treatment was associated with a reduced frequency of clinically significant postoperative ventricular dysrhythmias and an increased cardiac index (211).

Cardiac Arrhythmias and Magnesium

The contradictory findings of LIMIT-2 and ISIS-4 raise uncertainties about the effectiveness of intravenous magnesium in preventing deaths from serious arrhythmias in patients with acute myocardial infarction. Nevertheless, the intimate roles of Mg^{2+} in cellular biochemistry, including its functions in association with Na-K ATPase (213), Ca ATPase (214), transport via multiple-ion channels (29), and hormonal regulation, provide evidence for its importance in cardiac function. Its deficiency—often combined with that of potassium—may result in electrophysiologic and other abnormalities leading to arrhythmias that are reversible by magnesium (100). Magnesium has proven effective in suppressing a ventricular arrhythmia, torsade de pointes, which is potentially life threatening (212, 215).

MANAGEMENT OF DEPLETION

The physician should consider all predisposing factors in patients at risk, to anticipate hypomagnesemia and institute early treatments to *prevent* its occurrence or minimize its severity. These include instituting control of underlying disease, minimizing therapeutic insult, and initiating medical and dietary changes designed to maximize magnesium retention by the intestine and kidney. When magnesium depletion is evident, its cause must be determined (see Assessing Magnesium Nutriture above). Prior to initiating treatment, magnesium, calcium, potassium, and sodium levels in the blood and urine and the acid-base balance in blood must be determined. The amount, route, and duration of magnesium administration depend on the severity of depletion and its causes.

Adolescents and Adults. Seizures, acute arrhythmias, and severe generalized spasticity require immediate intravenous infusion with one of several protocols, depending on the state of renal function. One to 2 g $MgSO_4 \cdot 7H_2O$ (8.2–16.4 meq Mg^{2+}) is usually infused over 5 to 10 min, followed by continuous infusion of 6 g over 24 h or until the condition is controlled (93). Infusion of calcium gluconate should accompany the magnesium if blood levels are low. Alternatively, 2 g of the sulfate are given over 1 min, followed by 1.0 meq/kg (0.5 mmol) during the first 24 h, followed by 0.5 meq/kg for the next 3 days (215). A similar protocol (216) and others (217) have been used to suppress the ventricular arrhythmia torsade de pointes. In all instances, correction of electrolyte (especially potassium) and acid-base imbalances should accompany the magnesium therapy. Additionally, levels of serum and urine magnesium and other electrolytes should be determined at least twice daily in such patients.

Less severe manifestations (e.g., paresthesias with latent or active tetany associated with persisting intestinal or renal losses) are likewise best treated by the intravenous route, again in conjunction with appropriate therapy for the underlying condition and with correction of other electrolyte and acid-base abnormalities. When renal function is good, 3 g (25 meq) of magnesium sulfate may be given intravenously over 2 or 3 h in saline or dextrose solutions, with other nutrients as required. Another 3 or 4 g are then given by continuous infusion over the remaining 24 h. When the intravenous route cannot be used, equivalent periodic intramuscular injections can be given, although these are painful and may lead to fibrotic reactions. This regimen is continued for 2 or more days, and the situation is then reassessed. The dosages given must always exceed the daily losses as indicated by serum levels and urinary excretion. Intravenous calcium administration in the treatment of hypocalcemia secondary to magnesium deficiency is usually desirable for 1 or 2 days when tetany is initially apparent.

The return to the normal or slightly higher range of serum magnesium levels with any of these schedules is relatively rapid. However, repletion of magnesium lost from bone and other tissues requires more prolonged magnesium therapy at lower and/or less frequent doses, preferably by mouth. This regimen is continued until—or, if necessary, beyond—the time necessary to attain a persisting, relatively normal serum magnesium concentration and a urine output of 20% or more of the oral intake in the case of intestinal malabsorption. When intestinal absorption is normal and renal magnesium wasting is present, supplements should be added to the usual diet to maintain normal serum levels; this supplement should be 20% or more above the amount of magnesium lost in fecal water plus urine, as measured when only the diet is given.

For the asymptomatic patient with serum levels below approximately 0.5 mmol/L (1.0 meq/L), a trial of increased oral intake is prescribed, as tolerated and effective (see below); otherwise, injectable magnesium sulfate is given intramuscularly for a trial period. Those with continuing severe magnesium and potassium losses in the urine (as in cisplatin nephrotoxicity) may require long-term supplements. If this is not possible solely by increased oral intake, an alternative to painful intramuscular injections of magnesium salts is either intravenous infusion via an indwelling central catheter for home administration or a trial of the old-fashioned, but useful, hypodermic clysis. In the latter procedure, 2 g of 50% magnesium sulfate is diluted in 250 mL of 0.45% saline with potassium as indicated. This solution is then infused as rapidly as possible, through a very small bore needle inserted just under the abdominal skin, as often as is necessary to meet the patient's magnesium requirement.

When depletion is modest and persistent, initial efforts should be directed to increased intake of magnesium-rich foods. When necessary and feasible, supplementary oral magnesium may be taken as small gelatin capsules packed with the sulfate, chloride, acetate, citrate, or other salts with good solubility in enteric fluids. Several small capsules may be given 3 to 6 times per day, with a full glass of water to prevent or minimize magnesium-related diarrhea (60) and to ensure solubilization. For the individual on enteral feeding, one of these salts may be dissolved in the formula. Improvement of existing steatorrhea by dietary or other medical means will decrease fecal magnesium losses. Again, treatment of underlying disease and replacement of potassium deficits are essential.

Infants and Young Children. Symptomatic magnesium depletion in infants responds well to relatively small amounts of intravenous or intramuscular magnesium. When renal function is normal, parenteral administration is recommended: 3.6 to 6.0 mg (0.15–0.25 mmol or 0.3 to 0.5 meq)/kg body weight as 50% magnesium sulfate over the first several hours, followed by an equal amount, either intramuscularly or intravenously, over the remainder of the day (218). Calcium should also be infused initially, together with potassium and other electrolytes as indicated. When convulsions or arrhythmias are present in those beyond infancy, treatment may be initiated with an oral bolus of the 50% magnesium sulfate at a dose of 20 to 100 mg (1.65–8.25 meq/kg) over 1 min; this is followed by 1.0 meq/kg given continuously thereafter (219).

In patients with chronic malabsorption (e.g., primary hypomagnesemia), 12 to 18 mg/kg (0.5–0.75 mmol) in multiple, divided oral doses is suggested; this dosage schedule raises serum levels to near normal without inducing diarrhea (218).

HYPERMAGNESEMIA AND MAGNESIUM TOXICITY

Physiologic Effects of Hypermagnesemia

Magnesium at levels above normal relaxes vascular smooth muscle in vitro and reduces pressor responses (220). In humans, when serum magnesium levels were roughly twice normal, systolic and diastolic blood pressures fell by an average of 10 and 8 mm, respectively; renal blood flow increased significantly; and the pressor effect of angiotensin II was blunted (221). Urinary excretion of 6-keto-$PGF_{1\alpha}$ increased markedly. Cyclooxygenase inhibition with indomethacin or ibuprofen completely blocked the magnesium-induced fall in blood pressure, the rise in urinary 6-keto-$PGF_{1\alpha}$, and the rise in renal blood flow. The calcium-channel blocker nifedipine also prevented the magnesium-induced rise in 6-keto-$PGF_{1\alpha}$ and fall in blood pressure. These findings indicate that the effect of magnesium was mediated by prostacyclin release and increased Ca^{2+} flux. When magnesium chloride was infused acutely in healthy subjects to the point of doubling the plasma magnesium, PTH levels fell and plasma renin activity and renin levels increased (222).

Induced Hypermagnesemia As Therapy

Preeclampsia and Eclampsia

Preeclampsia and eclampsia are the most important causes of maternal death in the United States and many other countries (223). For many years, high-dose parenteral magnesium sulfate has been the drug of choice in North America for preventing eclamptic convulsions that may occur in association with severe hypertension and other problems in late pregnancy or during labor (224). Since 1995, magnesium sulfate has begun to replace phenytoin and diazepam in Europe and elsewhere (225). Despite many clinical trials and several metaanalyses suggesting that calcium supplements reduced the incidence of preeclampsia, a major double-blinded randomized study found that 2 g of elemental calcium given daily to healthy pregnant women did not prevent preeclampsia, pregnancy associated–hypertension, or adverse perinatal outcomes (225a). Magnesium is believed to reverse the cerebral vasospasm and ischemia that appear to be the genesis of eclampsia. A similar program of magnesium administration has been used in an effort to prevent premature labor (226); this use of magnesium as a tocolytic agent is disputed (see below). A loading dose and then maintenance doses are given to maintain a high serum level of approximately 2 to 3 mmol/L (4–6 meq/L) (224) or slightly above (226). With increased serum magnesium levels, circulating PTH levels may drop, with associated hypocalcemia (226, 227).

Patients with normal kidneys can excrete 40 to 60 g of magnesium sulfate · $7H_2O$ per day when it is given constantly by infusion. The high doses used are rarely associated with serious side effects, because patients are closely monitored with modification of dosage as indicated.

Fetuses delivered from mothers receiving high-dosage magnesium had hypermagnesemia of the umbilical vein and artery blood at about the elevated levels of the mother; however, serum levels fell progressively to normal levels in neonates by 48 hours (228). With maternal hypocalcemia, the fetus at delivery may have normal (228) or low serum calcium (229). Abnormal radiographic findings have been noted in the proximal humeral metaphysis in infants of mothers who were on high-dose magnesium therapy to delay labor; they resolved completely within the first few months (230).

Effect on Cerebral Palsy and Asthma

An increasing number of reports have associated prenatal exposure of the fetus to increased levels of magnesium sulfate (as in the treatment of preeclampsia) with a major reduction in the risk of cerebral palsy and, possibly, of mental retardation in very low birth-weight (VLBW) children (231). However, a preliminary report in a well-controlled randomized study is contradictory. Women in preterm labor at less than 34 weeks gestation who were not pre-eclamptic were given $MgSO_4$ as one of the randomized treatments. Its use was associated with increased pediatric mortality and the trial was stopped (231a). This observation "tilts the balance of evidence firmly away from magnesium use as a tocolytic or cerebroprotectant agent in preterm labour" (231b).

Induced hypermagnesemia may be potentially useful in the management of status asthmaticus in children (232).

Magnesium in Treatment of Suspected Drug Overdose

Magnesium-containing cathartics have been given orally with activated charcoal in single or multiple doses (each of 30 g $MgSO_4 \cdot 7H_20$ [245 meq Mg^{2+}]) in an effort to decrease blood levels of drugs, as part of the treatment of patients with suspected drug overdose. Despite initially normal serum creatinine concentrations (233), 9 of 14 patients were hypermagnesemic by the third dose at 8 hours, including 4 with magnesium levels of 3.0 meq/L and one of 5.0. The presence of drugs that decreased gut motility (e.g., anticholinergics or opioids) appeared related to the higher levels (231).

Disease-Related Hypermagnesemia

Hypermagnesemia may occur at symptomatic levels in patients with gastrointestinal disorders such as obstipation, severe constipation, ulceration, obstruction, or perforation when magnesium-containing cathartics or antacids are taken, even in moderate dosages, and renal insufficiency is mild or moderate (232).

Advanced Renal Failure with Exogenous or Endogenous Magnesium Load

In addition to the planned therapeutic hypermagnesemia noted above, elevated serum levels occur when magnesium-containing drugs, usually antacids or cathartics, are ingested chronically and in relatively large amounts by individuals with advanced renal insufficiency. Because 20% or more of Mg^{2+} from various salts may be absorbed, impaired renal clearance can induce significant hypermagnesemia. The common association of age or disease-related impairment of glomerular filtration, which may be exacerbated by ingestion of potentially nephrotoxic medications (such as steroidal antiinflammatory drugs for arthritic pain), and the chronic use of magnesium-containing antacids and/or laxatives, contribute to the danger of significant hypermagnesemia in such individuals. Uncommonly, *hypo*magnesemia may occur when there is tubulointerstitial nephropathy–induced magnesium wasting or severe intestinal malabsorption (235).

Magnesium Toxicity

The many potentially toxic and even lethal effects of magnesium excess are summarized in Figure 9.8 (236). One of the earliest effects is a fall in blood pressure, progressing with increasing hypermagnesemia; this appears to result from inhibition of Ca^{2+} flux and the vasoconstrictive action of norepinephine and angiotensin II (221). Some of the later effects, such as lethargy, confusion, and deterioration in renal function, may be related to the hypotension (234). ECG changes, such as prolongation of the P-R and Q-T intervals, occur at 5 meq/L (2.5 mmol). Tachycardia (probably secondary to hypotension) or bradycardia may occur. At 6 meq/L and above, muscle weakness and hyporeflexia may occur, presumably resulting from decreased release of acetylcholine and impaired transmission at the neuromuscular junction; hypocal-

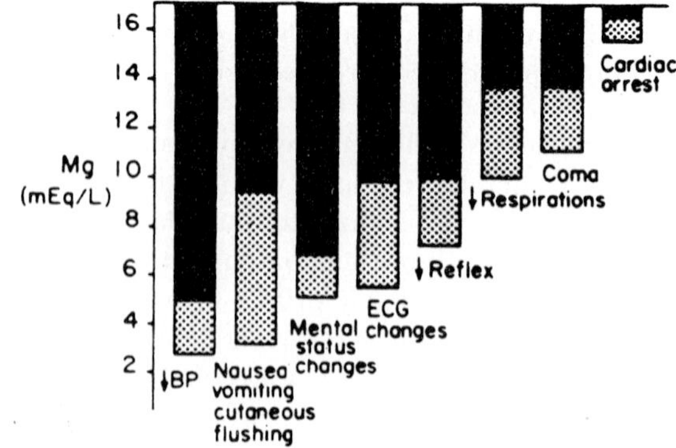

Figure 9.8. The progression in toxic effects as hypermagnesemia becomes more severe. An early sign is a lowering of blood pressure *(BP)*. Nausea, vomiting, and hypotension may occur in the range of 3 to 9 mEq/L; bradycardia and urinary retention also occur in this range. Electrocardiogram *(ECG)* changes, hyporeflexia, and secondary central nervous system depression may appear in the 5 to 10 mEq/L range, followed at higher concentrations by life-threatening respiratory depression, coma, and asystolic cardiac arrest. (From Mordes JP, Wacker EC. Pharmacol Rev 1978;29:274–300, with permission.)

cemia and hypokalemia may contribute to the progressive muscle weakness and respiratory difficulty. Complete heart block and cardiac arrest may occur at about 15 meq/L (236).

Management of Hypermagnesemia

Prevention or treatment of mild-to-moderate hypermagnesemia (≥1.5 mmol) requires reducing magnesium intake when absorption from all sources exceeds the renal excretory capability. At higher levels, when hemodynamic instability and muscle weakness are apparent, all magnesium intake should be stopped and an acute infusion of 5 to 10 meq of calcium should be given (234). Continued saline and calcium infusion will increase magnesium excretion. Dialysis will remove magnesium readily in the patient with poor renal function (234).

REFERENCES

1. Kruse HD, Orent ER, McCollum EV. J Biol Chem 1932;96:519–36.
2. Hirschfelder AD, Haury VG. JAMA 1934;102:1138–41.
3. Flink EB. J Am Coll Nutr 1985;4:17–31.
4. Cowan JA. Introduction to the biological chemistry of magnesium. In: Cowan JA, ed. The biological chemistry of magnesium. New York: VCH Publishers, 1995;1–24.
5. Ebel H, Gunther T. J Clin Chem Biochem 1980;18:257–70.
6. Black CB, Cowan JA. Magnesium dependent enzymes in nucleic acid biochemistry (chap 6) and Magnesium dependent enzymes in general metabolism (chap 7). In: Cowan JA, ed. The biological chemistry of magnesium. New York: VCH Publishers, 1995;137–58.
7. Mathews CK, van Holde KE. Biochemistry. Redwood City, CA: Benjamin/Cummings, 1990.
8. Vernon WB. Magnesium 1988;7:234–48.
9. Garfinkel D, Garfinkel L. Magnesium 1988;7:249–61.
10. Knighton DR, Zheng J, Ten Eyck LF, et al. Science 1991; 253:407–14.
11. Maguire ME. Trends Pharmacol Sci 1984;5:73–7.
12. Abe M, Sherwood LM. Biochem Biophys Res Commun 1972;48:396–401.
13. Rude RK, Oldham SB, Sharp CF Jr, et al. J Clin Endocrinol Metab 1978;47:800–6.
14. Smith D. Magnesium as the catalytic center of RNA enzymes. In: Cowan JA, ed. The biological chemistry of magnesium. New York: VCH Publishers, 1995;111–36.
15. Agris PF. Vitam Horm 1996;52:81–126
16. Kerrick WGL, Donaldson SKB. Biochim Biophys Acta 1972;272:117–24.
17. Elliott DA, Rizak MA. J Biol Chem 1974;249:3985–90.
18. Polimeni PI, Page E. Circ Res 1974:33:367–74.
19. Grubbs RD, Maguire ME. Magnesium 1987;6:113–27.
20. White RE, Hartzell HC. Biochem Pharmacol 1989;38:859–67.
21. Murphy E. Miner Electrolyte Metab 1993;19:266–76.
22. Smith DL, Maguire ME. Miner Electrolyte Metab 1993; 19:250–8.
23. Flatman PW. Annu Rev Physiol 1991;53:256–71.
24. Quamme GA, Rabkin SW. Biochem Biophys Res Commun 1990;167:1406–12.
25. Smith RL, Thompson LJ, Maguire ME. J Bacteriol 1995; 177:1233–8.
26. Quamme G. Miner Electrolyte Metab 1993;218–25.
27. Gunther T. Miner Electrolyte Metab 1993;19:259–65.
28. Romani A, Marfella C, Scarpa A. Miner Electrolyte Metab 1993;19:282–9.
29. Kelepouris E, Kasame R, Agus ZS. Miner Electrolyte Metab 1993;19:277–81.
30. Nichols CG, Shyng S-L, Nestorowicz A, et al. Science 1996;272:1755–87.
31. Burnstock G. Drug Dev Res 1993;28:195–206.
32. Burnstock G. Ciba Found Symp 1996;198:1–28.
33. Grzesiak JJ, Pierschbacher MD. J Invest Dermatol 1995;104:768–74.
34. Elin RJ. Magnesium Trace Elem 1991–92;10:60–6.
35. Toffaletti J, Alvarus B, Bird C, et al. Magnesium 1988;7: 84–90.
36. Nixon DE, Moyer TP, Johnson P, et al. Clin Chem 1986;32:1660–5.
37. Huijgen HJ, Van Ingen HE, Kok WT, et al. Clin Biochem 1996;29:261–6.
38. Cecco SA, Hristova EN, Niemela JE, et al. (Abstract 765) Clin Chem 1996;43:S279.
39. Csako G, Rehak N, Elin RJ. (Abstract 763) Clin Chem 1996:42:S279.
40. London RE. Annu Rev Physiol 1991;53:241–58.
41. Hoffenberg EF, Kozlowski P, Salerno TA, et al. J Surg Res 1996;62:135–43.
42. Golding EM, Dobson GP, Golding RM. Magn Reson Med 1996;35:174–85.
43. Kwack H, Veech LR. Curr Top Cell Regul 1992;33:185–207.
44. Aikawa JK, Gordon GS, Rhoades EL. J Appl Physiol 1960; 15:503–7.
45. Schwartz R. Fed Proc 1982;41:2709–13.
46. Schuette SA, Ziegler EE, Nelson SE, et al. Pediatr Res 1990;27:36–40.
47. Haigney MC, Silver B, Tanglao E, et al. Circulation 1995; 92:2190–7.
48. Gevens WB, Monnens LAH, Willems JL. Miner Electrolyte Metab 1993;19:308–13.
48a. Cook LA, Mimouni FB. J Am Coll Nutr 1997;16:161–3.
49. Wallach S. Magnesium Trace Elem 1990;9:1–14
50. Wenk C, Kohut M, Kunz G, et al. Z Ernahrungswiss 1993;32: 301–7.
51. Gupta RK, Moore RD. J Biol Chem 1980;255:3987–93.
52. Pennington JAT, Young B. J Am Diet Assoc 1991;91:179–83.
53. American Society for Experimental Biology, Life Sciences Research Office. Interagency Board for Nutrition Monitoring and Related Research. Third report on nutrition monitoring in the United States. Washington, DC: US GPO, 1995.
54. Pennington JAT, Wilson DB. J Am Diet Assoc 1990;90: 375–81.
55. US Department of Health and Human Services, Department of Agriculture. Nutrition Monitoring in the U.S. An update report on nutrition monitoring. DHHS publ. no. 89-1255. Washington, DC: US GPO, Sept, 1989.
56. Graham LA, Ceasar JJ, Burgen ASU. Metab Clin Exp 1960;9:646–59.
57. Fine KD, Santa Ana CA, Porter JL, et al. J Clin Invest 1991;88:396–402.
58. Roth P, Werner E. Int J Appl Radiat Isot 1979;30:523–6.
59. Milla PJ, Aggett, PJ, Wolff OH, et al. Gut 1979;20:1028–33.
60. Spencer H, Lesniak M, Gatza LA, et al. Gastroenterology 1980;79:26–34.
61. Lakshmann FL, Rao RB, Kim WW. Am J Clin Nutr 1984;40(Suppl 6):1380–9.

62. Hardwick LL, Jones MR, Brautbar N, et al. J Nutr 1991; 121:13–23.
63. Kayne LH, Lee DBN. Miner Electrolyte Metab 1993;19:210–7.
64. Karbach U, Rummel W. Gastroenterology 1990;98:985–92.
65. Spencer H, Osis D. Magnesium 1988;7:271–80.
66. Andon MB, Illich JZ, Tzagournis MA, et al. Am J Clin Nutr 1996;63:950–3.
67. Lewis NM, Marcus MSK, Behling AR, et al. Am J Clin Nutr 1989;49:527–33.
68. Greger JS, Smith SA, Snedeker SM. Nutr Res 1981;1:315–25.
69. Spencer H, Norris C, Williams D. J Am Coll Nutr 1994;13:479–84.
70. Turnlund JR, Betschart AA, Liebman M, et al. Am J Clin Nutr 1992;56:905–10.
71. Serfaty-Lacrosniere C, Wood RJ, Voytko D, et al. J Am Coll Nutr 1995;14:364–8.
72. Fine KD, Santa Ana CA, Fordtran JS. N Engl J Med 1991;324:1012–7.
72a. Kelsey JL, Behall KM, Prather ES. Am J Clin Nutr 1979; 32:1876–80.
72b. Siener R, Hesse A. Br J Nutr 1995;73:783–90.
72c. Wisker E, Nagel R, Tanudjaja TK, et al. Am J Clin Nutr 1991;54:553–9.
72d. Slavin JL, Marlett JA. Am J Clin Nutr 1980;33:1932–9.
73. Heaton FW, Hodgkinson A, Rose GA. Clin Sci 1964;27: 31–40.
74. Hodgkinson A, Marshall DH, Nordin BEE. Clin Sci 1979;57: 121–3.
75. Wilz DR, Gary RW, Dominquez JH, et al. Am J Clin Nutr 1979;32:2052–60.
76. Brannan PG, Vergne-Marini P, Pak YC, et al. J Clin Invest 1976;57:1412–8.
77. Norman DA, Fordtran JS, Brinkley LJ, et al. J Clin Invest 1981;67:1599–603.
78. Karbach U, Schmitt A, Hakan Saner F. Dig Dis Sci 1991;36:1611–8.
79. Rayssiguier Y, Thomasset M, Garel JM, et al. Horm Metab Res 1982;14:379–82.
80. Hemmingsen C, Staun M, Olgaard D. Miner Electrolyte Metab 1994;20:265–73.
81. Quamme GA, Dirks JH. The physiology of renal magnesium handling. In: Windhager EE, ed. Handbook of physiology, section 8, Renal physiology, vol 2. American Physiological Society. New York: Oxford University Press, 1992.
82. de Rouffignac C, Mandon B, Wittner M, et al. Miner Electrolyte Metab 1993;19:226–31.
83. Shafik IM, Quamme GA. Am J Physiol 1989;257:F974–7.
84. Francisco LL, Sawin LL, DiBona GF. Proc Soc Exper Biol Med 1981;168:382–8.
85. Wallach S. Magnesium 1988;7:262–70.
86. Drenick EG, Hung JF, Swendseid ME. J Clin Endocrinol 1969;29:1341–8.
87. Dunn MJ, Walser M. Metabolism 1966;15:884–95.
88. Altura BT, Altura BM. Magnesium Trace Elem (Abstract) 1990;9:311.
89. Shils ME. Medicine (Baltimore) 1969;48:61–85.
90. Rude RK, Stephen A, Nadler J. Magnesium Trace Elem 1991–92;10:117–21.
91. MacLean R, Dooley KL, Walter J, et al. (Abstract 782) Clin Chem 1996;42:S284.
92. Elin RJ, Hosseini JM. Clin Chem 1985;31:377–80.
93. Ryzen E. Magnesium 1989;8:201–12.
94. Ryan MF, Ryan MP. Ir J Med Sci 1979;148:108–9.
95. Ralston MA, Murname MR, Kelley RE, et al. Circulation 1989;80:573–80.
96. Elin RJ, Hosseini JM, Gill JR Jr. J Am Coll Nutr 1994;13:463–6.
97. Fleming CR, George L, Stoner GL, et al. Mayo Clin Proc 1996;71:21–4.
98. Sutton RAL, Domrongkitchaiporn. Miner Electrolyte Metab 1993;19:232–40.
99. Cadell JL, Reed GF. Magnesium 1989;8:65–70.
100. Rude RK. Magnesium disorders. In: Kokko JP, Tannen RL, eds. Fluids and electrolytes. 3rd ed. Philadelphia: WB Saunders, 1996.
101. Al Ghamdi SMG, Cameron EC, Sutton RAL. Am J Kidney Dis 1994;24:737–52.
101a. Food and Nutrition Board, Institute of Medicine. Dietary reference intakes for calcium, phosphorus, magnesium, vitamin D, and fluoride. Washington, DC: National Academy Press, 1997.
101b. Food and Nutrition Board, National Research Council. Recommended Dietary Allowances. 10th ed. Washington, DC: National Academy Press, 1989.
102. Berman BM, Larson DB, eds. Alternative medicine. Proceedings of a workshop on alternative medicine. Chantilly, VA: Sept 14–16, NIH publ. no. 94-066. Washington, DC: US GPO 1994;215.
103. Hathaway ML. Magnesium in human nutrition. Home economics research report no. 19. Agricultural Research Service, US Department of Agriculture. Washington, DC: US GPO, 1962.
104. Lowenstein FW, Stanton MF. J Am Coll Nutr 1986;5:399–414.
105. Shils ME, Rude RK. J Nutr 1996;126:2398S–403S.
106. Wood RJ, Suter PM, Russell RM. Am J Clin Nutr 1995;62: 493–505.
107. Shils ME. Magnesium. In: O'Dell BL, Sunde RA, eds. Handbook of nutritionally essential mineral elements. New York: Marcel Dekker, 1997;117–52.
108. Alcock NW, Shils ME. Proc Soc Exp Biol Med 1974;146: 137–41.
109. Shils ME. Magnesium deficiency and calcium and parathyroid hormone interrelations. In: Prasad A, ed. Trace elements in human health and disease, vol 2. New York: Academic Press, 1976;23–46.
110. Alcock NW, Shils ME, Lieberman PH, et al. Cancer Res 1973;33:2196–204.
111. Whang R, Oliver J, Welt LG, et al. Ann NY Acad Sci 1969;162:766–74.
112. Heggtveit HA. Ann NY Acad Sci 1969;162:758–65.
113. Morris ER, O'Dell BL. J Nutr 1963;81:175–81.
114. Bunce GE, Chiemchaisri V, Phillips PH. J Nutr 1962;76:23–9.
115. Fatemi S, Ryzen E, Endres DB, et al. J Clin Endocrinol Metab 1991;73:1067–72.
116. Yamamoto T, Kabata H, Yagi R, et al. Magnesium 1985;4: 153–64.
117. Johanneson AJ, Raisz LG. Endocrinology 1973;113:2294–8.
118. Freitag JJ, Martin KJ, Conrades E, et al. J Clin Invest 1979;64:1238–44.
119. Rude RK, Oldham SB, Sharp CF Jr, et al. J Clin Endocrinol Metab 1978;47:800–6.
120. Anast CS, Winnacher JL, Forte LR, et al. J Clin Endocrinol Metab 1976;42:707–17.
121. Ryan MP. Miner Electrolyte Metab 1993;19:290–5.
122. Shils ME. Ann NY Acad Sci 1980;355:165–80.
123. Mahaffey DD, Cooper CW, Ramp WK, et al. Endocrinology 1982;110:487–95.
124. Brown EM, Gamba G, Riccardi D, et al. Nature 1993;366: 575–80.

125. Anast CS, Mohs JM, Kaplan SL, et al. Science 1972; 177:606–8.
126. Rayssiguier Y, Thomaset M, Garel JM. Horm Metab Res 1982;14:379–82.
127. Anast CS, Forte LF. Endocrinology 1983;113:184–9.
128. MacManus J, Heaton FW. Biochim Biophys Acta 1970;215: 360–7.
129. Makgoba MW, Datta HK. Eur J Clin Invest 1992;22:692–6.
130. Reddy F, Sivakumar B. Lancet 1974;1:963–5.
131. Medalle R, Waterhouse C, Hahn TJ. Am J Clin Nutr 1976;29: 854–8.
132. Rosler A, Rabinowitz D. Lancet 1973;1:803–4.
133. Carpenter TO, Carnes DL Jr, Anast CS. Am J Physiol 1987;E253:E106–13.
134. Graber ML, Schulman G. Ann Intern Med 1986;104:804–5.
135. Rude RK, Adams JS, Ryzen E, et al. J Clin Endocrinol Metab 1985;61:933–40.
136. Fuss M, Cogan E, Gillet C, et al. Clin Endocrinol 1985;22:807–15.
137. Fuss M, Bergmann P, Bergans A, et al. Clin Endocrinol 1989;31:31–8.
138. Rudman D, Dedonis JL, Fountain MT, et al. N Engl J Med 1980;303:657–61.
139. Cunnane SC, Soma M, McAdoo KR, et al. J Nutr 1985;115:1498–503.
140. Geuex E, Mazur A, Cardot P, et al. J Nutr 1991;121:1222–7.
141. Nigam S, Averdunk R, Gunther T. Prostaglandins Leukotrienes Med 1986;23:1–10.
142. Rayssiguier Y, Geuex E, Bussiere L, et al. J Am Coll Nutr 1993;12:133–7.
143. Shils ME. Magnesium. In: Shils ME, Young VR, eds. Modern nutrition in health and disease. 7th ed. Philadelphia: Lea & Febiger, 1988;164–84.
144. Rudman E, Millekan WJ, Richardson TJ, et al. J Clin Invest 1975;55:94–104.
145. Baldwin D, Robinson PR, Zierler KL, et al. J Clin Invest 1952;31:850–8.
146. Whang R, Oei T, Aikawa JK, et al. Arch Intern Med 1984;144:1794–6.
147. Whang R, Hampton EM, Whang DD. Ann Pharmacother 1994;28:220–6.
148. Ryzen E, Wagers PW, Singer FR, et al. Crit Care Med 1985;13:19–21.
149. Chernow B, Bamberger S, Stoiko M, et al. Chest 1987;955: 391–7.
150. Fiaccadori E, del Canale S, Coffrini E, et al. Crit Care Med 1988;16:751–60.
151. Meyer KB, Madias NE. Miner Electrolyte Metab 1994; 20:201–13.
152. Kristiansen JH, Mortensen JB, Petersen KO. Clin Endocrinol 1985;22:103–16.
153. Christianssen C, Basstrup PC, Lindgreen P, et al. Acta Endocrinol 1978;88:528–34.
154. Purkerson ML, Rolf DB, Chase LR, et al. Kidney Int 1974;5:325–36.
155. Gullner HG, Gill JR Jr, Barter FC. Am J Med 1981;71: 578–82.
156. Swartz R. Fluid, electrolyte, and acid-base changes during renal failure. In: Kokko JP, Tannen RL, eds. Fluids and electrolytes. 3rd ed. Philadelphia: WB Saunders, 1996;515–6.
157. Keller J, Slatopolsky E, Delmez JA. Am J Kidney Dis 1994;24:453–60.
157a. Delmez JA, Keller J, Norword RY, et al. Kidney Int 1996; 49:163–7.
158. Flink EB. Alcohol Clin Exp 1986;10:590–4.
159. Abbott L, Nadler J, Rude RK. Alcohol Clin Exp 1994;18: 1076–82.
160. Laitinen K, Lamberg-Allardt C, Tunniner R, et al. N Engl J Med 1991;324:721–7.
161. Ascherio A, Rinn EB, Giovannucci GA, et al. Circulation 1992;86:1475–84.
162. Witteman JC, Willett WC, Stampfer MJ, et al. Circulation 1989;80:1320–7.
163. Sheehan JP. Magnesium Trace Elem (Abstract) 1990;9:320.
164. Mimouni F, Miodovnik RC, Tsang J, et al. Obstet Gynecol 1987;70:85–8.
165. Sjogren A, Floren CH, Nilsson A. Diabetes 1986;35:458–63.
166. Saggese G, Frederico G, Beretelloni S, et al. J Pediatr 1991;118:220–5.
167. Sjogren A, Floren C-H, Nilsson A. Magnesium 1988;7: 117–22.
168. Motil KJ, Altschuler SI, Grand RJ. J Pediatr 1985;7:473–9.
169. Paolisso G, Sgambato S, Gambardella A, et al. Am J Clin Nutr 1992;55:1161–7.
170. Kumar D, Leonard E, Rude RK. (Letter) Arch Intern Med 1978;138:660.
171. Resnick LM, Altura BT, Gupta RK et al. Diabetologia 1993;36:267–70.
172. Simon JA, Obarzanek E, Frederick MM. Am J Epidemiol 1994;139:130–40.
173. Albert DG, Morita Y, Iseri T. Circulation 1958;17:761–3.
174. Bauer FK, Martin HE, Mickey MR. Proc Soc Exp Biol Med 1965;120:466–8.
175. Tillman DW, Semple PF. Clin Sci 1988;75:395–402.
176. Gadallah M, Massry SG, Bigazzi R, et al. Am J Hypertens 1991;4:404–9.
177. Dyckner T, Wester PO. Br J Med 1983;286:1847–9.
178. Reyes AJ, Leary WP, Acosta-Barrios TN, et al. Curr Ther Res 1984;36:332–40.
179. Henderson DG, Schierup J, Schodt T. Br Med J 1986;293: 664–5.
180. Cappucio FP, Markandur ND, Beymon GW, et al. Br Med J 1985;291:235–8.
181. Zemel, PC, Zemel MB, Urberg M, et al. Am J Clin Nutr 1990;51:665–9.
182. Witteman JCM, Grobbee DE, Derkx FHM, et al. Am J Clin Nutr 1994;60:129–35.
183. Patki PS, Singh J, Gokhale SV, et al. Br Med J 1990; 301:521–3.
184. Trials of Hypertension Prevention Collaborative Research Group. JAMA 1992;267:1213–20.
185. Yamamoto ME, Applegate WB, Klag MJ, et al. Ann Epidemiol 1995;5:96–107.
186. Lind L, Lithell H, Pollare T, et al. Am J Hypertens 1991; 4:674–9.
187. Resnick LM, Gupta RKD, Fabrio B, et al. J Clin Invest 1994;94:1269–76.
188. Paolisso G, Galzerano D, Gambardella A, et al. J Hum Hypertens 1995:9:199–203.
189. Rosen, EU, Campbell PG, Moosa GM. J Pediatr 1970;77: 709–14.
190. Nichols BL, Alvarado J, Hazelwood CF, et al. Am J Clin Nutr 1978;31:176–88.
191. Jones CT, Sellwood RA, Evanson JM. Br Med J 1973;3:391–2.
192. Marier JR. Magnesium 1982;1:3–15.
193. Rubenowitz E, Axelsson G, Rylander R. Am J Epidemiol 1996;143:456–62.
194. Hammer DO, Hayden S. JAMA 1980;243:2399–400.
195. Leoni V, Fabiani L, Tichiarelli L. Arch Environ Health 1985; 40:274–8.

196. Comstock GW. Am J Epidemiol 1979;110:375–400.
196a. Elwood PC, Fehily AM, Ising H, et al. Eur J Clin Nutr 1996; 50:694–7.
197. Dyckner T, Wester PO. Am Heart J 1979;97:12–8.
198. Boyd JC, Bruns EE, Wills MR. Clin Chem 1983;29:178–9.
199. Whang R. Magnesium 1985;40:274–8.
200. Rasmussen HS. Arch Intern Med 1988;148:329–32.
201. Teo KK, Yusuf S, Collins R, et al. Br Med J 1991;303: 1499–503.
202. Lau J, Antman EM, Jimenez-Silva J, et al. N Engl J Med 1992:327:248–54.
203. Woods KL, Fletcher S, Roffe C, et al. Lancet 1992;339: 1553–8.
204. Woods KL, Fletcher S. Lancet 1994;343:816–9.
205. ISIS-4 (Fourth International Study of Infarct Survival) Collaborative Group. Lancet 1995;345:669–85.
206. Woods KL. Lancet 1995;346:611–4.
207. Baxter GF, Sumeray MS, Walker JM. Lancet 1996;348: 1424–6.
207a. Correspondence. Lancet 1997;349:282–3.
208. Hennekens CH, Albert CM, Godfried SL, et al. N Engl J Med 1996;335:1660–7.
209. Galloe AM, Rasmussen HS, Rasmussen HS, et al. Br Med J 1993;307:585–7.
210. Greco B, Jacobson HR. Fluid and electrolyte management in cardiac surgery. In: Kokko JP, Tannen RL, eds. Fluids and electrolytes. 3rd ed. Philadelphia: WB Saunders, 1996;749.
211. England MR, Gordon G, Salens M, et al. JAMA 1992;268: 2395–402.
212. Diaz J, Acosta F, Parilla P, et al. Transplantation 1996;61: 835–7.
213. Dorup I, Clausen T. Am J Physiol 1993;264:C457–563.
214. Krause SM. Am J Physiol 1990;261:H229–31.
215. Flink E. Acta Med Scand Suppl 1981;647:125–37.
216. Ramee SR, White CJ, Savarinth JT, et al. Am Heart J 1985;109:164–6.
217. Tzivoni D, Keren A. Am J Cardiol 1990;65:1397–9.
218. Stromme JH, Steen-Johnson J, Harnaes K, et al. Pediatr Res 1981;15:1134–9.
219. Allen DB, Greer FR. Calcium and magnesium deficiency beyond infancy. In: Tsang RC, ed. Calcium and magnesium metabolism in early life. Boca Raton, FL: CRC Press, 1995.
220. Altura BM, Altura BT. Magnesium Bull 1986;8:338–50.
221. Rude RK, Mamoogian C, Ehrich P, et al. Magnesium 1989;8:266–73.
222. Dechaux M, Kindermans C, Labordek K, et al. Kidney Int 1988;34:(A-25)S12–3.
223. Roberts JM, Redman CWG. Lancet 1993;341:1447–51.
224. Cunningham FG, Lindheimer MD. N Engl J Med 1992; 326:927–32.
225. Saunders N, Hammersley B. Lancet 1995;346:788–9.
225a. Levine RJ, Hauth JC, Curet LB, et al. N Engl J Med 1997;337:69–76.
226. Cholst IN, Steinberg SF, Tropper PJ, et al. N Engl J Med 1984;310:1221–5.
227. Eisunbud E, LoBoe CL. Arch Intern Med 1976;136:688–91.
228. McGuinness GA, Weinstein MM, Cruikshank DP et al. Obstet Gynecol 1980;56:595–600.
229. Donovan EF, Tsang RC, Steichen JJ, et al. J Pediatr 1980;96:305–10.
230. Santi MD, Henry GW, Douglas GL. J Pediatr Orthop 1994;14:249–53.
231. Nelson KB. Editorial. JAMA 1996;276:1843–33.
231a. Mittendorf R, Covert R, Bowman J, et al. Lancet 1997;350:1517–8.
231b. Editorial. Lancet 1997;350:1491.
232. Kattan M. Editorial. J Pediatr 1996;129:783–5.
233. Smilkstein MJ, Steedle D, Kulig KW, et al. Clin Toxicol 1988;26:51–65.
234. Clark BA, Brown RS. Am J Nephrol 1992;12:336–43.
235. Torralbo A, Portoles J, Perez A-JP, et al. Am Kidney Dis 1993;21:167–71.
236. Mordes JP, Wacker EC. Pharmacol Rev 1978;29:274–300.

SELECTED READINGS

Cowan JA, ed. The biological chemistry of magnesium . New York: VCH Publishers, 1995;1–254.

Garfinkel D, Garfinkel L. Magnesium and regulation of carbohydrate metabolism at the molecular level. Magnesium 1988;7:249–61.

Romani A, Marfella C, Scarpa A. Cell management, transport, and homeostasis: role of intracellular compartments. Miner Electrolyte Metab 1993;19:282–9.

Vernon WB. The role of magnesium in nucleic acid and protein metabolism. Magnesium 1988;7:234–48.

10. Iron in Medicine and Nutrition

VIRGIL F. FAIRBANKS

HISTORY OF IRON IN MEDICINE AND NUTRITION

Iron was a familiar metal in most of the ancient civilizations of the Mediterranean littoral and was used in numerous tools and weapons. This familiarity with iron may also have led to its early medicinal use. In the earliest extant manuscript, the Ebers papyrus of Egypt, rust was prescribed in an ointment to prevent baldness. In early Greece, a solution of iron in wine was esteemed as a means of restoring male potency. In the 17th century of our era, the most important clinical application of iron was discovered: the treatment of chlorosis, a disorder later shown to be due to iron deficiency (1).

Even before the role of iron in nutrition was firmly established, the first clinical description of iron overload disease was reported in 1871 (2). The earliest objective study of iron in human nutrition, performed nearly a century ago and published in 1895, showed that the diets of young women with chlorosis only provided 1 to 3 mg of iron daily, whereas the average iron content of diets of normal persons ranged from 8 to 11 mg daily (3). Yet, it was not until 1932 that a centuries-long controversy concerning the value of iron for treatment of chlorosis was finally resolved beyond doubt (4). The major aspects of iron metabolism were elucidated before 1960. Thousands of subsequent investigations have filled in important details.

Biologic Importance

More than any other metal, iron is a key element in the metabolism of all living organisms. The iron-sulfur complex of ferredoxins is required for an early step of photosynthesis. The iron-sulfur complex of aconitase in the tricarboxylic acid (Krebs) cycle intimately links the iron content of cells with energy production via oxidative phosphorylation both in carbohydrate and in lipid metabolism. Iron is a part of heme, which is the active site of electron transport in cytochromes and cytochrome oxidase. Heme is also the site of oxygen uptake by myoglobin and hemoglobin, thereby providing the means of transporting oxygen to tissues and within muscle cells. Hemoglobin in the root nodules of legumes protects nitrogen-fixing enzymes of symbiotic bacteria from oxidative inactivation. The ammonia formed is important in the synthesis of amino acids and proteins. The amino acids and proteins of legumes are transferred through the food chain to herbivores and thence to humans; we depend on them. Heme is also the active site of peroxidases that protect cells from oxidative injury by reducing peroxides to water. Figure 10.1 shows the structure of heme, a molecule vital to energy metabolism, electron transfer, nitrogen fixation, and oxygen transport.

Aconitase, a key enzyme of the Krebs cycle, catalyzes the interconversion of citrate, *cis*-aconitic acid, and isocitrate. This is the first step in the Krebs cycle, after condensation of acetyl-CoA and oxaloacetate to form citrate. Without aconitase, energy production becomes inefficient. Aconitase has an iron-sulfur cluster at its active site (Fig. 10.2). When there is sufficient iron in mitochondria or in cytosol, the iron-sulfur cluster of aconitase has a cubane, or cubelike, structure, with four atoms of iron and four

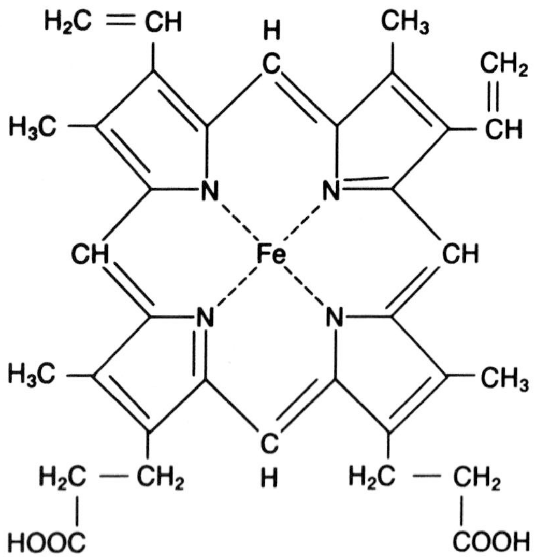

Figure 10.1. Structure of heme, showing iron at the center of a porphyrin ring. Heme is a component of hemoglobin, myoglobin, cytochromes, peroxidases, and cytochrome oxidase. In each of these, it is the functional site of the molecule, reversibly binding oxygen in hemoglobin and myoglobin, and serving as the site of the electron transfer in the oxidation-reduction reactions for which the other heme proteins are either enzymes or coenzymes.

atoms of sulfur at alternate apices (5, 6). This is the enzymatically active form of aconitase. On the other hand, when there is a deficiency of iron, the iron-sulfur complex is modified, with iron at only three apices (Fig. 10.2). In this form, aconitase is enzymatically inactive but becomes the iron-regulatory protein (IRP), binding to the iron-responsive elements of mRNA molecules for apoferritin, δ-aminolevulinic synthase, and transferrin receptor. By doing so, it inhibits synthesis of apoferritin but stimulates synthesis of the other two proteins. In this way, iron uptake and heme synthesis are regulated at the cellular level to meet the needs of oxidative phosphorylation via the Krebs cycle. Further details of this mechanism are presented below. Aconitase exists in both mitochondria and cytosol and both mitochondrial and cytosolic aconitase have the properties and functions described here.

Although iron is one of the most abundant metals on earth and in the universe, nearly all the iron in the environment is insoluble, existing as iron oxides or as metallic iron. Thus, little iron is available for biologic needs, and living organisms treasure iron as if it were a trace element. Our bodies zealously defend the few grams of iron that are within each of us—for iron, in its extraordinary variety of biologically active forms, is the metal of life.

IRON METABOLISM

Compartments

In humans, the total quantity of body iron varies with weight, hemoglobin concentration, sex, and size of the storage compartment. Table 10.1 shows approximate normal values for iron in various compartments. Of these, the largest is the iron in hemoglobin, contained within circulating erythrocytes. The size of this compartment varies considerably according to body weight, sex, and blood hemoglobin concentration. For example, a person weighing 50 kg (110 lb) whose blood hemoglobin concentration is 120 g/L (12.0 g/dL) would have a hemoglobin compartment iron content of 1.4 g. The size of the storage compartment, in which iron is contained in ferritin and hemosiderin, is also markedly influenced by age, sex, body size, and whether there has been excess iron loss (e.g., from bleeding or pregnancy) or iron overloading (e.g., hemochromatosis). Women and children often have very little storage iron. The tissue iron pool includes myoglobin and the tiny but essential fraction of iron in enzymes. The "labile pool," a rapidly recycling component defined by iron kinetic studies, does not have a definable anatomic or cellular location. The transport compartment is iron bound to transferrin, the iron-transport protein in plasma. This compartment is small but quite active; normally 20 to 30 mg cycles through the transport compartment daily. The main metabolic pathways of iron metabolism are illustrated in Figures 10.3 and 10.4. Further details concerning cellular iron metabolism and the proteins of the storage and transport compartments are given below.

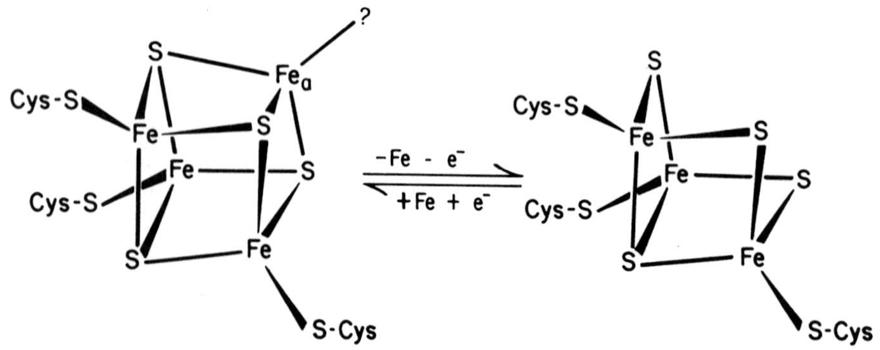

Figure 10.2. Iron-sulfur cluster of aconitase. This protein is involved both in glucose and fat metabolism and in regulation of iron metabolism. When iron is in abundance, it assumes the cubane structure shown on the *left;* when there is little iron in the cytosol, it loses an atom of iron, and it then has a more open structure as shown on the *right.* These changes in configuration are involved in its interaction with the stem-loop IREs shown in Figures 10.8 and 10.9. It functions in glucose and fat metabolism only in the iron-rich cubane configuration. (From Beinert H, Kennedy MC. FASEB J 1993;7:1442–9, with permission.)

Table 10.1
Iron Compartments in Normal Man[a]

Compartment	Iron Content (mg)	Total-Body Iron (%)
Hemoglobin iron	2000	67
Storage iron	1000	27
Tissue iron		
Myoglobin iron	130	3.5
Enzyme iron	8	0.2
Labile iron pool	80	2.2
Transport iron	3	0.08

[a]These values represent estimates for an "average" man: 70 kg, 177 cm (70 in). They are derived from data in several sources.

Intake

The average daily intake of iron in North American and Europe is between 10 and 20 mg, about 5 to 7 mg of iron per 1000 calories. A weight-conscious young woman who limits her intake to between 1000 and 1500 calories/day may consume only 6 to 9 mg of food iron, and if her diet consists largely of snack foods, pizza, and soft drinks, which have negligible iron content, it will be well below that.

Some natural fruit juices contain significant amounts of iron, but beer and soft drinks are generally quite poor in iron. Distilled alcoholic beverages are also iron poor. Some European ciders and wines may contain 16 mg of iron or more per liter. The iron content of city water supplies is usually less than 5 mg/L, but water from some deep wells may have a higher iron concentration. Table 10.2 shows the iron content of many commonly eaten foods (7–9). Since the quantity of food eaten is driven mostly by caloric need, it is most sensible to consider the iron content of foods as a function of their caloric value. The last column of the table shows this relationship. In this table, food groups are ranked according to their iron content per kilocalorie. Green vegetables and legumes provide the highest iron:calories ratios; milk products, snack foods, and soft drinks, the lowest. To the extent that the diet contains generous amounts of green vegetables or legumes, iron intake should be sufficient; to the extent that milk products, snack foods, and soft drinks predominate, iron nutrition will be poor.

In recent decades, there has been a marked shift in food consumption patterns in the United States, with progressive decline in consumption of meat or other sources of readily assimilable iron, and an increase in consumption of foods that are either low in iron content or contain iron in a form that is not readily assimilated. This trend since 1980 is shown in Figure 10.5 (10–12). For example, during the 25 years prior to 1995, the annual consumption

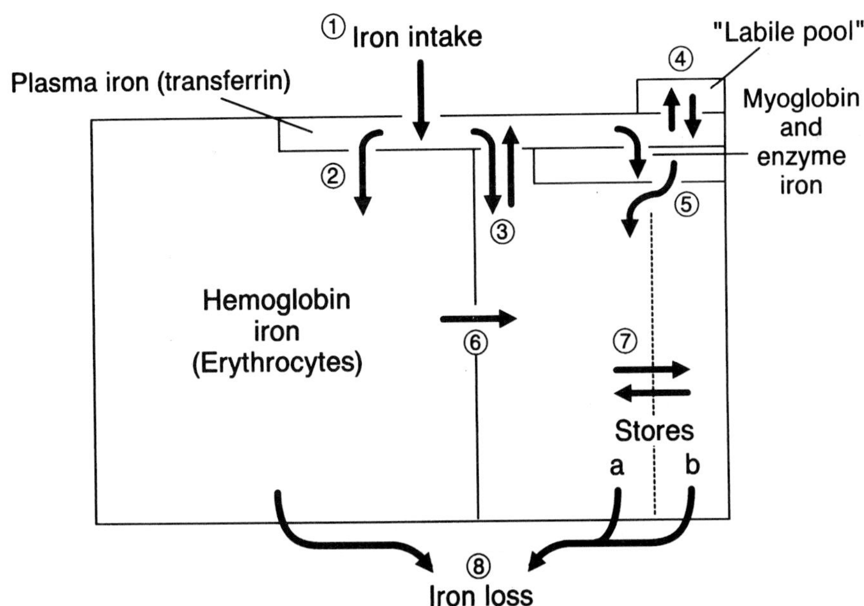

Figure 10.3. Scheme for the metabolic pathways of iron. Iron intake *(1)* is normally about 1 mg/day, by absorption from the upper intestinal tract, and is balanced by 1 mg of iron loss *(8)*, predominantly by exfoliation of epithelial cells of the intestinal mucosa. When iron loss exceeds 1 mg/day (e.g., during the reproductive years in women or from other blood loss), iron absorption must be proportionately increased. Iron absorbed by the small bowel is transported by transferrin in plasma predominantly (normally ~80% of absorbed iron) to hematopoietic bone marrow *(2)*, where hemoglobin is formed in erythrocytes later released into circulating blood. A smaller amount of iron enters other compartments, iron stores as ferritin and hemosiderin in many organs *(3)*, myoglobin in muscle cells, and enzyme iron in all cells *(5)*. A "labile pool" *(4)* may be iron that passes from plasma to lymph and then recycles into plasma via the lymphatic duct. When erythrocytes have completed their normal life span of 4 months in circulation, the metabolically "rundown," or senescent, red cells are phagocytized and digested by monocytes and macrophages of bone marrow, spleen, liver, lymph nodes, and other organs *(6)*. Some of the iron released in macrophages by hemoglobin catabolism is retained as storage iron, but most is reused by recycling to plasma and then to hematopoietic bone marrow (*3* to *2*), where this cycle begins anew. In the storage compartment *(7)*, iron exists in a rapidly exchanging pool *(a)* and a slowly exchanging pool *(b)*. The former corresponds to ferritin, and the latter to hemosiderin. A small amount of both hemosiderin and ferritin may be lost in feces as a result of exfoliation of intestinal epithelial cells *(8)*. Normally, a minute amount of blood is also lost in feces.

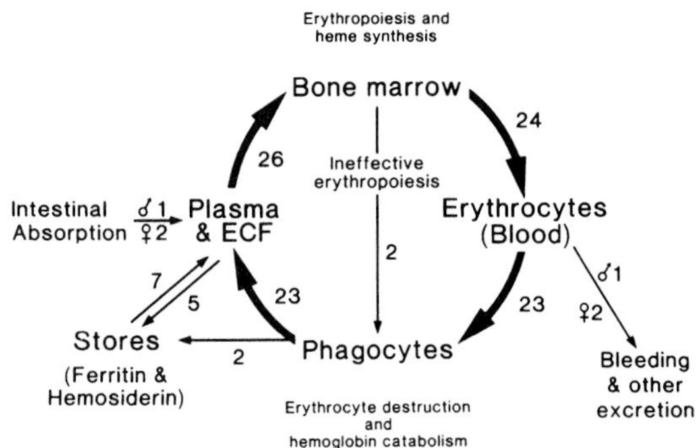

Figure 10.4. Iron cycle in humans. Iron is tightly conserved in a nearly closed system in which each iron atom cycles repeatedly from plasma and extracellular fluid *(ECF)* to *bone marrow,* where it is incorporated into hemoglobin. It then enters the peripheral blood within *erythrocytes* and circulates in the blood for 4 months. It then travels to *phagocytes* of the reticuloendothelial system, where senescent erythrocytes are engulfed and destroyed, hemoglobin is digested, and iron is released to *plasma,* where the cycle continues. With each cycle, a small proportion of iron is transferred to *stores,* where it is incorporated into ferritin or hemosiderin. A small proportion of storage iron is released to plasma; a small proportion is lost in urine, sweat, feces, or blood; and an equivalent small amount of iron is absorbed from the intestinal tract. In addition, a small proportion (about 10%) of newly formed erythrocytes normally is destroyed within the bone marrow and its iron released, bypassing the circulating blood part of the cycle *(ineffective erythropoiesis). Numbers* indicate the approximate amount of iron (in mg) that enters and leaves each of these iron compartments every day in healthy adults who do not have bleeding and other blood disorders.

of mozzarella cheese in the United States increased from 224 million pounds to 2.09 billion pounds, a compound rate of increase of 9.3% annually, and a 933% increase in mozzarella cheese consumption during this interval (13). At least 80% of the mozzarella cheese is consumed in the form of pizza. From 1985 to 1995, the consumption of pizza more than doubled. Pizza is now a major "fast food" in the American diet. It is predominantly a milk-and-flour product, with variable amounts of sausage. There is a negligible amount of iron in milk or cheese, and only a small amount of poorly absorbed metallic iron in flour. The same may be said of many other "fast food" products.

Surveys indicating that the total iron content of the average American diet has slightly increased during this decade must be considered in the context of the increasingly poor nutritional quality of the iron in the American diet. Approximately half the iron ingested in the average American diet is in the form of bread or other grain products from which it is poorly absorbed. In 1988 to 1991, median intakes of iron from food were less than recommended dietary allowance (RDA) values for children aged 1 to 2 years and for adolescent and adult women (13). Furthermore, for women aged 18 to 44 years, the population group most at risk of iron-deficiency anemia, the mean daily iron intake has been one-third less than the RDA of 15 mg. Non-Hispanic white women in this age group had a mean iron intake 24% below the RDA in 1989; African American and Hispanic women had mean iron intakes that were only 67 and 65% of the RDA, respectively (10–12, 14). During the reproductive years, most women cannot avoid negative iron balance, and many cannot avoid becoming anemic at these inadequate levels of iron intake.

Absorption

Mechanisms

In healthy persons who do not lose iron by bleeding, iron loss is very limited. Therefore, normal iron balance is maintained largely by regulation of iron absorption. Ingested inorganic iron is solubilized and ionized by acid gastric juice, reduced to the ferrous (FeII) form, and chelated. Iron absorption is promoted by substances that form low-molecular-weight iron chelates, such as ascorbic acid, sugars, and amino acids. The mucin of normal gastric juice chelates and stabilizes iron, thereby reducing its precipitation at the alkaline pH of the small intestine. Impaired iron absorption in achlorhydric or gastrectomized persons reflects decreased solubilization and chelation of the ferric iron in food.

Absorption may occur at any level of the small intestine, but it is most efficient in the duodenum. Prior to uptake by the brush border of the mucosal cell, the iron atom must first traverse the mucous layer. Passage of iron through this layer is facilitated by organic acids (15–16) or taurocholic acid (17) in normal bile or by polypeptides containing cysteine from digestion of meat, fish, or poultry (18–19). The divalent, or Fe(II), form of iron is more readily soluble than the trivalent, or Fe(III), form because of the low solubility of ferric hydroxides and phosphates at the alkaline pH of intestinal fluid. Thus, Fe(II) more readily traverses the mucous layer to reach the brush border of intestinal epithelial cells.

From mucin, iron is taken up by one or more proteins on the lumenal surface of the mucosal epithelium of the duodenum (20–21) (Fig. 10.6). Cell membrane proteins that have been postulated to function in this way are *(a)* an iron-binding protein that is a trimer of 54-kDa subunits (22); *(b)* a β_3-integrin of approximately 160 kDa that spans the cell membrane, and which consists of subunits of 150 kDa and 90 kDa (23); *(c)* the Hfe protein of approximately 44 kDa that also spans the cell membrane and functions together with β_2-microglobulin, a small protein of approximately 11 kDa (also see Fig. 10.14, in the section on hereditary hemochromatosis); *(d)* Nramp2, also a transmembrane protein. Each of these iron-binding proteins of the cell surface has been described by different investigators. It is not yet clear how they interact in determining the rate of iron absorption. It is also possible that different investigators have described the same iron-binding protein but given it different names. Integrins are known to bind cations and facilitate their absorption. By analogy with calreticulin, a related integrin, the β_3-integrin of the intestinal mucosal epithelium may interact in some man-

Table 10.2
Iron Content of Some Commonly Consumed Foods, Ranked by Food Group in Approximate Order of Iron Content per 1000 kcal

Food	Serving Size	Caloric Value (kcal)	Iron Content (mg/serving)	Iron Content (mg/1000 kcal)
Vegetables, cooked	1/2 cup			
Broccoli		25	0.9	36.0
Spinach		30	1.4	31.4
Lentils		115	3.3	28.7
Beans, red kidney		110	1.6	14.5
Beans, green		25	0.9	36.0
Peas		65	1.2	18.4
Cabbage		10	0.2	20.0
Beets		25	0.5	20.0
Corn		90	0.5	5.6
Potato, peeled, boiled	1 medium	115	0.4	3.5
Bread or flour-based foods (without butter or other spreads)				
Spaghetti, cooked	1 cup	155	1.7	11.0
Bagel, medium plain	1	200	1.8	9.0
Bread, white or whole wheat	1 slice	70	0.6	8.6
Croissant, medium (2 oz)	1	230	1.0	4.4
Meat, poultry, fish, eggs				
Beef, lean	3 oz.	215	0.9	4.2
Sausage				
Bologna	1 slice	90	0.4	4.4
Pepperoni	1 slice	25	0.1	4.0
Fish (nonbreaded)	3 oz	200	1.0	5.0
Chicken breast (skinless, roasted)		140	0.9	6.4
Egg, whole, boiled	1 large	75	0.7	9.3
Sandwiches				
Roast beef	1	345	4.0	11.6
Hamburger, regular	1	245	2.2	9.0
Cheeseburger, regular	1	300	2.3	7.7
Rice, brown, natural, cooked	1/2 cup	110	0.5	4.3
Fruits				
Grape	10	26	0.2	5.5
Avocado, Calif.	1 medium	305	0.3	5.0
Apples/pears	1 medium	100	0.3	3.0
Peaches/plums	1/2 cup	35	1.6	2.8
Bananas	1 medium	100	0.4	4.0
Oranges, raw	1 medium	40	0.1	2.5
Strawberries, raw	1/2 cup	40	0.3	7.5
Nuts				
Walnuts, English	14 halves	180	0.7	3.9
Pecans	1 oz	190	0.6	3.2
Peanut butter, natural	1 tb (15 mL)	95	0.3	3.2
Beverages				
Apple juice	1/2 cup	110	0.5	4.5
Orange juice	1/2 cup	55	0.2	3.6
Grape juice	1/2 cup	80	0.3	3.8
Cranberry juice	1/2 cup	75	0.2	2.7
Soft drinks	12 oz	125	0.2	1.6
Wine, dry, 12% ethanol	3.5 oz	87	0.4	4.6
Milk, whole	240 mL	150	0.1	0.7
City water, from well[a]	240 mL	0	0.1	—
Snack foods and pizza[b]				
Potato chips	1 oz	150	0.0	0.0
Fritos	1 oz	150	0.2	1.3
Chee-tos	1 oz	150	0.2	1.3
Tortilla chips	1 oz	150	0.2	1.3
Pretzels	1 oz	110	0.6	5.4
Popcorn (vegetable oil)	1 oz	160	0.4	2.5
Pizza (plain, sausage, or pepperoni)	1 slice	350	0.7	2.0
Dairy products				
Milk, whole	1 cup	150	0.1	0.7
Milk, skim	1 cup	85	0.1	1.2
Butter	1 tsp (4 mL)	90	trace	—
Cheese, mozzarella	1 slice (1 oz)	80	0.1	1.2

Data in this table are derived from several sources, including ref. 7–9.

[a]Municipal water, unsoftened, Rochester, MN.

[b]Data for snack foods and pizza are those shown on package labels. Pizza varies considerably between brands in calories per serving and iron content; the latter ranged from 0 to 15% of the RDA. The figures shown here represent average values for several brands.

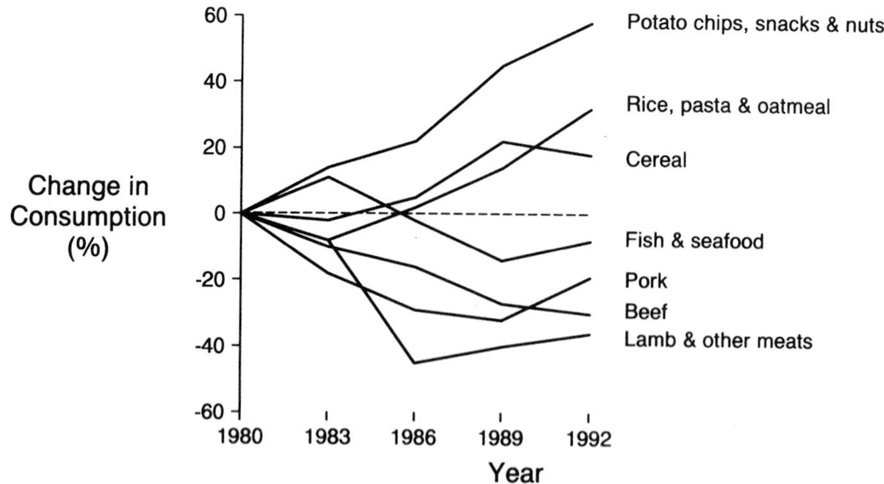

Figure 10.5. Changes in dietary patterns in the United States during the 12-year interval 1980–1992. (Based on data from ref. 10–13.)

ner with β_2-microglobulin and the Hfe protein to effect the uptake of iron from the intestinal lumen. This process remains to be elucidated.

Recently described is Nramp2, a transmembrane protein that is particularly expressed in epithelial cells of the upper duodenum but occurs also in most other cells, including the erythroblasts of bone marrow (24–25). Nramp2 is a member of a class of proteins designated *n*atural *r*esistance-*a*ssociated *m*acrophage *p*roteins. Nramp1 is responsible for resistance to mycobacterial and leishmanial infections, particularly by macrophages. However, the structurally similar protein Nramp2 is essential for iron absorption by intestinal epithelial cells and may also be the intracellular iron transport protein in the erythroblast. Inbred mice with hereditary microcytic anemia that are mk/mk homozygotes have a mutation in the Nramp2 gene that renders them unable to absorb iron from the diet. They also do not respond to parenterally administered iron, which implies impaired iron uptake by both intestinal epithelium and erythroblasts. Lack of this protein in erythroblasts causes hereditary microcytic anemia in Belgrade laboratory rats.

Once inside the mucosal epithelial cell, the iron is transferred successively to cytosolic proteins designated

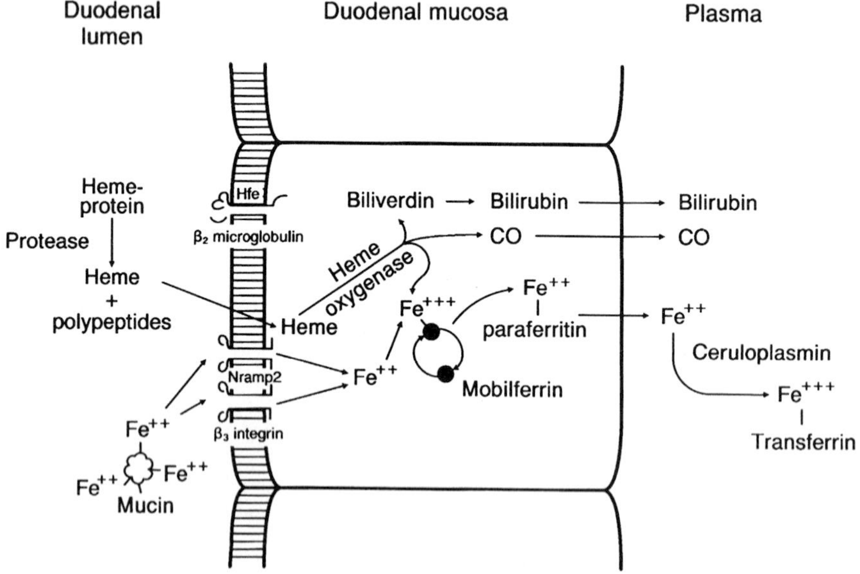

Figure 10.6. Scheme for the mechanism of iron uptake by duodenal epithelial cells and its transport across the epithelial cell to plasma of the subepithelial capillaries. At least eight proteins appear involved in this mechanism: *mucin* in the gastric and *duodenal lumen, β_3 integrin, Nramp2,* and *Hfe* proteins in cell membranes, *mobilferrin* and *paraferritin* within the cytosol, *ceruloplasmin* and *transferrin* in plasma. Either an iron-Nramp2 complex or an iron-integrin complex is internalized and complexed with mobilferrin; the iron is then transferred to paraferritin, which acts as the cytoplasmic iron-transport protein that delivers iron to the serosal side of the cell, where it is released as Fe(II), oxidized by ceruloplasmin to Fe(III), and taken up by transferrin in capillaries for transport to the rest of the body. Heme is also taken up by epithelial cells, but the iron must then be released by heme oxygenase before it is bound to paraferritin. It is not yet clear how the Hfe protein normally regulates this mechanism. Some of the complexities in this model may become better resolved in the next few years. (Based in part on Conrad ME, Umbreit JN, Raymond DA, et al. Blood 1993;81:517–21, with permission.)

mobilferrin (26) and paraferritin (27). It is then transported to the serosal surface of the epithelial cell, and it passes through this side of the cell membrane in the Fe(II) state. As it enters the blood of the subendothelial capillary network, it is oxidized by ceruloplasmin to Fe(III), and it is then bound to transferrin, which carries it in the portal venous system, first to the liver and then to all the tissues of the body.

A major source of iron in the diet is heme iron derived mostly from hemoglobin trapped in capillaries and myoglobin of muscle. Much lesser amounts of iron are obtained from peroxidases and cytochromes in the diet. To be absorbed, iron contained in heme proteins must be successively liberated, first by digestion of the protein, with liberation of heme (26–29). Heme is absorbed as such by the mucosal epithelium of the small bowel, although exactly how this occurs is not yet known. Within the cytosol, iron is liberated from protoporphyrin by the microsomal enzyme heme oxygenase, which breaks the porphyrin ring, yielding Fe(III), biliverdin, and CO. Fe(III) is then bound by paraferritin and transported to the serosal side of the cell, as described above. Biliverdin is converted to bilirubin, which is transported in plasma to the liver for excretion. The carbon monoxide released by heme catabolism is transported to the lungs for excretion in exhaled air.

Absorption of heme iron is not increased by ascorbic acid nor is it depressed by such substances as phytates and desferrioxamine. Its absorption is only slightly inhibited by simultaneous administration of inorganic iron and nonheme iron (30–32).

In mid-1996 the gene was identified for the major hereditary iron-overloading disorder, hereditary hemochromatosis (European or HLA-linked type) (33). This gene is responsible for synthesis of an MHC class I protein that spans the membranes of all cells that have been examined. On the cell surface it is associated with β_2-microglobulin, and together these proteins have homologies with immunoglobulins. This protein, which commonly is structurally altered in hereditary hemochromatosis, has been designated Hfe protein. It is presently unknown how it serves to regulate the absorption of iron by intestinal mucosal cells, although clearly, it must do so. As stated above, this mechanism may involve an interaction with β_3-integrin and Nramp2. Quite likely, this Hfe protein normally restricts uptake of iron when there is sufficient iron in the cytosol and permits iron uptake when there is not. The Hfe protein and its gene mutations are considered further in the section on hereditary hemochromatosis.

Intraluminal Factors

Intraluminal factors that decrease absorption include rapid transit time, achylia, malabsorption syndromes, precipitation by alkalinization, phosphates, phytates, and ingested alkaline clays or antacid preparations. Milk proteins, albumin, and soy proteins reduce iron absorption (34–36). However, ingestion of milk together with cereals neither enhances nor reduces the effect of cereal on iron absorption in humans. Tea and coffee both reduce iron absorption substantially, in proportion to the amount of tea or coffee ingested. Iron absorption is reduced about 60% by tea and about 40% by coffee (37–39). Phytate is inositol hexaphosphate, a substance that normally occurs in the fiber or bran component of wheat, rice, maize, psyllium, walnuts, peanuts, hazelnuts, and plant lignins, and which chelates iron, reducing its absorption (40–46). As little as 5 to 10 mg of phytate in bread can reduce nonheme iron absorption by 50% (42), and this effect of phytate on iron absorption can be maintained indefinitely (43). Addition of meat or ascorbic acid to the diet reverses the iron-chelating effect of phytate (42). Some other plant fibers such as that derived from yod kratin (leaves of the Southeast Asian lead tree) also reduce iron absorption (47), but cellulose does not (48). Beet fiber (β fiber) also does not appear to inhibit iron absorption (44). In contrast with the effect of phytate in retarding food iron absorption in humans, both rats and anemic pigs seem to absorb iron equally well from phytate-rich and phytate-poor diets (49). Concomitant ingestion of zinc and iron salts reduces iron absorption in humans (50).

As the ingested dose of iron increases, the total amount retained by the body rises steadily, although the percentage absorbed decreases. Plotting the logarithm of iron dosage against the logarithm of iron absorbed yields a straight line (51). For each twofold increment in iron dosage, a 1.6-fold increment in absorption can be anticipated. Uptake is increased by large oral doses of ascorbic acid, by certain weak chelating substances (e.g., citric acid, succinic acid, sugars, sulfur-containing amino acids) and by mucin. Digestion of meat or poultry enhances the absorption of iron by releasing cysteine or cysteine-containing small polypeptides (18, 19). The effects of ethanol ingestion and of deficient pancreatic exocrine function on iron absorption have been disputed. Whether ingested or administered parenterally, ethanol has little, if any, direct effect on iron absorption in humans and may even retard it (52). In rats, addition of alcohol to the diet increased iron absorption (53). In humans, acute or chronic alcohol consumption does not appear to increase iron absorption (54).

Systemic Regulation

The systemic regulatory mechanisms that influence iron absorption have never been identified despite intensive search. They operate to *(a)* increase absorption in iron deficiency and in hemochromatosis, during the latter half of pregnancy and when erythropoiesis is stimulated (including ineffective erythropoiesis) as in anemias or hypoxic states, and *(b)* decrease absorption in iron overload, in chronic disease such as rheumatoid arthritis, or in other circumstances when erythropoiesis is depressed.

With elucidation of Hfe and Nramp2 proteins, regulation of the rate of iron absorption may become better understood in the next few years.

Absorption of iron is modulated by intestinal mucosal cells. The columnar mucosal cells formed in crypts at the base of villi contain a variable amount of iron, which helps to regulate the quantity of intraluminal iron that enters cells. The iron in intestinal epithelial cells may enter the body according to need or may remain in ferritin within these cells to limit absorption and be lost when the cells are sloughed from the tips of villi at the end of their brief life spans. Little iron is incorporated into ferritin in the mucosal cells of iron-deficient subjects, and absorption is enhanced. Conversely, in iron-loaded subjects, the mucosal cells formed are well endowed with iron in ferritin; transport of iron into plasma is limited, and cellular iron is excreted when desquamation occurs.

Absorption from Foods

Healthy persons absorb about 5 to 10% of dietary iron, and those who are iron deficient absorb about 10 to 20%. The maximum amount of iron absorption expected from an average diet in the United States is about 1 to 2 mg in normal adults and 3 to 6 mg in iron-deficient patients.

The earliest measurements of iron absorption were made with balance techniques. The small difference between oral intake and fecal loss is difficult to measure with precision by chemical methods. Furthermore, such methods cannot distinguish excreted iron from iron contained in mucosal epithelial cells that have been desquamated into the intestinal lumen. Such balance studies were done using mixed diets fed over a period of several weeks; the effect of daily variation on results was minimized. Iron absorption, calculated on the basis of positive balance, ranged from 7.3 to 21% (55).

Table 10.3
Approximate Amount of Iron (mg) That May Be Absorbed from 10 mg of Iron Ingested in Various Foods

	Adult		Infant or Child	
Food	Normal	Fe Deficient	Normal	Fe Deficient
Liver	1.0	2.7		
Beef	1.0	3.0		
Veal	2.2			
Fish	1.2			
Eggs	0.3	0.8	0.7	
Soybeans	1.2	2.7		
Breakfast cereal and milk			1.2	
Lettuce	0.3	2.8		
Green vegetables	0.3	2.8		
Wheat	0.5	0.7		
Enriched bread	0.7	5.0		
Corn	0.4	0.8		
Milk	0.2		0.8	1.6
Beans	0.2			
Spinach	0.1			
Rice	0.08			

Based on data cited in ref. 56.

Single foods prepared or grown to contain a radionuclide of iron have been used to measure absorption of iron from these foods after they are prepared and fed as in a normal diet. Table 10.3 presents typical results (56). Overall absorption in 219 normal subjects approximated 10%, and that in 148 iron-deficient patients, 20%. Absorption of iron from food varies widely. It is greatest from meat of mammalian origin (e.g., beef), less from poultry or fish, and least from liver, muscle, eggs, milk, and cereals (57). It is generally greater in children than in adults.

Figure 10.7 summarizes results obtained in 520 subjects using seven foods of vegetable origin and five of animal origin (58). Iron absorption from meat exceeded 10%. Iron absorption from rice and spinach was poor, but that from soybeans exceeded iron absorption from other vegetable sources. Since radioiron-tagged foods were given as a single test dose, daily variations in absorption were not measured, nor was the effect of possible interactions between specific foods and iron absorption determined. For example, ascorbic acid increased, and eggs decreased, uptake of iron from some foods.

Polyphenols (e.g., plant tannins) and phytate retard absorption of food iron. The effects of organic acids, phytates, and polyphenols on absorption of dietary iron were studied by a radionuclide tag method in which $^{59}FeSO_4$ was mixed with food prior to ingestion by human subjects and the amount of ^{59}Fe retained was measured. Iron was poorly absorbed from wheat germ, lima beans, spinach, lentils, and beet greens, all foods with high phytate or oxalic acid content. In contrast, there was good-to-moderate iron absorption from carrots, potatoes, beet roots, pumpkin, broccoli, tomatoes, cauliflower, cabbage, turnips, and sauerkraut, all vegetables that contain substantial amounts of malic, citric, or ascorbic acids (59).

In Western-type whole meals, iron absorption is enhanced by inclusion of beef, poultry, or fish and by ascorbic acid. Meals that include principally pizza, hamburger, or spaghetti and cheese result in poor iron absorption, whereas those containing cod, beef, shrimp, or chicken result in good iron absorption. (It is not clear why iron absorption from the hamburger-based meal is poor; perhaps phytates in the bun or the milk in the milkshake inhibit iron absorption.) In one study, the best iron absorption resulted from an Italian meal of antipasto misto, spaghetti, meat, bread, oranges, and wine (60). In addition to the dietary factors enumerated above, soy flour proteins have been reported to retard (61) or enhance (62) iron absorption, while soy sauce enhances iron absorption (63).

The effects of food mixtures on iron absorption have also been investigated (64–66). One vegetable (maize or black beans) and one animal food (fish or veal muscle) tagged with different radionuclides (^{55}Fe and ^{59}Fe) were fed to the same subjects separately and mixed in the same meal. Iron absorption from veal was diminished about

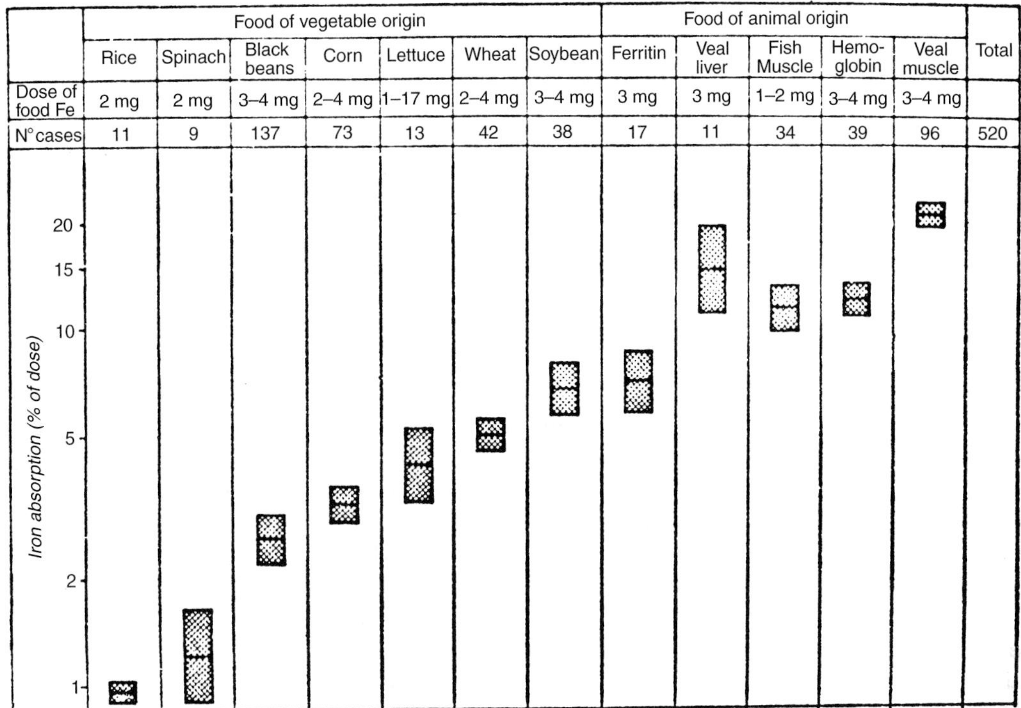

Figure 10.7. Absorption of iron from foods. (From Layrisse M, Cook JD, Martinez C, et al. Blood 1969;33:430–43, with permission.)

20% when veal was combined with vegetable foods; iron absorption from either maize or black beans was almost doubled when these foods were mixed with animal meat, such as veal, poultry, or fish. Furthermore, the enhancing effect could be duplicated by substituting amino acids in the same composition as in fish muscle. Cysteine seemed primarily responsible for the enhancing effect (19, 20).

Thus, overall iron absorption from a meal that contains many components cannot be estimated reliably from the percentage of iron absorption that would occur if single foods are separately fed. This is particularly true of attempts to estimate the adequacy of iron nutrition by tabulating iron content of foods without considering two facts: *(a)* some forms of iron, such as heme, are readily absorbed, whereas metallic iron and trivalent iron are not, and *(b)* phytates and other inhibitors of iron absorption are commonly present in foods and beverages and will significantly decrease iron absorption.

Table 10.4 shows the effect of various combinations of food on iron absorption. The authors of this study (67) thoughtfully observed, with respect to the amount of iron that could be absorbed daily from different diets, that

> a diet of low bioavailability supplies only about 0.7 mg of iron daily, which is insufficient to meet the normal physiological requirements of females and many males. The diet of intermediate bioavailability supplies about 1.4 mg daily, which is sufficient to meet the needs of more than 50% of women. The diet of high bioavailability supplies 2.1 mg daily, which meets the requirements of most adult members of the population . . . none of the diets is sufficient to match the daily requirements of 5–6 mg daily, which occur during the second and third trimesters of pregnancy.

Table 10.4
Relative Bioavailability of Iron in the Presence of Various Dietary Components

	Bioavailability of Iron		
Dietary Components	Low	Medium	High
Cereals	Maize	Corn flour	
	Oat meal	White flour	
	Rice		
	Sorghum		
	Whole wheat flour		
Fruits	Apple	Cantaloupe	Guava
	Avocado	Mango	Lemon
	Banana	Pineapple	Orange
	Grape		Pawpaw
	Peach		Tomato
	Pear		
	Plum		
	Rhubarb		
	Strawberry		
Vegetables	Eggplant	Carrot	Beets
	Lima beans	Potato	Broccoli
	Fava beans		Cabbage
	Lentils		Cauliflower
	Spinach		Pumpkin
			Turnip
Nuts	Almond		
	Brazil		
	Coconut		
	Peanut		
	Walnut		
High-protein foods	Egg		Fish
	Isolated soy protein		Meat
	Soy flour		Poultry

Adapted from Bothwell TH. J Intern Med 1989;226:357–65, with permission.

Transport

In blood or other body fluids, iron is transported by a protein called transferrin. Transferrin binds iron that either is released from intestinal epithelium into the blood or lymph or is secreted from macrophages following degradation of hemoglobin. It distributes transferrin iron throughout the body to wherever it is needed, mostly to erythrocyte precursors in the bone marrow for new hemoglobin synthesis.

Transferrins and lactoferrins comprise a group of iron transport proteins that are structurally and functionally quite similar. They are single polypeptide chains of approximately 679 amino acids, approximately 80 kDa in mass (68–71). Transferrin is the normal plasma protein that transports iron between various iron compartments. Lactoferrin occurs in a variety of body fluids including milk, semen, and the cytosol of granulocytes. It may function as an intracellular iron trap that protects the cytosol from potential superoxide injury induced by Fe(II).

Transferrins and lactoferrins are carbohydrate-rich globular proteins with single polypeptide chains. Each molecule has two binding sites for trivalent iron and two for bicarbonate. Each is bilobed, and within each lobe the iron-binding site is in a cleft between two domains designated N and C (for amino terminal and carboxy terminal) (70–72). Thus, each complete transferrin or lactoferrin molecule has two N domains and two C domains (e.g., N-C-hinge-N-C). The two lobes, or half molecules, consist of a complex of helices and β-pleated sheets, and the two lobes are connected by a "hinge" consisting of two linked helical segments. Within each lobe, Fe (III) is bound to both the N and C domains, which fold over the iron to bind it tightly. Each of the two C domains has a polysaccharide sialic acid side-chain that is so branched that it may be two-pronged or three-pronged, called *biantennary* or *triantennary*, respectively. Human transferrin is predominantly (80%) biantennary. The polysaccharide chains are bound to asparagine at amino acid positions 413 and 510. The polysaccharide chains may represent a signal for binding to the cell membrane. The transferrin gene is on chromosome 3. The complete DNA sequence of the gene has been determined (70).

Congenital deficiency of transferrin is extremely rare; only 9 cases are known worldwide (see below). Congenital inability to sialylate apotransferrin, the "carbohydrate-deficient transferrin syndrome," is associated with severe neurologic abnormalities, including seizures, hyperreflexia, peripheral neuropathy, and mental retardation (72, 73). Chronic alcoholics also have reduced sialylation of transferrin, but the alterations are difficult to demonstrate, so measurement of this analyte in serum is not a reliable test for chronic alcoholism.

One atom of Fe(III) can be bound, together with a bicarbonate ion, at each of the two binding sites. In humans, the two iron-binding sites seem to be functionally equivalent. When no iron is bound to the transferrin molecule, it is designated apotransferrin. Monoferric transferrin has one Fe(III), diferric transferrin, two. When all iron-binding sites are occupied by Fe(III), transferrin is said to be saturated. Normally, plasma transferrin is approximately one-third saturated; it is a mixture of monoferric and diferric transferrin.

The normal concentration of transferrin in plasma is about 2.2 to 3.5 g/L. Since iron is the natural ligand of transferrin, the plasma concentration of transferrin may be measured by the amount of iron that it will bind. This is called the total iron-binding capacity, or TIBC. The normal serum TIBC is about 45 to 80 μmol/L (250–450 μg/dL). The amount of iron actually bound to transferrin is measured as the serum iron concentration, or SI. The SI normally ranges from 12 to 31 μmol/L (70–175 μg/dL) in males and 11 to 29 μmol/L (60–165 μg/dL) in women. Percentage transferrin saturation (Tsat) is calculated as $(100 \times SI) \div TIBC$. The serum iron concentration normally exhibits diurnal variation. Highest values occur in midmorning (6–10 AM). Values are lower in midafternoon, and lower yet in the evening, with a nadir near midnight. In iron-deficiency anemia, SI is usually diminished, TIBC may be increased, and Tsat may be less than 15%. In iron-overload disorders, SI often exceeds 40 μmol/L, TIBC is usually normal or diminished, and Tsat may be 100%. In acute diseases (e.g., acute infections or myocardial infarction) and probably following immunizations, SI is diminished, TIBC is normal, and Tsat is diminished. In chronic disorders (e.g., chronic infections, rheumatoid arthritis, or malignancies), SI is diminished, TIBC is often diminished as well, and Tsat may be normal or low.

When transferrin is 100% saturated, iron absorbed by the intestinal mucosa cannot be bound by transferrin; most of this excess iron is deposited in hepatocytes of the liver, the first organ encountered by blood containing absorbed nutrients (including iron). In an extremely rare disorder called congenital atransferrinemia, there is no transferrin in plasma to carry the iron that enters plasma. Consequently, absorbed iron is rapidly deposited in hepatocytes of the liver and in other organs. In this condition, SI and TIBC are quite low, and transferrin cannot be measured. Because the normal mechanism for transport of iron to erythrocyte precursors is lacking, a severe microcytic anemia develops in addition to iron overload of many organs.

The normal plasma half-time for transferrin is 8 to 10.5 days. However, the transit time of iron through plasma is much shorter; the normal plasma iron clearance half-time for transferrin-bound radioiron is about 60 to 90 min. As shown in Table 10.1, only about 3 mg of iron is transferrin-bound at any time. Yet turnover is very rapid, as 25 to 30 mg of iron are transported daily from sites of absorption or release to cells where iron is needed. Normally, 70 to 90% of this iron is taken up by the erythropoietic cells of bone marrow for hemoglobin synthesis. Smaller quantities are delivered to other cells for formation of myoglobin, cytochromes, peroxidases, or other functional iron proteins and, in pregnant women, to the placenta for fetal needs. A small amount of iron is exchanged with iron released from ferritin and hemosiderin in macrophages.

Transferrin exhibits considerable heterogeneity. At least 19 molecular variants have been recognized in humans. All appear to be functionally identical.

Uptake by Cells

Cell membranes contain a protein called *transferrin receptor.* Early erythrocyte precursors have abundant transferrin receptors on their membranes; the number diminishes as these cells mature and fill with hemoglobin. On the cell membrane, diferric transferrin binds to transferrin receptors, and the iron-transferrin–transferrin receptor complex is internalized by endocytosis. Binding to transferrin receptors occurs in pits on the surface of the cell. Upon endocytosis, the pits become coated vesicles, within which iron is released from transferrin (74–85). Most other cells also have transferrin receptors on their membranes, although in smaller numbers. The same mechanism is involved in the internalization of iron in erythrocytes and other cells.

Transferrin receptor is a transmembrane glycoprotein with a molecular mass of approximately 90 kDa. It is 760 amino acids long and consists of two subunits linked by disulfide bonds. It is a group II membrane protein; that is, its amino terminus is on the cytoplasmic side of the membrane, and its carboxy terminus, on the outer surface (86–89).

The transferrin receptor gene is at the end of the long arm of chromosome 3. The gene has been cloned and much of its structure elucidated (90–92).

Belgrade laboratory rats are unable to remove iron rapidly from the internalized vesicles; most of the iron returns to the plasma still attached to transferrin. A somewhat similar disorder in an inbred strain of anemic mice is associated with a mutation in a gene called *Nramp2,* which may code for an intracellular iron-transporter protein. *Nramp2* is also deficient in Belgrade laboratory rats. Similar disorders have not yet been described in humans.

Regulation of Iron Metabolism in Cells

Cellular regulation of the iron balance depends on the effect of iron (or its lack) in stimulating or inhibiting synthesis of apoferritin within the cytosol, of transferrin receptors on the cell membrane, and of δ-aminolevulinic acid synthase (ALA-S) within mitochondria. These three proteins determine the availability of iron to meet the needs of cellular metabolism. Regulation of the rates of synthesis of these three critical proteins involves the interplay of iron and aconitase (also called iron responsive element–binding protein, or IREBP, or iron-regulatory protein, IRP-1) on iron-responsive elements (IREs) in the untranslated regions of transferrin receptor mRNA, apoferritin mRNA, and ALA-S mRNA. IREs are stem-and-loop structures in the mRNA. The loop is the short nucleotide segment CUGUG*X* on a short stem of nucleotides, where *X* can be C, A, G, or U (Fig. 10.8) (93). The IRE for transferrin receptor consists of as many as five loops and stems in the 3′ (downstream) untranslated portion of transferrin receptor mRNA (83–90). Synthesis of transferrin receptor is induced by iron deficiency or, experimentally, by incubation of cells with an iron-chelating agent such as desferrioxamine. Synthesis of transferrin receptor is inhibited by heme, and this inhibition can be blocked by desferrioxamine (89). Another locus in the 5′ (upstream) untranslated region of transferrin receptor mRNA also contributes to control of transferrin receptor synthesis (90).

Aconitase has been described as a "two-faced protein," because it both controls oxidation of glucose and fat in the Krebs cycle and regulates the iron economy of the cell. Thus, it fine-tunes cellular iron metabolism to meet the needs of energy metabolism. In the Krebs cycle, aconitase catalyzes the interconversion of citric acid, *cis*-aconitic acid, and isocitric acid. It can do this only when the cell contains enough iron to put the iron-sulfur cluster of aconitase in the cubane, or cubelike, configuration, with four atoms of iron and four atoms of sulfur alternating at the apices (5, 6, 94, 95) (see Fig. 10.2).

When iron is in short supply, the cubane structure

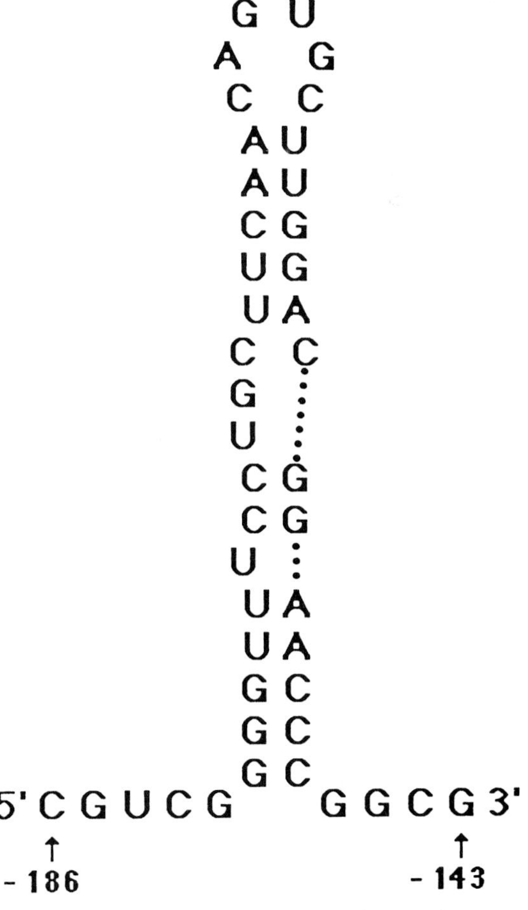

Figure 10.8. Stem-loop structure, the basic unit of the iron-responsive elements of mRNA. (From Hentze MW, Seuanez HN, O'Brien SJ, et al. Nucleic Acids Res 1989;11:6103–8, with permission.)

breaks open for lack of an iron atom at one apex (94, 95). Then aconitase loses its enzymatic function and becomes instead the IRP that binds to the stem-loop structures of the mRNAs for apoferritin, transferrin receptor, and ALA-S (Fig. 10.9). Here it prevents degradation of the mRNA by RNAase, and it accelerates synthesis of transferrin receptor on the cell membrane and of ALA-S within mitochondria. This results in increased iron uptake from transferrin in plasma and increased synthesis of protoporphyrin so that more heme, more cytochrome, and more hemoglobin can be formed, at least in bone marrow erythroblasts. Conversely, the binding of IRP to the IRE of apoferritin mRNA results in reduction of apoferritin synthesis. Thus, the iron that the cell takes up is less likely to be trapped in ferritin and rendered metabolically inactive.

When there is sufficient iron within the cytosol or mitochondria, IRP is displaced from the IREs, and the Fe-S cluster resumes the cubane configuration, again becoming the active enzyme aconitase that functions in the Krebs cycle ultimately to generate the high-energy bonds of ATP. These relationships are portrayed in Figures 10.2 and 10.9.

There are at least two structurally different aconitases in cells, c-aconitase in cytoplasm and m-aconitase in mitochondria. Both function as described above. Of course, m-aconitase regulates the synthesis of ALA-S, as the latter is a mitochondrial enzyme that catalyzes the first step in heme synthesis, and it is m-aconitase that is involved in energy metabolism. Aconitase is encoded by a gene in human chromosome 9.

Iron in the Erythroblast

Following endocytosis of the iron-transferrin–transferrin receptor complex in the coated vesicles, iron is released into the cytosol, and apotransferrin is returned to extracellular fluid. The release of iron from transferrin is stepwise: one atom may be released by low pH; the other may require mediation by ATP, hemoglobin, or other substances (96–101). Within the cytosol of the erythroblast, iron either is transported to mitochondria for incorporation into heme or is taken up by ferritin within siderosomes. Either transferrin itself or other iron-binding substances (101–104), such as the Nramp2 protein (24, 25), may participate in iron transport in the cytosol (Fig. 10.10). The mechanism of iron entry into mitochondria is unknown. In iron deficiency, sideroblasts almost disappear from the marrow. Conversely, in some states of iron overload, they may become more numerous and contain more siderotic granules than normally.

Within the mitochondria, iron is inserted into protoporphyrin to form heme in a reaction catalyzed by the enzyme heme synthetase (ferrochelatase). Heme inhibits release of iron from transferrin (105). This may be one of the feedback mechanisms for adjusting the iron supply to the rate of hemoglobin synthesis in the erythroblast.

Iron Utilization

A normal adult uses approximately 20 to 25 mg of iron per day for hemoglobin synthesis. These values can be calculated as follows: A man with a blood volume of 5000 mL

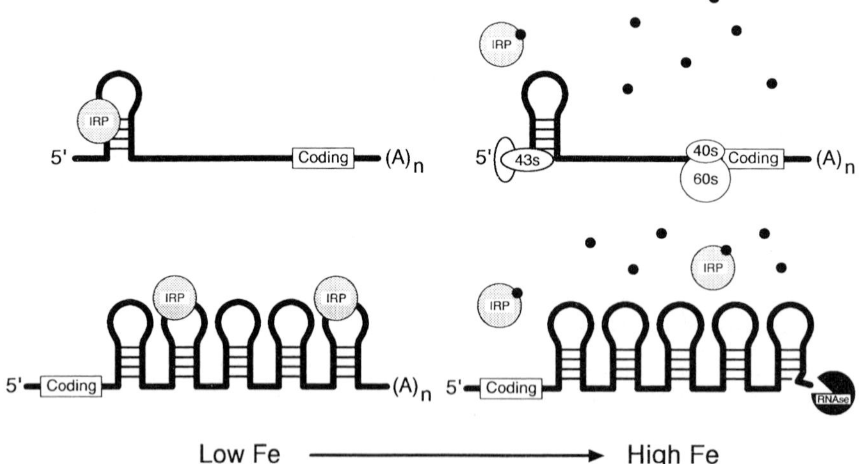

Figure 10.9. Regulation of iron metabolism within the cytosol by interaction of aconitase with iron response elements *(IREs)* on mRNA. IREs are stem-loop structures that are activated or inhibited by iron-depleted aconitase (iron-regulatory protein, or IRP, formerly called IRE-BP, or iron responsive element–binding protein) within the mitochondria or the cytosol. Synthesis of proteins critical to iron metabolism is regulated by the aconitase-IRE mechanism. (A similar mechanism may exist for Nramp2). The *upper panel* represents apoferritin mRNA, the *lower panel,* transferrin receptor mRNA. When there is little iron within the cytosol, desferriaconitase binds to the IREs of mRNA for each of these proteins, stabilizing the mRNA, to increase the number of transferrin receptor molecules on the cell surface, to decrease the synthesis of apoferritin, and to increase the synthesis of ALA-S, thus facilitating uptake of iron at the cell membrane and synthesis of protophorphyrin so more is available for heme synthesis. When iron is abundant within the cytosol, aconitase is displaced from the IREs, thereby stimulating apoferritin synthesis, inhibiting synthesis of transferrin receptor and ALA-S, and accelerating degradation of the mRNA. This results in enhanced synthesis of apoferritin and reduced synthesis of transferrin receptor, thus reducing iron uptake at the cell membrane and increasing storage capacity for the iron in the cytosol; there is also decreased synthesis of ALA-S and thus of heme. IRP, iron-regulatory protein, or desferriaconitase. (Modified from Knisely AS. Adv Pediatr 1992;39:383–403, with permission).

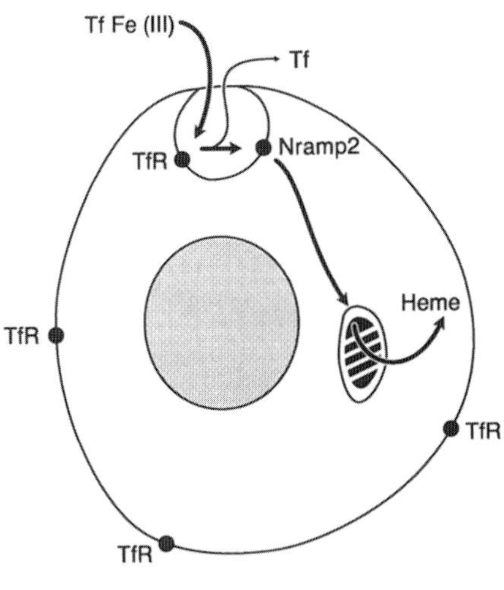

Figure 10.10. Cellular uptake of iron in an erythroblast in bone marrow. The Fe(III)-transferrin complex *[T_fFe(III)]* binds to transferrin receptor *(TfR)* on the cell membrane. The Fe(III)-transferrin TfR complex is then internalized in a pit that becomes an endosome. Within the acidic interior of the endosome, Fe(III) is released from transferrin and is transferred to *Nramp2,* which transports it to mitochondria, where Fe(III) is inserted into a porphyrin ring to form *heme.* The transferrin, now unburdened of Fe(III), is returned to the plasma ready to take up more Fe(III).

and a hemoglobin level of 150 g/L has 750 g of circulating hemoglobin or 2.55 g of circulating hemoglobin iron (total blood hemoglobin in grams multiplied by 0.34%). Since the normal life span of the red cell in circulating blood is about 120 days, 2.55 g ÷ 120, or 21 mg of iron, would be required daily to replace the catabolized hemoglobin. Iron use can also be determined after a tracer dose of radioiron is given intravenously. The amount of injected radioactive iron used for hemoglobin synthesis and delivered to the peripheral blood in newly formed erythrocytes is then measured. Normally, erythrocyte radioactivity rises for 7 to 14 days and then levels off at 75 to 90% of the injected amount. Iron-deficient persons typically use more than 90% of the injected ^{59}Fe.

Normally functioning bone marrow can effect a sixfold increase in its production of red blood cells and hemoglobin. Under maximal stimulation, therefore, as much as 100 to 125 mg of iron can be used for hemoglobin synthesis per day.

Iron Reutilization

The avid manner in which the body conserves and reutilizes iron is an important characteristic of iron metabolism. A normal adult catabolizes enough hemoglobin each day to release 20 to 25 mg of iron, most of which is promptly recycled by formation of new hemoglobin molecules. More than 90% of hemoglobin iron is repeatedly recycled by phagocytosis of old erythrocytes, which occurs chiefly in macrophages of the liver and spleen.

Phagocytized red cells are digested at a rate sufficient to release approximately 20% of the hemoglobin iron within a few hours, and the remainder more slowly. The iron released by the action of the monocyte-macrophage system is bound to transferrin and is ultimately redistributed. About 40% of the hemoglobin iron of nonviable erythrocytes reappears in circulating red cells within 12 days. The rate of reutilization varies considerably. In normal persons there is 19 to 69% reincorporation in 12 days. The rate of reutilization of iron is more variable in the presence of disease. The remainder of the iron derived from hemoglobin catabolism enters the storage pool as ferritin or hemosiderin and normally turns over very slowly: approximately 40% remains in storage after 140 days. When the rate of erythropoiesis increases, however, storage iron may be released more rapidly from the storage pools to plasma transferrin. Conversely, in the presence of chronic disease such as infection, rheumatoid arthritis, or malignancy, the storage iron derived from hemoglobin catabolism is reused much more slowly.

These alterations in the rate of iron reuse seem to be determined by the rate of iron release from cells of the monocyte-macrophage system to plasma transferrin. Thus, in the presence of chronic disease, the rate of release of iron by macrophages decreases, and iron storage in the monocyte-macrophage system increases. The effect is a reduced rate of iron delivery to developing erythroblasts, an accelerated rate of transport to the bone marrow of the iron available in the plasma pool, a reduced plasma iron concentration, and a reduced rate of erythropoiesis. Microcytic erythrocytes may result from the reduced flow of iron from the monocyte-macrophage system to the developing erythroblasts.

In addition to its role in regulating the size of iron stores, the monocyte-macrophage system appears to participate in regulation of the concentration of transferrin. Macrophages of this system can both synthesize apotransferrin and take up and degrade transferrin.

Storage Iron

Iron in excess of need is stored intracellularly as ferritin and hemosiderin, principally in the macrophage ("reticuloendothelial") system of liver, spleen, bone marrow, and other organs. Ferritin is the basic storage molecule for molecular iron; hemosiderin is aggregated ferritin partially stripped of its protein component. A complete ferritin molecule has an apoferritin protein shell that is 13 nm in outer diameter with an internal cavity 7 nm in diameter (106–113). The internal cavity holds one or more crystals of ferric oxyhydroxide (FeOOH) together with trace amounts of phosphate that may occur at imperfections or cleavage planes in the FeOOH crystals (Fig. 10.11). The cavity of each ferritin molecule can hold at maximum 4300 iron atoms as FeOOH crystals, although most ferritin molecules contain 2000 iron atoms.

The apoferritin protein shell is composed of 24 monomers, each with a molecular mass of approximately

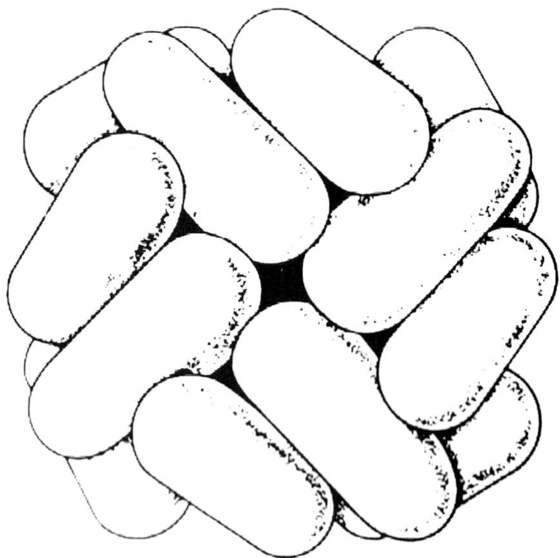

Figure 10.11. A scheme for the quaternary structure of the apoferritin molecule. It consists of 24 subunits, or apoferritin monomers, joined together to form a snubbed cube, or a cube with rounded apices. Four monomers comprise each facet of the cube, and at the center of the facet, where the ends of the monomers join, there is a pore through which may pass Fe(II), and possibly other small molecules, to enter the interior cavity of the molecule. Here, FeOOH forms one or more crystals, and it is in this crystalline form that iron is held in storage. (From Harrison PM, et al. In: Jacobs A, Worwood M, eds. Iron in Clinical Medicine. New York: Academic Press, 1980;131–171.)

20 kDa, and each formed in turn by four long, nearly parallel helical chains of amino acids, two short helical segments, and connecting nonhelical segments. The monomers are arranged in a nearly spherical structure—the apoferritin shell—with groups of four monomers aligned so that their short helices form pores. These six pores permit passage of small molecules to and from the interior of the apoferritin shell. The pores are large enough to permit iron, water, and possibly other small molecules, such as ascorbic acid, to enter the interior cavity (Fig. 10.10) (109–111). Furthermore, the pores appear to function as catalytic sites for the binding of Fe(II), its oxidation to FeOOH, and facilitated passage of the FeOOH to the interior, where it is added to the growing core crystal (Fig. 10.12) (111–112). Thus the apoferritin shell not only is an efficient iron trap but also functions enzymatically.

Oxidation and uptake of iron by apoferritin is very rapid. Similarly, the release of iron is rapid (113). Iron release from ferritin may be mediated by reduced flavin mononucleotide, although an enzymatic mechanism has not been excluded (111). Human ferritins may exist in multiple isomeric states (114). H and L monomers differ in mass, the former being about 20 kDa and the latter about 18 kDa. There are as many as 25 isoferritins, depending on the proportion of H and L monomers. Ferritin that contains mostly H monomers is relatively acidic, contains relatively more iron, and is found predominantly in heart. Ferritin that contains mostly L monomers is relatively basic, contains little iron, and is characteristically found in liver. Ferritin predominantly of the H type is increased in the serum, especially in patients with malignancies such as carcinoma of the breast, embryonal carcinomas, and lymphomas.

Hemosiderin, unlike ferritin, is insoluble in aqueous media. Hemosiderin contains slightly more iron (~30% by weight) than does ferritin. Immunologically, they appear to be identical. On electron microscopy, the apoferritin shell of ferritin is not seen, but the electron-dense FeOOH crystalline core appears as a tetrad because of its octahedral shape. Electron microscopy shows great numbers of ferritin core crystal tetrads in hemosiderin; thus, a molecular weight cannot be given for hemosiderin. The molecular mass of ferritin, which

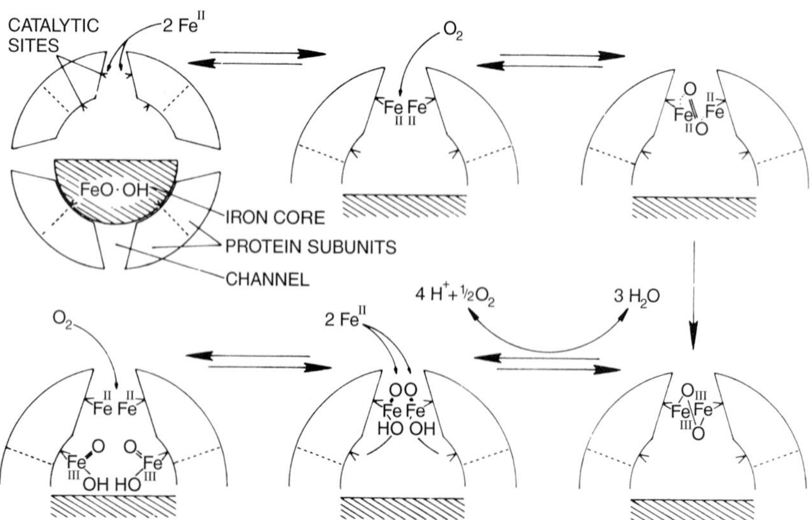

Figure 10.12. Scheme for uptake and deposition of iron by ferritin. Two pairs of iron-binding sites are envisioned, located near the intermonomeric pores of the apoferritin shell. See text for a more complete explanation. (From Crichton RR, Roman F. J Mol Catal 1978;4:75–82, with permission.) Currently it is believed that oxidation of iron from Fe(II) to Fe(III) involves sites only on the H monomer.

depends partly on its iron content, is usually stated as 620 kDa.

Within cells, apoferritin monomers are synthesized by ribosomes in response to the presence of iron. Regulation of apoferritin synthesis depends on the binding of IRP to the apoferritin mRNA. Iron in the cytosol relieves the inhibition of apoferritin synthesis by causing IRP to convert to aconitase with the iron-sulfur cluster in the cubane form. In this form it does not bind to the IRE. Iron also causes translocation of preformed ferritin messenger RNA to polyribosomes where ferritin synthesis occurs (115–119).

In the liver and spleen of normal animals, there is a slight preponderance of ferritin iron over hemosiderin iron. With increasing concentrations of tissue iron, this ratio is reversed, and at high levels, the additional storage iron is deposited as hemosiderin. Both forms can be mobilized for hemoglobin synthesis when the need for iron exists. Reducing substances such as ascorbate, dithionite, and reduced flavin mononucleotide ($FMNH_2$) cause rapid release of iron from ferritin. Thus, $FMNH_2$ might serve as the physiologic mediator of iron release (111–113).

Quantitation of normal iron stores has proved difficult, but reasonable estimates derived from available data are 300 to 1000 mg for adult women and 500 to 1500 mg for adult men. More individuals appear to fall into the lower half of these ranges than into the upper half, and many healthy women have virtually no iron reserves. Iron is released from ferritin as Fe(II) and as such traverses the cytosol and cell membrane to enter plasma, where it is again oxidized by ceruloplasmin to Fe(III) and is taken up by transferrin. The amount of stored iron may increase as a result of a shift of iron from the red cell mass to the stores. This occurs in all anemias except those due to iron deficiency. A true increase in total body iron is found in patients with hemochromatosis, transfusional hemosiderosis, or (rarely) after excessive and prolonged iron therapy. The total body burden of storage iron may exceed 30 g. An assessment of whether iron stores are deficient or excessive may be made from the serum iron, TIBC, serum ferritin, and stainable iron in bone marrow aspirates.

Enzyme Iron

It was once believed that iron enzymes were "inviolate" in iron-deficiency anemia. Extensive studies in experimental animals have shown that iron enzymes are in fact quite sensitive to iron deficiency. The degree of loss varies from enzyme to enzyme and from tissue to tissue. Cytochrome c and aconitase are quite readily depleted, cytochrome oxidase appears to be less susceptible, and catalase is the most resistant of all to depletion. Investigations of human leukocytes and buccal mucosa have shown depletion of cytochrome oxidase, however, even in relatively mild iron deficiency (120–121). Iron deficiency in rats is associated with marked (~70%) reduction in activity of the iron-sulfur enzymes succinate-ubiquinone oxidoreductase and NADH-ubiquinone oxidoreductase in rat skeletal muscle mitochondria. These important enzymes of the respiratory chain appear to be reduced in quantity rather than impaired in function, since both the peptide components and the flavin prosthetic groups were reduced (122).

Iron-deficient rats also have hyperphenylalaninemia that is directly proportional to the severity of anemia. The mechanism of this effect is uncertain, as the hepatic activity of the iron-containing enzyme phenylalanine hydroxylase is not reduced. It is suggested that iron deficiency results in metabolism of phenylalanine by an alternative pathway that might generate increased quantities of phenylpyruvic acid and thereby disturb brain function. Treatment of iron deficiency with iron dextran resulted in normal serum concentrations of phenylalanine within 1 week (123).

Poor work performance in iron-deficient rats has been attributed to reduced activity of muscle α-glycerophosphate dehydrogenase, as noted below (see "Clinical Manifestations"). Mitochondrial α-glycerophosphate dehydrogenase, a flavoprotein that contains nonheme iron, plays an important electron transport role in aerobic metabolism. That iron deficiency results in impairment of activities of cytochromes and of so many iron-containing enzymes is understandable. However, iron deficiency is also associated with reduced activity of many enzymes that do not contain iron. The activity of monoamine oxidase (MAO), a copper-containing enzyme important in the synthesis of neurotransmitters, is diminished in the liver and in platelets of iron-deficient humans (123–125). However, MAO activity was normal in the brains of iron-deficient rats (125).

Some diminution in the activities of other enzymes has also been reported in association with iron deficiency in rats. These include hepatic glucose-6-phosphate dehydrogenase, 6-phosphogluconate dehydrogenase, and various transaminases (126–128). These alterations appear to be minor and are probably of no physiologic import. Further, it is puzzling that activities of these enzymes should be affected, as none of them contains iron or requires iron as a cofactor.

Iron Loss

Excretion

The body has a limited capacity to excrete iron. Daily iron loss in adult men is between 0.90 and 1.05 mg, or approximately 0.013 mg/kg body weight, irrespective of climate-dependent variation in perspiration (130, 131). The daily external loss is distributed roughly as follows: gastrointestinal blood (hemoglobin), 0.35 mg; gastrointestinal mucosal (ferritin), 0.10 mg; biliary, 0.20 mg; urinary, 0.08 mg; and skin, 0.20 mg.

A slight increase in iron excretion—principally fecal, and not exceeding about 4 mg/day—may occur in persons with iron overload, in partial compensation for increased iron stores (132). Urinary iron excretion may be increased significantly in patients with proteinuria, hematuria, hemoglobinuria, and hemosiderinuria. Hemosiderinuria may cause iron deficiency in patients with artificial heart valves or calcific aortic stenosis. The iron excreted in feces is derived from blood lost into the alimentary canal (1.2 ± 0.5 mL whole blood/day) (133), from unabsorbed iron in bile, and from desquamated intestinal mucosal cells.

Menstruation

It is difficult to quantitate the "normal" iron loss due to menstruation or pregnancy, because of the wide variation encountered. While menstrual blood loss for any individual normal woman does not vary much from month to month, the difference between women is considerable. In studies of Swedish women, the mean menstrual loss was found to be 43 mL, equivalent to an average of about 0.6 to 0.7 mg of iron daily (134–136). The upper normal limit of menstrual loss was about 80 mL per period. However, women who consider their menses normal may lose more than 100 mL and occasionally more than 200 mL per period. Menstrual blood losses are increased by intrauterine devices and reduced by contraceptive pills.

Pregnancy

The iron "cost" of pregnancy is high. The external loss in urine, feces, and sweat amounts to about 170 mg for the gestational period. About 270 mg (200–370 mg) is contributed to the fetus, and another 90 mg (30–170 mg) is contained in the placenta and cord. The amount of iron lost in hemorrhage at delivery was underestimated in the past and is now believed to average about 150 mg (90–300 mg). Iron is required for the expansion of blood volume that occurs normally during the last half of pregnancy, but this amount is largely recovered when the circulating red blood cell volume is returned to normal after delivery. Lactation causes an additional drain of approximately 0.5 to 1 mg of iron daily. The volume of blood loss is roughly equal to a year's menstrual loss. Furthermore, the iron needed for the expanded blood volume and the enlarging uterus is mostly conserved. Therefore, the net iron "cost" of a normal pregnancy is in the range of about 420 to 1030 mg (Table 10.5), or an additional requirement of 1 to 2.5 mg/day, spread over the 15-month period of pregnancy and lactation.

Iron Transfer to the Fetus

The fetus has a highly effective acceptor system for assimilating iron. Iron from maternal transferrin is transferred to the placental tissue, to the plasma transferrin of the fetus, and then to the fetal tissues, by a unidirectional pathway that operates against increased maternal requirements for iron, even despite maternal iron deficiency. During the last trimester of pregnancy 3 to 4 mg of iron is transferred to the fetus each day.

Bleeding

Pathologic bleeding from any site constitutes an important form of iron loss: 1 mL of blood with a hemoglobin concentration of 150 g/L contains 0.5 mg of iron. A rough but useful rule-of-thumb is that 1 mL of packed red cells contains 1 mg of iron. The chronic loss of only a small volume of blood, therefore, may significantly increase iron requirements. For blood donors, each 500 mL of blood donated contains between 200 and 250 mg of iron. Spread equally over a year, that amounts to roughly 0.6 to 0.7 mg/day. A donor who gives blood every 2 months will have an increase in the average daily iron loss of 4 mg and will require at least a fourfold increase in iron intake to avoid becoming anemic. This is especially problematic for women who are blood donors. If they do not receive iron supplementation, many may cease being blood donors because of anemia. In a controlled study of the effects of iron supplementation for women blood donors, the dropout rate due to anemia was 32% for those not receiving iron supplements and only 4.5% for those given regular oral iron supplement. As little as 39 mg of iron daily (120 mg of ferrous sulfate) in a single dose sufficed to prevent anemia and allow 96% of adult women to donate blood at 8- to 12-week intervals (137). Despite this finding, many blood banks in the United States are unwilling to provide iron supplements to their regular blood donors.

IRON REQUIREMENTS

Growth

The iron required for growth and its attendant increase in circulating hemoglobin mass depends upon the rate of growth (i.e., the rapid growth during infancy and the growth spurt of adolescent males). The basis for estimating iron need is shown in Table 10.6. The average daily

Table 10.5
Iron "Cost" of a Normal Pregnancy (mg)

Iron contributed to fetus	200–370
In placenta and cord	30–170
In blood loss at delivery	90–310
In milk, lactation 6 months	100–180
Total	420–1030
Average per day (pregnancy, 9 months; lactation, 6 months)	1–2.5

Table 10.6
Minimum Daily Iron Requirements

	Amount That Must Be Absorbed for Hemoglobin Synthesis (mg)
Infants	1
Children	0.5
Young nonpregnant women	2
Pregnant women	3
Men and menopausal women	1

iron requirement is 0.35 to 0.7 mg/day for boys and 0.3 to 0.45 mg/day for girls prior to menarche. Other studies have shown a daily iron requirement of 38 mg/kg of optimal body weight, for both males and females between ages 4 and 14 years (138).

Nutritional Allowances

Estimates of the amount of iron required to maintain positive balance are shown in Table 10.7 (139). (See also Appendix Tables II-A-2 to A8 for U.S. and other national and international dietary recommendations for iron.) It is evident that men and nonmenstruating women, in the absence of pathologic bleeding, should have little difficulty obtaining the iron they need from diets customary in the United States (12–18 mg Fe per day). Iron balance is precarious, however, in many menstruating women and adolescent girls who, because of concern about weight, restrict their diets and frequently have iron intakes below 10 mg/day. Requirements during pregnancy frequently exceed the amount available from diet alone. Particularly in women with depleted stores, supplemental iron therapy is necessary during the latter half of pregnancy and for 2 to 3 months postpartum, if iron deficiency is to be prevented. Full-term neonates do not require iron supplementation for the first 3 months but should have iron supplementation thereafter as long as they are being formula- or breast-fed. Premature neonates should begin iron supplementation earlier.

IRON TOXICITY

Iron that is readily soluble, as ferrous salts in numerous medications, can be highly toxic or lethal to small children who ingest a small handful of iron tablets that look like candy. Such accidental ingestion by a child requires prompt and vigorous attention in a hospital emergency room. The small amounts of iron added to infant formula, to cereal, or given by dropper are quite safe and well tolerated. There has been much speculation in recent publications concerning a possible adverse effect in adults of either iron therapy or chronically high normal iron stores, since, by the well-known Fenton reaction, free ionic iron may catalyze generation of free radicals. It may be in part for this reason that iron in all biologic fluids, whether plasma or cytosol, is normally always protein bound.

Studies from Finland seemed to show that persons with high serum ferritin values had an increased risk of ischemic heart disease or acute myocardial infarction (140). The Finnish diet is high in meat (therefore in readily assimilated iron) and in saturated fats, and ischemic heart disease has quite a high prevalence in Finland irrespective of levels of serum ferritin. Studies reported both from Finland and from the United States have cast much doubt on the postulated adverse effect of iron in promoting ischemic heart disease (141–144). Further, patients with severe iron overload (hemochromatosis) appear to have a reduced risk of ischemic heart disease (144). The hemochromatosis allele that occurs with high frequency elsewhere in western Europe, however, appears to be rare in Finland.

Table 10.7
Recommended Daily Intake (RDI) of Iron

Category	Age	RDI (mg)
Infants (full term)	0–3 months	—
	3–6 months	6.6
	6–12 months	8.8
Children (male and female)	1–10 years	10
Males	10–18 years	12
	>18 years	10
Females		
Nonpregnant	10–45 years	15
Pregnant		45
Postmenopausal		10

Adapted from Herbert V. Am J Clin Nutr 1987;45:679–86.

IRON DEFICIENCY AND IRON-DEFICIENCY ANEMIA

Epidemiology

Worldwide, caloric insufficiency, manifested in hunger, famine, and starvation, appears to be the dominant nutritional problem. Iron deficiency, which affects an estimated 40% of the world's population, or two billion persons, is second only to hunger as a major nutritional problem worldwide. In tropical areas of Asia, Africa, and Central and South America, where intestinal helminthiasis such as hookworm infestation is common, iron-deficiency anemia has a particularly high prevalence. In India, where hookworm disease is prevalent and vegetarianism is mandated by religion, iron deficiency is nearly universal.

In the United States, where the dominant nutritional problem now seems to be obesity, iron deficiency is also the second most common nutritional problem. During the past few decades, it has been a common perception that iron deficiency and iron-deficiency anemia are no longer important nutritional problems in the United States. Clearly, this perception is in error. The prevalence rates for iron deficiency and iron-deficiency anemia have not diminished in the United States during the past 30 years; on the contrary, available evidence strongly suggests that iron deficiency and iron-deficiency anemia have gradually become more prevalent during this interval, while the quality of iron nutrition has declined.

Table 10.8 indicates the progressive declines in mean hemoglobin concentration and mean hematocrit values documented by the Centers for Disease Control since 1959 in successive Health and Nutrition Examination Surveys (145–147). Progressive declines in these values have been consistent in every age, sex and ethnic group examined, altogether in more than 50,000 persons surveyed. The observed declines have been most marked in women aged 18 to 44 years and in African Americans of every age group, both males and females. Part of the explanation may be that the earlier surveys were per-

Table 10.8
Changes (%) in Mean Values for Venous Hematocrit in Three National Surveys, 1959–1980

Group	Age (years)	% Change
White males	19–44	−4.9
White males	44+	−3.3
White females	19–44	−5.5
White females	44+	−2.4
Black males	19–44	−6.6
Black males	44+	−6.7
Black females	19–44	−5.4
Black females	44+	−6.5

Data from ref. 145–147. The First National Health Examination Survey conducted between October 1959 and December 1962 was taken as baseline in these calculations. National Health and Nutrition Examination Surveys (NHANES) 1 and 2 were conducted in the years 1971–1974 and 1976–1980, respectively. Declines were consistently observed and were approximately proportional between the first and second of these studies and the second and third. Analyses of the data from NHANES-3, conducted in 1988–1994, were not available at the time of preparation of this table. Preliminary evaluations of NHANES-3 data are alleged to indicate no further declines in hemoglobin concentration or hematocrit between NHANES-2 and NHANES-3, although the data have not been released. Equivalent declines have been demonstrated in hemoglobin concentration during these 21 years.

formed with specimens obtained from sitting persons and the later surveys from recumbent persons. Fluid shifts with recumbency are known to reduce hemoglobin concentration and hematocrit values. Part of the explanation may also be a change in the anticoagulant used to collect blood specimens; a dry powder was used in the earlier studies, and a liquid anticoagulant in 0.05 mL volume in the later studies. However, it is unlikely that either or both of these differences in sampling methods can account for the threefold difference in rates of decline in hemoglobin concentration and hematocrit for specimens obtained from African Americans or white females of ages 20 to 44 compared with those obtained from white males of the same age range.

Figure 10.13 shows the prevalence of anemia in one prosperous, largely middle-class, predominantly white, Midwestern U.S. community during the years 1987 to 1989 (148). A similarly high prevalence of both anemia and iron deficiency was reported in 1994 from a survey of 617 apparently healthy school children in Georgia (149). In that survey, the prevalence of iron deficiency was 30% among African American children and 33% among white children, although only 2% of the children were frankly anemic. St. Paul, Minnesota, a prosperous community with high employment, has a high incidence rate for iron-deficiency anemia in infants and children of economically disadvantaged status who are eligible for the WIC (Women, Infant and Children) program of nutritional supplementation. The incidence rates of anemia in children aged 18 months to 5 years who were previously nonanemic were 24% for white children, 22% for African American children, 24% for Asian children (predominantly Hmong), 16% for Hispanics, and 7.9% for Native American children (150). Incidence is specified for this group rather than prevalence because none of the children in this study had previously been anemic.

In northern Europe, with a well-fed population and a lifestyle not unlike that of middle-class white Americans, surveys have shown high prevalence rates for anemia and iron deficiency despite longstanding efforts to improve iron nutrition by addition of iron to wheat flour and bread. Conversely, no harm seems to have been done by this practice. In recognition of the lack of benefit from this practice, flour and bread are no longer iron fortified in Sweden and much of Europe.

As represented in Figure 10.13 and Table 10.9, the prevalence of anemia increases markedly in persons above age 70, because of chronic illness, chronic blood loss, or both. Acute or chronic blood loss (i.e., iron deficiency)

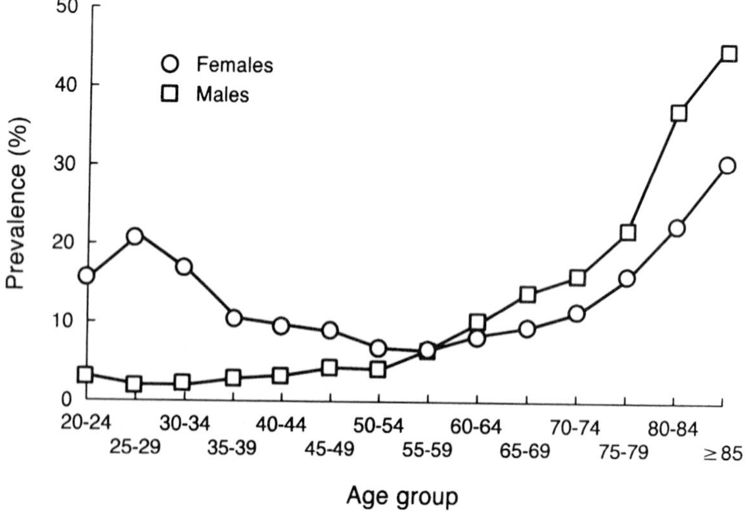

Figure 10.13. Prevalence of anemia in a prosperous community in Minnesota, predominantly of European derivation. Because pregnant women were not excluded, approximately half the prevalence of anemia in the age range 20–39 years may be due to the normal hydremia of pregnancy. Half of the other cases of anemia were due to blood loss, acute or chronic. Prevalence of anemia increases markedly after age 59 in both sexes; iron deficiency is the most common cause of anemia in this population. These observations refute the widely held view that at present, iron deficiency is a minor problem in North America. (Adapted from Anía BJ, Suman VJ, Fairbanks VF, Melton LJ III. Mayo Clin Proc 1994;69:730–5.)

Table 10.9
Prevalence of Anemia in an Affluent Midwestern U.S. Community, 1985–1989[a]

Ages (years)	White Males % Anemic	White Females % Anemic
20–39	3	10
40–44	3	10
45–59	5	7
60–64	10	8
65–69	12	8
70–74	15	11

[a]Data shown are for Olmsted County, MN, with a population of slightly more than 100,000, >95% Caucasian, with high employment and ready access to medical care. The table is from the same database as Fig. 10.13 but has been corrected by assuming that approximately half the "anemia" prevalence in women in the age range 20–39 may be attributed to the "dilutional anemia" of pregnancy. Data were obtained in 53,887 Olmsted County residents above age 20 and are considered to represent 78% of the population above age 20.[148] Anemia was defined as Hb concentration <13 g/dL in males or <12 g/dL in females (World Health Organization criteria, which also correspond to values below the 2.5 percentiles in NHANES-2). The prevalence of anemia increases rapidly for both males and females over age 74 years.

accounts for approximately half of the rapidly escalating frequency of anemia in the elderly. Some clinicians and some nutritionists have assumed that the anemia that is particularly common in elderly males is part of the normal process of aging. There is, however, no evidence to support this assumption.

Anemia is not a sensitive indicator of the prevalence of iron deficiency, nor is anemia solely due to iron deficiency. However, iron deficiency is by far the commonest cause of anemia. In most populations, the prevalence of iron deficiency may be estimated at 3 or 4 times the prevalence of anemia. One may reasonably assume that most of the economically deprived children of St. Paul, Minnesota, are iron deficient. Indeed, free erythrocyte protoporphyrin, a relatively sensitive indicator of iron deficiency (or of lead poisoning) was elevated in nearly half the white children, in nearly half the African American children, and in nearly 80% of Asian children who were admitted to the WIC program (150).

Poverty Remains a Major Determinant of Iron Malnutrition in the United States. Iron-deficient children are likely to become iron-deficient teenagers and adults and to have a higher prevalence of iron-deficiency anemia as women, both during the reproductive years and specifically in pregnancy. Declining values for hemoglobin concentrations in women and in African American males, shown in successive NHANES studies, may thus be preconditioned by iron-poor nutrition during childhood. Indeed, this is evident from recent nutritional monitoring in the CATCH survey (151, 152), the Bogalusa, Louisiana, Heart study (153), and in reports from the Nutrition Monitoring Study of the Federation of American Societies for Experimental Biology (10–12). In the first of these surveys, which was based on 24-h recalls of what middle-school students of northern states and California had eaten, nearly 90% of students were thought to have had iron intakes of at least 75% of the RDA (10 mg). The other two studies found that African American and Mexican American children were much less likely to have adequate iron nutrition. In low-income households, hunger was common and iron intake inadequate.

African Americans are particularly at risk of iron malnutrition because of the economic catastrophe that resulted from accelerating levels of unemployment since the 1950s (154). In the United States, the income gap between rich and poor has dramatically widened during the past few decades; poverty is increasing in the United States, although a small subset of the population is acquiring extreme wealth. Poor people have diets rich in fat and carbohydrate but poor in vegetables, fruits, and meat. The First (U.S.) Health and Nutrition Examination Survey, conducted between 1971 and 1974, found that the mean iron intake of American women of nearly every age group, irrespective of race or economic status, was less than optimal; for those below the poverty income level, dietary iron insufficiency was nearly universal (155). In that study, most males over 24 years of age had adequate iron intake.

In the 1980s, the U.S. federal government released large quantities of cheese and butter that had been stored by the Department of Agriculture (USDA) to the poor—a gift of calories, saturated fat, and protein that was nearly devoid of iron. Revision of the public welfare system of the United States will further worsen the nutritional status of poor children and young adults, who are mostly African American, Native American, and Hispanic. In early 1997, the USDA ruled that school lunch programs, primarily intended to improve the nutrition of poor children, can now substitute iron-poor yogurt for meat. This ruling will also adversely affect the iron nutrition of disadvantaged children.

By almost imperceptible steps, the diet of a large part of the U.S. population has come to consist predominantly of iron-poor dairy products, iron-poor snack foods and potato products, white bread and flour with only a little added iron that is poorly absorbed, and iron-poor soft drinks.

Prevalence of Iron Deficiency in the United States

The overall prevalence of iron-deficiency anemia in the United States in the last few years of the 20th century cannot be stated with certainty, but conservative estimates for middle-class white Americans are approximately 5% for children of ages 1 to 14 years, 10 to 20% for young women during the reproductive years, 30 to 60% for pregnant or postpartum women, 5 to 10% for postmenopausal women, 1 to 5% for males of ages 20 to 44 years, 5 to 10% for males of ages 45 to 70 years, and 10 to 30% for both males and females over 70 years of age (146). African Americans of both sexes, Mexican Americans, Native Americans, and poor people of any ethnic group have a higher prevalence of iron-deficiency anemia. A particularly high prevalence of iron deficiency that occurs among the Inuit people of Alaska and Canada has been related to a high prevalence of duodenal infestation with *Helicobacter pyloris*.

African Americans have a high prevalence of α-thalassemia, which is associated with slight microcytosis of the erythrocytes and may be responsible for slightly lower mean hemoglobin concentrations in non-iron-deficient persons than in Caucasians and Asians. The prevalence of α-thalassemia-2 trait in African Americans is 28%, and the prevalence of homozygous α-thalassemia-2 is about 3%. The mean hemoglobin concentration is approximately 7 g/L lower in African Americans than in Caucasians or Asians. There is a proportionately lower mean packed-cell volume (PCV or hematocrit). This systematically lower mean hemoglobin concentration in African Americans is considered in estimating prevalence rates for anemia.

Despite the long recognition of iron deficiency as a major nutritional problem in the United States and despite limited efforts to ameliorate it, the prevalence of iron-deficiency anemia seems to have remained essentially unchanged or perhaps increased during the past 30 years. Further reduction in the quality of iron nutrition seems inevitable.

Effect of Iron "Fortification" of Bread and Flour

Efforts to improve the iron nutrition of the U.S. population have been based mostly on iron fortification of cereal. These efforts have had little effect to date, because the principal means selected to increase iron intake was addition of "reduced" (i.e., finely powdered, metallic) iron to cereal. Metallic iron is poorly assimilated because it must be oxidized to Fe(III) and then reduced to Fe(II) while still in the upper small intestine, before it is absorbed (Table 10.10). Since the duodenum is the main site of iron absorption, most of the metallic iron in iron-fortified bread or other cereal products must arrive in the colon unchanged. Furthermore, whatever fraction of the metallic iron becomes oxidized, at any level of the intestinal tract, is likely to be chelated by phytate in cereal and thus be rendered nonabsorbable. In Sweden, where white flour was "enriched" by addition of reduced iron for several decades, neither harm nor benefit was demonstrated, and the practice was discontinued (156, 157). In Germany, the practice is illegal. Some major American flour-milling corporations are aware that the iron used to fortify flour is poorly absorbed.

Table 10.10
Iron Fortification of White Flour, White Bread, Rolls, and Buns in the United States

Form of Iron	Absorbability	Amount Added
Ferrous sulfate	Fair	None[a]
Metallic ("reduced")	Poor	20 mg/lb (44.1 ppm)

[a]Some local bakeries may fortify flour with ferrous sulfate. In this form, iron accelerates rancidification of fat, creating undesirable flavors and colors in bread, causing bread to spoil more quickly. Some frozen flour products may also contain ferrous sulfate rather than metallic iron. The major flour mills (General Mills, Pillsbury, ADM, and Conagra) fortify white flour with insoluble metallic iron. Whole wheat flour does not contain iron as an additive but has a small amount of iron as a natural component (about 20 mg/lb).

IRON OVERLOAD

An excessive body burden of iron can be produced by greater-than-normal absorption from the alimentary canal, by parenteral injection, or by a combination of both. Excess iron is deposited largely as hemosiderin in reticuloendothelial cells or in the parenchymal cells of certain tissues. The site of deposition depends in part on the portal of entry. Excess iron derived from intestinal absorption is carried to tissues, bound by plasma transferrin, and transferred to parenchymal and reticuloendothelial cells and developing erythroblasts. On the other hand, parenterally administered iron, given usually as transfused blood, accumulates largely in reticuloendothelial cells where the transfused erythrocytes are eventually destroyed and their hemoglobin degraded. In iron overload, serum iron concentration and transferrin saturation are usually increased, and the TIBC may be depressed. A simple classification based on the mechanism of iron overloading follows.

I. Excessive gastrointestinal absorption of iron
  A. Hereditary hemochromatosis
    1. Hereditary European (HLA-linked) hemochromatosis
    2. African hemochromatosis (once called "Bantu siderosis")
    3. Hereditary sideroblastic anemia
    4. Congenital atransferrinemia
    5. Congenital aceruloplasminemia
  B. Iatrogenic (from prolonged therapeutic administration of iron to subjects not iron deficient)
  C. Chronic alcoholism or chronic liver disease (usually alcoholic cirrhosis) and possibly pancreatic insufficiency
  D. "Shunt hemochromatosis"
  E. Certain types of severe chronic anemia, usually associated with ineffective erythropoiesis and increased hemolysis
II. Transfusional hemosiderosis or hemochromatosis

Traditionally, the term *hemosiderosis* has denoted an increase in iron storage without associated tissue damage; *hemochromatosis* has indicated that such damage is present, particularly in the liver, that the iron overload is generalized, and that the amount of iron is greatly increased (usually 20–40 g). In present usage, however, *hemochromatosis* has come to mean a severe or potentially severe iron-overload disorder with or without evidence of tissue injury.

Hereditary Hemochromatosis (European or HLA-Linked Type)

Hereditary hemochromatosis (HH) is a relatively common, autosomal recessive, inborn error of metabolism in which increased intestinal absorption of iron results in slowly progressive accumulation of the metal throughout life.

Genetics

Efforts by several groups of investigators to identify the gene for hemochromatosis culminated in the observation in mid-1996 that the gene is located approximately 4 Mb

(4 million nucleotide base pairs) telomeric to the major histocompatibility (MHC) complex on the short arm of chromosome 6. The gene has a sequence of 1029 base pairs arranged in 7 exons, of which 6 encode a protein, termed *Hfe,* that contains 343 amino acids. On the basis of the nucleotide sequence, the protein is quite similar to MHC class I molecules, including a signal sequence, a peptide-binding region, an immunoglobulin-like domain, a transmembrane region, and a small cytoplasmic portion (Fig. 10.14) (33). The extracellular portion of the molecule, as in other MHC class I proteins, has three domains, designated $\alpha 1$, $\alpha 2$, and $\alpha 3$. Each of these contains several β-pleated sheets. The $\alpha 3$ domain is closely associated with β_2-microglobulin, which is encoded by a gene on chromosome 15. The Hfe protein appears to be expressed in nearly all cell lines tested.

The function of Hfe protein is presently unknown. Since it spans the cell membrane, it may have a role in sensing iron content in cytosol and thus in controlling uptake or exclusion of iron or iron-carrier protein complexes at the cell surface. The complex of the $\alpha 3$ domain with β_2-microglobulin is structurally homologous with the constant region of immunoglobulin, and in MHC class I proteins, it is the site of binding to antigen. Thus, it is reasonable to conjecture that the postulated protein may bind another protein (possibly heme or mucin or another as yet unidentified protein) that carries iron and presents it to the cell membrane. The function of the Hfe protein might be to bind the iron-protein complex and exclude it from uptake by cells that have sufficient iron in the cytosol. Structural alteration of Hfe protein would then permit unregulated uptake of iron by intestinal epithelial cells as well as by hepatocytes and other parenchymal cells.

Mutations in the Hfe Protein. Two mutations have been identified, at nt (nucleotide) 845, G→A and at nt 187, C→G. These correspond to amino acid substitutions 282 Cys→Tyr (C282Y) and 63 His→Asp (H63D), respectively (33, 157, 158). The cysteinyl residue normally present at amino acid position 282 is involved in a disulfide bridge; replacement by a tyrosinyl residue at this position would significantly alter the quaternary structure of the protein and thus its function.

Identification of these two mutations indicates that three genotypes can be defined:

Wild type (normal) with 187 C and 845 G	Genotype 845 G (or 282C)
Mutant allele with 187 C, 845 A	Genotype 845 A (or 282Y)
Mutant allele with 187 G, 845 G	Genotype 187 G (or 63D)

Of 178 U.S. patients from numerous medical centers who were believed to be homozygous for HH, 5 of every 6, or 83%, were homozygous for genotype 845 A (282Y/282Y); thus, their Hfe proteins would have the substitution 282, Cys→Tyr. For a population in which there are three alleles for a gene, which occur together two at a time (because chromosomes are in pairs), six combinations may be predicted: there will be three sets of homozygotes and three sets of heterozygotes. These are shown in Table 10.11, together with the genotype frequencies observed in a study of 193 control subjects who did not have iron overload and 147 subjects who had been diagnosed by other means as having hemochromatosis (157). In this study, no instances were observed in the control population of homozygotes for the 282Y mutation, an observation that indicates very strong penetrance of this hemochromatosis gene. Compound heterozygotes who had the major hemochromatosis allele 282Y on one chromosome and the minor hemochromatosis allele 63D on the other also were at high risk of having full expression of hemochromatosis, although a fifth of these compound heterozygotes were in the control group. No cases were observed of homozygotes for the minor hemochromatosis allele 63D, probably reflecting only that they are relatively uncommon (the expected 63D homozygote frequency in this population would be only about 3/100 to have a

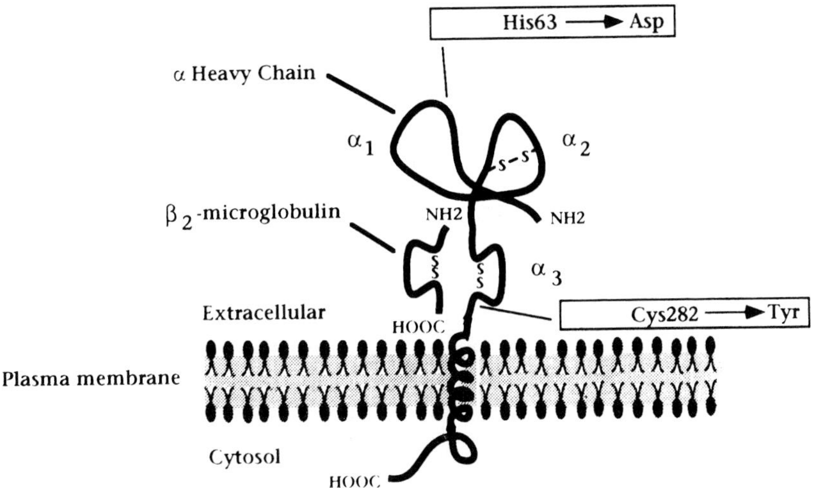

Figure 10.14. Postulated structure of the hemochromatosis protein. *Note:* The hemochromatosis protein and its gene are now designated Hfe rather than HLA-H. (From Feder JN, Gnirke A, Thomas W, et al. Nature Genet 1996;13:399–408, with permission.)

Table 10.11
Genotype Frequencies for the Hfe Alleles in Normal and Hemochromatosis Subjects

	Controls		Hemochromatosis	
Genotypes[a]	*N*	(%)	*N*	(%)
Homozygotes				
282C/282C	112	(58.0)	10	(7.8)
282Y/282Y	0		121	(82.3)
63D/63D	0		0	
Heterozygotes				
282C/282Y	27	(14.0)	2	(1.4)
282C/63D	52	(26.9)	6	(4.1)
282Y/63D	2	(1.0)	8	(5.4)

Data from Beutler E, Gelbart T, West C, et al. Blood Cells Mol Dis 1996;184:1975–85.
[a]As indicated in the text, the following are equivalent designations for the Hfe alleles. 282C = 845G, the normal or "wild type" allele; 282Y = 845A, the major hemochromatosis allele; 63D = 187G, a minor hemochromatosis allele.

282C/63D heterozygote frequency of 27%; no instances of 63D/63D homozygotes, in a sample of 193, is consistent with a homozygote frequency of 3%).

Clearly, elucidation of the molecular genetics of hemochromatosis has only begun. Genotypes 845A (282Y) and 187C (63D) account for 90% of cases of homozygous hemochromatosis. The other 10% of cases may represent iron overloading without a genetic basis or may be due to other mutations of this gene that remain to be identified. Furthermore, the molecular genetics of non-HLA-linked African hemochromatosis has yet to be elucidated. A strain of mice that lacks β_2-microglobulin has iron overload that closely resembles human HH (158). Absence of the Hfe $\alpha 3$ domain–β_2-microglobulin complex on the cell surface apparently results in loss of ability to prevent absorption of iron. An analogous mutation of the β_2-microglobulin gene has not been described in humans. However, if it does occur, it might account for some of the cases of hereditary hemochromatosis that appear not to be HLA linked. A constitutive mutation in the Nramp2 gene, might also lead to excessive absorption of iron (23, 24).

Geographic Distribution of HH. Extensive studies of the prevalence of HH indicate that the homozygous condition occurs with a frequency of about 3 to 5/1000 in Iceland, Norway, Denmark, Ireland, the United Kingdom, Sweden, France, the Netherlands, western and southern Germany, northern Spain, Canada, and the United States and in persons of predominantly European origin in South Africa, New Zealand, and Australia (159–171). HH appears to be quite rare in Finland, North Africa, Greece, Turkey, and the Middle East and in people of Asian origin. These prevalence rates imply a gene frequency of about 0.04 to 0.09 and a carrier rate of 10 to 15% for Caucasians of northern European derivation.

Furthermore, it implies that most cases of hemochromatosis are not correctly diagnosed during life. Very likely, many such cases are diagnosed as diabetes mellitus, rheumatoid arthritis, or idiopathic cardiomyopathy, without the underlying iron storage disease being recognized.

The occasional observation of apparent autosomal dominant inheritance of hemochromatosis now appears to result from homozygote-heterozygote matings. The homozygous state may be manifest any time after puberty in males, but it is unusual prior to menopause in women, since iron loss through menstruation provides a "safety valve."

The mechanism of increased iron absorption in hemochromatosis remains a puzzle. The mucosal epithelial cells themselves do not appear to have increased iron content, although the macrophages of the subendothelial layers do, as do nearly all other cells of the body. Furthermore, although, in HH, the mucosal epithelial cells are capable of markedly reducing their uptake of inorganic iron, they exhibit an increased rate of absorption of heme iron despite systemic iron overload.

Linkage between Hfe and HLA-A Genes. Because of the tight linkage to the HLA-A gene, there is a linkage disequilibrium between HLA genotypes in persons with HH of the European type; 70% have the HLA-A3 specificity, which is observed in only 28% of the general Caucasian population. Some physicians may be tempted to use HLA typing as a screening test for hemochromatosis or in the attempt to differentiate it from alcoholic cirrhosis. Either application is illogical, wastes resources, and is meaningless, because any patient with alcoholic cirrhosis has nearly a 30% likelihood of having the HLA-A3 antigen and 30% of patients with hemochromatosis do not have HLA-A3. The odds are nearly 100:1 that any person in the United States whose cells have the HLA-A3 antigen is not homozygous for, and will never develop, hemochromatosis. Furthermore, HLA testing is time consuming and costly. However, the procedure has merit for examining siblings of a known patient with hemochromatosis, since siblings who are genotypically identical to an affected patient may be presumed also to be homozygous for hereditary hemochromatosis. As a consequence, those who are not genotypically identical may be reassured. In this application, it does not matter what the HLA type is—A3 or any other type. However, now that the HH gene has been identified, DNA methods can be used to test for homozygous HH.

Clinical Features. The classical "triad" of hemochromatosis—cirrhosis, diabetes, and hyperpigmentation of the skin—are only the most striking clinical features of a far-advanced state of this disorder. The other major clinical features of hemochromatosis are fatigue, cardiac arrhythmias, dilated or restrictive cardiomyopathy (due to iron deposition in heart muscle cells), cardiac failure, arthropathy that may mimic rheumatoid arthritis, hypothyroidism, gonadal failure secondary to marked reduction in pituitary hormone secretion, and testicular atrophy. Arthritis has most often affected the second and third metacarpophalangeal joints, the knee, or the hip joint. The diabetes, arthropathy, and sterility are usually irreversible, but cardiac function and hepatic function commonly improve following removal of excess iron. Patients with hemochromatosis have a substantially increased risk of hepatocellular carcinoma. Overall, about one of every seven hemochromatosis patients dies of hepatoma. Of those who have liver cirrhosis, approximately 30% develop hepatoma (hepatocellular carcinoma) (172, 173). If cirrhosis is avoided by timely diagnosis and aggressive phlebotomy therapy, the risk of hepatoma becomes minuscule. The risk of hepatoma is not affected by phlebotomy therapy once cirrhosis has developed. Aberrations in mental function may be observed in about a third of patients with hemochromatosis. These aberrations include marked lethargy, somnolence, confusion, and disorientation.

Patients with hereditary hemochromatosis manifest increased susceptibility to infection. Sudden onset of overwhelming sepsis and shock was once a common cause of death in patients with this disorder. Persons with iron overload of any cause are especially susceptible to septicemia from the marine bacterium *Vibrio vulnificus,* a microorganism that grows rapidly when iron is readily available (174–176). The infection is usually acquired by handling or eating raw shellfish such as oysters. Septicemia is rapidly progressive and commonly fatal. Cases have also been reported of peritonitis and of septicemia due to *Yersinia enterocolitica* in patients with hereditary hemochromatosis, thalassemia major, or oral iron overdosing. This microorganism appears to be an "opportunistic pathogen," causing severe or fatal infections in persons debilitated from a variety of disorders. Sudden onset of, and death from, septicemia from *Escherichia coli,* a normal inhabitant of the gastrointestinal tract, has also been observed.

Diagnosis. Screening tests for hemochromatosis should include assay of serum iron concentration, TIBC, transferrin saturation (in %), and ferritin concentration. These should be performed on serum specimens from *everybody,* beginning at age 20. Extensive studies have proven universal screening for hemochromatosis to be highly cost effective in reducing the long-term costs of medical care, preventing morbidity, and saving lives.

The tests need to be repeated every few decades, since they may be falsely negative during early decades because iron overload develops very gradually. Taken together, these tests, when abnormal, provide a high level of confidence for identification of persons likely to have hemochromatosis, although many cases are missed even with these tests. Persons with serum iron concentrations above 32 μmol/L and transferrin saturation above 60% on repeated assays (at least twice) must be assumed to be at risk of hemochromatosis until proven otherwise. The observation of persistently elevated SI and transferrin saturation is a hallmark of the homozygous state for HH; these findings may be present for years before elevation of serum ferritin or other clinical or laboratory features of HH are manifest. Elevations in SI and transferrin saturation may persist despite vigorous phlebotomy therapy and normalization of iron stores and serum ferritin (177). Very often, serum activity of aspartate aminotransferase (AST, SGOT) is elevated early in the course of HH. Alanine aminotransferase (ALT, SGPT) may also be elevated. Serum bilirubin concentration is normal.

Examination of bone marrow iron content is often misleading in HH, as the iron content may be normal. Noninvasive methods for demonstrating iron overload in liver, such as computer-assisted tomography (CAT) or magnetic resonance imaging (MRI) scans have had a limited role in diagnosis. However, recent development of MRI techniques seems to offer promise for a sensitive noninvasive method of assessing the degree of iron excess in the liver. They do not document presence or absence of cirrhosis.

The definitive diagnostic test is usually liver biopsy. The specimen should be sectioned and stained with hematoxylin and eosin and with Perls' Prussian blue stain for iron. It is also useful to divide the specimen and measure the iron content in one portion.

Microscopic examination of iron content generally correlates well with the chemical assay. In normal liver, the iron content is estimated to be 0 to 1+ histologically and less than 50 μmol/g (2.8 mg/g) dry weight. In persons with alcoholic liver disease, the iron content of liver is not more than 0 to 2+ microscopically and less than 100 μmol/g (5.6 mg/g) dry weight. In hemochromatosis, liver iron content is 3 to 4+ by microscopic estimation and usually exceeds 100 μmol/g by chemical assay. Most patients with cirrhotic hemochromatosis have a liver iron content of at least 200 μmol/g (11 mg/g) dry weight. Since the iron content of liver normally increases slowly with age, a "hepatic iron index" (HII) can be calculated by dividing hepatic iron content in μmol/g by age in years (178, 179). Persons who are homozygous for HH have HII values above 1.9 but rarely above 20. There is a little overlap in HII values between some persons with homozygous HH and some heterozygotes, but patients are clearly distinguished from normal controls and alcoholic cirrhotics.

Treatment. Hereditary hemochromatosis is treated by a vigorous program of phlebotomy: removal of 500 mL of blood one to three times weekly over the course of 1 to 2 years. Since each 500 mL of blood contains 200 to 250 mg of iron, such treatment removes, in time, 10 to 40 g of iron. The phlebotomy program must be continued until the iron excess has been removed. This is first evidenced by a falling venous hemoglobin concentration that does not return to 110 g/L (women) or 120 g/L (men) within a week. The serum ferritin concentration should then be below 20 μg/L. When this point has been reached, the initial phase of treatment has been completed. Thereafter, patients should have a 500-mL phlebotomy once every 2 to 6 months for the remainder of their lives, with the objective of keeping the serum ferritin concentration at 20 μg/L or below. Measurement of SI, TIBC and Tsat in phlebotomy-treated patients is not warranted. The SI and Tsat will likely be high (172). These abnormalities are characteristic of hemochromatosis irrespective of the size of iron stores; SI and Tsat should not be used as guides to treatment.

The required phlebotomy frequency following the initial phase of treatment varies and must be determined individually. The dramatic improvement in longevity and reduction in complications that attend this treatment have been amply documented. If this program is undertaken before hepatic cirrhosis or diabetes mellitus has developed, survival is indistinguishable from age- and sex-matched normal subjects (180).

In addition to iron removal, the endocrine, cardiac, and joint manifestations of HH may require appropriate treatment. Patients with HH must abstain absolutely from alcohol consumption. However, attempts to reduce iron intake by reducing meat or bread consumption are rarely indicated. An ordinary well-balanced diet should be recommended.

Iron chelators such as desferrioxamine have no rational place in treatment of HH. In secondary hemochromatosis, as in transfusion-dependent thalassemia major, however, parenteral administration of iron chelators is essential.

African Hemochromatosis ("Bantu Siderosis")

Iron overload in black people of South Africa (first recognized in those of the Bantu linguistic stock, although not limited or predetermined by language) appears also to have a genetic basis, but it is usually associated with long-continued exposure to diets containing too much iron, derived largely from cooking pots and from the steel barrels used in preparation of fermented alcoholic beverages. The prevalence of the carrier state in sub-Saharan African populations has been reported as 30%. This gene presumably also occurs in African Americans, but no prevalence data are available.

In adult males, the iron intake from beer brewed in steel drums may exceed 100 mg iron per day. The condition frequently becomes manifest in late adolescence and reaches its greatest severity between the ages of 40 and 60 years. It is usually more severe in males, whose alcoholic consumption tends to be greater. The histologic pattern of the iron overload is initially one of deposition of iron in reticuloendothelial cells, such as Kupffer cells of the liver. Portal cirrhosis becomes evident in most patients (but not in all) when the hepatic concentration of iron reaches 2 g or more per 100 g dry weight. Redistribution of iron takes place, so that parenchymal deposits of hemosiderin are found in epithelial cells of many organs, particularly pancreas and the myocardium. Approximately 20% of these subjects develop clinical diabetes, but myocardial failure has not been described. To what extent these changes are caused by iron alone, by chronic alcoholism, or by associated nutritional disturbances is unknown.

Hereditary Sideroblastic Anemia

Hereditary sideroblastic anemia, a rare sex-linked disorder, is typically associated with anemia that may be mild to severe. The disorder is rarely seen in its complete form in women. In the erythroblasts of the bone marrow one may demonstrate, by Perls' stain, the presence of large blue granules encircling the nuclei like a necklace. These are "ringed sideroblasts." The granules are mitochondria stuffed with iron, which is the reason for the blue stain. Iron accumulates in the mitochondria because of a deficiency of ALA-S, the first enzyme in heme synthesis. This metabolic "bottleneck" in mitochondrial metabolism results in accumulation of heme precursors, most conspicuously iron. The gene has been identified on the X chromosome. All of the features of organ injury from iron overload in liver, pancreas, joints, pituitary, etc., are encountered in this disorder.

Congenital Atransferrinemia

Congenital atransferrinemia is an exceedingly rare disorder (the author's patient is the only one known to be living in the Western hemisphere at present). It is due to an inability to synthesize transferrin. The nature of the mutation is as yet unknown, but since it has occurred in two pairs of siblings (in Japan and Mexico), it appears to be an autosomal recessive disorder. There is a moderate-to-severe anemia. Serum iron concentration and total iron binding capacity are near zero. Serum ferritin may be very high as a result of excessive iron absorption from the gastrointestinal tract. All manifestations of severe generalized hemochromatosis may be observed, including hypogonadism due to absence of pituitary gonadotropins. Since patients have no transferrin to bind iron, they are unusually susceptible to overwhelming bacterial infections, which are the usual cause of death. The author's patient has responded well to monthly administrations of plasma (to provide transferrin) preceded by removal of 500 mL of blood (to remove iron). Replacement hormonal therapy is also required, since there is hypothalamic, hypogonadotrophic hypogonadism, as often occurs in severe iron overloading of any cause.

Congenital Aceruloplasminemia

Congenital aceruloplasminemia is a rare autosomal recessive disorder that leads to excessive iron accumulation in the brain, liver, and pancreas, with the clinical features of mental slowing or dementia and diabetes mellitus–induced retinal degeneration, dysarthria, blepharospasm, and "cogwheel" rigidity of the extremities. In contrast with Wilson's disease, a Kayser-Fleischer ring has not been observed. Serum iron concentration is low, total iron binding capacity is normal, and serum ferritin concentration is elevated (e.g., 1500 μg/L). There is a mild microcytic anemia. Ceruloplasmin is absent in serum; serum copper concentration is low, urinary copper excretion is normal; liver copper is normal. Liver biopsy specimens have shown 3+ deposition of iron in hepatocytes, indistinguishable from the pattern observed in European (HLA-linked) hemochromatosis (182).

Ceruloplasmin functions as ferroxidase in iron metabolism, catalyzing the interconversion of Fe(II) and Fe(III). It appears that in aceruloplasminemia, the divalent iron that enters plasma cannot be oxidized to trivalent iron, an essential conversion prior to uptake of trivalent iron by transferrin. Therefore, divalent iron is taken up by apoferritin in the cytosol of various tissues, and iron overloading ensues.

Because of the microcytic anemia and low serum iron and low transferrin saturation, such patients are at risk of being diagnosed as having iron deficiency and being treated with iron—clearly a therapy that is contraindicated. If clinicians rely on serum ferritin assay to diagnose iron deficiency, as they should, they will not make this mistake. It would be reasonable to treat these patients by phlebotomy to reduce the iron overload. However, such treatment has not yet been reported.

Alcoholic Cirrhosis, Chronic Alcoholism, and Pancreatic Insufficiency

Patients with alcoholic or nutritional portal cirrhosis of the liver frequently have slightly increased amounts of stainable iron in their livers. The total amount present rarely exceeds 1 g. Clinical similarity to hemochromatosis is accentuated by the occurrence also in alcoholic cirrhosis of increased skin pigmentation, a higher incidence of diabetes mellitus than can be ascribed to coincidence, testicular atrophy, and increased risk of hepatoma. Cardiac failure, when it occurs, can usually be accounted for on other grounds. More males than females are affected, and clinical manifestations are most prominent in late middle life.

A number of possible explanations for the iron overload have been cited. Patients with hepatic cirrhosis are frequently wine drinkers and may consume several liters daily. European wines may contain significant quantities of iron (although American wines may not), and several milligrams per day may be derived from that source alone. Patients with chronic liver disease or chronic pancreatitis may have greater than normal intestinal absorption of iron.

While the controversy over the genetic basis of "idiopathic" hemochromatosis has been resolved, there remains the issue of whether alcoholic cirrhosis per se can lead to serious iron overload. Seventy percent of cirrhotic patients with marked iron overload have the HLA-A3 allele, a frequency identical with that in hereditary hemochromatosis, whereas the frequency of HLA-A3 is 30% in cirrhotics without iron overload, identical to that in the general population (183). Thus, studies of HLA antigen frequencies in HH and in alcoholic cirrhosis show that all or most alcoholic cirrhosis patients with iron overload in fact have hereditary hemochromatosis, and ethanol abuse increases the risk of hepatic cirrhosis but is not the primary cause of iron overload.

Shunt Hemochromatosis

Many cases have been observed of "shunt hemochromatosis" that appears within a few years of establishment of a shunt between the portal and systemic venous systems. The shunt has usually been created surgically to relieve pressure in esophageal varices, and in most instances, iron loading has followed end-to-side anastomoses. However, the disorder has also developed spontaneously, presumably from formation of collateral channels between portal and systemic veins. Iron accumulation is astonishingly rapid. The mechanism is unknown. The manifestations are the same as those of hemochromatosis from other causes.

Prolonged Iron Therapy

A few cases have been reported in which inappropriate administration of iron, orally or parenterally, for decades, to non-iron-deficient patients has led to typical hemochromatosis. Since iron preparations are advertised widely in the United States, are available without prescription, and are consumed in large quantities, it is astonishing that so few cases have been reported. Therefore, the potential of iron preparations to cause iron overload deserves special attention. One can estimate mathematically the amount of iron that might accumulate in the body of normal persons when different amounts of medicinal iron are administered over long periods of time. These estimates, for which the calculations were shown in the seventh edition of *Modern Nutrition in Health and Disease,* are illustrated in Figure 10.15. As can be seen from the uppermost curve of

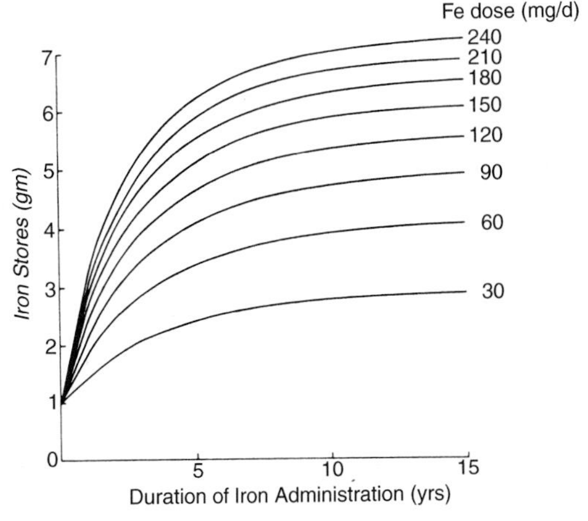

Figure 10.15. Expected accumulation of iron in menstruating women receiving single daily doses of 30 to 240 mg. Data are based on the assumptions that iron absorption in females is $D^{0.668}$, where D is the dose of iron in grams, that iron absorption is modified by stores to the extent of $3^{-0.196(F-1)}$, and that excretion is $0.0009\sqrt{F} + 0.0005$, where F is the iron stores in grams. 1 g Fe = 17.9 mmol.

this illustration, even at a daily dose of 240 mg of iron (e.g., four ferrous sulfate tablets daily), which amounts to a total ingested dose of 1.3 kg in 15 years, the increase in body iron content is still well below that commonly encountered in HH. These facts emphasize the remarkable way in which modulation of iron absorption by the intestinal mucosa tends to protect normal persons from the adverse effects of excessive iron ingestion. In view of the high prevalence of hereditary hemochromatosis, the widespread use of iron supplements, and the rarity of cases in which hemochromatosis is attributed to chronic ingestion of iron, some of these patients may be homozygous for hereditary hemochromatosis.

Clearly, there is some hazard from prolonged administration of large doses of iron to persons who are not iron deficient. This is particularly a problem for patients with thalassemias and other chronic anemias, for whom the ultimate development of hemochromatosis is a very serious complication of treatment. For premenopausal women who have normal menses and do not have thalassemia or other chronic anemias, the hazard of serious iron overload resulting from exogenous iron is slight. However, inappropriate and prolonged administration of iron, by oral or parenteral route, to adults who are not bleeding and not iron deficient needlessly exposes them to the risk of hemochromatosis with all its serious complications.

Severe Chronic Anemia

The amount of iron found in the tissues of patients with refractory anemia, particularly those with hypercellular marrows and ineffective erythropoiesis, is occasionally greater than can be accounted for by the transfusions they have received. In some cases, little blood was given during the course of the illness, yet excess iron was present. Some, but not all, of these subjects have been inappropriately treated with iron. Excessive absorption of dietary iron must have occurred, presumably because of the accelerated but ineffective erythropoiesis. Patients at risk include those with sideroblastic anemia, thalassemia major, pyruvate kinase deficiency, and paroxysmal nocturnal hemoglobinuria. The cardiac and hepatic complications of hemochromatosis are common causes of death in patients with sideroblastic anemias or β-thalassemia major.

Severe iron overload may occur in patients with congenital dyserythropoietic anemia. Hereditary spherocytosis and thalassemia minor are not usually associated with iron overload, except in patients misdiagnosed as having iron deficiency and given copious amounts of iron over many years. However, some cases have been reported in which these disorders coexisted with hereditary hemochromatosis. In view of the high prevalence of the latter disorder in persons of European ancestry, the concurrence of these disorders is hardly surprising. In such patients, large amounts of hemosiderin are found in both parenchymal and reticuloendothelial cells.

Transfusional Hemosiderosis

Whenever chronic anemia that has been treated by numerous transfusions over many years is found in a patient who does not have chronic bleeding, iron overload is likely to occur. These patients may experience all the consequences described above for HH. This complication is most often found in severe thalassemias such as β-thalassemia major, in some sideroblastic anemias, and in hypoplastic or other refractory anemias. For many of these patients, long-term treatment with the iron chelating agent desferrioxamine is essential. The desferrioxamine must be administered daily by subcutaneous infusion for 12 to 16 h, a treatment that is cumbersome and expensive. Effective oral iron chelating agents are being developed and may become available within a few years. They should supplant parenteral desferrioxamine therapy for these patients.

Surprisingly, some patients with marked iron overload resulting from transfusion never manifest severe organ damage. However, some persons with HH and marked iron overload also do not exhibit evidence of organ damage. These paradoxes may reflect the fact that serious organ injury is more likely to occur in patients subjected to toxic substance(s) or hepatitis in addition to iron excess.

OTHER DISORDERS RELATED TO IRON METABOLISM

Porphyria Cutanea Tarda

Porphyria cutanea tarda is typified by hepatic dysfunction, neuropathy, behavioral aberrations, and cutaneous sunlight hypersensitivity. It is related to iron metabolism in an as yet unknown manner. Most patients exhibit moderate iron overload. The manifestations of this disease are ameliorated by phlebotomy therapy.

Congenital Cataract with Hyperferritinemia

A few families have been described in which congenital nuclear cataracts were associated with hyperferritinemia without iron overload. The condition is inherited as an autosomal dominant disorder. The serum iron, TIBC, and transferrin saturation are normal, but serum ferritin concentration may be several thousand micrograms per liter. The ferritin contains only the L subunit. Hyperferritinemia is due to mutations in the IRE of the mRNA for apoferritin, such that normal regulation of apoferritin synthesis by the IRP-IRE mechanism cannot occur. So far as is known, there is no iron deposition in the affected lenses. However, unbridled constitutive synthesis of a protein within cells of the crystalline lens that should only contain lens protein may have an adverse colloid osmotic effect. There is, as yet, no report that any other cells or organs are adversely affected (184–186).

Superficial Hemosiderosis of the Central Nervous System

Superficial hemosiderosis of the central nervous system is a rare disorder that results from recurrent subarachnoid hemorrhages with deposition of iron in the meninges. It may be associated with ataxia and other central nervous system manifestations. It is not related in any way to disorders of iron metabolism (187).

REFERENCES

1. Fairbanks VF, Fahey JL, Beutler E. Clinical disorders of iron metabolism. 2nd ed. New York: Grune & Stratton, 1971;1–41.
2. Troisier E. Diabete sucre. Bull Soc Anat (Paris) 1871;46: 231–5.
3. Stockman R. J Physiol (London) 1895;18:484–9.
4. Heath CW, Strauss MB, Castle WB. J Clin Invest 1932; 11:1293–312.
5. Beinert H, Kennedy MC. FASEB J 1993;7(15):1442–9.
6. Haile DJ, Tracey AR, Harford JB, et al. Proc Natl Acad Sci USA 1992;89:11735–9.
7. Leveille GA, Zabik ME, Morgan KJ. Nutrients in foods. Cambridge, MA: Nutrition Guild, 1983.
8. Watt BK, Merrill AL. Composition of foods. Agriculture handbook no. 8. Washington, DC: Consumer and Food Economics Research Division, Agricultural Research Service, United States Department of Agriculture, 1963.
9. Adams CF. Nutritive value of American foods. Agriculture handbook no. 456. Washington, DC: Agricultural Research Service, United States Department of Agriculture, 1975.
10. Federation of American Societies for Experimental Biology, Life Science Research Office, Interagency Board for Nutrition Monitoring and Related Research. Third report on nutrition monitoring in the US, vol I. Washington, DC: U.S. Government Printing Office, 1995.
11. Federation of American Societies for Experimental Biology, Life Science Research Office, Interagency Board for Nutrition Monitoring and Related Research. Third report on nutrition monitoring in the US, vol II. Washington, DC: U.S. Government Printing Office, 1995.
12. Federation of American Societies for Experimental Biology, Life Science Research Office, Interagency Board for Nutrition Monitoring and Related Research. Third report on nutrition monitoring in the US. Executive summary. Washington, DC: U.S. Government Printing Office, 1995.
13. Anon. Cheese facts. Washington, DC: International Dairy Foods Association, 1995.
14. Kennedy E, Goldberg J. Nutr Rev 1995;53:111–26.
15. Simpson RJ, Moore R, Peters TJ. Biochim Biophys Acta 1988;941:39–47.
16. Simpson RJ, Venkatesan S, Peters TJ. Cell Biochem Funct 1989;7:165–71.
17. Sanyal AJ, Hirsch JI, Moore EW. J Lab Clin Med 1990; 116:76–86.
18. Slatkavitz CA, Clydesdale FM. Am J Clin Nutr 1988;47:487–95.
19. Taylor PG, Martinez-Torres C, Romano EL, et al. Am J Clin Nutr 1986;68–71.
20. Conrad ME, Umbreit JN, Moore EG. Gastroenterology 1991;100:129–36.
21. Teichmann R, Stremmel W. J Clin Invest 1990;86:2145–53.
22. Conrad ME, Umbreit JN, Raymond DA, et al. Blood 1993; 81(2):517–21.
23. Fleming MD, Trenor CC III, Su MA, et al. Nature Genet 1997;16:383–6.
24. Vulpe C, Gitschier J. Nature Genet 1997;16:319–20.
25. Conrad ME, Umbreit JN, Moore EG, et al. J Biol Chem 1994;269:7169–73.
26. Conrad ME, Umbreit JN, Moore EG. Gastroenterology 1993;104:1700–4.
27. Hallberg L, Sölvell L. Acta Med Scand 1965;181:335.
28. Weintraub LR, Weinstein, MB, Huser HJ, et al. J Clin Invest 1968;47:531–9.
29. Raffin SB, Woo CH, Roost KT, et al. J Clin Invest 1974; 54:1344–52.
30. Brown EB, Hwang YF, Nicol S, et al. J Lab Clin Med 1968;72:58–64.
31. Turnbull A, Cleton F, Finch CA. J Clin Invest 1962;41: 1897–907.
32. Hallberg L, Sölvell L. Acta Med Scand 1967;181:335–54.
33. Feder JN, Gnirke A, Thomas W, et al. Nature Genet 1996;13: 399–408.
34. Turnlund JR, Smith RG, Kretsch MJ, et al. Am J Clin Nutr 1990;52:373–8.
35. Hurrell RF, Lynch SR, Trinidad TP, et al. Am J Clin Nutr 1989;49:546–52.
36. MacFarlane BJ, van der Riet WB, Bothwell TH, et al. Am J Clin Nutr 1990;51:873–80.
37. Morck TA, Lynch SR, Cook JD. Am J Clin Nutr 1983; 37:416–20.
38. Munoz LM, Lonnerdal B, Keen CL, et al. Am J Clin Nutr 1988;48:645–51.
39. Fairweather-Tait SJ, Piper Z, Fatemi SJ, et al. Br J Nutr 1991;65:61–8.
40. MacFarlane BJ, Bezwoda WR, Bothwell TH, et al. Am J Clin Nutr 1988;47:270–4.
41. Hallberg L, Rossander L, Skonberg AB. Am J Clin Nutr 1987;45:988–96.
42. Hallberg L. Scand J Gastroenterol Suppl 1987;129:73–9.
43. Brune M, Rossander L, Hallberg L. Am J Clin Nutr 1989; 49:542–5.
44. Fairweather-Tait SJ, Wright AJ. Br J Nutr 1990;64:547–52.
45. Siegenberg D, Baynes RD, Bothwell TH, et al. Am J Clin Nutr 1991;53:537–41.
46. Fernandez R, Phillips SF. Am J Clin Nutr 1982;35:107–12.
47. Tuntawiroon M, Sritongkul N, Brune M, et al. Am J Clin Nutr 1991;53:554–7.
48. Rossander L. Scand J Gastroenterol Suppl 1987;129:68–72.
49. Frølich W, Lysø A. Am J Clin Nutr 1983;37:31–6.
50. Crofton RW, Gvozdanovic D, Gvozdanovic S, et al. Am J Clin Nutr 1989;50:141–4.
51. Beutler E, Kelly BM, Beutler F. Am J Clin Nutr 1962;11: 559–67.
52. Celada A, Rudolf H, Donath A. Am J Hematol 1978;5: 225–37.
53. Mazzanti R, Srai KS, Debnam ES, et al. Alcohol 1987; 22:47–52.
54. Chapman RW, Morgan MY, Boss AM. Dig Dis Sci 1983; 28:321–7.
55. Marx JJ, Gebbink JA, Nishisato T, et al. Br J Haematol 1982;52:105–10.
56. Moore CV. The absorption of iron from foods. In: Blix A, ed. Symposium on occurrence, causes and prevention of nutritional anaemias. Swedish Nutrition Foundation, Tylösand, 1967, Symposia 6. Uppsala: Almqvist and Wiksells, 1968.
57. Layrisse M, Martinez-Torres C. Prog Hematol 1971;7:137–60.
58. Josephs HW. Blood 1958;13:1–54.

59. Gillooly M, Bothwell TH, Torrance JD, et al. Br J Nutr 1983;49:331–42.
60. Hallberg L, Rossander L. Scand J Gastroenterol 1982;17:151–60.
61. Cook JD, Morck TA, Lynch SR. Am J Clin Nutr 1981;34:2622–9.
62. Morris ER, Bodwell CE, Miles CW. Plant Foods Hum Nutr 1987;37:377–89.
63. Baynes RD, Macfarlane BJ, Bothwell TH, et al. Eur J Clin Nutr 1990;44:419–24.
64. Layrisse M, Cook JD, Martinez C, et al. Blood 1969;33:430–43.
65. Martinez-Torres C, Layrisse M. Blood 1970;35:669–82.
66. Layrisse M, Martinez-Torres C, Cook JD, et al. Blood 1973;41:333–52.
67. Bothwell TH. J Intern Med 1989;226:357–65.
68. Bailey S, Evans RW, Garratt RC, et al. Biochem 1988;27:5804–12.
69. März L, Hatton MWC, Berry LR, et al. Can J Biochem 1982;60:624–30.
70. Yang F, Lum JB, McGill JR, et al. Proc Natl Acad Sci USA 1984;81:2752–6.
71. van Haerigen B, de Lange F, van Stokkum IH, et al. Proteins 1995;23:233–40.
72. Jaeken J, Hagberg B, Stromme P. Acta Paediatr Scand Suppl 1991;375:6–13.
73. Stibler H, Jaeken J. Arch Dis Child 1990;65:107–11.
74. Sly DA, Grohlich D, Bezkorovainy A. Biochim Biophys Acta 1975;385:36–40.
75. Sullivan AL, Grasso JA, Weintraub LR. Blood 1976;47:133–43.
76. Hemmaplardh D, Morgan EH. Biochim Biophys Acta 1974;373:84–99.
77. Morgan EH, Appleton TC. Nature 1969;223:1371–2.
78. Martinez-Medellin J, Schulman HM. Biochim Biophys Acta 1972;264:272–4.
79. Cheng TPO. Cell Tissue Res 1986;244:613–9.
80. Dautry-Varsat A. Biochimie 1986;68:375–81.
81. Schneider C, Williams JG. J Cell Sci Suppl 1985;3:139–49.
82. Zerial M, Melancon P, Schneider C, Garoff H. EMBO J 1986;5:1543–50.
83. Cox TM, O'Donnell MW, Aisen P, London IM. J Clin Invest 1985;76:2144–50.
84. Morgan EH, Baker E. Ann NY Acad Sci 1988;526:65–82.
85. Ajioka RS, Kaplan J. Proc Natl Acad Sci USA 1986;83:6445–9.
86. Casey JL, Di Jeso B, Rao KK, et al. Nucleic Acids Res 1988;16:629–46.
87. Casey JL, Di Jeso B, Rao KK, et al. Ann NY Acad Sci 1988;526:54–64.
88. Müllner EW, Kühn LC. Cell 1988;53:815–25.
89. Rouault T, Rao K, Harford J, et al. J Biol Chem 1985;260:14862–6.
90. Casey JL, Di Jeso B, Rao K, et al. Proc Natl Acad Sci USA 1988;85:1787–91.
91. Enns CA, Snomaleinin HA, Gebhart JE, et al. Proc Natl Acad Sci USA 1982;79:3241–5.
92. Miller YE, Jones C, Scoggin C, et al. Am J Hum Genet 1983;35:5783.
93. Hentze MW, Seuanez HN, O'Brien SJ, et al. Nucleic Acids Res 1989;11:6103–8.
94. Knisely AS. Adv Pediatr 1992;39:383–403.
95. Kim HY, LaVaute T, Iwai K, et al. J Biol Chem 1996;271:24226–30.
96. Young SP, Roberts S, Bomford A. Biochem J 1985;232:819–23.
97. Soda R, Tavassoli M. J Ultrastruct Res 1984;88:18–29.
98. Bergamaschi G, Eng MJ, Huebers HA, et al. Proc Soc Exp Biol Med 1986;183:66–73.
99. Larrick JW, Enns C, Raubitschek A, Weintraub H. J Cell Physiol 1985;124:283–7.
100. Stoorvogel W, Geuze HJ, Griffith JM, Strous GJ. J Cell Biol 1988;106:1821–9.
101. Blight GD, Morgan EH. Eur J Cell Biol 1987;43:260–5.
102. Nunez MT, Coles ES, Glass J. Blood 1980;55:1051–5.
103. Pollack S, Campana T, Weaver J. Am J Hematol 1985;19:75–84.
104. Funk F, Lecrenier C, Lesuisse E, et al. Eur J Biochem 1986;157:303–9.
105. Ponka P, Neuwirt J, Borova J. Enzyme 1974;17:91–9.
106. Harrison PM, Clegg GA, May K. Ferritin structure and function. In: Jacobs A, Worwood M, eds. Iron in biochemistry and medicine, II. New York: Academic Press, 1980;131–71.
107. Harrison PM. Semin Hematol 1977;14:557–70.
108. Clegg GA, Stansfield RFD, Bourne PE, et al. Nature 1980;288:298–300.
109. Harrison PM, Treffry A, Lilley TH. J Inorg Biochem 1986;27:287–93.
110. Fischbach FA, Gregory DW, Harrison PM, et al. J Ultrastruct Res 1971;37:495–503.
111. Crichton RR, Roman F, Roland F, et al. J Mol Catal 1980;7:267–76.
112. Crichton RR, Roman F. J Mol Catal 1978;4:75–82.
113. Hoy TG, Harrison PM, Shabbir M. Biochem J 1974;139:603–7.
114. Arosio P, Adelman TG, Drysdale JW. J Biol Chem 1978;253:4451–8.
115. Casey JL, Hentze MW, Koeller DM, et al. Science 1988;240:924–8.
116. Rogers J, Munro H. Proc Natl Acad Sci USA 1987;84:2277–81.
117. Zähringer J, Baliga BS, Munro HN. Proc Natl Acad Sci USA 1976;73:857–61.
118. Hentze MW, Rouault TA, Wright-Caughman S, et al. Proc Natl Acad Sci USA 1987;84:6730–4.
119. Mack U, Storey EL, Powell LW, et al. Biochim Biophys Acta 1985;843:164–70.
120. Beutler E. Ill Med J 1959;116:16–9.
121. Jacobs A. Lancet 1961;2:1331–33.
122. Ackrell BAC, Maguire JJ, Dallman PR, et al. J Biol Chem 1984;259:10053–9.
123. Symes AL, Sowkes TL, Youdim MBH, et al. Can J Biochem 1969;47:999–1002.
124. Youdim MBH, Green AR. CIBA Found Symp 1977;51:201–21.
125. Youdim MBH, Green AR. Proc Nutr Soc 1978;37:173–9.
126. Srivastava SK, Zaheer N, Krishnan PS. (Letter) Arch Biochem Biophys 1964;105:446–7.
127. Bailey-Wood R, Blayney LM, Muir JR, et al. Br J Exp Pathol 1975;56:193–8.
128. Dhur A, Galan P, Hercberg S. J Nutr 1989;119:40–7.
129. Kyaw A, Win T, Pe UH. Biochem Med 1974;11:194–7.
130. Green R, Charlton R, Seftel H, et al. Am J Med 1968;45:336–53.
131. Bothwell TH, Seftel H, Jacobs P, et al. Am J Clin Nutr 1964;14:47–51.
132. Crosby WH, Conrad ME Jr, Wheby MS. Blood 1963;22:429–40.
133. Ebaugh FG Jr, Clemens T Jr, Rodnan G, et al. Am J Med 1958;25:169–81.
134. Hallberg L, Nilsson L. Acta Obstet Gynecol Scand 1964;43:352–9.
135. Hallberg L, Högdahl AM, Nilsson L, et al. Acta Obstet Gynecol Scand 1966;45:320–51.
136. Rybo G. In: Menstrual blood loss. Hallberg L, Harwerth HG, Vannotti A, eds. Iron deficiency: pathogenesis, clinical aspects, therapy. New York: Academic Press, 1970.

137. Simon TL, Hunt WC, Garry PJ. Transfusion 1984;24:469–72.
138. Taylor PG, Mendez-Castellano H, Lopez-Blanco M. J Am Diet Assoc 1988;88:454–8.
139. Herbert V. Am J Clin Nutr 1987;45:679–86.
140. Salonen JT, Nyyssonen K, Korpela H, et al. Circulation 1992;86:803–11.
141. Manttari M, Mannin V, Huttunen JK, et al. (Abstract) Eur Heart J 1994;15:1599–1603.
142. Baer DM, Tekawa IS, Hurley LB. Circulation 1994;89:2915–8.
143. Solymoss BC, Marcil M, Gilfix BM, et al. Coronary Artery Dis 1994;5:231–5.
144. Miller M, Hutchins GM. JAMA 1994;272:231–3.
145. Vital Health Stat 1967, series 11, no. 24.
146. Vital Health Stat 1982, series 11, no. 229.
147. Vital Health Stat 1982, series 11, no. 232.
148. Anía BJ, Suman VJ, Fairbanks VF, Melton LJ III. Mayo Clin Proc 1994;69:730–5.
149. Adekile AD, Yuregir TZ, Walker EL III, et al. South Med J 1994;87:1132–7.
150. Moertel C, Braddock M, Henry P, et al. Blood (Abstract 2778) 1996;88:13b.
151. Lytle LA, Stone EJ, Nichaman MZ, et al. Prev Med 1996;25:465–77.
152. Nicklas TA, Dwyer J, Mitchell P, et al. Prev Med 1996;25: 478–85.
153. Frank GC, Farris RP, Cresanta JL, et al. Prev Med 1985;14: 123–39.
154. Rifkin J. The end of work. New York: GP Putnam's Sons, 1995.
155. Vital Health Stat 1979, series 11, no. 209.
156. Olsson KS, Safwenberg J, Ritter B. Ann NY Acad Sci 1988; 526:1–370.
157. Beutler E, Gelbart T, West C, et al. Blood Cells Mol Dis 1996;22:187–94.
158. Santos M, Schilham MW, Rademakers LH, et al. J Exp Med 1996;184:1975–85.
159. Witte DL, Crosby WH, Edwards CQ, et al. Clin Chim Acta 1996;125:139–200.
160. Merryweather-Clarke AT, Pointon JJ, Shearman JD, et al. J Med Genet 1997;34:275–8.
161. Powell LW, Ferluga J, Hallida JW, et al. Hum Genet 1987; 77:55–6.
162. MacSween RNM, Scott AR. J Clin Pathol 1973;26:936–42.
163. Edwards CQ, Griffen LM, Dadone MM, et al. Am J Hum Genet 1986;38:805–11.
164. Edwards CQ, Griffen LM, Goldgar D, et al. N Engl J Med 1988;318:1355–62.
165. Simon M, Le Midnon L, Fauchet R, et al. Am J Hum Genet 1987;41:89–105.
166. Borwein ST, Ghent CN, Flanagan PR, et al. Clin Invest Med 1983;6:171–9.
167. Meyer TE, Ballot D, Bothwell TH, et al. J Med Genet 1987; 24:348–56.
168. Olsson KS, Ritter B, Rosen U, et al. Acta Med Scand 1983;213:145–50.
169. Hallberg L, Bjorn-Rasmussen E, Juner I. J Intern Med 1989;225:249–55.
170. Lindmark B, Eriksson S. Acta Med Scand 1985;218:299–304.
171. Wiggers P, Dalhoj K, Kiaer H, et al. J Intern Med 1991;51: 143–8.
172. Tiniakos G, Williams R. Appl Pathol 1988;6:128–38.
173. Fargion S, Fracanzani AL, Piperno A, et al. Hepatology 1994; 21:1426–31.
174. Blake PA, Merson MH, Weaver RE, et al. N Engl J Med 1979;300:1–5.
175. Wright AC, Simpson LM, Oliver JD. Infect Immunol 1981; 34:503–7.
176. McManus R. JAMA 1984;251:323–5.
177. Edwards CQ, Griffen LM, Kaplan J, et al. J Int Med 1989; 226:373–9.
178. Bassett ML, Halliday JW, Powell LW. Hepatology 1986;6:24–9.
179. Adams PC. Dig Dis Sci 1990;35:690–2.
180. Niederau C, Fischer R, Sonnenberg A, et al. N Engl J Med 1985;313:1256–62.
181. Harris ZL, Takahashi Y, Miyajima H, et al. Proc Natl Acad Sci USA 1995;92:2539–43.
182. Logan JI, Harveyson KB, Wisdom GB, et al. Q J Med 1994;87:663–70.
183. LeSage G, Baldus WP, Fairbanks VF, et al. Gastroenterology 1983;84:1471–7.
184. Aguilar-Martinez P, Biron C, Masmejean C, et al. Blood 1996;88:1895–903.
185. Girelli D, Olivieri O, Gasparini P, et al. Blood (Letter) 1997;87:4912–3.
186. Girelli D, Corrocher R, Bisceglia L, et al. Blood 1995;86: 4050–3.
187. River Y, Honigman S, Gomori JM, et al. Movement Disorders 1994;9:559–62.

SELECTED READINGS

Crichton RR, Ward RJ. Biochemistry 1992;31:11255–11264.
Harrison PM, Arosio P. Biochim Biophys Acta 1996;1275:161–203.
Hentze MW, Kuhn LC. Proc Nat Acad Sci (USA) 1996;93:8175–8182.
Richardson DR, Ponka P. Biochim Biophys Acta 1997;1331:1–40.
Ponka P. Blood 1997;89:1–25.
Ponka P, Beaumont C, Richardson DR. Hemato 1998;35:35–54.

11. Zinc

JANET C. KING and CARL L. KEEN

HISTORICAL ASPECTS

Zinc (Zn) was recognized as a distinct element in 1509. Evidence of its essentiality was demonstrated in plants in 1869 and in animals in 1934 (1). Because of its wide prevalence in foodstuffs, naturally occurring Zn deficiency was considered unlikely until 1955, when swine parakeratosis was shown to be a Zn deficiency disease. That humans could suffer from Zn deficiency was suggested by observations that malnourished Chinese patients during World War II had low concentrations of plasma Zn. In 1956, a conditioned Zn deficiency syndrome in humans was demonstrated. Since 1961, when the endemic hypogonadism and dwarfism of rural Iran was suggested to be derived from Zn deficiency, there has been increasing appreciation of the magnitude of both the clinical and the public health significance of Zn deficiency states (1–3).

CHEMISTRY

Zn is a IIB element with a completed d subshell and two additional s electrons. Zn has an atomic number of 30, an atomic weight of 65.37 (isotopic mean), and in pure form is a bluish white metal. Zn occurs naturally as five stable isotopes: ^{64}Zn, 48.89%; ^{66}Zn, 27.91%; ^{67}Zn, 4.11%; ^{68}Zn, 18.57%; and ^{70}Zn, 0.62%. Six radioisotopes have been identified, of which three, ^{65}Zn, ^{69m}Zn, and ^{63}Zn are used often in tracer studies (half-lives of 245 days, 13.8 hours, and 38 minutes, respectively). In biologic systems, Zn is virtually always in the divalent state. Zn typically forms complexes with a coordination number of 4, with tetrahedral disposition of ligands around the metal. Zn readily complexes to amino acids, peptides, proteins, and nucleotides. Zn has an affinity for thiol and hydroxy groups and for ligands containing electron-rich nitrogen as a donor. Zn does not exhibit any direct redox chemistry.

BIOLOGIC ACTIVITY

Net delivery of Zn to an organism is a function of the bioavailability and the total amount of Zn in the diet. Bioavailability is defined as the proportion of Zn (or any other nutrient) in food that is absorbed and used. As with most minerals, Zn absorption typically exceeds the amount actually used; the excess absorbed is rapidly excreted.

Food Sources

Foods differ widely in their Zn content. Zn concentrations range from 0.02 mg/100 g for egg white to 1 mg/100 g for light chicken meat to 75 mg/100 g for oysters. Shellfish, beef, and other red meats are good Zn sources. Whole-grain cereals are relatively rich in total Zn. Most of the Zn is contained in the bran and germ portions, and nearly 80% of the total Zn is lost in the wheat milling process (2). There is no standard enrichment policy for Zn, but some breakfast cereal manufacturers fortify the Zn content of their product in amounts ranging from 25 to

100% of the United States recommended dietary allowance (RDA). Nuts and legumes are relatively good plant sources of Zn. Plant Zn concentrations may be enhanced if grown in Zn-rich soil or treated with Zn-rich fertilizers (4).

Zinc Intakes

Total dietary Zn intakes are influenced greatly by food choices. Animal products provide about 70% of the Zn consumed by people in the United States, with about half coming from meat (beef, veal, pork, lamb) (5, 6). Cereals are the primary plant source. Frequently, Zn intakes are correlated with protein intake, but the exact relationship is influenced by protein source. Diets consisting primarily of eggs, milk, poultry, and fish have a lower Zn:protein ratio than those composed of shellfish, beef, and other red meats. Similar variations occur in vegetarian diets. Diets with a rich Zn:protein ratio have liberal quantities of legumes, whole grains, nuts, and cheese, whereas those with a low ratio contain primarily fruits and vegetables. Drinking water is typically low in Zn, providing only 2% of the daily zinc intake (7). The mean daily intake from adult self-selected mixed diets in the United States ranges from 8.6 to 14 mg Zn (2). The mean or median intakes reported in 171 studies summarized by the International Atomic Energy Agency ranged from 4.2 to 19 mg/day; the 10th, 50th, and 90th percentiles of intake were 7, 10, and 14 mg/day, respectively (7). During the first 6 months of life, Zn intake varies with the mode of feeding. Reported intakes of breast-fed infants range from 0.03 mmol/day (1.9 mg/day) at 1 month of age to 0.04 mmol/day (2.7 mg/day) at 6 months (8); bottle-fed infants consumed 0.055 and 0.07 mmol/day (3.6 and 4.6 mg/day) at 1 and 6 months, respectively. The Zn content of commercial infant formulas depends on the fortification policy of the manufacturer. Typical zinc intakes of various population groups are reported in Table 11.1.

Factors Affecting Zinc Bioavailability

Zn bioavailability is defined as the fraction of zinc intake that is retained and used for normal physiologic functions. Zn absorption is a function of the solubility of Zn compounds at the absorption site and the body "status" or need. Zn in foods is relatively easily extractable at gastric pH; it tends to bind to organic compounds at higher pH (9). Small-molecular-weight ligands, such as amino acids and other organic acids, can increase solubility and facilitate absorption; larger-molecular-weight compounds, such as phytic acid, form poorly soluble compounds and reduce absorption. Competition between Zn and other elements for binding sites on the mucosal cell can influence absorbability.

Meats, liver, eggs, and seafood are considered good sources of Zn because of the relative absence of compounds that inhibit Zn absorption and the presence of certain amino acids that improve Zn solubility. For example, the absolute amount of zinc absorbed was about 80% higher when a high meat diet (280 g meat/day) was consumed than with a low meat (42 g meat/day) diet (10). Cysteine and methionine enhance Zn absorbability by forming stable complexes with Zn (11). Whole-grain cereal products and plant proteins, such as soy protein, contain Zn in a less available form. The phytic acid (myoinositol hexaphosphate) content of plant foods explains, at least in part, the lower availability of Zn from these foods. Fermentation of whole-meal bread reduces the phytic acid content and significantly improves Zn absorption, indicating that dietary fiber has little or no effect on zinc availability. Fermentation and enzymatic treatments gradually degrade the hexaphosphate form. The penta form depresses absorption like the hexa form, but lower inositol phosphates are less depressing (9). Extrusion cooking, which is used for breakfast cereals, seems to inhibit degradation of phytic acid in the gut and causes less efficient absorption of Zn (12). Millimolar phytate:Zn ratios above 10 increase the risk of poor Zn utilization.

Table 11.1
Daily Zinc Intakes of Various Population Groups

Group	No. of Studies	Percentile of Intake 10	50	90
Children	39	4.9	7.9	13.0
Males	36	6.6	12.0	15.4
Females	46	5.7	8.5	10.9
Pregnancy and lactation	17	8.1	9.6	12.9
Vegetarians	10	—	9.5	—
All adults	171	7.0	10.0	14.3

Modified from World Health Organization. Trace elements in human nutrition and health. Geneva: WHO, 1996. Based on a database maintained by the International Atomic Energy Agency.

Zinc-Nutrient Interactions

Transport mechanisms into cells for cations are in part determined by their configuration and coordination properties (13). Thus, elements with similar physicochemical characteristics compete for common pathways. Zn, with a preferred coordination number of 4, competes with copper (Cu) and cadmium (Cd). Mutual affinity for a carrier protein can also result in metal competition. This type of interaction may underlie reported Zn-iron (Fe) interactions.

Zinc-Copper

Large quantities of ingested Zn can interfere with Cu bioavailability (12). One explanation is that a high intake of Zn induces synthesis of the Cu-binding ligand metallothionein (MT) in the mucosal cell. This protein sequesters Cu, making it unavailable for serosal transfer, and thus decreases Cu absorption. Clinical signs of Cu deficiency developed in individuals taking 2.3 mmol/day (150 mg/day) of Zn for 2 years. Pharmacologic doses of

Zn (3–4.6 mmol/day; 200–300 mg/day) are used to treat Wilson's disease, a rare inborn error of Cu metabolism that causes excessive tissue accumulation of Cu (14). Lower, more typical Zn intakes do not affect copper absorption (15). A high Cu intake does not inhibit Zn absorption (2).

Zinc-Iron

Fe given as a supplement or in a liquid solution inhibits Zn absorption (2). Ferrous Fe has a greater impact than ferric Fe, and heme Fe does not cause any intestinal manifestation, suggesting that Fe and Zn compete at the same site for uptake into mucosal cells. Several studies showed that supplemental Fe lowers plasma Zn concentrations during pregnancy (2). The Institute of Medicine recommends that all pregnant women receiving more than 60 mg Fe/day also take supplemental Zn (16).

Zinc–Other Elements

High levels of dietary calcium impair Zn absorption in animals, especially from phytate-rich diets (12). Whether this occurs in humans is uncertain. High calcium intakes (34 mM or 1360 mg) reduced Zn absorption and balance in postmenopausal women but not in adolescent girls (17, 18). High intakes of tin (50 mg) increased fecal Zn excretion in a human balance study (19); but since the usual intake of tin is less than 8 μmol/day (<l mg/day), it is unlikely to have an adverse effect on Zn absorption from typical diets. Although high levels of dietary Cd can influence the distribution of Zn in the body, Cd does not seem to have a major effect on dietary Zn absorption.

Zinc–Folic Acid

Hydrolysis of dietary folates to their monoglutamate form requires the Zn-dependent enzyme pteroylpolyglutamate hydrolase (20). Administration of an oral dose of pteroylheptaglutamate to a group of Zn-depleted men prevented the usual rise in serum folic acid, whereas the serum response to an oral dose of pteroylmonoglutamate was normal (21). Several clinical studies show the converse, that folic acid supplementation impairs zinc use when zinc status is compromised (22). Supplementation with 800 μg folic acid/day for 25 days, however, did not alter zinc status in a group of students fed low-zinc diets (3.5 mg/day) (23). The interaction between zinc and folic acid needs further clarification.

METABOLISM

Zinc in the Human Body

Based on a total body concentration of about 0.3 μmol Zn/g (20 μg), it is estimated that the newborn contains approximately 0.9 mmol (60 mg) Zn (24). During growth and maturation, the Zn concentration of the human body increases to approximately 0.46 μmol/g (30 μg/g) (2). The adult total body Zn content ranges from about 2.3 mmol (1.5 g) in women to 3.8 mmol (2.5 g) in men.

Zn is present in all organs, tissues, fluids, and secretions of the body. Zn is primarily an intracellular ion, with well over 95% of total-body Zn found within cells. Zn is associated with all organelles of the cell, but about 60 to 80% of the cellular Zn is found in the cytosol. The Zn concentration and content of various tissues and the proportion of total-body Zn found in them are described in Table 11.2.

Zinc Uptake

Sites of Absorption. Zn is absorbed all along the small intestine; only small amounts are absorbed in the stomach and large intestine. Considering the length and surface area of the various segments of the small bowel, the transit time of digestion, and the endogenous secretion of Zn, most Zn is probably absorbed in the jejunum (25). After intake of a meal, the intraluminal quantity of Zn increases to about 1.5 to 3 times the amount ingested at the distal duodenum, presumably because of secretion of Zn-containing digestive juices. The luminal content of Zn declines substantially in the jejunum (26). In the postabsorptive state, Zn absorption was not affected by the quantity of Zn ingested until this exceeded 77 μmol (5 mg); Zn absorption from a meal providing 46 and 77 μmol (3

Table 11.2
Approximate Zinc Content of Major Organs and Tissues in a Normal Adult Man

Tissue	Approximate Zn Concentration		Total Zn Content		Percentage of Body Zn (%)
	Wet Weight μM/g	(μg/g)	mM	(g)	
Skeletal muscle	0.78	(51)	24	(1.53)	57 (approx.)
Bone	1.54	(100)	12	(0.77)	29
Skin	0.49	(32)	2	(0.16)	6
Liver	0.89	(58)	2	(0.13)	5
Brain	0.17	(11)	0.6	(0.04)	1.5
Kidneys	0.85	(55)	0.3	(0.02)	0.7
Heart	0.35	(23)	0.15	(0.01)	0.4
Hair	2.30	(150)	<0.15	(<0.01)	0.1 (approx.)
Blood plasma	0.02	(1)	<0.15	(<0.01)	0.1 (approx.)

Modified from Mills CF, ed. Zinc in human biology. London: Springer-Verlag, 1989.

and 5 mg) was less than that from a 15-μmol (1 mg) meal (27).

Intraluminal Factors. During the process of digesting a meal, digestive enzymes release dietary Zn from food matrices and endogenous Zn from various binding ligands. As such, this free Zn can form coordination complexes with various exogenous and endogenous ligands, such as amino acids, phosphates, and other organic acids (9). Histidine and the sulfur-containing amino acids methionine and cysteine are the preferred amino acid ligands. Zn-histidine and Zn-methionine complexes are absorbed more efficiently than Zn sulfate (28, 29). Although widely discussed, citric acid and picolinic acid do not appear to enhance zinc absorption.

Cellular Factors. The mechanism by which Zn enters mucosal cells is unknown. Presumably, it traverses the unstirred water layer in an exchangeable or diffusible form. Zn uptake across the brush border surface occurs by both a carrier-mediated (saturable) mechanism and a nonmediated (nonsaturable) component. At low-normal luminal concentrations of Zn (less than about 80 μmol/L), the carrier mechanism predominates. This carrier-mediated uptake by the cell does not require energy. Specific receptor proteins for Zn have not been characterized. When the dietary supply of Zn is low, the carrier affinity for Zn is not changed, but the capacity for carrier-mediated transport is greater, presumably due to a rise in the number of receptor sites (30). With high Zn intakes, the nonsaturable mechanism becomes prominent. This mechanism may involve passive diffusion and/or movement between mucosal cells. The positive, nonspecific effect of lactose and glucose polymers on Zn absorption may represent an increase in paracellular Zn movement.

Disposition of Zn within the cell is diverse. Intracellular Zn may be used by the cell for Zn-dependent processes, become bound firmly to MT and held within the cell, or pass through the cell. Cysteine-rich intestinal protein (CRIP) is associated with Zn absorption, but it is not likely to be involved in transcellular movement. MT gene expression is directly related to dietary Zn intake, however. Zn absorption declines as MT synthesis rises in response to dietary Zn (31). A vesicular transfer mechanism has also been proposed for transcellular Zn movement (32). Zn trapped within the cell is eventually lost in the feces in the normal course of mucosal cell turnover. Transport of Zn across the serosal membrane is carrier mediated and occurs by an adenosine triphosphate (ATP)-driven mechanism (33).

Portal Transport

Zn is released by the intestinal cells at the basolateral-serosal surface into the mesenteric capillary and is carried by the portal blood to the liver (33). The absorbed Zn is initially albumin bound.

Homeostatic Regulation

Total-body Zn content is controlled in part by regulating the efficiency of intestinal absorption and excretion from endogenous Zn pools. An inverse relationship between plasma Zn concentration and fractional Zn absorption has been reported (34, 35). As intestinal luminal concentrations of Zn rise, the fractional absorption of Zn decreases, but the actual amount of Zn absorbed rises. Thus, at high Zn intakes, regulation of intestinal absorption only provides "coarse control" of total-body Zn. Increased fecal excretion of endogenous Zn appears to provide the "fine control" needed to balance net retention of Zn with metabolic needs. Endogenous fecal Zn losses may increase severalfold to maintain Zn homeostasis with high intakes (36).

Homeostatic regulation of Zn is altered with changes in physiologic need. Experimental Zn deficiency in animals and humans enhances gastrointestinal Zn uptake (37, 38). In the rat, a specific increase in the efficiency of Zn absorption is observed in late pregnancy, possibly because of an increase in receptor sites (39). A similar increase has not been observed in pregnant women (34). Zinc absorption is enhanced during lactation, however, in both humans and experimental animals (34, 39).

The age of the individual influences absorptive capacity. Newborn animals absorb Zn to a higher degree than do older animals, perhaps because of a transport system with a higher affinity for Zn (40). Several studies show that Zn absorption decreases with age (41). Most report that Zn absorption in the elderly is approximately half that of young people, but one group found no difference in fractional Zn absorption in the elderly compared with young men. Moreover, old age does not appear to impair the ability of the intestine to increase the efficiency of Zn absorption in response to ingesting a low-Zn diet. Among the elderly with lower Zn absorption, balance was maintained, suggesting a decline in endogenous Zn losses.

Hormonal influences associated with stress (corticosteroids and select cytokines) can increase the efficiency of Zn absorption (38). Acute bacterial infection and endotoxemia in the rat significantly increase Zn absorption (38).

Zinc Turnover and Transport

Kinetic modeling using stable isotopes of Zn provides information about Zn pools and their turnover in humans. A two-component model best explains the elimination of absorbed Zn from the body (2). The initial rapid phase has a half-life in humans of 12.5 days, and a slower turnover phase has a half-life of about 300 days. The initial rapid half-life primarily represents liver uptake of circulating Zn and its release. The slower turnover rate reflects differing rates of Zn turnover in various tissues other than liver (2). Zn uptake by the central nervous system and bones is relatively slow; the pancreas, liver, kidney, and spleen have the most rapid rates of accumulation and turnover; uptake and exchange of Zn in red cells and muscle are slower than in the viscera.

Kinetic data suggest an exchangeable zinc pool whose size depends on zinc intake (42). Size of this pool was estimated to be 2.4 to 2.8 mmol (157–183 mg) Zn, which decreases by 26 to 32% with severe Zn restriction for 1 week. The size of this exchangeable pool may provide a good measure of tissue zinc status.

About 0.05 mmol (3 mg) of Zn is normally circulating in the plasma at any given moment. This Zn is partitioned among α-2-macroglobulin (40%), albumin (57%), and amino acids (3%) (43). These loosely bound albumin and amino acid fractions of circulating Zn provide the transport and delivery of Zn to tissues. The amino acid–bound fraction determines the amount filtered by the kidneys. Because the total amount of Zn present in the major tissues is much larger than the total present in plasma, relatively small variations in the Zn content of tissues, such as the liver, can dramatically affect plasma Zn. For example, a 1% increase of liver Zn, caused by enhanced retention of Zn, could cause a 40% decline in plasma Zn. Because all absorbed Zn passes through the plasma to the tissues, the flux of Zn through the plasma is replaced approximately 130 times/day (44). Figure 11.1 illustrates the metabolism of Zn.

Storage

There is no specific Zn "store." In all species studied, a marked reduction in dietary Zn intake is quickly followed by signs of Zn deficiency. Nonetheless, growing chicks fed a high-Zn diet prior to depletion took longer to develop a deficiency than chicks fed a low-Zn diet previously (45). High Zn intakes increase bone, liver, and intestinal Zn. Release of Zn from those tissues during depletion may slow the rate of onset of Zn deficiency symptoms. Reduced food intake associated with Zn deficiency causes catabolism of muscle tissue and release of Zn into the plasma (46).

Excretion

The major route for endogenous Zn excretion is into the gastrointestinal tract, with ultimate loss in the feces. When tracer doses of Zn are given either orally or intravenously, only about 2 to 10% is recovered in the urine; the remainder is lost in the feces (2).

Fecal Zn losses are a combination of unabsorbed dietary Zn and endogenous Zn secretions. Pancreatic secretions are a major source of endogenous Zn. Other sources include biliary and gastroduodenal secretions, transepithelial flux of Zn from the mucosal cells, and sloughing of old mucosal cells into the gut (2). Perfusion studies show that about 0.04 to 0.07 mmol (2.5–4.8 mg) Zn is secreted into the duodenum following intake of a meal, presumably as meal-stimulated pancreatic secretions. Much of the Zn secreted into the gut lumen is absorbed and returned to the body. Maintenance of an intact enteropancreatic Zn circulation is important for maintenance of body Zn. The amount of Zn secreted into the gut varies with Zn intake. In humans, endogenous fecal losses may range from 15 μmol/day (<1 mg/day) with extremely low intakes to over 80 μmol/day (>5 mg/day) with extremely high intakes (37, 47).

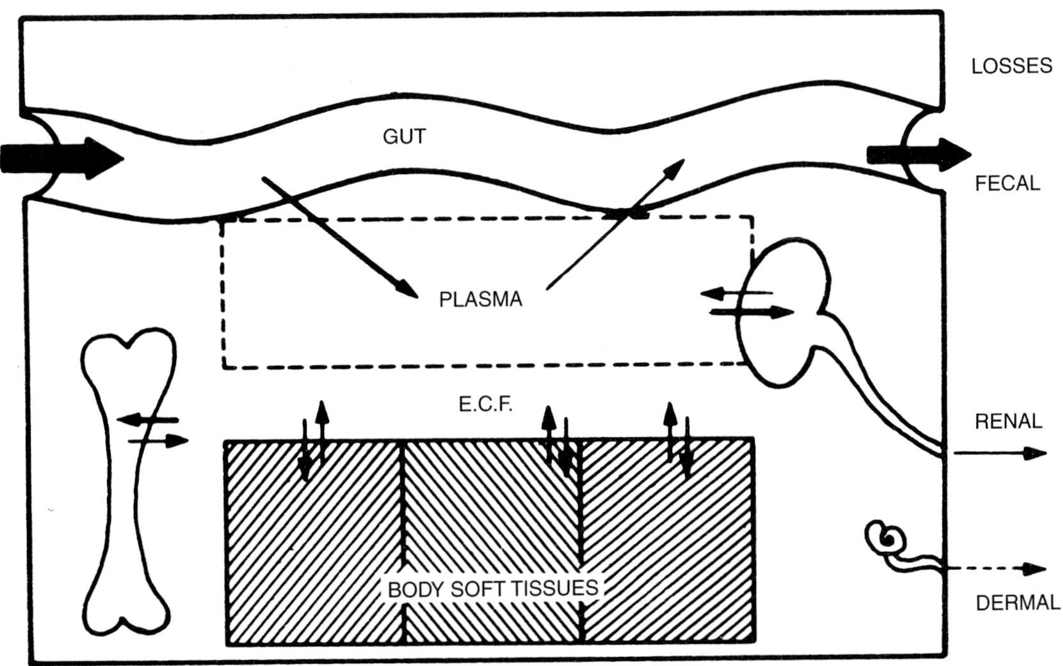

Figure 11.1. Schematic representation of the metabolism of zinc in mammals. (From Beisel WR, Pekarek RS, Wannamacher RW Jr. Homeostatic mechanisms affecting plasma zinc levels in acute stress. In: Trace elements in human health and disease, vol 1. New York: Academic Press, 1976.)

Normally, about 6 to 9 μmol (400–600 μg) of Zn is excreted daily in the urine. Urinary Zn arises largely from the ultrafilterable portion of the plasma Zn (2). Dietary Zn only influences urinary losses if intake is extremely low or extremely high. Under basal conditions, up to 95% of the filtered Zn is reabsorbed in the distal parts of the renal tubule (48). The amount of Zn excreted in urine is correlated highly with the rate of urine production (or urine volume) and creatinine excretion. Muscle catabolism, such as occurs with severe burns, major surgery, other trauma, or starvation, causes clinically significant increases in urinary Zn losses. Chelating agents, such as ethylenediaminetetraacetic acid (EDTA), also elevate urinary Zn levels (2).

Surface losses through desquamation of skin, outgrowth of hair, and sweat contribute up to 15 μmol (1 mg) of Zn daily. A marked reduction or marked increase in dietary Zn intake causes a concomitant change in surface losses (49). Other sources of loss include semen and menstrual secretions. An ejaculum of semen contains up to 15 μmol (1 mg) of Zn (37). Total menstrual loss is approximately 1.5 to 8.0 μmol (0.1–0.5 mg) per menstrual period (50).

BIOCHEMICAL AND PHYSIOLOGIC FUNCTIONS

Zn, the most abundant intracellular trace element, is involved in a multitude of diverse catalytic, structural, and regulatory functions. For example, Zn is found in numerous enzymes, is a component of biomembranes, is thought to be necessary for RNA, DNA, and ribosome stabilization, is involved in the binding of a number of transcription factors, stabilizes some hormone-receptor complexes, and may have a regulatory role in tubulin polymerization. Given its many functions, it is not surprising that a deficit of this element can pose serious physiologic challenges.

Biochemistry

With regard to metalloenzymes, Zn can have a catalytic, structural, or regulatory role. Examples are carbonic anhydrase, Cu,Zn–superoxide dismutase, and fructose bisphosphatase, respectively. Over 200 Zn enzymes have been found in biologic systems, and Zn enzymes are found in all six International Union of Biochemistry (IUB) classes (2, 51). An enzyme is considered to be a zinc metalloenzyme if removal affects activity without irreversibly altering the enzyme protein, and zinc replacement restores activity. It is not known how zinc is donated to apometalloenzyme proteins, but posttranslational modification may be involved. For additional details on Zn enzymes, the reader is directed to several reviews (2, 51, 52).

A critical function of Zn is its role in the structure and function of biomembranes. Some investigators have argued that a reduction in the concentration of Zn in biomembranes underlies some of the disorders associated with Zn deficiency (53), with a loss of Zn from the membrane resulting in increased susceptibility to oxidative damage, structural strains, and alterations in specific receptor sites and transport systems. The influence of Zn on biomembrane structure and function may be due in part to its ability *(a)* to stabilize thiol groups and phospholipids, *(b)* to occupy sites that might otherwise contain transition metals with redox potential (such as Fe), and *(c)* to be involved in the quenching of free radicals through its association with MT (54). Biomembrane accumulation of Zn can also alter membrane structure and function; for example, release of histamine from mast cells is reduced when Zn accumulates and blocks receptor sites for histamine-releasing agents (55).

The zinc-finger motif in proteins represents another extremely important structural role for zinc. Zinc fingers enable polypeptides that are too small to fold by themselves to fold stably when stabilized by bound zinc. The general structure of a zinc finger is repeated cysteine- and histidine-containing domains that bind Zn in a tetrahedral configuration. Several transcription factors have been reported to contain "Zn finger" regions (56). Up to 1% of the human genome (300–700 human genes) codes for these proteins. More than 10 classes of zinc fingers have been discovered and biochemically characterized. Zinc-finger proteins include transcription factors for DNA (i.e., retinoic acid and calcitriol receptors), the steroid-thyroid hormone–receptor superfamily, and the RING finger–protein family, which includes the breast and ovarian cancer susceptibility gene BRCA1. Zinc-finger proteins have also been found among signal transduction factors and may play a role in cell adhesion.

Zn also serves as a stimulator of *trans*-acting factors responsible for regulating gene expression (57). This function has been studied most extensively for the expression of MT or MT-like proteins. The metal-binding transcription factor for MT acquires Zn in the cell cytosol or nucleus and then can interact with the metal-response element to stimulate transcription. Dietary Zn is taken up by the cell nucleus in proportion to the Zn intake level, suggesting a close relationship between nuclear Zn and the dietary Zn supply.

Another regulatory role for Zn is in the polymerization of tubulin. Zn stabilizes neurotubules in vitro, possibly through formation of Zn mercaptide bridges between the tubulin dimer subunits. The rate of tubulin polymerization is decreased in brain extracts of Zn-deficient rats and pigs; Zn deficiency–induced reductions in the rate of tubulin polymerization have been postulated to underlie some of the developmental defects associated with Zn deficiency (58).

Physiologic Functions

To a great extent the appreciation of the physiologic roles of Zn is based on observations of signs of Zn deficiency in experimental animals and humans. Surprisingly, despite the long list of described Zn enzymes and nonenzymatic Zn-dependent processes, little consensus has been achieved on the precise biochemical lesions underlying development of the numerous signs of Zn deficiency. The following sections consider some of the signs of Zn deficiency, first in experimental animals and then in humans, and discuss some potential mechanisms that may underlie their development. At present, however, these mechanisms must be considered speculative.

ZINC DEFICIENCY IN EXPERIMENTAL ANIMALS

A Zn deficiency develops *differently* from most nutrient deficiencies. With most nutrients, insufficient dietary intake first causes mobilization of stores or functional reserves. Thereafter, tissue concentrations of the nutrient decline, and eventually, one or more specific functions or metabolic pathways that depend on the nutrient deteriorate. Thus, reduction in growth is a *late* manifestation of deficiency. In contrast, when dietary Zn intake is insufficient, the first responses are a reduction in growth by growing organisms and a decrease in endogenous losses of Zn to conserve tissue Zn. The important role of zinc in maintaining the structure of transcription factors and regulating gene expression provides a strong rationale for the avid conservation of tissue zinc. If the dietary deficiency is mild, Zn homeostasis may be reestablished after adjusting the rates of growth and excretion, and no further functional or biochemical changes occur. However, with a markedly deficient diet, the organism cannot reestablish homeostasis through adjustments in endogenous losses and growth, and as a consequence, generalized tissue dysfunction develops quickly. The prompt appearance of Zn deficiency signs in animals fed essentially Zn-free diets is attributed to loss of a small labile pool of Zn located within various tissues (59).

Zn deficiency can be induced rapidly. For example, within 12 hours of consuming a Zn-deficient meal, plasma Zn concentrations in the rat decrease by as much as 50% (60). Evidence that this reduction in plasma Zn is functionally significant is provided by the observation that feeding a Zn-deficient diet to pregnant rats for only a few days during the first trimester causes embryonic abnormalities (61). Administration of an excessive amount of dietary zinc to growing chickens permitted Zn accumulation in bone, liver, and intestine that was subsequently released for use during Zn deficiency (45). This was not true when the chicks were fed the minimum requirement of Zn. Although all species appear to lack any appreciable Zn stores or reserves that can be mobilized when needed, some reserves may be deposited in tissues when large quantities of Zn are fed. A homeostatic mechanism for release of that zinc is unknown; it may only become available when released in conjunction with cell turnover.

Early effects of Zn deficiency in many species are anorexia and cyclic feeding. Increased levels of norepinephrine and alterations in its receptor function in the hypothalamus of Zn-deficient animals have been suggested as mechanisms underlying the anorexia (62). Regardless of the biochemical explanation for the anorexia, the cyclic food pattern of Zn-deficient animals may represent adaptation of the animal to the low-Zn diet, because during periods of low food intake, the substantial muscle catabolism releases Zn into the plasma pool that can be used by hepatic and extrahepatic tissues for Zn-dependent processes (63).

If the period of Zn deficiency is prolonged, additional hallmarks of Zn deficiency are impaired growth, dermatitis, a compromised immune system, and decreased efficiency of food utilization. Although the lesions underlying these signs have not been defined, reduced cell replication is an early event in Zn deficiency. This reduced cell division has been related in part to the role of Zn in protein and nucleic acid synthesis, in chromatin decondensation, and in assembly of the mitotic spindle through its effect on microtubule polymerization (63).

Associated with Zn-deficiency-induced reduction in cell division is impaired growth, which has been demonstrated for numerous species including humans (63). It has been suggested that a reduced growth rate may represent accommodation by the animal to the Zn deficit, thus making more Zn available for Zn-dependent metabolic processes. An alternative explanation is that the slower growth rate is secondary to the anorexia and the concomitant reduction in food intake. However, animals fed diets adequate in Zn, in amounts equivalent to those consumed by Zn-deficient animals, gain considerably more weight than the Zn-deficient animals. Thus, the lower weight gain observed with Zn deficiency cannot be ascribed solely to reduced food intake (62).

In addition to an overall reduction in body size, Zn-deficiency-associated reductions in cell division may also contribute to abnormal bone growth and maturation. Both the number of osteoblasts and the chondrocyte number in epiphyseal cartilage are reduced in Zn deficiency (64). A reduction in cell division rates may also underlie some of the effects of Zn deficiency on the immune system; deficient animals often have a small thymus and spleen, with resultant reductions in their capacity for T- and B-lymphocyte production (65). Zn-deficiency-induced reductions in cell replication rates may also underlie the teratogenicity of embryonic Zn deficiency, because an interruption in normal replication rates and patterns could lead to asynchrony in cell and tissue maturation.

As already indicated, a deficiency of Zn during early development can be highly teratogenic. Typical malformations associated with Zn deficiency in experimental animals include brain and eye defects, spina bifida, cleft lip and palate, and numerous malformations of the heart, lung, skeleton, and urogenital system (61). Biochemical lesions proposed to contribute to the teratogenicity of Zn deficiency include abnormal nucleic acid and protein synthesis, alterations in the differential rates of cellular growth needed for normal morphogenesis, impaired tubulin polymerization with resultant reductions in cell motility and division, chromosomal defects, excessive cell death in areas adjacent to regions where programed cell death occurs, and excessive peroxidation of cell membrane lipids (61). Thus, the mechanisms leading to Zn-deficiency-associated abnormal development are probably multifactorial. In addition to its impact on the fetus, Zn deficiency during late gestation can result in parturition difficulties with delayed deliveries and excessive bleeding (61, 66). In Zn-deficient rats, the delay in delivery has been linked to an abnormally low normal activity of ovarian 20-α-hydroxysteroid dehydrogenase, an enzyme that catalyzes the degradation of progesterone, which is inhibitory to parturition (67). The subcellular distribution and metabolism of uterine estrogen-receptor complexes are altered in Zn-deficient rats. A poor response to estrogen priming may contribute to the delivery problems associated with Zn deficiency.

The influence of Zn on the reproductive process is not restricted to females. In Zn-deficient males, the testes are reduced in size with atrophy of the seminiferous epithelium. The resulting testicular dysfunction impairs spermatogenesis and the output of testosterone. It is thought that the primary defect underlying the effect of Zn deficiency on testicular function may involve impaired Leydig cell function, with a secondary effect on the pituitary-gonadal axis (68).

Zn can induce as well as block apoptosis, or programed cell death. High concentrations (500–1000 μM) block DNA fragmentation, whereas lower concentrations (80–200 μM) induce cell death (69). Although many mechanisms are likely to be involved, one pathway entails inhibiting the death signal by blocking binding of steroids to the glucocorticoid receptor. The significance of these effects is clouded by the fact that Zn does not provide long-term protection to cell survival.

A consequence of Zn deficiency can be marked alterations in several components of the immune system. Immune defects associated with Zn deficiency include reduced thymic hormone production and activity; impaired function of lymphocytes, natural killer cells, and neutrophils; impaired antibody-dependent cell-mediated cytotoxicity; altered immunologic ontogeny; and defective lymphokine production (65). As discussed above, Zn-deficient animals can be characterized by thymic atrophy and small spleens. Significantly, Zn deficiency reduces the mass of lymphoid tissues more than that of other tissues. The particular sensitivity of lymphoid tissue to Zn deficiency has not been clarified (65).

Impaired glucose tolerance has been reported by some investigators to occur in Zn deficiency. The impairment has been related to reduced insulin output, increased insulin degradation by glutathione insulin transhydrogenase, and increased peripheral insulin resistance (2).

Lipid metabolism is also affected by Zn deficiency. Reduced glucose use in Zn deficiency has been linked to an overall increased rate of lipid oxidation. Zn-deficient animals can be characterized by hypocholesterolemia (primarily caused by reduction in high-density-lipoprotein (HDL) cholesterol) and by an HDL fraction that is enriched in apo-E and low in apo-C content (2, 70). Moderate Zn deficiency in pregnant rats increased the use of linoleate for de novo lipogenesis and impaired whole body accumulation of polyunsaturated fatty acids (71). These changes in fatty acid metabolism explain why many of the signs of Zn deficiency are similar to those of essential fatty acid deficiency (72).

In addition to its putative effects on insulin and testosterone, the metabolism of several other hormones has been reported to be influenced by Zn. The synthesis, release, and binding of growth hormone, somatomedin, prolactin, thyroid hormone, corticosterone, luteinizing hormone–releasing hormone (LHRH), follicle-stimulating hormone (FSH), and luteinizing hormone (LH) have all been reported to be affected by Zn deficiency, although these findings are not universal (2, 67).

ZINC DEFICIENCY IN HUMANS

Mild Deficiency

Although severe Zn deficiency in humans is well documented, whether a physiologically significant mild Zn deficiency exists in humans is controversial. It is inherently unlikely, however, that human Zn deficiency is an "all-or-none" phenomenon. The concept of a graded response to progressive degrees of deficiency is supported by animal studies; for example, when weanling rats were fed graded amounts of dietary Zn ranging from 1 to 12 ppm, the 12-ppm diet supported normal growth, but impairment was increasingly severe with more severe dietary Zn restriction (73).

Demonstrating mild Zn deficiency is not as straightforward in humans as in experimental animals. If it is accepted that impaired growth velocity is the primary clinical feature of mild Zn deficiency, several studies in Denver, Colorado, provide convincing evidence (74, 75). Apparently healthy children with low height-for-age percentiles were selected for a double-blind, controlled trial of Zn supplementation. The treatment group received a small (0.08-mmol, 5-mg) Zn supplement. In all studies of these growth-retarded children, Zn supplementation increased the mean height increment and height-for-age percentile increment compared with those of placebo controls. Boys frequently had a greater response than girls. In one study, supplemental Zn improved the calculated energy and protein intake (76). Concurrently with these studies, Zn supplementation in children who were unselected with respect to growth percentiles did not increase their growth velocity (75).

Mild Zn deficiency may also affect the quality of growth. Zn supplementation of malnourished infants reduced the energy cost of growth, which was probably related to improved synthesis of lean body tissue (77). Idiopathic dysgeusia was improved in a single-blind trial of Zn therapy, but a subsequent double-blind trial failed to confirm this observation (78). Other functions that have responded to Zn supplementation include immune function in the elderly (79), oligospermia (80), and complications of pregnancy, such as pregnancy-induced hypertension, prematurity, prolonged labor, and intrapartum hemorrhage (81). However, these responses were generally to pharmacologic quantities of Zn and thus do not necessarily indicate a Zn deficiency. The response of these conditions to physiologic Zn doses (0.15–0.23 mmol/day, 10–15 mg/day) needs to be tested using double-blind, controlled designs.

Severe Deficiency

Severe Zn deficiency has been seen in patients with acrodermatitis enteropathica (AE), in patients fed total parenteral nutrition (TPN) solutions lacking Zn, and in experimental human Zn depletion. The clinical features of severe Zn deficiency in the three situations are similar. The symptoms of Zn deficiency in an individual depends on the severity of the deficiency and other factors.

Clinical Manifestations

The primary clinical manifestations of severe Zn deficiency are listed in Table 11.3. In severe deficiencies, growth ceases, whereas a less severe deficiency state causes decreased growth velocity. If growth retardation is mild, the response to Zn supplementation is modest. Persons suffering from more severe reduction in growth velocity, as those with AE or Middle Eastern adolescents consuming high-phytate diets, show a greater response to Zn supplementation. The original observations of human Zn deficiency in Persian and Egyptian dwarfs included hypogonadism and delayed sexual maturation (3). The effect of severe Zn deficiency on hypogonadism among patients with AE is unclear (82).

The skin lesions of severe Zn deficiency have a characteristic distribution, primarily at the extremities and adjacent to the body orifices. Lesions may occur elsewhere and can become generalized. Often the rashes are erythematous, vesiculobullous, and pustular (2, 82). Changes in the hair usually become apparent after the onset of dermatitis. The hair may become hypopigmented and acquire a reddish hue (82). Patchy loss of hair is common.

Table 11.3
Clinical Manifestations of Severe Human Zinc Deficiency[a]

Growth retardation
Delayed sexual maturation and impotence
Hypogonadism and hypospermia
Alopecia
Acroorificial skin lesions
Other epithelial lesions, including glossitis, alopecia, and nail dystrophy
Immune deficiencies
Behavioral disturbances, including impaired hedonic tone
Night blindness
Impaired taste (hypogeusia)
Delayed healing of wounds, burns, and decubitus ulcers
Impaired appetite and food intake
Eye lesions, including photophobia and lack of dark adaptation

[a]Features depend on the severity of the deficiency and other factors.

Diarrhea is a complication in AE and in patients receiving TPN. The mechanism(s) for diarrhea in Zn deficiency is unknown. Decreased mucosal disaccharidase activity and related carbohydrate malabsorption have been suggested (83), but the diarrhea seen in patients receiving TPN who are not ingesting meals clearly has a different origin. Other possible explanations include increased synthesis of prostaglandins, especially PGE_2, which can cause diarrhea, and a defect in enterocyte transport function.

Consistent with experimental animal data, Zn deficiency in humans alters several aspects of immune function. Thymic hypoplasia has been seen in patients with AE and in individuals suffering from protein-energy malnutrition. Impaired cutaneous responses to mitogens and in vitro lymphoblast responses have been noted, as have defects in monocyte and neutrophil chemotaxis (65).

The cornea, the tissue with the highest Zn concentration in the body, is affected by Zn deficiency. Corneal edema occurs and may progress to corneal clouding and opacities (82). Healing of more advanced lesions may leave residual scarring, but minor lesions may heal completely. A mild dry conjunctivitis may also occur and may progress to bilateral xerosis and keratomalacia. Vitamin A is ineffective in the treatment of these disorders.

Behavioral changes can occur with Zn deficiency. Irritability, lethargy, and depression are common in children with AE (82). Administration of large doses of histidine to induce zincuria caused anorexia and dysfunction of smell and taste in adult subjects (78). The subjects then became irritable, depressed, easy to anger, lethargic, and sleepy. Some developed a fine tremor, ataxic gait, and slurred speech. Supplementation with 0.8 mmol (50 mg) of Zn quickly reversed these symptoms.

Biochemical Correlates

Although information on the biochemical functions of Zn is extensive, the biochemical correlates of the clinical features of Zn deficiency have not been determined satisfactorily. Disturbances in nucleic acid metabolism and protein synthesis may account for some of the features of Zn deficiency in humans. Elevated blood ammonia and reductions in circulating proteins with short half-lives have been reported in human Zn deficiency (84). It has been suggested that a relative excess of dietary nitrogen in subjects fed a Zn-deficient diet can cause anorexia (77).

As in experimental animal models, some of the effects of Zn deficiency in humans appear to be mediated through effects on hormonal function. Hormones reported to be affected by Zn status in humans include growth hormone, the gonadotropins and sex hormones, prolactin, thyroid hormones, corticosteroids, insulin, and the hormonelike substances, prostaglandins.

CONDITIONS PREDISPOSING TO ZINC DEPLETION

Mild-to-marginal states of Zn deficiency may go undetected because those individuals do not display the specific clinical features of Zn depletion. Individuals at risk include those with decreased absorption, increased losses, or increased needs caused by growth or reproduction, particularly if their dietary Zn intake is also low.

Primary and Diet-Induced Zinc Deficiency

The occurrence of isolated Zn deficiency in normal, healthy free-living adults has not been, and is unlikely to be, documented because of the remarkable ability of individuals to reduce Zn losses and to reestablish homeostasis when the dietary supply is low (85). However, if Zn need is increased, as in growing infants and children or in pregnant and lactating women, the potential for Zn deficiency may be increased. This is especially true if the dietary supply is inadequate. Although the increase in metabolic requirements for Zn during pregnancy appear to be modest (about 1.5 mmol, 100 mg) (24), certain complications of pregnancy have been linked to poor Zn status, as discussed below. Moreover, physiologic Zn supplements have improved growth velocity rates in growth-retarded infants who appeared otherwise healthy (86). A reliable, sensitive laboratory index of Zn deficiency is needed before the incidence of Zn deficiency in these vulnerable groups can be documented.

Patients receiving TPN have developed the clinical features of Zn deficiency. In many cases, patients who became Zn deficient had conditions that predisposed them to the problem, such as diarrhea, inflammatory bowel disease, or other conditions that increased Zn loss. Patients receiving TPN often have increased urinary Zn loss because of release of Zn from catabolized tissues (87) or because of increased levels of glycosylated amino acid–Zn complexes (88).

Conditions of semistarvation, such as anorexia and protein-energy malnutrition (PEM), may cause Zn deficiency. Insufficient intake combined with poor digestibility and absorbability caused by the effects of malnutrition on gastrointestinal function are precipitating factors. Poor bioavailability of Zn in the food supply, due to high levels of dietary phytate, may contribute to Zn deficiency with marginal diets. Other contributory factors include dermal loss caused by excessive sweating and Zn loss through chronic gastrointestinal hemorrhage among populations in developing countries. Because of high phytate intake, vegetarianism is considered a risk factor for Zn deficiency among individuals subsisting on cereal-based diets.

Inborn Errors of Zinc Metabolism: Acrodermatitis Enteropathica

AE is a rare, inherited, autosomal recessive disease affecting both sexes (82). The basic defect in AE is thought to be impaired intestinal uptake and transfer of Zn, although it has been hypothesized that poor absorption is secondary to impaired cellular processing (89). In young patients with AE, intestinal Zn absorption was reduced, as assessed by whole-body retention of an orally administered dose of ^{65}Zn (90). The basic defect in Zn absorption is unknown, but the mucosal mechanism for Zn uptake and transfer at customary luminal concentrations seems to be defective (82). The beneficial therapeutic effect of large oral doses of Zn may result from net uptake and transfer of Zn by a less specific mechanism.

Diagnosis of AE is made from the clinical features. Hyperpigmented skin lesions over the acral surfaces of elbows and knees, often also involving the face, buttocks, and other surfaces, are characteristic (76). The rash usually first occurs in early infancy, but onset of the disease usually does not occur until solid foods are started or breast-feeding is completely discontinued. Secondary infection is common. Intestinal disturbances and growth failure are usually present. Psychologic and behavioral abnormalities are prominent, with irritability, lethargy, and depression occurring even during relatively mild stages of the disease (91). Plasma and serum Zn concentrations are typically below 6 mmol/L (40 mg/dL).

Oral Zn therapy causes a rapid and complete remission of the clinical and biochemical symptoms of AE and must be continued indefinitely to sustain remission and normal Zn status. The quantity of Zn required is 0.5 to 0.7 mmol/day (30 to 45 mg/day); smaller quantities may be used initially in the very young child or infant (91).

Another syndrome of altered Zn metabolism is found in lactating women. This condition results from inability of the mother's mammary gland to secrete normal quantities of Zn into her milk. Apart from low milk Zn concentrations, maternal Zn status is normal. Zn supplementation does not increase milk Zn concentrations (91). Infants who are entirely breast-fed by these mothers do not develop clinical features of severe Zn deficiency unless they were born prematurely. Temporary management with Zn supplements is required until breast-feeding is supplemented with other foods.

Secondary Acquired Zinc Deficiency

The major pathophysiologic abnormalities contributing to secondary Zn deficiency are Zn malabsorption and excessive urinary Zn loss. Any disease or condition altering the integrity of the mucosa cell can affect the efficiency of Zn absorption. Chelating agents and drugs can exacerbate the impact of a disease state on Zn metabolism. Penicillamine in the treatment of Wilson's disease and diethylenetriamine pentaacetate (DTPA) in the treatment of Fe overload in thalassemia patients have caused severe Zn deficiency (82). Moreover, anticonvulsant drugs, especially sodium valproate, may precipitate Zn deficiency. The antituberculous drug ethambutol has chelating properties and has been shown to increase Zn turnover rates in rats (92).

EVALUATION OF ZINC STATUS

Despite our knowledge of the biology of Zn and of factors promoting or predisposing persons to Zn depletion, assessment of the incidence of Zn deficiency in humans is impaired by the lack of sensitive, specific indicators of poor Zn nutriture. Approaches to assessing nutritional status in the laboratory involve measurement of static indices (e.g., concentration in tissues or fluids of Zn or surrogates for Zn, such as metal-containing enzymes and proteins) or functional indices (Zn-dependent physiologic functions). The problem is that many measurements do not accurately reflect nutritionally available Zn pool sizes.

Static Indices

Plasma/serum Zn concentration has been denigrated as a measure of Zn status because it does not fall with changes in Zn intake unless the dietary Zn levels are so low that homeostasis cannot be reestablished (59). Plasma Zn represents about 2% of a labile, or nutritionally available, total-body Zn pool that exchanges with isotopic Zn tracers in 24 hours (59). Because plasma Zn is the source of Zn for all tissues, plasma concentrations are maintained longer than other components of this labile body Zn pool. Plasma Zn kinetics or turnover tends to rise with Zn depletion. Thus, the rate of Zn turnover in the plasma compartment or in the total labile pool of the body might indicate Zn status (42, 93).

Metabolic states other than a change in Zn status alter plasma Zn concentrations. Stress, infection, food intake, short-term fasting, and the hormonal state all appear to influence the distribution of labile Zn among the tissues and thereby alter the amount in the plasma (94). Thus, plasma Zn can only be useful for assessment of Zn status if the effect of poor Zn nutriture can be differentiated from these other metabolic conditions. Erythrocyte metallothionein was suggested as a useful marker of tissue Zn distribution (95), but analytic difficulties prevent widespread use.

Other static measures of Zn status hold little promise. Erythrocyte Zn is little affected by Zn deficiency and is not a sensitive index. The response of leukocyte Zn to changes in Zn status is not consistent among laboratories, and the assay is laborious. Hair Zn levels may be depressed in mild Zn-deficiency states, but they may remain normal in severe states when hair growth is arrested. Urinary excretion rates are diminished in severe deficiency states, but this measurement is not sensitive to less dramatic changes and is confounded by many clinical disorders that increase urinary Zn losses.

Functional Indices

Several different in vitro and in vivo tests of physiologic function have been used to evaluate Zn status. Zn is a constituent of over 200 metalloenzymes and other proteins involved in immune function, antioxidant protection, and membrane stabilization. Zn-dependent enzymes proposed as biomarkers of status include serum or erythrocyte alkaline phosphatase (96), serum superoxide dismutase (97), and lymphocyte 5′ nucleotidase. The validity of these measurements as markers of Zn status needs further study. Many of the other functional tests are not routine and lack specificity. Dark adaptation requires a high degree of the subject's cooperation and time. Impaired taste acuity, immune function, and glucose tolerance tests lack specificity and must be combined with other biochemical indices of Zn status.

REQUIREMENTS AND RECOMMENDED INTAKES

Human nutrient requirements may be based on one of the following criteria: *(a)* the lowest intake required to support balance; *(b)* the amount of absorbed zinc required to replace endogenous losses; or *(c)* the intake needed to maintain normal function. The amount of absorbed zinc that replaces endogenous losses, or the factorial approach, is generally used. This approach is used because a good functional test for Zn status has not been identified, and balance can be achieved over a wide range of intakes, from 0.05 mmol (3 mg) to above 0.46 mmol (30 mg) (85).

The 1989 RDA (98) and the 1996 World Health Organization (WHO) (7) standards for Zn intake are shown in Table 11.4. The WHO Expert Committee set standards for high-, moderate-, and low-availability diets (7); the standards for high- and moderate-availability diets are shown in Table 11.4. In a highly available diet about 50% of the zinc is assumed to be available. This diet is composed of refined cereal fiber and phytate, with adequate protein principally from nonvegetable sources such as meat and fish. In a moderately available diet about 30% of the zinc is available, and it is supplied either by a mixed diet containing fish or animal protein or a lacto-ovo, ovovegetarian, or vegan diet not based principally on unrefined cereal grains. Only 15% of the zinc is available in a diet of low zinc availability; the diet is high in unrefined, unfermented, and ungerminated cereal grain.

Although typical U.S. diets are either of high or moderate availability for zinc, the RDAs are always greater than the WHO standards. In some cases a three-fold difference exists between the two sets of recommendations. The WHO Expert Committee cautioned that their standards should be considered provisional until further experimental or epidemiologic testing is completed.

HIGH-RISK CLINICAL SITUATIONS

Pregnancy

Zn is essential for normal growth and development. The requirement for Zn increases during pregnancy. Adverse effects of Zn deficiency in experimental animals are discussed above in this chapter. Studies of rhesus monkeys provide information about the effect of a marginal Zn deficiency on pregnancy outcome in a primate model (99, 100).

Table 11.4
Recommended Zinc Intakes (mg/day)

	Age (years)	Males RDA	Males WHO High[a]	Males WHO Moderate[a]	Females RDA	Females WHO High[a]	Females WHO Moderate[a]
Infants	0–0.5	5	—	—	5	—	—
	0.5–1	5	3.3	5.6	5	3.3	5.6
Children	1–3	10	3.3	5.5	10	3.3	5.5
	4–6	10	3.9	6.5	10	3.9	6.5
	7–10	10	4.5	7.5	10	4.5	7.5
Adolescents	11–14	15	6.5	10.7	12	5.5	9.3
	15–18	15	7.8	13.1	12	6.2	10.2
Adults	19–24	15	5.6	9.4	12	4.0	6.5
	25–50	15	5.6	9.4	12	4.0	6.5
	51+	15	5.6	9.4	12	4.0	6.5
Pregnancy					15	8.0	13.3
Lactation	0–6 months				19	7.3	12.2
	7–12 months				16	5.8	9.6

From Food and Nutrition Board, National Research Council. Recommended dietary allowances. 10th ed. Washington, DC: National Academy Press, 1989 and the World Health Organization. Trace elements in human nutrition and health. Geneva: WHO, 1996.
[a]High availability (50%) or moderate availability (30%).

The total incremental Zn need for pregnancy is modest in humans, about 1.5 mmol (100 mg), or an additional daily demand of 9 μmol (0.6 mg) of Zn during late gestation (24). Women may increase their Zn intake a modest amount if total food intake increases. The RDA is 0.23 mmol (15 mg) Zn per day; the WHO Expert Committee recommends 13.3 mg/day from a moderately available diet. The average daily intake is between 0.15 and 23 mmol (10–15 mg). If the increase in Zn intake is small, adequate delivery of Zn to the developing fetus must be achieved by adjustments in Zn use. No significant increase in Zn absorption has been reported in human pregnancies (34). Endogenous fecal Zn loss has not been measured. Urinary Zn loss increases in late pregnancy after a small decline in the first trimester. By late pregnancy, the concentration of circulating Zn in the plasma is about 15 to 35% lower in pregnant women than in nonpregnant women (24). The decline occurs as early as the first gestational month, stabilizes in the second trimester, and then declines further in the third trimester. The fall in plasma Zn may be attributed to expansion of the plasma volume, fetal uptake, and hormonal adjustments in the distribution of Zn from the circulation to other tissues, such as the liver.

In 1976, Jameson observed that low maternal serum Zn was associated with congenital malformations, fetal dysmaturity, prematurity, and maternal complications in otherwise healthy women (101). That report stimulated further research to examine the relationship between Zn status and pregnancy outcome. Several detailed reviews of this topic are available (24, 61, 66, 81, 102). Human studies indicate that some pregnant women who deliver infants with congenital abnormalities used Zn differently than women who delivered healthy infants. Several groups reported that mothers of infants with congenital anomalies had lower plasma Zn concentrations than other mothers (61). Zn deficiency has been implicated specifically in development of two neural tube defects, anencephaly and spina bifida. Association of plasma Zn concentrations with congenital malformations does not imply causation. Perhaps Zn status simply varies with and reflects the real, but unknown, causal factor(s), or perhaps the association between Zn and congenital abnormalities reflects poor or inefficient Zn use. Double-blind supplementation trials starting prior to conception and continuing through embryogenesis are needed to identify the causal relationship between zinc and congenital anomalies in humans.

Poor maternal Zn status may also cause intrauterine growth retardation. Results are available from 41 studies of the association between infant birth weight and maternal zinc nutriture from various parts of the world (81). Of these 41 studies, 22 claimed maternal zinc nutriture influenced birth weight; 19 did not. Zinc supplementation trials also provide mixed results. Nine supplementation trials have been completed; five provided evidence of a positive relationship. A recent double-blind study of 580 African American women in Alabama provides convincing evidence that maternal zinc nutriture may limit fetal growth and development in some populations. Administration of 25 mg of supplemental zinc from midpregnancy to term increased birth weight by 126 g and head circumference by 0.4 cm above that of infants born to mothers receiving placebo (103). This study is unique in that only mothers with plasma zinc concentrations below the 50th percentile were chosen for study. Possibly, zinc supplementation is only effective among populations with relatively low plasma zinc concentrations early in pregnancy.

Although many investigators have evaluated the relationship between zinc nutriture and infant birth weight, few have studied its association with gestational age at birth. In an epidemiologic study of 818 pregnant women, Scholl et al. found that women with zinc intakes in the lowest quartile (≤6 mg/day) had about a twofold increase in the risk of preterm delivery after controlling for calories and other confounding variables (104). Adequate zinc nutriture is important for immune function; recent studies suggest that upper genital tract infection is responsible for early-preterm delivery (81).

Poor Zn status also is associated with increased maternal morbidity including preeclampsia or pregnancy-induced hypertension, prolonged labor, and atonic bleeding (81). Results are not consistent, however.

Old Age

The mean intake of Zn by individuals over 65 years of age in the United States is less than two-thirds of the RDA for Zn (105). Analysis of the Second National Health and Nutrition Examination Survey (NHANES II) showed that white men and women over 65 years of age consumed 72 and 81%, respectively, of the Zn RDA; black men and women consumed 61 and 59%, respectively. The black individuals tended to report diets with lower Zn densities. Approximately two-thirds of the Zn was supplied by animal food sources for all groups.

Several factors may increase the risk of Zn deficiency in the elderly: reduced capacity to absorb Zn (106), increased likelihood of disease states that alter Zn utilization, use of drugs such as diuretics that increase urinary Zn excretion, and consumption of fiber, calcium, or Fe supplements that may alter Zn bioavailability.

Assessment of Zn nutriture in the elderly is confounded by the effects of age itself on both functional and static indicators of status. Elderly subjects tend to have lower plasma Zn levels than younger adults (107). Analysis of the results of the NHANES-II survey showed that serum Zn levels of 65- to 74-year-old individuals were lower than those of young adults, and the difference was more obvious among men than women (7). Generally, the average concentration of Zn in hair samples from elderly subjects is lower than that in hair samples from younger adults and adolescents. Nonetheless, only a few elderly subjects had less than 70 μg of Zn/g hair, a concentration often used to define low hair Zn levels (108).

Several clinical conditions associated with poor Zn status also are problems commonly reported by the elderly, such as slow wound healing, anorexia, dermatitis, depressed taste acuity, and impaired immune function (108). Double-blind or single-blind trials of Zn supplementation failed to improve these functions. Further evaluation of the supplements is warranted. If Zn absorption is compromised in the elderly, administration of a larger Zn supplement together with a Zn-binding ligand such as histidine or methionine may be beneficial.

Diarrhea and Other Malabsorptive Disorders

Diseases of the gastrointestinal tract are frequently complicated by Zn deficiency. Breakdown of the integrity of the gastrointestinal tract reduces normal absorption of dietary Zn and disrupts the enteropancreatic Zn circulation. Recent studies show that supplemental Zn reduces the duration of acute, severe diarrhea in children by 9 to 23%; this rose to 22 to 33% in children with lower initial Zn status (109). Persistent diarrhea is more prevalent than severe diarrhea and causes higher rates of morbidity and mortality. Supplemental Zn reduced the incidence of persistent diarrhea by one-half in children over 1 year of age; there was no effect on younger children (110). Zn supplementation could affect the incidence and duration of diarrheal disorders in children by improving immune status or by correcting pathologic changes in gut integrity.

There is evidence that patients with Crohn's disease, sprue, or short bowel syndrome may develop Zn deficiency. Crohn's disease, or regional enteritis, is a type of inflammatory bowel disease. Many investigators have reported low serum Zn concentrations in patients with Crohn's disease, and it is not unusual to find depressed urinary Zn excretion (83). Other clinical features of Zn deficiency reported in these patients include growth retardation, abnormal taste acuity, delayed sexual maturation, skin lesions, and retinal dysfunction (111–113). Zn absorption is probably impaired in these patients. For example, 3 mmol (200 mg) supplemental Zn/day restored plasma Zn concentrations in patients with Crohn's disease, but 0.9 mmol (60 mg) did not (114). Also, patients with Crohn's disease had a 35% reduction in the area under the serum concentration curve after a large oral dose, compared with healthy controls (112). Large gastrointestinal losses may result from the diarrhea common in these patients (115), and urinary losses may be elevated because of catabolism of skeletal muscle. Plasma Zn concentrations of these patients may be low because of the release of the cytokine interleukin-1.

Decreased plasma Zn levels have been reported in patients with celiac sprue (116). The area under the serum concentration curve for the Zn tolerance test is depressed in untreated sprue patients and improves when a gluten-free diet is fed, indicating that Zn absorption is impaired.

Patients with short bowel syndrome have a double defect in Zn absorption. First, the absorptive surface of the small bowel is decreased and the transit time is increased. Second, intestinal reabsorption of Zn from pancreatic juice is impaired if much of the distal bowel is removed (83). Patients with short bowel syndrome have developed acrodermatitis, abnormal protein metabolism, and impaired immune function, all of which were corrected with Zn supplementation.

Patients who have had intestinal bypass surgery frequently have depressed serum Zn levels (83). The capacity to absorb Zn is probably reduced, as these patients have a two-thirds reduction in the area under the serum Zn concentration curve after an oral load, compared with healthy controls (117). Poor Zn status may contribute to the high incidence of opportunistic infections following jejunoileal bypass surgery.

Alcoholism

Patients with alcoholic cirrhosis often have hyperzincuria, hypozincemia, and lower liver Zn concentrations than controls or patients without cirrhosis (118). Potential mechanisms underlying the hyperzincuria include shifting Zn in plasma to ligands that are easily excreted and that inhibit tubular reabsorption of Zn (118, 119). Although hypozincemia is most prevalent (70%) in alcoholics with liver disease (118), it is also observed in some alcoholics (30–50%), with no evident liver disease. Consistent with human data, long-term alcohol feeding resulted in lower liver Zn concentrations in monkeys, rats, and pigs (118, 120).

Alcoholism-associated changes in Zn metabolism may well be functionally significant. Several studies have linked Zn deficiency and altered vitamin A metabolism in alcoholism (118). As discussed above, Zn deficiency can result in reduced serum retinol concentrations and elevated liver vitamin A stores, presumably because of reduced synthesis of retinol-binding protein in the liver. Zn deficiency can also result in low retinol-alcohol dehydrogenase activity in the retina. Zn administration to alcoholic patients can improve dark adaptation, a retinol dehydrogenase-dependent function (119). Zn supplementation of patients with alcoholic cirrhosis has been reported to improve their immune responsivity and reduce hepatic lipid peroxidation (119, 121). Zn supplementation of alcoholics with low plasma Zn levels and hypogonadism can result in a return of normal gonadal function (122).

Because the teratogenic expression of Zn deficiency is similar to that of fetal alcohol syndrome (FAS), one hypothesis is that FAS develops by an alcohol-induced embryonic Zn deficiency. Consistent with this suggestion, plasma and umbilical cord blood Zn concentrations are often lower in pregnant women who drink than in controls (123). Although maternal alcohol feeding in rats is associated with reduced placental Zn transfer in the second trimester and with lower than normal fetal liver Zn concentrations, dietary Zn supplementation has not been effective in reducing FAS expression in animal models (124). A direct role for altered Zn metabolism in development of FAS in humans has not been established. Nonetheless, given the negative consequences associated with inadequate Zn delivery to the embryo/fetus, close monitoring of the Zn status of pregnant alcoholic women is prudent.

Diabetes

Altered Zn metabolism occurs in both diabetic humans and experimental animals. Adult rats with genetically or chemically induced diabetes are characterized by Zn accumulation in the liver and kidney and by hyperzincuria (125, 126). Both type 1 and type 2 diabetic patients often exhibit hyperzincuria, which increases with the severity of the diabetes (127). Hyperzincuria may cause a conditioned Zn deficiency in some individuals, but clinical symptoms of Zn depletion are not common among diabetics (128). Hypozincemia, however, is common among diabetics (127). Zn supplementation of diabetic patients has been reported to improve their immune function, but supplementation also caused an increase in hemoglobin A_{1c}, a marker of abnormal glucose tolerance (65, 128, 129). The influence of Zn supplementation on glucose metabolism in diabetic patients needs further study. In the rat, diabetes during pregnancy can result in fetal Zn depletion and poor reproductive performance (126). Whether altered Zn metabolism is a factor underlying the increased risk of birth defects associated with diabetes in humans remains to be established. The mechanisms underlying altered Zn metabolism in the diabetic have not been firmly identified.

Patients with Chronic Infections and/or Trauma

As mentioned above, tissue-specific hormonal induction of metallothionein can occur during periods of acute disease (infection), stress, and inflammation. One consequence of metallothionein induction is a redistribution of body Zn, and plasma Zn concentrations are often markedly reduced (33). The long-term implications of low plasma Zn concentrations secondary to recurring acute-phase reactions have not been well defined, although potentially they could lead to Zn deficiency in select extrahepatic tissues. Although it is tempting to suggest that these individuals should be provided with Zn supplements, at present it is not clear whether the reduction in plasma Zn may actually represent a positive response of the patient to some insults. This issue clearly needs clarification.

AIDS

Because patients with acquired immunodeficiency syndrome (AIDS) often exhibit immunologic abnormalities similar to those associated with Zn deficiency, Zn deficiency has been postulated to underlie the development of some of the disorders associated with AIDS. Although low plasma Zn concentrations have been reported in a number of AIDS patients, individuals with AIDS-related complex (ARC) and asymptomatic human immunodeficiency virus (HIV)-positive subjects have been reported to have normal plasma Zn concentrations (130). Thus, there is no clinical evidence that Zn deficiency is a common contributory factor of HIV infectivity or its clinical expression. In vitro studies show, however, that Zn ions inhibit HIV-1 protease (131). In the late stages of AIDS, excessive Zn loss from diarrhea, as well as from cytokine-directed redistribution of the element, may be expected to further lower plasma Zn concentrations.

ZINC TOXICITY

Acute Toxicity

Although rare, incidences of acute Zn toxicity in humans resulting from high intakes of Zn have been reported. Isolated outbreaks of Zn toxicity have occurred as a result of consumption of foods and beverages contaminated with Zn released from galvanized containers. Typical signs of acute Zn toxicosis include epigastric pain, diarrhea, nausea, and vomiting (106, 107). Doses above 200 mg/day are typically emetic. A fatal outcome occurred in a woman who was inadvertently given 1.5 g of Zn intravenously over a 3-day period (132). Metal fume fever has been reported following inhalation of Zn oxide fumes. Signs develop within 8 hours and include hyperpnea, profuse sweating, and general weakness (133). Signs of toxicity disappear 12 to 24 hours after the individual is removed from the Zn-contaminated environment.

Chronic Toxicity

The major consequence of long-term ingestion of excessive Zn supplements is induction of a secondary Cu deficiency caused by competition between these elements for intestinal absorption. Levels of Zn supplements as low as 50 mg/day have influenced copper status, as indicated by a decline in erythrocyte Cu,Zn–superoxide dismutase (7). Long-term consumption of Zn supplements in excess of 150 mg/day has also been reported to result in low serum HDL levels, gastric erosion, and depressed immune function (134).

The U.S. Environmental Protection Agency has established an oral reference dose (RfD) for Zn of 0.3 mg/kg/day (135). An RfD for a substance represents an estimate of a daily exposure to the human population that is likely to be without appreciable risk of deleterious effects over a lifetime. Increasing the level of intake and frequency of exposure above the RfD increases the probability of seeing adverse effects. Although the RfD for Zn is below the RDA for all age groups below 15 years of age, no health hazards are known to result from ingesting the RDA for Zn at any age.

REFERENCES

1. Todd WR, Elvehjem CA, Hart EB. Am J Physiol 1934;107:146–56.
2. Hambidge KM, Casey CE, Krebs NF. Zinc in trace elements. In: Mertz W, ed. Human and animal nutrition, vol 2. 5th ed. Orlando, FL: Academic Press, 1986;1–137.
3. Prasad AS, Halsted JA, Nadimi M. Am J Med 1961;31:532–46.
4. Welch RM, House WA, Van Campen D. J Nutr 1977;107:929–33.
5. Welsh SO, Marston RM. Food Technol 1982;36:70–6.
6. Committee on Technological Options to Improve the Nutritional Attributes of Animal Products, National Research Council. Designing foods. Washington, DC: National Academy Press, 1988;18–44.
7. World Health Organization. Trace elements in human nutrition and health. Geneva: WHO, 1996.
8. MacDonald LD, Gibson RS, Miles JE. Acta Paediatr Scand 1982;71:785–9.
9. Sandström B. Eur J Clin Nutr 1997;51:S17–9.
10. Hunt JR, Gallagher SK, Johnson LK, et al. Am J Clin Nutr 1995;62:621–32.
11. House WA, Van Campen DR, Welch RM. Nutr Res 1997;17:65–76.
12. Sandström B, Lönnerdal B. Promoters and antagonists of zinc absorption. In: Mills CF, ed. Zinc in human biology. London: International Life Sciences Institute, 1989;57–78.
13. Hurley LS, Keen CL, Lönnerdal B. Fed Proc 1983;42:1735–9.
14. Brewer GJ, Hill GM, Prasad AS. Ann Intern Med 1983;99:314–20.
15. Turnlund JR. J Am Diet Assoc 1988;88:303–8.
16. Institute of Medicine, Food and Nutrition Board. Nutritional status during pregnancy and lactation. Washington, DC: National Academy Press, 1990.
17. McKenna AA, Ilich JZ, Andon MB, et al. Am J Clin Nutr 1997;65:1460–4.
18. Wood RJ, Zheng JJ. Am J Clin Nutr 1997;65:1803–9.
19. Johnson MA, Baier MJ, Greger JL. Am J Clin Nutr 1982;35:1332–8.
20. Chandler CJ, Wang TTY, Halsted CH. J Biol Chem 1986;261:928–33.
21. Tamura T, Shane B, Baer MT, et al. Am J Clin Nutr 1978;31:1984–7.
22. Milne DB. J Trace Elements Exp Med 1989;2:297–304.
23. Kauwell GP, Bailey LB, Gregory JF III, et al. J Nutr 1995;125:66–72.
24. Swanson CA, King JC. Am J Clin Nutr 1987;46:763–71.
25. Weigand E. Int J Vitam Nutr Res 1983;25(Suppl):67–81.
26. Matseshe JW, Phillips SF, Malagelada J-R, et al. Am J Clin Nutr 1980;33:1946–53.
27. Sian L, Hambidge KM, Westcott JL, et al. Am J Clin Nutr 1993;58:533–6.
28. Schölmerich J, Freudemann A, Köttgen E, et al. Am J Clin Nutr 1987;45:1480–6.
29. Wedekind KJ, Hortin AE, Baker DH. J Anim Sci 1992;70:178–87.
30. Hoadley JE, Leinart AS, Cousins RJ. Am J Physiol 1987;252:G825–31.
31. Cousins RJ, Lee-Ambrose LM. J Nutr 1992;122:56–64.
32. Fleet JC, Turnbull AJ, Bourcier M, et al. Am J Physiol 1993;264:G1037–45.
33. Cousins RJ. Clin Physiol Biochem 1986;4:20–30.
34. Fung EB, Ritchie LD, Woodhouse LR, et al. Am J Clin Nutr 1997;66:80–8.
35. Morgan PN, Costa FM, King JC, et al. FASEB J 1990;4:A648.
36. Coppen DE, Davies NT. Br J Nutr 1987;57:35–44.
37. Baer MT, King JC. Am J Clin Nutr 1984;39:556–70.
38. Cousins RJ. Physiol Rev 1985;65:238–309.
39. Davies NT, Williams RB. Br J Nutr 1977;38:417–23.
40. Lönnerdal B. Intestinal absorption of zinc. In: Mills CF, ed. Zinc in human biology. London: International Life Sciences Institute, 1989;33–58.
41. Wood RJ, Suter PM, Russell RM. Am J Clin Nutr 1995;62:493–505.
42. Miller LV, Hambidge KM, Naake VL, et al. J Nutr 1994;124:268–76.
43. Harris WR, Keen CL. J Nutr 1989;119:1677–82.
44. Lowe NM, Shames DM, Woodhouse LR, et al. Am J Clin Nutr 1997;65:1810–9.
45. Emmert JL, Baker DH. Poult Sci 1995;74:1011–21.
46. Masters DG, Keen CL, Lönnerdal B, et al. J Nutr 1983;113:905–12.
47. Jackson MJ, Jones DA, Edwards RHT, et al. Br J Nutr 1984;51:199–208.
48. Victery W, Smith JM, Vander AJ. Am J Physiol 1981;241:F532–9.
49. Milne DB, Canfield WK, Mahalko JR, et al. Am J Clin Nutr 1984;39:535–9.

50. Hess FM, King JC, Margen S. J Nutr 1977;107:1610–20.
51. Vallee BL. Zinc in biology and biochemistry. In: Spiro TG, ed. Zinc enzymes. New York: John Wiley, 1983;1–24.
52. Chesters JK. Biochemistry of zinc in cell division and tissue growth. In: Mills CF, ed. Zinc in human biology. London: International Life Sciences Institute, 1989;109–18.
53. Bettger WJ, Fish TJ, O'Dell BL. Proc Soc Exp Biol Med 1978;158:279–82.
54. Wilson RL. Zinc and iron in free radical pathology and cellular control. In: Mills CF, ed. Zinc in human biology. London: International Life Sciences Institute, 1989;147–72.
55. Kazimierczak W, Adamas B, Maslinski C. Biochem Pharmacol 1978;27:243–9.
56. Berg JM, Shi Y. Science 1996;271:1081–5.
57. Cousins RJ. Annu Rev Nutr 1994;14:449–69.
58. Oteiza PI, Cuellar S, Lönnerdal B, et al. Teratology 1990;41:97–104.
59. King JC. J Nutr 1990;120:1474–9.
60. Hurley LS, Gordon P, Keen CL, et al. Proc Soc Exp Biol Med 1982;170:48–52.
61. Keen CL, Hurley LS. Zinc and reproduction: effects of deficiency on foetal and postnatal development. In: Mills CF, ed. Zinc in human biology. London: International Life Sciences Institute, 1989;183–220.
62. O'Dell BL, Reeves PG. Zinc status and food intake. In: Mills CF, ed. Zinc in human biology. London: International Life Sciences Institute, 1989;173–82.
63. Clegg MS, Keen CL, Hurley LS. Biochemical pathologies of zinc deficiency. In: Mills CF, ed. Zinc in human biology. London: International Life Sciences Institute, 1989;129–46.
64. Bergman B, Friberg U, Lohmander S, et al. Scand J Dent Res 1972;80:486–92.
65. Keen CL, Gershwin ME. Annu Rev Nutr 1990;10:415–31.
66. Apgar J. Annu Rev Nutr 1985;5:43–68.
67. Bunce GE. Zinc in endocrine function. In: Mills CF, ed. Zinc in human biology. London: International Life Sciences Institute, 1989;249–58.
68. McClain CJ, Gavaler JS, Van Thiel DH. J Lab Clin Med 1984;104:1007.
69. Fraker PJ, Telford WG. Proc Soc Exp Biol Med 1997;215: 229–36.
70. Koo SI, Lee CC. Am J Clin Nutr 1988;47:120–7.
71. Cunnane SC, Yang J. Can J Physiol Pharmacol 1995;73:1246–52.
72. Bettger WJ, Reeves PG, Moscatelli EA, et al. J Nutr 1979;109:480–8.
73. Williams RB, Mills CF. Br J Nutr 1970;24:989–1003.
74. Walravens PA, Hambidge KM, Koepfer DM. Pediatrics 1989;83:532–8.
75. Hambidge KM, Walravens PA, Casey CE, et al. J Pediatr 1979;94:607–8.
76. Krebs NF, Hambidge KM, Walravens PA. Am J Dis Child 1984;138:270–3.
77. Golden MHN, Golden BE. Am J Clin Nutr 1981;34:900–8.
78. Henkin RI. Biol Trace Element Res 1984;6:263–80.
79. Bogden JD, Oleske JM, Munves EM, et al. Am J Clin Nutr 1987;45:101–9.
80. Abbasi AA, Prasad AS, Rabbani P, et al. J Lab Clin Med 1980;96:544–50.
81. Tamura T, Goldenberg RL. Nutr Res 1996;16:139–81.
82. Aggett PJ. Severe zinc deficiency. In: Mills CF, ed. Zinc in human biology. London: International Life Sciences Institute, 1989;259–80.
83. McClain CJ. J Am Coll Nutr 1985;4:49–64.
84. Wada L, King JC. J Nutr 1986;116:1045–53.
85. King JC. J Am Diet Assoc 1986;86:1523–7.
86. Hambidge KM. Mild zinc deficiency in human subjects. In: Mills CF, ed. Zinc in human biology. London: International Life Sciences Institute, 1989;281–96.
87. Fell GS, Cuthbertson DP, Morrison C, et al. Lancet 1973;1:280–2.
88. Freeman JB, Stegink LD, May PD, et al. J Surg Res 1975;18:463–9.
89. Sandström B, Cederblad A, Lindblad BS, et al. Arch Pediatr Adolesc Med 1994;148:980–5.
90. Weismann K, Hoe S, Nikkelsen HI, et al. Br J Dermatol 1979;101:573–9.
91. Hambidge KM, Walravens PA. Clin Gastroenterol 1982; 11:87–117.
92. King AB, Schwartz R. J Nutr 1987;117:704–8.
93. Yokoi K, Alcock NW, Sandstead HH. J Lab Clin Med 1994;124:852–61.
94. Cousins RJ. Systemic transport of zinc. In: Mills CF, ed. Zinc in human biology. London: International Life Sciences Institute, 1989;79–94.
95. Grider A, Bailey LB, Cousins RJ. Proc Natl Acad Sci USA 1990;87:1259–62.
96. Miller CF, ed. Zinc in human biology. London: International Life Sciences Institute. 1989;371–81.
97. Olin KL, Golub MS, Gershwin ME, et al. Am J Clin Nutr 1995;61:1263–7.
98. Food and Nutrition Board, National Research Council. Recommended dietary allowances. 10th ed. Washington DC: National Academy Press, 1989.
99. Keen CL, Lönnerdal B, Golub MS, et al. Pediatr Res 1989;26:470–7.
100. Leek JC, Vogler JB, Gershwin ME, et al. Am J Clin Nutr 1984;40:1203–12.
101. Jameson S. Acta Med Scand 1976;593(Suppl):1–89.
102. Apgar J. J Nutr Biochem 1992;3:266–78.
103. Goldenberg RL, Tamura T, Neggers Y, et al. JAMA 1995;274: 463–8.
104. Scholl TO, Hediger ML, Schall JI, et al. Am J Epidemiol 1993;137:1115–24.
105. Mares-Perlman JA, Subar AF, Block G, et al. J Am Coll Nutr 1995;14:349–57.
106. Turnlund JR, Durkin N, Costa F, et al. J Nutr 1986;116: 1239–47.
107. Chooi MK, Todd JK, Boyd ND. Nutr Metab 1976;20:135–42.
108. Greger JL. Potential for trace mineral deficiencies and toxicities in the elderly. In: Bales CW, ed. Mineral homeostasis in the elderly. Current topics in nutrition and disease, vol 21. New York: Marcel Dekker, 1989;171–200.
109. Sazawal S, Black RE, Bhan MK, et al. J Nutr 1996;126:443–50.
110. Sazawal S, Black RE, Bhan MK, et al. N Engl J Med 1995;333:839–44.
111. McClain CJ, Su L-C, Gilbert H, et al. Dig Dis Sci 1983;28:85–7.
112. McClain CJ, Soutor C, Zieve L. Gastroenterology 1980;78: 272–9.
113. Nishi Y, Lifshitz F, Bayne MA, et al. Am J Clin Nutr 1980;33:2613–21.
114. Brignola C, Belloli C, De Simone G, et al. Aliment Pharm Ther 1993;7:275–80.
115. Sturniolo GC, Molokhia MM, Shields RR, et al. Gut 1980;21:387–91.
116. Elmes M, Golden MK, Love AHS. Q J Mol Med 1978;55:293–306.
117. Andersson KE, Brat L, Dencker H, et al. Eur J Clin Pharmacol 1976;9:423–8.
118. Halsted CH, Keen CL. Eur J Gastroenterol Hepatol 1990;2: 399–405.

119. McClain CJ, Su LC. Alcohol Clin Exp Res 1983;7:5–10.
120. Zidenberg-Cherr S, Halsted CH, Olin KL, et al. J Nutr 1990;120:213–7.
121. Cabre M, Folch J, Gimenez A, et al. Int J Vitam Nutr Res 1995;65:45–50.
122. McClain CH, Van Thiel JH, Parker S, et al. Alcohol Clin Exp Res 1979;3:135–41.
123. Flynn A, Martier SS, Sokol RJ, et al. Lancet 1981;1:572–4.
124. Zidenberg-Cherr S, Benak PA, Hurley LS, et al. Drug Nutr Interact 1988;5:257–74.
125. Failla ML, Kiser RA. Am J Physiol 1983;244:E115–21.
126. Uriu-Hare JY, Stern JS, Keen CL. Diabetes 1989;38:1282–90.
127. Walter RM, Uriu-Hare JY, Olin KL, et al. Diabetes Care 1991;14:1050–6.
128. Cunningham JJ, Fu A, Mearkle PL, et al. Metabolism 1994;43: 1558–62.
129. Niewoehmer E, Allen JI, Boosalis M, et al. Am J Med 1986;81: 63–8.
130. Walter RM, Oster MH, Lee TJ, et al. Life Sci 1990;46:1597–600.
131. York DM, Darden TA, Pedersen LG, et al. Environ Health Perspect 1993;101:246–50.
132. Brocks A, Ried H, Glazer G, et al. Br Med J 1977;1:1390–1.
133. Bertholf RL. Zinc. In: Seiler HG, Sigel H, eds. Handbook on toxicity of inorganic compounds. New York: Marcel Dekker, 1988.
134. Fosmire GM. Am J Clin Nutr 1990;51:225–7.
135. Mertz W, Abernathy CO, Olin SS. Risk assessment of essential elements. Washington, DC: ILSI Press, 1994.

SELECTED READINGS

Cousins RJ. Metal elements and gene expression. Annu Rev Nutr 1994;14:449–69.

Hambidge KM, Casey CE, Krebs NF. Zinc. In: Mertz W, ed. Trace elements in human and animal nutrition, vol 2. 5th ed. Orlando, FL: Academic Press, 1986;1–137.

Keen CL, Gershwin ME. Zinc deficiency and immune function. Annu Rev Nutr 1990;10:415–31.

King JC. Assessment of zinc status. J Nutr 1990;120:1474–9.

Mills CF, ed. Zinc in human biology. London: International Life Sciences Institute, 1989.

12. Copper

JUDITH R. TURNLUND

HISTORICAL INTRODUCTION

Copper has been used therapeutically since at least 400 BC, when Hippocrates prescribed copper compounds for pulmonary and other diseases (1). The use of copper compounds in the treatment of diseases reached its peak in the 19th century and subsequently declined when the treatments were not successful.

Copper was identified as a normal constituent of blood and its toxicity was described in the late 19th century. By 1900, an anemia that could not be prevented by iron supplements had been observed in animals kept on a whole-milk diet. In 1928, Hart reported that this anemia in rats responded to iron only when copper supplements were also given (2). Experiments in several animal species produced similar results and suggested that copper-deficiency anemia occurs in all species. Detailed reviews of the early history of copper have been published (1, 3).

Human disease was first linked to copper metabolism shortly after Wilson's disease was described in 1912 and long before the condition was recognized as an inborn error of metabolism in 1953 (1). As early as 1930, a relationship between anemia in humans and copper deficiency was suspected, but copper supplements only improved hemoglobin synthesis in some instances, so the hypothesis was not well accepted. Conclusive evidence of copper deficiency in humans was not reported until 1964 (4). Menkes' disease, another genetic disorder, was described in 1962 and recognized as a disorder of copper absorption in 1972. Since about 1950, an increasing number of diseases that are not specifically disorders of copper metabolism have been associated with altered, usually increased, levels of copper in blood or other tissues.

An official dietary copper recommendation, an estimated safe and adequate daily dietary intake, was first introduced in 1979 and modified in 1989 (3).

CHEMISTRY

Copper, a transition metal with an atomic mass of 63.54 daltons (Da), has two stable isotopes, ^{63}Cu and ^{65}Cu, with natural abundances of 69.2 and 30.8%, respectively. There are seven radioisotopes of copper, most with half-lives of seconds or minutes. The two with the longest half-lives, ^{67}Cu (61.9 h) and ^{64}Cu (12.9 h), and either the stable isotopes ^{65}Cu or ^{63}Cu are used as tracers of copper metabolism.

Copper has two oxidation states, Cu^{+} and Cu^{2+}, and may shift back and forth between the two during enzyme action. It may occur rarely as Cu^{3+} (6). Only minute quantities of Cu^{+} ions can exist in solution; thus Cu^{+} compounds are highly insoluble and strongly complexed (7). Copper is most often found in biologic systems as Cu^{2+}. At least three types of bound Cu^{2+}, each with distinctly different physicochemical properties, are found in copper-containing enzymes. Type 1 is a deep blue protein; many copper-containing oxidases are of this type. Type 2, characteristic of many multicopper oxidases, is not blue but is detectable by electron paramagnetic resonance (EPR). Type 3, neither blue nor detectable by EPR, is also found in a number of enzymes. A single protein may contain one or more types of copper (6, 8).

DIETARY CONSIDERATIONS

Estimates of dietary intake by Americans prior to 1970 were considerably higher than current estimates. This reflects marked improvements in analytical techniques for measuring copper and awareness of the importance of avoiding copper contamination of analytical samples. The usual diet was thought to contain 2 to 5 mg (30 to 80 μmol) of copper, but studies, including one study of 132 diet composites, now show that few diets contain over 2 mg (30 μmol) per day (9, 10). As with all nutrients, copper intake can vary widely, depending on food choices. Diets in countries where more whole-grain products, legumes, and organ meats are eaten contain more copper.

Food Sources

The richest sources of dietary copper contain from 0.3 to over 2 mg/100 g (50 to >300 nmol/g). These include shellfish, nuts, seeds (including cocoa powder), legumes, the bran and germ portions of grains, liver, and organ meats. Most grain products; most products containing chocolate, fruits and vegetables, such as dried fruits, mushrooms, tomatoes, bananas, grapes, and potatoes; and most meats have intermediate amounts of copper, from 0.1 to 0.3 mg/100 g (20–50 nmol/g). Other fruits and vegetables, chicken, many fish, and dairy products contain relatively low concentrations (<0.1 mg/100 g [20 nmol/g)]) of copper (11). Cow's milk is particularly low in copper. The major sources of copper in the US diet are meat, nuts, beans/peas, and main dishes (12).

Because information on the copper content of foods is incomplete and databases often contain missing values, copper intake is underestimated unless missing values are replaced with imputed values (9). A table of the copper content of foods compiled when much of the available data were from the 1930s and 1940s reported consistently higher copper concentrations (13) than tables that exclude pre-1960 data, suggesting that early values are too high. However, a critical evaluation of the reliability of post-1960 published values for the copper content of foods demonstrated that improvement is still needed (11). The copper content of foods can vary because of a combination of factors, including analytical method, sampling procedure, recipe, cooking method, and part of the country from which the foods are collected. Careful analysis of the copper content of high-copper foods from the FDA total diet study varied by an average CV (coefficient of variation) of 24%, which is in the middle of average variation of other minerals in the same foods (9, 12).

Bioavailability

Estimates of the bioavailability of dietary copper to humans are usually based on absorption (14). The amount of copper in the diet appears to influence bioavailability more than the composition of the diet or specific dietary components unless the levels are extremely high or low or diet composition is unusual. Absorption is discussed under "Metabolism."

Interactions

Interactions with Other Nutrients

Nutrients known to affect the bioavailability of copper when included in the diet of humans or animals in extreme amounts are iron, zinc, molybdenum, ascorbic acid, and carbohydrates. In addition, high or low levels of dietary copper may affect metabolism of some of these nutrients. Interactions between dietary copper and other nutrients or dietary components have been reviewed (15, 16).

Iron. Copper and iron may interact in a number of ways. As discussed under "Copper Deficiency," copper deficiency alters iron metabolism. Anemia, often accompanied by accumulation of iron in the liver, has been reported in all species studied, including humans. An excess of copper has produced anemia in the pig. Excessive iron in the form of inorganic iron salts decreased copper status and, in time, resulted in clinical signs of copper deficiency in several animal species (16).

Zinc. When the diet contains excessive zinc over a sufficient period, the copper status of animals and humans is impaired; the effect is reversed by copper supplements. One explanation for this interaction is that high dietary zinc induces intestinal metallothionein (MT). Copper does not play an important role in the induction of MT, but it has a stronger affinity for MT than does zinc. It displaces zinc in intestinal MT and is trapped (3, 17). Copper depletion was observed in humans when supplements of 50 mg (280 μmol) or more of zinc were given for extended periods. This caused concern that dietary zinc intake slightly above the recommended level might affect copper status, but copper absorption was not affected by 16.5 mg (250 μmol) of zinc per day. High doses of copper have in some cases reduced the effects of zinc deficiency in animals, but these effects were inconsistent (18). In one study, a high-copper diet reduced zinc absorption slightly and increased the excretion of zinc in young men but did not impair zinc status (19).

Molybdenum. Interactions between copper and molybdenum have been observed frequently in ruminants (3). Slight excesses of molybdenum in the presence of sulfide produce molybdenum toxicity and secondary copper deficiency. A similar response in rats requires much more molybdenum and is independent of sulfur. A single report of a high-molybdenum diet in humans increasing urinary copper excretion suggests that a similar interaction could occur in humans. The toxicity of molybdenum in ruminants is ameliorated when dietary copper is increased.

Ascorbic Acid. Ascorbic acid supplements have produced copper deficiency in laboratory animals and may affect the copper status of humans. Plasma ascorbic acid concentrations in premature infants are negatively correlated with plasma ceruloplasmin concentrations and plasma antioxidant activity (20). Daily ascorbic acid supplements of 1500 mg (8.5 mmol) given to young men caused ceruloplasmin activity to decline. Copper absorption was not impaired by 600 mg (3.4 mmol) of ascorbic acid, but ceruloplasmin declined, and the results suggested that the oxidase activity of ceruloplasmin may be impaired by excessive ascorbic acid (15).

Carbohydrates. The type of carbohydrate in the diet affects the rate and severity of copper depletion in rats. They are more resistant to copper deficiency when the carbohydrate source is cornstarch than when it is sucrose or fructose. The interaction between carbohydrate source and copper in humans is not clear. Erythrocyte superoxide dismutase (SOD) levels of humans in one study were lower with a high-fructose diet than with a high-cornstarch diet, but copper retention increased (21). In addition, research in young pigs, whose cardiovascular and gastrointestinal systems are similar to those in humans, suggests that the interaction observed in rats may not apply to humans (22, 23).

Interactions with Drugs and Nonnutrient Components of the Diet

Relatively little is known about interactions of copper with drugs. Penicillamine is used to chelate endogenous copper in the treatment of Wilson's disease. Its use results in excretion of up to 5 mg/day (79 mmol/day) of copper in the urine (24). Antacids may interfere with copper absorption (15) when used in very high amounts. Fiber and phytate in the diet influence the bioavailability of several minerals, but their effect on copper absorption and metabolism is not clear. Rat studies have demonstrated both inhibition and enhancement of copper absorption by phytate (15). Copper use may be influenced by both phytate and fiber in the diets of humans.

Adequacy of Intake by Various Population Groups

Dietary copper intake in the United States and other countries is usually below the currently recommended 1.5 mg/day (1). The new World Health Organization (WHO) estimated minimum requirements are 0.6 mg/day (9 mmol/day) for women and 0.7 mg/day (11 μmol/day) for men (10). The estimated usual dietary copper intake in the United States, after correcting for missing values in the USDA database, was 0.96 mg/day (15 μmol/day) for women and 1.4 mg/day (22 μmol/day) for men. A total diet study estimated intake at 0.92 mg/day (14 μmol/day) for women and 1.2 mg/day (19 μmol/day) for men (9). Frank copper deficiency in humans is very rare, which suggests that the current dietary intake usually suffices to prevent copper deficiency. It has been suggested that the usual copper intake is marginal and may not support optimal health, but data in this area conflict and do not yet suffice to support that hypothesis.

METABOLISM

Mammalian copper metabolism is depicted schematically in Figure 12.1. Some copper in the diet is absorbed into the body through the intestinal mucosa, transported via the portal blood to the liver, and incorporated into ceruloplasmin. Ceruloplasmin is released into the blood and delivers copper to tissues throughout the body. Albumin-bound copper exchanges with tissue copper and a number of low-molecular-weight moieties also supply copper to the tissues (25). Most endogenous copper is secreted into the gastrointestinal tract, where it combines with unabsorbed dietary copper and is eliminated from the body. A small amount of copper is eliminated through other excretory routes.

Absorption

Studies conducted with laboratory animals have begun to provide some basic information on the mechanism of copper absorption (3, 26). Copper is absorbed primarily in the small intestine, with a small amount absorbed in the stomach. Absorption is probably by a saturable, active transport mechanism at lower levels of dietary copper; at high levels of dietary copper, passive diffusion plays a role. Absorption may be regulated by the need for copper, with MT in intestinal cells involved in the regulation.

The recent development of methods for using a stable isotope of copper to investigate copper metabolism in humans has improved the reliability of copper absorption measurement (14). Early estimates of copper absorption in humans ranged from 15 to 97% (1). Estimates of copper absorption varied widely in part because of inadequate methods and because the level of dietary copper was not known or controlled. A series of stable isotope studies of copper absorption have since demonstrated that the level of dietary copper strongly influences absorption (14, 27). As dietary copper increases, the fraction absorbed declines and the amount absorbed increases. Absorption declined from 75% at 0.4 mg (6 μmol) Cu per day to 12% at 7.5 mg (120 μmol) Cu per day. The amount absorbed increased from 0.3 to 0.9 mg (5 to 15 μmol), or only tripled with 20 times the amount of dietary copper. This suggests that copper homeostasis is maintained in part by regulation of absorption.

Storage

The adult human body contains only about 50 to 120 mg (0.79–1.9 mmol) of copper (3), very little compared with other trace elements such as iron and zinc. Animal data suggest that copper is stored in the liver, bound to MT-like proteins. Ruminants and a few other animal species can store much more copper in the liver than can humans or most other animal species. Copper may also be held, at least temporarily, bound to intestinal MT.

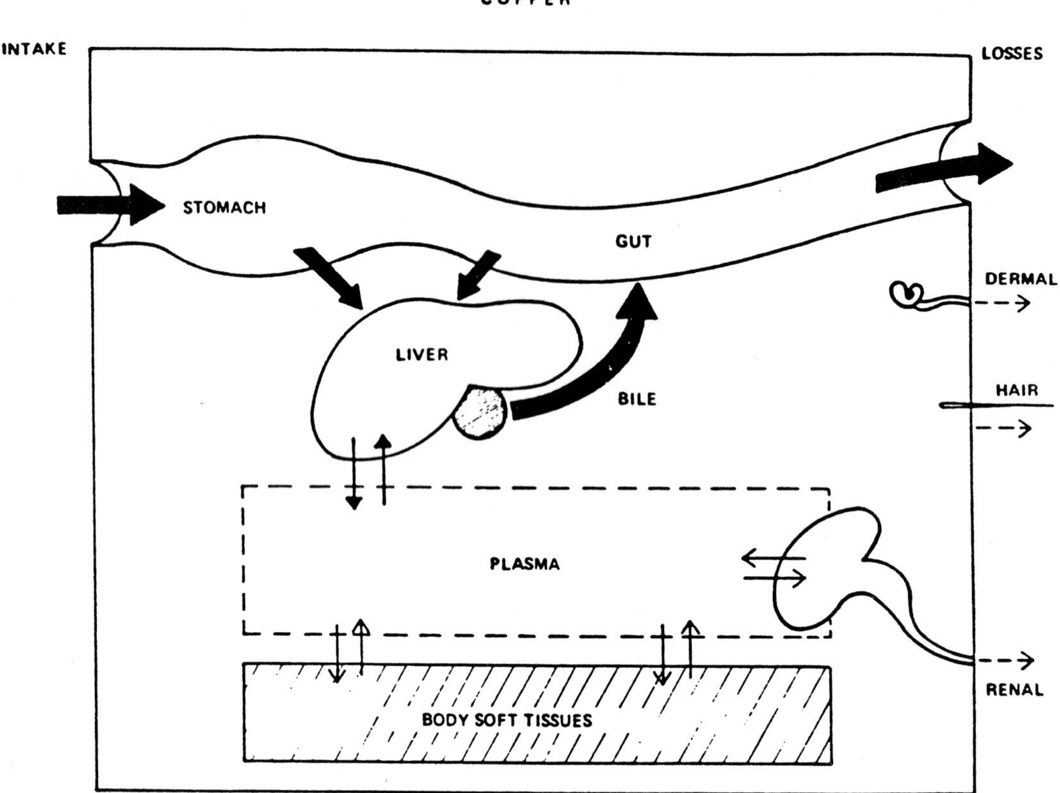

Figure 12.1. Schematic representation of the metabolism of copper in mammals. (From Solomons NW. Zinc and copper. In: Shils ME, Young VR, eds. Modern nutrition in health and disease. 7th ed. Philadelphia: Lea & Febiger, 1988.)

Transport

Following absorption, copper is transported bound primarily to albumin and to transcuprein and low-molecular-weight ligands (26, 28). The newly absorbed copper disappears rapidly from the plasma. Most is taken up by the liver; some is taken up by the kidney. Once in the liver, copper is incorporated into ceruloplasmin within hours. Some is incorporated into MT in the liver of animals, particularly when copper intake is high; a role for MT in cellular detoxification has been proposed (29). A role for copper in the kidney is not known, but copper is probably filtered by the glomerulus and reabsorbed in the tubules (30).

Copper bound to ceruloplasmin is released from the liver into the blood and delivered to cells with specific ceruloplasmin receptors on their surface. Ceruloplasmin binds to these receptors; the copper is reduced, dissociates from ceruloplasmin, and is released into the cells (31).

One suggested sequence leading to excretion of copper in bile is that ceruloplasmin with part of the copper removed may return to the liver, where it is partially degraded (26) and transferred to the bile accompanied by ceruloplasmin fragments. Glutathione, although not a cuproenzyme, may play a role in the rapid transfer of excessive copper to bile (32).

Excretion

The primary route of copper excretion is via bile into the gastrointestinal tract. Little of this copper is reabsorbed. It combines with a small amount of copper from intestinal cells, from pancreatic and intestinal fluids, and unabsorbed dietary copper and is then eliminated in the feces. Other routes of excretion contribute little to total copper losses. Healthy humans excrete only 10 to 30 μg (0.2–0.5 μmol) of copper in the urine (33, 34), but urinary losses can increase markedly in some conditions, such as renal tubular defects (30). Sweat and integumentary losses are usually less than 50 μg (0.8 mmol) per day (33).

Homeostatic Regulation

Absorption of ingested copper is regulated and is much more efficient when dietary copper is low. The importance of an individual's copper status in absorption is not understood. A low-copper diet increases the efficiency of absorption rapidly, but absorption does not become more efficient after several weeks on a low-copper diet (27). This suggests that the dietary content is more important than copper status in regulation of absorption. Another point of regulation in the homeostatic control of total body copper is the excretion of copper into the bile and from there into the gastrointestinal tract. Animals and humans increase endogenous copper excretion when the diet is high in copper and excrete little during copper deficiency or when dietary copper is low (26, 35, 36). When a stable isotope of copper was administered, tissue copper was conserved in copper-restricted rats. Intravenous doses of a stable isotope of copper were administered to human subjects. When dietary copper was 2.5 mg/day (39 μmol/day), 20% of the dose was excreted and eliminated in the stools in 6 days, while only 7% of the dose was eliminated when the diet contained 0.4 mg/day (6 μmol/day). The homeostatic regulation of copper absorption and excretion protects against copper deficiency and toxicity over a broad range of dietary intakes.

FUNCTIONS

Biochemical

Copper functions in vivo as a part of a number of proteins, including many important enzymes. Detailed descriptions of these proteins and their functions have been published (6, 8, 26). The copper proteins known to be present in humans are listed in Table 12.1 and described briefly below. Many other copper-containing proteins are found in plants, lower organisms, and some animal species. Some of the better known of these include ascorbate oxidase, carboxypeptidase A, hemocyanin, laccase, and uricase.

Copper-Containing Enzymes Found in Humans

Amine Oxidases. Several important amine oxidases are cuproproteins. Relatively small amounts of these enzymes are found circulating in blood plasma, where they inactivate and catabolize physiologically active amines such as histidine, tyramine, and polyamines. They are found in tissues throughout the body. Their activity is elevated in conditions in which connective tissue activation and deposition take place, including liver fibrosis, congestive heart failure, hyperthyroidism, childhood, and senescence (26).

Table 12.1
Copper-Containing Proteins in Humans

Copper-containing enzymes
Amine oxidases
Amine oxidase (flavin-containing)[monoamine oxidase, tyramine oxidase] (EC 1.4.3.4)[a]
Amine oxidase (copper-containing)[diamine oxidase, histaminase] (EC 1.4.3.6)
Lysyl oxidase (EC 1.4.3.13)
Peptidlyglycine-α-amidating monooxygenase (PAM)
Ferroxidases
Ferroxidase I [ceruloplasmin] (EC 1.16.3.1)
Ferroxidase II
Cytochrome *c* oxidase [cytochrome oxidase](EC 1.9.3.1)
Dopamine β-monooxygenase [dopamine β-hydroxylase] (EC 1.14.17.1)
Superoxide dismutase [hemocuprin, erythrocupin] (EC 1.15.1.1)
Extracellular superoxide dismutase
Copper/zinc superoxide dismutase
Monophenol monooxygenase [tyrosinase] (EC 1.14.18.1)
Copper-binding proteins
Metallothionein
Albumin
Transcuprein
Blood clotting factor V
Low-molecular-weight ligands
Amino acids
Peptides

[a] *The recommended names of enzymes are followed by other common names in brackets and by the code numbers assigned by the Nomenclature Committee of the International Union of Biochemistry (65) in parentheses.*

Monoamine Oxidase. Involved in inactivation of catecholamines, monoamine oxidase reacts with substances, such as serotonin, norepinephrine, tyramine, and dopamine, and is inhibited by tricyclic antidepressant drugs.

Diamine Oxidase. A number of copper-dependent diamine oxidase enzymes are found in cells throughout the body. Diamine oxidase inactivates histamine, acting in the small intestine, where histamine stimulates acid secretion, and in allergic reactions throughout the body, where histamine is released in response to exposure to antigens. It also inactivates polyamines involved in cell proliferation, which suggests that diamine oxidase may play a role in limiting excessive growth. Diamine oxidase activity is highest in the small intestine. Activity is also high in the kidney, where diamine oxidase inactivates diamines filtered from the blood, and in maternal placenta, where it may inactivate amines produced by the fetus.

Lysyl Oxidase. Lysyl oxidase, a unique amine oxidase, acts on lysine and hydroxylysine side chains of collagen and elastin. It deaminates the lysine of newly formed, immature elastin and collagen, after which cross-links are formed. The enzyme functions in the formation of connective tissue, including bone, blood vessels, vasculature, skin, lungs, and teeth. The concentrations are highest during development. Long-term estrogen treatment increases the activity of lysyl oxidase, and malignant transformation decreases activity.

Peptidylglycine-α-Amidating Monooxygenase. A newly identified cuproenzyme, peptidylglycine-α-amidating monooxygenase, is involved in the synthesis of many bioactive peptides and may be influenced by copper deficiency (37).

Ferroxidases. *Ceruloplasmin.* Ceruloplasmin, also called ferroxidase I, is an α_2 glycoprotein with a molecular weight of about 150,000. It contains six (possibly seven) atoms of copper per molecule, including Cu^{2+} atoms of all three types described under "Chemistry." Four copper atoms appear to be involved in the oxidation/reduction reactions the enzyme catalyzes. The role of the other atoms is not yet understood. This enzyme catalyzes the oxidation of ferrous iron and plays a role in the transfer of iron from storage to sites of hemoglobin synthesis. Ceruloplasmin also oxidizes aromatic amines and phenols.

Most of the copper in blood plasma is bound to ceruloplasmin. Estimates of the ceruloplasmin fraction range from 60 to 95% (26). The fraction of plasma copper associated with ceruloplasmin appears to be relatively constant within an individual but varies considerably among individuals (33).

Ferroxidase II. Ferroxidase II also catalyzes the oxidation of ferrous iron. It accounts for only about 5% of the ferroxidase activity in human plasma, but plays a more important role in some animal species.

Cytochrome *c* Oxidase. Cytochrome *c* oxidase enzyme, present in the mitochondria of cells throughout the body, is the terminal link in the electron transport chain. It reduces O_2 to form water and permits formation of adenosine triphosphate (ATP) in mitochondrial energy production. Cytochrome *c* oxidase is considered the single most important enzyme of the mammalian cell, because it is rate limiting in electron transport (28). It contains two or three copper atoms per molecule. The activity of this enzyme is highest in the heart and high in brain, liver, and kidney tissues.

Dopamine β -Hydroxylase. Dopamine β-hydroxylase catalyzes the conversion of dopamine to the neurotransmitter norepinephrine in the brain. Estimates of the copper content of dopamine β-hydroxylase range from two to eight atoms per molecule, with the most recent estimates being the higher amount (38). Dopamine β-hydroxylase concentration is two to three times higher in gray matter of the brain than in white matter, and it is present in the adrenal gland, where it is required for epinephrine production.

Superoxide Dismutase. *Extracellular Superoxide Dismutase (EC-SOD).* EC-SOD, a copper-containing enzyme, is present in high amounts in the lungs, thyroid, and uterus and in small amounts in blood plasma. It functions as a scavenger of superoxide radicals and protects against oxidative damage.

Copper/Zinc Superoxide Dismutase (SOD). Copper/zinc SOD, which contains two copper atoms per molecule, is present within most cells of the body, primarily within the cytosol. It protects intracellular components from oxidative damage, converting the superoxide ion to hydrogen peroxide. It requires both zinc and copper for catalytic function (39). High concentrations are found in brain, thyroid, liver, pituitary, erythrocytes, and kidney of humans. Erythrocyte levels of SOD are high in alcoholics and individuals with Down's syndrome.

Tyrosinase. Tyrosinase catalyzes the conversion of tyrosine to dopamine and the oxidation of dopamine to dopaquinone, steps in the synthesis of melanin. It is present in the melanocytes of the eye and skin and is responsible for the color in hair, skin, and eyes. Deficiency of tyrosinase in skin leads to albinism.

Copper-Binding Proteins

Metallothionein (MT). MTs are small nonenzymatic proteins, rich in cysteine, that are responsible for binding copper. Each molecule can bind 11 or 12 copper atoms as well as zinc and cadmium. They appear to play a role in metal storage and sequester excess metal ions, preventing toxicity. The concentration is highest in the liver, where metals accumulate in MT fractions. MTs are found in many other human tissues, including small amounts in the blood plasma. The presence in blood plasma has prompted the suggestion that MTs also play a role in copper transport, but if so, the role would be minor (26).

Albumin. Albumin, a protein with a molecular weight of 68,000, is the most prevalent protein in blood plasma and interstitial fluids. Albumin binds and transports copper and may also play a role in binding excess copper that would otherwise be toxic. Estimates of the fraction of copper in blood plasma that is bound to albumin range from 5 to 18% (26).

Transcuprein. Transcuprein, a recently isolated plasma protein with a molecular weight of about 270,000, binds copper and is found in humans. It has not yet been completely characterized and its functions are not clear, but it may play a role in copper transport. Considerably less serum copper is bound to transcuprein than to albumin (26).

Blood-Clotting Factor V. Blood-clotting factor V, a nonenzymatic component of the blood-clotting process, has recently been found to contain one atom of copper per molecule (40). Although this indicates that copper is required for blood clotting, impaired blood clotting is not among the reported manifestations of copper deficiency.

Low-Molecular-Weight Ligands

Amino acids and small peptides also carry a small fraction of the copper in the blood plasma. Estimates range from less than 1% to 4% (26). Histidine, glutamine, threonine, and cystine are examples of amino acids that bind copper in the plasma, and at least one copper peptide complex, glycyl-histidine-lysine, has been isolated from human plasma. The role of these complexes is not known, but the copper carried by low-molecular-weight ligands is thought to exchange with nonceruloplasmin copper in the blood. The ligands may carry copper to cells (25).

Physiologic

Many of the physiologic functions of copper can be deduced from reactions the cuproenzymes catalyze. Others are based on symptoms of copper deficiency. Detailed reviews of the physiologic functions of copper have been published (1, 3).

Connective Tissue Formation. Copper, through the enzyme lysyl oxidase, is essential for cross-linking of collagen and elastin, which are required for formation of strong, flexible connective tissue. Thus, copper plays a role in bone formation, skeletal mineralization, and the integrity of the connective tissue in the heart and vascular system. Lysyl oxidase activity declines during severe copper deficiency in weanling rats, and the resulting defects in connective tissue formation may be responsible for the multiple effects of copper deficiency on cardiac system integrity and bone formation (41). Copper depletion in humans also results in modest changes in lysyl oxidase activity in the skin (42), but the degree of change does not compromise function, as there is a large excess present.

Iron Metabolism. Several mechanisms have been proposed for the role of copper in iron metabolism and erythropoiesis (43). Ceruloplasmin and ferroxidase II oxidize ferrous iron, so it can be transported from the intestinal lumen and storage sites to sites of erythropoiesis. This may explain why anemia develops with copper deficiency, yet iron accumulates in the intestinal lumen and liver. Copper may also be required for formation of normal bone marrow cells, necessary for formation of red blood cells.

Central Nervous System. Copper plays more than one role in the central nervous system. It is required for formation or maintenance of myelin, a protective layer covering neurons, composed primarily of phospholipids. Phospholipid synthesis depends on cytochrome *c* oxidase activity, which may explain why copper deficiency leads to poor myelination, necrosis of nerve tissue, and neonatal ataxia in copper-deficient animals. The role of cuproenzymes in catecholamine metabolism (conversion of dopamine to norepinephrine by dopamine β-hydroxylase and the degradation of serotonin, norepinephrine, tyramine, and dopamine by monoamine oxidase) implies a function in normal neurotransmission (37).

Melanin Pigment Formation. The role of copper in the pigmentation of skin, hair, and eyes is related to the requirement for tyrosinase in melanin synthesis. Depigmentation of hair and skin is observed with copper deficiency in several animal species and in Menkes' disease.

Cardiac Function and Cholesterol Metabolism. The role of copper in cardiac function has been explored in a number of laboratory animal experiments (44). Cardiac myopathy and a variety of other conditions appear when weanling, but not older, rats are deprived of copper. Cardiac symptoms have not been reported in the few frankly copper-deficient humans, though links to heart irregularities in humans have been suggested (45). Blood cholesterol levels increase in animals fed copper-deficient diets, but results of studies on the effects of low-copper diets on blood cholesterol in humans are not consistent. Levels have increased in some and declined in others, and copper supplementation increased low-density lipoprotein (LDL) in a study in adult males (46).

Other Functions. Other physiologic functions suggested for copper are not as well understood as those described above. These include roles in thermal regulation and glucose metabolism. A role in blood clotting through factor V is known but has not yet been clearly associated with clinical manifestations of copper deficiency. Copper is known to be both prooxidant and antioxidant. Two key antioxidant enzymes, ceruloplasmin and superoxide dismutase, decrease in copper deficiency and may result in impaired antioxidant status (47). Recent evidence suggests a role for copper in immune function. Both low- and high-copper intake influenced immune function in laboratory animals (48). Some indices of immune function declined with copper depletion of humans, but they were not reversed by a higher copper intake (49). The effect of dietary copper on these functions warrants further investigation.

CAUSES AND MANIFESTATIONS OF DEFICIENCY

Copper Deficiency in Animals

Copper deficiency has been produced experimentally and observed in areas with copper-deficient soil in rats, mice, guinea pigs, rabbits, chicks, pigs, dogs, cattle, goats, and sheep. Detailed descriptions of deficiency symptoms and comparisons among species have been published (1, 3, 50). Animal studies have provided definitive information on the manifestations of copper deficiency. However, the deficiencies produced in animals were more severe than those reported in humans, and species differences make extrapolation to humans difficult.

Anemia, neutropenia, and osteoporosis are observed with copper deficiency in all species. Other well-established manifestations of copper deficiency observed in animal species are skeletal abnormalities, fractures, and spinal deformities; neonatal ataxia; depigmentation of hair and wool; impaired keratinization of hair, fur, and wool; reproductive failure, including low fertility, fetal death, and resorption; cardiovascular disorders including myocardial degeneration, cardiac hypertrophy and failure, rupture of blood vessels, and electrocardiographic changes; and impaired immune function. Changes in lipid and cholesterol metabolism, increased lipid peroxidation, and impaired glucose metabolism have been observed in some studies. Hypercholesterolemia may be linked to glutathione metabolism (32). Some of the manifestations of copper deficiency are considered controversial because they have only been observed in one or two species or under specific dietary conditions such as unusually high levels of fructose or zinc (3).

Copper Deficiency in Humans

For years following the discovery of copper deficiency in laboratory animals it was considered unlikely that copper deficiency could occur in humans. Although copper deficiency in humans is relatively rare, it has been reported a number of times since 1964 under special circumstances. Reviews of copper deficiency in humans have been published (30, 43).

Copper deficiency has been clearly documented in infants recovering from malnutrition, in premature and low-birth-weight infants fed milk diets, and in patients receiving prolonged total parenteral nutrition. In established cases, blood was sampled for determination of serum copper and ceruloplasmin levels prior to administration of copper supplements, and manifestations of copper deficiency were reversed following copper supplementation.

Frank copper deficiency is accompanied by hypocupremia and low ceruloplasmin levels. Levels fall to 30% of normal and below. Serum copper values as low as 0.5 μmol/L (3 μg/dL) and ceruloplasmin values as low as 35 mg/L (3.5 mg/dL) have been reported (50). Usual features of copper deficiency are anemia, leukopenia, and neutropenia. The anemia is most often described as normocytic and hypochromic but is sometimes normochromic and sometimes microcytic. Osteoporosis is often observed when bones are still growing and may be accompanied by metaphysial flaring and fractures at the margins of the metaphyses.

The possibility of mild copper deficiency because of marginal copper intake over a long period has been suggested. Possible manifestations, in addition to the features of severe deficiency, are conditions such as arthritis, arterial disease, loss of pigmentation, myocardial disease, and neurologic effects (30). Diminished glucose tolerance, increased serum cholesterol, and heart beat irregularities have been linked to marginal copper intake (3). These conditions were not accompanied by the low ceruloplasmin or serum copper levels or other features of severe deficiency, but serum copper levels declined in one individual with these symptoms. Dietary copper intake in these studies was within the range of intakes consumed by a large segment of the population, 0.8 to 1 mg (13–16 μmol) per day, and these effects were not produced in other studies at this level of dietary copper (33). Further research is required to establish whether these conditions are related to copper status or not, but this is complicated by ethical considerations related to feeding very low copper intakes, the possibility that some individuals may have a higher copper requirement than others, and possible nutrient interactions.

CLINICAL CONDITIONS

Clinical Conditions with Increased Risk of Copper Depletion

Most severe copper deficiency cases reported to date have been associated with other clinical conditions (30). Copper deficiency has been documented during total parenteral nutrition, in premature infants fed milk formulas, in infants recovering from malnutrition (usually associated with chronic diarrhea), in infants undergoing chronic peritoneal dialysis, and in severely handicapped patients (51). Two cases of copper deficiency were observed in full-term infants fed only cow's milk. Increased gastrointestinal losses due to diarrhea or fistulas increase copper losses and the risk of copper depletion. Diseases of malabsorption, such as celiac disease and nontropical sprue, increase the risk of copper depletion because of both malabsorption and increased losses, and it appears that the copper status of cystic fibrosis patients may be compromised (52). Prolonged use of antacids and long-term therapy with very high doses of zinc in treatment of sickle cell anemia have resulted in hypocupremia and some manifestations of copper deficiency.

Parenteral Nutrition. The realization that trace element deficiencies sometimes follow prolonged parenteral nutrition prompted recommendations that several trace elements, including copper, be added to the solutions. Guidelines for their preparation and addition were established in 1979, and these elements are now added routinely in the United States. Copper deficiency usually develops after months of parenteral nutrition without added copper; the risk of deficiency developing is increased substantially in individuals with excessive gastrointestinal losses. Free amino acid solutions increase urinary copper losses, adding to the risk. Adults receiving total parenteral nutrition (TPN) who did not have excessive gastrointestinal fluid losses could maintain balance and normal serum and ceruloplasmin levels on only 0.25 mg (3.9 μmol) Cu per day. These values did not increase after supplementation with copper. In contrast, serum copper and ceruloplasmin values declined steadily in others receiving a TPN solution in which copper was not detectable, and these indices increased when oral feeding was resumed. Stable adult patients receiving TPN need about 0.3 mg (4.7 μmol) Cu daily to maintain balance. The requirements are increased to 0.4 to 0.5 mg (6–8 μmol) daily with excessive gastrointestinal losses and should be reduced in patients with cholestasis and impaired biliary excretion (53).

Clinical Conditions Accompanied by Copper Accumulation

Copper can accumulate in the liver in any disease that causes impaired biliary excretion. Two of these, Wilson's disease and Indian childhood cirrhosis (ICC), are discussed below. Liver copper level is very high in primary biliary cirrhosis and biliary atresia. Copper chelation rather than dietary copper restriction is recommended to reduce the liver copper stores in these diseases (54).

Conditions with Increased Serum Copper

Serum copper and ceruloplasmin levels rise progressively during pregnancy, usually reaching twice-normal levels by term. This is partly due to redistribution of copper, and the change is accompanied by increased total body copper (55). Serum copper and ceruloplasmin levels rise, often to two to three times normal values, in inflammatory conditions, infectious diseases, hematologic diseases, diabetes, coronary and cardiovascular diseases, uremia, and malignant diseases and following surgery (1, 3). Smoking and some drugs also increase serum copper concentrations. Ceruloplasmin is an acute-phase reactant, and the rise in ceruloplasmin is probably responsible for the increase in serum copper in the above conditions, because the increases parallel one another. The mechanism for the increase or the role for ceruloplasmin is not understood but is under investigation in several laboratories (26).

Genetic Defects in Copper Metabolism

The two best-known defects in copper metabolism in humans are Menkes' disease and Wilson's disease. Several defects in production of cuproenzymes have been identified, including overproduction of SOD in Down's syndrome, absence of tyrosinase in albinism, changes in lysyl oxidase in cutis laxa (Ehlers-Danlos syndrome), and myopathy due to reduction in cytochrome *c* oxidase. Genetic defects in copper metabolism have also been observed in mice and dogs. The reader is referred to reviews of genetic diseases of copper metabolism (24, 56).

Menkes' Disease. Menkes' disease is a fatal X-linked disorder characterized by mental retardation, abnormal hair, and maldistribution of copper (56). It occurs in 1 in 50,000 to 100,000 live births and is usually fatal by the age of 3 years. Serum copper and ceruloplasmin levels are low, as are levels in liver and brain, but copper accumulates in intestinal mucosa, muscle, spleen, and kidney. Synthesis of ceruloplasmin, SOD, and cytochrome oxidase is impaired. Abnormalities in connective tissue cross-linking because of dysfunction of lysyl oxidase result in defective arteries in the brain and elsewhere, and in osteoporosis. Progressive nerve degeneration in the brain results in intellectual deterioration, hypotonia, and seizures. Hypothermia is common. Skin and hair are poorly pigmented, and hair is characteristically "kinky." The anemia and neutropenia common to nutritional copper deficiency are not found in Menkes' disease, a difference that cannot be explained. Administration of parenteral copper increases serum copper and ceruloplasmin levels but does not improve brain function or slow the progressive deterioration.

Wilson's Disease. Wilson's disease is an autosomal recessive disease of copper storage. The prevalence of the defect is uncertain but has been estimated at approximately 1 in 200,000 in the United States. Copper accumulates in the liver, the brain, and the cornea of the eye (Kayser-Fleischer rings). Urinary copper excretion is abnormally high, but ceruloplasmin values are usually low. There appears to be a defect in the catabolism and excretion of ceruloplasmin copper into the bile. If the disease goes untreated, copper accumulation in the liver and brain results in neurologic damage and cirrhosis. Hepatitis, hemolytic crisis, and hepatic failure may ensue. (An excellent clinicopathologic exercise of a case of Wilson's disease can be found in reference 57.)

Early diagnosis and treatment can prevent the severe consequences of the disease. Dietary copper restriction was advocated for Wilson's disease at one time, but chelation therapy, usually using D-penicillamine, is much more effective in reducing copper stores (54). Avoidance of large quantities of foods rich in copper may also be recommended, but diets very low in copper are not necessary. D-Penicillamine is an antimetabolite of pyridoxine, so daily pyridoxine supplements of 12.5 to 25 mg (75–150 nmol) are recommended. The treatment induces removal of excess copper and prevents reaccumulation through excretion of 1 to 5 mg (16–79 μmol) copper daily in the urine. As an alternative to penicillamine, tetrathiomolybdate, 20 mg six times per day, followed by oral zinc supplements of 150 mg/day is sometimes used to eliminate excess copper accumulation (24).

Childhood Cirrhosis. Indian childhood cirrhosis, a hereditary disease accompanied by rapid copper accumulation in the liver, was fatal but now can be treated with chelators, with improved chances of recovery. A genetic defect is present, but high copper intake is required for symptoms to appear. The incidence of ICC in India has decreased markedly in recent years, but diseases mimicking ICC have appeared in other parts of the world (58).

EVALUATION OF COPPER STATUS

Biochemical Indices

Currently used indices of copper status easily detect severe copper deficiency. Serum copper and ceruloplasmin concentrations fall to levels far below the normal range and respond quickly to copper supplementation (30). Ceruloplasmin concentration has generally been considered the most reliable index of copper status (15), but some consider red cell superoxide dismutase activity equally or more sensitive (59). SOD values have not yet been reported in cases of severe copper deficiency in humans, and a level that would indicate copper deficiency has not been established. The normal ranges of these indices vary between laboratories but are approximately as follows: 10.0 to 24.6 μmol/L (64–156 μg/dL) for serum copper; 180 to 400 mg/L (18–40 mg/dL) for ceruloplasmin; and 0.47 ± 0.067 mg/g for erythrocyte SOD (15).

Although serum copper and ceruloplasmin levels clearly reflect severe deficiency, they may not be sensitive to marginal copper status. In addition, ceruloplasmin is an acute-phase reactant and, as a result, serum copper and ceruloplasmin levels are elevated in a variety of conditions. Serum copper and ceruloplasmin levels could be within the normal range or even elevated, masking copper deficiency when one of these conditions occurs at the same time.

The search for a reliable index of marginal copper status has been unsuccessful, though a number of possibilities have been suggested (30). Copper levels in hair, nails, or saliva do not appear to reflect copper status. Urinary copper varies greatly between individuals and declines only when dietary copper is very low (27). Cytochrome C oxidase in red cells, or possibly in platelets or white cells (45), may be sensitive to copper status, but more data are needed. A single index is not sufficient to assess copper nutriture. Other indices may potentially provide information on copper status, such as leukocyte copper content (34) and changes in lysyl oxidase activity (42).

Functional Tests

Most functional tests that might be of value in assessing copper status, such as assessment of immune function or antioxidant status, lack the necessary specificity to diagnose copper deficiency. However, in conjunction with the more established indices of copper status, they may be valuable. Stable isotope measurements of total body copper, the exchangeable copper pool size, or copper turnover may prove useful in evaluating copper status, but research in this area has just begun (60). Compartmental models of copper metabolism should aid in evaluating copper status (61).

REQUIREMENTS AND RECOMMENDED INTAKES

Laboratory Animals

The copper requirements of laboratory animals are influenced by other components of the diet, including those discussed under "Interactions." They differ between species as well. Approximately 6 μg Cu/g diet appears to be adequate for young animals of most species (3), including pigs, rats, and guinea pigs. This amount can be lower under optimal conditions and higher with confounding factors or for specific functions.

Humans

Copper depletion/repletion studies to establish the minimum requirements of healthy humans were not done until recently with a copper intake low enough to produce systematic reduction in copper status. Recent studies have been conducted under highly controlled and closely monitored conditions. Relatively few cases of frank copper deficiency have been reported, and these were accompanied by confounding factors, such as malnutrition, malabsorption, and excessive gastrointestinal losses, limiting their value in establishing a minimum requirement for healthy individuals.

The most relevant example of a long-term diet containing less than the minimum copper requirement may be the following: An enteral diet containing 15 μg Cu/100 kcal (0.56 pmol/J) produced copper deficiency in six of six severely handicapped patients between the ages of 4 and 24 years after they had consumed the diet for 12 to 66 months. Serum copper values of 1.8 to 7.2 μmol/L (11.7–45.7 μg/dL) and ceruloplasmin values of 30 to 125 mg/L (3–12.5 mg/dL) were discovered, accompanied by other manifestations of copper deficiency. These values increased to within the normal range after 3 months of copper supplementation (62). By extrapolation (though it may not be valid to extrapolate from these growing, severely handicapped individuals to healthy adults), copper deficiency could be expected to develop eventually if the diet contained 15 μg Cu/100 kcal, or 0.44 mg Cu/2900 kcal for men and 0.29 mg Cu/1900 kcal for women (0.56 pmol/J). The above example, combined with one study in which healthy young men maintained copper balance and status at 0.79 mg/day (12 μmol/day) (14) and another in which young men did not maintain status at 0.37 mg/day (6 μmol/day) (27), suggests that the minimum copper requirement of men is somewhere between 0.4 and 0.8 mg/day (6–12 μmol/day). An adult basal copper requirement within that range, 0.6 mg/day (9 μmol/day) for women and 0.7 mg/day (11 μmol/day) for men, was suggested by WHO (10).

The daily dietary copper intake recommended by the National Research Council of the United States is now 1.5 to 3 mg (24–47 μmol) for adults. Recommended daily ranges for children are 0.4 to 0.6 mg (6–9 μmol) for infants 0 to 6 months of age, increasing to 1.5 to 2.5 mg (24–39 μmol) for children over 11 years of age (5) (see also Appendix Tables II-A-2-a-3 and II-A-2-b). WHO (10) estimated the normative requirement for individuals, which includes a factor of safety to include additional increment for almost all dietary conditions, to be 0.7 mg/day (11 μmol/day) for women and 0.8 mg/day (12.5 μmol/day) for men. After adding margins of safety to the individual requirement to include all dietary conditions, variations in usual intakes, and individual variability, a recommendation of 1.25 mg/day (19 μmol/day) was derived.

CAUSES AND MANIFESTATIONS OF TOXICITY

Copper toxicity can occur in all animal species. It has been observed in sheep, cattle, pigs, rats, and poultry, as well as in humans. The effects of copper poisoning and the levels required for deleterious effects to develop have been reviewed (3).

Copper Toxicity in Animals

Tolerance to high levels of copper differs greatly from one species to another, with sheep being the most susceptible to copper poisoning and rats having high tolerance to excessive copper. Because of species differences and the effects of the levels of zinc, iron, and molybdenum in the diet, the minimum toxic copper level varies. Deleterious effects were observed in pigs at 250 μg Cu/g (4 μmol/g) diet but could be avoided by increasing dietary iron and zinc. Poultry exhibit slowed growth and egg production at 500 μg/g (8 μmol/g), and fatality can occur at 1200 μg/g (19 μmol/g). Sheep have developed copper toxicosis from diets containing 12 μg/g (0.19 μmol/g), and some breeds of sheep are more susceptible to excess copper than others. Copper chloride is more toxic than copper sulfate; lower levels of copper are toxic when the molybdenum content of the diet is low. Single doses of 20 to 100 mg (0.31–1.8 mmol) copper per kilogram body weight have been toxic. Cattle are susceptible to toxicity when diets contain 3 to 12 times the required level of copper.

Ruminants can store more copper in their livers than other animals, and symptoms of toxicity appear when the capacity of the liver to sequester copper has been exceeded. Manifestations of copper toxicity include weakness, tremors, anorexia, and jaundice. Tissue copper levels increase, producing liver, kidney, and brain damage, and hemolytic crisis may follow. The immune function of mice was impaired following supplements of 100 ppm of copper in the drinking water (63).

Copper Toxicity in Humans

Acute copper poisoning has been observed to occur in the following ways: accidental consumption by children, ingestion of several grams in suicide attempts, application of copper salts to burned skin, drinking water from contaminated water supplies, or consumption of acidic food or beverages that had been stored in copper containers. Excessive copper produces epigastric pain, nausea, vomiting, and diarrhea, which usually prevents the more serious manifestations of copper toxicity. Serious manifestations include coma, oliguria, hepatic necrosis, vascular collapse, and death. Chronic copper toxicosis has been observed in dialysis patients following months of hemodialysis when copper tubing was used and in vineyard workers using copper compounds as pesticides. The amount of oral copper required to produce toxic effects is not well established, but liver damage in two infants may have been related to consuming water with 2 to 3 mg Cu/L (31–47 μmol Cu/L) in early infancy (58). An extremely wide range of oral copper, beginning at 0.07 mg/kg (1.1 μmol/kg) per day, has been associated with gastrointestinal effects. Wilson's disease, a genetic disorder described above, and certain liver and biliary diseases are associated with accumulation of toxic levels of copper in the liver and other tissues, without excessive intake. Subtle deleterious effects of high dietary copper have been observed. LDL cholesterol increased when copper supplements were given to men (46). Copper has a critical role in neurologic diseases and there is speculation that copper-induced production of hydroxy radicals may contribute to the neurodegeneration in Alzheimer's disease (64). The WHO recommends intakes below 10 mg/day for women and 12 mg/day for men (10).

REFERENCES

1. Mason KE. J Nutr 1979;109:1979–2066.
2. Hart EB, Steenbock J, Waddell J, et al. J Biol Chem 1928;77: 797–812.
3. Davis GK, Mertz W. Copper. In: Mertz W, ed. Trace elements in human and animal nutrition, vol 1. 5th ed. San Diego: Academic Press, 1987;301–64.
4. Cordano A, Baerti JM, Graham GG. Pediatrics 1964; 34:324–36.
5. National Research Council. Recommended dietary allowances. 10th ed. Washington, DC: National Academy Press, 1989.
6. Owen CA Jr. Biochemical aspects of copper. Copper proteins, ceruloplasmin, and copper protein binding. Park Ridge, NJ: Noyes Publications, 1982.
7. Dyer FF, Leddicotte GW. The radiochemistry of copper. Washington, DC: National Academy of Sciences, National Research Council, 1961.
8. Weser U, Schubotz LM, Younes M. Chemistry of copper proteins and enzymes. In: Nriugu JO, ed. Copper and the environment. Part II, Health effects. New York: John Wiley & Sons, 1979;197–239.
9. Pennington JAT, Wilson DB. J Am Diet Assoc 1990;90:375–81.
10. World Health Organization. Copper. In: Trace elements in human nutrition and health. Geneva: World Health Organization, 1996;123–43.
11. Lurie DG, Holden JM, Schubert A, et al. J Food Comp Anal 1989;2:298–316.
12. Pennington JAT, Schoen SA, Salmon GD, et al. J Food Comp Anal 1995;8:171–217.
13. Pennington JT, Calloway DH. J Am Diet Assoc 1973;63:143–53.
14. Turnlund JR, Keyes WR, Anderson HL, et al. Am J Clin Nutr 1989;49:870–8.
15. Turnlund JR. J Am Diet Assoc 1988;88:303–10.
16. Gawthorne JM. Copper interactions. In: Howell JM, Gawthorne JM, eds. Copper in animals and man, vol 1. Boca Raton: CRC Press, 1987;79–100.
17. Luza SC, Speisky HC. Am J Clin Nutr 1996;63:812S–20S.
18. Kirchgessner M. Interactions of copper with other trace elements. In: Nriugu JO, ed. Copper and the environment. Part II. Health effects. New York: John Wiley & Sons, 1979;433–72.
19. Turnlund JR, Keyes WR, Anderson HL. High dietary copper decreases zinc absorption, as determined with the stable isotope ^{67}Zn. In: Momcilovic B, ed. Trace elements in man and animals. 7th ed. Zagreb, Yugoslavia: Institute for Medical Research and Occupational Health, University of Zagreb, 1991;5/13–15.
20. Powers HJ, Loban A, Silvers K, et al. Free Rad Res 1995;22:57–65.
21. Reiser S, Smith JC, Mertz W, et al. Am J Clin Nutr 1985;42: 242–51.
22. Schoenemann HM, Failla ML, Steele NC. Am J Clin Nutr 1990;52:147–54.
23. O'Dell BL. Nutr Rev 1990;48:425–34.
24. Brewer GJ, Yuzbasiyan-Gurkan V. Medicine 1992;71:139–64.
25. Cousins RJ. Physiol Rev 1985;65:238–309.
26. Linder MC. The biochemistry of copper. New York: Plenum Press, 1991.
27. Turnlund JR, Keyes WR, Peiffer GL. (Abstract) Am J Clin Nutr 1995;61:908.
28. Frieden E. Clin Physiol Biochem 1986;4:11–9.
29. Bremner I. J Nutr 1987;117:19–29.
30. Danks DM. Annu Rev Nutr 1988;8:235–57.
31. Harris ED, Percival SS. Copper transport: insights into a ceruloplasmin-based delivery system. In: Kies C, ed. Copper bioavailability and metabolism. New York: Plenum Press, 1990;95–102.
32. Bunce GE. Nutr Rev 1993;51:305–7.
33. Turnlund JR, Keen CL, Smith RG. Am J Clin Nutr 1990;51: 658–64.
34. Turnlund JR, Scott KC, Peiffer GL, et al. Am J Clin Nutr 1996, in press.
35. Levenson CW, Janghorbani M. Anal Biochem 1994;221:243–9.
36. Turnlund JR, Keyes WR, Peiffer GL. (Abstract) FASEB J 1995;9:A725.
37. Prohaska JR. J Nutr Biochem 1990;1:452–61.
38. McCracken J, Desai PR, Papadopoulos NJ, et al. Biochemistry 1988;27:4133–7.
39. Harris ED. J Nutr 1992;122:636–40.
40. Mann KG, Lawler CM, Vehar GA, et al. J Biol Chem 1984;259:12949–51.
41. Werman MJ, Barat E, Bhathena SJ. J Nutr 1995;125:857–63.

42. Werman MJ, Bhathena SJ, Turnlund JR. J Nutr Biochem 1997;8:201–4.
43. Williams DM. Semin Hematol 1983;20:118–27.
44. Medieros DM, Davidson J, Jenkins JE. Proc Soc Exp Biol Med 1993;203:262–73.
45. Milne DB. Clin Chem 1994;40:1479–84.
46. Medeiros DM, Milton A, Brunett E, et al. Biol Trace Element Res 1991;30:19–35.
47. Johnson MA, Fisher JG. Crit Rev Food Sci Nutr 1992;32:1–31.
48. Prohaska JR, Failla ML. Copper and immunity. In: Klurfeld DM, ed. Human nutrition—a comprehensive treatise. New York: Plenum Press, 1993;309–32.
49. Kelley DS, Daudu PA, Taylor PC, et al. Am J Clin Nutr 1995;62:412–6.
50. Fujita M, Itakura T, Takagi Y, et al. JPEN 1989;13:421–5.
51. Shaw JCL. Copper deficiency in term and preterm infants. In: Fomon SJ, Zlotkin S, eds. Nutritional anemias. New York: Vevey/Raven Press, 1992;105–17.
52. Percival SS, Bowser E, Wagner M. Am J Clin Nutr 1995;62: 633–8.
53. Fleming CR. Am J Clin Nutr 1989;49:573–9.
54. Smithgall JM. J Am Diet Assoc 1985;85:609–11.
55. McArdle HJ. Food Chemistry 1995;54:79–84.
56. Bankier A. J Med Genet 1995;32:213–5.
57. Anonymous. Case Record of the Massachusetts General Hospital (case 1-1997). N Engl J Med 1997;336:118–25.
58. Muller-Hocker J, Meyer U, Wiebecke B, et al. Pathol Res Pract 1988;183:39–45.
59. Uauy R, Castillo-Duran C, Fisberg M, et al. J Nutr 1985; 115:1650–5.
60. Turnlund JR. J Nutr 1989;119:7–14.
61. Scott KC, Turnlund JR. J Nutr Biochem 1994;5:342–50.
62. Higuchi S, Higashi A, Nakamura T, et al. J Pediatr Gastroenterol Nutr 1988;7:583–7.
63. Pocino M, Baute L, Malave I. Fundam Appl Toxicol 1991;16: 249–56.
64. Multhaup G, Schlicksupp L, Hesse L, et al. Science 1996;271: 1406–9.
65. International Union of Biochemistry. Enzyme nomenclature. Recommendations (1978) of the Nomenclature Committee of the International Union of Biochemistry. New York: Academic Press, 1979.

SELECTED READINGS

Davis GK, Mertz W. Copper. In: Mertz W, ed. Trace elements in human and animal nutrition, vol 1. San Diego: Academic Press, 1987;301–64.

Howell JM, Gawthorne JM, eds. Copper in animals and man, vols 1 and 2. Boca Raton, FL: CRC Press, 1987.

Kies C, ed. Copper bioavailability and metabolism. New York: Plenum Press, 1990.

Linder MC. The biochemistry of copper. New York: Plenum Press, 1990.

Mason KE. A conspectus of research on copper metabolism and requirements of man. J Nutr 1979;109:1979–2066.

World Health Organization. Copper, chap 7. In: Trace elements in human nutrition and health. Geneva: World Health Organization, 1996;123-43.

13. Iodine

BASIL S. HETZEL and GRAEME A. CLUGSTON

HISTORY

Iodine, with an atomic weight of 127 and a molecular weight of 254, is an essential constituent of the thyroid hormones thyroxine, 3,5,3′,5′-tetraiodothyronine (T_4), and 3,5,3′-triiodothyronine (T_3). The major role of iodine in nutrition arises from the importance of thyroid hormones to growth and development (1–5).

Iodine was discovered by Courtois in 1811 during the course of making gunpowder. Some seaweed ash was being used from which the iodine vaporized as a violet vapor. The element was discovered in the thyroid gland by Baumann in 1895.

The relation of iodine deficiency to enlargement of the thyroid gland, or goiter, was first shown by David Marine, who found that hyperplastic changes occurred regularly in the thyroid when the iodine concentration fell below 0.1% (3). Subsequently, Marine and Kimball in 1922 demonstrated in school children in Akron, Ohio, U.S.A., that endemic goiter could be both prevented and substantially reduced by administration of small amounts of iodine (5). Mass prophylaxis of goiter with iodized salt was first introduced in Switzerland and in Michigan, U.S.A. (5). In Switzerland, the widespread occurrence of a severe form of mental deficiency and deaf mutism (endemic cretinism) was a heavy charge on public funds. However, following the introduction of iodized salt in 1922, goiter incidence fell rapidly and new cretins were no longer born. Goiter also disappeared from Army recruits (5).

A further major development was administration of injections of iodized oil in Papua New Guinea for people living in inaccessible mountain villages. The successful prevention of goiter and subsequently cretinism was shown in controlled trials over the period 1959 to 1972 (1–5).

Major attention is now focused on the effects of iodine deficiency on brain development in the fetus and in infancy. Iodine deficiency is now accepted as the most common cause of preventable mental defect in the world today (6). More details on the historical aspects can be found in the reviews cited (1–5).

ECOLOGY OF IODINE DEFICIENCY

There is a cycle of iodine in nature. Most of the iodine resides in the ocean. It was present during the primordial development of the earth, but large amounts were leached from the surface soil by glaciation, snow, or rain and were carried by wind, rivers, and floods into the sea. Iodine occurs in the deeper layers of the soil and is found in oil well and natural gas effluents. Water from such deep wells can provide a major source for iodine. In general, the older an exposed soil surface, the more likely it is to be leached of iodine (1, 5).

The most likely areas to be leached are the mountainous areas of the world. The most severely deficient areas are those of the Himalayas, the Andes, the European Alps, and the vast mountains of China. But iodine deficiency is likely to occur in all elevated regions subject to glaciation and higher rainfall, with runoff into rivers. However, it also occurs in flooded river valleys such as the Ganges in India.

Iodine occurs in soil and the sea as iodide. Iodide ions are oxidized by sunlight to elemental iodine, which is volatile, so that every year some 400,000 tons of iodine escape from the surface of the sea. The concentration of iodide in sea water is about 50 to 60 μg/L and in air is approximately 0.7 $\mu g/m^2$. The iodine in the atmosphere is returned to the soil by rain, which has concentrations in the range 1.8 to 8.5 μg/L. In this way, the cycle is completed.

However, the return of iodine to the soil is slow and limited in amount compared with the original loss of iodine, and subsequent repeated flooding ensures continuation of iodine deficiency in the soil. Because no "natural correction" can take place, iodine deficiency persists in the soil indefinitely. All crops grown in these soils will be iodine deficient. As a result, human and animal populations that are totally dependent on food grown in such soil become iodine deficient. The iodine content of plants grown in iodine-deficient soils may be as low as 10 μg/kg dry weight, compared with 1 mg/kg dry weight in plants grown in an iodine-sufficient soil. This low content of soil iodine accounts for the occurrence of severe iodine deficiency in vast populations in Asia who are living within systems of subsistence agriculture in flooded river valleys (India, Bangladesh, Burma).

An indication of the iodine content of the soil can be given by the local drinking water concentration. In general, iodine-deficient areas have water iodine levels below 2 μg/L, as in Nepal and India (0.1–1.2 μg/L), compared with levels of 9.0 μg/L in the city of Delhi, which is not iodine deficient.

Iodine deficiency will persist unless a supplement is provided, or alternatively, diversification of the diet occurs, with increased iodine intake derived from food sources outside the iodine-deficient areas. This process has occurred progressively in Europe during the 19th century. However, substantial areas of iodine deficiency remain in some countries (Germany, Italy, and Spain) as well as more localized areas in others (see below).

In developing countries, the World Health Organization (WHO) (6) in 1990 estimated that 1 billion persons were at risk of iodine-deficiency disorders (IDD), of whom 211 million are suffering from goiter and more than 5 million are suffering from mental retardation as gross cretins, while three to five times this number suffer from lesser degrees of mental defect (Table 13.1). In 1993 the WHO increased the estimate of the population at risk to 1.6 billion (7).

PHYSIOLOGY OF IODINE DEFICIENCY

The healthy human adult body contains 15 to 20 mg of iodine, of which about 70 to 80% is in the thyroid gland (1, 2). The thyroid gland, which weighs only 15 to 25 g, possesses a remarkable concentrating power for iodine. The amount of iodine in the gland is closely related to the iodine intake. The content may be reduced to 1 mg or less in the iodine-deficient enlarged thyroid (goiter).

Iodine is rapidly absorbed through the gut. The normal

Table 13.1
Prevalence of Iodine Deficiency Disorders in Developing Countries and Numbers of Persons at Risk (in millions)

	At Risk	Goiter	Overt Cretinism
Africa	227	39	0.5
Latin America	60	30	0.3
Southeast Asia	280	100	4.0
Asia (other countries including China)	400	30	0.9
Eastern Mediterranean	33	12	—
Total	1000	211	5.7

From World Health Organization. Report to 43rd World Health Assembly, Geneva, 1990;1–17.

intake and requirement are 100 to 150 μg per day. Excess iodine is excreted by the kidney. The level of excretion correlates well with the level of intake, so it can be used to assess the level of iodine intake (see below).

Iodine exists in the thyroid as inorganic iodine, the iodine-containing amino acids (monoiodothyronine [MIT], diiodothyronine [DIT], triiodothyronine [T_3], and thyroxine [T_4]), polypeptides containing thyroxine, and thyroglobulin. Thyroglobulin, a protein that contains iodinated amino acids in a peptide linkage, is the chief constituent of the colloid that fills the thyroid follicle. It is a glycoprotein (contains glucose) with a molecular weight of 650,000. It is the storage form of the thyroid hormones and contains approximately 90% of the total iodine in the gland.

The thyroid must trap about 60 μg of iodine per day to maintain an adequate supply of thyroxine. This is accomplished by a very active iodide-trapping mechanism, which maintains a gradient of 100:1 between the thyroid cell and the extracellular fluid. In iodine deficiency, this gradient may exceed 400:1 to maintain the output of thyroxine.

This increased trapping of iodine in iodine deficiency can be well demonstrated with radioiodine. In the Argentinean Andes of South America, Stanbury and his colleagues first showed that urinary radioiodine excretion was inversely related to the severity of iodine deficiency (5). Concomitantly, the percentage retention of administered ^{131}I was directly related to the severity of iodine deficiency (5).

Iodide trapping by the thyroid depends on an active transport mechanism (i.e., requires energy) called the *iodine pump*. This mechanism is regulated by the thyroid-stimulating hormone (TSH), which is released from the pituitary to regulate thyroid secretion.

Other ions can compete with iodide, including thiocyanate (SCN^-). Thiocyanate is derived from the metabolism of hydrogen cyanide (HCN), which is found in foods such as cassava. Cassava is a dietary staple in Zaire and in many other countries. The occurrence of goiter and severe hypothyroidism in Zaire (1, 2) is associated with the use of cassava, particularly when it is not well cooked.

Iodide is released by the thyroid cells into the colloid follicle phase between the cells and there is oxidized by hydrogen peroxide from the thyroid peroxidase system (Fig. 13.1). It then combines with tyrosine in the thyroglobulin to form MIT and DIT. The oxidation process then continues with the coupling of MIT and DIT to form the iodotyrosines. This oxidation process can be readily blocked by various drugs, including propylthiouracil and carbimazole, which are widely used for the treatment of hyperthyroidism. There may also be a congenital defect in the formation of iodinated tyrosine; this is a cause of congenital goiter and hypothyroidism that may run in families. Such a defect does not, however, occur in iodine-deficient goiter; the reason why iodine deficiency causes goiter in some people and not in others ingesting the same diet is not known.

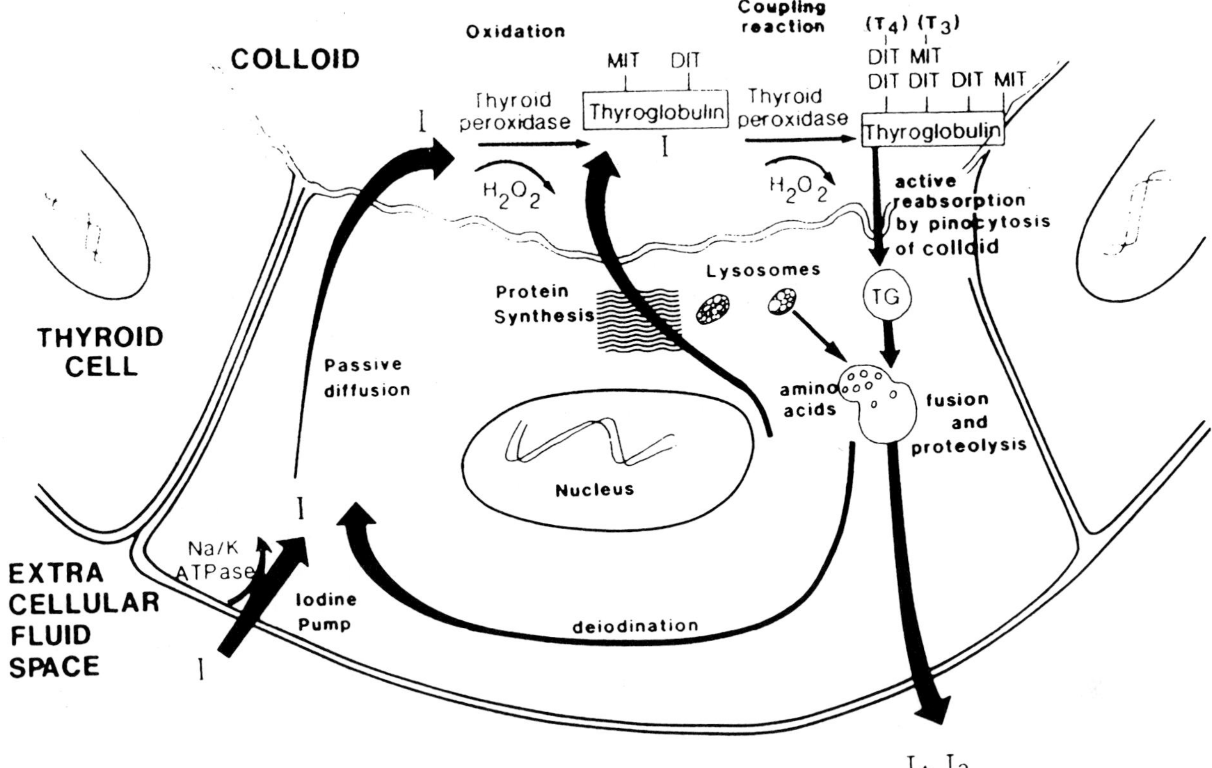

Figure 13.1. Diagram showing pathways of synthesis of thyroid hormones from iodine within the thyroid gland. (From Hetzel BS, Maberly GF. Iodine. In: Mertz W, ed. Trace elements in human and animal nutrition. 5th ed. New York: Academic Press 1986;2: 139–208.)

Finally, the iodinated thyroglobulin, including the iodinated amino acids, is absorbed back into the thyroid cells by pinocytosis. It is then exposed to proteolytic enzymes that break it down to release the T_4 and T_3 into the blood. The unused iodotyrosines are conserved for incorporation into a subsequent cycle of the biosynthetic process. With repeated thyroid stimulation, this reincorporation process may not be able to keep pace with the production of free iodotyrosines, which leak into the circulation but have no biologic effect.

The regulation of thyroid hormones is a complex process involving not only the thyroid, but also the pituitary, the brain, and the peripheral tissues. Secretion of T_3 and T_4 is under the control of the pituitary gland, through TSH. TSH is a glycoprotein with a molecular weight of approximately 28,000. There are two subunits: the X subunit has virtually the same structure as other pituitary hormones; the B subunit is specific for TSH but essentially the same across different species.

TSH secretion is controlled by a feedback mechanism closely related to the level of T_4 in the blood. As the blood T_4 falls, pituitary TSH secretion is increased to increase thyroid activity and the output of T_4 into the circulation, thus maintaining the necessary level of circulating hormone. If this is not possible because of severe iodine deficiency, then the level of T_4 remains lowered and the level of TSH rises. The critical factor in this control is the level of free T_4, the small fraction (less than 1%) not bound to the carrier protein.

The site of thyroid hormone action in regulating metabolic events is the nucleus, where binding of T_3 to a nuclear receptor (TR) initiates a cascade of changes in gene transcription rates (or messenger RNA stability), which eventuate in the phenotypic expression of thyroid hormone effects. When thyroid hormone enters the cell, it is rapidly bound to proteins in the cytosol but also rapidly enters the nuclear compartment. Within the cell, approximately 10% of the T_3 is in the nuclear compartment, for all tissues except anterior pituitary. In this tissue, the balance between mechanisms leading to nuclear T_3 accumulation and the concentration and affinity of the cytosolic binding proteins are such that roughly equal fractions of T_3 are found in the nuclear and extranuclear compartments.

Both tracer equilibrium and direct radioimmunoassay studies have demonstrated that in most tissues (e.g., the liver, kidney, and heart) receptors are approximately 50% occupied at physiologic plasma T_3 concentrations. There are exceptions; brain and pituitary nuclei have a higher degree of occupancy (80 to 90%) because of the T_3 produced locally from cellular T_4 by the type-2 deiodinase.

These predictions were verified by direct radioimmunoassay of brain cytosol. The free cytosolic T_3 concentrations were approximately 40 pM, three to four times that in the liver, kidney, and heart. That this increment in T_3 over that present in plasma was derived from local T_4 to T_3 conversion was established by showing that the concentration ratio of isotopic T_3 between cytosol and plasma was 1:1. Thus, these results independently verify the significant contribution of locally produced hormone to the nuclear T_3 in the central nervous system. A similar verification has been performed for pituitary tissue using direct radioimmunoassay of nuclear T_3. More detailed descriptions of the biochemistry of thyroid hormones can be found elsewhere (8).

Blood thyroid hormones and TSH are determined with radioimmunoassay (RIA). In RIA, known amounts of radioactively labeled hormones compete with the unknown amount of hormone in the blood in binding to a specific antibody. The technology for these determinations is still advancing.

Typical normal ranges of values for thyroid-related components of blood are shown in Table 13.2. The values given for TSH were obtained by the enzyme-linked immunoabsorbent (ELISA) assay (8).

DEVELOPMENT OF GOITER

The preceding discussion on the production and regulation of thyroid hormones provides the framework for understanding the development of goiter as a result of iodine deficiency. Iodine deficiency is the primary, although not sole, cause of goiter. Goitrogens, such as thiocyanates that can enhance the effect of iodine deficiency, are referred to as secondary factors (1, 2).

Iodine deficiency interferes with the production of thyroid hormones, T_4 and T_3 molecules. Lower hormone output from the thyroid leads to a fall in the blood levels of T_4 but some increase in T_3 (the less iodinated hormone is produced preferentially in iodine deficiency).

The fall in the level of T_4 leads to increased TSH output from the pituitary. TSH increases the uptake of iodide by the thyroid, with increased turnover of iodine associated with hyperplasia of the cells of the thyroid follicles. Because reserves of colloid-containing thyroglobulin are gradually used up, the gland appears more cellular than usual. The size of the gland increases, with formation of a goiter. Enlargement is regarded as significant in the human when the lateral lobes are larger than the terminal phalanx of the thumb of the person examined. More precise measurements can now be made by ultrasound (4).

Extensive reviews of the global geographic prevalence of goiter have been published (1–4).

Table 13.2
Normal Ranges of Thyroid-Related Components in Plasma and Blood

Test Factor	Standard Units	SI Units	Conversion
T_4	5–12 μg/mL	64–154 nmol/L	12.87
T_3	80–190 ng/dL	1.2–2.9 nmol/L	0.01536
Free T_4	0.8–2.0 ng/dL	10–26 pmol/L	12.87
Free T_3	2.6–5.2 pg/mL	4.0–8.0 pmol/L	0.01536
TSH[a]	0.17–2.9 μU/mL	0.17–2.9 mU/L	1

Modified from DeGroot LJ, Larsen PR, Henneman G. The thyroid and its diseases. 6th ed. New York: Churchill Livingstone, 1996;1–793.

[a]ELISA method (see text).

IODINE DEFICIENCY DISORDERS

The effects of iodine deficiency on growth and development are now denoted by the term *iodine deficiency disorders.* These effects are evident at all developmental stages but are particularly acute in the fetus, neonate, and infant, in the periods of rapid growth. The term *goiter* has been used for many years to describe the effect of iodine deficiency, and goiter is indeed the most obvious and familiar feature of iodine deficiency. Because knowledge has greatly expanded in the last 25 years about the wide spectrum of effects of iodine on growth and development, particularly on brain development (Table 13.3) (3–5), it is not surprising that a new term, *IDD,* has been coined.

The Fetus

Iodine deficiency in the fetus results from iodine deficiency in the mother. The condition is associated with a greater incidence of stillbirths, abortions, and congenital abnormalities, which can be reduced by provision of

Table 13.3
The Spectrum of Iodine Deficiency Disorders (IDD)

Fetus	Abortions Stillbirths Congenital anomalies Increased perinatal mortality Increased infant mortality Neurologic cretinism (mental deficiency, deaf mutism, spastic diplegia, squint) Hypothyroid cretinism (dwarfism, mental deficiency) Psychomotor defects Increased susceptibility of the thyroid gland to nuclear radiation (after 12 weeks)
Neonate	Neonatal goiter Neonatal hypothyroidism Increased susceptibility of the thyroid gland to nuclear radiation
Child and adolescent	Goiter Juvenile hypothyroidism Impaired mental function Retarded physical development Increased susceptibility of the thyroid gland to nuclear radiation
Adult	Goiter with its complications Hypothyroidism Impaired mental function Iodine-induced hyperthyroidism Increased susceptibility of the thyroid gland to nuclear radiation

Modified from Hetzel BS, Potter BJ, Dulberg EM. World Rev Nutr Diet 1990;62:59–119.

iodine. Many of the effects are similar to those observed with maternal hypothyroidism and can be reduced by thyroid hormone replacement therapy (9), which provides both hormone and iodine to mother and fetus.

Another major effect of fetal iodine deficiency is endemic cretinism. This condition occurs when iodine intake is below 25 μg/day (normal intake is 100–150 μg/day) and is still widely prevalent, affecting up to 10% of those living in severely iodine-deficient areas in India, Indonesia, and China as well as elsewhere (10). In its most common form, it is characterized by mental deficiency, deaf mutism, and spastic diplegia and is referred to as the "nervous" or neurologic-type cretin. The less common "myxedematous" type is characterized as hypothyroidism with dwarfism (Fig. 13.2).

Cretinism also occurs in Africa and in the Andean region (Ecuador, Peru, and Bolivia) of South America. In all these locations, with the exception of Zaire, neurologic features predominate. In Zaire, the myxedematous form is more common, probably because of the high intake of cassava (manioc or tapioca) (11). Clinically, neurologic cretinism varies considerably, including isolated deaf mutism and mental defects of varying degrees. The common neurologic form of endemic cretinism is not usually associated with severe clinical hypothyroidism, as is myxedematous cretinism, although mixed forms with both neurologic and myxedematous features do occur. Furthermore, the neurologic features are not reversed by administration of thyroid hormones (12).

Although isolated instances of cretinism can still be found, the apparent spontaneous disappearance of classic endemic cretinism in most of southern Europe during the 19th and early 20th centuries raised considerable doubt about the relation of iodine deficiency to the condition (5). To determine whether iodine deficiency and cretinism were related, a controlled trial was conducted in the western highlands of Papua New Guinea to see whether endemic cretinism could be prevented by correcting iodine deficiency with injection of iodized oil, then recently available (13). Injection of iodized oil before pregnancy prevented the occurrence of the neurologic syndrome of endemic cretinism in the infant (Fig. 13.3). The syndrome occurred in infants of women known to be pregnant at the time of oil injection, indicating that the damage probably occurred during the first half of pregnancy (14). This controlled trial also revealed a significant reduction in recorded fetal and neonatal deaths in the treated group (Table 13.4), which is consistent with other

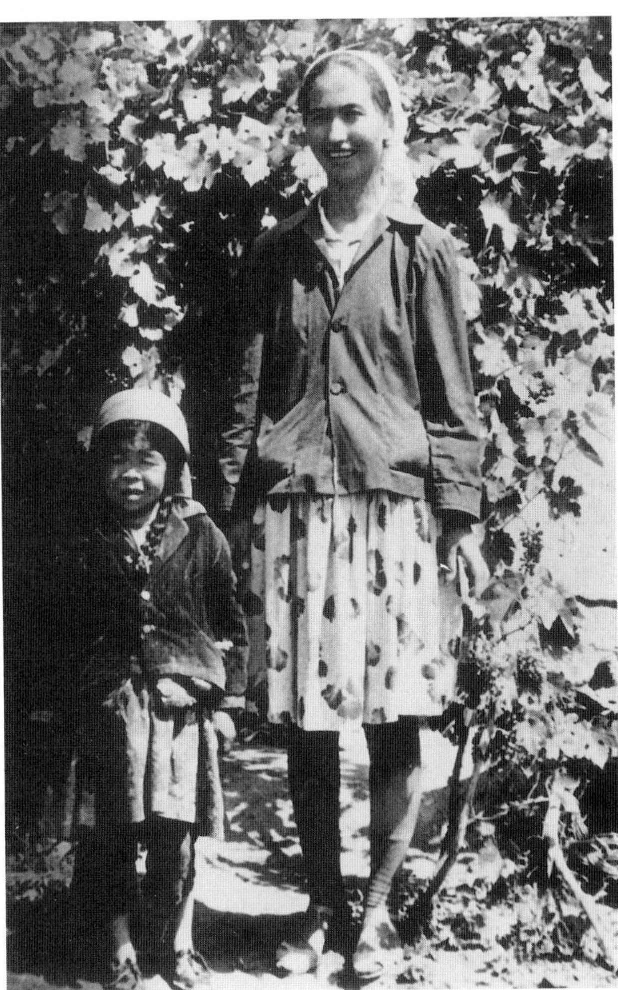

Figure 13.2. *Left,* A myxoedematous cretin from Sinjiang, China, who is also deaf mute. This condition is completely preventable. *Right,* the barefoot doctor of her village. Both are about 35 years of age. (From Hetzel BS. The story of iodine deficiency—an international challenge in nutrition. Oxford: Oxford University Press, 1989;1–236; with permission of Dr. T Ma of Tianjin, China.)

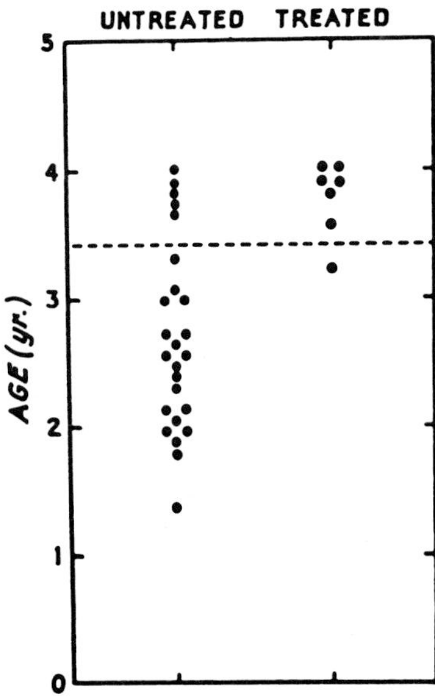

Figure 13.3. Results of a controlled trial of iodized oil injection in the Jimi River district of the highlands of Papua New Guinea. Alternate mothers were given a single injection of iodized oil or saline in September 1966. All newborn children were followed up for the next 5 years. Each dot represents a cretin child. The figure shows that by comparison with their persistence in the untreated group, mothers given iodized oil injections do not have subsequent cretin children, except for those known to be pregnant at the time of injection. (From Pharoah POD, Buttfield IH, Hetzel BS. Lancet 1971;1:308–10; with permission from Pharoah et al. 1971.)

Table 13.4
Controlled Trials of Iodized Oil in Iodine-Deficient Pregnant Women

Location	Characteristic	Untreated	Treated
Papua New Guinea	Total no. of children	406	412
	Normal	380	405
	Stillborn	97	66[a]
	Cretins	26	7[a,b]
Zaire[c]		2634	2837[a]
Birth-weight (g)	Perinatal mortality/1000	188	98[a]
	Infant mortality/1000	250	167[a]
	Development quotient	104	115[a]

Zaire data from Thilly CH. Bull Acad Med Belg 1981;136:389–412. Papua New Guinea data from Pharoah POD, Buttfield IH, Hetzel BS. Lancet 1971;1:308–10.
[a] $P < 0.05$ or more.
[b] At least six of the seven mothers were pregnant when treated.
[c] Data from Zaire were made on a variable number (66–263) of children in each group.

evidence indicating that iodine deficiency affects fetal survival (14). In a recent study in China, administration of iodine to iodine-deficient pregnant women up to the end of the second trimester protected the fetal brain from the effects of iodine deficiency. Treatment later in pregnancy or after delivery may improve brain growth and developmental achievement slightly but does not improve neurologic status (15).

A relationship between the level of maternal thyroxine and the outcome of current and recent past pregnancies, including mortality and the occurrence of cretinism was also found in Papua New Guinea. There were proportionally more perinatal (i.e., stillbirths and neonatal) deaths and cretins among the offspring of women with the lowest levels of serum thyroxine (16).

The demonstrated importance of maternal thyroid function to fetal survival and development is complemented by more recent studies. Studies in experimental animal models and, more recently, in man (17) indicate that maternal thyroxine is transferred to the fetus early in pregnancy. It would seem likely, therefore, that the effects of iodine deficiency on the fetus are mediated by reduced transfer of maternal thyroxine before the onset of fetal thyroid function and are not solely due to fetal deficiency of elemental iodine as originally suggested because of the lack of evidence of transfer of T_4 at that time (14).

The earlier "spontaneous" disappearance of endemic cretinism in Europe is now attributed to increased dietary iodine from dietary diversification and use of iodine supplements associated with economic development (18).

The Neonate

Increased perinatal mortality due to iodine deficiency has been shown in Zaire in a controlled trial of iodized oil injections alternated with a placebo injection given in the latter half of pregnancy (19). Following the iodized oil injection, infant mortality fell substantially, with improved birth weights (Table 13.4). Low birth weight of any cause is generally associated with a higher rate of congenital anomalies and a higher risk through childhood. This has been demonstrated by long-term follow-up of the controlled trial in Papua New Guinea, in children up to the age of 12 years (20).

Apart from mortality, the state of thyroid function in the neonate is important because the brain of the human infant at birth is only about one-half its full size and continues to grow rapidly until the end of the second year (21). Thyroid hormone, which depends on an adequate supply of iodine, is essential for normal brain development, as is confirmed by the animal studies cited above. Severe iodine deficiency that affects neonatal thyroid function and hence poses a threat to early brain development is still found in Europe (22). A series of 1076 urine samples was collected and analyzed in 16 centers from 10 different countries in Europe along with an additional series from Toronto, Canada (22). Because the distribution of urinary iodine is skewed, results were expressed in percentiles rather than as arithmetic means. Some very high values of urinary iodine were seen, which could be attributed to the use of iodinated contrast media for radiologic investigation of the mother during pregnancy. There was a marked difference in the results from the various European cities. The high levels of urinary iodine excretion in Rotterdam, Helsinki, and Stockholm differed from the low levels in Gottingen, Heidelberg, Freiburg, and Jena by a factor of more than 10. Intermediate levels were seen in Catania, Zurich, and Lille.

Data on neonatal thyroid function were analyzed for four European cities where data were available from enough newborns (30,000–102,000) to test the incidence of permanent congenital hypothyroidism (approximately 1/3500 in the absence of iodine deficiency) (22). The incidence of permanent congenital hypothyroidism was very similar in the four cities, but the rate of transient hypothyroidism was much higher in Freiburg (associated with the lowest level of urinary iodine excretion) than in Stockholm, with intermediate findings from Rome and Brussels. These data confirm the significance of iodine intake for neonatal thyroid function and therefore brain development.

In developing countries with more severe iodine deficiency, observations were made on blood taken from the umbilical vein just after birth. Neonatal chemical hypothyroidism was defined as a T_4 level below 3 μg/dL and a TSH value above 50 mU/L (23). In the most severely iodine deficient environments in northern India, where more than 50% of the population shows urinary iodine levels below 25 μg/g creatinine, the incidence of neonatal hypothyroidism was 75 to 115 per thousand births (23). By contrast, in Delhi, where only mild iodine deficiency is present with low prevalence of goiter and no cretinism, the incidence drops to six per thousand. In control areas without goiter, the level was only one per thousand.

In Zaire, the rate of chemical hypothyroidism among neonates is 10% (24). If the deficiency is not corrected, hypothyroidism persists into infancy and childhood with resultant retardation of physical and mental development (25). These observations indicate that a much greater risk of mental defect exists in severely iodine-deficient populations than is indicated by the presence of cretinism. They provide strong evidence for the need to correct the iodine deficiency in Europe as well as in developing countries.

Another important aspect of iodine deficiency in the neonate and child is an increased susceptibility of the thyroid gland to radioactive fallout. Delange (26) showed that thyroidal uptake of radioiodine reaches its maximum value in the earliest years of life and then declines progressively into adult life. The apparent thyroidal iodine turnover rate was much higher in young infants than in adults and decreased progressively with age. To provide the normal rate of T_4 secretion, Delange estimated that the turnover rate for intrathyroidal iodine must be 25 to 30 times higher in young infants than in adolescents and adults. In iodine deficiency, a further increase in turnover rate is required to maintain normal thyroid hormone levels. This is the reason for the greatly increased susceptibility of the neonate and fetus to iodine deficiency. Iodine deficiency also causes increased uptake of radioiodide resulting from exposure to nuclear radiation, as occurred in the Chernobyl disaster. Protection against this increased uptake can only be provided by correction of iodine deficiency, a further strong indicator for correction of iodine deficiency in Europe as well as in developing countries in view of the possibility of a recurrence of the Chernobyl disaster from other, similar power plants in Eastern Europe and Asia.

The Child

Iodine deficiency in children is characteristically associated with goiter. The classification of goiter, which has been standardized by the WHO, is discussed below. The goiter rate increases with age and reaches a maximum in adolescence. Girls have a higher prevalence than boys. Goiter rates in school children from 8 to 14 years of age provide a convenient indication of the presence of iodine deficiency in a community.

School children living in iodine-deficient areas from a number of countries show lower school performance and IQs than matched groups from iodine-sufficient areas. These studies are difficult to do because of the problem of the control group. The many possible causes for impaired performance in school and on IQ tests make interpretation of any observed differences difficult. Compared with the iodine-sufficient area, the iodine-deficient area is likely to be more remote and to have poorer school facilities. Its inhabitants usually suffer more social deprivation, have a lower socioeconomic status, and are in a poorer nutritional state. All such factors must be taken into account in evaluating the effects of iodine deficiency in addition to the problem of adapting tests developed in Western countries for use in Third World countries. In a metaanalysis of 18 studies in which comparisons were made between iodine-deficient and normal children, mean scores differed by 13.5 IQ points, which is highly significant ($P < .00001$) (27, 28).

The Adult

Iodine administration in the form of iodized salt, iodized bread, or iodized oil, is effective in the prevention of goiter in adults. Iodine administration may also reduce existing goiter in adults. This is particularly true of iodized oil injections (1, 4, 5), and this obvious effect leads to ready acceptance of the measure by people living in iodine-deficient communities. A rise in circulating thyroxine can be readily demonstrated in adult subjects following iodization by various means.

A more subtle effect in the adult is cerebral hypothyroidism (28) that is manifested by slow responses and by slow reaction times. Because the brain is especially sensitive to hypothyroidism, impaired brain function occurs before the functions of other organs are demonstrably affected. Recent advances in thyroid physiology and biochemistry explain this clinical observation. The major determinant of brain (and pituitary) T_3 is serum T_4, not serum T_3 (as is true of the liver, kidney, and muscle) (29). Low levels of brain T_3 have been demonstrated in iodine-deficient rats in association with reduced levels of serum T_4 and have been restored to normal with correction of iodine deficiency (30). These findings explain suboptimal brain function in subjects with endemic goiter and lowered serum T_4 levels and its improvement following correction of iodine deficiency.

In northern India, a high degree of apathy has been noted in populations living in iodine-deficient areas. This deficiency may even affect domestic animals such as dogs! This reduced mental function is due to cerebral hypothyroidism. Elimination of the iodine deficiency in these communities reverses the cerebral hypothyroidism and improves the capacity for initiative and decision making. Iodine deficiency is a major block to human and social development in communities in an iodine-deficient environment. Correction of the iodine deficiency makes a major contribution to development and also reduces susceptibility to nuclear radiation.

EFFECTS OF IODINE DEFICIENCY IN ANIMALS

Naturally occurring iodine deficiency in farm animals causes reproductive failure and thyroid insufficiency (31). In iodine-deficient areas, fetal development is retarded or arrested in gestation, resulting in early death or resorption, abortion, stillbirth, or birth of weak, hairless offspring associated with prolonged gestation and parturition and retention of placental membranes. Subnormal thyroid hormone levels in herds of cattle have been accompanied by a high incidence of aborted, stillborn, and weak calves (31).

In recent experimental work with animal models (3, 21, 31, 32), severe iodine deficiency has been established prior to and during pregnancy. Iodine deficiency in sheep (5–8 μg iodine per day for sheep weighing 40 kg) is associated with increased incidence of abortions and stillbirths. At the end of pregnancy, the fetus shows reduced body weight, complete absence of wool growth, deformation of the skull, and retarded bone development. Retarded brain development is indicated by reduced brain weight and a reduced number of cells (as measured by DNA) (Fig. 13.4). Similar effects have been observed in the marmoset monkey (0.3 μg iodine per day for 340 g body weight).

These data indicate that the effects of severe iodine deficiency on fetal development involve a combination of maternal and fetal hypothyroidism, with the effect of maternal hypothyroidism preceding the onset of fetal thyroid secretion. This implies an effect on neuroblast multiplication, which occurs from 40 to 80 days of gestation in the sheep and 11 to 18 weeks in the human (3, 21, 32, 33). In the rat (a postnatal brain developer in which neuroblast multiplication occurs in the last one-third of fetal life), maternal hypothyroidism early in pregnancy results in reduced weight and number of embryos, reduced brain weight, and reduced transfer of maternal T_4 to the fetus (3, 32). The findings indicate that iodine deficiency has an early effect on neuroblast multiplication; this could be important in the pathogenesis of the neurologic form of endemic cretinism (3, 32, 33).

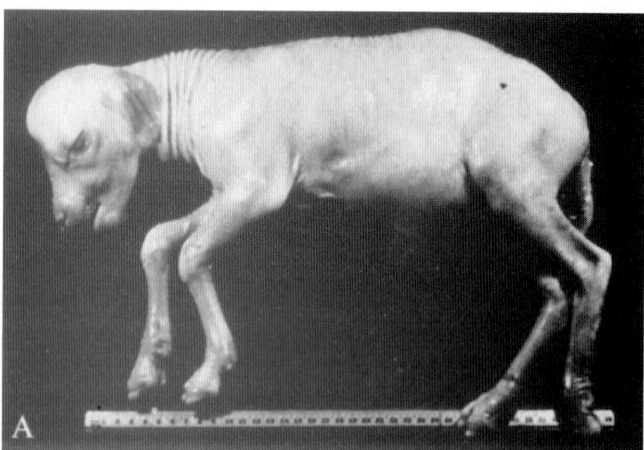

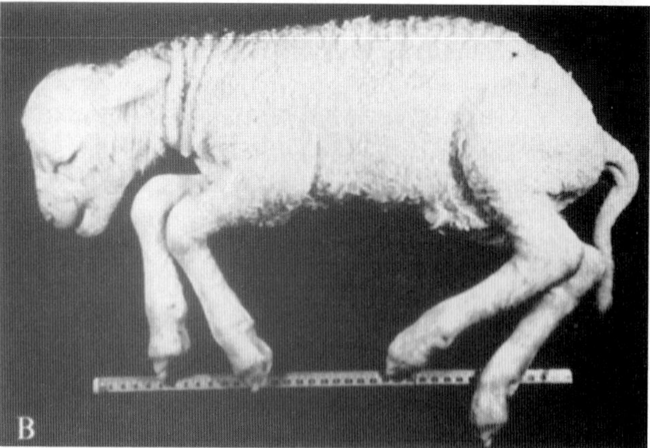

Figure 13.4. Effect of severe iodine deficiency during pregnancy on lamb development. **A.** A 140-day-old lamb fetus was subjected to severe iodine deficiency by feeding the mother an iodine-deficient diet (5–8 μg/day) for 6 months prior to and during pregnancy (full-term, 150 days). **B.** A control lamb of the same age fed the same diet with addition of an iodine supplement. The iodine-deficient lamb showed absence of wool coat, subluxation of the leg joints, and a domelike head caused by skeletal retardation and a smaller brain. (From Hetzel BS. The story of iodine deficiency—an international challenge in nutrition. Oxford: Oxford University Press, 1989;1–236.)

ASSESSMENT OF IODINE STATUS

The assessment of iodine status is important for public health programs that carry out iodine supplementation. The problem is therefore one of assessing a population or group living in an area suspected of being iodine deficient. The methods recommended are discussed below.

Goiter Rate

The goiter rate includes the rate of both palpable and visible goiter. A classification of goiter severity has recently been adopted by the WHO (Table 13.5), but there are still minor differences in technique between different observers. In general, visible goiter is more readily verified than palpable goiter. Observations in Tanzania (4) indicate that palpation of the thyroid generally overestimates the size of the gland as determined by ultrasonography, particularly in children. Determination of thyroid size by ultrasonography has now become standardized and, because it is an objective measure, is preferred when this technology is available (34).

Urinary Iodine Excretion

Urinary iodine determinations can be carried out on casual samples from a group of subjects, with iodine levels expressed as μg/L. Because the distribution is skewed, the median level is used for quick reference. Urinary iodine excretion is a good index of the level of iodine nutrition.

Table 13.5
Proposed Classification of Goiter

Grade 0	No palpable or visible goiter
Grade 1	A mass in the neck that is consistent with an enlarged thyroid that is palpable but not visible when the neck is in the normal position; it moves upward in the neck as the subject swallows; nodular alteration(s) can occur even when the thyroid is not enlarged
Grade 2	A swelling in the neck that is visible when the neck is in a normal position and is consistent with an enlarged thyroid when the neck is palpated

From Joint WHO/UNICEF/ICCIDD Consultation—Indicators for assessing iodine deficiency disorders and their control through salt iodization. Geneva: World Health Organization, 1994.

Recently simplified methods now allow processing of many more samples in a given period (35).

The range of levels include <20 μg/L (severe IDD), 20–49 μg/L (moderate IDD), and 50–99 μg/L (mild IDD). Values between 100 and 200 μg/L are considered satisfactory. Excessive iodine intake can also be most conveniently monitored by determination of urinary iodine excretion. The median level should not exceed 20 μg/dL in an iodine-deficient population following salt iodization programs.

Blood Thyroid-Stimulating Hormone

Particular attention is now focused on levels of TSH in neonatal blood because of the important influence of thyroid function on early brain development. Determination of the TSH level provides an indirect measure of iodine status. The availability of radioimmunoassay and immunometric methods with automated equipment enables large numbers of samples to be processed in a given period, and TSH determinations are now preferred to T_4 because of better stability under tropical conditions and easier methodology. The mean normal levels with the ELISA assay are given in Table 13.2.

In an increasing number of developed countries, mass screening is currently conducted with heel-prick blood samples from neonates (3–4 days after birth), which are spotted onto filter paper, dried, and sent to a regional laboratory. Blood levels of T_4, TSH, or both are measured by immunoassay techniques. As mentioned, the detection rate of neonatal hypothyroidism requiring treatment is about 1 per 3500 babies screened and varies little among developed countries (36).

In developing countries, severe biochemical hypothyroidism (T_4 concentrations <3 μg/dL) has been reported in up to 10% of neonates (36) in northern India and in Zaire (4). These data indicate the massive threat to brain development posed by severe iodine deficiency.

To summarize, iodine status is best determined initially by measuring urinary iodine excretion. Then, thyroid size and blood TSH in the neonate should be measured. The criteria adopted for monitoring progress toward the elimination of IDD as a public health problem are discussed below.

IODINE REQUIREMENTS

In 1989, the Food and Nutrition Board of the U.S. National Academy of Sciences, National Research Council, confirmed the previous 1980 recommendations for a daily iodine intake of 40 μg for children aged 0 to 6 months, 50 μg from 6 to 12 months, 70 to 120 μg from 1 to 10 years, and 120 to 150 μg from 11 years onward. The recommended rates during pregnancy and lactation were, respectively, 175 and 200 μg. The recommendations applied equally to both sexes (37) (See also Appendix Table II-A-2-a-2).

Participants in a series of recent WHO/ICCIDD (International Council for the Control of Iodine Deficiency Disorders) meetings suggested that requirements for infants and for pregnant and lactating women be increased. Their counsel has influenced the recent recommendations of the WHO (1996) (Table 13.6) (38).

IODINE TOXICITY

Iodine toxicity has been critically studied in man, laboratory species, poultry, pigs, and cattle. Wolff (39) has suggested that human intakes of 2000 μg I/day should be regarded as excessive or potentially harmful. Normal diets composed of natural foods are unlikely to supply 2000 μg I/day, and most would supply less than 1000 μg I/day, except those exceptionally high in marine fish or seaweed or containing foods contaminated with iodine from adventitious sources.

Inhabitants of the coastal regions of Hokkaido, the northernmost island of Japan, whose diets contain large amounts of seaweed, have remarkably high intakes of 50,000 to 80,000 μg I/day (40). Urinary excretion in five patients exhibiting clinical signs of iodide goiter exceeded 20 mg I/day, about 100 times the normal intake.

In Japan (41) it has been shown that

1. Healthy subjects can maintain normal thyroid function even when they are taking several milligrams/day of dietary iodine
2. High dietary iodine levels markedly decrease the incidence of nontoxic diffuse goiter and toxic nodular goiter
3. High dietary iodine levels do not affect the incidence of Graves' disease and Hashimoto's disease
4. High dietary iodine may induce hypothyroidism in autoimmune thyroid diseases and may inhibit the effects of thionamide drugs

Significant species differences exist in tolerance to high iodine intakes. In all well-nourished species studied, the tolerance is high (i.e., relative to normal dietary iodine intakes, a wide margin of safety exists for this element). The same tolerance does not apply to iodine-deficient populations.

Iodine-Induced Hyperthyroidism (IIH)

An increased incidence of hyperthyroidism has been described since introduction of iodized salt programs in Europe and South America and following the use of iodized bread in Holland and Tasmania (42, 43). A few cases were noted following administration of iodized oil in South America. The condition is easily overlooked in developing countries because the population is scattered and there are limited opportunities for observation (44).

Table 13.6
Recommended Intakes of Iodine (Population Requirements)

Age Range or State	Intake (μg/day)
0–12 months	50
1–6 years	90
7–12 years	120
12 years to (and through) adulthood	150
Pregnancy	200
Lactation	200

From Trace elements in human nutrition and health. Geneva: World Health Organization, 1996.

Natural remission occurs. The condition is largely confined to those over 40 years of age, and a smaller proportion of the population in developing countries is affected than in developed countries. Detailed observations are available from the island of Tasmania (43, 45) and, more recently, from Zimbabwe (46).

In Zimbabwe, careful investigation revealed the occurrence of IIH from excessive levels of iodine in the salt that resulted from faulty mixing at the factory. Thus, suitable monitoring procedures for salt iodization and urinary iodine excretion are essential to prevent excessive iodine intake and IIH. Monitoring is also essential to ensure an adequate intake that corrects iodine deficiency, which has been a greater problem than iodine excess in Asia and Latin America.

Joseph et al. (47) reported that daily iodine intakes below 0.10 mg pose no risk for patients with autonomous thyroids due to iodine deficiency but that critical daily intakes are probably between 0.10 and 0.20 mg (47). Iodization of bread in Tasmania resulted in hyperthyroidism for some individuals at iodine intakes of about 0.20 mg/day (43, 45). The use of iodized bread in Holland, which contributed an additional 0.12 to 0.16 mg of iodine per day, increased the incidence of hyperthyroidism. The spring-summer peak of thyrotoxicosis (related to winter milk) in England occurred with average daily iodine intakes of 0.24 mg for women and 0.32 mg for men (48). The lack of iodine deficiency in the Japanese population accounts for the absence of IIH (41).

IIH is accompanied by some morbidity and mortality in older age groups. It is readily controlled with antithyroid drugs or radioiodine. Spontaneous remission also occurs. Risk of hyperthyroidism (1, 2, 4), even with an increase to normal levels of intake, arises because an autonomous thyroid can develop independence from TSH control and continue its high rate of secretion despite increased iodine intake. To minimize IIH, the medium urinary iodine level should not exceed 20 μg/dL. Adequate facilities for diagnosis and treatment are also required.

The occurrence of IIH with consequent morbidity and mortality is not regarded as a contraindication to iodization programs in view of the enormous benefits that correction of iodine deficiency has for the whole population, particularly reduced child mortality, improved child learning, improved health of women, greater economic productivity, and improved quality of life (Table 13.4). Furthermore, correction of iodine deficiency prevents formation of an autonomous thyroid and thereby minimizes IIH. Hence, IIH is included as an "iodine deficiency disorder" (Table 13.3).

CORRECTION OF IODINE DEFICIENCY

Iodized Salt

Iodized salt has been the major method of correcting iodine deficiency since the 1920s, when it was first successfully used in Switzerland (1, 4, 5). Since then, many successful programs have been reported, including those in the U.S., Central and South America (e.g., Guatemala, Colombia), Finland, China, and Taiwan (5).

The difficulties in production, maintenance of quality, and consumption of iodized salt for the millions who are iodine-deficient, especially in Asia, were vividly demonstrated in India, where there was a breakdown in supply. These difficulties led to adoption of a universal salt iodization (USI) policy for India and many other countries. This policy requires access to iodized salt for 80% of the population. It has been promoted by WHO and UNICEF since 1993 to ensure that only iodized salt is available for human and animal consumption. In Asia, iodized salt production and distribution at present costs approximately 3 to 5 cents per person per year (4), which must be considered cheap in relation to the social benefits that accrue, as described above.

However, the problem still exists of ensuring that the salt actually reaches the iodine-deficient subject. There may also be a problem with distribution or with preservation of the iodine content (e.g., it may be left uncovered for long periods or exposed to heat). Salt should be added after cooking, to reduce the loss of iodine. Present recommendations for salt iodine content are in the range of 20 to 40 mg/kg (48a).

Finally, there is the difficulty of ensuring the actual consumption of iodized salt. While addition of iodine makes no difference to the taste of the salt, introduction of a new variety of salt to an area in which brands of noniodized salt are already available and much appreciated as a condiment is likely to be resisted. In the Chinese provinces of Sinjiang and Inner Mongolia, for example, the strong preference of the people for desert salt of very low iodine content led to a program of mass iodized oil injection to prevent cretinism rather than introduction of competing brands of salt (49).

Iodized Oil by Injection

The value of iodized oil injection in the prevention of endemic goiter and endemic cretinism was first established in New Guinea with controlled trials involving the use of saline injection as a control (4, 14). Experience in South America, Zaire, and China has confirmed the value of this measure. Quantitative correction of severe iodine deficiency by a single intramuscular injection can last for more than 4 years (13). Iodized oil is singularly appropriate for isolated mountainous village communities that are commonly endemic goiter areas. The striking regression of goiter following iodized oil injection ensures general acceptance of the measure.

In a high-risk area, until an effective iodized salt program is in place, the oil (1 mL of poppyseed oil contains 480 mg of iodine) should be administered to all females up to the age of 40 years and all males up to the age of 20 years. A repeat injection is required in 3 to 5 years, depending on the dose given and the age of the subject. Children have a greater need than adults do, and the recommended dose should be repeated in 3 years if severe iodine deficiency persists (4).

Iodized walnut oil and iodized soya bean oil were developed in China since 1980, and Indonesia has now developed iodized peanut oil for oral use (4).

Iodized Oil by Mouth

Because of the hazards associated with injections, there has been a strong recent trend toward oral administration of iodized oil. Recent studies in India and China reveal that oral iodized oil lasts only half as long as a similar dose given by injection (4). A recent study in children indicates that 1 mL (480 mg of iodine) of oral oil provides coverage of iodine deficiency for 1 year (50). Iodized salt and iodized oil are major mass supplementation measures that have been used on a large scale. More than 50 million doses of iodinated oil have been given with evidence of successful prevention of IDD.

Table 13.7
Criteria for Monitoring Progress Toward Eliminating IDD as a Public Health Problem

Indicator	Goal
1. Salt iodization	>90%
Proportion of households consuming effectively iodized salt	
2. Urinary iodine	
Proportion below 100 μg/L	<50%
Proportion below 50 μg/L	<20%
3. Thyroid size	
In school children 6–12 years of age:	<5%
Proportion with enlarged thyroid, by palpation or ultrasound	
4. Neonatal TSH	
Proportion with levels >5 mU/L whole blood	<3%

From Joint WHO/UNICEF/ICCIDD Consultation—Indicators for assessing iodine deficiency disorders and their control through salt iodization. Geneva: World Health Organization, 1994.

INTERNATIONAL ACTION

New knowledge of the causes of IDD and its impact on brain development, as well as the application of this new knowledge in national IDD control programs, particularly in developing countries, led to formation in 1985 of the ICCIDD (4, 5, 51). The inaugural meeting of this multidisciplinary group of epidemiologists, nutritionists, endocrinologists, chemists, public health planners, and economists was held in Kathmandu, Nepal, in March 1986. A series of papers on all aspects of IDD control programs presented in Kathmandu has been published as a monograph (4). The ICCIDD has established a global multidisciplinary network of some 400 professionals from more than 80 different countries with expertise relevant to IDD and IDD control programs. More than half of the members are from developing countries. The ICCIDD works closely with WHO, UNICEF, and national governments within the UN system in the development of national programs (4, 5, 51). Because major concentrations of populations at risk are in Asia, IDD control programs in the last 10 years have escalated in India, Indonesia, Nepal, Bangladesh, and more recently China.

In Latin America, earlier efforts have produced a large measure of control in such countries as Argentina, Brazil, Colombia, and Guatemala. The problem recurred in Colombia and Guatemala, however, largely associated with political and social unrest. Nonetheless, the combination of national government initiatives and support from international agencies through the USI policy has induced remarkable progress in the last 5 years (51).

In Africa, development of IDD control programs has lagged by comparison with the other continents. New initiatives began after a Joint WHO/UNICEF/ICCIDD Regional Seminar held in Yaounde, Cameroon, in March 1987. This seminar set up a joint IDD Task Force that initiated comprehensive planning for prevention and control of IDD in Africa (5).

In September 1990, the World Summit for Children held at the United Nations in New York was attended by 71 heads of state and 80 other government representatives. The World Summit signed a declaration and approved a plan of action that included the elimination of IDD as a public health problem by the year 2000. The criteria adopted for monitoring progress toward this goal are summarized in Table 13.7.

These meetings have led to a new era of political support at the country level. For example, China has made rapid progress since the World Summit for Children. Forty percent of the Chinese population lives in an iodine-deficient environment, either mountainous terrain or flooded river valleys. In 1993, a national advocacy meeting was held in the Great Hall of the People, sponsored by Premier Li Peng. Both the Chinese government and major international agencies made commitments to upgrading the national program with adoption of a USI policy and effective iodization of salt. The Chinese government recognized the major hazard presented by iodine deficiency as a cause of brain damage for the next generation. This concern was accentuated by the government's one-child family policy.

Recent data indicate remarkable progress with USI in developing countries. By mid-1996, WHO estimated that approximately 56% (2.4 billion) of the population in 83 developing countries with a significant IDD public health problem now has access to iodized salt. At the recent (1996) Joint WHO/UNICEF/ICCIDD Meeting in Africa attended by 45 countries, most reported good progress with the USI policy. This remarkable progress encourages confidence that IDD as a public health problem may be largely eliminated by the year 2000, with incalculable benefits to the quality of life of the many millions at risk (51).

REFERENCES

1. Stanbury JB, Hetzel BS. Endemic goiter and endemic cretinism. New York: Wiley, 1980.
2. Dunn JT, Pretell EA, Daza CH, eds. Towards the eradication of endemic goiter, cretinism, and iodine deficiency. Washington, DC: Pan American Health Organization, 1986.
3. Hetzel BS, Potter BJ, Dulberg EM. World Rev Nutr Diet 1990;62:59–119.
4. Hetzel BS, Dunn JT, Stanbury, JB, eds. The prevention and control of iodine deficiency disorders. Amsterdam: Elsevier, 1987.

5. Hetzel BS. The story of iodine deficiency—an international challenge in nutrition. Oxford: Oxford University Press, 1989.
6. World Health Organization. Report to 43rd World Health Assembly, Geneva, 1990;1–17.
7. World Health Organization. Micronutrient deficiency information system (MDIS) working paper no. 1. Global prevalence of iodine deficiency disorders. Geneva: WHO/UNICEF/ICCIDD, 1993;1–80.
8. DeGroot LJ, Larsen PR, Henneman G. The thyroid and its diseases. 6th ed. New York: Churchill Livingstone, 1996.
9. McMichael AJ, Potter JD, Hetzel BS. Iodine deficiency, thyroid function, and reproductive failure. In: Stanbury JB, Hetzel BS, eds. Endemic goiter and endemic cretinism. New York: Wiley, 1980;445–60.
10. Pharoah POD, Delange F, Fierro-Benitez R, Stanbury JB. Endemic cretinism. In: Stanbury JB, Hetzel BS, eds. Endemic goiter and endemic cretinism. New York: Wiley, 1980;395–421.
11. Delange F, Iteke FB, Ermans AM. Nutritional factors involved in the goitrogenic action of cassava. Ottawa: IDRC, 1982.
12. Fierro-Benitez R, Stanbury JB, Querido A, et al. J Clin Endocrinol Metab 1970;30:228–36.
13. Buttfield IH, Hetzel BS. Bull WHO 1967;36:243–62.
14. Pharoah POD, Buttfield IH, Hetzel BS. Lancet 1971;1:308–10.
15. Cao X-Y, Jiang X-M, Dou, Z-H, et al. N Engl J Med 1994; 331:1739–42.
16. Pharoah POD, Ellis SM, Ekins RP, Williams ES. Clin Endocrinol 1976;5:159–66.
17. Vulsma T, Gons MT, De Vijlder JJM. N Engl J Med 1989;321:13–6.
18. Burgi H, Supersaxo Z, Selz B. Acta Endocrinologica 1990;123:577–90.
19. Thilly CH. Bull Acad Med Belg 1981;136:389–412.
20. Pharoah POD, Connolly KC. Int J Epidemiol 1987;16:68–73.
21. Dobbing J. The later development of the brain and its vulnerability. In: Davis K, Dobbing J, eds. Scientific foundations of paediatrics. London: Heinemann Medical, 1974;565–77.
22. Delange F, Heidemann P, Bourdoux P, et al. Biol Neonate 1986;49:322–30.
23. Kochupillai N, Pandav CS. Neonatal chemical hypothyroidism in iodine deficient environments. In: Hetzel BS, Dunn JT, Stanbury JB, eds. The prevention and control of iodine deficiency disorders. Amsterdam: Elsevier, 1987;85–93.
24. Ermans AM, Bourdoux P, Lagasse R, et al. Congenital hypothyroidism in developing countries. In: Burrow BN, ed. Neonatal thyroid screening. New York: Raven Press, 1980;61–73.
25. Vanderpas J, Rivera MT, Bourdoux P, et al. N Engl J Med 1986;315:791–93.
26. Delange F. Iodine nutrition and risk of thyroid irradiation from nuclear accidents. In: Rubery E, Smales E, eds. Iodine prophylaxis following nuclear accidents. Oxford: Pergamon Press, 1990;45–50.
27. Bleichrodt N, Born M. A metaanalysis of research on iodine and its relationship to cognitive development. In: Stanbury JB, ed. The damaged brain of iodine deficiency. New York: Cognizant Communication Corporation, 1994;195–200.
28. Hetzel BS. Historical development of the concepts of the brain—thyroid relationships. In: Stanbury JB, ed. The damaged brain of iodine deficiency. New York: Cognizant Communication Corporation, 1994;1–7.
29. Crantz FR, Larsen PR. J Clin Invest 1980;65:935–38.
30. Obregon MJ, Santisteban P, Rodriguez-pena A, et al. Endocrinology 1984;115:614–24.
31. Hetzel BS, Maberly GF. Iodine. In: Mertz W, ed. Trace elements in human and animal nutrition. 5th ed. New York: Academic Press 1986;2:139–208.
32. Hetzel BS, Mano M. J Nutr 1989;119:145–51.
33. DeLong R. Neurological involvement in iodine deficiency disorders. In: Hetzel BS, Dunn JT, Stanbury JB, eds. The prevention and control of iodine deficiency disorders. Amsterdam: Elsevier, 1987;49–63.
34. Vitti P, Martino E, Aghini-Lombardi F, et al. J Clin Endocrinol Metab 1994;79:600–3.
35. Dunn JT, Crutchfield HE, Gutekunst R, Dunn AD, eds. Methods for measuring iodine in urine. The Netherlands: ICCIDD/UNICEF/WHO, 1993;1–71.
36. Burrow GN, ed. Neonatal thyroid screening. New York: Raven Press, 1980.
37. Food and Nutrition Board, National Academy of Sciences, National Research Council. Recommended dietary allowances. 10th ed. Washington, DC: National Academy of Sciences Press, 1989.
38. World Health Organization. Trace elements in human nutrition and health. Geneva: WHO/FAO/IAEA, 1996.
39. Wolff J. Am J Med 1969;47:101.
40. Suzuki H. Etiology of endemic goiter and iodide excess. In: Stanbury JB, Hetzel BS, eds. Endemic goiter and endemic cretinism. New York: John Wiley & Sons, 1980;237–54.
41. Nagataki S. Effects of iodide supplement in thyroid diseases. In: Vichayanrat A, Nitiyanant W, Eastman C, Nagataki S, eds. Recent progress in thyroidology. Bangkok: Crystal House Press, 1987;31–7.
42. Connolly RJ, Vidor GI, Stewart JC. Lancet 1970;1:500–2.
43. Stewart JC, Vidor GI, Buttfield IH, et al. Aust NZ J Med 1971;3:203–11.
44. Larsen PR, Silva JE, Hetzel BS, et al. Monitoring prophylactic programs: general consideration. In: Stanbury JB, Hetzel BS, eds. Endemic goiter and endemic cretinism. New York: John Wiley & Sons, 1980;551–66.
45. Vidor GI, Stewart JC, Wall JR, et al. J Clin Endocrinol Metab 1973;37:901–9.
46. Todd C, Allain T, Gomo ZAR, et al. Lancet 1995;342:1563–4.
47. Joseph K, Mayhlstedt J, Gonnermann R, et al. J Mol Med 1980;4:21–37.
48. Nelson M, Phillips DIW. Hum Nutr Appl Nutr 1985;39:213–6.
48a. WHO/UNICEF/ICCIDD. Recommended iodine levels in salt and guidelines for monitoring their adequacy and effectiveness. Micronutrient series WHO/NUT/96.13. 1996.
49. Ma T, Lu T, Tan U, et al. Food Nutr Bull 1982;4:13–9.
50. Benmiloud M, Chaouki ML, Gutekunst R, et al. J Clin Endocrinol and Metab 1994;79:20–4.
51. Hetzel BS, Pandav CS, eds. SOS for a billion: the conquest of iodine deficiency. Delhi: Oxford University Press, 1996.

SELECTED READINGS

General

Hetzel BS. The story of iodine deficiency: an international challenge in Nutrition. Oxford/Delhi: Oxford University Press, 1989.

Scientific

DeGroot LJ, Larsen PR, Hennemann G, eds. The thyroid and its diseases. 6th ed. New York: Churchill Livingstone, 1996.
Stanbury JB, ed. The damaged brain of iodine deficiency. New York: Cognizant Communication Corporation, 1994.

Public Health

Hetzel BS, Dunn JT, Stanbury JB, eds. The prevention and control of iodine deficiency disorders. Amsterdam: Elsevier, 1987.
Hetzel BS, Pandav CS, eds. SOS for a billion: the conquest of iodine deficiency disorders. Delhi: Oxford University Press, 1996.

14. Selenium

RAYMOND F. BURK and ORVILLE A. LEVANDER

Selenium first attracted biologic interest in the 1930s when it was found to cause alkali disease, a chronic poisoning of livestock resulting from the consumption of plants that grow on high-selenium soils (1). In 1957, Schwarz and Foltz reported that traces of selenium prevented liver necrosis in vitamin E–deficient rats, indicating that selenium was an essential nutrient and not only a toxin (2). Soon thereafter, deficiencies of selenium and vitamin E were shown to be involved in several economically important nutritional diseases of cattle, sheep, swine, and poultry (3). The first demonstration of a biochemical function for selenium in animals came in 1973, when it was shown to be a constituent of the enzyme glutathione peroxidase (4).

The importance of selenium in human nutrition was shown in 1979, when Chinese scientists reported that selenium supplementation prevented development of a cardiomyopathy known as Keshan disease in children living in low-selenium areas (5), and New Zealand workers reported a clinical response to selenium in a selenium-depleted patient (6). Information about the role of selenium in human nutrition increased rapidly in the 1980s, and a recommended dietary allowance (RDA) for selenium was established in 1989 (7). Dietary recommendations from the World Health Organization (WHO) were issued in 1996 (8). Over the last decade, research has provided extensive new information on selenoproteins and the molecular biology of selenium.

CHEMICAL FORMS

Most selenium in biologic systems is present in amino acids as constituents of proteins. The chemistry of selenium is similar to that of sulfur, reflecting its position in the oxygen series of the periodic table of elements. The three amino acids serine, cysteine, and selenocysteine contain, respectively, oxygen, sulfur, and selenium in the same carbon skeleton. Their differences in biochemical activity arise from the chemical reactivity of the element in each of them. Selenocysteine is the most reactive of the three, and its selenol (Fig. 14.1) performs catalytic functions in proteins. Selenomethionine, on the other hand, contains selenium bound to two carbon atoms and is not known to have a biologic function distinct from methionine.

A selenoprotein is a protein that contains stoichiometric amounts of selenium. Selenocysteine is the form in the primary structure of all the animal selenoproteins identified so far and all but one of the bacterial selenoproteins. Selenium occurs in an unidentified form (not selenocysteine) that is coordinated with molybdenum in nicotinic acid hydroxylase from *Clostridium barkeri* (9), indicating that selenoproteins exist containing forms of the element other than selenocysteine.

Numerous proteins contain selenium in nonstoichiometric amounts and may be referred to as selenium-containing proteins. This designation has low utility, because virtually all proteins that contain methionine will contain selenomethionine in proportion to the relative abundance of these two amino acids in the organism (see below).

Selenium enters the food chain through plants that incorporate it into compounds that usually contain sulfur. Thus plant selenium is in the form of selenomethionine and, to a lesser extent, selenocysteine and other analogues of sulfur amino acids. No evidence has been presented that plants require selenium incorporation into a specific molecule necessary for their existence.

Selenophosphate, an important intermediate compound in selenium metabolism, is produced by

Abbreviations: **RfD**—reference dose; **TPN**—total parenteral nutrition.

selenophosphate synthetase and serves as the selenium donor for production of selenium-containing transfer RNAs as well as for selenocysteine destined for incorporation into selenoproteins (10). Methylated forms of selenium are produced as excretory metabolites and rapidly appear in the urine and breath (11). A putative transport form of the element has been detected in blood plasma, but its identity has not been established (12).

DIETARY CONSIDERATIONS

Food Sources

Although SI units (Système International d'Unités, or International System of Units) are increasingly used to express concentrations of nutrients in body fluids and tissues, food composition tables primarily express values in micrograms per gram (μg/g). In this regard, 1 μg Se equals 0.0127 μmol Se. The richest food sources of selenium are organ meats and seafood, 0.4 to 1.5 μg/g fresh weight; followed by muscle meats, 0.1 to 0.4; cereals and grains, less than 0.1 to more than 0.8; dairy products, less than 0.1 to 0.3; and fruits and vegetables, less than 0.1 (13). The wide variation in the selenium content of cereals and grains is due to the fact that plants do not appear to require selenium and thus contain variable amounts, depending upon how much soil selenium is available for uptake (phytoavailability). For example, one study showed that the selenium content of corn collected in the People's Republic of China ranged from 0.005 to 8.1 μg/g, depending on whether the samples came from areas with soils that were poor or rich in phytoavailable selenium (14). The importance of geographic origin in determining the selenium content of grains was also recently indicated by the reported decline in the selenium content of the British diet from 65 to 31 μg/day after Britain switched its source of wheat from North America to Europe (15). Foods from animal sources vary somewhat in selenium content, but the variation is less because of the tendency toward homeostatic control of selenium under different conditions of exposure. Drinking water generally contributes negligible selenium to the overall intake, except perhaps in some localized highly seleniferous areas (16).

The Total Diet Study conducted by the U.S. Food and Drug Administration showed that a typical diet in the United States provided an average daily selenium intake of 100 and 70 μg for adult men and women, respectively, between 1982 and 1986 (17). Lower daily selenium intakes, 30 μg or less, have been reported in countries with selenium-poor soils, such as New Zealand (18). Because of the increasing evidence that good selenium status may confer human health benefits, the government of Finland decided to start adding selenium to the fertilizers used in that low-selenium country in 1984 as a way of improving the selenium status of the general population (19). Although daily dietary intakes increased from 39 μg in 1984 to 92 μg in 1986, resulting in an increase in plasma selenium concentrations from 0.95 to 1.52 μmol/L after 1.5 years of the intervention, no reduction has been observed in the incidence of cancer or cardiovascular disease to date (20). Extremely low dietary selenium intakes have been reported in Keshan disease–affected areas of China, from 3 to 22 μg/day (14). On the other hand, very high dietary intakes (up to 6690 μg/day) were observed in a region of China with endemic human selenosis (14). Food in this area was grown on soil contaminated with selenium leached from a highly seleniferous coal fly ash.

Bioavailability

Only a limited number of investigations have been carried out to determine the nutritional bioavailability of selenium in foods consumed by humans. Commonly, the experimental procedure to estimate selenium availability follows increases in hepatic glutathione peroxidase activity after feeding various food sources of selenium to rodents previously depleted of selenium (21). On this basis, selenium fed as mushrooms, tuna, and wheat was 5%, 57%, and 83% as available to rats, respectively, as sodium selenite (21, 22). A human bioavailability trial performed in Finland with men of moderately low-selenium status showed significant differences among various forms of selenium tested (e.g., selenate, wheat, yeast), depending on the criterion of availability used (increase in platelet glutathione peroxidase activity, elevation of plasma or red blood cell selenium content, retention of selenium) (23). This study pointed out the need to consider several variables in such trials, including short-term increases in glutathione peroxidase activity, long-term tissue retention of selenium, and metabolic conversion of retained selenium to biologically active forms.

Nutrient-Nutrient Interrelationships

Because of its role in the glutathione peroxidases and thioredoxin reductase, selenium probably interacts with any nutrient that affects the antioxidant/prooxidant balance of the cell. For example, the selenium requirement of chicks is inversely proportional to the dietary vitamin E intake (24). Selenium also protects against the toxicities of mercury, cadmium, and silver (25), and a physiologic role for selenium in counteracting heavy metal pollutants has been proposed (26). The low bioavailability of the selenium in tuna may be due to complex formation with mercury, but this issue needs further investigation (21).

METABOLISM

Selenium enters the body in several forms (Fig. 14.2). The two major ones are selenomethionine, derived ultimately from plants, and selenocysteine in animal selenoproteins. Selenomethionine does not appear to be specifically recognized as a selenium compound and is metabolized in the methionine pool. It is measured as tissue selenium because it occurs in methionine-containing proteins in tissues. The selenium in selenomethionine is

H
|
H_2N-C-COOH
|
CH_2
|
SeH

selenocysteine

H
|
H_2N-C-COOH
|
CH_2
|
CH_2
|
Se
|
CH_3

selenomethionine

Figure 14.1. Selenium-containing amino acids found in animals. Selenocysteine is the biologically active form of the element found in selenoproteins. Its selenol is largely ionized at physiologic pH and is a stronger nucleophile than the thiol of cysteine. These chemical properties contribute to its catalytic function in selenoenzymes. Selenomethionine contains selenium covalently bound to two carbon atoms. Thus, its selenium is shielded and not as chemically active as the selenium in selenocysteine. Selenomethionine appears to be distributed nonspecifically in the methionine pool.

made available for specific use when the amino acid is catabolized (Fig. 14.2). The selenium then enters regulated selenium metabolism and can be incorporated specifically into macromolecules, transported to other organs, or excreted.

Figure 14.3 outlines selenium metabolism in the cell. Selenomethionine catabolism occurs via the transsulfuration pathway and yields selenocysteine. Free selenocysteine, whether derived from selenomethionine or from selenoprotein catabolism, is degraded by selenocysteine β-lyase (28). The resulting selenide can enter the anabolic pathway by conversion to selenophosphate or be methylated for excretion (11, 29). The further metabolism of selenide is the likely point of homeostatic regulation of selenium in the body. The mechanism by which this form of selenium is directed into the anabolic pathway or into the excretory pathway has not been determined.

Absorption

Absorption appears to play no role in the homeostatic regulation of selenium. Virtually complete absorption occurs when the element is supplied as selenomethionine (30), and other forms are generally well absorbed. However, absorption of inorganic forms varies widely because it is influenced by luminal factors. Thus, selenium absorption is usually in the range of 50 to 100% and is not affected by selenium nutritional status.

Transport

Little is known about the extracellular transport of selenium. Two selenoproteins, selenoprotein P and extracellular glutathione peroxidase (GSHPx-3), have been identified in plasma, but both contain the element as selenocysteine in their primary structures, making them unlikely candidates for transport forms. Small-molecular-weight forms of the element recognized as minor components of the plasma selenium (12) might serve transport functions. Chemical identification of these forms has not yet been made.

Incorporation into Protein

The animal selenoproteins characterized so far contain selenocysteine in their primary structures. The mechanism by which selenocysteine, the 21st amino acid, is synthesized and then incorporated into selenoproteins is complex. Figure 14.4 outlines selenoprotein synthesis in animals. $tRNA^{[ser]sec}$, a unique transfer RNA with the anticodon for UGA, is charged with serine by seryl-tRNA ligase. The serine in the resulting $ser\text{-}tRNA^{[ser]sec}$ is then converted to selenocysteine by a process requiring selenophosphate synthesized by selenophosphate synthetase (Fig. 14.3). Two isoforms of selenophosphate synthetase have been identified (31, 32), and one is itself a selenoprotein. In prokaryotes, a pyridoxal phosphate enzyme catalyzes the selenophosphate-dependent conversion of

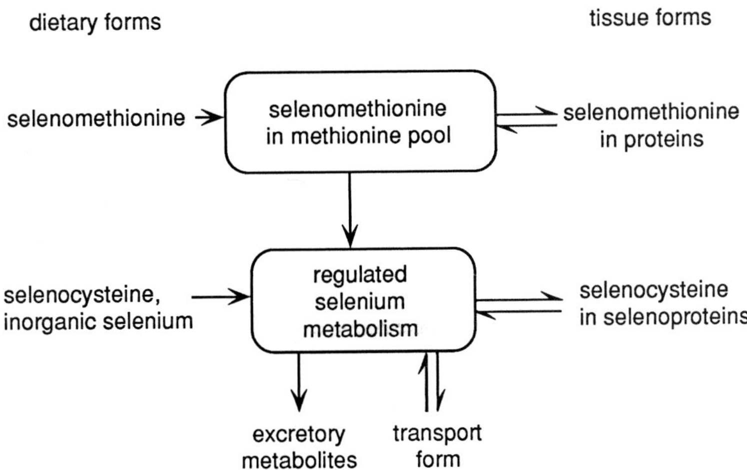

Figure 14.2. Relationships of dietary forms of selenium with tissue forms. Dietary forms of the element are shown on the *left* and tissue forms on the *right*. Excretory metabolites and the transport form are also present in tissues but only in relatively small quantities. (From Levander OA, Burk RF. Selenium. In: Ziegler EE, Filer LJ, eds. Present knowledge in nutrition. Washington, DC: ILSI Press, 1996;320–8, with permission.)

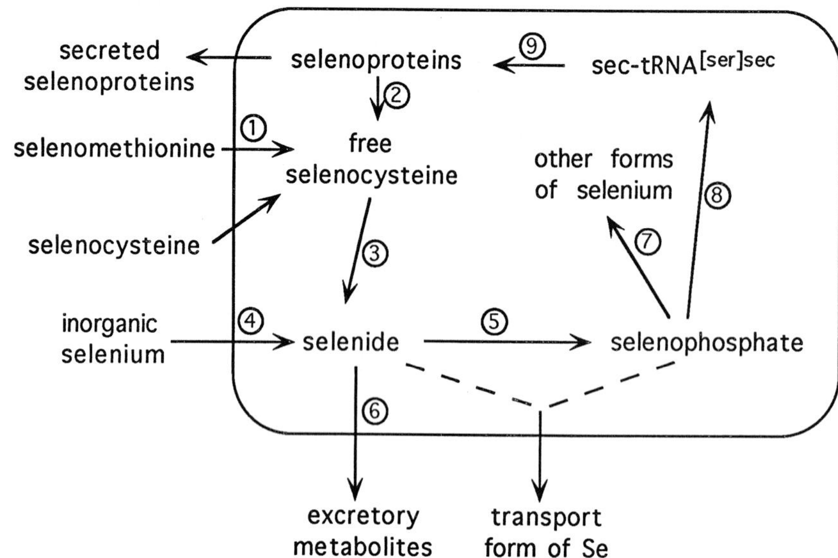

Figure 14.3. Regulated selenium metabolism. An outline of selenium metabolism based on reactions known to take place. The *box* represents the cell. Circled numbers indicate *(1)* the transsulfuration pathway, *(2)* proteolytic breakdown of proteins, *(3)* selenocysteine β-lyase, *(4)* reduction by glutathione, *(5)* selenophosphate synthetase, *(6)* methylation, *(7)* replacement of sulfur in tRNA by selenium, *(8)* replacement of oxygen in serine with selenium to produce selenocysteine, *(9)* decoding of UGA in mRNA with insertion of selenocysteine into primary structure of protein. The origin and identity of the transport form of selenium is unknown; it might arise from selenide or selenophosphate as indicated by the *broken lines*. (From Levander OA, Burk RF. Selenium. In: Ziegler EE, Filer LJ, eds. Present knowledge in nutrition. Washington, DC: ILSI Press, 1996;320–8, with permission.)

serine to selenocysteine (33). The corresponding enzyme has not yet been characterized in animals.

Figure 14.4*B* represents a typical selenoprotein messenger RNA (mRNA). UGA in the open reading frame codes for insertion of selenocysteine. A stem-loop structure with several conserved features is present in the 3′ untranslated region. Absence of the stem loop or modification of its essential features results in the UGA in the open reading frame functioning as a termination codon instead of designating selenocysteine insertion (34). The stem loop in prokaryotes is adjacent to the UGA codon (33). It binds a complex consisting of a unique elongation factor and sec-tRNA$^{[ser]sec}$ and approximates them to the UGA codon, facilitating selenocysteine insertion into the protein at that point. The precise mechanism by which the animal stem loop facilitates UGA readthrough as selenocysteine has not been determined, but evidence has been presented that an elongation factor is involved (35). It has been proposed that a complex of the putative elongation factor and sec-tRNA$^{[ser]sec}$ binds to the stem loop and that the mRNA then loops back to the ribosome so that the complex can prevent termination at the UGA and effect selenocysteine incorporation into the growing peptide chain (36).

Excretion

Homeostasis of selenium in the body is achieved through regulation of its excretion. As dietary intake increases from the deficient range into the adequate range, urinary excretion of the element increases and accounts for maintenance of homeostasis (37). At very high intakes, volatile forms of selenium are exhaled and the breath becomes a significant route of excretion. There is no evidence that fecal selenium is regulated. Thus, under physiologic conditions, urinary excretion is the primary site of body selenium regulation.

Most excretory metabolites of selenium appear to be methylated. A recent study indicates that a large fraction of urinary selenium is methylselenol (38). A smaller percentage is trimethylselenonium ion (11). Selenium in the breath is largely dimethylselenide (11). How formation of these metabolites is regulated is not known. However, a logical point of regulation would be at the level of selenophosphate synthetase (Fig. 14.3).

BIOCHEMICAL FUNCTIONS

Eleven selenoproteins have been characterized in animals (Table 14.1), and evidence has been presented that additional ones exist. A tRNA that contains selenium has also been described (10). Enzymatic functions have been described for most of the selenoproteins, but the biochemical functions of several have not been discovered.

Glutathione Peroxidases

The glutathione peroxidases use reducing equivalents from glutathione to catabolize hydroperoxides. Four selenium-containing glutathione peroxidases, all separate gene products, have been characterized (for reviews see [47, 48]). The cellular glutathione peroxidase, GSHPx-1, is the most abundant member of the group and is present in all cells. GSHPx-2, originally designated GSHPx-GI, is also a cellular enzyme but is found predominantly in tissues of the gastrointestinal tract (39). Extracellular glu-

A

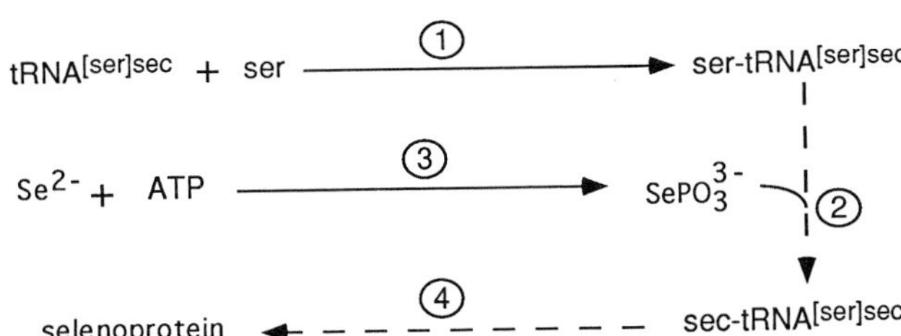

B

UGA
AAAAAAA
ORF
3'UTR

Figure 14.4. *Panel A.* Outline of selenoprotein synthesis. *Solid lines* indicate reactions that have been characterized and *broken lines* indicate ones that have not yet been characterized. The *circled numbers* indicate *(1)* seryl-tRNA ligase, *(2)* selenocysteine synthetase function (enzyme characterized in bacteria but not in animals), *(3)* selenophosphate synthetase, *(4)* elongation factor (characterized in bacteria but not in animals), and SECIS motif in selenoprotein mRNA. *Panel B.* Representation of a selenoprotein mRNA. The open reading frame *(ORF)* contains a UGA codon that is decoded as selenocysteine. The 3′ untranslated region (3′UTR) contains a stem-loop structure necessary for the decoding of the UGA as selenocysteine. The *asterisks* on the stem loop indicate the locations of conserved nucleotide sequences. One of these is present on the loop and the other two are present on bulges from the stem. The stem loop with its conserved sequences constitutes the SECIS motif. (From Levander OA, Burk RF. Selenium. In: Ziegler EE, Filer LJ, eds. Present knowledge in nutrition. Washington, DC: ILSI Press, 1996;320–8, with permission.)

tathione peroxidase, GSHPx-3, is present in plasma and milk (49). Phospholipid hydroperoxide glutathione peroxidase, GSHPx-4, is present inside cells and differs in several respects from other members of the group. It can catalyze reduction of fatty acid hydroperoxides that are esterified in phospholipids (48) and alternative processing can produce a form with a signal that localizes the protein to mitochondria (50).

Table 14.1
Animal Selenoproteins

Protein	Reference
Glutathione peroxidase family	
GSHPx-1 (cytosolic or classical)	(4)
GSHPx-2 (GI)	(39)
GSHPx-3 (extracellular or plasma)	(40)
GSHPx-4 (phospholipid hydroperoxide)	(41)
Iodothyronine deiodinase family	
Type I (liver, kidney, thyroid)	(34)
Type II (brain)	(42)
Type III (inactivating)	(43)
Thioredoxin reductase	(44)
Selenophosphate synthetase	(32)
Selenoprotein P	(45)
Selenoprotein W	(46)

Selenium deficiency causes a decrease in the activity of all glutathione peroxidases. However, the effect varies according to tissue and enzyme. Brain glutathione peroxidase is relatively well preserved in selenium deficiency as is GSHPx-4 in all tissues. Glutathione peroxidase activities in plasma and liver are very sensitive to selenium supply and are used as indices of selenium nutritional status.

The glutathione peroxidases catabolize hydrogen peroxide and fatty acid–derived hydroperoxides. They have been generally considered to protect cells from these oxidant molecules. However, many oxidant molecules have functions in metabolism and in signaling pathways. Thus, the glutathione peroxidases have regulatory roles in the cell because they affect the concentrations of oxidant molecules. Moreover, the four glutathione peroxidases have different localizations and different substrate specificities that could be part of a regulatory strategy.

Iodothyronine Deiodinases

The iodothyronine deiodinases, types I–III, are all selenoproteins (34, 42, 43). These enzymes catalyze the deiodination of thyroxine, triiodothyronine, and reverse triiodothyronine and thereby regulate the concentration of the active hormone triiodothyronine. Several thiols can serve as the reducing substrate for these enzymes, but glutathione is likely to be the physiologic substrate (34).

Thioredoxin Reductase

Thioredoxin reductase is an NADPH-dependent flavoenzyme that reduces the internal disulfide of thioredoxin (51). The prokaryotic enzyme is highly specific for thioredoxin as a substrate and interacts with it through a redox-active thiol pair. The animal enzyme has a broader substrate range that includes a number of small molecules, and the animal enzyme is considerably larger than the prokaryotic one. Animal thioredoxin reductase has recently been shown to contain selenocysteine (52), and evidence has been presented that selenium forms part of the active site. It regenerates ascorbic acid from dehydroascorbic acid (52a). The hepatic activity of the enzyme declines in selenium deficiency (53).

Selenoprotein P

Selenoprotein P was identified in plasma about two decades ago but resisted purification and characterization for many years (54). It has now been purified (45) as well as characterized at the nucleic acid level (55). Selenoprotein P is an extracellular glycoprotein that is found in plasma and also associated with endothelial cells (56). Its cDNA indicates that it has a typical signal peptide for secretion from the cell and that its open reading frame contains 10 to 12 UGAs that designate selenocysteine incorporation (55, 57). Thus, it and the type II iodothyronine deiodinase, which apparently has two selenocysteine residues, are the only selenoproteins known to contain more than one selenocysteine residue per polypeptide chain. Isoforms of the protein have been identified in rat plasma. A full-length form and a form that terminates at the second in-frame UGA have been isolated and characterized (58).

Selenoprotein P contains a large fraction of the plasma selenium, about 45% in a typical North American (59). The concentration of selenoprotein P declines in selenium deficiency and can be used as an indicator of selenium status (59).

The function of selenoprotein P is not known but it has been associated with the oxidant defense properties of selenium. Selenium-deficient rats are susceptible to diquat-induced lipid peroxidation and liver necrosis, and protection by selenium correlates with selenoprotein P concentration in plasma (60). It has been speculated that its endothelial cell location indicates that selenoprotein P protects those cells from oxidant molecules generated by inflammation or by xenobiotic metabolism (56).

Selenoprotein W

Selenoprotein W was originally identified in muscle and postulated to play a role in development of white muscle disease, a selenium deficiency condition in sheep. It has now been identified in many other tissues and shown to exist in several forms (46). One form has glutathione bound to it, suggesting that selenoprotein W undergoes redox changes. However, its biochemical function is unknown. Selenoprotein W concentration decreases in selenium deficiency (61).

Selenophosphate Synthetase

Two selenophosphate synthetases have recently been identified in animals. One contains a selenocysteine residue in its primary structure, and the other contains a cysteine residue at the same position (31, 32). Because regulation of selenium homeostasis appears to reside at the level of this activity, work on the function of these enzymes may reveal the mechanism of selenium regulation.

BIOLOGIC ACTIVITY

Selenium deficiency leads to marked changes in many biochemical systems. A number of drug-metabolizing enzymes, including the cytochrome P-450 system, are affected, some with activities increased and others with activities decreased (62). Glutathione S-transferase activities in rat liver, kidney, and lung rise in selenium deficiency. The underlying causes of these changes have not been established, but they are presumably related to changes in selenoproteins. Glutathione metabolism is affected by selenium deficiency. In the rat, plasma glutathione concentration is increased two to three times above the concentration in selenium-replete animals (63). This has been traced to increased hepatic synthesis of GSH and release of it into the plasma (63).

Changes in thyroid hormone metabolism were characterized many years ago in selenium-deficient animals (64) and are now explained by the discovery that the iodothyronine deiodinases are selenoenzymes. Other metabolic effects, such as changes in glucose metabolism, have not yet been traced to a selenoprotein (65).

Pure selenium deficiency does not usually cause clinical illness in free-living humans or animals. Only when laboratory animals are raised through several generations on a selenium-deficient regimen do they exhibit pathologic changes from selenium deficiency alone. However, first-generation selenium-deficient animals exhibit heightened sensitivity to certain stresses, which is the basis of most naturally occurring conditions of selenium deficiency. One of these stresses is vitamin E deficiency. Simultaneous selenium and vitamin E deficiencies lead to a number of pathologic conditions in animals (3). Selenium-deficient animals are more susceptible to injury by certain chemicals such as the redox cyclers paraquat, diquat, and nitrofurantoin. These injuries are generally oxidative and might be related to decreased levels of the selenoenzymes that defend against oxidative injury.

Selenium can influence the outcome of infections. The increased virulence of coxsackievirus B3 in selenium-deficient mice is described below. Additionally, potential selenocysteine-incorporation codons have been described in a number of viral genomes, including that of HIV (66). This points to a viral strategy of appropriating the selenium of the cell or of disrupting selenium-dependent functions in it. Research in this area is very active.

DEFICIENCY IN HUMANS AND ANIMALS

A combined deficiency of both selenium and vitamin E causes liver necrosis in rats and swine, exudative diathesis in chickens, and white muscle disease in sheep and cattle (3). In animals fed a selenium-deficient diet containing adequate levels of vitamin E, signs attributable to selenium deficiency included hair loss, growth retardation, and reproductive failure in rats fed a deficient diet for two generations (67) and pancreatic degeneration in chicks fed amino acid–based diets severely deficient in selenium (68). This pancreatic atrophy in the chick, however, can be prevented by feeding high levels of vitamin E or other antioxidants (69). Pancreatic atrophy can be induced in chicks fed practical rations from a selenium-deficient zone of China, but its severity is less than that seen with the amino acid diet, suggesting the presence of partially protective factors in the practical diet (70). In one study, adult squirrel monkeys fed a low-selenium diet for 9 months lost weight and developed alopecia, myopathy, nephrosis, and hepatic degeneration (71). However, in another study, consistent signs of selenium deficiency proved more difficult to produce in rhesus monkeys, even in offspring born to mothers fed a selenium-deficient diet (72). It was hypothesized that elevated glutathione transferase activity in the tissues of rhesus monkeys might account for their relative resistance to selenium deficiency.

Several lines of evidence indicate that selenium is a nutritionally essential trace element for humans. First, selenium is a component of the enzyme glutathione peroxidase isolated from human red blood cells (73). Secondly, favorable responses have been obtained after selenium supplementation of depleted patients undergoing long-term total parenteral nutrition (TPN) (see section below on high-risk clinical situations). Finally, selenium deficiency has been implicated in certain human diseases.

In 1979, Chinese scientists first described in English the relationship of selenium to Keshan disease, an endemic cardiomyopathy affecting children and young women that occurs in a long belt running from northeastern to southwestern China (5). The acute form is characterized by sudden onset of insufficient heart function, whereas individuals with chronic disease exhibit moderate-to-severe heart enlargement with varying degrees of heart insufficiency (74). The histopathologic features include multifocal necrosis, fibrous replacement of the myocardium, and myocytolysis. Keshan disease is related to a low dietary selenium intake and low blood and hair selenium levels (75). A series of intervention trials encompassing more than a million subjects demonstrated the protective effects of selenium supplements (76). However, selenium cannot reverse the cardiac failure once it occurs. Marginal-to-deficient vitamin E status has also been observed in subjects residing in endemic areas (77), and other complicating nutritional deficiencies (e.g., protein) may exacerbate the condition. Nonetheless, selenium deficiency appears to be the fundamental underlying condition predisposing individuals to development of Keshan disease. With improved living conditions in China, the disease has disappeared from endemic areas.

Because certain features of the disease could not be explained solely on the basis of selenium status (e.g., seasonal variation), it was suggested that a cardiotoxic agent, such as a virus, might also be necessary for the disease to occur (78). Scientists in Beijing provided evidence for a nutrition/infection interaction in the etiology of Keshan disease, since a coxsackievirus B4 isolated from a Keshan disease patient caused more severe cardiopathology when inoculated into selenium-deficient mice than when inoculated into normal mice (79). Beck et al. (80) also found that a myocarditic strain of coxsackievirus B3 (CVB3/20) produced more heart damage in selenium-deficient mice than in normal mice. Likewise, normal mice infected with a benign (amyocarditic) strain of coxsackievirus B3 (CVB3/0) suffered no heart damage, whereas moderate heart damage was observed in infected, selenium-deficient mice (81). Virus isolated from the selenium-deficient mice infected with originally benign CVB3/0 retained its cardiotoxicity when subsequently inoculated into normal mice, thus indicating that the avirulent virus had converted to a virulent strain via a genotypic change. Sequence analysis of the genome of this newly virulent virus revealed that six of the seven virulence-determining sites had been altered (82). To the authors' knowledge, this was the first report of an effect of host nutritional status on the genetic composition of a pathogen. At the present time, the extent to which these observations can be generalized to other RNA viruses, such as polio, hepatitis C, influenza, or HIV, is unknown.

Another disease that has been associated with poor selenium status in China is Kashin-Beck disease, an endemic osteoarthritis that occurs during preadolescence or adolescence (83). Necrotic degeneration of the chondrocytes is the most striking pathologic feature of this disease. Dwarfism and joint deformation result from these cartilage abnormalities. Aside from selenium deficiency, a number of other etiologic factors have been suggested for this condition (e.g., mycotoxins in grain, mineral imbalance, organic contaminants in drinking water) (84).

Numerous attempts have been made to associate selenium status with various chronic degenerative human diseases, especially cancer. However, the epidemiologic evidence linking low-selenium status and an increased incidence of cancer is conflicting (85) and is often based on small differences in plasma selenium levels between controls and subjects who later developed cancer (86). Some animal experiments show that high levels of dietary selenium can protect against certain chemically or virally induced cancers, but in some cases, selenium itself can stimulate tumorigenesis in rodent models (87).

Nonetheless, recent nutritional intervention studies suggest that selenium supplements may have some beneficial effects against cancer. For example, a study with about 30,000 poorly nourished rural Chinese subjects found that overall cancer mortality could be reduced 13% by giving a supplement containing selenium, vitamin E, and β-carotene (88). However, these results may not be directly applicable to Western populations of better nutritional status. In the United States, Clark et al. (89) recently reported the effect of selenium supplementation on development of basal or squamous cell carcinoma of the skin in subjects with a history of this disease. A total of 1312 patients representing a follow-up of 8271 person-years were enrolled in this multicenter, double-blind, randomized, placebo-controlled cancer prevention trial. The intervention consisted of oral administration of 200 μg of selenium as selenized yeast per day or placebo. Although no effect of selenium was seen on the primary end points for the trial (incidence of basal and squamous cell carcinoma of the skin), significant reductions were observed in several secondary end points, including a 37% reduction in total cancer incidence; 63, 58, and 46% declines in the incidence of prostate, colorectal, and lung cancers, respectively; and a 50% decrease in total cancer mortality. On the other hand, all-cause mortality declined insignificantly by 21%, suggesting that selenium treatment may have increased mortality from diseases other than cancer (90).

The study population used in this trial was unusual and consisted largely of male cotton and tobacco farmers with a history of arsenic exposure and skin cancer who were residing in a low-selenium area (20). It was concluded that the data were promising but that it would be "premature to change individual behavior, to market specific selenium supplements, or to modify public health recommendations based on the results of this one randomized trial" (91).

EVALUATION OF NUTRIENT STATUS

Selenium status can be evaluated by dietary and biochemical means.

Analytical Evaluation

Random urine samples are of little use in assessing selenium status because they are affected by dilution and the selenium content of the previous meal (92). Blood selenium levels, which vary widely in different countries, are thought to reflect dietary intakes (13), although a direct relation of dietary selenium to muscle levels or total body selenium content has yet to be established (92). Average blood selenium levels reported in different areas of the United States range between 2.03 and 3.29 μmol/L (93), whereas extreme values of 0.10 and 95.0 μmol/L have been reported in areas of China affected by Keshan disease and endemic selenosis, respectively (10). Plasma selenium levels, which respond to selenium supplementation more rapidly than whole blood levels, are an index of short-term status (92). Average plasma selenium levels observed in areas with marginally adequate (Maryland) or low (Ohio) levels of soil selenium in the United States were 1.70 and 1.51 μmol/L, respectively (94, 95). Levels below 0.63 μmol/L are often seen in healthy residents of the south island of New Zealand (18). Serum selenium concentrations fall soon after birth and then gradually increase to adult values (92). Response to selenium supplementation was observed in a New Zealand patient on TPN who had a plasma level of 0.11 μmol/L (6).

Measurement of plasma, serum, or whole blood selenium concentrations became much easier with the recent introduction of graphite furnace atomic absorption spectrometry with Zeeman background correction (96). This procedure lends itself to large-scale epidemiologic surveys because no pretreatment of the samples is required other than dilution (i.e., no wet ashing is needed). This method was used to measure serum selenium concentrations in the Third National Health and Nutrition Examination Survey (NHANES III, 1988–1994) as a way of helping to establish normal selenium ranges in the U.S. population. Determination of total selenium in blood or blood fractions provides no information about the speciation of selenium in blood. Compartmentalization of selenium can influence the interpretation of blood selenium levels (Fig. 14.2). Intake of diets rich in selenomethionine can raise blood selenium concentrations markedly, because this form of selenium is not subject to homeostatic regulation. Also, serum selenium does not reflect the buildup of selenium in the skeletal muscle of animals when high levels of selenomethionine are fed (97). Hair selenium was used in China to evaluate selenium status (76) but may not be valid in Western countries where shampoos containing selenium are used. Toenail selenium has been suggested as a convenient noninvasive index of selenium status (98). However, hair and nail selenium levels, at least in rats, are influenced by the form of selenium fed and the methionine content of the diet (97).

Assessment of selenium status by calculating the dietary intake from food composition tables is a risky procedure because of the wide variation in the selenium content of foods. Unless one is certain that the database used applies to the diet in question, the safest approach is direct chemical analysis of the diet. Nonetheless, it is possible to obtain reasonable agreement between calculated and analyzed selenium intakes if the appropriate database is available (99).

Biochemical and Clinical Evaluation

A direct relationship exists between blood glutathione peroxidase activity and blood selenium level up to 1.27 μmol selenium/L (100). Beyond that point, the activity of the enzyme plateaus and cannot be used to evaluate selenium nutriture. Moreover, numerous other factors can affect glutathione peroxidase activity (101). Nonetheless, glutathione peroxidase activity remains an extremely useful index of selenium status in the nutritional range of dietary intake, and automated enzyme assays suitable for large-scale surveys have been devised (96). At present, there are no suitable clinical methods for evaluating selenium status.

REQUIREMENTS AND RECOMMENDED INTAKES

In 1980, the National Research Council established an estimated safe and adequate daily dietary selenium intake for adults of 50 to 200 μg (102). This recommendation was the first dietary standard for selenium and was based primarily on extrapolation from animal experiments because few human data were available at that time. A nutritionally generous level of selenium for most animals appears to be about 0.1 μg/g dry diet. If it is assumed that humans consume 500 g of diet (dry basis) daily, then based on the animal results, humans would need 50 μg/day of selenium. Because of uncertainties about the bioavailability of selenium from different diets and possible individual variations in requirements, the dietary recommendation was given as a range.

In the past 15 years, results from a number of human studies have greatly increased our understanding of human selenium requirements. Some of the first attempts to delineate human selenium requirements more precisely involved balance studies, but comparison of international balance data revealed that people could maintain selenium balance over a broad range of intake (86). Thus, the balance method was not especially useful in clarifying human selenium requirements. Another approach was to conduct dietary surveys in areas with and without human selenium deficiency (i.e., with and without Keshan disease). Such surveys showed that Keshan disease was not present in areas where the selenium intake was at least 19 and 13 μg per day for men and women, respectively (78). These values can be considered minimum dietary requirements for selenium.

Human selenium requirements have also been estimated by determining the dietary selenium intake needed to maximize the activity of the selenoenzyme glutathione peroxidase. In these studies, the diets of Chinese men of very low selenium status (residents of an area with Keshan disease) were supplemented with graded doses of selenomethionine (103). Plasma glutathione peroxidase activity tended to be greatest in individuals who received 30 μg/day or more of supplemental selenium over a period of several months. That intake plus their habitual dietary intake (11 μg/day) yielded 41 μg/day as the lowest amount tested that resulted in a plateau in enzyme activity.

Maximization of plasma glutathione peroxidase activity was accepted by the U.S. National Research Council as the basis for its RDA for selenium in 1989 (7) (see also Appendix Table II-A-2-a-2). The Chinese value of 41 μg/day was multiplied by body weight and safety factors to come up with recommendations of 70 and 55 μg/day for adult men and women, respectively. Recommendations for children were extrapolated from the adult values on the basis of body weight. Infant requirements are estimated to be 4 to 7 μg/day, depending on the basis of the estimate (104). The selenium RDA for infants was set at 10 and 15 μg/day for the first and second 6 months of life, respectively, to allow for growth. Increased allowances for women during pregnancy and lactation were 10 and 20 μg/day, respectively, and were based either on fetal demand or lactation losses (see Appendix Table II-A-2-b).

Although North Americans should easily achieve the selenium RDA through consumption of a typical mixed diet, persons living in countries with selenium-poor soils would have difficulty in attaining such intakes (see above section on dietary considerations). For that reason, a recent expert consultation of the WHO produced dietary selenium standards that were considerably lower than the RDAs produced in the United States (8) (see also Appendix Table II-A-2-a-2). Moreover, the WHO advisory group presented the values in their report in the form of safe ranges of population mean intakes, which meant that their recommendations were applicable only to large groups of people and not to individual persons. The purpose of this was to make the WHO document more relevant from the public health point of view (diet planning for large groups and/or diagnostic assessment of dietary intakes of populations). Also, there was a two-tiered system of population mean intake based on two distinct levels of requirement: basal and normative. The basal requirement referred to the "intake needed to prevent pathologically relevant and clinically detectable signs of impaired function attributable to inadequacy of the element," whereas the normative requirement referred to the "intake that serves to maintain a level of tissue storage or other reserve that is judged . . . to be desirable."

The population minimum mean intake of selenium likely to meet basal requirements was given as 21 and 16 μg/day for adult males and females, respectively, with lower values for children and infants extrapolated on the basis of basal metabolic rate. These figures were calculated from Chinese epidemiologic dietary survey data that showed the selenium consumption necessary to protect against Keshan disease. The population mean intake of selenium that would meet the normative requirements was given as 40 and 30 μg/day for adult males and females, respectively. Again, lower values for children and infants were extrapolated on the basis of basal metabolic rate. These figures were calculated from Chinese experimental data that showed the amount of ingested selenium needed to achieve two-thirds of the maximum attainable activity of plasma glutathione peroxidase. This is in contrast to the RDA approach in the United States, which favored the dietary intake needed to achieve full activity of the enzyme. The decision to use two-thirds of maximal glutathione peroxidase activity was based on the observation that "abnormalities in the ability of blood cells to metabolize hydrogen peroxide became apparent only when the glutathione peroxidase activity in these cells declines to one-quarter or less of normal."

TOXICITY IN HUMANS AND ANIMALS

The level of dietary selenium needed to cause chronic selenium toxicity in animals is 4 to 5 μg/g (3). In livestock, chronic selenosis (alkali disease) is characterized by cirrhosis, lameness, hoof malformations, hair loss, and emaciation (3). Laboratory rats chronically poisoned with selenium exhibit growth depression and cirrhosis. The mechanism of selenium toxicity is not known, and the toxic effects of selenium may be modified by adaptation and certain dietary factors (13). No sensitive and specific biochemical test is currently available to indicate overexposure to selenium (105).

Public health surveys carried out in seleniferous areas of the United States failed to establish any symptom specific for selenium poisoning (106–108). Field studies conducted in Venezuela showed a higher incidence of dermatitis, loose hair, and diseased nails in children from a seleniferous area than in those from Caracas, a nonseleniferous area, but no differences were seen in the various biochemical tests performed (109). A report from China described an outbreak of endemic selenium poisoning in humans (14); the most common sign of intoxication was loss of hair and nails. In high-incidence areas, lesions of the skin, nervous system, and possibly teeth were observed. Biochemical analyses showed a change in the ratio of plasma selenium to erythrocyte selenium at selenium intakes over 750 μg/day (110). Signs of selenosis (nail changes) were seen in susceptible patients at intakes of 910 μg/day or more, corresponding to a blood selenium level of 13.3 μmol/L or higher. No signs or symptoms of selenium overexposure were observed among residents of seleniferous ranches in South Dakota or Wyoming whose dietary intake was as high as 724 μg/day (108). However, an episode of human selenium poisoning was reported in the United States in 1984 involving 13 persons who consumed a "health food" supplement that contained 182 times the selenium content listed in the label declaration, because of a manufacturing error (111, 112). The total amount of selenium consumed by these subjects was thought to have been between 27 and 2387 mg. Signs and symptoms of poisoning included nausea, diarrhea, irritability, fatigue, peripheral neuropathy, hair loss, and nail changes.

Based on the Chinese data discussed above, the U.S. Environmental Protection Agency formulated a reference dose (RfD) for selenium (113). The RfD is a toxicologic standard defined (114) as "an estimate (with uncertainty spanning perhaps an order of magnitude) of a daily exposure to the human population (including sensitive subgroups) that is likely to be without an appreciable risk of deleterious effects during a lifetime" and is calculated by the following formula:

$$RfD = (NOAEL \text{ or } LOAEL)/(UF \times MF)$$

where *NOAEL* is the no-observed-adverse-effect level, *LOAEL* is the lowest-observed-adverse-effect level, and *UF* and *MF* are various uncertainty factors and modifying factors, respectively (114). For selenium, an NOAEL of 0.853 mg/day was used, which for 55-kg persons would yield a value of 0.015 mg/kg/day. The NOAEL was calculated from whole-blood selenium concentrations measured in residents of the high-selenium area who exhibited no clinical signs of selenosis. Then the RfD was calculated using a UF of 3:

$$\text{RfD} = 0.015/3 = 0.005 \text{ mg/kg/day}$$

The UF of 3 was selected to take into account sensitive individuals via intraspecies extrapolation. For the standard 70-kg male, the RfD would be 0.005 × 70 or 350 μg/day. Chinese investigators familiar with the episodes of selenosis in their country suggested 400 μg/day as the maximum safe dietary selenium intake (115). Similarly, the WHO Expert Consultation proposed 400 μg/day as the upper limit of the safe range of adult population mean intake of selenium (8).

HIGH-RISK CLINICAL SITUATIONS

Subjects who are proved selenium deficient by biochemical testing can be considered to be at risk for developing pathologic conditions in response to certain stresses. Unfortunately, the particular stresses concerned are not well characterized. They may be nutritional, chemical, or infectious. Keshan disease is thought to be such a condition that occurs only in selenium-deficient subjects, perhaps triggered by oxidative stress or viral infection. Several patients who were selenium deficient as a result of receiving TPN were reported to have developed a cardiomyopathy similar to Keshan disease (116). Such selenium-deficient individuals might be sensitive to injury by drugs and chemicals, such as nitrofurantoin, in the same way as selenium-deficient animals are.

TPN solutions now contain selenium, so selenium deficiency in patients depending on this type of alimentation is now rare. Semipurified medical diets used to treat conditions such as phenylketonuria are often low in selenium and can produce deficiency of the element. Thus, specialized diets to be fed for protracted periods need to be evaluated for selenium to prevent development of selenium deficiency. Selenium deficiency does not occur in free-living healthy individuals in the United States. Because of food distribution patterns, people living in areas with very low soil selenium eat foods that are produced elsewhere and thus escape becoming deficient. Only populations living in selenium-deficient areas and eating local foods can be expected to develop biochemical selenium deficiency. Those populations are found in small countries that are almost entirely low in selenium or in low-selenium areas of large countries that do not distribute food among their regions.

REFERENCES

1. Moxon AL, Rhian MA. Physiol Rev 1943;23:305–37.
2. Schwarz K, Foltz CM. J Am Chem Soc 1957;79:3292–3.
3. National Research Council. Selenium in nutrition. (Revised) Washington, DC: National Academy of Sciences, 1983.
4. Rotruck JT, Pope AL, Ganther HE, et al. Science 1973;179:588–90.
5. Keshan Disease Research Group. Chin Med J 1979;92:471–6.
6. van Rij AM, Thomson CD, McKenzie JM, et al. Am J Clin Nutr 1979;32:2076–85.
7. National Research Council. Recommended dietary allowances. 10th ed. Washington, DC: National Academy of Sciences, 1989.
8. World Health Organization. Trace elements in human nutrition and health. Geneva: WHO, 1996.
9. Gladyshev VN, Khangulov SV, Stadtman TC. Proc Natl Acad Sci USA 1994;91:232–6.
10. Stadtman TC. Annu Rev Biochem 1996;65:83–100.
11. Bopp BA, Sonders RC, Kesterson JW. Drug Metab Rev 1982;13:271–318.
12. Kato T, Read R, Rozga J, Burk RF. Am J Physiol 1992;262: G854–8.
13. International Programme on Chemical Safety. Environmental health criteria 58. Selenium. Geneva: WHO, 1987.
14. Yang GQ, Wang S, Zhou R, et al. Am J Clin Nutr 1983;37:872–81.
15. Rayman MP. Br Med J 1997;314:387–8.
16. National Research Council. The contribution of drinking water to mineral nutrition in humans. In: Drinking water and

health, vol 3. Washington, DC: National Academy of Sciences, 1980.
17. Pennington JAT, Young BE, Wilson DB. J Am Diet Assoc 1989;89:659–64.
18. Robinson MF. Nutr Rev 1989;47:99–107.
19. Varo P, Alfthan G, Huttunen JK, Aro A. Nationwide selenium supplementation in Finland—effects on diet, blood and tissue levels, and health. In: Burk RF, ed. Selenium in biology and medicine. New York: Springer-Verlag, 1994;197–215.
20. Patterson BH, Levander OA. Cancer Epidemiol Biomarkers Prev 1997;6:63–9.
21. Levander OA. Fed Proc 1983;42:1721–5.
22. Chansler MW, Mutanen M, Morris VC, et al. Nutr Res 1986;6:1419–28.
23. Levander OA, Alfthan G, Arvilommi H, et al. Am J Clin Nutr 1983;37:887–97.
24. Thompson JN, Scott ML. J Nutr 1969;97:335–42.
25. Levander OA, Cheng L. Ann NY Acad Sci 1980;355:1–372.
26. Parizek J, Ostadalova I, Kalouskova A, et al. The detoxifying effects of selenium: interrelations between compounds of selenium and certain metals. In: Mertz W, Cornatzer WE, eds. Newer trace elements in nutrition. New York: Marcel Dekker, 1971;85–122.
27. Levander OA, Burk RF. Selenium. In: Ziegler EE, Filer LJ, eds. Present knowledge in nutrition. Washington, DC: ILSI Press, 1996;320–8.
28. Esaki N, Nakamura T, Tanaka H, et al. J Biol Chem 1982;257:4386–91.
29. Mozier NM, McConnell KD, Hoffman JL. J Biol Chem 1988;263:4527–31.
30. Swanson CA, Patterson BH, Levander OA, et al. Am J Clin Nutr 1991;54:917–26.
31. Low SC, Harney JW, Berry MJ. J Biol Chem 1995;270:21659–64.
32. Guimaraes MJ, Peterson D, Vicari A, et al. Proc Natl Acad Sci USA 1996;93:15086–91.
33. Böck A. Incorporation of selenium into bacterial selenoproteins. In: Burk RF, ed. Selenium in biology and human health. New York: Springer-Verlag, 1994;9–24.
34. Berry MJ, Larsen PR. Endocr Rev 1992;13:207–19.
35. Shen Q, McQuilken PA, Newburger PE. J Biol Chem 1995;270:30448–52.
36. Low SC, Berry MJ. Trends Biochem Sci 1996;21:203–8.
37. Burk RF, Brown DG, Seely RJ, et al. J Nutr 1972;102:1049–55.
38. Suzuki KT, Itoh M, Ohmichi M. Toxicology 1996;103:157–65.
39. Chu F-F, Doroshow JH, Esworthy RS. J Biol Chem 1993;268:2571–6.
40. Takahashi K, Cohen HJ. Blood 1986;68:640–5.
41. Ursini F, Maiorino M, Gregolin C. Biochim Biophys Acta 1985;839:62–70.
42. Salvatore D, Bartha T, Harney JW, et al. Endocrinology 1996;137:3308–15.
43. Croteau W, Whittemore SL, Schneider MJ, et al. J Biol Chem 1995;270:16569–75.
44. Tamura T, Stadtman TC. Proc Natl Acad Sci USA 1996;93:1006–11.
45. Yang J-G, Morrison-Plummer J, Burk RF. J Biol Chem 1987;262:13372–5.
46. Vendeland SC, Beilstein MA, Chen CL, et al. J Biol Chem 1993;268:17103–7.
47. Burk RF. Selenium-dependent glutathione peroxidases. In: Guengerich FP, ed. Comprehensive toxicology, vol 3. Biotransformation. Oxford: Pergamon, 1997;229–42.
48. Ursini F, Maiorino M, Brigelius-Flohe R, et al. Methods Enzymol 1995;252B:38–53.
49. Chu F-F, Esworthy RS, Doroshow JH, et al. Blood 1992;79:3233–8.
50. Pushpa-Rekha TR, Burdsall AL, Oleksa LM, et al. J Biol Chem 1995;270:26993–9.
51. Holmgren A, Björnstedt M. Methods Enzymol 1995;252:199–208.
52. Gladyshev VN, Jeang K-T, Stadtman TC. Proc Natl Acad Sci USA 1996;93:6146–51.
52a. May JM, Mendiratta S, Hill KE, et al. J Biol Chem 1997;272:22607–10.
53. Hill KE, McCollum GW, Boeglin ME, et al. Biochem Biophys Res Comm 1997;234:293–5.
54. Herrman JL. Biochim Biophys Acta 1977;500:61–70.
55. Hill KE, Lloyd RS, Yang J-G, et al. J Biol Chem 1991;266:10050–3.
56. Burk RF, Hill KE, Boeglin ME, et al. Histochem Cell Biol 1997;108:11–5.
57. Saijoh K, Saito N, Lee MJ, et al. Mol Brain Res 1995;30:301–11.
58. Himeno S, Chittum HS, Burk RF. J Biol Chem 1996;271:15769–75.
59. Hill KE, Xia Y, Åkesson B, et al. J Nutr 1996;126:138–45.
60. Burk RF, Hill KE, Awad JA, et al. Hepatology 1995;21:561–9.
61. Yeh J-Y, Gu Q-P, Beilstein MA, et al. J Nutr 1997;127:394–402.
62. Reiter R, Wendel A. Biochem Pharmacol 1983;32:3063–7.
63. Hill KE, Burk RF, Lane JM. J Nutr 1987;117:99–104.
64. Beckett GJ, MacDougall DA, Nicol F, et al. Biochem J 1989;259:887–92.
65. Fischer WC, Whanger PD. J Nutr 1977;107:1493–1501.
66. Taylor EW, Ramanathan CS, Jalluri RK, et al. J Med Chem 1994;37:2637–54.
67. McCoy KEM, Weswig PH. J Nutr 1969;98:383–9.
68. Thompson JN, Scott ML. J Nutr 1970;100:797–809.
69. Whitacre ME, Combs GF Jr, Combs SB, et al. J Nutr 1987;117:460–7.
70. Combs GF Jr, Liu CH, Lu ZH, et al. J Nutr 1984;114:964–76.
71. Muth OH, Weswig PH, Whanger PD, et al. Am J Vet Res 1971;32:1603–5.
72. Butler JA, Whanger PD, Patton NM. J Am Coll Nutr 1988;7:43–56.
73. Awasthi YC, Beutler E, Srivastava SK. J Biol Chem 1975;250:5144–9.
74. Ge K, Xue A, Bai J, et al. Virchows Arch [A] 1983;401:1–15.
75. Keshan Disease Research Group. Chin Med J 1979;92:477–82.
76. Yang G, Chen J, Wen Z, et al. Adv Nutr Res 1984;6:203–31.
77. Xia Y, Hill KE, Burk RF. J Nutr 1989;119:1318–26.
78. Yang G, Ge K, Chen J, et al. World Rev Nutr Diet 1988;55:98–152.
79. Ge KY, Bai J, Deng XJ, et al. The protective effect of selenium against viral myocarditis in mice. In: Combs GF Jr, Spallholz JE, Levander OA, et al., eds. Selenium in biology and medicine, part B. New York: Van Nostrand Reinhold, 1987;761–8.
80. Beck MA, Kolbeck PC, Rohr LH, et al. J Infect Dis 1994;170:351–7.
81. Beck MA, Kolbeck PC, Rohr LH, et al. J Med Virol 1994;43:166–70.
82. Beck MA, Shi Q, Morris VC, Levander OA. Nature Med 1995;1:433–6.
83. Allander E. Scand J Rheum 1994;23:1–6.
84. World Health Organization. Kashin Beck disease and non-communicable diseases. Beijing: Chinese Academy of Preventive Medicine, 1990.
85. Willett WC, Stampfer MJ. Br Med J 1988;297:573–4.
86. Levander OA. Annu Rev Nutr 1987;7:227–50.
87. Birt DF, Pour PM, Pelling JC. The influence of dietary sele-

nium on colon, pancreas, and skin tumorigenesis. In: Wendel A, ed. Selenium in biology and medicine. Berlin: Springer-Verlag, 1989;297–304.
88. Blot WJ, Li JY, Taylor PR, et al. J Natl Cancer Inst 1993;85: 1483–92.
89. Clark LC, Combs GF, Turnbull BW, et al. JAMA 1996;276: 1957–63.
90. Herbert V. JAMA 1997;277:880.
91. Colditz GA. JAMA 1996;276:1984–5.
92. Thomson CD, Robinson MF. Am J Clin Nutr 1980;33:303–23.
93. Allaway WH, Kubota J, Losee F, et al. Arch Environ Health 1968;16:342–8.
94. Levander OA, Morris VC. Am J Clin Nutr 1984;39:809–15.
95. Snook JT, Palmquist DL, Moxon AL, et al. Am J Clin Nutr 1983;38:620–30.
96. McMaster D, Bell N, Anderson P, et al. Clin Chem 1990;36:211–6.
97. Salbe AD, Levander OA. J Nutr 1990;120:200–6.
98. Morris JS, Stampfer MJ, Willett WC. Biol Trace Elem Res 1983;5:529–37.
99. Welsh SO, Holden JM, Wolf WR, et al. J Am Diet Assoc 1981;79:277–85.
100. Thomson CD, Rea HM, Doesburg VM, et al. Br J Nutr 1977;37:457–60.
101. Ganther HE, Hafeman DG, Lawrence RA, et al. Selenium and glutathione peroxidase in health and disease—a review. In: Prasad AS, ed. Trace elements in human health and disease, vol 2. Essential and toxic elements. New York: Academic Press, 1976;165–234.
102. National Research Council. Recommended Dietary Allowances. 9th ed. Washington, DC: National Academy of Sciences, 1980.
103. Yang GQ, Qian PC, Zhu LZ, et al. Human selenium requirements in China. In: Combs GF Jr, Spallholz JE, Levander OA, et al., eds. Selenium in biology and medicine. New York: Van Nostrand Reinhold, 1987;589–607.
104. Levander OA. J Nutr 1989;119:1869–73.
105. Levander OA. Selenium: biochemical actions, interactions and some human health implications. In: Prasad AS, ed. Clinical, biochemical and nutritional aspects of trace elements. New York: Alan R Liss, 1982;345–68.
106. Smith MI, Franke KW, Westfall BB. Public Health Rep 1936;51:1496–505.
107. Smith MI, Westfall BB. Public Health Rep 1937;52:1375–84.
108. Longnecker MP, Taylor PR, Levander OA, et al. Am J Clin Nutr 1991;53:1288–94.
109. Jaffe WG. Effect of selenium intake in humans and in rats. In: Proceedings of the symposium Selenium-Tellurium in the Environment. Pittsburgh: Industrial Health Foundation, 1976;188–93.
110. Yang G, Yin S, Zhou R, et al. J Trace Elem Electrolytes Health Dis 1989;3:123–30.
111. Jensen R, Clossen W, Rothenberg R. MMWR 1984;33:157–8.
112. Helzlsouer K, Jacobs R, Morris S. Fed Proc 1985;44:1670.
113. Poirier KA. Summary of the derivation of the reference dose for selenium. In: Mertz W, Abernathy CO, Olin SS, eds. Risk assessment of essential elements. Washington, DC: ILSI Press, 1994;157–66.
114. Dourson ML. Methods for establishing oral reference doses. In: Mertz W, Abernathy CO, Olin SS, eds. Risk assessment of essential elements. Washington, DC: ILSI Press, 1994;51–61.
115. Yang GQ, Xia YM. Biomed Environ Sci 1995;8:187–201.
116. Lockitch G, Taylor GP, Wong LTK, et al. Am J Clin Nutr 1990;52:572–7.

15. Chromium

BARBARA J. STOECKER

HISTORICAL INTRODUCTION

In 1959, chromium was identified as an element that potentiates insulin action and restores normal glucose tolerance in rats (1). Subsequently, infants recovering from malnutrition responded to an oral supplement of 250 μg (4.8 μmol) chromium as chromium chloride with improved glucose removal rates. In a patient receiving total parenteral nutrition (TPN), Jeejeebhoy et al. demonstrated that infusing 250 μg (4.8 μmol) chromium as chromium chloride markedly reduced exogenous insulin requirements as well as lowering circulating glucose and free fatty acid levels (2). Other investigators have confirmed benefits of supplementation with chromium chloride in two additional TPN patients. (For citations to additional references concerning chromium, the reader is referred to several reviews [3–7]).

CHEMISTRY AND NOMENCLATURE

Chromium (MW, 52 g/mol) occurs in multiple valence states, and marked differences based on valence characterize absorption, tissue distribution, and potential toxicity of chromium (5, 8, 9). Most chromium in the food supply is in the trivalent state (8). Any chromium (VI) in food or water as a contaminant should be reduced to chromium (III) by the acidic environment of the stomach (9). Chromium (III) can bind with a number of ligands to form complexes. Chromium is exchanged slowly from these complexes, which makes it unlikely that chromium functions at the active site of a metalloenzyme (8).

Chromium (VI), which usually occurs as chromate or dichromate, is a strong oxidizing agent. Because of their oxidative ability, chromium (VI) compounds are irritating and are potential health hazards.

BIOLOGIC ACTIVITY

Chromium salts differ substantially in solubility (8, 9), and these solubility differences are important in determining the absorption and use of chromium. In addition, chromium (III) can be complexed with many different ligands, which may enhance or hinder both its absorption and tissue retention.

A "glucose tolerance factor" form of chromium was hypothesized originally by Mertz (8) to contain chromium bound to nicotinic acid and the amino acids glycine, cysteine, and glutamic acid. The complex enhanced glucose tolerance and was a low-molecular-weight, dialyzable compound. It has not been possible to purify this particular compound, although some of the low-molecular-weight chromium compounds isolated from biologic fluids do show an ultraviolet-absorbing peak corresponding to nicotinic acid. Furthermore, certain other extracted compounds potentiated insulin activity to a greater extent than chromium chloride alone.

DIETARY CONSIDERATIONS

Food Sources

Chromium is widely distributed, albeit in small quantities, throughout the food supply. Whole grains and cereals contain higher concentrations of chromium than fruits or vegetables (10). Chromium may be added or removed during food processing (11). Refined sugars and flour usually are lower in chromium than less refined products (10); however, acidic foods take up chromium from contact with stainless steel (11). Processed meats are quite high in chromium (10).

Bioavailability

Because of the very low chromium concentrations in biologic tissues, its bioavailability is difficult to assess in humans. However, the solubility of chromium salts varies, and chromium absorption is sensitive to physiochemical reactions within the gastrointestinal tract (8, 9, 12). Several studies in rats examined the tissue distribution of chromium-51 (^{51}Cr) that was chelated to different ligands. Anderson et al. (13) reported that chromium concentrations in kidney were significantly higher after feeding a complex containing chromium dinicotinic acid, diglycine, cysteine, and glutamic acid for 3 weeks than after feeding eight other chromium compounds. However, the identified complex did not produce such clear concentration differences in liver, spleen, muscle, lung, and heart (13).

High-fiber intakes raise concerns about the bioavailability of dietary trace minerals. One study in rats indicated that phytate impaired, and oxalate enhanced, absorption of ^{51}Cr. Two other studies in rats found no reduction in ^{51}Cr absorption with lower concentrations of phytate in the diet.

The bioavailability of chromium from human milk is important because breast-fed infants have chromium intakes well below (14) the current estimated safe and adequate daily dietary intake (ESADDI) recommendations. No studies in humans have compared the bioavailability of chromium from human milk and formulas. The extremely low chromium concentrations in biologic fluids and tissues would make chromium bioavailability studies in human infants very difficult.

Nutrient-Nutrient Interrelationships

Chromium uptake is enhanced by simultaneous administration with ascorbate in both human beings and experimental animals. Offenbacher (15) administered 1 mg (19.2 μmol) chromium as chromium chloride with and without 100 mg (0.56 mmol) ascorbate and monitored plasma chromium concentrations for 8 hours. The plasma chromium concentration was consistently enhanced by the presence of ascorbate. In rats dosed with $^{51}CrCl_3$, oral supplementation with ascorbate increased [^{51}Cr] in urine without reducing tissue concentrations, which also suggests that ascorbate enhanced ^{51}Cr absorption (16).

Absorption of ^{51}Cr from $^{51}CrCl_3$ was enhanced in zinc-deficient rats, and oral administration of zinc decreased ^{51}Cr absorption in zinc-deficient rats (reviewed in [6]). Chromium absorption was higher in iron-deficient mice than in iron-replete mice (reviewed in [6]). These observations raise the issue of mineral-mineral competition for absorption.

Tissue chromium concentrations generally were higher in mice fed starch as a carbohydrate source than in those fed sucrose, fructose, or glucose (17). Some 19 men and 18 women consumed a diet containing either 35% of total calories from complex carbohydrates and 15% from simple sugars (reference diet) or a diet containing 35% of total calories from simple sugars and 15% from complex carbohydrates (high-sugar diet). The high-sugar diet enhanced urinary chromium losses in 27 of 37 subjects, for a significantly increased mean excretion (18).

Nutrient-Drug Interrelationships

Some commonly used medications affect absorption of ^{51}Cr from $^{51}CrCl_3$ in rats. Administration by gavage of large doses of antacids composed of calcium carbonate or magnesium hydroxide significantly reduced [^{51}Cr] in blood, tissues, and urine 6 to 12 hours after oral dosing with $^{51}CrCl_3$ (16, 19). Aspirin and indomethacin, which block the synthesis of prostaglandins, increased ^{51}Cr absorption (19, 20), while oral dosing with 16,16-dimethyl prostaglandin E_2 decreased ^{51}Cr absorption (20). Total chromium administration was low (<180 ng [<3.5 nmol] per rat) in these studies but was consistent with the low intakes required to demonstrate signs of chromium depletion in rodents. However, in another study, rats were dosed with less than 1000 ng (19.2 nmol) of chromium, and several prostaglandins did not affect chromium retention (21). These relationships need to be clarified.

Adequacy of Intakes

Lack of an appropriate indicator of status makes assessment of adequacy of chromium intake problematic. Chromium balance was monitored for 12 days in a metabolic unit in two normal males consuming a mean of 36.9 and 36.7 μg (0.71 μmol) chromium per day from the diet. Apparent net retention was 0.6 and 0.2 μg (12 and 4 nmol)/day, respectively, indicating that the subjects were in equilibrium (22). Bunker et al. (23) conducted a 5-day balance study with 22 apparently healthy elderly people between 69 and 86 years of age. Mean daily intake was 24.5 μg (471 nmol), with a mean retention of 0.2 μg (4 nmol), again indicating apparent adequacy of less than 25 μg (<480 nmol) chromium intake per day. In another study, subjects with serum glucose concentrations below 100 mg/dL (<5.56 mmol/L) 90 minutes after an oral glucose load were fed diets containing less than 20 μg/day chromium for a total of 9 weeks without apparent change in their glucose tolerance (24). Their glucose, insulin, and glucagon values also did not change in response to 4 weeks of chromium supplementation. On the other hand, upon feeding the same diet to subjects who initially presented with glucose values between 100 and 200 mg/dL (5.57–11.1 mmol/L) 90 minutes after a glucose load, glucose, insulin, and glucagon sums (over a glucose tolerance test) showed significant reductions after 4 weeks of supplementation with 200 μg chromium as chromium chloride (24).

These three carefully conducted studies suggest that the actual need for chromium in many healthy adults is substantially less than current recommendations (50–200 μg/day). Unfortunately, long-term studies in which diets have been supplemented with doses such as 25 or 50 μg (0.48–0.96 μmol) chromium, which would double or triple usual dietary intakes (~15 μg/1000 kcal) (10), have not yet been conducted. Such studies would allow fine-tuning of dietary recommendations.

Another indication that the requirement for chromium may be quite low is that the mean breast milk chromium concentration is approximately 0.18 ng/mL (3.43 nmol/L) (14). Thus, exclusively breast-fed infants would receive approximately 130 ng/day (2.5 nmol) chromium (14) or less than 1.3% of the current lower limit of the ESADDI for infants (10–40 μg). No studies of the bioavailability of chromium from breast milk have been conducted in human infants.

METABOLISM

Digestion

Solubility of any mineral in food is affected by reduction potential, pH, and processing techniques as well as by complex formation. Transition-series minerals, including chromium, can form hydrates that may become hydroxides as gastrointestinal pH is increased. The hydroxides may precipitate or form large aggregates with reduced solubility (8, 12).

Absorption

Dowling and colleagues (reviewed in [6]) used an in situ double-perfusion technique in which both the intestinal vasculature and the intestinal lumen were perfused to investigate absorption mechanisms. Amino acids in the test meal and the presence of either albumin or transferrin in the vascular perfusate enhanced chromium absorption. On the basis of studies in rats perfused with 3.8 μg (73 nmol) chromium plus 3 μCi of ^{51}Cr as $^{51}CrCl_3$, the authors concluded that absorption was a nonmediated process of passive diffusion (6). However, they noted that other mechanisms might also operate under specific conditions.

Chromium-depleted guinea pigs dosed with less than 200 ng (<3.8 nmol) ^{51}Cr as $^{51}CrCl_3$ absorbed a higher percentage of ^{51}Cr than did controls fed adequate chromium diets (25). In humans, Anderson and Kozlovsky (26) similarly reported that a higher percentage of dietary chromium intake was absorbed when dietary intakes were low, which also indicates some homeostatic control of absorption.

Transport

Chromium is transported primarily by transferrin (27). Incubation of serum with iron reduced the amount of ^{51}Cr bound by transferrin (27).

Storage

Chromium is a bone-seeking element (28), and its uptake in bone appears to be rapid. Several investigators have noted that chromium accumulates in bone, spleen, liver, and kidney. O'Flaherty emphasized the need for physiologically based kinetic modeling to understand the behavior of bone-seeking minerals (28). Early modeling work using rats indicated three pools for chromium with half-lives of less than 1 day, approximately 1 week, and 7 to 12 weeks. A recent model in humans suggested four compartments, with different half-lives for diabetic and normal subjects in at least some of the compartments (29). The half-life of chromium in the compartment that turned over most slowly was 346 days. This compartment presumably is related to long-term tissue deposition (29).

Homeostatic Regulation

Studies in guinea pigs (25) and humans (26) indicate that chromium absorption is higher when chromium intakes are low. Specifically, in humans, Anderson and Kozlovsky (26) noted that when dietary chromium intakes reached 40 μg (0.77 μmol)/day, apparent absorption (measured by urinary excretion) dropped to 0.5% per day.

Excretion

Most ingested chromium is excreted in the feces. In balance studies, Offenbacher et al. recovered a mean of 98.1% of the dietary chromium in stools (22). Excretion via the bile does not appear to be a major contributor to fecal chromium (7). Urinary excretion increased fourfold following a supplemental dose of 200 μg (3.8 μmol) chromium as $CrCl_3$ (30). Also, tannery workers who were occupationally exposed to trivalent chromium had significantly higher urinary chromium excretion than controls, and their urinary chromium declined significantly during a weekend without exposure to chromium (31).

Increased chromium excretion induced by stress may be an important factor exacerbating chromium deficiency (32). Ascorbate-depleted guinea pigs had high circulating cortisol concentrations (33) and excreted more ^{51}Cr from an oral dose of $^{51}CrCl_3$ than controls (33). Patients who had experienced physical trauma excreted more chromium than normally in urine (34). Furthermore, the urinary chromium excretion of distance runners was approximately doubled on the day of a 6-mile run, compared with a rest day (35).

FUNCTIONS

Chromium potentiates the action of insulin in vitro and in vivo. Mertz (4) recently summarized the results of 15 controlled studies in which subjects with impaired glucose tolerance were supplemented with defined chromium (III) compounds. In 12 of these studies, chromium supplementation improved the efficiency of insulin or had beneficial effects on the blood lipid profiles. The reasons for lack of response to chromium in the remaining three studies are uncertain; however, chromium depletion is not the only cause of impaired glucose tolerance. Furthermore, chromium status of subjects in supplementation trials still cannot be adequately assessed; a nonpharmacologic response to chromium supplementation would be expected only if the subjects were chromium depleted. Recent preliminary reports suggest that chromium supplementation may benefit diabetics, but these studies have not yet been published in their entirety.

A number of beneficial effects of chromium on lipid profiles have been reported. Responses are not consistent from study to study, but total cholesterol, low-density-lipoprotein (LDL)-cholesterol, and triglyceride levels have decreased, while HDL-cholesterol and apolipoprotein A levels have increased. These studies have been reviewed recently (4–7).

Intense public interest has emerged in using chromium as an ergogenic (muscle-building) aid. Chromium is second only to calcium in mineral supplement sales at the present time (5). This enthusiasm is surprising, given the equivocal effects on body composition seen to date in human studies. Evans (36) first reported an effect of chromium on body composition: young men undergoing resistance training and taking chromium picolinate supplements (200 μg [3.8 μmol] Cr daily) increased lean body mass and decreased fat mass. Skinfold thickness measurements were used to estimate changes in lean body mass. Several additional studies with both positive and negative results have been reviewed (5–7).

Two recent studies have used very sensitive techniques to estimate body composition. Lukaski et al. (37) supplemented 36 young men with placebo, chromium chloride, or chromium picolinate as they participated in an 8-week weight-training program. Fat-free mass, mineral-free mass, and body fat were estimated by dual x-ray absorptiometry. While resistive exercise increased lean body mass, no effects of chromium supplementation on either fat-free mass or body fat were found. Hallmark et al. (38) likewise supplemented 16 untrained healthy males undergoing a 12-week resistive-exercise program with 200 μg (3.8 μmol)/day chromium as picolinate or with placebo. Based on food records, these men were consuming approximately 36 μg (0.7 μmol) chromium from their diets. The authors assessed body composition with hydrodensitometry and found no significant differences in lean body mass, percentage body fat, or strength measurements as a result of chromium supplementation.

Chromium supplementation trials have also been conducted in rapidly growing food animals. Barrows were fed a fortified, corn-soybean meal basal diet supplemented with 0 or 200 μg (3.8 μmol)/kg diet of chromium as chromium picolinate. In this study, addition of chromium picolinate to the diet increased the accretion of muscle tissue and decreased the total gain of fat (39). In a study using gilts of a similar size, basal diets were supplemented with 300 μg (5.8 μmol) chromium/kg diet as chromium picolinate and recombinant porcine somatotropin (rPST) was administered to half of the pigs in a 2 × 2 factorial design. All rPST-treated gilts demonstrated better growth than controls. Diets supplemented with chromium picolinate, however, produced no differences in growth performance (40).

Effects of chromium on morbidity in livestock stressed by shipping or disease exposure have received a great deal of recent attention. Chromium significantly decreased serum cortisol (41, 42) and increased serum immunoglobulin M and total immunoglobulins in stressed and growing calves (42). Supplemental chromium also lowered serum cortisol after a disease challenge (41, 42).

KEY CAUSES OF DEFICIENCY AND THEIR MANIFESTATIONS

Chromium deficiency has been reported in three patients who did not receive supplemental chromium in their TPN solutions. The first, a female who had received TPN for more than 3.5 years, developed unexplained weight loss and peripheral neuropathy. Glucose removal from the plasma was impaired and her respiratory quotient was low, indicating preferential use of fat for fuel. Addition of 250 μg (4.8 μmol) chromium to the daily TPN infusate for 2 weeks restored the glucose removal rate and increased her respiratory quotient (2). Another patient developed severe hyperglycemia and rapid weight loss after 5 months of TPN therapy without added chromium (see reviews). The third patient developed weight loss, glycosuria, and hyperglycemia after 7 months of TPN. This patient was receiving 6 μg (0.12 μmol)/day of chromium, but the situation was perhaps complicated by jejunostomy losses. The American Medical Association has recommended supplementing TPN solutions with chromium (43). However, a number of different TPN solutions contain a fairly high basal level of chromium (34, 44), and a recent report suggests that some TPN patients may be exposed to excessive amounts of trivalent chromium, primarily as a contaminant from amino acids in the solutions (44).

The hypothesis has been advanced by Nielsen (32) that alterations in metabolism secondary to malnutrition, disease, injury, or stress may be responsible for deficiencies of the ultratrace elements. A number of studies in animals and humans lend support to his hypothesis. Trauma patients excreted more urinary chromium than normal controls (34). Strenuous exercise causes "dumping" of chromium in the urine (35). Guinea pigs excreted more ^{51}Cr from $^{51}CrCl_3$ when they were stressed by ascorbate depletion (25). Many of the studies in farm animals that report beneficial effects of chromium supplementation also involved some type of stress: shipping, infectious agents, crowding, hot temperatures.

Finally, some commonly used medications may interfere with chromium absorption. Chronic effects of these medications have not been investigated in relation to chromium; however, studies have indicated a negative effect of antacids on iron and copper status.

EVALUATION OF NUTRIENT STATUS

Currently, there is no reliable indicator of chromium status. Chromium in blood is very difficult to measure because the extremely low concentrations approach the detection limits of even sensitive instruments. Furthermore, serum or plasma chromium may not be in equilibrium with other body pools. No enzyme has been identified for which chromium is specific. Thus, both nutritional and clinical assessments are difficult. In the absence of reliable indicators of chromium status, considerable diversity must exist in the chromium status of patients in supplementation trials.

REQUIREMENTS AND RECOMMENDED INTAKES

Humans

The current ESADDI for adults of 50 to 200 μg (0.96–3.8 μmol)/day for chromium, established in 1980, was not changed in the 10th edition of the recommended dietary allowances (RDAs), published in 1989 (45) (see also Appendix Table II-A-2-a-2). Until the late 1970s, techniques and instrumentation for measuring the very low concentrations of chromium in biologic materials were very limited, and many laboratories reported mean daily urinary chromium excretion substantially above 2 μg/day. There is consensus that chromium absorption is between 0.5 and 2%. Thus, the ESADDI for adults was established in line with the data available at that time, and values for infants (10–40 μg) and children were extrapolated.

Anderson and Kozlovsky (26) determined the chromium content of self-selected diets of 10 males and 22 females for 7 consecutive days. The 7-day average intake for males was 33 μg (0.63 μmol)/day (range, 22–48 μg) and for females was 25 μg (0.48 μmol)/day (range, 13–36 μg). Mean chromium intake per 1000 kcal was approximately 15 μg (0.29 μmol). They observed that when dietary chromium intake was 10 μg (0.19 μmol), urinary excretion (representing absorption) was approximately 2%. With increasing intake to 40 μg (0.77 μmol), however, chromium absorption decreased to 0.5% (26).

Today, average urinary chromium excretion is considered to be approximately 0.20 ng/mL or approximately 0.4 μg/day for the average person. If absorption of 0.5 to 2% is assumed, the current ESADDI would be lowered substantially.

Experimental Animals

In experimental animals, dietary concentrations below 50 μg (0.96 μmol) chromium/kg diet are necessary to produce symptoms associated with chromium deficiency. The American Institute of Nutrition (AIN)-93 diet includes addition of chromium at the level of 1 mg (19.2 μmol) chromium/kg diet as chromium potassium sulfate and defines it as a "potentially beneficial mineral element" (46). Many experimental animals get enough chromium in their unsupplemented feed, however, to prevent well-recognized symptoms of deficiency.

TOXICOLOGY

Risk assessment for chromium is affected by its oxidation state. Trivalent chromium, which is the predominant form in the food supply, has low oral toxicity, at least partially because it is very poorly absorbed (8).

A recent report has generated some controversy about the safety of chromium (III) supplements (47). Relatively high concentrations of chromium picolinate, chromium chloride, or chromium nicotinate were added to Chinese hamster ovary cells in culture. Chromium picolinate and picolinic acid tested positive in an assay used to predict mutagenicity, while chromium nicotinate and chromium chloride did not (47). There have been many supplementation trials in humans with chromium chloride and with chelated chromium compounds without reports of toxicity. However, because of the current widespread use of chromium supplements, more research would be appropriate to evaluate the risk and cost/benefit ratios of trivalent chromium supplements.

On the other hand, chromium (VI), a product of manufacturing, is included in health risk assessments at Environmental Protection Agency superfund sites (9). Fortunately, certain foods and substances in our gastrointestinal tract have substantial capacity for reduction of chromium (VI) to chromium (III). For example, Kuykendall et al. (48) gave volunteers 5 mg (96 μmol) of chromium (VI), alone or fully reduced to chromium (III) with orange juice (prior to ingestion). They demonstrated no DNA-protein cross-links in leukocytes due to acute ingestion of either chromium (III) or (VI) and suggested that all of the chromium (VI) was reduced to chromium (III) intragastrically prior to absorption (48).

To evaluate further the in vivo genotoxicity of chromium (VI), Mirsalis et al. (49) administered chromium (VI) to mice at concentrations of 1, 5, or 20 mg (19.2, 96, or 384 μmol)/L in drinking water. These levels represent the range from a relevant human exposure level to the upper limit of palatability in rodents. They concluded that animals either had sufficient reductive capacity in their gastrointestinal tracts to prevent uptake of chromium (VI) or that even these high doses were insufficient to exert a genotoxic effect via oral administration (49).

Route of exposure has an impact on toxicity. Chromium (VI) is known to be a human pulmonary carcinogen. Stainless steel welding may be the most common source of occupational exposure to chromium. Various research groups have suggested that products formed during intracellular reduction of chromium (VI) to chromium (III) may be responsible for the DNA damage ascribed to chromium (VI) (50).

REFERENCES

1. Schwarz K, Mertz W. Arch Biochem Biophys 1959;85:292–5.
2. Jeejeebhoy KN, Chu RC, Marliss EB, et al. Am J Clin Nutr 1977;30:531–8.

3. Anderson RA. Chromium. In: Mertz W, ed. Trace elements in human and animal nutrition. 5th ed. New York: Academic Press, 1987;225–44.
4. Mertz W. J Nutr 1993;123:626–33.
5. Nielsen FH. Nutr Today 1996;31:226–33.
6. Offenbacher EG, Pi-Sunyer FX, Stoecker BJ. Chromium. In: O'Dell BL, Sunde RA, eds. Handbook of nutritionally essential mineral elements. New York: Marcel Dekker, 1997;389–411.
7. Stoecker BJ. Chromium. In: Ziegler EE, Filer LJ Jr, eds. Present knowledge in nutrition. 7th ed. Washington, DC: ILSI Press, 1996;N44–352.
8. Mertz W. Physiol Rev 1969;49:163–239.
9. O'Flaherty EJ. Comparison of reference dose with estimated safe and adequate daily dietary intake for chromium. In: Mertz W, Abernathy CO, eds. Risk assessment of essential elements. Washington, DC: ILSI Press, 1994;213–8.
10. Anderson RA, Bryden NA, Polansky MM. Biol Trace Elem Res 1992;32:117–21.
11. Offenbacher EG, Pi-Sunyer FX. J Agric Food Chem 1983;31: 89–92.
12. Clydesdale FM. Mineral interactions in food. In: Bodwell CE, Erdman JW, eds. Nutrient interactions. New York: Marcel Dekker, 1988;73–113.
13. Anderson RA, Bryden NA, Polansky MM, et al. J Trace Elem Exp Med 1996;9:11–25.
14. Anderson RA, Bryden NA, Patterson KY, et al. Am J Clin Nutr 1993;57:519–23.
15. Offenbacher EG. Trace Elem Elect 1994;11:178–81.
16. Seaborn CD, Stoecker BJ. Nutr Res 1990;10:1401–7.
17. Seaborn CD, Stoecker BJ. J Nutr 1989;119:1444–51.
18. Kozlovsky AS, Moser PB, Reiser S, et al. Metabolism 1986;35:515–8.
19. Davis ML, Seaborn CD, Stoecker BJ. Nutr Res 1995;15:202–10.
20. Kamath SM, Stoecker BJ, Davis-Whitenack ML, et al. J Nutr 1997;127:478–82.
21. Anderson RA, Polansky MM. Biol Trace Elem Res 1995;50:97–108.
22. Offenbacher E, Spencer H, Dowling HJ, et al. Am J Clin Nutr 1986;44:77–82.
23. Bunker VW, Lawson MS, Delves HT, et al. Am J Clin Nutr 1984;39:797–802.
24. Anderson RA, Polansky MM, Bryden NA, et al. Am J Clin Nutr 1991;54:909–16.
25. Seaborn CD, Stoecker BJ. Nutr Res 1992;12:1229–34.
26. Anderson RA, Kozlovsky AS. Am J Clin Nutr 1985;41:1177–83.
27. Hopkins LL Jr, Schwarz K. Biochim Biophys Acta 1964;90: 484–91.
28. O'Flaherty EJ. Toxicol Lett 1995;83:367–72.
29. Do Canto OM, Sargent T III, Liehn JC. Chromium (III) metabolism in diabetic patients. In: Sive Subrananian KN, Wastney ME, eds. Kinetic models of trace element and mineral metabolism. Boca Raton, FL: CRC Press, 1995;205–19.
30. Anderson RA, Polansky MM, Bryden NA, et al. Am J Clin Nutr 1982;36:1184–93.
31. Randall JA, Gibson RS. Proc Soc Exp Biol Med. 1987;185: 16–23.
32. Nielsen FH. Nutr Rev 1988;46:337–41.
33. Seaborn CD, Cheng NZ, Adeleye B, et al. Biol Trace Elem Res 1994;41:279–94.
34. Borel JS, Majerus TC, Polansky MM, et al. Biol Trace Elem Res 1984;6:317–26.
35. Anderson RA, Polansky MM, Bryden NA. Biol Trace Elem Res 1984;6:327–36.
36. Evans GW. Int J Biosocial Med Res 1989;11:163–80.
37. Lukaski HC, Bolonchuk WW, Siders WA, et al. Am J Clin Nutr 1996;63:954–65.
38. Hallmark MA, Reynolds TH, DeSouza CA, et al. Med Sci Sports Exerc 1996;28:139–44.
39. Mooney KW, Cromwell GL. J Anim Sci 1995;73:3351–7.
40. Myers MJ, Farrell DE, Evock-Clover CM, et al. Pathobiology 1995;63:283–7.
41. Kegley EB, Spears JW, Brown TT Jr. J Dairy Sci 1996;79: 1278–83.
42. Chang X, Mowat DN. J Anim Sci 1992;70:559–65.
43. Anonymous. JAMA 1979;241:2051–4.
44. Leung FY, Galbraith LV. Biol Trace Elem Res 1995;50:221–8.
45. National Research Council. Recommended dietary allowances. 10th ed. Washington, DC: National Academy Press, 1989; 241–3.
46. Reeves PG, Nielsen FH, Fahey GC Jr. J Nutr 1993;123:1939–51.
47. Stearns DM, Wise JP Sr, Patierno SR, et al. FASEB J 1995;9: 1643–9.
48. Kuykendall JR, Kerger BD, Jarvi EJ, et al. Carcinogenesis 1996;17:1971–7.
49. Mirsalis JC, Hamilton CM, O'Laughlin KG, et al. Environ Mol Mutagen 1996;28:60–3.
50. Stearns DM, Kennedy LJ, Courtney KD, et al. Biochemistry 1995;34:910–9.

SELECTED READINGS

Anderson RA. Chromium. In: Mertz W, ed. Trace elements in human and animal nutrition. 5th ed. New York: Academic Press, 1987;225–44.

Mertz W. Chromium in human nutrition: a review. J Nutr 1993;123:626–33.

Nielsen FH. Controversial chromium: does the superstar mineral of the mountebanks receive appropriate attention from clinicians and nutritionists? Nutr Today 1996;31:226–33.

Offenbacher EG, Pi-Sunyer FX, Stoecker BJ. Chromium. In: O'Dell BL, Sunde RA, eds. Handbook of nutritionally essential mineral elements. New York: Marcel Dekker, 1997;389–411.

Stoecker BJ. Chromium. In: Ziegler EE, Filer LJ Jr. eds. Present knowledge in nutrition. 7th ed. Washington, DC: ILSI Press, 1996;344–52.

16. Ultratrace Minerals[1]

FORREST H. NIELSEN

Ultratrace minerals are those elements with estimated dietary requirements usually less than 1 μg/g and often less than 50 ng/g of diet for laboratory animals (1). For humans, the term often is used for mineral elements with established, estimated, or suspected requirements below 1 mg/day, often expressed in micrograms per day. At least 18 elements could be considered ultratrace minerals: aluminum, arsenic, boron, bromine, cadmium, chromium, fluoride, germanium, iodine, lead, lithium, molybdenum, nickel, rubidium, selenium, silicon, tin, and vanadium. Two additional elements, cobalt and manganese, perhaps belong in the ultratrace category also. Although cobalt is required in ultratrace amounts, it has to be in the form of vitamin B_{12}; thus, it is usually discussed as a vitamin and is not considered here. An estimated safe and adequate daily dietary intake (ESADDI) for manganese of 2.5 to 5.0 mg/day has been established for adults (2); however, recent studies with humans suggest that the actual requirement may be near 1.0 mg/day. Even if it is above 1.0

[1]U.S. Department of Agriculture, Agriculture Research Service, Northern Plains Area is an equal opportunity/affirmative action employer and all agency services are available without discrimination.

mg/day, knowledge about the practical importance or beneficial actions of manganese is in a state similar to that for most of the ultratrace minerals; therefore it belongs in the discussion of the ultratrace minerals.

The quality of the experimental evidence for nutritional essentiality varies widely for the ultratrace elements. Evidence for the essentiality of the four elements iodine, manganese, molybdenum, and selenium is substantial and noncontroversial; specific biochemical functions have been defined for these elements. The nutritional importance of iodine and selenium are such that separate chapters have been devoted to them in this treatise. Manganese and molybdenum, however, are given less nutritional attention, apparently because deficiencies of these elements have only been unequivocally identified in a few individuals nourished by total parenteral nutrition (TPN) or with genetic defects causing metabolic disturbances involving these elements. Specific biochemical functions have not been defined for the other 15 elements; thus, their essentiality is based on circumstantial evidence, which most often is that dietary deprivation in some animal model results in a suboptimal biologic function that is prevented or reversed by an intake of physiologic amounts of the element in question. Often the circumstantial evidence includes biochemical actions suggesting a biologic role or beneficial actions in humans. The circumstantial evidence for essentiality is substantial for arsenic, boron, chromium, nickel, silicon, and vanadium; thus, except for chromium (discussed in Chapter 15), they are discussed in detail here. The evidence for essentiality of the other elements is generally limited to a few gross observations in one or two species by one or two research groups. Because it was judged premature to discuss these elements in detail here, they are only briefly mentioned at the end of the chapter. However, fluoride, which has a well-known beneficial pharmacologic property (anticariogenic), is discussed in detail.

ARSENIC

Historical Overview

For about 1100 years, through the 19th century, arsenic reigned as the king of poisons because some arsenic compounds were found to be convenient, scentless, and tasteless instruments for homicide. Although arsenic was considered synonymous with poison, by 1937, the pharmacologic actions of 8000 arsenicals had been recorded. Arsenicals were used at various times for the treatment of anorexia and other nutritional disturbances, syphilis, neuralgia, rheumatism, asthma, chorea, malaria, tuberculosis, diabetes, various skin diseases, and numerous hematologic abnormalities (3). The use of arsenicals for these disorders has either fallen into disrepute or been replaced by more effective alternatives. Although attempts to produce a nutritional arsenic deficiency first occurred in the 1930s, the first substantial evidence for arsenic essentiality appeared in 1975 and 1976 (4).

Chemistry

Both trivalent and pentavalent arsenic exists in biologic material. The most biochemically important organic arsenic compounds are those that contain methyl groups. Methylation of inorganic oxyarsenic anions occurs in organisms ranging from microbial to mammalian. The methylated end-products include arsenocholine, arsenobetaine, dimethylarsinic acid, and methylarsonic acid.

Other arsenic compounds of interest may be biologic molecules in which phosphate is replaced by arsenate. The relatively unstable nature of arsenyl esters is apparently why there is no direct evidence for the existence of compounds such as glucose-6-arsenate and adenosine diphosphate-arsenate. Nonetheless, an arsenate ester might be the form of arsenic that performs an essential function.

A comprehensive review of arsenic chemistry and biochemistry has been published (5).

Metabolism

Absorption of inorganic arsenic from the gastrointestinal tract correlates well with the solubility of the compound ingested (6). In humans and most laboratory animals, more than 90% of inorganic arsenate and arsenite fed in a water solution is absorbed (6). About 60 to 75% of inorganic arsenic ingested with food is absorbed (7). On the other hand, only 20 to 30% of arsenic in arsenic trioxide or lead arsenate, which are only slightly soluble in water, is absorbed by hamsters, rats, and rabbits.

The form of organic arsenic also determines how well it is absorbed. For example, when orally dosed, more than 90% of arsenobetaine was recovered in the urine of hamsters (8); 70 to 80% of arsenocholine was recovered in the urine of mice, rats, and rabbits (9); and 45% of dimethylarsinic acid was recovered in the urine of hamsters (10). In contrast, arsenosugars as found in seaweed are poorly absorbed from the gastrointestinal tract (10). They must be metabolized to another form before the arsenic can be absorbed.

Contrary to what once was believed, arsenate and phosphate, despite structural similarities, do not share a common transport pathway in the duodenum (12). The absorption of arsenate can be separated into two components. First, arsenate becomes sequestered primarily in or on the mucosal tissue. Eventually, the sites of sequestration become filled, with concomitant movement of arsenate into the body. The absorption of arsenate apparently involves a simple movement down a concentration gradient. In rats, some forms of organic arsenic are absorbed at rates directly proportional to their intestinal concentration over a 100-fold range. This finding suggests that organic arsenicals are absorbed mainly by simple diffusion through lipoid regions of the intestinal boundary.

Once absorbed, inorganic arsenic is transferred to the liver, where it is methylated with *S*-adenosylmethionine as the methyl donor (13). Before arsenate is methylated, it is reduced to arsenite in a reduction facilitated by glutathione (13). Arsenite methyltransferase is the enzyme that methylates arsenite. Methylation of the monomethylarsenic acid by monomethylarsenic acid methyltransferase, yields dimethylarsinic acid, the major form of arsenic in urine (14). The methylation of arsenic can be modified by changing the glutathione, methionine, and choline status of the animal (13).

The fate of absorbed organic arsenic depends on its form. For example, arsenobetaine passes through the body into the urine without biotransformation. Some orally ingested arsenocholine appears in the urine, and some is incorporated into body phospholipids in a manner similar to choline; however, most is transformed to arsenobetaine before being excreted in the urine.

Excretion of ingested arsenic is rapid, principally in urine. In some species, significant amounts of arsenic are excreted in the bile in association with glutathione (13). The usual proportions of the forms of arsenic in human urine is about 25% inorganic arsenic, 20% monomethylarsenic acid, and 55% dimethylarsinic acid (7). The proportions are quite different, however, with the consumption of organic arsenic. For example, an analysis of urine from 102 Japanese students who consumed luxuriant amounts of organic arsenic in seafood revealed 9.4% inorganic arsenic, 3.0% monomethylarsenic acid, 28.9% dimethylarsinic acid, and 58.2% trimethylated arsenic compound (15).

Functions and Mode of Action

The metabolic function of arsenic is not clearly defined. Recent findings suggest that arsenic has a biochemical role that affects the metabolism of the amino acid methionine or is involved in labile methyl-group metabolism. For example, arsenic deprivation has been found to slightly increase liver *S*-adenosylhomocysteine (SAH) and decrease liver *S*-adenosylmethionine (SAM) concentrations, thus resulting in a decreased SAM:SAH ratio (16); SAM and SAH are involved in methyl transfer. Also, arsenic deprivation depressed the concentration of the methionine metabolite taurine in plasma of hamsters and rats (17).

Arsenic possibly has a role in some enzymatic reaction. However, although arsenic has been found to activate some enzymes, this probably occurs because arsenate can act as a substitute for phosphate. Arsenic as arsenite inhibits many enzymes by reacting with key sulfhydryl groups.

Another possible role for arsenic is in the regulation of gene expression. Arsenite can induce the isolated cell production of certain proteins known as heat shock or stress proteins. Arsenite apparently has an effect at the transcriptional level, which may involve changes in the methylation of core histones (18). Recently, it has been shown that arsenic increases the methylation of the *p53* promoter, or DNA, in human lung cells (19). Also, arsenic enhances DNA synthesis in unsensitized human lymphocytes and in those stimulated by phytohemagglutinin (20).

Deficiency Signs

Arsenic deprivation has been induced in chickens, hamsters, goats, miniature pigs, and rats (4, 16, 17, 21). In the goat, miniature pig, and rat, the most consistent signs of arsenic deprivation were depressed growth and abnormal reproduction characterized by impaired fertility and increased perinatal mortality. Other notable signs of deprivation in goats were depressed serum triglyceride concentrations and death during lactation. Myocardial damage also occurred in lactating goats. The organelle of the myocardium most markedly affected was the mitochondrion at the membrane level. In advanced stages of deficiency, the membrane actually ruptured. Other reported signs of arsenic deprivation include changes in mineral concentrations in various organs. However, listing all signs may be misleading because the nature and severity of the signs of arsenic deprivation are affected by other factors. For example, female rats fed a diet conducive to kidney calcification have more severe calcification when dietary arsenic is low; kidney iron was also elevated (16). Male rats fed the same diet do not show these changes. Other factors that can affect the response to arsenic deprivation include variations in the dietary concentrations of zinc, arginine, choline, methionine, taurine, and guanidoacetic acid. Generally, the signs of arsenic deprivation can be changed and enhanced by nutritional stressors that affect sulfur amino acid or labile methyl-group metabolism.

Toxicology

Because mechanisms exist for homeostatic regulation of arsenic, its toxicity through oral intake is relatively low; it is actually less toxic than selenium, an ultratrace element with well-established nutritional value. Toxic quantities of inorganic arsenic generally are reported in milligrams. For example, reported estimated fatal acute doses of arsenic for humans range from 0.9 to 1.50 mmol (70–300 mg) or about 13 to 53 μmol (1.0–4.0 mg) As/kg body weight (22). These doses suggest that the human is more sensitive to the acute lethal effects of arsenic than are experimental animals. The ratio of the toxic to nutritional dose for rats apparently is near 1250. Some forms of organic arsenic are virtually nontoxic; a 56 mmol (10 g)/kg body weight dose of arsenobetaine depressed spontaneous motility and respiration in male mice, but these symptoms disappeared within 1 hour (23).

Briefly, the signs of subacute and chronic high exposure of arsenic in humans include the development of dermatoses of various types (hyperpigmentation, hyperkeratosis, desquamation, and hair loss); hematopoietic depression; liver damage characterized by jaundice, portal cirrhosis, and ascites; sensory disturbances; peripheral neuritis; anorexia; and loss of weight (24). A reference dose (RfD, lifetime exposure that is unlikely to cause adverse health effects) of 4.0 nmol (0.3 μg)/kg body weight/day has been suggested for arsenic (25).

Results of numerous epidemiologic studies suggest an association between chronic arsenic overexposure and the incidence of some forms of cancer, particularly skin cancer; however, the role of arsenic in carcinogenesis remains controversial. Arsenic does not seem to act as a primary carcinogen and is either an inactive or extremely weak mitogen.

Dietary Considerations

Only data from animal studies are available for estimating the possible arsenic requirement of humans. An arsenic requirement between 83 and 167 nmol (6.25 and 12.5 μg)/4.18 MJ (1000 kcal) was suggested for growing chicks and rats (26). Thus, a possible arsenic requirement for humans eating 8.37 MJ (2000 kcal) would be about 160 to 200 nmol (12–25 μg) daily. Reports from various parts of the world indicate that the average daily intake of arsenic is in the range of 160 to 800 nmol (12–60 μg) (26, 27). In the United States, the individual mean total arsenic intake from all food, excluding shellfish, has been estimated to be 400 nmol (30 μg)/day (27). Fish, grain, and cereal products contribute the most arsenic to the diet. Clarification of the need for arsenic for optimal health and performance is needed so that a safe and adequate intake of the element can be established.

Clinical Considerations

Until more is known about the biochemical and physiologic functions of arsenic, it is inappropriate to associate specific disorders with deficient arsenic nutriture. However, it has been suggested that arsenic could play an essential role in humans because injuries of the central nervous system, vascular diseases, and cancer were correlated with markedly decreased serum arsenic concentrations (28). Perhaps the most important consideration at present is recognizing the likelihood that arsenic is essential for humans. The belief that any form or amount of arsenic is unnecessary, toxic, or carcinogenic is unrealistic, if not potentially harmful.

BORON

Historical Overview

In the 1870s it was discovered that borax (sodium borate) and boric acid could be used to preserve foods. For about the next 50 years, borates were considered among the best of preservatives for extending the palatability of foods such as fish, meat, cream, and butter. In 1904, however, it was reported that human volunteers consuming over 500 mg of boric acid per day for 50 days displayed disturbed appetite, digestion, and health. After this report, the opinion that boron posed a risk to health gained momentum; by the middle 1950s, boron was essentially banned throughout the world as a food preservative.

In 1923 boron was shown to be essential for plants. About 15 years later, attempts to demonstrate boron essentiality for higher animals began; these attempts were unsuccessful. Thus, before 1980 students of biochemistry and nutrition were taught that boron was a unique element because it was essential for plants but not for higher animals. In 1981, it was reported that boron stimulated growth and partially prevented leg abnormalities present in marginally cholecalciferol-deficient chicks. Since then, evidence has been accumulating indicating that boron has an essential function in higher animals, including humans.

Chemistry

Boron biochemistry is essentially that of boric acid, which exists as $B(OH)_3$ and $B(OH)_4^-$ in dilute solutions at the pH of blood (7.4); because the pK_a of boric acid is 9.2, the abundance of these two species in blood should be 98.4 and 1.6%, respectively.

Boric acid forms ester complexes with hydroxyl groups of organic compounds; this occurs preferentially when the hydroxyl groups are adjacent and *cis*. Boron complexes with many substances of biologic interest, including sugars and polysaccharides, adenosine-5-phosphate, pyridoxine, riboflavin, dehydroascorbic acid, and pyridine nucleotides. To date, five naturally occurring biologic boron esters synthesized by various bacteria have been characterized, the latest being tartrolon B isolated from the myxobacterium *Sorangium cellulosum* (30). All of these boron esters are antibiotics. One of them, boromycin, reportedly can encapsulate alkali metal cations and increase the permeability of the cytoplasmic membrane to potassium ions (31).

Metabolism

Food boron, sodium borate, and boric acid are rapidly absorbed and excreted mostly in the urine. Based on urinary recovery findings, more than 90% of ingested boron is usually absorbed (32, 33). Most ingested boron probably is converted into, and transported through the body as, $B(OH)_3$, the normal hydrolysis end product of most boron compounds and the dominant inorganic species at the pH of the gastrointestinal tract.

Boron is distributed throughout the tissues and organs of animals and humans at concentrations mostly between 4.6 and 55.5 nmol (0.05 and 0.6 μg)/g fresh weight (29, 34). Bone, fingernails, and teeth usually contain several times these concentrations (34).

Evidence that boron is homeostatically controlled includes the rapid urinary excretion of absorbed boron, the lack of accumulation of boron in tissues, and the relatively narrow range of boron concentrations in blood of apparently healthy individuals. For example, mean plasma boron concentrations ranged from 1.85 to 6.2 nmol (20–67 ng)/mL in 44 perimenopausal women; upon supplementation with 3.0 mg of boron a day, this range increased to 2.8 to 6.9 nmol (28–75 ng)/mL (35). In some parts of the world where the daily intake of boron is very high because of environmental exposure (1.6 to 2.5 mmol [17–27 mg]/day), blood boron concentrations have been found to be much higher (41.7–65.9 nmol [450–659 ng]/mL) (36). As with other mineral elements, overcoming homeostatic mechanisms by high boron intakes elevates tissue boron concentrations.

Functions and Mode of Action

A biochemical function for boron has not been elucidated, even for plants for which boron has been known to be essential for 70 years. Its deficiency in plants, as in humans, has multiple effects. Two hypotheses, which accommodate a large and varied response to boron deprivation and the known biochemistry of boron, have recently been advanced for the biochemical function of boron in higher animals. One hypothesis is that boron acts as a metabolic regulator by complexing with a variety of substrate or reactant compounds that have hydroxyl groups in favorable positions (37). Because this complexing usually results in competitive inhibition of enzymes in vitro, the regulation is hypothesized to be mainly negative. The second hypothesis is that boron has a role in cell membrane function or stability such that it influences the response to hormone action, transmembrane signaling, or transmembrane movement of regulatory cations or anions (38). This hypothesis is supported by the findings that boron influences the transport of extracellular calcium and the release of intracellular calcium in rat platelets activated by thrombin (39) and that boron influences redox actions involved in cellular membrane transport in plants (40).

Deficiency Signs

Listing the signs of boron deficiency for animals is difficult because most studies used stressors such as magnesium or cholecalciferol deficiency to enhance the response to deprivation. However, although the nature and severity of the signs varied with the stressor used, many of the findings indicated that boron deprivation impairs calcium metabolism, brain function, and energy metabolism (37, 39). Recent studies also suggest that boron deprivation impairs immune function and exacerbates adjuvant-induced arthritis in rats (41).

Findings involving boron deprivation of humans come mainly from two studies in which men over the age of 45, postmenopausal women, and postmenopausal women on estrogen therapy were fed a low-boron diet (23 μmol/8.37 MJ [0.25 mg/2000 kcal]) for 63 days and then fed the same diet supplemented with 278 μmol (3.0 mg) of boron/day for 49 days (39). The major differences between the two experiments were the intakes of copper and magnesium: in one experiment they were marginal or inadequate; in the other they were adequate. Some effects of boron supplementation after 63 days of boron depletion found in these experiments are summarized in Table 16.1. Boron supplementation after depletion also enhanced the elevation in serum 17β-estradiol and plasma copper caused by estrogen ingestion (42), altered encephalograms to suggest improved behavioral activation (e.g., less drowsiness) and mental alertness, and improved psychomotor skills and the cognitive processes of attention and memory (43).

Toxicology

In a recent symposium (44), boron was described as having low toxicity when administered orally. Toxicity signs in animals generally occur only after dietary boron exceeds 9.25 μmol (100 μg)/g diet. In humans, the signs of acute toxicity include nausea, vomiting, diarrhea, dermatitis, and lethargy (45). In addition, high-boron intake induces riboflavinuria (46). The signs of chronic boron toxicity have been described as including poor appetite, nausea, weight loss, and decreased sexual activity, seminal volume, and sperm count and motility. Two infants who had their pacifiers dipped into a preparation of borax and honey for a period of several weeks exhibited scanty hair, patchy dry erythema, anemia, and seizures (47). The seizures stopped and the other abnormalities were alleviated when use of the borax and honey preparation was discontinued. Recently, it was suggested that an acceptable safe intake of boron could well be 13 mg/day (48).

Dietary Considerations

In the human studies just described, the subjects responded to a boron supplement after consuming a diet

Table 16.1
Responses of Boron-Deprived (23 μmol/8.37 MJ [0.25 mg/2000 kcal] for 63 days) Men over Age 45, Postmenopausal Women and Postmenopausal Women on Estrogen Therapy to a 278 μmol (3 mg) Boron per Day Supplement for 49 Days[a]

Metabolism Affected	Evidence for Effect
Macromineral and electrolyte	Increased serum 25-hydroxycholecalciferol Decreased serum calcitonin[b]
Energy	Decreased serum glucose[b] Increased serum triglycerides[c]
Nitrogen	Decreased blood urea nitrogen Decreased serum creatinine Decreased urinary hydroxyproline excretion
Oxidative	Increased erythrocyte superoxide dismutase Increased serum ceruloplasmin
Erythropoiesis/ hematopoiesis	Increased blood hemoglobin[c] Increased mean corpuscular hemoglobin[c] Decreased hematocrit[c] Decreased platelet number[c] Decreased red cell number[c]

[a]See review (39) for references to original articles.
[b]Found when dietary copper was marginal and magnesium was inadequate.
[c]Found when dietary copper and magnesium were adequate.

supplying boron at only about 23 μmol/8.37 MJ (0.25 mg/2000 kcal) for 63 days. Thus, humans apparently have a dietary requirement above this. On the bases of both human and animal data, an acceptable safe range of daily mean intakes of boron for adults could well be 0.09 to 1.2 mmol/day (1.0–13 mg/day) (48).

Foods of plant origin, especially noncitrus fruits, leafy vegetables, nuts, pulses, and legumes are rich sources of boron. Wine, cider, and beer are also high in boron. Meat, fish, and dairy products are poor sources of boron (49). Using food analyses included in the U.S. Food and Drug Administration total diet studies, the mean adult male daily intake has been determined to be 141 μmol (1.52 mg)/day (50) or 112 μmol (1.21 mg)/day (49).

Clinical Considerations

Knowledge about boron nutrition, biochemistry, and metabolism is growing, but more is needed before clinical disorders can be attributed to subnormal boron nutrition. Thus, reports such as those suggesting that low boron status may enhance the susceptibility or exacerbate some forms of arthritis (51) must be viewed with caution. Nonetheless, boron clearly is a biologically dynamic ultratrace element in higher animals, including humans. Thus, boron deprivation may have a role in some disorders of uncertain cause (e.g., osteoporosis, arthritis).

FLUORINE (FLUORIDE)

Historical Overview

Fluorine first attracted nutritional attention when its ion form, fluoride, was identified in the 1930s as causing mottled enamel of teeth known as "Colorado brown stain" or other such descriptive terms. It was also noted at this time that fewer dental caries occurred in areas with mottled enamel and subsequently that fluoride intakes could be achieved that resulted in caries reduction without mottling of teeth (52). In 1945, water fluoridation began as a public health measure. In the 1960s, an association was made between high fluoride intakes and reduced incidence of osteoporosis (53). Although the use of pharmacologic amounts of fluoride to prevent bone loss is still being investigated, its usefulness in this regard seems limited. In the early 1970s, scientists suggested that fluoride is necessary for hematopoiesis, fertility, and growth in mice and rats (53), but this suggestion was based on experiments in which animals were not fed optimal diets. It was later concluded that fluoride affected hematopoiesis, fertility, and growth through pharmacologic mechanisms (53), and thus no substantive evidence exists to support essentiality.

Chemistry

The biochemistry of fluoride has been briefly reviewed (53). Fluorine exists as the fluoride ion or as hydrofluoric acid (HF) in body fluids. However, approximately 99% of total body fluorine is found in mineralized tissues as fluorapatite. Fluoride is incorporated into apatite, a basic calcium phosphate mineral with a theoretical formula of $Ca_{10}(PO_4)_6(OH)_2$, by substituting for the OH^- moiety. This substitution occurs because F^- and OH^- have similar ionic radii and share the same charge and primary hydration number.

Metabolism

Several reviews of fluoride metabolism (52–55) indicate that about 75 to 90% of ingested fluoride is absorbed from the gastrointestinal tract. Generally, less than 20% of ingested fluoride is excreted in the feces. Absorption of fluoride is rapid; about 50% of a moderate dose of soluble fluoride is absorbed in 30 minutes, and complete absorption occurs in 90 minutes. The rapidity of absorption verifies that a significant portion of ingested fluoride is absorbed from the stomach; absorption also occurs throughout the small intestine.

Fluoride absorption is generally considered to occur by passive diffusion and to be inversely related to pH; thus, factors that promote gastric acid secretion increase the rate of absorption. The pH dependence of absorption is consistent with the generally accepted view that HF (pK_a = 3.4), and not ionic fluoride, is the form that is absorbed from the stomach. Diffusion as HF in the small intestine because of its high pH is less likely. In the small intestine, the HF concentration would be very low and the gradient small. In contrast, the concentration and gradient of F^- would be high.

Soluble fluorides, such as sodium fluoride, are almost completely absorbed. Less soluble sources, such as bone meal, are relatively poorly absorbed (less than 50%). Aluminum hydroxide, widely used as an antacid, markedly inhibits fluoride absorption.

The rapid absorption of fluoride following oral ingestion leads to a prompt rise in its plasma concentration. Fluoride in plasma exists in ionic form; it is not bound by plasma proteins or by any other constituent of plasma. However, HF, not ionic fluoride, apparently is the form that is in diffusion equilibrium across cell membranes.

Removal of fluoride from the circulation occurs principally through two mechanisms: renal excretion and calcified tissue deposition. Approximately 50% of fluoride absorbed each day is deposited in the calcified tissues (bone and developing teeth) within 24 hours, which results in about 99% of the body burden of fluoride being associated with these tissues. The rate of uptake by bone is affected by the stage of skeletal development. Renal excretion is the major route for removal of fluoride from the body; about 50% of the daily intake is cleared by the kidney. Urinary excretion of fluoride is directly related to urinary pH; thus, factors that affect urinary pH, such as diet, drugs, metabolic or respiratory disorders, and altitude of residence, can affect how much absorbed fluoride is excreted.

Functions and Mode of Action

The major known function of fluoride is its role in protecting against pathologic demineralization of calcified tissues. This is not an essential function in the true sense, but a beneficial action, described elsewhere in this treatise (Chapters 66 and 85). An essential function has not been described for fluoride.

Deficiency Signs

In the early 1970s, it was reported that mice fed low fluoride diets (as low as 0.26 nmol [5 ng]/g) exhibited anemia and infertility, compared with mice supplemented with 2.6 μmol (50 μg) F/mL of drinking water (53). These findings were obtained with diets that were iron deficient, however, and high dietary fluoride (similar to that fed to the supplemented controls) was shown to improve iron absorption or use. Thus, mice fed low-fluoride diets containing sufficient iron exhibited neither anemia nor infertility. Relatively high fluoride supplementation (130–395 nmol [2.5–7.5 μg]/g to a diet containing 2.1 to 24.2 nmol [0.04–0.46 μg]/g) slightly improved the growth of suboptimally growing rats (56) and (1.3 μmol [25 μg]/g diet) enhanced growth in chicks (57). These growth-promoting effects were probably pharmacologic. High or pharmacologic amounts of fluoride have also been found to depress lipid absorption (53) and to alleviate nephrocalcinosis induced by phosphorus feeding (58). Recently, it was reported that a fluoride deficiency in goats decreased life expectancy and caused pathologic histology in the kidney and endocrine organs (59, 60). These findings need to be confirmed in a nonruminant species before being accepted as evidence for essentiality in higher animals. In summary, unequivocal or specific signs of fluoride deficiency have not been described for higher animals including humans. However, fluoride still must be recognized as a trace element with beneficial properties.

Toxicology

The toxicity of fluoride has received much attention since it was discovered to cause mottled teeth. Reviews of fluoride toxicity (52, 53, 55) indicate that chronic toxicity through excessive intake, mainly through water supplies and industrial exposure, has been reported in many parts of the world. Ingestion of water and food containing in excess of 0.1 mmol (2 mg) F/kg results in dental fluorosis or mottled enamel, ranging from barely discernible to stained and pitted enamel. Crippling skeletal fluorosis apparently occurs in people who ingest 0.53 to 1.32 mmol F (10–25 mg) per day for 7 to 20 years (55). The asymptomatic preclinical stage of skeletal fluorosis is characterized by slight increases in bone mass that are detectable radiographically. As skeletal fluorosis progresses, symptoms range from occasional stiffness or pain in the joints to chronic joint pain and osteoporosis of long bones. In severe cases of chronic fluorosis, muscle wasting and neurologic defects occur.

The signs and symptoms of acute fluoride toxicity are nausea, vomiting, diarrhea, abdominal pain, excessive salivation and lacrimation, pulmonary disturbances, cardiac insufficiency and weakness, convulsions, sensory disturbances, paralysis, and coma (55). The probably acute toxic dose or the minimum dose of fluoride that could cause toxic signs and symptoms, including death, is 0.26 mmol (5 mg) per kg body weight (52).

Dietary Considerations

Although fluoride is not generally considered an essential element for humans, it is still considered a beneficial element. The Food and Nutrition Board (2) has established the following ESADDIs for fluoride: infants aged 0 to 0.5 years, 5.3 to 26.3 μmol or 0.1 to 0.5 mg; infants aged 0.5 to 1 years, 10.5 to 52.6 μmol or 0.2 to 1.0 mg; children and adolescents aged 1 to 3 years, 26.3 to 78.9 μmol or 0.5 to 1.5 mg, aged 4 to 6 years, 52.6 to 131.6 μmol or 1.0 to 2.5 mg, aged 7 years and older, 78.9 to 131.6 μmol or 1.5 to 2.5 mg; adults, 78.9 to 210.5 μmol or 1.5 to 4.0 mg. These ESADDIs are based on amounts that protect against dental caries and generally do not result in any mottling of teeth.

The major source of dietary fluoride in the United States is drinking water; about 52% of the population uses water with a fluoride concentration adjusted between 36.8 to 63.2 μmol (0.7–1.2 mg)/L (55). The richest dietary sources of fluoride are tea and marine fish that are consumed with their bones. Fluoride is ubiquitous in foodstuffs, but similar products can vary greatly with source. Thus, estimating fluoride intakes is difficult. For an adult male residing in a community with fluoridated water, estimates of daily fluoride intake range from 52.8 to 157.9 μmol (1–3 mg) per day. This range is reduced to less than 52.8 μmol (1.0 mg) per day in nonfluoridated areas (55). Foods marketed in different parts of the United States contribute only 15.8 to 31.6 μmol (0.3–0.6 mg) to the daily intake of fluoride (2).

Clinical Considerations

At present, the clinical importance of fluoride is not through its nutritional effects but through its beneficial pharmacologic (anticariogenic and possibly antiosteoporotic) or toxicologic (dental and skeletal fluorosis) actions. However, the possibility that fluoride is an essential nutrient should not be dismissed. It seems possible that fluoride could have a role in biologic mineralization.

MANGANESE

Historical Overview

Although manganese was known to be a constituent of animal tissues as early as 1913, it was not until 1931 that manganese deficiency signs were described for experimental animals. Manganese deficiency has since been induced in numerous species of animals. A few cases of possible manganese deficiency in humans have recently been reported. The importance of manganese in health and disease is the focus of a recent book (61).

Chemistry

A brief review of manganese biochemistry (62) indicated that the characteristic oxidative state of manganese in solution, in metal-enzyme complexes, and in metalloenzymes is Mn^{2+}. Mn^{3+} also is important in vivo; it is the oxidative state in the enzyme manganese superoxide dismutase, the form that binds to transferrin, and probably the form that interacts with Fe^{3+}. Ingested Mn^{2+} is thought to be converted into Mn^{3+} in the duodenum. In manganese-activated biologic reactions, the enzyme-manganese interaction involves either chelation of the metal ion with a phosphate-containing substrate (particularly adenosine triphosphate [ATP]) or a direct interaction with the protein. The chemistry of Mn^{2+} is similar to that of Mg^{2+}. Therefore, for most enzymatic reactions activated by Mn^{2+}, the activation is nonspecific; Mg^{2+} can also act as the activator.

Metabolism

For the adult human, absorption of manganese from the diet has long been assumed to be near 5%. This estimate is complicated, however, by the fact that endogenous manganese is almost totally excreted through biliary, pancreatic, and intestinal secretions into the gut. If manganese status is adequate, endogenous excretion of absorbed manganese into the gut is so rapid that it is difficult to determine the portion of fecal manganese not absorbed from the diet and the portion endogenously excreted. Thus, the true absorption of manganese by humans probably remains to be determined. Absorption efficiency apparently declines as dietary intake of manganese increases (63) and increases with low manganese status (64). On the other hand, endogenous excretion of manganese does not seem to be markedly influenced by dietary intake or status (64). Thus, the often cited hypothesis that manganese homeostasis is regulated mainly by variable excretion through the digestive tract probably needs to be replaced with one that has the control of absorption in the gut as a major factor.

Absorption of manganese, through an unestablished mechanism, apparently occurs equally well throughout the small intestine. Some findings indicate that manganese is absorbed through an active transport mechanism that is a rapidly saturable process involving a high-affinity, low-capacity, active-transport system (65). On the other hand, diffusion has been implicated because studies with brush border membrane vesicles indicated that mucosal transport of manganese occurs through a nonsaturable, simple diffusion process (66). Perhaps both processes are involved in manganese movement across the gut; studies using CACO-2 cells, which mimic many of the actions of enterocytes, showed that apical to basolateral manganese uptake and transport were strictly concentration dependent, but basolateral to apical uptake and transport were saturable (67). Manganese might well be absorbed by a two-step mechanism: initial uptake from the lumen followed by transfer across the mucosal cells. The two kinetic processes operate simultaneously, with manganese competing with iron and cobalt for common binding sites in both processes. Thus, one of these metals, if present in a high amount, can exert an inhibitory effect on absorption of the others.

The form of manganese entering the portal blood from the gastrointestinal tract is also controversial. In addition to hydrated manganese complexes, Mn^{2+} bound both to plasma α_2-macroglobulin (68) and to albumin (64) have been suggested to be the form. Regardless of the form, manganese is removed rapidly from the blood by the liver. A fraction is oxidized to Mn^{3+} and is bound to the plasma transport protein transferrin or possibly to a specific transmanganin protein. Transferrin-bound manganese is taken up by extrahepatic tissue.

Within cells, manganese is found predominantly in mitochondria, and thus organs rich in mitochondria, such as liver, kidney, and pancreas, have relatively high manganese concentrations; in contrast, plasma manganese in humans is extremely low (68).

As indicated above, manganese is almost totally excreted in feces; only trace amounts are found in urine. Excretion of absorbed manganese into the gut is rapid and apparently occurs in two waves. The first wave results from the clearance of initially absorbed manganese; the second represents a combination of initially absorbed manganese and that arising from the enterohepatic circulation.

Functions and Mode of Action

Manganese is known to function in enzyme activation and be a constituent of several metalloenzymes (69). The numerous enzymes that can be activated by manganese include oxidoreductases, lyases, ligases, hydrolases, kinases, decarboxylases, and transferases. Most enzymes activated by manganese can also be activated by other metals, especially magnesium; exceptions are the manganese-specific activation of glycosyltransferases and possibly of xylosyltransferase (62). There are only a few manganese metalloenzymes; these include arginase, pyruvate carboxylase, glutamine synthetase, and manganese superoxide dismutase (62, 69).

Deficiency Signs

Manganese deficiency (reviewed in refs. 70, 71) has been induced in many species of animals. Signs of deficiency include impaired growth, skeletal abnormalities, disturbed or depressed reproductive function, ataxia of the newborn, and defects in lipid and carbohydrate metabolism.

A review of studies reportedly describing manganese

deficiency in humans finds that most are not conclusive. One frequently cited case concerns a man who, after consuming a semipurified formula diet for an extended period, developed weight loss, depressed growth of hair and nails, dermatitis, and hypocholesterolemia. Also, his black hair developed a reddish tinge, and his clotting-protein response to vitamin K supplementation was abnormal. After these symptoms appeared, it was realized that manganese had been left out of his diet. The subject responded to a mixed hospital diet containing manganese (72). Unfortunately, supplementation with manganese alone was not tried. In another study (73), men were fed a purified diet containing only 2.0 μmol (0.11 mg) manganese per day for 39 days. They exhibited decreased serum cholesterol concentrations and a fleeting dermatitis. Calcium, phosphorus, and alkaline phosphatase activity increased in blood. Short-term manganese supplementation (10 days), however, did not reverse these changes. More recently, 14 young women consumed a conventional diet providing 18.2 μmol (1.0 mg) or 101.8 μmol (5.6 mg) manganese per day each for 39 days (74). Low dietary manganese slightly increased plasma glucose concentration during an intravenous glucose tolerance test (IVGTT) and increased menstrual losses of manganese, calcium, iron, and total hemoglobin. These intriguing findings need to be confirmed before they are accepted as signs of manganese deprivation because the subjects did not exhibit negative manganese balance during manganese deprivation, nor were the changes highly significant. Probably the most convincing case of manganese deficiency is that of a child on long-term parenteral nutrition who exhibited diffuse bone demineralization and poor growth that were corrected by manganese supplementation (75).

Manganese deprivation may contribute to disease processes. Low dietary manganese or low blood and tissue manganese has been associated with osteoporosis, diabetes, epilepsy, atherosclerosis, and impaired wound healing (61).

Toxicology

Manganese is often considered to be among the least toxic of the trace elements through oral intake. However, manganese may be of more toxicologic concern than believed in the past, especially for people with compromised homeostatic mechanisms or infants whose homeostatic control of manganese is not fully developed. In the past, the most common form of manganese toxicity identified in humans resulted from chronic inhalation of large amounts of airborne manganese as found in mines, steel mills, and some chemical industries. In these cases of toxicity, the principal organ affected was the brain. In miners intoxicated by manganese, the initial signs of toxicity were severe psychiatric abnormalities including hyperirritability, violent acts, and hallucinations, which were referred to as "manganic madness." As toxicity progressed, a permanent crippling neurologic disorder of the extrapyramidal system resulted that displayed morphologic lesions similar to those associated with Parkinson's disease (76). Although there is no conclusive report of oral toxicity of manganese in humans, many suggestive findings have recently appeared. High brain manganese concentrations have been associated with neurologic dysfunction (77). High manganese concentrations in hair have been associated with violent behavior (78). An RfD (safe daily intake over a lifetime) of 2.6 μmol (0.14 mg) per kg of body weight per day has been determined (79); for a 70-kg man this is a daily intake of 0.18 mmol (9.8 mg).

Dietary Considerations

The current United States ESADDIs for manganese (2) (see Tables of RDI [RDA] in the Appendix) are the following: infants aged 0 to 0.5 years, 5.5 to 10.9 μmol or 0.3 to 0.6 mg, and aged 0.5 to 1 years, 5.5 to 18.2 μmol or 0.6 to 1.0 mg; children and adolescents aged 1 to 3 years, 18.2 to 27.3 μmol or 1.0 to 1.5 mg, aged 4 to 6 years, 27.3 to 36.4 μmol or 1.5 to 2.0 mg, aged 7 to 10 years, 36.4 to 54.6 μmol or 2.0 to 3.0 mg, and aged 11 years and older, 36.4 to 91.0 μmol or 2.0 to 5.0 mg; adults, 36.4 to 91.0 μmol or 2.0 to 5.0 mg. Few data are available to support these estimates.

The above-cited values apparently were set mainly through the reasoning that most dietary intakes fall in this range and do not result in deficiency or toxicity signs. Other evidence used was balance data of questionable value. Thus, the ESADDIs of manganese may need modification as additional data become available. One recent study indicated a minimal requirement for manganese of 13.5 μmol (0.74 mg) per day for young men, based on obligatory losses while consuming a semipurified, manganese-deficient formula diet (73). However, this amount probably did not allow for storage of manganese for use at times of enhanced need nor for the possible inhibition of manganese absorption by dietary substances such as fiber. A requirement near 18 μmol (1.0 mg) per day was indicated in another study in which 14 young women were fed that amount for 39 days without negative manganese balance occurring (74). Five men who received varying amounts of manganese in a diet of conventional foods for 105 days exhibited negative retention of manganese with daily dietary intakes of 22.0, 37.5, and 52.6 μmol (1.21, 2.06, and 2.89 mg), but positive retention was found at daily dietary intakes of 48.2 and 69.0 μmol (2.65 and 3.79 mg). Regression analysis of intake versus balance yielded a recommended daily intake of 63.7 μmol (3.5 mg) (79). This value is difficult to reconcile with the fact that most diets contain less manganese, and no evidence that manganese deficiency is a problem has appeared. Also, attempts to produce manganese deficiency by feeding diets containing as little as 13.5 to 18.2 μmol (0.74 or 1.0 mg) per day resulted in no conclusive or significant effects on the health of adults. These studies show that no firm data are available to establish the lower value of the ESADDI of manganese.

The upper level of acceptable intake probably should be the amount encountered in a diet high in manganese-rich foods that allows positive balance if the diet contains large quantities of substances that inhibit manganese absorption. Thus, increasing the upper value to 182 μmol (10 mg) per day needs to be considered, especially since an RfD has been set at that level.

Unrefined cereals, nuts, leafy vegetables, and tea are rich in manganese; refined grains, meats, and dairy products contain small amounts (80). Most reported daily mean intakes of manganese throughout the world fall between 9.5 and 196 μmol (0.52 and 10.8 mg) (79).

Clinical Considerations

Determination of the importance of manganese in human nutrition is urgently needed. Key issues are whether or not low manganese status is an important clinical consideration for osteoporosis, atherosclerosis, epilepsy, diabetes, and wound healing and whether or not manganese toxicity is a significant factor in abnormal brain function.

MOLYBDENUM

Historical Overview

Reviews of molybdenum (81, 82) state that evidence for the essentiality of this element first appeared in 1953, when xanthine oxidase was identified as a molybdenum metalloenzyme. However, molybdenum deficiency signs appeared in rats and chickens only when the diet contained massive amounts of tungsten, an antagonist of molybdenum metabolism. These studies showed that the dietary requirement to maintain normal growth of animals was less than 10.4 nmol (1 μg) molybdenum/g diet, an amount substantially lower than requirements for other trace elements recognized essential at the time. Thus, molybdenum was not considered of much practical importance in animal and human nutrition. Consequently, over the past 35 years, relatively little effort has been devoted to studying the metabolic and pathologic consequences of molybdenum deficiency in monogastric animals or humans.

Chemistry

Molybdenum is a transition element that readily changes its oxidation state and can thus act as an electron transfer agent in oxidation-reduction reactions. In the oxidized form of molybdoenzymes, molybdenum is probably present in the 6+ state. Although the enzymes during electron transfer are probably first reduced to the 5+ state, other oxidation states have been found in reduced enzymes. Molybdenum is present at the active site of enzymes as a small nonprotein cofactor containing a pterin nucleus (82). Almost all molybdenum in liver exists as this cofactor, with about 60% of the total amount in sulfite oxidase and xanthine oxidase. In addition to the molybdenum cofactor and "enzymatic" molybdenum, the other important form of molybdenum is the molybdate ion (MoO_4^{2-}) (83), which is the main form in blood and urine.

Metabolism

Molybdenum (except as MoS_2) in foods and in the form of soluble complexes is readily absorbed. Humans absorbed 88 to 93% of the molybdenum fed as ammonium molybdate in a liquid formula component of a diet (84). In another study, about 57% of intrinsically labeled molybdenum in soy and 88% in kale were absorbed (85). Molybdenum absorption occurs rapidly in the stomach and throughout the small intestine, with the rate of absorption being higher in the proximal than in the distal parts (83). Whether an active or a passive mechanism is more important in the absorption of molybdenum is uncertain. One study indicated that at low concentrations, molybdenum absorption is carrier mediated and active (86). Another study showed that in vivo absorption rates were essentially the same over a 10-fold range of molybdenum concentrations, which suggests that molybdate was absorbed by diffusion only (87). Molybdate possibly is moved both by diffusion and by active transport, but at high concentrations, the relative contribution of active transport to molybdenum flux is small.

Molybdate is absorbed and transported loosely attached to erythrocytes in the blood; it tends to bind specifically to α_2-macroglobulin (88). Organs that retain the highest amounts of molybdenum are liver and kidney (81, 83, 88).

After absorption, most molybdenum is turned over rapidly and eliminated as molybdate through the kidney (84); this elimination is increased as dietary intake is increased. Thus, excretion rather than regulated absorption is the major homeostatic mechanism for molybdenum. Nonetheless, significant amounts of this element are excreted in the bile (88).

Functions and Mode of Action

Molybdenum functions as an enzyme cofactor (81, 82). Molybdoenzymes catalyze the hydroxylation of various substrates (89). Aldehyde oxidase oxidizes and detoxifies various pyrimidines, purines, pteridines, and related compounds. Xanthine oxidase/dehydrogenase catalyzes the transformation of hypoxanthine to xanthine and of xanthine to uric acid. Sulfite oxidase catalyzes the transformation of sulfite to sulfate.

Molybdate might also be involved in stabilizing the steroid-binding ability of unoccupied steroid receptors (90, 91). During isolation procedures, molybdate protects steroid hormone receptors, such as the glucocorticoid receptor, against inactivation. It is hypothesized, however, that molybdate affects the glucocorticoid receptor because it mimics an endogenous compound called "modulator."

Deficiency Signs

The signs of molybdenum deficiency in animals have been reviewed (81). Deficiency signs in goats and minipigs are depressed feed consumption and growth, impaired reproduction characterized by increased mortality in both mothers and offspring, and elevated copper concentrations in liver and brain. A molybdenum-responsive syndrome found in hatching chicks is characterized by a high incidence of late embryonic mortality, mandibular distortion, anophthalmia, and defects in leg bone development and feathering. Skeletal lesions, subsequently detected in older birds, include separation of the proximal epiphysis of the femur, osteolytic changes in the femoral shaft, and lesions in the overlying skin that ultimately were attributed to intense irritation in these areas. The incidence of this syndrome was particularly high in commercial flocks reared on diets containing high concentrations of copper (a molybdenum antagonist) as a growth stimulant. These apparently dissimilar pathologic changes could possibly be explained by a defect in sulfur metabolism.

Recognition that molybdenum is a component of sulfite oxidase whose deficiency disrupts cysteine metabolism has resulted in identification of human disorders caused by a lack of functioning molybdenum. A lethal inborn error in metabolism resulting from a sulfite oxidase deficiency is characterized by severe brain damage; mental retardation; dislocation of ocular lenses; increased urinary output of sulfite, *S*-sulfocysteine, and thiosulfate; and decreased urinary output of sulfate (82). A patient receiving prolonged TPN therapy acquired a syndrome described as "acquired molybdenum deficiency." This syndrome, exacerbated by methionine administration, was characterized by hypermethioninemia, hypouricemia, hyperoxypurinemia, hypouricosuria, and low urinary sulfate excretion. In addition, the patient suffered mental disturbances that progressed to coma. Supplementation with ammonium molybdate improved the clinical condition, reversed the sulfur-handling defect, and normalized uric acid production (92).

Toxicology

Large oral doses are necessary to overcome the homeostatic control of molybdenum (81, 83). Thus, molybdenum is a relatively nontoxic element; in nonruminants, an intake of 1.04 to 52.1 mmol (100–5000 mg)/kg of food or water is required to produce clinical symptoms. Ruminants are more susceptible to elevated amounts of dietary molybdenum. The mechanism of molybdenum toxicity is uncertain. Most toxicity signs are similar or identical to those of copper deficiency (i.e., growth depression and anemia). In humans, both occupational and high dietary exposures to molybdenum have been linked by epidemiologic methods to elevated uric acid concentrations in blood and an increased incidence of gout.

Dietary Considerations

The current United States ESADDIs for molybdenum (2) (see Tables of RDI [RDA] in the Appendix) are the following: infants aged 0 to 0.5 years, 0.16 to 0.31 μmol or 15 to 30 μg, and aged 0.5 to 1.0 years, 0.21 to 0.42 μmol or 20 to 40 μg; children and adolescents aged 1 to 3 years, 0.26 to 0.52 μmol or 25 to 50 μg, aged 4 to 6 years, 0.31 to 0.78 μmol or 30 to 75 μg, aged 7 to 10 years, 0.52 to 1.76 μmol or 50 to 150 μg, and aged 11 years or older, 0.78 to 2.08 μmol or 75 to 200 μg; adults, 0.78 to 2.61 μmol or 75 to 250 μg. Data to support these estimates are scant. These values apparently were set by using balance data (which may be questionable) and the reasoning that usual dietary intakes are within this range without apparent signs of deficiency or toxicity. Recent studies indicate that the requirement for molybdenum in adults is actually close to 0.26 μmol (25 μg) per day (93).

The daily intake of molybdenum ranges between 0.52 and 3.65 μmol (50 and 350 μg) (94–96). Most diets, however, apparently supply about 0.52 to 1.04 μmol (50–100 μg) molybdenum per day. The richest food sources of molybdenum include milk and milk products, dried legumes or pulses, organ meats (liver and kidney), cereals, and baked goods. The poorest sources of molybdenum include nonleguminous vegetables, fruits, sugars, oils, fats, and fish (95, 96).

Clinical Considerations

Except for the molybdenum-responsive patient with "acquired molybdenum deficiency" resulting from long-term use of TPN, there is no indication that molybdenum deficiency is of clinical importance. Nonetheless, the search for possible molybdenum-responsive syndromes in humans is still warranted because situations may be occurring where molybdenum nutriture is important. For example, low dietary molybdenum might be detrimental to human health and well-being through an effect on the detoxification of xenobiotic compounds. The molybdenum hydroxylases apparently are as important as the microsomal monooxygenase system in the metabolism of drugs and foreign compounds (89). This may be why molybdenum has an inhibitory effect on some forms of cancer in animal models (97).

NICKEL

Historical Overview

An earlier review of nickel (98) stated that although nickel was first suggested to be nutritionally essential in 1936, strong evidence for essentiality did not appear until 1970. Studies between 1970 and 1975, however, gave inconsistent signs of nickel deprivation, probably because of suboptimal experimental conditions. Since 1975, diets and environments that allow optimal growth and survival of laboratory animals have been used in studies of nickel nutrition and metabolism. Thus, most of the significant biochemical, nutritional, and physiologic studies of nickel appeared after 1975.

Chemistry

Books devoted to nickel have extensive reviews of the biochemistry of this element (99, 100). These reviews indicate that monovalent, divalent, and trivalent forms of nickel apparently are important in biochemistry. Like other ions of the first transition series, Ni^{2+} can complex, chelate, or bind with many substances of biologic interest. This binding, particularly by amino acids (especially histidine and cysteine), proteins (especially albumin), and by a macroglobulin called nickeloplasmin, probably is important in the extracellular transport, intracellular binding, and urinary and biliary excretion of nickel. Ni^{2+} in a tightly bound form is required for the activity of urease, an enzyme found in plants and microorganisms. In the microbial enzyme, methyl coenzyme M reductase, nickel is present in a chromophore called factor F430, which is a tetrapyrrole similar in structure to that in vitamin B_{12}. Ni^{3+} apparently is essential for enzymatic hydrogenation, desulfurization, and carboxylation reactions in mostly anaerobic microorganisms. In some of these reactions, the redox action of nickel may involve the 1+ oxidation state, especially in that of methyl coenzyme M reductase. Nickel is also a structural component of some enzymes.

Metabolism

When nickel in water is ingested after an overnight fast or in low quantities, as much as 50%, but usually closer to 20 to 25%, of the dose is absorbed (101, 102). Certain foodstuffs and simple substances, including milk, coffee, tea, orange juice, and ascorbic acid, however, depress this high absorption (101). Foods such as those found in a typical Guatemalan meal or in a North American breakfast suppress absorption of nickel to less than 1%. Thus, nickel is often poorly absorbed (less than 10%) when ingested with typical diets. Nickel absorption is enhanced by iron deficiency, pregnancy, and lactation (103, 104).

The mechanisms involved in transport of nickel through the gut are not conclusively established. Persuasive evidence indicates that no specific nickel carrier mechanism exists at the brush border membrane (104); this means that absorption probably depends on the efficiency of mucosal trapping via charge neutralization on the membrane. In other words, nickel crosses the basolateral membrane via passive leakage or diffusion, perhaps as an amino acid complex or some other low-molecular-weight complex. Passage as a lipophilic complex is a possibility, because these types of complexes markedly increase the nickel concentrations in tissues of experimental animals (106). However, there is also some evidence for energy-driven transport of nickel across the mucosal epithelium (104, 107).

Nickel transported in blood is principally bound to serum albumin (108). Small amounts of nickel in serum are associated with the amino acid L-histidine and with α_2-macroglobulin (108, 109). No tissue or organ significantly accumulates orally administered physiologic doses of nickel. In humans, the thyroid and adrenal glands apparently have relatively high nickel concentrations, with reported values of 2.40 and 2.25 μmol (141 and 132 μg)/kg dry weight, respectively (110). Most organs contain less than 0.85 μmol (50 μg) nickel/kg dry weight.

Although fecal nickel excretion (mostly unabsorbed nickel) is 10 to 100 times as great as urinary excretion, most of the small fraction of nickel absorbed is rapidly and efficiently excreted through the kidney as urinary low-molecular-weight complexes. Measurable amounts of nickel are also lost in sweat and bile. The nickel content in sweat is high (about 1.19 μmol or 70 μg/L), which points to active nickel secretion by the sweat glands (111). Biliary loss of nickel has been estimated at 34 to 85 nmol (2–5 μg) per day (110).

Functions and Mode of Action

No biochemical function for nickel has been clearly defined for higher animals or humans. Nickel may, however, function as a cofactor or structural component in specific metalloenzymes in higher organisms, because such enzymes have been identified in bacteria, fungi, plants, and invertebrates. These nickel-containing enzymes include urease, hydrogenase, methyl coenzyme M reductase, and carbon monoxide dehydrogenase (99, 100). Nickel may have a function in higher animals that involves a pathway using vitamin B_{12} and/or folic acid. Both these vitamins affect signs of nickel deprivation in rats (112, 114). The interaction between nickel and folic acid affects the vitamin B_{12}– and folic acid–dependent pathway of methionine synthesis from homocysteine (114). Nickel might also have a very basic function, because nickel in vitro is a calcium channel blocker (115) and can activate the Ca^{2+} "receptor" on the osteoclast to elicit cytosolic Ca^{2+} signals (116).

Deficiency Signs

Signs of nickel deficiency have not been described for humans. The reported signs of nickel deprivation for six animal species—chick, cow, goat, pig, rat, and sheep—are extensive and have been listed in several reviews (98, 103, 117). Unfortunately, many of the reported signs may have been misinterpreted manifestations of pharmacologic actions of nickel (118). High dietary nickel, used in some experiments, may have alleviated an abnormality caused by something other than a nutritional deficiency of nickel (many diets were apparently low in iron). However, recent studies with rats and goats indicate that nickel deprivation depresses growth, reproductive performance, and plasma glucose and alters the distribution of other elements in the body, including calcium, iron, and zinc. As with other ultratrace elements, the nature and severity of signs of nickel deprivation are affected by diet composition. For example, both vitamin B_{12} and folic acid affect the response to nickel deprivation (112–114).

Toxicology

Life-threatening toxicity of nickel through oral intake is unlikely. Because of excellent homeostatic regulation, nickel salts exert their toxic action mainly by gastrointestinal irritation and not by inherent toxicity (117). Generally, concentrations of Ni above 4.26 μmol (250 μg)/g of diet are required to produce signs of nickel toxicity (such as depressed growth and anemia) in animals; by weight extrapolation, a daily oral dose of 4.26 mmol (250 mg) of soluble nickel should produce toxic symptoms in humans. However, more moderate doses of nickel may have adverse effects in humans. An oral dose in water as low as 10.2 μmol (0.6 mg) nickel as nickel sulfate, which is well absorbed, given to fasting subjects produced a positive skin reaction in some individuals with nickel allergy (119). That dose is only a few times higher than the human daily requirement postulated on the basis of results from animal studies.

Dietary Considerations

Because of the strong circumstantial evidence indicating that nickel is essential for several animals, a reasonable hypothesis is that nickel is required by humans also. Moreover, knowledge about the nickel requirements of animals is helpful in estimating the amount of nickel possibly required by humans. Most monogastric animals have an apparent nickel requirement of less than 3.41 μmol (200 μg)/kg diet. On the basis that adult humans usually consume 500 g of a mixed diet daily (dry basis), a dietary requirement for humans of 426 to 596 nmol (25–35 μg) per day has been suggested (120). Total dietary nickel intakes of humans vary greatly with the amounts and proportions of foods of animal (nickel-low) and plant (nickel-high) origin consumed. Rich sources of nickel include chocolate, nuts, dried beans, peas, and grains (95, 120, 121); diets high in these foods could supply more than 15.33 μmol (900 μg) nickel per day. Conventional diets, however, often provide less than 2.55 μmol (150 μg) daily (some much less than 1.70 μmol [100 μg] daily). Examples of reported intakes are 1.18 to 2.76 μmol (69–162 μg) per day in the United States (95) and 2.21 μmol (130 μg) per day (range of 1.02–4.43 μmol or 60–260 μg) in Denmark (121).

Clinical Considerations

Until more is known about the physiologic function of nickel and its dietary requirement, it is inappropriate to suggest specific disorders other than nickel dermatitis as wholly or partially attributable to abnormal nickel nutrition. However, be aware that nickel status affects the functions of vitamin B_{12} and folic acid, two nutrients receiving increasing clinical attention.

SILICON

Historical Overview

As early as 1911, researchers (122) suggested that silicon might have an antiatheroma action. A review of silicon in nutrition (123) indicated that until 1972, silicon was generally considered nonessential, except for some lower classes of organisms (diatoms, radiolarians, and sponges), in which silica serves a structural role. Most of the limited studies on the biochemical, nutritional, and physiologic roles of silicon have been published since 1974.

Chemistry

The chemistry of silicon is similar to that of carbon, its sister element (124). Silicon forms silicon-silicon, silicon-hydrogen, silicon-oxygen, silicon-nitrogen, and silicon-carbon bonds. Thus, organosilicon compounds are analogues of organocarbon compounds. However, substitution of silicon for carbon, or vice versa, in organocompounds results in molecules with different properties, because silicon is larger and less electronegative than carbon.

In animals, silicon is found both free and bound. Silicic acid probably is the free form. The bound form has never been rigorously identified. Silicon might be present in biologic material as a silanolate, an ether (or esterlike) derivative of silicic acid. Bridges of R_1-O-Si-O-R_2 or R_1-O-Si-O-Si-O-R_2 possibly play a role in the structural organization of some mucopolysaccharides or collagen.

Metabolism

Little is known about the metabolism of silicon. Increasing silicon intake increases urinary silicon output up to fairly well defined limits in humans, rats, and guinea pigs. The upper limits of urinary silicon excretion, however, apparently are not set by the excretory ability of the kidney, because urinary excretion can be elevated above these upper limits by peritoneal injection of silicon (125). Thus, the upper limits apparently are set by the rate and extent of silicon absorption from the gastrointestinal tract. The form of dietary silicon determines whether it is well absorbed. In one study, humans absorbed only about 1% of a large single dose of an aluminosilicate compound but absorbed more than 70% of a single dose of methylsilanetriol salicylate, a drug used in the treatment of circulatory ischemias and osteoporosis (126). Some dietary forms of silicon must be well absorbed, because daily urinary silicon excretion in humans can be a high percentage (close to 50%) of daily silicon intake (127). The mechanisms involved in intestinal absorption and blood transport of silicon are unknown.

Silicon is not protein bound in plasma, where it is believed to exist almost entirely in the undissociated monomeric silicic acid form, $Si(OH)_4$ (123–128). Connective tissues, including aorta, trachea, tendon, bone, and skin and its appendages contain much of the silicon that is retained in the body (123). Absorbed silicon is mainly eliminated via the urine, where it probably exists as magnesium orthosilicate (123, 128).

Functions and Mode of Action

The distribution of silicon in the body and the biochemical changes in bone caused by silicon deficiency indicate that silicon influences bone formation by affecting cartilage composition and ultimately cartilage calcification. In bone (123, 129, 130), silicon is localized in the active growth areas or osteoid layer and within the osteoblasts. In bone of silicon-deficient animals, hexosamine (glycosaminoglycans) and collagen concentrations are depressed, but macromineral composition is not markedly affected. Silicon apparently affects collagen formation, because it is required for maximal bone prolylhydroxylase activity (130), and silicon deficiency decreases ornithine aminotransferase (131); both enzymes are involved in collagen formation. Silicon also apparently is involved with phosphorus in the organic phase in the series of events leading to calcification (129). Thus, silicon possibly has a function that facilitates association between phosphoprotein-mucopolysaccharide macromolecules and collagen, which plays a role in the initiation of calcification and the regulation of crystal growth. The finding that silicon affects gene expression in some diatoms suggests that a similar role might also exist in higher animals (132).

Deficiency Signs

Silicon deficiency signs have not been defined for humans. Most of the signs of silicon deficiency in chickens and rats indicate aberrant metabolism of connective tissue and bone (123, 129, 130, 133). Chicks fed a semisynthetic, silicon-deficient diet exhibit structural abnormalities of the skull and long-bone abnormalities characterized by small, poorly formed joints, defective endochondral growth and depressed contents of articular cartilage, water, hexosamine, and collagen. Silicon deprivation can affect the response to other dietary manipulations. Rats fed a diet low in calcium and silicon and high in aluminum accumulated high amounts of aluminum in the brain; silicon supplements prevented the accumulation (134). Also, high dietary aluminum intakes depressed brain zinc concentrations in thyroidectomized rats fed low dietary silicon; silicon supplements prevented the depression (135). The effects of silicon and aluminum were not seen in nonthyroidectomized rats.

Toxicology

Silicon is essentially nontoxic when taken orally. Magnesium trisilicate, an over-the-counter antacid, has been used by humans for more than 40 years without obvious deleterious effects. Other silicates are food additives used as anticaking or antifoaming agents. However, ruminants consuming plants with a high silicon content may develop siliceous renal calculi. Renal calculi in humans may also contain silicates (123).

Dietary Considerations

Postulating a silicon requirement is difficult because only limited data are available. Rats fed about 0.16 mmol (4.5 mg) silicon/kg diet, mostly as the very available sodium metasilicate, do not differ from rats fed about 1.25 mmol (35 mg) silicon/kg diet; both prevent, equally well, silicon deficiency signs exhibited by rats fed about 36 μmol (1.0 mg) silicon/kg diet (133). Thus, if dietary silicon is highly available, as animal data suggest, the human requirement for silicon is quite small, perhaps in the range of 0.07 to 0.18 mmol (2–5 mg) per day. However, much of the silicon found in most diets probably is not absorbable or as available as sodium metasilicate; significant amounts probably occur as aluminosilicates and silica, from which silicon is not readily available. Thus, the recommended intake of silicon probably should be higher than the estimated requirement. On the basis of balance data, a silicon intake of 1.07 to 1.25 mmol (30–35 mg) per day was suggested for athletes, which was 0.18 to 0.36 mmol (5–10 mg) higher than that for nonatheletes (136).

Total dietary silicon intake of humans varies greatly with the amount and proportions of foods of animal (silicon-low) and plant (silicon-high) origin consumed and with the amounts of refined and processed foods in the diet (137, 138). Normally, refining reduces the silicon content of foods. However, in recent years, silicate additives have been used increasingly as anticaking or antifoaming agents in prepared foods and confections. Although this increases total dietary silicon, most of it is not bioavailable. The silicon content of drinking water and beverages made thereof shows geographic variation; silicon is high in hard-water and low in soft-water areas. The richest sources of silicon are unrefined grains of high fiber content and cereal products (137, 138).

Average daily intakes of silicon apparently range from about 0.71 to 1.79 mmol (20–50 mg) per day. The calculated silicon content of the FDA total diet was 0.68 mmol (19 mg) per day for women and 1.42 mmol (40 mg) for men (138). A human balance study indicated that oral intake of silicon could be about 0.75 to 1.64 mmol (21–46 mg) per day (127). The average British diet has been estimated to supply 1.10 mmol (31 mg) silicon per day (137).

Clinical Considerations

Ample circumstantial evidence indicates that silicon is an essential nutrient for higher animals, including humans. However, more work is needed to clarify the consequences of silicon deprivation in humans. A severe lack of dietary silicon could have detrimental effects on brain and bone function and composition.

VANADIUM

Historical Overview

Findings reported between 1971 and 1974 by four different research groups led many to conclude that vanadium is an essential nutrient. However, many of these findings may have been the consequence of high vanadium supplements (10 to 100 times the amount normally found in natural diets) that induced pharmacologic changes in animals fed imbalanced diets (118, 139, 140). A surge of interest in vanadium started in 1977 when it was rediscovered that vanadate inhibits ATPases (141) and has been maintained by the finding that vanadium is an insulin-mimetic agent (142). The first vanadium-containing enzyme, a bromoperoxidase from a marine alga, was isolated in 1984 (143). These findings have stimulated speculation about the nutritional importance of vanadium, for which the most substantive evidence has appeared only since 1987.

Chemistry

The chemistry of vanadium is complex because the element can exist in at least six oxidation states and can form polymers. In higher animals, the tetravalent and pentavalent states apparently are the most important forms of vanadium (144). The tetravalent vanadyl cation, VO^{2+}, behaves like a simple divalent aquo ion and competes well with Ca^{2+}, Mn^{2+}, Fe^{2+}, etc., for ligand-binding sites. Thus, VO^{2+} easily forms complexes with proteins, especially those associated with iron, such as transferrin and hemoglobin, which stabilize the vanadyl ion against oxidation. The pentavalent form of vanadium is known as vanadate ($H_2VO_4^-$ or more simply VO^{3-}). Vanadate forms complexes, including those that result in its being a phosphate transition-state analogue, and thus competes with or replaces phosphate in many biochemical processes. Vanadate is easily reduced nonenzymatically by relatively small molecules such as ascorbate and glutathione.

Another form of vanadium, the peroxo form, might be responsible for many biologic actions of vanadium, including its insulin-mimetic action and haloperoxidase role (145). Vanadate can interact with O^- formed by NADPH oxidase to generate the peroxovanadyl (V-OO) radical. Peroxovanadyl can in turn remove a hydrogen atom from NADPH to yield vanadyl hydroperoxide (V-OOH). Peroxo (heteroligand) vanadate adducts represent a useful model for the active-site vanadium involved in bromide oxidation in haloperoxidases (145).

Metabolism

Recent reviews of vanadium metabolism (140, 146) found that most ingested vanadium is unabsorbed and is excreted in the feces. Based on the very low concentrations of vanadium normally found in urine compared with the estimated daily intake and fecal content of vanadium, less than 5% of vanadium ingested is absorbed. Animal studies generally support the concept that vanadium is poorly absorbed. However, two studies with rats indicated that vanadium absorption can exceed 10% under some conditions, which suggests caution in assuming that ingested vanadium always is poorly absorbed from the gastrointestinal tract.

Most ingested vanadium is probably transformed in the stomach to VO^{2+} and remains in this form as it passes into the duodenum (147). However, in vitro studies suggest that vanadate can enter cells through phosphate- or other anion-transport systems. This may explain why VO_3^- is absorbed 3 to 5 times more effectively than VO^{2+}. Thus, apparently the different absorbability rates, the effect of other dietary components on the forms of vanadium in the stomach, and the rate at which it is transformed into VO^{2+} markedly affect the percentage of ingested vanadium absorbed (147). Supporting this concept are the reviewed findings showing that a number of substances can ameliorate vanadium toxicity, including EDTA, chromium, protein, ferrous ion, chloride, and aluminum hydroxide (140).

If vanadate appears in the blood, it is quickly converted into the vanadyl cation, most likely in erythrocytes. The vanadyl cation, either absorbed as such or formed in vivo, complexes with transferrin and ferritin in plasma and body fluids (148). It remains to be determined whether vanadyl-transferrin can transfer vanadium into cells through the transferrin receptor or whether ferritin is a storage vehicle for vanadium. Vanadium is rapidly removed from the blood plasma and is retained in highest amounts in the kidney, liver, testes, bone, and spleen. However, little of the absorbed vanadium is retained under normal conditions in the body; most tissues contain less than 196 pmol (10 ng) V/g fresh weight (140). Bone apparently is a major sink for excessive retained vanadium.

Excretion patterns after parenteral administration indicate that urine is the major excretory route for absorbed vanadium (148, 149). However, a significant portion of absorbed vanadium may be excreted through the bile. Human bile contains measurable vanadium (about 20 pmol [1.0 ng]/g) (150), and about 10% of an injected dose of ^{48}V was found in the feces of rats (149).

Both high- and low-molecular-weight complexes of vanadium have been found in urine (148, 149); one of these may be the vanadyl-transferrin complex. The form of vanadium in bile has not been determined.

Functions and Mode of Action

A defined biochemical function for vanadium in higher animals and thus for humans has not been described. Numerous biochemical and physiologic functions for vanadium have been suggested on the basis of its in vitro and pharmacologic actions; these have been reviewed (144, 151, 152) and are too extensive to discuss in detail here. Briefly, in vitro studies with cells and pharmacologic studies with animals have shown that vanadium has insulin-mimetic properties; numerous stimulatory effects on cell proliferation and differentiation; effects on cell phosphorylation-dephosphorylation; inhibitory effects on the motility of sperm, cilia, and chromosomes; effects on glucose and ion transport across plasma membranes; interfering effects on intracellular ionized calcium movement; and effects on oxidation-reduction processes. Vanadium inhibits numerous ATPases, phosphatases, and phosphoryl transfer enzymes in in vitro cell-free systems. The pharmacologic action of vanadium receiving the most attention recently is its ability to mimic insulin (142).

Enzymatic roles for vanadium have been defined for some algae, lichens, fungi, and bacteria (143, 145, 153). Vanadium enzymes include nitrogenase in bacteria, which reduces nitrogen gas to ammonia, and bromoperoxidase, iodoperoxidase and chloroperoxidase in algae, lichens, and fungi, respectively. The haloperoxidases catalyze the oxidation of halide ions by hydrogen peroxide, thus facilitating the formation of a carbon-halogen bond. The best known haloperoxidase in animals is thyroid peroxidase. Vanadium deprivation in rats affects the response of thyroid peroxidase to changing dietary iodine concentrations (154).

Deficiency Signs

Most of the early reported deficiency signs for vanadium are questionable. The diets used in early vanadium deprivation studies had widely varying contents of protein, sulfur amino acids, ascorbic acid, iron, copper, and perhaps other nutrients that affect, or can be affected by, vanadium (139). Also, vanadium supplemention in these experiments was relatively high compared with apparent need. As a result, it is difficult to determine whether the deficiency signs in early experiments were true deficiency signs, indirect changes caused by an enhanced need for vanadium in some metabolic function, or manifestations of a pharmacologic action of vanadium. Vanadium deficiency signs for humans have not been described.

The uncertainty about vanadium deficiency signs prompted new efforts to characterize a consistent set for animals. In these studies, goats fed diets apparently containing adequate and balanced amounts of all known nutrients exhibited an elevated abortion rate and depressed milk production when deprived of vanadium. About 40% of kids from vanadium-deprived goats died between days 7 and 91 of life, with some deaths preceded by convulsions; only 8% of kids from vanadium-supplemented goats died during the same time. Also, skeletal deformations were seen in the forelegs, and forefoot tarsal joints were thickened (155). In a rat study, vanadium deprivation increased thyroid weight and the thyroid weight:body weight ratio and decreased growth (154). Stressors that change thyroid status or iodine metabolism enhanced the response of rats to vanadium deprivation.

Toxicology

Vanadium is a relatively toxic element. Acute toxicity studies indicate that vanadium is a neurotoxic and hemorrhagic-endotheliotoxic poison with nephrotoxic, hepatotoxic, and probably leukocytotactic and hematotoxic components (156). Apparently, this breadth of toxic effects is the reason for the large number of signs of vanadium toxicity described for animals that vary among species and with dosage (157). Some of the more consistent signs include depressed growth, elevated organ vanadium, diarrhea, depressed food intake, and death. Animal data indicate that long-term daily intake above 196 μmol (10 mg) vanadium might lead to toxicologic consequences. Limited studies with humans support this contention. When 12 subjects were given 265 μmol (13.5 mg) vanadium daily for 2 weeks and then 442 μmol (22.5 mg) vanadium daily for 5 months, five patients exhibited gastrointestinal disturbances and five patients exhibited green tongue (158). In another study, six subjects were fed 88 to 353 μmol (4.5–18 mg) vanadium daily for 6 to 10 weeks; green tongue, cramps, and diarrhea were observed at the higher doses (159).

Dietary Considerations

If vanadium is essential for humans, its requirement most likely is small. The diets used in animal deprivation studies contained only 39 to 491 pmol (2–25 ng) V/g diet; these amounts often did not markedly affect the animals. Vanadium deficiency has not been identified in humans, yet diets generally supply less than 589 nmol (30 μg) vanadium daily and most supply only 294 nmol (15 μg) daily (95, 96, 150). Thus, a daily dietary intake of 196 nmol (10 μg) vanadium probably will meet any postulated requirement. Foods rich in vanadium include shellfish, mushrooms, parsley, dill seed, black pepper, and some prepared foods (150, 161, 162). Beverages, fats and oils, and fresh fruits and vegetables contain the least vanadium (less than 20 to 98 pmol [1–5 ng]/g).

Clinical Considerations

The clinical importance of vanadium is uncertain. It will be necessary to disentangle pharmacologic from nutritional observations to assess the nutritional importance of vanadium and to determine its safe and adequate intakes. Because vanadium is so pharmacologically active, a beneficial clinical role for this element may be found.

OTHER ULTRATRACE ELEMENTS

As indicated above, the evidence for essentiality of aluminum, bromine, cadmium, germanium, lead, lithium, rubidium, and tin is quite limited. Nonetheless, because beneficial claims for the elements are sometimes made in health magazines, newsletters, books, special publications, announcements, and advertisements, they should be considered here. Most likely none of these mineral elements are of nutritional or toxicologic concern if intakes are near those in a typical well-balanced diet.

Aluminum

A dietary deficiency of aluminum in goats reportedly results in increased abortions, depressed growth, incoordination and weakness in hind legs, and decreased life expectancy (163). Aluminum deficiency has been reported to depress growth in chicks (164). Aluminum toxicity is not a concern for healthy individuals. Cooking foods in aluminum cookware does not lead to toxic intakes of aluminum. Ingestion of high dietary amounts of aluminum is no longer believed to cause Alzheimer's disease. However, high intakes of aluminum from such sources as buffered analgesics and antacids by susceptible individuals (e.g., those with impaired kidney function, including the elderly and low-birth-weight infants) may lead to pathologic consequences and thus should be avoided. Aluminum toxicity is of most concern when contaminated solutions are used for parenteral feeding or for kidney dialysis (165). Aluminum toxicity caused in this manner results in neurotoxicity and adverse skeletal changes. Severe neurotoxicity, called dialysis dementia, is characterized by speech disturbances, disorientation, seizures, and hallucinations. Aluminum skeletal toxicity is characterized by bone pain and fractures. The typical daily dietary intake of aluminum is 74 to 371 μmol (2–10 mg). Rich sources of aluminum include baked goods prepared with chemical leavening agents (e.g., baking powder), processed cheese, grains, vegetables, herbs, and tea (166).

Bromine (Bromide)

It has been reported that a dietary deficiency of the bromide anion results in depressed growth, fertility, hematocrit, hemoglobin, and life expectancy, and in increased milk fat and abortions in goats (167). Also, insomnia exhibited by some hemodialysis patients has been associated with bromide deficiency (168). The bromide anion has a low order of toxicity; thus, it is not of toxicologic concern in nutrition. The typical daily intake of bromide ion is 25 to 100 μmol (2–8 mg). Rich sources of bromide are grains, nuts, and fish (169).

Cadmium

Cadmium deficiency reportedly depresses growth of rats (170) and goats (171). Although cadmium might be an essential element at very low intakes, it is of more concern because of its toxicologic properties (172). Cadmium is a potent antagonist of several essential minerals, including zinc, copper, iron, and calcium. Cadmium has a long half-life in the body and thus high intakes can lead to accumulation resulting in damage to some organs, especially the kidney. The typical daily dietary intake of cadmium is 89 to 178 nmol (10–20 μg). Rich sources of cadmium include shellfish, grains (especially those grown on high-cadmium soils), and leafy vegetables (172).

Germanium

A low germanium intake alters the mineral composition of bone and liver and decreases tibial DNA in the rat (173). Germanium is also touted as having anticancer properties because some organic complexes of this element inhibit tumor formation in animal models (174). High intakes of inorganic germanium, which is more toxic than organic forms of germanium, causes kidney damage (174). Some individuals consuming high amounts of organic germanium supplements contaminated with inorganic germanium have died from kidney failure. The typical daily dietary intake of germanium is 5.5 to 20.7 μmol (0.4–1.5 mg). Rich sources of germanium include wheat bran, vegetables, and leguminous seeds (169).

Lead

A large number of findings from one research group (175, 176) suggest that low dietary intake of lead has adverse effects in pigs and rats. Apparent deficiency signs found include depressed growth; anemia; elevated serum cholesterol, phospholipids, and bile acids; disturbed iron metabolism; decreased liver glucose, triglycerides, LDL-cholesterol and phospholipid concentrations; increased liver cholesterol; and altered blood and liver enzymes. Although lead might have beneficial effects at low intakes, lead toxicity is of more concern than lead deficiency. Lead is considered a major environmental pollutant because of past use of lead-based paints and the combustion of fuels containing lead additives. Lead toxicity (177) results in anemia, kidney damage, and central nervous system abnormalities ranging from ataxia and stupor to coma and convulsions. Ingestion of high amounts of lead from the environment by children has been associated with reduced intelligence and impaired motor function. The typical daily dietary intake of lead is 72 to 483 nmol (15–100 μg). Rich sources of lead include seafood and plant foodstuffs grown under high lead conditions (178).

Lithium

Lithium deficiency reportedly results in depressed fertility, birth weight, and life span and in altered activity of several liver and blood enzymes in goats (179). In rats, lithium deficiency apparently depresses fertility, birth weight, litter size, and weaning weight (180, 181). Lithium is best known for its pharmacologic antimanic properties (182). Its ability to affect mental function perhaps explains the report that incidence of violent crimes is higher in areas with low-lithium drinking water (183). The principal disadvantage in the use of lithium for psychiatric disorders is the narrow safety margin between therapeutic and toxic doses. Mild lithium toxicity results in gastrointestinal disturbances, muscular weakness, tremor, drowsiness, and a dazed feeling (182). Severe toxicity results in coma, muscle tremor, convulsions, and even death (182). The typical daily dietary intake of lithium is 28.8 to 86.5

μmol (200–600 μg). Rich sources of lithium include eggs, processed meat, fish, milk, milk products, potatoes, and vegetables (179).

Rubidium

Rubidium deficiency in goats reportedly results in depressed food intake, growth, and life expectancy and increased spontaneous abortion (184). Rubidium is relatively nontoxic and thus not of toxicologic concern. The typical daily dietary intake of rubidium is 12 to 59 μmol (1–5 mg). Rich sources of rubidium include coffee, black tea, fruits, vegetables (especially asparagus), and poultry (185).

Tin

A dietary deficiency of tin has been reported to depress growth, response to sound, and feed efficiency; to alter the mineral composition of several organs; and to cause hair loss in rats (186, 187). Inorganic tin is relatively nontoxic. However, routine consumption of foods packed in unlacquered tin-plated cans may result in excessive exposure to tin, which could adversely affect the metabolism of other essential trace elements including zinc and copper (188). The typical daily dietary intake of tin is 8 to 337 μmol (1–40 mg). A rich source of tin is canned foods (188).

REFERENCES

1. Nielsen FH, Hunt CD, Uthus EO. Ann NY Acad Sci 1980;355:152–64.
2. Food and Nutrition Board, National Research Council. Recommended dietary allowances. 10th ed. Washington, DC: National Academy Press, 1989;230–5 (Mn);235–40 (F);243–6 (Mo).
3. Gorby MS. Arsenic in human medicine. In: Nriagu JO, ed. Arsenic in the environment. Part II: Human health and ecosystem effects. New York: John Wiley & Sons, 1994;1–16.
4. Nielsen FH, Uthus EO. Arsenic. In: Frieden E, ed. Biochemistry of the essential ultratrace elements. New York: Plenum, 1984;319–40.
5. Dhubhghaill OMN, Sadler PJ. Struct Bond 1991;78:129–90.
6. Vahter M. Metabolism of arsenic. In: Fowler BA, ed. Biological and environmental effects of arsenic. Amsterdam: Elsevier, 1983;171–98.
7. Hopenhayn-Rich C, Smith AH, Goeden HM. Environ Res 1993;161–77.
8. Yamauchi, H, Kaise T, Yamamura Y. Bull Environ Contam 1986;36:350–5.
9. Marafante E, Vahter M, Dencker L. Sci Total Environ 1984;34:223–40.
10. Yamauchi H, Yamamura Y. Toxicol Appl Pharmacol 1984;74:134–40.
11. Le X-C, Cullen, WR, Reimer KJ. Clin Chem 1994;40:617–24.
12. Fullmer CS, Wasserman RH. Environ Res 1985;36:206–17.
13. Vahter M. Species differences in the metabolism of arsenic. In: Chappell WR, Abernathy CO, Cothern CR, eds. Arsenic. Exposure and health. Northwood, UK: Science and Technology Letters, 1994;171–9.
14. Zakharyan R, Wu Y, Bogdan GM, et al. Chem Res Toxicol 1995;8:1029–38.
15. Yamato N. Bull Environ Contam Toxicol 1988;40:633–40.
16. Uthus EO. Arsenic essentiality and factors affecting its importance. In: Chappell WR, Abernathy CO, Cothern CR, eds. Arsenic. Exposure and health. Northwood, UK: Science and Technology Letters, 1994;199–208.
17. Uthus EO. Environ Geochem Health 1992;14:55–8.
18. Desrosiers R, Tanguay RM. Biochem Cell Biol 1986;64:750–7.
19. Wang L, Roop BC, Mass MJ. Toxicologist 1996;30–87.
20. Meng Z, Meng N. Biol Trace Elem Res 1994;42:201–8.
21. Anke M. Arsenic. In: Mertz W, ed. Trace elements in human and animal nutrition, vol 2. Orlando: Academic Press, 1986;347–72.
22. Abernathy CO, Ohanian EV. Environ Geochem Health 1992;14:35–41.
23. Kaise T, Watanabe S, Itoh K. Chemosphere 1985;14:1327–32.
24. Morton WE, Dunnette DA. Health effects in environmental arsenic. In: Nriagu JO, ed. Arsenic in the environment. Part II: Human health and ecosystem effects. New York: John Wiley & Sons, 1994;17–34.
25. Abernathy CO, Dourson ML. Derivation of the inorganic arsenic reference dose. In: Chappell WR, Abernathy CO, Cothern CR, eds. Arsenic. Exposure and health. Northwood, UK: Science and Technology Letters, 1994;295–303.
26. Uthus EO. Estimation of safe and adequate daily intake for arsenic. In: Mertz W, Abernathy CO, Olin SS, eds. Risk assessment of essential elements. Washington, DC: ILSI Press, 1994;273–82.
27. Adams MA, Bolger PM, Gunderson EL. Dietary intake and hazards of arsenic. In: Chappell WR, Abernathy CO, Cothern CR, eds. Arsenic. Exposure and health. Northwood, UK: Science and Technology Letters, 1994;41–9.
28. Mayer DR, Kosmus W, Pogglitsch H, et al. Biol Trace Elem Res 1993;37:27–38.
29. Woods WG. Environ Health Perspect 1994;102(Suppl 7): 5–11.
30. Schummer D, Irschik H, Reichenbach H, et al. Liebigs Ann Chem 1994;283–9.
31. Dunitz JD, Hawley DM, Miklos D, et al. Helv Chim Acta 1971;54:1709–13.
32. Vanderpool RA, Hoff D, Johnson PE. Environ Health Perspect 1994;102(Suppl 7):13–20.
33. Hunt CD, Stoecker BJ. J Nutr 1996;126:2441S–51S.
34. Ward NI. Boron levels in human tissues and fluids. In: Anke M, Meissner D, Mills CF, eds. Trace elements in man and animals—TEMA 8. Gersdorf: Verlag Media Touristik, 1993; 724–8.
35. Nielsen FH. Proc ND Acad Sci 1996;50:52.
36. Barr RD, Clarke WB, Clarke RM, et al. J Lab Clin Med 1993;121:614–9.
37. Hunt CD. Environ Health Perspect 1994;102(Suppl 7):35–43.
38. Nielsen FH. FASEB J 1991;5:2661–7.
39. Nielsen FH. Environ Health Perspect 1994;102(Suppl 7):59–63.
40. Blevins DG, Lukaszewski KM. Environ Health Perspect 1994;102(Suppl 7):31–3.
41. Hunt CD. J Trace Elem Exp Med 1996;9:185–213.
42. Nielsen FH, Gallagher SK, Johnson LK, et al. J Trace Elem Exp Med 1992;5:237–46.
43. Penland JG. Environ Health Perspect 1994;102(Suppl 7):65–72.
44. Anonymous. Health effects of boron. Environ Health Perspect 1994;102(Suppl):87–141.
45. Linden CH, Hall AH, Kulig KW, et al. Clin Toxicol 1986;24:269–79.
46. Pinto J, Huang YP, McConnell RJ, et al. J Lab Clin Med 1978;92:126–34.

47. Gordon AS, Prichard JS, Freedman MH. Can Med Assoc J 1973;108:719–21.
48. WHO/FAO/IAEA. Trace elements in human nutrition and health. Geneva: World Health Organization, 1996;175–9.
49. Anderson DL, Cunningham WC, Lindstrom TR. J Food Comp Anal 1994;7:59–82.
50. Iyengar GV, Clarke WB, Downing RG, et al. J Trace Elem Electrolytes Health Dis 1991;5:128–9.
51. Newnham RE. Environ Health Perspect 1994;102(Suppl 7):83–5.
52. Whitford GM. J Dent Res 1990;69(Spec iss):539–49.
53. Messer HH. Fluorine. In: Frieden E, ed. Biochemistry of the essential ultratrace elements. New York: Plenum, 1984; 55–87.
54. Jenkins GN. The metabolism and effects of fluoride. In: Priest ND, Van de Vyver FL, eds. Trace metals and fluoride in bones and teeth. Boca Raton, FL: CRC Press, 1990;131–73.
55. Phipps KR. Fluoride. In: Ziegler EE, Filer LJ Jr, eds. Present knowledge in nutrition. 7th ed. Washington, DC: ILSI Press, 1996;239–33.
56. Schwarz K, Milne DB. Bioinorg Chem 1972;1:331–8.
57. Carlisle EM, Everly JA. FASEB J 1991;5:A1646.
58. Fransbergen AJ, Lemmens AG, Beynen AC. Biol Trace Elem Res 1991;31:71–8.
59. Anke M, Groppel B, Krause U. Fluorine deficiency in goats. In: Momcilovic B, ed. Trace elements in man and animals 7. Zagreb: IMI, 1991;26.28–26.29.
60. Avtsyn AP, Anke M, Zhavoronkov AA, et al. Pathological anatomy of the experimentally-induced fluorine deficiency in she-goats. In: Anke M, Meissner D, Mills CF, eds. Trace elements in man and animals—TEMA 8. Gersdorf: Verlag Media Touristik, 1993;745–6.
61. Klimis-Tavantzis DJ, ed. Manganese in health and disease, Boca Raton, FL: CRC Press, 1994;1–212.
62. Keen CL, Lönnerdal B, Hurley LS. Manganese. In: Frieden E, ed. Biochemistry of the essential ultratrace elements. New York: Plenum, 1984;89–132.
63. Wiegand E, Kirchgessner M, Helbig U. Biol Trace Elem Res 1986;10:265–79.
64. Davis CD, Wolf TL, Greger JL. J Nutr 1992;122:1300–8
65. Garcia-Aranda JA, Wapnir RA, Lifshitz F. J Nutr 1983;113:2601–7.
66. Bell JG, Keen CL, Lönnerdal B. J Toxicol Environ Health 1989;26:387–98.
67. Finley JW, Monroe P. J Nutr Biochem 1997;8:92–101.
68. Hurley LS, Keen CL. Manganese. In: Mertz W, ed. Trace elements in human and animal nutrition. 5th ed. San Diego: Academic Press, 1987;185–223.
69. Wedler FC. Biochemical and nutritional role of manganese: an overview. In: Klimis-Tavantzis DJ, ed. Manganese in health and disease. Boca Raton, FL: CRC Press, 1994;1–37.
70. Finley JW, Johnson PE. Manganese deficiency and excess in rodents. In: Watson RR, ed. Trace elements in laboratory rodents. Boca Raton, FL: CRC Press, 1996;85–106.
71. Freeland-Graves J, Llanes C. Models to study manganese deficiency In: Klimis-Tavantzis DJ, ed. Manganese in health and disease. Boca Raton, FL: CRC Press, 1994;59–86.
72. Doisy EA Jr. Trace Subs Environ Health 1972;6:193–9.
73. Friedman BJ, Freeland-Graves JH, Bales CW, et al. J Nutr 1987;117:133–43.
74. Johnson PE, Lykken GI. J Trace Elem Exp Med 1991;4:19–35.
75. Norose N. J Trace Elem Exp Med 1992;5:100–1.
76. Mena I. Manganese. In: Bronner F, Coburn JW, eds. Disorders of mineral metabolism, vol 1: Trace minerals. New York: Academic Press, 1981;233–70.
77. Hauser RA, Zesiewicz TA, Rosemurgy AS, et al. Ann Neurol 1994;36:871–5.
78. Gottschalk LA, Rebello T, Buchsbaum MS, et al. Comp Psychiatry 1991;32:229–37.
79. Freeland-Graves J. Derivation of manganese estimated safe and adequate daily dietary intakes. In: Mertz W, Abernathy CO, Olin SS, eds. Risk assessment of essential elements. Washington, DC: ILSI Press, 1994;237–52.
80. Pennington JAT, Young B. J Food Comp Anal 1990;3:166–84.
81. Mills CF, Davis GK. Molybdenum. In: Mertz W, ed. Trace elements in human and animal nutrition, vol 1. San Diego: Academic Press, 1987;429–63.
82. Rajagopalan KV. Annu Rev Nutr 1988;8:401–27.
83. Winston PW. Molybdenum. In: Bronner F, Coburn JW, eds. Disorders of mineral metabolism, vol 1: Trace minerals. New York: Academic Press, 1981;295–315.
84. Turnland JR, Keyes WR, Pfeiffer GL. Am J Clin Nutr 1995;62:790–6.
85. Turnland JR, Weaver CM, Kim SK, et al. FASEB J 1996;10:A818.
86. Cardin CJ, Mason J. Biochim Biophys Acta 1976;455:936–46.
87. Kosarek LJ, Winston PW. Fed Proc 1977;36:1106.
88. Lener J, Bibr B. J Hyg Epidemiol Microbiol Immunol 1984;28:405–19.
89. Beedham C. Drug Metab Rev 1985;16:119–56.
90. Bodine PV, Litwack G. Proc Natl Acad Sci USA 1988;85:1462–6.
91. Barsony J, McKoy W. J Biol Chem 1992;267:24457–65.
92. Abumrad NN, Schneider AJ, Steel D, et al. Am J Clin Nutr 1981;34:2551–9.
93. Turnland JR, Keyes WR, Pfeiffer GL, et al. Am J Clin Nutr 1995;61:1102–9.
94. Evans WH, Read JI, Caughlin D. Analyst 1985;110:873–7.
95. Pennington JAT, Jones JW. J Am Diet Assoc 1987;87:1644–50.
96. Anke M. Lösch E, Glei M, et al. Der Molybdängehalt der Lebensmittel und Getränke Deutschlands. In: Anke M, Bergmann H, Bitsch R, et al., eds. Mengen- und Spurenelemente. Gersdorf: Verlag Media Touristik, 1993;537–53.
97. Seaborn CD, Yang SP. Biol Trace Elem Res 1993;39:245–56.
98. Nielsen FH. Nickel. In: Frieden E, ed. Biochemistry of the essential ultratrace elements. New York: Plenum, 1984;293–308.
99. Sigel H, Sigel A, eds. Metal ions in biological systems, vol 23. Nickel and its role in biology. New York: Marcel Dekker, 1988;1–488.
100. Lancaster JR Jr, ed. The bioinorganic chemistry of nickel. New York: VCH Publishers, 1988;1–337.
101. Solomons NW, Viteri F, Shuler TR, et al. J Nutr 1982;112:39–50.
102. Sunderman FW Jr, Hopfer SM, Swift T, et al. Nickel absorption and elimination in human volunteers. In: Hurley LS, Keen CL, Lönnerdal B, et al., eds. Trace elements in man and animals 6. New York: Plenum, 1988;427–8.
103. Kirchgessner M, Roth-Maier DA, Schnegg A. Progress of nickel metabolism and nutrition research. In: Howell J McC, Gawthorne JM, White CL, eds. Trace element metabolism in man and animals—TEMA 4. Canberra: Australian Academy of Science, 1981;621–4.
104. Tallkvist J, Wing AM, Tjalve H. Pharmacol Toxicol 1994;75:244–9.
105. Foulkes EC, McMullen DM. Toxicology 1986;38:35–42.
106. Borg-Neczak K, Tjalve H. Arch Toxicol 1994;68:450–8.
107. Tallkvist J, Tjalve H. Pharmacol Toxicol 1994;75:233–43.
108. Tabata M, Sarkar B. J Inorg Biochem 1992;45:93–104.

109. Nomoto S, Sunderman FW Jr. Ann Clin Lab Sci 1988;18:78–84.
110. Rezuke WN, Knight JA, Sunderman FW Jr. Am J Ind Med 1987;11:419–26.
111. Omokhodion FO, Howard JM. Clin Chim Acta 1994;231:23–8.
112. Nielsen FH, Zimmerman TJ, Shuler TR, et al. J Trace Elem Exp Med 1989;2:21–9.
113. Nielsen FH, Uthus EO, Poellot RA, et al. Biol Trace Elem Res 1993;37:1–15.
114. Uthus EO, Poellot RA. FASEB J 1994;8:A430.
115. Shibuya I, Douglas WW. Endocrinology 1992;131:1936–41.
116. Shankar VS, Bax CR, Bax BE, et al. J Cell Physiol 1993;155:120–9.
117. Nielsen FH, Nickel. In: Mertz W, ed. Trace elements in human and animal nutrition. 5th ed. San Diego: Academic Press, 1987;245–73.
118. Nielsen FH. J Nutr 1985;115:1239–47.
119. Cronin E, Di Michiel AD, Brown SS. Oral challenge in nickel-sensitive women with hand eczema. In: Brown SS, Sunderman FW Jr, eds. Nickel toxicology. New York: Academic Press, 1980;149–52.
120. Anke M, Angelow L, Müller M, et al. Dietary trace element intake and excretion of man. In: Anke M, Meissner D, Mills CF, eds. Trace elements in man and animals—TEMA 8. Gersdorf: Verlag Media Touristik, 1993;180–8.
121. Veien NK, Anderson MR. Acta Derm Venerol (Stockh) 1986;66:502–9.
122. Gouget MA. La Presse Medicale 1911;97:1005–6.
123. Carlisle EM. Silicon. In: Frieden E, ed. Biochemistry of the essential ultratrace elements. New York: Plenum 1984;257–91.
124. Wannagat U. Nobel Symp 1978;40:447–72.
125. Sauer F, Laughland DH, Davidson WM. Can J Biochem Physiol 1959;37:183–91.
126. Allain P, Cailleux A, Mauras Y. Therapie 1983;38:171–4.
127. Kelsay JL, Behall KM, Prather E. Am J Clin Nutr 1979;32:1876–80.
128. Berlyne GM, Adler AJ, Ferran N, et al. Nephron 1986;43:5–9.
129. Carlisle EM. Silicon in bone formation. In: Simpson TL, Volcani BE, eds. Silicon and siliceous structures in biological systems. New York: Springer, 1981;69–94.
130. Carlisle EM. Sci Total Environ 1988;73:95–106.
131. Seaborn CD, Nielsen FH. FASEB J 1996;10:A784.
132. Reeves CD, Volcani BE. J Gen Microbiol 1985;131:1735–44.
133. Seaborn CD, Nielsen FH. Nutr Today 1993;28:13–8.
134. Carlisle EM, Curran MJ. Alzheimer Dis Assoc Disorders 1987;1:83–9.
135. Carlisle EM, Curran MJ, Duong T. The effect of interrelationships between silicon, aluminum and the thyroid on zinc content in brain. In: Momcilovic B, ed. Trace elements in man and animals 7. Zagreb: IMI, 1991;12.16–12.17.
136. Nasolodin VV, Rusin VY, Vorob'ev VA. Vopr Pitan 1987;(4)37–9.
137. Bowen HJM, Peggs A. J Sci Food Agric 1984;35:1225–9.
138. Pennington JAT. Foods Addit Contam 1991;8:97–118.
139. Nielsen FH, Uthus EO. The essentiality and metabolism of vanadium. In: Chasteen ND, ed. Vanadium in biological systems. Physiology and biochemistry. Dordrecht: Kluwer, 1990;51–62.
140. Nielsen FH. Vanadium in mammalian physiology and nutrition. In: Sigel H, Sigel A, eds. Metal ions in biological systems, vol 31: Vanadium and its role in life. New York: Marcel Dekker, 1995;543–73.
141. Cantley LC Jr, Josephson L, Warner R, et al. J Biol Chem 1977;252:7421–3.
142. Orvig C, Thompson KH, Battell M, et al. Vanadium compounds as insulin mimics. In: Sigel H, Sigel A, eds. Metal ions in biological systems, vol 31: Vanadium and its role in life. New York: Marcel Dekker, 1995;575–94.
143. Vilter H. Vanadium-dependent-haloperoxidases. In: Sigel H, Sigel A, eds. Metal ions in biological systems, vol 31: Vanadium and its role in life. New York: Marcel Dekker, 1995;325–62.
144. Boyd DW, Kustin K. Adv Inorg Biochem 1984;6:311–65.
145. Wever R, Kustin K. Adv Inorg Chem 1990;35:81–115.
146. Nielsen FH. Vanadium absorption. In: Berthon G, ed. Handbook of metal-ligand interactions in biological fluids. Bioinorganic medicine, vol 1. New York: Marcel Dekker, 1995;425–7.
147. Chasteen ND, Lord EM, Thompson HJ. Vanadium metabolism. Vanadyl (IV) electron paramagnetic resonance spectroscopy of selected tissues in the rat. In: Xavier AV, ed. Frontiers in bioinorganic chemistry. Weinhein: VCH Verlagsgesellchaft, 1986;133–41.
148. Sabbioni E, Marafante E. J Toxicol Environ Health 1981;8:419–29.
149. Hopkins LL Jr, Tilton BE. Am J Physiol 1966;211:169–72.
150. Byrne AR, Kosta L. Sci Total Environ 1978;10:17–30.
151. Nechay BR. Annu Rev Pharmacol Toxicol 1984;24:501–24.
152. Willsky GR. Vanadium in the biosphere. In: Chasteen ND, ed. Vanadium in biological systems. Physiology and biochemistry. Dordrecht: Kluwer, 1990;1–24.
153. Eady RR. Vanadium nitrogenases of *Azotobacter*. In: Sigel H, Sigel A, eds. Metal ions in biological systems, vol 31: Vanadium and its role in life. New York: Marcel Dekker, 1995;363–405.
154. Uthus EO, Nielsen FH. Magnesium Trace Elem 1990;9:219–26.
155. Anke M, Groppel B, Gruhn K, et al. The essentiality of vanadium for animals. In: Anke M, Baumann W, Bräunlich H, et al., eds. 6th International Trace Element Symposium, vol 1. Jena: Friedrich-Schiller-Universitat, 1989;17–27.
156. Proescher F, Seil HA, Stillians AW. Am J Syph 1917;1:347–405.
157. Nielsen FH. Vanadium. In: Mertz W, ed. Trace elements in human and animal nutrition, vol 1. San Diego: Academic Press, 1987;275–300.
158. Somerville J, Davies B. Am Heart J 1962;64:54–6.
159. Dimond EG, Caravaca J, Benchimol A. Am J Clin Nutr 1963;12:49–53.
160. Myron DR, Zimmerman TJ, Shuler TR, et al. Am J Clin Nutr 1978;31:527–31.
161. Myron DR, Givand SH, Nielsen FH. Agric Food Chem 1977;25:297–300.
162. Illing H, Anke M, Müller M. Der Vanadiumgehalt Tierishcher Lebensmittel. In: Anke M., Meissner D, Bergmann H, et al., eds. Defizite und Überschüsse an Mengen- und Spurenelementen in der Ernährung. Leipzig: Verlag Harald Schubert, 1994;257–63.
163. Angelow L, Anke M, Groppel B, et al. Aluminum: an essential element for goats. In: Anke M, Meissner D, Mills CF, eds. Trace elements in man and animals—TEMA 8. Gersdorf: Verlag Media Touristik, 1993;699–704.
164. Carlisle EM, Curran MJ. Aluminum: an essential element for the chick. In: Anke M, Meissner D, Mills CF, eds. Trace elements in man and animals—TEMA 8. Gersdorf: Verlag Media Touristik, 1993;695–8.
165. Allfrey AC. Aluminum toxicity in humans. In: Tomita H, ed. Trace elements in clinical medicine. Tokyo: Springer-Verlag, 1990;459–64.
166. Greger JL. Annu Rev Nutr 1993;13:43–63.

167. Anke M, Groppel B, Angelow L, et al. Bromine: an essential element for goats. In: Anke M, Meissner D, Mills CF, eds. Trace elements in man and animals—TEMA 8. Gersdorf: Verlag Media Touristik, 1993;737–8.
168. Oe PL, Vis RD, Meijer JH, et al. Bromine deficiency and insomnia in patients on dialysis. In: Howell J McC, Gawthorne JM, White CL, eds. Trace element metabolism in man and animals—TEMA 4. Canberra: Australian Academy of Science, 1981;526–9.
169. Nielsen FH. Other elements: Sb, Ba, B, Br, Cs, Ge, Rb, Ag, Sr, Sn, Ti, Zr, Be, Bi, Ga, Au, In, Nb, Sc, Te, Tl, W. In: Mertz W, ed. Trace elements in human and animal nutrition, vol 2. Orlando: Academic Press, 1986;415–63.
170. Schwarz K, Spallholz JE. The potential essentiality of cadmium. In: Bolck F, Anke M, Schneider H-J, eds. Kadmium-Symposium. Jena: Friedrich-Schiller-Universitat, 1979;188–94.
171. Anke M, Hennig A, Groppel B, et al. The biochemical role of cadmium. In: Kirchgessner M, ed. Trace element metabolism in man and animals—3. Freising-Weihenstephen: Tech Univ Munchen, 1978;540–8.
172. Kostial K. Cadmium. In: Mertz W, ed. Trace elements in human and animal nutrition, vol 2. Orlando: Academic Press, 1986;319–45.
173. Seaborn CD, Nielsen FH. Biol Trace Elem Res 1994;42: 151–64.
174. Schauss AG. Biol Trace Elem Res 1991;29:267–80.
175. Reichlmayr-Lais AM, Kirchgessner M. Lead—an essential trace element. In: Momcilovic B, ed. Trace elements in man and animals 7. Zagreb: IMI, 1991;35.1–35.2.
176. Kirchgessner M, Plass DL, Reichlmayr-Lais AM. Lead deficiency in swine. In: Momcilovic B, ed. Trace elements in man and animals 7. Zagreb: IMI, 1991;11.20–11.21.
177. Skerfving S, Gerhardsson L, Schütz A, et al. Toxicity of detrimental metal ions. Lead. In: Berthon G, ed. Handbook of metal-ligand interactions in biological fluids. Bioinorganic medicine, vol 2. New York: Marcel Dekker, 1995;755–65.
178. Müller M, Anke M, Thiel C, et al. Exposure of adults to lead from food estimated by analysis and calculation-comparison of methods. In: Anke M, Meissner D, Mill CF, eds. Trace elements in man and animals—TEMA 8. Gersdorf: Verlag Media Touristik, 1993;241–2.
179. Anke M, Arnhold W, Groppel B, et al. The biological importance of lithium. In: Schrauzer GN, Klippel K-F, eds. Lithium in biology and medicine. Weinheim: VCH Publishers, 1990;148–67.
180. Patt EL, Pickett EE, O'Dell BL. Bioinorg Chem 1978;9: 299–310.
181. Pickett EE, O'Dell BL. Biol Trace Elem Res 1992;34:299–319.
182. Birch NJ. Lithium in medicine. In: Berthon G, ed. Handbook of metal-ligand interactions in biological fluids. Bioinorganic medicine, vol 2. New York: Marcel Dekker, 1995;1274–81.
183. Schrauzer GN, Shrestha KP, Flores-Arce MF. Biol Trace Elem Res 1992;34:161–76.
184. Anke M, Angelow L, Schmidt A, et al. Rubidium: an essential element for animal and man? In: Anke M, Meissner D, Mills CF, eds. Trace elements in man and animals—TEMA 8. Gersdorf: Verlag Media Touristik, 1993;719–23.
185. Anke M, Angelow L, Fresenius J. Anal Chem 1995;352:236–9.
186. Schwarz K, Milne DB, Vinyard E. Biochem Biophys Res Commun 1970;40:22–9.
187. Yokoi K, Kimura M, Itokawa Y. Biol Trace Elem Res 1990;24:223–31.
188. Greger JL. Tin and aluminum. In: Smith KT, ed. Trace minerals in foods. New York: Marcel Dekker, 1988;291–323.

SELECTED READINGS

Arsenic

Chappell WR, Abernathy CO, Cothern CR, eds. Arsenic. Exposure and health. Northwood: Science and Technology Letters, 1994.

Boron

Environmental health perspectives supplement. Health effects of boron, vol 102 (Suppl 7), 1994.

Manganese

Klimis-Tavantzis DJ, ed. Manganese in health and disease. Boca Raton, FL: CRC Press, 1994.

Nickel

Sigel H, Sigel A, eds. Metal ions in biological systems, vol 23. Nickel and its role in biology. New York: Marcel Dekker, 1988.

Silicon

Evered D, O'Conner M, eds. Ciba Foundation. Silicon biochemistry. Chichester: John Wiley & Sons, 1986.

Vanadium

Sigel H, Sigel A, eds. Metal ions in biological systems, vol 31. Vanadium and its role in life. New York: Marcel Dekker, 1995.

Molybdenum, Fluoride, and Other Trace Elements

Frieden E, ed. Biochemistry of the essential ultratrace elements. New York: Plenum Press, 1984.
WHO/FAO/IAEA. Trace elements in human nutrition and health. Geneva: World Health Organization, 1996.

17. Vitamin A and Retinoids

A. CATHARINE ROSS

HISTORICAL OVERVIEW

Historical research provides evidence that Egyptian and Greek physicians in ancient times may have understood the curative value of liver, a rich source of vitamin A, for night blindness, an early ocular manifestation of vitamin A deficiency (1). The first scientific reports of an essential dietary component with vitamin A activity were published in 1913 by E. V. McCollum and M. Davis and by T. B. Osborne and L. V. Mendel. These investigators noted that certain "lipins" extracted from butter, eggs, or cod liver oil were essential for the growth of young rats fed diets with lard or olive oil as the only fat. McCollum and Davis first referred to this then-unknown growth factor as "fat-soluble A," and later as "vitamin A." Steenbock and others soon recognized that a factor present in yellow vegetables had similar activity. Moore drew the prescient inference that the latter yellow substance, now recognized as carotene, might be a precursor of the nearly colorless vitamin A.

During the 1920s, several investigators made several fundamental discoveries regarding the relationship of vitamin A deficiency to growth, xerophthalmia, normal tissue differentiation, and resistance to infection. In the 1920s to 1930s, Karrer and his colleagues in Switzerland elucidated the chemical structure of vitamin A as all-*trans*-retinol, and in the late 1940s, Arens and van Dorp (2) reported the synthesis of vitamin A acid, now known as retinoic acid (RA). These investigators and others showed that RA restores growth in vitamin A–deficient animals. During the 1950s, the role of vitamin A in vision was elucidated by the work of Wald, Hubbard, and others, which showed that "retinene" (now retinal) is the essential visual pigment of the photoreceptor cells (3).

Other milestones in vitamin A research include a series of discoveries of proteins essential for transport and metabolism of retinoids. The plasma transport protein for retinol, retinol-binding protein (RBP), was isolated from human plasma in the late 1960s (4). A number of cellular retinoid-binding proteins were first identified in the 1970s and have been extensively characterized since then (5). Simultaneously, it became clear that RA is the most potent metabolite of vitamin A, possessing most, if not all, of vitamin A's biologic activities apart from the activity of retinal in vision.

The first members of a new family of nuclear retinoid receptors were described in 1987 and shown to be highly homologous in structure and mechanism of action to the previously described superfamily of steroid/thyroid hormone receptors. This area of retinoid receptor research has expanded extremely rapidly with the recognition of two main subfamilies of nuclear retinoid receptors (RAR and RXR) (6, 7). Through the use of molecular biologic techniques much has been learned about the nuclear retinoid receptors with respect to their physical characteristics, ligand specificities and interactions, patterns of expression in tissues and cells, and interactions with co-regulatory molecules and the DNA of retinoid-responsive

Abbreviations: **APL**—acute promyelocytic leukemia; **CRBP**—cellular retinol-binding protein; **CRABP**—cellular retinoic acid–binding protein; **RA**—retinoic acid; **RAR**—retinoic acid receptor; **REH**—retinyl ester hydrolase; **RXR**—retinoid X receptor; **RBP**—retinol-binding protein; **RARE**—RAR response element; **RPE**—retinal pigment epithelium; **RXRE**—RXR response element; **TTR**—transthyretin; **UV**—ultraviolet.

genes. The stage is now set for understanding molecular regulation of gene expression by retinoids under nutritionally relevant conditions and the therapeutic action of retinoids used as pharmacologic agents.

CHEMISTRY

Vitamin A is a nutritional term that describes a family of essential, fat-soluble dietary compounds that are structurally related to the lipid alcohol retinol and share its biologic activity. Vitamin A in its various forms is required for vision, growth, reproduction, cell proliferation, cell differentiation, and the integrity of the immune system. Formally, the term *vitamin A* includes those provitamin A carotenoids that serve as dietary precursors of retinol (see Chapter 33). The term *retinoids* refers both to retinol and its natural metabolites as well as to a large number of synthetic analogues that have structural similarities to retinol but may subserve only some (or none) of the functions of natural vitamin A.

Properties

Retinol (Fig. 17.1*A*) is a pale yellow crystalline solid of molecular mass 286.46. The molecule comprises a substituted cyclohexenyl (*β*-ionone) ring, a tetraene side chain, and a primary hydroxyl group at C-15. Retinol and its metabolites exist in nature as several geometric isomers including all-*trans*, 9-*cis*, 11-*cis*, and 13-*cis* retinoids (8). The system of five conjugated double bonds in retinol confers characteristic spectral properties (ultraviolet (UV) absorption and fluorescence absorption and emission) that are used in the detection, identification, and quantification of retinoids (9, 10). All-*trans*-retinol (vitamin A_1) has a characteristic UV spectrum with a maximum near 325 nm ($E^{1\%}_{1cm}$ in alcohol of 1835 [10]). The UV maximum of vitamin A_2 (all-*trans*-3,4-didehydroretinol), which has a second double bond within the *β*-ionone ring, is red-shifted to 351 nm.

Retinol's hydroxyl group may be esterified with a fatty acid. In nature, retinol is esterified with long-chain fatty acids (mainly palmitate and stearate), whereas pharmaceutical preparations may include short-chain esters. Long-chain esters are yellow viscous oils at room and body temperatures. Esterification confers greater stability on retinol, but the UV absorption maxima and molar extinction coefficients of unesterified and esterified retinol are nearly identical.

The hydroxyl group of retinol undergoes successive

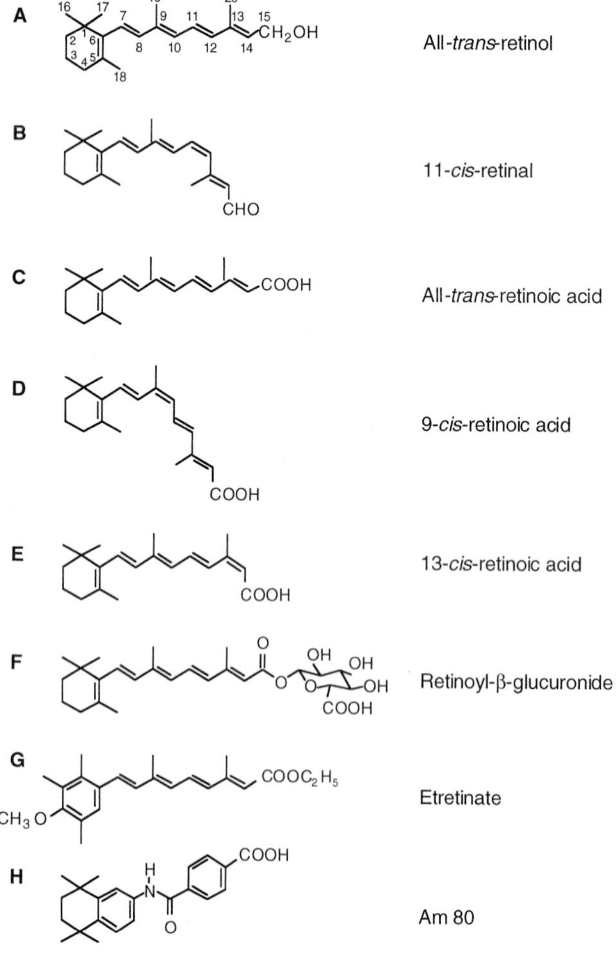

Figure 17.1. Structures of common biologic *(A–F)* and representative synthetic *(G, H)* retinoids.

oxidation to produce, first, an aldehyde (retinaldehyde, or retinal) which may be further oxidized to a carboxylic acid, RA. In the retina, 11-*cis*-retinal (Fig. 17.1*B*) plays a specific role through binding to proteins (opsins) to form the visual pigments rhodopsin (in rod cells) and iodopsins (in cone cells). (See "Vision" below.) Unbound 11-*cis*-retinal absorbs light maximally at 365 nm. RA (molecular mass, 300.4) exists as all-*trans*-RA (Fig. 17.1*C*), 9-*cis*-RA (Fig. 17.1*D*), and 13-*cis*-RA (Fig. 17.1*E*), as well as some di-*cis* isomers. All-*trans*-RA has a UV absorption maximum (in alcohol) of about 351 nm (10).

As analytical methods have improved, additional retinoids have been isolated and characterized. These include a number of more polar metabolites with keto, hydroxyl, or epoxide functional groups. Several water-soluble retinoids such as the glucuronide conjugates of retinol and RA (Fig. 17.1*F*) have been isolated from plasma, bile, and other tissues or have been synthesized. Water solubility is accompanied by marked reduction in most indices of toxicity, as well as differences in transport and metabolism, compared with lipophilic retinoids (11).

A large number of retinoid analogues have been synthesized (8). Naturally occurring retinoids are of limited use as pharmaceutical products because of their potential toxicity. Therefore, a principal goal of retinoid synthesis has been creation of new molecules with a higher therapeutic ratio, e.g., greater beneficial potency and/or less toxicity. Some synthetic retinoids have greater stability (conformationally restricted forms [12]) than the natural retinoids and/or bind selectively to certain retinoid receptors as agonists or antagonists. Figure 17.1*G* illustrates a synthetic retinoid, acitretin, an analogue of RA that is used in dermatology. Figure 17.1*H* illustrates a retinobenzoic acid, Am80, which binds selectively to the nuclear receptor RAR-α (13). Some retinoids (e.g., all-*trans*- and 13-*cis*-RA) belong to both the biologic and pharmaceutical categories of retinoids. A discussion of retinoid properties and routes of synthesis can be found in (8).

Most natural retinoids are soluble in body fat, oils, and most organic solvents but not in water. They are sensitive to isomerization, oxidation, and polymerization; therefore, they must be protected from light, oxygen, and high temperature. However, retinoids are usually quite stable when stored in crystalline form, oil, or some organic solvents, in the absence of light and oxygen, and at low temperature. In tissue specimens that have been kept sealed and deep-frozen (preferably at −70°C), retinol and its esters have been stable for several years (9).

Methods of Analysis

Most modern methods of retinoid analysis are based on solvent extraction of samples followed by chromatographic separation of molecular species, usually by high-performance liquid chromatography (HPLC), with detection by UV absorption at a single or multiple wavelengths (14). Some metabolic and biochemical studies have used forms labeled with deuterium or carbon-13. The proteins involved in retinoid transport and function have been analyzed spectrophotometrically, immunologically, and by the use of molecular biologic methods (5, 15).

NUTRITIONAL SOURCES

Plants and some lower organisms (e.g., algae) synthesize the carotenoids that serve as precursors of vitamin A (see Chapter 33), but they do not synthesize retinoids directly (the halobacteria, however, provide an interesting exception). Humans and other animals convert carotenoids to retinol and its metabolites, or they obtain preformed vitamin A in foods of animal origin or in nutritional supplements. It is possible to obtain an adequate intake of vitamin A from diets of diverse types, ranging from strictly vegetarian (see Chapter 106) to strictly carnivorous. Preformed vitamin A comprises over two-thirds of dietary vitamin A in the United States and Europe (16), whereas provitamin A predominates in many other parts of the world.

Vitamin A in the U.S. diet comes mainly from liver, yellow and green leafy vegetables, eggs, and whole-milk products (16). Liver and fish liver oils constitute the most concentrated sources of preformed vitamin A. Nutritional supplements contain vitamin A as retinol, esterified retinol, and/or β-carotene in doses that generally equal and sometimes exceed the recommended dietary allowances (RDAs). 3,4-Didehydroretinol, found in freshwater fish, has about 40% of the bioactivity of crystalline vitamin A_1. Foodstuffs contain very little retinal or RA.

The commonly used nutritional unit for vitamin A is the μg *retinol equivalent* (μg RE), equal to 1 μg of all-*trans* retinol. The USP unit or International Unit (IU) is still sometimes used to quantify vitamin A activity in pharmaceutical preparations. One USP unit or IU equals 0.30 μg of retinol, 0.344 μg of retinyl acetate, and 0.55 μg of retinyl palmitate, all as their all-*trans* isomers. Because preformed and provitamin A differ in biologic activity, it has been necessary to develop factors to equate the biologic activity of carotenoids and retinol in foods (9, 16). Generally, it is assumed that 6 μg of all-*trans*-β-carotene or 12 μg of other all-*trans* provitamin A carotenoids are equivalent nutritionally to one RE (μg) of all-*trans*-retinol (see refs. 16 and 17 and Chapter 33 for discussion). Système International d'Unités (SI) units are preferred for expressing vitamin A concentrations in tissues (see Appendix Tables I-A-1-a and b). Conversion factors are 1 μmol retinol/L equals 286.46 μg retinol/L of fluid or per g of tissue. One μmol/L of retinyl palmitate equals 524.86 μg/L of retinyl palmitate or 286.46 μg/L of retinol.

Recommended Dietary Allowance

The RDA for vitamin A (16), expressed in RE/day, ranges from 375 μg RE/day for infants to 1000 μg RE/day for male adults. A complete table of U.S. RDAs is found in Appendix Table II-A-2-b. The Appendix also contain tables of nutrient recommendations issued by Canada, the United Kingdom, Japan, Korea, and the World Health Organization (WHO).

RETINOID-BINDING PROTEINS AND RECEPTORS

Retinoid-binding proteins provide solubility to retinoids and serve as specific chaperones during their transport and metabolism. Three principal classes of transport or receptor proteins have been identified. In plasma, RBP functions to solubilize retinol and deliver it to cells. Within cells, cytosolic (cellular) retinoid-binding proteins limit the concentration of "free," unbound retinoid and channel retinoids to specific enzymes responsible for metabolic transformations. In the nuclei of cells, specific retinoid-receptor proteins bind RA and regulate the activity of retinoid-responsive genes (Table 17.1).

Retinol-Binding Protein (RBP)

Plasma RBP is the principal carrier of all-*trans*-retinol, which typically constitutes more than 90% of plasma vitamin A. RBP is a single polypeptide chain of molecular mass 21.2 kDa in humans, which circulates in association with a cotransport protein, transthyretin (TTR, also called prealbumin, molecular mass approximately 55 kDa). RBP and TTR have been well conserved during evolution, and homologous forms of these proteins exist in the plasma of all vertebrate species that have been examined (15). RBP binds retinol with high affinity ($K_a = \sim 1.5 \times 10^{-6}$ M · L^{-1}); furthermore, the binding affinity of retinol to RBP is approximately doubled by association of RBP with TTR (18).

Protein Structure and Genomic Characteristics. RBP is a member of a family of relatively low-molecular-weight proteins that bind small hydrophobic ligands (15). The tertiary structure of RBP is described as a "*β*-barrel." The barrel is formed from eight antiparallel *β*-sheets positioned in two orthogonal arrays. The interior of the RBP barrel provides a binding cavity into which one molecule of retinol fits with its hydroxyl group oriented toward the surface of RBP (15).

The gene for RBP has been cloned and partially characterized. The RBP gene exists as a single copy per haploid genome, is located on human chromosome 10q23-24, and comprises 10 kb of genomic DNA having six exons and five introns. Based on a comparison of the genomic and protein crystalline structures, each exon encodes a defined unit of protein structure. The human RBP cDNA is approximately 1000 bp long with a 600-bp open reading frame that encodes a 199–amino acid protein, including a 16–amino acid signal peptide and a 183–amino acid mature protein. The relative abundance of RBP mRNA is highest in liver (defined as 100%), less than 10 to more than 35% in various adipose beds, about 5 to 10% in kidney, and lower in a number of other tissues (15). RBP mRNA is also expressed at high relative abundance in the embryonic visceral yolk sac (~50%) and fetal liver (~25%). RBP protein is expressed by liver parenchymal cells, the eye, and visceral yolk sac, and perhaps by other RBP mRNA–containing organs (15). An RBP-like protein has been isolated from uterine/allantoic fluid (19).

RBP is present in plasma at a concentration of approximately 2 to 3 μmol/L (0.42–0.64 mg/mL). Regulation of RBP synthesis, secretion, plasma concentration, and turnover is discussed below.

Table 17.1
Properties of Major Retinoid-Binding Proteins

Name	Abbreviation	Size (kDa)	Major Ligand	Location	Physiologic Role	Mode of Regulation
Retinol-binding protein	RBP	21.2	All-*trans*-retinol	Plasma (complexed with TTR)	Plasma transport	Secretion of holo-RBP; renal catabolism
Cellular retinol-binding	CRBP-I	14.6	All-*trans*-retinol	Cytoplasm of many cell types	Delivers retinol to enzymes; controls free retinol concentration	Modest transcriptional regulation
Cellular retinol-binding II	CRBP-II	14.6	All-*trans*-retinol; retinal	Cytoplasm, mainly of intestinal absorptive cells	Delivers retinol to enzymes involved in vitamin A absorption	Possible regulation through RXRE and by fatty acids
Cellular retinoic acid–binding protein I	CRABP-I	14.6	All-*trans*-RA	Cytoplasm of many cells, at low levels	Controls RA concentration; facilitates catabolism	Unknown
Cellular retinoic acid–binding protein II	CRABP-II	14.6	All-*trans*-RA	Cytoplasm; mainly in skin	Controls RA concentration; related to RA catabolism?	Transcription induced by binding RA
Retinoic acid receptors	RAR-α, RAR-β, RAR-γ	~50	All-*trans*-RA (9-*cis*-RA)	Spatially and temporally varied expression patterns; nuclear location	Binds with RXR to RAREs	Developmentally regulated; RAR-β regulated by RA
Retinoid X receptors	RXR-α, RXR-β, RXR-γ	~50	9-*cis*-RA	Spatially and temporally varied expression patterns; nuclear location	Binds with RARs to RAREs, as homodimers to RXREs, and as the heterodimeric partner of other receptors	Developmentally regulated

Cellular Retinoid-Binding Proteins

The first cellular retinoid-binding protein was identified in 1973 (5) when a 14.6-kDa cytosolic protein that specifically binds all-*trans*-retinol, but otherwise is distinct from RBP, was identified in the cytoplasm of several tissues (e.g., testis, liver). Four main cellular retinoid-binding proteins are now known that bind either retinol or RA: cellular retinol-binding protein (designated CRBP or CRBP-I), CRBP-type II (CRBP-II), and two forms of cellular RA-binding protein designated CRABP-I and CRABP-II. Each of these proteins is a member of a gene family whose basic structural motif is a "β-clam" composed of a clamshell-like arrangement of two nearly orthogonal arrays of antiparallel β strands that enclose an interior pocket that binds a single molecule of ligand. In contrast to RBP, the retinoid ligand of the CRBP or CRABPs is oriented with its functional (hydroxyl or carboxylic acid) group innermost within the protein's binding cavity (5, 20). Each form of CRBP and CRABP is a unique gene product with distinct tissue and cellular distribution (5, 21); nearly all cells and organs contain one or more of these proteins. Each of the CRBP and CRABP genes is similarly arranged in four exons and three introns (5).

Cellular Retinol-Binding Proteins (CRBP-I and CRBP-II)

The principal endogenous ligand of CRBP-I is all-*trans*-retinol (5); however, some other ligands may also bind (20). CRBP-I is widely distributed, with greatest expression in liver, kidney, and the male reproductive tract. In liver, CRBP-I mRNA is expressed by gestational day 16, increases during the suckling and weaning periods, and then declines gradually to adult levels (22). In adult rat liver, CRBP-I is expressed in both parenchymal cells (hepatocytes) and stellate (vitamin A–storing) cells but is found in highest concentration in stellate cells, especially in animals fed vitamin A–enriched diets (23). CRBP-I expression is modestly regulated by retinoid status. Liver CRBP-I protein and mRNA levels were reduced somewhat in vitamin A–depleted rats, but they did not rise significantly in rats fed elevated levels of retinol or RA (24). The gene for CRBP-I does, however, contain an RA response element (RARE, below), and induction of CRBP-I mRNA by RA has been demonstrated in the lung (25).

CRBP-II was first isolated from neonatal rats and subsequently shown to be abundant (~1% of soluble mucosal protein) in the small intestine of young and adult rats and humans (5). Although CRBP-I and CRBP-II are nearly identical in size and structure, only 56% of their amino acids are identical. And, although all-*trans*-retinol is an endogenous ligand of both CRBP-I and CRBP-II, CRBP-II also binds all-*trans*-retinal (26). These differences in protein composition and ligand binding may be related to the proposed function of CRBP-II in vitamin A absorption (see below).

CRBP-II is expressed mainly in villus-associated enterocytes (5). During development, mRNA for CRBP-II is first detectable in the rat intestine between 16 and 19 days of gestation, a time corresponding to appearance of the absorptive epithelial cells (27). In adult rat jejunum, fatty acids modestly regulate CRBP-II expression (28). During the perinatal period, CRBP-II is also expressed transiently in the liver. The mouse CRBP-II gene was shown to be closely linked to the gene for CRBP-I on chromosome 9; both the CRBP-I and CRBP-II genes are located on human chromosome 3 (5).

Cellular Retinoic Acid–Binding Proteins (CRABP-I and CRABP-II)

The principal endogenous ligand for CRABP-I and CRABP-II is all-*trans*-RA. The tissue distributions of the CRABPs differ somewhat, and both are different from, and more restricted than, those of CRBP. Most organs of the adult rat express CRABP-I at very low levels, whereas neonatal rats and some adult organs (e.g., eye, some reproductive organs) express CRABP-I at a level similar to that of CRBP-I (5). Vitamin A status has little effect on expression of CRABP-I. CRABP-I is expressed in the skin of neonatal and adult mice (29), but not in human skin (30).

CRABP-II is expressed strongly in a number of tissues during embryogenesis but is largely restricted to skin (mouse and human [31]). The expression of CRABP-II, but not CRABP-I, mRNA was markedly induced by all-*trans*-RA in adult human skin, but not in lung fibroblasts (30). In developing mouse embryos and cultured embryonal stem cells, increased expression of CRABP was associated with a lower differentiation response to RA (32). Consistent with these data and as noted below, one function of CRABP-I may be to sequester all-*trans*-RA, thereby limiting its distribution to the nucleus and controlling RA's biologic effects. CRABP-I–associated RA also is a substrate for metabolism (33) (see "Metabolism" below).

The genes for CRABP-I and CRABP-II have been cloned (34), and their regulation studied. The promoter region of the mouse CRABP-I gene contains several positive and inhibitory elements that respond in a cell type–specific fashion. These elements may be responsible for the specificity of CRABP-I expression during development (35).

Other Retinoid-Binding Proteins. Variant forms of RBP, CRBP, and CRABP have been identified and characterized from certain tissues, particularly reproductive organs (5, 19). Additionally, at least two distinctly different types of retinoid-binding proteins are restricted almost entirely to the eye (which also has CRBP and CRABP). A binding protein of 45 kDa, known as cellular retinal-binding protein (CRALBP), is located in the retina; this protein can bind one molecule of either retinol or retinal (36). The primary structure of CRALBP (37) and its cDNA have been described (36). A larger protein (~145 kDa, 1264 amino acids) is located in the interphotoreceptor space between the photoreceptor cells and the retinal pigment epithelium (RPE). This interphotoreceptor (interstitial) retinoid-binding protein (IRBP) is a lipoglycoprotein with two binding sites for various isomers of retinol and retinal, but it can also bind other small lipid ligands (36, 38). IRBP is synthesized by photoreceptor cells and the pineal gland (38). The functions of CRALBP and IRBP in retinoid transport within and between cells of the visual system (36) are discussed in the section on vision.

Nuclear Retinoid Receptors

The fundamental mechanism of action of RA in cell differentiation was clarified with the discovery of the first retinoic acid receptor, RAR (now RAR-α1), a nuclear transcription factor shown to be activated by all-*trans*-RA. The six retinoid receptors of the RAR and RXR gene subfamilies are each a unique gene product; these receptors belong to the larger superfamily of steroid/thyroid hormone nuclear transcription factors. Numerous reviews of the RAR/RXR provide detailed information on the structure, expression, and function of these receptors (6, 7, 39). Each of the retinoid receptors is a protein of approximately 48 kDa, located in the nucleus, and organized similarly into four major functional domains: a DNA-binding domain (DBD) and a ligand-binding domain (LBD) separated by a hinge region; a heterodimerization domain; and one or more ligand-dependent transcription-activation domains (activation functions, AF). The mechanism of action of each receptor is thought to involve its interaction with a receptor partner (dimer formation); binding of a specific ligand; binding to specific DNA nucleotide sequences (response elements, RARE or RXRE); and interacting through one or more AF regions with other nuclear proteins that collectively regulate gene transcription, either positively or negatively. Although RAR and RXR are present in the nuclei of all retinoid-responsive cells, each receptor is regulated independently and has a unique spatial and temporal pattern of expression. Nearly all cells express at least one member of the RAR and RXR subfamilies.

Several other proteins of the steroid/thyroid/retinoid-receptor superfamily bear considerable homology to the RAR-RXR and are termed *orphan receptors* because their ligands, if they exist, are unknown. Examples are the ROR, LXR, and LOR. These receptors may function through interaction with the RXR to regulate retinoid-mediated signaling indirectly (40).

RARs

The RAR subfamily includes RAR-α, RAR-β, and RAR-γ (6, 7, 39). Each of these receptors exists in two or more isoforms (caused by differential usage of each gene's promoter region, which results in different amino-terminal [DNA-binding] ends). RAR-α is expressed nearly ubiquitously. As noted below (see "Cancer Chemoprevention and Treatment"), a chromosomal translocation affecting the gene for RAR-α is related to a specific disease, acute promyelocytic leukemia (APL). RAR-β is unusual in having an RARE in its promoter region. This RARE permits "autoregulation" of the expression of RAR-β by RA. RAR-γ is expressed mainly in connective tissue, skin, and the embryo at critical stages of development. Structurally, the three RARs are highly homologous within their DBD (zinc-finger) regions. The amino acid sequences of the DBDs of RAR-β and RAR-γ are 97% identical to the DBD of RAR-α, implying very similar abilities to bind to RAREs. In contrast, the LBDs of human RAR-β and RAR-γ are only 90 and 84%, respectively, identical to the LBD of RAR-α (41). Recently, a form of human holo-RAR-γ containing the LBD has been crystallized with all-*trans*-RA in the binding pocket, and its structure, analyzed by x-ray crystallography, has been compared with crystals of human apo-RXR-α (7). From this structural analysis it can be inferred that an α-helical portion of the RAR and RXR between their DBD and LBD domains serves as a molecular hinge that allows a significant change in receptor conformation. The conformational change induced by retinoid binding is thought to create one or more new "interaction surfaces" that are necessary for RAR-RXR to interact with cognate DNA response elements (see below) and with a complex of coactivator or repressor molecules and basal transcription factors (7).

RXRs

Shortly after discovery of the first RAR, another distinct yet homologous gene subfamily was identified and named the RXR. All-*trans*-RA was subsequently recognized to be a specific ligand only for the RAR, whereas 9-*cis*-RA can activate through binding to both the RAR and RXR (42). Although two RXRs may bind to one another as homodimers, they appear to function most often as the heterodimeric partner of RAR. Equally important, the RXRs bind as heterodimers with several other nuclear transcription factors, including the receptors for vitamin D (see Chapter 18) and thyroid hormone, the peroxisome proliferator–activated receptors (PPARs), and others (43). Through these "promiscuous" interactions with multiple partners, the RXRs mediate "cross-talk" among different signaling pathways that collectively may affect expression of a large number of genes (6). The RARs and RXRs also differ in that the RARs appear to be active only in the presence of RA (or an active analogue), whereas heterodimers of RXR need not bind RA as long as their partners are activated by their respective ligands (e.g., they may function as "silent," yet biologically active, partners).

The three RXRs are highly homologous to one another within their LBDs and DBDs. However, homology between RARs and RXRs is much lower, especially in their LBDs, consistent with their ligand specificity for all-*trans*-RA only (the RARs) and for all-*trans*-RA or 9-*cis*-RA (the RXRs). Indeed, the LBD of the RARs is more homologous to that of the thyroid hormone receptors than to the LBD of RXRs (41).

Levels of Expression

Information is still relatively scarce regarding the natural regulation of the retinoid receptor genes under most physiologic conditions. Receptor expression has been studied by in situ hybridization and analysis of extracted mRNA. In embryos (see "Development"), the expression of the RARs and RXRs follows unique temporal and spatial patterns. In most tissues of the adult rat, RAR-α predominates, especially in the intestinal tract, although many tissues express two or even three forms of RAR at different levels (44). RAR-γ is highest in reproductive and epidermal tissues (44). During vitamin A deficiency, expression of RAR-β mRNA is low (45, 46) but increases following administration of retinol or RA, especially in lung and skin (45). Further studies are needed to elucidate the regulation of the RARs and RXRs in vivo and to define new retinoid-responsive genes.

Chromosomal Abnormalities. Given the regulatory roles of retinoid receptors, it was to be expected that mutations would be associated with disorders of cell proliferation and differentiation (cancer) or development. Mutations in the receptors RAR-α and RAR-β have been found in cell lines that have become resistant to the action of RA and in certain human cancers. These are discussed below in the section "Cancer Chemoprevention and Treatment."

RAR and RXR Response Elements

Retinoid response elements—RAREs and RXREs—have been identified in the promoter regions of numerous genes that encode proteins with diverse functions. This is consistent with retinoids being pleiotropic regulators that affect development, cell proliferation, and differentiation. The strongest RAREs are direct repeats (DRs) of the consensus sequence *AGGTCA,* or slight variants thereof, which are spaced apart by either five or two nucleotides, denoted *N* (e.g., *AGGTCANNNNNAGGTCA* is a response element of the DR-5 type) (6). Response-element spacing is critical for receptor-DNA recognition and/or the appropriate alignment and intercalation of the receptor-protein complex into the major groove of DNA. The context (flanking regions) around the RARE or RXRE also affects the strength of receptor interaction (6, 47). Some of the retinoid-binding proteins and receptors discussed above have RARE or RXRE sequences within their own promoters, a feature that provides a mechanism for their autoregulation by retinoids. The gene promoters for RAR-β, CRBP-I, and CRABP-II have been shown to contain RAREs. The promoters for CRBP-II and CRABP-II-2 contain RXREs (6); however, their physiologic significance is not yet clear (7).

METABOLISM

Dietary vitamin A is first processed in the intestine. The overall absorptive efficiency for physiologic amounts of preformed vitamin A is high (70–90%) and remains high (60–80%) as intake increases. Over 90% of retinol enters the body as retinyl esters in the lipid core of chylomicra. The liver acts as a central clearinghouse and bank: it clears chylomicron vitamin A, is the principal organ of vitamin A storage, is a major site of retinoid oxidation and catabolism, and is responsible for regulated secretion of retinol bound to RBP. The target tissues for retinol and/or RA include nearly all organ systems of the body, and most can further metabolize these retinoids. The retinoid form present in greatest concentration in most tissues, esterified retinol, serves as a concentrated storage pool that can be readily hydrolyzed. As noted above, most cells contain one or more cellular retinoid-binding proteins and two or more RARs or RXRs. Figure 17.2 provides a schematic overview of some of these processes and their interrelationships. Retinol, RA, and a large number of more polar metabolites (e.g., with hydroxyl groups at carbons 4, 14, or 18; keto groups; or epoxide groups) have been isolated from various tissues. A schema of the metabolic relationships among some of the major retinoids is shown in Figure 17.3. Retinoid metabolism occurs in many organs

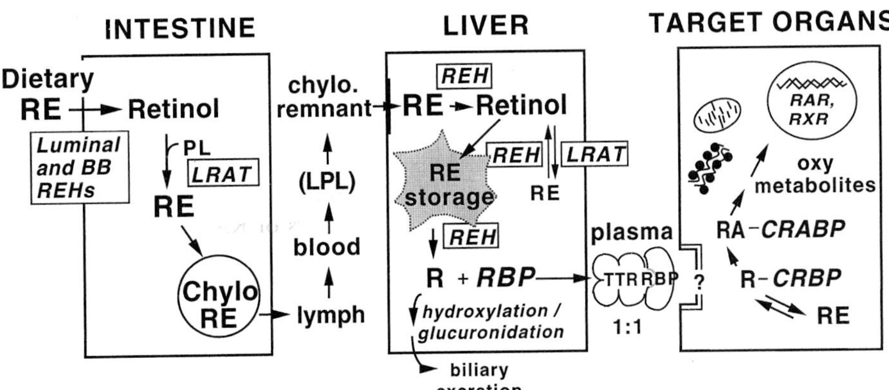

Figure 17.2. Schematic overview of intraorgan transport and cellular metabolism. PL, phospholipid; BB, brush border; RE, retinyl ester; LPL, lipoprotein lipase; Chylo, Chylomicron; LRAT, lecithin retinol acetyltransferase.

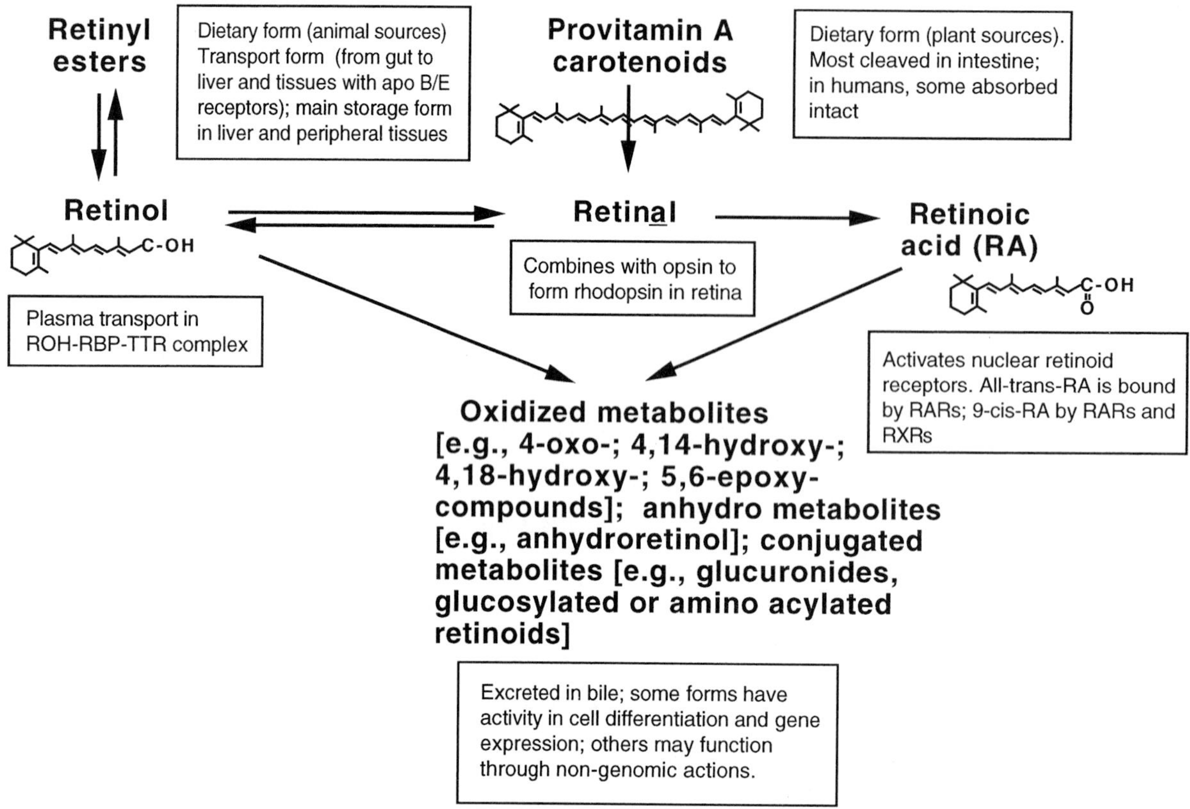

Figure 17.3. Simplified schematic of retinoid conversion reactions.

(liver, intestine, kidney, skin, etc.) in a manner specific to the tissue or cell type.

Digestion and Absorption

Vitamin A assimilation involves, first, processing of dietary retinyl esters, retinol, or carotenoids (see Chapter 33) in the lumen of the small intestine, followed by uptake of these molecules or their products into intestinal absorptive cells (48). Vitamin A is packaged along with newly absorbed lipids into chylomicra for transport through lymph and plasma to the liver. Numerous cycles of hydrolysis and reesterification are characteristic of the metabolism of vitamin A in the intestine, liver, and other tissues.

Luminal Processing. Dietary retinol must be released from foodstuffs by digestion and then emulsified with bile salts and lipids before being absorbed. Retinyl esters must be hydrolyzed. Several retinyl ester hydrolases (REHs) have been described (see [49] for review). The importance of luminal pancreatic cholesteryl ester hydrolase (also called carboxyl ester lipase, which is capable of retinyl ester hydrolysis in vitro [49]), has been challenged by new information that the small intestine contains microvillus-associated enzymes capable of hydrolyzing retinyl esters. Two REH activities are located in brush border membranes of rat small intestine (50): one of these preferentially hydrolyzes short-chain retinyl esters and apparently is derived from the pancreas; the other preferentially hydrolyzes long-chain retinyl esters and is an intrinsic component of the brush border (50). The hydrolytic activity of the latter enzyme, calculated for the rat small intestinal mucosa, is more than sufficient to process the daily requirement for vitamin A (50).

Factors that interfere with lipolysis or emulsification reduce intestinal absorption of vitamin A (51). Uptake of retinol is reduced by a lack of bile salts or too little dietary fat and significantly enhanced by micellar solubilization. It is thought that at physiologic concentrations retinol absorption is saturable, carrier mediated, and passive, whereas at high (pharmacologic) concentrations retinol absorption is nonsaturable (52). The latter feature is likely to contribute to the toxicity of preformed vitamin A.

Intracellular Retinol Metabolism and Chylomicron Formation. Regardless of whether β-carotene or retinol is ingested, the predominant form of vitamin A present in rat or human lymph is esterified retinol (53, 54). Vitamin A absorption is rapid, reaching a maximum by 2 to 6 hours. Cleavage of β-carotene (see Chapter 33) within the enterocytes yields retinal, which CRBP-II also binds. An enzyme in rat intestinal membranes, retinal reductase, can reduce retinal to retinol (55). Thus, retinol is a common intracellular product of the hydrolysis of preformed vitamin A and cleavage of provitamin A. Furthermore, CRBP-II is a common carrier for retinol and retinal. Analysis of the composition of chylomicron retinyl esters has shown a strong predominance of long-chain saturated fatty acids (palmitate and stearate), regardless of the fatty acid composition of the fat fed with the vitamin A. Years ago, palmitate and stearate were noted to also predominate at the *sn*-1 position of lymph lecithin (phosphatidyl choline) (56).

Esterification. Two different enzymatic activities present in the microsomal fraction (endoplasmic reticulum) can esterify retinol. Acyl-CoA-retinol acyltransferase (ARAT) has been assayed in rat and human intestinal microsomes (53). This activity does not recognize retinol bound to CRBP-II but does esterify unbound retinol. ARAT derives its fatty acid from fatty acyl-CoA (57). The reaction characteristics of ARAT suggest its involvement in esterifying retinol when retinol is present at relatively high concentrations. A second microsomal enzyme, lecithin:retinol acyltransferase (LRAT), esterifies retinol at physiologic concentrations. As substrates, LRAT uses retinol bound to CRBP-II and the *sn*-1 fatty acid of phosphatidyl choline, present in the same membranes. The newly formed retinyl esters are deposited in the endoplasmic reticulum where they are assembled with triglycerides, cholesteryl esters, and other neutral lipids into the chylomicron's lipid core. Thus, the quantity of retinyl ester in each chylomicron particle is directly related to recently absorbed vitamin A. CRBP-II apparently has two roles: to *solubilize* and sequester retinoids (either retinal or retinol) and to *direct* them to specific enzymes (e.g., retinal reductase and LRAT). As discussed below, a similar model applies to the role of CRBP in hepatic retinol esterification and oxidation and to the role of CRABP in further metabolism of RA (58). These models imply that the surfaces of the binding proteins must be recognized by the specific enzymes with which they interact (5).

Under physiologic circumstances, nearly all vitamin A is absorbed in chylomicra in the lymphatics and rapidly transported to the circulation (see Chapter 4). However, alternate absorptive pathways apparently may be used by patients with abetalipoproteinemia (absent or low levels of apolipoprotein B, which is essential for chylomicron assembly) because their plasma vitamin A is low without vitamin A treatment but normal after oral vitamin A supplementation (59).

Hepatic Metabolism of Vitamin A

Initial Processing of Chylomicron Vitamin A. As discussed in Chapter 4, chylomicron triglycerides are first metabolized in the periphery through the action of lipoprotein lipase, forming chylomicron remnants that are taken into hepatocytes by receptor-mediated endocytosis. Chylomicron retinyl esters remain in the chylomicron core during lipolysis and are rapidly cleared with chylomicron remnants into the liver (54). In kinetic studies, the half-life of vitamin A in lipoproteins with densities below 1.006 g/mL (containing chylomicron remnants) was less than 20 minutes in normal human subjects (60). Some factors that delay remnant clearance include familial dysbetalipoproteinemia (see Chapter 75) and low lipoprotein lipase activity (e.g., caused genetically or suppressed during inflammation). When remnant circulation is prolonged, retinyl esters may transfer to other lipoproteins such as low- and high-density lipoproteins, presumably through the action of the plasma cholesteryl ester–transfer protein (61). Thus, retinyl esters are associated with longer-lived lipoproteins that enter cells through their own receptor-mediated pathways.

Although most chylomicron vitamin A is rapidly taken up into liver parenchymal cells, other tissues may also assimilate some retinyl esters from chylomicra. The ability of human macrophage-like cells to take up chylomicron retinyl esters in vitro has been demonstrated (62), and uptake into bone marrow has been reported (63); however, the quantitative importance of these processes in humans is unknown.

In rats, the efficiency of uptake of vitamin A–labeled chylomicra into liver is very high (85–90%). Parenchymal cells are the initial site of processing of chylomicron vitamin A (Fig. 17.2). When vitamin A–labeled chylomicra were injected intravenously into recipient rats, retinyl esters of intestinal origin underwent rapid hydrolysis, followed by synthesis of new retinyl esters (54). Chylomicron remnant vitamin A apparently is not directed to lysosomes for processing (64). An REH associated with the plasma membrane (49) may function, either at the surface of the hepatocyte and/or within endocytic vesicles, to hydrolyze newly absorbed retinyl esters. This hydrolysis and reesterification resulted in even greater proportions of retinyl palmitate and stearate in liver, compared with those in chylomicra.

Blomhoff et al. (53) first showed that within a few hours of chylomicron uptake by parenchymal cells, chylomicron-derived vitamin A is transferred to hepatic stellate cells, the principal site of retinyl ester storage. Transfer was specific for vitamin A, as cholesteryl esters in the same chylomicra remained within hepatocytes. The mechanism of intercellular movement of vitamin A as well as the form of the retinoid at time of transfer is still uncertain. It has been suggested that retinol is transferred by RBP because injection of anti-RBP serum inhibited vitamin A transfer (65). It is also possible that some vitamin A transfers as retinyl ester or as a water-soluble retinoid (9). Collectively, these initial steps result in remodeling of dietary retinyl esters and intercellular transfer of vitamin A from hepatocytes to stellate cells for storage.

Hepatic Vitamin A Storage. When vitamin A status is adequate, approximately 50 to 85% of total body retinol is stored in the liver, more than 90% as retinyl esters (66, 67). Electron microscopy reveals that the perisinusoidal stellate cells contain numerous lipid droplets (68). The size and number of these droplets appear to increase with liver vitamin A content (69). In normally nourished rats, liver stellate cells contain approximately 30 times more total retinol per cell than parenchymal cells; neither liver endothelial nor Kupffer cells contain appreciable vitamin

A (70). Taking the number of rat liver parenchymal and stellate cells into account, it was estimated that 80 to 90% of vitamin A is contained within stellate cells (71).

Comparable figures for humans are not available. Species differences in stellate cells may be considerable, as the very high level of vitamin A in polar bear liver (sufficient to produce vitamin A toxicity in arctic explorers who consumed it) has been linked to an abundance of vitamin A–enriched hepatic stellate cells in this species (72).

Both hepatic stellate cells and parenchymal cells contain the plasma transport proteins RBP and TTR, as well as CRBP, a low level of CRABP, and several enzymes thought to be important in retinol esterification and retinyl ester hydrolysis. In isolated rat liver cells, the plasma retinoid-transport proteins were highly enriched in the parenchymal cell-enriched fraction. In contrast, CRBP, CRABP, and retinyl palmitate hydrolase were more nearly evenly distributed on a per cell basis (73, 74). When expressed per total liver, nearly 98% of RBP, 91% of CRBP, and 90% of the REH activity were associated with parenchymal cells (74).

As in the intestine, LRAT in liver is thought to be the principal enzyme involved in retinol esterification (54). Hepatic LRAT uses retinol bound to CRBP. LRAT activity is enriched in the stellate cell–rich fraction of liver (75, 76) in proportion to stored retinyl esters; in contrast, REHs are nearly equally distributed between parenchymal and stellate cells (76). Two mechanisms are likely to regulate the overall balance between retinol esterification (storage) and retinyl ester hydrolysis (mobilization). First, the activity of hepatic (not intestinal) LRAT is under very sensitive nutritional regulation; LRAT activity is reduced markedly in rats undergoing vitamin A depletion (77). However, hepatic LRAT activity is rapidly induced by dietary retinol or administration of RA (78). A reduction in hepatic LRAT activity may serve to reduce the esterification and storage of retinol, presumably sparing it for oxidation and/or other processes that take priority. Second, apo-CRBP, which increases in concentration as retinol falls, can stimulate hydrolysis of retinyl esters by a microsomal REH (79). When dietary vitamin A does not meet requirements, liver vitamin A stores can be almost totally mobilized. Kinetic studies have shown that both parenchymal and stellate cells lose their vitamin A nearly in proportion to their initial vitamin A contents (67).

Acute and chronic liver inflammation induces stellate cells to proliferate and to change their appearance into myofibroblast-like cells (71, 80). A gradual loss of vitamin A has been reported to accompany this morphologic change (81, 82) and to be partly reversed by supplementation with retinoids (80). In alcoholic liver disease, liver vitamin A is markedly reduced even though serum retinol, RBP, and TTR levels are still normal (6, and below).

Plasma Transport

Plasma Retinol and RBP Concentrations. The concentration of plasma (or serum) vitamin A may be determined as *total* retinol (measured after hydrolysis, i.e., saponification) or as *unesterified* retinol (measured without saponification). The difference is considered a valid estimate of *esterified retinol.* In fasting plasma samples, unesterified and total retinol values usually are nearly identical because more than 95% of plasma total retinol is unesterified. However, in postprandial plasma, the concentration of total vitamin A (or of retinyl esters measured separately) may be elevated. As noted above, these retinyl esters are associated with chylomicra or their remnants, and their concentration in plasma depends on the rates of vitamin A absorption and chylomicron clearance.

In healthy humans, plasma retinol concentrations are quite constant both within and between individuals, usually in the range of about 1.5 to 3 μmol/L (43–86 μg/dL). Plasma vitamin A levels in the U.S. population were measured in several national surveys (NHANES I, II, III, and Hispanic HANES, spanning 1976 to 1984 [83, 84]). Mean vitamin A levels were lowest in young children, increased in adolescence, and continued to increase throughout adulthood. Male adolescents and adults had higher mean serum retinol levels than premenopausal females, whereas values were similar after menopause (84). For all age groups, black Americans had slightly lower mean levels than white Americans. Retinyl esters were present at 2 to 20% of the serum retinol concentration (84). In NHANES I (conducted from 1976 to 1980), data for males and females between the ages of 3 and 74 years were used to form a reference sample that excluded individuals with factors known to alter plasma retinol (vitamin/mineral supplement users, women using oral contraceptives, and pregnant women). The 50th percentiles for male and female children were similar, near 35 μg/dL (1.23 μmol/L). For adult men and women (18 to 44 years), the 50th percentiles equaled 57 and 45 μg/dL (2.00 and 1.58 μmol/L), respectively (83). Significantly lower levels of plasma RBP and retinol have been observed in premature infants (<36 weeks gestation) than in term neonates (85).

Plasma levels of vitamin A and RBP may (86) or may not (87, 88) be depressed in chronic alcoholics. In chronic liver disease, regardless of cause, plasma concentrations of retinol and RBP are usually reduced in proportion to disease severity (89, 90). In a study of liver transplantation, the diseased liver was directly implicated in these low concentrations (91).

Nonlinear Relationship between Liver Vitamin A Storage and Plasma Vitamin A. Whereas hepatic vitamin A concentrations may vary widely within and between individuals, most plasma retinol concentrations fall within a narrow, regulated range, decreasing only when liver vitamin A stores are nearly exhausted. Thus, in the absence of inflammation, a low serum retinol level usually indicates that hepatic vitamin A stores are depleted. A useful theoretical curve (Fig. 17.4) (92) illustrates the relationship between plasma and liver vitamin A. Low hepatic stores (less than ~20 μg total retinol/g) are associated with low plasma

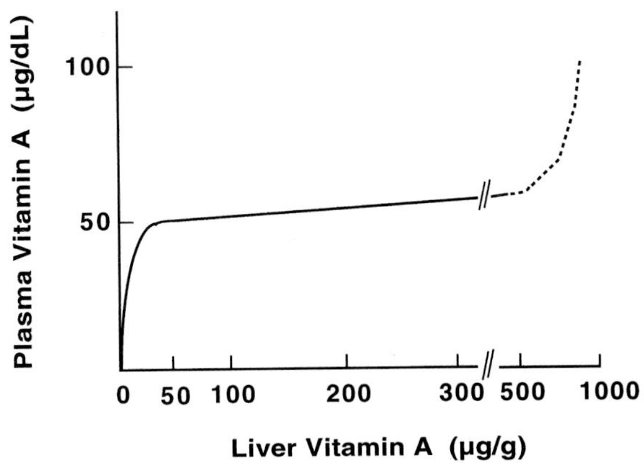

Figure 17.4. Relationship of plasma retinol to liver vitamin A stores. (Modified from Olson JA. J Natl Cancer Inst 1984;73:1439–44, with permission.

retinol concentration. From about 20 to 300 μg total retinol/g liver, plasma retinol is maintained at a relatively constant value. Above approximately 300 μg total retinol/g liver, circulating retinyl esters are likely to increase and be detectable by HPLC. Although total retinol concentration rises, unesterified retinol and RBP concentrations are still normal (92). If delayed chylomicron clearance is ruled out as a possible cause of the circulating retinyl esters, then this elevation in esterified retinol may indicate a state of hypervitaminosis A (see below).

Synthesis, Secretion, and Turnover of Holo-RBP-TTR

RBP

RBP is synthesized as a 24-kDa preprotein on ribosomes in the rough endoplasmic reticulum of hepatocytes. The amino-terminal signal sequence is cleaved cotranslationally, and the mature 21-kDa protein then progresses through the secretory pathway to the Golgi apparatus (15), where some of the newly synthesized RBP apparently combines, in a manner not yet fully understood, with retinol. Several hepatic REHs have been identified (49), but it still is unclear exactly how retinyl esters in stellate cells yield the retinol that, following combination with RBP in hepatocytes, is released into the circulation. Apparently not all newly synthesized RBP is secreted, and the RBP that does not complex with retinol undergoes proteolytic degradation (93). Hepatocytes also synthesize TTR. The synthesis and plasma concentrations of RBP and TTR depend on an adequate supply of amino acids and energy, and both are reduced during protein-energy malnutrition (94, 95). The level of mRNA for RBP and its translation are normal in vitamin A deficiency (96); however, secretion is markedly reduced, and apo-RBP builds up in liver. When retinol is provided, retinol combines with RBP and the holo-RBP complex is rapidly secreted (97). This retinol-regulated secretion of holo-RBP forms the basis for the relative dose-response tests described below (see "Assessment of Vitamin A Status"). Inflammation reduces the biosynthesis of RBP and TTR, which behave as negative acute-phase proteins (98, 99).

Transport and Kinetics. Holo-RBP (~21 kDa) and TTR (~55 kDa) interact strongly to form a 1:1 molar complex. Association of TTR with RBP stabilizes the binding of retinol to RBP, and the complex is too large for free filtration through the renal glomeruli. Plasma concentrations of retinol and RBP are highly correlated (4) and are nearly equal when expressed on a molar basis. Besides being reduced in vitamin A deficiency (4), RBP and TTR have been reported to be low during infections and inflammation (acute-phase response) (100) and trauma (101). A significant reduction in plasma retinol concentration (but still within the normal range) was reported to accompany successful reduction of hypercholesterolemia (102). Vitamin A and RBP concentrations (usually 1.9–2.4 μmol/L [40–50 μg/dL] [9]) are significantly increased (15–35%) in women using oral contraceptives (83, 103). Due to the relatively short plasma half-life of RBP and TTR (~0.5 day and 2–3 days, respectively [4]), a comparatively high rate of protein synthesis is necessary to maintain their concentrations. For this reason, RBP and TTR are used as indicators in clinical assessment of protein status (reflecting recent protein synthesis). Plasma also contains a small amount of apo-RBP, calculated to be 3.8% of total RBP (4). "Free" RBP is readily filtered in the kidneys, and its plasma half-life is only about 4 hours (4).

Kinetic studies have shown that the plasma half-life of retinol is longer than that of RBP. Kinetic modeling of turnover data has led to the understanding that retinol undergoes extensive recycling between the liver, plasma, and peripheral tissues before it is catabolized (4, 104). In contrast, RBP apparently is not reused after retinol dissociates (4). The relationship of whole-body retinol turnover to vitamin A status has been studied in rats with varying vitamin A reserves. In animals whose liver vitamin A contents differed more than 400-fold, the rate of irreversible vitamin A disposal differed by less than 10-fold (105). Therefore, although the body's capacity for vitamin A storage is high, its ability to degrade and eliminate vitamin A is quite limited. The low rate of catabolism together with efficient absorption seems to explain the propensity for vitamin A to accumulate in tissues. Plasma retinol and retinol kinetics are altered by drugs, including RA and synthetic retinoids (106–108; also see "Cancer Chemoprevention and Treatment"), and certain environmental toxins (109).

Most literature concerning retinoid transport and metabolism is based on studies conducted in humans or in rats, which have generally proved to be a good animal model. However, dogs and other carnivores differ significantly in transporting a large proportion of preprandial vitamin A as esterified retinol and in excreting significant quantities of vitamin A in urine (110).

Vitamin A Uptake by Tissues. Retinol from holo-RBP is taken into many tissues of the body, but the uptake mechanism is still uncertain. Two mechanisms have been proposed: *(a)* RBP may be bound by a plasma membrane receptor on target cells that facilitates retinol uptake, although not necessarily that of RBP (23, 111), or *(b)* retinol may dissociate from RBP in the aqueous environment, producing free retinol that then diffuses and partitions into cells. A third possibility, that the holo-RBP complex is taken up by cells, is unlikely, based on double-labeling experiments. By binding retinol, CRBP within cells may provide the driving gradient for continued uptake (112). Similarly, retinoid metabolism may function to keep the concentration of retinol low and to regenerate apo-CRBP.

More-polar retinoids such as RA and the retinoid glucuronides are presumed to enter cells by diffusion. Lipoprotein-associated retinyl esters may be assimilated as the result of lipoprotein internalization through cell-surface receptors (apo E, low-density lipoprotein, low-density lipoprotein-related protein (LRP), or scavenger receptors) (113).

Retinoic Acid in Plasma and Tissues

Several more-polar retinoids, including all-*trans*-RA, 13-*cis*-RA, and 13-*cis*-4-oxo-RA, are present in plasma at much lower concentrations than retinol. The acidic retinoids are transported in association with serum albumin, not RBP (114). Mean plasma concentrations of 4 to 14 nmol/L for all-*trans*-RA, 4 to 5 nmol/L for 13-*cis*-RA, and 11 to 12 nmol/L for 13-*cis*-4-oxo-RA have been reported for healthy males (115, 116). Concentrations of 13-*cis*-RA and 13-*cis*-4-oxo-RA increased two- to four-fold after daily doses of retinyl palmitate well in excess of dietary levels (116) or after consumption of liver (117). Other acidic metabolites, including 9-*cis*-RA and 9,13-di-*cis*-RA, have been reported (117) but not yet studied systematically.

The in vivo half-life of RA is quite short. In pharmacokinetic studies conducted in nonhuman primates, the initial decline in plasma all-*trans*-RA concentration following a large intravenous dose was described by a first-order (terminal) half-life averaging 19 minutes (118). However, a dose-dependent plateau in plasma concentration suggested that the clearance of all-*trans*-RA is capacity limited; no such plateau was observed after dosing with 9-*cis*-RA (119). All-*trans*-RA can induce its own catabolism (120; and see below). Thus, following RA administration, the rate of clearance increases as dosing is repeated (120). There is rapid interconversion between the all-*trans* and 9-*cis* isomers, and of all-*trans*-RA to 13-*cis*-RA in cultured cells and in vivo (121), but mechanisms have not been established.

Relatively few data are available on tissue concentrations of endogenous RA, but they appear to be greater than plasma levels (~40–580 pmol/g for kidney, liver, lung, and pancreas of normal rats vs. ~8–16 pmol/mL of plasma [122]). In liver and kidney, 9-*cis*-RA was present at concentrations of 13 and 100 pmol/g of tissue, respectively (123). In rats given oral ^{14}C-all-*trans*-RA for 8 days, less than 10% of the label remained in the body, and of this, the highest concentrations were present in the liver, kidney, and intestine. In liver, 58% of ^{14}C behaved as acidic lipid, presumably unchanged RA, and 23% was more polar than RA (114). RA metabolism in various tissues includes conversion between the all-*trans*, 9-*cis*, and 13-*cis* isomers (124–126), which may be concentration dependent (126); however, no enzymatic mechanism has yet been characterized except in the retina (see "Vision"). The relative contributions of plasma uptake of RA and synthesis of RA vary considerably among organs (127).

Glucuronide conjugates of retinol and RA also are present in human serum at low nanomolar concentrations (128). Retinoyl-β-glucuronide (11) has been described as a major metabolite of all-*trans*-RA administered at high dosage (126).

Mechanisms of Oxidative Metabolism

All-*trans*-RA is the most potent of the biologic retinoids in assays of cell differentiation and gene expression. The concentration of RA is closely regulated through both synthesis and degradation. Numerous enzymes have been implicated in RA formation and oxidation, but it is still uncertain which ones are most important in physiologic settings. Oxidation of retinol to RA is a two-step process involving a retinol dehydrogenase (RDH) and a retinal dehydrogenase. Several distinct enzymes in the membranous or soluble tissue fractions can oxidize retinol to retinal (129–131). It is proposed that CRBP acts as a "cassette" to direct retinol to one or more RDHs in the membrane fraction of liver and other tissues (129). Similarly, numerous aldehyde dehydrogenases use retinal as a substrate (129, 132–135). Once RA is formed, CRABP can facilitate its further metabolism to more-polar products (129). Several isoforms of the cytochrome P450 enzyme family hydroxylate various isomers of retinal (31, 136) or RA (132). Microsomes of several tissues catalyze β-glucuronidation of several isomers of RA (124, 136a). Side-chain-shortened metabolites have been found in excreta (137). In all, a large number of oxidative metabolites with varied structures are formed by metabolism of retinol and RA.

Renal Metabolism and Excretion

The kidneys are the principal organ of RBP loss and catabolism. Glomerular filtration and renal catabolism are estimated to account for metabolic clearance of RBP equivalent to about 7/8 L of plasma per day in a 70-kg human (4). Chronic renal disease is typically associated with abnormal elevations of plasma retinol and RBP (4). In 26 patients with chronic renal disease of various etiologies, plasma RBP averaged 116 μg/mL (5.5 μmol/L), versus 46.2 μg/mL (2.2 μmol/L) in 109 controls (138). The molar ratios of RBP to vitamin A and of RBP to TTR were both elevated. In a rat model of acute renal failure, serum retinol increased up to 70% within 2 hours of nephrectomy (139), whereas injection of apo-RBP caused a rapid and significant increase in plasma retinol (140). The latter result suggests that free apo-RBP, which is readily filtered, may provide a feedback signal to liver that stimulates output of holo-RBP. Urinary retinol excretion may be detected in some infections causing diarrhea (141) or proteinuria (142). Fex et al. (143) have proposed that an "acute vitamin A deficiency" may exist during inflammation and may contribute to the excess mortality associated with certain infectious diseases.

FUNCTIONS

Vision

Vitamin A is required in the eye in two distinct forms for two distinct processes: *(a)* as 11-*cis*-retinal, vitamin A functions in the retina in transduction of light into the neural signals necessary for vision and *(b)* as RA, vitamin A maintains normal differentiation of the cells of the conjunctival membranes, cornea, and other ocular structures, preventing xerophthalmia. Detailed reviews are available on phototransduction (36) and xerophthalmia (144).

The photoreceptor cells of the retina include the rods, which are specialized for motion detection and vision in dim light, and the red-, green-, and blue-sensitive cones, specialized for color vision in bright light. The essential light-absorbing unit consists of 11-*cis*-retinal bound to a protein (an opsin). Each cell type possesses specialized plasma membrane structures (outer segment disks) that contain a high concentration of a "visual pigment" (e.g., rhodopsin in rods and iodopsins in cones). Whereas unbound retinal maximally absorbs light of 365 nm, the absorption spectrum is shifted to longer wavelengths (the "opsin shift") by formation of a protonated Schiff base between the aldehyde of retinal and a lysine amino group in opsin and by additional conformational changes. As noted by Saari (36), "opsin is tailor-made to shift the absorption spectrum of the retinoid into the visible range, increase its quantum efficiency of photoisomerization, and trigger further biochemical responses." Thus, human rods absorb maximally at 509 nm, blue-sensitive cones at 420 nm, green-sensitive cones at 530 nm, and red-sensitive cones at 565 nm (36). As shown schematically in Figure 17.5, absorption of a photon of light catalyzes photoisomerization of a molecule of 11-*cis*-retin*al* to all-*trans*-retin*al*, followed by its release from opsin. This isomerization triggers a reaction cascade that involves G proteins, phosphorylation, and decreased sodium conductance across the photoreceptor cell's plasma membrane; the latter event initiates signaling to neuronal cells that communicate to the brain's visual cortex. Although this process is described for a single retinal molecule, in reality, signals from thousands of rods, each containing millions of molecules of rhodopsin (which reaches a concentration of 2.5 mmol/L in rod outer-segment membranes) are triggered simultaneously, and their signals integrated.

For vision to continue, 11-*cis*-retinal must be regenerated. In vertebrates this occurs through thermal—not light-catalyzed—processes ("dark reactions") in the supporting RPE cells that are adjacent to the rods and cones but separated by an interphotoreceptor space. The time constant for regeneration of rhodopsin is on the order of minutes (36). This process requires, first, reduction of all-*trans*-retinal to retinol and its movement across the photoreceptor space to the RPE cells by IRBP (38), a

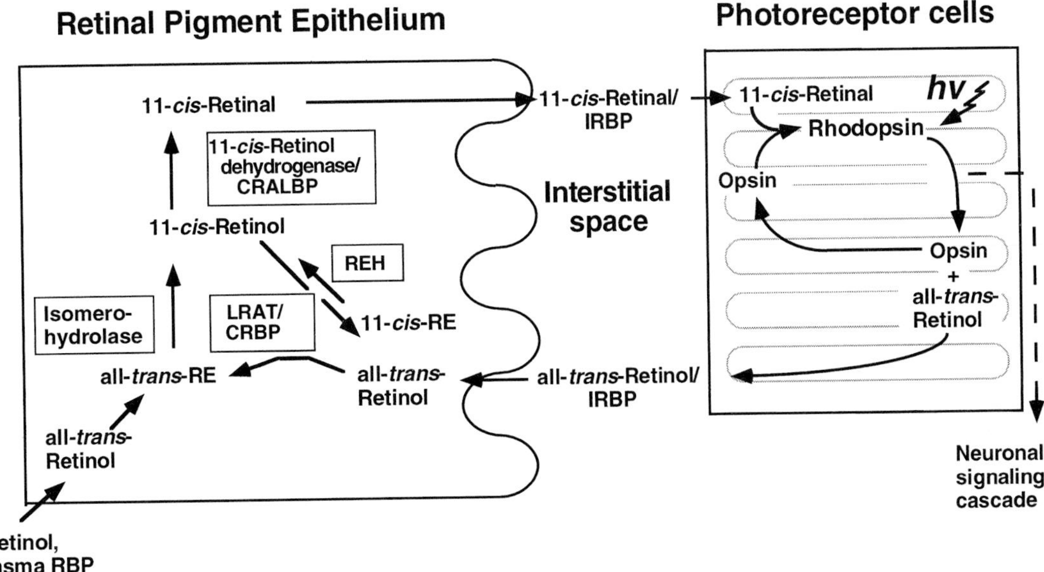

Figure 17.5. Retinoid metabolism in vision. CRALBP, cellular retinol-binding protein; RE, retinyl ester; LRAT, lecithin:retinol acyltransferase; IRBP, interstitial retinoid-binding protein; hr, light.

protein present in the photoreceptor space (36). In the RPE cells, all-*trans*-retinol is esterified through an LRAT-mediated reaction, providing a local storage pool of retinyl esters that, when needed, are hydrolyzed and isomerized to form 11-*cis*-retinol. This unusual reaction is coordinately catalyzed by isomerohydrolase, an enzyme unique to the retina. 11-*cis*-Retinol may then be esterified by LRAT or oxidized by a specific dehydrogenase (145) to form 11-*cis*-retinal. This retinoid is then shuttled by IRBP back across the interstitial space to the photoreceptor cells for recombination with opsin, thus beginning another photo cycle. Although the pool of retinyl esters in the RPE is small in comparison to total body reserves, this pool provides a highly concentrated source of vitamin A for immediate re-formation of 11-*cis*-retinal after bleaching. Thus, in a "conveyor belt"–like fashion, as molecules of 11-*cis*-retinal are bleached, other molecules are released from storage for rapid regeneration of the visual pigments. The phenomenon of poor dark adaptation after exposure to bright light (night blindness) results from light-stimulated depletion of rhodopsin, a normal event, *together with* a failure to resynthesize 11-*cis*-retinal rapidly; this latter failure is due to depletion of the RPE cells' retinyl ester storage pool. In a recent report, night blindness in Sorsby's fundus dystrophy, an autosomal dominant retinal degeneration, disappeared within a week after provision of 50,000 IU (~15,000 μg RE) of vitamin A to patients in early stages of disease (146).

The various cell types in the retina, cornea, and conjunctival epithelium contain several cellular retinoid-binding proteins and nuclear retinoid receptors whose presence implies that these structures depend on RA in the same manner as the epithelia of other tissues. The structural integrity of the cornea, an avascular tissue, depends on vitamin A delivered via tear fluid. The lacrimal gland can synthesize and secrete RBP, which is proposed to be important in solubilizing the retinol in tears (147).

The corneal pathology observed in vitamin A deficiency (see color plate in Chapter 30) appears to result from a lack of RA. Vitamin A deficiency appears as dryness of the conjunctival membranes and cornea (xerosis) (144) and the presence of Bitôt's spots (foamy-appearing deposits of cells and bacteria in the outer quadrant of the eye). These changes are reversible by vitamin A. If, however, vitamin A deficiency continues and the cornea softens (keratomalacia) and ulcerates, blindness is irreversible (144).

Cellular Differentiation

The first evidence that vitamin A is required for the integrity of epithelial tissues was reported in the mid-1920s by Wolbach and Howe (148). While examining the tissues of vitamin A–deficient rats under the light microscope, these investigators observed that epithelia normally composed of columnar or cuboidal mucus-secreting cells were, instead, flat (squamous), dry, and keratinized. Later studies with cultured cells showed that RA may induce undifferentiated stem cells to cease proliferation and to assume a differentiated, mature phenotype (149). It is now appreciated that all-*trans*- and 9-*cis*-RA, through activation of RAR and RXR, regulate expression of a large number of genes. Because the various forms of RAR and RXR, like other transcriptional regulators, are expressed in time and location-specific patterns, gene regulation can be finely tuned. Examples of genes with RARE include those encoding structural proteins (skin keratins), extracellular matrix (laminin), enzymes (alcohol dehydrogenases, transglutaminases), and retinoid-binding proteins and receptors (CRBP-I, CRABP-II, and RAR-β) (see [39] and [150] for reviews).

Retinoid-induced cell differentiation is often accompanied by an inhibition of cell proliferation. Retinoid receptors may form inhibitory complexes with nuclear factors known to promote proliferation, such as the AP-1 complex (151). Retinoid ligands with selective anti-AP-1 activity have been described (151). Retinoids may also stimulate apoptosis (programed cell death) (152). Induction of differentiation, inhibition of proliferation, and induction of apoptosis are either known or hypothesized to be related to the actions of retinoids as anticancer agents and in normal embryonic development.

Development

Both a deficiency and an excess of vitamin A cause fetal malformations. Association of vitamin A deficiency with failure of embryonic development and congenital abnormalities was well established during the 1940s to 1950s by the work of Wilson and others (153). Offspring of vitamin A–deficient mice and rats show a variety of abnormalities including microphthalmia, craniofacial abnormalities, umbilical hernia, edema, and spongy tissue structures of the thymus, liver, and heart (154). The teratogenic effects of vitamin A, especially of acidic retinoids, are well demonstrated in several models of vertebrate development (amphibian, avian, rodent, primate). Retinoids have been implicated in the development of the central nervous system, limbs, cardiovascular system, and eyes (see [154] for review).

RA does not appear to be involved in vertebrate embryogenesis prior to the stage of gastrulation (155). Following gastrulation, specific genes of the *Hox* family (homologues of the *Drosophila melanogaster HOM-C* genes that regulate body segmentation) are expressed in a wave, beginning about 7.5 days postcoitus in the mouse embryo, from the hindbrain posteriorly (154, 156). The *Hox* family consists of 38 genes arranged in four chromosomal clusters, *Hox A, B, C,* and *D,* which code for transcription factors that regulate development along the posterior axis. Some *Hox* genes (e.g., *Hoxa1, Hoxb1, Hoxd4*) possess a functional RARE and are subject to direct regulation by RA (155, 157). Therefore, it is proposed that RA functions as a posterior transformation signal that alters the identity of trunk mesoderm through regulation of 3′ members of the *Hox* gene family and perhaps additional genes (155, 157). Studies using RA-sensitive reporter genes have shown that RA, as well as RAR and RXR, CRBP, CRABP-I, and CRABP-II, is present in embryonic regions known to have organizing activity for development of structures posterior to the hindbrain (e.g., the spinal cord and vertebrae) (154). The presence of retinoids together with their binding proteins and receptors in a temporally precise manner provides strong circumstantial evidence that RA-activated RARs regulate *Hox* gene expression. Loss-of-function mutations of *Hox* and RAR result in similar phenotypic abnormalities affecting the anterior (cervical) vertebral region and, conversely, overexpression of *Hox* genes and provision of excess RA produce similar abnormalities in the posterior vertebral region, which are reciprocal to those above (155). Not all *Hox* genes are regulated by RA, and other mechanisms may well refine the boundaries established by *Hox* genes and RA (155). The concepts that RARs are involved in normal development at certain critical periods and that RA plays a role as a posteriorizing hormone are supported by recent work on the effect of RAR-β and RA on neural tube closure in the *curly tail* mouse, a genetic model of neural tube defects (154).

RA also functions in limb development and formation of the heart, eyes, and ears. Although the concept that RA itself is an endogenous morphogen in vertebrate limb development (158) has been challenged (155), substantial evidence indicates that RA can respecify undifferentiated regions of the limb buds (154, 157). RA is needed for normal development of the heart (159, 160). In the regions that form the eyes, specific isoforms of retinal dehydrogenase, which mediates RA biosynthesis, are expressed at appropriate times during development in tissue that will differentiate into the ventral and dorsal portions of the eye (161). Development of the otic vesicle (ear) is also sensitive to a deficiency or excess of vitamin A (154).

Using the technique of homologous recombination to delete specific genes (see Chapter 36), mice lacking one or more of the retinoid receptors or binding proteins have been created. The need for retinol transport in the fetus is inferred from the lethal effect of suppressing expression of RBP in the fetal yolk sac (162). However, mice lacking CRBP, which is expressed in many embryonic tissues, unexpectedly appeared normal at birth, and even double mutants lacking CRABP-I and CRABP-II showed only mild limb abnormalities. Similarly, the embryos of mice lacking RAR-α1 (the RAR-α1 homozygous null mutation, denoted RAR-$\alpha 1^{-/-}$) survived in utero and appeared normal at birth (154), and even embryos lacking all of the isoforms of RAR-α or RAR-β (total RAR-α or RAR-β knockouts) survived in utero and showed nearly normal development. Of the single RAR null mutations, only RAR-$\gamma^{-/-}$ mice were born with obvious congenital malformations of the type expected if RAR-γ is involved in *Hox* gene expression in the cervical spinal region (154). Mice lacking RXR-α showed abnormalities of the eye and heart, while mice lacking RXR-β appeared normal (although males were sterile). In general, single null mutations of RAR or RXR have resulted in abnormalities of differentiation that resemble those seen in vitamin A deficiency, rather than in the severe morphologic abnormalities that might have been expected. Most of these results are difficult to reconcile with the precise expression of retinoid-binding proteins and receptors during embryogenesis and the evidence for RA-induced gene expression. Functional redundancy among homologous receptors or binding proteins has been offered as a possible explanation. Mice bearing compound mutations show more severe abnormalities; e.g., mice lacking both RAR-α and RAR-γ (RAR-$\alpha^{-/-}$, RAR-$\gamma^{-/-}$) displayed multiple abnormalities of craniofacial, ocular, and limb structures, resembling those seen in wild-type embryos with severe vitamin A deficiency (163).

Requirement for Retinol. Most work has focused on understanding the functions and teratogenicity of RA during early development in the mouse or chick. However, studies conducted in pregnant, retinoid-depleted rats provide evidence that provision of RA alone is not sufficient for fetal development beyond day 15. To prevent later fetal resorption, it was necessary to provide a small quantity of retinol to pregnant dams by day 10 (164). These data imply that there are different retinoid signals—RA, retinol, or another metabolite (164)—with separate and necessary roles at different stages of gestation.

In summary, recent studies have clarified that vitamin A in the form of retinol must be transported within the embryo and that RA produced locally is necessary for normal postgastrulation development. Retinoid receptors interact with *Hox* and other regulatory genes to control morphogenesis. This regulatory system apparently has many built-in safeguards, as evidenced by the lack of severe defects in null mutants lacking a single type of retinoid receptor.

Immunity

Researchers in the 1920s to 1930s first recognized that vitamin A deficiency is associated with decreased resistance to infection. In the late 1960s, Scrimshaw et al. (165) reviewed over 50 clinical, experimental, and observational studies concerning vitamin A as part of an extensive review for the WHO and concluded that no nutritional deficiency is as likely to be associated with infection as a lack of vitamin A. Nevertheless, they also emphasized that not all infections appear to be exacerbated by vitamin A deficiency. It is now appreciated that immunity to pathogens is exquisitely specific; thus, it is not surprising that depending on the pathogen and type of host immune response that it elicits, vitamin A may or may not be a critical determinant in the host's response. In randomized, controlled community studies and hospital-based studies, interventions with vitamin A reduced the severity of some infections, especially measles and diarrhea (see [166–168] and

Chapter 97 for discussions of the impact of vitamin A in reducing child morbidity and mortality). In contrast, however, the severity of respiratory infections has not been reduced by vitamin A supplementation (169–171).

In experimental vitamin A deficiency, both cell-mediated immunity and antibody-mediated responses are generally reduced (see Chapter 45). Responses are generally poor to immune stimuli that depend on T cells for the host's response. Alterations are evident in the numbers of lymphocytes and their subset distribution (172) and in cytokine production (173). Nonspecific immunity, assessed by the microbicidal or cytotoxic functions of neutrophils, macrophages, and natural killer cells, has also been reported to be reduced or abnormal (174). In nearly all studies in which vitamin A has been provided to vitamin A–deficient hosts, immune functions have been restored, often quite rapidly. These observations and other evidence (175) suggest that the cellular "machinery" for an adequate response is intact but that the signaling pathways necessary for normal immune responses are impaired during retinoid deficiency and rapidly reestablished when vitamin A is provided.

PHARMACOLOGIC USE OF RETINOIDS

Dermatology

Nowhere has the clinical impact of retinoids been greater than in the treatment of diseases of the skin. Natural and synthetic retinoids influence epithelial cell proliferation and epidermal differentiation and have been used increasingly as systemic or topical agents in the treatment of hyperkeratotic disorders (e.g., etretinate and acitretin for psoriatic disease), acne and acne-related disorders (13-*cis*-RA, and retinoyl-β-glucuronide), and certain skin cancers (11, 176, 177). Acitretin (Fig. 17.1*G*) normalizes hyperproliferative states and induces differentiation of basal cells in the dermis toward a less keratinized, more epithelial phenotype. 13-*cis*-RA is a potent suppressor of sebocyte proliferation and sebum production. Retinoids most likely induce and modulate expression of dermal growth factors and their receptors (176, 177). Recent reviews provide detailed information on the indications for therapeutic use of retinoids in dermatology (176), characteristics of their metabolism (176), adverse reactions and tolerability (176), and retinoid metabolism and molecular biology of the skin (31, 177). The profile of adverse effects of oral retinoids is dose dependent and closely related to hypervitaminosis A (see below).

Other Treatments. In the near future, retinoids may prove beneficial for treatment of other diseases. A recent study reported significant improvement in the lungs of rats with experimentally induced emphysema after treatment for 25 days with RA (178). This result is consistent with a critical role of RA in lung development (25) and suggests that differentiation can be modulated by RA in the alveoli of adults.

Cancer Chemoprevention and Treatment

Epidemiologic (179, 180) and experimental data (180, 181) support a role for vitamin A and retinoids in decreasing the risk of certain cancers, especially those of epithelial origin. Some epidemiologic studies, many of the case-control design, have implicated total vitamin A as a beneficial dietary factor in reducing cancer risk (179, 182). Few studies, however, have shown a significant beneficial association between intake of preformed vitamin A and cancer risk (179, 180). In comparison, studies conducted in numerous rodent and other animal models have documented the ability of natural and synthetic retinoids to reduce carcinogenesis significantly in the skin, breast, liver, colon, prostate, lung, and other sites (181). The toxicity of natural retinoids precludes their long-term use in chemoprevention of human cancers, but some synthetic retinoids are better tolerated (180, 181), and some of these may prevent or delay cancer recurrence (180). Possible mechanisms of retinoid action in cancer chemoprevention are likely to include induction of cell differentiation, inhibition of proliferation, and/or induction of apoptosis (152, 183). The outcomes of clinical trials testing retinoids for cancer chemoprevention or therapy have been reviewed (11, 180, 184, 185).

Cancer Treatment: Acute Promyelocytic Leukemia

Experiments first conducted with the human promyelocytic cell line HL-60 implicated retinoids in myeloid differentiation (186). The chromosomal translocations observed in leukemias may contribute to carcinogenesis through enhanced expression of an oncogene or formation of chimeric fusion proteins with new functional properties (187). Also, cytologic analysis has shown that virtually all patients with a specific form of acute myeloid leukemia, acute promyelocytic leukemia (APL), bear a specific chromosomal abnormality characterized as a balanced reciprocal translocation between the long arms of chromosomes 15 and 17 (t15,17). In 1987, the gene for RAR-α was mapped to the long arm of chromosome 17 (17q21). In 1988, Chinese scientists reported that APL patients treated with high-dosage all-*trans*-RA (generally 45 mg/m^2/day) showed remarkable clinical improvement, with complete remission in about 90% of patients (188). At the same time, molecular genetic analysis revealed that in virtually all APL patients, the gene for RAR-α is severed in intron 2 and fused with a previously unknown gene now named *PML* (for promyelocytic leukemia) on chromosome 15 (187). This reciprocal chromosomal exchange results in two abnormal genes that are expressed in APL patients as the chimeric fusion proteins PML-RAR-α (always present) and RAR-α-PML (present in about two-thirds of cases) (187).

Although the effectiveness of all-*trans*-RA in inducing remission was rapidly confirmed, the reasons for the success of this "differentiation therapy" are still not fully understood. To date, APL is the only example of differentiation therapy of human cancer, and all-*trans*-RA is the only anticancer drug targeted to a defined genetic location (187). The abnormal fusion protein PML-RAR-α, which is expressed at higher abundance than RAR-α in APL cells, contains all of the putative or known functional domains of PML and the DBD and LBD of RAR-α (187). It therefore is possible that this chimeric receptor functions as a dominant negative competitor of the normal RAR-α allele. PML-RAR-α can bind to RXR. Thus, it is possible that this abnormal complex blocks normal hematopoietic differentiation at the promyelocytic stage, enabling leukemogenic transformation to occur. Treatment with all-*trans*-RA rapidly induces expression of the remaining normal RAR-α allele (188), which may rebalance the receptor system toward normal differentiation. Because all-*trans*-RA alone cannot eliminate the leukemogenic clone, standard chemotherapy is used with, or following, treatment with RA, as consolidation therapy.

In treating APL patients with high doses of RA, it rapidly became clear that this treatment is associated with a high-risk syndrome, the "retinoic acid syndrome" (188, 189), a combination of fever, respiratory distress, hypotension, and renal failure, which has led to death of a significant percentage of patients. Consequently, therapy has been modified so that high-dose all-*trans*-RA is strictly administered for only a short period, followed by conventional chemotherapy for consolidation (188, 190). Furthermore, APL patients treated with all-*trans*-RA become refractory to its differentiating activity, so patients who relapse after its withdrawal are resistant to further treatment with all-*trans*-RA (120, 188). Resistance appears to be due at least in part to an increase in the rate of RA catabolism (see "Metabolism").

DEFICIENCY AND TOXICITY

Vitamin A Deficiency

Nutritional vitamin A deficiency still exists in parts of the developing world, especially in young children (191). Deficiency leads to dedifferentiation (metaplasia), epithelial keratinization (e.g., trachea, skin), appetite changes that contribute to poor growth, and xerophthalmia. Animal and human studies have shown that the liver vitamin A content is low at birth because of limited placental transfer of fat-soluble vitamins, even in the offspring of well-nourished mothers (9, 192, 193). Hepatic vitamin A storage can increase significantly during the nursing period if milk vitamin A (related to maternal dietary vitamin A) is adequate (193). The liver vitamin A stores of children and young animals also depend on the adequacy of their postweaning diets (194). Provision of vitamin A to breast-feeding Indonesian women early in lactation increased their breast-milk vitamin A significantly and reduced the frequency of low serum retinol concentrations among their infants (195). Once liver vitamin A reserves are established, they can supply retinol to other tissues for several months or even longer. Vitamin A deficiency in children occurs most often in the postweaning period and thus is likely to reflect inadequate vitamin A both during the suckling period and in the postweaning diet.

The WHO criteria for a vitamin A public health problem now include not only the prevalence of traditional eye signs of severe deficiency (e.g., corneal xerosis, Bitôt's spots [see Fig 10.1]) but also population-based cutoff levels for subclinical indicators (e.g., low serum retinol, low breast-milk retinol [196]). It is estimated that each year, some 3 to 10 million children, most living in developing countries, become xerophthalmic, and between 250,000 and 500,000 go blind (144, 196). International public health programs to eradicate vitamin A deficiency and xerophthalmia continue to have high priority. Providing vitamin A supplements of 50,000 to 200,000 IU (15,000–60,000 μg RE, depending on age) to young children at risk of vitamin A deficiency is considered to protect for 4 to 6 months (196). Improved dietary intakes are clearly required for long-term solution to vitamin A deficiency (196).

Retinoid Toxicity and Teratogenicity

Hypervitaminosis A. The condition hypervitaminosis A results from acute or chronic overconsumption of preformed vitamin A (not carotenoids). The presence of esterified retinol in *fasting* plasma (in association with plasma lipoproteins) is an early indicator of hypervitaminosis A. However, the plasma concentration of holo-RBP remains near normal (197). Generally, signs of toxicity are associated with chronic consumption of doses in excess of 10 times the RDA resulting from food faddism (e.g., excessive consumption of liver [198]) or self-medication with high-dose vitamin A preparations (199). (See [198] and [197] for typical case reports of nutritionally induced vitamin A toxicity.) Even among healthy users of vitamin/mineral supplements (in quantities approximately one to two times the RDA for vitamin A), significant increases in fasting plasma retinyl esters were observed (200). In elderly men and women, an elevation of plasma retinyl esters was associated with long-term vitamin A supplement use (>5 years) and, in some, with biochemical evidence of liver damage (elevated serum transaminases) (200). These data raise the possibility that even moderate, chronic vitamin A supplementation may cause mild hypervitaminosis A in some individuals (199).

Dose-dependent manifestations of retinoid toxicity include headache, vomiting, diplopia, alopecia, dryness of the mucous membranes, desquamation, bone and joint pain, liver damage, hemorrhage, and coma (9, 16, 201, 202). Mechanisms that plausibly explain the etiology of hypervitaminosis A and vitamin A toxicity (203) include first, that retinoids may insert into, expand, and destabilize membranes (204). Symptoms such as joint and bone pain may be explained by rupture of membranes of cells and intracellular organelles such as lysosomes. Second, as intracellular retinoids accumulate, RA may induce inappropriate expression of genes. Several reviews (201, 203, 205, 206) provide information on structure-activity relationships associated with the clinical pharmacology, toxicology, and teratogenicity of retinoids.

Teratogenic Effects. A high incidence (>20%) of spontaneous abortions and birth defects has been observed in the fetuses of women ingesting therapeutic doses of 13-*cis*-RA (as prescribed for skin disorders, see above) during the first trimester of pregnancy (16), and similar retinoid-induced birth defects are well documented in several animal models (see [206] for review). Three retinoids are currently approved for oral use in the United States and many other countries (13-*cis*-RA [isotretinoin, Accutane]; etretinate [Tegison, Tigason] and acitretin [Neotigason]). Because 13-*cis*-RA is known to be teratogenic in humans, it is marketed in the United States as contraindicated during pregnancy (206). Tegison is currently approved for treatment of psoriasis. However, the risk for fetal dysmorphogenesis by these retinoids may persist for many months after use ceases (206). The dysmorphogenic effects caused by retinoids depend on dosage (exposure), the form of retinoid, its rate of metabolism, the species studied, and the stage of fetal development at the time of retinoid intake. Retinoids are teratogenic during the period of fetal organogenesis (first trimester). Human and other primate embryos are considerably more sensitive to retinoid-induced congenital malformations than are those of rabbits, rats, and mice, although the types of congenital malformations (exencephaly, craniofacial malformations, eye defects, and cardiac abnormalities [206]) are similar across species (201). Each of the main isomers of RA (9-*cis*, 13-*cis*, and all-*trans*-RA) is teratogenic in animals. Structure-activity analysis indicates that retinoids with stabilized structures, an acidic group at C-15 or the ability to form one in vivo, and a high rate of transplacental transfer are more teratogenic (206). In this regard, retinoyl-β-glucuronide, which lacks a free carboxyl group, shows little, if any, teratogenicity when given orally (11). The greater teratogenicity of 13-*cis*-RA in humans (1 mg/kg/day) versus rodents (75 mg/kg/day in rats and mice) is likely to be explained by a higher rate of placental transfer, a longer plasma half-life (10–20 h in humans vs. 1 h in rodents), and differences in metabolite formation, with more 4-oxo-all-*trans*-RA and 4-oxo-13-*cis*-RA produced in humans (206).

A recent epidemiologic study by Rothman et al. (207) investigated the relationship of dietary vitamin A intake to birth defects. Birth records and dietary interviews for 22,748 pregnant American women were reviewed. Of 339 babies with birth defects, 121 were in sites that originated from the embryonic cranial neural crest. From logistic-regression analysis these authors concluded that the risk of birth defects was significantly greater in women who consumed more than 10,000 IU/day of vitamin A from supplements (1.4% of the group studied) and was related to vitamin A consumption in the periconceptual period. Rosa (207a) has reviewed published case reports and reports to the U.S. Food and Drug Administration of birth defects associated with maternal vitamin A exposures in excess of 20,000 IU/day during early pregnancy. Concerns have also been raised about the frequent consumption by pregnant or potentially pregnant women of very high vitamin A foods such as liver (>100,000 IU [33,000 mg RE]/100 g) (117, 208).

Safe Upper Limit of Intake. A generally recognized safe upper limit of intake for vitamin A is 8,000 to 10,000 IU (~3,000 mg RE)/day (201, 209).

ASSESSMENT OF VITAMIN A STATUS

Vitamin A status comprises a continuum from overt, clinically evident deficiency to overt, clinically evident toxicity (Table 17.2). In between, the range of marginal, adequate, and excessive vitamin A covers a broad range of body vitamin A reserves. This range is not associated with clinical signs, and plasma retinol is quite constant (Fig. 17.4). The lack of sensitivity of plasma retinol to changes in body reserves has led to the quest for other indicators of status, particularly of marginal vitamin A status, which may be useful in clinical and population-based studies. In the 8th edition of *Modern Nutrition in Health and Disease,* Olson (9) dealt with several tests of vitamin A status in detail. This chapter focuses on recent results and on those tests most often used.

Clinical Assessment

Eye Signs. Conjunctival xerosis with Bitôt's spots in young children (WHO classification X1B) is strongly associated with vitamin A deficiency (9, 144). A prevalence above 0.5% X1B in young children is one of the criteria used by the WHO to identify vitamin A deficiency as a public health problem (see below). Questioning children and their parents on the child's ability to see in dim light (i.e., probing about night blindness) may be useful in revealing subclinical manifestations of vitamin A deficiency for which further tests may be indicated. Night blindness has also been reported during pregnancy in regions of low vitamin A intake.

Public Health Assessment. Although the serum retinol level is not considered a strong indicator of the vitamin A status of an individual, low values in populations have greater significance. In 1987, WHO identified 37 countries, most in Africa, whose populations had vitamin A deficiency of varying degrees of severity, based largely on the prevalence of xerophthalmia (210). In 1994, criteria were updated for determining whether vitamin A deficiency is a public health problem in children 6 to 71 months old (196). These criteria combine ocular, biochemical (including serum retinol), and nutritional indicators. Even when the prevalence of xerophthalmia is very

Table 17.2
Vitamin A Status: Typical Findings

Category	Serum Retinol	Serum Retinyl Esters in the Fasting State	Liver Stores	Clinical Signs	Vulnerable Groups/ Most Common Situations
Deficient	Generally, <0.35 μmol/L[a]	Very low, if at all detectable	Severely depleted (<5 μg/g)	Night blindness; other ocular manifestations (see "Vision"); dryness of skin	Preschool-age children and pregnant or lactating women with low VA intakes; chronic alcoholics; chronic liver diseases
Marginal	Generally 0.35–0.7 μmol/L	Low (<2%)	Severely depleted (5–20 μg/g)	None (however, responsive to provision of vitamin A)[b]	Large proportions of children and women living in poverty with poor diets; populations with high rates of infectious diseases[c]
Adequate	Generally >0.7–3 μmol/L	2–20%[d]	~20–300 μg/g	None	Typical of a well-nourished general population
Excessive	High normal to >3 μmol/L[e]	Significantly present in fasting plasma; carried on lipoproteins	High (>300 μg/g)[f]	Not apparent or very mild; elevated liver enzymes in plasma	Chronic supplement use; frequent intake of foods (e.g., liver) high in preformed VA
Toxic	Higher than the above concentration	May exceed retinol in its concentration	Very high in liver and increased in peripheral tissues	Headache; bone/joint pain; elevated liver enzymes in plasma and clinical signs of liver disease	Food faddists and users of high-dose VA supplements; patients treated with retinoids[g]

[a]Very rarely due to hereditary familial low retinol-binding protein (219); 0.35 μmol/L = 10 μg retinol/dL.
[b]Positive relative dose or modified relative dose-response test, an indicator that the secretion of RBP is limited by a lack of vitamin A.
[c]In infection/inflammation, low plasma retinol may represent the acute-phase response and low RBP production, not lack of vitamin A stores.
[d]Based on NHANES III data for U.S. population (83).
[e]Retinol and RBP normal; total retinol elevated due to retinyl esters.
[f]Based on data from rats fed a high vitamin A diet for 8 months (194); human values may be lower (~300 μg/g, see ref. 92).
[g]Retinoid treatment typically reduces, not increases, plasma retinol (106), and plasma retinyl esters are not observed; however, the clinical signs of retinoid toxicity resemble those for a nutritional excess of vitamin A.

low, the presence of other indicators—low serum retinol, low breast-milk retinol, abnormal cytology (see below)—still warns that mild, moderate, or severe vitamin A deficiency may be significant (Table 17.2). One impetus for this change is the growing awareness of an association between marginal vitamin A deficiency and increased child morbidity and mortality (see Chapter 97).

Biochemical

Vitamin A concentration in serum (plasma), breast milk, or tear fluid may indicate vitamin A deficiency. Of these, only serum retinol has generally accepted cutoff values for classification of vitamin A status. Liver vitamin A concentrations (which seldom are obtainable) below 5 μg total retinol/g have been associated with deficiency, and from 5 to 20 μg/g with marginal status (9).

Response assays have been developed to assess indirectly the adequacy of liver vitamin A stores. Based on the findings that RBP accumulates in the livers of vitamin A–deficient animals and is rapidly released when vitamin A is provided, the relative dose response (RDR) and the modified relative dose response (MRDR) were developed to assess the adequacy of liver stores in children and other vulnerable groups. In the RDR (9, 211), plasma is sampled for a baseline retinol concentration, and a small dose of retinol (1.6–3.5 μmol [450 to 1000 μg RE]) is given orally in oil. The larger dose (3.5 μmol) gives more reproducible results. Plasma is collected again about 5 hours later. An increase in retinol in excess of 20% of baseline is generally considered a positive result (although other values have been used [212]), which indicates that hepatic vitamin A reserves are not adequate to maximize secretion of holo-RBP. To reduce the blood requirement to a single sample, the MRDR test takes advantage of the low level of vitamin A_2 (3,4-didehydroretinol) normally present in plasma and the similarity of vitamin A_2 to retinol during absorption and in formation of holo-RBP in liver. A dose of 0.35 μmol vitamin A_2/kg body weight, recently revised to a 5.3 μmol dose for preschool children (213), is administered orally, and a single blood sample is collected 5 hours later (9, 214). A serum ratio of 3,4-didehydroretinol:retinol of 0.060 or above is generally considered to indicate inadequate status, and a value below 0.030, adequate status. For both the RDR and the MRDR, intermediate values suggest marginal deficiency but are harder to interpret. When the MRDR was used in a study of 57 pregnant Iowan women of low socioeconomic status, 26% had values between 0.030 and 0.060, interpreted as indicating marginal vitamin A deficiency, and 9% had values of 0.060 or above (214). Recent validation and comparison studies provide comparisons to other measures of status and references to earlier studies (212, 215).

Histologic. Evaluation of conjunctival histology (conjunctival impression cytology, CIC) has been proposed as a field-operative test. CIC is based on the lack of normal goblet cells and the presence of enlarged epithelial cells in the conjunctiva of vitamin A–deficient children or adults. Cells are transferred from the conjunctiva to filter paper with gentle pressure, stained, examined microscopically, and scored by a trained observer. The test requires patient cooperation. Recently, CIC has been compared with the RDR, serum retinol, and RBP measurements in a group of 2- to 8-year-old children in Belize, Central America (212). Some 49% of children in this population had an abnormal CIC test, compared with 24% with low serum retinol (<0.87 μmol/L) and 17% with a positive RDR test. The response of the corneal epithelium to vitamin A supplementation is typically slow, and several months may be required for the eye to appear normal (144, 215a).

Dietary Assessment

Because vitamin A is concentrated in relatively few foods and is well conserved in the body, short-term dietary recall (e.g., for 24 h) is not useful for individuals, but it may be useful in population studies. Food-frequency questionnaires have been used in numerous case-control clinical or epidemiologic studies, both with and without assessment of food portion size. As noted previously (9), dietary data are of greatest value in assessing the food habits of populations at risk of vitamin A deficiency.

Assessment Tools Now Limited to Research. Methods to assess body vitamin A reserves have been developed using stable isotopes that equilibrate with tissue retinoids. A test of the retinol isotope-dilution method in rats showed that liver stores could be predicted well over a wide range of vitamin A nutriture (mean liver vitamin A from 0.17 to 1885 nmol/g [216]). In human volunteers consuming different levels of vitamin A, a deuterated-retinol dilution test was both useful in estimating total body reserves of vitamin A and was responsive to differences in daily retinol consumption (217).

Ocular tests requiring specialized equipment have been used to assess visual acuity in relationship to vitamin A status. Pupillary response and visual threshold were tested in assessment of vitamin A status in young children and correlated with serum retinol and results of the RDR test (218). Children with abnormal pupillary thresholds had significantly higher RDRs and lower serum retinol concentrations than normal children.

SUMMARY

Vitamin A is essential for growth and life, taking part not only in vision but in developmental processes that begin early in embryogenesis. Vitamin A continues to be necessary to maintain normal cellular differentiation throughout life. The basic mechanism of action of vitamin A, in the form of RA and as a potent modulator of gene expression, is now well understood. However, much less is known of the physiologic and pharmacologic situations in which specific genes are regulated in vivo. This understanding will be necessary if vitamin A–like molecules are to be used over an extended time for cancer prevention and control. The value of synthetic retinoids or natural compounds used pharmacologically has been demonstrated dramatically in the treatment of dermatologic diseases and in the specific leukemia APL. At the same time, the inherent potential of most retinoids to be toxic or teratogenic has been observed anew or under new circumstances. Vitamin A thus remains an essential nutrient with an unusually broad range of activities, and it is likely that much more remains to be revealed.

ACKNOWLEDGMENTS

The author wishes to acknowledge research support from NIH grants DK-46869 and DK-41479 and the generous support of Dorothy Foehr Huck to the Pennsylvania State University.

REFERENCES

1. Wolf G. FASEB J 1996;10:1102–7.
2. Arens JF, van Dorp DA. Nature 1946;157:190–1.
3. Wald G. Science 1968;162:230–9.
4. Goodman DS. Plasma retinol-binding protein. In: Sporn MB, Roberts AB, Goodman DS, eds. The retinoids, vol 2. New York: Academic Press, 1984;42–88.
5. Ong DE, Newcomer ME, Chytil F. Cellular retinoid-binding proteins. In: Sporn MB, Roberts AB, Goodman DS, eds. The retinoids: biology, chemistry and medicine. New York: Raven Press, 1994;283–317.
6. Mangelsdorf DJ, Umesono K, Evans RM. The retinoid receptors. In: Sporn MB, Roberts AB, Goodman DS, eds. The retinoids: biology, chemistry and medicine. New York: Raven Press, 1994;319–49.
7. Chambon P. FASEB J 1996;10:940–54.
8. Dawson MI, Hobbs PD. The synthetic chemistry of retinoids. In: Sporn MB, Roberts AB, Goodman DS, eds. The retinoids: biology, chemistry and medicine. New York: Raven Press, 1994;5–178.
9. Olson JA. Vitamin A, retinoids and carotenoids. In: Shils ME, Olson JA, Shike M, eds. Modern nutrition in health and disease, 8th ed. Philadelphia: Lea & Febiger, 1994;287–307.
10. Merck Index. Whitehouse Station, NJ: Merck & Co, 1996.
11. Formelli F, Barua AB, Olson JA. FASEB J 1996;10:1014–24.
12. Muccio DD, Brouillette WJ, Alam M, et al. J Med Chem 1996;39:3625–35.
13. Hashimoto Y, Kagechika H, Shudo K. Biochem Biophys Res Commun 1990;166:1300–7.
14. Furr HC, Barua AB, Olson JA. Analytical methods. In: Sporn MB, Roberts AB, Goodman DS, eds. The retinoids: biology, chemistry, and medicine. New York: Raven Press, 1994;179–209.
15. Soprano DR, Blaner WS. Plasma retinol-binding protein. In: Sporn MB, Roberts AB, Goodman DS, eds. The retinoids: biology, chemistry, and medicine. New York: Raven Press, 1994;257–81.
16. Committee on the 10th edition of the RDAs. Fat-soluble vitamins. In: Food and Nutrition Board, National Research Council, eds. Recommended dietary allowances. Washington, DC: National Academy of Sciences Press, 1989;78–92.
17. Hathcock JN, Hattan DG, Jenkins MY, et al. Am J Clin Nutr 1990;52:183–202.
18. Noy N, Xu Z-J. Biochemistry 1990;29:3878–83.

19. Vallet JL. Domes Anim Endocrinol 1996;13:127–38.
20. Li E, Norris AW. Annu Rev Nutr 1996;16:205–34.
21. Gordon JI, Sacchettini JC, Ropson IJ, et al. Curr Opin Lipidol 1991;2:125–37.
22. Levin MS, Li E, Ong DE, et al. J Biol Chem 1987;262:7118–24.
23. Blomhoff R, Green MH, Green JB, et al. Physiol Rev 1991;71:951–90.
24. Rajan N, Blaner WS, Soprano DR, et al. J Lipid Res 1990;31:821–9.
25. Chytil F. FASEB J 1996;10:986–92.
26. Levin MS, Locke B, Yang N-C, et al. J Biol Chem 1988;263: 17715–23.
27. Li E, Demmer LA, Sweetser DA, et al. Proc Natl Acad Sci USA 1986;83:5779–83.
28. Suruga K, Suzuki R, Goda T, et al. J Nutr 1995;125:2039–44.
29. Bailey JS, Siu C-H. J Biol Chem 1988;263:9326–32.
30. Elder JT, Åström A, Pettersson U, et al. J Invest Dermatol 1992;98:673–9.
31. Fisher GJ, Voorhees JJ. FASEB J 1996;10:1002–13.
32. Boylan JF, Gudas LJ. J Cell Biol 1991;112:965–79.
33. Fiorella PD, Napoli JL. J Biol Chem 1991;266:16572–9.
34. Åström A, Tavakkol A, Pettersson U, et al. J Biol Chem 1991;266:17662–6.
35. Wei L-N, Chang L. J Biol Chem 1996;271:5073–8.
36. Saari JC. Retinoids in photosensitive systems. In: Sporn MB, Roberts AB, Goodman DS, eds. The retinoids: biology, chemistry, and medicine. New York: Raven Press, 1994;351–85.
37. Crabb JW, Johnson CM, Carr SA, et al. J Biol Chem 1988;263:18678–87.
38. Liou GIH, Geng L, Baehr W. Molecular biology of the retina: basic and clinically relevant studies. New York: Wiley-Liss, 1991;115–37.
39. DeLuca LM. FASEB J 1991;5:2924–33.
40. Mangelsdorf DJ, Evans RM. Cell 1995;83:841–50.
41. Lipkin SM, Rosenfeld MG, Glass CK. Genet Eng 1992; 14:185–209.
42. Levin AA, Sturzenbecker LJ, Kazmer S, et al. Ann NY Acad Sci 1992;669:70–86.
43. Mangelsdorf DJ, Thummel C, Beato M, et al. Cell 1995;83: 835–9.
44. Wan Y-JY, Wang L, Wu T-CJ. J Mol Endocrinol 1992;9:291–4.
45. Kato S, Mano H, Kumazawa T, et al. Biochem J 1992;286: 755–60.
46. Verma AK, Shoemaker A, Simsiman R, et al. J Nutr 1992;122:2144–52.
47. Nagpal S, Saunders M, Kastner P, et al. Cell 1992;70:1007–19.
48. Levin MS. Intestinal absorption and metabolism of vitamin A. In: Johnson LR, ed. Physiology of the gastrointestinal tract. New York: Raven Press, 1994;1957–77.
49. Harrison EH. Biochim Biophys Acta 1993;1170:99–108.
50. Rigtrup KM, Ong DE. Biochemistry 1992;31:2920–6.
51. Underwood BA. Vitamin A in animal and human nutrition. In: Sporn MB, Roberts AB, Goodman DS, eds. The retinoids, vol 1. Orlando, FL: Academic Press, 1984;281–392.
52. Hollander D, Muralidhara KS. Am J Physiol 1977;232:E471–7.
53. Blomhoff R, Green MH, Norum KR. Annu Rev Nutr 1992;12:37–57.
54. Ross AC. Vitamin A metabolism. In: Zakim D, Boyer T, eds. Hepatology: a textbook of liver disease. Philadelphia: WB Saunders, 1995;215–43.
55. Kakkad BP, Ong DE. J Biol Chem 1988;263:12916–9.
56. Huang HS, Goodman DS. J Biol Chem 1965;240:2839–44.
57. Helgerud P, Petersen LB, Norum KR. J Clin Invest 1983;71:747–53.
58. Ross AC. FASEB J 1993;7:317–27.
59. Kayden HJ. Annu Rev Med 1972;23:285–96.
60. Berr F. J Lipid Res 1992;33:915–30.
61. Zilversmit DB, Morton RE, Hughes LB, et al. Biochim Biophys Acta 1982;712:88–93.
62. Skrede B, Olafsdottir AE, Blomhoff R, et al. Scand J Clin Lab Invest 1993;53:515–9.
63. Hussain MM, Mahley RW, Boyles JK, et al. J Biol Chem 1989;264:17931–8.
64. Harrison EH, Gad MZ, Ross AC. J Lipid Res 1995;36: 1498–506.
65. Blomhoff R, Berg T, Norum KR. Proc Natl Acad Sci USA 1988;85:3455–8.
66. Goodman DS, Blaner WS. Biosynthesis, absorption and hepatic metabolism of retinol. In: Sporn MB, Roberts AB, Goodman DS, eds. The retinoids, vol 2. Orlando, FL: Academic Press, 1984;1–39.
67. Green MH, Balmer Green J, Berg T, et al. J Nutr 1988; 118:1331–5.
68. Geerts A, Bouwens L, Wisse E. J Electron Microsc Tech 1990;14:247–56.
69. Matsuura T, Naramori S, Hasumura S, et al. Exp Cell Res 1993;209:33–7.
70. Hendriks HFJ, Verhoofstad AMM, Brouwer A, et al. Exp Cell Res 1985;160:138–49.
71. Blomhoff R, Wake K. FASEB J 1991;5:271–7.
72. Leighton FA, Cattet M, Norstrom R, et al. Can J Zool 1988;66:480–2.
73. Hendriks HFJ, Blaner WS, Wennekers HM, et al. Eur J Biochem 1988;171:237–44.
74. Blaner WS, Hendriks HFJ, Brouwer A, et al. J Lipid Res 1985;26:1241–51.
75. Blaner WS, van Bennekum AM, Brouwer A, et al. FEBS Lett 1990;274:89–92.
76. Matsuura T, Gad MZ, Harrison ER, et al. J Nutr 1997;127: 218–24.
77. Randolph RK, Ross AC. J Biol Chem 1991;266:16453–7.
78. Matsuura T, Ross AC. Arch Biochem Biophys 1993;301:221–7.
79. Boerman MHE, Napoli JL. J Biol Chem 1991;266:22273–8.
80. Pinzani M, Gentilini P, Abboud HE. J Hepatol 1992;14:211–20.
81. Friedman SL, Wei S, Blaner WS. Am J Physiol 1993;264: G947–52.
82. Leo MA, Lieber CS. N Engl J Med 1982;307:597–601.
83. Life Science Research Office. Assessment of the vitamin A nutritional status of the U.S. population based on data collected in the health and nutrition examination surveys. Bethesda, MD: FASEB, 1985.
84. Sowell A, Briefel R, Huff D, et al. FASEB J 1996;10:A813.
85. Shenai JP, Rush MG, Stahlman MT, et al. J Pediatr 1990;116:607–14.
86. Chapman KM, Prabhudesai M, Erdman JW Jr. J Am Coll Nutr 1993;12:77–83.
87. Lecomte E, Grolier P, Herbeth B, et al. Int J Vitam Nutr Res 1994;64:170–5.
88. Ahmed S, Leo MA, Lieber CS. Am J Clin Nutr 1994;60:430–6.
89. Bell H, Nilsson A, Norum KR, et al. J Hepatol 1989;8:26–31.
90. Bankson DD, Rifai N, Silverman LM. Ann Clin Chem 1988;25:246–9.
91. Janczewska I, Ericzon BG, Ericksson LS. Scand J Gastroenterol 1995;30:68–71.
92. Olson JA. J Natl Cancer Inst 1984;73:1439–44.
93. Tosetti F, Ferrari N, Brigati C, et al. Exp Cell Res 1992;200:467–72.
94. Smith FR, Goodman DS, Arroyave G, et al. Am J Clin Nutr 1973;26:982–7.

95. Smith FR, Goodman DS, Zaklama MS, et al. Am J Clin Nutr 1973;26:973–81.
96. Soprano DR, Smith JE, Goodman DS. J Biol Chem 1982;257:7693–7.
97. Smith JE, Muto Y, Milch PO, et al. J Biol Chem 1973;248:1544–9.
98. Aldred AR, Schreiber G. The negative acute phase proteins. In: Mackiewicz A, Kushner I, Bauman H, eds. Acute phase proteins. Molecular biology, biochemistry, and clinical applications. Boca Raton, FL: CRC Press, 1993;21–37.
99. Rosales FJ, Ritter SJ, Zolfaghari R, et al. J Lipid Res 1996;37:962–71.
100. Thurnham DI, Singkamani R. Trans R Soc Trop Med Hyg 1991;85:194–9.
101. Felding P, Fex G. Acta Physiol Scand 1985;123:477–83.
102. Smith DK, Greene JM, Leonard SB, et al. Am J Med Sci 1992;304:20–4.
103. Vahlquist A, Johnsson A, Nygren K-G. Am J Clin Nutr 1979;32:1433–8.
104. Lewis KC, Green MH, Balmer Green J, et al. J Lipid Res 1990;31:1535–48.
105. Green MH, Balmer Green J, Lewis KC. J Nutr 1987;117:694–703.
106. Berni R, Clerici M, Malpeli G, et al. FASEB J 1993;7:1179–84.
107. Adams WR, Smith JE, Green MH. Proc Soc Exp Biol Med 1995;208:178–85.
108. Lewis KC, Zech LA, Phang JM. Cancer Res 1994;54:4112–7.
109. Nilsson CB, Hanberg A, Trossvik C, et al. Eur J Pharmacol Environ Toxicol Pharmacol 1996;2:17–23.
110. Schweigert FJ, Thomann E, Zucker H. Int J Vitam Nutr Res 1991;61:110–3.
111. Pfeffer BA, Clark VM, Flannery JG, et al. Invest Ophthalmol Vis Sci 1986;27:1031–40.
112. Noy N, Blaner WS. Biochemistry 1991;30:6380–6.
113. Wathne K-O, Norum KR, Smeland E, et al. J Biol Chem 1988;263:8691–5.
114. Smith JE, Milch PO, Muto Y, et al. Biochem J 1973;132:821–7.
115. Blaner WS, Olson JA. Retinol and retinoic acid metabolism. In: Sporn MB, Roberts AB, Goodman DS, eds. The retinoids: biology, chemistry, and medicine. New York: Raven Press, 1994;229–55.
116. Eckhoff C, Collins MD, Nau H. J Nutr 1991;121:1016–25.
117. Arnhold T, Tzimas G, Wittfoht W, et al. Life Sci 1996;59:PL169–77.
118. Adamson PC, Balis FM, Smith MA, et al. J Natl Cancer Inst 1992;84:1332–5.
119. Adamson PC, Murphy RF, Godwin KA, et al. Cancer Res 1995;55:482–5.
120. Rigas JR, Francis PA, Muindi JRF, et al. J Natl Cancer Inst 1993;85:1921–6.
121. Urbach J, Rando RR. Biochem J 1994;299:459–65.
122. Napoli JL, Posch KP, Fiorella PD, et al. Biomed Pharmacother 1991;45:131–43.
123. Heyman RA, Mangelsdorf DJ, Dyck JA, et al. Cell 1992;68: 397–406.
124. Sass JO, Forster A, Bock KW, et al. Biochem Pharmacol 1994;47:485–92.
125. Kraft JC, Eckhoff C, Kochhar DM, et al. Teratogen Carcinog Mutagen 1991;11:21–30.
126. Tzimas G, Nau H, Hendricks AG, et al. Teratology 1996;54:255–65.
127. Kurlandsky SB, Gamble MV, Ramakrishnan R, et al. J Biol Chem 1995;270:17850–7.
128. Barua AB, Batres RO, Olson JA. Am J Clin Nutr 1989;50:370–4.
129. Napoli JL. FASEB J 1996;10:993–1001.
130. Duester G. Biochemistry 1996;35:12221–7.
131. Kedishvili NY, Stone CL, Popov KM, et al. Adv Exp Med Biol 1997;414:321–9.
132. Roberts ES, Vaz ADN, Coon MJ. Mol Pharmacol 1992;41: 427–33.
133. Chen M, Achkar C, Gudas LJ. Mol Pharmacol 1994;46:88–96.
134. LaBrecque J, Dumas F, Lacroix A, et al. Biochem J 1995;305:681–4.
135. Zhao D, McCaffery P, Ivins KJ, et al. Eur J Biochem 1996;240:15–22.
136. Raner GM, Vaz ADN, Coon MJ. Mol Pharmacol 1996;49: 515–22.
136a. Genchi G, Wang W, Barua A, et al. Biochim Biophys Acta 1996;1289:284–90.
137. Roberts AB, DeLuca HF. Biochem J 1967;102:600–5.
138. Smith FR, Goodman DS. J Clin Invest 1971;50:2426–36.
139. Gerlach TH, Zile MH. J Lipid Res 1991;32:515–20.
140. Gerlach TH, Zile MH. FASEB J 1991;5:86–92.
141. Alvarez JO, Salazar-Lindo E, Kohatsu J, et al. Am J Clin Nutr 1995;61:1273–6.
142. Stephensen CB, Alvarez JO, Kohatsu J, et al. Am J Clin Nutr 1994;60:388–92.
143. Fex GA, Larsson K, Nilsson-Ehle I. J Nutr Biochem 1996;7: 162–5.
144. Sommer A, West KP Jr. Vitamin A deficiency: health, survival, and vision. New York: Oxford University Press, 1996.
145. Simon A, Lagercrantz J, Bajalica-Lagercrantz S, et al. Genomics 1996;36:424–30.
146. Jacobson SG, Cideciyan AV, Regunath G, et al. Nature Genet 1995;11:27–32.
147. Lee S-Y, Ubels JL, Soprano DR. Exp Eye Res 1992;55:163–71.
148. Wolbach SB, Howe PR. J Exp Med 1925;42:753–77.
149. Strickland S, Mahdavi V. Cell 1978;15:393–403.
150. Gudas LJ, Sporn MB, Roberts AB. Cellular biology and biochemistry of the retinoids. In: Sporn MB, Roberts AB, Goodman DS, eds. The retinoids: biology, chemistry, and medicine. New York: Raven Press, 1994;443–520.
151. Pfahl M. Endocr Rev 1993;14:651–8.
152. Lotan R. J Natl Cancer Inst 1995;87:1655–7.
153. Wilson JG, Roth CB, Warkany J. Am J Anat 1953;92:189–217.
154. Morriss-Kay GM, Sokolova N. FASEB J 1996;10:961–8.
155. Conlon RA. Trends Genet 1995;11:314–9.
156. Marshall H, Morrison A, Studer M, et al. FASEB J 1996;10: 969–78.
157. Hofmann C, Eichele G. Retinoids in development. In: Sporn MB, Roberts AB, Goodman DS, eds. The retinoids: biology, chemistry, and medicine. New York: Raven Press, 1994; 387–441.
158. Hoffman M. Science 1990;250:372–3.
159. Dickman ED, Smith SM. Dev Dyn 1996;206:39–48.
160. Gruber PJ, Kubalak SW, Pexieder T, et al. J Clin Invest 1996;98:1332–43.
161. McCaffery P, Dräger UC. Retinoic acid synthesizing enzymes in the embryonic and adult vertebrate. In: Weiner H, Holmes RS, Wermuth B, eds. Enzymology and molecular biology of carbonyl metabolism 5. New York: Plenum Press, 1995;173–83.
162. Båvik C, Ward SJ, Chambon P. Proc Natl Acad Sci USA 1996;93:3110–4.
163. Krezel W, Dupé V, Mark M, et al. Proc Natl Acad Sci USA 1996;93:9010–4.
164. Wellik DM, DeLuca HF. Arch Biochem Biophys 1996; 330:355–63.
165. Scrimshaw NS, Taylor CE, Gordon JE. Interactions of nutrition and infection. Geneva: World Health Organization, 1968.
166. Kirkwood BJ. Epidemiology of interventions to improve

vitamin A status in order to reduce child mortality and morbidity. In: Garza C, Haas JD, Habicht J-P, et al., eds. Beyond nutritional recommendations: implementing science for healthier populations. Ithaca: Cornell University, 1995;97–112.
167. Beaton GH. Basic biology of interventions: a synthesis review. In: Garza C, Haas JD, Habicht J-P, et al., eds. Beyond nutritional recommendations: implementing science for healthier populations. Ithaca: Cornell University, 1995;87–96.
168. Vitamin A and the immune function: a symposium. Binghamton, NY: Haworth Medical Press, 1996.
169. Dibley MJ, Sadjimin T, Kjolhede CL, et al. J Nutr 1996;126:434–42.
170. Kjolhede CL, Chew FJ, Gadomski AM, et al. J Pediatr 1995;126:807–12.
171. Dowell SF, Papic Z, Bresee JS, et al. Pediatr Infect Dis J 1996;15:782–6.
172. Ross AC, Hämmerling UG. Retinoids and the immune system. In: Sporn MB, Roberts AB, Goodman DS, eds. The retinoids: biology, chemistry, and medicine. New York: Raven Press, 1994;521–44.
173. Cantorna MT, Nashold FE, Hayes CE. Eur J Immunol 1995;25:1673–9.
174. Ross AC. Clin Immunol Immunopathol 1996;80:S36–72.
175. Ross AC. The relationship between immunocompetence and vitamin A status. In: Sommer A, West KP Jr, eds. Vitamin A deficiency: health, survival, and vision. New York: Oxford University Press, 1996;251–73.
176. Orfanos CE, Zouboulis CC, Almond-Roesler B, et al. Drugs 1997;53:358–88.
177. Peck GL, DiGiovanna JJ. Synthetic retinoids in dermatology. In: Sporn MB, Roberts AB, Goodman DS, eds. The retinoids: biology, chemistry, and medicine. New York: Raven Press, 1994;631–58.
178. Massaro GDC, Massaro D. Nature Med 1997;3:675–7.
179. Ross AC. Vitamin A and cancer. In: Carroll KK, Kritchevsky D, eds. Nutrition and disease update. Cancer. Champaign, IL: AOCS Press, 1994;27–109.
180. Hong WK, Itri LM. Retinoids and human cancer. In: Sporn MB, Roberts AB, Goodman DS, eds. The retinoids: biology, chemistry, and medicine. New York: Raven Press, 1994;597–630.
181. Moon RC, Mehta RG, Rao KVN. Retinoids and cancer in experimental animals. In: Sporn MB, Roberts AB, Goodman DS, eds. The retinoids: biology, chemistry, and medicine. New York: Raven Press, 1994;573–96.
182. Ziegler RG. Am J Clin Nutr 1991;53:251S–9S.
183. Lotan R. FASEB J 1996;10:1031–9.
184. Decensi A, Formelli F, Torrisi R, et al. J Cell Biol 1993;17G:226–33.
185. Lippman SM, Gilsson BS, Kavanagh JJ, et al. Eur J Cancer 1993;29A:S9–13.
186. Collins SJ, Tsai S. Curr Top Microbiol Immunol 1996;211:7–15.
187. de Thé H. FASEB J 1996;10:955–60.
188. Chomienne C, Fenaux P, Degos L. FASEB J 1996;10:1025–30.
189. Frankel SR, Eardley A, Lauwers G, et al. Ann Intern Med 1992;117:292–6.
190. Warrell RP Jr, de Thé H, Wang Z-Y, et al. N Engl J Med 1993;329:177–89.
191. Underwood BA. Vitamin A in human nutrition: public health considerations. In: Sporn MB, Roberts AB, Goodman DS, eds. The retinoids: biology, chemistry, and medicine. New York: Raven Press, 1994;211–27.
192. Dann WJ. Biochem J 1932;26:1072–80.
193. Davila ME, Norris L, Cleary MP, et al. J Nutr 1985;115:1033–41.
194. Zolfaghari R, Ross AC. Arch Biochem Biophys 1995;323:258–64.
195. Stoltzfus RJ, Hakimi M, Miller KW, et al. J Nutr 1993;123:666–75.
196. Underwood BA, Arthur P. FASEB J 1996;10:1040–8.
197. Smith FR, Goodman DS. N Engl J Med 1976;294:805–8.
198. Mahoney CP, Margolis T, Knauss TA, et al. Pediatrics 1980;65:893–6.
199. Kowalski TE, Falestiny M, Furth E, et al. Am J Med 1994;97:523–8.
200. Krasinski SD, Russell RM, Otradovec CL, et al. Am J Clin Nutr 1989;49:112–20.
201. Biesalski HK. Toxicology 1989;57:117–61.
202. Olson JA. Vitamin A. In: Machlin LJ, ed. Handbook of vitamins. New York: Marcel Dekker, 1990;1–57.
203. Armstrong RB, Ashenfelter KO, Eckoff C, et al. General and reproductive toxicology of retinoids. In: Sporn MB, Roberts AB, Goodman DS, eds. The retinoids: biology, chemistry, and medicine. New York: Raven Press, 1994;545–72.
204. Bangham AD, Dingle JT, Lucy JA. Biochem J 1964;90:133–40.
205. Muindi JRF, Young CW, Warrell RP Jr. Leukemia 1994;8:1807–12.
206. Soprano DR, Soprano KJ. Annu Rev Nutr 1995;15:111–32.
207. Rothman KJ, Moore LL, Singer MR, et al. N Engl J Med 1995;333:1369–73.
207a. Rosa FW. Retinoid embryopathy in humans. In: Koren G, ed. Retinoids in clinical practice. The risk-benefit ratio. New York: Marcel Dekker, 1993;77–109.
208. van den Berg H, Hulshof KFAM, Deslypere JP. Eur J Obstet Gynecol Reprod Biol 1996;66:17–21.
209. Biesalski HK, Hemmes C, Hanafy ME, et al. J Nutr 1996;126:973–83.
210. Underwood BA. J Nutr 1994;124:1467S–72S.
211. Loerch JD, Underwood BA, Lewis KC. J Nutr 1979;109:778–86.
212. Makdani D, Sowell AL, Nelson JD, et al. J Am Coll Nutr 1996;15:439–49.
213. Tanumihardjo SA, Cheng JC, Permaesih D, et al. Am J Clin Nutr 1996;64:966–71.
214. Duitsman PK, Cook LR, Tanumihardjo SA, et al. Nutr Res 1995;15:1263–76.
215. Apgar J, Makdani D, Sowell AL, et al. J Am Coll Nutr 1996;15:450–7.
215a. Chowdhury S, Kumar R, Ganguly NK, et al. Br J Nutr 1997;77:863–9.
216. Duncan TE, Green JB, Green MH. J Nutr 1993;123:933–9.
217. Haskell MJ, Handelman GJ, Peerson JM, et al. Am J Clin Nutr 1997;66:67–74.
218. Congdon N, Sommer A, Severns M, et al. Am J Clin Nutr 1995;61:1076–82.
219. Matsuo T, Matsuo N, Shiraga F, et al. Jpn J Ophthalmol 1988;32:249–54.

SELECTED READINGS

Chambon P, Olson JA, Ross AC, eds. The retinoid revolution. FASEB J 1996;10:939–1106.

Orfanos CE, Zouboulis CC, Almond-Roesler B, et al. Current use and future potential role of retinoids in dermatology. Drugs 1997;53:358–88.

Sommer A, West KP Jr. Vitamin A deficiency: health, survival and vision. New York: Oxford University Press, 1996.

Soprano DR, Soprano KJ. Retinoids as teratogens. Annu Rev Nutr 1995;15:111–32.

Sporn MB, Roberts AB, Goodman DS, eds. The retinoids: biology, chemistry, and medicine. New York: Raven Press, 1994.

18. Vitamin D

MICHAEL F. HOLICK

Vitamin D has existed on Earth for at least 500 million years. It was first produced in ocean-dwelling phytoplankton while they were exposed to sunlight for photosynthesis. Although the physiologic function of vitamin D in these lower life forms is unknown, vitamin D and its precursors may have acted either as a natural sunscreen to absorb high-energy ultraviolet radiation, thus protecting ultraviolet-sensitive organelles and macromolecules, or as a photochemical signal (1). For reasons that are not understood, terrestrial vertebrates during evolution became dependent on vitamin D for the development and maintenance of their ossified skeletons. The principal physiologic function of vitamin D in all vertebrates including humans is to maintain serum calcium and phosphorus concentrations in a range that supports cellular processes, neuromuscular function, and bone ossification. Vitamin D accomplishes this goal by enhancing the efficiency of the small intestine to absorb dietary calcium and phosphorus and by mobilizing calcium and phosphorus stores from bone.

Vitamin D is inherently biologically inactive and requires successive hydroxylations in the liver and kidney to form 1,25-dihydroxyvitamin D ($1,25(OH)_2D$), the biologically active form of vitamin D (2–4). $1,25(OH)_2D$ interacts with a specific nuclear receptor in its target tissues that results in a biologic response. Recent evidence suggests that $1,25(OH)_2D$ may also have rapid actions on intracellular calcium, phosphatidylinositol metabolism, and cyclic guanosine triphosphate (GTP) metabolism (2–4).

The identification of vitamin D metabolites led to development of assays for them. These assays have become valuable diagnostic tools for evaluating patients with hypocalcemic, hypercalcemic, and metabolic bone disorders.

The major target tissues for $1,25(OH)_2D$ are the intestine and bone; however, nuclear receptors for $1,25(OH)_2D$ have been identified in several other tissues and in cultured tumor cells. $1,25(OH)_2D$ inhibits the proliferation and induces terminal differentiation of many tumor and normal cultured cells that possess its receptor (2–4). These observations have been the impetus for a reevaluation of the physiologic and pharmacologic actions of $1,25(OH)_2D$.

HISTORY OF RICKETS

Although historians state that rickets occurred in humans as early as the 2nd century AD, the disease was not considered a significant health problem until the industrialization of northern Europe. In the 17th century, Whistler, DeBoot, and Glissen independently recognized that many of the children who lived in the crowded and polluted cities in northern Europe (Fig. 18.1) developed a severe bone-deforming disease characterized by enlargement of the epiphyses of the long bones and rib cage, bowing of the legs, bending of the spine, and weak and toneless muscles (Fig. 18.2) (5). The incidence of this debilitating bone disease increased dramatically in northern Europe and North America during the industrial revolution, and by the latter part of the 19th century, autopsy studies done in Leiden, the Netherlands, showed evidence that about 90% of the children had rickets (6). This disease was especially devastating for young women of childbearing age who often had a deformed pelvis, resulting in a high incidence of infant and maternal morbidity and mortality. This high incidence led to the development and widespread use of cesarean sections in Great Britain.

From the earliest recognition of rickets in 1650, scientists and physicians throughout Europe began what would be a 270-year search for the cause and cure of this unfortunate childhood malady. In 1822, Sniadecki observed that children living in Warsaw had a high incidence of rickets, whereas children living in rural areas outside

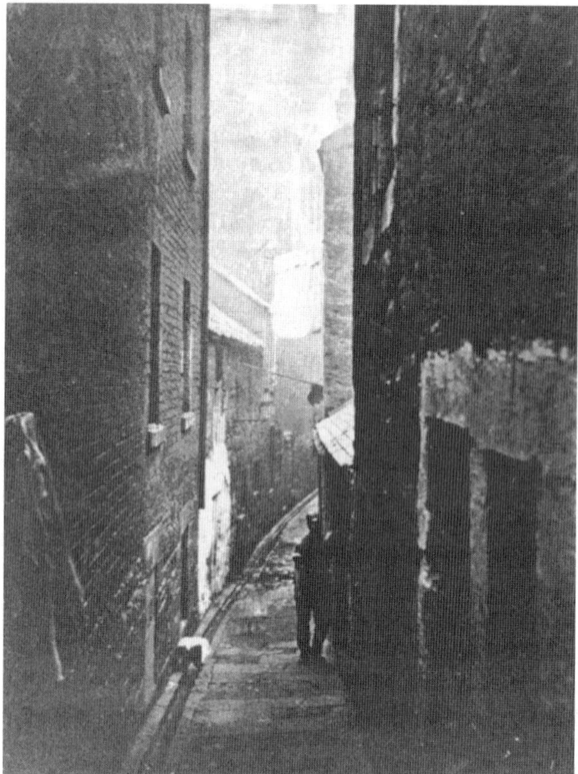

Figure 18.1. A typical scene in Glasgow in the mid-1800s is captured by this photograph taken by Thomas Annan. (From Thomas Annan. Photographs of the old closes and streets of Glasgow 1868/1877. New York: Dover, 1977, with permission.)

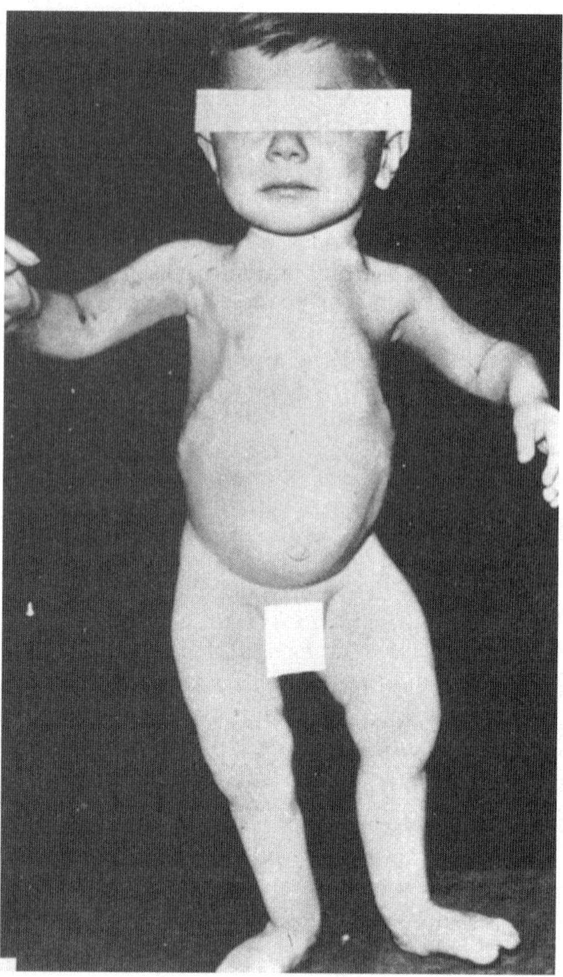

Figure 18.2. Child with rickets showing rachitic rosary of the rib cage, bowed legs, deformity of the long bones, and muscle weakness. (From Fraser D, Scriver CR. Hereditary disorders associated with vitamin-D resistance or defective phosphate metabolism. In: DeGroot L, ed. Endocrinology, vol 2. New York: Grune & Stratton, 1979, with permission.)

Warsaw did not (7). Based on this observation, he advocated exposure to sunlight as a means of curing this disease. Little attention was focused, however, on the environment as the cause of this disorder. In 1889 (8), the British Medical Society conducted an epidemiologic survey and confirmed previous observations that the incidence of rickets was extremely high in the industrialized cities in Great Britain and was less frequent in rural districts of the British highlands. This differed from the incidence of rheumatism and malignant disease, which were common in all districts in the British Isles (9). Unfortunately, they were unable to relate the lack of exposure to sunlight with their observations. One year later, however, Palm published an extensive epidemiologic survey and came to the same conclusion as Sniadecki (10). Observations he collected from a number of physicians throughout the British Empire and the Orient revealed that rickets was rare in children living in impoverished cities in China, Japan, and India where people received poor nutrition and lived in squalor, whereas the children of middle class and poor who lived in industrialized cities in the British Isles had a high incidence of rickets. Based on this survey, he urged systematic sunbathing as a preventive and therapeutic measure in rickets and other diseases. He also advocated educating the public to appreciate sunshine as a means of health.

Unfortunately, little attention was paid to the insightful observations of Sniadecki and Palm, and another 30 years passed before Huldschinski demonstrated that exposure of rachitic children to radiation from a mercury vapor arc lamp was effective in curing this bone disease (11). When he exposed one arm of a rachitic child to the ultraviolet radiation, he demonstrated that rickets in the other arm was cured to the same degree as in the exposed arm. He concluded that phototherapy was not a local effect and speculated that something made in the skin could be transported to distal sites to carry out its antirachitic activity. Two years later, Hess and Unger exposed seven rachitic children on a roof of New York City Hospital to varying periods of sunshine and reported that radiographic examinations showed improvement of rickets in each child as evidenced by calcification of the epiphyses (12).

THE ANTIRACHITIC FACTOR: VITAMIN D

During the 18th and 19th centuries, cod liver oil was used as a common folklore medicine for the prevention and cure of rickets. As early as 1827, Bretonneau treated acute rickets in a 15-month-old child with cod liver oil and noted the incredible speed with which the patient was cured. His student Trousseau advocated the use of oils from fish and sea mammals accompanied by exposure to sunlight for a rapid cure of rickets (13). This knowledge prompted intense investigation to determine what nutritional factor in cod liver oil was responsible for preventing rickets. In 1918, Mellanby reported that he could produce rickets in dogs by feeding them oatmeal and could cure the disease by adding cod liver oil to their diet (14). Two years later, McCollum et al. examined whether the antirachitic factor in cod liver oil was identical to or distinct from vitamin A (15). Cod liver oil was heated and oxidized to destroy all vitamin A activity. When the oil was administered to rachitic rats, it maintained its antirachitic properties. Thus, the antirachitic factor present in cod liver oil clearly was not vitamin A but a new fat-soluble vitamin that was called vitamin D.

Powers et al. showed that exposure to radiation from a mercury arc lamp had the same antirachitic potency as cod liver oil (16). At the same time, Hess and Weinstock (17) and Steenbock and Black (18) found that exposure of food and a variety of other substances such as rat liver; human serum; cotton, olive, and linseed oils; lettuce; growing wheat; and rat chow to ultraviolet radiation resulted in their having antirachitic properties. This led Steenbock to patent use of the addition of provitamin D to foods followed by ultraviolet irradiation to impart antirachitic activity. Addition of provitamin D_2 to milk followed by ultraviolet irradiation became widely practiced in the United States and Europe in the 1930s. This vitamin D–fortification process eradicated rickets as a significant health problem in countries that used it. Today, fortification of milk and infant formula with 400 IU (10 μg) of vitamin D_2 or vitamin D_3 has eliminated rickets as a health problem in the United States and Canada. In Europe, vitamin D fortification of milk is prohibited because of severe vitamin D intoxication that resulted from the indiscriminate addition of excessive amounts of vitamin D to infant formulas in the 1940s and 1950s. Today, some foods, including cereals and margarine, are fortified with vitamin D in many European countries.

PHOTOBIOLOGY

History

The first vitamin D isolated was a photoproduct from irradiation of the fungal sterol ergosterol. This vitamin D was known as vitamin D_1 until it was realized that it was a combination of substances. Further purification of the irradiation mixture yielded a single compound, which was called ergocalciferol, or vitamin D_2 (19) (Fig. 18.3). At the time of its identification, it was assumed that the vitamin D made in human skin during exposure to sunlight was vitamin D_2 (20). In the 1930s, however, it was reported that vi-

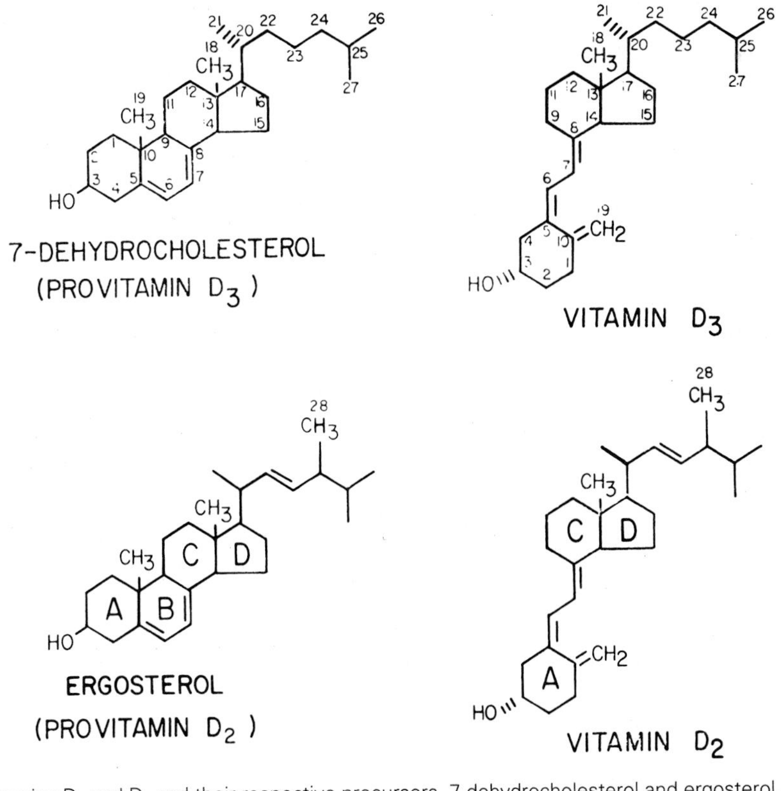

Figure 18.3. Structure of vitamins D_3 and D_2 and their respective precursors, 7-dehydrocholesterol and ergosterol. The only structural difference between vitamins D_3 and D_2 is their side chains; the side chain for vitamin D_2 contains a double bond between C_{22} and C_{23} and methyl group on C_{24}. (From MacLaughlin JA, Holick MF. Mediation of cutaneous vitamin D_3 synthesis by UV radiation. In: Goldsmith LA. Biochemistry and physiology of the skin. New York: Oxford University Press. 1983, with permission.)

tamin D obtained from irradiation of ergosterol had little antirachitic activity in chickens, whereas vitamin D isolated from irradiation of cholesterol-like sterol yielded a potent antirachitic substance (21–24). The confusion about whether vitamin D_2 was identical to the substance produced in human skin was resolved when Windaus and Bock reported the synthesis of a new provitamin D analogue that was similar to ergosterol except that the side chain was cholesterol (Fig. 18.3) (25). This provitamin D was called provitamin D_3, or 7-dehydrocholesterol, and on irradiation, it gave rise to vitamin D_3 (cholecalciferol) (Fig. 18.3). Vitamin D_3, unlike vitamin D_2, had equal antirachitic activity in chicks and rats and was identical to the vitamin D found in fish liver oils and mammalian skin. Therefore, it was concluded that 7-dehydrocholesterol rather than ergosterol was the parent compound in the skin and its resulting photoproduct was vitamin D_3.

Because of the availability of large quantities of ergosterol, vitamin D_2 was the vitamin D used for fortification of milk in the United States and Canada and for pharmaceutical preparations. During the past two decades, vitamin D_3 has also been used to fortify milk and other food substances worldwide.

Originally, it was believed that during exposure to sunlight, provitamin D_3 was directly converted to vitamin D_3. This concept was challenged by Velluz et al., who reported that exposure of provitamin D_3 in an organic solvent to ultraviolet radiation at 0°C did not yield any vitamin D_3 (26). They reported the isolation of a new photoproduct, which they called previtamin D_3 (27), that was thermally labile and underwent rearrangement of its double bonds to form vitamin D_3 in a temperature-dependent process.

Photosynthesis of Previtamin D_3 in Human Skin

The sun emits a broad spectrum of electromagnetic radiation. The high-energy photons that are most damaging to life on Earth (below 290 nm) are absorbed by the thin layer of ozone that envelops the planet. The small band of radiation between 290 and 315 nm (UV-B radiation) is responsible for the photolysis of provitamin D_3 in the epidermis and dermis. During exposure to sunlight, the 5,7-diene of provitamin D_3 absorbs radiation with energies between 290 and 315 nm (28), causing the cleavage of ring B between carbons 9 and 10 (Fig. 18.3) and the formation of a 6,7-*cis* conjugated triene to form a 9,10-seco (seco from the Greek word for split) sterol known as previtamin D_3 (Fig. 18.4). In adult skin, approximately 60% of the cutaneous stores of provitamin D_3 are found in the epidermis; the other 40% resides in the dermis (29). When white and black adults are exposed to sunlight, approximately 70 to 80% and 95 to 98% of the UV-B photons are absorbed by the epidermis, respectively (30). Therefore, approximately 80 to 90% of the previtamin D_3 that is formed in the skin occurs in the actively growing layers of the epidermis, including the stratum basale and stratum spinosum, and less than 20% occurs in the dermis (31). In neonates, approximately 50% of the provitamin D_3 stores are found in both the epidermis and dermis. Because the thin neonatal epidermis transmits more UV-B photons into the dermis, the dermis is also a major site for previtamin D_3 synthesis.

Once previtamin D_3 is made in the skin, it immediately begins to isomerize to vitamin D_2 in a temperature-dependent process (Fig. 18.4). This thermal equilibration would take approximately 1 to 2 days to reach completion at body temperature (37°C) in humans. However, because previtamin D_3 is made in the plasma membrane of skin cells, it is trapped in an *s-cis,s-cis* conformation. Once it isomerizes to vitamin D_3, its conformation is altered, resulting in vitamin D_3 being jettisoned from the plasma membrane into the extracellular space. The vitamin D–binding protein in the circulation in turn attracts vitamin D_3 into the dermal capillary bed (32).

Regulation of Previtamin D_3 Synthesis in Human Skin

Photochemical Regulation

Loomis speculated that melanin pigmentation evolved in humans who lived near the equator as a mechanism for preventing sunlight-induced vitamin D intoxication (33). Although melanin is an excellent natural sunscreen that competes with provitamin D_3 for UV-B photons, thereby limiting the cutaneous production of previtamin D_3 (29, 34), firm evidence exists that sunlight itself is responsible for regulating the total production of vitamin D_3 in human skin (29). Loomis based his theory on the concept that exposure to prolonged intense sunlight would result in a time-dependent increase in production of vitamin D_3 in the skin. Once previtamin D_3 is photosynthesized in the skin, however, it can either thermally isomerize to vitamin D_3 or, during exposure to sunlight, absorb ultraviolet radiation and isomerize to the biologically inert isomers lumisterol and tachysterol (Fig 18.4). Thus, if a white individual is exposed to sunlight at the equator, provitamin D_3 is rapidly converted to previtamin D_3 during the initial few minutes of exposure. Prolonged exposure to sunlight, however, does not increase previtamin D_3 production; rather, previtamin D_3 is photodegraded to biologically inert isomers (Fig 18.4) (29, 35).

Vitamin D_3 is exquisitely sensitive to photodegradation when exposed to sunlight (Fig. 18.4). The principal photoisomers that are formed are 5,6-*trans*-vitamin D_3 and supersterols I and II (Fig 18.4). Thus, once vitamin D_3 is made from previtamin D_3, it must exit the epidermis into the dermal capillary bed; otherwise, it is rapidly photodegraded during exposure to sunlight (36).

Effect of Age

Photoproduction of previtamin D_3 in any layer of skin depends on the concentration of provitamin D_3, the presence of chromophors that compete with provitamin D_3 for UV-B photons, and the quanta of UV-B photons that can

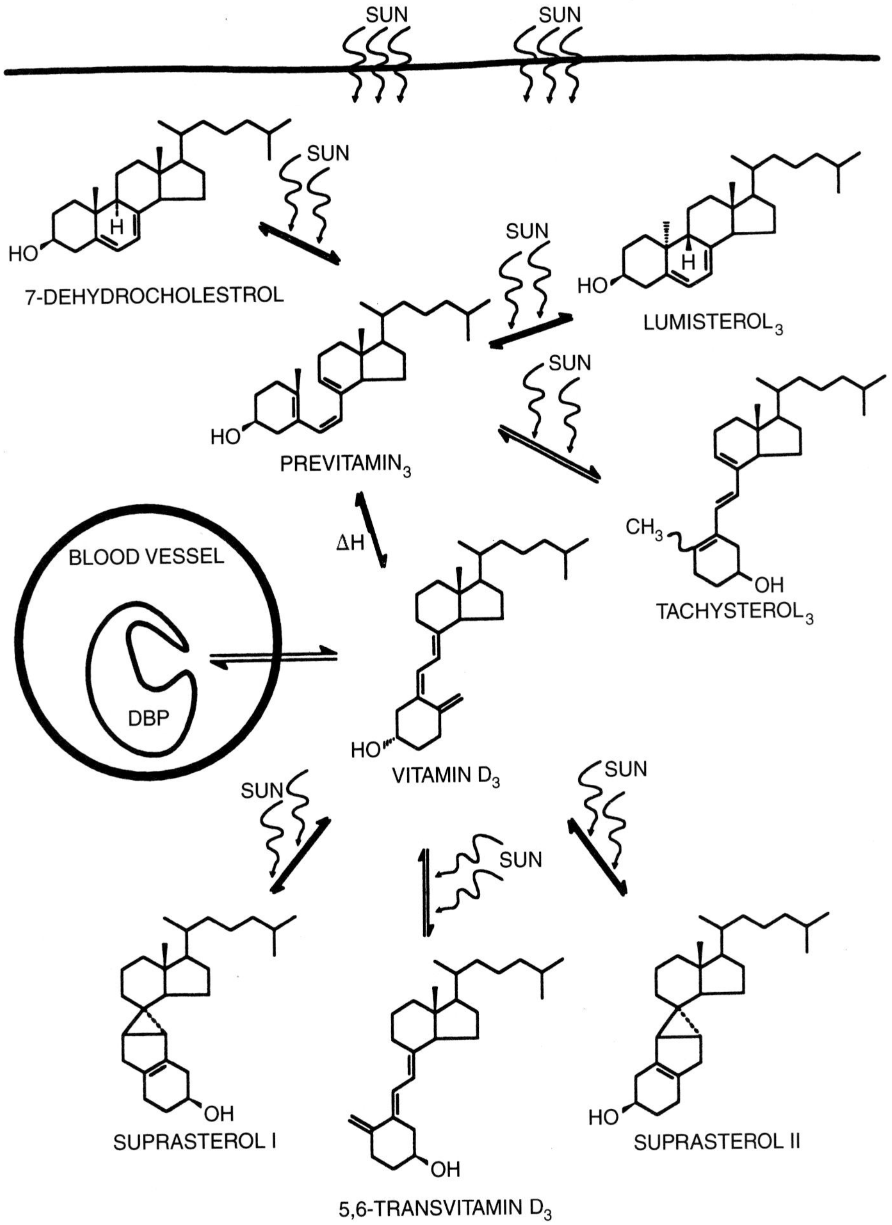

Figure 18.4. Photochemical events that lead to the production and regulation of cholecalciferol (vitamin D_3) in the skin. (From Holick MF. Am J Clin Nutr 1994;60:619–30, with permission.)

penetrate the skin and be absorbed by provitamin D_3. The average concentration of provitamin D_3 in 1 cm^2 of young adult skin is approximately 0.8 μg for the epidermis and 0.15 to 0.5 μg for the dermis (31). The concentrations of provitamin D_3 in the epidermis are inversely related to age (Fig. 18.5) (37). The net effect of this age-related decrease is demonstrated in Figure 18.6. Circulating concentrations of vitamin D were measured in healthy young and elderly subjects exposed to the same amount of whole body ultraviolet radiation. Peak circulating concentrations of vitamin D in the elderly were about 30% of those in young adults (38).

Sunscreens

Awareness that the alarming increase in the incidence of skin cancer is related to chronic exposure to sunlight has led to the recommendation that people apply sunscreen before going outdoors (39). The solar radiation responsible for causing wrinkles and skin cancer, however, is the same radiation responsible for producing previtamin D_3 in the skin. Thus, application of a sunscreen with a sun protection factor of only 8 can markedly reduce (~95%) cutaneous production of previtamin D_3 (Fig. 18.7) (40). The use of sunscreens by children and young adults should not affect their vitamin D status, because it is unlikely that they will always apply a sunscreen before going outdoors. The elderly, however, are often more conscious of their health and apply a sunscreen before going outdoors. Evidence exists that chronic use of sunscreens by the elderly can decrease circulating concentrations of 25-hydroxyvitamin D (25-OH-D), which is a hallmark for

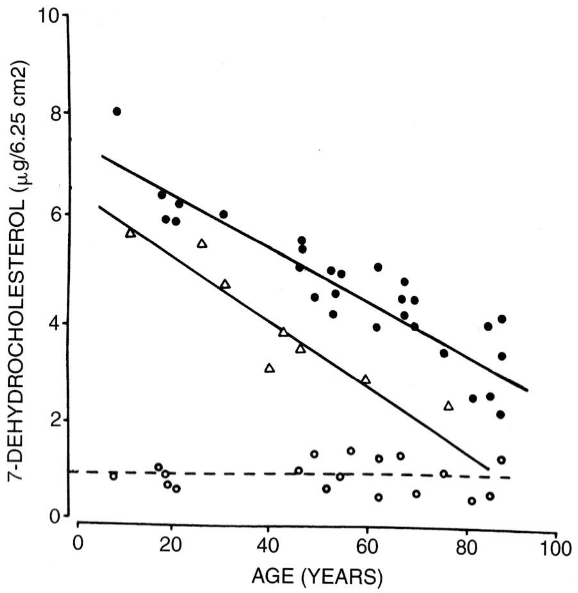

Figure 18.5. Effect of aging on 7-dehydrocholesterol concentrations in human epidermis and dermis. Concentrations of 7-dehydrocholesterol (provitamin D_3) per unit area of human epidermis *(open circles)* were obtained from surgical specimens from donors of various ages. Linear regression analysis gave slopes of −0.05, −0.06, and −0.0005 for epidermis (r = −0.89), stratum basale (r = −.92), and dermis (r = −0.04), respectively. The slopes for epidermis and stratum basale differ significantly from the slope for dermis (P <.001). (From MacLaughlin JA, Holick MF. J Clin Invest 1985;76:1536–8, with permission.)

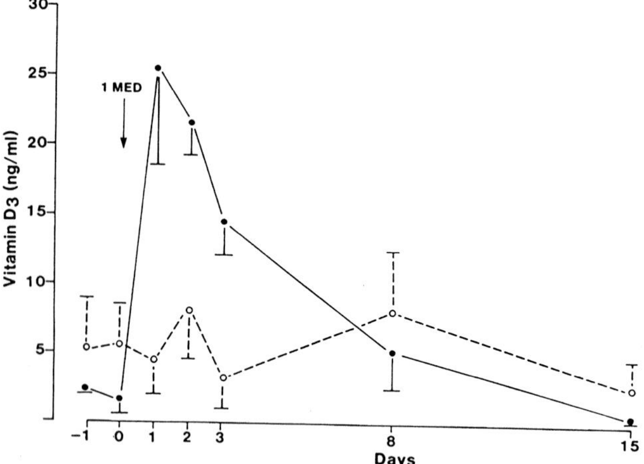

Figure 18.7. Mean (±SEM) serum vitamin D_3concentrations in eight normal subjects. Four subjects *(open circles)* applied *p*-aminobenzoic acid and four applied vehicle *(closed circles)* to the entire skin before exposure to ultraviolet B (UV-B). On day 0, all subjects underwent total body exposure to 1 MED of UV radiation. To convert nanograms of vitamin D per milliliter to nanomoles per liter, multiply by 2.60. (From Matsuoka LY, Ide L, Wortsman J, et al. J Clin Endocrinol Metab 1987;64:1165–8, with permission.)

determining vitamin D deficiency. As shown in Figure 18.8, almost one-half of subjects in Springfield, Illinois, who always wore a sunscreen before going outdoors had overt vitamin D deficiency as determined by low circulating concentrations of 25-OH-D (41).

Season, Latitude, and Time of Day

At the turn of the century, a seasonal incidence of rickets was recognized in the industrialized cities of the United States and Europe. Rickets was seen less frequently in children at the end of summer and more frequently at the end of winter and in early spring (9). As winter approaches, the solar zenith angle of the sun becomes more oblique. This configuration causes the UV-B photons to be absorbed more efficiently by the stratospheric ozone layer, thereby decreasing the total number of photons that reach the Earth's surface. As a result, cutaneous synthesis of previtamin D_3 is affected by the time of day, season of the year, and latitude. As shown in Figure 18.9, exposure to sunlight in Boston (42° N) promoted cutaneous photosynthesis of previtamin D_3 in human skin from March through October. By November, however, the number of 290- to 315-nm photons that penetrated the stratospheric layer into Boston was insufficient for significant conversion of provitamin D_3 to previtamin D_3. Just 10° north, in Edmonton (Alberta), Canada, this period ran from mid-October through mid-March. Farther south, in Los Angeles (34° N) and Puerto Rico (18° N), production of previtamin D_3 occurred throughout the year (Fig. 18.9) (42).

In Boston in summer, exposure to sunlight from 5:30 Eastern Standard Time (EST) to 18:30 EST resulted in cutaneous production of previtamin D_3. By October, however, most of the UV-B photons were absorbed by the ozone layer, and as a result, exposure to sunlight before 10:00 EST and after 15:00 EST was ineffective in producing previtamin D_3 in the skin (43) (Fig. 18.10). These observations are beginning to provide guidelines for recommendations regarding the use of sunlight as a means of providing people with their vitamin D requirement. For example, it is reasonable to advise people, especially elderly individuals, that exposure to morning or late afternoon sunlight in the summer is a good source for their vitamin D requirement. At these times, sunlight exposure is less damaging to the skin.

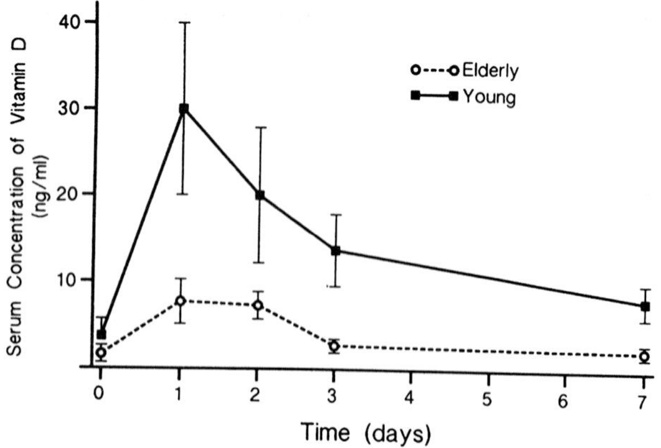

Figure 18.6. Circulating concentrations of vitamin D in healthy young and elderly volunteers exposed to ultraviolet radiation. To convert nanograms per milliliter to nanomoles per liter, multiply by 2.60. (From Holick MF, Matsuoka LY, Wortsman J. Lancet 1989;2:1104–5, with permission.)

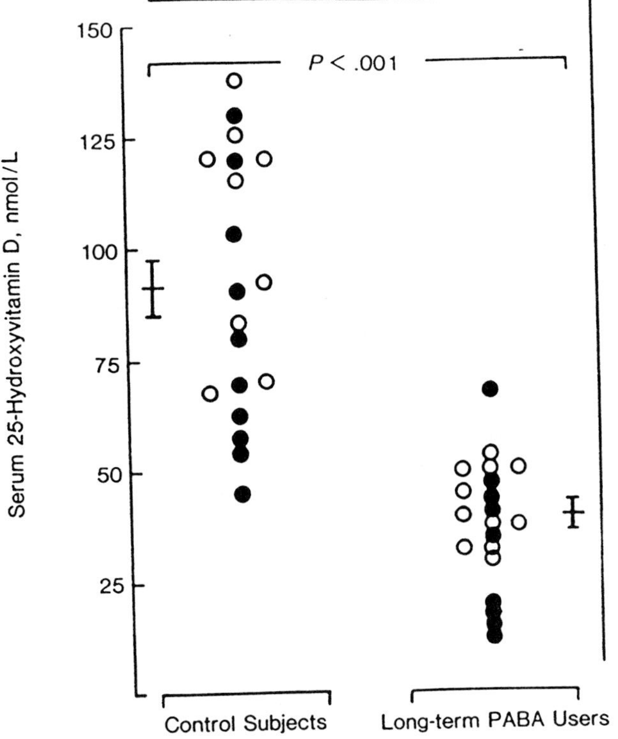

Figure 18.8. Serum concentration of 25-hydroxyvitamin D in long-term sunscreen users and in age- and sex-matched controls simultaneously. The mean serum 25-hydroxyvitamin D level was significantly lower in long-term sunscreen users ($P < .001$). Two long-term sunscreen users had absolute vitamin D–deficiency 25-hydroxyvitamin D levels below 20 nmol/L. PABA, *p*-aminobenzoic acid; *open circles,* subjects from Philadelphia; *closed circles,* subjects from Springfield, IL. (From Matsuoka LY, Wortsman J, Hanifan N, et al. Arch Dematol 1988;124:1802–4, with permission.)

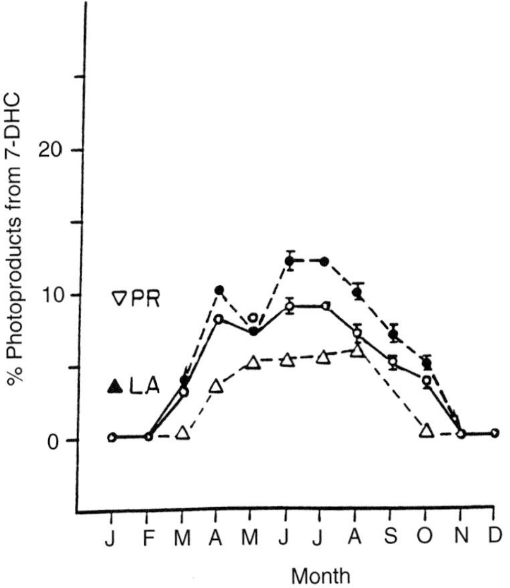

Figure 18.9. Photosynthesis of previtamin D_3 after exposure of 7-dehydrocholesterol *(7-DHC)* to sunlight in Boston (42° N) for 1 h *(open circles)* and 3 h *(closed circles)* and in Edmonton, Canada (52° N) after 1 h *(open triangles)* each month for 1 year, Los Angeles (34° N) *(closed triangle)* and Puerto Rico (18°) in January *(inverted triangle).* (From Webb AR, Kline L, Holick MF. J Clin Endocrinol Metab 1988;67:373–8, with permission.)

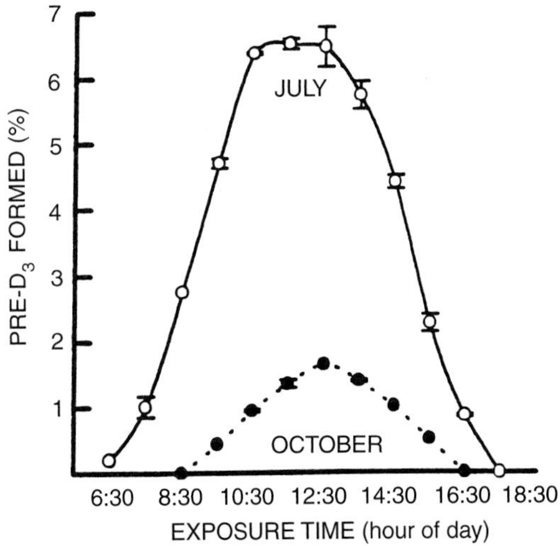

Figure 18.10. Photosynthesis of previtamin D_3 at various times on cloudless days in Boston in October *(closed circles)* and July *(open circles).* (From Lu Z, Chen T, Holick MF. Influences of season and time of day on the synthesis of vitamin D_3. In: Holick MF, Kligman A, eds. Proceedings, Biologic Effects of Light Symposium. Berlin: Walter De Gruyter, 1992;53–6, with permission.)

INTESTINAL ABSORPTION

In nature, only a few foods contain vitamin D: fish liver oils and fatty fish. Several countries fortify some foods with vitamin D. In the United States, milk is the principal dietary component subject to fortification with either vitamin D_2 or vitamin D_3. Some cereals, breads, and infant formulas are also fortified with vitamin D. However, the amount of vitamin D in milk can vary. Studies have found that up to 80% of milk samples tested did not contain 80 to 120% of the vitamin D, and about 14% had no detectable vitamin D (44–46). In other countries, some cereals, margarine, and breads have small quantities of vitamin D added to them.

When vitamin D is ingested, this fat-soluble compound is incorporated into the chylomicron fraction, and about 80% is absorbed into the lymphatic system (4). After ingestion of a single dose of 50,000 IU of vitamin D_2, circulating concentrations of vitamin D begin to increase within hours, peak at 12 hours, and gradually decline to near baseline by 72 hours (Fig. 18.11) (47). This provocative vitamin D absorption test has been useful in determining whether a patient with an intestinal malabsorption syndrome can absorb this fat-soluble vitamin. A blood sample is drawn just before and 12 to 24 hours after a single oral dose of 50,000 IU of vitamin D_2 (Fig. 18.11). If no elevation in the circulating concentration of vitamin D is observed, complete malabsorption of vitamin D should be suspected; however, any increase in the circulating concentration of vitamin D reflects vitamin D absorption. The dose of vitamin D can, therefore, be tailored accordingly.

Patients who suffer from chronic intestinal malabsorption syndromes caused by chronic liver disease, cystic fibrosis, Crohn's disease, Whipple's disease, and sprue are more likely to develop vitamin D deficiency because the

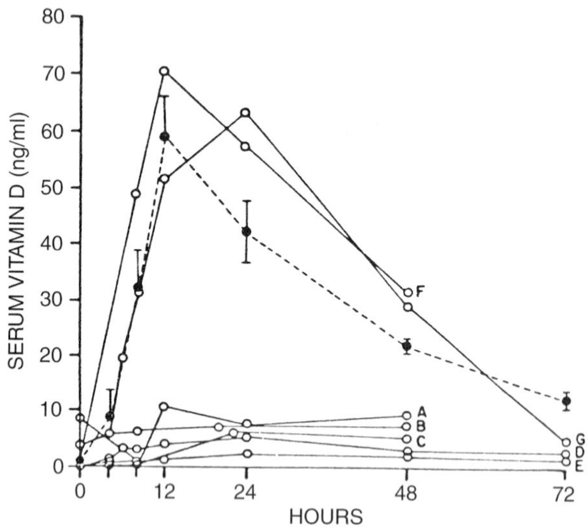

Figure 18.11. Serum vitamin D concentrations in seven patients with intestinal fat malabsorption syndromes after a single oral dose of 50,000 IU (1–25 mg) of vitamin D_2. The means and standard errors of vitamin D concentrations measured in seven normal control subjects after a similar dose are indicated by the *closed circles and dotted line.* Note that two patients, one with Crohn's ileocolitis (patient F) and one with ulcerative colitis (patient G), had essentially normal absorption curves. Five patients showed a dramatic lack of response, with no values above 25–2 nmol/L (10 ng/mL). (From Lo CW, et al. Am J Clin Nutr 1985;42:644–9.)

small intestine cannot absorb this fat-soluble vitamin. Diseases that affect the more distal small intestine and large intestine, such as ileocolitis caused by Crohn's disease and ulcerative colitis, have little effect on absorption of vitamin D (Fig. 18.11).

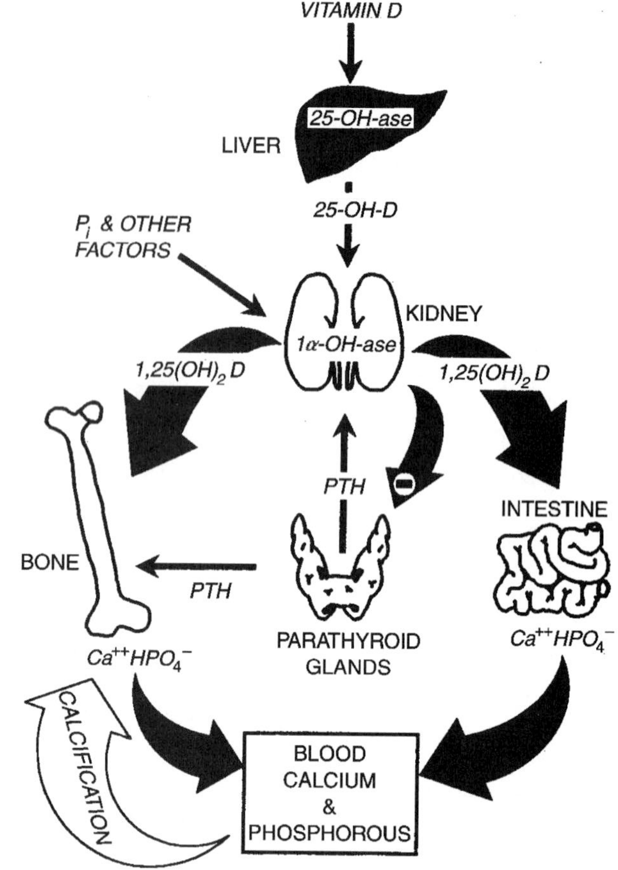

Figure 18.12. Metabolism of vitamin D and the biologic actions of 1,25-dihydroxyvitamin D ($1,25(OH)_2D$). (From Holick MF. Am J Clin Nutr 1994;60:619–30, with permission.)

METABOLISM

Vitamin D to 25-Hydroxyvitamin D

Once vitamin D (the term *vitamin D* without a subscript relates to either vitamin D_2, vitamin D_3, or both and their metabolites) enters the circulation, it is bound to the group-specific protein (Gc) commonly known as the vitamin D–binding protein. Vitamin D is transported to the liver, where it undergoes its first hydroxylation on carbon 25, resulting in formation of the major circulating form of vitamin D, 25-hydroxyvitamin D (25-OH-D) (Fig. 18.12) (2–4, 21, 48). Production of 25-OH-D by the liver is regulated by a negative feedback mechanism controlled by vitamin D, 25-OH-D, and $1,25(OH)_2D$ (49). This negative feedback control is not regulated tightly, inasmuch as an increase in exposure to sunlight or dietary intake of vitamin D results in increased circulating concentrations of 25-OH-D (Fig. 18.13) (50, 51). Although the liver is the major site of 25-OH-D production, some extrahepatic sites are capable of this hydroxylation. It is likely that cholesterol-25-hydroxylase can recognize vitamin D and hydroxylate the side chain on carbon 25 to produce 25-OH-D (4).

Circulating concentrations of 25-OH-D often are low in patients with severe parenchymal and cholestatic liver disease (52), in part because of the associated intestinal malabsorption of vitamin D as well as the decrease in the reservoir of the vitamin D-25-hydroxylase in the liver. Although low circulating concentrations of 25-OH-D can cause vitamin D–deficiency bone disease, it is unlikely that these low levels are responsible for the debilitating osteoporosis-like bone disease associated with severe liver failure. Little correlation exists between the severity of osteopenia and fractures in patients with primary biliary cirrhosis and other chronic liver disorders with circulating levels of 25-OH-D. Furthermore, treatment of these patients with 25-OH-D or its metabolites does not provide any significant benefit (53). Because these patients are more prone to developing vitamin D deficiency as a result of associated fat malabsorption, however, it is prudent to increase their vitamin D intake and monitor circulating concentrations of 25-OH-D.

25-Hydroxyvitamin D to 1,25-Dihydroxyvitamin D

Although 25-OH-D is the major circulating form of vitamin D, it is biologically inert at physiologic concentrations. For it to become active, it must be hydroxylated on carbon 1 by a specific 25-OH-D-1α-hydrolase, present in the kidney (see Fig. 18.12) (1–4, 21). Although the kidney

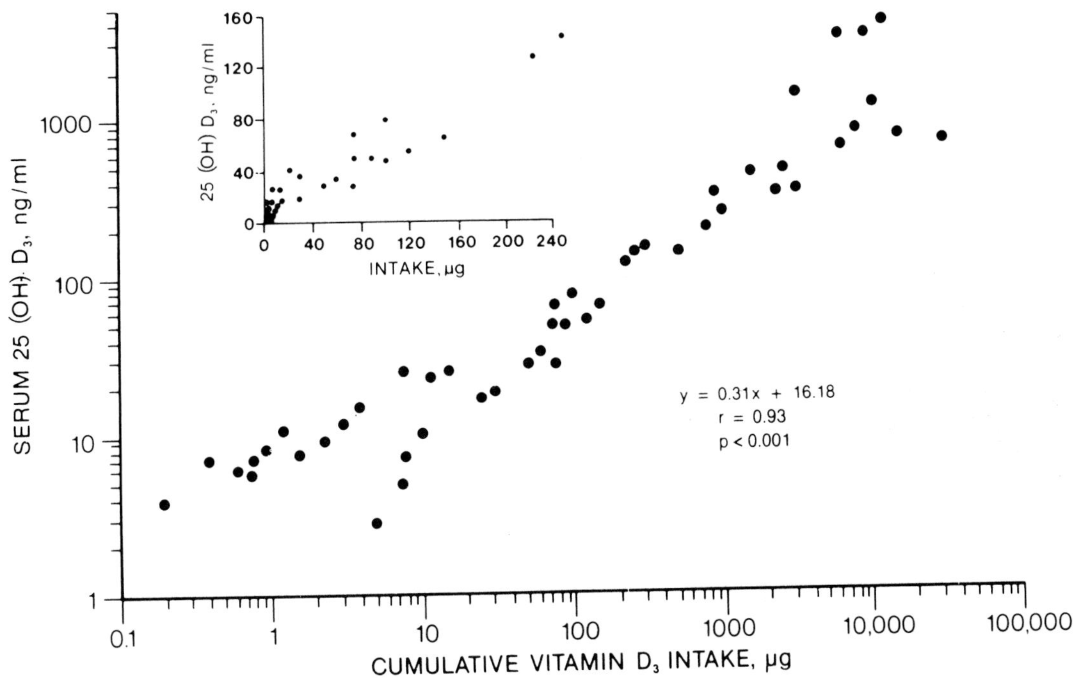

Figure 18.13. Serum levels of 25-OH-D_3 observed in response to various oral doses of vitamin D_3 given to vitamin D–deficient rats. A clear linear correlation extends well into the pharmacologic range for both parameters. To convert nanograms per milliliter to nanomoles per liter, multiply by 2.50. (From Holick MF. Vitamin D: relevance for clinical medicine. Los Angeles: Nichols Institute, 1981.)

is the principal site for the production of 1,25$(OH)_2$D under most circumstances, the placenta also appears to play a role in producing 1,25$(OH)_2$D at a time of increased requirement for calcium by the fetus (54–56). A variety of authors report extrarenal sites for production of 1,25$(OH)_2$D. Most of these studies were conducted in vitro. Certain cultured cells, such as placental cells, human bone cells, keratinocytes, and stimulated monocytes, also produce 1,25$(OH)_2$D (3, 4, 57–59). Some people speculate that 1,25$(OH)_2$D may be produced locally in cells to act in an autocrine or paracrine manner. In patients who have had bilateral nephrectomy or have chronic renal failure, the concentrations of 1,25$(OH)_2$D in the circulation usually are low or undetectable. Thus, the kidney is the principal organ responsible for activating vitamin D for the regulation of calcium metabolism.

Alternative Metabolism of 25-Hydroxyvitamin D

25-OH-D and its biologically active metabolite 1,25$(OH)_2$D are substrates for a variety of hydroxylases. The principal site of metabolism is the side chain, where carbons 23, 24, and 26 undergo hydroxylation and oxidation to yield a plethora of metabolites of 25-OH-D and 1,25$(OH)_2$D (2–4, 21). Although the metabolic importance of these side-chain modifications is uncertain, most likely they are related to the deactivation and rapid clearance of 1,25$(OH)_2$D. This is particularly true for the C-23 and C-24 oxidations, which ultimately yield a biologically inactive, water-soluble metabolite 1α-OH-24,25,26,27-tetranor-23-COOH-vitamin D_3 (calcitroic acid) (2, 50). In addition to the multiple hydroxylations in the side chain, 25-OH-D_3 can have its A ring oxidized, whereby a keto group replaces C-19. This reaction occurs in vivo in ruminants and in vitro in chick kidney homogenates, resulting in conversion of 25-OH-D_3 to the *cis* and *trans* isomers of 10-keto-19-nor-25-hydroxyvitamin D_3 (2, 4, 60). Although this keto metabolite is biologically inactive, it is of interest because it comigrates on many chromatographic systems with 1,25$(OH)_2D_3$ and can be mistaken for 1,25$(OH)_2D_3$. Additional chromatography with methylene chloride as one of the solvents separates these metabolites (4, 61).

To date, more than 40 metabolites of vitamin D have been structurally identified (62). On a weight basis, all of these metabolites are biologically less active than 1,25$(OH)_2$D. At present, many people believe that most of the side-chain and A-ring metabolites exist only in intoxicated states and are not relevant to the physiologic actions of vitamin D.

Regulation of Vitamin D Metabolism

Synthesis of vitamin D in the skin and its metabolism to 1,25$(OH)_2D_3$ are regulated carefully in the body. Sunlight regulates the total production of previtamin D_3 and vitamin D_3 in the skin. Once vitamin D enters the circulation, it can be stored in the fat for later use or metabolized in the liver to 25-OH-D. This hydroxylation step is feedback regulated. The most critical step in vitamin D metabolism is the production of 1,25$(OH)_2$D by the kidney. During periods of calcium deprivation, circulating ionized calcium concentrations decline. The parathyroid glands immediately detect this decrease and increase production and secretion of parathyroid hormone (63). The principal role of parathyroid hormone in calcium metabolism is to increase tubular reabsorption of calcium and renal production of $1,25(OH)_2D$. $1,25(OH)_2D$ travels to the small intestine where it increases the efficiency of intestinal calcium absorption. $1,25(OH)_2D$, along with parathyroid hormone, acts synergistically on osteoclasts, which in turn mobilize calcium stores from bone (Fig. 18.12).

It is generally believed that parathyroid hormone does not directly regulate the renal 25-OH-D-1α-hydroxylase. Evidence suggests that the hypophosphatemic effect of parathyroid hormone is ultimately responsible for enhancing the renal 1α-hydroxylase activity (64). In healthy men, phosphorus restriction caused an increase in circulating concentrations of $1,25(OH)_2D$ to 80% above control values; this increase was related to an increase in the production rate without any change in the metabolic clearance of this hormone (Fig. 18.13). With phosphorus supplementation, serum concentrations of $1,25(OH)_2D$ decreased abruptly, reaching a nadir within 2 to 4 days. After 10 days of supplementation, the mean concentration of $1,25(OH)_2D$ was 29% lower than the value measured when phosphorus intake was normal (Fig. 18.13).

Under certain physiologic circumstances, factors other than calcium, phosphorus, and parathyroid hormone may also modulate the activity of 25-OH-D-1-hydroxylase (4). The efficiency of intestinal calcium transport is enhanced when calcium demands are increased during pregnancy, lactation, and skeletal growth. Because $1,25(OH)_2D$ is the principal hormone responsible for regulation of calcium absorption in the small intestine, it is not surprising that growth hormone, estrogen, and prolactin can directly or indirectly enhance renal production of $1,25(OH)_2D$ in various in vitro and in vivo animal models (65–69). Although estrogen appears to play a significant role in regulating production of $1,25(OH)_2D$ (70–73) in laying hens, it does not have that same effect in women. This statement is based on the observation that circulating free concentrations of $1,25(OH)_2D$ do not change in women before, during, and after menopause. Furthermore, circulating concentrations of $1,25(OH)_2D$ are not altered in young women with estrogen deficiency caused by anorexia nervosa (71). A few authors have suggested that circulating concentrations of $1,25(OH)_2D$ are slightly lower in osteoporotic women than in age-matched control subjects. Estrogen replacement in postmenopausal women increased circulating concentrations of $1,25(OH)_2D$ (71).

The responsiveness of the renal 25-OH-D-1α-hydroxylase to parathyroid hormone may be affected by either age or osteoporosis (74–76). When osteoporotic women were infused with a synthetic fragment of parathyroid hormone, circulating concentrations of $1,25(OH)_2D$ doubled within 24 hours in healthy young control subjects; no significant increase was observed in older osteoporotic patients (Fig. 18.14). Whether the moment-to-moment regulation of renal 25-OH-D-1α-hydroxylase by parathyroid hormone is altered by aging or osteoporosis, and its role in the disease process, remain to be determined.

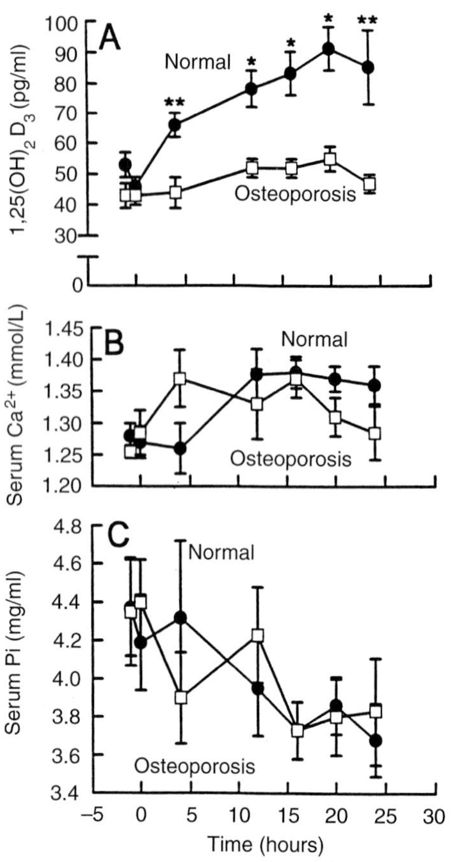

Figure 18.14. Effect of synthetic parathyroid hormone [hPTH-[1–34)] on levels of $1,25(OH)_2D$ in normal subjects *(closed circles)* and patients with untreated osteoporosis *(open squares)*. **A.** All values are expressed as the mean ± SEM; * denotes significant differences at $P < .01$, and ** at $P < .05$, between the level in the patients and that in the controls at corresponding time points. Asterisks also refer to significant differences between the preinfusion baseline levels on ionized calcium (Ca^{2+}) (**B**), and inorganic phosphate (P_i) (**C**) in normal subjects *(closed circles)* and patients with osteoporosis *(open squares)*. All values are expressed as means ± SEM. There was no significant difference between the levels in the two groups. (Modified from Slovik DM, Adams JS, Neer RM, et al. N Engl J Med 1981;305:372–4, with permission.)

One study has suggested that the number of vitamin D receptors (VDRs) in the small intestine decreases in the elderly (77). This may help explain why the efficiency of intestinal calcium absorption is decreased in elderly persons.

BIOLOGIC FUNCTIONS

Role in Calcium and Phosphorus Metabolism

The principal physiologic function of vitamin D in vertebrates, including humans, is to maintain intracellular and extracellular calcium concentrations within a physiologically acceptable range. Vitamin D accomplishes this goal through the action of $1,25(OH)_2D$ on regulating calcium and phosphorus metabolism in the intestine and bone. 1,25(OH)$_2$D interacts with a specific high-affinity receptor in its respective target tissue (2–4). This rare intracellular protein has been cloned and belongs to the superfamily of the steroid-hormone zinc-finger receptors (78). It selectively binds 1,25(OH)$_2$D and retinoic acid X receptor (RXR) to form a heterodimeric complex that interacts with specific DNA sequences, known as vitamin D–responsive elements (62, 76, 79).

This nuclear binding activity results in transcription of hormone-specific mRNA, which in turn governs the translation of several proteins, including the calcium-binding protein (Fig. 18.15) (80). This protein is thought to be important in the transcellular transport of calcium in the intestine. The net result is increased absorption of calcium and phosphorus from intestinal contents into the circulation (Fig.18.12).

1,25(OH)$_2$D has a variety of effects on bone cells. In keeping with its principal physiologic function in maintaining serum calcium levels within an acceptable physiologic range for cellular activity, it enhances mobilization of calcium and phosphorus stores from bone at times of calcium deprivation. 1,25(OH)$_2$D induces stem cell monocytes to become mature osteoclasts (81). Once mature, osteoclasts lose their nuclear receptors for 1,25(OH)$_2$D and, therefore, are no longer responsive to this hormone (82).

Osteoblasts have nuclear receptors for 1,25(OH)$_2$D (1–4). In vitro studies have suggested that 1,25(OH)$_2$D increases alkaline phosphatase activity and gene expression of osteocalcin and osteopontin (83, 84). Although vitamin D is regarded as essential for the development and maintenance of a healthy skeleton, evidence is minimal to suggest an active role for 1,25(OH)$_2$D in bone mineralization. Studies in vitamin D–deficient rats either maintained on a high-calcium, high-phosphorus, vitamin D–deficient diet or infused with calcium and phosphorus to maintain serum calcium and phosphorus concentrations within the normal range showed that they could mineralize their bones in a fashion similar to that of rats maintained on a normal-calcium, normal-phosphorus, vitamin D–sufficient diet (85, 86). Thus, vitamin-D and its metabolites are not absolutely required for the bone ossification process. Instead, vitamin D is responsible for maintaining extracellular calcium and phosphorus concentrations in a supersaturated state that results in the mineralization of bone (87).

Other Biologic Actions of 1,25(OH)$_2$D

Much effort has been directed toward identifying actions of 1,25(OH)$_2$D that are not directly related to maintenance of calcium and phosphorus homeostasis because a variety of tissues that are not related to calcium

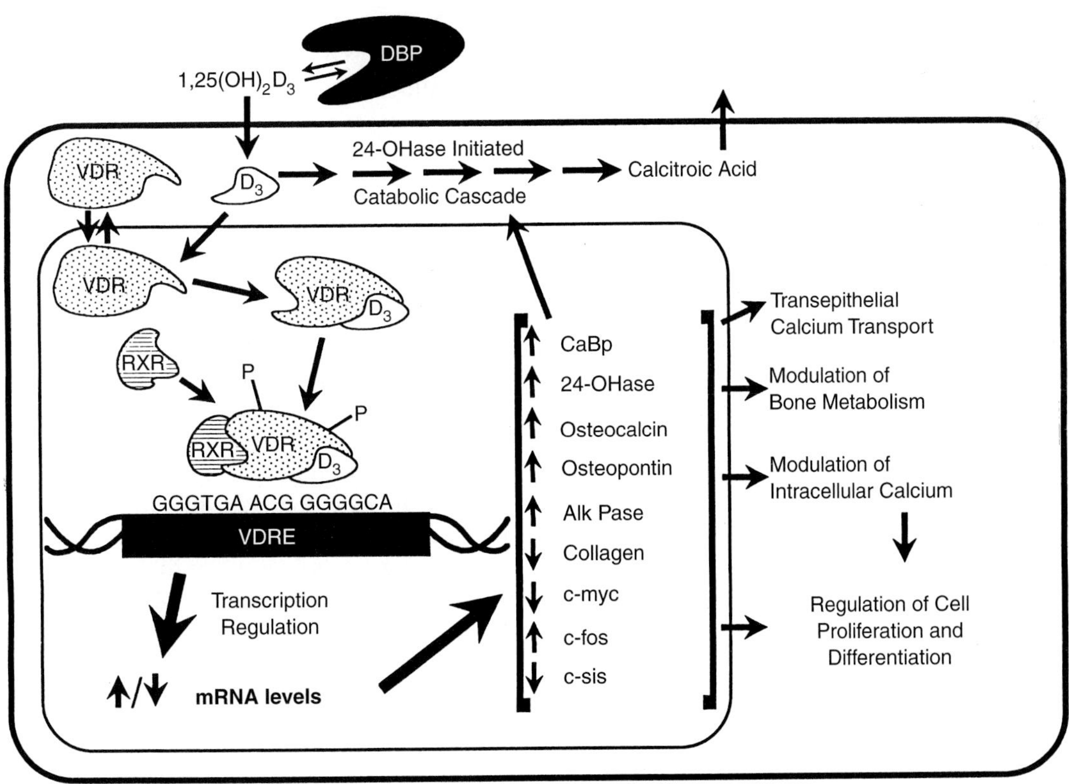

Figure 18.15. Proposed mechanism of action of 1,25(OH)$_2$D$_3$ in target cells, resulting in a variety of biologic responses. The free form of 1,25(OH)$_2$D$_3$ *(D$_3$)* enters the target cell and interacts with its nuclear vitamin D receptor *(VDR)*, which is phosphorylated *(P)*. The 1,25(OH)$_2$D$_3$-VDR complex combines with the retinoic acid X receptor *(RXR)* to form a heterodimer, which in turn interacts with the vitamin D–responsive element *(VDRE)* to enhance or inhibit transcription of vitamin D–responsive genes such as 25(OH)D-24-hydroxylase *(24-Ohase)*.

metabolism possess nuclear receptors for 1,25$(OH)_2$D (Table 18.1) (2–4, 88). Careful analysis has shown that these tissues as well as activated B and T lymphocytes (89, 90) and several cultured normal and tumor cell lines possess high-affinity, low-capacity 1,25$(OH)_2$D receptor–like proteins that are quantitatively similar to the intestinal receptor (2–4).

The first insight into a noncalcemic action of 1,25$(OH)_2D_3$ came when promyeloid leukemic cells (line M-1) that had nuclear receptors for 1,25$(OH)_2D_3$ responded to this hormone by differentiating into macrophages (91). 1,25$(OH)_2D_3$ induced time- and dose-dependent phagocytic activity and expression of cell surface antigens, including Fc and C3 receptors and lysozyme activity. Similar studies were done in a human promyelocytic leukemic cell line (HL-60). Cell growth was inhibited by as little as 10^{-9} M 1,25$(OH)_2D_3$ (92). 1,25$(OH)_2D_3$ was also found to be an effective antiproliferative agent for cultured tumor cells, such as tumor breast cells and melanoma cells, that possessed its nuclear receptor (93). The effect of 1,25$(OH)_2D_3$ on leukemia cells is reversible. When clones of HL-60 cells that possessed less than 10% of nuclear binding activity for 1,25$(OH)_2D_3$ were incubated with 1,25$(OH)_2D_3$, little difference in their proliferative activity was noted (94).

The effect of pharmacologic doses of 1,25$(OH)_2D_3$ on the immune system has been dramatically demonstrated in animal models for autoimmune diseases. 1,25$(OH)_2D_3$ markedly decreased the incidence of type I diabetes in NOD mice (Fig. 18.16) (95, 96). This calciotropic hormone also reduces development of thyroiditis and encephalomyelitis and prolongs the survival of transplanted skin allografts in mice (97–99).

Human epidermal cells have nuclear receptors for 1,25$(OH)_2D_3$, which inhibited the proliferation and induced terminal differentiation of cultured murine and human keratinocytes in a dose-dependent manner (100, 101). These laboratory observations were put to practical use by development of 1,25$(OH)_2D_3$ and its analogues as safe and effective treatment for the hyperproliferative epidermal disorder psoriasis (102–107).

Table 18.1
1,25$(OH)_2D_3$ Receptor Distribution in Mammalian Tissues

Bone
Brain
Breast
Embryonic liver
Embryonic muscle
Intestine
Kidney
Lymphocytes
Monocytes-macrophages
Ovary
Pancreas
Parathyroid
Parotid
Pituitary
Placenta
Skin
Stomach
Testes
Thymus
Uterus

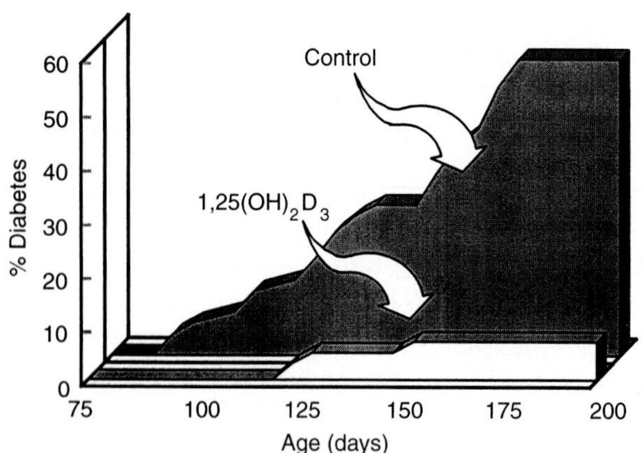

Figure 18.16. The effect of 1,25$(OH)_2D_3$ on reducing the incidence of diabetes mellitus type I in NOD mice. (From Mathieu C, Waer M, Laureys J, et al. Endocrinology 1994;136:866, 872, with permission.)

USE AND INTERPRETATION OF ASSAYS FOR VITAMIN D AND ITS METABOLITES

Vitamin D and 25-OH-D Assays

The first assays for vitamin D were chick and rat bioassays (108, 109). The rat bioassay, commonly known as the line-test, was used widely to determine the concentration of vitamin D in fortified foods such as milk (109). Development of specific assays for vitamin D and its biologically important metabolites made these bioassays obsolete.

A specific assay that measures circulating concentrations of vitamin D_2 and vitamin D_3 (110, 111) has been of great value in evaluating circulating concentrations of vitamin D after exposure to quantitative doses of UV-B radiation (50). It has also been useful as a provocative test for determining which patients with intestinal malabsorption syndromes are at risk for developing vitamin D deficiency (47). In this assay, the half-life of circulating vitamin D is approximately 24 hours. The serum concentration of vitamin D at any time depends on both the most recent ingestion of vitamin D and the last exposure to sunlight. The normal range of serum vitamin D is 0 to 310 nmol/L (0–120 ng/mL). Consequently, serum vitamin D_2 and vitamin D_3 concentrations are of little value in determining the vitamin D status of a patient.

Circulating concentrations of 25-OH-D are measured by a specific competitive protein-binding assay using the vitamin D-binding protein (112–115). Because the half-life of circulating 25-OH-D is approximately 3 weeks, the steady-state concentration of 25-OH-D in the circulation sums the concentrations of vitamin D derived from diet and photoproduction over several weeks to several months

(108). 25-OH-D_2 and 25-OH-D_3 can be measured separately (115, 116). Originally, it was thought that 25-OH-D_2 reflected the dietary component of vitamin D and 25-OH-D_3 reflected exposure to sunlight. Because milk is fortified with either vitamin D_2 or vitamin D_3, however, the separate measurement of these metabolites is of little value.

Measurement of the circulating concentration of 25-OH-D is most valuable for determining the vitamin D status of an individual. The normal circulating concentration of 25-OH-D is usually reported to be between 20 and 150 nmol/L (8–60 ng/mL). Serum values below 25 nmol/L (10 ng/mL) are considered to indicate impending or overt vitamin D deficiency. Although most diagnostic laboratories report the upper limit of the normal range for 25-OH-D to 150 nmol/L (60 ng/mL), a circulating concentration of 250 nmol/L (100 ng/mL) in lifeguards after a full summer of exposure to sunlight is not surprising and is considered normal. Vitamin D intoxication is usually associated with 25-OH-D concentrations above 375 nmol/L (150 ng/mL) with attendant hypercalcemia and hyperphosphatemia (63, 108).

The assay for serum 25-OH-D is clinically useful for determining vitamin D deficiency in patients with intestinal malabsorption syndromes, severe hepatic failure, and the nephrotic syndrome. It is the hallmark assay for determining vitamin D deficiency in very young and elderly individuals.

1,25-Dihydroxyvitamin D Assays

1,25$(OH)_2$D levels in serum and plasma can be specifically measured with a competitive receptor-binding assay using a nuclear/cytosolic receptor for 1,25$(OH)_2$D. The assay involves use of a bovine thymus 1,25$(OH)_2$D receptor that recognizes 1,25$(OH)_2D_2$ and 1,25$(OH)_2D_3$ equally well (76, 108, 117–119). A bioassay was developed that uses cultured calvaria (120). This assay, which is tedious to conduct, measures directly the biologic activity of 1,25$(OH)_2$D in serum.

The half-life of circulating 1,25$(OH)_2$D has been estimated to be between 4 and 6 hours. Normal serum values range between 38 and 144 pmol/L (16–60 pg/mL). As vitamin D deficiency develops, the body responds by increasing production and secretion of parathyroid hormone (Fig. 18.12). Parathyroid hormone in turn enhances the 1-hydroxylation of 25-OH-D. Thus, secondary hyperparathyroidism associated with vitamin D deficiency accelerates the conversion of 25-OH-D to 1,25$(OH)_2$D. Because the circulating concentration of 25-OH-D is about three orders of magnitude higher than that of 1,25$(OH)_2$D, even low levels of 25-OH-D in the blood can provide enough substrate for the formation of 1,25$(OH)_2$D. Thus, a patient who is becoming vitamin D deficient will still have enough 25-OH-D substrate for the renal 25-OH-D-1α-hydroxylase. As a result, a patient who has low stores of vitamin D and is becoming vitamin D deficient can have low, normal, or even high circulating concentrations of 1,25$(OH)_2$D (63). For example, if a patient who is vitamin D deficient is taken from his or her dwelling and exposed to sunlight on the way to the hospital or obtains vitamin D from dietary sources in the hospital, the vitamin D is rapidly metabolized to 25-OH-D and then to 1,25$(OH)_2$D. As a result, circulating levels of 1,25$(OH)_2$D can be elevated to twice normal levels for several months (50). Thus, serum 1,25$(OH)_2$D concentrations are of little value in evaluating vitamin D deficiency. In an absolute vitamin D deficiency state, no circulating 1,25$(OH)_2$D is detected.

Measurement of circulating 1,25$(OH)_2$D levels has been of great value to clinicians for evaluating patients with inherited and acquired disorders of 25-OH-D metabolism. Patients with chronic renal failure, hyperphosphatemia, hypoparathyroidism, pseudohypoparathyroidism, tumor-induced osteomalacia, hypercalcemia of malignancy (in most cases), or vitamin D–dependent rickets type I (an inborn error reducing the conversion of 25-OH-D to 1,25$(OH)_2$D) often have low circulating concentrations of 1,25$(OH)_2$D (2–4, 35, 63, 108). Serum concentrations of 1,25$(OH)_2$D are above normal in some patients with primary hyperparathyroidism; vitamin D–dependent rickets type II (an inborn error in which the recognition of 1,25$(OH)_2$D by target tissue receptors is defective); chronic granulomatous disorders such as sarcoidosis, tuberculosis, and silicosis; and lymphoma. Patients with chronic granulomatous disorders and some lymphomas that activate macrophages and lymphoma cells, respectively, can 1α-hydroxylate 25-OH-D, a process that is inhibited by glucocorticoids and ketoconazole (2–4, 63, 76, 108).

RECOMMENDATIONS

Exposure to Sunlight

It is not often appreciated that casual exposure to sunlight during everyday activities provides most humans with their vitamin D requirement (121). Increased awareness from scientific and lay press reports about the causal relationship between long-term exposure to sunlight and skin cancer and skin wrinkling has made sunscreen use more prevalent (10). Children and young active adults are often outdoors for short periods of time at least two or three times per week, and this casual exposure to sunlight will provide their vitamin D requirement.

Elderly persons, on the other hand, have a decreased capacity to produce vitamin D in their skin. In addition, they are likely to heed the warnings about the damaging effects of sunlight and use a sunscreen and wear more clothing, thus preventing cutaneous synthesis of vitamin D_3. Because many elderly individuals do not drink milk because of a lactase deficiency or because they believe that they no longer need milk (it is only for growing children), their only source of vitamin D is from either a multivitamin pill containing vitamin D or exposure to sunlight. If elderly persons do not take advantage of the beneficial effect of sunlight, they can develop vitamin D deficiency, which can result in secondary hyperparathyroidism. This condition accelerates osteoporosis and can cause a mineralization defect in bones, resulting in adult rickets or osteomalacia. The net effect of this process is to weaken bones and increase the risk of fracture (121–126), and several studies indicate that vitamin D deficiency does put elderly individuals at risk of developing hip fractures. An epidemiologic survey in a controlled nursing-home environment revealed that of both free-living and institutionalized elderly persons who took a vitamin supplement or drank two to three glasses of milk per day, approximately 80% were overtly to borderline vitamin D deficient by the end of the winter (Fig. 18.17) (127). Thus, especially for elderly people, exposure to sunlight in the morning or afternoon in the spring, summer, and fall (depending on skin sensitivity to sunlight) will provide the recommended vitamin D requirement and will permit them to store any excess vitamin D in fat for use during the winter months. Elderly individuals need not be exposed to prolonged periods of sunlight, because the amount they can produce in this period of time should satisfy their body's requirement.

Therefore, I recommend 5 to 30 minutes of exposure of hands, forearms, and face two or three times a week to a suberythemal amount of sunlight for elderly persons in Boston (depending on their sensitivity to sunlight). This is based on our observation that a healthy individual whose whole body is exposed to one minimal erythemal dose of simulated sunlight will have circulating vitamin D concentrations comparable to those from ingestion of 10,000 to 25,000 IU of vitamin D. After exposure to sunlight for a short period, elderly individuals should apply a sunscreen with a protection factor of at least SPF-8; this will protect them from the chronic damaging effects of excessive exposure to sunlight (10).

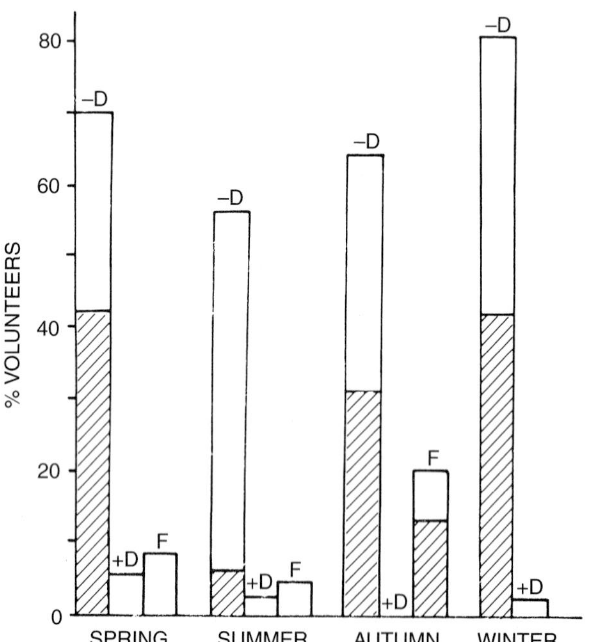

Figure 18.17. Seasonal averages of the percentage of volunteers with circulating concentrations of 25(OH)D > 37.5 nmol/L *(unshaded areas)* and 25(OH)D > 25.0 nmol *(shaded areas)*. Volunteers include those with *(+D)* and without *(–D)* vitamin D supplements and free-living subjects *(F)*, who were without supplements. (From Webb AR, Pilbeam C, Hanafin N, et al. J Clin Nutr 1990;51:1075–81.)

Vitamin D Supplements

A variety of pharmaceutical preparations are available by prescription, including a capsule that contains 50,000 IU of vitamin D_2 and an oil preparation that contains 100,000 IU/mL. Pharmaceutical preparations containing 50,000 IU of vitamin D_2 have been of value in treating vitamin D deficiency in elderly patients and in patients with intestinal malabsorption syndromes, hepatic failure, and nephrotic syndrome. The dose is generally 50,000 IU once per week for 8 weeks. Circulating concentrations of 25-OH-D usually increase into the midnormal range (~100 nmol/L, 40 ng/mL). For those unable to ingest a capsule containing vitamin D, an alternative source is an oil-based preparation. I usually recommend that patients take 800 IU each day until circulating concentrations of 25-OH-D are in the midnormal range. Once these concentrations have returned to normal, I recommend an over-the-counter multivitamin containing 400 IU of vitamin D. Because most pharmaceutical companies put in 1.5 to 2 times the amount of vitamin D stated on the label, patients often receive up to 800 IU of vitamin D per day. This amount usually suffices to maintain adequate circulating concentrations of 25-OH-D (Fig. 18.18).

Recommended Dietary Allowance of Vitamin D for Humans

Beginning in the 1930s, milk was fortified with 400 IU (10 μg of vitamin D_2 per quart). This fortification eliminated rickets as a significant health problem in the United States and other countries that used it. During the 1940s and early 1950s, milk in Great Britain was supplemented with up to 2000 IU of vitamin D to compensate for wartime nutritional deprivation that British children had undergone. Manufacturers often put 1.5 to 2 times as much vitamin D in the food preparations to compensate for anticipated vitamin D breakdown during shelf storage. As a result, an epidemic of hypercalcemia in neonates appeared (128). Although the hypercalcemia was easily reversible, some of the infants were thought to have suffered from hypercalcemia-induced brain damage. As a result, even though there was little scientific documentation, laws were passed in many European countries preventing fortification of milk and infant formulas with vitamin D. In August 1997, the Institute of Medicine in conjunction with the National Academy of Sciences recommended that the recommended requirement for vitamin D should be as an adequate intake (AI) rather than an RDA (129) (see Appendix Table II-A-2-b-4).

In the United States, infant formula is fortified with 400 IU of vitamin D per quart. It has been estimated that a

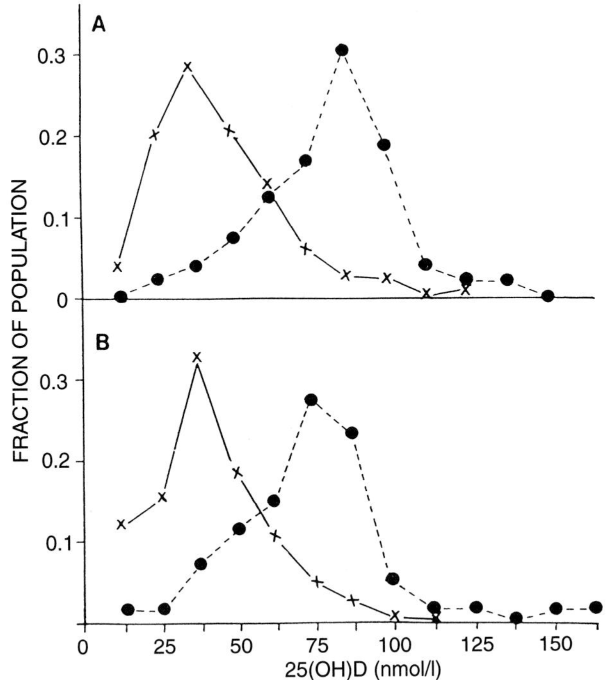

Figure 18.18. Distribution of circulating concentrations of 25(OH)D for residents with *(closed circles)* and without *(x)* vitamin D supplements in September (**A**) and February (**B**). Each data point represents *n* −10 to *n*; e.g., 75 represents all samples between 65 and 75.0 nmol/L. (From Webb AR, Pilbeam C, Hanafin N, et al. J Clin Nutr 1990;51:1075–81, with permission.)

minimum of 100 IU of vitamin D daily is required to prevent rickets in infants. To provide a margin of safety, the recommended AI was set at 5 μg (200 IU) for infants from birth to 6 months of age, which is approximately the amount consumed by formula-fed normal infants. Because human milk contains little vitamin D, it has been recommended that breast-fed infants be exposed to sunlight or ingest formula supplemented with vitamin D. The recommended allowance for children older than 6 months has been set at 5 μg (200 IU) to satisfy their requirement during rapid periods of bone growth and mineralization.

In the mid-1960s, studies in infants fed either 300 IU, 350 to 550 IU, or 1380 to 2170 IU daily demonstrated no differences in growth in length or weight or in serum calcium concentrations. Earlier studies, however, suggested that daily ingestion of 2000 to 5000 IU of vitamin D in the diet caused hypercalcemia and all of its clinical features (128).

Vitamin D–deficiency osteomalacia is associated with intakes below 100 IU of vitamin D per day. The recommended AI of 5 μg (200 IU) for adults is reasonable as long as there is adequate sun exposure. Otherwise, 400 to 800 IU/day may be needed to prevent vitamin D deficiency (35).

Aging does not alter vitamin D absorption (121). Most studies, however, have been conducted in otherwise healthy older individuals who received some exposure to sunlight. Thus, the combination of exposure to sunlight and 200 IU of vitamin D will suffice for adults under 50 years of age. However, the vitamin D requirement for older adults appears from the available literature to be higher. The newly recommended AIs for ages 51 to 70 and 71+ years are 10 μg (400 IU) and 15 μg (600 IU), respectively. The exact amount of vitamin D required by adults who are not exposed to sunlight is less well understood.

Since there was no supporting literature that there is an increased vitamin D requirement during pregnancy and lactation, the recommended AI for both was 5 μg (200 IU). However, in the absence of adequate exposure to sunlight, an intake of 400 IU is prudent.

The Institute of Medicine also provided guidelines for tolerable upper intake levels. For infants and neonates 0 to 12 months, the limit was set at 25 μg/day. For those older than 1 year and for pregnancy and lactation, the upper intake level was set at 50 μg/day.

ACKNOWLEDGMENTS

This work was supported in part by the following NIH grants: AR36963, DK43690, AG04390, M01RR005-3327.

REFERENCES

1. Holick MF. Phylogenetic and evolutionary aspects of vitamin D from phytoplankton to humans. In: Pang PKT, Schreibman MP, eds. Vertebrate endocrinology: fundamentals and biomedical implications, vol 3. Orlando, FL: Academic Press, 1989;7–43.
2. DeLuca H. FASEB J 1988;2:224–36.
3. Reichel H, Koeffler HP, Norman AW. N Engl J Med 1989;320:981–91.
4. Holick MF. Vitamin D: biosynthesis, metabolism, and mode of action. In: DeGroot LJ, ed. Endocrinology, vol 2. New York: Grune & Stratton, 1989;902–26.
5. Fraser D, Scriver CR. Hereditary disorders associated with vitamin-D resistance or defective phosphate metabolism. In: DeGroot LJ, ed. Endocrinology, vol 2. New York: Grune & Stratton, 1979;797–807.
6. Schmorl G. Med U Kinderh 1909;4:403.
7. Sniadecki J (1840), cited in Mozolowski W. Nature 1939;143:121.
8. Owen I. Br Med J 1889;1:113–6.
9. Holick MF. Vitamin D_3: synthesis and biologic functions in skin. In: Mukhtar H, ed. Pharmacology of the skin. Boca Raton, FL: CRC Press, 1991;183–202.
10. Palm TA. Practitioner 1890;45:270–9, 321–42.
11. Huldschinsky K. Dtsch Med Wochenschr 1919;45:712–3.
12. Hess AF, Unger LF. JAMA 1921;77:39.
13. Mayer J. Nutr Rev 1957;15:321–3.
14. Mellanby T. J Physiol 1918;52:11–4.
15. McCollum EF, Simmonds N, Becker JE, et al. J Biol Chem 1922;53:293–312.
16. Powers GF, Park EA, Shipley PG, et al. Proc Soc Exp Biol Med 1921;19:120–1.
17. Hess AF, Weinstock M. J Biol Chem 1924;62:301–13.
18. Steenbock H, Black A. J Biol Chem 1924;61:408–22.
19. Holick MF, MacLaughlin JA, Parrish JA, et al. The photochemistry and photobiology of vitamin D_3. In: Regan JD, Parrish JA, eds. The science of photomedicine. New York: Plenum Press, 1982;195–218.

20. Fieser LD, Fieser M. Vitamin D. In: Steroids. New York: Reinhold 1959;90–168.
21. Holick MF. Vitamin D and the skin: photobiology, physiology and therapeutic efficacy for psoriasis. In: Heersche J, Kanis J, eds. Bone and mineral research. 7th ed. Amsterdam: Elsevier Science, 1990.
22. Massengale ON, Nussmeier M. J Biol Chem 1930;87:423–5.
23. Steenbock H, Kletzien SWF. J Biol Chem 1932;97:249–64.
24. Waddell J. J Biol Chem 1934;105:711–39.
25. Windaus A, Bock F. Hoppe-Seyler's Z Physiol Chem 1937;245:168.
26. Velluz L, Petit A, Amiard G. Bull Soc Chim Fr 1948;15:1115–20.
27. Velluz L, Amiard G, Petit A. Bull Soc Chim Fr 1949;16:501–8.
28. MacLaughlin JA, Holick MF. Mediation of cutaneous vitamin D_3 synthesis by UV radiation. In: Goldsmith LA, ed. Biochemistry and physiology of the skin. Oxford: Oxford University Press, 1983.
29. Holick MF, MacLaughlin JA, Doppelt SH. Science 1981;211:590–3.
30. Anderson RR, Parrish JA. Optical properties of human skin. In: Regan JD, Parrish JA, eds. The science of photomedicine. New York: Plenum Press, 1982;147–94.
31. Holick M, MacLaughlin J, Clark M, et al. Science 1980;210:203–5.
32. Holick MF, Tian XQ, Allen M. Proc Natl Acad Sci USA 1995;92:3124–6.
33. Loomis F. Science 1967;157:501–6.
34. Clements TL, Henderson SL, Adams JS, Holick MF. Lancet 1982;74–6.
35. Holick MF. Am J Clin Nutr 1994;60:619–30.
36. Webb AR, DeCosta BR, Holick MF. J Clin Endocrinol Metab 1989;68:882–7.
37. MacLaughlin JA, Holick MF. J Clin Invest 1985;76:1536–8.
38. Holick MF, Matsuoka LY, Wortsman J. Lancet 1989;2:1104–5.
39. Montagna W, Carlisle MS. J Invest Dermatol 1979;73:47–53.
40. Matsuoka LY, Ide L, Wortsman J, et al. J Clin Endocrinol Metab 1987;64:1165–8.
41. Matsuoka LY, Wortsman J, Hanifan N, et al. Arch Dermatol 1988;124:1802–4.
42. Webb AR, Kline L, Holick MF. J Clin Endocrinol Metab 1988;67:373–8.
43. Lu Z, Chen T, Holick MF. Influences of season and time of day on the synthesis of vitamin D_3. In: Holick MF, Kligman A, eds. Proceedings, Biologic Effects of Light Symposium. Berlin: Walter De Gruyter, 1992;53–6.
44. Tanner JT, Smith J, Defibaugh P, et al. J Assoc Off Anal Chem 1988;71:607–10.
45. Holick MF, Shao Q, Liu WW, Chen TC. N Engl J Med 1992;326:1178–81.
46. Chen TC, Health H III, Holick MF. N Engl J Med 1993;329:1507.
47. Lo CW, Paris PW, Clemens TL, et al. Am J Clin Nutr 1985;42:644–9.
48. Holick MF. Kidney Int 1987;32:912–29.
49. Bell NH. J Clin Invest 1985;76:1–6.
50. Adams JA, Clemens TL, Parrish JA, et al. N Engl J Med 1981;306:722–5.
51. Holick MF, Clark MB. Fed Proc 1978;37:2567–74.
52. Long RG, Skinner RK, Meinhard E, et al. Gut 1976;17:824–7.
53. Kaplan MM, Goldberg MJ, Matloff DS, et al. Gastroenterology 1981;81:681–5.
54. Gray TK, Lester GE, Lorenc RS. Science 1979;204:1311–3.
55. Weisman Y, Vargas A, Duckett G, et al. Endocrinology 1978;103:1992–6.
56. Tanaka Y, Halloran B, Schnoes HK, et al. Proc Natl Acad Sci USA 1979;76:5033–5.
57. Mason RS. Extra-renal production of $1,25(OH)_2D_3$, the metabolism of vitamin D by non-traditional tissues. In: Norman AW, ed. Vitamin D: a chemical, biochemical and clinical update. Berlin: Walter de Gruyter, 1985;23–32.
58. Howard GA, Turner RT, Sherrard DJ, et al. J Biol Chem 1981;256:7738–40.
59. Bikle DD, Nemanic MD, Whitney JO, et al. Biochemistry 1986;25:1545–8.
60. Napoli J, Horst R. Vitamin D metabolism. In: Kumar R, ed. Vitamin D: basic and clinical aspects. Boston: Martinus Nijhoff, 1984;91–124.
61. Gray TK, Millington DS, Maltby DA, et al. Proc Natl Acad Sci USA 1985;82:8218–21.
62. Bouillon R, Okamura WH, Norman AW. Endocr Rev 1995;16:200–57.
63. Holick MF, Potts JR Jr, Krane SM. Calcium phosphorus and bone metabolism. In: Isselbacher KJ, Braunwald E, Wilson JD, et al. Harrison's principles of internal medicine. 12th ed. New York: McGraw-Hill, 1990;2137–51.
64. Portle AA, Halloran BP, Murphy MM, et al. J Clin Invest 1986;77:7–12.
65. Fraser D. Physiol Rev 1980;60:551–663.
66. Adams ND, Garthwite TL, Gray RW, et al. J Clin Endocrinol Metab 1979;49:628–30.
67. Kumar R, Abboud CF, Riggs BL. Mayo Clin Proc 1980;55:51–3.
68. Kumar R, Merimee TJ, Silva P, et al. The effect of chronic growth hormone excess or deficiency on plasma 1,25-dihydroxy vitamin D levels in man. In: Norman AW, et al., eds. Vitamin D, basic research and its clinical application. Berlin: Walter de Gruyer 1979;1005–9.
69. Turner RT. 1,25-Dihydroxyvitamin D-1-hydroxylase, measurements and regulation. In: Kumar R, ed. Vitamin D: basic and clinical aspects. Boston: Martinus Nijhoff, 1984;175–96.
70. Krabbe S, Hummer L, Christiansen C. J Clin Endocrinol Metabol 1986;62:503–7.
71. Rigotti NA, Nussbaum SR, Herzog DB, et al. N Engl J Med 1984;311:1601–6.
72. Sowers MF, Wallace RB, Hollis BW. Bone Miner 1990;10:139–48.
73. Hartwell D, Ruis BJ, Christiansen C. J Clin Endocrinol Metab 1990;71:127–32.
74. Riggs BL, Gallagher JC, Deluca HF, et al. Mayo Clin Proc 1978;53:701–6.
75. Slovik DM, Adams JS, Neer RM, et al. N Engl J Med 1981;305:372–4.
76. Holick MF. Vitamin D: photobiology, metabolism, mechanism of action, and clinical application. In: Favus MJ, ed. Primer on the metabolic bone diseases and disorders of mineral metabolism. 3rd ed. Philadelphia: Lippincott-Raven 1996;7481.
77. Ebeling PR, Sandren ME, DiMagno EP, et al. J Clin Endocrinol Metab 1992;75:176–82.
78. Pike JW. Nutr Rev 1985;43:161–8.
79. Darwish H, DeLuca HF. Crit Rev Eukaryotic Gene Express 1993;3:89–116.
80. Wasserman RH, Fullmer CS, Shimura F. Calcium absorption and the molecular effects of vitamin D_3. In: Kumar R, ed. Vitamin D: basic and clinical aspects. Boston: Martinus Nijhoff, 1984.
81. Bar-Shavit Z, Teitelbaum SL, Reitsma P, et al. Proc Natl Acad Sci USA 1983;80:5907–10.
82. Merke J, Klaus G, Hugel U, et al. J Clin Invest 1986;77:312–4.
83. Haussler MR, Donaldson CA, Kelly MA, et al. Functions and mechanism of action of the 1,25-dihydroxyvitamin D recep-

tor. In: Norman AW, ed. Vitamin D: a chemical, biochemical and clinical update. Berlin: Walter de Gruyter, 1985;83–92.
84. Demay MB, Roth DA, Kronenberg HM. J Biol Chem 1989;264:2279–82.
85. Underwood B, DeLuca HF. Am J Physiol 1984;246:E493–8.
86. Holtrop ME, Cox KA, Carnes DL. Am J Physiol 1986;251:E20.
87. Holick MF. J Nutr 1996;126:11595–645.
88. Stumpf WE, Sar M, Reid FA, et al. Science 1979;206:1188–90.
89. Bhalla AK, Clemens T, Amento E, et al. J Clin Endocrinol Metab 1983;57:1308–10.
90. Provvedine DM, Tsoukaas CD, Deftos LJ, et al. Science 1983;221:1181.
91. Abe E, Miyaura C, Sakagami H, et al. Proc Natl Acad Sci USA 1981;78:4990–4.
92. Tanaka H, Abe E, Miyaura C, et al. Biochem J 1982;204:713–9.
93. Eisman JA. 1,25-Dihydroxyvitamin D_3 in human cancer cells in vitamin D. In: Kumar R, ed. Vitamin D: basic and clinical aspects. Boston: Martinus Nijhoff, 1984;365–82.
94. Bar-Shavit Z, Kahn AJ, Stone KR, et al. Endocrinology 1986;118:679–86.
95. Mathieu C, Waer M, Laureys J, et al. Endocrinology 1994;136:866, 872.
96. Holick MF. Bone 1990;7:60–72.
97. Fournier C, Gepner P, Sadouk MB, Charreire J. Immunol Immunopathol 1990;54:53–63.
98. Holick MF. Photobiology and noncalcemic actions of vitamin D. In: Bilezikian JP, Raisz LG, Rodan GA, eds. Principles of bone biology. New York: Academic Press, 1996;447–60.
99. Binderup L. Biochem Pharmacol 1992;43:1885–92.
100. Hosomi J, Hosoi J, Abe E, et al. Endocrinology 1983;113: 1950–7.
101. Smith EL, Walworth ND, Holick MF. J Invest Dermatol 1986;86:709–14.
102. Smith EL, Pincus SH, Donovan L, et al. J Am Acad Dermatol 1988;19:516–28.
103. Holick MF. Arch Dermatol 1989;125:1692–7.
104. Morimoto S, Kumahara Y. Med J Osaka Univ 1985;35:51.
105. Kragballe K. Arch Dermatol 1989;125:1642–52.
106. Kato T, Rokugo M, Terui T, et al. Br J Dermatol 1986;115:431–3.
107. Perez A, Chen C, Turner A, et al. Br J Dermatol 1996;134:238–46.
108. Holick MF. J Nutr 1990;120:1464–9.
109. Steenbock H, Black A. J Biol Chem 1924;61:408–22.
110. Clemens TL, Adams JS, Holick MF. Clin Chim Acta 1982;121:301–8.
111. Chen T, Turner A, Holick MF. J Nutr Biochem 1990;1:272–6.
112. Haddad JG, Chuy KJ. J Clin Endocrinol Metab 1971;33:992–5.
113. Belsey R, Clark MB, Bernat M, et al. Am J Med 1974;57:50–6.
114. Hollis BW, Burton JH, Draper HH. Steroids 1977;30:285–93.
115. Chen TC, Turner AK, Holick MF. J Nutr Biochem 1990;1:315–9.
116. Jones G. Clin Chem 1978;24:287–98.
117. Hollis BW. Clin Chem 1986;32:2060–3.
118. Horst R. Recent advances in the quantitation of vitamin D and vitamin D metabolites. In: Kumar R, ed. Vitamin D: basic and clinical aspects. Boston: Martinus Nijhoff, 1984;423–38.
119. Chen TC, Turner AK, Holick MF. J Nutr Biochem 1990;1:320–7.
120. Stern PH, Hamstra AJ, DeLuca HF, et al. J Clin Endocrinol Metab 1978;46:891–6.
121. Holick MF. Clin Nutr 1986;5:121–9.
122. Krane SM, Holick MF. Metabolic bone disease. In: Isselbacher KJ, Braunwald E, Wilson JD, et al. Harrison's principles of internal medicine. 13th ed. New York: McGraw-Hill, 1994;2172–83.
123. Chalmers J, Conacher DH, Gardner DL, et al. J Bone Joint Surg (Br) 1967;49:403–23.
124. Doppelt SH, Neer RM, Daly M, et al. Orthop Trans 1983;7:512–3.
125. Sokoloff L. Am J Surg Pathol 1978;2:21–30.
126. Kavookjian H, Whitelaw G, Lin S, et al. Orthop Trans 1990;14:580.
127. Webb AR, Pilbeam C, Hanafin N, et al. J Clin Nutr 1990;51:1075–81.
128. Chesney RW. J Clin Nutr 1990;119:1825–8.
129. Food and Nutrition Board, Institute of Medicine. Dietary reference intakes for calcium, phosphorus, magnesium, vitamin D, and fluoride. Washington, DC: National Academy Press, 1997;S1–13.

19. Vitamin E

MARET G. TRABER

Vitamin E is unique in human nutrition because for decades it was "a vitamin looking for a disease" (1). Most water-soluble vitamins are enzyme cofactors; fat-soluble vitamins, such as vitamins A, D, and K, have specific roles in vision, bone formation, and blood clotting, respectively. Thus, it was anticipated that vitamin E would have a specific role in some metabolic function. But in 75 years of study, this has not proven to be the case. The literature is replete with studies describing a variety of vitamin E–deficiency symptoms in various species, leading to confusion about its function in humans. But, this range of symptoms is not surprising given that its major function is as an antioxidant. Consequently, vitamin E–deficiency symptoms in target tissues depend not only upon vitamin E content, uptake, and turnover, but also on the degree of oxidative stress and polyunsaturated fatty acid (PUFA) content. Furthermore, vitamin E activity depends upon an "antioxidant network" involving a wide variety of antioxidants and antioxidant enzymes, which maintains vitamin E in its unoxidized state, ready to intercept and scavenge radicals (2). In addition, vitamin E being fat-soluble is transported in plasma lipoproteins and partitions into membranes and fat-storage sites, where it has the unique role of protecting PUFAs from oxidation.

The antioxidant function of vitamin E cannot be fulfilled by just any antioxidant. Plasma vitamin E is apparently regulated by the liver α-tocopherol transfer protein (α-TTP) (3), and in humans, a genetic defect in α-TTP results in severe vitamin E deficiency (4). α-TTP is necessary for hepatic intracellular α-tocopherol transfer and likely is necessary for α-tocopherol incorporation into nascent very low density lipoproteins (VLDLs) (5).

This chapter describes the structure-function relationships of vitamin E, its antioxidant properties, its lipoprotein transport and delivery to tissues, and its role in human health and disease.

HISTORICAL PERSPECTIVE

The first two decades of vitamin E history were reviewed by Mason (6), a pioneer in studies of vitamin E. Vitamin E deficiency was first described by Evans and Bishop (7) at the University of California in Berkeley in 1922 during their investigations of infertility in rats fed rancid lard. In 1936, Evans et al. (8) isolated a factor from wheat germ with the biologic activity of vitamin E. They named this factor, "α-tocopherol" a name derived from the Greek *tokos* (offspring) and *pherein* (to bear) with an "ol" to indicate that it was an alcohol. Two other tocopherols, *β*- and *γ*-, were isolated from vegetable oils in the subsequent year, with lower biologic activities than α-tocopherol (9). This was the first description of different naturally occurring forms of vitamin E and demonstration that α-tocopherol is the most effective form in preventing vitamin E–deficiency symptoms.

These early observations formed the basis for determining the "biologic activity" of vitamin E. As defined by Machlin (10), the biologic activity of vitamin E is based on its ability to prevent or reverse specific vitamin E–deficiency symptoms (e.g., fetal resorption, muscular dystrophy, and encephalomalacia). The most popular, though most tedious and time-consuming, assay for the biologic activity of vitamin E is the fetal resorption assay (10). Here, vitamin E–depleted virgin female rats are mated with normal males. After successful mating, various levels of single vitamin E forms are fed in several divided doses to the females, which are killed 20 to 21 days after mating. The number of living, dead, and resorbed fetuses are counted, and the percentage of live young determined. Thus, vitamin E biologic activity depends on the amount necessary to maintain the maximum number of live fetuses.

Vitamin E–deficiency symptoms in various animal species were described by Machlin (10) in his comprehensive chapter on vitamin E. Necrotizing myopathy has been observed in vitamin E–deficient monkeys, pigs, rats, dogs, rabbits, goats, guinea pigs, horses, cows and calves, sheep and lambs, mink, chicken, ducks, turkeys, salmon, catfish, antelope, and elephants. Fetal death and resorption was a symptom of vitamin E deficiency in rats, mice, guinea pigs, cows, pigs, sheep, and chickens. Anemia has been observed in rats, pigs, monkeys, salmon, catfish, and chickens. Lipofuscin (a fluorescent pigment of "aging") frequently accumulates in tissues of vitamin E–deficient animals. Based on the symptoms observed in animals, attempts were made to treat humans with muscular dystrophy or anemia by supplementation with vitamin E. Except for anemia of prematurity (11), infants fed formulas high in PUFAs and iron (12), or children with anemia associated with protein-calorie malnutrition (13), these vitamin E trials were largely unsuccessful. These negative findings gave credence to the viewpoint, which we now know is incorrect, that vitamin E deficiency does not occur in humans.

Horwitt (14, 15) attempted to induce vitamin E deficiency in men by feeding a diet low in vitamin E for 6 years to volunteers at the Elgin State Hospital in Illinois. After about 2 years, their serum vitamin E levels decreased into the deficient range. Although their erythrocytes were more sensitive to peroxide-induced hemolysis, anemia did not develop. In 1968, the Food and Nutrition Board of the U.S. National Academy of Sciences (16) set for the first time a recommended daily allowance (RDA) for vitamin E: 30 mg for adult males and 25 mg for adult females. Subsequently, the RDA was reduced on the basis of observations that vitamin E intakes for most of the U.S. population were below these amounts and that PUFA intakes were not as high as in these experimental diets (10).

Not until the mid-1960s was vitamin E deficiency described in children with fat malabsorption syndromes, principally abetalipoproteinemia and cholestatic liver disease, as reviewed by Sokol (17). By the mid-1980s, it was clear that the major vitamin E–deficiency symptom in humans was a peripheral neuropathy characterized by degeneration of the large caliber axons in the sensory neurons (17). Subsequently, vitamin E–deficient patients with peripheral neuropathies without fat malabsorption were described (18). Studies in such patients opened new avenues in vitamin E investigations because they were found to have a genetic defect in hepatic α-TTP (4).

STRUCTURES AND NOMENCLATURE

Vitamin E is the collective name for molecules that exhibit the biologic activity of α-tocopherol, including all tocol and tocotrienol derivatives, as reviewed by Sheppard et al. (19). Vitamin E occurs naturally in eight different forms: four tocopherols and four tocotrienols, which have similar chromanol structures: trimethyl (α-), dimethyl (*β*- or *γ*-), and monomethyl (*δ*-) (Fig. 19.1). Tocotrienols differ from tocopherols in having an unsaturated side chain.

Unlike most other vitamins, chemically synthesized α-tocopherol is not identical to the naturally occurring form. α-Tocopherol synthesized by condensation of trimethyl hydroquinone with racemic isophytol (20) contains eight stereoisomers, arising from the three chiral centers (Fig. 19.1: 2,4′, and 8′) and is designated *all-rac*-α-tocopherol (incorrectly called *d,l*-α-tocopherol). The naturally occurring and most biologically active form, *RRR*-α-tocopherol (formerly called *d*-α-tocopherol) constitutes only one of the eight stereoisomers present in *all rac*-α-tocopherol. The other stereoisomers have lower biologic activity than *RRR*-α-tocopherol, with the 2*S*-forms generally having lower activity than the 2*R*-forms (21, 22).

Vitamin E supplements often contain esters of α-tocopherol, such as α-tocopheryl acetate, succinate, or nicotinate. The ester form prevents oxidation of vitamin E and prolongs its shelf life. Except in individuals with malabsorption syndromes, these esters are readily hydrolyzed in the gut and are absorbed in the unesterified form (23).

BIOLOGIC FUNCTION

Vitamin E functions in vivo as a chain-breaking antioxidant that prevents propagation of free radical damage in biologic membranes (24–27). In vitamin E deficiency, anemia occurs as a result of free radical damage (28). Similarly, peripheral neuropathy likely occurs because of free radical damage to the nerves (29).

Vitamin E is a potent peroxyl radical scavenger and especially protects PUFAs within phospholipids of biologic membranes and in plasma lipoproteins (26). When lipid hydroperoxides are oxidized to peroxyl radicals ($ROO^{\bullet}$), these react 1000 times faster with vitamin E (Vit E-OH) than with PUFA (RH) (2). The phenolic hydroxyl group

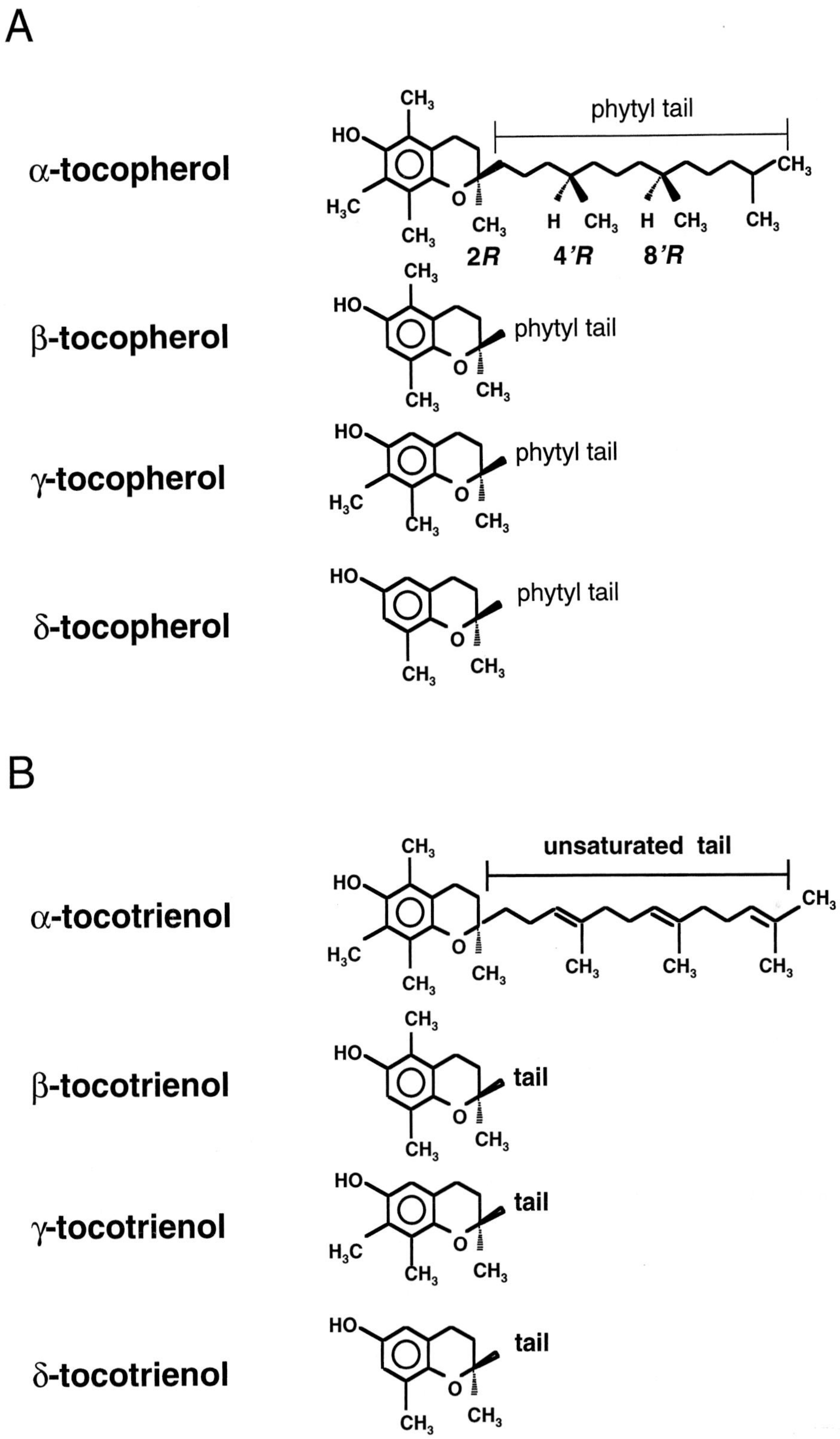

A

α-tocopherol

β-tocopherol

γ-tocopherol

δ-tocopherol

B

α-tocotrienol

β-tocotrienol

γ-tocotrienol

δ-tocotrienol

Figure 19.1. Structures of tocopherols and tocotrienols. There are 8 naturally occurring forms of vitamin E, the 4 tocopherols are shown in **A** and the 4 tocotrienols in **B**. Shown is the natural *RRR*-α-tocopherol stereochemistry; the three chiral centers give rise to 8 different stereoisomers in synthetic vitamin E (*all rac*-α-tocopherol): *RRR*-, *RRS*-, *RSR*-, *RSS*-, *SRR*-, *SSR*-, *SRS*-, *SSS*-.

of tocopherol reacts with an organic peroxyl radical to form the corresponding organic hydroperoxide and the tocopheroxyl radical (Vit E-O$^\bullet$) (30):

In the presence of vitamin E: $ROO^\bullet$ + Vit E-OH $\rightarrow$ ROOH + Vit E-O$^\bullet$

In the absence of vitamin E: $ROO^\bullet + RH \rightarrow ROOH + R^\bullet$
$R^\bullet + O_2 \rightarrow ROO^\bullet$

In this way vitamin E acts as a chain-breaking antioxidant, preventing the further autooxidation of lipids. Further information concerning the reactions of tocopherols and tocotrienols in vivo and in vitro can be found in the extensive review by Kamal-Eldin and Appelqvist (31).

Antioxidant Network

The tocopheroxyl radical (Vit E-O$^•$) formed in membranes emerges from the lipid bilayer into the aqueous domain. Here the tocopheroxyl radical reacts with vitamin C (or other reductants serving as hydrogen donors, AH), thereby oxidizing the latter and returning vitamin E to its reduced state.

$$\text{Vit E-O}^{\bullet} + \text{AH} \rightarrow \text{Vit E-OH} + \text{A}^{\bullet}$$

Biologically important hydrogen donors, which have been demonstrated in vitro to regenerate tocopherol from the tocopheroxyl radical, include ascorbate (vitamin C) and thiols (32), especially glutathione (33–36). Subsequently, the vitamin C and thiyl radicals can be reduced via metabolic processes. This phenomenon has led to the idea of "vitamin E recycling," in which the antioxidant function of oxidized vitamin E is continuously restored by other antioxidants (2). This antioxidant network depends upon the supply of aqueous antioxidants and the metabolic activity of cells.

Structure-Function Relationships of Vitamin E Forms

The biologic activities of the various vitamin E forms correlate roughly with their antioxidant activities; the order of relative peroxyl radical scavenging reactivities of α-, β-, γ-, and δ-tocopherols (100, 60, 25, 27, respectively) (37) is similar to the relative order of their biologic activities (1.5, 0.75, 0.15, 0.05 mg/IU, respectively), as determined by the classical fetal resorption assay in rats (38). However, biologic activities are unlikely to depend solely on antioxidant activity; indeed, some forms of vitamin E show high antioxidant activities but rather poor biologic activities. For example, α-tocotrienol has only one-third the biologic activity of α-tocopherol (38, 39), yet it has higher (40) or equivalent (41) antioxidant activity. A vitamin E analogue (2,4,6,7-tetramethyl-2-(4′,8′,12′-trimethyltridecyl)-5-hydroxy-3,4-dihydrobenzofuran), while showing equivalent biologic activity to *RRR*-α-tocopherol, has 1.5 times the antioxidant activity (43). Furthermore, the eight different stereoisomers of synthetic vitamin E (*all rac*-α-tocopherol) have equivalent antioxidant activity but different biologic activities (21).

Overall, the highest biologic activity is found in molecules with three methyl groups and a free hydroxyl group on the chromanol ring in which the phytyl tail meets the ring in the *R*-orientation (Fig. 19.1). This specific requirement for biologic, but not chemical, activity can best be rationalized by the preferential interactions of *RRR*-α-tocopherol with some stereospecific ligands in cells. One such ligand clearly is the hepatic protein α-TTP.

Hosomi et al. (43a) have demonstrated that the relative affinities of α-TTP towards the various forms of vitamin E (calculated from the degree of competition with RRR-α-tocopherol) were RRR-α-tocopherol = 100%; β-tocopherol = 38%; γ-tocopherol = 9%; δ-tocopherol = 2%; α-tocopheryl acetate = 2%; α-tocopheryl quinone = 2%; SRR-α-tocopherol = 11%; α-tocotrienol = 12%; and Trolox = 9%. They concluded that the affinity of vitamin E analogs for α-TTP is one of the critical determinants for the biological activity of vitamin E.

In addition to its antioxidant function, α-tocopherol shows structure-specific effects on several enzyme activities and membrane properties (44). The most convincing work in this respect is on the regulation of vascular smooth muscle cell proliferation and protein kinase C activity (45–47) and on the suppression of arachidonic acid metabolism via phospholipase A_2 inhibition (48).

Thus, Clement et al. (48a) report that α-tocopherol, but not β-tocopherol, prevents the phosphorylation of protein kinase Cα (PKCα) and suggest that α-tocopherol decreases PKCα-activity by this mechanism.

γ-, β- or δ-Tocopherols, unlike α-tocopherol, can be nitrated (48b–48d) in vitro, a potentially important reaction with nitric oxide (48d). The physiologic significance of the nitration of tocopherols, however, remains to be demonstrated.

Only one of the vitamin E forms, γ-tocotrienol, enhances the degradation of the enzyme 3-hydroxy-3-methyl glutaryl coenzyme A (HMGCoA) reductase, which is the rate-controlling step in cholesterol biosynthesis (48e–48g). Furthermore, the addition of γ-tocotrienol and lovastatin (a drug that competitively inhibits HMGCoA reductase) to the incubation medium of HepG2 cells decreased both the amount and the activity of HMGCoA reductase (48f). In this regard, γ-tocotrienol shows potent hypocholesterolemic effects in hypercholesterotemic humans in some studies (48h) but not in others (48i–48k). Because the presence of α-tocopherol reduces the inhibitory effect of γ-tocotrienol on HMGCoA reductase (48i, 48l), a possible explanation of these disparate findings may be the higher α-tocopherol/γ-tocotrienol ratio of the preparations used in the latter studies (48i–48k). On the other hand, when mixed tocopherols and tocotrienols (16 mg α-tocopherol, 40 mg γ- and α-tocotrienols) were given to patients with hyperlipemia and carotid stenosis, carotid atherosclerotic plaques significantly regressed in the treated group relative to matched controls (48m).

Thus, various forms of vitamin E show specific physiologic effects not directly related to their antioxidant activities.

DIETARY CONSIDERATIONS

The richest dietary sources of vitamin E are edible vegetable oils (19). These oils contain all four homologues: α-, β-, γ-, and δ-tocopherols in varying proportions. *RRR*-α-tocopherol is especially high in wheat germ oil, safflower oil, and sunflower oil. Soybean and corn oils contain predominantly γ-tocopherol, as well as some tocotrienols. Cottonseed oil and palm oil contain both α- and γ-tocopherols in equal proportion. In addition, palm oil contains large amounts of α- and γ-tocotrienols (49). Unprocessed cereal grains and nuts are also good sources of vitamin E; fruits and vegetables contain smaller amounts. Meats, especially animal fat, also contain vitamin E.

An important source of vitamin E in the American diet is the supplement pill. Many Americans believe that supplemental antioxidants, especially vitamin E, are beneficial. Vitamin E supplements are sold as esters (acetate, succinate, nicotinate, etc.) of either natural (RRR-) or synthetic forms (all rac-) of α-tocopherol. The vitamin E pills containing natural vitamin E (RRR-α-tocopherol) are labeled "d α-tocopherol," while those containing synthetic vitamin E (all rac-α-tocopherol), which consist of 8 different stereoisomers, are labeled "dl α-tocopherol." Because the relative bioactivities of RRR-α-tocopheryl acetate and all-rac-α-tocopheryl acetate by the resorption-gestation assay in rats in 1.36:1 (see Appendix Table IV-A-23-b), pills made with "natural" vitamin E need contain only 74% by weight of those made with synthetic vitamin E.

The biopotency of RRR-α-tocopherol relative to all-rac-α-tocopherol may well be considerably higher. When acetate esters of RRR-α-tocopherol labeled with 3 deuterium atoms and all-rac-α-tocopherol labeled with 6 were administered orally to human subjects, the relative bioavailability of the d_3/d_6 labeled compounds was 2.0 ± 0.06, determined by comparing the areas-under-the-curves of the plasma response with time (49a).

Kiyose et al. (48b, 49c) demonstrated that 2R-isomers, but only small amounts of 2S-isomers, were detectable in the serum of human subjects administered all-rac-α-tocopheryl acetate. Furthermore, the increase in the plasma concentration of RRR-α-tocopherol after daily doses of 100 mg RRR-α-tocopheryl acetate for 28 days was similar to the increase in plasma α-tocopherol after daily doses of 300 mg of all-rac-α-tocopheryl acetate for the same period. They suggest that the ratio of bioavailabilities is closer to 3 (49b).

Therefore, in view of the current availability of isotopically labeled tocopherol compounds and chiral HPLC columns, the relative bioavailabilities of various tocopherol species in humans clearly warrant reinvestigation.

INTESTINAL ABSORPTION

Vitamin E Absorption Requires Bile and Pancreatic Secretions

Absorption of vitamin E from the intestinal lumen depends upon processes necessary for fat digestion and uptake into enterocytes. Pancreatic esterases are required for release of free fatty acids from dietary triglycerides. Bile acids, monoglycerides, and free fatty acids are important components of mixed micelles (50).

Esterases are also required for the hydrolytic cleavage of tocopheryl esters (51), a common form of vitamin E in dietary supplements. Generally, these esterases are quite effective; the apparent absorption of deuterated *RRR*-α-tocopherol was similar whether administered as α-tocopherol, α-tocopheryl acetate, or α-tocopheryl succinate (23).

Bile acids, which are needed for the formation of mixed micelles, are essential for vitamin E absorption (52, 53). In the absence of either pancreatic or biliary secretions, vitamin E absorption and secretion into the lymphatic system is poor. In the absence of both, only negligible amounts of vitamin E are absorbed (52–55). Thus, vitamin E deficiency occurs as a result of malabsorption in patients with biliary obstruction, cholestatic liver disease, pancreatitis, or cystic fibrosis (18).

Vitamin E Absorption Requires Chylomicron Synthesis and Secretion

Movement of vitamin E through the absorptive cells is not well understood; no intestinal tocopherol-transfer proteins have been described. In the intestinal mucosa, chylomicrons containing triglycerides, free and esterified cholesterol, phospholipids, and apolipoproteins (especially apolipoprotein (apo) B-48) are synthesized. In addition, fat-soluble vitamins, carotenoids, and other fat-soluble dietary components are incorporated into chylomicrons. Subsequently, chylomicrons containing these fats are secreted by the intestine into the lymph (56). Even in healthy individuals, the efficiency of vitamin E absorption is low (~15–45%), estimated by using radioactively labeled α-tocopherol (57). The relative uptake decreases as the amount of vitamin E ingested increases, as shown in thoracic-duct–cannulated rats (58).

Differences in plasma concentrations of various forms of vitamin E are often assumed to result from differences in intestinal absorption, but this is not the case. Studies using deuterated tocopherols have shown that discrimination between forms of vitamin E does not occur during their absorption by the intestine and their secretion in chylomicrons (59, 60). Various forms of vitamin E, such as α- and γ-tocopherols (61, 62), or *RRR*- and *SRR*-α-tocopherols (59, 60), showed similar apparent efficiencies of intestinal absorption and secretion in chylomicrons. As shown in Figure 19.2, all dietary forms of vitamin E are absorbed and secreted into chylomicrons.

PLASMA TRANSPORT

Distribution of Vitamin E to Tissues During Triglyceride-Rich Lipoprotein Lipolysis

During chylomicron catabolism in the circulation, some of the newly absorbed vitamin E is transferred to circulating lipoproteins and some remains with the chylomicron remnants. Chylomicron catabolism is quite rapid—when rats were injected with [^{3}H]-tocopherol-labeled chylomicrons, the radioactivity disappeared from the circula-

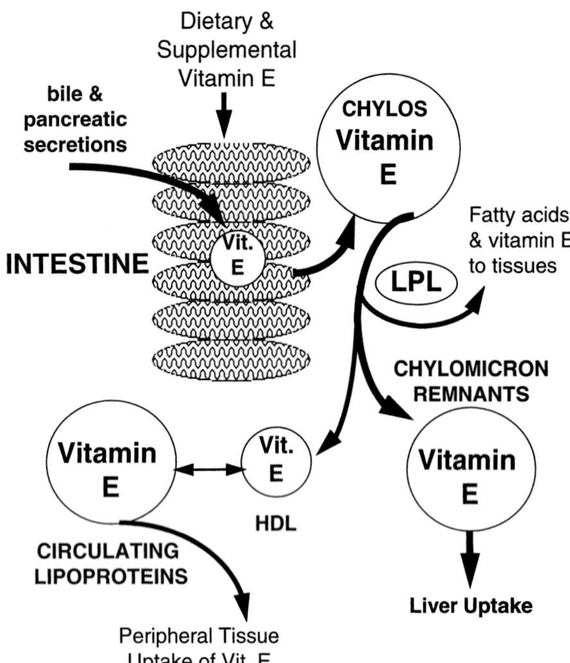

Figure 19.2. Pathways for absorption of vitamin E and its delivery to tissues during chylomicron catabolism. Vitamin E absorption requires bile acids (secreted from the liver) and fatty acids and monoglycerides (released from dietary fat by pancreatic enzymes) for micelle formation. Following uptake into enterocytes of the intestine, all forms of dietary vitamin E are incorporated into chylomicrons (chylos). These triglyceride-rich lipoproteins are secreted into the circulation where lipolysis by lipoprotein lipase *(LPL)* bound to the endothelial lining of capillary walls takes place. The resultant chylomicron remnants are mainly taken up by the liver. During lipolysis, various forms of vitamin E can be transferred to tissues or to high-density lipoproteins *(HDL)*. Vitamin E can exchange between HDL and other circulating lipoproteins, which can also deliver vitamin E to peripheral tissues.

tion in about 5 minutes (63, 64). During delipidation of chylomicrons by lipoprotein lipase, the size of the chylomicron triglyceride core is reduced, and excess surface is created. This excess surface is transferred to high-density lipoproteins (HDLs) (65). During this process, vitamin E is also transferred to HDLs. Because HDLs readily transfer vitamin E to other lipoproteins (66–70), vitamin E is distributed to all circulating lipoproteins (Fig. 19.2). Previously, this was thought to be a spontaneous process. However, Kostner et al. (71) demonstrated that the phospholipid transfer protein (PLTP) isolated from human plasma catalyzed vitamin E exchange between lipoproteins. The transfer activity was 2.45 ± 0.88 nmol/mL/h, a rate that represents transfer of approximately 10% of the plasma vitamin E per hour.

Requirement for VLDL Synthesis in the Preferential Secretion of α-Tocopherol from the Liver

Following partial delipidation by lipoprotein lipase and acquisition of apo-E, chylomicron remnants are taken up by the liver parenchymal cells. The precise mechanisms for chylomicron remnant uptake remain under intense investigation; several pathways involving lipoprotein lipase, apo-E, LDL-receptor-related protein (LRP), as well as the LDL receptor have been proposed (72, 73). The remnants taken up by the liver likely contain a major portion of absorbed vitamin E.

Once chylomicron remnants reach the liver, the dietary fats are repackaged and secreted into the plasma in VLDLs (65). Like chylomicrons, VLDLs have a triglyceride-rich core, but they have apolipoprotein B-100 (apo-B-100) as a major apolipoprotein instead of apo-B-48 (65). Vitamin E is secreted from hepatocytes in VLDL, as demonstrated in rats and in isolated rat hepatocytes (74, 75). In the circulation, VLDLs are delipidated to form LDLs, which retain apo-B-100. LDLs then interact with receptors for apo-B-100 in peripheral tissues as well as in the liver. During VLDL delipidation, which is similar to the lipoprotein interactions described above for chylomicron delipidation, vitamin E is transferred to HDL, which can transfer vitamin E to all of the circulating lipoproteins.

Unlike other fat-soluble vitamins, which have specific plasma transport proteins, vitamin E is transported nonspecifically in lipoproteins in the plasma. However, plasma vitamin E concentrations do depend upon secretion of vitamin E in VLDL from the liver (5, 59, 76). Remarkably, only one form of vitamin E, *RRR*-α-tocopherol, is preferentially secreted by the liver, as illustrated in Figure 19.3. In nascent VLDL isolated from perfusates of livers from cynomolgus monkeys fed 24 hours previously with various deuterated tocopherols, *RRR*-α-tocopherol represented about 80% of the total deuterated tocopherols (77). Thus, the liver, not the intestine, discriminates between tocopherols. The liver contains a mechanism by which *RRR*-α-

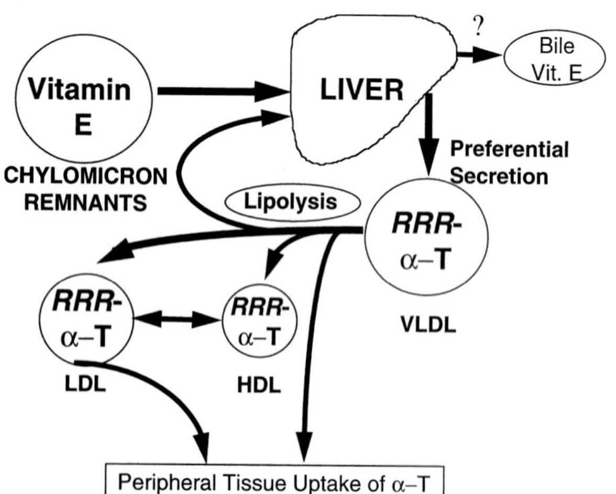

Figure 19.3. Pathways for the preferential delivery of α-tocopherol to peripheral tissues. Chylomicron remnants containing various forms of vitamin E are taken up by the liver. In the liver, the α-tocopherol-transfer protein preferentially incorporates α-tocopherol into nascent very low density lipoproteins *(VLDL)*. Following VLDL secretion into plasma, lipolysis of VLDL by lipoprotein lipase and hepatic triglyceride lipase results in the preferential enrichment of circulating lipoproteins with *RRR*-α-tocopherol. The metabolism of these lipoproteins results in the delivery of *RRR*-α-tocopherol to peripheral tissues.

tocopherol is specifically inserted into nascent VLDL. α-TTP is a likely candidate for this function.

Plasma Vitamin E Kinetics

A kinetic model of vitamin E transport in plasma was developed using data from studies with deuterium-labeled stereoisomers of α-tocopherol (*RRR*- and *SRR*-) (78). The mathematical model assumes that intestinal absorption and secretion of the two deuterated tocopherols (*RRR*- and *SRR*-α-tocopherols) into chylomicrons are similar and that the initial inputs into the plasma occur simultaneously for the two labels. In three patients with both ataxia and vitamin E deficiency (AVED), who have genetically defective α-TTP, the fractional disappearance rates of deuterium-labeled *RRR*- and *SRR*-α-tocopherols in plasma were measured. The disappearance rates (1.4 ± 0.6 and 1.3 ± 0.3 pools/day, respectively) were similar for the two stereoisomers, with a half-life of approximately 13 h for both α-tocopherols. Thus, in AVED patients both *RRR*- and *SRR*-α-tocopherols leave the plasma rapidly. In control subjects, the fractional disappearance rate of deuterium-labeled *RRR*-α-tocopherol (0.4 ± 0.1 pools/day) was significantly ($P < .01$) slower than that of *SRR*-α-tocopherol (1.2 ± 0.6). The apparent half-life of *RRR*-α-tocopherol in normal subjects was approximately 48 h, consistent with the "slow" disappearance of *RRR*-α-tocopherol from the plasma (78).

The similarity in the fractional disappearance rates for *RRR*- and *SRR*-α-tocopherols in the nondiscriminator patients, along with the similarity in *SRR*-α-tocopherol fractional catabolic rates between patients and controls, support the idea that *SRR*-α-tocopherol can be used in normal subjects to trace the irreversible loss of vitamin E from the plasma. The differences (0.8 ± 0.6 pools/day) between the *RRR*- and *SRR*-α-tocopherol rates in controls estimate the rate that *RRR*-α-tocopherol, which had left the plasma, was returned to the plasma. Although plasma labeled *RRR*-α-tocopherol concentrations in controls appear to change slowly, both *RRR*- and *SRR*-α-tocopherols leave the plasma rapidly. Because *RRR*-α-tocopherol is returned to the plasma, its apparent turnover is slow. This recirculation of *RRR*-α-tocopherol results in daily replacement of nearly all of the circulating *RRR*-α-tocopherol.

HEPATIC A-TOCOPHEROL TRANSFER PROTEIN

α-TTP (30–35 kDa) was first identified (79), purified, and characterized (80, 81) from rat liver cytosol. It has also been isolated from human liver cytosol (82) and its cDNA sequence reported. The human protein has 94% homology to the rat protein, and some homology both to the retinaldehyde-binding protein in the retina and to sec14, a phospholipid-transfer protein (83). The gene has been localized to the 8q13.1–13.3 region of chromosome 8 (83, 84). It is present only in the liver, not in other tissues; of the various liver cells, it has only been identified in hepatocytes (81). Purified α-TTP transfers α-tocopherol between liposomes and microsomes (80). Both α- and β-tocopherols are effective competitors, γ-tocopherol is about half as effective, and δ-tocopherol is about one-third as effective; α-tocopheryl acetate, tocopherol quinone, and cholesterol were ineffective competitors (80). Thus, α-TTP preferentially transfers *RRR*-α-tocopherol (77). Hypothetically, this ability to transfer tocopherol is necessary for the action observed in vivo, because nascent VLDL is secreted from the liver preferentially enriched in *RRR*-α-tocopherol. It remains to be demonstrated that the purified protein transfers α-tocopherol to nascent VLDL during its assembly in hepatocytes.

Other Tocopherol-Binding Proteins

Dutta-Roy et al. (85, 86) reported that both the liver and the heart contain an α-tocopherol-binding protein with a mass of 14.2 kDa. This protein is present in the liver in addition to α-TTP. The 14.2-kDa protein also transfers α-tocopherol in preference to γ- or δ-tocopherol. They suggest that the 14.2-kDa tocopherol-binding protein might regulate cellular α-tocopherol concentrations. Nalecz et al. (87) also reported the existence of various α-tocopherol-binding proteins in cultured smooth muscle cells. No function has been proposed for these proteins.

DISTRIBUTION TO TISSUES

Vitamin E is transported in plasma lipoproteins in a nonspecific manner. No plasma specific vitamin E–transport proteins have been described. It is likely that the mechanisms of lipoprotein metabolism determine the delivery of vitamin E to tissues. There are at least two major routes by which tissues likely acquire vitamin E: *(a)* via lipoprotein lipase–mediated lipoprotein catabolism and *(b)* via the LDL receptor (Figs. 19.2 and 19.3). In addition, vitamin E rapidly exchanges between lipoproteins and between lipoproteins and membranes and may enrich membranes with vitamin E.

Vitamin E Delivery to Tissues

During chylomicron catabolism, peripheral tissues can acquire vitamin E from lipoproteins, which contain all of the forms of vitamin E that were consumed. Following hepatic secretion of VLDL enriched with α-tocopherol, peripheral tissues take up primarily α-tocopherol. Delivery from both chylomicrons and from VLDL, likely mediated by lipoprotein lipase (88), is important for vitamin E delivery, based on tissue tocopherol concentrations. Patients with abetalipoproteinemia, who malabsorb vitamin E, provide an interesting illustration. In these patients, adipose tissue γ-tocopherol is usually undetectable (89, 90). One patient, however, who was treated with an intravenously administered lipid emulsion made from soybean oil, had adipose tissue γ-tocopherol concentrations equal to those of α-tocopherol (90). Thus, lipoprotein lipase presumably catabolizes the lipid emulsion and delivers both α- and γ-tocopherols to adipose tissue. This mechanism may be particularly important for tissues that express lipoprotein lipase, such as adipose tissue, muscle, and brain (88).

One other important mechanism for the delivery of tocopherols to tissues is via the LDL receptor. Using fibroblasts with and without LDL-receptor activity, Traber and Kayden (91) demonstrated that LDL containing vitamin E is taken up more effectively by the fibroblasts with functional LDL-receptor activity. Cohn et al. (92) demonstrated that in vivo both LDL-receptor-dependent and -independent pathways are important for tissue uptake of tocopherols.

Circulating blood cells likely obtain their vitamin E by transfer of tocopherols from lipoproteins, especially HDL. Patients with abetalipoproteinemia, who have HDL (66, 67) but do not have chylomicrons, VLDL, LDL, and other lipoproteins containing apolipoprotein B, have only about 1/10th the normal plasma vitamin E concentrations, and their erythrocytes contain about two–thirds of that found in controls (90). Thus, HDLs have an important role in delivering vitamin E to circulating cells. In addition, *RRR*-α-tocopherol-membrane-binding proteins (major component, kDa 65, and a minor component, kDa 125) on human erythrocytes were described by Kitabchi and Wimalasena (93, 94). Specific binding of α-tocopherol to erythrocyte membranes may be involved in the prevention of hemolysis, because α-tocopherol is more effective than other tocopherols in preserving erythrocytes (95).

Vitamin E concentrations were measured in lymphocytes and monocytes in normal subjects and in patients with lymphocyte leukemia (96). The cancer cells had lower concentrations of vitamin E, likely a result of the rapid growth of the cells. Alternatively, the oxidant/antioxidant balance of these cells may be altered.

Tissues with Slow- versus Fast-Turning-over Vitamin E Pools

Deuterated α-tocopherol was used to assess the kinetics and distribution of α-tocopherol into various tissues in rats and in guinea pigs (97, 98). These studies showed that a group of tissues is in rapid equilibrium with the plasma α-tocopherol pool. Tissues, such as erythrocytes, liver, and spleen, quickly replace "old" with "new" α-tocopherol (99). Other tissues, such as heart, muscle, and spinal cord, have slower α-tocopherol turnover times. The brain has the slowest α-tocopherol turnover time by far.

In general, the vitamin E content of the nervous system is spared during vitamin E depletion (100–102). Studies in adult beagle dogs demonstrated that the peripheral nerve is the most responsive of the nervous system to vitamin E concentrations in the diet (103). In dogs fed a vitamin E–deficient diet for nearly 2 years, the vitamin E concentrations in peripheral nerves were lower than those in any other nervous tissues and were as low as in most non-nervous tissues. By contrast, in dogs fed a vitamin E–supplemented diet, peripheral nerve concentrations were higher than in other nervous tissues. Thus, it is not surprising that in humans the peripheral nerves (18), albeit the sensory neurons, are the most susceptible to vitamin E deficiency (29). Furthermore, in vitamin E–deficient humans, the vitamin E concentration of sural nerve decreases prior to the appearance of histologic or functional defects (29).

Storage Sites of Vitamin E

The mechanisms for the release of tocopherols from tissues are unknown; no organ functions as a storage organ for α-tocopherol, releasing it on demand. The bulk of vitamin E in the body is localized in the adipose tissue (104). More than 90% of the human body pool of α-tocopherol is located in the adipose tissue, and more than 90% of adipose tissue α-tocopherol is in fat droplets, not membranes (104). Handelman et al. (105) estimated that 2 years or more are required for ratios of α:γ tocopherols to reach new steady-state levels in response to changes in dietary intake. Thus, analysis of adipose tissue α-tocopherol content yields a useful estimate of the long-term vitamin E status (89, 106).

Although triglyceride, but not vitamin E or cholesterol, is released from adipose tissue during weight reduction in humans (107), the α-tocopherol content is reduced in vitamin E–deficient patients (29, 58, 89, 90). In adult dogs, the adipose tissue also provides a source of vitamin E to the rest of the body (108), while tocopherol depletion from adipose tissue in guinea pigs is extremely slow (109). Thus, the degree of availability of adipose tissue α-tocopherol in humans remains controversial.

METABOLISM AND EXCRETION

Since the tocopheroxyl radical can be reduced back to tocopherol by ascorbate or other reducing agents, the flux through the cyclic radical pathway may be much larger than the flux through the pathway of further metabolism. Liebler and Burr et al. (110, 111) suggest that biologically relevant oxidation products formed from α-tocopherol include 4a,5-epoxy- and 7,8-epoxy-8a(hydroperoxy)tocopherones and their respective hydrolysis products, 2,3-epoxy-tocopherol quinone and 5,6-epoxy-α-tocopherol quinone. However, these products are formed during in vitro oxidation; their importance in vivo is unknown.

Excretion of Vitamin E and Its Metabolites via Bile, Urine, and Feces

The primary oxidation product of α-tocopherol is α-tocopheryl quinone, which can be conjugated to yield the glucuronate after prior reduction to the hydroquinone. The glucuronate can be excreted into bile or further degraded in the kidneys to α-tocopheronic acid, which is excreted in the urine (112). Further oxidation products, including dimers and trimers, as well as other adducts have also been described (31).

Schultz et al. (113) described a novel urinary metabolite of α-tocopherol (2,5,7,8-tetramethyl-2(2′carboxyethyl)-6-hydroxychromane), which is excreted in the urine when large supplemental doses of *RRR*-α-tocopherol are fed to humans. Doses in excess of 50 mg vitamin E result in excretion of this metabolite. Thus, excretion of this metabolite may indicate saturation of the plasma binding capacity for α-tocopherol (113). Surprisingly, a similar metabolite of γ-tocopherol has been proposed as a natriuretic factor and has been given the name LLU-α (114).

The major route of excretion of ingested vitamin E is fecal elimination, because of its low intestinal absorption. Forms of vitamin E not preferentially used, such as synthetic racemic mixtures or γ-tocopherol (115), are eliminated during the process of nascent VLDL secretion in the liver and are probably excreted in bile (61).

Excretion of Vitamin E via Skin

The skin may be an important route of vitamin E excretion. In the early 1970s, Shiratori (116) infused chylomicrons labeled with [^{3}H]-α-tocopherol into rats and found that nearly 40% was associated with the pelt. Application of these data to humans seemed questionable, since humans do not have fur. However, recent studies in hairless mice show that skin contains various forms of vitamin E similar to those in the diet, while the brain has virtually only α-tocopherol (117). Thus, skin vitamin E may be derived from chylomicrons containing dietary vitamin E. Furthermore, skin sebaceous glands may secrete vitamin E to provide antioxidants to protect cutaneous lipids. If so, this route could be important for vitamin E excretion in humans.

CAUSES OF DEFICIENCY

Vitamin E deficiency occurs only rarely in humans and virtually never results from dietary deficiencies because of the nearly ubiquitous distribution of tocopherols in foods, especially oils and fats (19). Vitamin E deficiency does occur as a result of genetic abnormalities in α-TTP and as a result of various fat malabsorption syndromes, as shown in Table 19.1.

Table 19.1
Disorders Requiring Administration of Supplemental Vitamin E to Prevent Deficiency

Genetic abnormalities
- α-Tocopherol-transfer protein (AVED, ataxia with vitamin E deficiency)
- Apolipoprotein B (homozygous hypobetalipoproteinemia)
- Microsomal triglyceride-transfer protein (abetalipoproteinemia)

Fat malabsorption syndromes
- Chronic cholestasis in children and adults
  - Idiopathic neonatal hepatitis
  - Familial cholestatic syndrome
  - Alagille syndrome
  - Paucity of interlobular bile ducts
  - Extrahepatic biliary atresia
  - Primary biliary cirrhosis
- Cystic fibrosis and pancreatic insufficiency
- Short bowel syndromes
  - Crohn's disease
  - Mesenteric vascular thrombosis
  - Intestinal pseudoobstruction
- Chronic steatorrhea
  - Blind loop syndrome
  - Intestinal lymphangiectasia
  - Celiac disease
  - Chronic pancreatitis
- Total parenteral nutrition

Vitamin E Deficiency Caused by Genetic Defects in the α-Tocopherol Transfer Protein

Genetic defects in α-TTP are associated with a characteristic syndrome, AVED (previously called familial isolated vitamin E [FIVE] deficiency). AVED patients have neurologic abnormalities that are similar to those of Friedreich's ataxia (118, 119). The symptoms are characterized by a progressive peripheral neuropathy with a specific "dying back" of the large-caliber axons of the sensory neurons, resulting in ataxia (120).

These patients respond to oral vitamin E supplements. A dose of 800 to 1200 mg/day usually suffices to prevent further deterioration of neurologic function, and in some cases, improvements have been noted, as reviewed by Sokol (18). Untreated patients have extraordinarily low plasma vitamin E concentrations (as low as 1/100 of normal), but if they are given vitamin E supplements, then plasma concentrations reach normal within hours (120). However, if supplementation is halted, then plasma vitamin E concentrations fall within days to deficient levels.

Traber et al. (5, 76) used deuterated tocopherols to determine the biochemical defect in AVED patients. Based on kinetic data, it appeared that *(a)* an hepatic α-TTP that preferentially incorporates *RRR*-α-tocopherol into VLDL is required to maintain plasma *RRR*-α-tocopherol concentrations via secretion in nascent VLDL by hepatocytes, *(b)* nondiscriminators either lack this protein or have a marked defect in the *RRR*-α-tocopherol-binding region of the protein, and *(c)* patients who discriminate, but have difficulty maintaining plasma *RRR*-α-tocopherol concentrations, have a less severe defect, perhaps a defect in transfer function.

Studies in patients with Friedreich's ataxia led to the characterization of genetic defects in α-TTP. The most common autosomal recessive ataxia is Friedreich's ataxia, which is linked to a defect on chromosome 9 and is characterized by absent tendon reflexes, deep sensory loss, and cerebellar and Babinski signs (121). From a large number of inbred Tunisian families, Ben Hamida et al. (118, 119) identified a small group of patients with ataxia who had defects on chromosome 8, not 9. Subsequent investigation revealed that these patients also had extraordinarily low plasma vitamin E concentrations (119). Ouahchi et al. (4) mapped their genetic defect to chromosome 8q13.1–13.3, the same chromosomal location as α-TTP (83, 84). Most of the patients described by Ouahchi et al. were found to have a truncation of the C-terminal portion of α-TTP.

The genetic defect in α-TTP has now been identified in some of the same patients who were analyzed using deuterium-labeled tocopherols. A truncation of the terminal portion of α-TTP (4, 122) causes an inability to discriminate between *RRR*- and *SRR*-α-tocopherols (123). However, patients who are heterozygous for the α-TTP truncation mutation (4, 122) can discriminate between stereoisomers (4, 122). In addition to truncation mutations, defective transfer function of α-TTP has also been described. A patient who experienced neurologic difficulties only after reaching about 50 years of age (124) preferentially incorporated *RRR*-α-tocopherol into lipoproteins, but at a reduced rate (5). This patient was found to be homozygous for a thymine-to-guanine transversion in the α-TTP gene that causes the histidine at position 101 to be replaced with glutamine (125). Gotoda et al. (125) screened 801 inhabitants near the patient's home on an isolated Japanese island, where 21 heterozygotes were found with this mutation. These heterozygotes had significantly lower serum vitamin E concentrations than a control population. The mutated gene, when expressed in COS-7 cells, produced a functionally defective α-TTP with approximately 11% of the activity of the wild-type α-TTP (125). Thus, the region around histidine 101 must be important for transfer activity. This region has a high degree of homology with both the retinaldehyde-binding protein present in retina and the yeast sec14 protein (83). Because these latter two proteins are also lipid-binding/transfer proteins, this region of all three proteins may be important for their lipid transfer roles.

Retinitis pigmentosa, a symptom of vitamin E deficiency in humans (126), has been described in patients with AVED (127, 128). Recently, the defective α-TTP gene in three AVED patients with retinitis pigmentosa was described; they all had the histidine 101–transfer defect (128). It is unknown whether the homology with the retinaldehyde-binding protein in the retina is important for α-TTP function in the eye or whether vitamin E deficiency itself causes retinitis pigmentosa. Vitamin E supplementation stops or slows the progression of retinitis pigmentosa caused by vitamin E deficiency (128). This is in contrast to results from a trial of vitamin E and A supplements in patients with retinitis pigmentosa without vitamin E deficiency (129), which showed a beneficial effect of 15,000 IU/day of vitamin A and a possible adverse effect of vitamin E. Therefore, the plasma vitamin E concentrations should be measured in patients with retinitis pigmentosa to evaluate their vitamin E nutriture before supplementation with vitamin E.

Vitamin E Deficiency Caused by Genetic Defects in Lipoprotein Synthesis

Studies of patients with hypobetalipoproteinemia or abetalipoproteinemia (low to nondetectable circulating chylomicrons, VLDL, or LDL) demonstrated that lipoproteins containing apo-B are necessary for effective absorption and plasma transport of lipids, especially vitamin E. These patients have steatorrhea from birth, because of their impaired ability to absorb dietary fat, which also contributes to their poor vitamin E status. Clinical features include steatorrhea, retarded growth, acanthocytosis, retinitis pigmentosa, and a chronic progressive neurologic disorder with ataxia.

Although the two groups of patients both lack apo-B-containing lipoproteins, their underlying genetic defects differ. Homozygous hypobetalipoproteinemia patients have a defect in the apo-B gene and thus any apo-B-containing lipoproteins that are secreted into the circulation turn over rapidly (130, 131). Abetalipoproteinemic patients have genetic defects in MTP (microsomal triglyceride-transfer protein) that prevent normal lipidation of apo-B (132). Thus, the secretion of apo-B-containing lipoproteins is virtually nonexistent. Indeed, apo-B does not leave the endoplasmic reticulum in the absence of lipidation by MTP (133).

Clinically, both groups of subjects become vitamin E deficient and develop a characteristic neurologic syndrome—a progressive peripheral neuropathy—if they are not given large vitamin E supplements (90, 134). Daily doses of 100 to 200 mg/kg, or about 5 to 7 g of vitamin E are recommended (18). In fact, plasma concentrations of vitamin E never reach normal levels. Studies using deuterated tocopherols in five patients with abetalipoproteinemia demonstrated that even with large doses of vitamin E (2 g), plasma concentrations remained less than 1% of normal (90). Despite low plasma concentrations, adipose tissue α-tocopherol concentrations are raised to normal levels in some patients given large vitamin E doses (90).

Vitamin E Deficiency as a Result of Fat Malabsorption Syndromes

Vitamin E deficiency occurs secondary to fat malabsorption because vitamin E absorption requires biliary and pancreatic secretions. Failure of micellar solubilization and malabsorption of dietary lipids lead to vitamin E deficiency in children with chronic cholestatic hepatobiliary disorders, including disease of the liver and anomalies of intrahepatic and extrahepatic bile ducts (18). Children with cholestatic liver disease who have impaired secretion of bile into the small intestine have severe fat malabsorption. Neurologic abnormalities, which appear as early as the 2nd year of life, become irreversible if the vitamin E deficiency is uncorrected (18, 53, 135).

Children with cystic fibrosis can also become vitamin E deficient, because the impaired secretion of pancreatic digestive enzymes causes steatorrhea and vitamin E malabsorption, even when pancreatic enzyme supplements are administered orally (18). More severe vitamin E deficiency occurs if bile secretion is impaired (55, 136–138). Winklhofer-Roob et al. (139) proposed that cystic fibrosis patients be supplemented with a daily 400-mg dose of vitamin E so that their plasma α-tocopherol concentrations increase above 26 to 28 μM. This higher plasma vitamin E concentration protects LDL from in vitro oxidation (139).

Any disorder that causes fat malabsorption can lead to vitamin E deficiency. The list of disorders associated with acquired vitamin E deficiency, assembled by Sokol (18), includes chronic dysfunction or resection of the small bowel, Crohn's disease, mesenteric vascular thrombosis or intestinal pseudoobstruction, blind loop syndrome, intestinal lymphangiectasia, celiac disease, and chronic pancreatitis. The development of neurologic symptoms of vitamin E deficiency in adults who acquire these disorders, however, takes decades. Serum vitamin E levels may fall within 1 to 2 years of acquired lipid malabsorption in adolescents and adults; however, a 10- to 20-year interval between the identification of biochemical vitamin E deficiency and the onset of neurologic symptoms is generally observed in adults (18). The prolonged time for onset of symptoms results from the prior accumulation of vitamin E in most tissues and its relatively slow release from nervous tissues.

Vitamin E supplementation is very difficult to achieve in patients with fat malabsorption syndromes because they malabsorb vitamin E. Sokol (18) suggests treatment with *RRR*-α-tocopherol (not the ester) at 25 to 50 mg/kg/day, advancing by 50 mg/kg/day up to 150 to 200 mg/day if the ratio of serum α-tocopherol to total lipids does not normalize (>0.8 mg/g). The dose should be given at the time of maximal bile flow, several hours before administration of any medication that may interfere with vitamin E absorption (e.g., cholestyramine, large doses of vitamin A or ferrous sulfate). In cases of severe cholestasis, intraluminal bile acid concentrations are well below the critical micellar concentration, which results in failure of vitamin E absorption. Here intramuscular injections of vitamin E, such as Viprimol (Hoffmann-LaRoche, Inc., Nutley, NJ) can be used to provide 1 to 2 mg/kg/day (18). A water-soluble ester of vitamin E, such as *d*-α-tocopherol polyethylene glycol-1000 succinate (TPGS, Eastman Chemical Products, Kingsport, TN), is absorbed when administered orally, appears to be nontoxic, and reverses or prevents neurologic dysfunction (18). However, products like TPGS should not be used if the patient suffers from renal failure or dehydration, because the excretion of absorbed polyethylene glycol may be impaired (140).

Vitamin E Deficiency in Patients Receiving Total Parenteral Nutrition

Patients receiving total parenteral nutrition (TPN) ideally are provided with all of their required nutrients—vitamin E (10 mg) is given as part of a vitamin mix and as a component of a lipid emulsion that also provides essential fatty acids and calories. Most intravenous preparations of lipid emulsions are made with soybean oil to provide PUFAs. However, the soybean oil emulsions contain high levels of γ, but not α-tocopherol (141). Evaluation of the vitamin E status of TPN patients receiving lipid emulsions suggests that they may be receiving inadequate amounts of α-tocopherol. They have elevated levels of exhaled pentane and ethane-markers of lipid peroxidation in vivo (142) and adipose tissue α-tocopherol concentrations that are half of normal, suggesting depletion of tissue stores of vitamin E (143).

Infusion of PUFAs may lead to an increased requirement for vitamin E in TPN patients. In normal subjects, infusion of lipid emulsions raised γ-tocopherol levels only during the infusion; by 24 hours postinfusion, γ-tocopherol concentrations had returned nearly to baseline (141). Furthermore, patients on long-term TPN may be depleting tissue vitamin E because the lipid emulsions remove α-tocopherol from the plasma lipoproteins, returning it to the liver (141). Thus, lipid emulsions currently used in TPN provide a high intake of PUFAs, which results in increased requirements for lipid-soluble antioxidants without providing sufficient α-tocopherol. These concerns have largely gone unnoticed, probably because of the lengthy interval required for development of vitamin E–deficiency symptoms.

PATHOLOGY OF HUMAN VITAMIN E DEFICIENCY

The primary manifestations of human vitamin E deficiency include spinocerebellar ataxia, skeletal myopathy, and pigmented retinopathy (18). Similarly, when raised on experimental vitamin E–deficient diets, rats and rhesus monkeys develop ataxia and neuroaxonal degeneration in the brainstem, spinal cord, and peripheral nerves, as well as pigmentary degeneration of the retina (18). Hence, the vitamin E–deficiency symptoms observed in humans are similar to those in experimental animals.

A distinct pattern in the progression of neurologic symptoms resulting from vitamin E deficiency in humans has been described (18). Hypo- or areflexia is the earliest symptom observed. By the end of the first decade of life, untreated patients with chronic cholestatic hepatobiliary disease have a combination of spinocerebellar ataxia, neuropathy, and ophthalmoplegia. The progression of neurologic symptoms is slower in children with cystic fibrosis and abetalipoproteinemia. The symptoms of vitamin E deficiency in AVED are similar to those found in these latter patients (120, 144). These observations suggest that there is increased oxidative stress in patients with cholestatic liver disease.

Deficiency in children and adults results in a progressive peripheral neuropathy with a dying back of the large caliber axons in the sensory neurons, as reviewed (120). The large-caliber, myelinated axons in peripheral sensory nerves are the predominant target in vitamin E deficiency in humans. In deficient humans, diminished amplitudes in sensory nerve action potential are common, whereas delayed conduction velocity, an indicator of demyelination, is unusual. Thus, axonal degeneration rather than demyelination is the primary sensory nerve abnormality; that is, the axons degenerate first, then demyelination occurs.

Axonal dystrophy has been observed in the posterior columns of the spinal cord and the dorsal and ventral spinocerebellar tracts, as reviewed (120). Specifically, swollen, dystrophic axons (spheroids) have been observed in the gracile and cuneate nuclei of the brainstem. Lipofuscin accumulation has been observed in dorsal sensory neurons and peripheral Schwann cell cytoplasm. Electromyographic studies show denervation injury of muscles in patients with advanced vitamin E deficiency. Somatosensory-evoked potential testing has shown a central delay in sensory conduction, correlating with degeneration of the posterior columns of the spinal cord.

REQUIREMENTS AND RECOMMENDED INTAKES

Vitamin E Units

According to the U.S. Pharmacopoeia (145), 1 international unit (IU) of vitamin E equals 1 mg *all-rac*-α-tocopheryl acetate, 0.67 mg *RRR*-α-tocopherol, or 0.74 mg *RRR*-α-tocopheryl acetate. These conversions were based on their relative biologic activities. The current recommended dietary allowance (RDA) for vitamin E is 8 mg for women and 10 mg for men of *RRR*-α-tocopherol or *RRR*-α-tocopherol equivalents (α-TEs) (146) (see also Appendix Table II-A-2-a-2).

For the purpose of calculating vitamin E intakes in α-TEs, γ-tocopherol is assumed to substitute for α-tocopherol with an efficiency of 10%, β-tocopherol of 50%, and α-tocotrienol of 30%. However, functionally, these forms of vitamin E are not equivalent to α-tocopherol. Deuterated γ-tocopherol concentrations decrease rapidly, compared with deuterated α-tocopherol, suggesting that the metabolic fate of γ-tocopherol is quite unlike that of α-tocopherol (60). Thus, sources of PUFAs that have high concentrations of γ-tocopherol and low concentrations of α-tocopherol, such as corn or soybean oils, may increase the potential for in vivo lipid peroxidation. That is, the PUFAs that are protected from lipid peroxidation by γ-tocopherol in the oil are not protected after they have been consumed because γ-tocopherol is not retained by the body (141). Thus, PUFA may more easily "turn rancid" in the body.

Adequacy of Vitamin E Intakes in Normal U.S. Populations

King (147) defined three different approaches to determining normal human nutrient requirements: *(a)* balance studies, in which nutrient losses are measured in relation to intake; *(b)* depletion-repletion studies, in which subjects are maintained on diets low or deficient in a nutrient, followed by correction of the deficiency with measured amounts of the nutrient; and *(c)* the observed intakes of a nutrient by healthy people. Because vitamin E turns over slowly and there are no functional biomarkers exquisitely sensitive to vitamin E, the intakes of healthy people are the general guideline for establishing adequacy of vitamin E status (146).

The adequacy of vitamin E intakes is often estimated by measurements of plasma concentrations of apparently healthy people in the U.S. The preliminary report of the Third National Health and Nutrition Examination Survey (NHANES III) has just been released (148). The α-tocopherol concentrations (5th to 95th percentiles) in people from age 6 to 80+ ranged from 6.10 to 19.02 μg/mL (14.2–44.2 μM). There was an increase in serum α-tocopherol concentrations associated with puberty that was not entirely normalized by expressing the data per mg serum cholesterol. Cholesterol-adjusted α-tocopherol concentrations (5th to 95th percentiles) were 3.76 to 8.53 μg/mg (3.41–7.67 μmol/mmol). The National Research Council estimated that the average daily intakes of α-TEs range from 7 to 11 mg for men, 7.1 for women, and 5.5 mg for children 1 to 5 years of age (146). The RDA was based on these intake data and an estimated average PUFA intake. The committee assumed that if the PUFA intake increases, the vitamin E will increase concomitantly.

Low-Fat Diets

Often patients with elevated cholesterol levels are encouraged to change their dietary habits, increasing PUFA-containing fat intake and decreasing saturated fat intake. Changes in dietary habits to lower plasma lipid levels in patients with elevated lipids or with diabetes may have deleterious effects on vitamin E intakes, because most dietary vitamin E is present in fats (19). This is especially true in subjects who change their diets to lower serum cholesterol by decreasing intake of saturated fats and increasing intake of PUFA-containing fats, usually corn oil or soybean oil, which contain high levels of γ-tocopherol but much less α-tocopherol (19). Intake of oxidizable lipids is thus increased, while intake of α-tocopherol is decreased. To avoid excessive intakes of PUFA, ingestion of monounsaturated fats, such as olive or canola oils, is currently recommended (149).

Supplemental vitamin E may be recommended to prevent inadequate intakes in patients with chronic diseases associated with free radical damage due to oxidative stress. After doses of 400 IU are administered to patients, for example, their LDLs are less susceptible to oxidative stress during subsequent in vitro testing (150).

Assessment of Vitamin E Status in Patients at Risk for Vitamin E Deficiency

As shown in Table 19.2, several parameters can be measured in patients who may be vitamin E deficient. Although low serum or plasma vitamin E concentrations indicate vitamin E deficiency, measurement of plasma levels are insuf-

Table 19.2
Techniques for Assessment of Vitamin E Status

Measurements of plasma vitamin E concentrations
Normal values are >10 nmol α-tocopherol/mL (or μM) or 5 μg/mL
Normal values are >0.8 mg α-tocopherol/g total lipid or 2.8 mg/g cholesterol
Measurements of adipose tissue vitamin E concentrations
>100 μg α-tocopherol/mg triglyceride
Functional signs of vitamin E deficiency
Increased red cell hemolysis
Increased lipid peroxidation
Increased expired ethane or pentane
Clinical signs of vitamin E deficiency
Neurologic testing—abnormal sensory nerve function
Histopathology of peripheral nerves
Electrophysiologic measurements
Gene testing
Genetic defects in α-tocopherol-transfer protein
Genetic defects on chromosome 8

ficient for patients with various forms of lipid malabsorption. Calculation of effective plasma vitamin E concentrations needs to take into account plasma lipid levels. Patients with elevated cholesterol or triglyceride concentrations may have vitamin E levels in the "normal" range, but these may not suffice to protect tissues. For example, Sokol et al. (151) showed that plasma vitamin E concentrations were in the normal range in patients with vitamin E deficiency as a result of cholestatic liver disease, which was also characterized by extraordinarily high lipid levels.

Patients with peripheral neuropathies or retinitis pigmentosa should be assessed for vitamin E deficiency. The ataxia of Friedreich's ataxia is so remarkably similar to that of AVED patients that plasma concentrations of vitamin E in all patients with ataxia should definitely be measured.

Controversial Topics

Epidemiologic studies and some intervention trials indicate a beneficial role of vitamin E supplements in decreasing risk of degenerative diseases, such as cardiovascular disease and atherosclerosis (152, 153), cancer (154), and cataract formation (155). Furthermore, large supplements of vitamin E have been proposed to be beneficial in preventing or decreasing the risk of chronic diseases or slowing the ravages of aging. Table 19.3 lists various disorders in which supplemental vitamin E has been proposed to have beneficial effects. Despite the virtual safety of large intakes of vitamin E (156, 157), the use of vitamin E in amounts beyond those that can be consumed in the diet remains controversial.

There is also concern about the potential role of vitamin E as a prooxidant. Vitamin E in LDL oxidized in vitro in the absence of aqueous antioxidants is a prooxidant (31, 158, 159). The relatively long lived tocopheroxyl radical acts as a chain-transfer agent, causing the oxidation of LDL core lipids. Thus far, however, there is no evidence that vitamin E has a proantioxidant activity in vivo. But this remains an important issue with respect to the use of vitamin E supplements in humans.

Table 19.3.
Disorders in Which Supplemental Vitamin E May Be Beneficial

Premature infants—retinopathy of prematurity (126)
Protection from retrolental fibroplasia
Possible protection of intraventricular hemorrhage
Increased risk of necrotizing enterocolitis or sepsis
Anemia of prematurity (160)
Protection from vitamin E deficiency caused by inappropriate formulas
May be beneficial in physiologic jaundice-anemia of newborn
Cardiovascular disorders
Decreased risk of coronary heart disease (152, 153, 161)
Decreased in vitro LDL oxidation (150, 162)
Decreased in vitro platelet aggregation (163)
Ischemia-reperfusion injury (164)
Immune response
Improved responses in elderly (165)
Cataract (126)
Tardive dyskinesia (166, 167)

CONCLUSIONS

Nearly 75 years from the time of its discovery, vitamin E remains an elusive molecule. Its potential for decreasing the risks of acquiring chronic disease have spurred the interest of scientists and clinicians worldwide. The description of vitamin E deficiency in patients with genetic abnormalities in human α-TTP has opened new avenues of investigation of α-tocopherol-transfer/binding proteins in various tissues. We are returned to the age-old questions, "What is the function of vitamin E?" and "Why do we need a specific protein that only recognizes α-tocopherol if all of the naturally occurring forms of vitamin E have nearly similar antioxidant functions?"

ACKNOWLEDGMENTS

I wish to express my sincere appreciation both to Professor Lester Packer for his guidance and support as well as to the many people who are listed in the cited joint publications, without whose collaboration those studies could not have been accomplished.

This work was supported in part by the University of California Tobacco Related Disease Research Program (4RT-0065), the Palm Oil Research Institute of Malaysia (PORIM, Kuala Lumpur, Malaysia), the Natural Source Vitamin E Association (NSVEA), and the Henkel Corporation (LaGrange, IL).

REFERENCES

1. Mason KE. Fed Proc 1977;36:1906–10.
2. Packer L. Sci Am Sci Med 1994;1:54–63.
3. Traber MG. Free Radic Biol Med 1994;16:229–39.
4. Ouahchi K, Arita M, Kayden H, et al. Nature Genet 1995;9:141–5.
5. Traber MG, Sokol RJ, Kohlschütter A, et al. J Lipid Res 1993;34:201–10.
6. Mason KE. The first two decades of vitamin E history. In: Machlin LJ, ed. Vitamin E: a comprehensive treatise. New York: Marcel Dekker, 1980;1–6.

7. Evans HM, Bishop KS. Science 1922;56:650–1.
8. Evans HM, Emerson OH, Emerson GA. J Biol Chem 1936;113:319–32.
9. Emerson OH, Emerson GA, Mohammed A, et al. J Biol Chem 1937;122:99–107.
10. Machlin LF. Vitamin E. In: Machlin LJ, ed. Handbook of vitamins. New York: Marcel Dekker, 1991;99–144.
11. Oski FA, Barness LA. J Pediatr 1967;70:211–20.
12. Williams ML, Shoot RJ, O'Neal PL, et al. N Engl J Med 1975;292:887–90.
13. Whitaker JA, Fort EG, Vimokesant S, et al. Am J Clin Nutr 1967;20:783–9.
14. Horwitt MK, Harvey CC, Duncan GD, et al. Am J Clin Nutr 1956;4:408–19.
15. Horwitt MK. Am J Clin Nutr 1960;8:451–61.
16. Food and Nutrition Board, National Research Council. Recommended dietary allowances. Washington, DC: National Academy of Sciences, 1968.
17. Sokol RJ. Annu Rev Nutr 1988;8:351–73.
18. Sokol RJ. Vitamin E deficiency and neurological disorders. In: Packer L, Fuchs J, eds. Vitamin E in health and disease. New York: Marcel Dekker, 1993;815–49.
19. Sheppard AJ, Pennington JAT, Weihrauch JL. Analysis and distribution of vitamin E in vegetable oils and foods. In: Packer L, Fuchs J, eds. Vitamin E in health and disease. New York: Marcel Dekker, 1993;9–31.
20. Kasparek S. Chemistry of tocopherols and tocotrienols. In: Machlin LJ, eds. Vitamin E: a comprehensive treatise. New York: Marcel Dekker, 1980;7–65.
21. Weiser H, Vecchi M, Schlachter M. Int J Vitam Nutr Res 1986;56:45–56.
22. Weiser H, Vecchi M. Int J Vitam Nutr Res 1982;52:351–70.
23. Cheesemen KH, Holley AE, Kelly FJ, et al. Free Radic Biol Med 1995;19:591–8.
24. Tappel AL. Vitam Horm 1962;20:493–510.
25. Burton GW, Ingold KU. Acc Chem Res 1986;19:194–201.
26. Burton GW, Joyce A, Ingold KU. Arch Biochem Biophys 1983;221:281–90.
27. Ingold KU, Webb AC, Witter D, et al. Arch Biochem Biophys 1987;259:224–5.
28. Kayden HJ, Silber R. Trans Assoc Am Physicians 1965;78:334–41.
29. Traber MG, Sokol RJ, Ringel SP, et al. N Engl J Med 1987;317:262–5.
30. Burton GW, Doba T, Gabe EJ, et al. J Am Chem Soc 1985;107:7053–65.
31. Kamal-Eldin A, Appleqvist LA. Lipids 1996;31:671–701.
32. Wefers H, Sies H. Eur J Biochem 1988;174:353–7.
33. McCay PB. Annu Rev Nutr 1985;5:323–40.
34. Niki E. Chem Phys Lipids 1987;44:227–53.
35. Sies H, Murphy ME. Photochem Photobiol 1991;8:211–24.
36. Sies H, Stahl W, Sundquist AR. Ann NY Acad Sci 1992;669:7–20.
37. Burton GW, Ingold KU. J Am Chem Soc 1981;103:6472–7.
38. Bunyan J, McHale D, Green J, et al. Br J Nutr 1961;15:253–7.
39. Weimann BJ, Weiser H. Am J Clin Nutr 1991;53:1056S–60S.
40. Serbinova EA, Tsuchiya M, Goth S, et al. Antioxidant action of α-tocopherol and α-tocotrienol in membranes. In: Packer L, Fuchs J, eds. Vitamin E in health and disease. New York: Marcel Dekker, 1993;235–43.
41. Suarna C, Food RL, Dean RT, et al. Biochim Biophys Acta 1993;1166:163–70.
42. Ingold KU, Burton GW, Foster DO, et al. FEBS Lett 1990;267:63–5.
43. Burton GW, Hughes L, Ingold KU. J Am Chem Soc 1983;105:5950–1
43a. Hosomi A, Arita M, Sato Y, et al. FEBS Letters 1997;409: 105–8.
44. Traber MG, Packer L. Am J Clin Nutr 1995;62(Suppl): 1501S–9S.
45. Boscoboinik D, Szewczyk A, Hensey C, et al. J Biol Chem 1991;266:6188–94.
46. Stauble B, Boscoboinik D, Tasinato A, et al. Eur J Biochem 1994;226:393–402.
47. Tasinato A, Boscoboinik D, Bartoli G, et al. Proc Natl Acad Sci USA 1995;92:12190–4.
48. Pentland AP, Morrison AR, Jacobs SC, et al. J Biol Chem 1992;267:15578–84.
48a. Clement S, Tasinato A, Boscoboinik D, et al. Euro J Biochem 1997;246:745–9.
48b. Green J, McHale D, Marcinkiewicz S, et al. J Chem Soc 1959;3362–73.
48c. Cooney RW, France AA, Harwood PJ, et al. Proc Natl Acad Sci USA 1993;90:1771–5.
48d. Christen S, Woodall AA, Shigenaga MK, et al. Proc Natl Acad Sci USA 1997;94:3217–22.
48e. Pearce BC, Parker RA, Deason ME, et al. J Med Chem 1992;35:3595–606.
48f. Parker RA, Pearce BC, Clark RW, et al. J Biol Chem 1993;268:11230–8.
48g. Pearce BC, Parker RA, Deason ME, et al. J Med Chem 1994;37:526–541.
48h. Qureshi AA, Qureshi N, Wright JJ, et al. Am J Clin Nutr 1991;53:1021S–26S.
48i. Qureshi AA, Bradlow BA, Brace L, et al. Lipids 1995;30:1171–7.
48j. Nazaimoon WMW, Sakinah O, Gapor A, et al. Nutr Res 1996;16:1901–11.
48k. Wahlqvist ML, Krivokuca-Bogetic Z, Lo CS, et al. Nutr Res 1992;12:S181–S201.
48l. Qureshi AA, Pearce BC, Nor RM, et al. J Nutr 1996;126:389–94.
48m. Tomeo AC, Geller M, Watkins TR, et al. Lipids 1995; 30:1179–83.
49. Dial S, Eitenmiller RR. Tocopherols and tocotrienols in key foods in the U.S. diet. In: Ong ASH, Niki E, Packer L, eds. Nutrition, lipids, health, and disease. Champaign, IL: AOCS Press, 1995;327–42.
49a. Acuff RV, Thedford SS, Hidiroglon NN, et al. Am J Clin Nutr 1994;60:397–402.
49b. Kiyose C, Muramatsu R, Kameyama Y, et al. Am J Clin Nutr 1997;65:785–9.
49c. Kiyose C, Muramatsu R, Fujiyama-Fujiwara Y, et al. Lipids 1995;30:1015–8.
50. Traber MG, Goldberg I, Davidson E, et al. Gastroenterology 1990;98:96–103.
51. Nakamura T, Aoyama Y, Fujita T, et al. Lipids 1975;10:627–33.
52. Gallo-Torres H. Lipids 1970;5:379–84.
53. Sokol RJ, Heubi JE, Iannaccone S, et al. Gastroenterology 1983;85:1172–82.
54. Harries JT, Muller DPR. Arch Dis Child 1971;46:341–44.
55. Sokol RJ, Readon MC, Accurso FJ, et al. Am J Clin Nutr 1989;50:1074–1.
56. Cohn JS, McNamara JR, Cohn SD, et al. J Lipid Res 1988;29:925–36.
57. Blomstrand R, Forsgren L. Int J Vit Nutr Res 1968;38:328–44.
58. Traber MG, Kayden HJ, Green JB, et al. Am J Clin Nutr 1986;44:914–23.
59. Traber MG, Burton GW, Ingold KU, et al. J Lipid Res 1990;31:675–85.

60. Traber MG, Burton GW, Hughes L, et al. J Lipid Res 1992;33:1171–82.
61. Traber MG, Kayden HJ. Am J Clin Nutr 1989;49:517–26.
62. Meydani M, Cohn JS, Macauley JB, et al. J Nutr 1989;119:1252–8.
63. Bjørneboe A, Bjørneboe G-EA, Bodd E, et al. Biochim Biophys Acta 1986;889:310–5.
64. Bjørneboe A, Bjørneboe G-EA, Drevon CA. Biochim Biophys Acta 1987;921:175–81.
65. Havel R. Am J Clin Nutr 1994;59:795–9.
66. Kayden HJ, Bjornson LK. Ann NY Acad Sci 1972;203:127–40.
67. Bjornson LK, Gniewkowski C, Kayden HJ. J Lipid Res 1975;16:39–53.
68. Massey JB. Biochim Biophys Acta 1984;793:387–92.
69. Granot E, Tamir I, Deckelbaum RJ. Lipids 1988;23:17–21.
70. Traber MG, Lane JC, Lagmay N, et al. Lipids 1992;27:657–63.
71. Kostner GM, Oettl K, Jauhiainen M, et al. Biochem J 1995;305:659–67.
72. Herz J, Qiu SQ, Oesterle A, et al. Proc Natl Acad Sci USA 1995;92:4611–5.
73. Strickland DK, Kounnas MZ, Argraves WS. FASEB J 1995;9:890–8.
74. Cohn W, Loechleiter F, Weber F. J Lipid Res 1988;29:1359–66.
75. Bjørneboe A, Bjørneboe G-EA, Hagen BF, et al. Biochim Biophys Acta 1987;922:199–205.
76. Traber MG, Sokol RJ, Burton GW, et al. J Clin Invest 1990;31:397–407.
77. Traber MG, Rudel LL, Burton GW, et al. J Lipid Res 1990;31:687–94.
78. Traber MG, Ramakrishnan R, Kayden HJ. Proc Natl Acad Sci USA 1994;91:10005–8.
79. Catignani GL, Bieri JG. Biochim Biophys Acta 1977;497: 349–57.
80. Sato Y, Hagiwara K, Arai H, et al. FEBS Lett 1991;288:41–5.
81. Yoshida H, Yusin M, Ren I, et al. J Lipid Res 1992;33:343–50.
82. Kuhlenkamp J, Ronk M, Yusin M, et al. Protein Exp Purific 1993;4:383–9.
83. Arita M, Sato Y, Miyata A, et al. Biochem J 1995;306:437–43.
84. Doerflinger N, Linder C, Ouahchi K, et al. Am J Hum Genet 1995;56:1116–24.
85. Dutta-Roy A, Gordon M, Leishman D, et al. Mol Cell Biochem 1993;123:139–44.
86. Dutta-Roy AK, Leishman DJ, Gordon MJ, et al. Biochem Biophys Res Commun 1993;196:1108–12.
87. Nalecz K, Nalecz M, Azzi A. Eur J Biochem 1992;209:37–42.
88. Traber MG, Olivercrona T, Kayden HJ. J Clin Invest 19985;75:1729–34.
89. Kayden HJ, Hatam LJ, Traber MG. J Lipid Res 1983;24:652–6.
90. Traber MG, Rader D, Acuff R, et al. Atherosclerosis 1994;108:27–37.
91. Traber MG, Kayden HJ. Am J Clin Nutr 1984;40:747–51.
92. Cohn W, Goss-Sampson M, Grun H. Biochem J 1992;287: 247–54.
93. Kitabchi AE, Wimalasena J. Biochim Biophys Acta 1982;684: 200–6.
94. Wimalasena J, Davis M, Kitabchi AE. Biochem Pharmacol 1982;31:3455–61.
95. Urano S, Inomori Y, Sugawara T, et al. J Biol Chem 1992;267:18365–70.
96. Kayden HJ, Hatam L, Traber MG, et al. Blood 1984;63:213–5.
97. Ingold KU, Buron GW, Foster DO, et al. Lipids 1987;22: 163–72.
98. Burton GW, Wronska U, Stone L, et al. Lipids 1990;25: 199–210.
99. Burton GW, Traber MG. Annu Rev Nutr 1990;10:357–82.
100. Bourre J, Clement M. J Nutr 1991;121:1204–7.
101. Vatassery GT. Lipids 1978;13:828–31.
102. Meydani M, Macauley JB, Blumberg JB. Lipids 1986;21: 786–91.
103. Pillai SR, Traber MG, Steiss JE, et al. Lipids 1993;28:1101–5.
104. Traber MG, Kayden HJ. Am J Clin Nutr 1987;46:488–95.
105. Handelman GJ, Epstein WL, Peerson J, et al. Am J Clin Nutr 1994;59:1025–32.
106. Handelman GL, Epstein WL, Machlin LJ, et al. Lipids 1988;23:598–604.
107. Schafer EJ, Woo R, Kibata M, et al. Am J Clin Nutr 1983;37:749–54.
108. Pillai SR, Traber MG, Steiss JE, et al. Lipids 1993;28:1095–9.
109. Machlin LJ, Keating J, Nelson J, et al. J Nutr 1979;109: 105–9.
110. Liebler DC, Burr JA. Lipids 1995;30:789–93.
111. Liebler DC, Burr JA, Philips L, et al. Anal Biochem 1996;236:27–34.
112. Drevon CA. Free Radic Res Commun 1991;14:229–46.
113. Schultz M, Leist M, Petrzika M, et al. Am J Clin Nutr 1995;62(Suppl):1527S–34S.
114. Wechter WJ, Kantoci D, Murray EDJ, et al. Proc Natl Acad Sci USA 1996;93:6002–7.
115. Traber MG, Kayden HJ. Ann NY Acad Sci 1989;570:95–108.
116. Shiratori T. Life Sci 1974;14:929–35.
117. Podda M, Weber C, Traber MG, et al. J Lipid Res 1996;37:893–901.
118. Ben Hamida M, Belal S, Sirugo G, et al. Neurology 1993;43:2179–83.
119. Ben Hamida C, Doerflinger N, Belal S, et al. Nature Genet 1993;5:195–200.
120. Sokol RJ, Kayden HJ, Bettis DB, et al. J Lab Clin Med 1988;111:548–59.
121. Belal S, Hentati F, Ben Hamida C, et al. Clin Neurosci 1995;3:39–42.
122. Hentati A, Deng H-X, Hung W-Y, et al. Ann Neurol 1996;39:295–300.
123. Traber MG. Regulation of human plasman vitamin E. In: Sies H, ed. Antioxidants in disease mechanisims and therapeutic strategies. San Diego: Academic Press, 1996;49–63.
124. Yokota T, Wada Y, Furukawa T, et al. Ann Neurol 1987;22:84–7.
125. Gotoda T, Arita M, Arai H, et al. N Engl J Med 1995;333:1313–8.
126. Trevithick JR, Robertson JM, Mitton KP. Vitamin E and the eye. In: Packer L, Fuchs J, eds. Vitamin E in health and disease. New York: Marcel Dekker, 1993;873–926.
127. Matsuya M, Matsumoto H, Chiba S, et al. Brain Nerve (Tokyo) 1994;46:989–94.
128. Yokota T, Shiojiri T, Gotoda T, et al. N Engl J Med 1996;335:1769–70.
129. Berson EL, Rosner B, Sandberg MA, et al. Arch Ophthalmol 1993;111:761–72.
130. Young SG, Bertics SJ, Curtiss LK, et al. J Clin invest 1987;79:1842–51.
131. Farese RV Jr, Linton MF, Young SG. J Intern Med 1992;231:643–52.
132. Wetterau JR, Aggerbeck LP, Bouma ME, et al. Science 1992;258:999–1001.
133. Du E, Wang SL, Kayden HJ, et al. J Lipid Res 1996;37: 1309–15.
134. Rader DJ, Brewer HB. JAMA 1993;270:865–9.
135. Sokol RJ, Heubi JE, Butler-Simon N, et al. Gastroenterology 1987;93:975–85.
136. Elias E, Muller DPR, Scott J. Lancet 1981;ii:1319–21.

137. Cynamon HA, Milov DE, Valenstein E, et al. J Pediatr 1988;113:637–40.
138. Stead RJ, Muller DPR, Matthews S, et al. Gut 1986;27:714–8.
139. Winklhofer-Roob BM, Ziouzenkova O, Puhl H, et al. Free Radic Biol Med 1995;19:725–33.
140. Sokol RJ, Butler-Simon N, Conner C, et al. Gastroenterology 1993;104:1727–35.
141. Traber MG, Carpentier YA, Kayden HJ, et al. Metabolism 1993;42:701–9.
142. Lemoyne M, Van Gossum A, Kurian R, et al. Am J Clin Nutr 1988;48:1310–5.
143. Steephen AC, Traber MG, Ito Y, et al. JPEN 1991;15:647–52.
144. Amiel J, Maziere J, Beucler I, et al. J Inherit Metab Dis 1995;18:333–40.
145. Anonymous. 1979. The United States Pharmacopeia. The National Formulary. The United States Pharmacopeial Convention.
146. Food and Nutrition Board NRC. Recommended dietary allowances. 10th ed. Washington, DC: National Academy of Sciences Press, 1989.
147. King J. Am J Clin Nutr 1996;63:s983–4.
148. Sowell A, Briefel R, Huff D, et al. FASEB J 1996;10:A813.
149. Reaven P, Parthasarathy S, Grasse BJ, et al. Am J Clin Nutr 1991;54:701–6.
150. Jialal I, Fuller CJ, Huet BA. Arterioscler Thromb Vasc Biol 1995;15:190–8.
151. Sokol RJ, Heubi JE, Iannaccone ST, et al. N Engl J Med 1984;310:1209–12.
152. Rimm EB, Stampfer MJ, Ascherio A, et al. N Engl J Med 1993;328:1450–6.
153. Stampfer MJ, Hennekens C, Manson JE, et al. N Engl J Med 1993;328:1444–9.
154. Blot WJ, Li J-Y, Taylor PR, et al. J Natl Cancer Inst 1993;85:1483–92.
155. Packer L. Vitamin E: biological activity and health benefits: overview. In: Packer L, Fuchs J, eds. Vitamin E in health and disease. New York: Marcel Dekker, 1993;977–82.
156. Bendich A, Machlin LJ. Am J Clin Nutr 1988;48:612–9.
157. Bendich A, Machlin LJ. The safety of oral intake of vitamin E: data from clinical studies from 1986 to 1991. In: Packer L, Fuchs J, eds. Vitamin E in health and disease. New York: Marcel Dekker, 1993;411–6.
158. Ingold KU, Bowry VW, Stocker R, et al. Proc Natl Acad Sci USA 1993;90:45–9.
159. Thomas SR, Neuzil J, Stocker R. Arterio Thromb Vasc Biol 1996;16:687–96.
160. Sinha S, Chiswick M. Vitamin E in the newborn. In: Packer L, Fuchs J, eds. Vitamin E in health and disease. New York: Marcel Dekker, 1993;861–70.
161. Stephens NG, Parsons A, Schofield PM, et al. Lancet 1996;347:781–6.
162. Jialal I, Grundy SM. J Lipid Res 1992;33:899–906.
163. Richardson PD, Steiner M. Adhesion of human platelets inhibited by vitamin E. In: Packer L, Fuchs J, eds. Vitamin E in health and disease. New York: Marcel Dekker, 1993; 297–311.
164. Steiner M, Glantz M, Lekos A. Am J Clin Nutr 1995;62: 1381S–4S.
165. Meydani SN, Hayek M, Coleman L. Ann NY Acad Sci 1992;669:125–39.
166. Dabiri LM, Pasta D, Darby JK, et al. Am J Psychiatry 1994;151:925–6.
167. Lohr JB, Caligiuri MP. J Clin Psychiatry 1996;57:167–73.

SELECTED READINGS

Krinsky NI, Sies H, eds. Antioxidant vitamins and β-carotene in disease prevention. Am J Clin Nutr 1995;62(Suppl):1299S–540S.

Ouahchi K, Arita M, Kayden H, et al. Ataxia with isolated vitamin E deficiency is caused by mutations in the alpha-tocopherol transfer protein. Nature Genet 1995;9:141–5.

Packer L, Fuchs J, eds. Vitamin E in health and disease. New York: Marcel Dekker, 1993.

Traber MG, Sies H. Vitamin E in humans: demand and delivery. Annu Rev Nutr 1996;16:321–47.

20. Vitamin K

ROBERT E. OLSON

Long periods of time may elapse between the discovery of a given vitamin deficiency disease, isolation and determination of the structure of the vitamin, and final elucidation of its metabolic function. This is true of vitamin K: its deficiency disease, fatal hemorrhage, was discovered in 1929, its isolation and structural determination was accomplished in 1939, and its metabolic function was suspected only after a new amino acid, γ-carboxyglutamic acid (Gla), was discovered in bovine prothrombin in 1974. It is now established that vitamin K is part of a membrane-bound carboxylase system that participates in the posttranslational carboxylation of a number of vitamin K–dependent proteins. The γ-glutamyl carboxylase has been isolated and sequenced, its gene cloned, and progress has been made in determining its transmembrane segments and active site. It is now clear that vitamin K–dependent proteins include not only those involved in coagulation, but others with functions in bone, kidney, and other tissues.

HISTORICAL OVERVIEW

Vitamin K was discovered by Henrik Dam in Copenhagen in 1929 in studies of sterol metabolism in chicks fed fat-free diets. He observed quite unexpectedly that some of the chicks developed hemorrhages under the skin, in muscle, and in other tissues and that blood, occasionally taken for laboratory examinations, showed delayed coagulation. The antihemorrhagic factor was found to be fat soluble. Similar observations were made in 1931 by MacFarlane and his coworkers in Canada and in 1933 by Holst and Halbrook at the University of California.

By 1934, Dam and coworkers had extended their work to show that none of the established vitamins could prevent the hemorrhagic disease they had described, and they named the new vitamin "K" (for *K*oagulation). They demonstrated that vitamin K was distributed in liver, hemp seeds, and green leafy vegetables. In Dam's laboratory, Schonheyder discovered in 1936 that the hemorrhagic disease was due to the absence of prothrombin activity in the plasma. About the same time, Almquist and Stokstad discovered that fish meal, particularly after putrefaction, was a good source of the vitamin. Efforts were then initiated to isolate the new factor from both alfalfa and putrefied fish meal.

In 1939, Doisy and his colleagues and Dam and his colleagues announced the isolation of vitamin K_1 from alfalfa. It was identified as 2-methyl-3-phytyl-1,4-naphthoquinone. In addition, Doisy's group reported the isolation of a related but not identical vitamin K from putrefied fish meal, which they named vitamin K_2.

In 1941, Campbell and Link discovered that the active agent in spoiled clover that caused a hemorrhagic disease in cattle, first described by Schofield in 1922, was bishydroxycoumarin (dicumarol) and that this compound was antagonistic to vitamin K. The availability of 4-hydroxycoumarin drugs also provided new tools for investigation of the complexities of blood coagulation. In the next decade, three additional vitamin K–dependent coagulation factors were discovered: proconvertin (factor VII), Stewart factor (factor X), and Christmas factor (factor IX) (1). During the past 25 years, four more vitamin K–dependent coagulation factors (protein C, protein S, protein Z, and a new growth-arrest-specific factor [Gas 6]) have been discovered. Two of these (proteins C and S) are anticoagulants, and Gas 6 is homologous to protein S (2).

In 1968, studies at the University of Lund by Ganrot and Nilehn showed that when the concentration of prothrombin was measured immunochemically in normal and coumarin-anticoagulated human subjects, the antigenic equivalents in coumarin-treated subjects did not decrease in proportion to the biologic activity as measured by the clotting time. They concluded that coumarin anticoagulant therapy (and by inference, vitamin K deficiency) interfered with the normal synthesis of prothrombin and produced an abnormal prothrombin, modified in some way to make it biologically inactive but immunologically reactive.

The study of the chemical properties of bovine prothrombin from normal and anticoagulated cows was then undertaken in several laboratories. In 1974, Stenflo et al. (3) in Sweden, Nelsestuen et al. (4) in the United States, and Magnusson and coworkers (5) in Denmark independently reported that the difference between normal and abnormal prothrombin was the presence of a new amino acid in normal prothrombin, γ-carboxyglutamic acid (Fig. 20.1). This carboxylated glutamic acid was not present in the prothrombin of animals given coumarin drugs or on vitamin K–deficient diets. It was therefore concluded that vitamin K acts to alter the structure of the vitamin K–dependent proteins posttranslationally by facilitating carboxylation of selected glutamate residues in their primary structures. This discovery revolutionized ideas about the function of vitamin K and led to studies of the enzymology of the vitamin K–dependent γ-glutamyl carboxylase and related vitamin K enzymes in the microsomes of liver, bone, and other tissues. The early history of vitamin K research has been extensively reviewed elsewhere (1, 6) and citations to all of the above discoveries are documented.

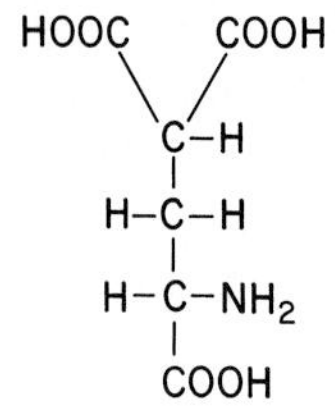

HOOC COOH
C–H
H–C–H
H–C–NH_2
COOH

Figure 20.1. Structure of γ-carboxyglutamic acid (Gla). Gla is a tricarboxylic acid that is stable in strong base but decomposes with γ-decarboxylation in strong acid. Its isoelectric point is pH 3.0.

CHEMISTRY AND NOMENCLATURE

Compounds with vitamin K activity all contain the 2-methyl-1,4-napthoquinone nucleus with a lipophilic side chain at position 3. Vitamin K_1, now known as phylloquinone, was identified as 2-methyl-3-phytyl-1,4-naphthoquinone (Fig. 20.2). It is the only homologue of vitamin K synthesized by plants. Vitamin K_2, isolated from fish meal, was identified as menaquinone-7. The menaquinone family of vitamin K_2 homologues is a large series of vitamins containing unsaturated isoprenyl side chains, which vary in length and are designated MK-*n*. Menaquinone-4 (MK-4) is synthesized in animals and birds from the provitamin menadione (2-methyl-1,4-naphthoquinone, formerly known as vitamin K_3) by enzymatic alkylation with digeranyl pyrophosphate (7). The alkylating enzyme has been partially purified and characterized from chick and rat liver microsomes. The other menaquinones are products of bacterial biosynthesis and range from menaquinone-7 to menaquinone-13 (8). Partially saturated menaquinones, menaquinone-9-H and menaquinone-8-H, are known. The molecular weight of vitamin K_1 is 450.68 g/mol and of vitamin MK-7 is 648.97 g/mol.

FOODS AS A SOURCE OF VITAMIN K

Phylloquinone is widely distributed in both animal and vegetable foods and varies from less than 2 nM (<0.1 μg/100 g) in citrus fruits, to 22 nM (1 μg/100 mL) in cow's milk, and to more than 8.8 μmol/kg (400 μg/100 g) in spinach, kale, and turnip greens. Menaquinones, on the other hand, are absent from most ordinary foods but are present to the extent of 200 nmol/kg (13 μg/100 g) in

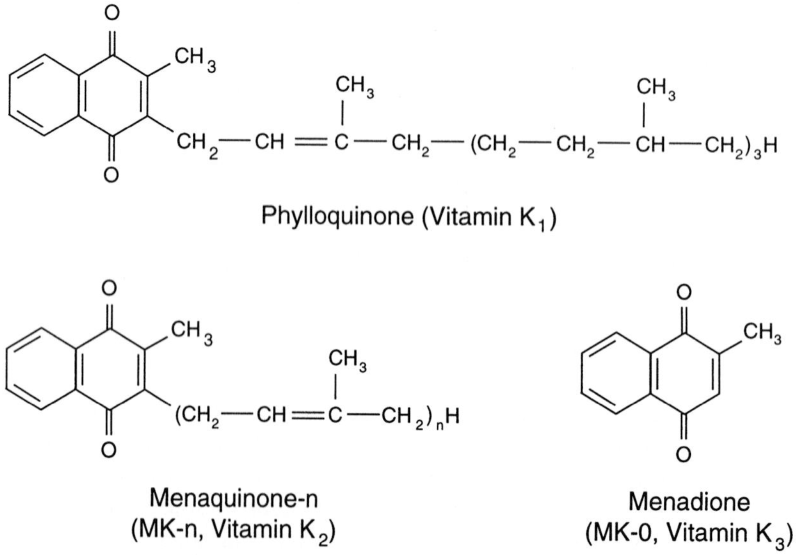

CH_3 CH_3 CH_3
CH_2—CH=C—CH_2—(CH_2—CH_2—CH—$CH_2)_3$H

Phylloquinone (Vitamin K_1)

CH_3 CH_3
(CH_2—CH=C—$CH_2)_n$H

Menaquinone-n
(MK-n, Vitamin K_2)

CH_3

Menadione
(MK-0, Vitamin K_3)

Figure 20.2. Structures of vitamin K homologues that are derivatives of 2-methyl-1,4-naphthoquinone: phylloquinone (vitamin K_1), menaquinone (vitamin K_2), and menadione (vitamin K_3).

liver and 300 nmol/kg in certain cheeses (9) The principal components are MK-8, MK-9, and MK-10. Natto, a fermented soybean preparation consumed by Asians, can contain 10 to 20 μmol/kg (1–2 mg/100 g) of MK-7 (10). Various methods have been used to measure vitamin K in foods. Because of the sensitivity of vitamin K to light, however, precautions must be taken to protect the vitamin during extraction and analysis.

Methods of Assay

For many years the only satisfactory procedure for determination of vitamin K activity of foods was a curative bioassay based on the response of deficient chicks to the added food. In this method, the prothrombin level was measured with Russell's viper venom and the response of unknowns was compared with the dose-response curve using phylloquinone as a standard. The sensitivity of the chick bioassay is 0.22 μmol (0.1 mg) phylloquinone per kilogram of food. Such assays, however, did not identify the form of vitamin K present in the material assayed and tended to overestimate the concentration of phylloquinone (11). Furthermore, the various homologues vary in their biologic activity when fed. Matschiner and Doisy found that menaquinone-1 had only 1% of the biologic activity of phylloquinone, whereas MK-4, MK-5, and MK-7 were identical to phylloquinone in activity. MK-2 and MK-10 each gave about 25% of the activity of phylloquinone. These data demonstrated that the very short chain and very long chain homologues were less active by mouth than phylloquinone, although MK-6, MK-7, MK-8, and MK-9 were as much as 25 times more potent than K_1 when injected intracardially.

More recently, vitamin K has been determined by chemical methods in which fat-solvent extraction of desiccated tissues is followed by column and thin-layer chromatography, and then by high-pressure liquid chromatography (HPLC) using both direct and reverse-phase columns. Vitamin K homologues are detected in the HPLC effluents by ultraviolet absorption, electrochemical techniques, or fluorescence of hydroquinone derivatives (12). Such methods have improved both the sensitivity and accuracy of vitamin K measurement. Use of combined gas chromatography (GC)-mass spectrometry allows measurements of vitamin K homologues in the femtomole range.

Analytical Values

The new set of values presented in Table 20.1 is based on two recent studies using advanced techniques for the measurement of phylloquinone. The first is the Total Diet Study (TDS) conducted annually by the FDA/USDA to monitor the safety and nutritional quality of the U.S. food supply. Some 264 core foods were identified from the 1987–1988 National Food Survey and analyzed at the USDA Human Nutrition Research Center at Tufts University (11). This work was complemented by a parallel study in Great Britain conducted by Shearer et al. (9, 13). These compilations are the most complete ever and provide the physician and dietitian with a suitable database for estimating vitamin K_1 intake.

Table 20.1
Average Vitamin K Content (μg/100 g) of Ordinary Foods

Food		Food	
Milk and milk products		Vegetables	
Butter	30.0	Asparagus	70
Cheese	2.8	Beans, green	46
Milk (cow)	1.0	Broccoli	147
Milk (human)	0.2	Brussels sprouts	250
Eggs		Cabbage	110
Hens (whole)	11.0	Celery	5
Meat and meat products		Collards	440
Bacon	0.1	Kale	726
Beef liver	3.0	Lettuce	75
Chicken liver	0.3	Peas, green	33
Ground beef	2.4	Potato	1
Ham	0.1	Spinach	415
Lamb chop	4.6	Tomato	5
Pork tenderloin	0.1	Turnip	1
Fats		Turnip greens	650
Olive oil	56	Fruits	
Soy bean oil	198	Applesauce	0.6
Corn oil	3	Banana	0.2
Safflower oil	10	Orange	0.1
Margarine	30	Peach	2.5
Cereal and grain products		Pear	4.0
Bread	2.5	Strawberry	1.5
Maize	0.1	Beverages	
Oatmeal	2.0	Coffee	<0.1
Rice	0.1	Cola	<0.1
Cornflakes	0.1	Tea	<0.1
Granola	1.8	Lemonade	0.1
Shredded wheat	1.5	Beer	<0.1
		Tobacco	
		Cigarettes	5000

Data from references 9, 12, 13, 98.

The variation in vitamin K_1 content of foods within food groups is conspicuous. For example, foods within the cereal and bread and meats groups can vary from 2.2 to 220 nmol/kg (0.1–10 μg/100 g). Fruits vary in their phylloquinone content from 2.2 nmol/kg (0.1 μg/100 g) in oranges to 88 nmol/kg (4.0 μg/100 g) in pears. Fats and oils also vary greatly, from 66 nmol/kg (3 μg/100 g) in corn oil to 4.4 mol/kg (198 μg/100 g) in soybean oil. Vegetables also vary, from 22 nmol/kg (1 μg/100 g) in turnips to 16.1 μmol/kg (726 μg/100 g) in kale.

Human milk contains about 6 nM (2–3 μg/L) phylloquinone; cow's milk contains about 22 nM (6–17 μg/L). Tobacco (not a typical food) is one of the richest sources of phylloquinone and contains 0.11 mmol/kg (5000 μg/100 g). When smoked, a small percentage of vitamin K is volatilized and can be absorbed through the mucous membranes, the nasopharynx, bronchi, and alveoli. The values for fruits, vegetables, and cereals shown in Table 20.1 are subject to significant variation depending on the soil and climatic conditions where the plant was grown. Table 20.2 compares the recommended mean dietary intakes of vitamin K_1 as stratified by age and gender with actual intakes measured in the Total Diet Study of the

USDA. The estimated vitamin K_1 intake of about 100 μg/day is much lower than previously estimated (150–500 μg) (11) and closer to the recommended dietary allowance (RDA). There is, however, no doubt that some persons ingest more vitamin K than indicated in Table 20.2 (14).

ABSORPTION, DISTRIBUTION, AND METABOLISM

Absorption of phylloquinone and the menaquinones requires bile and pancreatic juice for maximum effectiveness. Dietary vitamin K is absorbed in the small bowel, is incorporated into chylomicrons, and appears in the lymph. The efficiency of absorption varies widely depending on the source of the vitamin K and the vehicle in which it is administered and may be as low as 10% or as high as 80% (5). When isotopically labeled phylloquinone was administered to animals (16) or man by mouth in doses ranging from the physiologic to the pharmacologic, the vitamin appeared in the plasma within 20 minutes, peaked at 2 hours, and then declined exponentially to low values over 48 to 72 hours, reaching fasting levels of 1 to 2 nM (0.5–1.0 ng/mL). During this period, the vitamin K was transferred from chylomicron to chylomicron remnants. Vitamin K in these remnants can be taken up into hepatic, bone, and spleen cells. In the liver, some of the phylloquinone is stored, some oxidized to inactive end products, and some resecreted with very low density lipoprotein (VLDL), after which the phylloquinone appears in low-density lipoprotein (LDL) and high-density lipoprotein (HDL). In fasting persons, Kohlmeier et al. (16) found that approximately 50% of plasma phylloquinone is carried in the VLDL, about 25% in LDL, and about 25% in HDL.

Table 20.2
Estimated Versus Recommended Mean Dietary Intakes of Vitamin K_1 Stratified by Age and Gender

		Vitamin K_1 Intake (μg/day)	
Group	*N*	Estimate of 1990 TDS[a]	RDA[b]
Infants			
6 months	141	77	10
Children			
2 years	152	24	15
6 years	154	46	20
10 years	119	45	30
14–16 years			
Girls	188	52	45–55
Boys	174	64	45–65
Younger adults			
25–30 years			
Women	492	59	65
Men	386	66	80
40–45 years			
Women	319	71	65
Men	293	86	80
Older adults			
60–65 years			
Women	313	76	65
Men	238	80	80
70+ years			
Women	402	82	65
Men	263	80	80

From Booth SL, Pennington JAT, Sadowski JA. J Am Diet Assoc 1996;96:149–54, with permission.

[a]Total Diet Study (12).

[b]Recommended Dietary Allowance (96).

Between 8 and 30% of administered radioactive phylloquinone in animals and man (17) is recovered in the urine, and 45 to 60% of the administered dose is excreted in the feces over a 5-day period. One-third of the fecal radioactivity was unchanged vitamin K_1 and the remainder were oxidized products. Administration of nonabsorbable lipids, such as mineral oil or squalene, or malabsorption of fat because of disease of the bowel greatly reduces absorption of vitamin K (18).

In hyperlipidemias, the turnover of lipoproteins is reduced and transfer of vitamin K to tissues impaired. As a result, vitamin K levels are increased in fasting plasma. A mutant form of apolipoprotein E (E2), a component of chylomicron remnants that binds poorly to hepatic receptors, reduces the delivery of vitamin K to tissues (9). Similar observations have been made with respect to other hyperlipidemias (8).

The distribution of phylloquinone in the plasma of healthy adults has been studied by several investigators. Sadowski et al. (19) studied 326 fasting individuals: 131 ranged in age from 20 to 49 years, and 195 from 65 to 92 years. The range of phylloquinone concentrations was 0.29 to 2.64 nM (0.13–1.2 ng/mL). Age was not a significant variable. The raw data were skewed to the high side (median, 0.86 nM; mean, 1.01 nM), but the skewed curve was made to conform to a normal distribution by logarithmic transformation. Since the diet is a major determinant of the fasting phylloquinone level, values on the high side may reflect high intakes of phylloquinone and values on the low side may reflect low intakes of phylloquinone. It is difficult, however, to set a level that represents "vitamin K deficiency," since levels required to maintain normal levels of the coagulation factors are extremely low. Furthermore, the level required for maintenance of normal bone metabolism has not been determined. Similar data on plasma phylloquinone in normal humans were obtained by Shearer et al. (13).

As techniques for measuring vitamin K homologues improved, the high-molecular-weight menaquinones (MK-6, MK-7, and MK-8) as well as phylloquinone could be detected in plasma. In addition to MK-6, MK-7, and MK-8, even higher-molecular-weight menaquinones (MK-9 to MK-13) of bacterial origin *(Staphylococcus aureus, Bacteroides vulgatus, Bacillus subtilis,* and the actinomycetes) are absorbed from the terminal ileum and are found in the liver. Table 20.3 shows average values for phylloquinone and the menaquinones in plasma and liver. Early analysis (29) showed that phylloquinone made up about 50% of hepatic vitamin K, but more recent data show that

Table 20.3
Distribution of Vitamin K Homologues in Human Plasma and Liver (pmol/g)

	Plasma	Liver
K_1	1.24 ± 0.84	18 ± 9
MK-5		12 ± 8
MK-6		12 ± 13
MK-7	0.62 ± 0.39	71 ± 44
MK-8	0.71 ± 0.45	40 ± 54
MK-9		3 ± 2
MK-10		79 ± 32
MK-11		94 ± 39
MK-12		17 ± 7
MK-13		6 ± 3

Data from Suttie JW. Annu Rev Nutr 1995;15:399–417.

phylloquinone makes up only 10% of hepatic vitamin K (10, 16, 19).

Wiss et al. observed that the principal excretory metabolite of phylloquinone in the rat is a γ-lactone that appears to be excreted as a glucuronide. Vitamin K-2,3-epoxide has also been identified as a metabolite of vitamin K in animals and is metabolized to a homologous lactone (21, 22).

The turnover of vitamin K in the animal body is rapid, and the total body pool is surprisingly small. Bjornsson et al. (23) infused 300 μg of ^{3}H-phylloquinone into human volunteers with and/or without previous drug loading with warfarin or clofibrate. The initial half-time ($t_{1/2\alpha}$) for the first exponential phase was 26 ± 8 minutes, and the average terminal half-time ($t_{1/2\beta}$) was 166 ± 9 minutes under all conditions. Shearer et al. (24) obtained similar results with a 2.2-μmol (1.0-mg) intravenous dose of ^{3}H-phylloquinone in that $t_{1/2\alpha}$ equaled 20 to 24 minutes and $t_{1/2\beta}$ equaled 120 to 150 minutes. From data on the volume of distribution and clearance rate, Bjornsson et al. (25) calculated the turnover rate to be 0.4/hr, suggesting that the body pool turned over every 2.5 hours. More recently, Olson et al. (26), using 0.66 nmol (0.3 μg, 10 μCi) of ^{3}H-phylloquinone and longer periods of observation, reported that the phylloquinone pool turned over metabolically about once per day. From daily intakes of vitamin K of about 0.22 μmol/day (100 μg/day) and the turnover time of 24 hours, the body pool sizes were estimated to be 0.22 μmol (100 μg) or 3.1 nmol/kg (1.5 μg/kg) body weight. This body pool of vitamin K is smaller than that for vitamin B_{12} and is exceptionally low for a fat-soluble vitamin.

A rapid turnover of phylloquinone in humans is also supported by the studies of Usui et al. (10), who observed the changes in the concentration of plasma and hepatic phylloquinone in 22 surgical patients, half of whom were placed on a diet containing 5 μg of vitamin K for 3 days prior to surgery. During this period, plasma phylloquinone declined from 1.19 to 0.47 nM in patients on the low-K_1 diet and from 1.44 to 1.16 nM in those on the house diet. Liver biopsies showed that hepatic phylloquinone was 6.8 nM/kg on the low-K_1 diet, while the controls had a value of 28 nM/kg. Assuming a liver size of 1.2 kg, the authors calculated that during the time patients were on the low-K_1 diet, their total liver phylloquinone declined from 15 to 5 μg, or a fall of 66% in 3 days. A logarithmic plot of their data against time gives a $t_{1/2}$ of 1.5 days, in fairly good agreement with the findings of Olson et al. (26). Total menaquinones in the liver of patients before and after receiving the low-K_1 diet were not significantly changed (238 vs. 274 nmol/kg). Kindberg and Suttie (27) also observed a rapid turnover of phylloquinone in the livers of rats ($t_{1/2}$ = 24 h).

If the body pool is of the order of 3.1 nmol/kg (1.4 μg/kg) as calculated by Olson et al. (26), about 80 μg would be present in the patients studied by Usui et al. (10). If, further, only 15 μg (less than 20%) is present in the liver, the remaining body phylloquinone must be distributed among all the tissues containing γ-glutamyl carboxylase. Hodges et al. (28) measured the vitamin K content of bone with respect to both phylloquinone and menaquinones and found levels as high as those in liver. Since bones make up 8.6% of the body weight (about four times that of the liver), it follows that about 60 μg of vitamin K (75%) would be found in the skeletal system, and the remaining 7% would, no doubt, be found in other tissues containing γ-glutamyl carboxylases.

When menadione (2-methyl-1,4-naphthoquinone) is administered to animals or man, only a small amount (0.05–1.0%) is converted to MK-4 (29). The principal metabolites of menadione are the sulfate and glucuronide of dihydromenadione. The claim that phylloquinone may be converted to MK-4 in animal tissues is based on indirect evidence (30) and requires further study.

PHYSIOLOGIC FUNCTION

Regulation of Clotting-Protein Synthesis

The seven vitamin K–dependent coagulation proteins shown in Table 20.4 (with one exception, protein S) are proenzymes that are converted to serine proteases during coagulation. All require calcium for activation, a phenomenon mediated by their γ-carboxyglutamate residues. The

Table 20.4
Characteristics of the Vitamin K–Dependent Coagulation Proenzymes

	Factor				Protein		
Characteristic	II	X	IX	VII	C	S	Z
Plasma concentration (μg/L)	100	10	3	1	5	25	3
Molecular weight (kDa)	71.6	58.8	56.8	50.0	62.0	70.7	62.0
Carbohydrate (%)	8	15	17	13	11	8	10
Number of chains	1	2	1	1	2	1	1
Number of Gla residues	10	11	12	10	9	11	13

Data from references 1, 22, 33.

vitamin K–dependent procoagulant factors (II, VII, IX, and X) form the core of the proteolytic cascade leading to fibrin formation in hemostasis as shown in Figure 20.3. The intrinsic system, which is operative within the circulation, is activated by surface-mediated reactions involving high-molecular-weight kininogen and prekallikrein. They initiate a series of reactions that result in activation of factor XII to XIIa, the activation of XI to XIa, and the conversion of factor X to Xa. The extrinsic system, which is switched on by cell injury, requires tissue factor (TF, 46 kDa), which is an intrinsic membrane glycoprotein tightly associated with phospholipid. TF also has a high affinity for plasma factor VII, which it converts to factor VIIa. The factor VIIa-TF complex then converts factor X to Xa by limited proteolysis.

The final common pathway begins with the prothrombinase complex (factor Xa, Va, calcium, and phospholipid) on the platelet membrane that converts prothrombin (factor II) to thrombin (IIa), which in turn converts fibrinogen to fibrin. Two cofactors not dependent on vitamin K, factor VIII (the antihemophilic globulin) and factor V (accelerator globulin), are important in the middle stages of the cascade. Factor V is a peptide (290 kDa) that is cleaved by thrombin to factor Va, a carbohydrate-rich two-chain fragment (163 kDa). Factor VIII is a glycoprotein (330 kDa) that circulates in a complex with von Willebrand factor and is also cleaved to yield a two-chain VIIIa (140 kDa).

Protein C is an anticoagulant that serves as a brake on the speed of the intrinsic cascade through a feedback loop involving thrombin. When thrombin is made from prothrombin, thrombomodulin, a 75-kDa thrombin receptor on the surface of endothelial cells, combines with thrombin. As a result, the affinity of thrombin for fibrinogen, factor V, and platelets is reduced and its affinity for protein C is increased, which results in the activation of protein C. Activated protein C_a inhibits factors VIIIa and Va and the conversion of prothrombin to thrombin, thus slowing its own production. A recently discovered mutation in factor V (Leiden) in some persons prevents activation of protein C, which can lead to thrombosis (31). Protein S, another vitamin K–dependent protein, enhances the activity of protein C_a in the presence of phospholipid. This system normally provides feedback control and balance in the coagulation cascade. The other antagonist to thrombin is antithrombin III (58 kDa), for

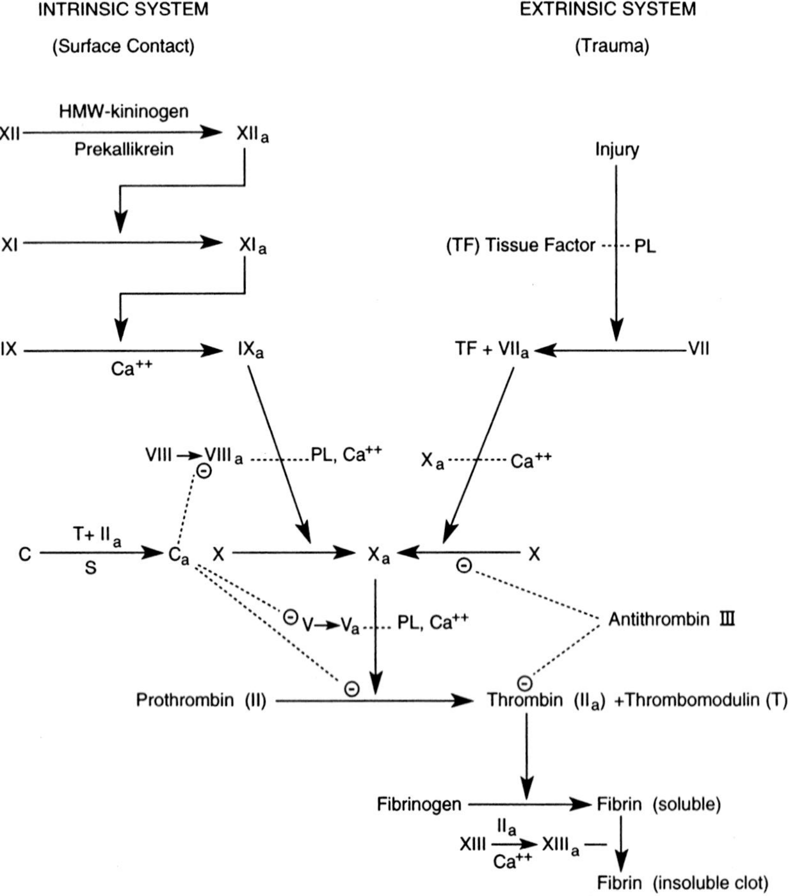

Figure 20.3. The clotting factor cascade. Factors II, VII, IX, and X and proteins C and S contain Gla and are vitamin K dependent. The first four factors occupy the core of the clotting scheme; protein C is an anticoagulant protein that inactivates factors Va and VIIIa and inhibits the conversion of factor II to IIa. Protein S is a cofactor for protein C and enhances its rate of activation by thrombin. Thrombomodulin further enhances the activation of protein C by thrombin. Antithrombin III also inhibits the intrinsic cascade. Ca^{2+} is required to activate Gla-containing factors. Factors V (accelerator globulin) and VIII (antihemophilic globulin) are cofactors. Factor XIII is a transpeptidase.

which heparan sulfate in the endothelium is a cofactor. Antithrombin III has a wide spectrum of antiprotease activities inhibiting thrombin as well as coagulation factors XIIa, XIa, IXa, and Xa.

Clearly, the coagulation cascade is tightly regulated by both procoagulants and anticoagulants, some of which are vitamin K dependent. Because most vitamin K–dependent coagulation factors are synthesized in the liver, hepatectomy (or severe liver disease) results in lowered plasma levels of these factors and reduced renal sensitivity to administration of vitamin K. Kemkes-Matthis and Matthis recently reported that protein Z promotes the association of thrombin with phospholipid surfaces (32). They observed that protein Z is not synthesized in patients with severe liver disease, which may contribute to the hemorrhage suffered by such patients.

All the genes that code for the seven vitamin K–dependent plasma coagulation factors have been cloned, and the complementary DNA (cDNA) sequences have been determined for all but protein Z (33). The size, composition, and location of each gene are shown in Table 20.5. Typical of the genes for vitamin K–dependent proteins is the gene for prothrombin, which is located on chromosome 11 at p11-q12. It is approximately 24 kilobases long and contains 13 introns (which are not translated) and 14 exons. The messenger RNA (mRNA) for prothrombin is about 2000 nucleotides long and contains a noncoding region of 97 base pairs and a poly A tail of 27 base pairs. As shown in Figure 20.4, mature prothrombin contains 579 amino acids and three carbohydrate chains at residues 78, 100, and 373, accounting for 8.2% of the 71.6-kDa molecule. As synthesized, however, prothrombin has a 43-amino acid leader sequence containing both signal and propeptide residues. The prosegment, which contains 18 amino acids, is the recognition site for the γ-glutamyl carboxylase and is similar in sequence to prosegments in other vitamin K–dependent proteins.

Table 20.5
Genes of Vitamin K–Dependent Proteins and Their Chromosome Locations

Factor	Gene (kb)	Exons	Introns	Chromosome
II	21	14	13	11
VII	13	8	7	13
IX	34	8	7	X
X	25	8	7	13
C	11	9	8	2
S	80	15	14	3

Data from Reiner AP, Davie EW. Introduction to hemostasis and the vitamin K–dependent coagulation factors. In: Scriver CR, Beaudet AL, Sly WS, Valle D, eds. The metabolic and molecular bases of inherited disease. 7th ed. New York: McGraw-Hill 1995;3181–221.

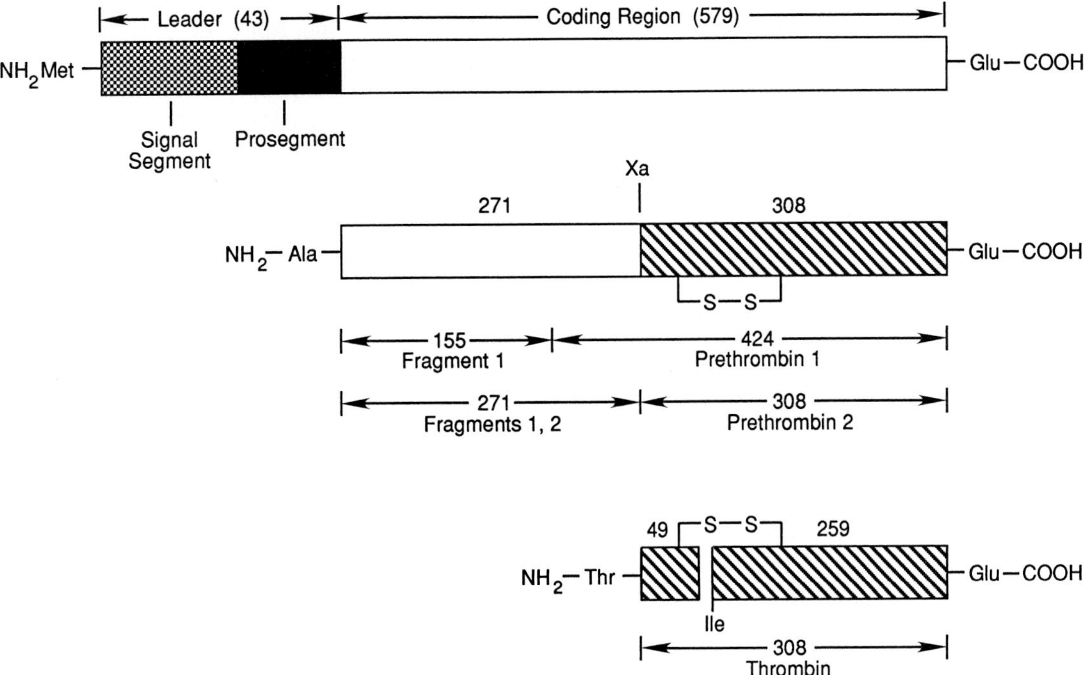

Figure 20.4. Structure of human prothrombin. A linear model of the nascent peptide is shown at the *top*. It has three components, a signal segment of 25 amino acids, a basic prosegment of 18 amino acids *(in black),* and a coding portion of 579 amino acids. The signal segment is cleaved by a signal peptidase on the luminal side of the rough endoplasmic reticulum (RER). After carboxylation of 10 N-terminal Gla residues in the mature peptide, the prosegment is cleaved in the Golgi apparatus before secretion. The *second linear drawing* shows the mature prothrombin secreted into plasma, which has an N-terminal alanine and a C-terminal glutamic acid. The thrombin portion is *crosshatched.* Prothrombin is split at arginine 271 by activated factor X to generate prethrombin-2, which is converted into an active two-chain, disulfide-linked thrombin by a second factor X_a clip at arginine 320. The thrombin formed autocatalytically splits prothrombin and fragment 1,2 at arginine 156 to yield prethrombin-1 and fragments 1 and 2. The 10 Gla residues in fragment 1 are at positions 7, 8, 15, 17, 20, 21, 26, 27, 30, and 33, and the carbohydrate moieties are at positions 78, 100, and 373.

Vitamin K–Dependent γ-Glutamyl Carboxylase

The vitamin K–dependent γ-glutamyl carboxylase is a membrane-bound component of the endoplasmic reticulum. It has been solubilized (34, 35) by various detergents and, in the soluble form, retains most of the properties of the microsomal system. The system requires a Glu-containing peptide substrate, O_2, CO_2, and either vitamin K plus NADH (the reduced form of nicotinamide adenine dinucleotide) or a vitamin K hydroquinone. CO_2, not HCO_3^-, is the active form of carbon dioxide incorporated into the γ-carboxyl group of peptide-bound glutamate (Gla_p) (36). Adenosine triphosphate (ATP) is not required, and biotin is not involved. Reduced vitamin K functions as a cosubstrate in the carboxylation reaction, but also as a cofactor because it is regenerated by two reductases in separate reactions. The overall carboxylation reaction is

$$KH_2 + O_2 + CO_2 + Glu_p \xrightarrow{Mn^{2+}} KO + Gla_p + H_2O$$

Under physiologic conditions, the oxidation of KH_2 to KO (vitamin K-2,3 epoxide) is coupled to the fixation of CO_2 in the γ position of peptide-bound glutamate to form Gla_p. Coupling depends upon the availability of CO_2 in the reaction mixture; in its absence, the enzyme functions as an epoxidase. The K_m for bicarbonate is between 0.2 and 0.4 mM (about 1% of the bicarbonate concentration in the plasma), in equilibrium with 0.01 to 0.02 mM CO_2 at intracellular pH. The rate of γ-carboxylation in vitro is conveniently measured by adding $H^{14}CO_3^-$ to the reaction medium and determining the radioactivity incorporated into peptide-bound glutamic acid. Artificial substrates such as Phe-Leu-Glu-Glu-Leu are CO_2 acceptors in this reaction, although at much higher concentrations than the physiologic substrates.

Efforts to purify the vitamin K–dependent γ-glutamyl carboxylase began in 1974 in several laboratories. By 1987, the best purification of the carboxylase from liver microsomes was 400 times. In 1989, Hubbard et al. (37) claimed they had purified the vitamin K–dependent carboxylase (77 kDa) to homogeneity (about 10,000 times from bovine microsomes) using synthetic propeptides as affinity columns, but alas, this carboxylase preparation was later shown to be extensively contaminated with a ubiquitous microsomal binding protein (BiP) also known as GRP-78.

In 1991, Wu et al. (38) reported purification of the γ-glutamyl carboxylase (94 kDa) to near homogeneity (about 70,000 times from bovine microsomes) by affinity chromatography and shortly thereafter cloned the human gene for the carboxylase (39). Starting with a nucleotide coding for a 37-amino acid sequence from the bovine γ-glutamyl carboxylase, these investigators screened a cDNA library from bovine liver and found three partial clones. An *Eco*RI cDNA fragment of 280 bp from the bovine library was then used to screen a human erythroleukemia (HEL) cDNA library, and one clone of the gene for the human carboxylase with an internal *Eco*RI site was obtained.

Several observations indicate that the entire coding sequence was contained within that cDNA: *(a)* the methionine identified as the first amino acid is the only in-frame methionine between a stop codon 27 nucleotides upstream and the first tryptic peptide 195 nucleotides downstream; *(b)* the open reading frame codes for 758 amino acids and predicts a molecular weight of 87,542, which, if one takes into account that the protein is glycosylated, agrees with the 94 kDa estimated by its mobility in SDS-polyacrylamide gel electrophoresis; and *(c)* the cDNA codes for functional carboxylase in mammalian cells.

The enzyme activity coded for by the human cDNA was expressed in human kidney 293 cells using the vector pCMV5 with/without the enzyme cDNA. Forty-eight hours after transfection, cells were harvested, microsomes prepared, and γ-glutamyl carboxylase activity determined by standard techniques using $^{14}CO_2$ and phe-leu-glu-glu-leu (FLEEL) as substrates. Under all conditions, including activation by $(NH_4)_2SO_4$ and a 19-residue peptide from profactor IX, the microsomes programed by enzyme cDNA resulted in an increase in activity of 9- to 27-fold over the mock-transfected cells.

In 1992, Berkner et al. (40) reported the isolation of a γ-glutamyl carboxylase with high activity and an apparent molecular mass of 98 kDa measured on SDS-polyacrylamide gels. In the same year, Kuliopulos et al. (41) reported that by use of the affinity label *N*-bromoacetyl-FLEEL-[^{125}IY] for the carboxylase, the molecular mass of 94 kDa was confirmed. It is likely that the enzyme isolated by Berkner et al. (40), alleged to have a molecular mass of 98 kDa (a 4% error in estimation), is identical with the carboxylase first isolated by Wu et al. (38), but cloning and functional analysis of the 98-kDa protein will be necessary to prove it.

The nucleotide sequence of the human γ-glutamyl carboxylase gene is 88% homologous to the gene for the bovine carboxylase (42), which also has a 758-amino acid reading frame. Eight of nine potential *N*-glycosylation sites are in the hydrophilic carboxyl-terminal half of the carboxylase, which projects into the lumen of the endoplasmic reticulum. There is a minimum of three hydrophobic transmembrane sites in the N-terminal portion of the protein and maybe as many as seven. The carboxylase and soybean lipoxygenase share 19.3% identity over a space of 198 amino acids from residues 468 to 666 (38).

In 1995, Roth et al. (43) produced a series of mutants of recombinant γ-glutamyl carboxylase with progressively larger COOH-terminal deletions. Recombinant wild type (residues 1–758) and mutants of the carboxylase terminating at residues 711, 676, and 572 were expressed in baculovirus-infected Sf9 cells. The kinetic behavior of mutant carboxylase, Cbx 711, was unchanged from the wild type. The mutant Cbx 676, however, retained a normal propeptide binding site, but the K_m for KH_2 had risen 23-fold and rate of epoxidase activity had fallen to 10%. The shortest mutant, Cbx 572, lacked both carboxylation and epoxidation activities. These results suggest that all but 47 residues at the C-terminal end contribute to the enzymatic activity of γ-glutamyl carboxylase.

Finally, Wu et al. (44), by using chemical cross-linking reactions, limited trypsin digestion, and polyclonal antibodies against synthetic polypeptides, localized the propeptide binding site on the lumenal lipoxygenase-like domain of γ-glutamyl carboxylase. Their limited tryptic digestion resulted in a 60-kDa C-terminal peptide and a 30-kDa N-terminal peptide joined by a disulfide bond. A tryptic fragment that cross-links to the propeptide substrate is immunochemically specific to the 60-kDa portion. They conclude that the propeptide binding site lies carboxyl-terminal to residue 438.

Thus, the location of the active site on the γ-glutamyl carboxylase is currently controversial. All laboratories have identified a range of sites from residues 218 to 676 that contribute to the overall activity of the carboxylase. The location of cysteines required for activity, however, is still unsolved. Figure 20.5 presents a hypothesis that might account for these disparate findings. The N-terminal end of the molecule is clearly the zone of the transmembrane segments. Figure 20.5 shows five such segments, although the incomplete data support a range of three to seven such segments. The C-terminal end clearly projects into the lumen where the carboxylation occurs, and the present data indicate that only the terminal 47 residues are dispensable. It is likely that the C-terminal portion folds to provide an area of confluence of several residues necessary for γ-glutamyl carboxylation. Since epoxidation is required for carboxylation, these reactions must be linked around a single active site. Finally, it must border the membrane because of the lipid solubility of vitamin K.

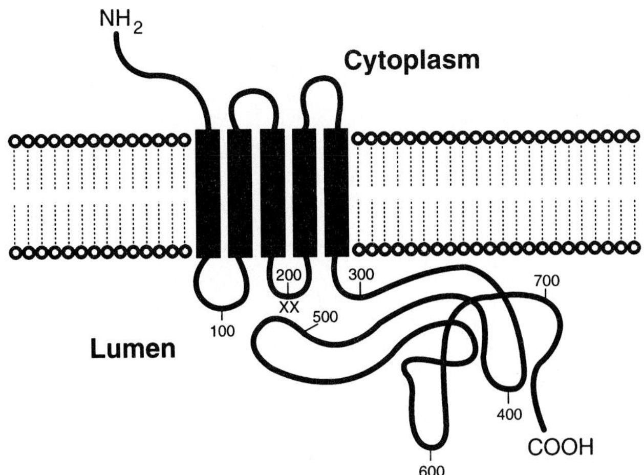

Figure 20.5. A proposed cellular location of γ-glutamyl carboxylase. Several N-terminal transmembrane segments of the enzyme span the membrane of the endoplasmic reticulum (ER) and then project into the lumen where carboxylation of peptide-bound glutamate occurs. Attempts to localize the "active site" of this enzyme have led to the view that most of the C-terminal part of the enzyme contributes residues to a cooperative site that is near the lumenal membrane.

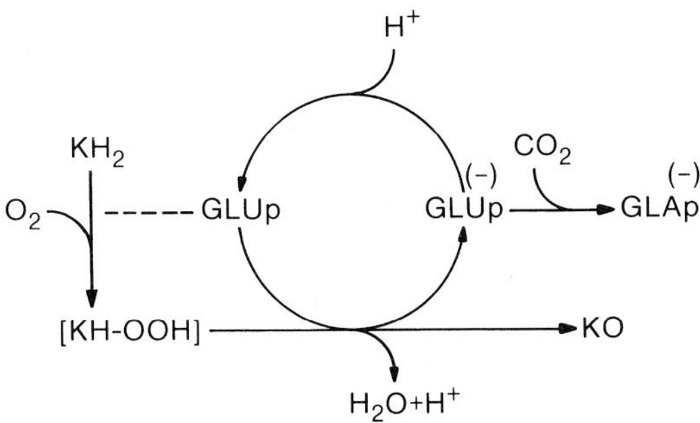

Figure 20.6. Mechanism for the coupling of carboxylation and epoxidation in vitamin K–dependent Gla synthesis. *KH_2*, vitamin K hydroquinone; *KH-OOH*, vitamin K hydroperoxide (which rearranges to an alkoxide moiety); *KO*, vitamin K-2,3-epoxide; *GLUp*, peptide-bound glutamate; *GLAp*, peptide-bound γ-carboxyglutamate.

The biochemical mechanism of the vitamin K–dependent carboxylation is still under study. A mechanism proposed by Larson and Suttie for the coupling of carboxylation and epoxidation in the vitamin K–dependent carboxylase is shown in Figure 20.6 (45). The reaction is presented as an ordered mechanism with three partial reactions. The first event is the combination of the enzyme with KH_2 and O_2 to yield a ternary enzyme-substrate complex that forms KHOOH, a hydroperoxide of vitamin K hydroquinone. This was initially visualized as the product of a reaction with oxygen at position 2 of the naphthoquinone ring, although now it appears that the initial attack is on the 1-carbon. This step is inhibited competitively by chlorophylloquinone and tetrachloropyridinol. The propeptide binds to the enzyme and provides the substrate for proton abstraction. Epoxidation can occur in the absence of peptide and CO_2, but peptide addition stimulates carboxylation and enhances epoxidation.

Larson and Suttie (45) proposed that the hypothetical vitamin K-hydroperoxy anion was sufficiently basic to remove the γ-methylene proton from peptide-bound glutamate. Olson's group, however, argued that the organic hydroperoxy anion was insufficiently basic ($pK_a = 9$) to remove a proton from the γ-methylene group and suggested an inductive mechanism for the labilization of the γ-methylene proton (46). On the basis of the study of a model system, Dowd and Ham suggested that the oxygen addition to reduced vitamin K results in formation of an extremely basic epoxy alkoxide anion ($pK_a = 27$) (47). This phenomenon, known as *base strength amplification,* provides a base of sufficient strength to remove a proton from the γ-carbon of peptide-bound glutamate. The proposed sequence of metabolic steps is shown in Figure 20.7. The first postulated step is ionization of the hydroquinone to give vitamin KH^-, followed by reaction with oxygen to form a peroxide that in turn rearranges via the K-dioxetane to the alkoxide. After removal of a proton from the γ position of peptide-bound glutamate, vitamin K-2,3-epoxide and water are formed.

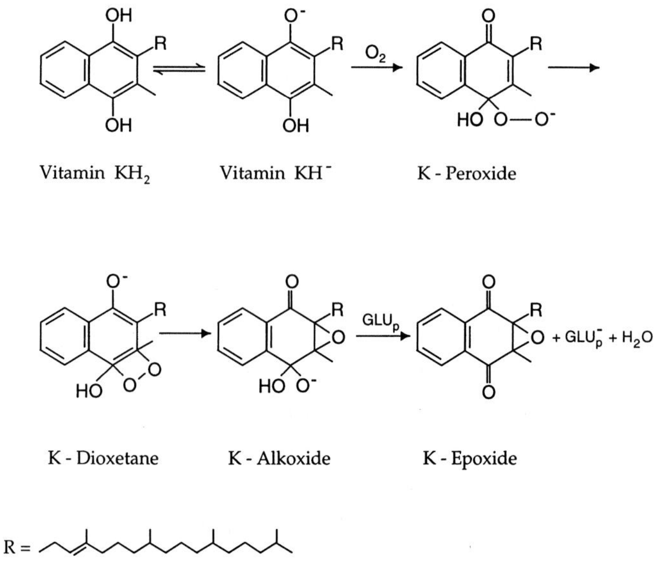

Vitamin KH_2 Vitamin KH^- K - Peroxide

K - Dioxetane K - Alkoxide K - Epoxide

R =

Figure 20.7. Proposed intermediates in the rearrangement of the initial vitamin K peroxide derivative to "achieve base amplification" and promote proton abstraction from peptide-bound glutamate.

Vitamin K Cycle

The vitamin K cycle is shown in Figure 20.8. In essence it is a salvage pathway for vitamin K, a vitamin present in only nanomolar quantities in liver and other tissues. In this cycle, vitamin K-2,3-epoxide, a product of the carboxylation reaction, is reduced to the quinone by a dithiol-dependent epoxide reductase. The regenerated vitamin K is then reduced to vitamin K hydroquinone by one of several enzymes, at least one driven by a dithiol and several by reduced forms of NADPH. The dithiol-dependent reductases for both the epoxide and the quinone are strongly inhibited by warfarin; the NADPH-dependent dehydrogenases are relatively insensitive to warfarin (48). The net effect of the cycle is the conversion of vitamin K-2,3-epoxide formed in the carboxylation reaction to vitamin K hydroquinone, which becomes available as a substrate for another round of carboxylation. In this way, vitamin K acts catalytically for Gla synthesis. Because of the low level of vitamin K in tissues and the relatively low intake of vitamin K (~60–100 μg/day), the cycle is vital to maintain the integrity of the vitamin K system.

Adult humans excrete about 40 μmoles of γ-carboxyglutamic acid (Gla) per day. Gla is liberated during the catabolism of K-dependent proteins and appears in the urine unchanged. For every mole of Gla formed in the body, 1 mole of vitamin K must be converted to its 2,3-epoxide. Since the daily intake of vitamin K is normally about 0.22 μmol (100 μg) per day, it follows that the cycle must make 200 revolutions per day under usual conditions. If, on the other hand, vitamin K intake is reduced to 0.01 μmol (5 μg) per day, the cycle must make 4000 revolutions per day to maintain normal Gla synthesis in K-dependent proteins. The K_m of γ-glutamyl carboxylase for KH_2 must be of the order of 10 nM in vivo to accomplish Gla synthesis under conditions of minimum intake of vitamin K and much below the K_m of 20 to 30 μM reported for the purified carboxylase.

Differences in vitamin K requirements may have more to do with the integrity of the vitamin K cycle than metabolic transformations of vitamin K. The difference between the requirements for vitamin K in the rat and

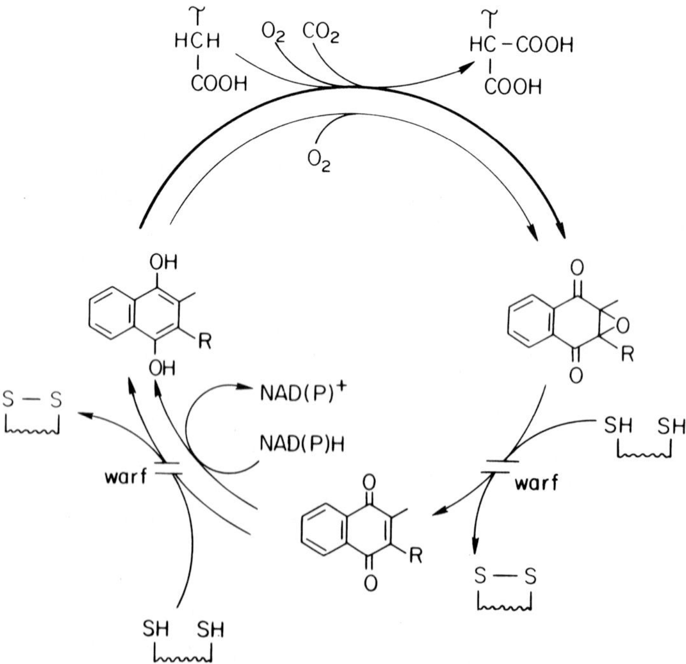

Figure 20.8. The vitamin K cycle occurs in the hepatic endoplasmic reticulum. Carboxylation and epoxidation are catalyzed by the same enzyme. The dithiol-dependent reductions of vitamin K epoxide and vitamin K are extremely sensitive to the action of coumarin anticoagulants such as warfarin (warf). NADPH-dependent dehydrogenases are not inhibited by warfarin.

chick (which is higher) is due to the activity of the vitamin K cycle (49).

Bone and Kidney Proteins Containing γ-Carboxyglutamate

Two vitamin K–dependent bone proteins have been discovered in the last 20 years. The first is bone Gla protein (BGP, or osteocalcin) secreted by osteoblasts and discovered independently by Hauschka et al. (50) and Price et al. (51) in 1975. The second is the matrix Gla protein (MGP) discovered in bone, dentin, and cartilage by Price et al. in 1985 (52). BGP, a water-soluble 49-residue protein with a molecular weight of 5700, contains three Gla residues at positions 17, 21, and 24 and one disulfide bond.

BGP is one of the most abundant noncollagenous proteins in bone, accounting for 15 to 20% of noncollagen proteins in most vertebrates, and appears to be derived from osteoblasts. The concentration in bone is about 5 mg/g. Small amounts of BGP are found in plasma: about 8 ng/mL in men and 5 ng/mL in women. These values are increased in patients with metabolic bone disease (53). In vitro, BGP binds strongly to hydroxyapatite and inhibits its formation. Both of these properties are lost when the Gla residues are decarboxylated. The nascent peptide of BGP contains a 23-residue leader sequence, a 26-residue propeptide, and, as indicated, a 49-residue mature protein that is not homologous with the coagulation proteins. The 26-residue propeptide, however, appears to serve as the recognition site for the γ-glutamyl carboxylase.

BGP occurs in both fully carboxylated and undercarboxylated (ucBGP) forms in plasma, which presumably represents the state of BGP in bone. Knapen et al. (54) compared the BGP concentration in pre- and postmenopausal women. They found that although the total immunoreactive BGP was the same in both groups, the hydroxyapatite-binding capacity (HAB) was 80 to 100% in normal young women but significantly reduced in older women (~50%). Both groups were given vitamin K_1 (1 mg per os), and BGP was measured 14 days later. In the postmenopausal group, vitamin K increased the level and the HAB capacity of BGP, decreased calcium excretion, and caused a decrease in urinary hydroxyproline excretion. Hodges et al. (55) observed depressed levels of both phylloquinone and menaquinones in the plasma of patients with osteoporotic fractures of the spine and femoral neck. Phylloquinone was reduced from a normal value of 1.1 to 0.21 nM (0.5–0.1 ng/mL), and the menaquinones (MK-7 and MK-8) from 0.70 to 0.06 nM (0.45–0.04 ng/mL). Hodges et al. (56) observed a fall in both plasma and bone levels of phylloquinone and menaquinones in elderly women with hip fracture.

MGP is a 79-residue protein with a molecular weight of 8700 that contains Gla residues at position 2, 37, 41, 48, and 52. It is only 20% homologous with BGP and has different properties, being highly insoluble in neutral salt solutions. This insolubility reflects a strong tendency to self-associate. MGP is found in the organic matrix of bone, dentine, and cartilage and does not react with hydroxyapatite. The nascent peptide of MGP contains a 19-residue signal sequence but no propeptide. It does, however, have an internal sequence of amino acids in the mature protein from residues 15 to 30 that is homologous with the propeptide in the other vitamin K–dependent proteins. This sequence appears to serve as the recognition site for the γ-glutamyl carboxylase (53).

Protein S, a cofactor for protein C, is also synthesized in osteoblasts and plays an undefined role in bone metabolism. Protein S, unlike the other vitamin K–dependent coagulation factors, does not yield a protease on limited proteolysis. In fact, its C-terminal portion resembles a steroid-binding protein. Children with inherited protein S deficiency not only suffer from the complications of thrombosis, but also have osteopenia with reduced mineral density and even vertebral compression fractures (57).

Microsomes from embryonic chick bone contain a vitamin K–dependent γ-glutamyl carboxylase that can carboxylate endogenous bone protein and Glu-containing pentapeptides (58). Warfarin inhibits the synthesis of both BGP and MGP. Unlike the coagulation proteins synthesized in the liver, however, vitamin K does not overcome the effect of warfarin on BGP and MGP synthesis (53). This appears to result from the lack of an NADP-linked reductase for vitamin K in bone tissue. This nonresponsiveness of bone tissue to vitamin K in animals on warfarin permits study of the role of the vitamin K–dependent proteins in bone without risk of hemorrhage. Synthesis of both BGP and MGP, furthermore, is regulated by 1,25-dihydroxyvitamin D_3 in cultured osteosarcoma cells (59). More recently, it has been demonstrated that both retinoic acid receptors and vitamin D hormone receptors may form heterodimers that bind to the osteocalcin promoter in MCF-7 cells (60). This permits a synergy between retinoic acid and 1,25-dihydroxyvitamin D_1 in cultured osteocarcinoma cells. These findings suggest that BGP and MGP mediate some actions of vitamin D on bone. Although the present data show that deficiency of BGP does not affect bone structure repairs or fractures, plasma BGP is elevated in metabolic bone disease (53). It is concluded that BGP may stimulate bone remodeling and mobilization of calcium, whereas MGP is associated with the inhibition of growth-plate mineralization.

Several cases of the Conradi-Hünermann teratogenic type of chondrodysplasia punctata were reported in infants born to mothers taking warfarin during the first trimester (61). This defect appears to result from a deficiency of BGP and MGP during embryogenesis.

At present it is known that γ-glutamyl carboxylase occurs in liver, bone, cartilage, dentin, kidney, placenta, pancreas, spleen, lung, testis, smooth muscle, fibroblasts, atherosclerotic plaques, and a wide variety of tumor cells (62). All of these extrahepatic Gla-proteins appear to resemble the bone type more than the liver type.

COUMARIN ANTICOAGULANT DRUGS

The coumarin anticoagulant agents (Fig. 20.9) inhibit the biosynthesis of prothrombin and other vitamin K–dependent factors in the liver and others in extrahepatic tissues and thus cause factor deficiencies in the plasma and elsewhere. Bell and Matschiner (63) first proposed that warfarin inhibited the vitamin K epoxide reductase and prevented the operation of the vitamin K cycle, a view that has been extensively confirmed. The S(2) enantiomer of warfarin is five times more active than the R(+) enantiomer and binds more intensely to vitamin K epoxide reductase (64). The dithiothreitol (DTT)-driven vitamin KO reductase is not the only reductase blocked by warfarin; a similar DTT-dependent vitamin K reductase also is inhibited (65). This combined attack by coumarin anticoagulants reduces KH2 to ineffective levels and stops carboxylation. The warfarin receptor, first described by Searcey et al. (66) in pharmacologic studies, has been identified as the vitamin K epoxide reductase (67). The DTT-driven vitamin K reductase has a very low Km compared with the NADPH-dependent vitamin, and under physiologic conditions is the pathway used. DTT is used in the laboratory as a reductant for the vitamin KO reductase, but several physiologic dithiols may serve as reductants including thioredoxin, reduced lipoic acid, and a protein disulfide isomerase (132). It is somewhat surprising that the vitamin KO reductase has never been isolated and characterized.

Overdosage can occur in patients who receive coumarin drugs to prevent thrombosis in coronary artery disease or pulmonary embolic disease. Intravenous administration of pharmacologic doses of vitamin K_1 reinitiates prothrombin and other vitamin K–dependent factor synthesis in the liver within minutes by bypassing the blocked DTT-dependent vitamin K reductase in the liver. As noted above, this does not occur in bone. Water-soluble derivatives of menadione (e.g., Synkayvite) are largely ineffective against the coumarin anticoagulant drugs because, as mentioned above, the rate conversion to MK-4 is so slow that pharmacologically effective levels of the alkylated vitamin are not obtained.

VITAMIN K DEFICIENCY

Primary vitamin K deficiency is uncommon in healthy adults. Several factors protect adults from a lack of vitamin K: *(a)* widespread distribution of vitamin K in plant and animal tissues, *(b)* the vitamin K cycle, which conserves the vitamin, and *(c)* the microbiologic flora of the normal gut, which synthesizes menaquinones that can contribute to the requirement for vitamin K, although the exact contribution is still uncertain. On the other hand, vitamin K deficiency in the breast-fed newborn remains a major worldwide cause of infant morbidity and mortality (68). Reduced levels of the vitamin K–dependent coagulation factors in adults are largely secondary to disease or drug therapy. Bleeding is the major manifestation of vitamin K deficiency, whether the cause is genetic deletion, inadequate dietary intake, or antagonism of vitamin K by drugs. Easy bruisability and mucosal bleeding (especially epistaxis, gastrointestinal hemorrhage, menorrhagia, and hematuria) occur in vitamin K deficiency. Blood may ooze from puncture sites or incisions following trauma, and life-threatening intracranial hemorrhage can occur in infants.

The gene for γ-glutamyl carboxylase is located on chromosome 2 (69). The rare hereditary lack of all the vitamin K–dependent coagulation factors, which is presumed to be due to lack of the carboxylase, has been described in seven patients in the world literature. The victims of this genetic disorder demonstrate all of the signs of vitamin K deficiency.

The causes of acquired vitamin K deficiency are discussed below.

Hemorrhagic Disease of the Newborn

Newborn infants represent a special case of vitamin K nutrition because *(a)* the placenta is a relatively poor organ for the transmission of lipids, *(b)* the neonatal liver is immature with respect to prothrombin synthesis, *(c)* breast milk is low in vitamin K, and *(d)* the infant gut is sterile during the first few days of life. As a result, a sizable number of infants develop hemorrhagic disease of the newborn (HDN). In normal infants, plasma concentrations of prothrombin and the other vitamin K–dependent factors are about 20% of adult values at birth, and they rise slowly to adult values at 3 weeks if vitamin K intake is adequate. If prothrombin values fall below 10%, HDN appears. HDN generally occurs 1 to 7 days postpartum and may be manifested by cutaneous, gastrointestinal, intrathoracic, or, in

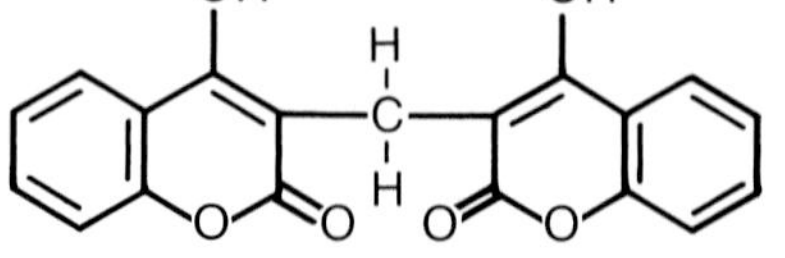

DICUMAROL 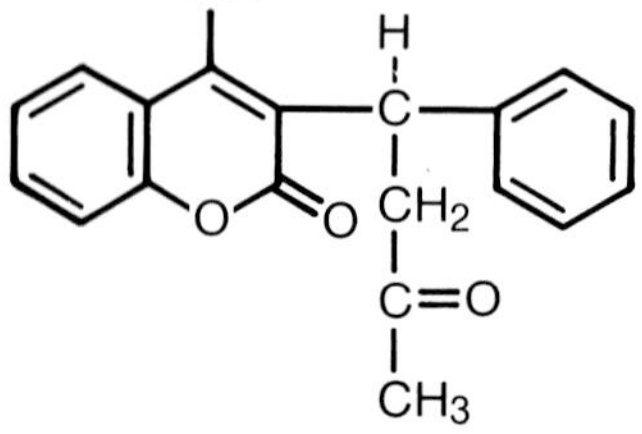 WARFARIN

Figure 20.9. Structures of two 4-hydroxycoumarin drugs.

the worst cases, intracranial bleeding. Late hemorrhagic disease (LHD) occurs 1 to 3 months postpartum and has the same clinical manifestations as HDN. It is usually associated with malabsorption or liver disease. If the mother has ingested hydantoin anticonvulsants, cephalosporin antibiotics, or coumarin anticoagulants, the incidence of all types of HDN is increased. About 30% of full-term infants have descarboxyprothrombin (PIVKA II) in their plasma during the first week of life (70). The level of phylloquinone in the plasma of newborn infants is less than 0.22 nM (0.1 ng/mL). As food is taken, the levels gradually climb to normal adult values over a period of weeks. Some infants, however, who are breast-fed and who have received no prophylactic vitamin K at birth develop late HDN during the 3rd to the 8th weeks of life (68). These infants may have some abnormality of liver function in addition to low vitamin K levels. In any event, they require intensive vitamin K therapy. Premature infants are even more susceptible to vitamin K deficiency than are full-term ones. Because the requirement for vitamin K in the newborn is estimated to be 11.1 nmol/day (5 μg/day), the very low content of vitamin K in human milk (2.2 to 4.4 nM [1–2 μg/L]) accounts for the predisposition of breast-fed infants to develop the hemorrhagic syndrome (71). Because breast milk is sterile and delays colonization of the gut with bacteria, it is recommended that breast-fed babies receive 2.2 μmol (1 mg) of phylloquinone (AquaMEPHYTON) intramuscularly at birth.

Infants of mothers on hydantoin anticonvulsants should have prophylactic vitamin K because diphenylhydantoin is an antagonist to vitamin K (72). Neonatal complications such as diarrhea, malabsorption, cystic fibrosis, idiopathic cholestasis, atresia of the bile duct, and prolonged parenteral nutrition are all indications for intramuscular or intravenous vitamin K administration to infants.

Dietary Inadequacy

Healthy adult subjects fed low–vitamin K diets (11–89 nmol/day; 5–40 μg/day) for several weeks demonstrate a fall in plasma vitamin K levels from 2.2 to 1.1 nM (1.0 to 0.5 ng/mL) but no significant change in plasma prothrombin values. In unusual cases, self-imposed dietary restriction may induce hypoprothrombinemia with hemorrhage responsive to oral vitamin K. Dietary deficiency of vitamin K is manifested more quickly following surgery and in debilitated patients, with or without antibiotics (73).

In protein-calorie malnutrition, amino acid deprivation may cause hypoprothrombinemia that is not responsive to vitamin K but that does respond to protein feeding. Aging per se does not seem to increase the vitamin K requirement or alter the vitamin K cycle (14).

Total Parenteral Nutrition

With the advent of subclavian vein catheterization in 1968 for long-term total parenteral nutrition (TPN) of both surgical and medical patients unable to eat, new nutritional deficiency syndromes have been reported, including hemorrhage due to vitamin K deficiency. It is advisable to give doses of 2.2 μmol (1 mg) of phylloquinone per week (equivalent to about 0.3 μmol, or 150 μg, of vitamin K per day) to patients on TPN.

Malabsorption Syndrome

Depression of the vitamin K–dependent coagulation factors is frequently found in the malabsorption syndromes and in other gastrointestinal disorders (e.g., biliary obstruction, cystic fibrosis, sprue, celiac disease, ulcerative colitis, regional ileitis, and short bowel syndrome) (74). Severe abnormalities of coagulation with extensive bleeding are common in biliary obstruction, but they do occur with sufficient frequency in other forms of malabsorption to be a concern of physicians caring for these patients. One complication of ileojejunostomy for morbid obesity is hemorrhage due to vitamin K deficiency. Patients with malabsorption should be treated with all the fat-soluble vitamins. Vitamin K should be given orally in doses of 2.2 to 4.4 μmol/day (1–2 mg/day) or parenterally in doses of 2.2 to 4.4 μmol/week (1–2 mg/week).

Liver Disease

Patients with parenchymal liver disease may have hypoprothrombinemia and an elevation in plasma descarboxyprothrombin (75). They are unable to use vitamin K in the biosynthesis of vitamin K–dependent clotting factors, usually because of destruction of the rough reticulum in the hepatocyte. Patients with liver disease should be challenged with vitamin K to determine the extent of the blockade of prothrombin synthesis; however, there is no need to give repetitive high doses of vitamin K if the patient is refractory to a single intravenous dose of 22 μmol (10 mg) of vitamin K (76).

Drug Therapy

Various drugs, including the 4-hydroxycoumarins, salicylates, certain broad-spectrum antibiotics, and vitamins A and E in pharmacologic doses, antagonize the action of vitamin K.

Coumarin- and Salicylate-Induced Hemorrhagic Disease

The coumarin anticoagulant drugs can induce serious hypoprothrombinemia and even hemorrhage by blocking the vitamin K epoxide and vitamin K reductases. Some of the contributory causes are reduction in dietary intake of vitamin K, ingestion of interfering drugs, and inadvertent alteration of the anticoagulant dosage schedule. Coumarin drugs, in rare cases, may cause coumarin skin necrosis. This condition probably occurs because coumarin drugs inhibit biosynthesis of the anticoagulant protein C before they affect the levels of the procoagulant factors, II, XII, IX, and X. The temporary imbalance may in fact stimulate local coagulation in venules, with resulting thrombosis (77). Salicylates in large doses may also depress vitamin K–dependent factors by inhibiting the vitamin K epoxide reductase. When overdosage with or without bleeding occurs, the anticoagulant should be discontinued, 22 μmol (10 mg) of vitamin K_1 should be given parenterally, and prothrombin times should be monitored until they are in a satisfactory range.

Broad-Spectrum Antibiotics

One source of vitamin K in humans is their own intestinal bacteria. Vitamin K, however, is not well absorbed from the colon. It is unclear whether the microorganisms synthesizing absorbable menaquinones in the intestine reside in the ileum or reside in the colon with reflux into the ileum where absorption of vitamin K is possible.

Sulfaquinoxaline, neomycin, and other broad-spectrum antibiotics can sterilize the bowel, which may contribute to vitamin K deficiency. Certain broad-spectrum cephalosporin antibiotics (moxalactam, cefamandole) cause vitamin K-reversible hemorrhage in man (77, 78). Lipsky (79) reported that the N-methylthiotetrazole moiety of these antibiotics blocks vitamin K–dependent peptide carboxylation in Triton-solubilized rat liver microsomes in a dose-dependent manner. However, Shearer et al. (80) concluded that those antibiotics oppose vitamin K by inhibiting hepatic vitamin K epoxide reductase.

Megadoses of Vitamins A and E

Megadoses of the fat-soluble vitamins A and E antagonize vitamin K. It has been recognized since 1944 that hypervitaminosis A in the rat leads to hypoprothrombinemia that can be prevented by the administration of vitamin K (81). A close relationship between the amount of dietary retinol (or retinoic acid) given and the severity of vitamin K deficiency was observed (82). The effect of vitamin A is more severe in males than in females, and retinoic acid is more effective than vitamin A acetate. Because parenterally administered retinoic acid failed to increase the vitamin K requirement, it was concluded that excess vitamin A reduced the absorption of vitamin K. Reduced plasma prothrombin levels have been reported in humans intoxicated with vitamin A (83).

Large amounts of vitamin E also antagonize the action of vitamin K in animals (84). Olson and Jones (85) observed that high dietary intakes of vitamin E in rats increased the vitamin K requirement. Vitamin E does not appear to affect vitamin K uptake or distribution from the gut, nor does vitamin E directly affect the vitamin K–dependent carboxylase in vitro. Bettger et al. (86) found α-tocopherolquinone to be a more potent antagonist of vitamin K activity in the rat than is *d*-α-tocopherol.

Dowd and Zheng (87) have proposed that the methene isomer of α-tocopherol quinone forms a covalent linkage with a thiol within the active site of γ-glutamyl carboxylase. Vitamin K deficiency in a human subject taking megadoses of vitamin E was reported by Corrigan and Marcus (88). Bleeding was observed in a middle-aged man taking 5 mg warfarin and 1200 IU vitamin E each day. Upon discontinuation of megavitamin E therapy, the bleeding tendency disappeared and the prolonged prothrombin time normalized.

EVALUATION OF NUTRITIONAL STATUS

Evaluation of individual persons for vitamin K status requires proper application of the classical medical approach to a patient, namely, take a history, do a physical examination, and conduct appropriate laboratory tests.

History

The medical history should include questions about hemorrhage in the mouth or from the nose, from the stomach and intestinal tract (hematemesis and melena), kidney (hematuria), and beneath the skin (ecchymoses). Persons at risk for vitamin K deficiency include newborn infants and adults who are on diets devoid of green, leafy vegetables and animal foods or who have malabsorption, osteoporosis, injury, or renal disease. A careful medical history should include questions about these risk factors and use of coumarin anticoagulant drugs. In addition, the diet history should include a list of foods frequently eaten, a 24-hour recall of foods eaten, and occasionally a 3-day diary.

Physical Examination

Evidence should be sought for a bleeding tendency, the cardinal sign of vitamin K deficiency. This can present in one or more of the following ways: bleeding from the nose or mouth; ecchymoses in the groin, around the collar line, or in the legs; splinter hemorrhages under the nails or in the conjunctiva; melena (gross or occult); hematuria; and hematemesis. Pallor may be a sign of previous bleeding. The perifollicular hemorrhages in the skin characteristic of scurvy are not seen in vitamin K deficiency.

Laboratory Tests

Reduction in prothrombin and other vitamin K–dependent factors (X, IX, VII, and protein C) below 50% in the plasma is an accepted indicator of vitamin K deficiency. Measurement of plasma phylloquinone, which requires reverse-phase high-pressure liquid chromatography, does not correlate too well with vitamin K status (18). The range of normal is 0.3 to 2.6 nM (0.15–1.0 ng/mL), with a mean of 0.9 nM (12). Restriction of vitamin K may lower plasma vitamin K levels about 50% in given individuals, usually without altering the level of plasma coagulation proteins. The most sensitive indicator of vitamin K deficiency is the amount of des-γ-carboxyprothrombin (DCP) in the plasma measured by a specific antibody (89). In healthy persons, the DCP concentration is zero; in persons with vitamin K deficiency, liver disease, or both, the values can rise to 30% of the total prothrombin (~0.5 μM). Other, more indirect methods measure the ratio of prothrombin activity to total immunochemical equivalents of prothrombin (II:Ag ratio) or the ratio of a thromboplastin-activated (Simplastin) prothrombin time to that activated by *Echis carinatus* venom (S:E ratio). In vitamin K deficiency, these ratios fall. Recently, the measurement of uncarboxylated osteocalcin has been used to verify the diagnosis of vitamin K deficiency (62, 90).

Finally, urinary Gla can be measured as an index of vitamin K–dependent protein catabolism. A single value of Gla in the urine has little significance, although a given individual may show a lower urinary Gla level when put on a vitamin K–restricted diet (14).

NUTRITIONAL REQUIREMENTS

The vitamin K requirement of mammals is met by a combination of dietary intake and microbiologic biosynthesis in the gut. Genetic factors influence the vitamin K requirement in both animals and humans, because males require more vitamin K per kilogram of body weight than females do. As regards the intestinal flora, in conventional rats, the vitamin K requirement is about 22 nmol (10 μg) per kg of body weight per day, whereas in germ-free rats the requirement is more than doubled, to about 56 nmol (25 μg) per kg per day (91).

Over the past 30 years, several attempts have been made to estimate the vitamin K requirement in humans. In 1967, Frick et al. (92) studied 10 patients victimized by stroke who were unable to take food by mouth and were given intravenous fluids containing electrolytes, dextrose, and water-soluble vitamins together with parenteral antibiotics to suppress intestinal flora. Seven of these patients developed vitamin K deficiency 21 to 28 days after interruption of oral nutrition, as indicated by a decline in vitamin K–dependent factors II, VII, and X to levels of 10 to 15% of normal. They were given intravenous doses of phylloquinone between 0.015 and 1.5 μg/kg body weight. Although small responses in factor levels were observed at levels below 0.24 μg/kg, physiologically significant changes required 0.5 to 1.0 μg/kg/day.

In 1971, O'Reilley (93) reported a study of four volunteers maintained on a purified diet containing 55 nmol vitamin K_1 per day (about 25 μg) and given antibiotics to suppress bacterial synthesis of menaquinones for 5 weeks. These subjects maintained their plasma prothrombin activity in the range of 70 to 100%, which led to the conclusion that the human requirement for vitamin K was of the order of 0.5 μg/kg/day.

In 1984, Olson et al. (26) fed four healthy young males an elemental diet (Vivonex) containing less than 10 μg phylloquinone per day for 8 weeks, during which time no change in factors II, VII, IX, and X or prothrombin antigen activity was observed. Neomycin or vitamin E was given to two of the four subjects during the second 4-week period without effect on vitamin K–dependent factors. Their average plasma phylloquinone level decreased from 2.2 nM (1.0 ng/mL) to 1.1 nM (0.5 ng/mL) over that period. It was concluded that their short-term vitamin K requirement was of the order of 0.2 μg/kg day.

In 1987, Allison et al. (94) reported on the results of a study of 33 normal volunteers fed a vitamin K–deficient diet containing from 2 to 5 μg of phylloquinone for 13 days. Starting on the 4th day, 10 groups of three volunteers each were given a range of antibiotics (which included therapeutic doses of two aminopenicillins, a macrolide antibiotic, a trimethoprim-sulfamethiazole, and six cephalosporins). Three of the cephalosporins contain the N-methylthiotetrazole (NMTT) moiety reported to induce vitamin K deficiency. Although 12 of the 33 persons complained of diarrhea during the experimental period, there were no other adverse effects. No significant changes in prothrombin time (11.5–13 sec) or factor VII levels were noted. Plasma phylloquinone levels declined 66% from 3.1 ± 2.0 nM (SD) to 0.88 ± 0.66 nM (1.4 ± 0.9–0.4 ± 0.3 ng/mL), both values within the normal range for plasma phylloquinone. The Simplastin:Ecarin (S:E) clotting ratios were found to be 1.03 ± 0.20 in a normal population (range, 0.64–1.42). Seventeen of the volunteers had S:E ratios below 0.6 and nine were above 0.6 after 13 days on the vitamin K–dependent diet with antibiotics. There appeared to be no difference between the effects of various types of antibiotics, including those cephalosporins with the NMTT side chains. The authors concluded that 5 μg of dietary vitamin K was adequate to maintain coagulation homeostasis during this relatively short period and suggested that the RDA of 1 μg/kg in healthy persons was too high.

In 1988, Suttie et al. (95) studied 10 college-aged nonsmoking males who modified their diets by avoiding vitamin K–rich foods for 3 weeks. Their vitamin K intake dropped from 178 nmol/day (80 μg/day) to about 89 nmol/day (40 μg/day), with a change in plasma phylloquinone from 2.00 ± 0.44 nM (0.90 ± 0.20 ng/mL) to 1.1 ± 0.44 nM (0.50 ± 0.20 ng/mL) during a 3-week period. There was no change in prothrombin time, although there was a 10% change in S:E clotting ratio and a 20% decrease in urinary Gla excretion.

The claim of Suttie et al. (95) that they induced a vitamin K deficiency in healthy college students on diets containing 40 μg of phylloquinone for 27 days is questionable. Furthermore, the S:E ratio was within normal limits (0.911 ± 0.09) according to the criteria given by Allison et al. (1.03 ± 0.20) (94).

In 1993, Ferland et al. (14) reported that a subclinical vitamin K deficiency was produced in 32 healthy subjects consisting of groups of male and female subjects ages 20 to 40 years and 60 to 80 years. All volunteers were initially fed a baseline diet of ordinary foods containing 100 μg of phylloquinone per day. This baseline period was followed by a 13-day depletion period during which the subjects were fed a weighed diet containing less than 10 μg of vitamin K_1 per day. After depletion, each subject entered a 16-day repletion period consisting of four stages, lasting 4 days each, during which they were fed supplements of 5, 15, 25, and 45 μg of vitamin K_1 per day.

On the house diet, the plasma phylloquinone values of both young and elderly subjects declined 30 to 40%, from initial values of 1.25 to 0.77 nM (0.56–0.35 ng/mL) in the older group and 1.08 nM to 0.45 nM (0.48–0.2 ng/mL) in the younger group. It appears that both groups were taking considerably more vitamin K than 100 μg/day during their ad libitum period. On the deficient diet, plasma phylloquinone declined further, from 0.77 nM (0.35 ng/mL) to 0.22 nM (0.1 ng/mL) in the elderly and from 0.45 nM (0.2 ng/mL) to 0.15 nM (0.07 ng/mL) in the young group. Both plasma K_1 levels were below the normal range. Gla excretion declined only 10% in the young and not at all in the elderly. There was no change in factor VII and protein C levels. A change in descarboxyprothrombin (PIVKA II) was detected by one antibody (but not a second one), which showed an infinitesimal rise in PIVKA II (about 2 ng/mL) equivalent to 0.002% of the prothrombin level. The addition of 5, 15, and 25 μg of vitamin K to the basal diet showed no significant change in plasma prothrombin levels, although 45 μg gave a positive response. These investigators calculated that the total expected turnover of known vitamin K–dependent coagulation factors could account for only 64% of the total Gla excreted, suggesting that bone Gla-proteins plus others must account for the difference. The greater lability of phylloquinone levels and Gla synthesis in young persons suggests that they have a higher turnover rate for vitamin K_1 and (as the authors mention) lower hepatic concentrations of phylloquinone than elderly persons.

Table 20.6
Food and Nutrition Board (NAS/NRC) Recommended Dietary Allowances for Vitamin K (1989)

Category	Age (years) or Condition	Weight (kg)	Vitamin K[a] (μg)
Infants	0.0–0.5	6	5
	0.5–1.0	9	10
Children	1–3	13	15
	4–6	20	20
	7–10	28	30
Males	11–14	45	45
	15–18	66	65
	19–24	72	70
	25–50	79	80
	51+	77	80
Females	11–14	46	45
	15–18	55	55
	19–24	58	60
	25–50	63	65
	51+	65	65
Pregnant			
Lactating	1st 6 months		65
	2nd 6 months		65

From Food and Nutrition Board, National Research Council. Recommended dietary allowances. 10th ed. Washington, DC: National Academy Press, 1989, with permission.

[a] 1 μg Vitamin K_1 = 2.2 nmol.

The available data do not conclusively establish the requirement for vitamin K in humans, mostly because none is a long-term study. These studies are also complicated by the fact that the coagulation factors do not respond to reduction of vitamin K intakes from more than 1 μg/kg to 0.2 μg/kg. The other feature not well studied is the requirement of bone cells for vitamin K. Plasma BGP is partially uncarboxylated in older persons and appears to respond to large doses of vitamin K. Further studies are needed to quantify the response as a function of dose.

NUTRITIONAL ALLOWANCES

The RDAs for vitamin K were set by the Food and Nutrition Board for children and adult men and women for the first time in the 10th edition of *Recommended Dietary Allowances* (1989) (96). RDAs are defined as the levels of intake of essential nutrients that, on the basis of current scientific knowledge, are judged to be adequate to meet the needs of all healthy persons.

Because the database for setting requirements for vitamin K in man is small, and because the RDA should be at least two standard deviations above the mean requirement, the values presented in Table 20.6 are considerably higher than the estimated requirements. This is appropriate because the available data do not include information about the requirements for bone and kidney metabolism.

TOXICITY

There are no reports of toxic effects of phylloquinone at 500 times its RDA. Although this lack of toxicity is true for phylloquinone, it is not true of the vitamin precursor, menadione (2-methyl-1,4-naphthoquinone) unsubstituted in the 3 position, and its water-soluble derivatives such as Synkayvite. Menadione can combine with sulfhydryl groups in membranes and cause hemolytic anemia, hyperbilirubinemia, and kernicterus in infants (97). Menadione should no longer be used as a therapeutic form of vitamin K.

REFERENCES

1. Olson RE. Annu Rev Nutr 1984;4:281–337.
2. Manfioletti G, Brancolini C, Avanzi G, et al. Mol Cell Biol 1993;13:4976–85.
3. Stenflo J, Fernlund P, Egan W, et al. Proc Natl Acad Sci USA 1974;71:2730–3.
4. Nelsestuen GL, Zytokovicz TH, Howard JB. J Biol Chem 1974;249:6347–50.
5. Magnusson S, Sottrup-Jensen L, Peterson TE, et al. FEBS Lett 1974;44:189–93.
6. Suttie JW. Annu Rev Biochem 1985;54:459–77.
7. Yekundi KG, Olson RE. Biochim Biophys Acta 1970;223:332–8.
8. Pennock JF. Vitam Horm 1966;24:307–29.
9. Shearer MJ, Bach A, Kohlmeier M. J Nutr 1996;126(Suppl):1181S–86S.
10. Usui Y, Tanimura H, Nishimura N, et al. Am J Clin Nutr 1990;51:846–52.
11. Olson RE. Vitamin K. In: Shils ME, Olson JA, Shike M, eds.

Modern nutrition in health and disease. 8th ed. Philadelphia: Lea & Febiger, 1994;342–57.
12. Booth SL, Sadowski JA, Pennington JAT. J Agric Food Chem 1995;43:1574–9.
13. Shearer MJ, Allan V, Haroon Y, et al. Nutritional aspects of vitamin K in man. In: Suttie JW, ed. Vitamin K metabolism and vitamin K–dependent proteins. Baltimore: University Park Press, 1980;317–27.
14. Ferland G, Sadowski JA, O'Brien WE. J Clin Invest 1993; 91:1761–8.
15. Vermeer C, Gijsbers BLMG, Craciun AM, et al. J Nutr 1966;126:1187S–91S.
16. Kohlmeier M, Salomon A, Saupe J, et al. J Nutr 1996;126: 11925–65.
17. Shearer MJ, Barkham P, Webster GR. Br J Haematol 1970;18:297–308.
18. Shearer MJ, McCarthy PT, Crampton OE, Mattock MB. The assessment of human vitamin K status from tissue measurements. In: Suttie JW, ed. Current advances in vitamin K research. New York: Elsevier, 1988;437–52.
19. Sadowski JA, Hood SJ, Dallal GE, et al. Am J Clin Nutr 1989;50:100–8.
20. Matschiner JT, Amelotti JM. J Lipid Res 1968;9:176–9.
21. Matschiner JT, Bell RG, Amelotti JM, et al. Biochim Biophys Acta 1970;201:309–15.
22. Olson RE. Vitamin K. In: Coleman RW, Hirsch J, Marder VJ, Salzman EW, eds. Hemostasis and thrombosis. 2nd ed. Philadelphia: JB Lippincott, 1987;846–60.
23. Bjornsson TD, Meffin PJ, Swezey SE, Blaschke TF. Disposition and turnover of vitamin K in man. In: Suttie JW, ed. Vitamin K metabolism and vitamin K–dependent proteins. Baltimore: University Park Press 1980;328–32.
24. Shearer MJ, McBurney A, Barkhan P. Vitam Horm 1974;32: 513–42.
25. Bjornsson TD, Meffin PJ, Swezey SE, et al. Pharmacol Exp Ther 1979;210:322–6.
26. Olson RE, Meyer RG, Chao J, et al. Circulation 1984;70:97.
27. Kindberg CG, Suttie JW. J Nutr 1989;119:175–80.
28. Hodges SJ, Bejui J, Leclercq M, et al. J Bone Miner Res 1993;8:1005–8.
29. Taggart WV, Matschiner JT. Biochem J 1969;8:1141–6.
30. Thijssen HHW, Drittij-Reijnders MJ, Fischer MAJG. J Nutr 1996;126:537–43.
31. Bertina RM, Koeleman BPC, Koster T, et al. Nature 1994; 369:64–7.
32. Kemkes-Matthis B, Matthis K. Haemostasis 1995;25:312–6.
33. Reiner AP, Davie EW. Introduction to hemostasis and the vitamin K–dependent coagulation factors. In: Scriver CR, Beaudet AL, Sly WS, Valle D, eds. The metabolic and molecular bases of inherited disease. 7th ed. New York: McGraw-Hill 1995;3181–221.
34. Giradot JM. J Biol Chem 1982;257:15008–11.
35. Larson AE, Suttie JW. FEBS Lett 1980;118:95–8.
36. Jones JP, Gardner EJ, Cooper TG, et al. J Biol Chem 1977;252: 7738–42.
37. Hubbard BR, Ulrich MMW, Jacobs M, et al. Proc Natl Acad Sci USA 1989;86:6893–7.
38. Wu S-M, Morris DP, Stafford DW. Proc Natl Acad Sci USA 1991;88:2236–40.
39. Wu S-M, Cheung W-F, Frazier D, et al. Science 1991;254: 1634–8.
40. Berkner KL, Harbeck M, Lingenfelter S, et al. Proc Natl Acad Sci USA 1992;89:6242–6.
41. Kuliopulos A, Cieurzo E, Furie B, et al. Biochemistry 1992;31:9436–44.
42. Rehemtulla A, Roth DA, Warley LC, et al. Proc Natl Acad Sci USA 1993;90:4611–15.
43. Roth DA, Whirl ML, Valasquez-Estades LJ, et al. J Biol Chem 1995;270:5305–11.
44. Wu S-M, Mutucumarana P, Geromanos S, et al. J Biol Chem 1997;272:401–6.
45. Larson AE, Suttie JW. Proc Natl Acad Sci USA 1978; 75:5413–6.
46. Hall AL, Kloepper R, Zee-Cheng RK-Y, et al. Arch Biochem Biophys 1982;214:45–50.
47. Dowd P, Ham SW, Geib SJ. J Am Chem Soc 1991;113: 7734–43.
48. Fasco MJ, Hildebrandt EF, Suttie JW. J Biol Chem 1982; 257:11210–2.
49. Will BH, Usui I, Suttie JW. J Nutr 1992;122:2354–60.
50. Hauschka PV, Lian JB, Gallop PM. Proc Natl Acad Sci USA 1975;72:3925–9.
51. Price PA, Otsuka AS, Poser JW, et al. Proc Natl Acad Sci USA 1976;73:1447–51.
52. Price PA, Urist MR, Otawara Y. Biochem Biophys Res Commun 1983;117:765–71.
53. Price PA. Annu Rev Nutr 1988;8:565–83.
54. Knapen MHJ, Hamulyak K, Vermeer C. Ann Intern Med 1989;111:1001–5.
55. Hodges A, Pilkington MJ, Stamp TCB, et al. Bone 1991;12:387–89.
56. Hodges SJ, Akesson K, Vergnaud P, et al. J Bone Miner Res 1993;8:1241–5.
57. Pan EY, Gomperts ED, Millen R, et al. Thromb Res 1990;58:221–31.
58. Lian JB, Gundberg CM. Clin Orthop 1988;226:267–91.
59. Price PA, Baukol SA. J Biol Chem 1980;255:11660–63.
60. Schräder M, Bendik I, Becker-Andre M, et al. J Biol Chem 1993;268:17830–6.
61. Warkany J. Am J Dis Child 1975;129:287–8.
62. Vermeer C, Jie K-SG, Knapen MHJ. Annu Rev Nutr 1995;15:1–22.
63. Bell RG, Matschiner JT. Arch Biochem Biophys 1969;141: 473–6.
64. O'Reilly R. Annu Rev Med 1976;27:245–61.
65. Fasco MJ, Hildebrandt EF, Suttie JW. J Biol Chem 1982; 257:11210–12.
66. Searcey MT, Graves CB, Olson RE. J Biol Chem 1977;252: 6260–7.
67. Thijssen HAW, Baars LGM. J Pharmacol Exp Ther 1987;243: 1082–8.
68. Lane PA, Hathaway WE. J Pediatr 1985;106:351–9.
69. Kuo W-L, Stafford DW, Cruces J, et al. Genomics 1995;25: 746–8.
70. Motohara K, Endo F, Matsuda I. Lancet 1985;2:242–4.
71. Sutherland JM, Glueck HI, Gleser G. Am J Dis Child 1967;113:524–33.
72. Evans AR, Forrester RM, Discombe C. Lancet 1970;1: 517–8.
73. Ansell JE, Kumar R, Deykin D. JAMA 1977;238:40–2.
74. Savage D, Lindenbaum J. Clinical and experimental human vitamin K deficiency. In: Lindenbaum J, ed. Nutrition in hematology. New York: Churchill Livingstone, 1983;271–319.
75. Blanchard RA, Furie BC, Jorgenson M, et al. N Engl J Med 1981;305:242–8.
76. Mehta R, Reilley JJ, Olson RE. JPEN 1991;15:350–3.
77. McGehee WG, Klotz TA, Epstein DJ. Ann Intern Med 1984;101:59–60.
78. Hooper CA, Harvey BB, Stone HH. Lancet 1980;1:39–40.
79. Lipsky JJ. Lancet 1983;2:192–3.

80. Shearer MJ, Bechtold H, Andrassy K, et al. J Clin Pharmacol 1988;25:88–95.
81. Light RF, Alsher RP, Frey CN. Science 1940;100:225–30.
82. Matschiner JT, Doisy EA Jr. Proc Soc Exp Biol Med 1962;109:139–42.
83. Smith FR, Goodman DW. N Engl J Med 1976;294:805–8.
84. March BE, Wong E, Seier L, et al. J Nutr 1973;103:371–7.
85. Olson RE, Jones JP. Fed Proc 1979;38:2542.
86. Bettger WJ, Jones JP, Olson RE. Fed Proc 1982;41:344.
87. Dowd P, Zheng ZB. Proc Natl Acad Sci USA 1995;92:8171–5.
88. Corrigan JJ, Marcus FI. JAMA 1974;230:1300–1.
89. Blanchard RA, Furie BC, Kruger SF, et al. J Lab Clin Med 1983;101:242–55.
90. Sokoll LJ, Sadowski J. Am J Clin Nutr 1966; 63:566–73.
91. Gustafsson BE, Daft FS, McDaniel, et al. J Nutr 1962;78:461–8.
92. Frick PG, Riedler G, Brogli H. J Appl Physiol 1967;23:387–9.
93. O'Reilley RA. Am J Physiol 1971;221:1327–30.
94. Allison PM, Mummah-Schendel LL, Kindberg CG. J Lab Clin Med 1987;110:180–8.
95. Suttie JW, Mummah-Schendel LL, Shah DV, et al. Am J Clin Nutr 1988;47:475–80.
96. Food and Nutrition Board, National Research Council. Recommended dietary allowances. 10th ed. Washington, DC: National Academy Press, 1989.
97. DiPalma JR, Ritchie DM. Annu Rev Pharmacol Toxicol 1977;17:133–48.
98. Ferland G, MacDonald DL, Sadowski JA. J Am Diet Assoc 1992;92:593–7.
99. Booth SL, Pennington JAT, Sadowski JA. J Am Diet Assoc 1996;96:149–54.
100. Suttie JW. Annu Rev Nutr 1995;15:399–417.

SELECTED READINGS

Olson RE. The function and metabolism of vitamin K. Annu Rev Nutr 1984;4:281–337.

Shearer MJ, Bach A, Kohlmeier M. Chemistry, nutritional sources, tissue distribution and metabolism of vitamin K with special reference to bone health. J Nutr 1996;126:1181S–86S.

Suttie JW. Vitamin K. In: Brown M, ed. Present knowledge in nutrition. 7th ed. Washington, DC: Int Life Science Institute, 1996;122–31.

Vermeer C, Jie K-SG, Knapen MHJ. Role of vitamin K in bone metabolism. Annu Rev Nutr 1995;15:1–22.

21. Thiamin

VICHAI TANPHAICHITR

HISTORICAL LANDMARKS

Although Neiching, the Chinese medical book, mentioned beriberi in 2697 BC it was not known for centuries that this illness was due to thiamin deficiency. In 1884, Takaki, a surgeon general of the Japanese navy, concluded beriberi was caused by a lack of nitrogenous food components in association with excessive intake of nonnitrogenous food. In 1890, Eijkman, a Dutch physician working in Java, discovered that fowl fed boiled polished rice developed polyneuritis that resembled beriberi in man and this polyneuritis could be prevented by rice bran or polishings. In 1911, Funk, a chemist working at the Lister Institute in London, was convinced that he had isolated the antiberiberi principle possessing an amine function from rice bran extracts. He named it "vitamine." His crystalline substance was shown later to have little antineuritic activity. In 1926, Jansen and Donath, Dutch chemists working in Java, succeeded in isolating and crystallizing antiberiberi factor from rice bran extracts. By 1934 Williams, a U.S. chemist, had isolated a sufficient quantity of thiamin so that its structure could be determined. Its synthesis was accomplished in 1936. In 1937, Lohman and Schuster discovered that the active coenzyme form of thiamin was thiamin pyrophosphate (TPP; cocarboxylase) (Fig. 21.1) (1–3).

CHEMISTRY AND NOMENCLATURE

The chemical name of thiamin, formerly known as vitamin B_1, vitamin F, aneurine, or thiamine, is 3-(4-amino-2-methylpyrimidin-5-ylmethyl)-5-(2-hydroxyethyl)-4-methylthiazolium (Fig. 21.1) (4). The free vitamin is a base. It is isolated or synthesized and handled as a solid thiazolium salt, i.e., thiamin hydrochloride or thiamin mononitrate. The synthesis of thiamin is accomplished by either the pyrimidine and thiazole rings being prepared separately and condensed via the bromide or the pyrimidine ring being synthesized and the thiazole ring formed in situ on it. The molecular weight of thiamin hydrochloride is 337.28 g/mol (1, 3), whereas that of the free base is 265.36 g/mol. The molecular weight of the free base is used in calculating molar amounts from mass units.

Thiamin hydrochloride is a white crystalline substance. It is readily soluble in water, only partly soluble in alcohol and acetone, and insoluble in other fat solvents. In the dry form it is stable at 100°C. Thiamin in aqueous solutions is quite stable below pH 5 to heat and to oxidation; above pH 5 it is destroyed relatively rapidly by autoclaving and at pH 7.0 or above by boiling. Thiamin is readily cleaved at the methylene bridge by sulfite treatment at pH 6.0 or above into 2-methyl-4-amino-5-methyl-pyrimidylsulfonate and 4-methyl-5-(2-hydroxyethyl) thiazole. At pH 8.0 or above, thiamin turns yellow and is destroyed by a complex series of irreversible reactions. In strong alkaline solution in the presence of oxidizing agents such as potassium ferricyanide, thiamin is converted to thiochrome, a fluorescent derivative that is used to determine thiamin content. Thiamin is precipitated by iron and ammonium citrate,

---

Abbreviations: **ATP**—adenosine triphosphate; **ATPase**—adenosine triphosphatase; **CSF**—cerebrospinal fluid; **ETKA**—erythrocyte transketolase activity; **FAD**—flavin adenine dinucleotide; **RDAs**—recommended dietary allowances; **TMP**—thiamin monophosphate; **TPD**—thiamin propyl disulfide; **TPP**—thiamin pyrophosphate; **TPPE**—thiamin pyrophosphate effect; **TTFD**—thiamin tetrahydrofurfural disulfide; **TTP**—thiamin triphosphate.

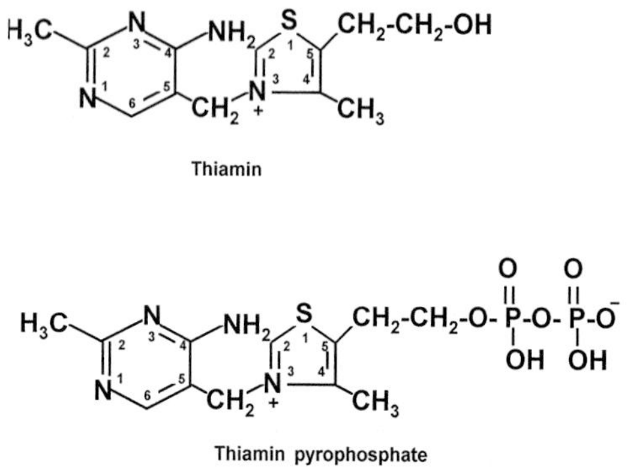

Thiamin

Thiamin pyrophosphate

Figure 21.1. Structural formulas of thiamin and thiamin pyrophosphate.

tannin, and various alkaloids. Thiamin forms esters at the hydroxethyl side chain with various acids. The most important esters are thiamin monophosphate (TMP), TPP, and thiamin triphosphate (TTP) (1–3).

BIOLOGIC ACTIVITY

Both pyrimidine and thiazole moieties are needed for its vitaminic activity, which is maximal when only one methylene group bridges the two moieties. In the thiazole portion, the quaternary nitrogen and a hydroxyethyl group at carbon 5 are needed, as is the amino group at carbon 4 in the pyrimidine portion. Several thiamin antagonists, including oxythiamin, pyrithiamin, and amprolium, produce thiamin deficiency in animals (1–3).

DIETARY CONSIDERATIONS

Thiamin status is affected by diet and a variety of other factors.

Food Sources

Thiamin, although found in a large variety of animal and vegetable products, is abundant in only a few foods. Excellent sources of thiamin are yeast, lean pork, and legumes, which contain 22.6 to 90.5, 2.7 to 3.9, and 2.0 to 3.8 μmol (6–24, 0.72–1.04, and 0.53–1.00 mg) of thiamin per 100 g edible portion, respectively. In cereal grains, thiamin is low in the endosperm but high in the germ. The thiamin contents in rice bran, home-pounded rice, and milled rice are 7.5 to 15.1, 0.3 to 0.5, and 0.1 to 0.15 μmol/100 g (2–4, 0.08–0.14, and 0.02–0.04 mg/100 g), respectively. Thiamin is absent from fats, oils, and refined sugars. Milk and milk products, seafood, fruits, and vegetables are not good sources (1, 3, 5).

Factors Affecting Thiamin Status

Thiamin status depends on its bioavailability in food products, ethanol consumption, the presence of antithiamin factors (ATFs) in the diet, and folate and protein status (3).

Thiamin Losses Resulting from Food Processing

pH. Thiamin is rapidly destroyed above pH 8. Thus, addition of sodium bicarbonate to green beans and peas to retain their green color or to dried beans to soften their skins inactivates thiamin (1, 3).

Temperature. Thiamin is also destroyed at high temperature. Thiamin losses during meat cooking and canning, bread baking, and vegetable cooking are 25 to 85%, 5 to 35%, and 0 to 60%, respectively. In pasteurization, sterilization, spray-drying, roller-drying, and condensation of milk, thiamin losses are 9 to 20%, 30 to 50%, 10%, 15%, and 40%, respectively. Freezing does not affect the thiamin content of foods. Processing foods at higher temperatures and under alkaline conditions in the presence of oxygen or other oxidants leads to formation of thiamin sulfides and disulfides, thiochrome, and other oxidation products. Only thiamin sulfides and disulfides still retain the biologic activity of thiamin (1, 3).

Solubility. Since thiamin is highly water soluble, significant amounts are lost in discarded cooking water (3, 5, 6).

Other Factors. Thiamin is also destroyed by x-rays, γ-rays, UV irradiation, and sulfites that form in treating dehydrated fruits with SO_2 (1, 3).

Ethanol Ingestion

Thiamin deficiency in chronic alcoholics is caused by multiple factors, including a low thiamin intake, impaired intestinal absorption, defective phosphorylation, and an apotransketolase deficiency. Ethanol given orally or intravenously also inhibits intestinal thiamin uptake (3, 7).

ATFs

Two types of ATFs exist: thermolabile and thermostable.

Thermolabile ATFs. The thermolabile ATFs include thiaminase I (EC 2.5.1.2) and II (EC 3.5.99.2). Thiaminase I is found in the viscera of freshwater fish, in shellfish, in ferns, in a limited number of sea fish and plants, and in several microorganisms, including *Bacillus thiaminolyticus* and *Clostridium thiaminolyticus*. Thiaminase I cleaves thiamin by an exchange reaction with an organic base or a sulfhydryl compound via a nucleophilic displacement on the methylene group of the pyrimidine moiety of thiamin. Thiaminase II is found in several microorganisms, including *Bacillus aneurinolyticus, Candida aneurinolytica, Trichosporon,* and *Oospora.* It hydrolyzes thiamin to 2-methyl-4-amino-5-hydroxymethyl pyrimidine and 4-methyl-5-(2-hydroxyethyl)thiazole. Thiamin is accessible to thiaminases when tissues are broken up at pH 4 to 8 or when excreted from cells. Thiaminases act during food storage or preparation prior to ingestion or during passage through the gastrointestinal tract. Thus, habitual intakes of raw freshwater fish, with or without fermentation, raw shellfish, and ferns are risk factors for the development of thiamin deficiency (3, 5, 6).

Thermostable ATFs. Thermostable ATFs have been demonstrated in ferns, tea, betel nut, some vegetables, other plants, and even in some animal tissues. In animal tissues, myoglobin, hemoglobin, and hemin may be involved. The ATFs found in plants and vegetables are related to *ortho-* and *para-*polyphenolic compounds such as caffeic acid (3,4-dihydroxycinnamic acid), chlorogenic acid [3-(3,4-dihydroxycinnamoyl)quinic acid], and tannic acid (tannin). The antithiamin activity of polyphenols requires a pH of 6.5 or above and oxygen. At high pH, polyphenols ionize, and the thiazole moiety of thiamin is ruptured at carbon 2 to yield the SH form of thiamin. In the presence of oxygen, polyphenols oxidize and polymerize to yield active quinones and relatively less active polymerized products. Quinones interact with the SH form of thiamin to give thiamin disulfide. Further hydrolysis and oxidation yield inactive products. Ascorbic acid and other reducing agents prevent formation of these quinones and thiamin disulfide.

Divalent cations, such as Ca^{2+} and Mg^{2+}, augment precipitation of thiamin by tannin, thereby making thiamin less bioavailable. Consequently, ascorbic, tartaric, and citric acids present in many fruits and vegetables protect thiamin, presumably by sequestering the divalent cations. Drinking tea, coffee, or decaffeinated coffee and chewing tea leaves or betel nut deplete thiamin in humans. Ascorbic acid intake improves the thiamin status of subjects (3, 5).

Folate and Protein Status

Subjects with folate or protein deficiency show a significant reduction in the maximum absorption of ^{35}S-thiamin. Thus the maximum absorption of ^{35}S-thiamin is increased after correction of the protein-energy malnutrition of alcoholics (7).

METABOLISM

Ingested thiamin is fairly well absorbed, rapidly converted to phosphorylated forms, stored poorly, and excreted in the urine as a variety of hydrolyzed and oxidized products.

Absorption

The small intestine absorbs thiamin by two mechanisms: active transport (<2 μmol/L) and passive diffusion (>2 μmol/L). A specific sodium- and energy-dependent carrier seems to exist. In this regard, a specific thiamin-binding protein is associated with thiamin transport across the cell membrane of *Escherichia coli.* Active thiamin absorption is greatest in the jejunum and ileum. The exit of thiamin from the serosal side of the mucosal cell depends on Na^+ and on adenosine triphosphatase (ATPase) at the serosal pole of the cell (1, 3). The intestinal transport of ^{35}S-thiamin in humans is rate limiting, with a V_{max} of 31.5 μmol (8.3 mg) and a K_m of 45.6 μmol (12.0 mg) (7).

Transport

Thiamin is carried by the portal blood to the liver. In normal adults, 20 to 30% of thiamin in the plasma is protein bound, all of which appears to be TPP (8). The transport of thiamin into erythrocytes seems to be a facilitated diffusion process, whereas it enters other cells by an active process (1, 3). Erythrocytes contain mainly TPP (8).

Tissue Distribution and Storage

The average total amount of thiamin in a normal adult is approximately 0.11 mmol (30 mg). High concentrations are found in the skeletal muscles, heart, liver, kidneys, and brain. About 50% of the total thiamin is present in muscles. The biologic half-life of ^{14}C-thiamin in the body is 9 to 18 days. Because thiamin is not stored in large amounts in any tissue, a continuous supply of thiamin is necessary (1, 3).

Metabolic Modification

Of the total thiamin in the body, about 80% is TPP, 10% is TTP, and the remainder is TMP and thiamin. The three tissue enzymes known to participate in formation of the phosphate esters are thiamin pyrophosphokinase, which catalyzes the formation of TPP from thiamin and ATP; TPP-ATP phosphoryl transferase, which catalyzes the formation of TTP from TPP and adenosine triphosphate (ATP); and thiamin pyrophosphatase, which hydrolyzes TPP to form TMP. Of 25 to 30 urinary metabolites of thiamin in rats and humans, pyrimidine carboxylic acid, thiazole acetic acid, and thiamin acetic acid predominate (Fig. 21.2) (1, 3).

Excretion

Thiamin and its metabolites are mainly excreted in the urine. Very little thiamin is excreted in the bile. Early milk contains a low thiamin level. Thiamin administered by oral or parenteral routes is rapidly converted to TPP and TTP in the tissues. Thiamin in excess of tissue needs and storage capacity is rapidly excreted in the urine in the free form (1, 3, 8).

FUNCTIONS

Thiamin, in the form of TPP, serves biochemically as the coenzyme of α-keto acid decarboxylation and transketolation. In a more physiologic context, thiamin functions in neurophysiologic processes (1–3).

Biochemical Functions

In mammalian systems, TPP functions as the Mg^{2+}-coordinated coenzyme for the active aldehyde transfers, which include the oxidative decarboxylation of α-keto acids and the transketolase reaction. The key feature of TPP is that the carbon atom between the nitrogen and sulfur atoms in the thiazole ring is much more acidic than most CH groups. It ionizes to form a carbanion, which readily adds

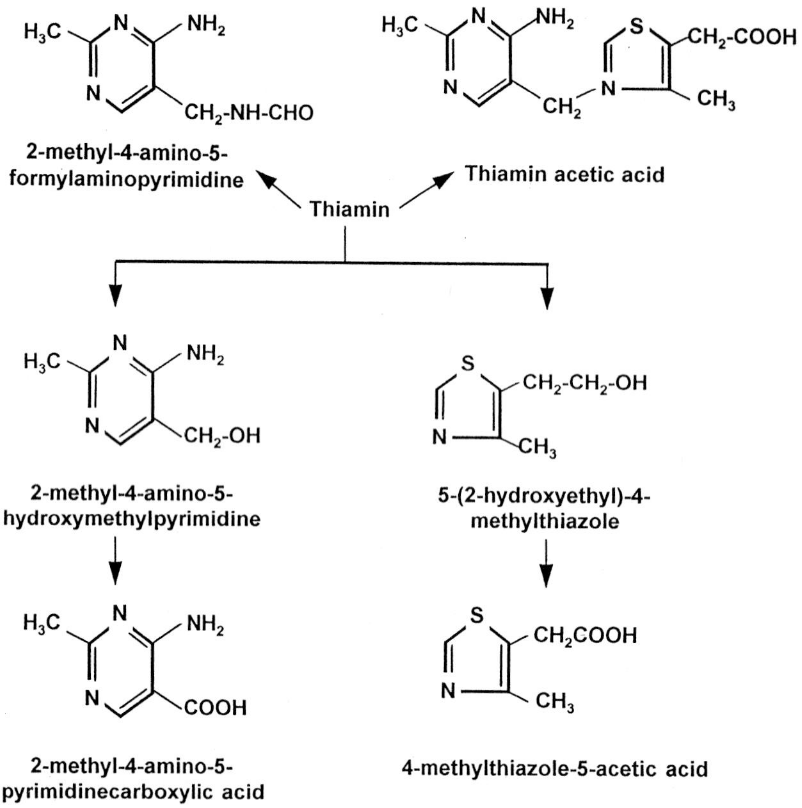

2-methyl-4-amino-5-formylaminopyrimidine

Thiamin acetic acid

Thiamin

2-methyl-4-amino-5-hydroxymethylpyrimidine

5-(2-hydroxyethyl)-4-methylthiazole

2-methyl-4-amino-5-pyrimidinecarboxylic acid

4-methylthiazole-5-acetic acid

Figure 21.2. Thiamin catabolism and its catabolites.

to the carbonyl group of α-keto acids or ketoses. The positively charged ring nitrogen of TPP then acts as an electron sink to stabilize formation of a negative charge, which is necessary for decarboxylation. Protonation then gives hydroxyethyl TPP (1, 3, 5).

Oxidative Decarboxylation of α-Keto Acids

Pyruvate, α-ketoglutarate, and branched-chain α-keto acids undergo oxidative decarboxylation. The net reaction of the oxidative decarboxylation of pyruvate catalyzed by the pyruvate dehydrogenase complex is

$$\text{Pyruvate} + \text{CoA} + \text{NAD}^+ \rightarrow \text{AcetylCoA} + \text{CO}_2 + \text{NADH} + \text{H}^+$$

In addition to CoA and NAD^+, TPP, lipoic acid, and flavin adenine dinucleotide (FAD) also serve as coenzymes. The pyruvate dehydrogenase complex, which is an organized assembly of three enzymes localized in the mitochondria, sequentially catalyzes the conversion of pyruvate into acetylCoA (1, 3, 5).

The net reaction in the oxidative decarboxylation of α-ketoglutarate, which takes place in the tricarboxylic acid cycle and is catalyzed by the α-ketoglutarate dehydrogenase complex, is

$$\alpha\text{-Ketoglutarate} + \text{CoA} + \text{NAD}^+ \rightarrow \text{SuccinylCoA} + \text{CO}_2 + \text{NADH} + \text{H}^+$$

The coenzyme requirements and the steps in the formation of succinylCoA are analogous to the oxidative decarboxylation of pyruvate (1, 3, 5).

Oxidative decarboxylation of the three branched-chain α-keto acids, α-ketoisocaproate, α–keto-β-methylvalerate, and α-ketoisovalerate, yield isovalerylCoA, α-methylbutyrylCoA, and isobutyrylCoA, respectively. These reactions are catalyzed by the branched-chain α–keto acid dehydrogenase complex, which is analogous to those for pyruvate and α-ketoglutarate (1, 3, 5).

Transketolase Reaction

A TPP-dependent transketolase found in the cytosol catalyzes the reversible transfer of a glycolaldehyde moiety from the first two carbons of a donor ketose phosphate to the aldehyde carbon of an aldose phsophate in the pentose phosphate pathway. These reactions are (1, 3)

$$\text{Xyl-5-P} + \text{Rib-5-P} \leftrightarrow \text{Glyc-3-P} + \text{Sedo-7-P}$$
$$\text{Xyl-5-P} + \text{Ery-4-P} \leftrightarrow \text{Glyc-3-P} + \text{Fruc-6-P}$$

Neurophysiologic Functions

Thiamin has been implicated in neurotransmission and nerve conduction (1–3).

Neurotransmission

In thiamin-deficient rats, acetylcholine turnover and acetylcholine utilization are reduced in the cerebral cortex, midbrain, diencephalon, and brainstem; the synthesis of catecholamines decreases in brain, including significant reductions in the norepinephrine content of cortex, hippocampus, and olfactory bulbs; the uptake of serotonin by cerebellar synaptosomes decreases; 5-hydroxyindoleacetic acid, a serotonin catabolite, significantly increases without alteration of tryptophan levels; and brain levels of glutamate, aspartate, γ-aminobutyrate, and glutamine are reduced (2).

Nerve Conduction

As originally postulated by von Muralt, thiamin may play a role in neurophysiology independent of its coenzyme function. Some evidence supporting this view follows: *(a)* thiamin antagonists adversely affect impulse conduction in peripheral nerves; *(b)* thiamin and thiamin pyrophosphatase are localized in nerve cell membranes but not in the axoplasm; *(c)* thiamin is released from membrane preparations of brain, spinal cord, and sciatic nerves by electrical stimulation; and *(d)* phosphorylated derivatives of thiamin are associated with sodium channel proteins. Thus, TTP may play a fundamental role in the control of sodium conductance at axonal membranes (1–3) as well as in other neurologic processes.

Functional Consequences of Thiamin Deficiency

The lack of thiamin in animals and humans affects the cardiovascular, muscular, nervous, and gastrointestinal systems. Cardiac failure, muscle weakness, peripheral and central neuropathy, and gastrointestinal malfunction have been observed in both animals and humans on diets restricted in thiamin. Although the precise biochemical defects responsible for the pathophysiologic manifestations of thiamin deficiency are not established, thiamin may well play three major roles at the cellular level. The first involves energy metabolism, largely related to the oxidative decarboxylation of α-keto acids, the inhibition of which leads to a failure in ATP synthesis. The second is concerned with synthetic mechanisms, as reflected by the importance of the transketolase reaction for the formation of NADPH and pentoses. The third deals with the functions of neurotransmitters and nerve conduction, as described above. In Wernicke's disease, failure of energy metabolism predominantly affects neurons and their functions in selected areas of the central nervous system. Glial changes may be caused by biochemical lesions that affect transketolase and nucleic acid metabolism. Membranous structures are visibly altered and secondary demyelination ensues (3, 5).

PATHOGENESIS OF THIAMIN DEFICIENCY AND CLINICAL MANIFESTATIONS

Thiamin deficiency in free-living populations and hospitalized patients can be caused by inadequate intake, decreased absorption, defective transport of thiamin, impaired biosynthesis of TPP, an increased requirement, and enhanced loss of thiamin. These mechanisms may reinforce each other.

High-Risk Situations

Populations vulnerable to the development of beriberi are breast-fed infants whose nursing mothers are thiamin deficient; adults who have high carbohydrate intake derived mainly from milled rice, with or without consumption of ATFs; and chronic alcoholics. Dietary factors are major causes of thiamin deficiency in Asia, whereas alcoholism is of greatest concern in the West. An increase in thiamin requirement because of strenuous physical exertion, fever, pregnancy, lactation, or adolescent growth may precipitate clinical manifestations in persons with marginal thiamin status. Other persons at risk are renal patients on dialysis, patients receiving parenteral nutrition, hypermetabolic patients, and patients with congestive heart failure treated with furosemide (1–3, 5–7, 9–13).

Clinical Manifestations

The clinical manifestations of beriberi vary with age and with the organ systems involved. The disease is divided into infantile and adult forms (3, 6, 10, 11).

Infantile Beriberi

Infantile beriberi most commonly occurs between the ages of 2 and 3 months. Infants may present with cardiac (acute fulminating), aphonic, or pseudomeningitic forms or a combination thereof. Infants with cardiac beriberi usually experience an acute attack that includes a loud piercing cry, cyanosis, dyspnea, vomiting, tachycardia, and cardiomegaly; death may occur within a few hours after the onset unless thiamin is administered. The striking feature in aphonic beriberi is the tone of the child's cry, which varies from hoarseness to complete aphonia. Infants with pseudomeningitic beriberi exhibit vomiting, nystagmus, purposeless movement of the extremities, and convulsion accompanied by a normal cerebrospinal fluid (CSF) (3, 6, 10).

Adult Beriberi

Children and adults may present with dry (paralytic or nervous), wet (cardiac), or cerebral (Wernicke-Korsakoff syndrome) forms of beriberi.

Dry Beriberi. The predominant features in dry beriberi are peripheral neuropathy, which is characterized by a symmetric impairment of sensory, motor, and reflex functions affecting the distal segments of limbs more severely than the proximal ones, calf muscle tenderness, and difficulty in rising from a squatting position (3, 6, 10, 11).

Wet Beriberi. In addition to peripheral neuropathy, common signs found in wet beriberi include edema, tachycardia, wide pulse pressure, cardiomegaly, and congestive heart failure. Some patients have abnormal electrocardiograms, including a prolonged OT interval, flat or inverted T waves in the precordial leads, and relatively low QRS-complex voltage. Typical hemodynamic findings in wet beriberi include high cardiac output and low peripheral and pulmonary vascular resistances. However, low cardiac output does not exclude the diagnosis of wet beriberi. Some patients experience sudden onset of a cardiac manifestation known as acute fulminant, or "shoshin," beriberi. The predominant features are tachycardia, dyspnea, cyanosis, cardiac enlargement, and circulatory collapse (3, 6, 10, 11).

Wernicke-Korsakoff Syndrome. Although alcoholism is the major cause of thiamin deficiency in Wernicke-Korsakoff syndrome, iatrogenic causes, including parenteral glucose administration and chronic dialysis, can aggravate the syndrome in patients with marginal thiamin status. The diagnosis of Wernicke's disease or encephalopathy is based on the triad of ocular motor signs, ataxia, and derangement of mental functions (2, 3, 5, 14). (See also Chapter 95.)

The ocular motor signs are the most readily recognized abnormalities and include a paresis or paralysis of abduction that is accompanied by horizontal diplopia, strabismus, and nystagmus; in advanced cases, there may be complete loss of ocular movement, and the pupils may become miotic and nonreactive. The ocular motor signs are attributable to lesions in the brainstem affecting the abducens nuclei and in the eye movement centers of the pons and rostral midbrain.

The ataxia affects stance and gait. The persistent ataxia is related to the loss of neurons in the superior vermis of the cerebellum; extension of the lesion into the anterior parts of the anterior lobes accounts for the ataxia of individual movements of the legs.

A derangement of mental function is found in about 90% of patients and takes one of the following three forms: *(a)* a global confusional-apathetic state, the most common form, characterized by profound listlessness, inattentiveness, indifference to the surroundings, and disorientation; *(b)* a disproportional disorder of retentive memory, i.e., Korsakoff amnesic state; or *(c)* the symptoms of alcohol withdrawal, found in a relatively small number of patients. The amnesic defect is related to lesions in the diencephalon, more specifically to those in the medial dorsal nuclei of the thalamus.

Wernicke's disease and Korsakoff's psychosis are not separate diseases. Korsakoff's psychosis is the psychic component of Wernicke's disease. Thus the clinical manifestations should be called Wernicke's disease when the amnesic state is not evident and the Wernicke-Korsakoff syndrome when both the ocular-ataxic and the amnesic manifestations are present (2, 3, 14).

Although the specific role of thiamin in Wernicke-Korsakoff syndrome is established and most of the patients with Wernicke-Korsakoff syndrome are alcoholics, only a few alcoholics are affected. Genetic abnormalities in erythrocyte transketolase (ETK) may underlie a predisposition to Wernicke-Korsakoff syndrome (2, 3, 5, 14). However, investigation of the hysteretic properties of human transketolase with emphasis on its dependency on TPP concentration has revealed a substantial lag in the formation of active holotransketolase as well as interindividual differences and cell type variation from the same individual in the lag period. These individual differences in the loss of transketolase activity during thiamin deficiency may explain, at least in part, the differential sensitivity to deficiency demonstrated by tissues and individuals (15).

Treatment

Thiamin should be promptly administered to beriberi patients. The daily dosage usually ranges from 0.19 to 0.38 mmol (50–100 mg) given intravenously or intramuscularly for 7 to 14 days, after which 0.04 mmol (10 mg)/day should be administered orally until the patient fully recovers. To prevent recurrence of beriberi, patients should be advised to change their dietary habits and to stop drinking alcohol (3, 6, 11).

The rationale underlying administration of a large dose of thiamin is to *(a)* replenish thiamin stores, which is consistent with the positive correlation between thiamin concentration in serum and CSF (16); *(b)* stimulate the TPP-dependent reactions maximally, which is consistent with the aforementioned thiamin-dependent hysteretic behavior of human transketolase (15); and *(c)* improve cardiovascular disorders. In regard to the latter, thiamin treatment reduces cardiac output and increases vascular resistance in beriberi patients who show high cardiac output and low peripheral and pulmonary vascular resistance. Similarly, thiamin treatment increases cardiac output in those showing low cardiac output (17). The parenteral route is used initially to ensure the bioavailability of thiamin.

Several thiamin derivatives, especially thiamin propyl disulfide (TPD) and thiamin tetrahydrofurfural disulfide (TTFD), are useful for oral administration to beriberi patients because they produce a significantly higher thiamin level in the blood, erythrocytes, and CSF than does thiamin hydrochloride or TPP at the same oral dose of 50 mg. Indeed, given orally, they are as effective as parenteral administration of thiamin hydrochloride or TPP to healthy subjects (18). Patients with cardiac beriberi also respond dramatically to daily intravenous administration of 50 mg of TTFD (19).

Response to Thiamin Administration

In wet beriberi, improvement within 6 to 24 hours after thiamin administration is characterized by reduced restlessness; the disappearance of cyanosis; reduction in heart rate, respiratory rate, and cardiac size; and clearing of pulmonary congestion. Dramatic improvement after thiamin treatment is also observed in infants with cardiac beriberi (3, 6, 10, 11).

It is difficult to use the response to thiamin administration as a criterion for immediate diagnosis in dry beriberi or in infants with aphonia because more time elapses before improvement is observed. Disappearance of impaired sensation and recovery of motor weakness occur 7 to 120 days and within 60 days, respectively, after thiamin treatment (3, 6, 10, 11).

The response of patients with Wernicke's disease to thiamin treatment follows a characteristic course. Ocular palsies may begin to improve within hours to several days after administration of thiamin. Sixth nerve palsies, ptosis, and vertical gaze palsies recover completely within 1 to 2 weeks in most cases, but vertical gaze–evoked nystagmus may persist for months. Ataxia improves only slowly and approximately half of patients recover incompletely. Apathy, drowsiness, and confusion also recede gradually (14).

Effects of thiamin treatment on the Korsakoff amnesic state vary. Recoveries range from complete or almost complete in less than 20% of patients to slow and incomplete in the remainder. The residual state is characterized by large gaps in memory, usually without confabulation, and an inability of the patient to sort out events in their proper temporal sequence (14).

EVALUATION OF THIAMIN STATUS

The subject's history, laboratory tests, and physical examination are the basis for evaluating thiamin status in humans (20).

Subject's History

Dietary assessment, demographic data, medical history, family history, and psychosocial history should be recorded for each subject, because all of these factors can affect thiamin status. Several dietary methods, including dietary scan, dietary record, and/or 24-hour dietary recall, have been used to assess thiamin intakes in various populations. Comparisons are then made between mean thiamin intakes and the recommended dietary allowances (RDAs) for thiamin. For instance, northern Thai villagers and the male North American population aged 65–75 years had mean daily thiamin intakes of 2.1 and 5.3 μmol, (0.56 and 1.40 mg), respectively (21, 22), which are 51% and 116% of the RDAs for thiamin for the North American population (23).

Laboratory Tests

Various biochemical tests have been developed to detect thiamin deficiency and assess the adequacy of thiamin status in humans. These include the measurement of urinary thiamin excretion; blood thiamin level; thiamin concentration in the CSF; blood pyruvate, lactate, and α-ketoglutarate levels; erythrocyte transketolase activity (ETKA); and the thiamin pyrophosphate effect (TPPE) on ETKA (1–3, 5, 6, 9–12, 16).

At present the most reliable and feasible method of evaluating human thiamin adequacy is the measurement of ETKA and the percentage enhancement resulting from added TPP, which is known as the TPPE. The diagnostic criterion for human thiamin inadequacy consists of a low ETKA, usually accompanied by a TPPE of 16% or above. However, in chronic thiamin deficiency, the TPP added in vitro cannot restore ETKA fully; under such conditions, TPPE may be in the normal range of 0 to 15%. Thus both ETKA and TPPE must be considered in assessing the adequacy of thiamin status (3, 6, 10–12). However, thus far there is no general agreement on the normal levels of ETKA because different methods are used to determine ETKA in various laboratories. The reference range of ETKA in our laboratory is 126 to 214 International Units, which is equivalent to the number of moles of sedoheptulose-7-phosphate formed per minute per liter of erythrocytes (12).

Physical Examination

Although physical signs of beriberi appear in the last stage of thiamin deficiency, physicians should be able to detect such developing abnormalities in patients for immediate and long-term nutritional management (20). Delay in diagnosing beriberi affects the morbidity and mortality rates of patients. Beriberi should be suspected in breast-fed infants of thiamin-deficient mothers. Infants with beriberi have a loud piercing cry, dyspnea, cyanosis, cardiac failure, and aphonia (3, 6, 10).

Common suggestive signs in dry beriberi include glove and stocking hypoesthesia of pain and touch sensations, loss of ankle and/or knee reflexes, tenderness at the calf muscle, difficulty in rising from the squatting position, and aphonia. However, other possible known causes of peripheral neuropathy must be carefully ruled out (3, 10, 11).

Patients with wet beriberi exhibit both peripheral neuropathy and edema. Those with severe cases show tachycardia, wide pulse pressure, cardiac enlargement, and pulmonary congestion (3, 10, 11).

Wernicke's disease must be suspected in chronic alcoholics presenting with the triad of ocular motor signs, ataxia, and derangement of mental functions. The diagnosis of Wernicke-Korsakoff syndrome should be made in those having both the ocular-ataxic and amnesic manifestations (14).

SUBCLINICAL THIAMIN DEFICIENCY

There is concern about the impact of persisting subclinical or borderline thiamin deficiency on the health status of a population. Subjects with subclinical thiamin deficiency show an increased risk of beriberi when stressed with extreme physiologic or pathologic conditions, including pregnancy, lactation, high physical activity, infection, and surgery. The presence of subclinical deficiency is well illustrated in a study of Japanese university students (24).

Routine physical examination of 766 students revealed irritability with mild cardiovascular signs in 42. Of these 42 students, 15 (35.7%) had whole blood thiamin levels below 190 nmol/L (<50 ng/mL). In review of 2754 chest x-ray films, 93 students had cardiothoracic ratios over 50%; of these 93 students, 44 had whole blood thiamin levels below 50 ng/mL. Analysis of the lifestyles of 59 students with low whole blood thiamin levels revealed that 50 to 60% ate their meals in restaurants and 39 to 47% did not eat breakfast. Furthermore, 86% of students with cardiac enlargement and low blood thiamin levels undertook strenuous exercise daily; only 20% were aware of their own abnormalities. Cardiothoracic ratios were improved in 63% of 83 subjects by limiting their strenuous exercise and providing nutritional advice.

More studies are needed to verify subclinical thiamin deficiency in those having psychologic, cardiovascular, and neurologic symptoms. Dietary assessment and laboratory tests should be conducted in populations with chronically low thiamin intake, and appropriate dietary guidelines should be implemented to improve their thiamin status.

REQUIREMENTS AND RECOMMENDED INTAKES

Since thiamin is essential for the metabolism of carbohydrates and branched-chain amino acids, the recommended thiamin intake is expressed in terms of total caloric intake. The current RDAs for thiamin in the United States are 1.9 μmol/4184 kJ (0.5 mg/1000 kcal) for children, adolescents, and adults, and 1.5 μmol/4184 kJ (0.4 mg/1000 kcal) for infants. These recommendations are based on assessment of the effects of varying levels of dietary thiamin on the occurrence of deficiency signs, on the excretion of thiamin or its metabolites, and on ETKA. A minimal thiamin intake of 3.8 μmol/day (1.0 mg/day) is recommended for adults, even though they might consume less than 8368 kJ (2000 kcal) daily. An additional thiamin intake of 1.5 μmol/day (0.4 mg/day) is recommended throughout pregnancy to accommodate maternal and fetal growth and increased maternal caloric intake. To account for both the thiamin secretion in milk and increased energy consumption during lactation, an increment of 1.9 μmol/day (0.5 mg/day) is recommended throughout lactation (23) (see also Appendix Table II-A-2-a-2). The 1989 recommended dietary intakes of thiamin in Thailand agree with values in the United States (25).

The 1988 United States recommended daily intakes vary from the 1989 RDA by only a few tenths of a mg (see Appendix Tables II-A-2-c-1 and related tables II-A-c-2 and 3) (26).

Patients with thiamin deficiency can be treated with physiologic doses of thiamin. However, patients with thiamin-responsive disease only respond to pharmacologic doses of thiamin. These disorders include thiamin-responsive megaloblastic anemia, thiamin-responsive lactic acidosis, thiamin-responsive branched-chain ketoaciduria, and subacute necrotizing encephalopathy (3, 5, 9).

TOXICITY

Excessive amounts of ingested thiamin are rapidly cleared by the kidneys. No evidence exists of thiamin toxicity by oral administration (3, 23).

REFERENCES

1. Gubler CJ. Thiamin. In: Machlin LJ, ed. Handbook of vitamins: nutritional, biochemical, and clinical aspects. New York: Marcel Dekker, 1984;245–97.
2. Haas RH. Annu Rev Nutr 1988;8:483–515.
3. Tanphaichitr V. Thiamin. In: Shils ME, Olson JA, Shike M, eds. Modern nutrition in health and disease. 8th ed. Philadelphia: Lea & Febiger, 1994;359–65.
4. International Union of Nutritional Sciences Committee on Nomenclature. J Nutr 1990;120:7–14.
5. Tanphaichitr V, Wood B. Thiamin. In: Olson RE, Broquist HP, Chichester CO, et al., eds. Present knowledge in nutrition. 5th ed. Washington, DC: Nutrition Foundation, 1984; 273–84.
6. Tanphaichitr V. Epidemiology and clinical assessment of vitamin deficiencies in Thai children. In: Eeckels RE, Ransome-Kuti O, Kroonenberg CC, eds. Child health in the tropics. Dordrect: Martinus Nijhoff, 1985;157–66.
7. Leevy CM. Ann NY Acad Sci 1982;378:316–26.
8. Davis RE, Icke JC, Thom J, et al. J Nutr Sci Vitaminol 1984;30:475–82.
9. Davis RE, Icke G. Adv Clin Chem 1983;23:93–140.
10. Chaithiraphan S, Tanphaichitr V, Cheng TO. Nutritional heart disease. In: Cheng TO, ed. The international textbook of cardiology. New York: Pergamon Press, 1986;864–70.
11. Tanphaichitr V, Vimokesant SL, Dhanamitta S, et al. Am J Clin Nutr 1970;23:1017–26.
12. Tanphaichitr V, Lerdvuthisopon N, Dhanamitta S, et al. Intern Med 1990;6:43–6.
13. Brady JA, Rock CL, Horneffer MR. J Am Diet Assoc 1995;95:541–4.
14. Victor M, Martin JB. Nutritional and metabolic diseases of the nervous system. In: Isselbacher KJ, Braunwald E, Wilson JD, et al., eds. Harrison's principles of internal medicine, vol 2. New York: MacGraw Hill, 1994:2328–39.
15. Singleton CK, Pekovich SR, McCool BA, et al. J Nutr 1995;125:189–94.
16. Tallaksen CME, Bohmer T, Bell H. Am J Clin Nutr 1992;56:559–64.
17. Sukumalchantra Y, Tongmitr V, Tanphaichitr V, et al. Mod Med Asia 1976;12:7–10.
18. Baker H, Thomson AD, Frank O, et al. Am J Clin Nutr 1974;21:676–80.
19. Djoenaidi W, Notermanus H, Dunca G. Eur J Clin Nutr 1992;46:227–34.
20. Tanphaichitr V. Evaluation of nutritional status. In: Wahlqvist ML, Vobecky JS, eds. Medical practice of preventive nutrition. London: Smith-Gordon, 1994:33–42.
21. Kimura M, Sato N, Itokawa Y. Trace Nutr Res 1988;(4):163–70.
22. Iber FL, Blass JP, Brain M, et al. Am J Clin Nutr 1982;6:1067–82.
23. Food and Nutrition Board, National Research Council. Recommended dietary allowances. 10th ed. Washington, DC: National Academy Press, 1989;125–32.
24. Hatanaka Y, Ueda K. J Osaka Univ 1981;(31):83–91.
25. Committee on the Second Edition of the Recommended Daily Dietary Allowances, Department of Health. Recommended daily dietary allowances and dietary guidelines for healthy Thais. Bangkok: Ministry of Public Health, 1989:65–8.

26. Food and Nutrition Board—Institute of Medicine. Dietary reference intakes. Thiamin, riboflavin, niacin, vitamin B_6, folate, vitamin B_{12}, pantothenic acid, biotin, and choline. Washington DC: National Academy Press, 1998.

SELECTED READINGS

Chaithiraphan S, Tanphaichitr V, Cheng TO. Nutritional heart disease. In: Cheng TO, ed. The international textbook of cardiology. New York: Pergamon Press, 1986:864–70.

Gubler CJ. Thiamin. In: Machlin LJ, ed. Handbook of vitamins: nutritional, biochemical, and clinical aspects. New York: Marcel Dekker, 1984:245–97.

Haas RH. Thiamin and the brain. Annu Rev Nutr 1988;8:483–515.

Tanphaichitr V. Thiamin. In: Shils ME, Olson JA, Shike M, eds. Modern nutrition in health and disease. 8th ed. Philadelphia: Lea & Febiger, 1994;359–65.

Rindi G. Thiamin. In: Ziegler EE, Filer LJ Jr, eds. Present knowledge in nutrition. 7th ed. Washington, DC: ILSI Press, 1996:160–6.

22. Riboflavin

DONALD B. McCORMICK

The "water-soluble B" fraction, reported by McCollum and Kennedy in 1916 to contain an antiberiberi substance (1), was subsequently shown by Emmett and Luros (1920) (2) and Smith and Hendrick (1926) (3) to contain at least a second more heat-stable antipellagra factor, which was termed B_2. It soon became apparent that this B_2 fraction was a complex containing a yellow growth factor called riboflavin in England and vitamin G in the United States, as well as the subsequently identified pellagra-preventive factor (niacin) and the rat antidermatitis factor (vitamin B_6). Although a water-soluble, yellow fluorescent compound was known in the latter part of the 19th century (4) to occur in such natural materials as whey, association of the pigment with vitaminic properties was not secured until its isolation in 1933 by several groups (5–7). Terms applied to riboflavin indicated the origin (e.g., lactoflavin [milk], ovoflavin [egg], hepatoflavin [liver], and uroflavin [urine]). Meanwhile, by 1932 Warburg and Christian in Germany had isolated a yellow respiratory ferment (now called "old yellow enzyme") from yeast (8). This flavoprotein was soon dissociated into a protein apoenzyme and a yellow prosthetic coenzyme that was clearly similar to riboflavin (9). Stern and Holiday (1934) found that the coenzyme was an alloxazine derivative (10), and Theorell (1934) demonstrated that it was a phosphate ester (11).

By 1935, the groups of Kuhn at Heidelberg (12, 13) and Karrer in Zurich (14, 15) had synthesized the vitamin. Theorell, in 1937, secured the structure of the simpler coenzyme as riboflavin 5′-phosphate (flavin mononucleotide, or FMN) (16). By 1938, Warburg and Christian had isolated and characterized the more abundant but complex prosthetic group, flavin-adenine dinucleotide (FAD), and showed its participation as the coenzyme of D-amino acid oxidase (17–20). More recently, diverse natural flavins have been found that have alterations in the side chain or ring system of the basic flavin structures (21). No fewer than four 8α-modified forms of FAD occur covalently attached to important flavoproteins in the mammal: the *N*(3)-histidyl-linked succinate and sarcosine dehydrogenases of the inner mitochondrial membrane, *S*-cysteinyl-linked monoamine oxidase of the outer mitochondrial membrane, and the *N*(1)-histidyl-linked L-gluconolactone oxidase of the liver microsomal fraction.

CHEMISTRY, INCLUDING PRINCIPAL ANALOGUES

Riboflavin (vitamin B_2) was chemically specified as 6,7-dimethyl-9-(1′-D-ribityl)isoalloxazine, but with evolution of systematic nomenclature is now correctly given as 7,8-dimethyl-10-(1′-D-ribityl)isoalloxazine. The free vitamin is a weak base normally isolated or synthesized as a yellowish orange amorphous solid. The 5′-hydroxymethyl terminus of the ribityl side chain in the vitamin is reacted to become an orthophosphate ester in the simpler coenzyme, FMN, which can be further enlarged to the more complex and frequently encountered FAD with a pyrophosphate-bridged adenylate moiety (Fig. 22.1). The molecular weight of riboflavin is 376.4; thus, 1 mg riboflavin equals 2.66 μmol.

There are some natural variations on the parent vitaminic structure, such as the 8-dimethylamino group of roseoflavin produced by *Streptomyces davawensis* (22, 23), the side-chain aldehyde and acid products (schizoflavins [24]) resulting from oxidation of the 5′-hydroxymethyl of riboflavin by a fungal enzyme narrowly specific for the vitamin (25, 25a), and 5′-glycosides of riboflavin, which can be formed by plant and animal species (26). Several natural variants of the coenzyme forms are listed in Table 22.1.

Chemical syntheses of riboflavin and similar isoalloxazines have been accomplished by several routes (27), most of which were adapted from the earlier procedures of Kuhn and Karrer and from modifications introduced by Tishler, Massey, and their associates (28, 28a).

Riboflavin is only modestly soluble in aqueous solutions, though strong acid flavinium salts formed at low pH (<1) and flavin anion formed at alkaline pH (>10) are considerably more soluble. Neutral and slightly alkaline solutions are yellow with a long-wavelength absorption band near 450 nm. Strongly acidic flavin solutions are paler, because their primary absorbance shifts with intensification to about 385 nm. Solutions of the neutral oxidized

Abbreviations: FAD—flavin adenine dinucleotide; **FMN**—flavin mononucleotide.

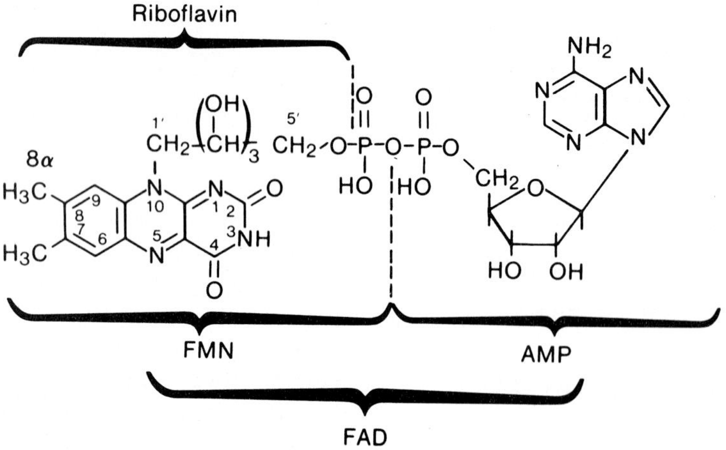

Figure 22.1. Riboflavin and flavin mononucleotide (FMN) as components of flavin-adenine dinucleotide (FAD).

(quinoid) form of the vitamin are strongly fluorescent, with an emission wavelength at 525 nm. Riboflavin also has phosphorescent character reflecting triplet state reactivity following light excitation. One consequence of flavin photochemistry is the photolability of the side chain. Riboflavin is photodegraded ultimately to yield vitaminically inactive lumiflavin (7,8,10-trimethyl-isoalloxazine) under alkaline conditions and lumichrome (7,8-dimethylalloxazine) at all pH values, especially in neutral to acidic solutions. Flavins are chemically and biologically reduced, often through the radical (semiquinone) forms, to the nearly colorless, nonfluorescent 1,5-dihydro forms that rapidly reoxidize upon exposure to air (oxygen).

Chemical syntheses of flavocoenzymes involve phosphorylation of riboflavin (29), commonly with chlorophosphoric acid, to form crude FMN, which is purified chromatographically. Conversion of FMN to FAD usually involves condensation of activated AMP, such as adenosine-5′-phosphoromorpholidate, with an FMN salt (30, 31). Extension of these techniques has been useful in forming coenzyme analogues (32).

BIOLOGIC ACTIVITY RELATING TO STRUCTURE

Numerous analogues of riboflavin and the coenzyme derivatives have been tested in whole organisms (33) and with apoflavoproteins (21, 28a, 34), respectively. In general, the full D-ribityl side chain is needed, though weak vitaminic activity has been found with the D-arabo configuration. Interestingly, flavin-dependent alcohol oxidase from methylotropic yeasts contains an araboflavin adenine dinucleotide (a-FAD) that is autocatalytically derived from the accompanying FAD (35). D-Galactoflavin is an antagonist. In addition to a normal pyrimidinoid portion, both 7- and 8-methyl substituents are required for optimal vitaminic activity, though sparing with corresponding monoethyl analogues has been reported. The 7,8-dihaloflavins are inhibitors, as is isoriboflavin with a 6,7-dimethyl structure. The 5′-phosphate, commonly occurring as the dianionic ester, is needed for binding in FMN-dependent systems, and an additional 5′-AMP moiety is needed with FAD-dependent enzymes.

ABSORPTION, TRANSPORT, METABOLISM, AND EXCRETION

The processes by which riboflavin and lesser amounts of natural derivatives are released by digestion of complexes with food proteins and then absorbed, transported, and metabolically altered have been reviewed fairly comprehensively (21). Salient features are that coenzyme forms of the vitamin (mainly FAD and less FMN) are released from noncovalent attachment to proteins as a consequence of gastric acidification. Nonspecific action of pyrophosphatase and phosphatase on the coenzyme forms occurs in the upper gut. Several percent of 8α-(amino acid)riboflavins originally in covalent attachment to certain enzymes, such as mitochondrial succinate dehydrogenase or monoamine oxidase, and traces of other ring and side-chain substituted flavins are also released by these actions following proteolysis. The vitamin is primarily absorbed in the human in the proximal small intestine by a saturable transport system that is rapid and proportional to dose before leveling off at 66.5 μmol (25 mg) of riboflavin. Bile salts appear to facilitate uptake, and a modest amount of the vitamin circulates via the enterohepatic system. Active transport at lower levels of intake may be Na^+ dependent and involve phosphorylation. An Na^+-dependent active transport process was suggested by studies on riboflavin uptake in rat intestine in vivo (36) and in vitro (37, 38); however, recent studies using Caco-2 human intestinal epithelial cells indicate that the uptake is Na^+ independent (39).

In the human, some of the riboflavin circulating in blood plasma is loosely associated with albumin, though significant amounts complex with other proteins. A subfraction of IgG binds avidly to a small portion of the total free flavin in blood (40), and several immunoglobulins contribute significantly to the circulatory transport of the vitamin (41). As found earlier in other mammals such as the cow (42), pregnancy increases the level of a riboflavin

Table 22.1.
Naturally Occurring Variants of Flavin Mononucleotide (FMN) and Flavin-Adenine Dinucleotide (FAD)

Name	Enzyme (source)
Arabo-FAD	Alcohol oxidase *(Hansenula polymorpha)*
6-Hydroxy-FMN or -FAD	Glycolate oxidase (porcine liver)
	Electron-transferring flavoproteins *(Megasphaera elsdenii)*
8-Hydroxy-FAD	Electron-transferring flavoprotein *(Megasphaera elsdenii)*
6-*S*-Cysteinyl(peptide)-FMN	Di- and trimethylamine dehydrogenases (bacterium W3A1, *Hyphomicrobium* X)
8α-*S*-Cysteinyl(peptide)-FAD	Monoamine oxidase A and B (mitochondria)
	Cytochromes c-532 and c-533 *(Chromatium* strain D, *Chlorobium thiosulfatophilum)*
8α-*O*-Tyrosyl(peptide)-FAD	*p*-Cresol methylhydroxylase *(Pseudomonas putida)*
8α-*N*(1)-Histidyl(peptide)-FAD	L-Glucono-γ-lactone oxidase (rat liver microsomes)
	L-Galactonolactone oxidase *(Saccharomyces cerevisiae)*
	Cholesterol oxidase *(Schizophyllum commune, Gleocystidium chrysocreas, Pseudomonas)*
	β-Cyclopiazonate oxidocyclase *(Penicillium cyclopium)*
	Thiamin dehydrogenase (soil bacterium ATCC 25589)
8α-*N*(3)-Histidyl(peptide)-FAD	Succinate dehydrogenase (bacteria, yeast, mitochondria)
	Sarcosine dehydrogenase/oxidase (bacteria, mitochondria)
	D-6-Hydroxynicotine oxidase *(Arthrobacter oxidans)*
	Fumarate reductase *(Escherichia coli)*
	Choline oxidase *(Alcaligenes* spp., *Arthrobacter globiformis)*
	D-Gluconate dehydrogenase *(Pseudomonas aeuginosa, P. fluorescens)*
Coenzyme F_{420} (5-deaza-5-carba-7,8-didemethyl-8-hydroxy; 5′-phospholactyldi-glutamyl)	Methane synthetase *(Methanobacterium)*

Updated from Edmondson DE, De Francesco R. Structure, syntheses, and physical properties of covalently bound flavins and 6- and 8-hydroxyflavins. In: Müller F, ed. Chemistry and biochemistry of flavoenzymes, vol I. Boca Raton, FL: CRC Press, 1991;73–103.

carrier protein in humans as well (43), and there are differential rates of uptake for the vitamin at the maternal and fetal surfaces of the placenta (44). Entry of riboflavin into mammalian cells appears to be carrier mediated (facilitated) at physiologic concentrations, but diffusion contributes to entry at higher levels (45, 46). Uptake exhibits relative specificity, and a riboflavin-binding protein has been found in the plasma membrane of rat liver cells (47). The parenchymal hepatocyte does not depend on Na^+ for riboflavin import (48) as does the renal proximal tubular cell (49). In all cases, metabolic trapping dependent on cytosolic flavokinase follows passage of the vitamin through the plasma membrane, which also contains nonspecific alkaline phosphatase that can catalyze release of vitamin from its internal phosphate ester (45).

Metabolic interconversions of flavins at the cellular level are outlined in Figure 22.2. Conversion of riboflavin to coenzymes occurs within the cellular cytoplasm of most tissues, but particularly in the small intestine, liver, heart, and kidney (21, 45, 50). The obligatory first step is the adenosine triphosphate (ATP)-dependent phosphorylation of the vitamin catalyzed by flavokinase. The FMN product can be complexed with specific apoenzymes to form several functional flavoproteins, but most is further converted to FAD in a second ATP-dependent reaction catalyzed by FAD synthetase (pyrophosphorylase). It seems likely that the biosynthesis of flavocoenzymes is tightly regulated and dependent on riboflavin status (51). Thyroxine and triiodothyroxine stimulate FMN and FAD synthesis in mammalian systems (52, 53), which seems to involve a hormone-mediated increase in an active form of flavokinase (54). As a product of the synthetase, FAD is also an effective inhibitor at this step and may regulate its own formation (55). FAD is the predominant flavocoenzyme in tissues, where it is mainly complexed with numerous flavoprotein dehydrogenases and oxidases. Interaction between coenzyme and apoenzyme usually involves a characteristic dinucleotide-binding fold with the amino acid fingerprint of GXGXXG (56). Less than 10% of the FAD can also become covalently attached to specific amino acid residues of a few important apoenzymes. Examples include the 8α-*N*(3)-histidyl FAD within succinate dehydrogenase and 8α-*S*-cysteinyl FAD within monoamine oxidase, both of mitochondrial localization. Turnover of covalently attached flavocoenzymes requires intracellular proteolysis, and further degradation of the coenzymes involves nonspecific pyrophosphatase cleavage of FAD to adenosine monophosphate (AMP) and FMN and action by nonspecific phosphatases on FMN. A 5′-nucleotidase purified from human placenta possesses specific FAD pyrophosphatase activity when stimulated with cobalt (57).

Because little riboflavin is stored as such, the urinary excretion reflects dietary intake and catabolic and photodegradative events (45). The diverse flavin-related products identified in the urine of humans and other mammals are shown in Figure 22.3. Both 7- and 8-hydroxymethylflavins appear in urine from the human and rat and are the result of microsomal mixed-function oxidases (58). 7-Hydroxymethylriboflavin (7α-hydroxyriboflavin) also appears as the only significant catabolite of the vitamin in human plasma (59). Smaller amounts of side-chain degradation products such as lumichrome, 10-formylmethylflavin, and 10-(2′-hydroxyethyl)flavin are also excreted and may largely result from intestinal microorganisms (60–62). Traces of 8α-flavin peptides and catabolites are found in urine and feces (62, 63). The α-D-gluco-

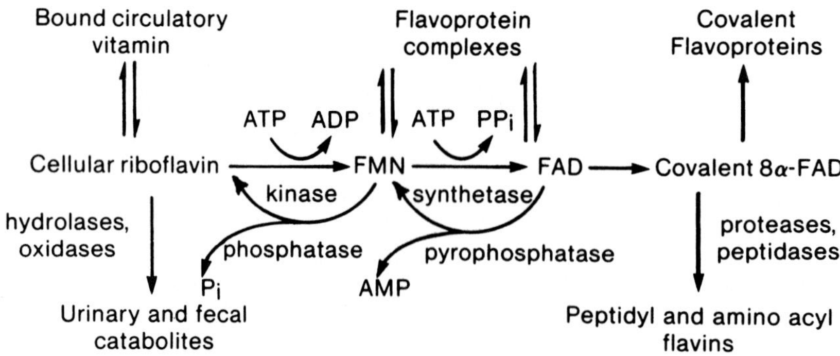

Figure 22.2. Cellular interconversions of flavins.

side attached to the side-chain 5′-position of riboflavin has been detected in liver (26) and urine (64), even though it is easily taken in and hydrolyzed by hepatocytes to liberate the free vitamin (65). A 5′-riboflavinyl peptide ester also occurs in human urine (66). For normal adults eating varied diets, riboflavin accounts for 60 to 70% of urinary flavin, 7-hydroxymethylriboflavin for 10 to 15%, 8α-sulfonylriboflavin for 5 to 10%, 8-hydroxymethylriboflavin

Lumichrome + Lumiflavin

10-Hydroxyethyl-flavin ⇌ 10-Formylmethyl-flavin

5′- Riboflavinyl-peptide and Riboflavin 5′-α-D-glucoside

Catabolites ← 8α-N[3]-Histidyl-FAD ← Riboflavin → 8α-S-Cysteinyl FAD → 8α-Sulfonyl-riboflavin

8-Carboxy- ← 8-Formyl- ← 8-Hydroxymethyl-riboflavin ← Riboflavin → 7-Hydroxymethyl-riboflavin → 7-Formyl- → 7-Carboxy-

8-Carboxylumichrome

7-Carboxylumichrome

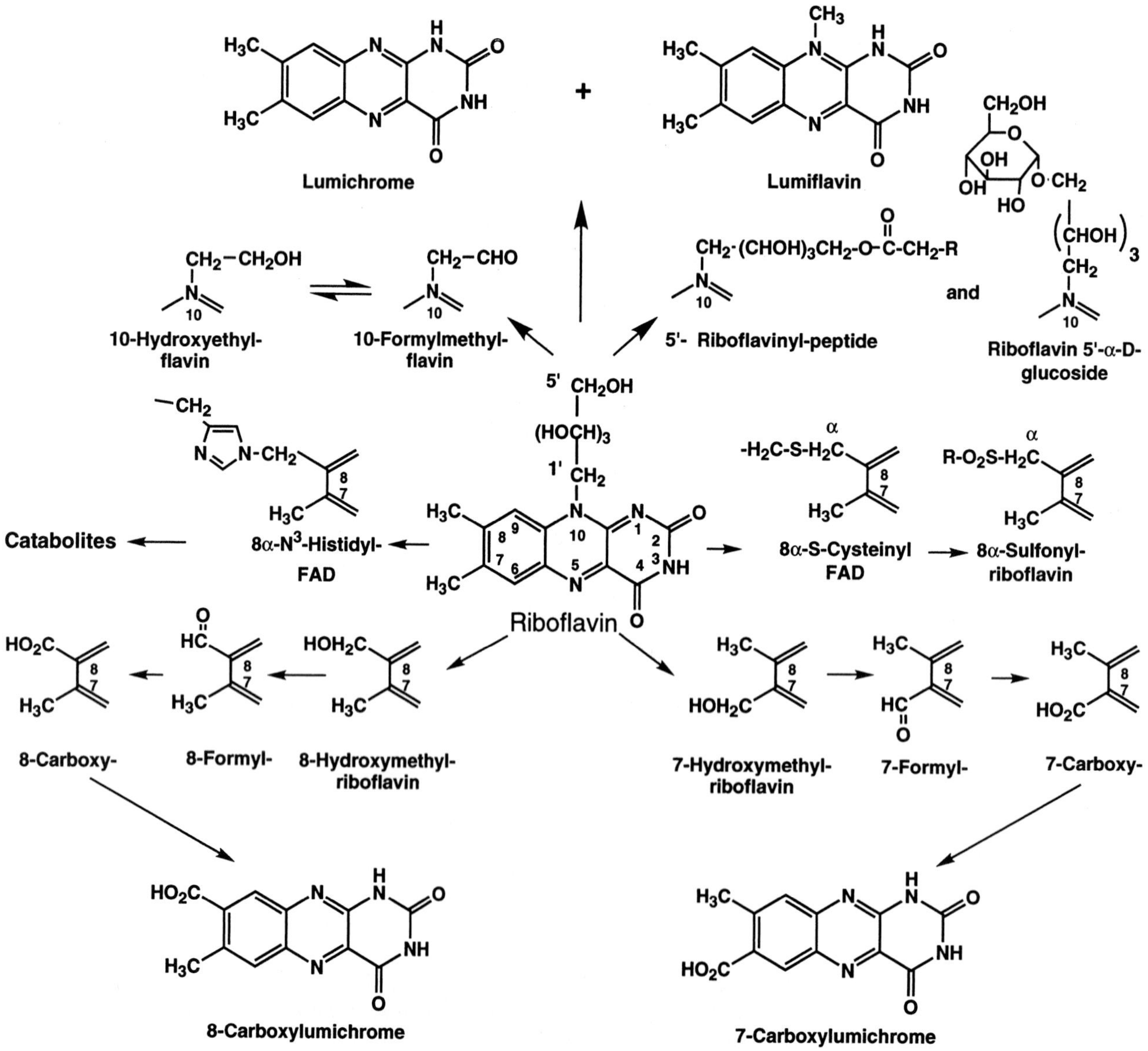

Figure 22.3. Urinary flavins and products related to riboflavin and 8α-flavocoenzymes.

for 4 to 7%, riboflavinyl peptide ester for 5%, and 10-hydroxyethylflavin for 1 to 3%, with traces of lumiflavin and varyingly the 10-formylmethylflavins and carboxymethylflavins (45).

Secretion of flavin into milk, an early recognized source (4) that came to be called lactoflavin, has been reexamined with better techniques for separation and identification. In milk from both cows (67) and humans (68), the flavin in highest concentration other than the free vitamin is FAD, which can account for over a third of total flavin. Much of this is hydrolyzed to FMN during pasteurization. Fairly significant quantities of the 10-(2′-hydroxyethyl)-flavin are notable, because this catabolite has antivitaminic activities as reflected in competitive inhibition of both cellular uptake (48) and subsequent flavokinase-catalyzed phosphorylation of riboflavin (69). Hence, this catabolite, which may reach 10 to 12% of flavin in cow's milk, subtracts from the biologic activity of the food. Several percent of both 7- and 8-hydroxymethylriboflavins are also present, with more of the former. Smaller amounts of other catabolites, including the 10-formylmethylflavin and lumichrome, account for most of the rest.

BIOCHEMICAL AND PHYSIOLOGIC FUNCTIONS

In bound coenzymic form, riboflavin participates in oxidation-reduction reactions in numerous metabolic pathways and in energy production via the respiratory chain. A variety of chemical reactions are catalyzed by flavoproteins (21, 50, 70). The redox functions of a flavocoenzyme, illustrated in Figure 22.4, include one-electron transfers, during which the biologically encountered, neutral, oxidized quinone level of flavin is half reduced to the radical semiquinone, which can exist in natural pH ranges as a neutral or anionic species. Further electron transfer can lead to a fully reduced hydroquinone. Additionally, a single-step two-electron transfer from substrate to flavin can occur with hydride ion transfer, as from reduced pyridine nucleotide, or by base abstraction of a substrate proton together with carbanion addition (21).

There are flavoprotein-catalyzed dehydrogenations that are both pyridine nucleotide-dependent and -independent, reactions with sulfur-containing compounds, hydroxylations, oxidative decarboxylations, dioxygenations, and reduction of O_2 to hydrogen peroxide. The

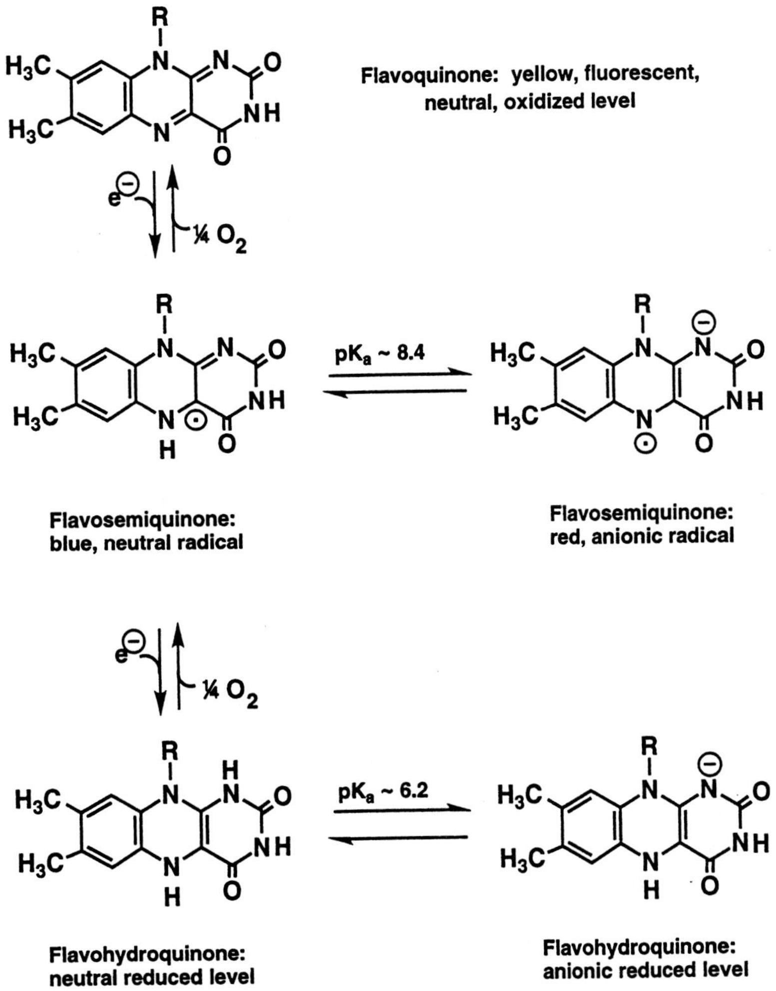

Flavoquinone: yellow, fluorescent, neutral, oxidized level

$e^{\ominus}$ ⇅ ¼ O_2

pK$_a$ ~ 8.4

Flavosemiquinone: blue, neutral radical

Flavosemiquinone: red, anionic radical

$e^{\ominus}$ ⇅ ¼ O_2

pK$_a$ ~ 6.2

Flavohydroquinone: neutral reduced level

Flavohydroquinone: anionic reduced level

Figure 22.4. Physiologically relevant redox states of flavocoenzymes.

intrinsic abilities of flavins to be varyingly potentiated as redox carriers upon differential binding to proteins, to participate in both one- and two-electron transfers, and in reduced (1,5-dihydro) form to react rapidly with oxygen permit wide scope in their operation.

DEFICIENCY AND EXCESS

Though riboflavin has a wide distribution in foodstuffs, many people live for long periods on low intakes; consequently, minor signs of deficiency are common in many parts of the world (71). Moreover, the deficiency encountered almost invariably occurs in combination with deficiency of other water-soluble vitamins (45). Clinical deficiency of riboflavin has been induced by feeding a riboflavin-deficient diet, by administration of an antagonist such as galactoflavin, or both. The deficiency syndrome is characterized by sore throat, hyperemia and edema of the pharyngeal and oral mucous membranes, cheilosis, angular stomatitis, glossitis (magenta tongue), seborrheic dermatitis, and normochromic, normocytic anemia associated with pure red cell cytoplasia of the bone marrow (72). However, some of these symptoms, such as glossitis and dermatitis, when encountered in the field may have resulted from other complicating deficiencies. Severe riboflavin deficiency can also affect the conversion of vitamin B_6 to its coenzyme and even curtail conversion of tryptophan to niacin (45).

Toxicity from ingestion of excess riboflavin by experimental animals or humans is doubtful. The human gastrointestinal tract may be able to absorb less than 30 mg of riboflavin from a single dose orally administered (73, 74). Pharmacokinetic analysis of riboflavin dynamics in healthy humans reflects the expected saturability of plasma levels, with excretion enhanced by renal tubular secretion (75). The limited solubility and absorptivity of this vitamin as encountered in multivitamin preparations and in natural foodstuffs and its ready excretion (which is typical of water-soluble vitamins) normally preclude a health risk. There is one report of electroencephalogram (EEG) abnormalities in two patients during long-term treatment with riboflavin and niacin (76).

CAUSES OF DEFICIENCY

Pure, uncomplicated riboflavin deficiency is probably never encountered in patients but is accompanied by multiple nutrient deficiencies. Ariboflavinosis can result from primary and secondary factors that commonly affect supply or use of other nutrients as well (77). Inadequate dietary intake, most commonly related to limited availability of food but sometimes exacerbated by poor storage or processing, remains the major cause. Anoretic persons rarely ingest adequate amounts of riboflavin and other nutrients.

Decreased assimilation results from abnormal digestion, absorption, or both. Lactose intolerance as a result of lactase insufficiency, mostly encountered among blacks and Asians, argues against consuming milk, which is a good source of the vitamin. Malabsorption can result from tropical sprue, celiac disease, malignancy and resection of the small bowel, and gastrointestinal and biliary obstruction. Poor absorption also results from disorders that increase motility and decrease gastrointestinal passage time, such as diarrhea, infectious enteritis, and irritable bowel syndrome.

Rarely encountered, but usually significantly improved by therapeutic treatment with riboflavin, are certain inborn errors in which the genetic defect affects formation of a normal flavoprotein. This category includes fatty acid desaturases in which specific defects have been found for the mitochondrial FAD-dependent dehydrogenases for short-chain (78), long-chain (79), and multichain acyl-CoAs (80). The young patients have a lipid storage myopathy, often accompanied by carnitine insufficiency, and exhibit glutaric aciduria (81–85). Low FMN-dependent pyridoxine-5′-phosphate oxidase activity caused by erythrocytic deficiency of FMN, confirmed by response to oral riboflavin, was reported in most patients with D-glucose-6-phosphate dehydrogenase deficiency in two studies (86, 87). Such cases seem to involve an accelerated conversion of FMN to FAD so that glutathione reductase is saturated. This contrasts with heterozygous β-thalassemia, in which there is an inherited slow erythrocytic conversion of riboflavin to FMN, a decrease in subsequent FAD, and high stimulation of the erythrocytic glutathione reductase by extraneous FAD (86, 88, 89).

Defective use can result from disturbances in hormonal production, certainly as related to thyroid hormone (52, 53), but is less likely to be affected by oral contraceptives (90). Phenothiazine derivatives appear to impair use of riboflavin (91).

Increased destruction of riboflavin occurs during treatment of neonatal jaundice with phototherapy (92, 93). In this case, the side chain of the vitamin is photochemically destroyed, as it is involved in the photosensitized oxidation of bilirubin to more polar excretable compounds (94, 95). The finding that phenobarbital induces microsomal oxidation of the 7-methyl function of the vitamin (58) lends credence to the belief that long-term use of barbiturates may jeopardize flavin status.

Enhanced excretion of riboflavin occurs in catabolic patients undergoing nitrogen loss. The relationship of the vitamin to protein status has long been recognized. Certain antibiotics and phenothiazine drugs also increase excretion of riboflavin (96, 97).

Increased requirements can, of course, result from one or more of the factors mentioned above. For example, protein-calorie malnutrition commonly accompanies diminution in both absorption and use of riboflavin. Systemic infections even without gastrointestinal involvement sometimes lead to increased requirements that can result from decreased intake, defective absorption, poor utilization, and increased excretion.

DIETARY CONSIDERATIONS

The requirement for riboflavin, in contrast to thiamin, does not increase when energy use is increased (98). Because of the interdependence of protein, energy intake, and metabolic body size, however, recommended dietary allowances (RDAs) calculated on these three bases do not differ significantly. Because RDA values are given in milligrams (98a), this mass unit has been used here. Nonetheless, 1 μmol riboflavin equals 0.376 mg, or inversely, 1 mg riboflavin equals 2.66 μmol. Thus, 0.4, 0.6, 1.2, and 1.7 mg riboflavin can be expressed as 1.06, 1.6, 3.2, and 4.5 μmol, respectively. Clinical signs of deficiency in adults can be prevented with intakes of riboflavin above 0.4 mg/1000 kcal, but more than 0.5 mg/1000 kcal may be required to maintain tissue reserves in adults and children, as reflected in urinary excretion, red cell riboflavin, and erythrocytic glutathione reductase. From these considerations, the riboflavin allowances are now computed as 0.6 mg/1000 kcal for people of all ages. 1989 RDAs ranged from 0.4 mg/day for early infants to 1.7 mg/day for young adult males (see Appendix Table II-A-2-a-2). However, for elderly people and others whose daily calorie intake may be less than 2000 kcal, a minimum of 1.2 mg per day was recommended. Because pregnancy imposes extra demands, as reflected by decreased excretion and elevated FAD stimulation of erythrocytic glutathione reductase activity, an additional 0.3 mg/day was recommended. The lactating woman secretes approximately 35 μg/100 mL of milk for an output of about 0.26 mg/day (750 mL) during the first 6 months and 0.21 mg/day (600 mL) during the second 6 months. Because the utilization of additional riboflavin for milk production is assumed to be 70%, an additional intake of 0.5 mg was recommended for the first 6 months and 0.4 mg for the second.

The 1998 RDAs for riboflavin are less (0.2–0.5 mg/day) than the 1989 RDAs for those ages 14 and above (see Appendix Table II-A-2-c-1) (98a).

Small amounts of riboflavin, occurring largely as digestible coenzymes, are present in most plant and animal tissue. Especially good sources are eggs, lean meats, milk, broccoli, and enriched breads and cereals (99). Such losses as occur during cooking are largely due to leaching of the heat-stable but light-sensitive flavins into water. (See Appendix Table IV-A-23-a for the riboflavin content of common foods.)

When supplementation or therapy with riboflavin is warranted, oral administration of 5 to 10 times the RDA usually is satisfactory (96).

METHODS FOR ASSAY AND STATUS DETERMINATION

Numerous biochemical methods are aimed at the separation and quantitation of the diverse natural flavins (100, 101). Among the more sensitive are those that invoke specific binding, such as riboflavin with egg white riboflavin–binding protein, FMN with apoflavodoxin, and FAD with apoproteins for D-amino acid oxidase or glucose oxidase. However, nutritional status is commonly assessed by measuring urinary excretion of the vitamin in fasting, random, or 24-hour specimens or by load return tests, measurement of erythrocyte riboflavin concentration, and determination of the erythrocyte glutathione reductase activity coefficient (77, 102).

Urinary riboflavin can be measured by fluorometric as well as by microbiologic procedures. Under conditions of adequate intake, the amount excreted per day is more than 0.32 μmol (120 μg), or at least 0.21 μmol (80 μg) are excreted per gram of creatinine. The rate of excretion expressed as mg/g creatinine is greater for children than for adults, who normally have 80 μg/g or more but fall below 27 μg/g when deficient. Conditions causing negative nitrogen balance and the administration of antibiotics and certain psychotropic drugs (phenothiazine) increase urinary riboflavin as a consequence of tissue depletion and displacement, respectively. A load return test augments the applicability to a given case. Only high-performance liquid chromatography (HPLC) of suitable extracts followed by specific identification of each flavin can distinguish the natural vitamin from other urinary flavins (62).

Erythrocytic riboflavin can also be determined either fluorometrically or microbiologically. Because changes are rather small, there is some problem with sensitivity and interpretation of results. Nevertheless, values below 27 nmol (10 μg)/dL cells should be considered to reflect a deficient status, compared with 40 nmol/dL or more ($\geq$15 μg/dL) for an acceptable status. Again, HPLC has been used to monitor more exactly the riboflavin composition of human blood (75, 103).

Currently, riboflavin status is most commonly assessed by determination of FAD-dependent glutathione reductase activity in freshly lysed red cells, as detailed for routine clinical use (104) from the procedure described by Sauberlich et al. (105). Activities of holo and apo forms of glutathione reductase in erythrocyte hemolysates are measured before and after addition of FAD, respectively, by spectrophotometric determinations of NADPH (the reduced form of nicotinamide-adenine dinucleotide phosphate) oxidation. Values obtained are expressed in terms of "activity coefficients," or ACs, (AC = ΔA_{340} with FAD/ΔA_{340} without FAD), which represent the degree of stimulation of apoenzyme resulting from addition of FAD in vitro. An AC of 1.0 indicates no stimulation and only the presence of holoenzyme as a result of excess FAD (and riboflavin) in the original erythrocytes. Guidelines suggested for such coefficients are <1.2, acceptable; 1.2 to 1.4, low; >1.4, deficient. Though it is currently the biochemical method of choice for assessing riboflavin status, the erythrocyte glutathione reductase assay has some drawbacks (77). The test cannot be used in persons with glucose 6-phosphate deficiency because of an increased avidity in the reductase for FAD in this disease, which occurs in about 10% of black Americans. In vitro treatment of blood with inosine and adenine elevates activity coefficients (106).

REFERENCES

1. McCollum EV, Kennedy C. J Biol Chem 1916;24:491–502.
2. Emmett AD, Luros GO. J Biol Chem 1920;43:265–86.
3. Smith MI, Hendrick EG. US Public Health Rep 1926;41: 201–7.
4. Blyth AW. J Chem Soc 1879;35:530–9.
5. Kuhn R, Gyorgy P, Wagner-Jauregg T. Ber Dtsch Chem Ges 1933;66B:317, 576–80, 1034–8.
6. Ellinger P, Koschara W. Ber Dtsch Chem Ges 1933;66B:315–7.
7. Booher LE. J Biol Chem 1933;102:39–46.
8. Warburg O, Christian W. Biochem Z 1932;254:438–58.
9. Warburg O, Christian W. Biochem Z 1933;266:377–411.
10. Stern KG, Holiday ER. Ber Dtsch Chem Ges 1934;67:1104–6, 1442–52.
11. Theorell H. Biochem Z 1934;272:155–6.
12. Kuhn R, Reinemund K, Kaltschmitt H, et al. Naturwissenschaften 1935;23:260.
13. Kuhn R, Reinemund K, Weygand F, et al. Chem Ber 1935;68:1765–74.
14. Karrer P, Schöpp K, Benz F. Helv Chim Acta 1935;18:426–9.
15. Karrer P, Salomon H, Schöpp K, et al. Helv Chim Acta 1935;18:1143–6.
16. Theorell H. Biochem Z 1937;290:293–303.
17. Warburg O, Christian W. Biochem Z 1938;295:261.
18. Warburg O, Christian W. Biochem Z 1938;296:294.
19. Warburg O, Christian W, Griese A. Biochem Z 1938;297:417.
20. Warburg O, Christian W. Biochem Z 1938;298:150–68.
21. Merrill AH Jr, Lambeth JD, Edmondson DE, et al. Annu Rev Nutr 1981;1:281–317.
22. Otani S, Takatsu M, Nakano M, et al. J Antibiot 1974;27:88–9.
23. Otani S. Studies on roseoflavin: isolation, physical, chemical, and biological properties. In: Singer TP, ed. Flavins and flavoproteins. Amsterdam: Elsevier, 1976;323–7.
24. Tachibana S, Murakami T. Isolation and identification of schizoflavins. In: McCormick DB, Wright LD, eds. Vitamins and coenzymes. Methods in enzymology, vol 66, pt E. New York: Academic Press, 1980;333–8.
25. Kekelidze T, Edmondson DE, McCormick DB. Arch Biochem Biophys 1994;315:100–3.
25a. Chen H, McCormick DB. J Biol Chem 1997;272:20077–81.
26. Whitby LG. Glycosides of riboflavin. In: McCormick DB, Wright LD, eds. Vitamins and coenzymes. Methods in enzymology, vol 18, pt B. New York: Academic Press, 1971;404–13.
27. Lambooy JP. The alloxazines and isoalloxazines. In: Elderfield RC, ed. Heterocyclic compounds, vol 9. New York: John Wiley & Sons, 1967;118–223.
28. Tishler M, Pfister K, Babson RD, et al. J Am Chem Soc 1947;69:1487–92.
28a. Murthy YVSN, Massey V. Syntheses and applications of flavin analogs as active site probes for flavoproteins. In: McCormick DB, Suttie JW, Wagner C, eds. Vitamins and coenzymes: methods in enzymology, vol. 280, pt J. New York: Academic Press, 1997.
29. Flexer LA, Farkas WG. (Abstract) XIIth International Congress Pure Applied Chemistry. New York: Sept. 1951;71.
30. Moffatt JG, Khorana HG. J Am Chem Soc 1958;80:3756–61.
31. Moffatt JG, Khorana HG. J Am Chem Soc 1961;83:649–58.
32. Föry W, McCormick DB. Chemical synthesis of flavin coenzymes. In: McCormick DB, Wright LD, eds. Vitamins and coenzymes. Methods in enzymology, vol 18, pt B. New York: Academic Press, 1971;458–64.
33. McCormick DB. NY State J Med 1962;62:2842–4.
34. McCormick DB. Metabolism of riboflavin. In: Rivlin RS, ed. Riboflavin. New York: Plenum Press, 1975;153–98.
35. van Berkel WJH, Eppink MHM, Schreuder HA. Protein Sci 1994;3:2245–53.
36. Rivier DA. Experientia 1973;29:1443–6.
37. Meinen M, Aeppli R, Rehner G. Nutr Metab 1977;21(Suppl 1):264–6.
38. Daniel H, Wille U, Rehner G. J Nutr 1982;113:636–43.
39. Said HM, Ma TY. Am J Physiol 1994;266:G15–21.
40. Merrill AH Jr, Froehlich JA, McCormick DB. Biochem Med 1981;25:198–206.
41. Innis WSA, McCormick DB, Merrill AH Jr. Biochem Med 1985;34:151–65.
42. Merrill AH Jr, Froehlich JA, McCormick DB. J Biol Chem 1979;254:9362–4.
43. Natraj U, George S, Kadam P. J Reprod Immunol 1988; 13:1–16.
44. Dancis J, Lehanka J, Levitz M. Am J Obstet Gynecol 1988; 158:204–10.
45. McCormick DB. Physiol Rev 1989;69:1170–98.
46. Bowman BB, McCormick DB, Rosenberg IH. Annu Rev Nutr 1989;9:187–99.
47. Nokubo M, Ohta M, Kitani K, et al. Biochim Biophys Acta 1989;981:303–8.
48. Aw T-Y, Jones DP, McCormick DB. J Nutr 1983;113:1249–54.
49. Bowers-Komro DM, McCormick DB. Riboflavin uptake by rat kidney cells. In: Edmondson DE, McCormick DB, eds. Flavins and flavoproteins. New York: Walter de Gruyter, 1988;449–53.
50. McCormick DB. Riboflavin. In: Brown ML, ed. Present knowledge in nutrition. 6th ed. Washington, DC: International Life Sciences Institute Nutrition Foundation, 1990;146–54.
51. Lee SS, McCormick DB. J Nutr 1983;113:2274–9.
52. Rivlin RS, ed. Riboflavin. New York: Plenum Press, 1975.
53. Rivlin RS. Nutr Rev 1979;37:241–5.
54. Lee SS, McCormick DB. Arch Biochem Biophys 1985;237: 197–201.
55. Yamada Y, Merrill AH Jr, McCormick DB. Arch Biochem Biophys 1990;278:125–30.
56. Wierenga RK, De Maeyer MCH, Hol WGJ. Biochemistry 1985;24:1346–57.
57. Lee RS, Ford HC. J Biol Chem 1988;263:14878–83.
58. Ohkawa H, Ohishi N, Yagi K. J Biol Chem 1983;258:5623–8, 5629.
59. Zempleni J, Galloway JR, McCormick DB. Int J Vitam Nutr Res 1996;66:151–7.
60. Oka M, McCormick DB. J Nutr 1985;115:496–9.
61. Chastain JL, McCormick DB. J Nutr 1987;117:468–75.
62. Chastain JL, McCormick DB. Am J Clin Nutr 1987;46:8 30–4.
63. Chia CP, Addison R, McCormick DB. J Nutr 1978;108:373–81.
64. Ohkawa H, Ohishi N, Yagi K. J Nutr Sci Vitaminol 1983;29: 515–22.
65. Joseph T, McCormick DB. J Nutr 1995;125:2194–8.
66. Chastain JL, McCormick DB. Biochim Biophys Acta 1988;967: 131–4.
67. Roughead Z, McCormick DB. J Nutr 1990;120:382–8.
68. Roughead Z, McCormick DB. Am J Clin Nutr 1990;52:854–7.
69. McCormick DB. J Biol Chem 1962;237:959–62.
70. Edmondson DE, McCormick DB, eds. Flavins and flavoproteins. New York: Walter de Gruyter, 1987.
71. Bates CJ. World Rev Nutr Diet 1987;50:215–67.
72. Wilson JA. Disorders of vitamins—deficiency, excess and errors of metabolism. In: Petersdorf RG, et al., eds. Harrison's principles of internal medicine. 10th ed. New York: McGraw-Hill, 1982;461–70.
73. Stripp B. Acta Pharmacol Toxicol 1965;22:353–62.
74. Mayersohn M, Feldman S, Gibaldi M. J Nutr 1969;98:288–96.

75. Zempleni J, Galloway JR, McCormick DB. Am J Clin Nutr 1996;63:54–66.
76. Santanelli P, Gobbi G, Albani F, et al. Neurophysiol Clin 1988;18:549–53.
77. Nichoalds GE. Riboflavin. Symposium in laboratory medicine. In: Clinics in laboratory medicine, vol 1, no 4. Philadelphia: WB Saunders, 1981;685–98.
78. DiDonato S, Gellera C, Peluchetti D, et al. Ann Neurol 1989; 25:479–84.
79. Amendt BA, Moon A, Teel L, et al. Pediatr Res 1988;23:603–5.
80. Gilkeson GS, Caldwell DS. Arthritis Rheum 1988;31:695–6.
81. Iafolla AK, Kahler SG. J Pediatr 1989;114:1004–6.
82. Mandel H, Africk D, Blitzer M, et al. J Inherited Metab Dis 1988;11:397–402.
83. Turnbull DM, Bartlett K, Eyre JA, et al. Dev Med Child Neurol 1988;30:667–72.
84. Turnbull DM, Shepherd IM, Ashworth B, et al. Brain 1988;111:815–28.
85. Lipkin PH, Roe CR, Goodman SI, et al. J Pediatr 1988; 112:62–5.
86. Anderson BB, Clements JE, Perry GM, et al. Eur J Haematol 1987;38:12–20.
87. Powers HJ, Bates CJ. Hum Nutr Clin Nutr 1985;39:107–15.
88. Anderson BB, Perry GM, Clements JE. Br J Haematol 1984;57:711–4.
89. Anderson BB, Perry GM, Clements JE, et al. Eur J Haematol 1989;42:354–60.
90. Roe DA, Boguzz S, Sheu J, et al. Am J Clin Nutr 1982;35:495–501.
91. Horvath C, Szonyi L, Mold K. Teratology 1976;14:167–70.
92. Rublatelli FF, Allegri G, Costa C, et al. J Pediatr 1974;85: 865–7.
93. Gromisch DS, Lopez R, Cole HS, et al. J Pediatr 1977;90: 118–22.
94. Knobloch E, Mandys F, Hodr R. J Chromatogr 1988;428: 255–63.
95. Knobloch E, Hodr R. Czech Med 1989;12:134–44.
96. Goldsmith GA. Prog Food Nutr Sci 1975;1:559–609.
97. Pinto J, Huang YP, Rivlin RS. Clin Res 1979;27:444A.
98. Food and Nutrition Board, National Research Council. Riboflavin. In: Recommended dietary allowances. 10th ed. Washington, DC: National Academy Press, 1989;132–7.
98a. Food and Nutrition Board—Institute of Medicine. Dietary reference intakes. Thiamin, riboflavin, niacin, vitamin B_6, folate, vitamin B_{12}, pantothenic acid, biotin, and choline. Washington DC: National Academy Press, 1998.
99. Watt BK, Merrill AL. Composition of food: raw processed, prepared. In: Agriculture handbook no. 8. Washington, DC: US Department of Agriculture, 1963.
100. McCormick DB, Wright LD, eds. Vitamins and coenzymes. Methods in enzymology, vol 18, pt B. New York: Academic Press, 1971.
101. McCormick DB, Wright LD, eds. Vitamins and coenzymes. Methods in enzymology, vol 66, pt E. New York: Academic Press, 1980.
102. Briggs M, ed. Vitamins in human biology and medicine. Boca Raton, FL: CRC Press, 1981.
103. Ishida T, Horiike K. Nippon Rinsho 1989;48:589–91.
104. McCormick DB, Greene HL. Vitamins. In: Burtis CA, Ashwood ER, eds. Tietz textbook of clinical chemistry. Philadelphia: WB Saunders, 1994;1275–316.
105. Sauberlich HE, Judd JH Jr, Nichoalds GE, et al. Am J Clin Nutr 1972;25:756–62.
106. Trout GE. Proc Soc Exp Biol Med 1989;191:12–17.

SELECTED READINGS

McCormick DB. Two interconnected B vitamins: riboflavin and pyridoxine. Physiol Rev 1989;69:1170–98.

McCormick DB. Riboflavin. In: Brown ML, ed. Present knowledge in nutrition. 6th ed. Washington, DC: International Life Sciences Institute-Nutrition Foundation, 1990;146–54.

Müller F, ed. Chemistry and biochemistry of flavoenzymes, vols I, II. Boca Raton, FL: CRC Press, 1991.

Yagi K, ed. Flavins and flavoproteins. Berlin: Walter de Gruyter, 1993.

23. Niacin

DANIEL CERVANTES-LAUREAN, N. GERARD McELVANEY, and JOEL MOSS

HISTORICAL BACKGROUND

Niacin (also known as nicotinic acid), a member of the B group of vitamins, was initially studied because of its association with pellagra. This nutritional deficiency disease was first described by Casal (1) in 1735 as "mal de la rosa," with the classic symptoms of dermatitis, diarrhea, and dementia, with death as the eventual outcome. Early this century, an epidemic of pellagra in the southern United States (2), initially thought to be of infectious origin, was noted to be associated with poor nutrition, inadequate meat and milk intake, and use of corn as the principal constituent of the diet. This disease seems now to be endemic in India and parts of China and Africa (3).

In 1922, Goldberger and Tanner (4) suggested that pellagra was an amino acid deficiency. Later, Elvehjem et al. (1937) demonstrated that nicotinic acid and nicotinamide (5) isolated from liver cured black tongue, the canine counterpart of pellagra, and in the same year, Fouts et al. (6) reported that niacin cured human pellagra. In 1949, tryptophan was shown to reverse the symptoms of pellagra (7). In 1961, Goldsmith et al. (8) quantified the conversion of tryptophan to niacin by monitoring such niacin metabolites as N^1-methylnicotinamide and N^1-methyl-5-carboxamide-2-pyridone. They found that, on average, 60 mg of tryptophan was equivalent to 1 mg of the vitamin. Elucidation of the biochemical pathway for conversion of tryptophan to nicotinic acid mononucleotide (NicMN) (Fig. 23.1) took more than 10 years, from 1950, when Knox and Mehler (9) showed that the first step in the biodegradation of tryptophan to *N*-formylkynurenine was catalyzed by tryptophan pyrrolase, to 1963, when Nishizuka and Hayaishi (10) showed that quinolinic acid reacts with phosphoribosepyrophosphate (PRPP) to form NicMN, a reaction catalyzed by the enzyme quinolinic acid phophoribosyltransferase. In this period of time, it was also shown (11) that NicMN was the substrate for NMN:ATP adenylyltransferase, which catalyzed its conversion to nicotinic acid adenine dinucleotide (NicAD). NicAD is the immediate precursor of nicotinamide adenine dinucleotide (NAD) (Fig. 23.2), which plays a critical role in redox and ADP-ribose transfer reactions. The pathway that synthesizes niacin from tryptophan is primarily found in the liver but has also been reported in the kidney (12).

Nicotinamide can be recycled to nicotinic acid by nicotinamidase (Fig. 23.2). Metabolically, nicotinic acid cannot, however, be directly converted to nicotinamide, which is rather produced from NAD in ADP-ribose transfer or NAD glycohydrolase reactions (13).

CHEMISTRY AND NOMENCLATURE

The structures of niacin, also known as nicotinic acid or pyridine-3-carboxylic acid, and nicotinamide, which is also termed niacinamide, are shown in Figure 23.3. The pyridine ring is substituted at position 3 by a carboxylic acid group in nicotinic acid and by a carboxamide moiety in nicotinamide. The nitrogen in the pyridine ring of niacin is positively charged when it is a component of NAD. This cationic nitrogen confers unique chemical properties to NAD (Fig. 23.4). For example, in oxidation-reduction reactions catalyzed by dehydrogenases, addition at position 4 of the pyridine ring of a hydride derived from a reduced substrate yields reduced NAD (NADH) and an oxidized substrate (12) (Fig. 23.5).

The positive charge on the nitrogen of the pyridine ring in NAD makes the glycosylic bond (Figs. 23.6 and 23.7) that links the ribose to nicotinamide a target for

Abbreviations: **ADP-ribose**—adenosine 5-diphosphoribose; **ADPRTases**—ADP-ribosyltransferases; **ARF**—ADP-ribosylation factor; **GPI**—glycosylphosphatidylinositol; **GTP**—guanosine 5-triphosphate; **GTPases**—GTP hydrolases; **HDL**—high-density lipoprotein; **IDDM**—insulin-dependent diabetes mellitus; **LDL**—low-density lipoprotein; **NAD**—nicotinamide adenine dinucleotide; **NADases**—NAD glycohydrolases; **NicADP**—nicotinic acid adenine dinucleotide-2′-phosphate; **NicMN**—nicotinic acid mononucleotide; **PARP**—poly(ADP-ribose) polymerase.

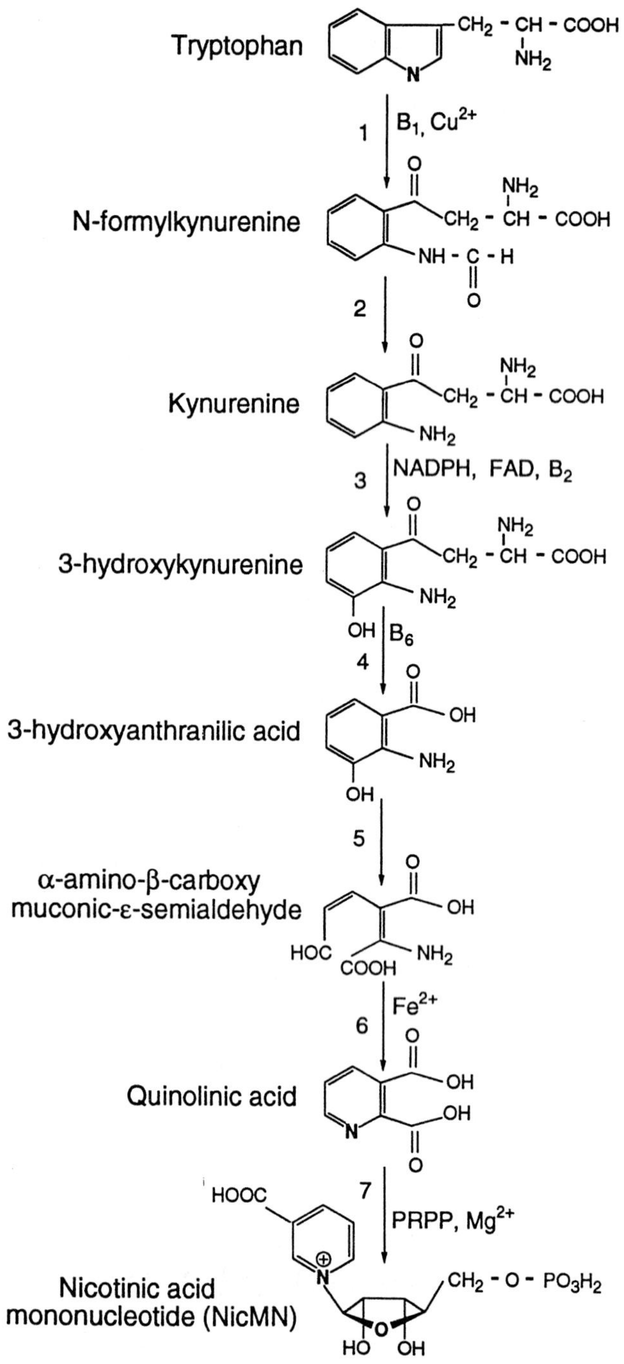

Figure 23.1. Metabolic conversion of tryptophan to nicotinic acid mononucleotide (12). *1*, tryptophan pyrrolase; *2*, kynurenine formamidase; *3*, kynurenine 3-monoxygenase; *4*, kynureninase; *5*, 3-hydroxyanthranilic acid oxygenase; *6*, nonenzymatic; *7*, quinolinic acid phophoribosyltransferase.

nucleophilic attack, leading to nicotinamide release and substitution at the electrophilic ribose 1″ carbon. These reactions are carried out by enzymes that replace the nicotinamide of NAD with nucleophilic acceptor molecules. The acceptors can be amino acids in target proteins, as in reactions catalyzed by monoadenosine diphosphate ribosyltransferases (ADPRTases) (13). In the substitution reaction, the ADP-ribose moiety of NAD is transferred to an acceptor amino acid, hence the name transferase. When the acceptor is the nitrogen at position 1 of the adenine moiety of NAD, cyclic ADP-ribose (Fig. 23.6) is formed in a reaction catalyzed by ADP-ribosyl cyclase (14, 15). In cells, cyclic ADP-ribose is believed to regulate Ca^{2+} influx (15). For the nuclear enzyme poly(ADP-ribose) polymerase (PARP), the acceptor nucleophile is the hydroxyl group in the 2′ position of a ADP-ribose monomer (forming 1″ to 2′ glycosidic linkages), already attached to a protein (this reaction is also catalyzed by PARP, which transfers ADP-ribose from NAD to a carboxylate group of an acceptor protein). Sequential additions of ADP-ribose molecules produce a long polymer with branches occurring, on average, every 40 to 50 residues (Fig. 23.8), which may have a role in DNA repair (16) and chromatin structure (17). Finally, the acceptor nucleophile may be water, a reaction catalyzed by NAD glycohydrolases (NADases) (18) that yields free ADP-ribose and nicotinamide.

DIETARY CONSIDERATIONS

Significant amounts of niacin are found in meat (especially red meat), liver, legumes, milk, eggs, alfalfa, cereal grains, yeast, fish, and corn (19). Although milk and eggs contain small amounts of preformed niacin, their content of tryptophan provides more than sufficient niacin equivalents. Red meat is reported to be one of the best sources of niacin equivalents because of its abundance of preformed niacin and tryptophan. As mentioned, tryptophan can provide niacin nutriture and it is generally believed that 60 g of the amino acid is converted to 1 g of the vitamin. Assuming that 1% (wt/wt) of proteins is tryptophan, 60 g of protein could provide 600 mg of tryptophan or 10 niacin equivalents (NE, 1 niacin equivalent equals 1 mg of either nicotinic acid or nicotinamide, which in turn corresponds to 8.13 mmol). Quantitatively, the major use of this amino acid is in protein biosynthesis. In humans, the amount of tryptophan converted to niacin depends on nutritional history (20) and hormonal factors (21). If there is a deficiency of tryptophan and niacin in the body, tryptophan is used primarily to maintain protein synthesis rather than to replenish niacin pools. Oral contraceptives and pregnancy may somewhat increase tryptophan conversion to niacin (21).

The role of dietary corn in causing pellagra led to the concept of amino acid imbalance as a potential cause of niacin deficiency (22). Corn, which contains significant amounts of niacin and tryptophan, also contains a high proportion of leucine, which inhibits the synthesis of NAD in isolated red blood cells (23), an effect counteracted by isoleucine and valine. Niacin and tryptophan requirements are also increased by threonine, cystine, methionine, and, to a lesser extent, phenylalanine (24). Although mature cereal grains are reported to contain 70% of niacin in a biologically unavailable form (3), in Mexico and Central America, populations with diets based on

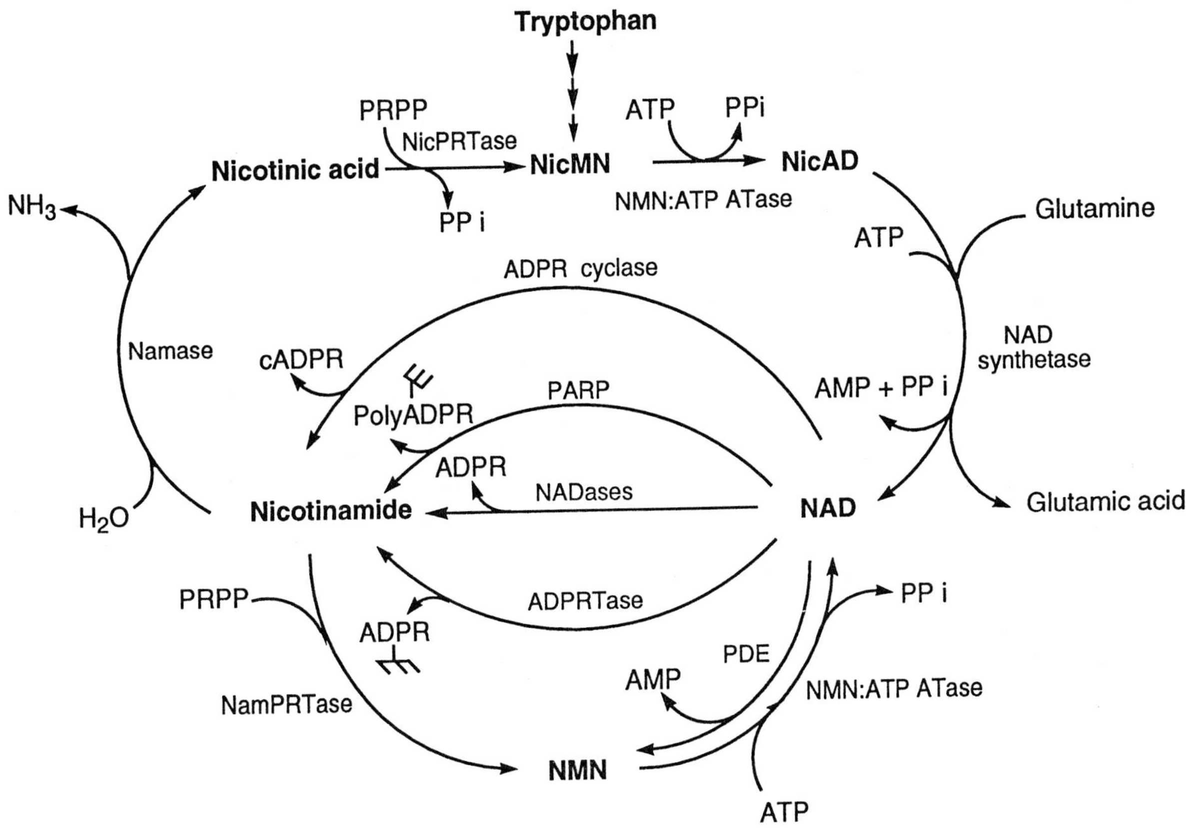

Figure 23.2. Biochemical pathways of niacin and nicotinamide metabolism. *NicPRTase,* nicotinic acid phosphoribosyltransferase; *NMN:ATP ATase,* nicotinamide-5′-mononucleotide adenosine-5′-triphosphate adenylyltransferase; *ADPRTase,* adenosine diphosphate ribosyltransferase; *PARP,* polyadenosine diphosphate ribosylpolymerase; *NamPRTase,* nicotinamide-5′-phosphoribosyltransferase; *NAD synthetase,* nicotinamide adenine dinucleotide synthetase; *PDE,* phosphodiesterase; *NADase,* nicotinamide adenine dinucleotide glycohydrolase; *ADPR cyclase,* adenosine diphosphate ribosyl cyclase; *Namase,* nicotinamidase; -E represents a bond to a protein.

corn do not suffer from pellagra. This may be related to the fact that in the preparation of tortillas, treatment of corn with alkali increases niacin availability (25).

Coffee, another common dietary constituent, is reported to contain an alkaloid known as trigonelline (N^1-methylnicotinic acid) that, in the presence of heat and acid, can form nicotinic acid. This reaction occurs during coffee bean roasting, leading to a 30-fold increase in niacin content (26).

METABOLISM: ABSORPTION, DISTRIBUTION, AND EXCRETION

Niacin and its amide adduct are absorbed through the intestinal mucosa by simple diffusion. Fifteen to 30% of niacin is bound to protein, and this vitamin-protein complex is taken up by tissues. Adipose tissue is responsible for the rapid clearance of niacin after an intravenous dose. Metabolic trapping, in which niacin and nicotinamide are converted to NAD, accounts for retention of these vitamins (27). Neutral niacin as a zwitterionic species with a carboxylic anion (pK_a = 4.5) and quaternary nitrogen cation may partition as a lipid-soluble molecule. In contrast, nicotinamide is lipid soluble only in the neutral form (i.e., with an uncharged nitrogen in the pyridine ring). Receptor-mediated uptake of nicotinamide has, however, been reported recently (28).

Niacin and nicotinamide are metabolized via different pathways. In liver, the major product of pharmacologic doses of niacin is the glycine conjugate, nicotinuric acid (Fig. 23.3), whereas the main metabolites of nicotinamide are N^1-methylnicotinamide and its oxidized products, 2- and 4-pyridones (29) (Fig. 23.3). Niacin and nicotinamide metabolites formed in the liver are excreted in urine. Quantification of excretion of nicotinuric acid and N^1-methylnicotinamide and its pyridones is useful in evaluating niacin nutriture. Since metabolism of niacin is a saturable process, the rate of niacin and nicotinamide ingestion affects their plasma levels.

FUNCTIONS

Niacin, nicotinamide, and tryptophan are precursors of NAD and NADP. These nucleotides are key components of oxidation-reduction reactions, ATP synthetic pathways, and ADP-ribose transfer reactions. In oxidation-reduction reactions, dehydrogenases use NAD/P(H) as coenzymes to oxidize or reduce a substrate. Position 4 of the pyridine ring, which in the reduced form contains two proquiral hydrogens, is the site of oxidation or reduction (12).

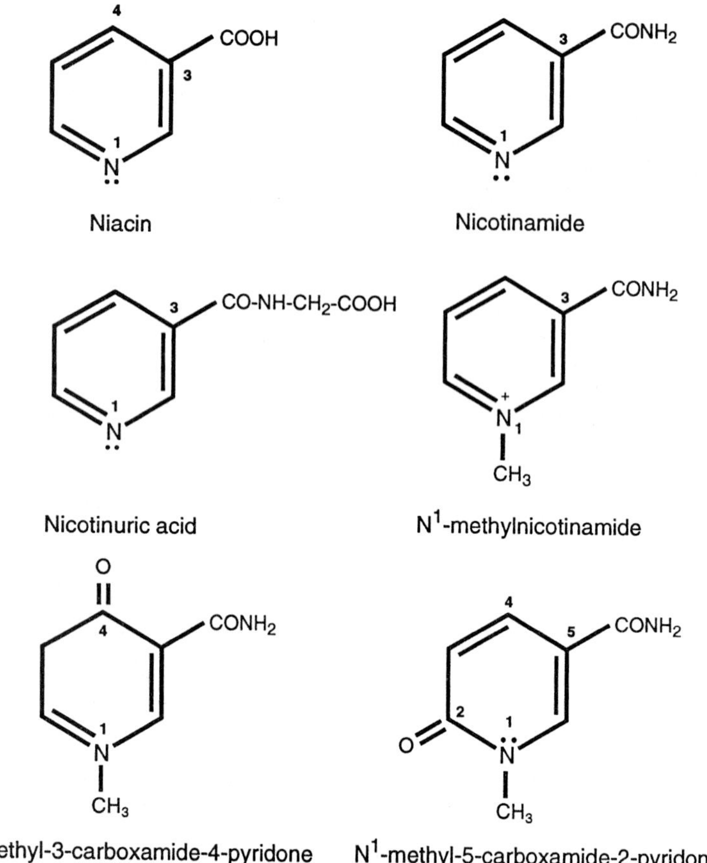

Figure 23.3. Chemical structures of niacin and nicotinamide and their metabolites. A unique metabolite of niacin is nicotinuric acid (glycine conjugate of niacin). The main metabolites of nicotinamide are N^1-methylnicotinamide and its 2- and 4-pyridone analogues.

Dehydrogenases use specifically one of the two hydrogens of the reduced NAD (see Fig. 23.5). For example, alcohol dehydrogenase from yeast and the cardiac isoenzyme of lactate dehydrogenase (LDH) use hydrogen H_b (Fig. 23.5), whereas hepatic glucose dehydrogenase and yeast glucose-6-phosphate dehydrogenase only use hydrogen H_a (30). The difference in wavelengths of maximal absorbance by NAD/P (254 nm) and NADH/PH (340 nm) is used in many assays involving dehydrogenases. NADP is directly formed from NAD by phosphorylation catalyzed by a specific kinase found in mammalian liver (12). A phosphatase has also been described that converts NADP to NAD (12).

NADP dehydrogenases are preferentially involved in anabolic reactions (e.g., synthesis of fatty acids and cholesterol [31]). In contrast, NAD is used in catabolic reactions to transfer the potential free energy stored in macronutrients such as carbohydrates, lipids, and proteins to NADH, which is then used to form ATP, the primary energy currency of the cell.

NAD Glycohydrolases

In the last 30 years, the importance of the high-energy glycosylic bond between the anomeric carbon of ribose

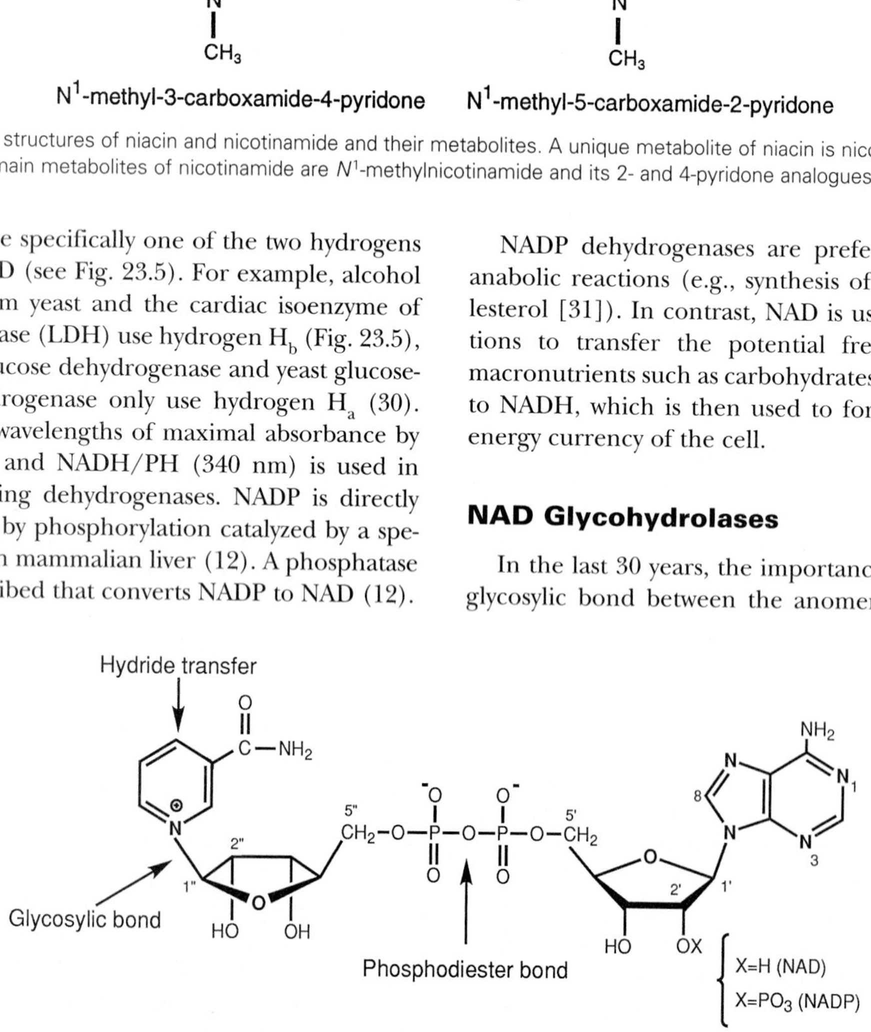

Figure 23.4. Structure of nicotinamide adenine dinucleotide.

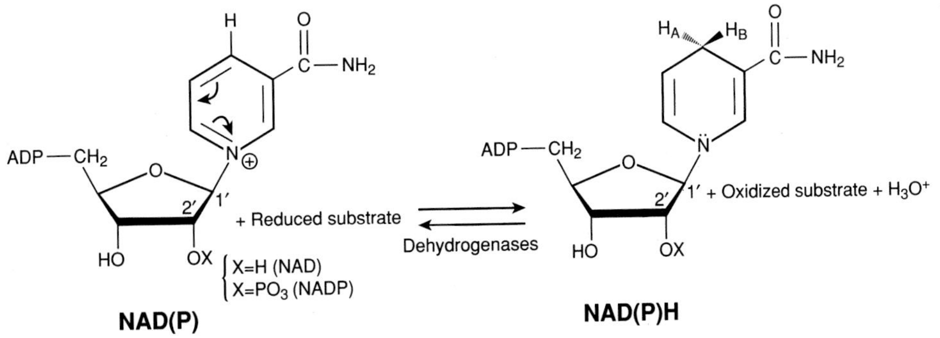

ADP—CH_2 + Reduced substrate ⇌ Dehydrogenases + Oxidized substrate + H_3O^+

X=H (NAD)
X=PO_3 (NADP)

NAD(P) NAD(P)H

Figure 23.5. General reaction of oxidation-reduction of NAD(P) by dehydrogenases.

and the quaternary nitrogen of the pyridine moiety of NAD and NADP (Fig. 23.4) in the biologic function of pyridine nucleotide coenzymes has been recognized. Early attempts to elucidate the role of NADases in vivo were fueled by the observation that isoniazid, which is a pyridine derivative used for tuberculosis treatment (2), could inhibit many NADases (32) and that this treatment could precipitate pellagra, especially in malnourished populations (33). The studies on NADases originally focused on their ability to catalyze transglycosylation reactions in vitro (18). In 1989, Lee et al. (34) reported that a metabolite of NAD, cyclic ADP-ribose (Fig. 23.6), could release Ca^{2+} from endoplasmic reticulum in sea urchins by use of ryanodine receptors. In 1993, Kim et al. (35) showed that NADases from canine spleen and from *Bungarus fasciatus* have dual activity (Fig. 23.7): *(a)* ADP-ribosyl cyclase and *(b)* cyclic ADP-ribose hydrolase, resulting in the net hydrolysis of NAD to ADP-ribose and nicotinamide. These findings raised the possibility that the elusive role of NADases could be related to signal transduction by formation of a second messenger, cyclic ADP-ribose. It is unclear whether all NADases possess this dual activity. Cyclic ADP-ribose formation and degradation by some NADases and the observation that CD38 (36) (a cell-surface antigen of T and B lymphocytes) possesses NADase and ADP-ribosyl cyclase activities renewed interest in the biologic function of NADases. The fact that CD38 is an ectoenzyme also raises the question of availability of NAD in the extracellular milieu.

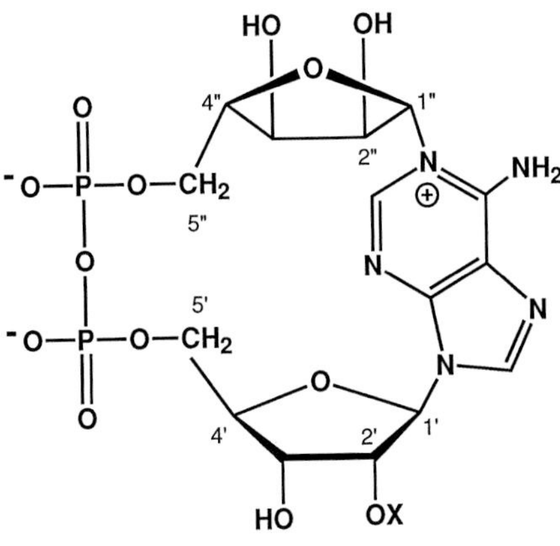

Figure 23.6. Structure of cyclic ADP-ribose (cADPR) and its 2′-phosphate analogue (14, 35, 38).

In 1996, two newly recognized products of the NADases/ADP-ribosyl cyclases (e.g., canine spleen enzyme and CD38) were shown to release Ca^{2+} from the endoplasmic reticulum. One of these products is nicotinic acid adenine dinucleotide-2′-phosphate (NicADP) (37), which is more potent than cyclic ADP-ribose; the second is cyclic ADP-ribose-2′-phosphate (38), which is as potent as cyclic ADP-ribose in releasing Ca^{2+}. Thus, NADases/ADP-ribosyl cyclases are among the few enzymes that can use both NAD and NADP as substrates. NicADP could be formed by the transglycosylation reaction of NADP with nicotinic acid catalyzed by NADases. This product may be involved in the physiologic responses to pharmacologic doses of niacin.

Mono ADP-Ribosyltransferases

NAD functions also in mono-ADP-ribosylation, the transfer of ADP-ribose from NAD to target proteins. This posttranslational modification was first characterized by use of bacterial toxins that possess intrinsic ADP-ribosyltransferase (ADPRTase) activity as well as receptor-binding components that target them to specific cells. The first toxin ADPRTase described was diphtheria toxin (39), which inhibits protein synthesis by ADP-ribosylating elongation factor 2, thereby inhibiting protein synthesis (Table 23.1). Later, it was demonstrated that *Pseudomonas aeruginosa* exotoxin A (40) catalyzes the same reaction. Cholera toxin and *Escherichia coli* heat-labile enterotoxin (41) ADP-ribosylate $G_{s\alpha}$, the α subunit of the heterotrimeric guanine nucleotide–binding (G) protein, which couples cell surface receptors that activate adenylyl cyclase to the cyclase catalytic unit. Cholera toxin–catalyzed ADP-ribosylation inhibits the GTPase activity of G_α, resulting in stabilization of an active $G_\alpha \cdot$ GTP form and persistent activation of the cyclase. ADP-ribosyltransferase activity of cholera toxin is enhanced by ADP-ribosylation factor (ARF) (42), a GTP-dependent eukaryotic protein that functions in intracellular vesicular trafficking (43). Pertussis toxin modifies the G_i, G_o, and $G_{t\alpha}$ subunits (44), proteins involved in regulating adenylyl cyclase, phospholipid turnover, and photore-

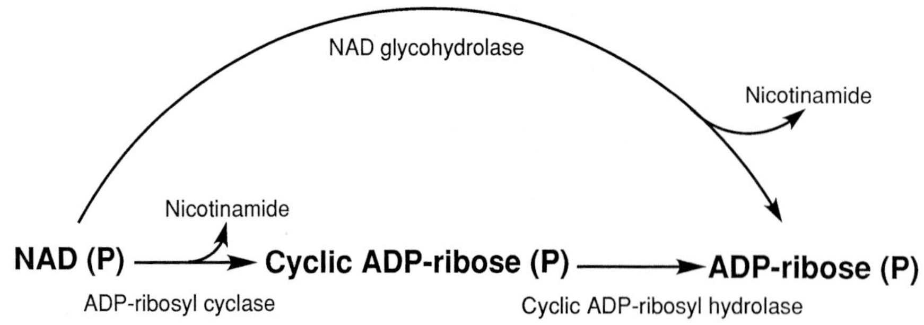

Figure 23.7. Formation of ADP-ribose from NAD. NADases can hydrolyze NAD to form ADP-ribose; some of them catalyze cyclic ADP-ribose formation first and subsequently ADP-ribose, via their intrinsic ADP-ribosyl cyclase and cyclic ADP-ribosyl hydrolase activities, respectively (35).

ceptor activation, respectively. ADP-ribosylation by pertussis toxin results in uncoupling of the modified G_α from receptor, thereby stabilizing the inactive heterotrimeric G protein.

Some strains of *Clostridium botulinum* produce a C3 ADP-ribosyltransferase (45) that ADP-ribosylates the ~20-kDa guanine nucleotide–binding protein, Rho, and a C2 toxin that ADP-ribosylates the cytoskeletal protein nonmuscle actin (46) (Table 23.1). Modification by either toxin abolishes the biologic activity of the proteins. *Clostridium perfringens* (46) produces a toxin similar in function to C2, named iota toxin, which also ADP-ribosylates actin. *P. aeruginosa* exotoxin S (47) uses as substrates Ras, Ral, Rap 1A, Rab3, and Rab4, all ~20-kDa guanine nucleotide–binding proteins (48). ADP-ribosylation by exotoxin S requires members of the 14-3-3 family of eukaryotic proteins (49). These proteins are very well conserved through evolution with biologic functions that involve signal transduction (e.g., protein kinase C activity), cellular proliferation (e.g., binding protooncogene products), Ca^{2+}-dependent exocytosis, and activation of tyrosine and tryptophan hydroxylase, enzymes involved in the synthesis of the neurotransmitters catecholamine and serotonin, respectively (50).

Eukaryotic ADPRTase counterparts of the toxins have been found, although their physiologic functions are not clear. A unique ADP-ribosyltransferase attached to the surface of skeletal and cardiac muscle cells through a glycosylphosphatidylinositol (GPI) anchor has recently been described by Zolkiewska et al. (51). Its substrate, integrin $\alpha7$, is part of a heterodimer ($\alpha7\beta1$) that interacts with extracellular matrix protein, laminin, and is regulated

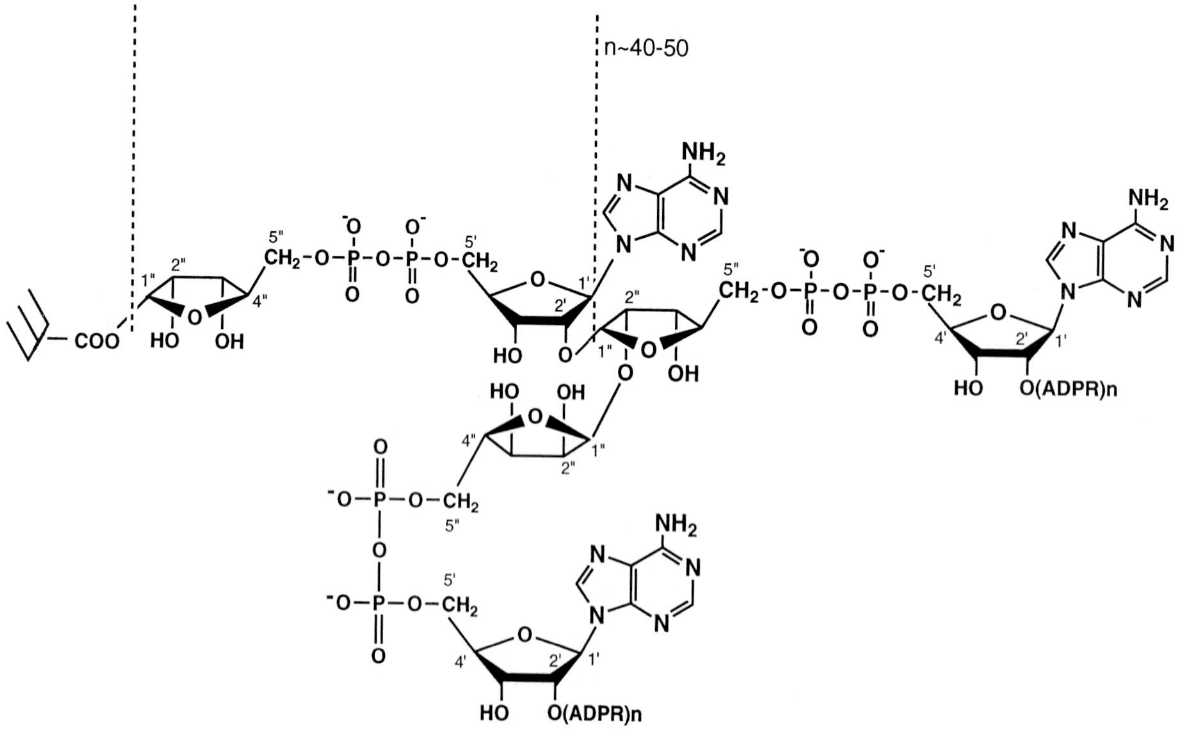

Figure 23.8. PolyADP-ribose polymer (56). The first monomer unit of ADP-ribose is linked to an acceptor protein through an α-glycosidic linkage on a carboxylate group. The linear polymer is formed with ADP-ribose units linked via α-1″-2′-glycosidic linkages and branches occurring, on average, every 40 to 50 residues via α-1″-2″-glycosidic linkages. Chemically, the glycosidic linkages attaching ADP-ribose units correspond to acetal bonds, which are acid sensitive (99); -E represents a bond to a protein.

Table 23.1
ADP-Ribosylation of Endogenous Proteins by Bacterial Toxins

Source of ADPRT Toxin	Target Protein	Protein Function
Corynebacterium diphtheriae and *Pseudomonas aeruginosa*	Elongation factor 2	Peptide translocation in protein synthesis
Vibrio cholerae and *Escherichia coli* heat-labile enterotoxin	Gsα	GTP binding subunit of heterotrimeric (α, $\beta\gamma$) complex involved in transmembrane signal transduction
Clostridium botulinum C3 *Clostridium limosum* exoenzyme *Bacillus cereus* exoenzyme Epidermal differentiation inhibitor (strain E1 of *Staphylococcus aureus*)	Rho p21	Small GTP-binding protein that regulates formation of actin stress fibers in response to growth factors
C. botulinum C2 *Clostridium perfringens* iota toxin *Clostridium spiroforme* *Clostridium difficile* (different from toxin A and B)	Nonmuscle G actin (β and γ isoforms)	Components of the cytoskeleton that form actin polymers (F actin)
P. aeruginosa exotoxin S	c-Ha-Ras, Ral, Rap 1A, Rab3, and Rab4	Key components of signaling pathways regulating cell proliferation, differentiation, and intracellular vesicle trafficking (all bind GTP)
Bordetella pertussis	$G_{\alpha i}$, $G_{\alpha o}$, and $G_{\alpha t}$	Subunit of heterotrimeric (α, $\beta\gamma$) involved in transmembrane signal transduction (all bind GTP)

developmentally. Another GPI-anchored ADPRTase, reported by Wang et al. (52), may regulate the response of cytotoxic T cells.

To date, the amino acids known to be modified by different mono-ADPRTases are arginine, cysteine, asparagine, diphthamide, histidine, and hydroxyl-containing amino acids (serine, threonine, and tyrosine) (53).

Poly(ADP-Ribose) Polymerase

Poly(ADP-ribose) polymerase (PARP), first described in 1966 by Chambon et al. (54), also uses NAD as a substrate. It is a nuclear enzyme that is activated by DNA strand breaks and synthesizes very large polymers of up to 200 ADP-ribose molecules, with branches approximately every 40 to 50 residues (55). PARP protein targets are histones and PARP itself (13). The carboxylate of glutamate, aspartate, and a C-terminal lysine can serve as ADP-ribose acceptors (13). Extensive studies with inhibitors of PARP showed its importance in DNA repair (56). Additional evidence comes from studies with PARP antisense mRNA (17) and mutant PARP cell lines (57). Cytotoxicity due to PARP activation may result from NAD reduction, i.e., energy depletion and cell death (58). More recent studies also implicate PARP in apoptosis (59), possibly via upregulation of the tumor suppressor gene p53 (60). Surprisingly, after disruption of the PARP gene, mice did not show a widespread appearance of tumors (61). Cells with this genotype were able to repair methylation damage caused by *N*-methyl-*N*′-nitro-*N*-nitroguanidine, MNNG, an alkylating agent (base excision repair) and photoproduct damage induced by UV radiation (nucleotide excision repair). Spontaneous skin cancer appeared in older PARP-knockout mice, however, which may be related to lack of the PARP protective mechanism, allowing mutated cells to survive and go through the stages of carcinogenesis. These findings suggest that the role of PARP might be related to the cellular response to environmental stress (62). Curiously, pellagra, which could limit PARP activity as a result of NAD deficiency, is characterized by a dermatitis similar to the "skin disease" of the knockout mice.

NAD also plays an important role in the ligation step during maturation of eukaryotic tRNA, in which a unique product is ADP-ribose 1″,2″-cyclic-phosphate (63).

DEFICIENCY AND MANIFESTATIONS

Niacin deficiency causes pellagra. The classic symptoms of this disease in the late stages are *dermatitis*, characterized by pigmented rash, especially in areas exposed to sunlight; *diarrhea*; and *dementia*, with symptoms including anxiety, insomnia and, in advanced stages, disorientation, hallucinations, and delirium (64). "Necklace" lesions on the lower neck, described by Casal (1), indicate advanced disease. Early stages of the dermatitis include skin thickening, scaling, and hyperkeratinization in sun-exposed areas. Inflammation of mucous membranes also occurs, with soreness of the tongue, stomatitis, esophagitis, urethritis, proctitis, and vaginitis. Intestinal inflammation leads to diarrhea. Advanced stages of pellagra can be cured with nicotinamide in intramuscular doses of 50 to 100 mg three times a day for 3 to 4 days, followed by similar quantities orally supplemented with 100 g protein per day.

Since the biotransformation of tryptophan to nicotinic acid requires several vitamins and minerals (Fig. 23.1), diets lacking these nutrients can predispose to pellagra (1). Vitamin B_6 is involved in several steps of tryptophan catabolism and increases production of tryptophan metabolites in animals and humans. As noted, isoniazid therapy of tuberculosis can cause niacin deficiency by depletion of pyridoxal phosphate (65) (vitamin B_6). Deficiency of copper, required for the conversion of tryptophan to *N*-formylkynurenine, can block niacin synthesis (66), and lack of riboflavin, required for the conversion of kynurenine to 3-hydroxykynurenine, increases excretion of kynurenine and kynurenic acid after a tryptophan load (67). It is not surprising, therefore, that riboflavin deficiency results in some of the same symptoms as niacin deficiency (e.g., stomatitis, cheilosis, and raw tongue) (26).

Hartnup's syndrome (an autosomal recessive disorder) is characterized by impaired synthesis of niacin from tryptophan, which results in pellagra-like symptoms (68). The disease results from defective absorption of tryptophan in the intestine and/or increased renal excretion (69). Treatment with nicotinamide in large doses (40–250 mg/day) markedly improves the dermatitis and neurologic problems (70).

EVALUATION OF NUTRIENT STATUS

Niacin nutriture has been assessed in several ways by a variety of methods. Bernofsky (71) described the use of Dowex-1 formate chromatography to separate pyridine nucleotides and N^1-methylnicotinamide.

Other methods used to assess niacin intake include quantification of pyridine nucleotides, (NAD/H) and (NADP/H), accurate determination of which depends on the method of extraction, since acid destroys NADH and NADPH and alkali degrades NAD and NADP. A method devised by Lowry et al. (1961) (72) to measure NAD and NADP is based on the sequential use of two dehydrogenases. The oxidized product is measured by adding extra pyridine nucleotide and an appropriate dehydrogenase, and the resulting pyridine nucleotide is finally quantified fluorometrically. A modification of this method by Slater and Sawyer (73) in 1961 and later by Nisselbaum and Green (74) in 1969 replaced one of the dehydrogenases with thiazolyl blue, which is reduced by NADH and NADPH, via phenazine methosulfate, to form a purple compound, formazan, in an amount proportional to the concentration of the coenzymes (oxidized and reduced). This assay uses appropriate dehydrogenases specific for either NAD or NADP. This method has been used to measure these pyridine nucleotides in tissue and blood.

Measurement of N^1-methylnicotinamide and its 2-pyridone derivative in urine (75) has been used to monitor niacin nutriture. Urinary levels of N^1-methylnicotinamide below 0.8 mg/day indicate niacin deficiency (76). A ratio of N^1-methyl-5-carboxamide-2-pyridone to N^1-methylnicotinamide of 1.3 to 2 is considered normal; it is less than 1 in niacin deficiency (77). Niacin status can also be assessed by measuring its physiologically active forms, NAD(H)/NADP(H).

Fu et al. (78) investigated possible markers of niacin nutriture in erythrocytes. The study spanned 12 weeks and was divided into four periods: stabilization, depletion, repletion, and high intake. Like the results in cultured cells (79), NADP levels were the same in all four periods, while NAD levels decreased significantly during the depletion period. It was proposed that an NAD:NADP ratio higher than 1 reflects adequate niacin nutriture and a ratio below 1, niacin deficiency. Since tryptophan concentrations in blood fell very rapidly from 11.5 to 6.1 mg/mL during the depletion period, it was suggested that the combination of NAD:NADP ratio and tryptophan concentration in erythrocytes could be used to assess severe niacin deficiency. In this study, leucine given with tryptophan did not affect blood levels of NAD and NADP, a finding inconsistent with the proposal that leucine interferes with tryptophan use in NAD biosynthesis.

REQUIREMENTS AND RECOMMENDED INTAKE

Prevention of pellagra requires 11.3 to 13.3 NE/day. The recommended dietary allowance (RDA) of 1989 was 15 to 20 NE/day in adult males and 13 to 15 in females, with caloric intake of no less than 2000 kcal (3) (see also Appendix Table II-A-2-a-2). The 1998 RDAs for niacin for children and adults are 1 to 3 mg/day less than the 1989 RDAs (100). The use of NE is based on the fact that dietary tryptophan can replace niacin. There is significant controversy about the correct ratio of tryptophan to niacin; it has been reported that 60 mg of tryptophan provides 1 mg of niacin, with a variation of about 30% (SD) among individuals (80).

There are no data concerning relevant niacin requirements in pregnancy and lactation. Based on an average increase in energy expenditure of 300 kcal/day during pregnancy, the niacin RDA for pregnant women was increased by 2 units. During lactation, women who breast feed provide 750 mL/day of milk that contains 1.0 to 1.3 NE. Taking this into consideration, as well as the increase in caloric expenditure during lactation, the niacin RDA may be increased by 5 NE/day. Although there are no data for infants and children, 5 to 9 NE/1000 kcal intake are assumed to suffice in infants, and 18 NE/1000 kcal in adolescents (3).

American women, 19 to 50 years old, consume, on average, 700 mg of tryptophan daily, whereas men in the same age range consume 1100 mg. These amounts represent 16 and 24 NE for women and men, respectively (3). After addition of preformed niacin in the diet, the values are 27 NE for women and 41 NE for men.

NIACIN AS PHARMACOLOGIC AGENT

Niacin in large doses (1–3 g/day) is antihyperlipidemic (81). Nicotinamide is being investigated as preventive therapy for insulin-dependent diabetes and is used currently to treat Hartnup's syndrome (69). Different pharmacologic responses to niacin and nicotinamide are consistent with the fact that these compounds, although obviously related, are metabolized differently by cells. Niacin and tryptophan share two common intermediates in pathways leading to NAD (Fig. 23.2). The first is NicMN, a substrate for NMN:ATP adenylytransferase, which catalyzes synthesis of the second common intermediate, NicAD. NicAD requires transamination to form NAD. In contrast, NMN is used directly for NAD synthesis via the nuclear enzyme NMN:ATP adenylyltransferase (which also can use NicMN as a substrate) (12). Fewer metabolic reactions are needed to convert nicotinamide than nicotinic acid to NAD, which may explain why nicotinamide is more effective in restoring NAD pools in niacin deficiency (Fig. 23.2).

Niacin decreases triglyceride levels in blood by lowering very low density lipoproteins (VLDL) (82). It is also effective in increasing high-density lipoprotein (HDL), while usually reducing low-density lipoprotein, LDL (83). Niacin treatment can result in a regression of atherosclerotic plaques and overall reduction in patient mortality (84, 85).

In 1990, the Familial Atherosclerosis Treatment Study (84) compared two lipid-lowering treatments. The first included lovastatin (an inhibitor of hydroxymethylglutaryl CoA reductase, a rate-limiting enzyme in the biosynthesis of cholesterol) and colestipol (which sequesters bile acids and interferes with lipid absorption). The second regimen included niacin with colestipol. In the control group, LDL levels fell slightly (7%); those in the niacin/colestipol group decreased by 32%, and those in the lovastatin/colestipol group, by 46%. Increases of 5% in HDL levels in the control group, 15% in the lovastatin/colestipol group, and 43% in the niacin/colestipol group were observed. The lovastatin/colestipol- and niacin/colestipol-treated groups showed a 50% decrease in the frequency of stenosis progression, a dramatic increase in stenosis regression, and a 73% decrease in frequency of cardiovascular events. Another landmark study, the Cholesterol-Lowering Atherosclerosis Study (CLAS I and II) (85), reported the effects of niacin/colestipol therapy on coronary atherosclerosis over a span of 6 years. The findings included significant differences in nonprogression (52% drug vs. 15% control) and regression (18% drug vs. 6% control) of coronary artery lesions.

Nicotinamide can prevent macrophage- (86) or interleukin 1β–induced β-cell damage in vitro (87), and treatment of mice with nicotinamide significantly decreased development of alloxan- and streptozotocin-induced (88) or spontaneous (89) insulin-dependent diabetes mellitus (IDDM). Nicotinamide protection appears to result, at least in part, from inhibition of interleukin 1β–induced nitric oxide production and from serving as a radical scavenger (90). In 1994, evidence for a role of nitric oxide activation of PARP in neurotoxicity was reported (91). This background provided the rationale for investigation of the effect of nicotinamide on prevention of the onset of IDDM in humans. IDDM is an autoimmune disease associated with β-cell destruction in the pancreatic islets of Langerhans and appearance of circulating antibodies long before the manifestation of insulin deficiency (92). Two marker antibodies can be used to identify people at risk. The one against glutamic acid decarboxylase and the other against islet cell antigen (ICA) were associated with risks of 17 and 20%, respectively, for onset of IDDM within 5 years (93). When both antibodies are present, the risk is 90%.

Compelling evidence of the effectiveness of nicotinamide in preventing or delaying the onset of IDDM was obtained in a study in Auckland, New Zealand (94). Of 81,993 children aged 5 to 7 years, 33,658 were selected randomly, and 20,195 of these agreed to be tested for ICA antibodies. Children with 20 units or more of ICA and those with 10 units of ICA plus first-phase insulin release (a measure of β-cell function) below 100 mmol/L were treated with nicotinamide. The incidence of IDDM was compared in those two groups (the 20,195 children who accepted ICA screening and the 13,463 who were randomly chosen but were not screened) as well as a third (termed random control) group. Incidence rates per 10^5 exposure years in the three groups were 20.1 for the control, 8.1 for those treated, and 15.1 for the chosen group that refused to be tested. A large trial of nicotinamide for prevention or delay in onset of IDDM is now in progress, with Canada and 18 European countries participating.

Nicotinamide and nicotinic acid have also been postulated to be important in carcinogenesis (95). The proposed role is based on the requirement for NAD to support proper functioning of PARP. It is suggested that proper repair of DNA damage by involvement of functional PARP, which requires abundant NAD, would prevent or retard, in the long term, the multistage process of carcinogenesis. The current hypothesis for cancer prevention is that if small amounts of DNA damage occur, optimal PARP activity in the presence of adequate NAD pools would be efficiently involved in repairing it (the precise role of PARP in DNA repair has not been defined) so that mutation is limited. If more DNA damage occurs, a functional PARP would trigger apoptosis, probably via increased p53, or cause cell death by NAD depletion, thus preventing survival of a putative mutated, and perhaps eventually carcinogenic, cell.

AVAILABLE FORMULATIONS OF NIACIN

As described above, niacin is used in large doses to treat hyperlipidemia. These doses are provided in two different formulations: modified-release niacin and regular crystalline niacin (96). Recommended doses are 1.5 to 2 g/day of modified niacin or up to 3 g/day of regular niacin. The advantage claimed for modified-release niacin over regular niacin is absence of the flushing that occurs in some patients after ingestion of large doses of unmodified niacin, but there is evidence that modified-release niacin is more likely to lead to gastrointestinal problems and hepatotoxicity. Since the flushing reaction caused by regular niacin can be prevented by acetylsalicylic acid or by starting therapy with lower doses of niacin and since the gastrointestinal and hepatotoxicity side effects of niacin may necessitate stopping therapy, regular niacin is recommended for treating hyperlipidemia.

TOXICOLOGY

Nicotinamide is excreted in urine as N^1-methylnicotinamide and its 2- and 4-pyridone derivatives. With the large doses of nicotinamide used to prevent onset of IDDM, the hepatic pathways involved in formation of its metabolites become saturated. This has raised concern that diversion of methylation equivalents required for anabolic pathways to nicotinamide methylation may lead to growth retardation in children (97). Side effects of pharmacologic doses of niacin used to treat hyperlipidemia are cutaneous flushing, pruritus, urticaria, nausea, vomiting, diarrhea, bloating, and constipation. Premedication with aspirin is used to control the flushing reaction. Caution is recommended in patients with unstable angina and in gout-predisposed patients. Some elevation in concentrations of liver enzymes (e.g., aspartate aminotransferase and alkaline phosphatase) may occur in the circulation (98). In some instances, hepatotoxicity may require stopping niacin treatment. Niacin may cause insulin resistance, which requires compensatory insulin secretion and, in patients with dysfunctional pancreatic β cells, may cause hyperglycemia. Patients with diabetes mellitus, therefore, require special monitoring during niacin treatment.

REFERENCES

1. Casal G. In: Martin M, ed. Obra Postuma. Madrid, 1762. (Cited in: Weiner M, Van Eys J. The discovery of nicotinic acid as a nutrient. In: Weiner M. Nicotinic acid: nutrient-cofactor-drug, clinical pharmacology. New York: Marcel Dekker, 1983;3–16.)
2. Follis RM. Deficiency disease. Springfield, IL: Charles C Thomas, 1958;316. (Cited in: Weiner M. Nicotinic acid: nutrient-cofactor-drug, clinical pharmacology. New York: Marcel Dekker, 1983;4.)
3. National Research Council. Recommended dietary allowances. 10th ed. Washington, DC: National Academy Press, 1989;137–142.
4. Goldberger J, Tanner WF. Public Health Rep 1922;37:462–86.
5. Elvehjem CA, Madden RJ, Strong FM, et al. J Am Chem Soc 1937;59:1767–8.
6. Fouts PJ, Helmer OM, Lepkovsky S, et al. Proc Soc Exp Biol Med 1937;37:405–7.
7. Vilter RW, Mueller JF, Bean WB. J Lab Clin Med 1949;34:409–13.
8. Goldsmith GA, Miller ON, Unglaub WG. J Nutr 1961;73:172–6.
9. Knox WE, Mehler AH. J Biol Chem 1950;187:419–30.
10. Nishizuka Y, Hayaishi O. J Biol Chem 1963;238:3369–77.
11. Preiss J, Handler P. J Biol Chem 1958;233:488–92.
12. Weiner M, Van Eys J. Assessment of the adequacy of niacin nutriture. In: Weiner M, ed. Nicotinic acid: nutrient-cofactor-drug, clinical pharmacology. New York: Marcel Dekker, 1983;57.
13. Althaus FR, Richter C, eds. ADP-Ribosylation of proteins: enzymology & biological significance. New York: Springer-Verlag, 1987;1–230.
14. Kim H, Jacobson EL, Jacobson MK. Biochem Biophys Res Commun 1993;194:1143–47.
15. Lee HC, Aarhus R. Cell Regul 1991;2:203–9.
16. Benjamin RC, Gill DM. J Biol Chem 1980;255:10493–501.
17. Ding R, Pommier Y, Kang VH, et al. J Biol Chem 1992;267:12804–12.
18. Kaplan NO. The pyridine coenzymes. In: Boyer PD, Lardy H, Myrback K, eds. The enzymes. New York: Academic Press, vol III. 1960;105–69.
19. The Merck Index. 12th ed. Rahway, NJ: Merck, 1996;1120.
20. Nakagawa I, Takahashi T, Sasaki A, et al. J Nutr 1973;103:1195–9.
21. Horwitt MK, Harper AE, Henderson LM. Am J Clin Nutr 1981;34:423–7.
22. Gopalan C, Rao KSJ. Vitam Horm 1975;33:505–28.
23. Gopalan C. Lancet 1969;1:997–9.
24. Hankes LV, Henderson LM, Elvehjem CA. J Biol Chem 1949;180:1027–35.
25. Goldsmith GA, Gibbens J, Unglaub WG, et al. Am J Clin Nutr 1956;4:151–60.
26. Zapsalis C, Beck RA. Food chemistry and nutritional biochemistry. New York: John Wiley & Sons, 1985;226–32.
27. Stein J, Daniel H, Whang E, et al. J Nutr 1994;124:61–6.
28. Olsson A, Olofsson T, Pero RW. Biochem Pharmacol 1993;45:1191–200.
29. Shibata K. J Nutr 1989;119:892–95.
30. San Pietro A, Kaplan NO, Colowick SP. J Biol Chem 1955;212:941–52.
31. Mayes PA. Structure function of water soluble vitamins. In: Murray KR, Granner DK, Mayes PA, et al., eds. Harper's biochemistry. 23th ed. East Norwalk, CT: Appleton & Lange, 1993;573–87.
32. Zatman LJ, Kaplan NO, Colowick SP. J Biol Chem 1954;209:453–84.
33. Shankar PS. Br J Tuberc 1955;49:20–2. (Cited in: Weiner M, Van Eys J. Nutritional biochemistry. In: Weiner M, ed. Nicotinic acid: nutrient-cofactor-drug, clinical pharmacology. New York: Marcel Dekker, 1983;29.)
34. Lee HC, Walseth TF, Bratt GT, et al. J Biol Chem 1989;264:1608–15.
35. Kim H, Jacobson EL, Jacobson MK. Science 1993;261:1330–33.
36. Takasawa S, Tohgo A, Noguchi N, et al. J Biol Chem 1993;268:26052–54.
37. Chini EN, Beers KW, Dousa TP. J Biol Chem 1995;270:3216–23.
38. Vu CQ, Lu P-J, Chen C-S, et al. J Biol Chem 1996;271:4747–54.
39. Collier RJ. J Mol Biol 1967;25:83–98.
40. Iglewski BH, Kabat D. Proc Natl Acad Sci USA 1975;72:2284–8.
41. Moss J, Vaughan M. Annu Rev Biochem 1979;48:581–600.
42. Moss J, Vaughan M. J Biol Chem 1995;270:12327–30.
43. Serafini T, Orci L, Amherdt M, et al. Cell 1991;67:239–53.
44. Moss J, Vaughan M. Adv Enzymol 1988;61:303–79.
45. Aktories K, Rosener S, Blaschke U, et al. Eur J Biochem 1988;172:445–50.
46. Aktories K, Wegner AJ. Cell Biol 1989;109:1385–7.
47. Iglewski BH, Sadoff J, Bjorn MJ, et al. Proc Natl Acad Sci USA 1978;75:3211–5.
48. Coburn J, Wyatt RT, Iglewski BH, et al. J Biol Chem 1989;264:9004–8.
49. Fu H, Coburn J, Collier RJ. Proc Natl Acad Sci USA 1993;90:2320–4.
50. Isobe T, Ichimura T, Sunaya T, et al. J Mol Biol 1990;217:125–32.
51. Zolkiewska A, Nightingale M, Moss J. Proc Natl Acad Sci USA 1992;89:11352–6.

52. Wang J, Nemoto E, Kots AY, et al. J Immunol 1994;153: 4048–58.
53. Jacobson MK, Aboul-Ela N, Cervantes-Laurean D, et al. ADP-ribose in animal cells. In: Moss J, Vaughan M, eds. ADP-Ribosylation toxins and G proteins: insights into signal transduction. Washington, DC: American Society for Microbiology, 1990;24:479–92.
54. Chambon P, Weil JD, Doly J, et al. Biochem Biophys Res Commun 1966;25:638–43.
55. Alvarez-Gonzalez R, Jacobson MK. Biochemistry 1987;26: 3218–24.
56. Moss J, Vaughan M, eds. ADP-Ribosylation toxins and G proteins: insights into signal transduction. Washington, DC: American Society for Microbiology, 1990.
57. Chatterjee S, Cheng MF, Berger NA. Cancer Commun 1990;2:71–5.
58. Heller B, Wang Z-Q, Wagner EF, et al. J Biol Chem 1995;270:11176–80.
59. Yoon YS, Kim JW, Kang KW, et al. J Biol Chem 1996;271: 9129–34.
60. Whitacre CM, Hashimoto H, Tsai M-L, et al. Cancer Res 1995;55:3697–701.
61. Wang Z-Q, Auer B, Stingl L, et al. Genes Dev 1995;9:509–20.
62. Gaal JC, Smith KR, Pearson CK. Trends Biochem Sci 1987;12:129–30.
63. Culver GM, McCraith SM, Zilmann M, et al. Science 1993;261:206–8.
64. Spies TD. In: Joliffe N, Tisdall F, Cannon PR, eds. Clinical nutrition. Hoeber, 1950;531. (Cited in: Weiner M, Van Eys J. The discovery of nicotinic acid as a nutrient. In: Weiner M, ed. Nicotinic acid: nutrient-cofactor-drug, clinical pharmacology. New York: Marcel Dekker, 1983;4.)
65. DiLorenzo PA. Acta Derm Venereol 1967;47:318–20. (Cited in: Weiner M, Van Eys J. Assessment of the adequacy of niacin nutriture. In: Weiner M, ed. Nicotinic acid: nutrient-cofactor-drug, clinical pharmacology. New York: Marcel Dekker, 1983;29.)
66. Jaffe IA. Ann NY Acad Sci 1969;166:57–60.
67. Henderson LM, Weinstock IM, Ramasarma GB. J Biol Chem 1951;189:19–29.
68. Baron DN, Dent CE, Harris M, et al. Lancet 1956;2:421–8.
69. Levy HL. Hartnup disorder. In: Stanbury JB, Wyngaarden JB, Frederickson DS, eds. The metabolic basis of inherited disease. 6th ed. New York: McGraw-Hill, 1989;101:2515–27.
70. Swenseid ME, Jacob RA. Niacin. In: Shils ME, Olson JA, Shike M, eds. Modern nutrition in health and disease. 8th ed. Philadelphia: Lea & Febiger, 1994;381.
71. Bernofsky C. Methods Enzymol 1980;66:23–39.
72. Lowry OH, Passonneau JV, Schulz DW, et al. J Biol Chem 1961;236:2746–55.
73. Slater TF, Sawyer B. Nature 1962;193:454–6.
74. Nisselbaum JS, Green S. Anal Biochem 1969;27:212–7.
75. Lee YC, Gholson RK, Raica N. J Biol Chem 1969;244:3277–82.
76. Sauberlich HE, Dowdy RP, Skala JH. Laboratory tests for the assessment of nutritional status. Boca Raton, FL: CRC Press, 1974;70–4.
77. Delange DJ, Joubert CP. Am J Clin Nutr 1964;15:169–74.
78. Fu CS, Swenseid ME, Jacob RA, et al. J Nutr 1989;119: 1949–55.
79. Jacobson EL, Lange RA, Jacobson MK. J Cell Physiol 1979;99:417–26.
80. Horwitt MK, Harper AE, Henderson LM. Am J Clin Nutr 1981;34:423–7.
81. Altschul R, Hoffer A, Stephen JD. Arch Biochem Biophys 1955;54:558–9.
82. Grundy SM, Mok HYL, Zech I, et al. J Lipid Res 1981;22:24–36.
83. Alderman JD, Pasternak RC, Sacks FM, et al. Am J Cardiol 1989;64:725–9.
84. Brown G, Albers JJ, Fisher LD, et al. N Engl J Med 1990;323(19):1289–98.
85. Cashin-Hemphill L, Mack WJ, Pogoda J, et al. JAMA 1990;264(23):3013–7.
86. Rabinovitch A, Suarez-Pinzon WL, et al. Diabetologia 1994;37: 733–8.
87. Buscema M, Vinci C, Gatta C, et al. Metabolism 1992;41:296–300.
88. Uchigata Y, Yamamoto H, Nagai H, et al. Diabetes 1982;32:316–8.
89. Yamada K, Nonaka K, Hanafusa T, et al. Diabetes 1982;31:749–53.
90. Pociot F, Reimers JI, Anderson HU. Diabetologia 1993;36:574–6.
91. Zhang J, Dawson VL, Dawson TM, et al. Science 1994;263:687–9.
92. Bingley PJ, Christie MR, Bonifacio E, et al. Diabetes 1994;43:1304–10.
93. Behme MT. Nutr Rev 1995;53:137–9.
94. Elliot RB, Pilcher CC, Steward A, et al. Ann NY Acad Sci 1993;696:333–41.
95. Jacobson EL, Dame AJ, Pyrek JS, et al. Biochimie 1995;77:394–8.
96. Kreisberg RA. Am J Med 1994;97:313–6.
97. Petley A, Macklin B, Renwick AG, et al. Diabetes 1995;44:152–5.
98. DiPalma JR, Thayer WS. Annu Rev Nutr 1991;11:169–87.
99. Panzeter PL, Zweifel B, Althaus FR. Biochem Biophys Res Commun 1992;184:544–48.
100. Food and Nutrition Board—Institute of Medicine. Dietary reference intakes. Thiamin, riboflavin, niacin, vitamin B_6, folate, vitamin B_{12}, pantothenic acid, biotin, and choline. Washington DC: National Academy Press, 1998.

SELECTED READINGS:

DiPalma JR, Thayer WS. Use of niacin as a drug. Annu Rev Nutr 1991;169–87.
Moss J, Vaughan M, eds. ADP-Ribosylation toxins and G proteins: insights into signal transduction. Washington, DC: American Society for Microbiology, 1990.
Sidney S. ADP-Ribosylation reactions. Biochimie 1995;77:313–8.
Weiner M, Van Eys J, eds. Nicotinic acid: nutrient-cofactor-drug, clinical pharmacology. New York: Marcel Dekker, 1983.

24. Vitamin B_6

JAMES E. LEKLEM

Since the discovery and identification of the structure of vitamin B_6 some 50 years ago, our knowledge of the functions of vitamin B_6 and the quantitative need for this vitamin has advanced significantly (1). Gyorgy and Lepkovsky were among the first to isolate vitamin B_6 in crystalline form. In the subsequent decade, Snell and coworkers were instrumental in elucidating the various forms of vitamin B_6 and developing microbiologic analytical techniques for measuring these forms in biologic systems (1, 2). Vitamin B_6 is recognized for its importance in diverse metabolic reactions and physiologic actions important for overall well-being.

CHEMISTRY

Vitamin B_6 is the name for derivatives of 3-hydroxy-5-hydroxymethyl-2 methyl pyridine (3). The four position can be found as the methylhydroxy (pyridoxine), the aldehyde (pyridoxal), or the methylamine (pyridoxamine). Each of these forms can also be phosphorylated at the five position (Fig. 24.1). Pyridoxal 5′-phosphate (PLP) and pyridoxamine 5′-phosphate (PMP) are the active coenzyme forms, with PLP being the primary form of biologic interest.

The free forms of vitamin B_6 are considered to be relatively labile, with the degree of lability influenced by pH. All three forms are relatively heat stable in an acid medium but heat labile under alkaline conditions (4). The hydrochloride and base forms are readily soluble in water and only minimally soluble in common organic solvents. In aqueous solution, the forms are light sensitive, but this sensitivity is also pH dependent. Pyridoxine hydrochloride is the form of vitamin B_6 most commonly found in vitamin pills and used in fortification of foods.

The coenzyme forms of vitamin B_6 are PLP and PMP. The PLP form is found covalently bound to enzymes via a Schiff base with the ϵ-amino group of lysine. In the formation of the Schiff base, the strong electron-attracting character of the pyridine ring and the subsequent withdrawal of electrons from one of the three substituents (R group, hydrogen, or carboxyl group) attached to the α-carbon of the amino acid substrate are key features in most enzymatic reactions (5). Nearly 100 enzymatic reactions (6) have been reported in which PLP plays a coenzyme role (6, 7). Although transamination reactions account for 40% of the PLP-catalyzed reactions, several other classes of reactions involve the α-, β, or δ carbon of amino acids.

FOOD SOURCES AND FORMS

An understanding of the various forms and the quantities of these forms in foods is important in the evaluation of the bioavailability and metabolism of vitamin B_6. The methods used to determine the amount of vitamin include microbiologic (8) and high-performance liquid chromatography (9) techniques. The relative proportion of each of the three forms in foods varies considerably. Table 24.1 contains data on the total amounts (see also Appendix Table IV-A-23-a), the relative proportion of the three forms, and the level of the pyridoxine glucoside form of vitamin B_6 in selected foods. This latter form of vitamin B_6 has been isolated from plant foods such as rice bran and identified as 5′-O-(β-D-glycopyranosyl) pyridoxine (10). To date only plant foods have been found to contain this interesting form of vitamin B_6 (11). The absence of the glucoside form in animal products suggests it does not have a biologic function. In plants it may be a storage form of vitamin B_6. In general, plant foods contain predominately pyridoxine, while animal products contain primarily pyridoxal and pyridoxamine (mainly as the phosphorylated forms (4)).

Food processing and storage may affect the vitamin content of foods (12, 13). Losses of 10 to 50% have been reported for a wide variety of foods and processing techniques. Pyridoxine added to flour and baked into bread is stable (14). Thermal processing (15) and low-moisture storage of certain foods results in reductive binding of the

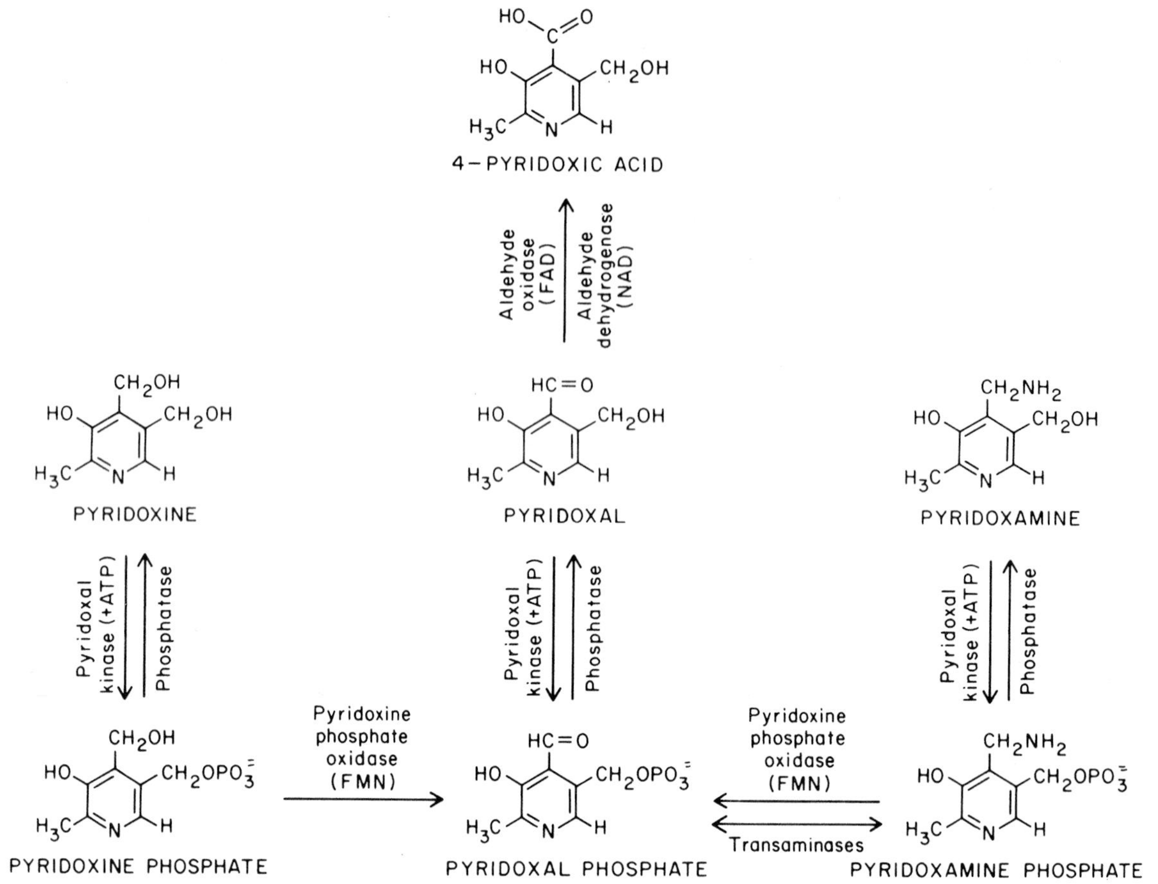

Figure 24.1. Forms, interconversion, and metabolism of vitamin B_6. (From Leklem JE. Nutr Today 1988;Sept/Oct:5, with permission.)

two aldehydes, pyridoxal and pyridoxal 5′-phosphate, to proteins via ε-amino groups of their lysyl residues. Such derivatives possess low or even antivitamin B_6 activity (16). Conversion of pyridoxine to 6-hydroxypyridoxine in the presence of ascorbic acid has been reported (17).

ABSORPTION AND BIOAVAILABILITY

Absorption

A proper assessment of the requirement of vitamin B_6 requires an understanding of how much vitamin B_6 is biologically available (i.e., absorbed and usable). Absorption of the several forms of vitamin B_6 has been examined primarily in animals (18) and to a limited extent in humans (19). The three primary forms of vitamin B_6 are absorbed to a major extent by a nonsaturable passive process (20), mainly in the jejunum (21). After hydrolysis of the phosphorylated forms by alkaline phosphatase and their uptake into the intestine, each can be phosphorylated and thus retained (a process referred to as metabolic trapping). However, forms of vitamin B_6 exit from the basolateral membrane side of the intestine, mainly nonphosphorylated.

Bioavailability

Studies in both animals and humans (22, 23) have provided information on the relative availability of vitamin B_6. A summary of the studies in humans is given in Table 24.2. Generally, more than 75% of vitamin B_6 is available in most foods studied (22). Human studies show an inverse relationship between the amount of pyridoxine glucoside (PNG) in the diet and bioavailability (24). However, PNG is absorbed and partially converted to 4-pyridoxic acid. In human studies, about 58% of the PNG was found to be bioavailable (25). PNG also appears to alter metabolism of coingested pyridoxine in rats (26) and may have a similar effect in humans. Food processing (formation of α-pyridoxyl-lysine) and fiber may also limit availability.

TRANSPORT AND METABOLISM

Vitamin B_6 is transported in the blood both in plasma and in red cells. PLP and PL are both bound to albumin (27), with PLP binding more tightly. In the red cell, both PLP and PL are bound to hemoglobin (28, 29). The extent of red cell involvement in vitamin B_6 transport, however, remains to be determined (30).

The liver is the primary organ responsible for metabolism of B_6 vitamers (27, 31). As a result, the liver supplies the active form of vitamin B_6, PLP, to the circulation and other tissues. Figure 24.1 depicts the interconversion of the B_6 vitamers and the enzymes involved. The three nonphosphorylated forms are converted to their respective phosphorylated forms by pyridoxine kinase, with zinc and ATP as cofactors (32). Pyridoxamine 5′-phosphate and

Table 24.1
Vitamin B_6 and Pyridoxine Glucoside (PNG) Content of Commonly Consumed Foods[a]

Food	Vitamin B_6 (mg/100 g)	PNG (mg/100 g)
Vegetables		
Carrots, raw	0.170	0.087
Cauliflower, frozen	0.084	0.069
Broccoli, frozen	0.119	0.078
Spinach, frozen	0.208	0.104
Cabbage, raw	0.140	0.065
Sprouts, alfalfa	0.250	0.105
Potatoes, cooked	0.394	0.165
Beans/legumes		
Soybeans, cooked	0.627	0.357
Beans, navy, cooked	0.381	0.159
Beans, lima, frozen	0.106	0.039
Peas, frozen	0.122	0.018
Peanut butter	0.302	0.054
Beans, garbanzo	0.653	0.111
Lentils	0.289	0.134
Animal products		
Beef, ground, cooked	0.263	n.d.[b]
Tuna, canned	0.316	n.d.
Chicken breast, raw	0.700	n.d.
Milk, skim	0.005	n.d.
Nuts/seeds		
Walnuts	0.535	0.038
Cashews, raw	0.351	0.046
Sunflower seeds	0.997	0.046
Almonds	0.086	—0—
Fruits		
Orange juice, fresh	0.043	0.016
Tomato juice, canned	0.097	0.045
Blueberries, frozen	0.046	0.019
Banana	0.313	0.010
Pineapple, canned	0.079	0.017
Peaches, canned	0.009	0.002
Avocado	0.443	0.015
Raisins, seedless	0.230	0.154
Cereals/grains		
Wheat bran	0.903	0.326
Shredded wheat, cereal	0.313	0.087
Rice, brown	0.237	0.055

[a]All values given as milligrams of pyridoxine per 100 g of food. 1 mg B_6 = 5.91 μmol.
[b]n.d., none detected.

Table 24.2
Studies in Which Bioavailability of Vitamin B_6 from Foods Has Been Assessed in Humans

Food	Estimated Bioavailability
Whole wheat bread	>85%
Cooked wheat bran	>85%
Wheat, rice, corn brans	60–65%
Peanut butter	63%, compared with tuna
Bananas	98%, compared with tuna
Hazelnuts	96%, compared with tuna
Soybeans	41%, compared with tuna
Orange juice	50%, compared with pyridoxine

From Leklem JE. Vitamin B_6 In: Machlin LJ, ed. Handbook of vitamins. 2nd ed. New York: Marcel Dekker, 1991;341–92, with permission.

pyridoxine 5′-phosphate can then be converted to PLP via a flavin mononucleotide (FMN) oxidase (33).

Phosphorylated forms can be hydrolyzed by alkaline phosphatases (31, 32). The pyridoxal that results from this dephosphorylation, as well as that derived from dietary sources, can then be converted to 4-pyridoxic acid (4-PA) in a nonreversible reaction involving FAD and an aldehyde oxidase (32). This reaction occurs in human liver, but the extent to which it occurs in other tissues is not known. Based on studies using human liver preparations, rates for the major reactions of vitamin B_6 metabolism have been determined and indicate that conversion of PL to 4-PA is favored (34). PL kinase is more active than PLP phosphatase. Because of the role of riboflavin coenzymes in the pathway, riboflavin status may affect vitamin B_6 metabolism (35).

Because PLP is a highly reactive molecule and readily forms a Schiff base with proteins, high cellular concentrations of PLP may be detrimental. The activity of the aldehyde (pyridoxal) oxidase in human liver appears to suffice, however, to convert excess PL to 4-PA and thus prevent high levels of PLP from accumulating (32).

In the circulating plasma, PLP and PL comprise nearly 75–80% of the total vitamin B_6 (4, 36, 37). Pyridoxine (PN) is the next most common form, and while PN is taken up into tissues and can be converted to PNP, many tissues lack sufficient oxidase activity to convert PNP to PLP (38). While information on kinetics of vitamin B_6 metabolism in humans is limited, studies in pigs (biochemically similar to humans) found that little PLP and PL from the circulation is recycled by the liver back to PLP in the plasma (39). PL is extensively recycled, probably in muscle and other tissues, via conversion to PLP and subsequent binding to protein.

Several body pools of B_6 exist (40). The major pool is in muscle, where most of the vitamin B_6 is present as PLP bound to glycogen phosphorylase (41). The total body pool of vitamin B_6 is estimated to be 1000 μmol, of which 800 to 900 μmol is present in muscle (42). Turnover of the various pools varies, depending on the metabolic state and nutritional well-being of the organism (4). Turnover of PLP in the plasma has been associated with a two-compartment model (4, 43), and turnover of the slowly turning over pool is estimated to be 25 to 33 days.

FUNCTIONS

The numerous functions of vitamin B_6 in humans are complex, multifaceted, and interrelated. Because of the reactivity of PLP with amino acids and several nitrogen-containing compounds, the biochemical functions of vitamin B_6 center around these molecules (44). In these biochemical functions, PLP serves as a versatile catalyst in a diverse number of reactions; a review of the mechanism of PLP-catalyzed reactions is available (45). In the case of glycogen phosphorylase, the phosphate group of PLP probably is involved in the coenzyme role (46). The role of PLP can be viewed from a systems/cellular perspective. These systems/cellular processes are listed in Table 24.3. A brief description and other highlights of each of these follows.

Table 24.3
Systems or Cellular Processes in Which Pyridoxal 5′-Phosphate Functions

Cellular Process of Enzyme System	System/Function
1-Carbon metabolism, steroid modulation	Immune
Transaminases, glycogen phosphorylase	Gluconeogenesis
Tryptophan metabolism	Niacin formation
Heme synthesis, O_2 affinity, transaminases	Red cell metabolism
Lipid and neurotransmitter synthesis	Nervous system
Binding of PLP to lysine of steroid receptor	Steroid (hormone) function

From Leklem JE. Vitamin B_6. In: Machlin LJ, ed. Handbook of vitamins. 2nd ed. New York: Marcel Dekker, 1991;341–92, with permission.

Gluconeogenesis

PLP is involved in gluconeogenesis via its role in transamination reactions (44) and in the action of glycogen phosphorylase (41, 46). However, a low intake of vitamin B_6 (0.2 mg/day, vs. "normal" intake of 1.8 mg/day) in humans for 4 weeks did not adversely affect fasting plasma glucose levels but did result in impaired glucose tolerance (47). Glycogen phosphorylase activities in liver and muscle are reduced in vitamin B_6–deficient rats (41, 48), but a deficiency of the vitamin, per se, does not result in mobilization of the vitamin B_6 (PLP) stored in muscle (49). However, in rats, a caloric deficit does lead to decreased muscle phosphorylase content (50). Thus, the reservoir of vitamin B_6 in muscle seems to be used only when gluconeogenesis increases.

Niacin Formation

Direct conversion of tryptophan to niacin involves a PLP-requiring enzyme, kynureninase. After 4 weeks of feeding women a diet containing 0.2 mg/day of vitamin B_6, the total urinary excretion of the two major niacin metabolites, *N*′-methyl-2-pyridone-5-carboxamide and *N*′-methylnicotinamide, in response to a tryptophan load test (2 g) was moderately less than that excreted when 1.8 mg of vitamin B_6 was fed (44, 51). Thus, a low intake (<1.0 mg/day) of vitamin B_6 had only a slight effect on the conversion of tryptophan to niacin.

Lipid Metabolism

The role of vitamin B_6 in lipid metabolism remains controversial. Animals fed diets deficient in either polyunsaturated fatty acids or vitamin B_6 showed similar visual signs and symptoms (52). Vitamin B_6–deficient rats fed high-protein (70%) diets developed fatty livers in some studies (53) but not in others. Increased levels of linoleic and δ-linolenic acid and decreased levels of arachidonic acid in liver phospholipids have been observed in B_6-deficient rats (54, 55). The changes in fatty acid levels may be related to altered phospholipid levels due to high levels of *S*-adenosylmethionine inhibiting methylation of phosphoethanolamine (56). This latter effect would tie together altered amino acid metabolism (homocysteine) and the changes in phospholipids and associated fatty acids.

The relationship between vitamin B_6 and cholesterol also remains controversial (57). In humans, a deficiency of vitamin B_6 is not associated with a significant change in serum cholesterol (4). Although supplemental intakes of vitamins in general or vitamin B_6 per se alter serum cholesterol levels (either decrease or prevent an increase) (4), there are no definitive studies on the effect of supplemental vitamin B_6 on serum cholesterol level. Nonetheless, plasma PLP levels are positively correlated with plasma HDL-cholesterol levels and negatively correlated with total cholesterol and LDL-cholesterol levels in monkeys (58).

Erythrocyte Metabolism and Function

In the erythrocyte, PLP is a coenzyme for transaminases. Both PLP and PL bind to hemoglobin. PL binds to the α-chain of hemoglobin and increases O_2 binding affinity, while PLP binds tightly to the β-chain and lowers O_2 binding affinity, a situation that may be important in sickle-cell anemia (59). A severe chronic deficiency of vitamin B_6 can lead to hypochromic, microcytic anemia. In addition, some patients with sideroblastic anemia and other anemias do respond favorably to PN therapy (60, 61).

Nervous System

Several in-depth reviews on the functions of vitamin B_6 in the nervous system are available (62, 64). PLP is a coenzyme for enzymatic reactions that lead to the synthesis of several neurotransmitters, including serotonin (from tryptophan), taurine, dopamine, norepinephrine, histamine, and δ-aminobutyric acid. Neurologic abnormalities in human infants (65) and animals (62) deficient in vitamin B_6 have been seen. Infants fed a formula in which the vitamin B_6 was destroyed during processing showed abnormal EEG tracings and convulsions (65). Treatment with 100 mg of vitamin B_6 corrected the EEG abnormalities. Adults fed a diet low in vitamin B_6 and high in protein (for 3, 4 weeks) also had abnormal EEGs (66), while those fed similar diets for a shorter period of time (<21 days) had no abnormal EEGs.

Extensive studies in animals fed varying intakes of vitamin B_6 showed that the progeny of vitamin B_6–deficient dams had altered fatty acid levels in the cerebellum and cerebrum of the brain (64, 67). Other changes in nerve cells, including reduced γ-aminobutyric acid levels (68) and altered amino acid levels, have been observed. These findings point to a need for adequate vitamin B_6 during nervous system development.

Immune Function

Vitamin B_6 intake has a significant impact on immune function (69). In both animal (70) and human studies (71, 72), a low intake of vitamin B_6 or decreased status is associated with impaired immune function. Decreased interleukin-2 production and lymphocyte proliferation are seen with vitamin B_6 depletion in humans (72). These effects on the immune system are probably mediated via altered 1-carbon metabolism, particularly the activity of serine hydroxymethyltransferase (73) and/or hormone modulation.

Hormone Modulation

Litwack et al. demonstrated that PLP binds to steroid receptors (74). PLP also binds to a second site on the steroid receptor and inhibits the binding of the steroid receptor to DNA (75). In further studies, the level of mRNA for liver cytosolic aspartate aminotransferase was sevenfold higher in vitamin B_6–deficient rats than in control rats. Furthermore, the DNA-binding activity of the glucocorticoid receptor was enhanced by vitamin B_6 deficiency (76). The increased amount of mRNA for cytosolic aspartate aminotransferase in vitamin B_6–deficient animals suggests that this steroid-responsive enzyme is regulated in part by the intracellular PLP concentration. Thus, in B_6-sufficient animals, steroid responsiveness is lower than that in B_6-deficient animals. Reactions between PLP and receptors for estrogen, androgen, progesterone, and glucocorticoid at physiologic concentrations of PLP suggest that the vitamin B_6 status of an individual may have significance in endocrine-mediated diseases.

VITAMIN B_6 STATUS

Determination of the vitamin B_6 status of an individual is of paramount importance in understanding the relationship between health and nutrient intake, factors that influence the requirement for vitamin B_6, and factors that affect the overall metabolism of vitamin B_6. Vitamin B_6 status can be assessed in three ways: direct methods, indirect methods, and dietary intake (77). Table 24.4 lists several indices used to evaluate vitamin B_6 status and suggested values for adequate status. A recent review of vitamin B_6 status is available (78).

Table 24.4
Indices Used to Assess Vitamin B_6 Status and Suggested Minimal Values for Adequate Status

Index	Adequate Status[a]
Direct	
Plasma pyridoxal 5′-phosphate	>30 nmol/L
Plasma total vitamin B_6	>40 nmol/L
Urinary 4-pyridoxic acid	>3.0 μmol/day
Urinary total vitamin B_6	>0.5 μmol/day
Indirect	
Erythrocyte alanine transaminase index	<1.25
Erythrocyte aspartic transaminase index	<1.80
2-g L-Tryptophan load; urinary xanthurenic acid	<65 μmol/day
3-g L-Methionine load; urinary cystathionine	<350 μmol/day
Diet intake	
Vitamin B_6 intake; weekly average	>1.25–1.5 mg/day
Vitamin B_6: protein ratio (mg/g)	≥0.016

From Leklem JE. J Nutr 1990;120:1503–7, with permission.
[a]1 μmol B_6 = 169 mg.

Direct Methods

Direct methods measure one or more of the metabolites of the B_6 vitamers. Currently, the most frequently used direct measure is plasma PLP concentration. Support for its use comes from both animal models (79) and human studies (4). However, use of PLP as a status index is controversial (78). Proper evaluation of plasma PLP concentration requires an understanding of factors that influence this level. Table 24.5 lists several such factors and the qualitative change that has been observed (4). Ideally, one would prefer to measure PLP in tissues. Erythrocyte PLP level may be useful as an additional index (78, 80). Until methodologic problems are resolved and further data are available, the use of this measure as an index of vitamin B_6 status is open to question. Plasma total vitamin B_6 and plasma PL concentrations are additional direct measures that have utility. Since PL is the form that enters the cell, its measurement may be more relevant than that of PLP.

Urinary direct methods include measurement of the major metabolic product 4-PA and of total vitamin B_6 (the sum of the nonphosphorylated and phosphorylated forms). Under normal conditions, 40 to 60% percent of the daily vitamin B_6 intake is excreted as 4-PA (81). Similarly, urinary B_6 vitamers represent 8 to 10% of the daily intake (19). Urinary 4-PA excretion is considered a short-term indicator of status. Excretion reflects and is influenced by vitamin B_6 intake over a 1- to 4-day period. To use urinary total vitamin B_6 properly as an indicator of status requires several 24-h urine collections during 1 to 3 weeks. Our knowledge of the factors (dietary and physiologic) that affect urinary 4-PA and total vitamin B_6 is limited primarily to the effect of protein intake (82, 83). As protein intake increases, urinary 4-PA excretion decreases (4).

Indirect Methods

The indirect measures of vitamin B_6 status currently used are based on products of metabolic pathways or specific enzymes that require PLP. Thus, they indirectly reflect PLP levels in certain tissues. Therefore, they do not

Table 24.5
Factors Influencing Plasma PLP Concentration

Factor	Effect on Plasma PLP
Diet	
↑ Vitamin B_6	↑
↑ Protein	↓
↑ Glucose	↓, acute
↓ Bioavailability	↓
Physiologic	
↑ Exercise, aerobic	↑, acute
↑ Age	↓
Pregnancy	↓
↑ Alkaline phosphatase activity	↓
Smoking, chronic	↓

From Leklem JE. J Nutr 1990;120:1503–7, with permission.

necessarily reflect the total vitamin B_6 content in tissues, nor do they always reflect circulating levels of PLP or B_6 vitamers. The most common indirect measures used are *(a)* urinary metabolites of the tryptophan pathway or the methionine pathway and *(b)* erythrocyte transaminase activity and stimulation (77). Other, less common tests are urinary oxalate excretion and EEG patterns.

Tryptophan and Methionine Load Tests

The tryptophan load test, one of the most widely used indices of vitamin B_6 status (84), is based on the fact that several steps in the major catabolic pathway of tryptophan are PLP dependent. A 2-g oral load of L-tryptophan is administered, and the urinary excretion of metabolites such as xanthurenic acid and kynurenic acid is determined. Brown has questioned the use of this test on the basis of an adverse effect on tryptophan metabolism by factors independent of vitamin B_6 intake (85).

The methionine load test has also been used as an indirect measure of vitamin B_6 status. Like the tryptophan load test, this test is considered primarily to reflect hepatic levels of vitamin B_6. The methionine pathway has four PLP-dependent steps. The step catalyzed by cystathionase, in which cystathionine is cleaved to form homoserine and cysteine, appears to be especially sensitive to vitamin B_6 deficiency. Indeed, this metabolite is excreted in elevated amounts following a 3-g methionine load (86). There may be a protein effect similar to that seen for tryptophan. With the recent interest in plasma homocysteine levels and coronary heart disease, there have been several studies of the effect of vitamin B_6 on plasma homocysteine (87, 88). While vitamin B_6 deficiency increases plasma homocysteine following a methionine load (89), it appears that folic acid is relatively more important than vitamin B_6 in modifying plasma homocysteine levels (88).

Erythrocyte Transaminase (Aminotransferases)

Measurements of erythrocyte alanine aminotransferase (EALT, or EGPT) and aspartic acid aminotransferase (EAST, or EGOT) transaminase activity and/or stimulation are commonly used indirect indices of vitamin B_6 status. They are considered long-term measures of vitamin B_6 status because of the life span of erythrocytes (77). Activities of the respective transaminases are measured in vitro in the presence and absence of excess PLP (90). From this the percentage stimulation is calculated:

$$\% \text{ Stimulation} = [(A_s - A_u)/A_u] \times 100\%$$

where A_s is stimulated activity and A_u is unstimulated activity.

Based on studies in women, EALT activity (index and percentage stimulation) is more sensitive to vitamin B_6 intake (91). However, the relative activity of EALT is only 5% of that of EAST. The EALT enzyme is also more likely to lose activity when erythrocytes are frozen. Because no long-term studies (>6 weeks) have measured transaminase activities after different levels of vitamin B_6 were fed, the utility of transaminase activity measures as an index of a specific vitamin B_6 intake is unknown. Also, the temporal relationship between enzyme activity measurement and intake of vitamin B_6 is little understood. A further consideration in using transaminase data as a status indicator is the existence of three phenotypes of EALT (92).

Dietary Intake of Vitamin B_6 and Protein

A proper assessment of vitamin B_6 status and interpretation of blood or urinary measures requires determination of both vitamin B_6 and protein intakes. Because carbohydrates may also play a role in B_6 utilization, intake of carbohydrate should also be documented (77). Vitamin B_6 status in a healthy population is best assessed by using a direct measure, an indirect measure, and appropriate dietary information. While these measures may be useful in certain clinical conditions, numerous factors that can influence metabolism of vitamin B_6 may preclude proper assessment (93).

VITAMIN B_6 DEFICIENCY

Any vitamin deficiency can be assessed by both outward clinical signs and biochemical/functional tests. Clinical signs usually occur in the later stages of deficiency. Table 24.6 lists the signs commonly seen with rather severe and chronic vitamin B_6 deficiency (4). Those seen in infants were first observed because of an error in food processing of formula that was subsequently fed to infants (65). In the earlier stages of vitamin B_6 deficiency, direct measures of vitamin B_6 status would be expected to become lower and indirect measures to become abnormal. EAST and EALT activity (and % stimulation) do change in vitamin B_6 deficiency (91) but only with chronic deficiency.

REQUIREMENTS

Since vitamin B_6 is involved in so many areas of metabolism and physiologic functions, establishing proper and adequate requirements is imperative. Numerous factors can influence a vitamin B_6 requirement (4), and for most of these we lack adequate information on their quantitative effect. The 1989 version (93) of the recommended dietary allowance (RDA) for vitamin B_6 for various age groups is summarized in Table 24.7 (see also Appendix

Table 24.6
Clinical Signs of Vitamin B_6 Deficiency

Signs Occurring Primarily in Infants	Signs Occurring Primarily in Adults
Abnormal electroencephalogram pattern	Stomatitis
Convulsions	Cheilosis
	Glossitis
	Irritability
	Depression and confusion

Adapted from Leklem JE. Vitamin B_6 metabolism and function in humans. In: Leklem JE, Reynolds RD, eds. Clinical and physiological applications of vitamin B_6. New York: Alan R Liss, 1988;3–28.

Table II-A-2-a-2). These RDAs are generally lower than prior RDAs for vitamin B_6 (i.e., 1974, 1980 versions), especially for adult men and women. The 1998 RDAs are even lower for children (0.5–0.8 mg/day), for adults (0.1–0.8 mg/day), and for pregnant and lactating women (0.1–0.3 mg/day) (see Appendix Table II-A-2-c-1 and related tables II-A-2-c-2 to 4.) (93a).

Of the factors affecting vitamin B_6 need, protein has been studied in greatest detail. Protein intake is inversely correlated with plasma PLP concentration and urinary 4-PA excretion, in both men (82) and women (83). Under conditions of low intakes of vitamin B_6, protein intake is directly correlated with excretion of tryptophan metabolites (83). Bioavailability of vitamin B_6 would be expected to affect its requirement. Vitamin B_6 status decreases in women fed a diet high in PNG (27% of intake), reflecting an increased vitamin B_6 requirement of about 15% (24). Exercise may also increase vitamin B_6 requirement (94). Since the vitamin B_6 content of human milk has been determined (4) and found to be influenced by intake (95), the vitamin B_6 needs of infants can be assessed. The current RDA for infants up to 0.5 years old is 0.3 mg (1.8 μmol), which would require an intake of 1.5 to 2 L of milk (assuming a vitamin B_6 content of 0.75 to 1.0 μmol/L). Based on a normal breast milk volume of 650 to 750 mL/day, an infant would receive only 30 to 50% of the current RDA. However, infants in the U.S. do not show signs of vitamin B_6 deficiency, which suggests that the current RDA for vitamin B_6 for infants is too high. Intake of 0.10 to 0.16 mg/day appears adequate (96).

The effect of sex and age (4) on vitamin B_6 requirements has received only minimal attention. In studies of vitamin B_6 metabolism in males and females, plasma PLP levels tend to be lower in females than in males. Several studies suggest that vitamin B_6 status decreases with age (4, 97), especially plasma PLP levels. However, the application of such findings to requirements is not known. The vitamin B_6 RDAs for adult males and females are based on metabolic studies, vitamin B_6 intake data, and protein intakes of populations (92). Metabolic studies in older adults (98), as well as those in younger adult women (83, 99), suggest that the current RDA is too low and that at least 2.0 mg/day (or 0.020 mg/g protein) may be more appropriate. The current RDAs are based primarily on the protein–vitamin B_6 interrelationship. For adults, a value of 0.016 mg of vitamin B_6 per gram of protein has been set.

Table 24.7
Recommended Dietary Allowances (1989) for Vitamin B_6 and Associated Vitamin B_6 Protein Ratios[1,2]

Age Group (in years) or Condition		Vitamin B_6 (mg/day)		Vitamin B_6 Protein[a] (mg/g)	
Infants	0.0–0.5	0.3		0.023	
	0.5–1.0	0.6		0.043	
Children	1–3	1.0		0.063	
	4–6	1.1		0.046	
	7–10	1.4		0.050	
		Males	Females	Males	Females
Adults	11–14	1.7	1.4	0.038	0.030
	15–18	2.0	1.5	0.034	0.030
	19–24	2.0	1.6	0.034	0.035
	25–50	2.0	1.6	0.032	0.032
	51+	2.0	1.6	0.032	0.032
Pregnant			2.2		0.036
Lactating	1st 6 months		2.1		0.032
	2nd 6 months		2.1		0.034

From Food and Nutrition Board, National Research Council. Recommended dietary allowances. 10th ed.

[a]This ratio was derived by dividing the RDA for vitamin B_6 by the RDA for protein for the respective age group. The RDA for vitamin B_6 for adults was established by using twice the RDA for protein (126 g/day for males and 100 g/day for females) and a vitamin B_6:protein ratio of 0.016 mg/g. 1 mg B_6 = 5.91 μmol.

CLINICAL CONDITIONS

Several reviews have examined the relationship between vitamin B_6 nutrition and disease states (100, 101). In a number of disease states, an apparent alteration of vitamin B_6 metabolism is reflected in altered tryptophan metabolism or decreased plasma PLP concentration. For example, tryptophan metabolism has been found to be altered in asthma (103), diabetes (104), breast and bladder cancer (85), and rheumatoid arthritis (105); plasma PLP concentration is decreased in asthma (106), renal disease (107), alcoholism (108), coronary heart disease (109), breast cancer (110), Hodgkin's disease (111), sickle-cell anemia (53), diabetes (112), and smoking (113). Many of these studies determined only one measure of vitamin B_6 status; thus, the extent to which the true status is compromised is unknown.

Vitamin B_6 (as pyridoxine hydrochloride) has been used as a preventive agent or as a therapeutic agent for several diseases. Papers from conferences on this aspect of vitamin B_6 are available (102, 114). Disorders treated with PN include Down's syndrome, autism, hyperoxaluria, gestational diabetes, carpal tunnel syndrome, depression, and diabetic neuropathy (101). In nearly every case, there has been limited therapeutic benefit. However, the dose of PN and length of administration has varied from study to study, making evaluation of efficacy difficult.

DRUG-VITAMIN B_6 INTERACTION AND TOXICITY

The widespread use of clinical drugs in our society necessitates understanding the effect of drug use on vitamin B_6 metabolism. Table 24.8, taken in part from a review by Bhagavan (114), lists several drugs that affect vitamin B_6 metabolism. In many cases, the drugs either react with PLP, induce PLP-dependent enzymes, or interfere with vitamin B_6 metabolism (115, 116). In most cases, administration of PN corrects altered vitamin B_6 metabolism. The effect of excess vitamin B_6 (>10 mg/day) on drug efficacy remains to be determined but should be considered in cases in which the drug reacts directly with PLP.

The use of high doses of PN (500–1000 mg/day) to treat certain disorders, such as premenstrual syndrome

Table 24.8
Drug-Vitamin B_6 Interactions

Drug	Effect on Vitamin B_6 Metabolism/Function
Iproniazid (hydrazines)	Reacts with PL and PLP
Cycloserine	Reacts with PLP, forms oxime
L-3,4-Dihydroxyphenylalanine	Reacts with PLP, forms tetrahydroquinoline derivative
Penicillamine	Reacts with PLP, forms thiazolidine
Ethinylestradiol, mestranol	Increased enzyme levels and retention of PLP in tissue
Ethanol	Increased catabolism of PLP
Theophylline, caffeine	Inhibition of pyridoxal kinase

Adapted from Dakshinamurti K, ed. Ann NY Acad Sci 1990;585, with permission.

and other neurologic diseases, has resulted in a small number of instances of neurotoxicity (117) and photosensitivity (4). These symptoms are rarely if ever seen with doses of 2 to 250 mg and usually are seen only with chronic use (118).

REFERENCES

1. Leklem JE, Reynolds RD, eds. Methods in vitamin B_6 nutrition. New York: Plenum Press, 1981.
2. Snell EE. Vitamin B_6 analysis: some historical aspects. In: Leklem JE, Reynolds RD, eds. Methods in vitamin B_6 nutrition. New York: Plenum Press 1981;1–19.
3. IUPAC-IUB Commission on Biochemical Nomenclature. Eur J Biochem 1973;40:325–7.
4. Leklem JE. Vitamin B_6. In: Machlin LJ, ed. Handbook of vitamins. 2nd ed. New York: Marcel Dekker, 1991;341–92.
5. Leussing DL. Model reactions. In: Dolphin D, Poulson R, Avramovic O, eds. Coenzymes and cofactors, vol 1. Vitamin B_6 pyridoxal phosphate. New York: John Wiley & Sons, 1986;69–115.
6. Sauberlich HE. Interaction of vitamin B_6 with other nutrients. In: Reynolds RD, Leklem, JE, eds. Vitamin B_6: its role in health and disease. New York: Alan R Liss, 1985;193–217.
7. Coburn SP. Vitam Horm 1994;48:259–300.
8. Polansky M. Microbiological assay of vitamin B_6 in foods. In: Leklem JE, Reynolds RD, eds. Methods in vitamin B_6 nutrition. New York: Plenum Press, 1981;31–44.
9. Gregory JF. J Food Comp Anal 1988;1:105–23.
10. Yasumoto K, Tsuji H, Iwami K, et al. Agric Biol Chem 1977;41:106–7.
11. Kabir H, Leklem JE, Miller LT. J Food Sci 1983;48:1422–5.
12. Richardson LR, Wilkes S, Ritchey SJ. J Nutr 1961;73:363–8.
13. Woodring MJ, Storvick CA. J Assoc Off Agric Chem 1960;43:63–80.
14. Perera AD, Leklem JE, Miller LT. Cereal Chem 1970;56:577–80.
15. Gregory JF, Kirk JR. J Food Sci 1977;42:1554–61.
16. Gregory JF. J Nutr 1980;110:995–1005.
17. Tadera K, Arima M, Yoshino F, et al. J Nutr Sci Vitaminol 1986;32:267–77.
18. Henderson LM. Intestinal absorption of B_6 vitamers. In: Reynolds RD, Leklem JE, eds. Vitamin B_6: its role in health and disease. New York: Alan R Liss, 1985;11–53.
19. Wozenski JR, Leklem JE, Miller LT. J Nutr 1980:110:275–85.
20. Roth-Maier DA, Zinner PM, Kirchgessner M. Int J Vitam Nutr Res 1982;52:272–9.
21. Middleton HM. J Nutr 1985;115:1079–88.
22. Leklem JE. Food Technol 1988;Oct:194–6.
23. Gregory JF, Kirk JR. The bioavailability of vitamin B_6 in foods. In: Reynolds RD, Leklem JE, eds. Vitamin B_6: its role in health and disease. New York: Alan R Liss, 1985;3–23.
24. Hansen CM, Leklem JE, Miller LT. J Nutr 1996;126:2512–18.
25. Gregory JF, Trumbo PR, Bailey LB, et al. J Nutr 1991;121: 177–86.
26. Nakano H, Gregory JF. J Nutr 1995;125:926–32.
27. Lumeng L, Brashear RE, Li T-K. J Lab Clin Med 1974;84: 334–43.
28. Mehansho H, Henderson M. J Biol Chem 1980;255:11901–7.
29. Benesch RE, Yung S, Suzuki T, et al. Proc Natl Acad Sci USA 1973;70:2595–9.
30. Anderson BB, Perry GM, Clements JE, et al. Am J Clin Nutr 1989;50:1059–63.
31. Lumeng L, Li T-K. Mammalian vitamin B_6 metabolism: regulatory role of protein-binding and the hydrolysis of pyridoxal 5′-phosphate in storage and transport. In: Tryfiates GP, ed. Vitamin B_6 metabolism and role in growth. Westport, CT: Food and Nutrition Press, 1980;27–51.
32. Merrill AH, Henderson JM, Wang E, et al. J Nutr 1984;114: 1664–74.
33. Wada H, Snell EE. J Biol Chem 1961;236:2089–95.
34. Merrill AH, Henderson JM. Ann NY Acad Sci 1990;585: 110–7.
35. Perry GM, Anderson BB, Dodd N. Biomedicine 1980;33:36–8.
36. Coburn SP, Mahuren JD. Anal Biochem 1983;129:310–7.
37. Hollins B, Henderson JM. J Chromatogr 1986;380:67–75.
38. Pogell BM. J Biol Chem 1958;232:761–6.
39. Coburn SP, Mahuren JD, Kennedy MS, et al. J Nutr 1992;122:393–401.
40. Coburn SP. Ann NY Acad Sci 1990;585:76–85.
41. Krebs EG, Fischer EH. Vitam Horm 1964;322:399–410.
42. Coburn SP, Lewis DL, Fink WJ, et al. Am J Clin Nutr 1988;48:291–4.
43. Shane B. Vitamin B_6 and blood. In: Human vitamin B_6 requirements. Washington, DC: National Academy Press, 1978;111–28.
44. Leklem JE. Vitamin B_6 metabolism and function in humans. In: Leklem JE, Reynolds RD, eds. Clinical and physiological applications of vitamin B_6. New York: Alan R Liss, 1988;3–28.
45. Hayashi H. J Biochem 1995;118:463–73.
46. Helmreich EJM, Klein HW. Angew Chem Int Ed Engl 1980;19:441–55.
47. Rose DP, Leklem JE, Brown RR, et al. Am J Clin Nutr 1975;28:872–8.
48. Angel JF, Mellor RM. Nutr Rep Int 1974;9:97–107.
49. Black AL, Guirard BM, Snell EE. J Nutr 1977;107:1962–8.
50. Black AL, Guirard BM, Snell EE. J Nutr 1978;108:670–7.
51. Leklem JE, Brown RR, Rose DP, et al. Am J Clin Nutr 1975;28:146–56.
52. Birch TW. J Biol Chem 1938;124:775–93.
53. Abe M, Kishino Y. J Nutr 1982;112:205–10.
54. Cunnane SC, Manku MS, Horrobin DF. J Nutr 1984;114: 1754–61.
55. Delrome CB, Lupien PJ. J Nutr 1976;106:169–80.
56. Loo G, Smith JT. Lipids 1986;21:409–12.
57. Chi MS. Nutr Res 1984;4:359–62.
58. Fincham JE, Faber M, Weight MJ, et al. Atherosclerosis 1987;66:191–203.
59. Reynolds RD, Natta CL. Vitamin B_6 and sickle cell anemia. In: Reynolds RD, Leklem JE, eds. Vitamin B_6: its role in health and disease. New York: Alan R Liss, 1985;301–6.
60. Bottomley SS. Iron and vitamin B_6 in the sideroblastic anemias. In: Lindenbaum J, ed. Nutrition in hematology. New York: Churchill Livingstone, 1983; 203–23.

61. Horrigan DL, Harris JW. Vitam Horm 1968;26:549–68.
62. Dakshinamurti K. Adv Nutr Res 1982;4:143–79.
63. Bender DA. J Neurochem 1971;18: 2407–16.
64. Kirksey A, Morre DM, Wasynczuk AZ. Ann NY Acad Sci 1990;585:202–18.
65. Coursin DB. JAMA 1954;154:406–8.
66. Canham JE, Baker EM, Harding RS, et al. Ann NY Acad Sci 1969;166:16–29.
67. Thomas MR, Kirksey A. J Nutr 1976;106:1415–20.
68. Wasynczuk A, Kirksey A, Morre DM. J Nutr 1983;113:746–54.
69. Rall LC, Meydani SN. Nutr Rev 1993;51:217–25.
70. Robson LC, Schwarz MR. Cell Immunol 1975;16:135–44.
71. Talbot MC, Miller LT, Kerkvliet NI. Am J Clin Nutr 1987;46: 659–64.
72. Meydani SN, Ribaya-Mercado JD, Russell RM, et al. Am J Clin Nutr 1991;53:1275–80.
73. Eichler H-G, Hubbard R, Snell K. Biosci Rep 1981;1:101–6.
74. Litwack G, Miller-Diener A, DiSorbo DM, et al. Vitamin B_6 and the glucocorticoid receptor. In: Reynolds RD, Leklem JE, eds. Vitamin B_6: its role in health and disease. New York: Alan R Liss, 1985;177–91.
75. Bender DA. World Rev Nutr Diet 1987;51:140–88.
76. Oka T, Komori N, Kuwahata M, et al. J Nutr Sci Vitaminol 1995;41:363–75.
77. Leklem JE. J Nutr 1990;120:1503–7.
78. Reynolds RD. Biochemical methods for status assessment. In: Raiten DJ, ed. Vitamin B_6 metabolism in pregnancy, lactation, and infancy. Boca Raton, FL: CRC Press, 1995;41–59.
79. Lumeng L, Ryan M, Li T-K. J Nutr 1978;108:545–54.
80. Leklem JE, Reynolds RC. Challenges and directions in the search for clinical applications of vitamin B_6. In: Leklem JE, Reynolds RD, eds. Clinical and physiological applications of vitamin B_6. New York: Alan R Liss, 1988;437–54.
81. Shultz TD, Leklem JE. Urinary 4-pyridoxic acid, urinary vitamin B_6, and plasma pyridoxal phosphate as measures of vitamin B_6 status and dietary intake in adults. In: Leklem JE, Reynolds RD, eds. Methods in vitamin B_6 nutrition. New York: Plenum Press, 1981;389–92.
82. Miller LT, Leklem JE, Shultz TD. J Nutr 1985;115:1663–72.
83. Hansen CM, Leklem JE, Miller LT. J Nutr 1996;126:1891–901.
84. Brown RR. The tryptophan load test as an index of vitamin B_6 nutrition. In: Leklem JE, Reynolds RD, eds. Methods in vitamin B_6 nutrition. New York: Plenum Press, 1981;321–340.
85. Brown RR. Possible role for vitamin B_6 in cancer prevention and treatment. In: Leklem JE, Reynolds RD, eds. Clinical and physiological applications of vitamin B_6. New York: Alan R Liss, 1988;279–302.
86. Linkswiler HM. Methionine metabolite excretion as affected by a vitamin B_6 deficiency. In: Leklem JE, Reynolds RD, eds. Methods in vitamin B_6 nutrition. New York: Plenum Press, 1981;373–81.
87. Vanden Berg M, Franken DG, Boers HJ, et al. J Vasc Surg 1994;20:933–40.
88. Ubbink JB, Vermaak WJH, Van der Merwe A, et al. J Nutr 1994;124:1927–33.
89. Miller JW, Nadeau MR, Smith D, et al. Am J Clin Nutr 1994; 59:1033–9.
90. Woodring MJ, Storvick CA. Am J Clin Nutr 1970;23:1385–95.
91. Brown RR, Rose DP, Leklem JE, et al. Am J Clin Nutr 1975;28:10–9.
92. Ubbink JB, Bissbort S, Van den Berg I, et al. Am J Clin Nutr 1989;50:1420–8.
93. Food and Nutrition Board, National Research Council. Recommended dietary allowances. 10th ed. Washington, DC: National Academy Press, 1989.
93a. Food and Nutrition Board—Institute of Medicine. Dietary reference intakes. Thiamin, riboflavin, niacin, vitamin B_6, folate, vitamin B_{12}, pantothenic acid, biotin, and choline. Washington DC: National Academy Press, 1998.
94. Manore MM, Leklem JE, Walter MC. Am J Clin Nutr 1987;46:995–1004.
95. Styslinger L, Kirksey A. Am J Clin Nutr 1985;41:21–31.
96. Borschel MW. Vitamin B_6 in infancy: requirements and current feeding practices. In: Raiten DJ, ed. Vitamin B_6 metabolism in pregnancy, lactation and infancy. Boca Raton, FL: CRC Press, 1995;109–24.
97. Lee CM, Leklem JE. Am J Clin Nutr 1985;42:226–34.
98. Ribaya-Mercado JD, Russell RM, Sahyoun N, et al. J Nutr 1991;121:1062–74.
99. Kretsch MJ, Sauberlich HE, Skala JH, et al. Am J Clin Nutr 1995;61:1091–101.
100. Reynolds RD, Leklem JE, eds. Vitamin B_6: its role in health and disease. New York: Alan R Liss, 1985.
101. Merrill AH Jr, Henderson JM. Annu Rev Nutr 1987;7:137–56.
102. Leklem JE, Reynolds RD, eds. Clinical and physiological applications of vitamin B_6. New York: Alan R Liss, 1988.
103. Collip PJ, Goldzier S, Weiss N. Ann Allergy 1975;35:93–7.
104. Musajo L, Benassi CA. Adv Clin Chem 1964;7:63–135.
105. Flinn JH, Price JM, Yess N, et al. Arthritis Rheum 1964;7: 201–10.
106. Reynolds RD, Natta CL. Am J Clin Nutr 1985;41:684–8.
107. Stone WJ, Warnock LG, Wagner C. Am J Clin Nutr 1975;28: 950–7.
108. Lumeng L, Li T-K. J Clin Invest 1974;53:693–704.
109. Serfontein WJ, Ubbink JB, DeVilliers LS. Atherosclerosis 1985;55:357–61.
110. Potera C, Rose DP, Brown RR. Am J Clin Nutr 1977;30: 1677–9.
111. Devita VT, Chabner BA, Livingston DM, et al. Am J Clin Nutr 1971;24:835–40.
112. Hollenbeck CB, Leklem JE, Riddle MC, et al. Am J Clin Nutr 1983;38:41–51.
113. Serfontein WJ, Ubbink JB, DeVilliers LS, et al. Atherosclerosis 1986;59:341–6.
114. Dakshinamurti K, ed. Ann NY Acad Sci 1990;585.
115. Bhagavan HN. Interaction between vitamin B_6 and drugs. In: Reynolds RD, Leklem JE, eds. Vitamin B_6: its role in health and disease. New York: Alan R Liss, 1985,401–15.
116. Ubbink JB, Bissbort S, Vermaak WJH, et al. Enzyme 1990;43:72–9.
117. Schaumburg H, Kaplan J, Windebank A, et al. N Engl J Med 1983;309:445–8.
118. Cohen M, Bendich A. Toxicol Lett 1986;34:129–39.

SELECTED READINGS

Dakshinamurti K, ed. Vitamin B_6. Ann NY Acad Sci 1990;585.

Leklem JE, Reynolds RD, eds. Clinical and physiological applications of vitamin B_6. New York: Alan R Liss, 1988.

Merrill AH Jr, Henderson JM. Diseases associated with defects in vitamin B_6 metabolism or utilization. Annu Rev Nutr 1987;7:137–56.

Raiten DJ, ed. Vitamin B_6 metabolism in pregnancy, lactation, and infancy. Boca Raton, FL: CRC Press, 1995.

Reynolds RD, Leklem JE, eds. Vitamin B_6: its role in health and disease. New York: Alan R Liss, 1985.

25. Pantothenic Acid

NORA PLESOFSKY-VIG

HISTORICAL INTRODUCTION

Independent research paths in microbiology and medicine led to the isolation and characterization of pantothenic acid (1, 2). Components of the vitamin B_2 complex, derived from liver, were separated and individually tested for their effects on specific animal disorders. One of the last purification steps was the separation of pantothenic acid from vitamin B_6; this was accomplished by adsorption chromatography in which pyridoxol and its derivatives (vitamin B_6) adsorbed to fuller's earth, while pantothenic acid remained in the filtrate. Whereas vitamin B_6 cured rats of the dermatitis produced by vitamin B_2 deficiency, dermatitis in chicks was cured only by the filtrate component, subsequently known as the "chick antidermatitis factor." This factor was identical, by biochemical and physiologic criteria, to the pantothenic acid that R. J. Williams had earlier demonstrated to be essential for the growth of yeast.

R. J. Williams and R. T. Major successfully synthesized pantothenic acid in 1940 (2). It was not until 1947, however, that F. Lipmann and colleagues (3) demonstrated that its biologically functional form was coenzyme A (CoA), an essential cofactor for biologic acetylation reactions, such as acetylation of sulfonamide in the liver and of choline in the brain. Pantothenate-containing CoA has since been shown to be essential to the respiratory tricarboxylic acid cycle, fatty acid synthesis and degradation, and many other metabolic and regulatory processes. The accepted biochemical structure of CoA was published in 1953 (4).

CHEMISTRY

Microorganisms synthesize pantothenic acid (1, 2, 5) by an amide linkage between pantoic acid and β-alanine (Fig. 25.1). Pantetheine, an essential growth factor for the yogurt-producing bacterium *Lactobacillus bulgaricus*, consists of a β-mercaptoethylamine group added to pantothenate in humans. CoA (Fig. 25.1) is composed of 4′-phosphopantetheine linked by an anhydride bond to adenosine 5′-monophosphate, which is modified by a 3′-hydroxyl phosphate. The sulfhydryl group of pantetheine is the active site of esterification to acetate and acyl groups.

In addition to functioning within CoA, 4′-phosphopantetheine is also found covalently linked to certain proteins (6), especially those involved in fatty acid metabolism. Fatty acid synthetase and the acyl carrier protein of bacteria and mitochondria are linked to 4′-phosphopantetheine by a phosphodiester bond via serine. Phosphopantetheine is also linked to citrate lyase of anaerobic bacteria and to enzymes involved in the nonribosomal synthesis of the peptide antibiotics tyrocidin and gramicidin S.

CoA and pantothenate-modified proteins participate in acyl group transfer and condensation reactions (5). In acyl group transfer, nucleophilic addition to the carbonyl group that is thioesterified to CoA leads to new ester bond formation and displacement of CoA. As a leaving group, CoA facilitates the transfer of acetyl or acyl groups. In condensation reactions, the α-carbon of the acyl group is acidified by its proximity to the thioester with CoA, and it attaches to an electrophilic center, leading to carbon-carbon bond formation or cleavage. Both types of reactions occur during fatty acid synthesis (7). Malonate is transferred from CoA to the enzyme-linked phosphopantetheine and acetate is transferred to an enzyme sulfhydryl group. After these acyltransferase reactions, there is condensation between the pantetheine-linked malonate and the introduced acetate or the growing fatty acid chain. In the tricarboxylic acid cycle of respiratory metabolism, acetyl-CoA condenses with oxaloacetic acid to yield citric acid.

DIETARY CONSIDERATIONS: FOOD SOURCES

Pantothenic acid is widely distributed in cells and tissues, being essential to all forms of life. Rich dietary sources are liver, kidney, yeast, egg yolk, and broccoli, which contain more than 50 μg pantothenate/g dry weight (2). Especially high levels of pantothenate are found in royal bee jelly (511 μg/g) and in ovaries of tuna and cod (2.32 mg/g). The pantothenate content of human milk increases fivefold within 4 days after parturition (2) from 2.2 to 11.2 μmol/L (48–245 μg/dL), a level similar to that in cow's milk. Pantothenic acid is relatively stable at neutral pH. However, cooking is reported to

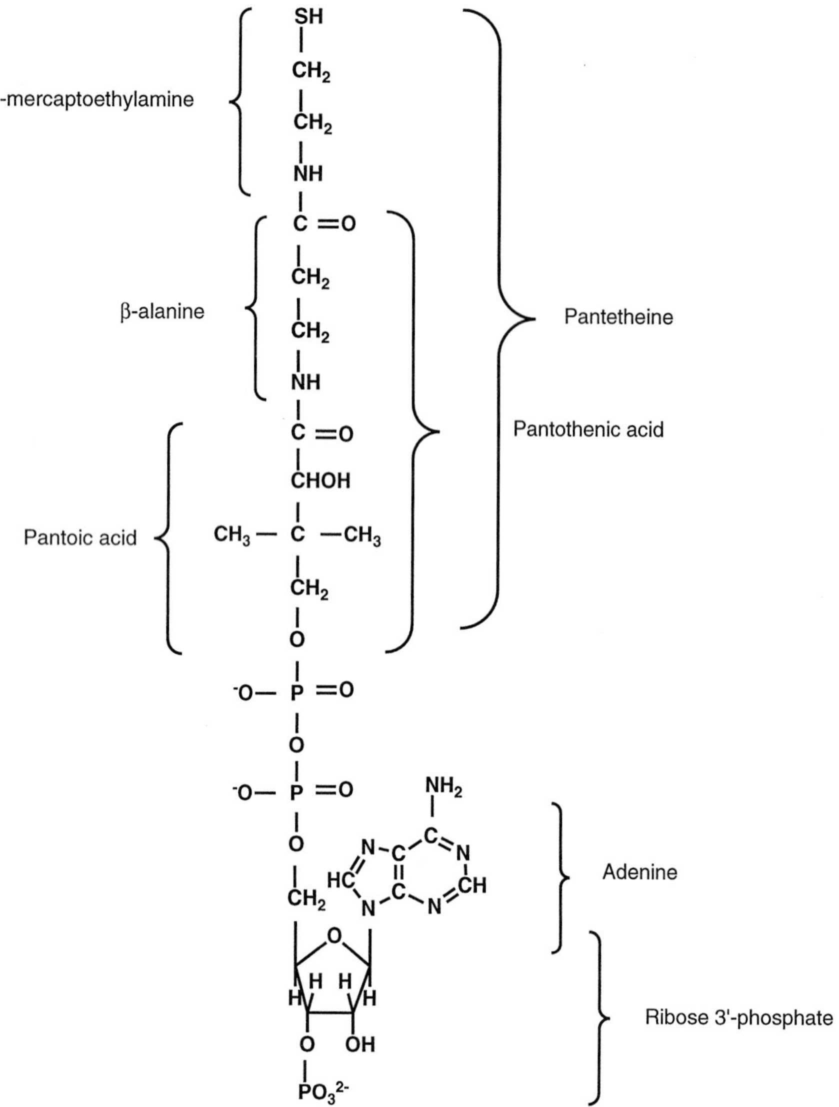

Figure 25.1. Coenzyme A and intermediates.

destroy 15 to 50% of the vitamin present in raw meat (2), and processing of vegetables causes pantothenate losses of 37 to 78% (8).

The average American diet has been estimated to provide 5.8 mg pantothenate/day. A study of adolescents (9) showed that despite a pantothenate intake of less than 4 mg/day by some subjects, blood concentrations of the vitamin were in the normal range (0.91–2.74 μmol/L). Excess pantothenate appeared to be eliminated by excretion, which was highly correlated with dietary intake.

Synthetic D-pantothenate, the active enantiomer, is available as a calcium or sodium salt. However, multivitamin preparations commonly contain its more stable alcohol derivative, panthenol, which is converted by humans to pantothenic acid (10).

METABOLISM

After ingestion in dietary sources, CoA is hydrolyzed in the intestinal lumen to pantothenic acid, which is absorbed into the bloodstream by sodium-dependent transport (11). Sodium cotransport is also the mechanism by which pantothenate is subsequently taken up from the plasma by most cells.

The first step in the synthesis of CoA is phosphorylation of pantothenic acid (Fig. 25.1), which is catalyzed by pantothenate kinase; this constitutes the primary regulatory site of CoA synthesis in bacteria and rat heart (12). Phosphorylation is followed by the ATP-dependent condensation of 4′-phosphopantothenic acid with cysteine, whose product, 4′-phosphopantothenoylcysteine, is decarboxylated to yield 4′-phosphopantetheine (13). CoA is formed by sequential transfers of adenosine monophosphate and phosphate from ATP to 4′-phosphopantetheine. All the enzymes required for CoA synthesis are present in the cytoplasm. Nevertheless, mitochondria must also be a final site of synthesis, since 95% of CoA is found in mitochondria and CoA does not cross the mitochondrial membranes (12).

Multiple hydrolytic steps liberate pantothenic acid

from CoA, with the unique, final reaction being the hydrolysis of pantetheine to cysteamine and pantothenate, which is excreted in urine (14).

FUNCTIONS

Cellular Metabolism

Pantothenate, usually in the form of CoA, performs multiple roles in cellular metabolism (5), being central to the energy-yielding oxidation of glycolytic products and other metabolites through the mitochondrial tricarboxylic acid cycle. In the first step of the cycle, acetyl-CoA condenses with oxaloacetate to yield citrate, and subsequently, succinyl-CoA provides energy for GDP phosphorylation. The β-oxidation of fatty acids and the oxidative degradation of amino acids also depend on CoA, which makes the catabolic products available to the respiratory tricarboxylic acid cycle.

Pantothenic acid is required for synthesis of many essential molecules. Synthesis of fatty acids and membrane phospholipids, including regulatory sphingolipids, requires pantothenate, and synthesis of the amino acids leucine, arginine, and methionine includes a pantothenate-requiring step. CoA is required for synthesis of isoprenoid derivatives, such as cholesterol, steroid hormones, dolichol, vitamin A, vitamin D, and heme A. Succinyl-CoA is essential to the synthesis of δ-aminolevulinic acid, which is the precursor of both the corrin ring in vitamin B_{12} and the porphyrin rings in hemoglobin and the cytochromes. CoA contributes an essential acetyl group to the neurotransmitter acetylcholine and to serotonin in its conversion to melatonin, as well as to the sugars *N*-acetylglucosamine, *N*-acetylgalactosamine, and *N*-acetylneuraminic acid, components of glycoproteins and glycolipids.

Protein Modification

Acetylation of Proteins

Amino-Terminal Acetylation. Most soluble proteins are N-terminally modified with an acetate group that is donated by CoA (15). The terminal methionine is usually cleaved and the second amino acid, typically alanine or serine, becomes acetylated cotranslationally on its α-amino group. It was proposed earlier that acetylation protected cellular proteins from degradation, based on in vitro assays. More recent experiments showed that N-acetylated proteins were also subject to ubiquitin-dependent degradation, if the assay mixtures included EF-1α, the translation elongation factor (16). Nevertheless, the importance of N-terminal acetylation was demonstrated genetically in *Saccharomyces cerevisiae,* in which a defect in N-terminal acetyltransferase activity disrupted cell cycle progression and sexual development (17). There was no evidence of protein instability due to the lack of acetylation. N-terminal acetylation appears to alter the structure of certain proteins. For example, it increases the N-terminal α-helical content of calpactin I, a calcium-binding protein that requires acetylation to assemble with its regulatory subunit (18).

Mammalian peptide hormones become N-terminally acetylated as they are processed from polyprotein precursors (6). This type of posttranslational addition of acetate strongly affects hormone activity. Pro-opiomelanocortin is the precursor of both adrenocorticotropin (ACTH), a steroidogenic hormone, and β-lipotropin, a lipolytic hormone. ACTH is processed in turn to α-melanocyte-stimulating hormone (MSH), and β-lipotropin is processed to the opioid β-endorphin. The products α-MSH and β-endorphin both become acetylated, but they differ in the tissues in which they are acetylated. Both become N-terminally acetylated in the intermediate pituitary, but only MSH is acetylated in brain, and neither is acetylated in the anterior pituitary. Acetylation has different effects on the activities of these two hormones, stimulating the activity of α-MSH but inactivating β-endorphin, which becomes unable to bind to opioid receptors. A single *N*-acetyltransferase activity has been identified in the intermediate, but not the anterior, lobe of rat and bovine pituitary. This activity may modify both hormones, providing a mechanism for differentially activating two products of a single precursor.

Internal Acetylation. Two major classes of proteins undergo reversible acetylation on the ϵ-amino group of internal lysine residues: histones and α-tubulin. In addition, protamines and the high-mobility-group proteins HMG1 and HMG2, which bind DNA, are subject to acetylation. The nucleosome is composed of the core histones, a tetramer of histones H3 and H4 and two dimers of histones H2A and H2B, around which is wrapped 146 bp of DNA. All these core histones of the octamer become acetylated within their amino-terminal regions; the internucleosomal histone H1 has no internal acetylation sites. Histones H3 and H4 each have four possible acetylation sites. In mammalian histone H3, lys-14 is the preferred acetylation site, followed by lys-23 and lys-18 (19). H4 becomes monoacetylated at lys-16, with further modification at lys-12, followed by lys-8 and lys-5. In histone H2B, lys-12 and lys-15 are acetylated before lys-5 and lys-20. There is only one acetylation site in histone H2A.

Histone acetylation, which neutralizes the charge of lysine residues, appears to weaken interactions between nucleosomes that depend on histone N-terminal tails. The presence of highly acetylated H3 and H4 affects nucleosomal structure. Acetylated chromatin has a more open, unfolded conformation, as indicated by its increased sensitivity to nucleases and its increased salt solubility (20). Gel electrophoresis shows that acetylation leads to decompaction of the chromatin fiber (21). Hyperacetylation of H3 and H4 decreases the negative supercoiling within nucleosomes, as indicated by reduction in the linking number change per nucleosome (22).

Histones that are highly acetylated tend to be associated with newly synthesized DNA or with DNA that is transcriptionally active, but different sites on the histones may become acetylated during these two processes. Furthermore, there is only transient acetylation of newly synthesized histones as they assemble with replicating chromatin, whereas the histones of transcriptionally active chromatin are continually and dynamically acetylated.

The acetylated chromatin fraction from chick embryo erythrocytes was immunoselected and found to be strongly enriched in actively transcribed α-D-globin gene sequences (23). There is not a strict correspondence, however, between acetylated chromatin and transcribed DNA. The presence of acetylated histones extended from the transcribed region into the interspersed, nontranscribed DNA of the β-globin locus (24). Furthermore, acetylated histones were contemporaneously associated with two globin genes that are expressed at different times during development (23). Similarly, association of acetylated chromatin with the platelet-derived growth factor B gene occurred prior to its induction by phorbol esters (25). These findings suggest that histone acetylation may be a precondition for transcription but does not specify which genes are expressed. Binding of transactivating factors is necessary for specific gene transcription, and in vitro experiments suggest that histone acetylation is required for proteins to bind to chromatin, for example, binding of TFIIIA to the 5S RNA gene (26). A transcriptional regulator of yeast, GCN5p, was shown to be a histone acetyltransferase. Its association with other transcriptional factors may account for targeting of the acetyltransferase to specific chromatin sites (27).

Mutation of acetylatable lysines in either histone H3 or H4 of yeast produced contrasting effects on gene transcription. A neutral replacement of lys-16 in H4 led to derepression of the silent mating locus, suggesting that this locus may be activated by H4 acetylation at lys-16 (28). In contrast, transcription of the *GAL1* and *PHO5* genes was inhibited by similar mutations in H4 (29). However, when acetylatable lysines in H3 were mutated, *GAL1* was strongly activated. These different effects on *GAL1* transcription are mirrored in the effects of mutated H3 and H4 N termini on chromatin structure of the *GAL1* promoter, since mutation of H4, but not of H3, made chromatin in the promoter region assume a more closed conformation (30).

During DNA replication, newly synthesized histones become transiently acetylated on their N-terminal tails. Deposition of histones onto DNA is a two-step process: H3/H4 tetramers are deposited first, followed by H2A/H2B dimers. H4 is diacetylated before it is deposited onto DNA and before it assembles with the other newly synthesized core histones (31). In the absence of DNA synthesis, newly synthesized H3 and H4 remain cytosolic, whereas H2A and H2B exchange preferentially into acetylated chromatin regions. Histone acetylation during deposition inhibits binding of the linker histone H1 to newly assembled chromatin, thereby reducing higher-order nucleosome interactions (32).

Microtubules are essential components of the cellular cytoskeleton, affecting cell shape and motility, and are central to chromosome segregation in nuclei. They are also the major structure within flagella and cilia. Microtubules are assembled from α- and β-tubulin dimers that polymerize and depolymerize dynamically. A subset of the α-tubulin within microtubules becomes acetylated on lys-40 (33). α-Tubulin acetylation occurs in the assembled microtubule, which is a better substrate than the tubulin dimer for acetylation (6). Deacetylation appears to be coupled to depolymerization of microtubules. Several observations suggest that acetylation may stabilize microtubules: *(a)* the acetylated microtubules are more stable to depolymerizing agents such as colchicine and *(b)* drugs that stabilize microtubules, like taxol, induce α-tubulin acetylation (6). Tubulin turnover in neurons was found to be much slower in the neurite shafts, where acetylated α-tubulin was concentrated, than in the cell body and growth cones (34).

Acetylated microtubules, detected by an antibody against the modified tubulin, are not distributed randomly in cells (6). They tend to be excluded from growing, motile regions of cells. In dorsal root ganglion neurons, acetylated α-tubulin is absent from growth cones at neurite tips, and it is excluded from the leading-edge microtubules of migrating 3T3 cells. In chick muscle fibers, acetylated microtubules underlie motor endplates, where they contribute to vesicle and organelle transport, but they are absent from the growing regions of cells (35). Individual axonal microtubules actually have separate regions of acetylated and unacetylated α-tubulin along their length, with the older regions corresponding to the acetylated domains (36). There is also nonrandom distribution of acetylated microtubules during mitosis and meiosis. In unfertilized mouse oocytes, for example, acetylated α-tubulin was mainly at the poles during meiotic metaphase; the spindle became acetylated at anaphase; and by telophase only the midbody microtubules were acetylated (37). The nonrandom distribution of acetylated microtubules is also associated with cell differentiation. In developing mouse embryos, acetylated microtubules that were associated with the cell cortex before differentiation relocated to the basal part of the cell cortex as cellular asymmetry developed. After asymmetric cell division, acetylated microtubules concentrated in the inside, rather than the outside, cells (38).

Acylation of Proteins

A wide variety of cellular proteins are covalently modified with long-chain fatty acids donated by CoA. This type of modification affects the location and activity of many central proteins, including those involved in signal transduction. The two fatty acids commonly added to proteins are myristic acid, a rare 14-carbon saturated fatty acid, and the more abundant 16-carbon palmitic acid (Table 25.1). These two fatty acids are attached to proteins by distinct

Table 25.1
Proteins (in text) That are Modified with Fatty Acids or Isoprenyl Groups

Myristate	Palmitate	Isoprenyl
G_o,G_i protein α subunits	G protein α subunits	Ras^v, Ras^c
transducin	$p56^{lck}$, $p59^{fyn}$	Rab proteins
ARF proteins	ecNOS	G protein γ subunits
Src^v, Src^c	Ras^v, Ras^c	nuclear lamins A and B
protein kinase A	receptors:	phosphorylase kinase
calcineurin	CD-mannose-6-phosphate	rhodopsin kinase
MARCKS	rhodopsin	
recoverin	dopamine (D_1,D_2)	
NADH-cytochrome b_5 reductase	α_{2A}-, β_2-adrenergic	
ecNOS	thyrotropin-releasing hormone	
gag, VP2, VP4	choriogonadotropin	
IgM heavy chain	iron-transferrin	
interleukin-1α, -1β,	insulin	
TNF α	nicotinic acetylcholine	
cytochrome *c* oxidase, su 1	asialoglycoprotein	
Band 4.2	CD4, CD44, CD36, P-selectin	
	HLA-B heavy chain	
	Band 3	
	ankyrin, spectrin, vinculin	
	fibronectin	
	actin	
	gap junction proteins	
	myelin proteolipid subunit	
	cysteine string proteins	
	acetylcholinesterase	
	glutamic acid decarboxylase$_{65}$	
	GAP-43, SNAP-25	

mechanisms, and they affect proteins differently. The myristoylation reaction that has been best characterized is irreversible and occurs cotranslationally through amide linkage to the α-amino group of an N-terminal glycine. In contrast, palmitate is added posttranslationally, forming a reversible ester bond with a cysteine or serine residue. The hydrophobicity of palmitate results in strong membrane association of the acylated protein, whereas the less hydrophobic myristoylation leads either to weak membrane association or to protein interactions.

Myristoylation. There are strict sequence requirements for N-terminal myristoylation of a protein (39). An N-terminal glycine, originally in the second position, is absolutely required, and a small, neutral subterminal residue and a sixth-position serine are preferable. Myristoyl-CoA is strongly preferred by the myristoyltransferase over other acyl-CoA donors (39). Disruption of the gene for *N*-myristoyl transferase in yeast was recessively lethal, demonstrating that myristoylation is essential for cell viability (40). Myristoylated proteins are located in the cytoplasm, as well as associated with various membranes, including the plasma membrane, the endoplasmic reticulum, and the nuclear membrane. Myristoylation, which is irreversible, commonly combines with other protein modifications to regulate a protein's localization or activity. These other modifications may include palmitoylation, isoprenylation, phosphorylation, and GTP or calcium binding.

Small GTP-binding proteins comprise an extensive group of cellular proteins that become modified by myristate and palmitate, as well as by isoprenyl groups. Among these proteins, the heterotrimeric G proteins, composed of α, β, and γ subunits, mediate transmembrane signaling from membrane receptors to effector proteins, in response to hormone, neurotransmitter, and other agonists. The α subunits of the G_i and G_o subfamilies are N-terminally myristoylated, a modification reported to affect interaction of α with the $\beta\gamma$ subunits and to be required for signal transduction by α_{i2} (41). Prior myristoylation increases the protein's membrane affinity, which is required for the addition of palmitate to α subunits (42). By separate mutations, it was determined that each of the lipid modifications contributes to the association of α_o with membranes. Furthermore, myristoylation appears to independently increase the affinity of α_i for adenylyl cyclase, the effector protein (43). The α subunit of transducin, the rhodopsin-stimulated G protein of photoreceptors, is heterogeneously modified at its N terminus with myristate, laurate, and unsaturated 14-carbon fatty acids. The nature of the attached fatty acid affects the strength of the interaction of transducin α with $\beta\gamma$ and may influence the speed of visual excitation (44).

ADP-ribosylation factors (ARFs) are small monomeric GTP-binding proteins involved in vesicular transport that are N-terminally myristoylated. ARFs cycle between soluble and membrane-associated forms, regulated by GTP hydrolysis and guanine nucleotide exchange. The mammalian ARF protein is the principal coat component of non-clathrin-coated vesicles, and its binding to Golgi membranes marks the site of vesicle budding. A comparison of myristoylated and nonmyristoylated ARF5 indicated that acylation is essential for ARF5 to bind to Golgi membranes in a GTP- and temperature-dependent manner and to function in transport (45). Myristoylation appeared to stabilize the N terminus of ARF1 in an amphipathic α helix, conducive to membrane binding, and it also stabilized the interaction of ARF1 with GTP, thereby integrating membrane and GTP binding with protein activation (46).

Another large family of proteins that are N-terminally myristoylated are the Src and Src-related tyrosine kinases. The Src protein from Rous sarcoma virus is responsible for cell transformation by the oncogenic virus, and the protein requires N-terminal myristoylation to associate with the plasma membrane and to transform cells. Addition of a less hydrophobic analogue of myristic acid prevented v-Src association with membranes (47). The cellular Src protein requires myristoylation for its activity in mitosis, presumably because c-Src is activated by a membrane-bound phosphatase (48).

The catalytic subunit of cAMP-dependent protein kinase is also myristoylated at its N terminus. Membrane association of the catalytic subunit is independent of myristoylation, instead being dependent on the regulatory subunit until dissociation by cAMP. However, myristoylation appears to increase the thermal structural stability of the kinase, possibly by stabilizing an intramolecular interaction between the N-terminal domain and an internal hydrophobic surface (49). The B subunit of calcineurin, the calmodulin-dependent phosphatase targeted by cyclosporine, is also N-terminally myristoylated. This modification at least partially contributes to the protein's membrane association (50).

The myristoylated alanine-rich C kinase substrate protein (MARCKS) cross-links actin filaments and likely is involved in cytoskeletal rearrangements during neuronal transmitter release, leukocyte activation, and growth factor–induced mitosis. The binding of MARCKS to the plasma membrane is regulated by a phosphoryl-myristoyl switch. N-terminal myristoylation provides one of the two initial membrane binding sites, but upon cell activation, phosphorylation occurs within the second, basic binding site, leading to dissociation of MARCKS from the membrane (51). Recoverin is an N-myristoylated protein of retinal cells that regulates the light excitation of rhodopsin by responding to changing levels of calcium. In a calcium-myristoyl switch, the binding of calcium to recoverin exposes the N-myristoyl group, which can then bind to membranes (52). Recoverin is heterogeneously acylated, like the retinal transducin α subunit. The more hydrophobic the N-terminal acyl group, with myristate being the most hydrophobic, the more recoverin inhibits the light-dependent phosphorylation of rhodopsin at high calcium concentrations (53).

Enzymes that are N-terminally modified with myristate include NADH-cytochrome b_5 reductase, which is located at the outer membrane of microsomes and mitochondria (54). The endothelial nitric oxide synthase (ecNOS), which functions in smooth muscle relaxation, requires myristoylation to localize to membranes and become modified with palmitate (55).

N-Terminal myristoylation of viral structural proteins, such as the gag polyprotein precursor, VP2, and VP4, is required for formation of mature mammalian retroviruses, papovaviruses, and picornaviruses, respectively (6). Fos and Jun are transcriptional activators that dimerize to form the AP-1 complex that activates genes containing the phorbol response element (TRE). An interesting functional conversion of Fos has resulted from substituting its N-terminus with the gag N-terminus to produce the oncogenic viral FBR v-fos. FBR v-fos has lost the ability to activate genes from the TRE promoter, but it has gained the ability to activate unique genes in chondroosseous sarcomas (56). This oncogenic change in function is due to the N-terminal myristoylation inherited from gag, since mutation at the myristoylation site converted FBR v-fos activation specificity to the original c-fos specificity.

A small number of proteins are internally myristoylated on the ϵ-amino group of lysine residues. This modification has been characterized especially for proteins of the immune system. The heavy chain of μ immunoglobulins becomes myristoylated during transport to the surface of developing B cells (57). Precursors of the cytokines interleukin (IL)-1α and -1β and the precursor of tumor necrosis factor (TNF)-α are all myristoylated on lysine residues. The mature processed forms of IL-1α and -1β are secreted, but a portion of the IL-1α myristoylated precursor remains as a plasma membrane–associated protein (58). Similarly, a portion of the acylated precursor of TNF-α remains unprocessed and membrane associated and is active in mediating inflammation, like the mature TNF-α (59).

Cytochrome *c* oxidase is the terminal electron carrier of the respiratory chain in the inner mitochondrial membrane. Its subunit 1, the core catalytic subunit, is modified by myristic acid on an internal lysine (60). There likely is an N-myristoylating activity in mitochondria, since the cytochrome oxidase subunit 1 is encoded by mitochondrial genes and synthesized within mitochondria.

Palmitoylation. In contrast to the *N*-myristoyl transferase, enzymes that transfer palmitate to proteins show little substrate specificity, either for the fatty acyl-CoA donor or for the peptide sequence at the site of acylation. The reversibility of palmitate addition, unlike that of myristate, allows palmitoylation to have a regulatory function.

All heterotrimeric G protein α subunits, except α_t, are thioesterified to palmitate near their N termini, frequently at the subterminal cysteine. The $G_{s\alpha}$ subunit, which transmits hormonal stimulation to adenylyl cyclase, requires palmitate modification to bind to the plasma membrane and to stimulate cAMP synthesis (61). Palmitoylation provides a mechanism for regulating α_s activity; following hormonal activation and GTP binding, α_s is rapidly depalmitoylated and dissociates from the membrane. Palmitoylation of α_i and α_o subunits, which are also myristoylated, is required for their strong association with membranes and contributes to their binding to $\beta\gamma$ subunits (42). Dual acylation of these G protein α subunits appears to target them to plasma membrane caveolae, via association with glycosylphosphatidylinositol (GPI)-anchored membrane proteins (42).

Although Src itself is not palmitoylated, several Src-related tyrosine kinases are acylated with palmitate near their N termini, as well as being myristoylated. This dual acylation is necessary for the kinases' association with GPI-anchored proteins in the outer plasma membrane. When palmitoylated cys-3 and cys-6 in p59^{fyn} and cys-3 and cys-5 in p56^{lck} were mutated to serines, the kinases no longer associated with decay-accelerating factor (DAF), a GPI-anchored protein (62). The reverse mutations in p60^{src}, from serines to cysteines, caused the Src protein to associate uncharacteristically with DAF.

Nitric oxide synthases (NOS) produce the signaling molecule nitric oxide. The endothelial form of NOS (ecNOS), which has a role in smooth muscle relaxation, is dually acylated with palmitate and N-terminal myristate (55). Addition of the agonist bradykinin leads to depalmitoylation of ecNOS and its simultaneous dissociation from membranes, which is followed by ecNOS phosphorylation. Palmitoylation likely regulates this change in localization of ecNOS.

Most viral and cellular Ras proteins, monomeric GTP-binding proteins, are esterified to palmitate. Palmitoylation near the carboxyl terminus is required for oncogenic viral Ras proteins to bind to the plasma membrane and transform cells; palmitoylation strengthens the weak membrane affinity conferred on Ras by C-terminal modification with an isoprenyl group (63). The mammalian Ras protein is an essential component of the mitogen-activated protein (MAP) kinase signaling cascade. The function of Ras is to direct the protein kinase Raf to the plasma membrane, and palmitoylation or a polybasic domain is required for this localization and the activation of MAP kinase (64). Palmitoylation of the Ras2 protein of yeast is also required for its efficient membrane localization but not for its interaction with adenylyl cyclase (65).

Palmitate modification also occurs on proteins associated with intracellular membranes. Palmitoyl-CoA is required in vitro to reconstitute vesicular transport through the Golgi stacks (66). Addition of acyl-CoA was necessary both for budding of vesicles from donor Golgi and for fusion of vesicles with acceptor Golgi cisternae. Furthermore, vesicle budding was inhibited by addition of a nonhydrolyzable analogue of palmitoyl-CoA or an acyl-CoA synthetase inhibitor. The cation-dependent mannose 6-phosphate receptor (CD-MPR) transports acid hydrolases from the trans-Golgi network to a prelysosomal compartment. Palmitoylation of cys-34 in the cytoplasmic tail prevents receptor movement from the prelysosomal endosomes to the lysosomes (67). Mutation of cys-34 caused the receptor to accumulate in dense lysosomes and impaired its ability to sort cathepsin D to lysosomes.

Many plasma membrane-anchored receptors are acylated with palmitate. One prominent group of palmitoylated receptors are those that are coupled to heterotrimeric G proteins. These receptors have a similar domain structure consisting of an extracellular N terminus, seven transmembrane α-helices, and an intracellular C terminus, leading to three intracellular and three extracellular loops. The C-terminal tail has a conserved cysteine whose palmitoylation has been characterized in many of these receptors, including rhodopsin, the dopamine (D_1 and D_2) receptors, β_2-adrenergic receptor, α_{2A}-adrenergic receptor, thyrotropin-releasing hormone receptor, and the choriogonadotropin receptor. Acylation appears to lead to formation of a fourth intracellular loop. Palmitoylated cys-322 and cys-323 of the retinal photoreceptor rhodopsin were shown by fluorescence quenching to be integrated into the cell membrane (68). The regulatory functions of palmitate addition vary for these receptors. For both the dopamine D_1 receptor (69) and the β_2-adrenergic receptor (70), palmitate is attached to the receptor shortly after its exposure to agonist, and acylation contributes to agonist-dependent desensitization of the receptor. It is also important for coupling of the β_2-adrenergic receptor with G_s. Palmitoylation contributes to downregulation of the number of α_{2A}-adrenergic receptors (71), but it slows internalization of thyrotropin-releasing hormone and choriogonadotropin receptors after prolonged exposure to agonist (72).

Other transmembrane receptors that are palmitoylated are the iron-transferrin receptor, the insulin receptor, and the nicotinic acetylcholine receptor (6). Palmitate addition to the asialoglycoprotein receptor was found to activate the receptor for ligand binding; it is suggested that receptor deacylation leads to ligand dissociation (73). A membrane glycoprotein of rat adipocytes becomes palmitoylated on an extracellular domain in response to insulin and energy depletion (74). Two cysteines become acylated at the cytoplasmic-membrane junction of CD4, the surface glycoprotein of T lymphocytes and macrophages that is involved in antigen recognition and serves as receptor for the human immunodeficiency virus (75). Palmitoylation of a CD44-related lymphoma glycoprotein was shown to be required for its binding to ankyrin, which connects the cell membrane to the cytoskeleton (76). The heavy chain of the human histocompatibility antigen HLA-B is thioesterified to palmitate (6), and platelet P-selectin is palmitoylated on a cysteine in its cytoplasmic tail (77).

Palmitate is attached to several membrane proteins that are linked to the cytoskeleton. In erythrocytes, the anion transport protein Band 3 is palmitoylated (78) and is linked to Band 4.2, a major myristoylated membrane protein (79). Band 4.2, in turn, is linked to ankyrin, which is palmitoylated. The palmitate-modified population of the spectrin β subunit is more tightly membrane-associated than the unmodified spectrin (80). Vinculin, fibronectin, a subpopulation of actin (6), and gap junction proteins of heart and eye lens (81) also become palmitoylated.

Several neuronal proteins are modified with palmitate. The proteolipid subunit of brain myelin, which is acylated on a threonine residue, was the first palmitoylated protein to be identified (6). Acylation of multiple cysteines in the cysteine string proteins (csp) appears to be a mechanism for attaching csp to vesicles, where they interact with presynaptic calcium channels (82). Acetylcholinesterase, which degrades the neurotransmitter acetylcholine, is anchored in the cell membrane by palmitoylation (83). Glutamic acid decarboxylase (GAD_{65}), which is located in synaptic vesicles of γ-aminobutyric acid (GABA)-secreting neurons and in microvesicles of pancreatic β cells, may also be anchored in the membrane by palmitoylation (84).

Protein palmitoylation appears to play an important role during neuronal development. In elongating axons, GAP-43 is a major component of growth cone membranes, and SNAP-25 is a synaptic protein involved in later stages of axon growth. The reversible palmitoylation of both these proteins is proposed to influence growth cone motility and process outgrowth in developing brains (85). Palmitoylation of GAP-43, at two cysteines near its N terminus, keeps GAP-43 membrane bound and inhibits its stimulation of G_o. Nitric oxide has been found to inhibit acylation of neuronal proteins, including GAP-43 and SNAP-25 (85). This inhibition is likely the mechanism by which nitric oxide causes growth cone collapse in cultured neurites and in vivo.

Isoprenylation of Proteins

Like synthesis of other isoprenoid compounds, farnesyl and geranylgeranyl synthesis requires CoA. One of these two isoprenoids is added to the mature carboxyl-terminal cysteine of specific proteins (Table 25.1). All Ras proteins have an isoprenyl and a methyl group added to the mature C terminus and have a second modification nearby, either palmitoylation of a cysteine or a polybasic region (63). Both modifications are required for viral Ras proteins to transform cells. The Ras proteins themselves are modified with a 15-carbon farnesyl group, and inhibitors of farnesyltransferase are effective antitumor agents in Ras-transformed cells. Farnesylation of yeast Ras2p appears to be important for adenylyl cyclase activation (86). A critical function of the mammalian Ras protein in the MAP kinase signaling cascade is to direct the protein kinase Raf to the plasma membrane. When Raf itself was engineered to have a farnesylation site, Ras proved to be unnecessary for signal transduction (87). Normal Ras function requires the farnesyl moiety specifically. Substitution of the more hydrophobic geranylgeranyl, while not interfering with transformation by viral Ras, caused cellular Ras proteins to become strong inhibitors of cell growth (88).

In contrast to Ras, Ras-related proteins are isoprenylated with the 20-carbon geranylgeranyl group, frequently on two neighboring cysteines (89). The multiple Ras-related mammalian Rab proteins help to regulate specific stages of vesicular transport to the cell surface (89). Through binding to vesicles, Rab proteins appear to target them to specific acceptor membranes. The cycling of Rab proteins between membranes and cytosol is related to membrane budding and fusion. Association of Rab proteins with organellar membranes requires their modification with geranylgeranyl. This isoprenylation is also needed for Rab to interact with its GDP dissociation inhibitor (GDI), which releases Rab from membranes (90). The Rab escort protein (REP), a protein with sequence homology to GDI, assists in the geranylgeranylation of Rab, and a defect in REP has been implicated in retinal degradation or choroideremia (91).

The γ subunit of heterotrimeric G proteins is also modified by geranylgeranyl, except for the γ subunit of retinal transducin, which is farnesylated. Isoprenylation of γ is not required for its dimerization with the β subunit, but it is required for membrane targeting of the $\beta\gamma$ dimer and for productive interactions of the dimer with α subunits, receptors, and effector proteins (92).

Other cellular proteins that are isoprenylated include the nuclear lamins A and B (93). Both the α and β subunits of phosphorylase kinase, the activator of glycogen phosphorylase, are modified with farnesyl (94). The retinal rhodopsin kinase is also farnesylated, a modification necessary for its membrane association in response to photon stimulation (95).

DEFICIENCY

Pantothenic acid deficiency in humans is rare. Naturally occurring deficiency has been detected only under conditions of severe malnutrition. In World War II, prisoners of war in the Philippines, Japan, and Burma experienced numbness in their toes and painful burning sensations in their feet. These symptoms of nutritional melalgia were relieved specifically by pantothenic acid (96). Pantothenate deficiency has been experimentally induced in humans by administering analogues of pantothenic acid, in combination with a pantothenate-deficient diet. The antagonist ω-methylpantothenate produced headache, fatigue, insomnia, intestinal disturbances, and paresthesia of hands and feet. There was also a decrease in the eosinopenic response to ACTH, loss of antibody production, and increased sensitivity to insulin (97). Effects of a pantothenate-restricted diet have been studied in many animals (2). Rats developed hypertrophy of the adrenal cortex, followed by hemorrhage and necrosis; monkeys showed depressed heme synthesis and became anemic. Chickens developed dermatitis and poor feathering, and they also displayed axon and myelin degeneration within the spinal cord.

Administration of pantothenate antagonists to humans has also occurred unintentionally, with deleterious side effects. Hopantenate is an analogue of pantothenic acid, in which GABA replaces β-alanine. Hopantenate was used in Japan, as an agonist of GABA, to cerebrally stimulate retarded individuals and to alleviate tardive dyskinesia symptoms induced by tranquilizers. Treatment with hopantenate produced severe side effects in patients, including lactic acidosis, hypoglycemia, and hyperammonemia, ultimately leading to acute encephalopathy (98). These effects were replicated in dogs given hopantenate and were shown to be due to induction of pantothenic acid deficiency. Dogs given an equivalent amount of pantothenic acid along with the calcium hopantenate did not develop the disorders (99).

Pantothenic acid has beneficial effects in cases not clearly related to pantothenate deficiency. Addition of pantothenate increased skeletal muscle energy metabolism in the murine model of Duchenne muscular dystrophy (100). It also protected rats against peroxidation and liver damage produced by carbon tetrachloride (101). Furthermore, in vitro, pantothenate dampened neutrophil (PMN) response to stimulatory peptides and cytokines (102). Apparently because of its antiinflammatory properties, pantothenic acid improved surgical wound healing.

EVALUATION OF NUTRIENT STATUS

Hydrolytic enzymes are required to release the pantothenate component of CoA for assays of pantothenic acid in biologic material other than urine. Microbiologic assays with yeast and lactobacilli have been used to determine the pantothenic acid content of blood, urine, and tissues (10). The exchange of radioactive β-alanine into pantothenic acid, which is catalyzed by pantothase, is one technique for measuring pantothenate concentration in food sources (103), and a radioimmunoassay has also been used for quantitation (104).

RECOMMENDED INTAKES FOR HUMANS

Formal recommended dietary allowances (RDAs) have not been established for pantothenic acid, but the estimated safe and adequate dietary intakes of pantothenate are 18 to 32 μmol (4–7 mg) for adults (Appendix Table II-A-2-a-3). Among younger age groups, 9 μmol (2 mg) were recommended daily for infants, and 18 to 23 μmol (4–5 mg) for children 7 to 10 years of age (105) in the 1989 RDA (Appendix Table II-A-2-a-2). The 1998 levels are presented as Adequate Intakes rather than RDAs. They are in the range of 1.7 to 3 mg/day for infants and children, 5 mg/day for adults, and 6 and 7 mg/day, respectively, for pregnant and lactating women (Appendix Table II-A-2-c-1) (106).

REFERENCES

1. Wagner AF, Folkers K. Vitamins and coenzymes. New York: John Wiley & Sons, 1964;93–112.
2. Robinson FA. The vitamin co-factors of enzyme systems. Oxford: Pergamon Press, 1966;406–86.
3. Lipmann F, Kaplan NO, Novelli GD, et al. J Biol Chem 1947;167:869–70.
4. Baddiley J, Thain EM, Novelli GD, et al. Nature 1953;171:76.
5. Metzler DE. Biochemistry. New York: Academic Press, 1977.
6. Plesofsky-Vig N, Brambl R. Annu Rev Nutr 1988;8:461–82.
7. Wakil SJ, Stoops JK, Joshi VC. Annu Rev Biochem 1983;52:537–79.
8. Tahiliani AG, Beinlich CJ. Vitam Horm 1991;46:165–228.
9. Eissenstat BR, Wyse BW, Hansen RG. Am J Clin Nutr 1986;44:931–7.
10. Bird OD, Thompson RQ. Pantothenic acid. In: Gyorgy P, Pearson WN, eds. The vitamins, vol 7. 2nd ed. New York: Academic Press, 1967;209–41.
11. Fenstermacher DK, Rose RC. Am J Physiol 1986;250:G155–60.
12. Robishaw JD, Berkich D, Neely JR. J Biol Chem 1982;257: 10967–72.
13. Brown G. J Biol Chem 1959;234:370–8.
14. Wittwer CT, Burkhard D, Ririe K. J Biol Chem 1983;258: 9733–8.
15. Driessen HPC, deJong WW, Tesser GI, et al. CRC Crit Rev Biochem 1985;18:281–306.
16. Gonen H, Smith CE, Siegel NR, et al. Proc Natl Acad Sci USA 1994;91:7648–52.
17. Mullen JR, Kayne PS, Moerschell RP, et al. EMBO J 1989;8:2067–75.
18. Johnsson N, Marriott G, Weber K. EMBO J 1988;7:2435–42.
19. Thorne AW, Kmiciek D, Mitchelson K, et al. Eur J Biochem 1990;193:701–13.
20. Ridsdale JA, Hendzel MJ, Delcuve GP, et al. J Biol Chem 1990;265:5150–6.
21. Krajewski WA, Panin VM, Razin SV. Biochem Biophys Res Commun 1993;196:455–60.
22. Norton VG, Marvin KW, Yau P, et al. J Biol Chem 1990;265:19848–52.
23. Hebbes TR, Thorne AW, Clayton AL, et al. Nucleic Acids Res 1992;20:1017–22.
24. Hebbes TR, Clayton AL, Thorne AW, et al. EMBO J 1994;13:1823–30.
25. Clayton AL, Hebbes TR, Thorne AW, et al. FEBS Lett 1993;336:23–6.
26. Lee DY, Hayes JJ, Pruss D. Cell 1993;72:73–84.
27. Brownell JE, Zhou J, Ranalli T, et al. Cell 1996;84:843–51.
28. Johnson LM, Fisher-Adams G, Grunstein M. EMBO J 1992;11:2201–9.
29. Durrin LK, Mann RK, Kayne PS, et al. Cell 1991;65:1023–31.
30. Fisher-Adams G, Grunstein M. EMBO J 1995;14:1468–77.
31. Perry CA, Dadd CA, Allis CD, et al. Biochemistry 1993;32:13605–14.
32. Perry CA, Annunziato AT. Exp Cell Res 1991;196:337–45.
33. LeDizet M, Peperno G. Proc Natl Acad Sci USA 1987;84:5720–4.
34. Lim SS, Sammak PJ, Borisy GG. J Cell Biol 1989;109:253–63.
35. Jasmin BJ, Changeux J-P, Cartaud J. Nature 1990;344:673–5.
36. Brown A, Li Y, Slaughter T, et al. J Cell Sci 1993;104:339–52.
37. Schatten G, Simerly C, Asai DJ, et al. Dev Biol 1988;130:74–86.
38. Houliston E, Maro B. J Cell Biol 1989;108:543–51.
39. Towler DA, Adams SP, Eubanks SR, et al. Proc Natl Acad Sci USA 1987;84:2708–12.
40. Duronio RJ, Towler DA, Heuckeroth RO, et al. Science 1989;243:796–800.
41. Gallego C, Gupta SK, Winitz S, et al. Proc Natl Acad Sci USA 1992;89:9695–9.
42. Mumby SM, Kleuss C, Gilman AG. Proc Natl Acad Sci USA 1994;91:2800–4.
43. Wilson PT, Bourne HR. J Biol Chem 1995;270:9667–75.

44. Kokame K, Fukada Y, Yoshizawa T, et al. Nature 1992;359:749–52.
45. Haun RS, Tsai S-C, Adamik R, et al. J Biol Chem 1993;268:7064–8.
46. Franco M, Chardin P, Chabre M. J Biol Chem 1995;270:1337–41.
47. Heuckeroth RO, Gordon JI. Proc Natl Acad Sci USA 1989;86:5262–6.
48. Bagrodia S, Taylor SJ, Shalloway D. Mol Cell Biol 1993;13:1464–70.
49. Yonemoto W, McGlone ML, Taylor SS. J Biol Chem 1993;268:2348–52.
50. Zhu D, Cardenas ME, Heitman J. J Biol Chem 1995;270:24831–8.
51. Taniguchi H, Manenti S. J Biol Chem 1993;268:9960–3.
52. Ames JB, Tanaka T, Stryer L, et al. Biochemistry 1994;33:10743–53.
53. Sanada K, Kokame K, Yoshizawa T, et al. J Biol Chem 1995;270:15459–62.
54. Borgese N, Longhi R. Biochem J 1990;266:341–7.
55. Robinson LJ, Buscone L, Michel T. J Biol Chem 1995;270:995–8.
56. Jotte RM, Kamata N, Holt JT. J Biol Chem 1994;269:16383–96.
57. Pillai S, Baltimore D. Proc Natl Acad Sci USA 1987;84:7654–8.
58. Stevenson FT, Bursten SL, Fanton C, et al. Proc Natl Acad Sci USA 1993;90:7245–9.
59. Stevenson FT, Bursten SL, Locksley RM, et al. J Exp Med 1992;176:1053–62.
60. Vassilev AO, Plesofsky-Vig N, Brambl R. Proc Natl Acad Sci USA 1995;92:8680–4.
61. Wedegaertner PB, Bourne HR. Cell 1994;77:1063–70.
62. Shenoy-Scaria AM, Gauen LKT, Kwong J, et al. Mol Cell Biol 1993;13:6385–92.
63. Hancock JF, Magee AI, Childs JE, et al. Cell 1989;57:1167–77.
64. Cadwallader KA, Paterson H, Macdonald SG, et al. Mol Cell Biol 1994;14:4722–30.
65. Kuroda Y, Suzuki N, Kataoka T. Science 1993;259:683–6.
66. Pfanner N, Orci L, Glick BS, et al. Cell 1989;59:95–102.
67. Schweizer A, Kornfeld S, Rohrer J. J Cell Biol 1996;132:577–84.
68. Moench SJ, Moreland J, Stewart DH, et al. Biochemistry 1994;33:5791–6.
69. Ng GYK, Mouillac B, George SR, et al. Eur J Pharmacol 1994;267:7–19.
70. Mouillac B, Caron M, Bonin H, et al. J Biol Chem 1992;267:21733–7.
71. Eason MG, Jacinto MT, Theiss CT, et al. Proc Natl Acad Sci USA 1994;91:11178–82.
72. Kawate N, Menon KMJ. J Biol Chem 1994;269:30651–8.
73. Zeng F-Y, Weigel PH. J Biol Chem 1995;270:21388–95.
74. Jochen A, Hays J. J Lipid Res 1993;34:1783–92.
75. Crise B, Rose JK. J Biol Chem 1992;267:13593–7.
76. Bourguignon LYW, Kalomiris EL, Lokeshwar VB. J Biol Chem 1991;266:11761–5.
77. Fujimoto T, Stroud E, Whatley RE, et al. J Biol Chem 1993;268:11394–400.
78. Kang D, Karbach D, Passow H. Biochim Biophys Acta 1994;1194:341–4.
79. Risinger MA, Dotimas EM, Cohen CM. J Biol Chem 1992;267:5680–5.
80. Mariani M, Maretzki D, Lutz HU. J Biol Chem 1993;268:12996–13001.
81. Manenti S, Dunia I, Benedetti EL. FEBS Lett 1990;262:356–8.
82. Mastrogiacomo A, Parsons SM, Zampighi GA, et al. Science 1994;263:981–2.
83. Randall WR. J Biol Chem 1994;269:12367–74.
84. Christgau S, Aanstoot H-J, Schierbeck H, et al. J Cell Biol 1992;118:309–20.
85. Hess DT, Petterson SI, Smith DS, et al. Nature 1993;366:562–5.
86. Bhattacharya S, Chen L, Broach JR, et al. Proc Natl Acad Sci USA 1995;92:2984–8.
87. Stokoe D, Macdonald SG, Cadwallader K, et al. Science 1994;264:1463–7.
88. Cox AD, Hisaka MM, Buss JE, et al. Mol Cell Biol 1992;12:2606–15.
89. Farnsworth CC, Seabra MC, Ericsson LH, et al. Proc Natl Acad Sci USA 1994;91:11963–7.
90. Araki S, Kaibuchi K, Sasaki T, et al. Mol Cell Biol 1991;11:1438–47.
91. Alexandrov K, Horiuchi H, Steele-Mortimer O, et al. EMBO J 1994;13:5262–73.
92. Wedegaertner PB, Wilson PT, Bourne HR. J Biol Chem 1995;270:503–6.
93. Sinensky M, Lutz RJ. BioEssays 1992;14:25–31.
94. Heilmeyer LMG, Serwe M, Weber C, et al. Proc Natl Acad Sci USA 1992;89:9554–8.
95. Inglese J, Koch WJ, Caron MG, et al. Nature 1992;359:147–50.
96. Glusman M. Am J Med 1947;3:211–23.
97. Hodges RE, Ohlson MA, Bean WB. J Clin Invest 1958;37:1642.
98. Otsuka M, Akiba T, Okita Y, et al. Jpn J Med 1990;29:324–8.
99. Noda S, Haratake J, Sasaki A, et al. Liver 1991;11:134–42.
100. Even PC, Decrouy A, Chinet A. Biochem J 1994;304:649–54.
101. Nagiel-Ostaszewski I, Lau-Cam CA. Res Commun Chem Pathol Pharmacol 1990;67:289–92.
102. Kapp A, Zeck-Kapp G. Allerg Immunol 1991;37:145–50.
103. Airas RK. Methods Enzymol 1986;122:33–35.
104. Wittwer C, Wyse B, Hansen RG. Anal Biochem 1982;122:213–22.
105. Food and Nutrition Board, National Research Council. Recommended dietary allowances. 10th ed. Washington, DC: National Academy Press, 1989.
106. Food and Nutrition Board—Institute of Medicine. Dietary reference intakes. Thiamin, riboflavin, niacin, vitamin B6, folate, vitamin B_{12}, pantothenic acid, biotin, and choline. Washington DC: National Academy Press, 1998.

SELECTED READINGS

Clarke S. Protein isoprenylation and methylation at carboxyl-terminal cysteine residues. Annu Rev Biochem 1992;61:355–386.

Johnson DR, Bhatnagar RS, Knoll LJ, et al. Genetic and biochemical studies of protein N-myristoylation. Annu Rev Biochem 1994;63:869–914.

Loidl P. Histone acetylation: facts and questions. Chromosoma 1994;103:441–9.

Milligan G, Parenti M, Magee AI. The dynamic role of palmitoylation in signal transduction. Trends Biochem Sci 1995;20:181–6.

Tahiliani AG, Beinlich CJ. Pantothenic acid in health and disease. Vitam Horm 1991;46:165–228.

26. Folic Acid

VICTOR HERBERT

HISTORY

Early reports of disease now recognizable as probable folate deficiency include those of Channing (1), Barclay (2), and Osler (3). In 1937, Wills and her associates described a macrocytic anemia in Hindu women in Bombay, usually associated with pregnancy (4), that responded to therapy with a commercial preparation of autolyzed yeast called Marmite; these workers produced a similar macrocytic anemia in monkeys, which responded to a "Wills factor" present in crude, but not in purified, liver extracts.

The more-purified liver extract was found to be a fairly pure solution of vitamin B_{12}, whereas Wills factor from the crude liver extract was found to be folic acid. This was clarified by advances in knowledge of folic acid (e.g., purification of pteroylglutamic acid in 1943 [5], its crystallization in the same year [6], and its synthesis and structural identification in 1946 [7]).

Folic acid has proved to be the same as the Wills factor; the "vitamin M" contained in dried brewers' yeast that corrected the deficiency anemia, leukopenia, diarrhea, and gingivitis of monkeys (8); the "vitamin Bc" contained in yeast that corrected the deficiency syndrome in chicks, characterized by anemia and growth failure; and the Norite eluate factor of liver, essential to the growth of *Lactobacillus casei* (9) (and therefore also called "*L. casei* factor") (10, 11). Sulfanilamide was shown to act by competitive inhibition of a bacterial metabolite, *para*-aminobenzoic acid. This metabolite was later found to be an essential component of *L. casei* factor (11, 12), that is, of folic acid.

The term *folic acid* was coined in 1941 by Mitchell et al. because they found this material in a leafy vegetable (spinach) (13). At that time, it was not recognized that vitamin B_{12}, not folic acid, was the active ingredient in the oral liver therapy that Minot and Murphy reported in 1926 as successful in treating pernicious anemia (for which work they received the Nobel Prize in Medicine in 1934) (14). Considerable progress has since been made in our understanding of the metabolic role of folic acid in health and disease and of the use of folate antimetabolites in the treatment of some infectious diseases and cancers.

CHEMISTRY

Pteroylglutamic acid (PGA), the common pharmaceutical form of folic acid, is not present *as such* in significant quantity in either the human body or the various foods from which folates were isolated. Folates are present in various reduced, metabolically active, coenzyme forms, often conjugated in peptide linkage. During the extraction procedures, these labile active forms are either destroyed by oxidation or oxidized and converted to PGA, the most stable form of the vitamin. Not until they are reduced by metabolic systems present within gut and other tissue cells do these stable forms become metabolically active folates. The Trinity College (Dublin, Ireland) group has shown that consumption of more than 266 μg of synthetic folic acid (PGA) results in absorption of unreduced PGA, which may interfere with folate metabolism over a period of years (15, 16, 16a).

Figure 26.1 (17) presents the structural formula of folic acid (PGA, PteGlu or $PteGlu_1$; PGA), the reference compound of the folate vitamin forms. The major subunits of the molecule are the pteridine moiety linked by a methylene bridge to *p*-aminobenzoic acid, which is joined by peptide linkage to glutamic acid. Because of its unique stability, it is the synthetic pharmaceutical form used for folate food fortification and in folate-containing supplements.

Crystalline folic acid is yellow (molecular weight, 441.4

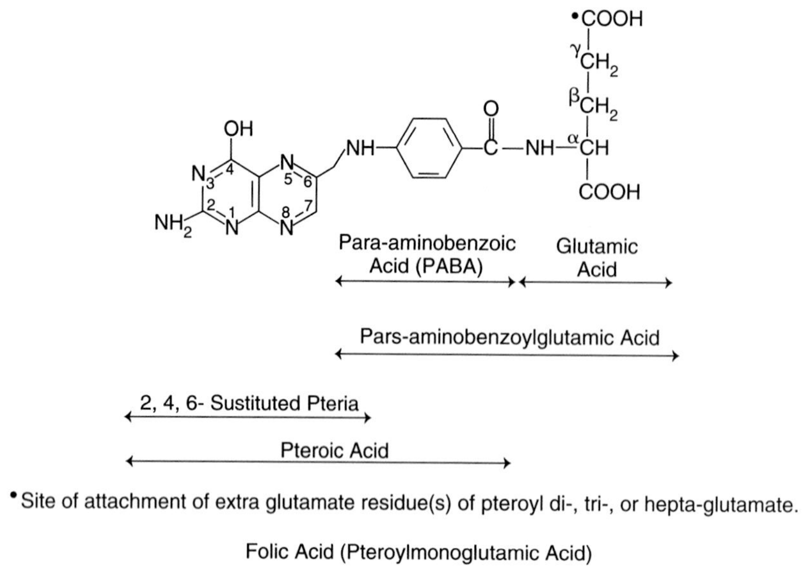

Figure 26.1. Structural formula of folic acid (PGA). (From Herbert V. Drugs effective in megaloblastic anemia: vitamin B_{12} and folic acid. In: Goodman LS, Gilman A, eds. The pharmacological basis of therapeutics. 5th ed. New York: Macmillan, 1975;1324–49, with permission of Macmillan Publishing.)

g/mol). The free acid is almost insoluble in cold water; the disodium salt is more soluble—about 1.5 g/dL (34.0 nmol/L). Injectable solutions are prepared by dissolving folic acid in isotonic sodium bicarbonate solution or by using the disodium salt. Folic acid is destroyed at a pH below 4 but is relatively/stable above pH 5, with no destruction in 1 hour at 100°C. The molecule usually splits into pteridine and *p*-aminobenzoyl glutamate.

Recommendations of an advisory panel to several commissions on nomenclature are as follows: "Folate and folic acid are the preferred synonyms for pteroylglutamate and pteroylglutamic acid, respectively. The term folates may also be used in a generic sense to designate any member of the family of pteroylglutamates, or mixtures of them, having various levels of reduction of the pteridine ring, one-carbon substitutions, and numbers of glutamate residues (18)." The term *folacin* is obsolete and no longer used.

PGA, an oxidized compound, is not normally found as such in foods or in the human body in significant concentrations. The forms that are found in such sources are the reduced forms indicated in Figure 26.2. They differ from the parent compound by virtue of one to three structural modifications. First, all are reduced folates and, except for 7,8-dihydrofolate, all are 5,6,7,8-tetrahydrofolates (THF). Second, as indicated in Figure 26.2, various one-carbon adducts may be linked to THF at the N-5, N-10, or N-5,10 positions, conferring on folates their role as one-carbon carriers. *N*5-Formyl THF (folinic acid, citrovorum factor) represents nonenzymatic conversion of folate during processing of natural materials (19). Third, the number of glutamate residues may vary from one to seven, and sometimes up to 11, each linked by peptide bonds between its amino group and the γ-carboxyl group of the preceding glutamate (Fig. 26.1).

UNITS OF MEASUREMENT AND METHODS OF ASSAY

Normal human serum contains 5 to 16 ng/mL (11.33–36.25 nmol/L) of folic acid activity (i.e., PteGlu equivalents) (1 ng = 10^{-9} g). These tiny quantities could be measured only microbiologically, as originally described

	R	OXIDATION STATE
N^5 formyl THFA	–CHO	formate
N^{10} formyl THFA	–CHO	formate
N^5 formimino THFA	–CH=NH	formate
$N^{5,10}$ methenyl THFA	>CH	formate
$N^{5,10}$ mthylene THFA	$>CH_2$	formaldehyde
N^5 methyl THFA	$–CH_3$	methanol

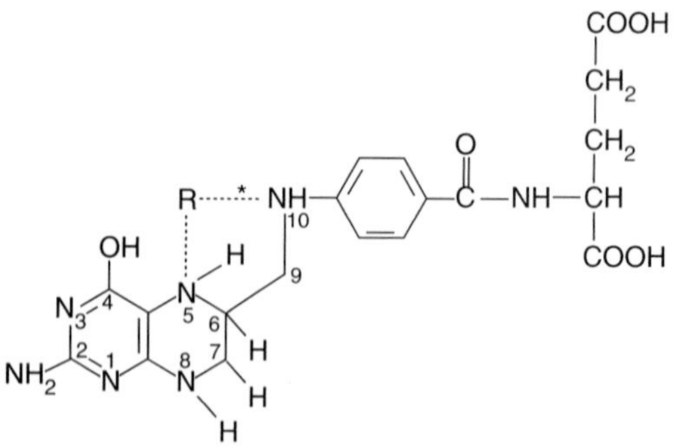

*Broken lines indicate the N^3 and/or N^{10} site of attachment of various 1-carbon units for which THFA acts as a carrier.

5, 6, 7, 8-Tetrahydrofolic Acid (THFA)(FH_4)(R=–H)

Figure 26.2. Structures and nomenclature in the folate field. The table above the formula lists some of the possible one-carbon adducts formed with THFA. (From Herbert V. Drugs effective in megaloblastic anemia: vitamin B_{12} and folic acid. In: Goodman LS, Gilman A, eds. The pharmacologic basis of therapeutics. 5th ed. New York: Macmillan, 1975;1324–49, with permission of Macmillan Publishing.)

in 1959 (20), until a radioisotopic assay was described in the 1970s (21, 22). The dominant form of folate in serum and red cells is 5-methyl THF (Fig. 26.2); folate assays must thus be able to measure this derivative. The only microbiologic assay that adequately measures serum and red cell folate uses *L. casei.* Similarly, the only radioassays that accurately measure serum folate are those that measure 5-methyl THF. Simultaneous radioisotope determinations of serum vitamin B_{12} and folate can be done in the same sample (23). The results correlate well with those of other radioassays.

Because serum folate is labile, falsely low values for serum folate activity occur if the serum has not been protected against oxidative destruction before assay, by storing the serum frozen, storing it in the absence of a reducing agent such as ascorbate, or both. (However, ascorbate may destroy B_{12} in storage.) Larger quantities of folate activity than those normally present in human serum may be measured chemically, fluorometrically, by paper and thin-layer chromatography, enzymatically, or by animal assay (24).

ABSORPTION

Food folate is absorbed primarily from the proximal third of the small intestine, although it can be absorbed from the entire length of the small bowel (25). Folate in food is primarily in polyglutamate form. Before absorption, the "excess" glutamates must be split off the side chain of the vitamin molecule by enzyme conjugases (pteroylpolyglutamate hydrolase). The products of conjugase action are detectable in the intestinal lumen before absorption and are due to a surface-active brush border conjugase that is functionally and chromatographically distinguishable from intracellular conjugase. The bioavailability of ingested folate monoglutamates (PteGlu) is significantly greater than that of folate polyglutamate ($PteGlu_n$) in humans, presumably because the latter must be hydrolyzed (25). The folate hydrolase (conjugase) in the brush border of small intestinal enterocytes, though much less abundant than intracellular folate hydrolase, is more than adequate for digestion of the 1989 recommended dietary allowance (RDA) of 3 μg (6.8 nmol) folate/kg body weight, simplified as 200 μg/day for adult males and 180 μg/day for fertile females (25a). Conjugase action may be specifically inhibited by food factors described in yeast and beans and may be nonspecifically impaired at acid pH. The altered activity of the brush border folate hydrolase in certain diseases and following exposure to drugs such as salicylazosulfapyridine, alcohol, and diphenylhydantoin appears to play a significant role in causing malabsorption and deficiency of folate (25, 26). The discovery that jejunal folate hydrolase shares gene homology with a prostate-tumor–specific protein and a neuronal enzyme implies folate hydrolase may relate to both brain development and carcinogenesis (26a).

Impaired mucosal transport of monoglutamyl folates after deconjugation probably accounts for most instances of folate malabsorption. Active mucosal transport is accelerated by glucose and galactose and impaired by unidentified factors present in many foods. However, studies using mild folate binder (see below) suggest that folate uptake in the gut is facilitated by prior binding. A small but relatively unchanging percentage of ingested folate is absorbed by passive diffusion after deconjugation (15, 16, 16a), as is the case with vitamin B_{12}. Passive diffusion may also account for absorption of unreduced synthetic PGA eaten as a bolus in excess of 266 μg (15, 16, 16a).

Folic acid absorbed from the intestine at physiologic concentrations is largely converted in the gut lumen and enterocytes (26) to reduced forms and then methylated or formylated; at higher concentrations, it is transported through the enterocytes without such modification (15, 16, 16a, 27). However, reduced and formylated or methylated forms of folate are transferred faster from the intestine to the circulation than is folic acid (28). How folate is transported from the enterocytes to the lamina propria of the villi or the circulation is poorly understood; a carrier-mediated system was suggested and is now identified (see next section) (29).

TRANSPORT, DISTRIBUTION, STORAGE, AND EXCRETION

Binding Proteins and Transport

Folate in plasma appears to be distributed in three fractions; free folate and that loosely bound to low-affinity binders are similar in magnitude; much less is bound to high-affinity binders (Fig. 26.3 [30]). Low-affinity binding is a nonspecific property of many different plasma proteins, including albumin, and is similar to nonspecific binding of bilirubin and various drugs. It was detected many years ago using ultrafiltration, equilibrium dialysis, and gel filtration. The potential binding capacity is several hundred times greater than the amount of folate in serum. Early data showing failure to half-saturate these binders at high concentrations of free folate indicate that the affinity constant (K_a) of the system is less than 104 L/mol, which might be compared with the 106 L/mol affinity constant of the carrier-mediated cell transport system for folate (31).

Study of the high-affinity serum folate binders was initiated by the discovery of such binders in chronic myeloid leukemia cells and in serum of the same patients (32). These binders are also demonstrable in granulocytes from some nonleukemic subjects and are released into the serum by these cells. Although their release has not yet been detected in most normal subjects, all human (and animal) serum contains these binders, which more often than not are largely saturated (33).

Only one class of high-affinity serum folate binders is thought to exist. These binders are glycoproteins with a molecular weight of about 40,000; they are probably syn-

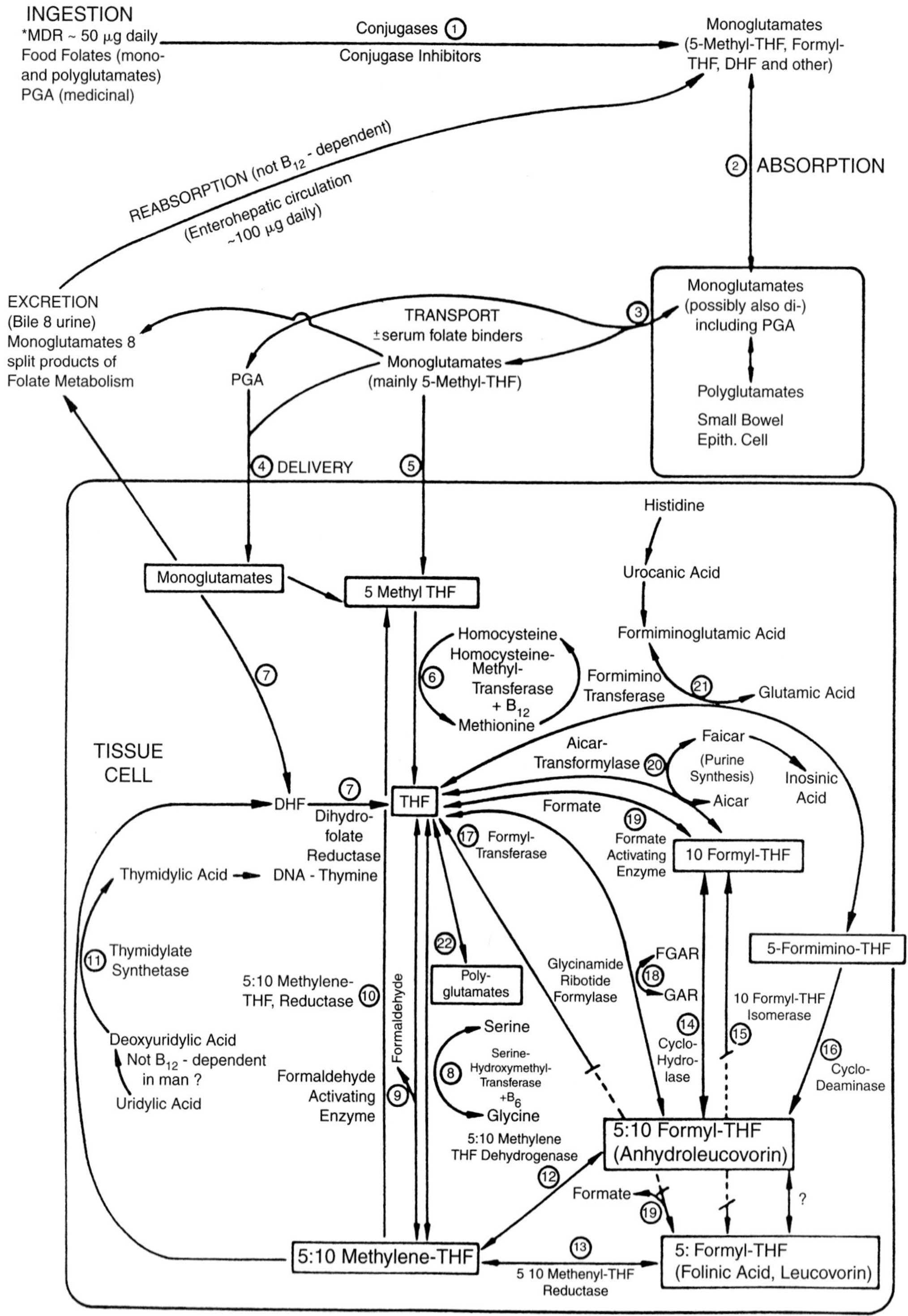

Figure 26.3. Flow chart of folate metabolism in man. *Circled numbers* identify individual steps in folate metabolism. In mammals, the same enzyme catalyzes reactions 12, 14, and 19, and another single enzyme catalyzes both steps 16 and 21. *THF,* tetrahydrofolate; *DHF,* dihydrofolate. (From Herbert V. In: Beeson PB, McDermott W, eds. Textbook of medicine. 14th ed. Philadelphia: WB Saunders, 1975.)

thesized in, and released from, granulocytes but are modified in liver and perhaps in kidney (33). They have binding constants (K_d) of approximately 10^{-10} mol/L of folic acid and of the order of 10^{-8} mol/L of 5-methyl THF, the main forms of folate present in serum. Although these affinities indicate that binder would be only half saturated at usual serum methyl THF concentrations, saturation normally averages 67%. This higher-than-expected saturation may be due to the binding of small quantities of nonmethyl unsubstituted folates on binders. Because of their low concentration in plasma, these binders carry less than 5% of serum folate.

Their physiologic function has not yet been demonstrated, but they may play a role in *(a)* delivering folate to liver, similar to the role of haptocorrin in vitamin B_{12} transport; *(b)* controlling folate distribution, breakdown, and excretion in deficient states; and *(c)* transporting oxidized folates from cerebrospinal fluid to blood. They are also present in milk, where they may enhance folate absorption from gut, and they may be related to membrane protein–mediated folate uptake. High-affinity folate-binding protein found in human serum appears to have a higher affinity for folic acid (PteGlu) than for reduced folate (34). Folate-binding proteins in several tissues closely resemble the serum binders (31).

Folate is delivered to bone marrow cells, reticulocytes, liver, cerebrospinal fluid, and renal tubular cells against a concentration gradient in a manner that suggests energy-dependent carrier-mediated transport (35). The transport constant (K_m) of these systems is about 10^{-6} M. Methyl THF, which accounts for almost all serum folate, appears to be transported more efficiently than folic acid across the intestinal cells and into the cells of the body. A cell membrane folate receptor protein identified in 1992 by Antony (36) and shown by Anderson et al. (37) to produce, by potocytosis, epithelial cell accumulation of methyl THF, is involved in folate transport into many cell types and across intestine, placenta, and choroid plexus barriers. A soluble form of the receptor has been identified in plasma, saliva, milk, seminal fluid, and amniotic fluid (38, 39).

Storage

Normal total-body folate stores range from 5 to 10 mg (11.3–22.6 μmol), of which approximately half is in the liver. It has been suggested that the enterohepatic circulation, which transports about 0.1 mg (0.226 μmol) of biologically active folate daily, is important in the maintenance of serum folate levels.

Most stored folate is present as polyglutamates (19), which have far greater molecular size and charge than monoglutamates. Transport across cell walls probably requires hydrolysis to monoglutamates, and the enzymes responsible for polyglutamate synthesis and hydrolysis are thus thought to play a major role in folate storage. These enzymes are known, respectively, as polyglutamate synthetase and conjugase (pteroylpolyglutamate hydrolase; γ-glutamyl-carboxypeptidase) (26). Conjugase is under partial hormonal control. Some of the folate-dependent reactions shown in Figure 26-3 are altered by varying glutamyl chain lengths. Folate polyglutamate synthetase has been purified from human liver and organs of other mammals; the enzyme is relatively unstable and is found in low quantity. Folate monoglutamates are the circulating and transport forms, whereas polyglutamates are the main intracellular storage forms of this vitamin. Recent evidence indicates that folate polyglutamates are the preferred substrates and active coenzyme forms in various one-carbon metabolism pathways and thereby regulate these metabolic processes (31). Excesses of oral synthetic PGA, if absorbed intact as the oxidized form, may interfere with folate metabolism (15, 16, 16a, 39).

Excretion

Folate is excreted in urine and bile in metabolically active and inactive forms. Urinary excretion of the biologically active material occurs after glomerular filtration of the free fraction and reabsorption of some filtered folate by active transport across the tubular cell wall. The principal breakdown product of folate in urine, acetamidobenzoylglutamate, suggests that the principal route of folate catabolism occurs through oxidative cleavage of the folate molecule at the 9-10 bond, with acetylation of the *p*-aminobenzyl moiety in the liver before excretion (40). Some workers believe that scorbutic patients may lose large amounts of folate through irreversible oxidation of 10-formylfolate and excretion of the latter in the urine (41). We agree.

As mentioned above, about 100 μg of biologically active folate is excreted in the bile daily. Studies with radioactive tracer folates indicate that a large proportion of injected radioactivity is excreted in the bile as a biologically inactive compound that is not a product of 9-10 cleavage but which is not well characterized. Alcohol interferes with the folate enterohepatic cycle. In chronic alcoholics, all six major causes of folate deficiency (see "Causes of Nutritional Deficiency") may occur simultaneously (42). For these reasons, nearly all alcoholics are in negative balance, and about 80% are clinically folate deficient.

NUTRITIONAL REQUIREMENTS IN HEALTH

The term *minimal daily requirement* (MDR), as used in this chapter, means the minimum *from exogenous sources* required to sustain normality, with *normality* defined as the absence of any biochemical hypofunction that is correctable by addition of greater quantities of the vitamin. By this definition, the MDR for folate is approximately 50 μg (113.3 nmol) for adults.

The MDR can be reduced to a formula: $MDR = UBS \div D$, where *MDR* is the minimal daily requirement of nutrient from exogenous sources, *UBS* is the usable body stores of nutrient, and *D* is the number of days required to develop tissue deficiency after cessation of absorption from exogenous sources of nutrient (with appropriate correction for incomplete cessation of absorption) (42, 43). Utilization rate is constant in the normal person but becomes first-order as negative balance progresses. As suggested previously, one can predict the time needed for any given nutrient deficiency to develop in any given person after reduction or cessation of absorption of the nutrient if one knows (or can reasonably estimate) the MDR for the nutrient and its utilizable body stores.

The RDA for folate intentionally greatly exceeds the MDR to produce some measurable amount of body stores to allow for normal variation in use and transiently increased requirements (see below). There is a tendency to err on the side of larger body stores when information is incomplete. Small storage surpluses of nutrients are rarely detrimental, whereas small deficits may result in deficiency over a long period of subtle negative balance.

The Food and Agricultural Organization (FAO) and World Health Organization (WHO) Expert Group in 1987 recommended a daily dietary intake of folate for adults of 3.1 μg (2.3 nmol)/kg of body weight, to equal a daily intake of 200 μg (453.33 nmol) for a 65-kg man and 170 μg (128 nmol) for a 55-kg woman (44) (Appendix Table II-A-8-a). This amount provides sufficient stores to prevent deficiency for 3 to 4 months of zero intake. To meet the added needs of pregnant women, FAO/WHO recommends a supplement from day zero of pregnancy of 200 to 300 μg (453.33–680.0 nmol) daily, so that the daily folate intake is no less than 350 μg (793.33 nmol) (or 7 μg/kg body weight), and a supplement of 100 μg (226.67 nmol) daily during lactation (i.e., a total of 5 μg, or 11.33 nmol, per kilogram body weight). The 1989 RDA (see Appendix Table II-A-2-a-2) ranged from 25 μg (56.7 nmol) for young infants to 35 μg for those 6 to 12 months old; and 50, 75, and 100 μg (227 nmol) for those 1 to 3, 4 to 6, and 7 to 10 years old, respectively. Recommendations were 150 μg for males and females from 11 to 14 years of age; thereafter, the recommendations were 200 μg for males and 180 μg for females. (The basic figure of the 1989 RDA was approximately 3 μg/kg body weight for adolescents and nonpregnant adults. This is the same figure as was recommended by Herbert [45, 45a].) The recomendation for pregnant women was 400 μg; for lactating women it was 280 μg for the first 6 months and 260 μg for the second 6 months (25a). On a percentage basis these values were appreciably below the 1980 RDAs.

The 1998 recommended intakes of folate of the Food and Nutrition Board—Institute of Medicine (Appendix Table II-A-2-c-1) (45b) are appreciably greater than those of the 1989 RDA (Appendix Table II-A-2-a-2) (45c). In comparison to the latter, the 1998 recommendations are approximately double for infants, three times or so for children, two to three times for all males of age 9 years or older, more than double for nonpregnant females, and appreciably more for pregnant and lactating women. The increases stem from the recent evidence indicating the need for more folate to minimize neural tube defects in pregnant women and other vascular changes induced by hyperhomocysteinemia (see also new data in Appendix Tables II-A-2-c-3 and 4).

The daily folate requirement is increased by factors that increase metabolic rate (e.g., infection and hyperthyroidism) and those that increase cell turnover (e.g., hemolytic anemia, rapid tissue growth in the fetus, and malignant tumors). Folate consumption by individual cells is proportional to their rate of one-carbon-unit transfer. As noted above, alcohol interferes with folate use and thus increases folate requirement.

Natural Sources of Folate

Unlike vitamin B_{12}, which is present only in animal protein, folates are ubiquitous in nature, being present in nearly all natural foods (see Appendix Table IV-A-23-a). Again unlike vitamin B_{12}, folate is highly susceptible to oxidative destruction: 50 to 95% of the folate in food may be destroyed by protracted cooking or other processing, such as canning, and all folate is lost from refined foods such as sugars, hard liquor, and hard candies. Foods with the highest folate content per unit of dry weight include yeast, liver and other organ meats, fresh green vegetables, and some fresh fruits.

The naturally occurring folates are active metabolic forms, usually in polyglutamate linkage (19) (with pteroylheptaglutamates dominant in yeast). Conjugases present in vegetable and mammalian tissues (46) (including human intestine) liberate pteroyldiglutamates and pteroylmonoglutamates from the conjugates, thereby making the folate available for absorption. As mentioned above, about 90% of the monoglutamate is absorbed by humans when ingested alone, but this percentage is markedly decreased in the presence of many foods, irrespective of whether the folate was derived from or added to the food (47).

CAUSES OF NUTRITIONAL DEFICIENCY

In the final analysis, nutritional deficiency means that the amount of a biologically active nutrient in one or more intracellular systems is inadequate to sustain normal biochemical functions. Such inadequacy presents in one or more of six basic categories: inadequate ingestion, inadequate absorption, inadequate utilization, increased requirement, increased excretion, and increased destruction. Any one or combination of these three inadequacies and three excesses may result in nutritional deficiency. Table 26.1 presents the currently known possible etiologic factors in each of these six categories that may produce a nutritional deficiency of folic acid. The ensuing sections will discuss in more detail mechanisms of inadequate absorption and utilization of folic acid.

FOLATE DEPLETION: PROGRESSION AND DETECTION

The sequence of events in developing folate deficiency in man is depicted in Figures 26.4 and 26.5. The stages are as follows (42):

Stage 1: Early negative nutrient balance is characterized by a fall in serum folate to below 3 ng/mL (6.8 nmol/L). Body folate stores are not detectably affected; red cell folate level is above 200 ng/mL (453.3 nmol/L).

Stage 2: Folate depletion is indicated by low serum folate and characteristically by a fall in erythrocyte folate below 160 ng/mL (362.67 nmol/L) (and pari passu by a fall in hepatic folate content).

Stage 3: Folate-deficient erythropoiesis is indicated by

Table 26.1
Causes of Folic Acid Deficiency

I. Inadequate ingestion
  A. Poor diet (lacking unprocessed fresh, uncooked, or slightly cooked food or fruit juices—folates are heat-labile)
    1. Nutritional megaloblastic anemia
      a. Tropical
      b. Nontropical
      c. Scurvy (diets low in vitamin C are low in folate)
    2. Chronic alcoholism with or without cirrhosis
II. Inadequate absorption (affecting upper third of small intestine, which is the main site of folate absorption; because most food folates are in polyglutamate forms, biliary and intestinal γ-glutamyl conjugates are necessary to split off excess glutamates to make folates absorbable)
  A. Malabsorption syndromes
    1. Gluten-induced enteropathy (childhood and adult celiac disease; idiopathic steatorrhea, nontropical sprue; coincident B_{12} malabsorption)
    2. Any other chronic functional or structural disorder involving the upper small intestine
      a. Tropical sprue (coincident B_{12} malabsorption almost invariably present; vicious cycle: B_{12} malabsorption further damages gut, which accelerates folate malabsorption and B_{12} malabsorption, etc.)
      b. Associated with herpetic and other skin disorders
    3. Drugs
      a. Anticonvulsants (e.g., phenytoin, primidone)
      b. Barbiturates
      c. Cycloserine
      d. Ethanol
      e. Metformin
      f. Amino acid excess (glycine or methionine)
      g. Nitrofurantoin? (antimicrobial)
      h. Glutethimide? (sedative)
      i. Cholestyramine
      j. Salicylazosulfapyridine (Azulfidine)
  B. Specific malabsorption for folate
    1. Congenital nonconjugase defects (four cases published)
    2. Acquired nonconjugase defects
    3. Inadequate biliary or intestinal conjugates
    4. Conjugase inhibitors (such as are contained in some beans)
  C. Blind loop syndrome (more commonly, bacteria make folate and actually raise serum folate level of host)
III. Inadequate use (metabolic block)
  A. Folic acid antagonists (dihydrofolate reductase inhibitors)
    1. 4-Amino-4-deoxyfolates (i.e., methotrexate—chemotherapy [especially with antifols like Methotrexate], immunosuppression, psoriasis)
    2. 2,4-Diaminopyrimidine (e.g., pyrimethamine, trimethoprim; malaria, toxoplasmosis; antibacterial)
    3. Triamterene (diuretic)
    4. Diamidine compounds (i.e., pentamidine, isothionate—[*Pneumocystis carinii,* protozoicidal])
  B. Diphenylhydantoin and possibly other anticonvulsants (which compete with folate for intestine, brain, and other cell surface folate receptors)
  C. Enzyme deficiency
    1. Congenital
      a. Formiminotransferase
      b. Dihydrofolate reductase
      c. Methyltetrahydrofolate transmethylase
      d. Other enzymes (some secondarily affect folate)
    2. Acquired
      a. Liver disease
        i. Formiminotransferase
        ii. Other enzymes
  D. Vitamin B_{12} deficiency (reduced folate uptake across gut and other cell walls and reduced cell retention of folate)
  E. Alcohol (both specific and nonspecific damage to stomach, gut, and other cells and cell receptors)
  F. Ascorbic acid deficiency (ascorbate is protective against oxidative destruction of folates)
  G. Dietary amino acid excess (glycine, methionine)
IV. Increased requirement
  A. Extra tissue demand
    1. By fetus
    2. By malignant tissue (especially lymphoproliferative disorders)
    3. By breast-fed infant
  B. Infancy
  C. Increased hematopoiesis
  D. Increased metabolic activity
  E. Lesch-Nyhan syndrome
  F. Drugs (L-dopa?)
V. Increased excretion
  A. Vitamin B_{12} deficiency (obligatory excretion of folate in urine and bile reduce ability to reabsorb methylfolate excreted in bile because B_{12} is required for its reabsorption)
  B. Liver disease
  C. Kidney dialysis
  D. Chronic exfoliative dermatitis
VI. Increased destruction
  A. Excessive "antioxidant" (actually redox) supplements

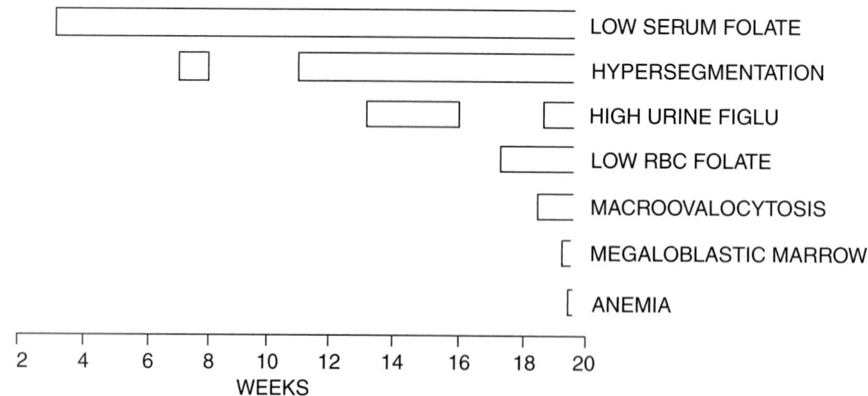

Figure 26.4. Biochemical and hematologic sequence of events in developing dietary folate deficiency in man. (From Herbert V. Trans Assoc Am Physicians 1962;75:307.)

defective DNA synthesis, abnormal diagnostic deoxyuridine (dU) suppression test results correctable in vitro by folates, and granulocyte nuclear hypersegmentation.

Stage 4: Clinical folate deficiency is manifested by gross macroovalocytosis, elevated mean corpuscular volume (MCV), and anemia.

More than half of folate-depleted individuals who have not yet reached the stage of anemia are missed by screening tests that do not recognize that folate depletion may precede anemia by months.

METABOLIC FUNCTIONS AND INTERRELATIONSHIPS

DNA Synthesis

As illustrated in Figure 26.3, both vitamin B_{12} and folic acid are required for synthesis of thymidylate and thus of DNA. A vitamin B_{12}–containing enzyme removes a methyl group from methyl folate and delivers it to homocysteine, thereby converting homocysteine to methionine (methylhomocysteine) and regenerating THF, from which the 5,10-methylene THF involved in thymidylate synthesis is made. Methyl folate is the predominant form of folate in human serum and liver and probably also in other body storage depots for folate. Because methyl folate may only return to the body's folate pool via a vitamin B_{12}–dependent step, patients with vitamin B_{12} deficiency have much of their folate "trapped" as methyl folate, which is metabolically inactive. This "folate trap" hypothesis helps explain the hematologic damage of vitamin B_{12} deficiency that is not clinically distinguishable from that of folate deficiency (48). In both instances, the hematologic defect results from lack of adequate 5,10-methylene THF, whose methyl group is transferred in the conversion of

SEQUENTIAL STAGES OF FOLATE STATUS

	POSITIVE BALANCE		NORMAL	NEGATIVE BALANCE: DEPLETION		NEGATIVE BALANCE: DEFICIENCY	
	STAGE II Excess*	STAGE I Early Positive Folate Balance	Normal	STAGE I Early Negative Folate Balance	STAGE II Folate Depletion	STAGE III Damaged Metabolism: Folate Deficiency Erythropoiesis	STAGE IV Clinical Damage: Folate Deficiency Anemia
Liver Folate / Plasma Folate / Erythron Folate	Excess						
Serum Folate (ng/ml)	>10	>10	>5	<3	<3	<3	<3
RBC Folate (ng/ml)	>400	>300	>200	>200	<160	<120	<100
Diagnostic dU Suppression	Normal	Normal	Normal	Normal	Normal	Abnormal*	Abnormal*
Lobe Average §	<3.5	<3.5	<3.5	<3.5	<3.5	>3.5	>3.5
Liver Folate (μg/g)	>5	>400	>3	>3	<1.6	<1.2	<1
Homocysteine ⌿	Normal	Normal	Normal	Normal	Normal	High	High
Erythrocytes	Normal	Normal	Normal	Normal	Normal	Normal	Macroovalocytic
MCV	Normal	Normal	Normal	Normal	Normal	Normal	Elevated
Hemoglobin (g/dL)	>12	>12	>12	>12	>12	>12	<12
Plasma Clearance of Intravenous Folate	Normal	Normal	Normal	Normal	Normal	Increased	Increased

* Dietary excess of folate reduces zinc absorption.

Due to hormonal effects (on receptors?), there may be folate deficiency (i.e. Stage III-IV negative balance) in cervical epithelial cells (a reversible lesion) (sometimes precancerous) when there is only folate depletion (i.e. Stage II negative balance) in the erythron (Ran et al, Blood, November 1990).

⌿ In serum and urine.

Figure 26.5. Sequence of events in developing folate deficiency. Earliest abnormalities in each stage are *boxed.*

deoxyuridylate to thymidylate used for DNA synthesis during the S (synthesis) phase. In either deficiency, inadequate DNA synthesis causes many hematopoietic cells to die in the bone marrow, possibly without ever completing the S phase of cell replication (i.e., a form of "ineffective erythropoiesis") (49).

The DNA damage caused by folate (or vitamin B_{12}) deficiency increases the risk of cancer (50–52). Megaloblastosis (the presence of giant germ cells) results from slowed DNA synthesis of any cause. The finely stippled sievelike open chromatin in megaloblasts suggests a defect in nuclear maturation. The precise molecular basis of megaloblastic maturation is obscure. Poor thymidylate synthesis (due to folate and/or vitamin B_{12} deficiency) may fail to promote elongation of DNA chains in the presence of a relatively normal capacity to initiate DNA synthesis. This process occurs, presumably, because the lowered thymidylate concentrations suffice for "initiation" but not for "elongation" of the DNA chain by polymerase (53). Alternatively, the defect may permit "illicit" incorporation of thymidylate precursors (such as deoxyuridylate) into DNA, with subsequent cleavage of the DNA containing the illicit nucleotide (54). Decreased synthesis and methylation of arginine-rich nuclear histone may contribute to megaloblastic maturation in pernicious anemia.

Morphologic changes are most striking in bone marrow cells, with the "ineffective hematopoiesis" resulting in peripheral blood pancytopenia (anemia, leukopenia, and thrombopenia) (55). However, megaloblastosis occurs in all duplicating cells of the body (56) and may be strikingly noted in the epithelial cells of the entire alimentary tract, producing glossitis and variable degrees of megaloblastosis along the entire alimentary tract epithelium. It is not yet clear why gut changes associated with vitamin B_{12} deficiency are often related to constipation, whereas those associated with folate deficiency are more commonly related to diarrhea. These differences may be connected to phenomena other than the nutrient deficiency per se.

"Packaging" Folate in Cells

Another important interrelationship of these two vitamins is the involvement of vitamin B_{12} in the transport and storage of folate in cells. In vitamin B_{12} deficiency, transport of methyl THF into both bone marrow cells and transformed lymphocytes is impaired, a defect that is corrected by addition of vitamin B_{12} (57). Similarly, humans and experimental animals with vitamin B_{12} deficiency have low erythrocyte folate and decreased liver folate stores. These defects are probably due to failure of vitamin B_{12}–dependent homocysteine:methionine transmethylation (see Chapters 27 and 34). Failure to remove the methyl group from folate, which causes an intracellular "methyl trap," may interfere with dissociation of the carrier-folate complex at the inner cell wall and may impair transport into the cell. It does impair folate storage, because THF is preferred over methyl THF as a substrate for polyglutamate synthetase (58, 59).

This "heat-labile" form of 5,10-methylene-THF reductase, an enzyme present in one of several forms depending on an individual's genetic blueprint, has become of central importance in studies of hyperhomocysteinemia (see Chapter 34). "Heat-labile" forms of this enzyme result in abnormal folate metabolism; that is, a biochemically induced deficiency of intracellular folate. More information on this rapidly developing area of research can be found in references 60–63, and in abstracts of papers presented at the Second International Conference on Homocysteine Metabolism (64).

Nerve Damage

Folate deficiency does not damage myelin, as does vitamin B_{12} deficiency, but it is associated with a high frequency of irritability, forgetfulness, and often hostile and paranoid behavior. These phenomena often strikingly improve within 24 hours of the start of therapy with folic acid. Other neurologic sequelae attributed by some to folate deficiency have been reviewed elsewhere (65), but the association has not been convincingly demonstrated. Homocysteine, which builds up in folate deficiency, may be a neurotoxin as well as a vasculotoxin.

SELECTIVE NUTRIENT DEFICIENCY

An important area of nutrition research concerns selective nutrient deficiency in one cell line or one tissue but not another in the same patient. This condition can result from one tissue obtaining food folate first, as do intestine cells when food folate is decreased. Another cause may be the presence of a more effective mechanism for folate uptake and a less effective one for folate rejection and relative loss in one cell line compared with another. Selective folate deficiency can occur, for example, in white cells but not in red cells (66). Therefore, lymphocytes (which in their resting form in the human blood appear impervious to vitamin B_{12} and folic acid, and to other nutrients such as nicotinamide) can be used to measure past nutrient deficiency up to 2 months after therapy; they can also reveal covert folate deficiency in patients who lack macroovalocytosis because of coincident iron deficiency or hemoglobinopathy (48, 67). Only when lymphocytes are making DNA do they appear to be pervious to nutrients (48, 65).

FOLATE IN NUTRIENT METABOLISM

Protein and Fat

Folate is involved in protein synthesis through its role in the synthesis of the amino acid methionine, and possibly in other ways as well. Because methionine is involved in making available more of the lipotropic substances choline and betaine, this is another area in which folate may play a role in lipid metabolism.

FOLATE IN ONE-CARBON-UNIT TRANSFERS

Folate coenzymes are concerned with mammalian metabolic systems involving transfer of a one-carbon unit (Fig. 26.3). These reactions include *(a)* de novo purine synthesis (formylation of glycinamide ribonucleotide [GAR] and 5-amino-4-imidazole carboxamide ribonucleotide (AICAR)]; *(b)* pyrimidine nucleotide biosynthesis (methylation of deoxyuridylic acid to thymidylic acid); *(c)* conversions of three amino acids—the interconversion of serine and glycine (which also requires vitamin B_6), catabolism of histidine to glutamic acid, and conversion of homocysteine to methionine (which also requires vitamin B_{12}); *(d)* generation of formate into the formate pool (and formate use, which relates to the formate starvation hypothesis of Chanarin et al. [49]); and *(e)* methylation of small amounts of transfer RNA. Folate is not involved in the physiologic methylation of biogenic amines (68).

There is no evidence of ascorbate involvement in reduction of PGA to tetrahydrofolic acid, a reaction mediated by folate reductases, but it may protect tetrahydrofolic acid against further oxidative destruction in vivo as it does in vitro.

With wide recognition of the vasculotoxicity of homocysteine, much folate (and vitamin B_{12}) research is focused on homocysteine metabolism (64, 69–71). The Hordaland Homocysteine Study (71a) of 18,043 middle-aged subjects found 67 with very high (>40 μmol/L) plasma homocysteine, of whom 73.1% had homozygosity for the C 677T mutation in the methylene tetrahydrofolate reductase gene (73.1% of cases versus 10.2% of controls). All also had lower plasma folate and cobalamin levels than controls; 10% had overt vitamin B_{12} deficiency. Flynn et al. (71b) found 49% of 171 "healthy" elderly, mean age 65, had malabsorption of vitamin B_{12}, and, of these, 60% had serum homocysteine greater than 17.5 μmol/L. An excellent review was recently published (71c).

ROLES IN THERAPY

The only established therapeutic use of folic acid is in treating deficiency of the vitamin. Prophylactic use can prevent about 2000 neural tube defect babies in the U.S. annually (72). Claims made for nutritional value in clinical situations in which deficiency of the vitamin does not clearly exist are without established foundation, except with respect to neural tube defects (72, 73, 73a, 74).

When the deficiency is only of folate, only that vitamin should be used for therapy. Use of folic acid to treat a patient whose deficiency is of vitamin B_{12} often produces temporary hematologic improvement, but does not adequately lower toward normal vasculotoxically elevated serum homocysteine levels due to vitamin B_{12} deficiency (71). Furthermore, it allows the neurologic damage of the underlying vitamin B_{12} deficiency to progress, often to an irreversible state (75). Folate supplementation produces unpredictable intra-individual variations in serum homocysteine levels (75a). The causes of folate deficiency in humans are listed in Table 26.1, and Table 26.2 lists the symptoms and signs of megaloblastic anemia.

In malaria zones, moderate folate deficiency may actually be desirable. Das et al. (76) have shown that mild folate deficiency protects against malaria in primates by making it impossible for malaria parasites to double their DNA and divide in red cells (77). Currently, Herbert and colleagues are studying the possible prevention of malaria in Africa by producing chronically low red cell folate without anemia with daily oral phenytoin in alternate new cases of epilepsy (65).

Critically Ill Patients

It is rarely necessary to institute immediate therapy before determining whether the cause of megaloblastic anemia is folate deficiency, vitamin B_{12} deficiency, both, or neither. Major indications for *emergency* therapy include severe thrombocytopenia (platelet count ≤50,000/mm^3) associated with bleeding, severe leukopenia (white cell count ≤3000/mm^3) associated with infection, infection itself, coma, severe disorientation, marked neurologic damage, severe hepatic disease, uremia, or other debilitating illness complicating the anemia. The anemia itself is not a problem because the dyspnea and occasional angina that may accompany a hematocrit below 15 volumes % are relieved by transfusion of one or two units of packed erythrocytes. Transfusion is unwarranted in the absence of *symptoms* of anemia. When venous pressure is elevated, transfusion of packed erythrocytes should be accompanied by withdrawal of equivalent or slightly smaller quantities of whole blood, which will reduce rather than raise the venous pressure. Transfusion of whole blood without withdrawal of blood has been responsible for acute rises in venous pressure with resultant irreversible congestive failure in elderly patients with megaloblastic anemia and unrecognized elevated venous pressure. Ideally, venous pressure should be determined before transfusion and monitored during both the transfusion of packed cells and the simultaneous withdrawal of whole blood. An alternative to exchange transfusion is parenteral injection of a diuretic before the administration of blood.

When, for one of the reasons discussed above, immediate vitamin therapy is necessary before etiologic diagnosis, a sample of blood is drawn to determine baseline status with respect to both vitamins, and then 100 μg (76.0 nmol) of vitamin B_{12} and 15 mg (34 μmol) of folic acid are given intramuscularly, followed by 100 μg (75.0 nmol) of vitamin B_{12} intramuscularly and 5 mg (11.3 μmol) of folic acid by mouth daily for 1 week. Such treatment produces excellent hematologic response except in patients whose hematopoiesis is suppressed by infection, uremia, chloramphenicol administration, or some other factor.

By producing megaloblastic enterocytes resulting in malabsorption, folate deficiency can produce secondary vitamin B_{12} deficiency, and vitamin B_{12} deficiency can pro-

Table 26.2
Clinical Picture of the Megaloblastic Anemias

Symptoms
- Weakness, tiredness
- Dyspnea
- Sore tongue
- Paresthesia (B_{12} deficiency only)
- Diarrhea (especially folate deficiency)
- Constipation (especially B_{12} deficiency)
- Irritability and forgetfulness (especially folate deficiency)
- Anorexia
- Syncope
- Headache
- Palpitation

Signs
- Megaloblastic bone marrow (orthochromatic megaloblasts, giant metamyelocytes)
- Anemia, leukopenia, thrombocytopenia, with macroovalocytes (normal MVC, 87 ± 5 μm^3) and "hypersegmented polys" (normal Arneth count 2 lobes, 20–40%; 3 lobes, 40–50%; 4 lobes, 15–25%; 5 lobes, 0–5%; 6 lobes, 0–0.1%; >6 lobes, 0) (normal "lobe average," 3.17 lobes ± 0.25). (Rule of fives: when 100 neutrophils are counted, the presence of more than 5% containing 5 or more lobes means hypersegmentation)
- Morphologic red herrings: congenital hypersegmentation (approximately 1% of population), hypersegmentation with renal disease; twinning deformities; macrocytes of pyruvate kinase deficiency, aplastic anemia, reticulocytosis, hypothyroidism, neoplasia
- Fever
- Icterus plus pallor (lemon-yellow skin)
- Glossitis
  - Acute
  - Chronic atrophic
- Neurologic damage (only B_{12} deficiency damages myelin; hyperhomocysteinemia, regardless of cause, is neurotoxic)
  - Vibration sense diminished
  - Position sense diminished, ataxia, "combined systems disease"
  - Impaired mentation, paranoid ideation (seen in both deficiencies)
- Malabsorption
- Slowly progressive gastric atrophy (primary with B_{12} deficiency or helicobacter pylori, secondary with folate deficiency)
- Splenomegaly (in approximately one-third of cases, if sought radiologically)
- Weight loss (especially folate deficiency)
- Pigmentation: vitiligo
- Postural hypotension (especially B_{12} deficiency)
- Low serum vitamin B_{12} or folate level
- Low or absent vitamin B_{12} in TCII (low holo-TCII)
- Low red cell B_{12} or folate level: low lymphocyte B_{12} or folate
- Elevated serum lactic dehydrogenase (LDH) and homocysteine
- Elevated urine formiminoglutamate and homocysteine
- Methylmalonic acidemia and aciduria (B_{12} deficiency only)
- High serum iron, increased saturation of iron-binding capacity of serum, increased bone marrow iron stores, normal free erythrocyte protoporphyrin (findings that may obscure occult Fe deficiency)
- Low red cell folate is present in either deficiency
- Circulating antibody to intrinsic factor in two-thirds of pernicious anemia (vitamin B_{12} deficiency) patients
- Circulating antibody to gastric parietal cells in most patients with gastric damage, regardless of cause (genetics; Helicobacter)
- Abnormal "dU suppression test" (corrected by adding missing vitamin or vitamins in vitro)
- Abnormal liver function test results
- Subnormal intestinal absorption

duce secondary folate deficiency (78). Many recent studies finding relatively low red cell folate in elderly persons along with "normal" serum total vitamin B_{12} erroneously diagnosed folate deficiency whereas the correct diagnosis was vitamin B_{12} deficiency (69). Had they measured holotranscobalamin II (69, 78), they would have correctly diagnosed inability to absorb vitamin B_{12}, with low red cell folate because vitamin B_{12} is necessary both to get folate into red cells and to keep it there (78).

Folate Deficiency

For combined differential diagnosis and therapy, the patient is treated with 100 μg (226.67 nmol) of folic acid orally daily (if the suspected diagnosis is folate malabsorption). This dosage produces a maximal hematologic response in patients with folate deficiency but does not produce hematologic response in patients with vitamin B_{12} deficiency (79). As in treated vitamin B_{12} deficiency, treatment of folate deficiency returns subnormal leukocyte and platelet levels to normal within 1 week of the start of therapy, at approximately the time of the reticulocyte peak.

Therapy with doses of folic acid above 0.1 mg (226.67 nmol) daily is desirable when the folate deficiency state is complicated by conditions that may suppress hematopoiesis (e.g., unrelated systemic diseases), conditions that increase folate requirement (e.g., pregnancy, hypermetabolic states, alcoholism, hemolytic anemia), and conditions that reduce folate absorption. Therapy should then consist of 0.5 to 1 mg (1.33–2.266 μmol) daily. There is no evidence that doses greater than 1 mg (2.266 μmol) daily have any greater efficacy; additionally, loss of folate in the urine becomes roughly logarithmic as the amount administered exceeds 1 mg (2.266 μmol). In fact, there is evidence that doses above 1 mg daily for a sustained period of time may be harmful (15–16a, 39).

Maintenance therapy is normally 0.1 mg (226.67 nmol) of folic acid daily for 1 to 4 months, which then should be discontinued only if the diet contains at least one fresh fruit or fresh vegetable daily. If the daily folate requirement is increased by increased metabolic or cell turnover, the daily maintenance dose should be 0.2 to 0.5 mg (0.453–1.133 μmol).

Ideal nutritional therapy for dietary folate deficiency is the ingestion of one fresh fruit or one fresh vegetable daily. Such a diet would probably eliminate nutritional folate deficiency from the earth (80). At present, nutritional folate deficiency probably affects approximately a third of all the pregnant women in the world (81).

Prevention of Folate Deficiency

Pregnant women should receive folate supplements from day zero of pregnancy. Supplements have also been recommended in clinical disorders that increase the risk of folate deficiency. However, major problems have been encountered in the delivery of such supplements to patients. Because of resultant gastrointestinal upsets, significant numbers of pregnant women do not ingest iron tablets given to them. Tablets containing both iron and folate may be better tolerated, inasmuch as the adverse gastrointestinal effects of iron ingestion may be decreased when folic acid is simultaneously ingested (82). However, the iron in the mixed supplement should not exceed the 30 mg (0.54 mmol) daily iron pregnancy supplement. The largest component of the problem is that antenatal care is not available for, or taken advantage of by, large numbers of pregnant women, particularly in populations in which folate deficiency is common.

As an alternative approach to alleviating the problem, a series of studies was devised to determine the feasibility of fortifying staple foods with folic acid. When the data generated in these studies were judged against criteria delineated by an Expert Committee of the FAO/WHO (83), such fortification appeared feasible, inexpensive, effective, and safe in populations with a demonstrable need for increased dietary levels of folic acid. Fortification by preventing megaloblastic anemia can mask vitamin B_{12} deficiency until there is neurologic damage (78, 84, 85). The WHO and other bodies have recommended that authorities concerned with populations in which folate deficiency is common should initiate trials to determine the feasibility and effectiveness of food fortification with folate (86).

Since the fetal neural tube (see Chapter 95) is formed early in pregnancy, all fertile nonblack females should ensure themselves of a diet adequate to provide 0.3 to 0.4 mg of folic acid daily or take such a supplement (72, 85). To eliminate neural tube defects that are due to a genetic defect in handling folate (72–74), the Food and Drug Administration (FDA) has mandated that folate be added to grain fortification, effective January 1, 1998 (74, 75, 85). Because African American fertile females do not have the gene defect that causes folate-treatable neural tube defects but do have a gene for early pernicious anemia, the FDA has been petitioned to mandate that vitamin B_{12} also be added (85). Another reason to add vitamin B_{12} is that, in the elderly, vitamin B_{12} deficiency is much more common than deficiency of folate (71).

TOXICITY

Folic acid ingested in the reduced forms active in humans is nontoxic in man, not only in small doses but also in doses that exceed the minimal daily adult human requirement (50 μg) by 20 times. Being water soluble, excesses tend to be excreted in the urine rather than, like fat-soluble vitamins, being stored in tissues. Folic acid appears to require binding to polypeptides as a precondition of storage; amounts that exceed the limited binding capacity in serum and tissues tend to be excreted rather than retained.

Daily doses of up to 15 mg (34 μmol) in healthy humans without convulsive disorders are without clear toxic effects; this daily dose is well below the amount that could lead to precipitation of crystalline folic acid in the kidneys (such precipitation produces renal toxicity in rats given massive doses of folic acid). One questionable instance of an allergic reaction to folic acid has been reported in man (87). Very large amounts of folic acid in its pharmaceutical oxidized form (PGA) may be noxious to the nervous system; can reverse the antiepileptic effects of phenobarbital, phenytoin, and primidone; and have provoked seizures in patients otherwise under control on anticonvulsant therapy (65, 88).

Although no such effect has been observed in controlled studies using oral doses of 15 mg (34 μmol) folic acid daily, experimental and clinical evidence demonstrates that very high concentrations of folic acid can have a convulsant effect (89). The convulsant dose in normal rats was shown in one study to be 45 to 125 mg (102 to 283.3 μmol) if administered intravenously and 15 to 30 mg (34 to 68 μmol) if preceded by induction of a focal cortical lesion. Convulsions have been reported in one of eight epileptics given parenteral folic acid under electroencephalographic monitoring. This reaction occurred after rapid intravenous infusion of 14.4 mg (32.64 μmol) of folic acid, which presumably elevated serum folate concentration in the cerebral vessels several times higher than folic acid ingestion would have (65). Anticonvulsant drugs and folic acid compete for absorption across the intestinal epithelial cells and at the brain cell wall (88). Evidence in uncontrolled studies suggests increased fit frequency in epileptics given oral therapeutic doses of folic acid. To date, no such effect of oral folic acid has been demonstrated in carefully conducted controlled trials. Being a physician-attorney aware of malpractice law, I recommend giving it only if absolutely necessary.

Oral folic acid supplements of 350 mg (793.3 μmol) daily reduce zinc absorption and may be a problem where maternal zinc depletion and intrauterine growth retardation are common (90).

REFERENCES

1. Channing W. N Engl Q J Med Surg 1824;1:157–80.
2. Barclay AW. Cited in: Castle WB. Trans Am Clin Climatol Assoc 1961;73:54–80.
3. Osler W. Br Med J 1919;1:1–4.
4. Wills L, Clutterbuch P, Evans BDF. Biochem J 1937;31: 2136–47.
5. Stokstad ELR. J Biol Chem 1943;149:573–4.
6. Pfiffner JJ, Binkley SB, Bloom ES, et al. Science 1943;97: 404–5.
7. Angier RB, Boothe JH, Hutchings BL, et al. J Am Chem Soc 1946;103:667–72.
8. Day PL, Mims V, Totter JR, et al. J Biol Chem 1945;157: 423–4.
9. Snell EE, Peterson WH. J Bacteriol 1940;39:273–80.
10. Stokstad ELR, Hutchings BL, Subba Row Y. J Am Chem Soc 1948;70:3–8.
11. Woods DD. Br J Exp Pathol 1940;21:74–83.
12. Rubbo SD, Gillespie JM. Nature 1940;146:838–9.
13. Mitchell HK, Snell EE, Williams RJ. J Am Chem Soc 1941;63:2284–90.
14. Minot GR, Murphy WP. JAMA 1926;87:470–6.
15. Kelly P, McPartlin J, Goggins M, et al. Am J Clin Nutr 1997;65:1790–5.
16. McPartlin J, Kelly P, Goggins M, et al. Am J Clin Nutr 1997;66:1481.
16a. Markle HV. Am J Clin Nutr 1997;66:1480–1.
17. Herbert V. Drugs effective in megaloblastic anemia: vitamin B_{12} and folic acid. In: Goodman LS, Gilman A, eds. The pharmacological basis of therapeutics. 5th ed. New York: Macmillan, 1975;1324–49.
18. IUPAC-IUB Commission on Biochemical Nomenclature. Nomenclature of vitamins, coenzymes and related compounds. Tentative rules. In: Blakely RL, Benkovic SJ, eds. Folates and pterins, vol I. Chemistry and biochemistry of folates. New York: John Wiley & Sons, 1984;29.
19. Herbert V. Am J Clin Nutr 1968;21:743–52.
20. Herbert V, Wasserman LR, Frank O, et al. Fed Proc 1959;18:246.
21. Waxman S, Schreiber C, Herbert V. Blood 1971;37:142–51.
22. Rothenberg SP, da Costa M, Rosenberg Z. N Engl J Med 1971;286:1335–9.
23. Gutcho S, Mansbach L. Clin Chem 1977;23:1609–14.
24. Herbert V, Colman C. Vitamin B_{12} and folacin radioassays in blood serum. In: Augustin J, Klein BP, Becker D, et al., eds. Methods of vitamin assays. 4th ed. New York: John Wiley & Sons, 1985;515–34,
25. Halsted CH. Intestinal absorption of dietary folates. In: Picciano MF, Stokstad ELR, Gregory JF III, eds. Folic acid metabolism in health and disease. New York: Wiley-Liss, 1990;23–45.
25a. Recommended Dietary Allowances. 10th ed. Washington DC: National Academy Press, 1989.
26. Halsted CH. Folylpoly-γ-glutamate carboxypeptidase. In: Barrett A, Woessner F, eds. Handbook of proteolytic enzymes. San Diego: Academic Press, 1998; in press.
26a. Halstead CH, Ling E-H, Villanuera JA, et al. FASEB J 1998;12:A550.
27. Strum WB. Biochim Biophys Acta 1979;554:249–57.
28. Darcy-Villon B, Selhub J, Rosenberg H. Am J Physiol 1988;255:361–6.
29. Said HM, Redha R. Biochem J 1987;247:141–6.
30. Herbert V. In: Beeson PB, McDermott W, eds. Textbook of medicine. 14th ed. Philadelphia: WB Saunders, 1975:1404–1413.
31. Ratnam M, Freisheim JH. Proteins involved in the transport of folates and antifolates by normal and neoplastic cells. In: Picciano MF, Stokstad ELR, Gregory JF III, eds. Folic acid metabolism in health and disease. New York: Wiley-Liss, 1990;91–120.
32. Rothenberg SP. Proc Soc Ex Biol Med 1970;133:428–32.
33. Colman N, Herbert V. Blood 1976;48:911–21.
34. Colman N, Herbert V. Annu Rev Med 1980;31:433–9.
35. Goldman ID. Ann NY Acad Sci 1971;186:400.
36. Antony AC. Blood 1992;79:2807–20.
37. Anderson RG, Kamen BA, Rothberg KG, et al. Science 1992;255:410–1.
38. Zittoun J. Congenital errors of folate metabolism. In: Wickramasinghe SN, ed. Megaloblastic anemia. London: Ballière Tindall, 1995;603–16.
39. Antony AC. Annu Rev Med 1996;16:501–21.
40. Murphy M, Keating M, Boyle P, et al. Biochem Biophys Res Commun 1976;71:1017–21.
41. Stokes PL, Melikian V, Leeming RL, et al. Am J Clin Nutr 1975;28:126–9.
42. Herbert V. Development of human folate deficiency. In: Picciano MF, Stokstad ELR, Gregory JF III, eds. Folic acid metabolism in health and disease. New York: Wiley-Liss, 1990;195–210.
43. Jadhav M, Webb JKG, Vaishava S, et al. Lancet 1962;2:903–7.
44. FAO/WHO Expert Group. Requirements of vitamin A, iron, folate and vitamin B_{12}. Geneva: FAO/WHO, 1987.
45. Herbert V. Am J Clin Nutr 1987;45:661–70.
45a. Tidwell F. *Victor Herbert, MD, JD v. United States,* no. 92-6726, Slip op. (CTCl. August 9, 1996).
45b. Food and Nutrition Board—Institute of Medicine Dietary reference intakes. Thiamin, riboflavin, niacin, vitamin B_6, folate, vitamin B_{12}, pantothenic acid, biotin, and choline. Washington, DC: national Academy Press, 1998.
45c. Food and Nutrition Board, National Research Council. Recommended dietary allowances. 10th ed. Washington, DC: National Academy Press, 1989.
46. Reed B, Weir DG, Scott JM. Am J Clin Nutr 1976;29:1393–6.
47. Colman N, Green R, Metz J. Am J Clin Nutr 1975;28:459–64.
48. Herbert V. Lab Invest 1985;52:3–19.
49. Wickramasinghe SN. Morphology, biology, and biochemistry of cobalamin- and folate-deficient bone marrow cells. In: Wickramasinghe SN, ed. Megaloblastic anemia. London: Ballière Tindall, 1995;441–59.
50. Herbert V. Advances in experimental biology and medicine. In: Poirier LA, Newberne PM, Pariza MW. Essential nutrients in carcinogenesis. New York: Plenum Press. 1986;206: 293–311.
51. Ran JY, Dou P, Wang LY, et al. Blood 1992;82(Suppl 1):532a.
52. Blount BC, Ames BN. DNA damages of folate deficiency. In: Wickramasinghe SN, ed. Megaloblastic anemia. London: Ballière Tindall, 1995;461–78.

53. Hoffbrand AV, Ganeshaguru K, Hooton JWL, et al. Clin Haematol 1976;5:727–45.
54. Luzzatto L, Falusi AO, Joju EA. N Engl J Med 1981;199: 1156–7.
55. Sarode R, Garewal G, Marwah N, et al. Trop Geogr Med 1989;41:331–6.
56. Herbert V. The megaloblastic anemias. New York: Grune & Stratton, 1959.
57. Tisman G, Herbert V. Blood 1973;41:465–9.
58. Allen RH. Prog Hematol 1975;9:57–84.
59. Pearson AG, Turner AJ. Nature 1975;258:173–4.
60. Guttormsen AB, Ueland PM, Nesthus I, et al. J Clin Invest 1996;98:2174–83.
61. Molloy AM, Daly S, Mills JL, et al. Lancet 1997;349:1591–3.
62. Wilcken DEL. Lancet 1997;350:603–4.
63. Blom HJ. Am J Clin Nutr 1998;67:188–9.
64. Second International Conference on Homocysteine Metabolism. April 26, 1998. Netherlands J Med Sci, May 1998.
65. Colman N, Herbert V. Folate metabolism in brain. In: Kumar S, ed. Biochemistry of brain. Oxford: Pergamon Press, 1979;127–42.
66. Das KC, Herbert V. Br J Haematol 1978;38:219–33.
67. Green R, Kuhl W, Jacobsen R, et al. N Engl J Med 1982;307:1322–5.
68. Meller E, Rosengarten H, Friedhoff A, et al. Science 1975;187:171–3.
69. Colloquium: homocysteine, vitamins and arterial occlusion diseases. J Nutr 1996;26(Suppl 4S):1235S–1300S.
70. First International Conference on Homocysteine Metabolism. From basic science to clinical medicine (abstracts). Ir J Med Soc 1995;164(Suppl 1):1–36.
71. Flynn MA, Herbert V, Nolph GB, et al. J Am Coll Nutr 1997;16:258–67.
71a. Nygard O, Refsum H, Ueland PM, Vollset SE. Am J Clin Nutr 1998;67:263–70.
71b. Flynn MA, Herbert V, Nolph GA, Krause G. FASEB J 1998; 12(4, part I):A246.
71c. Welch GN, Luscalzo J. New Engl J Med 1998;338:1042–50.
72. Herbert V. Nutr Today 1992;27(6):30–3.
73. Scott JM, Weir DG, Kirke PN. Folate and neural tube defects. In: Bailey LB, ed. Folate and health and disease. New York: Marcel Dekker, 1995;329–60.
73a. Butterworth CE Jr, Bendich A. Ann Rev Nutr 1996;16:73–97.
74. Oakley GP Jr. Am J Clin Nutr 1997;65:1889–90.
75. Herbert V. Am J Clin Nutr 1997;66:1478.
75a. Santhosh-Kumar CR, Deutsch JC, Ryder JW, Kolhouse JF. Eur J Clin Nutr 1997;51:188–92.
76. Das KC, Virdi JS, Herbert V. Blood 1992;80(Suppl 1):291a.
77. Herbert V. N Engl J Med 1993;328:1127.
78. Herbert V. Vitamin B_{12}. In: Ziegler EE, Filer LJ Jr, eds. Present knowledge in nutrition. 7th ed. Washington DC: ILSI Press, 1996;191–205.
79. Herbert V. N Engl J Med 1963;268:201–368.
80. Colman N, Demartino L, McAleer E. Blood 1986;68:45A.
81. Herbert V. Public issues and nutrition research opportunities. In: Doberenz AR, Milner JA, Schweigert BS, eds. Food and agricultural research opportunities to improve human nutrition for the 21st century. Newark, DE: University of Delaware College of Human Resources Press, 1986;1313–22.
82. Sood SK, Ramachandran K, Mathur M, et al. Q J Med 1975;44:241–50.
83. FAO/WHO. WHO Tech Rep Ser No. 477. Geneva 1981.
84. Herbert V. JAMA 1997;277:880–1.
85. Herbert V, Bigaouette J. Am J Clin Nutr 1997;65:572–3.
86. Nutritional Anemias. WHO. WHO Tech Rep Ser No. 580. Geneva, 1975.
87. Chanarin I. In: The megaloblastic anaemias. Oxford: Blackwell Scientific Publications, 1979.
88. Colman N, Herbert V. Folates and the nervous system. In: Blakely RL, ed. Folates and pterins, vol 3. New York: John Wiley & Sons, 1986;339–58.
89. Marcus A, Ullman HL, Saffer LB, et al. J Clin Invest 1962;41:2198–203.
90. Herbert V. Am J Clin Nutr 1987;45:671–8.

SELECTED READINGS

Bailey LB, ed. Folate in health and disease. New York: Marcel Dekker, 1995.

Eskes T, et al. Rc neural tube defects. Research progress report 1997 on prevention of birth defects. Nijmegen University, Nigmagen, The Netherlands, 40 pages.

Herbert V. Nutrition science as a continually unfolding story: the folate, vitamin B_{12} paradigm. The 1986 Herman Award Lecture. Am J Clin Nutr 1987;46:387–402.

Picciano MF, Stokstad ELR, Gregory JF III, eds. Folic acid metabolism in health and disease. New York: Wiley-Liss, 1990;1–277.

Rosenblatt DS. Inherited disorders of folate transport and metabolism. In: Scriver CR, Beaudet AL, Valle D, eds. The metabolic basis of inherited diseases. 6th ed. New York, McGraw-Hill, 1989;2049–64.

Selhub J, Rosenberg IH. Folic acid. In: Ziegler EE, Filer LJ Jr, eds. Present knowledge in nutrition. 7th ed. Washington, DC: ILSI Press, 1996;206–19.

Wickramasinghe SN, ed. Megaloblastic anaemia. Ballière's clinical haematology: international practice and research. London: Ballière Tindall, 1995 (see especially p. 271).

27. Vitamin B_{12} "Cobalamin"

DONALD G. WEIR and JOHN M. SCOTT

HISTORICAL INTRODUCTION

The early history of the chemistry and biochemistry of the corrinoid cobalamin (vitamin B_{12}) has recently been reviewed by Linnell and Bhatt (1) and by Stubbe (2) and can be summarized as follows. Vitamin B_{12} was isolated in 1948, simultaneously in the United States and in England. Discovery of its extraordinary three-dimensional structure by x-ray crystallography and the deep red color of the oxidized corrin ring subsequently led to identification of the carbon-cobalt bond in the two active cofactor forms of the vitamin, namely, adenosylcobalamin (adoCbl) and methylcobalamin (methyl Cbl). In 1958, adoCbl was identified as the coenzyme for glutamate mutase in microorganisms and, in the next year, for methylmalonyl-CoA mutase in mammals. Methyl Cbl was first synthesized and shown to be the main form of vitamin B_{12} in the plasma in 1963. Later in 1963, methyl Cbl was demonstrated to be the cofactor required for methylation of homocysteine to methionine by N^5-methyltetrahydrofolate (N^5-methyl-THF-glu$_{1-5}$) via methionine synthase. By 1979 the biosynthetic pathways of vitamin B_{12} had been elucidated and its synthesis was achieved.

The history of the clinical relevance of vitamin B_{12} deficiency has been reviewed by Weatherall (3) and Wickramasinghe (4). Deficiency of vitamin B_{12} produces two diseases in man, megaloblastic anemia and a specific neuropathy called vitamin B_{12}–associated neuropathy or subacute combined degeneration of the cord. These complications are seen mainly in pernicious anemia, the first description of which has been variously ascribed to James Coombe (1824), Thomas Addison (1855), and Anton Biermer (1872) (4). Paul Ehrlich first described megaloblastosis in the bone marrow (1880) (4). German physicians described the neuropathic appearance of the spinal cord as a *lachen felden* (field of holes), and in 1990, the clinical syndrome was described in detail.

The disease was universally fatal in 1 to 3 years following diagnosis. The therapeutic breakthrough came in 1926 when George Minot, working with William Murphy, demonstrated that feeding a daily diet of lightly cooked beef liver induced a remission of the anemia within months. Subsequently, beef was shown to contain an extrinsic factor (vitamin B_{12}) that required an intrinsic factor (IF) for its normal absorption. IF was produced by the gastric secretion of normal stomachs but not those of patients with pernicious anemia. IF was shown to complex with vitamin B_{12} to produce an "anti pernicious anaemia principle" that was required for its uptake and transport by a specific receptor on the ileal enterocytes in the terminal ileum in man.

CHEMISTRY AND NOMENCLATURE

Vitamin B_{12} is a member of a family of related molecules called corrinoids, a term used for all compounds that contain a corrin nucleus made up of a tetrapyrrolic ring structure (Fig. 27.1). The corrinoids and their related compounds are discussed elsewhere (5).

The center of the tetrapyrrole contains a cobalt ion that can be variously attached to methyl, deoxyadenosyl, hydroxy, or cyano groups. The former two are the naturally active forms, the latter two are converted into them in

Abbreviations: **adoCbl**—adenosylcobalamin; **adoHcy**—S-Dadenosyl-Dhomocysteine; **adoMet**—S-adenosylmethionine; **Cob I, II, III**—cobalamin with 1, 2, or 3 positive charges on cobalt; **Hc**—haptocorrins; **tHcy**—total of homocysteine and homocystine; **IF**—intrinsic factor; **IFCR**—intrinsic factor ileal enterocyte cell wall receptor; methionine synthase, N^5-methyltetrahydrofolate:homocysteinemethyltransferase; methyl Cbl, methylcobalamin; **MMA**—methylmalonic acid; N^5-methyl-THF-glu1, N^5-methyltetrahydrofolate monoglutamate; N^5-methyl-THF-glu5, N^5-methyltetrahydrofolate pentaglutamate; N^5,N^{10}-methylene-THF reductase, N^5,N^{10}-methylenetetrahydrofolate reductase, "methylene reductase"; OH-Cbl, hydroxycobalamin; **THF-glu$_1$**—tetrahydrofolate monoglutamate; **THF-glu$_5$**—tetrahydrofolate pentaglutamate; **TC I**—transcobalamin 1; **TC II**—transcobalamin 2; **TC III**—transcobalamin 3

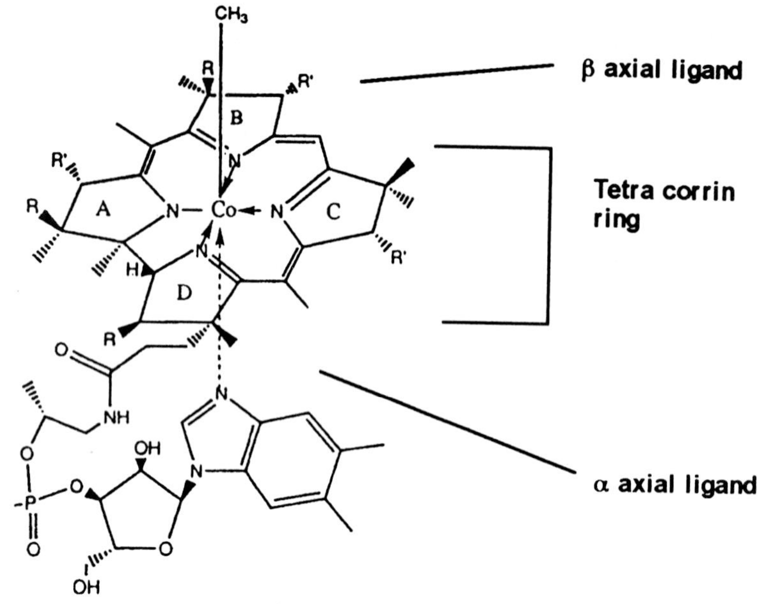

β axial ligand

Tetra corrin ring

α axial ligand

R = CH_2CONH_2

R' = $CH_2CH_2CONH_2$

Figure 27.1. Structure of vitamin B_{12}.

vivo. The methyl form attaches to methionine synthase, and the adenosyl form to methylmalonyl CoA mutase.

NUTRITION/DIETARY CONSIDERATIONS

Vitamin B_{12} is synthesized by bacteria, which is its only source. It is present in virtually all forms of animal tissues, which acquire the vitamin indirectly from bacteria. Thus, vitamin B_{12} is not present in plants and thus does not occur in vegetables or fruit. The dietary intake of vitamin B_{12} is about 5 μg/day when it is complexed with IF, which is the maximum capacity of the ileal receptors (5). When pharmacologic doses are used, 1% of the dose is absorbed by passive diffusion.

The highest levels of dietary vitamin B_{12} occur in animal liver, reflecting the fact that 50% of the body stores are in this organ. Levels in excess of 100 μg/100 g occur in beef and mutton. Dietary meat and fish are also good sources of the vitamin (5). By contrast, the level of the vitamin is 0.36 μg/100 mL in cow's milk and is 0.04 μg/100 mL in human milk from Caucasian mothers on a mixed diet. This level falls by a factor of 3 to 4 in mothers on a strict vegetarian diet (5).

The vitamin B_{12} dietary requirements for children, adult males, and females, and during pregnancy and lactation are described elsewhere (6) (Table 27.1) (see also Appendix Tables II-A-2-a and II-A-2-c-1 [U.S.A.], II-A-3-b [Canada], and II-A-7-a to c [Australia]). Dietary intake may be low in elderly patients and in strict vegetarians (also termed *vegans*). This can produce low serum vitamin B_{12} levels and raised levels of the substrates of the two mammalian enzymes for which vitamin B_{12} is a coenzyme, namely, methylmalonic acid (MMA) and the total of homocysteine and homocystine (tHcy). The evidence that these plasma changes induce significant megaloblastic anemia or neuropathy remains tentative. These changes may signal the presence of cobalamin-responsive neuropsychiatric symptoms (7).

ABSORPTION AND TRANSPORTATION

The cobalamins are bound with high affinity by glycoproteins, a group of proteins with varying carbohydrate component that have similar antigenic properties and occur in all mammalian tissues. One of them, IF, is required for normal absorption of vitamin B_{12}. The other

Table 27.1
Recommended Dietary Intakes for Vitamin B_{12} (μg/day)

	Reference Nutrient Intakes UK (6)	USA RDA 1989 (38)	USA RDA 1998 (39)
Age			
0–6 months	0.3	0.3	0.4[a]
6–12 months	0.4	0.5	0.5[a]
1–3 years	0.5	0.7	0.9
4–6 years	0.8	1.0	1.2 (4 to 8 years)
7–10 years	1.0	1.4	—
Males			
11–14 years	1.2	2.0	1.8 (9 to 13 years)
15–18 years	1.5	2.0	2.4
19–50 years	1.5	2.0	2.4
50 + years	1.5	2.0	2.4 (51 to >70 yr)
Females			
11–14 years	1.2	2.0	1.8 (9 to 13 years)
15–18 years	1.5	2.0	2.4
19–50 years	1.5	2.0	2.4
50 + years	1.5	2.0	2.4 (51 to >70 years)
Pregnancy	No increment	2.2	2.6
Lactating	—	2.6	2.8

[a]*Adequate intake values.*

glycoproteins include haptocorrins (Hc) (also called R binders, TC I and III, or cobalaphilin) and TC II. TC II binds to vitamin B_{12} in the terminal ileal cells and transports it in the plasma to the cells of the body (8). Absorption of vitamin B_{12} via IF and its specific IF ileal enterocyte cell-wall receptor (IFCR), and its transport by TC II in the body, summarized in Figure 27.2 is discussed in detail elsewhere (9, 10).

Characterization of the cDNA on chromosome II encoding IF synthesis demonstrated both its source and structure. Human IF is secreted by gastric parietal cells but is also present in fundal chief cells and antral G cells of the gastric mucosa and in the salivary glands (9). IF secretion depends on a variety of stimuli, including gastric histamine and acetylcholine. Both IF and TC II bind to the *α*-axial ligand of cobalamin. For cobalamins to bind IF and TC II requires a rearrangement of their Co-N bond. Thus IF and TC II cannot bind noncobalamin corrinoids. Haptocorrins are more nonspecific because they bind to the corrin ring of the corrinoid.

In the stomach, dietary vitamin B_{12} is initially released from its organic binding by the action of gastric acid and pepsin. The vitamin, which is predominantly methyl Cbl and adoCbl, is then bound by Hc, which has a markedly higher affinity for Hc than for IF at acid pH. In the intestine, however, the pH rises and this in combination with the partial proteolytic digestion of the Hc binder by pancreatic enzymes that do not affect IF, leads to vitamin B_{12} being released and transferred to IF. Only IF-bound Cbl is absorbed by the IFCR.

Hc-bound cobalamins are not absorbed and are excreted in the feces. The function of Hc in the intestinal lumen may well be to remove cobalamin analogues produced by food preservative techniques, cooking, and intestinal microflora, which might otherwise interfere with transfer of vitamin B_{12} to IF or have toxic effects if absorbed.

The IFCR consists of two b units situated in the ileal cell wall, with two flanking a units that bind to IF glycoprotein and lock the IF-Cbl complex into the receptor (9). Up to 0.2% of the total body pool of cobalamin is excreted per day in bile, bound to Hc. Also, apoptosis of intestinal mucosal cells containing cobalamin occurs at a constant rate. The partial proteolytic removal of Hc from cobalamin and subsequent reabsorption of the latter by the IFCR in the terminal ileum may constitute an enterohepatic cycle of the vitamin that amounts to more than 1.0 μg vitamin B_{12} per day. This may explain why vitamin B_{12} absorption specifically occurs in the final 60 cm of the ileum.

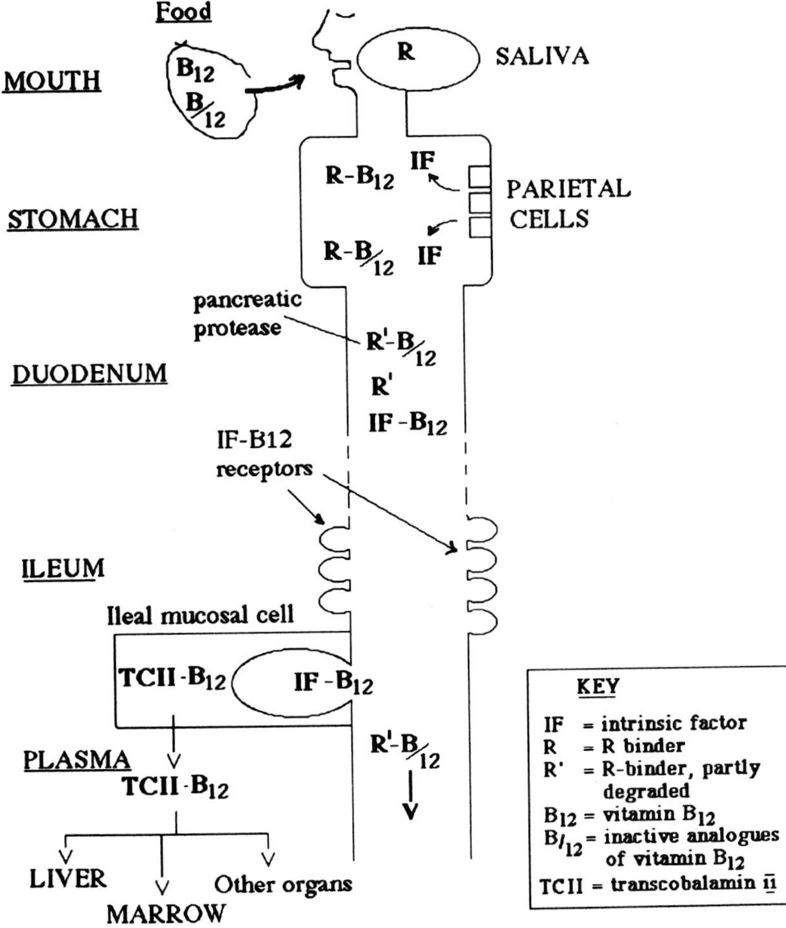

Figure 27.2. Mechanism of vitamin B_{12} absorption.

IF-bound OH-cobalamin uptake by the IFCR in the brush border microvilli of the ileal mucosal cells depends on the presence of calcium, a pH above 6, and components in bile. Once internalized in the ileal cell by endocytosis, cobalamin is liberated and IF degraded by separate mechanisms related to the prelysosomal acidic region. The absorbed cobalamin is converted to methyl Cbl and adoCbl, probably within the mitochondria of the ileal cell, and appears in the portal blood bound to TC II approximately 3 hours after absorption (9). TC II, whose half-life is only 6 minutes (11), is essential for physiologic transport of cobalamins to all cells in the body where it is endocytosed by specific cell wall receptors (10). In man, in contradistinction to other animals, 90% of cobalamin circulating in the blood is bound to TC I, whose half-life is 9.3 to 9.8 days. TC I–bound Cbl is probably only available to vitamin B_{12} storage cells such as liver and reticuloenothelial cells (11).

METABOLISM

The TC II–Cbl complex is internalized by adsorptive endocytosis using a specific high-affinity cell surface receptor, as discussed by Fenton and Rosenberg (10). TC II is then degraded by lysosomal proteases, releasing the cobalamin, which exits from the lysosome and is converted to either methyl Cbl in the cytosol, where it binds to methionine synthase, or to adoCbl in the mitochondria, where it binds to methylmalonyl-CoA mutase. Methionine synthase and methylmalonyl-CoA mutase are synthesized by the endoplasmic reticulum. The former remains in the cytosol, and the latter in the mitochondria. Both are 90 to 100% in the holo form. A potential alternative mechanism of taking up TC I–Cbl into haptocytes is reviewed elsewhere (10).

The total body content of vitamin B_{12} in adults is 3 to 5 mg, of which 50% is in the liver (5). AdoCbl accounts for more than 70% of cobalamin in liver, erythrocytes, brain, and kidney; methyl Cbl accounts for only 1 to 3%. Plasma cobalamin is mainly methyl Cbl (60–80%); the remainder is OH-Cbl and adoCbl. Since 90% of circulating cobalamin is bound to TC I, most of the methyl Cbl must travel with this Hc. The significance of these dramatic differences in distribution is unclear.

Excretion of cobalamin occurs via cellular apoptosis into the gastrointestinal tract, kidney, and skin. This is exceedingly slow, since total gastrectomy, which reduces physiologic cobalamin absorption to virtually zero, only produces a cobalamin deficiency sufficient to induce megaloblastic anemia after a period of 4 to 7 years (5). As explained above, this is due to the reabsorption of secreted vitamin B_{12} by the IFCR, forming an enterohepatic circulation.

FUNCTIONS

The two enzymes for which vitamin B_{12} is a coenzyme in mammalian cells are methylmalonyl-CoA mutase and methionine synthase.

Mechanisms of Action of Methionine Synthase

Crystallization of *Escherichia coli* methionine synthase by Ruma Banerjee and colleagues has allowed description of how one 27-kDa domain of its total 136kDa binds to methyl Cbl (12) (Fig. 27.3) (see [2] for references and discussion). This protein binds dimethylbenzimidazole, the *a* ligand of vitamin B_{12}, in a hydrophobic pocket that is displaced away from the cobalt ligand to the edge of the tetracorrin plate. In its place His^{759} from methionine synthase acts as an axial cobalt ligand. The methyl group on the *b* ligand, which is itself protected by hydrophobic residues on methionine synthase, is now transferred to homocysteine by a suggested protonation/deprotonation shuttle that converts six-coordinate Cob (III) to four-coordinate Cob (I). Cob (I) is then remethylated back to Cob (III) either by N^5-methyl-THF-Glu, which is the usual sequence, or in the event of Cob (I) becoming oxidized to Cob (II), which occurs every 100 to 2000 cycles in vitro, by the universal methylator AdoMet (2). The interesting potential for methionine synthase to shuttle both Cob (II) and Cob (I) to Cob (III) may also explain how the 5′-deoxyadenosyl B ligand of cobalamin is used by the mutase enzymes that use the Cob (II) cofactor form (2). The ability of Cob (II) to shuttle to Cob (III) suggests that methionine synthase might have a similar ligand to the adoCbl-requiring mutase enzymes, since recent evidence suggests a similar linkage of the dimethylbenzimidazole a ligand–binding pocket and His^{759} to the *a* Cob-N ligand (2).

Mechanism of Action of Methylmalonyl-CoA Mutase

Methylmalonyl-CoA mutase requires adoCbl as a cofactor. The associated disturbances caused by adoCbl deficiency and defects of methylmalonyl-CoA mutase function have been reviewed elsewhere (10, 13). A series of compounds, including the amino acids, valine, isoleucine, methionine, and threonine, along with cleavage products of cholesterol, thymine, and odd-chain fatty acids, is then metabolized via propionyl-CoA or methylmalonyl semialdehyde to methylmalonyl-CoA. At high concentrations propionyl-CoA can, in association with oxaloacetic acid and citrate synthase, produce 2-methylcitric acids I and II. *S*-Methylmalonyl-CoA is usually converted to succinyl-CoA via *S,R*-methylmalonyl-CoA racemase, and subsequently the adoCbl-dependent *R*-methylmalonyl-CoA mutase. In the context of vitamin B_{12} deficiency, methylmalonyl-CoA mutase function is impaired and *S*-methylmalonyl-CoA is then converted to MMA via a non-vitamin-B_{12}-dependent enzyme, *S*-methylmalonyl-CoA hydrolase. MMA is in turn converted to unknown metabolites. Consequently, in vitamin B_{12} deficiency, levels of methylmalonyl-CoA, its hydrolytic product MMA, and 2-methylcitric acids I and II are elevated in both plasma and urine (14).

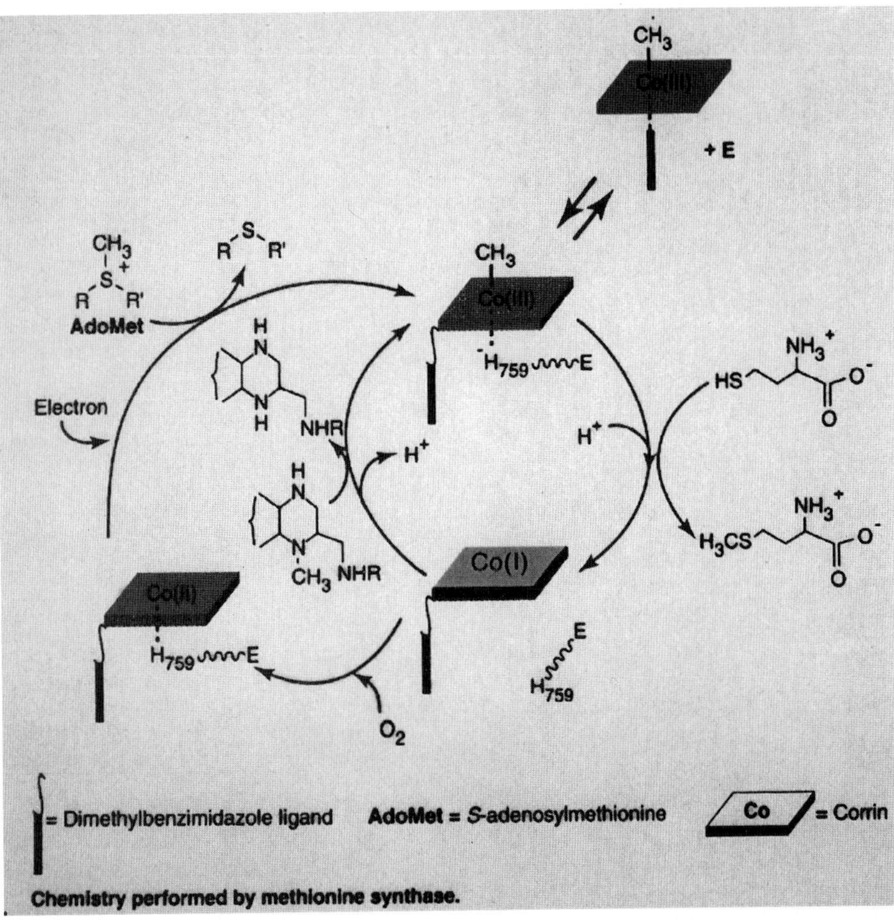

Figure 27.3. Mechanism of cobalamin involvement in methionine synthase. Reprinted from Stubbe J. Science 1994;266:1663–4, with permission.

Biochemistry of Methylcobalamin and Methionine Synthase

Methionine synthase stands at the junction between two important metabolic processes of internal metabolism: the synthesis of DNA and RNA via purine and pyrimidines and the methylation reactions via AdoMet (15, 16) (Fig. 27.4). These processes are achieved in the main via passage of carbon moieties from serine, which is easily synthesized from glucose. The β carbon of serine via serine hydroxymethyltransferase and THF-glu$_5$ synthesizes N^5,N^{10}-methylene-THF-glu$_5$ and glycine in the cytoplasm. The glycine carbon 2 can also be used to produce N^5,N^{10}-methylene-THF-glu$_5$ via a complex reaction that is only found in mitochondria (16). N^5,N^{10}-methylene-THF-glu$_5$ then stands at a metabolic crossroads. It can *(a)* synthesize thymidylate from deoxyuridylate monophosphate, which in turn produces one of the pyrimidine bases of DNA, *(b)* be converted to N^{10}-formyltetrahydrofolate pentaglutamate, which is used for the insertion of carbons 2 and 8 into the purine ring, or *(c)* be reduced via methylene reductase to N^5-methyl-THF-glu$_5$, which is used to remethylate homocysteine to produce first methionine via methionine synthase and then adoMet via the *S*-adenosylmethionine synthetase (see Chapter 26).

The other function of methionine synthase is to act as the gatekeeper for entry of folate into the cell. Folate circulates in the plasma as N^5-methyl-THF-glu$_1$. When it enters a cell, it can only remain inside if it is immediately demethylated by conversion of homocysteine to methionine and THF-glu$_1$ via methionine synthase. THF-glu$_1$ is then converted to THF-glu$_5$ via folyl-γ-glutamate synthetase. This enzyme has been synthesized and cloned; its function is described in detail elsewhere (17) (see Chapter 1). Since the avidity of methionine synthase for N^5-methyl-THF-glu$_1$ is orders of magnitude lower than for N^5-methyl-THF-glu$_5$, N^5-methyl-THF-glu$_1$ is only demethylated by methionine synthase if there is no N^5-methyl-THF-glu$_5$ available. This occurs on two occasions: *(a)* during cell division, when the cell reduces its intracellular folate content by 50% and the daughter cells must take up plasma folate to bring the intracellular folate level back to normal, and *(b)* when deficiency, inhibition, or impaired function of methylene reductase reduces synthesis of N^5-methyl-THF-glu$_5$.

Control of Methionine Synthase Function

The relative availability of the substrates of methionine synthase, tHcy and N^5-methyl-THF-glu, and of its cofactor

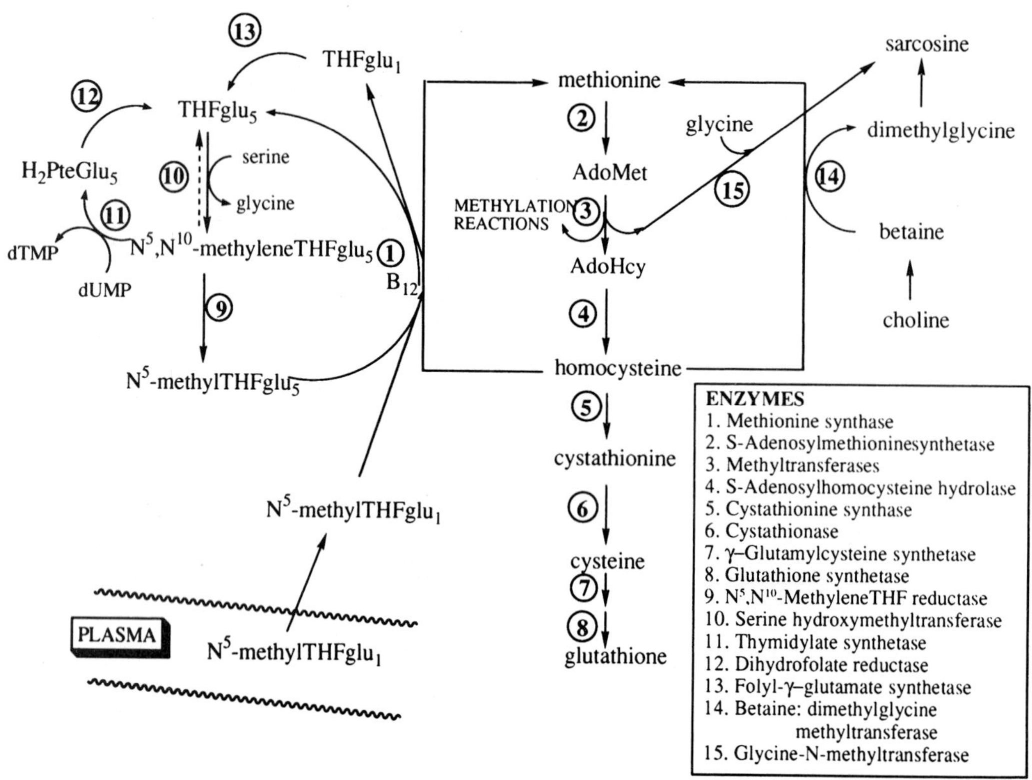

Figure 27.4. Biochemistry of methyl Cbl and methionine synthase.

methyl Cbl control its activity. These in turn are strictly regulated by the amount of dietary methionine and its product, Adomet, in the cell (15) (see Chapter 34).

At times of dietary methionine excess, the level of Adomet, the universal methylator, is high. This maintains the methylation reactions that are essential for internal metabolism, especially in the liver, pancreas, kidney, and brain. So far, 35 methylation reactions have been described in mammalian cells. These methylation reactions are controlled by the product of the methylation process, AdoHcy, which is a competitive inhibitor of AdoMet. Thus, the ratio of AdoMet to AdoHcy, the so-called methylation ratio, controls these methylation reactions to varying extents. The one exception is glycine-*N*-methyl transferase, which converts glycine to sarcosine via AdoMet. This enzyme is controlled not by AdoHcy but by N^5-methyl-THF-glu (16). So, in the liver, when methionine and AdoMet are in excess, AdoMet is demethylated by glycine-*N*-methyltransferase to form AdoHcy and sarcosine. AdoHcy is then converted to adenosine and tHcy by AdoHcy hydrolase. tHcy, when present in high concentrations, is catabolized via cystathionine synthase, the so-called transulfuration pathway, to cystathionine, cysteine, and glutathione. It is important for the cell to maintain the normal concentration of tHcy. Homocysteine, if it accumulates, will tend to re-form AdoHcy via AdoHcy hydrolase, since the equilibrium constant of the reaction strongly favors the back reaction (16a).

These events are controlled by the level of Adomet. Adomet in excess causes *(a)* inhibition of methylene reductase, the enzyme responsible for conversion of N^5,N^{10}-methylene-THF-glu$_5$ to N^5-methyl-THF-glu$_5$ (the latter is therefore not available either to remethylate homocysteine back to methionine via methionine synthase or to inhibit glycine-*N*-methyl transferase) and *(b)* activation of hepatic cystathionine synthase which controls the transulfuration pathway. In other cells such as nerve cells the catabolic pathway is less important.

When dietary methionine is lacking, the reverse occurs. AdoMet is now reduced, threatening the methylation reactions, and inhibition of methylene reductase is released, allowing synthesis of N^5-methyl-THF-glu$_5$ which is then available *(a)* to remethylate whatever tHcy is available to maintain methionine levels and *(b)* to inhibit glycine-*N*-methyl transferase and accordingly prevent removal of the now scarce AdoMet. Furthermore, AdoMet deficiency reduces cystathionine synthase induction, which is necessary for the catabolic transulfuration pathway described above, to retain available tHcy for remethylation and methionine synthesis. tHcy conversion to cystathionine occurs via cystathionine synthase, which has a high K_m, while remethylation of Hcy to methionine via methionine synthase has a low K_m. The result is that under normal circumstances Hcy is remethylated rather than catabolized at a ratio of 3:1(18). The catabolic pathway may only become dominant postprandially following a high cellular influx of exogenous methionine (19). A high tHcy concentration also enhances methionine synthase activity, all available N^5-methyl-THF-glu$_5$ being used to synthesize methionine (20).

Pathogenesis

In contradistinction to the checks and counterchecks that exist to control the supply of AdoMet via folate and methionine (described above), the body has no mechanisms to control the effects of vitamin B_{12} deficiency. This results in a series of clinical complications:

Definite association
1. Megaloblastic anemia
2. Neuropathy associated with vitamin B_{12}

Possible association

3. Atheroma causing coronary thrombosis, strokes, and peripheral vascular disease
4. Neural tube defects
5. Hepatic steatosis

DISEASES ASSOCIATED WITH METHYLCOBALAMIN DEFICIENCY

Megaloblastic Anemia

The inhibition of methionine synthase resulting from vitamin B_{12} deficiency leads to reduced synthesis of methionine and THF-glu_5 and accumulation of tHcy and N^5-methyl-THF-glu_5 (21) (see Chapter 88). The reduction in THF-glu_5 leads to reduced availability of N^5,N^{10}-methylene-THF-glu_5 for conversion of deoxyuridine monophosphate to thymidylate for DNA synthesis. The deficiency is further exacerbated by reductions in methionine and Adomet levels. This, as explained above, leads to reduced suppression of methylene reductase, which causes whatever N^5,N^{10}-methylene-THF-glu_5 was available for thymidylate synthesis to be converted to N^5-methyl-THF-glu_5, which under physiologic conditions is an irreversible reaction. This forms the basis of the "methyl trap" hypothesis for production of megaloblastic anemia in vitamin B_{12} deficiency.

Since N^5-methyl-THF-glu_1, the form of folate taken up by the cell from the plasma, is a poor substrate for folyl-γ-glutamate synthetase (17), N^5-methyl-THF-glu_1 is very poorly incorporated into the methyl Cbl–deficient cell. The resultant cellular THF-glu_5 deficiency in turn causes intracellular folate deficiency. The *megaloblastic anemia* induced by vitamin B_{12} deficiency is caused by this intracellular folate deficiency. It is thus not surprising that it is morphologically identical to that associated with folate deficiency, as described elsewhere (4) (see also Chapter 88).

Neuropathy Associated with Vitamin B_{12} Deficiency

The neuropathy associated with vitamin B_{12} deficiency has been described elsewhere ([7, 22] and Chapter 95). The pathogenesis of the neuropathy relates to changes in the methylation ratio (23). As explained above, the ratio of AdoMet to AdoHcy in brain tissue is usually greater than 4:1. When methionine synthase is inhibited because of vitamin B_{12} deficiency, homocysteine and AdoHcy accumulate, and methionine and AdoMet synthesis is impaired, causing the methylation ratio to fall. The methylation reactions are inhibited, inducing a state of hypomethylation and impaired synthesis of (among others) myelin basic protein. Other organs such as the liver and kidney can remethylate homocysteine to methionine via betaine methyltransferase at the same time as it converts betaine to dimethylglycine (Fig. 27.4). However, the brain does not possess betaine methyltransferase and relies on methionine synthase for endogenous synthesis of methionine and AdoMet at times of dietary methionine deprivation. Evidence that this complication is related to a derangement of the relationship between AdoMet and AdoHcy is discussed in detail elsewhere (23).

Neuropathy Induced in Animals by Nitrous Oxide (N_2O) Inhalation. Chronic inhalation of N_2O leads to a neuropathy in the monkey that is histologically similar to the neuropathy associated with vitamin B_{12} deficiency in the human. N_2O irreversibly inhibits methionine synthase, and oral methionine given prophylactically significantly ameliorates the lesion. N_2O-induced neuropathy in the pig is associated with a fall in the brain methylation ratio, which in turn reduces brain O and N protein methylation. The particular protein hypomethylation that leads to the neuropathy remains to be determined.

Neuropathy Associated with N_2O Inhalation in Humans. Acute N_2O inhalation produces megaloblastic anemia, while chronic intermittent N_2O inhalation induces a neuropathy similar to vitamin B_{12} deficiency (7). Patients who are already vitamin B_{12} deficient are at particular risk of N_2O-induced neuropathy, which can be prevented by pretreatment with methionine (24).

Congenital Deficiency of Enzymes Concerned with AdoMet Synthesis. Congenital deficiency of methylene reductase, methionine synthase, and AdoMet synthase (25, 26) and inborn errors of methylcobalamin synthesis (Cbl E and G) (26) lead to changes similar to those in the vitamin B_{12}–deficient brain. Methylene reductase malfunction in particular causes AdoMet deficiency and the neuropathy, because the ensuing deficiency of N^5-methyl-THF-glu_5 would (as explained above) lead to enhanced glycine methyl transferase activity. Thus AdoMet would continue to be demethylated, producing AdoHcy and sarcosine, even when AdoMet levels were low. The absence of any anemia in methylene reductase–deficient patients who get the neuropathy is strong clinical evidence in favor of the methyl trap hypothesis. The clinical presentation of the neuropathy has been described elsewhere (7).

Atheroma

Raised levels of tHcy in the blood and urine are a risk factor for vascular disease, whether affecting coronary, carotid, or peripheral artery and peripheral veins. The raised tHcy levels are usually caused by an abnormality in, or impaired function of, one of the three enzymes that control homocysteine metabolism (27). Cystathionine synthetase deficiency blocks the transsulfuration pathway, which produces the classical form of homocysteinemia. Reduced activity of methylene reductase induces a deficiency in N^5-methyl-THF-glu$_5$ and impairs remethylation of tHcy as do cobalamin mutants (Cbl C, D, E, and G) that impair the function of methionine synthase (Fig. 27.4) (26).

Dietary deficiency of the vitamins folate, cobalamin, and pyridoxine (Chapter 24) also raises homocysteine levels (14), especially in the elderly, since these vitamins are essential for the normal function of methylene reductase, methionine synthase, and cystathionine synthase, respectively. It seems probable that elevating tHcy levels long enough to induce atheromatous changes in the arterial endothelium may require both a genetic variant relating to one of three enzymes and a deficiency of the relevant vitamin. In particular, this is probably true of folate deficiency in association with the thermolabile variant of methylene reductase (27). Pernicious anemia patients do not have an increased incidence of atherosclerosis at autopsy, for reasons that are currently obscure. It may relate to the relative duration of the raised tHcy before diagnosis and treatment (28).

Neural Tube Defects

One study has suggested that deficiency of vitamin B_{12}, as well as folic acid, is a risk factor for neural tube defects (29). (See discussion elsewhere [30] and Chapters 34 and 95.)

Hepatic Steatosis

The pathogenesis of hepatic steatosis is associated with methionine and choline deficiency, and ethanol is also known to inhibit methionine synthase (31).

Mechanisms of Cobalamin Deficiency/Malfunction

Dietary Deficiency

Vegans who eat no animal-derived food develop vitamin B_{12} deficiency (5). Functional deficiency of vitamin B_{12} is common in the elderly, especially those living in institutions. The effect of dietary deficiency in the pathogenesis of vitamin B_{12}–related diseases remains uncertain, especially since (as explained above) the enterohepatic circulation preserves vitamin B_{12} that would otherwise be lost by gastrointestinal secretion and apoptosis.

Disorders of Cobalamin Absorption

The methods whereby vitamin B_{12} is malabsorbed have been discussed elsewhere (9, 10).

Malabsorption of Food Cobalamin. Patients with hypochlorhydria, such as occurs in the elderly and post-gastrectomy patients, may exhibit malabsorption of dietary cobalamin. Gastric acid releases cobalamin from its organic setting in food before it is taken up by Hc binders in the acidic pH of the stomach (32). Nevertheless, there is a discrepancy between patients who have low plasma vitamin B_{12} levels and those with impaired absorption. Patients with Hc deficiency and myelopathy have been reported, but the pathogenesis is not understood (10).

Pancreatic Insufficiency. Reduced secretion of pancreatic enzymes and bicarbonate leads to impaired digestion of Hc and elevation of intestinal pH, both of which are necessary for transfer of cobalamin from Hc binders to IF. This is the mechanism of the cobalamin malabsorption that characterizes chronic pancreatic diseases (9).

Pernicious Anemia. The amount of IF secreted by normal subjects exceeds what is required to capture the Hc-bound B_{12} released in the alkaline milieux of the duodenum. The number of upper intestinal sites now known to synthesize and secrete IF means that gastric atrophy alone probably cannot suffice to reduce the luminal IF concentration below a critical level. Antibodies to IF, which inhibit the function of any remaining IF produced by sites outside the gastric mucosa, are also necessary. Two types of antibodies, "blocking" and "binding," occur both in the serum, where they are innocuous, and in the intestinal lumen. These antibodies adhere to different sites on the IF-cobalamin complex and interfere differently with its uptake by the ileal IFCR, thus causing cobalamin malabsorption.

Congenital forms of impaired IF secretion also occur. One fails to produce an immunologically recognizable IF. Another produces a binder that is immunologically reactive to IF antibodies but is physiologically inactive because of a lack of affinity with the ileal IFCR.

Grasbeck-Immerslund Syndrome. The Grasbeck-Immerslund syndrome is associated with a low serum vitamin B_{12} level, megaloblastic anemia, and normal gastric and intestinal function; it usually presents between 1 and 5 years of age. Cobalamin absorption is not corrected by the addition of normal human IF with vitamin B_{12}. This syndrome is likely to be due to a series of defects in receptor uptake, enzymatic removal of IF, transfer to TC, and export to the portal venous system (8).

Infestation of the Intestinal Lumen. An abnormal connection between the colon and the small intestine or stagnation in diverticula, blind loops, or strictures leads to contamination of the small intestine with colonic bacteria at concentrations greater than 10^5 organisms per dL. This constitutes the "contaminated small bowel syndrome," characterized by steatorrhea and vitamin B_{12} deficiency. The latter is caused by competitive uptake of cobalamins by the microorganisms.

Diphyllobothrium latum, a fish tapeworm that infests the upper intestine, is a further example of competition for the vitamin between host and parasites. It occurs particularly in Scandinavian countries.

AIDS. Patients with AIDS are known to develop plasma vitamin B_{12} deficiency, thought to be due to a failure of IF-B_{12} complex uptake by the ileal IFCR. The pathogenic significance, if any, remains to be determined (33).

Disorders of Transport

Transcobalamin II deficiency usually presents within the 1st or 2nd month of life. It is potentially lethal and is associated with vomiting, weakness, failure to thrive, and megaloblastic anemia. Neurologic complications ensue associated with immunological deficiencies. The defect in TC II takes different forms: it may be absent, may be immunologically normal but fail to bind cobalamin, or may bind cobalamin but not be taken up by cell-wall receptors. The level of circulating serum vitamin B_{12} is normal, since in humans 90% is bound to TC I(9).

Transcobalamin I deficiency may also occur, but since it has no significant physiologic function, it is not associated with any known disease state.

Inherited Disorders of Cobalamin Metabolism

The inherited disorders of cobalamin metabolism, described elsewhere (1, 9) (Fig. 27.5), may be of particular interest because milder variants similar to those described for methylene reductase may exist but be undiscovered. Any cyano- or hydroxycobalamin in the diet or intestinal lumen that is not converted to adenosyl- or methylcobalamin during absorption and transport is rapidly metabolized to these forms in the cell. Defects in conversion to the active forms of the vitamin produce nine distinct mutant forms of the vitamin (discussed in detail elsewhere [1, 9, 13]).

Disorders of Adenosylcobalamin (Cbl A and Cbl B) and Methylmalonyl-CoA Mutase. Two distinct genetic loci are responsible for synthesis of two defective forms of adoCbl, Cbl A and Cbl B. Cbl A and Cbl B differ in the intramitochondrial conversion of OH-Cbl to adoCbl. There are also two distinct variants of methylmalonyl-CoA mutase, one has no mutase in the cells (mut^0) and the other is abnormal (mut^-). The only clinical difference between mut^0 and mut^- and adoCbl A and B is that the former presents within weeks, while Cbl A and Cbl B present later (months to 1 year).

The major metabolic changes are methylmalonic aciduria, metabolic acidosis, ketonemia, hyperammonemia, hyperglycinemia, and hypoglycemia. Bone marrow suppression in the form of anemia, leukopenia, and thrombocytopenia may also be present. Neither megaloblastic anemia nor neurologic disease occur (9, 13).

Defects of Cellular Methyl Cbl and AdoCbl Synthesis. Three mutant cobalamins (Cbl C, Cbl D, and Cbl F) are characterized by methylmalonic acidemia, homocysteinemia with or without hypercystathionemia and hypomethionemia, and megaloblastic anemia. Patients may present early with failure to thrive or in early adulthood with neurologic disorders such as dementia and myelopathy. In contrast to Cbl A and Cbl B mutants, hyperglycinemia and hyperammonemia does not occur. Cbl C, the commonest and most severe of these mutations, may also result in muscular hypotonia, developmental delay, microcephaly, seizures, and ocular retinal changes (9). Cbl D, a rarer and less severe mutant, is associated with neuromuscular abnormalities, and Cbl F has a similar clinical picture, which is occasionally associated with

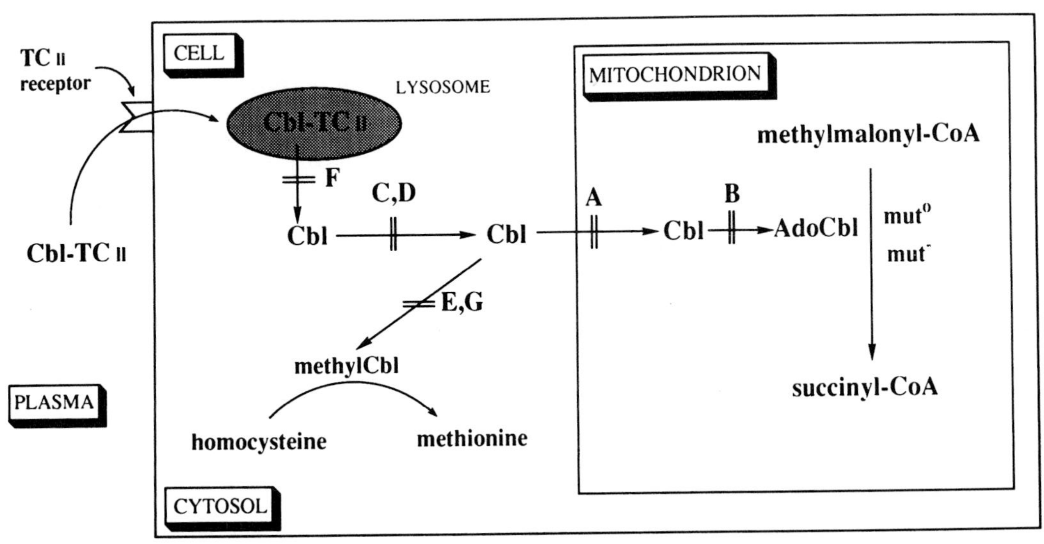

Figure 27.5. Defects of cobalamin metabolism.

abnormal vitamin B_{12} absorption and a low serum cobalamin level. Cbl C and D are due to defects in cytosolic metabolism, and Cbl F to a defect in lysosomal efflux. Treatment of these disorders with parenteral hydroxycobalamin produces a variable response.

Defects in Methyl Cbl Synthesis. Cbl E and Cbl G (1, 9, 26) represent defects in methyl Cbl synthesis. Patients exhibit failure to thrive and vomiting. They have marked neurologic abnormalities that take the form of microcephaly, seizures, impaired development, and hypotonia. Megaloblastic anemia occurs in association with raised homocysteine levels, hypomethioninemia, and no methylmalonic aciduria.

One 21-year-old patient with the Cbl G mutant presented with gait disturbances and progressively impaired sensation, closely resembling the changes found in the neuropathy associated with cobalamin deficiency. These defects appear to reflect a mutation affecting the maintenance of cobalamin I in the reduced state (Cbl E) and in the cobalamin-binding domain of methionine synthase (Cbl G).

STANDARD TECHNIQUES FOR DIAGNOSIS OF COBALAMINE DEFICIENCY

Hematologic Parameters

The classical textbook features of Cbl deficiency include anemia with macrocytosis and a megaloblastic anemia. However, it is now appreciated that significant Cbl deficiency can occur leading to neurologic dysfunction in the absence of any of these parameters (7).

Serum Cobalamin Assay

In most laboratories the serum Cbl assay remains the standard method for diagnosing deficiency, defined as less than 150 pg/mL. However, significant deficiency may occur in the face of low normal, or only marginally reduced, levels of serum Cbl, especially in the elderly. Objective evidence of Cbl deficiency has been found in patients whose available serum Cbl ranges from 200 to 300 pg/mL and even on occasions more than 300 pg/mL.

Whether the radioimmunoassay used in most laboratories is as specific or sensitive as the bioassay using *Leishmanii donovani* remains controversial. The radioassay, by its nature, must include Cbl bound to TC I, which is biologically inactive. This gives a falsely high reading for the serum Cbl. Recent improvements in the stability, reproducibility, and efficiency of the microbiologic assay by using cryopreservation, a colistin sulfate–resistant organism and β-lactamase to hydrolyze interfering antibiotics have made it the assay of choice (34). It is suggested that measuring holo TC II is a better method of assessing early cobalamin deficiency (35). Measurement of the substrates of the two Cbl-dependent enzymes, MMA and Hcy, is a new and more accurate method of assessing the presence of intracellular cobalamin deficiency (14, 28).

Methylmalonic Acid

The factors controlling MMA levels in the plasma are not well understood. Normal variations in dietary intake do not affect the plasma levels. Since intestinal organisms can produce propionic acid, a source of MMA in the body, antibiotics may lower plasma MMA levels (7). MMA is excreted in the urine, which results in a good correlation between plasma and urine concentrations. However, plasma MMA levels rise in the presence of renal failure. Plasma MMA levels rise in cobalamin deficiency but not in folate deficiency. In cobalamin deficiency, the plasma levels rise from normal levels of 0.1 to 0.4 μmol/L to 50 to 100 μmol/L (36). These high levels may result in both MMA and propionate being incorporated into odd-carbon branched-chain fatty acids and 2-methylcitrate (36). MMA in urine or plasma is thus a sensitive measure of absolute and/or functional cobalamin deficiency, especially in the diagnosis of subclinical cobalamin deficiency in the elderly.

Plasma MMA levels appear to be more specific than homocysteine levels and are significantly better than serum cobalamin levels. Apparently normal individuals with normal serum cobalamin have had elevated MMA levels that fell following a single injection of cyanocobalamin. Furthermore, elevated MMA and homocysteine levels have been observed to predate the drop in serum cobalamin (36).

Homocysteine

Plasma homocysteine is derived in the main from dietary methionine, although the levels obtained are also affected by dietary cobalamin, folate, and pyridoxine, the vitamin cofactors associated with its metabolism (see above). Normal plasma homocysteine levels are higher in men than in women up to the menopause and increase with age, especially after the age of 60 (37). Erect posture also gives significantly higher homocysteine levels than being prone, which probably reflects changes in plasma albumin binding (C. Cronin and colleagues, unpublished data). Renal excretion of homocysteine accounts for only 1% of the total homocysteine synthesized; nevertheless, plasma homocysteine rises in chronic renal failure.

Plasma homocysteine levels rise in *(a)* deficiency states of folate, cobalamin, and pyridoxine, *(b)* inborn errors of the enzymes associated with homocysteine metabolism, namely cystathionine synthetase, methylene reductase, and methionine synthase, and *(c)* defects associated with the synthesis of the cobalamin coenzymes required for normal function of methionine synthase (see also Chapters 26, 34, and 61). High plasma homocysteine levels have also been reported in hypothyroidism. Low levels occur in insulin-dependent diabetics without renal complications (C. Cronin and colleagues, unpublished data) and in Down's syndrome patients, who have an extra copy of the genes that produce cystathionine synthase (36). Some 7 to 9% of the normal population have raised plasma homocysteine levels due to genetic abnormalities associated with methylene reductase. The normal range for plasma homocysteine depends on the method used and the sex, age, and posture of the patient as described above; women have 6 to 12 μmol/L and men 8 to 14 μmol/L (subjects less than 60 years old).

Methionine loading tests (100 μg/kg body weight) have been used to accentuate abnormalities of the homocysteine metabolic pathways. This technique is mainly used to detect patients with obligate heterozygous cystathionine β-synthase deficiency, since the K_m for this enzyme is relatively high. As the K_m for methionine synthase is low, methionine loading adds little to the standard plasma homocysteine level in diagnosing those with defective remethylation.

Other Metabolites

Cobalamin deficiency is also associated with elevated levels of 2-methyl citrate, *N*-methylglycine, *N,N*-dimethylglycine, and cystathionine (14). What place these metabolites will have in the routine diagnosis of deficiency or defective function has yet to be determined.

SUMMARY

Vitamin B_{12} is an essential cofactor for two enzymes of internal metabolism. Methylmalonyl-CoA mutase is involved in the conversion of propionic to succinic acid, which is required for fatty acid metabolism. High levels of MMA are associated with low levels of vitamin B_{12} and are diagnostic of functional deficiency.

Methionine synthase controls two important processes in internal metabolism: nucleic acid synthesis and the methylation reactions of the body. Deficiency leads to two major clinical complications: megaloblastic anemia and cobalamin-associated neuropathy. Increased levels of a substrate (tHcy) of this enzyme have recently been shown to be associated with early atheromatous disease and may also induce birth defects such as spina bifida, and hepatic steatosis.

The mechanisms by which cobalamin deficiency occurs and the pathogenesis of the complications induced by such deficiency are described above.

REFERENCES

1. Linnell JC, Bhatt HR. Inborn errors of B_{12} metabolism and their management. In: Wickramasinghe SN, ed. Megaloblastic anaemias, clinical haematology. London: Bailliere Tindall, 1995;567–601.
2. Stubbe J. Science 1994;266:1663–4.
3. Weatherall D. Early successes breed new problems. In: Weatherall D, ed. Science and the quiet art. Oxford: Oxford University Press, 1995;55–88.
4. Wickramasinghe SN. Preface to megaloblastic anaemia. In: Wickramasinghe SN, ed. Clinical haematology. London: Bailliere Tindall, 1995;ix.
5. Chanarin I. The megaloblastic anaemias. Oxford: Blackwell, 1979.
6. Vitamin B_{12}. Dietary reference values for food energy and nutrients for the United Kingdom. Report on health and social subjects. London: HMSO, 1991;106–8.
7. Savage DG, Lindenbaum J. Neurological complications in cobalamin deficiency. In: Wickramasinghe SN, ed. Megaloblastic anaemias, clinical haematology. London: Bailliere Tindall, 1995;657–8.
8. Rothenberg SP, Quadros EV. Transcobalamin II and the membrane receptor for the transcobalamin II-cobalamin complex. In: Wickramasinghe SN, ed. Megaloblastic anaemias, clinical haematology. London: Bailliere Tindall, 1995;499–514.
9. Nicolas J-P, Guéant J-L. Gastric intrinsic factor and its receptor. In: Wickramasinghe SN, ed. Megaloblastic anaemias, clinical haematology. London: Bailliere Tindall, 1995; 515–31.
10. Fenton WA, Rosenberg LE. Inherited disorders of cobalamin transport and metabolism. In: Scriver CR, Beaudet AL, Sly WS, Valle D, eds. The metabolic basis of inherited disease. 7th ed. New York: McGraw-Hill, 1995;3129–49.
11. Herbert V, Fong W, Gulle V, Kasdan TS. Am J Hematol 1990;34:132–9.
12. Banerjee RV, Johnston NL, Sobaska JK, et al. J Biol Chem 1989;266:13888–95.
12a. Drennan CL, Huang S, Drummond JT, et al. Science 1994; 266:1669–74.
13. Fenton WA, Rosenberg LE. Disorders of propionate and methylmalonate metabolism. In: Scriver CR, Beaudet AC, Sly WS, Volke D, eds. The metabolic basis of inherited disease. 7th ed. New York: McGraw-Hill, 1995;1423–49.
14. Allen RH, Stabler SP, Savage DG, et al. FASEB J 1993;7: 1344–52.
15. Scott JM, Weir DG. Folate/vitamin B_{12} inter-relationships. In: Tipton KF, ed. Essays in biochemistry. London: Portland Press, 1994;28:63–72.
16. Wagner C. Biochemical role of folate in cellular metabolism. In: Bailey LB, ed. Folate in health and disease. New York: Marcel Dekker, 1995;23–42.
16a. De la Haba G, Cantoni GL. J Biol Chem 1959;234:603–8.
17. Shane B. Folate: chemistry and metabolism. In: Bailey LB, ed. Folate in health and disease. New York: Marcel Dekker, 1995;1–22.
18. Storch KJ, Wagner DA, Burke JF, Young VR. Am J Physiol 1988;255:E322–31.
19. Finkelstein JD. J Nutr Biochem 1990;1:228–37.
20. Selhub J, Miller JW. Am J Clin Nutr 1992;55:131–8.
21. Horne DW. BioFactors 1989;2:65–8.
22. Scott JM, Molloy AM, Kennedy DG, et al. Acta Neurol Scand (Suppl) 1994;154:27–31.
23. Weir DG, Scott JM. Biochemical basis of neuropathy in cobalamin deficiency. In: Wickramasinghe SN, ed. Megaloblastic anaemias, clinical haematology. London: Bailliere Tindall, 1995;479–97.
24. Christensen B, Guttormsen AB, Schneede J, et al. Anaesthesiology 1994;80:1046–56.
25. Surtees R, Leonard J, Austin S. Lancet 1991;338:1550–4.
26. Rosenblatt DS. Inherited disorders of folate transport and metabolism. In: Scriver CR, Beaudet AL, Sly WS, Valle D, eds. The metabolic and molecular basis of inherited disease. New York: McGraw Hill, 1995;3011–128.
27. Scott JM, Weir DG. Q J Med 1996;89:561–3.
28. Green R, Jacobsen DW. Clinical implications of hyperhomocysteinaemia. In: Bailey LB, ed. Folate in health and disease. New York: Marcel Dekker, 1995;75–122.
29. Kirke PN, Molloy AM, Daly LE, et al. Q J Med 1993;86: 703–8.
30. Scott JM, Weir DG, Kirke PN. Folate and neural tube defects.

In: Bailey LB, ed. Folate in health and disease. New York: Marcel Dekker, 1995;329–60.

31. Trimble KC, Molloy AM, Scott JM, Weir DG. Hepatology 1993;18:984–89.
32. Carmel R. Malaborption of food cobalamin. In: Wickramasinghe SN, ed. Megaloblastic anaemias, clinical haematology. London: Bailliere Tindall, 1995;533–66.
33. Trimble KC, Goggins MG, Molloy AM, et al. AIDS 1993;7: 1132–3.
34. Kellegher BP, Scott JM, O'Broin SD. Clin Lab Haematol 1990;12:87–95.
35. Herbert V. Am J Clin Nutr 1994;59(Suppl):1213S–22S.
36. Green R. Metabolite assays in cobalamin and folate deficiency. In: Wickramasinghe SN, ed. Megaloblastic anaemias, clinical haematology. London: Bailliere Tindall, 1995;533–66.
37. Brattstrom L, Lindgren A, Israelsson B, et al. J Intern Med 1994;236:633–41.
38. Natural Reseach Council. Recommended dietary allowances. 10th ed. Washington, DC: National Academy of Science Press, 1989.
39. Food and Nutrition Board—Institute of Medicine. Dietary reference intakes. Thiamin, riboflavin, niacin, vitamin B_6, folate, vitamin B_{12}, pantothenic acid, biotin, and choline. Washington, DC: National Academy Press, 1998.

SELECTED READINGS

Bailey LB, ed. Folate in health and disease. New York: Marcel Dekker, 1995.

Chanarin I. The megaloblastic anaemias. Oxford: Blackwell, 1979.

Scriver CR, Beaudet AL, Sly W, Valle D, eds. Basis of inherited disease. 7th ed. New York: McGraw-Hill, 1995.

Wickramsinghe SN, ed. Megaloblastic anaemias, clinical haematology, vol 8. London: Bailliere Tindall, 1995.

28. Biotin

DONALD M. MOCK

HISTORY OF DISCOVERY

Although a growth requirement for the *bios* fraction had been demonstrated in yeast, Boas first demonstrated the mammalian requirement for a factor, biotin, in rats fed egg white protein. The severe dermatitis, hair loss, and neuromuscular dysfunction was termed *egg-white injury* and was cured by a factor present in liver. The critical event in this egg-white injury of both humans and rats is the highly specific and very tight binding ($K_d = 10^{-15}$ M) of biotin by avidin, a glycoprotein found in egg white. Native avidin is resistant to intestinal proteolysis in both the free and biotin-combined forms. Thus, dietary avidin (e.g., in diets containing uncooked egg white) binds and prevents the absorption of both dietary biotin and any biotin synthesized by intestinal bacteria.

STRUCTURE, CHEMISTRY, AND BIOCHEMISTRY OF BIOTIN

Structure

The structure of biotin (Fig. 28.1) was elucidated independently by Kogl and du Vigneaud in the early the 1940s (1). Eight stereoisomers exist, but only one (designated *d*-(+)-biotin or, simply, biotin) is found in nature and is enzymatically active. Biocytin (ϵ-*N*-biotinyl-L-lysine) is about as active as biotin on a molar basis in mammalian growth studies.

Biotin is a bicyclic compound. One of the rings contains a ureido group (-N-CO-N-). The tetrahydrothiophene ring contains sulfur and has a valeric acid side chain. The Goldberg/Sternbach synthesis or modifications thereof is the method by which biotin is synthesized commercially (1). Additional stereospecific methods of synthesis have been published recently (2, 3).

Regulation

In mammals, biotin is an essential cofactor for four carboxylases, each of which catalyzes a critical step in intermediary metabolism—incorporation of bicarbonate as a carboxyl group into a substrate. All four use a similar catalytic mechanism. Attachment of biotin to the apocarboxylase (Fig. 28.1) is a condensation reaction catalyzed by holocarboxylase synthetase. An amide bond is formed between the carboxyl group of the valeric acid side chain of biotin and the ϵ-amino group of a specific lysyl residue in the apocarboxylase; these apocarboxylase regions contain sequences of amino acids that tend to be highly conserved within and between species for the individual carboxylases.

Regulation of intracellular mammalian carboxylase activity by biotin remains to be elucidated; however, the interaction of biotin synthesis and production of holoacetyl-CoA carboxylase in *Escherichia coli* has been studied extensively (4, 5). The biotin-protein ligase (specifically a holoacetyl-CoA carboxylase synthetase) catalyzes formation of the covalent bond between biotin and a specific lysine residue in the biotin carboxylase carrier protein (BCCP) of acetyl-CoA carboxylase. As with the four mammalian carboxylases, biotinylation of the apocarboxylase proceeds in two steps. First, the holocarboxylase synthetase reacts with biotin and ATP to form a complex between the synthetase and biotinyl-AMP, releasing pyrophosphate. If a suitable amount of apo-BCCP is present, the holocarboxylase is formed and AMP is released. If insufficient apo-BCCP is present, the holocarboxylase synthetase:biotinyl-AMP complex acts to repress

Abbreviations: **ACC**—acetyl-CoA carboxylase; **BCCP**—biotin carboxylase carrier protein; **MCC**—methylcrotonyl-CoA carboxylase; **PCC**—propionyl-CoA carboxylase.

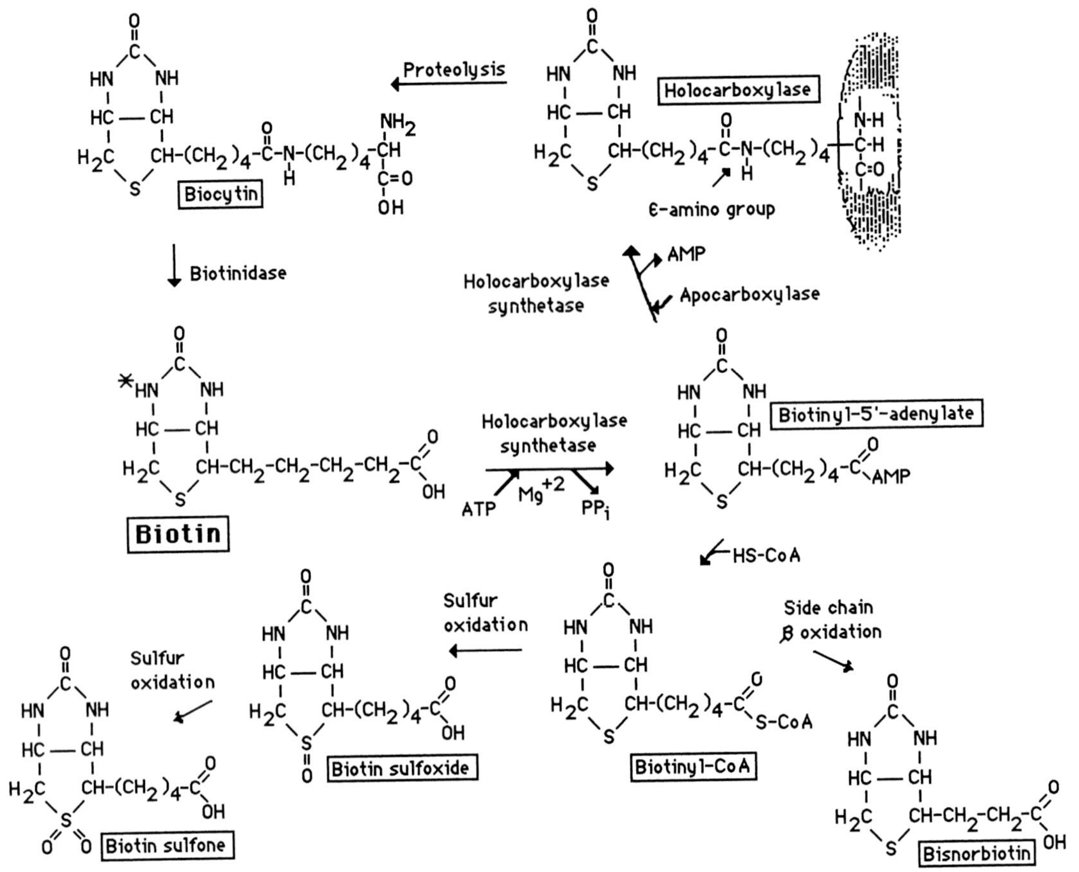

Figure 28.1. Biotin metabolism. The specific systems leading to the sulfoxides have not been defined. *HS-CoA*, coenzyme A; *, site of attachment of carboxyl moiety.

further synthesis of biotin by binding to the promoter regions of the biotin operon ("bio"). These promoters control a cluster of genes encoding enzymes that catalyze biotin synthesis, including biotin synthetase, the enzyme complex that converts dethiobiotin to biotin. Biotinyl-AMP acts as a corepressor through its role in the holocarboxylase synthetase:biotinyl-AMP complex. Thus, the rate of biotin synthesis is responsive to both the supply of apo-BCCP and the supply of biotin as reflected in the biotinyl-AMP concentration.

Chemistry

In the carboxylase reaction, the carboxyl moiety is first attached to biotin at the ureido nitrogen opposite the side chain; then the carboxyl group is transferred to the substrate. The reaction is driven by hydrolysis of ATP to ADP and inorganic phosphate. Subsequent reactions in the pathways of the four mammalian carboxylases release CO_2 from the product of the carboxylase reaction. Thus, these reaction sequences rearrange the substrates into more useful intermediates but do not violate the classic observation that mammalian metabolism does not result in the *net* fixation of carbon dioxide.

The common mechanism for the carboxylase reaction begins with tautomerization of the ureido ring, enhancing the nucleophilicity at the two nitrogens in the ureido ring (6, 7). Because of steric hindrance at the 3′-N (same side of the molecule as the valeric acid side chain that joins biotin to the protein backbone of the carboxylase), the 1′-N uniquely reacts with a carbonyl phosphate that was previously formed by the reaction between bicarbonate and ATP. The product of this reaction is the 1′-*N*-carboxybiotinyl enzyme. This reactive carboxylate group then is incorporated into the substrate, typically at a carbon with incipient carbanion character.

Carboxylases

Three of the four biotin-dependent carboxylases are mitochondrial; the fourth (acetyl-CoA carboxylase, ACC) is found in both mitochondria and the cytosol. Allred and coworkers (1) have postulated that an inactive mitochondrial form of ACC (EC 6.4.1.2) serves as storage for biotin. ACC catalyzes the incorporation of bicarbonate into acetyl-CoA to form malonyl-CoA (Fig. 28.2). This three-carbon compound then serves as a substrate for the fatty acid synthetase complex; the net result is elongation of the fatty acid substrate by two carbons and the loss of the third carbon as CO_2.

Pyruvate carboxylase (PC, EC 6.4.1.1) catalyzes the incorporation of bicarbonate into pyruvate to form oxaloacetate, an intermediate in the Krebs tricarboxylic acid cycle (Fig. 28.2). Thus, PC catalyzes an anaplerotic reaction. In gluconeogenic tissues (i.e., liver and kidney), oxaloacetate can be converted to glucose.

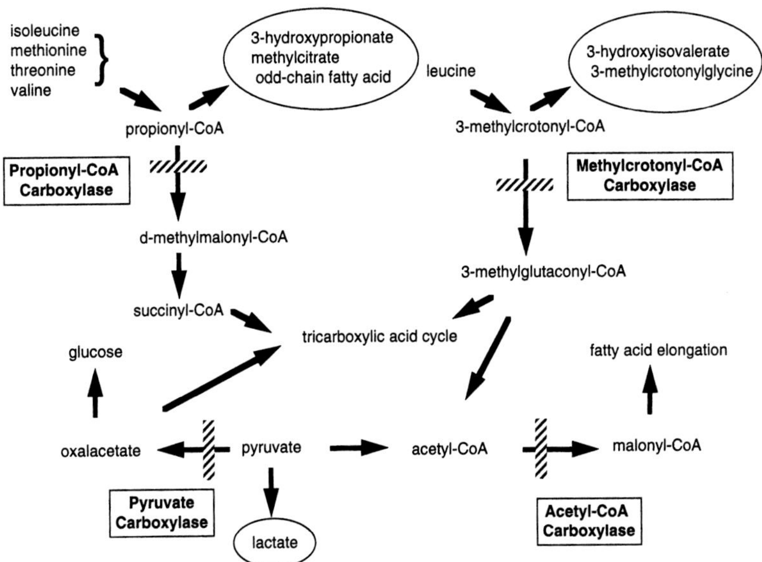

Figure 28.2. Pathways with biotin-dependent enzymes. Deficiencies *(hatched bar)* of PC, PCC, MCC, and ACC lead to increased blood concentrations and urinary excretion of characteristic organic acids denoted by *ovals*.

Methylcrotonyl-CoA carboxylase (MCC, EC 6.4.1.4) catalyzes an essential step in the degradation of the branched-chain amino acid leucine (Fig. 28.2). Deficient activity of this enzyme leads to metabolism of 3-methylcrotonyl-CoA to 3-hydroxyisovaleric acid and 3-methylcrotonylglycine by an alternate pathway (1). Thus, increased urinary excretion of these abnormal metabolites reflects deficient activity of MCC.

Propionyl-CoA carboxylase (PCC, EC 6.4.1.3) catalyzes the incorporation of bicarbonate into propionyl-CoA to form methylmalonyl-CoA, which undergoes isomerization to succinyl-CoA and enters the tricarboxylic acid cycle (Fig. 28.2). In a fashion analogous to MCC deficiency, deficiency of PCC leads to increased urinary excretion of 3-hydroxypropionic acid and 3-methylcitric acid (1).

In the normal turnover of cellular proteins, holocarboxylases are degraded to biocytin or biotin linked to an oligopeptide containing at most a few amino acid residues (Fig. 28.1). Because the amide bond between biotin and lysine is not hydrolyzed by cellular proteases, the specific hydrolase biotinidase (biotin amide hydrolase, EC 3.5.1.12) is required to release biotin for recycling.

Genetic deficiencies of holocarboxylase synthetase and biotinidase cause the two distinct types of *multiple carboxylase deficiency* that were previously designated the neonatal and juvenile forms. Biotinidase deficiency is particularly relevant to understanding biotin deficiency because the clinical manifestations appear to result largely from a secondary biotin deficiency. The gene for human biotinidase has been cloned, sequenced, and characterized (8, 9).

Metabolism and Measurement

Instead of being incorporated into carboxylases after entering the pools of biotin and its intermediary metabolites, biotin may be metabolized. About half of biotin undergoes metabolism before excretion. Biotin, bisnorbiotin, and biotin sulfoxide (Fig. 28.1) are present in molar ratios of approximately 3:2:1 in human urine and plasma (1). Two additional minor metabolites, bisnorbiotin methylketone and biotin sulfone, have recently been identified in human urine. Biotin metabolism is induced in some individuals by anticonvulsants and during pregnancy, thereby increasing the ratio of biotin metabolites to biotin (10, 11).

A variety of assays have been proposed for measuring biotin at physiologic concentrations (i.e., 100 pmol/L to 100 nmol/L), and a limited number have been used to study biotin nutriture. For a more detailed review, see Mock (12). All published studies of biotin nutriture have used one of three basic types of biotin assays: *(a)* bioassays (most studies), *(b)* avidin-binding assays (several recent studies), or *(c)* fluorescent derivative assays (two published studies).

Bioassays generally have adequate sensitivity to measure biotin in blood and urine, especially with recent modifications using injected agar plates or metabolic radiometry. However, the bacterial bioassays (and perhaps the eukaryotic bioassays as well) suffer interference from unrelated substances and variable growth response to biotin analogues. Bioassays give conflicting results if biotin is bound to protein (12).

Avidin-binding assays generally measure the ability of biotin *(a)* to compete with radiolabeled biotin for binding to avidin (isotope dilution assays), *(b)* to bind to avidin coupled to a reporter and thus prevent the avidin from binding to a biotin linked to solid phase, or *(c)* to prevent inhibition of a biotinylated enzyme by avidin. A variety of novel reporter systems have recently been described (1). Avidin-binding assays generally detect all avidin-binding substances, although the relative detectabilities of biotin and analogues vary between analogues and between assays, depending on how the assay is conducted. Chromatographic separation of biotin analogues with subsequent avidin-binding assay of the chromatographic fractions appears to be both sensitive and chemically specific.

A problem in the area of biotin analytical technology that remains unaddressed is the disagreement among the various bioassays and avidin-binding assays concerning the true concentration of biotin in human plasma. Reported mean values range from approximately 500 pmol/L to more than 10,000 pmol/L.

ABSORPTION OF BIOTIN

Digestion of Protein-Bound Biotin

Neither the mechanisms of intestinal hydrolysis of protein-bound biotin nor the determinants of bioavailability have been clearly delineated. The content of free biotin and protein-bound biotin in foods is variable, but most biotin in meats and cereals appears to be protein bound. Wolf et al. (13) have postulated that biotinidase plays a critical role in releasing biotin from covalent binding to protein. In patients with biotinidase deficiency, doses of free biotin that do not greatly exceed the estimated dietary intake (e.g., 50–150 μg/day) appear adequate to prevent the symptoms of biotinidase deficiency, suggesting that biotinidase deficiency causes biotin deficiency through impaired intestinal digestion of protein-bound biotin or impaired renal salvage or both.

Intestinal Absorption

Based on the work of Said, Bowman, McCormick, and others (1), a biotin transporter has been demonstrated to be present in the intestinal brush border membrane. Transport is highly structurally specific, temperature dependent, and electroneutral. In the presence of an Na^+ gradient, biotin transport occurs against a concentration gradient. However, at higher (pharmacologic) concentrations, diffusion predominates.

In rats, biotin transport is upregulated with maturation and by biotin deficiency. Although carrier-mediated transport of biotin is most active in the proximal small bowel of the rat, absorption of biotin from the proximal colon is still significant, supporting the potential nutritional significance of biotin synthesized by enteric flora. Clinical studies have also provided some evidence that biotin is absorbed from the human colon, but studies in swine indicate that absorption of biotin from the lower gut is much less efficient than from the upper intestine; further, biotin synthesized by enteric flora is probably not present at a location or in a form in which bacterial biotin contributes importantly to absorbed biotin (14, 15). Exit of biotin from the enterocyte (i.e., transport across the basolateral membrane) is also carrier mediated, but basolateral transport is independent of Na^+, is electrogenic, and does not transport biotin against a concentration gradient.

TRANSPORT OF BIOTIN

Transport in Blood from the Intestine

Biotin is probably transported in blood from the site of absorption in the intestine to the peripheral tissues and the liver, but little has been definitively established concerning the mechanism(s) of transport (1). Wolf et al. (16) originally hypothesized that biotinidase might serve as a biotin-binding protein in plasma or perhaps even as a carrier protein for the transport of biotin into the cell. Based on protein precipitation or equilibrium dialysis after incubation with ^{3}H-biotin, Chuahan and Dakshinamurti (17) concluded that biotinidase is the only protein in human serum that specifically binds biotin. However, using ^{3}H-biotin, centrifugal ultrafiltration, and dialysis to assess reversible binding in plasma from the rabbit, pig, and human, Mock and coworkers (18) found that less than 10% of the total pool of free plus reversibly bound biotin is reversibly bound to plasma protein; the biotin binding observed could be explained by binding to human serum albumin. Using acid hydrolysis and ^{3}H-biotinyl-albumin, Mock and Malik (19) found additional biotin covalently bound to plasma protein. The percentages of free, reversibly bound, and covalently bound biotin in human serum are approximately 81%, 7%, and 12%, respectively.

The results of the two approaches discussed above apparently conflict (1). The importance of either type of biotin binding to the transport of biotin from the intestine to the peripheral tissues is not yet clear.

Transport into the Liver

The uptake of biotin by liver and peripheral tissues from mammals has been the subject of several investigations (1). Studies in a variety of cell lines indicate that uptake of free biotin is mediated both by diffusion and by a specialized carrier system that is dependent upon an Na^+ gradient and temperature. Transport is electroneutral and specific for a free carboxyl group, though not as strongly specific for structure as the intestinal transporter.

Additional studies demonstrated the importance of metabolic trapping, presumably as covalently bound biotin in holocarboxylase enzymes (20). After entering the hepatocyte, biotin diffuses into the mitochondria via a pH-dependent process (21).

Transport into the Central Nervous System

A variety of animal and human studies suggest that biotin is transported across the blood-brain barrier (1). The transporter is saturable and structurally specific for the terminal carboxylate group on the valerate side chain. Transport into the neuron also appears to involve a specific transport system as well as subsequent trapping of biotin by covalent binding to brain proteins, presumably carboxylase.

Renal Handling

Specific systems for the reabsorption of water-soluble vitamins from the glomerular filtrate may contribute importantly to conservation of water-soluble vitamins (22). Animal studies indicate that biotin is reclaimed from the glomerular filtrate against a concentration gradient by a saturable, Na^+-dependent, structurally specific system. Subsequent egress of biotin from the tubular cells occurs via a basolateral membrane transport system that is not Na^+ dependent. Studies in patients with biotinidase deficiency suggest a possible role for biotinidase in the renal handling of biotin.

Placental Transport

Specific systems for transport of biotin from mother to fetus have recently been reported (23–25). Studies using microvillus membrane vesicles and cultured trophoblasts detected a saturable transport system for biotin that is Na^+ dependent and actively accumulates biotin within the placenta, with slower release into the fetal compartment. However, in the isolated, perfused, single cotyledon, net transport of biotin across the placenta was slow compared with placental accumulation. Little accumulation on the fetal side suggests that the overall placental transfer of biotin is most consistent with a passive process.

Transport into Human Milk

Using an avidin-binding assay, Mock and coworkers have concluded that more than 95% of the biotin is free in the skim fraction of human milk (26). The concentration of biotin in human milk varies substantially in some women (27) and exceeds the concentration in serum by one to two orders of magnitude, suggesting a transport system into milk. Bisnorbiotin accounts for approximately 50% and biotin sulfoxide about 10% of the total biotin plus metabolites in early and transitional human milk (28). With postpartum maturation, the biotin concentration increases, but the bisnorbiotin and biotin sulfoxide concentrations still account for 25 and 8%, respectively, at 5 weeks postpartum. Current studies provide no evidence for a predominant trapping mechanism or for a soluble biotin-binding protein.

BIOTIN DEFICIENCY

Circumstances Leading to Deficiency

The fact that normal humans have a requirement for biotin has been clearly documented in two situations: prolonged consumption of raw egg white and parenteral nutrition without biotin supplementation in patients with short gut syndrome and other causes of malabsorption (1). Biotin deficiency also has been clearly demonstrated in biotinidase deficiency. The mechanism by which biotinidase deficiency leads to biotin deficiency probably involves several processes: *(a)* gastrointestinal absorption of biotin may be decreased because deficiency of biotinidase in pancreatic secretions leads to inadequate release of protein-bound biotin; *(b)* salvage of biotin at the cellular level may be impaired during normal turnover of proteins to which biotin is linked covalently; and *(c)* renal loss of biocytin and biotin is probably abnormally increased.

The clinical findings and biochemical abnormalities caused by biotinidase deficiency are quite similar to those of biotin deficiency; the common findings include periorificial dermatitis, conjunctivitis, alopecia, ataxia, and developmental delay (1). These clinical similarities suggest the pathogenesis of biotinidase deficiency involves a secondary biotin deficiency. However, the reported signs and symptoms of biotin deficiency and biotinidase deficiency are not identical. Seizures, irreversible neurosensory hearing loss, and optic atrophy have been observed in biotinidase deficiency but have not been reported in human biotin deficiency.

Based on lymphocyte carboxylase activity and plasma biotin levels, Velazquez and coworkers have reported that biotin deficiency occurs in children with severe protein-energy malnutrition (1). These investigators have speculated that the effects of biotin deficiency may be responsible for part of the clinical syndrome of protein-energy malnutrition.

Accumulating data provide evidence that long-term anticonvulsant therapy in adults can lead to biotin depletion and that depletion at the tissue level can be severe enough to interfere with amino acid metabolism (1).

Biotin deficiency has also been reported or inferred in several other circumstances:

1. *Leiner's disease,* a severe form of seborrheic dermatitis that occurs in infancy: Although a number of studies have reported prompt resolution of the rash with biotin therapy (12), biotin was ineffective in the only double-blind therapeutic trial (29).
2. *Sudden infant death syndrome:* Biotin deficiency in the chick produces a fatal hypoglycemia dubbed "fatty liver-kidney syndrome"; impaired gluconeogenesis due to deficient activity of PC is the cause of the hypoglycemia. Johnson et al. (30) and Heard et al. (31) have proposed that biotin deficiency may cause sudden infant death syndrome (SIDS) by an analogous pathogenic mechanism. They supported their hypothesis by demonstrating that hepatic biotin is significantly lower at autopsy in SIDS infants than in infants dying from other causes. Additional studies (e.g., levels of hepatic PC, urinary organic acids, and blood glucose) are needed to confirm or refute this hypothesis.
3. *Pregnancy:* Concerns about the teratogenic effects of biotin deficiency led to studies of biotin status during human gestation. Some of these studies detected low plasma concentrations of biotin; others did not (1). Recent studies detected increased 3-hydroxyisovaleric acid in more than half of normal women by the third trimester of pregnancy, and urinary excretion of biotin was abnormally low in about 50% of the women studied (10).
4. *Dialysis:* Patients undergoing chronic hemodialysis have been

reported to have reduced (32) or increased plasma concentrations of biotin (33). Yatzidis et al. (34) reported nine patients on chronic hemodialysis who developed either encephalopathy (four patients) or peripheral neuropathy (five patients); all responded to biotin therapy. The etiologic role of biotin in uremic neurologic disorders remains to be determined.

5. *Gastrointestinal diseases or alcoholism:* Reduced blood or liver concentrations of biotin or urinary excretion of biotin have been reported in alcoholism, gastric disease, and inflammatory bowel disease (1).
6. *Brittle nails:* Colombo et al. treated women with brittle fingernails with 2.5 mg biotin per day orally (35) and observed a 25% increase in nail thickness and improved morphology by electron microscopy.

Clinical Findings of Frank Deficiency

Whether caused by egg-white feeding or omission of biotin from total parenteral nutrition, the clinical findings of frank biotin deficiency in adults, older children, and infants are similar. Typically, the findings appear gradually after weeks to several years of egg-white feeding or parenteral nutrition. Hair thinning and progression to loss of all hair including eyebrows and lashes have been reported. A scaly (seborrheic), red (erythematous) rash was present in most; in several, the rash was distributed around the eyes, nose, mouth, and perineal orifices. The appearance of the rash was similar to that of cutaneous candidiasis; typically, *Candida* could be cultured from the lesions. These cutaneous manifestations, in conjunction with an unusual distribution of facial fat, have been dubbed "biotin deficiency facies." Depression, lethargy, hallucinations, and paresthesias of the extremities were prominent neurologic symptoms in most adults. The most striking neurologic findings in infants were hypotonia, lethargy, and developmental delay.

Laboratory Findings of Biotin Deficiency

Although commonly used to assess biotin status in a variety of clinical populations, the putative indices of biotin status in humans had not been previously studied during progressive biotin deficiency. Mock and coworkers (36) induced progressive biotin deficiency by feeding egg white. Urinary excretion of biotin declined dramatically with time on the egg-white diet, reaching frankly abnormal values in 9 of 10 subjects by the 20th day of egg-white feeding. Bisnorbiotin excretion declined in parallel, providing evidence for regulated catabolism of biotin. By day 14 of egg-white feeding, 3-hydroxyisovaleric acid excretion was abnormally high in all 10 subjects providing evidence that biotin depletion decreased the activity of MCC and altered leucine metabolism earlier in biotin deficiency than previously appreciated. Plasma concentrations of free biotin fell to abnormal values in half of the subjects, providing confirmation of the impression (37) that blood biotin concentration is not an early or sensitive indicator of impaired biotin status.

Odd-chain fatty acid accumulation, a marker of biotin deficiency (1), is thought to result from PCC deficiency (Fig. 28.2); the isolated genetic deficiency of PCC results in accumulation of odd-chain fatty acids in plasma, red blood cells, and liver. Apparently, accumulation of propionyl-CoA leads to substitution of propionyl-CoA moiety for acetyl-CoA in the ACC reaction and to the incorporation of a three- (rather than two) carbon moiety during fatty acid elongation.

Biochemical Pathogenesis

The mechanisms by which biotin deficiency produces specific signs and symptoms remain to be completely delineated. However, several studies have given new insights into the biochemical pathogenesis of biotin deficiency. The tacit assumption of most of these studies is that the clinical findings of biotin deficiency result directly or indirectly from deficient activities of the four biotin-dependent carboxylases.

Sander et al. (38) initially suggested that the central nervous system effects of biotinidase deficiency (hypotonia, seizures, ataxia, and delayed development) might be mediated through deficiency of brain PC and the attendant central nervous system lactic acidosis. Support for the central nervous system lactic acidosis hypothesis has come from direct measurements of cerebral spinal fluid lactic acid in children with either biotinidase deficiency or isolated PC deficiency. The work of Suchy, Wolf, and Rizzo (39, 40) has provided evidence *against* an etiologic role for disturbances in brain fatty acid composition.

Several studies demonstrated abnormalities in metabolism of fatty acids in biotin deficiency and suggested that these abnormalities are important in the pathogenesis of the rash and hair loss. Significant abnormalities of the n-6 phospholipids are detectable in blood, liver, and heart, leading to speculation that n-6 abnormalities might result in abnormalities of the prostaglandins and related substances derived from n-6 fatty acids. Supplementation of n-6 polyunsaturated fatty acids (PUFA) prevented development of the cutaneous manifestations of biotin deficiency in a group of rats who were as biotin deficient (based on biochemical measurements) as a control biotin-deficient group that did not receive the supplemental n-6 fatty acids and that did develop the classic rash and hair loss; Mock (41) concluded that an abnormality in n-6 PUFA metabolism does play a pathogenic role in the cutaneous manifestations of biotin deficiency and that the effect of n-6 PUFA cannot be attributed to biotin sparing.

Other Effects of Deficiency

Subclinical biotin deficiency has been shown to be teratogenic in several species including chicken, turkey, mouse, rat, and hamster (1, 42–44). Differences in teratogenic susceptibility among rodent species have been reported; a corresponding difference in biotin transport from mother to fetus has been proposed as the cause (45).

Bain et al. (46) hypothesized that biotin deficiency affects bone growth via effects on the synthesis of prostaglandins derived from n-6 fatty acids. This effect on bone growth might be the mechanism for the teratogenic effects of biotin deficiency.

Diagnosis of Biotin Deficiency

Biotin deficiency can be diagnosed by demonstrating reduced urinary excretion of biotin, increased urinary excretion of the characteristic organic acids, and resolution of the clinical and laboratory abnormalities with biotin supplementation. Plasma or serum levels of biotin, whether measured by bioassay or avidin-binding assay, have not uniformly reflected biotin deficiency.

The clinical response to administration of biotin has been dramatic in all well-documented cases of biotin deficiency. Healing of the rash was striking within a few weeks, and growth of healthy hair generally occurred by 1 to 2 months. Hypotonia, lethargy, and depression generally resolved within 1 to 2 weeks, followed by accelerated mental and motor development in infants. Pharmacologic doses of biotin (e.g., 1–10 mg) have been used to treat most patients.

REQUIREMENTS AND ALLOWANCES

Data providing an accurate estimate of the dietary and parenteral biotin requirements for infants, children, and adults are lacking (47). Oral "safe and adequate intakes" for various age groups of healthy individuals were presented in the 1989 Food and Nutrition report (47) (see also Appendix Table II-A-2-a-3). The 1998 report gives suggested "adequate intakes," which are at lower levels than in the 1989 report (47a) (see also Appendix Table II-A-2-c-1). Oral and parenteral intake of biotin were suggested for preterm infants (48), and for parenteral intake in infants through adults (49).

DIETARY SOURCES OF BIOTIN

There is no published evidence that biotin can be synthesized by mammals; thus, higher animals must derive biotin from other sources. The ultimate source of biotin appears to be de novo synthesis by bacteria, primitive eucaryotic organisms such as yeast, molds, and algae, and some plant species.

The great majority of measurements of biotin content of foods have used bioassays. Despite the limitations due to interfering substances, protein binding, and lack of chemical specificity discussed above, there is reasonably good agreement among the published reports (50–54), and some worthwhile generalizations can be made. Biotin is widely distributed in natural foodstuffs, but the absolute content of even the richest sources is low when compared with that of most other water-soluble vitamins. Foods relatively rich in biotin include egg yolk, liver, and some vegetables. Based on the data of Hardinge and Crooks (50), the average dietary biotin intake was estimated to be approximately 70 μg/day for the Swiss population. This result is in reasonable agreement with the estimated dietary intake in Canada of 60 μg/day (55) and Britain of 35 μg/day (56, 57).

TOXI CITY

Daily doses up to 200 mg orally and up to 20 mg intravenously have been given to treat biotin-responsive inborn errors of metabolism and acquired biotin deficiency; toxicity has not been reported.

ACKNOWLEDGMENTS

Many thanks to Nell Mock for the artwork and Gwyn Hobby for typing this manuscript.

REFERENCES

1. Mock DM. Biotin. In: Ziegler EE, Filer LJ Jr, eds. Present knowledge in nutrition. Washington, DC: International Life Sciences Institutes Nutrition Foundation, 1996;220–35.
2. Miljkovic D, Velimirovic S, Csanadi J, et al. J Carbohydr Chem 1989;8:457–67.
3. Deroose FD, DeClercq PJ. J Org Chem 1995;60:321–30.
4. Brandsch R. J Nutr Sci Vitaminol 1994;40:371–99.
5. Cronan JE Jr. Cell 1989;58:427–9.
6. Knowles JR. Annu Rev Biochem 1989;58:195.
7. McCormick DB. Bio-organic mechanisms important to coenzyme functions. In: Handbook of vitamins. 3rd ed. 1998, in press.
8. Cole H, Reynolds TR, Lockyer JM, et al. J Biol Chem 1994;269:6566–70.
9. Pomponio RJ, Reynolds TR, Cole H, et al. Nature Genet 1995;11:96–8.
10. Mock DM, Stadler D, Stratton SL, et al. J Nutr 1997;27:710–6.
11. Mock DM, Dyken ME. Neurology 1997;49:1444–7.
12. Mock DM. Biotin. In: Brown M, ed. Biotin. 6th ed. Blacksburg, VA: International Life Sciences Institute Nutrition Foundation 1989;189–207.
13. Wolf B, Heard G, McVoy JRS, et al. J Inherited Metab Dis 1984;7:121–2.
14. Kopinski JS, Leibholz J, Bryden WL. Br J Nutr 1989;62:767–72.
15. Kopinski JS, Leibholz J, Bryden WL. Br J Nutr 1989;62:773–80.
16. Wolf B, Grier RE, McVoy JRS, et al. J Inherited Metab Dis 1985;8:53–8.
17. Chuahan J, Dakshinamurti K. Biochem J 1988;256:265–70.
18. Mock DM, Lankford GL. J Nutr 1990;120:375–81.
19. Mock DM, Malik MI. Am J Clin Nutr 1992;56:427–32.
20. McCormick D, Zhang Z. Proc Soc Exp Biol Med 1993;202: 265–70.
21. Said HM, McAlister-Henn L, Mohammadkhani R, et al. Am J Physiol 1992;263:G81–6.
22. Bowman BB, McCormick DB, Rosenberg IH. Annu Rev Nutr 1989;9:187–99.
23. Karl P, Fisher SE. Am J Physiol 1992;262:C302–8.
24. Schenker S, Hu Z, Johnson RF, et al. Alcoholism: Clin Exp Res 1993;17:566–75.
25. Hu Z-Q, Henderson GI, Schenker S, et al. Proc Soc Biol Exp Med 1994;206:404–8.
26. Mock DM, Mock NI, Langbehn SE. J Nutr 1992;122:535–45.
27. Mock DM, Mock NI, Dankle JA. J Nutr 1992;122:546–52.
28. Mock D, Mock N, Stratton S. J Pediatr 1997;131:456–8.

29. Erlichman M, Goldstein R, Levi E, et al. Arch Dis Child 1981;567:560–2.
30. Johnson AR, Hood RL, Emery JL. Nature 1980;285:159–60.
31. Heard GS, Hood RL, Johnson AR. Med J Aust 1983;2:305–6.
32. Livaniou E, Evangelatos GP, Ithakissios DS, et al. Nephron 1987;46:331–2.
33. DeBari V, Frank O, Baker H, et al. Am J Clin Nutr 1984;39:410–5.
34. Yatzidis H, Koutisicos D, Agroyannis B, et al. Nephron 1984;36:183–6.
35. Colombo VE, Gerber F, Bronhofer M, et al. J Am Acad Dermatol 1990;23:1127–32.
36. Mock N, Malik M, Stumbo P, et al. Am J Clin Nutr 1997;65:951–8.
37. Bonjour J-P. Biotin in human nutrition. In: Dakshinamurti K, Bhagavan H, eds. New York: New York Academy of Sciences, 1985;97–104.
38. Sander JE, Packman S, Townsend JJ. Neurology 1982;32: 878–80.
39. Suchy SF, Rizzo WB, Wolf B. Am J Clin Nutr 1986;44:475–80.
40. Suchy SF, Wolf B. Am J Clin Nutr 1986;43:831–38.
41. Mock DM. J Pediatr Gastroenterol Nutr 1990;10:222–9.
42. Watanabe T, Endo A. Teratology 1990;42:295–300.
43. Watanabe T. J Nutr 1993;23:2101–8.
44. Watanabe T, Dakshinamurti K, Persaud TVN. J Nutr 1995;125:2114–21.
45. Watanabe T, Endo A. Am Inst Nutr 1989;119:255–61.
46. Bain SD, Newbrey JW, Watkins BA. Poult Sci 1988;67:590–5.
47. National Research Council. Recommended dietary allowances. 10th ed. Washington, DC: National Academy Press, 1989.
47a. The Food and Nutrition Board—Institute of Medicine. Dietary reference intakes. Thiamin, riboflavin, niacin, vitamin B_6, folate, vitamin B_{12}, pantothenic acid, biotin, and choline. Washington, DC: National Academy press, 1998.
48. Greene HL, Smidt LJ. Water soluble vitamins: C, B1, B2, B6, niacin, pantothenic acid, and biotin. In: Tsang RC, Lucas A, Uauy R, et al., eds. Nutritional Needs of the Preterm Infant. Baltimore: Williams & Wilkins, 1993;121–33.
49. Greene HL, Hambridge KM, Schanler R, et al. Am J Clin Nutr 1988;48:1324–42.
50. Hardinge MG, Crooks H. J Am Diet Assoc 1961;38:240–5.
51. Wilson J, Lorenz K. Food Chem 1979;4:115–29.
52. Hoppner K, Lampi B. Nutr Rep Int 1983;28:793–8.
53. Pennington JAT, Church HN. Biotin. 14th ed. New York: Harper & Row, 1985.
54. Guilarte TR. Nutr Rep Int 1985;32:837–45.
55. Hoppner K, Lampi B, Smith DC. Can Inst Food Sci Technol J 1978;11:71–4.
56. Bull NL, Buss DH. Hum Nutr Appl Nutr 1982;36A:125–9.
57. Lewis J, Buss DH. Br J Nutr 1988;60:413–24.

SELECTED READING

Bonjour J-P. Biotin in human nutrition. In: Dakshinamurti K, Bhagavan H, eds. Biotin. New York: New York Academy of Sciences, 1985;97–104.

Bowman BB, McCormick DB, Rosenberg IH. Epithelial transport of water-soluble vitamins. Annu Rev Nutr 1989;9:187–99.

McCormick DB. Bio-organic mechanisms important to coenzyme functions. In: Handbook of vitamins. 3rd ed. 1998, in press.

Mock DM. Biotin. In: Ziegler EE, Filer LJ JR, eds. Present knowledge in nutrition, Washington, DC: International Life Sciences Institutes Nutrition Foundation, 1996;220–35.

29. Vitamin C

ROBERT A. JACOB

HISTORY

Among specific nutritional deficiency diseases, scurvy has ranked with the highest in its toll of human suffering and death. The symptoms are rather characteristic and appear to be described as far back as the ancient civilizations of the Egyptians, Greeks, and Romans. The disease was rampant in the sea explorers of the 16th to 18th centuries, AD, in whom typical physical symptoms of bleeding and rotting gums, swollen and inflamed joints, dark blotches on the skin, and muscle weakness occurred within months of departure. Throughout this period, the British expeditions suffered greatly because of scurvy. Of Admiral Anson's six ships circling the globe in 1740 to 1744, only the flagship returned, and 1051 men died. The carnage prompted the British Admiralty to seek the cure for scurvy, and in 1747, the Scottish surgeon James Lind performed an early clinical nutrition experiment on board ship. Six different diet supplements were given to six pairs of scorbutic sailors, and the results demonstrated the efficacy of oranges and lemons (and to a lesser extent apple cider) in curing scurvy. Lind published the results in his famous 1753 *Treatise of the Scurvy* wherein he also reasoned that scurvy was due to blocked perspiration resulting from damp salty sea air, resulting in "putrid humors" that had poisonous and noxious qualities when retained in the body. Captain James Cook in voyages from 1768 to 1775 first proved that long sea voyages did not necessarily result in scurvy. Throughout these voyages, he required that the crew eat local greens and grasses at every opportunity, maintain cleanliness, and practice fastidious personal hygiene. The British Admiralty was beset by inconsistent and conflicting accounts of scurvy cures, and it was not until 48 years after Lind's experiment that lemon or lime juice was made a part of routine British naval provisions.

The lessons of the Renaissance explorers were poorly learned by succeeding generations, however. Scurvy besieged 19th century populations on land, including much of Europe during the Great Potato Famine, armies of the Crimean and United States Civil War, arctic explorers, and California gold rush communities. In 1907, scurvy was produced experimentally in the guinea pig, and from 1928 to 1930, Albert Szent-György in Hungary and Glen King in the U.S. independently published their isolations of vitamin C or "hexuronic acid." This pure substance alone prevented and cured scurvy in guinea pigs. It was later named ascorbic acid for its antiscorbutic properties. The molecular structure was determined and an effective laboratory synthesis was developed in 1933. The history of scurvy and vitamin C has been summarized in a well-annotated volume (1).

CHEMISTRY AND ANALYSIS

Ascorbic acid (AA) is the enolic form of an α-ketolactone. The molecular structure (Fig. 29.1) contains two ionizable enolic hydrogen atoms that give the compound its acidic character (pK_{a1} at carbon 3 = 4.17; pK_{a2} at carbon 2 = 11.57). The asymmetric carbon 5 atom allows two enantiomeric forms, of which the L form is naturally occurring. Ascorbic acid is a stable, odorless white solid, formula $C_6H_8O_6$ (176.13 g/mol), which is soluble in water, slightly soluble in alcohol, and insoluble in organic solvents. In aqueous solution, the compound is easily oxidized to the diketo form, dehydroascorbic acid (DHAA), and then further transformed to diketogulonic, oxalic,

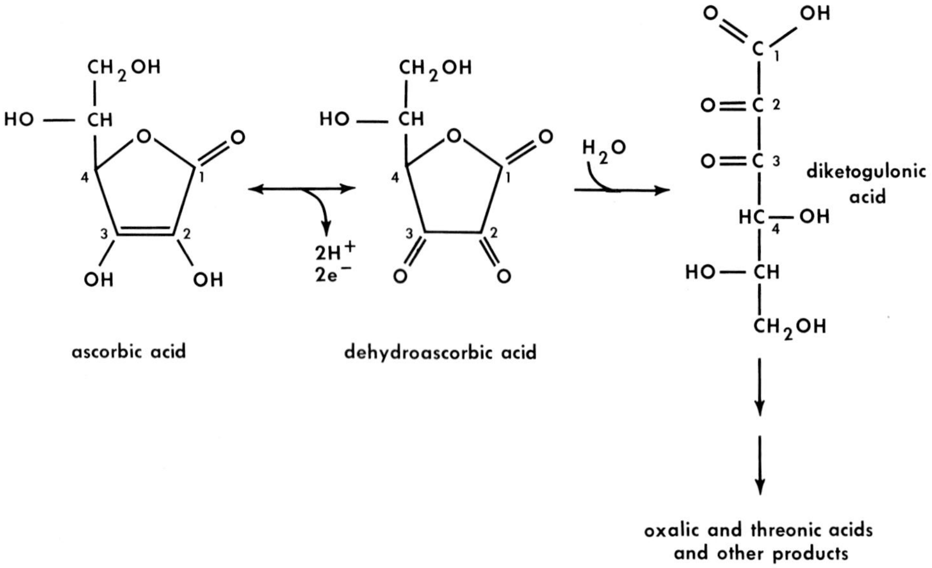

Figure 29.1. Metabolic pathway of ascorbic acid.

and threonic acids, as well as other minor products (Fig. 29.1). The oxidation of AA to DHAA is reversible, but catabolism beyond DHAA is irreversible and is enhanced by alkaline pH and metals, especially copper and iron. Hence, procedures for stabilizing the vitamin in biologic specimens require acidification and sometimes include addition of a reducing agent or metal chelator. Because DHAA is readily reduced in vivo, it possesses vitamin C (antiscorbutic) activity, whereas diketogulonic acid has no activity.

The chemical name for AA is 2,3-didehydro-L-threo-hexano-1, 4-lactone; other terms have included hexuronic acid, cevitamic acid, L-xyloascorbic acid, and vitamin C. Currently, vitamin C is used as the generic descriptor for all compounds exhibiting qualitatively the biologic activity of AA. Therefore, this term refers to both of the common biologically active forms, AA and DHAA.

A variety of analytical procedures for determining the amount of vitamin C in biologic specimens, foods, and pharmaceutical products have been described in which spectrophotometric, fluorometric, chromatographic, and electrochemical techniques are used (2, 3). Total vitamin C, AA, or DHAA can be determined depending on the particular assay technique selected. For example, AA may be determined by colorimetric techniques based on its ability to reduce chromogens such as 2,6-dichloroindophenol or an α,α-dipyridyl-iron complex. Methods that measure the total amount of vitamin C (AA + DHAA) involve oxidation of AA to DHAA and/or diketogulonic acid with copper, iodine, or ascorbate oxidase, followed by derivatization to form colored (e.g., hydrazones with 2,4-dinitrophenylhydrazine) or fluorescent (*o*-phenylenediamine) products. Total vitamin C content has also been determined as AA after reduction of sample DHAA with dithiothreitol or homocysteine. AA or DHAA can be determined by difference after measurements with and without sample pretreatment with exogenous oxidizing or reducing agents (2–4). Recently, automated and microtiter plate spectrophotometric methods for determining plasma and leukocyte AA have been developed to increase assay speed and sensitivity (5, 6).

Although spectrophotometric methods are convenient, high-performance liquid chromatography (HPLC) methods generally provide better specificity and sensitivity. A variety of chromatographic conditions have been used, and AA or DHAA can be determined by the use of ultraviolet, electrochemical or fluorescent detection modes (2, 3, 7, 8). Isoascorbic (erythorbic) acid, the epimer of L-ascorbic acid, can also be determined by HPLC. Its presence in the diet (added as an antioxidant) may result in erroneously high plasma AA values determined by some non-HPLC analytical methods (9).

BIOLOGIC ACTIVITY AND DIETARY INTAKE

AA and DHAA provide biologic vitamin C activity (antiscorbutic), whereas their immediate oxidation product diketogulonic acid and the AA epimer isoascorbic (erythorbic) acid do not. Erythorbic acid, however, is used as a food preservative because it possesses antioxidant properties similar to those of L-ascorbic acid. In this sense, the presence of erythorbic acid in biologic tissues or fluids provides some vitamin C–like activity, analogous to the role of AA as a biologic antioxidant.

Dietary intake surveys estimate U.S. per capita vitamin C intakes at approximately 95 and 107 mg/day for adult women and men (10), and 83 mg/day for children age 1 to 5 years (11). Approximately 90% of the vitamin C in Western diets comes from fruits and vegetables, with citrus fruits and their juices, green vegetables, tomatoes and tomato juice, and potatoes being major contributors (Table 29.1) (10, 12). The mean total vitamin C intake may be higher because of AA added in some processed foods as an antioxidant, and because of the consumption

Table 29.1
Reported Vitamin C Contents of Selected Foods

Food	mg/100 g[a]
Black currants	200
Broccoli	70–163
Brussels sprouts	90–150
Cauliflower	50–90
Strawberries	40–90
Lemons	50–80
Cabbage	31–83
Oranges	40–78
Spinach, fresh	6–70
Spinach, frozen	5–44
Grapefruit	28–48
Pineapple	20–40
Turnips	15–40
Liver, kidney	10–40
Potatoes	10–30
Tomatoes	9–30
Peaches	5–25
Beans	10–22
Bananas	7–19
Peas	10–15
Cucumber	5–14
Apples	5–10
Lettuce	1–7
Cow's milk	1–2
Apple juice	Up to 2
Meat, beef, and pork	Up to 2

From Agricultural Research Service. Composition of foods: raw, processed and prepared. Revision of Agricultural handbook no. 8-9 and 8-11. U.S. Department of Agriculture, Science and Education Administration, 1984, 1986. (Also see Appendix IV-A-23 for additional data.)

[a]mg/100 g × 56.8 = μmol/kg.

of vitamin C supplements by about 35% of the adult U.S. population (11). Consumption of five servings per day of fruits and vegetables as recommended by the USDA and the National Cancer Institute provides more than 200 mg/day of vitamin C.

Values for vitamin C content of food items listed in tables of food composition may represent either AA or total vitamin C, depending on the particular method of analysis. The DHAA content of fresh fruits and vegetables as a percentage of total vitamin C is on the order of 5 to 10%; storage and/or processing may increase the proportion to 30% or greater (10). The AA content of fresh fruits and vegetables may vary appreciably, even among different samples of the same item. The amount of available vitamin C in foods may be significantly reduced because of destruction that occurs during cooking and loss in cooking water. (See also Appendix Table IV-A-21 for the vitamin C content of common foods.)

METABOLISM

Absorption and Bioavailability

AA is absorbed in the human intestine through an energy-dependent active process that is saturable and dose dependent. Intestinal absorption of AA and its entry into cells are facilitated by conversion into DHAA, which is transported across cell membranes more quickly than AA (13). After its entry into the intestinal epithelium or tissue cells, DHAA is readily reduced to AA. At relatively low intakes (below 30 mg per day), AA is nearly completely absorbed, and 70 to 90% of the usual dietary intake of AA (30–180 mg/day) is absorbed (14, 15). However, absorption falls to about 50% with doses of 1 to 1.5 g and to 16% with a 12-g dose (14, 16). Single AA doses above 200 mg that contained ^{14}C-labeled AA resulted in postabsorptive degradation of AA in the intestine to carbon dioxide, which was expired in the breath (17). The amount of label recovered in CO_2 increased from 1 to 30% with increasing amounts of AA ingested, indicating greater postabsorptive AA degradation with the larger doses. The presence of large amounts of unabsorbed AA in the intestine may account for the diarrhea and intestinal discomforts sometimes reported by persons ingesting large doses of AA. Maximal AA absorption is attained by ingestion of several spaced doses of less than 1 g throughout the day rather than ingestion of a single megadose. A saturable absorption mechanism also explains the greater bioavailability sometimes seen for sustained-release forms of AA compared with equivalent pure doses (18). The bioavailability of vitamin C in food and "natural form" supplements is not significantly different from that of pure synthetic AA, despite claims to the contrary by manufacturers of "natural form" vitamin C supplements (19, 20).

Distribution and Transport

As seen in Table 29.2, vitamin C content in body tissues and fluids varies widely, with the highest levels in pituitary, adrenals, leukocytes, eye lens, and brain, and the lowest levels in plasma and saliva (21, 22). Vitamin C concentrations also vary widely in different blood cell types (22–24).

The total AA body pool in adults has been determined experimentally by feeding isotopically (^{13}C, ^{14}C, ^{3}H) labeled AA as a tracer (25–27). Pharmacokinetic data

Table 29.2
Vitamin C Content of Human Tissues and Fluids

Specimen	Vitamin C (μmol/100 g wet)[a]
Pituitary gland	227–284
Adrenal glands	170–227
Leukocytes	40–800
Eye lens	142–176
Brain	74–85
Liver	57–91
Spleen and pancreas	57–85
Kidneys	28–85
Heart muscle	28–85
Semen (whole)	20–60
Lungs	40
Skeletal muscle	17
Testes	17
Cerebrospinal fluid	13–26
Thyroid	11
Plasma	1.7–8.5
Saliva	0.01–0.5

[a]μmol/100 g wet × 0.176 = mg/100 g wet.

from healthy men given doses of 1-^{14}C-labeled AA along with steady-state AA intakes of 30 to 180 mg/day showed that the body half-life of AA was inversely related to intake and that the total body pool of AA increased to a maximum of about 20 mg/kg body weight or about 1500 mg for an average-sized man (25). The maximum body pool was reached at a plasma AA concentration of 57 μmol/L (1.0 mg/dL), attained by 95% of the male population with an AA intake of 100 mg/day (25). In experimental vitamin C depletion studies with healthy male prisoners, clinical symptoms of scurvy appeared at a total body AA pool below 300 mg/day, and disappeared when larger body pools were present (27). In other studies, which did not involve direct isotopic techniques, the estimated AA body pool was 22 mg/kg body weight and 32 to 34 mg/kg fat-free weight (28).

The high concentrations of intracellular AA relative to the plasma are due to an energy-driven cellular transport process. The vitamin is actively transported into human leukocytes by a saturable, temperature-dependent process that exhibits stereospecific preference for L-form over D-form epimers and shows different transport kinetics depending on the cell type (13, 22, 29, 30). Evidence suggests that DHAA is the form of the vitamin that primarily crosses the membranes of intestinal epithelial cells, erythrocytes, and leukocytes, after which it is reduced intracellularly to the active reduced form (29, 31, 32). Both chemical and enzymatic reduction of intracellular DHAA has been reported, with glutathione being the principal source of reducing equivalents (32, 33). Accumulation of AA into isolated human neutrophils and lymphocytes is mediated by both high- and low-affinity transporters, and the vitamin is localized mostly to the cytosol (30, 34). As in plasma (35), intracellular vitamin C exists predominately in reduced form and is not protein bound (30, 34).

Homeostasis

The dose-dependent intestinal absorption of AA discussed above provides a mechanism whereby whole body status of AA is regulated. A second important mechanism involves renal action to conserve or to excrete unmetabolized AA. As the amount of plasma AA increases, the ability of the renal tubules to reabsorb AA reaches a maximum and the unresorbed excess AA is excreted in the urine. This point, called the renal threshold, occurs in humans at plasma AA levels of about 68 μmol/L (1.2 mg/dL). Renal clearance of AA was found to depend on plasma concentrations, linearly between plasma levels of 57 and 227 μmol/L (1.0 and 4.0 mg/dL) and sigmoidally over a larger range (36). Hence, renal regulation of AA conserves body AA stores during low AA intakes through renal tubular reabsorption and limits plasma AA levels by excretion of AA loads that exceed the renal threshold. Plasma AA concentration-time profiles were similar for subjects ingesting AA doses of 0.5, 1.0, or 2.0 g/day for 1 week, and the percentage of the dose recovered in the urine decreased significantly with increasing dosage (36). This indicates that at high AA intakes, saturable intestinal absorption of AA results in a shift of the excess AA load toward the gastrointestinal route relative to urinary excretion. AA concentrations are regulated at the cellular level by controlled cellular transport (29) and enzymatic regeneration of cellular AA from DHAA (32, 33).

Turnover and Catabolism

In healthy nonsmoking men, the half-life of radioisotope-tracer AA was inversely related to the dosage, the average half-life being about 16 to 20 days (25). The half-life decreased from 40 to 8 days with increasing steady-state AA intakes from 30 to 180 mg/day, along with increased total AA turnover (14–134 mg/day) and increased AA body pool (11–22 mg/kg body weight) (25). In healthy prisoners depleted of AA, the whole body turnover of vitamin C, or catabolic rate, depended on the AA body pool size (27). The catabolic rate decreased from 45 mg/day at an initial body pool of 1500 mg to 9 mg/day at a pool size of 300 mg, below which, frank symptoms of scurvy appeared in all subjects. Overall, the body turnover of AA was about 3% of the existing body pool per day (27). At very low or zero intakes of AA, essentially no unmetabolized AA is excreted, yet an obligatory metabolic loss of several milligrams per day occurs. Intake of 8 to 10 mg/day of the vitamin is sufficient to compensate for obligatory catabolism and provide enough AA to satisfy critical functions and prevent overt scurvy symptoms.

In humans, AA is catabolized through oxidation to DHAA, hydrolysis of DHAA to diketogulonate, and decomposition of diketogulonate to a variety of compounds including oxalic and threonic acids, L-xylose, and ascorbate-2-sulfate (Fig. 29.1). The principal route of AA elimination is urinary excretion, with unmetabolized AA and all of the above-named metabolites being eliminated. Initial oxidation of AA to DHAA proceeds through a partially oxidized free radical intermediate, monodehydroascorbate (ascorbyl radical), which is unstable but can be detected by electron paramagnetic resonance spectroscopy. Metabolism of AA to exhaled CO_2 is a minor route of AA catabolism in humans consuming normal dietary intakes of the vitamin (17). Negligible amounts of AA or its metabolites are excreted in feces. The percentage of unmetabolized AA excreted in urine relative to catabolic products increases greatly with increasing dietary intake of AA. Oxalic acid constitutes a minor fraction (5–10%) of AA metabolites, but it seems to be an obligatory product in that it is found even at very low dietary AA intakes. With increasing AA intakes, conversion of AA to oxalate is limited (16, 37).

BIOCHEMICAL FUNCTIONS

The functions of AA are based primarily on its properties as a reversible biologic reductant. As such, it provides reducing equivalents for a variety of biochemical reac-

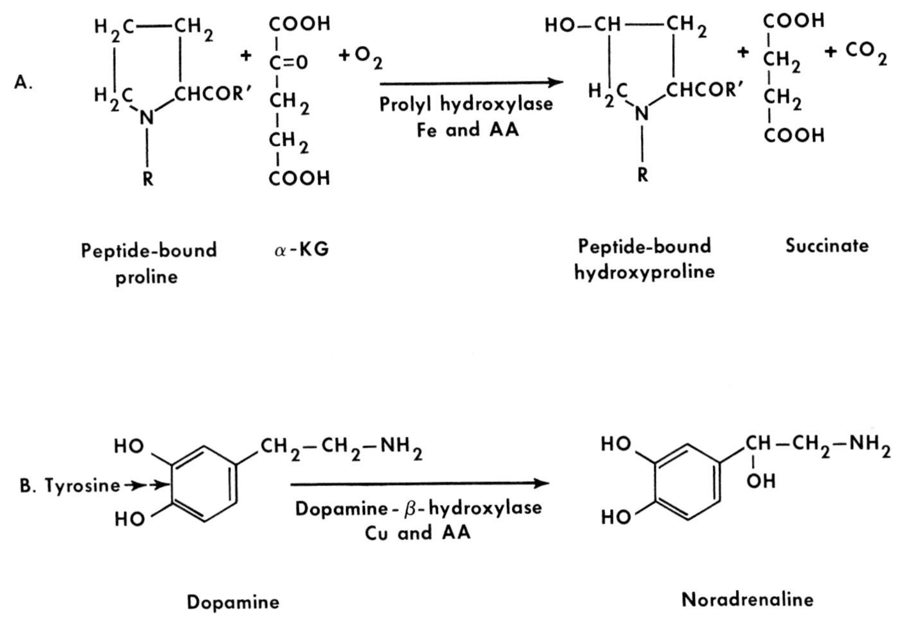

Figure 29.2. Reactions that require ascorbic acid as a cofactor with metals for hydroxylations of proline (**A**) and dopamine (**B**). *AA,* Ascorbic acid; *α-KG,* α-ketoglutarate; noradrenaline (norepinephrine).

tions, is essential as a cofactor for reactions requiring a reduced metal ion (Fe^{2+}, Cu^{1+}), and serves as a protective antioxidant that operates in the aqueous phase and can be regenerated in vivo when oxidized. Few of the roles of AA have been established on a definitive molecular basis. Its roles in metal-catalyzed hydroxylations that use molecular oxygen are best defined (Fig. 29.2). In such cases, AA is believed to act to reduce the metal catalyst, allowing reactivation of the metal-enzyme complex, and/or as a cosubstrate involved in reduction of molecular oxygen. The biochemical roles of AA have been reviewed (28, 38, 39).

Collagen and Connective Tissue

One of the best established roles of AA is as a reductive cofactor for posttranslational hydroxylation of peptide-bound proline and lysine residues during formation of collagen (38, 40). The hydroxyproline and hydroxylysine units allow cross-linking to stabilize the triple helical structure of tropocollagen, an essential subunit of procollagen. The enzyme involved in proline hydroxylation, prolyl hydroxylase, requires molecular oxygen, AA, iron, and α-ketoglutarate (Fig. 29.2*A*). During the hydroxylation reaction, the enzyme-bound iron is oxidized to Fe^{3+} and AA is involved in reactivating the enzyme by reduction of iron back to the ferrous state. In an analogous reaction, AA participates as a cofactor in the hydroxylation of lysine residues catalyzed by copper-dependent lysyl hydroxylase.

Considerable evidence suggests AA involvement in collagen gene expression and related mRNA processing, but specific in vivo mechanisms have not been established (40, 41). AA also influences cellular procollagen secretion and the biosynthesis of other connective tissue components, including elastin, fibronectin, proteoglycans, bone matrix, and elastin-associated fibrillin (40). Although not all details of the processes are clearly resolved, the absolute requirement for AA in formation of mature connective tissue explains the primary physical symptoms of scurvy. The importance of AA for connective tissue formation during in utero development is illustrated by the vascular and skeletal abnormalities observed in the uterus and fetuses of ascorbate-requiring swine made vitamin C deficient (42).

Antioxidant Functions

AA is believed to be the most versatile and effective of the water-soluble dietary antioxidants. AA can readily donate electrons to quench a variety of reactive free radical and oxidant species and is easily returned to its reduced state by such ubiquitous electron donors as glutathione and NADPH (32, 33). The vitamin efficiently scavenges hydroxyl, peroxyl, and superoxide radicals, as well as reactive peroxide, singlet oxygen, and hypochlorite species (43, 44). In addition, AA protects against plasma lipid and low-density lipoprotein (LDL) peroxidation (43, 45). AA appears to protect against lipid peroxidation by scavenging peroxyl radicals in the aqueous phase before they can initiate lipid peroxidation and by regenerating the active form of vitamin E, the important lipophilic antioxidant.

The high levels of AA in the eye provide antioxidant protection against photolytically generated free radicals in various ocular fluids and tissues, including the lens, cornea, vitreous humor, and retina. Concentrations of AA in seminal fluid some 8- to 10-fold higher than blood levels are believed to protect against oxidative damage to sperm proteins. Oxidative stress has been associated with sperm agglutination and decreased male fertility (see discussion of eye disorders and fertility under "Other Clinical and Therapeutic Aspects).

The high AA levels in neutrophils provide cellular and host tissue protection during the respiratory burst in which reactive oxidants and free radicals are produced. Myeloperoxidase-derived hypochlorous acid is scavenged by AA, and lack of sufficient vitamin at sites of inflammation such as the rheumatoid joint may well facilitate proteolytic damage (30).

As an intracellular antioxidant, AA appears to be important in protecting DNA from oxidative damage linked to mutagenesis and the initiation of carcinogenesis. Oxidative damage to sperm DNA, as measured by the oxidatively modified DNA base 8-hydroxydeoxyguanosine, was increased in healthy men given an AA-deficient diet of 5 mg/day and was returned to baseline upon repletion with either 60 or 250 mg/day of AA (46). AA supplementation decreased gastric mucosal DNA damage in gastritis patients as measured by ^{32}P-postlabeling assay and lymphocyte chromosome damage induced by in vitro exposure to bleomycin (47).

Indirect Antioxidant Protection. AA can provide indirect antioxidant protection by supplying electrons to regenerate the active reduced form of other biologic antioxidants such as glutathione, tocopherol, and flavonoids (48). Studies with guinea pigs show that AA regenerates the important endogenous antioxidant glutathione from its oxidized form and that reduced glutathione can regenerate ascorbate from its oxidized form. Thus AA can ameliorate the consequences of induced glutathione deficiency, such as cataracts, and glutathione can delay or prevent the symptoms of scurvy (48). In healthy adult humans supplemented with AA, red cell glutathione rose nearly 50%, and a decrease in red cell lytic sensitivity indicated improved oxidant defense (49). These results indicate that ascorbate functions as a secondary antioxidant by maintaining reduced glutathione, a primary cellular antioxidant.

Considerable in vitro evidence indicates that AA protects lipids indirectly by regenerating the active (reduced) form of tocopherol (50). However, studies in guinea pigs and humans have not shown a biologically significant "sparing" of vitamin E by AA in vivo, although some trends toward protection of human tissue tocopherol by higher AA intakes have been reported (51). Clearly, AA can regenerate some forms of oxidized tocopherol, and this likely occurs to some extent in vivo. However, this interaction may be difficult to demonstrate in vivo because oxidized tocopherol in the cell membrane and lipid-rich tissue is likely regenerated also by other biologic reductants, such as the lipid-soluble ubiquinol, and/or glutathione.

The synergistic antiproliferative effect of AA and flavonoids on carcinoma cells in culture has been attributed to the effect of AA in protecting the flavonoids against oxidation (52).

Neurotransmitter Synthesis and the Nervous System

The importance of AA in neurotransmitter synthesis and metabolism likely underlies the high concentrations and homeostatic control of AA found in adrenal and brain tissue and the relative resistance of these organs to AA depletion (28, 38, 53). AA is a required cofactor for the copper-containing dopamine-β-hydroxylase enzyme that catalyzes hydroxylation of the dopamine side chain to form norepinephrine (Fig. 29.2*B*). In guinea pigs, synthesis of biogenic amines has been shown to be AA dependent. AA is a cofactor for α-amidating monooxygenase enzymes in the biosynthesis of neuropeptides in the adrenals. AA also appears to be involved in the hydroxylation of tryptophan to form serotonin in the brain.

Activity of glutamatergic and dopaminergic neurons has been closely linked to changes in extracellular AA concentration in the brain. Aspects of neural activity modulated by AA concentrations include neurotransmitter membrane receptor synthesis and functions and neurotransmitter dynamics (53). Animal model and cell culture experiments indicate that AA is an important factor in the developing nervous system, particularly for the growth and maturation of glial cells and myelin.

Mixed-Function Oxygenase System

The microsomal drug-metabolizing system operates in liver microsomes and reticuloendothelial tissues to inactivate and metabolize a wide variety of substrates, such as endogenous hormones or xenobiotics (e.g., drugs and carcinogens). The systems operate with oxygenase enzymes, flavoproteins, cytochrome P450 protein, oxygen, and reducing agents such as NAD(P)H. The activity of the system is often affected by AA concentrations, although specific roles for the vitamin have not been elucidated (28). Results of animal studies indicate that AA depletion reduces the activity of system enzymes and the integrity of cytochrome P450 electron transport. Studies in animals and humans show that drug-metabolizing activity is reduced during AA deficiency and that stress (from steroid hormone activation) and/or use of drugs may alter AA metabolism and lower AA body status. Users of oral contraceptives have been shown to have reduced levels of plasma and leukocyte AA. Exposure of rats and guinea pigs to polychlorinated biphenyls (PCBs) increased their requirement for AA and the activity of cytochrome P450 enzymes. The mRNA of these enzymes was increased when mutant ascorbate-requiring rats exposed to PCBs were supplemented with AA (41).

AA is involved in the synthesis of corticosteroids and aldosterone in the adrenal cortex, apparently supplying reducing electrons to mitochondrial P450 enzymes (54). The vitamin is also involved in the hepatic cytochrome P450–dependent microsomal hydroxylation of cholesterol in the conversion of cholesterol to bile acids. Studies with guinea pigs showed that marginal AA deficiency reduces the activity of this rate-limiting step in cholesterol degradation. Animal studies on the effect of increased AA intakes on lipid metabolism have been inconsistent; some indicate no direct effect, whereas another reports an increased rate of cholesterol conversion and decreased blood and liver lipid levels as the ascorbate dose increased (28).

Iron Absorption and Metabolism

AA is involved in the regulation of iron metabolism at a number of points. Ascorbate reduction of iron to the ferrous state is required in iron transfer and storage pathways involving transferrin and ferritin. AA deficiency in guinea pigs results in low serum iron concentrations, iron deficiency, and changes in genetic expression of iron-related proteins (55).

Measurement of iron absorption from single meals by use of isotopic iron tracers shows that dietary AA enhances intestinal absorption of nonheme iron. The mechanism of action is believed to involve the ability of AA to reduce intraluminal iron to the more absorbable ferrous state and/or to counteract the effect of dietary iron absorption inhibitors. However, controlled human studies in which the vitamin is added to meals over long periods have not shown significant improvement of body iron status, indicating that AA has less effect on iron bioavailability than has been predicted from tests with single meals (56).

AA can increase iron absorption and interact with iron to promote oxidative damage, raising concern that high supplemental intakes of AA, a common occurrence in developed countries, exacerbate iron overload and its related pathology. A review of studies assessing iron status during high AA intakes concluded that high intakes are not a significant factor in iron overload (57). Nevertheless, the strong prooxidant nature of the iron-ascorbate couple has been convincingly demonstrated in vitro (58), and reports suggesting a prooxidant effect of high ascorbate concentrations in premature babies (59) and children with cystic fibrosis (60) have recently appeared. In the former case, high levels of serum AA were suggested to inhibit the ferroxidase activity of ceruloplasmin and therefore exacerbate oxidative damage via increased ferrous iron (59). The relevance of possible prooxidant AA-iron interactions to human health warrants further study, especially in cases of iron overload and where free iron may be released into tissues because of inflammation or tissue trauma.

Animal and human studies indicate that AA also affects copper metabolism in a variety of ways, including inhibition of intestinal absorption and ceruloplasmin oxidase activity, and labilization of ceruloplasmin-bound copper for cellular transport (61).

Other Functions

Carnitine Biosynthesis. Carnitine transports long-chain fatty acids across the mitochondrial membrane wherein β-oxidation provides energy to cells, especially for cardiac and skeletal muscle. Carnitine can be considered a conditionally essential nutrient for humans since we obtain carnitine from the diet and also biosynthesize carnitine from lysine and methionine. Ascorbate is required along with iron at two steps in the pathway of carnitine biosynthesis, in reactions similar to the hydroxylation of proline during collagen formation. Muscle carnitine concentrations are significantly decreased in scorbutic guinea pigs, suggesting that loss of carnitine-related β-oxidation energy may explain the fatigue and muscle weakness observed in human scurvy. Studies with guinea pigs and humans indicate that decreased tissue carnitine levels and increased urinary carnitine excretion in AA deficiency are due to defective renal reabsorption of carnitine rather than decreased carnitine synthesis (62, 62a). Increased free plasma carnitine in human AA deficiency was attributed to impaired carnitine transport into tissues because of a rise in δ-butyrobetaine, the immediate biosynthetic precursor to carnitine (63). Although vitamin C deficiency appears to alter carnitine metabolism, the specific interactions and their relevance to functional carnitine status in humans is unclear.

Miscellaneous Functions. AA exerts vasodilatory and anticlotting effects by altering the production of prostacyclin and other prostaglandins (64). The apparent stimulation by AA of prostaglandin synthesis has been hypothesized as a mechanism to explain a variety of reported effects of the vitamin, such as antihistaminic and hypocholesterolemic actions, modified bronchial and vascular tone, immune and insulin responses, and collagen synthesis. Some recent evidence suggests that AA may protect neural and endothelial tissue and affect vascular tone via interactions with nitrite ions, nitric oxide, and/or nitrogen dioxide (65). In some studies, AA increased cellular levels of cyclic nucleotides (cAMP and cGMP), but the mechanism and physiologic significance of this effect is not clear (38). AA prevents uroporphyrin accumulation in hepatocyte cultures and in ascorbate-requiring rats by inhibiting the oxidation of uroporphyrinogen, suggesting a role for the vitamin in preventing uroporphyria in humans (66). Vitamin C, as ascorbate-2-sulfate, has been suggested to serve as a sulfating agent, both of cholesterol as part of its catabolism and of mucopolysaccharides during formation of connective tissue. Evidence relating AA to immune function, risk of degenerative diseases, respiratory function, and other clinical conditions is discussed under "Clinical and Therapeutic Aspects."

DEFICIENCY

Due to a lack of the enzyme required to convert L-gulonolactone to AA, humans are among the few species unable to synthesize AA from glucose. When dietary intake of AA is insufficient, humans exhibit a set of reproducible conditions termed *scurvy.* The scurvy symptoms listed in Table 29.3 have been observed in both naturally occurring and experimentally induced scurvy (27). The mesenchymal symptoms result primarily from defects in connective tissue formation. A variety of hemorrhagic manifestations occur, including bleeding into joints, the peritoneal cavity and/or pericardial sac, and the adrenals

Table 29.3
Clinical Manifestations of Vitamin C Deficiency

Mesenchymal
Petechiae
Ecchymoses
Coiled hairs
Perifollicular hemorrhages
Inflamed and bleeding gums
Hyperkeratosis
Sjögren's syndrome
Dyspnea
Joint effusions
Arthralgia
Edema
Impaired wound healing
Systemic
Weakness
Fatigue
Lassitude
Psychologic and neurologic
Depression
Hysteria
Hypochondriasis
Vasomotor instability

in severe cases. A decrease in the ability of the gingiva to resist inflammation and bleeding seems to be an early physical sign of AA deficiency. As seen in Figure 29.3, even moderate (nonscorbutic) experimental AA depletion increased gingival bleeding in healthy men (67). In infants, AA deficiency may result in bone abnormalities, including impaired bone growth and disturbed ossification. Hemorrhagic symptoms may occur, such as retrobulbar and subperiosteal hemorrhages, epistaxis, hematuria, purpura, and resultant hypochromic anemia because of blood loss. The hemorrhagic manifestations of AA deficiency are presumed to be related to defective vascular tissue integrity, although no specific histologic defect has been identified. Adverse effects of AA deficiency on blood clotting are indicated by recent evidence that oxidative degradation of some blood coagulation factors is inversely related to plasma AA concentration (68).

A molecular basis for the weakness and fatigue associated with scurvy has not been established; alterations of iron or carnitine metabolism may be involved. Psychologic symptoms are likely related to altered neurotransmitter synthesis and metabolism. Some historically reported symptoms of scurvy may be attributable to coexisting nutrient deficiencies in thiamine, "wet beriberi" (edema), vitamin A (night blindness), vitamin D (rickets), and folic acid (megaloblastic anemia).

Prevalence

Clinical scurvy is rare in developed countries but is still occasionally seen in individuals with exceptionally poor

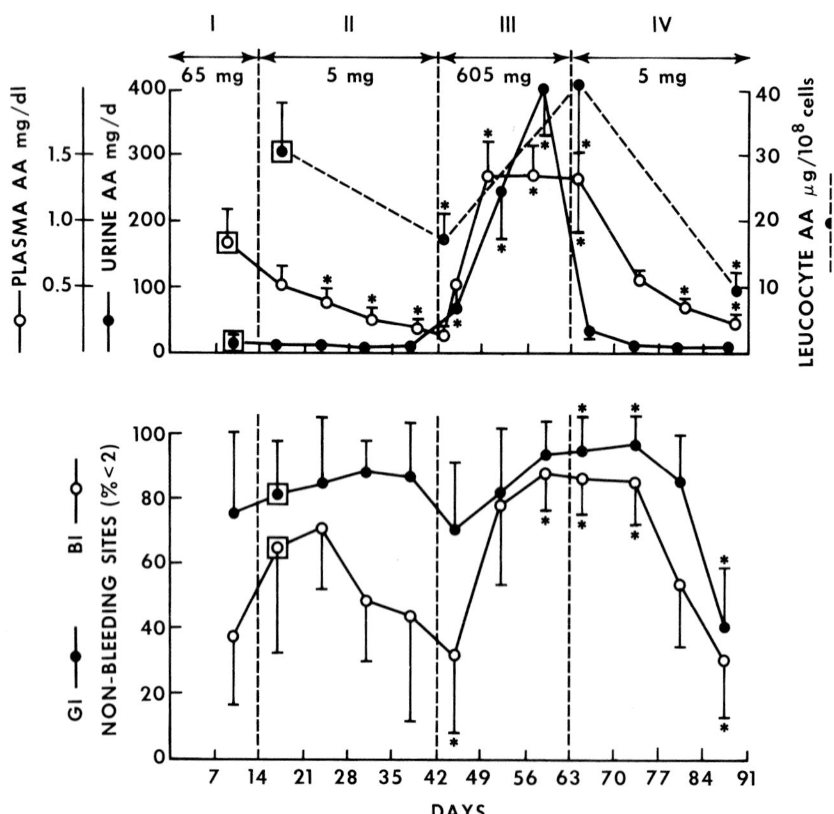

Figure 29.3. Blood and urine ascorbic acid levels and gingival bleeding indices in 11 healthy adult men receiving various ascorbic acid intakes between 5 and 605 mg/day as shown at *top*. *GI*, gingival index; *BI*, bleeding index (mg/dL × 56.8 = μmol/L). (From Leggott PJ, Robertson PB, Rothman DL, et al. J Periodontol 1986;57:480–5, with permission.)

diets (e.g., in alcoholism and drug abuse), peculiar or restricted diets, or diets with a near total lack of AA-containing foods. Most often, it is noted in elderly men who live alone and eat a diet frequently low in fruits and vegetables. Because breast milk provides adequate AA and infant formulas are fortified with AA, infantile scurvy is rarely seen.

Among U.S. population groups, the prevalence of low blood AA concentrations is higher in men than in women, higher in groups with lower socioeconomic status, and highest (about 20%) in poor elderly men (11). A greater proportion of low blood AA levels is observed in elderly persons who are institutionalized, housebound, or chronically sick (69). The trend to lower plasma and leukocyte AA levels observed in the elderly is not explained by differences in renal handling of AA (70). Although many factors related to aging have been postulated to explain lower AA levels in elderly individuals, no convincing evidence that any of these factors results in deficient AA status or an increased AA requirement in healthy elderly persons has been reported.

STATUS ASSESSMENT

Since no reliable functional tests of AA deficiency have been established, measurement of plasma and leukocyte AA levels remain the most practical and reliable tests for assessing human vitamin C status. Assessment of the total body AA pool provides a good integrated measure of status, but practical methods for making this determination have not been devised. Lack of increase in serum or urinary AA excretion after an oral vitamin C load can provide a useful test of AA tissue deficit in individuals, but this type of test is not practical for use in nutrition surveys (71).

Plasma and Leukocyte Tests

Plasma AA levels have generally been shown to correlate with dietary AA intake and with leukocyte AA in both epidemiologic and experimental studies (9, 24, 72, 73). The direct response of plasma and leukocyte AA levels to experimental changes in AA intake is shown in the top half of Figure 29.3 for 11 healthy adult men housed in a metabolic unit for 14 weeks (72). Plasma AA levels are most responsive to recent dietary intake, whereas leukocyte levels change more slowly but reflect AA tissue contents and the body pool more closely. Studies with monkeys and guinea pigs have confirmed that of a variety of blood AA measures, leukocyte AA levels correlate best with liver AA and AA body pool (24). Mixed leukocytes (e.g., the "buffy coat") constitute a heterogeneous mixture of blood cells for which interpretation of results is not standardized (see "Interpretive Guidelines"). Plasma AA tests are preferred for large population studies because the test requires less blood, is easier to perform, and yields results that are interpreted easily and reliably.

The typical relationship between plasma AA and dietary vitamin C intake is shown in Figure 29.4 for a healthy elderly population (74). The curve is similar to those published from a variety of other studies, both experimental and population based, in which steady-state plasma AA levels rise steeply from low vitamin C intakes below 20 mg/day and plateau between 68 and 102 μmol/L (1.2–1.8 mg/dL) at intakes above 200 mg/day (16, 72, 74).

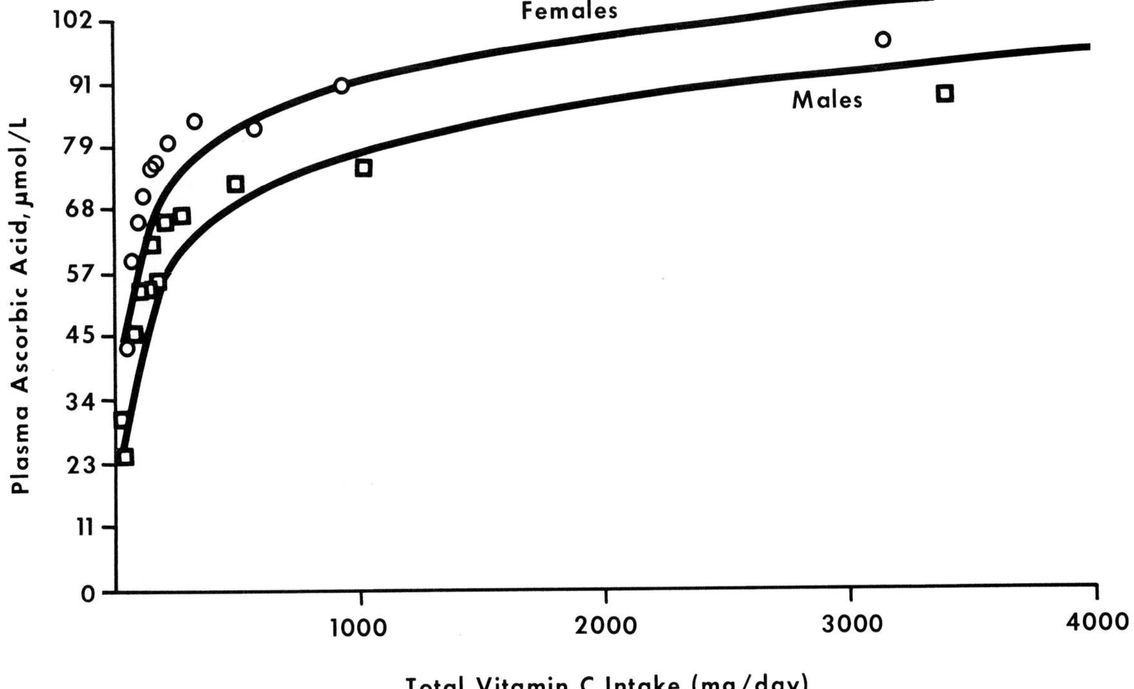

Figure 29.4. Plasma ascorbic acid versus total vitamin C intake (diet plus supplements) for elderly males (*N* = 235) and females (*N* = 442). Median plasma ascorbate values plotted at the median intakes for 12 percentiles of intake. (From Jacob RA, Otradovec CL, Russell RM, et al. Am J Clin Nutr 1988;48:1436–42, with permission.)

Other Tests

The pattern of changes in whole blood and erythrocyte AA levels after AA depletion in humans is qualitatively the same as for plasma levels, because of a relatively rapid exchange of the vitamin between plasma and red cells. Whole blood or erythrocyte AA levels are considered a less sensitive indicator of AA deficiency, however, because they do not change as much or fall as low as plasma levels during AA deficiency. In subjects nearly depleted of the vitamin, in whom scurvy symptoms exist or are imminent (AA body pool less than 300 mg), whole blood AA levels will fall to 17 μmol/L (0.3 mg/dL) or below, whereas plasma AA levels are less than 5.7 μmol/L (0.1 mg/dL).

The rate of excretion of AA in urine is not linear with AA intake because of efficient renal reabsorption at low AA intakes and renal clearance at high intakes. Healthy adults ingesting a normal Western diet containing 40 to 100 mg/day of AA would be expected to excrete some 5 to 50 mg/day of unmetabolized AA. At plasma AA levels exceeding the renal reabsorption threshold, about 68 μmol/L (1.2 mg/dL), excretion of AA increases abruptly with increased AA intake (Fig. 29.3). At AA intakes below 40 mg/day, urine AA excretion falls dramatically to less than 10 mg/day and to nearly undetectable levels in scurvy or in severe AA depletion. Hence, urinary AA content can be used to affirm a diagnosis of frank AA deficiency but is not useful for differentiating between subjects with normal or low but nonscorbutic AA status. Direct measurement of the AA body pool has been accomplished by radioisotope dilution techniques (25, 27), but no practical tests for the AA body pool have been developed. Salivary AA content does not appear to be a good measure of vitamin C status, as low or undetectable levels of salivary AA have been reported in nonscorbutic subjects, and salivary AA levels generally have not been found to correlate well with AA intake, plasma AA, or leukocyte AA levels (72).

Interpretive Guidelines

The reference ranges listed in Table 29.4 are general guidelines for interpreting biochemical AA measures. The guidelines for interpreting plasma AA levels are relatively well established. Few data on AA body pool measurements are available, however, and reported ranges of leukocyte AA vary greatly, in part because of the heterogeneous nature of blood cells and technical difficulties in their separation and analysis. Generally, the "deficiency" category represents frank vitamin C deficiency, in which clinical symptoms are either apparent or imminent. The "low" category represents a state of moderate risk for developing overt vitamin deficiency symptoms because of low AA intake and/or depleted body pool.

Unlike plasma levels, interpretation of leukocyte AA levels is complicated by differing AA concentrations among the various cell types. Mononuclear cells have AA levels two to three times those of polymorphonuclear (PMN) cells. Other clinical and physiologic factors (e.g., infection, drugs, and glycemic state) affect leukocyte AA levels because of alterations in either cell populations or their AA uptake. Similarly, AA concentrations of the heterogeneous "buffy coat" may be affected by diverse factors unrelated to AA nutriture, especially in clinical conditions (24). For leukocyte assay, determination of AA in isolated fractions of mononuclear or PMN cells appears to be the best choice; data are insufficient to recommend one over the other.

The oxidized form of the vitamin, DHAA, is present in negligible amounts in the plasma of healthy subjects (35). In leukocytes, however, a dynamic relationship exists between AA and DHAA, especially in phagocytic cells in which AA is active as an antioxidant and free radical scavenger attendant to the respiratory burst and DHAA is rapidly converted back to AA. Reported levels of DHAA in human leukocytes range from zero to nearly half of the total cellular content of vitamin C, although the vitamin exists in isolated human neutrophils solely in the reduced form (30). How much of the reported leukocyte levels of DHAA truly exists in vivo and how much results from methodologic (oxidative) artifacts is not clear.

Effects of Gender, Smoking, and Age

Results from a nutrition survey of healthy elderly Boston area residents shown in Figure 29.5 illustrate typical effects of gender (higher in women than men) and

Table 29.4
Guidelines for Interpreting Biochemical Measures for Ascorbic Acid Status[a]

	Plasma (μmol/L [mg/dL])[b]	Body Pool (mg)	Mixed Leukocytes (nmol/10^8) cells [μg/10^8 cells])[c]	Mononuclear Leukocytes (nmol/10^8 cells [μg/10^8 cells])
Adequate	>23 [>0.4]	>600	>114 [>20]	>142 [>25]
Low	11.4–23 [0.2–0.4]	300–600	57–114 [10–20]	114–142 [20–25]
Deficient	<11.4 [<0.2]	<300	<57 [<10]	<114 [<20]
Normal range	23–84 [0.4–1.5]	500–1500 [10–22 mg/kg]	114–301 [20–53]	142–250 [25–44]

[a]Upper end of ranges may be higher in subjects taking vitamin C supplements.
[b]μmol/L ÷ 56.8 = mg/dL.
[c]nmol/10^8 cells ÷ 5.68 = μg/10^8 cells; mixed leukocytes are buffy coat or mixed cell fraction containing neutrophils and mononuclear cells; 10^8 cells ~ 100 μL.

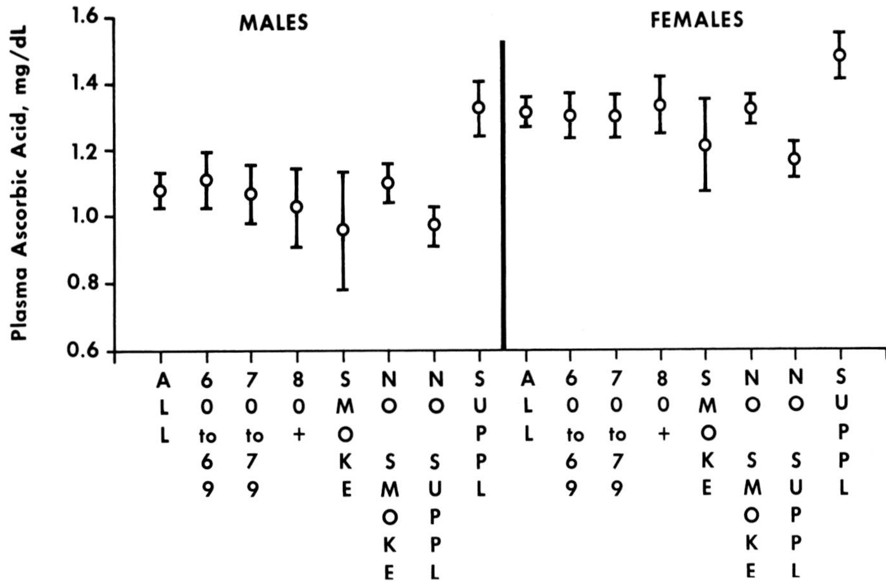

Figure 29.5. The 95% confidence intervals of the mean for plasma ascorbic acid in 677 healthy elderly by gender, age decade, cigarette smoking, and ascorbic acid supplement use (mg/dL × 56.8 = μmol/L). (From Jacob RA, Skala JH, Omaye ST, et al. Biochemical methods for assessing vitamin C status of the individual. In: Livingston GE, ed., Nutritional status assessment of the individual. Trumbull CT: Food & Nutrition Press, 1989;323–38, with permission.)

smoking (lower in smokers) on plasma AA concentrations (74). Women had higher plasma AA levels than men for all subgroups of age, smoking, or AA supplement use, even though dietary AA intakes were approximately the same. The gender-related differences in plasma AA concentrations are not explained by differences in renal handling of AA but are apparently due to such gender-related differences as lean body mass and hormonal influences (70). In nearly all studies, smokers show lower AA levels in plasma and leukocytes than nonsmokers, and lower dietary AA intake by smokers only partially explains the difference (24, 75). These findings suggest a higher AA dietary requirement for smokers, as discussed below. No significant relationship between age and plasma AA levels exists in the data presented in Figure 29.5, although the mean values for men tend to decrease with age. The AA status of the elderly population is discussed above.

DIETARY REQUIREMENTS

Beyond the absolute requirement of 5 to 10 mg/day to prevent scurvy, the human dietary requirement for vitamin C remains controversial. Current worldwide recommendations for vitamin C intake vary from 30 to 100 mg/day. The increases in the allowances over that required to prevent scurvy are based primarily on providing a total body pool of ascorbate (e.g., 900–1500 mg) that will ensure against scorbutic symptoms even after weeks of low ascorbate intake or periods of physiologic or exogenous stress that may increase the vitamin turnover or requirement. Given an AA turnover of about 3% of the body pool per day and development of the first scorbutic symptoms and/or reduction of total AA body pool to 300 mg or less in 24 to 30 days for both men and women, the RDA (recommended dietary allowance) in the United States was set in 1989 at 60 mg/day for adult men and women (see Appendix Table II-A-2-b-2) (75). To cover 95% of the population, the 60 mg/day value is 2 SD above the mean intake estimated to provide adequate vitamin C reserves. The 60 mg/day intake precludes appearance of scorbutic symptoms for at least 4 weeks, even in the face of deficient AA intakes and/or increased use and needs and also provides plasma and leukocyte AA levels above the "at risk" or low levels listed in Table 29.4 for most of the population. An AA intake of 60 mg/day is easily achieved in normal Western diets; median intakes of vitamin C in the U.S. in 1989–91 were above the RDA for all major population subgroups (76). The United Kingdom (Appendix Table II-A-4-d) and World Health Organization (Appendix Table II-A-8-a) value of 30 mg/day is deemed adequate for the population because it is about three times that needed to prevent scurvy.

Special Requirements

The lower plasma and leukocyte AA levels found in *smokers* (compared with nonsmokers) are explained only in part by their lower AA intakes. Radioisotope-labeled AA dilution studies showed that the metabolic turnover of AA in smokers averaged about twice that of nonsmokers (70.0 vs. 35.7 mg/day) (26). The reason for this difference has not been established, although increased AA catabolism caused by the oxidative stress of smoking has been suggested. The lower levels of AA and decreased AA half-life in smokers puts them at comparatively greater risk for development of AA deficiency. Hence the RDA in the United States is set at 100 mg/day for smokers, 40 mg higher than that for nonsmokers (75).

Despite frequently observed low blood AA levels as well as possible increased needs because of sickness and therapeutic drug use, no increase in the vitamin C allowance for the *elderly* has been established because convincing evidence of an increased requirement or AA turnover related to aging alone has not been reported (see discussion above of elderly AA status under "Deficiency"). As discussed above, additional dietary AA may significantly enhance nonheme iron absorption. This effect may be important in vegetarians or individuals with limited heme iron intakes, but the uncertain benefit of this effect to most omnivorous individuals does not justify increasing recommended AA intakes on a population basis.

Plasma AA levels of women decrease during *pregnancy*, primarily because of hemodilution. However, the plasma AA levels of the fetus and neonate are some 50% higher than those of the mother, indicating active transplacental transport and a relatively higher body pool of the vitamin. Based solely on the weight of a near-term fetus, the increased maternal requirement for AA would be about 3 to 4 mg/day, although AA turnover in the fetus is believed to be greater than that for adults. The RDA therefore includes an additional intake of 10 mg/day for pregnant women to compensate for AA losses during pregnancy and to maintain an adequate body pool (75).

Human breast milk contains 170 to 568 μmol/L (3–10 mg/dL) of AA, and average milk volumes are 750 mL/day (first 6 months) and 600 mL/day (7–12 months). To allow for variation in AA level and milk production, the RDA for lactating women includes an additional increment of 35 mg/day during the first 6 months of *lactation* and 30 mg/day thereafter (75).

On the basis of a complete lack of reports of scorbutic symptoms in breast-fed *infants* receiving 7 to 12 mg/day of AA and in formula-fed infants receiving about 7 mg/day, an intake of 30 mg/day is recommended to provide adequate vitamin C reserves plus a margin of safety in 95% of the population of infants during the first 6 months of life (75). Beyond 6 months, the requirements gradually increase to the adult level.

Evidence for Benefits of Higher Intakes

A great deal of evidence, covered briefly below, suggests that AA intake beyond that required to prevent scurvy may reduce the risk of developing chronic diseases such as cancer, coronary heart disease, age-related eye diseases, and neurodegenerative diseases. These results raise questions as to whether the goal of recommendations for AA intake should be plasma and/or tissue ascorbate saturation rather than prevention of scurvy symptoms. For example, authors of a recent pharmacokinetic study of AA intakes from 30 to 2500 mg/day in healthy men recommended an increase in the RDA to 200 mg/day, based partly on determination of AA plasma saturation (16). However, because body ascorbate accumulation is limited by homeostatic mechanisms including saturable absorption and renal excretion, ascorbate intakes required to maximize the body pool are only 100 to 150 mg/day in healthy nonsmoking adult men and about 150 and 80 mg/day for healthy elderly men and women, respectively (47).

The limitation on increasing the body ascorbate pool by higher intakes is one reason why recommended intakes for the vitamin have not been increased significantly. Otherwise, much of the evidence suggesting health benefits for higher intakes of AA is based on in vitro and animal studies whose results may or may not be relevant to humans and epidemiologic studies that show *associations* of the vitamin with reduced disease risk but cannot sort out what factors may be the responsible agents. Increasing evidence indicates that a wide variety of dietary substances besides AA contributes to reduced disease risk. The evidence that higher AA intakes alone provide health benefits to humans is mixed. While higher AA intakes may be recommended for certain groups such as smokers and those under a variety of stresses, the current data suggesting health benefits for consumption of higher doses are controversial and not widely accepted as a justification for recommending higher intakes as a public health measure.

CLINICAL AND THERAPEUTIC ASPECTS

Over the past three decades, a great deal of evidence suggesting health benefits for AA intake beyond that needed to prevent scurvy has been reported. While much of the evidence derives from in vitro, animal, and limited human studies, the few controlled human intervention trials have provided mixed results. A brief review of proposed extrascorbutic and clinical roles follows. The reader is referred to other sources for expanded and detailed coverage (28, 77–82).

Immune Function

Various immune-related functions are altered by ascorbate nutriture, including neutrophil chemotaxis, lymphocyte proliferation, antimicrobial and natural killer cell activities. The vitamin also affects many immune system modulators such as blood histamine, serum complement, prostacyclin, prostaglandins, and B- and T-cell cyclic nucleotides (83–86).

Results from studies of the effects of AA supplements on immune functions have not been consistent, perhaps because of methodologic problems in assessing immunocompetence and extrapolating the results of animal model and isolated cell studies to steady-state immune function in humans. Many studies suggest that the vitamin has beneficial effects, while other studies show no effects, or negative effects. Because of active transport of AA into leukocytes, attempting to increase leukocyte AA levels via increased dietary intake is questionable. For example, in a double-blind study of 24 healthy free-living women, ingestion of 1 or 4 g of AA daily produced increases in serum AA levels relative to the placebo group, but no differences were evident in leukocyte AA levels or leukocyte function (87).

AA inactivates or inhibits a wide range of viruses in vitro, including HIV (85), yet no clinical efficacy has been demonstrated. A review of 21 controlled human trials of megadose ascorbate intake and the common cold showed no consistent effect on reducing the incidence of colds, although the duration of episodes and severity of symptoms was reduced by an average of 23% (85). The basis for the reported decreases in severity of colds may lie in the antihistaminic action of the vitamin and/or its ability to reduce inflammation associated with reactive oxidants produced by phagocytic leukocytes. Results from a study of healthy adults supplemented with AA indicated that the vitamin may enhance neutrophil chemotaxis indirectly by reducing the immunosuppressive effects of histamine in vivo (86).

Controlled experimental depletion of ascorbate in healthy men, short of scurvy, decreased delayed skin hypersensitivity responsiveness but had no effect on lymphocyte proliferation capability (88). AA supplementation reduced the incidence of upper respiratory tract infection in marathon runners, suggesting similar benefits for the sedentary; however, interpretation of the study results has been criticized (79). As for many questions relating to the health benefits of vitamin C, claims of improved immunocompetence with high vitamin intake are controversial.

Cancer

Evidence suggesting a role for AA in cancer prevention is derived primarily from cell culture, animal model, and human epidemiologic studies (79, 89–93). Possible anticarcinogenic effects of AA likely involve its ability to block carcinogenic processes through antioxidant activity, to detoxify carcinogens, and/or to enhance immunocompetence. AA has been shown to prevent formation of carcinogenic substances, such as nitrosamines, in foods and in the gastrointestinal tract. The vitamin has also been reported to detoxify chemical mutagens and carcinogens, including anthracene, benzpyrene, organochlorine pesticides, and heavy metals. As a free-radical scavenger, the vitamin is believed to be important in preventing oxidative damage to proteins, DNA, and cell membranes. Oxidative damage to human sperm DNA, as determined by levels of 8-hydroxy-2′-deoxyguanosine, was increased in men consuming low dietary intakes of AA and was inversely related to semen AA levels (46). Lymphocytes can effectively destroy some types of cancer cells, and certain immune functions such as chemotaxis and natural killer cell activity may be augmented by AA.

Evidence that AA provides an antitumorigenic effect in animals exposed to carcinogens is seen in many but not all animal studies (mice, rat, and hamster). Some protective effects of AA have also been seen in tumor cell transplant and cell culture experiments, but results have been inconsistent. Some experimental studies have indicated that AA may enhance carcinogenesis and tumor formation (92).

Epidemiologic studies show strong associations of AA nutriture with reduced risk for cancers of the oral cavity, esophagus, stomach, and pancreas, somewhat less strong evidence for protection against cancers of the lung, cervix, rectum, and breast, and weak or no evidence for protection against cancers of the colon, bladder, ovaries, and prostate (90, 91). However, associations of AA-containing foods and decreased cancer occurrence cannot be attributed to the actions of AA alone, as numerous other putative anticarcinogenic micronutrients and dietary/lifestyle factors may be involved.

AA is actively secreted into the gastric juice, where it is postulated to reduce cancer risk by reduction of carcinogenic nitrosamines or prevention of oxidative damage in the gastric mucosa (93, 94). Increased oxidative damage to the gastric mucosa has been reported in patients with *Helicobacter pylori*–associated gastritis, a condition that predisposes to gastric cancer (94). The evidence suggests that increasing gastric juice AA concentrations by eradication of *H. pylori* and/or by AA supplementation may reduce the risk of developing gastric cancer.

Evidence for a chemopreventive effect of AA from controlled intervention trials is also limited by study design factors, such as study of multiple nutrients, high-risk populations, small numbers of subjects, and measurement of surrogate cancer markers over relatively short time periods. To date, the few controlled clinical intervention trials have generally shown no benefit of AA supplementation toward reduced cancer risk. Whereas experimental and epidemiologic evidence suggests a protective effect of AA nutriture on esophageal and gastric cancer (93), results from the 6-year Linxian, China, micronutrient intervention trial showed no benefit from a vitamin C–molybdenum supplement in a population having low AA status and a high rate of esophageal and stomach cancer (95). Overall, the present data do not provide strong support for the claim that high AA intakes protect against human cancer.

Studies reporting a therapeutic use of AA for treatment of cancer have been neither abundant nor consistent. Prolongation of survival, even cures, of cancer patients by AA megadosing has sometimes been claimed but has not been corroborated by controlled studies. Current data suggest no utility for AA as a cancer treatment agent.

Heart Disease

AA has been reported to affect a variety of factors associated with heart disease risk, including vascular tissue integrity, vascular tone, lipid metabolism, and blood pressure (96–98). The elasticity and structural integrity of the vascular matrix depends on ascorbate as an essential cofactor for molecular cross-linking of collagen; hence the connective tissue–related defects found in scurvy likely result from aberrant cross-linking. AA has beneficial effects on the human cardiovascular system beyond collagen formation. The vitamin inhibits plasma LDL oxidation, an in vivo event linked with initiation of atherosclerosis in the vascular intima (45). Ascorbate also exerts vasodilatory and anticlotting effects by altering the production of prostacyclin and other prostaglandins (64).

Human studies have shown mixed results as to the efficacy of AA in reducing heart disease risk and occurrence. Increased vitamin C intake has been linked with an improved blood lipid profile of total and HDL cholesterol, and with decreases in blood pressure (96, 97). However, treatment of elderly hypertensives for 6 weeks with 500 mg/day of AA provided no significant improvement in blood pressure compared with placebo (99). While in vitro studies suggest that ascorbate is an effective antioxidant against plasma lipid and LDL oxidation, results from the Nurses and Health Professionals prospective cohort studies showed that consumption of vitamin E, but not vitamin C, was associated with reduced coronary disease (45, 97). Furthermore, a 20-year follow-up cohort study of elderly persons in Britain showed that AA status was strongly associated with decreased risk of subsequent stroke but not of coronary heart disease (100). A review summarizes evidence linking vitamin C to reduced heart disease risk as largely circumstantial but suggesting an association (96). More recent reviews state that limited results from controlled intervention trials of antioxidant vitamins, including vitamin C, do not presently support the hypothesis of heart disease protection suggested by experimental and epidemiologic evidence and that the hypothesis is promising but unproven until corroborated by results from randomized trials designed specifically to answer this question (101, 102).

Other Clinical and Therapeutic Aspects

Evidence linking AA nutriture to a variety of other physiologic functions and disease conditions is briefly reviewed below. The cited references are recommended for comprehensive and detailed coverage (28, 77, 79, 80–82). As for the vitamin's links with degenerative diseases and immunocompetence, the evidence is not sufficiently convincing to recommend vitamin-based therapies or widespread increases in AA dietary intakes as prophylactic measures.

Improvement in a variety of *pulmonary functions* has been related to increased AA nutriture, possibly because of the vitamin's actions in degrading histamine, in attenuating free radical–related inflammation, and in modulating smooth muscle contractility via prostaglandin syntheses (103–105). Human studies have found AA-related improvements in forced expiratory volume, forced vital capacity, acute respiratory infections, and bronchial reactivity. Clinical studies relating AA status to the occurrence of asthma have provided conflicting results, however.

High AA levels in the humors and tissues of the eye protect against damage from photolytically generated free radicals that may result in *cataracts and macular degeneration.* Some human studies show that AA nutriture is directly associated with reduced risk of age-related eye diseases, cataracts, and macular degeneration; however, the evidence linking ascorbate alone to reduced eye disease is neither consistent nor conclusive. In recent studies, dietary carotenoids, vitamin E, or a combination of antioxidants showed stronger associations with reduced risk for these eye disorders than did AA alone (106–108). In contrast to evidence that AA protects against cataract formation, a variety of studies suggest that AA can facilitate lens opacities via the Maillard reaction or by the actions of AA breakdown products (109).

Ascorbate has been suggested to play various roles in *glucose metabolism and diabetes* (110). The metabolism and cellular transport of ascorbate is disturbed in animals made hyperglycemic and in diabetics, possibly because of the structural similarity of the glucose molecule to ascorbate. Low serum ascorbate levels often seen in diabetics are not explained by decreased dietary intake of the vitamin nor by increased urinary ascorbate loss (in subjects without renal pathology). Increased in vivo destruction of antioxidants because of free radical stress may provide an alternative explanation, as increased oxidative stress and decreased serum antioxidant capacity have been hypothesized as factors in the complications of diabetes. In human studies, AA nutriture has been associated with improvement in some aspects of glycemic control and vascular health and with decreased protein glycosylation and erythrocyte sorbitol (a glucose metabolite linked to diabetic complications). However, effects of AA supplementation on serum glucose and glycosylated hemoglobin (a time-integrated measure of blood glucose levels) have been inconsistent. Megadose supplements (2 g/day) of AA given to healthy adults delayed the insulin response to a glucose challenge, possibly by competitive inhibition by AA of glucose uptake into pancreatic β cells (111).

AA nutriture has been postulated to affect *fertility* via roles in cellular oxidant defense and hormone and collagen production (112). Some evidence suggests that the high levels of AA in the brain are important for protection against iron-related oxidant damage linked to *senile dementias and Parkinson's disease.* On the other hand, AA also exerts an in vitro prooxidant effect in brain tissue under certain conditions. AA is important to *wound healing,* presumably because of its role in biosynthesis of mature cross-linked collagen, and in maintaining healthy gingival tissue (Fig. 29.3) (67). AA has been shown to ameliorate *heavy metal toxicity* effects, in some cases because of reductive action that decreases metal absorption or converts metals to less toxic forms. Supplements of AA have been reported to alleviate pain and provide clinical benefit to patients suffering from acute *pancreatitis* and from some *bone diseases,* including osteoarthritis, bone metastases, Paget's disease, and osteogenesis imperfecta. Low plasma concentrations of the vitamin found in critically ill patients suggest compromised antioxidant protection, wound healing, and recovery in these patients. Other conditions linked to AA status include anemia, mental depression, idiopathic thrombocytopenic purpura, gastrointestinal ulcers and hemorrhage, menorrhagia, habitual abortion, premature birth, and premature rupture of fetal membranes (28, 77, 82).

PHARMACOLOGIC INTAKES

Possible harmful effects of pharmacologic intakes of AA in the range of 1 to 15 g/day have been suggested; however, literature reviews of controlled studies involving supplementation with large doses of AA show no related toxicity (81, 82, 113, 114). The paucity of reported AA-related harmful effects in a U.S. population in which some 1/3 of individuals consumes supplementary AA suggests that the vitamin is nontoxic for healthy adults even in large amounts. Homeostatic mechanisms—saturation of absorption at 2 to 3 g/day intake and renal clearance of excess unmetabolized vitamin—probably play the most important roles in preventing AA toxicity. Nausea and diarrhea that sometimes accompany megadose intakes are ascribed to osmotic effects of unabsorbed vitamin passing through the intestine.

The fact that oxalic acid is a metabolite of AA catabolism prompts concerns of hyperoxaluria and contributions to kidney stones, although excess AA is mostly excreted into the urine unchanged, and the amount metabolized to oxalate is limited regardless of intake. Urinary oxalate and urate excretion were higher in healthy volunteers receiving 1 g/day of AA than with lower doses (16). However, most studies show that increased AA intakes do not significantly increase body oxalate concentrations, and reports of stone formation linked directly to excess AA intake are limited to rare cases of individuals with renal disease (82, 115). Therefore, patients with kidney stones or renal disease are advised to avoid excess intake of AA.

The possible role of high dietary AA in facilitating intestinal iron absorption, exacerbating iron overload, and interacting with iron to promote in vivo oxidative damage warrants further study as discussed above in the "Biochemical Functions" section. Hemolysis has been reported in patients with glucose-6-phosphate dehydrogenase deficiency receiving high-dose AA therapy (82). The proposed toxic effects of high-dose AA ingestion, such as antagonism toward copper absorption and metabolism of vitamins B_6 and B_{12}, and systemic conditioning, are unconfirmed and appear to be unimportant (37, 61).

The reductive action of large amounts of AA in urine and feces can interfere with certain laboratory diagnostic tests such as those for glycosuria and fecal occult blood. A variety of blood tests based on redox chemistries, (e.g., cholesterol, glucose, uric acid) are biased by high plasma AA levels that result from supplement consumption (116). Large doses of AA may interfere with heparin or coumarin anticoagulant therapy.

REFERENCES

1. Carpenter KJ. The history of scurvy and vitamin C. New York: Cambridge University Press, 1986.
2. Pachla LA, Reynolds DL, Kissinger PT. J Assoc Off Anal Chem 1985;68:2–12.
3. Washko PW, Welch RW, Dhariwal KR, et al. Anal Biochem 1992;204:1–14.
4. Moeslinger T, Brunner M, Volf I, et al. Clin Chem 1995;41:1177–81.
5. Benzie IFF. Clin Biochem 1996;29:111–6.
6. Wei Y, Ota RB, Bowen HT, et al. J Nutr Biochem 1996;7:179–86.
7. Manoharan M, Schwille PO. J Chromatogr B Biomed Appl 1994;654:134–9.
8. Behrens WA, Madere R. J Liq Chromatogr 1994;17:2445–55.
9. Sauberlich HE, Kretsch MJ, Taylor PC, et al. Am J Clin Nutr 1989;50:1039–49.
10. Sinha R, Block G, Taylor PR. Am J Clin Nutr 1993;57:547–50.
11. Life Sciences Research Office, Federation of American Societies for Experimental Biology. Nutrition monitoring in the United States—an update report on nutrition monitoring. Prepared for the U.S. Department of Agriculture and the U.S. Department of Health and Human Services. DHHS publ. no. (PHS) 89-1255, Public Health Service. Washington, DC: U.S. Government Printing Office, September 1989.
12. Agricultural Research Service. Composition of foods: raw, processed and prepared. Revision of Agricultural handbook no. 8-9 and 8-11. U.S. Department of Agriculture, Science and Education Administration, 1984, 1986.
13. Welch RW, Wang YH, Crossman A, et al. J Biol Chem 1995;270:12584–92.
14. Kubler W, Gehler J. Int J Vitam Nutr Res 1970;40:442–53.
15. Kallner A, Hartmann D, Hornig D. Int J Vitam Nutr Res 1977;47:383–8.
16. Levine M, Conry-Cantilena C, Wang YH, et al. Proc Natl Acad Sci USA 1996;93:3704–9.
17. Kallner A, Hornig D, Pellikka R. Am J Clin Nutr 1985;41:609–13.
18. Sacharin R, Taylor T, Chasseaud LF. Int J Vitam Nutr Res 1977;47:68–74.
19. Mangels AR, Block G, Frey CM, et al. J Nutr 1993;123:1054–61.
20. Johnston CS, Luo B. J Am Diet Assoc 1994;94:779–81.
21. Hornig D. Ann NY Acad Sci 1975;258:103–18.
22. Schorah CJ. Proc Nutr Soc 1992;51:189–98.
23. Evans RM, Currie L, Campbell A. Br J Nutr 1982;47:473–82.
24. Jacob RA. J Nutr 1990;120:1480–5.
25. Kallner A, Hartmann D, Hornig D. Am J Clin Nutr 1979;32:530–9.
26. Kallner AB, Hartmann D, Hornig DH. Am J Clin Nutr 1981;34:1347–55.
27. Baker EM, Hodges RE, Hood J, et al. Am J Clin Nutr 1971;24:444–54.
28. Basu TJ, Schorah CJ. Vitamin C in health and disease. Westport, CT: AVI Publishing, 1982.
29. Goldenberg H, Schweinzer E. J Bioenerg Biomembr 1994;26:359–67.
30. Levine M, Dhariwal KR, Wang Y, et al. Ascorbic acid in neutrophils. In: Frei B, ed. Natural antioxidants in health and disease. San Diego: Academic Press, 1994;469–88.
31. Washko PW, Wang YH, Levine M. J Biol Chem 1993;268:15531–5.
32. May JM, Qu ZC, Whitesell RR, et al. Free Radic Biol Med 1996;20:543–51.
33. Xu DP, Washburn MP, Sun GP, et al. Biochem Biophys Res Commun 1996;221:117–21.
34. Bergsten P, Yu R, Kehrl J, et al. Arch Biochem Biophys 1995;317:208–14.

35. Dhariwal KR, Hartzell WO, Levine M. Am J Clin Nutr 1991;54:712–6.
36. Melethil S, Mason WD, Chang Y, et al. Int J Pharmacol 1986;31:83–9.
37. Jacob RA, Omaye ST, Skala JH, et al. Ann NY Acad Sci 1987;498:333–46.
38. Englard S, Seifter S. Annu Rev Nutr 1986;6:365–406.
39. Harris JR, ed. Subcellular biochemistry, vol 25, Ascorbic acid: biochemistry and biomedical cell biology. New York: Plenum Press, 1996;1–435.
40. Ronchetti IP, Quaglino D Jr, Bergamini G. Ascorbic acid and connective tissue. In: Harris JR, ed. Subcellular biochemistry, vol 25, Ascorbic acid: biochemistry and biomedical cell biology. New York: Plenum Press, 1996;249–64.
41. Hitomi K, Tsukagoshi N. Role of ascorbic acid in modulation of gene expression. In: Harris JR, ed. Subcellular biochemistry, vol 25, Ascorbic acid: biochemistry and biomedical cell biology. New York: Plenum Press, 1996;41–56.
42. Wegger I, Palludan B. J Nutr 1994;124:241–8.
43. Sies H, Stahl W. Am J Clin Nutr 1995;62(Suppl):1315S–21S.
44. Bendich A, Machlin LJ, Scandurra O, et al. Adv Free Radic Biol Med 1986;2:419–44.
45. Fuller CJ, Grundy SM, Norkus EP, et al. Atherosclerosis 1996;119:139–50.
46. Fraga CG, Motchnik PA, Shigenaga MK, et al. Proc Natl Acad Sci USA 1991;88:11003–6.
47. Jacob RA. Introduction: three eras of vitamin C discovery. In: Harris JR, ed. Subcellular biochemistry, vol 25, Ascorbic acid: biochemistry and biomedical cell biology. New York: Plenum Press, 1996;1–16.
48. Jacob RA. Nutr Res 1995;15:755–66.
49. Johnston CS, Meyer CG, Srilakshmi JC. Am J Clin Nutr 1993;58:103–5.
50. Niki E, Noguchi N, Tsuchihashi H, et al. Am J Clin Nutr 1995;62(Suppl):1322S–6S.
51. Jacob RA, Kutnink MA, Csallany AS, et al. J Nutr 1996;126:2268–77.
52. Kandaswami C, Perkins E, Soloniuk DS, et al. Anti-Cancer Drugs 1993;4:91–6.
53. Katsuki H. Vitamin C and nervous tissue: In vivo and in vitro aspects. In: Harris JR, ed. Subcellular biochemistry, vol 25, Ascorbic acid: biochemistry and biomedical cell biology. New York: Plenum Press, 1996;293–311.
54. Yanagibashi K, Kobayashi Y, Hall PF. Biochem Biophys Res Commun 1990;170:1256–62.
55. Gosiewska A, Mahmoodian F, Peterkofsky B. Arch Biochem Biophys 1996;325:295–303.
56. Hunt JR, Gallagher SK, Johnson LK. Am J Clin Nutr 1994;59:1381–5.
57. Bendich A, Cohen M. Toxicol Lett 1990;51:189–201.
58. Buettner GR, Jurkiewicz BA. Radiat Res 1996;145:532–41.
59. Powers HJ, Loban A, Silvers K, et al. Free Radic Res 1995;22:57–65.
60. Langley SC, Brown RK, Kelley FJ, et al. Pediatr Res 1993;33:247–50.
61. Harris ED, Percival SS. Am J Clin Nutr 1991; 54(Suppl):1193S–7S.
62. Rebouche CJ. Metabolism 1995;44:1639–43.
62a. Jacob RA, Pianalto FS. J Nutr Biochem 1997;8:265–9.
63. Johnston CS, Solomon RE, Corte C. J Am Coll Nutr 1996;15:586–91.
64. Horrobin DF. Ascorbic acid and prostaglandin synthesis. In: Harris JR, ed. Subcellular biochemistry, vol 25, Ascorbic acid: biochemistry and biomedical cell biology. New York: Plenum Press, 1996;109–15.
65. Millar J. Med Hypotheses 1995;45:21–6.
66. Sinclair PR, Gorman N, Sinclair JF, et al. Hepatology 1995;22:565–72.
67. Leggott PJ, Robertson PB, Rothman DL, et al. J Periodontol 1986;57:480–5.
68. Parkkinen J, Vaaranen O, Vahtera E. Thromb Haemost 1996;75:292–7.
69. Monget AL, Galan P, Preziosi P, et al. Int J Vitam Nutr Res 1996;66:71–6.
70. Oreopoulos DG, Lindeman RD, VanderJagt DJ, et al. J Am Coll Nutr 1993;12:537–42.
71. Sauberlich HE, Dowdy RP, Skala JH. Laboratory tests for the assessment of nutritional status. Boca Raton, FL: CRC Press, 1974.
72. Jacob RA, Skala JH, Omaye ST. Am J Clin Nutr 1987;46:818–26.
73. Jacob RA, Pianalto FS, Agee RE. J Nutr 1992;122:1111–8.
74. Jacob RA, Otradovec CL, Russell RM, et al. Am J Clin Nutr 1988;48:1436–42.
75. Food and Nutrition Board, National Research Council. Water-soluble vitamins. In: Recommended dietary allowances. 10th ed. Washington, DC: National Academy Press, 1989;115–23.
76. Life Sciences Research Office, Federation of American Societies for Experimental Biology. J Nutr 1996; 126(Suppl):1907S–36S.
77. Clemetson CAB, ed. Vitamin C (vols. I–III). Boca Raton, FL: CRC Press, 1989.
78. Burns JJ, Rivers JM, Machlin LJ. Ann NY Acad Sci 1987;498:1–538.
79. Gershoff SN. Nutr Rev 1993;51:313–26.
80. Weber P, Bendich A, Schalch W. Int J Vit Nutr Res 1996;66:19–30.
81. Bendich A, Langseth L. J Am Coll Nutr 1995;14:124–36.
82. Sauberlich HE. Annu Rev Nutr 1994;14:371–91.
83. Siegel BV. Vitamin C and the immune response in health and disease. In: Nutrition and immunology series: human nutrition: a comprehensive treatise. New York: Plenum Press, 1993;8:167–96.
84. Vojdani A, Ghoneum M. Nutr Res 1993;13:753–64.
85. Jariwalla RJ, Harakeh S. Antiviral and immunomodulatory activities of ascorbic acid. In: Harris JR, ed. Subcellular biochemistry, vol 25, Ascorbic acid: biochemistry and biomedical cell biology. New York: Plenum Press, 1996;215–31.
86. Johnston CS, Martin LJ, Xi C. J Am Coll Nutr 1992;11:172–6.
87. Hamilton Smith C, Hansson LO, Stendahl O. Int J Vitam Nutr Res 1979;49:160–5.
88. Jacob RA, Kelley DS, Pianalto FS, et al. Am J Clin Nutr 1991;54(Suppl):1302S–9S.
89. Block G, Schwarz R. Ascorbic acid and cancer: animal and cell culture data. In: Frei B, ed. Natural antioxidants in health and disease. San Diego: Academic Press, 1994;129–55.
90. Fontham ETH. Vitamin C, vitamin C-rich foods and cancer: epidemiologic studies. In: Frei B, ed. Natural antioxidants in health and disease. San Diego: Academic Press, 1994;157–97.
91. Block G. Am J Clin Nutr 1991;53(Suppl)270S–82S.
92. Shklar G, Schwartz JL. Ascorbic acid and cancer. In: Harris JR, ed. Subcellular biochemistry, vol 25, Ascorbic acid: biochemistry and biomedical cell biology. New York: Plenum Press, 1996;233–47.
93. Cohen M, Bhagavan H. J Am Coll Nutr 1995;14:565–78.
94. Drake IM, Davies MJ, Mapstone NP, et al. Carcinogenesis 1996;17:559–62.
95. Blot WJ, Li JY, Taylor PR, et al. J Natl Cancer Inst 1993;85:1483–92.

96. Simon JA. J Am Coll Nutr 1992;11:107–25.
97. Lynch SM, Gaziano JM, Frei B. Ascorbic acid and atherosclerotic cardiovascular disease. In: Frei B, ed. Natural antioxidants in health and disease. San Diego: Academic Press, 1994;331–67.
98. Ness AR, Khaw KT, Bingham S, et al. J Hypertens 1996;14:503–8.
99. Ghosh SK, Ekpo EB, Shah IU, et al. Gerontology 1994;40:268–72.
100. Gale CR, Martyn CN, Winter PD, et al. Br Med J 1995;310:1563–66.
101. Jha P, Flather M, Lonn E, et al. Ann Intern Med 1995;123:860–72.
102. Hennekens CJ, Gaziano JM, Manson JE, et al. Am J Clin Nutr 1995;62(Suppl):1377S–80S.
103. Maritz GS. Ascorbic acid protection of lung tissue against damage. In: Harris JR, ed. Subcellular biochemistry, vol 25, Ascorbic acid: biochemistry and biomedical cell biology. New York: Plenum Press, 1996;265–91.
104. Britton JR, Pavord ID, Richards KA, et al. Am J Respir Crit Care Med 1995;151:1383–7.
105. Hatch GE. Am J Clin Nutr 1995;61(Suppl):625S–30S.
106. Seddon JM, Ajani UA, Sperduto RD, et al. JAMA 1994;272:1413–20.
107. Seddon JM, Christen WG, Manson JE, et al. Am J Public Health 1994;84:788–92.
108. West S, Vitale S, Hallfrisch J, et al. Arch Ophthalmol 1994;112:222–7.
109. Delamere NA. Ascorbic acid and the eye. In: Harris JR, ed. Subcellular biochemistry, vol 25, Ascorbic acid: biochemistry and biomedical cell biology. New York: Plenum Press, 1996;313–29.
110. Hunt JV. Ascorbic acid and diabetes mellitus. In: Harris JR, ed. Subcellular biochemistry, vol 25, Ascorbic acid: biochemistry and biomedical cell biology. New York: Plenum Press, 1996;369–404.
111. Johnston CS, Yen MF. Am J Clin Nutr 1994;60:735–8.
112. Luck MR, Jeyaseelan I, Scholes RA. Biol Reprod 1995;52:262–6.
113. Diplock AT. Am J Clin Nutr 1995;62(Suppl):S1510–16.
114. Meyers DG, Maloley PA, Weeks D. Arch Intern Med 1996;156:925–35.
115. Curhan GC, Willett WC, Rimm EB, et al. J Urol 1996;155:1847–51.
116. Young DS. Lab Med 1983;14:278–82.

SELECTED READINGS

Englard S, Seifter S. The biochemical functions of ascorbic acid. Annu Rev Nutr 1986;6:365–406.

Gershoff SN. Vitamin C (ascorbic acid): new roles, new requirements? Nutr Rev 1993;51:313–26.

Harris JR, ed. Subcellular biochemistry, vol 25, Ascorbic acid: biochemistry and biomedical cell biology. New York: Plenum Press, 1996;1–435.

Packer L, Fuchs J, eds. Vitamin C in health and disease. New York: Marcel Dekker, 1997;1–552.

Sauberlich HE. Pharmacology of vitamin C. Annu Rev Nutr 1994;14:371–91.

30. Clinical Manifestations of Human Vitamin and Mineral Disorders: A Resumé

DONALD S. McLAREN

Nutritional disorders result from an imbalance between the body's requirements for nutrients and energy sources and the supply of these substrates of metabolism. This imbalance may take the form of either deficiency or excess and may be attributable to an inappropriate intake or to defective utilization or, frequently, a combination of both.

Despite our extensive understanding of human nutritional requirements for maintenance of health, malnutrition continues to be one of the main causes of morbidity and mortality in developing countries, especially in young children. In technologically advanced societies, undernutrition due to dietary restriction no longer constitutes a major hazard to health, but it continues to occur in hospitalized patients and in other especially vulnerable groups. The special nutritional needs in patients receiving total parenteral nutrition (TPN) and chronic renal dialysis are now much better recognized than in previous years. However, deficiency states continue to arise in patients with long-term alcohol or drug abuse problems and in food fadism. Secondary undernutrition resulting from malabsorption, failure in transport, storage, or cellular utilization, or excessive losses requires constant vigilance in clinical practice. The improper usage of nutrient supplements has led to numerous instances of vitamin and element toxicity, often because of ignorance on the part of the user or inadequate or improper information by the supplier.

This chapter is confined to a consideration of clinical manifestations of nutritional disorders related to vitamins and essential trace elements. Disorders of protein and energy are considered elsewhere. A number of vitamin-dependency states have been identified and their symptomatology relates to the metabolic abnormalities produced by the respective apoenzyme disorders and not to the vitamin per se. Consequently, they are considered elsewhere under the appropriate vitamin.

The clinical manifestations of vitamin and essential element disorders consist of the relevant symptoms expressed by the patient and the signs observed by the physician on general physical examination. The present intention is to provide a comprehensive, yet reasonably brief, resumé of clinical nutrition for the physician practicing medicine within a highly specialized context. The particular clinical circumstances within which the various nutritional disorders tend to arise are indicated to help prevent their being missed as so often happens when they are "out of sight out of mind."

VITAMINS

Vitamin A (Retinol)

Deficiency

The symptoms and signs of vitamin A deficiency have been studied in greater detail than those of any other nutritional deficiency disorder (1, 2). The eye is primarily involved and the condition, given the general name of xerophthalmia, predominantly affects young children. In a cooperative subject impaired dark adaptation of the retinal rods can be detected by instrumental means, scotometry or electroretinography. In young children night blindness can be elicited by a careful history and some simple tests in a poorly illuminated room (3). Photopic and color vision, mediated by the retinal cones, is usually unaffected.

Dryness (xerosis) and unwettability of the bulbar conjunctiva follow. Conjunctival impression cytology is abnormal at this stage. Bitot's spot is advanced conjunctival epithelial cell keratinization, a heaping up of desquamated cells most commonly seen in the interpalpebral fissure on the temporal aspect of the conjunctiva (Fig. 30.1*A*). In older children and adults, Bitot's spots may be stigmata of past deficiency or may be entirely unrelated to vitamin A deficiency, when local trauma may be responsible. Corneal involvement, starting as a superficial punctate keratopathy (4) and proceeding to xerosis (Fig. 30.1*B*) and varying degrees of "ulceration" and liquefaction (keratomalacia) (Fig. 30.1*C*), frequently results in blindness. Punctate degenerative changes in the retina (xerophthalmic fundus) are a rare sign of chronic deficiency usually seen in older children (5). Corneal scars may have many causes, but those that are bilateral in the lower and outer part of the cornea of a person with a history of past malnutrition and/or measles often signal earlier vitamin A deficiency. They may appear as fine nebulae or denser leukomata, or there may be total scarring of a shrunken globe (phthisis bulbi) or corneal ectasia or anterior staphyloma.

Extraocular manifestations include perifollicular hyperkeratosis, a heaping up of hyperkeratinized skin epithelium around hair follicles. This condition is most commonly seen on the outer aspects of the upper arms and the thighs. It is also seen in starvation and has been attributed to B complex vitamin or essential fatty acid deficiency. Other changes, which include impaired taste, anorexia, vestibular disturbance, bone changes with pressure on cranial nerves, increased intracranial pressure, congenital malformations and infertility, have been best demonstrated in animals (6) (see also Chapter 17).

In recent years, clinical and community trials of vitamin A supplementation of young children have demonstrated a significant decrease in all-cause mortality and morbidity (6a) (see also Chapter 97).

Toxicity (Hypervitaminosis A)

Acute toxicity is more common in children. Most of the features relate to a rise in intracranial pressure: nausea, vomiting, headache, vertigo, irritability, stupor, fontanel bulging (in infants), papilledema and pseudotumor cerebri (mimicking brain tumor) (7). There is also pyrexia and peeling of the skin.

Chronic poisoning produces a bizarre clinical picture that is often misdiagnosed because of failure to consider excessive vitamin A intake (7). It is characterized by anorexia, weight loss, headache, blurred vision, diplopia, dry and scaling pruritic skin, alopecia, coarsening of the hair, hepatomegaly, splenomegaly, anemia, subperiosteal new bone growth, cortical thickening (especially bones of hands and feet and long bones of the legs), and gingival discoloration.

X-ray appearance may assist in making a correct diagnosis (Figs. 30.3, 30.4). Cranial sutures are widened in the young child. Dense lines that appear at the metaphyses of all long bones represent cortical hyperostoses. These cortical thickenings usually stop short of the ends of the shafts. Premature fusion of hypertrophied epiphyseal ossification centers with their shafts is most often seen at the distal ends of the femurs. There may also be metaphyseal cupping and splaying of the affected end of the shaft. Cortical hyperostosis of the ribs may also occur.

Vitamin A and other retinoids are powerful teratogens in both pregnant experimental animals and women (7). Birth defects have been reported in the offspring of women receiving 13-cis-retinoic acid (isotretinoin) during pregnancy (8). An increased risk of birth defects is present in infants of women taking more than 10,000 IU of supplementary preformed vitamin A per day before the 7th week of gestation (9); other reports indicate that birth defects are likely to occur at levels several times higher.

Hypercarotenosis

Excessive intake of carotenoids can cause hypercarotenosis. Yellow or orange discoloration of the skin (xanthosis cutis, carotenoderma) affects areas where sebum secretion is greatest—nasolabial folds, forehead, axillae, and groin—and keratinized surfaces such as the palms and soles. The sclerae and buccal membranes are not affected, which distinguishes it from jaundice, in which they are stained (see Chapter 33).

Vitamin D (Calciferol)

Deficiency

Vitamin D deficiency is manifested as rickets in children and osteomalacia in adults. Those forms not due to primary nutrient deficiency—previously termed *metabolic rickets*—also exhibit signs and symptoms of the underlying disease and hypocalcemia.

Rickets. The rachitic infant is restless and sleeps poorly. Consequently, the occipital hair is denuded. Craniotabes, softening of the bones of the skull and their ready depression on palpation, is often the earliest sign, but it must be present away from the suture lines to be diagnostic of rickets. Frontal bossing occurs and the fontanels close late. Sitting, crawling, and walking are all delayed. If the disease is active when these activities occur, weight bearing results in bowing of the arms (Fig. 30.2*A*), knock-knees (genu valgum), or outward bowing (genu varum).

The characteristic x-ray appearance usually precedes clinical signs (Fig. 30.5). The diaphyseal ends of the bones, most characteristically the lower ends of the radius and ulna, lose their sharp, clear outline, become cup shaped, and show a spotty or fringelike rarefaction. Due to failure of calcification the distance between the radius and ulna and the metacarpals appears increased. Shadows cast by the shaft decrease in density, and the network formed by laminae becomes coarse. As healing begins, a thin white line of calcification appears in the epiphysis, becoming thicker and denser as calcification proceeds. Lime salts are deposited beneath the periosteum, the shaft casts a

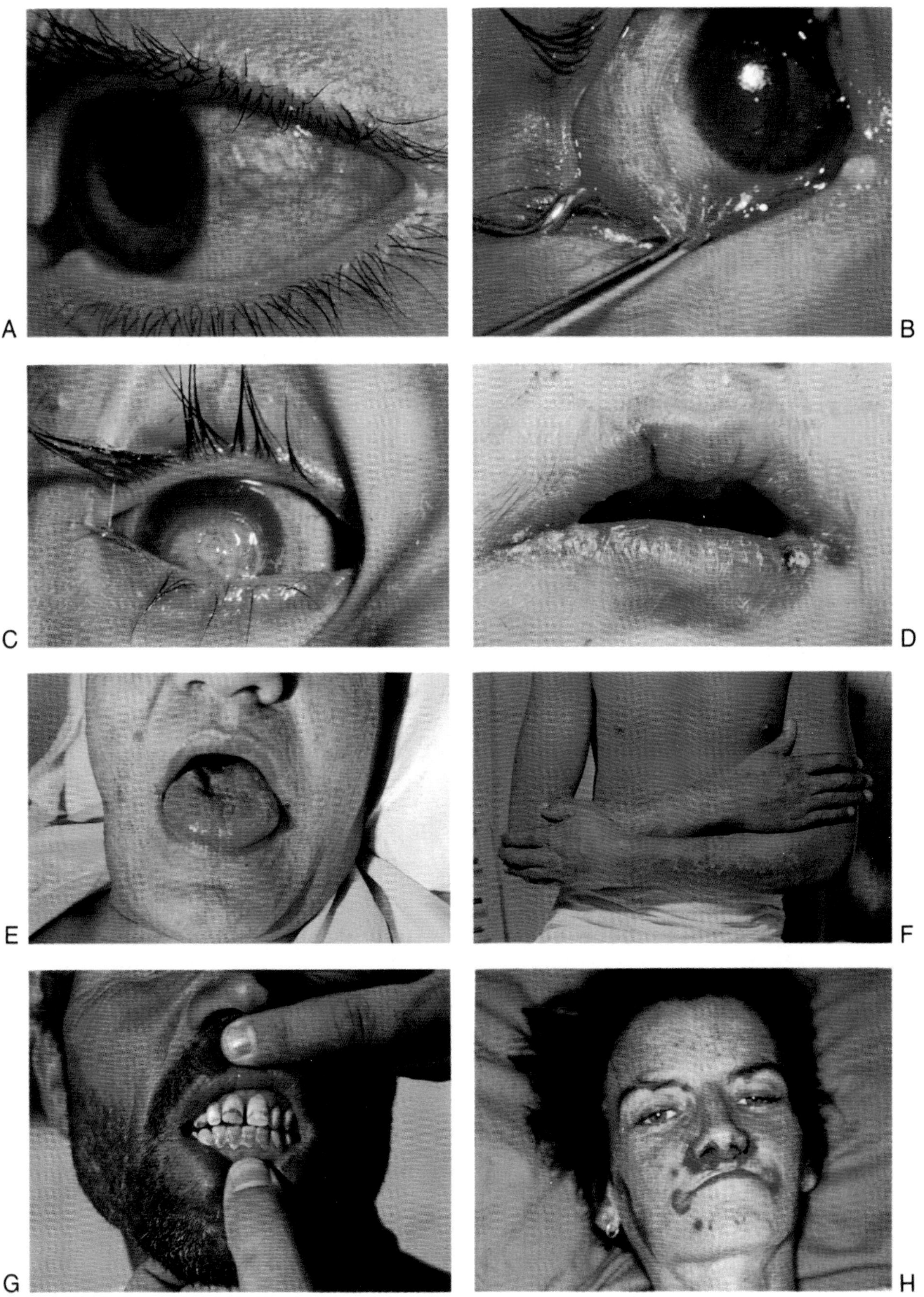

Figure 30.1. A. Vitamin A deficiency. Bitot's spot in temporal interpalpebral fissure. **B.** Vitamin A deficiency. Conjunctival and corneal xerosis. **C.** Vitamin A deficiency. Keratomalacia. **D.** Riboflavin deficiency. Cheilosis and angular stomatitis. **E.** Riboflavin deficiency. Magenta tongue. **F.** Niacin deficiency. Symmetric dermatosis of pellagra. **G.** Fluorosis. Early stage with brown mottling that is most marked on upper central incisors. **H.** Zinc deficiency. Typical dermatosis associated with alcoholic cirrhosis in this patient. (From Ilchyshyn A, Mendelsohn Z. Br Med J 1982;284:1676.)

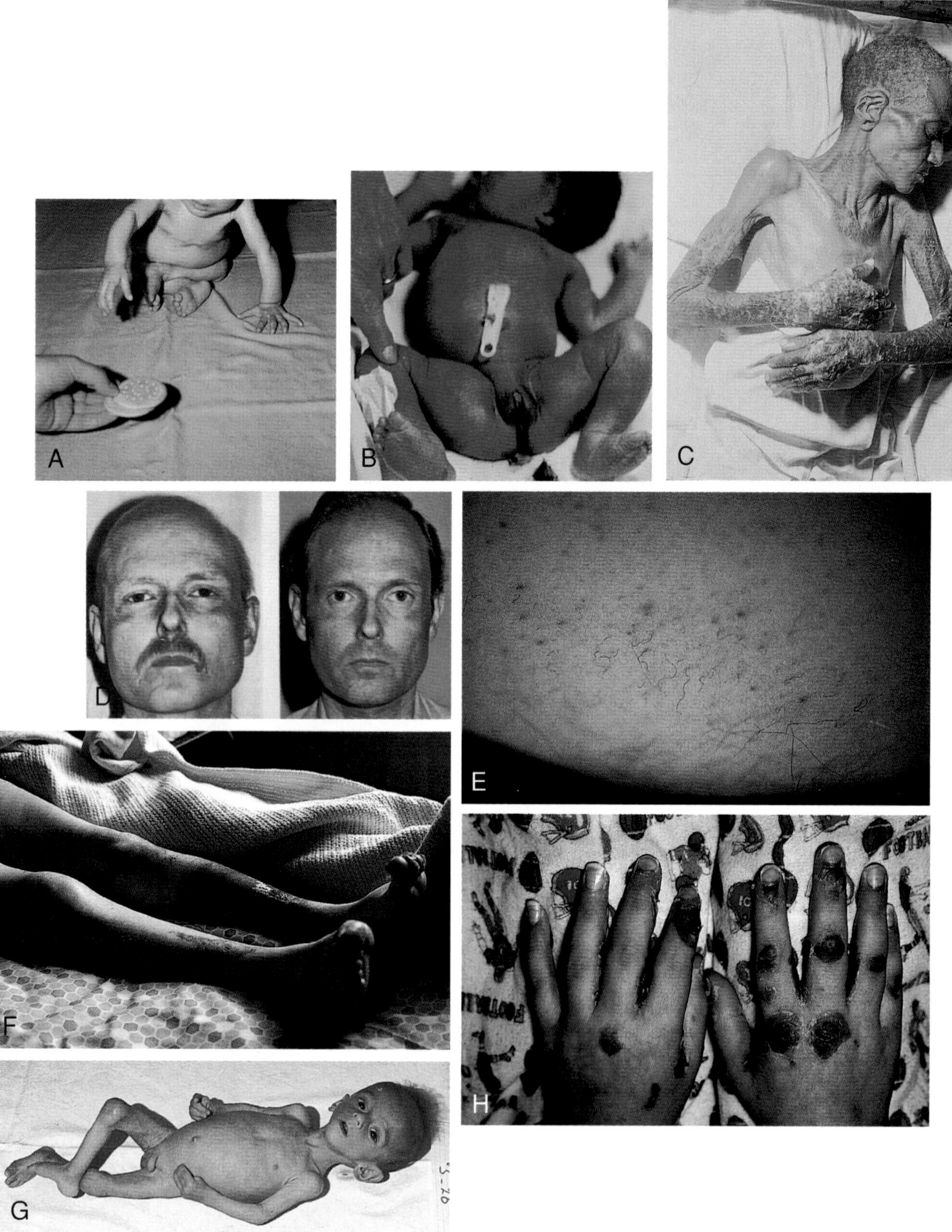

Figure 30.2. A. Rickets. An infant with nutritional rickets at the crawling stage, demonstrating the role of pressure in causing bowing of the bones, in this case of the arms. **B.** Vitamin K deficiency. Hemorrhagic disease of the newborn secondary to vitamin K deficiency. Hemorrhage around the genitalia is a common site. **C.** Pellagra. Casal's necklace, a broad band or collar of dermatosis, induced by exposure to sunlight, is a classic sign of pellagra. The patient was an elderly female in Tanzania. **D.** Biotin deficiency. Adult on prolonged parenteral nutrition devoid of biotin with alopecia, dermatitis, and conjunctivitis *(left)*. Slit lamp examination revealed corneal lesions. All were corrected by inclusion of 60 μg of biotin daily *(right)*. (From McClain et al. JAMA, 1982:247:3116, with permission.) **E.** Scurvy. "Swan neck" or "corkscrew" deformities of the hairs characteristic of the early stages of adult scurvy. **F.** Scurvy. In adult scurvy, petechiae are characteristically perifollicular and usually precede larger extravasations, termed *ecchymoses*. The thighs and shins are common sites. **G.** Hypocalcemia. The characteristic contraction of the hands (tetany) in this marasmic infant is associated with the presence of marked hypocalcemia often secondary to magnesium depletion. **H.** Zinc deficiency. Lesions on pressure areas on the back of the hands in a child on prolonged parenteral nutrition who had rapidly depleted zinc stores through loss of large volumes of intestinal contents following an intestinal fistula. Similar lesions occurred on the elbows and knees. Sterile pustules were present on the palms, and lesions were present about the mouth. All responded to increased zinc administration. (Courtesy of M. E. Shils.)

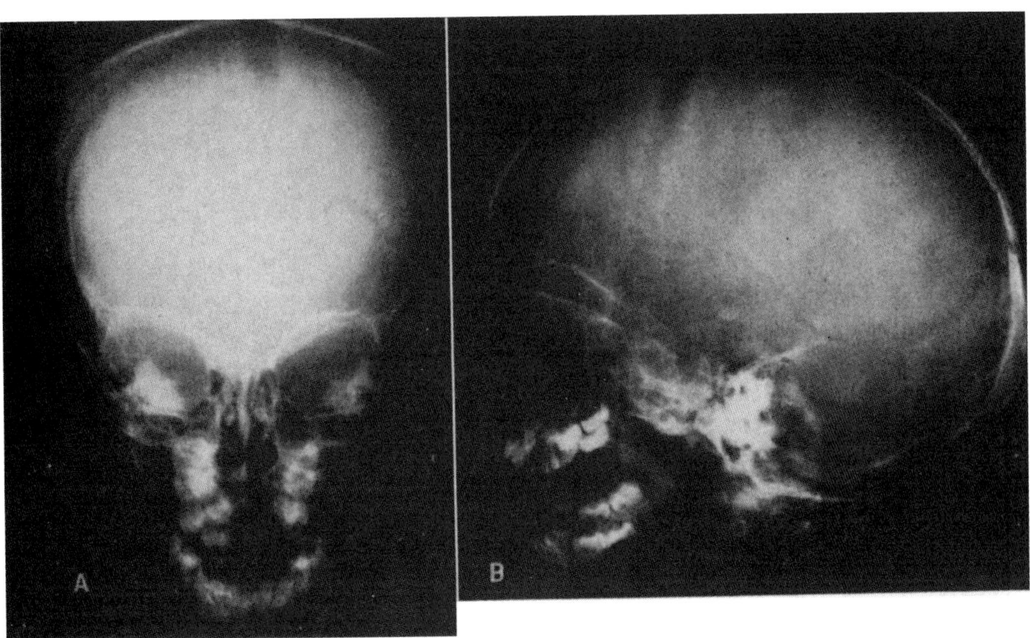

Figure 30.3. A. and **B.** Frontal and lateral projections of skull of a 2-year-old girl with hypervitaminosis A showing wide sagittal and coronal sutures. (From Watson RC, Grossman H, Meyers MA. Radiologic findings in nutritional disturbances. In: Shils ME, Olson JA, Shike M. Modern nutrition in health and disease. 8th ed. Philadelphia: Lea & Febiger, 1994, with permission.)

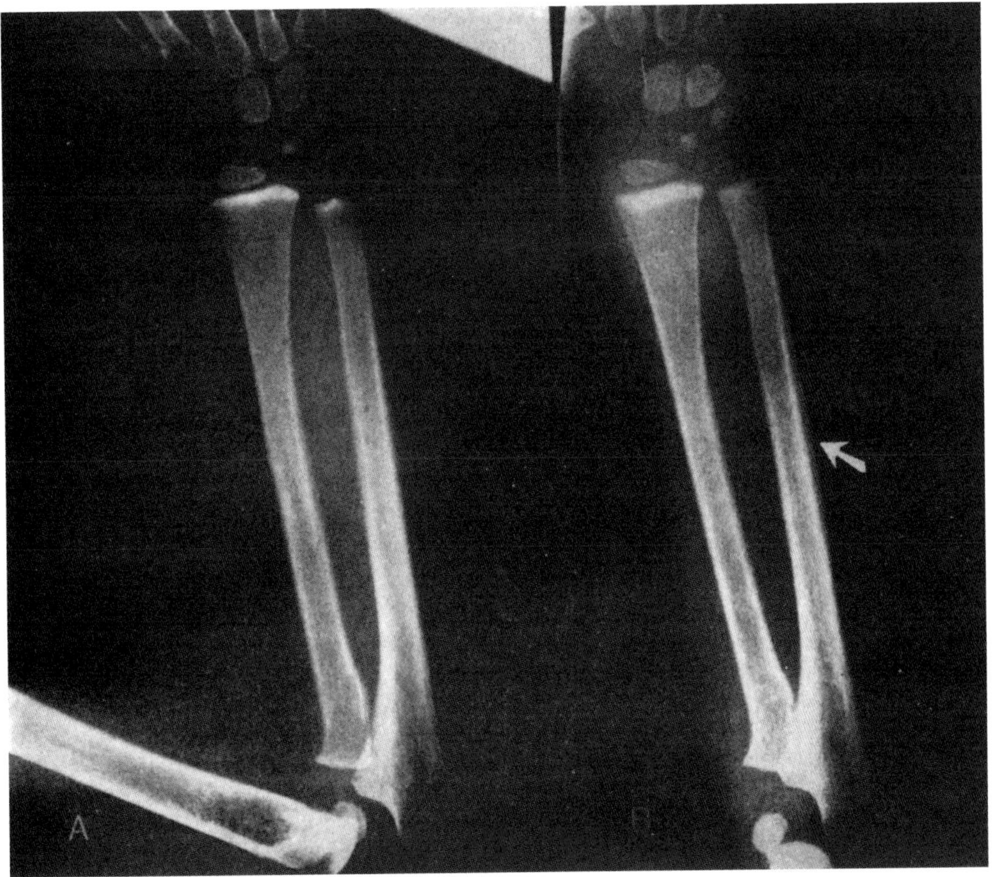

Figure 30.4. Same patient as in Figure 30.3. **A.** Dense line occurs at the distal end of radius and ulna. No subperiosteal new bone is present. **B.** Three weeks later, periosteal new bone is seen on the lateral aspect of the ulna. (From Watson RC, Grossman H, Meyers MA. Radiologic findings in nutritional disturbances. In: Shils ME, Olson JA, Shike M. Modern nutrition in health and disease. 8th ed. Philadelphia: Lea & Febiger, 1994, with permission.)

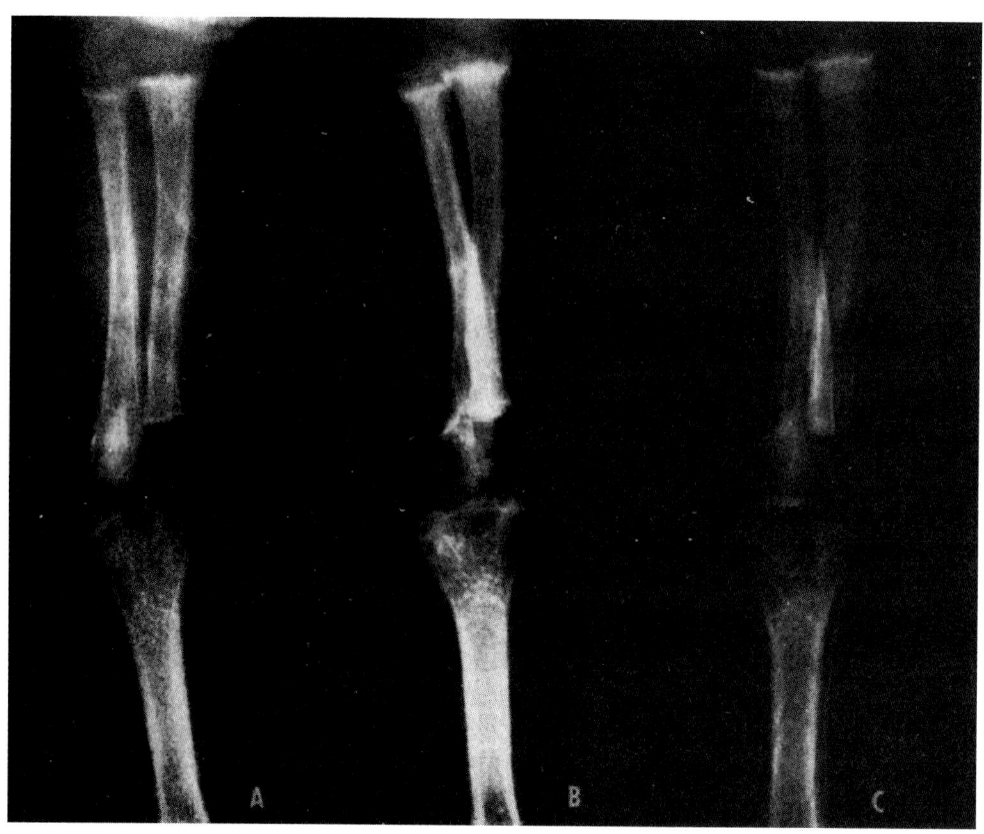

Figure 30.5. A 10-month-old boy during various stages of rickets. **A.** Noncalcified provisional zone and fraying of the distal humerus are evident. Strands of calcified osteoid project from the sides of the bone. **B.** Cupping, spread metaphysis, fraying, and cortical spurs occur. Transverse linear recalcified density develops in rachitic metaphysis. A fracture is present in the midshaft of the radius. Greenstick fractures are common in the long bones. **C.** Metaphyseal spongiosum recalcifies and fuses with that of the provisional zone of calcification. Diffuse layer of racalcified cortex is present. (From Watson RC, Grossman H, Meyers MA. Radiologic findings in nutritional disturbances. In: Shils ME, Olson JA, Shike M. Modern nutrition in health and disease. 8th ed. Philadelphia: Lea & Febiger, 1994, with permission.)

denser shadow, and the lamellae disappear. Bone morphology is also discussed in Chapter 83.

The rachitic rosary, caused by enlargement of the costochondral junctions of the ribs, is said to be smoother than that due to scurvy (see discussion of vitamin C). The chest may be deformed to give Harrison's sulcus or groove, which consists of a bilateral indentation of the lateral parts of the lower ribs (see also Chapter 18). Other deformities of the chest, such as depression (funnel chest or pectus excavatum) of the sternum, are now considered to be congenital and not rachitic in origin.

Occasionally, stridor and intermittent sudden airway obstruction due to laryngospasm may present in infancy as a result of hypocalcemia accompanying biochemical and x-ray evidence of rickets but without the classical bony physical signs. A few instances of congenital cataract appear to be due to vitamin D deficiency in the mother (10).

Osteomalacia. The main features of osteomalacia are bone pains and tenderness, skeletal deformity, and weakness of the proximal muscles. In severe cases, all the bones are painful and tender, often enough to disturb sleep. Tenderness may be particularly marked over Looser's zones (Milkman lines), usually occurring in the long bones, pelvis, ribs, and around the scapulae in a bilaterally symmetric pattern. These radiotranslucent zones are sometimes termed "pseudofractures." True fractures of the softened bones are common. The proximal muscle weakness, the cause of which is uncertain, is more marked in some forms of osteomalacia than in others. Osteomalacia usually results in a waddling gait and difficulty going up and down stairs. In the elderly it may simulate paraplegia; in younger persons it may simulate muscular dystrophy. Immigrant women to Europe and North America from Asia and the Middle East are especially susceptible.

Toxicity (Hypervitaminosis D)

Some of the symptoms and signs are related to hypercalcemia and are common to all causes of that condition. Anorexia, nausea, vomiting, and constipation are usually present. Weakness, hypotonia, stupor, and hypertension are less common. Polyuria and polydipsia are caused by hypercalciuria. Renal colic due to stone formation may result.

X-ray of the skeleton may assist diagnosis. There is increased epiphyseal bone density due to excessive calcium deposition.

Vitamin D excess has been reported to take two forms:

to 6 months of age, and the symptoms and signs are those already described. In the severe form, also seen in infants, in addition to the manifestations of hypercalcemia, there is mental retardation, stenosis of the aorta and the pulmonary arteries, and a characteristic facial appearance termed *elfin facies* (11).

Vitamin E (Tocopherol)

Deficiency

In recent years clinical disease responsive to vitamin E has attracted considerable attention. Low-birth-weight infants are particularly susceptible, especially if fed formulas high in polyunsaturated fatty acids after occurrence of hemolytic anemia; the condition is made worse by iron supplements (12, 13). Defective vitamin E status of premature infants may also contribute to their greater susceptibility to platelet dysfunction, intraventricular hemorrhage, retinopathy of prematurity, and bronchopulmonary dysplasia. Lipofuscin deposition within muscle cells has been reported to account for the brown bowel syndrome (14).

Recently, the molecular basis has been discovered of two conditions in which vitamin E deficiency has long been known to figure prominently (15). In *spinocerebellar ataxias* of the Friedreich's ataxia type there is a defect in the α-tocopherol-transfer protein (α-TTP), and in *abetalipoproteinemia* (Bassen-Kornzweig syndrome, acanthocytosis) there are mutations in the gene coding for one subunit of the microsomal triglyceride-transfer protein. Friedreich's ataxia presents in childhood with progressive ataxia of gait, dysarthria, areflexia, extensor plantar signs, and impaired vibratory and positional sense. In abetalipoproteinemia there is steatorrhea, acanthocytes (erythrocytes with spiny projections of the membrane), retinitis pigmentosa–like changes in the retina, ataxia, and mental retardation. (See also Chapter 19.)

Toxicity

In the early 1980s, use of an intravenous vitamin E product (E-Ferol), a drug that had not been approved by the United States Food and Drug Administration (FDA), led to pulmonary deterioration, thrombocytopenia, liver and renal failure, and a high mortality in newborn premature infants (16). Its toxicity may have been related to non–vitamin E constituents of the formulation (16a). Reports that low-birth-weight infants receiving pharmacologic doses of vitamin E had a high incidence of sepsis and necrotizing enterocolitis (17) have not been confirmed (see also Chapter 19 concerning safety).

Vitamin K

Deficiency (Hypoprothrombinemia)

Understanding of the pathogenesis of vitamin K deficiency in the neonate has increased considerably. Hemorrhagic disease of the newborn (HDN) is usually classified into three syndromes: early, classic, and late (18). The early form presents within 0 to 24 hours of birth and the most common bleeding sites are cephalohematoma, within the gut (producing melena neonatorum), and around the genitalia (Fig. 30.2*B*). Classical HDN presents on day 1 to 7, and the bleeding is usually gastrointestinal, dermal, nasal, or from circumcision. The peak incidence of late HDN is from the 3rd to 6th week, and intracranial hemorrhage (rare in classical HDN) accounts for about 50% of the bleeding episodes at presentation. Late HDN may occur over weeks 2 to 12 and also commonly affects the skin and gastrointestinal tract.

In the adult, bleeding from this cause is most common in chronic liver disease, obstructive jaundice, and in patients receiving anticoagulants, prolonged antibiotic therapy, or certain cephalosporin antibiotics, such as moxalactam disodium.

Rare instances of deficiency have been attributed to dietary restriction (19) or inadequate TPN (20). Large doses of vitamin E may induce deficiency of vitamin K (21).

Toxicity

Kernicterus (bilirubin encephalopathy) has occurred in low-birth-weight infants receiving large doses of menadione (75 mg) or its water-soluble derivatives; it has not occurred when vitamin K itself has been given. Lethargy, hypotonia, and loss of sucking reflex are followed by opisthotonos, generalized spasticity, and frequently death from pulmonary complications. Survivors may develop the postkernicterus syndrome: high-frequency nerve deafness, athetoid cerebral palsy, and dental enamel dysplasia.

Thiamin (Vitamin B_1, Aneurin)

Deficiency

Beriberi in the adult occurs in two distinct forms, wet and dry beriberi, in which the cardiovascular and the nervous systems, respectively, are affected. Both may be involved in the same patient, but one or the other tends to predominate. Infantile beriberi is described separately (see also Chapter 21).

Cardiovascular beriberi usually manifests as chronic high-output right- and left-sided heart failure with tachycardia, rapid circulation time, elevated peripheral venous pressure, sodium retention, and edema (22). A much less common acute fulminating form of heart failure (sometimes called "shoshin") is characterized by severe metabolic lactic acidosis, intense dyspnea, thirst, anxiety, and cardiovascular collapse. Signs also include stocking-glove cyanosis, extreme tachycardia, cardiomegaly, hepatomegaly, and neck vein distension. Edema is usually absent (23). This highly fatal form is not uncommon as a cause of sudden death in young migrant laborers in the Orient subsisting on rice.

Beriberi of the Nervous System (24). *Cerebral Beriberi (Wernicke-Korsakoff Syndrome).* Cerebral beriberi in its most severe form, mental confusion, accompanied by ophthalmoplegia due to paralysis of the 6th cranial nerve, leads to coma. Korsakoff's psychosis consists of loss of memory for distant events, inability to form new ones, and loss of insight and initiative. The patient is alert and can converse, think, and solve problems. Response to thiamin is complete in only 25% of cases and partial in 50%. Ethanol is thought to have a direct part in neurotoxicity (25, 26). Wernicke encephalopathy is most likely to occur in chronic alcoholics given carbohydrates without adequate thiamin replacement or in nonalcoholic depleted patients given infusions high in glucose without adequate thiamin. It is reported as a complication of vertical-banded gastroplasty for morbid obesity (27). (See Chapter 95.)

Peripheral Neuropathy. The most characteristic features of peripheral neuropathy are symmetric footdrop, associated with marked tenderness of the calf muscles, and a mild disturbance of sensation over the outer aspects of the legs and thighs and in patches over the abdomen, chest, and forearms. Ataxia with loss of position and vibration sense, burning paresthesias in the feet, and amblyopia are less common.

Infantile Beriberi. Early manifestations of infantile beriberi are anorexia, vomiting, pallor, restlessness, and insomnia. The disease progresses typically to *(a)* an acute cardiac form in infants 2 to 4 months of age, *(b)* a subacute aphonic form in those 5 to 7 months old, and *(c)* a chronic, pseudomeningeal form in those between 8 and 10 months of age. The acute form presents with dyspnea, cyanosis, a rapid thready pulse, and other signs of acute heart failure. In the subacute form, aphonia or a characteristic hoarse cry, dysphagia, vomiting, and convulsions predominate. The chronic form is characterized by neck retraction, opisthotonos, edema, oliguria, constipation, and meteorism (28).

Subacute Necrotizing Encephalomyopathy (SNE, Leigh's Disease). SNE may be related to a defect in thiamin metabolism. About 100 cases have been reported (29). Onset is usually before 1 year of age. Hypoventilation and apnea, cranial neuropathies, and hypotonia are the most common features.

Possible Toxicity

Large doses of thiamin have been given to alcoholics as a part of their therapy. A survey of the U.S. literature revealed a significant number of reports of adverse effects in the late 1930s to early 1940s. From 1943 to 1973 there were six reports of sensitization of an anaphylactic nature, with nothing similar until 1992. At that time a case was reported of an alcoholic with a high blood alcohol level given 100 mg of thiamin-HCl intravenously, which was associated with onset of nausea, anxiety, arrhythmia, moderate hypotension, and wheezing; improvement occurred with epinephrine, antihistamines, and steroids (30). In contrast, 9 deaths were reported in the European literature between 1965 and 1985. Of note is the absence of reports of anaphylactic reactions with multivitamins containing thiamin used in TPN solutions.

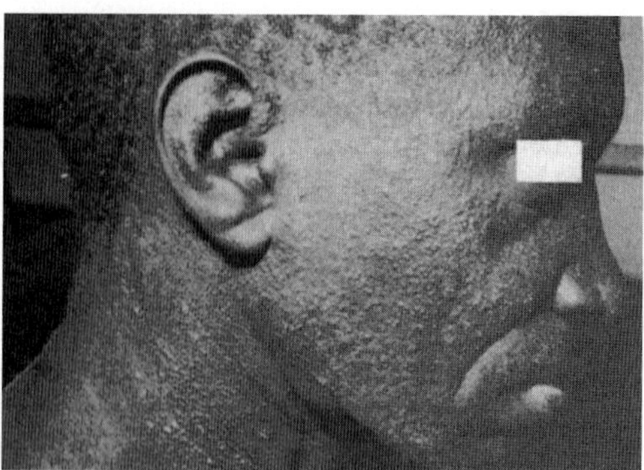

Figure 30.6. Dyssebacea associated with riboflavin deficiency.

Riboflavin

Deficiency

The skin and mucous membranes are affected in what is known as the orooculogenital syndrome. Areas of skin involved are usually those containing many sebaceous glands: mainly the nasolabial folds, alae nasi, external ears, eyelids, scrotum in the male, and labia majora in the female. They become reddened, scaly, greasy, painful, and pruritic. Plugs of inspissated sebum may accumulate in the hair follicles and give the appearance known as dyssebacia, or sharkskin (Fig. 30.6).

At the angles of the mouth there are painful fissures known as angular stomatitis when active (see Fig. 30.1*B* and *D*). When chronic, these fissures give rise to one form of rhagades. Vertical fissures of the vermilion surfaces of the lips constitute cheilosis. These and the angular lesions may become infected with *Candida albicans,* giving rise to the appearance known as perleche. The tongue may be painful, swollen, and magenta colored (Fig. 30.1*E*). These mucocutaneous changes may also be seen in other nutrient deficiencies or in elderly edentulous individuals with chronically moist angles. Because deficiency is often multiple, it is rarely possible in clinical practice to demonstrate the precise cause.

Other signs that have been described include photophobia, lacrimation, and conjunctival injection. Corneal neovascularization, so common in experimental animals, is rarely seen in man. The hemopoietic and nervous systems are occasionally affected. A normocytic normochromic anemia, reticulocytopenia, leukopenia, thrombocytopenia from marrow hypoplasia, and peripheral neuropathies with hyperesthesia, altered temperature sensation, and pain have been reported (31).

Niacin

Deficiency

Pellagra affects primarily the skin, gastrointestinal tract, and nervous system. Dermatosis is usually the earliest and most prominent manifestation. It is symmetric and appears on parts exposed to sunlight or trauma. Erythema progresses to keratosis and scaling with pigmentation. The back of the hands, wrists, forearms, face, and neck (Casal's necklace) are typically affected (Figs. 30.1*F* and 30.2*C*). The skin and mucous membrane changes of riboflavin deficiency are also commonly present (see above).

The tongue often has a "raw beef" appearance, is bright red, swollen, and painful. Symptoms of gastritis, bouts of diarrhea, and signs of malabsorption suggest similar changes in the gastrointestinal tract.

Nervous system involvement is suggested in the early stages by periods of depression with insomnia, headaches, and dizziness. Later, tremulous movement or rigidity of the limbs occurs with loss of tendon reflexes, numbness, and paresis of the extremities, ultimately incapacitating the patient. In profound deficiency, an encephalopathy has been described that resembles that of acute cerebral beriberi (see section on thiamin) but responds to some extent to niacin. Mental disturbance is so prominent in some patients that there is a real danger that the true diagnosis might be missed and the patient be incarcerated in a mental institution.

Toxicity

Side effects of megadoses (e.g., 3 g/day) include vasodilatation, flushing, pruritus, blistering of the skin with brown pigmentation, nausea, vomiting, and headache (32).

Pyridoxine (Vitamin B_6)

Deficiency

Pyridoxine deficiency is rarely severe enough to produce signs or symptoms. Volunteers receiving a deficient diet and a pyridoxine antagonist became irritable and depressed. Seborrheic dermatosis affected the nasolabial folds, cheeks, neck, and perineum. Several subjects also developed glossitis, angular stomatitis, blepharitis, and a peripheral neuropathy.

An uncommon form of sideroblastic anemia, often severe, has been reported to respond in some instances to pyridoxine, but most cases appear to be due to dependency rather than deficiency (33). Some years ago convulsions occurred in infants fed a milk formula in which the pyridoxine had been destroyed during processing (34).

Toxicity

A sensory neuropathy has been attributed to the abuse of pyridoxine in megadoses (35). Seven adults developed gradually progressive sensory ataxia and profound lower limb impairment of position and vibration sense. Touch, temperature, and pain perception were less affected. The motor and central nervous systems were unaffected. One review suggested that an impurity in the pharmacologic product might have been responsible (36).

Two patients with encephalitis suffered intensification of symptoms after dosing with pyridoxine and improved after its discontinuation (37).

Biotin

Deficiency

Biotin deficiency has occasionally been induced in patients who consumed large amounts of raw egg white over a prolonged period. Egg white contains avidin, which antagonizes the action of biotin. The skin of the face and hands becomes dry, shining, and scaling. The oral mucosa and tongue are swollen, magenta, and painful.

The most clear-cut cases of biotin deficiency occurred in children and adults maintained on long-term TPN in the early days before biotin was included in commercial vitamin formulations. An infant with short gut syndrome received TPN from 5 months of age. Five months later the infant lost all body hair and developed a waxy pallor, irritability, lethargy, mild hypotonia, and an erythematous rash. Biotin deficiency was confirmed biochemically, and all signs were reversed by supplementation (38). Two adult patients receiving home parenteral nutrition after extensive gut resection developed hair loss that was reversed by 200 μg biotin given intravenously daily (39). Another adult with alopecia, rash, and metabolic acidosis responded to 60 μg of biotin added to parenteral fluids (30.2*D*) (see also Chapter 28).

Vitamin B_{12} (Cobalamin)

Deficiency

Deficiency may be primary or secondary, as in pernicious anemia.

Pernicious Anemia. Pernicious anemia usually manifests after middle age. There is a slight female preponderance. It may be associated with signs of other autoimmune diseases. The most common complaints—those associated with anemia—ordinarily do not arise until the anemia is well advanced. Neurologic changes may long precede the hematologic changes. The tongue may be red, smooth, shining, and painful. Anorexia, weight loss, indigestion, and episodic diarrhea are all usually present (see Chapters 27 and 88).

The typical patient has prematurely gray hair and blue eyes. A few patients have widespread brownish pigmentation affecting nail beds and skin creases but sparing the mucous membranes (in contrast to Addison's disease). In advanced cases there is usually pyrexia, enlargement of the liver and spleen, and occasionally bruising due to thrombocytopenia. Older patients may present with congestive cardiac failure.

A distal sensory neuropathy with "glove and stocking" sensory loss, paresthesias, and areflexia may occur in isolation or more commonly together with a myelopathy known as subacute combined degeneration of the cord. In this condition the initial symptom is symmetric paresthesias of the feet or, occasionally, of the hands. A combination of weakness and loss of postural sense makes walking increasingly difficult. Psychiatric disturbances, especially mild dementia, may be the presenting or only feature. Visual loss from optic atrophy is not uncommon.

Congenital lack of intrinsic factor presents before the age of 2 years with irritability, vomiting, diarrhea, weight loss, and anemia. It was reported that an infant exclusively breast fed by a mother with latent pernicious anemia developed megaloblastic anemia and neurologic abnormalities (40).

Primary Dietary Deficiency. When dietary lack or malabsorption is the cause of deficiency, anemia is usually the most prominent feature, but glossitis, optic atrophy, and subacute combined degeneration of the cord have also been described. Hyperpigmentation of the skin of the forearms has been reported. Megaloblastic anemia developed in an infant exclusively breast fed by a vegan mother (41).

Folic Acid

Deficiency

The anemia of folic acid deficiency has morphologic features similar to those of vitamin B_{12} deficiency (see Chapter 26 and 88), but it develops much more rapidly. Subacute combined degeneration of the cord does not occur, but about 20% of patients may have peripheral neuropathy. The tongue may be red and painful in the acute stage. In chronic deficiency, the tongue papillae atrophy, leaving a shiny, smooth surface. Hyperpigmentation of the skin similar to that occasionally seen in vitamin B_{12} deficiency has been noted.

Folic acid therapy before conception is now accepted as protective against neural tube defects in infants of families in which these abnormalities have previously arisen (42). Inadequate one-carbon metabolism in conditions associated with genetic mutations and hyperhomocysteinemia is described in Chapters 26, 27, and 34).

Folate deficiency has been described in TPN with certain amino acid mixtures in the absence of supplementary folic acid (43). There is a single report of an infant, exclusively breast fed by a mother taking estrogen-progestogen contraceptive pills, who developed megaloblastic anemia responsive to folic acid (44).

Pantothenic Acid

Deficiency

Researchers reported "burning feet syndrome" in adult volunteers on a deficient diet and claimed that this condition responded to pantothenic acid. In clinical practice this distressing condition has rarely responded to this treatment, and there is at present no certain clinical manifestation of pantothenic acid deficiency.

Vitamin C (Ascorbic Acid)

Deficiency

Scurvy tends to affect either the very young or the elderly. The clinical picture differs in these two groups.

Infantile Scurvy (Barlow's Disease). The onset of infantile scurvy, usually in the second half of the 1st year of life, is preceded by a period of fretfulness, pallor, and loss of appetite. Localizing signs are tenderness and swelling, most marked at the knees or ankles. These signs result from characteristic bone changes demonstrable by radiograph (Figs. 30.7–30.9).

The earliest x-ray changes appear at the sites of most

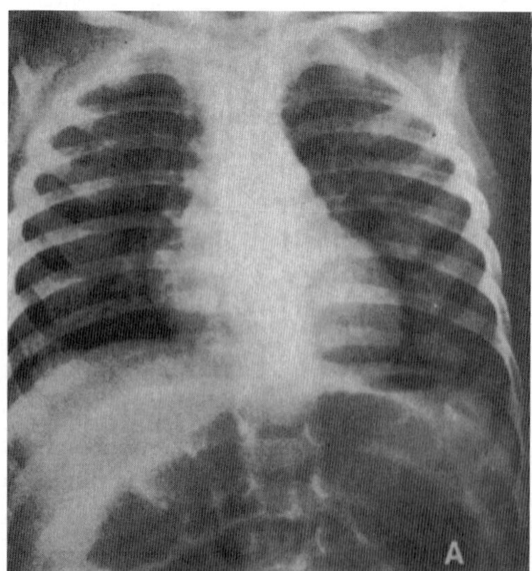

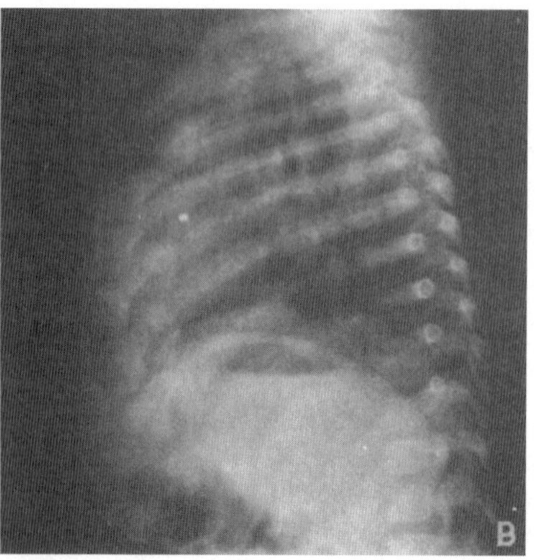

Figure 30.7. A 27-month-old boy with scurvy. Frontal (**A**) and lateral (**B**) chest roentgenograms demonstrate bony swelling at the costochondral junctions of the ribs. (From Watson RC, Grossman H, Meyers MA. Radiologic findings in nutritional disturbances. In: Shils ME, Olson JA, Shike M. Modern nutrition in health and disease. 8th ed. Philadelphia: Lea & Febiger, 1994, with permission.)

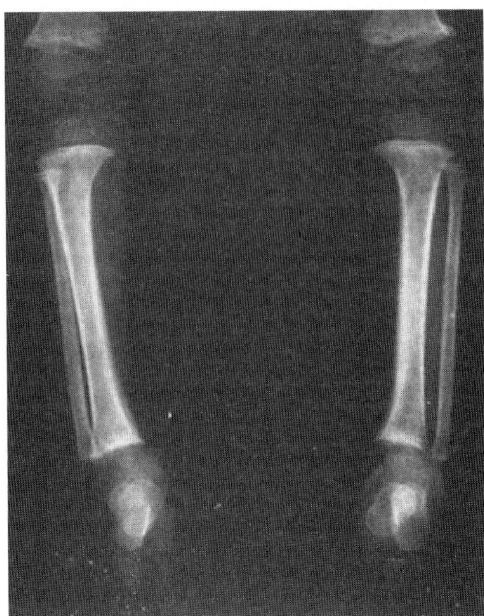

Figure 30.8. A 10-month-old boy with scurvy. A thick white line occurs at the metaphyses of the long bones of the knees. Linear breaks are present in the bones proximal and parallel to the white lines of the distal femur. Spurs are present and best seen at the ends of the femurs and medial aspect of the right tibia. The ossification centers have central rarefaction with heavy ring shadows on the margins. Periosteal new bone is along the medial aspects of the tibias. (From Watson RC, Grossman H, Meyers MA. Radiologic findings in nutritional disturbances. In: Shils ME, Olson JA, Shike M. Modern nutrition in health and disease. 8th ed. Philadelphia: Lea & Febiger, 1994, with permission.)

active growth; the sternal end of the ribs, distal end of the femur, proximal end of the humerus, both ends of the tibia and fibula, and distal ends of the radius and ulna. A zone of rarefaction immediately shaftward of the zone of provisional calcification gives rise to the "corner fracture" sign. Atrophy of trabecular structure and blurring of trabecular markings cause a "ground glass" appearance. Widening of the zone of provisional calcification causes a dense shadow at the end of the shaft which is also seen at the periphery of the centers of ossification. This ringlike appearance is seen best at the knee and is very characteristic of scurvy. As the deficiency proceeds, fractures may occur in areas of extending rarefaction. The overlying zone of provisional calcification may be comminuted with the shaft, and spur formation may occur. Epiphyses may separate and be displaced. Temporary healing often modifies the radiologic appearance. With treatment, even the grossest deformities resolve, although radiologic evidence may persist for several years.

Enlargement of the costochondral junctions produces the scorbutic rosary, which has a sharper feel than that due to rickets (see section on vitamin D). The infant often adopts the "pithed frog" position of maximum comfort, with the legs flexed at the knees and the hips partially flexed and externally rotated. The arms are less commonly involved. Hemorrhage and spongy changes in the gums are confined to the sites of teeth that have recently erupted or are about to do so. Bleeding may occur anywhere in the skin (the orbit is a frequent site) or from mucous membranes, including the renal tract. In infancy, intracranial hemorrhages are rapidly progressive if treatment is delayed, and death may occur. Petechiae and ecchymoses, usually found in the region of the bone lesions, are less common than in the adult. Microcytic hypochromic anemia is common, a normochromic normocytic picture less so. Older children may develop characteristic perifollicular hemorrhages and hair changes seen in the adult.

Adult Scurvy. Early symptoms of adult scurvy are weakness, easy fatigue, and listlessness, followed by shortness of breath and aching bones, joints, and muscles, especially at night. These symptoms are followed by characteristic changes in the skin (45). Acne, indistinguishable from that of adolescence, precedes defects in the hairs of the body. These defects consist of broken and coiled hairs and a "swan-neck" deformity resulting from their being flat instead of round in cross section (Fig. 30.2*E*). A salient feature of scurvy in the adult is perifollicular hemorrhages and perifollicular hyperkeratosis, most commonly affecting the anterior aspects of the thorax, forearms, thighs, and legs and the anterior abdominal wall (Fig. 30.2*F*).

Frank bleeding is a late feature of scurvy. The classic gum changes are only associated with natural teeth or buried roots and are enhanced by poor dental hygiene and advanced caries. The interdental papillae become swollen and purple and bleed with trauma. In advanced scurvy, the gums are spongy and friable, bleeding freely. Secondary infection leads to loosening of the teeth and to gangrene. Patients who are edentulous or whose teeth are in good repair have little or no evidence of scorbutic gingivitis. Hemorrhage commonly occurs deep in muscles and into joints as well as over large areas of the skin in the form of ecchymoses (Fig. 30.10). Multiple splinter hemorrhages may form a crescent near the distal ends of the nails. Old scars break down, and new wounds fail to heal. Bleeding into viscera or the brain leads to convulsions and shock; death may occur abruptly.

ESSENTIAL FATTY ACIDS (EFAS)

Although EFAs are not vitamins in the ordinary sense, it is convenient to consider symptoms of deficiency of these fatty acids here.

ω-6 EFA Deficiency

Growth retardation, sparse hair growth, branlike desquamation of the skin of the trunk, poor wound healing, and increased susceptibility to infection have been observed in infants receiving a formula deficient in essential fat or in children and adults receiving long-term, lipid-free parenteral nutrition (46).

Sometimes there is only dry, flaky skin, but more advanced deficiency results in scaling, eczematoid dermatosis, usually starting on the nasolabial folds and eye-

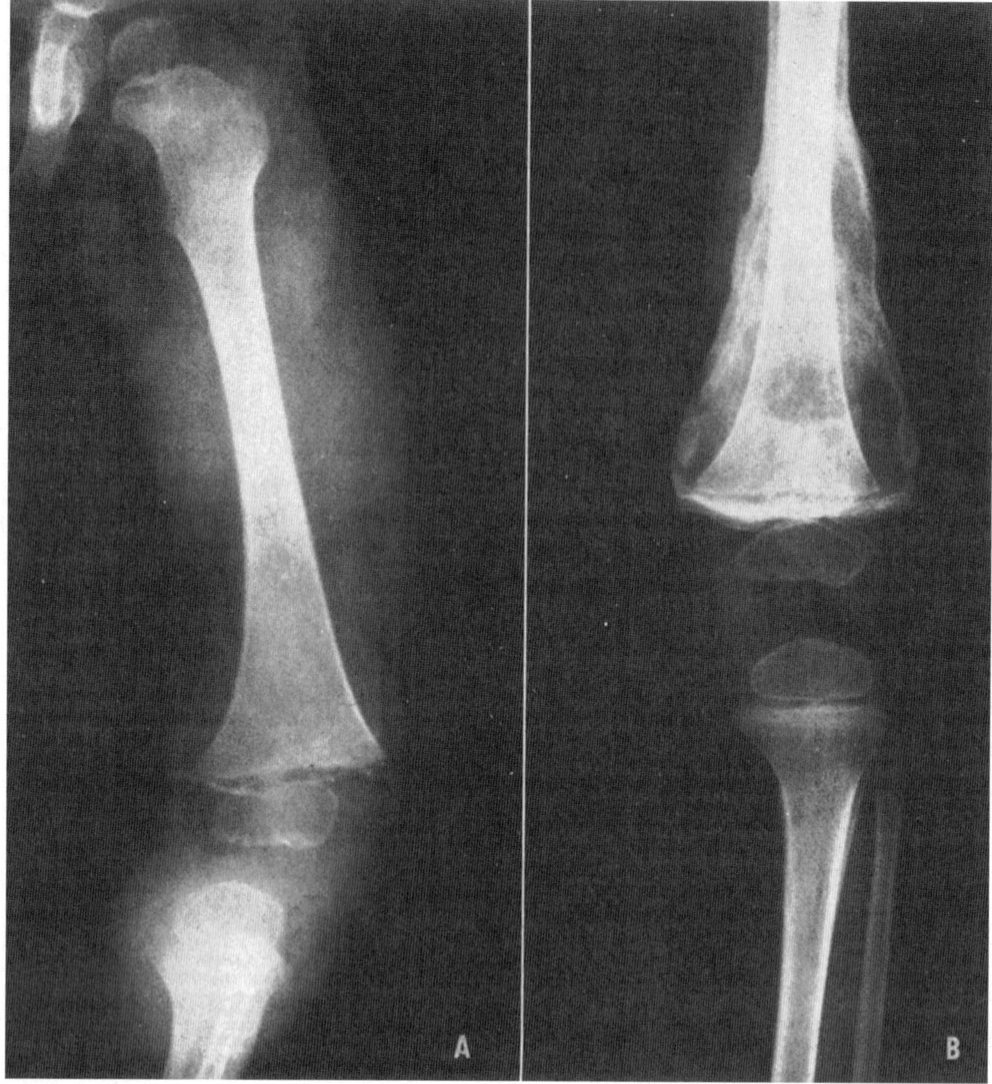

Figure 30.9. A 12-month-old boy with healing scurvy. **A.** Fracture of the provisional zone of the calcification of the distal femur with early calcification is apparent. Displacement of the soft tissues is due to hematoma that has not begun to calcify. **B.** Extensive calcification of elevated periosteum occurs after 2 weeks of vitamin C therapy. (From Watson RC, Grossman H, Meyers MA. Radiologic findings in nutritional disturbances. In: Shils ME, Olson JA, Shike M. Modern nutrition in health and disease. 8th ed. Philadelphia: Lea & Febiger, 1994, with permission.)

brows and spreading across the face and neck (Fig. 30.11). Anemia and enlarged fatty liver have also been reported.

ω-3 EFA Deficiency

The first human report of ω-3 EFA deficiency was of a 7-year-old girl with extensive gut resection who received TPN rich in ω-6 but very low in ω-3 fatty acids. Neurologic changes included paresthesias, weakness, inability to walk, pain in the legs, and blurred vision (47). These are reported to have responded to change of treatment, but it is possible that other deficiencies, including that of vitamin E, might have been responsible. Other possible cases have since been reported, and the subject has been reviewed (48). It now appears that the symptoms of the two kinds of fatty acid deficiency are quite distinct.

MINERALS

Calcium

Hypocalcemia

Symptoms and signs of underlying disorders are present in hypocalcemia. True hypocalcemia (i.e., subnormal ionized calcium) in clinical conditions is rarely caused by inadequate calcium ingestion but rather by disorders of calcium metabolism or use. It affects the nervous system with depression and psychosis, progressing to dementia or encephalopathy. The most characteristic syndrome is tetany, consisting of *(a)* paresthesias about the lips, tongue, fingers, and feet; *(b)* carpopedal spasm, resulting in "obstetrician's hand," or Trousseau's sign, a deformity that may be painful and prolonged (Fig. 30.2*G*); *(c)* generalized muscle aching; and *(d)* spasm of the facial muscles. At the earlier stage of latent tetany, neuromuscular irritability may be

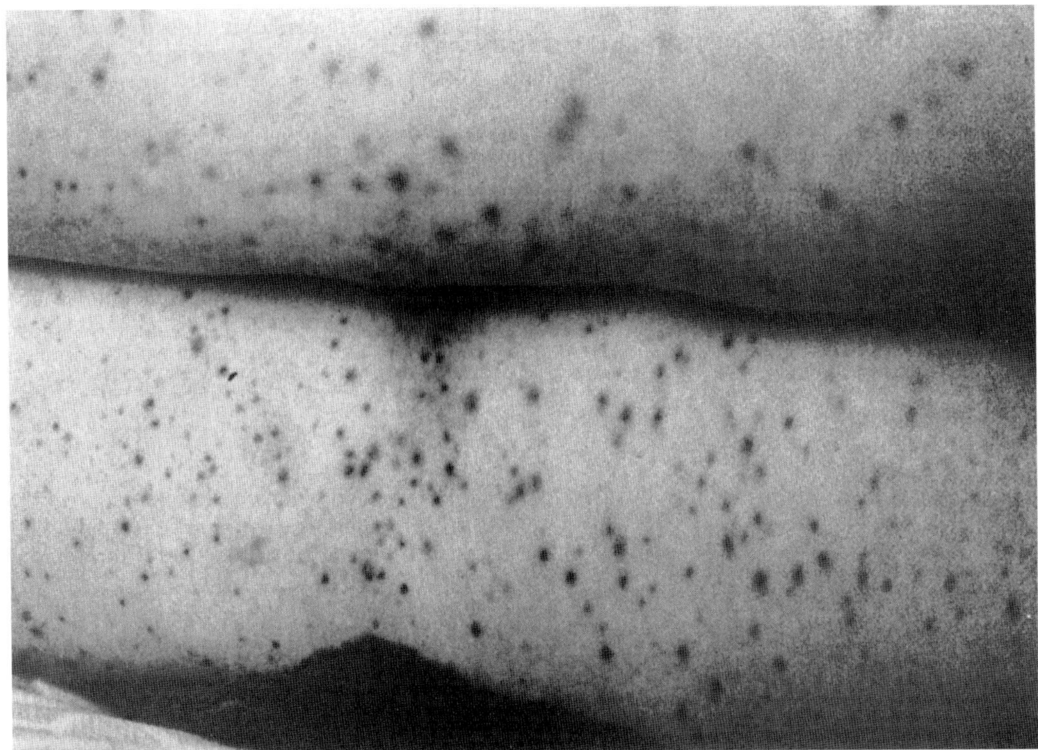

Figure 30.10. Perifollicular hemorrhages of the legs in adult scurvy.

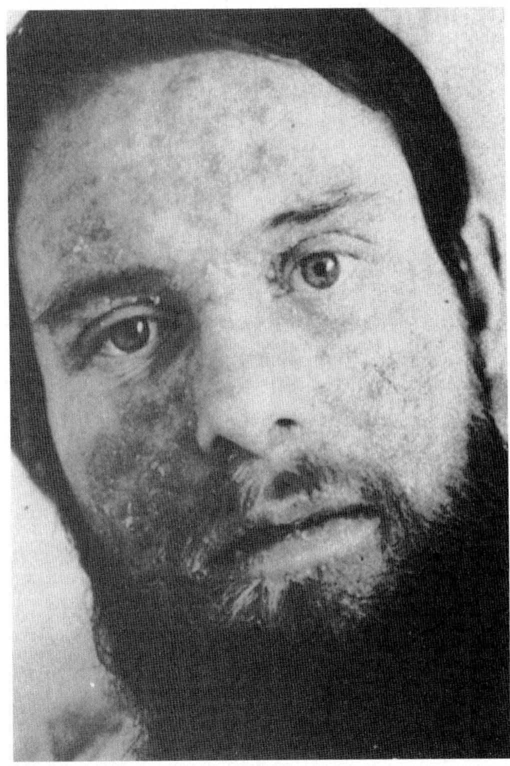

Figure 30.11. Dermatosis of essential fatty acid deficiency associated with total parenteral nutrition. (Courtesy of Dr. R. E. Hodges.)

elicited by provocative tests. Chvostek's sign is contraction of the facial muscles on light tapping of the facial nerve. Trousseau's sign is carpopedal spasm induced by restriction of the blood supply to a limb by a tourniquet or elevation above systolic pressure with a blood pressure cuff applied for 3 minutes or less. Rarely, cataract is the earliest feature.

In about 80% of very low birth weight infants, osteopenia can be diagnosed radiologically, and rickets is much less common (49). In the neonate and older infant, tetany may manifest as rhythmic, focal myoclonic jerks, sometimes followed by convulsions, cyanosis, and heart failure. Muscular spasms and laryngismus stridulus may occur in young children.

Osteoporosis

Calcium insufficiency plays an ill-defined role in this condition of loss of bone mass (see Chapters 83 and 85). It is common in the elderly, especially in postmenopausal white women. There is bone deformity, localized pain, and fractures. Osteomalacia may coexist. The most common deformity is loss of height caused by vertebral collapse, which accounts for most of the pain. Fractures of the neck of the femur and Colles' fracture above the wrist are most commonly precipitated by trauma, which may be trivial, in elderly persons with osteoporosis.

Calcium-Deficiency Rickets

Reports from South Africa suggested that true rickets can be produced by dietary calcium deficiency in the presence of normal vitamin D status (50). The histologic changes of rickets were confirmed by biopsy and responded to calcium therapy alone (51).

Hypercalcemia

Hypercalcemia has a variety of causes and produces a symptom complex that is, to some extent, characteristic. Gastrointestinal symptoms include anorexia, nausea, vomiting, constipation, abdominal pain, and ileus. Renal system involvement produces polyuria, nocturia, polydipsia, stone formation, and sometimes hypertension and signs and symptoms of uremia. Muscle weakness and myopathy occur. More advanced disease, which causes psychosis, delirium, stupor, and coma, may be fatal.

Phosphorus

Hypophosphatemia

Hypophosphatemia is defined as lowered inorganic phosphate level (<0.71 mmol/L, or 2.2 mg/dL) with or without a significant decrease in the total body phosphate in relation to total body nitrogen. The latter situation usually occurs in any situation stimulating anaerobic glycolysis, such as infusion of hypertonic glucose continuously without adequate phosphate replacement; this results in a shift of serum inorganic phosphate into cells and a fall in serum phosphate levels. The markedly depressed serum phosphate (usually <0.30 mmol/L, or 0.93 mg/dL) is associated in 3 to 4 days with circumoral and extremity paresthesias and red cell fragility and hemolysis.

Total Body Phosphate Depletion

Total body phosphate depletion occurs with total body nitrogen loss as the result of various diseases that lead to excessive loss of both in the stool (e.g., malabsorption, vitamin D deficiency) or in the urine (e.g., hyperparathyroidism, congenital or drug-induced renal tubular acidosis, severe potassium depletion). In the management of advanced renal disease, administration of phosphate-binding gels intended to reduce phosphate absorption in association with restricted phosphate in the diet may lead to symptomatic phosphate deficiency (52, 53) (Table 30.1) (see also Chapter 8).

Table 30.1
Manifestations of Phosphate Depletion and/or Hypophosphatemia

Organ System Affected	Manifestation
Constitutional	Anorexia, malaise, debility, lethargy
Neuropsychiatric	Altered sensorium, confusion, seizures, coma, decreased motor and sensory nerve conduction
Hematologic	Erythrocyte deformity, hemolysis, impaired phagocytosis, thrombocytopathy, hemorrhage
Metabolic	Insulin resistance and glucose intolerance
Gastrointestinal	Dysphagia, ileus, impaired liver function
Musculoskeletal	Rickets (osteomalacia), arthralgia, muscle weakness, rhabdomyolysis
Renal	Glycosuria, magnesuria, renal tubular acidosis

From Berner YM, Shike M. Annu Rev Nutr 1988;8:121–48.

Potassium

Deficiency

Potassium deficiency is usually due to excessive losses in urine or stool, less commonly to decreased intake, as in starvation or failure to give potassium in intravenous solutions, and losses in sweat as in cystic fibrosis.

Severe hypokalemia (serum K <3 mmol/L, or <3 mEq/L) may cause muscle weakness leading to respiratory failure, paralytic ileus, hypotension, and tetany. Potassium nephropathy results in polyuria with secondary polydipsia. Cardiac effects are particularly likely in patients receiving digitalis. The electrocardiogram (ECG) is characteristic with S-T segment depression, increased U wave amplitude, and T wave amplitude less than that of U wave in the same lead. Premature ventricular and atrial contractions and ventricular and atrial tachyarrhythmias occur.

Toxicity (Hyperkalemia)

Acute oliguric states are often responsible for hyperkalemia, but excessive ingestion or infusion may produce symptoms even in the presence of normal renal function.

Cardiac toxicity, of serious import, starts with shortening of the Q-T interval of the ECG and tall, peaked T waves. Progressive toxicity with serum K levels above 6.5 mmol/L (>6.5 mEq/L) causes nodal and ventricular arrhythmias, widening of the QRS complex, PR interval prolongation and disappearance of the P wave, and finally degeneration of the QRS complex with ventricular asystole or fibrillation and death.

Magnesium

Deficiency

In depletion studies in humans as well as in clinical practice, when hypomagnesemia (defined as serum Mg <1.5 mEq/L, <1.9 mg/dL) progresses below 1.0 mEq/L, it is often accompanied by hypocalcemia and hypokalemia.

The symptoms and signs of both experimental and clinical deficiency are primarily neuromuscular: Trousseau and Chvostek signs, muscle fasciculations, tremor, muscle spasm, personality changes, anorexia, nausea, and vomiting. Recently, low dietary intake of magnesium was associated with impaired lung function and wheezing (54). Convulsions or coma in infancy is not infrequently associated with magnesium deficiency.

Magnesium depletion has been associated with malabsorption syndromes, renal tubular abnormalities, endocrine dysfunction, and genetic and familial conditions (55). In some clinical situations, serum magnesium may be within normal limits despite evidence of cellular or tissue depletion (see also Chapter 9).

Toxicity (Hypermagnesemia)

Elevated serum magnesium levels (>2.1 mEq/L, >2.5 mg/dL) are not uncommon in patients with renal failure who are receiving magnesium-containing drugs and in children with chronic constipation treated with magnesium sulfate enemas. With higher levels, deep tendon reflexes disappear and ECG abnormalities (prolonged PR interval, widening of QRS complex, and increased T wave amplitude) occur. Hypertension, respiratory depression, narcosis, and ultimately cardiac arrest may occur with very high blood magnesium levels (see Chapter 9).

Iodide (Iodine)

Deficiency

Enlargement of the thyroid gland is the most common clinical sign of iodide deficiency. When it is due to iodine lack, this condition is termed simple, colloid, endemic, or euthyroid goiter. It is more common in women and is often noted at the onset of puberty, during pregnancy, or at the menopause. Early on, the enlargement is soft, symmetric, and smooth; later, multiple nodules and cysts may appear. Most patients are euthyroid, a few have hyperthyroidism, and rarely hypothyroidism occurs.

Severe endemic goiter is often accompanied by cretinism. Endemic cretinism occurs in two distinct forms, the myxedematous and the neurologic, which may coexist (56). In most areas of the world, the neurologic form is by far the more common. The clinical manifestations of the two conditions are listed in Table 30.2 (see also Chapter 13).

In recent years attention has been focused on the effects of iodine deficiency in early life (57). It is responsible for a proportion of stillbirths, spontaneous abortions, congenital malformations, and neonatal deaths. Physical growth and mental development are impaired in early childhood.

Toxicity

Prolonged excessive intake of iodine leads eventually to iodide goiter and myxedema, especially in patients with preexisting Hashimoto's thyroiditis.

Iron

Deficiency

Iron deficiency has its major impact on many systems via reduction in tissue oxygenation due to decreased hemoglobin concentration. The clinical picture depends on the rapidity of development of anemia and on its severity (see Chapters 10 and 88).

The typical microcytic hypochromic anemia of insidious onset manifests as increasing fatigue and slight pallor, best seen in the mucous membranes. Later, cardiorespiratory signs and symptoms include exertional dyspnea, tachycardia, palpitations, angina, claudication, night cramps, increased arterial and capillary pulsation, cardiac bruits, reversible cardiac enlargement and, if cardiac failure occurs, basal crepitations, peripheral edema, and ascites. Neuromuscular involvement is evidenced by headache, tinnitus, vertigo, cramps, faintness, increased cold sensitivity, and retinal hemorrhage. Gastrointestinal symptoms include anorexia, nausea, constipation, and diarrhea. Low-grade fever, menstrual irregularity, urinary frequency, and loss of libido may occur.

Iron deficiency per se has certain characteristics not usually associated with other forms of anemia. A nonspecific glossitis with almost complete loss of filiform papillae is common. Angular stomatitis is less frequent. Spoon-shaped nails (koilonychia) are characteristic of longstanding iron deficiency. The Patterson-Kelly (Plummer-Vinson) syndrome is the association of iron deficiency anemia, glossitis, dysphagia, and achlorhydria, usually seen in middle-aged women, but much less commonly than was formerly the case. In severe cases, postcricoid webs and malignant change in this region may occur. Signs of deficiency of some B group vitamins are also often present. Pica (geophagia) is an occasional feature. Even mild iron deficiency is considered important in decreased work efficiency (58). In infants and young children, certain aspects of learning ability are impaired.

Toxicity

Acute poisoning causes vomiting, upper abdominal pain, pallor, cyanosis, diarrhea, drowsiness, and shock.

Table 30.2
Comparative Clinical Features in Myxoedematous and Neurologic Cretinism

Feature	Myxedematous Cretin	Neurologic Cretin
Mental retardation	Present, often severe	Present, often severe
Deaf-mutism	Absent	Usually present
Cerebral diplegia	Absent	Often present
Stature	Severe growth retardation	Usually normal, occasionally slight growth retardation
General features	Coarse dry skin, protuberant abdomen with umbilical hernia, large tongue	No physical signs of hypothyroidism
Reflexes	Delayed relaxation	Excessively brisk
ECG	Small-voltage QRS complexes and other abnormalities of hypothyroidism	Normal
X-ray limbs	Epiphyseal dysgenesis	Normal
Effect of thyroid hormones	Improvement	No effect

From Hetzel BS, Hay ID. Clin Endocrinol 1979;11:445–60.

Death may occur in children mistaking iron tablets for sweets.

Chronic toxicity (hemochromatosis, iron overload) affects many tissues (see Chapter 10). Diabetes, often the presenting feature, eventually develops in about 80% of patients. The skin is a characteristic slate-gray color. The liver becomes enlarged and then cirrhotic, and hepatoma may develop. Cardiomyopathy leads to heart failure in about 50% of patients. Pituitary failure may cause testicular atrophy and loss of libido. Focal hemosiderosis damages the lungs and kidneys.

Copper

Deficiency

The principal features of copper deficiency are a hypochromic anemia unresponsive to iron therapy, neutropenia, and osteoporosis. Early radiologic findings are osteoporosis of the metaphyses and epiphyses and retarded bone age. Typical findings are increased density of the provisional zone of calcification and cupping with sickle-shaped spurs in the metaphyseal region. Other skeletal abnormalities include periosteal layering and submetaphyseal and rib fractures (Fig. 30.12).

Premature infants are especially vulnerable and have shown the following signs: pallor, decreased pigmentation of the skin and hair, prominent superficial veins, skin lesions resembling seborrheic dermatitis, failure to thrive, diarrhea, and hepatosplenomegaly. Some have features suggesting central nervous system damage, including hypotonia, apathy, psychomotor retardation, apparent lack of visual responses, and apneic episodes.

The most extreme form is seen in Menkes' steely hair disease (59), a complex X-linked disease of male infants in which there is both failure to absorb copper and then failure to form functional cuproproteins. Interference with cross-linking of elastin and collagen can be held responsible for many of the features: premature rupture of the membranes leading to premature birth, lax skin and joints, elongation and dilatation of major arteries resulting in rupture and hemorrhage, subintimal thickening with partial occlusion of major arteries, hernias, and diverticula of bladder and ureters causing recurrent infection or rupture. Osteoporosis, flaring of metaphyseal edges, and Wormian bones in cranial sutures may all be secondary to collagen abnormalities. Lack of pigmentation of the skin and hair and abnormal spiral twisting (pili torti) and fragility of hair add to the characteristic appearance of affected babies. Neurologic development rarely progresses beyond 6 to 8 weeks, and even these functions are lost during the ensuing months. Ataxia is striking in mild cases.

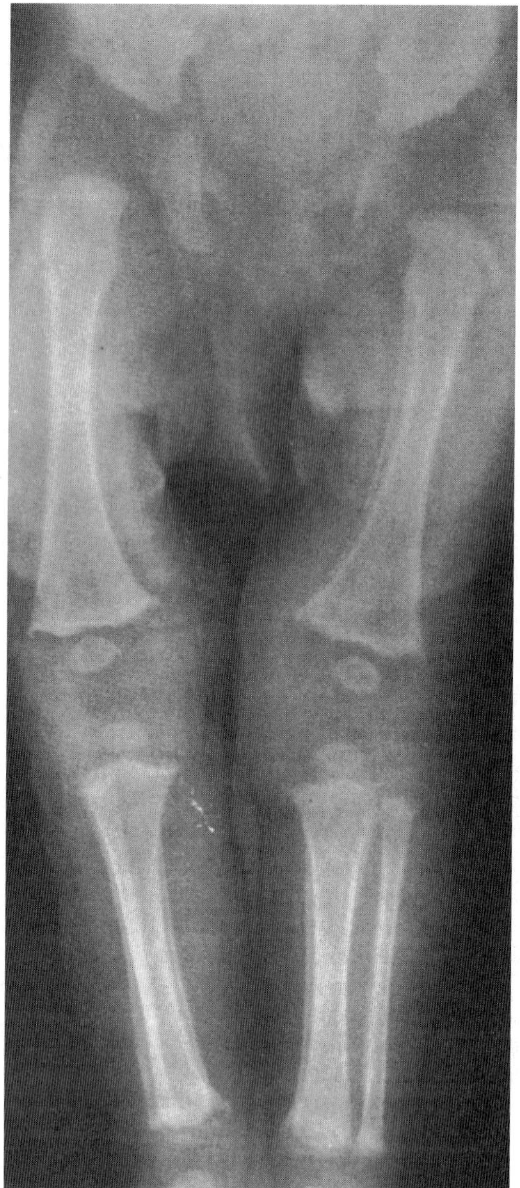

Figure 30.12. Bone changes due to copper deficiency. (From Bennani-Smires C, Medina J, Young LW. Am J Dis Child 1980;134:1155.)

Toxicity

In Wilson's disease (hepatolenticular degeneration) accumulation of copper in the liver leads to cirrhosis and signs of liver failure. Deposits in the brain result in tremors, choreoathetoid movements, rigidity, dysarthria, and eventually dementia. Anemia and signs of renal failure are common. Characteristic changes in the eye are the Kayser-Fleischer ring, a brown or green ring near the limbus of the cornea, and a "sunflower" cataract. Childhood cirrhosis has been common on the Indian subcontinent and is reported to occur in Indian children living elsewhere (60). It has been attributed to copper accumulation in the liver. The suggestion that the source of the copper is milk contaminated by boiling and storage in brass and copper pots has not been confirmed (61).

Acute poisoning has resulted from ingestion of solutions of copper salts or contaminated water supplies or dialysis fluid. In severe cases, evidence of hepatic or renal failure (or both) is found.

Zinc

Deficiency

The first report of human zinc deficiency was from Iran, consisting of a syndrome of dwarfism, hypogonadism, anemia, hepatosplenomegaly, rough dry skin, and lethargy associated with geophagia (62). In a similar picture in Egypt, parasitism appears to play an important role (63). Hypogeusia (impaired taste) and growth retardation in otherwise healthy children have been found to respond to zinc supplementation in parts of North America (64).

Clinical cases of zinc deficiency have been reported with various manifestations, depending on the severity of depletion and other factors. In addition to those mentioned above they include dermatoses, immune deficiencies, glossitis, photophobia, lack of dark adaptation, and delayed wound healing. Precipitating factors include short bowel syndrome, alcoholism with pancreatic and liver disease (Fig. 30.1*H*), sickle cell anemia, certain chelating medications, the acrodermatitis enteropathica genotype, intestinal losses via fistula, and inadequate amounts of zinc in parenteral nutrition fluids (see Chapter 11).

TPN with inadequate zinc supplementation has occasionally caused an acute deficiency syndrome consisting of diarrhea, mental depression, alopecia, and dermatosis, usually around the orbits, nose, and mouth (65) (Fig. 30.1*H*). Loss of zinc through an intestinal fistula was responsible for development of skin lesions about the mouth, palms (sterile pustules), and pressure points on hands and elbows in a 6-year-old child with non-Hodgkin's lymphoma (Fig. 30.2*H*); they responded rapidly to additional zinc.

Acrodermatitis enteropathica, an autosomal recessive disorder manifested in artificially fed infants, caused by a defect in zinc absorption, is characterized by extensive dermatitis, growth retardation, diarrhea, hair loss, and paronychia (see Chapter 11). The skin changes somewhat resemble those seen in kwashiorkor (66), but the skin changes of zinc deficiency have a typical appearance: the distribution is often acro-orificial, commonly also involving the flexures and friction areas, and may become generalized. Eczematoid, psoriaform, vesiculobullous, and pustular lesions may be present. The earliest skin lesions are bright reddish, nonscaly macules and patches.

Toxicity

Ingestion of large amounts of zinc, usually from an acid food or drink from a galvanized container, has caused vomiting and diarrhea. Excessive zinc intake, as in large daily doses (30–150 mg) for several weeks, interferes with copper absorption and leads to copper deficiency. Severe lethargy in dialysis patients has been attributed to excessive zinc in dialysis fluids. Accidental intravenous administration of 1.5 g has proven fatal.

Fluoride

Deficiency

Fluorine has not yet been proved an essential element for man, but it has a role in bone mineralization and hardening of tooth enamel. Areas with a low fluorine content in the water supply have high rates of dental caries. Fluoridation of the water or use of supplemented tooth paste is associated with a significant fall in dental caries rates (see also Chapter 16).

Toxicity (Fluorosis)

Fluorosis is associated with high levels (>10 ppm) in the drinking water. It is most evident in permanent teeth that develop during high fluorine intake. Deciduous teeth are affected only at very high levels. The earliest changes, chalky white, irregularly distributed patches on the surface of the enamel, become infiltrated by yellow or brown staining, giving rise to the characteristic "mottled" appearance (Fig. 30.1*G*). More severe fluorosis also causes pitting of the enamel.

Chronic ingestion of very large amounts of fluoride (>5 mg/day) for years may lead to crippling skeletal fluorosis progressing from occasional stiffness or joint pain to chronic pain and osteoporosis of long bones. This rare condition in the United States is associated with drinking high-fluoride well water (66a).

Selenium

Deficiency

Two syndromes have been described from China in which selenium deficiency is believed important. The first is Keshan disease, named for its place of origin, which consists of a highly fatal cardiomyopathy affecting mainly young children and women of childbearing age. Good response to selenium supplementation has been reported (67). The other, known as Kashin-Beck disease, features osteoarthritis during preadolescence or adolescence that results in dwarfing and joint deformities from cartilage abnormalities (68) (see Chapter 14).

In the United States, some patients have been reported to develop selenium deficiency on TPN with no added selenium (69). Features have included a severe cardiomyopathy, muscle pain and tenderness, dyschromotrichia, white fingernail beds, and macrocytosis.

Toxicity

Endemic selenosis, long recognized in animals, has been suspected in some human communities, most convincingly from China (70). The most frequently observed signs were loss of hair and nails. Skin lesions and polyneuritis were less certainly attributed to selenium toxicity.

Alopecia and nail changes occurred in New York City from consumption of a "health store" supplement containing excessive amounts of selenium (71). In eight reported cases of criminal poisoning, four were fatal (72). Symptoms and signs were distinctive: metallic taste, odor of garlic caused by methylation of selenium, mucosal irritation, gastroenteritis, paronychia, and red pigmentation of nails, hair, and teeth.

Chromium

Deficiency

A patient receiving total parenteral nutrition for more than 5 years unexpectedly developed 15% weight loss, peripheral neuropathy, and glucose intolerance after 3.5 years of nutritional support (73). These conditions were all reversed with chromium therapy. Two further cases have been reported, both with weight loss and hyperglycemia that responded to chromium (74, 75). In some parts of the world, protein-energy malnutrition appears to be complicated by chromium deficiency (76).

Toxicity

Toxicity usually results from direct contact or inhalation in industry. Chrome ulcers on the hands or perforation of the nasal septum may result. Lung cancer can occur, but only with hexavalent compounds.

Cobalt

There is little evidence of a role for cobalt in human nutrition other than as part of the vitamin B_{12} molecule.

Toxicity

Cobalt at one time was recommended for treatment of anemia of nephritis and infection in addition to the usual hemopoietic agents. In this context, it was reported to cause goiter, myxedema, and congestive heart failure in five patients (77). A cardiomyopathy with a high mortality has been described after industrial exposure, during maintenance dialysis, and after drinking beer that was contaminated with cobalt during processing (78).

Molybdenum

Deficiency

An autosomal recessive molybdenum cofactor deficiency resulting in deficiencies of xanthine oxidase and sulfite oxidase was reported in more than 20 patients in the past decade (79). There is severe brain damage, convulsions are frequent, and about half the patients failed to survive beyond early infancy.

Only one clear-cut case related to prolonged TPN has been reported to date (80), involving tachycardia, tachypnea, headache, night blindness, central scotomas, nausea, vomiting, lethargy, disorientation, and coma. These signs and symptoms were reversed by 300 μg/day of molybdenum, and the urinary excretion of abnormal amounts of methionine metabolites was dramatically decreased.

Toxicity

Elevated blood levels of molybdenum were associated with a goutlike syndrome in Armenia in 1961 (81). Other symptoms and signs mentioned suggested some involvement of liver, gastrointestinal tract, and kidney. The pathogenesis was unclear.

Manganese

Deficiency

One unsubstantiated case of human deficiency was reported to have occurred when manganese was inadvertently omitted from an experimental diet fed to a volunteer. Clinical sings included weight loss, transient dermatitis, nausea and vomiting, changes in hair color, and slow growth of hair (82).

Toxicity

Manganese toxicity is usually reported in those who mine or refine ore. Prolonged exposure has caused neurologic changes resembling those of parkinsonism or Wilson's disease. In an area in Greece, well water with a high manganese content may be responsible for occurrence of a parkinsonian syndrome (83). Recently, it has been reported that manganese accumulates in the basal ganglia of patients with cirrhosis of the liver, and it is suggested that this may be associated with the occurrence of encephalopathy in these patients (84). Toxicity has been reported in children given 0.8 to 1.0 mmol of manganese ion per kilogram body weight in long-term TPN (85). This level is about 50 times greater than the recommendations in Chapter 101.

REFERENCES

1. McLaren DS. Nutritional Ophthalmology. New York: Academic Press, 1980.
2. Sommer A. Nutritional blindness: xerophthalmia and keratomalacia. New York: Oxford University Press, 1982.
3. Sommer A, Hussaini G, Muhilal, et al. Am J Clin Nutr 1980;33:887–91.
4. Sommer A, Emran N, Tamba T. Am J Ophthalmol 1979;87: 330–3.
5. Teng KH. Ophthalmologica 1959;137:81–5.
6. International Vitamin A Consultative Group. The symptoms and signs of vitamin A deficiency and their relationship to applied nutrition. Washington, DC: IVACG, 1981.
6a. Sommer A, West KP Jr. Vitamin A deficiency: health, survival and vision. New York: Oxford University Press, 1996.
7. Hathcock JN, Hattan DG, Jenkins MY, et al. Am J Clin Nutr 1990;52:183–202.
8. Lammer EJ, Chen DT, Hoar RM, et al. N Engl J Med 1985;313:837–41.
9. Rothman KJ, Moore LL, Singer MR, et al. N Engl J Med 1995;333:1369–73.
10. Blau EB. Lancet 1996;347:626.
11. Black JA, Bonham Carter JE. Lancet 1963;2:745–9.
12. Melhorn DK, Gross SJ. Pediatr 1971;79:569–80.
13. Melhorn DK, Gross SJ. Pediatr 1971;79:581–8.
14. Foster CS. Histopathology 1979;3:1–17.
15. Rosenberg RN. N Engl J Med 1995;333:1351–2.
16. Lorch V, Murphy D, Hoersten LR, et al. Pediatrics 1985;75:598–602.

16a. Rivera A Jr, Abdo KM, Bucher JR, et al. Dev Pharmacol Ther 1990;14:231–237.
17. Johnson L, Bowen FW Jr, Abbasi S, et al. Pediatrics 1985;75: 619–38.
18. Shearer MJ. Lancet 1995;345:229–34.
19. Kark R, Lozner EL. Lancet 1939;2:1162–3.
20. Berthoud M, Bouvier CA, Krahenbuhl B. Schweiz Med Wochenschr 1966;96:1522–4.
21. Corrigan JJ, Marcus FI. JAMA 1974;230:1300–1.
22. Campbell CH. Lancet 1984;2:446–9.
23. Jeffrey FE, Abelmann WH. Am J Med 1971;50:123–8.
24. Haas RH. Annu Rev Nutr 1988;8:483–515.
25. Editorial. Lancet 1990;2:912–3.
26. Victor M, Adams RD, Collins GH. The Wernicke -Korsakoff syndrome. Oxford: Blackwell, 1971.
27. Seehra H, MacDermott N, Lascelles RG, et al. Br Med J 1996;312:434.
28. Jelliffe DB. Infant nutrition in the tropics and subtropics. 2nd ed. Geneva: WHO, 1968.
29. Pincus JH. Dev Med Child Neurol 1972;14:87–101.
30. Stephens JM, Grant R, Yeh CS. Am J Emerg Med 1992;10:61–3.
31. Lopez R, Cole HS, Montoya MF, et al. J Pediatr 1975;87:420–2.
32. Hankes LV. Nicotinic acid and nicotinamide. In: Machlin LJ, ed. Handbook of vitamins. New York: Marcel Dekker 1984; 329–77.
33. Weintraub LR, Conrad ME, Crosby WH. N Engl J Med 1966;275:169–76.
34. Coursin DB. Vitam Horm 1964;22:756–86.
35. Schaumberg H, Kaplan J, Windebank A, et al. N Engl J Med 1983;309:445–8.
36. Rudman D, Williams PJ. N Engl J Med 1983;309:488–9.
37. Hottinger A, Berger H, Krauthammer W. Schweiz Med Wochenschr 1964;94:221–8.
38. Mock DM, DeLorimer AA, Leberman WM, et al. N Engl J Med 1981;304:820–3.
39. Innis SM, Allardyce DB. Am J Clin Nutr 1983;37:185–7.
40. Johnson PR, Roloff JS. J Pediatr 1982;100:917–9.
41. Higginbottom MC, Sweetman K, Nyhan WL. N Engl J Med 1978;299:317–20.
42. MRC Vitamin Study Research Group. Lancet 1991;338:131–7.
43. Anonymous. Nutr Rev 1983;41:51–3.
44. Mandel H, Berant M. Arch Dis Child 1985;60:971–2.
45. Hodges RE, Hood J, Canham JE, et al. Am J Clin Nutr 1971;24:432–43.
46. Fleming CR, Smith LM, Hodges RE. Am J Clin Nutr 1976;29:976–83.
47. Holman RT, Johnson SB, Hatch TF. Am J Clin Nutr 1982;35:617–23.
48. Anderson GJ, Connor WE. Am J Clin Nutr 1989;49:585–7.
49. Bentur L, Alon U, Berant M. Pediatr Rev Commun 1987;1:291–310.
50. Pettifor JM, Ross P, Wang J, et al. J Pediatr 1978;92:320–4.
51. Marie PJ, Pettifor JM, Ross FP, et al. N Engl J Med 1982;307:584–8.
52. Knochel JP. N Engl J Med 1985;313:447–9.
53. Berner YM, Shike M. Annu Rev Nutr 1988;8:121–48.
54. Britton J, Pavord I, Richards K, et al. Lancet 1994;344: 357–62.
55. Shils ME. Annu Rev Nutr 1988;8:429–60.
56. Hetzel BS, Hay ID. Clin Endocrinol 1979;11:445–60.
57. Hetzel BS, Dunn JT. Annu Rev Nutr 1989;9:21–38.
58. Andersen HT, Barkve H. Scand J Clin Lab Invest 1970;25: (Suppl 114):1–62.
59. Danks DM. Annu Rev Nutr 1988;8:235–57.
60. Portmann B, Tanner MS, Mowat AP, et al. Lancet 1978;2:1338–40.
61. Report of ICMR Multicultural Collaborative Study on Indian Childhood Cirrhosis. New Delhi: Indian Council of Medical Research, in press.
62. Prasad AS, Halsted JA, Nadimi M. Am J Med 1961;31:532–46.
63. Prasad AS, Miale A Jr, Farid Z, et al. Arch Intern Med 1963;111:407–28.
64. Hambidge KM, Krebs NF, Walravens PA. Nutr Res 1985;1: 306–16.
65. Younaszai HD. JPEN 1983;7:72–4.
66. Golden MHN, Golden BE. Am J Clin Nutr 1981;34:900–8.
67. Chen X, Yang G, Chen J, et al. Biol Tr El Res 1980;2:91–107.
68. Mo D. Pathology and selenium deficiency in Kashin -Beck disease. In: Combs GF Jr, Lavandar OA, Oldfield JE, eds. Selenium in biology and medicine. New York: Van Nostrand Reinhold, 1987;924–33.
68a. National Research Council. Health effects of ingested fluoride. Washington, DC: National Academy Press, 1993.
69. Vinton NE, Dahlstrom KA, Strobel CT, et al. J Pediatr 1987;111:711–7.
70. Yang G, Wang S, Zhou R, et al. Am J Clin Nutr 1983;37:872–81.
71. Centers for Disease Control. MMWR 1984;33:157–8.
72. Ruta DA, Haider S. Br Med J 1989;299:316–7.
73. Jeejeebhoy KN, Chu RC, Marliss EB, et al. Am J Clin Nutr 1977;30:531–8.
74. Freund H, Atamian S, Fischer JE. JAMA 1979;241:496–8.
75. Brown RO, Forloines-Lynn S, Cross RE, et al. Dig Dis Sci 1986;31:661–4.
76. Gurson CT, Saner G. Am J Clin Nutr 1971;24:1313–9.
77. Kriss JP, Carness WH, Gross RT. JAMA 1955;157:117–21.
78. Sullivan JF, Egan JD, George RP, et al. J Lab Clin Med 1966;68:1022–3.
79. Rajagopalan KV. Annu Rev Nutr 1988;8:401–27.
80. Abumrad NN, Schneider AJ, Steele D, et al. Am J Clin Nutr 1981;34:2551–9.
81. Kovalskii VV, Yatovaya GA, Shmavonyau DM. Zh Obshch Biol 1961;22:179.
82. Doisy EA Jr. Effects of deficiency in manganese upon plasma and cholesterol in man. In: Hoekstra WG, Suttie JW, Ganther HE, et al., eds. Trace element metabolism in animals, vol 2. Baltimore: University Park Press, 1974;668–70.
83. Kondakis XG, Makris N, Leotsinidis M, et al. Arch Environ Health 1989;44:175–8.
84. Krieger D, Krieger S, Jansen O, et al. Lancet 1995;346:270–4.
85. Fell JME, Reynolds AP, Meadows N, et al. Lancet 1996;347:1218–21.

SELECTED READING

McLaren DS. A colour atlas and text of diet-related diseases. New ed. London: Wolfe, 1992.

31. Carnitine

CHARLES J. REBOUCHE

HISTORICAL INTRODUCTION

Carnitine was first discovered in muscle extracts independently by Gulewitsch and Krimberg and by Kutscher in 1905, and the correct structure was assigned in 1927 by Tomita and Sendju (1). Between 1948 and 1952, Fraenkel and colleagues demonstrated the essential nature of this compound for the mealworm, *Tenebrio molitor,* and assigned the term *vitamin* B_T to carnitine (1). A function for carnitine in fatty acid oxidation was first discovered independently by Bremer and by Fritz and Yue between 1962 and 1963 (2). The origin of the methyl groups of carnitine was identified by Wolf and Berger and Bremer in 1961 (2), and the origin of the carbon chain of carnitine from the essential amino acid lysine was first reported by Tanphaichitr and colleagues (3) in 1971. Clinical syndromes associated with carnitine deficiency were first reported by Engel and colleagues in 1973 (4) and 1975 (5), and carnitine deficiency was associated specifically with a defect in carnitine transport by Treem et al. in 1988 (6).

CHEMISTRY AND NOMENCLATURE

Carnitine (β-hydroxy-γ-*N,N,N*-trimethylaminobutyric acid) is a zwitterionic quaternary amine (Fig. 31.1) with molecular weight 161.2 g/mol (inner salt). Only the L isomer is biologically active. L-Carnitine participates in transesterification reactions (Fig. 31.1) in which short-chain organic acids or medium- or long-chain fatty acids are transferred from coenzyme A to the hydroxyl group of carnitine. These reversible reactions are catalyzed by a group of enzymes termed *carnitine acyltransferases.* Thus, carnitine exists in biologic systems in both nonesterified and esterified forms. Under normal conditions, the predominant ester of carnitine in cells and biologic fluids is acetylcarnitine.

FUNCTIONS

Mitochondrial Long-Chain Fatty Acid Oxidation

Long-chain fatty acids enter mitochondria only as acylcarnitine esters (Fig. 31.2). Carnitine palmitoyltransferase I (EC 2.3.1.21) on the inner surface of the outer mitochondrial membrane catalyzes transesterification of long-chain fatty acids from coenzyme A to carnitine. The acylcarnitine esters traverse the inner mitochondrial membrane via a carnitine-acylcarnitine translocase, and the acyl moieties are transesterified to intramitochondrial coenzyme A by the action of carnitine palmitoyltransferase II, located on the matrix surface of the inner mitochondrial membrane. Thus, carnitine is essential for mitochondrial use of long-chain fatty acids for energy production.

Modulation of Acylcoenzyme A:Coenzyme A Ratio

Coenzyme A is a required cofactor in many cellular reactions. If nonesterified coenzyme A is not available in a cellular compartment (e.g., cytosol, mitochondria, peroxisomes) because it is completely esterified, the flux through pathways that require this cofactor will diminish. Carnitine is a reservoir for excess acyl residues, generated, for example, by high rates of β-oxidation in mitochondria, in which the acyl residue is transesterified from coenzyme A to carnitine, thus freeing coenzyme A to participate in other cellular reactions (Fig. 31.2). The acylcarnitine ester formed in this process may remain in the organelle or cell of origin for use when needed, or may be exported out of the cell for use by other cells or tissues or for excretion. Because acetyl-CoA is a major product of cellular metabolism (e.g., β-oxidation of fatty acids, oxidation of pyruvate), the primary enzyme involved in this function is carnitine acetyltransferase (EC 2.3.1.7).

This function has important implications for cellular energy metabolism. For example, carnitine facilitates oxidation of glucose in working hearts by relieving inhibition of pyruvate dehydrogenase by fatty acids (7). The mechanism involves removal of acetyl groups generated from fatty acid β-oxidation by transesterification from acetyl-CoA to carnitine, thus freeing coenzyme A to participate in the pyruvate dehydrogenase reaction sequence.

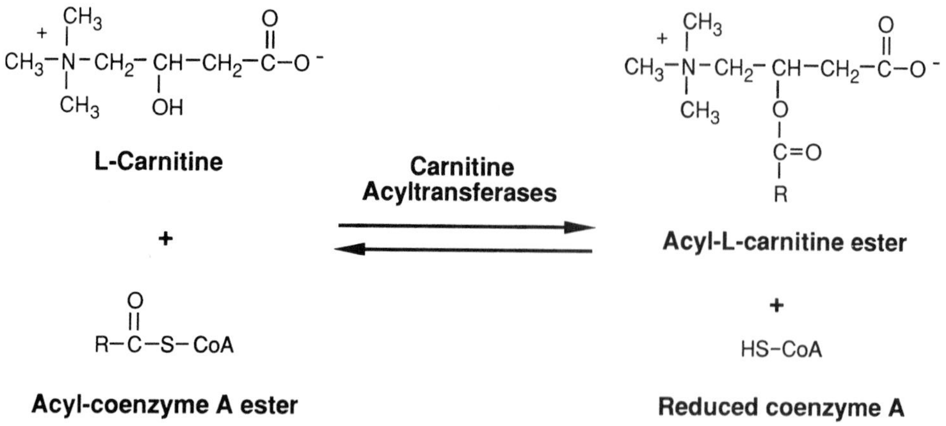

$CH_3-N^{+}(CH_3)_2-CH_2-CH(OH)-CH_2-C(=O)-O^{-}$

L-Carnitine

\+

$R-C(=O)-S-CoA$

Acyl-coenzyme A ester

Carnitine Acyltransferases ⇌

$CH_3-N^{+}(CH_3)_2-CH_2-CH(O-C(=O)-R)-CH_2-C(=O)-O^{-}$

Acyl-L-carnitine ester

\+

HS–CoA

Reduced coenzyme A

Figure 31.1. Carnitine structure and metabolic interconversions.

The role of carnitine in modulation of the acyl-CoA:CoA ratio also is important in long-chain fatty acid use for membrane remodeling (8). Carnitine acts as a reservoir for long-chain fatty acids destined for incorporation into membrane phospholipids, as, for example, during repair after oxidative insult. This role for carnitine, facilitated by extramitochondrial carnitine palmitoyltransferase activity, has been demonstrated in erythrocytes but presumably occurs in nucleated cells as well (8).

The ability of carnitine to act as a reservoir for activated acyl residues is important in abnormal cellular metabolism, in particular, in genetic diseases associated with defects in organic and fatty acid metabolism. For example, in propionyl-CoA carboxylase deficiency, propionyl-CoA is an end-product that, if not cleared, would starve the cellular energy-producing machinery of nonesterified coenzyme A. In patients with this disease, large amounts of propionylcarnitine are excreted, indicating that cells and tissues adapt to the demand for nonesterified coenzyme A by transesterification of excess propionyl residues to carnitine (9). Pharmacologic amounts of carnitine are often prescribed for treatment of this disease.

Other Actions in Cellular Metabolism

Carnitine and its esters may have other functions in mammalian cells. Pharmacologic administration of carnitine reduces the mortality and metabolic consequences of acute ammonium intoxication in mice (10). The mechanism for this effect may have two components: L-carnitine administration normalizes the redox state of the brain (perhaps by increasing the availability of β-hydroxybutyrate to the brain), and it increases the rate of urea synthesis in the liver. At least part of the protective effect of carnitine is associated with flux through the carnitine acyltransferases, as analogues of carnitine that are competitive inhibitors of carnitine acyltransferases enhance toxicity of acute ammonium administration (11). It has been proposed that carnitine increases urea synthesis in the liver by facilitating fatty acid entry into mitochondria, leading to increased flux through the β-oxidation pathway, an

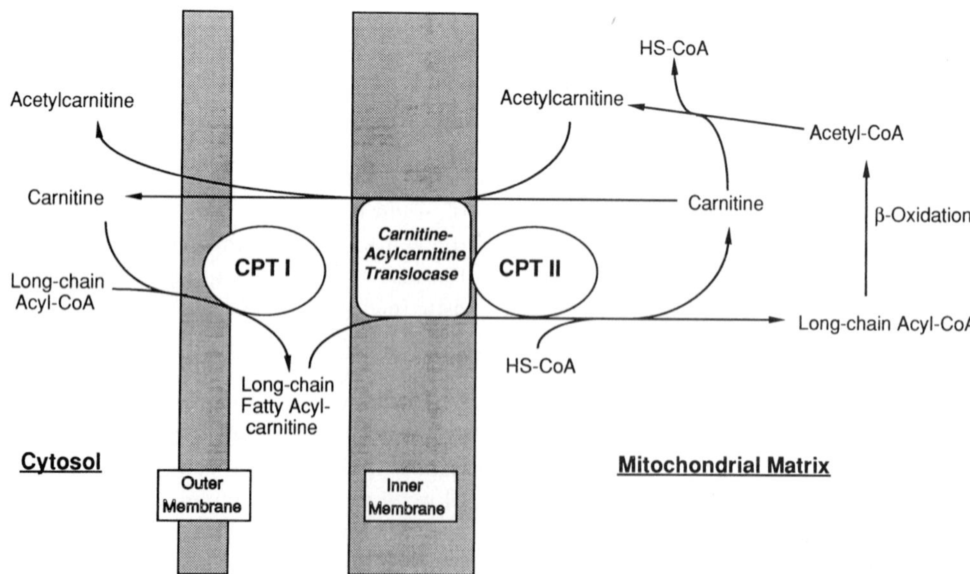

Figure 31.2. Carnitine function in facilitation of mitochondrial long-chain fatty acid oxidation and modulation of intramitochondrial acyl-CoA:CoA ratio.

increase of intramitochondrial reducing equivalents, and enhanced ATP production (10).

Propionyl-L-carnitine protects the ischemic heart from reperfusion injury, perhaps by scavenging free radicals or by preventing their formation by chelating iron necessary for generation of hydroxyl radicals (12). Propionyl-L-carnitine also improves contractile function of rat hearts, presumably by increasing the supply of four-carbon intermediates, thus increasing the flux through the citric acid cycle (13). The same effects were not achieved by propionate or carnitine alone. These mechanisms may be responsible for beneficial effects of propionyl-L-carnitine on ischemia-induced myocardial dysfunction in humans with angina pectoris (14).

L-Carnitine regulates the transcriptional response to triiodothyronine of genes for malic enzyme (EC 1.1.1.40) and fatty acid synthase (EC 2.3.1.85) in chick embryo hepatocytes (15). Acetyl-L-carnitine corrected the impaired mitochondrial DNA expression in brain and heart of senescent rats, restoring these rates to those seen in normal adult rats (16). This treatment had no effect on the rates of mitochondrial DNA expression in normal adult (nonsenescent) rats. Pharmacologic treatment with acetyl-L-carnitine improved the ability of patients with Alzheimer's disease to handle tasks requiring attention and concentration (17). Acetyl-L-carnitine may improve the mental ability of these patients by inhibiting apoptosis of nerve cells in the brain. In this regard, acetyl-L-carnitine inhibited apoptosis induced by serum deprivation in a teratocarcinoma cell line (18). The latter effect was shown not to involve the putative antioxidant effects (19) of acetyl-L-carnitine.

L-Carnitine greatly increased the survival rate of rats treated with *Escherichia coli* lipopolysaccharide, independent of any changes in activity of enzymes that metabolize fatty acids, coenzyme A, or carnitine derivatives in liver (20). Circulating cytokine (interleukin-1β, interleukin-6, and tumor necrosis factor-α) concentrations were reduced by carnitine treatment in this model as well as in a methylcholanthrene-induced sarcoma model of cachexia in rats (21). L-Carnitine prevented cardiac toxicity associated with interleukin-2 cancer immunotherapy (22).

Carnitine (either the L or D isomer) and to a lesser extent γ-butyrobetaine inhibit clustering of erythrocytes by fibrinogen or clusterin (23). The mechanism involves binding of carnitine to sulfhydryl groups on the erythrocyte membrane but not to fibrinogen or clusterin. The possible physiologic significance of these findings is unknown. Further investigation of these observations may identify new general roles for carnitine in cellular metabolism.

Proteins Associated with Carnitine Function

Carnitine Palmitoyltransferase

Two major forms of carnitine palmitoyltransferase have been identified, carnitine palmitoyltransferase I (CPT I) and carnitine palmitoyltransferase II (CPT II). CPT I is located on the inner surface of the outer mitochondrial membrane, whereas CPT II is found on the matrix surface of the inner mitochondrial membrane. CPT I, but not CPT II, is potently inhibited by malonyl-CoA. This reversible inhibition is a primary metabolic regulator that partitions fatty acids to mitochondrial oxidation or to triglyceride formation. There are at least two isoenzymes of CPT I, a "liver" isozyme of approximately 88 kDa, and a "muscle" isozyme of approximately 82 kDa (24). These isozymes differ in their affinities for carnitine and malonyl-CoA.

CPT II is synthesized as a 74-kDa proenzyme. The N-terminal 25 residues are cleaved following import into mitochondria, resulting in a mature protein of 71 kDa. CPT I and CPT II are distinct enzymes, coded by different genes (24). Moreover, the liver and muscle variants of CPT I also arise from separate genes.

Carnitine palmitoyltransferase activity is found extramitochondrially, in peroxisomes and endoplasmic reticulum. The activity present in peroxisomes is generally attributed to carnitine octanoyltransferase (see below) present in this organelle. Carnitine palmitoyltransferase activity in endoplasmic reticulum has been observed (e.g., in erythrocytes [8]) but has not been well characterized.

Carnitine Acetyltransferase (CAT)

CAT catalyzes reversible transesterification of short-chain organic acids (two to eight carbons, with maximal activity directed to acetyl and propionyl residues) between coenzyme A and carnitine. CAT is found in soluble form in mitochondria and peroxisomes and membrane-associated in endoplasmic reticulum (25). The enzyme has been purified from different tissues of various species. Reported molecular masses range from 51 to 75 kDa. On the basis of enzyme kinetics and specificity, it is generally accepted that carnitine acetyltransferase in the various subcellular compartments provides for efficient synthesis, use, and/or disposal of short-chain organic acids generated by mitochondrial or peroxisomal metabolism of both physiologic and xenobiotic compounds.

Carnitine Octanoyltransferase (COT)

COT is a broad-specificity enzyme with highest affinity for medium-chain fatty acids (highest activity with hexanoyl-CoA as substrate). It is found mostly in peroxisomes, and its activity in liver is increased by peroxisomal proliferating agents. Peroxisomes generally oxidize very long chain fatty acids that are not metabolized in mitochondria. Chain-shortened products, primarily medium-chain fatty esters of coenzyme A, are transesterified to carnitine and are subsequently oxidized in mitochondria. Peroxisomal COT has a molecular mass of approximately 62 kDa and is immunologically distinct from mitochondrial carnitine palmitoyltransferases and carnitine acetyltransferase (26). Like mitochondrial CPT I, it is inhibited by malonyl-CoA. COT accounts for the carnitine palmitoyltransferase activity observed in peroxisomal preparations.

COT activity is also found in rough and smooth endoplasmic reticulum. This 53-kDa protein is immunologically distinct from peroxisomal COT (27). Like mitochondrial CPT I, crude (membrane-bound) microsomal COT is inhibited by malonyl-CoA, but after solubilization with detergents, inhibition by malonyl-CoA is lost. Microsomal COT probably accounts for the carnitine palmitoyltransferase activity in endoplasmic reticulum. Like peroxisomal CAT and COT, reversible reaction kinetics of this enzyme favor formation of acylcarnitine esters at normal intracellular concentrations of its substrates (27).

Carnitine-Acylcarnitine Translocase

Entry of long-chain fatty acylcarnitine esters into mitochondria occurs by rapid-exchange diffusion (28), facilitated by a 32.5-kDa carnitine-acylcarnitine translocase in the inner mitochondrial membrane. This protein has been purified and functionally reconstituted into liposomes (29). It is inhibited by sulfhydryl-reactive reagents and some analogues of carnitine (e.g., sulfobetaines). The translocase has several other important functions in addition to its role in facilitating entry of long-chain fatty acylcarnitine esters into mitochondria. It facilitates entry into mitochondria of short- and medium-chain acylcarnitine esters formed in peroxisomes from oxidation of very long chain fatty acids. It also facilitates removal of short-chain acylcarnitine esters from mitochondria, freeing coenzyme A to recycle through the various pathways in the mitochondrial matrix.

BIOSYNTHESIS

Pathway

Carnitine ultimately derives from the essential amino acids lysine and methionine (Fig. 31.3). Lysine provides the carbon chain and nitrogen atom of carnitine, whereas three methionine molecules provide the methyl groups for one molecule of carnitine (30). Methylation of the epsilon amino group of lysine is catalyzed by one or more protein:lysine methyltransferases. Lysine residues destined for carnitine synthesis must be peptide linked; there is no evidence that free lysine is enzymatically methylated in mammals. ε-*N*-Trimethyllysine is released for carnitine synthesis via normal mechanisms of protein hydrolysis. In the pathway to carnitine synthesis, ε-*N*-trimethyllysine undergoes four sequential enzymatic reactions: hydroxylation at position two of the carbon chain, catalyzed by ε-*N*-trimethyllysine hydroxylase (EC 1.14.11.8); aldol cleavage between carbons two and three of the carbon chain, catalyzed by serine hydroxymethyltransferase (EC 2.1.2.1); oxidation of the resulting aldehyde by any of several NAD^+-requiring aldehyde dehydrogenases; and a second hydroxylation, catalyzed by γ-butyrobetaine hydroxylase (EC 1.14.11.1).

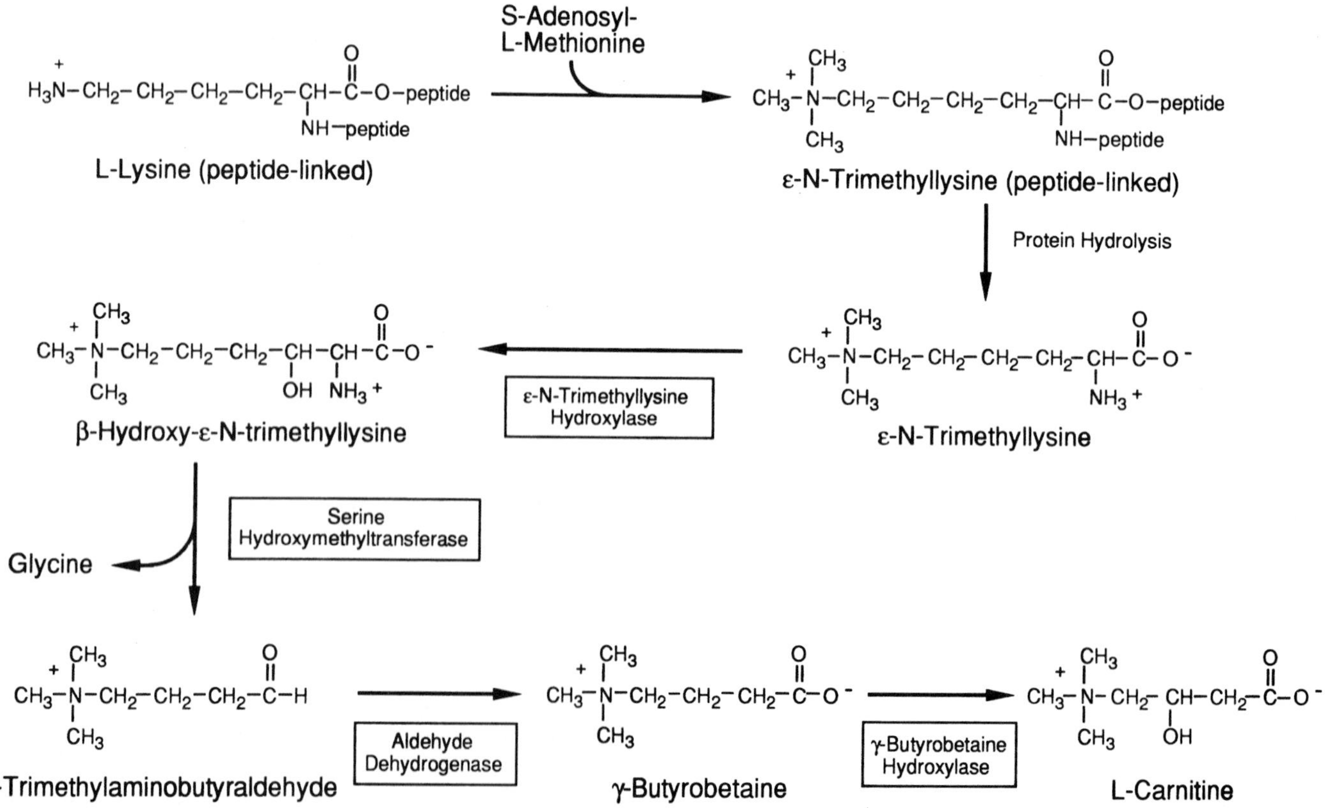

Figure 31.3. Pathway of carnitine biosynthesis in mammals. (Modified from reference 33: Rebouche CJ. Am J Clin Nutr 1991;54(Suppl): 1147S–52S, with permission.)

All enzymes in the pathway except γ-butyrobetaine hydroxylase are ubiquitous in mammalian tissues. The last enzyme in the pathway is not found in cardiac and skeletal muscle (30). γ-Butyrobetaine hydroxylase activity is highest in liver and testes, and in some species, including humans, it is abundant in kidney.

Rate and Regulation

The normal rate of carnitine synthesis in humans is approximately 1.2 μmol · kg body weight^{-1} · day^{-1} (31). This estimate is obtained from normal rates of urinary carnitine excretion by strict vegetarians, who obtain very little carnitine (generally less than 0.1 μmol · kg body weight^{-1} · day^{-1}) from dietary sources. Direct measurement of the rate of carnitine synthesis by, for example, isotope incorporation from labeled precursors, is not technically feasible (31).

The rate of carnitine synthesis in mammals is regulated by the availability of ε-*N*-trimethyllysine, which in turn is determined by the extent of peptide-linked lysine methylation and by the rate of protein turnover. ε-*N*-Trimethyllysine destined for carnitine synthesis probably is derived from the general protein pool and not from any single or small group of proteins. Provision of excess lysine in the diet may increase carnitine synthesis modestly (32), but the evidence is indirect, and the mechanism (e.g., increased flux through protein synthesis, methylation, and turnover; or stimulation of a putative vestigial capability to methylate free lysine) has not been identified.

DIETARY SOURCES, ABSORPTION, AND METABOLISM

Carnitine is generally abundant in food products of animal origin (Table 31.1). Fruits, vegetables, grains, and other plant-derived foods contain relatively little carnitine. Thus, a normal omnivorous diet provides approximately 2 to 12 μmol · kg body weight^{-1} · day^{-1} of carnitine, whereas a strict vegetarian diet contains about 0.1 μmol · kg body weight^{-1} · day^{-1} (31). Carnitine is available commercially as a diet supplement. Carnitine consumed orally in large quantities (about 5 g/day by an adult) may cause diarrhea or fish odor syndrome. No other toxic properties have been identified.

Approximately 63 to 75% of carnitine is absorbed from the normal omnivorous diet (34). The remainder is degraded by bacteria in the large intestine. The percentage of carnitine absorbed from supplements may be much lower; for example, from a 2-g daily supplement, approximately 20% is absorbed (35). Principal organic degradation products of carnitine are trimethylamine (excreted in

Table 31.1
Carnitine Content of Selected Foods

Food Item	Carnitine Content[a]	Food Item	Carnitine Content
Meat products		*Fruits*	
Beef steak	592 ± 260 (4)	Bananas	0.0056
Ground beef	582 ± 32 (3)	Apples	0.0002
Pork	172 ± 32 (3)	Strawberries	ND
Canadian bacon	146 ± 52 (3)	Peaches	0.0060
Bacon	145 ± 24 (3)	Pineapple	0.0063
Fish (cod)	34.6 ± 11.7 (3)	Pears	0.0107
Chicken breast	24.3 ± 8.0 (3)		
		Grains	
Dairy products		White bread	0.912
Whole milk	20.4	Whole-wheat bread	2.26
American cheese	23.2	Rice (cooked)	0.090
Ice cream	23.0	Macaroni	0.780
Butter	3.07	Corn Flakes	0.078
Cottage cheese	6.96		
		Nondairy beverages	
Vegetables		Grapefruit juice	ND
Broccoli (fresh)	0.0228	Orange juice	0.012
(cooked)	0.0111	Tomato juice	0.030
Carrots (fresh)	0.0408	Coffee	0.009
(cooked)	0.0393	Cola	ND
Green beans (cooked)	0.0189	Grape juice	0.093
Green peas (cooked)	0.0369		
Asparagus (cooked)	1.21	*Miscellaneous*	
Beets (cooked)	0.0195	Eggs	0.075
Potato (baked)	0.0800	Peanut butter	0.516
Lettuce	0.0066		

Adapted from Rebouche CJ, Engel AG. J Clin Invest 1984;73:57–67.

[a]Units are μmol/100 g (solid foods) or μmol/100 mL (liquids). ND, not detectable. Values for meat products are mean ± SD (number of observations in parentheses) and are based on precooked weight. Values reported are for total (nonesterified plus esterified) carnitine.

urine as trimethylamine oxide) and γ-butyrobetaine (excreted primarily in feces). Carnitine is not degraded by enzymes of animal origin (31).

Carnitine is concentrated in most tissues of the body. In humans, the intracellular concentrations of carnitine in skeletal muscle and liver are approximately 90 and 75 times higher, respectively, than that in extracellular fluid. Approximately 97% of all carnitine in the body is in skeletal muscle. Carnitine homeostasis is maintained by a low rate of carnitine synthesis and efficient reabsorption of carnitine by the kidney. Approximately 95% of filtered carnitine is reabsorbed in normal humans. Genetic diseases associated with reduced carnitine reabsorption efficiency (e.g., medium-chain acyl-CoA dehydrogenase deficiency) are characterized by carnitine depletion in skeletal muscle and extracellular fluid.

NUTRIENT-NUTRIENT AND DRUG-NUTRIENT INTERACTIONS

Carnitine status and/or metabolism are affected by several nutrients and drugs. For example, rates of carnitine excretion by humans supplemented with choline are lower than corresponding rates of unsupplemented individuals (36). Experimental vitamin C deficiency in guinea pigs is associated with decreased plasma carnitine levels and increased rate of urinary carnitine excretion (37).

Valproic acid and pivalic acid–containing prodrugs (antibiotics) negatively affect carnitine status in humans (38). Valproic acid administration lowers circulating carnitine concentrations in some patients. The mechanism for this effect has not been identified. Pivalic acid is conjugated to some antibiotics to improve their rates of absorption. In the intestinal mucosa, pivalic acid is cleaved by nonspecific esterases. Pivalic acid is conjugated to carnitine and is quantitatively excreted in urine as pivaloylcarnitine. Prolonged treatment with these antibiotics leads to depletion of the circulating carnitine pool and presumably tissue carnitine pools as well.

DEFICIENCY AND DEPLETION

Distribution and Diet

Carnitine has been described as a "conditionally essential" nutrient for some segments of the human population. Infants (both term and preterm) fed formulas lacking carnitine have very low circulating carnitine concentrations (31). Schmidt-Sommerfeld and Penn (39) estimated that the amount of carnitine in skeletal muscle of very premature infants, indexed to whole-body weight, is about 10 times less than that in adults. A number of investigators have observed various biochemical differences, with or without a lipid challenge, in preterm infants provided exogenous carnitine compared with those with no exogenous carnitine administration (31). Results of these studies have not provided clear evidence for a requirement for carnitine by preterm infants.

Fomon and Ziegler (40) summarized energy intake and growth of 204 normal term infants participating in designed growth studies and fed milk-based (70–230 μmol/L carnitine concentration) or soy protein–based (<2 μmol/L carnitine concentration) formulas from 8 to 111 days of age. They found no differences, with respect to formula fed, in energy intake, weight gain, or growth in length from 8 to 41 days, 42 to 111 days, or 8 to 111 days, in either male or female infants. In other studies, term infants fed soy protein–based formulas without added carnitine had lower serum carnitine concentrations, higher serum-free fatty acid concentrations, and higher rates of excretion of medium-chain dicarboxylic acids than did infants whose formulas were supplemented with carnitine. But growth (length and weight gain) was not different for infants consuming the unsupplemented and carnitine-supplemented soy protein–based formulas (31). Thus, it is reasonable to conclude that infants who do not acquire carnitine from their diet are not deficient in carnitine but that the demands of growth create a condition of carnitine depletion in these infants.

There is no evidence that carnitine deficiency occurs in the general population (children and adults) of strict vegetarians, whose diet generally provides a very minimal amount of carnitine. Strict vegetarian children have plasma carnitine concentrations about 70% of those in age- and sex-matched omnivores (31). Likewise, in strict vegetarian adults, plasma carnitine concentrations are about 10% lower than those in corresponding omnivores (31).

Genetic Disorders

Primary carnitine deficiency due to a genetic disorder in carnitine transport has been identified (6). Features of this disease include progressive cardiomyopathy, skeletal muscle weakness, and episodes of fasting hypoglycemia (41). The disease most often presents in the first 5 years of life. Circulating and skeletal muscle carnitine concentrations in affected individuals are generally less than 10 and 20%, respectively, of normal. No primary carnitine deficiency due to a defect in carnitine biosynthesis has been identified.

Carnitine deficiency or depletion occurs secondary to a large number of genetic and acquired disorders and conditions (see Chapter 62, this volume; and ref. 42). At least two basic mechanisms are responsible for these effects on carnitine status. In some disorders, the efficiency of carnitine reabsorption is impaired (e.g., medium-chain acyl-CoA dehydrogenase deficiency). In others, abnormal amounts of short-chain organic acids are produced, which are removed from the body by urinary excretion as acylcarnitine esters (e.g., propionylcarnitine in propionyl-CoA carboxylase deficiency). In these disorders, the rate of excretion of carnitine as short-chain acylcarnitine esters exceeds the combined rates of endogenous synthesis and dietary carnitine intake, leading to a state of carnitine depletion.

EVALUATION OF STATUS

Carnitine status most often is reported as a function of circulating carnitine concentration, and the ratio of esterified to nonesterified carnitine. In general, plasma-free carnitine concentration of 20 μmol/L or less, or total carnitine concentration of 30 μmol/L or less, is considered abnormally low. However, these values only demarcate the lower range of normal plasma carnitine concentrations; they do not reflect points at which functional carnitine deficiency is observed. A ratio of esterified to free carnitine of 0.4 or greater in plasma or serum (but not urine) is considered indicative of abnormal carnitine metabolism. This ratio is elevated primarily when mitochondrial energy metabolism is impaired, resulting in increased load of short-chain organic acids esterified to coenzyme A, which are transesterified to carnitine for export from tissues into the circulation. Thus, in genetic disorders of fatty acid and organic acid oxidation (see Chapter 62, this volume), the ratio of esterified to free carnitine in the circulation often is elevated. This elevated ratio is associated with carnitine depletion caused by either hyperexcretion of acylcarnitine esters or decreased ability of the kidneys to reabsorb carnitine and its esters. Rates of carnitine excretion in urine do not provide a particularly useful measure of carnitine status, because these rates vary considerably with dietary carnitine intake and other physiologic parameters. No validated tests or measures of functional carnitine deficiency are available to assess carnitine status in humans.

Carnitine concentration in body fluids and tissues is measured most accurately and efficiently by the radioenzymatic technique described by Cederblad and Lindstedt (43). Qualitative and quantitative methods are available for analysis of individual acylcarnitine esters and acylcarnitine ester profiles. These include liquid chromatography/mass spectrometry (44), radioisotope exchange/liquid chromatography (45), and derivatization/liquid chromatography (46). These methods are useful for detection and/or quantification of specific acylcarnitine esters that are diagnostic for various metabolic disorders.

REQUIREMENTS AND RECOMMENDED INTAKES FOR HUMANS

Carnitine is not a required nutrient for children and adults. Supplementation of formulas for infants (particularly premature infants) is recommended at a level normally found in human milk (28–95 μmol/L). These recommendations are based on observations of very low plasma and tissue carnitine concentrations and other biochemical differences observed in infants not fed exogenous carnitine (31). Exogenous carnitine is recommended for treatment in some genetic and acquired disorders (e.g., anticonvulsant polytherapy that includes valproic acid in children), but for these purposes, use of exogenous carnitine is pharmacologic rather than nutritional.

REFERENCES

1. Fraenkel G, Friedman S. Vitam Horm 1957;15:73–118.
2. Bremer J. Physiol Rev 1983;63:1420–80.
3. Tanphaichitr V, Horne DW, Broquist HP. J Biol Chem 1971;246:6364–6.
4. Engel AG, Angelini C. Science 1973;173:899–902.
5. Karpati G, Carpenter S, Engel AG, et al. Neurology 1975;25:16–24.
6. Treem WR, Stanley CA, Finegold DN, et al. N Engl J Med 1988;319:1331–6.
7. Broderick TL, Quinney HA, Lopaschuk GD. J Biol Chem 1992;267:3758–63.
8. Ramsay RR, Arduini A. Arch Biochem Biophys 1993; 302:307–14.
9. Roe CR, Millington DS, Maltby DA, et al. J Clin Invest 1984;73:1785–8.
10. O'Conner JE, Costell M, Miguez MP, et al. Biochem Pharmacol 1987;36:3169–73.
11. Ohtsuka Y, Griffith OW. Biochem Pharmacol 1991;41:1957–61.
12. Packer L, Reznick AZ, Kagan VE, et al. (Abstract) FASEB J 1992;6:A1369.
13. Russell RR III, Mommessin JI, Taegtmeyer H. Am J Physiol 1995;268:H441–7.
14. Bartels GL, Remme WJ, Pilay M, et al. Am J Cardiol 1994;74:125–30.
15. Roncero C, Goodridge AG. Arch Biochem Biophys 1992;295:258–67.
16. Gadaleta MN, Petruzzella V, Renis M, et al. Eur J Biochem 1990;187:501–6.
17. Spagnoli A, Kucca U, Menasce G, et al. Neurology 1991;41:1726–32.
18. Galli G, Fratelli M. Exp Cell Res 1993;204:54–60.
19. Shigenaga MK, Hagen TM, Ames BN. Proc Natl Acad Sci USA 1994;91:10771–8.
20. Takeyama N, Takagi D, Matsuo N, et al. Am J Physiol 1989;256:E31–8.
21. Winter BK, Fiskum G, Gallo LL. Br J Cancer 1995;72:1173–9.
22. Lissoni P, Galli MA, Tancini G, et al. Tumori 1993;79:202–4.
23. Fritz IB, Wong K, Burdzy K. J Cell Physiol 1991;149:269–76.
24. McGarry JD, Brown NF. Eur J Biochem 1997;244:1–14.
25. Colucci WJ, Gandour RD. Bioorg Chem 1988;16:307–34.
26. Farrell SO, Fiol CJ, Reddy JK, et al. J Biol Chem 1984;259:13089–95.
27. Chung CD, Bieber LL. J Biol Chem 1993;268:4519–24.
28. Pande SV, Murthy MSR. Biochim Biophys Acta 1994;1226: 269–76.
29. Indiveri C, Tonazzi A, Palmieri F. Biochim Biophys Acta 1990;1020:81–6.
30. Rebouche CJ. Am J Clin Nutr 1991;54(Suppl):1147S–52S.
31. Rebouche CJ. FASEB J 1992;6:3379–86.
32. Rebouche CJ, Bosch EP, Chenard CA, et al. J Nutr 1989;119:1907–13.
33. Rebouche CJ, Engel AG. J Clin Invest 1984;73:857–67.
34. Rebouche CJ, Chenard CA. J Nutr 1991;121:539–46.
35. Rebouche CJ. Metabolism 1991;40:1305–10.
36. Daily JW III, Sachan DS. J Nutr 1995;125:1938–44.

37. Rebouche CJ. Metabolism 1995;44:1639–43.
38. Melegh B, Pap M, Bock I, et al. Pediatr Res 1993;34:460–4.
39. Schmidt-Sommerfeld E, Penn D. Biol Neonate 1990;58(Suppl 1):81–8.
40. Fomon SJ, Ziegler EE. Isolated soy protein in infant feeding. In: Steinke FH, Waggle DH, Volgarev MN, eds. New protein foods in human health: nutrition, prevention and therapy. Boca Raton, FL: CRC Press, 1992;75–83.
41. Stanley CA, DeLeeuw S, Coates PM, et al. Ann Neurol 1991;30:709–16.
42. Di Donato S. Disorders of lipid metabolism affecting skeletal muscle: carnitine deficiency syndromes, defects in the catabolic pathway, and Chanarin disease. In: Engel AG, Franzini-Armstrong C, eds. Myology. 2nd ed. New York: McGraw Hill, 1994, 1587–609.
43. Cederblad G, Lindstedt S. Clin Chim Acta 1972;37:235–43.
44. Millington DS, Norwood DL, Kodo N, et al. Anal Biochem 1989;180:331–9.
45. Schmidt-Sommerfeld E, Penn D, Duran M, et al. J Pediatr 1993;122:708–14.
46. van Kempen TATG, Odle J. J Chromatogr 1992;584:157–65.

SELECTED READINGS

Bieber LL. Carnitine. Annu Rev Biochem 1988;57:261–83.

McGarry JD. The mitochondrial carnitine palmitoyltransferase system: its broadening role in fuel homeostasis and new insights into its molecular features. Biochem Soc Trans 1995;23:321–4.

Ramsay RR, Arduini A. The carnitine acyltransferases and their role in modulating acyl-CoA pools. Arch Biochem Biophys 1993;302:307–14.

Rebouche CJ. Carnitine function and requirements during the life cycle. FASEB J 1992;6:3379–86.

32. Choline and Phosphatidylcholine

STEVEN H. ZEISEL

Choline is a quaternary amine that is widely distributed in foods (1) and is essential for normal function of all cells. Choline ensures the structural integrity and signaling functions of cell membranes; it is the major source of methyl groups in the diet; it directly affects cholinergic neurotransmission; and it is required for lipid transport/metabolism (reviewed in [1]). Most choline in the body is found in phospholipids such as phosphatidylcholine and sphingomyelin. Phosphatidylcholine is the predominant phospholipid (>50%) in most mammalian membranes. Though representing a smaller proportion of the total choline pool, important metabolites of choline include platelet-activating factor, acetylcholine, choline plasmalogens, lysophosphatidylcholine, phosphocholine, glycerophosphocholine, and betaine.

First discovered by Strecker in 1862, choline was chemically synthesized in 1866 (2). It was known to be a component of phospholipids, but the pathway for its biosynthesis was first described in 1941 by duVigneaud (3). The route for its incorporation into phosphatidylcholine (lecithin) was not elucidated until 1956 (4). The importance of choline as a nutrient was first appreciated during the pioneering work on insulin (5). Depancreatized dogs maintained on insulin developed fatty infiltration of the liver and died. Administration of raw pancreas prevented hepatic damage; the active component was the choline moiety of pancreatic phosphatidylcholine. In 1935, the association between a low-choline diet and fatty infiltration of the liver in rats was recognized (6). The term *lipotropic* was coined to describe choline and other substances that prevented deposition of fat in the liver. Subsequently, researchers suggested that the liver disease associated with alcoholism might respond to choline therapy. However, few data supported this hypothesis until recently, when Lieber showed that phosphatidylcholine supplementation prevented fibrosis and fatty liver caused by ethanol ingestion in baboons (7).

In 1975, several laboratories reported that administration of choline accelerated synthesis and release of acetylcholine by neurons (reviewed in [8]). A revival of interest in choline ensued, resulting in a plethora of publications characterizing the metabolism, physiologic effects, and pharmacology of choline.

Our understanding of choline phospholipid–mediated signal transduction has vastly improved during the last decade. Breakdown products of choline phospholipids can amplify external signals or can terminate the signaling process by generating inhibitory second messengers (9). These signals are a matter of life and death for cells. Recently we found that choline deficiency activates an internal program for cell suicide called apoptosis (10). Apoptosis is involved in normal cell turnover, hormone-induced tissue atrophy, embryogenesis, and elimination of cancer cells.

Choline has not been considered an essential nutrient for humans because an endogenous pathway exists for de novo biosynthesis of choline (11). However, the presence of a pathway for endogenous synthesis does not make a nutrient dispensable; vitamin D is an excellent example. In the last few years, several investigators have identified choline-deficiency syndromes in humans (12–16). This review discusses the expected biochemical and physiologic uses for choline and the expected effects of choline deficiency.

DIETARY SOURCES OF CHOLINE

Many foods eaten by humans contain significant amounts of choline and esters of choline (Table 32.1). Some of this choline is added during food processing (especially when preparing infant formula (17). Average dietary intake of choline and choline esters in the adult human is estimated to be 7 to 10 mmol/day (18). When humans were switched from a diet of normal foods to a

Table 32.1
Choline Content of Some Common Foods

	Concentration (μmol/kg)[a]		
Food	Choline	Phosphatidylcholine	Sphingomyelin
Apple	27	280	15
Banana	240	37	20
Beef liver	5831	43500	1850
Beef steak	75	6030	506
Butter	42	1760	460
Cauliflower	1306	2770	183
Corn oil	3	12	5
Coffee	90	34	23
Cucumber	218	76	27
Egg	42	52000	2250
Ginger ale	2	4	3
Grape juice	475	15	5
Iceberg lettuce	2930	132	50
Margarine	30	450	15
Milk (bovine, whole)	150	148	82
Orange	200	490	24
Peanut butter	3895	3937	9
Peanuts	4546	4960	78
Potato	511	300	26
Tomato	430	52	32
Whole wheat bread	968	340	11

Modified from Zeisel SH. Biological consequences of choline deficiency. In: Wurtman R, Wurtman J, eds. Choline metabolism and Brain Function. New York: Raven Press, 1990;75–99.

[a]Choline, phosphatidylcholine and sphingomyelin were measured using a gas chromatography/mass spectrometry assay in foods prepared in the form that they would normally be consumed.

defined diet containing 5 mmol/day, plasma choline and phosphatidylcholine concentrations decreased in most subjects (13). Evidently, the average dietary intake of choline exceeds 5 mmol/day in adults. Human milk is rich in choline and choline esters (19, 20). Assuming that a newborn infant drinks 800 mL milk/day, daily choline intake (all forms) would be approximately 1.2 mmol/day. Per kilogram body weight, this intake is two to three times that ingested by the adult human.

Where does all of this choline in milk come from? Mammary epithelial cells are capable of concentrative uptake of choline from maternal blood (21)(Fig. 32.1). There are two uptake processes: one is saturable and obeys Michaelis-Menten kinetics; the other is nonsaturable and linear. Mammary epithelial cells can synthesize choline de novo (22) via phosphatidylethanolamine *N*-methyltransferase activity; this is the only pathway for synthesis of the choline moiety.

Rat pups denied access to milk have lower serum choline concentrations than do their milk-fed litter mates (23). Thus, dietary intake of choline contributes to the maintenance of high serum choline concentrations in the neonate. In the rat, supplemental choline is concentrated into the dam's milk (24). In lactating women eating a low-choline diet, milk choline content is lower than in those eating a more adequate diet (25). Dietary variation causes a 4-fold change (comparing choline-deficient and choline-supplemented diets) in milk phosphocholine content (19, 20).

Human milk, commercially available infant formulas, bovine milk, and rat milk contain approximately 1 to 2 μmol/L choline and choline esters (20). The free choline content of human milk is very high at the start of lactation and diminishes to approximate that in commercial formulas by 30 days postpartum (19). Human milk has significantly higher phosphocholine concentration and the same or lower glycerophosphocholine concentration than either bovine milk or bovine-derived infant formulas; phosphatidylcholine and sphingomyelin concentrations are similar. Soy-derived infant formulas have lower glycerophosphocholine and sphingomyelin concentrations and higher phosphatidylcholine concentrations than do either human milk or bovine milk–derived formulas.

METABOLISM

Intestinal Absorption

The extent to which dietary choline is bioavailable depends upon the efficiency of its absorption from the intestine. In adults, some ingested choline is metabolized before it can be absorbed from the gut. Gut bacteria degrade it to form betaine and to make methylamines (26). The free choline surviving these fates is absorbed all along the small intestine (reviewed in [1]). At this time, no other component of the diet has been identified as

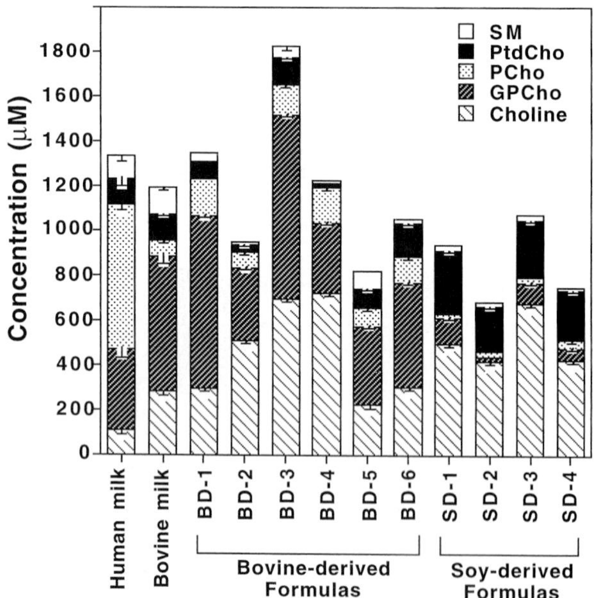

Figure 32.1. Forms of choline in milk and infant formulas. Human and bovine milks and infant formulas were analyzed for choline content by GC/mass spectrometry. Data are expressed as mean concentration (μmol/L) in human milk (N = 33), bovine milk (N = 3), and infant formulas (N = 3). Commercial powdered formulas are either bovine-derived *(BD)* or soy-derived *(SD)*. Abbreviations: *GPCho,* glycerophosphocholine; *PCho,* phosphocholine; *PtdCho,* phosphatidylcholine; *SM,* sphingomyelin. Variability of data is indicated as SEM within the stacked bar for the data. Error bars are not shown when they essentially coincided with the compound division line. (From Holmes-McNary M, Cheng WL, Mar MH, et al. Am J Clin Nutr 1996;64:572–6, with permission.)

competing with choline for transport by intestinal carriers. Both pancreatic secretions and intestinal mucosal cells contain enzymes (phospholipases A_1, A_2, and B) capable of hydrolyzing dietary phosphatidylcholine. The free choline that is formed enters the portal circulation of the liver (27).

In infants, there are differences in the bioavailability of the water-soluble, choline-derived compounds (choline, phosphocholine, and glycerophosphocholine) and the lipid-soluble compounds (phosphatidylcholine and sphingomyelin) present in milk (28). Liver tissue metabolizes the glycerophosphocholine ingested in milk differently than it does either choline or phosphocholine. In addition, phosphatidylcholine-derived label is metabolized very differently from other choline esters, with most remaining as phosphatidylcholine in liver and probably being incorporated into liver membranes. The various dietary sources of choline available in milk are, therefore, used differently by the liver in the rat pup. While the data obtained from the rat pup model cannot be directly extrapolated to the human infant, these variations in bioavailability and use should be considered when milk substitutes are developed. Human milk serves as a useful model for safe and effective provision of choline to the neonate from milk substitutes.

Increased Availability of Choline to Tissues during the Perinatal Period

During development, there is a progressive decline in blood choline concentration that begins in utero. In fact, plasma or serum choline concentrations are 6- to 7-fold higher in the fetus and neonate than they are in the adult (1). This decline in serum choline concentration occurs during the first weeks of life (29). High levels of choline circulating in the neonate presumably ensure enhanced availability of choline to tissues. Neonatal rat brain efficiently extracts choline from blood (30), and increased serum choline in the neonatal rat is associated with a 2-fold higher choline concentration in neonatal brain than is present later in life. Supplementing choline during the perinatal period further increases choline metabolite concentrations in blood and brain (31).

Large amounts of choline are delivered to the fetus across the placenta, where choline transport systems pump it against a concentration gradient (32). The placenta is one of the few nonneuronal tissues to store large amounts of choline as acetylcholine (33). Perhaps this is a special reserve storage pool that ensures delivery of choline to the fetus.

Uptake of Choline by Tissues

All tissues accumulate choline by diffusion and mediated transport, but uptake by liver, kidney, mammary gland, placenta, and brain are of special importance (reviewed in [1]). A specific carrier mechanism transports free choline across the blood-brain barrier at a rate proportional to serum choline concentration, and in the neonate, this choline transporter has especially high capacity (30). Hepatectomy increases the half-life of choline and the blood choline concentration. The rate at which liver takes up choline suffices to explain the rapid disappearance of choline injected systemically. The kidney also accumulates choline (34). Some of this choline appears in the urine unchanged, but most is oxidized within the kidney to form betaine (35). Betaine serves as an important intracellular osmoprotectant within kidney (36). Mean free choline concentrations in the plasma of azotemic humans are several times greater than those in normal controls. Hemodialysis rapidly removes choline from the plasma (37). Renal transplantation in humans lowers plasma choline from 30 μmol/L in the azotemic patient to 15 μmol/L within 1 day (38).

Tissue Distribution and Transformation

Only a small fraction of dietary choline is acetylated, catalyzed by the activity of choline acetyltransferase (reviewed in [8]). This enzyme is highly concentrated in the terminals of cholinergic neurons but is also present in the placenta. The availability of choline and acetyl-CoA influences choline acetyltransferase activity. In the brain, it is unlikely that choline acetyltransferase is saturated with either of its substrates, so choline (and possibly acetyl-CoA) availability determines the rate of acetylcholine synthesis. Increased brain acetylcholine synthesis is associated with an augmented release into the synapse of this neurotransmitter. Choline taken up by brain may first enter a storage pool (perhaps the phosphatidylcholine in membranes) before being converted to acetylcholine. The choline-phospholipids in cholinergic neurons are a large precursor pool of choline available for use in acetylcholine synthesis. This may be especially important in neurons with increased demands for choline to sustain acetylcholine release (e.g., when particular cholinergic neurons fire frequently, or when the supply of choline from the extracellular fluid is inadequate) (39). Human nerve cells in culture use choline from phosphatidylcholine as a source of choline for acetylcholine synthesis (40, 41).

Methyl Group Transfer

The methyl groups of choline can be made available from one-carbon metabolism, upon conversion to betaine (reviewed in [1]). This process requires two steps. First, choline is oxidized to betaine aldehyde by the enzyme choline dehydrogenase, which is present in the inner mitochondrial membrane (42). The oxidation of betaine aldehyde, catalyzed by betaine aldehyde dehydrogenase or by a nonspecific aldehyde dehydrogenase, takes place in both mitochondria and the cytosol. Liver and kidney are the major sites for choline oxidation. In kidney, betaine serves as an osmolyte (43). Betaine:homocysteine methyltransferase catalyzes the methylation of homocysteine, using betaine as the methyl donor. Betaine cannot be reduced back to choline. Thus, the oxidation pathway diminishes the availability of choline to tissues as it scavenges some methyl groups.

Phosphatidylcholine Biosynthesis

Elegant regulatory mechanisms control phosphatidylcholine biosynthesis and hydrolysis, many of which have been elucidated during the last decade (44). Synthesis occurs by two pathways. In the first, choline is phosphorylated, then converted to cytidine diphosphocholine (CDP-choline). This high-energy intermediate, in combination with diacylglycerol, forms phosphatidylcholine and cytidine monophosphate. In the alternative pathway, phosphatidylethanolamine is sequentially methylated to form phosphatidylcholine, using *S*-adenosylmethionine as the methyl donor.

Choline kinase, the first enzyme in the CDP-choline pathway, has been purified, and its properties have been reviewed elsewhere (45, 46). It is a cytosolic enzyme that also catalyzes the phosphorylation of ethanolamine. There are three isoforms of choline kinase in liver (45).

The second step in the pathway, catalyzed by CTP:phosphocholine cytidylyltransferase, is the rate-limiting (47) and regulated step of phosphatidylcholine biosynthesis (48). Deficient activity of this enzyme in the lungs of prematurely born human infants contributes to the respiratory distress syndrome (49). Cytidylyltransferase is present in the cytosol and probably within the nucleus (50) as an inactive dimer of two 42-kDa subunits; in the endoplasmic reticulum, the Golgi apparatus, and the nuclear envelope it is in an active membrane-bound form (48, 51). The presence of significant cytidylyltransferase activity in the nuclear membranes is remarkable because phosphatidylcholine synthesis was previously thought to occur exclusively in the endoplasmic reticulum and Golgi apparatus.

The state of phosphorylation of cytidylyltransferase, as well as membrane phosphatidylcholine and diacylglycerol content, regulates the reversible translocation of the enzyme between cytosol and membranes (48). When cytidylyltransferase is phosphorylated by a cAMP-dependent protein kinase it translocates from membranes into the cytosol and becomes inactivated. This process reverses when the enzyme is dephosphorylated by protein phosphatase (50). The phosphatidylcholine content of the membrane also regulates the amount of enzyme bound to membranes. Cytidylyltransferases bind to membranes more avidly when their phosphatidylcholine content decreases, whereas the reverse occurs when membrane phosphatidylcholine content increases (51, 52). This may explain why cytidylyltransferase activity increases in choline-deficient hepatocytes (53).

Diacylglycerol also regulates cytidylyltransferase. Treatments that increase intracellular diacylglycerol levels (exposure to oleate [54] or that mimic the actions of diacylglycerol (exposure to phorbol ester [55]) activate cytidylyltransferase. Fatty acids and diacylglycerol may be acting indirectly on cytidylyltransferase by modulating protein kinase C and protein phosphatase activities (50).

The third enzyme in the CDP-choline pathway (CDP-choline:1,2-diacylglycerol choline-phosphotransferase) is present in the membranes of the endoplasmic reticulum. Its properties were reviewed recently (56). Because it is not the rate-limiting enzyme in the pathway, CDP-choline does not accumulate in significant concentrations within cells. The efficacy of CDP-choline as a treatment for ischemia and memory disorders is currently being tested in clinical trials (57–59).

An alternative pathway for phosphatidylcholine biosynthesis (via methylation of phosphatidylethanolamine by phosphatidylethanolamine *N*-methyltransferase) is most active in liver but occurs in many other tissues, including brain (60, 61) and the mammary gland (22). This is the major (perhaps only) pathway for de novo synthesis of the choline moiety in adult mammals. However, plants (62) and perhaps embryonic neurons (from chicken or rat) (63) are capable of methylating phosphoethanolamine to form phosphocholine. The properties of phosphatidylethanolamine-*N*-methyltransferase were reviewed recently (64).

There are no accurate estimates of the activity of phosphatidylethanolamine-*N*-methyltransferase in vivo; the enzyme is membrane bound, and at least two isoforms exist (65). In adult liver, the availability of phosphatidylethanolamine, the *S*-adenosylmethionine:*S*-adenosylhomocysteine concentration ratio, and the composition of the boundary lipids that surround phosphatidylethanolamine-*N*-methyltransferase regulate its activity. *S*-Adenosylhomocysteine, a product of the reactions, inhibits the methyltransferase. The availability of *S*-adenosylmethionine in the liver of choline-deficient animals limits the activity of this pathway.

Interactions among Choline, Homocysteine, and Folate

The demand for choline as a methyl donor is probably the major factor that determines how rapidly a choline-deficient diet will induce pathology. The metabolism of choline, methionine, and methylfolate is closely interrelated (Fig. 32.2). The pathways intersect at the formation of methionine from homocysteine. Betaine:homocysteine methyltransferase catalyzes the methylation of homocysteine, using the choline metabolite betaine as the methyl donor (66). In an alternative pathway, 5-methyltetrahydrofolate:homocysteine methyltransferase regenerates methionine, using a methyl group derived de novo from the 1-carbon pool (66). Perturbing the metabolism of one of the methyl donors results in compensatory changes in the other methyl donors because of the intermingling of these metabolic pathways (67, 68). Rats ingesting a choline-deficient diet showed diminished tissue concentrations of methionine and *S*-adenosylmethionine (69) and diminished total folate (68).

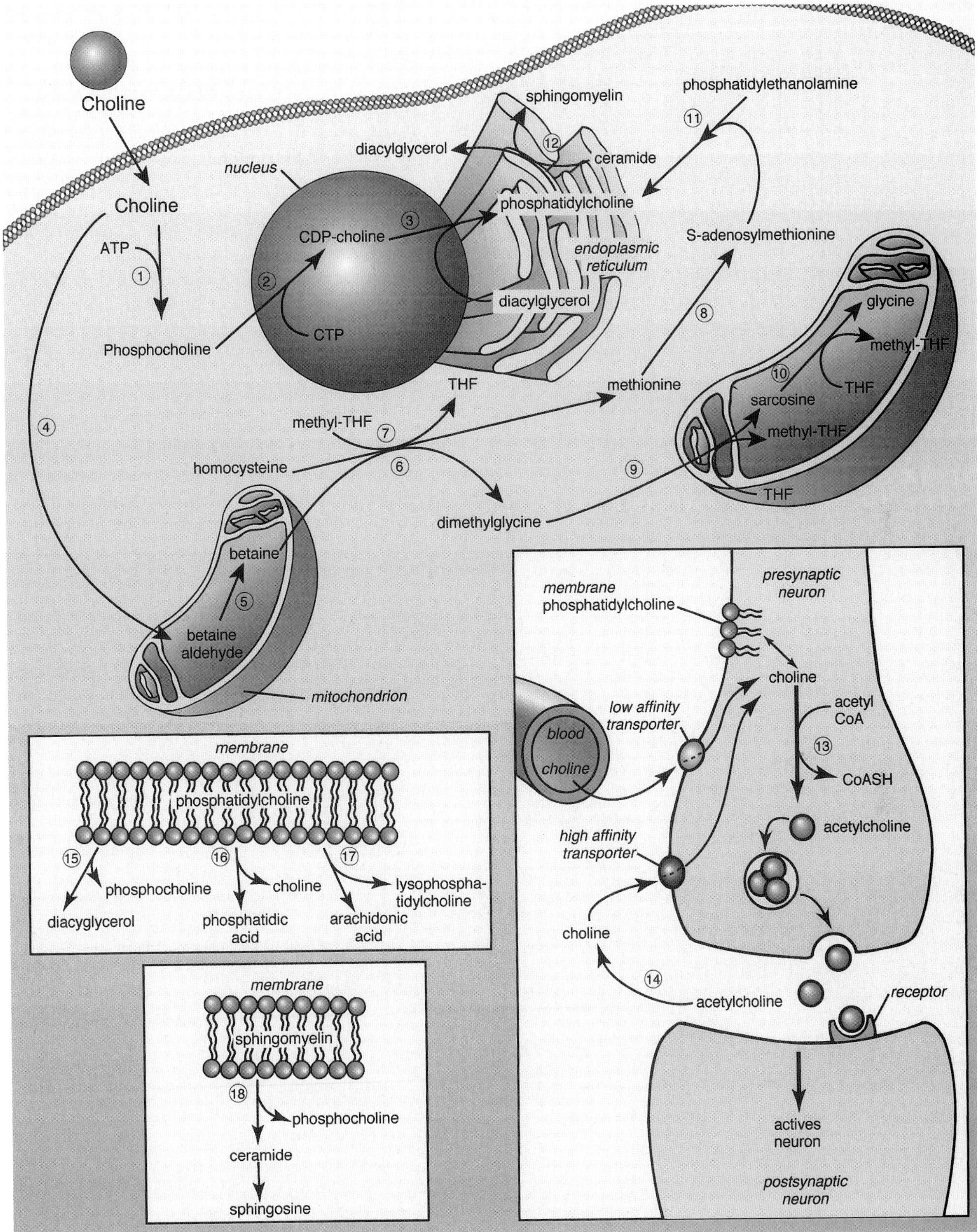

Figure 32.2. Metabolism of choline. The three major metabolic uses for choline are as a precursor for phosphatidylcholine biosynthesis, as a methyl donor, and as a precursor for acetylcholine biosynthesis. (From Cheng W-L, Holmes-McNary MQ, Mar M-H, et al. J Nutr Biochem 1996;7:457–64, with permission.)

Methotrexate, which is widely used in the treatment of cancer, psoriasis, and rheumatoid arthritis, limits the availability of methyl groups by competitively inhibiting dihydrofolate reductase, a key enzyme in intracellular folate metabolism. Rats treated with methotrexate have diminished pools of all choline metabolites in liver (70). Choline supplementation reverses the fatty liver caused by methotrexate administration (71–73).

The interrelationship between choline and folate is especially interesting because multiple studies in humans have demonstrated that individuals with diminished folate status are much more likely to have babies with neural tube defects (74), and the progeny of pregnant mice with folate deficiency show increased rates of exencephaly (75). Also, the intermingling of choline and homocysteine metabolism is important because increased plasma homocysteine concentration is an independent risk factor for cardiovascular disease (76).

BIOCHEMICAL AND PHYSIOLOGIC CONSEQUENCES OF CHOLINE DEFICIENCY

Chronic ingestion of a diet deficient in choline has major consequences, including hepatic, renal, pancreatic, memory, and growth disorders (reviewed in [1]). In most animals (except ruminants), choline deficiency results in liver dysfunction. Large amounts of lipid (mainly triglycerides) can accumulate in liver, eventually filling the entire hepatocyte. Fatty infiltration of the liver starts in the central area of the lobule and spreads peripherally. This process differs from that occurring in kwashiorkor or essential amino acid deficiency, in which fatty infiltration usually begins in the portal area of the lobule. Lipid accumulation within hepatocytes begins within hours after rats are started on a choline-deficient diet, peaks within the first 6 months (at >2000 mg/liver; control rats, 28 mg/liver), and then diminishes as the liver becomes fibrotic. Fatty liver occurs because triacylglycerol must be packaged as very low density lipoprotein (VLDL) to be exported from liver. Phosphatidylcholine is an essential component of VLDL (77, 78); other phospholipids cannot substitute. Methionine can substitute for choline only as long as phosphatidylethanolamine-*N*-methyltransferase (see above discussion) was fully active. Secretion of high-density lipoprotein (HDL) from hepatocytes does not require synthesis of new phosphatidylcholine molecules (79). Choline-deficient humans have diminished plasma low density lipoprotein cholesterol (LDL; derived from VLDL) (13). This observation is consistent with the hypothesis that in humans, as in other species, choline is required for VLDL secretion.

Renal function is also compromised by choline deficiency (reviewed in [1]), with abnormal concentrating ability, free water reabsorption, sodium excretion, glomerular filtration rate, and renal plasma flow. Gross renal hemorrhage also results. Infertility, growth impairment, bony abnormalities, decreased hematopoiesis, and hypertension have also been reported to be associated with diets low in choline (1).

CHOLINE AND THE DEVELOPING BRAIN

Nature has developed a number of mechanisms to ensure that a developing animal gets adequate amounts of choline. As discussed above, the placenta regulates transport of choline to the fetus. In this regard, the choline concentration in amniotic fluid is 10 times that in maternal blood (Zeisel, unpublished observations). The capacity of brain to extract choline from blood is greatest during the neonatal period. Neonatal rat brain has a novel phosphatidylethanolamine-*N*-methyltransferase that is extremely active (80); this enzyme is not present in adult brain. Furthermore, in the brains of newborn rats, *S*-adenosylmethionine concentrations are 40 to 50 nmol/g of tissue (81), which probably allows the neonatal phosphatidylethanolamine-*N*-methyltransferase to maintain high activity. As mentioned above, human and rat milk provide large amounts of choline to the neonate. These multiple mechanisms to ensure availability of choline to the fetus and neonate support the view that choline supply is crucial during this period.

There are two sensitive periods in the development of rat brain during which treatment with choline results in long-lasting enhancement of spatial memory. The first occurs during embryonic days 12 to 17; the other during postnatal days 16 to 30 (82–84). These two sensitive periods for responsiveness to supplemental choline correlate with the formation of cholinergic neurons (neurogenesis; prenatal) and nerve-nerve connections (synaptogenesis; postnatal) in the memory area of brain (hippocampus and basal forebrain), respectively. Choline supplementation during these critical periods elicits major improvement in memory performance at all stages of training on a 12-arm radial maze. The choline-induced spatial memory facilitation correlates with altered distribution and morphology of neurons involved in memory storage within brain (septal neurons) (83). A dam eating 50 g/day ingests 0.5 mmol of choline/day. The choline-supplemented dams in these memory studies consumed an additional 1 mmol/day of choline in drinking water. The progeny appeared normal in weight and showed no symptoms of choline deficiency. Note that the improvement in memory is detected months after the short exposure to choline. These effects of perinatal choline treatment on memory appear to be permanent, as both working and reference memory performance continued to show facilitation relative to controls even at 26 months of age (W. Meck, personal communication).

How a choline supplement supplied to the dam yields a permanent memory change in the offspring has not been elucidated. Our initial hypothesis was that the effects of neonatal choline supplementation on memory are mediated by increased brain choline levels with subsequent increased acetylcholine release. However, the amount of choline that accumulates in fetal brain after treatment of the pregnant dam is not enough to enhance acetylcholine release (31). Rather, supplementing choline to dams results in significantly greater accumulation of phosphorylcholine and betaine in fetal brain than in fetuses of controls (31). This leaves open the possibility that changes in these metabolites mediate these long-term effects on brain and behavior.

Whether these findings in rats also apply to humans is not known. Of course human and rat brains mature at different rates, with the rat brain comparatively more mature at birth than is the human brain. In humans, synaptogenesis may continue for months after birth. Should there be a recommended intake for choline in pregnant women? Are we varying the availability of choline when we feed infant formulas instead of milk? Does the form and amount of choline ingested contribute to variations in memory observed between humans? All these questions are worthy of additional research.

CARCINOGENESIS

Choline deficiency, alone among those of single nutrients, causes development of hepatocarcinomas in the absence of any known carcinogen (85). Choline-deficient rats not only have a higher incidence of spontaneous hepatocarcinoma but also are markedly sensitized to the effects of administered carcinogens (85). Choline deficiency is therefore considered to have both cancer-initiating and cancer-promoting activities.

Several mechanisms have been suggested to explain the cancer-promoting effect of a choline-devoid diet (86). These include *(a)* hepatic damage and regeneration, causing greater sensitivity to chemical carcinogens, *(b)* hypomethylation of DNA, causing abnormal repair of DNA, and *(c)* increased lipid peroxidation, which could be a source of free radicals that could modify DNA. As discussed below, we have proposed that choline deficiency perturbs protein kinase C (PKC; serine/threonine kinase) signal transduction and perturbs regulation of apoptosis, thereby promoting carcinogenesis.

FUNCTIONS

How Might Choline Influence Organ Function and Development

Cholinergic Neurons

Choline's relationships to acetylcholine synthesis have been thoroughly reviewed elsewhere (8). "Autocannibalism" of membrane phospholipid to supply choline for acetylcholine synthesis may explain the extensive degeneration of cholinergic neurons (which project to the brain cortex and hippocampus) in Alzheimer's disease (87). Abnormal phospholipid metabolism in this disease (88) results in reduced levels in brain (at autopsy) of phosphatidylcholine, phosphatidylethanolamine, choline, and ethanolamine and increased levels of glycerophosphocholine and glycerophosphoethanolamine.

Signal Transduction

Our understanding of choline phospholipid–mediated signal transduction has been vastly improved during the last decade. Stimulation of membrane-associated receptors activates neighboring phospholipases, resulting in formation of breakdown products that are signaling molecules per se (i.e., they stimulate or inhibit the activity of target macromolecules) or are converted into signaling molecules by specific enzymes. Much signaling research has focused on minor phospholipid components of membranes, particularly phosphatidylinositol derivatives (extensively reviewed elsewhere [89, 90]). However, choline phospholipids, especially phosphatidylcholine and sphingomyelin, are concerted biologically active molecules that can amplify external signals or terminate the signaling process by generating inhibitory second messengers (9).

In these signaling processes, activation of receptors at the plasma membrane leads to altered conformation of the receptor so that it can activate a guanosine triphosphate (GTP)-binding protein (G-protein). Activation of the G-protein results in the subsequent activation of phospholipase C activity within the plasma membrane. The phospholipases C are a family of phosphodiesterases that hydrolyze the glycerophosphate bond of intact phospholipids to generate 1,2-*sn*-diacylglycerol and an aqueous soluble head group.

The action of phospholipase C triggers the next event in the signal cascade, the activation of PKC. Products generated by phospholipid hydrolysis include diacylglycerol, which is both a messenger molecule and an intermediate in lipid metabolism. Normally, PKC is folded so that an endogenous "pseudosubstrate" region on the protein is bound to the catalytic site, thereby inhibiting activity. Diacylglycerol causes a conformational change in PKC, causing flexing at a hinge region, which withdraws the pseudosubstrate and unblocks the PKC catalytic site. The appearance of diacylglycerol in membranes is usually transient, so that PKC is activated only for a short time after a receptor has been stimulated.

There is also evidence that receptors with intrinsic tyrosine kinase activity (e.g., EGF or PDGF receptors) stimulate phosphatidylcholine hydrolysis (91). Sustained activation of PKC is essential for triggering cell differentiation and proliferation (92). Other products of phosphatidylcholine hydrolysis, such as phosphatidic acid, lysophosphatidylcholine, and free fatty acids also are second messengers (91, 93). Phosphatidic acid can also act as a mitogen (94). Lysophosphatidylcholine stimulates PKC activity (92) but is a membranolytic detergent with potential toxic effects. Lysophosphatidylcholine generation is important in chemotaxis, relaxation of smooth muscle, and activation of T lymphocytes (92). That modulation of

PKC isozymes by phosphatidylcholine may be isoform specific (95).

As discussed above, choline deficiency causes massive fatty liver in which 1,2-*sn*-diacylglycerol accumulates (96). In plasma membranes from livers of choline-deficient rats, diacylglycerol reaches levels higher than those occurring after stimulation of a receptor linked to phospholipase C activation (e.g., vasopressin receptor). This results in a stable activation of PKC and/or an increase in the total PKC pool in the cell (96, 97).

Characterization of events that occur downstream from PKC is just beginning. Serine-threonine kinases and tyrosine kinases catalyze phosphorylation of target proteins distal to PKC. Phosphorylation alters the biochemical properties of these substrates, resulting in a range of cellular responses. These phosphorylation cascades enhance amplification of the original signal. PKC signals impinge on several known intracellular control circuits (98), including receptors for insulin, epidermal growth factor, and many proteins involved in control of gene expression (99, 100). Accumulation of diacylglycerol and subsequent activation of PKC within liver during choline deficiency may contribute to the development of hepatic cancer in these animals (96, 97).

Although choline sphingolipids are ubiquitous components of mammalian cells, they have only recently been shown necessary for cellular survival and growth (101). Hydrolysis of sphingomyelin generates messengers that terminate the PKC signaling cascade. Sphingomyelin, sphingomyelinase, and ceramidase, which produces sphingosine and fatty acid from ceramide, are present in the outer leaflet of the plasma membrane. Ceramide is a potent inhibitor of cell growth as well as a promoter of cell differentiation. Its metabolite sphingosine is a potent inhibitor of PKC that acts by blocking diacylglycerol-mediated activation (102). Sphingosine concentrations in cells are in the micromolar range, perhaps high enough to inhibit PKC (103). Sphingosylphosphocholine (lysosphingomyelin) has recently been described as a potent mitogen (104).

Apoptosis

Apoptosis is a regulated form of cell suicide that is involved in such physiologic conditions as normal cell turnover, hormone-induced tissue atrophy, and embryogenesis (105). Cells undergoing apoptosis show internucleosomal DNA fragmentation and characteristic morphologic changes such as marked decrease in cell volume, nuclear condensation, nuclear fragmentation, and formation of apoptotic bodies consisting of membrane-enclosed pieces of condensed chromatin and well-preserved organelles (106, 107). Another characteristic change often occurring in apoptosis results from endonuclease activity that cleaves transcriptionally active nuclear DNA (106) (but not mitochondrial DNA) into 200-bp internucleosomal fragments that form a ladder on gel electrophoresis.

DNA strand breaks are an early consequence of choline deficiency (108, 109). DNA damage is important in the induction of morphologic changes associated with apoptosis (106). Rat hepatocytes maintained in a choline-deficient medium undergo apoptosis (10), and choline deficiency is a potent apoptosis inducer in neuronal cells as well. In PC12 cells (a neuronal cell line derived from a rat pheochromocytoma), choline deficiency could initiate apoptotic death, with characteristic DNA strand breaks and apoptotic body formation (109a). If choline availability modulates apoptosis in nerve cells, might it also alter the amount of apoptosis occurring in developing fetal brain? Could this explain why maternal intake of choline modulates the structure and function of their offspring's brains? In this regard, the amount of apoptosis in fetal brain inversely correlates with maternal choline intake (Holmes-McNary, unpublished observations). Thus, the behavioral effects of dietary choline could be due to changes in the relative survival of different groups of hippocampal cells at a critical period in brain development.

The process of carcinogenesis involves an initiating event that induces genetic damage, followed by survival and progression of selected clones of the mutant cells able to form tumors. Little is understood about the mechanisms that drive initiated cells to progress to carcinomas. As discussed above, something peculiar to the choline-deficient environment enhances tumor progression. Hepatocytes adapt and survive in a low-choline medium by becoming resistant to choline deficiency–induced apoptosis (110). Adapted hepatocytes may be resistant to choline deficiency–induced apoptosis because they have developed a defect in the apoptosis pathway involved. Perhaps prolonged choline deficiency creates a selective pressure that favors survival of cells with such defects. Adaptation to a choline-deficient environment is associated with cell transformation (increase in anchorage-independent growth and tumorigenic potential) (110). Thus, mutations that permit tumorigenesis may escape elimination because apoptosis is defective in adapted cells.

Is the apoptosis induced by choline deficiency due to a lack of choline moieties or to a methyl-group deficiency? Choline deficiency and methyl deficiency are often considered the same phenomenon, in which choline deficiency decreases methyl-group availability (85, 111). Methyl supplementation with betaine, methionine, folate, or vitamin B_{12}, however, did not prevent apoptotic death induced by choline-deficiency in hepatocytes (112). Thus, there are specific and important functions for choline that are not met when alternative methyl donors are substituted.

CHOLINE DEFICIENCY IN HUMANS

Humans require choline to sustain normal life. Is a dietary source of choline required? As discussed above, normal diets deliver sufficient choline. When healthy humans were fed a choline-deficient diet for 3 weeks, however, they developed biochemical changes consistent with choline deficiency (13). These changes included diminished plasma choline and phosphatidylcholine concentrations, as well as diminished erythrocyte membrane phosphatidylcholine concentrations. Serum alanine transaminase (ALT) activity, a measure of hepatocyte damage, increased significantly during choline deficiency.

Hepatic complications associated with total parenteral nutrition (TPN), which include fatty infiltration of the liver and hepatocellular damage, have been reported by many clinical groups. Frequently, TPN must be terminated because of the severity of the associated liver disease. Some liver disease associated with TPN is related to choline deficiency. Amino acid–glucose solutions used in TPN of humans contain no choline (14, 113). The lipid emulsions used to deliver extra calories and essential fatty acids during parenteral nutrition contain choline in the form of phosphatidylcholine (20% emulsion contains 13.2 mmol/L). Humans treated with parenteral nutrition required 1 to 1.7 mmol of choline-containing phospholipid/day during the first week of parenteral nutrition therapy to maintain plasma choline levels (14). Plasma choline concentrations decreased in parenteral nutrition patients at the same time that liver dysfunction was detected (114).

Clinical trials support the requirement for supplemental choline during TPN (15, 16). Patients were treated with TPN (average duration 7 years) including 4 kcal/kg/day as 20% Intralipid (delivering approximately 50 μmol/kg/day choline as phosphatidylcholine). These patients had low plasma choline concentrations (average, 6.3 μmol/L). In a double-blind protocol, investigators administered either 20 g lecithin (30% phosphatidylcholine; delivering approximately 300 μmol choline moiety/kg/day) or placebo (soybean oil) orally twice a day for 6 weeks. At the end of this experimental period, plasma choline had risen by more than 50% in the lecithin group, while in the placebo group it had decreased by 25%. Fatty liver was defined by computed tomography. In the treated group, liver density increased (fat decreased) by approximately 30% ($P < .05$); in the placebo group, liver density increased by only 8% (nonsignificant). Thus, choline seems to be an essential nutrient during long-term TPN.

PREGNANT ANIMALS DEPLETE THEIR CHOLINE RESERVES

Transport of choline from mother to fetus depletes maternal stores of choline and degrades tissue choline content (the choline concentration of maternal liver falls from a mean of 130 μmol/L in adult nonpregnant rats to 38 μmol/L in late pregnancy [115]). Pregnant rats eating a standard rat diet (AIN-76A diet) with and without choline for 6 days (days 12–18 gestation) were compared with nonmated female and male rats eating the same diets (116). Nonmated female rats eating the control diet had higher hepatic choline metabolite concentrations than did male rats (choline, 98% higher; betaine, 96% higher; phosphocholine, 55% higher) or pregnant rats (betaine, 42% higher; phosphocholine, 47% higher). Nonmated females eating a choline-deficient diet showed only a modest decrease (33%) in the labile choline metabolite phosphocholine in liver, compared with similar rats eating a control diet. Phosphocholine concentration in liver is the most reliable marker for changes in choline status. It was most sensitive to modest dietary choline deficiency in male adult rats, decreasing to 10 to 20% of control values after a short period of consuming a deficient diet (70). Pregnant rats had significantly greater diminution of hepatic phosphocholine (83% decrease) when fed a choline-deficient diet than did nonmated females (116). The depletion of choline stores evident in pregnant rats indicates that demand for choline exceeds the capacity of the combination of dietary intake and de novo synthesis during pregnancy. Even though female rats are more resistant to choline deficiency than are male rats, pregnancy renders them more vulnerable to deficiency than males are. Decreased demands for methylation and an enhanced capacity to form the choline moiety de novo may explain the relative resistance of nonmated females to choline deficiency. A major sink for methyl groups is formation of creatinine. In males this demand is much higher (because of greater muscle mass) than in females (117); therefore, females may use less choline (betaine) as a methyl donor. Phosphatidylethanolamine-*N*-methyltransferase activity in some tissues is influenced by sex hormones (118). Females have 10% (119) to 50% (120) greater phosphatidylethanolamine-*N*-methyltransferase activity in liver than do males. In addition, young women incorporate methylmethionine into phosphatidylcholine significantly faster than do postmenopausal women (121).

LACTATION EXACERBATES THE CHOLINE DEPLETION THAT STARTS IN PREGNANCY

Most of the choline moiety in human milk (2 mmol/L) is derived from maternal plasma. Thus, transport of choline from mother to infant via the mammary gland constitutes an appreciable drain on maternal choline stores and makes the lactating female even more vulnerable to the effects of choline deficiency. After eating a defined control diet for 25 days (gestation day 12 to postpartum day 15), lactating rats had lower hepatic choline metabolite concentrations (phosphocholine, 67%; phosphatidylcholine, 73%; and betaine, 37%) than similarly fed, nonmated females (116). These lactating rats clearly were highly sensitive to choline deficiency, inasmuch as their liver phosphocholine decreased 88% during the 25-day feeding period compared with a 12% decrease in nonmated females (116).

SUMMARY

Choline is crucial for sustaining life. It modulates the basic signaling processes within cells, is a structural element in membranes, and is vital during critical periods in brain development. Choline metabolism is closely interrelated with the metabolism of methionine and folate. Although the normal human diet provides sufficient choline to sustain healthy organ function, populations vulnerable to choline deficiency exist, including the growing infant, the pregnant or lactating woman, the cirrhotic patient, and the patient fed by TPN. Studies of choline requirements in these groups need to be pursued vigorously.

The 1998 Reference Dietary Intakes of the Food and Nutrition Board—Institute of Medicine include suggested "adequate intake" levels for healthy individuals of various age groups (123) (see also Appendix Tables II-A-2-c-1 and c-4).

ACKNOWLEDGMENTS

Some of the work described in this review was supported by a grant from the National Institutes of Health (AG09525).

REFERENCES

1. Zeisel SH, Blusztajn JK. Annu Rev Nutr 1994;14:269–96.
2. Strecker A. Ann Chem Pharm 1862;123:353–60.
3. duVigneaud V, Cohn M, Chandler JP, et al. J Biol Chem 1941;140:625–41.
4. Kennedy EP, Weiss SB. J Biol Chem 1956;222:193–214.
5. Best CH, Huntsman ME. J Physiol 1932;75:405–12.
6. Best CH, Huntsman ME. J Physiol 1935;83:255–74.
7. Lieber CS, Robins SJ, Li J, et al. Gastroenterology 1994;106:152–9.
8. Blusztajn JK, Wurtman RJ. Science 1983;221:614–20.
9. Zeisel SH. FASEB J 1993;7:551–7.
10. Albright CD, Lui R, Bethea TC, et al. FASEB J 1996;10:510–6.
11. Bremer J, Greenberg D. Biochim Biophys Acta 1961;46:205–16.
12. Chawla RK, Wolf DC, Kutner MH, et al. Gastroenterology 1989;97:1514–20.
13. Zeisel SH, daCosta K-A, Franklin PD, et al. FASEB J 1991;5:2093–8.
14. Sheard NF, Tayek JA, Bistrian BR, et al. Am J Clin Nutr 1986;43:219–24.
15. Buchman AL, Moukarzel A, Jenden DJ, et al. Clin Nutr 1993;12:33–7.
16. Buchman AL, Dubin M, Jenden D, et al. Gastroenterology 1992;102:1363–70.
17. FASEB Life Sciences Research Office. Evaluation of the health aspects of choline chloride and choline bitartrate as food ingredients. Report #PB-223 845/9. Bureau of Foods, Food and Drug Administration, Department of Health, Education, and Welfare, Washington, DC. 1975.
18. FASEB Life Sciences Research Office. Effects of consumption of choline and lecithin on neurological and cardiovascular systems. Report #PB-82-133257. Bureau of Foods, Food and Drug Administration, Department of Health, Education, and Welfare, Washington, DC. 1981.
19. Zeisel SH, Char D, Sheard NF. J Nutr 1986;116:50–8.
20. Holmes-McNary M, Cheng WL, Mar MH, et al. Am J Clin Nutr 1996;64:572–6.
21. Chao CK, Pomfret EA, Zeisel SH. Biochem J 1988;254:33–8.
22. Yang EK, Blusztajn JK, Pomfret EA, et al. Biochem J 1988;256:821–8.
23. Zeisel SH, Wurtman RJ. Biochem J 1981;198:565–70.
24. Zeisel SH. Choline availability in the neonate. In: Dowdall MJ, Hawthorne JN, eds. Cellular and molecular basis of cholinergic function. Chichester: Horwood, 1987;709–19.
25. Zeisel SH, Stanbury JB, Wurtman RJ, et al. N Engl J Med 1982;306:175–6.
26. Zeisel SH, Wishnok JS, Blusztajn JK. J Pharmacol Exper Ther 1983;225:320–4.
27. Lekim D, Betzing H. Hoppe Seylers Z Physiol Chem 1976;357:1321–31.
28. Cheng W-L, Holmes-McNary MQ, Mar M-H, et al. J Nutr Biochem 1996;7:457–64.
29. McMahon KE, Farrell PM. Clin Chim Acta 1985;149:1–12.
30. Cornford EM, Cornford ME. Fed Proc 1986;45:2065–72.
31. Garner SC, Mar M-H, Zeisel SH. J Nutr 1995;125:2851–8.
32. Sweiry JH, Page KR, Dacke CG, et al. J Dev Physiol 1986;8:435–45.
33. Leventer SM, Rowell PP. Placenta 1984;5:261–70.
34. Acara M, Rennick B. Am J Physiol 1973;225:1123–8.
35. Rennick B, Acara M, Glor M. Am J Physiol 1977;232:F443–7.
36. Grossman EB, Herbert SC. Am J Physiol 1989;256:F107–112.
37. Rennick B, Acara M, Hysert P, et al. Kidney Int 1976;10:329–35.
38. Acara M, Rennick B, LaGraff S, et al. Nephron 1983;35:241–3.
39. Ulus IH, Wurtman RJ, Mauron C, et al. Brain Res 1989;484:217–27.
40. Blusztajn JK, Liscovitch M, Richardson UI. Proc Natl Acad Sci USA 1987;84:5474–7.
41. Lee HC, Fellenz M, Maloney M, et al. Proc Natl Acad Sci USA 1993;90:10086–90.
42. Lin CS, Wu RD. J Protein Chem 1986;5:193–200.
43. Garcia-Perez A, Burg MB. J Membrane Biol 1991;119:1–13.
44. Vance DE. Biochem Cell Biol 1990;68:1151–65.
45. Ishidate K, Nakazawa Y. Methods Enzymol 1992;209:121–34.
46. Porter TJ, Kent C. J Biol Chem 1990;265:414–22.
47. Pelech S, Vance D. Biochim Biophys Acta 1984;779:217–51.
48. Vance DE. Biochem Cell Biol 1990;68:1151–65.
49. Farrell PM, Epstein MF, Fleischman AR, et al. Biol Neonate 1976;29:238–46.
50. Wang Y, MacDonald JI, Kent C. J Biol Chem 1993;268:5512–8.
51. Watkins JD, Kent C. J Biol Chem 1992;267:5686–92.
52. Jamil H, Hatch GM, Vance DE. Biochem J 1993;291:419–27.
53. Yao ZM, Jamil H, Vance DE. J Biol Chem 1990;265:4326–31.
54. Hatch GM, Jamil H, Utal AK, et al. J Biol Chem 1992;267:15751–8.
55. Utal AK, Jamil H, Vance DE. J Biol Chem 1991;266:24084–91.
56. Cornell R. Cholinephosphotransferase. In: Vance DE, ed. Phosphatidylcholine metabolism. Boca Raton, FL: CRC Press, 1989;47–65.
57. Cacabelos R, Alvarez X, Franco-Maside A, et al. Ann NY Acad Sci 1993;695:321–3.
58. Hamdorf G, Cervos-Navarro J, Muller R. Arzneimittelforschung 1992;42:421–4.
59. Spiers P, Myers D, Hochanadel G, et al. Arch Neurol 1996;53:441–8.
60. Blusztajn JK, Zeisel SH, Wurtman RJ. Brain Res 1979;179:319–27.
61. Crews FT, Calderini G, Battistella A, et al. Brain Res 1981;229:256–9.
62. Mudd SH, Datko AH. Plant Physiol 1989;90:306–10.
63. Andriamampandry C, Freysz L, Kanfer JN, et al. J Neurochem 1991;56:1845–50.
64. Vance DE, Ridgway ND. Prog Lipid Res 1988;27:61–79.
65. Cui Z, Vance JE, Chen MH, et al. J Biol Chem 1993;268:16655–63.

66. Finkelstein JD, Martin JJ, Harris BJ, et al. J Nutr 1983;113:519–21.
67. Varela-Moreiras G, Selhub J, da Costa K, et al. J Nutr Biochem 1992;3:519–22.
68. Selhub J, Seyoum E, Pomfret EA, et al. Cancer Res 1991;51:16–21.
69. Zeisel SH, Zola T, da Costa K, et al. Biochem J 1989;259:725–29.
70. Pomfret EA, da Costa K, Zeisel SH. J Nutr Biochem 1990;1:533–41.
71. Freeman-Narrod M, Narrod SA, Custer RP. J Natl Cancer Inst 1977;59:1013–7.
72. Custer RP, Freeman-Narrod M, Narrod SJ. J Natl Cancer Inst 1977;58:1011–5.
73. Aarsaether N, Berge RK, Aarsland A, et al. Biochim Biophys Acta 1988;958:70–80.
74. Rush D. Am J Clin Nutr 1994;59:511S–5S.
75. Trotz M, Wegner CHR, Nau H. Life Sci 1987;41:103–10.
76. Malinow MR. Clin Chem 1995;41:173–6.
77. Yao ZM, Vance DE. J Biol Chem 1988;263:2998–3004.
78. Yao ZM, Vance DE. J Biol Chem 1989;264:11373–80.
79. Yao ZM, Vance DE. Biochem Cell Biol 1990;68:552–8.
80. Blusztajn JK, Zeisel SH, Wurtman RJ. Biochem J 1985;232: 505–11.
81. Hoffman DR, Cornatzer WE, Duerre JA. Can J Biochem 1979;57:56–65.
82. Meck WH, Smith RA, Williams CL. Dev Psychobiol 1988;21:339–53.
83. Loy R, Heyer D, Williams CL, et al. Adv Exp Med Biol 1991;295:373–82.
84. Meck WH, Smith RA, Williams CL. Behav Neurosci 1989;103:1234–41.
85. Newberne PM, Rogers AE. Annu Rev Nutr 1986;6:407–32.
86. Zeisel SH, da Costa KA, Albright CD, et al. Adv Exp Med Biol 1995;375:65–74.
87. Blusztajn JK, Holbrook PG, Lakher M, et al. Psychopharmacol Bull 1986;22:781–6.
88. Nitsch RM, Blusztajn JK, Pittas AG, et al. Proc Natl Acad Sci USA 1992;89:1671–5.
89. Berridge MJ. JAMA 1989;262:1834–41.
90. Taylor CW, Marshall I. Trends Biochem Sci 1992;17:403–7.
91. Exton JH. J Biol Chem 1990;265:1–4.
92. Nishizuka Y. Science 1992;258:607–14.
93. Besterman JM, Duronio V, Cuatrecasas P. Proc Natl Acad Sci USA 1986;83:6785–9.
94. Wakelam MJO, Cook SJ, Currie S, et al. Biochem Soc Trans 1991;19:321–4.
95. Sasaki Y, Asaoka Y, Nishizuka Y. FEBS Lett 1993;320:47–51.
96. da Costa K-A, Garner SC, Chang J, et al. Carcinogenesis 1995;16:327–34.
97. da Costa K, Cochary EF, Blusztajn JK, et al. J Biol Chem 1993;268:2100–5.
98. Stabel S, Parker PJ. Pharmacol Ther 1991;51:71–95.
99. Nishizuka Y. Science 1986;233:305–12.
100. Weinstein IB. Adv Second Messenger Phosphoprotein Res 1990;24:307–16.
101. Hanada K, Nishijima M, Kiso M, et al. J Biol Chem 1992;267:23527–33.
102. Hannun YA. J Biol Chem 1994;269:3125–8.
103. Merrill AH, Jones DD. Biochim Biophys Acta 1990; 1044:1–12.
104. Desai NN, Spiegel S. Biochem Biophys Res Commun 1991;181:361–6.
105. Kerr JFR, Wyllie AH, Currie AR. Br J Cancer 1972;26:239–57.
106. Arends MJ, Morris RG, Wyllie AH. Am J Pathol 1990;136: 593–608.
107. Wyllie AH. Int Rev Cytol 1987;17(Suppl):755–85.
108. Wilson RB, Kula NS, Newberne PM, et al. Exp Mol Pathol 1973;18:357–68.
109. Rushmore TH, Farber E, Ghoshal AK, et al. Carcinogenesis 1986;7:1677–80.
109a. Holmes-McNary MQ, Loy R, Mar M-H, et al. Dev Brain Res 1997, in press.
110. Zeisel SH, Albright CD, Shin O-K, et al. Carcinogenesis 1997;18:731–8.
111. Christman JK. Adv Exp Med Biol 1995;375:97–106.
112. Shin OH, Mar MH, Albright CD, et al. J Cell Biochem 1997;64:196–208.
113. Chawla RK, Berry CJ, Kutner MH, et al. Am J Clin Nutr 1985;42:577–84.
114. Burt ME, Hanin I, Brennan MF. Lancet 1980;2:638–9.
115. Gwee MC, Sim MK. Clin Exp Pharmacol Physiol 1978;5: 649–53.
116. Zeisel SH, Mar M-H, Zhou Z-W, et al. J Nutr 1995;125: 3049–54.
117. Mudd SH, Poole JR. Metab Clin Exp 1975;24:721–35.
118. Drouva SV, LaPlante E, Leblanc P, et al. Endocrinology 1986;119:2611–22.
119. Lyman RL, Sheehan G, Tinoco J. Can J Biochem 1971;49:71–9.
120. Bjornstad P, Bremer J. J Lipid Res 1966;7:38–45.
121. Lindblad L, Schersten T. Scand J Gastroenterol 1976;11: 587–91.
122. Zeisel SH. Biological consequences of choline deficiency. In: Wurtman R, Wurtman J, eds. Choline metabolism and brain function. New York: Raven Press, 1990;75–99.
123. Food and Nutrition Board—Institute of Medicine. Dietary reference intakes. Thiamin, riboflavin, niacin, vitamin B_6, folate, vitamin B_{12}, pantothenic acid, biotin, and choline. Washington, DC: National Academy Press, 1998.

33. Carotenoids

JAMES ALLEN OLSON

The carotenoids consist of more than 600 compounds, exclusive of isomers, all of which are polyisoprenoids, possess an extensive system of conjugated double bonds, usually contain 40 carbon atoms, commonly show internal symmetry, and often have one or two cyclic structures at the ends of their conjugated chains. They are found in some species of most types of living organisms, including animals, plants, and microorganisms. They are required for survival in a few, but not many, life forms. They and their metabolites perform many useful functions in nature, including their involvement as accessory light-gathering pigments and as protective agents in photosynthesis, their conversion to vitamin A in animals and in some microorganisms, and the involvement of a metabolite in leaf abscission. They are prominent in the coloration of birds and other organisms, which is often related to mating cycles, and in flowers, possibly as an attractant for insects that enhance pollination. They are colorful, yielding a spectrum of compounds from yellow to red. Besides their above-cited functions, they delight the eye and raise human spirits.

This treatment of carotenoids, however, appropriately for a treatise devoted largely to human nutrition, focuses on their physiology and metabolism in animals and humans and on their potentially beneficial and adverse effects in human disease. Because they are easily extracted, brightly colored compounds, they have interested chemists and biologists for a century and a half (1). The term *carotenoids* was coined by Tswett in 1911 during his early elegant studies on their separation by chromatographic procedures.

CHEMISTRY

Some carotenoids commonly found in foods are shown in Figure 33.1. Although the most prevalent and stable form of each carotenoid is the all-*trans* isomer, many *cis* isomers exist. Indeed, the symmetric reference compound, β-carotene, can theoretically form 272 different isomers, whereas its asymmetric analogue, α-carotene, can form 512. Other than possibly the 9-*cis* isomer, however, few of the *cis* isomers currently are considered important in animal nutrition.

The carotenoids in large part are hydrophobic molecules and consequently interact with lipophilic parts of the cell; namely, membranes and lipid globules. The hydrocarbon carotenoids tend to be solubilized in the lipid cores of bilayer membranes. Being rigid molecules, they align themselves parallel to the surfaces of the membrane. The oxocarotenoids (xanthophylls) such as lutein and zeaxanthin (Fig. 33.1) tend to expose their hydroxyl groups at the membrane surface. They may align themselves perpendicular to the surface and even serve as transmembrane entities (2). Thus, dihydroxycarotenoids may affect both the fluidity and the function of membranes.

In nature, hydroxylated carotenoids are often present as esters with long-chain fatty acids (making them more hydrophobic) or as glycosides (making them more polar). Ketocarotenoids, such as canthaxanthin (Fig. 33.1) and its 3,3′-dihydroxy analogue, astaxanthin, can form discrete complexes with proteins by making Schiff bases with specific lysine residues. This interaction, as in α-crustacyanin of the lobster, shifts the spectrum of the carotenoid 144 nm toward the red to give a blue complex. Most free carotenoids in solution, however, absorb between 440 and

Abbreviations: **ARMD**—age-related macular degeneration; **CARET**—Carotene and Retinol Efficacy Trial; **FAD**—flavin adenine dinucleotide; **GI**—gastrointestinal; **HDL**—high-density lipoprotein; **LDL**—low-density lipoprotein; **MST**—mean sojourn time; **NAD**—nicotinamide adenine dinucleotide; **NADPH**—reduced nicotinamide adenine dinucleotide phosphate; **VLDL**—very low density lipoprotein.

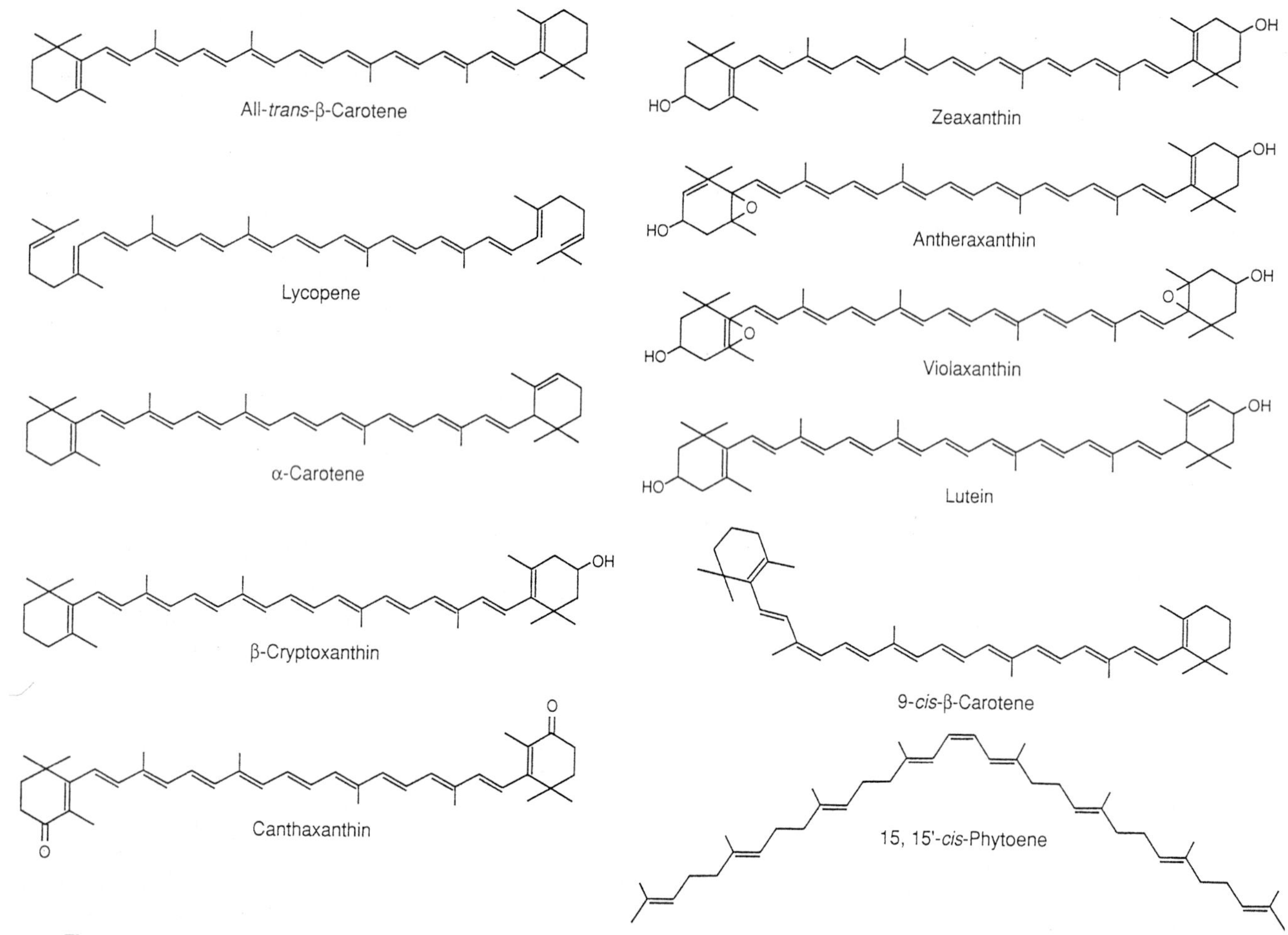

All-*trans*-β-Carotene

Zeaxanthin

Antheraxanthin

Lycopene

Violaxanthin

α-Carotene

Lutein

β-Cryptoxanthin

9-*cis*-β-Carotene

Canthaxanthin

15, 15'-*cis*-Phytoene

Figure 33.1. Some carotenoids commonly found in foods. (From Olson JA, Krinsky NI. FASEB J 1995;9:1547–50, with permission.)

490 nm, depending primarily on the number of conjugated double bonds present and the solvent used.

The C40 carotenoids can be oxidatively cleaved, both chemically and biologically, to yield a family of *β*-apocarotenoids with fewer than 40 carbon atoms. These derivatives usually absorb at wavelengths of 350 to 430 nm, depending primarily on the number of conjugated double bonds present.

Various isotopically labeled analogues, primarily *β*-carotene, have been synthesized both chemically and biologically from precursors containing ^{14}C, ^{13}C, ^{3}H, and ^{2}H. These labeled compounds have been very useful in studying the metabolism and in vivo kinetics of these compounds.

Carotenoids show two other important chemical characteristics: *(a)* an ability to quench singlet oxygen and *(b)* antioxidant/prooxidant properties. Singlet oxygen, which is much more reactive than the triplet oxygen present in the air, can interact with many components of the cell to yield oxidized inactive products. Carotenoids also interact with singlet oxygen to yield triplet oxygen and an excited triplet carotenoid, which in turn releases its energy harmlessly into the ambient solution (1, 2). Carotenoids also form both radical cations and radical anions under suitable conditions (2). These highly reactive molecules can interact with other free radicals, such as peroxy or hydroxy radicals, to give nonradical products, or they can interact with other molecules to restore the carotenoid to the ground state while producing a new free radical (2). Removal of free radicals from cells is usually considered beneficial, and generation of free radicals in cells is usually considered harmful. Thus, depending on circumstances, carotenoids can show either antioxidant or prooxidant actions. Under physiologic conditions, however, their antioxidant actions seem to predominate (2, 3).

In addition to the "mediator"-type reactions cited above, carotenoids can also be oxidized, both chemically and biologically, by strong oxidants to give a variety of products (4). In a physiologic context, these reactions can be beneficial (removal of strong oxidants from cells where they can cause oxidative damage), indifferent (not of sufficient importance to influence cell metabolism), or adverse (provitamin A carotenoids are destroyed).

The most-used methods for separation and quantitation of carotenoids involve high-performance liquid chromatography (HPLC) on reverse-phase or straight-phase columns, combined with spectrophotometric detection and peak integration (5). A so-called C30 HPLC column gives improved resolution (6). *β*-Carotene labeled with deuterium is detected by mass spectrometry combined with a variety of separation methods (7).

DIGESTION, ABSORPTION, AND TRANSPORT

Digestion and Absorption

Dietary carotenoids in foods exist in two major forms: *(a)* as true solutions in oil, as in red palm oil, or *(b)* as parts of matrices within the vegetable or fruit. The matrix is usually complex, consisting of fiber, digestible polysaccharides, and proteins. Because the matrix often is not fully disrupted during food preparation and during its passage through the intestine, the bioavailability of carotenoids can vary from less than 10%, such as in largely intact raw carrots, to more than 50% in oily solutions or in synthetic, gelatin-based, commercial preparations (8–10). Hydrocarbon carotenoids such as β-carotene and lycopene are solubilized in the lipid core of micelles in the gut lumen or alternatively form small clathrate complexes with conjugated bile acids, of which deoxycholate and cholate are the most effective (8, 11). Xanthophyll esters must be hydrolyzed before absorption. As in membranes, xanthophylls and carotenes associate differently with micelles (12). The absorption process does not seem to involve special epithelial transporters.

Apart from an incomplete release of carotenoids from the matrices of foods, other factors that lower carotenoid bioavailability include the presence of fiber, particularly pectins, in the diet; a lack of fat in the diet; the presence of nondigested lipids, including fat substitutes; inadequate bile flow; various clinical conditions involving lipid malabsorption; and reduced gastric acidity (10). The absorption efficiency of carotenoids decreases as the amount ingested increases (8–10).

Furthermore, carotenoids in substantial amounts interfere with each other's absorption (13, 14). The action is not mutually competitive, however, inasmuch as β-carotene inhibits canthaxanthin and lutein absorption, whereas the latter have little or no effect on β-carotene absorption (10, 13, 14). Vitamin E and carotenoids also interact. Vitamin E supplements tend to lower plasma carotenoid concentrations, although small amounts of vitamin E may prevent carotenoid oxidation in the gastrointestinal (GI) tract (10). β-Carotene supplements have been reported to decrease, increase, or not affect plasma tocopherol concentrations (10).

Bioavailability and Nutritional Equivalency

In a nutritional context, the great range of bioavailabilities of carotenoids makes any definition of their general equivalence as precursors of vitamin A difficult. Indeed, the retinol molar equivalency of small amounts of β-carotene in oil is approximately 0.5 (15), whereas that of carotenoids in rapidly stir-fried vegetables is very poor indeed (<0.05) (16). Carotenoids in fruits seem to be better utilized. Past bioavailability studies, which are often inconclusive and conflicting, have been reviewed (17).

The problem in defining a general factor for converting provitamin A carotenoids to vitamin A is not new. The World Health Organization (WHO) suggested in 1967 that 6 μg of all-*trans* β-carotene or 12 μg of all-*trans* provitamin A carotenoids in foods is equivalent to 1 μg of all-*trans* retinol (18). In the absence of precise information and because of the complexity of the problem, most national and international committees have used the same value.

Isomeric Forms

The 9-*cis* isomer of β-carotene is absorbed from the human intestinal lumen but, unlike the all-*trans* isomer, is not transported in significant amounts in plasma (19, 20). Thus, the 9-*cis* isomer may well be isomerized to the all-*trans* form in the intestinal mucosa before being released into lymph (9) or be cleaved in the intestinal mucosa to all-*trans* and 9-*cis* retinal (21, 22). In contrast, the *cis* isomers of lycopene seem to be absorbed better than the all-*trans* isomer in humans (23). Absorption, transport, and storage in the liver of isomeric forms of carotenoids seem to be species specific. Thus, in monkeys, relative to the all-*trans* form, 13-*cis* isomers of lutein and zeaxanthin seem to be preferentially absorbed and transported, whereas the 9-*cis* isomer seems to be more poorly absorbed (10). Thus, just as some vertebrates (humans, other primates, the preruminant calf, ferrets, and birds) absorb and transport appreciable amounts of carotenoids in the plasma whereas others (most rodents) do not, differential absorption and storage of isomeric forms seem to vary markedly from one species to another.

Relative Rates of Absorption of Different Carotenoids

In general, polar carotenoids seem to be absorbed better by humans than nonpolar ones. Thus, by using the area under the absorption curve (AUC) of plasma as an indicator, lutein seems to be absorbed about twice as well as β-carotene in humans (14). β-Apocarotenals and β-apocarotenols also seem to be absorbed better than less polar carotenoids (24). Relative to their proportions in a carotenoid mixture ingested by humans, lutein and zeaxanthin are enriched in the chylomicra (10). These deductions are based on the assumption that metabolism of carotenoids in the intestinal mucosa is only a minor part of their transfer into plasma and that their relative rates of clearance from plasma are similar. These assumptions may not hold for all-*trans* β-carotene and possibly for other provitamin A carotenoids.

Responders and Nonresponders

When a moderate to large dose of β-carotene is administered orally to humans, some subjects respond with a marked increase in the β-carotene concentration in plasma that peaks at 6 h, decreases, and then rises to higher concentrations with a second peak at approximately 24 h (8–10). This is considered a normal response. Other subjects, termed *nonresponders,* show little or no increase in the plasma concentration of β-carotene after dosing (10). Several explanations can be given for this unexpected observation: *(a)* β-carotene is absorbed, but at a much slower rate; *(b)* β-carotene may be cleared from the plasma at a much faster rate; and *(c)* β-carotene may be converted very rapidly to vitamin A in the intestinal mucosa. Although all of these factors may play a role, the rate of cleavage of β-carotene to vitamin A in the intestinal mucosa seems to be a key factor. In human lymph, the ratio of retinyl ester derived from β-carotene to intact β-carotene in several subjects was 2 or more (10). In addition, nonresponders to β-carotene responded normally to lutein (14) or to canthaxanthin (10), neither of which is appreciably metabolized in the intestinal mucosa. All subjects given carotenoid analogues such as 4,4′ dimethoxy β-carotene and ethyl β-apo-8′-carotenoate, responded normally (24). Finally, the rates of clearance of lutein and β-carotene from human plasma after dosing did not differ significantly (14). Thus, "nonresponders" to a dose of β-carotene may rather be "efficient converters" of β-carotene into vitamin A in the intestinal mucosa. Likewise, many animal species that do not transfer intact β-carotene into the plasma are efficient in converting β-carotene to vitamin A.

Plasma Transport

Newly absorbed carotenoids, together with retinyl ester and small amounts of retinol, are transported on chylomicra from the intestinal mucosa via lymph into the general circulation. Lipoprotein lipase hydrolyzes much of the triglyceride in the chylomicron, resulting in a chylomicron remnant (8–10). The latter, which retains apolipoproteins B48 and E on its surface, will interact with receptors for them on hepatocytes and be taken up by those cells. Small amounts of chylomicron remnants may also be taken up by other tissues.

The hepatocyte then incorporates much dietary carotenoid into lipoproteins. Hydrocarbon carotenoids predominate in very low density lipoproteins (VLDLs) and low-density lipoproteins (LDLs), whereas the xanthophylls are distributed more or less equally between high-density lipoproteins (HDLs) and LDLs (8–10). This distribution accords with the hydrophobicity of the carotenoids and lipoproteins. Specific mechanisms of incorporation, such as the α-tocopherol-transport protein of liver for *RRR*-α-tocopherol, have not been identified for carotenoids. A recently characterized β-carotene-binding protein of liver (25), however, may play some role in this process. HDLs may arise both from de novo synthesis in the liver and from pinching off of excess surface components from chylomicra in the plasma during triglyceride hydrolysis. It seems likely, however, that xanthophylls are primarily incorporated into HDLs in the liver.

In the plasma, VLDLs are rapidly converted by lipoprotein lipase to LDLs, which retain the carotenoids and apolipoprotein B100. Receptors for the latter are present on cells of many peripheral tissues as well as the liver. HDLs pick up cholesterol and possibly xanthophylls from peripheral tissues as well as apolipoprotein E from other plasma lipoproteins before being taken up by the liver. Except as noted above, carotenoids do not seem to be transferred from one lipid class to another, at least during in vitro incubation (10, 26).

Thus, carotenoids are involved in a complex and probably cyclic metabolic pathway involving the intestine, chylomicra, the liver, plasma lipoproteins, and peripheral tissues.

Plasma Carotenoids

In the fasting state, carotenoids are commonly found in human plasma. Of the 30 or more carotenoids present, six comprise 60 to 70% of the total (27, 28): lutein, lycopene, zeaxanthin, β-cryptoxanthin, β-carotene, and α-carotene. Because carotenoids are noncovalently bound to lipoproteins and apparently are not homeostatically controlled, their concentrations in plasma depend highly on the diet. In a more physiologic context, their steady-state plasma concentrations depend on the amounts in the diet, their intestinal absorption efficiencies, their uptake by tissues, their release from tissues back into plasma, and their catabolic rates. Because the distribution of carotenoids in a population is skewed toward lower values, median concentrations are generally used in data analysis. A preliminary report (29) of median values from NHANES III (1988–1994) for the six major carotenoids and their reference ranges in the United States population is summarized in Table 33.1. The reference ranges are expectedly broad, as they include individuals ingesting various amounts of carotenoids in the diet. Lutein and zeaxanthin, which tend to run closely together on HPLC, are grouped in this analysis. In general, the lutein:zeaxanthin ratio in plasma is 4 or 5:1 (30). Although the distribution and amounts of carotenoids in individuals differ markedly, each person maintains a fairly constant pattern for at least a month (30), probably reflecting a fairly uniform diet during that period, abetted by the presumed buffering effect of tissue carotenoid concentrations. Some key find-

Table 33.1
Median Concentrations (μmol/L) of Serum Carotenoids in 40-Year Old Humans in the United States, 1988–1994

Carotenoid	Men	Women	Reference Ranges[a] 5th–95th Percentile
Lycopene	0.47	0.41	0.13–0.82
Lutein + zeaxanthin	0.35	0.35	0.16–0.72
β-Cryptoxanthin	0.13	0.13	0.05–0.38
β-Carotene	0.22	0.28[b]	0.09–0.91
α-Carotene	0.065	0.081[b]	0.02–0.22

Unpublished NHANES III data, CDC, 1996. Summarized by Briefel R, Sowell A, Huff D, et al. FASEB J 1996;10:A813.

[a]For subjects ≥4 (n = 22,949). Ranges for 40-year-old adults were not available.

[b]Extrapolated from values for nonsmoking subjects.

ings that emerge from these surveys (29, 30) are that men show higher lycopene concentrations than women, women show higher β-carotene and α-carotene concentrations than men, and that smoking depresses carotenoid concentrations (except, oddly enough, for lycopene) by approximately 30% in all subjects. Median carotenoid concentrations also vary with age, but not in the same way for all carotenoids (29). Lycopene generally is the most common carotenoid in plasma, followed by lutein/zeaxanthin, β-carotene, β-cryptoxanthin, and α-carotene, in that order (29).

When subjects are fed a diet containing few, if any, carotenoids, plasma carotenoids expectedly decrease (31–33). Under these conditions, plasma carotenoid concentrations decrease in approximately a first-order manner for 14 to 30 days and then reach slowly declining plateau values (31). Estimated initial half-lives ($t_{1/2}$) in a 30-day study (32) and those calculated from the first 14 days of a 64-day study (31) are lycopene (9, 16 days), β-carotene (10, 12 days), lutein/zeaxanthin (12, 19 days), β-cryptoxanthin (16, 11 days) and α-carotene (17, 8 days). Serum concentrations of the above-cited carotenoids in subjects on a low-carotenoid diet for 64 to 72 days were 51% or less of their baseline concentrations (31, 33).

Tissue Carotenoid Content

Carotenoids are found in all tissues of the body (30, 34–38) (Table 33.2). On the basis of the relative weights of tissues in the adult human body (39), they clearly are mainly present in fat, liver, and plasma. Some relatively small tissues (e.g., testes and adrenal) and parts of some tissues (e.g., the corpus luteum [112 nmol/g]) show very high concentrations of carotenoids, whereas some major organs (e.g., muscle and brain) show very low concentrations. The only major human organs not cited in Table 33.2 are the skeleton and the GI tract. The former does not seem to have been studied in this regard and the latter, which deteriorates rapidly after death, also has not been examined in human autopsy specimens.

The total amount of carotenoid in the body varies greatly, depending largely on dietary intake. Thus, it is not surprising that the mean concentrations of carotenoids in fat and liver in various studies (34–37) differ markedly.

Inasmuch as 90% or more of the carotenoids in the body are found in tissues and less than 10% in plasma, the carotenoid patterns in various tissues are of interest. In nearly all tissues cited in Table 33.2, lycopene and β-carotene were in highest concentrations, lutein/zeaxanthin were intermediate, and cryptoxanthin and α-carotene were lower (30, 34–38). Tissue concentrations in most instances reflected the distribution pattern of carotenoids in plasma from the same population group. Some exceptions are the preferential accumulation of β-carotene in the pineal gland (40) and the corpus luteum (41) and of lutein/zeaxanthin in the macula of the eye (42).

Table 33.2
Estimated Total Carotenoid Content (nmol/g) of Selected Human Tissues

Organ	Mean Concentration[a]	Approximate Percentage of Body Weight[b]	Mean Total Amount (μmol)[c]	Percentage Total Amount[d]
Fat	3.3 (15.6)[e] (0.8)[f]	18.8	42.2	65.39
Liver	5.0 (14.1)[d] (5.1)[e] (21.0) }[f]	2.3	7.8	12.09
Muscle	ND[g] (0.07)[k]	42.8	2.04	3.16
Adrenal	33.7 (9.4)[f]	0.02	0.46	0.71
Plasma	ND[h] (1.1)[b] (1.6)[j]	4.9	4.5	6.97
Pancreas	3.7	0.16	0.40	0.62
Spleen	0.96 (5.9)[e]	0.25	0.16	0.25
Kidney	0.98 (1.2)[e] (0.9)[f] (3.1)[g]	0.41	0.27	0.42
Heart	0.81 (0.84)[e]	0.42	0.23	0.36
Testes	26.3 (7.6)[f]	0.04	0.72	1.12
Lung	ND[b] (1.9)[g]	0.73	0.94	1.46
Thyroid	0.79	0.04	0.021	0.03
Ovary	2.6 (0.9)[f]	0.01	0.018	0.03
Prostate	ND[h] (1.3)[i]	0.024	0.021	0.03
Skin	ND[h] (0.98)[i]	7.0	4.7	7.28
Brain	ND[h] (<0.04)[f]	2.0	0.054	<0.08
Total	—	79.9%	64.54 μmol	100%

[a]Mean concentrations, unless otherwise noted, are taken from ref. 34. An average molecular weight of mixed carotenoids in tissues is assumed to be 543. Thus, 1 μg = 1.84 nmol.
[b]From ref 39. Major unlisted organs are the stomach and intestines (7–10%) and the skeleton (12–15%).
[c]Based on a reference body weight of 68 kg.
[d]Based primarily on ref. 34.
[e]From ref. 35.
[f]From ref. 36. The plasma concentration is in nmol/mL.
[g]From ref. 37.
[h]ND, not determined in ref. 34.
[i]From ref 38. Lycopene and β-carotene only.
[j]From ref. 30.
[k]From ref. 145.

In Vivo Kinetics

The in vivo kinetics of an orally administered dose (73 μmol) of octadeuterated β-carotene has been carefully analyzed, albeit only in one male adult (43, 44). A model consisting of 11 compartments and a GI delay parameter has been devised on the basis of measurements of octadeuterated β-carotene and tetradeuterated retinol in the plasma at various times from 0 to 57 days, although measurements were made to 113 days. Compartments are 1 and 2, slow and fast pools of β-carotene in the liver; 3 and 4, slow and fast pools of retinol in the liver; 5, β-carotene in the enterocyte; 6, β-carotene in extrahepatic tissues; 7, β-carotene in plasma chylomicra; 8, retinyl ester in plasma chylomicra; 9, β-carotene in plasma lipoproteins other than chylomicra; 10, retinol bound to retinol-binding protein in plasma; and 11, β-carotene in the GI tract. By using several feasible assumptions, a set of fractional transfer coefficients (FTCs) were defined by use of SAAM 31 software (43, 44). The model predicts that 22% of the β-carotene dose was absorbed; that liver reserves of β-carotene and vitamin A were 7.5 and 324 μmol, respectively; and that 57% of the β-carotene conversion into vitamin A took place in the liver and 43% in the intestinal mucosa (43, 44). With average dietary intakes of β-carotene (7 μmol/day), however, the intestine may well play a larger role in the conversion process.

The mean sojourn time (MST), or residence time, is defined as the mean time that tracer molecules spend in the system from first entry to irreversible exit (10, 43, 44). The MST values of β-carotene and retinol (vitamin A) in the *body* were 51 days and 474 days, respectively, which agree well with estimates based on other data. Empirical MST values for β-carotene and retinol in *plasma* were much shorter; namely, 9 to 13 days and 26 days, respectively (43, 44). These differences between the MST values for plasma and the body may well reflect efficient recycling of retinol (see Chapter 17) and probably of carotenoids as well, in and out of tissue depots.

Plasma MST values for other carotenoids, based on empirical treatments, are similar to that of β-carotene: namely, dimethoxy-β-carotene, 6 days; ethyl β-apo-8′-carotenoate, 9 days; and canthaxanthin, 8 days (10, 24). Experimentally, MST values for carotenoids are not much affected by the dose given (10).

METABOLISM

Biosynthesis

Carotenoids are formed in microorganisms and plants but not in mammals. As polyisoprenoids, the initial rate-limiting step is conversion of β-hydroxy-β-methylglutaryl-CoA into mevalonic acid. Two C5 isoprene intermediates condense to form successively C10, C15, and C20 (geranylgeranyl-pyrophosphate) addition products. Two of the latter compounds condense in a tail-to-tail fashion to yield the first C40 carotenoid, 15,15′-*cis*-phytoene (Fig. 33.1) (45). The latter is successively dehydrogenated to give neurosporene, a C40, acyclic carotenoid with 12 double bonds. Depending on the bacterium or plant, neurosporene can be further dehydrogenated to lycopene, which either cyclizes to give β-carotene or α-carotene or is methoxylated and oxidized to give the ketocarotenoid, spheroidenone, an important accessory pigment in bacterial photosynthesis (45). Molecular oxygen is then introduced into hydrocarbon carotenoids to give mono- and dihydroxycarotenoids, the xanthophylls α- and β-cryptoxanthin, zeaxanthin, and lutein (Fig. 33.1) and, subsequently, a set of epoxy derivatives, such as antheroxanthin, violaxanthin (Fig. 33.1), and neoxanthin, an interesting allenic species commonly found in plants. Oxocarotenoids, such as canthaxanthin (Fig. 33.1), are formed from β-carotene by action of an oxygenase (45). A variety of other biologic transformations of these structures can also occur.

In addition to their roles as accessory pigments in photosynthesis, the epoxy xanthophylls play an important role in protecting plants from absorbing excessive amounts of energy from light. The intricacies of this so-called xanthophyll cycle in higher plants have been carefully reviewed (46).

Carotenoids are oxidized to a variety of compounds with fewer carbon atoms in plants and microorganisms, including β-apocarotenals, abscissic acid, trisporic acid, bixin, and crocetin (47, 48). Some of these breakdown products have important physiologic functions (47). Thus, nature can modify carotenoids in a variety of ways at almost every carbon atom in the molecule.

Vitamin A Formation

Physiologic Pathways

That β-carotene is converted biologically into vitamin A in mammals was first shown in 1930 (41). For many years, the pathways for its conversion were unclear, largely because the conversion rate is relatively slow, and cell-free preparations of tissues were inactive, β-carotene was rapidly oxidized chemically to various derivatives, and the resolving power and/or sensitivity of available methods was limited.

In 1960, John Glover (49) suggested that two pathways might exist for cleavage of carotenoids into vitamin A: *(a)* central cleavage to yield two molecules of retinal or *(b)* asymmetric cleavage to yield a shorter and a longer β-apocarotenal, the latter of which was sequentially shortened by removal of C2 and C3 fragments to yield retinal. The C2 and C3 fragments were subsequently presumed to be oxidized to CO_2 (49). While favoring asymmetric cleavage, Glover found, however, that the amounts of radioactive CO_2 produced by metabolism of ^{14}C-β-carotene and ^{14}C-retinol in the rat were the same, not at all in keeping with asymmetric cleavage as a major pathway. A few years later, ^{14}C-β-carotene was shown to yield labeled retinal as the sole detectable product (50, 51). Indeed, the stoichiometry of the reaction, the ratio of moles of retinal formed to moles of β-carotene consumed, was found to be 1.1 to 1.5. Any value greater than 1.0, of course, favors central cleavage. The enzyme, called carotenoid 15,15′-dioxygenase (EC 1.13.11.21), was found to require molecular oxygen. The issue thus seemed to be resolved; central cleavage was deemed to be the major, if not sole, pathway in mammals.

In 1979, Dmitrovskii reported the existence of an NADPH-dependent carotenoid dioxygenase in the nuclear membrane fraction of chick intestinal mucosa that preferentially cleaved β-carotene at the 11,12 double bond (52). This interesting observation, however, did not become widely known.

An interesting challenge to central cleavage appeared in 1988 (53); Hansen and Maret (53), although unable to repeat earlier studies (50, 51), showed that β-carotene could be converted to β-apocarotenals chemically in the presence of oxygen under normal incubation conditions. They repeated Glover's earlier arguments that asymmetric cleavage was a more logical reaction than central cleavage

(53). Their paper refocused attention on the mechanism of cleavage. In a careful reexamination of the cleavage reaction, Lakshman et al. (54) showed that retinal was the primary, if not sole, product of β-carotene cleavage catalyzed by a partially purified enzyme preparation of rabbit and rat intestinal cytosol.

The extent to which asymmetric cleavage occurred in mammals then became a key query. Wang and colleagues subsequently showed that whole intestinal homogenates converted β-carotene to a group of β-apocarotenals in the presence of oxygen (55, 56). Of particular interest in this regard was formation of a pair of β-apocarotenals that are counterparts in a 13′:14′ oxidative cleavage reaction (56). Inasmuch as retinal was a relatively minor product of the reaction in their studies, they concluded that sequential asymmetric cleavage was a major pathway for conversion of β-carotene to vitamin A. Possible pathways for conversion of all-*trans* β-carotene to retinal, retinol, and retinoic acid are summarized in Fig. 33.2.

The most appropriate way to resolve the relative importance of the two pathways clearly is an examination of the stoichiometry of the reaction. Central cleavage will yield 2 moles of retinal per mole of β-carotene consumed, whereas asymmetric cleavage will yield, via β-apocarotenals, a maximum of 1 mole of retinal. By using whole intestinal homogenates like those used by Wang et al. (55), Devery and Milborrow (57) reported a mean molar ratio of 1.72, and Nagao et al. (58) a molar ratio of 1.88 ± 0.08 (SD). After correcting for the efficiency of solvent extraction, the molar ratio was 2.07 ± 0.09 (SD) (58). β-Apocarotenals were detected, if at all, only in trace amounts in these latter studies (57, 58) as well as in others (59, 60). Furthermore, β-apo-8′-carotenal was converted to retinal very slowly, if at all, under the same incubation conditions in vitro (58). Thus far, no stoichiometric studies that favor asymmetric cleavage as the major pathway have been conducted. Thus, the total available information indicates that central cleavage is the predominant reaction in mammals.

Carotenoid Cleavage Enzymes

Although many of the enzymes involved in biosynthesis of carotenoids from mevalonic acid in plants and microorganisms have been characterized (45), much less attention has been given to mammalian enzymes that act on carotenoids. The only exception is carotenoid 15,15′-dioxygenase, which shows similar properties in various tissues and species (61, 62). It is localized in the cytosol, requires molecular oxygen, shows a K_M value for β-carotene of 1 to 10 μmol/L, has a slightly alkaline pH optimum (7.5–8.5), is inhibited by metal ion chelators and sulfhydryl-binding reagents, and is activated by glutathione (62). A possible mechanism for cleavage of all-*trans* β-carotene into molecules of retinal is presented in Figure 33.3. The activity of the intestinal mucosal enzyme

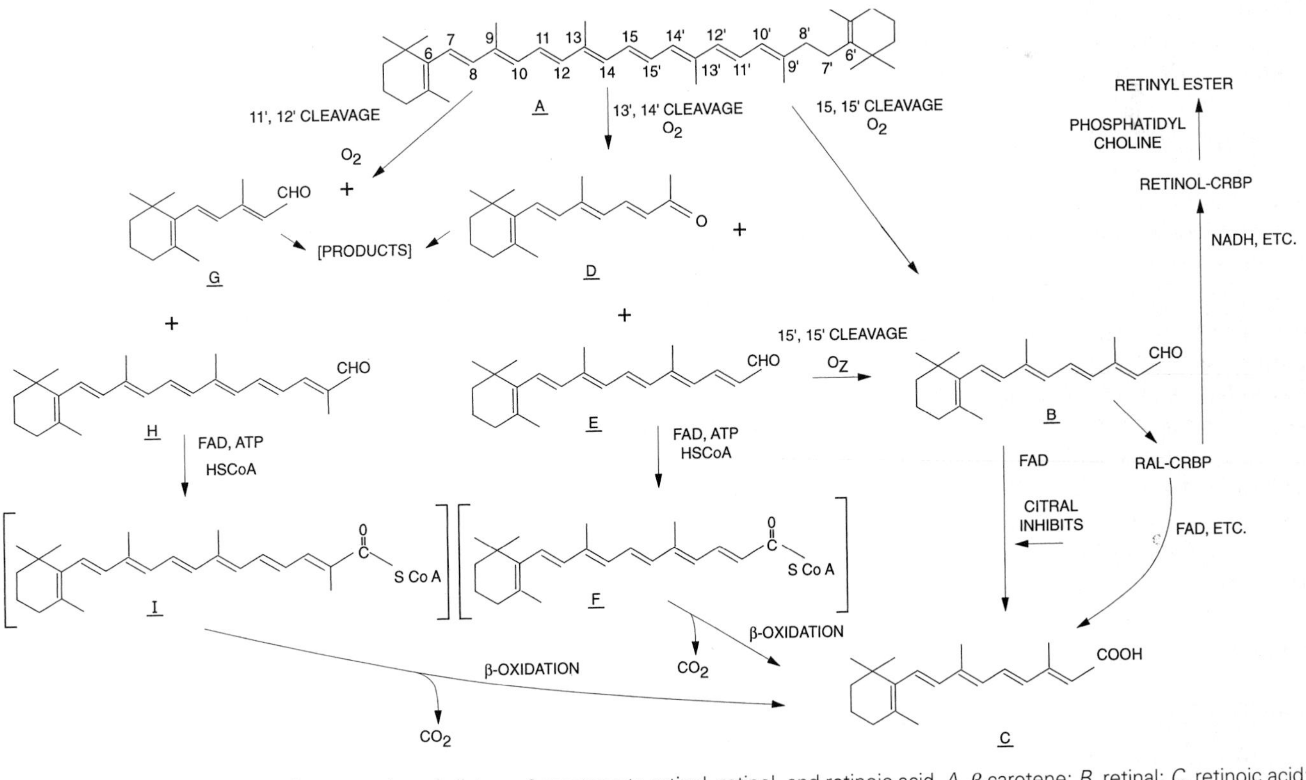

Figure 33.2. Possible pathways in conversion of all-*trans* β-carotene to retinal, retinol, and retinoic acid. *A*, β-carotene; *B*, retinal; *C*, retinoic acid; *D*, β-apo-13-carotenal; *E*, β-apo-14′-carotenal; *F*, β-apo-14′-carotenoyl-coenzyme A; *G*, β-apo-11-carotenal; *H*, β-apo-12′-carotenal; *I*, β-apo-12′-carotenoyl-coenzyme A; *CRBP*, cellular retinol-binding protein. All polyenes are in the *trans* configuration. Items in brackets have *not* been isolated or identified as essential components of the pathway. Cofactors other than NADH may be used in conversion of retinal to retinol and other than FAD in oxidation of retinal to retinoic acid.

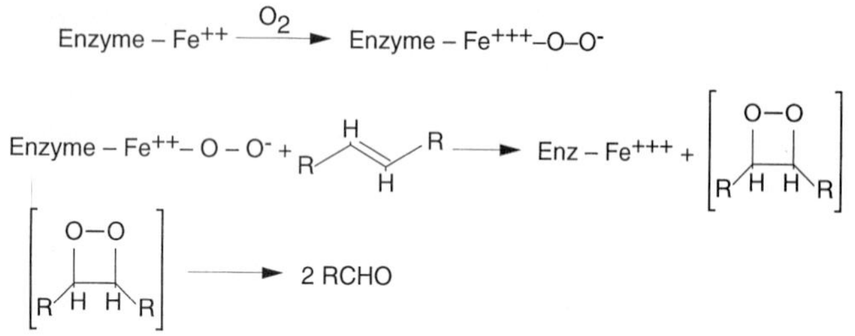

Enzyme – Fe^{++} $\xrightarrow{O_2}$ Enzyme – Fe^{+++}–O–O^-

Enzyme – Fe^{++}– O – O^- + RCH=CHR ⟶ Enz – Fe^{+++} + [dioxetane: O–O, R H H R]

[dioxetane: O–O, R H H R] ⟶ 2 RCHO

Figure 33.3. Postulated mechanism for cleavage of all-*trans* β-carotene into two molecules of all-*trans* retinal. Cleavage at other sites in carotenoids might proceed in a similar fashion. The highly unstable dioxetane (shown in parenthesis) would spontaneously break down to yield two molecules of retinal.

is enhanced in vitamin A deficiency (59, 63, 64) and by treatment with polyunsaturated fatty acids (PUFAs) (65), but is depressed by treatment with β-carotene (64). The activity of the liver enzyme, although seemingly less sensitive to vitamin A status (64), is increased by treatment with either β-carotene (64) or PUFAs (65).

An enzyme catalyzing excentric cleavage of carotenoids in mammalian tissues has been only partially characterized (52). NADPH-dependent carotene dioxygenase, which is present in the nuclear membrane fraction of chicken intestinal mucosa, acts both on xanthophylls and on β-carotene, preferentially cleaves carotenoids at the 11,12 double bond, requires NADPH or ascorbate, uses molecular oxygen, and is inhibited by iron chelators and sulfhydryl binding agents (52). Inasmuch as the stoichiometry of β-carotene cleavage to retinal and the appearance of β-apo-carotenals were not detectably affected by incubations with whole homogenates or cytosolic fractions of pig and guinea pig intestine (57, 58), however, the excentric cleavage enzyme seems to be much less active in these species than β-carotenoid-15,15′-dioxygenase.

An enzyme catalyzing an excentric cleavage reaction in *Cyanobacterium microcystis* has also been studied (66). β-Carotene 7,8;7′8′-dioxygenase cleaves β-carotene into two molecules of β-cyclocitral and crocetindial, presumably by acting first on one 7,8 double bond and then on the other. It requires molecular oxygen, is membrane bound, and is inhibited by metal ion chelators, sulfhydryl-binding reagents, and antioxidants (66). Iron is probably involved in the reaction, inasmuch as *o*-phenanthroline inhibits the enzyme. Zeaxanthin is also a substrate for this enzyme. Thus, not surprisingly, many properties of the three dioxygenases are similar, except for their preferential sites of cleavage, localization in the cell, and substrate specificities.

Other Pathways

Other pathways may exist for cleavage of β-carotene into retinoids. Lipoxygenases, which exist in animal cells, convert PUFAs to a *cis,trans*-peroxyacid in the presence of oxygen. β-Carotene can serve as an acceptor of the peroxide group, yielding a group of oxidized products and losing absorption at 450 nm (67). Neither retinal nor retinoic acid have been identified, however, as products of this reaction or of other peroxidative processes (68).

Formation of retinoic acid from β-carotene might proceed by central cleavage followed by conversion of the resultant retinal to retinoic acid by one of several aldehyde dehydrogenases (69). The diisoprenoid aldehyde citral inhibits formation of retinoic acid from retinal. Thus, citral should inhibit formation of retinoic acid from β-carotene if retinal is indeed a free intermediate in the reaction. Following earlier observations that retinoic acid might be produced directly from β-carotene (70), β-carotene, but not retinal, was found to be converted into retinoic acid in the presence of citral in whole intestinal homogenates (56) and was formed in portal blood derived from ferret intestine perfused with these substrates (71).

Several possible explanations might be given for these findings. One is that retinoic acid, probably initially as its coenzyme A derivative, is derived from β-apo-14′-carotenoyl-CoA by a β-oxidation pathway, presumably in the mitochondria (Fig. 33.2). Another is that retinal derived from β-carotene is immediately bound tightly to cellular retinol-binding protein type II (CRBP-II) (72). Oxidation of the retinal–CRBP-II complex to retinoic acid might possibly be much less affected by citral. A third is that retinal dehydrogenase and carotenoid dioxygenase form a tight complex in vivo, such that the cleavage and dehydrogenation reactions are concerted events on the interface between the two proteins that is not readily accessible to citral. These possibilities should be explored.

Metabolism of β-Apocarotenoids

β-Apocarotenals can be converted, albeit slowly in some cases (58), directly to retinal and to an uncharacterized short-chain aldehyde by the carotenoid 15,15′-dioxygenase (73). The rates of cleavage have been reported both to be higher (73) and to be considerably lower (58, 74) than that of all-*trans* β-carotene. β-Apo-8′-carotenal and presumably other analogues can be reduced to alcohols and then esterified in the human intestine as well as being oxidized to their corresponding acids (24). Several β-apocarotenoic acids can also be converted to retinoic acid in ferret liver mitochondria, presumably by β-oxidation (75). Ethyl β-apo-8′-carotenoate, however, was not detectably metabolized in humans (24), thus metabolically resembling etretinate, the ethyl ester of acitretin, which is stored in the body for long periods (76).

Metabolism of Other Carotenoids

Besides all-*trans* β-carotene, the carotenoid 15,15′-dioxygenase cleaves the all-*trans* isomers of 3,4,3′,4′-tetradehydro-β-carotene, 5,6-epoxy-β-carotene, 5,8-epoxy-β-carotene, α-carotene, 5,6-epoxy-α-carotene, 5,8-epoxy-α-carotene, and 3′,4′-dehydro-β-ψ-caroten-16′-al (62), but usually at rates considerably lower than that of all-*trans* β-carotene. The dioxygenase also cleaves 9-*cis*-β-carotene and possibly

13-*cis*-β-carotene, but again at lower rates than the all-*trans* isomer (21, 22). Carotenoids cleaved either at very low rates (<5% that of all-*trans* β-carotene) or not detectably include 5,6,5′,6′- and 5,8,5′,8′-diepoxy-β-carotene, 3′,4′-didehydro-β-cryptoxanthin, zeaxanthin, lutein, the 5,6 epoxides of several β-apocarotenals, and β-apocarotenoic acids (62). The dioxygenase has recently been reported to cleave β-cryptoxanthin, a fairly common dietary constituent and an active provitamin (77). The lack of activity of the dioxygenase toward β-apocarotenoic acids accords with the demonstrated β-oxidation of the latter to retinoic acid in mitochondria (75).

In humans, 4,4′-dimethoxy-β-carotene is converted to canthaxanthin (4,4′-diketo-β-carotene), to a monoketo-monohydroxylated product, and to a more polar, unidentified metabolite (24). α-Carotene is cleaved to retinal and α-retinal, presumably by carotenoid 15,15′-dioxygenase (77). Lycopene, although absorbed well from oily solutions and taken up by the liver and other organs, is metabolized by poorly understood pathways (78, 79). Radiolabeled lycopene is not converted to detectable products in rats and squirrel monkeys (78), although hydroxylated derivatives of lycopene have been detected in human plasma (79, 80). These derivatives or immediate precursors of them are also found in tomato products. Many isomers of lycopene are present in human plasma and tissues, of which the major ones are all-*trans* and 5-*cis* lycopene (79). Because a similar pattern of isomers is found in tomato products, however, the extent of isomerization of lycopene in vivo is not known.

Canthaxanthin, like lycopene, is not metabolized to detectable products in rats, squirrel monkeys, or humans (13, 78, 81). In chickens, however, a portion is reduced to the mono- and dihydroxy derivatives, which in turn are acylated (82).

Lutein may be oxidized in vivo in humans to its 3′-keto derivative, isomerized from the 6′*R* to the 6′*S* form, or converted to 3′-epilutein and zeaxanthin (80). Although the enzymatic reactions have not been clarified, such derivatives appear in human plasma after lutein supplementation.

Capsanthin, a major carotenoid in paprika, is a dihydroxymonoketo-carotenoid with one 5-carbon cyclic ring. When orally administered to men, capsanthin is well absorbed, is associated equally with HDL and LDL in plasma, and is cleared rapidly from the circulation (83). No metabolites were identified.

9′-*cis*-Bixin, a monomethylester of an acylic C25 dicarboxylic acid, and its congeners are found in seeds of the annatto plant. Extracts of these seeds are used as a common food coloring in Spain and Latin America. When ingested by human volunteers, 9-*cis*-bixin is well absorbed but rapidly cleared from the plasma (84). 9-*cis*-Bixin is both demethylated to the dicarboxylic acid norbixin and isomerized to all-*trans* bixin in vivo (84).

Little is known about the metabolism in mammals of other carotenoids, such as neoxanthin, violaxanthin, and astaxanthin. Although found in foods, these carotenoids have not been detected in human plasma (85).

CAROTENOIDS IN FOODS

Food composition tables traditionally expressed the carotenoid content of individual foods in IU/unit weight, in which 1 IU = 0.6 μg all-*trans* β-carotene or 1.2 μg of mixed other provitamin A carotenoids, or more recently in μg retinol equivalents, in which 6 μg all-*trans* β-carotene = 1 μg all-*trans* retinol (see Appendix Table I-A-1-b). Because 1 IU of retinol = 0.3 μg, the conventions for IU and for μg retinol equivalents clearly do not agree. The confusion caused by these two systems of units is only slowly being resolved. Factors and formulas used in interconverting units of vitamin A and carotenoids are summarized in Appendix I-A-1-b). In the last several years, analysis of individual carotenoids in foods has much improved (85, 86). The carotenoid patterns of some common foods are presented in Table 33.3 (86). In this analysis, the six major dietary carotenoids, with lutein and zeaxanthin pooled, were measured. The richest sources of carotenoids are the palm oils, which primarily contain β-carotene (4.7 mg/100 mL), α-carotene (3.7 mg/100 mL), and smaller amounts of other carotenoids. As already indicated, the bioavailability of carotenoids in vegetables, and to a lesser extent in fruits, is a key consideration in assessing the actual amount of carotenoids absorbed.

BIOLOGIC EFFECTS OF CAROTENOIDS

Carotenoids play many roles in nature. In mammals and in mammalian cells, they clearly serve as precursors of vitamin A. But can they, and do they, serve any other roles in mammals? In the past two decades, carotenoids have been implicated in a large number of biologic processes (87). In considering these effects, it is useful to categorize them as functions, actions, or associations.

Functions

A *function* is an essential role played by the nutrient in growth, development, and maturation. Because carotenoids are not needed by mammals with adequate preformed vitamin A in the diet, they cannot be considered essential. But, in the absence of adequate preformed vitamin A in the diet, they become essential or, more aptly, "conditionally essential," as in the case of certain amino acids. Because carotenoids are a major dietary source of vitamin A for much of humanity, however, their role as "conditionally essential" nutrients is highly important.

Actions

Actions are demonstrated effects in various biologic systems that may or may not have general physiologic significance.

Table 33.3
Carotenoid Composition of Typical Fruits and Vegetables (μg/100 g portion)

Item	β-Carotene	α-Carotene	Lutein/Zeaxanthin	Lycopene	Cryptoxanthin
Apricot, dried	17600	0	0	864	0
Beet greens	2560	3	7700	0	0
Broccoli, cooked	1300	1	1800	0	0
Cantaloupe	3000	35	0	0	0
Carrot, cooked	9800	3700	260	0	0
Corn, yellow	51	50	780	0	0
Greens, collard	5400	0	16300	0	0
Lettuce, leaf	1200	1	1800	0	0
Mango	1300	0	0	0	54
Orange	39	20	14	0	149
Papaya	99	0	0	0	470
Spinach, cooked	4100	0	10200	0	0
Tomato juice, canned	900	0	330	8580	0
Tomato, raw	520	0	100	3100	0

Adapted from Mangels AR, Holden JM, Beecher GR, et al. J Am Diet Assoc 1993;93:284–96.

Cell-to-Cell Communication

A good example of an action is enhancement of cell-to-cell communication in tissue culture (88, 89). Because both provitamin A (β-carotene) and nonprovitamin A (canthaxanthin) molecules show such effects, the action is not linked to formation of vitamin A. Whether 4-oxoretinal and 4-oxoretinoic acid (which also enhances cell-to-cell communication) play roles in this process as a result of cleavage of canthaxanthin is yet unclear (88, 89). Because retinoic acid is a more effective enhancer of cell-to-cell communication than the carotenoids, the physiologic significance of the carotenoid action in vivo is also unclear.

Cell Differentiation

5,6-Epoxy-β-carotene enhances differentiation of NB4 cells in vitro better than β-carotene does but less well than all-*trans* retinoic acid or 5,6-epoxyretinoic acid (90). Although the preferential action of an epoxycarotenoid relative to its parent hydrocarbon in mammalian cells is of interest, the physiologic significance is uncertain.

The Immune Response

Carotenoids, like retinoids, can also modulate the immune response in rats (91), mice (92), and lymphocytes in culture (93). In vivo, astaxanthin, canthaxanthin, lutein, and β-carotene stimulate the response (91, 92). In cultures of Th1 clones and primed spleen cells in vitro, astaxanthin, but not other carotenoids, stimulates antibody production and depresses production of interferon-γ (93). Under similar conditions with Th2 clones, only astaxanthin stimulates antibody production. In contrast, lycopene suppresses antibody production in Th2 clones incubated together with unprimed spleen cells (92). The key points are that *(a)* xanthophylls are more active enhancers than β-carotene, *(b)* various carotenoids differ in their activities in different immune systems, and *(c)* a primary site of action in humoral immune responses, as in the case of the retinoids, seems to be the T-helper cell. Again, the physiologic significance of these observations is not clear. Indeed, in female subjects fed a β-carotene-free diet for 68 days and then supplemented with β-carotene, mitogen-induced proliferation of blood lymphocytes was unaffected (33). In a similarly treated group of female subjects, however, mixed carotenoids did elicit a response (94). Furthermore, in healthy male nonsmokers, β-carotene supplementation (15 mg/day) significantly increased the percentage of blood monocytes expressing the major histocompatibility complex class II molecule HLA-DR, intercellular adhesion molecule–1, and leukocyte function-associated antigen–3, as well as secretion of tumor necrosis factor–α (95). These actions merit further attention.

Reproduction

Carotenoids might affect reproductive performance in animals and humans in two ways: *(a)* by being converted into vitamin A, which is essential for a successful outcome of pregnancy, and *(b)* by modulating per se one or several of the complex events associated with the reproductive process (96).

In dairy cattle, oral β-carotene supplements (100 mg/day) were reported in 1976 to offset various abnormalities found in unsupplemented cows, namely, delayed ovulation, increased incidence of ovarian cysts, lower progesterone production, reduced growth rate of corpora lutea, increased embryonic mortality, and increased diarrhea in calves (97). In subsequent studies conducted elsewhere, however, these positive effects of supplementation could not be confirmed (98–100). Indeed, large β-carotene supplements (500 mg/day) actually reduced the insemination rate (98).

Female pigs (gilts), when injected with, but not when fed, β-carotene (228 mg/week) during the breeding period, showed lower embryonic mortality, larger litter size, and heavier litter weight than unsupplemented gilts (96). Injection of an equivalent amount of vitamin A, however, showed similar benefits (101). Oral supplements of β-carotene also did not improve reproductive performance of vitamin A–sufficient female rabbits (102). In a more mechanistic sense, β-carotene was reported to induce progesterone formation by luteal cells in vitro better than vitamin A (96) and to enhance vitamin A formation from β-carotene locally in bovine follicular cells (103).

Of women who ingested an essentially carotenoid-free diet (10–66 μg RE/day) for 42 to 120 days, 63% showed delayed ovulation or anovulatory cycles, altered luteal phase length, and prolonged menstrual periods, whereas only 5% who ingested a carotenoid-containing diet showed such abnormalities (104, 105). Supplementation with a small amount of β-carotene (83 μg RE/day), however, did *not* correct these abnormalities (105). Possible dietary factors that may prevent these abnormalities include other carotenoids, phytoestrogens, and yet other components of the foods that were eliminated in the "carotenoid-free" diet. Alternatively, higher supplements of β-carotene might be required. These studies, presented thus far only in abstract form, should soon be published in full.

The upshot of these studies, both in animals and in women, is that carotenoids may modulate some facets of the reproductive process but clearly are not required nutrients. In some of the studies, the initial vitamin A status may have been impaired, in which case the most feasible explanation is that β-carotene is serving as a provitamin. In other cases, positive, albeit elusive, effects have been noted in animals and subjects who clearly were vitamin A sufficient. Thus, the situation is not yet fully resolved.

Other Effects

In various biologic systems, carotenoids inhibit a variety of processes: photoinduced neoplasm, mutagenesis, cell transformation, sister-chromatid exchange, and micronuclei formation induced in buccal epithelia by several stresses (87). These interesting observations also fall in the category of actions that may or may not have physiologic importance in well-nourished individuals.

Associations

The third category is *associations*. Such potential interactions are largely derived from epidemiologic studies of the relationships between specific dietary components and chronic diseases. Carotenoids as a whole, as well as specific compounds of the class, have been implicated in many such relationships. Many other dietary constituents, such as α-tocopherol, ascorbic acid, selenium, flavonoids, phenolic acids, polyphenols, and other phytochemicals have been similarly implicated. The key point is that these associations do not imply causal relationships but rather serve primarily as markers of a dietary pattern, lifestyle, or genetic makeup that is conducive to good health. They may, of course, contribute specifically to protective processes, but the association does not "prove" that they do.

The design and conduct of rigorous epidemiologic studies are difficult and complex, and their interpretation is subject to a variety of confounding factors (106). When the agreement among various similar studies is poor, the thrust of a given relationship clearly is weakened. Nonetheless, epidemiologic studies provide an analysis of important relationships in health and disease that cannot be obtained by other approaches. Their findings, particularly when agreement is good among various studies, serve as a first step in clarifying causal relationships.

Carotenoids, α-tocopherol, vitamin C, glutathione, and selenium are often termed *antioxidant nutrients*. Clearly, all of these compounds, as well as many others, can serve this chemical function. Antioxidants, by their very nature, prevent oxidation of important cellular structures, usually by being preferentially oxidized, i.e., by providing one or two electrons to some active cellular oxidant. Under different circumstances, such compounds can also accept electrons from a donor and thereby become prooxidants. Whether they serve as antioxidants or prooxidants in a given reaction depends both on their initial redox state and the chemical nature of the other interacting molecule. Thus, an emphasis solely on the ability of these molecules to serve as antioxidants is constraining. Furthermore, carotenoids, as well as these other compounds, may well act in ways that do not involve oxidation/reduction. The actions of carotenoids, for example, in cell-to-cell communication (88, 89) and in the immune response (91–93) apparently do not involve redox reactions. Furthermore, the interactions of carotenoids with membranes, which can influence membrane structure and potentially membrane function, do not inherently involve redox reactions (2). Thus, carotenoids, as well as many of these other so-called antioxidants, might better be called "nutritional modulators" (107). This terminology does not imply a mechanism of action, and the actions themselves, which might be either beneficial or adverse, are not presumed from the outset to be favorable.

RELATIONSHIP OF CAROTENOIDS TO CHRONIC DISEASES

Cancer

Lung Cancer

One of the most dramatic and consistent observations in epidemiologic studies is the inverse association between β-carotene intake and the incidence of lung cancer (108, 109). These findings have stimulated intervention trials in two high-risk groups, asbestos workers in Tyler, Texas (n = 755), and middle-aged male smokers (n = 29,133, 50–69 years old) in Finland. The results of these intervention trials were unexpected. In asbestos workers, no difference in the prevalence of sputum atypia was noted between treated (50 mg β-carotene + 25,000 IU retinol every other day) and control groups over a 5-year period. In the Finnish study (110), the group (n = 14,564) treated daily with β-carotene (20 mg) for 5 to 8 years, with or without α-tocopherol, showed a significantly higher incidence of lung cancer (relative risk (RR) = 1.18; 95% confidence interval (CI) = 1.03–1.36) and of total mortality (RR = 1.08; 95% CI = 1.01–1.16) than the placebo group (n = 7287 men). Supplemental β-carotene did not affect the incidence of other major cancers found in this population (109, 110).

The findings of the Finnish study have been confirmed in a similar large study (n = 18,314), the Carotene and Retinol Efficacy Trial (CARET), conducted in the northwestern United States (111). In this case, supplements of β-carotene (30 mg/day) and retinyl ester (25,000 IU/day) were given to smokers and asbestos workers. The trial was terminated after 4 years because lung cancer incidence was increased by 28% (RR = 1.28; 95% CI = 1.04–1.57; P = .02), and total mortality was 17% higher (RR = 1.17; CI = 1.03–1.33) in the supplemented group than in the placebo group (n = 8894) (111).

In another large study (n = 22,071 male physicians, 40–84 years old), the so-called Physicians' Health Study, β-carotene capsules (50 mg every other day) were ingested by physicians, of whom only 11% were current smokers, for 12 years (112). No differences in total cancer deaths or in deaths from specific types of cancer between supplemented (n = 11,036) and nonsupplemented (n = 11,035) groups were noted (RR = 0.98; 95% CI = 0.91–1.06) (112).

The unexpected enhancement of lung cancer in the Finnish and CARET studies has several possible explanations: *(a)* Supplemental β-carotene might be interfering with intestinal absorption of other possible chemopreventive nutrients. For example, β-carotene inhibits absorption in humans of lutein and canthaxanthin, which show good antioxidant activity (13, 14). In that same vein, α-carotene, which shows chemopreventive properties, might be similarly affected. The effects of β-carotene supplementation on serum concentrations of other carotenoids, however, were relatively minor, except for an increase in α-carotene, a contaminant in the β-carotene preparation (113, 114). *(b)* Supplemental β-carotene may be serving as a prooxidant in the well-oxygenated ambient of the lung (115). *(c)* Populations of middle-aged male smokers and asbestos workers are not representative of other groups, who might well benefit from a higher intake of carotenoids. *(d)* Vitamin C, which is low in the plasma of most Finns, may have played some role in the outcome of the Finnish study but not the CARET study. *(e)* Alcohol intake clearly plays an important role in the outcome. Indeed, in the Finnish study, the lung cancer incidence in abstemious smokers was not enhanced by β-carotene supplementation (RR = 1.03; 95% CI = 0.85–1.24), whereas the incidence in those who drank clearly was (RR = 1.35; 95% CI = 1.01–1.81) (116).

In a matched case-control study of nonsmoking men and women (n = 413 matched pairs, 31–81 years old), increased consumption of green vegetables and fruits was most closely associated with a reduced risk of lung cancer (RR = 0.61; 95% CI = 0.43–0.85; P for trend < .01) (117). Use of supplements of vitamin E was also associated with reduced risk (RR = 0.55; 95% CI = 0.35–0.85) (117). Males and females showed similar responses (117). A thoughtful analysis of the relationship between nutrition and lung cancer has recently appeared (118). The authors conclude that increased fruit and vegetable intake is strongly associated with a reduced risk of lung cancer in both men and women, but that the totality of epidemiologic evidence is not persuasive for specific effects of any single micronutrient (118).

Head and Neck Cancers

Development of head and neck cancers, including those of the oral cavity, pharynx, and larynx, is influenced by many factors including smoking, other uses of tobacco, alcohol, and diet (109, 119). Serum carotene concentrations, adjusted for smoking, are inversely related to the incidence of these carcinomas. Supplements of β-carotene can markedly reduce leukoplakia, although the lesion returns upon cessation of treatment (109). Several chemoprevention trials designed to assess the effect of daily supplements of β-carotene (50 mg), with or without vitamin E, on the recurrence of head and neck cancer are currently under way (109).

Esophageal and Stomach Cancers

The effects of various nutrient combinations on esophageal cancer and stomach cancer were evaluated in a large population (n = 30,000, 40–69 years old, both genders) living in Linxian, China, where the incidence of esophageal cancer is 100 times that in the United States (109). Of four nutrient treatments administered for 5 years, only one (involving supplements of β-carotene, selenium, and α-tocopherol) showed a positive effect; the reductions in total deaths, cancer deaths, esophageal cancer deaths, and gastric cancer deaths were 9% (RR = 0.91; 95% CI = 0.84–0.99), 13% (RR = 0.87; 95% CI = 0.75–1.00), 4% (RR = 0.96; 95% CI = 0.78–1.18), and 21% (RR = 0.79; 95% CI = 0.64–0.99), respectively (109). Although these results support the concept that diet influences cancer incidence, the general nutritional status of the population was poor. Thus, whether the mixed supplement or one component of it was protective as a result of generally improved health or of a more specific anticancer effect is not clear (109).

Colorectal Cancer

Dietary intake and serum concentrations of carotenoids are often inversely associated with colorectal cancer risk (109, 120). By using adenomas as an indicator in a 4-year clinical trial, however, supplemental β-carotene (25 mg/day) was found ineffective in the treated group (n = 184, 61 ± 8 years old, both genders) (RR = 1.01; 95%

CI = 0.85–1.20) relative to a similar placebo group in preventing recurrence of this lesion (109, 120).

Breast Cancer

β-Carotene intake has been associated with an improved survival rate in breast cancer patients (109). Whether supplements of carotenoids reduce the incidence of breast cancer in a well-designed clinical trial is not known. An ongoing trial is exploring the effect of hydroxyphenylretinamide on the recurrence of breast cancer (121, 122).

Cervical Cancer

The risk of cervical cancer has been correlated with prediagnostic serum levels of α-, β-, and total carotenoids (RR = 2.7–3.1; 95% CI = 1.1–8.1) (109). On the other hand, invasive cervical cancer among white women in the United States was not related to any specific dietary food group nor to use of supplements of vitamins A, C, and E or folic acid (123). However, cervical dysplasia, considered to be a precancerous lesion, did respond to β-carotene supplements (30 mg/day) (109).

Prostate Cancer

Lycopene is primarily found in tomato products (Table 33.3) and is also present in watermelon, guava, and to a lesser degree in pink grapefruit (79). Thus, the association of ingestion of tomato-based products with a reduced risk of a given disease raises the possibility that lycopene itself is protective. Just such an epidemiologic relationship exists with prostate cancer (124). While intake of other carotenoids was not associated with reduced risk, dietary lycopene was (RR = 0.79; 95% CI = 0.64–0.99; *P* for trend = 0.04). However, no correlation was found with tomato juice ingestion, possibly because of poor bioavailability (79). Lycopene inhibits cell proliferation in several cancer cell lines in vitro and tumor growth in mice in vivo (79). Furthermore, lycopene scavenges radicals and quenches singlet oxygen somewhat better than β-carotene does (79). Thus, a possible mechanism exists for its protective action. In malignant and nonmalignant prostate tissue, lycopene and β-carotene were the major carotenoids found, with most of the lycopene present as a large number of *cis* isomers (38). Despite these interesting relationships, the risk of prostate cancer, in a broader context, has been primarily associated with genetic makeup, androgenic hormones, and fat intake (125). Indeed, the association of prostate cancer with intake of fruits, vegetables, and their individual components is much less convincing (125). Nonetheless, current studies of this relationship will be followed with interest.

Skin Cancer

Recurrence of skin cancer in a group (n = 913, <85 years old, both genders) treated with a β-carotene supplement (50 mg/day) over a 5-year period was not affected (RR = 1.05; 95% CI = 0.91–1.22) (109, 126) relative to a similarly structured placebo group (n = 892).

Summation

Thus, a dichotomy exists. Most associations found between diseases and dietary or plasma levels do not agree with the results of intervention trials. The former tend to show strong significant correlations and the latter largely do not. Possible explanations are: *(a)* β-Carotene, which is only one of approximately 600 known carotenoids, might not be the most active one, or indeed, might inhibit the absorption of other more chemopreventive carotenoids and other nutrients. *(b)* Carotenoids might be only one of a group of chemopreventive agents in foods that act synergistically in preventing carcinogenesis. The fact that the relative risk (RR) values for colored fruits and vegetables usually are lower (i.e., are more protective) than those for carotenoids or for any other component of the food supports this viewpoint. *(c)* Carotenoid levels may serve solely as a useful *marker* for a healthful lifestyle or a protective genetic makeup. *(d)* The preventive action of carotenoids might occur very early in disease progression but be ineffective later. Thus, subjects in identified high-risk groups, who often have had a primary tumor, may be resistant to nutritional supplements. *(e)* The associations found in observational epidemiology are not causal and can be confounded by a variety of unanticipated and unmeasured factors (106). In essence, the intervention trials may well be providing more-valid answers (109).

Photosensitivity Disorders

Patients with erythropoietic porphyria and similar diseases benefit by ingesting supplements (180 mg/day) of β-carotene (109, 127). Canthaxanthin, although also protective, is no longer used because of the reversible retinopathy that results (128). Although concentrations of β-carotene and vitamin A are elevated in the livers of these patients, the side effects of β-carotene ingestion over a period of years are minimal (109, 127).

Cardiovascular Disease

Carotenoid intake has often been associated with a reduced risk of both coronary events and stroke (108, 109). In an extensive study in Europe (WHO/MONICA), mortality from ischemic heart disease correlated inversely with serum vitamin E concentrations (r^2 = 0.63) but not with β-carotene levels (r^2 = 0.04) (129). If the 3 Finnish sites (which were outliers) of the 16 examined were excluded, however, the inverse correlation with β-carotene concentrations markedly improved (r^2 = 0.50). A mean serum β-carotene concentration in populations of 0.4 μmol/L or higher was associated with good health in the European studies, whereas a concentration below 0.25 μmol/L in populations was related to an increased risk of coronary disease, stroke, and cancer (129). The risk of myocardial infarction was inversely related to adipose β-carotene content in smokers (RR = 2.62; 95% CI = 1.79–3.83) but not in nonsmokers (RR = 1.07) (109).

In a preliminary report from the Physicians' Health Study, subjects with stable angina or prior coronary revascularizations, who were supplemented with β-carotene for 5 years, showed a 51% reduction in the risk of major coronary events (130). β-Carotene supplements did not show any beneficial effects on the risk of cardiovascular disease (RR = 1.0; 95% CI = 0.80–1.43), however, in the total population enrolled in this study (112). In contrast, the incidence of cardiovascular deaths, including angina pectoris, in the Finnish lung cancer study was increased 11% by β-carotene supplementation (109, 110), 16% in a smaller (n = 1720) trial focused on skin cancer (RR = 1.16; 95% CI = 0.82–1.64) (131), and 26% (RR = 1.26; 95% CI 0.99–1.61) in the CARET study (111). These findings cannot be readily explained by any known physiologic mechanism. Inasmuch as the 95% confidence intervals all included 1.0, the observations may well be attributed to chance. On the other hand, in a group of men (n = 1862, 50–69 years old) who had a previous myocardial infarction in the Finnish study, the β-carotene group (n = 461) had 75% more deaths from coronary heart disease during a 5.3-year period (RR 1.75; 95% CI = 1.16–2.64, P = .007) than the placebo group (n = 438) (132).

The overall results, therefore, are somewhat mixed. The most likely mechanism of protective action of carotenoids (but by no means the only one) is reduced oxidation of LDLs, which seem to play a key role in atherogenesis (108). Of various antixoidants studied both in vivo and in vitro, however, β-carotene does not seem protective (133). On an opposite tack, β-carotene can serve as a prooxidant under appropriate conditions (115). Thus, as indicated in a recent review, the relationship among dietary intakes of carotenoids, their plasma and tissue concentrations, and cardiovascular disease remains unclear (134).

Age-Related Macular Degeneration (ARMD)

The macula of the eye predominantly contains two pigments, lutein and zeaxanthin (42, 135). In the eye, these carotenoids are associated with tubulin (136). Because these two pigments account for less than 25% of plasma carotenoids, their uptake from plasma and deposition in the macula show specificity. These pigments might consequently play a role in protecting the macula from damage caused by blue light. In a recent study comparing patients suffering from ARMD with matched controls, subjects in the highest quintile of carotenoid intake had a 43% lower risk (RR = 0.57; 95% CI = 0.35–0.92) of suffering from ARMD than those in the lowest quintile (109, 137). Of various carotenoid-containing foods, intake of spinach and collard greens, rich in lutein and zeaxanthin, was most strongly associated with reduced risk. Several other studies, however, do not support the association between ARMD and intake or serum levels of lutein and zeaxanthin (138).

ARMD, like most chronic diseases in the elderly, is a spectrum of related conditions with similar clinical symptoms. Thus, a variety of nutrients, such as zinc and several antioxidants, as well as other factors, such as smoking and exposure to sunlight, have been associated with the condition (139, 140). Nonetheless, current studies on the possible protective role of supplements of lutein and zeaxanthin will be followed with interest.

Cataracts

Cataract consists of gradual opacification of the lens with aging, which may in part result from oxidative stress. Carotenoid intake, as well as that of vitamins C and E, has been associated with a reduced risk of cataract (109, 139). In the Linxian, China, trial, however, combined supplements of β-carotene, selenium, and α-tocopherol were not associated with a reduced incidence of cataracts, and inconclusive results have been reported by others (109, 139). Thus, whereas the concept that antioxidant and light-absorbing nutrients such as the carotenoids might prevent oxidative damage to a fairly exposed structure such as the lens is highly feasible, the data supporting a protective role of dietary components in the process are mixed.

HIV Infection

In HIV infection, T-helper (CD4) cells are destroyed, thereby impairing the immune response. In humans as well as in experimental animals, both β-carotene (a provitamin A carotenoid) and canthaxanthin (which is not) enhance the immune response (141). Indeed, in HIV-infected patients, large doses of β-carotene increased the CD4:CD8 ratio, which is usually depressed in HIV infection, as well as improving the response to vaccines (141). Ultraviolet light tends both to activate human HIV expression, at least in transgenic mice, and to reduce plasma carotenoid concentrations in humans. In phase II HIV-infected subjects, plasma carotenoid concentrations are reduced by 50%. AIDS patients treated daily with a combination of β-carotene supplementation (120 mg) and whole-body hyperthermia (42°C, 1 h) showed a better and longer-lasting response than those treated either with β-carotene or with hyperthermia (142). Thus, carotenoids seem to ameliorate the condition of AIDS patients, probably at least in part by enhancing the immune response.

Another quite different effect of a carotenoid has also been reported, namely, that halocynthiaxanthin (5,6-epoxy-3,3′-dihydroxy- 7′,8′-didehydro-5,6,7,8-tetrahydro-β,β-carotene-8-one) strongly and rather specifically inhibits RNA-dependent polymerase of the HIV virus (141). The use of carotenoids in the treatment of patients with HIV infections clearly merits further attention.

TOXICITY

Orally ingested hydrocarbon carotenoids, such as β-carotene, show no detectable toxicity, even at very large doses (143). The reasons for their lack of toxicity are that *(a)* carotenoids, because of their rigid polyene structure, are not very well absorbed from the intestine; *(b)* the absorption efficiency of carotenoids decreases markedly with increasing intake; and *(c)* the rate of conversion of provitamin A carotenoids to vitamin A, while fully adequate to meet nutritional needs, is relatively slow in an enzymatic sense. Thus, hypervitaminosis A does not result from ingestion of large doses of β-carotene. The only adverse effect is the benign condition hypercarotenosis, in which the plasma contains high carotenoid concentrations, and parts of the skin assume a yellowish hue. This condition is distinguished from jaundice in that the whites of the eyes remain untinted. After the intake of large doses of carotenoids is terminated, hypercarotenosis slowly disappears.

The xanthophylls may be less benign. For example, when given in large doses for long periods as therapy for photosensitivity disorders, the diketocarotenoid canthaxanthin precipitates in a crystalline array in the retina (128). This canthaxanthin retinopathy, however, slowly resolves after the cessation of dosing (128). The effects of very high doses of other xanthophylls have not yet been carefully explored.

SUMMARY

Carotenoids are interesting molecules, both chemically and biologically. Nature uses them in a variety of functional roles in many organisms, from microbes to humans. Nutritionally, in humans and other vertebrates, approximately 50 of them are converted into vitamin A in the intestinal mucosa, liver, and other organs. The major pathway of conversion is central cleavage of the provitamin A carotenoid, although excentric cleavage also contributes to formation of vitamin A and particularly of retinoic acid. Because more than 600 carotenoids exist in nature, the question arises whether the 550 nonprovitamin A carotenoids have any effect on biologic processes in humans. Under various circumstances, not only β-carotene but also several non–provitamin A carotenoids show many biologic actions, including effects on cell-to-cell communication and the immune response. The extent to which these actions have significant impact on the health of well-nourished persons, however, is still unclear.

On the basis of epidemiologic studies of diet and chronic diseases, carotenoids, as well as many other phytochemicals and some minerals, have been implicated as protective agents. However, intervention trials with supplements of β-carotene have not shown beneficial effects. Indeed, in some instances, β-carotene supplementation yielded adverse outcomes. The current relationship of carotenoids with health and disease has recently been thoughtfully analyzed (144). In an epidemiologic sense, attention has now been focused on other carotenoids, such as α-carotene, lycopene, lutein, and zeaxanthin. Whether these carotenoids will be more effective than β-carotene in supplementation trials is uncertain. Indeed, the protective effect of diets rich in fruits and vegetables seems to exceed that of any single micronutrient (118).

In the evolution of life, nature must certainly have included both redundancy and flexibility as key factors in the competition for survival. Thus, panaceas in the form of single nutrients are not an attractive option. In a similar vein, amulets and magical potions were used in the distant past to ward off evil. The role of genetic makeup in susceptibility to disease is now being actively explored. In specific cases, therefore, we may find that a genetic subgroup of a given disease does respond to dietary intervention with a single nutrient, probably as a result of a specific metabolic defect.

Carotenoids, as found in foods, are nontoxic to humans. Even large oral supplements of β-carotene cause no harm, although canthaxanthin, when given in large oral doses for a long time, causes a reversible retinopathy. In general, however, toxicity is not worrisome with carotenoids.

The biologic roles and actions of carotenoids and their metabolites remain a fascinating field of study. New facets of their activities are constantly being revealed. Probing nature's well-kept secrets is always rewarding and diverting, and there is still much to be learned about this interesting class of compounds.

ACKNOWLEDGMENTS

The author is indebted to Professor John Dietschy for a valuable exposition of the formation of high-density lipoproteins in vivo and to Dr. Anne Sowell for providing unpublished NHANES-III data, CDC, 1996. The writing of this review, as well as some of the studies on which it is based, was supported by USDA-CDFIN 96-34115-2835. This is Journal Paper no. J-17602 of the Iowa Agriculture and Home Economics Experiment Station, Ames, IA; Project no. 3335, and supported by Hatch Act and State of Iowa funds.

REFERENCES

1. Olson JA, Krinsky NI. FASEB J 1995;9:1547–50.
2. Britton G. FASEB J 1995;9:1551–8.
3. Krinsky NI. Pure Appl Chem 1994;66:1003–10.
4. Liebler DC, McClure TD. Chem Res Toxicol 1996;9:8–11.
5. Furr HC, Barua AB, Olson JA. Retinoids and carotenoids. In: Nelis HJ, Lambert WE, DeLeenheer AP, eds. Modern chromatographic analysis of the vitamins. 2nd ed. New York: Marcel Dekker, 1992;1–71.
6. Sander LC, Sharpless KE, Craft NE, Wise SA. Anal Chem 1994;66:1667–74.
7. Dueker SR, Jones AD, Clifford AJ. Anal Chem 1994;66:4177–85.
8. Erdman JW Jr, Bierer TL, Gugger ET. Ann NY Acad Sci 1993;691:76–85.

9. Parker RS. FASEB J 1996;10:542–51.
10. Furr HC, Clark RM. J Nutr Biochem 1997;8:364–77.
11. El-Gorab MI, Underwood BA, Loerch JD. Biochim Biophys Acta 1975;401:265–77.
12. Borel P, Grolier P, Armand M, et al. Lipid Res 1996;37:250–61.
13. White WS, Stacewicz-Sapuntzakis M, Erdman JW Jr, Bowen PE. J Am Coll Nutr 1994;13:665–71.
14. Kostic D, White WS, Olson JA. Am J Clin Nutr 1995;62: 604–10.
15. Sauberlich HE, Hodges RE, Wallace DL, et al. Vitam Horm (USA) 1974;32:251–75.
16. de Pee S, West CE, Muhilal, et al. Lancet 1995;346:75–81.
17. de Pee S, West CE. Eur J Clin Nutr 1996;50(Suppl 3):S38–53.
18. FAO/WHO. Requirements of vitamin A, thiamine, riboflavine, and niacin. FAO Nutr Rep Ser no. 41, WHO Tech Rep Ser no. 360. Geneva: WHO Press 1967;1–86.
19. Morinobu T, Tamai H, Murata T, et al. J Nutr Sci Vitaminol (Tokyo) 1994;40:421–30.
20. Stahl W, Schwarz W, von Laar J, Sies H. J Nutr 1995;125: 2128–33.
21. Nagao A, Olson JA. FASEB J 1994;8:968–73.
22. Wang XD, Krinsky NI, Benotti PN, Russell RM. Arch Biochem Biophys 1994;313:150–5.
23. Stahl W, Sies H. J Nutr 1992;122:2161–6.
24. Zeng S, Furr HC, Olson JA. Am J Clin Nutr 1992;56:433–9.
25. Rao MN, Ghosh P, Lakshman MR. J Biol Chem 1997;272: 24450–60.
26. Romanchik JE, Morel DW, Harrison EH. J Nutr 1995; 125:2610–7.
27. Barua AB, Kostic D, Olson JA. J Chromatog 1993;617:257–64.
28. Khachik F, Beecher GR, Goli MB, et al. Anal Chem 1992;64: 2111–22.
29. Briefel R, Sowell A, Huff D, et al. FASEB J 1996;10:A813.
30. Peng Y-M, Peng Y-S, Lin Y, et al. Nutr Cancer 1995;23:233–46.
31. Rock CL, Swendseid ME, Jacob RA, McKee RW. J Nutr 1992;122:96–100.
32. Berzy D, Bowen PE, Stacewicz-Sapuntzakis M, et al. FASEB J 1997;11:A391.
33. Daudu PA, Kelley DS, Taylor PC, et al. Am J Clin Nutr 1994;60:969–72.
34. Kaplan LA, Lau JM, Stein EA. Clin Physiol Biochem 1990; 8:1–10.
35. Blankenhorn DH. J Biol Chem 1957;229:809–16.
36. Stahl W, Schwartz W, Sundquist AR, et al. Arch Biochem Biophys 1992;294:173–7.
37. Schmitz HH, Poor CL, Wellman RB, Erdman JW. J Nutr 1991;121:1613–21.
38. Clinton SK, Emenhiser C, Schwartz SJ, et al. Cancer Epidemiol Biomarkers Prev 1996;5:823–33.
39. Long C, ed. Handbook of biochemistry. Cleveland: CRC Press, 1961;639.
40. Shi HL, Furr HC, Olson JA. Brain Res Bull 1991;26:235–9.
41. Moore T. Vitamin A. Amsterdam: Elsevier 1957;1–645.
42. Handelman GJ, Dratz EA, Reay CC, et al. Invest Ophthalmol Vis Sci 1988;29:850–5.
43. Novotny JA, Dueker SR, Zech LA, Clifford AJ. J Lipid Res 1995;36:1825–38.
44. Novotny JA, Zech LA, Furr HC, et al. Adv Food Nutr Res 1996;40:25–54.
45. Armstrong GA, Hearst JE. FASEB J 1996;10:228–37.
46. Demmig-Adams B, Gilmore AM, Adams WW III. FASEB J 1996;10:403–12.
47. Olson JA. Ann NY Acad Sci 1993;691:156–66.
48. Pfander H, ed. Key to carotenoids. 2nd ed. Basel: Birkhäuser 1987;1–296.
49. Glover J. Vitam Horm (USA) 1960;18:371–86.
50. Goodman DS, Huang HS. Science 1965;149:879–80.
51. Olson JA, Hayaishi O. Proc Natl Acad Sci USA 1965;54: 1364–70.
52. Dmitrovskii A. Metabolism of natural retinoids and their functions. In: Ozawa T, ed. New trends in biological chemistry. Tokyo: Japan Scientific Societies Press 1991;297–308.
53. Hansen S, Maret W. Biochemistry 1988;27:200–6.
54. Lakshman MR, Mychkovsky I, Attlesey M. Proc Natl Acad Sci USA 1989;86:9124–8.
55. Wang X-D, Tang G-W, Fox JG, et al. Arch Biochem Biophys 1991;285:8–16.
56. Krinsky NI. Ann NY Acad Sci 1993;691:167–76.
57. Devery J, Milborrow BV. Br J Nutr 1994;72:397–414.
58. Nagao A, During A, Hoshino C, et al. Arch Biochem Biophys 1996;328:57–63.
59. van Vliet T, van Vlissingen MF, van Schaik F, et al. J Nutr 1996;126:499–508.
60. Duszka C, Grolier P, Azim E-M, et al. J Nutr 1996;126:2550–6.
61. During A, Nagao A, Hoshino C, et al. Anal Biochem 1996; 241:199–205.
62. Olson JA. Formation and function of vitamin A. In: Porter JW, Spurgeon SL, eds. Biosynthesis of isoprenoid compounds, vol 2. New York: John Wiley & Sons, 1983;371–412.
63. Villard L, Bates CJ. Br J Nutr 1986;56:115–22.
64. van Vliet T, van Schaik F, van den Berg H. Neth J Nutr 1992; 53:186–90.
65. During A, Nagao A, Terao J. Proc 11th Int Symp Carotenoids, Leiden, 1996;69.
66. Jüttner F, Höflacher B. Arch Microbiol 1985;141:337–43.
67. Canfield LM, Valenzuela JG. Ann NY Acad Sci 1993;691: 192–9.
68. Liebler DC. Ann NY Acad Sci 1993;691:20–31.
69. Blaner WS, Olson JA. Retinol and retinoic acid metabolism. In: Sporn MB, Roberts AB, Goodman DS, eds. The retinoids: biology, chemistry, and medicine. 2nd ed. New York: Raven Press, 1994;229–55.
70. Napoli JL, Race KR. J Biol Chem 1988;263:17372–7.
71. Hébuterne X, Wang X-D, Smith DEH, et al. J Lipid Res 1996;37:482–92.
72. Napoli JL. FASEB J 1996;10:993–1001.
73. Lakshmanan MR, Pope JL, Olson JA. Biochem Biophys Res Commun 1968:33:347–52.
74. Singh H, Cama HR. Biochim Biophys Acta 1974;370:49–61.
75. Wang X-D, Russell RM, Liu C, et al. J Biol Chem 1996; 271:26490–8.
76. Di Giovanna JJ, Zech LA, Ruddel ME, et al. Arch Dermatol 1989;125:246–51.
77. Sivakumar B, Parvin SG. Abstracts, 16th Int Congr Nutr, Montreal, Canada, 27 July–1 Aug, 1997;127.
78. Mathews-Roth MM, Welankiwar S, Sehgal PK, et al. J Nutr 1990;120:1205–13.
79. Stahl W, Sies H. Arch Biochem Biophys 1996;336:1–9.
80. Khachik F, Beecher GR, Smith JC Jr. J Cell Biochem Suppl 1995;22:236–46.
81. White WS, Peck KM, Bierer TL, et al. J Nutr 1993;123: 1405–13.
82. Tyczkowski JK, Yagen B, Hamilton PB. Poult Sci 1988;67: 787–93.
83. Oshima S, Sakamoto H, Ishiguro Y, et al. J Nutr 1997;127: 1475–9.
84. Levy LW, Regalado E, Navarrete S, et al. Analyst 1997;122: 977–80.
85. Khachik F, Beecher GR, Goli MG. Pure Appl Chem 1991;63:71–80.

86. Mangels AR, Holden JM, Beecher GR, et al. J Am Diet Assoc 1993;93:284–96.
87. Bendich A, Olson JA. FASEB J 1989;3:1927–32.
88. Bertram JS. Pure Appl Chem 1994;66:1025–32.
89. Stahl W, Sies H. Proc 11th Int Symp Carotenoids, Leiden, 1996;89.
90. Duitsman PK, Becker B, Barua AB, Olson JA. FASEB J 1996; 10:A732.
91. Bendich A, Shapiro SS. J Nutr 1986;116:2254–62.
92. Jyonouchi H, Zhang L, Gross M, et al. Nutr Cancer 1994;21:47–58.
93. Jyonouchi H, Sun S, Mizokami M, et al. Nutr Cancer 1996; 26:313–24.
94. Kramer TR, Burri BJ. Am J Clin Nutr 1997;65:871–5.
95. Hughes DA, Wright AJ, Finglas PM, et al. J Lab Clin Med 1997;129:309–17.
96. Chew BP. J Anim Sci 1993;71:247–52.
97. Lotthammer KH, Ahlswede L, Meyer H. Dtsch Tieraerztl Wochenschr 1976;83:353–8.
98. Folman Y, Ascarelli I, Kraus D, et al. J Dairy Sci 1987;70: 357–66.
99. Wang JY, Hafi CB, Larson LL. J Dairy Sci 1988;71:498–504.
100. Wang JY, Owen FG, Larson LL. J Dairy Sci 1988;71:181–6.
101. Coffey MT, Britt JH. J Anim Sci 1993;71:1198–202.
102. Besenfelder U, Solti L, Seregi J, et al. Theriogenology 1996; 1583–91.
103. Schweigert FJ, Wierch W, Rambeck WA, et al. Theriogenology 1988;30:923–30.
104. Fong AKH, Kretsch MJ, Burri BJ, et al. FASEB J 1993;7:A521.
105. Kretsch MJ, Fong AKH, Burri BJ, et al. FASEB J 1995;9: A171.
106. Feinstein AR. Science 1988;242:1257–63.
107. Olson JA. J Nutr 1996;126:1208S–12S.
108. Canfield LM, Krinsky NI, Olson JA. Ann NY Acad Sci 1993;691:1–300.
109. Mayne ST. FASEB J 1996;10:690–701.
110. Heinonen OP, Huttunen JK, Albanes D, et al. N Engl J Med 1994;330:1029–35.
111. Omenn GS, Goodman GE, Thornquist MD, et al. N Engl J Med 1996;334:1150–5.
112. Hennekens CH, Buring JE, Manson JE, et al. N Engl J Med 1996;334:1145–9.
113. Albanes D, Virtamo J, Taylor PR, et al. Am J Clin Nutr 1997; 66:366–72.
114. Mayne ST. FASEB J 1997;11:A448.
115. Burton GW. J Nutr 1989;119:109–11.
116. Albanes D, Heinonen OP, Taylor PR, et al. J Natl Cancer Inst 1996;88:1560–70.
117. Mayne ST, Janerich DT, Greenwald P, et al. J Natl Cancer Inst 1994;86:33–8.
118. Ziegler RG, Mayne ST, Swanson CA. Cancer Causes Control 1996;7:151–77.
119. Khuri FR, Lippman SM, Spritz MR, et al. J Natl Cancer Inst 1997;89:199–211.
120. Greenberg ER, Baron JA, Tosteson TD, et al. N Engl J Med 1994;331:141–7.
121. Formelli F, Barua AB, Olson JA. FASEB J 1996;10:1014–24.
122. Hong WK, Itri LM. Retinoids and human cancer. In: Sporn MB, Roberts AB, Goodman DS, eds. The retinoids: biology, chemistry, and medicine. 2nd ed. New York: Raven Press, 1994;597–630.
123. Ziegler RG, Brinton LA, Hamman RF, et al. Am J Epidemiol 1990;132:432–45.
124. Giovannucci E, Ascherio A, Rimm EB, et al. J Natl Cancer Inst 1995;87:1767–76.
125. Kolonel LN. Cancer Causes Control 1996;7:83–94.
126. Greenberg ER, Baron JA, Stukel TA, et al. N Engl J Med 1990;323:789–95.
127. Matthews-Roth MM. Ann NY Acad Sci 1993;691:127–38.
128. Weber U, Georz G, Baseler H, Michaelis L. Klin Monatsbl Augenheilkd 1992;201:174–7.
129. Gey KF, Moser UK, Jordan P, et al. Am J Clin Nutr 1993;57:787S–97S.
130. Gaziano JM, Hennekens CH. Ann NY Acad Sci 1993; 691:148–55.
131. Greenberg ER, Baron JA, Karagas MR, et al. JAMA 1996; 275:699–703.
132. Rapola JM, Virtamo J, Ripatti S, et al. Lancet 1997;349: 1715–20.
133. Princen HMG, van Poppel G, Vogelezang C, et al. Arterioscler Thromb 1992;12:554–62.
134. Kohlmeier L, Hastings SB. Am J Clin Nutr 1995;62:1370S–6S.
135. Bone RA, Landrum JT, Hime GW, et al. Invest Ophthalmol Vis Sci 1993;34:2033–40.
136. Bernstein PS, Balashor NA, Tsong ED, et al. Invest Ophthalmol Vis Sci 1997;38:167–75.
137. Seddon JM, Ajani U, Sperduto RD, et al. JAMA 1994;272: 1413–20.
138. Mares-Perlman JA, Brady WE, Klein R, et al. Arch Ophthalmol 1995;113:1518–23.
139. Schalch W, Weber P. Vitamins and carotenoids—a promising approach to reducing the risk of coronary heart disease, cancer and eye disease. In: Armstrong D, ed. Free radicals in diagnostic medicine. New York: Plenum Press, 1994;335–50.
140. Snodderly DM. Am J Clin Nutr 1995;62(Suppl):1448S–61S.
141. Bendich A. Pure Appl Chem 1994;66:1017–24.
142. Pontiggia P, Santamaria AB, Alonso K, Santamaria L. Biomed Pharmacother 1995;49:263–5.
143. Bendich A. Nutr Cancer 1988;11:207–14.
144. Erdman JW Jr, Russell RM, Rock CL, et al. Nutr Rev 1996;54:185–8.
145. Dimitrov NV, Ullrey DE. Bioavailability of carotenoids. In: Krinsky NI, ed. Carotenoids: chemistry and biology. New York: Plenum Press, 1990;269–77.

SELECTED READINGS

Britton G, ed. Tenth international symposium on carotenoids. Pure Appl Chem 1994;66:931–1076.

Britton G, Liaaen-Jensen S, Pfander H. Carotenoids, vol 1A, Isolation and analysis, 1995; vol 1B, Spectroscopy, 1995; vol 2, Synthesis, 1996. Basel: Birkhäuser Verlag.

Canfield LM, Krinsky NI, Olson JA, eds. Carotenoids in human health. Ann NY Acad Sci 1993;691:1–300.

Furr HC, Clark RM. Intestinal absorption and tissue distribution of carotenoids. J Nutr Biochem 1997;8:364–77.

Olson JA, Krinsky NI, eds. Carotenoid serial reviews. FASEB J 1995;9:1547–50, 1551–8, 1996;10:228–37, 403–12, 542–51, 690–701.

34. Homocysteine, Cysteine, and Taurine

MARTHA H. STIPANUK

Abbreviations: **Cys**—cysteine (any form), with thiol and disulfide forms indicated as CySH, CySSCy, and CySSR; **tCys**—sum of all forms of Cys including that present as thiol, half-disulfide, mixed disulfide, and protein-bound disulfide; **Cyst(e)ine**—cysteine and/or cystine; **Hcy**—homocysteine (any form) with thiol and disulfide forms indicated as HcySH, HcySSHcy, and HcySSR; **tHcy**—sum of all forms of Hcy; **Homocyst(e)ine**—homocysteine and/or homocystine; **Glu**—glutamate; **Gly**—glycine; GSH, glutathione; **SCMC**—*S*-carboxymethylcysteine; THF, tetrahydrofolate.

HISTORICAL INTRODUCTION

The importance of sulfur amino acids for growth or protein synthesis has been recognized since 1915 when Osborne and Mendel (1) demonstrated that addition of cystine to a low-casein diet restored rapid growth of rats. The amino acid methionine was identified almost two decades after most amino acids in protein had been discovered (2) and was subsequently shown to also be an effective supplement to low-casein diets (3). Womack et al. (4) demonstrated that cyst(e)ine was not essential for rats when dietary methionine was adequate and that the effect of cyst(e)ine was due to its ability to replace part, but not all, of the methionine in the diet. Rose and Wixom (5) demonstrated the same relation of methionine and cyst(e)ine requirements in their studies of amino acid requirements of adult men. Thus, only methionine is considered an essential amino acid, but in practice, the methionine or total sulfur amino acid requirement is usually met by a combination of methionine and cyst(e)ine.

More recently, the nutritional importance of taurine, a metabolite of cysteine, and the clinical significance of homocysteine, a metabolite of methionine, have been recognized. Homocysteine was discovered by du Vigneaud in 1932 (6) as the product of methionine demethylation. The role of homocyst(e)ine in the conversion of methionine sulfur to cysteine (the transsulfuration pathway) was studied in the following years, and homocyst(e)ine was shown to support growth of animals fed diets deficient in cysteine, methionine, or choline. Homocystinuria, an inborn error of metabolism, was identified in 1962 when mentally retarded individuals were screened for abnormal urinary amino acid patterns (7). During the past decade, it has been recognized that small increases in plasma homocysteine concentrations are associated with increased risk of vascular disease and neural tube defects in the general population (8–11).

Taurine is an end product of cysteine catabolism, first isolated from the bile of the ox *(Bos taurus)* in 1827 (12). Interest in taurine surged following the discovery in 1975 that cats fed diets containing little or no taurine suffered retinal degeneration accompanied by low retinal and plasma taurine concentrations (13). This was soon followed by the observation that infants fed purified formulas lacking taurine had lower plasma and urine taurine levels than did infants fed pooled human milk (14, 15). Because of increasing evidence of a possible role of taurine in development, taurine has been added to most human infant formulas since the mid-1980s.

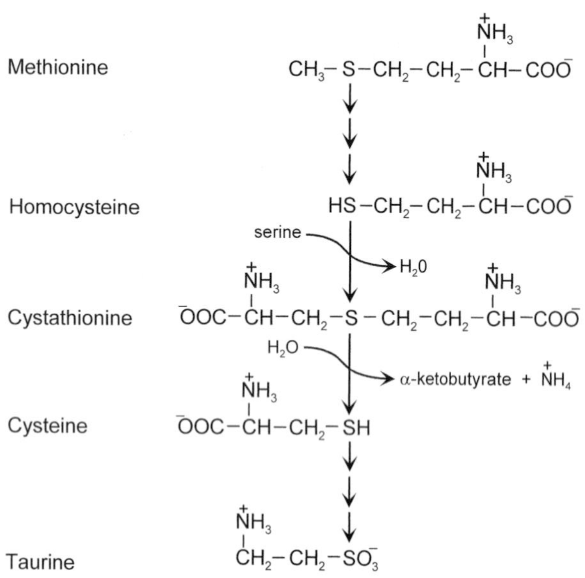

Figure 34.1. Structures and metabolic relations of sulfur amino acids.

CHEMISTRY, NOMENCLATURE, AND CELLULAR/EXTRACELLULAR FORMS

The structures of cysteine, homocysteine, and taurine and their relations with precursor amino acids (methionine and serine) are shown in Figure 34.1. Like other amino acids with an asymmetric carbon atom, the L-isomers of methionine, homocysteine, and cysteine are the biologically active forms. Both homocysteine and cysteine have a free sulfhydryl group. The carbon skeleton of homocysteine, which is derived from methionine, has one more carbon than the carbon chain of cysteine, which is derived from serine. Taurine, 2-aminoethane sulfonate, is formed from cysteine by removal of the carboxyl group and oxidation of the sulfur to form a sulfonic acid group. The carboxyl ($pK_a \approx 1.7$), sulfonic ($pK_a \approx 1.5$), sulfhydryl ($pK_a \approx 8.3$), and amino ($pK_a \approx 9–11$) groups all undergo ionization; the zwitterionic forms shown in Figure 34.1 are the dominant species at physiologic pH.

Technically, the terms cysteine and homocysteine refer to the thiol or reduced form (RSH) of these amino acids. However, cysteine (Cys) and homocysteine (Hcy), like other aminothiols, also exist in free oxidized forms, including the disulfide (RSSR) and mixed disulfides (RSSR′), and in the protein-bound oxidized form (via formation of disulfides with cysteinyl residues of proteins; PSSR) (16, 17). The thiol form of Cys (CySH) dominates intracellularly, whereas disulfide forms of Cys (protein-bound cysteine, PSSCy, and cystine, CySSCy) dominate in the more oxidized extracellular environment. Intracellularly, low concentrations of Hcy are present in free (HcySH) and protein-bound (PSSHcy) forms. Extracellularly, Hcy is present predominantly as mixed disulfides of Hcy with protein (PSSHcy) or Cys (HcySSCy). High levels of the disulfide of Hcy (homocystine, HcySSHcy) are excreted by individuals with the inborn error of metabolism known as homocystinuria.

The distribution of Cys and Hcy in plasma of healthy adults is shown in Figure 34.2. Cys is the major plasma thiol, with total Hcy (tHcy) present at 10% or less of the concentration for total Cys (tCys). Both Cys and Hcy are predominantly present as protein-bound disulfides, with intermediate concentrations of disulfides (predominantly CySSCy and HcySSCy) and with very low concentrations of free thiols. The Cys-containing peptides, cysteinylglycine (CysGly), γ-glutamylcysteine (γGluCys), and glutathione (GSH, or γGluCysGly), are also present in plasma and tissues.

The protein binding and redox status of different plasma aminothiols are interactive because of presumed ongoing redox cycling and disulfide exchange reactions. For example, Hcy will displace protein-bound Cys or CysGly (18). After ingestion of a methionine load or a protein-containing meal, protein-bound Cys tends to decrease, probably because of displacement of protein-bound Cys by Hcy (16, 19).

Measures of tHcy or tCys are useful in clinical studies because they are not affected in vitro by disulfide exchange reactions and redistribution between forms. Mean fasting plasma tHcy was 11.9 μmol/L (median, 11.6) with a range of 3.5 to 66.8 μmol/L in 1160 subjects aged 67 to 95 years (20); mean plasma tHcy is slightly

Reduced	Oxidized		Total Concentration
	Free	Protein-Bound	
CySH 13.9 μmol/L	RSSCy 88.1μmol/L	PSSCy 196.3 μmol/L	Cys 298 μmol/L
HCySH 0.05 μmol/L	RSSHCy 1.28 μmol/L	PSSHCy 10.06 μmol/L	Hcy 11.4 μmol/L
CySHGly 3.9 μmol/L	RSSCyGly 5.5 μmol/L	PSSCyGly 17.7 μmol/L	CysGly 27.1 μmol/L

Figure 34.2. Concentrations of various forms of the major aminothiols in human plasma. *Cys,* cysteine; *Hcy,* homocysteine; *CysGly,* cysteinylglycine; *PS,* sulfhydryl group of cysteinyl residue in protein; *RS,* unspecified thiol, usually Cys in plasma. The designation *RSH* is used to represent the reduced thiol form, *RSSR* or *RSSR′* to represent the disulfide of the thiol with itself or another thiol, and PSSR to represent protein-bound disulfides. Mean fasting values for plasma thiols are based on the data of Manssoor et al. (16) for 34 male and 31 female control subjects. Other plasma thiols include glutathione (total GSH ≈ 7 μmol/L) and γ-glutamylcysteine (total γ-GluCys ≈ 3 μmol/L) (17).

lower for younger adults than for older ones and for women than for men (21–23). Mean fasting plasma tCys concentrations in healthy adults range from about 220 to 320 μmol/L (16–19).

A wide range of plasma taurine concentrations has been reported for human subjects. Trautwein and Hayes (24) reviewed values reported in the literature and found the reported mean plasma concentration of taurine in human subjects ranged from 39 to 116 μmol/L. Whole blood taurine ranged between 160 and 320 μmol/L with a mean of 225 μmol/L in a small sample of adults (24). Plasma taurine concentrations change more rapidly in response to changes in taurine intake than do whole blood concentrations, and whole blood taurine concentrations are not correlated with plasma taurine concentrations except during periods of depletion or excess intake. Plasma taurine concentrations are somewhat lower in vegans than in omnivores and somewhat lower in females than in males (25, 26).

Careful handling of blood samples is essential for measurement of plasma concentrations of aminothiols and taurine. Plasma tHcy concentrations may increase with storage of blood because of transsulfuration in blood cells unless the blood is rapidly cooled and processed (27). Hemolysis or contamination of the plasma fraction with platelets or white cells interferes with analysis of plasma taurine but not with measures of whole blood taurine (24).

DIETARY CONSIDERATIONS AND TYPICAL INTAKES

Methionine and Cyst(e)ine

The sulfur amino acids, methionine and cyst(e)ine, are normally consumed as components of dietary proteins. Normal Western diets provide 15 to 20 mmol (~2.25–3 g) of sulfur amino acids per day. Mixtures of proteins consumed in the United States contain about 35 mg methionine plus cyst(e)ine per gram of protein (28). Sulfur amino acids tend to be more abundant in animal and cereal proteins than in legume proteins, and the ratio of methionine to cysteine tends to be higher in animal proteins than in plant proteins (Table 34.1) (29).

The 1989 RDA committee recommended a sulfur amino acid intake of 13 mg/kg/day, a protein intake of 0.75 g/kg/day, and a desirable amino acid pattern for adults that includes at least 17 mg methionine plus cyst(e)ine per gram of protein (28). This suggested intake of sulfur amino acids is easily met by mixtures of protein commonly consumed in the United States. However, Young et al. (30) and Storch et al. (31) have proposed that the sulfur amino acid allowance set by the FAO/WHO (32) and the NRC (28) at 13 mg/kg/day (0.087 mmol/kg/day, or 6 mmol/day for a 70-kg adult) represents the average requirement of healthy adults rather than the upper end of the normal distribution of requirements (mean + 2 SD). Their studies indicated that an intake of 25 mg/kg/day (0.17 mmol/kg/day or 12 mmol/day for a 70-kg adult) was necessary to ensure an adequate intake for the entire population.

Table 34.1
Methionine and Cysteine Content of Selected Foods

	Amount		Pattern	
	Met (mg/100 g edible portion)	Cys (mg/100 g edible portion)	Met (mg/g protein)	Cys (mg/g protein)
Cheese, cheddar	652	125	26	5
Milk, whole	83	30	25	9
Egg, whole, chicken	392	289	32	24
Chicken, flesh only, cooked roasted	800	370	28	13
Beef, round, separable lean only	557	224	26	11
Wheat flour, whole meal	186	278	14	21
Corn grits, regular, dry	196	237	22	22
Oats, regular, dry	266	398	17	25
Peanut butter	292	365	10	13
Soybean, green cooked	150	113	12	9
Brown rice, dry	142	152	19	21

Data from or calculated from values in USDA handbook no. 8 (29).

Despite the availability of food proteins that provide ample amounts of sulfur amino acids, some individuals probably have inadequate intakes because of either inadequate intake of total protein or selection of a restricted variety of proteins that provide inadequate sulfur amino acids. Analysis of diets of long-term vegans living in California indicated an average protein intake of 64 g/day and a sulfur amino acid intake of 1.04 g (7.6 mmol) per day (26); this is equivalent to an intake of ~15 mg/kg/day of sulfur amino acids and an amino acid pattern of 16 mg methionine plus cyst(e)ine per gram protein. This level of intake would meet but not exceed the average requirement as estimated by Young et al. (30) and Storch et al. (31) and would be marginal for adults with higher-than-average requirements. Careful selection of plant proteins to ensure an adequate intake of sulfur amino acids may be very important for strict vegan adults and even more so for children fed a strict vegan diet.

Taurine

Although taurine is an end product of sulfur amino acid metabolism, it is usually obtained from the diet as well. Food taurine content has not been widely determined, but data from several reports (33–36) are summarized in Table 34.2. Taurine is present in most animal foods and is either absent or present in very low levels in most plant foods. Relatively high concentrations of taurine have been reported for some lower plants such as seaweeds (36, 37). Analysis of the diets of strict vegans living in England yielded no detectable taurine, whereas the

Table 34.2
Taurine Content of Selected Foods

Animal foods	
Poultry	89–2445 μmol/100 g wet wt
Beef and pork	307–489 μmol/100 g wet wt
Processed meats	251–981 μmol/100 g wet wt
Seafood	84–6614 μmol/100 g wet wt
Cow's milk	18–20 μmol/100 mL
Yogurt, ice cream	15–62 μmol/100 mL
Cheese	Not detected
Plant foods	
Most fruits, vegetables, seeds, cereals, grains, beans, peanuts	Not detected
Soybean, chick peas, black beans, pumpkin seeds, some nuts[a]	≤1–4 μmol/100 g wet wt
Seaweeds (marine algae)	1.5–100 μmol/100 g wet wt

Data from Laidlaw et al. (33), Pasantes-Morales et al. (34), Roe and Weston (35), and Kataoka and Ohnishi (36).

[a]Low reported values should be regarded as upper limits because contamination of food or methodologic interference by compounds that coelute with taurine could account for these low concentrations of taurine.

diets of omnivores contained 463 ± 156 (SE) μmol/day (25). The analyzed taurine intake of adults fed omnivorous diets in a clinical study center in the U.S. was 1000 to 1200 μmol/day (33).

The taurine content of milk from lactating women was 41.3 ± 7.1 (SE) μmol/100 mL for early milk (1–7 days) and 33.7 ± 2.8 μmol/100 mL for later milk (>7 days) (38). Taurine is added to infant formulas at levels comparable to those in human milk or at somewhat higher levels in formulas for premature infants (33). The mean taurine content of milk of lactating vegan women is lower than that of lactating omnivores, but values overlap considerably between the two groups, and the taurine concentration in milk of vegan mothers is still about 30 times the level in the cow's milk–based infant formulas used prior to the mid-1980s (25).

ABSORPTION, TRANSPORT, AND EXCRETION

Absorption of the products of protein digestion across the intestinal epithelium is highly efficient (~95–99%). Dietary methionine, a precursor of Cys, is transported by neutral amino acid transport systems ($B^{0,+}$, ASC, and L), and as methionine-containing peptides by peptide transport systems. Dietary Cys is absorbed as CySH, CySSCy, and Cys-containing peptides by a variety of L-amino acid and peptide transport systems in the small intestinal mucosa. Cysteine is transported by neutral amino acid transporters including system B in the apical (brush border) membrane and system ASC in both the apical and basolateral plasma membranes of the intestinal mucosa cells; cysteine uptake is largely Na^+ dependent. Cystine is transported by system $b^{0,+}$, a Na^+-independent system present in the apical membranes of the intestinal mucosa, which serves cationic amino acids as well as zwitterionic amino acids. Efficient absorption of taurine is facilitated by the β-amino acid or taurine transport system, a Na^+ and Cl^--dependent carrier that serves taurine, β-alanine, and γ-aminobutyric acid, which is present in the apical membrane of intestinal mucosa cells.

Amino acids enter the plasma and circulate as free amino acids until they are removed by tissues. The liver removes a substantial proportion of the sulfur-containing amino acids from the portal circulation and uses them for synthesis of protein and glutathione or for catabolism to taurine and sulfate. GSH is exported into plasma, and this cysteine-containing tripeptide as well as its metabolites, CysGly and γ-GluCys, can be a source of cysteine to tissues. Hcy is not normally present in the diet, and only very low amounts are normally released from tissues into the plasma.

The reabsorptive epithelium of the kidney proximal tubule has transport systems similar to those of the absorptive epithelium of the intestine, and the kidney efficiently reabsorbs amino acids from the filtrate. Renal reabsorption of Cys and methionine is normally very high (≥94%), and the loss of amino acids in the urine is normally negligible (39). Urinary methionine excretion has been reported to be 22 to 41 μmol/day (25, 40). Urinary cyst(e)ine excretion by adults has been reported to be 63 to 285 μmol/day (25, 40).

Cystinuria is an inherited disorder of cystine and dibasic amino acid transport. One cause of cystinuria is a defect in the gene that encodes the rBAT (related to $b^{0,+}$ amino acid transporter) protein, a subunit of the system $b^{0,+}$ transporter that is expressed by the kidney and small intestine (41–43). Urinary cystine excretion exceeding 1.2 mmol/day (~2.5 mmol Cys/day) is usually diagnostic of homozygous cystinuria (44). Cystine is very insoluble and can cause cystine stones if it is present above its aqueous solubility limit (250 mg/L, or 1 mmol/L).

Urinary excretion of extracellular Hcy is limited, even in individuals with defective Hcy metabolism, because the extensive binding of plasma Hcy to proteins limits filtration and because of the normally active renal reabsorption of free Hcy. Of the plasma Hcy filtered by the kidney, only about 1 to 2% is excreted in the urine (45). Normal urinary Hcy excretion ranges from 3.5 to 9.8 μmol/day (45). Higher levels of Hcy in urine indicate very high plasma tHcy concentrations and an inborn error of metabolism. For example, Hcy excretion in urine of patients with $N^{5,10}$-methylenetetrahydrofolate reductase deficiency ranged from 15 to 667 μmol/day (46).

Unlike most amino acids, taurine is not usually completely reabsorbed, and fractional excretion may vary over a wide range. Normally, the kidney regulates the body pool size of taurine and adapts to changes in dietary taurine intake by regulation of the proximal tubule brush-border membrane transporter for taurine (β system). During periods of inadequate dietary intake of taurine or its sulfur amino acid precursors, more taurine is reabsorbed from the filtrate because of enhanced taurine transporter activity, less taurine is excreted in the urine, and more of the tissue taurine stores are maintained. The renal taurine concentration seems to be the signal for changes in renal taurine transporter activity (47, 48).

Consistent with differences in taurine intake and with adaptive regulation of taurine reabsorption, urinary taurine levels vary widely. Urinary taurine levels of 250 μmol/day have been reported for adult vegans consuming diets with no preformed taurine, whereas excretion of taurine by adult omnivores usually exceeds 600 μmol/day, and values above 1000 μmol/day are not uncommon (25, 26, 40).

METHIONINE/HOMOCYSTEINE METABOLISM AND CYSTEINE FORMATION

Metabolic Pathways

Transmethylation

The essential amino acid methionine is activated by ATP to form *S*-adenosylmethionine in a reaction catalyzed by *S*-adenosylmethionine synthetase (EC 2.5.1.6). *S*-Adenosylmethionine serves primarily as a methyl donor via reactions catalyzed by a variety of methyl transferases and involving a variety of acceptors. These *S*-adenosylmethionine-dependent methylations are essential for the biosynthesis of a variety of cellular components including creatine, epinephrine, carnitine, phospholipids, proteins, DNA, and RNA (Fig. 34.3).

S-Adenosylhomocysteine, the byproduct of these methyl transfer reactions, is hydrolyzed by *S*-adenosylhomocysteine hydrolase (EC 3.3.1.1), thus generating adenosine and homocysteine. Although the equilibrium of *S*-adenosylhomocysteine hydrolase actually favors formation of *S*-adenosylhomocysteine, the reaction is normally driven forward by rapid removal of the products.

The homocysteine generated by hydrolysis of *S*-adenosylhomocysteine has two likely metabolic fates, remethylation or transsulfuration. In remethylation, homocysteine acquires a methyl group from N^5-methyltetrahydrofolate or betaine to form methionine. In transsulfuration, the sulfur is transferred to serine to form cysteine, and the remainder of the homocysteine molecule is catabolized to α-ketobutyrate and ammonium.

Remethylation

The remethylation pathway allows methionine to be regenerated from homocysteine by use of new methyl groups synthesized in the folate coenzyme system or preformed methyl groups, both of which may subsequently be transferred to acceptors via *S*-adenosylmethionine-

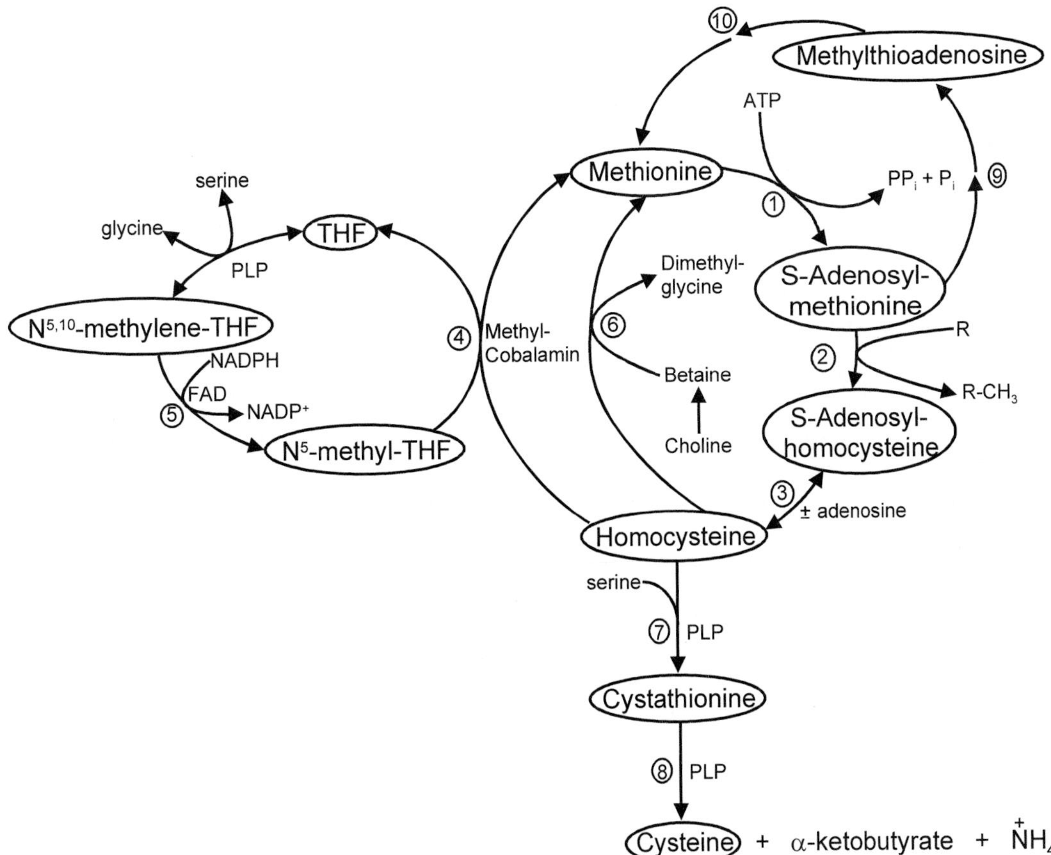

Figure 34.3. Methionine metabolism. Numbered reactions are catalyzed by the following enzymes: *(1)* methionine adenosyltransferase; *(2)* various methyltransferases; *(3)* adenosylhomocysteine hydrolase; *(4)* N^5-methyltetrahydrofolate-homocysteine methyltransferase; *(5)* $N^{5,10}$-methylenetetrahydrofolate reductase; *(6)* betaine-homocysteine methyltransferase; *(7)* cystathionine β-synthase; *(8)* cystathionine γ-lyase; *(9)* enzymes involved in polyamine synthesis; and *(10)* enzymes involved in methylthioadenosine salvage pathway.

dependent methyltransferase reactions. The remethylation of homocysteine by transfer of a methyl group from N^5-methyltetrahydrofolate is catalyzed by N^5-methyltetrahydrofolate-homocysteine methyltransferase (EC 2.1.1.13), commonly called methionine synthase. Methionine synthase is widely distributed in mammalian tissues and contains methylcobalamin as an essential cofactor. The methyl group of N^5-methyltetrahydrofolate is synthesized de novo in the folate coenzyme system. The final step of N^5-methyltetrahydrofolate synthesis is the irreversible reduction of $N^{5,10}$-methylenetetrahydrofolate, which is catalyzed by the flavoenzyme, $N^{5,10}$-methylenetetrahydrofolate reductase (EC 1.1.1.68), using NADH as the electron donor.

The other homocysteine methyltransferase, betaine-homocysteine methyltransferase (EC 2.1.1.5), is present only in liver and kidney of humans and requires betaine as the methyl donor (49). This reaction uses preformed methyl groups because betaine is derived from choline, which is either obtained from the diet or synthesized through successive *S*-adenosylmethionine-dependent methylations of phosphatidylethanolamine.

Transsulfuration

The transsulfuration of homocysteine to cysteine is catalyzed by two pyridoxal 5′-phosphate (PLP)-dependent enzymes, cystathionine β-synthase (EC 4.2.1.22) and cystathionine γ-lyase (EC 4.4.1.1; cystathionase). Cystathionine β-synthase catalyzes the condensation of homocysteine and serine to form cystathionine. Cystathionine is then hydrolyzed by cystathionine γ-lyase to form cysteine and α-ketobutyrate plus ammonium. Thus, the transsulfuration pathway is responsible for both the catabolism of homocysteine derived from methionine and the transfer of methionine sulfur to serine to synthesize cysteine.

Regardless of the extent of remethylation, in the steady-state metabolic condition, intake of methionine sulfur is balanced by metabolism of an almost equivalent amount of homocysteine sulfur through the transsulfuration pathway (50, 51). Although some methionine (via decarboxylated *S*-adenosylmethionine acting as a donor of aminopropyl groups) is used for polyamine synthesis, the methylthioadenosine that is a byproduct of this pathway is effectively recycled to methionine. The sulfur and methyl carbon of methionine and the carbon chain of ribose are reused in methionine synthesis by the methylthioadenosine salvage pathway (51, 52). Hence, little sulfur is oxidized or lost during methionine metabolism, and essentially all methionine sulfur is transferred to cysteine prior to oxidation/excretion of the sulfur atom.

Regulation of Remethylation versus Transsulfuration

Response to Changes in Methionine Intake

The remethylation and transsulfuration pathways can be considered to be competing for available homocysteine. Studies of whole body methionine kinetics demonstrated that in young adult men fed a diet with adequate methionine (~14 mmol/day), about 17 mmol/day of homocysteine was formed by transmethylation; approximately 38% of this homocysteine was remethylated to methionine, and 62% was catabolized by transsulfuration (31). In another study, transmethylation or homocysteine formation decreased markedly in subjects fed a sulfur amino acid–free diet, from approximately 20 mmol/day in men on an adequate diet to 6 mmol/day in men on a sulfur amino acid–free diet; the percentage of homocysteine remethylated to methionine increased from 36% in men on the adequate diet to 67% in men on the sulfur amino acid–free diet (53). As a result of decreased transmethylation or homocysteine formation and the greater percentage remethylation of homocysteine, transsulfuration or oxidation of methionine was reduced from 12 mmol/day in men fed the methionine-adequate diet to 2 mmol/day in subjects fed the sulfur amino acid–free diet.

Response to *S*-Adenosylmethionine as an Effector

Whether homocysteine is metabolized by remethylation or transsulfuration seems to be coordinated in response to cellular *S*-adenosylmethionine concentrations or the need to generate methionine methyl groups (54). *S*-Adenosylmethionine is both an allosteric inhibitor of $N^{5,10}$-methylenetetrahydrofolate reductase and an activator of cystathionine β-synthase. Hence, when the cellular *S*-adenosylmethionine concentration is low, synthesis of N^5-methyltetrahydrofolate proceeds uninhibited and cystathionine synthesis is suppressed, which conserves homocysteine for methionine synthesis. Conversely, when the *S*-adenosylmethionine concentration is high, inhibition of N^5-methyltetrahydrofolate synthesis is accompanied by diversion of homocysteine through the transsulfuration pathway because of stimulated cystathionine synthesis. This coordinate control results in both regulation of cellular *S*-adenosylmethionine concentration and maintenance of a homocysteine concentration that is compatible with the need for methyl groups synthesized de novo.

Methionine-Sparing Effect of Cyst(e)ine

Cyst(e)ine is said to have a "methionine-sparing" effect by reducing methionine catabolism via the transsulfuration pathway. The effect of supplemental cyst(e)ine added to a sulfur amino acid–free diet or a low-methionine diet may be at least partially due to promotion of methionine incorporation into protein so that less methionine is catabolized (53, 55). The effect of cyst(e)ine used to replace part of the dietary methionine (keeping total sulfur amino acid level the same) may be explained by a reduction in the hepatic concentrations of methionine and *S*-adenosylmethionine and, hence, less activation and reduced activity of hepatic cystathionine β-synthase. Less homocysteine catabolism by transsulfuration would result in increased recycling of homocysteine to methionine, using methyl groups generated by the folate coenzyme system.

Response to Supplemental Betaine

Normal adult subjects given a control diet with a betaine supplement had increased rates of methionine transmethylation and transsulfuration (56), suggesting that an increased dietary supply of methyl groups may increase methionine catabolism. A high dietary intake of betaine when coupled with a marginal intake of methionine could interfere with the normal coordinated regulation of remethylation versus transsulfuration by increasing *S*-adenosylmethionine concentration and stimulating methionine catabolism (56). Presumably, increased remethylation induced by betaine increases *S*-adenosylmethionine concentrations, resulting in inhibition of N^5-methyltetrahydrofolate-dependent remethylation and stimulation of homocysteine catabolism.

HOMOCYSTINURIA AND HYPERHOMOCYSTEINEMIA

Homocystinuria Due to Inborn Errors of Metabolism

Severe forms of hyperhomocysteinemia result in excretion of homocysteine, homocystine, and mixed disulfides of homocysteine in the urine. Homocystinuria (urinary Hcy > 10 μmol/24 h) is rare and results from severe hyperhomocysteinemia caused by several inborn errors of metabolism. The most common inborn error of sulfur amino acid metabolism and the most common cause of homocystinuria is a lack of cystathionine β-synthase activity, which is commonly associated with plasma tHcy concentrations above 200 μmol/L in untreated patients. Two clinical forms have been described: one not responsive to treatment with the coenzyme precursor pyridoxine and a pyridoxine-responsive form that improves with a high intake of vitamin B_6. The latter is usually associated with residual cystathionine β-synthase activity and milder disease (57). Based on newborn-screening programs, the estimated incidence of cystathionine β-synthase deficiency is 1:170,000 (58). The actual incidence of cystathionine β-synthase deficiency is thought to be closer to 1:340,000, however, because newborn-screening programs fail to detect most infants with the pyridoxine-responsive form of the disease. Cystathionine β-synthase deficiency is inherited as an autosomal recessive disorder and results in dislocation of optic lenses, skeletal abnormalities, mental retardation, neurologic disorders, and widespread thromboembolic phenomena. This disorder has been shown to be due to heterogeneous mutations, and most patients are compound heterozygotes; more than 18 mutations have been identified in patients with cystathionine β-synthase deficiency (59, 60).

A second inborn error of metabolism that causes homocystinuria is a lack of $N^{5,10}$-methylenetetrahydrofolate reductase activity. This is the major known inborn error affecting folate metabolism and the second leading known cause of homocystinuria. $N^{5,10}$-Methylenetetrahydrofolate reductase deficiency is inherited as an autosomal recessive disorder with an incidence about 1/10th that of cystathionine β-synthase deficiency. Individuals with severe deficiencies have residual activity that ranges from undetectable to 20% of normal activity. At least nine different mutations have been identified in patients with a severe lack of $N^{5,10}$-methylenetetrahydrofolate reductase activity (61, 62). Homocystinuria and hyperhomocysteinemia in these patients are usually less severe than in patients with cystathionine β-synthase deficiency, and a wide range of neurologic and vascular disturbances have been observed in these patients (see Chapters 26 and 95).

A third group of inborn errors giving rise to homocystinuria are those affecting various steps in the synthesis of methylcobalamin, an essential cofactor for methionine synthase (63). Cobalamin metabolism loci C, D, E, F, and G have been shown to result in reduced activity of methionine synthase and homocystinuria (see Chapter 27).

Hyperhomocysteinemia and Its Genetic, Nutritional, and Metabolic Bases

Milder forms of hyperhomocysteinemia have been recognized more recently and are much more prevalent than is homocystinuria. Heterozygosity for one of the inborn errors of metabolism resulting in homocystinuria may be one cause of milder hyperhomocysteinemia. However, the predicted incidence of heterozygosity for these inborn errors is too small to account for a large proportion of the observed hyperhomocysteinemia.

A milder form of $N^{5,10}$-methylenetetrahydrofolate reductase deficiency that results in approximately 50% residual enzyme activity in homozygotes is caused by a point mutation (677C→T) in the $N^{5,10}$-methylenetetrahydrofolate reductase gene (62, 64, 65). This genetic deficiency of $N^{5,10}$-methylenetetrahydrofolate reductase is also described as the "thermolabile variant" because of the marked thermolability of the altered enzyme in vitro (66). Approximately 5% of subjects studied by Kang et al. (66) and 12% of those studied by Rozen et al. (67) were homozygous for this 677C→T mutation in the $N^{5,10}$-methylenetetrahydrofolate reductase gene. This mutation is hypothesized to be an underlying cause of much of the hyperhomocysteinemia and associated increased risk for vascular disease and neural tube defects (62, 64, 68, 69).

Nutritional disorders that potentially lead to hyperhomocysteinemia, particularly in individuals with underlying genetic predispositions, are deficiencies of folate, vitamin B_{12}, and vitamin B_6 (20, 70–72). Selhub et al. (20) estimated that 67% of cases of hyperhomocysteinemia are at least partially due to inadequate B-vitamin status. As noted above, de novo synthesis of methionine methyl groups requires both vitamin B_{12} and folate coenzymes, whereas transsulfuration requires PLP. Evidence for an inverse correlation between vitamin intake or status and hyperhomocysteinemia is stronger and more consistent for folate than for vitamin B_{12} or vitamin B_6 (20, 21, 71–75). The thermolabile variant of $N^{5,10}$-methylenetetrahydrofolate reductase is very responsive to folate status; hyperhomocysteinemia is observed most frequently in homozygotes who also have a low folate intake and rarely in homozygotes who have a higher folate intake (65, 75).

Mild-to-moderate hyperhomocysteinemia and increased incidence of atherosclerotic disease are also observed in patients with renal disease. Plasma tHcy levels are significantly increased in patients with moderate renal failure and rise steeply in terminal uremia (76, 77). The rise in plasma tHcy levels in patients with renal failure is attributed to loss of renal parenchymal uptake and metabolism of plasma Hcy rather than to decreased urinary excretion of Hcy.

Clinical Significance of Hyperhomocysteinemia

Apparent associations of mild hyperhomocysteinemia with atherosclerotic disease, venous thromboses, neural tube defects, placental abruption/infarction, and unexplained pregnancy loss have been reported (8–11, 22, 69, 74, 77–82). In populations of individuals with arteriosclerotic disease, mild hyperhomocysteinemia is observed about as frequently as hypercholesterolemia or hypertension. Hyperhomocysteinemia is now considered an independent risk factor for vascular disease of the coronary, cerebral, and peripheral arteries, with an increase in plasma tHcy of only 5 μmol/L estimated to result in a 50 to 80% increase in risk for cerebrovascular or coronary artery disease (73).

The basis of the association of hyperhomocysteinemia with vascular disease is not clear (9, 83–86). Hypotheses related to a direct adverse effect of homocysteine (endothelial cell damage, oxidative damage, promotion of thrombogenesis via alterations in the coagulation and fibrinolytic systems, impaired regulation of vasoconstriction, stimulation of vascular smooth muscle cell proliferation) are currently being investigated. It is also possible that a decreased intracellular ratio of *S*-adenosylmethionine to *S*-adenosylhomocysteine or reduced availability of *S*-adenosylmethionine, either of which may be associated with hyperhomocysteinemia, interferes with essential methylation reactions and leads to the adverse effects associated with hyperhomocysteinemia. Similarly, impaired methylation of proteins has been implicated as a possible cause of neural tube defects (87, 88).

Detection of Homocystinuria and Hyperhomocysteinemia

Inborn errors giving rise to homocystinuria may be detected by newborn-screening programs (see Chapter 61). Most current screening programs detect individuals with cystathionine β-synthase deficiency by primary screening for hypermethioninemia and secondary screening for elevated urine and/or plasma tHcy levels, low plasma tCys concentration, and deficient cystathionine β-synthase activity in fibroblasts, leukocytes, or liver biopsy specimens. These screening programs fail to detect many pyridoxine-responsive forms of cystathionine β-synthase deficiency, which may not give rise to abnormal plasma Hcy or methionine concentrations in infants, especially if the protein intake is low or if testing is done within the first few weeks of life (58). Screening for hypermethioninemia will also not detect homocystinuria due to defects in folate or cobalamin metabolism because plasma methionine concentrations in these patients are either normal or low (46). Patients with defects in folate or cobalamin metabolism tend to have lower urinary Hcy levels than do patients with cystathionine β-synthase deficiency, and analysis of urine or plasma Hcy levels often yields a negative test result in affected newborns. Genotyping will likely be used more widely in the future to identify both homocystinuric individuals and heterozygous carriers.

Milder forms of hyperhomocysteinemia (heterozygotes for cystathionine β-synthase or $N^{5,10}$-methylenetetrahydrofolate reductase deficiency; B-vitamin deficiency; thermolabile $N^{5,10}$-methylenetetrahydrofolate reductase; renal failure; etc.) may be indicated by elevated fasting plasma tHcy concentrations ($\sim$16–30 μmol/L). Normal reference intervals for plasma tHcy vary, depending on methodology and the selection of reference individuals. Because as much as 40% of the population, including individuals with relatively low plasma tHcy values, may respond to folate or B-vitamin supplementation with a reduction in plasma tHcy (20, 71, 74, 80) and because even small elevations in plasma tHcy seem to be associated with increased risk of vascular disease, it has been difficult to establish exact desirable or reference values for the normal population. Use of 90th percentile values as cutoffs has resulted in use of plasma fasting tHcy values above 14 to 16 μmol/L as indicators of hyperhomocysteinemia (21, 89). A lower cutoff for the normal range may be appropriate, however, because the frequency distribution of plasma tHcy concentrations is positively skewed (74). Use of reference intervals based on presupplementation measurements of plasma tHcy in subjects who can be classified as weak responders to folate supplementation has been suggested. Rasmussen et al. (23) found a mean $\pm$ SD of 7.76 $\pm$ 1.54 μmol/L for these weak responders, compared with 12.33 $\pm$ 2.04 μmol/L for the high responders; they derived age- and gender-specific 95% confidence intervals including values between 4.5 and 11.9 μmol/L for the weak responders. Ubbink et al. (74) suggested using a mathematical model to predict the plasma tHcy that could be expected for a population with improved vitamin status; their calculated 95% reference range was 4.9 to 11.7 μmol/L for a population with improved folate, vitamin B_{12}, and vitamin B_6 status. Hence, about 12 μmol/L would seem to be the upper end of the normal "desirable" range for adult fasting plasma tHcy.

The use of both fasting and post–methionine load measurements may have benefits in screening for mild forms of hyperhomocysteinemia (54, 90). In one study, fasting plasma tHcy determination alone failed to identify more than 40% of persons classified as hyperhomocysteinemic when both fasting and post–methionine load measurements were used (89). Measurement of plasma tHcy 2 or 4 hours after administration of an oral load dose of methionine (~0.1 g or 670 μmol/kg) yielded plasma tHcy concentrations (mean ± SD) of 29.2 ± 10.4 μmol/L, compared with 9.6 ± 4.2 μmol/L for fasting concentrations; the 90th percentile cutoff value used to define hyperhomocysteinemia was 41.4 μmol/L for post–methionine load values, compared with 13.6 μmol/L for fasting tHcy (89).

Dietary Treatment of Homocystinuria and Hyperhomocysteinemia

The goal of dietary treatment of homocystinuria is to decrease the biochemical abnormalities (reduce plasma Hcy, maintain normal concentrations of plasma methionine and Cys) and to minimize development of clinical complications. Treatment of individuals with inborn errors of transsulfuration (cystathionine β-synthase deficiency) usually involves restriction of dietary methionine intake while providing adequate cyst(e)ine intake (see Chapter 61). Small, frequent feedings are also recommended to minimize a methionine load effect. Newborns diagnosed with cystathionine β-synthase deficiency are fed low-protein formula in controlled quantities or formula low in methionine and supplemented with cystine in an effort to maintain normal plasma methionine concentrations (20–40 μmol/L) and very low plasma concentrations of tHcy. Inclusion of choline or betaine (25–165 mmol/day; 100–600 mg/kg/day) as a methyl donor is also beneficial (58, 91); these levels of betaine supplementation are very high compared with the normal total choline intake in the adult (5.0–8.3 mmol/day), of which only a portion becomes available as betaine (92). Pyridoxine at levels ranging from 150 to 1200 mg/day has been used successfully in treatment of cystathionine β-synthase-deficient adults; these levels greatly exceed the normal recommended intake of approximately 2 mg/day for adults.

In homocystinuria due to inborn errors in the methionine remethylation pathway, the goal of dietary treatment is to maintain sufficient levels of methionine methyl groups without elevating the plasma Hcy concentration; this usually involves relatively high levels of B-vitamin supplementation (folate, vitamin B_{12}) to stimulate the N^5-methyltetrahydrofolate-dependent homocysteine remethylation pathway, betaine or choline to stimulate the betaine-dependent homocysteine remethylation pathway, and in some cases methionine supplementation to ensure sufficient availability of *S*-adenosylmethionine (93).

Modest levels of vitamin supplementation (~0.6 mg folic acid, 0.4 mg cyanocobalamin, and 10 mg pyridoxine) reduce plasma tHcy concentrations in a proportion of individuals with mild hyperhomocysteinemia (74, 77, 94–96). Some individuals with plasma tHcy levels in the reference range (fasting values <12 μmol/L) also respond to folate or B-vitamin supplementation with a reduction in plasma tHcy (74, 94, 95). Although Hcy-lowering therapy reduces the vascular risk of patients with severe hyperhomocysteinemia due to inborn errors of metabolism, the outcome of treatment of mild hyperhomocysteinemia on atherosclerotic and thromboembolic disease is yet to be reported (97). Periconceptual supplementation with folate reduces the incidence of neural tube birth defects in newborns (79). To increase the folate intake of women of childbearing age, the U.S. Food and Drug Administration ruled in 1996 to require fortification of most breads and grain products as of 1998. Fortification of foods with folate may have some beneficial effects on additional pregnancy outcome measures and the incidence of vascular and thromboembolic disease.

METABOLISM OF CYSTEINE

Pathways of Cysteine Metabolism

Cysteine, whether formed from methionine and serine via transsulfuration or supplied preformed in the diet, serves as a precursor for synthesis of proteins and several other essential molecules as shown in Figure 34.4. These metabolites include GSH, coenzyme A, taurine, and inorganic sulfur.

At intakes near the requirement, a large proportion of available cysteine is used for synthesis of proteins and GSH. In addition to the specific metabolic functions of GSH, GSH serves as a reservoir of Cys and as a means for transporting Cys to extrahepatic tissues (86). A large proportion of the sulfur amino acid intake is converted to GSH by the liver and released into the circulation. γ-Glutamyl transpeptidase, an enzyme located on the outer surface of the plasma membrane of cells in a number of tissues, hydrolyzes GSH (or its disulfide) to yield CysGly (or its disulfide), which can be further degraded by peptidases to release cysteine (or cystine) into the plasma. The normal turnover of GSH in humans is estimated to be 40 mmol/day (99, 100), nearly two to three times the typical sulfur amino acid intake of 15 to 20 mmol/day and six to seven times the estimated sulfur amino acid requirement. This estimate suggests that the magnitude of turnover of the Cys pool as a result of GSH turnover may be slightly greater than that resulting from protein turnover in the body (~30 mmol/day; [31]).

Cysteine is also a precursor for synthesis of coenzyme A and for production of taurine and inorganic sulfate. These three fates of cysteine involve loss of the cysteine moiety as such. Cysteine is substrate for coenzyme A synthesis in that it donates the cysteamine (decarboxylated cysteine) moiety of the coenzyme A molecule and, hence, contributes the reactive sulfhydryl group. Coenzyme A turnover is thought to be slow, such that coenzyme A synthesis does

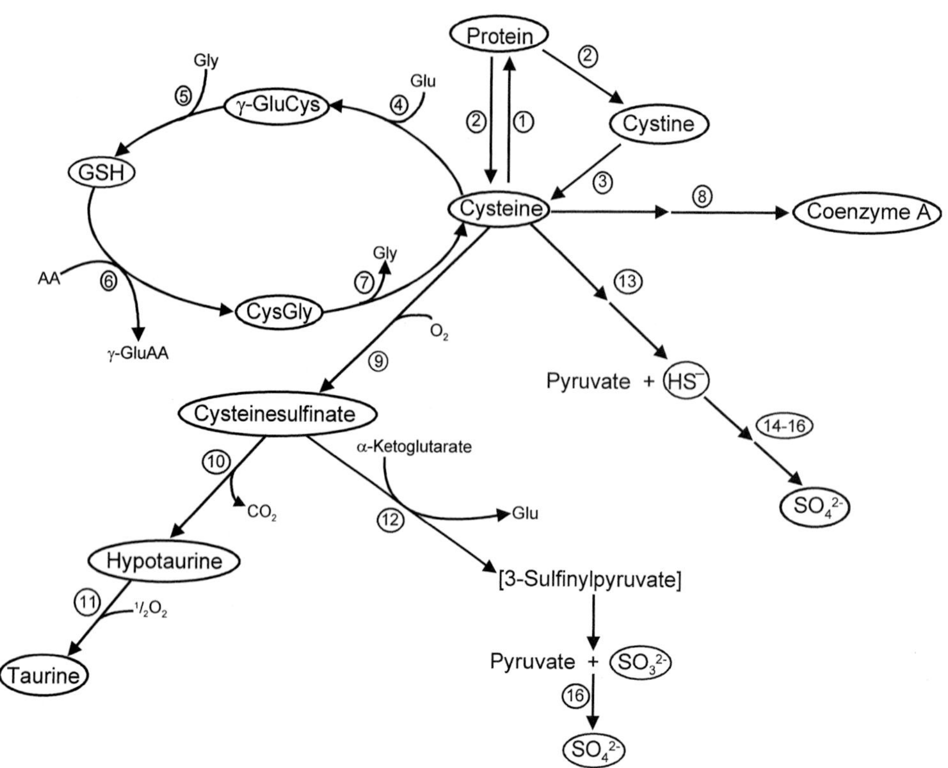

Figure 34.4. Pathways of cysteine metabolism. Numbered reactions are catalyzed by the following enzymes or pathways: *(1)* protein synthesis; *(2)* protein degradation; *(3)* GSH-thioltransferase or nonenzymatic thiol-disulfide exchange of cystine with GSH; *(4)* γ-glutamylcysteine synthetase; *(5)* glutathione synthetase; *(6)* glutathione transpeptidase; *(7)* dipeptidase; *(8)* pathway of coenzyme A synthesis; *(9)* cysteine dioxygenase; *(10)* cysteine sulfinate decarboxylase; *(11)* enzymatic or nonenzymatic oxidation of hypotaurine; *(12)* aspartate (cysteine sulfinate) aminotransferase; *(13)* cysteine sulfinate-independent or desulfhydration pathways of cyst(e)ine catabolism; *(14)* sulfide oxidase; *(15)* thiosulfate sulfurtransferase or GSH-dependent thiosulfate reductase; and *(16)* sulfite oxidase.

not consume a large amount of dietary cysteine. The functions of coenzyme A are discussed in Chapter 25.

Both taurine and inorganic sulfur are products of cysteine catabolism. As shown in Figure 34.4, there are several pathways for cysteine catabolism. Cysteine catabolism may occur by desulfuration of cysteine to yield pyruvate and reduced sulfur (often in the form of a persulfide such as thiocysteine, mercaptopyruvate, or thiosulfate). Cysteine desulfuration can be catalyzed by the β-cleavage of cyst(e)ine by cystathionine γ-lyase or by transamination of cysteine to β-mercaptopyruvate followed by de- or transsulfuration by mercaptopyruvate sulfurtransferase (51). Individuals with a rare inborn error of metabolism in which β-mercaptopyruvate sulfurtransferase is deficient excrete the mixed disulfide of cysteine and β-mercaptolactate, suggesting that transamination of cysteine to mercaptopyruvate occurs to some extent in humans (101). However, these patients excrete normal levels of urinary sulfate, indicating that overall cysteine catabolism is not impaired. The reduced sulfur may be used in synthesis of molecules requiring a source of reduced sulfur, or it may be oxidized to thiosulfate (inner sulfur), sulfite, and finally sulfate. Although most of the inorganic sulfur is eventually oxidized to sulfate, mammals depend upon the cysteine sulfinate–independent or desulfhydration pathways of cysteine metabolism as a source of reduced forms of inorganic sulfur because they cannot reduce sulfate or sulfite to thiosulfate or sulfide.

In animals fed high-protein or high sulfur amino acid–containing diets, the major pathway of cysteine catabolism involves oxidation of cysteine to cysteine sulfinate by cysteine dioxygenase (EC 1.13.11.20), which is an inducible enzyme in rat liver (51, 102). Cysteine sulfinate may be decarboxylated to hypotaurine, which is subsequently oxidized to taurine, or cysteine sulfinate may be transaminated (with α-ketoglutarate) to the enzyme-bound intermediate, β-sulfinylpyruvate, which gives rise to pyruvate and sulfite. Sulfite is further oxidized to sulfate by sulfite oxidase (EC 1.8.3.1).

In all catabolic pathways except that resulting in taurine formation, the carbon chain of cysteine is released as pyruvate, the sulfur is released as inorganic sulfur, and the amino group is released as ammonium or transferred to a keto acid acceptor. When taurine is the end product, only the carboxyl carbon of the cysteine is released, and the other three carbons as well as the nitrogen and sulfur atoms remain in the end product. Thus, the distribution of Cys among its catabolic pathways potentially affects the use of amino acid carbon chains for energy, the net production of acid or fixed anions (sulfate), and the synthesis of essential metabolites (inorganic sulfur and taurine). Although taurine and sulfate can be regarded as end products of cellular cysteine catabolism, both of these compounds participate in conjugation reactions and have a variety of essential physiologic functions prior to their ultimate excretion.

Adult human subjects remain in sulfur balance, with sulfur excretion essentially equivalent to sulfur intake (15–20 mmol/day). Both sulfate and taurine are excreted in the urine. In studies of total urinary sulfur excretion by children and adults, inorganic sulfate accounted for about 77 to 82%, ester sulfate about 8 to 9%, taurine about 3%, and cyst(e)ine about 0.6 to 0.7%. Other sulfur-containing compounds found in urine in trace amounts (<0.2% of total sulfur) include methionine, Hcy, cystathionine, *N*-acetylcysteine, mercaptolactate, mercaptoacetate, thiosulfate, and thiocyanate (40, 103).

Cysteine Oxidation and Taurine Synthesis in Humans

Relatively little is known about the specific pathways of cysteine metabolism in humans. Taurine synthesis requires both cysteine dioxygenase and cysteine sulfinate decarboxylase (EC 4.1.1.29). Significant expression of the cysteine dioxygenase gene was indicated by the presence of mRNA for cysteine dioxygenase in human liver, kidney, and lung (104). *S*-Carboxymethyl-L-cysteine (SCMC) has been used as a marker substrate for cysteine metabolism, presumably by cysteine dioxygenase, in vivo (105). Metabolism of SCMC is polymorphic, and about 20% of healthy individuals are poor S-oxidizers, based upon conversion of SCMC to urinary metabolites, SCMC sulfoxide, or methylcysteine sulfoxide. A low capacity to oxidize SCMC has been observed in some individuals with liver diseases or rheumatoid arthritis (105, 106). Individuals who exhibited low capacities for SCMC oxidation also had elevated cysteine:sulfate plasma ratios, excreted a smaller percentage of a dose of acetaminophen as the sulfate (vs. the glucuronide conjugate), and had a lower sulfate concentration in synovial fluid, all of which are consistent with impaired cysteine oxidation.

The human liver has been reported to have low cysteine sulfinate decarboxylase activity (107). Nevertheless, the adult human seems to have a significant ability to synthesize taurine. In vivo assessment of the ability of adults to synthesize taurine, based upon incorporation of ^{18}O (from inhaled $^{18}O_2$) into taurine, resulted in conservative estimates of synthesis in the range of 200 to 400 μmol/day (108). These estimates are equivalent to 1 to 3% of the total sulfur amino acid intake and compare favorably with the mean taurine excretion observed in strict vegans consuming an essentially taurine-free diet (approximately 250 μmol/day [25, 26]). Thus, the percentage of the sulfur amino acid intake or total urinary sulfur excretion that is represented by urinary taurine in humans fed taurine-free diets is similar to that observed in rats fed taurine-free diets (2–6%) (109), which seems to dispute the often-made statement that the rat has a high capacity for taurine synthesis whereas humans have a low capacity. Possibly, relatively high hepatic cysteine dioxygenase activity in man permits high rates of cysteine catabolism to cysteine sulfinate, and relatively high concentrations of cysteine sulfinate allow adequate rates of taurine synthesis despite relatively low cysteine sulfinate decarboxylase activity.

ESSENTIAL FUNCTIONS OF CYSTEINE AND ITS METABOLITES

Synthesis of Protein and Glutathione

Cysteine, either preformed or synthesized from methionine and serine, is required for protein synthesis and, hence, growth or nitrogen balance. Both the reactive sulfhydryl group of cysteinyl residues in proteins and the ability of these residues to form disulfide linkages play important roles in protein structure and function.

The Cys-containing tripeptide GSH has a number of essential functions in the body in addition to serving as a storage or circulating reservoir of Cys (110, 111). Because GSH has a reactive sulfhydryl group, it can readily form disulfides with itself (oxidized glutathione or GSSG) or with other thiol compounds (GSSR). The ratio of GSH to GSSG in most cells is greater than 500, so GSH serves as a supply of reducing equivalents or electrons. Glutathione is involved in protection of cells from oxidative damage because of its role in reduction of hydrogen peroxide and organic peroxides via glutathione peroxidases and because of its ability to inactivate free radicals by donating hydrogen to the radical; these processes result in oxidation of GSH to GSSG. GSSG and GSH can be interconverted via the glutathione reductase reaction, which uses $NADP^+$/NADPH as the oxidant/reductant; hence, glutathione plays a role in maintenance of the cellular redox state. GSH is an important source of reducing equivalents for the intracellular reduction of cystine to cysteine, which can occur by thiol-disulfide exchange or enzymatically via thioltransferase, with GSH providing the reducing equivalents.

GSH may participate in the transport of amino acids via the membrane-bound enzyme γ-glutamyl transpeptidase, the same enzyme responsible for extracellular hydrolysis of GSH. This enzyme catalyzes the transfer of the γ-glutamyl group of GSH to the α-amino group of an acceptor amino acid such as cystine or glutamine. The γ-glutamyl amino acid is transported into the cell, where the amino acid is released and the glutamyl moiety cyclizes to 5-oxoproline, which is then hydrolyzed to regenerate glutamate. The CysGly dipeptide that is the byproduct of γ-glutamyl-transpeptidation can be hydrolyzed to Cys and glycine either extracellularly or intracellularly by dipeptidases; hence, no net consumption of amino acids results from this transport cycle. The contribution of this proposed transport system to amino acid transport cannot exceed the rate of GSH turnover, which is ~40 mmol/day in an adult.

GSH also serves as a cosubstrate for several reactions,

including certain steps in leukotriene synthesis and melanin polymer synthesis. GSH is the substrate for a group of enzymes, glutathione S-transferases, that form GSH conjugates from a variety of acceptor compounds including various xenobiotics (112). These conjugates are normally degraded by the enzymes of the γ-glutamyl cycle to yield cysteinyl derivatives that may be acetylated using acetyl-CoA to mercapturic acids, which are excreted in the urine. This is usually a detoxification and excretion process.

Functions of Inorganic Sulfur

Reduced sulfur is required for synthesis of iron-sulfur proteins and other compounds. The activated form of sulfate, 3′-phospho-5′-phosphosulfate (PAPS), serves as the substrate for a variety of sulfotransferase reactions. Many structural compounds are sulfated; in particular, the oligosaccharide chains of proteoglycans contain many sulfated sugar residues. In addition, many compounds of both endogenous and exogenous origin are excreted as sulfoesters; sulfoesters of steroid hormones and the drug acetaminophen are examples. Inorganic sulfur is largely obtained from the metabolism of cysteine in the body, but animal studies have suggested that dietary inorganic sulfate may improve growth, feed efficiency, and sulfation of cartilage proteoglycans when sulfur amino acid intake is insufficient (113).

Functions of Taurine

The only physiologic function of taurine that is well understood is its role in bile acid conjugation (37). Taurine conjugates are the major metabolites of taurine formed in vertebrates. Taurocholate is a very efficient bile salt because of the low pK_a of the sulfonic acid group, which faciliates its ionization and hence detergent action, solubility, slower reabsorption, and higher intraluminal concentration. Taurine is also a conjugation substrate for certain other compounds, such as *all-trans*-retinoic acid, increasing polarity, aqueous solubility, and, in most cases, clearance from the body.

Humans can conjugate bile acids with both taurine and glycine. In adults, the taurocholate:glycocholate ratio is about 3:1, but this ratio varies from individual to individual and with changes in the hepatic concentration of taurine. In contrast, the human fetus and neonate are exclusive taurine conjugators. Glycine conjugation is not usually observed until about the 3rd week of life, but it appears sooner in infants deprived of dietary taurine (114). Taurine supplementation resulted in lower cholesterol synthesis and higher bile acid excretion and fatty acid absorption in preterm infants with a gestational age less than 33 weeks but not in older preterm or full-term infants (115).

Taurine is present in high concentrations in many human tissues (~25 μmol/g wet wt in retina and leukocytes), and a number of other physiologic actions of taurine in various tissues have been hypothesized (15, 37). Unfortunately, these actions are not well understood despite several decades of intensive work (15, 37, 48). Taurine is involved in osmoregulation in many marine invertebrates and fish and may also function as an organic osmolyte in mammals. Taurine seems to modulate many Ca^{2+}-dependent processes and to be involved in phospholipid/Ca^{+2} interactions. Taurine has been said to have "antioxidant or radioprotective" functions, but these are probably largely secondary to its membrane-stabilizing actions. The metabolic precursor of taurine, hypotaurine, can function as an antioxidant; and the cysteine derivative, cysteamine, derived from coenzyme A catabolism, is a good radioprotectant. Additionally, taurine facilitates removal of hypochlorite, a strong oxidant generated from peroxide and Cl^- by myeloperoxidase. Taurine reacts with hypochlorite to form *N*-chlorotaurine, which can then be reduced to taurine and Cl^-. *N*-Chlorotaurine may itself have a regulatory role in the inflammatory process.

Taurine is involved in development, with substantial evidence supporting a crucial role during the pre- and postnatal development of the central nervous and visual systems. The specific manner in which taurine participates in these events is not clear. In primates deprived of taurine, retinal changes, impaired visual acuity, and degenerative ultrastructural changes in photoreceptor outer segments have been observed, with changes being more severe in younger animals (37, 48). Some human infants and children whose only nutrition was taurine-free parenteral infusion or taurine-devoid formulas have exhibited ophthalmoscopically and electrophysiologically detectable retinal abnormalities and immature brainstem auditory-evoked responses (37, 48).

POSSIBLE CAUSES OF DEFICIENCY OF CYSTEINE OR TAURINE

Inability to Synthesize or Conserve

Immaturity

Immaturity may be associated with a conditional requirement for both cysteine and taurine. Preterm infants (≤32 weeks gestation) have a low capacity for transsulfuration (low cystathionine γ-lyase activity), low plasma Cys concentrations, elevated plasma cystathionine concentrations, and a low rate of GSH synthesis from methionine in erythrocytes (116, 117). These observations all suggest that transsulfuration may be insufficient to meet the cysteine requirements of the very premature infant. Full-term formula-fed infants have also been observed to have increased cystathionine and decreased taurine levels in urine, suggesting a limited capacity for transsulfuration even in term infants (118).

In addition to a limited capacity to convert methionine to cysteine and hence to taurine (low synthetic rate), several other characteristics of premature infants contribute to their conditional requirement for taurine and/or cysteine (15, 48). First, the premature infant may have a greater requirement for cysteine because of more rapid growth and for taurine because of a likely role of taurine in development of the nervous and visual systems. The brain and retina of developing animals have high taurine concentrations, and morphologic and functional impairments have been observed in animals deprived of taurine during development. Second, premature infants are born with lower stores of taurine than are mature infants. Third, the β-amino acid transport system in the immature kidney does not adapt to poor taurine status by increasing reabsorption of taurine. The urinary taurine content of premature neonates is markedly elevated, with a fractional excretion ranging from 38 to 60%, compared with fractional excretion below 10% in term infants. Premature infants who received parenteral nutrition solutions devoid of taurine had high urinary taurine excretion rates despite very low plasma taurine values (47, 119, 120). By contrast, term neonates given a taurine-deficient parenteral nutrition solution can maintain plasma taurine concentrations by increased renal reabsorption of taurine with as little as 1% of the filtered taurine load being excreted. (See also Chapter 51 concerning taurine administration parenterally.)

Hepatic Dysfunction

Because liver is the major site for transsulfuration and taurine synthesis, hepatic dysfunction can adversely affect sulfur amino acid status. Patients with advanced forms of liver dysfunction or cirrhosis had low plasma taurine, Cys, and glutathione concentrations, an elevated plasma cystathionine concentration, decreased urinary taurine excretion, a decreased ratio of urinary sulfate to total sulfur, and increased urinary excretion of Cys and cystathionine (121, 122). These patients appeared to have a decreased ability to metabolize methionine (to cysteine, with cystathionine accumulation) and cysteine (to taurine and inorganic sulfate, with thiosulfate, Cys, and *N*-acetylcysteine accumulation).

Inadequate Supply Relative to Need

Total Parenteral Nutrition

Patients on long-term total parenteral nutrition (TPN) have experienced adverse effects on their sulfur amino acid status, both because of the route of administration and the composition of the TPN solutions. The amino acid mixtures used for TPN solutions usually contain little if any cysteine, because cysteine is rapidly converted to its disulfide, cystine, which is very insoluble in aqueous solution. Taurine is not routinely added to adult TPN solutions. Hence, patients on TPN must synthesize both cysteine and taurine from the methionine provided by TPN (see Chapter 101). However, synthesis of cysteine and taurine from methionine is restricted when first-pass metabolism by the liver is bypassed with parenteral alimentation. In adult subjects given parenteral alimentation solutions free of Cys via different routes, plasma Cys concentration dropped markedly when the feeding was via the parenteral route whereas it rose when feeding was switched to the oral route (123). The liver apparently removes much of the methionine on the first pass when solutions are administered by the oral route, thus facilitating cysteine and taurine synthesis from methionine.

Vegan Diets

Because strict vegan diets tend to be lower in total sulfur amino acid content and virtually free of taurine, adult vegans and particularly children consuming vegan diets are at somewhat greater risk of inadequate sulfur amino acid status. Adult humans who consume a strict vegetarian diet have been reported to have lower plasma taurine concentrations and greatly reduced urinary taurine excretion compared with omnivores. However, vegans consuming little or no preformed taurine are healthy, and the children born to and nursed by vegan mothers have normal growth and development (25). (See Chapter 106.)

Drug Metabolism

Various drugs and toxins are partially metabolized and excreted by conjugation with sulfate, glutathione (mercapturic acid synthesis), or even taurine. Rats fed up to 1 g (6.6 mmol) of acetaminophen per 100 g diet experienced dose-dependent inhibition of growth that was independent of hepatotoxicity and that could be overcome by addition of methionine or cyst(e)ine to the diet (99, 124). Lauterburg and Mitchell (99) found that therapeutic doses of acetaminophen (600 and 1200 mg, or 4 and 8 mmol) administered to healthy adult subjects markedly stimulated the rate of turnover of the pool of Cys available for synthesis of GSH. Patients and volunteers with prolonged ingestion of acetaminophen in doses of 2 to 4 g (13–26 mmol) per day had a decreased urinary output of inorganic sulfate but no decrease in plasma sulfate concentrations (125). Subjects produced a maximum of 0.6 mmol/h of acetaminophen sulfate, whereas total sulfur excretion was 7.5 to 26.7 mmol/24 h (0.3–1.1 mmol/h). A marginal sulfur amino acid intake accompanied by prolonged ingestion of high doses of drugs or toxins that are metabolized by sulfate and/or glutathione conjugation could have adverse effects on both sulfur amino acid status and drug metabolism.

MEASURES OF TAURINE STATUS AND OF CYSTEINE AND/OR SULFUR AMINO ACID STATUS

Sulfur amino acid adequacy has generally been assessed by measures of nitrogen balance or growth. Although growth and nitrogen balance have been used to define the nutritional requirements for amino acids, they are not necessarily good indicators of whether or not sulfur amino acid intake is sufficient for optimal rates of production of glutathione, inorganic sulfur, or taurine.

Plasma and blood taurine concentrations, plasma tCys concentration, and the plasma glutathione concentration have been used as indicators of sulfur amino acid status. Normal values for these measures are discussed above in this chapter.

Because most of the sulfur from sulfur amino acids is excreted in the urine, primarily as inorganic sulfate, measures of total urinary sulfur or of urinary sulfate are useful indicators of sulfur amino acid intake and/or metabolism. The urinary taurine level can also be used as an indicator of adequate supply of sulfur amino acids or taurine because taurine excretion increases as plasma taurine concentration and/or taurine intake increases.

RECOMMENDED INTAKES FOR HUMANS

The estimated upper-end requirement for sulfur amino acids (methionine plus cyst(e)ine) is 58 mg/kg/day for infants, 27 mg/kg/day for children (~age 2 years), 22 mg/kg/day for older children (~10–12 years), and 13 mg/kg/day for adults (28). A conservative estimate of methionine replacement by cyst(e)ine, up to 30% of the methionine requirement, is suggested (28). In cases of limited ability to convert methionine to cysteine (whether due to hepatic dysfunction, inborn errors of methionine metabolism to cysteine, or prematurity), the total amount of sulfur amino acids in the diet, the balance of cysteine and methionine, and the adequacy of taurine should all be considered.

By consensus, taurine is considered conditionally essential during infant development and probably for adults in some special circumstances. Because brain and retina of human infants are not fully developed at birth and may be vulnerable to the effects of taurine deprivation, it has been judged prudent to supplement human infant formulas and pediatric feeding solutions with taurine (15, 37). During the 1980s, manufacturers of infant formulas began adding taurine to their products, and taurine is presently added to virtually all human infant formulas and pediatric parenteral solutions throughout the world. The taurine content of human milk has been used as a guideline for supplementation levels.

TOXICITY

Large doses of cysteine or cystine are neuroexcitotoxic in several species. The effect of cysteine seems to involve the *N*-methyl-D-aspartate subtype of the glutamate receptor for which cysteine sulfinate and cysteic acid are agonists (125–129). Single injections of cysteine (0.6–1.5 g/kg) into 4-day-old rat pups resulted in massive damage to cortical neurons (130), permanent retinal dystrophy (131), atrophy of the brain (132), and hyperactivity (126). Cats fed a 5% cystine diet had no obvious immediate ill effects but exhibited acute neurotoxic symptoms after several months (133). The onset of symptoms in the cats was sudden, with rapid progression to a moribund state or death, usually within 48 hours. The morphologic changes observed in the retinas of cats fed the cystine-rich diets were comparable to those described in the retinas of young rodents treated with glutamate or certain other acidic or excitotoxic amino acids. It is not clear whether cysteine or a metabolite (cysteine sulfinate) is responsible for the cytotoxicity. These observations have given rise to concerns about administration of excess cyst(e)ine to humans, especially to infants.

Studies in rodents also demonstrated influences of dietary sulfur amino acids on lipid metabolism, with 2 to 5% (by wt) L-cystine resulting in elevated plasma cholesterol concentration, increased hepatic cholesterol biosynthesis, and depressed plasma ceruloplasmin activity (134, 135). Excess L-cysteine (0.8 or 2% of diet by wt) did not result in an elevation in plasma cholesterol whereas addition of 0.8% L-methionine did (135, 136).

Sturman and Messing (137) found no evidence of adverse effects of prolonged feeding of high taurine diets (up to 1 g [8 mmol]/100 g diet) on adult female cats or their offspring. In fact, taurine may protect against toxic effects of some other compounds. Taurine addition to cat diets provided some protection against the adverse effects of a high level of cystine, supporting a neuroprotective role of taurine against the excitotoxic damages in the mammalian nervous system (133). Studies in rodents have suggested that dietary taurine also has hypolipidemic and antiatherosclerotic effects (138, 139).

REFERENCES

1. Osborne TB, Mendel LR. J Biol Chem 1915;20:351–78.
2. Mueller JH. Proc Soc Exp Biol Med 1921;19:161–3.
3. Jackson RW, Block RJ. J Biol Chem 1932;98:465–77.
4. Womack M, Kemmerer KS, Rose WC. J Biol Chem 1937;121:403–10.
5. Rose WC, Wixom RL. J Biol Chem 1955;216:763–73.
6. du Vigneaud VE. Trail of research in sulfur chemistry and metabolism and related fields. Ithaca, NY: Cornell University Press, 1952.
7. Carson NAJ, Neill DW. Arch Dis Child 1962;37:505–13.
8. Clarke R, Daly L, Robinson K, et al. N Engl J Med 1991;324:1149–55.
9. Robinson K, Mayer E, Jacobsen DW. Cleve Clin J Med 1994;61:438–50.
10. Steegers-Theunissen RPM, Boers GHJ, Trijbels FJM, et al. Metabolism 1994;43:1475–80.
11. Wouters MCAJ, Boers GHJ, Blom HJ, et al. Fertil Steril 1993;60:820–5.
12. Tiedemann F, Gmelin L. Ann Physik Chem 1827;9:326–37.
13. Hayes KC, Carey RE, Schmidt SY. Science 1975;188:949–51.
14. Sturman JA, Rassin DK, Gaull GE. Life Sci 1977;21:1–22.
15. Sturman JA. Physiol Rev 1993;73:119–47.
16. Mansoor MA, Bergmark C, Svardal AM, et al. Arterioscler Thromb Vasc Biol 1995;15:232–40.
17. Andersson A, Isaksson A, Brattstrom L, et al. Clin Chem 1993;39:1590–7.
18. Mansoor MA, Ueland PM, Svardal AM. Am J Clin Nutr 1994;59:631–5.
19. Guttormsen AB, Schneede J, Fiskerstrand R, et al. J Nutr 1994;124:1934–41.
20. Selhub J, Jacques PF, Wilson PWF, et al. JAMA 1993;270: 2693–8.

21. Dalery K, Lussier-Cacan S, Selhub J, et al. Am J Cardiol 1995;75:1107–11.
22. Nygard O, Vollset SE, Refsum H, et al. JAMA 1995;274:1526–33.
23. Rasmussen K, Moller J, Lyngbak M, et al. Clin Chem 1996;42:630–6.
24. Trautwein EA, Hayes KC. Am J Clin Nutr 1990;52:758–64.
25. Rana SK, Sanders TAB. Br J Nutr 1986;56:17–27.
26. Laidlaw SA, Shultz TD, Cecchino JT, et al. Am J Clin Nutr 1988;47:660–3.
27. Malinow MR, Axthelm MK, Meredith MJ, et al. J Lab Clin Med 1994;123:421–9.
28. National Research Council. Recommended dietary allowances. 10th ed. Washington, DC: National Academy Press, 1989.
29. US Department of Agriculture. Agricultural handbook no. 8. Agriculture Research Service, United States Department of Agriculture, 1976–1986.
30. Young VR, Wagner DA, Burini R, et al. Am J Clin Nutr 1991;54:377–85.
31. Storch KJ, Wagner DA, Burke JF, et al. Am J Physiol 1988;255:E322–31.
32. FAO/WHO/UNI. Energy and protein requirements. WHO technical report #724. Geneva: World Health Organization, 1985.
33. Laidlaw SA, Grosvenor M, Kopple JD. JPEN 1990;14:183–8.
34. Pasantes-Morales H, Quesada O, Alcocer L, et al. Nutr Rep Int 1989;40:793–801.
35. Roe DA, Weston MO. Nature 1965;203:287–8.
36. Kataoka H, Ohnishi N. Agric Biol Chem 1986;50:1887–8.
37. Huxtable RJ. Physiol Rev 1992;72:101–63.
38. Rassin DK, Sturman JA, Gaull GE. Early Hum Dev 1978;2:1–13.
39. Paauw JD, Davis AT. Am J Clin Nutr 1994;60:203–6.
40. Martensson J, Hermansson G. Metabolism 1984;33:425–8.
41. Palacin M, Chillaron J, Mora C. Biochem Soc Trans 1996;24:856–63.
42. Mora C, Chillaron J, Calonge MJ, et al. J Biol Chem 1996;271:10569–76.
43. Chillaron J, Estevez R, Mora C, et al. J Biol Chem 1996;271:17761–70.
44. Sakhaee K. Miner Electrolyte Metab 1994;20:414–23.
45. Refsum H, Helland S, Ueland PM. Clin Chem 1985;31:624–8.
46. Erbe RW. Inborn errors of folate metabolism. In: Blakley RL, Whitehead VM, eds. Folates and pterins, vol 3. New York: John Wiley & Sons, 1986;413–65.
47. Jensen H. Biochim Biophys Acta 1994;1194:44–52.
48. Sturman JA, Chesney RW. Pediatr Nutr 1995;42:879–97.
49. McKeever MP, Weir DG, Molloy A, et al. Clin Sci 1991;81: 551–6.
50. Poole JR, Mudd SH, Conerly E, et al. J Clin Invest 1975;55:1033–48.
51. Stipanuk MH. Annu Rev Nutr 1986;6:179–209.
52. Backlund PS Jr, Smith RA. J Biol Chem 1981;256:1533–5.
53. Storch KJ, Wagner DA, Burke JF, et al. Am J Physiol 1990;258:E790–8.
54. Selhub J, Miller J. Am J Clin Nutr 1992;55:131–8.
55. Stipanuk MH, Benevenga NJ. J Nutr 1977;107:1455–67.
56. Storch KJ, Wagner DA, Young VR. Am J Clin Nutr 1991;54:386–94.
57. Shih VE, Fringer JM, Mandell R, et al. Am J Hum Genet 1995;57:34–9.
58. Mudd SH, Levy HL, Skovby F. Disorders of transsulfuration. In: Scriver CR, Beaudet AL, Sly WS, Valle D, eds. The metabolic and molecular bases of inherited disease, vol 1. New York: McGraw-Hill, 1995;1279–327.
59. Kraus JP. J Inherited Metab Dis 1994;17:383–90.
60. Sebastio G, Sperandeo MP, Panico M, et al. Am J Hum Genet 1995;56:1324–33.
61. Goyette P, Frosst P, Rosenblatt DS, et al. Am J Hum Genet 1995;56:1052–9.
62. Rozen R. Clin Invest Med 1996;19:171–8.
63. Fenton WA, Rosenberg LE. Inherited disorders of cobalamin transport and metabolism. In: Scriver CR, Beaudet AL, Sly WS, Valle D, eds. The metabolic and molecular bases of inherited disease, vol 3. New York: McGraw-Hill, 1995;3129–49.
64. Engbersen AMT, Franken DG, Bower GHJ, et al. Am J Hum Genet 1995;56:142–50.
65. Jacques PF, Bostom AG, Williams RR, et al. Circulation 1996;93:7–9.
66. Kang S-S, Wong PWK, Bock H-GO, et al. Am J Hum Genet 1991;48:546–51.
67. Rozen R, Jacques P, Bostom A, et al. Am J Hum Genet 1995;57S:A250.
68. Kang S-S, Wong PWK, Susmano A, et al. Am J Hum Genet 1991;48:536–46.
69. Van der Put NMJ, Steegers-Theunissen RPM, Frosst P, et al. Lancet 1995;346:1070–1.
70. Guttormsen AB, Schneede J, Ueland PM, et al. Am J Clin Nutr 1996;63:194–202.
71. Verhoef P, Stampfer MJ, Buring JE, et al. Am J Epidemiol 1996;143:845–59.
72. Ubbink JB, van der Merwe A, Delport R, et al. J Clin Invest 1996;98:177–84.
73. Boushey CJ, Beresford SAA, Omenn GS, et al. JAMA 1995;274:1049–57.
74. Ubbink JH, Becker PJ, Vermaak WJH, et al. Clin Chem 1995;41:1033–7.
75. Schmitz C, Lindpaintner K, Verhoef P, et al. Circulation 1996;94:1812–4.
76. Arnadotti M, Hultberg B, Nilsson-Ehle P, et al. Scand J Clin Invest 1996;56:41–6.
77. Chauveau P, Chadefaux B, Conde M, et al. Miner Electrolyte Metab 1996;22:106–9.
78. den Heijer M, Koster R, Blom HJ, et al. N Engl J Med 1996;334:759–62.
79. Mills JL, Scott JM, Kirke PN, et al. J Nutr 1996;126:756S–60S.
80. Selhub J, Jacques PF, Bostom AG, et al. N Engl J Med 1995;332:286–91.
81. Goddijn-Wessel TAW, Wouters MGAJ, Van de Molen EF. Eur J Obstet Gynecol Reprod Biol 1996;66:23–9.
82. Kluijtmans LAJ, van den Heuvel LPWJ, Boers GHJ, et al. Am J Hum Genet 1996;58:35–41.
83. Harpel PC, Zhang X, Borth W. J Nutr 1996;126:1285S–9S.
84. Blom HJ, Van der Molen EF. Fibrinolysis 1994;8(Suppl 2):86–7.
85. Lentz SR, Sobey CG, Piegors DJ, et al. J Clin Invest 1996;98:24–9.
86. Tsai JC, Wang H, Perrella MA, et al. J Clin Invest 1996;97:146–53.
87. Moephuli SR, Klein NW, Baldwin MT, et al. Proc Natl Acad Sci USA 1997;94:543–8.
88. Eskes TKAB. Eur J Obstet Gynecol Reprod Biol 1997;71: 105–11.
89. Bostom AG, Jacques PF, Nadeau MR, et al. Atherosclerosis 1995;116:147–51.
90. Tsai MY, Garg U, Key NS, et al. Atherosclerosis 1996;122: 69–77.
91. Dudman NPB, Guo X-W, Gordon RB, et al. J Nutr 1996;126:12295S–300S.
92. Zeisel J, Blusztajn JK. Annu Rev Nutr 1994;14:269–96.

93. Rosenblatt DS. Inherited disorders of folate transport and metabolism. In: Scriver CR, Beaudet AL, Sly WS, Valle D, eds. The metabolic and molecular bases of inherited disease, vol 3. 7th ed. New York, McGraw-Hill, 1995;3111–28.
94. Brattstrom LE, Israelsson B, Jeppsson JO, et al. Scand J Clin Lab Invest 1988;48:215–21.
95. Ubbink JB, Vermaak WJH, van der Merwe A, et al. J Nutr 1994;124:1927–33.
96. Kang S-S. J Nutr 1996;126:1273S–5S.
97. Fortin LJ, Genest J Jr. Clin Biochem 1996;28:155–62.
98. Lieberman MW, Wiseman AL, Shi ZZ, et al. Proc Natl Acad Sci USA 1996;93:7923–6.
99. Lauterburg BH, Mitchell JR. J Hepatol 1987;4:206–211.
100. Fukagawa NK, Ajami AM, Young VR. Am J Physiol 1996:270:E209–14.
101. Crawhall JC. Clin Biochem 1985;18:139–42.
102. Bella DL, Kwon YH, Stipanuk MH. J Nutr 1996;126:2179–87.
103. Martensson J. Metabolism 1982;31:487–92.
104. Koide T, Watanabe M, Shimada M. Acta Histochem Cytochem 1994;27:384.
105. Davies MH, Ngong JM, Pean A, et al. J Hepatol 1995;22:551–60.
106. Bradley H, Gough A, Sokhi RS, et al. J Rheumatol 1994;21:1192–6.
107. Gaull GE, Rassin DK, Raiha NCR, et al. J Pediatr 1977;90:348–55.
108. Irving CS, Marks L, Klein PD, et al. Life Sci 1986;38:491–5.
109. Bella DL, Stipanuk MH. Am J Physiol 1995;269:E910–7.
110. DeLeve LD, Kaplowitz N. Pharmacol Ther 1991;52:287–305.
111. Meister A. Pharmacol Ther 1991;51:155–94.
112. Hinchman CA, Ballatori N. J Toxicol Environ Health 1994;41:387–409.
113. Sasse CE, Baker DH. Dev Brain Dysfunct 1994;7:230–6.
114. Brueton MJ, Berger HM, Brown GA, et al. Gut 1978;19:95–8.
115. Wasserhess P, Becker M, Staab D. Am J Clin Nutr 1993;58:349–53.
116. Miller RG, Jahoor F, Jaksic T. J Pediatr Surg 1995;30:953–8.
117. Vina J, Vento M, Garcia-Sala F, et al. Am J Clin Nutr 1995;61:1067–9.
118. Martensson J, Finnstrom O. Early Hum Dev 1985;11:333–9.
119. Zelikovic I, Chesney RW, Friedman AL, et al. J Pediatr 1990;116:301–6.
120. Helms RA, Christensen ML, Storm MC, et al. J Nutr Biochem 1995;6:462–6.
121. Chawla RK, Berry CJ, Kutner MH, et al. Am J Clin Nutr 1985;42:577–84.
122. Martensson J, Foberg U, Fryden A, et al. Scand J Gastroenterol 1992;27:405–11.
123. Stegink LD, den Besten L. Science 1972;178:514–6.
124. McLean AEM, Armstrong GR, Beales D. Biochem Pharmacol 1989;38:347–52.
125. Blackledge HM, O'Farrell JO, Minton NA, et al. Hum Exp Toxicol 1991;10:159–65.
126. Mathisen GA, Fonnum F, Paulsen RE. Neurochem Res 1996;21:293–8.
127. Santucci AC, Spincola L-J. Dev Brain Dysfunct 1994;7:230–6.
128. Porter RHP, Roberts PJ. Neurosci Lett 1993;154:78–80.
129. Zerangue N, Kavanaugh MP. J Physiol 1996;493:419–23.
130. Sandberg M, Orwar O, Hehmann A. J Neurochem 1991;57:S152.
131. Pedersen OO, Lund-Karlsen R. Invest Ophthalmol Vis Sci 1980;19:886–92.
132. Lund-Karlsen R, Grofova I, Malthe-Sorenssen D, et al. Brain Res 1981;208:167–80.
133. Imaki H, Sturman JA. Nutr Res 1990;10:1385–400.
134. Serougne C, Ferezou J, Rukaj A. Biochim Biophys Acta 1987;921:522–30.
135. Yang B-S, Wan Q, Kato N. Biosci Biotech Biochem 1994;58:1177–8.
136. Sugiyama K, Akai H, Muramatsu K. J Nutri Sci Vitaminol 1986;32:537–49.
137. Sturman JA, Messing JM. J Nutr 1992;122:82–8.
138. Murakami S, Yamagishi I, Asami Y, et al. Pharmacology 1996;52:303–13.
139. Kamata K, Sugiura M, Kojima S, et al. Eur J Pharmacol 1996;303:47–53.

SELECTED READINGS

Boushey CJ, Beresford SAA, Omenn GS, et al. A quantitative assessment of plasma homocysteine as a risk factor for vascular disease. Probable benefits of increasing folic acid intakes. JAMA 1995;274:1049–57.
DeLeve LD, Kaplowitz N. Glutathione metabolism and its role in hepatotoxicity. Pharmacol Ther 1991;52:287–305.
Kang S-S. Treatment of hyperhomocyst(e)inemia: physiological basis. J Nutr 1996;126:1273S–5S.
Rozen R. Molecular genetic aspects of hyperhomocysteinemia and its relation to folic acid. Clin Invest Med 1996;19:171–8.
Stipanuk MH. Metabolism of sulfur-containing amino acids. Annu Rev Nutr 1986;6:179–209.
Sturman JA. Taurine in development. Physiol Rev 1993;73:119–47.

35. Glutamine and Arginine

STEVE F. ABCOUWER and WILEY W. SOUBA

The amino acids glutamine (GLN) and arginine (ARG) are of special interest because they have been recently classified as conditionally essential amino acids, indicating that they may be required in increased amounts by patients suffering from a catabolic insult such as injury, cancer, or severe infection (see Chapter 1). However, the utility of including glutamine or arginine in the nutritional support of patients recovering from surgery or suffering from trauma, infection, or cancer has yet to be conclusively demonstrated in clinical settings. Most studies examining the metabolism of these two amino acids have used cultured cells and animal models of trauma or infection. A wealth of experimental data proves the ability of glutamine-supplemented parenteral nutrition to support gut function, improve nitrogen balance, and alleviate catabolic demands upon muscle mass. In addition, limited clinical trials have found that glutamine feeding improves patient outcome in a number of settings (Table 35.1). Similarly, experimental data have shown that arginine can promote intestinal function and repair, promote wound healing, stimulate endocrine hormone production, and improve immune system function. Limited clinical trials have confirmed that inclusion of arginine in enteral and parenteral nutrition can improve nitrogen balance and immune defenses of patients (see [1] for a recent review). This chapter reviews a selection of these experimental and clinical studies and examines the limitations of these two nutrients as therapeutic adjuvants.

GLUTAMINE METABOLISM

Glutamine as a Nitrogen Carrier

The presence of two nitrogen atoms, an α-amino group and an amide group, as well as the abundance of glutamine in plasma combine to make this amino acid the most important "nitrogen shuttle" in the body. In fact, approximately one-third of all amino acid–derived nitrogen transported by the blood is in the form of glutamine. This amino acid serves as a vehicle for transportation of ammonia in a nontoxic form from peripheral tissues to visceral organs where it can be excreted as ammonium by the kidneys or converted to urea by the liver. The vast majority of nitrogen supplied by muscle in the postprandial period is exported as glutamine (2). Ammonia derived from glutamine in the mitochondria (by hydrolysis of glutamine to glutamate by the enzyme glutaminase or by hydrolysis of glutamate to α-ketoglutarate by the enzyme glutamate dehydrogenase) can combine with CO_2 to form carbamoyl phosphate that then enters the urea cycle (3). The amino group of glutamate can be used in the synthesis of aspartate from oxaloacetate. Through aspartate, the amino nitrogen of glutamine can also enter the urea cycle. In fact, glutamine is the major source of both nitrogen used in hepatic ureagenesis (4) and nitrogen excreted in urine (5). In addition, perfusion of isolated rat livers with glutamine greatly stimulated urea output (6, 7).

The liver has evolved an elegant mechanism for concerted ammonia detoxification and glutamine supply (8). In the periportal region, high incoming concentrations of ammonia from the splanchnic bed are utilized for urea synthesis while at the same time ammonia and glutamate are being generated from incoming glutamine by the hepatic isozyme of the enzyme glutaminase. In the perivenous portion of the liver, high levels of glutamine synthetase convert glutamate and excess ammonia into glutamine, effectively reducing the ammonia concentrations in hepatic venous blood to non-toxic levels. With this intraorgan glutamine cycle, the liver is able to effectively detoxify incoming blood of ammonia and control output of glutamine. In contrast, the kidney counteracts acidosis by utilizing a the "kidney-type" isozyme of glutaminase to generate ammonia from glutamine (9). The kidney disposes of excess nitrogen by consuming glutamine and excreting the ammonia produced (10).

Table 35.1
Clinical Studies Demonstrating Benefits of Supplementing TPN with Glutamine (GLN)

Population Studied	Type of Study	Endpoints Measured	Effect of GLN Supplementation	Comments/Criticisms
Postoperative cholecystectomy (63)	Randomized, controlled clinical trial	Nitrogen balance Muscle glutamine concentration Muscle ribosomal content	Improved nitrogen balance Diminished fall in muscle GLN Improved muscle protein synthesis	Cholecystectomy patients would not ordinarily receive postop TPN; no impact on surgical outcome
Postoperative, resection for colorectal cancer (62)	Randomized, controlled clinical trial	Nitrogen balance Muscle glutamine concentration	Improved cumulative nitrogen balance Preserved muscle GLN levels	These patients would not ordinarily receive TPN; no impact on outcome
Bone marrow transplant for hematologic malignancies (188)	Double-blind, randomized, controlled clinical trial	Extracellular water and total body water	Water retention and expansion of the extracellular fluid compartment were attenuated	Mechanism by which GLN-supplemented TPN restores normal body fluid distribution was not addressed
Bone marrow transplant for hematologic malignancies (189)	Double-blind, randomized, controlled clinical trial	Nitrogen balance Infectious incidence Length of stay	Improved nitrogen balance Diminished incidence of infection Shortened hospital stay by 7 days	Improvements observed despite no differences between groups in the incidence of fever, antibiotic requirements, or time to neutrophil engraftment
Bone marrow transplant (liquid/solid tumors) (190)	Randomized, double-blind clinical trial	Nitrogen balance Infectious complications Length of stay	Reduction in total body water Reduced length of stay	A 6-day reduction in hospital was associated with considerable cost savings
Gastrointestinal diseases (191)	Randomized, controlled clinical trial	Intestinal permeability Mucosal morphometrics	Prevented deterioration of gut permeability Preserved mucosal structure	Glutamine is a principal gut mucosal fuel; impact of preserving gut barrier function was not studied
Postoperative, resection for colorectal cancer (192)	Randomized, controlled clinical trial	Peripheral blood T-cell response Proinflammatory cytokine production	Enhanced T-cell DNA synthesis	These patients would not ordinarily receive TPN; impact on infectious complications not studied
Short gut (193)	Each patient served as own control	Nutrient absorption TPN requirements Costs	39% improvement in protein absorption 33% decrease in stool volume Reduction in TPN requirements $ savings	Growth hormone was administered in conjunction with glutamine
Premature infants (194)	Double-blind, randomized, controlled clinical trial	Days of TPN Time to full feeding Ventilator days Length of stay	In babies <800 g receiving GLN, there was a reduction in TPN days, ventilator days, time to full feeding and a trend toward a shortened hospital stay	A larger study with longer follow-up is necessary to fully evaluate the safety of this treatment

Glutamine as a Metabolic Intermediate

Glutamine also plays a key role in cellular energetics and metabolism by functioning as an important source of cellular fuel as well as a source of carbon and nitrogen for metabolic intermediates and macromolecular synthesis (Fig. 35.1). Glutamine acts as a fuel through its partial oxidation to form lactate or its complete oxidation to form CO_2. In fact, glutamine can serve as the primary respiratory substrate in enterocytes, lymphocytes, and cells in culture (discussed below). Glutamine plays a key role in regulating protein synthesis in tissues and cultured cells (11–13). Glutamine itself is used in peptide synthesis and is a precursor to many other amino acids. In addition, glutamine is converted to numerous metabolic intermediates and donates an amine group in many metabolic pathways including those leading to purine and pyrimidine nucleotide synthesis and the formation of glucosamine. Acetyl groups derived from glutamine are used in the synthesis of fatty acids and therefore incorporated into membrane phospholipids. In the kidney and liver, the carbon skeleton of glutamine is used for gluconeogenesis during times of starvation (14, 15). Thus, glutamine has many important metabolic and synthetic roles essential for cellular viability.

The first step in the use of glutamine as a respiratory fuel, metabolic precursor, and nitrogen donor is its conversion to glutamate (GLU). Glutamate is the most abundant intracellular amino acid in most tissues, with the notable exception of muscle, in which intracellular glutamine levels exceed those of glutamate (16, 17). Glutamate and ammonia are formed by hydrolysis of glutamine's amide group by the enzyme glutaminase. Glutamate is also formed by transfer of glutamine's amide group, catalyzed by a number of transaminase enzymes. Enzymatic transfer of glutamine's amide nitrogen occurs in various synthetic

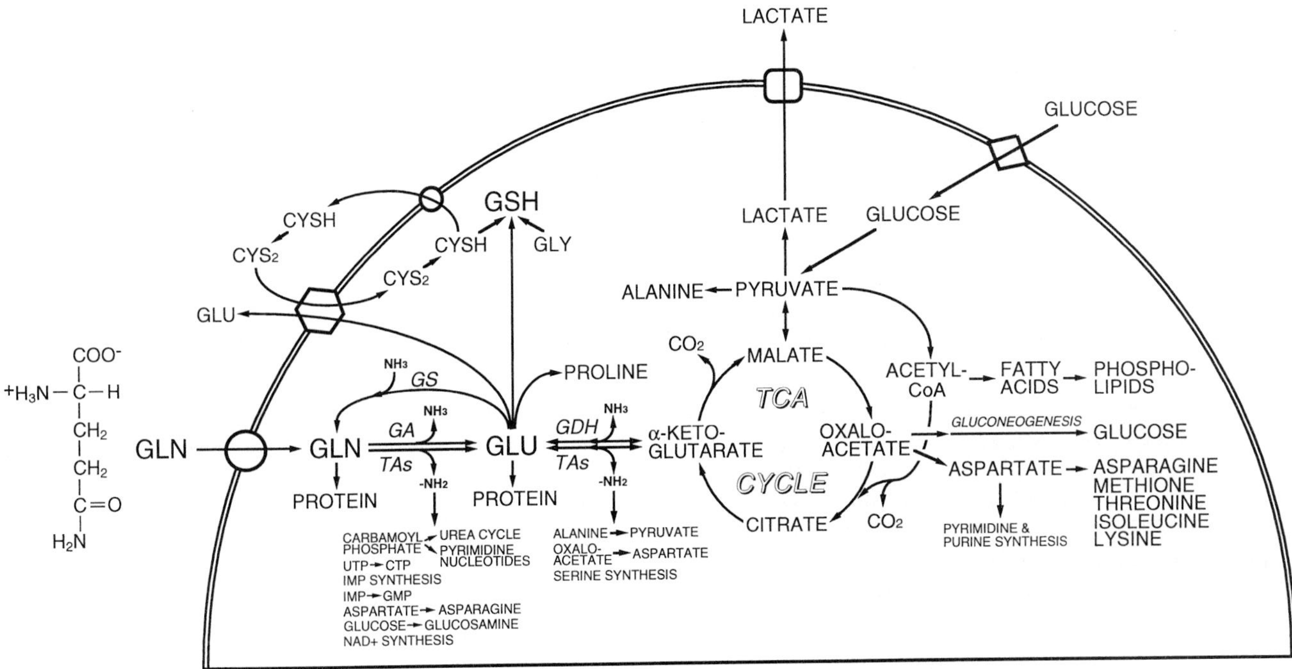

Figure 35.1. Metabolic functions of glutamine *(GLN)*. Glutamine enters the cell by an active carrier-mediated process. Most utilized glutamine is converted to glutamate *(GLU)* through hydrolysis catalyzed by the enzyme glutaminase *(GA)* and by a number of transaminase enzymes *(TAs)*. Glutamate is used in protein synthesis, used for glutathione *(GSH)* synthesis, and potentially converted back into glutamine by the enzyme glutamine synthetase *(GS)*. GLU is also exported from the cell in exchange for import of cystine *(CYS2)*. Imported cystine is converted to cysteine, which together with glutamate and glycine *(GLY)* form glutathione. GLU is converted to proline or converted to α-ketoglutarate by glutamate dehydrogenase *(GDH)* or transaminases. As α-ketoglutarate, the carbon backbone of glutamine enters the TCA cycle. Once in the TCA cycle the glutamine-derived carbons can be oxidized to CO_2 or serve as a backbone for formation of numerous metabolites and amino acids. In addition to glutamate and lactate, appreciable amounts of glutamine carbons are exported from the cell as aspartate, citrate, malate, pyruvate, alanine, and proline (16).

reactions. For example, glutamine is the nitrogen donor in formation of cytosolic carbamoyl phosphate, which is then used with aspartic acid in the committed step in pyrimidine synthesis (formation of *N*-carbamoylaspartate). Transamination from glutamine occurs in synthesis of the pyrimidine nucleotide CTP from UTP. In the purine biosynthetic pathway, glutamine contributes two amine groups in reactions leading to the synthesis of IMP and donates a third amine group in the conversion of IMP to GMP. Glutamine also provides an amide group for synthesis of asparagine, glucosamine, and nicotinamide adenine dinucleotide (NAD^+). Glutamate formed from glutamine can in turn be further deaminated, converted to proline or back into glutamine, used for glutathione synthesis, or exported. As glutamate, the α-amino group of glutamine is used in several transamination reactions including synthesis of alanine from pyruvate, synthesis of aspartate from oxaloacetate, and formation of phosphoserine, which is subsequently hydrolyzed to serine.

The five-carbon backbone of glutamine enters the tricarboxylic acid (TCA) cycle through conversion of glutamine-derived glutamate to α-ketoglutarate (2-oxoglutarate) by glutamate dehydrogenase or one of several transaminases. Via the TCA cycle, glutamine serves as a respiratory fuel source and the precursor of many synthetic intermediates. For example, through oxaloacetate, a TCA cycle intermediate, glutamine is used for gluconeogenesis or converted to aspartate or alanine. Aspartate can in turn be converted to asparagine, methionine, threonine, isoleucine, and lysine, be a precursor in pyrimidine synthesis, and again be an amine donor in purine synthesis (discussed above). Through malate and then pyruvate (the precursor of alanine), the carbon backbone of glutamine can be converted to lactate or acetyl-CoA. The acetyl group of acetyl-CoA can reenter the TCA cycle, eventually leading to the complete respiratory oxidation of glutamine carbons to CO_2. Acetyl-CoA also provides glutamine-derived carbon in the synthesis of fatty acids that can be used in production of phospholipids for cellular membranes.

Glutamine as a Supporter of Glutathione Metabolism

Considerable evidence suggests that glutamine may play a key role in the support of glutathione synthesis (Fig. 35.1) (see also Chapter 34). Glutathione, a tripeptide composed of glutamate, cysteine, and glycine, is the major store of cellular reducing equivalents and serves to protect cells from oxidative stress (18). As a source of intracellular glutamate, glutamine provides one of the constituents of glutathione. Glutamine carbons are incorporated into glutathione by rat kidney glomeruli (19), and the decline of hepatic glutathione levels during acetaminophen-induced liver injury was inhibited by treating rats with glutamine-supplemented parenteral nutrition (20). In fact, radioactive glutamine carbons are incorporated into glutathione in several animal tissues (20). Glutamine may also be essential for maintenance of cellular cysteine levels. Bannai and Ishii demonstrated a functional link between the use of glutamine and cystine (CYS2) by human diploid fibroblasts when they found that both the quantity of glutamine used and the quantity of glutamate released by these cells depended upon the concentration of cystine in the culture media (21). They concluded that approximately one-third of the glutamine used by these fibroblasts was used to produce extracellular glutamate. Tracer studies demonstrated that exported glutamate is a major end product of glutamine used by kidney cells (22) as well as several tumor cell lines (16). In our laboratory, we have found that approximately 40% of glutamine consumed by human breast cell lines and breast cancer cells is released as glutamate, and the rate of glutamate release by these cells also depends upon the extracellular concentration of cystine (16a). A working model predicts that glutamine, by serving as a source of glutamate, provides two of the three precursors for glutathione synthesis: glutamate itself, which is directly utilized in glutathione synthesis, and cysteine, which is derived from cystine imported via the export of glutamate. This role in glutathione synthesis suggests that glutamine availability may have profound effects upon cellular redox control and that glutamine utilization may be increased under conditions of oxidative stress.

Glutamine as an Energy Source

A substantial portion of glutamine can be used for cellular respiration. For example, HeLa and CHO cells each convert approximately 30% of catabolized glutamine carbons to CO_2 and 15% to lactate, while approximately 20% of its carbons are incorporated into macromolecules (23, 24). The total amount of cellular energy derived from glutamine depends upon the extent of oxidation and the rate of glutamine utilization. These factors in turn depend largely on the absolute amounts and relative proportions of glutamine and glucose available as well as the type and proliferative state of the cell. For example, glutamine is a primary fuel source for the intestine and for enterocytes in culture (25, 26). Likewise, thymocytes derive a large portion of their energy from glutamine oxidation, especially after mitogenic stimulation (27). Under physiologic conditions, glutamine oxidation can account for as much as one-third of the cellular ATP production in cultured cells of many types (28–30), and relative glutamine oxidation increases at lower glucose levels (24, 31). Cells survive and even grow in glucose-free media containing sufficient glutamine and nucleic acid precursors (32, 33). Thus, glutamine is an important source of cellular energy. However, little is known about what determines the rate of glutamine use or oxidation for a cell or tissue type.

GLUTAMINE IN CATABOLIC STATES

Interorgan Glutamine Transfer

During catabolic states, a combination of increased glutamine use and decreased nutrient uptake creates a glutamine demand that is met primarily by increased glutamine efflux from lung and muscle tissue (see also Chapter 98). Although plasma glutamine levels are usually maintained in septic rats and injured patients (34–36), lung and muscle glutamine stores can be rapidly depleted after injury or infection (34, 37–40). Muscle is a major producer of glutamine during normal and catabolic states. In the normal postabsorptive 200-g rat, glutamine is released from the hindquarter at a rate of approximately 0.4 mmol/min (35). Given that skeletal muscle glutamine concentrations are approximately 6 to 8 mmol/L intracellular water (41), even a normal rate of release cannot be sustained for long without de novo glutamine synthesis. During catabolic states the efflux of glutamine from rat and dog muscle increases markedly (34, 37, 42, 43), and increased net production rate must eventually compensate for this heightened release. The muscle can maintain a rapid efflux of glutamine in part by increasing the rate of proteolysis while decreasing the rate of protein synthesis (44). This increases the intracellular pool of amino acids for export and for production of glutamine, which can be derived from a large number of amino acids through their conversion to glutamate, either directly or through α-ketoglutarate (Fig. 35.1). Thus, any amino acid that can feed into the TCA cycle can support glutamine production. Glutamate can then be converted to glutamine by the action of glutamine synthetase (GS).

Muscle glutamine levels may be an indication of severe catabolic stress. Investigators have shown a significant correlation between survival in septic patients and skeletal muscle glutamine stores (45). In addition, an association between reduction of plasma and muscle glutamine levels and disease severity has been reported for pancreatitis patients (46). Presumably, muscle glutamine stores and glutamine supplied by muscle proteolysis do not suffice to meet demand for glutamine in some cases, because of either the magnitude of glutamine use or depletion of muscle mass.

Hormonal Influences on Glutamine Synthesis

Adrenocorticoids may play a pivotal role in regulation of glutamine metabolism in response to stress. Glucocorticoid hormones increase glutamine production and glutamine efflux from skeletal muscle, as well as GS mRNA levels in this tissue (47–49). In addition, the glucocorticoid receptor antagonist RU38486 reduces muscle glutamine content as well as the rate of glutamine release from muscle (50, 51). One established effect of glucocorticoids is augmentation of the GS transcription rate in muscle cells via the glucocorticoid receptor (52, 53).

Results from our laboratory have demonstrated that GS expression is induced in a tissue-specific fashion in rats following dexamethasone injection and major burn injury, with augmentation of GS mRNA levels in lung and muscle (54). In addition, we have found that the level of GS mRNA in rat skeletal muscle following burn injury and endotoxemia depends largely on the presence of the adrenal gland (55, 56). Although the adrenal glands produce other hormones (aldosterone and the sex steroids as well as epinephrine and norepinephrine), to our knowledge only glucocorticoids have been demonstrated to stimulate GS expression in skeletal muscle. However, glucocorticoids may not be the sole regulator of GS expression in catabolic states. We have found that GS expression in muscle does increase in response to injury and infection in adrenalectomized rats, although not to the levels observed in sham-operated animals with functional adrenal glands (55, 56).

The level of GS protein and activity is also influenced by posttranscriptional mechanisms. Depletion of glutamine in the media of cultured muscle cells causes a pronounced increase in GS activity and protein levels (57, 58). This effect is not due to an increase in GS mRNA levels, but instead, intracellular glutamine depletion causes the stability of GS protein to increase and thus the steady-state level to rise (59). Consistent with this mechanism, we have observed that the increase in GS protein levels observed in lung and muscle in response to glucocorticoids or sepsis is much lower than the increase in GS mRNA levels (54, 56).

Muscle-Sparing Effect of Glutamine

A major benefit of nutritional support including glutamine or glutamine precursors is to spare muscle mass. In the absence of nutritional support, the precursors for enhanced glutamine production by muscles of traumatized rats are derived from proteolysis of muscle protein (60, 61). Protein synthesis correlates with glutamine concentration in perfused rat muscles (41), and postoperative nutritional support including glutamine spares the muscle glutamine pool and stimulates muscle protein synthesis in both humans and animals (38, 62, 63). Provision of α-ketoglutarate (which can be converted to glutamate) can also help spare muscle glutamine pools in postoperative patients (64), demonstrating that synthesis of glutamine can keep pace with release if ample precursors are provided.

Glutamine Effect on Intestinal Repair and Function

Another clear benefit of glutamine supplementation during catabolic states is the promotion of gut structure and function. Several studies have found that enteral and parenteral glutamine reduces intestinal permeability and improves gut mucosal integrity in rat models of sepsis (65, 66). Intestinal sodium absorption in diarrheagenic *Escherichia coli*–infected rabbits can be enhanced by enteral administration of glutamine (67). Infusion of glutamine into the lumen of transplanted rat small intestine increases small bowel protein content and augments glucose absorption (68). Addition of glutamine to total parenteral nutrition (TPN) attenuated the endotoxin-induced damage to the jejunum and ileum in septic rats (69). In addition, enteral diets containing glutamine decreased bacterial translocation across the intestines of mice with major burn injuries (70). Inclusion of glutamine in parenteral nutrition formulations reduced the villous atrophy associated with long-term TPN administration to rats (71–73) and increased jejunal mucosal weight and DNA content (74). The intestine's dependence upon glutamine was also illustrated by the finding that depletion of plasma glutamine levels by intravenous injection of bacterial glutaminase caused diarrhea, mild villous atrophy, mucosal ulcerations, and intestinal necrosis in experimental animals (75). Work by Burke and colleagues suggested that addition of glutamine to TPN decreased bacterial translocation because of glutamine's ability to enhance the rat's gut immune function (76). Thus, glutamine may support gut function by a duel mechanism including stimulation of mucosal growth and intestinal immune surveillance.

Glutamine and Cancer

Numerous rodent studies have suggested that tumor burden creates an exaggerated glutamine demand that is met by increased glutamine production by host tissues (for examples see [77] and [78]). In light of the role of glutamine as a fuel for tumor cells, a pressing issue is whether glutamine-supplemented nutritional support will improve the outcome of cancer patients or accelerate tumor growth. Animal studies in which bacterial glutaminase was used to reduce plasma glutamine concentrations as well as those using glutamine antagonists have demonstrated the dependency of experimental tumors on glutamine for growth (for examples see [79] and [80]). Conversely, rodent studies also suggested that glutamine feeding benefits the tumor-bearing animals without enhancing tumor growth (81–83). It is conceivable that provision of glutamine can help alleviate glutamine depletion in muscle and thus reduce protein catabolism associated with cancer cachexia (83, 84). Recent studies found that glutamine enhanced the effectiveness of methotrexate in treatment of experimental tumors (85, 86). Glutamine also boosted the immune response to tumors implanted in rats by increasing killer cell activity (87).

Glutamine may be particularly useful for increasing tolerance to radiation and chemotherapy, thus allowing use of more effective dosages. For example, glutamine-supplemented nutritional support may accelerate healing of the intestinal injury that results from chemotherapy or radiation therapy. Addition of glutamine to an elemental enteral diet significantly reduced the severity of enterocolitis and mortality of rats given large doses of methotrexate (88). Addition of glutamine to this diet also reduced endotoxin transmigration from the gut lumen, caused by methotrexate. A glutamine-enriched intravenous diet accelerated healing of the gut mucosa in rats receiving 5-fluorouracil (5-FU) (89). Likewise, provision of oral glutamine following abdominal irradiation also supported gut glutamine metabolism and decreased the morbidity and mortality of rats subjected to abdominal radiation (90). Administration of a glutamine-enriched oral diet prior to abdominal radiation was equally beneficial to rats (91).

On balance, considerable evidence from rodent systems suggests that glutamine supplementation of the diets of cancer patients could provide benefits without increasing tumor proliferation. Theoretically, the impact of glutamine feeding on tumor growth would be determined by the actual impact upon plasma glutamine concentration, the effectiveness of glutamine delivery to the growing tumor, and whether or not growth of that particular tumor is indeed limited by glutamine availability. An examination of 65 human tumor xenografts found that only 20% exhibited appreciable net glutamine uptake, demonstrating that many tumors do not obtain sustenance from this nutrient (92). It is likely that many tumors ultimately become relatively glutamine-independent as they adapt to growth in the nutrient-deprived tumor microenvironment. These adapted tumors may not exhibit accelerated growth even if plasma glutamine supply is increased. It is conceivable that the benefits of glutamine-enriched nutrition upon muscle mass preservation, immune system function, and intestinal healing and function will consistently outweigh the risk that this nutrient might facilitate tumor growth.

ARGININE METABOLISM

Arginine and Nitrogen Balance

Although arginine contains four nitrogen atoms, it is not considered a major interorgan nitrogen shuttle. However, arginine does play an integral role in nitrogen metabolism as an intermediate in the urea cycle and is therefore essential for ammonia detoxification (Fig. 35.2). In the cytoplasm, arginine is hydrolyzed by arginase to form urea and ornithine. Ornithine is transported into the mitochondria where it is combined with carbamoyl phosphate to form citrulline. In contrast to cytosolic formation of carbamoyl phosphate, in which an amine group is derived by transamination from glutamine, mitochondrial carbamoyl phosphate is formed from carbon dioxide and ammonia derived largely from hydrolysis of glutamine. Citrulline then combines with aspartic acid in the cytosol to form arginosuccinate, which is then cleaved to form arginine and succinate. As arginine completes the cycle, two nitrogen molecules are shuttled into urea for excretion. One of these nitrogens is derived from mitochondrial ammonia and the other from cytosolic aspartate with the formation of fumarate. Fumarate enters the TCA cycle through malate and regenerates aspartate when oxaloacetate is transaminated via the conversion of α-amino acids to α-keto acids.

Arginine is not considered an essential amino acid because adult mammals can synthesize this amino acid de novo. However, plasma arginine levels are largely dictated by dietary intake, because arginine synthetic rates do not increase to compensate for inadequate supply (93, 94). In young rats and dogs, dietary arginine is essential and can be limiting for optimal growth (95, 96), and in mature animals, an arginine-free diet can cause ammonia toxicity (97). Arginine deficiency causes an increase in plasma ammonia levels by affecting function of the urea cycle. A large increase in orotic acid excretion in the urine is observed (98, 99), which may reflect use of carbamoyl phosphate for formation of carbamoyl aspartate (and subsequently orotate) rather than for synthesis of citrulline from ornithine. Arginine deficiency causes an increased flux of ornithine (but not of citrulline) across the portal-drained rat viscera (99). Arginine or ornithine supplementation alleviates ammonia toxicity while increasing liver citrulline and urea content as well as plasma urea levels in rats (100). This was interpreted as indicating that arginine increases ornithine decarboxyltransferase activity by increasing ornithine availability. Paradoxically, arginine deficiency in rats was alleviated by citrulline but not ornithine supplementation (101). Citrulline supplementation elevated plasma levels of arginine in the absence of increased splanchnic output of this amino acid, suggesting that arginine was produced from citrulline in nonsplanchnic organs such as the kidney. In fact, in the rat, citrulline, either infused or produced by the liver, is converted to arginine by the kidneys (102).

Arginine as a Metabolic Intermediate

Aside from its role in protein synthesis and as an intermediate in the urea cycle, arginine is a substrate for nitric oxide production (discussed below) and phosphocreatine synthesis as well as a precursor to glutamate, proline, and putrescine via ornithine (Fig. 35.2). Arginine is rapidly converted to ornithine in vivo so that administration of arginine causes a large increase in plasma ornithine levels (103). Many (but not all) of the therapeutic effects of arginine can be attributed to elevated plasma ornithine levels. Ornithine can be converted to glutamate via glutamic semialdehyde (104); however, there is little evidence of an appreciable flux of arginine to glutamate or glutamine in vivo, with the possible exception of the lactating mammary gland (105). By the action of ornithine aminotransferase, ornithine can also be converted to 1-pyrroline 5-carboxylate, a precursor for proline synthesis (104). In fact, much of the proline in extracellular wound fluid may be derived from arginine via ornithine (106). Ornithine is also used in the polyamine synthesis pathway, in which the initial step is the conversion of ornithine to putrescine by ornithine decarboxylase (107, 108). Polyamines play a key

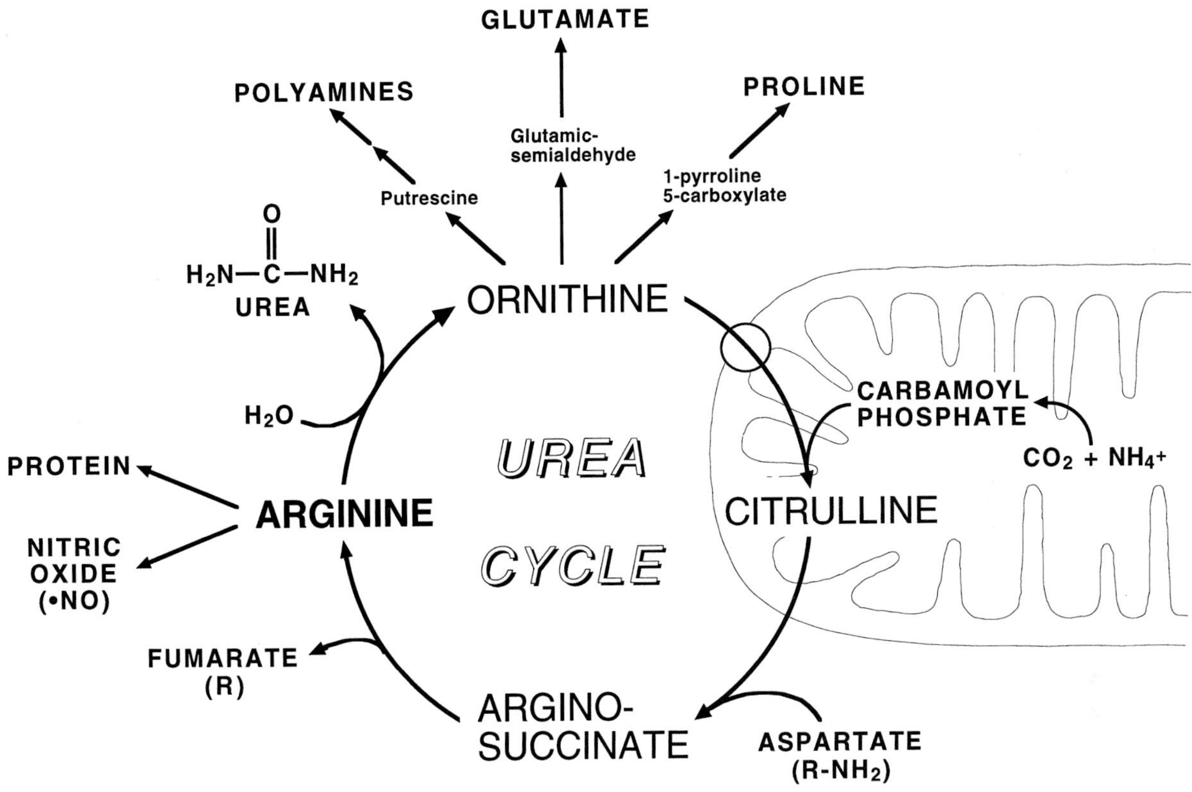

Figure 35.2. Metabolic functions of arginine. Arginine is used for protein synthesis, as an intermediate in the urea cycle, as a substrate for nitric oxide production and phosphocreatine synthesis as well as a precursor to glutamate, proline, and putrescine via ornithine. In the urea cycle, two nitrogen molecules are shuttled into urea for excretion. One of these nitrogens is derived from mitochondrial ammonia and the other from cytosolic aspartate with the formation of fumarate. In the cytoplasm, arginine is hydrolyzed by arginase to form urea and ornithine. Ornithine is transported into the mitochondria where it is combined with carbamoyl phosphate to form citrulline. Mitochondrial carbamoyl phosphate is formed from carbon dioxide and ammonia (as well as 2 ATPs and water). Citrulline then combines with aspartic acid in the cytosol to form arginosuccinate, which is then cleaved to form arginine and fumarate. Nitric oxide synthetase enzymes convert arginine to nitric oxide *(•NO)* and citrulline. Ornithine formed from arginine can be converted to glutamate via glutamic semialdehyde, to 1-pyrroline 5-carboxylate (a precursor for proline synthesis), or to the polyamine putrescine.

role in cellular proliferation for both normal and tumor cells (109). In fact, blockade of polyamine synthesis by inhibition of ornithine decarboxylase combined with limiting dietary intake of polyamines provides effective inhibition of experimental tumor growth (110).

Arginine as a Source of Nitric Oxide

An important role of arginine is as a substrate for nitric oxide (•NO). Nitric oxide has received considerable attention since its identification as endothelium-derived relaxation factor in 1987 (111, 112). Soon thereafter, arginine was shown to be the biologic precursor of nitric oxide (113, 114). This molecule and citrulline are formed from arginine by nitric oxide synthetase (Fig. 35.3). Three isoforms of this enzyme have been identified; two are constitutively expressed and one is inducible (115). An immense body of literature has been produced concerning the biologic roles and properties of nitric oxide (for recent reviews see [116] and [117]). This molecule plays a role in hypertension (118), myocardial dysfunction (119), inflammation (120), cell death (121), and protection against oxidative damage (122). Nitric oxide may mediate many of the effects of septic shock including vascular (123), myocardial (124), and hemodynamic instability (125). In fact, inhibition of nitric oxide synthesis (or specifically, inhibition of inducible nitric oxide synthetase, which is upregulated in many tissues during sepsis) has been explored as a therapy for septic shock. Inducible nitric oxide synthetase inhibitors increase blood pressure and vascular resistance and cause a decrease in cardiac output (126, 127). However, the utility of such treatments is still in question (125).

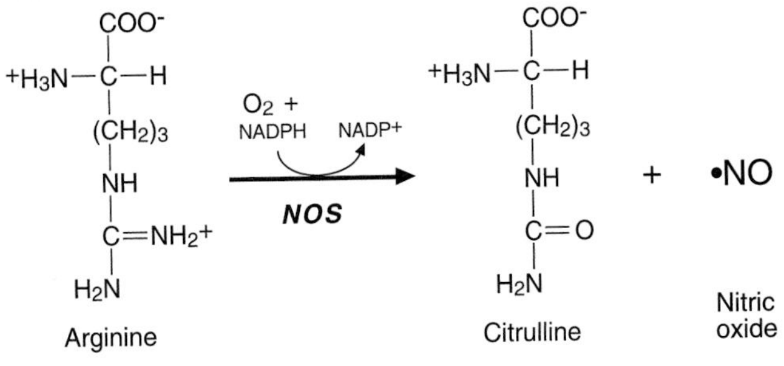

Arginine: $^{+}H_3N—CH(COO^-)—(CH_2)_3—NH—C(=NH_2^+)—H_2N$ → (O_2 + NADPH → $NADP^+$; NOS) → Citrulline: $^{+}H_3N—CH(COO^-)—(CH_2)_3—NH—C(=O)—H_2N$ + •NO (Nitric oxide)

Figure 35.3. Biosynthesis of nitric oxide *(•NO)* from arginine. One of three isoforms of nitric oxide synthase *(NOS)* combines nitrogen from arginine, oxygen from molecular oxygen *(O_2)* and electrons from NADPH to form •NO along with citrulline and $NADP^+$.

Nitric oxide synthesis provides protection to tissues after ischemia and reperfusion. During reperfusion, basal tissue nitric oxide synthesis is diminished, causing increased neutrophil adherence and infiltration (128–130). Numerous studies have demonstrated that inhibition of nitric oxide synthesis increases ischemia-reperfusion injury, whereas perfusion with nitric oxide or nitric oxide donors decreases injury and neutrophil accumulation (for recent reviews see [131] and [132]). In the lung, inhalation of nitric oxide gas can lower pulmonary vascular resistance after lung injury, surgery, and heart or lung transplant (133, 134). In other organs, arginine has been successfully used to increase basal nitric oxide synthesis and thus reduce ischemia-reperfusion injury (128, 135–138). This effect of arginine could also be due to increased vascular dilation. Extended oral supplementation of arginine to hypercholesterolemic young men with endothelial dysfunction increased endothelium-dependent dilation of the brachial artery during increased cardiac output (138a).

ARGININE IN CATABOLIC STATES

Arginine Deficiency in Catabolic States

During catabolic states, arginine may become a conditionally essential amino acid. This may be due to a number of contributing factors including an increased rate of arginine degradation (139), reduced dietary intake (140), and reduced gut absorption (141, 142), as well as reduced synthesis of citrulline by the gut (143).

Effect of Arginine upon Intestinal Function and Repair

Arginine has beneficial effects on gut function and repair following trauma or bowel resection. Bacterial translocation in septic rodents is reduced by arginine-supplemented diets (144, 145). This effect was largely abrogated by inhibition of nitric oxide synthesis, suggesting that arginine's beneficial effects may be due to support of the bactericidal function of immune cells. In rats, arginine promoted mucosal repair after intestinal ischemia (135) and relieved mucosal damage during endothelin-induced ulceration (146). Both of these effects were abrogated by inhibition of •NO synthesis. Arginine may also promote mucosal growth and repair by supporting polyamine synthesis (147). Brzozowski et al. found that intragastric injection of arginine accelerated healing of gastric ulcers in rats and that this effect could be attributed to stimulation of blood flow through increased nitric oxide synthesis, stimulation of mucosal growth though polyamine synthesis, and stimulation of plasma gastrin levels (148).

Effect of Arginine on Wound Healing

Arginine-supplemented diets and TPN can also promote wound healing. This supplementation increased both wound strength and collagen deposition in rats (106, 149, 150). Likewise, arginine-deficient diets reduced wound strength and collagen deposition in rats (151). Arginine promotes collagen synthesis by serving as a substrate for proline synthesis (106). Healing may also be stimulated by increased growth hormone secretion. This hypothesis is supported by the observation that the beneficial effect of arginine supplementation on wound healing was diminished in hypophysectomized rats (152).

Effect of Arginine on Endocrine Systems

Arginine administration has pronounced effects upon the adrenal and pituitary systems of humans. Arginine stimulates release of catecholamines (153), insulin (154, 155), glucagon (155, 156), growth hormone (157, 158), and prolactin (159). In addition, arginine increases insulin-like growth factor (IGF-1) levels in elderly patients (160, 161). However, little is known of how arginine exerts these effects upon endocrine systems. Regardless of the mechanisms involved, an increase in hormone levels may be key to some of arginine's positive metabolic effects following trauma and infection. As discussed above, stimulation of growth hormone secretion may play a key role in the support of wound healing by arginine. Stimulation of anabolic steroid levels may contribute to arginine's ability to increase the growth of rats following surgery or trauma (151, 162). Heightened growth hormone levels also counteract muscle glutamine depletion and preserve muscle protein synthesis rates in postoperative patients (163, 164). In addition, growth hormone replacement therapy positively affects natural killer cell activity levels in women (165).

Arginine and the Immune System

Arginine can alleviate posttraumatic immune depression as characterized by reduced lymphocyte function. Several studies by Barbul and colleagues have demonstrated that intravenous hyperalimentation including arginine abrogates the immune suppression observed in rats after bilateral femoral fractures (see [166] and references therein). A study of 30 cancer patients demonstrated that enteral supplementation with arginine can prevent immune depression following major gastrointestinal operations (167). In addition, enteral feeding with arginine, in combination with RNA and ω-3 fatty acids, attenuated immune depression and improved recovery of cancer patients undergoing major gastrointestinal surgery (168, 169). Similar TPN formulas containing arginine, RNA, and ω-3 fatty acids improved the immune function and outcomes of ICU patients suffering from persistent sepsis syndrome (170). Elderly patients and those suffering from chronic infections may also benefit from immune stimulation by arginine supplementation (160, 171).

The mechanism by which arginine stimulates the immune system has not been defined (172). However, arginine increases thymic weight and cellularity in rats as well as lymphocyte responsiveness to mitogenic stimulation in both rats and humans (166, 167, 173, 174). Arginine also seems to improve neutrophil function (171), and arginine promotes the bactericidal capability of rat and murine macrophages by supporting nitric oxide synthesis (145, 175, 176). However, this may not be the case for human macrophages, which have not consistently produced nitric oxide in culture (177).

Arginine in Cancer

In several studies using rodent experimental tumor models, arginine-supplemented diets suppressed tumor incidence, growth, and metastasis (178–180). In contrast, some experimental tumors are stimulated by arginine-containing diets or inhibited by arginine-free diets (181, 182). Arginine's ability to inhibit tumor growth has been attributed to its effect on immune function. In fact, the inhibitory effect of arginine-supplemented diets may depend upon stimulation of the host's immune system and the immunogenicity of the experimental tumor (183, 184). Arginine-supplemented diets improve nitrogen balance and increase protein synthesis in muscle of tumor-bearing rats (185). In breast cancer patients, arginine has been reported to increase protein synthesis rate in the tumor (186); however, arginine stimulates lymphocyte and killer cells activity in breast cancer patients as well (186, 187).

REFERENCES

1. Heys SD, Gough DB, Khan L, Eremin O. Br J Surg 1996;83:608–19.
2. Elia M, Folmer P, Schlatmann A, et al. Am J Clin Nutr 1989;49:1203–10.
3. Welbourne TC, Joshi S. Proc Soc Exp Biol Med 1986;182:399–403.
4. Nissim I, Cattano C, Nissim I, Yudkoff M. Arch Biochem Biophys 1992;292:393–401.
5. Nissim I, Yudkoff M, Segal S. J Biol Chem 1985;260:13955–67.
6. Pastor CM, Morris SM Jr, Billiar TR. Am J Physiol 1995;269:G861–6.
7. Bode AM, Nordlie RC. J Biol Chem 1993;268:16298–301.
8. Haussinger D. Adv Enzyme Regul 1986;25:159–80.
9. Deferrari G, Garibotto G, Robaudo C, et al. Contrib Nephrol 1994;110:144–9.
10. Dejong CH, Deutz NE, Soeters PB. J Clin Invest 1993;92:2834–40.
11. Higashiguchi T, Noguchi Y, Meyer T, et al. Clin Sci (Colch) 1995;89:311–9.
12. Yoshida S, Yunoki T, Aoyagi K, et al. J Surg Res 1995;59:475–81.
13. Jepson MM, Bates PC, Broadbent P, et al. Am J Physiol 1988;255:E166–72.
14. Curthoys NP, Watford M. Annu Rev Nutr 1995;15:133–59.
15. Watford M. FASEB J 1993;7:1468–74.
16. Lanks KW, Li PW. J Cell Physiol 1988;135:151–5.
16a. Collins CL, Wasa M, Souba WW, et al. J Cell Physiol, in press.
17. Bergstrom J, Furst P, Noree LO, Vinnars E. J Appl Physiol 1974;36:693–7.
18. Meister A, Anderson MA. Annu Rev Biochem 1983;52:711–60.
19. Welbourne TC. Can J Biochem 1979;57:233–7.
20. Hong RW, Rounds JD, Helton WS, et al. Ann Surg 1992;215:114–9.
21. Bannai S, Ishii T. J Cell Physiol 1988;137:360–6.
22. Nissim I, States B, Nissim I, et al. Kidney Int 1995;47:96–105.
23. Reitzer LJ, Wice BM, Kennell D. J Biol Chem 1979;254:2669–76.
24. Wu P, Ray NG, Shuler ML. Ann NY Acad Sci 1992;665:
25. Darcy-Vrillon B, Posho L, Morel MT, et al. Pediatr Res 1994;36:175–81.
26. Kimura RE. Pediatr Res 1987;21:214–7.
27. Brand K, Fekl W, von Hintzenstern J, et al. Metabolism 1989;38:29–33.
28. Lazo PA. Eur J Biochem 1981;117:19–25.
29. Mares-Perlman JA, Shrago E. Cancer Res 1988;48:602–8.
30. Spolarics Z, Lang CH, Bagby GJ, Spitzer JJ. Am J Physiol 1991;261:G185–90.
31. Krutzfeldt A, Spahr R, Mertens S, et al. J Mol Cell Cardiol 1990;22:1393–404.
32. Barbehenn EK, Masterson E, Koh SW, et al. J Cell Physiol 1984;118:262–6.
33. He Y, Chu SH, Walker WA. J Nutr 1993;123:1017–27.
34. Ardawi MS, Majzoub MF. Metabolism 1991;40:155–64.
35. Austgen TR, Chakrabarti R, Chen MK, Souba WW. J Trauma 1992;32:600–6; discussion 606–7.
36. Zunic G, Savic J, Ignjatovic D, Taseski J. J Trauma 1996;40:S152–6.
37. Ardawi MS. Clin Sci (Colch) 1988;74:165–72.
38. Furst P, Albers S, Stehle P. Kidney Int Suppl 1989;27:S287–92.
39. Ardawi MS. Clin Sci (Colch) 1991;81:603–9.
40. Austgen TR, Chen MK, Salloum RM, Souba WW. J Trauma 1991;31:1068–74; discussion 1074–5.
41. MacLennan PA, Brown RA, Rennie MJ. FEBS Lett 1987;215:187–91.
42. Parry-Billings M, Leighton B, Dimitriadis G, et al. Int J Biochem 1989;21:419–23.
43. Kapadia CR, Colpoys MF, Jiang ZM, et al. JPEN J Parenter Enteral Nutr 1985;9:583–9.
44. Rennie MJ, MacLennan PA, Hundal HS, et al. Metabolism 1989;38:47–51.
45. Roth E, Funovics J, Muhlbacher F, et al. Clin Nutr 1982;1:25–41.
46. Roth E, Zoch G, Schulz F, et al. Clin Chem 1985;31:1305–9.
47. Ardawi MS, Jamal YS. Clin Sci (Colch) 1990;79:139–47.
48. Max SR, Mill J, Mearow K, et al. Am J Physiol 1988;255:E397–402.
49. Max SR. Med Sci Sports Exerc 1990;22:325–30.
50. Leighton B, Parry-Billings M, Dimitriadis G, et al. Biochem J 1991;274:187–92.
51. M, Leighton B, Dimitriadis GD, et al. Biochem Pharmacol 1990;40:1145–8.
52. Feng B, Hilt DC, Max SR. J Biol Chem 1990;265:18702–6.
53. Max SR, Thomas JW, Banner C, et al. Endocrinology 1987;120:1179–83.
54. Abcouwer SF, Bode BP, Souba WW. J Surg Res 1995;59:59–65.
55. Abcouwer SF, Lohmann R, Bode BP, et al. J Trauma 1996;42:421–8.
56. Lukaszewicsz G, Souba WW, Abcouwer SF. Shock 1997;7:1–7.
57. Feng B, Shiber SK, Max SR. J Cell Physiol 1990;145:376–80.
58. Tadros LB, Willhoft NM, Taylor PM, Rennie MJ. Am J Physiol 1993;265:E935–42.
59. Arad G, Kulka RG. Biochim Biophys Acta 1978;544:153–62.

60. Mermel VL, Wolfe BM, Hansen RJ, Clifford AJ. JPEN J Parenter Enteral Nutr 1991;15:128–36.
61. Downey RS, Monafo WW, Karl IE, et al. Surgery 1986;99: 265–74.
62. Stehle P, Zander J, Mertes N, et al. Lancet 1989;1:231–3.
63. Hammarqvist F, Wernerman J, Ali R, et al. Ann Surg 1989;209:455–61.
64. Wernerman J, Hammarkvist F, Ali MR, Vinnars E. Metabolism 1989;38:63–6.
65. Chen K, Okuma T, Okamura K, et al. JPEN J Parenter Enteral Nutr 1994;18:167–71.
66. Gianotti L, Alexander JW, Gennari R, et al. JPEN J Parenter Enteral Nutr 1995;19:69–74.
67. Nath SK, Dechelotte PDD. et al. Am J Physiol 1992;262: G312–8.
68. Frankel WL, Zhang W, Afonso J, et al. JPEN J Parenter Enteral Nutr 1993;17:47–55.
69. Yoshida S, Leskiw MJ, Schluter MD, et al. Am J Physiol 1992;263:E368–73.
70. Zapata-Sirvent RL, Hansbrough JF, Ohara MM, et al. Crit Care Med 1994;22:690–6.
71. Platell C, McCauley R, McCulloch R, Hall J. JPEN J Parenter Enteral Nutr 1993;17:348–54.
72. Grant JP, Snyder PJ. J Surg Res 1988;44:506–13.
73. Inoue Y, Grant JP, Snyder PJ. JPEN J Parenter Enteral Nutr 1993;17:165–70.
74. Hwang TL, O'Dwyer ST, Smith RJ, et al. Surg Forum 1987;38:56.
75. Baskerville A, Hambleton P, Benbough JE. Br J Exp Pathol 1980;61:132–138.
76. Burke DJ, Alverdy JC, Aoys E, Moss GS. Arch Surg 1989; 124:1396–9.
77. Sauer LA, Stayman JW, Dauchy RT. Cancer Res 1986;46: 3469–75.
78. Le Bricon T, Cynober L, Field CJ, Baracos VE. J Nutr 1995;125:2999–3010.
79. Yoshioka K, Takehara H, Okada A, Komi N. Tokushima J Exp Med 1992;39:69–76.
80. Chance WT, Cao L, Nelson JL, et al. Surgery 1987;102:386–94.
81. Bartlett DL, Charland S, Torosian MH. Ann Surg Oncol 1995;2:71–6.
82. Austgen TR, Dudrick PS, Sitren H, et al. Ann Surg 1992;215:107–13.
83. Klimberg VS, Souba WW, Salloum RM, et al. J Surg Res 1990;48:319–23.
84. Kaibara A, Yoshida S, Yamasaki K, et al. J Surg Res 1994;57:143–9.
85. Rouse K, Nwokedi E, Woodliff JE, et al. Ann Surg 1995; 221:420–6.
86. Klimberg VS, Nwokedi E, Hutchins LF, et al. JPEN J Parenter Enteral Nutr 1992;16:83S–7S
87. Fahr MJ, Kornbluth J, Blossom S, et al. JPEN J Parenter Enteral Nutr 1994;18:471–6.
88. Fox AD, Kripke SA, De Paula J, et al. JPEN J Parenter Enteral Nutr 1988;12:325–31.
89. Jacobs DO, Evans DA, O'Dwyer ST, et al. Surg Forum 1987;38:45–74.
90. Klimberg VS, Salloum RM, Kasper M, et al. Arch Surg 1990;125:1040–5.
91. Klimberg VS, Souba WW, Dolson DJ, et al. Cancer 1990;66:62–8.
92. Kallinowski F, Runkel S, Fortmeyer HP, et al. J Cancer Res Clin Oncol 1987;113:209–15.
93. Castillo L, Chapman TE, Sanchez M, et al. Proc Natl Acad Sci USA 1993;90:7749–53.
94. Castillo L, Ajami A, Branch S, et al. Metabolism 1994;43: 114–22.
95. Milner JA, Wakeling AE, Visek WJ. J Nutr 1974;104:1681–9.
96. Ha YH, Milner JA, Corbin JE. J Nutr 1978;108:203–10.
97. Milner JA. J Nutr 1985;115:516–23.
98. Gross KL, Hartman WJ, Ronnenberg A, Prior RL. J Nutr 1991;121:1591–9.
99. Hartman WJ, Prior RL. J Nutr 1992;122:1472–82.
100. Goodman MW, Zieve L, Konstantinides FN, Cerra FB. Am J Physiol 1984;247:G290–5.
101. Hartman WJ, Torre PM, Prior RL. J Nutr 1994;124: 1950–60.
102. Dhanakoti SN, Brosnan JT, Herzberg GR, Brosnan ME. Am J Physiol 1990;259:E437–42.
103. Castillo L, Sanchez M, Vogt J, et al. Am J Physiol 1995;268: E360–7.
104. Jones ME. J Nutr 1985;115:509–15.
105. Mezl VA, Knox WE. Biochem J 1977;166:105–13.
106. Albina JE, Abate JA, Mastrofrancesco B. J Surg Res 1993;55:97–102.
107. Allen JC. Cell Biochem Funct 1983;1:131–40.
108. Gopalakrishna R, Nagarajan B. Anal Biochem 1980;107: 318–23.
109. Luk GD, Casero RA Jr. Adv Enzyme Regul 1987;26:91–105.
110. Quemener V, Blanchard Y, Chamaillard L, et al. Anticancer Res 1994;14:443–8.
111. Ignarro LJ, Buga GM, Wood KS, et al. Proc Natl Acad Sci USA 1987;84:9265–9.
112. Palmer RM, Ferrige AG, Moncada S. Nature 1987;327:524–6.
113. Schmidt HH, Nau H, Wittfoht W, et al. Eur J Pharmacol 1988;154:213–6.
114. Sakuma I, Stuehr DJ, Gross SS, et al. Proc Natl Acad Sci USA 1988;85:8664–7.
115. Forstermann U, Gath I, Schwarz P, et al. Biochem Pharmacol 1995;50:1321–32.
116. Gross SS, Wolin MS. Annu Rev Physiol 1995;57:737–69.
117. Wink DA, Hanbauer I, Grisham MB, et al. Curr Top Cell Regul 1996;34:159–87.
118. Umans JG, Levi R. Annu Rev Physiol 1995;57:771–90.
119. Hare JM, Colucci WS. Prog Cardiovasc Dis 1995;38:155–66.
120. Lyons CR. Adv Immunol 1995;60:323–71.
121. Brune B, Messmer UK, Sandau K. Toxicol Lett 1995; 82–83:233–7.
122. Wink DA, Cook JA, Pacelli R, et al. Toxicol Lett 1995;82–83:221–6.
123. Rees DD. Biochem Soc Trans 1995;23:1025–9.
124. Brady AJ. Int J Cardiol 1995;50:269–72.
125. Wolfe TA, Dasta JF. Ann Pharmacother 1995;29:36–46.
126. Booke M, Meyer J, Lingnau W, et al. New Horiz 1995;3: 123–38.
127. Thiemermann C. Prog Clin Biol Res 1995;392:383–92.
128. Engelman DT, Watanabe M, Engelman RM, et al. J Thorac Cardiovasc Surg 1995;110:1047–53.
129. Ma XL, Weyrich AS, Lefer DJ, Lefer AM. Circ Res 1993; 72:403–12.
130. Fukuda H, Sawa Y, Kadoba K, et al. Circulation 1995;92:II413–6.
131. Vinten-Johansen J, Zhao ZQ, Sato H. Ann Thorac Surg 1995;60:852–7.
132. Lefer AM. Ann Thorac Surg 1995;60:847–51.
133. Fullerton DA, McIntyre RC Jr. Ann Thorac Surg 1996;61:1856–64.
134. Date H, Triantafillou AN, Trulock EP, et al. J Thorac Cardiovasc Surg 1996;111:913–9.

135. Raul F, Galluser M, Schleiffer R, et al. Digestion 1995;56:400–5.
136. Hiramatsu T, Forbess JM, Miura T, et al. Ann Thorac Surg 1996;61:36–40; discussion 40–1.
137. Jin JS, D'Alecy LG. Hypertension 1995;26:406–12.
138. Dagher F, Pollina RM, Rogers DM, et al. J Vasc Surg 1995;21:453–8; discussion 458–9.
138a. Clarkson P, Adams MR, Powe AJ, et al. J Clin Invest 1996;97:1989–94.
139. Yu YM, Young VR, Castillo L, et al. Metabolism 1995;44: 659–66.
140. Barbul A. JPEN J Parenter Enteral Nutr 1986;10:227–38.
141. Sarac TP, Souba WW, Miller JH, et al. Surgery 1994;116: 679–85; discussion 685–6.
142. Gardiner KR, Gardiner RE, Barbul A. Crit Care Med 1995;23:1227–32.
143. Wakabayashi Y, Yamada E, Yoshida T, Takahashi H. J Biol Chem 1994;269:32667–71.
144. Adjei AA, Yamauchi K, Nakasone Y, et al. Nutrition 1995;11:371–4.
145. Gianotti L, Alexander JW, Pyles T, Fukushima R. Ann Surg 1993;217:644–53; discussion 653–4.
146. Lazaratos S, Kashimura H, Nakahara A, et al. J Gastroenterol 1995;30:578–84.
147. McCormack SA, Johnson LR. Am J Physiol 1991;260: G795–806.
148. Brzozowski T, Konturek SJ, Drozdowicz D, et al. Digestion 1995;56:463–71.
149. Barbul A, Lazarou SA, Efron DT, et al. Surgery 1990;108:331–6; discussion 336–7.
150. Chyun JH, Griminger P. J Nutr 1984;114:1697–704.
151. Seifter E, Rettura G, Barbul A, Levenson SM. Surgery 1978;84:224–30.
152. Barbul A, Rettura G, Levenson SM, Seifter E. Am J Clin Nutr 1983;37:786–94.
153. Imms FJ, London DR, Neame RLB. J Physiol (London) 1969;200:55P–6P.
154. Iversen J. J Clin Invest 1971;50:2123–36.
155. Palmer JP, Walter RM, Ensinck JW. Diabetes 1975;24:735–40.
156. Weir GC, Samols E, Loo S, et al. Diabetes 1979;28:35–40.
157. Knopf RF, Conn JW, Fajans SS, et al. J Clin Invest 1965;25: 1140–4.
158. Merimee TJ, Lillicrap DA, Rabinowitz D. Lancet 1965; 668–70.
159. Rakoff JS, Siler TM, Sinha YN, Yon SSC. J Clin Endocrinol Metab 1973;37:641–4.
160. Kirk SJ, Hurson M, Regan MC, et al. Surgery 1993;114:155–9; discussion 160.
161. Hurson M, Regan MC, Kirk SJ, et al. JPEN J Parenter Enteral Nutr 1995;19:227–30.
162. Pui YM, Fisher H. J Nutr 1979;109:240–6.
163. Hammarqvist F, Stromberg C, von der Decken A, et al. Ann Surg 1992;216:184–91.
164. Mjaaland M, Unneberg K, Larsson J, et al. Ann Surg 1993;217:413–22.
165. Crist DM, Peake GT, Mackinnon LT, et al. Metabolism 1987;36:1115–7.
166. Barbul A, Wasserkrug HL, Yoshimura N, et al. J Surg Res 1984;36:620–4.
167. Daly JM, Reynolds J, Thom A, et al. Ann Surg 1988;208: 512–23.
168. Kemen M, Senkal M, Homann HH, et al. Crit Care Med 1995;23:652–9.
169. Daly JM, Lieberman MD, Goldfine J, et al. Surgery 1992;112:56–67.
170. Cerra FB, Lehmann S, Konstantinides N, et al. Nutrition 1991;7:193–9.
171. Azzara A, Carulli G, Sbrana S, et al. Drugs Exp Clin Res 1995;21:71–8.
172. Anonymous. Nutr Rev 1993;51:54–6.
173. Barbul A, Fishel RS, Shimazu S, et al. J Surg Res 1985;38: 328–34.
174. Barbul A, Sisto DA, Wasserkrug HL, Efron G. Surgery 1981;90:244–51.
175. Green SJ, Meltzer MS, Hibbs JB Jr, Nacy CA. J Immunol 1990;144:278–83.
176. Hrabak A, Idei M, Temesi A. Life Sci 1994;55:797–805.
177. Murray HW, Teitelbaum RF. J Infect Dis 1992;165:513–7.
178. Milner JA, Stepanovich LV. J Nutr 1979;109:489–94.
179. Tachibana K, Mukai K, Hiraoka I, et al. JPEN J Parenter Enteral Nutr 1985;9:428–34.
180. Rettura G, Padawer J, Barbul A, et al. JPEN J Parenter Enteral Nutr 1979;3:409–16.
181. Lea MA, Xiao Q, Klein KM, Grote-Holman E. Cancer Biochem Biophys 1993;13:171–9.
182. Grossie VB Jr, Nishioka K, Ajani JA, Ota DM. J Surg Oncol 1992;50:161–7.
183. Reynolds JV, Thom AK, Zhang SM, et al. J Surg Res 1988;45:513–22.
184. Chany C, Cerutti I. Int J Cancer 1982;30:489–93.
185. Oka T, Ohwada K, Nagao M, et al. JPEN J Parenter Enteral Nutr 1994;18:491–6.
186. Park KG, Heys SD, Blessing K, et al. Clin Sci (Colch) 1992;82:413–7.
187. Brittenden J, Park KG, Heys SD, et al. Surgery 1994;115: 205–12.
188. Scheltinga MR, Young LS, Benfell K, et al. Ann Surg 1991;214:385–93; discussion 393–5.
189. Ziegler TR, Young LS, Benfell K, et al. Ann Intern Med 1992;116:821–8.
190. Schloerb PR, Amare M. JPEN J Parenter Enteral Nutr 1993;17:407–13.
191. van der Hulst RR, van Kreel BK, von Meyenfeldt MF, et al. Lancet 1993;341:1363–5.
192. O'Riordain MG, Fearon KC, Ross JA, et al. Ann Surg 1994;220:212–21.
193. Byrne TA, Persinger RL, Young LS, et al. Ann Surg 1995;222:243–54; discussion 254–5.
194. Lacey JM, Crouce J, Benfell K, et al. JPEN J Parenter Enteral Nutr 1996;20:74–80.

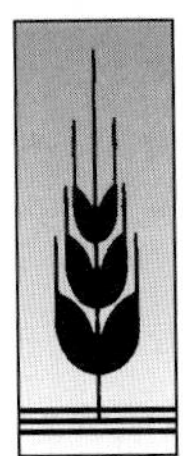

PART II.

Nutrition in Integrated Biologic Systems

36. Nutritional Regulation of Gene Expression

ROBERT J. COUSINS

Gene expression is a term that has different interpretations. These are dictated by the context in which the term is used. For example, exhibited phenotypes are manifestations of gene expression. Similarly, the mechanics of gene transcription and mRNA translation that influence which proteins are produced also constitute gene expression. From the standpoint of nutritional influences on gene expression, processes are envisioned in which dietary conditions, through either direct interaction of specific nutrients with transcription factors or, more commonly, through indirect means (e.g., hormones or signaling systems) produce changes in transcription of specific genes to yield proteins, including mediators and enzymes, that define phenotypic expression. Alternatively, nutrients can influence gene expression via control of mRNA translation. Again, this can be mediated by direct or indirect means.

HISTORICAL PERSPECTIVE

It is not possible to identify exactly when the fact that specific nutrients influence gene expression was first appreciated. It was clear by the 1950s that essential amino acids, when not available in sufficient amounts, limited the production of proteins. The classic experiments of the Nobelists François Jacob and Jacques Monod in 1961, although conducted in bacteria *(Escherichia coli)*, demonstrated that regulatory genes under nutrient control influence genes needed for the synthesis of enzymes involved in the metabolism of that nutrient. In the case studied, lactose (the nutrient inducer) increased the expression of three structural genes (lac operon) coding for lactose metabolizing enzymes (1).

Experiments with eukaryotic systems followed after the operon model was proposed. Classic experiments of particular note were those demonstrating that polyribosome formation depended upon the presence of essential amino acids in the diet (2). In addition, inhibitors of mRNA synthesis (actinomycin D and cordycepin) and translation (cycloheximide) were used in animal experiments to study, for example, the iron-induced synthesis of ferritin (3), regulation of phosphoenolpyruvic-carboxykinase by high carbohydrate intake and fasting (4), and biochemical and physiologic changes induced by vitamin D (5).

The area of nutrient regulation of gene expression is a well-recognized research emphasis in contemporary nutritional science. In this area of research, it is essential to be able to separate direct effects from those caused by nutrient-induced changes in secondary systems remote from the nutrient's initial effects. Unfortunately, it is difficult to separate direct effects of nutrients on gene expression from those produced indirectly through mediators (Fig. 36.1). Consequently, experiments at the level of individual cells are essential to identify clearly direct effects of nutrients. However, interpretation of cell-level findings must be kept within an integrative context of the whole multicellular organism to fully appreciate how dietary components influence the expression of genes in various tissues. How the external environment, including nutrients, hormones, cytokines, and growth factors, can influence the general process of protein synthesis as well as the differential expression of specific genes provides an excellent opportunity for investigators in the science of nutrition (6). Furthermore, the technical approaches described in this review are relatively low cost and do not require expensive or complex equipment or elaborate instrumentation.

GENOMIC ORGANIZATION AND REGULATION

Our understanding of the complexity of genomic organization has advanced considerably since the early experiments on nutrient influences on gene expression. The basics of gene expression include activation of the gene to

Abbreviations: **PCR**—polymerase chain reaction; **PAGE**—polyacrylamide gel electrophoresis; **RT**—reverse transcriptase; **AGE**—agarose gel electrophoresis.

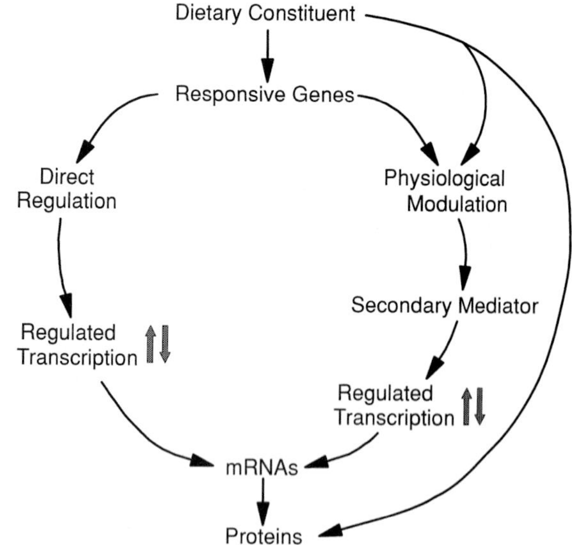

Figure 36.1. Direct and indirect effects of nutrition on regulation of gene expression.

a transcribable structure followed by transcription, transcript processing and splicing, translocation to the cytoplasm, mRNA translation and, for some proteins, posttranslational modification. The general scheme, as shown in Figure 36.2, has been described in exquisite detail (7, 8). The response to changes in nutrient intake likely influences expression of many genes. Since only about 30% of the genes in the total human genome have been identified, it would appear that dietary patterns influence unidentified genes of yet unknown function.

Transcription rates for individual genes can be altered by various mechanisms and represent the major point of gene regulation. Factors influencing the binding of RNA polymerase to DNA, specifically the promoter region of the gene (the 5′-flanking region) and other sequences in close proximity, control transcription. These factors (transcription factors) are proteins with domains that recognize a specific nucleotide sequence (response element) located in the promoter. Response elements are usually short sequences found within the first few hundred nucleotides upstream from the start site of the structural gene. There are exceptions, however. As more promoter sequence information is obtained for upstream (>1000 bases) sequences, it is clear that distant response elements may, through various mechanisms or interactions, influence basal-level transcription rates. Specific transcription factors form dimers or other complex combinations through protein-protein interactions among regulatory proteins or molecules to influence transcription. These aspects of transcription have been reviewed in detail (7).

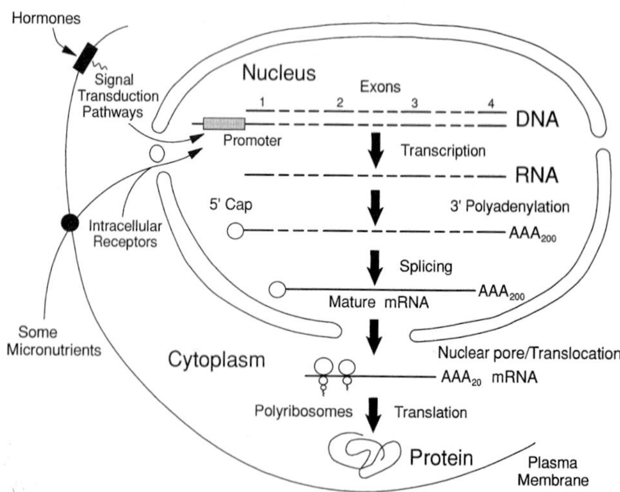

Figure 36.2. Basic aspects of gene expression and protein synthesis. Nutritional regulation of genes can occur directly or through hormones or other mediators that activate signaling systems.

The direct interaction of response elements and transcription factors with nutrients has been documented. Examples include the sterol response element for sterol-regulated genes (9), the calcitriol receptor-response elements for vitamin D–regulated genes (10), the retinoic acid receptor-response element combinations for vitamin A–regulated genes (11), fatty acids and some of their metabolites (11a, 11b) and the metal response elements for zinc-regulated genes (12) and associated transcription factors. The human genome contains approximately 100,000 genes, of which 10% may be transcriptionally active at any one time (13). Consequently, many unidentified response elements may be under nutrient control. In addition, cytokines and hormones act by altering gene expression, usually transcription (8), and response elements for these factors may exist at other locations within a gene's promoter that are also influenced by a specific nutrient or dietary pattern. Furthermore, the abundance of some transcription factors in cells can be regulated by physiologic processes that may be influenced by diet.

It is unlikely that a specific gene is regulated by a single response element or even multiple copies of a response element in a promoter. An example of the likely complexity is the phosphoenolpyruvate carboxykinase promoter which, within the first 1 kb of upstream sequence (5′ from the transcription start site), has five response-element sequences (cAMP, glucocorticoid, insulin, peroxisome proliferator–activated receptor, and thyroid hormone) and may interact with at least 10 transcription factors (14).

IDENTIFICATION OF GENES REGULATED BY INDIVIDUAL NUTRIENTS OR DIETARY PATTERNS

The following section describes some techniques and approaches of particular interest to investigators studying the effect of nutrition on gene expression. Examples of these techniques from the contemporary literature concentrate on the results of experiments with animals or human subjects fed diets that produce metabolic changes.

Polyacrylamide Electrophoresis of Proteins and Immunoblotting

Extremely valuable information can be obtained by measuring specific gene products (proteins) related to altered phenotypic expression. For such purposes, proteins are most frequently separated by sodium dodecyl sulfate (SDS) polyacrylamide gel electrophoresis (PAGE) using any of the innumerable variations of the PAGE format (15). To identify the proteins of interest, proteins are electroblotted to nitrocellulose (or another membrane) from the polyacrylamide gel for specific times to ensure that the proteins are retained on the nitrocellulose. The protein(s) of interest is usually detected immunologically by a process referred to as western blotting.

Immunodetection methods allow investigators to examine a specific protein among the thousands of tissue proteins transferred to the membrane. The spectrum of antibodies available for these applications (western blot) from commercial sources is substantial. Alternatively, many investigators working on newly identified or rare proteins use antibodies produced to chemically synthesized peptides corresponding to a specific region of the intact protein that is likely to be highly antigenic. These peptides usually correspond to 20 to 30 amino acids of the protein. Frequently, the amino acid sequence is deduced from the cDNAs of genes for which the gene product has not yet been isolated and sequenced (16). This approach allows examination of the nutritional regulation of proteins encoded by newly identified genes. Furthermore, the sensitivity of some immunodetection methods allows examination of proteins present in low abundance.

Small proteins or peptides used to elicit antibodies are conjugated to keyhole limpet hemocyanin or another protein to enhance antigenicity. Larger proteins are most frequently used without conjugation. Antibodies are most frequently raised in rabbits, but goats and sheep are often used (15). Immunization of chickens and recovery of antibodies from egg yolk is gaining in popularity (17). Mammalian polyclonal antibodies are usually purified by protein A or G chromatography to obtain the IgG fraction. Frequently, these are further selected by chromatography using a support to which the protein or peptide antigen has been coupled to yield a monospecific IgG population.

Monoclonal antibodies are also widely used in nutrition-related studies on gene expression. The availability of hybridoma facilities has greatly furthered production of monoclonal antibodies derived from proteins and peptides generated by the procedures described above.

Protocols for incubating the blotted proteins on nitrocellulose with the primary antibody (immunoblot) vary widely (15). Options for detection via a secondary antibody include colorimetric detection, binding of ^{125}I-labeled protein A, or the very sensitive method in which the secondary antibody provides a luminescent signal detected by x-ray film (or a luminescence detector). The latter approach has become very widely used. In Figure 36.3, GLUT4 (see Chapter 3) protein levels in transgenic mice are determined by ^{125}I-labeled protein A which binds to anti-GLUT4 antibody (18). The response to high-fat or high-carbohydrate diets shows that overexpression of the GLUT4 transgene results in considerably more transporter protein being produced.

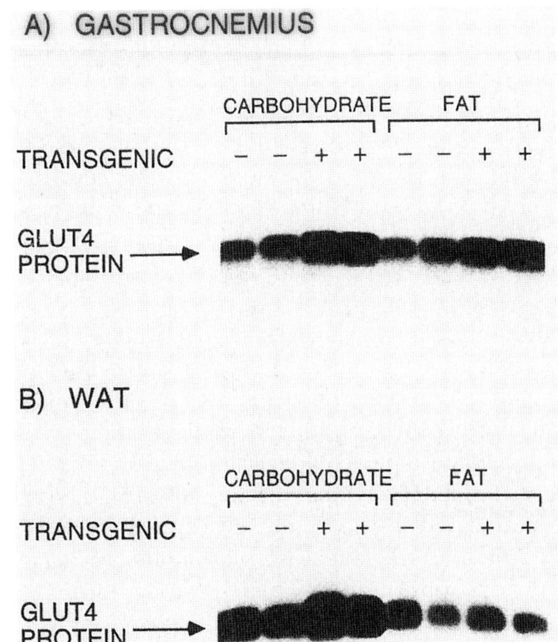

Figure 36.3. SDS polyacrylamide gel electrophoresis of proteins from muscle (gastrocnemius) or adipose (white adipose tissue) homogenates from transgenic mice that overexpress the *GLUT4* gene. Western blotting: proteins were transferred to membranes, incubated with antiserum against GLUT4 protein, and detected with ^{125}I-protein A. The transgenic mice were fed control (–), high fat or high carbohydrate (+) diets for 14 weeks. (From Ikemoto S, Thompson KS, Takahashi M, et al. Proc Natl Acad Sci USA 1995;92:3096–9, with permission.)

Immunohistochemistry and Immunocytochemistry

Advances in microscopy have dramatically increased the use of fluorescent antibodies for intracellular localization of specific proteins. Epifluorescence, confocal, and 3D deconvolution microscopic techniques can all take advantage of fluorescently tagged antibodies. Flow cytometry can also be used effectively in nutrition-related research, particularly that focused on immunology (19). In the future, these approaches will see further application in experiments focused on nutrition, especially in human studies in which sample sizes are small.

Northern Analysis

The universal availability of cloned gene sequences through computer-searchable databases provides the opportunity to use this information to identify nutritionally regulated genes (13). Northern analysis (northern blotting) gives researchers interested in examining genes that are nutritionally regulated a powerful experimental technique. Using DNA sequence information, it is possible to produce oligonucleotides (oligomers, oligos) that can be used directly for northern analysis or, as described below, as primers for production of complementary DNA (cDNA) probes by polymerase chain reaction (PCR) methods. Alternatively, there are commercially available probes for specific genes, and most investigators are willing to share cDNAs for use as probes for northern analysis studies.

The task of identifying which genes are regulated by nutrient intake level and specific diet formulations or consumption patterns is formidable indeed. Northern analysis has clearly been a workhorse for these studies to date. Hundreds of examples could be cited. The original method has been modified innumerable times (15). Similarly, tissue RNA extraction procedures have evolved, and currently, guanidinium isothiocyanate–based methods, some with proprietary formulations, are almost universally used.

The purpose of northern analysis is to detect a specific mRNA and determine its relative static abundance. The method involves agarose gel electrophoresis (AGE) of the RNA extract, transfer to a filter (nylon or nitrocellulose), binding the RNA to the filter by UV-induced cross-linking, and hybridization to a ^{32}P-labeled DNA probe (15). The hybridization is detected by autoradiography or phosphorimaging instrumentation, but nonradioactive alternatives are evolving. Intensity of the RNA-DNA hybridization is usually quantified by video densitometry. Another constitutively produced mRNA should be concurrently examined as a control for equal loading of the RNA extracts being compared. β-Actin and glyceraldehyde-3-phosphate dehydrogenase cDNAs are frequently used for comparative purposes. Ethidium bromide staining of RNA separated by AGE prior to transfer can also be used. Results of typical northern blot analyses are shown in Figure 36.4. In panel A, leptin mRNA levels (see Chapter 87) are lower in fasted rats than in those refed and/or given insulin (20). In panel B, metallothionein mRNA levels (see Chapter 11) are virtually undetectable in zinc-deficient rats compared with levels in rats fed adequate amounts of zinc (21). Here, northern blot data are used to assess nutritional status.

As described in the section on antisense techniques, solution hybridization and RNase protection assays provide an alternative to northern analysis for estimating the mRNA abundance of a gene suspected of being influenced by nutrition. Dot blots are occasionally used in screening experiments; however, since no size separation of the RNA is involved, the method requires that the probe used produces a signal specific for the mRNA of interest (15). Recent advances in the technique of in situ hybridization using fluorescent probes allow estimation of the intracellular abundance of a specific mRNA (22).

Polymerase Chain Reaction

The PCR technique has been used in experiments focused on nutrition and gene expression. PCR can pro-

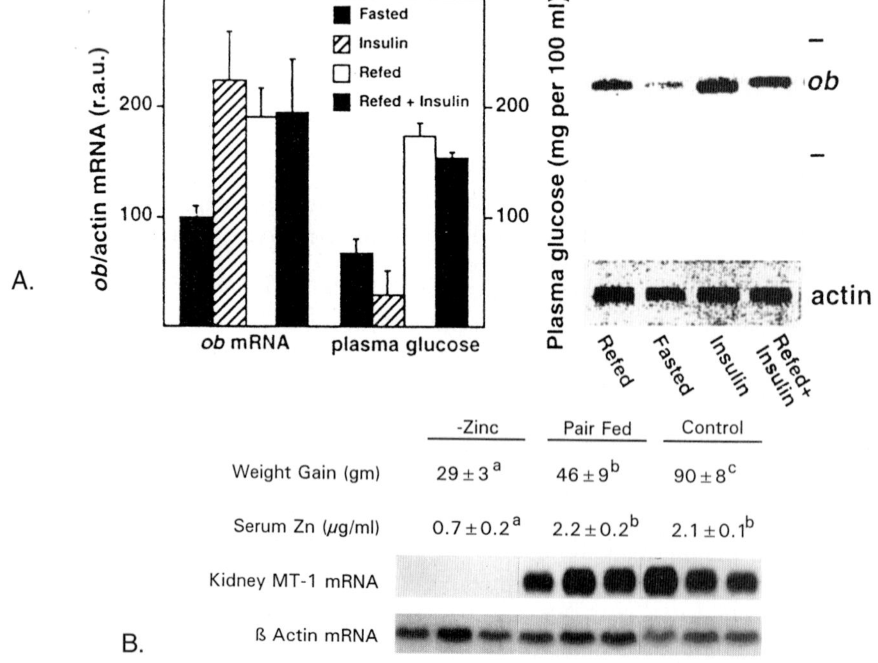

Figure 36.4. A. Northern analysis of total RNA from adipose tissue of rats showing the effects of food intake and insulin on leptin mRNA (*ob* gene) expression. β-Actin mRNA is the control for gel-loading efficiency. *Left panel* shows the relative abundance of the leptin mRNA as determined by densitometry as well as the plasma glucose concentration. *Right panel* shows the actual northern blot of leptin and β-actin mRNA. (From Saladin R, De Vos P, Guerre-Millo M, et al. Nature 1995;377:527–9, with permission.) **B.** Northern analyses of total RNA from rats showing the effect of zinc deficiency (−Zinc) on kidney metallothionein mRNA, compared with rats fed adequate amounts of zinc ad libitum (Control) or pair fed. β-Actin is the control mRNA. (From Blanchard RK, Cousins RJ. Proc Natl Acad Sci USA 1996;93:6863–8, with permission.)

vide multiple copies of a DNA or RNA sequence. Two oligonucleotide primers (a 5′ primer and a 3′ primer) that span the targeted sequence of interest must be synthesized (15, 23). Repeated sequential polymerase reactions of the target sequence in both directions under controlled temperatures with a thermocycler allow the targeted sequence to be amplified as a double-stranded cDNA copy in sufficient quantity for further use. Frequently, the amplified DNA is cloned by standard methods and purified by AGE as needed (15, 24).

Reverse transcriptase–PCR (RT-PCR) is used to produce cDNA copies of mRNA. The mRNA is first converted to cDNA with reverse transcriptase, using a specific 3′ primer for the target mRNA (25). PCR is then performed with another specific primer to provide sufficient quantities of the DNA sequence of interest for purification and/or analysis by AGE. RT-PCR is usually semiquantitative at best, since the amplification process is exponential and differences in mRNA levels usually encountered with nutritionally regulated genes are not large enough for the technique to be widely applicable. Nevertheless, RT-PCR is valuable for production of cDNAs for use in northern analysis experiments (26). Availability of cDNA sequence information allows development of primers for production of a specific cDNA by PCR and subsequent cloning to retain the cDNA for labeling and use in hybridizations as needed.

In contrast, competitive RT-PCR (C-RT-PCR) provides a measure of amplification efficiency and an internal control of known concentration so that the C-RT-PCR technique is quantitative (25, 27, 28). Consequently, this approach is very attractive for nutrition experimentation, particularly in human studies or others in which the number of available cells is very small (29). The steps in C-RT-PCR are shown in Figure 36.5 (30). C-RT-PCR requires construction of a third primer to generate a cDNA to act as the internal control competitor. In practice, prior to PCR, the mRNA is reverse transcribed soon after RNA isolation, since cDNA is more stable during storage. The method has been applied to zinc status assessment in humans (30).

PCR can be used to identify allelic differences in genotypes that may respond differently to nutrients. A notable example is the polymorphism in the human vitamin D receptor (VDR) gene and its corresponding link to bone mineral density (BMD) (31, 32). Expression of the osteocalcin gene is regulated by the VDR, a *trans*-acting transcription factor that requires 1,25$(OH)_2$ vitamin D_3 (calcitriol) as a ligand for binding to the vitamin D response element of the osteocalcin promoter. For these experiments, PCR was used to amplify genomic DNA from each subject. Subsequent AGE separation of the DNA, after restriction enzyme digestion, produced bands of different lengths for the two alleles of the VDR gene. The genotypes were differentiated in this way. This approach was also used to examine the positive effects of dietary fat modulation of plasma low-density-lipoprotein (LDL) cholesterol

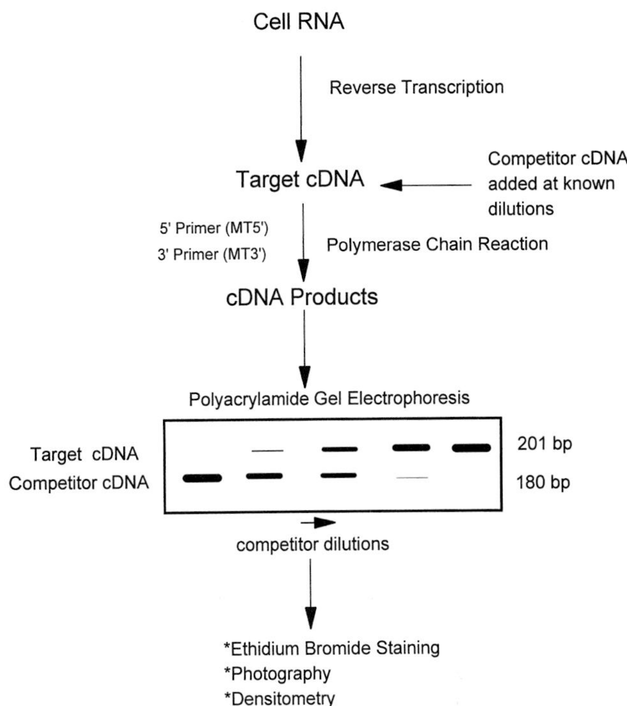

Figure 36.5. Competitive reverse transcriptase–polymerase chain reaction (C-RT-PCR). Extracted RNA is reverse transcribed to cDNA and, together with a competitor cDNA of known concentration, is amplified by PCR. Comparison of amplification to the competitor concentration allows determination of the relative abundance of the original mRNA. (Modified from Sullivan VK, Cousins RJ. J Nutr 1997;127:694–8, with permission.)

in individuals with the *apoE4* allele (33). The approach has wide application for genes that produce differences in the use or actions of nutrients and thus serve as biomarkers for differences in nutritional effects.

Promoter Analysis

A number of experiments within the past decade have shown direct interactions between specific nutrients and transcription factors regulating the expression of specific genes. Metabolites of fat-soluble vitamins, trace metals, sterols including cholesterol, and fatty acids are examples. In each case, an initial interaction between the nutrient and a receptor or transcription factor(s) is followed by a direct interaction of the transcription factor with specific nucleotide sequences within the nucleus. Typically, this occurs in the promoter/regulatory region located upstream from the start site of the coding sequence.

The approach taken to examine transcriptional regulation generally follows one of two techniques. The first is the nuclear run-on experiment. This requires generating purified nuclei from cells or tissues from animals fed a specific diet or provided a nutrient of interest. The nuclei are incubated in the presence of α-^{32}P-UTP to produce a radioactive RNA transcript. The transcript is then detected by hybridization to a specific probe (15). Since this ^{32}P-nucleotide is only incorporated into mRNA during transcription, the change in the rate of transcription produced in response to the nutrient is believed to reflect regulation at the level of transcription. A number of genes for hepatic proteins involved in carbohydrate and lipid metabolism have been shown by nuclear run-on assays to have altered transcription rates in response to a high carbohydrate diet (34, 35). However, these experiments provide little information about mechanisms involved in transcriptional regulation.

Another approach to promoter analysis enables determination of specific sequences involved in gene expression but requires sequence information about the genes of interest. In this technique, the promoter region, usually a few thousand bases (kb) of the 5′ flanking region, is excised with appropriate restriction enzymes and ligated to a reporter gene. Usually the chloramphenicol acyltransferase (CAT) or β-galactosidase (β-Gal) genes are used as reporters. The heterologous promoter-reporter construct must be transfected into a cell type of interest. The cell type is critical since transcription factors are specific to certain cells. Reporter genes generate products that may be analyzed by liquid scintillation counting or thin layer chromatography (for CAT) or colorimetrically (for β-Gal). The approach has been used for a number of nutritionally relevant genes (11a, 11b, 34, 36–38). Promoter/reporter gene systems can be used as an in vitro model for examining the responses of a promoter to specific nutrients, hormones, or drugs. The leptin gene promoter/reporter construct is an example of this potential (39).

Using deletion analysis with restriction enzymes, the location of the nucleotide sequence(s) of a promoter that is essential for the nutrient regulation can be identified. Mutational analysis of the promoter can define the exact nucleotides needed for specific regulation. Frequently, the latter analysis shows that the response element (sequence) is not always completely uniform. Consequently, response elements are usually reported as consensus sequences.

Differential Hybridization

The technique of differential hybridization, or plus-minus screening, allows comparison of a gene's expression with two dietary treatments or different periods of development (40, 41). A plasmid cDNA library is produced by reverse transcription of mRNA from one of the treatment groups. The cDNA is made double-stranded, ligated into a vector, and used to transform competent *E. coli*. In addition, a single-stranded cDNA probe is separately generated from mRNA of the other treatment groups. After *E. coli*-containing recombinant plasmids are grown with antibiotic selection, the plasmid DNA is cross-linked to nylon filters. The DNA-containing filters are hybridized separately with the single-stranded cDNA probes (after ^{32}P labeling). The signals generated in autoradiographs will be similar except in a few cases. The latter potentially represent differentially expressed genes. The colony hybridization procedure is usually repeated for confirmation that a signal is different with the two different probes. Finally, a northern analysis is carried out using cDNAs from the bacterial colonies in which differential signals originated. These cDNAs must then be sequenced and searches of genome databases (e.g., the BLAST search program for GenBank) carried out to identify what genes the recovered sequence represents. This procedure has been used for intestinal genes responsive to dietary zinc intake (41).

Differential mRNA Display

An elegant approach to examine differential gene expression was developed in 1992. Differential mRNA display is based on reverse transcription combined with PCR. It enables identification of mRNAs that increase or decrease in quantity in response to various conditions (42). Differential display was designed initially to identify genes differentially expressed in transformed and non-transformed cells. Recently, the technique has been used to identify genes regulated or influenced by micronutrients: zinc (21, 43, 44), selenium (45), and copper (46, 47).

Isolation of RNA from tissues is the first step in this technique. Reverse transcription of the RNA uses an oligo d(T) primer that has two non-T bases at the 3′ end. This is the "anchored primer" because it anchors cDNA synthesis at the end of the poly(A) tail and 3′ untranslated region. Four anchored primers, each with a different nucleotide, are used independently for cDNA synthesis to obtain the full array of sequences that can be displayed (Fig. 36.6). The anchored primer used for the RT reaction and one of 24 decanucleotide primers (arbitrary primers) are used for cDNA amplification by PCR. These constitute the 3′ and 5′ primers, respectively. A ^{32}P- or ^{33}S-labeled nucleotide is included in this PCR reaction. The resulting labeled cDNA then represents one of 24 possible subsets of mRNAs from the original RNA used for analysis. The four anchored primers, when used with the 24 arbitrary primers, require 96 separate PCR reactions to provide a thorough differential display from a given tissue or cell type. A few mRNAs may not be recognized because of a lack of sufficient poly(A) tail sequence or poor priming with the random primers used. As shown in Figure 36.6, differential mRNA display can be viewed as a library with four floors (one for each anchored primer) and 24 shelves with many books (one for each arbitrary primer). When all shelves on all floors have been read, all of the information has been viewed.

Denaturing polyacrylamide gel electrophoresis (PAGE) and autoradiography allow separation and isolation of individual cDNA bands (Fig. 36.7). Bands are usually up to 400 bp, but newer variations of the original method may significantly increase that size, thus increasing the probability of sequence identification. The cDNA bands resulting from mRNAs of animals fed under differing dietary conditions are resolved by PAGE and those that differ in intensity are considered manifestations of altered levels of

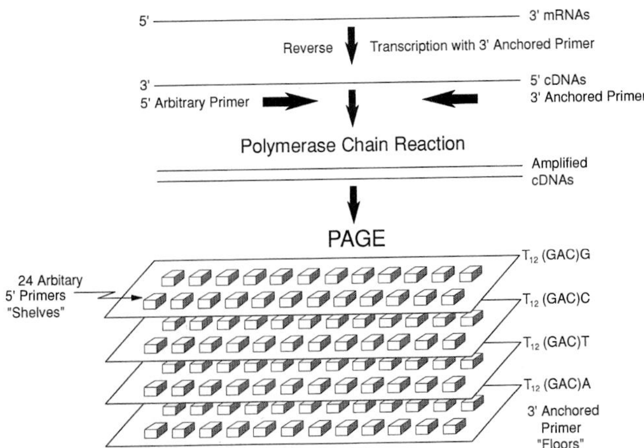

Figure 36.6. Differential mRNA display. Cell RNA is converted to cDNA, which is amplified by PCR using one anchored primer (3') and one arbitrary primer (5'). These are analogous to a floor and stack in a library, respectively. The cDNA products are then separated by polyacrylamide gel electrophoresis and compared as shown in Figure 36.7.

a specific mRNA (i.e., one that is differentially expressed). In the example, there are cDNAs that increase and decrease in relative abundance during zinc deficiency (21).

Subsequently, the cDNA band from a differentially expressed mRNA is cloned into a plasmid to maintain a renewable source of the cDNA. Verification of differential expression requires northern analysis using the cDNA in question (after ^{32}P labeling) and RNA from other experimental animals subjected to the same dietary conditions. If northern analysis confirms differential expression, this cDNA is sequenced, and its identity is determined through genome database searches as described above. Some searches do not reveal any previously reported sequences. Other searches identify a specific gene sequence, a gene of close homology, or an expressed sequence tag (EST). The latter represents a partial cDNA sequence of an unidentified gene. As more of the genomes of humans and experimental animals are sequenced, the EST data will become more useful.

Positional Cloning

An excellent example of positional cloning is that of the *ob* gene (48). This led to identification of a new peptide hormone, leptin, which, when secreted by adipocytes, regulates food intake and energy expenditure and influences non-insulin-dependent diabetes in obese individuals (49). This research was based on observations of mutations in mouse strains made over four decades earlier. (See Chapter 87 for more information.)

The first step in this approach is obtaining genetic maps to identify the locus of the mutation of interest. In many cases the chromosomal location of a mutation is known in the murine and human genomes. For genes that influence nutrition, phenotypic expression (i.e., the development of obesity) is used to segregate the mutant gene through specific genetic crosses. Linkage studies position the gene relative to molecular markers or known/identifiable areas of the genome. Establishing linkages to known genes helps greatly, particularly if they are "tightly linked" to the gene of interest. In the case of the *ob* gene, the region of chromosome 6 where the *ob* gene was located had been identified by two flanking markers. Using this location information, the appropriate region of the DNA is cloned. The use of yeast artificial chromosomes (YACs), specific restriction enzyme digests, and specific crosses refine the location. Subsequent screening of restriction digests will yield smaller sections of DNA, some of which will hybridize to RNA from a tissue in which the gene is expressed. Using this DNA as a probe, the mRNA of interest is identified, the cDNA sequence of the gene can then be established, and eventually, as in the case of leptin, the primary sequence of protein product deduced (48).

Experiments of this type are extremely time consuming and expertise in molecular genetics is essential. Nevertheless, the results have great benefit for understanding important aspects of nutrition. The fruits of such

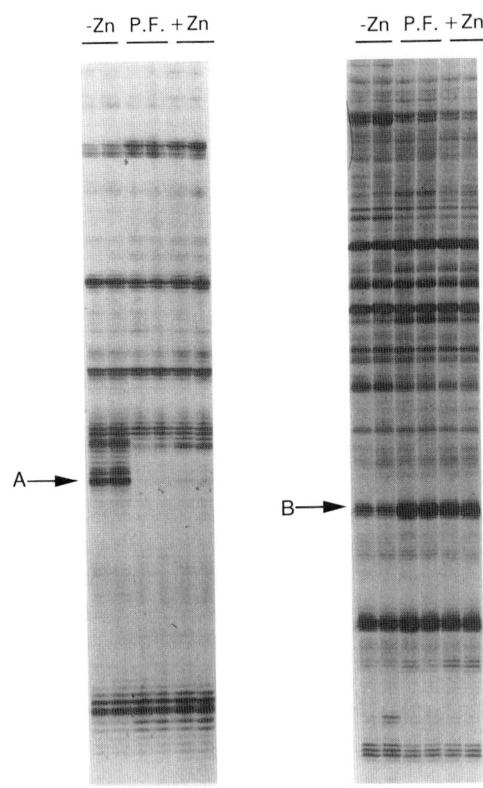

Figure 36.7. Differential display of intestinal mRNA from zinc-deficient rats. The mRNA is converted to cDNA by reverse transcription. cDNA is amplified by PCR with one of four anchored primers (3') and one of 24 arbitrary primers (5'), followed by PAGE of the cDNAs run in duplicate (as outlined in Fig. 36.6). RNA was from rats fed a zinc-deficient (−*Zn*) diet or zinc-adequate diet provided ad libitum (+*Zn*) or pair fed (*P.F.*). The display series to the *left* shows a cDNA **(A)** derived from an mRNA increased in −Zn while the display series to the *right* shows a cDNA **(B)** derived from an mRNA decreased in −Zn. (From Blanchard RK, Cousins RJ. Proc Natl Acad Sci USA 1996;93:6863–8, with permission.)

efforts are usually extensive, rapid, and enlightening. A database search for leptin reveals recent studies on the use of leptin protein and analytical assays (50), production of corollary animal models (51), therapeutic opportunities (49, 52), and additional components, such as neuropeptide Y (53), of the system of body composition regulation.

MANIPULATING GENES REGULATED BY INDIVIDUAL NUTRIENTS OR DIETARY PATTERNS

Transgenic Animals

The opportunity to overexpress a gene and thus increase production of a gene product has significant potential for nutrition research. Genes responsive to specific nutrients can be beneficial or deleterious when overexpressed.

The transgenic overexpression technique involves production of a construct consisting of a promoter and structural gene. The promoter can be the gene's normal promoter (homologous) or a different promoter (heterologous). A purified sample of the construct is injected into fertilized eggs (usually murine or porcine) and, if the construct DNA becomes integrated into the genome of some eggs, transgenic animals will be produced from them after full gestation in foster mothers. Southern (DNA) blotting or PCR is required for detection of the unique DNA construct to initially distinguish transgenic animals from their nontransgenic littermates. Selective breeding can produce homozygous lines of animals carrying transgenes.

A salient example of the transgenic approach used the metallothionein gene promoter to direct expression of the growth hormone (GH) gene in mice and pigs (54, 55). In pigs, additional GH was produced and secreted that greatly increased lean body mass. Since the metallothionein gene is induced by dietary zinc (56), adding extra zinc to the food or drinking water was used to increase expression of the transgene. This approach was used to produce transgenic animals with a construct composed of the metallothionein promoter and LDL receptor structural gene (57). Injection of the inducer metal activates the promoter and yields a lowered circulating cholesterol level within hours, coincident with increased production of the LDL receptor protein.

Other examples of the use of transgenic animals to address questions of nutritional interest are available. The glucose transporter (GLUT4) was overexpressed in mice using the aP2 fatty acid–binding protein promoter and a genomic DNA fragment containing the entire human GLUT4 gene as the construct (58). Overexpression was detected by increased GLUT4 protein in membranes from both white and brown fat (Fig. 36.8). These transgenic mice also had higher glucose transport rates, lower glucose tolerance curves, and more body fat than littermates. In contrast, overexpression of metallothionein, a zinc/copper-binding protein, did not produce very dramatic gross effects on body composition or growth (59) but influenced zinc homeostasis (60). The genes for phosphoenolpyruvate carboxykinase, copper/zinc superoxide dismutase, hepatic lipase, lipoprotein lipase, and several apolipoproteins (see Chapters 74 and 75) have been overexpressed in transgenic mice (61–67). Table 36.1 lists some genes of nutritional interest that have been overexpressed in transgenic mice.

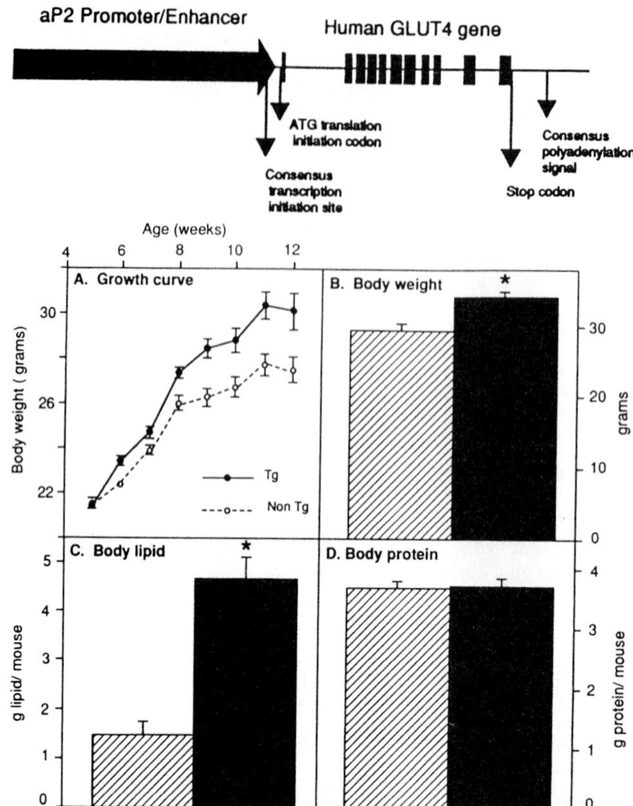

Figure 36.8. Overexpression of the human *GLUT4* gene in transgenic mice. *Top panel,* the transgene construct consisting of the mouse aP2 fatty acid–binding promoter ligated to 6.3 kb of human genomic DNA that includes all 11 exons of the glut4 transporter gene. *Bottom panels,* Growth and body composition comparisons for control *(cross-hatched bars)* and *GLUT4* transgenic mice *(solid bars)* fed a normal diet. (From Shepherd PR, Gnudi L, Tozzo E, et al. J Biol Chem 1993;268:22243–6, with permission.)

An encouraging aspect of the application of transgenic animals for nutrition research is that as these strains become more available through the Jackson Laboratory and other specialized distributors or from individual investigators, major new insights into nutrient metabolism and function will emerge.

Gene Knockout (Null Mutation) Animals

Gene knockout technology provides the opportunity to delete expression of a specific gene (null mutation). As a result, the normal gene product is not produced. Consequently, this technology is the engineered counterpart to spontaneous mutations that occur in laboratory animals and are propagated by selective breeding. The *ob* gene mutation of mice is an example of a spontaneous mutation.

Table 36.1
Transgenic Mice Overexpressing Genes of Interest in Nutrition Research—Examples

Gene Overexpressed	Ref.	Metabolic Consequences
Low-density-lipoprotein receptor	57	Increased disappearance of LDL from circulation
GLUT4 glucose transporter	18, 58	Increased body fat; glycemic control maintained with a high-fat diet
Metallothionein 1 and 2	59, 60	Protection against zinc deficiency and reduced zinc absorption
Phosphoenolpyruvate carboxykinase	61	Development of non-insulin-dependent diabetes mellitus
Copper/zinc superoxide dismutase	62	Enhanced tolerance of pancreatic β cells to oxidative stress
Hepatic lipase	63	Decreased total plasma cholesterol
Lipoprotein lipase	64	Reduced plasma VLDL
Apolipoprotein A-I	38, 65	Increased HDL cholesterol levels; increased HDL cholesterol and apoAI levels after fenofibrate treatment
Apolipoprotein C-III	66	Increased VLDL cholesterol and hypertriglyceridemia
Apolipoprotein B	67	Increased LDL cholesterol levels
Cellular glutathione peroxidase	67a	Increased GPX1 in RNA; normal lipid peroxidation

Knockout technology in animals has, thus far, been applied exclusively to murine genes. In some cases, the animals die prior to birth if a critical gene product is not produced. Numerous examples of this phenomenon have been reported. Deletion of the C/EBPα gene, which is required for energy (glucose) utilization, is an example relevant to nutrition (68). In some instances of deletion of a gene that may appear critical for nutrient metabolism (e.g., metallothionein for zinc metabolism), mice bearing the null mutation still reproduce and develop normally, albeit metabolic abnormalities can be demonstrated (60, 69). Similarly, a null mutation in the cellular retinoic acid–binding protein I gene (CRABPI), which is believed to be required for the function of vitamin A (retinol) via the metabolite retinoic acid, produces animals that appear to have a normal phenotype (71). These latter results indicate that, in some instances, another gene product provides the same phenotypic effect through redundancy of functional roles of specific genes or a gene family. Redundancy of function can obscure the true function of the deleted gene. Deletions of the genes for β_2-microglobulin, metallothionein, α-lactalbumin, Cu/Zn superoxide dismutase, cellular glutathione peroxidase, and apolipoprotein E have been reported to have metabolic consequences (72–78a). Table 36.2 shows examples of nutrient-related consequences detected in mice with null mutations.

In an interesting extension of the knockout technique, transgenic mice overexpressing apolipoprotein A-I were bred to apolipoprotein E null mice. The offspring had higher HDL levels and increased atherosclerotic lesions (79). Similarly, a mouse model with features of familial combined hyperlipidemia can be produced by crossing transgenic mice carrying the human apolipoprotein C-III to mice null for the LDL receptor (66).

The technique of creating a knockout animal model or null mutation is more correctly called "gene targeting by homologous recombination." Animal cells are diploid, i.e., they contain two copies (alleles) of a gene. The targeted gene is disrupted in one allele (producing heterozygotes with the null mutation), and homozygous genotypes are then produced by selective breeding of the heterozygous strain.

There are two approaches to developing knockout mice. The original approach is to isolate the murine gene under investigation, identify the exons by mapping, delete part of an exon, and replace it with the gene encoding neomycin resistance (thus producing a marker for selection). An entire exon can also be deleted. This construct is the gene targeting vector. The targeting vector is linearized and transfected into embryonic stem (ES) cells by microinjection or electroporation. The transfected cells are then injected into the blastocysts of mice at 3.5 days of pregnancy and introduced into pseudopregnant mice. Chimeric pups are often identified by the agouti coat color provided by genes from the ES cells. Selective breeding to obtain a null mutant (−/−) follows (15, 83).

Table 36.2
Knockout (Null Mutation) Mice with Deleted Genes of Interest in Nutrition Research—Examples

Gene Deletion	Ref.	Metabolic Consequence
C/EBPα	68	Hypoglycemia (lethal)
Metallothionein 1 and 2	60, 69, 70, 77, 78	Increased zinc absorption
Cellular retinoic acid–binding protein I	71	No effect
β_2-Microglobulin	72	Iron overload (increased absorption)
α-Lactalbumin	77	Increased milk viscosity; increased milk cholesterol; pups cannot remove milk from mammary gland
Copper/zinc superoxide dismutase	74	O_2 sensitivity
Apolipoprotein E	75, 76, 79–82	Severe hypercholesterolemia when fed low-fat, low-cholesterol diet; reduction of arteriosclerotic lesion development by estrogen; xanthomatous lesions in tissues; severe atherosclerosis resulting from impaired efflux of LDL cholesterol from macrophages
Low-density-lipoprotein receptors	66	Increased plasma LDL cholesterol levels
Cellular glutathione peroxidase	78a	Decreased tissue glutathione peroxidase activity and total liver selenium content

The second and more recent approach allows cell type–specific targeting of a gene deletion (84, 85). The gene is engineered to have specific sequences (lox P sites) on either side and, by ES cell technology, a transgenic line is created carrying the target gene and flanking lox P sites. Another transgenic strain is produced with a construct comprising the CRe recombinase gene and a promoter (e.g., Mx1) that can be activated by an inducer (e.g., Interferon-α [IFNα]) in a tissue-specific manner. These mouse strains are crossed and, when IFNα is injected into offspring, the CRe gene product (CRe recombinase; a bacteriophage enzyme) acts at one of the lox P sites, deleting the target gene in a specific tissue/cell type where the CRe gene product is produced (84, 85).

These techniques, while specialized, are yielding murine strains that will be generally available for nutritional and metabolic studies. As with transgenic overexpressing mice, commercial suppliers may act as a resource for such animals.

Inhibition of Specific Gene Expression by Antisense Oligonucleotides and Transgenes

Antisense RNA has recently been used as a research tool for questions of nutritional interest. There are three ways in which antisense sequences can be used. Computer searches of the literature usually do not differentiate between these uses.

The first is the use of antisense RNA as probes in solution hybridization/RNase protection assays. When sequence information is known, specific oligonucleotides can be generated and used to obtain information about the relative abundance of a specific mRNA. Tissue RNA is hybridized with the ^{32}P-labeled antisense RNA probe, treated with RNase to hydrolyze single-stranded RNA, and then the protected ^{32}P-labeled RNA (hybridized RNA) is precipitated and separated by electrophoresis followed by autoradiography. Abundance is measured by densitometry. Once the assay has been established, the precipitated ^{32}P-labeled hybrid is measured by liquid scintillation counting for comparison of mRNA abundance. This approach has been used to examine GLUT4 transporter expression and glucagon receptor expression (86, 87).

The second application of antisense oligonucleotides is selective permanent inhibition of a targeted RNA (88). Usually, oligonucleotides are at least 12 to 25 nucleotides long to provide the specificity needed for identification of a unique mRNA. Sites where targeting is most effective are the double-stranded regions of secondary mRNA structure. This approach has been used in experiments with cells. To address directly questions of nutritional interest, antisense sequences can be used to generate transgenic mice. The antisense sequences are introduced by the construct used for microinjection. Mice carrying the transgene continually produce antisense sequences that neutralize the effect of the targeted mRNA, thus preventing formation of the gene product. Consequently, these transgenics have altered phenotypes. This approach has received limited use in experiments focused on nutrition and gene expression (89, 90).

Table 36.3
Antisense Oligonucleotide–Inhibited Gene Expression—Examples

Gene	Ref.	Metabolic Consequence
Neuropeptide Y (NPY)-Y1 receptor	92	Increased food intake
Neuropeptide Y	93	Increased food intake and body weight
Corticotropin-releasing factor	94	Increased food intake
Oxytocin	95	Decreased salt intake

The third use of antisense sequence information is for transient inhibition of translation of specific mRNAs by hybridization. This approach has received attention because of the potential therapeutic use of antisense oligonucleotides. The exact mechanisms of their action are also actively investigated (reviewed in [88, 91]). These oligonucleotides appear to be taken up by cells in the brain and some tissues. The approach has been recently applied to inhibition of mRNAs for peptides involved in regulation of feeding behavior and body weight (92–95). In these cases, antisense DNA sequences are introduced into specific areas of the brain. Examples of use of this technique are shown in Table 36.3.

SUMMARY

The area of nutrition and gene expression is gaining interest rapidly and is now a recognized research discipline in nutritional sciences. As our knowledge of animal and human genomes expands, the technologies described here and new approaches still to be developed will have a profound impact on nutrition as a field and on our understanding of how the diet influences genetic expression.

ACKNOWLEDGMENTS

The author expresses his appreciation to Drs. Barbara A. Davis of Virginia Polytechnic Institute and State University and Cathy W. Levenson of Florida State University for their review of this chapter and valuable comments, and to Mr. Walter M. Jones for drawing some of the figures.

REFERENCES

1. Jacob F, Monod J. J Mol Biol 1961;3:318–56.
2. Baliga BS, Pronczuk AW, Munro HN. J Mol Biol 1968;34:199–218.
3. Zähringer J, Baliga BS, Munro HN. Proc Natl Acad Sci USA 1976;73:857–61.
4. Tilghman SM, Hanson RW, Reshef L, et al. Proc Natl Acad Sci USA 1974;71:1304–8.
5. Zull JE, Czarnowska-Misztal E, DeLuca HF. Science 1965;149:182–4.
6. Thomas PR, Earl R, eds. Opportunities in the nutrition and food sciences. Washington, DC: National Academy Press, 1994;47–97.

7. Lewin B. Genes V. New York: Oxford University Press, 1994.
8. Alberts B, Bray D, Lewis J, et al., eds. Molecular biology of the cell. New York: Garland Publishing, 1994.
9. Goldstein JL, Brown MS. Nature 1990;343:425–30.
10. Holick MF. Vitamin D. In: Shils ME, Olson JA, Shike M, eds. Modern nutrition in health and disease. 8th ed. Philadelphia: Lea & Febiger, 1994;308–25.
11. Pfahl M, Chytil F. Annu Rev Nutr 1996;16:257–83.
11a. Forman BM, Chen J, Evans RM. Proc Natl Acad Sci USA 1997;94:4312.
11b. Kliewer SA, Sundseth SS, Jones SA, et al. Proc Natl Acad Sci USA 1997;94:4318.
12. Cousins RJ. Annu Rev Nutr 1994;14:449–69
13. Schuler GD, Boguski MS, Stewart EA, et al. Science 1996;274:540–6.
14. Savon SP, Hakimi P, Crawford DR, et al. J Nutr 1997;127: 276–85.
15. Ausubel FM, Brent R, Kingston RE, et al., eds. Current protocols in molecular biology. New York: John Wiley & Sons, 1987, 3 volumes.
16. Palmiter RD, Findley SD. EMBO J 1995;14:639–49.
17. Gassmann M. Thömmes P, Weiser T, et al. FASEB J 1990;4: 2528–32.
18. Ikemoto S, Thompson KS, Takahashi M, et al. Proc Natl Acad Sci USA 1995;92:3096–9.
19. King LE, Osati-Ashtiani F, Fraker PJ. Immunology 1995;85: 69–73.
20. Saladin R, De Vos P, Guerre-Millo M, et al. Nature 1995;377: 527–9.
21. Blanchard RK, Cousins RJ. Proc Natl Acad Sci USA 1996;93: 6863–8.
22. Haugland RP. Handbook of fluorescent probes and research chemicals. 6th ed. Eugene, OR: Molecular Probes, 1996.
23. Kawasaki ES. Amplification of RNA. In: Innis MA, Gelfand DH, Sninsky JJ, et al., eds. PCR protocols, a guide to methods and applications. San Diego: Academic Press, 1990;21–7.
24. Sambrook J, Maniatis T, Fritsch EF. Molecular cloning: a laboratory manual. 2nd ed. Cold Spring Harbor, NY: Cold Spring Harbor Laboratory Press, 1989, 3 volumes.
25. Kohler T, Labner D, Thamm B, et al., eds. Quantitation of mRNA by polymerase chain reaction. Nonradioactive PCR methods. Berlin: Springer-Verlag, 1995;3–13.
26. Levenson CW, Shay NF, Lee-Ambrose LM, et al. Proc Natl Acad Sci USA 1993;90:712–5.
27. Celi FS, Zenilman ME, Shuldiner AR. Nucleic Acids Res 1993;21:1047.
28. Gilliland G, Perrin S, Blanchard K, et al. Proc Natl Acad Sci USA 1990;87:2725–9.
29. Klebe RJ, Grant GM, Grant AM, et al. BioTechniques 1996;21:1094–100.
30. Sullivan VK, Cousins RJ. J Nutr 1997;127:694–8.
31. Morrison NA, Qi JC, Tokita A, et al. Nature 1994;367:284–7.
32. Fleet JC, Harris SS, Wood RJ, et al. J Bone Miner Res 1995;10:985–90.
33. Lopez-Miranda J, Ordovas JM, Mata P, et al. J Lipid Res 1994;35:1965–75.
34. Lamers WH, Hanson RW, Meisner HM. Proc Natl Acad Sci USA 1982;79:5137–41.
35. Towle HC. J Biol Chem 1995;270:23235–8.
36. Jump DB, Clarke SD, MacDougald O, et al. Proc Natl Acad Sci USA 1993;90:8454–8.
37. Levenson CW, Shay NF, Hempe JM, et al. J Nutr 1994;124:13–7.
38. Schoonjans K, Peinado-Onsurbe J, Lefebre A-M, et al. EMBO J 1996;15:5336–48.
39. Miller SG, De Vos P, Guerre-Millo M, et al. Proc Natl Acad Sci USA 1996;93:5507–11.
40. Birkenmeier EH, Gordon JI. Proc Natl Acad Sci USA 1986;83:2516–20.
41. Shay NF, Cousins RJ. J Nutr 1993;123:35–41.
42. Liang P, Pardee AB. Science 1992;257:967–71.
43. Blanchard RK, Cousins RJ. FASEB J 1995;9:A866.
44. Blanchard RK, Cousins RJ. Am J Physiol 1997;272:G972–8.
45. Kendall SD, Christensen MJ. FASEB J 1995;9:A158.
46. Levenson CW. Am J Clin Nutr 1998, in press.
47. Wang YR, Wu JYJ, Reaves SK, et al. J Nutr 1996;126:1772–81.
48. Zhang Y, Proenca R, Maffei M, et al. Nature 1994;372:425–32.
49. Halaas JL, Gajiwala KS, Maffei M, et al. Science 1995;269: 543–6.
50. Considine RV, Sinha MK, Heiman ML, et al. N Engl J Med 1996;334:292–5.
51. Lönnqvist F, Arner P, Nordfors L, et al. Nat Med 1995;1:950–3.
52. Muzzin P, Eisensmith RC, Copeland KC, et al. Proc Natl Acad Sci USA 1996;93:14804–8.
53. Erickson JC, Hollopeter G, Palmiter RD. Science 1996;274: 1704–7.
54. Palmiter RD, Brinster RL, Hammer RE. Nature 1982;300: 611–5.
55. Pursel, VG, Pinkert CA, Miller KF, et al. Science 1989;244: 1281–8.
56. Cousins RJ, Lee-Ambrose LM. J Nutr 1992;122:56–64.
57. Hofmann SL, Russell DW, Brown MS, et al. Science 1988;239:1277–81.
58. Shepherd PR, Gnudi L, Tozzo E, et al. J Biol Chem 1993;268:22243–6.
59. Dalton T, Fu K, Palmiter RD, et al. J Nutr 1996;126:825–33.
60. Davis SR, McMahon RJ, Cousins RJ. J Nutr 1998, in press.
61. Valera A, Pujol A, Pelegrin M, et al. Proc Natl Acad Sci USA 1994;91:9151–4.
62. Kubisch HM, Wang J, Luche R, et al. Proc Natl Acad Sci USA 1994;91:9956–9.
63. Fan J, Wang J, Bensadoun A, et al. Proc Natl Acad Sci USA 1994;91:8724–8.
64. Zsigmond E, Scheffler E, Forte TM, et al. J Biol Chem 1994;269:18757–66.
65. Walsh A, Ito Y, Breslow JL. J Biol Chem 1989;264:6488–94.
66. Masucci-Magoulas L, Goldberg IJ, Bisgaier CL, et al. Science 1997;275:391–4.
67. Callow MJ, Stoltzfus LJ, Lawn RM, et al. Proc Natl Acad Sci USA 1994;91:2130–4.
67a. Chang WH, Ho YS, Ross DA, et al. J Nutr 1997;127:675.
68. Wang N, Fingold MJ, Bradely A, et al. Science 1995;269: 1108–12.
69. Kelly EJ, Quaife CJ, Froelick GJ, et al. J Nutr 1996;126:1782–90.
70. Coyle P, Philcox JC, Rofe AM. Biochem J 1995;309:25–31.
71. Gorry P, Lufkin T, Dierich A, et al. Proc Natl Acad Sci USA 1994;91:9032–6.
72. Rothenberg BE, Voland JR. Proc Natl Acad Sci USA 1996;93: 1529–34.
73. Stinnakre MG, Vilotte JL, Soulier S, et al. Proc Natl Acad Sci USA 1994;91:6544–8.
74. Carlsson LM, Jonsson J, Edlund, et al. Proc Natl Acad Sci USA 1995;92:6264–8.
75. Plump AS, Smith JD, Hayek T, et al. Cell 1992;71:343–53.
76. Bourassa P-AK, Milos PM, Gaynor BJ, et al. Proc Natl Acad Sci USA 1996;93:10022–7.
77. Michalska AE, Choo KHA. Proc Natl Acad Sci USA 1993;90:8088–92.

78. Masters BA, Kelly EJ, Quaife CJ, et al. Proc Natl Acad Sci USA 1994;91:584–8.
78a. Chang WH, Ho YS, Ross DA, et al. J Nutr 1997;127:1445.
79. Plump AS, Scott CJ, Breslow JL. Proc Natl Acad Sci USA 1994;91:9607–11.
80. van Ree JH, Gijbels MJJ, van den Broek WJAA, et al. Atherosclerosis 1995;112:237–43.
81. Hayek T, Oiknine J, Brook JG, et al. Biochem Biophys Res Commun 1994;205:1072–8.
82. Pászty C, Maeda N, Verstuyft J, et al. J Clin Invest 1994;94: 899–903.
83. Majzoub JA, Muglia LJ. N Engl J Med 1996;334:904–7.
84. Gu H, Marth JD, Orban PC, et al. Science 1994;265:103–6.
85. Kühn R, Schwenk F, Aguet M, et al. Science 1995;269:1427–9.
86. Woloschak M, Shen-Orr Z, LeRoith D, et al. Proc Soc Exp Biol Med 1993;203:172–174.
87. Svoboda M, Tastenoy M, Vertongen P, et al. Mol Cell Endocrinol 1994;105:131–7.
88. Wagner RW, Matteucci MD, Grant D, et al. Nature Biotech 1996;14:840–4.
89. Pepin M-C, Pothier F, Barden N. Nature 1992;355:725–8.
90. Moxham CM, Hod Y, Malbon CC. Science 1993;260:991–5.
91. Phillips MI, Gyurko R. Regul Pept 1995;59:131–41.
92. Heilig M. Regul Pept 1995;59:201–5.
93. Hulsey MG, Pless CM, White BD, et al. Regul Pept 1995;59:207–14.
94. Hulsey MG, Pless CM, Martin RJ. Regul Pept 1995;59:241–6.
95. Morris M, Li P, Barrett C, et al. Regul Pept 1995;59:261–6.

SELECTED READINGS

Berdanier CD, Hargrove JL, eds. Nutrition and gene expression. Boca Raton, FL: CRC Press, 1993.

Cousins RJ. Metal elements and gene expression. Annu Rev Nutr 1994;14:449–69.

Nizielski SE, Lechner PS, Croniger CM, et al. Animal models for studying the genetic basis of metabolic regulation. J Nutr 1996;126:2697–708.

Thomas PR, Earl R, eds. Opportunities in the nutrition and food sciences. Washington, DC: National Academy Press, 1994;47–97.

Towle HC. Metabolic regulation of gene transcription in animals. J Biol Chem 1995;270:23235–8.

37. Transmembrane Signaling: A Tutorial

ROBERT A. GABBAY and JEFFREY S. FLIER

The evolution of life forms from unicellular to multicellular organisms necessitated a mechanism for cells to communicate with each other. One of the primary modes of cellular communication is the release of soluble factors from one cell or organ to influence the metabolism and biology of another. These soluble factors—which include hormones, neurotransmitters, growth factors, and cytokines—are generally hydrophilic molecules that cannot cross the hydrophobic plasma membrane of cells. A system is therefore required to recognize these extracellular signals and transmit the information across the plasma membrane to direct appropriate changes in the intracellular environment. This tutorial focuses on the basic principles underlying this signaling system, with an emphasis on those mechanisms pertinent to physiology and nutrition. Then, we see how aberrations in this signaling system can result in diabetes, cancer, and a host of other metabolic disturbances.

Any transmembrane signaling system requires several features. First, there must be specificity in responding to a given extracellular signal. Recognition of this signal will then generate a specific response. This response should also be specific to the cell type or organ involved. Next, the response to a specific signal must be rapid. An efficient mechanism is required to shut off that signal when it is no longer needed. Finally, there must be a means of regulating a host of processes that will ultimately produce the biologic response desired (1).

Extracellular signals are recognized through their specific binding to cell surface *receptors.* These receptors, generally transmembrane proteins, interact with an intracellular effector system that often results in production of small soluble molecules *(second messengers)* that diffuse through the cell to mediate the actions of the given extracellular stimulus (Fig. 37.1). The concept of a second messenger was first proposed by Sutherland in 1959 when he identified cyclic AMP as a second messenger capable of mimicking the effects of the hormone epinephrine. Sutherland proposed that the hormone is the first messenger released into the bloodstream to interact with a specific membrane receptor on the target tissue. The specific binding of the hormone to its cell-surface receptor leads to generation of a second, intracellular messenger that then mediates the intracellular actions of the given hormone. This model of hormone action has been borne out for many different extracellular signals. Although there are few second messenger systems, they are used by a myriad of different extracellular stimuli. Along with cyclic AMP, the other main second messengers mediating hormone action include cyclic GMP, calcium, and diacylglycerol. In most cases, GTP-binding proteins *(G-proteins)* act as molecular switches to couple receptor binding to the enzymes that generate the specific second messenger. All these signaling pathways share a final common mechanism in activating *protein kinases* that alter subsequent enzyme activities through covalent addition of a phosphate group to serine, threonine, or tyrosine residues of various proteins. Although many hormones act through the generation of second messengers that then stimulate specific protein kinases, some directly lead to protein kinase activation by binding to receptors that have intrinsic tyrosine kinase activity. Regardless of the route leading to protein kinase activation, subsequent changes in protein phosphorylation alters the activity of proteins involved in nutrient flux, transcription of specific genes, protein synthesis, and cellular trafficking of proteins.

The steroid hormones are more hydrophobic and capable of crossing the plasma membrane. They bind specifically to a soluble receptor in the cytoplasm. The hormone-receptor complex then enters the nucleus to function as a DNA-binding protein that directly affects transcription of specific genes. We will not cover this nuclear hormone signaling mechanism here but, instead, will focus on transmembrane signaling at the plasma membrane. The prototypical signaling pathways through which the vast majority of other hormones act and, finally, how aberrations in these signaling mechanisms may underlie diseases from cancer to diabetes are described in detail below.

The rapid advances in understanding transmembrane signal transduction have been aided by the use of several powerful techniques. Recombinant DNA technology (see Chapter 36) has permitted the rapid cloning of members of signaling families, i.e., structurally and functionally related groups of proteins. The hundreds of different receptors can be grouped into only a few large families of receptor types. The introduction of several mutants and inhibitors of signaling pathways into cultured cells has allowed further dissection and understanding of the transmembrane signaling pathway. Finally, the development of transgenic animals in which a particular gene and protein can either be overexpressed or "knocked-out" allows integration of cellular signaling pathways with physiologic studies.

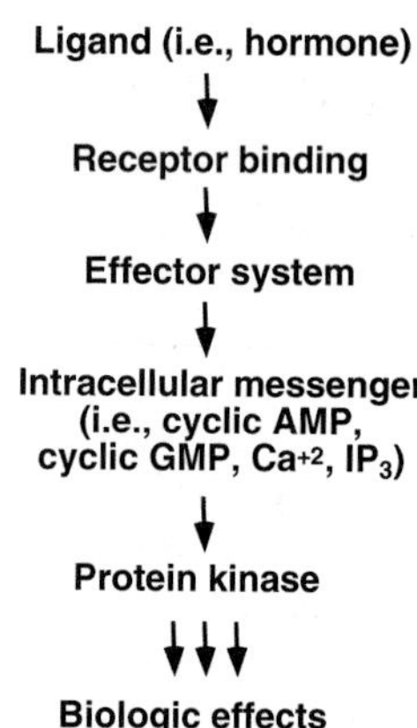

Figure 37.1. General schematic overview of ligand-receptor pathway of biologic effects.

RECEPTORS

The initial step in transmembrane signaling involves the binding of the extracellular signal or hormone to a cell-surface receptor. Receptors provide the first level of specificity by their presence on only certain tissues and cell types. These receptors have several characteristics that poise them for recognition of extracellular signals (2). First, they have *high affinity* for the *ligand* (hormone or other extracellular signal that binds to the receptor). This is necessary because most hormones circulate in the bloodstream at concentrations below 10^{-8} M. This high affinity enables cells to respond to small changes in hormone concentration. Receptors are also *specific* for their ligand or hormone. This means that insulin binds only to the insulin receptor, whereas glucagon binds only to the glucagon receptor. Various structural analogues of a given hormone bind to their receptor with differing affinities that correspond to their biologic activity. For example, insulin binds to the insulin receptor with 50 times higher affinity than proinsulin and is 50-fold more potent than proinsulin in stimulating glucose uptake. Receptor binding can be plotted as shown in Figure 37.2. Agents can be found that have higher affinity for a receptor (potent *agonists*), whereas others may bind to receptors with high affinity but not trigger the usual transmembrane signaling and biologic responses *(antagonists)*. These principles have led to the development of a large number of widely used pharmacologic therapies.

Hormone-receptor interactions can be studied by a variety of techniques. The receptor number and affinity on a particular target cell is classically measured using a *Scatchard analysis* (Fig. 37.3). By allowing labeled hormone to compete with unlabeled (cold) hormone for receptor binding, the amount of hormone bound to receptor is determined at a number of hormone concentrations. This amount of bound hormone is plotted against the ratio of bound to free hormone, typically yielding a straight line. The slope of this line is the negative value of the association constant ($^{-}K_a$), which indicates the receptor affinity for the hormone or ligand. The intercept on the abscissa represents the total receptor concentration (R_T).

A given hormone can bind to several different receptors, each of which communicates with a unique intracellular effector system. For example, epinephrine can bind to both α- and β-adrenergic receptors. β-Adrenergic receptors are coupled to a cyclic AMP–generating second-messenger system, whereas α-adrenergic receptors use calcium as their second messenger or act by decreasing the level of cyclic AMP (3). Further specificity of action is obtained by the presence of various receptor subtypes located in different tissues. For example, β_1-adrenergic receptors are present primarily in the heart, where they function to stimulate heart rate and increase the force of cardiac contraction. β_2-Receptors, on the other hand, are primarily located in the lungs, where they cause bronchial dilation. This specificity in receptor subtype tissue distribution has been used to develop specific pharmacologic agents with high affinity for particular receptor subtypes (e.g., β_1-adrenergic receptor–blocking agents that selectively decrease heart rate without causing bronchoconstriction or β_2-agonists that cause bronchial dilation with minimal effects on cardiac function).

The ligands that bind to receptors can take many forms. Initially, the study of receptors focused on protein hormones as the ligands of interest. Since that time, a variety of ligands including neurotransmitters, cytokines (proliferating and differentiating agents of the hematopoietic and immune systems), and various growth factors also

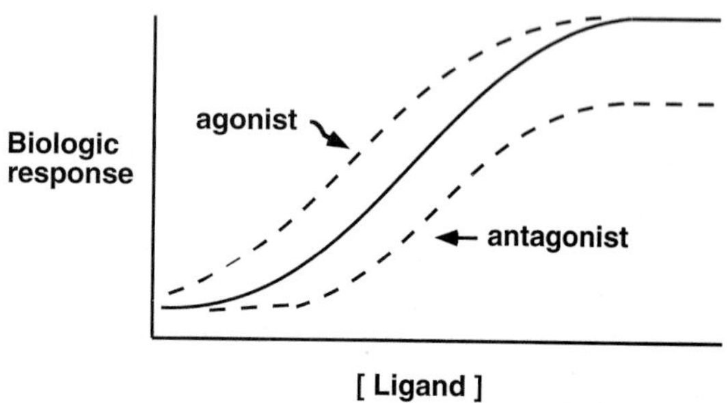

Figure 37.2. Concentration dependence of the effects of an agonist and an antagonist relative to native hormone on a typical biologic response.

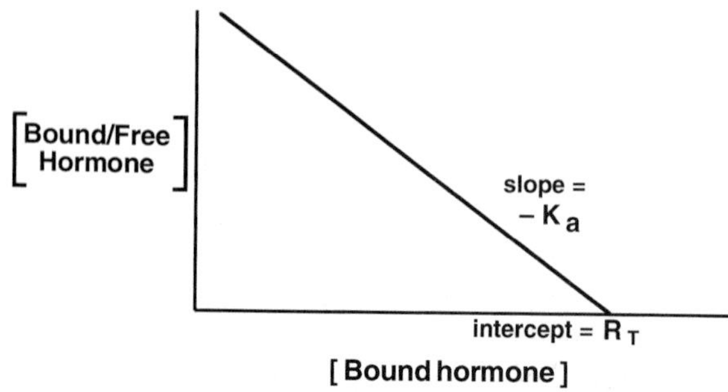

Figure 37.3. Diagram of Scatchard analysis, showing the relationship of slope to $-K_a$ and of the intercept to the total number of receptors.

have been shown to act through receptor binding to specific cell-surface receptors. Metabolites also can act as ligands through binding to specific receptors. For example, fatty acids released by fat metabolism can bind to a specific transcription factor receptor (peroxisome proliferator-activating receptor, PPARγ) to stimulate specifically adipose cell differentiation. Another "ligandlike" agent is light, which, through photoisomerization of 11-*cis*-retinal, stimulates a specific receptor in the eye to begin the transmembrane signaling cascade responsible for vision (see Chapter 17).

Receptor Types

Receptors can be divided into four major types: *(a)* G-protein-linked receptors; *(b)* enzyme-linked receptors; *(c)* ion-channel-linked receptors; and *(d)* steroid hormone receptors. *G-protein-linked receptors* use a GTP-binding protein to couple the receptor to the particular effector system that, typically, generates a second messenger (i.e., cyclic AMP, cyclic GMP, inositol trisphosphate, or diacylglycerol). *Enzyme-linked receptors* either have intrinsic enzyme activity or are tightly coupled to proteins with enzyme activity. As discussed above (see Chapters 17 and 18), steroid/retinoid hormone receptors are located in the cytoplasm and/or nucleus where they recognize steroid hormones that have diffused across the plasma membrane. These receptors still possess the same basic properties of receptors described above (i.e., high affinity and specificity), but they have several unique features as described in other chapters. Ion channel receptors, also termed *ligand-gated channels,* act to increase ion flux (usually calcium, potassium, or sodium) across the plasma membrane, either as direct conduits for ion flow or through coupling to ion channels (see Chapter 38). The following sections focus on the G-protein-linked and enzyme-linked receptors.

G-Proteins

Over the last 25 years, many receptors linked to effector systems by trimeric GTP-binding proteins (G-proteins) have been described. These proteins regulate the activity of a specific plasma membrane enzyme or ion channel in response to receptor binding. This transmembrane signaling pathway, first described by Gilman, uses a trimeric GTP-binding protein as a molecular switch to activate the appropriate effector system rapidly. Hormone binding leads to G-protein activation through the binding of GTP. The G-protein, which is active in the GTP-bound state, can then move through the plasma membrane to modulate the appropriate effector system. G-Proteins have an intrinsic GTPase activity that hydrolyzes the bound GTP to GDP, inactivating the G-protein. This permits both the rapid turning on (binding of GTP) and turning off (hydrolysis by GTPase) of the signal that is needed to respond to rapid fluctuations in hormone levels.

Several different types of G-proteins couple to specific plasma-membrane enzyme-effector systems leading to generation of soluble second messengers (5). Cyclic AMP was the first second messenger discovered. Subsequent research showed that a specific G-protein (G_s) couples receptor binding to the activation of the enzyme that generates cyclic AMP *(adenylate cyclase).* As a second messenger, the cyclic AMP that is generated mediates all the intracellular actions of the hormone. The rapid generation of cyclic AMP can be turned off by hydrolysis with phosphodiesterase, providing a transient response to a given signal (Fig. 37.4). In addition, the G protein has an intrinsic GTPase activity that hydrolyzes the GTP bound to G_s, restoring G_s to the inactive form. Finally, a different G-protein (G_i), when activated by other receptors, leads to direct inhibition of adenylate cyclase activity and, thus, cyclic AMP generation. A host of hormones act through this G_s–adenylate cyclase–cyclic AMP mechanism (Fig. 37.4).

Several naturally occurring bacterial toxins have been instrumental in unraveling the role of G-proteins in cyclic AMP signaling and disease processes. Cholera toxin was discovered to attach the ADP-ribose moiety from NAD to the G_s protein, thereby blocking its GTPase activity (also see Chapter 23). The resulting inability of the G_s protein to turn off its signal leads to prolonged elevation of cyclic AMP levels in the intestinal epithelium. In turn, this causes the large efflux of sodium ions and water into the gut that is responsible for the severe diarrhea of cholera. Similarly, pertussis toxin (from the bacteria causing whooping cough) transfers ADP-ribose from NAD to the G_i protein, thereby preventing interaction of G_i with its receptor, rendering G_i unable to lower cyclic AMP levels. In this situation, the prolonged elevation in cyclic AMP in the bronchial epithelium appears to contribute to cellular necrosis.

Different receptors are coupled to different G-proteins, and the same hormone sometimes can either decrease or increase cyclic AMP levels, depending on which receptor it binds to. For example, epinephrine can bind to both the α- and β-adrenergic receptors. The β receptor for epinephrine is coupled to G_s, and therefore, the binding of epinephrine increases cyclic AMP levels; whereas the α_2-adrenergic receptor is coupled to G_i, so that epinephrine binding leads to a decrease in cyclic AMP levels. The specificity of these responses is governed by the receptor and its specific localization in a particular tissue (Table 37.1).

Actions of Cyclic AMP. Cyclic AMP actions are mediated by the stimulation of *cyclic AMP–dependent protein kinase.* This protein kinase family phosphorylates a series of different proteins leading to activity changes that account for the hormone's biologic actions. Activation of protein kinases upon receptor binding is a fundamental aspect of hormone action. The first delineation of these protein phosphorylations responsible for hormone action was in the pathways for skeletal muscle glycogen metabolism.

The release of epinephrine in response to a threat to an

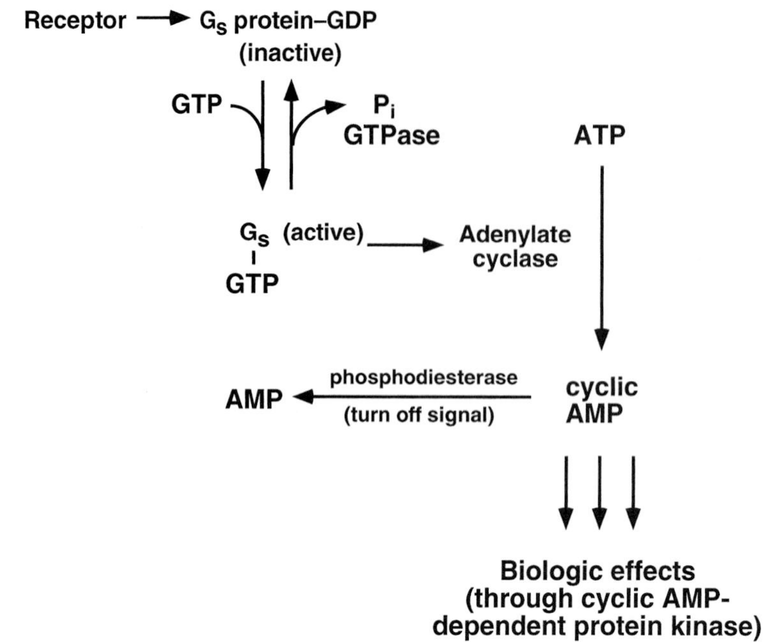

Figure 37.4. Schematic overview of the pathway from receptor through a G-protein signaling cascade involving formation of cyclic AMP.

animal (the fight-or-flight response) leads to rapid mobilization of muscle glycogen for fuel requirements. As illustrated in Figure 37.5, the binding of epinephrine to the β-adrenergic receptors on skeletal muscle leads to activation of G_s and adenylate cyclase. The cyclic AMP that is formed and released activates cyclic AMP–dependent protein kinase, which then phosphorylates phosphorylase kinase. This enzyme, upon the covalent addition of a phosphate group, becomes an active kinase that phosphorylates the enzyme phosphorylase. Phosphorylase is converted to the active form by this phosphorylation so that it may catalyze the hydrolysis of glycogen to glucose-1-phosphate, which can now enter the glycolytic pathway and the tricarboxylic acid cycle to provide metabolic energy for muscle activity. Knowledge of this phosphorylation cascade in muscle energy metabolism has served as the paradigm for hormone regulation of metabolic processes in other systems.

The different G-protein-coupled receptor signaling mechanisms (cyclic AMP, calcium, diacylglycerol) all share certain basic properties. In general, they involve the generation of mediators that initiate a cascade of intracellular reactions (well characterized in the example of epinephrine regulation of glycogen metabolism in Figure 37.5). One inherent advantage of this cascading signaling mechanism is *amplification* of the signal as it is relayed along the chain. For example, a single signaling molecule or hormone binds to one receptor that can then activate several G-proteins, each of which may activate its coupled enzyme (i.e., adenylate cyclase). Each adenylate cyclase may catalyze formation of multiple cyclic AMP molecules, each of which may activate one cyclic AMP–dependent protein kinase. This kinase can then phosphorylate multiple molecules of other kinases; thus, the cascade continues to amplify as it travels "downward" toward the ultimate target. The advantage of such an amplification system is that a very small amount of hormone (often in the nanomolar range) can lead to a thousandfold increase in the level of a second messenger, leading to a robust biologic response. The circulating concentration of hormone must be quite low to enable the organism to respond to small changes and to ensure that the given hormone does not bind to other, somewhat similar, but lower-affinity, receptors that may exist within a given receptor family. In addition, systems with multiple steps have the potential for additional regulation from other factors at each step in the pathway. The additional regulation allows fine-tuning of the signal as well as the ability to override a given stimulus under appropriate circumstances.

Table 37.1
Some Hormones That Act Through Cyclic AMP

Target Tissue	Hormone	Major Response
Heart	Epinephrine	Increase in heart rate; increase force of contraction
Liver	Glucagon	Glycogen breakdown; gluconeogenesis
Kidney	Vasopressin	Water reabsorption
Fat	Epinephrine	Triglyceride breakdown
Muscle	Epinephrine	Glycogen breakdown
Thyroid gland	TSH	Thyroid hormone synthesis and secretion
Adrenal gland	ACTH	Cortisol secretion
Ovary	LH	Progesterone secretion

Counterbalancing Mechanisms. For this exquisitely sensitive amplification system to be useful, there must be powerful counterbalancing mechanisms to shut off the signal and restore the resting state. This is accomplished at sev-

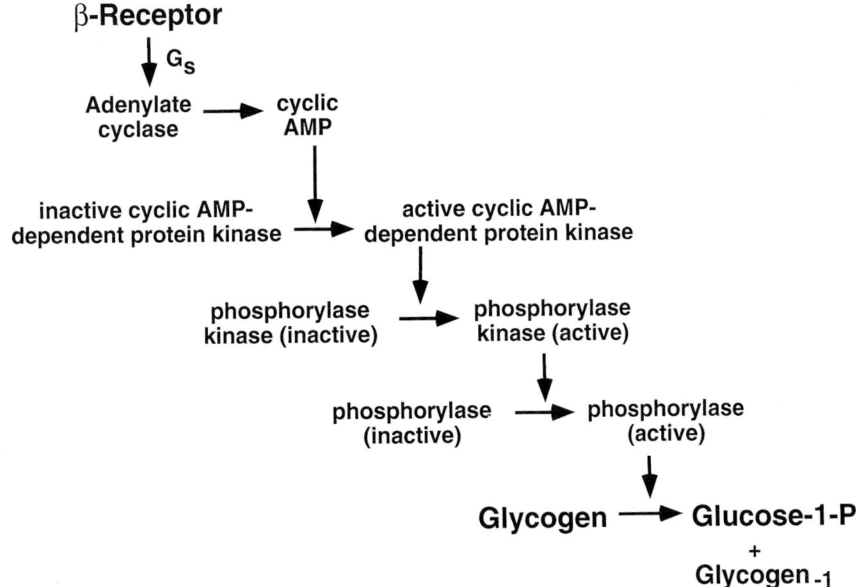

Figure 37.5. The glycogen cascade, illustrating the sequence of phosphorylation events that lead to glycogenolysis.

eral levels of the signal transduction system. First, after hormones bind to receptors they are often internalized for destruction of the ligand. Next, as described above, G proteins are inactivated by their intrinsic GTPase activity. In addition, second messengers such as cyclic AMP are rapidly hydrolyzed by phosphodiesterase. In the case of intracellular calcium as a second messenger, intracellular pumps exist to remove cytosolic calcium, thereby returning the cell to the resting state.

Organisms have also developed mechanisms to desensitize themselves to a continuous stimulus. Prolonged stimulation by a growth factor, for example, could have devastating effects on homeostasis. Desensitization mechanisms provide another level at which a signal can be shut off (4). The most common form of desensitization is through decreasing hormone receptor number (i.e., regulation of receptor number at the cell surface). Therefore, despite continued presence of the hormone in question, transmembrane signaling is blunted because there are fewer receptors to bind the hormone. Recently, a new mechanism of signal desensitization has been described for the *β*-adrenergic receptor. Prolonged receptor stimulation leads to activation of a *β*-adrenergic receptor kinase that phosphorylates the receptor, causing it to uncouple from the G_s protein.

The cyclic AMP signaling system can also control transcription of specific genes. Cyclic AMP–dependent protein kinase phosphorylation of the cyclic AMP response element–binding protein (CREB) enhances CREB's binding to a specific site on the promoter of a gene termed the *cyclic AMP response element* (CRE). This protein-DNA (CREB-CRE) interaction results in changes in transcription of the particular gene containing the CRE, altering gene expression (see Chapter 36).

Analogous to the cyclic AMP system, another enzyme, guanylate cyclase, produces cyclic GMP that specifically activates a cyclic GMP–dependent protein kinase. This system is particularly important in the response of the photoreceptors of the eye to light. As shown below, a related system is implicated in the actions of atrial naturetic factor—a regulator of renal fluid handling and vascular tone.

Calcium As a Second Messenger

The next major second-messenger system involves increases in *intracellular calcium*. Cells maintain an intracellular calcium concentration of about 10^{-7} M in the face of an extracellular calcium concentration of 10^{-3} M. This 10,000-fold concentration gradient is maintained by a number of plasma membrane–associated calcium-ATPase pumps that remove calcium from cells. These pumps can be either voltage-gated as in excitable cells (i.e., they release calcium in response to changes in cellular depolarization) or, in most cells, not regulated. The pool of intracellular calcium that is regulated in these cells resides in the endoplasmic reticulum and in a newly described calcium-storage site called the *calciosome*. The first evidence that calcium can serve a messenger role within the cell came from experiments in which injection of calcium into skeletal muscle cells resulted in muscle cell contraction. Since that time, an elegant transmembrane signaling system has been unraveled in which the turnover of phosphatidylinositides leads to a rise in intracellular calcium.

Hokin and Hokin (6) first suggested a role for phosphoinositide turnover in cellular signaling in 1953 when they observed that various extracellular signaling molecules stimulated incorporation of ^{32}P from ATP into plasma membrane phosphoinositides. This was later explained by the rapid breakdown and resynthesis of phosphatidylinositols in response to these stimuli (6). In particular, the breakdown of phosphatidylinositol bisphosphate generates two second messengers: *inositol 3,4,5-trisphosphate (IP_3)* and *diacylglycerol*. Analogous to the generation of cyclic AMP, a specific G-protein (G_q) couples receptor binding to activation of a phosphoinositide-specific phospholipase C that hydrolyzes phosphatidylinositol to generate these two intracellular messengers (7).

IP_3 is released into the cytoplasm where it binds to a receptor on the calciosome, leading to release of calcium into the cytoplasm. IP_3 is then dephosphorylated to shut off this calcium release signal. In addition, IP_3 can be phosphorylated to inositol 1,3,4,5-tetrakiphosphate, a molecule that has been implicated in the sustained release of calcium from the endoplasmic reticulum that is observed in response to stimulation by some hormones. *Calcium-binding proteins* within cells mediate the effects of increased intracellular calcium. For skeletal muscle contraction, troponin binds calcium to initiate actin-myosin-mediated contraction. A more ubiquitous mediator of intracellular calcium is the calcium-binding protein calmodulin. A family of serine/threonine protein kinase *(calmodulin-dependent protein kinases)* is stimulated by this calcium-binding protein. Analogous to the situation with cyclic AMP, some extracellular stimuli result in G-protein-mediated generation of an intracellular signal (calcium) that then activates a protein kinase (calmodulin-dependent protein kinase), leading to a host of biologic responses (8).

One of the first-described calmodulin-dependent protein kinases was phosphorylase kinase, the enzyme that activates phosphorylase in skeletal muscle glycogen breakdown. As described above (Fig. 37.5), this enzyme is part of the phosphorylation cascade, in which it acts as a substrate for cyclic AMP–dependent protein kinase, thereby mediating cyclic AMP effects on glycogenolysis. However, in addition, a rise in intracellular calcium from signal-initiated phosphatidylinositol breakdown and IP_3-mediated calcium release directly activates phosphorylase kinase by binding to the calmodulin subunit of this enzyme. In this way, the same calcium signal that initiates muscle contraction also ensures that there is adequate glucose to power the contraction. Smooth muscle also contracts in response to extracellular signal-mediated calcium release through activation of myosin–light chain kinase, another calmodulin-dependent protein kinase. Several other calmodulin-dependent protein kinases have been described, with varying tissue localization and substrate specificities.

Diacylglycerol and Protein Kinase C

G-protein-coupled phosphatidyl inositol hydrolysis leads to generation of another messenger besides IP_3, namely diacylglycerol. Diacylglycerol, in conjunction with calcium, stimulates another kinase, protein kinase C. This enzyme has several isoforms, some of which are translocated from the cytosol to the plasma membrane in response to hormone stimulation. Generation of diacylglycerol in the plasma membrane is crucial for activation of certain isoforms of protein kinase C. Protein kinase C phosphorylates various substrates, leading to a wide variety of biologic effects. Like most signaling molecules, diacylglycerol is short-lived, either being reincorporated into phosphoinositides as part of the phosphatidylinositol turnover process or hydrolyzed to arachidonic acid, the precursor of the prostaglandins (see Chapter 4). Prolonged stimulation of protein kinase C appears to mediate some of the proliferative and differentiation responses that are observed for some cells. It appears, however, that sustained levels of diacylglycerol are supplied by a second pathway involving stimulation of phosphatidylcholine hydrolysis.

Table 37.2
Hormones That Act, with Calcium, through Phosphatidylinositol Phosphate Breakdown

Target Tissue	Signaling Molecule	Major Response
Pancreas	Acetylcholine	Amylase secretion
Smooth muscle	Acetylcholine	Contraction
Liver	Vasopressin	Glycogen breakdown
Blood platelets	Thrombin	Aggregation
Mast cells	Antigen	Histamine release

The list of hormones and extracellular signals that act through the IP_3/diacylglycerol signaling system is extensive (Table 37.2). Just as the effects of hormones that use cyclic AMP as their second messenger can be reproduced by exogenous addition of this small molecule, diacylglycerol effects are mimicked by the protein kinase C activator, phorbol ester, while the calcium ionophore A23187 mimics the effects of IP_3 release. Using A23187 and phorbol esters, many of the effects of the hormones in Table 37.2 can be mimicked in cell culture.

Crosstalk among Signals

An increased level of complexity exists whereby one signaling mechanism or messenger system can interact with another—this is termed *crosstalk* (Figure 37.6). As examples, several interactions between the cyclic AMP and cal-

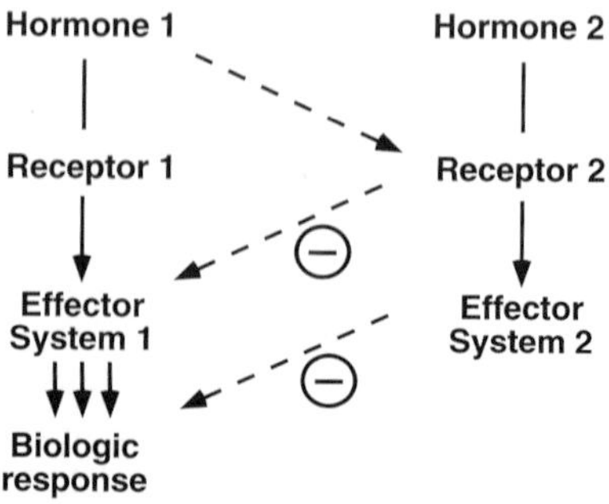

Figure 37.6. Schematic overview of potential crosstalk between two hormone-responsive receptor-mediated pathways.

cium messenger systems have been discovered, and some forms of the enzyme that hydrolyzes cyclic AMP (phosphodiesterase) are regulated by calcium/calmodulin interactions. Cyclic AMP–dependent protein kinase can also phosphorylate the IP_3 receptor, altering its sensitivity to IP_3-induced calcium release. More than one signal may influence the same downstream kinase. We have mentioned above how the enzyme of glycogen metabolism, phosphorylase kinase, is activated by both cyclic AMP–dependent protein kinase phosphorylation and through the binding of calcium to its calmodulin subunit. It appears that the cyclic AMP–dependent phosphorylation of phosphorylase kinase makes the enzyme more sensitive to calcium, allowing skeletal muscle glucose metabolism to respond more robustly to the initiation of muscle contraction in response to a fight-or-flight stimulus. Recently, interactions within the same signaling cascade have been uncovered. As we will see below, it now appears that insulin stimulation of the signaling protein ras (see below) also can lead to some effects on phosphatidylinositol-3-kinase that were initially believed to represent a separate pathway activated in response to insulin receptor binding.

G-Proteins Linked to Ion Channels Directly

As discussed in more detail in the next chapter (see Chapter 38), many receptors directly activate ion channels; however, in some cases G-proteins can link receptor binding to the opening of ion channels. For example, acetylcholine, through the muscarinic receptor, activates G_i, which along with lowering cyclic AMP levels, directly opens potassium ion channels. Other cyclic nucleotide–regulated channels (through adenylate cyclase or calmodulin-dependent protein kinase) similarly are coupled to ion channels; some of these play a crucial role in the chemical senses, vision and smell.

RECEPTORS AS ENZYMES

Not all extracellular signals mediate their responses through the classic mechanism of G-protein-coupled generation of intracellular messengers. Some receptors bypass the G-proteins and second messengers and directly initiate the final common pathway that transduces the signals for the vast majority of extracellular stimuli; this common pathway involves protein phosphorylation. The best studied receptors in this group are the *tyrosine kinase receptors.* A large family of different growth factors uses this transmembrane signaling system (Table 37.3). Several mutations in the signaling molecules described below lead to unrestrained cellular growth and cancer. The tyrosine kinase receptors have an extracellular surface (domain) that contains a hormone-binding site and an intracellular domain with tyrosine kinase activity. In each case, receptor binding by its cognate ligand causes dimerization of the plasma membrane receptor, which activates the intrinsic tyrosine kinase activity, leading the receptor to phosphorylate itself *(autophosphorylation).* These tyrosine phosphorylated sites then act as high-affinity binding sites for various intracellular signaling molecules that contain specific protein sequences called an SH2 domain (*src homology* 2, based on their initial identification in the *src* cancer gene) (1). Different receptors bind different combinations of these signaling molecules, providing one level of signal specificity. Autophosphorylation functions as a switch for the transient assembly of intracellular signaling molecules. Insulin and insulin-like growth factor–1 (IGF-1) (8) differ somewhat from other hormones in that activation of their receptor tyrosine kinases leads to phosphorylation of other proteins (primarily insulin receptor substrates, IRS-1 and IRS-2) which then, similar to one another, function as assembly anchors for a variety of other signaling molecules. The identification of some extremely insulin resistant patients whose disease results from mutations in the insulin receptor that block tyrosine kinase activity has helped confirm the central role of tyrosine phosphorylation in insulin action.

Table 37.3
Protein Ligands That Signal through Tyrosine Kinases

Insulin
IGF-1 (insulin-like growth factor–1; somatomedin-C)
Epidermal growth factor (EGF)
Platelet-derived growth factor (PDGF)
Colony-stimulating factor–1 (CSF-1)
Fibroblast growth factor (FGF)

The phosphotyrosine anchor, in the form of the autophosphorylated receptor or IRS-1, binds a variety of signaling molecules through its SH2 domains. The ras/MAP kinase system is one of the best studied pathways integral to cell growth that is activated by the phosphotyrosine anchor binding described above. *Ras* is a small, monomeric, GTP-binding protein that, like the trimeric G-proteins discussed above, is active in the GTP-bound state and inactive when GDP is bound. Ras plays a central role in the regulation of cell differentiation and growth. In fact, the ras proteins were first discovered based on mutations that promote cancer by disrupting the normal controls on cell proliferation and differentiation (9, 10). About 30% of human cancers have mutations in the *ras* gene. Two intermediate proteins function to couple receptor binding and tyrosine phosphorylation to the activation of ras. Sos (son-of-sevenless, named on the basis of its original identification in *Drosophila* development) is a guanine nucleotide–releasing protein, which results in the release of GDP from ras. Since ras is present on the cytoplasmic side of the plasma membrane and the cytosol contains 10 times more GTP than GDP, once ras has lost its GDP, it is activated by binding GTP. A second protein, Grb-2, binds to both the phosphotyrosine group on either the tyrosine kinase receptor or IRS-1 and the Sos-Ras complex to bring them together. In this way, tyrosine kinase receptor binding leads to activation of ras (Fig. 37.7*A*).

As discussed above, the final mechanism through which

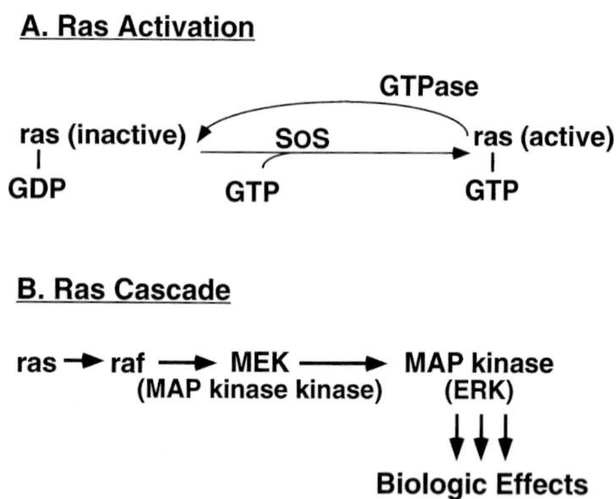

Figure 37.7. *A.* The *ras* activation pathway. *Sos,* son-of-sevenless, an intermediate protein that functions to couple receptor binding and tyrosine phosphorylation to the activation of ras. *B.* The *ras* cascade leading through intermediate protein kinases to biologic effects. *raf,* a protein kinase also known as MAP kinase kinase kinase; *MAP,* mitogen-activated protein; MAP kinase and *ERK,* alternative nomenclatures.

transmembrane signaling leads to intracellular events involves activation of various protein kinases, and this is true for the tyrosine kinase receptors as well. Ras activation initiates another specific protein kinase cascade leading to activation of *MAP kinase* (*mitogen-activated protein kinase,* also sometimes called extracellular-regulated kinase [ERK]). Ras activates the protein kinase known as raf (or MAP kinase kinase kinase) which phosphorylates and activates MEK (MAP kinase kinase) which activates MAP kinase through phosphorylation. MAP kinase relays signals downstream by phosphorylating various proteins within the cell, including other protein kinases and nuclear DNA–binding proteins involved in gene regulation (Fig. 37.7*B*).

Several studies have indicated that the ras/MAP kinase pathway plays a central role in mediating the growth-promoting effects of the tyrosine kinase receptor family of hormones. As mentioned above, activated mutants of ras result in unrestrained cell growth and cancer. In general, it seems that activating mutations in any component of this signaling pathway results in uncontrolled growth. In fact, many of the signaling molecules just described were first identified as mutant forms in cancer cells or cancer-promoting tumor viruses. These mutant genes were called *oncogenes* (cancer genes) before their origins from normal genes were understood; therefore, the normal genes are now sometimes called *proto-oncogenes.*

Insulin, although capable of acting as a growth factor in cell culture, has a host of metabolic effects not shared by the growth factors in the tyrosine kinase receptor family. The signaling molecules mediating these effects are still incompletely understood. One signaling molecule that appears to play a central role is *phosphatidylinositol 3-kinase (PI 3-kinase).* PI 3-kinase catalyzes phosphorylation of the inositol ring of phosphatidylinositol at the 3 position. PI 3-kinase contains an SH2 domain that binds to a specific phosphorylated tyrosine group on IRS-1, leading to its activation. Growth factors other than insulin and IGF-1 whose autophosphorylation provides direct anchoring for SH2-containing molecules can bind PI 3-kinase directly. The mechanisms through which PI 3-kinase activation leads to biologic responses are still unclear. Recently, several possible downstream targets have been identified, including specific subtypes of protein kinase C and a newly identified protein kinase called Akt or protein kinase B (based on its intermediate homology to protein kinases A and C).

Much of the evidence implicating an important role for PI 3-kinase in insulin factor signaling has come from the use of specific inhibitors of the enzyme. It appears, for example, that PI 3-kinase activation is critical for both the growth-promoting effects of insulin and for many of the metabolic effects of insulin such as glycogen synthesis, glucose transport, and gluconeogenesis. In contrast, the ras/MAP kinase pathway appears to be involved primarily in the growth-promoting actions of insulin and is not necessary for many of the classic metabolic actions of this hormone.

In addition to the receptor tyrosine kinases described above, some receptors, although not containing an intrinsic kinase activity, rapidly associate with a tyrosine kinase upon receptor binding. Many of the cytokines (soluble factors involved in proliferation and differentiation of the hematopoietic and immune systems), the antigen-specific receptors of B and T lymphocytes, and certain protein hormones (growth hormone, prolactin, and possibly the adipostat, leptin [see Chapter 87]) act through such a pathway. The binding of cytokines, antigens, or hormones to these specific receptors leads to receptor aggregation and activation of specific tyrosine kinases that can then initiate the biologic responses directed by the given stimulus.

One important example of such a system is the *JAK-STAT* regulatory pathway. For certain cytokines, as well as the adipose tissue–signaling molecule leptin, receptor binding leads to the binding of JAK, a tyrosine kinase. JAK thus activated phosphorylates various proteins, perhaps the most important of which is the transcription factor family, STAT (*s*ignal *t*ransducer and *a*ctivator of *t*ranscription). STAT proteins then migrate to the cell nucleus where they influence the transcription of responsive genes.

Another group of enzyme-linked receptors are those receptors that are protein tyrosine phosphatases. When activated, these receptor enzymes remove phosphate groups from phosphotyrosine proteins. One example of this family of tyrosine phosphatase receptors is CD45, a transmembrane receptor protein that has an integral function in the immunologic activation of B and T lymphocytes by foreign antigens.

Enzyme-linked receptors can also be linked to guanylate cyclase. The prototype for this is the receptor for atrial naturetic factor (ANF). This hormone, released from the heart, stimulates the kidneys to excrete sodium ions and water, and thereby stimulates smooth muscle cell relaxation. The extracellular domain of the ANF receptor binds

ANF, leading to activation of the intracellular portion of the receptor that is a guanylate cyclase. The cyclic GMP that is formed then stimulates a cyclic GMP–dependent protein kinase, analogous to the actions of cyclic AMP on cyclic AMP–dependent protein kinase that were described above.

TRANSMEMBRANE SIGNALING DEFECTS LEADING TO DISEASE

Given the myriad physiologic responses that depend on transmembrane signaling, it is not surprising that disturbances in these signaling pathways lead to disease. In fact, one might expect that many mutations in signaling molecules would be lethal. There are, however, several well-described defects underlying specific diseases. What is even more intriguing is the evidence that aberrations in signaling may underlie many common diseases. Modern molecular biologic tools have only recently made it possible to investigate the role of discrete signaling defects in human disease. As discussed above, many of the signaling molecules involved in growth factor and insulin action were discovered on the basis of mutations that lead to cancer. We shall first discuss examples of defects in particular sites of transmembrane signaling and then focus on the possible involvement of signaling disturbances in some common diseases (Table 37.4).

Receptor Defects

Mutations may occur in receptors that affect the initial step in transmembrane signaling. These mutations often lead to decreased responsiveness or resistance of the cell to the stimulus in question. The first disorder discovered to be secondary to a defect in a G-protein-coupled receptor was color blindness, in 1989. Red and green cone opsins are essentially retinal light receptors. These light receptors, when stimulated by various light frequencies, are coupled to a specialized G-protein (transducin) that mediates stimulation of a specific cyclic AMP phosphodiesterase. A mutation has been found in the light receptor (opsin, see Chapter 17) that causes color blindness. Similarly, a mutation in the light receptor of the rod cells (rhodopsin) causes retinitis pigmentosa.

Table 37.4
Abnormal Transmembrane Signaling in Human Disease

- Receptor defects
  - Color blindness
  - Retinitis pigmentosa
  - X-Linked diabetes insipidus
- G-protein defects
  - Cholera
  - Pertussis
  - Pseudohyperparathyroidism
- Tyrosine kinase pathway defects
  - Many human cancers
- Postreceptor defects likely
  - Non-insulin-dependent diabetes mellitus (NIDDM)
  - Possibly congestive heart failure, obesity

Several other receptor mutations have been uncovered as the cause for disease. Mutations in the growth hormone receptor are responsible for Laron-type dwarfism. The characteristic phenotype of this disease is altered growth hormone transmembrane signaling in various tissues, including the musculoskeletal system, leading to short stature. In X-linked nephrogenic diabetes insipidus, a mutation in the vasopressin receptor makes the kidneys insensitive to the urine-concentrating effects of vasopressin. As mentioned above, several specific insulin receptor mutations have been found in a small subset of patients with severe insulin resistance and non-insulin-dependent diabetes mellitus (NIDDM). A characteristic of all the receptor defects described above is marked elevation in hormone levels in an attempt to compensate for the hormone resistance.

G-Protein Defects

As discussed above, the bacteria that cause cholera release a toxin that causes ADP-ribosylation of the G_s subunit and results in constitutive activation of adenylate cyclase. This constituitively elevated cyclic AMP signal leads to excessive transport of sodium and water across the intestinal lumen, culminating in severe diarrhea. G-protein abnormalities underlie other diseases as well. Pseudohypoparathyroidism (Albright's hereditary osteodystrophy) is a disorder in which the bones are resistant to the calcium-mobilizing effects of parathyroid hormone. Parathyroid hormone is coupled to G_s and adenylate cyclase activation. A genetic defect in G_s blocks parathyroid hormone action.

Diabetes

The most common form of diabetes mellitus, NIDDM, (type 2, or adult-onset diabetes), has long been known to result from a combination of resistance to the actions of insulin and a relative deficiency of insulin secretion. Early characterization of the insulin receptor indicated that a change in insulin receptor number or hormone-binding affinity could not explain this insulin resistance. This led to the concept that NIDDM results from a postreceptor defect in insulin action. Several sites in the newly discovered insulin signaling pathway have been examined as potential sites of this lesion. Adipose cells from diabetic patients have decreased tyrosine kinase activity; but, when tested in vitro, this does not seem to account for the insulin resistance observed clinically. Several families have been identified with mutations in the insulin receptor leading to blunted transmembrane signaling and profound insulin resistance. At present, many genes encoding signaling molecules are being screened in the hopes of discovering the central lesions in NIDDM.

Recently, an intriguing hypothesis has been proposed to explain the long-known clinical phenomenon whereby hyperglycemia itself exacerbates peripheral insulin resistance. Hyperglycemia, through a yet unexplained mechanism, appears to stimulate protein kinase C activity. In an example of crosstalk between signaling cascades, this protein kinase C can phosphorylate specific serines on either the insulin receptor or IRS-1, rendering it a poorer substrate for the tyrosine phosphorylation reaction involved in insulin signaling and, consequently, desensitizing the cell to insulin's action. To what extent this type of crosstalk can explain the pathogenesis of diabetes mellitus remains to be determined.

Obesity

Obesity is probably the most common disease in the Western world. A powerful link between obesity and insulin resistance has long been described. Obesity leads to hyperinsulinemia that—likely through receptor desensitization—causes a decrease in insulin receptor number. However, the mechanism through which obesity leads to insulin resistance (presumably a transmembrane signaling defect) remains to be established.

One possible receptor defect that may contribute to a genetic predisposition to obesity is alterations in the β_3-adrenergic receptor. This receptor appears to mediate the thermogenic effect of brown adipose tissue. Several new pharmacologic tools are currently under development to stimulate this receptor in the hopes of increasing fuel metabolism and weight loss. Recently, a mutation has been identified in this receptor that appears to be present in several population groups at high risk for development of obesity and insulin resistance. Whether altered β_3-adrenergic signaling significantly contributes to obesity awaits the results of further investigation.

An exciting new insight into the pathogenesis of obesity came with discovery of a new hormone, leptin, released from adipose tissues. Leptin appears to act as an adipostat by signaling the brain regarding the amount of adipose tissue stores. Administration of exogenous leptin to deficient rodents leads to decreased food intake, increased metabolic activity, and weight loss. However, in humans with obesity, leptin levels appear quite high, suggesting that obesity may represent a state of leptin resistance. With the recent cloning of a leptin receptor, studies are under way to determine what defects in leptin-receptor signaling may explain development of obesity.

Finally, as signaling pathways involving many hormones, neurotransmitters, cytokines, and growth factors are uncovered, searches for defects in human disease are moving rapidly. Congestive heart failure may result from a signaling defect. Several studies have suggested reduced β-adrenergic receptor function in these patients. Some data have suggested that an increase in the β-adrenergic receptor kinase, a serine kinase that phosphorylates the β-receptor leading to receptor desensitization, may be activated in congestive heart disease. The net result of this β-receptor desensitization would be a reduced response to the cardiostimulatory effects of epinephrine. Asthma has been linked with defects in β_2 receptors. Defects in brain transmembrane signaling systems have been implicated in several neuropsychiatric conditions including alcoholism, schizophrenia, and Alzheimer's disease. Clearly in the coming years, as our understanding of transmembrane signaling expands, new insights into several disease states will be on the horizon.

REFERENCES

1. Alberts B, Bray D, Lewis J, et al. Molecular biology of the cell. New York: Garland Publishing, 1994;721–82.
2. Kahn CR, Smith RJ, Chin WW. In: Wilson JD, Foster DW, eds. William's textbook of endocrinology. 8th ed. Philadelphia: WB Saunders, 1992;91–134.
3. Insel PA. N Engl J Med 1996;334:580–5.
4. Gershergorn MC. Endocrinology 1994;134:5–6.
5. Raymond JR. Am J Physiol 1995;269:F141–58.
6. Hokin MR, Hokin MR. J Biol Chem 1953;203:967–77.
7. Berridge MJ, Irvine RF. Nature 1989;341:197–201.
8. Saltiel AR. Am J Physiol 1996;270:E375–85.
9. Schnabel P, Bohm M. J Mol Med 1995;73:221–8.
10. Spiegel AM, Weinstein LS, Shenker A. J Clin Invest 1993;92:1119–25.

SELECTED READINGS

Caro JF, Sinha MK, Kolaczynski JW, et al. Leptin: the tale of an obesity gene. Diabetes 1996;45:1455–62.

Insel PA. Seminars in medicine of the Beth Israel Hospital, Boston. Adrenergic receptors—evolving concepts and clinical implications. N Engl J Med 1996;334:580–5.

Saltiel AR. Diverse signaling pathways in the cellular actions of insulin. Am J Physiol 1996;270:E375–85.

Spiegel AM, Weinstein LS, Shenker A. Abnormalities in G protein-coupled signal transduction pathways in human disease. J Clin Invest 1993;92:1119–25.

Speigelman BM, Flier JS. Adipogenesis and obesity: rounding out the big picture. Cell 1996;87:377–89.

38. Membrane Channels and Transporters: Paths of Discovery

DAVID ERLIJ

All nutrients have to cross one or more cell membranes before reaching their final destination in the organism. For more than 100 years, scientists have used a variety of approaches to inquire into the nature of these movements. The outcome has been nothing short of prodigious: detailed molecular mechanisms of membrane permeation are now well on their way to full elucidation.

This inquiry started with the realization that cells have an internal composition that differs markedly from their surrounding environment. Since both the intracellular and the extracellular environments are aqueous solutions, an envelope, the cell membrane, is necessary to prevent complete mixing of the two solutions. Moreover, cells are not static, impermeable structures; many substances continuously enter and leave the cytoplasm. Hence the membrane must be understood in terms of both the substances allowed to pass through and those that are held back.

Our understanding of selective movement of substances through biologic membranes stems from formulating biologic problems in terms of physical processes. A major step in such a formulation is establishing the relationship between the forces acting on a substance and its movement across the membrane. Such an approach reveals a great deal about the organization of the membrane and has provided the basis for definition of the several fundamentally different molecular mechanisms of membrane permeation.

This chapter attempts to provide the nonspecialized reader with an overview of the different types of mechanisms for membrane permeation and their regulation. Instead of a simple summary of current findings and theories, it describes how the major concepts in the field were developed. The purpose of this approach is not merely historical but to illustrate how new concepts originate from careful analysis of experimental observations.

STRUCTURE OF THE MEMBRANE

The first major insight into the chemical nature of the cell membrane dates from 1895, when the English physiologist Ernest Overton, working in Switzerland, compared the rates at which a large number of diverse compounds penetrated the cell membrane. He found that the ability of substances to penetrate the cell membrane correlates with their solubility properties (1).

The capacity of a substance to dissolve into a given solvent is a function of both the structure of the solvent and the solute. At one end of the spectrum is water and all the solutes that dissolve readily in it. Compounds that readily mix with water are called *hydrophilic.* This property arises because hydrophilic solutes have a molecular structure that strongly interacts with water molecules. At the other end of the spectrum we have *hydrophobic* compounds, so called because their molecules do not interact with water, and therefore they separate from it. Hydrophobic solutes dissolve well in hydrophobic solvents; extreme examples of hydrophobic solvents are oils, such as olive oil.

Overton discovered that the higher the solubility of a compound in oil, the faster it penetrates cell membranes, i.e., the higher is its membrane permeability. He reasoned that oil-soluble substances passed through the membrane faster because they can dissolve in the membrane; hence, the membrane must be made of lipids.

A second important insight emerged when other investigators, following Overton's original strategy, i.e., deducing membrane properties from measurements of the pattern of permeability of a great variety of compounds, discovered that a number of molecules that are very hydrophilic, i.e., lipid insoluble, also pass rapidly through biologic membranes (2). This observation appeared to contradict Overton's proposal, since it was difficult to explain how substances that do not dissolve in lipids could pass rapidly through the membrane. An acceptable explanation came when it was realized that the hydrophilic substances that pass the membrane are of low molecular volume. Urea and many ions, for instance, enter cells rapidly although they are practically lipid insoluble.

If substances of very different solubility properties can pass through the membrane, then the membrane is not a homogeneous structure. Separate pathways must exist for the movement of hydrophilic and hydrophobic substances. The concept of the membrane as a noncontinuous lipid barrier with pores that permit the passage of hydrophilic particles of small volume was proposed to reconcile all the observations. This concept of a heterogenous membrane composed of lipids that include multiple pathways for the movements of hydrophilic substances remains the basis of our current understanding of the structure and function of the membrane. Of course, the original model has been considerably refined and our understanding advanced since the model was proposed.

The first advance concerns the organization of the lipids. In agreement with Overton's original idea, it is now well established that most of the surface area of the membrane is composed of lipids. Chemical, biophysical, and structural analyses show that the membrane lipids form a continuous bilayer enveloping the cell. In biologic membranes, the lipids are mostly phospholipids and are packed in a regular pattern. Hydrophilic heads are aligned adjacent to each other along the cytoplasmic and external faces of the cell membrane while the hydrocarbon tails face each other inside the membrane (Fig. 38.1). Lipid-soluble solutes pass through this phospholipid bilayer (1).

The other important advance concerns the nature of the pathways for hydrophilic solutes. It turns out that membranes are not made solely of lipid; they contain large amounts of protein. An important number of these proteins, called *integral membrane proteins,* span the whole thickness of the membrane extending from the extracellular to the intracellular surface. Many integral membrane proteins exist in each cell, and quite a few of them form the pathways through which hydrophilic solutes permeate the membrane (3). The remainder of this chapter concerns the manners in which these proteins are involved in individual permeation processes.

To understand the permeation processes associated with different types of membrane proteins, we must first consider the forces driving the movement of substances across the membrane.

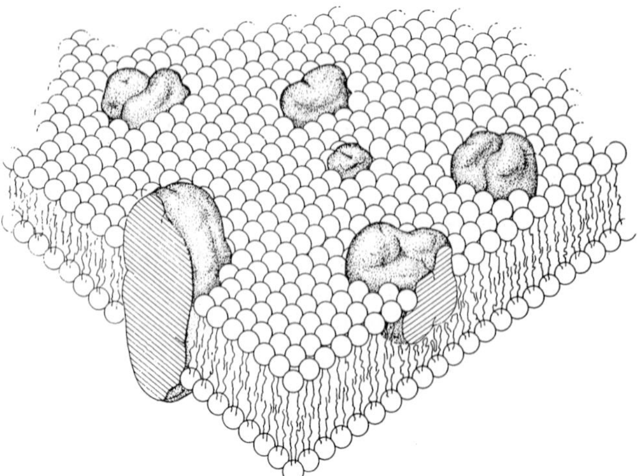

Figure 38.1 Schematic representation of the structure of the membrane. The lipid bilayer is depicted showing the polar heads of the phospholipids as *circles* and the fatty acid (hydrocarbon) tails as *wavy lines*. The proteins are shown as *solid bodies with stippled surfaces.* (Modified from Singer SJ, Nicholson GL. Science 1972;175:720–31, with permission.)

FORCES AND FLOWS: ACTIVE AND PASSIVE TRANSPORT

Gradients across Biologic Membranes

No movement can be understood unless the forces driving it are known. Hence, to understand how substances pass through a membrane, we must analyze the forces causing such flows. This approach has been extremely fruitful because it led to the realization that substances pass membranes by two fundamentally different mechanisms: passive and active transport.

The flow of a substance across a membrane occurs by passive transport when movement is caused by gradients of force that exist across the membrane. What forces can drive such flows across the membrane? The most common process for passive solute flow is diffusion.

Diffusion is a common, everyday phenomenon; molecules in a liquid or gas tend to distribute themselves uniformly throughout the vessel in which they are contained. A familiar example is the fate of a lump of sugar deposited in a cup of tea. If enough time is allowed to pass, the sugar will be distributed evenly throughout the tea solution.

The concentration difference generates the driving force for the movement of sugar molecules from a region of higher concentration to one of lower concentration; this movement ceases when the concentration is uniform throughout the cup. In other words, a concentration difference causes the net movement of molecules.

In addition to concentration gradients, voltage is a source of force driving solutes passively across the membrane. Of course, voltage only acts on charged particles, but an important number of solutes in an organism bear an electrical charge; the most abundant osmotically active solutes in extracellular fluid are Na^+ and Cl^- and in intracellular fluid, K^+. When a charged particle is placed in a region in which a voltage gradient exists, the positive particles will be pushed toward the negative pole and the negative particles toward the positive pole. There are important voltage gradients across almost every biologic membrane. Hence, ions in the organism are under the influence of two sources of force: the voltage gradient and the concentration gradient.

In which direction will a particle move when influenced by two forces? To intuitively understand this problem, consider a rather familiar situation in which two major forces are at work. A flying airplane's height is determined by two major forces: the gravitational pull of the earth and the upward driving force generated by the engines. When does a plane climb? When the upward force generated by the engines exceeds the gravitational field of the earth. When does it come down? When the opposite is true. Under what conditions does the aircraft maintain a constant height? When the two forces are opposite and equal.

Similarly, the movement of substances across membranes should be determined by the concentration gradient and, in the case of charged particles, the voltage gradient.

These considerations of how more than one force can affect the movement of a particle are important when considering the cell composition. When the forces driving solute movements across cell membranes are considered, one remarkable fact emerges: an important number of substances move, and are distributed in the organism, in a manner that obeys predictions based on *neither* the voltage nor the concentration gradient. For example, [Na^+] inside most cells is 10 mM and its concentration in extracellular fluid is about 140 mM, while the voltage inside the cell is negative relative to the outside, increasing further the inward force driving Na^+ into the cells. Regardless of these enormous inward-driving forces, Na^+ is kept low within the cell, being expelled almost as soon as it enters the cytoplasm. Therefore, some additional force must cause the difference in composition.

Active Transport and Ion Pumps

If the distribution and movement of certain solutes do not obey predictions based on concentration and voltage gradients across the membrane, what is causing them?

Early clues to solving this enigma came from work with erythrocytes, cells that are made almost exclusively of cell (plasma) membranes. By the time they reach maturity, all their intracellular organelles have degenerated, and they consist of a cell membrane surrounding a solution rich in hemoglobin and containing relatively few enzymes. The ionic composition of this solution is similar to most other intracellular fluids: high in K^+ and very low in Na^+, compared with extracellular fluid. This concentration difference is maintained indefinitely if erythrocytes are incubated under appropriate conditions, e.g., body temperature and an adequate supply of substrates. One remarkable property becomes apparent when they are incubated at 4°C. The ions in the interior of the erythrocyte equilibrate with the extracellular fluid; Na^+ and K^+ reach equal concentrations in the intracellular and extracellular solutions. More remarkably, when these erythrocytes are rewarmed to body temperature they regain their original ionic gradients, K^+ moves into the cell, and Na^+ moves out. Since these movements occur against concentration gradients, there must be a component in the erythrocyte membranes that moves ions against their concentration gradients (4).

Another interesting feature of this ion movement against the gradients is that it requires metabolic activity. In erythrocytes, use of glucose by the glycolytic pathway is the only way to generate energy. If glycolysis is interrupted by either incubating erythrocytes in a solution free of glucose or by specifically inhibiting glycolysis with poisons such as iodoacetate, the reaccumulation of K^+ in the cell and the extrusion of Na^+ are blocked. This means that these movements against gradients are coupled to the energetic metabolism of the cell. Glycolysis makes energy available to the cells because an end result of this process is the synthesis of adenosine triphosphate (ATP). This compound acts as a source of energy because it has a high-energy chemical bond that, when hydrolyzed, releases large amounts of energy. The release of energy by the breakdown of high-energy chemical bonds is a familiar phenomenon: gasoline is a substance with high-energy chemical bonds that, when broken down, can release energy explosively. That is why gasoline is useful in propelling car engines or manufacturing Molotov cocktails.

Once we stop glycolysis in the erythrocyte and interrupt, in turn, synthesis of ATP and movement of Na^+ and K^+ against their gradients, we can restore these ion movements by supplying ATP. The restored ion transport occurs as ATP is hydrolyzed. This means that the component in the membrane that moves Na^+ and K^+ against their gradients uses the hydrolysis of ATP as a source of energy. Such membrane components that use ATP as a source of energy and move ions against their concentration gradients are called *ion pumps,* by analogy with the device that brings water up from the bottom of a well against a pressure gradient by using energy from an external source.

Once it was known that membranes contained a structure that could pump ions against their concentration gradients, it was natural to try to purify this component to characterize it. An enormous advance in this process occurred when it was discovered that a class of substances, the cardiac glycosides, acting at low concentrations block the activity of the Na^+, K^+ pump, i.e., they selectively stop active transport of ions and ATP hydrolysis in the erythrocyte without blocking such other processes as glycolysis or passive ion movements (4).

To purify a component of the membrane, it is necessary to break down the membrane and then separate the desired component from the many other molecules that make up the membrane. If broken membranes yield many kinds of molecules, how is it possible to identify which one is the Na^+ pump? The answer was to use cardiac glycosides together with the physiologic properties of transport as markers. Since transport involves hydrolysis of ATP, membrane components that hydrolyze ATP, i.e., ATPases, were first targeted. Indeed, several ATPases could be purified from the membrane, but only one was inhibited by cardiac glycosides. Moreover, the activity of this enzyme required Na^+ and K^+ in the solution. This parallelism between the activity of the purified enzyme in a test tube and the pump in the whole cell provided the first credible evidence that the purified membrane protein was the ion pump of the whole cell (4). The Na^+ pump is not the only structure that pumps ions against concentration and voltage gradients using ATP as a source of energy. Two other ions, Ca^{2+} and H^+, are transported actively in many instances by the action of specific ATPases. A number of H^+ ATPases and Ca^{2+} ATPases have been isolated, identified, and sequenced.

Passive Movements: Ion Channels

The Early Revolution in Electrophysiology

A great deal of the progress in our understanding of how ions passively cross membranes was the result of analyzing the responses of excitable tissues. Excitable cells (e.g., nerve, cardiac, and muscle cells) respond by briefly changing the voltage across their membranes. These electrical signals are due to the movement of ions down their concentration and voltage gradients. The ions move through specialized membrane structures that are now called *ion channels.*

The first proposal that hinted at the existence of channels as we know them today was made by Bernstein in 1906 (2). He was trying to explain the origin of the continuous voltage difference that exists across the resting membrane of most cells, making their interior negative relative to the outside. He based his explanation on two points. One is a fact: the concentration of K^+ is much higher inside the cell than outside. This concentration gradient drives K^+ continuously out of the cell. The second was a brilliant conjecture that turned out to be correct: voltage is generated because the pathway by which K^+ leaves the cell is selective for K^+, that is, only K^+ passes through this pathway, other ions cannot go through. This conjecture has a solid physical basis: to generate a voltage, charges have to be separated. If other ionic species were moving together with K^+, they would neutralize the charge separation and there would be no voltage generated (2, 5).

Bernstein had a second important insight: if cells can change their voltage under different physiologic conditions, then the membrane can change the amount and nature of charges being separated at any time (i.e., charge separation is regulated). He went further and suggested that this regulation occurred because the membrane changed permeability under different physiologic conditions.

Bernstein's proposals were based on relatively scant evidence because the methodology of his time was extremely limited. Full experimental proof had to wait until after World War II, when Hodgkin, Huxley, and Katz (5) brought new and sophisticated technology to the analysis of these problems and provided extraordinary quantitative proof for the notion that membranes had a variety of individual pathways with selectivity for specific ions and that the passage of ions through them was regulated. Their studies on nerve and the nerve-muscle junction demonstrated an additional general property of the system: very different parameters in the cell environment can regulate the permeability of each specific pathway. The permeability of the pathways in nerve membrane is controlled mostly by the voltage across the membrane, while the permeability of the muscle membrane right at the junction with its nerve terminal is controlled not by the voltage across the membrane but by the action of a substance released by the nerve ending, acetylcholine. Thus, there are two major agents that control ion permeability. One is the voltage across the membrane, the other is the interaction of the membrane with a chemical agent that appears normally in its environment.

Hodgkin, Huxley, and Katz (2, 5) made their analysis on the basis of measurements of ion movements through large areas of the membrane. But they clearly understood that the behavior they observed corresponded to the responses of discrete areas of the membrane. For example, the property of selectivity raised an important problem already mentioned above: if charged hydrophilic particles such as ions pass through simple pores that only select on the basis of size, how can they permit the movement of K^+ while blocking other ions of similar size? Evidently, the pathway for hydrophilic substances cannot be such a simple structure as a pore. This view is further strengthened when one considers that ion permeability is precisely controlled by either chemicals or voltage acting on the membrane.

Channels and Poisons. Proof of the chemical nature of the pathways through which ions passively cross the membrane emerged from the use of specific poisons (2). The strategy involved was, in broad outline, similar to that discussed above for the purification of the sodium pump. It hinged on the discovery that some toxins are poisonous because they selectively block specific passive ion pathways; for example, tetrodotoxin, responsible for the poisoning caused by Japanese puffer fish, blocks the Na^+ channel with exquisite selectivity. Bungarotoxin, one of the most toxic components of the venom of the Siamese cobra snake *(Naja naja siamensis),* blocks the acetylcholine-regulated channel of the neuromuscular junction (2).

Once the specificity of these toxins was established, they were used to purify the components responsible for ion permeability from solubilized membranes. Because of their high affinity, they bind the proteins involved in the permeation process, which then are extracted and used to determine amino acid sequences.

Tetrodotoxin had another important use: it provided one of the first pieces of quantitative support for the existence of channels in the membrane. After it became evident that ions do not traverse the membrane through simple pores, two possible mechanisms for permeation were considered. One was that carriers with binding sites for specific ions ferried back and forth across the membrane. The other was that permeation was due to channels, i.e., continuous openings with walls of complex structure that could select among different ions and close and open in response to regulatory influences. The availability of radioactive tetrodotoxin permitted counting the number of Na^+ permeation sites in the membrane. Since the maximum number of Na^+ ions crossing the membrane was known from measurements of membrane ionic currents, it was a simple matter to calculate the speed at which Na^+ moved through a single site. It turned out that a carrier mechanism, shuttling back and forth across the membrane, was too slow to accommodate the large currents through each site, while a small number of open channels could easily pass the measured ion flows (2).

The Second Revolution: Patch Clamp and Molecular Biology

Two developments, the use of the patch clamp and the application of the methods of molecular biology, have permitted the observation and manipulation of molecules involved in the passive movement of ions across the membrane. The patch clamp permits recording and analysis of the activity of single channels in the membrane. The methods of molecular biology allow the analysis of the relationship between structure and function of the channels.

Patch Clamp and Gating in Single Channels. The patch clamp is a technique for making electrical recordings of very small patches of cell membrane, usually a few square microns in diameter. By recording from such small patches of membrane it is possible to record the behavior of single channels. The technique hinges on pushing a glass pipette with a polished tip diameter of about 1 μm against the cell membrane surface until the edge of the pipette makes a very high resistance seal with the membrane. In this manner only the electrical activity of the area within the pipette tip is recorded. Since this area is so small, it frequently contains only a single channel (6).

The passage of ions through the channel is detected by measuring the electrical current that passes through the membrane in the patch. Figure 38.2 shows recordings of the current measured when a single channel is within the pipette. In the absence of any additional experimental perturbation, the current shifts between two values: zero and some other fixed value. The transition between the two states is extremely rapid, because chemical transition states are very short lived. This behavior indicates that the channel structure spontaneously fluctuates through two major configurations, one in which it is closed and does not permit any ion flows and the other in which it is open and permits the passage of an ionic current. This spontaneous transition between open and closed states is termed *channel gating*. Channel function is mostly regulated by controlling the time that the channel spends in the open position (i.e., the probability that the channel is open at any moment). Agents that increase membrane permeability increase the open time of the channel, while the converse is true for agents that decrease it.

The size of the current passing through the open channel (i.e., the height of the current deflection between open and closed states) depends on two parameters. One is the driving forces for the ion moving through the channel, namely, voltage difference and concentration gradient. The other is the channel conductance, measured by comparing the ionic current forced through the channel by a driving force of fixed magnitude. Channel conductance is approximately proportional to channel diameter: more ions are forced by the same driving force through a channel of larger diameter than through a smaller one.

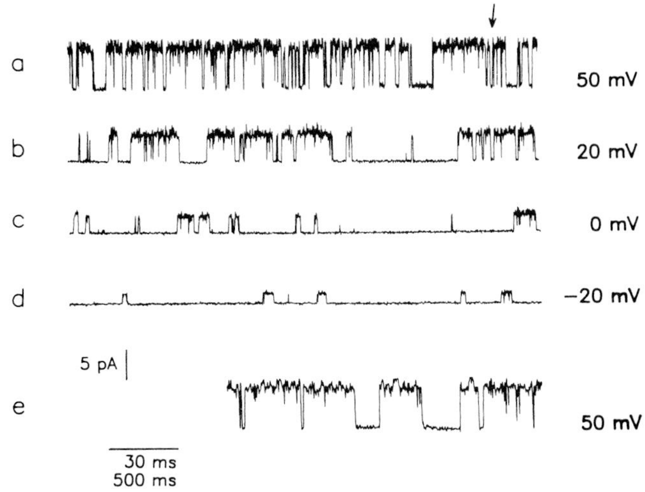

Figure 38.2. Patch-clamp recordings of a single channel. The records show the channel fluctuating spontaneously between open *(upper level of the tracing)* and closed *(lower level of the tracing)* positions and the effects of membrane voltage. Two effects of voltage are shown. First, as the voltage across the patch is changed from 50 to −20 mV (see voltage values at the right end of each tracing) the time that the channel spends in the open state is greatly reduced. Second, as the voltage is shifted from 50 mV to −20 mV the current passing through the open channel is reduced because the driving force for ion movements is reduced by the change in voltage. The lower tracing *(e)* shows the final portion of tracing *a* (from the *point marked* to the *arrow* to the end of the tracing) with an expanded time scale. The 500-msec bar is the time calibration for all tracings except tracing *e*, in which it is equivalent to 30 msec. (Modified from J Gen Physiol 1988;92:187, with permission.)

Voltage-Gated Channels. One of the most remarkable contributions of the Hodgkin-Huxley studies was the demonstration that the electrical responses of excitable cells are due to the existence of separate voltage-controlled pathways for Na^+ and K^+ in the nerve membrane. As indicated above, this means that the voltage across the membrane changes the time that a channel spends open (i.e., there are certain values of membrane voltage for which the channel will be mostly open and values at which it will be mostly closed).

With the aid of tetrodotoxin and the techniques of molecular biology, the Na^+ channel composition has been determined. Its main component is a glycosylated protein of 1820 amino acids (7). This protein contains four homologous domains, each containing about 300 amino acids. What is the shape of this protein within the membrane?

Depending on their amino acid composition, polypeptide chains arrange themselves in space to present a surface of different degrees of hydrophobicity. This is important because the hydrophobic surface of a polypeptide will separate itself from any aqueous or polar environment and become embedded in the lipid core of the membrane (8). It turns out that each of the four homologous domains of the sodium channel contains six hydrophobic regions that stay within the lipid phase of the membrane. These four domains arrange themselves to surround a pore, as shown in Figure 38.3.

The fact that membrane voltage changes channel gating implies that a portion of the channel molecule can sense the voltage across the membrane. One of the intramembrane domains of the channel proteins has a high number of positively charged amino acid residues that would be displaced when the voltage within the membrane is changed. Displacement of this portion is responsible for voltage-dependent gating. Quite a few voltage-gated channels that operate following similar principles have been identified: at least three Na^+ channels, four Ca^{2+} channels, and many types of K^+ channels (7, 9).

Ligand-Gated Channels. As mentioned above, gating in certain channels is not altered by modifying the membrane voltage, but the presence of specific substances in the extracellular space will markedly change gating. These substances, which act at very low concentrations, are called *ligands;* they bind to specific proteins of the cell membrane called *receptors.* The consequence of the interaction between ligand and receptor is a change in cell function (2).

Some types of channels are also receptors, that is, ligands bind directly to the channel. The interaction between ligand and receptor produces a conformational change that opens the channel and permits movement of ions across the cell membrane.

The best studied ligand-activated channel is the acetylcholine receptor of the vertebrate neuromuscular junction. Other transmitters directly activate postsynaptic channels in a variety of neurons. In many cases, these involve inhibitory responses in which the transmitters are amino acids such as glycine and GABA γ-aminobutyric acid), which act by opening anion-selective channels. There is a ubiquitous transmitter in the central nervous system, glutamic acid, that affects many synapses by directly opening channels that have selective permeability for monovalent cations.

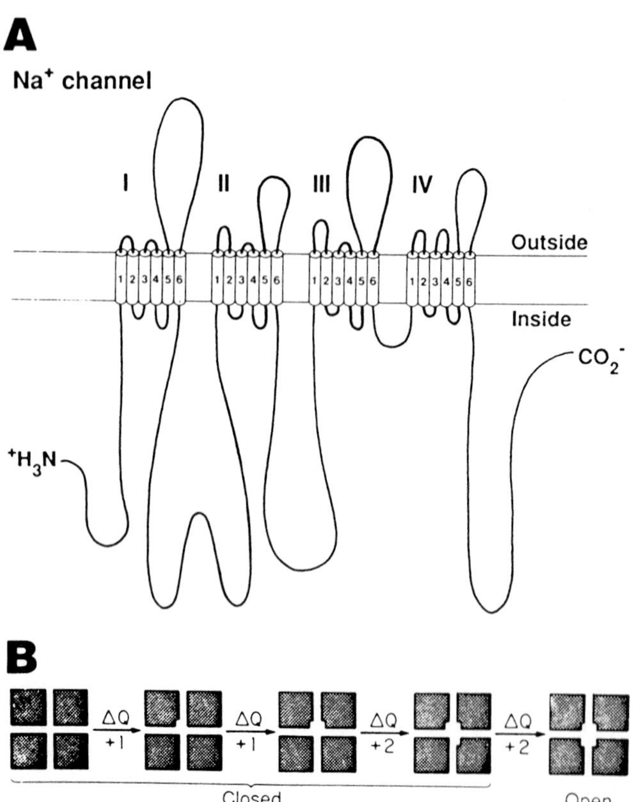

Figure 38.3. Schematic representation of the Na^+ channel protein. Panel *A* shows the complete channel polypeptide with four homologous domains (*I* to *IV*). Each domain has six hydrophobic regions *(cylinders labeled 1 to 6)* that are located within the lipid bilayer. Panel *B* shows the topologic arrangement of the channel viewed in a cross-section parallel to the surface of the membrane. Each of the four homologous domains is shown forming a quarter of the channel. Depolarization produces a sequential series of voltage-induced changes in channel conformation that result in an opening at the core of the channel. (From Catterall W. Science 1988;242:50–61, with permission.)

G-Proteins and Channel Control

Many channel types change gating in response to ligands in the extracellular environment, although the channels themselves are not receptors. These responses are initiated through receptors that are separate proteins in the membrane. When receptor-ligand interactions occur, a sequence of steps is initiated that finally modifies channel behavior (2, 9).

Two major steps follow the receptor-ligand interaction. The first is the coupling of the receptor-ligand complex with another type of intramembrane protein that binds guanine nucleotides, called for this reason a *G-protein.* The second step involves the coupling of G-proteins with other membrane proteins, the effectors, whose activity is in turn modified.

By now more than 10 different varieties of G-proteins have been identified. These G-proteins activate effector proteins when their guanine binding site is occupied by GTP. In the resting state, the site is occupied by GDP, when the receptor-ligand complex couples with the G-protein, the bound GDP is released and GTP takes its place. The activity of the GTP protein ceases when GTP is hydrolyzed to GDP (9).

Two major types of effector proteins are activated by G-proteins. In one type, G-proteins interact directly with the channel. The most typical example is the K^+ channel activated by acetylcholine in the heart. It is important to note that the receptor that mediates this response to acetylcholine is fundamentally different from the acetylcholine receptor described in the previous section that mediates the responses of skeletal muscle. In the second group of G-protein-mediated responses, the effector that is activated by a phosphorylated G-protein is an enzyme that generates a second messenger. This second messenger in turn activates a sequence of reactions whose products modify gating of a channel (9) (Fig. 38.4).

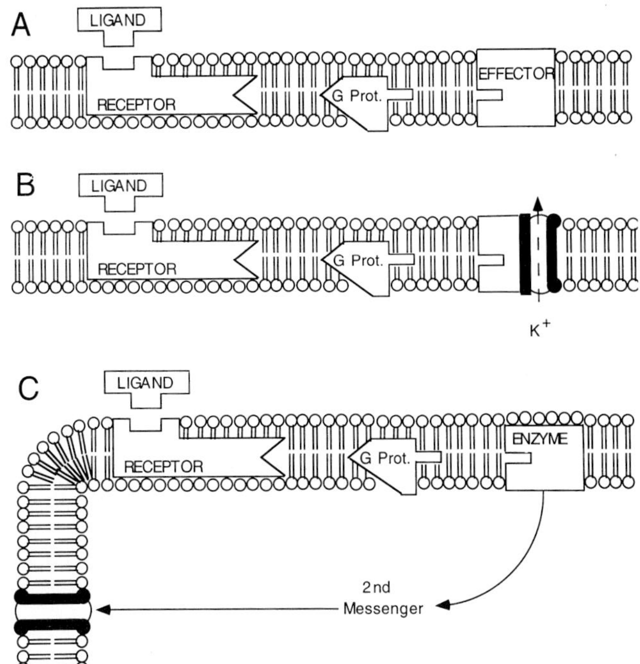

Figure 38.4. Schematic representation of the effectors for G-protein regulation of cell membrane function. *A.* General organization of the G-protein pathway. *B.* A channel as effector for G-protein action. *C.* An enzyme as effector for G-protein action. Synthesis of a second messenger initiates activity in a pathway whose products eventually will modify channel behavior.

There are four common ways in which G-proteins control the rate of second messenger production: *(a)* stimulation of adenyl cyclase; *(b)* inhibition of adenyl cyclase; *(c)* activation of phospholipase A; and *(d)* activation of phospholipase C. These four methods of control probably affect the greatest number of channels.

The multiplicity of ion channels and regulatory mechanisms allows for an enormous number of possible permutations. Indeed, channels and their regulatory mechanisms are being discovered in every cell type. A testimony to this variety is the latest edition (1996) of the "Receptor and Ion Channel Nomenclature Supplement" published by the journal *Trends in Pharmacological Sciences;* it has 80 pages filled with tables summarizing channel and receptor properties (10).

Facilitated Diffusion

In addition to the movement of lipid-soluble substances that pass through the lipid bilayer of the membrane driven by their concentration gradient and the movement of ions that move through specific channels driven by electrical and concentration gradients, there is a third modality of movement, also driven by the concentration gradient across the membrane (11). This modality is called *facilitated diffusion.* The concept of facilitated diffusion evolved when it was recognized that there is a group of organic solutes that pass cell membranes down their concentration gradient but are not lipid soluble. The most widely studied of these substances is glucose.

It was recognized very early that glucose diffuses through the membrane of most cells by interacting with a specific transporter in the cell membrane. Now, molecular techniques have shown the existence of a family of proteins, the GLUT transporters, which are responsible for glucose transport down its concentration gradient. Although ubiquitous, these transporters are notably absent from the microvilli of the small intestine and kidney where massive glucose transport takes place. At these locations glucose passes through a special active process called *cotransport* (see below). However, the GLUT transporters are essential to permit passage of glucose across almost all other cell membranes. In the case of the small intestine, they play a central role in allowing the exit of glucose from the intestinal cell into the interstitial spaces, after glucose has been absorbed into the cytoplasm by a specialized process in the apical microvilli.

Secondary Active Transport and the Absorption of Nutrients

Analysis of the mechanisms of absorption of carbohydrate and protein nutrients in the small intestine led to the recognition that these functions involve a unique process. This process is neither diffusion nor a form of active transport in which metabolic energy stored in a biochemical intermediary such as ATP is used directly to drive the movement of solutes.

For more than a century we have known that both carbohydrate and protein nutrients are completely absorbed from the intestinal lumen, where their concentrations fall to negligible levels. The precise mechanisms of such powerful absorption processes were unknown until quite recently. However, even before the detailed mechanisms were elucidated, it was clear that some form of active transport must be involved, because substrates moved from low- to high-concentration regions. The key discovery was that the specialized event in this active transfer occurs at the cell membranes that line the lumen of the small intestine (12).

The first indication that such a specialized event occurs in the luminal membrane of the epithelial cell of the small intestine came from studies in isolated sacs of intestine. In these studies the composition of the solution bathing the lumen of the intestine was compared with the composition of the cytoplasm of intestinal epithelial cells and of the solution in contact with the interstitial spaces of the intestine. As expected, both amino acids and monosaccharides were passed from luminal to serosal solution, raising substrate levels in the interstitial fluid. The unexpected and fascinating finding was that by far the highest concentrations of substrate were found in the cytoplasm of the intestinal cells. This means that the membrane of the intestinal cell facing the lumen contains a system or systems that can actively accumulate nutrients in the cytoplasm of the intestinal cell, and from there they can pass into the interstitial spaces, driven by their concentration gradients.

Other important findings followed. Foremost was the observation that nutrient absorption only occurred when sodium was present in the luminal solution. Active absorption of nutrients was abolished when the lumen was incubated with Na^+-free solutions; no other cation can substitute for Na^+.

The other major observation was that abolishing the gradient of $[Na^+]$ across the cell membrane, normally maintained by the Na^+, K^+ ATPase, also abolishes accumulation of nutrients within the intestinal cell. Crane (13) synthesized these apparently unrelated facts into an elegant explanation. He reasoned that nutrient uptake depends on Na^+ because the transporter allows the movement of glucose only when it occurs simultaneously with Na^+, i.e., the movements of Na^+ and glucose are strictly coupled by a single transporter molecule. In addition, he proposed that the force for nutrient accumulation is provided by the Na^+ gradient, and for this reason, dissipation of the Na^+ gradient interferes with nutrient accumulation.

Since Crane's original proposal, a great mass of data has accumulated supporting his fundamental concept that two different substrates move together through a single transporter, with the concentration gradient for one of them providing the energy to drive the active transport of the second. All forms of active transport that do not directly use energy derived from metabolism but rather use energy from a concentration gradient are now known as *secondary active transport*. The forms of active transport that derive their energy directly from metabolism through such compounds as ATP are called *primary active transports*.

Subsequently, it has been recognized that secondary transport occurs in two forms. In the first, described above and called *cotransport, or symport,* the transported solutes ride together in the same direction across the membrane. The second form of secondary transport, called *countertransport, or antiport,* involves exchange of a solute of one species on one side of the membrane for a solute of a different species on the other side of the membrane. A concentration gradient for at least one of the species involved is necessary to produce a net flow of solute. Again, in this case, the energy for moving one species against its gradient comes from the other species moving down its concentration gradient.

After these two forms of secondary active transport were identified, two major advances occurred in the field. One was recognition of the ubiquitous nature of secondary transport systems. The other was development of molecular techniques that revealed correlations between the structure of transporters and their function.

The number of substances transported through cotransport mechanisms is enormous; they range from nutrients in the small intestine and kidney to neurotransmitters in the nerve terminals of the brain. The most significant, from the nutritional point of view, are located in the small intestine where they are important in the absorption of free amino acids, di- and tripeptides, monosaccharides, and water-soluble vitamins. Operation of most of these cotransporters appeared to be coupled to the Na^+ gradient across the mucosal membrane. However, recent observations have revealed an important difference. Uptake of di- and tripeptides in the intestine and kidney is driven by the H^+ gradient that exists across the apical membrane of the epithelial cells and not by the Na^+ gradient; this is an exception to the more general situation in which the energy for cotransport comes from the transmembrane gradient for Na^+ (14).

The exception is important because, in the small intestine, absorption of di- and tripeptides is quantitatively more important than absorption of free amino acids. Moreover, a common cotransporter is responsible for transport of di- and tripeptides in the kidney and the intestine, and in both cases, the transport of peptides is not affected by the Na^+ gradient but is markedly affected by the H^+ gradient that exists across the brush border membrane (14).

As with all other types of transporters, the techniques of molecular biology are now being used to identify the relationship between molecular architecture and function of counter- and cotransporters (12). Although detailed strategies vary, the pattern established early for the sodium/glucose cotransporter of the intestinal brush border, SGLT1, has been repeated; after cloning and establishing a full amino acid sequence of the transporter, its arrangement across the membrane and the orientation of different moieties have been deduced. Then the clone and a variety of analogues have been functionally expressed in *Xenopus* oocytes, permitting determination of the role of specific amino acids in controlling the behavior of the molecule.

SUMMARY AND CONCLUSIONS

After more than a century of research, the study of membrane function has culminated in identification of a variety of specific modalities of permeation across the cell membrane. This chapter briefly describes the different modalities by which substances pass across cell membranes. Table 38.1 lists these modalities, with some selected examples of each that are of significance to nutrition. Since the major criteria that distinguish the different modalities are the relationship between fluxes and the forces that produce them, they are also listed in the table. It is now also clear that except for the movement of lipid-soluble compounds, each modality of permeation is due to the action of a specific intramembrane protein.

An outline of the strategies that initially permitted purification of the intramembrane proteins involved in the different forms of permeation is also included in the chapter to give the reader a glimpse of how individual components of the membrane were identified as subserving individual functions. The last two decades have seen great acceleration in this task with the introduction of the

Table 38.1
Distinct Modalities for Transmembrane Movements of Solutes with Selected Examples of Nutritional Relevance

Mechanism	Driving Force	Significant Examples
Passive		
Diffusion through lipid in membranes	Concentration gradient	Absorption of lipid-soluble compounds like oils and fats, fat-soluble vitamins, and drugs
Facilitated diffusion	Concentration gradient	Glucose movement across most cell membranes
Channel permeation	Electrochemical gradient	All passive movements; essential to maintain cell composition
Primary transporters		
Na-K ATPase	ATP or other high-energy intermediates	Extrusion of Na^+ and uptake of K^+ against electrochemical gradients; the formation of ion gradients serves in turn to drive cotransport and countertransport
Secondary transporters		
Cotransport (symport)	Na^+ or H^+ gradient	Na^+- or H^+-dependent absorption of most hydrophilic solutes in brush border of apical membrane of small intestine
Countertransport (antiport)	Na^+ or H^+ gradient	Na^+-H^+ exchange that maintains H^+ gradient across intestinal cells

patch clamp and molecular biology techniques. We now know so many channels and transporters in molecular detail that specific study of each family of transporters has become a subspecialty in itself.

REFERENCES

1. Overton E. Pfluger's Arch 1902;92:115–39.
2. Hille B. Ionic channels of excitable membranes. 2nd ed. Sunderland, MA: Sinauer, 1992.
3. Singer SJ, Nicholson GL. Science 1972;175:720–31.
4. Glynn IM. J Physiol 1993;462:1–30.
5. Katz B. Nerve, muscle and synapse. New York: McGraw Hill, 1996.
6. Neher E, Sackmann B. Sci Am 1992;266:28–35.
7. Catterall W. Science 1988;242:50–61.
8. Unwin N, Henderson R. Sci Am 1984;250:78–94.
9. Smith CUM. Membrane signaling systems. In: Lee AG. Biomembranes, vol I. General principles. 5th ed. Greenwich, CT: JAI Press, 1995;245–70.
10. Anonymous. TIPS 1996;(Suppl):1–81.
11. Thorens B. Annu Rev Physiol 1993;55:591–608.
12. Wright EM. Annu Rev Physiol 1993;55:575–89.
13. Crane RK. Rev Physiol Biochem Pharmacol 1977;78:99–159.
14. Leibach FH, Ganapathy V. Annu Rev Nutr 1996;16:99–119.

SELECTED READINGS

Aidley D, Stanfield P. Ion channels: molecules in action. Cambridge: Cambridge University Press, 1996.

Hall ZW. Introduction to molecular neurobiology. Sunderland, MA: Sinauer, 1992.

Hille B. Ionic channels of excitable membranes. 2nd ed. Sunderland, MA: Sinauer, 1992.

Katz B. Nerve, muscle and synapse, New York: McGraw Hill, 1966.

Smith CUM. Elements of molecular neurobiology. 2nd ed. Chichester: John Wiley & Sons, 1996.

39. The Alimentary Tract in Nutrition: A Tutorial

SAMUEL KLEIN, STEVEN M. COHN, and DAVID H. ALPERS

The alimentary tract is a tubular structure that extends from the posterior oropharynx to the anus. Its primary function is to digest and absorb ingested nutrients. This chapter reviews the structural and functional components of the alimentary tract and describes the interactions of these components in response to a meal. Gastrointestinal (GI) tract flora and the immune system are also reviewed briefly because of their importance in overall GI function.

GASTROINTESTINAL TRACT STRUCTURE

Substructures and Cells

The GI tract consists of four contiguous segments: the esophagus, stomach, small intestine, and colon (Fig. 39.1). The wall of each segment contains four distinctive layers: the mucosa, submucosa, muscularis propria, and serosa or adventitia (Fig. 39.2). The mucosa is composed of three distinct layers: the epithelium, lamina propria, and muscularis mucosae. The epithelial layer forms a barrier between the lumen and the underlying tissues. Many of the different region-specific secretory, absorptive, and barrier functions of the alimentary tract are accounted for by differences in the type and distribution of various differentiated epithelial cell populations along the length of the gut; thus, the epithelium shows the greatest variability among different regions of the GI tract. The lamina propria is a connective tissue space between the epithelium and the thin layer of muscle fibers, the muscularis mucosae, which forms the lower boundary of the mucosa. The lamina propria contains many cells involved in immunologic functions, including immunoglobulin-secreting plasma cells, macrophages, and lymphocytes. In addition, abundant lymphoid nodules that often extend through the muscularis mucosae into the underlying submucosa are present. Subepithelial fibroblasts produce collagen and many other extracellular matrix components that underlie the basal lamina of the epithelium. These fibroblasts and the extracellular matrix that they secrete have an important role in regulating cell proliferation and differentiation events within the overlying epithelium.

The mucosal epithelium contains numerous enteroendocrine cells in addition to cells with secretory, absorptive, and barrier functions. The enteroendocrine cells, found in gastric, intestinal, and colonic epithelium, are characterized by their polygonal shape, broad base, and the numerous membrane-bound secretory granules in their basilar portion. Enteroendocrine cells are joined to other adjacent cells in the epithelium via junctional complexes located near the apical pole. The regulatory peptides or bioamine products stored in the basally located secretory granules are secreted through the basolateral membrane and act through paracrine or endocrine mechanisms as mediators of gastrointestinal secretion, absorptive function, and motility in response to luminally and/or basolaterally derived signals.

The submucosa extends from the mucosa to the muscularis externa and contains numerous small- to moderate-sized veins, arteries, and lymphatic channels surrounded by connective tissue. Ganglion cells and autonomic nerve fibers of Meissner's plexus are also found in the submucosa. Fibers of this submucosal plexus together with the myenteric plexus form the enteric nervous system, which regulates and coordinates a number of intestinal functions including motility. Additionally, scattered lymphoid aggregates or nodules may be found in this layer of the gut wall.

The muscularis propria is organized into two layers of muscle: an inner circular layer, in which muscle cells circle the intestine, and an outer longitudinal layer, in which muscle cells run parallel to the long axis of the intestine. In the upper esophagus, skeletal muscle fibers interdigitate with smooth muscle fibers, whereas the muscularis of

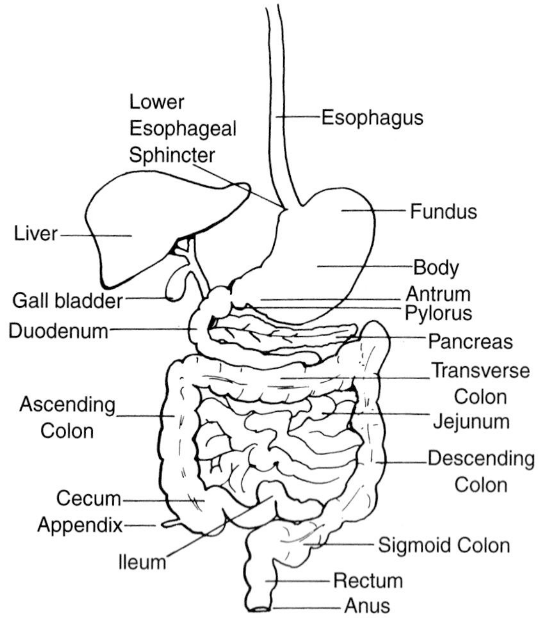

Figure 39.1. Diagram of the major parts of the gastrointestinal tract. Anatomy of the stomach, small intestine, and large intestine. The *duodenum* is located in the retroperitoneal space and bends around the head of the *pancreas*. The *jejunum* lies within the peritoneal cavity and begins at the ligament of Treitz. Jejunal bowel loops are predominately located in the left and middle upper abdomen. The proximal *ileum* lies in the middle abdominal region. The distal ileum lies in the right lower quadrant and joins the *colon* at the ileal cecal valve. The cutout reveals the duodenum and the ligament of Treitz, which lie behind the transverse colon. (From Greene HL, Moran JR. The gastrointestinal tract: regulatory nutrient absorption. In: Shils ME, Olson JA, Shike M, eds. Modern nutrition in health and disease. 8th ed. Philadelphia: Lea & Febiger, 1994; 551.)

the remaining alimentary tract is composed entirely of smooth muscle.

Esophagus

The adult esophagus is approximately 25 cm long and extends from the posterior oropharynx at the level of the cricoid cartilage to just below the diaphragmatic hiatus, where it enters the stomach at the esophagogastric junction. The esophageal mucosa is lined by a thick, incompletely keratinized, stratified squamous epithelium that provides protection against abrasion during passage of a swallowed food bolus and against refluxed stomach acid. The lamina propria contains occasional lymphoid aggregates and mucosal glands that secrete neutral mucus. Submucosal glands that secrete acidic mucus extend through the lamina propria and muscularis mucosae and are most abundant in the upper half of the esophagus.

In the upper esophagus, skeletal muscle fibers blend with the smooth muscle fibers found throughout the rest of the esophagus. The upper esophageal sphincter is formed by a thickened band of oblique muscle. These skeletal muscle fibers are under voluntary control and are involved in regulating initial passage of a swallowed bolus into the upper esophagus. The remaining smooth muscle of the muscularis is innervated by parasympathetic fibers originating from the vagus nerve. A thickened band of circular smooth muscle adjacent to the esophagogastric junction form the lower esophageal sphincter. Contraction of this specialized region of smooth muscle coupled with the abrupt angulation of the esophagus as it passes through the diaphragmatic hiatus where it joins the gastric cardia

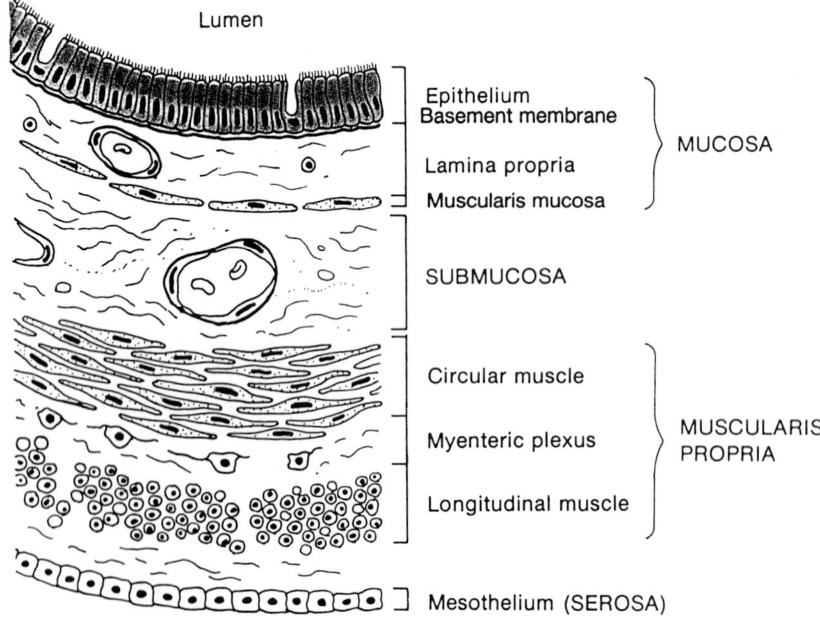

Figure 39.2. Schematic organization of the wall of the gastrointestinal tract. (From Yamada T, Alpers DH, Owyang C, et al., eds. Textbook of gastroenterology. 2nd ed. Philadelphia: JB Lippincott, 1991;142, with permission.)

provides a mechanism for preventing reflux of the acid contents of the stomach into the esophagus.

Stomach

The stomach is an asymmetric organ that extends from the gastroesophageal junction in the cardia to the duodenum (Fig. 39.3). The upper portion of the stomach, which lies under the left hemidiaphragm, is called the fundus. The gastric body comprises the largest portion of the stomach and extends to the angularis, where the stomach abruptly bends. The pyloric sphincter is a round band of muscle that forms the opening of the stomach into the duodenum. The flat glandular mucosa of the stomach changes to the villus epithelium seen in the duodenum at the pylorus. The gastric antrum lies between the angularis and the pylorus.

The entire stomach is lined by a simple columnar epithelium. The mucosa contains numerous invaginating gastric pits, or foveolae, which form glands at their base. Each glandular unit is composed of three regions: the upper pit region lined by surface mucus-secreting cells; a narrow isthmus or neck containing many immature undifferentiated cells and mucous neck cells; and a basilar gland that contains three cell types—parietal cells, chief cells, and enteroendocrine cells. Most of the gastric body and fundus is lined by oxyntic mucosa consisting of fundic-type glands responsible for secretion of acid pepsinogens and intrinsic factor. These glands contain abundant parietal cells in their upper half. Chief cells predominate near the base of glands in fundic-type mucosa. The cardiac glands found in the first 3 to 4 cm adjacent to the esophagogastric junction are primarily mucus-secreting glands, with few parietal or chief cells. Pyloric glands in the prepyloric antrum are coiled and remarkable for their fairly long foveolae and increased population of enteroendocrine cells.

Surface mucous cells form a uniform population of columnar epithelial cells lining the surface mucosa and gastric pits. These cells secrete a glycoprotein-rich neutral mucus layer that protects the epithelium from the acid environment of the stomach. Surface mucous cells are constantly shed into the gastric lumen and are replaced by replication of undifferentiated cells within the neck or isthmus region of each gastric gland, which differentiate during migration up the foveola and onto the gastric mucosal surface.

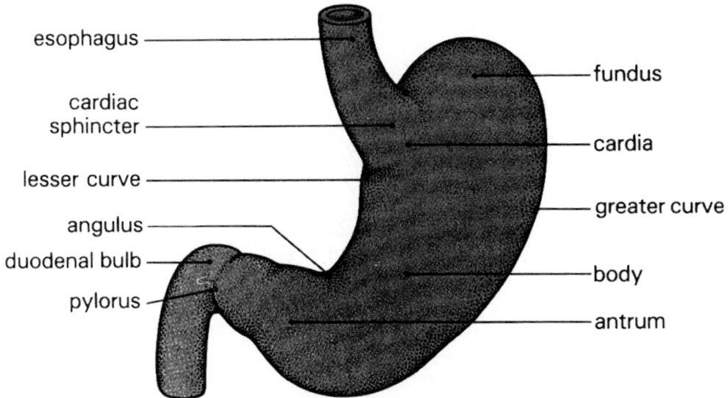

Figure 39.3. Regional organization of the stomach and proximal duodenum. (From Yamada T, Alpers DH, Owyang C, et al., eds. Textbook of gastroenterology. 2nd ed. Philadelphia: JB Lippincott, 1991;1304, with permission.)

Parietal cells secrete hydrochloric acid and are located in the middle and basilar portions of the gastric glands. These cells are large, with clear or acidophilic cytoplasm and abundant mitochondria. They have well-developed intracellular canaliculi containing a microvillus border that greatly expands the apical surface available for acid secretion. Receptors for histamine, gastrin, and acetylcholine located at the basolateral surface regulate parietal cell secretory function. Intrinsic factor, a binding protein for vitamin B_{12}, is secreted by parietal cells.

Chief cells, or zymogenic cells, are found near the base of the gastric glands. These cells are characterized by an extensive basilar rough endoplasmic reticulum and supranuclear zymogen granules, reflecting their role in the production of pepsinogens and other proteases. Pepsinogens are synthesized and secreted by these cells into the gastric lumen. Hydrochloric acid in the lumen converts the pepsinogen proenzyme to the active pepsins, which begin digestion of proteins to lower-molecular-weight polypeptides.

Enteroendocrine cells are most abundant in the prepyloric antrum and secrete many different neuropeptides and regulatory molecules discussed below. Gastrin-secreting G cells predominate in the antrum; enterochromaffin cells (ECs) are found throughout the gastric mucosa and secrete serotonin and either substance P or motilin; glucagon-secreting A cells are found in the proximal third of the stomach; and somatostatin-secreting D cells can be found in both the upper third of the stomach and the antrum but not in the midstomach. This complex web of enteroendocrine signals is important in integrating responses to both luminal conditions and basolateral signals.

Small Intestine

The small intestine extends from the gastric pylorus to the ileocecal valve and is divided into three regions—the duodenum, the jejunum, and the ileum.

Duodenum

The duodenum is approximately 30 cm long and is fixed in place, molded around the head of the pancreas. Histologically, the duodenum is characterized by the presence of abundant submucosal Brunner's glands that secrete alkaline mucus. The first portion of the duodenum, known as the bulb, is attached to a mesentery. The second (descending), third (transverse), and fourth (ascending) portions of the duodenum are retroperitoneal. Bile and pancreatic secretions enter the second portion of the duodenum from the common bile duct at the ampulla (papilla) of Vater. The junction of the duodenum and jejunum is defined by the position of the ligament of Treitz, where the duodenum reenters the peritoneal cavity. The histologic appearance of the small intestine does not change at this transition.

Jejunum and Ileum

The jejunum and ileum are mobile because of their attachment to an extensive mesentery. The proximal two-fifths of the small intestine beyond the ligament of Treitz is defined as jejunum, while the distal three-fifths are ileum. The jejunum is characterized by a larger diameter, more-prominent folds, and longer villi than the ileum. The ileum is characterized by the presence of abundant lymphoid follicles (Peyer's patches) in the submucosa.

The length of the jejunum and ileum in adults ranges from 320 to 846 cm. Several structural features of the small intestine amplify the mucosal surface area available for nutrient absorption to more than 200 m^2, which is larger than a doubles tennis court (Fig. 39.4).The surface area is magnified by a series of folds and invaginations. First, the cylinder of the intestine is heaped up into circular folds (plicae circulares) involving both submucosa and mucosa. These folds are particularly prominent in the jejunum. Second, the mucosal surface is further expanded by numerous villi, long fingerlike projections of mucosa containing an arteriole, vein, and central draining lacteal. Third, the apical surface of each small intestinal epithelial cell along the villi is covered by microvilli, providing thousands of hills and valleys for surface expansion. The folds, villi, and microvilli increase the surface area 600 times that of the surface area present in a simple cylinder.

Epithelium

The simple columnar epithelium that lines the small intestine is composed of four principal differentiated cell types: absorptive enterocytes, goblet cells, Paneth cells, and enteroendocrine cells. Cells are joined to adjacent cells by junctional complexes that regulate the paracellular movement of fluid and macromolecules (see "Fluid and Electrolytes"). Absorptive enterocytes are responsible for digestion of di- and tripeptides and disaccharides and for nutrient absorption. The microvilli of absorptive enter ocytes are supported by a central core of actin filaments that join with a dense terminal web of actin and myosin filaments oriented parallel to the apical surface of the enterocyte. The apical surface is covered by a glycoprotein-rich glycocalyx. Many enterocyte-encoded proteins important for digestive function are present at the apical surface, including dipeptidases, disaccharidases, enterokinase, and intestinal alkaline phosphatase. Goblet cells are flask-shaped cells with large apical vesicles that store and secrete mucus. This mucus forms a viscous gel that functions both as a lubricant and to protect the surface epithelium against adherence of invading pathogens. Paneth cells reside at the base of the intestinal crypts and produce proteins involved in antibacterial defenses, including lysozyme and a variety of defensins.

Enteroendocrine cells contain a large number of neuroendocrine mediators (see "Gastrointestinal Hormones"). The distribution of individual enteroendocrine cell subpopulations within the epithelium differs along the length of the small intestine. Although enteroendocrine cells arise from the same stem cell as the other differentiated cell types found in the small intestine, they have a much longer half-life than enterocytes or goblet cells. Thus, their migration onto and along the intestinal villi is uncoupled from the migration of the other epithelial cell types in the intestine.

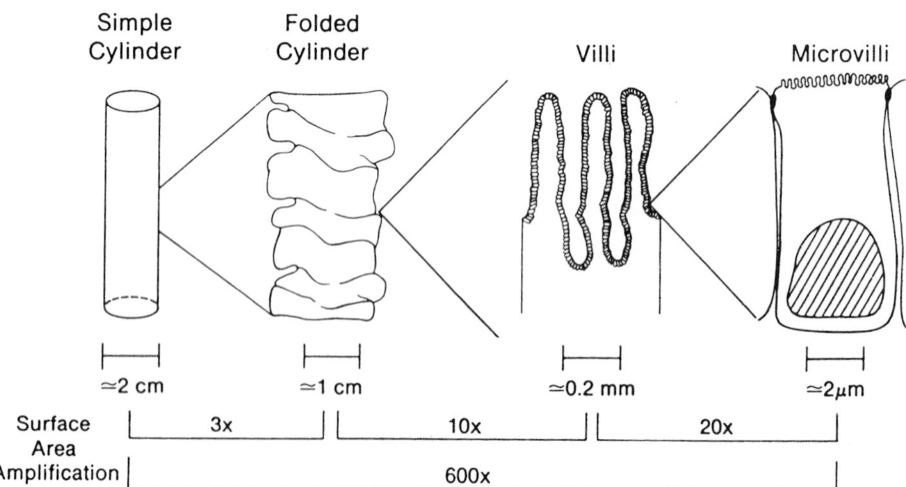

Figure 39.4. The intestinal surface area is expanded by intestinal folds (plicae conniventes) and villi. Microvilli further expand the surface area of epithelial cells in contact with luminal contents. These structural features taken together expand the surface area of the small intestine approximately 600-fold. (From Yamada T, Alpers DH, Owyang C, et al., eds. Textbook of gastroenterology. 2nd ed. Philadelphia: JB Lippincott, 1991;327, with permission.)

Renewal

Under normal physiologic circumstances, cells within the intestinal epithelium are continuously and rapidly replaced by migration of cells onto the villus from several adjacent crypts of Lieberkuhn or intestinal glands (Fig. 39.5). The four principal differentiated cell types of the small intestinal epithelium are all derived from multipotent stem cell(s) located near the base of each intestinal crypt. Under normal circumstances, these crypt stem cells divide rarely to produce a daughter stem cell (self-renewal) as well as a more rapidly replicating transit cell. Transit cells, in turn, undergo four to six rapid cell divisions in the proliferative zone located in the lower half of each crypt, and their progeny subsequently differentiate during a bipolar migration away from this zone. Goblet cells and enterocytes undergo terminal differentiation as they are rapidly translocated upward from the zone of proliferation to the apical extrusion zone (a process lasting 48 to 72 hours) located adjacent to the villus tip where they undergo apoptosis and are sloughed into the lumen. Paneth cells arise during downward migration to the crypt base, and enteroendocrine cells differentiate during migration from the zone of proliferation in either direction. Cell renewal, migration, and differentiation are interrelated processes regulated at multiple levels.

Colon

Structure

The colon is approximately 100 to 150 cm long, extending from the ileocecal valve to the proximal rectum (Fig. 39.1). The colon consists of the cecum, ascending colon, hepatic flexure, transverse colon, splenic flexure, descending colon, and sigmoid colon. The terminal ileum enters the cecum on its posteromedial border at the ileocecal valve. The cecum is a large blind pouch approximately 7.5 to 8.5 cm in diameter that projects from the antimesenteric side of the ascending colon. The appendix extends from a narrow opening in the base of the cecum. The diameter of the colon diminishes progressively; the sigmoid colon is approximately 2.5 cm in diameter and is the narrowest portion of the colon. The omentum is attached to the transverse colon on its anterior superior edge. The ascending colon, descending colon, rectum, and posterior surface of the hepatic and splenic flexures are fixed retroperitoneal structures. The cecum, transverse, and sigmoid colon are intraperitoneal and thus lack a complete serosal layer.

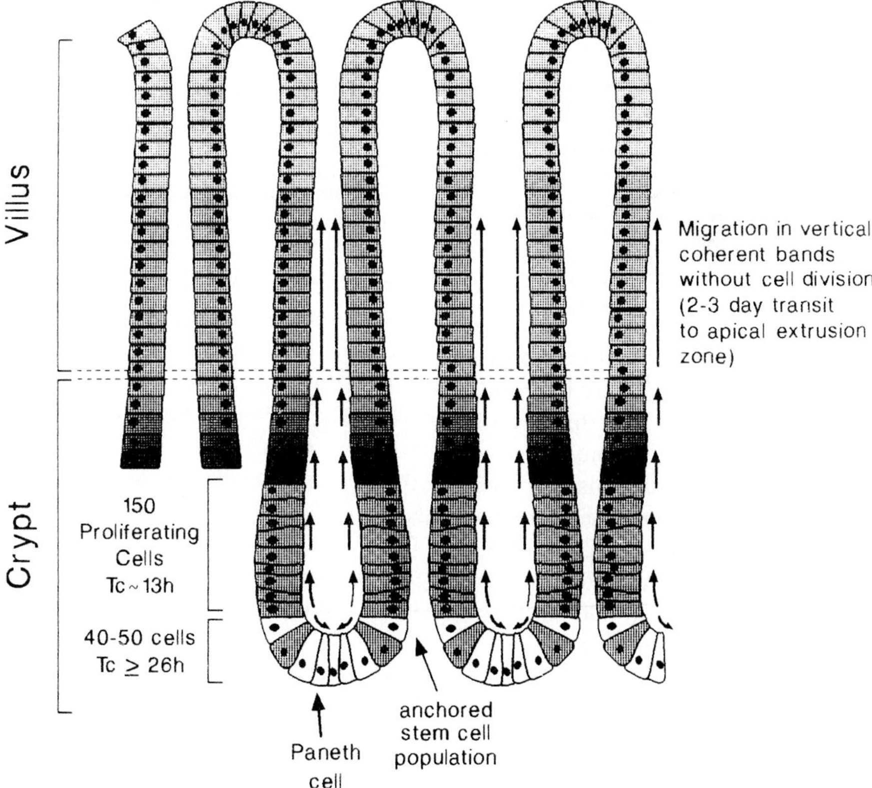

Figure 39.5. Schematic organization of the epithelium in the adult mouse small intestine. The small intestinal crypt contains approximately 250 cells. The lower five cell positions contain 40–50 cells that have an average cycle time (Tc) ≥26 hours. This region includes Paneth cells and is postulated to include undifferentiated, anchored stem cells at the fifth cell position above the base. The undifferentiated cells divide asymmetrically to give rise to proliferating transit cells (Tc ≈ 13 hours) that migrate upward toward the villus and subsequently differentiate into enterocytes, goblet cells, and enteroendocrine cells. Paneth's cells differentiate during downward translocation to the crypt base. Senescent cells are extruded near the villus tips. (From Yamada T, Alpers DH, Owyang C, et al., eds. Textbook of gastroenterology. 2nd ed. Philadelphia: JB Lippincott, 1991;1561, with permission.)

Epithelium. Three principal differentiated epithelial cell types are found in the adult colonic epithelium: absorptive colonocytes, goblet cells, and the enteroendocrine cells. All of these cell lineages appear to be derived from a common epithelial cell stem cell precursor. Undifferentiated cells, replicating cells, and enteroendocrine cells predominate near the base of each colonic gland (crypt). Cells belonging to each of the principal cell lineages differentiate as they migrate away from the zone of proliferation toward the surface epithelium. The average life span of goblet cells and absorptive cells, from their birth deep in the crypt until they are sloughed into the lumen, is approximately 6 days. As in the small intestine, some enteroendocrine cell subtypes appear to have a much longer life span than goblet cells or absorptive colonocytes.

As absorptive colonocytes differentiate during their migration up the crypt, they develop short microvilli and clear apically oriented vesicles containing a fibrillar, glycoprotein-rich secretory product that may contribute to a glycocalyx. These apical vesicles are lost, and microvilli elongate and increase in number as the maturing absorptive cells emerge onto the surface epithelium. At this point, alkaline phosphatase activity appears on the brush border, and the basolateral membranes have acquired a considerable amount of Na^+-K^+ ATPase activity, reflecting their function in water and electrolyte transport.

Many different enteroendocrine cell types are found within the colonic epithelium, including L cells, which contain both enteroglucagon and peptide YY (PYY); cells that secrete only PYY; EC_1 cells that secrete serotonin, substance P, and leu-enkephalin; pancreatic polypeptide-secreting cells; and rare somatostatin-secreting cells. Enteroendocrine cells are more numerous in the appendix and the rectum then in the rest of the colon.

Other Layers. The inner circular muscle fibers form a continuous layer around the colon. The outer longitudinal smooth muscle fibers are condensed into three bands (taeniae coli) equidistant around the circumference of the colon. Haustra are the bulging sacculations that form between adjacent taeniae coli. The serosa is a mesothelial derived cell layer that covers the peritoneal aspects of the colonic wall. Therefore, regions of the ascending colon, the descending colon, and rectum that do not lie within in the peritoneal cavity have no outer serosal layer.

Appendix

The appendix is similar in histologic organization to the rest of the colon. The mucosa of the appendix consists of deep folds lined by a columnar epithelium forming simple tubular or forked glands. This epithelium contains abundant goblet cells and enteroendocrine cells. Numerous lymphoid nodules are found in the lamina propria. The normal histologic architecture of the adult appendix is often replaced by fibrous scar tissue as a result of subclinical bouts of appendicitis.

Rectum

The rectum is approximately 12 to 15 cm long and extends from the sigmoid colon to the anal canal following the curve of the sacrum (Fig. 39.1). The rectal wall consists of mucosal, submucosal, inner circular, and outer longitudinal muscular layers. There is no serosal layer in the rectum. The anal canal is approximately 3 cm long. The anal verge is the junction between anal and perianal skin. Anal epithelium (anoderm) lacks hair follicles, sebaceous glands, or sweat glands. The dentate line is the true mucocutaneous junction located just above the anal verge. A 6- to 12-mm transitional zone exists above the dentate line where the squamous epithelium of the anoderm becomes cuboidal and then columnar epithelium.

VASCULATURE

Blood and lymphatic vessels provide the transportation system for delivering absorbed nutrients to other body tissues. In addition, the arterial blood supply provides nutrients to the alimentary tract itself. In the small intestine, each villus contains a single arteriole that breaks into a capillary network at the villous tip before anastamosing with a draining venule. Each villus contains a lymphatic vessel (lacteal) that drains into a submucosal plexus connected to larger lymphatics. In the colon, arterioles pass between crypts to the epithelial cell surface and form a network of capillaries around the crypts. Lymphatic vessels in the colon do not extend higher than the base of the crypts.

Blood from the small intestine and colon drains into the portal vein, which delivers absorbed water-soluble nutrients directly to the liver, where they can be metabolized or released directly into the hepatic veins and ultimately the systemic circulation. Bile salts absorbed in the terminal ileum travel through the portal vein to the liver where they can be secreted back into the small intestine, providing an enterohepatic circulation for bile salt recycling, which is critical for normal bile salt homeostasis and fat absorption. Intestinal lymphatic vessels, which are closely associated with arteries supplying the alimentary tract, carry absorbed fat-soluble nutrients to the thoracic duct, which drains into the left subclavian vein and the systemic circulation.

Adequate intestinal blood flow is critical because it provides oxygen necessary for intestinal cell survival. Therefore, GI tract blood flow is carefully regulated by metabolic, vascular, and hormonal factors to ensure adequate tissue oxygenation. Food ingestion increases intestinal blood flow and oxygen requirements.

ENTERIC NERVOUS SYSTEM AND MOTILITY

Many GI tract motor patterns have been described and involve complicated interactions between a series of stimulatory and inhibitory impulses from the enteric nervous system (ENS) to GI smooth muscle. Intestinal smooth muscle consists of circular and longitudinal muscle layers, so the interaction of muscular contraction between layers determines the pattern of motility. The two most important motility patterns are the migrating myoelectric complex (MMC) and peristalsis, which are programed by the ENS.

The MMC, the major complex motility pattern in mammals, is cyclical and passes from the stomach to the terminal ileum. During digestion this complex consists of irregular contractions that promote mixing and propulsion over moderate distances, modulated by distention and by chemical and mechanical stimulation of the mucosa. Sleeve contractions facilitate mixing of core and peripheral intestinal fluid contents and enhance nutrient contact with intestinal mucosa. During interdigestive periods, the MMC consists of coordinated activity that empties the stomach and sweeps down the intestine. The frequency of interdigestive ring contraction waves varies with location. Contractions occur at a rate of 3/min in the stomach and 11 to 12/min in the duodenum and decrease progressively down the small intestine to 7/min in the ileum. These interdigestive movements clear the gut for the next meal. The MMC also includes sleeve contractions that are also rhythmic, and their periodicity declines along the small intestine.

The regulation of peristalsis, the smallest unit of the propulsive reflex, is one of the simplest programed motor activities of the ENS but is still quite complex (Fig. 39.6). The reflex has two components: orad contraction and caudad relaxation, whose combination moves intestinal contents in a caudad direction. The propulsive movement is the end result of contractions and relaxations of the longitudinal and circular external muscles and of the muscularis mucosae. The circular muscle has the major role in mixing and propulsion by ring contractions that decrease the diameter of the intestine, whereas the longitudinal muscle shortens the segment by sleeve contractions, with little alteration in luminal diameter. Excitatory and inhibitory motor neurons supply the muscle, and inhibitory reflexes modulate these activities by monitoring luminal contents. Multiple chemical mediators are involved in this reflex (Fig. 39.7) (Table 39.1).

The presence of luminal nutrients can increase absorption by feedback regulation of intestinal motility. Fat or carbohydrate in the ileum and colon stimulates the release of PYY from ileal and colonic endocrine cells. PYY then enters the systemic circulation and inhibits gastric emptying and slows down small intestinal transit. Thus, this ileal and colonic brake mechanism enhances absorption by increasing the contact time between luminal nutrients and intestinal mucosa.

The ENS is able to regulate such complex and diffuse motility functions by its vast network throughout the GI tract. The ENS consists of approximately 100 million nerve cell bodies (neurons) and their processes, which are embedded in the wall of the GI tract. These neurons lie in clusters (ganglia) and are segregated largely into two layers: *(a)* the myenteric ganglia, which form a continuous plexus between the circular and longitudinal muscle layers of the muscularis propria and extend from the upper esophagus to the internal anal sphincter, and *(b)* the submucous plexus, which is located in the submucosa and is especially prominent in the small and large intestines. The processes from these ganglia form dense networks and innervate the muscularis propria, muscularis mucosae, epithelium, and other structures. Nonganglionated plexuses supply all the layers of the tubular GI tract, accompanying the arteries that supply the gut wall.

The ENS is connected to the central nervous system (CNS) by transmission along axons in both directions,

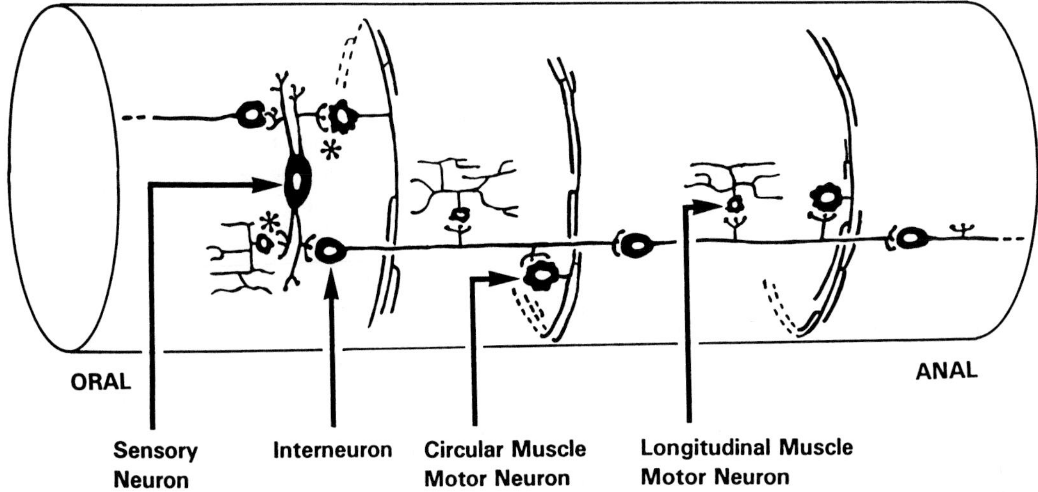

Figure 39.6. Pathways for propulsive reflexes in the intestine. A short segment of intestine is represented, on which the descending inhibitory reflex pathway and the first connections of the ascending pathway are depicted. They provide outputs to ascending and descending interneurons and monosynaptic connections to motor neurons (*). The interneurons form descending and ascending chains and provide outputs to motor neurons. In the descending pathway, some neurons excite the longitudinal muscle, and some neurons inhibit the circular muscle. Ascending reflex pathways supply inputs to excitatory longitudinal muscle motor neurons and excitatory circular muscle motor neurons (From Yamada T, Alpers DH, Owyang C, et al., eds. Textbook of gastroenterology, 2nd ed. Philadelphia: JB Lippincott, 1991;15, with permission.)

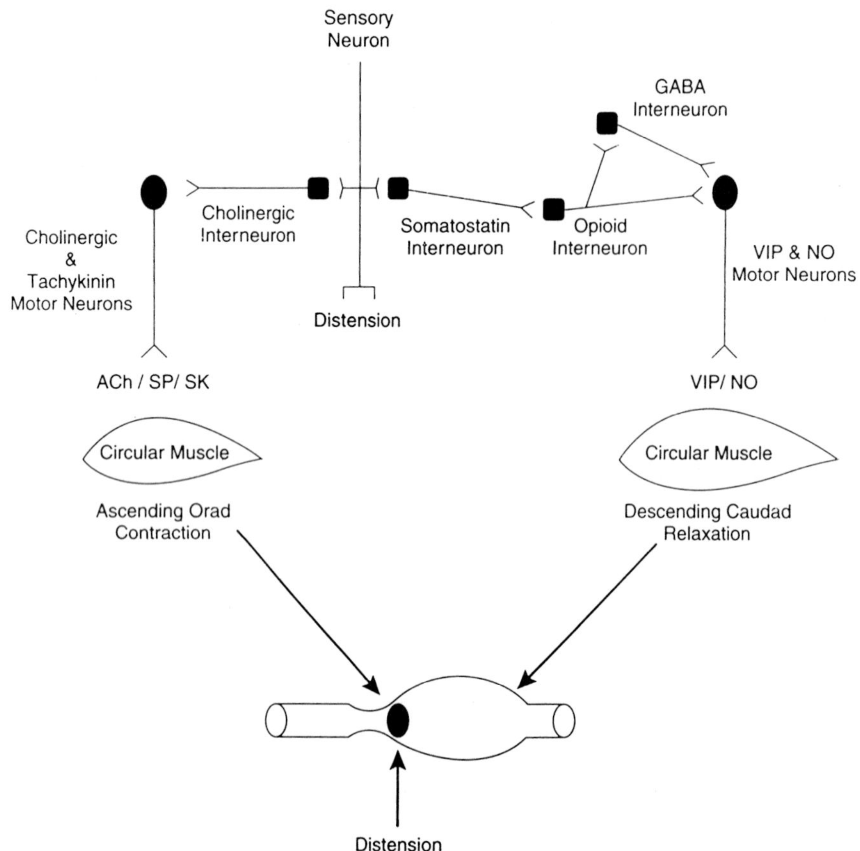

Figure 39.7. Regulation of peristaltic reflex by neurons of the myenteric plexus. The reflex has two components: ascending or orad contraction and descending or caudad relaxation. The stimulus (i.e., distension or mucosal stimulation) is relayed by sensory neurons to cholinergic interneurons coupled to vasoactive intestinal peptide *(VIP)* and nitric oxide *(NO)* synthase neurons caudad and acetylcholine *(Ach)* and tachykinin *(SP, SK)* neurons orad. Somatostatin, opioid, and γ-aminobutyric acid *(GABA)* neurons exert a modulatory influence on VIP and NO synthase neurons. (From Yamada T, Alpers DH, Owyang C, et al., eds. Textbook of gastroenterology, 2nd ed. Philadelphia: JB Lippincott, 1991;105, with permission.)

from GI tract to brain and from brain to ENS. The connections are largely due to the vagus nerve and to pathways leaving the spinal cord. Most vagal fibers (>90%) are afferents that interact with neurons in the nucleus tractus solitarius in the midbrain. Because there are relatively few efferent vagal fibers compared with the large number of ENS neurons, the vagus functions more to initiate activity of the integrated circuits in the ENS rather than to coordinate gut function by direct signaling. Efferent centers in the spinal cord can receive efferent signals from the CNS, which are relayed to the ENS. In addition, the spinal centers can process afferent signals from the gut.

The vagal and spinal components comprise the extrinsic branches of the autonomic nervous system, including the parasympathetic and sympathetic systems (Fig. 39.8). The striated muscles in the upper esophagus and external anal sphincter are directly innervated by cholinergic fibers, whereas the remaining gut is innervated by a variety of neural mediators, including acetylcholine, gut peptides, and nitric oxide (NO). These preganglionic fibers form synapses with the enteric plexuses, which in turn are connected with smooth muscle, secretory, and endocrine cells. The sympathetic nervous system contains preganglionic connections between prevertebral ganglia and the spinal cord, but the gut itself is innervated by postganglionic connections, mediated largely by epinephrine and norepinephrine. These postganglionic fibers innervate the plexuses of the ENS as do the parasympathetic fibers, but the sympathetic fibers also directly innervate blood vessels, smooth muscle layers, and mucosal cells.

The sympathetic nervous system affects intestinal secretion, blood flow, and motility. The sensory fibers that accompany the sympathetic nerves (intestinofugal neurons) are primary sensory neurons that are not part of the autonomic nervous system and are not really "sympathetic" sensory nerves. Sympathetic efferent neurons inhibit motility by decreasing contractile activity and by constricting sphincters. These various effects can be relayed along the gut to other regions before returning to the region of the initial stimulus by means of prevertebral ganglia connections. Examples of these inhibitory reflexes include slowing of gastric emptying by acidity or hypertonicity in the upper small intestine.

Intestinal smooth muscle is of unitary type and is characterized by spontaneous activity, including active tension to stretching, and activity that is not initiated by nerves but modulated by them. The circular muscle is innervated by both excitatory and inhibitory motor neurons and forms a thick syncytium surrounding the submucosa. Contraction

Table 39.1
Gastrointestinal Hormones*

Peptide[a]	Action	Site of Release	Releaser
Endocrine			
Gastrin	Stimulates Gastric acid secretion Growth of gastric oxyntic gland mucosa	Antrum (duodenum)	Peptides Amino acids Distention Vagal stimulation
CCK	Stimulates Gallbladder contraction Pancreatic enzyme secretion Pancreatic bicarbonate secretion Growth of exocrine pancreas Inhibits gastric emptying	Duodenum Jejunum	Peptides Amino acids Fatty acids >8C in length
Secretin	Stimulates Pancreatic bicarbonate secretion Biliary bicarbonate secretion Growth of exocrine pancreas Pepsin secretion Inhibits Gastric acid secretion Trophic effect of gastrin	Duodenum	Acid
GIP	Stimulates insulin release Inhibits gastric acid secretion	Duodenum Jejunum	Glucose Amino acids Fatty acids
Peptide YY	Ileal brake	Ileum	Fatty acids Glucose
Motilin[b]	Stimulates gastric and duodenal motility	Duodenum Jejunum	Unknown
Pancreatic polypeptide[b]	Inhibits Pancreatic bicarbonate secretion Pancreatic enzyme secretion	Pancreas	Protein
Enteroglucagon[b]	Unknown	Ileum	Glucose Fat
Neurocrines			
VIP	Relaxes sphincters Relaxes gut circular muscle Stimulates intestinal secretion Stimulates pancreatic secretion	Mucosa and smooth muscle of IG tract	
Bombesin or GRP	Stimulates gastrin release	Gastric mucosa	
Enkephalins	Stimulates smooth muscle contraction Inhibits intestinal secretion	Mucosa and smooth muscle of GI tract	
Paracrines			
Somatostatin	Inhibits Gastrin release Other peptide hormone release Gastric acid secretion	GI mucosa Pancreatic islets	Acid Vagus inhibits release
Histamine[c]	Stimulates gastric acid secretion	Oxyntic gland mucosa ECL cell	Unknown

*From references 11 and 12.
[a]CCK, cholecystokinin; GIP, glucose-dependent insulinotropic peptide; VIP, vasoactive intestinal polypeptide.
[b]Unknown physiologic function.
[c]Histamine is an amine, not a peptide.

shortens the radius but increases the length of each fiber and in turn the syncytium. In contrast, the longitudinal muscle layer surrounding the circular muscle is thin, is shortened by contraction (with enlarged radius), and is only innervated by excitatory neurons. Electrical slow waves derive from the muscle itself and trigger action potentials that lead to contractile activity. Action potentials in intestinal smooth muscle are propagated through gap junctions from cell to cell, creating an electrical syncytium.

GASTROINTESTINAL HORMONES

The mucosa of the GI tract contains an abundance of regulatory substances that are critical for precise coordination of activities necessary to handle a meal. These sub-

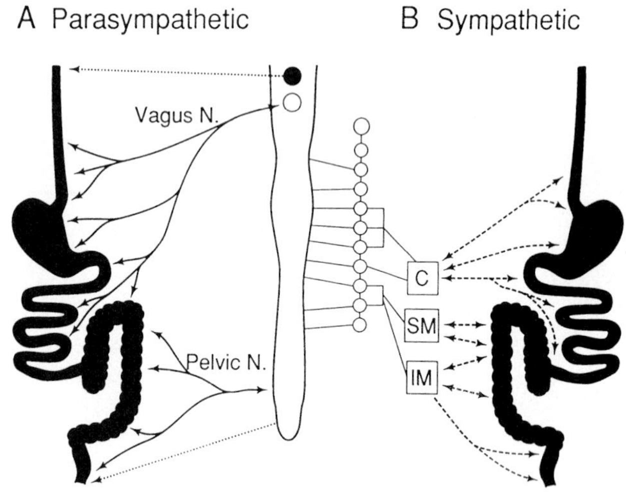

Figure 39.8. Extrinsic branches of the autonomic nervous system. *A.* Parasympathetic. *Dashed lines* indicate cholinergic innervation of the striated muscle in the esophagus and external anal sphincter. *Solid lines* indicate afferent and preganglionic innervation of the remaining gastrointestinal tract. *B.* Sympathetic. *Solid lines* denote the afferent and preganglionic efferent pathways between the spinal cord and the prevertebral ganglia (*C,* celiac; *SM,* superior mesenteric; *IM,* inferior mesenteric). *Dotted lines* indicate the afferent and postganglionic efferent innervation. (From Johnson LR, Alpers DH, Jacobson ED, et al., eds. Physiology of the gastrointestinal tract, vol 1. 3rd ed. New York: Raven Press, 1994;451, with permission.)

stances are mostly peptides that communicate by endocrine, neurocrine, and paracrine pathways (Fig. 39.9, Table 39.1), not all of them mutually exclusive. Endocrine peptides are hormones released from sensory cells in the intestine in response to a mechanical or chemical stimulus, which enter the bloodstream to act on a distant target organ. Gut neurocrine peptides are produced within the ENS and are located in nerves within the gut itself. Most of these peptides are also produced by the brain and represent a gut-brain axis. Paracrine peptides (and histamine) are produced by intestinal cells and act on adjacent or nearby cells, either by direct cellular extension to other cells or by release of the peptide (or histamine) into the mucosa (e.g., somatostatin, histamine) or the intestinal lumen (e.g., monitor peptide, CCK-releasing peptide, trefoil peptides).

Some of the hormones listed in Table 39.1 are especially important in the response to a meal (e.g., gastrin, CCK, secretin, motilin, glucose-dependent insulinotropic peptide [GIP], somatostatin) and all three major fuels (protein, carbohydrate, fat) are responsible for release of these substances. Other hormones are also released in response to a meal, but they do not act at the level of intestinal mucosal cells (e.g., insulin, glucagon) and are not considered further here. Because the coordination of function in the upper intestinal tract is so crucial, involving the stomach, duodenum, pancreas, and gallbladder, it is not surprising that these sites are most important in the release of GI hormones.

The specificity and coordination of action of GI hormones depend on three major factors: the multiple functions of each hormone, the paracrine actions between neuroendocrine and mucosal cells, and the regulatory functions of the ENS. Most GI hormones have multiple actions and mediate both stimulatory and inhibitory functions (e.g., gastrin, CCK, secretin, GIP, vasoactive intestinal polypeptide [VIP], enkephalins) (Table 39.1). Other GI

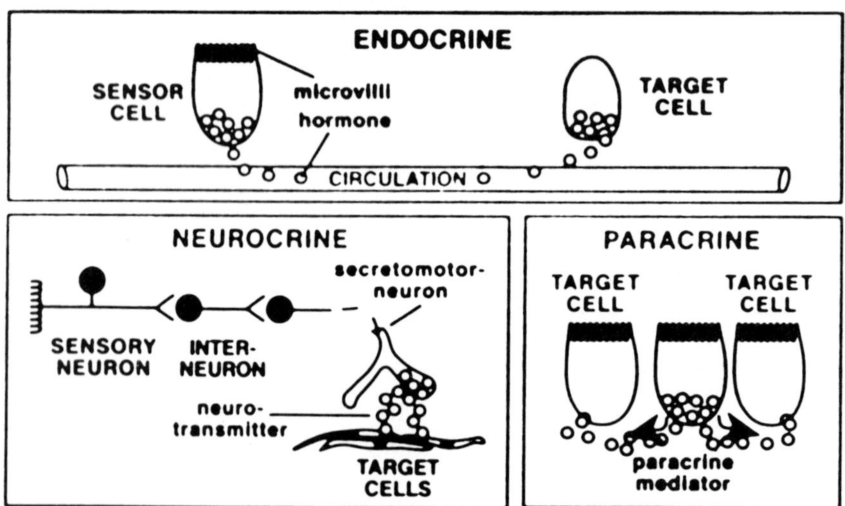

Figure 39.9. Three mechanisms of communication that mediate responses in the GI tract: endocrine, neurocrine, and paracrine. For the endocrine mechanism, sensory cells respond to stimuli by releasing transmitters that travel via the blood to their target cells or tissues. There are many examples of endocrine sensory cells in the GI tract that respond to either mechanical or chemical stimuli to release their hormones. Some types of endocrine cells respond to changes in pH or osmolality; others respond to changes in specific nutrients. For the neurocrine mechanisms, sensing and transmissions to the target tissue are completely mediated by nerves and neurotransmitters. Nerves sense stimuli such as nutrients, pH, and osmolality in the luminal contents, as well as movement of the contents and distention of the gut lumen. (From Raybould H, Pandol SJ. Integrated response to a meal, undergraduate teaching project, unit 29. Bethesda, MD: American Gastroenterological Association, 1995.)

hormones or amines are solely stimulatory (e.g., histamine, motilin, gastrin-releasing peptide [GRP], monitor peptide, CCK-releasing peptide) or inhibitory (e.g., somatostatin, pancreatic polypeptide). Thus, release of these hormones has the potential to create multiple effects on GI organs, coordinated in time. The presence of multiple cells in the mucosa, each possessing receptors to many of the GI hormones, also helps to create specificity of response. For example, in isolated cell systems, CCK stimulates acid production. However, CCK injected into the intact animal does not stimulate acid production because of a greater effect of CCK on the D cell producing somatostatin, an inhibitor of acid secretion, than on the parietal cell that produces acid. Gastrin, on the other hand, has the reverse effects on those two mucosal cells. In this way, the multiplicity of mucosal specific cells adds a layer of complexity and control to the multiple hormones present in the mucosa. Finally, the ENS with its many neuronal connections to mucosal cells, integrates the stimuli controlling GI hormone release. Both preganglionic parasympathetic cholinergic nerves and postganglionic fibers, mediated by neurocrine peptides, are important regulators of the gastrointestinal response to feeding. In addition, chemosensory neurons detect intraluminal events and regulate mucosal function by intrinsic mucosal reflexes.

INTEGRATED RESPONSE TO A MEAL

The integrated response of the GI tract to a meal represents a coordinated series of events, including regulation of food intake, stimulus-evoked responses in anticipation of the meal, ingestion and transfer of the meal to the stomach, digestion and absorption of the meal, and elimination of waste products of the meal, bringing into play all the individual regulatory controls reviewed above.

Regulation of Food Intake

The GI tract is involved in the earliest part of feeding beginning with the control of nutrient ingestion. Peptide hormones and other neurotransmitters in the gut have been implicated in the short-term regulation of energy intake (see Chapter 40). Olfactory and visual signals, along with mood and degree of physical activity can regulate intake via hypothalamic and brainstem centers (see Chapter 41). Taste buds in the tongue can affect energy intake during a meal. Gut hormones suggested to be regulators of food intake include insulin, glucagon, CCK, and GRP. Neurotransmitters possibly involved include serotonin, dopamine, epinephrine, opiates, and γ-butyric acid. Considerable evidence supports the role of CCK and GRP as satiety factors, both of them neurally released. Insulin probably stimulates the hunger drive. Recently, evidence has implicated two nonhormonal gut peptides as physiologically relevant satiety factors, enterostatin (the amino-terminal peptide of colipase) and apolipoprotein A-IV. The abundance of potential satiety agents makes it appear likely that the gut signals important in the short-term control of energy intake are multiple and perhaps additive.

Stimulus-Evoked Responses

The anticipatory responses to a meal are mediated by the CNS. Visual, olfactory, and auditory senses as well as the presence of food in the mouth can activate secretory responses from the salivary glands, stomach, and pancreas and can initiate relaxation in the stomach, contraction of the gallbladder, and relaxation of the sphincter of Oddi. These actions prepare the GI tract to initiate digestion when the meal arrives. This preparation is important, because digestive products of foodstuffs (e.g., amino acids, free fatty acids) are important stimuli in creating the maximum responses necessary to digest and absorb a meal. Thus, these nutrient products must be produced early in the meal. This cephalic phase of the meal is mediated through various brain centers, but the efferent signals all reach the gut through the vagus nerve. Once the meal enters the GI tract, the ENS becomes activated and works in concert with the CNS. For example, distention of the esophagus and/or stomach causes a contractile response mediated entirely by the ENS.

The best studied anticipatory CNS-mediated response is the cephalic phase of gastric secretion. Sensory input from the eye, nose, ear, and mouth sends afferent signals to the dorsal vagal complex in the midbrain where they are integrated and transmitted to GI organs by vagal efferent nerves. The stomach responds by producing acid and pepsin. Acetylcholine release from the vagus stimulates pepsinogen release into the lumen of the stomach. In the distal stomach, the vagal efferents activate the ENS to produce GRP to release gastrin, stimulating acid and pepsinogen production. Thus, when food enters the stomach, some of the protein is rapidly converted to oligopeptides by the action of pepsin, produced from pepsinogen and activated by the low pH. These oligopeptides stimulate release of more gastrin to perpetuate the digestive process. In this process, as well as in other anticipatory responses, appetizing meals elicit more response than bland or unappetizing meals. Thus, the higher centers of the CNS are important in regulating the initial response of the GI tract.

Although these anticipatory responses clearly occur at each meal, it is not certain to what degree they are essential for the assimilation of nutrients. For example, the stomach can be removed and digestion and absorption can proceed fairly completely. Anticipatory responses to a meal may be more important in determining the amount of food eaten at a meal than in the absorption of nutrients. The loss of anticipatory relaxation of the proximal stomach allows only small volumes to be consumed at one time, so that consuming enough food to maintain weight becomes difficult. Although this deficit can be overcome by cognitive training, the response to a meal is impaired. Impairment in the senses of sight, taste, and/or smell affects the cognitive drive that creates the desire to eat.

Mouth

Chewing and salivary secretion form the food into a round and smooth portion that can be swallowed. The mouth is the receptacle for two functions: secretion and motility. Secretion into the oral cavity originates from the salivary glands and consists of fluid, electrolytes, and proteins. The structure and function of salivary glands, which are composed of acini that secrete their products through ducts, are analogous to those of the pancreas. Chloride enters the lumen of the salivary gland through chloride channels, and sodium enters paracellularly to maintain electroneutrality. In the ducts, the fluid is modified as sodium and chloride leave the lumen; some sodium is exchanged for potassium and some chloride is exchanged for bicarbonate, producing a final salivary secretion rich in bicarbonate. Stimulation of the parasympathetic nerves is the major factor in regulating salivary secretion by direct acinar and duct cell innervation and by altering the blood supply. However, vasoactive peptides are also released to regulate blood flow. Sympathetic nerve input also stimulates secretion, but to a much lesser extent.

Proteins present in salivary secretions are important during the initial stages of nutrient assimilation. The influence of salivary amylase on starch digestion in the mouth and esophagus is small because of the short residence time of food in the mouth. However, in the stomach, attachment of amylase to its substrate protects the enzyme from inactivation at the slightly acid environment (pH 5–6) of the stomach when it is buffered by food. Thus, the enzyme achieves significant initial hydrolysis of dietary starch while still in the stomach. In addition, a non-bile-salt-dependent triglyceride lipase is produced by Ebner's glands at the base of the tongue. Although the oral production is relatively small, the gastric mucosa produces more of this lipase. As is the case with salivary amylase, the digestion of triglycerides due to this lingual/gastric lipase occurs primarily in the gastric lumen. The best dietary substrates for this enzyme are triglycerides that contain medium-chain fatty acids. The salivary glands also secrete haptocorrin (also known as R protein), a carrier protein that protects vitamin B_{12} from acid-peptic digestion in the stomach. Most of the other salivary proteins largely enhance lubrication, provide antibacterial action, and enhance mucosal integrity.

The motility functions of the oral cavity are coordinated with the upper esophageal sphincter to propel the food bolus into the esophagus. This action requires the coordination of extrinsic muscles to modify the shape of the pharyngeal cavity and to close the airways and of intrinsic muscles to propel the bolus caudally. These two groups work in succession, so that food does not reflux into the nose or larynx. These muscular units work in reverse order during the act of vomiting, again with the purpose of preventing luminal contents from entering the airways.

Esophagus

The esophagus carries the food bolus from the mouth to the proximal stomach. The upper esophageal sphincter relaxes immediately after swallowing, along with increased pharyngeal pressure. These pressure changes move the bolus into the esophagus. The esophagus is the first gut organ in which the phenomenon of peristalsis is encountered. Peristalsis along the length of the esophagus (primary peristalsis) is enhanced by esophageal distention produced by the food bolus (secondary peristalsis). The coordinated caudal movement of contraction and relaxation waves moves the food bolus along the length of the esophagus. The act of swallowing initiates both pharyngeal and esophageal peristalsis and relaxation of the lower esophageal sphincter (LES), allowing the swallowed bolus to enter the proximal stomach. Immediately after a swallow, the LES pressure falls to that of the stomach and remains low until the swallow is completed. At the end of the swallow, the LES contracts, stripping the end of the esophagus of any remaining food contents. The most important neurotransmitters for the motility pattern in the esophagus are acetylcholine (contraction) and VIP/NO (relaxation). Although the esophagus is often depicted as an open tube, the walls of the esophagus are actually approximated to each other during fasting conditions and in areas not distended by a food bolus during feeding. Thus, the bolus cannot travel down the esophagus in the absence of peristalsis. Surprisingly, gravity is not a significant factor in the function of the esophagus.

Stomach

Although the oral cavity initiates some changes in the food bolus, not until residence in the stomach are the physical and chemical characteristics of the meal altered. The food bolus enters the stomach as large particles, following chewing action in the mouth. In the stomach, the food is mixed and ground with secreted fluid and enzymes and converted to a suspension of particles small enough to pass the pylorus into the duodenum. In addition, fats are converted into an emulsion by mixing action, and small amounts of fatty acids and monoglycerides are formed. Protein and starch digestion also proceeds to create monomeric and oligomeric nutrients that can act further in the duodenum to potentiate the intestinal response to a meal. The two major components responsible for these overall actions of the stomach are motility and acid/peptic secretion.

The anticipatory cephalic phase and distention of the stomach by a meal both lead to receptive relaxation of the proximal stomach, thus accommodating the meal without increasing gastric pressure. Vagal afferent fibers in the gastric wall respond to changes in tension in the muscular coat of the stomach. These responses are processed in the dorsal vagal nucleus in the medulla and create vagal efferent responses that not only relax the proximal stomach but also increase gastrin, acid, and pepsinogen secretion, initiate antral and gallbladder contraction, relax the sphincter of Oddi, and stimulate pancreatic secretion. These vagovagal reflexes are important in the coordinated function of the organs of the upper GI tract (stomach,

the duodenum must either add or absorb fluid and electrolytes. Remarkably, this adjustment is made within the first 50 cm (20 in) of the duodenal bulb. Under normal circumstances, however, the maximum rate of gastric emptying is about 2 mL/min so the proximal duodenum is not presented with larger volumes than it can accommodate for isotonic adjustment.

Thus, passage through the duodenum changes the physical properties of the meal because of the contributions of the organs in the duodenal cluster unit. Large amounts of pancreatic hydrolases and bile salts are added, digesting nearly all ingested macromolecules (except dietary fiber) to oligomers or monomers solubilized in a form compatible with absorption. Intestinal fluid leaving the duodenum is more isoosmotic, and the pH is more neutral.

Biliary System

Bile salts are crucial for solubilization and absorption of lipid-soluble nutrients. Bile salts are synthesized and secreted by the liver, conjugated to either taurine or glycine to improve solubility, stored and concentrated in the gallbladder, and delivered to the duodenal lumen in response to a meal. Between meals, the gallbladder stores and concentrates the bile salts extracted by the liver from the blood. Two major factors regulate the supply of bile salts following a meal. First, contraction of the gallbladder and relaxation of the sphincter of Oddi releases the gallbladder contents into the upper duodenum. This provides the first and immediate load of bile salts to enhance pancreatic lipase digestion and fatty acid/monoglyceride and cholesterol solubilization. Second, bile salts subsequently move down the small intestine to the ileum, where they are absorbed by a receptor-mediated mechanism and returned to the liver via the bloodstream. The enterohepatic circulation (reabsorption in the ileum, uptake by the liver, and secretion back into the intestine) preserves bile salts and diminishes the need for new synthesis in the 1 to 2 hours after a meal. The entire body pool of bile salts (approximately 3–4 g) is recirculated two to four times after each meal, providing 6 to 16 g of bile salts to the upper duodenum during the first hours after a meal. With a total luminal volume from diet and secretions of 2 to 3 L after each meal, this provides a large margin of safety for maintaining a luminal concentration above the critical micellar concentration of 2 to 4 mM needed for lipid solubilization and activation of pancreatic lipase.

Pancreas

Three phases of pancreatic secretion follow a meal: cephalic, gastric, and intestinal (Table 39.4). These phases have been described in an attempt to classify the multitude of events that occur postprandially. As seen in the other organs described above, pancreatic secretion is mediated by neural (vagal) efferent responses and by gut hormones. The cephalic phase of secretion is largely, if

Table 39.4
Phases of Pancreatic Secretion after a Meal

Phases	Pancreatic Response (%)	Stimulants	Mediators
Cephalic	25	Sight, smell, taste, eating	Vagal innervation
Gastric	10	Distention	Vagal-cholinergic pathways
Intestinal	50–75		Cholecystokinin, secretin
		Amino acids	Enteropancreatic reflexes
		Fatty acids Ca^{2+},H^+	Other hormones (?)
		Distention	

Adapted from Yamada T, Alpers DH, Owyang C, et al., eds. Textbook of gastroenterology. 2nd ed. Philadelphia: JB Lippincott, 1991;2–110:158–278.

not exclusively in humans, mediated by the vagus nerve. In this and the gastric phase, the pancreas secretes mostly water and bicarbonate. Pancreatic polypeptide (PP), located in specific PP cells in the pancreatic islets, acts as a negative feedback mechanism for the vagally stimulated portion of pancreatic secretion. PP is released in response to vagal efferent stimulation and inhibits the vagal efferent effect on the pancreas.

In the intestinal phase, pancreatic enzymes are added to the large volume of fluid secreted. As noted above, products of proteolysis and lipolysis stimulate the CCK (endocrine I) cell to release CCK, which acts humorally on the pancreatic acinar cells to produce enzymes. At the same time, H^+ ions stimulate the S cell to release secretin, which acts humorally on the pancreatic duct cells to secrete a bicarbonate-rich fluid, necessary to neutralize gastric acid and allow pancreatic enzymes to be effective. In addition, enteropancreatic reflexes within the ENS, sensitive to distention, osmolarity, and various nutrients, stimulate pancreatic enzyme secretion mediated by acetylcholine, GRP, and VIP. Most of the hydrolases secreted by the pancreas are proteases, secreted in an inactive precursor form to prevent digestion within the pancreas (Table 39.5). Trypsinogen accounts for 40% of the pancreatic protein secreted. In the intestinal lumen, trypsinogen is activated to trypsin by the enzyme enterokinase, produced by duodenal enterocytes. Trypsin in turn converts trypsinogen and all other proenzymes to their active forms, and the intraluminal phase of intestinal digestion is initiated.

Pancreatic insulin secretion in response to a meal is

Table 39.5
Intestinal Brush Border Membrane Hydrolase Activity in Normal Human Biopsy Specimens

Hydrolase	Approximate Activity (units/g protein)
Glucoamylase	250
Sucrase	100
α-Dextrinase	100
Lactase	45

enhanced by the release of GIP from the GIP cell, a mucosal endocrine cell. Although GIP was first recognized for its ability to inhibit gastric acid secretion, it was later found that the major function of this peptide is to mediate meal-stimulated insulin release from the pancreas. This observation led to changing the name of GIP from "gastric inhibitory polypeptide" to "glucose insulinotropic polypeptide." Intraluminal glucose stimulates GIP release, which acts humorally to augment the glucose-mediated release of insulin from β cells in pancreatic islets. This action of GIP helps maintain blood glucose levels within a reasonable range after a meal and provides another example of the redundancy characteristic of the regulation of gastrointestinal function following a meal.

NUTRIENT ABSORPTION

Fluid and Electrolytes

The GI tract absorbs large volumes of fluid each day. Approximately 9 L of water is delivered to the upper small intestine daily from dietary intake (2000 mL), saliva (1500 mL), gastric secretions (2500 mL), bile (500 mL), pancreatic secretions (1500 mL), and small intestinal secretions (1000 mL). Some 98% of the daily fluid load is absorbed, while only 100 to 200 mL/day is excreted in stool; approximately 85% (7.5 L) of water is absorbed in the jejunum and ileum, and 13% (1.4 L) in the colon.

Water is absorbed passively throughout the intestine and is regulated primarily by active electrolyte absorption. Specific features of epithelial cells throughout the intestine are important in regulating fluid and electrolyte absorption. First, the apical (luminal) membrane contains specific electrolyte transporters and channels. Second, the basolateral (serosal) membrane contains a sodium pump that provides the drive for electrolyte absorption. Third, intestinal epithelial cells are linked to each other by tight junctions located close to the apical surface. The "permeability" of intestinal epithelium depends on the number of tight junctions. The permeability of these intercellular junctions to solute, ion, and water movement decreases distally through the intestine. Therefore, the jejunum is more permeable or "leaky" than the ileum, which is more "leaky" than the cecum, which is more "leaky" than the rest of the colon.

Fluid and electrolytes are absorbed from the intestinal lumen directly through (transcellular pathway) or between (paracellular pathway) epithelial cells. Passive transport does not require energy and can occur transcellularly or paracellularly. The lipid content of the epithelial cell membrane prevents passive diffusion of charged electrolytes. Specialized proteins present in the apical membrane form channels or pores that permit electrolyte transport (see Chapter 38). Passive transport through membrane channels is regulated by concentration and electrochemical gradients across the membrane. Ion channels are usually specific for certain ions and can be opened or closed by cellular "messages." In the open state, more than a million ions can pass through per second, but no ions pass when the channel is closed. Passive transport can also occur via carriers, which are proteins, located in the cell membrane. Carriers are specific for certain solutes or ions and facilitate their passive movement along a concentration or electrochemical gradient across the cell membrane. Carrier-mediated transport is much slower than movement through channels.

Active transport requires energy and permits movement of a solute or ion against a concentration or electrochemical gradient. Active transport only occurs transcellularly and is mediated by a "pump" that moves ions in and out of the cell. The most important epithelial cell pump is the Na^+ pump (also known as Na^+-K^+ ATPase), which moves three Na^+ ions across the basolateral membrane in exchange for two K^+ ions (Fig. 39.10). Thus, the Na^+ pump lowers intracellular sodium concentration and makes the intracellular potential difference negative compared with the extracellular environment.

Secondary active transport is transport that combines both passive and active processes. For example, the negative intracellular voltage of epithelial cells enhances cation entry and anion exit from the cell. Thus, ions may move passively against their concentration gradients because of the electrical potential difference across the cell generated by the active sodium pump. The use of oral rehydration therapy in patients with severe diarrhea, such as those with cholera or short bowel syndrome, takes advantage of secondary active transport and the Na-glucose cotransporter in small intestinal epithelium (Fig. 39.10). This transporter, present in the apical membrane, binds both sodium and glucose. Glucose is transported across the cell membrane into the cell against its concentration gradient because of the low sodium concentration and the negative potential difference present in the cell. As glucose accumulates in the cell, it moves along its concentration gradient across the basolateral membrane via a specific transport carrier. Similar sodium-cotransport mechanisms also facilitate absorption of amino acids, vitamins, and bile salts. The Na^+ pump also drives passive absorptive or secretory transport of hydrogen, chloride, potassium, and bicarbonate (Fig. 39.10). Transport regulation can occur at the channel, carrier, or pump levels.

Water is absorbed passively throughout the GI tract and follows the absorption of electrolytes and other osmotically active nutrients. As noted above, water moves both transcellularly and paracellularly in response to increased osmolarity of the intracellular and subepithelial spaces. Sodium absorption is the most important factor in regulating water absorption. The Na-nutrient cotransporter and electroneutral NaCl exchange transporter are responsible for most water absorption. Furthermore, water absorbed between epithelial cells can increase absorption of solutes present in water, a process known as "solvent drag" (Fig. 39.11). Both sodium and water movement in response to an osmotic gradient is much greater in the

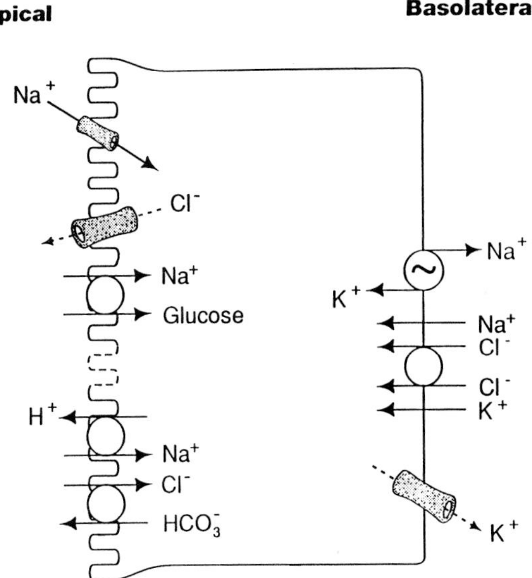

Figure 39.10. Electrolyte and solute absorption. Sodium can travel from the intestinal lumen into the epithelial cell by an ion channel *(apical side top)*, the Na^+-glucose cotransporter *(apical side middle)*, or a Na^+-H^+ exchanger *(apical side bottom)*. Release of H creates a favorable gradient for HCO_3 exit, which facilitates Cl entry via the Cl-HCO_3 exchanger. The Na-K-Cl cotransporter in the basolateral membrane also increases Cl uptake. Electrogenic Cl secretion occurs via a Cl channel on the apical membrane. Intracellular glucose accumulation favors glucose transport across the basolateral membrane via a specific carrier protein. The Na pump (Na-K-ATPase) provides the energy for these processes by generating low intracellular sodium concentrations and a transmembrane electrochemical gradient. (From Sleisenger MH, Fordtran JS, Scharschmidt BF, Feldman M, eds. Gastrointestinal disease. 5th ed. Philadelphia: WB Saunders, 1993;954–76.

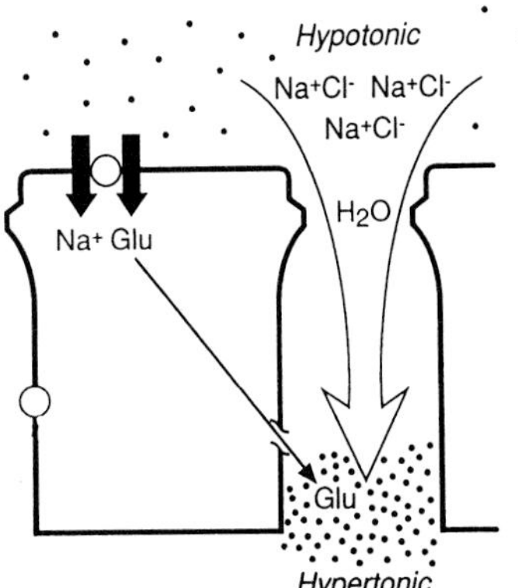

Figure 39.11. Electrolyte and water absorption in the jejunum. The Na-glucose cotransporter in the small intestinal binds both sodium and glucose and transports them across the epithelial cell membrane. As glucose accumulates in the cell, it moves along its concentration gradient across the basolateral membrane via a specific transport carrier. Water is absorbed passively by both transcellular and paracellular routes in response to increased osmolarity in the intracellular and subepithelial spaces. The Na-nutrient cotransporter shown in this figure and the electroneutral NaCl exchange transporter are responsible for most water absorption. Water absorbed between epithelial cells can increase the absorption of solutes present in water by "solvent drag."

jejunum than in the ileum because the junctions between epithelial cells are leakier in the jejunum than in the ileum. In the jejunum, sodium is primarily absorbed by uptake via the sodium-nutrient cotransporter and solvent drag. Therefore, ingestion of fluids or a meal with a low sodium content increases the osmolality in the upper small intestine and causes net secretion of water and sodium into the lumen. Patients with a jejunostomy and less than 100 cm of jejunum have difficulty maintaining fluid and electrolyte balance; thus, longer lengths of small intestine are often required for optimal fluid and electrolyte absorption. Balance studies performed after liquid ingestion by patients with a very short bowel ending in a jejunostomy demonstrate that drinking solutions with sodium concentrations below 90 mmol/L leads to net sodium and water losses, while drinking a solution with 90 mmol/L or more causes net sodium and fluid absorption. Although most water is absorbed in the small intestine, approximately 1 to 1.5 L enters the colon each day. Some 95% of the fluid that enters the colon is absorbed. Moreover, the colon can absorb up to approximately 5 L/day of fluid.

Lipid

Approximately 100 g of fat, equivalent to about 40% of total energy intake, is consumed daily in an adult Western diet. Most (95%) fat intake consists of long-chain triglycerides (LCTs); the remainder includes cell membrane phospholipids, cholesterol, other sterols, and fat-soluble vitamins. In addition, a large quantity of endogenous lipids (~60 g) is delivered into the intestinal lumen daily from bile (containing ~30 g bile salts, 10–15 g phospholipids, and 1–2 g cholesterol), desquamated intestinal cells (containing ~5 g membrane lipids), and dead bacteria (containing ~10 g membrane lipids). The upper limit of normal fecal fat output while consuming a 100-g fat diet is about 7 g/day. Therefore, at least 95% of fat delivered to the intestine is usually absorbed. Most dietary fat is absorbed before the fat contained in a meal reaches the ileum. However, even when no dietary fat is ingested, a small amount of fat can still be detected in stool because of the contribution from endogenous sources.

Assimilation of dietary fat provides a good general index of intestinal absorptive function because it involves most of the components involved in digestive and absorptive processes. Triglycerides are particularly difficult to digest and absorb because they are insoluble in water. Therefore, absorption requires *(a)* breakdown of ingested fat into an emulsion, which enhances contact between lipolytic enzymes and triglycerides; *(b)* enzymatic hydrolysis of triglycerides; *(c)* water-soluble micelle formation, which permits transport across the unstirred water layer to intestinal epithelial cells; *(d)* uptake of fatty acids by epithelial cells; *(e)* repackaging of fatty acids into water-soluble chylomicrons within the epithelial cell; and *(f)* secretion of chylomicrons into the systemic circulation by lymphatic vessels.

The stomach is important in initiating fat digestion. Approximately 20% of ingested triglycerides are hydrolyzed in the stomach by gastric lipase, which is produced by chief cells, functions in an acid environment, and is resistant to denaturation by pepsin. In addition, gastric muscle contractions, gastric acidity, and pepsin mash food particles and release dietary lipids from their protein interactions, generating an emulsion of small particles that is delivered into the duodenum.

In the duodenum, the emulsion particles are further stabilized by addition of bile salts and phospholipids secreted by the gallbladder. The presence of gastric acid in the duodenum stimulates secretin release from duodenal mucosa. Secretin enters the portal circulation and stimulates the pancreas to secrete bicarbonate, which raises the intraluminal pH above 6. The presence of fatty acids and amino acids in the duodenum stimulates CCK release from duodenal mucosa, which then enters the portal circulation and stimulates the pancreas to secrete lipase, colipase, and other digestive enzymes, and stimulates gallbladder contraction and bile flow into the duodenum. Lipase and colipase are secreted by the pancreas in a 1:1 molar ratio and act at the surface of the emulsion particles to hydrolyze triglycerides to monoglycerides and fatty acids. The near neutral pH of the duodenum maximizes lipase and colipase activity; pancreatic lipase is not functional in an acidic environment. Colipase is a critical cofactor for lipolysis, acting as a link between pancreatic lipase and triglycerides. In fact, pancreatic lipase cannot gain access to triglycerides within the emulsion without colipase because of interference from bile salts and phospholipids coating the emulsion particles. Although pancreatic lipase is responsible for most intestinal triglyceride lipolysis, the pancreas also secretes bile salt–activated lipase that hydrolyzes ester linkages in cholesterol, phospholipids, and fat-soluble vitamins. Fat digestion by gastric and pancreatic lipases is very effective, and most ingested triglycerides are hydrolyzed within the first 100 cm of jejunum.

Fatty acids, monoglycerides, and other lipids interact with bile salts to form water-soluble mixed micelles. Bile salts contain both water-soluble and lipid-soluble portions, allowing them to surround the digested lipid products—their hydrophobic side pointing toward the interior and the hydrophilic side toward the exterior. Thus, bile salts make fatty acids, monoglycerides, cholesterol, and other intraluminal lipids soluble in water by "hiding" them inside mixed micelles (Fig. 39.12). Although bile salts secreted in bile are diluted by luminal fluid, the intraduodenal concentration (10–20 mmol/L) is still well above the critical micellar concentration (2–3 mmol/L). The products of triglyceride digestion by pancreatic lipase can also coalesce to form vesicles. Lipid within vesicles is usually transferred to micelles but these vesicles can also transport lipid directly to the mucosa. Vesicle formation is believed to permit absorption of more than half of ingested triglycerides when bile salts are absent (e.g., in patients with severe cholestasis). However, vitamins D, E, and K are particularly insoluble and require micelle formation for adequate absorption.

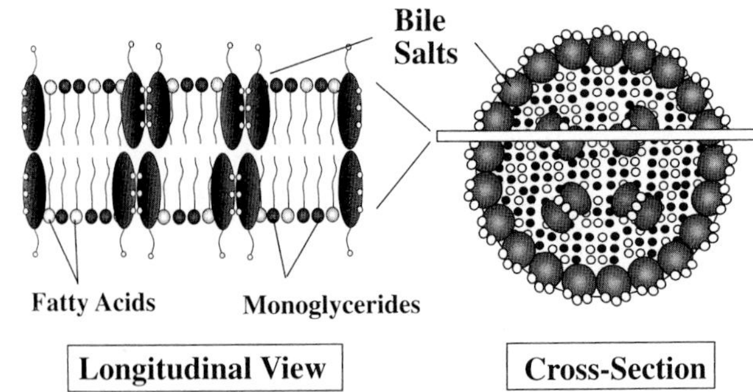

Figure 39.12. Structure of a mixed lipid–bile salt micelle. The products of lipolysis are solubilized in the interior of the particle. The bile salt molecules orient with their hydroxyl groups *(black circles)* facing the aqueous phase or, when they are in the interior of the micelle, facing each other. Fatty acids and monoglycerides orient in the micelle with their polar head groups in contact with the aqueous phase and their hydrocarbon tails in the interior of the micelle. (From Chang EB, Sitrin MD, Black DD, eds. Gastrointestinal, hepatobiliary, and nutritional physiology. Philadelphia: Lippincott-Raven, 1996;147, with permission.)

Mixed micelles must pass through a 40-μm deep unstirred water layer at the surface of intestinal epithelium to deliver their contents to the apical portion of the enterocytes. Quantitative diffusion of fatty acids through the unstirred water layer is enhanced more than 100-fold when fatty acids are carried within micelles rather than as monomeric fatty acids. Fatty acid and lipid uptake across the epithelial brush border membrane occurs by both passive diffusion, facilitated diffusion, and active transport. A membrane fatty acid–binding protein has been identified that may transport fatty acids, monoglycerides, and cholesterol across the enterocyte apical membrane.

After fatty acids and lipolytic products enter the intestinal epithelial cell, they are bound to cytosolic fatty acid–binding proteins. These binding proteins are found predominantly in villous cells in the jejunum; their expression declines progressively down the GI tract. Fatty acid–binding proteins are important for intracellular trafficking by directing fatty acids from the cell membrane to the smooth endoplasmic reticulum for triglyceride synthesis. Furthermore, this intracellular fatty acid–transport system enhances fatty acid uptake by maintaining a fatty acid concentration gradient and prevents potentially toxic interactions between fatty acids and intracellular organelles.

Fatty acids and monoglycerides present in smooth endoplasmic reticulum are used to produce triglycerides and phospholipids. Triglyceride, phospholipid, cholesterol, and fat-soluble vitamins are joined by apolipoproteins made in the rough endoplasmic reticulum to form chylomicrons, which consist of a core of triglyceride, cholesterol esters, fat-soluble vitamins and other lipids and a surface of phospholipids, free cholesterol, and apolipoproteins (apolipoproteins B-48, A-IV, and A-I) (Fig. 39.13). These nascent chylomicrons are transferred to the Golgi apparatus and incorporated into secretory vesicles that fuse with the basolateral membrane of the epithelial cell and are released by exocytosis into the extracellular space. These chylomicrons move through the lamina propria into the villous core, which contains a network of capillaries and a single lymph lacteal. Chylomicrons cannot enter the bloodstream directly because they are too large to pass through the fenestrations between capillary endothelial cells. Fat absorption stimulates lacteal distention, which produces gaps between endothelial cells and facilitates chylomicron uptake by the lymphatic system and ultimate delivery into the systemic circulation. Newly formed circulating chylomicrons interact with other circulating lipoproteins and exchange components, thereby acquiring additional apolipoproteins including apolipoproteins C-II and E, which have important functions in chylomicron metabolism.

Medium-chain triglycerides (MCTs) contain fatty acids with a chain length of 6 to 12 carbon atoms. A normal diet usually does not contain appreciable amounts of MCTs, but specialized diets for patients who have fat malabsorption or who require a low-LCT diet may include supplementation with MCT oil or MCT-enriched liquid formulas. Absorption of MCTs differs markedly from that of LCTs. MCTs are hydrolyzed more rapidly by lipases than are LCTs, do not require bile salts for absorption because they are water soluble, and can be absorbed as intact triglycerides. Once inside the intestinal epithelial cell, MCTs and medium-chain monoglycerides are rapidly hydrolyzed to medium-chain fatty acids (MCFAs) by specific cellular lipases. MCFAs do not bind to fatty acid–binding proteins, are not reesterified to triglycerides, and are not packaged in chylomicrons. After leaving the enterocyte, MCFAs enter the portal system where they are bound to albumin and transported to the liver.

Carbohydrate

A typical Western diet contains 200 to 300 g/day of carbohydrate (45% of total energy intake), which includes starch derived from cereals and plants (amylose, amylopectin), sugars derived from fruits and vegetables (glucose, fructose, sucrose), milk (lactose), and refined processed foods (sucrose, fructose, oligosaccharides, polysaccharides), and fiber derived from plant wall polysaccharides and lignin. Starch consists of long chains of glucose molecules joined together by α-1,4 linear linkages (amylose) or by both α-1,4 linear and α-1,6 branched linkages (amylopectin) (Fig. 39.14). Ingested sugars consist of monosaccharides (glucose, fructose) and disaccharides (sucrose, containing glucose linked with fructose; lactose, containing glucose linked with galactose). Approximately 10 to 20 g of dietary fiber is ingested daily in an average Western diet, consisting mostly of celluloses and hemicelluloses but also including pectin, gums, and lignin. Cellulose consists of glucose molecules joined together by β-1,4 linear linkages, whereas hemicellulose consists of pentose and hexose monomers joined together by both β-1,4 linear and branched linkages. Most dietary carbohydrates are completely digested and absorbed in the jejunum. However,

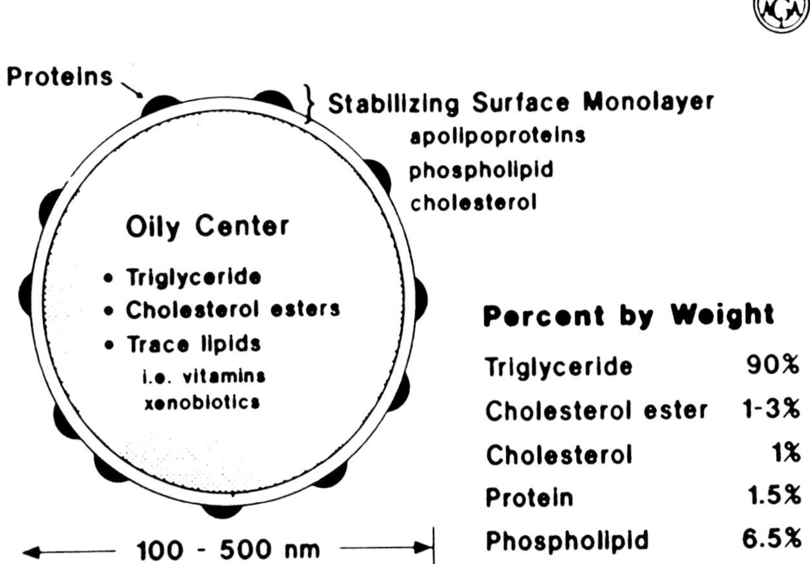

Figure 39.13. Chylomicrons are fat droplets that are coated with a monolayer of phospholipid and cholesterol. Dispersed in the monolayer are apoproteins (Apo)A-1, apoA-IV, and ApoB, and probably also some ApoC-11 and ApoC-111. These proteins help direct the tissue uptake and catabolism of the chylomicrons. In the circulation, chylomicrons acquire additional apoproteins. Although triglycerides are the major lipid carried in chylomicrons, they also carry cholesterol, fat-soluble vitamins, and small amounts of many other trace lipophilic molecules. (From Patton JS, Hoffman AF. Lipid digestion, undergraduate teaching project, unit 19. Bethesda, MD: American Gastroenterological Association, 1986, with permission.)

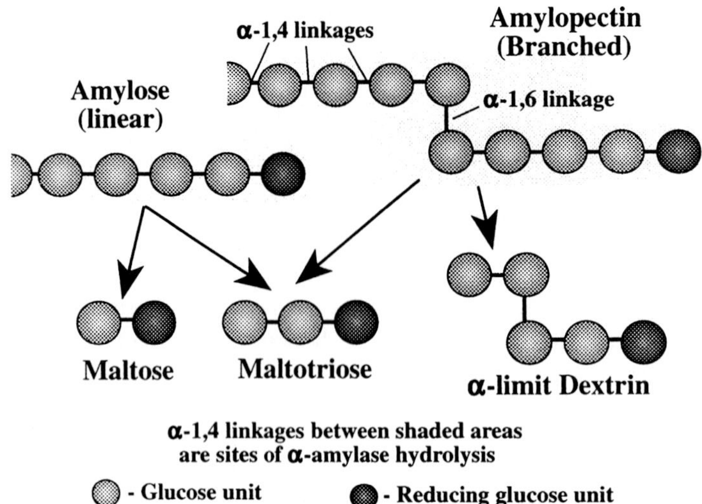

Figure 39.14. Starch (amylose and amylopectin) digestion by pancreatic amylase produces maltose, maltotriose, and α limit dextrins. (From Chang EB, Sitrin MD, Black DD, eds. Gastrointestinal, hepatobiliary, and nutritional physiology. Philadelphia: Lippincott-Raven, 1996;122, with permission.)

dietary fiber cannot be digested in the small intestine because the β-1,4 bond is resistant to amylase.

Amylases secreted by the salivary glands and pancreas cleave the α-1,4 bond but not the α-1,6 bonds of starch, generating linear oligosaccharides, branched α limit dextrins, maltotrioses, and maltoses (Fig. 39.14). Pancreatic amylase is responsible for most starch digestion. The contribution from salivary amylase is not clear and depends on the duration and amount of contact between salivary amylase and ingested starches. Presumably, slow and careful chewing increases starch digestion by salivary amylase. Furthermore, the physical interaction between salivary amylase and its substrate provides some protection from acid denaturation after ingested carbohydrates and amylase enter the stomach.

Brush border membrane hydrolases, glucoamylase (maltase), sucrase–α-dextrinase (sucrase-isomaltase), and lactose-phlorizin hydrolase (lactase), are required for complete hydrolysis of dietary disaccharides and the products of amylase starch digestion before they can be completely absorbed. Glucoamylase cleaves α-1,4 bonds, releasing one glucose molecule at a time from oligosaccharides containing up to nine residues. Sucrase–α-dextrinase represents two enzyme subunits with distinct properties. Sucrase hydrolyzes sucrose disaccharides to glucose and fructose and short-chain α-1,4 linked oligosaccharides to glucose. α-Dextrinase also hydrolyzes short-chain α-1,4 linked oligosaccharides to glucose and can also hydrolyze α-1,6 linked α limit dextrins. Lactase hydrolyzes lactose to glucose and galactose. Digestion of di-, tri-, and oligosaccharides at the surface brush border membrane usually exceeds the capacity of monosaccharide enterocyte transport. However, hydrolysis of lactose is the rate-limiting step for absorption because lactase activity is lower than that of all other brush border hydrolases, even in persons who have complete lactase activity (Table 39.5).

The brush border membrane hydrolases are glycoproteins produced by enterocytes. These hydrolases are secreted from the cell and inserted into the brush border membrane; the hydrophobic end attaches to the membrane while the oligosaccharidase component projects into the lumen. Brush border hydrolases are only expressed in villous enterocytes, predominantly in the duodenum and jejunum, with decreased expression distally. Enzyme expression and activity are regulated by transcriptional, translational, and posttranslational processes that are modified by dietary intake, pancreatic enzyme activity, trophic factors, and GI diseases.

Transport proteins known as "glucose transporters," present in the apical and basolateral cell membranes, facilitate monosaccharide absorption (Fig. 39.15). These transporters are expressed only in villous cells. Glucose and galactose absorption occurs principally by a Na-monosaccharide cotransporter, SGLT1, which delivers two Na molecules for every monosaccharide across the cell membrane. GLUT-5 facilitates Na-independent fructose absorption, but fructose is not as well absorbed as glucose. Glucose and fructose exit the enterocyte through the basolateral membrane into the portal circulation via the Na-independent GLUT-2 transporter.

Starches and dietary fiber not absorbed in the small intestine enter the colon, where colonic bacteria can metabolize these carbohydrates to short-chain fatty acids (SCFAs) (acetate, propionate, and butyrate), carbon dioxide, and hydrogen. Absorption of SCFAs allows the colon to salvage a considerable amount of energy that would otherwise be lost in stool; butyrate is a preferred large intestine fuel that provides about 70% of daily colonic fuel requirements, propionate may have important effects on hepatic metabolism, and acetate provides an important systemic fuel. Furthermore, SCFA absorption enhances colonic sodium and water absorption.

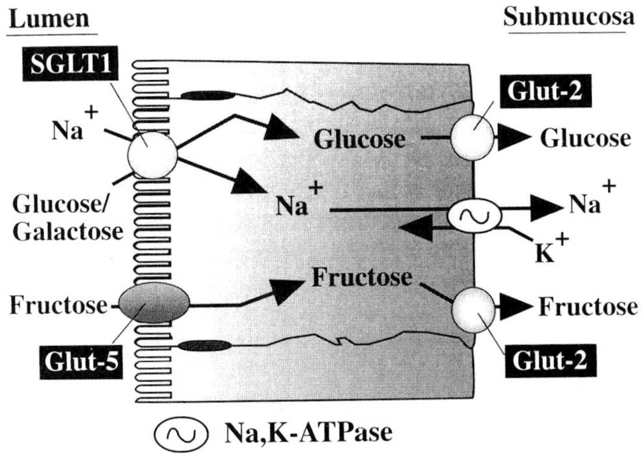

Figure 39.15. Monosaccharide absorption by the enterocyte occurs by active and passive processes. Glucose and galactose are absorbed by a Na-dependent glucose/galactose transporter ($SGLT_1$), driven by a Na^+ gradient generated by Na^+/K^+ ATPase at the basolateral membrane of the enterocyte. Fructose is absorbed by facilitated diffusion using a transporter called GLUT 5. All monosaccharides exit the enterocyte by facilitated diffusion via a carrier protein called GLUT 2. (From Chang EB, Sitrin MD, Black DD, eds. Gastrointestinal, hepatobiliary, and nutritional physiology. Philadelphia: Lippincott-Raven, 1996;125, with permission.)

Protein

Approximately 70 to 100 g of protein, representing about 15% of total energy intake, is ingested daily as part of a typical Western diet. Additional proteins are presented to the GI tract from salivary, gastric, biliary, pancreatic, and intestinal secretions (~35 g/day), desquamated intestinal cells (~30 g/day), and plasma protein (~2 g/day). Normally, more than 95% of the total protein load delivered to the gut is absorbed.

Protein digestion begins in the stomach, where a family of proteolytic enzymes (pepsins) hydrolyzes peptide bonds. Pepsins are generated from pepsinogens, which are inactive proenzymes produced mostly by chief cells. When exposed to the acidic environment of the stomach, pepsinogen undergoes a conformational change with loss of a terminal peptide to its active pepsin form. Pepsin is active at low pH and is inactivated in an alkaline environment. The stomach is not essential for protein digestion, and patients with atrophic gastritis and even a total gastrectomy can absorb protein normally. However, release of amino acids in the stomach triggers part of the initial GI response to a meal: gastric acid secretion, CCK secretion, gastrin secretion, and gastric emptying.

A significant amount of protein digestion occurs in the duodenum; 60% of protein is digested by the time it reaches the proximal jejunum. Several proteases (Table 39.6), in the form of inactive proenzymes, are secreted into the duodenal lumen by the pancreas. Enterokinase, a brush border enzyme that is released into the lumen by bile acids, cleaves the N-terminal peptide from trypsinogen to form trypsin. Trypsin activates additional trypsinogen molecules as well as the other pancreatic proenzymes.

Table 39.6
Pancreatic Proteases

Protease	Function
Endopeptidases	
Trypsin	Cleaves internal bonds at lysine or arginine residues and cleaves other pancreatic proenzymes
Chymotrypsin	Cleaves bonds at aromatic or neutral amino acid residues
Elastase	Cleaves bonds at aliphatic amino acid residues
Exopeptidases	
Carboxypeptidase A	Cleaves aromatic amino acids from carboxy-terminal end of protein and peptides
Carboxypeptidase B	Cleaves arginine or lysine from carboxy-terminal end of proteins and peptides

Pancreatic proteases act as either endopeptidases (trypsin, chymotrypsin, and elastase) or exopeptidases (carboxypeptidase A and B). Endopeptidases and exopeptidases work efficiently in concert to degrade protein into smaller subunits. However, proline-containing peptides are resistant to cleavage by pancreatic proteases. After pancreatic hydrolysis of proteins is complete, approximately 70% of amino nitrogen is present as oligopeptides containing 2 to 6 amino acids, and 30% is present as free amino acids.

The mucosal brush border membrane contains approximately 20 peptidases that cleave specific amino acids present in di-, tri, and oligopeptides, thereby generating free amino acids, dipeptides, and tripeptides. These peptidases are produced by enterocytes, released at the cell surface, and anchored to the cell membrane with the active site projecting into the lumen. Most brush border peptidases are aminopeptidases that sequentially cleave the N-terminal amino acid from oligopeptides. Several specific peptidases can hydrolyze proline-containing peptides, thus compensating for the inability of pancreatic proteases to cleave the proline–amino acid bond.

Amino acids, dipeptides, and tripeptides generated by intraluminal and brush border protein hydrolysis are transported across the enterocyte apical cell membrane by specific transport mechanisms. Amino acid transport is facilitated by several transport systems (Table 39.7). Some amino acids can use many different carriers because of

Table 39.7
Brush Border Membrane Amino Acid Transport Systems

Transport System	Amino Acids	Na-Dependent
Neutral amino acids		
NBB	Neutral amino acids	Yes
PHE	Phenylalanine, methionine	Yes
IMINO	Proline, hydroxyproline	Yes
β	β-Alanine	Yes
Acidic amino acids		
X^-_{GA}	Glutamate, aspartate	Yes
Basic		
Y^+	Basic amino acids	Yes
y^+	Basic amino acids	No

overlapping specificity between systems. Amino acid transport in most systems is coupled to sodium uptake (sodium dependent). However, amino acid uptake can also occur by sodium-independent processes by facilitated or passive diffusion. Di- and tripeptides are absorbed intact by intestinal epithelia by a sodium-independent process that involves hydrogen-peptide cotransport along a hydrogen gradient. Peptide transport is an important mechanism for amino acid absorption; in the jejunum, most amino acids are absorbed faster as peptides than as free amino acids.

Enterocyte absorption of digested dietary and intestinal proteins generates intracellular amino acids, dipeptides, and tripeptides. Peptides present in the enterocyte are hydrolyzed to individual amino acids by several cytosolic peptidases. In fact, dipeptidases and tripeptidases are much more abundant inside the cell than in the brush border membrane. Intracellular amino acids are transported out of the enterocyte through the basolateral membrane by active transport, facilitated diffusion, and simple diffusion. During meals, most amino acid transport out of the cell occurs by facilitated or simple diffusion because of the large amino acid concentration gradient across the cell membrane. Several amino acid transport systems have been identified. Passive diffusion and the L facilitated carrier system are principally involved in amino acid exit from the enterocyte, whereas the active Na^+-dependent A and ASC systems and the Na^+-independent asc and y^+ systems are principally involved in amino acid uptake.

Absorbed amino acids can have several fates: some provide fuel for the small intestine itself (particularly glutamate and glutamine), some are used for protein synthesis, and most are transported into the portal circulation for metabolism in the liver or for subsequent delivery to peripheral tissues via the bloodstream. Despite the presence of intracellular peptidases, approximately 10% of portal blood amino nitrogen is in the form of peptides that have escaped intracellular hydrolysis. After a meal, villous cells receive their amino acid requirements from absorption of luminal proteins. In contrast, crypt cells receive most of their amino acids from the bloodstream, as do villous cells during postabsorptive conditions.

Minerals

Mineral absorption involves three types of events: *(a)* intraluminal events that transform ingested minerals into absorbable forms, *(b)* mucosal events that govern mineral uptake by intestinal epithelium, and *(c)* postmucosal events that regulate mineral transport into the mesenteric and portal circulation for subsequent delivery to the liver and peripheral tissues. Although some general comments regarding intestinal mineral absorption are made in this section, specific absorptive processes for each mineral are reviewed in specific chapters in this book.

Minerals ingested in the diet are frequently bound to proteins within a matrix of organic molecules. Therefore, mechanical separation by mastication and dispersion and digestion by pancreatic enzymes are needed to convert ingested minerals into forms necessary for effective absorption. Unlike other nutrients, intestinal absorption of some minerals is regulated by body stores to prevent excessive uptake and toxicity. Furthermore, absorption of one mineral can decrease absorption of another. For example, there are absorptive interactions between calcium and magnesium and between iron, zinc, and copper. These interactions can be used therapeutically; oral zinc supplementation inhibits copper absorption in patients with Wilson's disease, who have excessive tissue copper loads.

Mineral absorption can be complicated because some minerals are released into the lumen as charged ions while others are part of an organic complex. For example, iron is ingested as a component of heme (animal sources) and nonheme (animal and plant sources) iron compounds (see Chapter 10). Dietary nonheme iron is usually present in the ferric (Fe^{3+}) form, which is soluble in the acid pH of the stomach but insoluble at a pH above 3. Other dietary compounds and intestinal secretions can either enhance iron absorption by making iron more soluble (by forming unstable chelates or reducing iron to the more soluble ferrous [Fe^{2+}] form) or decrease iron absorption by making iron less soluble (by precipitating iron or forming stable chelates). Heme iron is soluble at the alkaline pH of the small intestine and is more efficiently absorbed than nonheme iron. Iron is predominantly absorbed in the duodenum, while other minerals are predominantly absorbed throughout the small intestine. Absorption of macrominerals is discussed in Chapters 6 to 9 and that of trace minerals in Chapters 10 to 16.

Vitamins

Water-soluble vitamins (thiamin, riboflavin, niacin, pyridoxine, biotin, pantothenate, folate, cobalamin, and ascorbic acid) are usually present in foods as part of a coenzyme system and are often associated with proteins. This complex arrangement must be digested to a simpler form before the vitamins can be transported across the apical epithelial cell membrane. Vitamins are usually present in the diet in low concentrations and require active carrier systems for adequate absorption. However, water-soluble vitamins are also absorbed by passive diffusion. Therefore, oral vitamin supplementation with large doses can often overcome defects in normal vitamin transport by achieving high intraluminal concentrations. All water-soluble vitamins are absorbed primarily in the upper small intestine with the exception of vitamin B_{12}, which is absorbed principally in the terminal ileum. The specific mechanisms involved in absorption of each water-soluble vitamin are reviewed in Chapters 21 to 29.

Absorption of fat-soluble vitamins (vitamins A, D, E, and K) requires bile salts for solubilization within micelles, which enhances their delivery through the unstirred water layer to the enterocyte apical membrane. Thus, the absence of bile salts can seriously impair fat-soluble vitamin absorption, particularly that of the highly insoluble vitamins D and K. Vitamin K is unique in that body stores reflect absorption of both vitamin K_1 (phyloquinone) ingested in the diet and vitamin K_2 (menaquinone) produced by intestinal bacteria. Vitamin K of bacterial origin comes predominantly from vitamin K synthesized by small-intestinal bacteria or colonic bacteria, which refluxed into the small intestine because absorption by the colon is limited. Once inside the enterocyte, fat-soluble vitamins are incorporated within the core of chylomicrons for transport into intestinal lymphatics. Most ingested fat-soluble vitamins are absorbed in the proximal small intestine, although often less than 50% of total dietary intake is absorbed. The specific mechanisms involved in the absorption of each fat-soluble vitamin are reviewed in Chapters 17 to 20.

INTESTINAL MICROFLORA

The human gastrointestinal tract contains approximately 10^{14} bacteria representing more than 500 different species. The number of bacteria increases progressively down the gastrointestinal tract; the colon has more than 100 times more species and 100,000 times more organisms than any other intestinal area (Table 39.8). These organisms serve important metabolic and defense functions.

The mouth contains mostly anaerobic bacteria. However, the distribution of the oral flora is not uniform, and bacterial composition and density vary with location. The most densely populated areas are the gingival crevices. Poor oral hygiene and immunologic variations permit overgrowth of subgingival organisms, leading to gingivitis. Most bacteria that enter the stomach are killed by the acid environment. However, some species, such as *Lactobacillus, Streptococcus* viridans, *Staphylococcus, Peptostreptococcus,* and *Neisseria,* and the yeast *Candida* are found in the stomach because they are more acid-resistant than other organisms. *Helicobacter pylori,* an important cause of gastritis and ulcer disease, may be the only organism to truly colonize the stomach. The duodenum and proximal small bowel (jejunum) also contain few microorganisms, mostly aerobes and facultative anaerobes. In the ileum, bacterial numbers increase markedly and there is a shift from aerobic to anaerobic organisms. In the colon, the number of microorganisms increases a millionfold and the flora consists almost entirely of strict anaerobes such as *Bacteroides* spp., anaerobic lactobacilli, and clostridia. The ileocecal valve is a physical barrier between the small and large intestine. Resection of the ileocecal valve permits translocation of bacteria from the colon to the remaining ileum, where the bacterial population becomes similar to that of the colon.

The interaction between enteric microflora and the host is complex. The presence of enteric organisms enhances the defense against pathogenic bacteria by stimulating antibody production, increasing cell-mediated immunity, and preventing the overgrowth of more pathogenic organisms. Normal flora effectively compete for intraluminal fuels and adhere better to the intestinal wall, preventing pathogenic bacteria from establishing residence. The importance of this defense mechanism is illustrated by germ-free animals who cannot survive exposure to hostile microbes.

Intestinal bacteria also have important metabolic and nutritional functions, including hydrolysis of cholesterol esters, androgen, estrogen, and bile salts; utilization of carbohydrate, lipid, and protein; and consumption (vitamin B_{12} and folate) and production (biotin and vitamin K) of vitamins. All compounds that enter the alimentary tract by ingestion or intestinal secretion are potential substrates for bacterial metabolism (Table 39.9).

Table 39.8
Intestinal Microflora[a]

	Aerobes/Facultative Anaerobes	Anaerobes	Total Bacteria
Stomach	$0–10^3$	0	$0–10^3$
Jejunum	$0–10^4$	0	$0–10^4$
Ileum	$10^2–10^5$	$10^3–10^7$	$10^5–10^8$
Colon	$10^2–10^9$	$10^9–10^{12}$	$10^{10}–10^{12}$

Adapted from Toskes P, Donaldson RM. Enteric bacterial flora. In: Sleisenger MH, Fordtran JS, Scharschmidt BF, Feldman M, eds. Gastrointestinal disease. 5th ed. Philadelphia: WB Saunders, 1993;1106–18.

[a]Values are per milliliter or gram of contents.

Table 39.9
Biochemical Reactions by Intestinal Bacteria

Reaction	Representative Substrate
Hydrolysis	
Glucuronides	Estradiol-3-glucuronide
Glycosides	Cycasin
Sulfamates	Cyclamate, amygdalin
Amides	Methotrexate
Esters	Acetyldigoxin
Nitrates	Pentaerythritol trinitrate
Dehydroxylation	
C-hydroxy groups	Bile acids
N-hydroxyl groups	*N*-Hydroxyfluorenylacetamide
Decarboxylation	Amino acids
D-Demethylation	Biochanin A
Deamination	Amino acids
Dehydrogenase	Cholesterol, bile acids
Dehalogenation	DDT
Reduction	
Nitro groups	*p*-Nitrobenzoic acid
Double bonds	Unsaturated fatty acids
Azo groups	Food dyes
Aldehydes	Benzaldehydes
Alcohols	Benzyl alcohols
N-Oxides	4-Nitroquinoline-1-oxide
Nitrosamine formation	Dimethylnitrosamine
Aromatization	Quinic acid
Acetlylation	Histamine
Esterification	Galic acid

From Goldin BR, Lichtenstein AH, Gorbach SL. Nutritional and metabolic roles of intestinal flora. In: Shils ME, Olson JA, Shike M, eds. Modern nutrition in heatlth and disease. 8th ed. Philadelphia: Lea & Febiger, 1994;569–82.

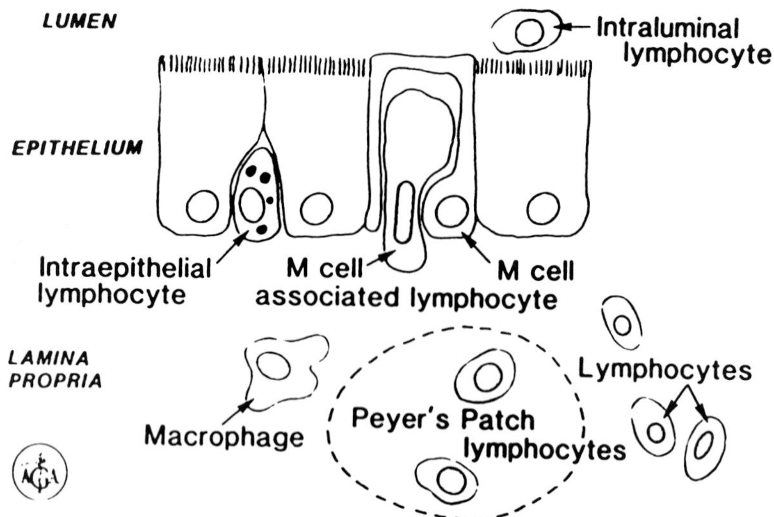

Figure 39.16. Gut-associated lymphoid tissue (GALT) including intraepithelial lymphocytes, M cells, and M cell–associated lymphocytes overlying the lymphoid follicles of a Peyer's patch. In addition, lymphocytes and macrophages are present within the lamina propria. (From Ernst PB, Befus AD, Bienenstock J Immunol Today 1985;6:50, with permission.)

IMMUNE SYSTEM

The alimentary tract houses a major portion of the body's immune system and is directed toward defending the host against bacterial, viral, parasitic, and food antigens that are constantly present in the intestinal lumen. The intestinal immune system consists of *(a)* T lymphocytes, *(b)* B lymphocytes, *(c)* natural killer cells, *(d)* myelomonocytic cells (monocytes, neutrophils, eosinophils, and basophils), *(e)* cytokines, *(f)* antibodies (IgG, IgM, and secretory IgA), and *(g)* gut-associated lymphoid tissue (GALT). (See also Chapter 45.)

Secretion of the dimeric immunoglobulin, IgA, is an important GI tract protective mechanism. Secretory IgA, the predominant intestinal immunoglobulin, is produced by B lymphocytes in the lamina propria. Secretory IgA binds dietary antigens, thereby preventing their absorption, and can bind to pathogenic microorganisms thereby preventing epithelial cell adherence and intestinal colonization.

GALT contains anatomically organized and nonorganized compartments within the submucosa, lamina propria, and epithelium to provide specialized host defense functions (Fig. 39.16). An important component of GALT is organized follicle-associated epithelium, which contains M cells that overlie Peyer's patches. M cells provide a selective site for sampling intraluminal antigens by permitting transport of large molecules and microorganisms. These antigens come into contact with lymphocytes and macrophages located within an indented space below the M cell before entering Peyer's patches. A Peyer's patch consists of a collection of lymphoid follicles that release lymphocytes after antigen processing (see Chapter 45). These lymphocytes migrate to mesenteric lymph nodes, the systemic circulation, and back to specific mucosal sites, where they provide protective immunity from the offending antigen. In addition, GALT contains a nonorganized distribution of intraepithelial T lymphocytes, lamina propria immune cells (T and B lymphocytes, plasma cells, and macrophages), and mucosal and submucosal mast cells.

REFERENCES

Gastrointestinal Tract Structure

1. Furness J, Costa M. Anatomy of the enteric nervous system. In: Johnson LR, ed. Physiology of the gastrointestinal tract. 2nd ed. New York: Raven Press, 1987.
2. Podalsky DK. Am J Physiol 1993;264:G179–86.
3. Neutra MR, Forstner JF. Gastrointestinal mucus: synthesis, secretion, and function. In: Johnson LR, ed. Physiology of the gastrointestinal tract, vol 1. 2nd ed. New York: Raven Press, 1987.
4. Gordon JI. Cell Biol 1989;108:1187.
5. Yamada T, Alpers DH, Owyang C, et al., eds. Textbook of gastroenterology. 2nd ed. Philadelphia: JB Lippincott, 1991; 141–57, 1303–17, 1555–76, 1735–47.
6. Greene HL, Moran JR. The gastrointestinal tract: regulatory nutrient absorption. In: Shils ME, Olson JA, Shike M, eds. Modern nutrition in health and disease. 8th ed. Philadelphia: Lea & Febiger, 1994;549–68.

Vasculature

7. Granger DN, Richardson PDI, Kvietys PR, Mortillaro NA. Gastroenterology 1980;78:837–63.
8. Chou CC. Fed Proc 1983;42:1658.

Enteric Nervous System and Motility

9. Johnson LR, Alpers DH, Jacobson ED, et al., eds. Physiology of the gastrointestinal tract, vol 1. 3rd ed. New York: Raven Press, 1994.
10. Yamada T, Alpers DH, Owyang C, et al., eds. Textbook of gastroenterology, 2nd ed. Philadelphia: JB Lippincott, 1991; 2–110, 158–278.

Gastrointestinal Hormones

11. Brand SJ, Schmidt WE. In: Yamada T, Alpers DH, Owyang C, et al., eds. Textbook of gastroenterology. 2nd ed. Philadelphia: JB Lippincott, 1991;25–71.

12. Walsh JH, Mayer EA. Gastrointestinal hormones. In: Sleisenger MH, Fordtran JS, Scharschmidt BF, Feldman M, eds. Gastrointestinal disease. 5th ed. Philadelphia: WB Saunders, 1993;18–44.

Integrated Response to a Meal

13. Pandol SJ, ed. Gastrointestinal system, section 6. In: West JB, ed. Physiological basis of medical practice. 12th ed. Baltimore: Williams & Wilkins, 1991;606–722.
14. Raybould H, Pandol SJ. Integrated response to a meal, undergraduate teaching project, unit 29. Bethesda, MD: American Gastroenterological Association, 1995.
15. Johnson LR, ed. Essentials of medical physiology, part V. Gastrointestinal physiology. New York: Raven Press, 1992; 449–530.
16. Sachs G, Prinz C. Gastric enterochromaffin-like cells and the regulation of acid secretion. News Physiol Sci 1996;11:57–62.

Nutrient Absorption

17. Anderson JM, Van Itallie CM. Am J Physiol Gastrointest Liver Physiol 1995;269:G467–76.
18. Horisberger J-D, Canessa C, Rossier BC. Cell Physiol Biochem 1993;3:283–94.
19. Semenza N, Kessler M, Schmidt U, et al. Ann NY Acad Sci 1985;456:83–96.
20. Ghisan FK. Pediatr Clin North Am 1988;35:35–51.
21. Spiller RC, Jones BJM, Silk DBA. Gut 1987;28:681–7.
22. Debognie JC, Phillips SF. Gastroenterology 1978;74:698–703.
23. Levitt M. Gastroenterology 1983;85:769–70.
24. Hopfer U. Membrane transport mechanisms for hexoses and amino acids in the small intestine. In: Johnson LR, ed. Physiology of the gastrointestinal tract. New York: Raven Press, 1987:1499–526.
25. Fine KD, Santa Ana CA, Porter JL, Fordtran JS. Gastroenterology 1993;105:1117–25.
26. Mueckler M, Caruso C, Baldwin SA, et al. Science 1985; 229:941.
27. Hunziker W, Spiess M, Semenza G, et al. Cell 1986;46:227–34.
28. Pappenheimer Jr, Reiss KZ. J Membr Biol 1987;100:123–36.
29. Ruppin H, Bar-Meir S, Soergel KH, et al. Gastroenterology 1980;78:1500–7.
30. Erickson RH, Kim YS. Annu Rev Med 1990;41:133–9.
31. Kim YS, Erickson RH. Gastroenterology 1985;88:1071–3.
32. Silk DBA, Grimble GK, Rees RG. Proc Nutr Soc 1985;44:63.
33. Tobey N, Heizer W, Yeh R, et al. Gastroenterology 1985;88:913.
34. Carey MC, Hernell O. Semin Gastrointest Dis 1992;3:189–208.
35. Lowe ME. Gastroenterology 1994;107:1524–36.
36. Staggers JE, Hernell O, Stafford RJ, et al. Biochemistry 1990;29:2028–40.
37. Hernell O, Staggers JE, Carey MC. Biochemistry 1990;29: 2041–56.
38. Chang EB, Sitrin MD, Black DD, eds. Gastrointestinal, hepatobiliary, and nutritional physiology. Philadelphia: Lippincott-Raven, 1996;91–210.
39. Sleisenger MH, Fordtran JS, Scharschmidt BF, Feldman M, eds. Gastrointestinal disease. 5th ed. Philadelphia: WB Saunders, 1993;954–76.
40. Patton JS, Hoffman AF. Lipid digestion, undergraduate teaching project, unit 19. Bethesda, MD: American Gastroenterological Association, 1986.

Intestinal Microflora

41. Goldin BR, Lichtenstein AH, Gorbach SL. Nutritional and metabolic roles of intestinal flora. In: Shils ME, Olson JA, Shike M, eds. Modern nutrition in health and disease. 8th ed. Philadelphia: Lea & Febiger, 1994;569–82.
42. Toskes P, Donaldson RM. Enteric bacterial flora. In: Sleisenger MH, Fordtran JS, Scharschmidt BF, Feldman M, eds. Gastrointestinal disease. 5th ed. Philadelphia: WB Saunders, 1993;1106–18.
43. Roediger WEW. Gut 1980;21:793–8.

Immune System

44. Brandtzaeg P, Sollid L, Thrane P, et al. Gut 1988;29:1116.
45. Underdown BJ, Schiff JM. Annu Rev Immunol 1986;4:389.
46. Perdue MH, Bienenstock J. Curr Opin Gastroenterol 1991;7:421.
47. Cooper M. N Engl J Med 1987;317:1452.
48. Wolf JL, Rubin DH, Finberg R, et al. Science 1981;212:471.
49. Ernst PB, Befus AD, Bienenstock J. Immunol Today 1985;6:50.
50. Banwell JG, Lake AM. Gut immunology and biology, undergraduate teaching project, unit 17. Bethesda, MD: American Gastroenterological Association, 1984.

40. Control of Food Intake

GERARD P. SMITH

Our understanding of the controls of food intake has been transformed during the past decade. The traditional view that intake was tightly controlled by hypothesized deficits of nutrient metabolism has been replaced by a neuroendocrine system that uses peptides, steroids, and amines to encode ingested food stimuli and metabolic state. This system depends on the brain to integrate the neural effects of these mediators to control intake and to coordinate it with the mechanisms of energy expenditure and storage to achieve energy balance. This transformation was driven by shifts in experimental strategies and new techniques.

There have been five shifts in experimental strategy. The first was to analyze neural control in terms of the integrated activity of forebrain (brain anterior to the brainstem, i.e., the cerebral cortex, basal ganglia, limbic system structures, and hypothalamus) and brainstem (brain between the hypothalamus and the spinal cord) networks rather than as reciprocal interactions of lateral and medial hypothalamic regions. This expanded neural system is capable of distributed processing (i.e., using neurons in different parts of the brain to transform and integrate incoming sensory information into appropriate motor commands), and thus can deal with the multiple stimuli that stimulate or inhibit a central pattern generator for control of the rhythmic movements of eating.

The second shift was to see the meal as the functional unit of eating and to concentrate on how the size of an individual meal is controlled. This revealed that meal size was determined by quantitative interaction between the positive- and negative-feedback effects of ingested food during a meal and led to identification of some of the underlying mechanisms.

The third shift in strategy was to search for controls of intake that transcend an individual meal and explicitly serve metabolic requirements. Investigating the endocrine controls of intake that operate after a prolonged period of food deprivation or during severe food restriction demonstrated that peripheral endocrine responses to deprivation-induced metabolic changes affect eating by changing the synthesis and release of brain peptides with reciprocal actions on food intake.

The fourth shift was to apply molecular genetics to the syndromes of genetic obesity in rodents. Besides yielding precise descriptions of genomic mutations and altered gene products, this strategy uncovered a peptide secreted from adipose tissue that decreases intake while activating neuroendocrine mechanisms for energy expenditure.

The fifth shift was to investigate the impact of learning on the controls of intake. This shift demonstrated that learned controls are potent and pervasive and account for the preferences and aversions observed in a variety of circumstances.

The shifts in experimental strategy exploited new techniques, including behavioral techniques such as computer-assisted lickometers, and videotape and electromyographic analysis (used to record the electrical activity associated with movements of muscles involved in eating and swallowing) that measure the rate and pattern of ingestive behaviors used during a meal; neurochemical, pharmacologic, and molecular techniques for measuring synthesis, storage, and release of steroids, peptides, and amines in the brain and periphery; molecular genetic techniques; and techniques for investigating learning and memory at the level of behavioral and synaptic plasticity (i.e., changes in behavior and the functional connections between neurons that result from prior experience).

This chapter considers these five areas of investigation in separate sections.

NEURAL CONTROL OF EATING

Eating refers to rhythmic oral movements elicited by food stimuli. The oral movements depend on the nature of the food stimuli: Solid food elicits mastication and liquid food elicits licking and lapping. Ingestion of either type of food is accomplished by lingual and palatal movements that move food to the oropharynx where the food stimulates the swallowing reflex. Thus, the control of food intake is fundamentally a problem in the sensory control of rhythmic movements. This is heuristic because it directs us to the extensive literature on the neural control of other rhythmic movements, such as locomotion.

The general plan of a neural system to control rhythmic movements consists of two categories of neurons. The first is a network (i.e., a group of neurons that interact to accomplish a function) that generates rhythmic motor output; such a network is termed a *central pattern generator*. The second category includes all of the afferent neural inputs that turn the central pattern generator on and off. In the case of locomotion, central pattern generators exist in the brainstem and the spinal cord. They are turned on and off by local afferent projections from segmental stimuli, as well as by long afferent projections from forebrain and brainstem sites that integrate information from visual, auditory, proprioceptive, tactile, and olfactory stimuli (1).

Recent work shows a similar arrangement of the components of the neural system that controls licking and mastication (2, 3). The central pattern generators are in the hindbrain, the part of the brainstem lying underneath the cerebellum. They are controlled by local afferent stimuli from the mouth, stomach, small intestine, and liver, and by forebrain stimuli carrying information about the current environment, metabolic state, and the effects of prior ingestive experience. Thus, the caudal brainstem's relation to the controls of eating is similar, if not functionally identical, to the spinal cord's relationship to limb movement and locomotion.

If the caudal brainstem is the spinal cord of eating, then disconnecting the caudal brainstem from the forebrain should reveal the potency of orosensory and postingestive afferent stimuli that project to the caudal brainstem below the level of the disconnection to control the central pattern generator in the absence of forebrain afferent stimuli. Grill and Kaplan (4) used this approach to investigate the control of liquid intake in the chronic decerebrate rat.

The chronic decerebrate rat is produced by cutting through the brainstem at the level of the superior colliculus just behind the hypothalamus. This lesion disconnects the forebrain from the brainstem because it completely severs the ascending and descending fiber connections between them (Fig. 40.1).

With appropriate care, such rats remain healthy for long periods of time. Most importantly for our purposes, this rat never initiates eating despite the presence of food in its environment. Thus, nutritional balance must be produced through periodic tube feedings. In contrast to this total lack of spontaneous eating, the decerebrate rat initiates eating and swallowing when milk or other liquid food stimuli are infused into its mouth through an implanted oral catheter. Ingestion continues until the decerebrate rat is satiated and allows the infused liquid to drip out of its mouth. Thus, the chronic decerebrate rat, like the neurologically intact rat, eats meals. Furthermore, the size of these meals varies with the food stimulus infused. For

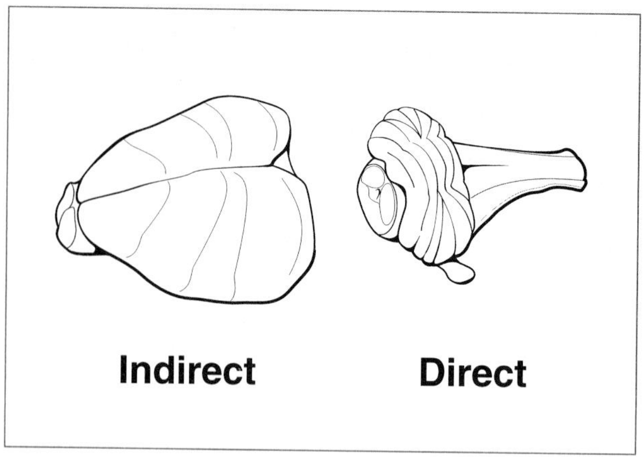

Figure 40.1. The space between the forebrain *(left)* and the hindbrain *(right)* emphasizes the disconnection produced by the chronic decerebrate lesion at the upper brainstem. Functional analysis of the controls of eating in such rats (4, 5) revealed that the direct controls of eating that are mediated by stimulation of orosensory and viscerosensory neurons by food are effective because these afferent neurons project to the hindbrain. The indirect controls that depend on distributed processing of diverse types of relevant information (see text) are not, however, because the efficacy of indirect controls depends upon connections between the forebrain and the hindbrain. When the connections are intact in the normal rat, eating is the integrated action of indirect and direct controls of the central pattern generator in the hindbrain that organizes the oral movements of eating.

example, the shape of the intake-response function to a series of concentrations of sucrose solutions is identical to that of intact rats. Furthermore, gastric preloads of nutrients given prior to an oral infusion of a liquid food reduces intake and decreases meal size. But even when liquid food is infused into the mouth, the chronic decerebrate rat does not change its meal size in response to the metabolic consequences of food deprivation (5), acute metabolic deficits produced by 2-deoxy-D-glucose or insulin hypoglycemia, or experimental toxic effects associated with prior ingestive experience (conditioned taste aversion).

These results demonstrate that the disconnected brainstem contains the central pattern generator for eating and that it has sufficient neural complexity to integrate orosensory and postingestive food stimuli into premotor commands that can turn the pattern generator on and off and produce a discrete bout of eating, i.e., a meal. Meal size is dynamic under these conditions. The size of the meal varies according to the type of food stimulus infused into the mouth and the amount of food loaded into the stomach.

The fact that metabolic state and the aversive consequences of prior ingestive experience have no effect on meal size suggests that normal control of meal size depends on the connections between the forebrain and brainstem that have been severed in these rats. Furthermore, because the central pattern generator is a "final common path" to the rhythmic movements of eating, controls that require the forebrain and controls for which the brainstem suffices must both affect this common path. This is the classic Sherringtonian analysis of movement and posture applied to eating.

A MEAL IS THE FUNCTIONAL UNIT OF EATING

A meal is the functional unit of eating because food intake over time is completely determined by the number and size of meals (6). A meal is a discrete bout of eating. Thus, it has three phases—initiation, maintenance, and termination. The functional analysis of a meal is concerned with the adequate stimuli and sufficient mechanisms for each of the three phases.

Initiation of Eating

Eating can be initiated by numerous external and internal stimuli. The external stimuli include visual, auditory, and olfactory stimuli related to food, diurnal cycle, temperature, temporal schedules of access to food, the relative density of predators and food in an environmental niche, social stimuli, and, in humans, culinary preferences, ethnic and religious rituals, and psychologic distress. Many of these external stimuli are conditioned by prior experience, and the ease of such conditioning has been clearly demonstrated in the rat (see "Learning and Eating," below) and experienced by us.

All internal stimuli for initiation of eating are related to metabolism. Food deprivation and acute decreases in the utilization of glucose and oxidation of fatty acids produced by specific metabolic inhibitors initiate eating. The effects of metabolic inhibitors have been viewed as emergency responses (7), and their relationship to the effects of food deprivation and nondeprived eating remains to be demonstrated.

Le Magnen, Campfield, and their colleagues discovered a new stimulus for initiation of eating in the rat (8, 9), namely, the pattern of plasma glucose changes that begin to occur about 10 minutes before a spontaneous meal. This pattern is characterized by a decline in plasma glucose concentration of approximately 12%, which is not sufficient to produce hypoglycemia. Eating is initiated when the glucose level is returning toward baseline after its nadir. The metabolic mechanism(s) responsible for this pattern is unknown and its presence in humans is controversial (10, 11).

Maintenance and Termination of Eating

Once initiated, the size of a meal is determined by the mechanisms that maintain and terminate eating. That these mechanisms are separate was demonstrated by using the sham-feeding rat (Fig. 40.2). In sham feeding, the ingested liquid food is withdrawn or drained continuously out of the stomach after eating is initiated (12–14). Sham feeding increases intake markedly. The increase is larger after longer deprivation or after repeated tests during which a conditioned inhibitory control extinguishes (see below). After overnight deprivation, sham feeding is almost continuous for hours, so that a meal never ends under these conditions (12). Thus, orosensory food stimuli in the absence of postingestive stimuli suffice to main-

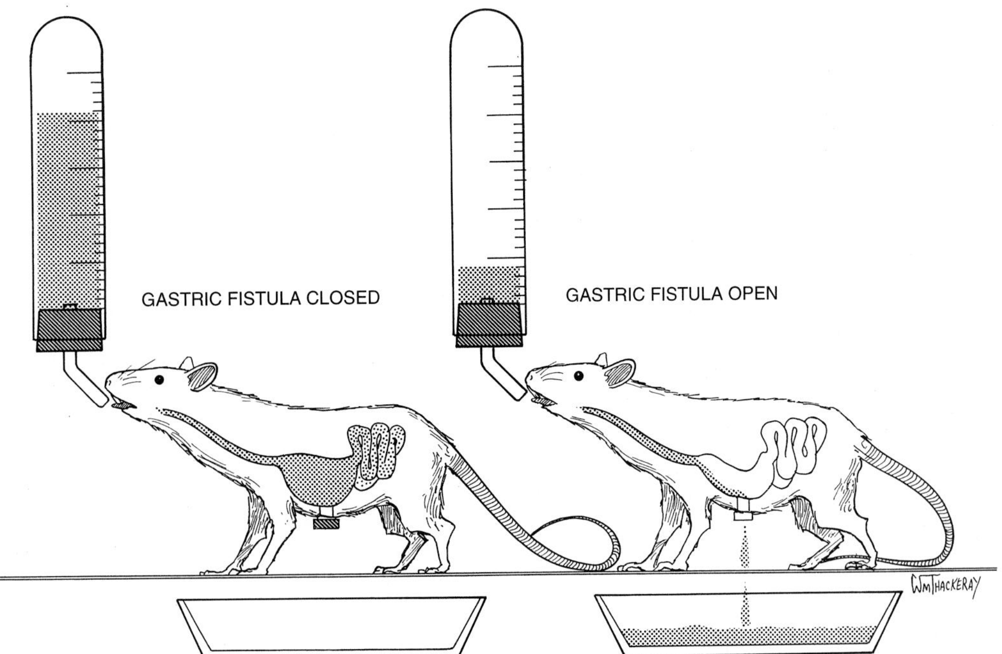

Figure 40.2. Chronic gastric fistula rat preparation for sham feeding. When the cannula is opened during a test *(right)*, ingested food drains out of the stomach so that the postingestive, negative-feedback effects of food are minimized or eliminated. Outside the test situation, the cannula is closed with a screw cap *(left)*, ingested food is digested and absorbed normally, and the rat maintains normal nutrition and body weight. (From Smith GP, Gibbs J, Young RC. Fed Proc 1974;33:1146–9, with permission.)

tain eating for much longer than the duration of the usual meal of the same diet under the same conditions.

This suggested that postingestive food stimuli are involved in terminating a meal rather than maintaining it, which was confirmed by a large number of experiments. Food stimuli in the stomach or small intestine terminate eating. Volume is the primary stimulus in the stomach (15), and chemical load is the primary stimulus in the small intestine (16). Although experiments showed that gastric or small intestinal stimuli acting alone suffice to terminate eating, they are synergistic when they are stimulated simultaneously by food stimuli during the normal meal (17).

Note that the small intestinal stimuli act prior to absorption into the portal blood, and most, if not all, probably act at the mucosal surface. Thus, a meal is terminated before significant amounts of nutrients are available for metabolism and storage. Thus termination of a meal is not primarily determined by *immediate* metabolic consequences, with the possible exception of rapid changes in the liver. In the rat (18), the metabolic consequences of one meal can affect the initiation of the next meal but not its size. This effect of metabolism on the timing of meals has not been observed in humans (19).

The demonstration that orosensory stimuli control the mechanisms that maintain eating, and postingestional, preabsorptive stimuli control the mechanisms that terminate eating facilitates investigation of these mechanisms. This has been exploited in the rat and to a less extent in the human.

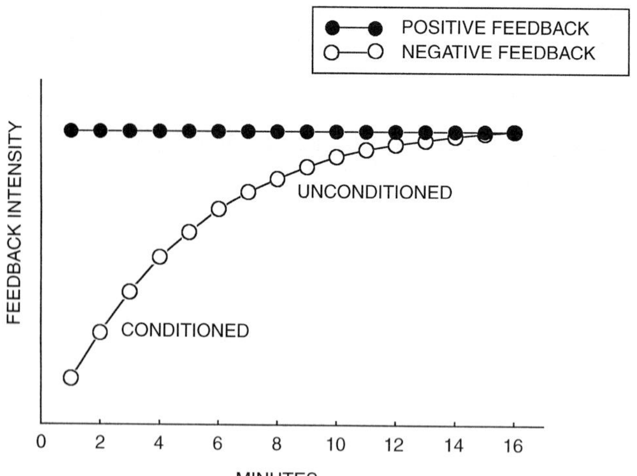

Figure 40.3. Temporal interaction of positive and negative feedback effects produced by ingested carbohydrate solutions during a scheduled meal. Eating stops and the meal ends when the potencies of the positive- and negative-feedbacks are judged to be equal by a comparator function(s) of the central networks for the control of eating. Note that the negative-feedback effect during the early part of the meal is a conditioned orosensory effect, and the unconditioned effect in the later part of the meal is an unconditioned postingestive effect (see text). The relative contributions of conditioned and unconditioned positive-feedback has not been analyzed yet. (From Smith GP, Davis JD, Greenberg D. The direct control of meal size in the Zucker rat. In: Bray GA, Ryan DH, eds. Molecular and genetic aspects of obesity. Pennington Biochemical Medical Center nutrition series, vol 5. Baton Rouge: Louisiana State University Press, 1996;161–74, with permission.)

Positive and Negative Feedbacks

Because orosensory and postingestive stimuli are the consequences of eating, they stimulate feedback mechanisms for the control of eating. The feedback effect of orosensory stimuli is positive; the feedback effect of gastric and small intestinal stimuli is negative (20). The duration and size of a meal is determined by the interaction of the positive and negative feedbacks activated by ingested food stimuli. Because the path of ingestion leads from the mouth through the stomach to the small intestine, positive feedback always occurs before negative feedback. Eating is maintained as long as the potency of positive feedback exceeds the potency of negative feedback as judged by a comparator function located somewhere in the brain (i.e., the function of a postulated neural network somewhere in the brain that compares the potency of positive- and negative-feedbacks). Eating ends when the potency of negative feedback equals or exceeds that of positive feedback (Fig. 40.3).

Microstructure of a Meal and Feedback Effects

Although the identification of orosensory positive feedback and postingestive negative feedback derived from sham feeding and other experimental preparations, the same feedback effects have been shown to operate when rats eat scheduled meals of carbohydrate solutions or oil emulsions (21, 22). Given access to a sucrose solution (0.8 M) after 4 hours of food deprivation, a rat begins to lick almost immediately (Fig. 40.3). The rate of licking is a monotonic function of sucrose concentration, and it is sustained for at least 1 minute. The number of licks during this interval is a measure of the orosensory stimulation by positive feedback of sucrose on the central network that controls licking.

The number of licks per minute then decreases at an approximately exponential rate over the next 15 minutes until licking stops. Because this exponential rate of decay of licking does not occur in a rat that has sham-feeding experience, it depends on postingestive negative feedback from gastric and small intestinal stimuli. Note that the exponential rate of decay is not a measure of the negative-feedback effect alone. Instead, it reflects the interaction of positive- and negative- feedback effects on the control of licking. As the meal proceeds, the potency of the negative feedback increases, and so licking slows and finally stops. The potency of negative feedback on licking increases because the amount of ingested sucrose in the stomach and small intestine is increased.

The early part of the curve of the potency of negative feedback in Figure 40.3 is labeled *conditioned* and the latter part is labeled *unconditioned.* Evidence for this distinction comes from experiments with the sham-feeding rat (21). The first time the postingestive effects of sucrose are prevented by having a rat sham feed 0.8 M sucrose, the number of licks increases significantly during the latter part of the meal, but the decay in the number of licks during the first 5 minutes does not change. In subsequent sham-feeding tests, the number of licks in the first 5 minutes gradually increases until there is little or no decrease in the rate of licking from the beginning to the end of the test. Thus, the decay of licking that occurs during the first 5 minutes of real feeding is due to a conditioned inhibitory control, because it does not change during the first sham-feeding test and it extinguishes gradually during subsequent sham-feeding tests. This conditioned negative feedback results from a learned association between the oral stimulus and its postingestive effects (23). This association can be formed within one or two meals, and two meals suffice to maintain it (21). In contrast, the decay of licking during the latter part of the meal appears to be unconditioned because the number of licks increases in the first sham-feeding test and does not increase further during subsequent sham-feeding tests (21).

The changes in the pattern of licking in meals of 0.8 M sucrose are assumed to be paradigmatic. Although similar changes were observed in a recent analysis of scheduled meals of corn oil (22), a different pattern has been observed in spontaneous meals or during meals in which rats must press a lever to obtain food (24, 25). No matter what pattern of licking occurs during a meal, however, that pattern and the size of the meal result from the interaction of the positive- and negative-feedback effects of the food that was eaten. We now consider the mechanisms of these feedback effects.

Mechanisms of Positive Feedback

Food in the mouth stimulates gustatory, thermal, tactile, and olfactory receptors (by the retronasal route). The receptors transduce these stimuli into afferent neural activity in cranial nerves 1, 5, 7, 9, and 10. With the exception of the olfactory projections to the anteroventral forebrain, all afferent neurons project directly to the caudal brainstem that contains the network for the control of licking. Second- and third-order neurons also carry this afferent information to the forebrain where it is processed and eventually influences forebrain neurons (especially in the amygdala, ventral striatum, and hypothalamus) that project back to the caudal brainstem (Fig. 40.4).

Substantial evidence indicates that dopaminergic and opioid neurons in the forebrain are important for normal processing of the orosensory feedback stimuli that maintain eating. For example, specific antagonists of dopamine and opioids decrease licking during sham feeding in a dose-related manner (26, 27). Furthermore, dopamine is released in the hypothalamus and nucleus accumbens during eating (26).

Microstructural analysis of the effect of a dopamine antagonist on sham feeding revealed that it decreases intake primarily by prolonging the intervals between bursts of licking. This suggests that central dopamine maintains eating by reinitiating licking during a meal (26). This hypothesis was confirmed by the observation that dopaminergic antagonists did not decrease intake when the need to reinitiate eating during a meal was abolished by continuously infusing sucrose into the mouth through a sublingual oral catheter (26). Because intact and decerebrate rats adjust their intake during sham feeding to the concentration of sucrose infused orally, neural mechanisms other than dopamine and opioids are clearly involved in the positive-feedback effect of orosensory stimuli that maintain eating. These mechanisms remain to be identified.

Mechanisms of Negative Feedback

Food stimuli in the stomach and small intestine activate mechanical and chemical receptors distributed along the mucosal membrane of these organs. Mechanical stimuli are most potent in the stomach, and chemical stimuli are most potent in the small intestine. Gastric mechanoreceptors receptors are well characterized and their activation of vagal afferent activity has been studied intensively (28, 29). However, the relationship of this mechanoreceptor-induced vagal afferent activity to the inhibitory effect of food stimuli in the stomach is not clear.

Splanchnic visceral afferent fibers are sensory fibers from the gut that have their cell bodies in the dorsal root ganglia, and project to neurons in the spinal cord that convey this sensory information to the caudal brainstem. These fibers are also activated by gastric mechanoreceptors (28), and they may carry important negative-feedback information from the stomach for the control of meal size. This function, however, has not been investigated.

Results with administration of the exogenous peptide gastrin-releasing peptide have repeatedly suggested a role for it and possibly the structurally related peptide neuromedin B in the genesis of nutrient-related, negative-feedback, afferent activity from the stomach (30). Attempts to demonstrate that the endogenous peptides produce this effect, however, have not been successful so far.

In contrast to the uncertain role of vagal afferent fibers in mediating the negative-feedback effect of gastric stimuli, extensive evidence supports the importance of vagal activity in the negative-feedback effect of digestive products of fats and carbohydrates in the small intestine. Vagal afferents are stimulated by nutrient stimuli directly (31, 32) and by cholecystokinin (29), pancreatic glucagon (33), and insulin (34) released by preabsorptive nutrient digestive products. Other peptides released by small intestinal nutrients, such as neurotensin (35), may also stimulate vagal afferents, but this remains to be demonstrated.

The negative-feedback effects of ingested food and cholecystokinin are mediated by the central serotonergic system, because pretreatment with serotonergic antagonists, particularly of the 5-HT_{2c} receptor subtype, de-

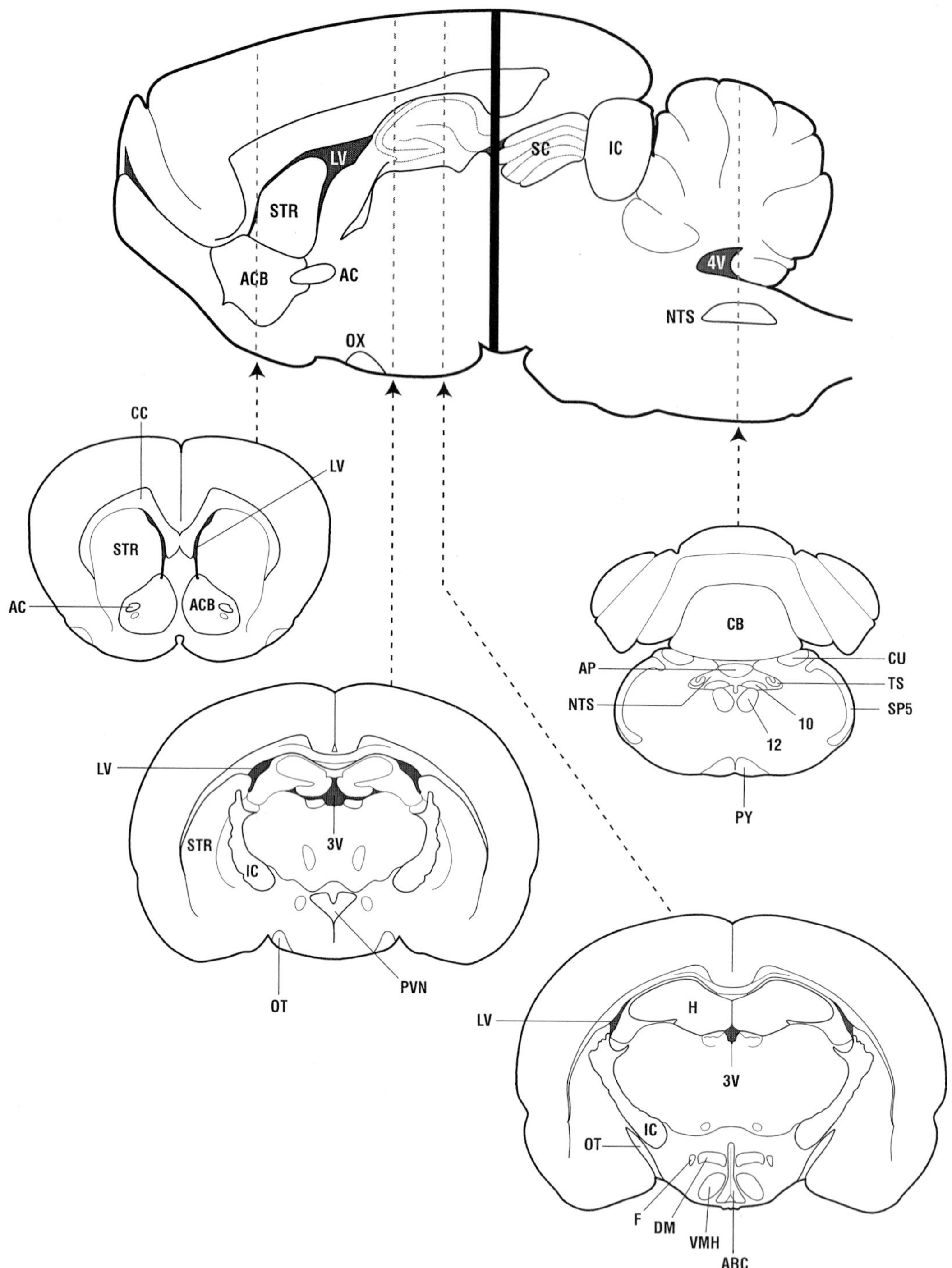

Figure 40.4. Schematic drawing of sagittal and coronal sections of the rat brain. The *black vertical line* marks the plane of the complete disconnection of the forebrain from the hindbrain that occurs in the chronic decerebrate rat. The *lines from the four coronal sections to the sagittal sections* indicate the site of each coronal section. *AC,* anterior commissure; *ACB,* nucleus accumbens; *AP,* area postrema; *ARC,* arcuate nucleus, *CB,* cerebellum; *CC,* corpus callosum; *CU,* cuneate nucleus; *DM,* dorsomedial hypothalamic nucleus; *F,* fornix; *H,* hippocampus; *IC,* inferior colliculus; *NTS,* nucleus of the solitary tract; *OT,* optic tract; *OX,* optic chiasm; *PVN,* paraventricular hypothalamic nucleus; *PY,* pyramidal tract; *SC,* superior colliculus; *SP5,* spinal tract of the trigeminal nerve; *STR,* striatum; *TS,* solitary tract; *VMH,* ventromedial hypothalamic nucleus; *LV,* lateral ventricle; *3V,* third ventricle; *4V,* fourth ventricle; *10,* dorsal motor nucleus of the vagus nerves; and *12,* hypoglossal nucleus. (Adapted from Paxinos G, Watson C. The rat brain in stereotaxic coordinates. New York: Academic Press, 1982.)

creases their inhibitory effects on intake (36). This may be the basis of the hyperphagia observed in mice with a genetic knockout lesion of the gene that encodes this receptor (37).

Direct and Indirect Controls

If meal size depended totally on the positive- and negative-feedback effects of the stimuli of ingested food, then the meal size for a specific food (e.g., 0.8 M sucrose) would be the same under all conditions. But meal size is dynamic; it varies over a relatively large range in response to changes in external conditions and metabolic states. The external conditions include the phase of the diurnal rhythm, environmental temperature, ecologic niche, and psychosocial stimuli that increase in complexity from animals to humans. The metabolic states include those produced by deprivation, overfeeding, obesity, growth, lactation, pregnancy, and ovarian steroid rhythms and the chronic effects of diets that differ in macronutrient composition.

Furthermore, animals and people readily associate metabolic states, environmental stimuli, and ingested food stimuli. Thus, external stimuli become conditioned stimuli (i.e., stimuli that control intake because of a prior association with eating or its consequences) for the effects of preabsorptive food stimuli and the pattern of stimuli produced by metabolic states. In this way, conditioned preferences and aversions are formed that influence the size of the meal (see "Learning and Eating").

Repeated attempts have been made to classify these various controls of meal size. Classification criteria have been derived from three perspectives: *(a)* presumed site of control (internal and external or central and peripheral); *(b)* presumed category of stimuli (physiologic and psychologic); and *(c)* the time over which a control was presumed to act (short term and long term). Although each of these perspectives provides a framework for discussion and investigation of some of the controls of meal size, none of them is comprehensive, and all of them are based on assumptions that are plausible but not proven.

Furthermore, none of these classifications provides a rationale for research on how to determine the relative potencies of the different controls in a specific situation. This is a crucial limitation, because the most urgent scientific need in this field is to understand how eating and metabolism are coordinated to determine body weight—the gap between the meal and the scale (6).

To attempt to close this gap, Smith (20) recently proposed a new classification, derived from an unambiguous criterion, which is comprehensive, provides a metric to measure the potency of different controls, and is heuristic for mechanistic research. The criterion of this new classification is direct contact of peripheral preabsorptive receptors by food stimuli. Controls that result from such contact are direct controls of meal size. Direct controls are stimulated by the chemical, colligative, and mechanical stimuli of ingested food as it passes from the mouth to the small intestine during a meal. The core of the direct controls consists of afferent neural activity from the gut to the brain and the central processing of this afferent input into efferent outputs for the control of licking, mastication, and other movements related to ingestion, as well as efferent outputs to the autonomic and endocrine controls of digestion and metabolism (Fig. 40.5).

All other controls of meal size are indirect controls, which differ from the direct controls in not having preabsorptive, peripheral receptors that are stimulated by ingested food during a meal. In addition to distinction by

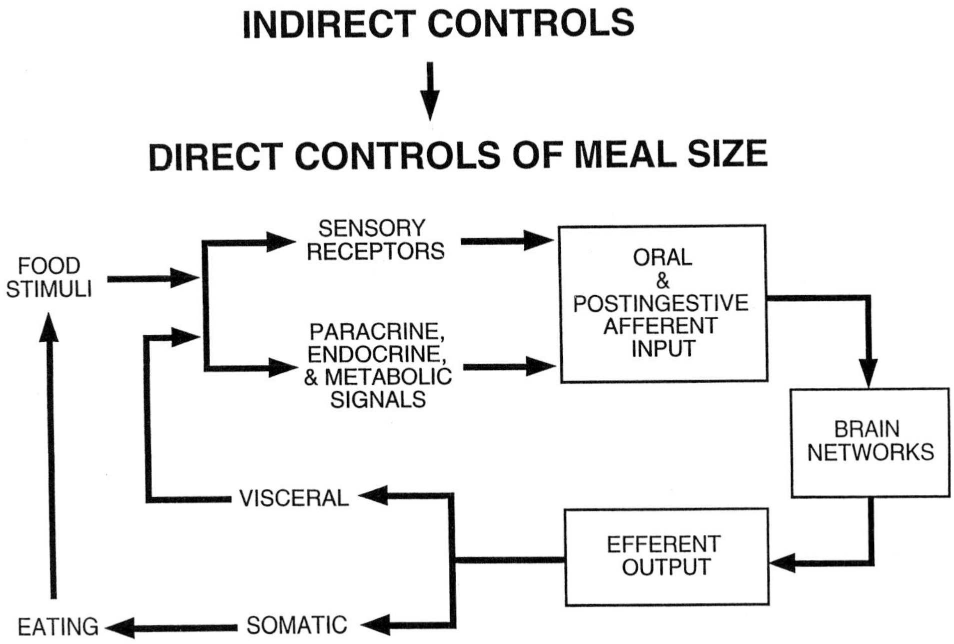

Figure 40.5. Flow diagram of the direct controls of meal size stimulated by ingested food acting on preabsorptive receptors of the gastrointestinal tract. Note that food stimuli activate afferent neurons directly and indirectly through effects on paracrine, endocrine, and metabolic signals and that the efferent output of the central networks for the control of eating is carried over visceral and somatic efferent fibers. Because some of the direct controls are stimulated by ingested food in every meal, indirect controls of meal size exert their effects by modulating direct controls. This is the reason for the unidirectional arrow between indirect and direct controls. (From Smith GP. Neurosci Biobehav Rev 1996;20:41–6, with permission.)

the physical criterion of receptor site, the duration of action of indirect controls is longer than a single meal, which makes the mechanisms of indirect controls the likely source of the information required to close the gap between the meal and the scale.

Three conclusions can be deduced from this classification. First, direct controls must operate every time eating occurs, but a specific indirect control may not. Second, because indirect controls are, by definition, not activated by the preabsorptive, peripheral stimulation of ingested food, indirect controls must exert their effect on meal size by modulating some elements of the direct controls. This is the basis for the unidirectional arrow between indirect controls and direct controls at the top of Figure 40.5. Indirect controls could modulate direct controls in a number of ways. The major modulation likely occurs in the brain networks that carry out the central processing of the afferent input of the direct controls and the comparator functions required to maintain the rate and duration of eating based on the relative potencies of the positive- and negative-feedback effects of ingested food (see above). It is also possible for indirect controls to modulate direct controls by changing the endocrine, metabolic, or paracrine responses to food stimuli; by changing the number or sensitivity of preabsorptive, afferent receptors; or by changing intracellular metabolism through effects on second messengers or genomic mechanisms. The site and kind of effect of a specific indirect control can only be determined by further investigation.

Measurement of the Potency of Direct and Indirect Controls

Because indirect controls of meal size produce their effects by modulating the direct controls of meal size, measurement of meal size does not provide quantitative information about the separate contributions of the direct or indirect controls that determined the size of the meal. This very significant problem is complicated further by the fact that an indirect control could modulate the positive- or negative-feedback effects of the direct controls. Increased meal size, for example, could be due to changes in potency of positive feedback, negative feedback, or both (Table 40.1).

The solution to this problem requires the following experimental sequence:

First, the change(s) in positive or negative feedback must be identified using measures listed in Table 40.2. The specific measures used depend on the experimental setting, but all of the measurement techniques have been reported in humans as well as animals.

After identifying the change(s) in feedback of the direct controls correlated with the abnormally large meal, curve-shift analysis is undertaken. This technique measures the potency of an indirect control by the amount that it shifts the potency of a direct control (Fig. 40.6) (see [20] for details). Examples of curve-shift analysis for the potency of indirect controls include *(a)* food deprivation for 17 hours shifted the eating-response functions for four carbohydrate solutions during sham feeding to the left by approximately one log in concentration (38) and *(b)* that the inhibitory potency of CCK was displaced to the left in the light compared with the dark in the rat (39), in a short photoperiod compared with a long one in hamsters (40), and by central administration of insulin in rats (41).

Curve-shift analysis not only measures the potency of indirect controls, it also provides a framework for evaluating putative mechanisms of indirect controls, such as insulin, the OB protein secreted by adipose tissue, neuropeptide Y, and corticotropin-releasing factor.

Table 40.1
Three Possible Combinations of Changes in Feedback Effects of Direct Controls Responsible for an Increase of Meal Size

Positive Feedback	Negative Feedback
Increase	No change
No change	Decrease
Increase	Decrease

Table 40.2
Measures of Positive and Negative Feedbacks

Positive Feedback	Negative Feedback
Sham feeding	Preload in stomach or small intestine
Initial rate of ingestion	Slope of the rate of decay of eating
"Sip and spit" psychophysics	

[a]Except for psychophysics involving linguistic reports of sensory and hedonic intensity, these measures can be made in animals and humans.

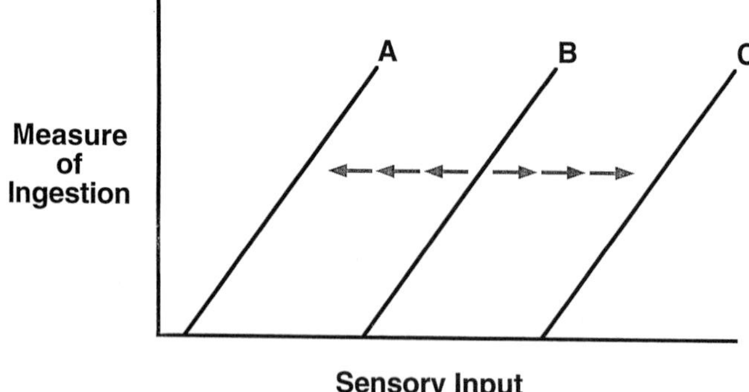

Figure 40.6. The method of curve-shift analysis used to measure the potency of a specific indirect control of meal size by measuring the displacement it causes of a direct control, preabsorptive sensory-eating response function *(B)*. If the indirect control increases the potency of the direct control, B will be displaced to the left *(A)*. If the indirect control decreases the potency of the direct control, B will be displaced to the right *(C)*. Note that the slope of function B is arbitrary and that indirect controls could also change it. Sensory input is inferred from the intensity of adequate stimulus. In most cases, this will be the load of the stimulus (concentration × volume) because afferent receptors in the gut are distributed over a relatively large area of the mucosal surface. (From Smith GP. Neurosci Biobehav Rev 1996;20:41–6, with permission.)

MECHANISMS OF INDIRECT CONTROLS

Insulin

Kennedy (42) first suggested that a humoral signal proportional to fat mass and acting in the brain in a negative-feedback manner was necessary for coordination of intake, energy storage, and body weight. A sustained search for this humoral signal revealed that pancreatic insulin and OB protein (leptin) have this function. Insulin is discussed here and the OB protein below in the context of genetic hyperphagia.

Insulin was suggested as a negative-feedback signal proportional to fat mass (43) because the resting concentration of plasma insulin is tightly correlated with the mass of fat tissue in humans. Proposed by Woods, Porte, and their colleagues in 1979, this hypothesis has been investigated in rats and to a lesser extent in baboons and dogs. The following statements summarize the major evidence for this hypothesis (43):

1. Insulin enters the brain from the plasma by a transmembrane uptake mechanism in the walls of cerebral capillaries.
2. Insulin administered into the third ventricle or into the medial hypothalamic tissue adjacent to that ventricle decreases intake (and body weight). This is the site of the negative-feedback effect.
3. The effect of insulin is in the brain because it is produced by doses of insulin that are too small to affect plasma glucose levels in the periphery.

Neuropeptide Y

Neuropeptide Y (NPY), a member of the pancreatic polypeptide family, contains 36 amino acids. Originally isolated from the porcine brain by Tatemoto (44), it has also been found in the brain of rats, humans, and other mammals (45). NPY is widely distributed in the brain and is colocalized in catecholaminergic cells in the hindbrain, some of which project to the paraventricular nucleus (PVN) (46). Although injection of NPY into a number of hypothalamic sites increases intake, the PVN (Fig. 40.4) has received the most experimental attention for two reasons: *(a)* the PVN appears to be a site of integration for peptide and monoamine controls of eating, and *(b)* neurons of the arcuate nucleus that synthesize NPY project to the PVN.

Injection of NPY into the PVN, lateral ventricle, or third ventricle increases food intake in a variety of situations (47). In fact, NPY is the most potent stimulant of food intake that has been discovered. Because rats do not show tolerance to its orexigenic effect, repetitive injections of NPY into the PVN produce sustained hyperphagia and obesity (48).

NPY has a major effect on initiation of eating and a variable effect on meal size. For example, Kalra et al. (49) noted that during a continuous infusion of NPY into the third ventricle, rats increased the number of meals, but meal size varied from small to large. The importance of the initiation of eating to the orexigenic effect of NPY was supported by the recent observation that bolus administration of NPY into the third ventricle increased intake when rats initiated eating by approaching liquid food and licking it, but NPY had no effect on intake when eating was passively initiated by infusing the same liquid food into the mouth through an intraoral catheter (50). Endogenous NPY is probably involved in the control of spontaneous eating, because NPY concentration and release in the PVN are correlated with eating (51, 52); injection of antibodies to NPY into the PVN decreased eating (53), and injection of antisense oligodeoxynucleotides into the arcuate nucleus to disrupt NPY synthesis also decreased eating (54).

Since NPY can increase intake, identification of the controls of its synthesis and release is crucial. There is evidence for a number of these controls, and most of them are inhibitory (55) (Table 40.3). Thus, disinhibition is the dominant process for stimulation of NPY (see below).

The orexigenic action of NPY is attenuated by an α_2-adrenergic antagonist (47), by haloperidol (a dopaminergic antagonist [56]), by fenfluramine (a 5-HT agonist and uptake blocker [57]), and by naloxone and naltrexone (58). The site of this opioid mediation is in the hindbrain, not in the hypothalamus, because injections of naltrexone in the nucleus tractus solitarius (NTS) in the hindbrain blocked the affect of NPY, while injection of naltrexone in the PVN was much less effective. This is a good example of how a stimulus in the forebrain depends on hindbrain mechanisms for its effect on eating.

Corticotropin-Releasing Factor

Just as NPY is a peptide in the hypothalamus that stimulates eating under a variety of conditions, corticotropin-releasing factor (CRF) is a neuropeptide that inhibits eating under a variety of conditions (59). First purified in 1981, CRF is a 41-amino acid peptide named for its action of stimulating corticotropic cells in the anterior lobe of the pituitary gland after being released from nerve terminals into the hypophyseal portal veins. The neurons that secrete CRF into the portal system are in the parvicellular part of the PVN. Neurons containing CRF in the PVN also project to other neural sites including the NTS, the site where visceral afferent stimuli also project.

Table 40.3
Reciprocal Effects of Stimuli That Control Food Intake on Hypothalamic NPY and CRF

Stimulus	Effect on Food Intake	NPY	CRF
Insulin	↓	Decrease	?[a]
OB protein	↓	Decrease	Increase
Estrogen	↓	Decrease	Increase
Serotonin	↓	Decrease	Increase
Glucocorticoids	↑	Increase	Decrease
Exercise	↓	Increase	Increase

[a]Effect of the stimulus is not clear or has not been reported.

Because of its critical role in stimulating release of adrenocorticotropic hormone (ACTH), which then stimulates release of adrenal glucocorticoids, the neuroendocrine signature of stress responses, the anorectic action of CRF was originally demonstrated in that context (60). The parallel effect of CRF to increase the activity of the sympathetic nervous system was consistent with that view. But subsequent work demonstrated that CRF mediated at least part of the inhibitory effect on eating of acute exercise, estrogen, serotonin, and the satiating action of peripherally administered bombesin (59). The peptide also appeared to mediate the inhibitory effect of adrenalectomy on intake in lean rats and genetically obese rats (61, 62). Most recently, increased CRF has been implicated in the anorexia that results from involuntary overfeeding (63). From these various results, CRF is now viewed as exerting an important inhibitory control on eating in a number of circumstances that are not simply a reaction to stress.

A major site for this inhibitory action is the PVN. Injections of CRF into the PVN decreased eating (64), and injections of α-helical CRF_{9-41}, an antagonist of CRF, blocked this effect. Although CRF neurons project from the PVN to the hindbrain, their role in the inhibition of eating is not clear. Oxytocinergic projections (i.e., efferent fibers of neurons that synthesize, store, and release oxytocin at their terminals) from the PVN to the hindbrain may be more important, because an oxytocin antagonist abolished the inhibitory effect of CRF on eating (65).

When the controls of NPY and CRF are compared (Table 40.3), most controls (exercise is an interesting exception) have reciprocal effects on NPY and CRF activity, measured primarily by in situ hybridization, less often by protein content, and occasionally by peptide release. CRF can block the effect of NPY on intake, NPY decreases CRF mRNA in the PVN, and CRF decreases NPY mRNA in the arcuate nucleus. Such reciprocal actions are consistent with major roles for NPY and CRF in the indirect control of eating. Because NPY and CRF also decrease and increase sympathetic nervous activity, respectively, their reciprocal interactions on intake and sympathetic activity are consistent with their coordinating the frequently observed inverse correlation between intake and sympathetic activity in lean and obese rodents (55, 59).

NPY, CRF, and the Eating Response to Food Deprivation

The importance of reciprocal changes in NPY and CRF has been tested in a situation of fundamental biologic interest—the increased eating that occurs after 24 to 48 hours of food deprivation. After deprivation, the eating response is robust and reproducible and, together with metabolic adjustments, restores body weight to normal with impressive precision. Such deprivation increases NPY mRNA in the arcuate nucleus and decreases CRF mRNA in the PVN (66). Food restriction, such as occurs in dieting, produces the same effect.

The changes in NPY and CRF are related to negative energy balance. Schwartz et al. (67) suggested that the low circulating insulin level (and resultant low level of central insulin) was the critical signal for the increase in NPY. Their idea predicted that the increased eating observed in insulin-deficient diabetes would be correlated with increased NPY levels, which proved to be the case (68). Furthermore, administration of insulin into the third ventricle in diabetic rats decreased NPY mRNA in the arcuate nucleus and decreased eating (69). Dallman has emphasized the importance of increased glucocorticoids in the eating response to deprivation (70). Glucocorticoids increase NPY and decrease CRF (71).

Further evidence for the reciprocal actions of NPY and CRF comes from involuntary overfeeding that produces increased body weight and decreased intake. The predicted effects occurred—NPY mRNA decreased and CRF mRNA increased (63). Although NPY appears to be important for the eating response to deprivation, it is not necessary, because mice with a knockout lesion of the NPY gene still show an eating response to deprivation (72). The non-NPY mechanisms and the changes of CRF that are involved in this mouse remain to be determined.

GENETICS OF HYPERPHAGIA

Increased eating is a characteristic phenotype of single gene mutations in rodents (73). These include four recessive mutations *(obese, diabetes, tubby,* and *fat)* and two dominant mutations (*yellow* and *Adipose*) in mice and the recessive Zucker *fatty* mutations in rats. Although there has been important progress in the molecular genetics of these mutations (Table 40.4), the functional analysis of how the gene products of these mutations result in increased eating is just beginning.

The functional analysis began with the discovery that a protein synthesized and secreted by white adipose tissue in lean mice was not present in obese mice *(ob/ob)* because of a nonsense mutation at codon 105 (74). Peripheral or central injection of recombinant OB protein (leptin) into *ob/ob* mice decreased food intake and body weight (75). Thus, the abnormal OB protein from *ob/ob* mice lacks the inhibitory effect of the normal molecule. This deficiency of normal OB protein accounts for the hyperphagia and obesity in *ob/ob* mice.

Table 40.4
Rodent Obesity Mutations[a]

Gene	Mutation	Gene Product	Rodent Chromosome
OB	*ob*	OB protein	Mouse 6
OB-R	*db/fa*	OB receptor	Mouse 4, rat 5
Cpe	*fat*	Carboxypeptidase E	Mouse 8
Tub	*tub*	TUB protein	Mouse 7
agouti	A^y	Agouti signaling protein	Mouse 2

[a]See (73) for details.

Normal OB protein administered to mice with the diabetes mutation *(db/db)* had no effect (74). This suggested that the hyperphagia and obesity in *db/db* mice was due to a defect in the receptor (OB-R) for OB protein, which is the case. The *db* mutation results in an alternatively spliced transcript of the long intracellular domain form of the OB-R (76, 77). These recent results confirm the hypothesis that *ob* encodes a ligand for *db,* proposed by Coleman in 1973 on the basis of parabiosis experiments (78).

Because genetic mapping studies indicated that *fa* and *db* are homologous loci in the rat and mouse genomes, respectively, the hyperphagia and obesity in *fa/fa* rats was also hypothesized to be a defect in the OB-R, which was confirmed (79). The missense mutation consisted of a nucleotide substitution at position 880 (A $\rightarrow$ C) that causes an amino acid substitution at position 269 (Glu-Pro). The mutant OB-R has greatly reduced binding of OB at the cell surface, which is correlated with a markedly reduced (80) or total lack of response (81) to OB in the *fa/fa* rat. The *fa/fa* rat also does not respond to central insulin (82). Thus, the hyperphagia of the *fa/fa* rat that is correlated with increased NPY (83) and can be reduced by increased CRF (84), is probably related to the lack of normal response to insulin and OB protein. The interaction between insulin and OB protein at the level of the hypothalamus will be interesting to define. In the periphery, insulin increases the synthesis of OB protein (85).

The inhibitory effect of OB protein on intake and body weight has now been extended to nondeprived and deprived rats (80, 81). The decreased intake after deprivation produced by OB protein is associated with decreased NPY mRNA and increased CRF mRNA (86). This is identical to the central effect of insulin and reinforces the importance of the reciprocal changes of these peptides for the eating response to food deprivation.

These new relationships between a gene product (OB) secreted in proportion to adipose mass in mice (87) and humans (88, 89), a hormone (insulin) sensitive to energy balance, adipose mass, and metabolic state, and two neuropeptides (NPY and CRF) with reciprocal actions on eating are a major advance that provides a heuristic framework for further analysis of these single-mutation syndromes of hyperphagia and obesity. This problem will be more complicated in humans, in whom the genetics of the hyperphagia involved in obesity is oligogenic or polygenic, except in such unusual cases as the Prader-Willi syndrome (90).

LEARNING AND EATING

Successful omnivores, such as rats and people, learn to identify foods from the various stimuli provided by their environment. Having succeeded in distinguishing nutrients from water and poisons, omnivores develop preferences and aversions to different foods.

With the exception of the unconditioned preference for sweet taste and the unconditioned aversion to bitter taste, all identification and selection is accomplished by forming associations between olfactory and orosensory stimuli and postingestive stimuli. The olfactory and orosensory (gustatory and texture) stimuli serve as conditioned stimuli (CS), and postingestive stimuli serve as unconditioned stimuli (UCS), that is, stimuli that control intake independent of a prior association with eating or its consequences. Because every meal provides olfactory, orosensory, and postingestive stimuli, there is ample opportunity for such learning to occur. In fact, learning is so pervasive in eating that specific protocols are required to distinguish learned and unconditioned controls, which has not been done much (see "Microstructure of a Meal and Feedback Effects," above, for the distinction between conditioned and unconditioned satiation). There have been three kinds of explanation for conditioned preferences and aversions—deficiency, reinforcement, and molecular.

Beginning with Curt Richter's insight that eating could serve nutrient homeostasis (91), preferences have been commonly ascribed to nutrient deficiencies. Salt appetite is an example of an appetite elicited by a specific deficiency, but salt appetite is innate, not learned (92). Experimental vitamin deficiency proved to be a better paradigm for investigating learning about eating in response to a deficiency (93). Certainly this learning can be demonstrated during acute deficiencies of carbohydrates and protein (94, 95); however, the sites and mechanisms of the recognition of these deficits and their repletions have never been identified.

Such deficiency-dependent appetites could occur in an environment that was nutritionally marginal but not in a nutritionally adequate environment. Preferences and aversions observed under that condition must arise by differential reinforcements of orosensory, olfactory, and postingestive stimuli. Two major kinds of mechanisms underlie conditioned preferences—flavor-flavor and flavor-postingestive (96). The flavor-postingestive mechanism is more potent and more interesting because it is clear that rats can distinguish among the postingestive stimuli of the type and quantity of nutrients. Some of this detection may occur preabsorptively in the stomach and small intestine, but most probably occurs in postabsorptive metabolic events. The site, mechanism, and detection of those events is under active investigation. Conditioned preferences endure for relatively long times without periodic reinforcement, while the effect of these associations on intake extinguish when the CS occurs in the absence of postingestive nutrient effects (96).

Conditioned aversions are also formed by associations between olfactory, orosensory, and postingestive stimuli, but the postingestive stimuli are aversive (nausea is commonly reported in humans). This appears to be involved in the anorexia observed in amino acid imbalances (97). This anorexia (smaller and less frequent meals) depends on a serotonergic mechanism, because 5-HT_3 antagonists abolish it. The same 5-HT_3 mechanism operates in the conditioned aversion observed in cancer patients undergoing chemotherapy (98).

Recent work has used the *c-fos* technique to map changes in the neural network that underlies the expression of a conditioned taste aversion. These changes center on the NTS in the hindbrain and in the amygdala in the forebrain (99). The NTS changes depend on the forebrain because they are abolished ipsilateral to hemidecerebration (surgical procedure) at the level of the superior colliculus (100). This is another example of an eating response being organized by forebrain and hindbrain interactions.

Finally, there have been repeated suggestions that preferences can be the direct effect of central neurotransmitters and neuromodulators, and there is some evidence for this form of molecular determinism. For example, NPY produces a preference for carbohydrates, galanin and opioids produce a preference for fats, and serotonin mediates the alternating preference for carbohydrates and protein (101). This evidence, however, is fragile, because small changes in experimental protocols produce different results (101, 102), which argues against any strong form of molecular determinism. The action of synaptic transmitters and modulators in food preferences is more reasonably understood as influencing a complex, central neural network that is processing food stimuli in a specific context of environment and experience.

CONCLUSIONS

Although the control of eating involves reflexes stimulated by ingested food, metabolic states, and a variety of environmental and neuroendocrine stimuli, this reflex control is augmented by rapid learning of associations between orosensory stimuli, viscerosensory stimuli, and metabolic effects.

All of the recent progress in understanding the controls of eating has come from investigation of rats and mice. This is encouraging because these omnivores have previously proven to be good models of human nutrition. The progress in rodents sets the problem for new human investigation. We must now move beyond measures of meal size to mechanisms of direct and indirect controls of eating. Because most measurements involve peripheral manipulations and sampling that are feasible in humans, we can expect to make real progress in our understanding of the controls of human eating and its contribution to normal nutrition.

ACKNOWLEDGMENTS

I thank Mr. Berkeley Cooley and Ms. Terri Popeil for expert processing of this manuscript. I am also grateful for the constructive criticism of Drs. J. Davis, N. Geary, R. Leibel, A. Sclafani, R. Seeley, K. Simansky, and S. Woods. This review was prepared while I was supported by a Research Scientist Award of the National Institutes of Mental Health (MH00149).

REFERENCES

1. Cohen AH. Evolution of the vertebrate central pattern generator for locomotion. In: Cohen AH, Rossignol S, Grillner S, eds. Neural control of rhythmic movements in vertebrates. New York: John Wiley & Sons, 1988;129–66.
2. Travers JB. Drinking: hindbrain sensorimotor neural organization. In: Ramsay DJ, Booth DA, eds. Thirst: physiological and psychological aspects. New York: Springer-Verlag, 1991;258–75.
3. Lund JP, Enomoto S. The generation of mastication by the mammalian central nervous system. In: Cohen AH, Rossignol S, Grillner S, eds. Neural control of rhythmic movements in vertebrates. New York: John Wiley & Sons, 1988;41–72.
4. Grill HJ, Kaplan JM. Caudal brainstem participates in the distributed neural control. In: Stricker EM, ed. Handbook of behavioral neurobiology, vol 10. Neurobiology of food and fluid intake. New York: Plenum Press, 1990;125–49.
5. Seeley RJ, Grill HJ, Kaplan JM. Behav Neurosci 1994;108:347–52.
6. Smith GP. The physiology of the meal. In: Silverstone T, ed. Drugs and appetite. New York: Academic Press, 1982;1–21.
7. Ritter S, Calingasan NY, Hutton B, et al. Cooperation of vagal and central neural systems in monitoring metabolic events controlling feeding behavior. In: Ritter S, Ritter RC, Barnes CD, eds. Neuroanatomy and physiology of abdominal vagal afferents. Boca Raton, FL: CRC Press, 1992;249–77.
8. Campfield LA, Smith FJ. Systemic factors in the control of food intake. In: Stricker EM, ed. Handbook of behavioral neurobiology, vol 10. Neurobiology of food and fluid intake. New York: Plenum Press, 1990;183–206.
9. Louis-Sylvestre J, Le Magnen J. Neurosci Biobehav Rev 1980;4:13–5.
10. Campfield LA, Smith FJ, Rosenbaum M, et al. Neurosci Biobehav Rev 1996;20:133–7.
11. Pollak CP, Green J, Smith GP. Physiol Behav 1989;46:529–34.
12. Young RC, Gibbs J, Antin J, et al. J Comp Physiol Psychol 1974;87:795–800.
13. Davis JD, Campbell CS. J Comp Physiol Psychol 1973;83:379–87.
14. Sclafani A, Nissenbaum JW. Am J Physiol 1985;248:R387–90.
15. Phillips RJ, Powley TL. Am J Physiol 1996;271:R766–79.
16. Liebling DS, Eisner JD, Gibbs J, et al. J Comp Physiol Psychol 1975;89:955–65.
17. McHugh PR, Moran TH. The stomach: a conception of its dynamic role in satiety. In: Sprague JM, Epstein AN, eds. Progress in psychobiology and physiological psychology, vol 11. New York: Academic Press, 1985;197–232.
18. LeMagnen J, Tallon S. J Physiol 1966;58:323–49.
19. Green J, Pollak CP, Smith GP. Physiol Behav 1987;41:141–7.
20. Smith GP. Neurosci Biobehav Rev 1996;20:41–6.
21. Davis JD, Smith GP. Am J Physiol 1990;259:R1228–35.
22. Davis JD, Kung TM, Rosenak R. Physiol Behav 1995;57: 1081–7.
23. Weingarten HP, Kulikovsky OT. Physiol Behav 1989;45:471–6.
24. Rushing PA, Houpt TA, Henderson R, et al. Physiol Behav 1997;62:1185–8.
25. Burton MJ, Cooper SJ, Popplewell DA. Br J Pharmacol 1981;72:621–33.
26. Smith GP. Dopamine and food reward. In: Fluharty S, Morrison AR, Sprague J, et al., eds. Progress in psychobiology and physiological psychology, vol 16. New York: Academic Press, 1995;83–144.
27. Kirkham TC, Cooper SJ. Physiol Behav 1988;44:491–4.
28. Grundy D, Scratcherd T. Sensory afferents from the gastroin-

testinal tract. In: Wood JD, ed. Handbook of physiology, section 6. The gastrointestinal system, vol 1. Motility and circulation, pt 1. New York: Oxford University Press, 1989;593–620.
29. Schwartz GJ, McHugh PR, Moran TH. Am J Physiol 1993;265:R872–6.
30. Gibbs J, Smith GP, Kirkham TC. Gastroenterology 1994;106: 1374–76.
31. Melone J. J Auton Nerv Syst 1986;17:331–41
32. Mei N. J Physiol 1978;282:485–506.
33. Geary N, Smith GP. Physiol Behav 1983;31:391–4.
34. VanderWeele DA. Physiol Behav 1993;54:477–85.
35. Rosell S, Rokaeus A. Acta Physiol Scand 1979;107:263–7.
36. Simansky KJ. Behav Brain Res 1996;73:37–42.
37. Tecott LH, Sun LM, Akana SF, et al. Nature 1995;374:542–8.
38. Joyner K, Smith GP, Shindledecker R, et al. Soc Neurosci Abstr 1985;11:1223
39. Kraly FS. Appetite 1981;2:177–92.
40. Bartness TJ, Morley JE, Levine AS. Peptides 1986;7:1079–85.
41. Riedy CA, Chavez M, Figlewicz DP, et al. Physiol Behav 1995;58:755–60.
42. Kennedy GC. Proc R Soc London (Biol) 1953;140:578–92.
43. Woods SC. Insulin and the brain: a mutual dependency. In: Fluharty S, Morrison AR, Sprague J, et al., eds. Progress in psychobiology and physiological psychology, vol 16. New York: Academic Press, 1995;53–81.
44. Tatemoto K. Proc Natl Acad Sci USA 1982;79:5485–9.
45. Tatemoto K. Neuropeptide Y: isolation, structure, and function. In: Mutt V, Füxe K, Hökfelt T, et al., eds. Neuropeptide Y. New York: Raven Press, 1989;23–32.
46. Everitt BJ, Hökfelt T. The coexistence of neuropeptide-Y with other peptides and amines in the central nervous system. In: Mutt V, Füxe K, Hökfelt T, et al., eds. Neuropeptide Y. New York: Raven Press, 1989;61–71.
47. Kalra SP, Kalra PS. Neuropeptide Y: a novel peptidergic signal for the control of feeding behavior. In: Ganten D, Pfaff D. Curr Top Neuroendocrinol 1990;10:191–220.
48. Stanley BG, Kyrkouli SE, Lampert S, et al. Peptides 1986;7:1189–92.
49. Kalra SP, Dube MG, Kalra PS. Peptides 1988;9:723–8.
50. Seeley RJ, Payne CJ, Woods SC. Am J Physiol 1995;272: R423–7.
51. Beck B, Jhanwar-Uniyal M, Burlet A, et al. Brain Res 1990;528:245–9.
52. Kalra SP, Dube MG, Sahu A, et al. Proc Natl Acad Sci USA 1991;88:10931–5.
53. Shibasaki T, Oda T, Imaki T, et al. Brain Res 1993;601:313–6.
54. Akabayashi A, Wahlestedt C, Alexander JT, et al. Mol Brain Res 1994;21:55–61.
55. Sahu A, Kalra SP. Trends Endocr Metab 1993;4:214–24.
56. Levine AS, Morley JE. Peptides 1984;5:1025–30.
57. Bendotti C, Garattini S, Samanin R. J Pharmacol 1987; 39:900–3.
58. Kotz CM, Grace MK, Briggs J, et al. J Clin Invest 1995;96: 163–70.
59. Richard D. New York Acad Sci 1993;697:155–72.
60. Morley JE, Levine AS. Life Sci 1982;31:1459–64.
61. Arase K, Shargill NS, Bray GA. Physiol Behav 1989;45:565–70.
62. Rohner-Jeanrenaud F, Walker CD, Greco-Perotto R, et al. Endocrinology 1989;124:733–9.
63. Seeley RJ, Matson CA, Chavez M, et al. Am J Physiol 1996;271:R819–23.
64. Krahn DD, Gosnell BA, Grace M, et al. Brain Res Bull 1986;17:285–9.
65. Olson BR, Drutarosky MD, Stricker EM, et al. Am J Physiol 1991;260:R448–52.
66. Brady LS, Smith MA, Gold PW, et al. Neuroendocrinology 1990;52:441–7.
67. Schwartz MW, Sipols AJ, Marks JL, et al. Endocrinology 1992;130:3608–16.
68. White JD. Regul Pept 1993;49:93–107.
69. Sipols AJ, Baskin DG., Schwartz MW. Diabetes 1994;44: 147–51.
70. Dallman MF, Strack AM, Akana SF, et al. Front Neuroendocrinol 1993;14:303–47.
71. Schwartz MW, Dallman MF, Woods SC. Am J Physiol 1995;269:R949–57.
72. Erickson JC, Clegg K, Palmiter R. Nature 1996;381:415–8.
73. Leibel RL, Chua SC Jr, Chung WK. Animal models of genetic obesity. In: Angel A, Anderson H, Bouchard C, et al., eds. Progress in obesity research: 7. London: John Libbey & Co. 1996;263–271.
74. Zhang Y, Porcina R, Maffei M, et al. Nature 1994;372:425–32.
75. Campfield LA, Smith FJ, Guisez Y, et al. Science 1995; 269:546–9.
76. Tartaglia LA, Dembski M, Weng X, et al. Cell 1995;83: 1263–71.
77. Chua SC, Chung WK, Wu-Peng S, et al. Science 1996;271: 994–6.
78. Coleman DL. Diabetologia 1973;9:294–8.
79. Chua S, White D, Wu-Peng X, et al. Diabetes 1996;45:1141–3.
80. Cusin I, Rohner-Jeanrenaud F, Stricker-Krongrad A. Diabetes 1996;45:1446–50.
81. Seeley RJ, van Dijk G, Campfield LA, et al. Horm Metab Res 1996;28:664–8.
82. Ikeda H, West DB, Pustek JJ, et al. Appetite 1986;7:381–6.
83. Beck B, Burlet A, Nicolas JP, et al. Physiol Behav 1990;47:449–53.
84. Bchini-Hooft OB, Rohner-Jeanrenaud F, Jeanrenaud B. J Neuroendocrinol 1993;5:381–6.
85. Trayhurn P, Rayner DV. Biochem Soc Trans 1996;24:565–70.
86. Schwartz MW, Seeley RJ, Campfield LA, et al. J Clin Invest 1996;98:1101–6.
87. Frederich R, Hamann A, Anderson S, et al. Nature Med 1995;1:1311–4.
88. Rosenbaum M, Nicolson M, Hirsch J, et al. J Clin Endocrinol Metab 1996;81:3424–7.
89. Maffer M, Halaas J, Ravussin E, et al. Nature Med 1995;1:1–7.
90. Reed P, Ding Y, Xu W, et al. Int J Obes 1995;19:599–603.
91. Richter CP. Harvey Lect 1943;38:63–103.
92. Epstein AN, Stellar E. J Comp Physiol Psychol 1955; 48:167–72.
93. Harris LJ, Clay J, Hargreaves F, et al. Proc R Soc Lond (Biol) 1933;113:161–90.
94. Mayer-Gross W, Walker J. Br J Exp Pathol 1946;27:297–305.
95. Baker BJ, Booth DA, Duggan JP, et al. Nutr Res 1987;7:481–7.
96. Sclafani A. Proc Nutr Soc 1995;54:419–27.
97. Gietzen DW. J Nutr 1993;123:610–25.
98. Costall B, Naylor RJ, Tyers MB. Rev Neurosci 1988;2:41–65.
99. Houpt TA, Philopena JM, Joh TH, et al. Learn Mem 1996;3:25–30.
100. Schafe GE, Seeley RJ, Bernstein IL. J Neurosci 1995; 15:6789–96.
101. York DA, Bray GA. Animal models of hyperphagia. In: Bouchard C, Bray GA, eds. Regulation of body weight: biological and behavioral mechanisms. Chichester: John Wiley & Sons, 1996;15–31.
102. Blundell JE. Food intake and body weight regulation. In: Bouchard C, Bray GA, eds. Regulation of body weight: biological and behavioral mechanisms. Chichester: John Wiley & Sons, 1996;111–33.

SELECTED READINGS

Booth DA, ed. Neurophysiology of ingestion. New York: Pergamon Press, 1993.

Bouchard C, Bray GA, eds. Regulation of body weight, biological and behavioral mechanisms. Chichester: John Wiley & Sons, 1996.

Leibel RL, Chua SC Jr, Chung WK. Animal models of genetic obesity. In: Angel A, Anderson H, Bouchard C, et al., eds. Progress in obesity research: 7. London: John Libbey & Co., 1996;263–71.

Schwartz MW, Dallman MF, Woods SC. The hypothalamic response to starvation: implications for the study of wasting disorders. Am J Physiol 1995;269:R949–57.

Smith GP. The direct and indirect controls of meal size. Neurosci Biobehav Rev 1996;20:41–6.

Travers JB. Drinking: hindbrain sensorimotor neural organization. In: Ramsay DJ, Booth DA, eds. Thirst: physiological and psychological aspects. New York: Springer-Verlag, 1991;258–75.

41. Metabolic Consequences of Starvation

L. JOHN HOFFER

Starvation is the physiologic condition that develops when macronutrient intake is inadequate. The manifestations of the disease that results from chronic starvation are due to protein and energy deficiency, hence the term *protein-energy malnutrition* (1). Since this chapter emphasizes both normal and pathologic responses to macronutrient deprivation, the broad concept of starvation is retained in the discussion that follows. Most human starvation results from deprivation of food, not selected nutrients, so the clinical disease that results from it is usually associated with micronutrient and macronutrient deficiencies (2–4).

The physiology of starvation is central to human nutrition and important for understanding many aspects of metabolism and medicine. Chapter 59 deals with the clinical presentation and treatment of protein-energy malnutrition. This chapter summarizes what is known about the metabolic consequences of protein and energy deficiency, as studied, for the most part, in human metabolic laboratories. The aim is to establish links between basic nutritional physiology and areas of applied clinical nutrition covered in other chapters in the text, including, among others, protein and energy metabolism, body composition, and nutritional assessment.

The chapter begins with an overview of water deprivation and describes metabolism during prolonged fasting and the effects of modifying a fast by selective carbohydrate or protein provision. There follows a description of the clinically more common forms of starvation in which protein or energy are consumed, but in deficient amounts. Finally, the metabolic effects of refeeding starving patients are discussed.

DEFINITIONS

Although detailed studies of human starvation physiology have been conducted for more than a century, there is little uniformity in the terminology used to describe it. In this chapter, *starvation* refers to prolonged inadequate intake of protein, energy, or both. A *fast* or a *total fast* is exclusion of all food energy. However, for other authors, starvation refers to complete deprivation of dietary energy (i.e., a fast), and *semistarvation* to the commoner condition of merely insufficient energy and protein provision. Yet other authors consider any diet restricted to only a few nutrients to be a fast, such as a "juice fast." The term *fast* is also commonly applied to the normal condition of any person after the overnight sleep (i.e., the period before "breakfast"). Terms such as *starvation, inanition, wasting,* and *cachexia* have, in the past, been used synonymously to describe the malnourished condition of famine victims, underfed prisoners, or patients with chronic disease and serious weight loss. However, in recent years some authors have used the term *cachexia* to refer specifically to the wasting that results from metabolic stress, also termed *cytokine-induced malnutrition* (5), and the term *starvation* to refer to wasting that results from simple food deprivation in the absence of stress.

The different forms of starvation have much in common, but they are not identical. Thus, metabolism during a fast longer than 2 to 3 days is dominated by the low-insulin state that develops once the liver's limited glycogen store is exhausted, a state characterized by lipolysis, ketone body production, and, at least in its initial phase, increased protein catabolism (6). Provision of as little as 150 g carbohydrate per day fully abolishes ketosis (7), so only rarely are patients with even advanced protein-energy malnutrition ketotic, nor do they manifest the hormonal and metabolic profile of prolonged fasting. Thus, when interpreting the results of biochemical studies of starvation, it is important to know whether the nutritional manipulations resulted in an extremely low insulin state (as in fasting or diabetes), protein deficiency in the presence of adequate carbohydrate energy, or gradations between these extremes.

WATER DEPRIVATION

Fluid deprivation occurs as extracellular volume deficiency, pure water deficiency (dehydration), or a combination of the two (see Chapter 6). Volume deficiency occurs when a combination of sodium and water loss depletes the extracellular fluid volume. The clinical presentation includes weight loss, poor skin turgor, dry mucous membranes, diminished sweat, and postural hypotension. The diagnosis is confirmed by the patient's response to appropriate treatment. Typical (but not invariable) biochemical findings are hyponatremia and an increased serum urea concentration, the latter due to reduced renal glomerular filtration and urea clearance. Thirst may be present or absent, and anorexia or even nausea are common (8).

Dehydration occurs when whole body water loss occurs with relative preservation of extracellular volume; its clinical hallmark is hypernatremia. The commonest cause of dehydration is failure to drink, and the earliest symptom is thirst (9). Symptoms of dehydration develop slowly when water is deprived, as long as urinary and insensible water losses are normal. In healthy persons denied food or water for 24 hours, plasma viscosity increases by about 15% (10), but serum sodium, albumin, and the hematocrit increase by only a few percent (9, 11). These small changes are predictable, since only about 4% of body water is normally lost in a day. With persistent water deprivation the serum sodium continues to rise, and the resulting hyperosmolality leads to confusion, weakness, lethargy, obtundation, coma, and ultimately death (12). The risk of dehydration is greater in elderly persons, who, for unknown reasons, have less appreciation of thirst during water deprivation than young adults (9).

It is common in hospice care not to supplement the voluntary fluid intake of dying patients (12, 13). As a result, dehydration commonly develops and is frequently the proximate cause of death. In one study, symptoms of thirst and hunger occurred in only a minority of such patients, and when it did occur, small amounts of food or fluid and moistening the mouth sufficed to alleviate it (13). Less commonly, dehydration may cause an agitated delirium that can be prevented or treated with rehydration (14).

From experiments in which a 40% depletion of body water caused death in animals, it has been estimated that a human adult could survive for 2 weeks if deprived of all water, while losing 1.3 L water daily from all sources (15). This calculation assumes that fat oxidation produces about 250 mL of water per day. It seems more likely that a 25% depletion would be fatal, since this would raise the serum sodium concentration from 140 to 180 mmol/L. If first-order kinetics are assumed and 4% of body water is lost per day, the predicted survival is 6 days. If 3% of body water is lost per day, survival is 8 days.

PROLONGED FASTING

Carbohydrate Metabolism

A lucid description of carbohydrate metabolism during prolonged fasting best proceeds from the last meal before the fast. Characteristic of the fed state are increased blood concentrations of glucose, fats, amino acids, and their metabolites. Insulin secretion is induced by the absorbed carbohydrates and amino acids, and it regulates their disposition within the tissues by stimulating glucose incorporation into glycogen in the liver, glucose transport and glycogen synthesis in muscle, triglyceride synthesis, and amino acid transport and synthesis into proteins in the insulin-sensitive peripheral tissues (mainly muscle). Glucagon levels are unchanged or decreased during meals containing carbohydrate, but a protein meal low in carbohydrate stimulates glucagon secretion (16). This directs the liver to continue glycogen breakdown and increase gluconeogenesis, thereby maintaining a normal blood glucose level despite the concurrent insulin-mediated glucose uptake by the peripheral tissues.

The fed state ends after the last nutrient has been absorbed and the transition to endogenous fuel consumption begins. The condition that exists after an overnight fast has been found convenient for study and is termed the *basal* or *postabsorptive* state. It is characterized by the release, interorgan transfer, and oxidation of endogenous fatty acids and the net release of glucose from liver glycogen and amino acids from muscle, all of these the results of relatively low levels of circulating insulin. Even with high carbohydrate diets, the body's predominant postabsorptive fuel is fat. As indicated by the characteristic nonprotein respiratory quotient (NPRQ) of 0.8, fat oxidation accounts for two-thirds of the body's postabsorptive resting energy expenditure (17).

Under postabsorptive conditions, glucose disappears into the tissues at a rate of 8 to 10 g/h; the free glucose pool of the body (about 16 g) must therefore be replaced every 2 hours (18). Glucose is normally the brain's only metabolic fuel; any reduction in the blood glucose concentration below a critical value promptly impairs consciousness and, if prolonged, results in neurologic damage. Given the brain's fixed and high metabolic requirement (more than half the total glucose production rate) there is no room for error in the delivery of adequate amounts of glucose from the liver into the circulation. The blood glucose concentration of healthy individuals is tightly regulated by the action of several physiologic control systems, chief of which are the insulin and glucagon systems.

As the blood glucose concentration is progressively lowered by tissue uptake, insulin levels fall in parallel, slowing further blood glucose lowering by reducing the rate of glucose transport into muscle and fat and by stimulating glycogenolysis and inhibiting glycogen synthesis in the liver. As a result, glycogen gradually releases its store of glucose into the circulation, while new glucose molecules synthesized from lactate, glycerol, and amino acids pass directly into the circulation instead of being sequestered in glycogen.

There is now good evidence that hepatic gluconeogenesis is continuous, even in the fed state. Starting very early in the postabsorptive period, approximately one-half of the glucose appearing in the circulation originates from gluconeogenesis, and one-half from glycogen breakdown (18–22). The precise amount of glucose each of these sources contributes to the circulating glucose pool in the early postprandial period must largely be determined by the carbohydrate and protein content of the preceding diet, for these would, respectively, determine the size of the liver's glycogen store and the amount of substrate presented to the liver for gluconeogenesis (23).

In a fast longer than 12 to 24 hours, the insulin concentration is further reduced, and this, together with an increasing glucagon concentration, results both in continuing gluconeogenesis and rapid mobilization of free fatty acids from adipose tissue triglyceride and of free amino acids from muscle (24), while the lowered insulin: glucagon ratio activates the liver for fatty acid oxidation. Once the liver is activated in this way, its rate of fatty acid oxidation is determined by the rate at which fatty acids are delivered to it (25). Thus, along with diminished conversion of glucose and glucose precursors to acetyl coenzyme A, the entry substrate for the Krebs cycle, acetyl coenzyme A production due to fatty acid oxidation increases. Some of the acetyl coenzyme A produced from fatty acid oxidation is terminally oxidized through the intrahepatic Krebs cycle, thus serving as the predominant energy source for the liver (26), but most of it is oxidized only as far as the 4-carbon molecule acetoacetic acid, which in turn is reversibly converted to its oxidoreduction partner, β-hydroxybutyric acid, and, to a lesser extent, irreversibly decarboxylated to form acetone.

A fast longer than 2 to 3 days exhausts the liver's glycogen reserve (20, 27) and about half the glycogen in muscle (27, 28). All glucose oxidized thereafter must be synthesized from endogenous glycerol, the glucogenic amino acids, and lactate and pyruvate produced by glycolysis of preexisting glucose via the Cori cycle. Consequently, the NPRQ falls to 0.7. An NPRQ of 0.7 and appearance in the circulation of large amounts of acetoacetate, β-hydroxybutyrate, and acetone, collectively known as the "ketone bodies," are the hallmarks of the low insulin:glucagon ratio and rapid hepatic fatty acid oxidation that characterize a prolonged fast.

During the period of glycogen depletion, gluconeogenesis from glucogenic amino acids (chiefly alanine and glutamine) accounts for a progressively larger fraction of total glucose output during the first 2 days of fasting (20, 22). The absolute rate of gluconeogenesis does not appear to increase during this period; rather, total glucose release into the circulation decreases by 40 to 50% within the first few days of fasting (20, 29–31).

The shortfall in glucose production during this period is matched by a corresponding reduction in glucose use. Only a part of this is due to a reduction in terminal glucose oxidation in muscle and fat or by reduced Cori cycle activity. Indeed, the Cori cycle seems not to change significantly even after a fast of several weeks (32). The reduction of plasma glucose disappearance that occurs both in the earliest phase and later, during prolonged fasting, can only be explained by a reduction in brain glucose metabolism, made possible by the concurrent availability of ketone bodies as an alternative fuel. This was recently confirmed in a study of short-term fasted humans that used a combination of positron emission tomography (to measure glucose metabolism) and arterial–internal jugular vein sampling (to measure β-hydroxybutyrate consumption). After a 3.5-day fast, brain glucose consumption was reduced by 25% (approximately 100 kcal/day), whereas ketone body consumption increased from approximately 16 to 160 kcal/day (33).

Ketosis

Even in the fed state, small amounts of acetoacetic acid are produced and oxidized in the liver (34), and under basal conditions, acetoacetic acid oxidation furnishes about 2 to 3% of the body's total energy requirement (26). Circulating ketone body concentrations are almost unmeasurably low under normal conditions (0.1 mmol/L or less), and ketone body export from the liver is negligible (35). Starvation ketosis is arbitrarily defined as being present when the blood acetoacetate concentration has risen to 1.0 mmol/L and β-hydroxybutyrate to 2 to 3 mmol/L, as typically occurs by day 2 or 3 of fasting (26). After an overnight fast, the urine of an adult is normally free of ketone bodies, but their appearance in the overnight urine of thin persons, especially women, is not uncommon and indicates their relatively low basal insulin state (36).

After release into the blood, acetoacetic acid and β-hydroxybutyric acid dissociate to become water-soluble anions. Acetone is a volatile molecule soluble both in water and lipids. After 3 or 4 days of fasting it appears in small amounts in the breath, imparting a characteristic sweet odor.

The circulating concentration of free fatty acids (and consequently their rate of delivery to the liver) is a major determinant of the ketogenic rate and the level of ketonemia. Another factor is the maximum rate of hepatic fatty acid β-oxidation, which cannot exceed the upper limit set by the liver's rate of energy use. All tissues with mitochondria oxidize ketone bodies, and ketone body oxidation provides 30 to 40% of the body's total energy use in the first 4 to 7 days of fasting. After about 2 weeks, however, muscle ketone body oxidation decreases, and this tissue returns to oxidizing fatty acids as its main resting fuel (18). Ketogenesis is maximal by about 3 days of fasting, but since its uptake into muscle is reduced after 2 weeks and renal tubular reabsorption increases, blood ketone body levels continue to rise steadily and, after about 3 weeks, reach a steady state double that found after 3 to 5 days of fasting. The brain's rate of ketone body use is determined by the blood ketone body concentration, so brain ketone body oxidation steadily increases over this period, and glucose oxidation is further reduced. After 3 to 5 weeks of fasting, brain glucose metabolism is globally reduced by about 50% (37). Moreover, only 60% of glucose taken up by the brain is now fully oxidized to CO_2 and water; the other 40% of glucose carbon is recycled to the general circulation as pyruvate and lactate for use in gluconeogenesis (38). This combined adaptation of reduced terminal oxidation and Cori cycling reduces irreversible glucose oxidation in the brain by 75%, with an equivalent reduction in the requirement for gluconeogenesis from amino acids and glycerol.

Metabolic Significance of Ketosis

Mention of ketosis or ketoacidosis (ketosis sufficient to reduce the blood bicarbonate, but within its normal buffering capacity) brings diabetes mellitus to mind. In the most severe form of diabetes, destruction of the β cells of the pancreas produces virtually complete insulin deficiency. The result is increased mobilization of fatty acids and priming of the liver for ketone body production and gluconeogenesis, as in simple fasting (25, 39). However, when carbohydrate is ingested but insulin is lacking, little of the resulting blood glucose is removed by muscle and adipose tissue, and the blood glucose concentration rises to high levels, exceeding the renal threshold for glucose reabsorption. The resulting glycosuria creates an osmotic diuresis that depletes the body of water and extracellular fluid. In fasting nondiabetic persons, ketone body levels seldom rise higher than 6 to 8 mmol/L, whereas in untreated diabetes they may rise to 12 to 14 mmol/L, imposing an acid load too great for the body's buffering system to absorb and causing a dangerous fall in pH (ketoacidemia).

Why is severe ketoacidemia common in untreated insulin-dependent diabetes but almost unheard-of in fasting, nondiabetic persons? One possibility is that sufficiently high ketone body concentrations are normally self-regulated. In some studies, ketone body infusions slightly stimulated insulin secretion, and this in turn increased peripheral ketone body use (35, 40). Against this, at least as a sole explanation, is the uncommon but well-recognized syndrome of "nondiabetic ketoacidosis." This usually occurs in alcoholic persons who, following an alcoholic binge with little or no food consumption, subsequently develop recurrent vomiting (41). The resulting fasting ketoacidemia may be as severe as diabetic ketoacidosis, but the blood glucose concentration is low, not high; appropriate treatment involves volume replacement and glucose, without insulin. Nondiabetic ketoacidosis also occurs in pregnancy, although rarely. In pregnancy, fasting hypoglycemia and mild ketosis develop rapidly because of the high glucose demands of the fetus (18). As with alcoholic nondiabetic ketoacidosis, gestational nondiabetic ketoacidosis has been reported in a setting of fasting, hypoglycemia, and volume depletion or metabolic stress (42).

A feature that distinguishes all forms of severe ketoacidosis from the benign ketoacidosis of fasting is hypermetabolism. Uncontrolled diabetes is characterized by hyperglucagonemia and increased norepinephrine secretion. These increase gluconeogenesis and the metabolic rate, whereas fasting is normally a hypometabolic state. Metabolic stress also stimulates gluconeogenesis and the delivery of free fatty acids and gluconeogenic precursors to the liver (43, 44). These factors act together to increase the liver's energy consumption and hence its ketogenic capacity (45). For nondiabetic fasting persons, a stress-induced increase in blood glucose would, under most conditions, stimulate insulin release sufficiently to restrain lipolysis and gluconeogenesis, thereby limiting ketogenesis (35), but in exceptional circumstances, this does not happen. The occasional development of severe nondiabetic ketoacidosis in a setting of combined fasting and hypermetabolism thus becomes understandable, and indeed, it is consistent with observations made in the preinsulin era. Prior to 1922, the only treatment that extended the life of insulin-dependent diabetic patients was a diet low in glucose, to prevent hyperglycemia, and low in total energy, which reduced the metabolic rate and hence the liver's ketogenic capacity (46).

In summary, prolonged fasting is characterized by a low blood glucose concentration, which leads to physiologic hypoinsulinemia and ketosis, whereas uncontrolled insulin-dependent diabetes is characterized by a high blood glucose concentration, hypermetabolism, and ketosis, all of which are the direct or indirect result of a pathologic insulin lack. Unlike diabetic ketoacidosis, fasting ketosis is physiologic and a manifestation of proper metabolic regulation. It will not develop into a severe condition similar to diabetic ketoacidosis (18, 25), except, potentially, in a setting of severe volume depletion and/or metabolic stress.

Ketosis during Pregnancy

While normally benign, ketosis is to be avoided during pregnancy because of possible adverse consequences to the fetus. Maternal ketonemia in pregnancy has been associated with a reduction in the intelligence of the offspring (18). Thus, periods of fasting or carbohydrate restriction are to be avoided during pregnancy.

Protein and Energy Metabolism

After an overnight fast, insulin levels drop enough to stimulate mild net muscle proteolysis, thereby releasing amino acids as an endogenous substrate for hepatic gluconeogenesis. In a fast longer than a day, insulin secretion drops yet further, muscle proteolysis is more strongly stimulated, and considerable skeletal muscle protein is lost. During the first 7 to 10 days of fasting, whole body N loss may be in the range of 10 to 12 g/day, excreted chiefly as urinary urea. Since mixed body protein is 16% N and the wet weight:dry weight ratio of lean tissue is about 3–4:1, this corresponds to the loss of 1 to 2 kg of lean tissue over this time (47, 48). If this rate of body N loss were to continue, the body's lean tissue reserve would be lethally depleted within 3 weeks of fasting. Instead, after 7 to 10 days an adaptation begins that, by the end of 2 to 3 weeks of fasting, has reduced the rate of body N loss to less than half of what it was during the first several days. This still incompletely understood adaptation is all the more remarkable since about 50% of urinary N by this time is in the form of ammonium excreted to buffer the protons generated by keto acid production, and it can be eliminated by simple bicarbonate administration (16, 49). Indeed, when ammonium excretion is reduced to normal by providing an exogenous buffer, the body N losses in late, "adapted" fasting are close to the "obligatory" rate of N loss considered to reflect the maximum attainable efficiency of body protein turnover (50, 51).

What accounts for the remarkable reduction in muscle protein catabolism that takes place in the face of the catabolic stimulus of persistent hypoinsulinemia? Metabolic investigations have, so far, been unable to explain this mystery.

In the first 1 to 3 days of fasting, plasma branched-chain amino acid concentrations double, and their release from whole-body proteins and subsequent oxidation increase by variable amounts from postabsorptive values (52, 53). Urinary 3-methylhistidine excretion, an indicator of myofibrillar protein breakdown, also increases in the first few days of fasting (52, 54). By 7 to 10 days, the early increase in amino acid turnover is superseded in most (52, 55) (although not all [53]) studies by a reduction of leucine or lysine (56) release due to proteolysis, in a setting of continued significant urinary N loss and leucine oxidation. By week 4, when N excretion has clearly diminished, protein turnover is reduced even further (57, 58), and 3-methylhistidine excretion is below the prefasting rate (57).

Even early in fasting, the liver is primed for gluconeogenesis (18), and its avidity for gluconeogenic precursors remains unchanged for the duration of the fast. The protein-sparing mechanism of prolonged fasting therefore resides in muscle, and indeed, muscle amino acid output, especially of alanine and glutamine, decreases at this time (18, 59). The reduced muscle protein synthesis and increased proteolysis that make free amino acids available for catabolism in early fasting are due to the combined effect of absent exogenous amino acids and insulin deficiency (24, 60). What reduces muscle proteolysis after 2 weeks of fasting? Most authorities regard the shift in muscle metabolism from ketone body oxidation to fatty acid oxidation and the resulting rise in blood ketone bodies and their delivery to the brain after 2 weeks of fasting as important factors. As ketone bodies increasingly displace glucose as the brain's oxidative fuel, the requirement for amino acid conversion to new glucose molecules is dramatically reduced.

Missing from this scheme, however, is the signal that "tells" muscle to reduce its catabolic rate (61). Some evidence suggests that hyperketonemia has a direct protein-sparing effect on skeletal muscle (62, 63), but clear proof is still lacking (53). Another possibility is that the process by which muscle metabolism switches from ketone body oxidation to fatty acid oxidation after approximately 2 weeks of fasting is responsible, in some manner, for the reduction in muscle proteolysis. Perhaps increased fatty acid oxidation in muscle spares the branched-chain amino acids (which have structural similarity to fatty acids), and they (or their metabolites) are responsible for the diminished proteolysis (16). This possibility is attractive because of evidence that these molecules, particularly leucine, have protein-sparing effects (64). Finally, ketone bodies may stimulate a rise in peripheral insulin too slight to be detected with currently available methods (25, 35, 65) but which still exerts a protein-sparing effect.

Resting energy expenditure decreases by approximately 15% after 2 weeks of fasting (66) and is 25 to 35% below normal after 3 to 4 weeks (67). This reduction is too great to be entirely due to lean tissue loss, although lean tissue loss is plainly responsible for further reductions as the fast continues.

Other Metabolic Effects

The serum albumin concentration remains normal both in short-term and prolonged fasting, but concentrations of the rapidly turning over liver secretory proteins, transthyretin (thyroid-binding prealbumin) and retinol-binding protein, promptly decrease, as they do in response to any form of carbohydrate restriction (68, 69). Serum total bilirubin may increase by 50% after a 24-hour fast, doubling by the end of day 2 and remaining constant thereafter (70). Hyperuricemia invariably occurs, the consequence of inhibition of renal tubular excretion of urate by ketone bodies (18) and increased renal tubular urate reabsorption when the extracellular volume is depleted (71). Gastric emptying slows after only 4 days of fasting (72). In therapeutic fasts longer than 4 weeks, postural hypotension and nausea become prominent problems. Other metabolic effects and medical complications of prolonged fasting are described in clinical reviews (18, 73, 74).

Weight Loss

Weight and body N loss occur in roughly direct proportion to the existing body weight and lean body mass (73, 75), exhibiting the characteristics of a biexponential "decay" process. The pattern of weight loss is highly variable. Nonobese men with free access to water may lose 4 kg over the first 5 days of a fast and a further 3 kg over the next 5 days (48, 67), whereas obese men lose about 50% more than this. In one extreme case, a patient initially weighing 245 kg lost 32 kg in the first 30 days of fasting (73).

Water, not fat, accounts for most of the initial weight loss during fasting (76). This can be demonstrated by a simple calculation. If total energy expenditure is assumed to be 2400 kcal/day during the initial week of a fast and N loss is 10 g/day (equivalent to the catabolism of 62.5 g body protein, and hence, to the provision of 250 kcal of endogenous energy), negative energy balance is 2400 − 250 or 2150 kcal/day. Stored fat provides 9.4 kcal/g, so 2150/9.4 or 229 g of fat is oxidized per day to make up the energy balance. The adipose tissue lost during weight reduction is 85% fat by weight (77, 78), so body weight loss directly due to fat loss will be 229/0.85 or 269 g/day or 1.9 kg/week. This represents only one-third or less of the total weight loss during this period; the other two-thirds is water unrelated to adipose tissue. Of all the water lost in the first 3 days of fasting, approximately 65% is from the extracellular compartment (67). This rapid mobilization of extracellular water and sodium is due to a combination of absent dietary sodium and the low insulin level, since insulin has an antinatriuretic action on the kidneys (79). The dissolution of liver glycogen (2–3 g water/g glycogen [80]) and to a lesser extent muscle glycogen (3–4 g water/g glycogen [81]) contribute to intracellular water loss over the first 3 days, as does lean tissue dissolution, which persists at a rate of at least 10 g N/day (19–25 g water/g N [47]) during the first 7 to 10 days. After 2 weeks of fasting, extracellular fluid loss has almost completely ceased (73), and by the third week, weight loss slows substantially, a consequence of slower lean tissue loss, reduced metabolic rate, and stabilization of glycogen and extracellular water balance. During this phase of fasting, weight loss is due to continuing adipose and lean tissue loss and amounts to about 300 g/day in moderately obese persons (82).

Nutritional Modifications of Fasting Metabolism

It has been known for most of this century that carbohydrate, but not fat, reduces protein catabolism during fasting (17, 55, 83). As described 50 years ago in Gamble's famous "experiences on a life raft" lecture (15), 100 to 150 g of glucose per day prevents the ketonuria of fasting and reduces urea N excretion and extracellular volume loss by half. For these reasons, hospitalized patients who cannot eat or drink are customarily administered 2 to 3 L/day of intravenous fluids containing 50 g dextrose/L.

The important protein-sparing effect of carbohydrate occurs in the first 7 to 10 days of a fast. When given later, even large amounts of carbohydrate are only modestly more effective at limiting N loss than is accomplished by this time by natural adaptation (7, 84). Moreover, prolonged carbohydrate administration without protein can have adverse consequences. Hypoalbuminemia and immune system dysfunction have been observed in acutely ill, hospitalized patients maintained for prolonged periods on intravenous dextrose solutions, a syndrome reminiscent of kwashiorkor, the disease of protein-malnourished children with free access to carbohydrate. This syndrome is attributed to a carbohydrate-induced high peripheral insulin concentration that, in the setting of protein deficiency, drives scarce circulating amino acids into muscle tissue at the expense of the visceral protein store. For this reason, patients who cannot obtain normal oral nutrition for periods longer than 7 to 10 days require parenteral amino acids as well as energy.

The timing of the protein-sparing effect of dietary protein is the reverse of that of carbohydrate. When given in the first 7 to 10 days of fasting, protein has little effect on the rate of body protein loss, but after 2 or more weeks of continuous high-quality protein feeding in doses of 50 to 80 g/day, N balance gradually improves and may even return to zero after 3 or more weeks (85, 86). When protein is introduced during the adapted phase of a total fast, N balance abruptly becomes positive (57, 87).

Survival

Depletion of 50% or more of the body's lean tissues is said to be incompatible with survival (88) and has commonly been claimed to signal impending death due to fasting (3). However fat, not protein, may determine survival in this unique form of starvation (89, 90). Nonobese adults die after approximately 60 days of fasting, in reasonable agreement with the estimated time required to lose all their body fat, but only one-third of their lean tissues. Perhaps fat depletion is lethal in fasting humans because it reduces the availability of fatty acids, which are necessary both for hepatic ketone body synthesis and as the energy substrate that sustains gluconeogenesis (90). Fasting, therefore, should be avoided by individuals with depleted fat stores even if their lean tissue stores are ample (91).

Obese individuals have tolerated fasts of astonishing length (92, 93). The longest monitored fast on record was by a 27-year-old man whose starting weight was 207 kg. He lost 60% of his body weight after 382 days of uninterrupted fasting (94). Despite such spectacular experiences, total fasts longer than about 4 weeks are potentially dangerous, even for very obese persons. Although minimized, lean tissue loss does not cease in prolonged fasting. In cases of extremely prolonged fasting in which lean tissue loss was measured, critical levels of depletion were observed (93). Acute thiamin deficiency can be a devastating complication of fasting (95–97) and could contribute to its lethality.

PROTEIN DEFICIENCY

Protein deficiency occurs when protein intake is chronically below the requirement level but energy intake is maintained. Severe protein deficiency has been relatively little studied in adults, since it rarely occurs without simultaneous energy deficiency. On the other hand, syndromes due to mild chronic protein deficiency are of considerable interest, for they have an important bearing on the definition of minimum protein or essential amino acid requirements. Considerable uncertainty continues to exist in this area (98–102).

Adaptation and Accommodation

The normal response to a reduction in protein intake is an adaptive reduction of dietary and endogenous amino acid oxidation to match the new lower intake and, after a few days, restoration of N balance. Consumption of less protein than the minimum nutritional requirement exceeds the limit of this adaptation and results in sustained body protein loss (50). In most cases, a new steady state occurs later in which N equilibrium is restored after a variable amount of lean tissue loss. Waterlow has drawn attention to the difference, when assessing the nutritional value of diets, between *adaptation,* which is a normal physiologic response to variations within the acceptable range of protein intakes, and the protein-sacrificing response to an inadequate protein intake, which he termed *accommodation* (103, 104). Other terms, such as *normal adaptation* and *pathologic adaptation* would serve the same purpose; what is important is the distinction. Adaptation is understood to be an aspect of normal physiology, whereas accommodation implies a physiologic compromise with adverse health consequences.

The phenomenon of accommodation is illustrated by the response of elderly but healthy women who were randomly assigned to diets that provided either surfeit (0.92 g/kg) or moderately inadequate (0.45 g/kg) protein, in the presence of adequate energy. After 9 weeks, the women consuming inadequate protein suffered no weight loss, and their N balance was only slightly negative, indicating approximate metabolic homeostasis. Moreover, their serum albumin (often considered a sensitive indicator of adequate protein nutrition) remained normal. Unlike the control subjects, however, their lean tissue mass was reduced, and muscle function and immune status were impaired (105). Similar abnormalities have been observed in patients with more severe or prolonged protein deficiency, but in these cases serum albumin is reduced (106), indicating more severe compromise. In all cases fat stores are normal.

When consumed by healthy persons for only a week or two, protein-free diets are without adverse effect; in fact, such diets were widely used in the past to estimate the minimum dietary protein requirement. When a normal adult is switched from a conventional diet high in protein (e.g., 100 g/day) to one that is protein free, urinary N decreases, and after about 7 days it reaches an apparent steady-state excretion of 37 mg N per kg body weight, accounting for almost 70% of total body N loss (the other sources of N loss, which do not change, are in the feces and secretions and from skin shedding) (50, 51, 107). This "obligatory" N loss indicates the lowest rate to which endogenous protein loss can be adaptively reduced and is considered to indicate the minimum dietary protein requirement (50, 108). The problem with this calculation of the minimum protein requirement is that it assumes no loss of dietary amino acids occurs during their absorption from the gut and resynthesis as new protein in the tissues. Gut absorption of amino acids is, in fact, normally highly efficient, but the biochemical steps leading to the conservation of dietary amino acids within newly synthesized endogenous proteins are not, and the degree of inefficiency varies under different conditions (109). When increasing amounts of high-quality protein are added to a protein-free diet, N balance improves steeply at low levels of intake (indicating highly efficient dietary protein retention) but more slowly at higher intakes (51). When the results of N balance studies that included many levels of dietary protein are analyzed and the lowest intake at which N equilibrium occurs is interpolated, the average daily intake of high-quality protein (0.6 g/kg) is substantially more than indicated from obligatory N loss (0.34 g/kg). Nevertheless, the precision of the protein-free diet method is such that it can still be useful for assessing the efficiency of basal protein metabolism in conditions in which only small numbers of subjects are available for study (110).

Protein and Energy Metabolism

Consumption of a severely protein deficient diet for 7 to 10 days reduces whole body protein turnover (110–112) and also the rate of albumin synthesis, although the serum albumin concentration does not change (107, 113). Essential amino acid deficiency also promptly reduces whole body protein turnover (114). In animals, severe protein deficiency reduces liver protein synthesis (115–117), consistent with the observation that protein synthesis in this organ fluctuates in close response to fluctuations in the amino acid supply comparable to those normally encountered during the ingestion of protein meals (118). Increased protein synthesis by delivery of amino acids can even be evoked in the isolated perfused liver, showing that the hormonal responses evoked during meal absorption are not essential for liver protein synthesis (118, 119).

Less clear, in the human, are the effects of acute changes in protein intake within the normal adaptive range. As expected, most studies carried out in the fed state indicate that a low protein intake reduces amino acid catabolism and a high intake increases it, since these responses would act to keep N balance close to zero. Some (120–122) but not all (123–125) studies indicate that the increased or decreased leucine oxidation evoked by high or low leucine intakes is carried over into the basal period between meals. Basal protein turnover has been found insensitive to changes of protein intake within the normal physiologic range in most (121, 122, 124, 125) but not all (111, 126, 126a) human studies.

In the study of chronic protein deficiency described above, 9 weeks of moderate protein deficiency did not reduce fed-state whole body protein synthesis and breakdown nor urinary 3-methylhistidine excretion (127). This is a surprising result that challenges current concepts about the adaptation to protein deficiency. Regrettably, basal protein turnover, which may have been more reliable for detecting an adaptive reduction in protein turnover in this setting, was not measured (105, 107). Serum albumin and the concentrations of the liver secretory proteins, retinol-binding protein and transferrin, remained normal (105). Evidently, plasma concentrations of these proteins provide less insight into the adaptation to protein deficiency than would knowledge of their actual synthesis, secretion, and removal rates. It also provides further evidence that plasma transthyretin, retinol-binding protein, and transferrin concentrations, often taken as indicators of the adequacy of protein nutrition, are far more sensitive to carbohydrate and total energy intake than to protein nutrition per se (68, 69).

What are the health implications of reduced whole body protein turnover, as observed during severe protein or essential amino acid deficiency? Protein synthesis is energetically expensive (128), so the continuous recycling of body proteins in a seemingly "futile cycle" presumably confers a biologic advantage. Newsholme and Stanley showed that substrate cycles at regulation points in metabolic pathways permit finely tuned control of metabolite flow (129). Does recycling of entire proteins similarly allow rapid remodeling of body protein distribution and function in times of need? If so, then slowed rates of protein turnover characteristic of severe or prolonged protein or essential amino acid deficiency could be bad for the organism (104). It appears that the greater the protein intake, the coarser (and perhaps, therefore, less efficient) the regulation (121, 122, 130). When protein is consumed above the requirement level, dietary protein conservation is inefficient, as indeed it must be to eliminate the excessive amino acids provided by the diet. When protein intake is severely reduced below the requirement level, protein turnover rates are reduced to maximize amino acid reuse, a state manifested by low fluctuations in N excretion (130, 131). Thus, according to this view, adaptation to significant protein deficiency necessarily involves reduction in the rate of cellular protein turnover, because rapid flux through the free amino acid pools is incompatible with the finest regulation (and efficiency) of amino acid oxidation (57, 114).

There is little information on energy expenditure in pure protein deficiency. The resting metabolic rate appears to remain normal, either when measured after 7 to 10 days of a protein-free diet (132) or when related to the metabolic mass after prolonged, moderate protein deficiency (127).

Labile Protein

In 1866, Carl Voit first demonstrated the existence of a small protein store whose amount was determined by the dietary protein content and which was excreted during the first several days of fasting or upon changing from a higher to a lower protein intake. This protein store is now known to be an example of a general phenomenon of rapid body protein gain or loss in response to variations in protein intake (83, 133). When a normal adult consumes a low-protein diet, urinary N excretion remains higher than intake for 3 to 5 days before diminishing to a new steady state. When the former protein intake is resumed, N balance becomes positive until the previous losses are made up (Fig. 41.1). Labile protein is said to constitute about 3% of body protein in well-nourished rats or humans (133), an insignificant amount in terms of total body N economy, but of potential importance to understanding adaptation to starvation.

Although small, the amount of labile protein in the body is larger than the free amino acid pool, which makes up only about 0.5 to 1.0% of the body's amino acids and an even smaller percentage of the essential ones (134–136). The free amino acid pool, because of its small size and rapid turnover, can be assumed to be essential to the regulation of tissue protein synthesis and breakdown (136). Since labile protein undergoes the most rapid

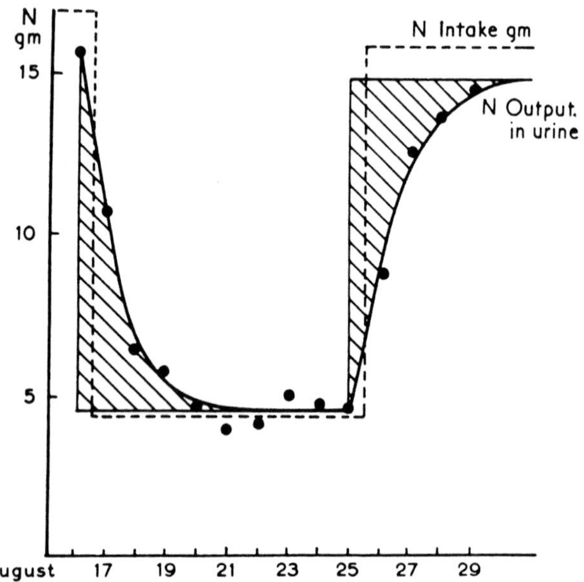

Figure 41.1. Labile protein. The *solid line* indicates the N excretion of a human subject abruptly changed to a low-protein diet. The *dashed line* indicates the level of N intake. Initially, N intake approximates its excretion, and the subject is close to N equilibrium. On switching to the lower N intake, N loss exceeds intake for several days until equilibrium is reestablished. The N lost from the body during this period is shown in the *first shaded area*. On resuming former intake, the subject stores N, as shown by the *second shaded area*. The two shaded areas are approximately equal. (From Munro HN. General aspects of the regulation of protein metabolism by diet and hormones. In: Munro HN, Allison JB, eds. Mammalian protein metabolism, vol 1. New York: Academic Press, 1964;381–481, with permission.)

exchange with the free amino acid pool, it is tempting to regard it as important in determining the extent of oxidation of amino acids, particularly those newly entering from the diet (133). In the protein-deficient or fasted rat, the greatest acute loss of protein is from the liver, with the other visceral organs making up large contributions as well, as might be predicted from the rapid turnover rates of proteins in these organs (107, 117).

A labile pool of rapidly turning over protein could help explain how the efficiency of dietary protein retention improves after reduction of protein intake within the normal adaptive range. To what extent does an increase or decrease in whole-body protein turnover represent a slight change in the rate of synthesis and breakdown of a large, slowly turning over protein pool of nearly constant mass, and to what extent a considerable increase or decrease in the size of a small, rapidly turning over pool, such as labile protein? The contributions of the different protein pools of the body to whole-body protein turnover are not well defined, so the notion that labile protein synthesis and breakdown contribute importantly to whole body protein turnover remains speculative (52). If a high protein intake increases the labile protein pool, then "basal" protein turnover ought to be more rapid in persons adapted to higher protein intakes and lower after they adapt to lower intakes within the normal range (137). The apparent insensitivity of basal whole-body protein turnover to variations in protein intake thus argues against a significant regulatory role for labile protein (122).

PROTEIN-ENERGY STARVATION

The commonest form of starvation results from a deficiency of all food, and hence represents the combined features of energy deficiency, protein deficiency, and, in all likelihood, deficiencies of certain micronutrients whose role in the pathogenesis of the clinical entity of protein-energy malnutrition is not yet elucidated (98, 138). In general, protein-energy starvation combines the hypometabolic adaptation of energy deficiency with the reduced whole-body protein turnover characteristic of severe or chronic protein deficiency; it is a far more variable entity than simple fasting or short-term protein deficiency. Metabolism during protein-energy starvation depends to a considerable degree on the composition and duration of the starvation diet, and it is frequently complicated by the medical or surgical condition that led to its development in the first place (see also Chapters 59, 96, and 98).

Weight Loss

The most detailed study of the effects of chronic energy and protein deficiency on human physiology was conducted between 1944 and 1946 by Keys and his coworkers, in an experiment in which 32 healthy young men volunteered to live on the campus of the University of Minnesota and consume a diet providing approximately 1600 kcal/day, about two-thirds of their normal energy requirement (139).

The Minnesota volunteers lost an average of 23% of their initial body weight. Body composition measurements indicated that they lost more than 70% of their body fat. Muscle was lost as well; in all, the volunteers lost 24% of their lean tissue mass (termed *active tissue mass* in the study), which accounted for 60% of their weight loss. Weight loss alone underestimated the sum of their fat and lean tissue losses, because their extracellular fluid volume increased. In extreme cases (and especially in the presence of other diseases associated with water retention), the increase in extracellular volume causes obvious fluid accumulation within the skin and interstitial tissues, called "hunger edema." When present, edema makes assessment of the severity of lean tissue depletion more difficult (140); midarm circumference takes on special usefulness in this situation (141).

Adaptation

As in fasting, weight loss early in semistarvation is rapid, but it gradually slows, even if there is no change in the starvation diet. Whereas weight loss can never slow to zero during fasting, a pathologic adaptation is commonly achieved in less extreme states of energy deficiency by which body weight stabilizes at a lower steady-state value. This occurred for the Minnesota volunteers after 24 weeks. Evidently it involved cessation of losses both of fat (energy) and lean tissue (protein).

Energy Expenditure

The resting energy expenditure (REE) of the Minnesota volunteers decreased by 40% after 24 weeks of starvation, thus coming approximately into line with their energy intake. This decrease in REE was largely the result of a diminished lean tissue mass, which is responsible for most of the metabolic processes that determine energy expenditure (142). REE was also reduced per unit of remaining lean tissue (Fig. 41.2). Total energy expenditure also decreased substantially, because smaller meals evoke a smaller thermic effect of food, and a lower body weight demands less work in moving (143). Moreover, the volunteers reduced their level of voluntary physical activity by more than half, a form of adaptation shown in other studies of chronic starvation (144, 145) and in some (146) but not all (147) short-term starvation studies. Such adjustments, when successful, bring starving individuals back into energy equilibrium.

Lean Tissue Loss

The energy-restricted organism can restore energy balance by reducing its lean tissue mass, but it cannot lose so much lean tissue that the adverse metabolic consequences of protein deficiency become intolerable. Successful adaptation is a process of controlled protein loss that should cease when just enough has been sacrificed to permit zero

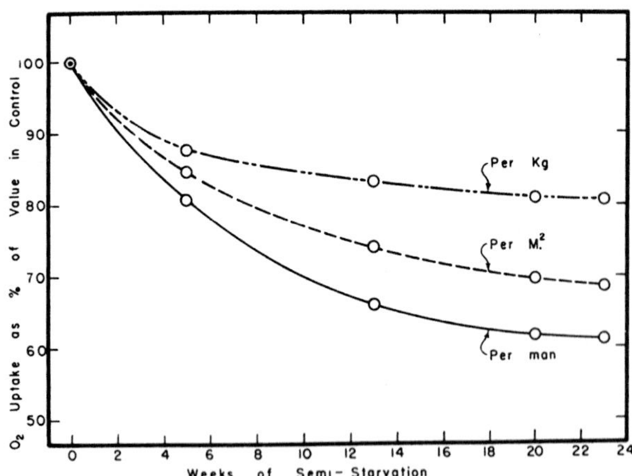

Figure 41.2. Mean basal metabolism for 32 men before and during 24 weeks of starvation. All values are expressed as percentage of the prestarvation values for the oxygen uptake per man, per square meter of body surface, and per kg of body weight. (From Keys A, Brozek J, Henschel A, et al. The biology of human starvation. Minneapolis, University of Minnesota Press, 1950, with permission.)

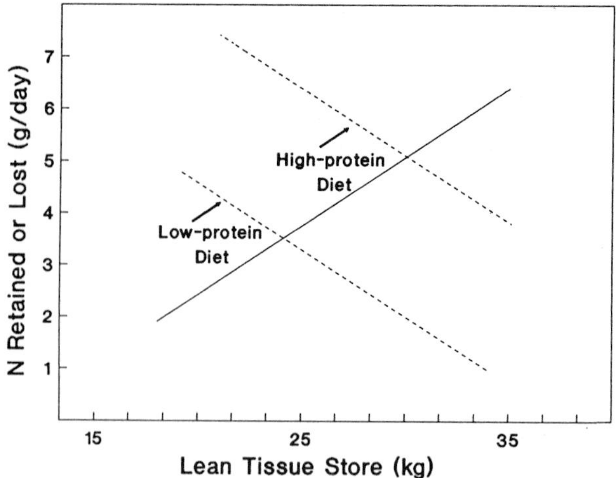

Figure 41.3. A hypothetic scheme to account for adaptation to starvation in the adult. A first-order (linear) relationship exists between the amount of lean tissue and the rate at which it is depleted. This is indicated by the *solid line*. An *inverse* relationship exists between the amount of lean tissue and the efficiency of retention of protein in the diet. This relationship is affected by the concentration of protein in the diet, resulting in a family of curves *(dashed lines)*. As starvation progresses and the lean tissue store diminishes, the rate of protein depletion slows as the amount of protein retained from each meal increases. At the crossover point a new equilibrium is established and lean tissue loss ceases. The "price" paid to achieve this physiologic adaptation is a diminished lean tissue store. This scheme illustrates that a high-protein diet may permit protein equilibrium after only moderate lean tissue wasting; a low-protein diet may also be compatible with protein equilibrium, but the cost, in terms of protein wasting, will be greater.

energy balance to be reestablished. N equilibrium is reestablished by an adaptation that can be separated conceptually into two components: *(a)* decreased endogenous N loss and *(b)* increased efficiency of dietary protein retention (Fig. 41.3). As starvation proceeds, the rate of continuing lean tissue loss is roughly proportional to the amount of lean tissue remaining, and hence it automatically slows as the lean tissue mass decreases (148). Simultaneously, cellular metabolism adjusts to reduce the rate of endogenous amino acid oxidation (149) and increase the efficiency of exogenous (dietary) protein retention. The increased avidity of starving tissues for dietary protein has long been recognized (150–152). Net body protein loss continues until the slowing of endogenous protein loss matches the increasing efficiency of dietary protein retention and a new state of protein equilibrium is established (Fig. 41.3).

Determinants of Lean Tissue Conservation

Because the starving individual must sacrifice a certain amount of protein to reestablish zero energy balance, protein loss can be regarded as a beneficial survival mechanism during prolonged starvation (153). However, energy intake is only one of several factors that affect the rate of N loss during starvation and the total amount of lean tissue that must be sacrificed to reestablish N equilibrium. These factors include energy balance, protein intake, protein-nutritional state, biologic individuality, and possibly obesity.

Energy Balance. The Minnesota volunteers consumed an amount of protein close to the amount regarded as safe for normal adults (0.75 g/kg body weight), but they still lost a large amount of body protein. Many studies have shown that N balance at a constant protein intake is improved by increased, and worsened by decreased, energy intake (133, 154). The energy effect is most potent in the modestly submaintenance range of both protein and energy intakes (155). Under most circumstances, the predominant energy source (carbohydrate or fat) is immaterial (156).

Kinney and Elwyn emphasized the importance of measuring the energy balance (the difference between exogenous energy ingested and energy expended), not simply energy intake (157, 158). Because it is the amount of dietary energy in surplus or in deficit after accounting for expenditure, energy balance is probably the specific physiologic variable that when negative worsens N balance and when positive improves it (159). Direct measurement of energy balance may be particularly important in hospitalized patients whose energy expenditure varies considerably (157).

Protein Intake. The combination of protein and energy deficiency results in a greater loss of body protein than is physiologically necessary to reduce energy expenditure. N balance is improved by increased protein intake over a wide range of energy intakes from deficient to maintenance (133); thus, increased protein intake may compensate for negative energy balance (133, 160–162). This interaction is illustrated in Figure 41.3. When the lean tissues are depleted, a greater fraction of the protein in a given meal is retained, so (over an appropriate range of protein intakes) a meal high in protein will be associated with greater absolute protein retention than one low in protein. This explains why a high-protein starvation diet may be associated with protein equilibrium after only moderate lean tissue wasting; a low-protein starvation diet may also be compatible with protein equilibrium, but the ultimate protein-wasting will be greater.

Thus, in the Minnesota study, fat-free mass (FFM, body weight minus pure fat) accounted for 71% of the weight loss after 12 weeks of starvation (139), whereas, in a recent 10-week study of normal-weight men whose energy intake was reduced by a not dissimilar margin, but whose protein intake (94 g/day) was nearly twice that of the Minnesota volunteers, only 17% of the weight lost was from FFM. This is close to the amount of extracellular fluid associated with adipose tissue (77, 78). Urinary creatinine excretion (an indicator of skeletal muscle mass) remained constant, further evidence that the high-protein diet effectively spared body protein in these normal starving men (163).

The sparing effect of a high protein intake is also demonstrated in most N balance studies of obese persons on weight reduction diets. N losses tend to be greater in men than women, and some body N and FFM loss appears inevitable when severely obese persons are starved. This occurs because adipose tissue has nonfat components that are measured as FFM (164) and because there is a reduced need for muscles after significant weight reduction (85, 165, 166). Most, but not all (86), studies have shown that a high-protein diet (at least 1.5 g protein per kg of normal body weight) maintains N balance (85) or FFM (167) better than lower intakes. The failure to find a difference in N balance between diets providing 50 and 70 g protein per day in a recent study (86) may have been because the protein levels were not sufficiently different to detect it.

Stage of Starvation. The efficiency of N retention at any protein and energy intake is increased by prior protein depletion (57). In part, this occurs simply because a smaller mass of active body protein requires less amino acid replacement than a larger one. However, cellular adaptations also improve the efficiency of amino acid use; these are described below. The influence of protein-nutritional status is implicit in the scheme shown in Figure 41.3, in which a given lean tissue mass (indicated on the horizontal axis) has an important effect on both endogenous protein loss and dietary protein avidity.

Obesity. It has been suggested that obesity confers a sparing effect on protein loss during starvation (76). In my view this is not well established, especially considering differences in sex, protein intake in relation to FFM, and the greater physical activity level of obese, weight-reducing persons than of nonobese starving ones. Indeed, to the extent that lean tissue mass is increased in severely obese individuals, their absolute rate of N loss is faster than that of less obese persons during starvation (73, 168). An analysis of the composition of weight loss by weight-reducing patients did not show any slower loss of FFM in those more obese (169).

Other Factors. When weight loss continues in spite of conditions conducive to adaptation, attention should be directed to such correctable factors as malabsorption, the adequacy of micronutrient provision (170, 171), or supervening physiologic stress (5) (see also Chapter 59). These factors are considered in detail below, but even when they are all controlled or considered, the variation in individual responses to starvation is wide (172). This is consistent with the scope of biochemical individuality (173) and, specifically, with the wide variation in individual amino acid requirements of normal men (174).

Characteristics of Successful Adaptation

Pathologic adaptation has "succeeded" when energy equilibrium is reestablished through reduction of total energy expenditure and a process of controlled lean tissue wasting that is arrested before the adverse consequences of lean tissue depletion become insupportable. The organism survives, but a metabolic and functional price must be paid (107). The most apparent deficits are loss of insulating fat and loss of muscle mass with its associated reduction of physical power. A hypometabolic state of "unwellness" is induced, reminiscent of (but not identical to) hypothyroidism (175). Starving patients are hypothermic and do not mount an appropriate thermic response to environmental cold (176). The loss of muscle mass diminishes the body's protein reserve and, together with slower protein turnover in the remaining muscle (177), reduces the body's options for protein remodeling in response to changing metabolic needs. Thus, starving patients mount a blunted rise in protein turnover and a smaller catabolic response during metabolic stress (178). The physical appearance of patients with protein-energy malnutrition is reminiscent of advanced aging, and indeed, some similarities of body composition exist (179).

In addition to the loss of peripheral proteins, deficits in central protein occur as well. The anatomic and functional consequences of severe human starvation are covered in clinical depictions (139, 180, 181) and medical reviews (3, 165, 182, 183). These effects include anemia, altered heart muscle mass and function, decreased pulmonary mechanical function and a diminished response to stimuli to breathe, altered gut anatomy and mildly impaired absorptive function, altered drug metabolism (184–186), and immunodeficiency (187, 188).

Immune competence is crucial for long-term survival, yet the precise nature of immune dysfunction in human starvation remains poorly understood. In both animals and humans, advanced protein-energy malnutrition results in a variety of immune deficits, especially of cell-mediated immunity (demonstrated clinically by anergy, the loss of delayed cutaneous hypersensitivity) (187, 188). However, the clinical importance of immune deficiency in moderate starvation and the possible additive effect of concurrent micronutrient deficiency have not been well studied (189). A potentially broad area of interaction is cytokine production or release, which is independently impaired in protein-energy malnutrition and in several micronutrient deficiencies (190).

Weight-stable anorexia nervosa in an otherwise healthy young individual is a useful clinical paradigm for well-adapted starvation (191). More complex examples can be observed daily in any outpatient chronic disease clinic and in segments of the population of many parts of the world. The defining features of successful adaptation are less-than-critical total lean tissue depletion, weight stability, normal plasma albumin level (in the absence of dehydration), normal peripheral blood total lymphocyte count, and intact delayed cutaneous hypersensitivity (192).

Central and Peripheral Protein Depletion

An important aspect of successful adaptation involves preferential visceral uptake of amino acids released from muscle. This results in relative preservation of the mass and function of critical "central" proteins despite large losses of "peripheral" skeletal muscle protein (192). When adaptation is unsuccessful, either because the food restriction is too severe, because of micronutrient deficiency, or for other reasons, the peripheral lean tissue depletion becomes too great and proteins are lost from both the central and peripheral compartments (Fig. 41.4). Metabolic stress frequently precipitates central protein deficiency. The hyperglycemia induced by stress hormones stimulates insulin release, which drives scarce amino acids into the insulin-sensitive peripheral proteins at the expense of the insulin-insensitive central proteins (133, 192). By contrast, moderate stress in the well-nourished organism is characterized by mobilization of peripheral proteins to the center (193, 194).

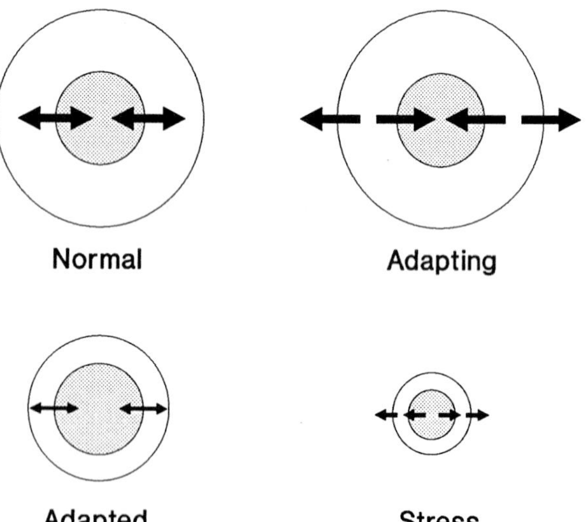

Figure 41.4. Adaptation to starvation. The *outer circles* represent the mass of peripheral, metabolically active proteins. The *inner circles* represent the central (visceral) proteins. The *arrows* represent N transfer. In normal life, protein equilibrium exists. During adaptation to starvation, N is lost from the body, but there is a relative sparing of the central proteins. When adaptation is successful, equilibrium is reestablished at a major cost to peripheral proteins but at a relatively minor cost to central proteins. Stress (or other reversal of adaptation) causes a loss of both central and peripheral N.

Development of central protein deficiency, as manifested by anergy and hypoalbuminemia (with resultant edema), indicates a dangerous condition (192). Parallels have been drawn between simple, adapted adult protein-energy malnutrition and childhood marasmus, on the one hand, and between central protein malnutrition in the adult and kwashiorkor (which may also be precipitated by stress or a high-energy, low-protein intake) on the other (195). However, starvation in the chronically ill adult is only approximately similar to childhood marasmus or kwashiorkor (176, 196), and there is uncertainty about the precise pathogenesis of kwashiorkor (195, 197, 198). Most often, advanced protein-energy malnutrition in the adult has a mixture of "central" and "peripheral" features that tends toward one end of a spectrum or the other (106, 199).

Failed Adaptation

Failed adaptation should be suspected when a starving patient develops metabolic stress, as indicated by fever or a rapid heart rate. However, these responses to stress may be blunted in starving patients, and their absence does not rule out stress nor does it exclude factors other than stress that reverse the adapted state. A more reliable sign of stress-induced protein wasting is an inappropriate rise in serum urea concentration and urinary urea excretion. By far, the simplest indicator of the reversal of accommodation from any cause is resumption of weight loss in a previously weight-stable, malnourished patient or the failure to gain weight despite development of edema. Either situation indicates new lean tissue loss. Factors that can impair adaptation and thus should alert the clinician to its possible failure, include further diminution of food intake, worsening of the primary disease or development of one of its complications, onset of a new disease that imposes a metabolic stress, or administration of a treatment that alters protein or energy metabolism.

Metabolic Stress. The hypermetabolic, protein-catabolic response to severe infection, trauma, or traumatic major surgery reverses the adaptation to starvation (5, 192, 200) (see also Chapters 96 and 98). Food intake previously compatible with homeostasis is now inadequate. Starving, stressed patients move rapidly into a state of central protein deficiency because their peripheral protein reserves have previously been depleted.

Mineral Deficiency. Mineral deficiencies, particularly of potassium (170, 171), phosphorus (170), zinc (201, 202), and presumably magnesium, prevent maximal protein-sparing and an appropriate anabolic response to refeeding.

Metabolic Disease or Administration of Hormones or Antimetabolites. Hyperthyroidism, pheochromocytoma, glucagonoma, poorly controlled diabetes mellitus, and states of glucocorticoid excess (203) are all associated with protein wasting. The existence of any of these diseases or its new development in starving patients calls for attention to the patient's nutritional status. In any of these situations, protein-energy malnutrition may rapidly develop, or the previously successful adaptation to existing starvation may be reversed, resulting in rapid progression to an advanced stage. Some evidence reveals that the efficiency of protein metabolism remains abnormal even with appropriate insulin treatment of insulin-dependent diabetes (204). Diabetic patients may therefore be at increased risk of severe protein depletion during starvation.

Glucocorticoids or antimetabolites used to treat inflammatory conditions, or chemotherapeutic agents and extensive radiotherapy used in cancer therapy, may impair the adaptation to starvation. Anorexia is a systemic manifestation of certain malignancies, including those of the pancreas, stomach, and liver (205), and may add to the anorexia induced by many chemotherapeutic agents (206), abdominal radiation, and psychologic factors. The combination of reduced food intake and metabolic stress is common in these patients.

Food Restriction Too Severe. The most common maladaptation to starvation should not be described as maladaptation at all but is merely the consequence of food deprivation too severe to allow adaptation. The result is continuous weight loss until death.

Chronic Energy Deficiency

Starvation in a ward or clinic patient is easily recognized, requiring only physician or nutritionist awareness and confirmation of the diagnosis on the basis of a food-intake and body-weight history, physical examination, and a record of weight over time (207). However, in societies where scarcity and low body weight are common, it can be difficult to define the minimum acceptable food intake and corresponding nutritional state (88, 153, 208). To address this, a form of adapted protein-energy starvation, "adult chronic energy deficiency" (CED), has been described (209, 210). This stable but malnourished condition is compatible with gainful employment, pregnancy, and other aspects of daily life and is thus clearly distinct from "acute energy deficiency," which corresponds to the weight-losing stage of poorly adapted starvation, or to the clinical condition of protein-energy malnutrition. CED is defined as a subnormal body mass index (BMI, body weight in kilograms divided by the square of height in meters), and classified into 3 grades of severity: grade I, 17.0–18.4; grade II, 16.0–16.9; and grade III, less than 16 (210).

BMI reflects the body's fat store both in obesity and underweight. A BMI between 20 and 25 is generally regarded as optimum (50). In the United States, Hungary, or Brazil, fewer than 5% of adults have a BMI below 18.5, whereas 10% of Chinese, 20% of Congolese, 25% of Pakistani or Philippino adults, and nearly 50% of Indian adults are in this category (209, 210). Only grades II and III CED have been associated with an increased probability of days of illness, reduced physical work capacity, poorer reproductive function, and poorer lactation performance. A measurable decrease in voluntary physical activity has been shown only in grade III CED. These observations suggest that a BMI of 17.0 to 18.5 may be compatible with normal health. Therefore, an appreciable number of normal persons (especially young adults) with BMIs in this range could be incorrectly diagnosed as malnourished (209, 210).

CED described in active young adults living in poor countries could well be the same condition as the successfully adapted protein-energy starvation of weight-stable anorexia nervosa patients or the wasting that commonly accompanies chronic disease. It is also possible that years or decades of CED induce long-term adaptations, including psychologic ones, that we do not yet understand (107, 199). The BMIs of the Minnesota volunteers fell from 21.4 to 16.3 after 6 months of starvation (139). If their 1.8 kg of extracellular fluid gain is subtracted, their BMI becomes 16.0, a value within the range associated with disability in CED. On the other hand, the BMI of patients described as severely malnourished in one detailed study (106) was 17.5. In that study, undernutrition was diagnosed on the basis of a combination of features that included serum albumin and urinary creatinine for height, as well as body weight for height.

In summary, it appears that young adults without intercurrent disease can tolerate a BMI as low as 17 without apparent physiologic dysfunction, despite their lack of nutritional reserves. Even a BMI below 17, while associated with disability, can be tolerated in well-adapted CED. This is in marked contrast to much medical experience, which dictates that a weight loss of more than 10% is sufficient to identify malnutrition (211, 212). At the other extreme, a BMI above 18.5 does not rule out severe malnutrition, since fat and extracellular fluid mass can greatly affect body weight. Evidently, better criteria than body weight or BMI alone are required to identify dangerous protein or protein-energy starvation. The best clinical criteria currently available are ones that point to failed adaptation to starvation. These include continuing weight loss, functional disability, and hypoalbuminemia, especially in the presence of physiologic stress (205, 213–215).

MECHANISMS GOVERNING ADAPTATION TO STARVATION

The above discussion highlighted nutritional factors that influence physiologic adaptation to starvation. This section deals with the biochemical mechanisms that could mediate this adaptation.

Energy Metabolism

The adaptive reduction in REE during energy restriction is caused by alterations in the peripheral metabolism of thyroxine (T_4), the hormone secreted by the thyroid gland, to its more active metabolite, triiodothyronine (T_3), and perhaps, to a lesser extent, by changes in sympathetic nervous system activity (85, 148, 175, 216, 217). Serum T_4 levels and those of thyrotropin (the pituitary hormone that regulates T_4 secretion) remain normal, but serum T_3 decreases within a few days (or even hours) of initiating a starvation diet. Serum levels of an inactive metabolite, reverse T_3, rise. Both energy intake and, specifically, the amount of carbohydrate consumed affect this conversion process, apparently through their effect on insulin secretion (175, 218). Although an association clearly exists between decreased circulating T_3 and lowered REE during starvation, its precise nature is not well understood (85, 175), nor is T_3 the only modulating factor. Thus, a carbohydrate-free diet that provides maintenance energy reduces T_3 levels, but the resting metabolic rate does not decrease (219). Poorly controlled diabetes mellitus is associated with decreased serum T_3 levels, but the metabolic rate is increased (220).

In uncomplicated starvation, and especially if volume depletion has been prevented (221), catecholamine secretion and turnover decrease, as measured in the blood and urine of humans and in the organs of laboratory animals (144, 153). The blood pressure, heart rate, and core temperature of starving patients are reduced as is their thermic response to cold or to a norepinephrine infusion. Pupil size, an indicator of basal sympathetic tone, is diminished (139, 144, 176). As with T_4 to T_3 conversion, both energy balance and carbohydrate intake, at least in part because they stimulate insulin release, are important regulators of these effects. The thyroid and catecholamine effects are interconnected (153). T_3 increases the number of tissue norepinephrine receptors, and in its absence, the number decreases (222).

It has been common, when attempting to identify the factors responsible for changes in energy metabolism, to divide the measured REE value by body weight or FFM, on the assumption that a change in REE/FFM implies a change in metabolism at the cellular level (Fig. 41.2). Unless FFM is constant, however, this procedure is prone to error. First, while normal resting (and total) energy expenditure can be accurately predicted from the FFM, the body's FFM is inhomogeneous with respect to its energy-producing elements (223, 224) and these are lost in different proportions in starvation (225). Secondly, even though FFM accurately predicts normal REE over a wide range of FFM, the equation is of the form REE = E(0) + B · FFM, where E(0) is a constant nonzero energy factor (the *y* intercept), and B is the proportionality factor relating increasing FFM and REE. Dividing REE by FFM incorrectly diminishes the effect of E(0) on REE and does so in biased fashion, since larger values of FFM diminish this constant more. As a result, REE/FFM increases as FFM decreases, even when REE is in precise agreement with the predictive equation (226, 227). The importance of the error introduced by this incorrect normalizing technique depends on the relative sizes of E(0) and B. In analyses in which FFM is appropriately adjusted for by use of covariate analysis, adjusted REE is reduced in adapted starving patients (228, 229).

Protein Metabolism

Tissue protein synthesis is regulated to a large extent by the supply of amino acids, whereas the kinetics of the enzymes that catabolize amino acids are such that transamination and oxidation increase linearly with increasing tissue concentrations. As a consequence, body protein synthesis is sensitive to amino acid intakes within the adaptation range of protein provision, while amino acids consumed in excess of synthesis are rapidly catabolized (116, 149). In confirmation, whole-body studies consistently find that leucine oxidation is roughly proportional to its plasma concentration when leucine or protein intakes are above the requirement level (230).

Few measurements of whole-body protein turnover have been carried out in chronically starved nonobese individuals. On the basis of these studies (127, 178), the results of animal experiments, and extrapolations from the literature on weight reduction and short-term protein deficiency, it may be concluded that adaptation to starvation reduces protein turnover in most body tissues (107, 116, 231, 232). It also appears that the major nutritional regulator of protein turnover is protein intake itself. Thus, very low energy (500 kcal) reducing diets that include generous amounts of high-quality protein (58, 233, 234) maintain protein turnover, whereas fasting (57, 58) or low-energy diets that are low in protein (or provide only low-quality protein) dramatically reduce it (55, 233).

As with energy expenditure, the contribution of a reduced lean tissue mass to slowing of whole-body protein turnover during starvation cannot be discerned simply by dividing a whole-body turnover parameter by body weight or FFM (235). Protein turnover proceeds at different rates in different lean tissue compartments (236), and these compartments are depleted to different extents during starvation (3). Also, as with energy expenditure, any equation relating body weight or FFM to basal protein turnover is likely to have a nonzero *y* intercept (226, 227). Thus, in a recent study of adults with chronic energy deficiency, whole-body protein turnover per kilogram FFM was higher than that of normal adults. This was attributed to the markedly greater loss of slowly turning over skeletal muscle than of rapidly turning over central proteins in these adapted starving persons (225).

Many hormonal changes occur in starvation (218, 237), but our understanding of how these changes govern adaptive changes in protein metabolism remains incomplete. T_3 plays a role in the regulation of muscle metabolism, but its precise effects in starvation are not yet well defined (162, 175). T_3 levels decrease early in starvation, and T_3 administration to fasting obese subjects increases their body N losses (175), suggesting that the decreased T_3 is important (at least permissively) for successful adaptation. However, the doses of T_3 administered in those studies were physiologically excessive (85). Moreover, the relationship between T_3 and N balance apparent in total fasting studies is less clear when patients on hypocaloric diets are studied (85).

Insulin stimulates protein synthesis and inhibits its breakdown in muscle and in liver, and the absence of insulin reduces protein synthesis and increases proteolysis (24, 59, 238). Even in advanced protein-energy malnutrition, carbohydrate intake stimulates enough insulin release to prevent ketosis and the acute catabolic state characteristic of early fasting (7, 151). A milder reduction of insulin effect does occur, however (239), and this (in combination with reduced dietary amino acid delivery) curtails tissue protein synthesis (116) and, secondarily, proteolysis (162). The combination of reduced insulin and amino acid cellular action could be expressed both directly on the cells and indirectly, by diminishing the peripheral action of thyroid hormone (162).

It has been known for many years that protein or energy restriction and catabolic states reduce circulating concentrations of the protein anabolic peptide hormone, insulin-like growth factor-1 (IGF-1). This occurs despite increased serum concentrations of growth hormone, which normally stimulates IGF-1 release (240, 241). Structurally related to insulin, IGF-1 stimulates net protein synthesis in cultured cells and in isolated muscle in a manner similar to insulin (24). Much information about IGF-1 and its nutritional interactions has become available in recent years (242–246). Despite the complexity implied by IGF-1's autocrine and paracrine functions and its six plasma binding proteins (IGFBP), IGF-1 is clearly important in the adaptation of protein metabolism to altered nutritional states, acting in combination with (and modulated by) insulin and thyroid hormone (247, 248).

IGF-1 is synthesized in many tissues, but most of the IGF-1 found in the bloodstream is released by the liver, where it circulates as part of a large ternary complex with IGFBP-3 (244, 245). Serum total IGF-1 thus corresponds closely to the serum IGFBP-3 concentration (245). The IGF-1–IGFBP-3 complex is too large to leave the circulation, but IGF-1 complexes with other binding proteins, notably IGFBP-1, which are much smaller and readily enter the extracellular space; presumably they deliver IGF-1 from the circulation to its tissue receptors (240, 245). The circulating half-life of the IGF-1–IGFBP-3 complex is more than 12 hours, and its plasma concentration changes only sluggishly, whereas IGFBP-1 turns over very rapidly in the circulation, and its serum levels increase dynamically in humans by as much as seven-fold (249) in response to short-term fasting or pathologic insulin deficiency and rapidly decrease following glucose or food consumption or in response to insulin administration in diabetic persons. These changes are due to both changes in hepatic release and clearance from the circulation (245).

In human studies, both energy and protein intake affect IGF-1 levels. When dietary energy is severely restricted, the amount of carbohydrate eaten is a major determinant of the circulating IGF-1 response to growth hormone stimulation (240, 250). In the rat, short-term protein restriction reduces hepatic IGF-1 mRNA (251) and increases its clearance from the circulation (246); serum IGF-1 levels decrease and IGFBP-1 levels increase in protein-restricted humans (240, 252). A specific role for IGFBP-2 in the metabolic adaptation to protein restriction has been suggested (251, 252).

In summary, the level (and quality) of protein intake appears to be the key external regulator of adaptation of protein metabolism to starvation, since it provides the substrate (or lack of it) for protein synthesis. Both energy and protein restriction evoke an intricate, coordinated hormonal response, mediated by insulin, growth hormone, IGF-1, and thyroid hormone, that reorganizes amino acid traffic to bring about an orderly adaptation to the altered nutritional environment (253). Under favorable conditions, this adaptation progressively reduces the maintenance protein requirement until it matches protein intake. The adaptation is partly automatic (because the lean tissue mass has decreased) and partly regulated, since a lower rate of protein synthesis and breakdown in the remaining lean tissues allows more efficient processing of dietary protein and recycling of endogenous amino acids.

DEATH

Adult body protein content is normally about 12 kg, half of it being structural, and the other half intracellular lean tissue protein. Lean tissue loss in the range of 50% is considered incompatible with survival (88, 182, 187, 254). BMI is a better predictor than body weight of the certainty of death. Data analyzed by Henry (255) suggest that death is certain when the BMI falls below about 13 in men and 12 in women, but more recent experience in Somalia indicates that a BMI of 10 is compatible with life in mature adults, and even lower BMIs can be tolerated by young adults (199). One-fifth of starving adults over age 25 and nearly one-half of those under age 25 admitted to a medical unit for treatment of terminal starvation had BMIs below 12. Survival with a BMI this low is rare on hospital wards, where advanced starvation typically occurs in older persons as the consequence of a primary medical or surgical condition. This further confirms the importance of the interaction among malnutrition, age, and disease in causing starvation-related death.

In developed countries where severe malnutrition is almost always associated with a primary medical or surgical disease, the immediate causes of death are infectious pneumonia (related to decreased ventilatory mechanical function and drive, lung stasis, and ineffective cough); skin breakdown with local and systemic infection (related to inactivity, skin thinning, and edema); sepsis spreading from intravenous infusion catheters; diarrhea with dehydration; or synergistic worsening of the primary disease.

Contributing to all these causes is starvation-induced immunodeficiency, itself the result of decreased mobilizable protein stores, hypothermia, anemia, and any of several possible micronutrient deficiencies (2, 3). In some patients, death is attributed to a cardiac arrhythmia (139, 256).

In summary, the nature and tempo of the primary disease strongly, but not solely, determine death in moderate starvation. As lean tissue depletion approaches and exceeds about 40%, death directly due to starvation becomes increasingly more certain. This thermodynamic law is unaffected by the number of diagnostic procedures, operative interventions, or antibiotic combinations administered to the patient, unless they are combined with nutritional therapy (257).

Descriptions of needless death from starvation evoke dismay in most commentators. Particularly moving are the writings of Fliederbaum, whose observations in the Warsaw ghetto probably provide the best clinical description of the effects of severe starvation ever published (181):

> Boys and girls from blooming like roses change into withered old people. One of the patients said, "Our strength is vanishing like a melting wax candle." Active, busy, energetic people are changed into apathetic, sleepy beings, always in bed, hardly able to get up to eat or to go to the toilet. Passage from life to death is slow and gradual, like death from physiological old age. There is nothing violent, no dyspnea, no pain, no obvious changes in breathing or circulation. Vital functions subside simultaneously. Pulse rate and respiratory rate get slower and it becomes more and more difficult to reach the patient's awareness, until life is gone. People fall asleep in bed or on the street and are dead in the morning. They die during physical effort, such as searching for food, and sometimes even with a piece of bread in their hands.

REFEEDING

The refeeding syndrome may develop in severely wasted patients during the first week of nutritional repletion (200, 258–262). Expansion of the extracellular fluid volume is rapid and considerable, frequently producing dependent edema; it results from increased sodium intake combined with the antinatriuretic effect of insulin stimulated by the increased carbohydrate consumption. This aspect of the syndrome can be minimized by limiting sodium intake during refeeding (263). Refeeding (especially with carbohydrate) can stimulate enough glycogen synthesis to lower serum phosphate and potassium concentrations. Refeeding also increases REE and, when combined with protein, stimulates N retention, new cell synthesis, and cellular rehydration (263, 264). Depletions of phosphate, potassium, magnesium, and vitamins occur commonly in this setting (200, 258, 261), and unless mineral status is judiciously monitored during refeeding, acute deficiencies, especially of phosphorus or potassium, may occur. Less apparent deficiencies may merely prevent an anabolic response to refeeding (170, 171, 201). Left heart failure may occur, especially in predisposed patients. The ingredients for heart failure are an abrupt increase of the intravascular volume, increased REE (which increases demand for cardiac output), an atrophic left ventricle with a poor stroke volume (139, 265), and myocardial deficiencies of potassium, phosphorus, or magnesium. Cardiac arrhythmias may occur (266). Acute thiamin deficiency is a potential hazard.

REE returns toward normal (and energy needs correspondingly increase) as the sum of two processes: *(a)* the hypometabolic state of adapted starvation reverses, causing an important increase in REE within the first week of refeeding (264, 267, 268), and *(b)* REE gradually increases as the lean tissue mass is rebuilt.

Circulating IGF-1 levels, which are reduced in all forms of starvation, increase rapidly within days to a week of refeeding in concert with improving N balance (240, 252, 269). Because T_3 potentiates growth hormone–induced expression of mRNA for IGF-1 (247) and stimulates IGF-1 release from the liver (270), the refeeding effect could be mediated by insulin-stimulated rises in T_3 (162).

The specific changes in body composition induced by refeeding are determined by the existing metabolic state and body composition and, importantly, by the composition of the refeeding diet (271–273). A diet high in sodium and carbohydrate predisposes to large increases in extracellular volume and edema. A low-protein, high-energy refeeding diet brings about fat gain without an increase in the lean tissue mass (263). A high-protein diet (e.g., 2 g/kg body weight/day) can arrest ongoing N losses, even when energy balance is negative (160). A high-energy, high-protein diet will replete both fat and lean tissue stores at a rate that can be predicted with reasonable accuracy from the resulting energy and N balances, both of which can be measured or estimated. Activity is a factor because it increases energy needs and, more importantly, exercises muscles. Malnourished patients with limited mobility will increase their central protein stores, which confers an important benefit, but they cannot be expected to gain muscle mass unless their muscles are exercised (272, 274, 275). The catabolic effect of metabolic stress reduces or prevents protein accretion during protein and energy provision, even if energy balance is positive; the patient will simply gain fat (276). For severely stressed patients, the best attainable objective of nutritional intervention is often cessation of ongoing protein catabolism; but this in itself may be life saving.

Several features of the refeeding process are illustrated by a clinical trial in which various protein levels were fed sequentially to severely starved men (263). When the diet was generous in energy (2250 kcal/day) but low in protein (27 g/day), the patients' weight, body fat, and serum cholesterol increased, but N balance remained nearly zero; their serum albumin, blood hematocrit, and urinary creatinine excretion failed to increase even after 45 days of refeeding. When the low-protein diet was replaced by one providing 100 g protein, daily N balance became positive by 7 g (equivalent to a daily lean tissue accretion of 200 g). After 45 days on this diet, BMI had increased to normal, serum albumin was nearly normal, and creatinine excretion had increased by 40%. Ninety days of the 100-g protein diet were required before serum albumin, BMI, and blood hemoglobin were fully normalized.

In general, the steps in refeeding severely malnourished patients are as follows. After normalizing fluid and electrolyte parameters and maintaining them, if necessary, by continuing supplementation, a mixed diet is provided at the maintenance energy level to establish tolerance and avoid the refeeding syndrome. Even at this level of energy provision N balance will become positive (157). Energy intake is then increased to create a positive energy balance to promote fat regain and accelerate protein accretion. A generous protein intake (1.5–2.0 g/kg of existing adult body weight) promotes the most rapid repletion of body protein at any energy level (157, 161). Protein intakes substantially greater than this confer no additional advantage to the adult and could be dangerous (199).

REFERENCES

1. Jelliffe DB. J Pediatr 1959;54:227–56.
2. Golden MHN, Jackson AA. Chronic severe undernutrition. In: Olson RE, Brosquist HP, Chichester CO, et al., eds. Present knowledge in nutrition. 5th ed. Washington, DC: The Nutrition Foundation, 1984;57–67.
3. Rivers JPW. The nutritional biology of famine. In: Harrison GA, ed. Famine. Oxford: Oxford University Press, 1988;57–106.
4. Bachrach LK, Katzman DK, Litt IF, et al. J Clin Endocrinol Metab 1991;72:602–6.
5. Beisel WR. Am J Clin Nutr 1995;62:813–9.
6. Cahill GF Jr. Diabetes 1971;20:785–99.
7. Aoki TT, Muller WA, Brennan MF, et al. Am J Clin Nutr 1975;28:507–11.
8. Billings JA. J Am Geriatr Soc 1985;33:808–10.
9. Phillips PA, Rolls BJ, Ledingham JGG, et al. N Engl J Med 1984;311:753–9.
10. Aronson HB, Horne T, Blondheim SH, et al. Isr J Med Sci 1979;15:833–5.
11. Horne T, Gutman A, Blondheim SH, et al. Isr J Med Sci 1982;18:591–5.
12. Sullivan RJ Jr. J Gen Intern Med 1993;8:220–7.
13. McCann RM, Hall WJ, Groth-Juncker A. JAMA 1994;272: 1263–6.
14. Fainsinger R, Bruera E. J Palliat Care 1994;10:55–9.
15. Gamble JL. Harvey Lectures 1947;43:247–73.
16. Cahill GF Jr. Clin Endocrinol Metab 1976;5:397–415.
17. Lusk G. The science of nutrition. 4th ed. Philadelphia: WB Saunders, 1928.
18. Felig P. Starvation. In: DeGroot LJ, Cahill GF Jr, Odell WD, et al., eds. Endocrinology. New York: Grune & Stratton, 1979;1927–40.
19. Nilsson LH, Hultman E. Scand J Clin Lab Invest 1973;32: 325–30.
20. Rothman DL, Magnusson I, Katz LD, et al. Science 1991;254:573–6.
21. Petersen KF, Price T, Cline GW, et al. Am J Physiol 1996;270:E186–91.
22. Landau BR, Wahren J, Chandramouli V, et al. J Clin Invest 1996;98:378–85.
23. Jungas RL, Halperin ML, Brosnan JT. Physiol Rev 1992;72: 419–48.
24. Kettelhut IC, Wing SS, Goldberg AL. Diabetes Metab Rev 1988;4:751–72.
25. Foster DW, McGarry JD. N Engl J Med 1983;309:159–69.
26. Owen OE, Caprio S, Reichard GA Jr, et al. Clin Endocrinol Metab 1983;12:359–79.
27. Hultman E, Nilsson LH. Nutr Metab 1975;18(Suppl 1):45–64.
28. Sugden MC, Sharples SC, Randle PJ. Biochem J 1976;160: 817–9.
29. Cahill GF Jr, Herrera MG, Morgan AP, et al. J Clin Invest 1966;45:1751–69.
30. Nair KS, Woolf PD, Welle SL, et al. Am J Clin Nutr 1987;46:557–62.
31. Eriksson LS, Olsson M, Bjorkman O. Metabolism 1988;37: 1159–62.
32. Streja DA, Steiner G, Marliss EB, et al. Metabolism 1977; 26:1089–98.
33. Hasselbalch SG, Knudsen GM, Jakobsen J, et al. J Cereb Blood Flow Metab 1994;14:125–31.
34. Endemann G, Goetz PG, Edmond J, et al. J Biol Chem 1982;257:3434–40.
35. Balasse EO, Fery F. Diabetes Metab Rev 1989;5:247–70.
36. Haymond MW, Karl IE, Clarke WL, et al. Metabolism 1982;31:33–42.
37. Redies C, Hoffer LJ, Beil C, et al. Am J Physiol 1989;256: E805–10.
38. Owen OE, Morgan AP, Kemp HG, et al. J Clin Invest 1967;46:1589–95.
39. McGarry JD, Woeltje KF, Kuwajmi M, et al. Diabetes Metab Rev 1989;5:271–84.
40. Robinson AM, Williamson DH. Physiol Rev 1980;60:143–87.
41. Fulop M. Diabetes Metab Rev 1989;5:365–78.
42. Mahoney CA. Am J Kidney Dis 1992;20:276–80.
43. Schade DS, Eaton RP. Diabetes 1979;28:5–10.
44. Miles JM, Haymond MW, Nissen SL, et al. J Clin Invest 1983;71:1554–61.
45. Halperin ML, Cheema-Dhadli S. Diabetes Metab Rev 1989;5: 321–36.
46. Bliss M. The discovery of insulin. Toronto: McLelland & Stewart, 1982.
47. Reifenstein ECJ, Albright F, Wells SL. J Clin Endocrinol 1947;5:367–95.
48. Krzywicki HJ, Consolazio CF, Matoush LO, et al. Am J Clin Nutr 1968;21:87–97.
49. Sapir DG, Chambers NE, Ryan JW. Metabolism 1976;25: 211–20.
50. FAO/WHO/UNU Expert Consultation. Energy and protein requirements. Technical report series no. 724. Geneva: World Health Organization, 1985.
51. Crim MC, Munro HN. Proteins and amino acids. In: Shils ME, Olson JA, Shike M, eds. Modern nutrition in health and disease. 8th ed. Philadelphia: Lea & Febiger, 1994;3–35.
52. Lariviere F, Wagner DA, Kupranycz D, et al. Metabolism 1990;39:1270–7.
53. Umpleby AM, Scobie IN, Boroujerdi MA, et al. Eur J Clin Invest 1995;25:619–26.
54. Giesecke K, Magnusson I, Ahlberg M, et al. Metabolism 1989;38:1196–200.
55. Vazquez JA, Morse EL, Adibi SA. J Clin Invest 1985;76:737–43.
56. Henson LC, Heber D. J Clin Endocrinol Metab 1983; 57:316–9.
57. Hoffer LJ, Forse RA. Am J Physiol 1990;258:E832–40.
58. Winterer J, Bistrian BR, Bilmazes C, et al. Metabolism 1980;29:575–81.

59. Abumrad NN, Williams P, Frexes-Steed M, et al. Diabetes Metab Rev 1989;5:213–26.
60. Jefferson LS. Diabetes 1980;29:487–96.
61. Cahill GF Jr. JPEN J Parenter Enteral Nutr 1981;5:281–7.
62. Palaiologos G, Felig P. Biochem J 1976;154:709–16.
63. Nair KS, Welle SL, Halliday D, et al. J Clin Invest 1988; 82:198–205.
64. May ME, Buse MG. Diabetes Metab Rev 1989;5:227–45.
65. Biden TJ, Taylor KW. Biochem J 1983;212:371–7.
66. Tracey KJ, Legaspi A, Albert JD, et al. Clin Sci 1988;74:123–32.
67. Drenick EJ. The effects of acute and prolonged fasting and refeeding on water, electrolyte, and acid-base metabolism. In: Maxwell MH, Kleeman CR, eds. Clinical disorders of fluid and electrolyte metabolism. New York: McGraw Hill, 1980;1481–501.
68. Shetty PS, Watrasiewicz KE, Jung RT, et al. Lancet 1979; 2:230–2.
69. Hoffer LJ, Bistrian BR, Young VR, et al. Metabolism 1984;33: 820–5.
70. Barrett PVD. JAMA 1971;217:1349–53.
71. Weinman EJ, Eknoyan G, Suki WN. J Clin Invest 1975; 55:283–91.
72. Corvilain B, Abramowicz M, Fery F, et al. Am J Physiol 1995;269:G512–7.
73. Drenick EJ. Weight reduction by prolonged fasting. In: Bray GA, ed. Obesity in perspective: John E. Fogarty International Center for Advanced Study in the Health Sciences. DHEW publ no. NIH 75-708. Bethesda, MD: NIH, 1973;341–60.
74. Stunkard AJ, Rush J. Ann Intern Med 1974;81:526–33.
75. Contaldo F, Presto E, Di Biase G, et al. Int J Obes 1982; 6:97–100.
76. Van Itallie TB, Yang M-U. N Engl J Med 1977;297:1158–61.
77. Grande F, Keys A. Body weight, body composition and calorie status. In: Goodhart RS, Shils ME, eds. Modern nutrition in health and disease. 6th ed. Philadelphia: Lea & Febiger, 1980;3–34.
78. Garrow JS. Am J Clin Nutr 1982;35:1152–8.
79. Hood VL. Fluid and electrolyte disturbances during starvation. In: Kokko JP, Tannen RL, eds. Fluids and electrolytes. Philadelphia: WB Saunders, 1986;712–41.
80. Nilsson LH. Scand J Clin Lab Invest 1973;32:317–23.
81. Olsson K-E, Saltin B. Acta Physiol Scand 1970;80:11–8.
82. Hoffer LJ. Starvation. In: Shils ME, Olson JA, Shike M, eds. Modern nutrition in health and disease. 8th ed. Philadelphia: Lea & Febiger, 1994;927–49.
83. Peret J, Jacquot R. Nitrogen excretion on complete fasting and on a nitrogen-free diet—endogenous protein. In: Bigwood EJ, ed. Protein and amino acid functions. Oxford: Pergamon Press, 1972;73–118.
84. O'Connell RC, Morgan AP, Aoki TT, et al. J Clin Endocrinol Metab 1974;39:555–63.
85. Gelfand RA, Hendler R. Diabetes Metab Rev 1989;5:17–30.
86. Vazquez JA, Kazi U, Madani N. Am J Clin Nutr 1995;62: 93–103.
87. Bolinger RE, Luker BP, Brown RW, et al. Arch Intern Med 1966;118:3–8.
88. James WPT, Ferro-Luzzi A, Waterlow JC. Eur J Clin Nutr 1988;42:969–81.
89. Goodman MN, Lowell B, Belur E, et al. Am J Physiol 1984;246:E383–90.
90. Leiter LA, Marliss EB. JAMA 1982;248:2306–7.
91. Friedl KE, Moore RJ, Martinez-Lopez LE, et al. J Appl Physiol 1994;77:933–40.
92. Thomson TJ, Runcie J, Miller V. Lancet 1966;2:992–6.
93. Barnard DL, Ford J, Garnett ES, et al. Metabolism 1969;18:564–9.
94. Stewart WK, Fleming LW. Postgrad Med J 1973;49:203–9.
95. Drenick EJ, Joven CB, Swendseid ME. N Engl J Med 1966;274:937–9.
96. Devathasan G, Koh C. Lancet 1982;Nov 13:1108–9.
97. Frommel D, Gautier M, Questiaux E, et al. Lancet 1984; 1:1451–2.
98. Carpenter KJ. Protein and energy: a study of changing ideas in nutrition. New York: Cambridge University Press, 1994.
99. Millward DJ, Pacy PJ. Clin Sci 1995;88:597–606.
100. Young VR. J Nutr 1994;124:1517S–23S.
101. Zello GA, Wykes LJ, Ball RO, et al. J Nutr 1995;125:2907–15.
102. Fuller MF, Garlick PJ. Annu Rev Nutr 1994;14:217–41.
103. Waterlow JC. What do we mean by adaptation? In: Blaxter K, Waterlow JC, eds. Nutritional adaptation in man. London: John Libbey, 1985;1–11.
104. Young VR, Marchini JS. Am J Clin Nutr 1990;51:270–89.
105. Castaneda C, Charnley JM, Evans WJ, et al. Am J Clin Nutr 1995;62:30–9.
106. Barac-Nieto M, Spurr GB, Lotero H, et al. Am J Clin Nutr 1978;31:23–40.
107. Waterlow JC. Annu Rev Nutr 1986;6:495–526.
108. Young VR, Bier DM, Pellett PL. Am J Clin Nutr 1989;50: 80–92.
109. Millward J. J Nutr 1994;124:1509S–16S.
110. Lariviere F, Kupranycz D, Chiasson J-L, et al. Am J Physiol 1992;263:E173–9.
111. Motil KJ, Matthews DE, Bier DM, et al. Am J Physiol 1981;240:E712–21.
112. Hoerr RA, Matthews DE, Bier DM, et al. Am J Physiol 1993;264:E567–75.
113. Kelman L, Saunders SJ, Frith L, et al. Am J Clin Nutr 1972;25:1174–8.
114. Marchini JS, Cortiella J, Hiramatsu T, et al. Am J Clin Nutr 1993;58:670–83.
115. Oratz M, Rothschild MA. The influence of alcohol and altered nutrition on albumin synthesis. In: Rothschild MA, Oratz M, Schreiber SS, eds. Alcohol and abnormal protein synthesis. New York: Pergamon Press, 1975;343–72.
116. Eisenstein RS, Harper AE. J Nutr 1991;121:1581–90.
117. McNurlan MA, Pain VM, Garlick PJ. Biochem Soc Trans 1980;8:283–5.
118. Munro HN, Hubert C, Baliga BS. Regulation of protein synthesis in relation to amino acid supply—a review. In: Rothschild MA, Oratz M, Schreiber SS, eds. Alcohol and abnormal protein biosynthesis. New York: Pergamon Press, 1975;33–66.
119. Jefferson LS, Flaim KE. Role of amino acid availability in the regulation of liver protein synthesis. In: Blackburn GL, Grant JP, Young VR, eds. Amino acids: metabolism and medical applications. Boston: John Wright PSG, 1983;167–82.
120. Brodsky IG, Robbins DC, Hiser E, et al. J Clin Endocrinol Metab 1992;75:351–7.
121. Pacy PJ, Price GM, Halliday D, et al. Clin Sci 1994;86:103–18.
122. Quevedo MR, Price GM, Halliday D, et al. Clin Sci 1994;86: 185–93.
123. Stuart CA, Shangraw RE, Peters EJ, et al. Am J Clin Nutr 1990;52:509–14.
124. Goodship THJ, Mitch WE, Hoerr RA, et al. J Am Soc Nephrol 1990;1:66–75.
125. Zello GA, Telch J, Clarke R, et al. J Nutr 1992;122:1000–8.
126. Pannemans LE, Halliday D, Westerterp KR, et al. Am J Clin Nutr 1995;61:69–74.
126a. Brodsky IG, Devlin JT. Am J Physiol 1996;270:E148–57.
127. Castaneda C, Dolnikowski GG, Dallal GE, et al. Am J Clin Nutr 1995;62:40–8.
128. Waterlow JC. Annu Rev Nutr 1995;15:57–92.

129. Newsholme EA, Stanley JC. Diabetes Metab Rev 1987; 3:295–305.
130. Price GM, Halliday D, Pacy PJ, et al. Clin Sci 1994;86:91–102.
131. Millward DJ, Rivers JPW. Eur J Clin Nutr 1988;42:367–93.
132. Scrimshaw NS, Hussein MA, Murray E, et al. J Nutr 1972; 102:1595–604.
133. Munro HN. General aspects of the regulation of protein metabolism by diet and hormones. In: Munro HN, Allison JB, eds. Mammalian protein metabolism, vol 1. New York: Academic Press, 1964;381–481.
134. Munro HN. Free amino acid pools and their regulation. In: Munro HN, ed. Mammalian protein metabolism, vol 4. New York: Academic Press, 1970;299–386.
135. Bergstrom J, Furst P, Noree L-O, et al. J Appl Physiol 1974;36:693–7.
136. Waterlow JC, Fern EB. Free amino acid pools and their regulation. In: Waterlow JC, Stephen JML, eds. Nitrogen metabolism in man. London: Applied Science Publishers, 1981;1–16.
137. Garlick PJ, McNurlan MA, Ballmer PE. Diabetes Care 1991;14:1189–98.
138. Golden BE, Golden MH. Eur J Clin Nutr 1992;46:697–706.
139. Keys A, Brozek J, Henschel A, et al. The biology of human starvation. Minneapolis: University of Minnesota Press, 1950.
140. Kotler DP, Wang J, Pierson RN Jr. Am J Clin Nutr 1985; 42:1255–65.
141. Collins S. JAMA 1996;276:391–5.
142. Ravussin E, Lillioja S, Anderson TE, et al. J Clin Invest 1986;78:1568–78.
143. Foster GD, Wadden TA, Kendrick ZV, et al. Med Sci Sports Exerc 1995;27:888–94.
144. Shetty PS, Kurpad AV. Eur J Clin Nutr 1990;44(Suppl 1):47–53.
145. Minghelli G, Schutz Y, Charbonnier A, et al. Am J Clin Nutr 1990;51:563–70.
146. Leibel RL, Rosenbaum M, Hirsch J. N Engl J Med 1995;332: 621–8.
147. Heyman MB, Young VR, Fuss P, et al. Am J Physiol 1992;263:R250–7.
148. Grande F. Man under caloric deficiency. In: Dill DB, ed. Handbook of physiology, section 4: Adaptation to the environment. Washington, DC: American Physiological Society, 1964;911–37.
149. Young VR, Moldawer LL, Hoerr R, Bier DM. Mechanisms of adaptation to protein malnutrition. In: Blaxter K, Waterlow JC, eds. Nutritional adaptation in man. London: John Libbey, 1985;189–217.
150. Lusk G. Physiol Rev 1921;1:523–52.
151. Smith SR, Pozefsky T, Chhetri MK. Metabolism 1974;23: 603–18.
152. Taveroff A, Hoffer LJ. Metabolism 1993;43:1338–45.
153. Shetty PS. Nutr Res Rev 1990;3:49–74.
154. Elwyn DH, Gump FE, Munro HN, et al. Am J Clin Nutr 1979;32:1597–611.
155. Calloway DH. Energy-protein relationships. In: Bodwell CE, Adkins JS, Hopkins DT, eds. Protein quality in humans: assessment and in vitro estimation. Westport, CT: Avi Publishing, 1981;148–68.
156. Munro HN. Physiol Rev 1951;31:449–88.
157. Elwyn DH. Repletion of the malnourished patient. In: Blackburn GL, Grant J, Young VR, eds. Amino acids: metabolism and medical applications. Boston: John Wright PSG, 1983;359–75.
158. Kinney JM, Elwyn DH. Annu Rev Nutr 1983;3:433–66.
159. Goranzon H, Forsum E. Am J Clin Nutr 1985;41:919–28.
160. Greenberg GR, Jeejeebhoy KN. JPEN J Parenter Enteral Nutr 1979;3:427–32.
161. Shaw SN, Elwyn DH, Askanazi J, et al. Am J Clin Nutr 1983;37:930–40.
162. Millward DJ. Clin Nutr 1990;9:115–26.
163. Velthuis-te Wierik EJM, Westerterp KR, van den Berg H. Int J Obes 1995;19:318–24.
164. Waki M, Kral JG, Mazariegos M, et al. Am J Physiol 1991;261:E199–203.
165. Owen OE. Starvation. In: DeGroot LJ, Besser GM, Cahill GF Jr, et al., eds. Endocrinology. 2nd ed. Philadelphia: WB Saunders, 1989;2282–93.
166. Deriaz O, Fournier G, Tremblay A, et al. Am J Clin Nutr 1992;56:840–7.
167. Piatti PM, Monti F, Fermo I, et al. Metabolism 1994;43: 1481–7.
168. Henry RR, Wiest-Kent TA, Scheaffer L, et al. Diabetes 1986;35:155–64.
169. Donnelly JE, Jacobsen DJ, Whatley JE. Am J Clin Nutr 1994;60:874–8.
170. Rudman D, Millikan WJ, Richardson TJ, et al. J Clin Invest 1975;55:94–104.
171. Knochel JP. Adv Intern Med 1984;30:317–35.
172. Passmore R, Strong JA, Ritchie FJ. Br J Nutr 1958;12:113–22.
173. Williams RJ. Biochemical individuality. New York: John Wiley & Sons, 1956.
174. Hegsted DM. Fed Proc 1963;22:1424–30.
175. Danforth E Jr, Burger AG. Annu Rev Nutr 1989;9:201–27.
176. Golden MHN. Marasmus and kwashiorkor. In: Dickerson JWT, Lee MA, eds. Nutrition and the clinical management of disease. 2nd ed. London: Edward Arnold, 1988;88–109.
177. Millward DJ. Proc Nutr Soc 1979;38:77–88.
178. Tomkins AM, Garlick PJ, Schofield WN, et al. Clin Sci 1983;65:313–24.
179. Lipschitz DA, Mitchell CO. Nutritional assessment of the elderly—special considerations. In: Wright RA, Heymsfield S, eds. Nutritional assessment. Boston: Blackwell Scientific Publications, 1984;131–9.
180. Helweg-Larsen P, Hoffmeyer H, Kieler J, et al. Acta Med Scand 1952;144(Suppl 274):1–460.
181. Fliederbaum J. Clinical aspects of hunger disease in adults. In: Winick M, ed. Hunger disease: studies by the Jewish physicians in the Warsaw ghetto. New York: John Wiley & Sons, 1979;11–44.
182. Grant JP. Clinical impact of protein malnutrition on organ mass and function. In: Blackburn GL, Grant JP, Young VR, eds. Amino acids: metabolism and medical applications. Boston: John Wright, 1983;347–58.
183. Silberman H. Parenteral and enteral nutrition. 2nd ed. Norwalk, CT: Appleton & Lange, 1989.
184. Albrecht R, Pelissier MA, Miladi N, et al. Ann Nutr Metab 1986;30:73–80.
185. Krishnaswamy K. Clin Pharmacokinet 1989;17(Suppl 1): 68–88.
186. Speerhas R. Cleve Clin J Med 1995;62:73–5.
187. Roubenoff R, Kehayias JJ. Nutr Rev 1991;49:163–75.
188. Fischer JE, Ghory MJ. Protein depletion and immunity in the hospitalized patient. In: Wright RA, Heymsfield S, eds. Nutritional assessment. Boston: Blackwell Scientific Publications, 1984;111–29.
189. Buzina R. Am J Clin Nutr 1989;50:172–6.
190. Grimble RF. Clin Sci 1996;91:121–30.
191. Wade S, Bleiberg F, Mosse A, et al. Am J Clin Nutr 1985;42:275–80.
192. Bistrian BR. Nutritional assessment of the hospitalized patient: a practical approach. In: Wright RA, Heymsfield S, eds. Nutritional assessment. Boston: Blackwell Scientific Publications, 1984;183–205.

193. Moldawer LL, Lowry SF. Annu Rev Nutr 1988;8:585–609.
194. Nair KS, Ford GC, Ekberg K, et al. J Clin Invest 1995;95: 2926–37.
195. Latham MC. Protein-energy malnutrition. In: Brown ML, ed. Present knowledge in nutrition. 6th ed. Washington, DC: International Life Sciences Institute–Nutrition Foundation, 1990;39–46.
196. Bistrian BR. JPEN J Parenter Enteral Nutr 1990;14:329–34.
197. Jelliffe DB, Jelliffe EF. Pediatrics 1992;90:110–3.
198. Mayatepek E, Becker K, Gana L, et al. Lancet 1993;342: 958–60.
199. Collins S. Nature Med 1995;1:810–4.
200. McMahon MM, Farnell MB, Murray MJ. Mayo Clin Proc 1993;68:911–20.
201. Wolman SL, Anderson GH, Marliss EB, et al. Gastroenterology 1979;76:458–67.
202. Khanum S, Alam AN, Anwar I, et al. Eur J Clin Nutr 1988;42:709–14.
203. Garrel DR, Delmas PD, Welsh C, et al. Metabolism 1988;37: 257–62.
204. Hoffer LJ, Taveroff A, Schiffrin A. Am J Physiol 1997;272: E59–67.
205. Nelson KA, Walsh D, Sheehan FA. J Clin Oncol 1994;12: 213–25.
206. Ollenschlaeger G, Konkol K, Wickramanayake PD, et al. Am J Clin Nutr 1989;50:454–9.
207. Jeejeebhoy KN, Detsky AS, Baker JP. JPEN J Parenter Enteral Nutr 1990;14:193S–6S.
208. Garby L. World Rev Nutr Diet 1990;61:173–208.
209. James WPT, Ralph A. Eur J Clin Nutr 1994;48(Suppl 3):S1–202.
210. Shetty PS, James WP. FAO Food Nutr Pap 1994;56:1–57.
211. Veterans Affairs Total Parenteral Nutrition Cooperative Study Group. N Engl J Med 1991;325:525–32.
212. ASPEN Board of Directors. JPEN J Parenter Enteral Nutr 1993;17:1SA–52SA.
213. Okabe K. Intern Med 1993;32:837–42.
214. Detsky AS, Smalley PS, Chang J. JAMA 1994;271:54–8.
215. American Dietetic Association. J Am Diet Assoc 1994;94: 902–7.
216. Palmblad J, Levi L, Burger A, et al. Acta Med Scand 1977;201:15–22.
217. Fricker J, Rozen R, Melchior J-C, et al. Am J Clin Nutr 1991;53:826–30.
218. Becker DJ. Annu Rev Nutr 1983;3:187–212.
219. Phinney SD, Bistrian BR, Wolfe RR, et al. Metabolism 1983;32:757–68.
220. Pittman CS, Suda AD, Chambers JB Jr, et al. Metabolism 1979;28:333–8.
221. Welle S. Am J Clin Nutr 1995;62:1118S–22S.
222. Bilezikian JP, Loeb JN. Endocr Rev 1983;4:378–88.
223. Weinsier RL, Schutz Y, Bracco D. Am J Clin Nutr 1992; 55:790–4.
224. Elia M. Nutr Res Rev 1991;4:3–31.
225. Soares MJ, Piers LS, Shetty PS, et al. Clin Sci 1994;86: 441–6.
226. Ravussin E, Bogardus C. Am J Clin Nutr 1989;49:968–75.
227. Allison DB, Paultre F, Goran MI, et al. Int J Obes 1995;19:644–52.
228. Luke A, Schoeller DA. Metabolism 1992;41:450–6.
229. Scalfi L, Di Biase G, Coltorti A, et al. Eur J Clin Nutr 1993; 47:61–7.
230. Young VR, Meredith C, Hoerr R, et al. Amino acid kinetics in relation to protein and amino acid requirements: the primary importance of amino acid oxidation. In: Garrow JS, Halliday D, eds. Substrate and energy metabolism in man. London: John Libbey, 1985;119–34.
231. Rennie MJ, Harrison R. Lancet 1984;1:323–5.
232. Wykes LJ, Fiorotto M, Burrin DG, et al. J Nutr 1996;126: 1481–8.
233. Garlick PJ, Clugston GA, Waterlow JC. Am J Physiol 1980;238:E235–44.
234. Hoffer LJ, Bistrian BR, Young VR, et al. J Clin Invest 1984;73:750–8.
235. Carbonnel F, Messing B, Darmaun D, et al. Metabolism 1995;44:1110–5.
236. Tessari P, Garibotto G, Inchiostro S, et al. J Clin Invest 1996;98:1481–92.
237. Crim MC, Munro HN. Protein-energy malnutrition and endocrine function. In: DeGroot LJ, Cahill GF Jr, Odell WD, et al., eds. Endocrinology. New York: Grune & Stratton, 1979;1987–2000.
238. Jefferson LS, Flaim KE, Peavy DE. Protein metabolism. In: Ellenberg M, Rifkin H, eds. Diabetes mellitus, theory and practice. 12th ed. New York: New Hyde Park: Medical Examination Publishing, 1983;47–59.
239. Hoogwerf BJ, Laine DC, Greene E. Am J Clin Nutr 1986;43:350–60.
240. Clemmons DR, Underwood LE. Annu Rev Nutr 1991; 11:393–412.
241. Sullivan DH, Carter WJ. J Am Coll Nutr 1994;13:184–91.
242. Langford KS, Miell JP. Eur J Clin Invest 1993;23:503–16.
243. Jones JI, Clemmons DR. Endocr Rev 1995;16:3–34.
244. Adamo ML. Diabetes Rev 1995;3:2–27.
245. Bach LA, Rechler MM. Diabetes Rev 1995;3:38–61.
246. Ketelslegers J-M, Maiter D, Maes M, et al. Metabolism 1995;44:50–7.
247. Tollet P, Enberg B, Mode A. Mol Endocrinol 1990;4:1934–42.
248. Fryburg DA, Barrett EJ. Diabetes Rev 1995;3:93–112.
249. Shishko PI, Dreval AV, Abugova IA, et al. Diabetes Res Clin Pract 1994;25:1–12.
250. Snyder DK, Clemmons DR, Underwood LE. J Clin Endocrinol Metab 1989;69:745–752.
251. Strauss DS, Takemoto CD. Endocrinology 1990;127:1849–60.
252. Smith WJ, Underwood LE, Clemmons DR. J Clin Endocrinol Metab 1995;80:443–9.
253. Millward DJ, Rivers JPW. Diabetes Metab Rev 1989;5:191–211.
254. Heymsfield SB, McManus CB III, Seitz SB, et al. Anthropometric assessment of adult protein-energy malnutrition. In: Wright RA, Heymsfield S, eds. Nutritional assessment. Boston: Blackwell Scientific Publications, 1984;27–82.
255. Henry CJK. Eur J Clin Nutr 1990;44:329–35.
256. Isner JM, Roberts WC, Heymsfield SB, et al. Ann Intern Med 1985;102:49–52.
257. Kotler DP, Tierney AR, Wang J, et al. Am J Clin Nutr 1989; 50:444–7.
258. Solomon SM, Kirby DF. JPEN J Parenter Enteral Nutr 1990;14:90–7.
259. Foxx-Orenstein A, Jensen GL. Nutr Rev 1990;48:406–13.
260. Graham GG. N Engl J Med 1993;328:1058–61.
261. Bowling TE, Silk DB. Nutrition 1995;11:32–4.
262. Mehler PS. Hosp Pract 1996;31:109–13.
263. Barac-Nieto M, Spurr GB, Lotero H, et al. Am J Clin Nutr 1979;32:981–91.
264. Grande F, Anderson JT, Keys A. J Appl Physiol 1958;12:230–8.
265. Webb JG, Kiess MC, Chan-Yan CC. Can Med Assoc J 1986;135:753–8.
266. Fisler JS. Am J Clin Nutr 1992;56:230S–4S.

267. Vaisman N, Rossi MF, Corey M, et al. Eur J Clin Nutr 1991;45:527–37.
268. Obarzanek E, Lesem MD, Jimerson DC. Am J Clin Nutr 1994;60:666–75.
269. Donahue SP, Phillips LS. Am J Clin Nutr 1989;50:962–9.
270. Ikeda T, Fujiyama K, Hoshino T, et al. Ann Nutr Metab 1990;34:8–12.
271. Heymsfield SB, Casper K. Am J Clin Nutr 1988;47:900–10.
272. Loprinzi CL, Schaid DJ, Dose AM, et al. J Clin Oncol 1993;11:152–4.
273. Royall D, Greenberg GR, Allard JP, et al. JPEN J Parenter Enteral Nutr 1995;19:95–9.
274. Russell JD, Mira M, Allen BJ, et al. Am J Clin Nutr 1994;59:98–102.
275. Gray-Donald K, Payette H, Boutier V. J Nutr 1995;125:2965–71.
276. Moldawer LL, Copeland EM III. Cancer 1997;79:1828–39.

SELECTED READINGS

Fliederbaum J. Clinical aspects of hunger disease in adults. In: Winick M, ed. Hunger disease: studies by the Jewish physicians in the Warsaw ghetto. New York: John Wiley & Sons, 1979;11–44.

Helweg-Larsen P, Hoffmeyer H, Kieler J, et al. Famine disease in German concentration camps: complications and sequels. Acta Med Scand 1952;144(Suppl 274);1–460.

Rivers JPW. The nutritional biology of famine. In: Harrison GA, ed. Famine. Oxford: Oxford University Press, 1988;57–106.

Waterlow JC. Metabolic adaptation to low intakes of energy and protein. Annu Rev Nutr 1986;6:495–526.

42. Nutrition and the Chemical Senses

RICHARD D. MATTES

During the Paleolithic era, the perpetual search for sustenance regularly presented humans the daunting challenge of distinguishing food from nonfood or suffering dire consequences. With the cultivation of plants, domestication of animals, and control of fire, Neolithic peoples had the luxury of expressing their sensory preferences. Decisions about an item's wholesomeness and palatability were, and still are, aided by the human chemosensory systems of taste, smell, and chemesthesis (chemically stimulated somatosensory sensation).

Much of the early interest in olfaction focused on its functions (1). In many cultures (e.g., Egyptian, Greek, Arab) odors were ascribed religious significance, thought to sway sexual behavior, and believed to reflect and influence health status. Theophrastus, a student of Aristotle, recognized that olfaction was both a means of locating food in the environment and a gatekeeper for its ingestion. Odors facilitate selection of nutritious and appealing items, prompt rejection of many others, and initiate digestive processes. Historically, Western interest in taste was primarily concerned with its physiology (e.g., the existence and number of taste primaries). The first treatise formally considering the mechanisms of taste dates back to the Greek physician Alcmaeon in the middle of the 6th century BC (2). It has long been recognized that taste is strictly a contact sense, with a limited repertoire of perceptual qualities (e.g., sweet, sour, salty, bitter) relative to olfaction, but it serves as the final checkpoint before a voluntary decision is made to internalize a substance.

U.S. interest in the sensory properties of foods expanded in the 1940s because of heightened concern about the morale and health of the military during the war effort as well as mounting complaints by consumers who indicated that changes in the food industry were compromising the sensory quality of products. Given the increased consumer demand for products with attributes (e.g., reduced fat, sugar, salt and/or energy) that facilitate attainment of various health goals without sacrificing sensory quality, there is an unprecedented level of activity in the fields of sensory evaluation (focus on the sensory properties of foods) and psychophysics (focus on the perceptual abilities of individuals). Nevertheless, understanding of the nutritional implications of the chemical senses remains wanting.

OVERVIEW OF THE ANATOMY AND PHYSIOLOGY OF THE CHEMICAL SENSES

The flavors of foods are an amalgam of input from all sensory systems. Each system is distinct anatomically, has different functional characteristics, and contributes unique information. Variations in any one source of input will alter the overall perceived flavor of a food, much as the loss of a single piece can alter the appearance of a jigsaw puzzle. Such variations may be innate or acquired. The prevalence of innate selective olfactory and gustatory deficits in individuals with otherwise normal senses of smell and taste is high (>50% of the population) (3). The incidence of acquired selective losses due to, for example, pathologies or medication use is not known. Temporary losses attributable to perceptual adaptation following exposure to selected sensory stimuli are common. These conditions contribute to individual perceptual variability and virtually ensure that no food is experienced in quite the same way by any two individuals. The mechanisms underlying these individual differences are not well characterized but probably involve alterations in the anatomy and/or physiology of the sensory systems as described below.

Gustation

In mammals, the gustatory system comprises specialized epithelial cells located on the tongue, soft palate, pharynx, epiglottis, larynx, and upper one-third of the esophagus, as well as the components of the peripheral and central nervous system (CNS) that transmit and decode electrical signals generated in the taste cells. On the tongue, taste cells coalesced in onion-shaped taste buds occur in fungiform, foliate, and circumvallate papillae. Combined, taste cells represent less than 1% of the lingual epithelium.

The fungiform papillae are mushroom-shaped structures (appearing as red bumps) on the anterior two-thirds of the tongue. There are typically 100 to 200 fungiform papillae on a tongue, each containing 0 to 20 taste buds, with a mean of about 3. Taste cells in these structures receive innervation from the chorda tympani nerve (lingual branch of the facial nerve, cranial nerve VII). Foliate papillae appear as 2 to 9 folds on the posterior lateral margins of the tongue and contain an average of 120 taste buds per papilla. These structures are innervated anteriorly by the chorda tympani nerve and by the glossopharyngeal nerve (lingual branch of cranial nerve IX) posteriorly. Eight to 12 circumvallate papillae are arranged in a "V" configuration on the posterior dorsal tongue. Each papilla is surrounded by a trench where 200 to 250 taste buds are arranged in tiers on the lower two-thirds of the papillae. These taste cells are innervated by the glossopharyngeal nerve. Taste buds on the epiglottis are innervated by the superior laryngeal branch of the vagus nerve (cranial nerve X). The greater superficial petrosal nerve subserves taste buds on the soft palate (4, 5). All gustatory neurons initially synapse in the nucleus of the solitary tract. Projections to other sites where additional coding occurs remain poorly characterized in humans.

The responsivity of taste cells to sapid stimuli varies in different regions of the oral cavity. However, subjective reports and electrophysiologic recordings following stimulation of single taste cells with varying taste qualities demonstrate that individual cells and regions respond to multiple taste qualities (6). Consequently, damage to a specific region of the tongue or to a specific gustatory nerve does not result in loss of responsivity to a specific taste quality.

Whether taste is a synthetic or analytic sense has yet to be resolved. The former view holds that there are taste primaries, commonly identified as sweet, salty, sour, and bitter (although the Japanese include *umami*, or "meat flavor"), which in combination can account for the full range of taste sensations. Vision is an example of a synthetic sense where combinations of three primaries result in all possible colors. The analytical view is that there are multiple tastes that, even in combination, are distinguishable. Audition is an example of an analytic sense.

Chemosensory transduction mechanisms are just being elucidated in humans. Perception of saltiness probably involves passage of sodium through amiloride-sensitive ion channels in the apical end of taste cells and other channels in the basolateral membrane. A role for voltage-dependent ion channels in the apical membrane remains a possibility as well.

Organic and inorganic acids are perceived as sour. The most widely accepted mechanism involves proton inhibition of outward-going potassium channels. Protons can also pass through amiloride-sensitive channels.

Sweet taste is elicited by a wide array of substances including sugars, glycosides and modified sugars, D-amino acids, peptides, proteins, coumarins, dihydrochalcones, ureas and other nitrogenous compounds, substituted aromatic substances, and selected salts. Whether a single transduction mechanism can account for the common sensation provided by this diversity of chemical structures is unresolved. The most widely accepted mechanism posits that all sweet compounds possess a hydrogen ion donor and a hydrogen ion acceptor group that form a double-hydrogen-bonded complex with a similarly configured system on the taste receptor. Amiloride-sensitive channels may also contribute to the sensation.

Multiple receptors and transduction mechanisms have been proposed for human bitter taste to account for the broad diversity of substances (e.g., quinine, urea, xanthines, divalent cations, certain amino acids and peptides, modified sugars) eliciting this sensation. Among the better substantiated mechanisms are *(a)* receptor-stimulated G-protein activation of phospholipase C leading to generation of inositol 1,4,5-triphosphate, which causes release of calcium from internal stores and subsequent neurotransmitter release, *(b)* gustducin activation of cAMP phosphodiesterase, which would lead to reduced intracellular cAMP and decreased phosphorylation of basolateral potassium channels, and *(c)* direct potassium-channel blockade (7).

Olfaction

A 2- to 4-cm^2 patch of olfactory epithelium is located at the apex of the superior turbinate. It contains approximately 10^7 receptor cells. These receptor cells are first-order neurons that merge into the olfactory nerve (cranial nerve I), pass through the cribriform plate, and synapse directly with the olfactory bulb. These first-order neurons are unique in two respects: first, they are in direct contact with both the external environment and the CNS, and second, they are capable of regeneration. Given the primacy of their location and susceptibility to damage by volatile environmental toxins, the latter characteristic reflects the importance of the sense and undoubtedly accounts for the preservation of function over much of the life cycle.

Olfactory stimuli consist of volatile molecules, but the characteristics responsible for quality discrimination remain elusive. There are presently two predominant hypotheses. One holds that quality is determined by specificity of receptors for the physicochemical properties of the myriad ambient olfactory stimuli. Recent work has identified a family of genes that appear to code for a large number of putative receptor proteins located on the cilia of olfactory neurons that could provide the basis for quality coding. The other theory argues that physicochemical properties of olfactory stimuli determine their temporal and spatial distribution across the olfactory epithelium and that the pattern of activation of neurons in different areas provides quality information. These views are not mutually exclusive, and human perception may reflect a combination of these mechanisms. Transduction mechanisms are not well characterized but likely involve receptor binding and activation of second-messenger systems (e.g., G proteins, cAMP, cGMP, IP_3) (7).

Chemesthesis

Sensitivity to chemical irritants (e.g., capsaicin, the burning compound in chili peppers) in the oral and nasal cavities is mediated by elements of the somatosensory system. This subpopulation of fibers is often referred to as the "common chemical sense." The primary somatosensory pathway in the nose and mouth is the trigeminal nerve (cranial nerve V), although in the oral cavity the chorda tympani, glossopharyngeal, and vagus nerves also contain fibers that respond to temperature, touch, and/or irritancy. The chemosensitive afferent sensory neurons of this sensory system are believed to comprise subsets of fibers associated with the senses of pain and temperature (8). Input from chemical stimuli is primarily transduced by polymodal nociceptors. However, cold fibers also respond to some chemical irritants such as menthol. Presently, there is only suggestive evidence that warm-sensitive fibers respond to chemical stimuli. While there may be specific protein receptors for some compounds, stimulation probably occurs nonspecifically when irritants disturb neural membranes or act directly upon ion channels.

CHEMOSENSORY DISORDERS

Manifestations

Disorders may present as lost, diminished, distorted, or, rarely, heightened sensation. Losses are termed *ageusia* (taste) or *anosmia* (smell) and may be complete or quality specific. Approximately one-third of individuals reporting to taste and smell centers are anosmic. Ageusia is rare, accounting for less than 1% of patient complaints. Hypogeusia and hyposmia (the most common disorders) are diminutions of sensation that may be generalized or quality specific. Dysgeusia and dysosmia (parosmia) are taste and smell distortions in which individuals experience inappropriate and/or obnoxious sensations to common stimuli. A variant of this problem is phantom tastes or smells—persistent and often unpleasant sensations in the absence of obvious stimuli. This type of problem may greatly affect quality of life. Olfactory and gustatory agnosia refer to an inability to identify or classify odor and taste stimuli, respectively. Hyperosmia and hypergeusia refer to heightened sensation and are rarely encountered.

These disorders may occur alone or in combination. Most patients with a primary chemosensory complaint report that both taste and smell are affected, but this is confirmed in less than 10% of cases. Most have only an olfactory disturbance. Patients are likely confused by their reduced ability to sense the odorous volatiles released from food in the oral cavity via retronasal stimulation. Since the oral cavity is the source of such stimuli, the sensation they evoke is often referred to as a "taste."

Etiologies

Chemosensory disorders have multiple etiologies. Extensive lists and references of implicated pathologies, medications, and toxins have been published (9–12), but over half of patients presenting to taste and smell centers have disorders with one of three causes. The most frequent finding is a link with an upper respiratory tract infection. Presumably, this leads to viral invasion of peripheral nerves, although damage to central structures is also possible. Symptoms may appear suddenly and be persistent or manifest gradually and spontaneously remit. There is no known treatment for abnormalities attributable to viral infection. Damage to peripheral and/or central structures following head trauma accounts for approximately 15 to 20% of patient visits. Aside from cases in which surgical reconstruction can eliminate mechanical barriers to odorant access to the olfactory epithelium, there are no known treatments for chemosensory abnormalities stemming from head trauma. Between 5 and 40% of patients recover olfactory function spontaneously, and the prognosis may be somewhat better for taste. Nasal or sinus disease resulting in obstruction of pathways for odorants to reach the olfactory epithelium accounts for another 15 to 20% of cases. Surgical procedures and steroid sprays to reduce swelling have proven effective in some patients (11). Another 15 to 20% of patient complaints are classified as idiopathic. Most chemosensory disturbances related to pathologies and medications resolve when the underlying illness is effectively treated or the offending medication is discontinued. Marked nutrient imbalances may adversely affect taste and smell but are rarely the primary cause of disorders.

Prevalence

The prevalence of chemosensory abnormalities in the general population is unknown. Data have not been systematically collected, in part due to a lack of standardized evaluation criteria, low awareness by health care workers who thus do not solicit information on these senses when evaluating patients, and incomplete reporting by many affected individuals who do not view the problem as life threatening. However, nearly everyone experiences at least a mild transient abnormality (e.g., reduced olfactory ability associated with a cold), and in some, the problem is severe and chronic.

Health Implications

Abnormalities of taste and/or smell can increase the risk of environmental toxin exposure (since the chemical senses provide an early warning system for such compounds), compromise quality of life, and adversely affect diet and nutritional status. Among individuals presenting at clinical taste and smell centers, approximately 75% report decreased enjoyment of food, and about half report a compensatory alteration of eating patterns. The latter response can be problematic if it involves less healthful dietary choices such as reliance on a limited array of foods or increased use of salt or fat. One recent study noted that elderly women with olfactory dysfunction adopted diets associated with increased cardiovascular risk (13). Fifteen to 20% experience an increase or decrease in body weight exceeding 10% of their predisorder weight (14). Approximately half gain weight owing to increased intake as a means of deriving the missed sensory pleasure foods provide or in an attempt to mask an unpleasant sensation. Others decrease intake, often because food has lost its appeal or is believed to exacerbate an unpleasant sensation. At present, no set of patient or symptom characteristics provides a reliable predictor of a specific dietary response. Thus, dietary intervention must be individualized.

ASSESSMENT OF CHEMOSENSORY FUNCTION

Threshold

The senses of taste and smell convey intensity and quality information about appropriate stimuli. The most traditional measure of function is threshold sensitivity, which may be determined as the "detection" or the "recognition" threshold. The former is the lowest concentration of a stimulus that can be detected in a given medium, and the latter is the lowest concentration that can be recognized with respect to its quality (e.g., NaCl is salty). Taste and odor thresholds are not innate, invariant characteristics of an individual. Rather, they are statistical concepts in which one arbitrarily determines a criterion level of performance (typically 50%) on a task requiring individuals to detect or recognize a stimulus in a given medium. Thresholds are also strongly influenced by methodologic factors.

Intensity and Identification

Intensity ratings reflect the strength of sensation elicited by suprathreshold stimulus concentrations. Assessments of this facet of sensory responsiveness in the oral cavity may be made with whole-mouth stimulation (e.g., sipping and swishing a solution) or by regional stimulation to explore the functional status of the various gustatory nerves. It is argued that intensity ratings are more nutritionally relevant than thresholds, since stimuli are presented at levels more commonly encountered under normal eating conditions. However, attempts to demonstrate associations between intensity ratings and either food preferences or intake have generally been unsuccessful. Suprathreshold concentrations of stimuli are also used in identification tasks in which subjects are asked to indicate the quality of unlabeled simple compounds or foods. Each of these measures provides unique functional information. Correlations between the measures are generally weak.

Time-Intensity

The above measures represent integrated information and fail to recognize that the time course of sensation following chemosensory stimulation varies across stimuli and for a given stimulus in different media. Sensation parameters that vary include onset time, rate of appearance, time to maximal intensity, rate of extinction, and total duration. They can be measured by tracking intensity responses over time. Temporal properties can markedly influence the appeal of foods.

Hedonics

Assessments of food acceptability rely upon higher-order processing of intensity and quality information from the periphery. Commonly evaluated hedonic dimensions include, but are not limited to, the preferred frequency of stimulus intake, preferred concentration of the stimulus in a medium, and preference for stimuli with a characteristic quality.

Hedonic responses to the odors and tastes of foods reflect innate and acquired characteristics. Knowledge of innate taste and odor preferences is rudimentary. Compelling data indicate the appeal of sweetness and saltiness is congenital, although for the latter, there is a postnatal lag of about 6 months before it is apparent (15). Data are less clear for responses to sour and bitter but suggest each is viewed negatively at an early age. Human neonates consistently exhibit a preferential orientation to breast odors from lactating females, suggesting early olfactory preferences. However, in light of recent evidence that maternal diet can influence the sensory qualities of amniotic fluid and breast milk (16), it is not clear whether such early preferences are congenital or attributable to fetal conditioning. The basis for the appeal of dietary fats has not been established. Differential sucking responses to formulas with varying fat content among newborns have been small and inconsistent (17, 18) as have hereditabilty estimates for fat preferences and intake in children and adults (19, 20).

The resistance of immigrants to abandoning the flavor principles of their native diet underscores the importance of culture and learning on flavor preferences. Multiple mechanisms are likely involved, including exposure effects and associative learning. Studies with children and adults demonstrate a direct association between frequency of exposure to novel items and their acceptance ratings (21). However, the time course and magnitude of the effect may reflect an innate bias, predominantly sweet and salty novel foods gain in acceptability more readily than sour or bitter items (22). Exposure frequency can also modify responses to familiar foods. A reduction in sensory exposure to dietary salt and fat leads to a heightened preference for foods with lower salt and fat levels, respectively, compared with ratings from individuals with comparable total intake of each food constituent but higher sensory exposure (23, 24). Preliminary evidence suggests hedonic shifts based on restricted sensory exposure require about 8 to 12 weeks to develop. The extent to which desired shifts in preferred levels of dietary constituents facilitate long-term compliance with therapeutic diets (e.g., reduced sodium or fat) has not been determined.

The flavors of foods also acquire positive and negative properties due to their association with metabolic cues stemming from ingestion. Illness following ingestion of a food can lead to subsequent rejection of the food based on its sensory characteristics. Approximately one-third of the population has held such a food aversion (25). Conditioned preferences have been shown in animals but have been more difficult to demonstrate in humans.

Whether early hedonic responses are innate or learned, the limited available data do not indicate that they predict preferences later in life. This has been documented for selected food constituents such as salt (26) as well as diets. Changes in flavor preferences are marked over the life cycle, as exemplified by early rejection of bitter or spicy foods; yet items with bitter notes (e.g., coffee, alcohol) become highly preferred, and globally, chili peppers are one of the most commonly used flavor principals. Indeed, family studies of food preferences generally reveal a low-order association between parents and offspring and a stronger relationship between peers (27).

Chemesthesis

Perception of chemical irritancy in the oral and nasal cavities is not routinely evaluated in clinical research centers because of the rarity of complaints about this component of the chemical senses. The appeal of chemesthetic stimuli is acquired and a principal component in many cuisines. Although there is a tendency to report diminished taste sensation for foods with a strong chemesthetic stimulus (e.g., capsaicin, piperine) psychophysical studies have yielded equivocal results.

RELATIONSHIPS BETWEEN NUTRIENT INTAKE AND THE CHEMICAL SENSES

There is a reciprocal relationship between nutrient intake and chemosensory function. Peripheral gustatory and olfactory tissues are composed of specialized epithelial cells with relatively high turnover rates (10–12 days for taste and 30–45 days for olfaction) and metabolic requirements. Provision of adequate nutrients is vital for proper function. At the same time, the functional status of these sensory systems can strongly influence food and nutrient intake. Despite longstanding recognition of this association, little is known about the nutrient requirements of these tissues (28).

Effects of Nutritional Status on Chemosensory Function

Vitamin A

Vitamin A deficiency leads to increased keratinization of the oral and nasal epithelia. In addition, decreased mucopolysaccharide synthesis leads to reduced cleansing of the perireceptor area and drying of the epithelia. Blockage of stimulus access to chemosensory receptors ensues (Fig. 42.1). Vitamin A depletion results in a gradual loss of taste in rats (29) that is reversible with vitamin repletion. Chemosensory deficits are not a common feature of vitamin A deficiency in areas where this problem is endemic. However, hypogeusia and hyposmia have been reported in normal adults made vitamin A deficient as well as in patients with cirrhosis, acute viral hepatitis, and malabsorption disorders who were depleted of the vitamin (30). Supplementation with vitamin A reverses these chemosensory losses. It is important to recognize the role of zinc in maintaining normal plasma vitamin A levels, especially among patients with liver disorders. Zinc administration may also reduce taste deficits in alcoholic cirrhosis patients (31). Given the potential toxicity of vitamin A, its probable etiologic role in a sensory disorder must be established before therapeutic supplementation is initiated.

B Vitamins

Studies in dogs reveal that diet-induced deficiencies of niacin, riboflavin, pyridoxine, pantothenic acid, and folic acid result in noninflammatory lesions of the oral mucosa, especially on the dorsal tongue surface (32). Papillary atrophy and degeneration are also observed, particularly on the anterior tongue, although in niacin deficiency, the entire tongue surface may be involved (Fig. 42.2). Fungiform papillae are the most severely affected. No abnormalities have been noted in circumvallate papillae. Pathologic changes worsen progressively with successive deficiency trials. Replacement therapy results in prompt restoration of the epithelium. Improvement is apparent in 2 to 3 days and is complete within a week. Recovery of connective tissue is slower. Distinct lesions are apparent in animals with specific vitamin deficiencies, and these identifiable lesions are superimposed in animals with multiple deficiencies.

Findings similar to those reported in dogs have been observed in humans (33). In addition, deficiencies of pyridoxine, riboflavin, and cobalamin may lead to peripheral

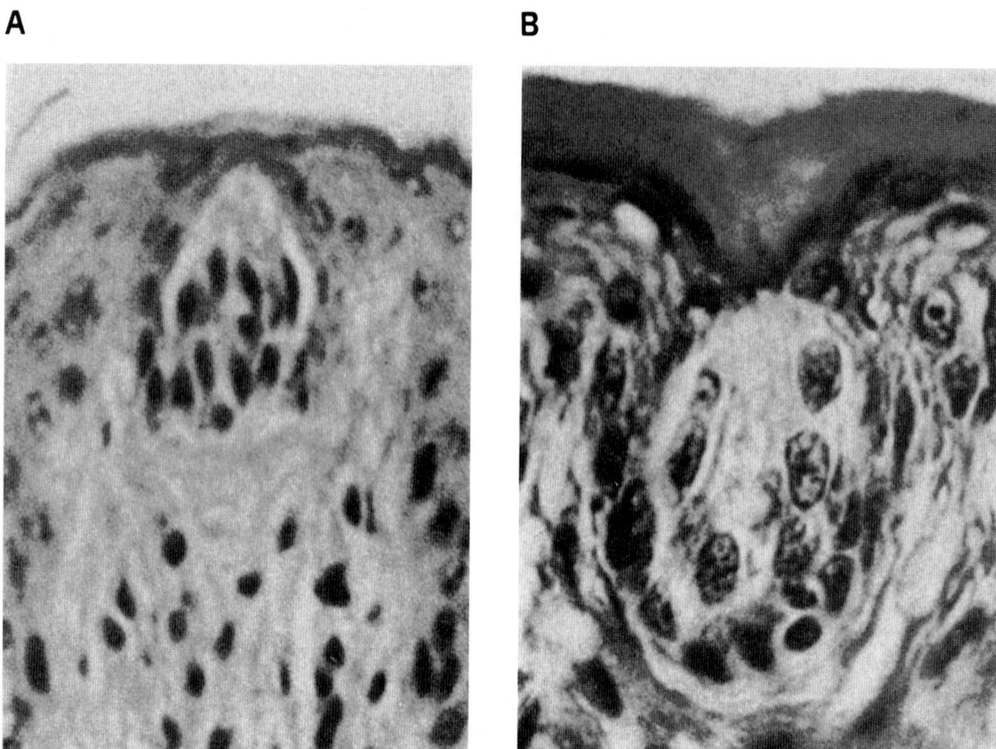

Figure 42.1. A. Longitudinal section of single taste bud in a fungiform papilla from a vitamin A–replete rat. **B.** Comparable section from a vitamin A–deficient rat. The taste bud pore is infiltrated with keratin. (From Bernard RA, Halpern BP. J Gen Physiol 1968;52:444–64, with permission.)

neuropathies. However, this has only been reported in case studies involving severe deficiency (34). Importantly, while repletion of pyridoxine has reportedly corrected chemosensory disturbances in patients with subclinical pellagra (34), high levels of pyridoxine have also been associated with peripheral neuropathy (35). In such patients, nonspecific axonal degeneration was observed, with a loss of sensory nerve action potentials in response to an electromyogram. Thus, indiscriminate use of high levels of B vitamins to treat chemosensory disorders is inappropriate.

Vitamin E

A direct association, but no causal relationship, between plasma vitamin E concentration and papillary atrophy was reported in one study of elderly patients with atrophic glossitis (36). There are no data linking vitamin E status to subjective reports of chemosensory function.

Copper

Reversible hypogeusia has been reported in humans with low ceruloplasmin levels during treatment with penicillamine (37). However, it is not clear that the effect of penicillamine is copper specific. The drug also binds zinc, nickel, and other cations, and zinc has also been reported to improve taste sensitivity in patients treated with this medication. Administration of penicillamine to patients with Wilson's disease does not lead to chemosensory complaints.

Iodine

Diminutions of taste and olfactory sensitivity, or dysgeusias, have been documented in hypothyroid patients (38). The reported incidence of sensory complaints in such patients ranges from a few percent to over 80%. This may be attributable to the generally slow onset of symptoms and consequent lack of subjective awareness. Replacement hormone therapy generally corrects the chemosensory disorder. Treatment of hyperthyroid patients with antithyroid agents (e.g., methimazole, methylthiouracil) has also led to partial or complete loss of taste and smell, which resolves upon cessation of drug use.

Iron

Hypogeusia has been reported in patients with iron deficiency anemia (39). Normalization of iron status with oral iron supplements (50 to 100 mg/day) led to restoration of taste within 2 weeks in most patients and improvement in others. Cravings and pica have been reported in iron-depleted individuals, but there is presently no evidence that this is related to shifts in chemosensory function.

Zinc

Marked zinc deficiency may lead to chemosensory abnormalities (i.e., hypogeusia, hyposmia, distortions) that resolve with zinc repletion (40). Whether sensory dis-

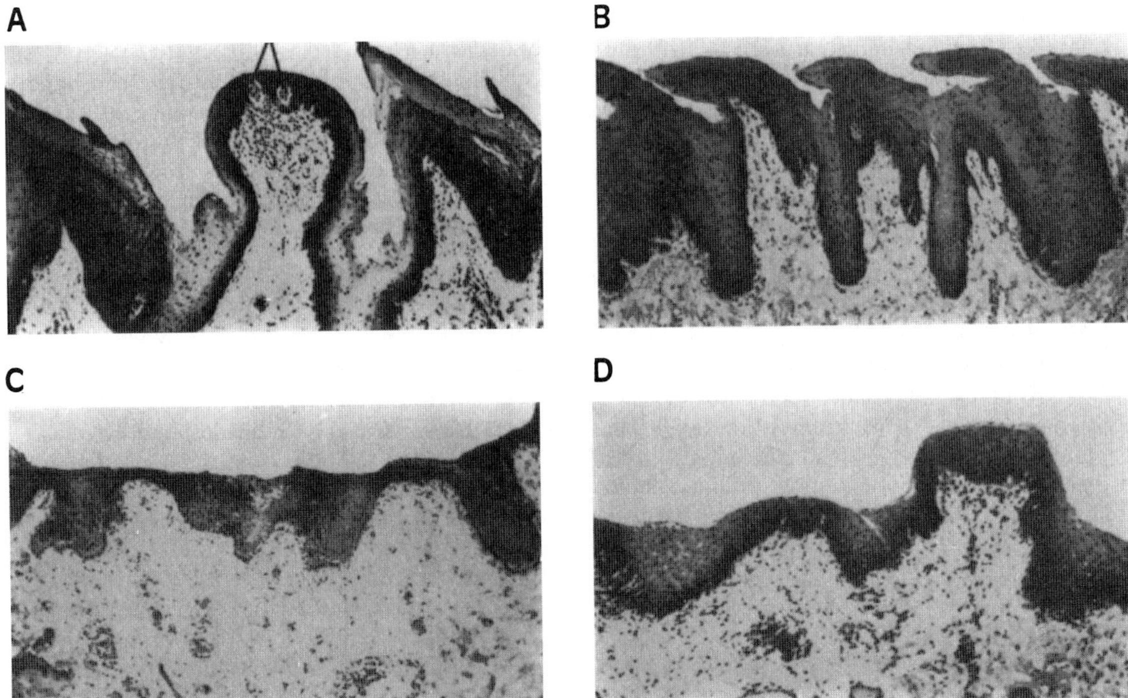

Figure 42.2. A. Longitudinal section of a canine normal fungiform papilla containing two taste buds. On either side of the fungiform papilla are filiform papillae. **B.** Papillary atrophy in a niacin-deficient dog. **C.** Late-stage papillary atrophy in a dog deficient in pyridoxine. **D.** Absence of filiform papillae and atrophied fungiform papillae of a dog made riboflavin deficient for the first time. (From Afonsky D. Ann NY Acad Sci 1960;85:362–7, with permission.)

turbances reported by patients with pathologies involving negative zinc balance or altered zinc metabolism (e.g., acute infectious hepatitis, chronic cirrhosis of the liver, Crohn's disease, chronic renal disease) are attributable to the change in zinc status or other factors remains largely unresolved. Double-blind crossover studies (41, 42) have not supported a causal role for zinc in most patients with chemosensory complaints. Evidence that levels of zinc recommended for use with chemosensory disorders (i.e., 100 mg/day) may lead to anemia, neutropenia, and impaired immune function (43) indicate that this therapeutic approach must only be used with caution.

Heavy Metals

Case studies in humans indicate that accidental exposure to mercury or lead as well as parenteral administration of gold can produce taste abnormalities. The mechanisms in these cases remain unexplored.

The Chemical Senses and Nutrient Utilization

A potential role of sensory stimulation on the digestion, absorption, and utilization of nutrients has been recognized since the work of Pavlov but remains poorly characterized. Sensory, especially chemosensory, stimulation elicits digestive, thermogenic, cardiovascular, and renal responses that anticipate the arrival of food in the gut. They are termed *preabsorptive- or cephalic-phase responses* (44). Examples of such responses are listed in Table 42.1. They are typically small and transient, with unknown nutritional significance. They may play an important priming role that determines the extent of postabsorptive events and the efficacy of nutrient metabolism.

THE CHEMICAL SENSES AND DIET IN SELECTED POPULATIONS

Aging

Statistically significant declines in taste and especially smell sensitivity have been reported in many, but not all, studies of the elderly (57). However, the functional significance of these changes is unclear because the absolute

Table 42.1
Cephalic Phase Responses

System	(Ref)	Increased Response
Salivary	(45)	Flow
Gastric	(46–48)	Acid, gastrin and gut peptide secretion, motility
Pancreatic exocrine	(49, 50)	Lipase, amylase, trypsin, chymotrypsin, total secretion
Pancreatic endocrine	(51–53)	Insulin, glucagon, pancreatic polypeptide
Thermogenic	(54)	Heat production
Cardiovascular	(55)	Heart rate, cardiac output, resistance of mesenteric vasculature
Renal	(56)	Urine volume (decreased osmolality) to hypotonic stimulus

magnitude of decline is small. Data in Figure 42.3, representing an age- and sex-stratified sample of healthy adults, reveal a statistically significant decline in salt taste and phenylethyl alcohol odor thresholds with age, but the more striking feature of these data is the number of elderly with normal function (58). To reconcile this observation with the high level of complaints of diminished sensory abilities by the elderly requires consideration of more subtle aspects of sensory function and testing.

Elderly persons exhibit slower recovery following adaptation to a stimulus, reduced retronasal olfaction (a large component of food flavor), and compromised ability to discriminate stimuli in complex foods. None of these measures is included in standard chemosensory testing regimens. Increased use of medications and a higher prevalence of health disorders that may influence sensory function may also contribute to the belief that aging is associated with marked declines in chemosensory function. Finally, age-related decrements in memory, cognition, and testing skills can result in poorer testing. The decline in taste bud number with age is small, and the number of taste buds is not closely correlated with taste function, since only a small number of buds may provide the full range of sensory experience (much as a small patch of skin can convey temperature information as well as a larger area). Further, receptive structures in one area of the oral cavity compensate for losses of sensation in other areas (59).

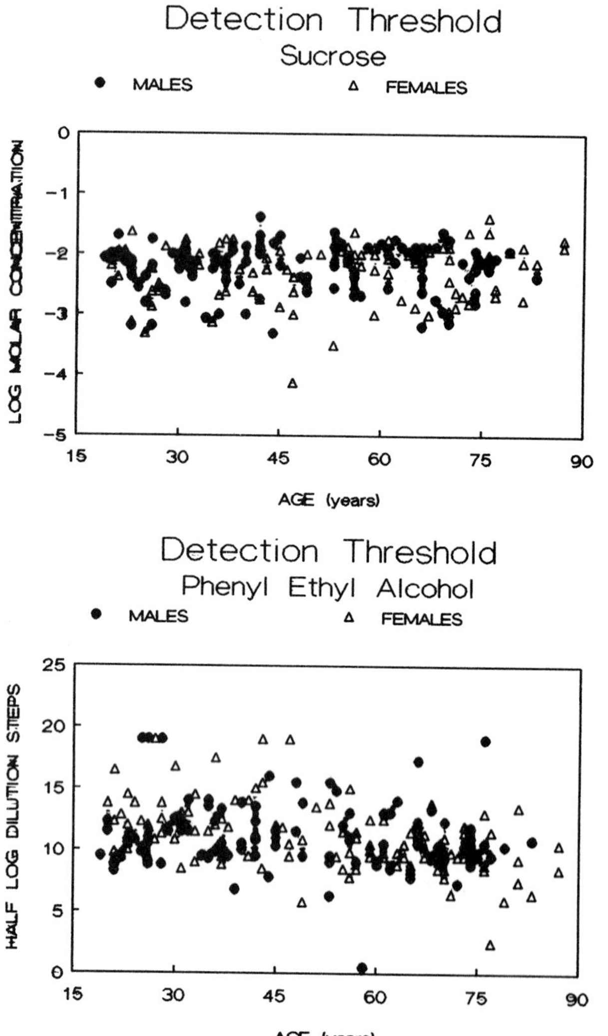

Figure 42.3. *Top,* Scatterplot of sucrose taste-detection thresholds for healthy adults 19 to 87 years of age. *Bottom,* Scatterplot of olfactory detection thresholds of healthy adults 19 to 87 years of age for phenyl ethyl alcohol.

The diversity of influences and variability of their effects on the different sensory systems preclude a standardized treatment approach. Flavor fortification may hold some benefit for individuals with sensory decrements (not loss or distortion), but it requires an individualized plan because changes are often quality-specific and a correct level of fortification for one individual will be excessive or inadequate for another.

Hypertension

The view that sodium intake is related to hypertension has prompted studies of salt taste in various high-risk populations including different classes of hypertensive patients (e.g., low vs. high renin, salt sensitive vs. salt insensitive) and normotensive offspring of hypertensive individuals. Small differences between some of these groups and control subjects on isolated measures of salt taste (i.e., recognition thresholds but not detection thresholds) have been noted. However, most work has failed to reveal any meaningful associations (60, 61). Further, there is no clear evidence for a heightened preference for salt by hypertensive patients. Normotensive and hypertensive individuals exhibit a comparable increment in hedonic responses to reduced-salt foods following adherence to a diet restricted in sensory exposure to the salty taste.

Diabetes

Disturbances of taste and smell have long been recognized in diabetics (62) and may affect over 60% of patients. The most consistent sensory changes involve alterations in glucose taste thresholds among non-insulin-dependent diabetics as well as their nondiabetic first-degree relatives. This suggests a general abnormality of glucose receptors. However, complications of hyperglycemia probably also contribute, since the severity of hypogeusia increases with progressing neuropathy (63). Macrovascular disease and peripheral neuropathy have also been implicated in olfactory disturbances (64, 65). The extent to which these chemosensory changes influence food selection and adherence to prescribed diets has not been established. Diabetic patients and healthy controls show similar decrements in hedonic responses to a sweet solution following a glucose load (66).

Cancer and Bone Marrow Transplantation

Changes of chemosensory function (sensitivity and preferences) are frequently reported by untreated patients with cancer. Systematic study of these complaints has failed to identify any consistent pattern of change with respect to the nature of the sensory complaint (e.g., quality specific vs. general loss, loss vs. distortion) and the site, severity, or duration of pathology. Similarly, no clear association between sensory function and anorexia has been established in this patient population (67, 68). Antineoplastic treatment may be more problematic for the sensory systems than the pathology. Radiotherapy involving gustatory and olfactory tissues results in a profound loss of function because of damage to sensory end organs as well as supporting tissues (e.g., salivary glands) (69, 70). Bitter and salty tastes are often more severely affected than sweet and sour. Impairment is first apparent following an accumulated dose of approximately 20 Gy. A total dose of 60 to 70 Gy may lead to elevated thresholds (i.e., decreased sensitivity) that persist for years (69), whereas suprathreshold function may be less severely affected (71). Among patients with head and neck cancer receiving radiotherapy, there is a strong association between loss of sensory function, anorexia, and weight loss. Altered chemosensory function may also result from chemotherapy regimens, but the impact of these changes on diet are less clear (72).

It is commonly argued that learned food aversions (LFA) contribute to anorexia and weight loss in cancer patients. In untreated cancer patients, the incidence of aversions is about 50%, but following the onset of either chemotherapy or radiotherapy, approximately 50 to 55% of patients form new LFAs. High-protein items are particularly problematic, but any item, including water, may be targeted (73). Typically, treatment-related aversions are specific (a mean of 3–4 items per individual) and transient (often less than 1 month duration); consequently, they hold little dietary significance. Several approaches aimed at preventing formation of LFAs have been explored. First, patients may be counseled to refrain from eating prior to treatments, but evidence that LFAs may form toward items consumed the day before or following treatment indicates such advice is often not practical. Antiemetics administered to reduce the adverse side effects of treatments (the purported conditioning stimulus) have also proven ineffective. One approach that appears promising involves exposing patients to a nutritionally inconsequential food just before their first treatment. This may interfere with formation of LFAs toward wholesome foods in the patient's customary diet. Such an approach has reduced the incidence of treatment-related LFAs by over 30% (74).

Taste sensitivity abnormalities have also been reported following allogeneic bone marrow transplantation (75, 76). Reports note quality-specific effects, with a salt hypogeusia being the most consistent finding. Abnormalities are most pronounced during the acute phase of graft-versus-host disease but may persist for months. The mechanism is not clear, since patients receiving autologous bone marrow transplants experience many of the same oral complications but have no gustatory complaints.

HIV Infection

The human immunodeficiency virus invades the CNS in a large number of infected individuals. This may lead to various neurophysiologic abnormalities, including disturbances of chemosensory function. Reported taste and smell complaints by infected individuals have led to speculation that such symptoms may provide an early index of CNS involvement and contribute to the anorexia often associated with advanced infection. However, assessments of olfactory ability reveal little or no decrement in patients who may or may not be immunocompromised but are otherwise healthy (77, 78). The severity of olfactory complications, most notably odor identification ability, is directly related to progression of disease. The most marked olfactory changes occur in patients with AIDS dementia complex (79). No changes of taste have been reported. Thus, chemosensory changes do not provide a reliable early hallmark of CNS infection. Further, the limited available data do not support a substantive role for chemosensory disturbances in the loss of appetite associated with infection, although this has not been systematically evaluated in patients with AIDS (77).

Obesity

While small differences in sensory responses to aqueous solutions of taste stimuli or experimentally prepared foods have been noted between obese and lean persons (80, 81), the preponderance of evidence fails to support an association between body weight and chemosensory responses (82–84). Differences in the importance and nature of food and flavor preferences are reported more consistently (85) and may lead to erroneous assumptions about sensory function. Few data indicate that sensory responses among the obese actually influence their eating behavior, so the assumption that sensory factors play an etiologic role in the onset or maintenance of obesity is not appropriate.

Chronic Renal Disease and Dialysis

Patient complaints of diminished chemosensory sensation are supported by evidence that taste detection and recognition thresholds are elevated in chronic renal disease (86) and worsen with advancing disease. Concomitant low levels of zinc in some studies and improved sensory function with zinc supplementation (87, 88) prompted hypotheses that this may be the underlying cause. However, additional data show no correlation between zinc status and sensory measures (86, 89, 90) and no therapeutic efficacy of zinc supplementation (91, 92). The conflicting observations may indicate that there is a subset of patients with compromised zinc status who will benefit from supplementation, but many will require alternative approaches. Dialysis typically has no effect on sensory deficits (89, 90, 93, 94). Chemosensory function may improve with renal transplantation but may require up to 1 year (95). The limited published data on hedonic shifts associated with uremia and dialysis are inconsistent (94, 96, 97). The influence of sensory changes on food selection and nutritional status remain poorly characterized.

Smoking

Most evidence indicates that smoking has little effect on taste. Studies of taste thresholds before and immediately after smoking a cigarette (98, 99) or following 2-week periods of enforced increased and decreased smoking frequency (100) reveal no significant differences. Comparisons of chronic smokers and nonsmokers, controlling for recent use, have yielded mixed findings (101–103). Perceived intensity ratings also show little difference between smokers and nonsmokers (100). Studies of taste hedonics have focused on sweetness and have yielded mixed findings (104, 105).

Early work on olfaction showed no significant general elevation of thresholds (98, 106), although sensitivity to pyridine, a substance in tobacco smoke, was lower in smokers (106). Small but significant differences in perceived intensity ratings (107, 108) and odor identification (106) have been reported more recently. Interestingly, for pyridine, the difference was marked only at low concentrations and resolved after 5 days of smoking abstinence (106). These findings indicate that decreased perception of pyridine may be an adaptation effect. Whether the more general effects can be attributed to smoking is questioned by evidence that smokers have elevated thresholds for other sensory modalities (e.g., audition [109]) presumably unaffected by smoking status. Cigar and pipe smoking do not alter test performance. At present there is no evidence supporting a causal role for smoking-related chemosensory changes in the lower body weight of smokers or their weight gain upon cessation of smoking.

REFERENCES

1. Cain WS. History of research on smell. In: Carterette EC, Friedman MP, eds. Handbook of perception. New York: Academic Press, 1978.
2. Bartoshunk LM. History of taste research. In: Carterette EC, Friedman MP, eds. Handbook of perception. New York: Academic Press, 1978.
3. Amoore JE. Chem Sens Flavor 1977;2:267–81.
4. Sandick B, Cardello AV. Chem Sens 1981;6:197–214.
5. Mistretta CM. Gerodontology 1984;3:131–6.
6. Nilsson B. Acta Odont Scand 1977;35:51–62.
7. Kinnamon SC, Getchell TV. Sensory transduction in olfactory receptor neurons and gustatory receptor cells. In: Getchell TV, Doty RL, Bartoshuk LM, Snow JB, eds. Smell and taste in health and disease. New York: Raven Press, 1991;145–72.
8. Green BG. Effects of thermal, mechanical, and chemical stimulation on the perception of oral irritation. In: Green BG, Mason JL, Kare MR, eds. Chemical senses, vol 2, Irritation. New York: Marcel Dekker, 1990.
9. Schiffman SS. Drugs influencing taste and smell perception. In: Getchell TV, Doty RL, Bartoshuk LM, Snow JB, eds. Smell and taste in health and disease. New York: Raven Press, 1991;845–50.
10. Doty RL, Bartoshuk LM, Snow JB Jr. Causes of olfactory and gustatory disorders. In: Getchell TV, Doty RL, Bartoshuk LM, Snow JB, eds. Smell and taste in health and disease. New York: Raven Press, 1991;449–62.
11. Mott AE, Leopold DA. Med Clin North Am 1991;75:1321–53.
12. Rankin KM, Mattes RD. Toxic agents, chemosensory function, and diet. In: Massaro EJ, ed. Handbook of human toxicology. Boca Raton, FL: CRC Press, 1997;347–67.
13. Duffy VB, Backstrand JR, Ferris AM. J Am Diet Assoc 1995;95:879–84.
14. Mattes RD, Cowart BJ. J Am Diet Assoc 1994;94:50–6.
15. Beauchamp GK, Cowart BJ, Moran M. Dev Psychobiol 1986;19:17–25.
16. Mennella JA, Beauchamp GK. Olfactory preferences in children and adults. In: Laing DG, Doty RL, Breipohl W, eds. The human sense of smell. Berlin: Springer-Verlag, 1992;167–80.
17. Chan S, Pollitt E, Leibel R. Infant Behav Dev 1979;2:201–8.
18. Nysenbaum AN, Smart JL. Early Hum Dev 1982;6:205–13.
19. Falciglia GA, Norton PA. J Am Diet Assoc 1994;94:154–8.
20. Oliveria SA, Ellison RC, Moore LL, et al. Am J Clin Nutr 1992;56:593–8.
21. Pliner P, Pelchat M, Grabski M. Appetite 1993;20:111–23.
22. Mattes RD. Physiol Behav 1994:6:1229–36.
23. Bertino M, Beauchamp GK, Engelman K. Am J Clin Nutr 1982;36:1134–44.
24. Mattes RD. Am J Clin Nutr 1993:57:373–81.
25. Mattes RD. Physiol Behav 1991;50:499–504.
26. Whitten CF, Stewart RA. Acta Pediatr Scand 1980;Suppl 279:1–17.
27. Borah-Giddens J, Falciglia GA. J Nutr Educ 1993;25:102–7.
28. Gershoff SN. The role of vitamins and minerals in taste. In: Maller O, Kare MR, eds. The chemical senses and nutrition. New York: Academic Press, 1977.
29. Bernard RA, Halpern BP. J Gen Physiol 1968;52:444–64.
30. Garrett-Laster M, Russell RM, Jacques PF. Hum Nutr Clin Nutr 1984;38C:203–14.
31. Weismann K, Christensen E, Dreyer V. Acta Med Scand 1979;205:361–6.
32. Afonsky D. Ann NY Acad Sci 1960;85:362–7.
33. Afonsky D, Changsha H. Oral Surg Oral Med Oral Pathol 1950;3:1299–327.
34. Green RF. JAMA 1971;218:1303.
35. Schaumburg H, Kaplan J, Windebank A, et al. N Engl J Med 1983;309:445–8.
36. Drinka PJ, Langer EH, Voeks SK, et al. J Am Coll Nutr 1993;12:14–20.
37. Henkin RI, Keiser HR, Jaffe IR, et al. Lancet 1967;II:1268–71.
38. Mattes RD, Heller AD, Rivlin RS. Abnormalities in suprathreshold taste function in early hypothyroidism in humans. In: Meiselman HL, Rivlin RS, eds. Clinical measurement of taste and smell. New York: Macmillan, 1986.
39. Osaki T, Ohshima M, Tomita Y, et al. J Oral Pathol Med 1996;25:38–43.
40. Henkin RI. Biol Trace Element Res 1984;6:263–80.
41. Henkin RI, Schecter PJ, Friedewald WT, et al. Am J Med Sci 1976;272:285–99.
42. Gibson RS, Vanderkooy PDS, MacDonald, AC, et al. Am J Clin Nutr 1989;49:1266–73.
43. Fosmire GJ. Am J Clin Nutr 1990;51:225–7.
44. Brand JG, Cagan RH, Naim M. Annu Rev Nutr 1982;2:249–76.
45. Richardson CT, Feldman M. Am Physiol Soc 1986;250: G85–91.
46. Feldman M, Richardson CT. Gastroenterology 1986;90: 428–33.
47. Katschinski M, Dahmen G, Reinshagen M, et al. Gastroenterology 1992;103:383–91.

48. Wisén O, Björvell H, Cantor P, et al. Regul Pept 1992;39:43–54.
49. Novis BH, Banks S, Marks IN. Scand J Gastroenterol 1971;6: 417–22.
50. Behrman HR, Kare MR. Proc Soc Exp Biol Med 1968;129: 343–6.
51. Teff KL, Levin BE, Engelman K. Am J Physiol 1993;265: R1223–30.
52. Louis-Sylvestre J, LeMagnen J. Neurosci Biobehav Rev 1980;4(Suppl 1):43–6.
53. Teff KL, Devine J, Engelman K. Physiol Behav 1995;57: 1089–95.
54. Diamond P, Brondel L, LeBlac J. Am J Physiol 1985;248: E75–9.
55. Vatner SF, Patrick TA, Higgins CB, et al. J Appl Physiol 1974;36:524–9.
56. Akaishi T, Shingai T, Miyaoka Y, et al. Chem Sens 1991;16:277–81.
57. Murphy C, Cain WS, Hegsted DM. Ann NY Acad Sci 1989;561.
58. Cowart BJ. Ann NY Acad Sci 1989;561:39–55.
59. Kveton JF, Bartoshuk LM. Laryngoscope 1994;104:25–9.
60. Mattes RD. J Chronic Dis 1984;37:195–208.
61. Mattes RD, Falkner B. Chem Sens 1989;14:673–9.
62. Settle RG. Diabetes mellitus and the chemical senses. In: Meiselman HL, Rivlin RS, eds. Clinical measurement of taste and smell. New York: Macmillan, 1986.
63. Abbasi AA. Geriatrics 1981;36:73–8.
64. Weinstock RS, Wright HN, Smith DU. Physiol Behav 1993;53:17–21.
65. Le Floch J-P, Le Lièvre G, Labroue M, et al. Diabetes Care 1993;16:934–7.
66. Bhatia S, Sharma KN. Diebetes Res Clin Pract 1991;12: 193–200.
67. Trant AS, Serin J, Douglass HO. Am J Clin Nutr 1982;36: 45–58.
68. Carson JAS, Gormican A. Research 1977;70:361–5.
69. Mossman K, Shatzman A, Chencharick J. Int J Radiat Oncol Biol Phys 1982;8:991–7.
70. Mossman KL. Br J Cancer 1986;53(Suppl VII):9–11.
71. Schwartz LK, Weiffenbach JM, Valdez IH, et al. Physiol Behav 1993;53:671–7.
72. Bruera E, Carraro S, Roca E, et al. Cancer Treat Rep 1984;68:873–6.
73. Mattes RD, Curran WJ, Alavi J, et al. Cancer 1992;70:192–200.
74. Mattes R. Nutr Cancer 1994;21:13–24.
75. Boock CA, Reddick JE. J Am Diet Assoc 1991;91:1121–2.
76. Marinone MG, Rizzoni D, Ferremi P, et al. Haematologica 1991;76:519–22.
77. Mattes RD, Wysocki CJ, Graziani A, et al. Laryngoscope 1995;105:862–6.
78. Lehrner JP, Kryspin-Exner I, Vetter N. Chem Sens 1995;20: 325–8.
79. Brody D, Serby M, Etieene N, et al. Am J Psychiatry 1991;148: 248–50.
80. Rodin J, Moskowitz HR, Bray GA. Physiol Behav 1976;17: 591–7.
81. Drewnowski A, Brunzell JD, Sande K, et al. Physiol Behav 1985;35:617–22.
82. Spitzer L, Rodin J. Appetite 1981;2:293–329.
83. Frijters JER, Rasmussen-Conrad EL. J Gen Psychol 1982;107:233–47.
84. Pangborn RM, Bos KEO, Stern JS. Appetite 1985;6:25–40.
85. Drewnowski A. Int J Obes 1985;9:201–12.
86. Burge JC, Park HS, Whitlock CP, et al. Kidney Int 1979;15:49–53.
87. Mahajan SK, Prasad AS, Lambujon J, et al. Am J Clin Nutr 1980;33:1517–21.
88. Atkin-Thor E, Goddard BW, O'Nion J, et al. Am J Clin Nutr 1978;31:1948–51.
89. Vreman HJ, Venter C, Leegwater J, et al. Nephron 1980;26: 163–70.
90. Ciechanover M, Peresecenschi G, Aviram A, et al. Nephron 1980;26:20–2.
91. Zetin M, Stone RA. Clin Neurol 1980;13:20–5.
92. Henkin RI, Schechter PJ, Friedewald WT, et al. Am J Med Sci 1976;272:285–99.
93. Conrad P, Corwin J, Katz L, et al. Nephron 1987;47:115–8.
94. Bellisle F, Dartois A-M, Kleinknecht C, et al. J Am Diet Assoc 1990;90:951–4.
95. Mahajan SK, Abraham J, Migdal SD, et al. Transplantation 1984;38:599–602.
96. Shepherd R, Farleigh CA, Atkinson C, et al. Appetite 1987;9:79–88.
97. Shapera MR, Moel DI, Kamath SK, et al. J Am Diet Assoc 1986;86:1359–65.
98. Pangborn RM, Trabue IM, Barylko-Pikielna N. Percept Psychophys 1967;2:529–32.
99. Krut LH, Perrin MJ, Bronte-Stewart B. Br Med J 1961;1:384–7.
100. Pangborn RM, Trabue IM. Percept Psychophys 1973;1: 139–44.
101. Sinnot JJ, Rauth JE. J Gen Psychol 1937;17:151–3.
102. Krut LH, Perrin MJ, Bronte-Stewart B. Br Med J 1961;1:384–8.
103. McBurney DH, Moskat LJ. Percept Psychophys 1975;18:71–3.
104. Perkins KA, Epstein LH, Stiller RL, et al. Pharmacol Biochem Behav 1990;35:671–6.
105. Pomerleau CS, Garcia AW, Drewnowski A, et al. Pharmacol Biochem Behav 1991;40:995–9.
106. Moncrieff RW. Am Perfumer 1957;72:40–3.
107. Ahlström R, Berglund B, Berglund U, et al. Am J Otolaryngol 1987;8:1–6.
108. Frye RE, Schwartz BS, Doty RL. JAMA 1990;263:1233–6.
109. Berglund B, Nordin S. Chem Sens 1992;17:291–306.

SELECTED READINGS

Doty RL. Handbook of olfaction and gustation. New York: Marcel Dekker, 1995.

Getchell TV, Doty RL, Bartoshuk LM, Snow JB, eds. Smell and taste in health and disease. New York: Raven Press, 1991.

Mott AE, Leopold DA. Med Clin North Am 1991;75:1321–53.

43. Fiber and Other Dietary Factors Affecting Nutrient Absorption and Metabolism

DAVID J. A. JENKINS, THOMAS M. S. WOLEVER, and ALEXANDRA L. JENKINS

The Roman God Janus has two faces. Similarly, two opposing treatment strategies have been developed that involve modifying nutrient absorption from the gut. In the treatment of gastrointestinal disease, emphasis has been placed on improving absorption of nutrients in conditions such as Crohn's disease, celiac disease, short bowel and stagnant loop syndromes, radiation enteropathy, postgastrectomy disorders, and Whipple's disease. Other situations, however, involve attempts to reduce the rate or amount of nutrient absorption, including the treatment of diabetes, hyperlipidemia, or obesity with, for example, high-fiber diets, enzyme inhibitors, nonabsorbable food substitutes, or gastric stapling.

Manipulations that increase or decrease the rate of absorption are likely to have certain physiologic consequences, as illustrated in Figures 43.1 and 43.2. When the absorption rate is reduced, a larger length of small intestine is likely to be exposed to the nutrient, with an increased proportion absorbed more distally (see Fig. 43.1*A*). On the other hand, rapidly absorbed foods are likely to be taken up more proximally in the small intestine and over a shorter segment (see Fig. 43.1*B*).

After oral intake, the consequences of a slower flux of nutrient into the system result in lower circulating nutrient levels and thus lower endocrine responses (Fig. 43.2*A*), as opposed to the sharper rises and falls seen with more rapid fluxes (Fig. 43.2*B*). In addition, differences can be expected in nutrient absorption characteristics (e.g., chylomicra synthesis), depending on where in the bowel it takes place. Regional specialization also occurs in terms of gut endocrine responses to nutrients absorbed in different parts of the bowel. For example, more gastric inhibitory polypeptide (GIP) is secreted when carbohydrates are absorbed proximally, and more enteroglucagon is secreted when they are absorbed distally.

The food factors that influence the absorption of nutrients relate not only to the nature of the nutrients themselves, but also to their interaction with each other and with the nonabsorbable components of the food, the complex of substances referred to collectively as dietary fiber, and associated antinutrients. All these factors (Table 43.1) combined produce the form or physical state of the food, which itself exerts a major influence on the handling of a food by the gastrointestinal tract. Some of these effects are short term, but food constituents also have long-term effects. They may influence the absorptive capacity of the gut either by enzyme induction or by effects that may be stimulatory, inhibitory, or toxic to mucosal cell growth, turnover, and villus structure.

EFFECTS OF MACRONUTRIENTS

Before discussing the effects of food form and so-called antinutrients on the absorbability of natural diets, it is useful to consider the similarities and differences within the three macronutrient groupings and their relationships to each other and to fiber.

Carbohydrates

Traditionally, it was held that "complex" carbohydrates (starches) are absorbed more slowly than "simple" carbohydrates (1). Meals containing a higher proportion of their carbohydrates as sugars were considered to result in more rapid absorption and higher increases in blood glucose levels (2). This view was challenged by several studies. Using solutions of starch (a glucose polymer), caloreen

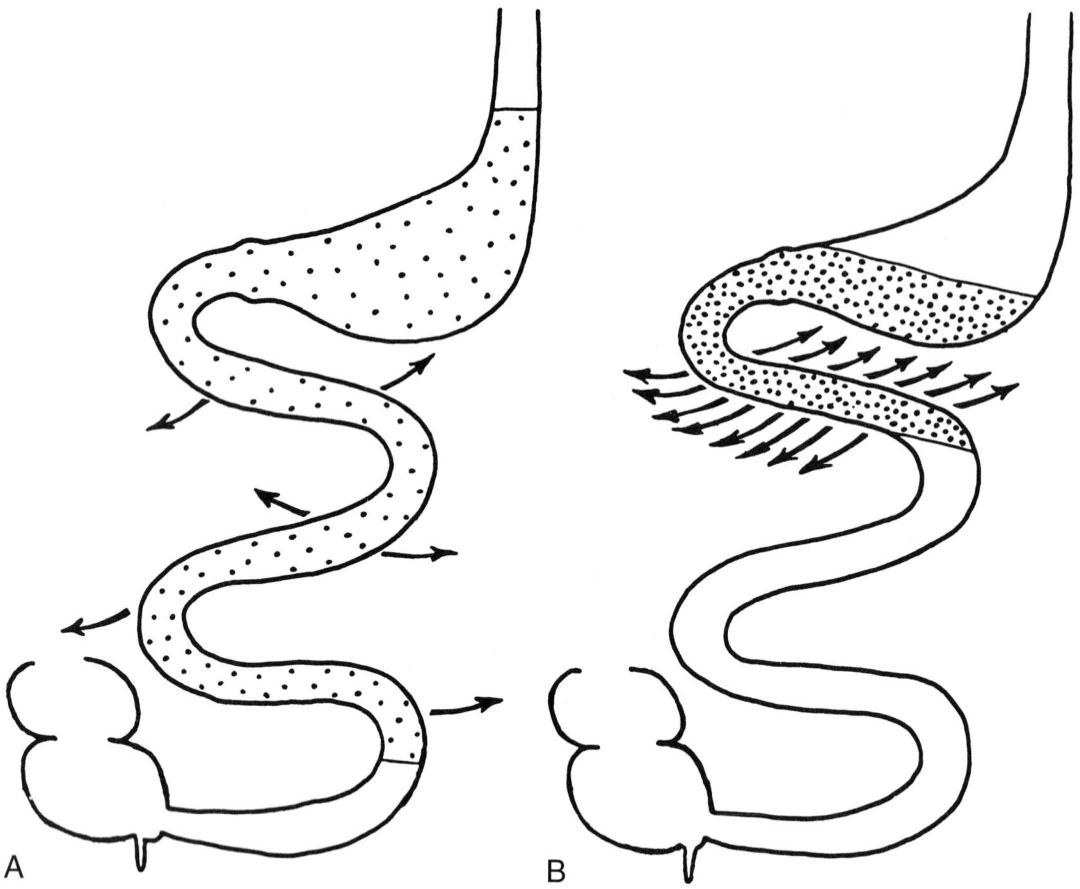

Figure 43.1. Schematic representation of stomach and small intestine showing (**A**) slow digestion and absorption of energy-dilute food in a "fiber-rich" diet and (**B**) rapid digestion and absorption of energy-dense food from a low-fiber diet.

(predominantly 5 glucose units), and glucose itself, Wahlquist et al. demonstrated similar glucose and insulin rises following consumption of 50-g carbohydrate loads of each of these glucose sources by healthy volunteers (3) (Table 43.2).

Starch

Such results should have been predictable because earlier work by Dahlquist and Borgstrom and Fogel and Gray showed that luminal hydrolysis of starch is not rate limiting for starch digestion (4, 5). Fogel and Gray found that even patients with chronic pancreatitis and significant exocrine pancreatic insufficiency (amylase secretion rate 10% of normal) hydrolyzed starch in vivo at a rate similar to that of normal subjects (5). Their studies involved feeding 50-g starch loads and aspirating the residual hydrolytic contents at the ligament of Treitz (duodenojejunal junction). This finding does not indicate that luminal events are unimportant in the digestion of foods of complex composition but that differences in absorption are unlikely among meals containing sugars or highly

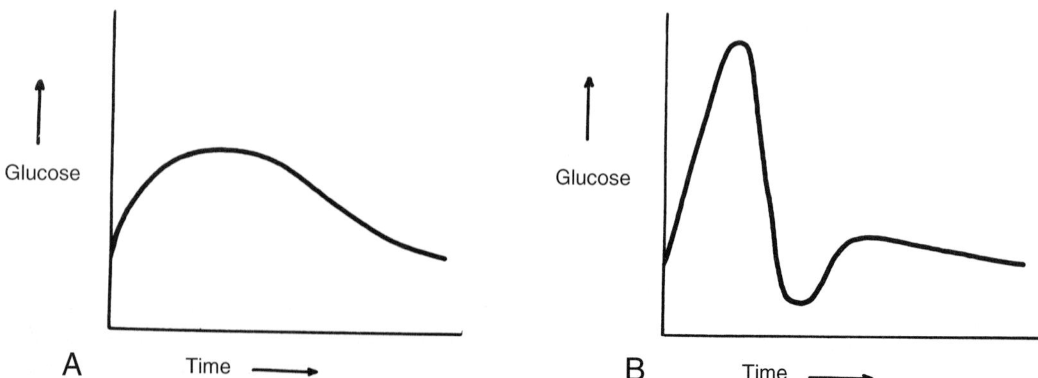

Figure 43.2. Schematic representation of the postprandial glycemia following (**A**) slow absorption of starchy fiber-rich meals and (**B**) rapid absorption with undershoot due to excessive insulin release following refined, fiber-depleted carbohydrate foods.

Table 43.1
Dietary Fiber Components

Classical Nomenclature	Solubility Characteristics	Classes of Polysaccharide
	Water Insoluble	
α-Cellulose	Insoluble in alkali	Cellulose (glucan)
Hemicelluloses	Insoluble in water	Arabinoxylans Galactomannans
	Soluble in alkali	Xyloglucans
Lignin	Insoluble in 12 *M* H_2SO_4 Water Insoluble	Polyphenolpropane Noncarbohydrate
Pectic substances	Water soluble	Galacturonans Arabinogalactans β-Glucans Arabinoxylans
Gums	Water soluble or dispersible	Galactomannans Arabinogalactans
Mucillages	Water soluble or dispersible	Wide range of branched and substituted galactans

After Southgate DAT. Dietary fiber parts of food plants and algae. In: Spiller GA, ed. CRC handbook of dietary fiber in human nutrition. Boca Raton, FL: CRC Press, 1992.

processed, low-amylose, or soluble starches (25–30% amylose and 70–75% amylopectin) (6).

Still, differences in food form or indigestible food components may profoundly affect the rate of luminal digestion. If proportions of amylose (1–4 linked straight-chain starch) and amylopectin (1–6 linked branched starch) vary in a food, alterations in digestibility may be seen. Traditionally, such branching was considered nutritionally significant because α-amylase has poor specificity for 1–6 branch points and produces α-limit dextrins (7). Digestion was considered to proceed more slowly for this reason. However, the brush border α-glucosidases are so efficient that it makes no difference in terms of rates of uptake whether the substrate for absorption is glucose, maltose, or α-limit dextrins (8). Some evidence even indicates that absorption rate increases with chain length up to 10 glucose units (8). Part of the explanation may be related to a reduced osmotic effect.

Table 43.2
Differences in Digestion Rates and Sugars Released from Common Foods[a]

Food	Sugar Concentration (mg/L at 3 h)	Percentage of Total as		
		Glucose	Maltose	Maltotriose
White bread standard	866	6.97	6.61	6.5
Whole wheat bread	811	6.21	7.21	7.2
Rice	652	3.97	1.72	4.4
Corn flakes	954	4.97	3.52	1.7
Porridge oats	424	6.37	6.51	7.3
Spaghetti	583	5.67	3.42	1.0
Potato	638	8.87	4.21	7.1
Mean	707	6.07	4.61	9.4
Kidney beans	263	6.97	9.8	13.3
Chick peas	263	8.77	9.1	12.3
Lentils	258	10.6	84.0	5.4
Mean	261	8.78	81.0	10.3
P[b]	.005	.05	.005	.005

Adapted from Jenkins DJA, Wolever TMS, Thorne MJ, et al. Am J Clin Nutr 1984;40:117.

[a]Mean concentrations and percentages of sugars released into 800 mL dialysate after 3 hours of salivary digestion of 2-g carbohydrate portions of 10 foods.

[b]Significance of difference between beans and other foods.

Differences do exist between amylose and amylopectin, but opposite to those originally expected, perhaps because of the more compact structure and hydrogen bonding of the glucose chains in amylose, which render it physically less accessible to amylolytic attack than the more open and branched amylopectin (9). Raw legume starch (higher in amylose) is less digestible in rats than cornstarch (higher in amylopectin), and the rate of hydrolysis of legume starch in vitro is less than that of cornstarch (10, 11). Possible differences in the nature of starches from different foods have been emphasized by Crapo and coworkers (12–15). In vivo studies of whole legumes (30–40% amylose) show lower glycemic responses than those with cereals (25 to 30% amylose) (16, 17). They are also digested less rapidly in vitro than other starchy foods (18, 19). As expected from their higher amylose content, they produce more glucose and less maltotriose on digestion. Studies with high-amylose long-grain rice demonstrated that the amylose content is related to the glycemic effect of the rice. The greater the amylose content, the flatter the response (20). High-amylose diets reduce insulin secretion and serum lipids in healthy volunteers (21).

The degree of hydration of the starch is a major determinant of digestibility (22), and hydration is a function of both cooking and other forms of processing. Cooked starch produced higher blood glucose responses than raw starch (Fig. 43.3) (23); perhaps because of the degree of gelatinization of starch. Uptake of water by the starch molecule may render it more accessible to enzymatic digestion. In addition, processing (milling) legumes prior to cooking increased digestibility more effectively than grinding after cooking (24), and damp heat was more effective than dry heat in making both the carbohydrate (24–26) and protein (27, 28) more easily absorbed.

Comparisons of legumes and cereal foods illustrate many facets of foods that influence absorbability. Studies have clearly demonstrated the slower digestibility of legumes by comparison with cereal products and the relationship of digestibility with the glycemic response in both normal and diabetic volunteers (19, 29). Such studies also highlight other factors of possible importance, including food form, fiber, and nonnutritive food factors (including the so-called antinutrients) in determining absorbability of carbohydrate from foods.

Today, it is probably useful to divide the starches that are resistant to digestion into three broad classes according to Cummings and Englyst (29a): RS1, RS2, and RS3. RS1 starches may increase starch malabsorption and may be produced by coarse milling or large particle size of

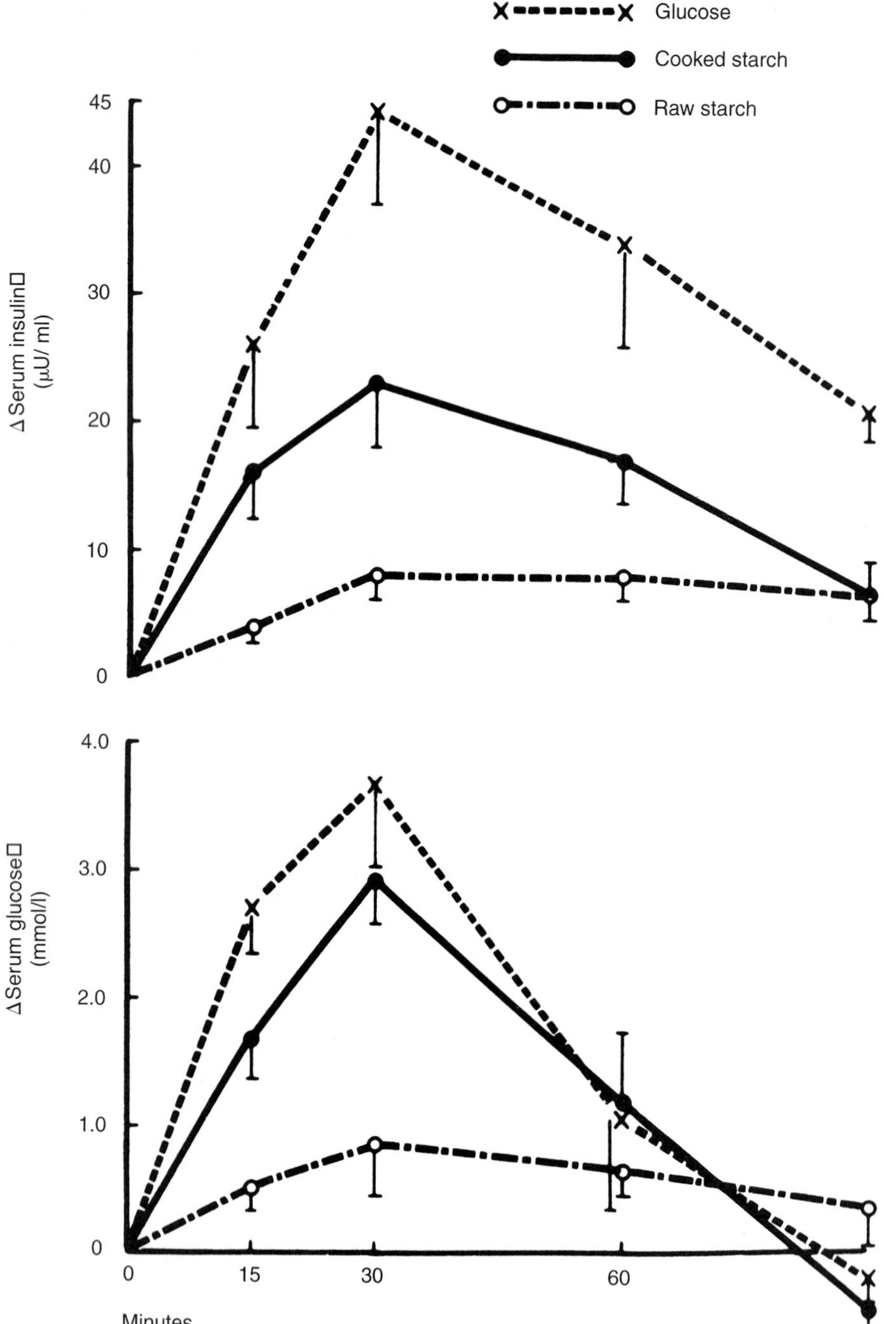

Figure 43.3. Mean serum insulin and glucose concentrations after ingestion of glucose monohydrate (1.1 g/kg body weight) and cooked and raw cornstarch (0.91 g/kg body weight) in healthy volunteers. Conversion (SI to traditional units): glucose, 1 mmol/L ≈ 18 mg/dL. (From Collings P, Williams C, MacDonald I. Br Med J 1981;282:1032.)

cereal grains (e.g., whole-grain pumpernickel bread or bulgar). RS2 starches, resistant starches that are crystalline and resist hydration, are found in green bananas, high-amylose corn, and relatively high amylose legumes (peas, beans, and lentils). Starches, especially high-amylose starches that are cooked and allowed to cool, undergo retrogradation with more-crystalline realignment. These starches are produced in common foods such as potato, rice, and bread and are termed RS3 starches. Resistant starches in this category are produced commercially from high-amylose corn starch (e.g., Novelose) by enzymatically debranching the remaining 1,4-linkages and allowing the resulting 1,6-linked starch to "retrograde" into a highly crystalline, digestion-resistant starch.

Sugars

Efficient transport systems exist for maltose, maltotriose, α-limit dextrins, sucrose, lactose, glucose, and galactose. Fructose absorption is less efficient, and the transport maxima may be exceeded with large amounts of this sugar. The pentose D-xylose is only approximately 50% absorbed, and considerable malabsorption is found with the sugar alcohols, or polyols, sorbitol and xylitol (30).

Therefore, great differences exist among sugars in absorption rate and proportions.

The comparative effects of sugars and starches on metabolic responses have generated much interest. Contrary to many previous assumptions, numerous studies showed a lower response to sucrose than to an equivalent amount of starch in both normal and diabetic volunteers (16, 31). Nevertheless, different sugars raise the blood glucose concentration to markedly different degrees: fructose causes a comparatively small rise, lactose and sucrose are intermediate, and glucose and maltose cause the highest rises (16, 32–35). This effect is apparently related to the proportion of glucose in the sugar molecule, with nonglucose components raising the blood glucose minimally. On the other hand, fructose may raise serum lipids higher than starch does, which may offset the advantage of slower absorption and flatter glycemic response (36).

Fats

Much work has been done on the absorption of fatty acids, but most fat in the human diet is in the form of triglycerides. Studies by Calloway et al. indicated comparable digestibility of many edible fats including butter, lard, and soybean, coconut, corn, and cottonseed oils (37). Butter, lard, shortening, and cod liver and corn oils appeared to be absorbed to the same extent, with maximum absorption occurring within 6 to 8 hours, at a time when the chylomicra rise would also have peaked (16, 31–35, 37–41). It was estimated that 24 to 41% of the fat was absorbed by 2 hours, 53 to 71% by 4 hours, 68 to 86% by 6 hours, and 97 to 99% after 12 hours (38). Comparing lymphatic absorption of long-chain fatty acids, including palmitic, oleic, linoleic, and stearic acids in man, showed a slight discrimination against triglyceride synthesis from stearic acid and favored cholesterol ester synthesis from oleic acid (42). Other studies suggest that triglycerides composed of the saturated dietary fatty acids (palmitic and stearic) are less well absorbed in the presence of high calcium, whereas triglycerides containing the unsaturated fats with lower melting points (oleic and linoleic) are unaffected (43, 44). Investigators have suggested that in general, either palmitic or stearic acid in the 1,3 positions of the triglyceride molecule reduced the absorption of that fat (45, 46).

Medium-chain triglycerides (MCTs) are being used in drinks, baked foods, and enteral feedings, however, in an attempt to increase the absorption of dietary fat. Their advantage lies in their direct absorption without micelle formation, with uptake as the fatty acid into the portal vein and clearance by the liver. They can therefore be absorbed even in the absence of bile salts or when lipoprotein synthesis necessary for chylomicra production is impaired or absent. Animal studies suggest that MCTs are absorbed four times as efficiently as long-chain triglycerides (47).

MCT use has been advocated in various situations, including small intestinal disease or damage, short bowel syndrome, pancreatic and biliary insufficiency (biliary atresia), and α-β-lipoproteinemia (Tangier disease); but they do not stimulate chylomicra formation, and fat-soluble vitamins are thus not transported out of the enterocyte (48). In addition, in rats, dietary substitution of MCTs for corn oil resulted in 20% less weight gain, largely through lack of deposition of carcass fat. In man, weight gain has been variable (42), and the early clinical use of MCTs was in the control of obesity (49, 50). The increased absorptive efficiency of the gut for MCTs was questioned on the grounds that the widely used solvent system for stool lipid extraction in the Van de Kamer method (51) only extracts up to 68% of the medium- to short-chain fatty acids (SCFAs) (52); however, the titrimetric determination assumes a mean molecular weight of 284 for fatty acids while MCTs have a mean molecular weight of 144, so the conversion factor used to derive the grams of fat malabsorbed is twice the number that should be applied to the MCTs. Thus, the two errors should balance out (53). However, cramping abdominal pain and increased diarrhea, together with increased steatorrhea, have been reported in the short bowel syndrome following MCT use (54). In addition, MCT should not be used in decompensated cirrhosis because poor clearance of short- and medium-chain fatty acids may exacerbate encephalopathy (55, 56). Further, in two instances, cirrhosis evolved in young patients with α-β-lipoproteinemia who were fed diets high in MCT on a long-term basis (57).

Thus, in terms of dietary fats, foods containing oleic or linoleic acid appear to be well absorbed. MCT may have an advantage in specific states, but it should be monitored cautiously. As dietary fat load is increased, fecal fat decreases proportionately (58).

Protein

Comparatively little is known about the intrinsic digestibility of proteins from different food sources independent of other factors in the food such as inhibitors. Some data suggest differences among common protein foods such as eggs, meats, poultry, fish, and cheeses that might favor their specific incorporation into the therapeutic diets of patients with limited absorptive capacity. In general, evidence indicates that animal proteins are more rapidly absorbed and metabolized than vegetable proteins (59). Surprisingly, in patients with cirrhosis, nitrogen balance studies showed no advantage of conventional animal protein foods over protein from cereal and legumes (60–62).

Although foods may be processed in ways that may influence the digestibility of their constituent proteins, studies have focused on the total amount absorbed or retained, rather than on how the rate of absorption may be modified. When protein foods are heated, cross-linking may occur among amino acids or between amino acid side chains and sugars. In the latter reaction, the free NH_2 groups on the lysine chains combine with the reducing groups of sugars, especially in the presence of heat, as in the baking of breads or cereal products and the manufacture of breakfast cereals. This synthesis (Maillard reaction) reduces the effectiveness of tryptic digestion and reduces the biologic value of the protein in experiments in animals. The effect on blood amino acid responses in man remains to be assessed.

In addition, much work is being done on modifying proteins such as those of soy (63), fish (64), casein, and whey (65) to improve such functional properties as solubility, emulsifying capacity, and heat stability, so they may be used in human foods. Their nutritional and digestibility properties will be reduced, however, because common methods involve succinylation or acetylation of the ϵ-amino group of lysine, the hydroxyl group of serine and threonine, the sulfhydryl group of cysteine, the phenol group of tyrosine, or the imidazole group of histidine (66). In vitro, succinylated proteins have low digestibility, owing to resistance of the succinyl-lysyl bonds to pancreatic digestion (66, 67).

Thus, processing generally reduces the digestibility of proteins. Nevertheless, these processes (e.g., heat) may be essential to remove the antinutrients from other food sources (e.g., legumes, cereals, and tubers) and to enhance digestibility, so that use of heat is likely to have a net positive nutritional impact.

DIETARY FIBER

Many of the differences in the digestibility of foods that cannot be explained by intrinsic differences in their macronutrient components are due to differences in their non-nutrient constituents, the plant materials that are resistant to small intestinal digestion, collectively known as dietary fiber.

Large differences exist in the physical form and the physiologic effect of various classes of dietary fiber. In general, purified viscous fibers such as gums, gels, and mucilages reduce the rate of nutrient absorption, whereas particulate fibers (e.g., cereal brans) have little effect on nutrient absorption in the small intestine but have a major impact on colonic function (see below in this section).

Definition

The definition of dietary fiber has always been controversial, and some feel the term is obsolete. One of the most widely accepted definitions is that of Trowell et al. (67a): "Fiber is composed of the plant polysaccharides and lignin which are resistant to digestion by the digestive enzymes of man." This is a physiologic rather than a chemical definition. Those who feel the term is obsolete favor such terms as plant cell wall nonstarch polysaccharides (NSPs) (67b), since dietary fibers were originally thought to be the structural elements responsible for maintaining the shape of plant cells via a cellulose-lignin lattice "waterproofed" with other NSP molecules. Cell wall NSPs can be directly measured, but focus on cell wall material exclusively may be deceptive, since nonstarch storage polysaccharides in foods such as legumes (e.g., galactomannan [guar] in the cluster bean *[Cyamopsis tatagonaloba]*), though analyzed as NSP, are not necessarily cell wall materials.

Classification

Dietary fiber was originally called crude fiber, a term from ruminant nutrition that referred to the fraction of plant material (forage) that was resistant to ruminant digestion and therefore of no nutritional value. It constituted the very resistant cellulose lignin fraction of what is now called dietary fiber. Van Soerst later developed analyses that gave greater definition to dietary fiber and classified fiber fractions as acid or neutral detergent fiber. Acid detergent fiber (ADF) was closer to the original crude fiber, and neutral detergent fiber (NDF) was closer to what we now term dietary fiber but without some of the water-soluble fiber fraction. These terms are still the standards used in animal nutrition. The chief dietary fiber components of interest are the water-insoluble celluloses, hemicelluloses, and lignins, and the water-soluble pectic substances, gums, and mucilages (Table 43.1). In general, dietary fiber and its components of interest are polymers of glucose or other sugars; the exception is lignin, which is polyphenol propane.

Dietary Fiber Hypothesis

The health benefits of eating cereal fiber and high-fiber plant foods in general were promoted in the 19th century by the well-known health advocates Graham and Kellogg in America and Allinson in Britain. However, much of the interest generated in the latter half of this century is the result of the work of Denis Burkitt and Hugh Trowell. From their experience of over 30 years, medical and surgical practice in Uganda, and subsequent studies of disease incidence in other countries, they proposed that many Western diseases resulted from maladaption to low-fiber diets. Diseases they attributed to a lack of dietary fiber included colonic disorders, constipation, diverticular disease, colon cancer, and such systemic disorders as hyperlipidemia, cardiovascular disease, diabetes, and obesity. Their theory, known as the dietary fiber hypothesis (67c), has been the stimulus for physiologic, clinical, and epidemiologic research since. A major focus of this research has been how fiber alters the absorption of macro- and micronutrients and bile acids along the length of the gastrointestinal tract and the biochemical consequences of these alterations.

Physiologic and Metabolic Effects (See Also Chapter 86)

Although dietary fibers have been divided into those that are water soluble (soluble fiber) and those that are not (insoluble fiber), there is concern that these terms should be discarded. Most foods contain both soluble and insoluble components in varying ratios, with the average for Western diets being about 1:3 soluble:insoluble fiber.

They have, however, proved useful conceptually. Insoluble fibers are considered to be those with the greatest effect on fecal bulk (68–68e) (e.g., cereal brans from wheat, rye, and rice). The soluble fibers, most importantly the viscous fibers, have metabolic effects (e.g., pectins from fruit and vegetables; β-glucan from oats and barley, gums from legumes, roots such as konjac, mucilages from the outer surface of plants such as sea weeds). They tend to flatten blood glucose and insulin levels postprandially (69) and reduce serum cholesterol in association with increased fecal bile acid losses (70–71b). The effects are related to viscosity, and in general, these fibers have little fecal bulking effect since they are rapidly fermented to gases and SCFAs by the colonic microflora. In fact, pectin may have a constipating effect. The fecal bulking and metabolic effects are therefore usually dissociated. A notable exception is psyllium husk, which has a high viscosity but is not well fermented by colonic microflora and thus also has a fecal bulking effect. The mechanisms of action for the metabolic effects of fibers in the small intestine and colon are discussed below.

Viscous Fibers and the Upper Gastrointestinal Tract

Dietary fibers of the viscous type, such as gums and pectic substances, delay gastric emptying (72–75) and slow small intestinal uptake of sugars, amino acids, (69, 76) and drugs such as acetaminophen and digoxin. Fiber is also associated with increased small intestinal (ileostomy) (71b) and fecal losses of bile acids (70–71a). As a result, increases in bile acid synthesis rates (especially of chenodeoxycholate) are seen (76a–76c). The effect of fiber on the small intestine is thought to be due to its ability to increase the thickness of the unstirred water layer, which acts as a barrier to diffusion of nutrients to the enterocyte brush border. Studies using pectin have supported this concept (77). It has also been suggested, however, that viscous fibers slow absorption simply by impeding diffusion in the bulk phase. The mechanism may also differ along the length of the small intestine as water is absorbed. Use of a triple-tube lumen and balloon tamponade to isolate a segment of human small intestine in vivo showed that adding guar to the perfusate reduces the rate of small intestinal absorption of glucose (78). Nevertheless, although slow absorption has been observed, malabsorption has not resulted, as judged by urinary recovery of xylose (69) and acetaminophen (72) and the lack of breath H_2 evolution (80). In addition, fat and protein losses increased minimally, as judged by the marginally increased output of protein and fat from the terminal ileum (80) after bran supplementation. Viscous fiber preparations are associated with enhanced chylomicronemia and higher postprandial fat-soluble vitamin levels, possibly because they stabilize lipid emulsions (81, 82). Similar enhanced vitamin A absorption has been seen with cholestyramine at a low level (74) but not at high levels at which fat absorption is depressed (84). Viscous fiber preparations have been used in the management of diabetes (85–88), as well as to reduce serum cholesterol levels in hyperlipidemia (89–91). These preparations also improve symptoms in the dumping syndrome following gastric surgery (70, 92, 93). Detailed studies demonstrated that added viscous fiber in test meals blunted the glucose, insulin, and GIP responses when taken with a glucose load (73) and decreased both the undershoot in blood glucose (72) and hemoconcentration, assessed by hematocrit (74a).

The viscosity of the fiber appears to determine its metabolic effects, especially in terms of postprandial glycemia. Hydrolysis of the viscous fibers guar or oat β-glucan renders them ineffective (69, 94a). The effects of hydrolysis on the cholesterol-lowering effect are less clear, since the one study reported with guar gum still used an hydrolyzed guar gum with significant residual viscosity (94b). Low-viscosity fibers (e.g., acacia gum) have proved ineffective in lowering serum cholesterol, as have some oat β-glucans, presumably related to their low viscosity (94c–94e). Indeed, standardization of oat β-glucan solubility and viscosity in foods may be of great importance now that health claims are permitted by the Food and Drug Administration (FDA) for foods containing more than 1 g β-glucan per serving, without requiring assessment of product efficacy (94f).

Indeed the effectiveness of fiber in foods in reducing the rate of absorption and altering associated metabolic events is generally less clear. No significant differences in glycemic response or digestibility were found between white bread, pasta, and rice and their wholemeal or bran equivalents (94, 95) (Fig. 43.4) (19). In addition, when over 50 foods of equivalent carbohydrate content were compared, the flattening in postprandial glycemia was significantly negatively related to their fat and protein contents, but not to fiber (Fig. 43.5) (16). This may have been due to the large number of high-cereal fiber foods examined. Because cereal fiber of medium-to-large particle size (500–1200 μm) appears to have little effect on small intestinal absorption, the effect of other types of fiber may have been obscured. The selection of particle size and fiber sources may be all important because this debate continues, with some (96), but not all (97), workers finding a fiber-glycemic index relationship.

Studies with purified fibers therefore indicate that certain types of fiber may affect the absorbability of foods. Fiber in unprocessed foods is also likely to influence the absorption of the macronutrient components in a Western diet through its effect on food form (discussed below).

NUTRIENT-NUTRIENT INTERACTIONS IN FOODS

Nutrient-nutrient interactions have a significant effect on the digestibility of foods. Studies using breath hydrogen measurement to assess carbohydrate malabsorption indicate significant (10–20%) malabsorption from white

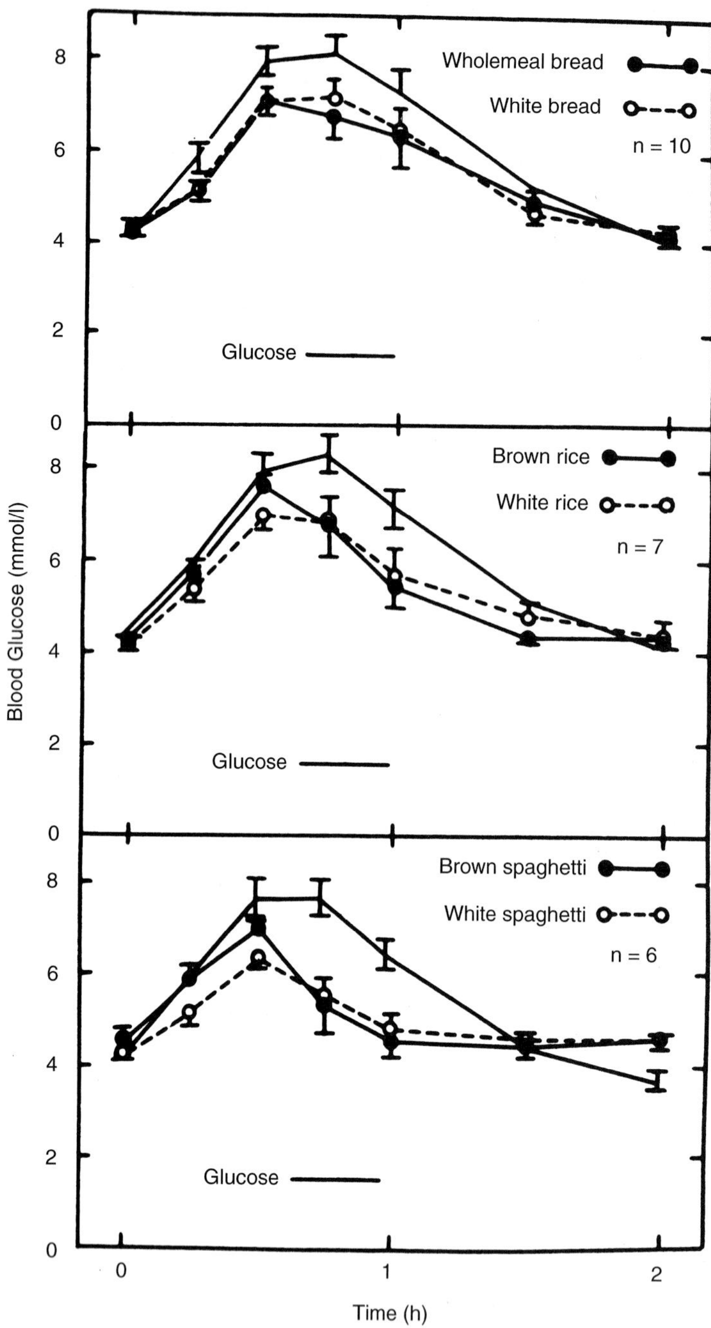

Figure 43.4. Effect of fiber depletion on the mean blood glucose curves after eating 50-g carbohydrate portions of bread, rice, and spaghetti compared with 50-g glucose tolerance tests. (From Jenkins DJA, Wolever TMS, Taylor RH, et al. Diabetes Care 1981;4:509–513.)

bread and other farinaceous products (98). When gluten-free flour was used, no malabsorption was seen, nor was malabsorption produced by adding back purified gluten to the same level as found originally in the white bread (Fig. 43.6). The investigators concluded that the natural physical interaction of the starch and protein in wheat limited its rate of digestion, resulting in some malabsorption (98). The implication is that patients without definite evidence of celiac disease who are placed on a gluten-free diet and appear to improve may do so because of the enhanced availability of dietary starch rather than elimination of the gliadin component of wheat protein. Such a measure may thus be generally applicable therapeutically when malabsorption of carbohydrate (starch) is a problem. Furthermore, the in vitro digestion rate of gluten-free or gluten-reconstituted bread was more rapid than that of regular bread and the in vivo glycemic response to feeding breads made of these flours (gluten reduced) was also higher (99).

Conversely, the presence of protein in the small intestine helps to stabilize fat emulsions and enhances micelle formation and fatty acid uptake (39, 100). This was demonstrated with casein given with olive oil to dogs (39, 100), in mixtures of proteins (bovine albumin and bovine hemaglobin/ovalbumin mixture), and in various digests of these administered to rats (100). In addition, the effect of fiber in reducing the glycemic response to carbohydrate

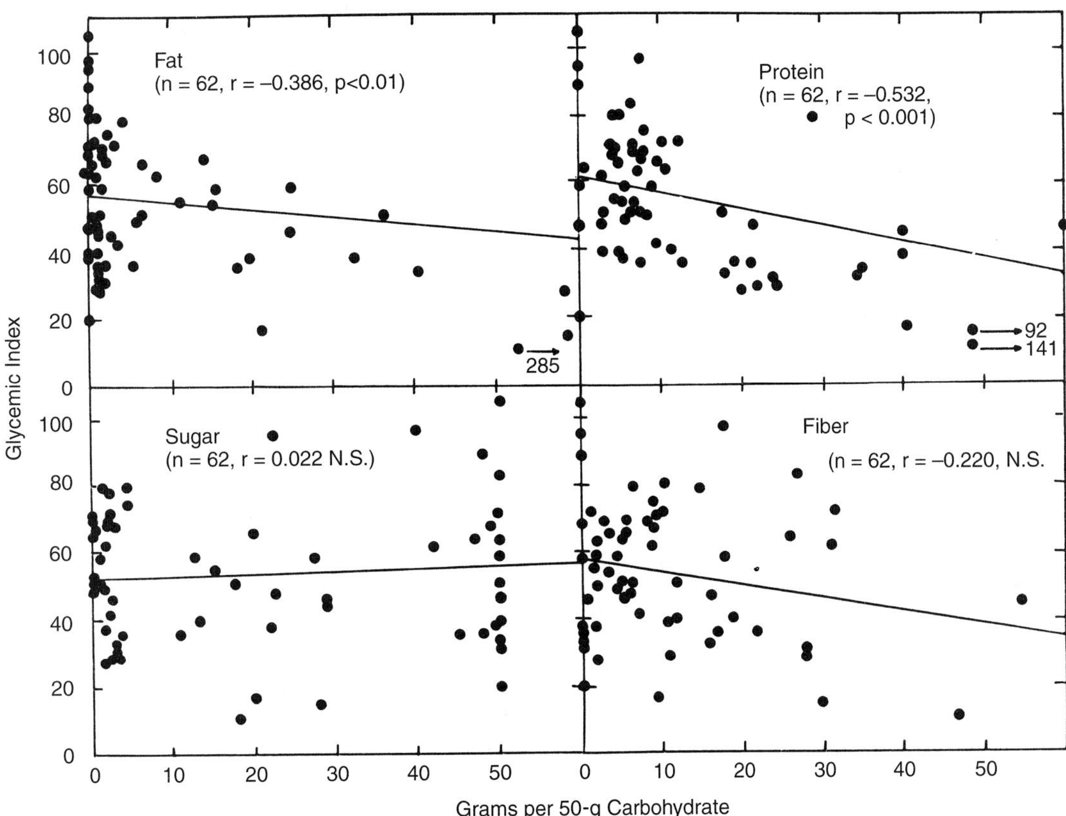

Figure 43.5. Relationship of fat, protein, and fiber content of 62 foods and sugars with the glycemic index of 50-g carbohydrate portions. (From Jenkins DJA, Wolever TMS, Taylor RH. Am J Clin Nutr 1981;34:362–366.)

was reported to diminish as dietary protein levels increased (101).

Fat, on the other hand, delays gastric emptying (102) and thus slows digestion and absorption of other nutrients. However, the extent of this delay may depend on the stability of the fat-food mixture, because separation of fat into an upper lipid phase may cause the fat to have little effect on the gastric emptying of the carbohydrate and protein lying below.

A starch-lipid interaction has been described in which the hydrocarbon chain of a monoglyceride becomes embedded within the relatively hydrophobic internal portion of the amylose α-helical structure (103). Investigators suggested that starch-lipid interactions may form in the upper part of the small intestine during fat ingestion and may slow the rate of starch digestion and reduce the glycemic response.

Lipid-lipid interactions are also important. For example, lecithin may enhance triglyceride absorption by facilitating micelle formation (39, 104). Similarly, owing to their effect in stimulating chylomicron formation, long-chain fatty acids increase cholesterol absorption (105) and, most importantly, absorption of fat-soluble vitamins (106).

MICRONUTRIENT INTERACTIONS

Our discussion has so far focused on the factors affecting absorption of the so-called macronutrients from foods, rather than the minerals, trace elements, and vitamins. This level has another series of interrelationships. Evidence indicates that fiber binds minerals in vitro (107). Various types of fiber to reduce the absorbability of calcium (Ca^{2+}), iron (Fe^{2+}), and magnesium (Mg^{2+}) (108–111). Phytate, a fiber-associated antinutrient, may also be important, although its relationship to deficiency states is not clear. Results are affected by the kind of fiber and by the presence of other agents in foods. Responses to test meals given to human subjects indicate that fiber may decrease absorption of iron and zinc (112). Responses were affected by amounts of fiber and minerals and by the presence of protein and phytate in test meals. Although fiber intakes by vegetarians have been reported to be higher than those for omnivores, studies reveal no differences in blood mineral levels between the two groups (112).

Results of human balance studies involving fiber and mineral bioavailability are controversial. Many factors influence the outcome of such studies, making them difficult to evaluate. Phytate and oxalate in food can also bind minerals and may contribute to decreased mineral balances (113). The relative levels of fiber, minerals, protein, and other substances in the diet are important and contribute to the confusion in attempts to compare different studies. The type of fiber is also a variable, and indications are that insoluble fibers are more likely than soluble fibers to have an adverse effect on mineral bioavailability.

The length of the study period is important in evaluating the results of human balance studies (114).

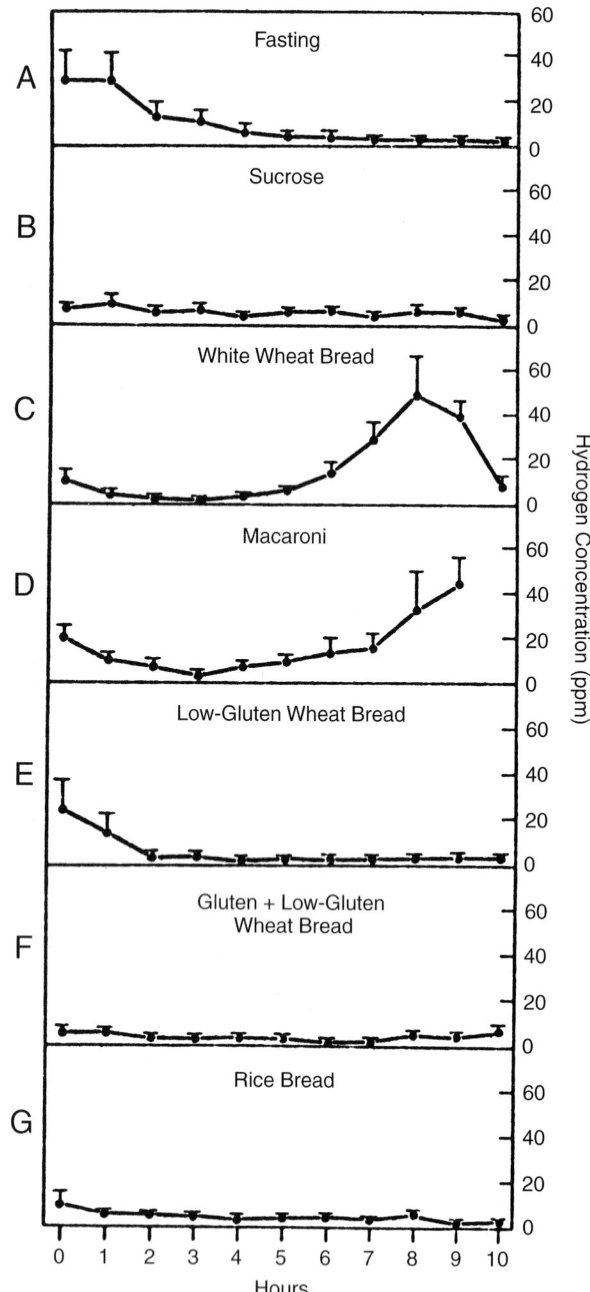

Figure 43.6. Breath hydrogen concentration as a measure of carbohydrate malabsorption in healthy volunteers during a 10-hour fast (**A**) and after ingestion of 100 g carbohydrate (**B** through **G**). (From Anderson IH, Levine AS, Levitt MD. N Engl J Med 1981;304:891–892, by permission of the New England Journal of Medicine.)

Adaptation to a different level of mineral intake or to a different level of availability may take considerable time, depending on the magnitude of the change. Thus, study subjects fed a lower level of a mineral than in their usual diets may develop negative mineral balance at the beginning of the study but become adapted to the new level if sufficient time is allowed. From reports of balance studies in the literature, it appears that an intake of 25 g per day of insoluble fiber does not adversely affect mineral nutrition if adequate mineral intake is maintained.

Consumption of long-chain fatty acids facilitates fat-soluble vitamin uptake. High levels of fat in the diet may increase Ca^{2+} losses in the feces (115). Raising dietary protein intake may diminish the absorption of zinc (Zn^{2+}), copper (Cu^{2+}), and Ca^{2+}, all in the presence of modest amounts of fiber (101). In the colon, reduction of pH by carbohydrate fermentation favors absorption of Mg^{2+} (116) and vitamin K (117). Many other such interrelationships are discussed in their respective sections of this book.

INFLUENCE OF FOOD FORM AND NONNUTRIENT FOOD COMPONENTS

Many of the studies showing differences in the absorbability of natural diets were carried out in relation to factors concerned with absorption of carbohydrate from foods; thus, much of the present discussion uses carbohydrate digestibility to illustrate general principles. Factors include food form, fiber content, and the presence of lectins, tannins, saponins, and phytates. The possible role of fiber is discussed above.

Food Form

The form in which a food is eaten is a major determinant of its rate of digestion and absorption. Apples eaten whole rather than blended produced flatter blood glucose and insulin responses, indicating a slower rate of absorption (118). Crapo and coworkers demonstrated differences in glucose and insulin responses to a range of starchy foods including baked potato, boiled rice, bread, and corn, which in part might be attributed to food form (12, 13). Maize and rice (whole seeds) produced the least response, whereas baked potato, a less "compact" food, approximated the blood glucose rise seen when the equivalent amount of carbohydrate was given as glucose (12–14). Furthermore, rice that was ground and then cooked evoked rises in blood glucose and insulin approximating those for glucose (119) and a more rapid rate of in vitro digestion than whole rice.

Particle size, an important aspect of food, is not detected by assessing the chemical composition of the diet. Many traditional foods with low glycemic indices have large particle sizes, including whole-grain barley, as used in traditional soups; cracked wheat or tabouli, a staple food in North Africa and throughout the Middle East; and pumpernickel bread with 80% whole rye grains, as commonly used in northern Europe. The proportion of whole grain (wheat or barley) in a bread mix determines the glycemic effect and the in vitro rate of digestion; more whole grain in the bread produces slower absorption and a flatter glycemic response (120). Heaton et al. used this concept to explain possible health benefits of traditionally milled flours, independent of their fiber content. Their studies showed that traditional coarse-milled flours with large particle sizes produce flatter postprandial glucose and insulin responses (121).

The digestibility of cereal grains also appears to be influenced by "parboiling," i.e., precooking a grain in its husk before dehusking. Possibly because of prevention of swelling and hence a reorganization of the starch molecule, subsequent cooking fails to hydrate the dehulled grain, which, although perfectly acceptable for consumption, produces a lower glycemic response (122). This is a traditional way of processing rice.

Although food form is a determinant of digestibility, application of this principle may not be universal. Studies with lentils indicated that blending to a smooth paste after cooking did not affect the in vitro digestion rate or the glycemic response (123), nor did boiling for an additional 40 minutes. Heat treatment for 12 hours was required to increase the digestibility of the lentils (123).

Enzyme Inhibitors

Enzyme inhibitors in foods, although common in storage organs such as seeds, cereal grains, and beans, are usually effectively destroyed by the heat treatment of conventional cooking practices (124). Their relevance to human nutrition is therefore likely to be limited. In terms of animal nutrition, however, the antitryptic activity of uncooked bean meal has attracted attention because it limits the protein quality of animal feeds. In rats, it was associated with impaired growth and pancreatic hypertrophy (102).

On the positive side, purified enzyme inhibitors are beginning to find a use in modifying small intestinal absorption. Inhibitors of carbohydrate absorption have been developed specifically to control the rate of carbohydrate absorption. An anti-α-amylase isolated from wheat was shown to reduce the rate of starch digestion and the glycemic response to a starch meal in rats, dogs, and man (125). Subsequently, a commercially developed α-glycoside hydrolase inhibitor with antisucrase, antimaltase, and antiamylase activity found application in the treatment of diabetes (126, 126a) and the dumping syndrome (127). In the dumping syndrome, relief was obtained despite enhanced carbohydrate losses (127). Presumably, the reduced glycemic excursions caused by dampening the carbohydrate flux offered a large measure of relief to patients and outweighed the discomfort of carbohydrate malabsorption to which they were already accustomed. Thus, although enzyme inhibitors may be of little relevance in the context of commonly eaten foods and dietetic manipulations, pharmacologic development of these agents may in the future provide a further means of modifying small intestinal absorption.

Saponins

Saponins, steroidal or triterpenoid amphiphilic glycosides with surface-active and emulsion-stabilizing properties, are relatively heat resistant; thus, their levels are maintained in fat-containing plant foods and oils. Under normal circumstances, they are not absorbed. They have attracted attention by possibly precipitating cholesterol and interfering with micelle formation in the small intestine by enhancing the binding of bile acids to fiber (128). There is no suggestion that they would induce major changes in fat absorption, but in view of their effects on cholesterol absorption, they may possibly interfere with fat-soluble vitamin uptake. The exact effect of these surface-active agents on the enterocyte or digestive enzymes is unknown.

Tannins

Tannins, large, condensed polyphenols, are powerful reducing agents widely distributed in plant food. Because they are heat stable, however, they survive cooking procedures and can complex with dietary proteins and reduce protein digestibility (129). They also reduce the activity of the digestive enzymes trypsin and amylase (130, 131). Tannins may therefore reduce the rate or total absorption of both dietary starch and protein from foods. Although tannins occur in high concentrations in certain natural diets, their effects have not been studied directly in man; however, their concentration in foods is inversely related to the digestibility and glycemic response of a wide range of foods tested (132).

Phytates

The most important phytate is *myo*-inositol 1,2,3,4,5,6 hexakis dihydrogen phosphate, which is found in relatively high concentrations in many high-fiber foods (cereals, legumes, and vegetables). Its levels are reduced by the action of yeast in the leavening of bread. Nevertheless, phytates can bind metal ions and bind to protein (133, 134) and possibly to starch, thereby reducing macro- and micronutrient digestibility. As a consequence, phytates were implicated in calcium and zinc deficiency in man (135). Their exact role in macronutrient absorption, however, seems to be less important than that of fiber (136). Nevertheless, phytates reduce carbohydrate digestibility when they are added to white bread in the same concentration as found in legumes (Fig. 43.7) (137). This effect is probably due to the binding of Ca^{2+}, which catalyzes the action of amylase (138), because addition of excess Ca^{2+} minimizes the effect (137).

Although phytate may also bind to proteins and so reduce protein digestibility (133, 134), the significance of this effect in commonly eaten foods is not clear. Phytates may possibly play a major role in determining starch digestibility in foods, because they have a highly significant negative relationship with digestibility and glycemic response to many foods tested in man (137). Their levels are especially high in legumes, which show some of the slowest rates of in vitro digestion (19).

Lectins

These substances are a diverse family of proteins and glycoproteins found ubiquitously in plant foods (139).

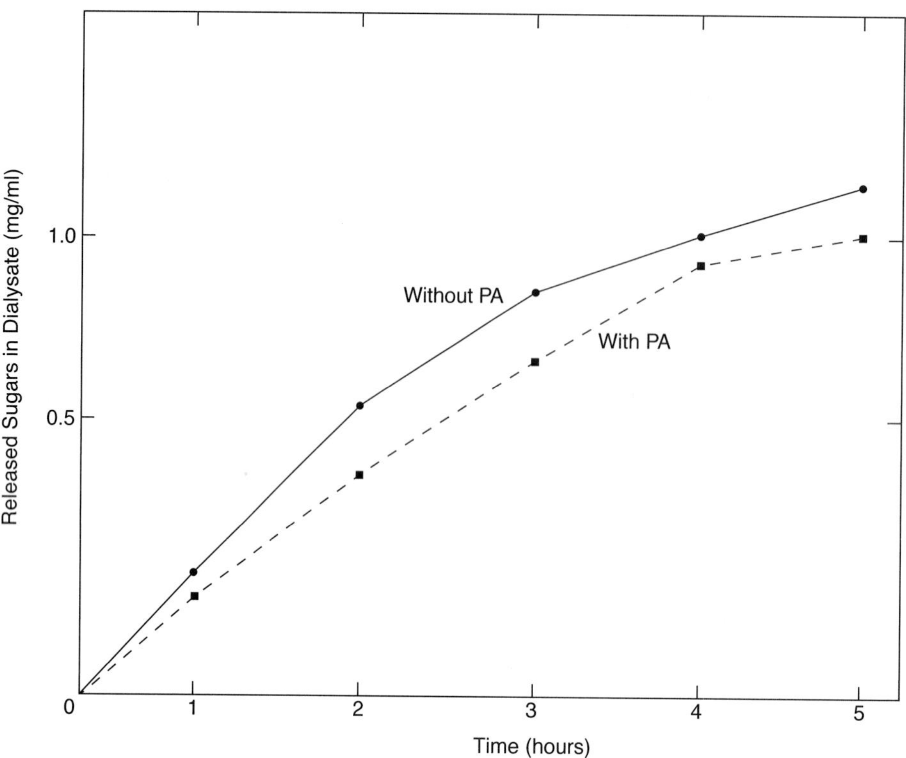

Figure 43.7. Rate of digestion of starch in unleavened breads with and without addition of sodium phytate (PA). (From Yoon JH, Thompson LU, Jenkins DJA. Am J Clin Nutr 1983;38:835–842.)

Lectins bind to carbohydrate receptors on cell surfaces and, in extremely high concentrations, have caused small intestinal mucosal damage in rats (140). Apart from retrospective studies by Noah et al. concerning raw kidney bean consumption (141), no toxic effects have been reported in man at levels commonly found in the diet; however, preliminary studies indicate that, as with many antinutrients, the lectin content of a food and its digestibility both in vitro and in vivo are related (142). The exact significance of this finding awaits further elaboration.

Rate of Food Ingestion and Meal Frequency

Finally, the rate of nutrient delivery to the organism can be slowed simply by reducing the rate and prolonging the time over which food is ingested (Fig. 43.8). In many ways, this also provides the least complicated model for examining the physiologic effects of reducing the rate of absorption. In short-term studies of glucose or mixed meals, possibly the most notable effect is the reduction in postprandial insulin levels (143–145). The possible benefits of increased meal frequency discussed here refer to isocaloric redistribution of food so that absorption of a defined material load is spread over a longer time. It is not intended to imply a benefit from ingesting more food. Lack of emphasis of this point has often resulted in a negative connotation for "snacking" or "eating between meals" when associated with increased caloric intake.

Over 50 years ago, Ellis noted the beneficial effect of frequent oral glucose administration in the management of insulin-dependent diabetes (145a). More recently, studies showed benefits on glycemia and insulinemia in non-insulin-dependent diabetes over the day from increased meal frequency (145, 145b). The most recent nutrition recommendations of the American Diabetes Association also draw attention to the possible advantages of increased meal frequency (145c).

Economy in insulin secretion has been seen in longer-term studies (Fig. 43.8*A*) and has been associated with reduced serum lipid and lipoprotein levels, notably LDL cholesterol and apolipoprotein B (Fig. 43.8*B*). Indeed, for over a quarter of a century, evidence has accumulated on the beneficial effect of meal frequency on serum lipids (146–148, 148a, 148b). Stable isotope studies in man showed that increased meal frequency reduced cholesterol synthesis; reduced insulin levels were also noted (148c). In addition to reduced insulin levels and hence lower stimulation of hydroxymethylglutaryl coenzyme A (HMGCoA) reductase, (149, 150) the rate-limiting step in cholesterol synthesis, alteration or expansion of the bile salt pool, secondary to more frequent enterohepatic cycling, may also be a factor in lowering serum lipid levels. These benefits of increased meal frequency on serum lipids and coronary heart disease (151) were not seen in relation to cancer; increased cancer incidence has been noted (152, 153). In the cancer studies, the determining factor may be the nature of the snack foods used (high fat, high salt, etc.) in uncontrolled diets. These findings highlight the need for more research into the physiologic and pathologic conse-

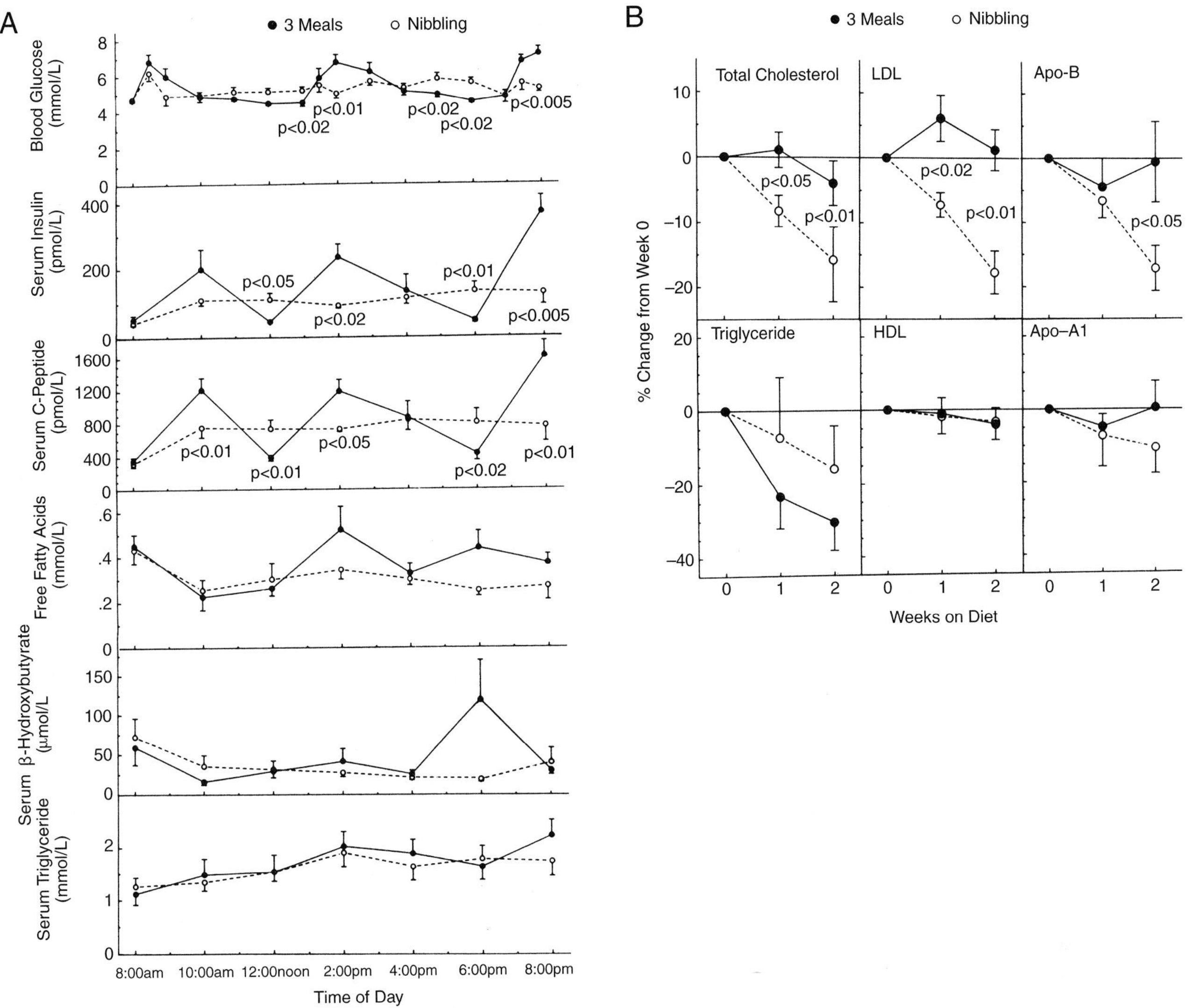

Figure 43.8. A. Mean (± SE) blood glucose levels and serum concentrations of insulin, C-peptide, free fatty acids, 3-hydroxybutyrate, and triglyceride in seven men on day 13. During the nibbling diet, meals were eaten hourly from 8 AM onward, and during the three-meal diet, 8 AM, 1 PM, and 7 PM. **B.** Mean (± SE) percentage of change from time 0 in serum lipid and apolipoprotein (apo) concentrations in seven men during the nibbling diet and the three-meal diet. (From Jenkins DJA, Wolever TMS, Vuksan V, et al. N Engl J Med 1989;321:929–34, with permission.)

quences of alterations in food frequency and, by inference, factors that prolong absorption time in general.

DIFFERENCES IN DIGESTIBILITY OF FOODS AND PHYSIOLOGIC IMPLICATIONS

General Considerations

Because many factors may alter the digestion and absorption of foods, we cannot predict the rate at which a food will be digested simply by knowing its constituents. Nevertheless, as illustrated by starch-containing foods, large differences are seen among different foods (Table 43.1) (28). Predictably, the legumes that are relatively high in soluble fiber and antinutrients are digested more slowly than cereal foods and potato (28). In addition, they release a greater proportion of glucose and maltose and a smaller proportion of maltotriose. As mentioned above, this effect may reflect their higher content of the less readily digested amylose form of starch. On the other hand, the content of cereal fiber in white and wholemeal bread demonstrates clearly that this form of fiber does not reduce the rate of digestion of bread.

Again, by contrast, foods of similar composition (e.g., white bread and white spaghetti) differ markedly, presumably because of differences in food form. Because the rate of digestion relates well to the glycemic response to foods (19), the physiologic implications of these differences are great. Flatter glycemic responses are seen (expressed as a glycemic index) in response to foods that are digested less rapidly (Fig. 43.9) (19). As data accumulate, it should be possible to select diets on the basis of rates of digestion to achieve the desired physiologic and metabolic effects.

Glycemic Index (See Also Chapter 86)

Because many factors in foods may influence their rates of digestion and glycemic responses and because most of

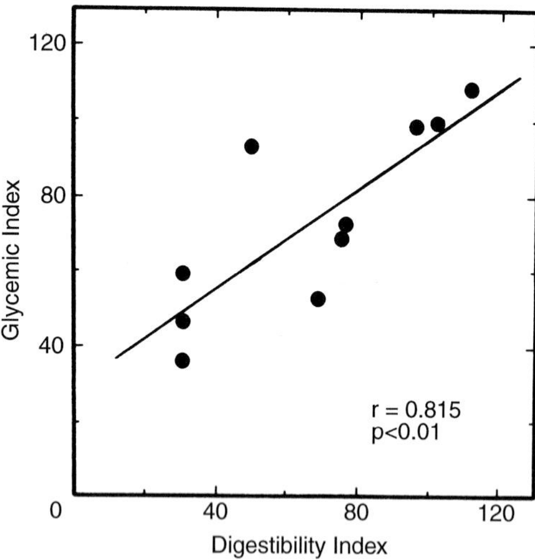

Figure 43.9. Relationship between the mean glycemic index and mean digestibility index for each of the 10 foods studied. The glycemic and digestibility indices were calculated by ascribing to white bread a value of 100, both for the glycemic response areas observed over 3 hours after consumption of the test foods and for the total sugars liberated at 3 hours during in vitro digestion (descending order of digestibility: cornflakes, white and wholemeal breads, rice, potato, spaghetti, porridge, kidney beans, chick peas, and lentils). (From Jenkins DJA, Ghafari H, Wolever TMS. Diabetologia 1982;22: 450–455.)

these factors are not listed in food tables and many have nothing to do with food composition, it is not possible to predict the physiologic effect of a food on the basis of its chemical composition. The glycemic index was developed as an index of the physiologic effect of foods to supplement information on chemical composition (16). It was reasoned that such information might allow a better understanding of the effects of carbohydrate foods and aid in the selection of appropriate foods for therapeutic diets. The glycemic index is defined as the blood glucose response to a 50-g available carbohydrate portion of a food expressed as a percentage of the response to the same amount of carbohydrate from a standard food, which has been either glucose or white bread. Bread is the preferred standard and gives glycemic index values 1.38 times greater than glucose (because glucose produces a glycemic response 138% that of white bread). The glycemic index value obtained also depends on the method of calculating the area under the glycemic response curve and, to a lesser extent, on other methodologic variables, discussed fully elsewhere (154). Relatively comprehensive tables of the glycemic indices of foods are now becoming available (154a).

A compilation of over 75 different foods tested in various centers is provided in Appendix Table IV-A-26-a (155). For most foods tested more than once in different centers there is reasonable agreement, with an average coefficient of variation of the mean glycemic index values of 16% (154). The variability of certain foods in many cases has been found subsequently to be due to subtle differences among foods, such as the method of rice processing (parboiled vs. polished) (122), different varieties of potato (154), and the ripeness of banana (156). Different individuals may have vastly different absolute glycemic responses to a food, depending upon their glucose tolerance status. The glycemic index normalizes each subject's response to that of a standard food, however, so differences among individuals are removed (157). Thus, the glycemic index values of foods are the same in normal and diabetic subjects.

In individual subjects, blood glucose responses vary from day to day. For this reason, the glycemic index cannot be applied quantitatively in individual subjects who test foods only once. One can predict the ranking of glycemic responses, however, with the chance of a correct prediction determined by the variation of glycemic responses within the subject tested, the expected glycemic index difference, and the number of times the subject repeats the tests (158). The glycemic index can be applied to mixed meals if appropriate methods are used (154, 159). Briefly, the meal glycemic index is the weighted average of the glycemic index value of all the individual carbohydrate foods in the meal, with the weighting based on the proportion of the total meal carbohydrate contributed by each food. The percentage differences among meal glycemic index values accurately predicts the percentage differences among the mean incremental glycemic response areas of mixed meals taken by groups of subjects, provided accurate glycemic index values are known for the individual foods. A reasonable correlation exists between the glycemic and insulinemic indices of different foods (159a).

The clinical relevance of the glycemic index was demonstrated in studies in which the types of starchy carbohydrate foods in the diet were altered without changing the overall dietary composition in terms of fat, protein, carbohydrate, and dietary fiber (see Chapter 85). A low-glycemic-index diet reduced blood lipids in hypertriglyceridemic subjects (160, 161); reduced insulin secretion (162); improved overall blood glucose control in insulin-dependent and non-insulin-dependent diabetic subjects (163–166); reduced abnormal blood glucose, insulin, and amino acid levels in patients with cirrhosis (167); and reduced urinary urea excretion, presumably by increasing nitrogen trapping by colonic bacteria (162). In addition, some evidence indicates that low-glycemic-index foods enhance satiety (168) and increase athletic endurance (169).

Studies appear to be confirming that low-glycemic-index foods may offer protection from development of non-insulin-dependent diabetes. Studies of 65,174 nurses (women) (169a) and 42,759 health professionals (men) (169b) followed up for more than 5 years, found that diabetes was less common in both sexes in those with low-glycemic-index and higher-cereal-fiber diets (Fig. 43.10).

Colonic Absorption

Food residues not completely absorbed in the small intestine may be absorbed in the colon. In terms of over-

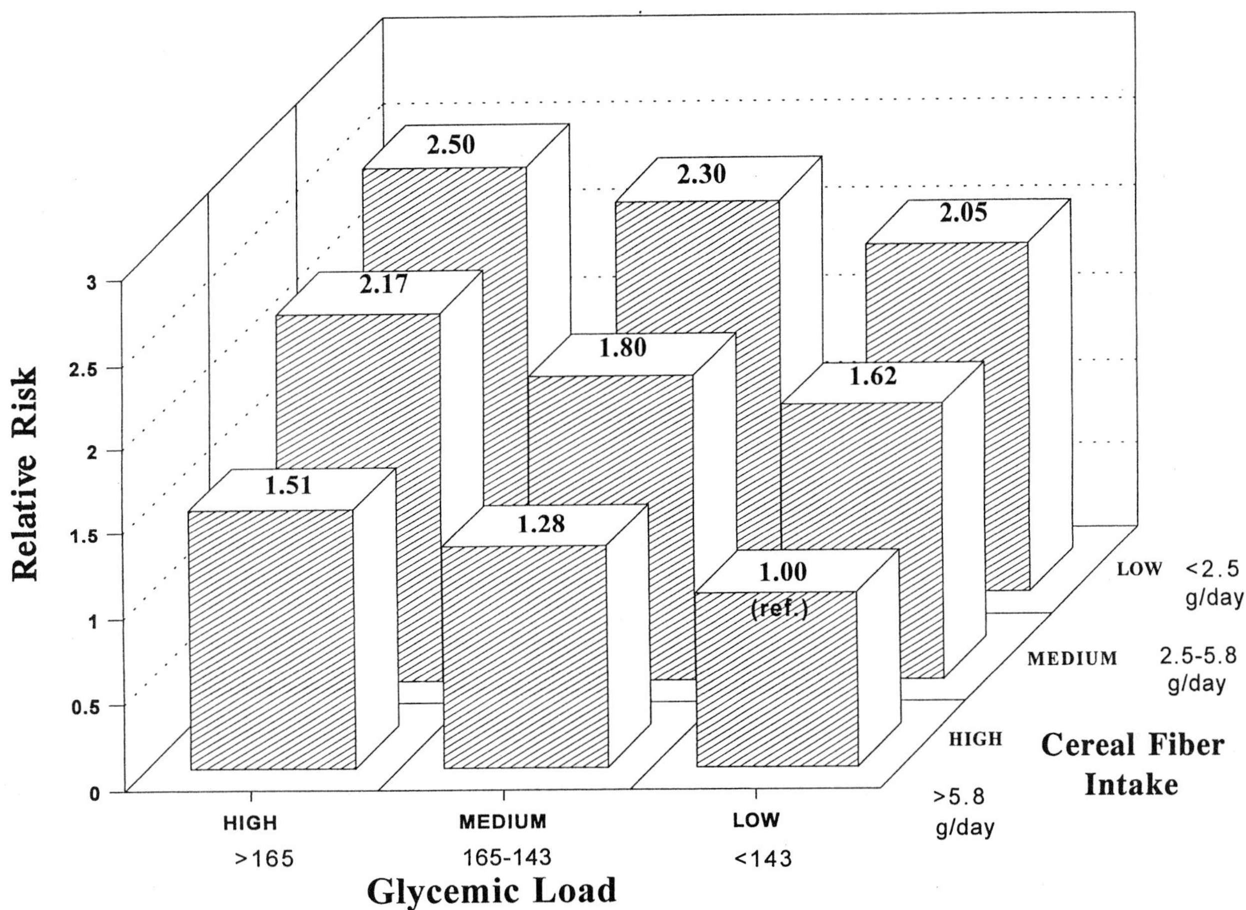

Figure 43.10. Relative risk of NIDDM by different levels of cereal fiber and glycemic load. (From Salmeron J, Stampfer MJ, Colditz GA, et al. JAMA 1997;277:472–77, with permission.)

all protein metabolism, ammonia and the bacterial metabolites of amino acids may have little impact apart from their deleterious effects in the genesis of encephalopathy in liver disease. In the case of malabsorbed carbohydrate, however, the situation differs. A small proportion of the starch in many commonly consumed foods escapes absorption in the small intestine and enters the colon. This is especially true for foods that are absorbed slowly. Breath H_2 (105, 123) and ileostomy studies (170, 171) indicate that 7 to 20% of the starch in bread enters the colon. With other foods, such as legumes, the percentage lost may be higher. Although these losses relate to the in vitro rate of digestion, the differences in the percentage of carbohydrate malabsorbed among foods are much smaller than the percentage differences in their glycemic responses (16, 17, 172). Carbohydrate losses thus do not appear to account for the flatter glycemic responses of starchy foods of low glycemic index.

In terms of energy losses from carbohydrate foods (starch, sugars, and fiber), much may be salvaged by colonic absorption of the resulting volatile fatty acids (173, 174), which have been estimated to contribute 10% or more of dietary calories (174). Therefore, factors that alter the rate of carbohydrate digestion may not be reflected in malabsorption so much as in an altered balance of nutrient absorption from different parts of the gut, including the colon.

Short-Chain Fatty Acids: Local and Systemic Metabolism

The major products of carbohydrate fermentation in the colon are the SCFAs, acetate, propionate, and butyrate. These anions are taken up rapidly from the colonic lumen and may exert local and systemic effects on metabolism. Studies indicate that SCFAs may enhance the uptake of divalent metal ions (175), and investigators have suggested that the colon may be a major organ for salvaging minerals and trace elements trapped by fiber fermented in the colon (176). In man, colonic Ca^{2+} absorption is enhanced by incorporating acetate and propionate into the perfusate. SCFAs are also considered valuable energy sources for the host. Butyrate is a preferred substrate for the colonocyte and has been suggested to have antineoplastic properties (177). Butyrate has been used in enemas to treat exclusion (diversion) colitis (178). Propionate is largely extracted by the liver. It is gluconeogenic and may have an inhibitory effect on cholesterol synthesis (179). Acetate is taken up by both liver and peripheral tissues. Of the three SCFAs mentioned, only acetate appears in significant quantities in the peripheral circulation.

Colonic SCFAs may influence systemic carbohydrate and lipid metabolism, but the exact effects are not fully known, and this is an area of current research. Acetate has no effect on intravenous or oral glucose tolerance or glucose turnover rates (180, 181). It may influence glucose use indirectly, however, by reducing serum free fatty acid levels. This effect was first described in studies suggesting that acetate accounted for the free fatty acid–lowering effect of alcohol (182). Recently, investigators have demonstrated that colonic acetate also has the same effect in reducing serum free fatty acids (183). Propionate has direct effects on carbohydrate metabolism. Evidence indicates that as in ruminants, propionate is gluconeogenic in humans (183). Feeding propionate improves carbohydrate tolerance, which may be related, in part, to an inhibitory effect of propionate on starch digestion (184).

The potential effects of colonic SCFAs on lipid metabolism have been of major interest, especially as a mechanism for the lipid-lowering effect of soluble fiber. In vitro, propionate inhibits cholesterol synthesis in slices of hepatic tissue (185); however, the concentration of propionate required may exceed that ever reached in the portal vein (186). In human feeding studies, propionate has no effect on serum cholesterol (184, 187). Nevertheless, propionate can inhibit incorporation of acetate into cholesterol and triglyceride by isolated hepatocytes (188). This may be significant in humans, because rectal infusion of acetate results in increased serum cholesterol within 1 hour, an effect partly blocked by addition of a physiologic amount of propionate (183). The serum cholesterol–raising effect of acetate was further suggested by the finding that feeding lactulose for 2 weeks to healthy subjects increased serum total and LDL cholesterol, apolipoprotein B, and triglyceride concentrations (Fig. 43.11) (189). Therefore, the influence of propionate on lipid metabolism cannot be determined until the importance of colonic acetate as a substrate for cholesterol synthesis is known.

Recent interest has focused on substrates that produce specific SCFA spectra. One goal has been to enhance butyrate synthesis to improve colonic health (189a–189d). There is growing evidence that colonic fermentation of resistant starches increases intracolonic levels of butyrate and propionate, depending on the starch source and the butyrate:SCFA ratio (189e, 189f). These findings raise the question of the possible use of resistant starches in the treatment of ulcerative colitis and in polyp and colonic cancer prevention.

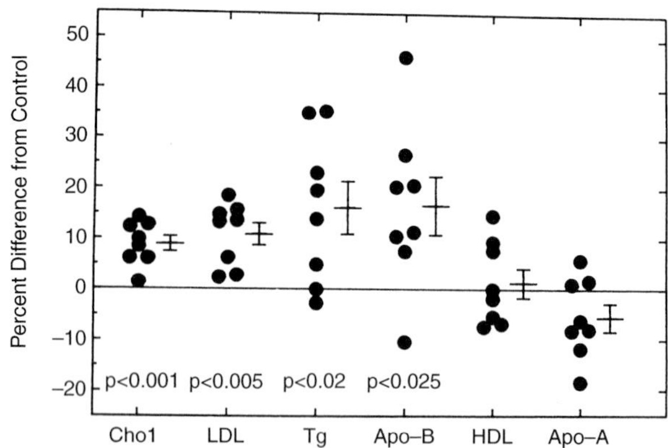

Figure 43.11. Mean 2-week lactulose values for blood lipids and apolipoproteins expressed as the percentage difference from the corresponding control values. *Bars* represent the mean ± SE of the lipid and lipoprotein categories for subjects. (Adapted from Jenkins DJA, Wolever TMS, Jenkins AL, et al. Am J Clin Nutr 1991;54:141–147.)

Long-Term Effects of Dietary Components

Not only can specific foods or food processes be identified with specific short-term effects in gastrointestinal function and absorption, important long-term effects may also be associated with specific diets and dietary components. For example, diets high in carbohydrate induce sucrase-isomaltase and enhance the absorption of sucrose, whereas removal of carbohydrate from the diet rapidly reverses this trend (190). Diets high in specific dietary fibers reduce sucrase levels in rats (191); pectin reduced sucrase and lactase, tannin and galactomannan reduced lactase, and cellulose was without effect (191). Other studies have demonstrated that increasing protein or carbohydrate in the diets of diabetic rats decreased or increased absorption of cholesterol, respectively (192).

Changes in small intestinal morphology may also be produced by diet. The broad, leaflike jejunal villi seen in inhabitants of areas where high-fiber diets are common but not associated with tropical sprue made researchers wonder what effect unprocessed vegetable material had on villous structure. Studies in rats showed that standard chow and pectin feeding resulted in a flattened villous structure not seen when cellulose or cholestyramine were the only unabsorbable component of the diet (193). An unexplored but possibly analogous situation might exist in subjects habitually consuming diets high in the glycoproteins (lectins). Certainly, this is evident in extreme form in susceptible individuals (with celiac) exposed to gliadin, the glycoprotein of wheat.

Dietary components apparently may be used to induce changes not only in morphology, enzyme levels, and absorptive function of the upper gastrointestinal tract but also in motor activity. After 4 weeks of pectin supplementation, gastric emptying of a pectin-free meal in healthy volunteers was half that of the original control. This, too, may have important nutritional and metabolic consequences. Cellulose supplementation was without effect (194).

In summary, the nature of dietary carbohydrates, fats, and proteins has an acutely important influence on the absorption of natural diets. Perhaps less well recognized is the role of food form and food preparation procedures, especially those that alter either the absolute amount of fiber and antinutrients within a food or their relationship with the macronutrients. Increasingly, factors that alter carbohydrate absorption can be viewed not simply as causing or reducing malabsorption, but as altering the rate of absorption. Thus, factors that reduce the rate of absorption result in absorption at sites further along the small intestine. Finally, carbohydrate that is not absorbed in the small intestine may still be salvaged as SCFAs in the colon. The endocrine and metabolic effects of these changes can be considerable, as are the effects on absorption of other nutrients. In addition, long-term adaptation of small intestinal and, indeed, colonic function to the maneuvers described is only beginning to be explored. Active modification of small intestinal absorption probably has the potential to become an important therapeutic technique in the future (195).

REFERENCES

1. Allen FM. J Exp Med Balt 1920;31:381–402.
2. Christakis G, Miridjanian A. In: Ellenberg M, Rifkin H, eds. Diabetes mellitus. Theory and practice. New York: McGraw-Hill, 1970;594–623.
3. Wahlquist ML, Wilmshurst EG, Richardson EN. Am J Clin Nutr 1978;31:1988–2001.
4. Dahlquist A, Borgstrom B. Biochem J 1961;81:411–8.
5. Fogel MR, Gray GM. J Appl Physiol 1973;35:263–7.
6. Wolfrom ML, Khoden HE. Chemistry and technology. New York: Academic Press, 1965;254.
7. Gray GM, Fogel MR. In: Goodhart RS, Shils ME, eds. Modern nutrition in health and disease. 6th ed. Philadelphia: Lea & Febiger, 1980;99–112.
8. Silk DBA, Sawson AM. In: Crane RH, ed. International reviews of physiology: gastrointestinal physiology III, vol 19. Baltimore: University Park Press, 1979;151–204.
9. Leach HW. Starch chemistry and technology. New York: Academic Press, 1965.
10. Geervani P, Theophilus F. J Food Sci 1981;46:817–28.
11. Shurpalekar KS, Sunderavalu DE, Rao MN. Nutr Rep Rev 1979;19:111–7.
12. Crapo PA, Reaven G, Olefsky J. Diabetes 1976;25:741–7.
13. Crapo PA, Reaven G, Olefsky J. Diabetes 1977;26:1178–82.
14. Crapo PA, Kolterman OG. Waldeck N, et al. Am J Clin Nutr 1980;33:1723–8.
15. Crapo PA, Insel J, Sperling M, et al. Am J Clin Nutr 1981;34:184–190.
16. Jenkins DJA, Wolever TMS, Taylor RH, et al. Am J Clin Nutr 1981;34:362–6.
17. Jenkins DJA, Wolever TMS, Jenkins AL, et al. Diabetologia 1983;24:257–64.
18. Jenkins DJA, Wolever TMS, Taylor RH, et al. Br Med J 1980;281:14–7.
19. Jenkins DJA, Ghafari H, Wolever TMS, et al. Diabetologia 1982;22:450–5.
20. Juliano BO, Goddard MS. Plant Foods Hum Nutr 1986;36: 35–41.
21. Behall KM, Scholfield DJ, Canary J. Am J Clin Nutr 1988;47: 426–32.
22. Bocher CE, Behan I, McNeans E. J Nutr 1951;45:75.
23. Collings P, Williams C, MacDonald I. Br Med J 1981;282:1032.
24. Kon S, Wagner JR, Booth AN, et al. J Food Sci 1971;36:635–9.
25. Geervani P, Theophilius F. J Sci Food Agric 1981;32:71–8.
26. Devados RP, Leela R, Chanchasilearan KN. J Nutr Diet 1964; 1:84–6.
27. Alli I, Baker RE. J Sci Food Agric 1980;31:1316–22.
28. Pak CW, Belea CS, Bartter FC. N Engl J Med 1974;290:175–8.
29. Jenkins DJA, Wolever TMS, Thorne MJ, et al. Am J Clin Nutr 1984;40:1125–91.

29a. Cummings JH, Englyst HN. Am J Clin Nutr 1995;61 (Suppl):938S–45S.

30. Felber J-P. Beta Release 1983;7:6–9.
31. Bantle JP, Laine DC, Castle GW. N Engl J Med 1983;309:7–12.
32. Schauberger G, Brinck UC, Guldner G, et al. Diabetes 1977;26:415.
33. Crapo PA, Scarlett JA, Kolterman OG, et al. Diabetes Care 1982;5:512–7.
34. Swan DC, Davidson P, Albrink MJ. Lancet 1966;1:60–3.
35. Bohannon NV, Karana JH, Forsham PH. Diabetes 1978;27(Suppl 2):438.
36. Swanson JE, Laine DC, Thomas W, et al. Am J Clin Nutr 1992;55:851–6.
37. Calloway DH, Kurtz GW, McMullen JJ, et al. Food Res 1956;21:621.
38. Steenbock H, Irwin MH, Weber J. J Nutr 1936;12:103–11.
39. Turner DA. Am J Dig Dis 1958;3:594–708.
40. Jenkins DJA, Gassull MA, Leeds AR, et al. Int J Vitam Nutr Res 1976;46:226–30.
41. Gassull MA, Blendis LM, Jenkins DJA, et al. Int J Vitam Nutr Res 1976;46:211–4.
42. Bloomstrand R, Gurtler J, Werner B. J Clin Invest 1965;44: 1766–77.
43. Werner M, Lutwak L. Fed Proc 1963;22:553–63.
44. Cheng ALS, Morehouse MG, Davel HJ. J Nutr 1949;37: 237–50.
45. Tomarelli RM, Meyer BJ, Waeber JR, et al. J Nutr 1968;95: 583–90.
46. Filer LJ, Mattson FH, Formon SJ. J Nutr 1969;99:293–8.
47. Bennett S. Q J Exp Physiol 1964;49:210–8.
48. Geliebter A, Torbay N, Braeco EF, et al. Am J Clin Nutr 1983;37:1–4.
49. Winawer SJ, Broitman SA, Wolochow DA. N Engl J Med 1966;274:72–8.
50. Kaunitz H, Slanetz CA, Johnson RE, et al. J Nutr 1958;64:513.
51. Van de Kamer JH, ten Bokkel Huinink H, Weyers HA. J Biol Chem 1949;177:347–55.
52. Saunders DR. Gastroenterology 1967;52:135–6.
53. Senior B. In: Senior B, Van Italie TB, Greenberger N, eds. Medium chain triglycerides. Philadelphia: University of Pennsylvania Press, 1968;38.
54. Greenberger NJ, Ruppert RD, Tzagousis M. Ann Intern Med 1967;66:727–34.
55. Muto Y, Takahaski Y. Postgrad Med 1965;37:A158.
56. Zieve L. Arch Intern Med 1966;118:211–23.
57. Partin JS, Partin JC, Schubert WK, et al. Gastroenterology 1974;67:107–18.
58. Cummings JH, Wiggins HS, Jenkins DJA, et al. J Clin Invest 1978;61:953–62.
59. Gannon MC, Nattall FG, Neil BJ, et al. Metabolism 1988;37: 1081–8.
60. Uribe M, Marquez MA, Ramos GG, et al. Dig Dis Sci 1982;27:1109–16.
61. de Bruijn KM, Blendis LM, Zilm DH, et al. Gut 1983;24: 53–60.
62. Shaw S, Wroner TM, Lieber CS. Am J Clin Nutr 1983; 38:59–62.
63. Franzen K, Kinsella JE. J Agric Food Chem 1976;24:788–95.
64. Mehychyn P, Stapley RB. United States Patent 3764711, 1973.
65. Creamer LK, Roeper J, Lahrey EN. NZ J Dairy Sci Technol 1971;6:107.
66. Siu M, Thompson LU. J Agric Food Chem 1982;30:743–7.
67. Matoba T, Doi E. J Food Sci 1979;44:537.

67a. Trowell H, Southgate DAT, Wolever TMS, et al. Lancet 1976;1:967.

67b. Englyst H, Wiggins HS, Cummings JH. Analyst 1982;107:307–18.
67c. Burkitt DP, Trowell HC. Refined carbohydrate and disease. New York: Academic Press, 1975.
68. Cowgill GR, Anderson WE. JAMA 1932;98:1866–75.
68a. Williams RD, Olmsted WH. J Nutr 1936;11:433–42.
68b. Cummings JH, Branch W, Jenkins DJA, et al. Lancet 1978;1:5–9.
68c. Wyman JB, Heaton KW, Manning AB, Wicks ACB. Am J Clin Nutr 1976;29:1474–9.
68d. Burkitt DP, Walker RP, Painter NS. Lancet 1972;2 (792):1408–12.
68e. Cummings J. The effect of dietary fiber on fecal weights and composition: In: Spiller GA, ed. Handbook of dietary fiber in human nutrition. Boca Raton, FL: CRC Press, 1993.
68f. Floch MH, Fuchs HM. Am J Clin Nutr 1978;31:S185–9.
69. Jenkins DJA, Wolever TMS, Leeds AR, et al. Br Med J 1978;1:1392–4.
70. Eastwood MA, Hamilton D. Biochim Biophys Acta 1968;152:165–73.
71. Kay RM, Truswell AS. Am J Clin Nutr 1977;30:171–5.
71a. Jenkins DJA, Wolever TMS, Roa AV. N Engl J Med 1993;239:21–6.
71b. Lia A, Hullmans G, Sandberg A-S, et al. Am J Clin Nutr 1995;239:1245–51.
72. Holt S, Heading RC, Carter DC, et al. Lancet 1979;1:636–9.
73. Leeds AR, Ralphs DNL, Boulos D, et al. Proc Nutr Soc 1978;37:33.
74. Kasper H, Zilly W, Fassl H, et al. Am J Clin Nutr 1979;32: 2436.
74. Leeds AR, Ralphs DNL, Ebied F, et al. Lancet 1981;1:1075–8.
75. Taylor RH. Lancet 1979;1:872.
76. Elsenhans B, Sufke V, Blume R, et al. Clin Sci 1980;59: 373–80.
76a. Everson GT, Daggy BP, McKinley C, et al. J Lipid Res 1992;33:1183–92.
76b. Marlett JA, Hosig KB, Vollendorf NW, et al. Hepatology 1994;20:1450–7.
76c. Jenkins DJA, Wolever TMS, Vidjen E, et al. Am J Clin Nutr 1997;65:1524–33.
77. Florie B, Vidon N, Florent CH, et al. Gut 1984;25:936–41.
78. Blackburn NA, Redfern JS, Jarjis H, et al. Clin Sci 1984;66:329–36.
79. Sandberg AS, Anderson H, Hallgren B, et al. Br J Nutr 1981;45:283–94.
80. Jenkins DJA. In: Carlson LA, Paoletti R, Sirtori CR, et al. International conference on atherosclerosis. New York: Raven Press, 1978;173–82.
81. Kasper H, Rabast U, Fassl H, et al. Am J Clin Nutr 1979;38: 1847–9.
82. Weintraub MS, Eisenberg S, Breslow JL. J Clin Invest 1987;79:1110–9.
83. Jenkins DJA, Leeds AR, Gassull MA, et al. Ann Intern Med 1972;86:20–3.
84. Barnard DL, Heaton KW. Gut 1973;14:316–8.
85. Jenkins DJA, Wolever TMS, Hockaday TDR, et al. Lancet 1977;2:779–80.
86. Jenkins DJA, Wolever TMS, Nineham R, et al. Br Med J 1978;2:1744–6.
87. Aro A, Uusitupa M, Voutilainen E, et al. Diabetologia 1981;21:29–33.
88. Doi K, Matsuura M, Kuwara A, et al. Lancet 1979;1: 987–8.
89. Fahrenbach MJ, Riccardi BA, Saunders JL, et al. Circulation 1965;31/32(Suppl 2):1141.
90. Miettinen TA, Tarpila S. Clin Chim Acta 1977;79:471–7.
91. Jenkins DJA, Reynolds D, Slavin B. Am J Clin Nutr 1980;33:575–81.
92. Jenkins DJA, Gassull MA, Leeds AR, et al. Gastroenterology 1977;73:215–7.
93. Jenkins DJA, Bloom SR, Albuquerque RH, et al. Gut 1980;21:574–9.
94. Jenkins DJA, Wolever TMS, Taylor RH, et al. Diabetes Care 1981;4:509–13.
94a. Wood PJ, Braaten JT, Scott FW, et al. Br J Nutr 1994;72: 731–43.
94b. Blake DE, Hambleth CJ, Frost PG, et al. Am J Clin Nutr 1997;65;107–13.
94c. Swain JF, Rouse IL, Curley CB, Sacks FM. N Engl J Med 1990;322:147–52.
94d. Leadbetter J, Ball MJ, Mann JI. Am J Clin Nutr 1991;54: 841–5.
94e. Noakes M, Clifton PM, Nestel PH, et al. Am J Clin Nutr 1996;64:944–51.
94f. FDA. Food labeling: health claims; oat and cardiovascular heart disease; final rule. Federal Register 62(15):358323601. Washington, DC: US Government, 1997.
95. Jenkins DJA, Wolever TMS, Jenkins AL, et al. Diabetes Care 1981;6:155–9.
96. Nishimune T, Yakushiji T, Sumimoto T, et al. Am J Clin Nutr 1991;54:414–9.
97. Wolever TMS. Am J Clin Nutr 1990;51:72–5.
98. Anderson IH, Levine AS, Levitt MD. N Engl J Med 1981;304:891–2.
99. Jenkins DJA, Thorne MJ, Wolever TMS, et al. Am J Clin Nutr 1987;45:946–51.
100. Meyer JH, Stevenson EA, Watts HD. Gastroenterology 1976;70:232–9.
101. Monoz JM. In: Vahouny GV, Kritchevsky D, eds. Dietary fiber in health and disease. New York: Plenum, 1982;85–9.
102. Thomas EJ. Physiol Rev 1957;37:453–74.
103. Holm J, Bjorck I, Ostrowska S, et al. Starch Staerke 1983;35: 294–7.
104. Augur V, Rollman HS, Deuel HJ. J Nutr 1947;33:177–86.
105. Sylven C, Borgstrom B. J Lipid Res 1969;10:351–5.
106. Roels DA, Trout H, Dujacquier R. J Nutr 1958;65:115–27.
107. Kelsay JL. Update on fiber and mineral availability. In: Vahouny GV, Kritchevsky D, eds. Dietary fiber in health and disease. New York: Plenum, 1985;361–72.
108. Reinhold JG, Faradji B, Abadi P, et al. J Nutr 1976;106: 493–503.
109. Cummings JH, Hill MJ, Jivraj T, et al. Am J Clin Nutr 1979;32:2086–93.
110. Jenkins DJA, Hill MJ, Cummings JH. Am J Clin Nutr 1975;28:1408–11.
111. Kelsay J. In: Vahouny GV, Kritchevsky D, eds. Dietary fiber in health and disease. New York: Plenum, 1985;361–72.
112. Pilch SM, ed. Physiological effects and health consequences of dietary fiber. Bethesda, MD: Federation of American Societies for Experimental Biology, 1985.
113. Kelsay JL. Am J Gastroenterol 1987;82:983–6.
114. Kelsay JL, Prather ES, Clark WM, et al. J Nutr 1988;118: 1197–204.
115. Nicolaysen R, Eeg-Larsen N, Malm OJ. Physiol Rev 1953;33: 424–44.
116. Rayssiguier Y, Remesy C. Ann Rech Vet 1977;8:105–10.
117. Hollander D, Rim E, Ruble PE. Gastroenterology 1977;72: A48/1071.
118. Haber EB, Heaton KW, Murphy D, et al. Lancet 1977;2: 679–82.

119. O'Dea K, Nestel PJ, Antionoff L. Am J Clin Nutr 1980;33:760–5.
120. Jenkins DJA, Wesson V, Wolever TMS, et al. Br Med J 1988;297:958–60.
121. Heaton KW, Marcus SN, Emmett PM, et al. Am J Clin Nutr 1988;47:675–82.
122. Wolever TMS, Jenkins DJA, Kalmunsky J, et al. Nutr Res 1986;6:349–57.
123. Jenkins DJA, Thorne MJ, Camelon K, et al. Am J Clin Nutr 1982;36:1093–101.
124. Leiner IE. Proc Nutr Soc 1979;38:109–13.
125. Puls W, Keup V. Diabetologia 1973;9:97–101.
126. Walton RJ, Sherif IT, Noy GA, et al. Br Med J 1979;1:220–1.
126a. Chiasson J-L, Josse RG, Hunt JA, et al. Ann Intern Med 1994;121:928–35.
127. Jenkins DJA, Barker HM, Taylor RH, et al. Lancet 1982;1:109.
128. Oakenfull DG, Fenwick DE. Br J Nutr 1978;40:299–309.
129. Bressani R, Elias LG. In: Hulse JH, ed. Polyphenols in cereals and legumes. Ottawa: International Development Research Centre, 1980.
130. Singh D, Jambunathan R. J Food Sci 1981;46:1364–7.
131. Griffiths DW, Moseley G. J Sci Food Agric 1980;31:255–9.
132. Thompson LU, Yoon JH, Jenkins DJA, et al. Am J Clin Nutr 1984;39:745–51.
133. Erdman JW. J Am Oil Chem Soc 1979;56:736–40.
134. Cheryan M. CRC Crit Rev Food Sci Nutr 1980;13:297–335.
135. Reinhold JG, Lahimgarzodeh A, Nasr K, et al. Lancet 1973;1:28–33.
136. James WPT. Dietary fiber and mineral absorption. In: Spiller GA, Kay RM, eds. Medical aspects of dietary fiber. New York: Plenum, 1980;239–59.
137. Yoon JH, Thompson LU, Jenkins DJA. Am J Clin Nutr 1983;38:835–42.
138. Alfonsky D. Saliva and its relation to oral health. Birmingham: University of Alabama Press, 1966.
139. Nachbar MS, Oppenheim JD. Am J Clin Nutr 1980;33:2338–45.
140. Puzstai A, Clarke EMW, King TP. Proc Nutr Soc 1979;38:115–20.
141. Noah ND, Bender AL, Reaidi GB, et al. Br Med J 1980;281:236–7.
142. Rea R, Thompson LU, Jenkins DJA. Nutr Res 1985;5:919–29.
143. Jenkins DJA, Wolever TMS, Vuksan V, et al. N Engl J Med 1989;321:929–34.
144. Jenkins DJA, Wolever TMS, Ocana AM, et al. Diabetes 1990;39:775–81.
145. Jenkins DJA, Ocana AM, Jenkins AL, et al. Am J Clin Nutr 1992;55:461–7.
145a. Ellis A. Q J Med 1934;27:137–53.
145b. Bertelsen J, Christiansen C, Thomson C, et al. Diabetes Care 1993;16:3–7.
145c. Franz MJ, Horton ES, Brantle JP, et al. Diabetes Care 1994;17:490–518.
146. Gwinup G, Byron RC, Roush W, et al. Am J Clin Nutr 1963;13:209–13.
147. Irwin MI, Feeley RM. Am J Clin Nutr 1967;20:816–24.
148. Young CM, Frankel DL, Scanlan SS, et al. J Am Diet Assoc 1971;59:473–80.
148a. Arnold LM, Ball MJ, Duncan AW, Mann J. Am J Clin Nutr 1993;57:446–51.
148b. McGrath SA, Gibney MJ. Eur J Clin Nutr 1994;48:402–7.
149c. Jones PJH, Leitch CA, Pederson RA. Am J Clin Nutr 1993;57:868–74.
149. Lakshmanan MR, Nepokroeff CM, Ness GC, et al. Biochem Biophys Res Commun 1973;50:704–10.
150. Jaganathan SN, Connon WF, Beveridge JMR. Am J Clin Nutr 1964;15:90–3.
151. Fabry P, Tepperman J. Am J Clin Nutr 1970;23:1059–68.
152. Potter JD, McMichael AJ. J Natl Cancer Inst 1986;76:557–69.
153. Young TB, Wolf DA. Int J Cancer 1988;42:167–75.
154. Wolever TMS, Jenkins DJA, Jenkins AL, et al. Am J Clin Nutr 1991;54:846–54.
154a. Foster-Powell K, Brand-Miller J. Am J Clin Nutr 1995;62:871S–93S.
155. Wolever TMS. World Rev Nutr Diet 1990;62:120–85.
156. Wolever TMS, Jenkins DJA, Jenkins AL, et al. J Clin Nutr Gastroenterol 1988;3:85–8.
157. Wolever TMS, Jenkins DJA, Vuksan V, et al. Diabetes Care 1990;13:126–32.
158. Wolever TMS, Csima A, Jenkins DJA, et al. J Am Coll Nutr 1989;8:235–47.
159. Wolever TMS, Jenkins DJA. Am J Clin Nutr 1986;43:167–72.
159a. Miller JB, Pang E, Broomhead L. Br. J Nutr 1995;73:613–23.
160. Jenkins DJA, Wolever TMS, Kalmusky J, et al. Am J Clin Nutr 1985;42:604–17.
161. Jenkins DJA, Wolever TMS, Kalmusky J, et al. Am J Clin Nutr 1987;46:66–71.
162. Jenkins DJA, Wolever TMS, Collier GR, et al. Am J Clin Nutr 1987;46:968–75.
163. Collier GR, Giudici S, Kalmusky J, et al. Diabetes Nutr Metab 1988;1:11–9.
164. Fontvieille AM, Acosta M, Rizkalla SW, et al. Diabetes Nutr Metab 1988;1:139–43.
165. Brand JC, Colagiuri S, Crossman S, et al. Diabetes Care 1991;14:95–101.
166. Wolever TMS, Jenkins DJA, Vuksan V, et al. Diabetes Care 1992;15:562–4.
167. Jenkins DJA, Thorne MJ, Taylor RH, et al. Am J Gastroenterol 1987;82:223–30.
168. Brand JC, Holt S, Saveny C, et al. Proc Nutr Soc Aust 1990;15:209.
169. Thomas DE, Brotherhood JR, Brand JC. Med Sci Sports Med Exerc 1990;22(Suppl):S121.
169a. Salmeron J, Stampfer MJ, Colditz GA, et al. JAMA 1997;277:472–7.
169b. Salmeron J, Ascherio A, Rimm EB, et al. Diabetes Care 1997;20:545–50.
170. Wolever TMS, Thorne MJ, Thompson LU, et al. Proc Nutr Soc 1985;5:919–29.
171. Stephen AM, Haddad AC, Phillips SF. Gastroenterology 1983;85:589–95.
172. Steinhart AH, Jenkins DJA, Mitchell S, et al. Am J Gastroenterol 1992;87:48–54.
173. Bond JA, Currier BE, Buchwald H, et al. Gastroenterology 1980;78:444–7.
174. Cummings JH. Gut 1981;22:763–79.
175. James WPT. Dietary fiber and mineral absorption. In: Spiller GA, McPherson-Kay R, eds. Medical aspects of dietary fiber. New York: Plenum 1980;237–59.
176. Thompson LU, Trinidad T, Wolever TMS. Calcium absorption in the colon. In: Seventh international symposium on Trace Elements in Man and Animals, Dubrovnik, May 20–25, 1990. Zagreb: Institute for Medical Research and Occupational Health, 1990.
177. Kruk J. Mol Cell Biochem 1982;42:65–82.
178. Haing JM, Soergel KH, Komorowski RA, et al. N Engl J Med 1987;320:23–8.

179. Thacker PA, Solomon MO, Aheme FX, et al. Can J Anim Sci 1981;61:969–75.
180. Scheppach W, Cummings JH, Branch WJ, et al. Clin Sci 1988;75:355–61.
181. Scheppach W, Wiggins HS, Halliday D, et al. Clin Sci 1988;75:363–70.
182. Crouse JR, Gerson CD, DeCarli LM, et al. J Lipid Res 1968;9:509–12.
183. Wolever TMS, Spadafora P, Eshuis H. Am J Clin Nutr 1991;53:681–7.
184. Todesco T, Rao AV, Bozello O, et al. Am J Clin Nutr 1991;54:860–5.
185. Chen W-JL, Anderson JW, Jennings D. Proc Soc Exp Biol Med 1984;175:215–8.
186. Illman RJ, Topping DL, McIntosh GH, et al. Ann Nutr Metab 1988;32:97–107.
187. Venter CS, Vorster HH, Cummings JH. Am J Gastroenterol 1990;85:549–53.
188. Nishina PM, Freedland RA. J Nutr 1990;120:668–73.
189. Jenkins DJA, Wolever TMS, Jenkins AL, et al. Am J Clin Nutr 1991;54:141–7.
189a. Weiner GA, Krause JA, Miller TL, Wolin MJ. Gut 1988;29: 1539–43.
189b. Candito EP, Reeves R, Davie JR. Cell 1978;14:105–13.
189c. Whitehead RH, Yong GP, Bhathal PS. Gut 1986;27: 1457–63.
189d. McIntyre A, Gibson PR, Yong GP. Gut 1993;34:386–91.
189e. Birket A, Muir J, Phillips J, et al. Am J Clin Nutr 1996;63:766–72.
189f. Cummings JH, Beatty ER, Kingman SM, et al. Br J Nutr 1996;75:733–47.
190. Rosensweig NS, Herman R. J Clin Invest 1968;47:2253.
191. Thomsen LL, Tasman-Jones C. Digestion 1982;23:253.
192. Thomson ABR, Rajotte R. Am J Clin Nutr 1983;37: 244–52.
193. Tasman-Jones C, Owne RL, Jones AL. Dig Dis Sci 1982;27:519.
194. Schwartz SE, Levine RA, Singh A, et al. Gastroenterology 1982;83:812–7.
195. Creutzfeldt W. Introduction. In: Creutzfeldt W, Folsch UR, eds. Delaying absorption as a therapeutic principle in metabolic diseases. New York: Thieme-Stratton, 1983;1.

44. Hormone, Cytokine, and Nutrient Interactions

IRWIN G. BRODSKY

This chapter examines the effects of various hormones on the metabolism of macronutrients. Defining hormones in a broad sense, the chapter examines the effects of humoral factors from classic endocrine organs such as pancreatic islets, thyroid, pituitary, gonads, and adrenals as well as from tissues not traditionally characterized as regulators of metabolic homeostasis. In particular, the chapter examines cytokine and eicosanoid elaboration by immune cells and growth factor production by a variety of tissues that contribute to nutrient disposition and mobilization during illness and tissue repair. The chapter examines the *endocrine* actions of hormones, in which hormones act at sites distant from their tissues of origin, generally traversing the circulation to reach their target tissues. It reports the *paracrine* actions of hormones, in which hormones act on neighboring cells within their tissues of origin. Finally, it identifies occasions in which a given hormone acts as an *autocrine* factor, acting to affect the cell from which it was secreted.

The chapter creates a context for understanding hormone-nutrient interactions that underscores the role of hormones in determining availability of nutritional substrates for immediate needs or long-term storage. There is interindividual variability in the response of tissues to hormones, and nutritional substrates may partially regulate their own use. Figure 44.1 and Table 44.1 distinguish the effects of hormones primarily affecting nutrient storage (Fig. 44.1) and those mediating nutrient mobilization (Fig. 44.2). Table 44.2 summarizes the influence of various hormones on circulating concentrations of glucose, free fatty acids, and amino acids.

PANCREATIC ISLET HORMONES (INSULIN, GLUCAGON, AND SOMATOSTATIN)

Carbohydrate Metabolism

Carbohydrate metabolism is finely regulated by interactions between insulin, the hormone promoting fuel storage, and the counterregulatory hormones such as glucagon, epinephrine, cortisol, growth hormone, and immune cell cytokines. Glucose homeostasis is maintained in the presence of widely varying quantities and compositions of food intake. Because the brain has a limited ability to vary its extraction of glucose with variation in glucose supply (1), the importance of these homeostatic mechanisms is apparent.

Insulin

Insulin has a central role in promoting glucose disposal into peripheral tissues and storage as glycogen, a characteristic of the fed state. Like other peptide hormones, insulin initiates its metabolic effects by binding to a cell-surface receptor. These effects depend on the activation of a tyrosine-specific protein kinase, which is contained in the β-subunit of the receptor (2, 3). After binding to the receptor, insulin accelerates membrane transport of sugars following initiation of a cascade of intracellular enzyme phosphorylation events (4). Increases in maximal glucose transport rates in response to insulin vary from 3.2-fold in skeletal muscle to 30-fold in adipocytes (5–7). This effect is produced by insulin-mediated translocation

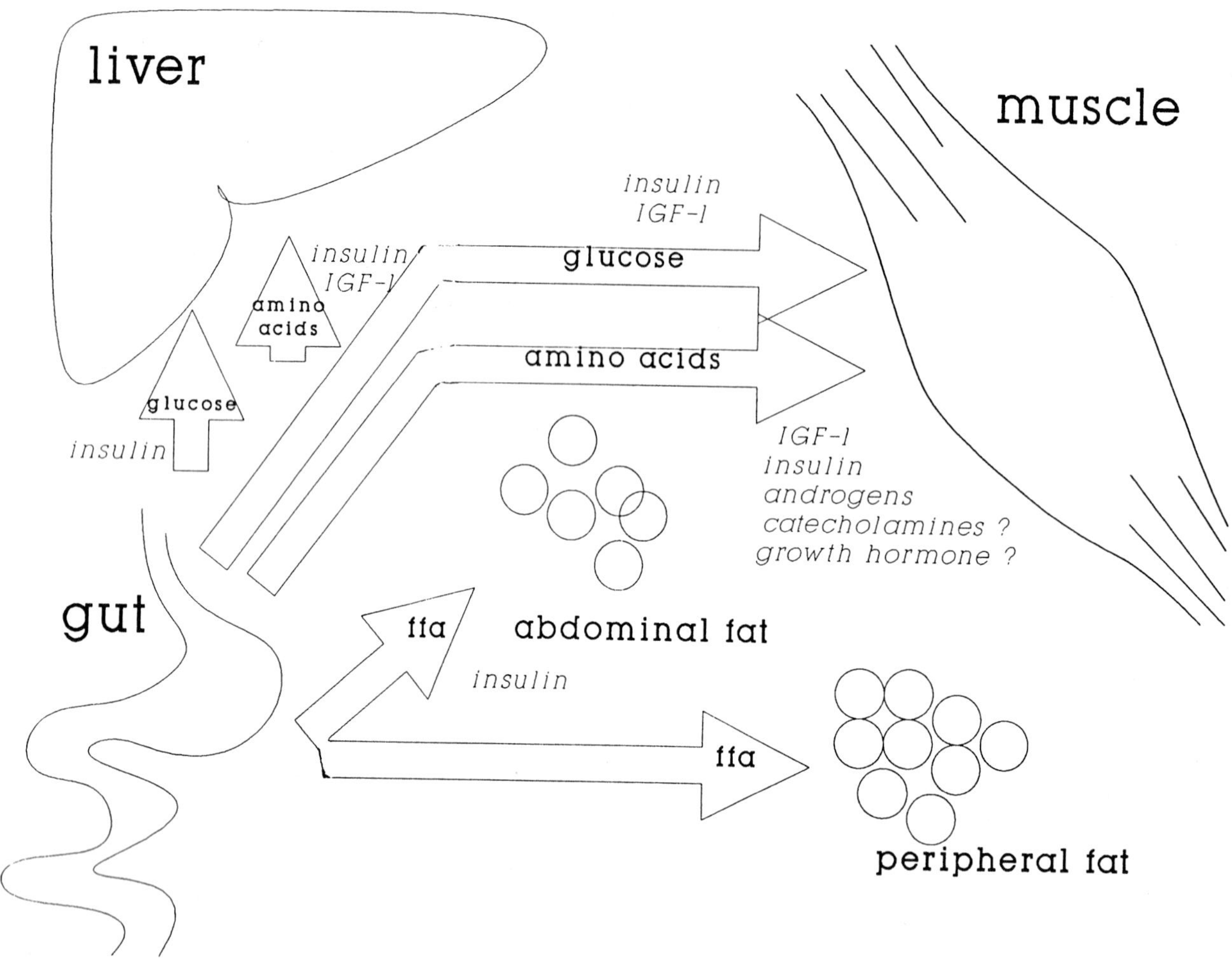

Figure 44.1. Hormones promoting nutrient storage. *Arrows* represent release of ingested nutrients from the gut to storage sites in liver, skeletal muscle, and adipose tissue. The hormones promoting storage of particular nutrients are presented in italics juxtaposed to the appropriate arrows. *IGF-1,* insulin-like growth factor; *ffa,* free fatty acids.

of glucose transporter proteins from intracellular membrane pools to plasma membrane in insulin-sensitive tissues (8, 9). Transporters located in the insulin-sensitive tissues (e.g., adipose tissue, skeletal muscle, and heart muscle) are sodium-independent, facilitative transporters named GLUT1 and GLUT4 (10). GLUT4 is the primary protein involved in insulin-stimulated translocation (11). Despite the pivotal role of GLUT4 in insulin-stimulated glucose transport, clinical resistance to the metabolic effects of insulin on glucose disposal, as seen in non-insulin-dependent diabetes, does not appear to be due to disorders of GLUT4 expression but is more likely due to impaired communication between the insulin receptor and GLUT4-containing intracellular vesicles (12).

Insulin rapidly increases membrane glucose transport, within 1 to 2 minutes, with a maximal effect in 15 to 20 minutes. Many tissues, including brain and liver, maintain glucose uptake independent of insulin concentrations (13). This ability corresponds to the predominance in those tissues of glucose transporters such as GLUT1 (a ubiquitous transporter) and GLUT3 (brain) or GLUT2 (liver), respectively, which have plasma membrane activities known to be independent of insulin concentrations (14). The hypothalamus may represent a brain region with some dependence on insulin for glucose use, particularly in the glucose-sensitive areas of the ventromedial and lateral nuclei (15, 16). Conversely, skeletal muscle (generally an "insulin-sensitive" tissue) may take up glucose without insulin stimulation under circumstances of contractile stimulation (17).

In addition to increasing glucose transport, insulin also has major effects on intracellular glucose metabolism (Fig. 44.3). In experimentally induced diabetes, activities of enzymes involved in glycolysis and glucose oxidation, such as glucokinase, phosphofructokinase, and pyruvate kinase, are decreased, and activities of gluconeogenic enzymes, such as glucose-6-phosphatase, fructose 1,6-bisphosphatase, phosphoenolpyruvate carboxykinase, and pyruvate carboxylase, are increased. These abnormalities are corrected by insulin replacement. Insulin also promotes glycogen synthesis, by promoting the conversion of glycogen synthase to its active, glucose-6-phosphate-independent ("I") form and by decreasing the activity of phosphorylase. Insulin causes rapid decreases in phosphorylase

Table 44.1
Effect of Hormones on Nutrient Stores

Hormones	Carbohydrate	Lipid	Protein
Pancreatic hormones			
Insulin	↑	↑	↑
Glucagon	↓	↓	↓
Somatostatin	*	*	*
Thyroid hormones			
Thyroxine (T_4)/triiodothyronine (T_3)	*	↓	*
Glucocorticoid/ACTH			
ACTH	•	↓	*
Cortisol	*	*	↓
Growth hormone/IGF-1			
Growth hormone	*	*	↑
Insulin-like growth factor-1 (IGF-1)	↑	↑	↑
Catecholamines			
Epinephrine/norepinephrine	↓($\alpha + \beta$)	↓(β)	*
Gonadal hormones/prolactin			
Estrogen	*	*	*
Progesterone	*	*	*
Testosterone	↓	*	↑
Prolactin	*	↓	*
Cytokines/eicosanoids			
Thromboxane A2 (TXA2)/prostaglandin E2, and F2α (PGE_2, $PGF_{2\alpha}$)	↓	*	*
Tumor necrosis factor-α (TNF-α)	*	↓	↓
Interleukin-6	*	*	↑

* No effect, variable effects, or unknown; see text.

activity and more gradual increases in synthase I activity, although the hormonal effect is brief in vivo (18).

Insulin generates an enzymatic profile that decreases glucose carbon recycling (seen during insulin deficiency) and promotes glucose use for energy storage (19). It stimulates glycolysis and lipogenesis in adipose tissue and both glycolysis and glycogen synthesis in skeletal muscle tissue and inhibits gluconeogenesis in the renal cortex and liver (20). Skeletal muscle glycogenolysis is very sensitive to inhibition by insulin according to studies in rats; it is inhibited by concentrations of insulin that inhibit hepatic glucose output—concentrations much lower than those required to stimulate circulating glucose uptake (21). Studies in humans suggest that both direct, hepatic effects of insulin (most potent when insulin is delivered in a typical manner through the portal vein) and indirect effects (from the influence of insulin on gluconeogenic substrate availability) operate in regulating hepatic glucose production (22). Some may be more important than insulin concentrations in activating glycogen synthase and glycogen deposition in the liver, whereas insulin has a key role in regulation of skeletal muscle glycogen metabolism (23). However, results of studies with cultured hepatocytes indicate that glucose-stimulated glycogen deposition plateaus within 2 hours of exposure to high-glucose medium, and insulin is required to continue glycogen accumulation beyond that time (24).

Ingestion of carbohydrate produces a prompt increase in plasma insulin and a decrease in glucagon concentrations (25). The rise in insulin occurs before the rise in arterial glucose concentrations comprising the so-called enteroinsular axis and cephalic-phase insulin release, which are mediated through hormonal (26, 27) and parasympathetic (28, 29) mechanisms. This early insulin release creates a "priming effect" in which the action of insulin begins concurrently with the absorption of glucose to minimize the extent of hyperglycemia after a meal. As glucose is absorbed, hepatic production of glucose is decreased through the hormonal changes mentioned above, and glucose uptake by the liver, muscle, and adipose tissues increases. Approximately 75% of glucose taken orally bypasses hepatic metabolism and is taken up peripherally (30). Skeletal muscle is the predominant tissue for disposal of an oral glucose load.

During periods of starvation, maintenance of euglycemia is critically important to the organism (see Chapter 41). In the nonketotic state, the energy needs of the brain can only be met by glucose, and its absence results in death of central nervous system tissues. Because the glucose pool can provide only 15 to 20 g in the adult, and glycogen that can be mobilized to provide circulating glucose (i.e., hepatic glycogen) averages 70 g, preformed glucose can provide less than an 8-h supply of glucose on average. Thus, gluconeogenesis is important for maintenance of postabsorptive plasma glucose concentrations and becomes the sole source of glucose production beyond a 24- to 48-h fast. Only the liver and kidneys contain glucose-6-phosphatase, the enzyme necessary for release of glucose into the circulation. The liver and kidneys also contain the enzymes necessary for gluconeogenesis (pyruvate carboxylase, PEP carboxykinase, and fructose 1,6-bisphosphatase). Except after prolonged starvation when renal gluconeogenesis becomes important, the liver is the sole source of *endogenous glucose production* (EGP). Starvation is associated with a decline in insulin and a rise in glucagon concentrations (31), which result in increased rates of gluconeogenesis. Decreased plasma insulin concentrations allow decreased glucose use by peripheral tissues and enhanced lipolysis; free fatty acids are thus more available for use as an oxidative fuel during starvation. These changes in serum insulin and glucagon concentrations also result in increased conversion of free fatty acids to the ketone bodies, acetoacetate and β-hydroxybutyrate, which can substitute for glucose as an energy supply for the brain (32). The change from a glucose- to a lipid-based (free fatty acids and ketone bodies) energy supply in prolonged starvation helps minimize skeletal muscle protein catabolism by reducing the need for amino acid–derived gluconeogenesis (33). β-Hydroxybutyrate also directly increases skeletal muscle protein synthesis in humans while simultaneously decreasing leucine oxidation (34). Similarly, studies in dogs demonstrated that increased free fatty acid availability decreases the whole-body leucine oxidation rate and leucine carbon flux (an estimate of protein degradation rate) (35).

The effects of insulin deficiency are exemplified by type

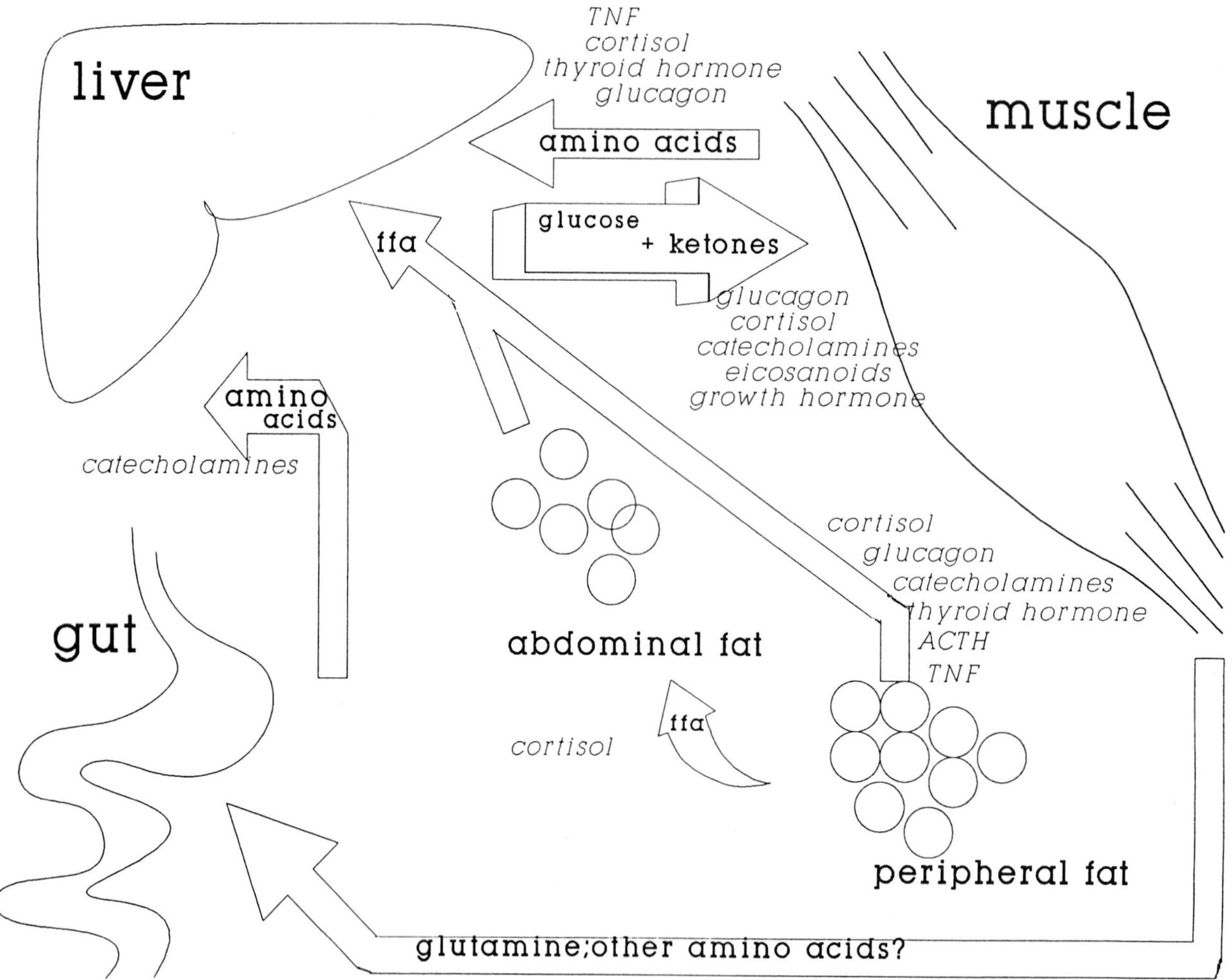

Figure 44.2. Hormones promoting nutrient mobilization from tissue stores. *Arrows* represent release of nutrients from storage sites in skeletal muscle, adipose tissue, gut, and liver. The hormones stimulating the release of particular nutrients are indicated in italics next to the appropriate arrows. *TNF,* tumor necrosis factor; *ACTH,* adrenocorticotropic hormone; *ffa,* free fatty acids.

1, insulin-dependent diabetes mellitus (IDDM). As stated above, this disorder is associated with increased activities of enzymes involved in gluconeogenesis, and decreased activities of glycolytic and oxidative enzymes. In addition, IDDM often is associated with relative or absolute hyperglucagonemia (36, 37), resulting from loss of the restraining influence of insulin (38) on the secretion of glucagon by the pancreatic α cell (39). An increase in glucose concentration also fails to inhibit glucagon secretion (40, 41) as it normally does and may paradoxically increase glucagon release (42). Glucagon responses to protein are also excessive in association with IDDM (20) and are not blunted by hyperglycemia (43). Control of the plasma glucose concentration to near normal levels with insulin therapy corrects the basal hyperglucagonemia (44) and the exaggerated response to protein ingestion (42).

Inappropriate hyperinsulinemia, as seen in insulin-producing islet cell adenomas or hyperplasia, results in postabsorptive hypoglycemia. In this condition, insulin secretion probably does not decrease as the plasma glucose declines in the postabsorptive state. The result is a low rate of EGP, with rates of glucose uptake that are not high in the absolute sense but are inappropriately high relative to the plasma glucose concentration. The hypoglycemic effect of insulin is potent. When insulin is present in sufficient quantity, it can cause hypoglycemia despite the actions of all known counterregulatory factors. Postabsorptive hypoglycemia may also occur when both glucagon and epinephrine are deficient and insulin is present (45). This situation occurs in some patients with IDDM (46, 47) but has not been demonstrated convincingly in other conditions.

Glucagon

Glucagon is secreted from the α cells of the pancreatic islets into the hepatic portal circulation and is thought to act predominantly on the liver under physiologic conditions. It exerts its effects through activation of adenylate cyclase (48) (Fig. 44.3*A*). Cyclic adenosine monophosphate (AMP) concentrations in liver rise within seconds after administration of glucagon. Glucagon is a potent activator of glycogenolysis and gluconeogenesis and is able to increase EGP within minutes, although the effect is

Table 40.2.
Effects of Hormones on Circulating Concentrations of Metabolites

Hormones	Glucose	Free Fatty Acids	Amino Acids
Pancreatic hormones			
Insulin	↓	↓	↓
Glucagon	↑	↑	↓
Somatostatin	↑	↑	*
Thyroid hormones			
Thyroxine (T_4)/triiodothyronine (T_3)	↑	↑	*
Glucocorticoid/ACTH			
ACTH	*	↑	*
Cortisol	↑	↑	↑
Growth hormone/IGF-1			
Growth hormone	*	*	*
Insulin-like growth factor-1 (IGF-1)	↓	↓	↓
Catecholamines			
Epinephrine/norepinephrine	↑	↑	↓
Gonadal hormones/prolactin			
Estrogen	*	*	*
Progesterone	*	*	*
Testosterone	↑	*	*
Prolactin	↑	↑	*
Cytokines/eicosanoids			
Thromboxane A2 (TXA2)/prostaglandin E2, and F2α (PGE_2, $PGF_{2\alpha}$)	↑	*	*
Tumor necrosis factor-α (TNF-α)	*	↑	↑
Interleukin-6	*	*	*

* No effect, variable effects, or unknown; see text.

transient. Glucagon decreases levels of fructose-2,6-bisphosphate, a key regulator of gluconeogenesis and glycolysis. Despite ongoing hyperglucagonemia, EGP decreases toward basal levels within 90 minutes. Glucagon-induced hyperglycemia is transient because the increase in glycogenolysis does not persist. This transient response is not the result of glycogen depletion, but more likely of glucagon-induced insulin secretion coupled with an autoregulatory effect of hyperglycemia to inhibit EGP. (See Chapter 37 for a more detailed discussion of cell signaling.)

During fasting in humans, about 75% of EGP is mediated by glucagon (49). In circumstances of combined glucagon and insulin deficiency, the decreased glucose production may not be balanced by decreased insulin-mediated glucose use because only about 40% of glucose use occurs in insulin-sensitive tissues. Therefore, plasma glucose concentrations would remain constant or even fall. The effect of insulin on the liver is to oppose the effect of glucagon (50). Insulin deficiency has a minimal influence on hepatic glucose and ketone metabolism in the absence of glucagon, and significant overproduction of glucose and ketones by the liver does not occur without glucagon (51).

Glucagon deficiency, produced experimentally by infusion of somatostatin with partial insulin replacement,

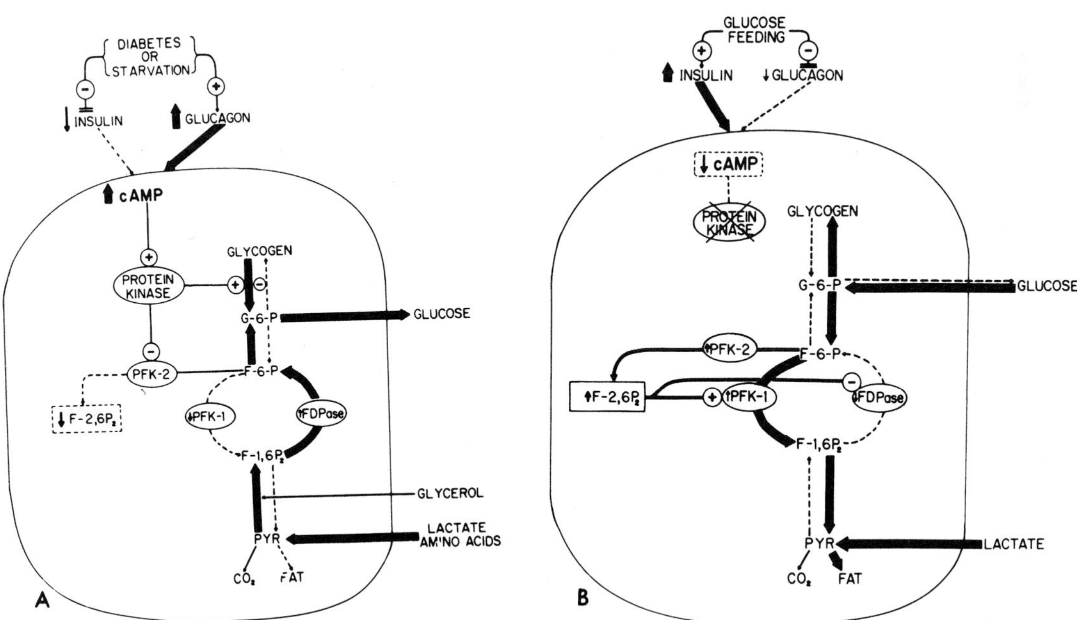

Figure 44.3. A. Enhancement of gluconeogenesis and glycogenolysis by glucagon in diabetes and starvation. Both processes are activated by increases in cyclic adenosine monophosphate *(cAMP)* in the hepatocyte. Phosphofructokinase-1 *(PFK-1)* catalyzes formation of fructose 1,6-bisphosphate *(F-1,6-P₂)* in the glycolytic pathway, whereas PFK-2 synthesizes fructose-2,6 biphosphate *(F-2,6-P₂)*, a regulator of PFK-1 activity; cAMP-induced phosphorylation of the enzyme decreases PFK-1 and increases PFK-2. Decreased F-2,6-P_2 decreases glycolysis and increases gluconeogenesis. **B.** Inhibition of gluconeogenesis and activation of glycogen synthesis and lipogenesis by insulin. Insulin decreases cAMP, deactivates protein kinase, and reverses changes in F-2,6-P_2 and substrate flux over the glycolytic-gluconeogenic pathway produced by glucagon. Glycogen synthesis and lipogenesis are also increased. (From Unger RH, Foster DW. In: Wilson J, Foster DW. Williams textbook of endocrinology. 7th ed. Philadelphia: WB Saunders, 1985.)

reduces nadir glucose concentrations after glucose ingestion by approximately 30%. Patients who have glucagon deficiency from pancreatectomy manifest decreased rates of glucose "recyling" (measured as the difference between 6-^{3}H-glucose and 1-^{14}C- glucose turnover rates, an index of gluconeogenesis) and increased serum concentrations of gluconeogenic precursors such as alanine and lactate (52). However, prolonged hypoglycemia does not occur because it is prevented by epinephrine secretion. As noted above, combined glucagon and epinephrine deficiency, as seen in some longstanding IDDM subjects, totally disrupts the counterregulatory process and results in hypoglycemia late after glucose ingestion. Diminished glucagon response to insulin-induced hypoglycemia is in part related to concomitant insulin-induced hypoaminoacidemia (53).

Exercise requires increased glucose production to counterbalance the increased glucose use that occurs with muscular work. Approximately 60 to 70% of the increased glucose production is mediated by increased glucagon secretion coupled with inhibited insulin release; another 30 to 40% is the result of epinephrine secretion (54, 55). The changes in glucagon and insulin are associated with decreased fructose-2,6-bisphosphate concentration in liver with resultant increased gluconeogenesis; simultaneous increases in epinephrine concentration produce increased concentrations of fructose-2,6-bisphosphate in nonexercising muscle with resultant stimulation of glycolysis and lactate production for use in gluconeogenesis (56). Combined glucagon deficiency and adrenergic blockade during exercise at 60% of maximal oxygen consumption produce profound hypoglycemia between 30 and 60 minutes of the exercise bout (54).

Glucagon excess, as seen in islet-cell glucagonoma, is associated with glucose intolerance, hypoaminoacidemia, and a characteristic rash, "necrolytic migratory erythema," thought to result from either the hyperglucagonemia or the decreased plasma amino acid levels (57, 58). The glycogenolytic and gluconeogenic actions of glucagon result in mild hyperglycemia that can usually be controlled by dietary therapy. The syndrome is also characterized by increased resting energy expenditure that is blunted by insulin infusion (59). The cause of the hypermetabolism is unknown.

Somatostatin

Somatostatin is a peptide hormone of 14 amino acids that originates from the δ cells of pancreatic islets. Its general effect is to inhibit cellular secretion of other peptides, particularly peptide hormones. In the somatostatinoma syndrome (60), seen in somatostatin-producing islet cell adenomas, suppression of both insulin and glucagon causes mild diabetes mellitus. Neither the hyperglycemia nor the hyperketonemia is severe, most likely because of glucagon and growth hormone suppression. The somatostatin analogue octreotide can similarly blunt postprandial glycemic excursions in IDDM patients and decrease prandial insulin requirements (61).

Lipid Metabolism

Insulin and glucagon also play important roles in lipid metabolism; increased insulin concentrations stimulate lipogenesis and lipid storage, and the decreased insulin and increased glucagon levels seen in fasting promote lipolysis and lipid oxidation (62). The major function of stored triglyceride in adipose tissue is to act as an efficient energy reserve. Triglyceride stores can serve as fuel to support many weeks of fasting, whereas stored carbohydrate can support a fast of only several hours. Stored triglyceride yields over twice as many calories per gram as either carbohydrate or protein and requires less than half as much intracellular water for storage.

In the fed state, insulin and glucose are required for lipogenesis. Glucose use is needed for fatty acid synthesis and esterification and supplies the following: *(a)* acetyl coenzyme A (CoA) as a precursor of long-chain fatty acids, *(b)* α-glycerophosphate for esterification to fatty acids to form triglycerides, and *(c)* nicotinamide adenine dinucleotide phosphate (NADPH). Insulin stimulates carrier-mediated glucose transport, and *(a)* activates pyruvate dehydrogenase for conversion of glucose to acetyl-CoA (63), and *(b)* inhibits lipolysis, thereby reducing concentrations of palmitoyl-CoA, an inhibitor of lipogenesis (64). In humans, however, less than 1% of ingested carbohydrate is converted to lipid (65). The mixed fat and carbohydrate intake of humans allows dietary fat to supply lipid for storage in a more energy efficient process than would be achieved if significant lipogenesis from carbohydrate occurred (i.e., 2 vs. 23% of ingested calories, the cost of storing these nutrients as lipid) (66). Nonetheless, recent studies suggest that consumption of a diet with very high carbohydrate and low fat content stimulates lipogenesis from carbohydrate in humans. Very low density lipoprotein (VLDL)-triglyceride produced from de novo synthesis increases from 0% on a high-fat diet (40% fat) to 44% on a very low fat, high-carbohydrate diet (10% fat) (67).

Fatty acids stored in adipose tissue as triglycerides are derived from either dietary (chylomicrons) or endogenous (hepatic VLDL) sources. Preformed triglycerides are transported from the gastrointestinal tract and liver to adipose tissue, where they are hydrolyzed by the enzyme lipoprotein lipase (LPL) on the cell surface of the capillary endothelium. Insulin has an important role in maintaining and stimulating the activity of LPL (68). In addition, insulin has a direct stimulatory effect on free fatty acid uptake by adipose tissue. During insulin deficiency, LPL activity is reduced, and uptake of free fatty acids by adipose tissue is diminished (69).

In humans, liver as well as adipose tissue is a major site of lipid synthesis, occurring when dietary fat is replaced by carbohydrate. The liver removes a large proportion of circulating free fatty acids delivered from adipose tissue in a concentration-dependent manner. Fatty acids synthesized in the liver are converted mainly to VLDLs, which are secreted into plasma and then cleared from the circulation within minutes to hours by mechanisms similar to those involved in the removal of chylomicron triglycerides (see Chapters 4 and 74). During insulin deficiency, hexose monophosphate shunt activity is impaired, and NADPH is not provided for fatty acid synthesis (70). In addition, decreased glucose use reduces the availability of acetyl-CoA and citrate, which retards lipogenesis.

Lipolysis, with a net release of free fatty acids and glycerol from adipose tissue, occurs during fasting, exercise, stress, and uncontrolled diabetes mellitus. Low levels of insulin and perhaps increased glucagon concentrations enhance this mobilization of lipid from adipose tissue (62). The latter effect of glucagon to increase lipolysis has been variable, may be influenced by the effect of glucagon to increase inhibitory insulin levels, and remains somewhat controversial (71). Insulin reduces catecholamine-stimulated cAMP concentrations in adipose tissue (72), by either decreasing adenylate cyclase and/or increasing phosphodiesterase activity (73). With lipolysis, glycerol diffuses out of the adipocyte, because adipose tissue lacks the enzyme glycerolkinase and cannot reuse glycerol. Free fatty acids can either be released into the circulation or reesterified with glycerol phosphates into triglycerides in adipose tissue. Part of the antilipolytic action of insulin is to stimulate reesterification of fatty acids.

After release from adipose tissue, glycerol and free fatty acids circulate briefly in the plasma. Glycerol is metabolized primarily in the liver and kidney, where it is phosphorylated and either reesterified to triglyceride or used for gluconeogenesis. Free fatty acids are taken up by tissues in proportion to local blood flow and plasma concentrations. The potential fate of those taken up by the liver includes reesterification to triglyceride, oxidation, or conversion to ketone bodies, depending on the hormonal milieu. In the absence of either glucose or insulin and in the presence of glucagon, only a small proportion of the free fatty acids taken up by the liver is reesterified to triglyceride and released as VLDL. The insulin:glucagon ratio (74) appears to be critical in regulating hepatic metabolism of free fatty acids.

Activated fatty acids must be transported into the mitochondria for oxidation or conversion to ketone bodies, and neither free fatty acids nor their CoA derivatives can penetrate the inner mitochondrial membrane. Carnitine palmitoyl transferase I, an enzyme present on the inner mitochondrial membrane, reversibly transfers fatty acyl groups from CoA to carnitine and allows entry into the mitochondria. A second enzyme, carnitine palmitoyl transferase II, irreversibly transfers the fatty acyl groups to mitochondrial CoA, allowing them to undergo either β-oxidation or conversion to the ketone bodies acetoacetate and β-hydroxybutyrate. The activity of the key enzyme, carnitine palmitoyl transferase I, is regulated via the effects of insulin and glucagon on malonyl-CoA concentrations (75). In addition to their effects on carnitine palmitoyl transferase I activity, low insulin and high glucagon concentrations also contribute to increased lipid oxidation and ketogenesis by increasing adipose tissue lipolysis and free fatty acid delivery. Ketone bodies circulate in plasma and are metabolized in skeletal muscle and heart and brain tissues.

Alterations in lipid metabolism are frequently present in subjects with diabetes mellitus, with hypertriglyceridemia occurring in approximately one-third of patients. This finding is related to the key role insulin plays in both hepatic triglyceride production and removal of triglyceride-rich lipoproteins (76). Insulin is essential for the normal function of LPL; in severe insulin deficiency, hypertriglyceridemia is secondary to acquired LPL deficiency. "Diabetic lipemia," with milky plasma and eruptive xanthoma, may result from coexistent poorly controlled IDDM and a familial form of hypertriglyceridemia (77). This defect is promptly reversed with appropriate insulin replacement. Withdrawal of insulin from subjects with IDDM can produce decreased LPL activity and hypertriglyceridemia within 48 hours.

Obese subjects, both with and without diabetes, have higher than normal rates of VLDL triglyceride production (78, 79), probably related to an increased flow of glucose and free fatty acids to the liver as part of an insulin resistance syndrome (80). Free fatty acid delivery to the liver is enhanced when adipose tissue is deposited in an intraabdominal depot. This form of hypertriglyceridemia responds dramatically to weight reduction (81).

The predominant insulin deficiency of IDDM and the predominant insulin resistance of NIDDM have other widespread effects on lipoprotein metabolism (82). In IDDM, this may include increased low-density lipoprotein (LDL) from decreased insulin-stimulated LDL-receptor activity. However, no consistent abnormalities are noted in the physicochemical properties of LDL or VLDL lipoproteins in IDDM patients (83). In NIDDM, abnormalities include *(a)* low levels of high-density lipoprotein (HDL) from decreased transfer of surface components of triglyceride-rich lipoproteins to HDL, *(b)* triglyceride enrichment of LDL and VLDL particles, and *(c)* accumulation of VLDL remnant particles, related perhaps in part to an increased ratio of apoprotein CIII to CII. Nonenzymatic glycosylation of lipoproteins in both forms of diabetes may further alter their clearance characteristics such that LDL catabolism is decreased and HDL catabolism is increased (84).

The effect of dietary composition on lipoprotein metabolism in diabetes remains controversial. Current recommendations maintain that less than 10% of energy should be consumed as saturated fat. The remaining nonprotein energy should be tailored to the patient's individual response to dietary carbohydrate (85). Some patients experience exacerbation of hypertriglyceridemia with high intake of dietary carbohydrate. Some investigators suggest that a moderate carbohydrate intake with expanded use of monounsaturated fats provides the most effective control of the VLDL elevation and low HDL of type 2 diabetes (81, 86, 87).

Protein Metabolism

Insulin and other hormones play an important role in protein metabolism. Within several hours of starvation, protein catabolism is increased to provide amino acids for gluconeogenesis. With more prolonged starvation, metabolic adjustments occur that spare muscle protein, such as increased reliance by the central nervous system on ketone bodies as an oxidative fuel (see Chapter 41). Nonetheless, muscle continues to yield a net release of amino acids as plasma insulin levels fall during prolonged starvation; the phenomenon can be reversed completely when insulin delivery is increased (88). When fuel supplies become plentiful, protein synthesis is restored.

Insulin lowers blood concentrations of several amino acids in both normal and diabetic subjects in a time pattern resembling that for glucose concentration. The serum insulin concentrations required to produce half-maximal suppression of plasma amino acid concentrations are similar to those required for half-maximal stimulation of peripheral glucose disposal (89). Plasma levels of the essential amino acids are lowered in a pattern that corresponds to their relative concentrations in muscle protein. Isolated muscle preparations incubated in vitro liberate amino acids; the rate of release is depressed by addition of insulin. The presence of glucose may be necessary for insulin-mediated inhibition of heart muscle proteolysis (90). Insulin also inhibits intracellular protein degradation in isolated hepatocytes, an effect that depends on internalization of insulin by the cells (90). In addition to inhibiting release, insulin also stimulates accumulation of amino acids in skeletal muscle. Of the seven identified amino acid transport systems, insulin most potently stimulates two, the A and the X_{sc} systems (transporters for neutral amino acids and long-chain anionic amino acids, respectively) (91). System A is similarly regulated by insulin in hepatocytes (92). The primary effect of insulin is to increase the V_{max} of transport, felt to represent an increase in plasma membrane transporter number. Other studies have shown that the ASC and N^m systems (system ASC shows preference for alanine, serine, and cysteine and is relatively pH insensitive; system N^m is a sodium-dependent transport system for amino acids with N-containing side chains, like Gln, His, Asn) are also stimulated by insulin, the latter more potently (93, 94). Though circulating concentrations of branched-chain amino acids such as leucine, isoleucine, and valine are dramatically decreased by insulin and their muscle uptake is stimulated, there is no evidence that insulin stimulates the branched-chain amino acid transport system (system L) (95). It is possible that the effect of insulin to decrease branched-chain amino acid concentrations is related to its ability to inhibit protein degradation, thereby decreasing intracellular concentrations of these essential amino acids and promoting their movement into cells down a concentration gradient.

Prior exercise may potentiate the ability of insulin to increase amino acid uptake by muscle tissues (96). Exercise additionally inhibits amino acid release from skeletal muscle protein, but the effect appears limited to nonmyofibrillar proteins (97). When added to isolated muscle preparations, insulin promotes incorporation of labeled amino acids into tissue protein (98). At the subcellular level, protein synthesis appears to be stimulated in both cytoplasm and mitochondria (99).

Insulin stimulates incorporation of labeled precursors into nucleic acid (100). Although insulin increases RNA synthesis in muscle, the increase does not appear requisite for hormone-mediated stimulation of protein synthesis; actinomycin, an inhibitor of RNA synthesis, does not impair the ability of insulin to increase protein synthesis (101). To the extent that insulin promotes protein synthesis, it appears to do so by stimulating translation rather than transcription. Specifically, insulin, through insulin-receptor-substrate-1 (IRS-1) and phosphatidylinositol-3-kinase (PI3K), dissociates regulatory peptides from eukaryotic initiation factor eIF-4E and phosphorylates eIF-4E itself, allowing it to initiate translation (102, 103).

The importance of insulin in regulation of protein balance was demonstrated most clearly in subjects with IDDM who rapidly develop negative nitrogen balance with cessation of insulin therapy. In heart and most skeletal muscles studied, the absolute protein content (i.e., the quantity of protein per tissue or organ) was significantly lower in diabetic, than in control, animals. In contrast, the protein content of liver was unaffected in those with diabetes (104). The most significant loss of protein in vivo, as the result of insulin deficiency, occurs in muscle. Studies using stable isotopes of amino acids to examine rates of whole-body protein turnover and oxidation demonstrated increased rates of protein degradation and leucine oxidation in insulin-deprived IDDM subjects, which could be decreased by insulin infusions (105). In vitro (106) and animal (107) studies have demonstrated decreased rates of protein synthesis in diabetes. In contrast, increased rates of protein synthesis were found in insulin-deprived IDDM human subjects, although protein breakdown was more accelerated (108). The postulated mechanism for this increase in protein synthesis in vivo, not found in vitro, is that accelerated protein degradation provides increased intracellular free amino acid concentrations as precursors for protein synthesis. Conversely, insulin administration to insulin-dependent diabetic patients decreases intracellular free amino acid concentrations through inhibition of protein degradation in skeletal muscle, resulting in an inability of insulin to increase muscle protein synthesis in vivo (109, 110).

A persistent theme in all of these hypotheses about the effects of insulin on protein metabolism in vivo in humans is that amino acid concentrations in the circulation are important for maintenance of protein synthesis, particularly in muscle, and that the effect of insulin to decrease amino acid concentrations may blunt its effect to stimulate protein synthesis. Recent reports indicate that local infusion of insulin into the legs of human subjects at rates that do not affect systemic amino acid concentrations augments extraction of several amino acids from the circulation by leg tissues and stimulates muscle protein synthesis (111).

Given the importance of insulin in maintaining nitrogen balance, inhibiting protein degradation, and stimulating protein synthesis, it is reasonable to speculate that the dietary protein requirements of patients with insulin-dependent diabetes might be increased to counterbalance the abnormal regulation of insulin as an anabolic hormone. Some authors have reported resistance to insulin-mediated suppression of branched-chain amino acid (BCAA) plasma concentrations (112), and rates of BCAA turnover and oxidation (113) in IDDM. Others have shown that IDDM patients following a diet containing the mean minimum adult requirement for protein experience decreases in muscle strength, persistently negative nitrogen balance, and increased adiposity (114). However, close examination of amino acid metabolism in IDDM patients consuming the minimum protein requirement reveals a normal adaptation to the dietary protein restriction as long as the subjects are euglycemic (115). Indeed, investigators have reported normalization of whole-body amino acid metabolism in IDDM with prolonged tight glycemic control (116). Protein requirements in IDDM appear to be determined by the chronic level of glycemic control (117).

Glucagon has three effects on amino acid metabolism: *(a)* increased membrane transport of amino acids, *(b)* decreased protein synthesis and increased catabolism (when accompanied by insulin deficiency, both protein degradation and amino acid oxidation rates increase), and *(c)* increased amino acid conversion into glucose (gluconeogenesis) (118, 119). Glucagon increases gluconeogenesis in perfused liver, an effect that can be reproduced by perfusion with cyclic AMP. Glucagon increases hepatic use of glycine, alanine, glutamate, and phenylalanine for gluconeogenesis. In addition, glucagon increases the rate of ureagenesis.

During early starvation, plasma glucagon and insulin concentrations increase and decrease, respectively, resulting in increased rates of gluconeogenesis and ureagenesis. Splanchnic extraction of alanine is increased from 43% in the postabsorptive state to 71% after 3 days of fasting, but this value decreases to 53% after 6 weeks of fasting (120). These effects of fasting are mimicked by glucagon infusion (121). With prolonged starvation, the brain adapts by developing the capacity to use ketone bodies as an energy source, thereby decreasing the need for increased rates of gluconeogenesis.

Glucagon can increase liver protein catabolism in the intact animal; liver protein content is decreased and branched-chain amino acid release from the liver is increased. This increased protein catabolism can be suppressed by administration of insulin or a mixture of amino acids. When protein is ingested without accompanying carbohydrate, insulin concentrations increase slightly, allowing skeletal muscle protein retention, with a parallel rise in glucagon (25) that prevents hypoglycemia (122).

As mentioned above, patients with glucagonoma syndrome commonly exhibit hypoaminoacidemia. When similar degrees of hyperglucagonemia are produced by infusions of glucagon in normal volunteers, reductions in blood amino acid concentrations are similar (123). High-protein diets can normalize the plasma amino acid profile and result in a positive nitrogen balance in patients with glucagonoma syndrome (124). When glucagon deficiency is produced by infusions of somatostatin with insulin replacement, amino acid concentrations increase (125). Urinary urea nitrogen and total nitrogen excretion rates are lower during glucagon deficiency than during glucagon excess, suggesting that alterations in the rate of gluconeogenesis constitute one mechanism by which glucagon influences blood amino acid levels.

GUT PEPTIDES: GLP-1, GIP, CCK

It is reasonable that the first organ to encounter nutritional substrate, the gut, should initiate anabolic stimuli for nutrient storage (see Chapter 39). Certain peptide hormones produced by the gut clearly contribute to general body anabolism. In particular, glucose-dependent insulinotropic peptide (GIP; previously known as gastric inhibitory polypeptide), cholecystokinin C-terminal octapeptide (CCK-8), and glucagon-like peptide 1 (GLP-1) enhance anabolism through their stimulation of insulin secretion in response to meal ingestion. GLP-1 is several times more potent as an insulin secretagogue than GIP (126). Its antagonism results in an important disturbance in glucose tolerance in baboons (127), and its supplementation results in improved glucose control in humans with type 2 diabetes (128).

Other gut hormones are likely to contribute to trophic phenomena specific to the gut itself; examples include peptide YY that is trophic for gut mucosa. Peptide YY preserves gut mass in rats receiving total parenteral nutrition, a circumstance that generally results in gut atrophy (129). Additionally, pentagastrin, neurotensin, and bombesin provide trophic stimuli to the intestine of rats, particularly the jejunum, during an atrophy-inducing elemental diet (130).

THYROID HORMONES

Carbohydrate Metabolism

Thyroid hormones exert multiple effects on carbohydrate metabolism. Patients with hyperthyroidism frequently (30–50%) display mild-to-moderate glucose intolerance (131–133). Part of this abnormality is due to more-rapid gastric emptying and intestinal absorption of glucose in hyperthyroidism (134), whereas glucose absorption is delayed in hypothyroidism. Additionally, insulin secretion is reduced in hyperthyroidism in response to oral, but not intravenous, administration of glucose (135) and may be accompanied by impaired processing of proinsulin to insulin (136).

Rates of hepatic glucose production are increased by 20% in the fasting state, and the liver is less sensitive to insulin infusions in hyperthyroid human subjects (137). Hepatic glycogen stores are reduced in states of thyroid hormone excess. Thyroid hormones appear to modulate the magnitude of the glycogenolytic and hyperglycemic actions of epinephrine and norepinephrine, possibly by enhancing the responsiveness of the adenylate cyclase–cyclic AMP system. In rats, thyroid hormone exerts a biphasic effect on liver glycogen. Small doses of thyroid hormone increase glycogen synthesis in the presence of insulin, whereas large doses augment hepatic glycogenolysis. Small doses of thyroid hormone enhance, and large doses depress, the glycogenolytic response to epinephrine (138). The glycogen content of liver and muscle tissues is decreased in hypothyroidism, possibly reflecting a new balance between simultaneously decreased rates of glycogen synthesis and degradation (139).

Rates of gluconeogenesis are also increased in hyperthyroidism, in part because of an increase in substrate supply from protein breakdown and lipolysis. Splanchnic uptake of gluconeogenic precursors is increased by 20 to 120% in hyperthyroidism (137). Gluconeogenesis is suppressed in hypothyroidism. In vitro, addition of T_3 to hypothyroid hepatocytes stimulates hepatic gluconeogenesis by approximately 80 to 90% within 30 to 40 minutes (139).

Rates of total glucose disposal during euglycemic, hyperinsulinemic clamp studies were normal, suggesting that skeletal muscle is not insulin resistant in hyperthyroidism (140). However, in vitro skeletal muscle preparations from hyperthyroid rats display rates of insulin-stimulated glucose oxidation that are significantly (twofold) increased, whereas rates of glycogen synthesis are reduced (141). Oxidative glucose use appears to be synergistically stimulated by exercise and thyroid hormones.

Total-body-glucose turnover rates are increased in thyrotoxicosis. Most of the increased glucose turnover is accounted for by increased glucose recycling. Recycling through both the Cori (glucose-lactate) and the glucose-alanine cycles increases in hyperthyroidism and decreases in hypothyroidism (138). In addition, patients with hyperthyroidism form hexose intermediates of both glycolysis and gluconeogenesis simultaneously at increased rates (i.e., glucose → glucose-6-P and fructose-6-P → fructose-1,6-di-P) (142). In part, thyroid hormone facilitates these cycling phenomena by stimulating glucose-transporter gene expression and enhancing glucose transport across the plasma membrane in muscle and liver cells (143, 144). Likewise, thyroid hormone increases insulin-stimulated glucose transport in skeletal muscle by increasing GLUT4 content (145) but produces a simultaneous increase in GLUT2 in the liver to facilitate hepatic glucose output (146).

Lipid Metabolism

Thyroid hormones also have an impact on multiple aspects of lipid metabolism, including lipid synthesis, mobilization, and degradation. Degradation is affected more than synthesis, so the net effect of excess thyroid hormone is decreased total body lipid stores and plasma concentrations. Thyroid hormones increase lipolysis in adipose tissue by both directly stimulating cyclic AMP production and increasing the sensitivity to other lipolytic agents (catecholamines, TSH, ACTH, growth hormone, glucocorticoids, and glucagon). Conversely, lipolysis is impaired in hypothyroidism.

Delivery of free fatty acids to peripheral tissues and the liver is increased in hyperthyroidism. Free fatty acid turnover rates are approximately doubled in thyrotoxicosis (147). Lipid oxidation rates are also increased in thyrotoxicosis, which may contribute to the calorigenic action of thyroid hormones.

Hepatic triglyceride synthesis increases in hyperthyroidism, in large part because of increased delivery of free fatty acids and glycerol to the liver. Synthesis and clearance of cholesterol and triglyceride are accelerated in hyperthyroidism, with the latter effect predominating. Serum cholesterol and triglyceride levels are usually modestly reduced (148). Conversely, serum lipid levels may increase in hypothyroidism because of impaired clearance. HDL-cholesterol levels decrease in hypothyroidism, even at a subclinical stage, and revert to normal with thyroxine therapy (149). Both hepatic and adipose tissue LPL activity has been reported to be low in hypothyroidism (150, 151).

At a cellular level, lipid transfer into and out of membranes is altered by thyroid hormone. Cholesterol is transferred out of erythrocyte plasma membranes into plasma in hyperthyroidism, resulting in a higher relative phospholipid content in the erythrocyte membrane (152). The hyperthyroidism-induced change in the lipid content of mitochondrial membranes allows increased phosphate transport (153)—teleologically, a favorable compensation for partially uncoupled electron transport in this condition.

Protein Metabolism

Short-term administration of thyroid hormones produces increases in liver protein and RNA content, with a concomitant decrease in muscle protein. With more prolonged administration, both liver and peripheral tissues decrease in size (154). Thyroid hormone increases amino acid uptake by the liver and increases incorporation of amino acids into protein by isolated liver microsomes and mitochondria (155). The latter does not occur in the presence of actinomycin, suggesting that these effects of thyroid hormone are mediated by DNA transcription and RNA translation (156).

Clinically, a great excess of thyroid hormone appears to have the opposite effect, with suppressed rates of protein synthesis (157), increased catabolism of collagen (158), and increased forearm amino acid release (159) in human subjects. Nitrogen excretion increases in thyrotoxicosis, and nitrogen balance may be normal or negative depending on whether intake meets the increased demand.

In hypothyroidism, rates of protein synthesis and degradation both decrease. Patients are usually in positive nitrogen balance. Treatment of myxedema is accompanied by mobilization of extracellular protein and a significant temporary negative nitrogen balance. Total serum protein concentrations are usually normal in hypothyroidism.

Thyroid hormone, particularly T_3 in the intracellular environment, regulates production of a wide range of proteins through its interaction with its nuclear receptor—a member of a family of hormone-responsive nuclear receptors. The interaction of thyroid hormone with its receptor and its actions on particular tissues has been reviewed in detail (160). Proteins that exhibit increased production and expression of their respective genes include myosin α-chain, Na^+-K^+ ATPase, Ca^{2+}-ATPase, malate dehydrogenase, glucose 6-phosphate dehydrogenase, fatty acid synthase, hepatic lipase, and LDL receptor of certain genotypes.

Taken together, the metabolic effects of thyroid hormone can be interpreted as indicating a role for thyroid hormone in maintaining substrate turnover. Maintaining activity in metabolic pathways that simultaneously produce and consume metabolic substrates, though energetically costly, may be beneficial in allowing the organism to produce or degrade a particular product rapidly in response to urgent need. The need may be particularly frequent during growth and development, when tissue remodeling might be expected. The role of thyroid hormone in simultaneously stimulating glycogen synthesis and glycogenolysis, lipogenesis and lipolysis, and protein synthesis and proteolysis is consistent with its importance for normal growth and development.

GLUCOCORTICOIDS

Carbohydrate Metabolism

Corticosteroids in excess produce increases in plasma insulin and glucose concentrations, i.e., a state of insulin resistance. This resistance is out of proportion to the degree of obesity seen in patients with Cushing's syndrome (161–163). Glucose intolerance in association with Cushing's syndrome has been reported in 80 to 90% of patients, although overt diabetes occurs in only 15 to 20% of subjects (164, 165).

Glucocorticoids counteract the effects of insulin at numerous steps in glucose homeostasis. First, rates of gluconeogenesis may be augmented by several mechanisms: *(a)* increased release of gluconeogenic precursors, i.e., amino acids (166) and lactate (167), from peripheral tissues; *(b)* increased activity of key gluconeogenic enzymes (168), including pyruvate carboxylase and phosphoenolpyruvate (PEP) carboxykinase, the unidirectional, rate-limiting enzyme in the initiation of the gluconeogenic cascade from pyruvate; and *(c)* stimulation of glucagon secretion by pancreatic α cells (166, 169). The latter effect may be the result of increased proteolysis and hyperaminoacidemia. Corticosteroids act in conjunction with glucagon to increase rates of gluconeogenesis in perfused rat liver (170).

The physiologic nocturnal increase in cortisol in humans contributes to maintenance of gluconeogenesis postprandially (171), perhaps in part due to increased lipolysis and fatty acid delivery to the liver as well as decreased insulin secretion with increased glucagon production during hypercortisolemia (172). However, other in vivo human studies implicate increased glucose-6-phosphatase activity rather than gluconeogenesis as the cause of increased hepatic glucose output in response to dexamethasone (173). Likewise, studies in insulin-deficient dogs indicate that cortisol does not increase gluconeogenesis (174), whereas insulin deficiency itself and epinephrine are potent promoters of gluconeogenesis. Thus, the subject remains controversial.

The second way in which glucocorticoids may affect glucose tolerance is by decreasing production of glucose transporters and promoting their sequestration in intracellular pools rather than at the plasma membrane, an effect reported in rat adipocytes (175) and fibroblasts (176). Third, glucocorticoids decrease insulin binding to its receptor through decreases in receptor affinity (177, 178) and number (175). Finally, glucocorticoids may induce postreceptor defects in insulin action that remain to be characterized (162, 179). The hyperglycemic action of glucocorticoids is amplified if increases in glucagon, catecholamines, or growth hormone exist (180, 181). However, in regard to epinephrine, this synergism may only occur when epinephrine levels are elevated briefly in the presence of increased cortisol and not during prolonged (72-h) elevation of levels of both hormones (182).

Glucocorticoids stimulate hepatic glycogen deposition and in this regard resemble insulin. The carbon for this new liver glycogen is derived from breakdown of muscle protein with release of amino acids. The activity of glycogen synthase, the rate-limiting enzyme for glycogen synthesis, is decreased in adrenalectomized rats and restored to normal by corticosteroid treatment.

Lipid Metabolism

Glucocorticoids appear to exert a permissive effect on lipolysis through activation of cyclic AMP–dependent hormone-sensitive lipase in the adipocyte. Epinephrine-induced lipolysis is promoted by cortisol (183), which appears necessary for full stimulation of lipolysis by catecholamines (184). Glucocorticoids are similarly required for maximal lipolytic action of growth hormone. The lipolytic action of cortisol is prevented by inhibitors of protein synthesis (185).

Prolonged treatment with glucocorticoids may result in increased plasma triglyceride concentrations (186). This effect is seen most often in the presence of diabetes mellitus and primarily reflects impaired triglyceride removal. However, hepatocytes in culture increase triglyceride production and VLDL-apoprotein synthesis when incubated with glucocorticoids (187). LDL uptake and degradation by cultured fibroblasts and smooth muscle cells are also impaired by high doses of glucocorticoids (188). Chronic glucocorticoid treatment may result in a "fatty liver," because of increased lipolysis and free fatty acid delivery associated with enhanced hepatic uptake of free fatty acids.

A chronic excess of corticosteroids also increases total body fat in humans and in laboratory animals. Pair-feeding experiments suggest that increased food intake is the major factor contributing to obesity in steroid-treated rats (189). Changes in body fat distribution are also characteristic of Cushing's syndrome, with accumulations of fat in the supraclavicular, truncal, and facial areas (190). Increased energy intake in excess of a small increase in energy expenditure has been confirmed as the cause of excess energy storage during glucocorticoid administration in humans (191). The mechanism by which this occurs is unknown but is speculated to be partly related to inhibition of corticotropin-releasing hormone (CRH)-stimulated neuropeptide Y (NPY) secretion in the hypothalamus. The altered fat distribution in humans with Cushing's syndrome is associated with enhanced adipocyte LPL activity and diminished lipolytic response to catecholamines in abdominal fat, compared with femoral-region fat (192). In addition, glucocorticoid receptor number and its mRNA are increased in abdominal region subcutaneous fat, compared with femoral region subcutaneous fat, and they are increased even more in omental adipose tissue (193).

Administration of ACTH stimulates lipolysis through cyclic AMP–mediated activation of adipose tissue hormone-sensitive lipase. This is a direct action of ACTH, because it is demonstrable in adrenalectomized animals (194).

Protein Metabolism

One of the major metabolic effects of glucocorticoids is to stimulate skeletal muscle protein breakdown. Many of the clinical features of Cushing's syndrome, such as loss of bone density, increased capillary fragility and dermal atrophy, muscle wasting, and growth retardation in children, are attributable in part to this augmented proteolysis. In addition to increasing protein breakdown, corticosteroids also appear to inhibit incorporation of amino acids into muscle protein (195, 196). Elevations of cortisol levels within the physiologic range increase muscle proteolysis, with increased activation of muscle branched-chain ketoacid dehydrogenase and BCAA oxidation (197, 198), de novo alanine synthesis (199), and muscle glutamine release (200). Corticosteroid inhibition of muscle protein synthesis is sustained during prolonged elevation of glucocorticoid levels in the rat, whereas muscle proteolysis shows adaptation toward normal levels within a few days (201). Thus, diminished protein synthesis rather than proteolysis may account for long-term effects of glucocorticoids that produce muscle wasting. The mechanism of adaptation of muscle myofibrillar protein breakdown is unknown; nonmyofibrillar muscle proteins may be spared by adaptive increases in insulin (202).

Administration of glucocorticoids results in increased protein and RNA content in liver and other viscera (203). Amino acids delivered as a result of enhanced muscle proteolysis and decreased peripheral use for protein synthesis are transported to the liver where they can be used for protein synthesis. Administration of cortisol to rats results in enhanced hepatic uptake of α-aminoisobutyric acid (196) and increased free amino nitrogen concentrations in the liver (204). These effects of glucocorticoids depend on the diet, with increased protein synthesis occurring when the caloric and protein contents of the diet are adequate. Under circumstances of systemic inflammatory processes, glucocorticoids increase hepatocyte receptors for interleukin 6, a potent stimulator of synthesis of acute-phase proteins such as C-reactive protein and fibrinogen (205).

The pattern of metabolic effects induced by cortisol (and other hormones with glucocorticoid effect) substantiates its role as a "stress hormone." Glucocorticoids produce not only catabolism with dissipation of nutritional substrate but also anabolism such that substrate is rearranged. The simultaneous stimulation of gluconeogenesis and glycogen deposition, lipolysis and abdominal lipid deposition, muscle proteolysis and visceral (e.g., hepatic) protein synthesis increases resting energy expenditure during glucocorticoid excess (206). One may speculate teleologically that the energy is well spent in rearranging substrate into depots most accessible during stress—liver glycogen, abdominal fat, and hepatic protein.

GROWTH HORMONE AND INSULIN-LIKE GROWTH FACTOR–1 (IGF-1)

In considering the metabolic effects of growth hormone, it is important to distinguish the direct effects of growth hormone from those of IGF-1. IGF-1 is synthesized by liver and other tissues in response to stimulation by growth hormone, although nutritional intake appears to have a direct effect on IGF-1 production. In normal human volunteers, IGF-1 levels decline 60 to 70% during a 5-day fast (207). Studies in the rat have shown that both adequate dietary protein and total energy content are necessary to produce IGF-1-stimulated cartilage growth (208). The "somatomedin hypothesis" states that many of the anabolic, growth-promoting effects of growth hormone are mediated by IGF-1 (previously known as somatomedin C), whereas growth hormone has direct catabolic effects on glucose and lipid metabolism. The somatomedin hypothesis may not be entirely correct, as evidence is accumulating that growth hormone may have direct, specific anabolic actions.

Carbohydrate Metabolism

Acute administration of growth hormone elicits a biphasic response. During the initial 2 hours after administration, growth hormone exhibits an insulin-like effect, lowering plasma glucose levels by directly stimulating β-cell insulin secretion (209) and also by stimulating glucose use in peripheral tissues. Nonetheless, growth hormone does not produce hypoglycemia in normal subjects. It does have such an effect, however, in hypophysectomized animals that also have an impaired pituitary-adrenal axis (210). From 2 to 12 hours after acute administration, growth hormone exhibits antiinsulin effects. This state of insulin resistance results from a postreceptor defect in peripheral glucose use, coupled with hepatic insulin resistance (211, 212).

With chronic administration in animals and humans, growth hormone results in an insulin-resistant state. Glucose intolerance in association with acromegaly has been reported in 60 to 70% of patients, although elevated fasting plasma glucose concentrations are reported to occur in only 6 to 25% of acromegalic patients (213–216). Even more striking than glucose intolerance is the hyperinsulinemia and resistance to insulin that occur in acromegaly (214) and in patients receiving growth hormone by injection (217). In most patients, increased insulin secretion can compensate for the insulin-resistant state. Chronic excess of growth hormone results in increased rates of hepatic glucose production and decreased glucose use by peripheral tissues (218, 219), largely the result of decreased glucose oxidation (220). Whether the insulin resistance of acromegaly derives from defects at the level of the insulin receptor or is entirely postreceptor is controversial. Decreased peripheral glucose use in acromegaly is associated with a decreased number of insulin receptors on peripheral blood monocytes (221). However, the defect is not reproduced by incubation of monocytes with acromegalic plasma or growth hormone. Furthermore, porcine adipocytes show no defects in insulin binding or insulin receptor tyrosine kinase activity with chronic growth hormone treatment (222). Elevations in the concentration of plasma free fatty acids and ketone bodies inhibit glucose use by muscle tissue and may in part explain the postreceptor defect seen in acromegaly (223). Successful treatment of acromegaly results in improved glucose tolerance and lower serum insulin concentrations in most patients (214, 224, 225). In contrast to acromegaly, chronic growth hormone deficiency produces increased insulin sensitivity.

Whereas chronic elevations in growth hormone concentrations produce antiinsulin effects, many of the actions of IGF-1 mimic those of insulin. This is not surprising given the structural similarities in tertiary configuration between IGF-1 and proinsulin (226). IGF-1 acts through a specific cell-surface receptor with substantial homology to the insulin receptor but can also stimulate the insulin receptor itself (227). IGF-1 increases glucose transport (228) and rates of glycolysis and glycogen synthesis (229) in heart and skeletal muscle tissues.

Lipid Metabolism

The acute effects of growth hormone administration on lipid metabolism are similar in their insulin-like nature to those described for glucose. Within the first few hours after growth hormone is given, plasma free fatty acid concentrations drop. In addition, reduced rates of epinephrine-stimulated lipolysis have been described in hypophysectomized rats during this early period after growth hormone administration (230).

Free fatty acid and ketone body levels increase as the result of longer-term growth hormone administration. Increased glycerol concentrations after in vivo administration of biosynthetic growth hormone in humans suggest stimulation of lipolysis (215). Growth hormone–mediated lipolysis is similar to that induced by glucocorticoids in that a lag time of at least 1 hour is required before the effect can be observed, and the lipolytic actions can be blocked by inhibitors of protein synthesis (231). Some investigators have shown significant growth hormone–mediated lipolysis to occur only in the presence of insulin deficiency (232–235). No lipolytic response to growth hormone is seen in vivo or in vitro in the growth hormone–deficient mouse (236). Rather, fatty acid synthesis is inhibited by growth hormone, suggesting a primary role for blunted lipogenesis in the deranged fat metabolism in this model. Ketogenesis occurs in response to increased free fatty acid delivery to the liver and as the result of a direct hepatic effect of growth hormone on ketone production (237).

Humans exhibit regional differences in the response of adipocyte lipolysis and lipogenesis to growth hormone: abdominal cells are more affected than are peripheral (e.g., gluteal) cells. This variation results in fat redistribution from "android" (truncal) to "gynoid" (hip/thigh) deposition in patients treated with growth hormone (238).

In contrast to the effects of growth hormone on lipid metabolism, IGF-1 increases lipogenesis and inhibits epinephrine-stimulated lipolysis in adipose tissue (239). IGF-1 infusion in humans decreases serum triglyceride levels and the ratio of total to HDL cholesterol (240).

Protein Metabolism

One of the major effects of growth hormone is promotion of linear growth and skeletal maturation. IGF-1 is responsible for these effects, producing increased synthesis of DNA, RNA, and protein in fibroblasts and chondrocytes (241). While circulating IGF-1, responsible for linear skeletal growth, depends on the presence of growth hormone, IGF-1 secretion occurs in multiple tissues and may serve as an anabolic factor independent of growth hormone in tissue hypertrophy and repair by autocrine and paracrine actions (242, 243).

The exact physiologic roles for the anabolic actions of growth hormone and IGF-1 and their physiologic interdependence are not yet completely defined. Growth hormone administration stimulates amino acid uptake and incorporation into protein in both liver and skeletal muscle tissues (244). The effect on muscle is underscored by the absence of an effect of systemically administered growth hormone on whole-body protein synthesis in humans, even while forearm (largely composed of muscle) protein synthesis is stimulated (245). In humans, local administration of growth hormone to forearm skeletal muscle stimulates amino acid uptake (246). This response may occur without increases in systemic IGF-1 levels, suggesting that growth hormone effects in muscle are not necessarily mediated by IGF-1. However, the extent to which growth hormone can stimulate protein anabolism directly and independently of IGF-1 paracrine or autocrine actions remains controversial. Recent studies in rats support an independent role for growth hormone on muscle anabolism. Comparing the effects of growth hormone and IGF-1 administration on organ-specific protein synthesis indicated that growth hormone specifically promotes protein synthesis in skeletal muscle, while IGF-1 specifically promotes protein synthesis in gut (247) but not muscle. However, to complicate matters, the importance of each hormone for anabolism may depend on how anabolic responses are defined under given study conditions. For example, certain investigators have noted that while IGF-1 does not stimulate muscle protein synthesis in fed rats, anti-IGF-1 antibody decreases it below control values, suggesting that IGF-1 serves a permissive or facilitative role for skeletal muscle protein synthesis rather than a stimulatory role (248)—a function that may be considered anabolic by some and not others.

Despite the data suggesting a specific role for growth hormone in promoting skeletal muscle anabolism, there appears to be an absence of growth hormone effect on muscle strength in healthy adults, suggesting that the effect of growth hormone supplementation may be to stimulate production of noncontractile muscle proteins in this group (249, 250). However, growth hormone may have a modest effect in increasing muscle protein synthesis and strength in growth hormone–deficient patients, implying that growth hormone may facilitate maintenance of normal rates of muscle contractile protein synthesis (251).

What may be most obvious about the effects of growth hormone and IGF-1 on protein metabolism is that the current understanding of their actions is inadequate and that their functions and interdependence are likely to be complex. This is particularly true because their actions vary with nutritional state and physiologic stress, circumstances in which growth hormone concentrations are often elevated in the face of catabolism.

INSULIN-LIKE GROWTH FACTOR–BINDING PROTEINS

Insulin-like growth factor–1 actions on nutrient substrates and nutrient stores cannot be completely understood without an examination of the binding proteins that largely sequester the growth factor. The biologic actions of these binding proteins and IGFs themselves have been reviewed in depth (252, 253). This section summarizes issues relevant to nutrient metabolism.

IGF-1 circulates with a high-molecular-weight (~150,000) binding complex consisting of a 46- to 53-kDa protein termed *insulin-like growth factor–binding protein–3* (IGFBP-3) complexed with an 88-kDa glycoprotein that does not bind IGF, called the acid labile subunit (ALS). IGFBP-3 production, like that of IGF-1, is stimulated by insulin. Its functions other than that of a carrier protein for IGF-1 are controversial. It is speculated to assist in delivery of circulating IGF-1 to the interstitium of peripheral tissues and to serve as a reservoir for IGFs during stress. The latter function may be activated by degradation of IGFBP-3 by specific proteases. The ability of IGFBP-3 to both stimulate and inhibit cellular functions independent of binding IGFs has been noted in cell culture, depending on the prevailing culture conditions. The physiologic relevance of these findings remains in question.

Another binding protein for IGF-1, IGFBP-1, is believed to either inhibit or stimulate its actions, depending upon whether it is phosphorylated (inhibitory) or nonphosphorylated (stimulatory). Its predominant action is believed to be inhibitory, which is consistent with the findings that IGFBP-1 is increased in the circulation during catabolic states such as uremia, insulinopenia, and starvation. IGFBP-1 may act directly to stimulate cellular anabolism (apart from IGF) by binding to a fibronectin-binding cellular integrin. The functional significance of integrin binding remains poorly described.

Other binding proteins believed to inhibit IGF-1 actions include IGFBP-2 and IGFBP-4. In contrast, IGFBP-5, largely associated with extracellular matrix, appears to potentiate IGF-1's actions. A sixth binding protein, IGFBP-6, remains poorly characterized in terms of its physiologic activity.

In summary, physiologic phenomena that raise or lower IGF-1 concentrations must be viewed in the context of the effect on the array of IGF-binding proteins. This may be particularly true when the effect of IGF-1 on a particular tissue is being examined, as the ability of IGFBPs to sequester IGFs and either inhibit or potentiate their actions may be particularly important within a local tissue milieu.

CATECHOLAMINES

The catecholamines are epinephrine, norepinephrine, and dopamine. Norepinephrine is secreted from the sympathetic neurons throughout the body and to a limited extent from the adrenal medulla. The principal secretory product of the adrenal medulla is epinephrine. Both epinephrine and norepinephrine have α- and β-agonist activities, although norepinephrine predominantly produces α-adrenergic effects. The major stimuli to sympathetic nervous system stimulation and adrenomedullary secretion are physical exercise, circulatory dysfunction, trauma, cold exposure, pain, emotional stress, and hypoglycemia. Although combined increases in epinephrine and norepinephrine secretion occur with most stresses, hypoglycemia predominantly augments epinephrine secretion (254). However, epinephrine appears to be critical for recovery from hypoglycemia only in the absence of glucagon (255).

Carbohydrate Metabolism

Catecholamines have multiple effects on carbohydrate metabolism. α-Adrenergic stimulation inhibits insulin secretion, whereas β-adrenergic stimulation augments insulin release. The α-adrenergic inhibitory effects on pancreatic β-cell function generally prevail under conditions of stress or sympathetic nerve stimulation. Both α- and β-adrenergic stimulation appear to augment pancreatic glucagon secretion (256, 257).

Catecholamines increase glycogen breakdown in liver and muscle tissues. β-Adrenergic stimulation activates phosphorylase and inhibits glycogen synthase through a cAMP-dependent mechanism. In addition, the α-adrenergic system can activate phosphorylase and inhibit glycogen synthase through a cAMP-independent mechanism involving membrane calcium transport (258–261). Liver glycogenolysis appears to be mediated predominantly through α-adrenergic, cAMP-independent mechanisms. This conclusion derives from in vitro data showing inhibition of catecholamine-mediated hepatic glycogenolysis (and gluconeogenesis) by α-adrenergic, but not β-adrenergic, blocking drugs (260–262). A study in conscious dogs, however, yielded contradictory findings (263). In contrast, skeletal muscle glycogenolysis is mediated by β-adrenergic stimulation of adenylate cyclase (264) and does not appear to be affected by α-adrenergic mechanisms (258, 265). The effects of catecholamines on muscle glycogen metabolism are antagonized by insulin and depend on glucocorticoids (266–268).

As mentioned, catecholamines also stimulate hepatic gluconeogenesis through α-adrenergic mechanisms. Catecholamines increase delivery of gluconeogenic precursors to the liver through their lipolytic (glycerol) and muscle glycogenolytic (lactate and pyruvate) actions. In addition, α-adrenergic agonists increase hepatic uptake of amino acids and possibly lactate (269, 270). The decreases in circulating insulin and increases in glucagon concentrations after sympathetic stimulation also promote glycogenolysis and gluconeogenesis. However, dose-related increases in such activity occur as the result of direct hepatic effects of epinephrine when plasma insulin and glucagon are maintained at fixed concentrations (271).

Infusions of epinephrine resulting in physiologic elevations of plasma concentrations inhibit insulin-stimulated glucose uptake by peripheral tissues, even when plasma glucose and insulin concentrations are controlled by use of the insulin clamp technique (272, 273). This effect is primarily associated with diminished insulin-stimulated glycogen deposition as glucose oxidation is slightly increased (274). In contrast to these *acute* responses, *chronic* administration of terbutaline, a β_2-adrenergic agonist, significantly increased peripheral insulin sensitivity through increased nonoxidative glucose use (glycogen deposition) during insulin clamp studies (275). Chronic infusion of norepinephrine, an α- and β_1-agonist, produces similar increases in peripheral insulin sensitivity in the rat (276). Finally, the argument that catecholamines promote insulin sensitivity as part of their chronic, long-term action is bolstered by the recent finding that people with mutations in the β_3-adrenergic receptor have reduced insulin sensitivity (277–279), increased capacity for weight gain (280), and earlier onset of non-insulin-dependent diabetes (281).

Taken together, the *acute* actions of catecholamines on carbohydrate metabolism promote increased availability of glucose in the circulation. The most common physiologic circumstance in which these functions are evident is in exercise, in which catecholamines are primarily responsible for the hepatic production of glucose to compensate for the increased glucose use during the exercise bout (282). The effect of catecholamines to inhibit glucose clearance during exercise seems counterintuitive when fuel is required for mechanical work, but it is an important protection that ensures adequate circulating glucose for brain function when muscle fuel needs are high. Following the end of a bout of exercise, glucose clearance remains impaired because of catecholamine effects and hyperglycemia develops (e.g., as may occur in insulin-deficient diabetic persons following exercise) unless there is an acute increase in insulin concentration (the normal physiologic response) to counteract the catecholamine effect (283). The *chronic* effect of catecholamines may be to promote glucose storage in the periphery.

Lipid Metabolism

The major effect of catecholamines on lipid metabolism is augmentation of lipolysis. Both epinephrine and norepinephrine activate hormone-sensitive lipase in adipose tissue, liver, heart, and skeletal muscle. Some studies have reported that stimulation of lipolysis is cAMP dependent and mediated through β_1-adrenergic stimulation of adenylate cyclase (284, 285). Other authors studying the increased lipolysis in burn patients have reported that it can be inhibited only by medications that antagonize the β_2-adrenergic receptor (286). Still others have reported that both β_1 and/or β_2 receptors in dogs may be involved in lipolysis, with β_3 receptors recruited only when catecholamines are present in very high concentration (287, 288). α_2-Adrenergic stimulation has an antilipolytic effect (284), although this may not be of physiologic importance. Many other hormonal factors affect catecholamine-induced lipolysis, with insulin producing a major opposing role. Thus, catecholamine inhibition of insulin secretion is important in promoting lipolysis.

Catecholamines increase lipogenesis and ketogenesis. Hepatic triglyceride synthesis is increased by adrenergic stimulation, although this effect is predominantly related to increased free fatty acid delivery resulting from enhanced lipolysis (264). Augmented ketogenesis is also partly the result of increased free fatty acid delivery to the liver, although other mechanism(s) coexist. Norepinephrine produces dose-dependent increases in ketogenesis in isolated rat hepatocytes, without increasing free fatty acid uptake (289).

Catecholamines increase in plasma lipid levels. Cholesterol synthesis and plasma levels increase after epinephrine administration, through activation of the rate-limiting enzyme controlling cholesterol synthesis, 3-hydroxy-3-methylglutaryl CoA reductase (290–292). Triglyceride levels increase acutely during catecholamine infusions (293) but are not elevated after chronic administration.

Thus, the combined effects of catecholamines on lipid metabolism increase the availability of lipids and ketones for peripheral use. This is accomplished through mobilization of lipids from storage sites and stimulation of triglyceride and ketone production.

PROTEIN METABOLISM

Catecholamines have insulin-like effects on plasma amino acid levels. Infusing epinephrine to produce plasma concentrations similar to those seen during acute stress result in a decrease in total amino acid levels, although alanine concentrations are unchanged (294). This effect occurs in the absence of insulin secretion (in type 1 diabetics) and can be prevented by β-adrenergic blockade with propranolol. Drugs with β_2 agonist activity increase body weight, body protein content, and weight of certain skeletal muscles (but not cardiac muscle weight) in guinea pigs with burn injuries (295). Likewise, lambs given β-agonists experience increased muscle protein content accompanying decreased rates of protein degradation while fat content decreases (296).

In contrast to insulin, epinephrine increases both splanchnic uptake of gluconeogenic amino acids and peripheral de novo alanine synthesis and hepatic alanine delivery (297, 298). As dogs recover from insulin-induced hypoglycemia, amino acids are released from the gut into the portal circulation, providing gluconeogenic precursors (299); the amino acid release is suppressed by α-adrenergic blockade and is associated with release of endogenous opioids, suggesting involvement of catecholamines and opioids in the response (300, 301). Stimulation of lactate uptake by liver during hypoglycemia occurs after α-adrenergic blockade and is inhibited by β-adrenergic blockade (302). Perhaps consistent with evidence suggesting a protein anabolic role for catecholamines, epinephrine has not been shown to increase nitrogen excretion despite the enhancement of gluconeogenesis.

SEX STEROIDS AND PROLACTIN

Carbohydrate Metabolism

Estrogen therapy as used in oral contraceptive preparations has been reported to exacerbate mild diabetes mellitus. However, some reports suggest that it is the progestogen component, specifically the 19-nortestosterone derivatives, of oral contraceptives that alters glucose tolerance. The effect is only seen with some of these compounds and is less prominent in low-dose formulations (303, 304). Administration of testosterone to female rats decreased insulin-stimulated glucose transport, increased plasma insulin levels, decreased muscle glycogen synthesis, and decreased capillarization and number of type 1 muscle fibers (associated with insulin resistance) (305).

Lipid Metabolism

Pharmacologic doses of estrogens influence the production and removal rates of plasma lipoproteins. Plasma concentrations of VLDL-cholesterol increase because of enhanced hepatic production rates (306). Certain estrogen-responsive apolipoproteins in avian models markedly elevate VLDL triglyceride levels in the presence of estrogen when overexpressed in transgenic mice, suggesting that estrogen may specifically stimulate production and secretion of certain hepatic VLDL proteins (307). These effects may be counterbalanced slightly by an effect of estrogen to produce a minor inhibition of lipolysis (308). However, estrogen also inhibits LPL activity and so estrogen may, on balance, reduce fat mass. The clinical importance of these effects and the particular adipose tissue depots most affected have not been determined.

Testosterone has biphasic effects on fat tissue. High concentrations of testosterone increase lipolysis, particularly in the abdominal fat depot, and inhibit LPL and fat deposition into the abdominal repository (309). The decrease in LPL activity may be due to production of estrogen from testosterone through testosterone aromatization (310). The summed effects of high levels of testosterone decrease the waist:hip ratio in testosterone-supplemented obese men and concomitantly increase insulin-induced glucose disposal (311). However, low levels of testosterone increase LPL activity (312). The dual effects of testosterone to promote fat storage at low concentration and inhibit fat accretion (particularly abdominal fat) at high concentrations may be related to the seeming paradox that men (and women displaying androgen excess) accumulate fat in the abdominal region from which originates the term "androgenic" obesity (i.e., male pattern, upper-body adiposity). The former effect may dominate at usual male and elevated female testosterone concentrations, while the latter effect may become manifest during androgen supplementation.

In contrast to the effect of estrogen in increasing VLDL, clearance of LDL is enhanced by estrogens, in part because of increased hepatic excretion of cholesterol in the bile (313). This effect has led to the therapeutic use of estrogens in some types of familial hypercholesterolemia, with the most striking results seen in women with familial dysbetalipoproteinemia (type III) and in some postmenopausal women with heterozygous familial hypercholesterolemia (type II) (314). Oral, but not transdermal, estrogen increases HDL apo-A1 production (315). Whereas oral estrogens produce significant increases in plasma HDL-cholesterol levels, the progestogens of the 19-nortestosterone series, often combined with estrogen in oral contraceptives, may lower HDL concentrations (316). A large-scale clinical study of the use of combined estrogen/progestin oral contraceptives indicated that levonogestrel produced a dose-dependent increase in LDL-cholesterol and a decrease in HDL-cholesterol (particularly the HDL2 subfraction) (317). In contrast, norethindrone had opposite effects, indicating that lipoprotein changes related to progestogens may vary with their molecular side-chain configurations. Testosterone lowers HDL-cholesterol concentrations during supplementation and at physiologically relevant levels, possibly because of enhanced HDL clearance by hepatic endothelial triglyceride lipase (312).

Despite the pharmacologic effects of sex hormones on plasma lipids, epidemiologic evidence does not support a major role for sex hormones as the cause of abnormalities of lipoprotein levels in otherwise healthy people (318, 319). However, relationships between sex hormones and lipids may be obscured by the fact that hyperinsulinemia and upper-body obesity, commonly associated with syndromes of hyperlipidemia, tend to decrease levels of sex hormone–binding globulin (SHBG), thereby decreasing the ratio of total to free hormone (320–322). An interesting corollary to this observation is that Western-style refined carbohydrate, low-fiber, high-fat diets, also associated with hyperlipidemia, appear to increase the availability of sex hormones, raising total concentrations while decreasing SHBG (323).

Protein Metabolism

Testosterone administration to hypogonadal or castrated men decreases urinary nitrogen excretion and results in weight gain (324) and increased body density (325, 326). The weight gain is largely composed of fat-free mass when testosterone is given in supraphysiologic doses to healthy, young men (327, 328) or to reproduce youthful doses in elderly men (329). Testosterone replacement in hypogonadal men increases fat-free mass in large part by producing increased muscle mass that results from increased rates of skeletal muscle protein synthesis (330). Attempts to use androgens to improve the rate of nitrogen repletion in patients suffering from catabolic illness have had little or no therapeutic benefit (331).

Estrogens in pharmacologic doses inhibit somatic growth. This effect may be mediated through suppression of IGF-1 generation, which has been demonstrated in growth hormone–treated hypopituitary subjects (332).

Prolactin has a weak stimulatory effect on IGF-1 generation in patients with prolactin-secreting pituitary tumors (333). Prolactin administration to growth hormone–deficient human subjects mimics many of the actions of growth hormone, producing nitrogen retention, lipid mobilization, glucose intolerance, and modest skeletal growth.

VASOACTIVE FACTORS (ANGIOTENSIN II AND BRADYKININ)

Hormones such as insulin that are known to stimulate certain patterns of intracellular nutrient metabolism may also be vasoactive. It is reasonable to think that delivery of nutrients to sites of potential use or storage may be nearly as important for substrate metabolism as processing the substrate once it arrives at the site. Indeed, the decreased ability of insulin in obese persons and those with non-insulin-dependent diabetes to dispose of glucose in peripheral tissues such as skeletal muscle is partially due to inhibition of an insulin-stimulated vasodilatory response (334). Angiotensin II, a vasoactive hormone, promotes insulin-stimulated glucose disposal in healthy humans. Some authors suggest that the angiotensin effect is independent of its effect on blood flow (335), but others state that the hemodynamic effects of angiotensin II to redirect blood flow to insulin-sensitive tissues may contribute to its metabolic actions (336).

The converse may also be true. It is now recognized that hormones typically considered important for maintenance of the circulation are also important for regulation of intracellular substrate metabolism. Angiotensin II stimulates glucose uptake into many cells including astroglia, cardiac muscle, and skeletal muscle of rats. It appears to mediate this effect in part by stimulating production of GLUT1 and GLUT4 glucose transporters (337, 338).

Though angiotensin II appears to stimulate glucose use, administration of angiotensin-converting-enzyme (ACE) inhibitors improves glucose disposal despite lowering angiotensin II levels. It has been hypothesized that bradykinin, a hormone degraded by ACE, may have even more potent effects on glucose disposal than angiotensin and that its accumulation during the use of ACE inhibitors may account for this increased glucose disposal. Bradykinin increases glucose transporter (GLUT1 and GLUT4) translocation to the plasma membrane of cardiac muscle (339). Antagonism of bradykinin-B2 receptors abolishes the effect of ACE inhibitors in enhancing insulin-mediated glucose transport in muscle. However, some authors have reported no effect of bradykinin in enhancing in vivo glucose disposal in humans (340), bringing into question the relevant mechanism for the effects of ACE inhibitors.

CYTOKINES AND EICOSANOIDS

The severely injured or infected patient shows dramatic metabolic responses characterized by mobilization of stored carbohydrate, fat, and protein substrates. Additionally, an "acute-phase" response is initiated in which certain, largely fast-turnover, proteins are created at the expense of other structural and functional proteins such as muscle, for reasons that are unknown but are expected to account for homeostasis of vital tissues during injury and infectious stress. As mentioned above, these phenomena occur in part because of elaboration of classic "stress hormones" such as cortisol and catecholamines from endocrine organs such as the adrenal. It is now recognized that cells of immune origin such as macrophages, monocytes, and lymphocytes, well known to mediate tissue repair and elimination of infecting organisms, also mediate some of the metabolic responses to injury and infection. (See Chapters 35, 37, 45, and 96 for more information on cytokines and growth factors.)

Carbohydrate Metabolism

Thromboxane A2 (TXA2) and prostaglandins $F_{2\alpha}$ ($PGF_{2\alpha}$) and PGE_2, derivatives of arachidonic acid (see Chapter 4), increase glycogenolysis when secreted by Kupffer cells in the liver (205). These prostanoids are released in response to stimulation by phagocytosis and bacterial lipopolysaccharide, explaining in part the glucose intolerance and insulin resistance associated with infection and inflammation. Likewise, interleukin-6 (IL-6) stimulates glucose production from the liver but appears to do so by increasing secondarily secretion of glucocorticoids and glucagon (341). Interleukin 1-α (IL-1-α) increases hepatic glucose production when infused peripherally in rats, an effect that can be blocked by IL-1 receptor antagonists (342). IL-1-α may provide another example of indirect effects of a cytokine on metabolism. IL-1-α acts on the central nervous system to enhance hepatic glucose production in excess of a smaller increase in peripheral glucose use, thus elevating plasma glucose. The effect is mediated by stimulation of the central nervous system adrenergic system that in turn stimulates peripheral secretion of both glucagon and insulin (343).

Tumor necrosis factor–α (TNF-α), also known as cachectin, promotes energy depletion in muscle by stimulating substrate cycling within the glycolytic pathway. Phosphofructokinase and fructose bisphosphate phosphatase activities are simultaneously enhanced in myocytes exposed to TNF-α, depleting ATP so that glycolysis and its resulting elevated glucose utilization, increased lactate production, decreased oxygen consumption, and decreased CO_2 production from glucose can continue unabated (344). However, these effects on cultured muscle cells may not be relevant to the in vivo situation in which TNF-α appears to produce insulin resistance with attendant decreased glucose use in rats and humans (345, 346). Some authors have concluded that the decreased glucose use and insulin sensitivity effected by TNF-α may represent either direct effects of TNF-α on tissues (i.e., TNF-α inhibits insulin receptor and/or insulin receptor substrate–1 phosphorylation in part by stimulating phosphotyrosine phosphatases) or indirect effects of TNF-α-induced increases in circulating free fatty acids (347, 348). Even such equivocating conclusions must be interpreted with caution, however, given the rudimentary current understanding of cytokine and stress hormone responses and actions.

It is becoming clear that conclusions based on models of injury or infections are clouded by the large array of hormones and cytokines elaborated in these conditions, and the metabolic effects of any one factor, such as TNF-α, are difficult to elucidate. Additionally, each factor may in turn stimulate production of others (Fig. 44.4). Models based on infusion of a given cytokine may attribute metabolic effects to the cytokine that in fact belong to a secondary hormone. Such is likely the case with TNF-α; those concluding that it decreases glucose use and increases lipolysis during physical stress may be mistakenly attributing the effects of simultaneously secreted catecholamines to TNF-α. Those concluding that TNF-α increases glucose production and lipolysis may be mistakenly attributing these responses to TNF when in fact they are due to TNF-stimulated production of glucagon (349). Even though some effects may be mediated indirectly by agents such as glucagon, this should not diminish the importance of TNF-α. The fact that glucagon concentrations can remain elevated for weeks during sepsis or severe injury and not be suppressed by glucose-related feedback may underscore the importance of TNF.

Lipid Metabolism

TNF-α has been implicated as the cytokine producing many of the metabolic and nutritional perturbations associated with the critically ill patient (346). Specifically with regard to lipid metabolism, it induces anorexia and lipolysis while inhibiting lipogenesis. These effects have been attributed to the ability of TNF-α to stimulate adipocyte hormone-sensitive lipase while suppressing expression of LPL, fatty acid–binding protein, and glycerol-3-phosphate dehydrogenase (350). As stated above, however, some of these apparent actions of TNF have not been reproduced by other authors. It should be assumed that apart from

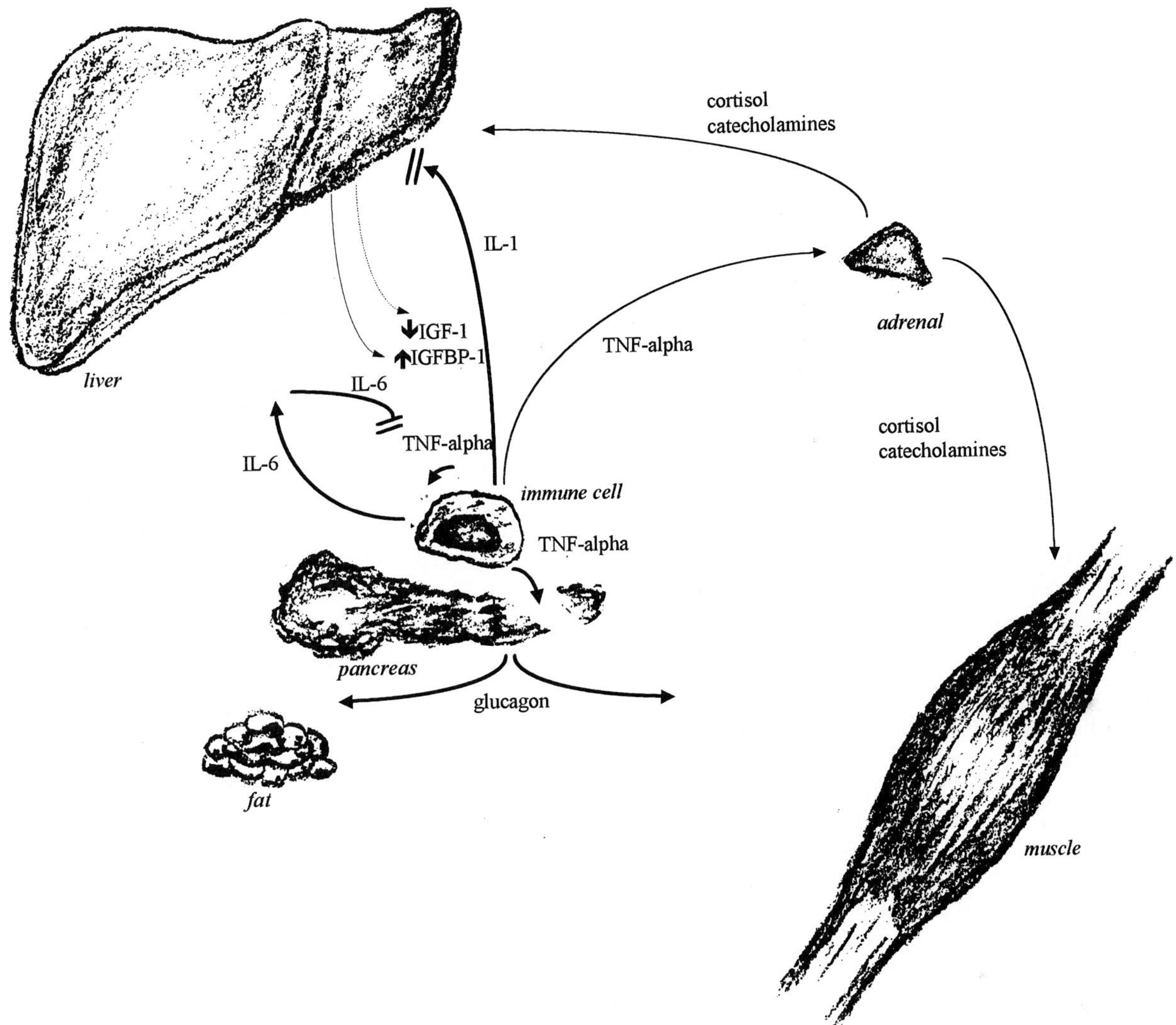

Figure 44.4. The stress response elicited by generation of immune cytokines: hormones induced by cytokines. *Arrows from an immune cell* (*IL-1:* macrophages, NK cells, T cells, tumors such as lung malignancy, *IL-6:* macrophages, fibroblasts, tumors such as melanoma and lung, *TNF-α*: macrophages, T cells, tumors such as breast) indicate cytokine stimulation of a secondary hormone from the indicated glands. *Arrows intersecting parallel lines* indicate inhibition of secretion of factors from the indicated organ. *Arrows from target glands* indicate stimulated secretion of the designated hormones. *Dotted lines/arrows* indicate decreased secretion of the designated factor. In some cases, immune cells may stimulate or inhibit other immune cells as indicated by *arrows directed toward the immune cell representation.*

obvious differences among studies (e.g., species differences in recipients of TNF-α), other differences in study conditions (e.g., duration of anorexia and starvation allowed during TNF administration or inhibition of secondary hormones such as glucagon and insulin) may account for differing interpretations of the effect of TNF-α on lipids. For the present, it suffices to say that TNF-α is at the center of a cytokine and hormonal response to severe stress that results in elevated free fatty acids. The elevation in fatty acids identified with increased concentrations of TNF-α may be accompanied by increased serum cholesterol and decreased HDL-cholesterol concentrations that in hamsters have been shown to result from increased transcription of HMG CoA reductase and decreased transcription of apo A-1 genes, respectively (351). The cholesterol effects are also induced by IL-1 and are additive to those of TNF-α.

Other cytokines have been implicated in the metabolic (lipid and glucose) effects of inflammatory stress in addition to TNF-α, most notably IL-6. Administration of IL-6 to humans increases energy expenditure, fatty acid and ketone production, fat oxidation, glucose production, lactate production, and glucose oxidation (352). Such effects account for many of the manifestations of inflammatory stress, implicating IL-6 as the direct cause of them, perhaps the mediator of some of the effects of TNF-α, which secondarily stimulates IL-6 production. However, like TNF, IL-6 in turn stimulates production of catecholamines, glucagon, and cortisol, which may mediate some or all of the effects of IL-6. In a fashion that resembles classic endocrine hormones, IL-6 provides feedback inhibition of the cytokine cascade that erupts during physical stress by inhibiting TNF-α and IL-1 production (353). Interestingly, IL-6 levels also increase during exercise, another circumstance beside injury in which nutrient mobilization is essential, and are inhibited by glucocorticoids, underscoring feedback on the cytokine cascade by the adrenal axis, which is potently stimulated by IL-6 (354).

Finally, two other cytokines described in the past decade and elaborated during sepsis have been shown to affect lipid metabolism. Ciliary neurotrophic factor (CNTF) and leukemia inhibitory factor (LIF) both produce hypertriglyceridemia and hepatic triglyceride synthesis (from free fatty acids released by lipolysis and produced de novo) through stimulation of a signal transducer, gp130, that is shared with IL-6 (355). The effects of CNTF and LIF to produce hypertriglyceridemia are only noted during the fasting state, but this may be common given that these cytokines produce anorexia in the same fashion as TNF.

The bulk of the effects of cytokines on lipid metabolism increase free fatty acid availability and induce the production of triglycerides. Some authors have concluded that the increase in circulating lipids is beneficial during stress because lipids are delivered to cells involved in the stress response or tissue repair and because lipoproteins, including VLDL, may bind endotoxin (356).

Protein Metabolism

TNF-α promotes catabolism of skeletal muscle protein, in large part by promoting anorexia with resultant starvation. TNF-α stimulates skeletal muscle proteolysis in vivo independent of starvation, an effect that may be mediated by another, undefined factor, as it does not occur when skeletal muscle is incubated with TNF-α in vitro (357). A similar effect is seen in rats in response to IL-1. The proteolysis and concomitantly decreased protein synthesis appear to be confined to fast-twitch muscle rather than slow-twitch or cardiac muscle (358, 359). The impaired protein synthesis induced by sepsis and particularly IL-1 in skeletal muscle and the seromuscular layer of the intestine, kidney, and potentially other organs (360) is likely due to poor availability of eukaryotic initiation factor-2B

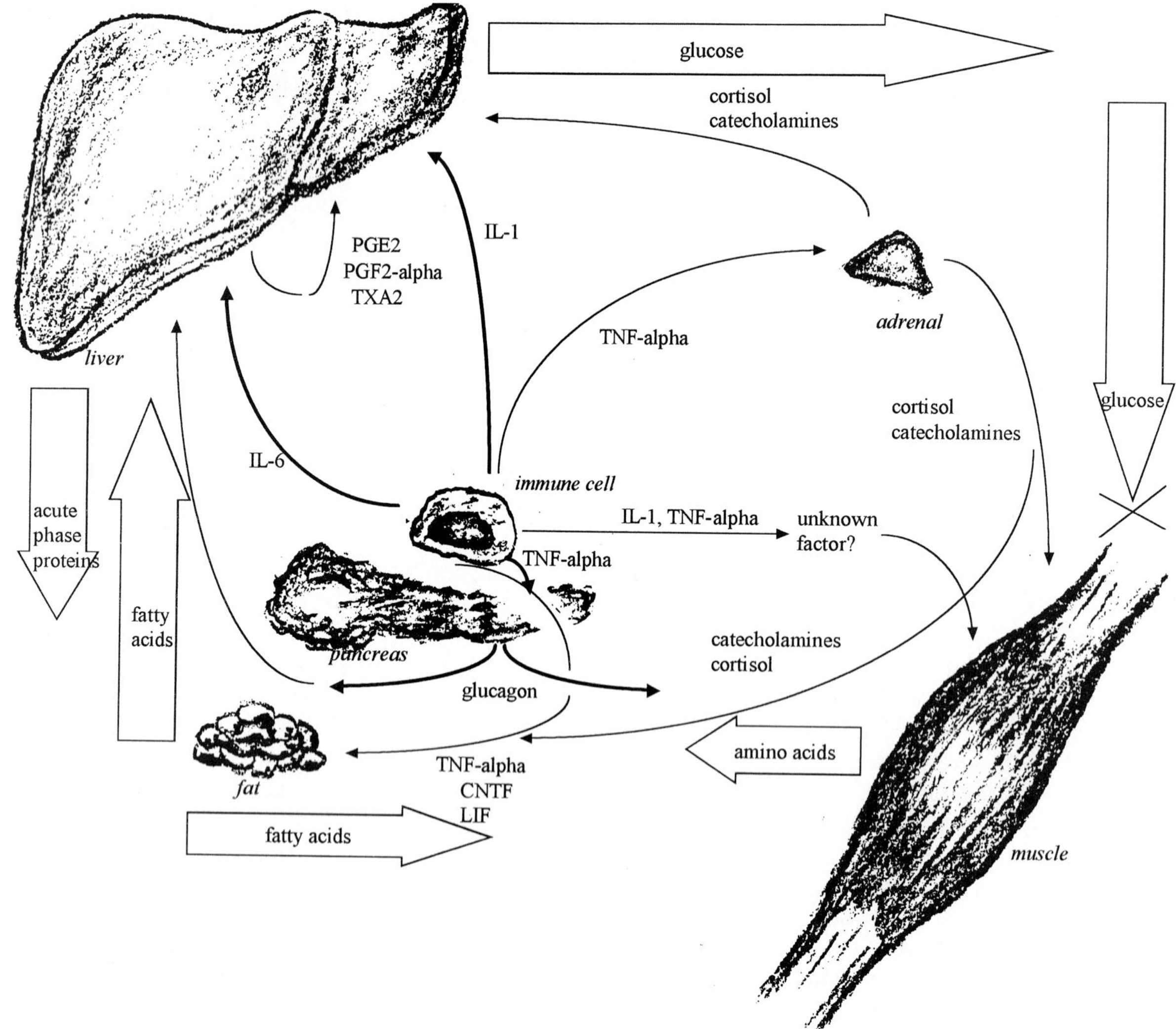

Figure 44.5. The stress response elicited by generation of immune cytokines: alteration in substrate release and use by cytokines. *Large arrows* indicate the net directional movement of the substrate noted within the arrow. *Large arrows intersecting crossed lines* indicate impaired disposal/use of the indicated substrate. *Small arrows* indicate relevant cytokine and hormone effectors of substrate release and use.

(eIF-2B) with impairment of peptide chain initiation (361, 362).

In contrast to skeletal muscle, visceral protein content and cell proliferation are enhanced by TNF-α such that liver, heart, and lung weight are all increased (363). Production of circulating proteins such as albumin and transferrin is depressed by TNF-α. Albumin gene transcription and steady-state albumin mRNA levels are decreased by TNF-α (364). However, acute-phase circulating proteins may be increased by TNF-α, probably resulting in large part from stimulation of IL-6 formation. IL-6 is the most potent stimulator of hepatic acute-phase protein synthesis currently known (365). IL-1 does not appear to be involved in stimulation of hepatic protein synthesis during the acute-phase reaction, as its receptor antagonist, known to preserve muscle protein synthesis from an acute-phase decrease, has no effect on hepatic proteins (360). Thus, elaboration of cytokines from immune cells helps to explain further the peripheral wasting and visceral preservation noted after prolonged critical illness. The effects are opposite to those seen during adequate nutrition and health, when insulin and IGF-1 promote peripheral storage of nutrients. Interestingly, some investigators have found that administration of insulin to TNF-α-treated rats may reverse the catabolic effects of that cytokine (366), and others have noted that IL-1 may mediate some of its effects in decreasing somatic protein synthesis via decreasing circulating and tissue levels of IGF-1 and increasing levels of the inhibitory IGF-binding protein IGFBP-1 (367) (Fig. 44.5).

Cytokines, in summary, are elaborated in a cascade in response to severe physical stress such as infection or injury. The accelerating cascade of interdependent immune factors such as IL-1 and TNF-α and hormones such as catecholamines and glucagon produces a redistribution of nutrients that largely sacrifices peripheral nutrient stores. Protein stores in muscle and fat stores in adipose tissue are mobilized in favor of circulating proteins and lipids that may protect the organism from infectious agents or assist in the repair of tissue. Some elements of the cascade that assist in the nutrient redistribution, such as IL-6 and glucocorticoids, also feed back to calm the inflammatory events. Indeed, macrophages that are integral components of many inflammatory phenomena secrete an IL-1 receptor antagonist so that the same cell simultaneously stimulates and retards inflammation (368).

REFERENCES

1. Kumagai AK, Kang YS, Boado RJ, et al. Diabetes 1995;44: 1399–404.
2. Kahn CR. Clin Res 1983;31:326–35.
3. Kasuga M, Zick Y, Blithe DL, et al. Nature 1982;298:667–9.
4. Kahn CR. Diabetes 1994;43:1066–84.
5. Sternlicht E, Barnard RJ, Grimditch GK. Am J Physiol 1988;254:E633–8.
6. Cushman SW, Wardzala LJ. J Biol Chem 1980;255:4758–62.
7. Suzuki K, Kono T. Proc Natl Acad Sci USA 1980;77:2542–5.
8. Wardzala LJ, Cushman SW, Salans LB. J Biol Chem 1978;253:8002–5.
9. Wardzala LJ, Jeanrenaud B. J Biol Chem 1981;256:7090–3.
10. Charron MJ, Brosius FC III, Alper SL, et al. Proc Natl Acad Sci USA 1989;86:2535–9.
11. Klip A, Paquet MR. Diabetes Care 1990;13:228–43.
12. Stephens JM, Pilch PF. Endoc Rev 1995;16:529–46.
13. Hertz MM, Paulson OB, Barry DI, et al. J Clin Invest 1981;67:597–604.
14. Bell GI, Kayano T, Buse JB, et al. Diabetes Care 1990;13: 198–208.
15. Debons AF, Krimsky I, From A, et al. Am J Physiol 1969;217: 1114–8.
16. Oomura Y, Kita H. Diabetologia 1981;20:290–8.
17. Goodyear LJ, King PA, Hirschman MF, et al. Am J Physiol 1990;258:E667–72.
18. Curnow RT, Rayfield EJ, George DT, et al. Am J Physiol 1975;228:80–7.
19. Benn JJ, Rai R, Sonksen PH. Diabetologia 1990;33:158–62.
20. Taunton OD, Stifel FB, Green HL, et al. J Biol Chem 1974;249:7228–39.
21. Rossetti L, Hu M. J Clin Invest 1993;92:2963–74.
22. Lewis GF, Zinman B, Groenwoud Y, et al. Diabetes 1996;45:454–62.
23. Parkes JL, Grieninger G. J Biol Chem 1985;260:8090–7.
24. Agius L, Peak M, Alberti KG. Biochem J 1990;266:91–102.
25. Muller WA, Faloona GR, Aguilar-Parada E, et al. N Engl J Med 1970;283:109–15.
26. Unger RH, Ketterer H, Dupre J, et al. J Clin Invest 1967;46:630–45.
27. Andersen DK, Elahi D, Brown JC, et al. J Clin Invest 1978;62:152–61.
28. Bloom SR, Vaughan NJA, Russell RCG. Lancet 1974;2:546–9.
29. Berthoud H, Bereiter DA, Trimble ER, et al. Diabetologia 1981;20:393–401.
30. Katz LD, Glickman MG, Rapoport S, et al. Diabetes 1983;32: 675–9.
31. Aguilar-Parada E, Eisentraut AM, Unger RH. Diabetes 1969;18:717–23.
32. Owen OE, Morgan AP, Kemp HG, et al. J Clin Invest 1967;46: 1589–95.
33. Cahill GF, Herrera MG, Morgan AP, et al. J Clin Invest 1966;45:1751–69.
34. Nair KS, Welle SL, Halliday D, et al. J Clin Invest 1988;82: 198–205.
35. Tessari P, Nissen SL, Miles JM, et al. J Clin Invest 1986;77: 575–81.
36. Aguilar-Parada E, Eisentraut AM, Unger RH. Am J Med Sci 1969;257:415–9.
37. Unger RH, Aguilar-Parada E, Muller WA, et al. J Clin Invest 1970;49:837–48.
38. Samois E, Tyler JM, Marks V. Glucagon-insulin interrelationships. In: Lefebvre PJ, Unger RH, eds. Glucagon: molecular physiology, clinical and therapeutic implications. New York: Pergamon Press, 1972;151–73.
39. Samols E, Weir GC, Bonner-Weir S. Intraislet insulin-glucagon-somatostatin relationships. In: Lefebvre PJ, ed. Glucagon, vol 2. Berlin: Springer, 1983;133–73.
40. Unger RH. Diabetologia 1981;20:1–11.
41. Unger RH, Madison LL, Muller WA. Diabetes 1972;21:301–7.
42. Buchanan KD, McCarroll AM. Lancet 1972;2:1394–5.
43. Raskin P, Aydin I, Yamamoto T, et al. Am J Med 1978;64: 988–97.
44. Raskin P, Pietri A, Unger RH. Diabetes 1979;28:1033–5.
45. Rosen SG, Clutter WE, Berk MA. J Clin Invest 1984;73:405–11.

46. White NH, Skor D, Cryer PE, et al. N Engl J Med 1983;308:485–91.
47. Santiago JV, White NH, Skor DA, et al. Am J Physiol 1984;247:E215–20.
48. Rodbell M. The actions of glucagon at its receptor: regulation of adenylate cyclase. In: Lefebvre PJ, ed. Glucagon, vol 1. Berlin: Springer, 1983;263–90.
49. Liljenquist JE, Mueller GL, Cherrington AD, et al. J Clin Invest 1977;59:369–74.
50. Boyd ME, Albright EB, Foster DW, et al. J Clin Invest 1981;68:142–52.
51. Dobbs S, Sakurai H, Sasaki H, et al. Science 1975;187:544–7.
52. de Kreutzenberg VS, Maifreni L, Lisato G, et al. J Clin Endocrinol Metab 1990;70:1023–9.
53. Nair KS, Welle SL, Tito J. Diabetes 1990;39:376–82.
54. Marker JC, Hirsch IB, Smith LJ, et al. Am J Physiol 1991;260:E705–12.
55. Hirsch IB, Marker JC, Smith LJ, et al. Am J Physiol 1991;260:E695–704.
56. Winder WW, Fisher SR, Gygi SP, et al. Am J Physiol 1991;260:E756–61.
57. Mallinson CM, Bloom SR, Warin AP, et al. Lancet 1974;2:1–5.
58. Wood SM, Polak JM, Bloom SR. Glucagonoma syndrome. In: Lefbvre PJ, ed. Glucagon, vol 2. Berlin: Springer, 1983; 411–30.
59. Devlin J, Calles-Escandon J, Poehlman E, et al. Diabetes 1989;38(Suppl 2):224A.
60. Krejs GJ, Orci L, Conlon JM, et al. N Engl J Med 1979;301:285–92.
61. Nosari I, Lepore G, Querci F, et al. J Endocrinol Invest 1989;12:413–7.
62. Felig P. N Engl J Med 1970;283:149–50.
63. Taylor SI, Mukherjee C, Jungas RL. J Biol Chem 1973;248: 73–81.
64. Weber G, Lea MA, Stamm NB. Lipids 1969;4:388–96.
65. Bjorntorp P, Sjostrom L. Metabolism 1978;27:1853–65.
66. Acheson KJ, Schutz Y, Bessard T, et al. Am J Physiol 1984;246:E62–70.
67. Hudgins LC, Hellerstein M, Seidman C, et al. J Clin Invest 1996;97:2081–91.
68. Bagdade JD, Porte D, Bierman EL. N Engl J Med 1967;276: 427–33.
69. Kessler JI. J Clin Invest 1963;42:362–7.
70. Siperstein MD, Fagan VM. J Clin Invest 1958;37:1185–95.
71. Miles JM, Jensen M. J Clin Endocrinol Metab 1993;77:5A–B.
72. Butcher RW, Baird CE, Sutherland EW. J Biol Chem 1968;243:1705–12.
73. Keirns JJ, Freeman J, Bitensky MW. Am J Med Sci 1964;268:62–91.
74. Unger RH. Diabetes 1971;20:834–8.
75. McGarry JD, Wright PH, Foster DW. J Clin Invest 1975;55: 1202–9.
76. Bierman EL. Isr J Med Sci 1972;8:303–8.
77. Chait A, Brunzell JD. Metabolism 1983;32:209–14.
78. Grundy SM, Mok HYI, Zech L, et al. J Clin Invest 1979;63:1274–83.
79. Kissebah AH, Alfarsi S, Evans DJ, et al. Diabetes 1982;31:217–25.
80. Dunn FL. Med Clin North Am 1988;72:1379–98.
81. Hollenbeck CB, Coulston AM. Diabetes Metab Rev 1987;3:669–89.
82. Betteridge BJ. Br Med Bull 1989;45:285–311.
83. Igau B, Lestavel S, Clavey V, et al. Atherosclerosis 1996;120: 209–19.
84. Steinbrecher UP, Witztum JL. Diabetes 1984;33:130–4.
85. American Diabetes Association. (Position statement) Diabetes Care 1997;20(Suppl 1):S14–7.
86. Garg A, Bonanome A, Grundy SM, et al. N Engl J Med 1988;319:829–34.
87. Franz MJ, Horton ES, Bantle JP, et al. Diabetes Care 1994;17:490–518.
88. Fryburg DA, Barrett EJ, Louard RJ, et al. Am J Physiol 1990;259:E477–82.
89. Fukagawa NK, Minaker KL, Young VR, et al. Am J Physiol 1986;250:E13–7.
90. Sugden PH, Smith DM. Biochem J 1982;206:467–72.
91. Longo N, Franchi-Gazzola R, Bussolati O, et al. Biochim Biophys Acta 1985;844:216–23.
92. Shotwell MA, Kilberg MS, Oxender D. Biochim Biophys Acta 1983;737:267–84.
93. Hundal HS, Rennie MJ, Watt PW. J Physiol (Lond) 1987;393:283–305.
94. Hundal HS, Rennie MJ, Watt PJ. J Physiol (Lond) 1989;408:93–114.
95. Flakoll P, Carlson MG, Cherrington A. Physiologic action of insulin. In: LeRoith D, Taylor SI, Olefsky JM, eds. Diabetes mellitus: a fundamental and clinical text. Philadelphia: Lippincott-Raven, 1996;121–32.
96. Zorzano A, Balon TW, Garetto LP, et al. Am J Physiol 1985;248:E546–52.
97. Rodnick KJ, Reaven GM, Azhar S, et al. Am J Physiol 1990;259:E706–14.
98. Jefferson LS, Robertson JW. Diabetes 1972;21(Suppl 1): 341.
99. McKee EE, Grier BL. Am J Physiol 1990;259:E413–21.
100. Wool IG. Am J Physiol 1960;199:719–21.
101. Davidson MB, Goodner CJ. Diabetes 1966;15:835–8.
102. Mendez R, Myers MG Jr, White MF, et al. Mol Cell Biol 1996;16:2857–64.
103. Pause A, Belsham GJ, Gingras AC, et al. Nature 1994;371:747–8.
104. Manchester KL. Sites of hormonal regulation of protein metabolism. In: Munro HN, ed. Mammalian protein metabolism, vol 4. New York: Academic Press, 1970;229–98.
105. Umpleby AM, Boroujerdi MA, Brown PM, et al. Diabetologia 1986;29:131–41.
106. Jefferson LJ, Rannels DE, Munger BL, et al. Fed Proc 1974;33:1098–104.
107. Sloan GM, Norton JA, Brennan MF. J Surg Res 1980;28:442–8.
108. Nair KS, Garrow JS, Ford C, et al. Diabetologia 1983;25:400–3.
109. Pacy PJ, Nair KS, Ford C, et al. Diabetes 1989;38:618–24.
110. Bennett WM, Connacher AA, Smith K, et al. Diabetologia 1990;33:43–51.
111. Biolo G, Fleming RYD, Wolfe RR. J Clin Invest 1995;95:811–9.
112. Trevisan R, Nosadini R, Avogaro A, et al. J Clin Endocrinol Metab 1986;62:1155–62.
113. Tessari P, Nosadini R, Trevisan R, et al. J Clin Invest 1986;77:1797–804.
114. Brodsky IG, Robbins DC, Hiser E, et al. J Clin Endocrinol Metab 1992;75:351–7.
115. Brodsky IG, Devlin JT. Am J Physiol 1996;270:E148–57.
116. Luzi L, Castellino P, Simonson D, et al. Diabetes 1990;39:38–48.
117. Lariviere F, Kupranycz DB, Chiasson J-L, et al. Am J Physiol 1992;263:E173–9.
118. Marliss EB, Aoki TT, Cahill GF. In: Lefebvre PJ, Unger RH, eds. Glucagon: molecular physiology, clinical and therapeutic implications. New York: Pergamon Press, 1972.
119. Nair KS, Halliday D, Matthews DE, et al. Am J Physiol 1987;253:E208–13.

120. Felig P, Owen OE, Wahren J, et al. J Clin Invest 1969;48: 584–94.
121. Boden G, Tappy L, Jadali F, et al. Am J Physiol 1990;259: E225–32.
122. Unger RH, Ohneda A, Aguilar-Parada E, et al. J Clin Invest 1969;48:810–22.
123. Liljenquist JE, Lewis SB, Cherrinton AD, et al. Metabolism 1981;30:1195–9.
124. Abraira C, DeBartolo M, Katzen R, et al. Am J Clin Nutr 1984;39:351–5.
125. Boden G, Rezvani I, Owen OE. J Clin Invest 1984;73:785–93.
126. Elahi D, McAloon-Dyke M, Fukagawa NK, et al. Regul Pept 1994;51:63–74.
127. D'Allesio DA, Vogel R, Prigeon R, et al. J Clin Invest 1996;97: 133–8.
128. Nauck MA, Kleine N, Orskov C, et al. Diabetologia 1993;36:741–4.
129. Chance WT, Zhang X, Balasubramaniam A, et al. Life Sci 1996;58:1785–94.
130. Evers BM, Izukura M, Townsend CM Jr, et al. Ann Surg 1990;211:630–6.
131. Kreines K, Jett M, Knowles HC. Diabetes 1965;14:740–4.
132. Doar JWH, Stamp TCB, Wynn V, et al. Diabetes 1984;188: 633–9.
133. Maxon HR, Kreines KW, Goldsmith RE, et al. Arch Intern Med 1975;139:1477–80.
134. Holdsworth CD, Besser GM. Lancet 1980;2:700–2.
135. Ikeda T, Fujiyama K, Hoshino T, et al. Metabolism 1990;39:633–7.
136. Beer SF, Parr JH, Temple RC, et al. Clin Endocrinol (Oxf) 1989;30:379–83.
137. Wennlund A, Felig P, Hagenfeldt L, et al. J Clin Endocrinol Metab 1986;62:174–80.
138. Ingbar SH. The thyroid gland. In: Wilson JD, Foster DW, eds. Textbook of endocrinology. Philadelphia: WB Saunders, 1985;682–815.
139. Muller MJ, Seitz HJ. Klin Wochenschr 1984;62:11–8.
140. Randin J-P, Tappy L, Scazziga B, et al. Diabetes 1986;35:178–81.
141. Dubaniewicz A, Kaciuba-Usciko H, Budohoski L. Biochem J 1989;263:243–7.
142. Shulman GI, Ladenson PW, Wolfe M, et al. J Clin Invest 1985;76:757–64.
143. Brodie C. J Neurochem 1990;55:186–91.
144. Weinstein SP, Watts J, Graves PN, et al. Endocrinology 1990;126:1421–9.
145. Weinstein SP, O'Boyle E, Haber RS. Diabetes 1994;43:1185–9.
146. Weinstein SP, O'Boyle E, Fisher M, et al. Endocrinology 1994;135:649–54.
147. Saunders J, Hall SEH, Sonksen PH, et al. Clin Endocrinol (Oxf) 1980;13:33–44.
148. Agdeppa D, Macaron C, Mallik T, et al. J Clin Endocrinol Metab 1979;49:726–9.
149. Caron P, Calazel C, Parra HJ, et al. Clin Endocrinol (Oxf) 1990;33:519–23.
150. Krauss RM, Levy RI, Fredrickson DS. J Clin Invest 1974;54:1107–24.
151. Pykalisto O, Goldbert AP, Brunzel JD. J Clin Endocrinol Metab 1976;43:591–600.
152. Ruggiero FM, Cafagna F, Quagliariello E. Lipids 1990; 25:529–33.
153. Paradies G, Ruggiero FM. Biochim Biophys Acta 1990; 1019:133–6.
154. Munro HN. General aspects of the regulation of protein metabolism by diet and hormones. In: Munro HN, ed. Mammalian protein metabolism, vol 1. New York: Academic Press, 1964;381–481.
155. Roche J, Dumazert C, Emond Y, et al. C R Soc Biol 1942;136:326.
156. Sokoloff L, Kaufman S, Gelboin HV. Biochim Biophys Acta 1961;52:410–2.
157. Crispell KR, Parson W, Hollifield G. J Clin Invest 1956; 35:164–9.
158. Kivirikko KI, Laitinen O, Aer J, et al. Endocrinology 1967;80: 1051–61.
159. Foley TH, London DR, Prenton MA. J Clin Endocrinol Metab 1966;26:781–5.
160. Brent GA. N Engl J Med 1994;331:847–53.
161. Wajchenberg BL, Leme CE, Lerario AC, et al. Diabetes 1984;33:455–9.
162. Nosadini R, Del Prato S, Tiengo A, et al. J Clin Endocrinol Metab 1983;57:529–36.
163. De Pirro R, Green A, Kao MY-C, et al. Diabetologia 1981;21:149–53.
164. Plotz CM, Knowlton AJ, Ragan C. Am J Med 1952;13:597–614.
165. Pupo AA, Wajchenberg BL, Schnaider J. Diabetes 1966;15: 24–9.
166. Wise JK, Hendler R, Felig P. J Clin Invest 1973;52:2774–82.
167. Issekutz B, Allen M. Metabolism 1972;21:48–59.
168. Wicks WD, Barnett CA, McKibbin JB. Fed Proc 1974;33: 1105–11.
169. Marco J, Calle C, Roman D, et al. N Engl J Med 1973;288: 128–32.
170. Eisenstein AB, Strack I. Endocrinology 1968;83:1337–48.
171. Dinneen S, Alzaid A, Miles J, et al. Am J Physiol 1995;268: E595–603.
172. Dinneen S, Alzaid A, Miles J, et al. J Clin Invest 1993;92: 2283–90.
173. Wajngot A, Khan A, Giacca A, et al. Am J Physiol 1990;259: E626–32.
174. Goldstein RE, Abumrad NN, Lacy DB, et al. Diabetes 1995;44:672–81.
175. Kahn BB, Flier JS. Diabetes Care 1990;13:548–64.
176. Horner HC, Munck A, Lienhard GE. J Biol Chem 1987;262: 17696–702.
177. Olefsky JM, Johnson J, Liu F, et al. Metabolism 1975;24: 517–27.
178. Kahn CR, Goldfine ID, Neville DM, et al. Endocrinology 1978;103:1054–66.
179. Olefsky JM. J Clin Invest 1975;56:1499–508.
180. Shamoon H, Hendler R, Sherwin RS. J Clin Endocrinol Metab 1983;52:1235–41.
181. Eigler N, Sacca L, Sherwin RS. J Clin Invest 1979;63:114–23.
182. Martin IK, Christopher MJ, Alford FP, et al. Am J Physiol 1991;260:E148–53.
183. Nayak RV, Feldman EB, Carter AC. Proc Soc Exp Biol Med 1962;111:682–6.
184. Shafrir E, Steinberg D. J Clin Invest 1960;39:310–9.
185. Fain JN. Science 1967;157:1062–4.
186. Bagdade JD, Porte D, Bierman EL. Arch Intern Med 1970;125:129–34.
187. Martin-Sanz P, Vance JE, Brindley DN. Biochem J 1990; 271:575–83.
188. Henze K, Chait A, Albers JJ, et al. Eur J Clin Invest 1983;13:171–7.
189. Kroteiwski M, Bjorntorp P. Acta Endocrinol (Copenh) 1975;80:667–75.
190. Lamberts SWJ, Birkenhager JC. J Clin Endocrinol Metab 1976;42:864–8.

191. Tataranni PA, Larson DE, Snitker S, et al. Am J Physiol 1996;271:E317–25.
192. Rebuffe-Scrive M, Krotiewski M, Elfverson J, et al. J Clin Endocrinol Metab 1988;67:1122–8.
193. Rebuffe-Scrive M, Bronnegard M, Nilsson A, et al. J Clin Endocrinol Metab 1990;71:1215–9.
194. Engel FL. Vitam Horm 1961;19:189–227.
195. Kostyo JL. Endocrinology 1965;76:604–13.
196. Noall MW, Riggs TR, Walker LM, et al. Science 1957;126: 1002–5.
197. Block KP, Richmond WR, Mehard WB, et al. Am J Physiol 1987;252:E396–407.
198. Block KP, Buse MG. Med Sci Sports Exerc 1990;22:316–24.
199. Simmons PS, Miles JM, Gerich JE, et al. J Clin Invest 1984;73:412–20.
200. Muhlbacher F, Kapadia CR, Colpoys MF, et al. Am J Physiol 1984;247:E75–83.
201. Kayali AG, Young VR, Goodman MN. Am J Physiol 1987;252:E621–6.
202. Kayali AG, Goodman MN, Lin J, et al. Am J Physiol 1990;259:E699–705.
203. Clark I. J Biol Chem 1953;200:69–76.
204. Weber G, Srivasta SK, Singhal RL. J Biol Chem 1965;240: 750–6.
205. Decker K. Eur J Biochem 1990;192:245–61.
206. Brillon DJ, Zheng B, Campbell RG, et al. Am J Physiol 1995;268:E501–13.
207. Isley WL, Underwood WE, Clemmons DR. J Clin Invest 1983;71:175–82.
208. Phillips LS, Orawski AT, Belosky DC. Endocrinology 1978;103:121–7.
209. Frohman LA, MacGillivray MH, Aceto T. J Clin Endocrinol Metab 1967;27:561–7.
210. Kostyo JL, Reagan CR. Pharmacol Ther (B) 1976;2:591–604.
211. Bratusch-Marrain PR, Smith D, DeFronzo RA. J Clin Endocrinol Metab 1982;55:973–82.
212. Ng SF, Storlien LH, Kraegen EW, et al. Metabolism 1990;39:264–8.
213. Beck P, Schalch DS, Parker ML, et al. J Lab Clin Med 1965;66:366–79.
214. Sonksen PH, Greenwood FC, Ellis JP, et al. J Clin Endocrinol Metab 1967;27:1418–30.
215. Boden G, Soeldner JS, Steinke J, et al. Metabolism 1968;17:1–9.
216. Emmer M, Gorden P, Roth J. Med Clin North Am 1971;55:1057–64.
217. Seng G, Galgoti C, Louisy P, et al. Am J Clin Nutr 1989;50:1348–54.
218. Weil R. Acta Endocrinol 1965;98(Suppl):7–92.
219. Kipnis DM. In: Leibel BS, Wrenshall GA, eds. The nature and treatment of diabetes. New York: Exerpta Medica, 1965;258.
220. Moller N, Jorgensen JO, Alberti KG, et al. J Clin Endocrinol Metab 1990;70:1179–86.
221. Muggeo M, Bar RS, Roth J, et al. J Clin Endocrinol Metab 1979;48:17–25.
222. Magri KA, Adamo M, Leroith D. Biochem J 1990;266:107–13.
223. Randle PJ, Garland PB, Hales CN, et al. Lancet 1963;1:785–9.
224. Luft R, Cerasi E, Hamberger CA. Acta Endocrinol 1967;56:593–607.
225. Eastman RC, Gordon P, Roth J. J Clin Endocrinol Metab 1979;48:931–40.
226. Blundell TL, Bedarkar S, Rinderknecht E, et al. Proc Natl Acad Sci USA 1978;75:180–4.
227. Nissley SP, Rechler MM. Clin Endocrinol 1984;13:43–68.
228. Meuli C, Froesch ER. Eur J Clin Invest 1975;5:93–9.
229. Froesch ER, Muller WA, Burgi H, et al. Biochim Biophys Acta 1966;121:360–74.
230. Goodman HM. Metabolism 1970;19:849–55.
231. Fain JN, Dodd A, Novak L. Metabolism 1971;20:109–18.
232. Gerich JR, Lorenzi M, Bier DM. J Clin Invest 1976;57:875–84.
233. Metcalfe P, Johnston DG, Nosadini R, et al. Diabetologia 1981;20:123–8.
234. Schade DS, Eaton RP, Peake GT. Diabetes 1978;27:916–24.
235. Luft R, Ikkos D, Gemzell CA, et al. Lancet 1958;1:721.
236. Ng FM, Adamafio NA, Graystone JE. J Mol Endocrinol 1990;4:43–9.
237. Villar-Pilasi C, Larner J. Annu Rev Biochem 1970;39:639–72.
238. Rosenbaum M, Gertner JM, Leibel RL. J Clin Endocrinol Metab 1989;69:1274–81.
239. Zapf J, Schoenle E, Waldvogel M, et al. Eur J Biochem 1981;113:605–9.
240. Guler HP, Schmid C, Zapf J, et al. Acta Paediatr Scand 1990;367(Suppl):52–4.
241. Zapf J, Schoenle E, Froesch ER. Eur J Biochem 1978,87: 285–96.
242. Daughaday WH, Rotwein P. Endocr Rev 1989;10:68–91.
243. Skottner A, Arrhenius-Nyberg V, Kanje M, et al. Acta Paediatr Scand 1990;367(Suppl):63–6.
244. Nutting DF. Endocrinology 1976;98:1273–83.
245. Fryburg DA, Barrett EJ. Metabolism 1993;42:1223–7.
246. Fryburg DA, Gelfand RA, Barrett EJ. Am J Physiol 1991;260: E499–504.
247. Lo H-C, Ney DM. Am J Physiol 1996;271:E872–8.
248. Svanberg E, Zachrisson H, Ohlsson C, et al. Am J Physiol 1996;270:E614–20.
249. Yarasheski KE, Zachwieja JJ, Campbell JA, et al. Am J Physiol 1995;268:E268–77.
250. Taafe DR, Jin IH, Vu TH, et al. J Clin Endocrinol Metab 1996;81:421–5.
251. Rutherford OM, Beshyah SA, Schott J, et al. Clin Sci 1995;88:67–71.
252. Jones JI, Clemmons DR. Endocr Rev 1995;16:3–34.
253. Mohan S, Pettis JL. J Clin Endocrinol Metab 1996;81:3817–21.
254. Garber AJ, Cryer PE, Santiago JV, et al. J Clin Invest 1976;58:7–15.
255. Clarke WL, Santiago JV, Thomas L, et al. Am J Physiol 1979;236:E147–52.
256. Smith PH, Madson KL. Diabetologia 1981;20:314–22.
257. Smith PH, Porte D. Annu Rev Pharmacol Toxicol 1976;16: 269–85.
258. Exton JH. Am J Physiol 1980;238:E3–12.
259. Kneer NM, Bosch AL, Clark MG, et al. Proc Natl Acad Sci USA 1974;71:4523–7.
260. Hutson NJ, Brumley FT, Assimacopoulos FD, et al. J Biol Chem 1976;251:5200–8.
261. Cherrington AD, Assimacopoulos FD, Harper SC, et al. J Biol Chem 1976;251:5209–18.
262. Tolbert MEM, Butcher FR, Fain JN. J Biol Chem 1973;248: 5686–92.
263. Steiner KE, Stevenson RW, Green DR, et al. Metabolism 1985;34:1020–3.
264. Himms-Hagen J. Effects of catecholamines on metabolism. In: Blaschko H, Muscholl E, eds. Catecholamines: handbook of experimental pharmacology, vol 33. Berlin: Springer, 1972;363–462.
265. Dietz MR, Chiasson J-L, Soderling TR, et al. J Biol Chem 1980;255:2301–7.
266. Shikama H, Chiasson J-L, Exton JH. J Biol Chem 1981;256: 4450–4.

267. Foulkes JG, Cohen P, Strada SJ. J Biol Chem 1982;257:12493–6.
268. Green GA, Chenoweth M, Dunn A. Proc Natl Acad Sci USA 1980;77:5711–5.
269. Exton JH, Park CR. J Biol Chem 1968;243:4189–96.
270. Le Cam A, Freychet P. Endocrinology 1978;102:379–85.
271. Stevenson RW, Steiner KE, Connoly CC, et al. Am J Physiol 1991;260:E363–70.
272. Abramson EA, Arky RA. Diabetes 1968;17:141–6.
273. Chiasson J-L, Shikama H, Chu DTW, et al. J Clin Invest 1981;68:706–13.
274. Raz I, Katz A, Spencer MK. Am J Physiol 1991;260:E430–5.
275. Scheidegger K, Robbins DC, Danforth E. Diabetes 1984;33:1144–9.
276. Lupien JR, Hirshman MF, Horton ES. Am J Physiol 1990;259:E210–5.
277. Urhammer SA, Clausen JO, Hansen T, et al. Diabetes 1996;45:1115–20.
278. Kadowaki H, Yasuda K, Iwamoto K, et al. Biochem Biophys Res Commun 1995;215:555–60.
279. Widen E, Lehto M, Kanninen T, et al. N Engl J Med 1995;333:348–51.
280. Clement K, Vaisse C, Manning B, et al. N Engl J Med 1995;333:382–3.
281. Walston J, Silver K, Bogardus C, et al. N Engl J Med 1995;333:343–7.
282. Sigal RJ, Fisher S, Halter JB, et al. Diabetes 1996;45:148–56.
283. Purdon C, Brousson M, Nyveen SL, et al. J Clin Endocrinol Metab 1993;76:566–73.
284. Fain JN, Garcia-Sainz JA. J Lipid Res 1983;24:945–66.
285. Belfrage P, Fredrickson G, Olsson H, et al. Control of adipose tissue lipolysis by phosphorylation/dephosphorylation of hormone-sensitive lipase. In: Angel A, Holberg CH, Ronicari DAK, eds. The adipocyte and obesity: cellular and molecular mechanisms. New York: Raven Press, 1983;217–24.
286. Herndon DN, Nguyen TT, Wolfe RR, et al. Arch Surg 1994;129:1301–4.
287. Galitzky J, Reverte M, Portillo M, et al. Am J Physiol 1993;264:E403–12.
288. Galitzky J, Reverte M, Carpene C, et al. J Pharmacol Exp Ther 1993;266:358–66.
289. Oberhaensli RD, Schwendimann R, Keller U. Diabetes 1985;34:774–9.
290. Edwards PA. Arch Biochem Biophys 1975;170:188–203.
291. Edwards P, Lemongello D, Fogelman AM. J Lipid Res 1979;20:2–7.
292. George R, Ramasarma T. Biochem J 1977;162:493–9.
293. Miller HI. Metabolism 1967;16:1096–105.
294. Shamoon H, Jacob R, Sherwin RS. Diabetes 1980;29:875–81.
295. Nelson JL, Chalk CL, Warden GD. J Trauma 1995;38:237–41.
296. del Barrio AS, Garcia-Calonge MA, Fernadez Quintela A, et al. Ann Nutr Metab 1995;39:317–24.
297. Miles JM, Nissen SL, Gerich JE, et al. Am J Physiol 1984;247:E166–72.
298. Del Prato S, DeFronzo RA, Castellino P, et al. Am J Physiol 1990;258:E878–87.
299. Hourani H, Williams P, Morris JA, et al. Am J Physiol 1990;259:E342–50.
300. Molina PE, Abumrad NN. JPEN J Parenter Enteral Nutr 1994;18:549–56.
301. Abumrad NN. Personal communication, 1991.
302. Hourani H, Lacy DB, Nammour TM, et al. J Trauma 1990;30:1116–23.
303. Spellacy WN, Ellingson AB, Tsibris JC. Adv Contracept 1990;6:185–91.
304. Brooks PG. J Reprod Med 1984;29(Suppl):539–46.
305. Holmang A, Svedberg J, Jennische E, et al. Am J Physiol 1990;259:E555–60.
306. Glueck CJ, Fallat RW, Scheel D. Metabolism 1975;24:537–45.
307. Zsigmond E, Nakanishi MK, Ghiselli FE, et al. J Lipid Res 1995;36:1453–62.
308. Jensen MD, Martin ML, Cryer PE, et al. Am J Physiol 1994;266:E914–20.
309. Marin P, Oden B, Bjorntorp P. J Clin Endocrinol Metab 1995;80:239–43.
310. Gray JM, Nunez AA, Siegel LI, et al. Physiol Behav 1979;23:465–9.
311. Marin P, Krotkiewski M, Bjorntorp P. Eur J Med 1992;1:329–36.
312. Mooradian AD, Morley JE, Korenman SG. Endocr Rev 1987;8:1–28.
313. Everson GT, McKinley C, Kern F. J Clin Invest 1991;87:237–46.
314. Tikkanen MJ, Nikkila EA, Vartiainen E. Lancet 1978;2:490–1.
315. Walsh BW, Li H, Sacks FM. J Lipid Res 1994;35:2083–93.
316. Wahl P, Walden C, Knopp R, et al. N Engl J Med 1983;308:862–7.
317. Godsland IF, Crook D, Simpson R, et al. N Engl J Med 1990;323:1375–81.
318. Duell PB, Bierman EL. Arch Intern Med 1990;150:2317–20.
319. Cauley JA, Gutai JP, Kuller LH, et al. Am J Epidemiol 1990;132:884–94.
320. Pasquali R, Casimirri F, Cantobelli S, et al. Metabolism 1991;40:101–4.
321. Nestler JE, Powers LP, Matt DW, et al. J Clin Endocrinol Metab 1991;72:83–9.
322. Weaver JU, Holly JM, Kopelman PG, et al. Clin Endocrinol (Oxf) 1990;33:415–22.
323. Adlercruetz H. Scand J Clin Lab Invest 1990;201(Suppl):3–23.
324. Kenyon AT, Knowlton K, Sandiford I, et al. Endocrinology 1940;26:26–45.
325. Hamilton JB. Recent Prog Horm Res 1948;3:257–322.
326. Wilson JD, Griffin JE. Metabolism 1980;29:1278–95.
327. Griggs RC, Kingston W Jozefowicz R, et al. J Appl Physiol 1989;66:498–503.
328. Welle S, Jozefowicz R, Forbes G, et al. J Clin Endocrinol Metab 1992;74:332–5.
329. Urban RJ, Bodenburg YH, Gilkison C, et al. Am J Physiol 1995;269:E820–6.
330. Brodsky IG, Balagopal P, Nair KS. J Clin Endocrinol Metab 1996;81:3469–75.
331. Tweedle D, Walton C, Johnston IDA. Br J Clin Pract 1972;27:130–2.
332. Wiedemann E, Schwartz E. J Clin Endocrinol Metab 1972;34:51–8.
333. Clemmons DR, Underwood LE, Ridgway EC, et al. J Clin Endocrinol Metab 1981;52:731–5.
334. Laakso M, Edelman SV, Brechtel G, et al. J Clin Invest 1990;85:1844–52.
335. Townsend RR, Di Pette DJ. Am J Physiol 1993;265:E362–6.
336. Buchanan TA, Thawani H, Kades W, et al. J Clin Invest 1993;92:720–6.
337. Tang W, Richards EM, Raizada MK, et al. Am J Physiol 1995;268:E384–90.
338. Hoenack C, Roesen P. Diabetes 1996;45(Suppl 1):S82–7.
339. Rett K, Wicklmayr M, Dietze GJ, et al. Diabetes 1996;45:S66–9.
340. Nuutila P, Raitakari M, Laine H, et al. J Clin Invest 1996;97:1741–7.
341. Stith RD, Luo J. Circ Shock 1994;44:210–5.

342. Ling PR, Istfan NW, Colon E, et al. Am J Physiol 1995;268: E255–61.
343. Petit F, Jarrous A, Dickinson RD, et al. Am J Physiol 1994;267:E49–56.
344. Zentella A, Manogue K, Cerami A. Cytokine 1993;5:436–47.
345. Lang CH, Dobrescu C, Bagby GJ. Endocrinology 1992; 130:43–52.
346. Van der Poll T, Romijn JA, Endert E, et al. Am J Physiol 1991;261:E457–65.
347. Hotamisligil GS, Spiegelman BM. Diabetes 1994;43:1271–8.
348. Kroder G, Bossenmaier B, Kellerer M, et al. J Clin Invest 1996;97:1471–7.
349. Sakurai Y, Zhang XJ, Wolfe RR. Am J Physiol 1996;270: E864–72.
350. Beutler B, Cerami A. Endocr Rev 1988;9:57–66.
351. Hardardottir I, Moser AH, Memon R, et al. Lymphokine Cytokine Res 1994;13:161–6.
352. Stouthard JML, Romijn JA, van der Poll T, et al. Am J Physiol 1995;268:E813–9.
353. Chrousos GP. N Engl J Med 1995;332:1351–62.
354. Papanicolaou DA, Petrides JS, Tsigos C, et al. Am J Physiol 1996;271:E601–5.
355. Nonogaki K, Pan X-M, Moser AH, et al. Am J Physiol 1996;271:E521–8.
356. Hardardottir I, Grunfeld C, Feingold KR. Curr Opin Lipidol 1994;5:207–15.
357. Goodman MN. Am J Physiol 1991;260:E727–30.
358. Vary TC, Kimball SR. Am J Physiol 1992;262:C1513–9.
359. Cooney R, Owens E, Jurasinski C, et al. Am J Physiol 1994;267:E636–41.
360. Cooney RN, Owens E, Slaymaker D, et al. Am J Physiol 1996;270:E621–6.
361. Voisin L, Gray K, Flowers KM, et al. Am J Physiol 1996;270: E43–50.
362. Vary TC, Voisin L, Cooney RN. Am J Physiol 1996;271: E513–20.
363. Hoshino E, Pichard C, Greenwood CE, et al. Am J Physiol 1191;260:E27–36.
364. Brenner DA, Buck M, Feitelberg SP, et al. J Clin Invest 1990;85:248–55.
365. Andus T, Geiger T, Hirano T, et al. Eur J Biochem 1988;173:287–93.
366. Fraker DL, Merino MJ, Norton JA. Am J Physiol 1989;256: E725–31.
367. Lang CH, Fan J, Cooney R, et al. Am J Physiol 1996;270: E430–7.
368. Dripps DJ, Brandhuber RC, Thompson RC, et al. J Biol Chem 1991;266:10331–6.

45. Nutrition and the Immune System

STEVEN H. YOSHIDA, CARL L. KEEN, AFTAB A. ANSARI, and M. ERIC GERSHWIN

The fundamental concept underlying the function of the immune system is the ability to distinguish, at the molecular level, the host from foreign materials. This "self/nonself discrimination" is responsible for selective destruction of microbial infectious agents, neutralization of chemical toxicants, rejection of foreign tissue grafts, and allergic responses to certain xenobiotics. Thus, the immune system has been deemed a sensory tissue that develops a sense of identity.

The study of nutritional influences on the immune system represents an area of growing concern to nutritionists, food scientists, and immunologists. This chapter summarizes basic information on the structure and function of the immune system. A brief section on the evolution of the immune system is followed by overviews of the two basic forms of immune defenses: the innate/natural and acquired/adaptive/specific immune systems. Subsequent sections provide more details on topics such as the cellular interactions necessary for generation and regulation of immune responses. These are followed by discussions of some of the known associations between nutrition and immunity.

Abbreviations: **APC**—antigen-presenting cell; **C**—complement component; **CD**—cluster of differentiation; **CRP**—C-reactive protein; **DTH**—delayed-type hypersensitivity; **EC**—endothelial cell; **IFN**—interferon; **Ig**—immunoglobulin; **IL**—interleukin; **MHC**—major histocompatibility complex; **NK**—cell, natural killer cell; **NO**—nitric oxide; **PMN**—polymorphonuclear leukocyte; **Tc**—cytotoxic T cell; **TCR**—T-cell receptor; **TGF**—transforming growth factor; **Th**—helper T cell; **TNF**—tumor necrosis factor.

FUNDAMENTALS OF IMMUNOLOGY

Innate Immunity

Innate, as opposed to acquired, immune responses are defined as those that are not qualitatively and quantitatively affected by repeated contacts with the same specific immunologic stimulus. Such responses are not customized for the offending stimulus, and there is no enhanced response following another exposure to the stimulus (there is no immunologic memory of past contacts). Thus, innate immunity is considered a more primitive, basal, or constitutional form of defense. On this foundation developed the more flexible acquired immune system that exhibits aspects of learning and memory (discussed below).

Phagocytes

The major phagocytes are the polymorphonuclear (PMN) leukocytes, or neutrophils, and the macrophages. Neutrophils are produced in the bone marrow and released into the blood where they constitute between one-half and two-thirds of all leukocytes. A typical adult human has about 50 billion neutrophils in the circulation, with a life span of 1 to 2 days; thus, the bone marrow uses much of its hematopoietic capacity for neutrophil production. A mature PMN is characterized by a multilobed nucleus and a large reservoir of cytoplasmic granules containing enzymes and other proteins used to degrade and digest phagocytosed particles. Sizable glycogen stores also support glycolytic anaerobic activity among PMNs.

Macrophages are produced in the bone marrow and circulate in the blood as monocytes (1). Although macrophages constitute a relatively minor (1–6%) percentage of circulating leukocytes, their frequency often increases during infections. Blood monocytes further mature to tissue macrophages or histiocytes. Collectively, these macrophages are widely distributed in the host as the mononuclear phagocyte system. Tissue macrophages attain distinct morphologic characteristics as Kupffer cells (liver), microglia (brain), mesangial cells (glomerulus), and osteoclasts (bone). Macrophages also reach substantial numbers in connective tissues and the lung (alveolar macrophages). The life span of tissue macrophages can extend into months.

A typical phagocytic event is initiated by adherence of a microbe to the phagocyte. Adherence mechanisms range from nonspecific hydrophobicity to specific receptor–ligand interactions. Intracellular contractile systems then extend pseudopods around the particle, followed by a "zippering" effect and encasement of the particle in a cellular vacuole called the phagosome. Cytoplasmic granules consisting of proteolytic enzymes then fuse with the phagosome and release their active constituents to begin bacterial digestion (Fig. 45.1).

There are two main granule types in the PMN: the primary azurophilic granules that contain myeloperoxidase, defensins, bactericidal/permeability increasing factor and cathepsin G and the secondary specific granules containing lactoferrin, lysozyme, alkaline phosphatase, and cytochrome b_{558}. The preformed antimicrobials of PMN granules perform a variety of functions depending on intraphagosomal conditions. Increased vacuolar pH, following the dismutation of superoxide anion and the consumption of hydrogen ions, activates peptides such as the defensins, which form voltage-regulated ion channels in bacteria, fungi, and some enveloped viruses. The neutral proteinase, cathepsin G, also increases bacterial permeability. Lysozyme degrades the peptidoglycan wall of certain bacteria, while lactoferrin chelates iron. Acidification of phagosomes promotes target hydrolysis and increases the activities of other enzymes (2).

Following phagocytosis by macrophages, phagosomes migrate to the perinuclear region where they fuse with lysosomes. These lysosomes contain acid hydrolases (proteases, nucleases, glycosidases, phosphatases, lipases, etc.) that are potentiated by the acidic environment produced by proton pumps located in the phagosome. The digested materials are then stored as "dense bodies" or expelled by

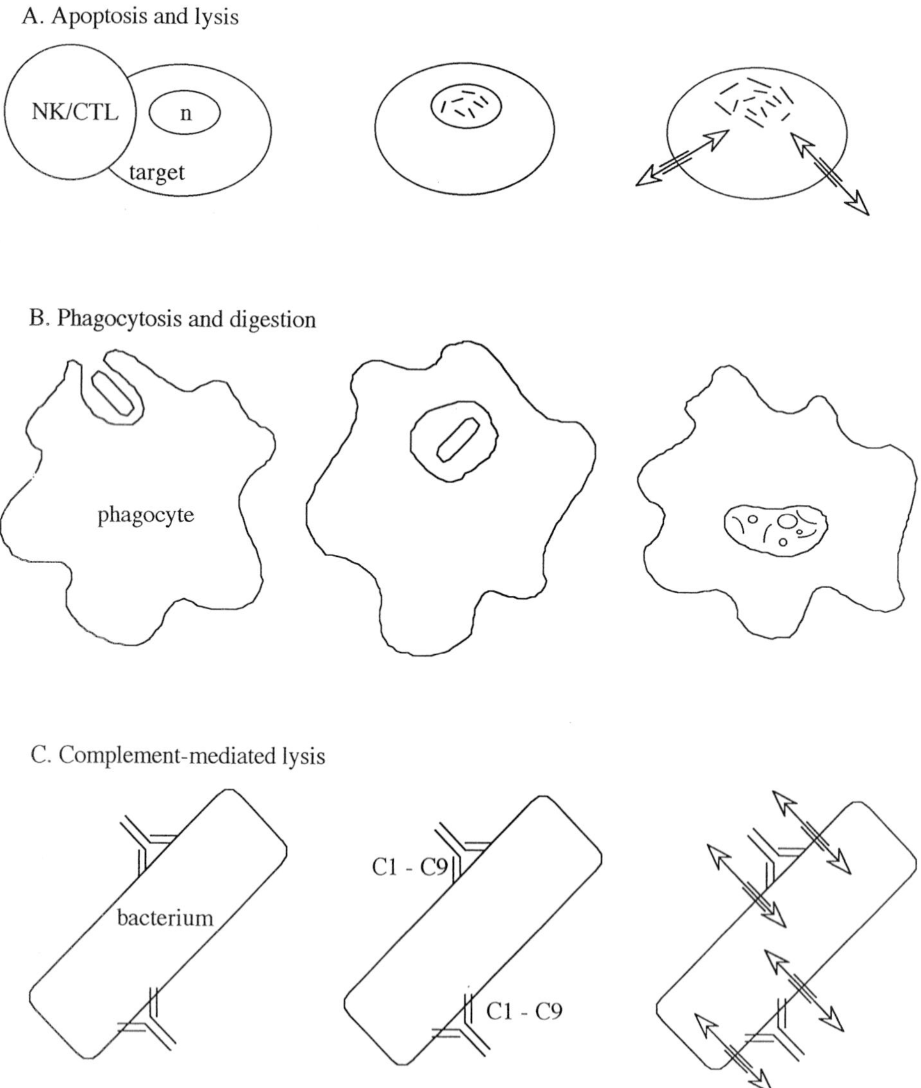

Figure 45.1. Three methods of killing cells by the immune system. *(A)* Both cytolytic T lymphocytes and NK cells induce apoptosis in their targets. Although apoptosis is illustrated by nuclear degradation, not all apoptotic cells exhibit DNA fragmentation. In addition to apoptosis, the plasma membrane is perforated by attack membrane complexes similar to complement-mediated lysis. *(B)* Phagocytes wholly engulf items and degrade them intracellularly with a variety of enzymes. If foreign materials are too large to phagocytize, enzymes and reactive oxygen species are released extracellularly. *(C)* The complement cascade activated by antibodies forms membrane attack complexes that result in cell membrane damage.

exocytosis. Importantly, some macrophage phagosomes (endosomes) can be recycled to the cell surface, a process that is important in antigen presentation (see below).

Phagocytes also generate reactive oxygen molecules for killing microorganisms in a process called the respiratory, oxidative, or metabolic burst because of the characteristic increase in oxygen consumption (3). An increase in the hexose monophosphate shunt results in enhanced NADPH synthesis, consuming glucose and producing lactate. Electron transfer leads to reduction of molecular oxygen to superoxide anion. Superoxide dismutase then catalyzes the conversion of superoxide anion to hydrogen peroxide. Neutrophilic myeloperoxidase combines with peroxides and halide ions (e.g., Cl^-, Br^-, I^-) to form hypohalites (e.g., HOCl), which oxidize a wide range of biomolecules, including thiols, nucleic acids, and proteins. The relative stability of H_2O_2 allows its diffusion to more distal sites and extends the range of antimicrobial action. Hydrogen peroxide may be further processed to form the highly reactive hydroxyl radicals that bind to targets more proximal to the phagocyte. Phagocytes are protected from their reactive oxygen by the sulfhydryl-containing tripeptide reduced glutathione and catalase, which enzymatically converts H_2O_2 to water and oxygen. Although release of these toxic materials to the extracellular space allows phagocytes to eliminate large parasites that cannot be ingested, this process can cause considerable damage to surrounding host tissues.

Nitric oxide (NO), a reactive nitrogen radical, is toxic to bacteria and tumor cells. The enzymatic activity of NO synthase on molecular oxygen and L-arginine generates citrulline and NO. The antibacterial mechanism of NO may involve degradation of Fe-S prosthetic groups of electron transport enzymes and the generation of hydroxyl radicals.

In general, phagocytosis by macrophages tends to be slower than that by PMNs, and the metabolic burst is less intense. In addition, the longer life span of macrophages is reflected in their more gradual and extended degradation of engulfed materials, compared with PMNs. This is partly a function of the relatively lower density of lysosomes present in macrophages. But unlike neutrophils, macrophages can synthesize new lysosomes and hydrolytic enzymes. Together, PMNs and macrophages provide both short- and longer-term phagocytic function for elimination of microbes and other particulate foreign materials.

Complement

Complement is a term for approximately 25 plasma proteins and protein fragments that are important in host defense (4). The functional roles of the complement system include lysis of cells and enveloped viruses, facilitation of phagocytosis, and phagocyte activation and chemotaxis. Many of these proteins are zymogens or proenzymes that require proteolytic cleavage to become active. The complement cascade is a series of such cleavages mediated in large part by the complement proteins themselves. There are two major cascade pathways; the innate alternative pathway and the antibody-dependent classical pathway have different initiation conditions, but eventually converge to a common series of reactions (Fig. 45.2). The alternative pathway is directly activated by the cell walls of certain microorganisms, while the classical pathway is initiated by antibodies.

The Acute-Phase Response

The acute-phase response is a rapid reaction to tissue damage that integrates the elimination of microbes, the control of further tissue damage, the cleanup of debris, and the initiation of repair processes (5). For example, microbial endotoxins induce macrophages to release cytokines interleukin-1 (IL-1), IL-6, and tumor necrosis factor (TNF). These are followed by changes in the concentrations of many plasma proteins, such as increased production of C-reactive protein (CRP) by the liver. CRP then attaches to the phosphorylcholine-containing membranes of certain microorganisms and activates the complement cascade. In addition, the binding of CRP to necrotic host tissues may protect against autoimmune responses by promoting the rapid removal of self molecules from the circulation. Other proteins that increase in the plasma include complement components B, C3, and C4; ceruloplasmin, the major copper-binding protein, which removes iron from inflammatory sites and may act as an oxygen radical scavenger; fibrinogen, a protein involved in coagulation and bacterial clumping; serum amyloid A and P, proteins that bind to the extracellular matrix and are possible components of amyloid deposits; and α_1-PI, a protease inhibitor important in modulating tissue damage.

Some plasma proteins decrease in concentration during the acute-phase response. The role of albumin as a "metabolic compensator" in maintaining an overall constant rate of protein synthesis is suggested by its decreased production during the acute-phase response. Albumin is also a transport protein and its sequestration may be important in minimizing nutrient delivery to microbes. In addition, decreases in circulating transferrin, concomitant with increased activity of intrahepatic ferritin, decreases iron availability at peripheral sites of infection.

Cytotoxic Cells

The process of cell killing by another cell type is termed *cytotoxicity*. One proposed function of the immune system is elimination of abnormal host cells that are thought to constantly appear throughout an individual's life. This process of immune surveillance is thought to be the prime function of the natural killer (NK) cell (6).

Morphologically, NK cells are categorized as large granular lymphocytes. Relative to other lymphocytes, they are large, are granular in appearance, and have low

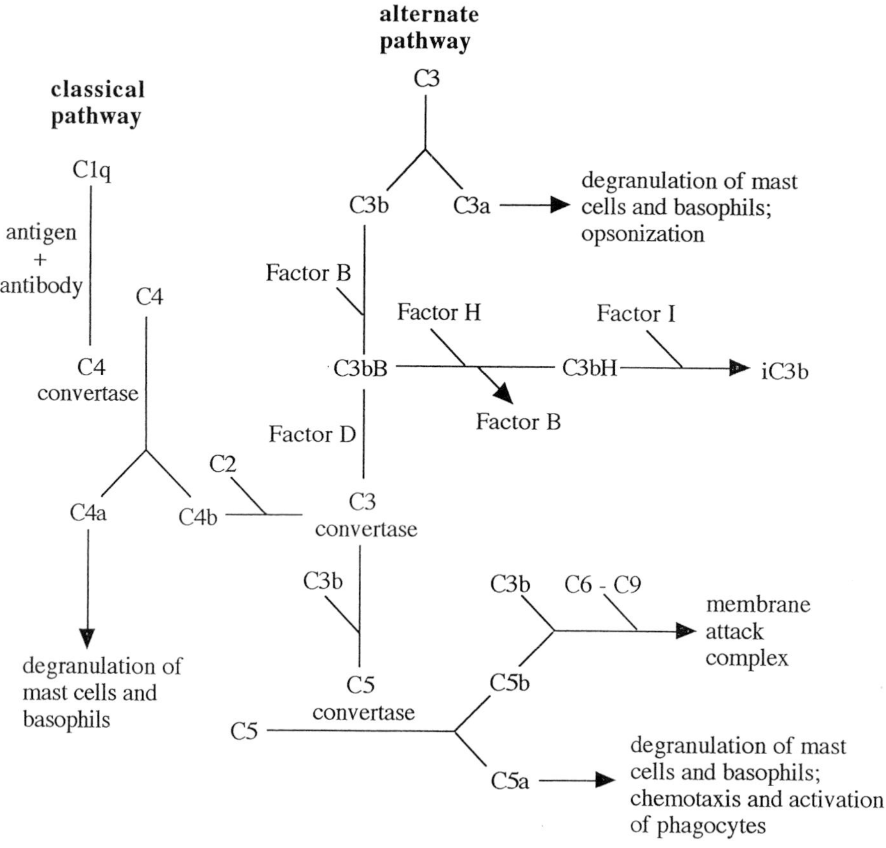

Figure 45.2. Schematic diagram of the classic and alternate complement pathways. The complement pathway is regulated by the instability of C3 convertase and the displacement of factor B by factor H. IC3b can be further degraded, or can act as an opsonin. C3 convertase is able to catalyze the cleavage of C3 to C3a and C3b.

nuclear:cytoplasmic ratios. NK cells normally constitute about 15% of circulating lymphocytes and 4% of splenic lymphocytes. These cells are distinct from T and B lymphocyte lineages. For example, certain immunodeficiency states are characterized by a lack of T and B cells but not NK cells. However, NK cells do share certain characteristics with T lymphocytes. NK cells, cytotoxic T (Tc) cells, and T cells that possess the $\gamma\delta$ T-cell receptor (TCR) exhibit similar cytotoxic activities and target cell specificities, surface protein markers, and cytokine production.

Although the means by which NK cells recognize their choice of target cells is controversial, binding of lectinlike NK receptors to carbohydrate ligands on target cells appears important (7). NK cells are known to kill syngeneic (genetically identical), allogeneic (same species but different genotype), and xenogeneic (different species) tumor cells. There is evidence that the expression of major histocompatibility complex (MHC) class I molecules on target cells is inversely related to susceptibility to killing.

NK cells can kill their chosen targets by cytolysis and/or by inducing apoptosis. Fragmentation of target cell DNA occurs early, suggesting that apoptosis is the principal mode of target cell destruction. Additionally, within minutes of NK–target cell contact, NK cell granules migrate to the regions of contact and release their contents (e.g., perforin or cytolysin, which are structurally and functionally similar to C9) to form transmembrane pores in the target cell's plasma membrane (Fig. 45.1). Other granule constituents include a family of serine proteases (granzymes) that function as perforin activators, and ionized ATP, which may initiate apoptosis. NK cells are protected from their own armaments by a lack of cell surface ATP receptors and the presence in their granules of chondroitin sulfate A, a protease-resistant, negatively charged proteoglycan that inhibits autolysis.

The eosinophil, another component of the innate immune system, is associated with allergic reactions and antihelminthic responses (8). Eosinophils normally constitute about 1 to 3% of circulating leukocytes, a frequency that may increase in atopic situations. The vast majority of eosinophils are sequestered in the bone marrow and connective tissues. Most helminths activate the alternate complement pathway and production of C3b, an eosinophil opsonin and activator. Activated eosinophils release a variety of bioactive materials such as eosinophil peroxidase to generate reactive oxygen intermediates, the lysophosphatase Charcot-Leyden crystal protein, major basic protein that induces release of histamine from mast cells and basophils, a C9-like amphipathic molecule, and the helminthotoxic eosinophil cationic protein. Eosinophils also release regulators of inflammatory mediators.

Histaminase inactivates histamine, while arylsulfatase A antagonizes the slow reactive substance of anaphylaxis (SRS-A) and leukotrienes C4, D4, and E4.

In summary, the innate immune system is composed of a network of cellular and humoral immune components that are able to respond to numerous microbial and cellular challenges. However, a constantly evolving infectious environment requires a more adaptable form of defense. This type of flexibility is provided by the adaptive immune system.

Adaptive Immunity

To generate effective responses to unique microbial challenges, the immune system developed the ability to recognize a large array of molecular shapes. Central to this recognition system are the antigen receptors of leukocytes: the cell surface–bound immunoglobulins of B cells and their soluble counterparts and the T-cell receptors.

Secreted Antibodies/Immunoglobulins

The monomeric antibody molecule (immunoglobulin, Ig) is a covalently linked complex of four polypeptide subunits: two smaller light chains and two larger heavy chains. Monomeric antibodies may be covalently linked to form dimeric or multimeric antibodies. The Ig molecule contains three major functional regions. The first is the antigen-binding site, the region with high interclonal variability that allows recognition of different antigens. An antigen-binding site is created from one heavy and one light chain; because of the presence of two identical heavy-light chain sets, each monomeric antibody has two identical antigen-binding sites for a specific epitope configuration. At the other end is the Fc region that binds to Fc receptors present on the surfaces of many leukocytes. This spatial arrangement gives immune cells an added form of antigen recognition through the use of antibodies as bridges or adaptors. Between these ends is a portion of the antibody that activates the classic complement pathway. Both Fc and complement-activating regions are functions of the heavy Ig chains. The antibody molecule is also separated into constant and variable regions. The antigen-binding site is contained within the variable region, while the complement-fixing and Fc portions are in the constant region.

There are five isotypes, or classes, of antibodies as defined by the structure of the constant region of the heavy chain: IgM, IgG, IgA, IgE, and IgD. Structural differences among heavy chain isotypes are limited to the constant regions where they influence the non-antigen-binding characteristics of antibodies. For example, secreted antibodies are not necessarily monomeric. IgM is released as a pentamer, and IgA may be secreted as a dimer. Functionally, only IgG crosses the placenta, while IgM is the most efficient activator of the classic complement pathway, and IgA is the major isotype found in mucosal secretions. As for the functions of antibodies as cellular bridges, mast cells and basophils have Fc receptors for IgE (Fcϵ) only, while neutrophils and macrophages express Fc receptors for IgG (Fcγ). Since the constant regions of the heavy and light chains are selected independently from the variable regions (more on this with the descriptions of generation of antibody diversity and isotype switching), antibodies that differ by isotype could have the same light and heavy chain variable regions and thus the same epitope specificity. As a result, different immunologic effector mechanisms could be mobilized to respond to the same antigen.

Heavy and light chain isotypes are coded for by distinct genetic loci, and these loci exist in different allelic forms within the population. These allotypes are relatively minor polymorphisms due to, at most, a few amino acid substitutions. In humans, allotypes have been found for the heavy chains γ, α, and ϵ, and the κ light chain. People may be allotypically heterozygous or homozygous; in heterozygous allotypes, the markers are expressed codominantly. Allotypic patterns have no significant effect on antibody function and are of interest primarily because of their immunogenicity in certain situations, such as blood transfusion and pregnancy. Additionally, patients with rheumatoid arthritis may produce rheumatoid factor or antibodies that recognize allotypic epitopes of IgG.

Idiotypic characteristics are determined by the variable regions of the antibody. The ability of an individual to produce specific immune responses to a large number of antigens requires an equally large number of antigen-binding sites. Therefore, idiotypic variations are quantitatively greater than isotype and allotype differences. Anti-idiotypic antibodies (antibodies that bind to the antigen-binding sites of other antibodies) have been useful reagents in characterizing the antigen-binding sites of immunoglobulins. Antiidiotype antibodies are also important in the regulation of the immune system, as they are normal constitutents in the pool of circulating antibodies.

B- and T-Cell Receptors

The B-cell antigen receptor is similar in structure to a secreted antibody (9). But there are important differences between secreted and membrane-bound Igs (sIg and mIg). Unlike sIgM and sIgA, mIg is monomeric. Also, an mIg has a hydrophobic transmembrane region that allows the antibody to sit on the membrane as a receptor. The production of sIg or mIg is determined by the differential splicing of the exon for the membrane-spanning region in the Ig transcript. The sIg molecule is coexpressed in association with a set of membrane-bound molecules that are involved in signal transduction.

The TCR is a heterodimer composed of disulfide-linked α and β chains (9, 10). The TCR is similar to the B-cell receptor in several respects. The amino-terminal antigen-binding regions of the TCRs are highly polymorphic, and an individual T cell expresses TCRs of only one antigenic specificity. Also, the TCR is associated with a set of nonpolymorphic accessory proteins, the CD3 complex, which is required for TCR expression and function. Aside from the $\alpha\beta$ isotype, there is also the $\gamma\delta$ TCR (11). These TCR isotypes differ in antigen specificity, MHC restriction, and appearance during ontogeny. T cells that express $\alpha\beta$ TCRs also differ in effector functions and anatomic locations from those with $\gamma\delta$ TCRs.

The most striking differences between Igs and TCRs are the nature of antigens they recognize. Receptors of both types bind to antigens via noncovalent molecular interactions: electrostatic, hydrogen bond, hydrophobic, and Van der Waals. While some Igs recognize linear sequences of amino acids within protein antigens, most immunoglobulins bind to native, as opposed to denatured or degraded, antigens. Thus, most antibodies recognize discontinuous or conformational molecular structures that are lost through denaturation. On the other hand, TCRs recognize linear epitopes, and quite unlike antibodies that bind ligands without the involvement of accessory molecules, TCRs only recognize antigen-derived peptide fragments in conjunction with MHC molecules on the surfaces of antigen-presenting cells.

Clonal Selection of Lymphocytes

Constituitive production of antibodies to every possible foreign antigen would be an inefficient use of resources. Instead, selected immune responses are generated in response to antigens via the activation and proliferation of lymphocyte clones that possess antigen receptors capable of recognizing these antigens. Antigens are responsible for the clonal selection of antigen-specific lymphocytes.

As described in more detail below, each B lymphocyte synthesizes antibodies with one antigen-binding specificity (12). The host is essentially a carrier of a large population of resting B-cell clones capable of responding to a wide range of immunogenic stimuli. Upon entering the host, a microbe encounters these B lymphocytes and activates those with the appropriate antigen-specific sIgs. A similar strategy is used in the clonal selection of antigen-specific T lymphocytes.

Affinity Maturation and Isotype Switching

During an antibody response, two properties of the secreted antibodies change (12, 13). First, the affinity, or strength of binding, of the antibodies to their antigens increases. Following B-cell activation and during their proliferation, the immunoglobulin genes undergo somatic hypermutation. Point mutations accumulate to alter the antigen specificity of the synthesized Igs. Concurrently, as antigens become limiting, B-cell clones with higher binding affinities for antigens are preferentially reactivated by antigens, compared with clones with lower affinities. Second, antibody isotypes switch from IgM to other isotypes (e.g., IgG, IgA, IgE) as directed by T-cell signals. This isotype switching increases the functional diversity of sIgs. IgE will bind to its respective Fc receptors on granulocytes, IgA is released into mucosal sites, and IgG passes through the placenta. Isotype switching is accomplished by alternate splicing of immunoglobulin primary RNA transcripts.

Classic Complement Pathway

Unlike the alternate pathway, the classic pathway is initiated by secreted antibodies (Fig. 45.2). C1q-binding sites within the constant regions of aggregated IgG or a single IgM are activated following antigen binding. As with the alternate pathway, opsonins are situated on the cell membrane to facilitate phagocytosis, chemotactic substances are released, and membrane attack complexes are formed.

Cell-Mediated Immunity

Many infectious microbes live within host cells, including immune cells, and thus are inaccessible for elimination by host humoral immune mechanisms. The inability of humoral immune components such as Ig and complement to neutralize intracellular parasites efficiently necessitates another strategy for their elimination. T lymphocytes are important in this respect because their antigen receptors can recognize foreign antigens present on the surfaces of host cells. For example, T helper (Th) cells of the type 1 variety (Th1) activated via the TCR-dependent recognition of infected cells release a variety of soluble signaling molecules, or cytokines (especially interferon-γ [IFN-γ]), into their immediate environment (1). These cytokines include those that are chemotactic for macrophages and activate their microbicidal processes. If macrophages themselves are the hosts of intracellular parasites, T cell–derived cytokines stimulate these phagocytes to kill their parasites.

Cytotoxic T cells (Tc) can kill infected cells directly (14). The mechanism of killing requires direct contact of Tc cells and their targets, recognition of target antigens by TCRs, and release of cytoplasmic granules in the vicinity of the target cell. The granular constitutents of Tc cells are similar to those of NK cells, and cytotoxicity is also accomplished by apoptosis and lysis (Fig. 45.1). Release of IFN-γ also aids in reducing the spread of virus particles to neighboring host cells.

Antibody/Cell Interactions

An effector mechanism exists that combines both humoral and cellular components, termed *antibody-dependent cell-mediated cytotoxicity* (ADCC). Unlike opsonization, in which immune cells recognize antigen-bound antibodies via their FcRs, ADCC denotes the "arming" of leukocytes with antibodies via Fc-FcR interactions. This facilitates leukocyte binding to antigen. Both macrophages and NK cells possess FcRs that can presumably link with antigen-specific IgG. Cellular contact with antigens expressed on the surface of an infected cell then results in phagocytosis and/or cytotoxic killing of the target cell.

Antibodies also enable granulocytes to recognize foreign antigens. FcRs for IgG and especially IgA are present on neutrophils. Of particular importance to those with immediate hypersensitivities are the Fcε receptors for IgE expressed by basophils and mast cells (15). IgE is the primary humoral mediator of anaphylaxis (16). The anaphylactic phenomenon is characterized by vasodilation and smooth muscle contraction and in its most severe form includes bronchiole/bronchi constriction and hypotension. Atopic people are prone to produce IgE to a variety of noninfectious xenobiotics (e.g., foods, pollen, drugs), which then arm circulating basophils and tissue mast cells via Fcε receptors. Contacts with these allergens result in the cross-linking of Fcε receptors by IgE and antigens, release of inflammatory mediators, and allergic responses such as anaphylaxis, asthma, gastrointestinal responses, and dermatitis.

Immunologic Memory

Immunologic memory distinguishes the adaptive immune system from innate immunity. This memory (enhanced secondary response) is evidenced by the protective effects of vaccination and the improbability of recurrence of certain diseases (e.g., measles) in normal individuals. The enhanced secondary response is based on the clonal expansion of lymphocytes by antigen and the subsequent generation of memory cells (17). When an individual first comes in contact with an immunogen (e.g., tetanus toxoid, inactivated virus), a primary immune response is initiated in which specific antibodies appear in several days to clear the foreign material. A second contact, even some time later, results in a reaction that is quantitatively and qualitatively different. Among other things, this secondary response is characterized by a shorter lag time, and a much higher concentration of antigen-specific immunoglobulin in the circulation is ultimately reached. Clonal selection of immunogen-specific lymphocytes occurs during the primary response, and this enlarged population of cells is responsible for the stronger second reaction. Memory of a specific immunogenic stimulus may be long-lived, on the order of years if not decades. Two hypotheses have been forwarded to define the means by which immunologic memory is retained: *(a)* long-lived memory cells are preserved in a dormant state until reactivated by antigen or *(b)* the antigen responsible for immunologic memory persists for the duration of the memory response, and/or restimulation is induced by subclinical infections or by cross-reactive antigens. The last stimulus set refers to close mimics of the original immunogen, which may not be able to activate naive or previously unstimulated cells but can reactivate these clones following prior stimulation with the original immunogen.

Phenotypic and functional differences readily distinguish memory from naive lymphocytes. In general, memory T and B lymphocytes are more easily stimulated by succeeding contact with antigens, principally through antigen receptors with higher affinity for the antigen. Among B cells, this is due to somatic hypermutation of antigen-receptor genes; an isotype switch (e.g., from mIgM to mIgG) is also considered a marker of memory B cells. For T cells, TCR affinity changes are probably due to a form of clonal selection for T-cell clones that bind the antigen efficiently. There are also changes in the expression of various T-cell surface markers, such as an increase in the relative density of adhesion molecules. Also, there is a change in the isoform of the leukocyte common antigen, CD45. Naive T cells are defined by the presence of CD45RA, while memory cells express the lower-molecular-weight CD45RO. Although these changes in surface molecules suggest an activated status and support the notion that memory cells are in a constant state of activity, there is the possibility that in the absence of antigenic stimulation, $CD45RO^+$ cells may revert to the CD45RA phenotype and join a resting pool of memory cells.

Inflammation

Inflammation is a complex and coordinated response by the host to eliminate foreign materials and enact tissue repair. It encompasses aspects of both innate and adaptive immunity and has traditionally been described as a progression from acute to chronic stages followed by healing and reconstruction. Chronic inflammation also accompanies a large number of pathologic states such as autoimmune diseases and allergies, although their etiologies are for the most part unclear. What is certain is that in these cases, inflammatory reactions become destructive to the host.

The overall function of the inflammatory response is to bring humoral and cellular defense and repair components to the area of injury. Following tissue injury, inflammation is initiated by release of soluble mediators from tissue mast cells and vascular cells. These signals contribute to an initial vasoconstriction of several seconds followed by dilation of precapillary arterioles. The observed redness is due to increased blood flow to the site. There is also an associated increase in the permeability of postcapillary venules because of retraction of endothelial cells and formation of intercellular gaps. This leads to leakage of plasma into the interstitial space and resultant swelling and edema. The combined directed channeling of blood and fluid leakage results in a decreased blood flow and accumulation of blood cells at the affected site. This facilitates adherence of leukocytes (particularly neutrophils and macrophages) to the vascular walls and their migration into the interstitial space. Thus, the classic symptoms of inflammation are localized redness or erythema, warmth, and swelling.

In addition to the phagocytes and granulocytes already mentioned, two other cell types are important in inflammation: endothelial cells and platelets. Endothelial cells (ECs) provide the boundary between the intra- and extravascular spaces and, under normal conditions, provide a nonsticky, impermeable conduit for the passage of blood components. ECs also contribute to the regulation of vascular tone via the release of vasodilators (prostaglandin I_2, adenosine, nitric oxide) and vasoconstrictors (endothelin). Disruption of EC function or integrity leads to alterations in mediator release, exposure of the basement membrane, eventual aggregation of platelets and leukocytes, and changes in blood flow patterns. Activation of ECs increases their surface expression of adhesion molecules that bind to counterparts on leukocytes and aids in the localized accumulation of inflammatory cells. Once this initial localization of leukocytes is accomplished, chemotactic factors guide the migration of leukocytes closer to the affected area.

Platelets provide several functions in the inflammatory reaction. In conjunction with the coagulation cascade, platelet aggregation forms plugs at sites of vessel damage. Platelet aggregation is promoted by contact with the extracellular matrix following vascular injury, as well as exposure to adenosine diphosphate (ADP), thromboxane A_2, or the coagulation cascade. Coagulation, in return, can be activated by the aggregation of platelets, the surfaces of ECs and monocytes, and various tissue-derived factors. These processes result in construction of a fibrin and platelet network that inhibits the outflow of blood from injured vessels. Aggregated platelets also release a number of primarily proinflammatory cytokines (eicosanoids, proteases, and ADP) that regulate the activities of ECs and leukocytes. In addition, platelet-derived growth factors are important in mobilizing fibroblasts and smooth muscle cells toward wound healing and scar formation.

The noncellular plasma components that infiltrate the inflammatory site include the immunoglobulins, complement, and acute-phase proteins discussed above. In addition, molecules of the "contact-activation system" function to generate bradykinin and activate the coagulation cascade. The proinflammatory consequences of bradykinin include increased vascular permeability, smooth muscle contraction, and with prostaglandins, induction of soluble mediator–induced pain. This system integrates with platelets and other cells and coagulation and inflammatory mediators to produce the fibrin thrombus.

Many pro- and antiinflammatory soluble factors are associated with the metabolism of arachidonic acid (AA) (18). Incidentally, these 20-carbon oxygenation products of AA, the "eicosanoids," may form only a fraction of existing "oxylipins," or signaling molecules, that can be derived from oxygenated polyunsaturated fatty acids (PUFAs); AA is one of many known PUFAs. (See Chapter 4 for AA metabolism and eicosanoid function.) The three classes of enzymes that use AA as a substrate for formation of eicosanoids are the cyclooxygenases (prostaglandins [PGs]), the lipoxygenases (leukotrienes [LTs], lipoxins [LXs], hydroxyeicosatetraenoic acids [HETEs]), and the epoxygenases (epoxyeicosatrienoic acids). There are two forms of cyclooxygenase (COX): COX1 is constitutively active, while COX2 is an inducible enzyme. Cyclooxygenase can catalyze two distinct reactions: the cyclization of AA and the hydroperoxidation of the cyclopentane ring, forming short-lived lipid hydroperoxide intermediates. Lipid hydroperoxides and hydroperoxyeicosatetraenoic acids (HPETEs) are the precursors of the various PGs and TXs and the array of LTs and LXs, respectively.

Platelet-activating factor (PAF), a term for a group of bioactive molecules that share the structure 1-*O*-alkyl-2-acyl-*sn*-glycero-3-phosphocholine, is produced by a large number of cells including phagocytes, granulocytes, and platelets, as well as endothelial and epithelial cells.

Histamine is an inflammatory mediator that composes up to 10% of the granule contents of basophils and mast cells. The consequences of histamine release are due to its binding to tissue histamine receptors.

Lymphocyte Development

As mentioned above, all leukocytes develop from a unique, self-renewing, pluripotential hematopoietic stem cell (19). From this cell type, different developmental signals and tissue microenvironments give rise to the known white blood cells.

T (thymus-ependent) lymphocytes develop from self-renewing progenitors that migrate from the bone marrow to become situated in the thymus (20, 21). Maturation of thymocytes is manifested by changes in the expression of cell surface molecules and the locations of these cells within the thymus. The surface markers most commonly used in staging the thymocytes are CD3, CD4, and CD8. The progenitors are initially $CD3^-CD4^-CD8^-$. In the thymic cortex, prothymocytes rearrange their TCR genes and express TCR and CD3. $\gamma\delta$ TCR^+ cells tend to remain $CD4^-CD8^-$ (doubly negative) while $\alpha\beta$ TCR^+ cells convert to a $CD4^+CD8^+$ (doubly positive) phenotype. Clonal selection through TCR binding with MHC results in positive selection of clones that are capable of MHC-restricted interactions. Doubly positive $\alpha\beta$ TCR^+ cells then develop into $CD4^-CD8^+$ or $CD4^+CD8^-$ (singly positive) cells. These thymocytes migrate to the thymic medulla where negative selection occurs. At this junction, clones that can recognize self-antigen–MHC complexes are eliminated to minimize the potential for autoreactivity. These mature cells are then released into the peripheral circulation. More than 90% of thymocytes initially produced are eliminated through the positive and negative selection processes, primarily by apoptosis (22).

Since the mammalian thymus begins to involute during puberty, there is much interest in the status of T-cell development in postpubertal years. Studies suggest that with age, T-cell development shifts to other tissues, in particular, the intestines (23, 24). These age-dependent changes in T-cell development are possibly related to increased susceptibility to various immunopathologic states. For example, the onset of most forms of autoimmune diseases occurs during or after puberty (25). Also, graft-versus-host disease is more frequent in adults than in children, which suggests that following bone marrow transplantation, the absence of a thymus in the adult results in abnormal redevelopment of the immune system.

Unlike the T cell, mammalian B cells are produced primarily in the bone marrow. Although the fetal liver is a source of B cells early in life, B-cell production eventually shifts to the bone marrow. As with T-cell development, the stages of B-cell lineage are noted by the rearrangement and expression of antibody genes, as well as by other cell surface markers. An interesting surface marker that distinguishes two separate B-cell lineages is CD5. As with $\alpha\beta$ and $\gamma\delta$ TCR^+ T cells, $CD5^+$ (B1) and $CD5^-$ (B2) B lymphocytes are separable by phenotype, appearance in ontogeny, distribution, and antigen specificity. Indeed, there is the notion of the existence of a two-layered immune system composed of evolutionarily older B1 cells and $\gamma\delta$ TCR^+ T cells and the more recently evolved B2 cells and $\alpha\beta$ TCR^+ T cells (26).

Generation of antibody diversity begins with the random combination of V, D, H, and J constant-region immunoglobulin genes. In a developing B cell, an immunoglobulin heavy-chain variable (V) region gene (of which there are hundreds) recombines with one diversity (D) region and one joining (J) region by excision of intervening genomic DNA. In addition, the terminal deoxyribonucleotidyl transferase enzyme inserts random nucleotides at these junctions prior to splicing. Diversity is increased through V-region exchange and transcription of D regions from one of three different reading frames. At the protein level, functional variation at the antigen-binding site is further enhanced by random combination of heavy and light chains. Finally, as mentioned above, somatic hypermutation in rapidly dividing B cells creates genetic variation. Except for the inability of T cells to undergo somatic hypermutation, these concepts apply to the TCR. The inhibition of T-cell, but not B-cell, somatic hypermutation is rationalized as the need to limit the random appearance of autoreactive T cells that could promote undesirable autoimmune reactions.

Cellular Interactions in Adaptive Immune Responses

Secondary Lymphoid Tissues

The adaptive immune response is generated from a network of cellular and subcellular components that are called into play following host contact with foreign material. These processes occur in specialized lymphoid tissues that provide the necessary environment for full expression of an adaptive response. In contrast, innate and inflammatory responses can be initiated and maintained in potentially any site in the body. The separation of primary and secondary lymphoid tissues is based on function. The bone marrow and thymus are the primary lymphoid tissues responsible for leukocyte production, whereas secondary sites (e.g., lymph nodes, spleen, mucosal tissues) generate adaptive immune responses.

The lymphatic and circulatory systems facilitate translocation of leukocytes and immunoactive molecules and the immunologic protection of tissues distant from the actual site of immunogen contact. There are numerous examples of this process: activated immune cells migrate from the gut to the lungs; following contact with microbial antigens, macrophage-like cells of the skin migrate to lymphatic tissues to initiate an antimicrobial response; systemic infections result in the trapping of microbes as they pass through the filtering activity of lymphoid tissues.

In lymph nodes, activity is noted by the appearance of lymphoid follicles—aggregations of lymphocytes and supporting follicular dendritic cells. Primary follicles contain mature resting B cells, suggesting a minimum of immune activity. Following an immunogenic challenge, a secondary follicle containing a germinal center of rapidly proliferating B cells is formed. T lymphocytes and antigen-presenting cells are found in the paracortex, an adjacent region downstream of the follicles. Lymph node swelling or lymphadenopathy indicates increased lymph node activity following immune stimulation.

The spleen is the major lymphoid tissue that filters the blood. Blood enters the spleen via the splenic artery and branches into finer arterioles, whereupon it contacts T cells, B cell–containing lymphoid follicles, and a spongy network of reticular cells and macrophages. Approximately half of the total blood volume passes through the spleen daily, where it is monitored for infectious agents and damaged red and white blood cells.

The mucosa is an ideal entry point for infectious microbes since it provides sites for transfer of materials between the internal and external environments. Lymphoid tissues lining mucosal regions are collectively termed the *mucosa-associated lymphoid tissues* (MALT) (27, 28). Unlike their systemic counterparts (e.g., spleen), these mucosal lymphoid regions are somewhat distinct in their lack of well-defined tissues. Instead, the mucosal epithelia of the lungs and gut are lined primarily by diffused masses of lymphocytes and phagocytes, with occasional lymphoid follicles. More-organized structures, such as the tonsils of the upper respiratory tract and the Peyer's patches of the gut, are constituents of the MALT. However, these structures are not composed of distinct capsules nor vessels, as are lymph nodes and spleens. The MALT also differs from the systemic immune system in the preferential formation of IgA and IgE, as well as the limited circulation of mucosa-derived lymphocytes to mucosal regions.

Antigen Processing and Presentation

Antigens must be processed and presented by antigen-presenting cells (APCs) to facilitate their recognition by lymphocytes (29). There are several such APCs, which differ in antigen-processing characteristics, anatomic location, the types of lymphocytes they interact with, and the stages of the immune response at which they are employed. There are two characteristics common to the process of antigen presentation. First, T cells recognize antigens in the form of 9- to 25–amino acid stretches of linear short peptides. Second, these peptides must be complexed to MHC molecules on the APC surface.

Major Histocompatibility Complex. The MHC is a set of genes whose extreme polymorphism accounts for much of the immunogenetic difference between individuals of the same species as well as problems associated with tissue allograft rejection. However, they are indispensable for generation of antigen-specific immune responses. Indeed, the survival of populations or species facing constantly evolving infectious challenges has been attributed to this polymorphism (30). The human MHC is termed the *human leukocyte antigen (HLA) system.* Other vertebrate species have genes analogous to the human MHC; for example, the murine counterpart is designated the H-2 system.

There are three major classes of MHC molecules encoded by the HLA genes: MHC-class I, II, and III. The cell-surface histocompatibility molecules are found in the class I and II loci, whereas class III codes for complement and other soluble proteins. Both MHC class I and II molecules are transmembrane heterodimers that contain structural domains formed by disulfide bridging. Similar domains are found in other molecules, and thus the MHC is included in the "immunoglobulin gene superfamily." However, there are very clear differences in the structure and function of these two classes of MHC molecules. These differences translate into interactions between class II molecules with $CD4^+$ "helper/inducer" T cells, and class I molecules with $CD8^+$ "cytotoxic/suppressor" T cells. MHC class I antigens are found on most, if not all, somatic nucleated cells, have recognition sites for CD8, and present endogenously processed (e.g., peptide products of viral proteins expressed by the host's cells) antigens. Thus, $CD8^+$ T cells are considered MHC class I restricted, and their immune responses constitute major defenses against virus-infected and tumor cells. MHC class II antigens are expressed by a more limited range of cell types; they are found primarily on macrophages, B and T lymphocytes, dendritic cells, and ECs. The density of the MHC class II molecules increases following cell stimulation. Class II^+ APCs activate $CD4^+$ T cells (class II restriction) and present exogenous antigens (e.g., phagocytosed bacteria). Class II-restricted responses promote antibacterial immunity and immunity to other exogenous protein antigens. These interactions involve the $\alpha\beta$ TCR. Other "nonclassic" MHC forms are less polymorphic and appear to activate T cells with the $\gamma\delta$ TCR (11).

Antigen-Presenting Cells. Since virtually all cells express MHC class I molecules, most cells can present endogenous antigens to $CD8^+$ T cells. Specialization among class II–restricted APCs implies a need to direct immune responses to exogenous antigens and not self antigens. Among APCs, macrophages historically received the most attention. The phagocytic activity of this ubiquitous scavenger cell is found among blood monocytes, liver Kupffer cells, brain glia, and macrophages in systemic and mucosal lymphoid tissues. Macrophages are especially important in generating primary immune responses, as their relatively non-antigen-specific phagocytic activity allows the processing and presentation of many types of exogenous antigens. Similarly, dendritic cells such as skin Langerhans' cells and blood dendritic cells are important APCs in the initiation of a primary response. B cells, on the other hand, are important APCs in secondary immune responses. Following a primary response, expanded populations of antigen-specific B cells capture and endocytose antigens via their sIg. These antigens are then processed and presented. Antigen uptake in the gut is accomplished by M cells, which are specialized transport cells with no MHC class II expression. These cells are interspersed among the gut epithelial cells and pass antigens to the underlying macrophage and dendritic APCs (31).

Adhesion and Accessory Molecules. There is a constantly growing list of receptor-ligand interactions that involve cell surface molecules known collectively as adhesion molecules (32, 33). Relevant interactions include those involving MHC, CD4, CD8, and surface-antigen receptors. Adhesion molecules bind cells together to mediate a number of different activities, including cell killing, phagocytosis, signal transmission, and cell migration. The expression of adhesion molecules often depends on the activation state of the cell and its microenvironment. For example, the density of lymphocyte function-associated antigen–1 (LFA-1) on T cells increases following contact with macrophages (Table 45.1).

Table 45.1
Selected Adhesion Molecules[a,b]

Family/Species	Distribution	Target Cell/Ligand Distribution
Immunoglobulin superfamily		
CD2	NK cells, T cells	LFA-3 (CD58)
CD4	T cell subset	MHC class II
CD8	T cell subset	MHC class I
CD28	T cells	B7
ICAM-1	EC, lymphocytes	LFA-1, Mac-1
ICAM-2	EC, lymphocytes	LFA-1
VCAM-1	EC, macrophages	VLA-4
Integrins		
VLA-4 (a4b1)	Eosinophils, lymphocytes	FN, VCAM-1
LFA-1 (CD11a/CD18)	PMNs, lymphocytes	ICAM-1, ICAM-2
Mac-1 (CD11b/CD18)	PMNs	ICAM-1, iC3b
gp 150,95	Myeloid cells	iC3b
Selectins		
E-Selectin (ELAM-1)	EC	Sialyl Lewis^x, others
L-Selectin (LAM-1)	Lymphocytes, PMNs	CD34, GlyCAM-1
P-Selectin	EC, platelets	Sialyl Lewis^x, PSGL-1

[a]( ) indicate alternate designations.
[b]EC, endothelial cells; FN, fibronectin; PSGL-1, P-selectin glycoprotein ligand.

Cell-surface accessory molecules also direct T-cell activation during antigen presentation (34). During generation of a primary immune response, the activation of T cells requires costimulatory signals in addition to that derived from the TCR-MHC binding. This costimulation is provided by the ligation of the T-cell CD28 molecule and the APCs B7 molecule. Interaction of the TCR with its cognate peptide–MHC molecule in the absence of CD28/B7 interaction renders the T cell anergic and unresponsive to further stimulatory signals. However, unlike a requirement for costimulation by resting T cells, T cells previously activated by antigens do not need costimulatory signals to be reactivated.

Cytokines. Cytokines are protein molecules, most of which have pleiotropic effects. They are produced by virtually all nucleated cells and include lymphocyte-derived lymphokines, monocyte-derived monokines, hematopoietic colony-stimulating factors, and connective tissue growth factors (35). Individual cytokine species may be secreted by more than one cell type, and the functional activity of a cytokine is mediated by typical ligand/receptor binding events. These factors differ from hormones in that they operate at short distances within tissues for paracrine and/or autocrine communication. Generally, cytokines are induced by infectious challenge or other stressors and are not constitutively released. The understanding of cytokine networks is complicated by their numerous cellular sources, their pleiotropic effects, synergisms and antagonisms engendered by cytokine mixtures, and their ability to alter the production of other cytokines and their receptors. This communication network is an important aspect of immune system regulation. Information on the major cytokines is summarized in Table 45.2.

Regulating the Immune System

Since the function of the immune response is the elimination of foreign parasites and abnormal host cells, regulatory mechanisms are needed to minimize destruction of normal host cells. These devices, most of which are not well understood because of the complexity of their interactions, are crucial to the maintenance of human health. Indeed, problems in immune regulation result in chronic autoimmune, allergic, and other inflammatory conditions.

Clonal Deletion and Anergy

T cells can be deleted (i.e., certain lymphocyte clones are physically eliminated) or anergized (i.e., clones are insensitive to stimulation, although they may still be present) (34). Several factors contribute to the selection of T cells for deletion or anergy, including the stage of development or activation; differences in the type of APCs, cytokines, and other signals; the affinity of TCR-antigen-MHC binding; and the presence of costimulatory signals. Costimulatory signals, exclusive of TCR-MHC interactions, include cytokines and other receptor-ligand interactions. Without such associated signals, TCR-MHC interactions tend to result in T-cell anergy rather than activation. The principles governing B-cell tolerance are similar to those of T cells, such as antigen-binding affinity and the developmental state of the B cell.

$CD8^+$ T Cytotoxic/Suppressor Cells

Mature $CD4^-CD8^+$, $\alpha\beta$ TCR^+ T cells are generally MHC class I restricted and traditionally fall into two major categories. Cytotoxic (Tc) $CD8^+$ T cells, which are well-described, are important in the killing of virus-infected and tumor cells. Suppressor T (Ts) $CD8^+$ cells, although less well characterized, are thought to inhibit the activation phase of immune responses (36–38).

Cytokines and Eicosanoids

Cytokines as promoters of cell growth and differentiation were described above. Cytokines may also inhibit immune responses or concurrently activate one immune component while downregulating another. For example, transforming growth factor–β (TGF-β) is produced by many hematopoietic cell types, including Ts cells, and is involved in embryonic development, tumorigenesis, inflammation, and immunoregulation. The functions of TGF-β include inhibition of T-cell proliferation and the cytotoxic activity of Tc and NK cells.

Distinctions between the cytokine-release profiles of type 1 and type 2 T helper (Th1, Th2) cells are noteworthy (39). Although these Th cells cannot be distinguished phenotypically (they are both $CD4^+CD8^-$), they are separable by cytokine production. Th1 cells release IFN-γ and induce cell-mediated immune responses. Th2 cells typically produce IL-4, IL-5, IL-6, and IL-10 and are primarily involved in stimulating antibody production. These cell types and the immune networks they promote can be mutually antagonistic. For example, IFN-γ blocks the growth of Th2 cells, while IL-4 inhibits some of the functions of macrophages activated by IFN-γ. In addition, $CD5^+$ B-1 cells release IL-10 and are activated by IL-5 (40). Another example of selective inhibitory function is shown by prostaglandin E_2 (PGE_2). Studies on Th1 and Th2 cells demonstrate the ability of PGE_2 to arrest the function of Th1, but not Th2, cells (41, 42).

Antibody Feedback

Antibodies can provide negative feedback to limit antibody responses. By eliminating or neutralizing immunogens that stimulate the immune system, antigen-specific antibodies contribute to limiting the extent of the immune response.

Of particular interest to researchers studying the relationships between immune networks and ontogeny are natural autoantibodies (NAs), their ligands, and the cells that produce NAs (43). NAs, their ligands, and NA-producing $CD5^+$ B-1 cells are thought to represent a phy-

Table 45.2
Cytokines

Name	Primary Sources	Primary Targets	Functions
Interleukin-1	Monocytes, macrophages	Leukocytes, hepatocytes, endothelial cells	Promotes: inflammation, fever, arachidonic acid metabolism, lymphocyte maturation and proliferation, colony-stimulating factor production Inhibits: vascular smooth muscle contraction
Interleukin-2	Th1 cells	B and T cells, NK cells, monocytes, macrophages	Promotes: growth and differentiation of target cells
Interleukin-3	Th1 and Th2 cells, mast cells	Myeloid and lymphoid lineage cells	Promotes: activation and differentiation of pluripotent hematopoietic stem cells, monocytes/macrophages, PMNs, eosinophils, basophils, mast cells, megakaryocytes, erythroid cells
Interleukin-4	Th2 cells	B cells, Th2 cells	Promotes: maturation of pre–B cells, differentiation of mature IgM^+ B cells to IgG1 and IgE producers, Th2 cell activity
Interleukin-5	Th2 cells	B cells, eosinophils	Promotes: proliferation of IgM^+ and IgG^+ B cells, differentiation of B lymphocytes to IgA production, eosinophil proliferation and activation
Interleukin-6	Th2 cells, monocytes, fibroblasts	Many leukocyte types, hepatocytes	Promotes: B- and T-cell growth and differentiation, growth of plasmacytomas and hepatocytes, acute-phase protein release, anterior pituitary hormone release Inhibits: growth of breast carcinoma and myeloleukemic cell lines
Interleukin-7	Bone marrow stroma	B and T cells, NK cells, monocytes	Promotes: proliferation of immature B-lineage cells, $CD4^-CD8^-$T cells, and mature NK cells; monocytes activation
Interleukin-8	Leukocytes, smooth muscle cells, epithelial cells, etc.	Neutrophils	Promotes: chemotaxis and activation of neutrophils
Interleukin-9	T helper cells	B and T cells, mast cells, erythroid cells	Promotes: mast cell and T cell proliferation, IgG1 and IgE release by B cells, erythropoiesis
Interleukin-10	Th2 cells	B and T cells, NK cells, macrophages, mast cells	Promotes: B cell proliferation and antibody production, mast cell proliferation Inhibits: macrophage activity; NK, Th1 and $CD8^+$ T-cell cytokine production; DTH, TNF-α effects
Interleukin-12	Macrophages, B cells	Th1 cells, Nk cells	Promotes: Th1 growth, NK cytolytic activity
Interleukin-13	Th2 cells	Monocytes, B cells	Promotes: IgE production by B cells Inhibits: inflammatory cytokine release by macrophages
Interleukin-14	B and T cells	B-lineage cells	Promotes: ?; IL-14 receptors found on B-lineage leukemic cells
Interleukin-15	Monocytes, epithelial cells	T cells	Promotes: T cell activity
Tumor necrosis factor-α	Monocytes, macrophages others	Many cell types	Promotes: fever, anorexia, acute-phase protein synthesis, cachexia, production of inflammatory cytokines (IL-1, IL-6, IL-8, IFN-γ), apoptosis of tumor cells
Tumor necrosis factor-β (Lymphotoxin-a)	B and T cells, NK cells, LAK cells	Many cell types	Promotes: apoptosis of tumor cells
Transforming growth factor-β	B and T cells, macrophages	Many cell types	Promotes: antiinflammatory effect, tumor development Inhibits: TNF-α effects, lymphocyte proliferation, cytotoxicity (T, NK, and LAK cells), respiratory burst by phagocytes
Type I interferon (α,ω,β)	Many cell types	Many cell types	Inhibits: viral replication, cell replication
Type II interferon (γ)	Th1 cells, $CD8^+$ cytotoxic T cells, NK cells	Macrophages, T and B cells	Promotes: TNF-α effects, macrophage activation, cytotoxic T cells and NK cells, IgG2a production by B cells Inhibits: Th2 cells

Table 45.2—*Continued*
Cytokines

Name	Primary Sources	Primary Targets	Functions
Granulocyte-macrophage colony-stimulating factor	T cells, macrophages endothelial cells, fibroblasts	Myeloid hematopoietic cells	Promotes: development of granulocytes and macrophages, macrophage activation; overproduction may promote leukemic states
Granulocyte colony-stimulating factor	Macrophages, endothelial cells, fibroblasts	Neutrophils	Promotes: neutrophil development
Macrophage colony-stimulating factor factor (CSF-1)	Epithelial cells, fibroblasts, bone marrow stromal cells	Macrophages	Promotes: macrophage differentiation and proliferation
CC Chemokines	B and T cells, monocytes, others	Monocytes, granulocytes, others	Promotes: chemotaxis (monocytes, T cells, eosinophils), activation (monocytes, basophils)

logenetically ancient immune recognition system (26). Although the function of NAs is controversial, they may be important in clearing cellular debris from the circulation. Their unusually broad antigen specificity could provide a constitutive immune defense against infectious agents, probably through recognition of common or ubiquitous antigenic structures. NAs may also be important for self-nonself discrimination and the generation of self-tolerance by the immune system.

Laboratory Tests of Immune Function

A large number of immunologic tests are routinely available to assess the immunologic status of any individual's immune system. This section summarizes representative assays.

Antibodies and Antigens

Enzyme-linked immunosorbent assays, or ELISAs, constitute one of the most commonly used techniques in immunology. There is often a need to quantify the levels of circulating antibodies and their antigen specificity and isotype. This assay is based on the binding of plasma/serum antibodies with defined antigens on a solid phase (typically plastic or glass) and the commercial availability of antibodies linked to reporter molecules.

Immunoblotting is a useful technique for detection of antibodies to relatively ill-defined antigens, such as antigens from a tissue homogenate. After separation by gel electrophoresis, antigens are transfered to a matrix (blotting strips) and incubated with patient sera. Antigen-specific antibodies can then be detected by a color reaction. The location and intensity of the color change provide information on the relative amounts of antibody and the molecular mass of its ligand.

Enumerating Antigen-Specific B Cells

The ELISPOT is used to quantify the number of antigen-specific B cells in a fashion similar to the ELISA. In this case, B cells are added to the wells of ELISA plates previously coated with a particular antigen; these B cells are then nonspecifically activated to produce antibodies. B cells that recognize the antigen will then bind to the solid phase and can be detected by a subsequent color reaction. These cells show as visible spots, representing individual antibody-producing B cells, which can be counted.

Leukocyte Function

The extent of proliferation following exposure to activation signals is frequently used as a general measure of lymphocyte health. Briefly, a predetermined number of purified lymphocytes in a cell culture medium are stimulated by mitogens or agents that activate cells in an antigen-nonspecific (non-sIg and -TCR) fashion. After a short period of culture (approximately 3 days), the cells are pulsed with ^{3}H-thymidine, which is incorporated into the newly synthesized DNA of the proliferating cells and detected by scintillation counting.

Proliferation is also induced by mixing leukocytes from genetically different sources. This form of activation is induced by TCR-MHC interactions and is thus antigen (MHC) specific. This test is used as one functional measure of MHC differences (histocompatibility) between individuals and is considered an in vitro counterpart to tissue mixing (e.g., tissue grafts, bone marrow transplants).

Cytotoxicity Assays

Cytotoxicity assays are used to determine the killing activity of cytotoxic cells, such as Tc and NK cells. Traditionally, tumor cell lines provide the sources of genetically consistent indicator or "target" cells used to measure NK cell function. Target cells are loaded with ^{51}Cr and incubated with their appropriate effector lymphocytes; release of this radiolabel is then used as a measure of target cell killing. More-recent innovations include the use of fluorescent, rather than radioactive, markers. DNA fragmentation (apoptosis) is also used as an endpoint.

Hypersensitivity Skin Tests

Hypersensitivity to exogenous antigens or allergens is a common problem in humans. The strategy of avoiding contact with allergens to minimize the frequency or intensity of allergic reactions first requires identification of these environmental agents. Skin tests are often used in this regard. Basically, samples of allergens are injected subcutaneously and a measure of reactivity is based on the size of the inflammatory skin reaction. Immediate hypersensitivities mediated by IgE (e.g., pollen extract) become evident in minutes. Delayed-type hypersensitivity (DTH) reactions (e.g., tuberculin test), which are due to T-cell recruitment of phagocytes to the injection site, require 24 to 48 hours.

Identification and Quantification of Leukocyte Subpopulations

Flow cytometry is the most reliable way to determine the frequencies of different leukocyte types in a sample. Flow cytometers use a hydraulic system to pass a single-cell suspension before a laser source. Information, in the form of light scatter and fluorescence, is collected to measure a variety of cell characteristics that serve to identify leukocytes as lymphocytes, macrophages, etc. The flexibility of the flow cytometer is greatly enhanced by the use of monoclonal antibodies that recognize specific cellular markers. These antibodies, which bind to specific cell-surface epitopes, are conjugated to fluoresceinated materials that, when excited by the laser, serve to identify cell types (e.g., $CD4^+$ vs. $CD8^+$ T cells). Flow cytometry is also used to measure other cellular parameters such as membrane fluidity, DNA content, and intracellular Ca^{2+}.

Cytokine Assays

Cytokines released by cells in vitro or present in plasma may be measurable by ELISA. However, because cytokines such as the interleukins tend to operate at very short intercellular distances, have very short half-lives, and/or are produced in minute quantities, ELISA detection may be impractical. Alternatively, Northern blot analysis or the polymerase chain reaction may be used to measure the levels of cytokine mRNA in cells, or intracellular cytokines may be detected by fluorescent anticytokine antibodies and quantified by flow cytometry.

EFFECTS OF NUTRITION ON IMMUNE RESPONSES

A survey of the literature shows that most nutritional deficits lead to suppressed immune responses. This is not surprising, since anabolic and catabolic pathways in the immune system require the same sort of building blocks and energy sources as other physiologic activities. Lipids seem to diverge from this generalization in that excess fatty acids and certain shifts in the balance of lipid species also lead to immunosuppressed states. Caloric restriction is another area of emerging interest, with important implications for human health. In general, moderate caloric restriction appears to have beneficial effects on longevity and disease resistance. However, these trends and generalizations must be approached with some care. Dietary manipulation can have selective effects on one portion of the immune system and not others. Also, factors such as ongoing chronic infections, gender, and age add more complexity to the study of immunonutrition.

Protein-Calorie Malnutrition

Protein-calorie malnutrition (PCM) is a major cause of immunodeficiency. Kwashiorkor (protein deficiency) and marasmus (generalized undernutrition or starvation) are the two clinical manifestations of PCM. Consequently, the immunologic manifestations of PCM are broad and include lymphoid tissue atrophy, decreases in lymphocyte numbers, and abnormally low cellular and humoral immune responses. As a result, PCM is associated with a high incidence of morbidity and mortality from infections (44, 45). Deficits in protein and energy may be accompanied by other nutrient deficits. The following sections focus on the better-defined forms of nutritional deficits.

Caloric Intake

Unlike the immunodeficiencies observed in severe PCM, moderate deprivation is associated with increased T-cell functions (46–48). Palmblad (49) showed that short-term starvation lowered T-cell responses to mitogens and reduced the levels of acute-phase reactants but had little effect on circulating leukocyte numbers or resistance to infection. In experimentally induced dietary fasts in mice, the ability of T cells to proliferate in vitro increased (50), while food restriction inhibited the progression of disease in a mouse model of systemic lupus erythematosus (51). These observations are of interest within the context of life span extension, improved immune function, and caloric restriction (Table 45.3).

The balance of energy intake relative to expenditure partially determines body weight and composition, which in turn influence immune characteristics. Indeed, leanness is associated with tumor and infection resistance. The diets of anorexics (anorexia and bulimia nervosa) are low in energy but may contain sufficient protein, vitamins, and minerals. Bowers and Eckert (52) reported that although patients with anorexia nervosa were leukopenic, they did not appear to be more susceptible to infectious disease than control subjects. Increased immunocompetence during mild anorexia was observed by Pertschuk et al. (53). Immunocompetence decreased when body weight dropped below 60% of ideal body weight.

Patients with bulimia nervosa consume large quantities of food, followed by fasting, vomiting, or laxative use. Generally, they are not severely emaciated and are considered in relatively good physical health. A study of bulimics by Marcos et al. (54) reported a 40% incidence of

Table 45.3
Moderate Food or Caloric Restriction and the Immune System

Effects of food restriction	
Mice:	Increases T-cell proliferative responses
	Inhibits progression of systemic lupus erythematosus
Humans:	Decreases immunocompetence when body weight drops below 60% of ideal weight
	Decreases CD4+ T cells, but not CD8+ T cells
	Increases frequency of circulating B cells
	Normal to enhanced plasma antibodies
	Decreases plasma complement
	Following weight reduction in obese people, increases mitogenic responses by peripheral blood leukocytes
Effects of caloric restriction	
Mice:	Inhibits immune-mediated diseases, tumor virus expression, and malignancies
	Decreases the proliferative ability of autoreactive B1 cells
	Decreases inflammatory cytokines Il-6 and TNF-α
	Decreases immunosuppressive cytokine TGF-β
	Increases T-cell proliferation to mitogens
	Decreases PGE2 release by spleen cells
Proposed mechanisms of these effects	
Reduction in accumulation of oxidant and radical damage	
Alterations in fat deposition, obesity, and hormones	

leukopenia. Decreases in circulating $CD4^+$ T cells without alteration in $CD8^+$ populations resulted in lowered CD4:CD8 ratios. Bulimics also had more circulating B lymphocytes and low complement but normal immunoglobulin levels. These authors hypothesized that cell-mediated immunity is selectively compromised (54). Similarly, PCM was associated with increased plasma immunoglobulin levels and complement deficiency (55). In addition, both $CD4^+$ and $CD8^+$ T-cell levels were depressed. Chronic infections or decreases in T-suppressor cells were suggested to be responsible for the elevations in antibodies.

A primary consideration among claims of enhanced immune responses with caloric restriction or mild malnutrition is the accurate determination of the nutritional intake of the subjects under study. Defining the sources of calories is important, since lipids provide functions other than energy (e.g., eicosanoid signaling), while certain amino acids (e.g., glutamine) are important energy sources for leukocytes. Subtle changes in other nutrients such as zinc may offset any gains produced by caloric restriction (56). Such changes could result in the reported declines in immune function associated with mild or moderate malnutrition (57). Opportunistic infections may also result from anorexia nervosa (58). Therefore, the alleged benefits of caloric restriction should be evaluated with care.

To address these issues, the effects of individual nutrients were studied in animal models of regulated caloric restriction without severe alteration of protein, vitamin, and mineral levels. Studies by Good et al. (56, 59) demonstrated that a 40% decrease in caloric intake, relative to ad libitum feeding, increased the life spans of several strains of mice. Such chronic energy restriction also inhibited or delayed development of immune-mediated renal disease, vasculitis, lymphoproliferative disease, tumor virus expression, and malignancies. Furthermore, some of these effects depended on the relative contributions of fat and carbohydrate to the caloric content; a high-carbohydrate component was more conducive to good health than high fat. Caloric restriction also downregulated the proliferative ability of lymphocytes, including $CD5^+$ B1 cells. More recently, caloric restriction in a mouse model of Sjögren's syndrome decreased the inflammatory cytokines IL-6 and TNF-α while enhancing the level of immunosuppressive TGF-β1.

Others also support the association of caloric moderation and immunologic benefits. A review of the literature by Newberne and Locniskar (44) shows general improvements in longevity and immune function with experimental caloric restriction in mice. Heightened T-cell proliferative responses to mitogen stimulation (with less effect on B cells) and increased splenic T-cell numbers were among the benefits.

Obesity is associated with a variety of immunologic disorders (44). Increased incidence of infections and abnormalities in cellular and humoral immune components are characteristic of obesity. In a study of obese humans, mitogenic responses among peripheral blood leukocytes increased following weight reduction (60). However, strong genetic influences in obesity are not easily attenuated by diet modification. In a study of genetically obese *(ob/ob)* C57Bl/6 mice, food restriction had no effect on the proliferative ability of spleen cells (61). However, food restriction reduced B-cell frequencies and increased CD4 and CD8 T-cell frequencies in both obese and lean mice. Although food restriction did not change the CD4:CD8 T-cell ratio in obese mice, this ratio was reduced in lean mice.

Proteins and Amino Acids

Inadequacies in generalized protein intake lead to suboptimal tissue repair and decreased resistance to infections and tumors. Studies on T lymphocytes do indicate that protein malnutrition can have selective effects on immune function (62). Chronic protein deprivation in mice resulted in diminished IgG and DTH responses after 3 weeks, followed by reinstatement of normal responses by 11 weeks. Perhaps this is another example of delayed maturation of immune function, as suggested for caloric restriction (44). Additionally, protein deprivation affects oral tolerance to ovalbumin. Increased humoral immune tolerance to ovalbumin was manifested by a decrease in antiovalbumin antibody synthesis. However, increases in DTH inflammatory responses suggested impaired T-cell suppression of the cell-mediated response (63).

Arginine. Arginine, a semiessential amino acid important to the urea cycle, supports the synthesis of other amino acids and of polyamines, urea, and NO (64, 65). Arginine is important for cell-mediated immunity, and exogenous sources are often required during sepsis. The growth and function of T lymphocytes in culture requires L-arginine. In vivo, arginine has the effect of retarding thymic involution by encouraging production of thymic hormones and thymocyte proliferation. The thymotropic effect of arginine depends on an intact hypothalamic-thymic axis, suggesting that the thymus is a target organ for growth hormone and prolactin release induced by arginine.

Arginine also promotes leukocyte-mediated cytotoxicity in a number of ways. Growth hormone receptors are widespread in the immune system, and arginine may increase the cytotoxic activities of macrophages, NK cells, cytotoxic T cells, and neutrophils by releasing growth hormone. A product of arginine metabolism, NO, has tumoricidal and microbicidal activities, induces blood vessel dilation, and influences leukocyte-endothelial cell adhesion.

Glutamine. Glutamine is the most abundant amino acid in the blood and in the body's free amino acid pool (66). Lymphocytes and macrophages use glutamine as a source of energy and molecular intermediates for purine and pyrimidine synthesis. As with arginine, glutamine is an essential component of leukocyte cell culture media. Following cellular uptake, a glutaminase in the inner mitochondrial membrane converts glutamine to glutamate and ammonia. Further processing results in production of aspartate and oxidation of about 25% of the glutamine to carbon dioxide. This "glutaminolysis" pathway works in conjunction with the glycolytic pathway to allow the combined use of glucose and glutamine as energy sources in lymphocytes and macrophages.

Infection and inflammation release glutamine from large (20 mM in normal humans) intracellular stores in skeletal muscles. An additional response is de novo production of glutamine by the lungs. The observation that glutamine transport from tissue stores to leukocytes, and not glutamine metabolism, is rate limiting suggests a role for skeletal muscle in regulating leukocyte metabolism. Thus, a deficiency in glutamine stores or nutritional support is likely to lead to poor immune responses.

The integrity of the intestinal immune system also relies heavily on sufficient glutamine intake. In animals, addition of glutamine to total parenteral nutrition inhibited the mucosal atrophy and leukocyte depletion normally associated with intravenous feedings, reduced bacterial translocation across the gut epithelium, and increased secretory IgA production.

In all, information on arginine and glutamine point to their potential uses in food supplementation to enhance wound healing, increase resistance to tumorigenesis and infections, and improve immune function in aged and immunocompromised persons (Table 45.4).

Table 45.4
Proteins, Amino Acids and the Immune System

Moderate protein deficiency		
	Mice:	Temporary reduction in DTH and plasma IgG in oral tolerance to ovalbumin, increases humoral (Th2?) tolerance, but decreases DTH (Th1?) tolerance
		Generalized decrease in tissue repair
Severe protein deficiency (kwashiorkor)		
	Humans:	Depresses both humoral and cell-mediated immune parameters
		Oxidant stress
Arginine		
	Important in the urea cycle and the synthesis of other amino acids, polyamines, urea, and nitric oxide	
	Secretagogue for pituitary, pancreatic, and adrenal hormones	
	Promotes T-cell development and growth and thymic integrity	
	Deficiency leads to decrease in immune competence	
	Exogenous sources important during sepsis	
Glutamine		
	Important energy source for lymphocytes and macrophages	
	Deficiency leads to poor immune responses	
	Skeletal muscles store glutamine	
	Supplementation in experimental parenteral feeding reduces gut mucosal atrophy and leukopenia	

Nucleic Acids

Preformed purines and pyrimidines in the diet appear necessary to maintain a number of cell-mediated immunologic mechanisms (67). A variety of T cell–associated processes declined when mice were fed nucleotide-free diets, including DTH responses, graft rejection, IL-2 and IFN-γ production, T-cell proliferation, splenic NK cell cytotoxicity, and impairments of PMN functions. Dietary restriction of nucleotides also slowed the maturation of T lymphocytes. On the other hand, nucleotide supplementation altered human immune responses by increasing NK cell activity in human infants (68). Among septic or critically ill patients, feeding commercial diets containing nucleotides resulted in shorter hospitalization than with a nucleotide-free diet (69).

Elements

Copper

In animal and human studies, copper (Cu) deficiency is associated with increased susceptibility to infections. Copper deficiency may impair phagocyte functions, decrease T lymphocyte numbers and activities, lower IL-2 production, and increase B cell numbers (44, 70, 71). Bala et al. (72) reported increased IL-2 receptor and transferrin receptor expression by T cells from Cu-deficient rats. A report on human responses to experimental Cu deficiency described a decrease in T-cell proliferation and increased numbers of B cells (73). Excess dietary Cu also results in reductions in phagocyte numbers and performance. Explanations for these effects include copper's involvement in complement function, cell membrane integrity, immunoglobulin structure, Cu-Zn superoxide dismutase, and interactions with iron (Fe).

Following observations that Cu-deficient male rats tended to show a more marked depression in lymphocyte proliferation and more severe anemia than their female counterparts, Kramer and Johnson (70) studied the interaction of Cu with Fe. Better Fe utilization in female rats was hypothesized. Indeed, Fe supplementation did not alleviate the anemia of Cu-deficient male rats. However, interestingly, spleen cells mitogenesis was greater in male rats deficient in both Cu and Fe.

Iron

A reduction in the concentration of plasma iron is considered an important host response to microbial infection. However, a number of T-cell and phagocyte abnormalities follow Fe deficiencies (45). Characteristic changes include reduced inflammatory responses such as the DTH reaction; impairments in neutrophil and macrophage cytotoxic activity; reductions in lymphocyte proliferation, T-cell numbers, cytokine release, and antibody production; and lymphoid tissue atrophy. Whitley et al. (74) noted decreased allograft rejection and changes in the migration patterns of T lymphocytes. Other parameters of immune function increase in activity (44, 75). These seeming inconsistencies may be due to complexities in Fe metabolism and its interactions with other nutrients.

The effects of Fe in immune function may be related to its involvement in folate metabolism, mitochondrial energy production, the respiratory burst, and/or its function as a component of many metalloenzymes including NO synthase, COX, lipoxygenase, and catalase (76). In addition, Fe metabolism and immune function are considerations in the "anemia of chronic disease" (77). Indeed, chronic inflammation is often associated with low serum Fe concentrations and increased Fe stores. There appear to be unique Th1-macrophage interactions in Fe metabolism; Th1, and not Th2, cells show hypoferremia-induced inhibition of DNA synthesis (78). Th1 cytokines such as IFN-γ and IL-2, as well as the inflammatory mediators IL-1 and TNF, induce NO synthesis in macrophages. Apparently, IFN-γ activity is inversely related to the availability of low-molecular-weight and transferrin-bound Fe, perhaps because of direct physical interactions between Fe and IFN-γ (79). Thus, high Fe levels tend to correlate with lower IFN-γ and NO production.

In cells, Fe and NO levels regulate translation of mRNA containing iron-responsive elements (IREs) posttranscriptionally, as high Fe and low NO interfere with the binding of Fe-regulatory protein (IRP) to IREs situated on the 5′ untranslated region of ferritin and erythroid 5-aminolevulinic acid synthase (ϵ-ALAS) mRNA and on the 3′ untranslated region of the transferrin receptor mRNA. Thus, depressed IRP-IRE binding encourages degradation of transferrin receptor mRNA and translation of ferritin and ϵ-ALAS mRNAs. Consequently, Fe is stored by the formation of Fe-ferritin complexes and heme synthesis. Conversely, lower Fe and higher IFN-γ, IL-2, and NO levels enhance transferrin-mediated Fe uptake by macrophages and lower Fe storage and erythropoiesis. Thus, activation of Th1 cells increases Fe storage, limits Fe availability for microbial agents, and promotes the antimicrobial and antitumor effects of NO. Because Fe consumption is but one of numerous factors that influence Fe status, the overt inconsistencies noted in the relationship of Fe status and immune function (44, 75) are, in hindsight, not surprising.

Magnesium

Animal studies have associated magnesium (Mg) deficiency with increases in thymic cellularity and inflammatory cells (especially eosinophils). Guinea pigs fed a Mg-deficient diet were at increased risk of anaphylactic shock, perhaps because of increased levels of tissue histamine. Also, release of histamine by mast cells may be regulated in part by the actions of Ca and Mg on cAMP formation. Magnesium deficits also elevate plasma concentrations of inflammatory cytokines such as IL-1, IL-6, and TNF-α. Conversely, Mg deficiency decreased concentrations of acute-phase molecules (45, 80). Relatedly, complement activity depends on an optimum Mg concentration range.

In vitro Tc cell–mediated lysis of target cells is directly proportional to Mg concentration, an effect possibly mediated via interactions with adhesion molecules (81). Since Tc cells may also induce target cell death by release of ATP, low Mg levels enhanced ATP-mediated killing of target cells. Maurois et al. (82) reported that experimental Mg deficiency in mice reduced parasitemia. Apparently, the increased oxidative environment caused by low Mg levels in red blood cells decreased the infectivity of these parasites for erythrocytes (82).

Manganese

Information on manganese (Mn) and immunity is relatively limited (44, 45). Manganese induces macrophages to spread on glass surfaces. Phagocytes incubated in medium supplemented with Mn salts showed reduced chemotaxis and uptake of amino acids. Manganese is also a constituent of the T-cell mitogen concanavalin A (con A). Manganese is a component of several metalloenzymes that may participate in immune functions, including arginase, peroxidases, catalase, and Mn superoxide dismutase (76).

Selenium

Selenium (Se) deficiency is associated with suppression of a large number of immunologic endpoints including resistance to infection, antibody synthesis, cytotoxicity, cytokine secretion, and lymphocyte proliferation; chronic Se deficiency in human populations is also associated with a high incidence of cancer. Conversely, experimental Se supplementation increases most immune parameters, suggesting that this element has adjuvant properties.

Selenium is an essential component of glutathione peroxidase (GPx), an antioxidant enzyme that, in conjunction with vitamin E, prevents peroxidation of cellular and membrane lipids (45, 57). As an example of their interaction, lowered antibody production caused by Se deficiency is reversible by vitamin E supplementation. Since phagocytes produce reactive oxygen species, limiting the potential for lipid peroxidation during immune and inflammatory processes is important to prevent autoxidation as well as damage to surrounding tissue. Indeed, excess H_2O_2 is neutralized by phagocyte-produced GPx. In addition, Taylor (83) reported that Se could mediate posttranslational modifications of important immune system proteins. A study of human mRNA sequences coding for CD4, CD8, and HLA-R suggested alternate reading frames that could code for selenoproteins. Taylor hypothesized that redox reactions and selenium availability at these selenocysteine sites may alter the conformation of these proteins.

Zinc

Insufficient zinc (Zn) intake may be the most common form of mineral deficiency, particularly among people consuming diets high in cereal and low in animal products (see Chapter 106). The best-documented immunologic consequences of Zn deficiency are low thymic weights and T-cell defects (44, 45, 84). Several T-cell abnormalities are related to Zn deficiency, including reductions in T-cell numbers and responsiveness to mitogenic stimuli, T-cell help toward antibody production, DTH reactions, thymic hormone production, Tc cell activity, and T-cell maturation. Interestingly, Zn deprivation does not affect T-cell responses to con A while the responses to phytohemagglutinin and pokeweed mitogen are reduced, suggesting differences in Zn dependency among T-cell subpopulations. Zinc-deprivation increases corticosteroid production and enlarges adrenal glands, which may be of interest in relation to corticosteroid-induced T-cell apoptosis. However, adrenalectomy does not prevent thymic involution. B-cell functions are relatively intact as tested by mitogen-induced proliferation. Other immune parameters such as NK cell activity and cytokine production have shown mixed results.

Zinc supplementation produces beneficial effects on thymic and T-cell characteristics. Zinc induces secretion of thymulin from cultured human thymic epithelial cells (85). In addition, in vitro Zn concentration is inversely related to susceptibility to apoptosis induced by dexamethasone or serum starvation (86).

The presence of Zn in many (>300) proteins (87) (see Chapter 11) complicates the understanding of Zn-related immune effects. Zn is a widely used structural component; Zn-finger structures are found in transcription factors and nuclear hormone receptors (88). Zn is known to influence endocrine function. Recently, prolactin was shown to bind Zn (89). The activity of thymulin is Zn dependent (90), as is the respiratory burst of macrophages (91). Obviously, a deficiency of Zn may cause numerous irregularities in the immune system.

Mineral Interactions

Studies of single-nutrient deficiencies face difficulties in interpretation because of the physiologic interactions among nutrients. Apart from those reported herein (Fe and Cu; Zn and other metals), numerous other examples were reviewed by Couzy et al. (92).

Vitamins

Taken as a whole, vitamins are important factors in a wide variety of metabolic processes such as gene transcription, enzymatic reactions, and redox reactions. Reviews of the literature present a correspondingly broad range of immunologic effects related to vitamin deficiencies and excesses (44, 45, 57, 93).

Vitamin A

A deficiency of vitamin A is associated with increased morbidity and mortality, most likely because of increased severity of infections (94). Vitamin A and related retinoids maintain the integrity of epithelial boundaries and the production of mucosal secretions. Some of the immunologic abnormalities that follow vitamin A inadequacies include a reduced number of leukocytes (except PMNs, which may increase), reduced lymphoid organ weights, reduced circulating levels of complement, impaired T-cell functions, and decreased resistance to immunogenic tumors. Vitamin A–deficient rats showed significant decreases in NK cell functions compared with controls (95). Vitamin A deficiency also decreased antigen-specific IgG responses and induced generalized hypergammaglobulinemia (96). Relatedly, vitamin A deficiency in rats somewhat increased IFN-γ production by leukocytes, lowered resistance to helminth infections, and decreased IgE synthesis (97). Studies confirm that Th1 cell activity precedes that of Th2 cells and that vitamin A supports Th2 development (98). Thus, vitamin A deficiency may lead to elevated Th1:Th2 ratios during an immune response.

Vitamin A supplementation studies showed decreases in respiratory infections and neutrophil counts and increases in reticuloendothelial system function, lymphocyte proliferation, tumor resistance, graft rejection, and cytotoxic T-cell activities. Supplementation above that required to maintain normal vitamin A stores results in adjuvant effects. Excess vitamin A increases antibody and cell-mediated immune responses, stimulates Kupffer cells, and potentiates some types of liver toxicity and gouty arthritis (99, 100). The inhibition of T-cell apoptosis by retinoic acid (101) may possibly contribute to its adjuvant effect. The use of vitamin A as an immunologic adjuvant was recently tested (102). Because of a high prevalence of subclinical vitamin A deficiency, some infants vaccinated for measles also received 100,000 IU of vitamin A. Infants who had at least a 1:8 titer of maternally transmitted antimeasles antibodies and received vitamin A showed a significantly lower frequency of seroconversion. The researchers hypothesized that vitamin A inhibited the replication of the measles virus which was necessary to provoke a protective immune response.

The vitamin A precursor *β*-carotene is generally considered an antioxidant with activities that are independent of its provitamin A function. Some of its reported benefits include protecting host cells and tissues from oxidation by the respiratory burst and promoting lymphocyte proliferation, T-cell functions, cytokine production, and cell-mediated cytotoxicity. However, Bates (103) cautioned that carotenoids can exhibit prooxidant as well as antioxidant activity. Also, their record in ameliorating chronic and degenerative diseases is not consistent. Bates suggested that in addition to antioxidant activity, beneficial carotenoids may also function by promoting gap junction communication and connexin synthesis.

B Complex Vitamins

Pyridoxine or vitamin B_6 deficiency induces lymphocytopenia with decreases in lymphoid tissue weights and reduced proliferative responses to mitogens. There are general deficiencies in cell-mediated immunity, including allograft rejection, IL-2 production, and the DTH response (93). Humoral immunity is also affected, as seen by lowered antibody responses and depressions in antigen-specific secondary responses. Macrophage and NK cell cytotoxicity toward target cell lines was unchanged by pyridoxine deficiencies. The pyridoxine requirement for nucleic acid and protein synthesis during lymphocyte proliferation is probably responsible for the greater effect on lymphocytes than on macrophages or NK cells. Appropriate vitamin B_6 supplementation readily restores these immunologic endpoints. Pyridoxine supplementation also protects mice from the immunosuppressive effects of UV-B radiation (104). Pyridoxine may compete with *cis*-urocanic acid, a mediator of photoimmunosuppression, for binding on histamine-like receptors on T cells.

Cyanocobalamin (vitamin B_{12}) deficiency and folate deficiency are clinically indistinguishable since they are both required for synthesis of thymidylate. They depress a number of immunologic parameters including the respiratory burst, phagocytosis by PMNs, DTH responses, and T-cell proliferation to phytohemagglutinin. Proliferating T cells from patients with pernicious anemia are "megaloblastoid" in character, being larger in size and with an abnormal chromatin pattern. The defect in nuclear maturation results from inadequate thymidylate synthesis.

Biotin deficiency is associated with humoral and cell-mediated immune deficiencies. Depressions in thymic weights, antigen-specific antibody responses, and reduced lymphocyte-mediated suppressor activity have been noted.

Deficiencies in pantothenic acid commonly lead to decreased antibody responses. The biochemical lesion may be an inability to secrete newly synthesized proteins to the extracellular space.

Immunologic abnormalities associated with thiamin deficiency include increased susceptibility to infectious disease agents, premature thymic atrophy, decreased antibody responses, and reduced PMN mobility.

Riboflavin deficiency in dogs increased PMNs with concurrent decreases in peripheral blood lymphocytes. In other animal studies, decreased antibody responses and thymic weights and increased susceptibility to challenge with infectious disease agents were observed.

Vitamin C

Vitamin C, another antioxidant vitamin, functions as a biologic reductant in regeneration of oxidized vitamin E (105). Apart from a sparing effect on Se, interactions between vitamin C and glutathione may be important for phagocyte microtubule function. Scavenging of extracellular superoxide anion and hydroxyl radicals by ascorbic acid minimizes autoxidation of phagocytes and damage to bystander host cells without compromising intracellular oxidant capacity. Immunologic problems associated with vitamin C deficits include decreases in resistance to infections and cancer, phagocyte mobility and phagocytosis, the DTH response, skin allograft rejection, and wound repair. Studies on people of various age groups demonstrated the ability of vitamin C supplementation to enhance many of these immunologic parameters, including the DTH and antibody responses (106). However, research does not support the use of megadoses (>1 g/day) of vitamin C to prevent common colds, although low doses may have minor prophylactic effects or reduce their symptoms. Indeed, high ascorbic acid levels arrested in vitro lymphocyte proliferation by mitogens (105).

Vitamin D

Vitamin D has both stimulatory and suppressive effects on immune responses because of its influence on mineral metabolism and its hormonal nature. For example, vitamin D stimulates maturation of normal and neoplastic myelomonocytic cells to more differentiated monocytes and macrophages. Certain tumors also reinforce myelopoiesis through the production of granulocyte-macrophage colony-stimulating factor (GM-CSF). Vitamin D_3 reduces tumor growth and its associated immunosuppression by blocking release of GM-CSF (107). The potential autocrine nature of vitamin D is suggested by its synthesis by activated macrophages and the presence of vitamin D receptors in mononuclear phagocytes. Tokuda and Levy (108) compared the effects of 1,25-dihydroxyvitamin D_3 ($1,25(OH)_2D_3$) and PGE_2 on monocyte function. While both cytokines increased phagocytosis, $1,25(OH)_2D_3$ also reduced HLA-DR expression. This suggests that both cytokines activate innate responses (phagocytosis) while $1,25(OH)_2D_3$ also inhibits an acquired immune response by downregulating MHC molecule expression required for antigen presentation.

Receptors for vitamin D, which are present on the surface of activated lymphocytes, probably mediate vitamin D's influence on lymphocyte proliferation and function. $1,25(OH)_2D_3$ inhibits $CD4^+$ T-cell activities such as IL-2 and IFN-γ production, Tc activation in mixed leukocyte reactions, and T-cell promotion of immunoglobulin production by B cells. NK cell generation is also reduced. However, $1,25(OH)_2D_3$ does not interfere with the cytotoxic function of already established T and NK cells (109). Interestingly, $1,25(OH)_2D_3$ preferentially inhibits Th1 functions and not those of Th2 (110) or $CD8^+$ T cells (111). This overall promotion of immunosuppression may be important in the reported modulation of autoimmune diseases (109, 112).

Vitamin E

Vitamin E deficiency is relatively rare in human populations and controversy exists about recommended intakes. However, its essential nature derives from its function as a radical scavenger to limit cell membrane peroxidation and its interactions with other antioxidants (113). Experimentally induced deficiency leads to depressed leukocyte proliferation, lower chemotaxis and phagocytosis by PMNs and macrophages, and decreased tumor resistance while leaving NK cell cytotoxicity either unchanged or enhanced. Vitamin E supplementation increased a number of immune parameters including lymphocyte proliferation, antibody levels, the DTH reaction, IL-2 and 6-keto $PGF_{1\alpha}$ production, and phagocytosis. Supplementation also reduced PGE_2 synthesis, levels of plasma lipid hydroperoxides, and oxidant damage induced by burns in lung tissues. The inverse relationship of PGE_2 and 6-keto $PGF_{1\alpha}$ production to changes in vitamin E level is evidence for redox influences on arachidonic acid metabolism and, consequently, immune function. Vitamin E supplementation also restored Th1 activity and IL-2 and IFN-γ production in murine AIDS (114). Finally, in human populations, high vitamin E intake increases resistance to infections among the elderly.

Lipids

FAs function as energy sources, as cell membrane components, and as mediators of cell signaling. Among the PUFAs, the most important dietary PUFAs are in the n-3 and n-6 classes. Since cell membrane composition is partially dependent on the FA species taken in through the diet (115), dietary lipids are an important influence on cell function.

Arachidonic acid (20:4 n-6) is an important constituent of plasma membrane phospholipids and a precursor of cell-derived eicosanoids (18). Eicosanoids are members of a family of 20-carbon PUFAs derived from oxygenation of arachidonic acid. Collectively, they contribute to an enormous range of physiologic and stress responses including inflammation, immunity, reproduction, blood flow, and temperature regulation. The evolution of signaling by eicosanoids may have its roots in the oxidation of membrane FAs during cellular damage. The disassembly and oxygenation of membrane components are an aspect of the stress response of cells and, indeed, the extent of membrane alterations may be proportional to the level of stress placed on a cell. The development of mechanisms to use these cellular responses to stress as cell signals could conceivably have driven the evolution of eicosanoid production. Within the context of the immune response, such signals are used in activation of immune cells during periods of host stress, such as microbial infection.

PGE_2 exhibits selective inhibitory function. Studies on Th1 and Th2 cells demonstrated the ability of PGE_2 to arrest the function of Th1, but not Th2, cells (41, 42, 116). The previously prescribed thesis of PGE_2 as an immunosuppressor was apparently based on studies of primarily cell-mediated not humoral immune functions. Thus, the downregulation of Th1 cells and the promotion of Th2 cells by PGE_2 may enhance antibody production.

The contribution of dietary lipids toward autoimmune disease is highlighted by the beneficial effects of experimental essential fatty acid (EFA) deficiency in animal models of diabetes and lupus (117). An important outcome of EFA deficiency is altered macrophage function related to arachidonic acid metabolism and eicosanoid synthesis (118, 119). As a result, there is interest in reducing the arachidonic acid content in the cell membranes of humans. Manipulation of eicosanoid synthesis often means replacing conventional vegetable oils with fish oils that are relatively rich in n-3 FAs, which can supplant membrane n-6 FAs and alter the eicosanoid species produced. As a result, ingesting fish oil leads to lower production of PGE_2 by spleen cells than an n-6-rich corn oil diet (120). Clinical studies demonstrated the effectiveness of fish oils in reducing autoimmune and other immunopathologic parameters. Fish oil supplementation on a mouse model of systemic lupus erythematosus, the NZB/NZW F1 strain, reduced levels of IL-1β, IL-6, and TNF-α and increased antioxidant enzyme activities (121). Sanderson et al. (122) reported that feeding rats fish oils increased graft survival while decreasing popliteal lymph node NK cells and $CD8^+$ T cells. Relative to safflower oil, fish oils decreased the frequency of $\gamma\delta TCR^+$ splenic T cells and the activity of lymphokine-activated killer (LAK) cells (123). Fish oil supplementation of multiple sclerosis patients similarly decreased IL-1, TNF-α, IL-2, and IFN-γ levels (124). However, fish oils from different sources possess different characteristics. Unlike menhaden and sardine oils, feeding rats cod liver oil decreased α-tocopherol levels in spleen cells (125), possibly because of antagonistic interactions between vitamin E and the vitamin A found in fish liver oil.

In addition, n-3 PUFAs are directly obtained from plant sources. Wu et al. (126) demonstrated the ability of plant-derived α-linolenic acid to reduce PGE_2 production by the peripheral blood leukocytes of cynomolgus monkeys. In this study, consumption of either marine- or plant-derived n-3 PUFAs led to a drop in the absolute numbers of circulating T cells but not B cells. Collectively, studies such as these demonstrate attenuation of a number of inflammatory states and immune-mediated diseases by dietary FA manipulation.

An alternative to both the n-3 and n-6 PUFAs are the monounsaturates. The monounsaturated FA, oleic acid (18:1 n-9), is abundant in olive and rapeseed oils, is not converted to eicosanoids, and is highly resistant to oxidation compared with PUFAs. These factors contribute to the widespread reputation of olive, and now canola, oil in minimizing coronary heart disease and possibly other chronic ailments. In experimental studies on the effects of edible oils on inflammation, olive and rapeseed oils are sometimes used as control or placebo oils (127). As caveats, the spectrum of biologic effects, particularly negative effects, that could result from the dominant use of these oils and the cellular enrichment of oleic acid is probably not known. Also, oleic acid is not highly competitive with arachidonic acid for incorporation into phospholipids.

Studies on experimental animals demonstrated associations between increasing consumption of dietary fats and immunosuppression (44, 45). High-PUFA diets decreased the proliferative capacity of mouse lymphocytes, while low-PUFA diets enhanced cell division. In addition, an examination of in vitro macrophage activity showed that supplementation of culture medium with saturated FAs decreased phagocytosis of zymosan particles (128). By comparison, PUFAs increased phagocytosis, with arachidonic acid giving the greatest response. Of practical concern, increased susceptibility to bacterial and tumor challenges may result from the immunosuppression caused by high-fat diets. Of course, the caveats to such studies include the extrapolation of in vitro studies to in vivo situations and the multiple effects of dietary fats (e.g., energy considerations vs. signaling).

This is not to say that a low-lipid diet is unequivocally advantageous. Enhancements in certain parameters of immune function with reductions in dietary fats may depend on the duration of food restriction. Long-term deficiency in EFAs (especially linoleic acid) in mice can result in reduced cell-mediated immune responses rather than enhancements. Unsaturated FAs are also not necessarily of better quality than saturates. In a study of hairless mice, dietary butter fat was more effective than vegetable oil or margarine in preventing the immunosuppression induced by UV-B radiation (129). The mechanism of protection may be related to differences in dietary FAs and the FA composition of the skin. Additionally, studies showed that mice on high-fat diets had prolonged tissue graft survival, while EFA-deficient diets accelerated skin graft rejection (44, 45). The latter observation coincides with the association of increased PGE_2 production by liver Kupffer cells with decreased heart allografts (130, 131). The downregulation of Th1 cells and cell-mediated immune responses is probably responsible for the PGE_2 effect.

The lipid composition of foods given to patients is a target of research and development (132, 133). Modification of the FA composition of medical foods is seen as one means of increasing resistance to infection following surgery. Triglycerides are fat molecules formed from the covalent attachment of three FAs to a glycerol moiety. Triglycerides in the enteral and parenteral diets of medical patients provide calories and linoleic acid and carry fat-soluble vitamins. Long-chain triglycerides, which generally contain FAs of 14 carbons or longer, were initially used in medical foods. Unfortunately, intravenously administered long-chain triglycerides tended to impair macrophage and neutrophil functions. Indeed, experiments in animals demonstrated that long-chain triglycerides reduced the efficiency of their livers to clear injected bacteria and increased their risk of lung infections. More-recent innovations include medium-chain triglycerides with FAs of 8 to 10 carbons, and structured lipids prepared by the hydrolysis and reesterification of FAs to form mixed-length triglycerides. Medium-chain triglycerides and structured lipids appear to avoid the negative side effects of long-chain triglycerides.

Collectively, such studies show that dietary lipids are important factors that influence the characteristics of an immune response. However, stronger immune responses are not advantageous in all situations. Allergies and autoimmune diseases are examples of hyperactive or misdirected immune reactions. Also, since the immune system is responsible for rejection of tissue grafts, an ability to selectively suppress this aspect of an immune response would be useful. Therefore, the specific manipulation of dietary lipids in response to one health problem may not be appropriate for other situations.

Antioxidants

Nutrition interfaces with oxidant balance and immunity through antioxidant vitamins, trace elements and superoxide dismutase, the effects of caloric restriction on life span, and the endogenous production of reactive oxygen and radical species by leukocytes (134–136). Of special interest to the present discussion are oxidized lipids, dietary antioxidants, and the effects of redox-related events on different lymphocyte subsets.

In terms of oxidant balance and the regulation of the immune system, some information is available from studies on inflammatory rheumatic diseases (137, 138) and allergies (139). Of more defined interest are the immunoregulatory effects of oxidants and associated signaling molecules on T-cell subpopulations. This is of immense importance as phagocytes are endogenous producers of reactive oxygen and T lymphocytes are central to the activation of specific immune reactions. There is evidence to suggest that $CD8^+$ T cells are more susceptible to prooxidant inhibition than $CD4^+$ T cells. Droge et al. (140) demonstrated the ability of an inhibitor of glutathione synthesis to lower in vitro proliferation of $CD8^+$ T cells without a similar effect on $CD4^+$ cells. In addition, human peripheral blood $CD8^+$ T cells have less intracellular superoxide dismutase than $CD4^+$ T cells, and this quantitative difference increases with age (141). These observations are relevant within the context of selective prooxidant-mediated apoptosis of T lymphocytes.

The selective inhibition of Th1 cells also suggests that this T helper subset may be an important site for feedback inhibition of cell-mediated immune responses. PGE_2 inhibits Th1 function without a similar reduction in Th2 activity (41, 42, 116). Relatedly, inflammatory signals, including reactive oxygen, activate cyclooxygenase (142). As mentioned above, interactions between circulating Fe and Th1 cells affect iron storage (77), DNA synthesis in Th1 cells (78), and IFN-γ activity (79). Iron sequestration also lowers Fe-mediated catalysis of hydroxyl radicals from H_2O_2 substrates. Furthermore, UV-B radiation mediates the conversion of provitamin D_3 to previtamin D_3. Interestingly, 1,25-dihydroxyvitamin D_3 preferentially inhibits Th1 functions and not Th 2 (121) or $CD8^+$ T cells (111). Of possible related interest, UV-B radiation causes release of Fe from transferrin (143). In addition, vitamin A downregulates the activity of Th1 and actively promotes development of Th2 cells (98, 144). Conversely, the antioxidant vitamin E is able to restore Th1 activity (113, 114). There is sufficient information to suggest that prooxidants and associated molecules and processes provide negative feedback signals to Th1 cells as a means of balancing cell (Th1)- and antibody (Th2)-mediated effector mechanisms. The rationale or significance of preferentially inhibiting Th1 cells is the modulation of cell-mediated immune responses. Cell-mediated reactions are responsible for the endogenous production of much of the reactive oxygen and radical effectors and, relatedly, the collateral tissue damage during inflammation.

Intracellular signaling pathways responsive to pro- or antioxidants are being defined and are likely to explain the effects of oxidant balance on T cells. Prooxidants are generally associated with the activation of the NF-κB transcription protein through dissociation of its inhibitor, IκB. Likewise, a response to antioxidants is the binding of fos-jun dimers to AP-1 binding sites that are found upstream of several T-cell interleukin genes (145). Promoter/enhancer regions often have sites for the cooperative binding of NF-κB, AP-1, and other transcription regulators, and the interactions among these transcription factors are yet to be resolved.

As mentioned above, Th1 cells are more sensitive to hypoferremia-induced inhibition of DNA synthesis than are Th2 cells (78). Thus, iron levels could be one component in an overall strategy toward managing the relative levels of different T-cell subpopulations in health and disease. Dietary manipulation of iron can affect the health of autoimmune mice (146); iron supplementation of MRL-lpr/lpr mice increased morbidity and mortality, possibly by enhancing the Fenton reaction and oxidant stress. Conversely, moderate iron deficiency improved the health status of these mice. Since autoimmune diseases are associated with Th1 and Th2 imbalances (147, 148), manipulation of dietary Fe may partially normalize T-cell functions.

Lipid oxidation is of immunologic interest because of the potential for oxidant-induced immune activation and cell apoptosis. Vitamin E is an important radical quencher that limits the peroxidation cascade among phospholipid FAs. However, cell membranes are also sites of reactive oxygen and radical production, including formation of lipid hydroperoxides via metabolism of arachidonic acid (149, 150) and synthesis of reactive oxygen during the respiratory burst (151). Metals such as Fe are also implicated in the oxidation of lipids by catalyzing the formation of hydroxyl radicals (152). In addition, scavenger receptors on phagocytes act as receptors for oxidized low-density lipoproteins that have platelet activating factor–like activity (153). Foods constitute a potentially major source of oxidized lipids that act to compromise the antioxidant capabilities of the consumer (152, 154).

Foods are an important source of antioxidant activity, which varies as a function of the quality of the diet. Apart from the vitamins and trace minerals already mentioned, plant sources contain other nutritional antioxidants; of particular significance are the polyphenolics (155, 156). However, the antioxidant nature of a compound depends highly on its chemical environment, and indeed many plant-derived antioxidants that inhibit lipid oxidation promote carbohydrate oxidation (155). Finding oxidant stress in kwashiorkor (157) and the use of glutathione and other cysteine-containing antioxidants in the treatment of protein-energy malnutrition (158) show that dietary antioxidants and adequate energy sources help to maintain antioxidant defenses.

Age

Schandler (159) recently reviewed the contributions of human milk toward immunologic defense in infants. In particular, comparisons between human and bovine milks indicate a higher quality of the former for infant development. Human milk passively transfers immunoglobulin, antibacterial proteins such as lactoferrin and lysozyme, and oligosaccharides with bacteria-binding activity. Additionally, the composition of protein and fat from human milk is more conducive for absorption. Lahov and Regelson (160) also described casein-derived proteins, casecidins, with antibacterial properties. A purified polypeptide of casein, isracidin, increases the survival of mice during bacterial challenge. Although its mechanism of action is not clear, it does increase phagocyte activity.

Immune function in the elderly undergoes immunosenescence. During this period, decreases in antigen-specific immune responses to infections and cell-mediated immunity and increases in autoantibodies and autoimmune conditions are common (25, 161, 162). A focus of much interest in immunosenescence is the T cell (24, 163, 164).

The start of thymic involution during puberty results in alterations in the developmental environment of T lymphocytes. Therefore, extrathymic sites for T-cell development, such as the gut, may become more important with increasing age. Changes in T-cell populations include declining IL-2 production, Th1/Th2 ratios, $CD8^+$ T cells, and lymphocyte mitogenic responses. Increases are noted in the proportion of memory T cells, in PGE_2 production, and in NK cell numbers. Age-related changes in membrane composition and function also accompany declines in leukocyte activity.

Nutrition is useful in delaying or partially reversing the progression of immunosenescence. Nutritional status in the elderly is often compromised by a combination of physiologic and environmental factors. Thus, caloric restriction is generally not considered a viable option, as malnutrition is of concern in the elderly (161). On the other hand, vitamin-mineral supplements do improve cell-mediated immune responses in older people (165). Most of the data on supplementation with specific nutrients are related to antioxidants, and the proposed mechanism by which caloric restriction appears to affect human health and aging (by limiting oxidant damage) is also considered important as a remedy for immunosenescence.

Several studies focused on the relationship of dietary Zn to immunocompetence. At least in aged mice that exhibited a negative Zn balance, supplementary Zn partially restored thymic architecture and function, as well as a number of immunologic parameters (166, 167). These authors noted normalization of the thymic epithelial cell network and increases in thymic hormone production and thymocyte numbers. Also enhanced were mitogen responses to phytohemagglutinin and concanavalin A, splenic T-cell numbers (particularly $CD8^+$ T cells), and target-cell killing by NK cells.

Meydani et al. (168) recently summarized the benefits of dietary antioxidants on immune function in the aged. Vitamin E supplementation has its greatest effect on cell-mediated Th1 immune responses as manifested by increases in DTH responses and IL-2 production and decreases in PGE_2 synthesis. However, antigen-specific antibody responses to influenza virus and killing of *Candida albicans* by PMNs were unchanged. Vitamin E also decreased plasma lipid peroxidation. β-Carotene supplementation increased NK cell cytotoxicity and DTH responses to recall antigens, probably as results of alterations in cytokine production.

Cellular and tissue levels of glutathione decline with age, a condition that is partially reversible in mice by dietary glutathione (168). In this situation, improvements in DTH reactions and mitogen responses were associated with increased tissue levels of glutathione. In vitro addition of glutathione to cultures of human peripheral blood leukocytes showed a curious biphasic effect on mitogen-induced proliferation. The designated optimum concentration (5 mmol/L) for proliferation was slightly higher than that found in vivo. Compared with controls with no added glutathione, 5 mmol/L enhanced IL-2 production and inhibited PGE_2 and LTB4. However, 0.5 and 1.0 mmol/L glutathione significantly decreased cell proliferation in comparison to controls. Meydani et al. (168) suggest that the lower levels (<1.5 mmol/L) of glutathione present in the extracellular medium actually enhanced hydroxyl radical production above that of controls. Therefore, glutathione, like other dietary antioxidants, can alter the release of cell metabolites as well as markers of oxidant stress.

EPILOGUE

This review supports the view that nutrients are an important environmental influence on the immune system. Advances in dietary and nutritional practices will contribute to an enhanced quality of life and, in particular, the prevention and improvement of immune-mediated degenerative conditions. Oxidant and radical balances appear to be important focal points for regulating the immune system, especially since the immune response is a major source of reactive oxygen species. In addition, the information suggests that nutrients may be useful tools for manipulating the proportions of T-cell subpopulations that are central to immune regulation. Food and nutritional sciences will continue to provide interesting insights into the working of the immune system as well as identify practical dietary applications for the enjoyment of life.

ACKNOWLEDGMENTS

The authors thank Dr. J. Bruce German for reviewing the content of the manuscript and Ms. Nikki Phipps for her help in preparing the manuscript. NIH National Research Service Award DK07355 to Steven Yoshida.

REFERENCES

1. Gordon S, Clarke S, Greaves D, et al. Curr Opin Immunol 1995;7:24–33.
2. Lloyd AR, Oppenheim JJ. Immunol Today 1992;13:169–72.
3. Rosen GM, Pou S, Ramos CL, et al. FASEB J 1995;9:200–9.
4. Roitt I. Essential immunology. 8th ed. Oxford: Blackwell Scientific Publications, 1994.
5. Baumann H, Gauldie J. Immunol Today 1994;15:74–80.
6. Klein E, Mantovani A. Curr Opin Immunol 1993;5:714–8.
7. Gumperz JE, Parham P. Nature 1995;378:245–8.
8. Gleich GJ, Adolphson CR, Leiferman KM. Eosinophils. In: Gallin JI, Goldstein IM, Snyderman R, eds. Inflammation: basic principles and clinical correlates. 2nd ed. New York: Raven Press, 1992.
9. DeFranco AL. Curr Opin Cell Biol 1995;7:163–75.
10. Hein WR. Semin Immunol 1994;6:361–672.
11. Havran WL, Boismenu R. Curr Opin Immunol 1994;6:442–6.
12. Klinman NR. Curr Opin Immunol 1994;6:420–4.
13. Banchereau J, Briere F, Liu YJ, et al. Stem Cells 1994;12: 278–88.
14. Podack ER. Curr Opin Immunol 1995;7:11–6.
15. Huntley JF. J Comp Pathol 1992;107:349–72.
16. Gounni AS, Lamkhioued B, Delaporte E, et al. J Allergy Clin Immunol 1994;94(6 pt 2):1214–6.

17. Gray D. Curr Opin Immunol 1994;6:425–30.
18. Goetzl EJ, An S, Smith WL. FASEB J 1995;9:1051–8.
19. Scott MA, Gordon MY. Br J Haematol 1995;90:738–43.
20. Kisielow P, Von Boehmer H. Adv Immunol 1995;58:87–209.
21. Jameson SC, Hogquist KA, Bevan MJ. Annu Rev Immunol 1995;13:93–126.
22. Sprent J, Gao EK, Webb SR. Science 1990;248:1357–63.
23. Abo T. Microbiol Immunol 1993;37:247–58.
24. Franceschi C, Monti D, Sansoni P, et al. Immunol Today 1995;13:12–6.
25. Beeson PB. Am J Med 1994;96:457–62.
26. Kantor AB, Herzenberg LA. Annu Rev Immunol 1993;11: 501–38.
27. Brandtzaeg P. APMIS 1995;103:1–19.
28. Dunkley M, Pabst R, Cripps A. Immunol Today 1995;16: 231–6.
29. Germain RN. Ann NY Acad Sci 1995;754:114–25.
30. Salter-Cid L, Flajnik MF. Crit Rev Immunol 1995;15:31–75.
31. Giannasca PJ, Neutra MR. Infect Agents Dis 1994;2:242–8.
32. Albelda SM, Smith CW, Ward PA. FASEB J 1994;8:504–12.
33. Postigo AA, Sánchez-Madrid F. Transplant Proc 1993;25:65–9.
34. LaSalle JM, Hafler DA. FASEB J 1994;8:601–8.
35. Thomson AW. The cytokine handbook. 2nd ed. San Diego: Academic Press, 1994.
36. Arnon R, Teitelbaum D. Int Arch Allergy Immunol 1993;100:2–7.
37. Kemeny DM, Noble A, Holmes BJ, et al. Immunol Today 1994;15:107–10.
38. Le Gros G, Erard F. Curr Opin Immunol 1994;6:453–7.
39. Anderson GP, Coyle AJ. Trends Pharmacol Sci 1994;15: 324–32.
40. O'Garra A, Howard M. Int Rev Immunol 1992;8:219–34.
41. Gold KN, Weyand CM, Goronzy JJ. Arthritis Rheum 1994;37:925–33.
42. Hilkens CM, Vermeulen H, van Neerven RJ, et al. Eur J Immunol 1995;25:59–63.
43. Coutinho A. Scand J Immunol 1995;42:3–8.
44. Newberne PM, Locniskar M. Nutrition and immune status. In: Rowland I, ed. Nutrition, toxicity, and cancer. Boca Raton, FL: CRC Press, 1991.
45. Myrvik QN. Immunology and nutrition. In: Shils ME, Olson JA, Shike M, eds. Modern nutrition in health and disease. 8th ed. Philadelphia: Lea & Febiger, 1994.
46. Cooper WC, Good RA, Mariani T. Am J Clin Nutr 1974;27:647–64.
47. Jose DG, Good RA. Nature 1971;231:323–5.
48. Kramer TR, Good RA. Clin Immunol Immunopathol 1978;11:212–28.
49. Palmblad J. Scand J Haematol 1976;17:217–24.
50. Weindruch RH, Gottesman SRS, Walford RL. Proc Natl Acad Sci USA 1982;79:898–904.
51. Urao M, Ueda G, Abe M, et al. J Nutr 1995;125:2316–24.
52. Bowers TK, Eckert E. Arch Intern Med 1978;138:1520–5.
53. Pertschuk MJ, Crosby LO, Bardot L, et al. Am J Clin Nutr 1982;35:968–72.
54. Marcos A, Varela P, Santacruz I, et al. Am J Clin Nutr 1993;57:65–9.
55. Özkan H, Olgun N, Sasmaz E, et al. J Trop Pediat 1993;39:257–60.
56. Good RA, Lorenz E. Int J Immunopharmacol 1992;14:361–6.
57. Kuvibidila S, Yu L, Ode D, et al. The immune response in protein-energy malnutrition and single nutrient deficiencies. In: Klurfield DM, ed. Nutrition and immunology. New York: Plenum Press, 1993.
58. Tenholder MF, Pike JD. South Med J 1991;84:1188–91.
59. Mizutani H, Engleman RW, Kurata Y, et al. J Nutr 1994;124:2016–23.
60. Tanaka S-I, Inoue S, Isoda F, et al. Int J Obes 1993;17:631–6.
61. Boissonneault GA, Harrison DE. J Nutr 1994;124:1639–46.
62. Ferguson A. Gut Suppl 1994;1:10S–2S.
63. Weiner HL, Friedman A, Miller A, et al. Annu Rev Immunol 1994;12:809–37.
64. Redmond HP, Daly JM. Arginine. In: Klurfield DM, ed. Human nutrition—a comprehensive treatise, vol 8: Nutrition and immunology. New York: Plenum Press, 1993.
65. Barbul A, Dawson H. Arginine and immunity. In: Forse RA, ed. Diet, nutrition, and immunity. Boca Raton, FL: CRC Press, 1994.
66. Dudrick PS, Alverdy JC, Souba WW. Glutamine and the immune system. In: Forse RA, ed. Diet, nutrition, and immunity. Boca Raton, FL: CRC Press, 1994.
67. Kulkarni AD, Rudolph FB, Van Buren CT. Nucleotide nutrition dependent immunosurveillance: natural killer cell cytotoxicity, gamma interferon production, and polymorphonuclear cell function. In: Forse RA, ed. Diet, nutrition, and immunity. Boca Raton, FL: CRC Press, 1994.
68. Carver JD. J Nutr 1995;124:144S–8S.
69. Van Buren CT, Kulkarni AD, Rudolph FB. J Nutr 1995;124: 160S–4S.
70. Kramer TR, Johnson WT. Copper and immunity. In: Cunningham-Rundles S, ed. Nutrient modulation of the immune response. New York: Marcel Dekker, 1993.
71. O'Dell BL. Nutr Rev 1993;51:307–9.
72. Bala S, Failla ML, Lunney JK. J Nutr 1991;121:745–53.
73. Kelley DS, Daudu PA, Taylor PC, et al. Am J Clin Nutr 1995;62:412–6.
74. Whitley WD, Hancock WW, Kupiec-Weglinski JW, et al. Transplantation 1993;56:1182–8.
75. Bryan CF, Stone MJ. The immunoregulatory properties of iron. In: Cunningham-Rundles S, ed. Nutrient modulation of the immune response. New York: Marcel Dekker, 1993.
76. Karlin KD. Science 1993;261:701–8.
77. Weiss G, Wacther H, Fuchs D. Immunol Today 1995;16: 495–500.
78. Thorson JA, Smith KM, Gomez F, et al. Cell Immunol 1991;134:126–37.
79. Weiss G, Lutton JD, Fuchs D, et al. Proc Soc Exp Biol Med 1993;202:470–5.
80. McCoy H, Kenney MA. Magnesium Res 1992;5:281–93.
81. Redegeld F, Filippini A, Sitkovsky M. J Immunol 1991;147: 3638–45.
82. Maurois P, Delcourt P, Slomianny C, et al. Magnes Res 1995;8:159–66.
83. Taylor EW. Biol Trace Element Res 1995;49:85–95.
84. Vruwink KG, Keen CL, Gershwin ME, et al. The effect of experimental zinc deficiency on development of the immune system. In: Cunningham-Rundles S, ed. Nutrient modulation of the immune response. New York: Marcel Dekker, 1993.
85. Saha AR, Hadden EM, Hadden JW. Int J Immunopharmacol 1995;17:729–33.
86. Provinciali M, Di Stefano G, Fabris N. Int J Immunopharmacol 1995;17:735–44.
87. Berg JM, Shi Y. Science 1996;271:1081–5.
88. Klug A, Schwabe JWR. FASEB J 1995;9:597–604.
89. Lorenson MY, Patel T, Liu J-W, et al. Endocrinology 1996;137:809–16.
90. Hadden JW. Int J Immunopharmacol 1995;17:697–701.
91. Cook-Mills JM, Fraker PJ. The role of metals in the production of toxic oxygen metabolites by mononuclear phagocytes.

In: Cunningham-Rundles S, ed. Nutrient modulation of the immune response. New York: Marcel Dekker, 1993.
92. Couzy F, Keen C, Gershwin ME, et al. Prog Food Nutr Sci 1993;17:65–87.
93. Blumberg JB. Vitamins. In: Forse RA, ed. Diet, nutrition, and immunity. Boca Raton, FL: CRC Press, 1994.
94. Ross AC, Hämmerling UG. Retinoids and the immune system. In: Sporn MB, Roberts AB, Goodman DS, eds. The retinoids: biology, chemistry, and medicine. 2nd ed. New York: Raven Press, 1994.
95. Naus KM, Newberne PM. J Nutr 1985;115:1300–24.
96. Cantorna MT, Nashold FE, Hayes CE. Eur J Immunol 1995;25:1673–9.
97. Carman JA, Pond L, Nashold F, et al. J Exp Med 1992; 175:111–20.
98. Cantorna MT, Nashold FE, Hayes CE. J Immunol 1994;152: 1515–22.
99. Watson RR, Earnest DL, Prabhala RH. Retinoids, carotenoids, and macrophage activation. In: Cunningham-Rundles S, ed. Nutrient modulation of the immune response. New York: Marcel Dekker, 1993.
100. Mawson AR, Ono GI. Semin Arthritis Rheum 1991;20: 297–304.
101. Iwata M, Mukai M, Nakai Y, et al. J Immunol 1992;149:3302–6.
102. Semba RD, Munasir Z, Beeler J, et al. Lancet 1995;345: 1330–2.
103. Bates CJ. Lancet 1995;345:31–5.
104. Reeve VE, Bosnic M, Boehm-Wilcox C, et al. Am J Clin Nutr 1995;61:571–6.
105. Muggli R. Vitamin C and phagocytes. In: Cunningham-Rundles S, ed. Nutrient modulation of the immune response. New York: Marcel Dekker, 1993.
106. Cunningham-Rundles WF, Berner Y, Cunningham-Rundles S. Interaction of vitamin C in lymphocyte activation: current status and possible mechanisms of action. In: Cunningham-Rundles S, ed. Nutrient modulation of the immune response. New York: Marcel Dekker, 1993.
107. Young MRI, Ihm J, Lozano Y, et al. Cancer Immunol Immunother 1995;41:37–45.
108. Tokuda N, Levy RB. Proc Soc Exp Biol Med 1996;211:244–50.
109. Lemire JM. J Cell Biochem 1992;49:26–31.
110. Lemire JM, Archer DC, Beck L, et al. J Nutr 1995;125: 1704S–8S.
111. Jordan SC, Sakai R, Koeffler HP, et al. Immunoregulatory and prodifferentiating effects of 1,25-dihydroxyvitamin D_3 in human mononuclear cells. In: Cunningham-Rundles S, ed. Nutrient modulation of the immune response. New York: Marcel Dekker, 1993.
112. Mathieu C, Laureys J, Sobis H, et al. Diabetes 1992;41:1491–5.
113. Meydani SN, Blumberg JB. Vitamin E and the immune response. In: Cunningham-Rundles S, ed. Nutrient modulation of the immune response. New York: Marcel Dekker, 1993.
114. Wang Y, Huang DS, Eskelson CD, et al. Clin Immunol Immunopathol 1994;72:70–5.
115. Taraszewski R, Jensen GL. n-6 Fatty acids. In: Forse RA, ed. Diet, nutrition, and immunity. Boca Raton, FL: CRC Press, 1994.
116. Katamura E, Shintaku N, Yamauchi Y, et al. J Immunol 1995;155:4604–12.
117. Wright JR, Lefkowith JB, Schreiner G, et al. Proc Natl Acad Sci USA 1988;85:6137–41.
118. Lefkowith JB, Morrison A, Lee V, et al. J Immunol 1990;145:1523–9.
119. Lefkowith JB, Rogers M, Lennartz MR, et al. J Biol Chem 1991;266:1071–6.
120. Chavali SR, Forse RA. The role of w-3 polyunsaturated fatty acids on immune responses during infection and inflammation. In: Forse RA, ed. Diet, nutrition, and immunity. Boca Raton, FL: CRC Press, 1994.
121. Chandrasekar B, Fernandes G. Biochem Biophys Res Comm 1994;200:893–8.
122. Sanderson P, Yaqoob P, Calder PC. Cell Immunol 1995;164: 240–7.
123. Berger A, German JB, Chiang B-L, et al. J Nutr 1993;123: 225–33.
124. Gallai V, Sarchielli P, Trequattrini A. J Neuroimmunol 1995;56:143–53.
125. Alexander DW, McGuire SO, Cassity NA, et al. J Nutr 1995;125:2640–9.
126. Wu D, Meydani SN, Meydani M, et al. Am J Clin Nutr 1996;63:273–80.
127. Hillier K, Jewell R, Dorrell L, et al. Gut 1991;32:1151–5.
128. Calder PC, Bond JA, Harvey DJ, et al. Biochem J 1990;269:807–14.
129. Cope RB, Bosnic M, Boehm-Wilcox C, et al. J Nutr 1996;126:681–92.
130. Swanson C, Morgon M, Erickson K, et al. Portal venous transfusion (PVT) up regulates Kupffer cell (KC) cyclooxygenase: a mechanism of immunosuppression (Abstract). Proc Assoc Acad Surg, Detroit, 1995;115.
131. Wanders A, Tufveson G, Gerdin B. Scand J Thorac Cardiovasc Surg 1992;26:33–7.
132. Blackburn GL. Proc Soc Exp Biol Med 1992;200:183–8.
133. Gollaher CJ, Bistrian BR. Structured lipids. In: Forse RA, ed. Diet, nutrition, and immunity. Boca Raton, FL: CRC Press, 1994.
134. Ames BN, Shigenaga MK, Hagen TM. Proc Natl Acad Sci USA 1993;90:7915–22.
135. Halliwell B. Nutr Rev 1994;52:253–65.
136. Chew BP. J Nutr 1995;125(Suppl):1804S–8S.
137. Yoshida SH, German JB, Fletcher MP, et al. Reg Toxicol Pharmacol 1994;19:60–79.
138. Yoshida SH, Teuber SS, German JB, et al. Food Chem Toxicol 1994;11:1089–1100.
139. Hatch GE. Am J Clin Nutr 1995;61(Suppl):625S–30S.
140. Droge W, Schulze-Osthoff K, Mihm S, et al. FASEB J 1994;8:1131–8.
141. Grigolo B, Borzi RM, Mariani E, et al. Mech Ageing Dev 1994;73:27–37.
142. Feng L, Xia Y, Garcia GE, et al. J Clin Invest 1995;95:1669–75.
143. Aubailly M, Salmon S, Morliere P, et al. Redox Rep 1996;2:41–5.
144. Cantorna MT, Nashold FE, Chun TY, et al. J Immunol 1996;156:2674–9.
145. Schulze-Osthoff K, Los M, Baeuerle PA. Biochem Pharmacol 1995;50:735–41.
146. Leiter LM, Reuhl DR, Racis SP Jr, et al. J Nutr 1995;125: 474–84.
147. Bach J-F. Immunol Today 1995;16:353–5.
148. Liblau RS, Singer SM, McDevitt HO. Immunol Today 1995;16:34–8.
149. Davies P, MacIntyre DE. Prostaglandins and inflammation. In: Gallin JI, Goldstein IM, Snyderman R, eds. Inflammation: basic principles and clinical correlates. 2nd ed. New York: Raven Press, 1992.
150. Lam BK, Austen KF. Leukotrienes. In: Gallin JI, Goldstein IM, Snyderman R, eds. Inflammation: basic principles and clinical correlates. 2nd ed. New York: Raven Press, 1992.
151. Eze MO. Med Hypotheses 1992;37:220–4.
152. Kubow S. Free Rad Biol Med 1992;12:63–81.

153. Zimmerman GA, Prescott SM, McIntyre TM. J Nutr 1995;125:1661S–5S.
154. Liu J-F, Huang C-J. J Nutr 1995;125:3071–80.
155. Aruoma OI. Food Chem Toxicol 1994;32:671–83.
156. Albrecht R, Pélissier MA. Food Chem Toxicol 1995;33: 1081–3.
157. Ramarathnam N, Osawa T, Ochi H, et al. Trends Food Sci Technol 1995;6:75–82.
158. Bray TM, Taylor CG. Biochem Pharmacol 1994;47:2113–23.
159. Schandler RJ. Clin Perinatol 1995;22:207–22.
160. Lahov E, Regelson W. Food Chem Toxicol 1996;34:131–45.
161. Burns EA, Goodwin JS. Aging: nutrition and immunity. In: Forse RA, ed. Diet, nutrition, and immunity. Boca Raton, FL: CRC Press, 1994.
162. Weksler ME. Ann Neurol 1994;35:S35–7.
163. Lesourd BM, Meaume S. Immunol Lett 1994;40:235–42.
164. Rose NR. Immunol Lett 1994;40:225–30.
165. Bogden JD, Bendich A, Kemp FW, et al. Am J Clin Nutr 1994;60:437–47.
166. Dardenne M, Boukaiba N, Gagnerault MC, et al. Clin Immunol Immunopathol 1993;66:127–35.
167. Mocchegiani E, Santarelli L, Muzzioli M, et al. Int J Immunopharmacol 1995;17:703–18.
168. Meydani SN, Wu D, Santos MS, et al. J Clin Nutr 1995;62(Suppl):1462S–76S.

SELECTED READINGS

Cunningham-Rundles S, ed. Nutrient modulation of the immune response. New York: Marcel Dekker, 1993.
Forse RA, ed. Diet, nutrition, and immunity. Boca Raton, FL: CRC Press, 1994.
Janeway CA Jr, Travers P. Immunobiology. London: Current Biology, 1994.
Klurfeld DM, ed. Human nutrition—a comprehensive treatise, vol 8: Nutrition and immunity. New York: Plenum Press, 1993.
Stites DP, Terr AI, Parslow TG. Basic and clinical immunology. 8th ed. Norwalk, CT: Appleton & Lange, 1994.

46. Oxidative Stress and Oxidant Defense

JAMES A. THOMAS

Oxidative stress has been implicated in human disease by a growing body of scientific evidence. However, cells have multiple protective mechanisms against oxidative stress and succeed in preventing cell damage to the extent that these protective mechanisms are effective. Many dietary constituents are important sources of protective agents that range from antioxidant vitamins and minerals to food additives that might enhance the action of natural antioxidants. Indeed, at least part of the benefit of a high fruit and vegetable diet is thought to derive from the variety of plant antioxidants that might act as beneficial supplements in humans. On the other hand, materials such as pesticides, polyunsaturated lipids, and a variety of plant and microorganism-derived toxins might produce prooxidant effects in man. This chapter deals with our current understanding of the molecules that cause oxidative stress at the cellular level, the antioxidant systems that function at the cellular and organismal level, and the role of dietary materials in oxidative stress and human disease. Other chapters in this volume present more detailed information about individual vitamins and minerals and their potential participation in oxidative stress.

Oxidative stress has been defined as a disturbance in the equilibrium status of prooxidant/antioxidant systems in intact cells (1). This definition implies that cells have intact prooxidant/antioxidant systems that continuously generate and detoxify oxidants during normal aerobic metabolism. When additional oxidative events occur, the prooxidant systems may outbalance the antioxidant, resulting in oxidative damage to lipids, proteins, carbohydrates, and nucleic acids, ultimately leading to cell death in severe oxidative stress. Oxidative stress may induce an alteration in the antioxidant systems by inducing or repressing proteins that participate in these systems and by depleting cellular stores of antioxidant materials such as glutathione and vitamin E.

A disturbance in prooxidant/antioxidant systems results from many different oxidative challenges, including radiation, xenobiotic metabolism of environmental pollutants and administered drugs, and challenges to the immune system in human disease or abnormal immune function. Clear evidence for the role of a variety of radical species in these processes has led to considerable interest in the reactions of partially reduced oxygen species and radical and nonradical species derived from them. Recently, it has also become clear that a variety of reactive nitrogen species derived from the reactions of nitric oxide play important roles as well. A radical species is specifically understood to be any atom that contains one or more orbital electrons with unpaired spin states. The radical may be a very small molecule, such as oxygen or nitric oxide, or part of a large biomolecule such as a protein, carbohydrate, lipid, or nucleic acid. Some radical species are very reactive with other biomolecules, and others, like the normal triplet state of molecular oxygen, are relatively inert.

RADICALS AND NONRADICALS IN OXIDATIVE STRESS

Oxygen Species

Radicals of oxygen (superoxide anion, hydroxyl radical, and peroxy radicals), reactive nonradical oxygen species such as hydrogen peroxide and singlet oxygen, as well as carbon, nitrogen, and sulfur radicals make up the variety of reactive molecules that can constitute an oxidative stress to cells (2, 3). It has been estimated that a maximum of 5% of the total oxygen metabolism of liver tissue results in production of partially reduced oxygen species such as those shown in Figure 46.1. This represents a significant stress by itself, but extracellular sources of these molecules may be even more significant sources of oxidative stress. Therefore, considerable attention centers on identification of oxyradical-generating processes.

Atmospheric oxygen, although a radical, is not particularly reactive with biologic molecules because the two orbital electrons participating in oxidation reactions have the same spin state. Thus, electrons that might be added

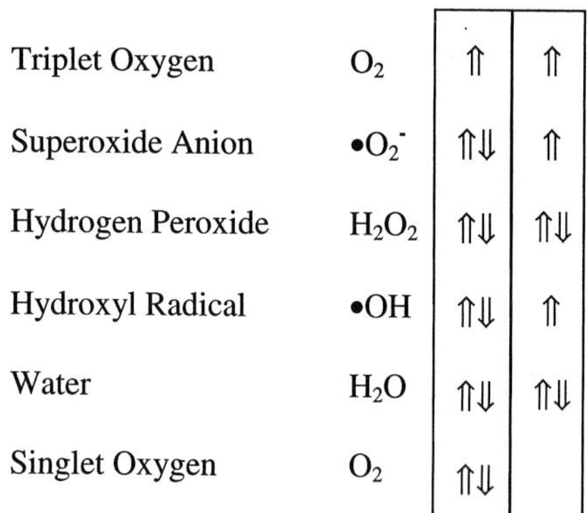

Figure 46.1. Molecular species of oxygen in oxidative stress. Each relevant orbital electron is indicated by an *arrow* showing its spin state. Each molecular species (except for singlet oxygen) is obtained by a one-electron reduction of the one above it in the table. In intact cells, singlet oxygen is formed by oxidation of one of the partially reduced states of oxygen.

to these orbitals during reduction of oxygen must be added singly rather than as a pair of electrons with paired spins. This spin restriction prevents rapid reactions with compounds that could easily react without the spin restriction. Any process that produces a one-electron reduction of oxygen produces the more reactive radical called superoxide anion. A second form of oxygen, singlet oxygen, is a much more reactive form with paired electrons. Reduction of this form of oxygen does not have the same spin state restriction. Singlet oxygen is formed by oxidation of the other reactive oxygen intermediates in Figure 46.1. It has been identified in tissues under oxidative stress and may be an important reactant in oxidative stress.

Superoxide anion is generated continuously by several cellular processes including the microsomal and mitochondrial electron transport systems. In addition, xanthine dehydrogenase/oxidase and other cellular oxidases may be important sources of this molecule. Myeloid cells have a special role in production of superoxide anion since they contain a plasma membrane–bound electron-transfer complex, NADPH oxidase, that reduces oxygen with NADPH to produce copious amounts of superoxide anion (4). The products of this reaction are essential for effective bacterial killing. Absence of this enzyme activity is responsible for an inherited human condition, chronic granulomatous disease, characterized by recurrent infections.

The universal presence of superoxide dismutase in both cytoplasm and mitochondria ensures that much superoxide anion is rapidly converted into hydrogen peroxide. Superoxide anion is not particularly reactive, and it can diffuse considerable distances from its site of production. It may combine with other reactive species such as nitric oxide, produced by macrophages, to yield a more reactive species. It must be transported across membranes (by an anion transport mechanism), and in the vicinity of membranes, it may be protonated to $HO_2\bullet$, a much more reactive substance.

Hydrogen peroxide is generated by the same sources that produce superoxide anion since both enzymatic (superoxide dismutase) and nonenzymatic destruction of superoxide anion produces hydrogen peroxide. A number of other specific enzymes produce hydrogen peroxide directly. These include peroxisomal enzymes associated with fatty acid metabolism and cytoplasmic enzymes responsible for oxidation of a variety of cell metabolites. Hydrogen peroxide can diffuse over considerable distances and may pass membranes readily in this process. Thus, pools of hydrogen peroxide equilibrate rapidly.

Hydrogen peroxide and superoxide anion can occur in the extracellular space and in blood plasma as a result of the membrane-associated reaction in myeloid cells such as neutrophils and macrophages (4). The membrane-associated NADPH-oxidase produces superoxide anion that rapidly dismutes to hydrogen peroxide as well.

In the presence of a transition cation such as iron or copper, superoxide anion can give rise to the highly reactive hydroxyl radical species (HO•) by the Haber-Weiss reaction (see below) (5, 6). Some forms of bound iron are more efficient than free iron in this process. Other complexes of iron prevent its participation in these reactions.

Haber-Weiss reaction

$$O_2\bullet^- + H_2O_2 \rightarrow O_2 + HO^- + HO\bullet$$

Iron-catalyzed Haber-Weiss reaction

$$Fe^{III} + O_2\bullet^- \rightarrow Fe^{II} + O_2$$
$$Fe^{II} + H_2O_2 \rightarrow Fe^{III} + HO^- + HO\bullet$$

Hydroxyl radical is considered a principal actor in the toxicity of partially reduced oxygen species since it is very reactive with all kinds of biologic macromolecules, producing products that cannot be regenerated by cell metabolism (Fig. 46.2). The rate of reaction of hydroxyl radical is diffusion controlled, and it reacts very close to its site of production. Therefore, damage by this radical is very site specific.

Peroxyl radicals occur during oxidation of lipids in oxidative stress and they are associated with the action of prostaglandin H synthase in prostaglandin synthesis (7). These radicals are formed by a one-electron transfer from a carbon-centered radical to oxygen (reaction 1 below). The peroxyl radical species, which are not very reactive, may diffuse a considerable distance. They react avidly with sulfhydryl groups (thiols) to generate the thiyl radical (reaction 2 below) (8).

(1) $R\text{—}\overset{|}{\underset{|}{C}}\bullet + O_2 \rightarrow R\text{—}\overset{|}{\underset{|}{C}}OO\bullet$

(2) $R\text{—}S^- + ROO\bullet \rightarrow R\text{—}S\bullet + ROO^-$
thiolate anion — thiyl radical

Singlet oxygen is formed by oxidation of other partially reduced oxygen species, resulting in an oxygen with paired electrons in the reactive orbital (2).

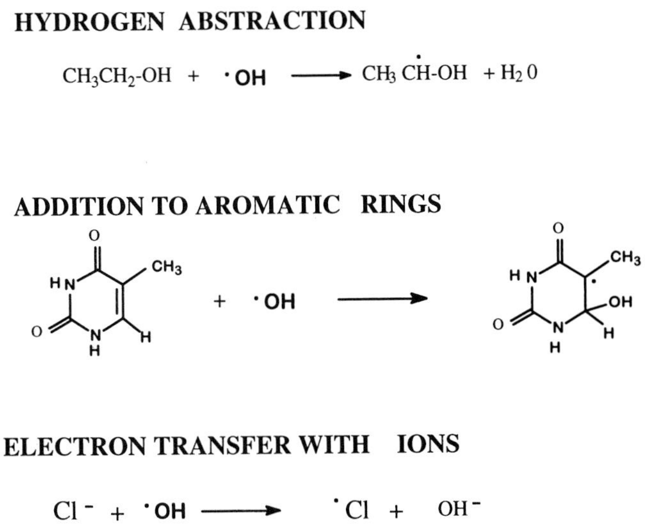

HYDROGEN ABSTRACTION

$$CH_3CH_2\text{-}OH + {}^\bullet OH \longrightarrow CH_3\dot{C}H\text{-}OH + H_2O$$

ADDITION TO AROMATIC RINGS

$$\text{Thymine} + {}^\bullet OH \longrightarrow \text{Thymine–OH adduct radical}$$

ELECTRON TRANSFER WITH IONS

$$Cl^- + {}^\bullet OH \longrightarrow {}^\bullet Cl + OH^-$$

Figure 46.2. Reaction of hydroxyl radicals with biologic molecules.

The variety of oxygen species described above indicates the complexity of the reactions that can result from oxidative stress. Factors such as the site of production, the availability of transition metals, and the action of enzymes determine the fate of each radical species and its availability for reaction with cellular molecules. The H_2O_2 concentration under steady-state conditions in liver has been estimated to be 10^{-7} to 10^{-9} M, while superoxide anion may be 10^{-11} M.

Nitrogen Species

Nitric oxide (NO•) is an abundant reactive radical that acts as an important oxidative biologic signal in a large variety of diverse physiologic processes, including smooth muscle relaxation, neurotransmission, and immune regulation (9). The nitric oxide synthase enzyme generates this nitrogen-based radical species by a five-electron oxidative reaction that uses arginine as its substrate. This enzyme is found in both constitutive and inducible forms in many different cell types, and its activity is highly regulated by Ca^{2+} and other factors. The reaction is a complex one that involves flavin and pterin molecules. Calcium sensitivity is dependent on calmodulin (Fig. 46.3*A*). Nitric oxide synthase is especially active in macrophages and neutrophils. Thus, these cells produce both superoxide anion and nitric oxide during the oxidative burst triggered during inflammatory processes. Under these conditions, nitric oxide and superoxide anion may react together to produce significant amounts of a much more oxidatively active molecule, peroxynitrite (10) (Fig. 46.3*B*). Peroxynitrite is a strong oxidant that attacks protein cysteines and methionines. It also adds an NO_2 to the ring of protein tyrosines. The protein modifications that result from peroxynitrite production may explain some of the observed biologic effects of NO•. Additionally, NO• adds to thiols to form *S*-nitrosothiols (11) (Fig. 46.3*B*). The sulfhydryl is formally oxidized by one electron in this reaction, and subsequent reaction with a reduced thiol leads to formation of a disulfide. *S*-Nitrosothiols may provide a mechanism for transport of NO• in the blood plasma where the low concentration of reduced thiol compounds prevents further reaction of the NO•/thiol adduct.

Production of nitric oxide can *(a)* trigger the production of cGMP through NO•-mediated stimulation of the guanylate cyclase enzyme; *(b)* produce adducts with thiols of various types (e.g., glutathione and protein thiols), generating *S*-nitrosothiols (Fig. 46.3*B*) as intermediates on the way to disulfide formation; *(c)* cause nitration of protein

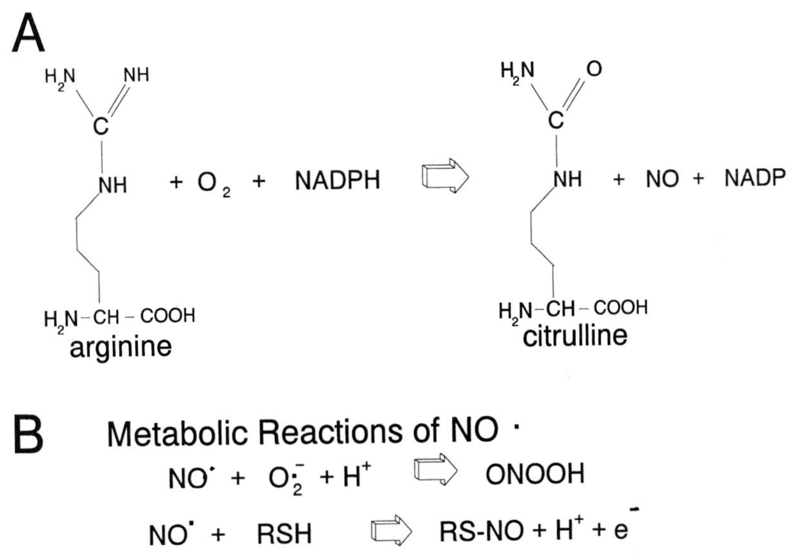

A

$$\text{arginine} + O_2 + NADPH \Rightarrow \text{citrulline} + NO + NADP$$

arginine: $H_2N\text{-}C(=NH)\text{-}NH\text{-}(CH_2)_3\text{-}CH(NH_2)\text{-}COOH$

citrulline: $H_2N\text{-}C(=O)\text{-}NH\text{-}(CH_2)_3\text{-}CH(NH_2)\text{-}COOH$

B Metabolic Reactions of NO ·

$$NO^\bullet + O_2^- + H^+ \Rightarrow ONOOH$$

$$NO^\bullet + RSH \Rightarrow RS\text{-}NO + H^+ + e^-$$

Figure 46.3. Formation and reactions of nitric oxide. *A.* The reaction catalyzed by nitric oxide synthase. The exact stoichiometry of the reaction is not known. The five-electron reaction generates nitric oxide and oxidizes NADPH in the process. *B.* Two important byproducts of nitric oxide generation are shown. In the *top reaction,* peroxynitrite is a simple addition product of superoxide anion and nitric oxide. No oxidation or reduction is necessary. In the *lower reaction, S*-nitrosothiols are formed by a reaction between thiols and nitric oxide that involves a one-electron oxidation. The reaction requires some electron-accepting species.

tyrosine residues through direct nitration reactions; and (*d*) increase oxidative stress through generation of peroxynitrite.

EFFECTS OF OXIDANTS ON MACROMOLECULES

Carbohydrates

Hydroxyl radicals react with carbohydrates by randomly abstracting a hydrogen atom from one of the carbon atoms, producing a carbon-centered radical (12). This leads to chain breaks in important molecules such as hyaluronic acid (Fig. 46.4) in a process that involves such intermediates as peroxyl radicals. In the synovial fluid surrounding joints, accumulation and activation of neutrophils during inflammation produces significant amounts of oxyradicals. This phenomenon apparently accounts for a significant decrease in the synovial fluid of affected joints.

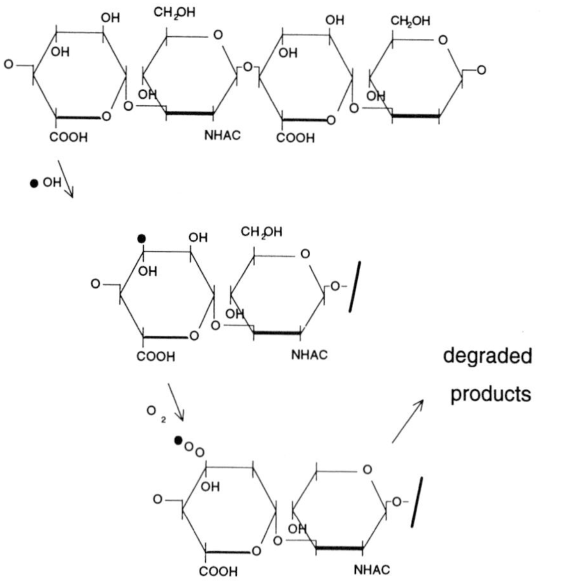

Figure 46.4. Reaction of hydroxyl radicals with polysaccharides (hyaluronic acid).

Nucleic Acids

Nucleic acids are pentose-phosphate polymers that can undergo reactions with hydroxyl radical like those depicted for hyaluronic acid (Fig. 46.4) (13). There are also several important examples of modifications to the base portion of the polymer (Fig. 46.5). In fact these base modifications may be responsible for genetic defects produced by oxidative stress. Recently, 8-hydroxyguanosine has generated considerable interest as a product of hydroxyl radical attack on DNA that can be used to estimate DNA damage in humans (14, 15). Oxidative damage to DNA in humans has been estimated as 104 hits per cell per day. Estimation of modified bases in urine is a useful means of assessing the amount of DNA damage in an animal. Products such as 8-hydroxyguanosine, thymidine glycol, and uric acid are used for these estimates. DNA damage has also been estimated by chain breaks and base modifications in cultured cells under oxidative stress. An important metabolic effect of DNA damage is rapid induction of polyadenosine diphosphate ribose synthesis (ADP-ribosylation) in nuclei, resulting in extensive depletion of cellular NADH pools. ADP-ribosylation has been associated with repair of damaged DNA.

Proteins

Proteins have many reactive sites that can be damaged during oxidative stress, but interest has centered on three measurable events. First, aggressive radicals such as hydroxyl radical can fragment proteins in plasma, and the fragmented products of specific proteins, if known, can be detected (16). This fragmenting is associated with reactions at specific amino acids such as proline (Fig. 46.6*A*) and histidine (17). Second, proteins may contain metal-binding sites that are especially susceptible to oxidative events through interaction with the metals. These reactions usually produce irreversible modifications in amino acids that might be involved in metal ion binding (e.g., histidine). These modifications may produce signal sequences that are recognized by specific cellular proteases that degrade such proteins (18, 19). Finally, many intracellular proteins have "reactive" sulfhydryl groups on specific cysteine residues (see "Cellular Antioxidants") that can be modified (oxidized) to specific forms (disulfides) that can be reduced again metabolically (20). Similarly, some proteins have a "reactive" methionine that can undergo reversible modification to methionine sulfoxide (Fig. 46.6*B*) (21, 22). The disulfide and sulfoxide

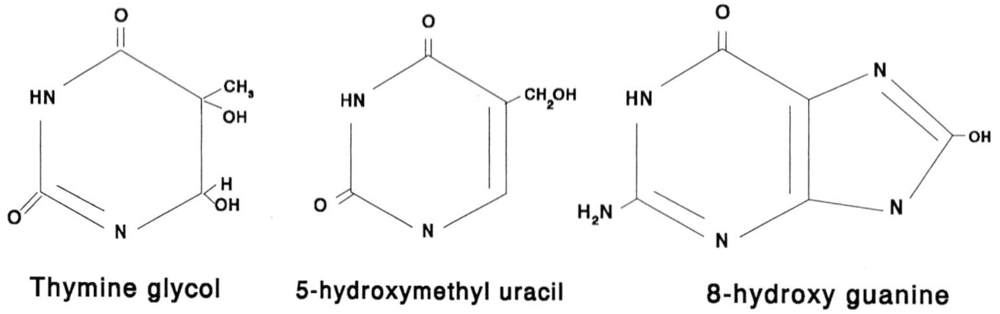

Figure 46.5. Selected modified bases found in DNA after oxidative stress.

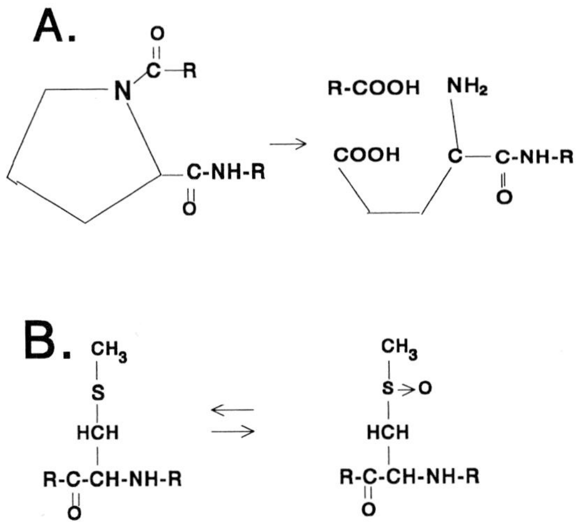

Figure 46.6. Methionine and proline oxidation. *A.* Irreversible oxidation of proline in a peptide. The result is a break in the polypeptide chain and introduction of new carboxyl groups that can be measured to quantitate these events. *B.* Reversible oxidation/reduction of methionine as it occurs in several proteins. The reduction is an enzymatic process that requires a reduced thiol such as glutathione.

forms of these two amino acids may actually serve a protective role, since metabolic reversibility of the protein modification effectually detoxifies the oxidative species that caused the modification. The reversible nature of the modifications of cysteine and methionine also suggests that oxidative modifications of this type may have a role in regulating metabolic events in cells under oxidative stress.

Lipids

Lipid peroxidation of polyunsaturated lipids is a facile process. This oxidation affects materials prevalent in dietary constituents and seriously affects the flavor of foods. In intact cells, these materials are major constituents of cellular membranes (23, 24), where peroxidation of membrane lipid seriously impairs membrane function. Most peroxidized membrane lipid results from oxidative stress in intact cells, but some dietary material may be directly incorporated into cell structures (25). Lipid peroxidation is a radical-initiated chain reaction that is self-propagating in cellular membranes. As a result, isolated oxidative events may have profound effects on membrane function. The reactions of this process are depicted in Figure 46.7.

The products of lipid peroxidation are easily detected in blood plasma and have been used as a measure of oxidative stress. The most commonly measured product is malondialdehyde (Fig. 46.7). In addition, the unsaturated aldehydes produced from these reactions have been implicated in modification of cellular proteins and other materials (26). The peroxidized lipid can produce peroxy radicals and singlet oxygen by reactions discussed above. Vitamin E is a particularly effective antioxidant in lipid-peroxidizing systems.

STEPS OF LIPID PEROXIDATION

(INITIATION) LIPID + R•/OH• → LIPID•

(PROPAGATION) LIPID• + O_2 → LIPID-OO•

LIPID-OO• + LIPID → LIPID-OOH + LIPID•

(TERMINATION) LIPID• + LIPID• → LIPID-LIPID

LIPID-OO• + LIPID• → LIPID-OO-LIPID

(SCAVENGING) LIPID• + VIT E → LIPID + VIT E•

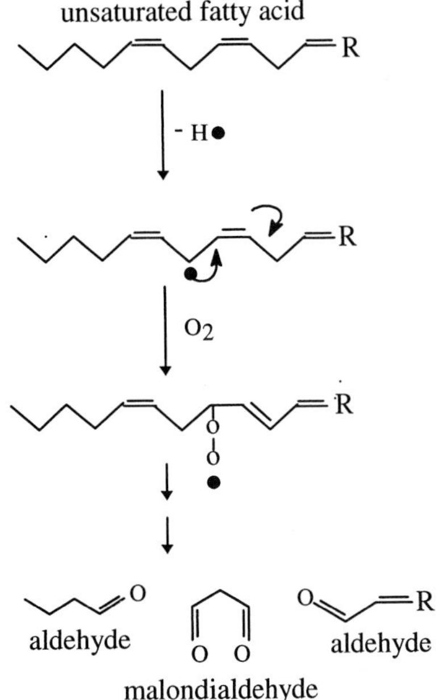

Figure 46.7. Reactions of lipid peroxidation.

CELLULAR ANTIOXIDANTS

The most effective antioxidant in oxidative stress depends on the specific molecules causing the stress (i.e., superoxide anion, lipid peroxides, iron-generated hydroxyl radical, etc.) and the cellular or extracellular location of the source of these molecules. For example, cell membrane damage occurs from both internally and externally generated oxidative stress. This damage is most effectively prevented by vitamin E, which reacts with peroxyl and hydroxyl radicals; carotenoids, which react with singlet oxygen; and possibly membrane-bound proteins. The chain-breaking antioxidant function of vitamin E in membranes results from its close association with polyunsaturated components of the membrane (27). It can be regenerated by reaction with cytoplasmic vitamin C and glutathione or by membrane-bound quinols. Vitamin C is subsequently reduced by glutathione through the glutathione cycle, described below. Thus, a specific attack on membranes results in participation of at least three different antioxidants. Similarly, when oxidative stress occurs in plasma, a variety of different antioxidants participates in the response. Many plasma proteins are affected by the process, causing either irreversible or reversible loss of functional protein activity. A good example is the oxidation of methionine residues in α-1-protease inhibitor (an inhibitor of elastase). The modification can be reversed by a specific reductase enzyme that restores the activity of the inhibitor (21) (Fig. 46.6).

Glutathione Redox Cycle and the Protein S-Thiolation Cycle

The low-molecular-weight thiol, glutathione, and "reactive" protein sulfhydryls (exposed cysteines in many proteins) are primary participants in cellular antioxidant systems. Glutathione (Fig. 46.8) is abundant (3 to 10 mM) in cytoplasm, nuclei, and mitochondria and is the major soluble antioxidant in these cell compartments (28). Reactive protein sulfhydryls are abundant in both soluble and membrane-bound proteins (29).

The sulfur atom in sulfhydryl groups easily accommodates the loss of a single electron (reaction 1 below). The resultant radical species of sulfur (e.g., a thiyl radical) may have significantly longer lifetimes than many other radicals generated during stress. Sulfhydryl groups also partially ionize at cellular pH values, producing the more reactive nucleophile, thiolate anion (reaction 2). The pK_a of the sulfhydryl group of glutathione is 9.3, and many other sulfhydryl groups, especially those on proteins, may have considerably lower pK_as because of local electronic effects. The thiolate anion is responsible for the reactivity of thiols with a variety of foreign materials in conjugation reactions during xenobiotic metabolism. Thus, the reactions of sulfhydryl groups during oxidative stress include examples in which both sulfur radicals and thiolate anions are important.

(1) Glutathione—SH → glutathione-S•
Protein-SH → protein-S•
(2) R—SH → R—S^- + H^+
Protein—SH → protein—S^- + H^+

The enzymes of the glutathione redox cycle and the protein S-thiolation cycle are shown in Figure 46.9*A*. The glutathione redox cycle is primarily mediated by enzyme-catalyzed reactions. Glutathione is oxidized by hydrogen peroxide to glutathione disulfide by the selenium-containing enzyme glutathione peroxidase and other enzymes that may use lipid peroxides rather than hydrogen peroxide as the oxidant. Thus, glutathione can detoxify both soluble and lipid peroxides. Glutathione disulfide is subsequently reduced by glutathione reductase, using NADPH as the reductant. Cellular NADPH, produced by the pentose-P pathway and other cytoplasmic sources, provides the major source of reducing power for detoxifying many peroxides.

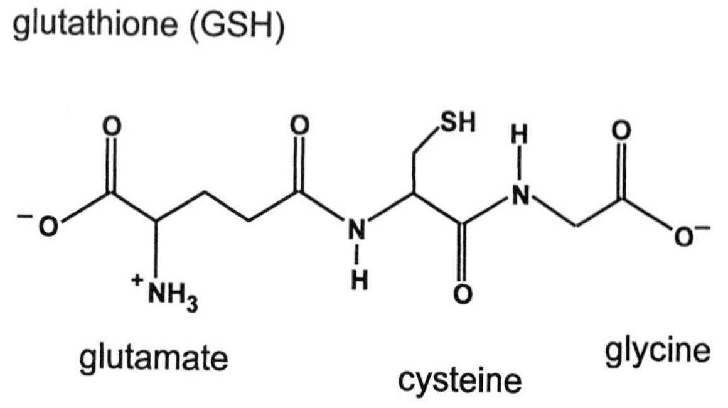

glutathione (GSH)

glutamate cysteine glycine

Figure 46.8. Structure of glutathione.

The concentration of cellular glutathione has a major effect on its antioxidant function, and it varies considerably as a result of nutrient limitation, exercise, and oxidative stress. Under oxidative conditions, the glutathione concentration can be considerably diminished through conjugation to xenobiotics and by secretion of both the glutathione conjugates and glutathione disulfide from the affected cells. Considerable glutathione may also become protein bound during severe oxidative stress. Recently, compounds have been developed that can both increase and decrease the glutathione concentration when administered to animals (30). Some of these compounds may provide the means to modify glutathione concentration in humans in the future. Experiments have already shown benefits in autoimmune disease in which glutathione concentrations are reduced.

The protein S-thiolation cycle (Fig. 46.9*A*) shows the effects of reactive oxidizing molecules on proteins that contain at least one reactive sulfhydryl. During oxidative stress, a large family of proteins that contain reactive sulfhydryls are modified by oxidation to mixed disulfides with attached glutathione (S-thiolation) (20). Other oxidized forms of protein sulfhydryls may occur in special circumstances. One such case may be when the glutathione concentration is too low for reaction with the protein sulfhydryl and reaction with molecular oxygen irreversibly oxidizes it to the sulfonic acid. Another case might be found in proteins in which adjacent protein sulfhydryls can react together to form a protein disulfide. The potential to form protein disulfides is not great for intracellular proteins, although these modifications are abundant in extracellular proteins. Figure 46.9*A* illustrates the protein oxidation cycle that involves formation of S-thiolated proteins. Figure 46.9*B* illustrates the mechanism for reduction of S-thiolated proteins by the low-molecular-weight protein glutaredoxin (31, 32). Glutaredoxin is kept reduced by the glutathione pool. It binds to, and reduces, proteins that have glutathione attached by S-thiolation, by virtue of the specific binding site for glutathione at the active site of the protein. This protein is uniquely designed to reduce S-thiolated proteins.

Vitamin E and Membrane Peroxidation

The term *vitamin E* refers to a family of related compounds (tocopherols) that have hydroxylated aromatic rings (chromanol rings) and isoprenoid side chains. These molecules are highly lipophilic and reside almost

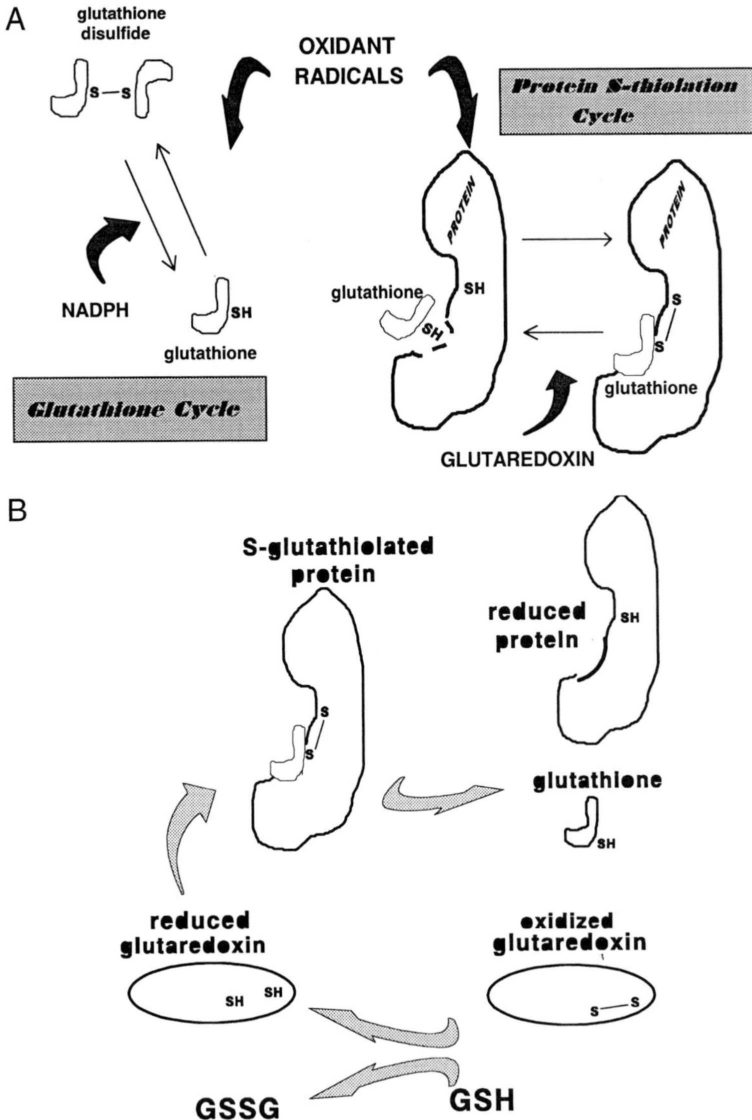

Figure 46.9. Redox cycles of cellular thiols. *A.* The figure on the *top* shows the glutathione and protein S-thiolation redox cycles. Glutathione is oxidized to glutathione disulfide primarily by hydrogen peroxide. It is reduced again by an enzyme, glutathione reductase, that requires NAPDH. Proteins are oxidized to S-thiolated forms by several oxidants and reduced again by the protein glutaredoxin. Glutaredoxin is kept reduced by glutathione. *B.* Molecular details of the reaction of glutaredoxin, a dithiol protein, with S-thiolated proteins.

exclusively in cell membranes, where the chromanol ring may be at the surface of the membrane, with the isoprenoid chain inserted into the bilayer (33). Since lipid peroxidation occurs on unsaturated fatty acid chains that reside within the lipid bilayer and the chromanol ring is the active radical-quenching part of the vitamin, the function of vitamin E as an antioxidant must involve considerable movement of lipids and vitamin E to promote molecular interaction (34). The reactions in which a chromanol ring can participate in these processes are shown in Figure 46.10. This figure shows that vitamin E is a chain-reaction-breaking antioxidant since it quenches the intermediate in the chain reaction. The ascorbate radical formed in this process reacts rapidly with the reduced glutathione pool or with a specific vitamin C reductase enzyme.

Enzymes As Antioxidants in Cells

Superoxide dismutase (SOD) is one of the most important enzymes that function as cellular antioxidants (35). It is present in cell cytoplasm (copper-zinc enzyme) and in mitochondria (manganese enzyme) to maintain a low concentration of superoxide anion. It catalyzes the dismutation of superoxide anion in the following manner.

$$2\ O_2\bullet^- + 2\ H^+ \rightarrow O_2 + H_2O_2$$

Absence of this enzyme is lethal. However, too much may also be detrimental, since an excess of this enzyme may produce hydrogen peroxide at a rate that is toxic to cells during oxidative stress. The amount of superoxide dismutase is controlled by specific redox-sensitive genes in cells (36). An extracellular form of superoxide dismutase exists

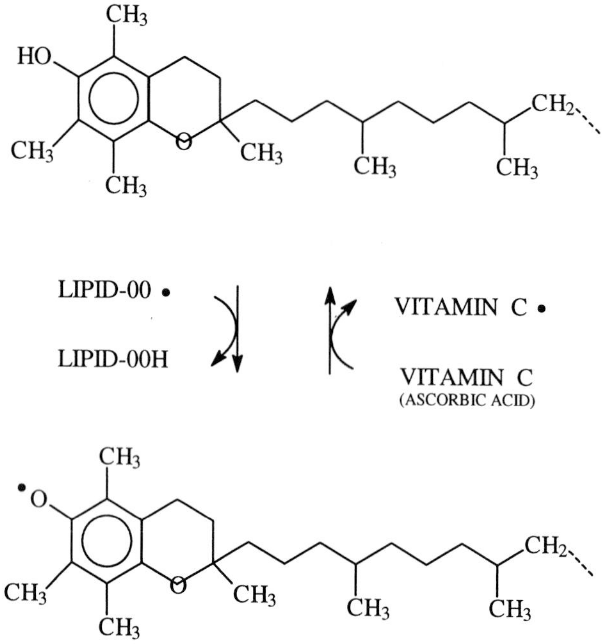

LIPID-00 •

LIPID-00H

VITAMIN C •

VITAMIN C
(ASCORBIC ACID)

Figure 46.10. Oxidation of vitamin E by lipid radicals and reduction by vitamin C.

in plasma, lymph, and synovial fluid that differs from the intracellular forms of the enzyme (37). This enzyme may function at cell surfaces.

Catalase is a heme protein that catalyzes the reaction shown below in which hydrogen peroxide is detoxified. It is usually found in peroxisomes, but in cells like erythrocytes that do not contain these organelles (38), it is a cytoplasmic enzyme. Catalase provides a protective role that is similar to that of glutathione peroxidase in that both remove hydrogen peroxide. The relative contributions of catalase and glutathione peroxidase to hydrogen peroxide detoxification may be quite variable (39).

$$2\ H_2O_2 \rightarrow O_2 + 2\ H_2O$$

PLASMA ANTIOXIDANTS

Human plasma contains little catalase, superoxide dismutase, glutathione, or glutathione peroxidase, but a number of small molecules and protein constituents contribute to the antioxidant properties of this important fluid. Plasma has been studied by use of artificially generated oxidants and with such natural oxidants a cigarette smoke. Plasma ascorbate is among the first compounds that become oxidized in stress (40, 41). Other materials may become oxidized only when ascorbate is depleted. Oxidation affects thiol groups (mostly on proteins), bilirubin, urate, and vitamin E. Bilirubin (bound to albumin) and uric acid, both considered to be waste products in plasma, are potentially good scavengers of oxyradicals. Transport in and out of erythrocytes may provide additional antioxidant potential, since the reductive processes of these cells are quite vigorous.

The most important antioxidant proteins of plasma include ceruloplasmin, albumin, transferrin, haptoglobin, and hemopexin. The first three proteins may sequester iron and copper ions in forms that prevent their participation in reactions that generate the aggressive hydroxyl radical. Haptoglobin and hemopexin bind free heme, a source of iron that can participate in lipid oxidation reactions.

A second aspect of oxidative stress in plasma fractions is the oxidation of lipid particles such as low-density lipoproteins (LDLs) (42). These materials contain proteins and lipids that are good targets for oxidation, and the oxidized forms of LDLs are strongly implicated in fatty lesions (atheromas) in artery walls. Oxidation of LDLs causes a fragmentation of the apoprotein B component of these particles and also producing a variety of lipid peroxidation products, including adducts between lipid and apoprotein B. LDL particles contain a significant amount of vitamin E, which serves as a primary antioxidant.

HUMAN DISEASE AND OXIDATIVE STRESS

The role of oxidative stress in human disease is a subject of intense interest in recent years. The human immune response makes extensive use of many of the oxidative molecules discussed here, generating both superoxide anion and nitric oxide as an integral part of the response to foreign materials. Clearly, this defense system is a two-edged sword that also increases the oxidative risk to its human host. Other foreign materials, including some medicines, also generate oxidative stress during metabolic events associated with their detoxification or excretion. The following paragraphs summarize research that points to the potential importance of oxidative stress in specific human diseases.

Cancer

Radicals of different kinds are potentially involved in both initiation and promotion in multistage cancer development (43, 44). In this process, DNA is damaged and cellular antioxidant systems are modified as a result of expression of different genetic components in precancerous and tumor cells. Since specific genes are apparently controlled by oxidation/reduction switching of important gene regulatory proteins, the effect of oxidative stress may be manifested directly by alterations in these specific proteins (36, 44). On the other hand, base modifications (Fig. 46.5) may also alter the response of certain genes during oxidative stress. Free-radical scavengers function as inhibitors at both the initiation and promotion stage of carcinogenesis, thus protecting cells from the oxidative damage that occurs (45). In tumors the enzymes involved in antioxidant systems are altered, i.e., tumors are low in manganese superoxide dismutase and possibly the copper-zinc enzyme, while glutathione peroxidase, reductase, and *S*-transferase are increased. In keeping with increased glutathione metabolism, one also finds increased glucose 6-P dehydrogenase, a source of NADPH for the glutathione and protein S-thiolation cycles (Fig. 46.9).

Some of the effective quinone-type anticancer drugs are promoters of oxyradical production (46). These drugs may be effective in part because of their ability to generate oxidative species that cause DNA, membrane, or enzyme damage in tumor cells.

Cataracts and Eye Injury

The crystallins, major proteins of the eye lens, are long-lived proteins that are abundant in methionine and cysteine. As discussed above, these amino acids are sensitive to oxidation, and much work has suggested that oxidation of these proteins is involved in development of lens opacities (47, 48). The lens is a highly susceptible target, since it is continually exposed to the effects of light and a number of oxidizing metabolic products. It has a high concentration of glutathione and glutathione reductase, and there is evidence that glutathione decreases substantially in lens lesions. The vitreous humor of the eye also contains hyaluronic acid that is depolymerized when exposed to oxyradicals. Dietary vitamin E helps to prevent eye damage in infants exposed to high oxygen concentrations.

Reperfusion Injury

There is growing evidence that oxyradicals can mediate tissue injury during ischemia and reperfusion (49). Accumulation of neutrophils in the damaged tissue produces a significant oxidant stress to the surviving tissue cells, leading to irreversible injury to those cells as a result of massive generation of superoxide anion and other neutrophil products (50). Much of this damage is preventable by inhibitors of oxyradical generation and by materials that destroy the radicals after generation (e.g., superoxide dismutase or mannitol.

Arthritis and Rheumatic Disorders

Arthritis and rheumatic disorders are characterized by inflammatory responses in which extensive tissue damage can occur through oxidative stress (51). In rheumatoid arthritis, the effects of oxyradicals on the function of synovial fluid have been well documented (see Fig. 46.4). In addition, extensive cellular damage results in release of clastogenic factors, and typical cellular damage products are detected in urine. Thus, materials such as peroxidized lipid or modified bases from cellular DNA have been found in patients suffering from these diseases. It has been postulated that antigens may be created by oxyradical attack on biomolecules, thereby instigating development of autoimmune antibodies and a continuing inflammatory response in affected tissue.

Amyotrophic Lateral Sclerosis

The motor neuron degeneration characteristic of amyotrophic lateral sclerosis has been related to genetic defects in the superoxide dismutase gene (52). Many of the patients with the familial form of this disease have defective superoxide dismutase enzymes. The mutations in the protein occur in many different locations, and apparently all can be related to a loss of enzymatic activity. Since nonhereditary forms of this disease do not contain these lesions, the exact role of oxidative stress in motor neuron degeneration is unclear.

Viral Autoimmune Disease

The autoimmune disease caused by retroviruses is characterized by a loss of specific circulatory immune cells and depression of the glutathione content of virus-infected cells (53). It has been suggested that glutathione deficiency is permissive for replication of the AIDS virus and that supplementation with agents that can increase glutathione is preventive for virus replication (54, 55). It has also been suggested that part of this effect may result from oxidation/reduction control of certain transcription factors, including NFκB.

REFERENCES

1. Sies H. Oxidative stress: introductory remarks. In: Sies H, ed. Oxidative stress. Orlando, FL: Academic Press, 1985;1–10.
2. Cardenas E. Annu Rev Biochem 1989;58:79–110.
3. Slater TF. Biochem J 1984;222:1–15.
4. Badwey JA, Karnovsky M.L. Curr Topics Cell Regul 1986;28: 183–208.
5. Halliwell B, Gutteridge JMC. Biochem J 1984;219:1–14.
6. Sutton HC. J Free Radic Biol Med 1985;1:195–202.
7. Marnett LJ. Carcinogenesis 1989;8:1365–73.
8. Willson RL. Organic peroxy free radicals as ultimate agents in oxygen toxicity. In: Sies H, ed. Oxidative stress. Orlando, FL: Academic Press, 1985;41–72.
9. Bredt DS, Snyder SH. Annu Rev Biochem 1994;63:175–95.

10. Radi R, Beckman JS, Bush KM, Freeman BA. J Biol Chem 1991;266:4244–50.
11. Gow AJ, Buerk DG, Ischiropoulos H. J Biol Chem 1997; 272:2841–5.
12. von Sonntag C. Adv Carbohydr Chem Biochem 1980;37:7–77.
13. Shulte-Frohlinde D, von Sonntag C. Radiolysis of DNA and model systems in the presence of oxygen. In: Sies H, ed. Oxidative stress. Orlando, FL: Academic Press, 1985;11–37.
14. Fraga CG, Shigenaga JP, Degan P, Ames BN. Proc Natl Acad Sci USA 1990;87:4533–7.
15. Floyd RA. FASEB J 1990;4:2587–97.
16. Wolff SP, Garner A, Dean RT. Trends Biochem Sci 1986;11: 27–31.
17. Dean RT, Wolff SP, McElligott MA. Free Radic Res Commun 1989;7:97–103.
18. Stadtman ER. Free Radic Biol Med 1990;9:315–25.
19. Davies KJA. J Biol Chem 1987;262:9895–901.
20. Thomas JA, Poland B, Honzatko R. Arch Biochem Biophys 1995;319:1–9.
21. Brot H, Weissbach H. Arch Biochem Biophys 1983;223:271–81.
22. Levine RL, Mosoni L, Berlett BS, Stadtman ER. Proc Natl Acad Sci USA 1997;93:15036–40.
23. Gutteridge JMC. Lipid peroxidation; some problems and concepts. In: Halliwell B, ed. Oxygen radicals and tissue injury. Bethesda, MD: FASEB for Upjohn Co., 1988;9–19.
24. Gardner HW. Free Radic Biol Med 1989;7:65–86.
25. Wills ED. The role of dietary components in oxidative stress in tissues. In: Sies H, ed., Oxidative stress. Orlando, FL: Academic Press, 1985;197–220.
26. Witz G. Free Radic Biol Med 1989;7:333–49.
27. Pascoe GA, Reed DJ. Free Radic Biol Med 1989;6:209–24.
28. Meister A. J Biol Chem 1988;263:17205–8.
29. Ziegler DM. Annu Rev Biochem 1985;54:305–30.
30. Anderson ME, Meister A. Anal Biochem 1989;183:16–20.
31. Jung CH, Thomas JA. Arch Biochem Biophys 1996;335:61–72.
32. Gravina SA, Mieyal JJ. Biochemistry 1993;32:3368–76.
33. Niki E, Yamamoto Y, Takahashi M, et.al., Ann NY Acad Sci 1989;570:23–31.
34. Wayner DDM, Burton GW, Ingold KU, et al. Biochim Biophys Acta 1987;924:408–19.
35. Fridovich I. J Biol Chem 1989;264:7761–4.
36. Storz G, Tartaglia LA, Ames BN. Science 1990;248:189–94.
37. Marklund SL. Proc Natl Acad Sci USA 1982;79:7634–8.
38. Jones DP. Arch Biochem Biophys 1982;214:806–14.
39. Thayer WS. FEBS Lett 1986;202:137–40.
40. Halliwell B, Gutteridge JMC. Arch Biochem Biophys 1990;280: 1–8.
41. Stocker R, Glazer AN, Ames BN. Proc Natl Acad Sci USA 1987;84:5918–22.
42. Steinbrecher UP, Zhang H, Lougheed M. Free Radic Biol Med 1990;9:155–68.
43. Sun Y. Free Radic Biol Med 1990;8:583–99.
44. Abate C, Patel L, Raucher FJ, Curran T. Science 1990; 249:1157–61.
45. Ito N, Hirose M. Adv Cancer Res 1989;53:247–303.
46. Powis G. Free Radic Biol Med 1989;6:63–101.
47. Bloemendal H. CRC Crit Rev Biochem 1982;14:1–38.
48. Mandel K, Chakrabarti B, Thomson J, Siezen RJ. J Biol Chem 1987;262:8096–102.
49. Simpson PJ, Fantone JC, Lucchesi BR. Myocardial ischemia and reperfusion injury: oxygen radicals and the role of the neutrophil. In: Halliwell B, ed. Oxygen radicals and tissue injury. Bethesda, MD: FASEB for Upjohn Co., 1988;63–80.
50. Warren JS, Yabroff KR, Mandel DM, et al. Free Radic Biol Med 1990;8:163–72.
51. Halliwell B, Gutteridge JMC. Free radicals in biology and medicine. 2nd ed. Oxford: Clarendon Press, 1989;422–38.
52. Deng HX, Hentati A, Tainer JA, et al. Science 1993;261: 1047–51.
53. Staal FJT, Roederer M, Israelski R, et al. AIDS Res Hum Retroviruses 1992;8:20–9.
54. Staal FJ, Roederer M, Herzenberg LA, Herzenberg LA. Proc Natl Acad Sci USA 1990;87:9943–7.
55. Kalebic T, Kinter A, Poli G, et al. Proc Natl Acad Sci USA 1991;88:986–90.

SELECTED READINGS

Halliwell B, Gutteridge JMC. Free radicals in biology and medicine. 2nd ed. Oxford: Clarendon Press, 1989.

Packer L. ed. Methods in enzymology; oxygen radicals in biological systems, part C. San Diego: Academic Press, 1994.

Packer L, ed. Methods in enzymology; oxygen radicals in biological systems, part D. San Diego: Academic Press, 1994.

Sies H, ed. Oxidative stress: oxidants and anti-oxidants. London: Academic Press, 1991.

Tarr M, Samson R, eds. Oxygen free radicals and tissue injury. Boston: Birkhauser, 1993.

Weir EK, Archer SL, Reeves JT, ed. Nitric oxide and radicals in the pulmonary vasculature. Armonk, NY: Futura Publishing, 1996.

47. Diet in Work and Exercise Performance

ERIC HULTMAN, ROGER C. HARRIS, and LAWRENCE L. SPRIET

Interest in the relationship between diet and activity, whether athletic, combative, or occupational, is not new, although the current explosion of literature in the field would suggest the opposite. An adequate intake of foodstuffs is fundamental to the maintenance of health and the survival of the individual. Reportedly, both the Greeks and Romans were interested in the best foodstuffs for maximal performance, but it would be surprising if even earlier, man did not have a similar interest. Understanding the significance of different foodstuffs and rationalization of this information to the energy requirements of different levels of activity, however, only really began in the last century with the work of the German physiologist von Liebig (1). He considered that muscle proteins were the main provider of energy in working skeletal muscle, although by the end of the 19th century, it was clear that this was incorrect and the main sources were in fact carbohydrate and possibly also fat (2, 3).

The first positive evidence of the importance of fat as a substrate for energy production during contraction of muscle was presented by Himwich and Rose (4). They measured respiratory quotients (RQs) of muscle in dogs, which in the well-fed state were 0.92 at rest and 0.94 during exercise. After 5 to 15 days of starvation, these values decreased to 0.80 both at rest and during exercise. Since oxidation of carbohydrates results in an RQ of 1.00 and fat one of 0.70, the results clearly indicated increased use of fat by the muscle after starvation. A decade later, Christensen and Hansen in their classic study of the influence of diet on work performance in man similarly observed lower RQs both at rest and during exercise after a high-fat diet and a 30% reduction in endurance time compared with that when a mixed diet was given (5). In contrast, a high-carbohydrate diet resulted in an increase in exercise RQ, and although this value decreased during exercise (showing an increase in fat use), it never went below the resting value measured after the mixed diet. Endurance time after the carbohydrate diet was about twice that after the mixed diet.

Today, we know that some energy expenditure during exercise can also be derived from protein use, especially when the work time is prolonged. The amount of energy covered, however, is only a few percent of the total, and in the isocaloric state, carbohydrate and fatty acids constitute the major energy sources. Final proof was eventually provided by direct measurement of the different substrates in the working muscles, using the needle biopsy technique introduced by Bergström and Hultman in the mid-1960s. Initially devised to study water and electrolytes in kidney patients (6), the biopsy technique was subsequently used to study muscle glycogen in diabetic patients (7) and local energy stores in normal muscle at rest and during exercise

---

Conversion of SI to traditional units: phosphate (as inorganic phosphorus), mmol/L × 3.097 = mg/dL; glucose, mmol/L × 18 = mg/dL; 1 kilojoule (kJ) = 4.18 kcal; 1 megajoule (MJ) = 1000 kJ.

(8–21). Introduction of the needle biopsy technique had a major, almost catalytic effect on the growth of exercise biochemistry and physiology as scientific disciplines. In 1970, the closely similar liver biopsy technique was used to measure the second major carbohydrate store in the body (22–26). In combination with muscle, blood, and respiratory measurements, an almost complete picture of substrate use in exercising man could be obtained.

An understanding of substrate use by the body during exercise and work is basic to a rational assessment of the nutritive needs of an individual. Today, with the immense popularity of recreational exercise, awareness of the effects of adequate nutrition on work performance is perhaps greater than ever before. However, even among the most fastidious—the elite athletes and their trainers—a plethora of nutritive practices exist that seem to owe more to the early work of von Liebig than to subsequent studies.

ENERGY SUBSTRATES AVAILABLE FOR WORK

When a muscle such as the quadriceps femoris is stimulated from rest to near maximal activity, the rate of energy expenditure increases approximately 300-fold. The energy used by the body to perform work is chemical, and the immediate energy source for muscle contraction is adenosine triphosphate (ATP). ATP, however, is stored in only small amounts in the muscle cells (approximately 5.5 mmol/kg) and must be continually resynthesized from adenosine diphosphate (ADP). The energy for rephosphorylation can be derived from several reactions that can be divided into those requiring oxygen (aerobic metabolism) and those that can proceed in its absence (anaerobic metabolism).

Aerobic resynthesis of ATP occurs only within the mitochondria, the rate of synthesis depending largely on the size and number of mitochondria per muscle cell and the rate of oxygen uptake. Basic fuels that can supply substrates for oxidation are glucose transported from the liver by the blood, locally stored glycogen, and free fatty acids (FFAs) taken up from the blood or to a limited extent derived from triglyceride depots within the muscle. Each of these fuels may be metabolized within the cytoplasm to smaller subunits that then enter the tricarboxylic cycle within the mitochondria.

When oxidative energy production is insufficient to cover the expenditure, as in the early stages of exercise before full readjustment of the blood supply or during high-intensity exercise, ATP is also resynthesized anaerobically, which involves two metabolic pathways. The first is from phosphocreatine (PCr), which in the presence of creatine kinase can directly rephosphorylate ADP to ATP. The second route is from glycogen or glucose with formation of lactate. This process is energetically far less efficient than metabolizing either substrate completely to CO_2 and H_2O; anaerobic metabolism generates only 2 to 3 ATPs compared with 38 to 39 ATPs per glucose unit when oxidized.

The contribution of the different fuel supplies to the total energy output by the muscle varies with both the intensity and duration of exercise and is influenced further by the fitness of the individual, the nutritional status both before and during exercise, the level of anxiety, and even the environment (altitude, temperature, and humidity). Morphologic differences in muscle fiber makeup between individuals may also affect their use of the different fuels available during a standard exercise.

The maximum theoretical rate of use of a particular fuel for muscle contraction is determined by the activity of the enzymes involved in its metabolism. Estimates of the maximum power available from PCr, carbohydrate, and fat use by muscle are presented here both as the maximum amount of high-energy phosphate (~P) that may be generated per kilogram of fresh muscle per second and as the maximum rate calculated for the whole muscle mass, assumed to be 28 kg in a 70-kg person. Values in this latter case are given as moles of ~P per minute.

$$\text{ATP, PCr} \rightarrow \text{ADP, Creatine} \quad (47.1)$$

a. Max. rate of degradation: 2.6 mmol ~P/kg muscle/sec, corresponding totally to 4.4 mol ~P/min
b. Amount available (quadriceps muscle): 24 mmol ~P/kg muscle, or totally, 0.67 mol/28 kg of muscle

The estimate of 2.6 mmol ~P/kg muscle/sec was calculated from direct measurements in needle biopsy samples obtained from human quadriceps muscle during near-maximum voluntary isometric contraction (27, 28) or during tetanic electrical stimulation (29). Other workers have suggested a figure nearer to 6 mmol ~P/kg muscle/sec on the basis of less-direct measurements (30–32). This is close to the maximum velocity of creatine kinase measured in human muscle (33).

$$\text{Glycogen} \rightarrow \text{lactate (anaerobic glucolysis)} \quad (47.2a)$$

a. Max. rate of ~P generation: 1.4 mmol ~P/kg muscle/sec, corresponding totally to 2.35 mol ~P/min
b. Amount available (quadriceps muscle): 240 mmol ~P/kg, or totally, 6.7 mol/28 kg of muscle

The estimate of 1.4 mmol ~P/kg muscle/sec was calculated from direct measurements of metabolite changes during near-maximum isometric contraction of the quadriceps muscle (27, 28). The total amount of ~P available from glycogen was calculated assuming that 90% of the normal store (i.e., 80 mmol glucose units/kg) is used (13) and that 3 mmol ~P is formed per mole of glucose in glucolysis. Total use of the muscle glycogen stores, however, never occurs, because of increased acidosis within the muscle. According to Margaria et al., accumulation of 1 mol of lactate is the maximum the body can tolerate (34). This amount would limit the total amount of ~P from anaerobic use of glycogen to 1.5 mol during heavy continuous work.

$$\text{Glycogen} \rightarrow CO_2 + H_20 \quad (47.2b)$$

a. Max. rate of ~P generation: 0.51 to 0.68 mmol ~P/kg muscle/sec, corresponding totally to 0.85 to 1.14 mol ~P/min.
b. Amount available (quadriceps femoris): 3000 mmol ~P/kg, or totally 84 mol/28 kg of muscle.

The limiting factor for the rate of glycogen oxidation is most probably mitochondrial electron transport determined by the activity of the oxygen transfer mechanisms. The rates of 0.51 to 0.68 were calculated assuming maximum rates of oxygen use available for glycogen oxidation of 3 L O_2/min in an untrained individual and 4 L/min in a marathon runner. Aerobic glycogen degradation gives 38 mol ~P/mol glucose.

$$\text{Glucose} \rightarrow CO_2 + H_2O \quad (47.2c)$$

a. Max. rate of ~P generation: 0.22 mmol ~P/kg muscle/sec, corresponding totally to 0.16 mol ~P/min.
b. Total amount available: 18 mol ~P.

The maximum rate of use is approximate and assumes maximum output from the liver of 5 mmol glucose/min, of which 4 mmol/min is available to the working muscles (calculated in this study as 11 kg) (20, 35). During a short period of exercise, most of this glucose is derived from liver glycogen, which corresponds to 500 mmol glucose totally in the resting state after a mixed diet (36). This quantity will amount to 18 mol ~P.

$$\text{Fatty acids} \rightarrow CO_2 + H_2O \quad (47.3)$$

a. Max. rate of ~P generation: 0.24 mmol ~P/kg muscle/sec, corresponding totally to 0.4 mol ~P/min
b. Amount available: in adipose tissues, about 4000 mol ~P.

The maximum rate of ~P generation, which was calculated by McGilvery (37), is based on experimental results published by Pernow and Saltin (38). As noted by McGilvery, the low rate of ~P generation from FFA oxidation must be the result of a limiting step located before formation of acetyl coenzyme A (acetyl-CoA), because the later steps are also used when carbohydrates are oxidized.

SUBSTRATE USE IN RELATION TO WORKLOAD

The mechanisms by which the muscle cells regulate the use of the different fuels are complex. In essence, FFAs constitute the main energy substrate at rest and are used in preference to carbohydrate; at supramaximal workloads, muscle glycogen and PCr are the major fuels. At no one workload, however, does muscle use just one fuel.

Some examples of energy demands during different types of exercise are given in Table 47.1. The rate of energy expenditure and the amount of energy needed for the activity determine the choice of substrate. Estimates of the energy requirement used in different activities are derived from Fox (39). Estimates of maximum rates available from the different fuel sources together with the total amount available are drawn from our own work based on direct measurements from biopsy studies, with the exception of the estimates for fat oxidation. Values for fat oxidation were recalculated by McGilvery from studies by Pernow and Saltin. The maximum rate during a 100-m sprint has been estimated to be 2.6 mol ~P/min. This value is below the maximum rate obtainable from PCr breakdown but above that from anaerobic glucolysis. On energetic grounds, therefore, ATP and PCr are obligatory fuels for this level of activity, although supply is augmented by anaerobic glucolysis. It was held previously that during intense exercise, an alactic acid period of up to 10 seconds occurred, but lactic acid accumulation begins within 1.3 sec (29). Other athletic activities that depend mainly on PCr breakdown are the shot-put, high jump, javelin, tossing the caber, and the hammer throw.

During a 400-m sprint, PCr breakdown is again used to meet the rate of ~P expenditure (2.3 mol/min) but alone cannot cover the total energy requirement of 1.72 mol ~P. To meet this demand, further energy is required from anaerobic glucolysis with, in practice, an increasing contribution from aerobic glucolysis as the race continues. The same is true both for 800- and 1500-m distances, but in these races, total expenditure exceeds even the combined total possible from PCr breakdown and tolerance from the accumulation of lactate. At these distances, energy demand necessitates oxidative use of muscle glycogen. At ultralong distances, such as the marathon, the ATP turnover rate in an elite athlete lies just below the rate sustainable by aerobic use of carbohydrate; however, the total demand requires considerable use of fat as well. When all available carbohydrate has been used, running speed is dictated by the maximum rate of fat use. Some marathon runners can reach this point (synonymous with "hitting the wall") at about 15 to 20 miles, depending on how the race is run. From then on, the race is run on oxidation of fat, the only fuel available, with little or no possibility for acceleration of pace.

The preceding calculations are drawn from athletic performances, but undoubtedly, the same spectrum of fuel use also exists in occupational work ranging from light office work to hard intermittent manual labor.

During exercise, PCr functions both as an energy buffer to ATP use, particularly when the ATP demand is momentarily increased and/or sustained above the level available from glucolysis and oxidation, and as a buffer to the release of free ADP (ADP_f) at the muscle contractile site. A fall in the PCr content below the critical threshold required to maintain ADP_f homeostasis will result in the onset of adenine nucleotide degradation to inosine monophosphate (IMP) as the adenosine monophosphate (AMP) concentration increases. In normal subjects undertaking strenuous exercise, the onset of adenine nucleotide degradation is linked to the decline in intracellular pH, possibly because of displacement of the equilibrium of the creatine kinase reaction. In other situations, adenine

Table 47.1
Energy Requirements for Different Activities and the Maximum Rate of Energy Provision and Amounts Available from Different Substrates (~P mol • min⁻¹ and ~P, respectively)

	Energy Requirement		Energy Available from Substrates		
Activity	Rate	Amount	Max. Rate	Amount	Source
100-m sprint	2.6	0.43	4.4	0.50	ATP + PCr
400-m sprint	2.3	1.72	—	—	
800-m run	2.0	3.43	2.35	1.50	Glucolysis[a] (anaerobic)
1000-m run	1.7	6.00	0.85–1.14	85	Glucose oxidation
Marathon	1.0	150.00	0.4–0.6	4000	All of the above plus fat oxidation
Rest	0.07	0.36	—	—	

[a]Calculated from the amount of lactate tolerated by the body, i.e., 1 mol total.

nucleotide degradation may be precipitated by an insufficient rate of glucolysis caused by a lack of available glycogen. In either case, a decline in the availability of PCr near the site of ATP use is seen as the primary cause of the increase in ADP_f. Accumulation of AMP and IMP within fibers may contribute to the activation of glycogenolysis during intense exercise (40).

Accumulation of lactate is, however, self-limiting, because the decrease in muscle pH in turn inhibits further glucolysis and/or muscle contraction at the end of work with maximum power output (41). Under these conditions, the glycogen store is never totally used. At work rates close to the subject's maximum oxygen uptake (VO_2max), total glycogen use in the working muscles can occur (Fig. 47.1), and the amount of glycogen initially present is a determinant of work capacity. If work continues beyond this point, the work rate will decline as the muscles become progressively more dependent on FFAs and blood-borne glucose for their supply of energy. As discussed above, the maximum rate of ~P production from these two sources is appreciably lower than that from local muscle glycogen degradation.

During any form of prolonged exercise in excess of 1 hour, the use of fat progressively increases with time because of the increased availability of FFAs. For instance, in a study by Ahlborg et al., a 4-hour exercise at a work load corresponding to 30% of VO_2max resulted in an energy contribution by FFAs of 37% during the first 40 minutes and 62% during the final hour (Fig. 47.2) (42).

The above estimates of maximal fuel use assume a mean muscle fiber composition of 50% type I and 50% type II fibers. Subjects with a higher type I fiber composition, are likely to have a lower maximum rate of glucolysis and increased oxidative capacity. The opposite will be observed when the fraction of type II fibers is higher than 50%. Superimposed on this is the effect of any physical training, which favors an increase in the oxidative capacity of both fiber types, resulting in a still higher maximum use of FFAs (43–46). The maximum power output sustainable by FFA use in trained subjects will increase from about 55 to 65% of the person's VO_2max. Above this level, however, work performance is still limited by the availability of muscle glycogen (47). The relationship between the glycogen degradation rate and work intensity is shown in Figure 47.3. The almost exponential rise in the rate of glycogen degradation with increased workload is consistent with *(a)* high use of other energy sources (predominantly fat) at low workloads; *(b)* principally oxidative use of glycogen at middle loads; and *(c)* rapid but energetically inefficient anaerobic use of glycogen at the highest workloads.

Use of Protein

The quantitative role of protein as an energy substrate in the isocaloric state is small, contributing at most about

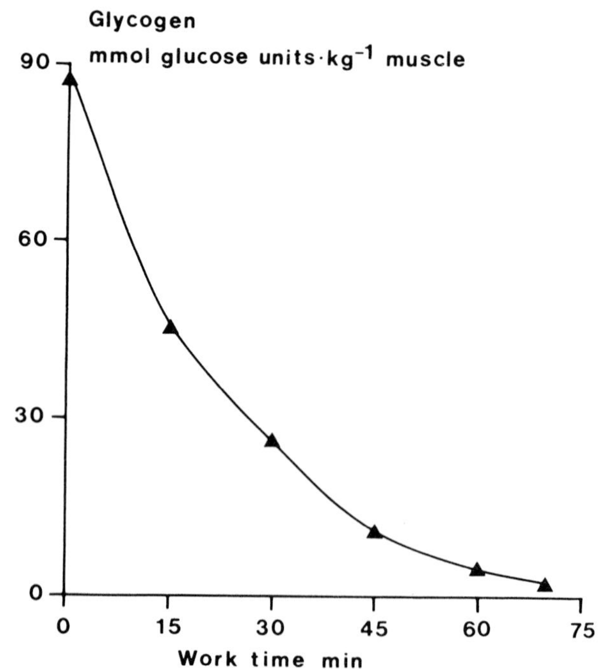

Figure 47.1. Glycogen content in the quadriceps femoris muscle during continuous bicycle exercise maintained at a load corresponding to 75% VO_2max (14). Each point is the mean value determined on 10 subjects. In each case the exercise was continued until exhaustion, at which time depletion of the muscle glycogen stores was virtually complete. (From Bergström J, Hultman E. Scand J Clin Lab Invest 1967;19:218–28, with permission.)

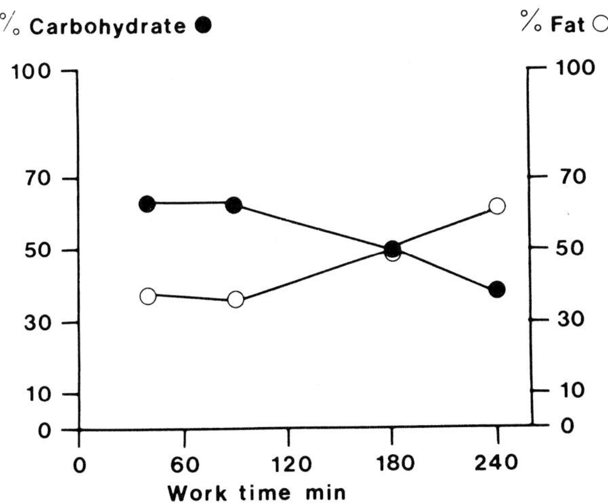

Figure 47.2. Use of carbohydrate and fat during prolonged bicycle exercise at a workload of 40% VO_2max. (From Ahlborg G, Felig G, Hagenfeldt L, et al. J Clin Invest 1974;53:1080–90, with permission.)

5 to 10% of the total energy turnover (48, 49). Nonetheless, during prolonged exercise or training, degradation of protein can be important with respect to whole body homeostasis.

Studies have shown that the extracellular level of urea nitrogen increases during prolonged exercise (48, 50–52), and urinary output of urea increases during the rest period immediately after exercise (51–54). In addition, measurements of the uptake and release of amino acids over the working muscles and over the splanchnic area and of the metabolism of isotopically labeled amino acids also indicate a significant contribution by protein to total energy turnover during exercise. Transport of amino acids from the working muscles as alanine and glutamine was first shown by Felig and coworkers (55–57). The carbon skeletons of alanine and glutamine apparently were derived from pyruvate and glutamate, and the amino groups from deamination of amino acids in the muscle. The alanine and glutamine are converted to glucose in the liver (55).

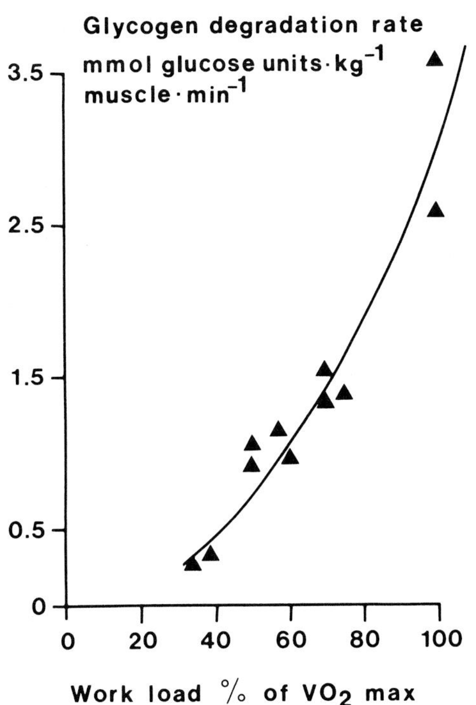

Figure 47.3. Rate of muscle glycogen degradation during bicycle exercise sustained at different workloads. (From Hultman E. Muscle glycogen store and prolonged exercise. In: Shephard EJ, ed. Frontiers of fitness. Springfield, IL: Charles C Thomas, 1971;30–9, with permission.)

Branched-chain amino acids are released from the liver and taken up by working muscle (42). Studies have also suggested that branched-chain amino acids are oxidized during prolonged exercise to exhaustion at 75% VO_2max and that a significant amount of the ammonia released from muscle is derived from amino acid degradation (58, 59). When a low-carbohydrate diet was ingested before exercise at 75% VO_2max, resting plasma branched-chain amino acid concentrations were elevated, and the exercise-induced decrease in levels of these amino acids was greater, suggesting that amino acid oxidation was higher (60). Plasma ammonia levels were also elevated during exercise, suggesting that a significant amount of the released ammonia was derived from amino acid metabolism.

The carbon skeleton of the branched-chain amino acid leucine is used for production of CO_2 during exercise (61–63) at a rate that is related to the work output (64, 65). Use of leucine, however, is modified by the amount of glycogen available in the muscles; a high glycogen content depresses the rate of leucine use (48). Glucose infusion during exercise also decreases the use of leucine (64), whereas increased availability of FFAs can have the opposite effect (66). Increased oxidation of fat as a result of increased availability of FFAs or decreased use of carbohydrate during prolonged exercise apparently increases oxidation of the carbon skeleton of branched-chain amino acids, possibly by direct stimulation of oxidative decarboxylation of the ketoacids formed (66).

Possible sources of amino acids for energy production are the free amino acid pools in muscle or plasma or those released from protein catabolism. A decreased level of amino acids in plasma is observed during prolonged exercise (53, 67, 68). Similarly, Rennie et al. found a lower free amino acid content in muscle at the end of prolonged exercise and calculated that the decrease in the amino acid pool in plasma and muscle corresponded to 20% of the total nitrogen loss (52). Thus, 80% of the nitrogen in this study must have been derived from degradation of body protein. The origin of this protein, however, is not known. Studies of 3-methyl-histidine excretion as a marker of muscle protein turnover have produced conflicting results (53, 64, 69), but they generally indicate that the contractile proteins are not broken down in exercise bouts if no apparent damage occurs to the muscle cells. Millward et al. indicated that the liver may be an important source of protein for use by the working muscles (64). Most probably, the use of protein as a fuel represents a general effect in which the normal protein synthesis rate (about 300 g/day) (70) is decreased, and part of the amino acids released by normal protein degradation supplies energy in working muscle cells. During recovery after prolonged exercise, the rate of protein synthesis increases (52).

ENERGY STORES AND EXERCISE CAPACITY

Phosphocreatine

At supramaximal power outputs with endurance times of just a few seconds, energy supply is mainly derived from the use of PCr, supplemented by anaerobic glucolysis. At maximum or near-maximum exercise intensities, performance may be limited by the ability of PCr to regulate the accumulation of ADP_f at the contraction site. Until recently it was commonly held that the PCr stores were essentially impervious to dietary manipulation and were unaffected by physical training (71, 72), despite earlier indirect data suggesting that creatine supplied in the diet was retained in the body. Confirmation that the muscle content was increased by oral administration of creatine (Cr) was obtained by Harris et al. (73). In addition, this study showed an increase in PCr content, demonstrating that the additional Cr taken up was fully assimilated into the general metabolic pool. Subsequent studies demonstrated that elevation of the muscle Cr content significantly increases work output during single or repeated bouts of maximal exercise (74–79). The increased work output is found only in short-duration exercise performed at maximum or near-maximum intensity; no effect on performance or metabolism has been recorded during prolonged submaximal exercise (80).

Carbohydrate

At work intensities close to or above the subject's VO_2max, lactate accumulation with an attendant decrease in muscle pH inhibits work output and energy production before depletion of the local glycogen stores. However, at work intensities corresponding to 65 to 85% VO_2max, the entire muscle store of glycogen may be used if the exercise is sufficiently prolonged, and power output from the muscle then declines. The onset of hypoglycemia can limit prolonged performance if the liver glycogen store at the start of exercise is low and no carbohydrate is taken during the work. In this range, any increase in the muscle glycogen store helps improve performance. Increased glycogen storage can, as discussed below, be achieved by one or more regimens of exercise and diet.

Fat

Because of the almost limitless stores of FFAs in the well-fed individual, no grounds exist for supposing that an increase in the lipid stores will increase endurance performance, even during excessively prolonged exercise periods. The limitation to work at low workloads appears to be related to factors other than the lack of substrate.

Protein

In contrast to fat and carbohydrates, no evidence exists of any specific body protein store available for exercise that can be increased by diet. A dietary effect related to protein, however, is the protein-sparing effect of carbohydrates shown by lower use of protein when blood glucose levels and muscle glycogen content are high (48, 64). Lemon and Mullin showed that the protein share of the energy substrates used during a 60-minute exercise was 4% if the glycogen store in the muscle was increased but 10% if it was depleted before the start of exercise (48). Therefore, athletes engaged in frequent training sessions should increase their total energy intake to meet the needs of training. Most of the increased energy intake should be carbohydrate.

NUTRITION FOR INCREASED WORK PERFORMANCE

Phosphocreatine Store and Diet

Only the Cr store in muscle can be increased directly through the diet; no dietary means to increase the ATP store is known. Dietary intake of creatine is highly variable, ranging from none in a vegetarian to 2 g/day with consumption of meat and fish. Cr in meat is relatively stable to storage but may be partially destroyed by cooking and processing (81). Even in the absence of a dietary source, biosynthesis of Cr from arginine, glycine, and methionine suffices to maintain a body store in the human of 120 to 160 g. A 20% increase in skeletal muscle Cr content can, however, be achieved through additional ingestion of 100 g Cr monohydrate taken as four 5-g doses/day for 5 days ("rapid"-loading regimen) (73). The resulting increase in Cr can then be maintained by continued supplementation of 2 g/day (82). A slower method of achieving a 20% increase in muscle Cr content uses consumption of 3 g Cr/day for 30 days ("slow"-loading regimen) (82). Elevation of the total Cr store is accompanied by an increase in PCr at rest (73), which is manifested also during recovery from intense exercise (83). Elevation of the muscle Cr store appears to increase work output significantly during single or repeated bouts of maximal exercise (74–79).

Muscle Glycogen Store and Diet

Initial studies on the influence of diet on muscle glycogen stores showed that feeding a carbohydrate-rich or carbohydrate-poor diet or even total starvation over a period of days had little effect on the stores at rest (Fig. 47.4) (16). However, a remarkable difference was noted between diets when feeding was preceded by depletion of

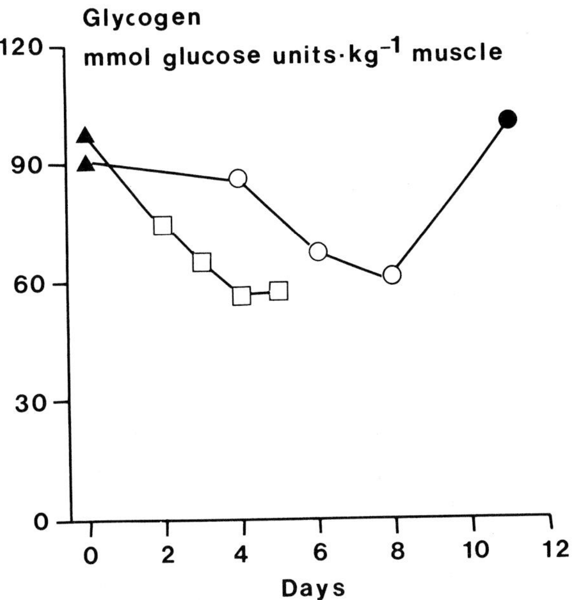

Figure 47.4. Glycogen content in the quadriceps femoris muscle after mixed diet *(solid triangles)*, during 5 days of total starvation *(open squares)*, and during 8 days of carbohydrate-free diet *(open circles)* followed by a carbohydrate-rich diet *(solid circle)*. (From Hultman E, Bergström J. Acta Med Scand 1967;182:109–17, with permission.)

the stores by exercise. Total starvation or a carbohydrate-free diet resulted in low rates of glycogen resynthesis, and normal values were not achieved for several days, whereas a carbohydrate-rich diet resulted in rapid resynthesis to values above the normal range (Fig. 47.5). Studies in which only one leg was exercised showed that rapid resynthesis of glycogen to supernormal values was a local phenomenon restricted to the exercised muscles (Figs. 47.6 and 47.7) (9).

How "supercompensation" in glycogen is brought about is not known. Enzyme studies revealed that glycogen synthetase, the enzyme responsible for glycogen formation, is transformed from the inactive D form to active I form when the glycogen store is depleted. After 1 day of carbohydrate refeeding, the I form falls to normal (84). Other forms of the enzyme, intermediate between active and inactive, however, have been described (85), and these forms could account for the continuation of glycogen synthesis to supernormal values.

The dramatic effect of increased muscle glycogen content on work capacity is illustrated in Figure 47.8. In this study, exhaustive exercise was repeated three times with an interval of 3 days between bouts. The diet given before the first exercise was a normal mixed diet, which was followed by a carbohydrate-free diet and finally (before the last exercise) by a carbohydrate-rich diet (18). The effect of the different diets was to increase work time from 1 hour after the carbohydrate-free diet to 3 hours or more after

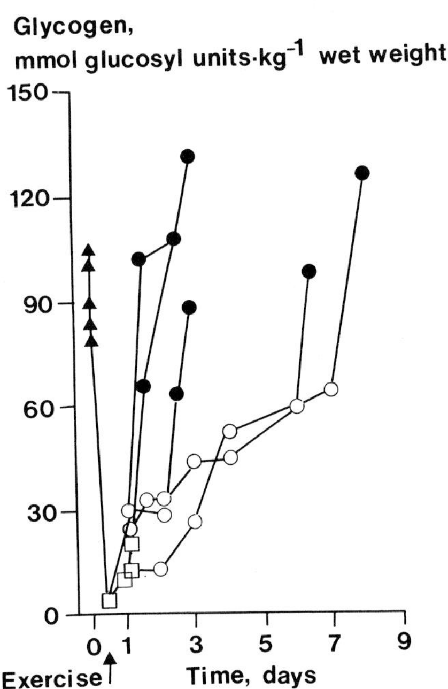

Figure 47.5. Muscle glycogen content before and after exercise. Before exercise the diet was normal mixed *(solid triangles)*, and on the following days either total starvation *(open squares)* or a carbohydrate-free diet *(open circles)* was followed by 1 or 2 days of carbohydrate-rich diet *(solid circles)* (16). Note the slow rate of glycogen resynthesis when the diet is carbohydrate free compared with the rate when the diet is rich in carbohydrate (see also Fig. 47.7).

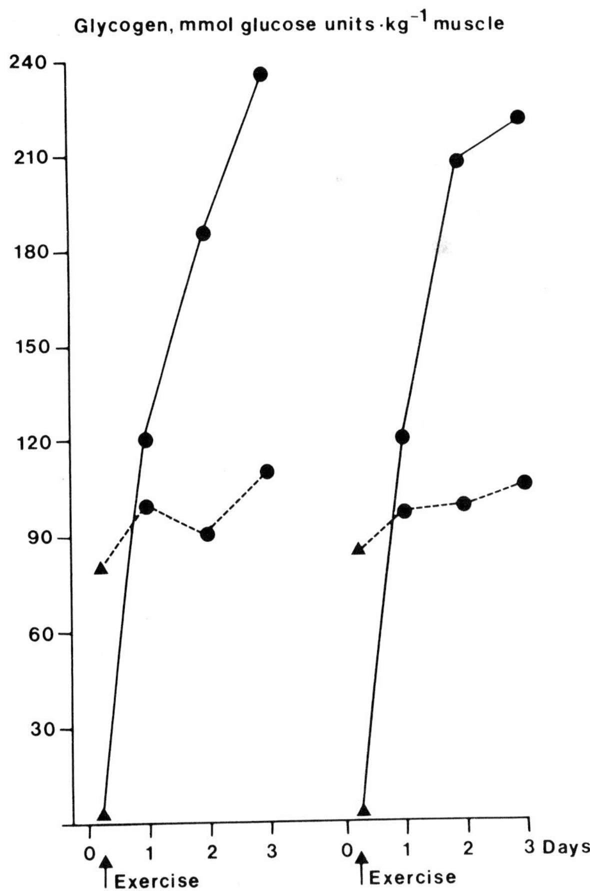

Figure 47.6. One-leg exercise study showing the glycogen content of the exercised *(solid lines)* and rested *(broken lines)* legs of two subjects (9). Biopsies were obtained immediately after the exercise and during 3 days when subjects were fed a carbohydrate-rich diet.

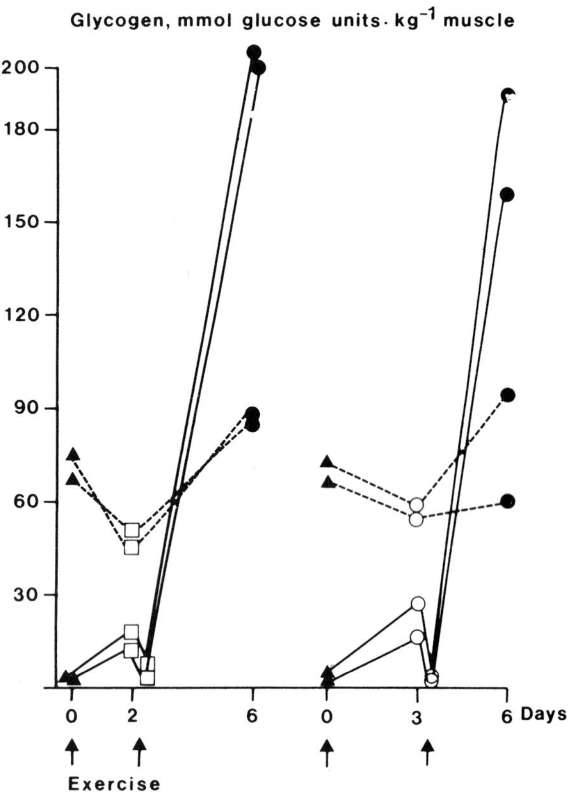

Figure 47.7. The same "one-leg exercise" procedure as in Figure 47.6 showing the glycogen content in the exercised *(solid lines)* and the rested leg *(broken lines)*. The diet was either total starvation *(open squares)* or carbohydrate free *(open circles)* during 2 and 3 days, respectively (16). This was followed by a second one-leg exercise, after which a carbohydrate-rich diet *(solid circles)* was given. The *solid triangles* represent a normal diet.

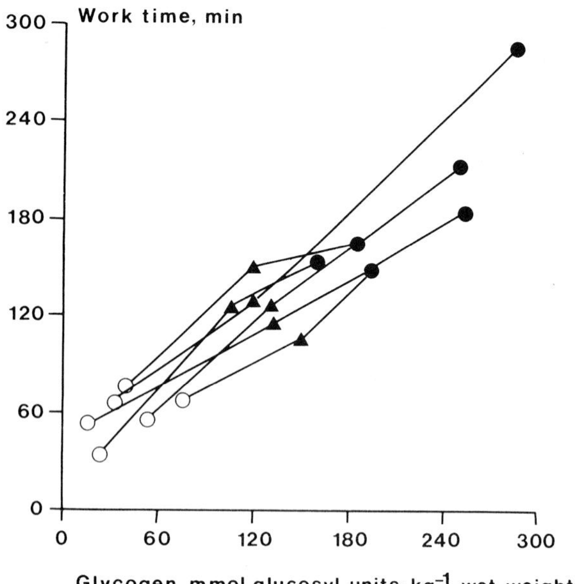

Figure 47.8. Relationship between the initial glycogen content in the quadriceps femoris muscle and work time. Bicycle work was performed to exhaustion at a workload corresponding to 75% of VO_2max. Each subject worked three times, and the experiments were preceded by 3 days of a dietary regimen: initially a mixed normal diet *(solid triangles)*, followed by a carbohydrate-free diet *(open circles)* and thereafter a carbohydrate-rich diet *(solid circles)*. The energy content of the diets was the same. (From Bergström J, Hermansen L, Hultman E, et al. Acta Physiol Scand 1967;71:140–50, with permission.)

the carbohydrate-rich diet. The study was done originally to demonstrate the relationship between work capacity and the size of the muscle glycogen stores, but the method used to increase the muscle glycogen content has since been adopted by athletes as a procedure to increase these stores.

A drawback to this regimen is that it leaves athletes with extremely low muscle glycogen stores for a period of 2 to 3 days, and this state could interfere with training. Sherman et al. proposed a modified regimen of diet and exercise that avoids any period of carbohydrate-free diet yet still results in equally high glycogen levels (86). For subjects in regular training, it is probably sufficient if they perform a depleting exercise twice during a period of mixed diet and thereafter change to a carbohydrate-rich diet during the final 3 days before competition. During the first two of these days, light exercise is possible, leaving only the last day for total rest.

Glycogen is stored in muscle together with water and potassium ions, 1 g (6 mmol) being associated with 2.7 g of water and 0.45 mmol of potassium (21, 87, 88). Consequently, glycogen supercompensation considerably increases muscle water content, which increases body weight and may induce feelings of heaviness and stiffness in the muscle. Supercompensation cannot, therefore, be recommended for athletes needing only limited supplies of glycogen, e.g., sprinters.

Liver Glycogen Store—Effect of Diet

In contrast to muscle, the liver glycogen store is extremely labile, even in the resting state. The glycogen content after an overnight fast varies from 90 to 500 mmol glucose units/kg liver tissue (about 14–80 g glycogen) (36). This value corresponds to a total glycogen store of 160 to 900 mmol glucose units in a 1.8-kg liver, which is the normal weight. Measurements of glycogen in repeated liver biopsy samples taken in the postprandial state showed a continuous decrease, amounting to 0.3 mmol glucose units/min/kg liver, from which it can be calculated that just 1 day of starvation would empty the liver glycogen stores (23). This situation was found in two subjects from whom biopsies were taken after 1 day without food: liver glycogen stores decreased from 155 to 24 and 345 to 48 mmol glucose units/kg. In one of the subjects, starvation was continued for a further 2 days, with biopsies performed each morning. Liver glycogen contents in these biopsy samples were 15 and 21 mmol glucose units/kg (Fig. 47.9) (23).

However, during even short periods of starvation, both fat and protein degradation increase, which results in an increase in gluconeogenic substrate brought to the liver.

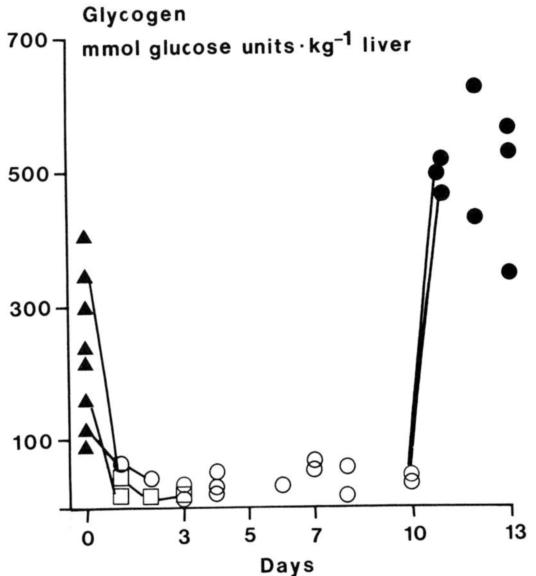

Figure 47.9. Glycogen content in the liver determined in needle biopsy specimens from normal subjects after different diets (23). A normal mixed diet *(solid triangles)* was followed by 1 or 3 days of starvation *(open squares)* or 1 to 10 days of a carbohydrate-free diet *(open circles)*. The period was ended by 1 or 3 days of a carbohydrate-rich diet *(closed circles)*.

Evidently, this increase does not suffice for de novo synthesis of glycogen in the liver. To increase the supply of gluconeogenic substrates, a diet consisting of protein and fat with a caloric content of 8400 kilojoules (kJ)/day was administered to subjects, but liver glycogen content showed no increase during a 10-day period (Fig. 47.9) (23). When the diet was changed to one rich in carbohydrates with the same caloric content, the liver glycogen content increased immediately (up to 500–600 mmol glucose units/kg). Dietary carbohydrate intake is obviously necessary to preserve the liver glycogen store. In these studies, the fat and protein diet consisted of bacon, eggs, meat, vegetable oils, butter, and small amounts of tomatoes and lettuce, and the carbohydrate-rich diet contained bread, spaghetti, potatoes, sugar, fruit, and juice such that 90% of the consumed energy was derived from carbohydrates. Spices and meat extract were added for taste.

The blood glucose concentration during fasting or during the period of carbohydrate-free diet decreased only marginally from 5.2 to 4.3 mmol/L after 10 days, with the lowest value being recorded on day 5 (3.8 mmol/L). Only light office work was done during the experimental period. Glucose output by the liver decreased, however, by 60%, which corresponds to the share normally derived from glycogen degradation (24). The fact that the blood glucose concentration shows only a small change is the result of various adaptations in body metabolism, including increased output of ketone bodies from the liver (24) and a shift from glucose use to ketone body oxidation by the brain (89, 90). Seemingly, the adaptation by the brain is a rapid process.

Liver Glycogen Store—Glucose Release and Effect of Exercise

During exercise, glucose output from the liver increases. In one study of intense bicycle exercise, a continuous increase in output was seen from 1 mmol/min before exercise to 5 mmol/min during the last minute of work (20). The average output over the entire exercise period was 2.4 mmol/min. In a further study in which liver biopsies were taken, 1 hour of intense bicycle exercise resulted in a mean glycogen degradation rate of 2.1 mmol glucose units/min/kg liver (25). This result means that up to one-half of the normal liver glycogen store is lost during 1 hour of heavy exercise, and most of the glucose output is derived from liver glycogen, with only a small fraction from gluconeogenesis.

If exercise is performed after a carbohydrate-free diet, glucose output from liver glycogen is decreased and is compensated only in part by increased gluconeogenesis from the precursors lactate, amino acids, and glycerol. The effect, therefore, is a decrease in the blood glucose concentration during exercise. This process is illustrated in the study of Bergström et al. mentioned above in which a pronounced decrease in blood glucose concentration occurred shortly after the start of exercise performed following a period of carbohydrate-free diet (18). The mean total glucose content decreased during the first hour of exercise from 5.0 to 2.8 mmol/L, and several subjects suffered from headache and dizziness during the later part of the exercise. One subject had to stop working because of hypoglycemic effects on the central nervous system. With a blood glucose concentration of 1.7 mmol/L, the subject could not continue the exercise because of severe dizziness and headache. The corresponding mean blood glucose level after the carbohydrate-rich diet was 4.4 mmol/L after 1 hour of exercise and 3.5 mmol/L at the end of the work (after 3 hours).

Glucose production through gluconeogenesis normally is not increased during short-term exercise, but it can increase during prolonged work to values nearly twice the resting level (42). An increased rate of gluconeogenesis, however, does occur during short intervals of hard exercise preceded by a period of carbohydrate-free diet (35, 91), although total glucose output, as mentioned above, is still lower than after a normal mixed diet. After a carbohydrate-free diet, about 50% of the glucose released from the liver can be accounted for by use of gluconeogenic substrates, whereas after a carbohydrate-rich diet, the corresponding share is only 5 to 10%. After the carbohydrate-free diet, increased oxygen uptake by the liver was observed (91), which is consistent with the increased rate of gluconeogenesis, an energy-consuming process.

In summary, dietary increase in liver glycogen stores would be beneficial in most types of continuous or prolonged intermittent exercise/work. During work of several hours duration, a high liver glycogen level buffers against development of hypoglycemia that may lead to deleterious effects on central nervous function and exhaustion. One day of a carbohydrate-rich diet before competition suffices to produce high levels of glycogen in the liver.

ENERGY REQUIREMENTS

During Occupational Work

The caloric need at rest has been calculated by Passmore and Durnin to be 105 kJ/kg body weight (BW)/day for men and 100 kJ/kg BW/day for women (92). The FAO/WHO recommendations on the energy needs for men and women in occupational work are indicated in Table 47.2 (93). These estimates are for subjects with body weights of 65 and 55 kg, respectively, and aged 20 to 39 years. Energy requirement decreases with increasing age; subjects aged 40 to 49 years require 95% of the preceding estimates; 50 to 59 years, 90%; 60 to 69 years, 80%; and above 70 years old, 70%. Energy needs increase with activity (Fig. 47.2). The numbers in Table 47.2 are similar to those presented by other authors such as Norgan and Ferro-Luzzi for Italian shipyard workers engaged in occupational work requiring light activity (94). The same authors also studied horticulturists in Papua New Guinea and found a similar requirement in dietary energy of 160 to 190 kJ/kg BW/day. Total energy requirements are obtained by multiplying the preceding estimates by body weight (in kg). Thus, for occupational work with light activity, total daily requirements for a 65-kg man and 55-kg woman would be 10.9 megajoules (MJ; 1 MJ = 1000 kJ) and 8.4 MJ, respectively (93). More-recent estimates of the energy costs of work are given in Appendix Tables III-A-11-d and e.

During Exercise

The energy requirement during athletic performance or training is determined by the type of activity and its duration. Several studies of the relative caloric costs of different sports have been published (92, 95). No details are given here, however, except to note that requirements vary from 12.5 to 25 MJ, the higher values associated with high-intensity endurance sports such as cross-country running or skiing and marathon running. High-energy intakes of the same order are also required in the course of sports requiring intense repetitive effort such as team sports (football, ice hockey, basketball), tennis, and fencing. In sports requiring sustained intense effort for shorter periods, such as swimming events over 100 m, wrestling, downhill skiing, and running for 1 to 2 miles, the average daily expenditure is on the order of 12.5 to 21 MJ. The lowest energy requirement, up to 16.7 MJ per day, is observed in low-intensity sports of long duration, such as baseball or golf, and when strenuous or maximal efforts are produced only during short periods, i.e., hurdles, long jump, 50- to 100-m swimming events, discus, hammer throw, high jump, and javelin.

The total caloric need is influenced also by body weight, the frequency of repetition of the event, and the length of practice during training. Training itself increases the daily caloric need by 5 to 40%, depending on the nature of the exercise and the length of practice (see [95]). The preceding estimates of energy expenditure were adapted from Buskirk and are calculated to cover the caloric needs of 75% of all male subjects (95). Women athletes require 10% fewer calories to cover the energy need for each type of sport or during training.

RECOMMENDED USE OF MACRONUTRIENTS DURING WORK

Estimates of energy expenditure during normal occupational work were given above. This energy can be derived from a variety of combinations of fat and carbohydrate. Protein is used as a significant energy source only when the carbohydrate stores have been exhausted and then only during prolonged work periods. Available free amino acids may be used, although as indicated above, their contribution to the total amount of energy used is probably small.

As seen in Table 47.3, much more energy is stored in the body as fat than is stored as carbohydrate. Theoretically, fat can sustain light work for long periods without supplementation. In contrast, the body's glycogen store would be exhausted within half a day if used exclusively. In practice, light occupational work relies mainly on fat use, delaying considerably exhaustion of the carbohydrate stores. At exceptionally high workloads, the capacity to oxidize fats is insufficient to meet energy needs, and at these work rates, carbohydrate plays the central role in energy provision. Only carbohydrate use can match the high rates of energy expenditure necessary to fulfill the work. In practice, intense labor is interspersed with peri-

Table 47.2
Energy Needs ($kJ \cdot kg^{-1} \cdot day^{-1}$)[a] for Occupational Work Activity

Activity	Men	Women
Light	167	157
Moderate	192	167
High	225	194
Exceptionally high	257	225

From FAO/WHO Expert Committee Report. WHO Tech Rep Ser 1973;52:1–118.
[a]1 kJ = 4.18 kcal.

Table 47.3
Fuel Stores in the Average Man

	Fuel Reserves		Days Reserves Last if Used As Exclusive Source	
Fuel	(g)	(kJ)	Light Exercise	Exceptionally High Activity
Adipose tissue	9000	337,570	29	18.8
Liver glycogen	100	1,600	0.14	0.09
Muscle glycogen	350	5,800	0.5	0.3
Blood glucose	3	48	—	—

ods of lighter activity with lower energy demand that can be sustained through fat oxidation. The limited availability of the carbohydrate store in the body (Table 47.3), however, ultimately determines the duration of the work. This fact emphasizes the importance of a regular intake of sufficient carbohydrate to keep the body's stores high.

Carbohydrate

Dietary carbohydrate is essential for both maintenance of the liver glycogen store and rapid resynthesis of muscle glycogen. A loss of liver glycogen results in decreased blood glucose content, and a lack of muscle glycogen decreases the work capacity. Omitting carbohydrate from the diet for more than 1 day results in increased production of ketone bodies, degradation of body protein, and loss of cations and water. These effects are counteracted by a minimum intake of about 100 g of carbohydrate (600 mmol glucose units) per day.

Generally, however, it is recommended that 60 to 65% of the energy content of the diet be carbohydrate. In a 70-kg person given a normal mixed diet, 70 to 150 g carbohydrate is stored as glycogen in the liver and 300 to 500 g in muscles. The energy equivalents of these stores are 1.25 to 2.5 MJ and 5.0 to 8.3 MJ, respectively. As discussed above, these stores may be greatly increased by a combination of diet and exercise. If the carbohydrate intake exceeds the capacity for storage and its immediate requirement as an energy source, transformation to fat and subsequent storage will occur.

For optimal use, carbohydrates should be included in the diet as complex saccharides, such as starch in bread, pasta, potatoes, rice, and cereals, and not as simple sugars, such as glucose and sucrose. Starch and other complex carbohydrates are digested more slowly in the intestine and are absorbed over a longer time so that a larger fraction is deposited in the glycogen stores and less as fat.

Fat

Fat in the form of FFAs can be used directly as an energy substrate by most of the tissues in the body. Exceptions are the cells in the central nervous system and the red blood cells. Central nervous system cells can use both carbohydrate and ketone bodies if available, but the red blood cells and some other small cell compartments rely totally on carbohydrate. FFAs constitute the largest energy reserve in the body and are stored as triglycerides in adipose tissue. The store in an average 70-kg person is about 9 kg, which corresponds to approximately 338 MJ. It is generally recommended that the diet contain 8 to 10% of the total energy in the form of polyunsaturated fatty acids and the total fat intake not exceed 30% of the dietary energy.

Protein

Dietary proteins provide amino acids for de novo synthesis of proteins and other tissue constituents in the body. Replacement of protein is an ongoing process in the body. The result is a daily loss of nitrogen in the form of urea and amino acids, which must be covered by the intake of nitrogen-containing nutrients.

Dietary amino acids are used primarily for protein synthesis, but in excess, they are degraded rapidly because the body has no protein or amino acid store. An intake in excess of the need for synthesis of proteins results in increased formation of urea, which is excreted in urine and sweat. The carbon skeleton of the amino acids, however, is retained and used as an energy substrate. The carbon skeleton in some cases can also be converted to glucose in the liver. If protein and energy intake is greater than required, the extra amino acids may be converted to fat and carbohydrate and stored.

Energy production by the body is fundamental to life, and amino acids are used preferentially as an energy source if the total energy intake is lower than the amount needed. Calculation of the minimum protein requirement in the diet thus requires that the caloric need is adequately met by other dietary sources. The mean daily use of body protein in a normal individual fed a protein-free diet is of the order of 0.45 g/kg BW (96). When a high-quality protein is given, such as egg protein, the efficiency of use is about 70%, which increases the estimate of protein required to 0.59 g/kg BW. For the North American diet, the average efficiency of use for the mixture of protein ingested is still lower, so that the recommended protein intake is increased to 0.8 g/kg BW (96). A 70-kg man would thus require 56 g protein per day, and a 55-kg woman would require 44 g. Further data on dietary protein are given in Appendix Tables II-A-2 through II-A-8.

Dietary Protein Intake in Different Diets

The actual protein intake in the average Swedish diet with an energy content of 11.7 MJ is 84 g, corresponding to 1.2 g/kg BW for a 70-kg man. This amount is 50% higher than the recommendations by the Committee on Dietary Allowances, Food and Nutrition Board (RDA) (96). The energy value of the protein intake corresponds to 12% of the total content in the Swedish diet. The corresponding value for protein intake for Italian shipyard workers is 12.5 to 12.8% (97), the mean Japanese diet is reported to contain 14.4% of the energy in the form of protein (98), the West German diet contains 11.1% (99), and the American diet about 12% (96).

PROTEIN REQUIREMENT IN TRAINING

As discussed above, the increase in the use of protein during exercise is only marginal. According to RDA, no increase in protein intake is needed when energy output is increased during training and competition or even during heavy exercise (96). The increased loss of protein during prolonged heavy exercise/work was estimated by Lemon and Mullin to be only 4% of the total energy expenditure when there were adequate levels of glycogen in both muscle and liver, but about 10% when these were depleted (48). Similar figures were presented by Rennie et al., who calculated the contribution of amino acid oxidation as 4 to 8% of the total energy expenditure during prolonged exercise (3 3/4 hours) (52). In studies examining the protein requirements of untrained subjects initiating a training program at 40 to 50% VO_2max, investigators found an initial decline in nitrogen balance that reached equilibrium within 2 weeks while ingesting 0.57 g egg white protein/kg BW/day (100, 101). The protein requirement for trained endurance runners maintained on an adequate energy intake and either 1.1 or 2.4 g mixed food protein/kg/day during alternate 10-day periods was measured and compared with that of a sedentary control group (102). The predicted nitrogen intake required for equilibrium was 1.37 and 0.73 g/kg/day in the athlete and sedentary group, respectively.

These results suggest that athletes engaged in endurance training require more protein than sedentary individuals. However, the requirement is still well within the amount that the average North American consumes, so extra protein supplements are not required. Also, the protein requirements derived from high protein intakes may result in inflated values; however, the relative relationship of protein requirements between sedentary and trained individuals appears valid (103). Thus, if protein is to be increased during heavy endurance training, it seems reasonable to limit the increase to 10% of the extra requirement of energy intake. Because the protein content of a normal diet constitutes 11 to 14% of the total energy, simply increasing the amounts consumed to comply with the increased energy requirement will suffice. No adjustment in the actual makeup of the diet is required. This recommendation is probably still valid when the daily energy requirement is far above that of normal athletes, as in ultraendurance events. For example, a study that simulated the 22-day Tour de France demonstrated that these cyclists require more than 1.5 g of protein/kg/day (104). This amount could be achieved by increasing the energy intake without altering the proportion of protein consumed.

In calculating the required increase in protein, however, it was assumed that no preferential loss of any one essential amino acid (possible exception, leucine) occurred. If such a loss did occur, it would result in a negative nitrogen balance during longer periods of training, because a lack of essential amino acids would decrease the normal protein synthesis rate. Although findings of a few studies support this hypothesis (50, 54), most results indicate that nitrogen balance is maintained during training (105–109) and may even be positive during heavy weight training (110), when subjects are given a moderate protein intake of 0.8 to 1.4 g/kg/day. Marable et al. observed an increase in lean body mass of 2 kg after 28 days of heavy weight training with a protein intake of 0.8 g/kg/day (110). A protein intake of 2.4 g/kg resulted in a large increase in urinary nitrogen loss but the same rate of body protein synthesis. Similarly, Toråun et al. found that total body potassium, an indicator of muscle mass, was unchanged or increased after 4 to 6 weeks of isometric exercise training when the subjects were given an egg protein intake of 1 g/kg/day (105).

Much higher intakes of protein, however, are often seen in athletes. A dietary survey of Italian athletes showed an intake of protein corresponding to 17 to 18% of the energy content of the food, or 2.2 to 2.8 g/kg BW (97). Laritcheva et al. reported a protein intake of 2.12 to 2.76 g/kg in weight lifters during training, although this amount decreased to 1.36 to 1.80 g/kg between training sessions (111). Russian athletes studied by Rogozkin had a recommended intake of 13% of the dietary nutrients as protein for a total intake of 18.8 to 21 MJ, 12% for 23 to 27 MJ, and 11% at about 33 MJ (112).

The excess of dietary protein of an athlete is often on the order of 100 g/day. If the protein were used for muscle protein synthesis, muscle mass would increase by 500 g/day. This of course is not the case. The extra dietary protein only increases production and release of urea and thus increases the metabolic and excretory work by the liver and kidney. The calculation shows that extra intake of protein concentrates and protein pills, which is common today among athletes and muscle builders, is of no value when the normal diet already contains protein in excess of that needed for both energy production and muscle protein synthesis.

Diet Composition

Depending on work rate, the recommended daily energy intake is 160 to 250 kJ/kg BW for men and 130 to 220 kJ/kg BW for women. Between 60 and 65% of the energy intake should be in the form of complex carbohydrates, 25% as fat (about half of which should be supplied as vegetable fat), and the remaining 10 to 15% in the form of high-quality protein. Athletes in training can use essentially the same diet but with increased energy intake to meet the increase in energy expenditure. Exceptions to this statement are long-distance runners, cyclists, and cross-country skiers, who need to especially increase their carbohydrate intake during prolonged bouts of training. For such individuals, 70 to 75% of the extra energy should be in the form of carbohydrate and a maximum of 10% as protein.

DIET IN PREPARATION FOR COMPETITION

Based on current published data, Creatine (Cr) may be given as a supplement when preparing for competition involving short-term intense exercise or repeated bouts of maximal or near-maximal exercise. Supplementation should be instituted at least 1 week before the start of competition when 20 g of Cr monohydrate may be given daily for 5 days (rapid-loading regimen). The 20 g of Cr should be taken as 5-g doses four times during the waking hours of the day. An additional increase in muscle Cr content will be obtained if supplementation is taken in conjunction with exercise training (73). It is also possible to increase muscle Cr content before competition in a slower manner by consuming 3 g of Cr/day for 30 days (slow-loading regimen) (82).

When the athlete is preparing for a competition involving prolonged heavy exercise for more than 60 minutes, the muscle glycogen stores may be increased to maximum by the following program of diet and exercise. On day 1 (i.e., 6 days before the competition), an exhausting exercise is performed, followed by 2 days of a low-carbohydrate diet with further bouts of exhausting exercise. Thereafter, a carbohydrate-rich diet (75–80% carbohydrate) is given for 3 days, during which no hard exercise is performed. To avoid excessive depletion of the muscle glycogen stores, Sherman et al. recommend a normal mixed diet for the first 3 days (50% carbohydrate) after which the carbohydrate-rich diet is given (86). At the same time, shorter periods of exercise are performed also on days 4 and 5, and rest is taken only on the day preceding the competition. This procedure is probably sufficient for athletes in regular training.

For competitions lasting less than 1 hour, a normal mixed diet is adequate during the final day of preparation. The protein intake recommended in the normal diet is sufficient for resistance sports, even during intensive training periods, provided the total caloric intake is adequate to meet energy needs.

On the day of competition, a carbohydrate-rich meal should be given, preferably at least 2 hours before the start of the event. Intake of rapidly absorbed sugars, notably glucose, within 1 hour before competition may result in increased release of insulin leading to decreased blood glucose levels, inhibition of FFA release (113), and eventually, greater use of muscle glycogen stores. In longer events of 2 hours or more, in which replacement of water and electrolytes also is necessary, repeated intake of a glucose polymer solution can delay the onset of fatigue (114, 115). These findings demonstrate that glucose ingestion is important to maintain the blood glucose concentration, a fall in which may inhibit sustained prolonged exercise because of the effect of hypoglycemia on the central nervous system and/or decreased carbohydrate availability in the working muscle. Hypoglycemia results from increased glucose use by exercising muscle when the local glycogen store is depleted and the liver glycogen store is emptied during prolonged exercise. The carbohydrate solution, taken in small amounts at frequent intervals, counteracts hypoglycemia and depletion of the liver glycogen store.

WATER AND ELECTROLYTE BALANCE IN PHYSICAL ACTIVITY

Water is of great importance to those performing physical activity. Indeed, it is the only nutrient whose lack presents an immediate and serious health risk or even the possibility of death to the participants (116, 117). Without question, dehydration can decrease performance (118–120). Water balance, therefore, should be of concern to all involved with physical activity.

Role of Water

The central role of water in the performance of exercise is a direct consequence of its involvement in the cardiovascular, metabolic, and thermoregulatory systems of the human body. During exercise, oxygen and fuel substrates must be delivered to the working cell, and metabolites must be removed. Consequently, a redistribution of cardiac output to the working muscles must occur. A consequence of the elevated rate of work is additional heat production. Heat production in contracting muscles during intense physical exercise can be 15 to 20 times that of basal metabolism. This rate of heat production is sufficient to raise core body temperature in an average person by 1°C every 5 to 8 minutes if no temperature-regulating mechanisms are activated (117, 121). The metabolic heat must be dissipated to prevent hyperthermia from occurring in 15 to 25 minutes. Fortunately, the body activates heat loss mechanisms. One of these mechanisms is to dilate the skin blood vessels and thus redistribute the cardiac output to the periphery (122). Skin temperature increases because of the increased skin blood flow that permits heat to be lost from the skin to the environment by radiation and convection. A second heat loss mechanism is the activation of sweating. Sweat glands secrete water onto the surface of the skin where it can evaporate. Because sweat rates can be as high as 2 to 2.8 L/h, nearly all of the heat produced during exercise can be dissipated through this mechanism under ideal conditions.

When the weather is cool, most of the required heat loss during exercise occurs through radiation and convection from the exposed skin. Extensive sweating is not needed and does not occur, making the risk of dehydration relatively low. As the environmental temperature increases and approaches the skin temperature, heat transfer by radiation and convection cannot occur to any great extent. This condition leaves evaporation of sweat as the only effective means of dissipating heat. Consequently, the sweat rate is high during exercise in hot environments, and the lost body fluids must be replenished to maintain exercise performance and to prevent fatigue and hyperthermia (123–125). The extent to which body fluid loss affects performance is governed by many factors, including the type and mode of exercise, the intensity and duration of the work, the environmental conditions under which the work is performed, and the physical characteristics of the athlete (age, sex, weight, height, state of nutrition, hydration, and training).

Water metabolism during activity cannot be separated from the body's mineral balance. Water shifts between intracellular and extracellular spaces are accompanied by shifts in sodium, potassium, magnesium, and chloride ions (Na^+, K^+, Mg^{2+}, Cl^-, respectively). Sweat losses also provide a means for electrolyte loss (119, 126, 127). Disturbance of water and electrolyte balance occurs not only during single exercise bouts but also over prolonged periods of training.

Types of Stress

Two different situations stress water balance. In "make weight" sports such as wrestling, the competitor deliberately restricts intake of food and fluid and strives to lose water by exercise, heat exposure, laxatives, and diuretics, ostensibly to meet a smaller and weaker opponent (128, 129). This practice has been rejected for health reasons by professional associations (118). Even so, the abuse continues and is prevalent in intense activities of brief duration that emphasize strength and coordination.

In contrast to such activities are endurance events such as road racing. These events may last for several hours, and the exertional and environmental heat load imposed on the body may produce rectal temperatures in excess of 40.6°C (117). Under such conditions, athletes may lose fluid at rates of 2.0 to 2.8 L/h, resulting in a water deficit of 6 to 8% of body weight (130, 131).

Effects of Dehydration

Numerous studies have been performed to assess the effects of dehydration on performance; the data reported include physiologic and biochemical variables and measures of muscular strength and endurance, anaerobic capacity, and aerobic power. Dehydration states have been produced thermally or in combination with exercise. The results depend on the extent of the dehydration, which is expressed as the percentage of body weight lost (%BWL).

As little as 2% BWL imposes an increased strain on the cardiovascular (132) and thermoregulatory systems (127). A 2.5% decrease in plasma volume and a 1% decline in muscle water typically occur for each 1% BWL. Plasma water accounts for 10 to 11% of the total water deficit (119). Rectal temperature increases 0.4 to 0.5°C for each 1% BWL (133). A 4% BWL results in an approximately 30% decline in isometric and isotonic strength, although peak isokinetic torque declined only 13% when an 8% BWL was induced by food and fluid restriction (129). However, 5% BWL was without effect in an anaerobic cycling test, and no impairment was noted at 8% BWL in an anaerobic running test (129). A 4 to 5% BWL produced no change in VO_2max, although a decrease in the maximal work time was seen (132). Similarly, during activities of long duration, dehydration has invariably been reported to result in a decreased ability to work (118, 124, 132, 134, 135). In other studies, a decreased capacity is strongly suggested (126, 133). No positive benefits of weight reduction by hypohydration have been shown.

Electrolyte losses occur together with water loss, but because sweat is hypotonic, the loss in water exceeds the loss of Na^+, K^+, Mg^{2+}, or Cl^-. The net result is that the plasma becomes hypertonic. The principal ions lost in sweat are Na^+ and Cl^- (119). A sweat loss causing a 5.8% BWL was found to produce a deficit of 5.7% in body Na^+ and Cl^-, but a 1% loss of K^+ and Mg^{2+} (124).

Replacement Strategies

Rehydration strategies to prevent, compensate for, or replace water loss are important in avoiding hypohydration. The aim of rehydration is either to replace water and reestablish water and electrolyte balance quickly, as in the case of dehydrated performer about to enter an event, or to prevent or retard water loss that occurs during an endurance event. Studies reveal that several factors are involved in fluid replacement, such as fluid composition, drinking frequency, volume intake, and fluid temperature (136, 137). The rate of gastric emptying provides a measure of rehydration efficiency, because almost all absorption of sugar, electrolytes, and water proceeds from the intestine (138).

Effect of Fluid Composition. It is often necessary during endurance exercise to supplement not only fluid stores but also carbohydrate stores through oral ingestion of glucose, fructose, sucrose, or carbohydrate polymers. These carbohydrate solutions can provide a slow release of energy substrate to the body over a prolonged period (124). However, results of initial studies revealed that carbohydrate concentrations above 140 mM (25 g/L) significantly retarded gastric emptying, which is detrimental for rapid rehydration (136). More-recent studies demonstrated that both carbohydrate and water were delivered to the duodenum at near-maximal rates when the carbohydrate concentration of the drink was 440 to 560 mM (80–100 g/L) (138–140). During these studies, subjects exercised for 2 hours and drank 120 mL every 15 minutes. Therefore, if water replacement is the major concern during exercise, solutions with lower carbohydrate content should be ingested, and if water replacement is not a priority, more-concentrated carbohydrate solutions can be ingested. Most sports beverages routinely contain carbohydrate concentrations of 280 to 560 mM (50–100 g/L).

Many fluid replacement drinks also contain small amounts of salt. The addition of 10 to 30 mM NaCl may help replace body stores of Na^+ and Cl^-, the major ions lost in sweat (119). Low levels of Na^+ are also reported to improve gastric emptying and to assist in maintaining the osmotic drive for drinking (141). Drinking water only rapidly dilutes the blood, removes the drive for drinking, and stimulates urine output. However, large amounts of NaCl increase the osmolality of the drink and may actually cause fluid shifts into the gastrointestinal tract, thereby hindering gastric emptying (134). Potassium supplements are not needed in replacement drinks because little K^+ is lost in sweat, and these supplements are considered dangerous (142).

Fluid Volume. Although large volumes of ingested fluid (up to 600 mL) increase the emptying rate, gastric discomfort may result. Drinking 100 to 200 mL every 10 to 15 minutes seems appropriate (137, 139, 140).

Fluid Temperature. Chilled fluids (6–12°C) leave the stomach more quickly than warm ones and can reduce body temperatures (133, 136).

Drinking Schedule. It is recommended that 400 to 500 mL of fluid be taken 10 to 15 minutes before competition, although this does not replace the need for drinking during the event (133). Hyperhydration 40 to 80 minutes before an event can precipitate diuresis, and rapid rehydration after exercise-induced dehydration can produce the same result (143).

The consensus of reviews on this topic is to drink 100 to 200 mL of solution containing 280 to 560 mM (50–100 g/L) carbohydrate and 10 to 30 mM NaCl every 15 to 20 minutes when engaging in exercise lasting longer than 1 hour (119, 137, 138, 144, 145). It is also beneficial if the solution is chilled to 6 to 12°C. Tremendous individual variation exists in the ability to tolerate carbohydrate-electrolyte drinks during prolonged strenuous exercise. This variation necessitates that individuals experiment with these drinks before competition to develop their own optimal strategy.

Efficacy of Rehydration

Rehydration before or during an event is of significant benefit. Consuming 150 mL of fluid every 10 minutes during a 2-hour cycling task in the heat dramatically limits the reduction in plasma volume, elevation of heart rate, and increase in body temperature (124). Rectal temperature was about 0.7°C lower at the end of 2 hours of exercise when 200 mL of fluid was consumed every 20 minutes (133).

The problems of dehydration may be alleviated in part during activity by the availability of water produced by metabolism and liberated during the breakdown of glycogen. Similarly, K^+ is released as glycogen is used (11, 21, 87). These effects should help maintain fluid and electrolyte balance during exercise. Glycogen degradation and oxidation provide more water than does fat metabolism because of the release of stored water as well as metabolic water. As the fuel source shifts in favor of muscle glycogen at higher workloads, plasma volume and thermoregulatory control are maintained. In practice, however, production of metabolic water plays only a minor role (146).

Unfortunately, rehydration often is only partially complete during exercise (131, 136). Inevitably, a delay in drinking sufficient fluid occurs because of increased exercise/thermal stress, termed *involuntary dehydration* (147). Rules of a given event may also impede drinking (114). Between 800 and 1500 mL/h of fluid can be replaced (134, 136), but fluid deficits of 400 to 800 mL during even light exercise (with free drinking) have been reported (147). Forced drinking before the onset of thirst may be used to minimize dehydration (124).

After thermal dehydration, even a 4-hour rehydration period is insufficient to restore fluid and electrolyte balances (143). During repeated, heavy exercise, normal fluid balance is regained within 12 hours, but sodium conservation by the kidneys continues for 24 hours.

Training Adaptation

In response to endurance training, heat-exposed athletes adapt and improve their work-heat tolerance (148). Hypervolemia develops over several days of prolonged training or with three or more bouts of intense, intermittent work. This expansion of plasma volume may contribute to the cardiovascular and thermoregulatory adaptations resulting from training (149–151). These adaptations reduce the extent of body fluid shifts during exercise in the trained person (123). Sweat rates increase as an adaptive response (147, 148, 151), but water and electrolyte balances appear to be maintained. Together with an increase in voluntary fluid ingestion, the effect is a reduced fluid deficit during work (147). Hormonal control mechanisms operate to cause renal conservation and minimize the disturbance of water and electrolyte balance (150, 152). Given free access to food and fluid, trained runners can maintain body weight and normal fluid balance during 20 days of severe prolonged exercise in warm temperatures (152).

IRON BALANCE IN PHYSICAL ACTIVITY

Iron balance and metabolism in humans at rest and during exercise has been the topic of several reviews (153–156). The subject is complex and still not fully understood. Its importance to persons engaged in physical activity derives from the central role of iron in cell metabolism. Iron is essential in the transport and delivery of O_2 to the mitochondria of the working cell through the proteins hemoglobin and myoglobin. It is also a component of many other protein systems, including the cytochromes and α-glycerophosphate oxidase (157) (see Chapter 10). Iron deficiency, with or without anemia, is frequent, especially in women in childbearing years, and is generally associated with decreased work performance and other discomforting symptoms (158).

Incidence of Iron Deficiency in Athletes

Surveys of athletic groups have shown that both males and females, particularly those involved in intense endurance sports, have hemoglobin concentrations in the low and midrange of the population norms (158–164). This state is often referred to as "sports anemia," but this term is imprecise and a misnomer (165). In most athletes, the lower hemoglobin concentration is caused by a training-induced increase in plasma volume that dilutes the red blood cells (149, 150). The increase in blood plasma is a beneficial adaptation to aerobic exercise and should be called dilutional pseudoanemia. Some athletes, however, develop true anemia (iron deficiency anemia), which is a deficiency in the total amount of circulating hemoglobin or red blood cells. The number of athletes with true anemia is low, although significant. In one study, 11% of the females in a small group were anemic (162), and in a second study, 10% of the males and none of the women had anemia (160).

Serum ferritin, transferrin saturation, and bone marrow iron levels are sensitive indicators of prelatent and latent iron deficiency and are used in assessing tissue iron stores (153). From these measurements it has been determined that many male and female endurance runners, although not anemic, are at risk for depletion of the iron stores. In studies including a range of sample sizes, investigators report 8 to 58% of male athletes and 40 to 80% of female athletes are iron deficient (160, 162, 166–169). The extent of iron deficiency in athletes appears to be far higher than in the general population (162). Without question, elite runners have lower plasma ferritin levels (protein-bound iron) than the general population. This difference may be related to hemodilution, transfer of stored iron into larger muscles and red blood cells, or altered iron metabolism, but regardless of the cause, this is the norm for these people. Comprehensive examinations of iron metabolism and dilutional pseudoanemia in male endurance athletes have concluded that no sports anemia or iron deficiency existed when all markers of iron status were considered (166, 170, 171).

Factors Influencing Iron Status

Several mechanisms have been proposed to account for iron deficiency anemia in athletes. This situation is most commonly caused by iron deficiency secondary to inadequate ingestion of iron to meet the body needs (155, 156). It typically occurs in rapidly growing adolescents involved in athletics, females involved in athletics, and those athletes engaged in activities that encourage low-energy intakes and low body weights (160, 162). A second and far less important cause is "footstrike" hemolysis (172, 173). Several other factors may also contribute to iron status and ultimately iron deficiency anemia, but most are considered minor. Exercise increases the elimination of iron and interferes with the normal increase in iron absorption when iron stores are depleted (164). Iron loss from gastrointestinal bleeding has been noted in some athletes associated with racing, but this condition is not a major cause of iron loss in most athletes (156). The focus of some studies has been on iron loss in sweat (164, 167), but findings of one detailed study suggest these losses are trivial (174).

Effects on Performance

Investigators have studied the ability to work aerobically over a wide range of hemoglobin concentrations, ranging from severe anemia to blood doping or induced erythrocythemia (175–177). It is clear that VO_2max and the capacity for intense endurance exercise are correlated with hemoglobin concentration when the hemoglobin levels are below the mean of the population, including when anemia is present. Blood doping and recombinant human erythropoietin injection studies have also shown that increasing the hemoglobin concentration by about 10%, without altering blood volume, increases VO_2max and aerobic performance (177–181). Reinfusion of red blood cells into trained athletes was first shown by Buick et al. to increase VO_2max by 5% and work performance by 35% (179). Also, some evidence shows that iron deficiency anemia has detrimental effects on the endurance and productivity of workers (175, 182).

Controversy exists regarding whether iron depletion without anemia adversely affects athletic performance. Results of some studies suggest that performance is adversely affected only when anemia is present. Iron deficiency induced without anemia in healthy males had no effect on VO_2max or endurance performance (183). In addition, iron therapy in female marathoners with low ferritin levels did not improve performance (184).

Treatment of Iron Deficiency

When iron deficiency anemia has been diagnosed in athletes, oral iron therapy has corrected the condition, and athletic performance has improved (161, 162). Oral iron treatment for iron deficiency without anemia has more inconsistent results. Hematologic variables of elite long-distance runners failed to show uniform improvement with iron therapy over 2 years during which a rich dietary source and supplemental iron were given. Iron stores remained depleted, although iron balance was maintained (164), suggesting again that iron metabolism in endurance athletes is unlike that of the normal population. Iron supplementation restored measures of mild iron deficiency to normal and lowered blood lactate levels during maximal exercise, but it had no effect on performance (185). When iron deficiency has not been diagnosed, iron supplementation has had little or no effect on hematologic measures or performance (158, 163).

Endurance athletes of both sexes, particularly runners who undergo prolonged, intense training, are susceptible to iron deficiency, with or without anemia. Impairment of performance may result. Iron status should be monitored regularly by serum ferritin and hemoglobin analyses. If latent or manifest iron deficiency is seen, supplemental oral iron treatments appear justified. When several measures of iron status reveal no true iron deficiency, routine iron supplementation is not indicated (171). Iron deficiency can be prevented in most athletes by manipulating the diet to increase iron intake, such as eating more lean red meat and dark meat of chicken; drinking a source of vitamin C instead of coffee or tea when eating bread and cereal to improve iron absorption; cooking in cast iron pans; and eating dried beans or peas with poultry or seafood to increase iron absorption from the vegetables.

VITAMINS, TRACE MINERALS, AND EXERCISE

The use of vitamins and minerals remains controversial. The conservative recommendations of most recognized scientific authorities contrast sharply with the practice of athletes and coaches who experiment with a wide range of diets and supplements in the hope of maximizing performance. Clearly, physical work capacity is reduced by deficient nutrition, and an adequate diet is an important base for optimal work performance.

Results of studies suggest that exercise increases the need for some vitamins and minerals and that certain groups of athletes have specific vitamin and mineral deficiencies (186, 187). However, findings also show that the increased need can be met and the deficiencies can be corrected by a well-balanced diet. The most common method of assessing vitamin and mineral status in athletes is to monitor dietary intake. Unfortunately, this method relies on the accuracy of the recollection of the subject and records from only a few days may not be representative for some minerals and vitamins. Clinical signs are also used in evaluating a vitamin and mineral status. However, the most accurate methods are direct biochemical assays of blood and, in many individuals, tissue vitamin and mineral levels.

Although controversy exists, few authors have documented any beneficial effect of vitamin and mineral supplementation in subjects who are not deficient. In addition, large doses of certain vitamins and minerals can be toxic. Reviews on this topic consistently agree with the above conclusions and note that most studies in this area have weak experimental designs and are poorly controlled (186–189). Some of the problems are lack of control and placebo groups, lack of double-blind and crossover designs, inappropriate measurements of performance for the vitamin or mineral studied, and lack of an initial assessment of subject fitness (186). Properly designed, well-controlled studies are difficult to perform in this area.

This chapter does not include an examination of all the vitamins and trace minerals that may relate to exercise for several reasons: the numerous reviews that exist in this area (186–189), the large number of poorly designed and controlled studies, and the lack of investigations examining the relationship between exercise and some vitamins and minerals.

Fat-Soluble Vitamins

The fat-soluble vitamins include vitamins A, D, and E. Vitamins A and E may be related to exercise as antioxidants and vitamin D is instrumental in bone mineral metabolism. No evidence exists that these compounds enhance performance in nutritionally adequate individuals. Overdoses of vitamin A may lead to anorexia, hypercalcemia, and liver and kidney damage, and overdoses of vitamin D can produce hypercalcemia and hypercalciuria (186, 190).

Water-Soluble Vitamins

Evidence suggests that exercise may affect the need for vitamin C, riboflavin, and thiamin (187, 191, 192). Vitamin C supplementation did improve the ability to train in subjects who were vitamin C depleted (193). However, in nutritionally balanced sedentary individuals and athletes, supplementation with thiamin, riboflavin, vitamin B_6 (pyridoxine), pantothenic acid, vitamin B_{12} (cobalamin), so-called vitamin B_{15} ("pangamic" acid), and vitamin C had no effect on performance (186, 194–199). No study has been made of the effects of folate and biotin supplementation on exercise performance. The intake of a niacin supplement is known to inhibit the release of FFAs from adipose tissue (200). The result is increased muscle glycogen degradation during prolonged exercise, which leads to an earlier onset of fatigue (201). Therefore, niacin supplements should be avoided.

TRACE MINERALS

Many trace elements are involved directly in energy metabolism or in other functions related to exercise or recovery from exercise. Zinc is involved in carbohydrate (e.g., lactate dehydrogenase), fat, and protein metabolism, and in tissue repair. Copper is involved in oxidative phosphorylation (e.g., cytochrome aa_3), erythropoiesis, and catecholamine regulation. Chromium potentiates the effect of insulin and is involved in carbohydrate and fat metabolism. Selenium is an antioxidant, and iron has a well-known role in oxygen delivery to tissues.

Iron status is examined above, and no studies have assessed the effects of chromium and selenium supplementation on athletic performance. Small amounts of zinc are known to be lost in sweat, and reports indicate that some athletes ingest inadequate amounts of zinc (202, 203). Some endurance athletes have low resting blood levels of zinc (202, 204), whereas others have adequate levels (205, 206). One investigation measured plasma and red blood cell concentrations of zinc and copper and reported no relationship with VO_2max in athletes (207). Surprisingly, few studies have examined the effect of zinc supplementation on exercise performance. However, this may be due to the negative effects of excessive zinc consumption: impaired copper absorption from the diet and hypocupremia, a reduction in levels of circulating high-density lipoproteins, and impaired immune responses (186, 208).

Several studies have also attempted to assess the potential benefits of supplementation with multivitamin/mineral combinations because several vitamins and minerals act synergistically. Two studies demonstrate no effects of 1 to 3 months of multivitamin/mineral ingestion on VO_2max and metabolic profiles during submaximal endurance tests to exhaustion in well-trained athletes (209, 210).

All athletes should eat a varied and well-balanced, nutrient-dense diet to ensure adequate vitamin and mineral intake. No evidence supports the idea that consuming large doses of vitamin and mineral supplements improves athletic performance and that some vitamins/minerals decrease performance or produce negative side effects. The most recent United States (96) and Canadian dietary recommendations (211) review data concerning needs for thiamin, riboflavin, and niacin in relation to energy expenditure (see also Appendix Tables A-2b and A-3a). If the demands of training increase the need for energy, the intake of vitamins and minerals also increases. Therefore, the most logical way to ensure that both of these conditions are met is simply to increase the daily energy intake. However, many groups of athletes limit their energy intake, including those concerned with the cosmetic and performance aspects of extra weight (gymnasts, dancers, figure skaters, and divers) and those who must "make weight" to compete (wrestlers, boxers, jockeys, and lightweight-class sports participants). For these people and any athletes who for a number of reasons do not consume an adequate diet, a basic daily multivitamin/mineral tablet is appropriate, but megadose supplements are not.

SUMMARY

The recent interest concerning nutrition and diet in work and exercise stems not so much from our interest in occupational work but from those of high-caliber training and competition in sports. It seems we have come full circle from the times of the Greeks and Romans. Elite athletes now experiment with a wide range of so-called ergogenic acids, including nutrients and foodstuffs, in what is often an irrational attempt to succeed (212). It is at this level of exercise, which in the modern world places the greatest degree of physical stress on the human body, that the relationship between nutrition and performance is best seen.

Scientific investigations have provided a sound understanding of the physiologic and biochemical events that occur in a variety of exercise situations; these studies form the basis for the recommendations on energy and fluid intake for optimization of performance and avoidance of exertional injury. Research has shown that dietary supplementation with vitamins and minerals above physiologic needs is both ineffective and unnecessary and, with abuse, may actually impair performance and health.

Results of studies have shown, however, that physical activity can make an individual susceptible to micronutrient deficiency states that may ultimately impair performance. Accompanying any increase in energy requirement is an increased need for thiamin, riboflavin, and niacin. Thus, the diet of an athlete must maintain a proper nutrient density as well as energy content. Exercise, by affecting absorption and/or elimination of nutrients, can upset the nutritional balance. Examples include riboflavin and minerals such as iron. At present, the risk of iron deficiency is best documented in young athletes. Continued research is needed in this area to better define the proper analytic measures as they relate to exercise performance, the effect of exercise on nutrient balance, and the means of preventing occurrence of a suboptimal nutritional state.

A factor complicating general recommendations on nutrition and diet for athletes is the variety of activities constituting what is known as sport. This variety is highlighted in a detailed 4-year study of the dietary intake of university athletes (213). At one extreme are strength sports (American football) in which one 118-kg player consumed 61.2 MJ in 1 day. At the other end of the continuum are lightweight wrestlers, gymnasts, and dancers with small bodies and dietary patterns that fluctuate widely in energy content but average 8.5 MJ daily. This extensive analysis of athletic diets across the range of sports revealed two points: that proper diet can provide the nutrition required for performance across the sports spectrum and that many athletes were at risk because of poor intake of one or more nutrients. Trends in these athletic diets reflect certain modern concerns, such as a high intake of saturated fat, cholesterol, and sodium and appreciable vitamin and mineral supplementation (214). Studies reveal the need for more education programs about nutrition for athletes, trainers, and coaches and show that these groups are eager for factual information (213, 215).

Nutritional advice must be tailored to the demands of the specific work and exercise (213). The statement by the American Dietetic Association provides a good model (216). Recommendations for the general public and for athletes involved in training or competition are separated, yet span the categories of athletic, combative, or occupational activity. The recommendations and overall viewpoint within the present review are in basic agreement with the succinct recommendations contained in the statement. The significance of diet, nutrition, work, and exercise are best summarized as follows:

1. An adequate, balanced diet is necessary for effective performance but does not guarantee it, because nutrition is but one aspect of performance.
2. A poor diet, on the other hand, guarantees substandard performance.
3. Being a fit, trained athlete does not alter the dietary requirements for most nutrients. Energy (carbohydrates), water, iron, and certain B vitamins are possible exceptions. These increased needs may, however, still be met through a balanced diet.
4. Ingestion of one or more nutrients in amounts much greater than body needs will not enhance performance and may actually impair it.

REFERENCES

1. von Liebig J. Animal chemistry or organic chemistry in its application to physiology and pathology. London: Taylor and Walton, 1842.
2. Zuntz N. Pflugers Arch 1897;68:191.

3. Zuntz N. Arch Gesamte Physiol Mens Tiere 1901;83:557–71.
4. Himwich HE, Rose MI. Am J Physiol 1927;81:485–6.
5. Christensen EH, Hansen O. Scand Arch Physiol 1939;81: 160–75.
6. Bergström J. Scand J Clin Lab Invest 1962;14(Suppl 68): 1–110.
7. Bergström J, Hultman E, Roch-Norlund AE. Nature 1963; 198:97–8.
8. Bergström J, Hultman E. Scand J Clin Lab Invest 1966;18: 16–20.
9. Bergström J, Hultman E. Nature 1966;210:309–10.
10. Hultman E, Bergström J, McLennan-Anderson N. Scand J Clin Lab Invest 1967;19:56–66.
11. Ahlborg B, Bergström J, Ekelund L-G, et al. Acta Physiol Scand 1967;70:129–42.
12. Hultman E. Circ Res 1967;20 & 21(Suppl 1):1–99.
13. Hultman E. Scand J Clin Lab Invest 1967;19:209–17.
14. Bergström J, Hultman E. Scand J Clin Lab Invest 1967;19: 218–28.
15. Bergström J, Hultman E. Acta Med Scand 1967;182:93–107.
16. Hultman E, Bergström J. Acta Med Scand 1967;182:109–17.
17. Hermansen L, Hultman E, Saltin B. Acta Physiol Scand 1967;71:129–39.
18. Bergström J, Hermansen L, Hultman E, et al. Acta Physiol Scand 1967;71:140–50.
19. Ahlborg B, Bergström J, Brohult J, et al. Försvarsmedicin 1967;3:85–100.
20. Hultman E. Scand J Clin Lab Invest 1967;19(Suppl 94):1–63.
21. Bergström J, Beroniade V, Hultman E, et al. Symposium über Transport und Funktion intracellulärer Elektrolyte. 3–4 Juni, Schüren/Saar, 1967;108–17.
22. Nilsson LH. Studies on liver glycogen metabolism in man with special reference to diet and sugar infusion. Thesis, Karolinska Institutet, Stockholm 1974.
23. Nilsson LH, Hultman E. Scand J Clin Lab Invest 1973;32: 325–30.
24. Nilsson LH, Fürst P, Hultman E. Scand J Clin Lab Invest 1973;32:331–7.
25. Hultman E, Nilsson LH. Adv Exp Med Biol 1971;11:143–51.
26. Nilsson LH, Hultman E. Scand J Clin Lab Invest 1974;33: 5–10.
27. Bergström J, Harris RC, Hultman E, et al. Adv Exp Med Biol 1971;11:341–55.
28. Harris RC. Muscle energy metabolism in man in response to isometric contraction. A biopsy study. Thesis, University of Wales, 1981.
29. Hultman E, Sjöholm H. Substrate availability. In: Knuttgen HG, Vogel JA, Poortmans J, eds. International series on sports sciences, vol 13. Champaign, IL: Human Kinetic, 1983:63–75.
30. Fletcher JGL, Lewis HK. Ergonomics 1959;2:114–5.
31. Wilkie DR. Ergonomics 1960;3:1–8.
32. Davies CTM. Ergonomics 1971;14:245–56.
33. Kleine TO. Z Klin Chem 1967;5:244–7.
34. Margaria R, Cerretelli P, Mangili F. J Appl Physiol 1964;19: 623–8.
35. Hultman E. Regulation of carbohydrate metabolism in the liver during rest and exercise with special reference to diet. In: Landry F, Orban WAR, eds. Third international symposium on biochemistry of exercise, vol 3. Miami: Symposia Specialists, 1979;99–126.
36. Nilsson LH. Scand J Clin Lab Invest 1973;32:317–23.
37. McGilvery RW. The use of fuels for muscular work. In: Howald H, Poortmans JR, eds. Metabolic adaptation to prolonged physical exercise. Basel: Birkhäuser Verlag, 1975;12–30.
38. Pernow B, Saltin B. J Appl Physiol 1971;31:416–22.
39. Fox EL. Sports physiology. 2nd ed. Philadelphia: WB Saunders, 1984.
40. Ren J-M, Hultman E. J Appl Physiol 1989;67:2243–8.
41. Spriet LL, Soderlund K, Bergstrom M, et al. J Appl Physiol 1987;62:616–21.
42. Ahlborg G, Felig G, Hagenfeldt L, et al. J Clin Invest 1974;53: 1080–90.
43. Holloszy JO. Biochemical adaptations to exercise: aerobic metabolism. In: Wilmore JH, ed. Exercise and sport science review. New York: Academic Press, 1973;45–71.
44. Holloszy JO, Booth FW. Annu Rev Physiol 1976;38:273–91.
45. Holloszy JO, Winder WW, Fitts RH, et al. Energy production during exercise. In: Landry F, Orban WAR, eds. Regulatory mechanisms in metabolism during exercise. Miami: Symposia Specialists, 1978;61–74.
46. Holloszy JO. Arch Phys Med Rehabil 1982;63:231–4.
47. Hultman E. Muscle glycogen store and prolonged exercise. In: Shephard EJ, ed. Frontiers of fitness. Springfield, IL: Charles C Thomas, 1971;30–9.
48. Lemon PWR, Mullin JP. J Appl Physiol 1980;48:624–9.
49 Brooks GA. Med Sci Sports Exerc 1987;19:S150–6.
50. Yoshimura H, Inoue T, Yamada T, et al. World Rev Nutr Diet 1980;35:1–86.
51. Refsum HE, Strömme SB. Scand J Clin Lab Invest 1974;33:247–54.
52. Rennie MJ, Edwards RHT, Krywawych S, et al. Clin Sci 1981;61:627–39.
53. Dåecombaz J, Reinhardt P, Anantharaman K, et al. Eur J Appl Physiol 1979;41:61–72.
54. Gontzea I, Sutsesco R, Dimitrache S. Nutr Rep Int 1975;11:231–6.
55. Felig PE, Wahren J. J Clin Invest 1971;50:2703–14.
56. Felig P. Metabolism 1973;22:179–207.
57. Felig P. Annu Rev Biochem 1975;44:933–55.
58. Graham TE, Pedersen PK, Saltin B. J Appl Physiol 1987;63: 1457–62.
59. MacLean DA, Spriet LL, Hultman E, et al. J Appl Physiol 1991;70:2095–103.
60. MacLean DA, Spriet LL, Graham TE. Can J Physiol Pharmacol 1992;70:420–7.
61. Young VR, Bier DM. Stable isotopes (^{31}C and ^{15}N) in the study of human protein and amino acid metabolism and requirements. In: Beers RF, Bassett EG, eds. Nutritional factors: modulating effects on metabolic processes. New York: Raven Press, 1981;241–63.
62. Hagg SA, Morse EL, Adibi SA. Am J Physiol 1982;242:407–10.
63. Wolfe RR, Goodenough RD, Wolfe MH, et al. J Appl Physiol 1982;52:458–66.
64. Millward DJ, Davies CTM, Halliday D, et al. Fed Proc 1982;41:2686–91.
65. White TP, Brooks GA. Am J Physiol 1981;240:155–65.
66. Buse MG, Biggers JF, Friedrici KH, et al. J Biol Chem 1972;247:8085–96.
67. Haralambie G, Berg A. Eur J Appl Physiol 1976;36:231–6.
68. Refsum HE, Gjessing LR, Strömme SB. Scand J Clin Lab Invest 1979;39:407–13.
69. Dohm GL, Williams RT, Kasparek GJ, et al. J Appl Physiol 1982;52:26–33.
70. Munro HN. Ciba Found Symp 1974;221:5–18.
71. Boobis LH, Williams C, Wootton SA. J Physiol 1983;342: 36P–7P.
72. Nevill ME, Boobis LH, Brooks S, et al. J Appl Physiol 1989;67: 2376–82.
73. Harris RC, Soderlund K, Hultman E. Clin Sci 1992;83:367–84.

74. Greenhaff PL, Casey A, Short A, et al. Clin Sci 1993;84: 565–71.
75. Harris RC, Viru M, Greenhaff PL, et al. J Physiol 1993; 467:74P.
76. Balsom PD, Ekblom B, Soderlund K, et al. Scand J Med Sci Sports 1993;3:143–9.
77. Birch R, Noble D, Greenhaff PL. Eur J Appl Physiol 1994;69:268–70.
78. Dawson B, Cutler M, Moody A, et al. Aus J Sci Med Sports 1995;27:56–61.
79. Casey A, Constantin-Teodosiu D, Howell S, et al. Am J Physiol 1996;271:E31–7.
80. Balsom PD, Harridge SDR, Soderlund K, et al. Acta Physiol Scand 1993;149:521–3.
81. Harris RC, Lowe JA, Warnes K, et al. Res Vet Sci 1996;62: 58–62.
82. Hultman E, Soderlund K, Timmons JA, et al. J Appl Physiol 1996;81:232–7.
83. Greenhaff PL, Bodin K, Soderlund K, et al. Am J Physiol 1994;266:E7225–30.
84. Hultman E, Bergström J, Roch-Norlund AE. Adv Exp Med Biol 1971;11:273–88.
85. Brown JH, Thompson B, Mayer SE. Biochemistry 1977;16: 5501–8.
86. Sherman WM, Costill DL, Fink WJ, et al. Int J Sports Med 1981;2:114–8.
87. Bergström J, Guarnieri G, Hultman E. J Appl Physiol 1971;30:122–5.
88. Bergström J, Guarnieri G, Hultman E. Changes in muscle water and electrolytes during exercise. In: Keul J, ed. Limiting factors of physical performance. Stuttgart: Georg Thieme, 1973;173–8.
89. Owen OE, Morgan AP, Kemp HG, et al. J Clin Invest 1967; 46:1589–95.
90. Owen OE, Felig P, Morgan AP, et al. J Clin Invest 1969; 48:574–83.
91. Hultman E, Nilsson L. Liver glycogen as a glucose-supplying source during exercise. In: Keul J, ed. Limiting factors of physical performance. Stuttgart: Georg Thieme, 1973;179–89.
92. Passmore JVGA, Durnin JV. Energy, work and leisure. London: Heineman, 1967.
93. FAO/WHO Expert Committee. Energy and protein requirements. WHO Tech Rep Ser 1973;52:1–118.
94. Norgan NG, Ferro-Luzzi A. Int Ser Sport Sci 1978;7:167–93.
95. Buskirk ER. Nutrition for the athlete. In: Ryan AJ, Allman FL Jr, eds. Sports medicine. New York: Academic Press, 1974; 141–59.
96. National Research Council, Food and Nutrition Board. Recommended dietary allowances. 10th ed. Washington, DC: National Academy of Sciences, 1989.
97. Ferro-Luzzi A, Venerando A. Int Ser Sport Sci 1978;7:145–54.
98. Suzuki S, Oshima S, Tsuji E, et al. Int Ser Sport Sci 1978;7: 194–214.
99. Wirths W. Int Ser Sport Sci 1978;7:227–35.
100. Butterfield GE, Calloway DH. Br J Nutr 1984;51:171–84.
101. Todd KS, Butterfield GE, Calloway DH. J Nutr 1984;114: 2107–18.
102. Tarnapolsky MA, MacDougall JD, Atkinson SA. J Appl Physiol 1988;64:187–93.
103. Butterfield GE. Amino acids and high protein diets. In: Lamb DR, Williams R, eds. Perspectives in exercise science and sports medicine, vol 4. Carmel, IN: Benchmark Press, 1991;87–122.
104. Brouns F, Saris WHM, Stroecken J, et al. Int J Sports Med 1989;10:S32–S40.
105. Toråun B, Scrimshaw NS, Young VR. Am J Clin Nutr 1977;30:1983–93.
106. Consolazio CR, Johnson HL, Nelson RA, et al. Am J Clin Nutr 1975;28:29–35.
107. Darling RC, Johnson RE, Pitts GC, et al. J Nutr 1944;28:273–81.
108. Pitts GC, Johnson RE, Consolazio FC, et al. Am J Physiol 1944;142:253–9.
109. Rasch PJ, Pierson WR. Am J Clin Nutr 1962;11:530–2.
110. Marable NL, Hickson JF Jr, Korslund MK, et al. Nutr Rep Int 1979;19:795–805.
111. Laritcheva KA, Yalovaya NI, Shubin VI, et al. Int Ser Sports Sci 1978;7:155–63.
112. Rogozkin VA. Int Ser Sports Sci 1978;7:119–23.
113. Koivisto VA, Karonen, S-L, Nikkilä EA. J Appl Physiol 1981;51:783–7.
114. Coyle EF, Hagberg JM, Hurley BF, et al. J Appl Physiol 1983;55:230–5.
115. Coyle EF, et al. J Appl Physiol 1986;61:165–72.
116. Canadian Association of Sports Sciences. Can J Appl Sport Sci 1981;6:99–100.
117. American College of Sports Medicine. Med Sci Sports Exerc 1987;19:529–33.
118. American College of Sports Medicine. Med Sci Sports Exerc 1983;15:ix–xiii.
119. Saltin B, Costill DL. Fluid and electrolyte balance during prolonged exercise. In: Horton ES, Terjung RL, eds. Exercise, nutrition, and energy metabolism. New York: Macmillan, 1988;150–8.
120. Sawka MN, Pandolf KB. Effects of body water loss on physiological function and exercise performance. In: Gisolfi CV, Lamb DR, eds. Perspectives in exercise science and sports medicine, vol 3. Carmel, IN: Benchmark Press, 1990;1–38.
121. Nadel ER, Wenger CB, Peters MF, et al. Ann NY Acad Sci 1977;301:98–109.
122. Rowell LB, Marx HJ, Bruce RA, et al. J Clin Invest 1966;45:1801–16.
123. Senay LC Jr. Med Sci Sports Exerc 1979;11:42–8.
124. Costill DL, Miller JM. Int J Sports Med 1980;1:2–14.
125. Sawka MN, Young AJ, Fransesconi RP, et al. J Appl Physiol 1985;59:1394–401.
126. Sjogaard G. Am J Physiol 1983;245:R25–31.
127. Senay LC Jr. J Appl Physiol 1979;47:1–7.
128. Brownell KD, Nelson Steen S, Wilmore JH. Med Sci Sports Exerc 1987;19:546–56.
129. Houston ME, Martin DA, Green HJ, et al. Phys Sportsmed 1981;9:73–8.
130. Costill DL. Ann NY Acad Sci 1977;301:175–89.
131. Myhre LG, Hartung GH, Nunneley SA, et al. J Appl Physiol 1985;59:559–63.
132. Saltin B. J Appl Physiol 1964;19:1125–32.
133. Gisolfi CV, Copping JR. Med Sci Sports Exerc 1974;6:108–13.
134. Bergström J, Hultman E. JAMA 1972;221:999–1006.
135. Armstrong LE, Costill DL, Fink WJ. Med Sci Sports Exerc 1985;17:456–61.
136. Costill DL, Saltin B. J Appl Physiol 1974;37:679–83.
137. American College of Sports Medicine. Med Sci Sports Exerc 1996;28:i–vii.
138. Costill DL. Gastric emptying of fluids during exercise. In: Gislofi CV, Lamb DR, eds. Perspectives in exercise science and sports medicine, vol 3. Carmel, IN: Benchmark Press, 1990;97–127.
139. Mitchell JB, Costill DL, Houmard JA, et al. Med Sci Sports Exerc 1988;20:110–5.
140. Mitchell JB, Costill DL, Houmard JA, et al. Med Sci Sports Exerc 1989;21:269–74.

141. Nose H, Mack WG, Schi X, et al. J Appl Physiol 1988;65: 325–31.
142. Knochel JP. Ann NY Acad Sci 1977;301:175–89.
143. Costill DL, Sparks KE. J Appl Physiol 1973;34:299–308.
144. Hultman E, Spriet LL. Dietary intake prior to and during exercise. In: Horton ES, Terjung RL, eds. Exercise, nutrition and energy metabolism. New York: Macmillan, 1988;132–49.
145. Maughan R. Carbohydrate-electrolyte solutions during prolonged exercise. In: Lamb DR, Williams M, eds. Perspectives in exercise science and sports medicine. vol 4. Carmel, IN: Benchmark Press, 1991;35–85.
146. Pivarnik JM, Leeds EM, Wilkerson JE. J Appl Physiol 1984;56: 613–8.
147. Greenleaf JE, Brock PJ, Kiel LC, et al. J Appl Physiol 1983;54:414–9.
148. Gisolfi CV, Wilson NC, Claxton B. Ann NY Acad Sci 1977;301:129–50.
149. Green HJ, Thomson JA, Ball ME, et al. J Appl Physiol 1984;56:145–9.
150. Convertino VA, Brock PT, Kiel LC, et al. J Appl Physiol 1980;48:665–9.
151. Convertino VA. Med Sci Sports Exerc 1983;15:77–82.
152. Wade CE, Dressendorfer RH, O'Brien JC, et al. J Appl Physiol 1981;50:709–12.
153. Conrad ME, Barton JC. Am J Hematol 1981;10:199–225.
154. Finch CA, Huebers H. N Engl J Med 1982;306:1520–8.
155. Haymes EM. Med Sci Sports Exerc 1987;19:S197–200.
156. Eichner ER. Other medical considerations in prolonged exercise. In: Lamb DR, Murray R, eds. Perspectives in exercise science and sports medicine, vol 1. Indianapolis, IN: Benchmark Press, 1988;35–85.
157. Finch CA, Gollnick PD, Hlastala MP, et al. J Clin Invest 1979;64:129–37.
158. Pate RR. Phys Sportsmed 1983;11:115–31.
159. Clement DB, Asmundson RC, Medhurst CW. Can Med Assoc J 1977;17:614–6.
160. Clement DB, Asmundson RC. Phys Sportsmed 1982;10:37–43.
161. Hunding A, Jordal R, Paulev PE. Acta Med Scand 1981;209: 315–8.
162. Nickerson HJ, Tripp AD. Phys Sportsmed 1983;11:60–6.
163. Brotherhood J, Brozovic B, Pugh LGC. Clin Sci 1975;48: 139–45.
164. Ehn L, Carlmark B, Högland S. Med Sci Sports Exerc 1980;12: 61–4.
165. Eichner ER. Phys Sportsmed 1986;14:122–30.
166. Magnusson B, Hallberg L, Rossander L, et al. Acta Med Scand 1984;216:149–55.
167. Paulev PE, Jordal R, Pedersen NS. Clin Chim Acta 1983;127: 19–27.
168. Par RB, Bachman LA, Moss RA. Phys Sportsmed 1984;12: 81–6.
169. Wishnitzer R, Vorst E, Berrebi A. Int J Sports Med 1984;4: 27–0.
170. Hallberg L, Magnusson B. Acta Med Scand 1984;216:145–8.
171. Magnusson B, Hallberg L, Rossander L, et al. Acta Med Scand 1984;216:157–64.
172. Yoshimura H. Nutr Rev 1970;10:251–3.
173. Eichner ER. Am J Med 1985;78:321–5.
174. Brune M, Magnusson B, Persson H, et al. Am J Clin Nutr 1986;43:438–43.
175. Gardner GW, Edgerton VR, Senewiratne B, et al. Am J Clin Nutr 1977;30:910–7.
176. Perkkiö MV, Jansson LT, Brooks GA, et al. J Appl Physiol 1985;58:1477–80.
177. Gledhill N. Med Sci Sports Exerc 1982;14:183–9.
178. Gledhill N. The influence of altered blood volume and oxygen transport capacity on aerobic performance. In: Terjung RL, ed. Exercise and sport science reviews. New York: Macmillan, 1985;75–93.
179. Buick FJ, Gledhill N, Froese AB, et al. J Appl Physiol 1980; 48:636–42.
180. Spriet LL, Gledhill N, Froese AB, et al. J Appl Physiol 1986;61:1942–8.
181. Ekblom B, Berglund B. Scand J Med Sci Sports 1991;1:88–93.
182. Edgerton VR, Gardner GW, Ohira Y, et al. Br Med J 1979;2:1546–9.
183. Celsing F, Blomstrand E, Werner B, et al. Med Sci Sports Exerc 1986;18:156–61.
184. Matter M, Stittfall T, Graves J, et al. Clin Sci 1987;72:415–22.
185. Schoene RB, Escourrou P, Robertson HT, et al. J Lab Clin Med 1983;102:306–12.
186. Clarkson PM. Vitamins and trace minerals. In: Lamb DR, Williams R, eds. Perspectives in exercise science and sports medicine, vol 4. Carmel, IN: Benchmark Press, 1991;123–82.
187. Belko AZ. Med Sci Sports Exerc 1987;19:S191–6.
188. Williams MH. Vitamins, iron and calcium supplementation: effect on human physical performance. In: Haskell W, Scala J, Whittan J, eds. Nutrition and athletic performance. Palo Alto: Bull, 1982;73–81.
189. Wilmore JH, Freund BJ. Nutr Abst Rev, Series A: Human and Experimental 1984;54:1–16.
190. DiPalma JR, Ritchie DM. Annu Rev Pharmacol Toxicol 1977;17:133–48.
191. Belko AZ, Obarzanek K, Kalkwarf HJ, et al. Am J Clin Nutr 1983;37:509–17.
192. Leklem JE, Schultz TD. Am J Clin Nutr 1983;38:541–8.
193. Buzina K, Buzina R, Brubacker G, et al. Int J Vitam Nutr Res 1984;54:55–60.
194. Montoye H, Spata PJ, Pinckney V, et al. J Appl Physiol 1955;7:589–92.
195. Tin-May-Than, Ma-Win-May, Khin-Sann-Aung, et al. Br J Nutr 1978;40:269–73.
196. Keren G, Epstein Y. J Sports Med Phys Fitness 1980;20:145–8.
197. Keith RE, Driskell JA. Am J Clin Nutr 1982;36:840–5.
198. Gray ME, Titlow LW. Med Sci Sports Exerc 1982;14:424–7.
199. Tremblay A, Boilard B, Breton MF, et al. Nutr Res 1984;4:201–8.
200. Herbert V, Jacob E. JAMA 1974;230:241–2.
201. Bergström J, Hultman E, Jorfeldt L, et al. J Appl Physiol 1969;26:170–6.
202. Deuster PA, Kyle SB, Moser PB, et al. Am J Clin Nutr 1986;44:954–62.
203. Peters AJ, Dressendorfer RH, Rimar J, et al. Phys Sportsmed 1986;14:63–70.
204. Dressendorfer RH, Sockolov R. Phys Sportsmed 1980;8: 97–100.
205. Weight LM, Noakes TD, Labadarios D, et al. Am J Clin Nutr 1988;47:186–91.
206. Bazzarre TL, Marquart LF, Izurietz M, et al. Med Sci Sports Exerc 1986;18:S90.
207. Lukaski HC, Bolonchuk WW, Klevay LM, et al. Am J Clin Nutr 1983;37:407–15.
208. McDonald R, Keen CL. Sports Med 1988;5:171–84.
209. Weight LM, Myburgh KH, Noakes TD. Am J Clin Nutr 1988;47:192–5.
210. Barnett DW, Conlee RK. Am J Clin Nutr 1984;40:586–90.
211. Health and Welfare Canada. Nutrition recommendations. Report of the Scientific Review Committee. Ottawa: Supply and Services, 1990.
212. Percy EC. Med Sci Sports Exerc 1978;10:298–303.

213. Short SH, Short WR. J Am Diet Assoc 1983;82:632–45.
214. Ellsworth NM, Hewitt BF, Haskell WL. Phys Sportsmed 1985;13:78–92.
215. Bedgood BL, Tuck MB. J Am Diet Assoc 1983;83:672–7.
216. American Dietetic Association. J Am Diet Assoc 1980;76: 437–43.

SELECTED READINGS

Hargreaves M, ed. Exercise metabolism. Champaign, IL: Human kinetics, 1995.

Horton ES, Terjung RL, eds. Exercise, nutrition, and energy metabolism. New York: MacMillan, 1988.

Parizkova J, Rogozkin VA, eds. Nutrition, physical fitness and health. Baltimore: University Park Press, 1978.

Perspectives in Exercise Science and Sports Medicine. Carmel, IN: Indiana Benchmark Press; Cooper Publishing Group.

Lamb DR, Murray R, eds. Vol 1: Prolonged exercise. 1988.

Gislofi CV, Lamb DR, eds. Vol 2: Youth, exercise and sport. 1989.

Gislofi CV, Lamb DR, eds. Vol 3: Fluid homeostasis during exercise. 1990.

Lamb DR, Williams M, eds. Vol 4: Ergogenics—enhancement of performance in exercise and sport. 1991.

Lamb DR, Gislofi CV, eds. Vol 5: Energy metabolism in exercise and sport. 1992.

Gislofi CV, Lamb DR, Nadel ER, eds. Vol 6: Exercise, heat and thermoregulation. 1993.

Lamb DR, Knuttgen HG, Murray R, eds. Vol 7: Physiology and nutrition for competitive sport. 1994.

Gislofi CV, Lamb DR, Nadel ER, eds. Vol 8: Exercise in older adults. 1995.

Bar-Or O, Lamb DR, Clarkson RM, eds. Vol 9: Exercise and the female—a life span approach. 1996.

Lamb DR, Murray R, eds. Recent advances in the science and medicine of sport, vol 10. 1997.

Rowell LB, Shepherd JT, eds. Handbook of physiology, section 12. Exercise: regulation and integration of multiple systems. Cary, NJ: Oxford University Press, 1996;1–1210.

Symposium. Maximizing performance with nutrition. Med Sci Sports Exerc 1987;19:S179–200.

Symposium. Nutritional ergogenic aids. Int J Sports Nutr 1995;5:S1–S130.

48. Nutrition in Space

HELEN W. LANE and SCOTT M. SMITH

Humans have been flying in space for more than 35 years (Table 48.1). In the early days of the space program concerns centered around crewmembers' ability even to swallow food in weightlessness. Now it is apparent that nutrition plays a critical role in the ability of humans to explore the solar system.

Although most medical research has been conducted before and after flight, short-term in-flight studies have been conducted, especially on missions in which a laboratory module is carried in the Shuttle's cargo bay. In the United States space program, the key opportunities for studying physiology and nutrition during long-term flights have been the Skylab missions and the joint U.S.-Russian missions on board the Russian space station, Mir. Studies of energy requirements, body composition, fluid homeostasis, protein metabolism, calcium/bone metabolism, and hematology have been conducted.

Ground-based models have been used to simulate the effects of microgravity (weightlessness) on humans. Bed rest, either horizontal or head-down (−6°) tilt, simulates the headward shift of fluids, disuse atrophy of muscle, and bone loss. Unfortunately, as more results from space flight become available, the limitations of bed rest as a model for nutritional studies have become apparent.

In this chapter, we review current knowledge regarding human nutrition during space flight, with emphasis on results from flight research. Spacecraft food systems and crew dietary intake patterns are reviewed, and suggestions for research are offered.

BODY MASS

Body composition changes with a 1 to 5% loss of total body mass during space flight (1–4). Decreases in total body water usually represent 0.5 to 1.0 kg, with the remainder from loss of muscle, bone, and adipose tissues. Results from Skylab, Space Shuttle, and Russian flights have shown that crewmembers lose body mass despite being provided adequate energy from food sources (1–4). In-flight energy intake, particularly during short flights, is often considerably less than preflight intake. During Shuttle flights, body weight loss in 13 crewmembers varied from none to 3.9 kg (5). Their mean energy consumption was 11.38 ± 2.06 MJ/day before flight, but only 8.76 ± 2.26 MJ/day during flight. This intake was less than the WHO standard (6) for people with moderate activity levels. The crew on the 84-day Skylab flight proved that people can consume enough food to maintain body weight during flight (7). Nevertheless, inadequate food consumption contributes to in-flight weight loss.

ENERGY UTILIZATION

Another potential reason for loss of body mass in space relates to energy utilization: is it different in space than on Earth? The work expended in aerobic exercise during flight generally is less than that on Earth, not only because of the absence of gravity but because of limitations on crew time and the habitable volume in spacecraft (8). Studies using a doubly labeled water technique showed energy expenditures of 13 Shuttle crewmembers to be 12.40 ± 2.83 MJ/day before flight and 11.70 ± 1.89 MJ/day during flight (5). Resting energy expenditure may increase during space flight as indicated by elevated plasma and urine cortisol concentrations (9). The combination of lesser energy expenditure from exercise and greater energy expenditure at rest may explain the finding that total energy expenditure is similar in space and on Earth. NASA uses the WHO calculation with moderate activity for estimating space flight energy requirements (Table 48.2).

Energy expenditure during extravehicular activities ("space walks"), which might be expected to be physically stressful, was found to be relatively low, i.e., 9–12 $kJ \cdot kg^{-1} \cdot h^{-1}$ during Shuttle flights (10). This finding, calculated from the CO_2 production and heart rate of spacesuited crewmembers, reflects the relative comfort and heat-dissipation capability of the current spacesuits (11), as well as the tendency for movements made during spacewalks to be slow and deliberate, requiring minimal exertion. No additional energy is required for extravehicular activities.

FLUID AND ELECTROLYTE REGULATION

The characteristic facial puffiness of space crewmembers (12) is related to the headward shift of fluids without significant loss of total body water (9). Plasma volume

Table 48.1
Chronology of Crewed U.S. Space Flights

Year	Flight Program	Flight Duration
1961–1963	Mercury	15 minutes–34 hours
1965–1966	Gemini	5 hours–14 days
1968–1972	Apollo	5–13 days
1973–1974	Skylab	28, 59, and 84 days
1981–present	Space Shuttle	4–16 days
1995–present	Joint U.S.-Russian [Mir]	90–180 days
2000	International Space Station Program	120–180 days

declines during the first 24 hours of space flight and levels off at about 15% less than preflight values. Glomerular filtration rate increases by about 15% during the first few hours of space flight and remains elevated. Also reductions in plasma aldosterone and atrial natriuretic peptide and sometimes increases in plasma antidiuretic hormone occurred with Shuttle crewmembers (9). Concurrent decreases in total plasma protein levels resulted in isotonic plasma with normal electrolyte composition. The mechanisms underlying these effects are unknown. After the initial decline in plasma volume, the body seems to adjust to a new homeostatic setpoint. Decreased plasma volume at landing probably contributes to orthostatic intolerance (13). Shuttle crewmembers are required to consume salt tablets with water (to equal 1 L of isotonic saline) immediately before landing, which replaces about half of the plasma volume decrement and seems to improve postflight orthostatic intolerance (14–15).

Table 48.2
Daily Nutritional Recommendations for 90- to 360-Day Space Flights

Nutrient	Recommendations[a]
Energy	WHO (moderate activity level)
Protein	12–15% of total energy consumed
Carbohydrate	50% of total energy consumed
Fat	30–35% of total energy consumed
Fluid	238–357 mL per MJ consumed
Fiber	10–25 g
Vitamin A	1000 μg retinol equiv.
Vitamin D	10 μg
Vitamin E	20 mg α-tocopherol equiv.
Vitamin K	80 μg (for men; 65 μg for women)
Vitamin C	100 mg
Vitamin B_{12}	2.0 μg
Vitamin B_6	2.0 mg
Thiamin	1.5 mg
Riboflavin	2.0 mg
Folate	400 μg
Niacin	20 mg
Biotin	100 μg
Pantothenic acid	5.0 mg
Calcium	1000–1200 mg
Phosphorus	1000–1200 mg
Magnesium	350 mg (for men; 280 mg for women)
Sodium	<3500 mg
Potassium	3500 mg
Iron	10 mg
Copper	1.5–3.0 mg
Manganese	2.0–5.0 mg
Fluoride	4.0 mg
Zinc	15 mg
Selenium	70 μg
Iodine	150 μg
Chromium	100–200 μg

[a]These recommendations were generated by two Nutritional Advisory Committees to NASA.

Fluid intake, in the form of food moisture and beverages, varies from 2000 to less than 1000 mL/day during flight, apparently because of reductions in thirst. Urine production is correspondingly low and ranges from 2800 mL to less than 500 mL/day. Crewmembers are encouraged to consume at least 2000 mL of fluids daily during flight (Table 48.2).

BONE AND CALCIUM HOMEOSTASIS

Bone metabolism is affected by weight-bearing ambulation, ultraviolet (UV) light, and stress, all of which are altered during space flight. All crewmembers lose bone mineral during flight, most notably in weight-bearing bones such as the calcaneus. Biochemical evidence of changes in bone homeostasis is present within the first hours to days of weightlessness (16–20).

Bone loss during space flight and accretion following return to a gravitational environment vary among crewmembers and among bones. Those Skylab crewmen who experienced significant loss in calcaneal density had not regained their preflight densities by 95 days after landing. Similar results have been demonstrated in Russian studies. Bed rest also produces bone loss, biochemical and endocrine changes, and bone resorption. Recovery of bone mass after bed rest is also slow and variable.

Serum concentrations of calcium do not seem to change during space flight. Small increases (<10%) were noted in the ionized calcium fraction during a 115-day Mir mission, but not on Shuttle missions. Both short and long space flights, however, are associated with increases in urinary calcium and in the risk of renal stone formation. All nine of the Skylab crewmen had higher urine calcium concentrations during flight than before, with the greatest difference occurring in those who also had significant loss in calcaneal density.

Insight into the mechanisms underlying bone loss comes from the study of factors known to regulate bone and calcium homeostasis, such as parathyroid hormone (PTH), calcitonin, alkaline phosphatase, and vitamin D. Plasma PTH concentrations decline during flight, which probably explains the corresponding decreases in serum calcitriol. Serum calcidiol concentrations after a 115-day mission aboard Mir were less than preflight values, probably because of low ambient UV light. After the 84-day Skylab-4 mission (but not after the two shorter missions), plasma calcidiol was slightly less than preflight concentrations, despite daily supplementation of vitamin D (12.5 mg) on all three missions. NASA's current recommendation for vitamin D is 10 μg/day (Table 48.2), which is provided as a supplement to ensure the adequacy of intake in the absence of adequate food sources and UV light.

Markers of bone metabolism have been studied to determine whether bone loss is associated with changes in bone resorption or formation (21–22). During a 115-day Mir mission, serum concentrations of bone-specific alkaline phosphatase dropped from preflight levels by 39% on flight day 14 and by 11% on flight day 110. Urine concentrations of collagen metabolites provide additional clues of bone turnover. In six of the Skylab crewmen, urinary hydroxyproline was 33% higher after flight than before. Urine concentrations of pyridinium cross-links and *n*-telopeptide (markers of bone resorption) were almost 40% higher during and after space flight (Shuttle) or bed rest, relative to their respective control periods. These results suggest that microgravity-related bone loss is associated with both increases in resorption and decreases in formation. Reductions in PTH and calcidiol shift the calcium balance toward the negative, because of a combination of reduced absorption and increased excretion of calcium. NASA recommendations for calcium and phosphorus are 1000 to 1200 mg/day for crewmembers on long-duration space flights (Table 48.2).

MUSCLE AND PROTEIN

Exposure to microgravity reduces muscle mass and performance, especially in the legs. Magnetic resonance imaging and manual measurements with tape measures have revealed decreases of 4 to 10% in calf-muscle volume, with the amount lost corresponding to flight duration (23). Leg strength, measured with a dynamometer, declines in similar fashion. Another study, in which five Space Shuttle crewmembers (3 men and 2 women) underwent biopsy of the vastus lateralis before and after an 11-day flight, showed decreased cross-sectional area only in type II (fast-twitch) myofibers, the fiber type that responds to resistive exercise (24).

Other assessments of muscle loss in space include nitrogen and potassium balances, urinary 4-pyridoxic acid excretion, creatinine clearance, and whole-body protein turnover, as well as records of protein and energy consumption (7, 25–28). Potassium and nitrogen balances became significantly negative throughout the Skylab flights, but urinary creatinine did not change, despite losses of muscle volume. Disuse atrophy of muscle in space may be related to changes in whole-body protein turnover. A comparison of whole-body protein turnover (^{15}N-alanine) to phenylalanine kinetics in leg tissue before, during, and after a 2-week $-6°$ bed-rest period showed that whole-body protein synthesis decreased by about 13% during bed rest and that half of that decrease could be accounted for by the leg muscles (26). Excretion of 4-pyridoxic acid increases during bed rest, possibly indicating a decrease in metabolically active muscle tissue (27). Whole-body protein turnover was measured in four crewmembers before and during a 9-day space flight (28). Unlike the bed-rest subjects, whose diet was controlled, crewmembers' ad lib consumption of protein and energy decreased during flight, and they lost an average of 0.5 kg of body mass. Urinary nitrogen in this group declined sharply, but whole-body protein turnover increased from 2.0–2.3 g $\cdot$ kg^{-1} $\cdot$ day^{-1} before flight to 3.0–3.1 g $\cdot$ kg^{-1} $\cdot$ day^{-1} during flight. Stein et al. (28) suggested that flight-induced muscle atrophy is caused by an increase in protein-turnover rate that may be related to stress.

Nutritional means of preventing disuse atrophy have been evaluated (29, 30). Oral doses of branched-chain amino acids had little effect on leg-muscle protein kinetics; however, feeding a bed-rest group adequate energy with excess protein reversed nitrogen losses. On the other hand, Skylab crewmen fed energy and protein equivalent to those in the bed-rest group still had negative nitrogen balance and lost muscle strength in their legs (21, 31). It remains unclear whether nutritional means beyond the consumption of adequate energy and protein would be beneficial in reducing muscle atrophy. NASA's current protein recommendation resembles the RDA (Table 48.2).

HEMATOLOGY

Anemia, manifested as a reduction in circulating red blood cell (RBC) mass, has been found after space flights (32–35). After a 115-day Mir mission, RBC mass was 93% of preflight values. On shorter Shuttle flights, RBC mass decreased at a rate of approximately 1%/day. Plasma erythropoietin levels decrease early in flight. The high partial pressure of oxygen in early spacecraft led some to propose that hyperoxia was inducing RBC membrane peroxidation; however, changes in erythropoiesis are still evident in Space Shuttle crews, even though the ambient air is normoxic (35). Radiochromate studies have shown that the rate at which RBCs are removed from circulation is unchanged during flight but that release of new red cells halts upon exposure to microgravity. Iron turnover does not change during flight, suggesting that synthesis of hemoglobin and RBCs is unchanged from preflight levels. These findings suggest that new RBCs are destroyed before they are released into circulation.

One consequence of a reduced RBC mass is increased iron storage (34). Serum ferritin concentrations are elevated during and after flight, and serum iron concentrations are normal to elevated as well. The implications of excess iron storage during long space flights are unknown. Current space food systems provide excessive amounts of dietary iron (approximately 20 mg/day), which may compound the potential for deleterious effects. Dietary iron absorption in space has not been studied; results from such studies may alleviate concerns about iron overload during long flights. The recommendation for future 90- to

360-day missions is for men and women to limit their iron intake to no more than 10 mg/day (Table 48.2).

Indices of iron metabolism and erythropoiesis quickly return to normal after landing. This efficient recovery suggests that in-flight anemia represents an adaptation to weightlessness, perhaps in response to easier delivery of oxygen to tissues in the absence of gravity or to the relatively high concentrations of RBCs during the first few days of flight, because of decreased plasma volume.

OTHER CONSIDERATIONS

Other flight-related circumstances that influence nutritional requirements and status are changes in gastrointestinal (GI) function and exposure to space radiation. Fluid shifts, in combination with reduced fluid intake and possibly space motion sickness, could be expected to slow GI motility. Although GI transit time has not been systematically studied in flight, 10 days of −6° head-down bed rest significantly extended the mouth-to-cecum transit time relative to ambulatory control periods (1). Russian scientists have reported that the bacterial count in the GI tract increases during flight, and the composition of the flora differs as well (36, 37). However, absorption of protein and total available dietary energy were no different during than before Skylab flights.

Radiation can be a major risk factor because of unavoidable encounters with various types and elevated levels of radiation that are not present on Earth (38–40). Radiation exposures up to 30 rem are possible during long-term space flight. Radiation can kill, mutate, or transform cells, either through direct interactions with nuclear DNA or through production of free radicals. Accumulated doses can significantly increase cancer incidence. Any means of mitigating the radiation health risk to crewmembers is desirable, including the use of antioxidants that have low toxicity. Protease inhibitors, retinoids, and selenium can suppress the promotion or progression of radiocarcinogenesis. Although the protective value of antioxidants has not been tested, their potential for mitigating radiation risk has been considered in establishing the dietary recommendations for vitamin C, selenium, vitamin E, and vitamin A (as carotene) (Table 48.2).

DIETARY INTAKE

Crewmembers in all U.S. space programs typically are provided with about 125% of the nutrient recommendations shown in Table 48.2, although actual intake can vary widely (1, 41–43). Figure 48.1 illustrates the relative intakes of crewmembers during Skylab (n = 9), Space Shuttle (n = 21), and Mir (n = 3) flights as percentages of the recommendations for energy, protein, carbohydrate, fat, and fluid. The Skylab group met all of their nutritional recommendations through consumption of adequate amounts of energy and fluid. Their diet was high in protein (114 ± 25 g/day), with 58% of their energy derived from carbohydrates and 15% from fat. In contrast, for Mir and Shuttle crewmembers, the dietary intakes were 49 to 76% of their recommended energy levels and their protein intakes were 55 ± 10 and 79 ± 20 g/day, respectively. Calcium and potassium intakes were adequate at 800 mg and over 2 g/day, respectively, but sodium intakes were generally high at about 4 g/day. Iron intakes tended to be above the 10 mg/day requirement, with the exception of the Mir crewmembers, who consumed only about 8 to 9 mg/day because of their low energy intakes.

Except for iron, consumption of micronutrients has not been adequately studied. However, given the menu available, if crewmembers had consumed adequate energy, they could have met most of the micronutrient recommendations, except for those for vitamin D and perhaps the antioxidants. For flights longer than 180 days, vitamin D supplements along with antioxidants are provided. Adequate levels of fiber have been available in the foods supplied. However, fluid intake (food moisture plus beverages) was sometimes below nutritional recommendations with 2829 ± 700, 2379 ± 750, and 1128 ± 315 mL/day, for Skylab, Shuttle, and Mir crewmembers, respectively.

The food intake by the Skylab crews was much greater than that of Shuttle or Mir crews (Fig. 48.1). The Skylab and Mir crewmembers participated in metabolic studies during flight, whereas most Shuttle crews did not. The importance of food intake was stressed to Skylab crews, and they received daily advice on their food and fluid intake for the metabolic studies. This is the only program in which such intense concern about diet occurred. The Skylab crews also ate fresh and frozen foods, whereas

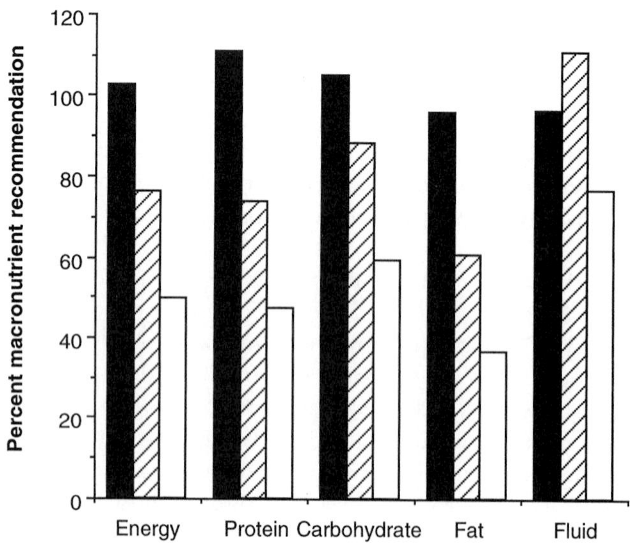

Figure 48.1. Macronutrient consumption by Skylab *(solid bar)*, Space Shuttle *(hatched bar)*, and Mir *(open bar)* crewmembers as a percentage of NASA nutrient recommendations. Energy requirements were derived from the WHO calculation for people engaged in moderate activity; macronutrient recommendations were calculated as percentage of calories as follows: protein, 12–15%; carbohydrates, 50%; and fat, 30–35%. 100% indicates that energy requirements or nutritional recommendations were met.

Shuttle and Mir crews ingested mostly dehydrated or canned foods. For Shuttle flights, no emphasis was placed on food intake nor was a specified time allowed for eating. Skylab crews probably ingested more food than other crews because *(a)* nutrition was emphasized, *(b)* fresh and frozen foods similar to those found on Earth were provided, and *(c)* adequate time was scheduled for meals.

Another potential explanation for inadequate food consumption in space is that food may taste different, perhaps because of nasal congestion from fluid shifts or the effects of a closed air system on odor perception. In the single controlled in-flight test completed to date, with one subject, taste perception during space flight and on Earth did not differ (44). A $-6°$ head-down bed-rest study with six subjects, designed to test whether headward fluid shifts would change perceptions of taste and odor, demonstrated no change in sensitivity to taste (sucrose, sodium chloride, citric acid, quinine, monosodium glutamate, and capsaicin), odor (isoamylbutyrate and menthone), or other trigeminal stimuli. Space foods are generally soft, and this lack of textural variety, in combination with a lack of food odors because of packaging and the presence of odors in recycled air, may confer taste-sensory monotony, which also would discourage adequate food consumption.

SPACE FOOD SYSTEMS

NASA has always strived to provide a palatable, nutritious diet in space; however, every space food system is subject to constraints on weight, volume, storage, preparation time and techniques, odors, and waste materials (41, 43). On the Mercury, Gemini, and early Apollo missions, many foods were provided in tubes that were squeezed directly into the mouth. Other foods were packaged in bite-size units to minimize formation of crumbs. The Gemini and early Apollo programs had no means of heating foods, while later Apollo missions had heated water (65°C) available.

Skylab is the only space program to date that included on-board freezers and refrigerators for food storage. Although refrigerators and freezers are costly in terms of stowage and power, they allow a greater variety of food during flight and reduce the need for salt or other preservatives.

Current space food systems attempt to emulate foods on Earth. Despite the lack of refrigeration for food on Space Shuttle flights, many items in the Shuttle food system are similar to standard American foods. The Shuttle galley includes a small convection oven for reheating entrees. Rehydratable foods are common; their packaging adds little weight, and forms a ready-to-use bowl when water is added. The inclusion of "off-menu" items has improved crew interest in meals. The advent of joint U.S.-Russian missions brought more variety to the food system, which tends to include about equal proportions of U.S. and Russian items. Menus for Shuttle-Mir missions consisted of 6-day menu cycles, with some additional food items provided for variety.

The International Space Station will include freezers and refrigerators for food storage and a combination microwave/convection oven. Many unique items are being developed for extended missions aboard this station, such as tortillas that have a 6-month shelf life. Current plans call for a 28-day menu cycle for 90- to 120-day missions. Facilities aboard the International Space Station are expected to provide a nutritious, appealing diet (Fig. 48.2) that can maintain crew nutritional status and confer the psychosocial sense of well-being associated with group mealtimes.

Future missions, such as those involved in establishing a permanent lunar base or traveling to Mars, undoubtedly will require some form of regenerative life-support system. The advantages of such a system would include the production of fresh food for crewmembers, as well as the opportunity for plants to be used in producing oxygen and recycling water.

SUMMARY

Food serves multiple roles during space flight, with perhaps the most obvious being the ingestion of recommended amounts of essential nutrients. Nutrition is an essential aspect of maintaining skeletal and muscle integrity, hydration status, and hematologic and endocrine function. All of these physiologic systems play essential roles in maintaining the health and safety of space crews, particularly during long missions. Group mealtimes can also build team morale and foster productivity. In summary, the realization of the full role of nutrition will be critical for the success of space exploration.

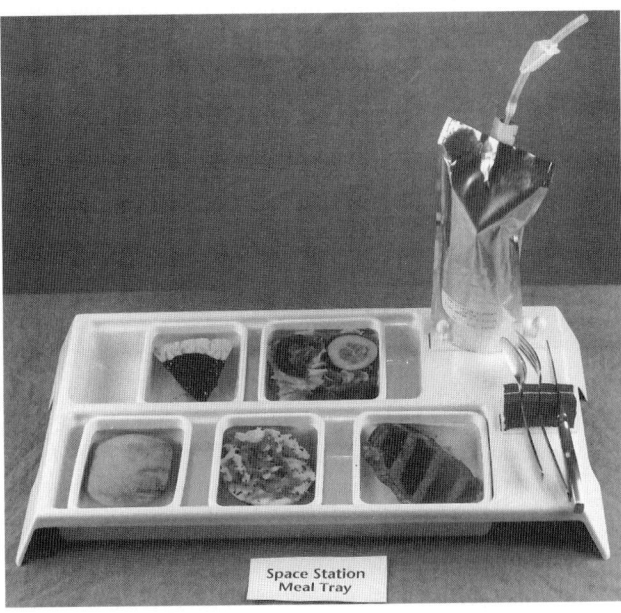

Figure 48.2. Space station food items.

REFERENCES

1. Lane HW, LeBlanc AD, Putcha L, et al. Am J Clin Nutr 1993;58:583–8.
2. Leonard JI, Leach CS, Rambaut PC. Am J Clin Nutr 1983;38:667–9.
3. Lane HW. J Nutr 1992;22:13–8.
4. Yegorov AD, Kasyan II, Zlatorunskiy AA, et al. Changes in body mass of cosmonauts in the course of a 140-day space flight. Kosm Biol Aviakosm Med 1981;15(1):34–6.
5. Lane HW, Gretebeck RJ, Schoeller DA, et al. Am J Clin Nutr 1997;65:4–12.
6. World Health Organization. Report of a joint FAO/WHO/UNU expert consultation, Technical Report Series 724, WHO, Geneva, 1985.
7. Leach CS, Rambaut PC. Biochemical responses of the Skylab crewmen: an overview. In: Johnston RS, Dietlein LF, eds. Biomedical results from Skylab, NASA SP-377. Washington, DC: National Aeronautics and Space Administration, 1977;204–16.
8. Michel EL, Rummel JA, Sawin CF, et al. Results of Skylab medical experiment M171—metabolic activity. In: Johnston RS, Dietlein LF, eds. Biomedical results from Skylab, NASA SP-377. Washington, DC: National Aeronautics and Space Administration, 1977;372–87.
9. Leach CS, Alfrey CP, Suki WN, et al. J Appl Physiol 1996;81:105–16.
10. Lane HW, Gretebeck RJ. Adv Space Res 1994;14:(11)147–55.
11. Powell MR, Horrigan DJ Jr, Waligora JM, et al. Extravehicular activities. In: Nicogossian AE, Huntoon CL, Pool SL, eds. Space physiology and medicine. 3rd ed. Philadelphia: Lea & Febiger, 1994;128–40.
12. Nicogossian AE, Sawin CF, Leach-Huntoon, CS. Overall physiologic response to space flight. In: Nicogossian AE, Huntoon CL, Pool SL, eds. Space physiology and medicine. 3rd ed. Philadelphia: Lea & Febiger, 1994;213–27.
13. Charles JB, Bungo MW, Fortner GW. Cardiopulmonary function. In: Nicogossian AE, Huntoon CL, Pool SL, eds. Space physiology and medicine. 3rd ed. Philadelphia: Lea & Febiger, 1994;286–304.
14. Charles JB, Lathers CM. J Clin Pharmacol 1991;31:1010–23.
15. Nicogossian AE, Sawin CF, Grigoriev AI. Countermeasures to space deconditioning. In: Nicogossian AE, Huntoon CL, Pool SL, eds. Space physiology and medicine. 3rd ed. Philadelphia: Lea & Febiger, 1994;447–67.
16. Oganov VS, Rakhmanov AS, Novikov VE, et al. Acta Astronaut 1991;23:129–33.
17. Smith MC, Rambaut PC, Vogel JM, et al. Bone mineral measurement—experiment M078. In: Johnston RS, Dietlein LF, eds. Biomedical results from Skylab, NASA SP-377. Washington, DC: National Aeronautics and Space Administration, 1977;183–90.
18. Whitson PA, Pietrzyk RA, Pak CYC, et al. J Urol 1993;150:803–7.
19. LeBlanc AD, Schneider VS, Evans HJ, et al. J Bone Miner Res 1990;5:843–50.
20. LeBlanc AD, Schneider VS, Spector ER, et al. Bone 1995;16:(Suppl)301–4.
21. Whedon GD, Lutwak L, Rambaut PC, et al. Mineral and nitrogen metabolic studies—experiment M072. In: Johnston RS, Dietlein LF, eds. Biomedical results from Skylab, NASA SP-377. Washington, DC: National Aeronautics and Space Administration, 1977;164–74.
22. Eyre DR. J Clin Endocrinol Metab 1992;74:470A–C.
23. LeBlanc AD, Rowe R, Schneider VS, et al. Aviat Space Environ Med 1995;66:1151–4.
24. Day MK, Allen DL, Mohajerani L, et al. J Gravitational Physiol 1995;2:47–50.
25. Thornton WE, Hoffler GW. Hemodynamic studies of the legs under weightlessness. In: Johnston RS, Dietlein LF, eds. Biomedical results from Skylab, NASA SP-377. Washington, DC: National Aeronautics and Space Administration, 1977;324–30.
26. Ferrando AA, Lane HW, Stuart CA, et al. Am J Physiol 1996;270:E627–33.
27. Coburn SP, Thampy KG, Lane HW, et al. Am J Clin Nutr 1995;62:979–83.
28. Stein TP, Leskiw MJ, Schluter MD. Am J Physiol 1993;264:E824–8.
29. Stuart CA, Shangraw RE, Prince MJ, et al. Metabolism 1988;37:802–6.
30. Ferrando AA, Williams BD, Stuart CA, et al. J Parenter Enteral Nutr 1995;19:47–54.
31. Thornton WE, Rummel JA. Muscular deconditioning and its prevention in space flight. In: Johnston RS, Dietlein LF, eds. Biomedical results from Skylab, NASA SP-377. Washington, DC: National Aeronautics and Space Administration, 1977;191–7.
32. Fischer CL, Johnson PC, Berry CA. JAMA 1967;200:579–83.
33. Leach CS, Johnson PC. Science 1984;225:216–8.
34. Udden MM, Driscoll TB, Picket MH, et al. J Lab Clin Med 1995;125:442–9.
35. Johnson PC. The erythropoietic effects of weightlessness. In: CDR Dunn, ed. Current concepts in erythropoiesis. New York: John Wiley & Sons, 1983;279–300.
36. Lizko NK. Microecol Ther (Germany) 1995;21:117–23.
37. Smirnov KV, Lizko NN, Sysoev AE. Microecol Ther (Germany) 1995;21:82–7.
38. Nachtwey DS, Yang TC. Acta Astronaut 1991;23:227–31.
39. Borek C. Nutritional, hormonal, and enyzymatic factors as modulators of radiation and chemical oncogenesis in vitro. In: Nygaard OF, Simic MG, eds. Radioprotectors and anticarcinogens. New York: Academic Press, 1983;495–513.
40. Troll W, Weisner R. Protease inhibitors as anticarcinogens and radioprotectors. In: Nygaard OF, Simic MG, eds. Radioprotectors and anticarcinogens. New York: Academic Press, 1983;567–74.
41. Lane HW, Rambaut PC. Nutrition. In: Nicogossian AE, Huntoon CL, Pool SL, eds. Space physiology and medicine. 3rd ed. Philadelphia: Lea & Febiger, 1994;305–16.
42. Lane HW, Rice B, Kloeris V, et al. J Am Diet Assoc 1994;94:87–8.
43. Lane HW, Smith SM, Rice BL, et al. Am J Clin Nutr 1994;60(Suppl):801–5.
44. Watt DGD, Money KE, Bondar RL, et al. Can Aeronaut Space J 1985;31:215–26.

SELECTED READINGS

Articles presenting results of experiments on Spacelab Life Sciences missions 1 and 2 are included in J Appl Physiol 1996;81:3–207.

Lane HW, Schulz LO. Nutritional questions relevant to space flight. Annu Rev Nutr 1992;257–78.

Nicogossian AE, Huntoon CL, Pool SL, eds. Space physiology and medicine. 3rd ed. Philadelphia: Lea & Febiger, 1994.

Nutrition and metabolism during spaceflight. Proceedings of an AIN/ASCN symposium, Experimental Biology, 1993. Am J Clin Nutr 1994; 60:801S–30S.

49. Body Composition: Influence of Nutrition, Physical Activity, Growth, and Aging

GILBERT B. FORBES

Der sehr fettarme Muskel eines verhungerten Tiers kann nicht ohne weiteres dem fettreichen bei normaler Ernährung gegenübergestellt werden. Zülassig ist nur der Vergleich fettfrei berechneter Organe.[1]

Adolph Magnus-Levy (1906)

The promulgation of the concept of fat-free tissue at the turn of the century paved the way for development of techniques for estimating body composition in vivo; and physiologists of that era spoke of the existence of an "active protoplasmic mass," to which various metabolic phenomena could be related. The 19th century continental chemists had established with some precision the composition of blood and tissue; now the 20th century investigators were to supply the concept of volume, first with blood and later with other body fluid compartments, and to conceive the idea of metabolic balance. Soon after the discovery of deuterium, Georg von Hevesy used this isotope to estimate total body water, and later Francis Moore introduced the concept of total exchangeable potassium and sodium. By applying Archimedes' principle, Albert Behnke showed us how to estimate the relative proportions of lean and fat in the human body. Rudolph Sievert found that the human body contained enough ^{40}K (a natural isotope) to be easily detectable and thus opened the way for the use of this technique to estimate lean and fat noninvasively. More recent years have seen the use of neutron activation, of special roentgenographic procedures (such as the CAT scan), of electrical conductivity and bioimpedance, and of nuclear magnetic resonance. Conceptualization and technical development both have played a role in this historical development, the one powerless without the other, to the point where we now possess a great deal of information on certain aspects of body composition throughout the age span of man.

The literature on body composition is vast. I have listed a number of books and review articles that contain a great deal of basic information (1–18). Individual references are limited for the most part to articles published in recent years.

BODY WEIGHT AND HEIGHT

Body weight and height measurements are easily done and are of great use in assessing growth and nutritional status. For the infant and child, growth velocity is truly a bioassay for energy balance and certain hormonal functions; in the adult, a change in weight suggests an abnormal process, nutritional or otherwise. See the Appendix for height-weight standards.

Normative values, despite what the adjective implies, cannot necessarily be construed as optimum. In an attempt to define optimum, tables of "desirable weight" for height have been developed from actuarial data gathered by the Metropolitan Life Insurance Company. Tables in the Appendices list such "desirable weights" for adults 25 years of age and older. While no provision is made for

[1]The fat-poor muscle of a starved animal cannot be compared directly to one normally nourished and rich in fat. It is permitted only to compare organs on a fat-free basis.

age, adults are categorized by body frame size, which is determined by inspection or by elbow width; the lack of precision in defining "desirable" is evident in the range of values given for each frame and height category. These ranges vary progressively from 2.7 kg for the shortest "small frame" category to 11.8 kg for the tallest "large frame" category of persons.

Body Mass Index

BMI is body weight divided by a power of height, usually (height)^2, which is said to be independent of stature. Calculations based on values for ideal body weight suggest that BMIs for normal men and women should be in the range of 20 to 27 kg/m^2. Indeed, this range roughly corresponds to the 10th to 75th percentile values recorded from adult individuals who participated in the 1971–74 National Health and Nutrition Survey. For infants and children, average BMI values change with age, from 13 kg/m^2 at birth, to a peak of 18 at about 1 year, a nadir of 15 at about age 6 years, and then a rise to adult values during adolescence. Individuals with high indices are classified as overweight, even obese, and those with subnormal indices as undernourished. However, such classifications cannot be applied, for example, to short muscular men or to tall asthenic women, and despite the sex difference in body fat, the average index is about the same for both sexes during the adolescent and young adult years.

The numerator of the index is total body weight, and the BMI provides a good approximation of body fat for population groups because most of the weight differential among adults is due to body fat. This is demonstrated in Figure 49.1, which is derived from body composition assays of adult females. Once a body weight of about 60 kg is reached, further increases in weight are principally due to increases in body fat.

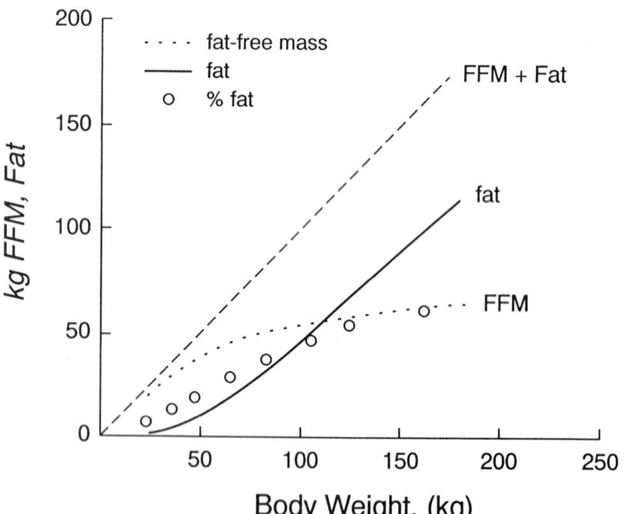

Figure 49.1. Plots of body fat, fat-free mass, and percentage fat in relation to weight for women. Author's observations on 164 women 156–170 cm in height, assayed by ^{40}K counting.

Andres has analyzed the relationship between BMI and mortality in adults (19). The curve is U-shaped: the lowest mortality rate is at a BMI of about 20 kg/m^2 for individuals 20 to 29 years old, and the nadir progressively increases with age to reach about 27 kg/m^2 for those 60 to 69 years old. Based on morbidity, the lowest rate for Japanese men and women aged 30 to 59 years is at a BMI of 22 kg/m^2 (20). Of interest is the lack of a sex difference for this ideal body mass index. Since males generally have more lean weight (fat-free mass, [FFM]) and less fat than females at any given BMI, FFM must be a factor in health risk as well as body fat.

Constancy of Body Weight

Support for the hypothesis that body weight is homeostatically controlled comes from the observation that many adults maintain their weight within narrow limits over long periods of time, and many children maintain their relative weight status as they grow. Indeed, following a period of weight loss, overweight individuals tend to return to their previous weight. Parizkova's (5) study of Olympic gymnasts showed that the gain in FFM and loss of body fat during training were completely reversed in time once the contests were finished. Individuals who gain FFM and lose body fat in response to anabolic steroids tend to revert in time to their previous body composition status and weight when the drugs are stopped (21, 22). Short-term fluctuations in weight can result from changes in water balance or changes in liver and muscle glycogen induced by diet and/or physical activity. Episodes of infection, serious trauma, enforced bed rest, malignancy, and nutritional inadequacy and surfeit lead to weight change; and many women state that they gain weight toward the end of the menstrual cycle.

The fluctuations noted above indicate that homeostatic control is not perfect; nevertheless, the absence of long-term change in healthy individuals suggests that energy balance oscillates around a mean value and that appetite (which controls intake) is geared in some mysterious manner to metabolic rate (which determines expenditure). When these homeostatic mechanisms fail, body weight changes significantly, and the result is obesity or anorexia nervosa.

Influence of Heredity

A significant influence on children's height is the height of their parents. Family resemblances in relative weight and in body build are readily appreciated, as is the tendency toward obesity. Monozygotic twins are more concordant for body size, even if reared apart, than are dizygotic twins (23). Genetic influence on metacarpal cortex thickness (24), bone density (25), skinfold thickness (26), body fat, FFM, BMI, and body fat distribution has been demonstrated (26–28). While family lifestyle and feeding practices may modulate the amount of body fat, studies of adopted children as well as animal models provide additional evidence for the role of heredity.

Racial differences in stature are well known; generally speaking, Oriental adults are shorter than Caucasians and have a smaller FFM, and southern Europeans are shorter than northern Europeans. North American blacks exhibit higher values for total body K and Ca than whites (29). The average Pygmy male is 144 cm tall, the female 137 cm, and the average birth weight is 2600 g.

Secular Changes

Today's children are taller and heavier and have an earlier puberty than those of previous generations, a phenomenon that has occurred in all countries in which it has been studied. While the reason(s) for this change is not known, the recorded increases in weight/height ratios suggest that improved nutrition is a prime factor.

Aging

Once middle age is reached, there is a progressive decline in stature, the result of thoracic kyphosis, compression of intervertebral discs, and change in angulation of the femoral neck. Borkan et al. (30) report a loss of 7.3 cm in males between age 22 and 82 years, and they estimate that 3.0 cm (41%) of the total change is secular in origin and 4.3 cm is due to aging. The longitudinal data of Flynn et al. (31) show a decline of 0.3 cm per decade in young adult males and 0.8 cm in females, with a gradual increase to 1.4 cm and 3.3 cm per decade, respectively, in those over 60 years of age.

BODY COMPOSITION

Body weight is the sum total of its parts. Modern techniques have made it possible to partition the body into several components, to carry out a "bloodless dissection."

In reports of animal experiments, the word *carcass* seems to have more than one definition: the entire animal body; body minus viscera, head, and hooves; body minus contents of the gastrointestinal tract. The first of these is comparable to the human situation, while the third is often used because of the comparatively large capacity of the gastrointestinal tract in many animals. The second is designed for the meat processor and is in no way comparable to the body composition situation for the living human.

The techniques used are listed in Table 49.1 and discussed in detail below. Most are considered *direct*, based on anatomic or chemical analysis. The last three in the list are considered *derivative* by comparison with other in vivo techniques; another example is intracellular fluid (ICF) volume.

Body Fluid Volumes

Body fluid volumes are based on the dilution principle: a known amount of material is injected intravenously (or in certain instances given by mouth) and after an interval for equilibration, a sample of blood, urine, or saliva is obtained for analysis (in the case of metabolizable substances, several such samples are required, with subsequent extrapolation to time zero). When urinary losses are appreciable, a correction is made for these; however, losses into the lumen of the gastrointestinal tract are usually neglected.

The general equation is

$$V_2 = C_1V_1/C_2$$

where V is volume, C is concentration, C_1V_1 is the quantity of material administered, C_2 is the concentration in body fluid at equilibrium, and V_2 is body fluid volume.

Since the body is not a static system, true equilibrium may never be achieved, particularly in the central nervous system and in bone, and there is always some question as to whether the apparent volume of distribution of the administered material coincides with that of the compartment in question. ICF volume cannot be determined directly, only by the difference between total body water and extracellular fluid (ECF) volume, and the value for the latter varies with the material used for its determination.

Plasma volume can be estimated with indocyanine green or Evans blue dye (T-1824) or ^{131}I-labeled albumin, and total red cell mass estimated with red blood cells (RBCs) tagged with ^{32}P, ^{51}Cr, ^{55}Fe, or ^{59}Fe or by carbon monoxide uptake. Materials for ECF volume are inulin, $^{35}S_2O_3^-$, $^{35}SO_4^{2-}$, SCN^-, Br^-, and $^{82}Br^-$. Cohn et al. (32) have used the ratio of total body Cl (by neutron activation) to serum Cl for this purpose. The first two materials in this list yield smaller values for ECF volume than the others. Appropriate corrections must be made for serum water, and in the case of ionized injectates, for the Donnan equilibrium.

Total body water is estimated by deuterium or tritium dilution or by dilution of urea, alcohol, or *N*-acetyl-4-aminopyrine. Water labeled with oxygen-18 is also used to estimate total body water (33). Administered deuterium and tritium undergo some exchange with nonaqueous hydrogen and thus overestimate total body water by 4 to 5%; this is not the case for oxygen-18. Bromide and SCN^- both overestimate ECF volume by about 10% because of penetration of erythrocytes.

Some of these materials can be given by mouth, others must be given intravenously; some readily penetrate the cerebrospinal fluid, and others do so very slowly. However, all appear in gastrointestinal secretions, which poses a problem in animals with a large gastrointestinal tract.

Repeat determinations in normal subjects show that the total error (i.e., biologic variation plus technical error) ranges from 2 to 9% for the various assay methods. It should be remembered that body weight, which can be measured quite accurately, varies by at least 1% during a 24-hour day, and individuals tend to be 1 to 2 cm (up to 1%) shorter in the evening than in the morning.

Table 49.1
Body Composition Techniques: Advantages and Disadvantages

	Advantages	Disadvantages
Density	Estimates FFM and fat simultaneously Nonhazardous	Subject cooperation necessary Unsuitable for young children and elderly people Error from intestinal gas
Dilution methods	Estimate body fluid volumes Great variety: determines Na, K, Cl (Br), H_2O, ECF	Radiation exposure (some materials) Blood samples needed (some materials) Incomplete equilibration of Na, K Overestimation by deuterium, tritium; value for extracellular fluid depends on method used; ^{18}O assay requires elaborate equipment
^{40}K counting	No hazard Minimal subject cooperation needed	Instrument expensive Proper calibration necessary Problem in interpretation in subjects with K deficiency
Metabolic balance	No hazard Suitable for many elements Can detect small changes in body content (<1%)	Measures only change in body composition Meticulous subject cooperation required Metabolic ward expensive Error from unmeasured skin losses
Anthropometry (skinfold thickness, circumferences)	Inexpensive Direct estimate of body fat and regional muscle, fat distribution	Poor precision in obese subjects and in those with firm subcutaneous tissue Regional variation in s.c. fat layer; uncertainty ratio s.c. fat:total fat
CAT scan	Delineates organ size; fat and muscle distribution; bone size	Instrument expensive Radiation exposure
Neutron activation	Minimal subject cooperation needed Body content of Ca, P, N, Na, Cl	Apparatus very expensive Calibration very difficult Radiation exposure, minimal
Nuclear magnetic resonance	Delineates organ size, muscle, fat, fat distribution, total body water	Apparatus very expensive
Dual-photon absorptiometry	Estimates bone mineral content, total and regional; body fat, soft tissue lean	Expensive Radiation exposure, minimal
Electrical conductivity (TOBEC)	No hazard Estimate of FFM	Apparatus expensive
Bioelectrical impedance	Apparatus inexpensive No hazard Estimate of total body H_2O	Many prediction formulas
Creatinine excretion	No hazard Estimate of muscle mass	Meticulous subject cooperation required Influenced by diet Collection time critical Day-to-day variation (c.v. 5–10%)

Total Body Content of Elements

The body content of a number of elements can now be assayed, by several methods. The isotope dilution technique can be applied to Na, K, and Cl as well as water by using the following equation:

$$Q = \frac{[Q^* \text{ admin} - Q^* \text{ excreted}]}{[Q^*/Q \text{ (serum, urine, saliva)}]}$$

where Q is body content (g, mmol) and Q* is the isotope (^{24}Na, ^{22}Na, ^{42}K, ^{82}Br, stable Br). Bromide is used because there is no convenient isotope of Cl. The result is expressed as total exchangeable content (Na_e, K_e, Cl_e), since this procedure underestimates total body content of both K and Na. Total exchangeable K (K_e) is 90 to 95% of total body K because of incomplete exchange with erythrocytes and brain. Total exchangeable Na is only 70 to 80% of total body Na, because of incomplete exchange with bone. However, Br dilution appears to be a good reflection of total body Cl.

Shizgal et al. (34) have devised a method for estimating total exchangeable K without the need to use the short-lived and inconvenient ^{42}K ($t_{1/2}$ = 12 h). Total body water and total exchangeable Na (Na_e) are measured together with Na, K, and H_2O in a sample of whole blood, and

$$K_e = [(Na + K)/H_2O \text{ (blood)} \times \text{body } H_2O] - Na_e$$

The correlation between measured K_e and K_e estimated by this method is high. Since Na_e is measured with long-lived ^{22}Na, some of which goes to bone, this method may not be suitable for children.

Francis Moore et al. (2) developed the concept of body cell mass (BCM), which they defined as "the working, energy-metabolizing portion of the human body in relation to its supporting structures." BCM consists of the cellular components of muscle, viscera, blood, and brain; and its size is estimated from total body K content, either as K_e from isotopic dilution or from ^{40}K counting. The BCM concept is useful because it encompasses those lean tissues most likely to be affected by nutrition, disease, or physical activity over relatively short intervals of time.

Neutron Activation

Neutron activation has been used to estimate total body Na, Cl, N, Ca, and P (8, 14). The subject is irradiated with neutrons, and the induced radioactivity determined by suitable gamma-ray detectors. The dose of radiation to the subject is about 30 millirads. However, the facilities required are very expensive and highly sophisticated, so only a very few are in existence. Total body N is proportional to FFM.

The possibility exists of determining total body Mg, H, C, O and individual organ content of I and Cd and possibly Pb. Details can be found in reviews by Cohn (6, 7).

^{40}K Counting

The body contains enough of the naturally occurring isotope ^{40}K ($t_{1/2} = 1.3 \times 10^9$ years; body content, 0.1 μCi) to permit its detection and quantitation by low-background scintillation counters. From the known abundance of ^{40}K (0.012%) one can then calculate total body K content, which provides an estimate of FFM. This technique is noninvasive and requires very little cooperation by the subject. Each instrument must be properly calibrated to account for absorption of ^{40}K gamma rays by subcutaneous fat and for subject geometry.

Body Density

Archimedes is credited with discovering that one can estimate the relative proportions of a two-component mixture, each of known density, by measuring the density of the whole system. Hence from a measurement of body density, the relative proportions of lean (D = 1.100 g/cm^3) and fat (D = 0.900 g/cm^3) can be calculated. Body density can be measured by underwater weighing, i.e., weight in air divided by loss of weight submerged, with corrections for the density of water and air and for the volume of air in the lungs. Body volume can also be estimated by water displacement, helium dilution, and special photographic and acoustic techniques. A new procedure in which the subject is seated in a closed chamber on land is now undergoing trials (35, 36); the pressure change induced by a known change in the volume of the chamber is used (Boyle's law) to calculate the volume of the subject. This technique has the great advantage of being quick and of requiring relatively little cooperation by the subject.

Metabolic Balance

The metabolic balance technique can detect small changes in body content and body composition. For example, a change in body N content of 16 g (1.1 mol), equivalent to 0.5 kg FFM, is easily detected, whereas such a change is well within the error of body composition techniques. However, the metabolic balance technique cannot provide data on actual body content, and it is actually rather expensive when one adds up the cost of running a metabolic ward and supporting laboratory facilities.

The usual procedure is to subtract urine and fecal excretions from intake, neglecting cutaneous losses since they are very difficult to measure. If the balance is strongly positive or negative, the introduced error is small, but it becomes appreciable as balance approaches zero. Cutaneous losses of N and K increase as their respective intakes rise, and many authors automatically subtract 5 or 8 mg N/kg/day. Another problem is the nonrandom nature of the intake and excretion variables; this results in positive balances being overestimated and negative balances underestimated, never the reverse. Corrections must be made for element content of blood samples and for menstrual losses. For elements such as Ca, Fe, and Pb whose main route of excretion is fecal, the balance periods must be long enough to account for day-to-day variation and to include intestinal transit time.

Anthropometry

Anthropometry includes measurement of skinfold thickness—really a double layer of skin and subcutaneous tissue measured with special calipers—and various body circumferences. The usual sites for skinfold measurements are the midtriceps region, the midbiceps region, at the inferior tip of the scapula, and just above the iliac crest. Since human skin is only 0.5 to 2 mm thick, subcutaneous fat contributes the bulk of the measured value. One grasps the tissue between thumb and forefinger, shaking it gently in hopes of excluding underlying muscle and stretching it just far enough to permit the jaws of the spring-activated caliper to impinge on the tissue. Since the jaws compress the tissue, the caliper reading diminishes for a few seconds and then the dial is read. (Satisfactory calipers include Harpenden Caliper, H. E. Morse Co., Holland, Michigan; Holtain-Harpenden Caliper, Holtain Ltd, Brynberian, Crymmych, Pembrokeshire, Wales; Lange Caliper, Cambridge Scientific Industries, Inc., Cambridge, Maryland.) In subjects with moderately firm, rather thin subcutaneous tissue, the measurement is easy to make, but those with flabby, easily compressible tissue and those with very firm tissue not easily deformable present a real problem. A recent comparison between caliper measurements and CAT scans of the midarm region showed that the former progressively underestimated subcutaneous tissue thickness as thickness increased (37).

Cross-sectional area of the muscle and bone (M + B) and fat components of the arm can be calculated from the arm circumference (circ, in cm) and skinfold thickness (SF, in cm) at the midpoint as follows (T is triceps skinfold, B is biceps):

$$\text{M + B area} = 1/4\pi\,[\text{circ} - (\pi/2)(\text{T + B})\text{SF}]^2$$

Subtraction of M+B area from total arm area ($\text{circ}^2/4\pi$) yields a value for arm fat area. Data on arm M+B area and arm fat area for 6- to 17-year-old children have been published by the National Center for Health Statistics (see

Appendices Tables III A 16a–d). The values were calculated using only arm circumference and TSF

$$M + B \text{ area} = 1/4\pi\ [\text{circ} - \pi \text{TSF}]^2$$

The problem here is that TSF often differs from BSF and hence is not representative of the entire subcutaneous mantle of the arm.

Extensive studies by many investigators have established relationships between various anthropometric measurements and FFM or body fat, and although the correlations are often not very high, the simplicity of the techniques allows them to be applied to large numbers of individuals in the field. Obviously such measurements as skinfold thickness and abdominal and buttocks circumference bear some relationship to body fat, and bisacromial, wrist, elbow, and knee diameters vary with FFM. The quantitative relationships between anthropometric measurements and body composition vary somewhat by age and sex.

Durnin and Womersley (38) measured skinfold thickness and body density in a large number of men and women and developed relationships between body density and the logarithm of the sum of four skinfolds (biceps, triceps, subscapular, and suprailiac). They present a table from which percentage body fat for various age and sex groups can be read from the sum of skinfold values (Appendix Table III-A-17-a). Pollock et al. (39) constructed a similar table from which percentage fat can be read from a sum of skinfold measurements (triceps, iliac, thigh for women; chest, abdomen, thigh for men) (Appendices Tables III-A-17-b and c. See also III-A-17-d for other measurements).

While these tables have been widely used, there are some problems. Durnin and Womersley's (38) gives rather high estimates of percentage fat for subjects with low values for skinfold thickness. Their estimates, as well as those of others using different anthropometric formulations, do not provide satisfactory values for subjects who are ill or who have lost considerable weight. The subcutaneous tissues in the elderly are easily compressed by the caliper jaws, which leads to falsely low readings.

Since FFM comprises 70 to 90% of body weight in normal children and adults, it is obvious that FFM and weight are related; and body fat and weight should also be related in subjects of widely varying fat content. As noted below, FFM is a function of stature at all ages. It was the failure of weight-height functions for individuals whose excess weight consisted of muscle that led Albert Behnke to develop the specific gravity technique.

There is now considerable interest in body fat distribution as a possible factor in adult health. Long-term studies have shown that men and women with high ratios of abdomen circumference to hip circumference (the "apple" configuration) have a higher mortality from cardiovascular disease and stroke than those with low ratios (the "pear" configuration) (references in [8, 14]).

Figure 49.2 shows a plot of abdomen:hip ratio against age for normal individuals studied in the author's laboratory (40). This ratio varies with age, and a definite sex difference develops by about age 12 years.

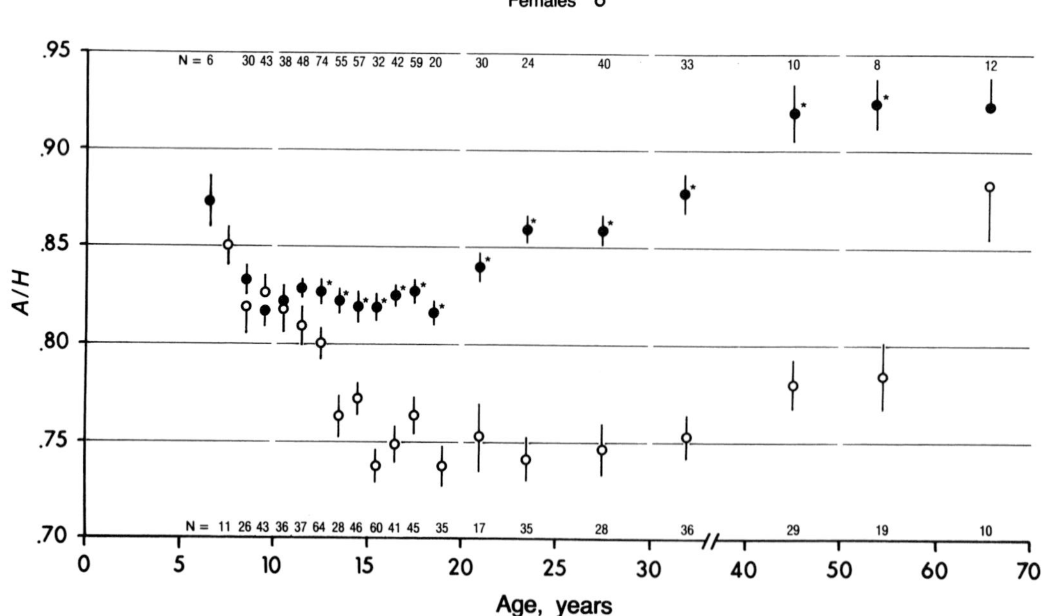

Figure 49.2. Normative data for abdomen:hip ratio derived from 661 normal males and 646 normal females (40). Abdominal circumference measured at the level of the umbilicus, hip circumference at maximum protuberance of the buttocks. *Vertical bars* are ±SEM. (From Forbes GB. Int J Obes 1990;14:149, with permission.)

Imaging Techniques

Computerized Axial Tomography (CAT Scan)

A CAT scan can differentiate lean soft tissue from fat and bone from soft tissue as well as determine organ size. However, assessment of visceral fat is hampered by intestinal peristalsis, and the use of the CAT scan to estimate total body FFM, fat, and bone is limited because of the radiation dose. This instrument is very expensive.

Tokunaga et al. (41), Kvist et al.(42) and Chowdhury et al. (42a) have made serial CAT scans of the body, from which they determined body fat volumes in both subcutaneous and internal sites. Of the total body fat volume in women, a large proportion is located in the pelvis, thigh, and hip regions. A variable relationship between visceral and subcutaneous fat has been noted in individuals with the same abdominal circumference. It is apparent that regional variations in adipose tissue sites exist, and there is now some interest in determining whether such variations influence health.

Magnetic Resonance Imaging (MRI)

MRI is a powerful tool that permits assessment of body fat, fat-free lean, bone, total body water, and the size of individual organs, large blood vessels, and muscles, all without radiation exposure. Estimates of adipose tissue at various sites in the pig correspond to chemical analysis, except in the abdominal region, where intestinal movement interferes (43). MRI facilities are expensive and very sophisticated.

Dual-Energy X-ray Absorptiometry (DEXA)

The body is scanned by two x-ray beams of different intensities, after which a complicated and as yet undisclosed computer program can be used to estimate bone mineral, soft tissue lean, and fat in the body. Pietrobelli et al. have reviewed the basic principles underlying this technique (43a). It is widely used to assess the bone mineral content and density of the pelvic region and hence the likelihood of hip fracture. There is some difficulty in estimating visceral fat and the soft tissue content of the head, and because a sizable portion of the soft tissue of the body lies in the shadow of bone, special compensatory maneuvers are needed to provide an estimate of total nonbone mass. Comparisons of DEXA-derived estimates of body fat and skeletal size with chemical analysis in pigs have shown some discrepancies (44, 45), and Jebb et al. (46) have found that DEXA readings are influenced by tissue thickness. The radiation dose is small, less than that acquired during a transcontinental airplane flight, but the instrument is expensive.

Creatinine Excretion

The assumption that urinary creatinine excretion is an index of muscle mass is supported by the work of Schutte et al. who found a good correlation between urinary creatinine excretion and dissectable muscle mass in dogs and a good correlation between creatinine (Cr) excretion and total plasma creatinine (plasma Cr concentration times plasma volume) (47). Urine collections must be timed accurately, and the excretion rate can be affected by diet. Studies of subjects of widely varying body size and both sexes have also shown a good relationship between creatinine excretion and lean weight (8). For subjects on *ad libitum intake,* this relationship is

$$\text{FFM (kg)} = 29.1\ \text{Cr (g/day)} + 7.38, \text{ with } r^2 = 0.97$$

and for those on meat-free diets it is

$$\text{FFM (kg)} = 24.1\ \text{Cr (g/day)} + 20.7, \text{ with } r^2 = 0.91$$

Welle et al. (48) found a similar relationship for older adults

$$\text{FFM (kg)} = 23.3\ \text{Cr (g/day)} + 21.1, \text{ with } r^2 = 0.87$$

They also found that creatinine excretion bore a good relationship (r^2 = 0.76–0.87) to arm and thigh cross-sectional muscle areas. Heymsfield et al. (49) concluded that the ratio of muscle mass to daily Cr excretion is in the range of 17 to 22 kg/g, which includes Schutte's earlier value (47) of 17.9 kg/g.

In a small group of adult males (n = 12) on a meat-free diet, Wang et al. (50) found that total muscle mass estimated by MRI was related to creatinine excretion

$$\text{Muscle mass (kg)} = 18.9\ \text{Cr (g/day)} + 4.1, \text{ with } r^2 = 0.85$$

It will be interesting to see whether this relationship holds for children and women. However, it seems that urinary Cr excretion can be used to estimate total fat-free weight and total muscle mass.

Electrical Conductivity Methods

Total Body Electrical Conductivity (TOBEC)

The subject is placed in a hollow cylinder containing a solenoid coil driven by a 2.5- to 5-MHz oscillating-radiofrequency current. The perturbation of the electromagnetic field by the subject is an index of electrical conductivity, which is a property of lean tissue. The instrument has been validated against carcass analysis of rabbits and pigs (8, 51), and DeBruin et al. (52, 52a) report an excellent correlation between TOBEC readings and total body water in infants. Studies of both static subjects (53) and those losing weight (54) give evidence of the usefulness of this instrument. The energy delivered to the subject is small enough (7 mW/cm^2) to pose no hazard. Unfortunately, the manufacturers have ceased production of this instrument.

Bioelectrical Impedance (BIA)

Electrodes are attached to the subject's wrist and ankle, a weak alternating current (800 μA, 50 kH$_z$) is applied, and the voltage drop is detected by electrodes placed proximal to those carrying the current. The hypothesis is that the resistance (impedance) to the electrical current is directly proportional to the length (L) of the conductor (lean tissue) and inversely proportional to its cross-sectional area (A), so that $R = pL/A$, where p is volume resistivity. Multiplying the right side of the equation by L/L, $R = pL^2/V$, or in terms of height (H), volume $= pH^2/R$ (for some unexplained reason, height is used instead of total length between the electrodes). Some investigators have used more than one frequency in an attempt to improve precision. Certain precautions (subject position, avoidance of recent food, etc.) are necessary to achieve reliable readings (14, 55), but the fact that the measurement is quick and without discomfort has made BIA very popular.

The problems are that the body is far from a perfect cylinder, that resistivity undoubtedly varies from tissue to tissue, and that the arms and legs contribute almost all of the resistance of the body (56). Reactance, a measure of cell membrane capitance, can also be recorded by the instrument; however, it is small in comparison to resistance and is usually neglected. A discussion of the principles of the technique can be found in reference 55a. A disturbing feature is that "the theoretical basis of the technique is ...unclear" (55a, p. 388S).

There are conflicting reports about the validity of this technique. Some report excellent correlations between BIA estimates of lean weight and density, total body water, and/or ^{40}K counting (53, 57, 58), while others (59, 60) claim it is no better than anthropometry. The failure (in some hands) of the BIA technique to predict body composition change accurately during diet-induced weight loss or gain (61, 62) is disturbing.

Precision of BIA estimates of lean weight is improved by adding weight, sex, and age to the basic H^2/R parameter. Several prediction equations have been devised. Unfortunately, the computerized analytic program provided by the manufacturer is a closely guarded secret. The inclusion of height and weight in the final calculation is bound to improve predictability because lean weight is related to both of these parameters.

Table 49.1 lists the advantages and disadvantages of the various techniques. Some are inexpensive, easy to use, and suitable for individuals in the field; others require a laboratory and rather expensive equipment; yet others are so sophisticated that few are actually in operation. Before proceeding, the investigator should determine the reliability and precision of the technique to be used. This is especially important in evaluating changes in body composition resulting from nutrition or disease.

Multicompartment Techniques

In the realization that the ratios of body water, body protein, and bone mineral are probably not constant throughout the life span, and that there are gender differences, some investigators have suggested that precision could be improved by making simultaneous measurements of total body water and body density; or body water, body nitrogen, and body calcium; or body water, density and DEXA (13, 14). The claim that such techniques yield more precise estimates of body composition than the simpler two-component models must be tempered by the realization that they place much more strenuous demands on the investigator.

Other Techniques

Other techniques are listed below. Some are not in common use because of expense, the need for special diet precautions, or lack of advantage over other techniques.

1. Uptake of fat-soluble gases (cyclopropane, xenon, radiokrypton) provides a direct estimate of total body fat (8)
2. Subcutaneous fat thickness by ultrasound (14), infrared interactance (63)
3. Urinary excretion of 3-methylhistidine as an index of muscle mass; a prerequisite is 3 days on a meat-free diet
4. Energy balance together with change in body weight yields a satisfactory estimate of body fat loss during weight reduction, according to Garrow (64); the formula is $\Delta\text{fat (kg)} = [\Delta E\ (\text{Mcal}) - \Delta W\ (\text{kg})]/8$, which assumes energy equivalents of fat and lean as 9 and 1 kcal/g, respectively
5. Estimates of body volume by special photographic techniques and by acoustic plethysmography (8); density then is W/V
6. Estimation of body fat from total body carbon (65)

Variables in Estimating Body Composition

Estimates of lean weight and total body fat from measurements of body density; total body K, N, and H_2O; electrical conductivity; and bioimpedance all assume that the composition of the lean body mass does not vary among normal adult individuals. The water, K, and N contents of the FFM do vary somewhat, as determined by carcass analysis (51, others in [8]). Of these, K exhibits the greatest variability, water the least. Bone has a low water content and a low K content but a high density in comparison to soft tissue; hence one must assume that bone:soft tissue ratios do not vary greatly among individuals. In neutron activation studies, Ellis and Cohn (66, 66a) found that the whole body Ca:K ratio is related to stature and so is a little lower in men than in women; nonetheless, the limited variability of this ratio indicates that the bone:soft tissue ratio does not vary a great deal among normal individuals.

In an extensive DEXA study of children and adolescents Ogle et al. (67) found a good correlation ($r = 0.98$) between soft tissue lean (i.e., total lean tissue minus bone) and total bone mineral content, as did Faulkner et al. (68) earlier. Indeed, the adolescent spurt in total bone mineral content is rather similar to that described for total FFM: bone mineral content reaches an apparent peak earlier in females and attains a value about three-quarters that of males. The ratio of bone mineral content to soft tissue lean weight was somewhat higher in girls, reminiscent of the earlier observation by Ellis and Cohn (66) that the total body Ca:K ratio is a little higher in women. From one point of view, males have more soft tissue lean per unit skeleton; alternatively, females have more skeleton per unit of soft tissue lean mass. These data pertain to young and middle-aged adults.

Assessment of individuals with massive obesity presents a problem. They cannot cooperate with the underwater weighing procedure, proper calibration of ^{40}K counters is difficult, skinfold measurements are imprecise, and the thickness may exceed the maximum jaw width of the usual calipers. Some patients have mild to moderate edema.

Another consideration stems from the fact that the ECF:total water ratio varies somewhat with age, being higher in neonates than in young adults and rising again in the elderly (8). Hence neither the K, N, or H_2O contents of the FFM nor its density can be considered constant throughout the human age span. The K:N ratio varies among body tissues, from a high of 24 mmol K/g N in erythrocytes, to 5.0 in brain, 2.8 in skeletal muscle, about 2.5 in viscera, to a low of 0.45 in plasma and skin (3). Hence the ratio of change in body K to change in body N resulting from a change in weight will depend on the particular tissue components involved. In states of under- or overhydration the density of the FFM will be altered, and in states of K deficiency the K content of the FFM will be subnormal. This is particularly important when dealing with diseased subjects.

The values for K, H_2O, and N content of the FFM listed in Table 49.2 are based on cadaver analyses (8), with the K:FFM ratio altered for females on the basis of the reported sex difference in the K_e:H_2O ratio. Some investigators prefer to derive values for FFM composition from a comparison of in vivo assays. Cohn et al. (69) have chosen values of 64.5 and 58 mmol K/kg FFM for males and females, respectively, while Womersley et al. (70) suggest 66.4 and 59.7. Lukaski et al. (71, 71a) derived a value of 62.6 mmol K/kg FFM for males. They also offer one of 746 mL H_2O/kg FFM; however, their values of 32.1 g N and 32.7 g N/kg FFM are close to the one derived from cadaver analysis. A number of values for total body K:N ratios (mmol/g) in living subjects have been reported: 1.88 to 1.95 for males; 1.67 to 1.78 for females. The average value from cadaver analysis is 2 mmol K/g N.

The variations noted above reflect the criteria used to assess FFM, differences in analytic techniques, or even biologic variability. Investigators tend to use the densitometric techniques as the "standard" with which results of other techniques should be compared. While densitometry is subject to less technical error than the other techniques, it is obviously impossible to determine its accuracy for living subjects, and it is likely that the density of the FFM (upon which the test implicitly depends) varies with age (it does change with growth) and perhaps with sex. There would seem to be no a priori reason to choose any one technique as a standard for comparison.

Table 49.2
Composition of Fat-Free Mass

Age	H_2O (%)	ECF/ICF Ratio	K (mmol/kg)	N (%)	Density (g/mL)
Fetus, 24 weeks	89	1.9	40	1.4	
Birth[a]	81	1.5	49	2.4	1.063
Adult	73	0.70	68 (64)[b]	3.3	1.10
Elderly		0.85			

[a]Fomon et al. (60a) provide estimates for ages birth to 10 years.
[b]Females in parentheses.

Effects of Age on Composition of FFM

Some effects of age on composition of FFM are shown in Table 49.2. Composition of the fetus and newborn is quite different, and changes occur with aging. Water content falls progressively during early life, as does the ratio of ECF volume to total body water, which rises again in old age. K and N contents rise, as does calculated density. Cross-sectional data on aging adults show that the ratio of N and K to total body water tends to decline with age; total body Ca declines faster in females, but the ratio of N decline to K decline is variable (14). Problems with the cross-sectional data include the relatively small number of subjects, the possibility of selection bias, and the failure to account for variations in height and weight, both of which influence total body K, N, and Ca.

Precision of Various Techniques

Two factors must be considered: technical error and biologic variability. These include such phenomena as the random nature of radioactive isotope emissions and the day-to-day fluctuations in urinary creatinine excretion. Body weight exhibits diurnal and day-to-day variations, and it is safe to assume that certain features of body composition also exhibit some variability. It is instructive to calculate the effect of adding or subtracting 500 mL H_2O from an adult subject, which will change the density and the K, N, and H_2O contents of the FFM slightly, as well as the ratio of element metabolic balance to weight change. A change in the ECF:ICF ratio will change the K:FFM ratio of the body as well as the density and H_2O content of the FFM. The *total* error—technical plus biologic—must be taken into account, and this can only be evaluated by replicate assays on individuals, which is not always feasible with assays involving radiation exposure.

The magnitude of the observed error will depend on the method used to express the results. When FFM is measured, fat is determined by subtraction, so in subjects in whom FFM exceeds 50% of body weight, the relative error for fat will be greater than that for FFM; the same is true for densitometry. The existence on rare occasions of individuals with an estimated body fat content of 1% or even a negative value proves that error can occur.

Published data show coefficients of variation (c.v.) of 2 to 4% for ^{40}K counting, 2.5 to 6.1% for total exchangeable K, 5.5% for body Ca, 3.5% for total body N, and 5 to 10% for urinary Cr excretion. Densitometry appears to be the most reproducible technique (c.v. 1.2%); skinfold thickness is the worst, with recorded c.v.'s of 6 to 24% (references in [8]). The c.v. for bioimpedance ranges from 1.3 to 7% (55a), for TOBEC is about 1% (54), and for DEXA about 1% (67). Error can be reduced somewhat by making two or more assays at the start of an experimental procedure (e.g., induced weight loss) and again at the end.

Not even the newer techniques are problem free. As noted above, DEXA readings are influenced by tissue thickness, and DEXA estimates of soft tissue and bone do not always correspond to chemically determined values in pigs. Inaccurate MRI readings of intraabdominal fat were mentioned above. Adipose tissue is not pure fat; it contains a variable amount of connective tissue, blood vessels, and adipocyte nuclei, and hence some water, nitrogen, and electrolytes (pork fat contains 18% water). While the total body K and H_2O methods do detect the fat-free portion of adipose tissue, DEXA, MRI, and CAT do not; hence their estimates of body fat may be a bit too high. However, both CAT and MRI can detect intramuscular adipose tissue.

CHANGES IN BODY COMPOSITION WITH GROWTH AND AGING

Reference Data by Gender and Age

Table 49.3 lists many of the elements found in the body of a male adult, the so-called reference man, as determined by the International Committee on Radiation Protection (72). Since the FFM of the average woman is about two-thirds that of the average man, her body content will be two-thirds to three-fourths of the amounts listed, with exception of O_2, C, and H_2, which are present in fat. Hence I have added some values for the average woman estimated from body composition assays of living subjects; the male values for Ca and P were also derived in this manner. The values listed are averages; for some, such as F, Se, and Fe, the quantities depend on diet.

Table 49.3
Reference Man and Woman: Total Body Content

Substance[a]	Amount (g)	
	Male	Female
Water	45,000 (2500 mol)	31,000 (1700 mol)
Hydrogen, nonaqueous	2,000 (1000 mol)	
Oxygen, nonaqueous	2,900 (90 mol)	
Carbon	16,000 (1333 mol)	
Nitrogen	1,800 (64 mol)	1,300 (46 mol)
Calcium	1,100 (27 mol)	830 (21 mol)
Phosphorus	500 (16 mol)	400 (13 mol)
Potassium	140 (3600 mmol)	100 (2560 mmol)
Sodium	100 (4350 mmol)	77 (3350 mmol)
Chlorine	95 (2680 mmol)	70 (2000 mol)
Sulfur	140 (4400 mmol)	
Magnesium	19 (780 mmol)	
Silicon	18 (640 mmol)	
Iron	4.2 (75 mmol)	
Fluorine	2.6 (140 mmol)	
Zinc	2.3 (35 mmol)	
Copper	0.07 (1.1 mmol)	
Manganese	0.01 (180 μmol)	
Iodine	0.01 (79 μmol)	

[a]Seventeen additional elements (all less than 330 mg) are listed in reference 72. For many the body content is a function of diet. The body also contains a number of radioactive elements: uranium (10^{-4} g), radium (10^{-11}), strontium-90, and cesium-137.

Average organ weights for an adult man are listed in Table 49.4 and compared with those for the newborn infant (8). The adult, who weighs 20 times as much as the newborn, has 33 times as much muscle, 23 times as much skeleton, 19 times as much heart, and 10 times as much skin, liver, and kidney; however, brain is only about 3 times as large. One-third of the newborn skeleton consists of cartilage, and relative organ size is different in the neonate: at this age muscle accounts for 22% of body weight, brain for 10%, and liver for 4%, compared with 40, 2, and 2.6%, respectively, in the adult.

FFM and Weight Variability Compared

Among individuals of the same age and sex, body fat exhibits much more variability than FFM; hence body fat accounts for most of the variability in body weight. However, FFM and fat are *not* completely independent entities. As shown below, a change in body weight that results from changes in energy balance usually involves both body components.

In women, the maximum FFM appears to be about 70 kg, in men, about 100 kg; although a few Japanese sumo wrestlers (73) and professional football players (74) have achieved values as high as 118 kg. Perhaps there is a limit to FFM as there is for stature, while body fat can increase enormously.

Age and Sex

Figures 49.3 and 49.4 show average values for FFM and fat from midgestation through the eighth decade, compiled from several sources. Note that the abscissa scale for Figure 49.3 is in postconception years. The fetus does not acquire appreciable amounts of body fat until the last trimester of gestation, and the human neonate has a larger percentage of body fat (14%) than other mammals at birth. Relative body fat continues to increase during the

Table 49.4
Reference Man and Neonate: Gross Organ Size (g)

	Adult	Newborn
Weight	70,000	3,400
Skeletal muscle	28,000	850
Adipose tissue (fat 12,000)	15,000	500
Skeleton (cortical bone 4,000, trabecular bone 1,000, marrow 3,000, cartilage 1,100, periarticular tissue 900)	10,000	440 (cartilage 140)
Skin	4,900	510
Liver	1,800	170
Brain	1,400	440
Heart	330	17
Kidneys	310	34

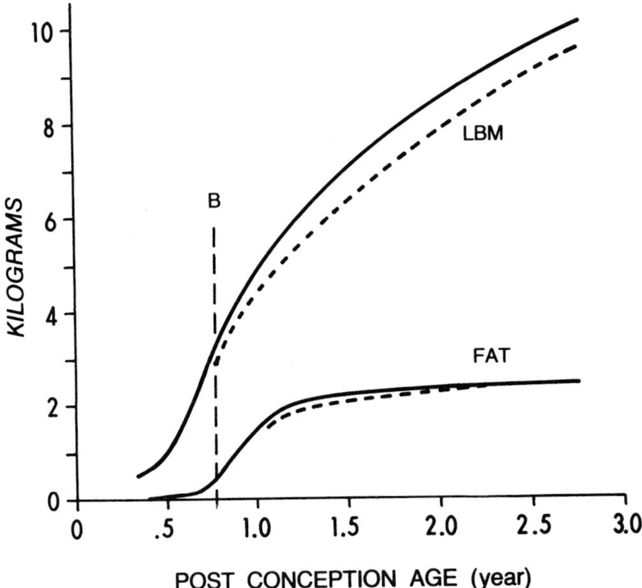

Figure 49.3. Average value for FFM and fat in fetus and infant. Age in postconception years. Boys *(solid line)*, girls *(dotted line)*. (From Forbes GB. Human body composition. New York: Springer-Verlag, 1987, with permission.)

first 6 months of postnatal life to a maximum of 25% and to a nadir of about 13% in boys and 19% in girls in late childhood (Table 49.5).

Sexual dimorphism in body composition is present in early life, well in advance of mature gonadal function. Once adolescence is under way, the sex difference becomes pronounced, the male spurt in FFM being much more rapid while females acquire more fat. Between the ages of 10 and 20 years the average increment in FFM is 33 kg in boys but only 16 kg in girls, and by age 20 years, the male:female FFM ratio is 1.45. This can be compared with a weight ratio of 1.25 and a height ratio of 1.08 at age 20. During the male adolescent spurt, the peak velocity for

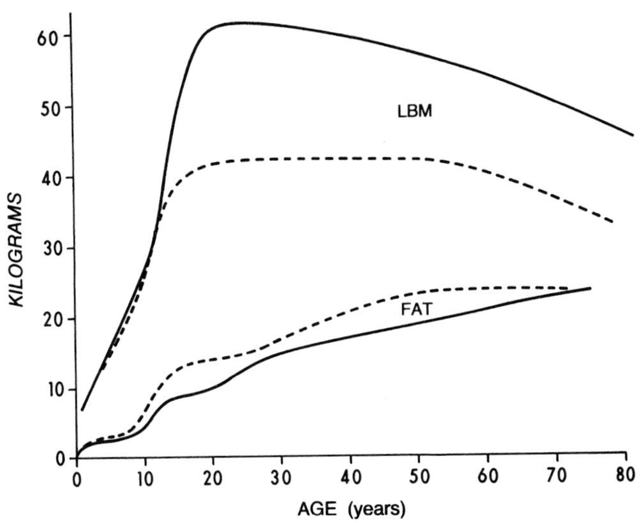

Figure 49.4. Average values for FFM and fat in child and adult. Males *(solid line)*, females *(dotted line)*. (Sources of data in reference [8].)

Table 49.5
The Reference Person

	Newborn	10-Year-Old Boy	10-Year-Old Girl	Adult Man	Adult Woman
Weight (kg)	3.4	31	32	72	58
FFM (kg)	2.9	27	26	61	42
Fat (%)	14	13	19	15	28

FFM coincides with peak height velocity (5). The sex difference in the magnitude of the adolescent spurt in FFM is likely due to the fact that the testosterone production rate in males is about 6 times that of females. Earlier mention was made of the good correlation between bone and soft tissue at this time of life; hence the sex difference in the former is similar to that of the FFM.

The adult years are characterized by a slow fall in FFM, which is somewhat more rapid in males. The data appear to indicate that female FFM is preserved until menopause. By age 75 years, FFM in males is roughly equivalent to that of the average 14-year-old boy, and in females to that of the average 13-year-old girl. So it appears that much of the FFM increment acquired during the adolescent growth spurt is dissipated by the aging process.

The cross-sectional studies of Cohn et al. (32, others in [14]) show a progressive decline in total body K, N, and Ca during the adult years. Between ages 25 and 75 years, body K declines by about 4.5% per decade and body N by about 3.5% per decade in both sexes. However, body Ca declines by 5.4% per decade in women and 2% per decade in men, which is consistent with observed decreases in the density of the spine and appendicular skeleton, especially in women, with advancing years. The decline in total body water is somewhat less than that for K and N, (14) which agrees with the age-associated increase in the ECF:ICF ratio. However, all of these values are derived from cross-sectional observations.

A few investigators have followed adults over extended periods of time, and such longitudinal observations tend to show a somewhat smaller age decline than do the cross-sectional data. Steen et al. (75) did repeat assays of total body water and body K in men and women from age 70 to age 81. An analysis of the individual data (kindly provided by Dr. Bertil Steen) showed that those who lost significant amounts of weight lost more total body water and K than those who had minimal weight loss or some weight gain. On average, the former group lost about 5 kg FFM/decade, the latter only 2 kg FFM/decade. Flynn et al. (76) did repeated ^{40}K assays on a large group of adults over an 18-year period. Those individuals under 51 years of age at the initial assay who gained weight tended to gain FFM, and those who lost weight tended to lose FFM. On the other hand, older individuals tended to lose FFM regardless of body weight change; the average loss was about 4 kg/decade for both sexes. I have made repeated ^{40}K assays on two adult males—one for 27 years, the other for 37 years, by which time both were in their early 80s.

The first subject lost an average of 0.5 kg FFM/decade, the second 1.0 kg/decade; the first tended to put on weight, the second did not. This observation taken in conjunction with those noted above makes it necessary to consider body weight change in evaluating longitudinal changes in FFM. Incidentally, in keeping with cross-sectional data, the decline in FFM as calculated from total body water was somewhat less, namely 0.6 kg/decade, for the second subject (77).

As shown in Figures 49.3 and 49.4, girls have slightly more body fat than boys from an early age; once adolescence is under way girls acquire much more body fat than boys, and this sex difference persists throughout the adult years. Figure 49.5 shows that these changes are reflected in triceps skinfold thickness; the great variability in this measurement is clearly evident.

Stature

At all ages studied, FFM is a function of height. On average, the regression slope is 0.69 kg/cm in adult males and 0.29 kg/cm in adult females (8). Skeletal size is also a function of height (80); and Ellis and Cohn's data (66, 66a) show that the same is true for total body Ca, whose regression slope is 20 g Ca/cm. Based on their findings a 186-cm male would be expected to have about 1370 g Ca in his body, a 154-cm woman only 730 g Ca.

Data such as these mean that comparisons of FFM and total body Ca among individuals are valid only if height, as well as age and sex, is controlled. Many athletes are taller than average, which is one reason why they tend to have a larger FFM.

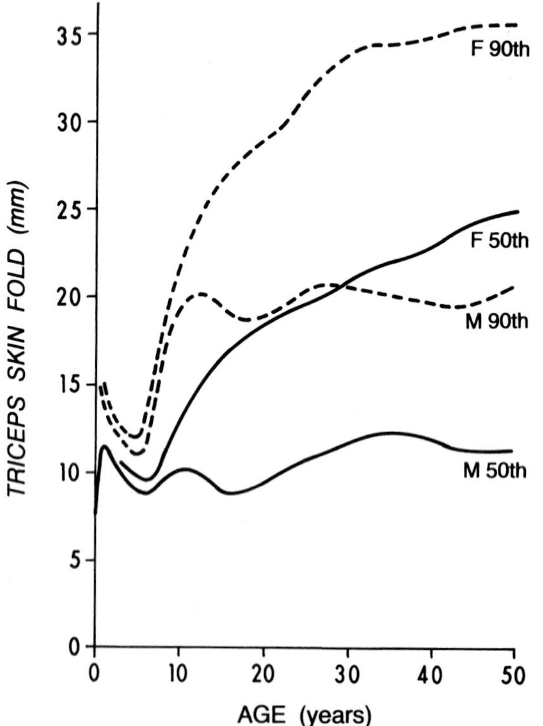

Figure 49.5. 50th and 90th percentiles for triceps skinfold thickness. Data for infants and children less than 6 years old from Tanner and Whitehouse (78), others from Cronk and Roche (79).

Pregnancy

Of the total weight gain during pregnancy, 12 to 13 kg on average, the fetus, placenta, and amniotic fluid together account for about 4.2 kg; the remaining 8 kg is maternal tissue. All components of body water increase—plasma, ECF, and ICF volumes—as well as total red cell mass, and since the ratio of body water:body K increases, the increase in ECF volume is proportionately greater than that of ICF volume, which is consistent with the observation that many pregnant women have mild edema. A portion of the weight gain, variously estimated at 2 to 4 kg, consists of fat (references in [8]).

Correlates of Body Composition

Since the adult female has on average only about 70% the amount of FFM of the average male, the requirements for energy and protein are correspondingly less. The recommended dietary allowances of the National Research Council reflect this sex difference (see Appendices Tables II A2a1 and 2). Both basal metabolic rate (BMR) and blood volume are more closely related to FFM than to body weight. Prentice et al. (81) found a fairly constant relationship between BMR and FFM during pregnancy. It would seem prudent to adjust the dose of various drugs on the basis of FFM rather than body weight. Some of the adult decline in such metabolic parameters as glucose tolerance and maximal oxygen consumption may possibly reflect the age-associated decline in FFM.

Studies of individuals consuming "essentially" protein-free diets (references in [8]) show a linear relationship between endogenous urinary N excretion and body cell mass. The dietary protein requirement is thus a function of body cell mass, and hence of FFM rather than body weight with its variable component of fat. On this basis, the need for protein—and perhaps other dietary nutrients as well—should be lower in the elderly than in the young adult and lower in women than in men.

INFLUENCE OF NUTRITION

Energy Deficit and Excess

Maintenance of body weight in the adult and satisfactory growth rate in the child depends on an adequate supply of energy. Subnormal intakes lead to a decline in the child's growth rate and the adult's body weight, and generally speaking, the rate of weight loss is a function of the magnitude of the energy deficit. After the first few days, fasting results in a loss of about 0.5 kg/day in the obese (82) and about 0.35 kg/day in the nonobese (83). Mathematical analysis shows that the weight loss during fasting is exponential (8), which suggests that the loss rate is proportional to weight itself (body tissues being the only source of energy) and so tends to diminish with time. The same phenomena has been described in fasting geese (84), although toward the end of the fast weight loss tends to increase, as fat reserves are exhausted. In thin rats this premortem phase is associated with increased urinary N loss in about 2 weeks of fasting; the obese rat can tolerate fasts for 2 months or more without such an occurrence (85). The fractional loss rate is lower in the obese human than in the nonobese (0.34 vs. 0.56%/day). Smaller energy deficits produce slower rates of weight loss.

Consumption of energy in excess of maintenance needs produces an increase in body weight; and close observation reveals that the increase is roughly proportional to the total excess energy consumed during the overfeeding period (86). The energy cost of weight gain has been computed for several types of human subjects. On average this turns out to be 5.0 kcal/g gain for infants recovering from malnutrition (87), 4.0 kcal/g gain for growing prematurely born infants (88), 4.7 kcal/g for adolescent girls recovering from anorexia nervosa (89), and 8.0 kcal/g for normal adults who are deliberately overfed (86, 90); the energy cost is about the same for women as for men.

Body Composition Changes

Nutrition can affect lean weight as well as body fat. Compared with normal individuals of the same stature, age, and sex, undernourished subjects have a lower FFM and less fat, and the obese have an increase in both (8, 91). Indeed, Keys and Brozek (1) spoke many years ago of "obesity tissue" consisting of protein and body fluid as well as fat.

When rats are systematically underfed from an early age they are smaller and thinner than ad libitum–fed controls, but they are longer-lived and have fewer neoplasms and degenerative lesions. Studies have shown that fat-free tissue accounts for one-half to two-thirds of the weight difference (92).

Young adult monkeys whose body weight is held fairly constant for many years by careful feeding (including some with frank diabetes) totally escape the glucose intolerance that affects about half of their ad libitum–fed controls. By age 18 years the former animals weigh about two-thirds as much as the latter, and about half of this 5-kg difference consists of lean tissue (93). The question is whether the enhanced life span and better health of the underfed animals is due to the smaller fat burden or the smaller FFM.

Careful studies of underfed subjects, using either nitrogen balance or body composition techniques or urinary creatinine excretion, have shown that significant weight reduction involves loss of both FFM and fat. Underfed animals, including hibernators, lose lean as well as fat. CAT scans of fasting seals clearly show a decrease in muscle tissue as well as fat (94). The relative contribution of lean and fat components to the total weight loss depends on two principal factors: the *initial body fat* content and the *magnitude of the energy deficit.*

During a fast, thin individuals lose twice as much body N per unit weight loss as do obese individuals (95); about two-thirds of their weight loss consists of lean tissues, while for the obese about two-thirds of the loss consists of fat. The same general trend holds for fasting animals, including hibernators. Figure 49.6 is a plot of the fraction of weight loss due to FFM as a function of initial body fat percentage for several species. It shows that the obese preferentially burn fat and so tend to conserve lean.

Even though hibernators lose weight very slowly, the composition of their weight loss for a given initial body fat percentage does not differ greatly from that of the nonhibernators. However, the hibernating black bear seems to be unusually efficient in this respect; the three animals studied by Lundberg et al. (101) (average body fat, 46%) did not on average lose any lean tissue during 60 days of winter sleep, despite a 13% weight loss. According to Nelson et al. (112), the animal achieves this by reabsorbing nitrogen and electrolytes through the wall of the bladder.

The other exception to the general trend is the obese fasting human, who appears to be less efficient at conserving lean weight at a given level of fatness than other species. A possible explanation could be the relatively large size of the human brain compared with that of animals. According to Brody (113), the human brain weighing 1300 g makes up 2 to 2.5% of body weight; the value for small animals is about 0.5% of body weight, and the ratio drops progressively to about 0.15% in animals as

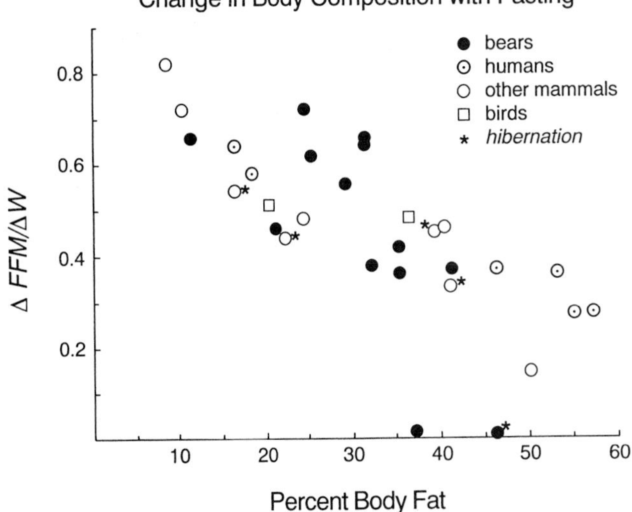

Figure 49.6. Relative contribution of FFM to weight loss during fasting plotted against initial percentage body fat. Symbols: humans *(circle with dot)*; bears *(solid circles)*; other mammals (rat, brown bat, marmot, arctic ground squirrel, seal) *(open circles)*; birds (antarctic penguin, great-winged petrel) *(open squares)*; hibernation *(*)*. Duration of fast 3 weeks or more, except for rat (13–15 days) and petrel (17 days). Unduly long fasts include hibernating arctic ground squirrel (6 months) and marmot (5 months); and female polar bears (207 days). (Data from references 84, 85, 95–111.)

large as the bear. The high demand of the brain for glucose means that the fasting human has a greater need for gluconeogenesis than most animals. Of additional interest is the situation for winged species such as the goose and the bat, in whom the pectoral muscles suffer a smaller weight loss during fasting than do other muscles (105, 114).

Henry (13) has described an interesting relationship between the BMR and the loss of body N during fasting. While this ratio is fairly constant for a given individual throughout a fast, it is 3 to 4 times higher in the obese than in the nonobese; hence the obese waste less nitrogen per basal calorie expended, which is consistent with the observation that the obese excrete less nitrogen per unit weight loss.

The second factor is equally important: for all categories of initial body fat content studied to date, the ΔFFM:ΔW loss ratio is inversely related to energy intake and thus directly related to the energy deficit. As Benedict et al. (115) showed many years ago, even modest energy deficits lead to some loss of body N, and densitometric techniques have confirmed the loss of FFM, as has the CAT scan (94). One searches in vain for well-controlled studies showing that body N and FFM can be preserved on low-energy diets. Nitrogen losses do tend to diminish with time, however, both on low-energy diets and during fasting, as do weight losses. Indeed, during fasting, N loss is exponential, and the fractional N loss is greater in the nonobese than in the obese (95), which may partly account for the greater tolerance of the obese for fasting.

The combined influence of initial body fat content and energy deficit on the composition of the weight lost during weight reduction is shown in Figure 49.7. Included are

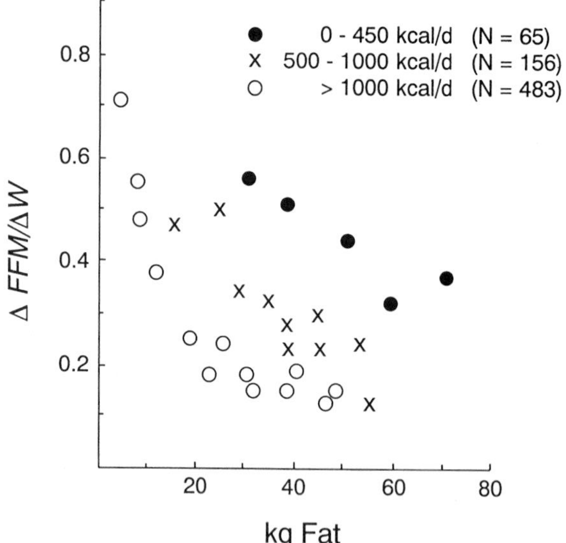

Figure 49.7. Plot of the ratio of FFM loss to total weight loss as a function of body fat content in individuals fed various energy-deficient diets. (Modified from Forbes GB. Human body composition. New York: Springer-Verlag, 1987 with additional data from references 86, 116–132.)

data on 704 men and women who had body composition assays both before and after at least several weeks or complete nitrogen balance on a weight-reduction diet. Except for those given 300 kcal or less daily, all had adequate protein intakes. Average values for the proportion of weight loss represented by FFM (the ΔFFM:ΔW loss ratio) are grouped in categories according to initial body fat content and reported energy intake. ΔFFM:ΔW is very high for thin subjects and falls progressively for all energy intake categories as initial body fat increases; and for any given value for body fat, the ratio progressively rises with decreasing energy intakes (and hence increasing energy deficits).

Obese patients subjected to intestinal bypass or gastric stapling operations also lose FFM as they lose weight. In various studies, 15 to 40% of the weight lost by these patients consisted of FFM (references in [8]).

When undernourished individuals are induced to gain weight, FFM and fat both increase (91), and the same is true for growing infants and children. Both components also increase when normal adults are deliberately overfed. For such subjects the energy cost of the weight gain averages 8 kcal/g, and about one-third of the gain consists of FFM (86, 90, 133). From their study of overfed twins, Bouchard et al. (134) concluded that genetic factors influenced the magnitude of the response. These data were collected from experiments lasting only a few weeks, the longest being 100 days. Since no controlled studies of longer duration in man exist, the situation over the long term is unknown.

The importance of adequate protein intake cannot be overemphasized. While undernourished men can gain weight on low-protein diets, some FFM is lost while body fat is gained. When adequate protein was given to these subjects without a change in energy intake, they gained FFM as well as fat (135). When Miller and Mumford (136) gave excess food low in protein to normal individuals, they lost FFM (as judged by body K content) as they gained weight, whereas excess food high in protein produced a gain in FFM and a greater total gain per excess calorie consumed. Hence low-protein diets are inefficient and even hazardous.

Reasons for FFM Change in Response to Nutritional Intervention

It is easy to understand why FFM declines during fasting: blood glucose must be maintained, and since the glycerol moiety of the mobilized lipids is not equal to this task, gluconeogenesis from protein becomes necessary. Low-energy diets containing carbohydrate do reduce nitrogen losses (137, 138). The detailed studies of Moore et al. (116) show that energy deficits are accompanied by reductions in plasma levels of testosterone, insulin-like growth factor, and insulin, all of which are anabolic. Moreover, the plasma levels of these three hormones rise when adult females are overfed (139).

Body Composition in Obesity

Human obesity can occur only in the face of a positive energy balance, so in this sense, it is a nutritional disease. It is fruitless to argue whether decreased physical activity or increased food intake is the prime factor; obesity results from a failure of the homeostatic mechanisms that balance energy intake and outgo in normal people. Studies of obese children, adolescents, and young adults show that 10 to 30% of their excess weight consists of FFM; however, a few have normal FFM values (91). Data on polar bears show a similar trend; very obese animals have a larger FFM than those with lesser fat burdens, and about one-third of the weight difference is lean tissue (99). Overfed rats acquire some additional lean weight as well as fat (140).

The situation is very different in animals rendered obese by experimentally produced hypothalamic lesions, for they tend to have a smaller FFM than controls. Children and adolescents with the Prader-Willi syndrome (obesity, hypogonadism, muscle hypotonia, and mild mental retardation) also have a subnormal FFM and smaller skeleton in the face of a supranormal body fat content (141, 141a).

Obese children tend to be taller than average and to have some advance in skeletal maturation, and obese girls have an earlier menarche. Such data indicate that most obese individuals are overnourished and that the foods eaten are nutritious. Autopsy observations show that the obese have larger hearts, kidneys, and livers (142). BMR is increased (143), as are blood hemoglobin levels (144), metacarpal cortex thickness (145), and total bone mineral content (141a). These observations speak against the hypothesis that the increased lean weight in obesity is due to muscle hypertrophy from greater weight-bearing; indeed they support the concept that the obese are simply overnourished.

One of the goals of obesity research should be to distinguish cosmetic fatness from fatness that is hazardous to health (13).

Body Composition in Undernutrition

Individuals with chronic energy deficits uncomplicated by significant infection or disease usually have normal, or only slightly reduced, serum protein levels and are not incapacitated. Patients with anorexia nervosa have very thin subcutaneous tissue, small heart and liver volumes, reduced blood volume, and even some reduction in renal function (146). There is a reduction in both FFM and body fat (89). The same is true of undernourished male laborers; however, ECF volume is not reduced, so the ratio of ECF/ICF volume is supranormal (135).

INFLUENCE OF PHYSICAL ACTIVITY

Exercise

The well-known phenomenon of work hypertrophy is nicely illustrated by the fact that the dominant arm of professional tennis players has larger muscles and thicker bones. Generally, athletes of both sexes have a larger FFM than their nonathletic peers and many have less body fat. The enlarged FFM is particularly true of weight lifters, "body builders," discus throwers, shot putters, and football players.

The question is whether the larger FFM is the result of training and/or exercise or is merely an inherent feature of the athletic individual. A number of studies have been done on individuals engaged in training and/or exercise programs of various types who have presumably not taken androgenic/anabolic steroids. These studies show a tendency for FFM to rise and for body fat to fall, but the documented changes are not great. Wilmore's (147) review of 55 such studies shows that FFM increased in 22 (maximum, 3.1 kg), decreased in 7, and was unchanged in 26. Parizkova (5) studied gymnasts in training for the Olympics and found that FFM increased by an average of 1.8 kg in the males and 1.2 kg in the females, with an equivalent loss of body fat. After the contests, body composition reverted in time to its pretraining status.

The experiments described by Oscai et al. (148, 149) are of interest in this regard. When rats are forced to swim daily for many weeks (about 20% of their life span), they acquire more lean tissue (+5%) and less fat (−16%) than their *paired-weight sedentary* controls; skeletal muscle accounts for one-third of the FFM increase. However, when the exercised animals were compared with sedentary controls *fed ad libitum*, the results were very different. Now the exercised animals weighed less than the controls and had a *smaller* FFM (by 14%) as well as less fat. The explanation is that the exercised animals ate less food and expended more energy and so incurred an energy deficit. A review of experiments conducted on exercising rats showed that they gained some FFM and lost some body fat if their body weight did not change much. However, if they lost more than about 30 g weight, there was some loss of FFM as well as fat (150a). On average, FFM contributed about one-third of the total weight loss.

The finding in experimental animals that exercise-induced increases in FFM depend on adequate intake of food has been confirmed in humans. An analysis of Wilmore's (147) compilation of body composition changes induced by exercise shows that subject groups that maintained their weight or gained little had a modest increase in FFM, while those who lost weight lost FFM as well as body fat (150). This phenomenon has recently been confirmed by an analysis of individual subjects, including athletes and sedentary individuals, who engaged in exercise programs (150a). Body fat content influenced the body composition response to exercise and/or training; individuals (of both sexes) with body fat burdens of 25 kg or more could sustain a greater weight loss without incurring a loss of FFM than those who were thin (150). Bouchard et al. (151) studied a group of males kept on a constant diet for 100 days while exercising vigorously. Their estimated energy deficit was 353 MJ (84,370 kcal);

average weight loss was 8 kg, of which 1.3 kg represented FFM.

Figure 49.8 shows the observed change in FFM as a function of change in body weight resulting from exercise programs. Adults of both sexes are included as well as a variety of exercise programs. Only subjects who had body composition assays at the beginning and at the end of the exercise period were included. There were 12 groups of males, 15 groups of females (1 group lactating), and 3 groups of mixed sexes. Exercise programs consisted of either aerobics, resistance training, or weight lifting, singly or in combination, and one group of Army Rangers (116). The two solid dots in the upper right quadrant of the illustration, at about +10 and +20 kg ΔW, represent the difference between body builders and Japanese sumo wrestlers, respectively, and control males of comparable stature. Individuals who maintain their body weight during exercise tend to gain FFM and lose body fat; those who gain weight also gain FFM; those who lose weight tend to lose FFM also, but those with larger body fat burdens tend to lose less FFM for a given weight loss than those who are thin. Exercise and/or training cannot sustain lean weight, much less increase it, in the face of an appreciable energy deficit. Athletes who have high energy expenditures must eat well if they want to augment, or even sustain, their lean weight.

Immobilization and Space Travel

Decreased muscle mass and bone density in immobilized or paralyzed limbs is a well-known phenomenon. Healthy young men placed in plaster spicas from the waist down for several weeks lost some body nitrogen, calcium, and phosphorus and had a reduction in blood volume, although body weight did not change (166). Ordinary bed rest also results in negative balance of Ca, K, and P.

Studies of astronauts have included estimates of FFM. The loss of FFM during the 84-day flight varied according to the method used: 3.4 kg by ^{42}K dilution, 1.2 kg by densitometry, 2.6 kg by nitrogen balance, and 1.1 kg by total body water. The average is 2.1 kg FFM loss in the face of 2.8 kg weight loss (167). Blood volume declined by 10% (168). Mild hyponatremia, suggesting a change in body fluid osmolality, the strong positive N balance prior to the flight, and the fact that body weight was rapidly regained on returning to Earth make interpretation of these results difficult. Pitts et al. (169) found an 8% drop in fat-free weight, a drop in total body Ca, and an increase in body fat in rats who had spent 18 days in space. (See also Chapter 48.) Thus, maintenance of normal body composition depends on gravity and normal physical activity as well as muscle innervation.

IMPORTANCE OF BODY FAT

Data now suffice to show that relative changes in body composition are influenced by the amount of body fat. Obese animals tolerate starvation better than thin ones, and the same is true of humans. Obese subjects can survive fasts of more than 100 days, while the Irish hunger strikers of some years ago (who did not appear obese) died in about 2 months. During fasting, obese humans and animals both lose proportionally less lean tissue than those with lower burdens of body fat (Fig. 49.6). Observations

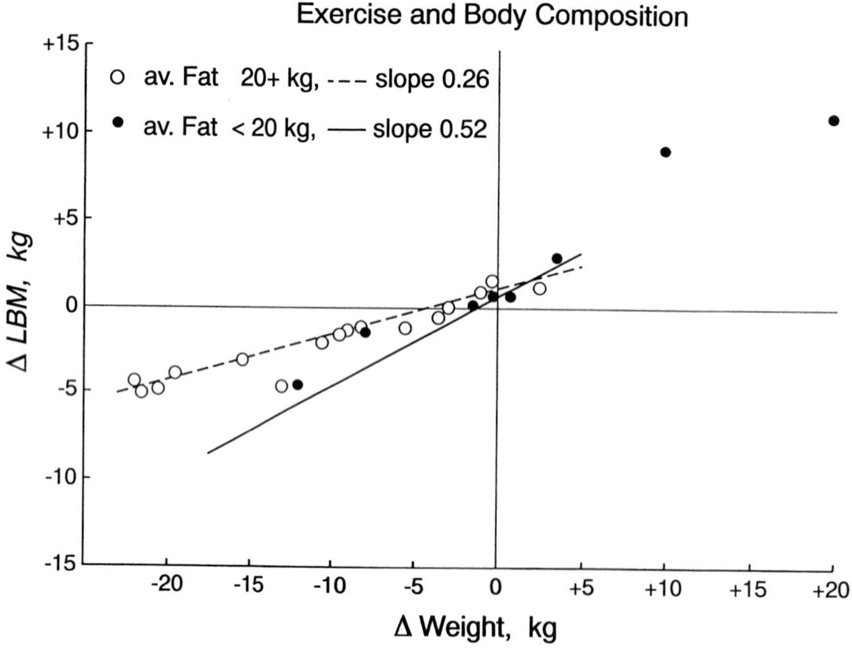

Figure 49.8. Plot of change in FFM against change in weight resulting from exercise programs. The regression lines are based on earlier data (150a) for 166 subjects with less than 20 kg body fat *(solid line)* and 248 subjects with larger burdens of body fat *(dotted line)*. More-recent data are indicated for 171 thin subjects *(solid circles)* and for 301 subjects with more body fat *(open circles)*. (From 73, 116–119, 123, 125, 126, 151–165.)

on individuals fed low-energy diets also show that the relative contribution of FFM to the total weight loss is an inverse function of body fat content. Animals are known to increase their body fat stores prior to hibernation. When weight is gained in response to nutritional surfeit, thin individuals tend to put on relatively more FFM than the obese, at least in the initial phase (170).

Studies of twins show that the intrapair difference in FFM is quantitatively relationed to the difference in body weight for both monozygous and dizygous like-sexed twins (28). Furthermore, the slope of the intrapair $\Delta FFM/\Delta W$ regression is about twice as steep for thin twins than for those with large body-fat burdens; hence for the latter, body fat accounts for more of the intrapair weight difference.

The body composition response to exercise is also influenced by body fat: those with generous fat burdens tend to lose less FFM and more fat when weight is lost during exercise than those who are thin (Fig. 49.8). The limited data on migrating birds suggest that fatter species conserve FFM better than thinner ones, in the face of what surely must be vigorous exercise (8).

INFLUENCE OF HORMONES

Large doses of adrenal corticosteroids act to decrease muscle and bone mass; hence individuals with Cushing's syndrome have subnormal total body K and Ca and an increased body Na:K ratio, and total body K increases with treatment. Excessive amounts of parathyroid and thyroid hormones result in negative Ca balance, and the latter in loss of body N as well. Treatment of children with hypopituitarism is associated with an increase in FFM and a decrease in body fat. Individuals with acromegaly have increased body K, N, Na, and Ca and an increase in ECF volume (references in [8]).

In normal individuals (including the elderly), growth hormone causes an increase in FFM and a loss of body fat (171). In cattle, the effect on nitrogen balance is dose related (172).

Striking effects are produced by the androgenic/anabolic steroids. Nitrogen balance becomes positive, and animal studies have shown an increase in amino acid uptake in muscle and an increase in muscle size. Large doses enhance muscle protein synthesis (173) and produce a significant increase in FFM and a fall in body fat in man (8, 22), and this effect is dose related. These effects are apparently perceived by athletes, among whom the use of such steroids is said to be widespread. Indeed, androgenic/anabolic steroids can enhance FFM in the absence of exercise, and large doses produce a greater effect than does exercise alone.

Insulin has both anabolic and lipotrophic activity, so deficiency of this hormone leads to negative nitrogen balance and fat dissolution. Normal pregnancy is associated with an increase in maternal FFM and fat, changes facilitated by the increased levels of testosterone, prolactin, progesterone, estrogen, and insulin that occur, as well as the increase in food intake.

Although vitamin D is now considered a hormone, its action on body tissues is presented in Chapter 18 on this vitamin.

INFLUENCE OF DISEASE

Cuthbertson showed many years ago that severe trauma to the limbs was accompanied by a significant loss of body nitrogen; the negative balance in his patients was as high as 137 g, equivalent to a loss of 4 kg FFM. Earlier, Shaffer and Coleman had found that N losses occurred during the course of typhoid fever and that addition of energy in the form of carbohydrate could minimize the N loss in such patients. Beisel et al. recorded significant N losses in other types of infections and showed that these losses exceeded those due to the decreased food intake that often accompanies infection. They also recorded losses of K, Na, P, and Mg in their subjects. It is now common practice to provide extra nutrients—often by the parenteral route—to patients with severe trauma or infection or who have had major surgery. The metabolic response to surgery also includes an increase in the $Na_e:K_e$ ratio (references in [8]).

Neuromuscular disease has a profound effect. Serial studies of boys with the Duchenne type of muscular dystrophy show a progressive departure from the normal total body K with age (8). Individuals with cirrhosis as well as those with cardiac failure have an increase in the ratio of Na space to total body water. As expected, individuals with osteoporosis have reduced total body Ca. The loss of weight in patients with cancer involves FFM as well as fat (references in [8]).

Severe malnutrition is associated with increases in the ECF:ICF ratio, the $Na_e:K_e$ ratio, and intracellular Na in muscle and a decrease in K. In such states, ECF volume appears to be better preserved than cell mass, the shrunken cells retaining their fluid covering. Picou et al. (174) evaluated the relative amounts of collagen and noncollagen protein in the bodies of malnourished infants. While the latter was reduced to about one-half the expected value, the former had not changed significantly. Skin and bone accounts for about 70% of the total body collagen.

The observations of Picou et al. (174) help to explain the difference in calculated changes in body composition produced by different techniques. Tendon has a higher density and a lower K concentration than muscle, so an increase in the ratio of collagen to noncollagen protein during weight loss would be expected to increase the density and decrease the K content of the FFM. Hence the use of standard values for each will result in a slight underestimation of the FFM contribution to the weight loss by densitometry and an overestimation by ^{40}K counting. The smaller contribution of FFM to total weight loss by density than by ^{40}K counting found by Garrow (15) during weight reduction and by Leonard et al. (167) during space flight is consistent with this hypothesis. Such inconsistencies serve as a reminder that body composition measurement techniques may not always yield precise results.

COMPANIONSHIP OF LEAN AND FAT

Modern body composition techniques have helped define the composition of the weight change induced by nutritional manuevers. As discussed above, nutritional surfeit produces an increase in FFM as well as fat both in animals and humans, and a portion of the excess weight in obese individuals consists of lean tissue; energy deficits lead to a decline in both lean and fat, even in hibernating animals (Figs. 49.6 and 49.7). Prehibernation fattening of arctic ground squirrels includes an increase in lean weight (106) as does premigratory fattening of birds (175, 176). Very obese polar bears have a larger FFM than those with lesser burdens of body fat (99). Hence, these two body components—lean and fat—are not independent of each other, but are linked together in some fashion, whose elucidation would seem most worthwhile.

However, there are situations in which this linkage is violated. The best example of discordant changes in FFM and fat is provided by the effect of androgen administration. Large doses of anabolic/androgenic steroids act to increase FFM (a proportion of which is muscle) and decrease body fat, changes that are welcomed by athletes, especially by body builders. Similar changes occur with administration of growth hormone in both normal and hypopituitary subjects. Another discordant situation involves obese patients with the Prader-Willi syndrome, who have a subnormal FFM despite their large burden of body fat, as do animals with experimental lesions of the hypothalamus. Hence these are not appropriate models for the usual type of human obesity.

Exercise and/or physical training can lead to a modest gain in FFM and a fall in body fat if body weight does not change much; however, if more than a few kilograms of weight are lost, FFM usually declines. As shown in Figure 49.8 exercisers who eat enough to produce a positive energy balance and hence gain weight show the largest increase in FFM. Bed rest and zero gravity cause a modest reduction in FFM.

Modern techniques have helped define a constellation of body composition changes that result from various stimuli. Inferences derived from work on animals can now be tested in man, and the investigator, now freed from the constraints of the metabolic balance method, can assess body content at any point in time as well as changes that occur over long periods.

ACKNOWLEDGMENT

Supported in part by NIH grants HD18454 and RR00044.

REFERENCES

1. Keys A, Brozek J. Physiol Rev 1953;33:245–345.
2. Moore FD, Olesin KH, McMurray LD, et al. The body cell mass and its supporting environment. Philadelphia: WB Saunders, 1963.
3. Widdowson EM, Dickerson JWT. Chemical composition of the body. In: Comar CL, Bronner F, eds. Mineral metabolism, vol 2, pt A. New York: Academic Press, 1964;2–247.
4. Cheek DB. Human growth. Philadelphia: Lea & Febiger, 1968.
5. Parizkova J. Body fat and physical fitness. The Hague: Martinus Nijhoff, 1977.
6. Cohn SH. Med Phys 1981;8:145–54.
7. Cohn SH, ed. Non-invasive measurements of bone mass and their clinical application. Boca Raton, FL: CRC Press, 1981.
8. Forbes GB. Human body composition. New York: Springer-Verlag, 1987.
9. Lukaski HC. Am J Clin Nutr 1987;46:537–56.
10. Shepard RJ. Body composition in biological anthropology. New York: Cambridge University Press, 1991.
11. Deurenberg P. The assessment of body composition: uses and misuses. Nestlé Foundation annual report. Lausanne, Switzerland: 1992;35–72.
12. Kreitzman SN, Howard AN, eds. The Swansea trial: body composition and metabolic studies with a very low calorie diet (VLCD). London: Smith-Cordon and Co, 1993.
13. Davies PSW, Cole TJ, eds. Body composition techniques in health and disease. Cambridge: Cambridge University Press, 1995.
14. Roche AF, Heymsfield SB, Lohman TG, eds. Human body composition. Champaign, IL: Human kinetics, 1996.
15. Garrow JS. Energy balance and obesity in man. Amsterdam: North-Holland Publishing, 1974.
16. Sutcliffe JF. Phys Med Biol 1996;41:791–883.
17. Whitehead RG, Prentice A, eds. New techniques in nutritional research. New York: Academic Press, 1991.
18. Ellis KJ, Eastman JD, eds. Human body composition: in vivo methods, models and assessment. New York: Plenum Press, 1993.
19. Andres R. Ann Intern Med 1985;103:1030–3.
20. Tokunga K, Matsuzawa Y, Kotani K, et al. Int J Obes 1991; 15:1–5.
21. Forbes GB. Some influences on lean body mass: exercise, androgens, pregnancy, and food. In: White PL, Mondeika T, eds. Diet & exercise: synergism in health maintenance. Chicago: American Medical Association, 1982;75–90.
22. Forbes GB, Porta CR, Herr BE, et al. JAMA 1992;267: 397–99.
23. Foch TT, McClearn GE. Genetics, body weight, and obesity. In: Stunkard AJ, ed. Obesity. Philadelphia: WB Saunders, 1980;48–71.
24. Smith DM, Nance WE, Kang KW, et al. J Clin Invest 1973; 52:2800–8.
25. Lutz J, Tesar R. Am J Clin Nutr 1990;52:872–7.
26. Bouchard C, Savard R, Després JP, et al. Hum Biol 1985; 57:61–75.
27. Stunkard AJ, Harris JR, Pedersen NL, et al. N Engl J Med 1990;322:1483–7.
28. Forbes GB, Procheska EP, Weitkamp LR. Metabolism 1995; 44:1442–6.
29. Cohn SH, Abesamis C, Zanzi L, et al. Am J Physiol 1977;232: E419–22.
30. Borkan GA, Hults DE, Glynn RJ. Hum Biol 1983;55:629–41.
31. Flynn MA, Nolph GB, Baker AS, et al. Am J Clin Nutr 1989;50:713–7.
32. Cohn SH, Vaswani AN, Yasumura S, et al. Am J Clin Nutr 1984;40:255–9.
33. Schoeller DA, Van Sauten DW, Peterson DW, et al. Am J Clin Nutr 1980;33:2686–93.

34. Shizgal HM, Spanier AH, Humes J, et al. Am J Physiol 1977;233:F253–9.
35. Dempster P, Aitkens S. Med Sci Sports Exerc 1995;27: 1692–7.
36. McCrory MA, Gomez TD, Bernauer EM, et al. Med Sci Sports Exerc 1995;27:1686–91.
37. Forbes GB, Brown MR, Griffiths HJL. Am J Clin Nutr 1988;47:929–31.
38. Durnin JVGA, Womersley J. Br J Nutr 1974;32:77–97.
39. Pollock ML, Wilmore JH, Fox SM III. Exercise in health and disease. Philadelphia: WB Saunders, 1984.
40. Forbes GB. Int J Obes 1990;149–57.
41. Tokunaga K, Matsuzawa Y, Ishikawa K, et al. Int J Obes 1983;7:437–46.
42. Kvist H, Sjöström L, Tylén U. Int J Obes 1986;10:53–67.
42a. Chowdhury B, Sjöström L, Alpsten M. Int J Obes 1994;219–234.
43. Fowler PA, Fuller MF, Glasbey CA, et al. Am J Clin Nutr 1992;56:7–13.
43a. Pietrobelli A, Formica C, Wang Z, et al. Am J Physiol 1996;271:E941–51.
44. Ellis KJ, Shypailo RJ, Pratt JA, et al. Am J Clin Nutr 1994;60:660–5.
45. Svendsen OL, Haarbo J, Hassager C, et al. Am J Clin Nutr 1993;57:605–8.
46. Jebb SA, Goldberg GR, Jennings G, et al. Clin Sci 1995;88:319–24.
47. Schutte JE, Longhurst JC, Gaffney FA, et al. J Appl Physiol 1981;51:762–6.
48. Welle S, Thornton C, Forbes GB. Am J Clin Nutr 1996;63:151–6.
49. Heymsfield SB, Arteaga C, McManus C, et al. Am J Clin Nutr 1983;37:478–94.
50. Wang Zi-M, Gallagher D, Nelson ME, et al. Am J Clin Nutr 1996;63:863–9.
51. Keim NL, Mayclin PL, Taylor SJ, et al. Am J Clin Nutr 1988;47:180–5.
52. DeBruin NC, Westerterp KR, Degenhart HJ, et al. Pediatr Res 1995;38:411–7.
52a. DeBruin NC, Van Velthoven KAM, deRidder M, et al. Arch Dis Child 1996;74:386–99.
53. Segal KR, Gutin B, Presta E, et al. J Appl Physiol 1985;58: 1565–71.
54. Van Loan MD, Belko AZ, Mayclin PL, et al. Am J Clin Nutr 1987;46:5–8.
55. Kushner RF. J Am Coll Nutr 1992;11:199–209.
55a. Yanovski SZ, Hubbard VS, Heymsfield SD, Lukaski HC, eds. Am J Clin Nutr (Suppl) 1996;64:3875–5325.
56. Baumgartner RN, Chumlea WC, Roche AF. Am J Clin Nutr 1989;50:221–6.
57. Lukaski HC, Bolonchuk WW, Hall CB, et al. J Appl Physiol 1986;60:1327–32.
58. Kushner RF, Schoeller DA. Am J Clin Nutrition 1986;44: 417–24.
59. Ross R, Léger L, Martin P, et al. J Appl Physiol 1989;67: 1643–8.
60. Deurenberg P, Smith HE, Kusters CSL. Eur J Clin Nutr 1989;6:247–55.
60a. Fomon SJ, Haschke F, Ziegler EF, et al. Am J Clin Nutr 1982;35:1169–75.
61. Tagliabue A, Cena H, Trentani C, et al. Int J Obes 1992;16:649–52.
62. Forbes GB, Simon W, Amatruda JM. Am J Clin Nutr 1992;56:4–6.
63. Conway JM, Norris KH, Bodwell CE. Am J Clin Nutr 1984;40:1123–30.
64. Garrow JS. Treat obesity seriously. London: Churchill Livingstone, 1981.
65. Kehayias JJ, Heymsfield SB, LoMonte AF, et al. Am J Clin Nutr 1991;53:1339–44.
66. Ellis KJ, Cohn SH J Appl Physiol 1975;38:455–60.
66a. Cohn SH. Personal communication.
67. Ogle GD, Allen JR, Humphries IRS, et al. Am J Clin Nutr 1995;61:746–53.
68. Faulkner RA, Bailey DA, Drinkwater DT, et al. Calcif Tissue Int 1993;53:7–12.
69. Cohn SH, Vartsky D, Yasumura S, et al. Am J Physiol 1980;239:E524–30.
70. Womersley J, Boddy K, King PC, et al. Clin Sci 1972;43:469–75.
71. Lukaski HC, Mendez J, Buskirk ER, et al. Am J Physiol 1981;240:E302–7.
71a. Lukaski HC, Mendez J, Buskirk ER, et al. Metabolism 30:777–82.
72. International Committee on Radiation Protection. Report of the Task Group on Reference Man for Purposes of Radiation Protection. Oxford: Pergammon, 1975.
73. Kondo M, Abe T, Ikegawa S, et al. Am J Hum Biol 1994; 6:613–8.
74. Torine J. Personal communication.
75. Steen B, Bruce A, Isaksson B, et al. Acta Med Scand 1977;611(Suppl):87–112.
76. Flynn MA, Nolph GB, Baker AS, et al. Am J Clin Nutr 1989;50:713–7.
77. Forbes GB. Unpublished observations.
78. Tanner JM, Whitehouse RH. Arch Dis Child 1975;50:142–5.
79. Cronk CE, Roche AF. Am J Clin Nutr 1982;35:351–4.
80. Borisov BK, Marei AN. Health Phys 1974;27:224–9.
81. Prentice AM, Goldberg GR, Davies, HL, et al. Br J Nutr 1989;62:5–22.
82. Drenick EJ, Swendseid ME, Blahd WH, et al. JAMA 1964;187:100–5.
83. Benedict FG. A study of prolonged fasting. Washington, DC: Carnegie Institute, 1915.
84. Deswasmes Y, LeMaho AC, Groscoles R, Cornet A, et al. J Appl Physiol 1980;49:888–96.
85. Cherel Y, Robin JP, Heitz A, et al. J Comp Physiol (B) 1992;162:305–13.
86. Forbes GB, Brown MR, Welle SL, et al. Br J Nutr 1986;56:1–9.
87. Spady DW, Payne PR, Picou D, et al. Am J Clin Nutr 1976;29:1073–88.
88. Reichman B, Chessex P, Putet G, et al. N Engl J Med 1981;305:1495–500.
89. Forbes GB, Kreipe RE, Lipinski BA, et al. Am J Clin Nutr 1984;40:1137–345.
90. Diaz E, Prentice AM, Goldberg GR, et al. Am J Clin Nutr 1992;6:641–55.
91. Forbes GB, Welle SL. Int J Obes 1983;7:99–108.
92. Yu BP, Masoro EJ, Murata I, et al. J Gerontol 1982;37:130–41.
93. Hansen BC, Bodkin NL. Diabetes 1993;42:1809–14.
94. Nordoy ES, Blix AS. Am J Physiol 1985;249:R471–6.
95. Forbes GB, Drenick EJ. Am J Clin Nutr 1979;32:1570–4.
96. Fisler JS, Drenick EJ, Blumfield DE, et al. Am J Clin Nutr 1982;35:471–86.
97. Drenick EJ. Personal communication.
98. Filer LE Jr. Personal communication.
99. Atkinson SN, Ramsay MA. Funct Ecol 1995;9:559–67.
100. Atkinson SN, Nelson RA, Ramsay MA, Physiol Zool 1996;69:304–16.
101. Lundberg DA, Nelson RA, Wahner HW, et al. Mayo Clin Proc 1976;51:716–22.
102. Benedict FG. A study of prolonged fasting. Washington, DC: Carnegie Institute, 1915.

103. Owen OE, Felig P, Morgan AP, et al. J Clin Invest 1969;48:574–83.
104. Margulis S. Fasting and undernutrition. New York: EP Dutton, 1923.
105. Yacoe ME. J Comp Physiol 1983;152:97–104.
106. Galster W, Morrison P. Can J Zool 1976;54:74–8.
107. Belkhou R, Cherel Y, Heitz A. Nutr Res 1991;11:365–74.
108. Ortiz CL, Costa D, LeBoeuf BJ. Physiol Zool 1978;51:166–78.
109. Groscalas R, Schreiber L, Marin F. Physiol Zool 1991;64:1217–33.
110. Boyd IL, Duck CD. Physiol Zool 1991;64:375–92.
111. Bowen WD, Oftedal OT, Boness DJ. Physiol Zool 1992;65:844–66.
112. Nelson RA, Jones JD, Wahner HW, et al. Mayo Clinic Proc 1975;50:141–6.
113. Brody S. Bioenergetics and growth. New York: Reinhold, 1945.
114. LeMaho HV, Van KHA, Koubi H, et al. Am J Physiol 1981;241:E342–54.
115. Benedict FG, Miles WR, Roth P, et al. Human vitality and efficiency under prolonged restricted diet. Washington, DC: Carnegie Institute, 1919.
116. Moore RJ, Friedl KE, Kramer TR, et al. Technical rep. no. T13-92. Natick, MA: US Army Research Institute of Environmental Medicine. 1992.
117. Racette SB, Schoeller DA, Kushner RF, et al. Am J Clin Nutr 1995;61:48–94.
118. Dengel DR, Hagberg JM, Coon PJ, et al. Metabolism 1994;43:867–71.
119. Frey-Hewitt B, Vranizan KM, Dreon DM, et al. Int J Obes 1990;14:327–34.
120. Behnke AR, Wilmore JH. Evaluation and regulation of body build and composition. Englewood Cliffs, NJ: Prentice-Hall, 1974.
121. Svendsen OL, Hassager C, Christiansen C. Am J Med 1993;95:131–40.
122. Van der Kooy K, Leenen R, Deurenberg P, et al. Int J Obes 1992;16:657–83.
123. Kempen K, Saris W, Westerterp KR. Am J Clin Nutr 1995;62:722–9.
124. Deurenberg, P, Weststrate JA, Hautvast JGAJ. Am J Clin Nutr 1989;49:33–6.
125. Donnelly JE, Pronk NP, Jacobson DJ, et al. Am J Clin Nutr 1991;54:56–61.
126. Whatley JE, Gillespie WJ, Honig J, et al. Am J Clin Nutr 1994;59:1088–92.
127. Fulco CS, Hoyt RW, Baker-Fulco CJ, et al. J Appl Physiol 1992;72:2181–7.
128. Stallone DD, Stunkard AJ, Wadden TA, et al. Int J Obes 1991;15:775–80.
129. Davies HJA, Baird IM, Fowler J, et al. Am J Clin Nutr 1989;49:745–51.
130. Belko AZ, Van Loan M, Barbieri TF, et al. Int J Obes 1987;11:93–104.
131. Morgan WD, Ryde S, Birks JL. Am J Clin Nutr 1992;56:2625–45.
132. Heyman MB, Young VR, Fuss P, et al. Am J Physiol 1992;263:R250–7.
133. Bandini LG, Schoeller DA, Edwards J, et al. Am J Physiol 1989;256:E357–67.
134. Bouchard C, Tremblay A, Després J-P, et al. N Engl J Med 1990;322:1477–82.
135. Barac-Nieto M, Spurr GB, Lotero H, et al. Am J Clin Nutr 1979;32:981–91.
136. Miller DS, Mumford P. Am J Clin Nutr 1967;20:1212–22.
137. Vasquez JA, Siamak A. Metabolism 1992;41:406–14.
138. Vasquez JA, Kazi V, Madami N. Am J Clin Nutr 1995;62:93–103.
139. Forbes GB, Brown MR, Welle SL, et al. Am J Clin Nutr 1989;49:608–11.
140. Pitts GC. Am J Physiol 1984;246:R495–501.
141. Schoeller DA, Levitsky LL, Bandini LG, et al. Metabolism 1988;37:115–20.
141a. Brambilla P, Bosio L, Manzoni P, et al. Am J Clin Nutr 1997;65:1369–74.
142. Naeye RL, Roode P. Am J Clin Pathol 1970;54:251–3.
143. James WPT, Bailes J, Davies HL, et al. Lancet 1978;1:1122–5.
144. Garn SM, Ryan AS. Am J Clin Nutr 1982;36:189–91.
145. Dalén N, Hallberg D, Lamke B. Acta Med Scand 1975;197:353–5.
146. Heymsfield SB, McManus CB. Cancer 1985;55:238–49.
147. Wilmore JH. Med Sci Sports Exerc 1983;15:21–31.
148. Oscai LB, Holloszy JO. J Clin Invest 1969;48:2124–8.
149. Oscai LB, Mole PA, Krusack LM, et al. J Nutr 1973;103:412–8.
150. Forbes GB. J Appl Physiol 1991;70:994–7.
150a. Forbes GB. Nutr Rev 1992;50:157–61.
151. Bouchard C, Tremblay A, Nadeau A, et al. Int J Obes 1990;14:57–73.
152. Reinhardt KF. Effects of diet on muscle and strength gains during resistive training. In: Garrett WE, Malone TR, eds. Ross Symposium on Muscle Development. Columbus, OH: Ross Laboratories, 1988;78–83.
153. Andersson B, Xu X, Rebuffé-Scrive M, et al. Int J Obes 1988;15:75–81.
154. Dewey KG, Lovelady CA, Rivers LA, et al. N Engl J Med 1994;330:449–53.
155. Coon PJ, Bleecker ER, Drinkwater DT, et al. Metabolism 1989;38:1201–9.
156. Ross R, Pedwell H, Rissanen J. Am J Clin Nutr 1995;61:1179–85.
157. Kirwan JP, Kohrt WM, Wojta DM, et al. J Gerontol 1993;48:M84–90.
158. Meijer GAL, Westerterp KR, Seyts GHP, et al. Eur J Appl Physiol 1991;62:18–21.
159. Van Loan MD, Keim NL, Barbieri TF, et al. Eur J Clin Nutr 1994;48:408–15.
160. Keim NL, Barbieri TF, Van Loan M, et al. Int J Obes 1991;15:283–93.
161. Campbell WW, Crim MC, Young VR. Am J Physiol 1995;268:E1143–53.
162. Ross R, Rissanen J. Am J Clin Nutr 1994;60:695–703.
163. Van Etten LMLA, Westerterp KR, Verstappen FTJ. Med Sci Sports Exerc 1995;27:188–93.
164. Welle SL, Forbes GB. Unpublished data.
165. Weltman A, Weltman JY, Schurrer R, et al. J Appl Physiol 1993;72:2188–96.
166. Deitrick JE, Whedon GD, Shorr E. Am J Med 1948;4:3–36.
167. Leonard JI, Leach CS, Rambaut PC. Am J Clin Nutr 1983;38:667–9.
168. Rambout PC, Smith MC Jr, Leach CS, et al. Fed Proc 1977;36:1678–82.
169. Pitts GC, Ushakov AS, Pace N, et al. Am J Physiol 1983;244:R332–7.
170. Forbes GB. Nutr Rev 1987;45:225–31.
171. Rudman D, Feller AG, Nagraj HS, et al. N Engl J Med 1990;323:1–6.
172. Crooker BA, McGuire MA, Cohick WS, et al. J Nutr 1990;120:1256–63.
173. Griggs RC, Kingston W, Jozefowicz RF, et al. J Appl Physiol 1989;66:498–503.

174. Picou D, Halliday D, Garrow JS. Clin Sci 1966;30:345–51.
175. Ellis HI, Jehl JR Jr. Physiol Zool 1991;64:973–84.
176. Marsch, RL. Physiol Zool 1984;57:105–17.

SELECTED READINGS

Ellis KJ, Eastman JD, eds. Human body composition: in vivo methods, models and assessment. New York: Plenum Press, 1993.

Forbes GB. Human body composition. New York: Springer-Verlag, 1987.

Garrow JS. Energy balance and obesity in man. Amsterdam: North-Holland Publishing, 1974.

Keys A, Brozek J. Body fat in adult man. Physiol Rev 1953;33: 245–345.

Roche AF, Heymsfield SB, Lohman TG, eds. Human body composition. Champaign, IL: Human kinetics, 1996.

Widdowson EM, Dickerson JWT. Chemical composition of the body. In: Comar CL, Bronner F, eds. Mineral metabolism, vol 2, pt A. New York: Academic Press, 1964;2–247.

50. Maternal Nutrition

WILLIAM J. McGANITY, EARL B. DAWSON, and JAMES W. VAN HOOK

Significant changes in the female life cycle have occurred over the past 150 years. The decline in the average age of the onset of menarche has apparently stabilized at about 12.5 years. The average age of menopause is now more than 50 years. Consequently, female reproductive potential has expanded to nearly 40 years of a female's 75-year life span (1).

During the last two decades, the number of live births to women younger than 20 years of age has decreased slightly, and the number of women delaying their first pregnancy until they are over 30 years of age has increased significantly. In the United States, of the more than 5 million pregnancies annually, only 75% result in live births. The remainder end in induced abortions or spontaneous miscarriages before the 20th week of pregnancy.

The ever-improving availability and quality of obstetric and neonatal care has produced a downward trend in perinatal and infant mortality in the United States; however, the rates among the black population remain twice those of the white or Hispanic populations. Little change has occurred in the incidence of low birth weight (LBW, <2500 g), which remains at 7%, also twice as high among the black population. The incidence of very LBW infants (weighing <1500 g) is three times higher in the black population. Unfortunately, between 25 and 30% of all pregnant patients do not enter into prenatal care before the second trimester of pregnancy. Few public-sector patients achieve the recommended standard of 14 prenatal visits. They average fewer than eight visits, most of which occur in the late second and third trimester of pregnancy (2).

Nationally, approximately 40% of all pregnant women receive their prenatal care and delivery services in the public sector. Health care insurance coverage, available

Abbreviations: **BMI**—body mass index; **CBC**—complete blood count; **LBW**—low birth weight; **MCHC**—mean corpuscular hemoglobin concentration; **MCV**—mean corpuscular volume; **NTD**—neural tube defect(s); **PE**—preeclampsia; **PIH**—pregnancy-induced hypertension; **PROM**—premature rupture of the membrane; **PSW**—percentage of standard weight; **RBC**—red blood cell(s); **RDA**—recommended dietary allowance; **WHO**—World Health Organization; **WIC**—Supplemental Feeding Program for Women, Infants, and Children.

through the expanded federal and state Medicaid program, covers most pregnant women with incomes below 185% of the poverty level. In many areas of the United States, medical manpower (particularly for public-sector patients) for prenatal and delivery services is being replaced by physician extenders—certified nurse midwives, clinical nurse practitioners, and physician assistants.

What are these mothers' expectations in the 1990s? The number of pregnancies per reproductive career has decreased by 25% in the past 30 years (from 3.2 to 2.3 children per reproductive career). The present-day American mother expects a perfect outcome to each pregnancy. If any question arises about the condition of her fetus, she is likely to exercise her option to interrupt the pregnancy. When the maternal and/or fetal outcome is not perfect, she is predisposed to blame her health care team for the failures that result and frequently seeks legal recourse.

Several reviews of the current state of prenatal nutrition emphasize that the goals for the mother and her offspring remain constant (3–5): *(a)* for the mother, freedom from complications and intercurrent diseases throughout pregnancy and postpartum and a return to her normal, healthy nonpregnant state free of sequelae; and *(b)* for the infant, a mature baby of normal gestational age and birth weight, free of any anomalies or disabilities, and able to thrive in the external environment.

OPTIMAL NEEDS FOR REPRODUCTIVE PERFORMANCE

Pregnancy should not be treated as a haphazard event. If the common goals of the mother and her health care team are to be achieved, one must identify and eliminate as many maternal risk factors as possible by careful evaluation and appropriate treatment, and prevent or ameliorate as many of the actual risks as possible before the pregnancy begins. Usual prenatal care in the United States consists of an initial visit for pregnancy confirmation and health examination after the individual's second missed menstrual period, followed by 12 periodic examinations at 4-, 2-, and 1-week intervals during the remaining course of the pregnancy, plus a minimum of one postpartum visit 4 to 6 weeks after delivery. A well-planned pregnancy in the late 1990s should include an initial health examination 8 to 12 weeks before conception. Those 60 to 90 days of preconceptional care are essential to controlling all maternal risk factors. Pregnancy preparation should start a year before the desired month of delivery, and care should extend at least 6 weeks after delivery. This regimen covers 54 weeks or more from the time that the prospective mother should have discontinued her nonbarrier forms of contraception. Two or more normal, spontaneous menstrual cycles are desirable before the barrier contraception is removed for the purpose of conceiving. Similarly, after delivery, time is required for reproductive involution and maternal nutritional repletion to occur.

Prerequisites for Optimal Performance

At least nine prerequisites for optimal maternal reproductive performance are recognized (Table 50.1).

Pregnancy Is Optimal When the Mother Is Biologically Mature

A biologically mature female is a young woman who is at least 5 years postmenarchal. This has greater impact on pregnancy performance than her chronologic age. Thus, if a 14-year-old girl began menstruating when she was 9 years old, she is 5 years postmenarchal and as biologically mature as she will ever become. Certainly, she may not be emotionally, economically, educationally, or psychosocially mature, but she is as biologically mature as her 20-year-old counterpart. If another 14-year-old girl were to become pregnant during the first year after menarche, however, she would be biologically immature. The growth demands of the pregnancy and fetus superimposed on the growth demands of an adolescent during the first year after menarche may result in undesirable reproductive outcomes.

Prevent Everything That You Possibly Can

The risk of German measles in the first trimester of pregnancy has been all but eliminated by an effective immunization program whereby all young girls are vaccinated against the disease before menarche. As discussed below, an intake of 400 μg folic acid/day (0.9 μmol/day; conversion factors to SI units for various nutrients are given in Appendix Table I-A-1-a), from diet and/or as a supplement before conception and throughout the first trimester of pregnancy, significantly reduces both the initial and recurrent risks of neural tube defects (NTDs) in the fetus.

Control of Maternal Chronic and Metabolic Disorders

Pregnancy in the diabetic mother requires enough dietary and insulin control so that throughout the pregnancy, blood levels of glucose fluctuate only within the normal range of the nondiabetic patient. If so, the expected perinatal mortality associated with diabetic mothers is now 4%, a fourfold reduction in the last 20

Table 50.1
Needs for Optimal Reproductive Performances

Biologic maturity of the prospective mother
Preparation begun at conception minus 60 days
Protection from all preventable diseases
Tight control of all chronic and metabolic disorders
Eradication of all habits harmful to the fetus
Early and frequent prenatal care
Body weight within an acceptable range
Adequate nutrient intake and transport system
Working placental transfer and lactation delivery system

years. The associated risk of fetal congenital malformations in the diabetic mother can be reduced by 50% only if her glycosylated hemoglobin (A_1C) is brought into the normal range prior to conception.

The young patient with a classical phenylalanine metabolism disorder (phenylketonuria, PKU) typically has been on a special diet from infancy until the age of 8 or 9 years, after which she may have been able to manage on a more regular diet. However, she needs to be back on strict dietary control before and throughout her pregnancy. Otherwise, the probability of offspring developing some form of congenital malformation and/or another developmental abnormality is greater than 80%. All female reproductive-aged patients must be asked specifically whether they have ever been on a special diet. If the maternal serum phenylalanine level prior to conception and throughout the first trimester is maintained below 6 to 10 ng/dL (<605 nmol/L), major congenital malformations can be essentially eliminated.

All pregnancies should be started with a maternal height/weight relationship between 90 and 120% of standard weight, equivalent to a body mass index (BMI) of 20 to 26, because maternal and fetal consequences occur at both extremes. BMI is more fully discussed in Chapter 87; a nomograph is given in Appendix Table II-A-13-b. A patient's percentage of standard weight (PSW) is calculated by first measuring her nude height and weight, then using the American Diabetes Association's formulas to calculate PSW. Based on 1983 height/weight standards (see Appendix Table III-A-12-a-2), 105 lb (48 kg) are allotted for the first 5 ft (175 cm) of height, and then 5 lb (2.3 kg) is added for every additional inch (2.5 cm) of height. This calculated weight defines the 100% value of PSW. The patient's actual weight is then divided by this calculated ideal weight to give her own PSW. When a woman is underweight (<90% standard weight) when her child is conceived, her infant is more likely to be of low birth weight, particularly if weight gain is also inadequate during her pregnancy. On the other hand, a prepregnant weight that is more than 135% of standard weight (BMI > 29) predisposes the patient to maternal hypertension, pregnancy-induced toxemia, diabetes, cesarean section, and other maternal complications. Also, the fetus of a significantly obese mother is twice as prone to central nervous system congenital malformations (6). Maternal weight gain targets for the patient during her pregnancy should be based on her prepregnancy PSW or BMI category, as discussed below.

Reduce and/or Eliminate All Substance Abuse, Be It Tobacco, Alcohol, or Drugs

Tobacco, alcohol, and drugs all have an impact on the maternal and/or fetal outcome of the pregnancy. The impact may be direct or indirect, through the pocketbook, through physiologic alterations, or by metabolic competition with nutrient intake.

PROVISION OF ADEQUATE NUTRITION

A pregnant woman can provide the nutrients for herself and her fetus to meet the demands during her pregnancy in three ways. The most common and desirable way is ingestion of an adequate, safe food intake by mouth, with normal digestion, absorption, and transport into maternal circulation, normal metabolism, and normal transfer of simple nutrient building blocks from mother to fetus across the placenta. Individual nutrients cross with the assistance of maternal transport carriers and are released within placental cell(s) to be picked up by their fetal counterparts (7). This transfer system requires a functioning maternal cardiovascular system and adequate uterine blood flow, with an ample concentration of nutrients on the maternal side to transfer the building blocks to the fetal side. Without these essential components, there will be some intrauterine fetal growth retardation. The same is true with respect to the normal lactation system in the nursing mother. Second, where necessary, provision of nutrients may be replaced or augmented by use of enteral (8) and/or parenteral (8, 9) feeding, even for prolonged periods of time. A third and less desirable pathway is mobilization of the mother's body reserves for the required calories, proteins, minerals, and vitamins needed for growth and development of mother and fetus.

To ensure the expectant mother an adequate diet, there must be an available, safe food supply and functioning food distribution system, as well as the necessary economic capacity to produce and/or procure the food. Without a safe, dependable, and abundant supply of all food needs, the woman has no way to provide the nutrients for her pregnancy. Two important supplemental food programs exist for public-sector patients: the Food Stamp Program, which serves millions of patients per month, and the Supplemental Feeding Program for Women, Infants, and Children (WIC), which serves over 7 million persons per month, of whom 22 to 25% are pregnant or lactating women.

Additional Risk Factors

Low Hemoglobin

A woman living at sea level should maintain her hemoglobin above 110 g/L (11 g/dL) or her hematocrit above 331 (33%). For an adequate oxygen transport system, this hemoglobin level should be above 110 g/L (11 g/dL), whether she is pregnant, not pregnant, or lactating. The odds of detecting any type of nutrient-deficiency anemia when hemoglobin is above 11 g/dL are less than 1%. This standard needs to be increased about 1 g/dL for every 5000 feet of elevation above sea level to provide for the needed expansion of the hemoglobin oxygen-carrying capacity of the red cells during pregnancy. This hemoglobin standard is 20 g/L (2 g/dL) higher than those used in many developing countries where mothers may have complicating diseases, such as malaria and other parasites in addition to an inadequate dietary intake of available hemopoietic nutrients—iron, folate, and vitamin B_{12}. These mothers may have some unique capacity to compensate for the lower levels of hemoglobin; however, their maternal risks are enhanced, and their margin of safety is compromised. One of the few illustrations of nutritional fetal parasitism is that the hematologic condition of the fetus may be protected during pregnancy and the early weeks of lactation (10–12).

Pregnancy is the occasion for the mother to gain weight. Maternal weight gain should be based on the prepregnant weight status and should occur in an orderly manner during the second and third trimesters of pregnancy. Of all the biologic factors that influence the birth weight of the fetus, maternal weight gain has the strongest influence.

Maternal weight gains above 1 kg/week are cause for concern. A weight gain above 1 kg/week solely from the ingestion of food would require an intake of 7000 kcal (1000 kcal/day) in excess of her need. This amount is unlikely because it represents almost 50% more than the usual total daily caloric intake during pregnancy. Hence, this level of weight gain suggests an abnormal accumulation of tissue fluid. Beware of any weight losses and/or weight gains of less than 1 kg/month. The impact of weight loss on the mother or the fetus is discussed below.

The decision and plans for breast-feeding should be made when the mother first feels her baby move, or at approximately 20 weeks of gestation, rather than at or after the actual delivery. Making the decision to nurse at this time allows time for weight gain to be targeted to accumulate body stores during the third trimester for use during lactation. If the expectant mother is not going to nurse, then her maternal weight gain goals need to be decreased modestly to facilitate her return to her prepregnant weight status. Under ideal circumstances, breast-feeding is the method of choice in both developed societies and the less-developed societies of the world. However, such is not the case in the United States. Most-recent data indicate a downward trend in breast-feeding among all segments of American society, being more pronounced in the black population (2). Only 50% of mothers are breast-feeding their babies at the time of hospital discharge, and only one-third of those continue breast-feeding for 6 months; but remember, the first 4 to 6 weeks of infant breast-feeding is a very important start of the newborn's nutrition.

PRENATAL HISTORY, PHYSICAL EXAMINATION, AND NUTRITIONAL ASSESSMENT OF THE EXPECTANT MOTHER

General obstetric care requires, at the initial visit, a thorough evaluation of the pregnant woman and a careful and complete history of her obstetric and medical characteristics followed by a comprehensive physical examination. Prior to this, the patient has been weighed, her pulse taken, respiration and blood pressure recorded, and a urine sample tested by dipstick for several items of diagnostic value. A series of blood samples are drawn for determination of any abnormalities that may exist in her hematologic, serologic, immunologic, and metabolic status. A few simple nutritional assessments can readily be added that are not time consuming and can be carried out by members of the health care team. Simply prescribing a mineral/vitamin prenatal supplement does not substitute for basic nutritional assessment.

Both height and weight measurements are an essential part of the initial clinical anthropometry. Together, these measurements permit calculation of PSW and BMI and proper targeting of weight gain throughout pregnancy. A detailed nutritional assessment requires

1. A physical examination of the appropriate exposed portions of the body including the arms, legs, face, and neck for clinical evidence of nutritional deficiencies
2. A dietary food intake assessment based on either a food frequency questionnaire or a dietary history of 3-, 5-, or 7-day food intake
3. Basic anthropometric measurements of height, weight, and, on occasion, skinfold thickness
4. A biochemical assessment of selected nutrients or their metabolites as measured in blood and urine

All of these measurements are usually not possible on an individual obstetric patient. However, a rapid nutritional assessment is needed for every pregnant patient to identify any significant nutritional problems that may exist. If evidence of depletion is found, further assessments by the dietitian and/or nutritionist are needed to develop recommendations for nutritional therapies.

The physician in solo, group, or clinic practice must be able to identify available personnel in the community who can provide a detailed nutritional assessment. Such individuals may be within the hospital setting as a part of its dietary department, they may be associated with the local health clinic and/or WIC program, or they may be in private practice.

Most expectant mothers are normal, healthy women without conditions that interfere with ingestion, digestion, absorption, metabolism, or use of a normal well-balanced diet. If all of the hematologic data and multiple biochemical items on the health screening profile are normal—among which are measurements of direct nutritional significance, namely, electrolytes, glucose, magnesium, calcium, cholesterol, serum lipids, liver enzymes, albumin, urea nitrogen, and ferritin—they are unlikely to have evidence of either biochemical or clinical manifestations of any nutritional disorder. Hence, a more detailed assessment by trained nutrition personnel is not necessary. However, if a person's intake is regularly below 70% of the recommended dietary intake levels (see Appendices Tables I-A-2-a and b), one anticipates detecting abnormally low biochemical levels such as hemoglobin, serum ferritin, or serum albumin. When the patient's dietary intake is consistently below 50% of the recommended dietary allowance (RDA), one should anticipate finding clinical manifestations of early nutritional disorders. These will not be the classical pictures of nutritional deficiency, but early manifestations of abnormalities such as

1. Lesions of the gums associated with low vitamin C
2. Fissures around the angles of the mouth associated with ariboflavinosis
3. Lesions of the eyes and the skin over the arms associated with inadequate vitamin A
4. Symmetric enlargement of the thyroid gland associated with the lack of iodine

National dietary goals suggest that 15% of total caloric intake come from protein, 30% from fat, and the remainder from carbohydrates, primarily starches. The United States Department of Agriculture (USDA) recently issued a food guide pyramid to guide choices of various food groups and to achieve the proper mix of foods (13). This system provides adequate calories and healthier sources of proteins, fats, and carbohydrates coupled with the necessary amounts of minerals, vitamins, and fiber. The prescription is fairly simple: an average daily intake of 6 to 11 servings of breads, cereals, rice, and pasta; 2 to 4 servings of various fruits; 3 to 5 servings of various vegetables; 2 to 3 servings of dairy products, and a similar number of servings of meats, fish, poultry, legumes, eggs, or nuts; fats, oils, and sweets are to be used sparingly.

It has been convenient to assume that the average prepregnant and pregnant woman in America has a more-than-adequate nutrient intake of calories, proteins, minerals, and vitamins, but the results of 1980 and 1986 market-basket surveys by the USDA give reason to question that assumption. This survey showed that 50 to 60% of the female population failed to ingest 70% or more of the recommended intake of several nutrients (14). Watch for the patient who seldom eats any vegetables, fruits, or dairy products. Such a patient is probably consuming less than half of her RDA of vitamins A and C, calcium, and riboflavin. She needs more than a supplemental mineral/vitamin pill; she needs nutritional counseling. Physicians and other members of the health care team should ensure that their obstetric patients have an adequate nutrient intake. The nutritional/biochemical assessment is designed to help in that determination. Needed help can be given in group education classes or, in specific circumstances, may require individual therapeutic dietary instruction.

PHYSIOLOGIC AND METABOLIC CHANGES IN PREGNANCY

Pregnancy is a normal physiologic process associated with major alterations affecting every maternal organ system and metabolic pathway. Every single blood and urine measurement—nutrients included—is significantly altered from nonpregnant values as a result of these changes. Values change as the pregnancy advances from first to third trimester and to delivery and then return toward normal during the postpartum period. The two major physiologic forces driving these changes are *(a)* the 50% expansion of plasma volume with a 20% increase in hemoglobin mass and *(b)* the ever-increasing levels of estrogen and progesterone as well as other placenta-related hormones. These have a particular impact on the maternal lipids, cholesterol, carotene, and vitamin E, as well as on blood-clotting factors. These two physiologic modifications result in two dominant patterns of change. The first leads to decreased biochemical levels of substances in the blood such as albumin and hemoglobin during pregnancy, with a return to normal 8 to 10 weeks postpartum. Second, the estrogen-progesterone placental hormone changes cause lipid levels to rise during pregnancy and return to baseline levels postpartum.

Nutritional Biochemical and Laboratory Measurements

The 50% expansion of plasma volume during the last trimester reaches a peak by weeks 28 to 32 of gestation. The red blood cell (RBC) and hemoglobin mass also increases about 20% and peaks at about the time of delivery (15). This physiologic dilution results in a mandatory decrease of over 20% in blood hemoglobin concentration and of about 15% in hematocrit. Despite these changes, the mean corpuscular volume (MCV) and mean corpuscular hemoglobin concentration (MCHC) remain relatively unchanged in the nonanemic patient throughout pregnancy.

Other adaptations include progressive increases in cardiac output to a peak at 28 weeks, accumulation of body water, and changes in renal, respiratory, gastrointestinal, and genitourinary functions (Table 50.2). These physiologic adaptations during pregnancy alter the blood levels of many nutritional components.

Generally, nutrients that are water-soluble follow the progressive decline of serum albumin level and ferritin, for example, the serum levels of vitamin C, folic acid, vitamin B_6, and vitamin B_{12} (Table 50.3). In addition, urinary excretion of the end products of folate, niacin, and pyridoxine metabolism, and of intact riboflavin increases. In contrast, the serum levels of several fat-soluble nutrients such as carotene and vitamin E increase as much as 50% during pregnancy; vitamin A levels, however, are relatively unchanged.

Proper interpretation of laboratory results of the pregnant patient with these normal physiologic changes

Table 50.2
Major Prenatal Physiologic Alterations

↑↑ Plasma volume
↑ Red blood cell volume
↑ Cardiac output
↑ Body water
↑↑ Renal glomerular filtration rate
↑ Respiratory tidal volume
↓ Gastrointestinal and genitourinary motility

Table 50.3
Calculated Percentage Ratios of Nutrients in Maternal and Fetal Serum by Gestational Age

	Maternal				Fetal	
Serum	NP/NL[a]	3rd Trimester	Delivery	Lactating	Birth	Infant
Glucose	100	90	85	100	105	118
Protein	100	90	90	88	77	77
Albumin	100	85	81	104	71	71
Globulin	100	95	122	108	67	92
Lipids	100	140	150	139	94	134
Metals						
Calcium	100	90	90	80	110	90
Iron	100	70	70	100	100	100
Zinc	100	70	100	100	100	80
Vitamins						
A	100	90	70	130	40	40
β-carotene	100	160	200	105	40	80
D	100	220	80	50	60	62
E	100	130	160	n/a	40	130
C	100	73	50	40	110	160
Thiamin	100	60	60	80	110	110
Riboflavin	100	40	90	100	190	170
Niacin	100	150	160	83	120	122
B_6	100	40	70	80	220	130
Folate	100	70	40	120	150	80
B_{12}	100	90	30	60	100	80
Hemoglobin	100	90	96	100	139	83
Mean corpuscular volume	100	100	100	100	116	89
Mean corpuscular hemoglobin concentration	100	100	100	100	92	97

Data compiled from 18 literature references.
[a]Nonpregnant, not lactating.

requires conducting biochemical assessments at suitable intervals throughout gestation and interpreting the results against gestational norms, not the nonpregnant female standards. By converting blood nutrient values to levels per unit hematocrit, one can partially adjust for expansion of maternal blood volume for a better measure of absolute nutrient change in gestation (16). Table 50.4 identifies major prenatal nutritional alterations.

The preferred initial assessment of maternal hematologic status is an automated complete blood count (CBC) profile that provides more information than a hemoglobin or hematocrit level. Such data allow detection of iron-deficiency anemia or macrocytic anemia. One of the first clues to macrocytic anemia, when associated with a low hemoglobin, is a decrease in the total number of RBCs. An erythrocyte count at or near the 3 million/mL level is due to only one of three possible problems: *(a)* macrocytic anemia, *(b)* hemolysis that is destroying red cells, or *(c)* a recent, significant acute blood loss. All of these abnormalities result in an MCV in excess of 100.

As noted above, a health screening biochemical profile will provide several different biochemical measurements for monitoring organ and hormonal functions. Table 50.5 identifies key metabolic alterations during pregnancy, including increased plasma levels of the thyroid hormones T_3 and T_4, resulting in a physiologic state of mild hyperthyroidism. Changes in plasma insulin result in variations in the metabolism of glucose and the occurrence of gestational diabetes. No other "stress test" can match the pronounced challenge of pregnancy for identification of subsequent onset of adult diabetes. Calcium, iron, and zinc are probably required in proportionally greater quantities because of the requirements of the fetal skeletal and blood-forming tissues and factors related to the efficiency of their placental transport systems early in pregnancy. As noted below, folate catabolism increases, with a resultant increase in the requirement for folate.

Table 50.4
Major Prenatal Nutritional Alterations

↓ Hematologic status
↑ White blood cells
↓↓ Serum albumin
↓ Serum vitamin C, folic acid, B_{12}
↑ Serum carotene
→ Vitamin A
↑ Serum tocopherol
↑ Urinary *N*′-methylnicotinamide
↑ Urinary riboflavin
↑ Urinary xanthuric-acid excretion

Table 50.5
Major Prenatal Metabolic Alterations

↑ Plasma T_3 and T_4
↑ Plasma insulin
↑ Abnormal glucose tolerance test
↑ Calcium and iron absorption
↑ Nitrogen retention (anabolic)
↑ Triglyceride, cholesterol, fibrinogen

The pregnant woman becomes anabolic for protein with significant nitrogen retention, particularly during the first 24 weeks of gestation. Enhanced alterations in the lipid metabolic pathways occur, and the serum levels of triglycerides and cholesterol double. Almost all blood-clotting factors increase. Intestinal absorption of all nutrients is enhanced to a degree that depends on the amount presented from the diet, the maternal body stores, and the progressively increasing maternal and fetal nutrient use.

PLACENTAL TRANSFER OF NUTRIENTS

All nourishment to the fetus is provided by the mother across the placental barrier during intrauterine life and, if the infant is fully breast-fed, by the mother and her mammary transfer system during extrauterine life. Both supply systems depend on an adequate maternal nutrient intake. These nutrient delivery systems are impeded and a fetal deficiency is created, if the mother cannot ingest, absorb, metabolize, use, and transport these nutrients to the placenta or breast. Maternal pregnancy complications, such as *(a)* chronic cardiovascular and renal disease, *(b)* diabetes, and *(c)* pregnancy-induced preeclampsia, compromise the maternal capacity to deliver essential nutrients, as well as oxygen, across the placenta to her fetus. Normal fetal growth increases rapidly and reaches a rate of 30 g/day during the last 16 weeks of gestation, which is 50% more than can be achieved at any time during the infant's neonatal period.

Placental transfer of nutrients depends on their concentration in the maternal plasma as well as the adequacy of the uterine blood flow perfusing the placenta. The transfer of nutrients increases up to sixfold as pregnancy advances and is fueled by maternal glucose. As shown in Table 50.6, most of the electrolytes, gases, and fat-soluble vitamins cross the placental syncytiotrophoblast by simple diffusion; carbohydrates cross by facilitated diffusion; and active transport is required for amino acids, water-soluble vitamins, and essential metal ions such as calcium and iron.

As a result of three pathways, gradients in nutrient concentration on the maternal and fetal side of the placenta establish a maternal/fetal nutrient ratio. Certain entities are lower in the fetus and higher in the mother; others are equal in concentration on both sides of the placenta barrier; and some are lower in concentration in the mother and higher in the fetus. Levels of the water-soluble vitamins

Table 50.6
Methods of Placental Transfer of Nutrients

Diffusion		
Simple	Facilitated	Active Transport
Gases Free fatty acids Electrolytes Fat-soluble vitamins Plus: Pinocytosis, solute drag, breaks in villi	Carbohydrates	Amino acids Water-soluble vitamins Sodium/calcium/iron

and some of the essential metals tend to be lower in the mother than in the fetus in the unsupplemented pregnant woman. Plasma levels of the fat-soluble vitamins, in contrast, are higher in the mother than in the fetus, maintaining the diffusion gradient. Maternal supplementation of some of the water-soluble vitamins, such as folic acid, pyridoxine, and vitamin B_{12} may significantly alter their plasma levels but not eliminate these maternal/fetal ratios (17).

Years ago, we reported seasonal variations in the placental concentration of nine cations that coincided with the concentrations in the water supply in Galveston, Texas. As of the onset of our tourist season (May to October), our well water supply had to use more brackish water from the deeper wells on the mainland. About 6 weeks later, we found significant changes in deposition of several metals in the placentae of our obstetric patients—high concentrations of sodium, potassium, copper, zinc, and lead. These levels remained elevated until mid-November, about 6 weeks after the secondary sources of our community's well water were shut off. This summer period also correlated with our peak incidence and frequency of pregnancy-induced toxemia of pregnancy (18, 19).

NUTRITION PROBLEMS AMONG THE YOUNG AND OLD

Pregnant Teenagers

As noted above, the onset of menses ranges between 9 and 16 years of age in the United States, with a mean of less than 13 years. Improved nutritional status, particularly increased calorie consumption, has contributed to the decrease of about 2.5 years that has occurred over many years. A difference in intake of 200 kcal/day between two groups of young girls resulted in a 1.5-year earlier onset of menarche in the group with the higher intake (20). Frisch's (21) study of 38 young female runners and swimmers in training for the 1980 Olympics also emphasizes the importance of adequate intake at this period.

The United States has the highest frequency of teenage pregnancy of all industrialized countries in the world, and Texas ranks second among the states. About 16% of all live births occur to young women who are younger than 20 years of age, with a little over one-third (6%) of those births occurring in women younger than 18 years of age, many of whom are less than 5 years postmenarchal. The results of the Texas section of the Ten State Nutrition Survey Report (1968 to 1970) provided convincing evidence that significant numbers of adolescent females failed to ingest 50% of the RDA of all nutrients excluding calories.

Evidence indicates no real improvement in the intervening years. In general, teenagers currently appear to be in poorer overall health and nutritional condition than their parents (22). They continue to have significant excesses and deficits in calories, fat, calcium, and iron; calcium intake remains below half the RDA, with 40% of the females not regularly ingesting dairy products. Their diets are high in fat, both as total fat and as saturated components. In 1968, 10% of the Texas teenage population were obese (over 120% of standard weight). In comparison, 1990 data indicate an obesity problem in the range of 15 to 25% (23).

All obstetric and fetal performance studies of teenage pregnancies, particularly among those younger than 18 years of age (less than 5 years postmenarchal), have reported three common trends: *(a)* a decrease in mean infant birth weight that results in an increased percentage of LBW newborns, *(b)* an increase in the perinatal mortality rate, and *(c)* an increase in pregnancy-induced toxemia. These pregnant teenagers are part of a population group that receives its health care primarily in the public sector. This issue was examined recently in a series of reports in a volume on adolescent nutritional disorders (23a).

Older Primigravidas

Over the past 25 years, we have seen a significant twofold increase in the number of women 30 years old or older who are delivering their first child. The older primigravida patient usually receives her health care in the private sector.

How nutritionally well prepared is the older patient for pregnancy? Upward of 40% of women in this age group are on, or have been on, some type of weight-reduction diet for the previous 5 to 6 months (24). Of the 10 most popular types of diets evaluated in 1987, 90% had fewer than 1500 calories, 70% had more than 20% of their calories coming from protein, and 60% had more than 30% coming from fat (25). Seven out of 10 of these diets were inadequate in essential minerals and vitamins. For many women, their nutritional status before their first pregnancy is not better than that of many teenagers. Pregnant women over 35 years of age have more chronic hypertension, a threefold increase in diabetes, and twice the incidence of third-trimester bleeding—placenta previa and abruptio placentae. They also have a higher rate of cesarean section that is not necessarily associated with obstructive labor problems and a higher incidence of LBW infants than women under 18 years old.

RECOMMENDED DIETARY ALLOWANCES FOR PREGNANCY AND LACTATION

During the half-century that successive editions of the United States RDAs have been published, changes have occurred in recommendations for nutrients, minerals, and vitamins based on the then-current status of nutritional knowledge. For example, energy recommendations for nonpregnant adult women have varied from a low of 2000 kcal/day in 1948 and 1968 to a high of 2300 kcal in 1953 and 1958. Data based on the 1983 revision of the Metropolitan Life Height, Age, and Weight Tables and on data derived from the National Health and Nutrition Examination Survey (NHANES) II indicate that women of reproductive age are about 2 cm taller and 2 kg heavier than the RDA reference woman of the 1960s (26). Since 1974, the recommendations for increased energy need during the second and third trimesters of pregnancy and the first 6 months of lactation have remained constant at 300 and 500 kcal/day, respectively.

The 1989 revision of the RDAs had several significant changes in the recommendation for the nonpregnant, pregnant, and lactating woman (Table 50.7); see also

Table 50.7
1989 Recommended Dietary Allowances for Pregnant and Lactating Women 15 to 25+ Years Old

Nutrient[a]	Nonpregnant	Pregnant	Percentage Change[b]	Lactating 1–6 Months	Percentage Change[b]
Energy (kcal)	2200	2500	114	2700	123
Protein (g)	44–50	60	120	65	130
Calcium (mg)	800	1200	150	1200	150
Phosphorus (mg)	800	1200	150	1200	150
Iron (mg)	15	30	200	15	100
Magnesium (mg)	280	320	114	355	127
Iodine (μg)	150	175	117	200	133
Zinc (mg)	12	15	125	19	158
Selenium (μg)	55	65	118	75	136
Vitamin A (μg RE)	800	800	100	1300	162
Vitamin D (μg)	10	10	100	10	100
Vitamin E (mg & TE)[c]	8	10	125	12	150
Vitamin K (μg)	55	55	100	65	118
Vitamin C (mg)	60	70	117	95	158
Thiamin (mg)	1.1	1.5	136	1.6	145
Riboflavin (mg)	1.3	1.6	123	1.8	138
Niacin (mg NE)	15	17	113	20	133
Folate (μg)	180	400	222	280	108
Vitamin B_6 (mg)	1.6	2.2	138	2.1	131
Vitamin B_{12} (μg)	2.0	2.2	110	2.6	130

From Food and Nutrition Board, National Research Council. Recommended dietary allowances. 10th ed. Washington, DC: National Academy Press, 1989.
[a]RE, retinol equivalents; NE, niacin equivalents.
[b]Allowances for pregnancy and lactation ÷ nonpregnant women 15 to 25+ years old.
[c]As milligrams of α-trocopherol.

Appendix Tables II-A-2-a-1 and 2. Compared with the 1980 RDAs (27), the 1989 RDAs for nonpregnant women recommended a small increase in protein and a decreased need for iron, zinc, folate, and vitamin B_6, in the face of a 5% increase of energy—100 kcal/day (4.2×10^5 joules), an increase from 2100 to 2200 kcal/day. The 1989 RDA for the pregnant woman included a 15 to 25% increase above the recommendations for the nonpregnant woman for calories, protein, magnesium, iodine, zinc, selenium, vitamin E, vitamin C, thiamin, and niacin. The recommendations also included a 50% increase in calcium and phosphorus to the same amount recommended for a growing teenager. Only the RDAs for iron and folic acid are more than 100% over those for nonpregnant women. The 1997 Food and Nutrition Board dietary reference intakes increase the RDAs for calcium, phosphorus, and magnesium, especially for female adolescents (see Appendix Tables II-A-2-b-1 to 3).

Essentials of Human Lactation

The nutritional requirements for successful human lactation have been reviewed (27a). During pregnancy, the breasts readied for the demands of the infant postdelivery. Stimulation of the ductal system by the ever-increasing production of estrogen, and the concurrent enhancement of alveolar growth by maternally produced progesterone, result in enlargement of the breasts and nipples, their increased blood supply, and development of skin striae. Colostrum can be expressed from the nipples throughout the latter half of pregnancy.

The alveoli produce the milk that flows along the ducts to the nipple; milk is then withdrawn by the infant's sucking and ejected secondary to the release of maternal oxytocin. Initiation of breast milk flow begins with the release of prolactin by the mother's pituitary gland; this is the byproduct of the sharp fall in maternal estrogen and progesterone levels that occurs following delivery of the infant and placenta.

Some 90% of infant breast milk feeding occurs in the first 3 to 5 minutes of suckling, as the milk letdown reflex comes into operation. A full-term infant will receive 90 to 270 mL/day from the first to third postdelivery day. By the end of the first week, milk production reaches 420 mL; and by days 28 to 30 it exceeds 600 mL/day.

Human breast milk is unique and quite different from cow's milk and soy-based formulas. In addition to the nutritional advantages, its immunologic characteristics provide essential protection during those critical 100 to 120 days postdelivery. In no way have our most sophisticated infant formulas been able to match human milk as the preferred food for all newborn infants, be they in developed or developing regions of the world.

Human breast milk, for the first 100 days, is a complete meal in itself (Table 50.8). Protein (1.5%) is in the form lactalbumin and a fine, digestible casein. Fat (3.5%) occurs as fine droplets. Carbohydrate (7.0%) is in the form of lactose. All the essential minerals and vitamins are included in adequate amounts except iron, which requires supplementation. Each 30 mL of breast milk provides 20 kcal, or about 600 to 750 kcal daily.

Table 50.8
Estimate of Mean Concentration of Nutrients per Liter of Mature Human Milk

	Units	Amount
Lactose	g	72.0
Protein	g	10.5
Fat	g	39.0
Minerals		
Calcium	mg	280
Phosphorus	mg	140
Magnesium	mg	35
Iron	mg	0.3
Zinc	mg	1.2
Copper	mg	0.25
Iodine	μg	110
Selenium	μg	20
Manganese	μg	6
Fluoride	μg	16
Chromium	μg	50
Vitamins		
A	RE	670
E	mg	2.3
D	μg	0.55
K	μg	2.1
C	mg	40
Thiamin	mg	0.21
Riboflavin	mg	0.35
Niacin	mg	1.5
B_6	mg	93
Pantothenic acid	mg	1.8
Folate	μg	85
B_{12}	μg	0.97

Adapted from Institute of Medicine. Nutrition during lactation—milk composition. Washington, DC: National Academy Press, 1991;116.

Maternal macronutrient dietary intake has little effect on the nutrient composition of human milk, except for its fatty acid content. Major minerals in the milk, such as calcium, phosphorus, magnesium, sodium, potassium, and iron, are not affected by maternal dietary intake. In contrast, content is positively correlated with intake of selenium and iodine. All essential water- and fat-soluble vitamins in milk depend on current maternal intake and stores. Chronically low maternal intake leads to low content in the milk. Infant parasitism is evidenced by iron, calcium, folate, and vitamin C—the milk content is maintained irrespective of the maternal concentration. If the maternal dietary intake consistently exceeds the RDA, only vitamin D, vitamin B_6, iodine, and selenium appear in higher than usual concentrations in breast milk.

Recent studies have added to our knowledge about the interaction between the mother's and infant's nutritional status as a result of full lactation during the 6 months following delivery. Among lactating Mexican Indian women with low BMI (21.4) at delivery, maternal weight and body fat declined during the first 6 months of nursing. However, their low-energy balance was not associated with significant changes in production and composition of breast milk or infant growth rate (27b). Investigators from Iowa reported a careful 10-week weight-reduction study of a small group of postpartum nursing mothers. They averaged a calorie deficit of 538 kcal/day. While maternal weight was reduced 4.8 kg, there was no significant decrease in breast milk production or infant growth rate (27c).

Michigan investigators examined prolonged lactation effects on maternal bone density among two groups of biologically mature postpartum women (mean age, 27 and 29 years) with a calcium intake of almost 1700 mg and 1600 mg/day, respectively, during pregnancy and lactation. They found no significant changes in bone density during the first 5 months of nursing, compared with nonnursing controls. Beyond 6 months of nursing, there was a significant decrease in maternal bone density, even with a maternal daily calcium intake in excess of 1200 mg (27d). We wonder what these effects would be among 17-year-old nursing mothers with a calcium intake below 800 mg/day.

Nutritional Requirements

During the first 6 months of lactation, the maternal requirements for protein, zinc, niacin, and vitamins A, E, and C increase above those in pregnancy. However, compared with the requirements of the pregnant woman, the requirements for iron and folic acid decrease.

Concern has been expressed that excessive calories during and after pregnancy and lactation may be a major contributor to obesity. Pregnant and lactating women *do* need additional energy, but whether the additional 300 and 500 kcal/day that are recommended for pregnancy and lactation are truly needed, on top of the nonpregnant recommendation of 1800 or 2200 kcal/day, remains unresolved.

In developing countries, pregnant and lactating women with caloric intakes of 60 to 80% and 50 to 72%, respectively, of the 1989 RDAs are supporting pregnancies and lactation (26, 28). Depressed basal metabolic rate during the first 18 weeks of gestation was noted in chronically and marginally undernourished Gambian women (29). In western and northern European and in Australian studies, actual caloric intakes for pregnant women averaged 78 to 100% (mean, 2140 kcal/day) per day of the RDAs and 85 to 109% (mean, 2480 kcal/day) of the RDAs for women during lactation, with superior maternal and fetal performance (28). However, this summary also included data from a study in the United States on lactating women (30), which had the lowest average of any of the studies listed. Appendix Table II-A-3-a shows that the 1990 Canadian recommendations for pregnant and lactating women averaged 200 and 250 kcal/day lower than those of the U.S. RDAs. United Kingdom standards are also appreciably lower than U.S. RDAs (see Appendix Table II-A-4-a).

Since the 1970s, the usual reference standard for the pregnant woman has been based on Hytten and Leitch's calculation that pregnancy requires an additional 80,000 kcal (31), believed to accumulate in the course of pregnancy, as illustrated in Fig. 50.1. This figure of 80,000 is based on a pregnancy in which the mother gained 12.5 kg (27.5 lb) and gave birth to an infant weighing 3.3 kg (7.3 lb). This estimate was used by the World Health Organization (WHO) in 1973 for the energy allowances for pregnancy, with an increase from an extra 150 kcal/day for the first trimester to 350 kcal/day for the sec-

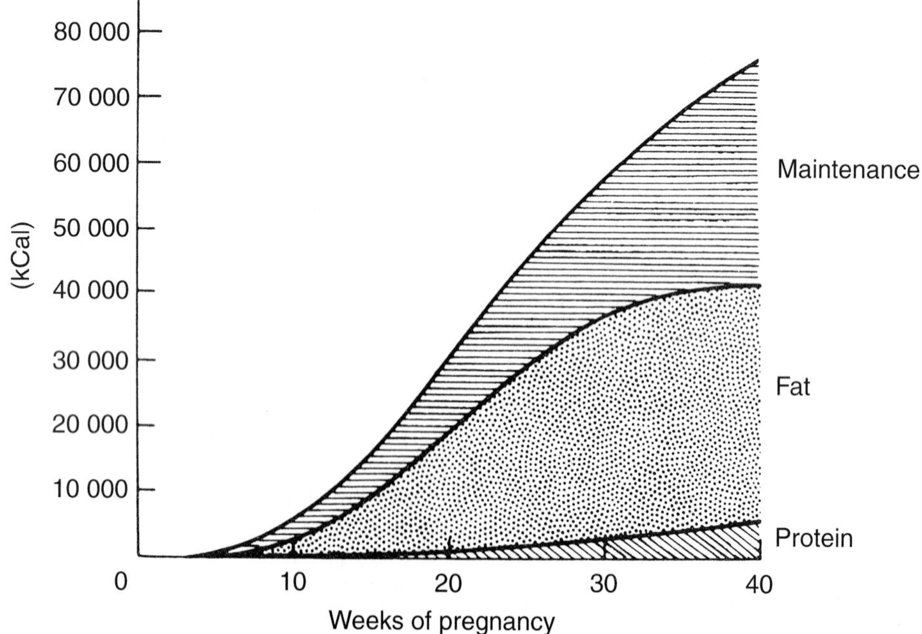

Figure 50.1. The cumulative energy cost of pregnancy and its components. (From Hytten F, Chamberlain G. Clinical physiology in obstetrics. Oxford: Blackwell Scientific Publications, 1980, with permission.)

ond and third trimesters. In the 1985 WHO revision, an additional 250 kcal/day was recommended throughout pregnancy, with a reduction to 200 kcal/day throughout pregnancy when the expectant mother can reduce physical activity proportionately (32). One of the major components of the energy cost is the accumulation of approximately 3.5 kg of fat, most of which is laid down by the 30th week. This accumulation occurs while the fetus and maternal reproductive organs are increasing slowly in weight and was considered protective against the high energy costs of the last trimester of pregnancy and lactation. The other major energy cost concerns the increased requirements for maintenance metabolism that occur in the latter half of pregnancy.

Alternative assumptions have been made on the basis of further analyses of composition of the new tissues and more detailed observations of both energy intakes and expenditures of pregnant women and of their resting metabolism. Such calculations have led to estimates of the cost of pregnancy in healthy, well-nourished women as low as 45,000 kcal (33) or 68,000 kcal (34), and as high as 110,000 kcal (35). The lower figures are based on the assumption of decreased activity of the pregnant woman during the third trimester of pregnancy.

For the healthy pregnant woman, an adequate intake (with supplementation of iron, folate, and perhaps zinc) is achieved by choosing among a variety of foods in the proportions recommended in the USDA pyramid. Weight gain management should follow appropriate weight targets, as described below. Individuals who prefer an ethnic diet (e.g., Far Eastern, Near Eastern, Hispanic, and vegetarian) can meet their nutrient needs with proper food selection. Food exchange lists for a variety of food patterns are given in Appendix Table V-A-25. A strict vegan has dietary deficits in nutrients important for hematologic well-being, particularly vitamin B_{12}. To maintain adequate nutritional status during pregnancy, strict vegans must regularly ingest a mineral/vitamin supplement that contains, at least, iron, zinc, folate, and vitamin B_{12}.

Not all family providers in our society have the economic means to support their family's needs for food, clothing, and shelter. Some 10% of the U.S. population receives food stamps, and their children participate in the school lunch and breakfast programs. Another 1.5 million women and over 5.5 million children are enrolled in the WIC program. The WIC Food Package V for pregnant and breast-feeding women provides more than 840 kcal/day, which is more than 30% of the total recommended caloric intake, 65% of protein needs, and 100% of almost all the mineral and vitamin requirements except for iron and zinc during pregnancy and lactation. Apparently, not all this supplemental food is ingested by the mother but is assimilated into the total food availability of the family unit. Evidence indicates an increase in mean infant birth weight of only 30 to 100 g for infants whose mothers receive the WIC supplement during pregnancy (2).

MATERNAL WEIGHT GAIN

In the last two decades, the prevalence of obesity among American women has increased greatly. Overall, 33 to 50% of potential American mothers are obese (>27 BMI or >120% PSW). Studies from the United States, United Kingdom, and France have all found excess perinatal mortality, hypertension, pregnancy-induced toxemia, gestational diabetes, cesarean section, and congenital malformations in the fetus. These obstetric complications all convert to a major increase in medical and hospital costs (36–39).

Maternal weight gain during pregnancy is an essential component of the normal growth and development of the mother and her fetus. Over the past 100 years, the medical profession has adopted acceptable/optimal weight gain guidelines. In the late 1890s, under the fear of maternal mortality associated with overly large infants and the risks of cesarean section delivery, our German predecessors initiated the pattern of trying to restrict maternal weight gain deliberately in an attempt to reduce infant size and weight, therefore expediting the vaginal birth process. This pattern existed in one form or another through the 1960s. In 1970, the National Research Council's report *Maternal Nutrition and the Course of Pregnancy* increased weight gain targets by a modest 5 to 8 lb/pregnancy (40).

Today, the pendulum has swung toward "ad libitum feeding" and further maternal weight gain, to the extent that it may be a major contributor to the ever-increasing incidence of obesity in the female population of the United States. Over 25% of young women below 20 years of age are obese, and one-third of all females in the United States weigh more than 120% of standard weight (24). On any given day, 40% of adult U.S. women are on diets and have been for 6 months or longer. The birth weight of the offspring depends on two major maternal weight–related factors: *(a)* how much weight did the mother gain during her pregnancy? and *(b)* what was her height/weight relationship (PSW or BMI) when she began her pregnancy?

In its 1990 report on maternal weight gain, the National Research Council (3) recommended that all pregnant women have a BMI calculation on entry into prenatal care. If a woman has a BMI below 20, her weight gain target should be 1.1 lb/week during the second and third trimester, leading to 31 lb (14 kg) of overall weight gain; the woman whose BMI is above 26, has a weight gain target of only 0.7 lb/week, requiring up to 20 lb (9 kg) of overall weight gain (2). As noted above, another method of weight/height expression of PSW, from the American Diabetes Association, equates a PSW below 90% of standard weight with a BMI below 20, and a PSW of 135 with a BMI above 29.

Components of Weight Gain

During normal pregnancy, the components of weight gain consist of the fetus, placenta, amniotic fluid, enlarged uterine and breast tissue, and expanded maternal blood components (Fig. 50.2). Together, they constitute the "obligatory" weight gain associated with pregnancy. In addition, there are highly variable accumulations of tissue fluid, adipose tissue, and protein stores. Studies from industrialized countries show obligatory weight gains of about 7.5 kg (16.5 lb). Among developing countries, obligatory maternal weight gain is about 20% less (6 kg, or 13.2 lb), with lesser accumulations of tissue fluid, adipose tissue, and protein stores (41).

If a woman 65 in (1.67 m) tall begins her pregnancy at 128 lb (58.2 kg), over the 40 weeks of pregnancy her PSW will increase 13% (16.5 lb = 7.5 kg) from the obligatory weight gain of pregnancy alone. If, instead, she gains 32 lb (15 kg), her PSW will increase almost 26%, of which 1 to 2 kg will be tissue fluid and 7 kg will be in the form of fat deposits. Returning to her prepregnant weight after delivery or nursing will require at least 12 weeks of reduced calories and increased exercise. It may well take a year for a primiparous, singleton mother who gains over 40 lb (18.2 kg) to return to her initial weight.

Individual Weight Gain Targets

No single maternal weight gain target meets the needs of all types of pregnant women. Individualized pattern(s) of maternal weight gain should be adjusted for *(a)* height and/or PSW, *(b)* biologic age, *(c)* plans to breast-feed, and *(d)* whether more than one fetus is being carried.

Does a biologically immature female need more weight gain during pregnancy to produce an equivalent-weight offspring? Garn et al. (42) examined the data from the National Perinatal Study and found that white and black women 14 years of age required almost 4 g of maternal weight to yield 1 g of baby. Their fully mature counterparts produced 200-g heavier infants on only 3 g of maternal weight for every 1 g of baby. These findings translate into a need for an additional 150 kcal/day (3 kg in overall weight gain) for the biologically immature pregnant woman.

General Targets of Appropriate Weight Gain

We have developed five maternal weight-gain targets (Fig. 50.3):

1. The woman who enters her pregnancy at more than 120% of standard weight, has an obligatory weight gain of 7 to 8 kg (15–18 lb) at a rate of no more than 300 g (0.7 lb) per week (target I)
2. The woman of normal PSW who is not going to nurse, has the target of 10 kg overall at a rate of 350 g (0.8 lb) per week (target II)
3. The woman who enters her pregnancy between 90 and 110% of standard weight and is planning to nurse her baby, has the target of 12 kg (26 lb) overall at a rate of 400 g (0.9 lb) per week during the second and third trimesters (target III)
4. The biologically immature adolescent and the woman less than 90% of standard weight have the target of 14 to 15 kg (32 lb) at a rate of 500 g (1.1 lb) per week (target IV)
5. The woman who is going to have twins has the target of 18 kg (40 lb) of weight gain, with a weekly rate of 650 g (1.4 lb) during the last 20 weeks of her pregnancy (target V)

Risks of Excessive Weight Gain

As noted above, the 1990 maternal nutrition report of the National Research Council (3, 126) recommended an additional 5- to 10-lb increase above the 1980 targets for

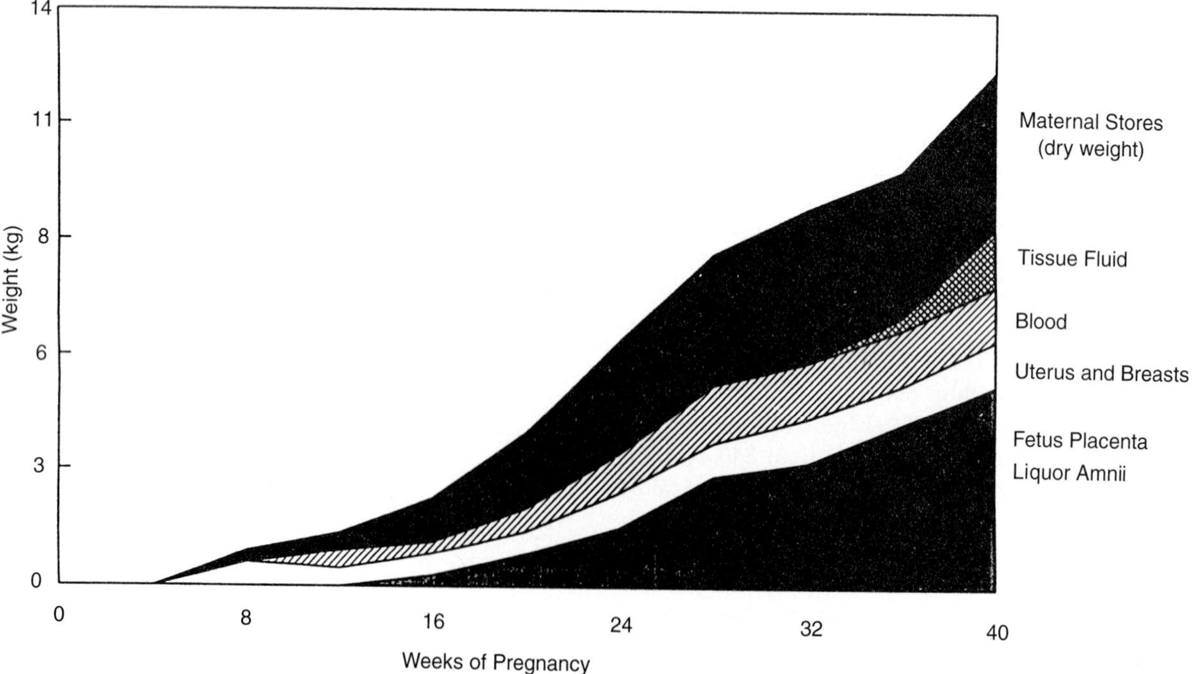

Figure 50.2. Components of weight gain in normal pregnancy. (From Hytten FE, Leith I. Physiology of human pregnancy. Oxford: Blackwell Scientific Publications, 1964, with permission.)

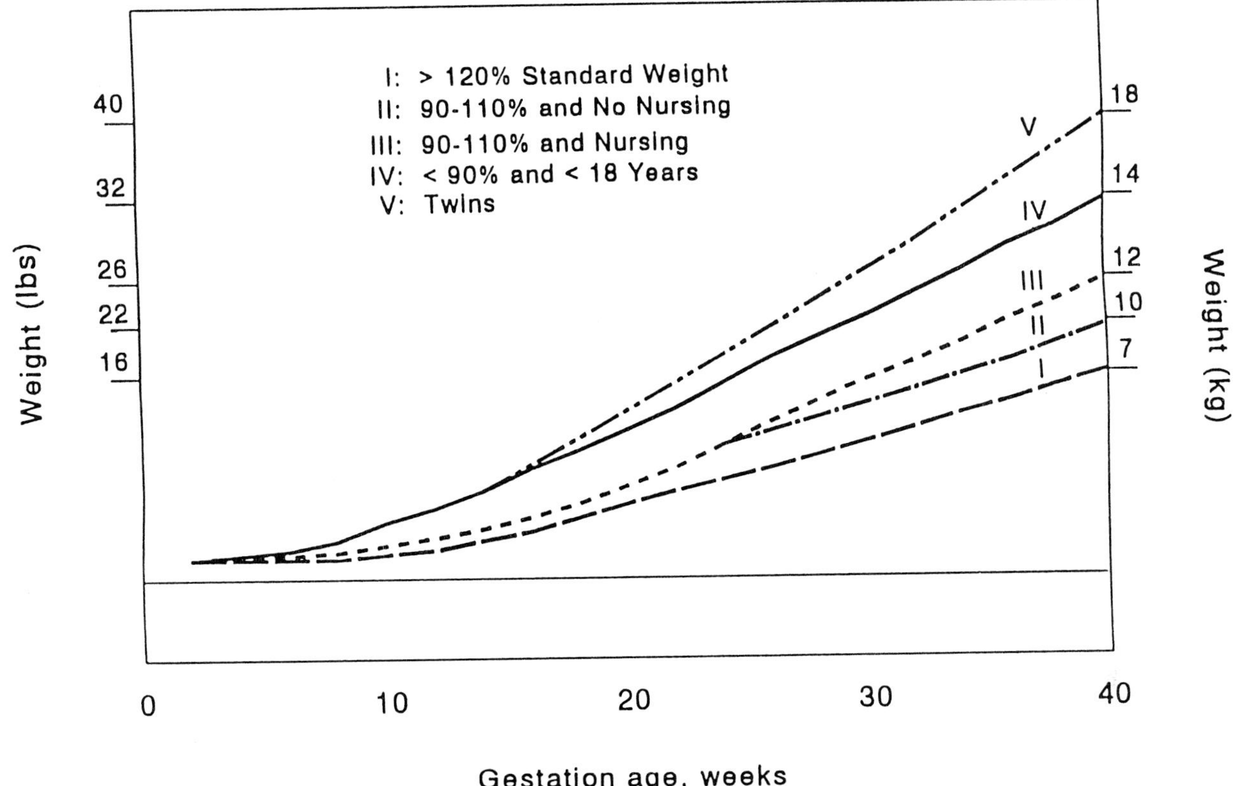

Figure 50.3. Maternal weight gain targets.

maternal weight gain to produce heavier, but not necessarily more biologically mature, newborns (31). This recommendation implies that the benefits of a heavier baby outweigh the costs associated with increased problems with delivery, as well as the maternal health costs associated with ever-increasing residual obesity. The wisdom of this recommendation merits discussion.

No convincing evidence indicates that an infant who is biologically mature at birth and who weighs over 3200 g would be better off or healthier if he or she were to weigh 3500 g. In contrast, there is tremendous difference with respect to neonatal morbidity and mortality if an infant, at birth, weighs 1000, 1250, 1500, or 2000 g. Here fetal weight status is far more important. A 300-g weight differential with its 10 days of additional biologic maturation may be crucial to the survival and well-being of the fetus. Furthermore, excessive maternal weight gain has been associated with increased rates of labor problems, cesarean section, fetal macrosomia, late delivery dates, and meconium staining of the fetus.

Obesity, Age, and Parity

Cross-sectional data from the Texas Nutritional Survey of 1968 showed a progressive increase in the incidence of female obesity associated with advancing maternal age, from 10% obesity in the 15- to 19-year-old age group to as much as 60% in 40- to 44-year-old women (43). Although obesity is directly related to advancing age, a much higher correlation exists between obesity and the number of times a woman has been pregnant (gravidity). Our data showed a 16% obesity rate among those who were never pregnant; this rate rose to 50 to 68% among grand multiparous women (Table 50.9). An average of 2.5 kg (5.5 lb) was added permanently to the woman's body for each of her pregnancies.

Longitudinal data from separate national collaborative studies of over 1200 and 600 women also found residual weight gain correlated with the number of prior pregnancies. Weiss and Jackson (44) reported a 3-lb increase in black mothers and 3.8-lb increase in white mothers from one pregnancy to the next. Garn et al. (42) found an

Table 50.9
Percentage Under and Overweight by Gravidity

Percentage of Standard Weight		<80	≥120
No. Pregnancy	N		
0	286	7.5	15.7
1	57	5.4	33.3
2	65	7.7	36.9
3	72	4.2	47.2
4	73	1.4	47.9
5	67	3.0	55.2
6	57	—	45.6
7	38	—	50.0
8	33	3.1	66.6
9	22	—	68.2
10	70	—	52.9

From McGanity WJ, Dawson EB. Unpublished data. Ten State Nutrition Survey, 1968–1970.

increase greater than 5 kg from the first to the third pregnancy, with lesser gains in smokers. More-recent reports confirm this trend and add that the weight increases are greater in multiparous women over 35 years of age and that black women have twice the relative risk of white women of adding to their obesity with successive pregnancies (45).

As described above, the pregnant woman has been encouraged to increase her dietary intake by 300 kcal/day for the last 200 days of prenatal care and by 500 kcal or more per day during her months of full lactation. However, once these needs end, she must be prepared to reduce her caloric intake and increase her activity. Otherwise, she will continue with a 2200- to 2700-kcal appetite and an energy expenditure of only 1800 to 2000 kcal/day. Remember, 250 excess calories per day will add over 2 lb (1 kg) of weight *per month* to her frame. In reality, a 500 kcal/day *deficit* is desired, so she will lose 1 lb/week until she returns to a normal BMI or PSW.

Lactation itself may or may not help the mother return to her prepregnant weight status. Some evidence suggests that the nonlactating female loses more weight and at a faster rate than the lactating mother (46). These data also suggest that greater prenatal weight gain is associated with greater weight loss. In a well-controlled study, Dewey et al. (45) demonstrated that the long-term, breast-feeding mother lost considerably more weight postpartum than the mother who fed less than 3 months.

IODINE

Iodine deficiency remains a major international public health problem (see Chapter 13). It is estimated that 800 million people may be at risk for the effects of iodine deficiency, known as iodine deficiency disorders (47). In humans, these effects occur at all stages of development: the fetus, the neonate, the child, and the adult. Low levels of dietary iodine, observed in endemic areas, decrease the synthesis of the thyroid hormones and result in maternal hypothyroidism, lowered maternal metabolism, and lowered fetal nutrition (48, 49). Overt or marginal hypothyroidism occurs in about 50% of pregnant women residing in areas of endemic iodine deficiency (50) when the iodine need is dramatically increased during the first 20 weeks of pregnancy (49, 51). The effects include miscarriages, stillbirths, and congenital anomalies, as well as goiter, cretinism, impaired brain function, and hypothyroidism in children and adults (47). Endemic areas of iodine deficiency are located in mountainous regions of Europe, the eastern Mediterranean, Asia, South and Central America, and Africa (52, 53). Indeed, iodine deficiency is considered the single most important and widespread nutrient deficiency (54) (also see Chapter 13).

Although North America is no longer a region of endemic iodine deficiency (50), the Ten State Nutrition Survey of 1971–1972 revealed a goiter rate of 3.1%, with a slightly higher rate among females than males (53). Apparently, the low incidence of iodine deficiency in the United States may be attributed to iodination of several commercial foodstuffs: salt, bread, cereal, etc. (50). However, marginal prenatal iodine deficiency remains a clinical problem in North America. It has been hypothesized that women relying heavily or solely on vegetable diets prior to pregnancy and in early pregnancy are at risk for prenatal iodine deficiency (55). No adverse effects on mother or fetus have been reported from prenatal iodine supplementation (56).

ANEMIA PREVENTION

"Low" hemoglobin is the most common nutritional biochemical problem encountered in everyday prenatal care. If not accounted for by the normal 12 to 20% decline due to hemodilution, 9 in 10 true hemopoietic nutrient deficit problems are related to iron, and 1 in 10 is related to folic acid. Except in those few individuals who are strict vegans (see Chapter 106) and the rare patients who have had a vitamin B_{12} problem diagnosed and treated before their pregnancy, it is essentially unknown for macrocytic anemia to develop during pregnancy because of inadequate vitamin B_{12}.

In the United States, the most common cause of a hemoglobin concentration below 110 g/L (11 g/dL) is an exaggerated hemodilution caused by the expansion of blood volume. A true nutritional anemia will develop when one or more of the following occur: *(a)* an inadequate dietary intake of hematopoietic nutrients, *(b)* an excess loss of blood, or *(c)* inadequate nutrient stores to maintain hemoglobin production and RBC maturation.

Iron

Iron is an essential trace metal that functions as a cofactor for transporting oxygen in the hemoglobin in RBCs, the myoglobin in muscle, and the cytochrome systems within mitochondria. Within each of these systems, the iron atom transfers the oxygen molecule for respiration of all maternal and fetal cells. However, the primary function of RBC hemoglobin is to transport oxygen from the lungs to the other respiratory systems, and it is critical for cellular metabolism. The oxygen requirement for cellular metabolism increases during pregnancy (with increased demands for maternal and fetal growth and development); the highest risk of nutritional inadequacy occurs during the last weeks of pregnancy. Consequently, maintaining the oxygen-carrying capacity of the pregnant woman is essential for her and for the developing fetus. The oxygen-carrying capacity is most conveniently estimated by the level of maternal hemoglobin, which in turn depends on the pregnant woman's plasma iron level.

The iron status (hemoglobin status, O_2 carrying capacity) depends on *(a)* the level of maternal hemopoietic stores, *(b)* intestinal absorption of iron, folate, vitamin B_{12}, etc., *(c)* acute or chronic loss of blood due to internal or external bleeding, *(d)* the absence of any hemolyzing agents, *(e)* an adequate supply of other essential hemopoietic nutrients to permit the synthesis of RBCs and to fill them with iron-containing hemoglobin, and *(f)* a working placental transfer system for iron, folate, vitamin B_{12}, etc., from mother to fetus.

The change from full iron stores with an adequate dietary intake to a classic, chronic iron-deficiency anemia (small, hemoglobin-poor RBCs) has many steps. An RBC distribution width of 15% or more, determined by the automated Coulter Counter CBC, is one of the earliest indicators of a developing iron-deficiency anemia. Another key is the level of plasma ferritin, which reflects the adequacy of the body's iron stores. Levels of 12 μg/L (ng/mL) or less have been considered deficient, and even levels below 35 μg/dL in the first trimester provide little margin of safety in meeting the later iron requirements of mother and fetus for optimal growth and development.

The typical American diet contains between 6 and 7 mg (0.5 and 0.6 nmol) of iron per 1000 kcal. An average of only 10% of the ingested iron is transported into the portal circulation. Table 50.10 lists the mean number of milligrams of iron per day that must be transported into the maternal circulation during the various stages of the reproductive cycle from nonpregnant, through the three trimesters of pregnancy, and during lactation. Cessation of menses decreases the amount of iron required in the first trimester. In response to maternal and fetal demands, however, the requirement increases throughout both the second and third trimesters. As long as total lactation continues, the mother will remain amenorrheic and her own postpartum iron requirement will remain low. In the third trimester of pregnancy, an average 4 mg/day of iron must cross into the maternal circulation. However, because of fetal demands this requirement may peak as high as 7 mg/day of iron for a short time during the middle (30–34 weeks) of the third trimester.

How much dietary iron is required to transport 4 to 7 mg iron across the intestinal barrier and into the maternal circulation? Based on the current RDA for pregnant women and usual dietary intakes, this might require an efficiency of iron absorption of 50%, if iron was available only from dietary sources. Various investigators have found that pregnant women have an enhanced ability to absorb iron across the intestinal mucosa (57). Maternal intestinal iron absorption increases from 10% to more than 50% during the last trimester of pregnancy. This ability to increase the efficiency of iron absorption may suffice to meet the increased maternal and fetal requirements of pregnancy, provided there are sufficient maternal stores of iron and an acceptable level of available iron is ingested and presented to the intestinal cells for mucosal transfer (58). If the pregnant woman ingests 15 mg of iron from dietary sources and another 30 mg is available as an iron supplement, she should have no difficulty meeting the iron requirements for pregnancy and her fetus during pregnancy, lactation, and the first 100 days postpartum. If the maternal hemoglobin level exceeds 110 g/L (11 g/dL) at sea level and the serum ferritin is 35 ng/dL or more, a 30-mg iron supplement is adequate. If a typical prenatal mineral/vitamin supplement containing 30 mg of iron and an additional three tablets of 325-mg ferrous sulfate (60 mg of Fe^{2+}) are prescribed, the patient will ingest over 200 mg of elemental iron to get 7 mg across the gut. This is iron excess, which leads to gastric irritation and patient noncompliance. If the pregnant woman's hemoglobin level is below 100 g/L (10 g/dL) and her serum ferritin is 12 ng/dL or less, with low MCV and MCHC—characteristic of classic iron-deficiency anemia—she will need a total of 120 to 150 mg/day of elemental iron to meet these demands until her hemoglobin exceeds 120 g/L (12 g/dL) and her serum ferritin level is again over 35 μg/L.

Maintaining optimal oxygen-carrying capacity requires almost 1 g/dL more hemoglobin for each 5000 feet of elevation for all persons, including prospective mothers, compared with those residing at sea level (1). For example, an acceptable hemoglobin level may be more than 11.0 g/dL in Galveston (sea level), while the standard needs to be more than 12.0 g/dL in Denver (1 mile high) and more than 13.0 g/dL in Leadville, Colorado (elevation above 10,000 feet).

The NHANES II and other studies found that hemoglobin and serum transferrin levels of black women are about 10% lower than those of either white or Hispanic women. Similarly, hemoglobin levels are 12% higher in the first trimester of pregnancy than in the third; they are also higher in obese pregnant women than in those who are underweight (59). In a therapeutic trial using a mineral/vitamin supplement containing three dosage levels of iron (0, 18, and 65 mg/day) and two levels of folate (400 and 1000 μg/day) (Table 50.11), young women were studied from the 16th week of pregnancy through the remainder of their pregnancy, at delivery, and for the first 12 weeks postpartum. Fig. 50.4 illustrates that the mean serum ferritin in each group dropped significantly from the initial values at entry into the study to the time of delivery, and all values recovered somewhat in the postpartum period. Only in group C, women who were receiving the 65-mg iron supplement, did values return to their initial entry levels by the 12th week postpartum. None of these

Table 50.10
Provisional Requirements of Dietary Iron in Women

Age	Daily Requirements (mg)	Iron Available in Daily Diet (mg)		
		10%	20%	30%
11–50 years, nonpregnant, nonlactating	1.8	18.0	9.0	6.0
Pregnant 1st trimester	1.0	10.0	5.0	3.0
2nd trimester	3.0	30.0	15.0	10.0
3rd trimester	4.0	40.0	20.0	13.0
Lactating	1.5	15.0	7.5	5.0

Table 50.11
Hematologic Outcome versus Serum Ferritin at 20 Weeks Gestational Age

Iron Supplementation Group	*N*	Gestational (*N* = 61)		Therapeutic Failure (*N* = 14)	
		Ferritin >35	Ferritin <35	Ferritin >35	Ferritin <35
A (0 mg)[a]	21	4	17	0	9
B (18 mg)[a]	19	11	8	1	4
C (65 mg)[b]	21	10	11	0	0
Total	61	25	36	1	13

[a] 1 mg iron = 18 μmol.
[b] +400 μg (0.91 μmol) folate.
[c] +800 μg (1.82 μmol) folate.

three levels of maternal iron supplementation sufficed to overcome the dilutional effect of blood volume expansion and/or the demands for iron by the mother and fetus during the second and third trimester of pregnancy. In contrast, the mothers' ability to lay down new iron stores occurred when the iron supplement was given before the pregnancy began and during the first weeks after delivery.

Women may be in a state of low or deficient iron at the beginning of pregnancy because of an inadequate diet, excessive menstrual losses, or other factors. Iron status should be determined very early in pregnancy or, even better, before conception. Unfortunately, many women don't enter prenatal care until after the first trimester of pregnancy, by which time nutrient inadequacy has already developed. Normal expansion of maternal blood volume has begun, which renders several maternal laboratory indices less diagnostic. The leading cause of low maternal hemoglobin (<11.0 g/dL) during the second and third trimesters of pregnancy is expansion of blood volume, particularly of the plasma component. The vital importance of an adequate expansion of maternal blood volume is emphasized by its positive correlations with low hemoglobin in the third trimester of pregnancy and with mean birth weight. When the lowest third-trimester hemoglobin levels in an iron-unsupplemented group of over 150,000 Englishwomen remained above 10.5 g/dL, there were increased risks of LBW and preterm delivery (60). Similar results have been reported for plasma ferritin, with high values in the late second trimester of pregnancy being associated with low birth weight and preterm delivery (61).

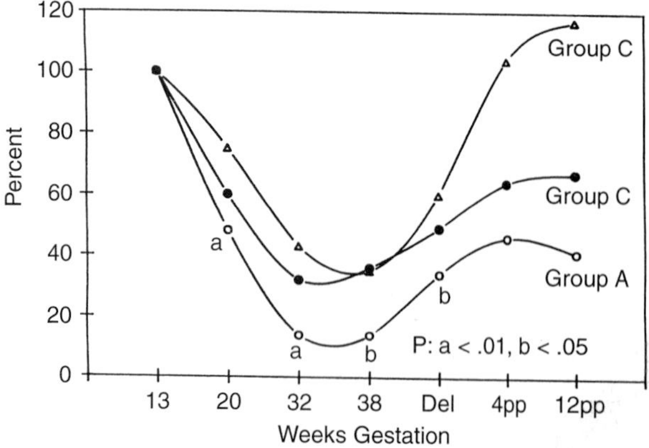

Figure 50.4. Mean relative percentage of change from prestudy baseline of serum ferritin levels (adjusted for serum volume) for groups *A*, *B*, and *C*, who were given an iron supplement of 0, 18, and 65 mg/day.

Table 50.11 also compares the adolescent pregnant groups by level of iron supplementation, initial serum ferritin level, and the number who failed to maintain their hemoglobin above 110 g/L (11 g/dL) throughout their pregnancy. Some 40% of group A, who were not receiving additional iron, dropped below the 11 g/dL lower limit; 20% of group B, receiving 18 mg of iron, were also in this category; but none of group C, receiving 65 mg/day, fell below 11 g/dL. Only 1 of 15 (7%) subjects receiving either 0 or 18 mg of iron fell below 11 g/dL when her serum ferritin level prior to 20 weeks of gestation was above 35 μg/L (ng/mL), whereas 13 of 25 (52%) of the subjects did so if their initial serum was below 35 μg/L (ng/mL).

Deficient serum ferritin levels (below 12 ng/mL) have been associated with a two- to threefold increase in the incidence of LBW and preterm deliveries. Our data (1, 63) suggest that pregnant women with serum ferritin levels below 35 ng/mL during the first trimester are also at risk unless they receive adequate iron supplementation during the last half of their pregnancy. Routine assessment of maternal serum ferritin before 20 weeks of gestation should indicate the need for an appropriate level of elemental iron supplementation throughout the remainder of the pregnancy and for 100 days postpartum.

In contrast to reports from Norway (62) and the United States (above), our counterparts in the United Kingdom do not believe that all pregnant women should routinely receive supplemental iron. A recent paper (58) concluded that a normal pregnant woman can maintain her hemoglobin level at 11.0 g/dL or above by using her natural ability to increase iron absorption as pregnancy advances and maternal and fetal demands expand. A comparison of our Galveston data of 1987 (1, 63) with their Newcastle data of 1994 (58) is summarized in Table 50.12. Our group of women who received no additional iron in their supplement is very similar to their group of women. If anything, our women's serum ferritin concentrations dropped more severely than those of the women from Newcastle. In the third trimester of pregnancy, 40% of our patients and 16% of theirs had Hb values below 11.0 g/dL. Only the Galveston group that received 65 mg/day of iron in their supplement had their mean serum ferritin values return to first-trimester levels by 12 weeks postpartum (63). We remain skeptical of iron sufficiency when published data from Newcastle reveal that their subjects' late third-trimester serum ferritin levels ranged from 5 to 6 ng/dL—almost 90% lower than their initial mean levels at

Table 50.12
Comparisons of Mean Iron Status among Pregnant Women Galveston 1987* versus Newcastle 1994†

	Mean Hb (g/dL)				Mean MCV				Mean Serum Ferritin (ng/dL)				Mean RDW (%)			
Weeks Gestation	12	24	36	PP[a]	12	24	36	PP[a]	12	24	36	PP[a]	12	24	36	PP[a]
Newcastle ($N = 12$)																
Iron content, mg 0	12.7	11.6	11.6	12.6	89.4	89.9	87.7	86.6	43.8	11.1	5.4	25.6				
Galveston ($N = 21$)																
Iron content, mg 0	12.4	11.5	11.4	12.9	87.3	86.6	85.2	84.2	44.8	6.6	6.6	16.8	13.6	13.9	14.1	15.3
18	12.5	11.9	12.0	12.9	86.4	89.6	88.6	85.2	58.3	17.9	19.9	35.7	13.3	13.1	14.0	14.4
65	12.7	12.0	12.4	13.1	87.7	87.3	90.1	86.4	48.1	20.8	17.1	53.4	13.5	13.7	14.0	14.1

Data from Dawson EB, McGanity WJ. J Reprod Med 1987;32:478–487 (Galveston) and Barrett JF, Whittaker PG, Williams JG, et al. Br Med J 1994;309:79–82 (Newcastle).
[a]PP, postparturition.

the end of the first trimester. Even at 12 weeks postpartum, the women in Newcastle had mean levels of iron stores 60% below the first trimester. What they consider as normal physiologic adaptation, we consider to be serious iron deficiency.

The Preventive Services Task Force of the U.S. Public Health Services issued, in late 1993, a policy statement on iron supplementation (64). It stated that iron supplementation can improve maternal hematologic indices; however, controlled clinical trials have not resulted in improvement in maternal or newborn outcomes. The task force acknowledged that 20 to 40% of all American pregnant women have hemoglobin levels of 10.0 g/dL or less and that many studies confirm an association between "anemia" during pregnancy and outcomes such as LBW and preterm delivery. These reports were dismissed by the task force for lack of control of other variables that might have directly affected the pregnancy. They carefully excluded from their conclusions pregnant women in developing countries. We wonder if our obstetric patients from the barrios of south Texas and the inner city of Camden, New Jersey, belong in the American or Third World groups. Somehow the fact that hemoglobin is the O_2 transport and transfer carrier to all maternal and fetal tissues seems to have been lost in the task force's statistical fury (64).

It is true that pregnant women and their infants, over the centuries and in the developing world today, have survived the consequences of even severe maternal chronic anemia (Hb < 7.0 g/dL). However, as we enter the 21st century, we contend that the standard of care should not be what a pregnant woman can tolerate, but what provides optimal nutritional health for her and her newborn offspring.

Folic Acid

Deficiency of folic acid (folate) is associated with an increased incidence of LBW babies and megaloblastic anemia in mothers (65). Because the calculated total fetal and placental folate content is about 800 μg at term, the increased demand for this vitamin is not likely to be due merely to fetal transfer, which represents a drain of less than 5 μg/day (66). In normal pregnant women, the urinary concentration of a breakdown product of folate (*p*-acetamidobenzoylglutamate) rose significantly in the second trimester and returned to baseline postpartum (67). The increased rate of folate metabolism during the second and third trimesters was estimated to produce an extra demand for dietary folate of about 200 to 300 μg/day in pregnant women.

Folate supplementation given to the same three groups of women noted in Table 50.11 increased levels of tissue storage in all three groups during gestation, measured as folate in the maternal RBC. The higher 800 μg/day folate supplement resulted in higher tissue levels throughout the pregnancy and beyond.

The role of folic acid and vitamin B_{12} in the prevention of NTDs is reviewed below.

Homeostasis of Iron Status in the Fetus and Newborn Infant

Over the last 60 years, various investigators have demonstrated the ability of the maternal hemopoietic system to protect the fetus in the face of a range of severe hematologic deficits (10–12). Hemoglobin, serum iron, and serum ferritin all can be low during pregnancy and lactation, yet the newborn infant's iron status and mother's breast-milk content remain unaffected.

As noted in Chapter 10, "Iron," Table 10.5, the total iron cost of an uncomplicated pregnancy, plus that lost in milk during lactation for 6 months, is in the broad range of 420 to 1030 mg or 1.2 to 2.5 mg/day over this 15-month period—with the major need in the third trimester, as noted above. Adequate maternal iron stores must be created before pregnancy, not by trying to do catch-up during gestation. Adequate dietary intake and/or iron supplementation should begin in the months before conception. The typical well-balanced American diet alone does not provide adequate iron to meet maternal and fetal needs during the last half of pregnancy, nor does it provide iron to replenish the 600 to 1000 mL of maternal blood lost at delivery. Even the nonlactating, postpartum woman needs iron supplementation for 100 days (12 weeks) after delivery to replenish her own body stores. And, even though the pregnant woman has an increased ability to absorb iron from her diet, a supplement of 30 mg/day is protective and preventative during the period from the 12th week of gestation through 12 weeks postdelivery and/or postweaning.

From these observations, we have concluded that for optimal maternal, fetal, and neonatal health, a woman should maintain 11.0 g/dL or more of hemoglobin throughout her reproductive years and 35 ng/dL or more of serum ferritin at the 20th week of pregnancy.

PERINATAL MORBIDITY AND MORTALITY

Over the past 100 years, the rate of infant mortality in the United States has dropped from 15% to less than 1%, as sanitation, immunizations, antibiotics, blood replacements, and the development of start-of-the-art neonatal care have become generally available.

Infant Mortality

Before the mid-1980s, the leading cause of infant mortality in the United States was associated with LBW and prematurity. Over the past 10 years, birth defects (at 25%) have replaced them. Both the infant and perinatal mortality rates in the United States and the percentage of LBW infants have decreased by over 20% since 1980 (2). This decrease has occurred to a greater extent in the white population than among African Americans. Among all developed countries, the United States ranks below 20th in overall infant and perinatal mortality.

Perinatal Mortality

Perinatal mortality (fetal deaths plus neonatal deaths), on the other hand, remains strongly associated with the fetus's birth weight and gestational age at the time of delivery. Birth defects contribute 25 to 30% of overall perinatal mortality. As noted in Chapter 51, approximately 7% of all infants born in the United States weigh less than 2500 g at birth. Newborn infants who weigh less than 700 g and have a biologic age below 24 weeks of gestation have the risk of perinatal mortality of 80% or more; whereas those weighing 2000 g and over 34 weeks gestational age have a perinatal mortality risk below 1.5%. How much of this improvement may be due to maternal nutritional status before and during pregnancy? Certainly the amount of maternal weight gain is inversely proportional to the rate of perinatal mortality. Poor maternal weight gain during pregnancy increases the risks to the fetus in utero. Increased perinatal mortality rates have also been associated with consistently low levels of serum vitamin C (68).

Pregnancy-Induced Hypertension

Pregnancy-induced hypertension (PIH) remains a significant cause of worldwide maternal and fetal morbidity and mortality. Approximately 6% of gravidas develop PIH (69). PIH is further subdivided into preeclampsia (PE), eclampsia, and late transient hypertension (70). Patients with preexisting hypertension are at increased risk for development of superimposed PE. PE is multisystem—including hypertension and concomitant proteinuria with or without edema. Patients with PE who exhibit seizure activity are classified as having eclampsia. Pregnant patients with severe PE may also exhibit hepatic failure, thrombocytopenia, coagulation disorder, renal failure, and pulmonary edema. The multisystem nature of PE suggests a complex etiology. It also suggests that hypertension is a symptom and manifestation rather than a causative factor in the underlying disease process (70, 71).

The precise etiology of PIH/PE remains unknown, but most data suggest that poor tissue perfusion is essential in development of PIH/PE. Placental "hypoplasia" in patients with PE implies at least a relationship between PE and placental homeostasis (72, 73). Hemodynamically, patients destined to develop PE display altered vascular responsiveness to angiotensin and catecholamines long before clinical development of PE (74). Theories abound concerning the pathogenesis of PE/PIH, but most involve alterations in placental or vascular vasoactive mediators producing endothelial tissue injury. Given the placenta's large arachadonic acid content, prostaglandins (see Chapter 4) have been at least partially implicated in the pathogenesis of PIH. Alterations in thromboxane and/or prostacyclin are also involved in the pathogenesis of the disease. Endothelium-derived relaxation factor has been more recently implicated in PIH/PE. Quite possibly, a complex set of mediator-driven events is central to development of PIH/PE (75, 76).

Over the past century, the influence of nutrition on PIH/PE has been investigated from several perspectives. Maternal weight and body mass are related to development of PIH/PE. After controlling for several confounding factors, excessive maternal weight appears to cause a graded, up to 12-fold risk on development of PIH/PE (74, 76) and to cause a 9-fold increase in the likelihood of becoming hypertensive (39).

Nutritional intake has been evaluated in patients at risk for development of PIH/PE. Patients with PIH/PE often have diminished protein stores, and while this was generally attributed to renal losses (proteinuria), Brewer (77, 78) postulated that consumption of adequate protein would prevent PIH/PE. Other investigators do not support this view (79, 80). A very compelling, but unproven, effect of renal hyperperfusion (as caused by excessive protein intake) also deserves investigation. Lipid supplementation has a theoretical influence on hypertension. Magness et al. (81) reported that daily supplementation with the n-6 polyunsaturated fatty acid linoleic acid reduced blood pressure and prolonged pregnancy in patients with PE. The lack of PIH/PE in pregnant patients receiving n-6 and/or n-3 polyunsaturated fatty acids through parenteral hyperalimentation has also been observed (81–83). Their effect on thromboxane or prostacyclin production has been postulated (75, 81–83). Further work in this area is necessary to elucidate a possible relationship between lipid supplementation and PIH/PE.

Because pregnancy is normally associated with an increased renin-angiotensin-aldosterone axis and since resistance to the pressor effects of angiotensin II is lost in pregnant patients destined to develop PIH/PE, salt restriction at one time was thought to play a role in prevention of the disease (84). Since most pregnant patients with PIH/PE are volume contracted, excessive salt restriction to less than 2 to 4 g/day is not recommended (75, 76, 85).

More compelling is the possible relationship between calcium and hypertension. Villar et al. (86) showed a hypotensive effect in a pregnant population supplemented with calcium. Other studies have reported this effect as well (87–89). Populations low in calcium intake have a higher incidence of PIH/PE than do those with calcium supplementation (90, 91). In contrast, based on a metaanalysis of 33 trials involving over 2400 nonpregnant subjects, a group from McMaster University found that calcium supplementation only modestly reduced systolic blood pressure and had an insignificant effect on the diastolic component (92). Based on a metaanalysis of 14 randomized trials involving almost 2500 pregnant women who received calcium supplementation of 1500 to 2000 mg/day, the same group from McMaster found significant reductions of 5.4 and 3.4 mm Hg in systolic and diastolic blood pressure, respectively. Of the various maternal and fetal outcomes of pregnancy, only mild PE was significantly reduced (93). A more recent randomized double-blind study in the United States of 4589 healthy women, 13 to 21 weeks pregnant, given either 2 g of elemental calcium or a placebo found that the calcium supplement did not prevent preeclampsia, pregnancy-associated hypertension, or adverse perinatal outcomes (93a).

Magnesium may also play a role in PIH/PE, although the interaction between magnesium and calcium may be the actual mechanism (75). For years, magnesium sulfate has been used in the United States as the first-line medication for the nutritionally unrelated pharmacologic indication of seizure prophylaxis in patients with PIH/PE (69) (see also Chapter 9).

Plasma zinc concentrations are reportedly lower in pregnant patients with PIH/PE (94, 95). The implications of this finding are presently uncertain. Furthermore, since plasma zinc competes with cadmium at biochemical binding sites, and cadmium toxicity is clinically very similar to the maternal manifestations of severe PIH/PE, an interaction between cadmium and plasma zinc has been postulated to play a role in PIH/PE pathogenesis (96). Whole blood lead levels may correlate with hypertension during pregnancy (97). We speculate a relationship between intracellular blood lead and PIH, albeit the precise mechanism of action between blood lead and PIH is not known. Finally, maternal multivitamin supplementation was shown to be associated with a lower incidence of PE, although the study design of the investigation limits any firm conclusions (76, 98).

In sum, pregnancy-induced hypertension/preeclampsia currently remains a mysterious disease with an uncertain etiology. The precise interaction between nutritional factors and PIH/PE is not well delineated. Poor maternal nutritional status appears to have at least some influence on the natural development of PIH/PE. Much more investigation into the interaction of nutritional factors on PIH/PE is certainly in order.

Congenital Malformations

Since 1986, almost one-fourth of all infant mortality in the United States has been associated with birth defects (99). As a percentage of infant deaths, congenital malformations have increased from 8 to 24% between 1916 and the early 1990s (95). In 1993, 1% of all live births and 11% of all fetal deaths in the state of Texas were reported to have a significant congenital malformation. Neural tube, cardiovascular, and pulmonary abnormalities, and chromosomal defects have proved the most lethal during the first year after birth (100).

We have known since the late 1940s that single maternal nutrient deficits or excesses in the experimental laboratory animal can result in an increased frequency of congenital malformations in their offspring. To date, deficiencies of seven essential minerals, five of eight water-soluble vitamins, and three of four fat-soluble vitamins are reported to cause neural, cardiac, or renal birth defects (101). In the human, it has taken over 40 years to confirm the role of a nutrient, folic acid, in the primary and secondary prevention of NTDs.

Congenital malformations have their origin, about 20% of the time, in mendelian errors; 10% are chromosomal problems, and 5% are due to environmental factors. The remaining 65% of malformations have multifactorial or "unknown" contributing factors. In normal intrauterine growth and development of the embryo from the time of conception through implantation and early fetal development, almost all the cell cleavages and fusions necessary in formation of the normal fetal architecture and their basic functions are established by the 10th week of gestation. In fact, the most critical period for neural tube closure occurs within the first 28 days of the fetus's gestational life. During this period, the pregnant woman is usually not being followed medically because entry into prenatal care usually occurs about the time of her second missed menstrual period, 45 to 60 days after conception. If we are to do anything about the prevention of congenital malformation, we must actively intervene in the 8 to 10 weeks before conception. In early pregnancy, certain vitamins (e.g., folic acid) (see also Chapters 26, 34, and 95) can prevent some birth defects, and others (e.g., vitamin A) can cause birth defects. Physicians and patients of reproductive age need to make sure that on the one hand, there is an adequate intake of folic acid (400 μg/day) in the preconceptional period, and on the other hand, the total daily intake of vitamin A from all sources (food and supplements) is less than 10,000 IU/day (see Chapter 17).

The following five examples further illustrate areas in

which nutrition intervention before conception can play a major role in preventing life-threatening birth defects.

Diabetes Mellitus

The level of glycosylated hemoglobin (A_1C) in the diabetic patient needs to be maintained within acceptable values by tight dietary control and insulin regulation as needed. Proper management can significantly improve overall reproductive well-being, decrease the rate of spontaneous abortions, and reduce by 50% the otherwise three-to-four times greater frequency of congenital malformations in the offspring of diabetic mothers. Tight control of maternal carbohydrate metabolism throughout pregnancy has reduced perinatal mortality from 16% to less than 4% over the last 20 years.

Phenylketonuria

Over 3000 American women now of reproductive age have a significant abnormality in phenylalanine metabolism. Three hundred affected newborns are delivered annually in the United States. Since about 70% of these mothers have classic PKU, this adds each year about 105 new female offspring to our pool of future PKU mothers.

Serum phenylalanine levels are normally 1.5 to 2.0 times higher on the fetal side of the placenta. With aggressive dietary management as developed by the National Maternal PKU Collaborative Project, elevated serum phenylalanine in the mother can be lowered from more than 20 to less than 2 ng/dL within 5 to 7 days.

If such a patient is returned to the required strict dietary control before she conceives a child, and if her serum phenylalanine level is kept below 605 nmol/L (10 ng/dL) during pregnancy, the risk of congenital and developmental abnormalities in her newborn offspring can be essentially eliminated (102). In contrast, the expectant mother with uncontrolled PKU faces an 80 to 90% chance that her baby will have some type of congenital defect or cranial maldevelopment.

Spina Bifida and Other Neural Tube Defects

Each year in the United States about 3000 infants are born with the NTDs hydrocephalus, spina bifida, and anencephaly. In addition, an estimated 800 to 900 fetuses affected by these birth defects are aborted or result in early fetal deaths. All infants born with anencephaly die shortly after birth, whereas most babies born with hydrocephaly and spina bifida grow into adulthood with, in severe cases, paralysis and varying degrees of neurologic damage including bowel and bladder incontinence.

Evidence has been accumulating for several years that supplementation of folic acid and vitamin B_{12} before conception can reduce the number of NTDs by 50 to 70%. Supplementation with 400 μg/day of folic acid alone reduced the recurrence rate by over 70%. Primary NTDs were reduced by 50% (103, 104). In combination with vitamin B_{12} in a multivitamin/mineral supplement, folate reduced the incidence of NTDs over 90% (105). Both of these vitamins are required by the enzyme methionine synthase, which methylates homocysteine to form methionine. Subsequent biochemical studies have confirmed that depressed methionine synthase activity is associated with NTDs (106–110). Whitehead et al. (111), investigating the gene that regulates one of the enzymes that regulate homocysteine concentrations, found that people with NTDs were three times as likely to be homozygous for this abnormal gene as control subjects without NTDs. The parents of children with NTDs also had an excess of this abnormal gene.

In the randomized controlled trials sponsored by the British Medical Research Council, relatively high-dose folic acid supplements (4.0 mg/day) were taken by women who had a prior pregnancy affected by an NTD. This vitamin supplement reduced the risk of a subsequent pregnancy being affected by NTD by 70% (103). The risk of NTD was also reduced for women without a prior pregnancy affected by NTD who consumed multivitamin/mineral supplements that included 400 to 800 μg of folic acid during pregnancy (112). The U.S. Centers for Disease Control have reviewed this literature (113). On the basis of such evidence, the U.S. Public Health Service recommended in 1992 that all women in the United States who are capable of becoming pregnant should consume 400 μg/day of folic acid to reduce their risk of having a pregnancy affected with spina bifida or another NTD. Because the effects of high folate intakes are not well known but include complicating the diagnosis of vitamin B_{12} deficiency, care should be taken to keep total folate consumption below 1 mg/day, except under the supervision of a physician.

Because women who have had a prior NTD-affected pregnancy are at high risk of having a subsequent affected pregnancy, when these women are planning to become pregnant they should consult their physicians for advice (114). Women who have had a pregnancy affected by an NTD are advised to consume 400 μg/day of folic acid unless they are planning a pregnancy; in that instance, they are advised to consult their physicians about the desirability of taking up to 4.0 mg/day of folic acid (114). After careful review, the U.S. Food and Drug Administration followed the United Kingdom's lead and announced, in early 1996, that it would require enrichment of all cereal grain products in an amount to provide 10% of the RDA per serving, with a maximum of 1 mg/day intake of folic acid (115).

The form in which folate should be consumed by reproductive-aged women was evaluated in a 3-month, four-pronged trial by Cuskelly et al. (116) from the University of Ulster. All groups were targeted to increase their daily folate intake by 400 μg. Only the two groups that either received folic acid in the form of a pill supplement or consumed folate-fortified foods had a significant increase in their RBC folate concentration. Women ingesting natural folate-rich foods or receiving dietary advice showed no such change. Another Irish research team concluded that an effective national fortification program that provides an additional 400 μg of folic acid could be expected to reduce the overall NTD rate by 48%—a figure very similar to that reported by the multicenter and Hungarian studies (104–106) that used a pill to provide the folate supplement (117).

Endemic Cretinism

A deficit in iodine intake by the mother will cause fetal iodine deficiency. When this occurs, one finds excess abortions, fetal deaths, and congenital malformations (55). Endemic cretinism results when maternal iodine intake falls below 25 μg/day (one-third to one-sixth the recommended intake). In the United States, prevention of iodine deficiency through iodination of salt in the Great Lakes region was begun in 1922. Iodination has essentially eliminated the development of goiters and birth of cretins among the U.S. population. Even today, however, 10% of the population in less developed mountainous regions of Africa, Asia, the western Pacific, and South America are severely iodine deficient. Development of enlarged thyroid glands (goiter; see Chapter 13) among females is higher than among males, with bursts of increased size occurring in the female with the onset of menses and during pregnancy.

Maternal Obesity

Beginning in the mid-1960s, Welsh case-control studies (118) were published that linked maternal obesity with a higher incidence of anencephalic infants. Since then, four additional American reports (119–122) have confirmed a twofold increased risk of NTDs in fetuses/infants of mothers who began their pregnancies with a BMI of 28 or above (PSW ≥ 135%). This is independent of the folate status and supplement intake. Trends over the past 25 years reveal an ever-increasing incidence of obesity among postmenarchal young women. This trend must be stopped. We need an all-out crusade to decrease caloric intake and increase physical activity among 12- to 35-year-old American women.

LOW-BIRTH-WEIGHT PREGNANCIES: PREVENTIVE ASPECTS

Low birth weight (less than 2500 g) in the newborn infant is a problem that has resisted solution. The percentage of LBW infants delivered in the United States between 1980 and 1994 has not changed, remaining around 7% of total live births. Twice as many such infants are born to African American mothers as to white or Hispanic mothers.

The rate of intrauterine fetal weight gain follows a straight-line progression between weeks 22 and 38 of pregnancy, with the infant gaining a daily average of about 30 g, or 0.21 kg (almost half a pound) per week (123). In the obstetric management of a patient in the third trimester with premature labor and intact membranes, every effort is made to quiet the contractions, to stabilize the uterus, and to allow the intrauterine fetal growth to continue as long as the placental transfer system is functioning well. The 30 g/day of fetal weight gain inside the uterus is 50% more than the best that can be accomplished after delivery, even with the newborn infant in an intensive neonatal care nursery. Perinatal survival improves to 50% between weeks 24 and 27 of gestation (700–1000 g in birth weight). By 34 weeks (2000 g), the perinatal survival rate is over 98%. It is critical that we use the best incubator and nutrient delivery system yet designed—called "the uterus and placenta"—until adequate fetal maturation has been achieved for normal extrauterine survival.

As obstetricians and nutritionists, can we intervene and prevent the occurrence of prematurity and LBW infants? We must remember that the target is the delivery of an undamaged infant who weighs more than 2500 g, whose biologic age is more than 37 weeks of gestation, and who will be able to survive in its external environment once the umbilical cord has been severed. Weiss and Jackson (44) identified over 30 obstetric-related factors that influenced the birth weight of both black and white infants. As further described below, the most important of these factors were *(a)* maternal age, *(b)* how much weight the mother gained during her pregnancy and her height/weight status (PSW or BMI) at the time she became pregnant, *(c)* whether she had ever given birth to an LBW infant before, *(d)* whether or not she smoked a package or more of cigarettes a day, *(e)* whether she had entered early into prenatal care and had frequent prenatal visits (up to 10–14 per pregnancy), and *(f)* avoidance of weight reduction during pregnancy. Independent of the mother's age, marital status or ethnic background, appropriate weight gain, 90 to 110% of PSW at conception, no previous LBW delivery, nonsmoking status, and early prenatal care and follow-up were all associated with improved mean infant birth weight and a reduced number of neonates weighing less than 2500 g at delivery.

Age and Maternal Weight

The highest incidence of LBW infants occurs in the youngest and oldest mothers—younger than 16 or 18 years of age or over 35 years of age—as a consequence of their biologic immaturity or advanced reproductive years, inadequate nutrient stores and/or dietary intake, and late entry into prenatal care.

Edwards et al. (124) found that when the mother was underweight at conception (less than 90% of standard weight or 20 BMI), the birth weight of the offspring was almost 230 g lower than that of matched controls. Women who were underweight (<90% PSW) at conception had an overall LBW rate twice as high as that of pair-matched controls, and the rate of gestational prematurity was nearly so.

A review of several studies indicates that the intake of energy, rather than protein, is probably the limiting prenatal factor in the reduced birth weight of LBW newborns. Apparently, the placenta can maintain an adequate concentration of the necessary amino acids in the fetal blood, even with low levels of amino acids in the maternal blood. In contrast, the concentration of glucose is always lower in fetal than in maternal blood. This implies that the fetoplacental unit is better able to compensate for a deficiency in maternal protein intake than a deficiency in energy intake. The lower limit of the protein:calorie ratio considered adequate to prevent LBW pregnancies is 11%, based on a requirement for 2200 kcal/day (125). Several longitudinal studies of maternal supplementation with 300 kcal/day during the third trimester found a relatively insignificant gain in fetal birth weight. However, when caloric supplementation was increased to 500 kcal/day, birth weight increased significantly. The total added energy cost of the pregnancy is approximately 55,000 kcal, based on 2115, 2275, and 2356 kcal/day for the three successive trimesters of pregnancy (126); this is only 70% of Hytten's old formula.

Smoking

One-third of single pregnant women and one-fifth of married pregnant women smoke at least a pack of cigarettes a day during pregnancy. Most of them are white, and they are spread evenly throughout the maternal age range. Stopping smoking completely is no easier for a pregnant woman than for one who is not. If usage can be reduced to fewer than five cigarettes per day, the nutritional and fetal consequences are likely to disappear, at least from a statistical point of view. Unpublished, fragmentary reports suggest that use of nicotine patches by the mother does not lead to adverse maternal or fetal outcomes.

Effect on Infant Birth Weight

Smoking one or more packs of cigarettes per day costs the infant's potential weight about 220 to 250 g (127). In addition, the number of abortions and preterm deliveries and the perinatal mortality rate all increase. This impact of cigarette smoking is dose related. How does cigarette smoking reduce an infant's birth weight at delivery? Smokers have up to a 10% reduction in their oxygen-carrying capacity because of the carboxyhemoglobin formed as a byproduct of smoking. Smoking causes vascular constriction, which decreases blood flow to the placenta and may well interfere with the fetal nutrient delivery system. Smokers require an intake of almost three times as much folate as nonsmokers to maintain the same serum folate concentration (128) and twice as much vitamin C per day to maintain the same serum ascorbate concentration (see Chapter 29 on vitamin C). Passive smokers have plasma ascorbic acid levels in between those of active smokers and uncontaminated individuals. When low vitamin C intake is combined with either active or passive smoking, one should expect reduced body pools of ascorbic acid. Scottish and Danish groups found that plasma vitamin C levels increased significantly after 4 weeks in subjects who successfully quit smoking. The vitamin C change was evident within days of discontinuing cigarettes and persisted for at least 26 weeks (129). Serum levels of carotene, vitamin B_{12}, and zinc also tend to be lower in smokers (130). Consistently low vitamin C intakes and serum levels throughout pregnancy have been associated with a higher frequency of LBW (69). A low dietary intake or low serum folate level during the second and third trimesters of pregnancy was found to be associated with LBW and preterm delivery (112). We should not forget that folate deficiency is the cause of the macrocytic anemia of late pregnancy that occurs throughout the world.

Association with Vitamin C

Recent studies have confirmed an association between low vitamin C and premature rupture of the membrane (PROM), causing premature delivery. Vitamin C is specifically required for synthesis and maintenance of collagen, a major component of the chorioamnionic membrane. Subjects with PROM were found to have weakened amniotic membranes associated with low levels of collagen (hydroxyproline), low amniotic fluid vitamin C levels (128, 129), and low maternal plasma vitamin C levels in the third trimester (131). In addition, a relationship was reported between maternal prenatal vitamin C status and PROM (68, 132), both inversely correlated with maternal smoking (133–136).

In a depletion-repletion study of seven male nonsmoking volunteers aged 20 to 26 years, researchers from the National Institutes of Health developed support for an RDA for vitamin C of 200 mg/day based on the result of kinetics, bioavailability, and plasma saturation data (137). This recommendation is three times higher than the 1989 RDA, but the findings require confirmation. How these results are related to the vitamin C requirements during pregnancy and lactation remains to be seen. Forty years ago, the Vanderbilt Maternal Nutrition Study showed that only when the vitamin C intake consistently exceeded 80 mg/day did the plasma level of vitamin C remain at or above 0.8 mg/dL, rather than declining as the mother's plasma volume expanded with advancing gestation (68). Additionally, women who nursed their infants during the first 10 weeks postpartum had lower plasma vitamin C levels, regardless of their vitamin C dietary intake.

Avoidance of Weight Reduction during Pregnancy

A weight-reduction regimen should not be instituted at any time during pregnancy or lactation. A dramatic demonstration of this severe risk to pregnant women and their offspring occurred with the semistarvation imposed by the siege of Rotterdam in 1944 and 1945. A reduction of almost 50% in the intake of calories and protein, especially during the second and third trimesters, interfered with normal intrauterine growth and development of the fetus (138). The result was a 10% (330 g) reduction in the mean birth weights of the newborns (Table 50.13). When the city was freed and maternal refeeding resumed, during the second and/or third trimester, partial fetal weight catch-up was attained.

The 1990s American equivalent of wartime intrauterine starvation is chronic cocaine abuse. Its impact is most severe on an infant's birth weight—causing as much as a 500-g deficit. In addition, the newborns of cocaine addicts have severely immature mental development. Whether these effects result from drug use alone or whether they are a byproduct of inadequate nutrient intake has not been fully determined.

As shown in Table 50.14, we have developed estimates of the cost to the potential birth weight of the fetus for each of seven nutrition-related maternal insults. Combinations of two or more have an additive (not concurrent) effect, which in total could reduce the potential weight of the developing infant as much as 2 lb. If identified in the months before conception, each of these maternal insults is correctable and the consequences to the fetus preventable.

OTHER NUTRITIONAL AND ENVIRONMENTAL FACTORS

Use of Mineral and Vitamin Supplements

Both calcium and zinc supplements have been reported to improve maternal reproductive outcome. An additional calcium intake of 2000 mg/day decreased systolic and diastolic blood pressure and development of mild pregnancy-induced PE (139). Supplemental zinc, 22 mg/day, has been associated with less abruptio placentae, fewer preterm deliveries, and a lower rate of perinatal mortality (140). Although clinicians and scientists in the United States and United Kingdom may argue about whether it is good public health policy to provide supplemental iron during the course of pregnancy, the need for increased iron intake among women and children in most developing countries cannot be challenged (141). The problem has been how to enrich local foods to benefit all of the population. In Guatemala (142) and Venezuela (143), sugar and cereal fortification programs are showing encouraging results. Under clinical study conditions, medicinal iron supplementation for pregnant women has also succeeded in improving maternal iron status and fetal outcome. However, under routine public health clinic application there has been very limited benefit. Problems are encountered in maintaining a continuous supply of pills at each clinic site, in providing adequate patient counseling, and in patient compliance. These problems are no different from those encountered in North American clinics. Daily ingestion of an iron pill(s) alone or as a prenatal mineral/vitamin tablet remains a problem. Gastrointestinal side effects are reduced with a lower dosage of iron. A recent clinical study from Indonesia demonstrated that among pregnant women—three-quarters of whom had a hemoglobin level below 11.0 g/dL at entry into prenatal care—therapeutic effectiveness of a 60-mg iron supplement daily or a 120-mg supplement once a week for 12 weeks did not differ, although patient compliance improved from 54 to 62% with the lower dose (144).

Table 50.13
Changes in Mean Birth Weight in Dutch Women before and after Famine Conditions

	Postpartum Maternal Weight (kg)	Birth Weight (g)
Before famine	59.0	3.338
Famine during third trimester	57.6	3.220
Famine during second and third trimester	56.5	3.011
Famine during first and third trimester	61.0	3.370
Famine during first trimester	61.6	3.312
After famine	62.0	3.308

Adapted from Stein Z, Suzzer M. Pediatr Res 1975;9:70–83.

Table 50.14
Estimated Impact of Maternal Risks on Birth Weight of Fetus

Maternal Factor	Fetal Effect
<5 years postmenarchal	↓ 100–130 g
<90% standard weight	↓ 230 g
Excessive work and/or exercise	↓ 200 g
50% ↓ in kcal in 2nd and 3rd trimesters	↓ 330 g
50% ↓ in kcal in 3rd trimester	↓ 120 g
>20 cigarettes per day	↓ 250 g
Chronic cocaine addiction	↓ 500 g

No evidence exists that daily ingestion of a prenatal mineral/vitamin supplement containing less than twice the RDA is hazardous to either the mother or her fetus/infant during pregnancy and/or lactation in at-risk groups of mothers. There is added nutritional protection with the ingestion of a daily prenatal mineral/vitamin supplement that contains no more than the RDA for only the essential minerals and vitamins. Such formulas are available "over the counter" at less than 3 cents/day. They are well tolerated, with a very high rate of patient compliance.

Antioxidants

The need for antioxidant vitamins during pregnancy changes with *(a)* changes in basal metabolic rate during pregnancy, being lower in the first trimester and gradually increasing toward labor and delivery; *(b)* the level of daily physical activity, which decreases in the last weeks of pregnancy; and *(c)* the type and degree of exposure of the mother and her intrauterine fetus to toxic substances in the environment, including carbon monoxide, formaldehyde, tobacco smoke, pesticides, polycyclic aromatic hydrocarbons, volatile organic compounds, nitrogen dioxide, phenylcyclohexane, radon, and asbestos (145). Normal metabolism and exposure to environmental pollution result in formation of molecular free radicals (discussed in Chapters 19 and 29) whose excess electrons react with and destroy essential cellular components. Vitamins A, E, and C are often classified as antioxidant nutrients that protect biologic lipid phases, such as cell membranes, or as low-density lipoproteins—β-carotene and vitamin E—and the aqueous compartments of the cytosol, plasma, and other body fluids by vitamin C (146).

Caffeine

Most pregnant women (approximately 74%) consume caffeine daily from multiple sources—coffee, tea, soft drinks, and chocolate. Average total daily intake ranges from 100 to 150 mg/day of caffeine. Caffeine, which acts as a central nervous system stimulant (see Chapter 99), has a greatly lengthened half-life during pregnancy and in oral contraceptive users; however, caffeine ingestion does not appear to affect a woman's fertility or her ability to conceive. Caffeine intake is not metabolized by the fetus or, if consumed during lactation, by the infant. Earlier reports raised concerns about its safe use, citing increased risk of birth defects and intrauterine growth retardation. More-recent studies, however, found that moderate caffeine intake (less than 300 mg/day) does not increase the risks of spontaneous abortion, fetal growth retardation, or birth defects (147). The amounts of caffeine in 12 ounces of a carbonated drink, 6 ounces of tea, and 6 ounces of nondecaffeinated brewed coffee are 37, 36, and 103 mg, respectively (148).

Alcohol

Half of all women have an occasional alcoholic drink during their pregnancy, and even more consume alcohol during lactation. Less than 5% of pregnant women have a drink every day, and another 3% have a drink three times a week. It is estimated that 2 to 3% of all pregnant women are chronic, heavy drinkers. Alcoholism is more prevalent in white women than in either Hispanic or black women, and the incidence is higher among older and more educated women. (The caloric content of various alcoholic beverages is given in Appendix Table IV-A-19).

Fetal alcohol syndrome is the end result of chronic alcohol abuse during pregnancy, but not all fetal outcomes are this severe. The consequences to the fetus range across a spectrum from no apparent sequelae, to intrauterine fetal growth retardation, to severely damaged infants. Acute maternal ethanol intoxication in late pregnancy results in suppressed fetal respiration and abnormal electrocorticographic and electrooculographic activity (149). Permanent residual effects of fetus alcohol exposure include *(a)* mental retardation, *(b)* a damaged immune system, and *(c)* abnormalities of the craniofacial and limb bones (150–152) (see also Chapter 60).

Alcoholic beverages provide calories that are more difficult for the expectant mother and her fetus to metabolize; moreover, they are devoid of protein, minerals, and vitamins. The pregnant woman who has ingested up to 1500 kcal/day as ethanol from a liter of whiskey or its alcohol equivalent as beer and/or wine cannot meet her other essential nutrient requirements from the remaining third of her calories. As a result, absorption, metabolism, and use of nutrients are impaired, maternal protein synthesis is decreased, placental transfer of amino acids is restricted, and the availability of zinc, vitamin A, folic acid, and thiamin is reduced. Although an occasional glass of wine with food has not been demonstrated to have maternal and/or fetal consequences, clinicians and nutritionists should be on the lookout for, and actively seek out, the chronic alcohol abuser and weekend binge drinker, for whom fetal consequences are most likely.

Drugs

Drug-nutrient interactions are discussed in detail in Chapter 99. Whether drugs enter the body by mouth or by injection, they reach equilibrium between mother, fetus, and infant within about 30 minutes of entry. Most are readily transferred across the placenta and carried in breast milk to the nursing infant. Pregnant women often have four or more prescription medications, several of which have drug-nutrient interactions that reduce the effectiveness of the drug and/or interfere with the availability of the nutrient(s).

Between 10 and 27% of pregnant women acknowledge using marijuana during pregnancy (153). The metabolites of marijuana cross the placenta, and because they are fat soluble, they are excreted extremely slowly. Like tobacco, marijuana tends to reduce the oxygen-carrying capacity of RBC hemoglobin. Marijuana also increases heart rate and blood pressure, resulting in decreased uterine blood flow and placental perfusion. Infant birth weights are lower, and preterm deliveries are increased. Direct drug-nutrient interference has not been confirmed.

No street drug has had as severe an impact on the maternal and fetal outcome of pregnancy as cocaine and crack cocaine. Various reports indicate that about 10% (3–17%) of all pregnant women have used these drugs during pregnancy (154). Use of these drugs is higher among Hispanic and black pregnant women, and in those who live in inner cities. Cocaine readily crosses the placenta, and once on the fetal side, it may be detected in the meconium for up to 8 weeks. Chronic cocaine users have decreased appetite, food intake, and uptake of tryptophan. The fetus and newborn of the cocaine abuser is likely to be growth retarded, and the mother is more susceptible to abruptio placentae and premature labor. These street drugs are not used in isolation, but their use is complicated further by other abuses and high-risk behaviors, of which practices associated with human immunodeficiency virus (HIV) infection are currently the most serious (see Chapters 60 and 97).

Exercise

The maternal and fetal effects of exercise during pregnancy have been comprehensively reviewed (155). Walking, cycling, climbing stairs, and swimming are excellent types of activity for the normal, healthy pregnant woman when done in moderation by time and cardiovascular response. If you cannot carry on a conversation while doing it, the level of exercise is too much! Severe exercise elicits a temperature response and circulatory redistribution that takes away from the uterus and placenta and directs blood to the lower extremities. The pregnant woman needs to build up her conditioning program gradually and specifically to avoid trauma-prone exercises, high altitudes, dehydration, and serious competition. For women with complicated pregnancies, rest, not exercise, may be the prescription of choice.

Postdelivery or postweaning exercise is essential along with caloric restriction in the woman regaining her prepregnant weight status (155).

YEAR 2000 GOALS FOR MATERNAL AND CHILD HEALTH

Ten years ago, the United States set goals to significantly improve maternal, infant, and children's health by the year 2000. Six of the goals have direct or indirect nutritional implications:

1. Reduce the rate of LBW births
2. Reduce fetal alcohol syndrome
3. Increase adequate maternal weight gain during pregnancy
4. Increase the number of mothers nursing their infants to 6 months of age
5. Decrease maternal use of tobacco, alcohol, and drugs
6. Increase early entry into prenatal care

For the late 1990s and the 2000s, we believe that the following additional goals, each having nutritional implications, should be added:

7. Prevent and reduce birth defects
8. Prevent and reduce maternal obesity prior to and following pregnancy and lactation

SUMMARY

Based on the previous discussion, our prescription for optimal maternal and fetal reproductive performance as we enter the 21st century includes

- A woman who is 5 years or more postmenarchal and under 35 years of age
- Entry into prenatal care 60 to 90 days prior to conception
- Adequate expansion of maternal blood volume
- Maintenance of hemoglobin concentration at or above 11.0 g/dL throughout gestation
- Ingestion of a safe, adequate diet that provides the necessary energy and nutrients to meet all requirements of the mother, fetus, and infant during pregnancy/gestation and lactation/nursing
- Maternal weight gain between 7.5 and 18 kg, depending on maternal age, BMI, and the number of fetuses
- Use of prenatal mineral-vitamin supplements that contain no more than the RDA for pregnant women for essential ingredients, with particular attention to the contents of iron, folate, calcium, zinc, and vitamin A
- Prevention of all nutrient-dependent causes of congenital malformations, which requires prevention of excessive weight gain; maintenance of immunizations; entry into pregnancy with diabetes and phenylketonuria in tight control; and an adequate intake of iodine, folate, and vitamin B_{12} throughout pregnancy
- Reduction, or even better elimination, of the nonnutritional hazards of excess—smoking, alcohol, and drugs

ACKNOWLEDGMENTS

For editorial and graphic assistance, we thank Mac McConnell and his Ob/Gyn Publications staff, Kristi Barrett, John Helms, and Steve Schuenke. The authors wish to gratefully acknowledge the technical assistance of Moni DeVora.

REFERENCES

1. McGanity WJ, Dawson EB, Fogelman, A. Nutrition in pregnancy and lactation. In: Shils ME, Olson JA, Shike M, eds. Modern nutrition in health and disease. 8th ed. Philadelphia: Lea & Febiger, 1994;705–27.
2. US Department of Health and Human Services. Child health USA 1991, publ. no. HRS-M-CH91-1. Washington, DC: US Department of Health and Human Services, 1991.
3. Institute of Medicine. Nutrition during pregnancy. Washington, DC: National Academy Press, 1990.
4. Worthington-Roberts B, Williams SR. Nutrition in pregnancy and lactation. 4th ed. St. Louis: Times Mirror/Mosby College, 1989.
5. Pitkin RM. Clin Obstet Gynecol 1994;37(3):449–500.
6. Prentice A, Goldberg G. Nutr Rev 1996;54(5):146–52.
7. Harris ED. Nutr Rev 1992;50:329–31.
8. Barclay BA. Nutr Clin Pract 1990;5:153–5.
9. Wolk RA, Rayburn WF. Nutr Clin Pract 1990;5:139–52.
10. Strauss MB. J Clin Invest 1933;12:345–53.
11. Woodruff CW, Bridgeforth EB. Pediatrics 1953;12:681–5.
12. Murray MJ, Murray AB, Murray NJ, et al. Br J Nutr 1978;39:627–30.
13. US Department of Agriculture, Human Nutrition Information Service. The food guide pyramid. Home and garden bulletin no. 252. Hyattsville, Md: US Department of Agriculture, 1992.
14. US Department of Agriculture. Nationwide food consumption survey, report no. 85-1. Hyattsville, Md: Nutrition Monitoring Division, Human Nutrition Information Service, US Department of Agriculture, 1985.
15. Whittaker PG, McPhails, Lind T. Obstet Gynecol 1996;88:33–9.
16. Dawson EB, Clark RR, McGanity WJ. Am J Obstet Gynecol 1969;104:953–8.
17. King JC. Nutrition in pregnancy. London: Royal College of Obstetricians and Gynaecologists, 1982.
18. Dawson EB, Croft HA, Clark RR, et al. Am J Obstet Gynecol 1968;120(3):354–61.

19. Dawson EB, Croft HA, Clark RR, et al. Am J Obstet Gynecol 1969;103(8):1144–7.
20. Mitchell HS, Reed RB, Valeadian I, et al. Proceedings of the 7th International Congress of Nutrition, vol 4. Oxford: Pergamon Press, 1966;132–9.
21. Frisch RE. Biol Rev Camb Philos Soc 1984;59:161–88.
22. Meredith CN, Dwyer JT. Annu Rev Public Health 1991; 12:309–33.
23. Story M, Alton I. Top Clin Nutr 1991;6:51–8.
23a. Jacobson MS, Rees JM, Golden NH, et al., eds. Adolescent nutritional disorders. Ann NY Acad Sci 1997;817:1–402.
24. Atkinson RL. Nutr Rev 1992;50:338–9.
25. Fisher MC, Lachance PA. J Am Diet Assoc 1985;85:450–4.
26. National Health and Nutrition Examination Survey II. Unpublished data. Hyattsville, Md: National Center for Health Statistics, Public Health Service, US Department of Health, Education and Welfare, 1976–1980.
27. National Research Council. Recommended dietary allowances. 10th ed. Washington, DC: National Academy Press, 1989.
27a. Institute of Medicine. Nutrition during lactation—milk composition. Washington, DC: National Academy Press, 1991:116.
27b. Barbosa L, Butle NF, Vallapando S, et al. Am J Clin Nutr 1997;66:575–83.
27c. Dusdieker LB, Hemingway DL, Steinbo PJ. Am J Clin Nutr 1994;59:833–40.
27d. Sowers M, Corton G, Shapiro B, et al. JAMA 1993;269: 3130–5.
28. Whitehead RG. Pregnancy and lactation. In: Shils ME, Young VR, eds. Modern nutrition in health and disease. 7th ed. Philadelphia: Lea & Febiger, 1988;931–43.
29. Poppitt SD, Prentice AM, Jequier E, et al. Am J Clin Nutr 1993;57:353–64.
30. Sims LS. J Am Diet Assoc 1978;73:139–46.
31. Hytten FE, Leitch I. The physiology of human pregnancy. 2nd ed. Oxford: Blackwell Scientific, 1971.
32. Food and Agriculture Organization/World Health Organization/United Nations University. Energy and protein requirements. WHO tech. rep. series no. 724. Geneva: WHO, 1985.
33. Durnin JVGA. Energy requirements of pregnancy: an integration of the longitudinal data from the 5-country study. In: Nestle Foundation annual report. Lausanne, Switzerland: Nestle Foundation, 1986;147–54.
34. van Raaij JM, Schonk CM, Vermaat-Miedema SH, et al. Am J Clin Nutr 1989;49:765–72.
35. Forsum E, Sadurkis A, Wager J. Am J Clin Nutr 1988;47: 942–7.
36. Garbaciak JA Jr, Richter M, Miller S, et al. Am J Obstet Gynecol 1985;152:238–45.
37. Abrams B, Parker J. Int J Obes 1988;12:293–303.
38. Galtier-Dereure F, Montpeyroux F, Boulot P, et al. Int J Obes 1995;19:443–8.
39. Edwards LE, Hellerstedt WL, Alton IR, et al. Obstet Gynecol 1996;87:389–94.
40. Committee of Maternal Nutrition. Maternal nutrition and the course of pregnancy. Washington, DC: National Academy of Sciences, 1970.
41. Hurley LS. Developmental nutrition. Englewood Cliffs, NJ: Prentice-Hall, 1980.
42. Garn SM, LaVelle M, Pesick SD, et al. Am J Dis Child 1984;138:32–34.
43. McGanity WJ, Dawson EB. Unpublished data, Ten State Nutrition Survey, 1968–1970.
44. Weiss W, Jackson EC. Maternal factors affecting birth weight. In: Perinatal factors affecting human development. Washington, DC: Pan American Health Organization, 1969;54–69.
45. Dewey KG, Heinig MJ, Nommsen LA. Am J Clin Nutr 1993;58:162–6.
46. Potter S, Hannum S, McFarlin B, et al. J Am Diet Assoc 1991;91:441–6.
47. Hetzel BS, Mano MT. J Nutr 1989;119(2):145–51.
48. Krzyczkowska-Sendrakowska M, Zdebski Z, Kaim I, et al. Endokrynol Pol 1993;44(3):367–72.
49. Vermiglio F, Lo Presti VP, Scaffidi Argentina G, et al. Clin Endocrinol 1995;42(4):409–15.
50. Thilly CH, Hetzel BS. An assessment of prophylactic programs: social, political, cultural, and economic issues. In: Stanbury JB, Hetzel BS, eds. Endemic goiter and endemic cretinism. New York: Wiley Medical Publications, 1980.
51. Nohr SB, Laurberg P, Borlum KG, et al. Acta Obstet Gynecol Scand 1993;72(5):350–3.
52. Centanni M, Scaccini C, Maiani G, et al. Nutrition 1991;7(6):417–20.
53. Trowbridge FL, Hand KE, Nichaman MZ. Am J Clin Nutr 1975;28:712–6.
54. DeLong GR. Am J Clin Nutr 1993;57(2 Suppl):286(S)–90(S).
55. Wada L, King JC. Clin Obstet Gynecol 1994;37(3):574–86.
56. Pharoah PO, Connolly KJ. Arch Dis Child 1991;66(1):145–7.
57. Hahn PF, Carothers EL, Darby MD, et al. Am J Obstet Gynecol 1951;61:477–86.
58. Barrett JF, Whittaker PG, Williams JG, et al. Br Med J 1994;309:79–82.
59. Garn SM, Ridella SA, Petzold AS, et al. Semin Perinatol 1981;5:155–62.
60. Steer P, Alam MA, Wadsworth J, et al. Br Med J 1995;310:489–91.
61. Goldenberg RL, Tamura T, Dubara M, et al. Am J Obstet Gynecol 1996;175(5):1356–9.
62. Romslo I, Haram K, Sagen N. Br J Obstet Gynaecol 1983;90:101–7.
63. Dawson EB, McGanity WJ. J Reprod Med 1987;32:478–87.
64. U.S. Preventive Services Task Force. JAMA 1993;270: 2846–54.
65. Sauberlich HE. Evaluation of folate nutrition in population groups. In: Picciano MF, Stokstad ELR, Gregory JF III, eds. Folic acid metabolism in health and disease. New York: Wiley-Liss, 1990;211–35.
66. Iyengar L, Apte SV. Br J Nutr 1972;47:313–7.
67. McPartlin J, Halligan A, Scott JM, et al. Lancet 1993;341: 148–9.
68. Martin MP, Bridgeforth E, McGanity WJ, et al. J Nutr 1957;62:201–25.
69. Cunningham FG, MacDonald PC, Gant NF, et al. Hypertensive disorders in pregnancy. In: Cunningham FG, MacDonald PC, Gant NF, et al., eds. Williams obstetrics. 19th ed. Norwalk, CT: Appleton & Lange, 1993;763–819.
70. Gifford RW, August P, Chesley LC, et al. Am J Obstet Gynecol 1990;163:1691–712.
71. Roberts JM. Pregnancy-related hypertension. In: Creasy RK, Resnik R, eds. Maternal-fetal medicine: principles and practice. 3rd ed. Philadelphia: WB Saunders, 1994;804–43.
72. Khong TY, De Wolf F, Robertson WB, Brosens I. Br J Obstet Gynaecol 1986;93:1049–59.
73. Zeek PM, Assali NS. Am J Clin Pathol 1950;20:1099–109.
74. Gant NF, Daley GL, Chand S, et al. J Clin Invest 1973;52:2682–9.

75. Newman V, Fullerton JT. J Nurse Midwifery 1990;35:282–91.
76. Green J. Diet and the prevention of preeclampsia. In: Chalmers I, Enkin M, Keirse MJNC, eds. Effective care in pregnancy and childbirth. Oxford: Oxford University Press, 1989;281–300.
77. Brewer TH. J Reprod Med 1974;13:175–6.
78. Brewer TH. Am J Obstet Gynecol 1976;125:281–3.
79. Chaudhuri SK. Am J Obstet Gynecol 1970;107:33–7.
80. Zlatnik FJ, Burmeister LF. Am J Obstet Gynecol 1983;147:345–6.
81. Magness RR, Cox K, Gant NF. Effects of low-dose aspirin (ASA) and lioleic acid (LA) on PGI2 and TXA2 and pregnancy outcome in preeclampsia (PE) (abstract). Proceedings of 38th annual meeting, Society for Gynecologic Investigation, San Antonio, Texas, March 20–23, 1991.
82. Hoffman DR, Favour S, Uauy R, et al. Prostaglandins Leukotrienes Essent Fatty Acids 1993;49:907–14.
83. Greenspoon JS, Safarik RH, Hayashi JT, et al. J Reprod Med 1994;39:87–91.
84. Robinson M. Lancet 1958;(i):178.
85. Brown JJ, Lever AF, Robertson JI, et al. Lancet 1984;(2):1333–4.
86. Villar J, Repke J, Belizan JM, et al. Obstet Gynecol 1987;70:317–22.
87. Belizan JM, Villar J, Repke J. Am J Obstet Gynecol 1988;158:898–902.
88. Repke JT, Villar J, Anderson C, et al. Am J Obstet Gynecol 1989;160:684–90.
89. Belizan JM, Pineda O, Sainz E. Am J Obstet Gynecol 1981;141:163–9.
90. Villar J, Belizan JM, Fisher P. Int J Gynaecol Obstet 1983;21:271–8.
91. Masoroni R, Koirtyohann SR, Pierce J, et al. Sci Total Environ 1976;6:41–53.
92. Bucher HC, Cook RJ, Guyatt GH, et al. JAMA 1996;275: 1016–22.
93. Bucher HC, Guyatt GH, Cook RJ, et al. JAMA 1996;275: 1113–7.
93a. Levine RJ, Hauth JC, Curet LB, et al. N Engl J Med 1997;337:69–76.
94. Cherry FF, Bennett EA, Bazzano GS, et al. Am J Clin Nutr 1981;34:2367–75.
95. Zimmerman AW, Dunham BS, Nochimson DJ, et al. Am J Obstet Gynecol 1984;149:523–9.
96. Chisolm JC, Handorf CR. Med Hypotheses 1985;17:231 –42.
97. Rabinowitz M, Bellinger D, Leviton A, et al. Hypertension 1987;10:447–51.
98. The People's League of Health. J Obstet Gynaecol Br Commonw 1946;53:498–509.
99. Centers for Disease Control. MMWR 1989;38:633–85.
100. Division of Vital Statistics. Personal communication, Texas Department of Health, 1995.
101. Basu TK. Int J Environ Stud 1981;17:31–5.
102. Platt LD, Koch R, Azen C, et al. Am J Obstet Gynecol 1992;166:1160–2.
103. MRC Vitamin Study Research Group. Lancet 1991;338:131–7.
104. Smithells RW, Nevin NC, Seller MJ, et al. Lancet 1983;1:1027–31.
105. Czeizel AE, Dudas I. N Engl J Med 1992;327:1832–5.
106. Schorah CJ, Smithells RW, Scott J. Lancet 1980;1:880.
107. Kirke PN, Molloy AM, Daly LE, et al. Q J Med 1993;86:703–8.
108. Scott J, Kirke P, Molloy A, et al. Proc Nutr Soc 1994;53:631–6.
109. Mills JL, McPartlin JM, Kirke PN, et al. Lancet 1995;345:149–51.
110. Willson JR, Carrington ER. Obstetrics and gynecology. 8th ed. St. Louis: Mosby, 1987;259.
111. Whitehead AS, Gallagher P, Mills JL, et al. Q J Med 1995;88:763–6.
112. Scholl TO, Hediger ML, Schall JI, et al. Am J Clin Nutr 1996;63:520–5.
113. Centers for Disease Control. MMWR 1992;41:81–5.
114. Smithells RW. Br Med J 1996;313:128–9.
115. Federal Register. Food additives permitted for direct addition to food for human consumption—folic acid. 1996;61(44): 8750–807.
116. Cuskelly GJ, McNutty H, Scott JM. Lancet 1996;334:657–9.
117. Daly LE, Kirke PN, Molloy A, et al. JAMA 1995;274:1698–702.
118. Richards IDG. Br J Prev Soc Med 1969;23:218–25.
119. Naeye RL. Am J Clin Nutr 1990;52:273–9.
120. Walter DK. Am J Obstet Gynecol 1994;170:541–8.
121. Shaw GM, Vilie EM, Schaffer D. JAMA 1996;275:1093–6.
122. Walters M. Am J Epidemiol 1994;139:Sii.
123. Widdowson EM. Biology of gestation. New York: Academic Press, 1968;1–49.
124. Edwards LE, Alton IR, Barrada MI, et al. Am J Obstet Gynecol 1979;135:297–302.
125. Lechtig A, Klein RE. In: Dobbing J, ed. Maternal nutrition in pregnancy. Eating for two. New York: Academic Press, 1981; 131–55.
126. National Academy of Sciences, Subcommittee on Nutritional Status and Weight Gain during Pregnancy. Nutrition during pregnancy. Washington, DC: National Academy Press, 1990:150–71.
127. Butler NR, Goldstein H, Ross EM. Br Med J 1972;2:127–30.
128. Smith JL, Hodges RE. Ann NY Acad Sci 1987;498:144–52.
129. Tribble DL, Giuliano LJ, Fortimann SP. Am J Clin Nutr 1993;58:886–90.
130. Lykkesfeldt J, Prieme H, Loft S, et al. Br Med J 1996;313:91–2.
131. Barrett BM, Sowell A, Gunter E, et al. Int J Vitam Nutr Res 1994;64:192–7.
132. Widman GL, Baird GH, Bolding OT. Am J Obstet Gynecol 1964;88:592–5.
133. Eryurek FG, Geuc S, Surmen E, et al. J Clin Biochem Nutr 1991;10:225–30.
134. Comstock GW, Shah FK, Meyer MB. Am J Obstet Gynecol 1971;111:53–9.
135. Norkus EP, Hsu H, Cehelsky MR. Ann NY Acad Sci 1987;489:580–1.
136. Caldwell EJ, Carlson SE, Palmer SM, et al. Int J Vitam Nutr Res 1988;58:319–25.
137. Levine M, Conry-Cantilena C, Wang Y, et al. Proc Natl Acad Sci USA 1996;93(8):3704–9.
138. Stein Z, Susser M. Pediatr Res 1975;9:76–83.
139. Anonymous. Nutr Rev 1992;50:233–6.
140. Kuhnert BR, Kuhnert PM, Groh-Wargo SL, et al. Am J Clin Nutr 1992;55:981–4.
141. Yip R. Am J Clin Nutr 1996;63:853–5.
142. Viteri FE, Alvarez E, Batres A. Am J Clin Nutr 1995;61:1153–63.
143. Layrisse M, Chaves JF, Mendez-Castellano M. Am J Clin Nutr 1996;64:903–7.
144. Ridwan E, Schultink W, Dillon D, et al. Am J Clin Nutr 1996;63:884–90.
145. US Environmental Protection Agency (EPA). EPA 400-F-94-004, 1991.
146. Sies H, Stahl W. Am J Clin Nutr 1995;62(Suppl):1315S–21S.

147. Mills JL, Holmes LB, Aarons JH, et al. JAMA 1993;269:593–7.
148. Cutrutelli R, Matthews RH. Agriculture handbook, no. 8-14, US Department of Agriculture, May 1986.
149. Brien JF, Smith GN. J Dev Physiol 1991;15(1):21–32.
150. Smith KJ, Eckardt MJ. Recent Dev Alcohol 1991;9:151–64.
151. Jerrells TR. Adv Exp Med Biol 1991;288:229–36.
152. Duester G. Alcohol Clin Exp Res 1991;15(3):568–72.
153. Zuckerman B, Frank DA, Hingson R, et al. N Engl J Med 1989;320:762–8.
154. Lutiger B, Graham K, Einarson TR, et al. Teratology 1991;44:405–14.
155. Revelli A, Durando A, Massobrio M. Obstet Gynecol Surv 1992;47:355–67.

SELECTED READINGS

Beard JL, Dawson HD, Piñero DJ. Iron metabolism: a comprehensive review. Nutr Rev 1996;54:295–317.

Institute of Medicine. Nutrition during pregnancy. Washington, DC: National Academy Press, 1990.

Institute of Medicine. Nutrition during lactation—milk composition. Washington, DC: National Academy Press, 1991:116.

Pitkin RM, guest ed. Nutrition in pregnancy. Clin Obstet Gynecol 1994;37(3):499–776.

Suitor CW. Maternal weight gain: a report of an expert work group. Arlington, VA: National Center for Education in Maternal and Child Health, 1997.

Worthington-Roberts B, Williams SR. Nutrition in pregnancy and lactation. 4th ed. St. Louis: Times Mirror/Mosby College, 1989.

51. Nutritional Requirements During Infancy

WILLIAM C. HEIRD

The nutritional requirements of infants and children reflect this population's unique needs for growth and developmental changes in organ function and body composition as well as their maintenance needs. Moreover, since the metabolic rate of infants and children is greater and the turnover of nutrients more rapid than in the adult, the unique nutritional needs for growth and development are superimposed upon higher maintenance requirements than those of the adult. In addition, the potential impact of intake during early life on later development and health must be considered. Finally, provision of these greater needs, particularly to the smaller members of this population, is hindered by their lack of teeth as well as their limited digestive and metabolic processes.

This chapter discusses the nutritional needs of normal infants as well as those of low-birth-weight (LBW) infants. Since nutritional management of LBW infants presents some of the most pressing problems encountered by those involved in feeding infants and children, nutritional needs of this subpopulation are discussed more fully. Nutritional needs of infants and children with acute or chronic diseases that affect nutritional needs and/or management are discussed in Chapter 64, which also includes a general discussion of approaches to providing the nutritional needs of compromised infants and a detailed discussion of parenteral nutrition in pediatric patients.

NUTRITIONAL REQUIREMENTS OF THE NORMAL INFANT

The nutritional requirements of the normal infant have been addressed by many investigators over a number of years, and both estimated requirements and recommended dietary allowances for most nutrients have been established. *Requirements* and *recommended allowances* must be distinguished. The former is the amount of a specific nutrient required to achieve some physiologic endpoint, most frequently the amount necessary to maintain a satisfactory rate of growth and development and/or prevent development of specific signs of deficiency. The requirement of a specific nutrient is usually defined experimentally, in a small, homogeneous study population. *Recommended allowance* is the intake of an essential nutrient deemed by a scientifically knowledgeable group of individuals to be adequate to meet the "requirement" of all healthy members of a population. In general, if the requirement of a specific population is normally distributed, the recommended allowance is set at the mean requirement of the population plus two standard deviations. Since the requirements of most nutrients are not normally distributed, other considerations of population variability frequently are necessary.

The most recent recommended dietary allowances (RDAs) of the National Research Council Food and Nutrition Board (1) are summarized in Table 51.1 See also Appendices Tables A 2a-1 to 3 for these data from the 1989 RDA. The 1997 U.S. dietary reference intakes for calcium, phosphorus, magnesium, vitamin D, and fluoride are presented in Appendices Tables A-2b 1 to 6. The requirements and recommended intakes of some nutrients are discussed briefly below.

Energy

Per unit of body weight, the energy requirement of the normal newborn infant is 3 to 4 times that of the adult: 90 to 120 kcal/kg/day versus 30 to 40 kcal/kg/day. This greater need reflects primarily the infant's relatively high resting metabolic rate and special needs for growth and development, but the somewhat inefficient intestinal absorption of infants, compared with that of adults, may contribute.

For some time there has been concern that the RDA for energy was excessive. This issue was reviewed recently by the International Dietary Energy Consultative Group (IDECG), which concluded that energy requirements of

Table 51.1
Recommended Daily Allowances of Nutrients for Normal Infants

Nutrient	Recommended Intake per Day 0–6 Months Weight = 6 kg	6–12 Months Weight = 9 kg
Energy (kcal)	650	850
Fat (g)		
Carbohydrate		
Protein (g)	13	14
Electrolytes and minerals		
Calcium (mg)	400	600
Phosphorus (mg)	300	500
Magnesium (mg)	40	60
Sodium (mg)[a]	120	200
Chloride (mg)[a]	180	300
Potassium (mg)[a]	500	700
Iron (mg)	6	10
Zinc (mg)	5	5
Copper (mg)[b]	0.4–0.6	0.6–0.7
Iodine (μg)	40	50
Selenium (μg)	10	15
Manganese (μg)[b]	0.3–0.6	0.6–1.0
Fluoride (mg)[b]	0.1–1	0.2–1
Chromium (μg)[b]	10–40	20–60
Molybdenum (μg)	15–30	20–40
Vitamins		
Vitamin A (μg RE)	375	375
Vitamin D (μg)	7.5	10
Vitamin E (μg α-TE)	3	4
Vitamin K (μg)	5	10
Vitamin C (mg)	0.3	0.4
Thiamin (mg)	0.3	0.4
Riboflavin (mg)	0.4	0.5
Niacin (mg NE)	5	6
Vitamin B_6 (μg)	0.3	0.6
Folate (μg)	25	35
Vitamin B_{12} (μg)	0.3	0.5
Biotin (μg)[b]	10	15
Pantothenic acid (mg)[b]	2	3

Data from Food and Nutrition Board, National Research Council. Recommended dietary allowances. 10th ed. Washington, DC: National Academy Press, 1989.
[a]Minimum requirements (mg/day) rather than recommended.
[b]Estimated safe and adequate daily intake.

infants should be estimated from measurements of energy expenditure and growth rather than from dietary intake data (2). Using available data, the group's estimated energy requirement was about 90 kcal/kg/day during the entire 1st year of life (ranging from 84 kcal/kg/day between 4 and 6 months of age to 94 kcal/kg/day between 2 and 3 months of age for breast-fed and formula-fed infants combined). However, more data on energy expenditure and body composition of infants was considered desirable.

Unlike the RDA for other nutrients, that for energy is the same as the estimated requirement. In other words, the RDA does not include an upward adjustment to account for individual variation. This is because the higher recommendation would likely result in excessive intakes for at least some individuals and, hence, further increase the prevalence of obesity. Individual energy requirements can, of course, vary considerably.

With respect to the source of energy, there is no evidence that either carbohydrate or fat is superior, provided total energy intake is adequate. Sufficient carbohydrate to avoid development of ketosis and/or hypoglycemia is required (<5.0 g/kg/day) as is enough fat to avoid development of essential fatty acid deficiency (0.5–1.0 g/kg/day of linoleic acid plus a smaller amount of α-linolenic acid). There is concern that infants may also require at least some of the longer-chain, more unsaturated derivatives of linoleic and α-linolenic acids (e.g., arachidonic and docosahexaenoic acids). These are present in breast milk but not in currently available formulas. Furthermore, formula-fed infants have less of these fatty acids in plasma and erythrocyte lipids than breast-fed infants (3, 4), and the brain content of docosahexaenoic, but not arachidonic, acid also is lower in formula-fed infants (5, 6). However, results of functional outcome studies comparing functional outcomes of breast-fed and formula-fed infants (7, 8) as well as infants fed formulas with and without arachidonic and docosahexaenoic acid (8, 9) are inconclusive. Overall, these studies provide no convincing evidence that the absence of these fatty acids in formulas is problematic, provided linoleic and α-linolenic acid intakes are adequate (10).

In concert with the recommendation that the dietary fat intake of the general population be reduced, particularly that of cholesterol and saturated fat, some agencies have suggested that this guideline be applied to infants. However, since fat is a major source of energy as well as a source of essential fatty acids, there is concern that such diets might limit growth. Thus, groups responsible for making recommendations for infants have not endorsed this recommendation for infants under 2 years of age (11).

Until recently, there were few data concerning this issue, but a recent Finnish study suggests that the fear of growth failure with such diets may be overrated (12). This study involved over a thousand infants; the caregivers for half of them were counseled to limit saturated fat and cholesterol intake, the others were not. There was no difference in growth between groups. Interestingly, although energy and fat intake of the intervention group was somewhat lower than that of the control group, the mean fat intake of both groups was lower than expected (~30% of total energy). The intervention group also had a lower serum cholesterol concentration at 3 years of age or upon termination of the study.

Protein

The protein requirement of the normal infant per unit body weight is also greater than that of the adult but not as great as the requirement of the LBW infant. The infant also requires a higher proportion of essential amino acids than the adult (Table 51.2). The minimal intakes of essential amino acids consistent with normal growth were determined some time ago under conditions of maximal nitrogen sparing (13). Thus, if the required intakes of the

Table 51.2
Essential Amino Acid Requirements of the Term Infant

Amino Acid	Minimum Requirement (mg/kg/day)
Leucine	76–229
Isoleucine	102–119
Lysine	88–103
Methionine (with cyst(e)ine)	33–45
Phenylalanine (with tyrosine)	47–90
Threonine	45–87
Tryptophan	15–22
Valine	85–105
Histidine	16–34

Adapted from Holt LE Jr, Snyderman SE. JAMA 1961;175:100–3.

essential amino acids are met, the total intake of nitrogen probably is more important than the particular mixture of amino acids provided. Indeed, the overall protein requirement is some two to three times the aggregate requirement for essential amino acids. Obviously, the required intake of a specific protein is a function of its quality, which usually is defined as how closely its amino acid pattern resembles that of human milk. It also follows that the overall quality of a specific protein can be improved by supplementing it with any missing essential amino acid(s). For example, soy protein in the native state has insufficient methionine but, when fortified with methionine, approaches or equals the overall quality of bovine milk protein (14).

While the amino acid composition of human milk is ideal, its overall protein content, approximately 1.0 g/dL, is such that ingestion of 180 to 200 mL/kg/day is required to ensure a protein intake equal to the current RDA (2.0–2.2 g/kg/day). This fact has led some to question the adequacy of the protein content of human milk and others to question the validity of the recommended intake. On balance, the high quality and easy digestibility of human milk protein appear to compensate for any quantitative deficiency. On the other hand, bovine milk protein, the protein source of most infant formulas, also is a very high quality protein and, if properly processed, is used nearly as well as human milk protein. Thus, the actual requirement for protein when bovine milk is the source may be very little higher, if at all, than when human milk is the source (15).

The IDECG also recently evaluated the protein and amino acid requirements of infants (16). Basing requirements on the needs for maintenance plus growth and assuming that the efficiency of nitrogen use for infant growth is 70%, the group concluded that the protein requirement during infancy ranges from about 2.0 g/kg/day during the 1st month of life to about 0.8 g/kg/day from 9 to 12 months of age. Estimates for the safe level of protein intake (equivalent to recommended daily allowance) ranged from 2.7 g/kg/day during the 1st month of life to approximately 1.0 g/kg/day from 9 to 12 months of age. The lower estimate is approximately one-third less than previous estimates. As with the revised estimates of energy requirements, the group pointed out that more research is needed.

Electrolytes, Minerals, and Vitamins

The electrolyte, mineral, and vitamin requirements of the normal infant are not as well defined as those for energy and protein. Nonetheless, RDAs for most have been established (Table 51.1), and infants who receive these intakes experience few problems. Recently, the concept that limitation of sodium intake may decrease the incidence of hypertension later in life has received some attention, but there are few data on which to base a definitive conclusion (17).

Iron deficiency is the most common nutrient deficiency syndrome in infancy. This is somewhat surprising since the normal infant has sufficient stores of iron at birth to meet requirements for 4 to 6 months. However, these stores as well as the absorption of iron are quite variable. Although human milk contains less iron than most formulas, iron deficiency is less common in breast-fed infants. To prevent development of iron deficiency, routine use of iron-fortified formulas is recommended (18). Whether breast-fed infants should receive iron supplements is controversial.

If protein intake is adequate, vitamin deficiencies are rare; if not, deficiencies of nicotinic acid and choline, which are synthesized, respectively, from tryptophan and methionine, may develop. In contrast, if bovine milk and bovine milk formulas were not supplemented with vitamin D, hypovitaminosis D would be endemic among formula-fed infants, particularly those with limited exposure to sunlight. The breast-fed infant may be relatively better protected from development of vitamin D deficiency (19), but vitamin D supplementation of breast-fed infants is also recommended. Routine perinatal administration of vitamin K is recommended for all infants as prophylaxis against hemorrhagic disease of the newborn. All currently available formulas contain adequate amounts of all vitamins for which a requirement has been established.

Water

The normal infant's absolute requirement for water probably is 75 to 100 mL/kg/day. However, because of higher obligate renal, pulmonary, and dermal water losses as well as a higher overall metabolic rate, the infant is more susceptible to developing dehydration, particularly with vomiting and/or diarrhea. Thus, provision of 150 mL/kg/day is recommended. Both breast-fed and formula-fed infants usually consume at least this volume for the first several weeks of life.

Human Milk versus Artificial Formula

The ready availability and safety of human milk coupled with the possibility that it may enhance intestinal development, resistance to infection, and bonding between mother and infant have led most to conclude that human milk is the perfect food for the normal infant (20). However, there are both theoretical and practical concerns about breast-feeding that deserve consideration.

The major nutritional concern is not that human milk contains too little protein (see above) but that its low content of calcium and phosphorus may not support optimal skeletal development. In this regard, breast-fed infants have a less well mineralized skeleton throughout the early months of life than formula-fed infants. However, since no major differences in bone density appear in older formerly breast-fed and formerly formula-fed infants, the lower calcium and phosphorus intakes of breast-fed infants do not seem to be detrimental.

Hyperbilirubinemia is more common in breast-fed than in formula-fed infants. This usually is a transient phenomenon limited to the first few days to weeks of life; thus, most feel that proscription of breast-feeding is not necessary unless hyperbilirubinemia persists or plasma bilirubin concentration is excessively high. Even in these situations, substituting formula at every other feeding and/or substituting formula for only 1 to 2 days usually resolves the problem.

Certain noxious or infectious agents (e.g., chemicals, drugs, foreign proteins, viruses) may be present in breast milk. However, the risk of infection secondary to mode of feeding is far greater in formula-fed than breast-fed infants, particularly if the artificial formula is prepared under less than optimal hygienic conditions.

As publicized recently in the lay press (21), it cannot automatically be assumed that maternal milk supply will be adequate and/or constant. Thus, breast-fed infants, particularly firstborn infants, must be followed closely over the first few days to weeks of life to ensure that growth and development are proceeding normally. With proper counseling, most problems can be corrected and/or avoided.

In large part, the problems historically associated with artificial feeding have been solved. The safety and easy digestibility of modern infant formulas, in fact, approach the safety and digestibility of breast milk. Furthermore, the clear economic advantages and microbiologic safety of breast-feeding are less important for affluent, developed societies with ready access to a clean water supply than for less-developed, less-affluent societies. Thus, a reasonable and conservative approach is to allow the mother to make an informed choice of how she wishes to feed her infant and support her in that decision. As Fomon (22) stated, "In industrialized countries, any woman with the least inclination toward breast feeding should be encouraged to do so, and all assistance possible should be provided by nurses, physicians, nutritionists and other health workers. At the same time, there is little justification for attempts to coerce women to breast feed. No woman in an industrialized country should be made to feel guilty because she elects not to breast feed her infant."

Evidence suggesting that breast-fed infants in affluent societies have fewer common and serious infections during early life than formula-fed infants is increasing. If this difference is shown to be due to breast-feeding rather than to a myriad of other possible factors (e.g., mother's competence, education, and/or socioeconomic status), the current emphasis on promoting breast-feeding is clearly warranted.

A number of formulas are available for feeding the normal infant. Compositions of those most commonly used are shown in Table 51.3. Most are available in both a "ready-to-use" and a concentrated liquid form. Powdered products, which are somewhat lower in cost, are being used with increasing frequency. These products usually are the only ones available in many parts of the world.

The most commonly used formulas contain either unmodified or modified bovine milk protein. The protein concentration of all is about 1.5 g/dL. Thus, the infant who receives from 150 to 180 mL/kg/day receives a protein intake of 2.25 to 2.7 g/kg/day. This is as much as 50% above the intake of the breast-fed infant and as much as 25% above the current RDA for protein.

Unmodified bovine milk protein has a whey:casein ratio of 18:82, whereas modified bovine milk protein has a whey:casein ratio of 60:40. Products containing the latter protein are prepared from either a mixture of bovine milk protein and bovine milk whey proteins or a mixture of bovine milk whey proteins and caseins. Modified and unmodified bovine milk protein appear to be equally efficacious for the normal term infant. Formulas containing soy protein and formulas containing partially hydrolyzed bovine milk proteins are available for feeding infants who are intolerant of bovine milk or soy protein (Table 51.4).

Although lactose-free bovine milk formulas have recently been introduced, the major carbohydrate of the most commonly used bovine milk formulas is lactose. The most commonly used soy protein formulas contain either sucrose or a glucose polymer; thus, these formulas or lactose-free bovine milk protein formulas are useful for the infant with either transient or congenital lactase deficiency.

The fat content of both bovine milk and soy protein formulas usually comprises about 50% of the nonprotein energy. In general, the blend of vegetable oils present in most formulas is quite easily absorbed; most studies suggest that intestinal absorption is at least 90%.

The electrolyte, mineral, and vitamin contents of most formulas are similar, and when fed in adequate amounts (150–180 mL/kg/day), all provide the RDAs for these nutrients. Both iron-supplemented (~12 mg/L) and nonsupplemented (~1 mg/L) formulas are available; as mentioned above, iron-supplemented formulas are recommended.

The goal of both breast-feeding and formula feeding is to deliver enough nutrients to support adequate growth. As a rule of thumb, the normal term infant's weight should double by 4 to 5 months of age and triple by 12 months of age. Demand feeding is considered preferable, particularly during the early weeks of life. However, most infants easily adjust to roughly an every 3 or 4 hour schedule and, after 2 months of age, rarely demand night feedings.

Table 51.3
Composition (amount/100 kcal) of Standard Formulas for Normal Infants

Component	Similac[a]	Enfamil[b]	Good Start[c]
Protein (g)	2.14 (bovine milk)	2.1 (bovine milk, whey)	2.4 (whey)
Fat (g)	5.4 (coconut and soy oils)	5.3 (palm-olein, soy, coconut, and high-oleic sunflower oils)	5.1 (palm-olein, soy, coconut, and high-oleic safflower oils)
Carbohydrate (g)	10.7 (lactose)	10.9 (lactose)	11.0 (lactose, maltodextrin)
Electrolytes and minerals			
Calcium (mg)	73	78	64
Phosphorus (mg)	56	53	36
Magnesium (mg)	6	8	6.7
Iron (mg)	0.22 (1.8)[d]	0.7 (1.81)[d]	1.5
Zinc (mg)	0.75	1	0.75
Manganese (μg)	5	15	7
Copper (μg)	90	75	80
Iodine (μg)	9	10	8
Selenium (μg)	2.2	2.8	—
Sodium (mg)	27	27	24
Potassium (mg)	105	108	98
Chloride	64	63	59
Vitamins			
Vitamin A (IU)	300	300	300
Vitamin D (IU)	60	60	60
Vitamin E (IU)	3.0	2	2
Vitamin K (μg)	8	8	8.2
Thiamin (μg)	100	80	60
Riboflavin (μg)	150	140	135
Vitamin B_6 (μg)	60	60	75
Vitamin B_{12} (μg)	0.25	30.3	0.22
Niacin (μg)	1050	1000	750
Folic acid (μg)	15	16	9
Pantothenic acid (μg)	450	500	450
Vitamin C (mg)	9	12	8
Biotin (μg)	4.5	3	2.2
Choline (mg)	16.0	12	12
Inositol (mg)	4.7	17	18

[a]Ross Laboratories, Columbus, Ohio.
[b]Mead-Johnson Nutritionals, Evansville, Indiana.
[c]Carnation Nutritional Products, Glendale, California.
[d]Content of iron-fortified formula shown in parentheses.

NUTRITIONAL REQUIREMENTS OF THE 6- TO 12-MONTH-OLD CHILD

Considerably less attention has been paid to the nutritional needs of the 6- to 12-month-old child than to those of the younger infant. In fact, the RDAs for the various nutrients for this age group (Table 51.1) rely heavily upon extrapolations from data obtained in younger infants, taking into account the developmental differences between the younger and the older infants as well as the greater activity and somewhat slower rate of growth of the 6- to 12-month-old child. Despite the lack of specific data, few participants in a symposium on the nutritional needs of the 6- to 12-month-old child held in 1989 felt that the most recent RDAs for this age group required extensive revision (23).

One exception concerns energy, the recommended intake of which is somewhat higher than the current energy intake of apparently normal infants (24). Infants receiving the lower intake exhibit lower rates of weight gain as well as lower rates of increase in skinfold thicknesses than the National Center for Health Statistics (NCHS) standard rates (see Appendices Tables III a14b), but the rates of increase in length and head circumference are not compromised. Thus, proponents of a lower energy intake (i.e., 85 vs. 95 kcal/kg/day) argue that the growth response of infants ingesting the lower energy intake reflects the current concepts of parents regarding appropriate body size and proportions and that these responses are appropriate for current feeding practices (e.g., delayed introduction of solid foods). As noted above, more data are needed concerning this issue, but currently there is no evidence that the lower energy intake apparently characteristic of many modern infants is harmful.

By 6 months of age, the infant's previously compromised capacity to digest and absorb a variety of dietary components as well as to metabolize, use, and excrete the absorbed products of digestion approaches the adult capacity (25). Moreover, these infants are more active and are beginning to explore their surroundings. Hence, during this interval, diet plays a variety of roles other than delivery of required nutrients. A variety of concerns also

Table 51.4
Composition of Soy and Hydrolyzed Protein Formulas

Component	Isomil[a]	Prosobee[b]	Nutramigen[b]	Pregestimil[b]	Alimentum[a]
Protein (g)	2.45 (soy) protein isolate, L-methionine)	3 (soy protein isolate, L-methionine)	2.8 (casein hydrolysate, L-cystine, L-tyrosine, L-tryptophan)	2.8 (casein hydrolysate, L-cystine, L-tyrosine, L-tryptophan)	2.75 (casein hydrolysate, L-cystine, L-tyrosine, L-tryptophan)
Fat (g)	5.59 (soy and coconut oils)	5.3 (palm-olein, soy, coconut, and high oleic sunflower oils)	5.0 (corn oil)	5.6 (medium-chain triglycerides, corn, soy, and high-oleic safflower oils)	5.54 (medium-chain triglycerides, safflower and soy oils)
Carbohydrate (g)	10.2 (corn syrup, sucrose)[d]	10 (corn syrup solids)	11 (corn syrup solids, solids, modified cornstarch)	10.3 (corn syrup solids, modified cornstarch, dextrose)	10.2 (sucrose, modified tapioca starch
Electrolytes and minerals					
Calcium (mg)	105	105	94	94	105
Phosphorus (mg)	75	83	63	63	75
Magnesium (mg)	7.5	11	11	10.9	7.5
Iron (mg)	1.8	1.8	1.8	1.88	1.8
Zinc (mg)	0.75	1.2	1	0.94	0.75
Manganese (μg)	30	25	95	31	30
Copper (μg)	75	75	75	94	75
Iodine (μg)	15	15	15	7	15
Selenium (μg)	2.1	2.8	1.8	—	2.8
Sodium (mg)	44	36	47	39	44
Potassium (mg)	108	120	110	109	118
Chloride	62	80	86	86	80
Vitamins					
Vitamin A (IU)	300	300	300	380	300
Vitamin D (IU)	60	60	60	75	45
Vitamin E (IU)	3	2	2	3.8	3
Vitamin K (μg)	15	8	8	18.8	15
Thiamin (μg)	60	80	80	78	60
Riboflavin (μg)	90	90	90	94	90
Vitamin B_6 (μg)	60	60	60	63	60
Vitamin B12 (μg)	0.45	0.3	0.3	0.31	0.45
Niacin (μg)	1350	100	1000	1250	1350
Folic acid (μg)	15	16	16	15.6	15
Pantothenic acid (μg)	750	500	500	470	750
Biotin (μg)	4.5	3	3	7.8	4.5
Vitamin C (mg)	9	12	12	11.7	9.0
Choline (mg)	8	12	12	13.3	8
Inositol (mg)	5	17	17	4.7	5

[a]Ross Laboratories, Columbus, Ohio.
[b]Mead Johnson Nutritionals, Evansville, Indiana.
[c]Isomil-SF (sucrose free) has a similar composition except that glucose polymers are substituted for corn syrup and sucrose.

emerge during this period. For example, with the eruption of teeth, the role of diet in development of dental caries must be considered (26). Consideration of the long-term effects of inadequate or excessive intakes during infancy also assumes greater importance as does consideration of the psychosocial role of foods during development.

These considerations are the basis for most of the recommendations for feeding during the second 6 months of life. While all nutrient needs during this period can clearly be met with reasonable amounts of currently available infant formulas, although perhaps not with exclusive breast-feeding, addition of weaning foods to the diet of infants over 4 to 6 months of age usually is recommended.

Weaning, or "follow-up," formulas that have a somewhat higher protein content than regular infant formulas are popular in Europe but not in the United States. This situation may change with the recent introduction of a second such formula. The first follow-up formula to become available in the United States (Carnation Follow-Up Formula, Carnation Nutritional Products, Glendale, CA) contains 3 g of bovine milk protein per 100 kcal; fat content is 3.9 g/100 kcal (a mixture of corn, palm, and high-oleic safflower oils), and carbohydrate content is 13.2 g/100 kcal (a mixture of lactose and corn syrup solids). The more recently introduced follow-up formula (Similac Toddler's Best, Ross Laboratories, Columbus, OH) contains 3.5 g of bovine milk protein per 100 kcal; fat and carbohydrate contents, respectively, are 4.7 g/100 kcal (a mixture of coconut, soy, and high-oleic safflower oils) and 11 g/100 kcal (a mixture of sucrose and lactose). As the name implies, the latter formula is intended for the slightly older infant.

Aside from the association of bottle feeding with dental caries, little is known about the various issues related to the nonnutritional role of diet during the second half of the 1st year of life. Thus, feeding practices vary widely during this period. Nonetheless, most recent surveys indicate that infants fed according to current practices receive the RDAs for most nutrients (27).

One current feeding practice, the increasing use of bovine milk, particularly low-fat bovine milk, deserves comment. Although current recommendations are to limit the intake of bovine milk and to avoid low-fat or skimmed milk before 1 year of age (28), recent surveys suggest that a sizable percentage of 6- to 12-month-old infants, albeit still fewer than 25 to 30 years ago, are fed bovine milk rather than infant formula (29, 30). More important, almost half of these infants are fed low-fat or skimmed milk. The consequences of this practice are not known with certainty. However, infants fed bovine milk ingest, on average, roughly three times the recommended daily allowance for protein and 1.5 times the upper limit of the "safe range" of sodium intake but only two-thirds of the recommended daily intake of iron and only half of the recommended intake of linoleic acid. The protein and sodium intakes of infants fed skimmed rather than whole bovine milk are even higher, iron intake is equally low, and, most important, intake of linoleic acid is less than half of that recommended. Interestingly, while the most common reason for substituting low-fat or skimmed milk for whole milk or formula is to reduce fat and energy intakes, the energy intake of infants fed skimmed milk is not lower than that of infants fed whole milk or formula (30). Rather, they appear to compensate for the lower energy density of low-fat or skimmed milk by increasing intake of other foods.

Current knowledge is insufficient to support definitive statements concerning the consequences of the high protein and sodium intakes associated with feeding either whole or skimmed milk. The low iron intake clearly is not desirable but probably can be overcome by use of medicinal iron supplementation. The low intake of linoleic acid is more problematic. While signs and/or symptoms of essential fatty acid deficiency appear to be uncommon in infants fed either whole or skimmed milk, no exhaustive search for such symptoms has been made. Moreover, since essential fatty acid deficiency develops in both younger and older infants fed formulas providing roughly the same linoleic acid intake, it would be very surprising if such a search did not uncover a reasonably high incidence of biochemical essential fatty acid deficiency. On the other hand, older infants who were breast-fed or fed formulas with a high linoleic acid content prior to 6 months of age could conceivably have accumulated sufficient body stores of this fatty acid to limit the consequences of a low intake between 6 and 12 months of age. However, simply assuming that this is true could have undesired consequences; although biochemical essential fatty acid deficiency may not result in clinically detectable symptoms, animal studies suggest that it may result in long-term deleterious effects on development (31).

Addressing the concerns raised by the practice of feeding bovine milk is important for practical as well as health reasons. For example, the cost of bovine milk is roughly one-third that of infant formula, a large enough difference to have important economic consequences for most families. In addition, if food supply programs for infants provided bovine milk rather than formula to infants over 6 months of age, the program's current funds would permit expanding benefits to many more of the country's most needy infants. While clearly desirable, this obviously cannot be done until the safety of feeding bovine milk during the second 6 months of life is substantiated.

The questions raised by the increasingly common practice of substituting skimmed or low-fat milk for whole milk or formula are even more complex. The suggestion that infants fed skimmed milk increase their intake of other foods raises the important question of whether food intake during infancy may in some way imprint intake patterns throughout life. If so, this apparent attempt to improve longevity or at least cardiovascular health, paradoxically, may be more detrimental to both than a less prudent diet during infancy.

NUTRITIONAL REQUIREMENTS OF THE 1- TO 10-YEAR-OLD CHILD

The 1-year-old child has several teeth, and the various digestive and metabolic systems are functioning at or near adult capacity. Thus, the earlier restrictions with respect to source of nutrients no longer apply. Indeed, by 1 year of age, most children tolerate table foods, either as presented to other family members or with minimal alterations. Although coordination remains poor until 3 to 4 years of age, most children begin at least attempting to feed themselves during the early part of their 2nd year of life. Until coordination improves, however, these attempts usually result in as much food on the table or floor as in the child's stomach.

Most children are walking or beginning to walk by 1 year of age. Hence, with improved coordination over the next few years, activity increases dramatically. This greater activity, in turn, increases energy needs. Concurrently, the rate of growth decreases; for example, while the birth weight triples over the 1st year of life, it does not quadru-

Table 51.5
Weight and Length of Male Children from One to Ten Years of Age

Age (years)	Weight (kg) 5th Percentile	Weight (kg) 50th Percentile	Weight (kg) 95th Percentile	Length (cm) 5th Percentile	Length (cm) 50th Percentile	Length (cm) 95th Percentile
1	8.43	10.15	11.99	71.7	76.1	81.2
2	10.49	12.34	15.50	82.5	86.8	94.4
3	12.05	14.62	17.77	89.0	94.9	102.0
4	13.64	16.69	20.27	95.8	102.9	109.9
5	15.27	18.67	23.09	102.0	109.9	117.0
6	16.93	20.69	26.34	107.7	116.1	123.5
7	18.64	22.85	30.12	113.0	121.7	129.7
8	20.40	25.30	34.51	118.1	127.0	135.7
9	22.25	28.13	39.58	122.9	132.2	141.8
10	24.33	31.44	45.29	127.7	137.5	148.1

ple until about 3 years of age (Table 51.5). Thus, although the energy requirement incident to activity increases dramatically after the 1st year of life, the requirement for nutrients stored during growth decreases. These changing nutrient needs are reflected in the RDAs for various nutrients for children from 1 to 3, 4 to 6, and 7 to 10 years of age (Table 51.6).

As demonstrated by Davis (32) almost 75 years ago and more recently by Birch et al. (33), most young children given access to a varied diet including items from each of

Table 51.6
Recommended Daily Allowances (RDA) of Nutrients for Normal Infants[a]

Nutrient	Recommended Intake Per Day: 1–3 Years (weight = 13 kg)	4–6 Years (weight = 20 kg)	7–10 Years (weight = 28kg)
Energy (kCal)	1300	1800	2000
Fat (g)			
Carbohydrate			
Protein (g)	16	24	38
Electrolytes and minerals			
Calcium (mg)	800	800	800
Phosphorus (mg)	800	800	800
Magnesium (mg)	80	120	170
Sodium (mEq)[b]	13	20	28
Chloride (mEq)[b]	13	20	28
Potassium (mEq)[b]	26	36	40
Iron (mg)	10	10	10
Zinc (mg)	10	10	10
Copper (mg)[c]	0.7–1.0	1.0–1.5	1–2
Iodine (μg)	70	90	120
Selenium (μg)	20	20	30
Manganese (μg)[c]	1–1.5	1.5–2	2–3
Fluoride (mg)[c]	0.5–1.5	1–2.5	1–2.5
Chromium (μg)[c]	20–80	30–120	50–200
Molybdenum (μg)	25–50	30–75	50–150
Vitamins			
Vitamin A (μg RE)	400	500	700
Vitamin D (μg)	0.10	10	10
Vitamin E (mg α-TE)	6	8	7
Vitamin K (μg)	15	20	30
Vitamin C (mg)	40	45	45
Thiamin (mg)	0.7	0.9	1.0
Riboflavin (mg)	0.8	1.1	1.2
Niacin (mg NE)	9	12	13
Vitamin B_6 (mg)	1	1.1	1.4
Folate (μg)6	50	75	100
Vitamin B_{12}	0.7	1.0	1.4
Biotin (μg)[c]	20	25	30
Pantothenic acid (mg)[c]	3	3–4	4–5

Data from Food and Nutrition Board, National Research Council. Recommended dietary allowances. Washington, DC: National Academy Press, 1989.
[a]For the 1997 Dietary Reference Intakes recommended by the Food and Nutrition Board see Appendix Table II-A-2-b1 to 4.
[b]Minimal requirements rather than recommended.
[c]Estimated safe and adequate daily intake.

the major food groups consume adequate amounts of all nutrients. However, most children, particularly those under 5 to 6 years of age, are very finicky eaters. Moreover, many tend to use eating (or not eating) to exert control over parents and/or caretakers. Thus, the intake of most children at a single meal, or even over an entire day, is not necessarily well balanced. Rather, a balanced intake is achieved over a period of several days.

The erratic eating pattern of most young children is usually of considerable concern to parents, particularly those who have not witnessed this behavior before. Unfortunately, their efforts to control the child's intake usually make matters worse. They should be reassured and instructed to present the child with well-balanced meals and snacks throughout the day, to remove the food after a reasonable period of time, and to avoid coaxing and cajoling, particularly offering preferred foods or treats as rewards.

The importance of providing items from most or all of the major food groups cannot be overemphasized. Obviously, if the child does not have access to items from all food groups on a regular basis, self-selection of a balanced diet, either in the same day or over several days, is impossible. It also is important to limit intake between regular meals and snacks. Otherwise, the child is unlikely to be hungry when the regularly scheduled meal or snack is offered. Alternatively, if the appetite is not dampened, intake between regular meals and snacks will increase total energy intake disproportionately and contribute to development of obesity. A major distinction between meals and snacks also should be avoided so that the child has access to an adequate amount and variety of food when he or she is hungry or willing to eat rather than only at conventional meal times.

As the child matures and begins to socialize more, it becomes increasingly difficult to control the content of snacks or meals. Many modern children, in fact, eat away from home as much or more than they eat at home—a practice that many think contributes to development of obesity. Perhaps the best that can be done, short of changing modern lifestyles, is to counsel parents concerning the potential problem and advise them to devise ways of assessing their children's intakes away from home. Regular monitoring of weight and height should alert the clinician to existence of a potential problem.

Perhaps the major controversy concerning the nutrient needs of the 1- to 10-year-old child concerns the extent to which the currently advocated dietary guidelines are appropriate for this population. Although the American Heart Association (34), the American Health Foundation (35), and the National Institutes of Health Consensus Development Panel (36) recommend that the current guidelines be applied to children over the age of 1 to 2 years, the Committee on Nutrition of the American Academy of Pediatrics (37) expresses a number of concerns. Chief among these concerns is the safety of a diet emphasizing lower intakes of fat, cholesterol, and salt along with higher intakes of bulky cereal grains and plant products. Such a diet, the committee points out, could result in lower than desired intakes of energy as well as many other essential nutrients (e.g., essential fatty acids, amino acids, calcium, vitamins, iron, and other trace minerals). On the other hand, as noted above, a recent study in Finland (12) provides little support for this concern.

The efficacy of such a diet during childhood in lowering serum cholesterol was confirmed by the Finnish study. However, the extent to which this reduces the risk of atherosclerosis later in life has been questioned. Although fatty streaks are present in the aortas of most 10-year-old children, the distribution of fibrous plaques, the characteristic lesion of atherosclerosis, is less ubiquitous (38). Moreover, it is not certain that fatty streaks progress to fibrous plaques (39). The committee also emphasizes that the frequency of atherosclerotic lesions in casualties of the Vietnam war was about 40% lower than the frequency of such lesions in casualties of the Korean war (45 versus 77.3%) and that this change occurred without a major change in childhood dietary habits (40, 41). The decreasing incidence of atherosclerotic disease over the past several decades (42) is cited as yet another example of the lack of compelling evidence for the necessity of the proposed dietary changes during childhood.

Nonetheless, the committee concludes that the current dietary trends toward decreased consumption of saturated fats, cholesterol, and salt and increased consumption of polyunsaturated fats, if followed in moderation, are sensible for children over 2 years of age. A total fat intake of 30 to 40% of calories is considered reasonable for adequate growth and development. The committee also advocates counseling children and their parents on maintaining ideal weight and adopting other lifestyle practices likely to reduce the risks of atherosclerosis (exercise, avoidance of tobacco, etc.). Screening children over 2 years of age with a family history of atherosclerosis is recommended. If serum cholesterol concentration is elevated and not due to high-density lipoprotein cholesterol, appropriate dietary therapy to lower serum cholesterol is endorsed.

NUTRITIONAL REQUIREMENTS OF THE LOW-BIRTH-WEIGHT (LBW) INFANT

Approximately 7% of all infants born in the United States each year weigh less than 2500 g at birth, and over the past few decades, their survival has improved steadily. Today, for example, at least 75% of even the smallest such infants (those weighing <1000 g at birth) survive, and survival of larger LBW infants approaches 100%. This increasing number of surviving LBW infants must be fed, thus heightening awareness of the problems encountered in meeting their nutritional needs.

The importance of adequate early nutritional management of the LBW infant can be illustrated by considering the energy metabolism of the fasted infant. As in the adult, energy to meet ongoing needs during fasting is derived from endogenous stores of various nutrients. Although hepatic glycogen stores are used initially, these are quite limited and hence soon depleted. Thus, fat stores become the major source of endogenous energy, although protein stores are also used to provide amino acids from which glucose can be synthesized (gluconeogenesis) for use by tissues with an absolute requirement for glucose. Therefore, if hydration is adequate, the available endogenous stores of fat and protein ultimately determine how long a fasting infant can survive.

As illustrated in Table 51.7, body content of both protein and fat, particularly fat, increases throughout gestation (43). Thus, an infant weighing 3500 g at birth has more-extensive endogenous nutrient reserves than one weighing 2000 g, and an infant weighing 1000 g has very limited reserves. In other words, the smaller the infant, the more marked is its inability to withstand starvation. Assuming on-going energy needs of 50 kcal/kg/day, the 1000-g infant who receives no exogenous nutrient intake has sufficient endogenous reserves to survive for only 4 to 5 days. The 2000-g infant has sufficient reserves to survive for approximately 12 days without exogenous nutrients, and the term infant has sufficient reserves to survive for approximately a month (44). Daily provision of glucose intravenously (e.g., 7.5 g/kg/day, the amount provided by 150 mL/kg/day of a 5% glucose solution or 75 mL/kg/day of a 10% glucose solution), theoretically, will prolong survival of the 1000-g, 2000-g, and 3500-g infant, respectively, by 7, 18, and 50 days (44).

These theoretical calculations depict in a semiquantitative manner the general clinical observations concerning the LBW infant's susceptibility to starvation and, hence, the necessity for careful attention to early nutritional management. In addition to this very practical role of early adequate nutrition, there is concern that inadequate nutrition at any time during the period of cellular proliferation of various organ systems, particularly the central nervous system, may result in nonrecoupable cellular deficits. This concern is based on evidence obtained primarily in rodents (45) but thought to be applicable to all species (46). If so, the prematurely born infant, whose brain would have grown considerably during the last trimester of intrauterine life, may be particularly vulnerable to inadequate nutrition. Although the period of cellular proliferation of the entire human brain encompasses at least the first 18 months of life (47) and transient cellular deficits apparently can be reversed if adequate nutrition is provided before the end of this period (48), little is known about the duration of cellular proliferation within specific regions of the brain. This uncertainty, coupled with the persistently high incidence of neurodevelopmental deficits in surviving LBW infants, suggests that better nutritional management not only might decrease mortality but also might improve neurodevelopmental outcome.

The factors discussed above are recognized by neonatologists, and the importance of early adequate nutritional management of the LBW infant is generally accepted. As a result, the general subject of the LBW infant's nutritional requirements is an area of active investigation. The discussion that follows attempts to summarize the present state of knowledge.

Table 51.7
Intrauterine Accretion Rates of Various Nutrients during the Last Trimester of Pregnancy

	Accumulation during Various Stages of Gestation[a]		
Component	26–30 Weeks	30–34 Weeks	34–38 Weeks
Weight (g)	600	750	930
Protein (g)	68	97	126
Fat (g)	60	95	145
Water (g)	459	539	627
Calcium (g)	3.4	5.12	8.7
Phosphorus (g)	2.2	3.3	5.4
Magnesium (mg)	93	131	193
Sodium (mEq)	46	53	64
Potassium (mEq)	25	31	39
Chloride (mEq)	35	37	37

Adapted from Ziegler EE, O'Donnell AM, Nelson SE, et al. Growth 1976;40:329–40.
[a]Body weight increases from 880 g at 26 weeks to 1480 g at 30 weeks, 2230 g at 34 weeks, and 3160 g at 38 weeks.

Goals of Nutritional Management

The most generally accepted goal for nutritional management of the LBW infant is to provide sufficient amounts of all nutrients to support, at a minimum, continuation of the intrauterine rate of growth (49). Thus, the LBW infant's minimal requirements for various nutrients are assumed to be the amounts necessary to allow their accumulation at intrauterine rates (Table 51.7). This concept figures prominently in the recommended nutrient intakes for LBW infants proposed by the Committee on Nutrition of the American Academy of Pediatrics (Table 51.8) as well as the composition of formulas designed for feeding the hospitalized LBW infant (Table 51.9).

Opposing views concerning the goals for nutritional management of LBW infants include, on one hand, the fear that failure to provide human milk will deprive the infant of factors needed for optimal development of the gastrointestinal tract and immune system and, on the other, the desire to produce the most rapid growth rate possible, thereby recouping as quickly as possible the roughly 10 to 15% of body weight usually lost over the first several days of life and also possibly reducing the duration and hence the cost of hospitalization. Proponents of the former view advocate feeding human milk because of its theoretical nonnutritional benefits: enhanced maternal infant bonding, protection against infection and necrotizing enterocolitis, and better neurodevelopmental outcome. They also point out that the lower protein content of human milk is less likely to overwhelm the LBW infant's limited capacity to catabolize excess protein. Proponents of the latter view stress the potential advantages of catch-

Table 51.8
Recommended Nutrient Intakes for Low-Birth-Weight Infants

Nutrient	Recommended Intake (amount/100 kcal)
Protein (g)	2.7–3.1
Fat (g)	4.3–5.4 (300 mg essential fatty acids)
Carbohydrate	—
Electrolytes and minerals	
Sodium (mEq)	2.3–2.7
Potassium (mEq)	1.8–1.9
Calcium (mg)	140–160
Magnesium (mg)	6.5–7.5
Phosphorus (mg)	95–108
Chloride (mEq)	2–2.4
Iron[a]	
Zinc (mg)	0.5
Copper (μg)	90
Manganese (μg)	5
Iodine (μg)	5
Vitamins	Amount/day
Vitamin A (IU)	1400
Vitamin D (IU)	500
Vitamin E (IU)	5–25 (1.0 IU/g linoleic acid)
Vitamin C (mg)	35
Thiamin (μg)	300
Riboflavin (μg)	400
Niacin (mg)	6
Vitamin B_6	300 (15 μg/g protein)
Folic acid (μg)	50
Vitamin B_{12} (μg)	0.3
Pantothenic acid (mg)	2
Biotin (μg)	35

American Academy of Pediatrics Committee on Nutrition. Pediatrics 1985;75:976–86. Lower values are the recommended intakes for larger infants; higher values are the recommended intakes for smaller infants (BW < 1250 g).
[a]See text.

up growth and point out that protein intakes well in excess of those from human milk do not appear to tax the LBW infant's ability to catabolize protein.

Results from a multicenter study conducted in the early 1980s in England (50) provide considerable insight into this longstanding controversy. In this study, infants whose mothers elected to provide milk for feeding their infants were assigned randomly to receive supplements of either banked human milk or formula, and infants whose mothers elected not to provide milk were assigned randomly, at some centers, to receive either a preterm formula or banked human milk and, at others, to receive a preterm or term formula. Thus, to some extent, the usual confounding factor of the mother's intent to breast feed or not breast feed her infant was controlled, and infants also received a variety of protein intakes. Results published to date indicate that infants fed human milk, either as the sole diet or with formula, have a lower incidence of necrotizing enterocolitis during the neonatal period and also appear to be more resistant to infection (51). In addition, while developmental indices at 18 months of age were higher in formula-fed infants who received preterm formula than in those who received term formula (i.e., higher vs. lower protein intake) during the neonatal period (52), those fed human milk were less adversely affected (53). Moreover, when all groups were combined, those fed human milk during hospitalization, either their mother's milk or banked milk, had a neurodevelopmental advantage at 7 to 8 years of age (54).

Energy Requirements

LBW infants are usually assumed to require approximately 120 kcal/kg/day, 75 kcal/kg/day for resting expenditure and the remainder for specific dynamic action (10 kcal/kg/day), replacement of inevitable stool losses (10 kcal/kg/day), and growth (25 kcal/kg/day). The usual allotment for resting needs (75 kcal/kg/day) includes the basal requirement (50–60 kcal/kg/day) as well as additional requirements imposed by activity and response to cold stress. However, LBW infants are relatively inactive, and with careful control of environmental temperature, energy expenditure in response to cold stress is minimal. In fact, studies in relatively inactive infants maintained in a strictly thermoneutral environment suggest that their resting energy requirement (i.e., the basal requirement plus requirements for activity and response to cold stress) is closer to 60 kcal/kg/day (55–59). The energy required for specific dynamic action, or the thermic effect of food (i.e., the difference between resting energy expenditure of the fed infant and that of the fasted infant), may be a function of the composition of the diet. Protein intake was once thought to be the primary determinant of this component, but more-recent studies suggest that energy intake may be equally important (57–59). Fecal loss of nutrients, especially fat, appears to be inevitable in the fed LBW infant. The extent of this loss is a function of the infant's stage of development and the nature of the fat intake (see "Fat Requirements"). In infants fed either human milk or modern formulas, stool fat losses rarely exceed 15% of the fat intake, or less than 7.5% of the total energy intake.

The precise energy requirement for growth is unknown. This requirement includes two components: the energy cost of synthesizing new tissue (which probably is small and included in the measurement of resting expenditure) and the energy value of stored nutrients. Values of 3 to 6 kcal/g weight gain have been reported for the latter component. Since this obviously depends upon the composition of the newly synthesized tissue (e.g., deposition of calorically dense fat tissue requires more calories than deposition of lean body mass), such a range is to be expected. The calculated energy value of tissue deposited by the fetus between the 30th and 38th weeks of gestation is 2.0 to 2.5 kcal/g (Table 51.7), whereas the calculated energy value of tissue deposited by the normally growing term infant between birth and 4 months of age is approximately 4.5 kcal/g (60).

Thus, the energy requirement of the LBW infant may range from 95 to 160 kcal/kg/day. Aside from growth, the

Table 51.9
Composition (amount/100 kcal) of Standard Formulas for Low-Birth-Weight Infants

Component	Similac Special Care[a]	Enfamil Premature[b]
Protein (g)	2.71 (bovine milk, whey)	3 (bovine milk, whey)
Fat (g)	5.43 (medium-chain triglycerides, soy and coconut oils)	5.1 (medium-chain triglycerides, soy and coconut oils)
Carbohydrate (g)	10.6 (lactose, glucose polymers)	11.1 (lactose, corn syrup solids)
Electrolytes and minerals		
Calcium (mg)	180	165
Phosphorus (mg)	100	83
Magnesium (mg)	12	6.8
Iron (mg)	1.8 (0.37)[c]	1.8
Zinc (mg)	1.5	1.5
Manganese (mg)	12	6.3
Copper (μg)	250	125
Iodine (μg)	6	25
Selenium (μg)	1.8	—
Sodium (mg)	43	39
Potassium (mg)	129	103
Chloride (mg)	81	85
Vitamins		
Vitamin A (IU)	680	1250
Vitamin D (IU)	150	270
Vitamin E (IU)	4	6.3
Vitamin K (μg)	12	8
Thiamin (μg)	250	200
Riboflavin (μg)	620	300
Vitamin B_6 (μg)	250	150
Vitamin B_{12} (μg)	0.55	0.25
Niacin (μg)	5000	4000
Folic acid (μg)	37	35
Pantothenic acid (μg)	1900	1200
Vitamin C (mg)	37	20
Biotin (μg)	37	4
Cholin (mg)	10	12
Inositol (mg)	5.5	17

[a]Ross Laboratories, Columbus, Ohio.
[b]Mead Johnson Nutritionals, Evansville, Indiana.
[c]Iron content of low-iron formula.

factors of greatest quantitative importance are the infant's activity state and the environmental conditions under which it is nursed. For most LBW infants, an energy intake of 120 kcal/kg/day is adequate.

Protein Requirements

The then-common practice of feeding LBW infants human milk was largely abandoned about 50 years ago after Gordon et al. (61) showed that higher protein intakes resulted in a greater rate of weight gain. However, the formulas used in this study also contained more electrolytes and minerals than human milk, and some attributed the greater weight gain to water retention secondary to the greater electrolyte/mineral intake rather than to the greater protein intake. This debate was finally settled when subsequent studies demonstrated that both total body water and extracellular fluid of infants fed high-protein, high-solute intakes exceeded those observed in infants fed low-solute formulas (62). Nonetheless, that there also is a direct relationship between protein intake and deposition of lean body mass, independent of its water content (62–64).

In general, a protein intake of approximately 3 g/kg/day appears to be adequate for the LBW infant (65). On the other hand, higher intakes are well tolerated metabolically and support a greater rate of weight gain (64, 65). The protein, of course, must provide sufficient amounts of all essential amino acids including, for the LBW infant, histidine (66), tyrosine (67), and cysteine (67, 68). In this regard, current LBW infant formulas contain "humanized" bovine milk protein (60% whey proteins and 40% caseins). However, despite a higher cyst(e)ine content, there is little evidence that this protein is more efficacious than unmodified bovine milk protein (18% whey protein and 82% caseins), particularly with respect to growth (69). Of theoretical interest is the fact that plasma threonine concentrations of infants fed "humanized" bovine milk formulas are approximately double those observed in infants fed unmodified bovine milk protein, while plasma tyrosine concentrations are higher in infants fed unmodified bovine milk formulas (69–71).

Fat Requirements

Although fat accounts for about half of the nonprotein energy content of human milk and most infant formulas, including those designed for LBW infants, the only known requirement for fat in human nutrition is to provide essential fatty acids. Formerly, it was thought that this requirement could be met by providing 2 to 4% of the total energy intake as linoleic acid, but it is now clear that some linolenic acid also is required (72). Some also feel that the LBW infant, and perhaps the term infant as well, also may require longer-chain, more-unsaturated ω-6 and ω-3 fatty acids, e.g., arachidonic acid and docosahexaenoic acid (73–76). These latter fatty acids rather than their precursors, linoleic and linolenic acids, accumulate in the central nervous system during development (77, 78). However, plasma and erythrocyte lipid levels of these polyunsaturated fatty acids (PUFAs) are lower in infants who do not receive an exogenous source of these fatty acids (79). Currently, formulas containing long-chain PUFAs are available in Europe and Asia, but to date, such formulas are not available in North America. Most available studies suggest that supplementation with these fatty acids may have at least transient benefits for visual function of LBW infants (80, 81). On the other hand, since these fatty acids are quite bioactive (e.g., precursors of eicosanoids), there is concern about the safety of supplemented products.

Carbohydrate Requirements

The central nervous system and the hematopoietic tissue depend primarily on glucose as a metabolic fuel. However, glucose can be produced from either exogenously administered protein or endogenous protein stores (gluconeo genesis). Thus, in contrast to requirements for specific amino acids and fatty acids, there appears to be no absolute requirement for carbohydrate. On the other hand, exogenous glucose often is necessary to prevent hypoglycemia, particularly during the immediate neonatal period.

Carbohydrates, like fat, make up approximately half of the nonprotein energy content of human milk and infant formulas, including those designed for LBW infants. Although the predominant carbohydrate of human milk is lactose, LBW infant formulas usually contain a mixture of lactose and glucose polymers (Table 51.9). Development of intestinal lactase activity lags behind development of other disaccharidases, but most viable infants tolerate lactose quite well. In fact, satisfactory clinical progress has been observed with formulas that contain only lactose, only sucrose, only glucose, only glucose polymers, and mixtures of these sugars.

Fluid Requirements

Several bases of reference have been suggested for estimating maintenance fluid requirements: for example, body weight, body surface area, and energy expenditure. Of these, energy expenditure, which focuses attention on the physiologic and nonphysiologic factors most likely to modify fluid requirements (e.g., body temperature, ambient temperature, ambient humidity, activity, and respiratory rate), seems most relevant. In the older infant, the maintenance fluid requirement is approximately 1 mL/kcal expended. This allotment replaces usual insensible water losses through the lungs and skin as well as obligatory renal and gastrointestinal losses.

Insensible water loss varies considerably among infants, particularly LBW infants. Moreover, both pulmonary and cutaneous components of insensible water loss are related inversely to ambient humidity. Under usual nursery conditions, the insensible water loss of term infants is approximately 30 mL/100 kcal. In the very small infant with altered skin permeability to water, cutaneous losses may be considerably greater, although nursing the infant in relatively high humidity tends to decrease both this component of insensible fluid loss and pulmonary losses. Phototherapy, a common modality for treating LBW infants with hyperbilirubinemia, also increases insensible water losses (82). Thus, the insensible water losses of LBW infants usually are at least twice those of the term infant, and those of the most immature LBW infants may be severalfold greater.

Obligatory renal losses of LBW infants also are quite variable. While even very immature infants can regulate the volume of urine excreted according to the solute load and the available water, renal concentrating and diluting mechanisms are both somewhat limited (83). In general, sufficient fluid to allow a urinary volume of 50 to 60 mL/100 kcal permits excretion of the usual range of solute loads at urinary concentrations of 150 to 450 mOsm/L, which are easily achieved, even by a very immature kidney.

In unfed infants, fluid losses via the gastrointestinal tract are minimal. If the infant is fed, however, approximately 10% of the fluid intake is lost in stool. Infants receiving phototherapy lose even more water in stool (82).

The fluid requirement for growth is a function of both the rate of growth and the water content of the newly synthesized tissue. The water content of tissue deposited during the last trimester of gestation is approximately 70% (Table 51.7), whereas the water content of the tissue deposited by the term infant between birth and 4 months of age is 40 to 45% (60). An estimate of 50 to 60% for the growing LBW infant seems reasonable.

The water requirements for insensible (30–60 mL/100 kcal) and obligatory losses (50–60 mL/100 kcal) as well as for growth (10–20 mL/100 kcal) are reduced by the endogenously produced water of oxidation, approximately 12 mL/100 kcal. Thus, the LBW infant, like the term infant, seems to have a minimum water requirement of about 1 mL/kcal used. The fasting infant thus requires at least 65 to 75 mL/kg/day, while the growing infant requires at least 120 mL/kg/day; however, the very immature infant and the infant undergoing phototherapy may require much more. In general, a fluid intake of 140 mL/kg/day is well tolerated by most infants after the first few days of life. Intakes above this amount are thought to increase the likelihood of developing patent ductus arteriosus.

Electrolyte Requirements

The estimated daily obligatory electrolyte losses of the term infant after the first several days of life are approximately 0.5 mEq/kg of both sodium and chloride and approximately 0.75 mEq/kg of potassium. Since renal reabsorption mechanisms are not fully developed in the LBW infant, their renal losses are likely to be greater. Electrolyte losses probably are greater also in infants with increased fluid losses secondary to phototherapy, etc.

The electrolytes required for tissue synthesis, of course, depend upon the rate of growth. Assuming continuation of the intrauterine growth rate (Table 51.7), the daily requirement of these nutrients for tissue synthesis would approximate the amounts that accumulate during the last trimester of gestation: 1.0 to 1.5 mEq/kg/day of sodium and 0.5 to 1.0 mEq/kg/day of both potassium and chloride. If the rate of weight gain is more or less than the intrauterine rate, or if the composition of weight gain is different, the requirements obviously change proportionally. In this regard, the neonate usually deposits less extracellular fluid than the fetus and, hence, less sodium.

The minimal daily sodium, potassium, and chloride requirements of the LBW infant receiving adequate protein and energy and growing at the intrauterine rate are, respectively, 1.5to 2.0 mEq/kg, 1.25 to 1.75 mEq/kg, and 1.0 to 1.5 mEq/kg. Enough potassium and chloride is present in the volumes of both human milk and commonly used formulas usually ingested to provide these requirements. However, the sodium content of human milk (approximately 1.2 mEq/100 kcal), even if completely absorbed, may be low. On the other hand, the growth rate of LBW infants fed human milk is somewhat lower than the intrauterine rate; therefore, their sodium requirement for growth probably is less than 1.5 mEq/kg/day. The intakes recommended by the Committee on Nutrition of the American Academy of Pediatrics are considerably higher than these minimal intakes (Table 51.8).

Mineral Requirements

Early studies of calcium and phosphorus needs were directed toward defining the intakes necessary to prevent hypocalcemia. Since this condition develops more commonly in infants fed formulas with a high content of phosphorus relative to calcium (i.e., a low calcium:phosphorus ratio), the calcium:phosphorus ratio rather than the absolute intakes of either mineral was emphasized. Experience has shown that a ratio of roughly 1.5 to 2.0 is satisfactory.

The amount of calcium retained during the latter part of normal intrauterine growth is approximately 5 mmol/kg/day. Human milk can provide only about 0.5 mmol/kg/day, and this is not completely absorbed. Thus, if the LBW infant's requirement for calcium is assumed to be the amount necessary to support continuation of the rate of accumulation that occurs in utero, human milk obviously contains inadequate calcium. The phosphorus content of human milk also is low. Moreover, LBW infants fed human milk have less dense skeletons radiographically than those fed formulas containing large amounts of calcium, and many develop rickets and/or fractures (84). Thus, LBW infants fed human milk, including those fed their own mother's milk, require supplemental calcium and phosphorus for optimal skeletal mineralization.

Iron requirements depend upon the existing body stores and the rate of growth. The LBW infant obviously has more-limited stores of iron than the term infant and, therefore, is more susceptible to development of iron deficiency, especially during periods of rapid growth. It has been estimated that the LBW infant's endogenous iron stores, in the absence of exogenous intake, would be depleted sometime during the 2nd or 3rd month of life rather than during the 4th or 5th month of life, as occurs in the term infant. However, most LBW infants experience further depletion of iron stores secondary to blood losses incident to biochemical monitoring during periods of clinical instability. Thus, it is recommended that the LBW infant receive iron supplements or iron-fortified formulas as early as possible. Such supplements, however, may increase the infant's need for vitamin E, especially when formulas high in PUFAs are fed (see below). In addition, the bactericidal properties of the iron-binding proteins of human milk (lactoferrin and lactoglobulin) are abolished if they are saturated with iron (85). Current LBW infant formulas contain moderate amounts of polyunsaturated fats, ample vitamin E, and 0.37 to 1.88 mg/100 kcal of iron (Table 51.9).

Little information is available concerning the LBW infant's requirements for other trace minerals. In general, the recommended intakes of these minerals are based on either the amounts provided by human milk or the amounts that accumulate in utero during the last trimester of pregnancy.

The amounts listed in Table 51.8 appear adequate. A zinc intake of 500 μg/100 kcal, assuming 50% absorption from the gastrointestinal tract, should allow accumulation of zinc at the intrauterine rate. The concentration of zinc in human milk is approximately 3 to 5 mg/L; thus, it provides minimally adequate zinc to allow accumulation at the intrauterine rate. On the other hand, zinc in human milk is absorbed more efficiently than that in bovine milk (86). The recommended copper intake (see Table 51.8) is approximately the amount present in human milk, which might not allow accumulation of copper at the intrauterine rate. Thus, some recommend a higher copper intake.

Since hepatic stores of copper are quite large, this probably is not necessary.

Vitamin Requirements

Specific recommendations concerning either requirements or advisable allowances of vitamins for LBW infants are not available; thus, it is usually suggested that the RDAs for term infants be given. Infants fed sufficient amounts of either human milk or artificial formulas to produce adequate growth usually receive sufficient amounts of all vitamins, although human milk may be deficient in vitamin D. Nonetheless, since consumption of sufficient volumes of formula to satisfy vitamin requirements may not be attained for several weeks, a supplement containing vitamins A, C, and D is often recommended. In addition, the LBW infant may have special needs for vitamin E.

Vitamin E functions as an antioxidant to prevent peroxidation of PUFAs in various cell membranes. Thus, it is not surprising that inadequate vitamin E intake results in erythrocyte hemolysis (87). Since the PUFA content of all membranes is related to intake of these fatty acids or their precursors, infant formulas containing vegetable oils with a high PUFA content impose a greater vitamin E requirement. Such formulas, therefore, should contain more vitamin E. In general, the aim should be to provide at least 1 IU of vitamin E per gram of PUFAs—an E:PUFA ratio of 1. This may need to be reevaluated if formulas are supplemented with long-chain PUFAs (see above).

LBW infants fed formulas containing PUFAs and given therapeutic doses of iron also have a greater incidence of erythrocyte hemolysis and lower serum vitamin E levels than infants fed formulas containing less iron and PUFAs (88). Thus, the relationship between the vitamin E and iron contents of the formula as well as the relationship between the vitamin E and polyunsaturated fat contents of the formula are important. For this reason, careful attention must be given to vitamin E intake if iron supplements are given. The fatty acid, iron; and vitamin E contents of current LBW infant formulas appear to be appropriate.

Large doses of vitamin E have been recommended to prevent both retrolental fibroplasia (89) and bronchopulmonary dysplasia (90). However, it is not clear that these recommendations are warranted, particularly considering the potential toxicity of the large doses recommended.

Delivery of Nutrient Requirements to LBW infants

For most LBW infants, the foregoing discussion of nutrient requirements is largely academic. Underlying illnesses as well as a number of neurophysiologic deficiencies (e.g., poor or unsustained suck, uncoordinated sucking and swallowing mechanisms, delayed gastric emptying, and poor intestinal motility) make delivery of enteral nutrition virtually impossible, particularly during the early neonatal period. During this time, a nutritional regimen that prevents catabolism and allows some increment in lean body mass probably is satisfactory. This more realistic goal for the first several days of life can be achieved in sick LBW infants with a parenteral regimen that provides as few as 60 kcal/kg/day, an amino acid intake of 2.0 to 3.0 g/kg/day, and necessary electrolytes, minerals, and vitamins (91, 92). A similar regimen delivered enterally should be equally efficacious if intestinal absorption is not severely compromised.

Various methods of delivering nutrients by the intravenous route (total parenteral nutrition) as well as methods of delivering feedings by the gastrointestinal tract (e.g., continuous nasogastric or transpyloric infusions) have been proposed as alternatives to more conventional feeding techniques. Although no one method is likely to be ideal for all situations, use of a combination of these methods of nutrient delivery, allowing the particular clinical problems of an individual infant to dictate the method of delivery, should improve nutritional management. In many infants, a combination of conventional as well as these less conventional methods of feeding permits delivery of sufficient nutrients to support "normal" growth by 1 to 2 weeks of age.

Within reason, every infant should be given a trial at conventional feeding, i.e., tolerated nipple or gavage feedings of either human milk or a standard formula, plus intravenous supplementation with 5 to 10% glucose solutions. If adequate nutrients cannot be delivered in this way, a trial of continuous nasogastric or transpyloric feedings is warranted. Tolerated enteral feedings delivered conventionally or by continuous infusion also can be supplemented by intravenous infusions of appropriate mixtures of glucose, amino acids, and/or lipid. If enteral feedings are not tolerated, parenteral administration of a balanced nutritional mixture is indicated. A regimen that provides 75 kcal/kg/day plus amino acids, electrolytes, minerals, and vitamins can be delivered by peripheral vein infusion without imposing an unreasonable fluid load. Such a regimen almost certainly maintains existing body composition and, hence, is particularly applicable for infants who are likely to tolerate enteral intake within a brief period of time. Use of a central vein catheter allows delivery of a more concentrated nutrient mixture and is particularly useful in situations associated with prolonged intolerance of enteral feedings.

Role of Human Milk in Feeding the LBW Infant

Although many advocate feeding the LBW infant human milk, evidence that it is nutritionally superior for this population is lacking. In fact, the growth rate of LBW infants fed human milk, even that of infants fed their own mother's milk, which has approximately 20% more protein than term human milk (93), is lower than that of infants fed LBW formulas (94). Moreover, plasma albumin and prealbumin (transthyretin) concentrations often fall to frankly low values (95). In addition, the low amounts of calcium and phosphorus do not support adequate skeletal mineralization.

In contrast to the nutritional disadvantages of human milk for the LBW infant, its immunologic properties may be a distinct advantage. These properties (i.e., cellular as well as humoral components), theoretically, may confer passive immunity and/or enhance immunologic maturation, thereby providing some protection against infections and perhaps necrotizing enterocolitis. Indeed, recent studies show that the incidence of both infection and necrotizing enterocolitis are lower in infants fed either banked human milk or their own mother's milk (see above). Clearly, these advantages of human milk, may far outweigh its nutritional disadvantages.

The steps involved in collecting, storing, and dispensing expressed human milk make inadvertent contamination likely. Thus, stringent hygienic techniques and bacterial screening are mandatory to ensure bacteriologic safety. Viral contamination also is a concern. For example, CMV excretion in the milk of seropositive women is relatively common (96), and CMV infection has been reported in infants fed CMV-positive milk (97). Moreover, one case of HIV infection transmitted by human milk has been reported (98). Herpes and rubella viruses and hepatitis B surface antigen also have been detected in human milk, but transmission of these viruses via milk has not been demonstrated.

Clearly, more research is necessary to elucidate the role of human milk, provided by either the infant's mother or a donor (or donors), in feeding the LBW infant. This research should be well under way before enormous expense and effort are spent in establishing milk banks to supply safe human milk for routine feeding of LBW infants. On the other hand, if an individual mother wishes to provide milk for her infant, the potential psychologic benefits of her involvement in the infant's care as well as the benefits with respect to eventual success in nursing are strong reasons for encouraging milk expression until the infant can be breast-fed. Moreover, two commercial preparations for supplementing human milk with protein, calcium, phosphorus, sodium, and vitamins are available, and use of these supplements appears to overcome many of the nutritional inadequacies of human milk for LBW infants (99, 100).

REFERENCES

1. Food and Nutrition Board, National Research Council. Recommended dietary allowances. 10th ed. Washington, DC: National Academy Press, 1989.
2. Butte NF. Eur J Clin Nutr 1996;S24–36.
3. Agostoni C, Riva E, Bell R, et al. J Am Coll Nutr 1994;13:658–64.
4. Ponder DL, Innis SM, Benson JD, Siegman JS. Pediatr Res 1992;32:683–8.
5. Farquaharson J, Jamieson EC, Abbasi KA, et al. Arch Dis Child 1995;72:198–203.
6. Makrides M, Neumann MA, Byard RW, et al. Am J Clin Nutr 1994;60:189–94.
7. Jorgensen MH, Hernell O, Lund P, et al. Lipids 1996; 31:99–105.
8. Auestad N, Montalto MB, Hall RT, et al. Pediatr Res 1997;41:1–10.
9. Carlson SE, Ford AJ, Werkman SH, et al. Pediatr Res 1996;39:882–8.
10. Heird WC, Prager TC, Anderson RE. Curr Opin Lipidol 1997;8:12–6.
11. Committee on Nutrition, American Academy of Pediatrics. Pediatrics 1992;89:525–7.
12. Niinikoski H, Lapinleimu H, Viikari J, et al. Pediatrics 1997;99:687–94.
13. Holt LE Jr, Snyderman SE. JAMA 1961;175:100–3.
14. Fomon SJ, Thomas LN, Filer LJ, et al. Acta Pediatr Scand 1973;62:33–45.
15. Räihä NCR. Pediatrics 1985;75:136–41.
16. Dewey KG, Beaton G, Fjeld C, et al. Eur J Clin Nutr 1996;50:S119–50.
17. Holliday MA. Do dietary factors in the 6 to 12 month period of life affect blood pressure later in life? In: Heird WC, ed. Nutritional needs of the six- to twelve-month-old infant. New York: Raven Press, 1991;283–95.
18. American Academy of Pediatrics Committee on Nutrition. Pediatrics 1976;58:765–8.
19. Lakdewala DR, Widdowson EM. Lancet 1977;1:167–8.
20. American Academy of Pediatrics Committee on Nutrition. Pediatrics 1980;65:657–8.
21. Wall Street Journal. 22 July 1994;1.
22. Fomon SJ. Recommendations for feeding normal infants. In: Craven L, Billus L, eds. Nutrition of normal infants. St. Louis: Mosby Year Book, 1993;455.
23. Heird WC, ed. Nutritional needs of the six- to twelve-month-old infant. New York: Raven Press, 1991.
24. Whitehead RG, Paul AA. Dietary energy needs from 6 to 12 months of age. In: Heird WC, ed. Nutritional needs of the six- to twelve-month-old infant. New York: Raven Press, 1991; 135–48.
25. Montgomery RK. Functional development of the gastrointestinal tract the small intestine. In: Heird WC, ed. Nutritional needs of the six- to twelve-month-old infant. New York: Raven Press, 1991;1–17.
26. Mandel ID. The nutritional impact on dental caries. In: Heird WC, ed. Nutritional needs of the six- to twelve-month-old infant. New York: Raven Press, 1991;89–107.
27. Purvis GA, Bartholmey SJ. Infant feeding practices: commercially prepared baby foods. In: Tsang R, Nichols B, eds. Nutrition during infancy. Philadelphia: Hanley & Belfus, 1988;399–417.
28. American Academy of Pediatrics, Committee on Nutrition. Pediatrics 1983;72:253–5.
29. Ryan AS, Martinez GA, Kreiger FW. Am J Phys Anthropol 1987;73:539–48.
30. Martinez GA, Ryan AS, Malec DJ. Am J Dis Child 1985;139:1010–8.
31. Crawford MA, Stassam AG, Stevens PA. Prog Lipid Res 1981;20:31–40.
32. Davis CM. Am J Dis Child 1928;36:651–79.
33. Birch LI, Johnson SI, Andersen G, et al. N Engl J Med 1991;324:232–5.
34. Weidman W, Kwiterovich P Jr, Jesse MJ, et al. Circulation 1983;67:1411A–4A.
35. Wynder EL, Berenson GS, Epstein FH, et al. Prev Med 1983;12:728–40.
36. Consensus Development Panel. JAMA 1985;253:2080–6.

37. American Academy of Pediatrics Committee on Nutrition. Pediatrics 1986;78:521–5.
38. Ross R, Glomset JA. N Engl J Med 1976;295:369–77; (Part II) 1976;295:420–5.
39. Small DM. N Engl J Med 1977;297:873–7; (Part II) 1977;297:924–9.
40. McNamara JJ, Molot MA, Stremple JF, et al. JAMA 1971;216:1185–7.
41. Enos WF, Holmes RH, Beyer J. JAMA 1953;152:1090–3.
42. Health United States 1984: US Department of Health and Human Services publ. no. 851232. Washington, DC: Government Printing Office, 1984.
43. Ziegler EE, O'Donnell AM, Nelson SE, et al. Growth 1976;40:329–40.
44. Heird WC. Nutritional support of the pediatric patient including the low birth weight infant. In: Winters RW, Greene HC, eds. Nutritional support of the seriously ill patient. New York: Academic Press, 1983;157–79.
45. Fish I, Winick M. Exp Neurol 1969;25:534–70.
46. Winick M, Rosso P. Pediatr Res 1969;3:181–4.
47. Winick M, Rosso P, Waterlow J. Exp Neurol 1970;26:293–300.
48. Grantham-McGregor SM, Powell CA, Walker SP, Himes JH. Lancet 1991;338:1–5.
49. American Academy of Pediatrics Committee on Nutrition. Pediatrics 1985;75:976–86.
50. Lucas A, Gore SM, Cole TJ, et al. Arch Dis Child 1984;59: 722–30.
51. Lucas A, Cole TJ. Lancet 1990;336:1519–23.
52. Lucas A, Morley R, Cole TJ. Lancet 1990;335:1477–81.
53. Lucas A, Morley R, Cole TJ, Gore SM. Arch Dis Chld 1994;70:F141–6.
54. Lucas A, Morley R. Lancet 1991;339:261–4.
55. Whyte RK, Haslam R, Vlainic L, et al. Pediatr Res 1983;17: 891–8.
56. Reichman BL, Chessex P, Putet G, et al. Pediatrics 1982;69:446–51.
57. Schulze KF, Stefanski M, Masterson J, et al. J Pediatr 1987;110:753–9.
58. Van Aerde J, Sauer P, Heim T, et al. Pediatr Res 1985; 13:215–20.
59. Brooke OG, Alvear J, Arnold M. Pediatr Res 1969;13:215–20.
60. Fomon SJ. Pediatrics 1967;40:863–70.
61. Gordon HH, Levine SZ, McNamara H. Am J Dis Child 1947;73:442–52.
62. Kagan BM, Stanicova V, Felix NS, et al. Am J Clin Nutr 1972;25:1153–67.
63. Davidson M, Levine SZ, Bauer CH, et al. J Pediatr 1967; 70:694–713.
64. Kashyap S, Forsyth M, Zucker C, et al. J Pediatr 1986;108:955–63.
65. Kashyap S, Schulze KF, Forsyth M, et al. J Pediatr 1988;113: 713–21.
66. Snyderman SE, Boyer A, Rothman E, et al. Pediatrics 1963;31:786–801.
67. Snyderman SE. The protein and amino acid requirements of the premature infant. In: Jonxis JHP, Visser HKA, Troelstra JA, eds. Metabolic processes in the fetus and newborn infant. Leiden: Steinfert Kruesse, 1971;128–41.
68. Sturman JA, Gaull GE, Räihä NCR. Science 1970;169:74–6.
69. Kashyap S, Okamoto E, Kanaya S, et al. Pediatrics 1987; 79:748–55.
70. Rassin DK, Gaull GE, Heinonen K, et al. Pediatrics 1977;59: 407–22.
71. Rassin DK, Gaull GE, Räihä NCR, et al. J Pediatr 1977; 90:356–60.
72. Holman RT, Johnson SB, Hateh TF. Am J Clin Nutr 1982;35:617–23.
73. ESPGAN Committee on Nutrition. Acta Paediatr Scand 1991;80:887–96.
74. British Nutrition Foundation Task Force on Unsaturated Fatty Acids. Unsaturated fatty acids and early development. In: Unsaturated fatty acids: nutritional and physiological significance. London: Chapman & Hall, 1992;63–67.
75. Food and Agriculture Organization/World Health Organization. Lipids in early development. In: Fats and oils in human nutrition: report of a joint expert consultation. Rome: FAO/WHO, 1994;49–55.
76. ISSFAL Board Statement. ISSFAL Newslett 1994;1:4–5.
77. Clandinin MT, Chappell JE, Leong S, et al. Early Hum Dev 1980;4:121–9.
78. Clandinin MT, Chappell JE, Leong S, et al. Early Hum Dev 1980;4:131–8.
79. Carlson SE, Rhodes PG, Ferguson MG. Am J Clin Nutr 1986; 44:798–804.
80. Uauy RD, Birch DG, Birch EE, et al. Pediatr Res 1990; 28:485–92.
81. Carlson SE, Cooke RJ, Rhodes PG, et al. Pediatr Res 1991;30(5):404–12.
82. Oh W, Kareoki H. Am J Dis Child 1972;124:130–232.
83. Aperia A, Broberger O, Herin P, et al. Acta Pediatr Scand (Suppl) 1983;305:61–5.
84. Steichen JJ, Gratton TL, Tsang RC. J Pediatr 1980;96:528–34.
85. Bullen JJ, Rogers HJ, Leigh L. Br Med J 1972;1:69–75.
86. Sanstrom B, Cedeblad A, Lonnerdal B. Am J Dis Child 1983;137:726–9.
87. Oski FA, Barness LA. J Pediatr 1967;70:211–20.
88. Williams ML, Shoot RJ, O'Neal PL, Oski FA. N Engl J Med 1975;292:887–90.
89. Mintz-Hittner H, Godio LB, Rudolph AJ, et al. N Engl J Med 1981;305:1366–71.
90. Ehrenkranz RA, Bonta BW, Ablow RC, Warshaw JB. N Engl J Med 1978;299:564–9.
91. Anderson TL, Muttart CR, Bieber MA, et al. J Pediatr 1979;94: 947–51.
92. Kashyap S, Heird WC. Protein requirements of low birthweight, very low birthweight, and small for gestational age infants. In: Räihä NCR, ed. Protein metabolism during infancy. Nestlé nutrition workshop series, vol 33, Nestlé Ltd. New York: Vevey/Raven Press, 1995;133–51.
93. Atkinson SA, Anderson GH, Bryan MH. Am J Clin Nutr 1980;33:811–5.
94. Gross SJ. N Engl J Med 1983;308:237–41.
95. Kashyap S, Schulze KF, Forsyth M, et al. Am J Clin Nutr 1990;52:254–62.
96. Stagno S, Reynolds DW, Pass RF, et al. N Engl J Med 1980;302:1073–6.
97. Ballard RA, Drew WL, Hufnagle KG, et al. Am J Dis Child 1979;133:482–5.
98. Ziegler JR, Cooper DA, Johnson RO, et al. Lancet 1985;1:896–7.
99. Schanler RJ, Hurst NM. Semin Perinatol 1994;18:476–84.
100. Schanler RJ, Burns PA, Abrams SA, et al. Pediatr Res 1992;31:583–6.

52. Diet, Nutrition, and Adolescence

FELIX P. HEALD and ELIZABETH J. GONG

The nutritional requirements of adolescents are influenced primarily by the normal events of puberty and the simultaneous growth spurt. Puberty is an intensely anabolic period, with increases in height and weight, alterations in body composition resulting from increased lean body mass and changes in the quantity and distribution of fat, and enlargement of many organ systems. Adolescence is a unique period of development of physiologic, psychosocial, and cognitive levels, all of which affect the nutritional needs of the adolescent. The teenager is a rapidly changing biologic organism, and so nutritional management of adolescents must consider the rapid growth, maturation, and psychosocial changes of each individual. Three aspects of growth must be emphasized: the intensity and extent of the pubertal growth spurt, the sexual differences in the timing of growth as well as the nature of change of body composition, and individual variation in the timing of the pubertal growth spurt.

The velocity of growth exerts a major influence on nutrient requirements. Adolescence is the only time in extrauterine life when growth velocity increases. The average American female experiences her most rapid spurt in linear growth between ages 10 and 13 years; the growth spurt of the average American male occurs about 2 years later, between 12 and 15 years. (See Appendix Tables III-A-14-e-1 and 2 for height velocity in centiles of girls and boys, respectively. Data from NHANES I and II for stature of girls and boys are given in Appendix Tables III-A-14-c-1-a and b by height, by age, and percentiles are given in Table A.15a.) This time is frequently termed *the period of maximum growth,* and for both height and weight, it is greatest in girls in the year preceding menarche. The linear spurt during adolescence contributes about 15% to final adult height; its contribution to the adult weight is approximately 50%. (NHANES I and II data on weight in girls and boys by percentiles are given in Appendix III-A-14-b-1 and 2, weight by age and percentiles in Appendix Table III-A-15-b, and weight by height in percentiles for males and females in Appendix Tables III-A-15-c and d, respectively.) Therefore, nutrition clearly plays a significant role in the doubling of body mass during pubescence. Because nutritional requirements are closely related to rapid increase in body mass, it is not surprising that peak nutritional requirements appear to occur during the year of maximum growth.

Although both adolescent males and females gain significant weight, gender-related differences exist with respect to the rate, quantity, composition, and distribution of tissues. During adolescence, boys tend to gain more weight at a faster rate, and their skeletal growth continues for a longer time than that of adolescent girls. Girls deposit relatively more total body fat; boys deposit more muscle mass (see Chapter 49). Patterns of body composition and distribution diverge during adolescence. Boys become leaner and paradoxically increase the number of actual adipose tissue cells while decreasing the percentage contribution of fat to total body mass. Girls have a steep rate of increase in actual fat deposition as well as increased percentage of fat to total body mass and increased lean body mass. As a result of pubertal changes, males have a larger lean body mass, a larger skeleton, and less adipose tissue as total body mass than females. As lean body mass has more active metabolic function than adipose tissue, sex differences in body composition produce sex differences in the nutritional requirements of adolescents (1, 2).

The large individual variance in the time at which the growth spurt begins, as well as the intensity of growth, makes chronologic age a poor index of nutritional requirements. Physiologic growth, or maturational age, is a better indicator for establishing requirements or evaluating intakes. Figure 52.1 illustrates three normal males and three normal females in prepubertal, midpubertal, and postpubertal stages of development (3). Although each group is at the same chronologic age, each individual is at different physiologic age; each adolescent has a different rate of growth and different body composition, both important determinants of nutrient needs. Standards for assessing physiologic age have been developed. Tanner's sexual maturity ratings are used widely clinically and are helpful in describing the stage of development of individual adolescents (4).

NUTRITIONAL REQUIREMENTS

Few actual data on adolescents are available on which to base recommendations for their nutrient needs. Most recommendations are based on estimates of intakes associated with good health and growth, extrapolations from animal research, or interpolation from studies on children

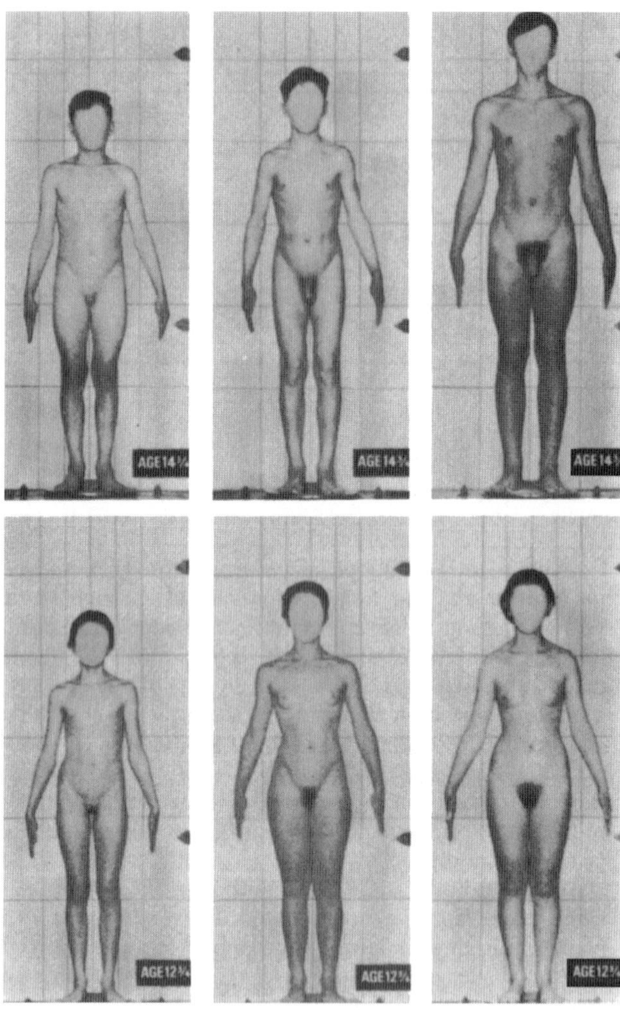

Figure 52.1. Differing degrees of adolescence at the same chronologic age. *Top,* Three boys all aged 14.25 years. *Bottom,* Three girls all aged 12.75 years. (From Tanner JM. Growth and endocrinology of the adolescent. In: Gardner LI, ed. Endocrine and genetic diseases of children and adolescents. Philadelphia: WB Saunders, 1975, with permission.)

and adults. The most recent recommended dietary allowances (RDAs) of the Food and Nutrition Board of the National Research Council (NRC) for adolescents are given in terms of weight, sex, and age (4-year intervals, except for the age group 19–24 years; this age class has been extended in the 1989 RDAs because peak bone mass probably is not attained before the age of 25 years) (5). (See also Appendix Tables II-A-2 to 8 for U.S. and other national and international dietary reference values for energy and various nutrients.)

Energy

The caloric requirements for the growing adolescent have not been studied enough to give an accurate expression of the energy needs of individual teenagers. Some of the best data come from a study done by Wait et al. (6). Energy intake data from bomb calorimetry determinations support the thesis that the relationship of total calories to height or calories per unit height per age are the preferred indices for determining caloric needs. From these observations, as well as supporting findings of Widdowson (7), it appears that increments in height during adolescence may best represent the anabolic effect of this growth period. The practical application of determining individual requirements using the kilocalorie per centimeter has been described. RDAs calculated on kilocalorie per centimeter of height for males and females are shown in Table 52.1.

In a group of normally growing teenagers followed longitudinally, Beal noted that actual energy intake for some teens fell outside the range of the RDA (8). Thus, even when using the parameter for calculating calories best supported by data (kilocalorie per centimeter height), the margin of error is considerable. Nevertheless, kilocalorie per centimeter height may represent the best way to calculate individual energy requirements of adolescents at the present time.

A review of studies of energy intake of children and adolescents in the United States shows that girls appear to consume their peak caloric intake, about 2550 kcal, at the time of menarche (around 12 years). This peak demand is followed by a slow decline. In boys, caloric intake appears to parallel the adolescent growth spurt, increasing until age 16 years to approximately 3400 kcal and then decreasing by 500 kcal by age 19 years (9).

The most accepted way of assessing adequacy of energy intake is to evaluate growth and body composition. The normal variability of pubertal growth patterns makes ideal weight during puberty an untenable concept. A common practice is to plot height and weight on the National Center for Health Statistics (NCHS) growth chart with the percentiles for each age group (10). This plot tells us the position of that teenager relative to the NCHS sample. Growth data gathered in the NCHS survey published in 1973 form the basis for the growth charts currently used in the United States (11) (see Appendix Tables III-A-12-d and e). If multiple measurements over time are available, any significant changes in rates of linear growth or body mass can be detected by percentile shifts. However, the teenager in the 90th percentile for height may or may not be appropriately in the 90th percentile for weight. For

Table 52.1
Recommended Energy Intakes for Adolescents

Age (years)	Average Allowance (kcal/cm height)	(kcal/day)
Males		
11–14	15.9	2500
15–18	17.0	3000
19–24	16.4	2900
Females		
11–14	14.0	2200
15–18	13.5	2200
19–24	13.4	2200

From Food and Nutrition Board, National Research Council. Recommended dietary allowances. 10th ed. Washington, DC: National Academy Press, 1989.

example, a male at the 90th percentile weight-for-height with a triceps skinfold in the lower percentiles would be muscular. Another teenager in the 90th percentile weight-for-height with a triceps skinfold in the 95th percentile would be classified as obese (survey data summarized in Appendix Tables III-A-14-a-1 through 4).

To determine appropriate weight-for-height for an adolescent and assess whether he or she has excess or deficient energy intake, the height and weight of youths 12–17 years, United States (11) tables (Appendix Tables III-A-14-c-1-b and 2-b, d-1-b and 2-b, and III-A-15.) are often used clinically. The data are problematic (such as sample size, lack of references to sexual maturity, ethnic differences, etc.), although the tables separate the percentiles of weight by age, sex, and height, providing a range of weights for a particular height and age. With the additional information gained from triceps percentiles (Appendix Tables III-A-14-b-1 and 2), overweight (triceps skinfold >95th percentile) or underweight (triceps skinfold <25th percentile) can be assessed.

The National Center for Health data have been analyzed in such a sophisticated way that accurate assessment of growth and simple measures of body composition are available to measure the impact of energy excess or scarcity on the growing teenager. However, the effects of marginal energy deficits have a subtle effect on growth. The work of Dreizen et al. (12) is one of the few studies in the United States of the long-term effect of chronic mild malnutrition on growth. The net effect over time was a diminished rate of growth during late childhood and adolescence and delay of puberty by 2 years, but ultimately, this group of malnourished youths in southeastern United States reached heights and weights similar to those of a comparison group. Keeping in mind the great variation in timing and intensity of growth seen in adolescents, we must emphasize the large variation in caloric intake in this group.

Physical activity also contributes significantly to the total energy requirement of an individual, as does previous growth and nutritional status. When considering the energy requirements of adolescents, the importance of individual variation from one adolescent to another must be recognized in making nutritional recommendations. Table 52.2 presents energy expenditure, expressed in three different body weights, for different activities (13). The different activities have highly variable energy costs and can be used to guide dietary advice or weight management.

Table 52.2
Energy Expenditure of Selected Activities (calories expended/min activity)

Activity	kcal/min/kg	45 kg	55 kg	65 kg
Basketball	0.138	6.2	7.6	9.0
Cycling				
5.5 mph	0.064	2.9	3.5	4.2
9.4 mph	0.100	4.5	5.5	6.5
Dancing (twist)	0.168	7.6	9.2	10.9
Football	0.132	5.9	7.3	8.6
Running				
11.5 min/mile	0.135	6.1	7.4	8.8
8 min/mile	0.208	9.4	11.4	13.6
Sitting quietly	0.021	0.9	1.2	1.4
Walking, normal pace	0.080	3.6	4.4	5.2
Writing, sitting	0.029	1.3	1.6	1.9
Vacuuming				
Females	0.045	2.0	2.5	2.9
Males	0.048	2.2	2.6	3.1
Ironing				
Females	0.033	1.5	1.8	2.1
Males	0.064	2.9	3.5	4.2

Adapted from McArdle WD, Katch FI, Katch VL. Exercise physiology: energy, nutrition, and human performance. Philadelphia: Lea & Febiger, 1991.

Protein

As with energy recommendations, protein needs for an adolescent are more useful when physiologic age is emphasized over chronologic age. Using the RDA for protein related to height is probably the most useful method for determining protein needs for adolescents (5). For adolescent males, the daily protein recommendations are 0.29, 0.34, and 0.33 g/cm height for the age groups 11 to 14, 15 to 18, and 19 to 24 years, respectively. For adolescent females, the daily recommendations are 0.29, 0.27, and 0.28 g/cm height for the age groups 11 to 14, 15 to 18, and 19 to 24 years, respectively. The protein requirement is determined by the amount needed for maintenance plus that needed for growth of new tissue, which during adolescence may represent a substantial portion of the total need. Unfortunately, data on either of these determinants of requirements are lacking for adolescents and have been interpolated from results of studies involving infants and adults (5, 14).

The RDA for daily protein intake for adolescents ranges from 44 to 59 g (5). Peak intakes of protein coincide with the peak energy intake. The proportion of total energy intake represented by protein remains fairly constant, between 12 and 14%, throughout childhood and adolescence (9).

Results of studies show that average intakes of protein in adolescents exceed the recommended levels (9, 15, 16). Although it appears that most adolescents in the United States have sufficient protein intake, some teenagers who restrict food intake because of a desire to lose weight, eating disorders such as anorexia nervosa and bulimia, or socioeconomic problems, may be at risk of poor protein intake. Without adequate caloric intake, protein is used in gluconeogenesis and is unavailable for tissue synthesis. Heald and Hunt demonstrated that in the rapidly growing adolescent, protein metabolism is particularly sensitive to caloric restriction (17).

Anthropometric measurements generally are a simple way to assess protein status. Height, weight, and midarm circumference measurements (used to assess lean body mass) can be used as growth indicators. Midarm circumference measurements and arm muscle area between the 25th and 75th percentiles probably indicate good nutritional status (18).

Biochemical assessments of protein nutriture include creatinine/height index and serum concentrations of certain proteins: albumin, transferrin, prealbumin, and retinol-binding protein (19–22). Determinations of prealbumin and retinol-binding protein are the most sensitive indicators of changes in diet that may indicate subclinical malnutrition (22). A detailed evaluation of assessment procedures is given in Chapter 56.

Minerals

Because of the adolescent growth spurt, the need for three minerals is of particular importance: calcium to sustain increased skeletal mass, iron to aid expansion of red cell and muscle mass, and zinc to generate new skeletal and muscle tissues. In addition to significant increases in need, intake of these nutrients has been shown to be below the recommended levels for adolescents (15, 16, 23–25).

Boys take in more calcium than do girls and are closer to achieving the recommended intakes (26). Daily iron intakes reported by the Ten State Nutrition Survey were relatively lower. Most (80%) girls 10 to 16 years of age were below the recommended 18 mg of iron per day (15). Some evidence shows an association between low concentrations of zinc in hair and poor growth. An analysis of food intake suggests poor eating habits (27). The full extent of zinc deficiency and its adverse effect on puberty needs more inquiry.

Calcium

With approximately 99% of total-body calcium in the skeleton (28), the adolescent growth spurt associated with increased skeletal length and mass obviously has a significant impact on dietary requirements for calcium. Skeletal growth during adolescence accounts for approximately 45% of the adult skeletal mass. Because the absolute amount of calcium in the skeleton of a boy in the 95th percentile for height and that for a boy in the 5th percentile for height will differ by 36%, the calcium needs of these two boys will differ sharply because of the difference in skeletal size. The problem is compounded further by the normal differences in pubertal development, making age and sex alone poor predictors of individual calcium needs. Lastly, growth of skeletal mass and gains in height and muscle mass continue until the third decade of life (29–31). Table 52.3 shows the average increments of body calcium for adolescence and the daily increments of body calcium at the peak of the growth spurt. At the peak of growth, daily deposition of calcium is approximately twice the average increment during the adolescent period. The daily peak increment of calcium during the growth spurt is greater, occurs later, and lasts longer in boys than in girls (28).

Table 52.3
Daily Increments in Body Content Due to Growth

Mineral		Average for Age 10–20 years (mg)	At Peak of Growth Spurt Period (mg)
Calcium	M	210	400
	F	110	240
Iron	M	0.57	1.1
	F	0.23	0.9
Nitrogen	M	320	610 (3.8 g protein)
	F	160	360 (2.2 g protein)
Zinc	M	0.27	0.50
	F	0.18	0.31
Magnesium	M	4.4	8.4
	F	2.3	5.0

From Forbes GB. Nutritional requirements in adolescence. In: Suskind RM, ed. Textbook of pediatric nutrition. New York: Raven Press, 1981, with permission.

The amount of calcium absorbed from different dietary sources varies. During peak periods of growth in adolescence, the average calcium retention is approximately 300 mg/day. Because the lower range of absorption is approximately 30%, a minimum of 900 mg/day of calcium would be necessary during active skeletal growth (32).

A wide difference exists in the daily allowances of calcium recommended by two expert committees. The WHO recommends intakes of 600 to 700 mg/day for 11- to 15-year-old adolescents and 500 to 600 mg/day for 16- to 19-year-old adolescents (30). The National Institutes of Health Consensus Conference recommended 1200 to 1500 mg/day for adolescents and young adults (11–24 years) (33). The Food and Nutrition Board's 1997 dietary reference intake value for ages 9 through 18 years is 1300 mg/day (33a) (see Appendix Tables II-A-2-b-1; see also Chapter 7). These differences in recommended intakes show that the amounts of dietary calcium needed to sustain growth and to provide maintenance require further study.

Establishing requirements for the teenage group is difficult because many individuals can achieve equilibrium on a wide range of dietary intakes. A large error is likely in calculating calcium balance because of errors in measuring intakes and excretions, individual differences in rate of biologic maturation; and effects on calcium metabolism of protein, vitamin D, phosphorus, fiber (31), caffeine, and sucrose (32).

Surveys in the United States reveal that adolescent girls are less likely to meet the recommended levels of calcium than are teenage boys (15, 16, 23). In addition, preliminary evidence suggests that adolescent females may need more calcium to reach optimal bone mass. In a recent study, 1500 mg/day of calcium was needed for maximal calcium retention in a small group of 14-year-old girls (34).

Data from retrospective studies indicate that low calcium intakes during adolescence are associated with lower bone densities in women (35, 36). In a recent study, bone density was correlated with calcium intake in a group of boys and girls 2 to 16 years of age. Those ingesting more than 1000 mg/day of calcium had greater bone density than those ingesting less. Most serum determinations of calcium, phosphate, magnesium, alkaline phosphate, parathyroid hormone, 25-hydroxyvitamin D and 1,25-dihydroxyvitamin D levels were normal and not correlated with bone mineral status (37). Decreased bone density may increase the risk of osteoporosis in later life (38, 39). Teen mothers who breast-feed may also be at risk for poor calcium balance. Lactating adolescents who consumed about 900 mg/day of calcium had a 10% decline in bone mineral content. Lactating teen mothers who consumed 1600 mg of calcium remained in calcium balance (40).

Iron

Iron deficiency is found in all races, both sexes, and all socioeconomic groups (see Chapters 10 and 88). Teenagers require additional iron to synthesize substantial amounts of new myoglobin and hemoglobin. As puberty is initiated, boys accumulate more lean body mass than girls. In fact, at the end of puberty, boys have twice the lean body mass of girls. Thus, Hepner calculated that for each additional kilogram of added tissue, males require 42 mg iron/kg body weight, compared with 31 mg iron/kg body weight for girls (41). In addition to the described sex differences, the normal biologic differences in body size make a tremendous difference in iron requirements. For example, a boy in the 97th percentile for body weight requires twice as much iron as a boy in the 3rd percentile.

Dietary intake of iron must suffice to account for losses in feces, urine, skin, and menstruation, as well as to provide for expansion of red cell volume and for tissue growth in adolescence. The NRC recommends an additional 2 mg/day for males during the pubertal growth spurt (between ages 10 and 17 years), for a total of 12 mg/day of iron (5). With menarche, the adolescent girl has additional iron loss from menstruation. The NRC recommends an additional 5 mg/day for females, starting with the pubertal growth spurt and menstruation, which begins at approximately 11 to 14 years. The iron recommendation for adolescent females is 15 mg/day (5).

In a comprehensive review of iron requirements, Bowering et al. could find only one report on a controlled study with adolescents (42). In the iron balance study of six adolescent girls, Schlaphoff and Johnson found that 0.62 to 1.82 mg/day (mean, 1.0 mg/day) was retained, which included iron required to replace menstrual losses (43). Assuming a rate of 10% absorption, they recommended a daily intake of 12 to 13 mg iron. Similar balance data are not available for boys. Finally, the amount of iron available in the American diet is estimated at 6 mg/1000 calories. Therefore, teenage girls whose caloric intake varies between 2000 and 2400 calories may find it difficult to ingest 15 mg of iron from dietary sources alone. Bioavailability of dietary iron is critical in iron nutrition. Diets high in lean meat and ascorbic acid and low in phytate cover the iron requirements of most nonpregnant women (44).

In the Ten State Nutrition Survey, between 5 and 10% of teenagers had hemoglobin or hematocrit levels below normal (15). Analysis of data from the Health and Nutrition Examination Survey (HANES) II showed the highest prevalence of impaired iron status (ferritin model) was in teenagers—14.2% of the 15- to 19-year-old females and 12.1% of the 11- to 14-year-old males (45). The results of other studies vary (46, 47), generally reporting more iron deficiency than iron deficiency anemia in adolescents.

Results of several large surveys—the Ten State Nutrition Survey (48), the HANES I (47), and the HANES II (49)—have shown a racial difference in hemoglobin level in adolescents. Blacks have approximately 1 g less hemoglobin than whites, which apparently is unrelated to socioeconomic level, education, diet, or obesity (50). These differences have led many authors to recommend race-specific standards in screening for anemia (48, 51–55). Although use of different standards for hemoglobin concentration has been proposed, the biochemical basis for the racial difference in hemoglobin is unknown. The factors affecting hemoglobin differences, including genetic, socioeconomic, and dietary, are complex. At the present time, no data indicate that iron needs of black and white adolescents are different. Clearly, the standards for "normal" values used in any study determine the amount of iron deficiency or anemia in any population. Measurements of hematocrit and hemoglobin, the most widely used screening procedures for anemia, are relatively insensitive indicators. The diagnosis of iron deficiency can be made by using the serum ferritin level, which provides the most accurate assessment of iron stores. The true nature of iron deficiency anemia in adolescents awaits more sophisticated studies.

Adolescent athletes may be at risk of iron deficiency caused by red blood cell destruction, increased need for red blood cell and tissue synthesis during puberty, or poor dietary intake (53, 54). Many (34–44%) teenage female runners have been found to be iron deficient, as assessed by low iron stores (53, 54). This deficiency is associated with abnormal gastrointestinal bleeding (54).

Sports anemia may also be common; increased destruction of erythrocytes and a transient drop in hemoglobin concentration in the adolescent athlete results from an acute stress-response to exercise training. However, because the causes and treatments of sports anemia remain controversial, no basis currently exists for recommending iron supplementation for this transient condition (55, 56).

Zinc

Zinc affects protein synthesis and is essential for growth. Zinc is particularly important in adolescence because of the rapid rate of growth and sexual maturation. Table 52.3 reveals that during the adolescent growth spurt, zinc retention in both males and females is much higher than the average for the adolescent period. This striking increase in zinc retention is related to the increase of lean body mass during this period (57).

The 1989 RDAs (5) reduced the daily zinc intake to 12 mg for adolescent females on the basis of their lower body weight. The recommendation for males remained at 15 mg/day.

Zinc deficiency has been associated with growth retardation and hypogonadism in adolescents (58, 59); zinc supplementation resulted in accelerated growth and sexual maturation (58, 60). Poor dietary zinc sources and inhibition of zinc absorption by phytates in high-cereal diets contributed to the evolution of zinc deficiency and were major factors in growth retardation and delayed sexual maturation (59).

Evidence that adolescents undergoing rapid growth may be highly susceptible to inadequate dietary zinc is provided by Butrimovitz and Purdy (61). These investigators found low plasma zinc concentrations during infancy and puberty, both periods of rapid growth. For adolescent girls and boys, plasma zinc levels were lowest at the ages when puberty was expected to occur.

Mild zinc deficiency has been reported in the United States. Hambidge et al. studied zinc status in apparently healthy children in Denver and found an association between low growth percentiles, diminished taste acuity, and low hair zinc levels (62). Apparently, marginal zinc status may be a health problem in American children. Adolescents undergoing rapid growth are at risk for inadequate zinc levels. Young pregnant teenagers may be particularly susceptible to zinc deficiency, because of the rapid cell division and growth of the developing fetus as well as continued growth of the biologically immature teenager. These teenagers should be encouraged to include such zinc-rich foods in their daily intake as poultry, lean meats, lowfat and nonfat dairy products, legumes, and grain products, particularly whole grains (63).

Vitamins

Data on vitamin requirements for adolescents are even more limited than those for mineral requirements. The vitamin requirements for youth are interpolated from data on infant and adult allowances; few data are derived directly from studies on adolescents. Emphasis should be placed on vitamins necessary for the additional nutrient requirements of the pubertal growth spurt.

Vitamin A is required for vision, growth, cellular differentiation and proliferation, reproduction, and immune system integrity. Vitamin A levels and intake in adolescents are considerably below the recommended amount (15, 16, 64, 65). Vitamin D is involved in maintaining homeostasis of calcium and phosphorus in the mineralization of bone. No controlled studies exist on vitamin D requirements for adolescents.

Vitamin C is essential for collagen synthesis, and intakes in adolescents are often below the recommended levels (66, 67). Added to the unknown demands of growth and changes in vitamin C status because of smoking (68, 69) and oral contraceptive use (70), some teenagers may have problems with vitamin C adequacy.

Because of its role in DNA synthesis, folate is important during periods of increased cell replication and growth. Folate status may be at risk in some adolescents, particularly those from low-income populations (71) and pregnant teenagers (72). The recent association of folate deficiency with neurotubal defects emphasizes the importance of adequate folate intake in teenage girls (73). The FDA has recently mandated fortification of standard enriched grain products with folate. Dietary intakes and serum folate levels have indicated poor folate status in adolescent girls (74–76) and boys (76).

Adolescents appear to have increased need for vitamin B_{12}, which is required for rapid cell growth, particularly during the growth spurt. Vitamin B_6 is involved in a large number of enzyme systems associated with nitrogen metabolism. The rapid growth of muscle mass, particularly in boys, makes vitamin B_6 adequacy important during puberty. Riboflavin, niacin, and thiamin are involved in energy metabolism and thus are also important during puberty.

SPECIAL NUTRITIONAL PROBLEMS

Effect of Nutrition during Adolescence on Adult Morbidity and Mortality

Prospective studies of adults who are overweight or obese generally show increased morbidity and mortality. Does any of the risk in morbidity and mortality result from obesity originating during childhood or adolescence? (For discussion of adolescent obesity see Chapter 63.) Or does the risk result from adult obesity? What about thinness during the juvenile period as a predictor of disease or increased mortality during maturity in adults? Is promotion of growth in height and weight during childhood and adolescence consistent with optimal adult health? The answers to these questions have significant implications for health professionals advising adolescents on nutritional matters. This discussion only applies to populations in which food supplies are adequate and available.

Many studies associate obesity in adults with increased morbidity and mortality from a variety of clinical disorders. As Bray indicates, cardiovascular disease, hypertension, diabetes mellitus, gallbladder disease, osteoarthritis, and colon cancer are major coconditions seen more frequently in obese adults (77). Bray goes on to say that in adults whose BMI exceeds 30 kg/m^2, more than 50% of all-cause mortality among those in the United States aged 20 to 74 years can be attributed to overweight.

Until recently, little was known about the effect of overweight during adolescence as a predictor of disease in adults. Subjects from the Harvard Growth Study (1922–1935) were followed for 55 years. They were then classified as overweight or lean. Morbidity and mortality data from this cohort clearly predicted additional health risks for adults who were overweight adolescents compared with those who were lean. The risk of death from all causes and of coronary heart disease is elevated in men who were overweight as adolescents. Men have a higher risk of atherosclerotic cerebrovascular disease and colon cancer. In contrast, in women overweight as adolescents, all cause or cause-specific mortality is not increased in adulthood.

Other studies have shown a risk of increased morbidity from coronary heart disease and atherosclerosis in men and women who were overweight as teenagers. Morbidity from colorectal cancer and gout was elevated in men overweight during adolescence. Arthritis was significantly higher in women who were overweight as adolescents. These risks were strongly predicted by overweight during adolescence, compared with adult-onset obesity (78). This concept is further supported by other long-term studies (79, 80).

There are no population studies on the effect of thinness during adolescence on adult morbidity and mortality. Waaler suggests that the excess morbidity and mortality associated with short stature and low weight may result from poor nutrition during growth (81). The one model that may give clues to the effect of thinness on adult health is anorexia or bulimia. These disorders are most common in adolescent girls when bone growth is at its peak. Once puberty is complete, very little bone growth occurs. Osteopenia is a common complication of anorexia nervosa during adolescence (82). The concern is raised that osteopenia developed by anorectic girls may not be reversible. Thus, osteoporosis may be the eventual outcome of this undernutrition during adolescence. Further research will determine whether this is true.

Brain mass is reduced in anorexia nervosa. Cognitive defects have been described during the acute phase of this disorder. Reduction in brain mass is important as it occurs during brain development. Long-term follow-up is necessary to determine whether these deficits result in significant brain malfunction as an adult.

The state of nutrition during adolescence is important in determining morbidity and mortality during adult life. How much and what kind of food is enough for growth compatible with optimal adult health? Is maximal growth the same as optimal growth? These important questions must await the results of more research.

Eating Disorders

As mentioned above, two major eating disorders, anorexia nervosa and bulimia (or bulimia nervosa), may pose major problems in adolescence (83–85) (see also Chapter 93). Most eating disorder patients develop the problem during adolescence. Some of the psychologic changes in adolescence may make it difficult to distinguish an adolescent with "normal" eating habits from one with an eating disorder. Adolescents may use food as a means of experimenting, gaining control, or establishing themselves as individuals. Dissatisfaction with body weight, fear of obesity (resulting in unhealthy eating behavior), and preoccupation with dieting are common among today's youth, particularly adolescent girls (86–89). Mellin et al. (90) found a high prevalence of disordered eating, particularly dieting; fear of fatness; and binge eating in a group of middle-class predominantly white girls and adolescents. Additional studies suggest that unhealthy weight-control behaviors occur in adolescents of other ethnic/racial subgroups (88, 91) and in adolescents with chronic illness (92).

Adolescents with eating disorders should be evaluated and treated by an interdisciplinary team of professionals with expertise in treating adolescents (93, 94). Interdisciplinary treatment should be appropriate for the teenager's developmental needs. Recent findings from a group of over 33,000 adolescents suggest that frequent dieting and eating-disordered behaviors should not be viewed in isolation. These eating-disordered behaviors occur in a broader social context of adolescent health and risk-taking behavior (95).

Pregnancy

Nutritional care of the pregnant adolescent must consider the health of both mother and infant. Knowledge of the role of nutrients is vital, as is consideration of the principles of adolescent growth and development. Physiologically, the adolescent is at risk if she has not completed her growth (96–99). Individual variability is great, but most growth occurs before menarche. Linear growth in the adolescent female typically is not completed until approximately 4 years after the onset of menarche. Although the rate of growth after menarche has decelerated considerably, growth allowances should still be considered.

Gynecologic age (the difference between chronologic age and age at menarche) can give some indication of physiologic maturity and growth potential. A young adolescent (gynecologic age, 2 years or less) who becomes pregnant may still be growing. Her own needs for growth and development, along with the extra demands of fetal growth, make the nutrient requirements of this young teen higher than those of a pregnant adult (96, 100) (see also Chapter 50).

The few studies that have focused on the energy needs of pregnant teenagers generally report that the teenagers frequently do not achieve the caloric intake recommended by the NRC (5). Naeye hypothesized that optimal weight gains for fetal survival may be higher in young teenagers because mother and infant compete for nutrients (101). Recent findings appear to support such a competition (102–104). Results of further studies (104–108) suggest that optimal weight gains for adolescents during pregnancy, particularly for girls who are biologically immature (104), are greater than the adult recommendations.

The Institute of Medicine (109) recommends (by prepregnancy weight-for-height) that young adolescents strive for weight gains at the upper end of the ranges suggested for adults. Young adolescents (<2 years postmenarche) may deliver smaller infants for a given weight gain than do older women (109, 110). Inadequate weight gain during pregnancy has been associated with low-birth-weight infants (111) and preterm delivery in pregnant teens (112). Inadequate weight gain during early stages of adolescent pregnancy was associated with significant deficits in infant birth weight and increased risk of low-birth-weight and small-for-gestational-age infants (112–114).

Recent studies have found that adolescents deliver a disproportionate number of very low birth weight infants (115) and low-birth-weight infants, compared with adult mothers (116). In addition, low-birth-weight infants of teen mothers were associated with higher neonatal mortality (116). Teenagers who smoke may be at increased risk of low prenatal weight gain and reduced infant birth weight (107, 117).

Preliminary data from our research using anthropometric measurements as predictors of low-birth-weight outcome in pregnant teenagers suggest that mothers of low-birth-weight infants tend to exhibit prenatal depletion of fat reserves (estimated from triceps skinfold measurements and from calculating arm fat area), while mothers of normal-birth-weight infants accumulate fat (118). In addition, prenatal protein stores of mothers of low-birth-weight infants changed little, whereas mothers delivering normal-birth-weight infants gained protein stores (estimated from midarm circumference measurements and arm muscle area calculations). Scholl et al. (104) found that despite weight gain and accumulation of fat stores during pregnancy, growing adolescents delivered infants with lower birth weights than those of nongrowing teenagers and adult women. Estimates of energy requirements indicate that sedentary adolescents needed at least 2400 to 2600 kcal/day. Physically active or rapidly growing adolescents needed additional energy, perhaps 50 kcal/kg pregnant body weight/day (119).

The issue of protein requirements for the pregnant adolescent is complex. Using careful nitrogen balance studies on pregnant teenagers, King et al. presented the best experimental data on which to base protein recommendations (120). Their data suggested greater nitrogen retention than was previously reported. In addition, maternal lean tissue of these adolescents increased during pregnancy, particularly during the last half of pregnancy.

Iron deficiency anemia in pregnancy has been associated with increased risk of preterm delivery and low birth weight (121–123). The recommended intake of iron for pregnant adolescents is 30 mg/day, which is twice the recommendation for the nonpregnant teenage girl (5).

Zinc metabolism is an important consideration during pregnancy. Data from a study of a small group of teenagers (124) are consistent with results of studies in adults, indicating that prenatal iron supplementation impairs zinc retention. However, these adolescents did not show lower serum zinc concentrations during the second and third trimesters, as observed in adults, implying differences in zinc metabolism between adolescent and adult pregnancy (124). Prenatal zinc supplementation in low-income teenagers was associated with improved pregnancy outcome and reduced numbers of premature births, compared with a placebo group (125).

On the basis of recent data, it appears pregnant teenagers, particularly those who may still be in their own growth phase, do have increased needs for nutrients during pregnancy. The pregnant adolescent needs an additional 300 calories and 14 to 16 more grams of protein daily, which can be supplied by addition of foods such as those shown on Table 52.4 (126).

Vegetarian Diets

During a time of increased independence and decision making and greater influence by peers and role models, adolescents may use food as part of the process of individuation. Because nutritional needs are high, vegetarian teenagers may be particularly at risk for nutritional deficiencies, especially at the time of the growth spurt (see also Chapter 106).

Growing adolescents who are vegetarians may have problems meeting their energy requirements because of the high-bulk content of vegetarian food patterns. In addition, vegetarian diets that are low in animal products are low in fat content (127, 128). Without sufficient energy intake, protein is used as an energy source and thus is unavailable for tissue synthesis and growth. Hence, protein quality, protein quantity, and energy intake of the individual must be assessed. Other nutrients of concern for the teenage vegetarian, particularly the strict vegetarian (who excludes all foods of animal origin), include calcium, iron, zinc, and vitamins D and B_{12} (127–131).

Conscious effort and careful planning are necessary to

Table 52.4
Foods to Increase Calories and Protein for the Pregnant Adolescent

Food	Calories	Protein (g)
Cereal (1 c), low-fat milk (8 oz), banana	330	
Peanut butter (2 tbsp) sandwich	320	
Cheese (2.5 oz) and 4 saltine crackers	320	
Cheeseburger (regular)	300	
Pizza, pepperoni (1/8 of 12" pizza)	180	
Baked or refried beans (1 c)		16
Meat or poultry (2 oz)		15
Peanut butter (2 tbsp) sandwich		13
Pizza, pepperoni (1/8 of 12" pizza)		10
Spaghetti with meat sauce (1 c)		12
Milk (12 oz)		12
Macaroni and cheese (3/4 c)		11

From Pennington JAT. Bowes and Church's food values of portions commonly used. 16th ed. New York: Harper & Row, 1994, with permission.

ensure adequacy of these nutrients. Supplements may be necessary to meet the recommended allowances. The vegetarian should carefully plan a diet from a variety of foods. Protein complementation (combining different plant foods so that low essential amino acids from one protein source are complemented by essential amino acids from another protein source, resulting in a complete protein) can ensure that the qualitative aspects of protein adequacy are met. Evaluation of the quantitative aspects of protein adequacy of the vegetarian is also necessary. The RDA for total protein intake during adolescence ranges from 44 to 59 g/day (5), providing energy requirements are met.

Vegetarian adolescents can generally meet their nutritional requirements for growth if they consume well-planned diets (129, 132). Vegetarian food guides for adolescents are available in such sources as reports by Marino and King (133), the University of California's *Creative Eater's Handbook* (134), Messina and Messina (130), and Johnston and Haddad (135). Haddad has developed daily dietary patterns for vegetarians at three different energy levels (136).

REFERENCES

1. Marshall WA, Tanner JM. Arch Dis Child 1969;44:291–303.
2. Marshall WA, Tanner JM. Arch Dis Child 1970;45:13–23.
3. Tanner JM. Growth and endocrinology of the adolescent. In: Gardner LI, ed. Endocrine and genetic diseases of children and adolescents. 2nd ed. Philadelphia: WB Saunders, 1975.
4. Tanner JM. Growth and adolescence. 2nd ed. Oxford: Blackwell Scientific, 1952.
5. Food and Nutrition Board, National Research Council. Recommended dietary allowances. 10th ed. Washington, DC: National Academy Press, 1989.
6. Wait B, Blair R, Roberts LJ. Am J Clin Nutr 1969;22:1383–96.
7. Widdowson EM. Medical Research Council special report series no. 257. London: His Majesty Stationery Office, 1947.
8. Beal VA. Nutritional intake. In: McCammon RW, ed. Human growth and development. Springfield, IL: Charles C Thomas, 1970.
9. Heald FP, Remmell PS, Mayer J. Caloric, protein and fat intake in children and adolescents. In: Heald FP, ed. Adolescent nutrition and growth. New York: Appleton-Century-Crofts, 1969.
10. National Center for Health Statistics. NCHS growth charts, 1976. Monthly vital statistics report 25(3) suppl. (HRA) 76-1120. Rockville, MD: National Center for Health, 1976.
11. National Center for Health Statistics. Vital Health Stat (11) 1973;124.
12. Dreizen S, Spirakis CN, Stone RE. J Pediatr 1967;70:256–63.
13. McArdle WD, Katch FI, Katch VL. Exercise physiology. Energy, nutrition, and human performance. Philadelphia: Lea & Febiger, 1991.
14. Johnson JA. Ann NY Acad Sci 1958;69:881–901.
15. Center for Disease Control. Ten State Nutrition Survey in the United States, 1968–1970. Atlanta, GA: Health Services and Mental Health Administration, 1972.
16. National Center for Health Statistics. Caloric and selected nutrient values for persons 1–74 years of age. First Health and Examination Survey, 1971–1974, DHEW publ. (PHS) 79-1657. Hyattsville, MD: National Center for Health, 1979.
17. Heald FP, Hunt SM. J Pediatr 1965;66:1035–41.
18. Frisancho AR. Am J Clin Nutr 1974;27:1052–8.
19. Jensen TG, Englert D, Dudrick SJ. Nutritional assessment. A manual for practitioners. Norwalk, CT: Appleton-Century-Crofts, 1983.
20. Ingenbleek Y, Van Den Schrieck HG, De Nayer P, et al. Clin Chim Acta 1975;63:61–7.
21. Ingenbleek Y, De Visscher M, De Nayer P. Lancet 1972;2: 106–9.
22. Shetty PS, Watrasiewicz KE, Jung RT, et al. Lancet 1979;2: 230–2.
23. Irwin MI, Kienholz EW. J Nutr 1973;103:1019–95.
24. Henkin RI. Trace elements in nutrition. New York: Marcel Dekker, 1971.
25. Committee on Nutrition, American Academy of Pediatrics. Pediatrics 1978;62:826–34.
26. Garn SM, Wagner B. The adolescent growth of the skeletal mass and its implications to mineral requirements. In: Heald FP, ed. Adolescent nutrition and growth. New York: Appleton-Century-Crofts, 1969.
27. Roche AF, Roberts J, Hamill PV. Vital Health Stat (11) 1978; 167:1–98.
28. Forbes GB. Nutritional requirements in adolescence. In: Suskind RM, ed. Textbook of pediatric nutrition. New York: Raven Press, 1981.
29. Greenwood CT, Richardson DP. World Rev Nutr Diet 1979; 33:1–41.
30. World Health Organization. Handbook on human nutritional requirements. Monograph series no. 61. Geneva: WHO, 1974.
31. Schuette SA, Linksweiler HM. Calcium. In: Present knowledge of nutrition. 5th ed. Washington, DC: Nutrition Foundation, 1984.
32. Hollinbery PW, Massey LK. (Abstract 1280) Fed Proc 1986;45:375.
33. Optimal calcium intake. NIH consensus statement. Bethesda, MD: National Institutes of Health, 1994.
33a. Food and Nutrition Board, Institute of Medicine. Dietary reference intakes for calcium, phosphorus, magnesium, vitamin D, and fluoride. Washington, DC: National Academy Press, 1997.
34. Matkovic V, Fontana D, Tominac C, et al. (Abstract 168) J Bone Miner Res 1986;(Suppl 1).
35. Sandler RB, Slemenda CW, LaPorte RE, et al. Am J Clin Nutr 1985;42:270–4.
36. Anderson JJB, Tylavsky FA, Lacey JM, et al. (Abstract 1841) Fed Proc 1987;46:632.
37. Chan GM. Am J Dis Child 1991;145:631–4.
38. Heaney RP, Gallagher JC, Johnston CC, et al. Am J Clin Nutr 1982;36(Suppl):986–1013.
39. Allen LH. Nutr Today 1986;21:6–10.
40. Chan GM, McMurry M, Westover K, et al. Am J Clin Nutr 1987;46:319–23.
41. Hepner RE. Nutrient requirements in adolescence. Cambridge: MIT Press, 1976.
42. Bowering J, Sanchez AM, Irwin MI. J Nutr 1976;106:985–1074.
43. Schlaphoff D, Johnson FA. J Nutr 1949;39:67–82.
44. Hulten L, Gramatkovski E, Gleerup A, et al. Eur J Clin Nutr 1995;49:794–808.
45. Expert Scientific Working Group. Am J Clin Nutr 1985; 42:1318–1330.
46. National Academy of Sciences, Food and Nutrition Board. Iron nutriture in adolescence. DHEW publ. no. (HSA) 77-5100. Washington DC: U.S. Department of Health, Education and Welfare, 1976.
47. Johnson CL, Abraham S. Hemoglobin and selected iron-

related findings of persons 1-74 years of age: United States, 1971–74. DHEW publication no. 46. Washington, DC: U.S. Department of Health, Education and Welfare, 1979.
48. Garn SM, Smith NJ, Clark DC. J Natl Med Assoc 1975;67:91–6.
49. Yip R, Johnson C, Dallman PR. Am J Clin Nutr 1984; 39:427–36.
50. Dallman PR, Barr GD, Allen CM, et al. Am J Clin Nutr 1978; 31:377–80.
51. Owen GM, Yanochik-Owen A. Am J Public Health 1977; 67:865–6.
52. Daniel WA Jr. Nutritional requirements of adolescents. In: Winick M, ed. Adolescent nutrition. New York: John Wiley & Sons, 1982.
53. Brown RT, McIntosh SM, Seabolt VR, et al. J Adolesc Health Care 1985;6:349–52.
54. Nickerson HJ, Holubets MC, Weiler BR, et al. J Pediatr 1989; 114:657–63.
55. Sports and Cardiovascular Nutritionists (SCAN) Dietetic Practice Group. Sports nutrition. In: Marcus JB, ed. A guide for the professional working with active people. Chicago: American Dietetic Association, 1986.
56. Position of the American Dietetic Association. J Am Diet Assoc 1987;87:933–9.
57. Sandstead HH. Am J Clin Nutr 1973;26:1251–60.
58. Prasad AS, Miale A Jr, Farid Z, et al. J Lab Clin Med 1963; 61:537–49.
59. Sandstead HH, Prasad AS, Schulert AR, et al. Am J Clin Nutr 1967;20:422–42.
60. Prasad AS, Halsted JA, Nadimi M. Am J Med 1961;31:532–46.
61. Butrimovitz GP, Purdy WC. Am J Clin Nutr 1978;31:1409–12.
62. Hambidge KM, Hambidge C, Jacobs M, et al. Pediatr Res 1972;6:868–74.
63. Moser-Veillon PB. J Am Diet Assoc 1990;90:1089–93.
64. Canada National Survey. Nutrition. A national priority. Ottawa: Department of National Health and Welfare, 1973.
65. Schorr BC, Sanjur D, Erickson EC. J Am Diet Assoc 1972; 61:415–20.
66. Huenemann RL, Shapiro LR, Hampton MC, et al. J Am Diet Assoc 1968;53:17–24.
67. Nelson M. Dietary practices of adolescents. In: Winick M, ed. Adolescent nutrition. New York: John Wiley & Sons, 1982.
68. Pelletier O. Am J Clin Nutr 1970;23:520–4.
69. Schectman G, Byrd JC, Gruchow HW. Am J Public Health 1989;79:158–62.
70. Rivers JM. Am J Clin Nutr 1975;28:550–4.
71. Daniel WA Jr, Gaines EG, Bennett DL. Am J Clin Nutr 1975;28:363–70.
72. Vande Mark MS, Wright AC. J Am Diet Assoc 1972;61:511–6.
73. Anon. MMWR 1991;40:513–6.
74. Kirksey A, Keaton K, Abernathy RP, et al. Am J Clin Nutr 1978;31:946–54.
75. Reiter LA, Boylan LM, Driskell J, et al. J Am Diet Assoc 1987; 87:1065–7.
76. Clark AJ, Mossholder S, Gates R. Am J Clin Nutr 1987; 46:302–6.
77. Bray GA. J Endocrinol Metab Clin North Am 1996;25:907–19.
78. Must A, Jacques PF, Dallal GE, et al. N Engl J Med 1992; 327:1350–5.
79. Nieto J, Szklo M, Comstock GW. Am J Epidemiol 1992; 136:201–13.
80. Hoffman MD, Kromhount D, de Lezenne Coulander C. The impact of body mass index of 78,612 18 year old Dutch men on 32 year mortalities from all causes. J Clin Epidemiol 1988; 41:749–56.
81. Waaler HT. Acta Med Scand Suppl 1984;64:1–56.
82. Katzman DK, Zipursky RB. Ann NY Acad Sci 1997;817:127–37.
83. Committee on Diet and Health, Food and Nutrition Board, National Research Council. Diet and health. Implications for reducing chronic disease risk. Washington, DC: National Academy Press, 1989.
84. Nussbaum MP. Anorexia nervosa. In: McAnarney ER, Kreipe RE, Orr DP, Comerci GD. Textbook of adolescent medicine. Philadelphia: WB Saunders, 1992.
85. Adams LB, Shafer MAB. J Nutr Educ 1988;20:307–13.
86. Moore DC. Am J Dis Child 1988;142:1114–8.
87. Moses N, Banilivy MM, Lifshitz F. Pediatrics 1989;83:393–8.
88. Emmons L. J Am Diet Assoc 1992;92:306–12.
89. Casper RC, Offer D. Am J Clin Nutr (Abstract 6) 1989; 49(Suppl):1128–9.
90. Mellin LM, Irwin CE, Scully S. J Am Diet Assoc 1992;92:851–3.
91. Story M, French SA, Resnick MD, et al. Int J Eating Disord 1995;18:173–9.
92. Neumark-Sztainer D, Story M, Resnick MD, et al. Arch Pediatr Adolesc Med 1995;149:1330–5.
93. Kreipe RE, Golden NH, Katzman DK, et al. J Adolesc Health Care 1995;16:476–9.
94. Rees JM. J Am Diet Assoc 1996;96:22–3.
95. French SA, Story M, Downes B, et al. Am J Public Health 1995; 85:695–701.
96. Jacobson MS, Heald FP. Nutritional risks of adolescent pregnancy and their management. In: McAnarney ER, ed. Premature adolescent pregnancy and parenthood. New York: Grune & Stratton, 1983.
97. Rees JM, Worthington-Roberts B. Adolescence, nutrition, and pregnancy interrelationships. In: Mahan LK, Rees JM, eds. Nutrition in adolescence. St. Louis: Times Mirror/Mosby College Publishing, 1984.
98. Gutierrez Y, King JC. Pediatr Ann 1993;22:99–108.
99. Position of The American Dietetic Association. J Am Diet Assoc 1994;94:449–50.
100. Gong EJ. Weight issues and management. In: Story M, ed. Nutrition management of the pregnant adolescent. A practical reference guide. March of Dimes Birth Defects Foundation. Washington, DC: U.S. Department of Health and Human Services, U.S. Department of Agriculture, 1990.
101. Naeye RL. Pediatrics 1981;67:146–50.
102. Scholl TO, Hediger ML, Ances IG. Am J Clin Nutr 1990;51:790–3.
103. Scholl TO, Hediger ML. J Am College Nutr 1993;12:101–7.
104. Scholl TO, Hediger ML, Schall JI, et al. Am J Clin Nutr 1994; 60:183–8.
105. Frisancho AR, Matos J, Flegel P. Am J Clin Nutr 1983;38: 739–46.
106. Meserole LP, Worthington-Roberts BS, Rees JM, et al. J Adolesc Health Care 1984;5:21–7.
107. Hediger ML, Scholl TO, Ances IG, et al. Am J Clin Nutr 1990;52:793–9.
108. Rees JM, Engelbert-Fenton KA, Gong EJ, et al. Am J Clin Nutr 1992;56:868–73.
109. Subcommittee on Nutritional Status and Weight Gain During Pregnancy, Food and Nutrition Board. Institute of Medicine. National Academy of Sciences. Summary. Nutrition during pregnancy. Part I. Weight gain. Washington, DC: National Academy Press, 1990.
110. Committee to Study the Prevention of Low Birthweight, Division of Health Promotion and Disease Prevention, Institute of Medicine. Preventing low birthweight. Washington, DC: National Academy Press, 1985.

111. Eastman NJ, Jackson E. Obstet Gynecol Surv 1968;23: 1003–25.
112. Hediger ML, Scholl TO, Belsky DH, et al. Obstet Gynecol 1989;74:6–12.
113. Scholl TO, Hediger ML, Ances IG, et al. Obstet Gynecol 1990;75:948–53.
114. Scholl TO, Hediger ML, Khoo CS, et al. J Clin Epidemiol 1991;44:423–8.
115. Miller HS, Lesser KB, Reed KL. Obstet Gynecol 1996;87: 83–8.
116. Rees JM, Lederman SA, Kiely JL. Pediatrics 1996;98:1161–6.
117. Muscati SK, Mackey MA, Newsom B. J Nutr Educ 1988;20:299–306.
118. Maso MJ, Gong EJ, Jacobson MS, et al. J Adolesc Health Care 1988;9:188–93.
119. Blackburn ML, Calloway DH. J Am Diet Assoc 1974;65: 24–30.
120. King JC, Calloway DH, Margen S. J Nutr 1973;103:772–5.
121. Rosso P. Nutrition and metabolism in pregnancy. Mother and fetus. New York: Oxford University Press, 1990.
122. Scholl TO, Hediger ML, Fischer RL, et al. Am J Clin Nutr 1992;55:985–8.
123. Scholl TO, Hediger ML. Am J Clin Nutr 1994;59 (Suppl):492S–501S.
124. Dawson EB, Albers J, McGanity WJ. Am J Clin Nutr 1989;50:848–52.
125. Cherry FF, Sandstead HH, Rojas P, et al. Am J Clin Nutr 1989;50:945–54.
126. Pennington JAT. Bowes and Church's food values of portions commonly used. 15th ed. New York: Harper & Row, 1989.
127. Raper NR, Hill MM. Nutr Rev 1974;32(Suppl):29–33.
128. MacLean WC Jr, Graham GG. Am J Dis Child 1980;134: 513–9.
129. Jacobs C, Dwyer JT. Am J Clin Nutr 1988;48:811–8.
130. Messina M, Messina V. The dietitian's guide to vegetarian diets. Issues and applications. Gaithersburg, MD: Aspen Publishers, 1996.
131. Carruth BR. J Curr Adolesc Med 1980;2:44–7.
132. Position of The American Dietetic Association. J Am Diet Assoc 1993;93:1317–9.
133. Marino DD, King JC. Pediatr Clin North Am 1980;27:125–39.
134. University of California. The creative eater's handbook. Better nutrition through vegetarian eating. Berkeley: University Student Health Service, 1982.
135. Johnston PK, Haddad EH. Vegetarian and other dietary practices. In: Rickert VI, ed. Adolescent nutrition: assessment and management. New York: Chapman & Hall, 1996.
136. Haddad EH. Am J Clin Nutr 1994;59(Suppl):1248S–54S.

53. Nutrition in the Elderly

LYNNE M. AUSMAN and ROBERT M. RUSSELL

Currently, 25 million Americans are over the age of 65; by the year 2030, 57 million will be 65 or older. The increasing numbers of elderly and aged, especially in Western societies, present challenges to those concerned with their physical and emotional well-being. An understanding of the role of both early and later nutrition in slowing or modulating the aging process and in providing adequate nutriture for the elderly is important. Further, nutrient needs may change with aging, and the interaction of drugs and nutrients may play a major role in the nutrient needs of some elderly persons. A thorough and comprehensive review of all aspects of nutrition, aging, and the elderly can be found in the work of Munro and Danford (1).

THEORIES OF AGING

Aging is a gradual process taking place over many decades. Most theories of aging relate to impaired DNA replication and loss of viability of the cell and hence of the body's organs. The most common theories of aging relate to one or more of the following: immunologic breakdown, cellular proliferation, basal metabolic rate, rate of DNA repair, free radical damage, and/or rate of protein synthesis and catabolism. One classification of general theories of aging is shown in Table 53.1.

Dietary Restriction Experiments with Animal Models

Animal studies yield the strongest evidence that diet plays a major role in longevity and the aging process (2). The most consistent finding from experimental rodent studies is that moderate dietary restriction markedly extends the life span of experimental animals, compared with control animals fed ad libitum. Dietary restriction also decreases the incidence of several chronic diseases such as glomerulonephritis, atherosclerosis, and tumors.

Dietary restriction by selective removal of individual macronutrients (fat, carbohydrate, or protein) has also been carried out. However, without a concomitant decrease in energy intake, little extension of life span has been found. Dietary excess of protein or fat, however, *(a)* increases the incidence of tumors and certain organ pathologies and *(b)* shortens the time of appearance of several physical, biochemical, and immunologic indices of early maturational development and aging.

The severity, age of initiation, and duration of the dietary perturbation are important in determining the eventual response to the dietary restriction. Many other factors, including the species and strain of laboratory animal used, are important variables in determining the outcome of these experiments. Individual micronutrients also have effects on life span and modulate the mechanisms of aging, at least to some extent. For example, increased levels of dietary antioxidants (ascorbic acid, α-tocopherol, carotenoids) may partially decrease cellular free-radical concentrations (3). It is yet unclear whether any of these changes are related to the mechanism of aging.

FACTORS AFFECTING NUTRITIONAL STATUS

The elderly are a more diverse population than any other age group; individuals have widely varying capabilities and levels of functioning. On the whole, elderly persons are more likely than younger adults to be in marginal nutritional health and thus to be at higher risk for frank nutritional deficiency in times of stress or health care problems. Physical, social, and emotional problems may interfere with appetite or affect the ability to purchase, prepare, and consume an adequate diet (4). These factors include whether or not a person lives alone, how many daily meals are eaten, who does the cooking and shopping and any physical impediments that would make this impossible, problems in chewing and denture use, adequate income to purchase appropriate foods, and alcohol and medication use.

Table 53.1
Selected Theories of Aging

Cellular
Free radical damage
Glycosylation and other cross-links
Changes in DNA or chromatin
Decreased accuracy or quantity of protein synthesis
Limited cell division capacity ("Hayflick limit")
Decreased DNA repair activity
Organ systems
Role of immune phenomena
Role of neuroendocrine phenomena
Population
Theories associating aging with differentiation or growth cessation
Rate of living
Theories based on the evolution of life span in mammals

Adapted from Weindruch RH, Walford RL. The retardation of aging and disease by dietary restriction. Springfield, IL: Charles C Thomas, 1988.

NUTRITIONAL REQUIREMENTS

A decline in organ function normally accompanies the aging process, especially in the older elderly (i.e., those above 80 years old). Many of these changes in normal function might reasonably be expected to influence nutrient needs of the individual (5–7) (Table 53.2).

Energy

Several studies have documented decreased energy needs in the elderly. In the Baltimore Longitudinal Study of Aging, energy intakes of a sample of males decreased from 11.3 MJ (2700 kcal) per day at age 30 years to 8.8 MJ (2100 kcal) per day for those about 80 years. Two-thirds of this reduction was attributable to decreased physical activity, and the remainder to decreased basal metabolism (8). These findings have generally been supported by other studies. In NHANES III (preliminary), young men and women, aged 20 to 29, consumed 12.6 and 8.2 MJ (3025 and 1957 kcal), whereas men and women aged 50 to 59 consumed 9.8 and 6.8 MJ (2341 and 1629 kcal), and those 80+ consumed 7.4 and 5.6 MJ (1776 and 1329 kcal), respectively.

The recommended energy intake from the 1989 *Recommended Dietary Allowances* (RDAs) is 9.6 MJ (2300 kcal) for the reference 77-kg elderly male and 7.9 MJ (1900 kcal) for the reference 65-kg female 51 years of age and older (9), both similar to the mean energy intake of the 50- to 59-year-old age group (see Appendix Table II-A-2-a-1). The RDAs and estimated intakes based on population studies both appear to underestimate total energy expenditure (TEE) for men, derived from using the excretion of administered $^2H_2^{18}$ to estimate the usual energy consumption of healthy elderly people. The TEE for men, aged 68 years, was 11.3 MJ (2700 kcal) (10) and for women, aged 74 years, was 7.6 MJ (1800 kcal) (11). The discrepancy between the RDA and the TEE for men could suggest that the small group studied in the TEE experiment was not an accurate subsample of the total population or that individuals actually are consuming more than they record. In either case, this higher TEE is not a recommendation for elderly men to consume more calories.

Protein

High-protein diets may be less well digested and absorbed in the elderly, judged by a minor increase in fecal nitrogen content in response to a protein load (12). However, little quantitative information is available regarding absorptive changes in the elderly for amino acids and peptides in more usual amounts.

Table 53.2
Changes in Organ Function with Aging That May Influence Nutrient Status

Organ Function	Physical Change	Importance to Nutrition
Taste and smell	Fewer taste buds and papilla on tongue Decrease in taste and olfactory nerve endings Change in taste and smell threshold	Loss of ability to detect salt and sweet Decreased palatability causing poor food intake
Saliva secretion	Saliva flow may be reduced	Doubtful clinical significance
Esophageal function and swallowing	Minor changes including disordered contractions	Doubtful clinical significance
Gastric function and emptying	Decreased secretion of hydrochloric acid, intrinsic factor, and pepsin in 20% of healthy population >60 years of age (atrophic gastritis) Rapid rate of emptying of liquids, increased pH in the proximal small bowel, bacterial overgrowth in bowel	Decreased bioavailability of minerals, vitamins, and proteins Decreased absorption of protein-bound vitamin B_{12} and folate Increase in bacterial folate synthesis to counteract malabsorption
Hepatic and biliary function	Decreased size and blood flow Minor structural and biochemical changes Activity of drug-metabolizing enzymes reduced	Rate of albumin synthesis may be decreased Drug dosages may need to be lower
Pancreatic secretion	Slightly lower bicarbonate and enzyme outputs	Doubtful clinical significance
Intestinal morphology and function	Insignificant changes in small bowel morphology	Doubtful clinical significance
Intestinal microflora	Bacterial overgrowth in proximal small bowel in atrophic gastritis	Functional significance unknown; influences supply of water-soluble vitamins and vitamin K

From Rosenberg IH, Russell RM, Bowman BB. Aging and the digestive system. In: Munro HN, Danford DE, eds. Nutrition, aging, and the elderly. New York: Plenum Press, 1989;43–60, with permission.

The current RDA for protein (0.8 g/kg/day) is adequate for the elderly when excessive energy intakes are observed (i.e., ≥167 kJ (40 kcal/kg) per day) (13) (see Appendix Table II-A-2-a-2). However, when an energy intake more usual for the elderly is used (e.g., 125 kJ (30 kcal/kg) per day), nitrogen balance is not attained in more than half of elderly subjects (14). The degree of adaptation of the individual to the lower energy or lower protein intake before the actual experimental trial began may account for many of the discrepancies in nitrogen needs reported in the literature (15). Furthermore, whereas 0.92 g/kg/day was needed to maintain nitrogen balance and tissue protein stores in sedentary elderly persons (16), possibly less suffices if resistance training is part of the daily routine (17). The average protein consumption among free-living elderly persons in Boston was 1.05 g/kg/day in one study, with no evidence that lower intakes were correlated with protein-energy malnutrition (18). On the whole, a daily intake of 1 g/kg (and probably less) meets the needs of this population (1).

Carbohydrate

Carbohydrate absorption (mannitol, xylose, 3-*O*-methyl glucose) may be slightly impaired with advanced aging, although decreased renal function may interfere with interpretation of "absorption" test results based on urinary excretion (19–21). In one study in elderly persons 65 to 89 years of age, breath hydrogen was measured in response to a 100- to 200-g carbohydrate challenge to estimate carbohydrate malabsorption (22). At the highest carbohydrate load, 80% had increased breath hydrogen. The increased breath hydrogen found in most elderly persons could result from carbohydrate malabsorption with age, increased bacterial enzyme activity in the small bowel, or both. Lactase activity decreases with age (especially in early life), but other brush border hydrolase activities appear to remain fairly constant (23–24). The diminished lactase activity with age may create only a minor problem because most lactose-intolerant individuals can tolerate the lactose present (12.5 g) in a glass of milk (25). Furthermore, in a double-blind study of healthy elderly persons given either lactose-containing or lactose-free products, about 30% of both groups showed bloating and discomfort associated with lactose intolerance. Although the elderly tend to avoid consumption of milk products (which are excellent sources of riboflavin, vitamin D, and calcium), the perceived bloating and discomfort may not be due to lactose intolerance. Therefore, the true prevalence of lactose intolerance in the elderly is difficult to define.

There is no RDA for dietary carbohydrate. However, the United States Department of Agriculture (USDA), American Heart Association, and American Cancer Society, among others, recommend a dietary carbohydrate component of 55 to 60% of calories, with an increase in the proportion of complex carbohydrates to simple sugars.

Fat

Fat digestion and absorption in the elderly is equivalent to that of young adults when measured at normal consumption levels (100 g) (21–26). At higher dietary levels (120 g/day), the elderly showed slightly less fat absorption than did the young adults (11), and institutionalized elderly persons may absorb even less (27). Although not too common, fat malabsorption in the elderly, when found, is most often due to bacterial overgrowth of the small intestine, causing deconjugation of bile salts. However, most bacterial overgrowth in hypochlorhydric subjects is not associated with clinical malabsorption of fat or carbohydrate, despite the presence of positive indicators such as abnormal ^{14}[C]-D-xylose absorption (28). Chylomicron appearance in blood after a 100-g fat meal is somewhat slower in elderly persons than in young adults; however, an observed difference in gastric emptying times might explain this apparently slower lipid hydrolysis and uptake (29).

There is no RDA for total fat. However, it is widely felt that a prudent diet with 30% or less of calories as fat (less than 10% saturated, 10 to 15% monounsaturated, and no more than 10% polyunsaturated fatty acids) may be just as important in the elderly as in young adults for preventing or ameliorating chronic diseases such as heart disease or cancer. At the same time, these amounts of polyunsaturated fat are consistent with a diet providing adequate amounts of essential fatty acids (linoleic and linolenic acid) (9).

Fiber

Little is known about dietary fiber requirements of either adults or elderly persons. However, the various classes of dietary fiber (see Chapter 43) found in a mixed diet have different mechanical and metabolic effects in the gastrointestinal tract. In population studies, increased consumption of dietary fiber is correlated with decreased rates of heart disease and cancer. Fiber is also included in a treatment regimen for a variety of diseases that particularly affect the elderly—constipation, hemorrhoids, diverticulosis, hiatal hernia, varicose veins, diabetes mellitus, hyperlipidemia, and obesity (30). Without evidence to the contrary, recommendations for fiber consumption for the elderly would be the same as for the adult, about 25 g/day, the recommended "Daily Value" on the new food label.

Fluid

Fluid balance is as important in the elderly as in other age groups. Nevertheless, it deserves particular attention because dehydration often goes unrecognized in the elderly. Indeed, a recent study indicated that dehydration was responsible for 6.7% of hospitalizations (31). Poor fluid balance may be due to both inadequate (lower then normal) intake and excessive losses (32). Chronically ill, immobilized, or demented patients and those with bladder control problems often fail to drink sufficient fluids. On the other hand, several clinical conditions such as fever, diarrhea, malabsorption, vomiting, and hemorrhage lead to excessive losses. Therapy with certain diuretics and laxative or hypertonic intravenous solutions also contribute to the problem. In the absence of severe clinical problems, consumption of 30 mL/kg/day is probably sufficient for the elderly.

Vitamins

Low-to-inadequate dietary intake may account for much of the poor vitamin nutriture observed in the elderly (33). In addition, physiologic changes associated with the aging gut may increase or decrease vitamin absorption, thereby influencing total dietary vitamin requirements. Table 53.3 lists the major water- and fat-soluble vitamins, the current RDA (Appendix Table II-A-2-a-2) or "safe and adequate daily dietary intake" (Appendix Table II-A-2-a-3), and an assessment of whether or not the current recommendation is appropriate for the elderly. Individual vitamins are discussed below.

Thiamin. The 1989 RDA for the elderly for thiamin is 1.2 mg/day for males and 1.0 mg/day for females. When corrected for caloric consumption, intake should not decrease below 0.5 mg/1000 kcal. The NHANES I, II, and III (preliminary) data indicate that the mean intake for the 65- to 75-year-old age group was above this amount. Aging appears to be associated with an increased erythrocyte transketolase-activation coefficient in a small percentage of normal, free-living elderly persons (34). It is not known whether this increase is normal for aging or represents nutritional inadequacy. There are no consistent changes in absorption of thiamin with age (35–36). Thiamin deficiency in the elderly is largely due to alcoholism accompanied by low thiamin intake. However, the RDA for thiamin appears to cover the needs of most well elderly persons.

Riboflavin. The 1989 RDA for riboflavin for the elderly is 1.4 and 1.2 mg/day for males and females, respectively. Deficiency of the vitamin as diagnosed by increased erythrocyte glutathione reductase activity coefficient (37–38) or decreased urinary riboflavin excretion (33) has been most often associated with low dietary intake of riboflavin. Little evidence exists for altered absorption of the vitamin (39) or for altered tissue concentration with age (40). However, Boisvert et al. (41) recently demonstrated that the riboflavin requirement for a group of elderly people does not differ from that previously reported for younger adults (42). Therefore, current RDAs are generous for the elderly.

Ascorbic Acid. The current 1989 RDA for vitamin C is 60 mg/day for both sexes. Although the vitamin is widely abundant in many foods, intakes in the elderly vary widely. Factors such as smoking, medications, and emotional and

Table 53.3
Estimate of Adequacy of 1989 RDA for Vitamins for the Elderly

Vitamin	Current RDA for Age 51+[a]	Adequacy of RDA for Elderly	Physiologic Reason for Change
Vitamin A	800–1000 μg RE	May be too high	Change in unstirred water layer may lead to increased absorption in elderly; decreased uptake by the liver of newly absorbed vitamin A
Vitamin D	5 μg	Is too low	Lack of sun exposure, decreased number of intestinal vitamin D receptors, reduced vitamin D absorption, reduced vitamin D_3 synthesis in skin and impaired renal 1-α hydroxylation suggest that the dietary requirement might be higher
Vitamin E	8–10 mg	I/C data[b]	—
Vitamin K	65–80 μg[c]	I/C data[b]	—
Thiamin	1–1.2 mg	Adequate	—
Riboflavin	1.2–1.4 mg	Adequate	—
Niacin	13–15 mg	I/C data[b]	—
Vitamin B_6	1.6–2.0 mg	Is too low	Serum homocysteine levels rise when dietary vitamin B_6 is less than 2.0 mg/day and poor response to B_6 supplements in normal range suggests altered absorption or metabolism
Folate	180–200 μg	May be too low	Serum homocysteine levels rise when dietary folate is less than 400 μg/day
Vitamin B_{12}	2.0 μg	May be too low	Atrophic gastritis and competition from bacterial overgrowth reduce availability of B_{12}
Ascorbate	60 mg	Adequate	—
Biotin	30–100 μg[c]	I/C data[b]	—
Pantothenate	4–7 mg[c]	I/C data[b]	—

From Russell RM, Suter PM, Am J Clin Nutr 1993;58:4–14, with permission.

[a]RDA for female and male elderly 51+ years of age.

[b]Insufficient or conflicting data.

[c]Estimated safe and adequate daily dietary intake (adapted from ref. 9).

environmental stress all adversely affect vitamin C nutriture (9, 43). Leukocyte and plasma vitamin C levels decline with age, although the significance of this is unclear (33–50). Maintenance of the plasma level at 1.0 mg/dL would require 75 mg/day for females and 150 mg/day for males (45); however, there is no evidence that saturating the body pool is advantageous for this age group. Changes in tissue concentration with age are not consistent, and there is little evidence that vitamin C absorption changes with aging (44, 46). There is no compelling evidence that vitamin C requirements per se change with age. However, evidence is accumulating that vitamin C in amounts above the RDA protects against cataract formation (47).

Niacin. The 1989 RDA for niacin is the same as for young adults, 15 mg/day for males and 13 mg/day for females. Individuals with low excretion of urinary *N*-methyl nicotinamide usually have a poor niacin intake or are very sick or very old (86 to 99 years) (38); in the latter case, decreased renal function should be considered. Little if any evidence indicates that niacin requirements change with age (33).

Vitamin B_6. Because the vitamin B_6 content of many foods is not known, dietary intakes calculated from food composition tables vary widely and may be low. Nevertheless, serum and plasma B_6 levels in the elderly tend to decrease with age. Studies indicating poor B_6 nutriture based on activity coefficient tests (response of whole blood B_6 enzymes to exogenous B_6 supplementation) show that with moderate oral supplementation, activity coefficients in some elderly persons still do not return to normal. The current RDA for vitamin B_6 in the elderly is 2.0 mg/day for men and 1.6 mg/day for women. However, the average requirement (without addition of 2 S.D. to ensure adequacy for most of the population) in both male and female elderly persons was recently shown to be about 2.0 mg/day (48). Further, in those above 67 years old, Selhub et al. showed that serum homocysteine levels rise when dietary vitamin B_6 drops below 2.0 mg/day (49). Therefore, the RDA for vitamin B_6 should be considerably higher in the elderly.

Folate. Despite low folate intake levels, only 3 to 7% of persons in NHANES I (50) or free-living elderly persons have low serum folate levels (i.e., <3.0 ng/mL). In a Swedish study of 35 elderly subjects (51), intake of only 100 to 200 μg/day normalized whole-blood folate concentrations. Furthermore, although atrophic gastritis with aging causes malabsorption of folic acid due to a rise in pH of the proximal gastrointestinal tract, this is more than offset by the production and subsequent absorption of folate synthesized by bacterial overgrowth in the proximal small bowel (52). The current RDA in the elderly is 200 μg/day for men and 180 μg/day for women. Serum homocysteine levels increase, however, when dietary folate drops below 400 μg/day (49). The reliability of the data on food folate content, however, has been questioned by Beecher and Matthews, who stress a need for development of alternative methods of measuring folate in foods (53). Given the uncertainties of food folate data and the emerging relevance of homocysteine as a marker for coronary artery and cerebral vascular disease, the current RDA for folate may be too low for elderly persons.

Vitamin B_{12}. Serum or plasma vitamin B_{12} levels in the elderly are often found to be low because of decreased body reserves (54–55). Low intake, especially among the poor, and impaired absorption of vitamin B_{12} may be important factors. Decreased digestive release of vitamin B_{12} from food and bacterial overgrowth in the small bowel (as found in atrophic gastritis) leading to competition for vitamin B_{12} seem important in reducing absorption (56). Atrophic gastritis per se, however, is not associated with significantly decreased production of intrinsic factor. The current RDA of 2.0 μg/day is sufficient for elderly persons without atrophic gastritis but may be too low for those with atrophic gastritis.

Vitamin A. Although vitamin A is not distributed widely in foods, excess daily amounts can be stored in the liver. Most individuals consume food rich in vitamin A one or two times per week. Estimates of vitamin A intakes derived from 24-hour recalls overestimate the number of individuals having low intakes.

After a dose of vitamin A, plasma retinyl ester values in the elderly remain higher than in young adults because of reduced clearance of the lipid-rich lipoproteins carrying the retinyl esters in the elderly (57–58). A change in the character of the luminal epithelium or a decrease in the thickness or character of the unstirred water layer, as demonstrated in elderly rats, might increase absorption. In addition, provitamin A carotenoids (e.g., β-carotene, α-carotene, cryptoxanthin) are also a source of vitamin A. Although still an unresolved question, these compounds, consumed as part of the daily diet, may help prevent cancer and cardiovascular disease. Therefore, although the need for preformed vitamin A may be lower for the elderly, it would be prudent to obtain a large fraction of the vitamin A requirement from carotene-containing fruits and vegetables.

Vitamin D. Because vitamin D is found in only a few foods, including seafood and fortified milk products, it is not surprising that over three-quarters of elderly persons have vitamin D intakes less than two-thirds of the RDA. The contribution of sunlight to the vitamin D status of the elderly is also reduced, because they receive less sun exposure and have a decreased efficiency of vitamin D synthesis in the skin (59). The diet may not provide sufficient vitamin D for institutionalized subjects with little access to sunlight (60). Moreover, when given in physiologic amounts, absorption of vitamin D from the gastrointestinal tract is reduced with age, (61) possibly because the number of vitamin D receptors decreases with advancing age (62). Thus, the dietary need for vitamin D may be greater in the elderly than in younger individuals. Supplementation with 10 μg (400 IU) per day (twice the RDA) is recommended for homebound elderly persons or those in nursing homes who are not exposed to sunlight.

In one study, although serum 25-OH-D levels were not decreased in elderly subjects, average 1,25-$(OH)_2$-D levels were significantly lower in elderly osteoporotic females than in younger females (63), suggesting impaired renal conversion (renal 1-α-hydroxylase) of vitamin D to its active form. 1,25-$(OH)_2$-D levels were significantly correlated with intestinal calcium absorption.

Changes in bone density have recently been used to determine vitamin D requirements of elderly persons. In one study of postmenopausal women, the experimental group received 400 IU/day of vitamin D, while those on placebo received no extra vitamin D (64). Both groups had an average dietary intake of 100 IU vitamin D. During the winter and early spring season, the placebo-fed group lost considerably more bone mineral density than did the group receiving the 400 IU supplement. This study showed that a total intake of 500 IU resulted in better bone density than only 100 IU, which is consistent with other data showing a greater need for vitamin D in the elderly. The study also illustrates the use of a disease endpoint (osteoporosis) for judging vitamin D adequacy rather than a static serum level of vitamin D.

The 1989 RDA for vitamin D of 5 μg of cholecalciferol has been modified in the 1997 adequate intake reference values to 10 μg for ages 51 through 70 and to 15 μg for older individuals (Appendix Table II-A-2-b-4).

Vitamin E. As for vitamin C, the antioxidative properties of vitamin E (tocopherol) may help to retard the aging process. The 1989 RDA for the elderly is 10 mg/day for males and 8 mg/day for females. Most populations consume adequate amounts, although in one study, 40% of a free-living population consumed less than 75% of the RDA from the diet alone (65). (Of note, one-third of this population took vitamin E supplements.) Because plasma α-tocopherol is carried passively in the lipid-rich lipoproteins (very low density lipoproteins [VLDLs] and low-density lipoproteins [LDLs]) (66–67), it is most accurate to express the vitamin E concentration in relation to blood lipid content (68). When this is done, the plasma vitamin E:lipid ratio is not related to age (69). The data on tissue concentrations (platelets, liver, adrenal glands, heart) of vitamin E with age are inconsistent, and the erythrocyte hemolysis test shows no evidence of increased vitamin E needs with age (33). Finally, there is no evidence for altered vitamin E absorption with aging (67).

Vitamin E given in pharmacologic amounts may have a protective effect against coronary artery disease due to inhibition of LDL oxidation. However, the doses required for such an effect appear to be well beyond the levels that are possible in a healthful diet. Vitamin E supplementation has also been reported to benefit the immune system (70). However, once again, the doses required are probably higher than can be achieved in a healthful diet. Thus, the present RDAs for vitamin E appear adequate.

Vitamin K. A new method of measuring vitamin K metabolites in plasma has revealed that serum phylloquinone levels vary as a function of gender, age, and serum lipid levels (71). Expressed per millimole of triglyceride, plasma phylloquinone concentrations in the young subjects were 0.82×10^{-6} mmol and in the elderly 0.62×10^{-6} mmol (72). The nutritional significance of this decrease in the elderly is not yet understood. When human volunteers were purposely depleted in vitamin K, elderly subjects appeared more resistant to acute vitamin K deficiency than younger subjects (73). However, the best way to judge vitamin K sufficiency is presently uncertain. Classically, blood coagulation parameters were used, but now, bone carboxylated proteins are measurable. In fact, carboxylation of bone protein may be more susceptible to vitamin K deficiency than are the various coagulation factors (74). Thus, a functional test (carboxylation of vitamin K–dependent protein) may be more useful for defining vitamin K deficiency than static vitamin K levels in serum. The 1989 RDA for vitamin K for the elderly is 80 μg/day for men and 65 μg/day for women.

Minerals

Table 53.4 lists current RDAs or safe and adequate daily dietary intakes and an assessment of whether or not the current recommendation is appropriate for elderly persons. Individual minerals are discussed below.

Calcium. Lifetime calcium intake appears to be a factor in the incidence of osteoporosis in the elderly, and laying down sufficient bone in early life is one of the most critical factors protecting against fracture in old age. In both men and women, absorption of calcium decreases with age (63, 75). Calcium carbonate absorption may also decrease with the achlorhydria observed in some elderly persons (76), although this may be overcome by taking the calcium with a meal (77). One study measured calcium absorption in 94 normal volunteers (aged 30 to 90) and 52 untreated women with postmenopausal osteoporosis (63). Although fractional calcium absorption decreased with age, it was not correlated with calcium intake. The elderly also appear less able than young adults to adapt to a low-calcium diet (78). Poor vitamin D nutriture and activity in the elderly is widely thought to be partially responsible for the decreased calcium absorption.

In the NHANES I and II studies, average calcium intakes for women were about 500 mg/day, below the 1989 RDA of 800 mg/day. NHANES III preliminary data show a slight improvement in calcium intakes in the older age groups, but median intakes are still below the present RDA of 800 mg/day. Studies in Yugoslavia found a greater metacarpal cortical thickness in a population that routinely consumed 1100 mg calcium per day than in a population with a typically low-calcium intake (500 mg/day)

Table 53.4
Estimate of Adequacy of 1989 RDA for Minerals for the Elderly

Mineral	Current RDA for Age 51+[a]	Adequacy of RDA for Elderly	Physiologic Reason for Change
Calcium	800 mg	Too low	Absorption decreases with age; calcium balance and improved bone density achieved at higher dietary levels
Iron	10 mg	Adequate	—
Zinc	12–15 mg	Adequate	—
Copper	1.5–3.0 mg[b]	Adequate	—
Selenium	55–70 μg	Adequate	—
Magnesium	280–350 mg	Too high	Efficient renal conservation at low intake levels; markedly low intake levels in elderly do not result in deficiency
Chromium	50–250 μg[b]	Too high	Balance achieved below RDA levels

[a]RDA for female-male elderly 51+ years of age.
[b]ESADDI, estimated safe and adequate daily dietary intake (adapted from ref. 9).

(79). Bone loss progressed with age in both districts, but the rate of hip fracture was higher in the group with low calcium intake, suggesting lower calcium reserves before osteoporosis became apparent. In another study, spinal bone loss in healthy postmenopausal elderly patients was lower in women consuming more than 777 mg calcium per day than in those consuming less than 405 mg/day. In this study, supplementation exceeding a total daily intake of 800 mg appears unnecessary (80).

Two other studies challenge these results (81, 82). In one study beneficial effects on lumbar spinal bone density were seen in individuals taking a calcium supplement of 1000 mg/day, even though the mean dietary intake of the calcium-supplemented group was in the range of 800 mg/day (the present RDA). Although the data are not clear on what the best RDA may be, these investigations show that bone density may be the most useful parameter for determining RDAs for calcium for the elderly population.

In 1994, an NIH consensus conference on optimal calcium intakes recommended 1000 mg of calcium per day for adult men and estrogen-sufficient women less than 65 years old, and 1500 mg of calcium per day for both men and women 65 years and older (83). Even greater amounts of dietary calcium may be needed in the medical management of women with established osteoporosis. However, there is a potential downside to increasing calcium in the diet too much—interference with absorption of other minerals. Such mineral-mineral interactions must be studied before fully rational and strong recommendations for calcium requirements can be made. In addition, more studies are needed on the effect of exercise on bone loss in the elderly, which could further modulate the calcium need (84).

The 1997 adequate intake reference value for calcium of the Food and Nutrition Board is 1200 mg/day for those 51 years and above. This is an increase of 400 mg/day above the 1989 RDA (see Appendix Tables A-2-a-2 and A-2-b-1).

Iron. The iron deficiency seen in the elderly is due to inadequate iron intake, blood loss due to chronic disease, and/or reduced nonheme iron absorption secondary to the hypohydria or achlorhydria of atrophic gastritis (85). Chronic use of antacids or other acid-lowering medications can also impair intestinal iron absorption. Iron absorption per se does not appear to decline significantly with age (86), although one study showed that red cell uptake of absorbed intestinal iron was reduced by about one-third (87). In the NHANES I and II studies, average iron intakes were 14 mg/day for men and 10 mg/day for women (88). In NHANES III (preliminary) data, median iron intakes for males and females over 80 years of age were 13.2 and 9.6 mg, respectively. In these studies, a 4% prevalence of anemia in men was more often due to chronic disease than to iron deficiency; iron-deficiency anemia without apparent disease was rare for women.

Some surveys have suggested that iron may accumulate in the body with age, as reflected by elevated serum ferritin levels (88, 90). However, these studies for the most part did not control for chronic inflammation or diseases known to alter ferritin levels. Although a ferritin level of 12 μg/L has been used as a cutoff to indicate depleted iron stores, two recent studies have reported that patients presenting with anemia had no stainable iron in their bone marrow despite apparently normal serum ferritin (91–92). Additional research is needed to define appropriate age-sensitive values for ferritin and other iron indices.

In the NHANES survey, iron overload was found in 0.2% of adults who were probably homozygous for the hereditary hemochromatosis gene (93). Although individuals who are heterozygous for this gene are more common (10% of the population of white northern Europeans), heterozygous individuals in Canada have normal serum ferritin and transferrin saturations (94). A reported direct relationship between iron intake, serum ferritin, and the risk of myocardial infarction (95) has not been confirmed by others. Therefore, the RDA of 10 mg/day for elderly persons seems adequate and appropriate.

Zinc. Zinc intakes of the elderly, 10 mg for males and 7 mg for females, are well below the 1989 RDA of 15 mg/day for men and 12 mg/day for women (65, 96). However, no consistent relationship has been found between dietary zinc and plasma zinc (97). Zinc absorption as measured by isotopic studies decreases with age, although zinc balance remains intact (98). There are conflicting data in the literature indicating normal or decreased plasma zinc concentrations in the elderly (99). The significance of any decrease in plasma levels is difficult to ascertain, however, because diagnosis of zinc deficiency is problematic.

Since zinc nutriture may affect immune competence, the question arises whether poor zinc status may partially explain decreased immune function in the elderly (97). Both immune suppression and immune stimulation by zinc supplementation have been reported in the elderly (100–101). The present RDAs for zinc for elderly men (15 mg) and women (12 mg) appear to be justified, at least until better measures of zinc status are available.

Copper. As determined by isotope studies, copper absorption in the elderly is similar to that in young adults (102). Copper absorption is affected by the presence of other trace minerals and factors in the diet that inhibit or enhance cation absorption (e.g., phytates, zinc, oxalates). A study in elderly males suggests that only 1.1 mg of copper is necessary for copper balance, less than the usual intake of 2 to 3 mg (also the RDA) observed in the elderly (102).

Selenium. The RDA for selenium for adults 51 years or older is 70 μg/day for men and 55 μg/day for women. Because age-related changes in absorption or metabolism of selenium have not been described, poor selenium intake is probably responsible for the prevalence of poor selenium indices reported among most elderly people. Nevertheless, in one study of housebound elderly people, the mean selenium intake of 37.5 μg/day did not result in a negative selenium balance (103). Further, although selenium is part of the body's antioxidant defense system, it is uncertain that higher selenium intakes would decrease the incidence of chronic disease. For now, the RDA for selenium appears adequate.

Magnesium. In 1989, the magnesium RDA for adults of both sexes was set at 4.5 mg/kg, which translates into an intake of 350 mg for a reference 76-kg male and 280 mg/day for a reference 62-kg female. Various surveys show that older men and women consume only about two-thirds of the current RDAs. Despite this low intake, there is no evidence that magnesium deficiency is prevalent in this age group. Further, little or no information suggests significant alteration in magnesium absorption or metabolism with advancing age. This may, in part, reflect efficient renal conservation on low dietary intakes of magnesium. Although the serum magnesium level has been criticized as a measure for total body magnesium status, tissue levels (e.g., red blood cell, white blood cell) of magnesium have not been shown to decline with age. Thus, it appears that the magnesium RDA is probably set too high for the elderly and is in need of reexamination. As noted in Appendix Table II-A-2-b-3, the RDAs for magnesium for those 51 years and above have been increased by 70 and 40 mg/day for men and women, respectively, above the 1989 RDA.

Chromium. The estimated safe and adequate daily dietary intake for chromium is set between 50 and 250 μg/day. However, accurate data on the chromium content of foods are scarce, and several studies indicate that the elderly have chromium intakes far below the recommended range (102). In fact, a chromium intake of 50 μg/day might well require an energy intake of 3000 kcal/day. Balance studies among elderly people have shown that positive chromium balance can be maintained at levels below the current RDA (102). Although chromium enhances the activity of insulin, glucose tolerance in the elderly is not consistently improved after chromium supplementation. In one study, chromium supplementation increased HDL cholesterol (104); however, the amounts needed could not be achieved by diet alone (i.e., the effect appeared to be pharmacologic rather than physiologic). One autopsy study reported apparent accumulation of chromium in various tissues with advancing age (105). Since chromium balance can be achieved at intakes quite a bit below 50 μg/day, the recommended lower limit appears too high for the elderly and should be reexamined.

Other Trace Minerals. The nutritional status and requirement of manganese, molybdenum, phosphorus, iodine, and fluoride in relation to aging have not been adequately studied.

NUTRITIONAL STATUS

Dietary Intake

Dietary intakes and nutritional status of the elderly have been examined in several studies over the last 25 years: the large nationwide NHANES I for 1971 to 1974 (106), NHANES II for 1976 to 1980 (107), NHANES III preliminary data for 1988–1991 (108–109), the Third Report on Nutrition Monitoring in the United States (110), the Continuing Survey of Food Intakes by Individuals, 1994 (111), and several smaller studies of specific populations of free-living and institutionalized elderly persons (112–119). The sample population studied, the type of dietary instrument used, and the standards used to interpret the actual intake data influence the results of the study.

Methodology of Diet History

Three instruments are currently in use: dietary food records, food recall, and food frequency. The food record requires that an individual record current food intake for 3 to 7 days. The recall method is used for consumption during the previous 24-h period but may be particularly inappropriate for older persons with short-term memory problems. Finally, food frequency methods cover usual food consumption patterns for a 3-, 6-, or 12-month period including seasonal variations. Each of these methods incorporates questions on the use of dietary supplements and alcohol. The various advantages and disadvantages of each method have been reviewed (120) (see also Chapter 58). Many of these methods tend to underestimate food intake. For some nutrients, especially vitamin B_6 and zinc, the actual content in foods is not well established.

Dietary Intake Standards

Standards used to interpret dietary data in the elderly range from the RDA in use at the time of the survey to a special standard set up for a particular study, such as two-thirds of the RDA. Since the RDAs of 1974, there have been separate categories for individuals 51 years of age or older.

Nutritional Evaluation

Biochemical Standards

The biochemical standards recommended for use for the elderly are currently the same as for adults (121). Although some studies had speculated that serum albumin concentrations declined with aging, a recent study of 1066 healthy elderly persons found only minimal decreases (122).

Hematologic Standards

Standards for interpreting hematologic data (e.g., red blood cells, white blood cells, hemoglobin) for the elderly are slightly lower than those for young and middle-aged adults (123). By convention, values below the tenth percentile for NHANES II are considered "at risk." There are no reliable standards to indicate significant ethnic differences in the elderly.

Anthropometric Standards

Body Weight. The correlation of obesity with increased morbidity and mortality is well known (124–129). The pattern of distribution of the body fat (higher risk with increased waist:hip girth) is also a factor in the excess morbidity and mortality (129–132). However, determination of obesity in the elderly is problematic, because few body weight standards specifically for the elderly are currently in use. One of the earliest standards is based on accumulated body weight data on 5600 elderly men and women (65–94 years of age) who reported on an ambulatory basis to their respective doctors (133).

Data on the elderly up through age 74 are also available from the NHANES I and II studies. (See Appendix Tables III-A-15-a to f [133a].) Using these data, Frisancho (134) established body weight standards for persons 25 to 54 and 55 to 74 years of age for sex, age, height, and frame size (estimated from elbow breadth) (135) (data are presented in Appendix Tables III-A-12-c and d). These standards agree closely with data from the Baltimore Longitudinal Aging Study (136–137) (see also Appendix Table III-A-12-b). Because the mean body mass index (BMI) in the NHANES I, NHANES II, and several other studies was approximately 22.5 kg/m^2 for both sexes, Frisancho's summary tables (134) were prepared in weight ranges according to height and age but not gender. NHANES I and II data for BMI by age and gender are given in Appendix Table III-A-13-a. There are also body weights in the USDA dietary guidelines (138) but no data showing that they apply to the elderly (139). BMI has been shown useful in predicting body fatness (140) or risk of morbidity in elderly women (141).

The Metropolitan Life Tables (127) (see Appendix) are based on persons aged 25 to 59 and do not account for possible changes in body weight and height with age; thus, they are probably not useful for the elderly. Furthermore, because these tables represent the experience of the insurance industry, they are certainly not a truly representative sample of the general population. Thus, the Metropolitan Life Tables are not accurate or desirable for use in persons over the age of 54.

Other Anthropometric Standards. Anthropometric data such as triceps skinfold have also been used to assess nutritional status of populations (142), as well as to monitor response to treatment of patients in a hospital setting (143). Lean body mass declines with aging whereas body fat stores increase (144). The increased body fat is stored intraabdominally and intramuscularly in the elderly rather than subcutaneously as in the young (145). Thus, triceps skinfold thickness alone and measures derived from it (e.g., midarm muscle area) do not accurately predict body fat content in the elderly. Several groups have addressed the problem of using anthropometry to study body composition of elderly persons (146–147).

Review of Studies of Institutional and Free-Living Elderly Populations

A review of 28 dietary surveys that included data from elderly persons concluded that the mean caloric intake was most often below the standard used (148). In several large surveys of note (65, 106–108, 110, 117–119), mean energy intakes (kcal/kg/day) averaged 1792 to 2171 for males and 1168 to 1770 for females, generally below the 1989 RDA of 2300 for males and 1900 kcal/day for females. Caloric intakes of sedentary elderly persons may indeed be below current estimates. The low intakes may also result from the tendency of many methods to underestimate food intake. Indeed, when the doubly labeled water method was used on an elderly population, TEE exceeded that estimated from food intake (10, 11).

Protein nutriture has been assessed in the elderly by dietary intake and accompanying biochemical parameters. The average protein intakes in NHANES I, II, and III (preliminary) as well as in other surveys of institutional and free-living elderly were above the 1989 RDA. Thus, protein nutriture, in the absence of chronic disease, appears adequate. In some studies, certain serum proteins (albumin, transferrin, prealbumin, retinol-binding protein) appear to decline with age (118, 149, 150). A lower serum albumin level is often not correlated with protein intake and may represent a normal decrease for the elderly (1, 15, 18). A study of serum albumin levels in healthy elderly persons appears to show minimal decreases with age (122).

The nutritional status of the elderly with respect to several vitamins and minerals has been assessed. Based on both dietary intake and/or biochemical measures in the NHANES I, II, and III (preliminary) studies as well as in other studies (60, 117, 118), low intakes of calcium and vitamin D appear most frequently and can be attributed to the low intake of dairy products among certain groups in this population.

The situation with vitamin B_6 nutriture is complex. Several studies show vitamin B_6 intakes well below the RDA and up to 28% of individuals with abnormal erythrocyte aspartate aminotransferase stimulation tests (117, 118, 151). However, reported vitamin B_6 intakes might be somewhat higher if the food table values for vitamin B_6 (as well as for zinc, folate, and vitamin B_{12}) were more complete. As for any nutrient, current standards for biochemical tests of nutrient status for vitamin B_6 may be inappropriate for the elderly. In addition, inferring deficiency on the basis of a single screening should be tempered by the fact that intraindividual variance in biochemical measures is large enough to account for a portion of the "deficiency" at any one measurement time (152).

Mean intakes of most other vitamins and minerals (with an adequate database) appear adequate, although in a few studies, biochemical tests indicate that 5 to 20% of elderly people may have low serum levels of thiamin, riboflavin, iron, zinc, and folate (109–153).

Supplement Use by the Elderly

In a study of a Meals on Wheels program, 14 of 33 subjects were considered at risk for protein-energy malnutrition. Supplementation with a liquid polymeric supplement for 4 months increased weight in most subjects; the weight gain was associated with increases in serum albumin, total iron-binding capacity, folate, vitamin C, and vitamin B_{12}, thus providing evidence of improved nutritional status (154).

Supplement use was also examined as part of the nutritional status survey of free-living elderly in Boston (155). Daily vitamin and mineral use was reported by about half of the elderly; use of vitamin C and E supplements was most common. Supplement use markedly decreased the number of individuals whose total daily intake (diet plus supplement) of vitamins B_6, B_{12}, and D, of folate, and of calcium would be considered low. Of concern, both elderly males and females consumed excessive levels (at least 10 times the RDA) of vitamin A. These results are consistent with other studies of supplementation in the elderly (156). However, an even greater prevalence of supplementation (72%) was observed in a survey of an affluent community of "health conscious" residents (157).

DRUG-NUTRIENT INTERACTION

Nutrients can affect drug action by altering the digestion, absorption, distribution, metabolism, and/or excretion of the drug. Less often recognized is that for all age groups, drugs may influence the nutritional status of the individual. Drugs may affect nutritional status in several ways: effects on food intake, alteration of nutrient absorption, alteration of nutrient metabolism, and alteration in nutrient excretion (158). This is particularly important for the elderly, who often have multiple chronic diseases and are taking several medications or drugs concurrently. Risk of adverse side effects increases with the number of drugs taken simultaneously and with the duration of exposure to the drugs.

Alcohol and Nutritional Status in the Elderly

Alcohol is the most common drug used by the population at large. In large amounts taken chronically, the overall nutritional status is adversely affected, including reduced appetite and impaired nutrient absorption, metabolism, and excretion. Ethanol is also associated with several serious medical and social problems such as hepatic cirrhosis, adenocarcinoma of the gastrointestinal tract (particularly mouth, pharynx, larynx, and esophagus) and liver, and impaired driving. Most elderly individuals who consume alcohol, however, consume small amounts (159). A survey of 554 nonalcoholic subjects who had participated in a nutritional status assessment of the elderly in the Boston area, classified alcohol use into three categories: less than 5 g/day, 5 to 14 g/day, or more than 15 g/day (160). The extent of alcohol use was related to nutritional, biochemical, and physical parameters of these individuals. Plasma retinol, ferritin, and high-density lipoprotein cholesterol concentrations were significantly higher, and serum copper, zinc, and potassium were significantly lower in those consuming more than 15 g/day than in those consuming less than 5 g/day. The statistically significant effects were small, however, and thus of questionable biologic significance, and alcohol only affected potassium and copper levels in patients using diuretics.

REFERENCES

1. Munro HN, Danford DE. eds. Nutrition, aging, and the elderly. New York: Plenum Press, 1989.
2. Weindruch RH, Walford RL. The retardation of aging and disease by dietary restriction. Springfield, IL: Charles C Thomas, 1988.
3. Halliwell B. Annu Rev Nutr 1996;16:33–50.
4. Russell RM, Sahyoun NR. The elderly. In: Paige EM, ed. Clinical nutrition. 2nd ed. Washington, DC: CV Mosby, 1988;110–6.

5. Bowman BB, Rosenberg IH. Am J Clin Nutr 1982;35:1142–51.
6. Thompson ABR, Keelan M. Can J Physiol Pharmacol 1986; 64:30–8.
7. Rosenberg IH, Russell RM, Bowman BB. Aging and the digestive system. In: Munro HN, Danford DE, eds. Nutrition, aging, and the elderly. New York: Plenum Press, 1989;43–60.
8. McGandy RB, Barrows CH, Spanias A, et al. J Gerontol 1966;21:581–7.
9. Food and Nutrition Board, National Research Council. Recommended dietary allowances. 10th ed. Washington, DC: National Academy Press, 1989.
10. Roberts SB, Fuss P, Heyman MB, Young VR. Am J Clin Nutr 1995;62(Suppl):1053S–8S.
11. Sawaya AL, Saltzman E, Fuss P, et al. Am J Clin Nutr 1995;62:338–44.
12. Werner I, Hambraeus L. The digestive capacity of elderly people. In: Carlson LA, ed. Nutrition in old age. Uppsala: Almquist and Wiksell, 1972;55–60.
13. Cheng AHR, Gomez A, Gergan JG, et al. Am J Clin Nutr 1978;31:12–22.
14. Gersovitz M, Motil D, Munro HN, et al. Am J Clin Nutr 1982;35:6–14.
15. Munro HN, Suter PM, Russell RM. Annu Rev Nutr 1987; 7:23–49.
16. Campbell WW, Crim MC, Dallal GE, et al. Am J Clin Nutr 1994;60:501–9.
17. Campbell WW, Crim MC, Young VR, et al. Am J Physiol 1995;268:E1143–53.
18. Munro HN, McGandy RB, Hartz SC, et al. Am J Clin Nutr 1987;46:586–92.
19. Beaumont DM, Cobden I, Sheldon WL, et al. Age Ageing 1987;16:294–300.
20. Guth PH. Am J Dig Dis 1968;13:565–71.
21. Arora S, Kassarjian Z, Krasinski SD, et al. Gastroenterology 1989;96:1560–5.
22. Feibusch JM, Holt PR. Dig Dis Sci 1982;27:1095–100.
23. Welsh JD, Russell LC, Walker AW Jr. Gerontology 1974; 66:993–7.
24. Welsh JD, Poley JR, Bhatia M, et al. Gastroenterology 1978;75:847–55.
25. Debongnie JC, Newcomer AD, McGill DB, Philips FS. Dig Dis Sci 1979;24:225–31.
26. Southgate DAT, Durnin JVGA. Br J Nutr 1970;24:517–35.
27. Pelz KS, Gottfried SP, Sooes E. Geriatrics 1968;23:149–53.
28. Saltzman JR, Kowdley KV, Pedrosa MC, et al. Gastroenterology 1994;106:615–23.
29. Webster SGP, Wilkinson EM, Gowland E. Age Ageing 1977;6:113–7.
30. Gray DS. Am Fam Physician 1995;51;419–25.
31. Warren JL, Bacon WE, Harris T, et al. Am J Public Health 1994;84:1265–9.
32. Rowe JW. Renal and lower urinary tract diseases in the elderly. In: Calkins E, Davis PJ, Ford AB, eds. The practice of geriatrics. Philadelphia: WB Saunders, 1986.
33. Suter PM, Russell RM. Am J Clin Nutr 1987;45:501–12.
34. Iber FL, Blass JP, Brin M, et al. Am J Clin Nutr 1982;36: 1067–82.
35. Thomson AD. Gerontol Clin 1966;8:345–61.
36. Breen KJ, Buttigier R, Iossifidis S, et al. Am J Clin Nutr 1985;42:121–6.
37. Chen LH, Fan Chiang WL. Int J Vitam Nutr Res 1981;51: 232–8.
38. Harrill I, Cervone N. Am J Clin Nutr 1977;30:431–40.
39. Said HM, Hollander D. Life Sci 1985;36:69–73.
40. Schaus R, Kirk JE. J Gerontol 1957;11:147–50.
41. Boisvert WA, Mendoza I, Castaneda C, et al. J Nutr 1993;123:915–25.
42. Horwitt MK, Harvey CC, Hills OW, et al. J Nutr 1950;41: 247–64.
43. Pelletier O. NY Acad Sci 1975;258:156–68.
44. Kirk JE, Chieffi M. J Gerontol 1953;8:305–11.
45. Garry PJ, Goodwin JS, Hunt WC, et al. Am J Clin Nutr 1982;36:332–9.
46. Cheng L, Cohen M, Bhagavan HN. Vitamin C and the elderly. In: Watson RR, ed. Handbook of nutrition in the aged. Boca Raton, FL: CRC Press, 1985.
47. Jacques PF, Chylack LT. Am J Clin Nutr 1991;53:352S–5S.
48. Ribaya-Mercado JD, Russell RM, Sahyoun N, et al. J Nutr 1991;121:1062–74.
49. Selhub J, Jacques PF, Wilson PWF. JAMA 1993;270:2693–8.
50. Senti FR, Pilch SM, eds. Assessment of the folate nutritional status of the U.S. population based on data collected in the second National Health and Nutrition Examination Survey, 1976–1980. Bethesda, MD: FASEB, 1984.
51. Jagerstad M, Westesson AK. Scand J Gastroenterol 1979; 14(Suppl 52):196–202.
52. Russell RM, Krasinski SD, Samloff IM, et al. Gastroenterology 1986;91:1476–82.
53. Beecher GR, Matthews RH. Nutrient composition of foods. In: Brown LM, ed. Present knowledge in nutrition. 6th ed. Washington, DC: International Life Sciences Institute, 1990;430–43.
54. Garry PJ, Goodwin JS, Hunt WC. J Am Geriatric Soc 1984;32:719–26.
55. Magnus EM, Bache-Wiig JE, Aanderson TR, et al. Scand J Haematol 1982;28:360–6.
56. Suter PM, Golner BB, Goldin BR, et al. Gastroenterology 1991;101:1039–45.
57. Krasinski S, Russell RM, Otradovec CL, et al. Am J Clin Nutr 1989;49:112–20.
58. Krasinski SD, Cohn JS, Schaefer EJ. J Clin Invest 1990;85: 883–91.
59. MacLaughlin J, Holick MF. J Clin Invest 1985;76:1536–8.
60. Webb AR, Pilbeam C, Hanafin N, et al. Am J Clin Nutr 1990;51:1075–81.
61. Barragry JM, France MW, Corless D, et al. Clin Sci Mol Med 1978;55:213–20.
62. Ebeling PR, Sandgrren E, DiMagno EP, et al. J Clin Endocrinol Metab 1992;75:176–82.
63. Gallagher JC, Riggs BL, Eisman J, et al. J Clin Invest 1979;64:729–36.
64. Dawson-Hughes B, Dallal GE, Krall EA, et al. Ann Intern Med 1991;115:505–12.
65. Garry PJ, Goodwin JS, Hunt WC, et al. Am J Clin Nutr 1982;36:319–31.
66. Horwitt MK, Harvey CC, Dahm CJ Jr. NY Acad Sci 1972;203:223–36.
67. Bjornson LK, Kayden HJ, Miller E, Moshell AN. J Lipid Res 1976;17:343–52.
68. Davies E, Kelleher J, Losowhy MS. Clin Chim Acta 1969;24: 431–6.
69. Vatassery GT, Johnson GJ, Krezowski AM, et al. J Am Coll Nutr 1983;4:369–75.
70. Meydani SN, Barklund MP, Liu S, et al. Am J Clin Nutr 1990;52:557–63.
71. Haroon Y, Bacon DS, Sadowski JA. J Chromatogr 1987;384: 383–9.
72. Sadowski JA, Hood SJ, Dallal GE, et al. Am J Clin Nutr 1989;50:100–8.

73. Ferland G, Sadowski JA, O'Brien ME. J Clin Invest 1993;91: 1761–8.
74. Shearer MJ. Lancet 1995;345:229–34.
75. Bullamore JR, Wilkinson R, Gallagher JC, et al. Lancet 1970;2:535–7.
76. Krasinski SD, Russell RM, Samloff IM, et al. J Am Geriatr Soc 1986;34:800–6.
77. Knox TA, Kassarjian Z, Dawson-Hughes B, et al. Am J Clin Nutr 1991;53:1480–6.
78. Ireland P, Fordtran JS. J Clin Invest 1973;52:2672–81.
79. Matkovic V, Kostial K, Simonovic I, et al. Am J Clin Nutr 1979;32:540–9.
80. Dawson-Hughes B, Dallal GE, Krall EA, et al. N Engl J Med 1990;323:878–83.
81. Aloia JF, Vaswani A, Yeh JK, et al. Ann Intern Med 1994;120: 97–103.
82. Reid IR, Ames RW, Evans MC, et al. N Engl J Med 1993;328: 460–4.
83. NIH Consensus Development Panel on Optimal Calcium Intake. JAMA 1994;272:1942–8.
84. Nelson M, Fiatarone MA, Morganti CM, et al. JAMA 1994;272:1909–14.
85. Lynch SR, Finch CA, Monsen ER, et al. Am J Clin Nutr 1982;36:1032–45.
86. Bunker VW, Lawson MS, Clayton BE. J Clin Pathol 1984; 37:1353–7.
87. Marx JJM. Blood 1979;53:204–11.
88. Pilch SM, Senti FR, eds. Assessment of the iron nutritional status of the U.S. population based on data collected in the second National Health and Nutrition Examination Survey, 1976–1980. Bethesda, MD: FASEB, 1984.
89. Cook JD, Finch CA, Smith N. Blood 1976;48:449–55.
90. Casale G, Bonora C, Migliavacca A, et al. Age Ageing 1981;10: 119–22.
91. Guyatt GH, Patterson C, Ali M, et al. Am J Hosp Med 1990; 88:205–9.
92. Holyoake TL, Stott DJ, McKay PJ, et al. J Clin Pathol 1993;46:857–60.
93. Expert Scientific Working Group. Summary of a report on assessment of the iron nutritional status of the United States population. Am J Clin Nutr 1985;42:1318–30.
94. Adams PC. Am J Hematol 1994;45:146–9.
95. Salonen JT, Nyyssonen K, Korpela H, et al. Circulation 1992;86:803–11.
96. Pilch SM, Senti FR, eds. Assessment of the zinc nutritional status of the U.S. population based on data collected in the second National Health and Nutrition Examination Survey, 1976–1980. Bethesda, MD: FASEB, 1984.
97. Bogden JD, Oleske JM, Munves EM, et al. Am J Clin Nutr 1987;46:101–9.
98. Turnlund JR, Durkin N, Costa F, et al. J Nutr 1986;116: 1239–47.
99. Jacob RA, Russell RM, Sandstead HH. Zinc and copper nutrition in aging. In: Watson R, ed. Handbook of nutrition in the aged. Boca Raton, FL: CRC Press, 1985;77–88.
100. Bogden JD, Oleske JM, Lavenhar MA, et al. J Am Coll Nutr 1990;9:214–25.
101. Bogden JD, Bendich A, Kemp FW, et al. Am J Clin Nutr 1994;60:437–47.
102. Wood RJ, Suter PM, Russell RM. Am J Clin Nutr 1995; 62:493–505.
103. Bunker VW, Lawson MS, Stansfield MF, et al. Br J Nutr 1988;59:171–80.
104. Abraham AS, Brooks BA, Eylath U. Metabolism 1992;41: 768–71.
105. Martin BJ, Lyon TDB, Fell GS. J Trace Elem Electrol Health Dis 1991;5:202–11.
106. Lowenstein FW. J Am Coll Nutr 1982;1:165–77.
107. National Center for Health Statistics, Carroll MD, Abraham S, Dresser CM. Vital and health statistics, series 11, no. 231. DHHS publ. no. (PHS) 83-1681. Public Health Service. Washington, DC: US Government Printing Office, 1983.
108. McDowell MA, Briefel RR, Alaimo K, et al. Energy and macronutrient intakes of persons ages 2 months and over in the United States: Third National Health and Nutrition Examination Survey, Phase 1, 1988–91. Advance data from vital and health statistics; no. 225. Hyattsville, MD: National Center for Health Statistics, 1994.
109. Alaimo K, McDowell MA, Briefel RR, et al. Dietary intake of vitamins, minerals, and fiber of persons ages 2 months and over in the United States: Third National Health and Nutrition Examination Survey, Phase 1, 1988–91. Advance data from vital and health statistics; no. 258. Hyattsville, MD: National Center for Health Statistics, 1994.
110. Federation of American Societies of Experimental Biology, Life Sciences Research Office. Prepared for the Interagency Board for Nutrition Monitoring and Related Research. Third report on nutrition monitoring in the United States, vol 1 and 2. Washington, DC: US Government Printing Office, 1995.
111. US Department of Agriculture. Continuing survey of food intakes by individuals. Food code and nutrient data base for CSFII 1994. Agricultural Research Service, CD-ROM, January 1996.
112. Attwood EC, Robey E, Kramer JJ, et al. Age Ageing 1978;7: 46–56.
113. Stiedemann M, Jansen C, Harrill I. J Am Diet Assoc 1978;73: 132–9.
114. Prothro J, Mickles M, Tolbert B. Am J Clin Nutr 1976;29: 94–104.
115. Barr SI, Chrysomilides SA, Willis EJ, et al. Nutr Res 1983;3:417–31.
116. Kohrs MB, O'Neal R, Preston A, et al. Am J Clin Nutr 1978;31:2186–97.
117. McGandy RB, Russell RM, Hartz SC, et al. Nutr Res 1986;6:785–98.
118. Sahyoun NR, Otradovec CL, Hartz SC, et al. Am J Clin Nutr 1988;47:524–33.
119. Mowé M, Bøhmer T, Kindt E. Am J Clin Nutr 1994;59:317–24.
120. Thompson FE, Byers T. Dietary assessment resource manual. J Nutr 1994;124:2245S–317S.
121. Morrow FD. Clin Nutr 1986;5:112–20.
122. Campion EW, DeLabry LO, Glynn RJ. J Gerontol 1988;43: M18–20.
123. National Center for Health Statistics, Fulwood R, Johnson CL, et al. Vital and health statistics, series 11, no. 232. DHHS publ. no. (PHS) 83-1682. Public Health Service. Washington, DC: US Government Printing Office, 1982.
124. Manson JE, Stampfer MJ, Hennekens CH, et al. JAMA 1987;257:353–8.
125. Simopoulos AP, Van Itallie TB. Ann Intern Med 1984;100: 285–95.
126. Chicago Society of Actuaries. Build study, 1979. Chicago: Society of Actuaries and Association of Life Insurance Medical Directors of America, 1980.
127. Metropolitan Height and Weight Tables. New York: Metropolitan Insurance Company, 1983.
128. Garrison RJ, Feinleib M, Castelli WP, et al. JAMA 1983;249: 2199–203.
129. Kissebah AH, Vydelingum N, Murray R, et al. J Clin Endocrinol Metab 1982;54:254–60.

130. Krotkiewski M, Björntorp P, Sjöström L, et al. J Clin Invest 1983;72:1150–62.
131. Lapidus L, Bengtsson C, Larsson B, et al. Br Med J 1984;289:1257–61.
132. Larsson B, Svärdsudd K, Welin L, et al. Br Med J 1984;288: 1401–4.
133. Master AM, Lasser RP. JAMA 1960;172:658–62.
133a. Frisancho AR. Anthropometric standards for assessment of growth and nutritional status. Ann Arbor: University of Michigan Press, 1990.
134. Frisancho AR. Am J Clin Nutr 1984;40:808–19.
135. Frisancho AR, Flegel PN. Am J Clin Nutr 1983;37:311–4.
136. Andres R, Elahi D, Tobin JD, et al. Ann Intern Med 1985;103: 1030–3.
137. Andres R. Mortality and obesity: the rationale for age-specific height-weight tables. In: Andres R, Bierman EL, Hazzard WR. Principles of geriatric medicine. New York: McGraw Hill, 1985;311–8.
138. USDA, US Department of Health and Human Services. Dietary guidelines for Americans. 4th ed. 1995.
139. Russell RM. Nutrition. JAMA 1966;275:1828–9.
140. Roubenoff R, Dallal GE, Wilson PWF. Am J Public Health 1995;85:726–8.
141. Launer LJ, Harris T, Rumpel C, et al. JAMA 1994;271:1093–8.
142. National Center for Health Statistics, Najjar MF, Rowland M. Vital and health statistics, series 11, no. 238. DHHS publ. no. (PHS) 87-1688. Public Health Service. Washington, DC: US Government Printing Office, 1987.
143. Blackburn GL, Thornton P. Med Clin North Am 1979;63: 1103–15.
144. Forbes GB. Hum Biol 1976;48:161–73.
145. Cohn SH, Ellis KJ, Sawitsky A, et al. Am J Clin Nutr 1981; 2839–47.
146. Visser M, van den Jeuvel E, Deurenberg P. Br J Nutr 1994;7: 823–33.
147. Chumlea WC, Baumgartner RN. Am J Clin Nutr 1989;50: 1158–66.
148. O'Hanlon P, Kohrs MB. Am J Clin Nutr 1978;31:1257–69.
149. Yearick ES, Wang M-SL, Pisias SJ. J Gerontol 1980;35:663–71.
150. Jansen C, Harrill I. Am J Clin Nutr 1977;30:1414–22.
151. Smith JL, Wickiser AA, Korth LL, et al. J Am Coll Nutr 1984;3:13–25.
152. Garry PJ, Hunt WC, VanderJagt D, et al. Am J Clin Nutr 1989;50:1219–30.
153. Garry PJ, Goodwin JS, Hunt WC. Am J Clin Nutr 1982;36: 902–9.
154. Lipschitz DA, Mitchell CO, Steele RW, et al. JPEN J Parenter Enteral Nutr 1985;9:343–47.
155. Hartz SC, Otradovec CL, McGandy RB. J Am Coll Nutr 1988;7:119–28.
156. Hale WE, Stewart RB, Cerda JJ, et al. J Am Geriatr Soc 1982; 30:401–3.
157. Gray GE, Paganini-Hill A, Ross RK. Am J Clin Nutr 1983;38:122–8.
158. Roe DA, ed. Drugs and nutrition in the geriatric patient. New York: Churchill Livingstone, 1984.
159. Russell RM. Drug Nutr Interact 1985;4:165–70.
160. Jacques PF, Hartz SC, Russell RM. FASEB J 1988;2:A1613.

SELECTED READINGS

Corti M-C, Guralnik JM, Salive ME, Sorkin JD. Serum albumin level and physical disability as predictors of mortality in older persons. JAMA 1994;272:1036–42.

Morley JE, Glick Z, Rubenstein LZ, eds. Geriatric nutrition: a comprehensive review. New York: Raven Press, 1990.

Russell RM, Suter PM. Vitamin requirements of elderly people: an update. Am J Clin Nutr 1993;58:4–14.

USDA Human Nutrition Research Center on Aging, Tufts University. Nutrition in the elderly. The Boston nutritional status survey. London: Smith-Gordon and Co., 1992.

Wood RJ, Suter PM, Russell RM. Mineral requirements of elderly people. Am J Clin Nutr 1995;62:493–505.

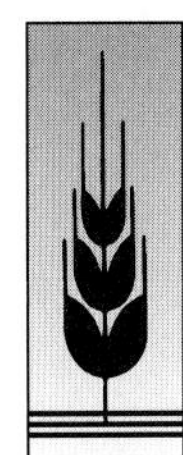

PART III.

Dietary and Nutritional Assessment of the Individual

54. Clinical Nutrition Assessment of Infants and Children

VIRGINIA A. STALLINGS and ELLEN B. FUNG

Nutritional status assessment in children is essential for identifying either the undernourished or overnourished state and estimating the optimum energy intake to promote growth and well-being. In children with moderate-to-severe disabilities or many of the chronic diseases, nutritional assessment is complicated by interaction of the primary disease process (i.e., muscle atrophy, contractures, chronic malabsorption), drug-nutrient interactions, and acute and/or chronic malnutrition.

This chapter aims to provide the reader with an appropriate knowledge base, current references, and methodology for assessing the nutritional status of healthy infants and children and the methodologic modification required for children with chronic disease. Nutritional assessment in children has several components, including evaluation of dietary intake, growth status, body composition, energy expenditure, and laboratory data in the context of the medical history, diagnoses, and current therapy. Dietary and biochemical assessment are important tools for evaluating the nutritional status of the child and are presented thoroughly in Chapters 57 and 58. Nutrition is a major determinant of growth patterns in infants and children; thus, this chapter focuses on assessment of growth, body composition, and energy expenditure.

ELEMENTS OF NUTRITIONAL ASSESSMENT

The elements of complete nutritional assessment are based on the standard pediatric medical evaluation that includes a medical history, a physical examination, and laboratory assessment. Children are usually assessed by the primary physician, pediatric caregiver, physician's assistant, or nurse practitioner, though others (dietitians, speech therapists, occupational and physical therapists, social workers) may also participate in the assessment, depending upon the setting. Because nutritional assessment of the child is multidisciplinary, cooperation of the interdisciplinary team is important. For example, the medical history and physical examination may be completed by the pediatric caregiver, the dietary history and anthropometry by the dietitian, and any effects of family structure on food availability and/or meal planning completed by the social worker. For children with special needs, other disciplines (e.g., speech and occupational therapy) may be involved in assessing oral motor function and/or proper positioning for feeding the child. No single test provides an adequate measure of overall nutritional status; instead evaluation is based on a variety of somewhat nonspecific indicators.

Medical History

The medical history includes assessing acute and chronic medical conditions, medications, allergies, activity pattern, and a diet history since infancy. The diet-intake history includes review of a typical day's food intake; past dietary history and recent changes in diet pattern; use of caloric, vitamin, or mineral supplements; general appetite; presence of pica; food aversions or special food practices by the child or family; food and/or formula preparation; behaviors that may interfere with feeding; and caregiver nutritional knowledge. Past growth patterns, growth charts, and pubertal history are reviewed. Pubertal rating, most commonly assessed by the Tanner stages (1), is divided into five anatomically defined stages based on

---

Abbreviations: **DXA**—dual-energy x-ray absorptiometry; **FFM**—Fat-free mass; **HC**—head circumference; **MAC**—mid-upper-arm circumference; **NCHS**—National Center for Health Statistics; **REE**—resting energy expenditure; **TSF**—triceps skinfold; **WHO**—World Health Organization.

phallus and pubic hair development in boys and breast and pubic hair development in girls (Table 54.1). For screening purposes, a self-assessment instrument has been devised using pictographs of Tanner's pubertal stages (2). The medical history also includes a review of systems with emphasis on the dental and oral motor function and the gastrointestinal tract (emesis, gastroesophageal reflux, diarrhea, and constipation).

Physical Examination

The nutritionally oriented physical examination may include the following measurements: current weight, height/length or alternative linear growth measure, head circumference, midarm circumference, and skinfold measurements. Details of anthropometric methodology and reference standards are presented in the next section. Reviews of physical findings associated with nutritional deficiencies are available (3, 4), and a summary is presented in Table 54.2. Though specific nutrient deficiencies are not as common in infants and children in the United States as in developing countries, deficiencies of certain nutrients (e.g., iron, vitamin A, and zinc) have been observed in otherwise healthy children; thus, primary care providers *must* be aware of the clinical presentations. Children with chronic diseases, syndromes, or developmental disabilities are at particular risk for developing specific nutrient deficiencies because of poor intake, feeding problems, food aversions/food specificity, altered nutrient or energy needs, and/or long-term medication use (5). Though not specifically listed in Table 54.2, obesity is a form of malnutrition that is increasingly prevalent in U.S. children and adults. The problem of obesity in children is reviewed thoroughly in Chapter 63.

Table 54.1
Typical Stages of Male and Female Pubertal Development

Pubic hair development for males and females
- Stage 1: There is no pubic hair
- Stagle 2: Sparse growth of lightly pigmented hair is usually straight or only slightly curled, primarily at either side of the base of the penis or along the labia
- Stage 3: The hair spreads over the pubic symphysis and is considerably darker and coarser and usually more curled
- Stage 4: The hair is now adult in character but covers an area considerably smaller than in most adults; there is no spread to the medial surface of the thighs
- Stage 5: The hair is distributed in an inverse triangle as in the female; hair is adult in quantity and type with extension to the thighs

Male genitalia
- Stage 1: The infantile state which persists from birth until puberty begins; during this time the genitalia increase slightly in overall size, but there is little change in general appearance
- Stage 2: Scrotum has begun to enlarge, and there is some reddening and change in texture of the scrotal skin
- Stage 3: The penis has increased in length, and there is a smaller increase in breadth; there has been further growth on the scrotum
- Stage 4: Further growth of testes and scrotum and increase in size of the penis especially in breadth
- Stage 5: The genitalia are adult in size and shape

Breasts
- Stage 1: The infantile stage persists, elevation of the papilla only
- Stage 2: This is the bud stage, a small mound is formed by the elevation of the breast and papilla; the areolar diameter enlarges
- Stage 3: Further enlargement of breasts and areola with no separation of their contours
- Stage 4: The areola and papilla are further enlarged and form a secondary mound projecting above the corpus of the breast
- Stage 5: This is the typical adult stage with a smooth rounded contour, the secondary mound present in stage 4 having disappeared

From Tanner JM. Growth at adolescence. 2nd ed. Oxford: Blackwell Scientific Publications, 1962, with permission.

Table 54.2
Summary of Clinical Signs of Nutritional Deficiency

Clinical Sign	Possible Nutrient Deficiency
Hair	
Alopecia	Protein, zinc
Menke's "steely" hair	Copper
Eyes	
Night blindness, xerophthalmia	Vitamin A
Keratomalacia, Bitôt's spot	Vitamin A
Oral area	
Glossititis	Folate, vitamin B_{12}
Magenta tongue	Riboflavin
Hypogeusia	Zinc
Angular stomatitis, cheilosis	Niacin, riboflavin
Poor dentition, dental caries	Fluoride
Inflamed, bleeding gums	Vitamin C
Skin/nails	
Petechiae	Vitamins C, K
Seborrheic dermatitis	Riboflavin, vitamin B_6, zinc
Dryness, xerosis	Biotin, linoleic acid, zinc
Pellagrous dermatosis	Niacin
Impaired wound healing	Vitamins A, C, zinc
Kiolonychia, spoon-shaped nails	Iron
Glands/endocrine	
Goiter, thyroid enlargement	Iodine
Cardiac	
Palpitations, tachycardia	Thiamin
Cardiomegaly	Selenium, thiamin
Arrhythmia	Potassium
Gastrointestinal	
Diarrhea	Niacin, zinc
Extremities	
Muscle wasting	Protein-calorie malnutrition
Peripheral edema	Protein, thiamin
Osteomalacia, osteoporosis	Calcium, vitamin D
Rickets, bowed legs	Vitamin D
Circulation	
Anemia, hemolytic	Vitamin E
Anemia, microcytic, hypochromic	Copper, iron
Anemia, megaloblastic	Folate, vitamin B_{12}
Prolonged clotting time	Vitamin K
Neurologic	
Mental confusion, irritability	Niacin, thiamin, vitamin B_{12}
Ataxia, loss of ankle/knee reflexes	Thiamin, vitamins B_{12}, E
Convulsions	Magnesium, vitamin B_6

Adapted from refs. 3, 4, and 36.

ANTHROPOMETRY

Anthropometric evaluation is an essential component in determining nutritional status and monitoring care. It is a rapid, inexpensive, noninvasive means of assessing both short- and long-term nutritional status. However, the assessment is only as good as the accuracy and reproducibility of the measurements; therefore, a well-trained anthropometrist is required. A variety of anthropometric measurements exist, each offering different information, and no single measure suffices for full characterization of nutritional status. Comparing the child with national reference norms for growth and nutritional status provides the means for interpreting these measurements. A description of measurement error and a summary of reference data are available for growth and body composition of normal children (6). A recent publication by Johnston and Ouyang (7) highlights the importance of the criteria selected to compare with reference data. Anthropometric measurements are most commonly recorded as percentiles above or below the mean reference data. However, when measurements for children are far below the 5th percentile or far above the 95th percentile, these rankings are difficult to interpret. Therefore, a z-score, or standard deviation score, is used frequently in some clinical and research settings to avoid these problems. The z-score is calculated as

$$\frac{\text{(the observed value)} - \text{(median value for the reference population)}}{\text{(standard deviation for the age and gender)}}$$

A z-score of -1 corresponds to the 16th percentile on the National Center for Health Statistics (NCHS) growth charts, whereas a z-score of -2 corresponds to the 2.5th percentile. Computer programs are available for these calculations (8). Methodology of anthropometry is reviewed thoroughly by Cameron (9) and Lohman et al. (10) (see also Chapter 56). Commonly used pediatric anthropometry is summarized below.

Weight

A single measurement of body weight cannot provide sufficient information to differentiate between acute and chronic malnutrition and may result in improper classification. Serial measurement of body weight is the most common assessment of growth in children. Weight should be measured on a calibrated, digital electronic or beam balance to the nearest 0.1 kg in older children and to the nearest 0.01 kg in infants; standard international units are preferred. Children should be weighed after voiding, wearing little or no outer clothing and no shoes; infants should be measured unclothed and without diapers.

Weight is plotted by age and gender and compared with the reference standards from the NCHS (see Appendix Tables III-A-14-b-1 and 2 and III-A-14-d-1 and 2). Tracking the weight of an individual over time in combination with his or her height improves the measurement as a diagnostic tool (see Appendices Tables IIIA 14b-1 and 2 and 14d2). Reference standards for weight (11) and 1-, 3-, or 6-month-interval weight-gain velocity are available (12, 13) (see also Appendix Tables III-1-A-4-e-1 and 2).

Height

Linear growth, as a component of a child's nutritional history, enables the clinician to distinguish between short- and long-term malnutrition. Length or stature measurements are appropriate for children who can be properly positioned as described below. For children less than 2 years of age, a supine length is taken. For children more than 2 years of age who cannot stand erect unsupported or have spinal curvature and/or contractures or other body habitus abnormalities precluding accurate length or height measurement, upper-arm length and lower-leg length are alternative stature measurements (described below) (see Appendix Tables III-A-14-f and g).

To measure supine length, an infantometer or an inflexible length board with a fixed headboard and movable footboard is used. Supine length measurement requires two people to position and hold the child. The infant's head is placed at the top of the board, knees are flattened to fully extend the legs, and feet are placed together and flexed to a 90° angle (9, 10). For stature, a stadiometer should be used with a head paddle that glides smoothly but is firmly perpendicular to the back of the stadiometer. Position the child with heels, buttocks, and back of the head against the stadiometer and arms down and relaxed. The head is positioned so that the Frankfort plane is parallel to the floor. The anatomic Frankfort plane extends from the lower margin of the orbit to the upper margin of the auditory meatus. Both length and stature measurements are accurate to 0.1 cm; three measurements are taken, and the mean is recorded. When comparing a supine length measurement with a growth chart for stature, the length is decreased approximately 2 cm to adjust for the known difference between length and stature due to gravity (14).

Length/height is plotted by gender and age and compared with NCHS growth charts (11) (Appendix Tables III-A-14-e-1 and 2). As with weight, multiple measurements taken over time are more useful than a single plot of height. Height velocity is more sensitive for determining delayed or accelerated growth. To calculate velocity, two height measurements are taken at least 6 months apart, preferably 12 months; shorter periods reflect seasonal variations in growth. The height difference is divided by the time between the two measurements, and a rate is calculated in centimeters per year. Height velocity charts are available for normal, early, and late-maturing children (15) (Appendix Tables III-A-14-e-1 and 2).

Whenever possible, the stature of both biologic parents is obtained and midparental stature is computed to identify the genetic potential for linear growth and make corrections when necessary (16). If the parents are stunted secondary to poor nutritional status during growth, it is not appropriate to use their statures for patient height adjustment.

Head Circumference

Brain growth is most rapid in the first 3 years of life, and head circumference (HC) is a good indicator of brain growth and malnutrition in otherwise healthy children. Of all anthropometric indicators, HC is best preserved in the presence of malnutrition and is included in the assessment of growth and nutritional status in children up to 36 months of age. In general, weight and then height are affected when a child is nutritionally compromised before brain and HC growth are slowed. HC is of limited use for nutritional assessment of patients with central nervous damage (micro- or macrocephalus of nonnutritional etiology) and of healthy patients with familial micro- or macrocephalus.

A flexible metal or nonstretchable plastic-coated measuring tape scaled to 0.1 cm is used. The tape is placed over the supraorbital ridge and around the occiput so that a maximum circumference is obtained. Care should be taken that the tape is evenly placed on all sides and flat against the skull. Three measurements are taken, and the mean is recorded. Reference data for HC are available by age from birth to 18 years of age (17).

Anthropometric Assessment of Body Composition

Anthropometric indicators of body composition are very useful in assessing clinical nutritional status because they are quick, inexpensive, clinically available indexes of energy and protein reserves that may reflect more subtle changes in nutritional status than measures of weight and height alone.

Midarm Circumference

Mid-upper-arm circumference (MAC) is a composite measure of muscle, fat, and bone in the arm. It is sensitive to current nutritional status and is used frequently in combination with the triceps skinfold thickness. The method is described in detail in Chapter 56 and reference data for MAC are available for children (18).

Skinfold Measurements

Skinfold thickness estimates subcutaneous fat stores at specified sites. The triceps and subscapular skinfold measures taken together generally indicate whole-body fat stores and are sensitive to changes in nutritional status. However, of all skinfold measures, the triceps skinfold appears clinically the most sensitive to changes in energy balance (25). The specific method of measurement and a description of how to optimize precision are presented in Chapter 56. References for skinfold thickness for children are available (19, 20). (See Appendix Tables III-A-16-a and b.)

Because of the variability of fat-free mass (FFM) density in infants and children, equations developed to estimate body fat from skinfold measurements in adults are inappropriate for the pediatric population. A variety of equations have been developed for use in children. The most reliable equations are those developed by Brook (21) for use in prepubescent children aged 1 to 11 years and by Durnin and Rahaman (22) for older children (Table 54.3) using four skinfold sites. For children aged 8 to 18 years, body fat can be estimated from two skinfold sites (triceps and subscapular) using the prediction equations of Slaughter et al. (23) (Table 54.4). These equations are specific to pubertal status, age, and ethnic background and correlate well with body composition measured by stable isotopes in normal children (23) as well as in children with cystic fibrosis (24) and cerebral palsy (25). Reilly et al. recently compared the most frequently used equations for estimating body fat from skinfolds in children (26).

NEONATAL NUTRITIONAL ASSESSMENT

Infants born preterm, less than 37 weeks gestation, are at increased risk for nutritional deficiency because of limited stores of energy and nutrients, confounded by decreased absorptive and digestive capacity. Rapid growth normally occurs between postconceptual ages 24 to 40 weeks. During this period there is increased muscle and fat accumulation, bone mineralization, micronutrient storage, brain myelination, and lung and gastrointestinal maturation. Interruption of these growth processes through suboptimal nutritional support may result in acute and/or chronic malnutrition and developmental repercussions. Infants born in the United States are not immune to malnutrition during the neonatal period; low birth weight and prematurity remain leading causes of infant mortality (Chapter 50). A thorough review of nutritional assessment for the neonate is available (27).

Methodology used to assess the neonate is similar to that used for the infant and child, with a few modifications. When completing a medical history for a premature or growth-retarded neonate, a review of the mother's preg-

Table 54.3
Anthropometric Equations for Predicting Percentage Fat from Four Skinfold Sites

a. Measure the following skinfolds in mm: triceps, biceps, subscapular, suprailiac.
b. Add the four skinfold measurements (Σ) and compute the log Σ.
c. For children between the ages 1 and 11 years, compute body density (D) using one of the following equations[a]:
  Males: $D = 1.169 - 0.0788 \times (\log \Sigma)$
  Females: $D = 1.2063 - 0.0999 \times (\log \Sigma)$
d. For children between the ages of 12 and 17 years, compute body density (D) using one of the following equations[b]:
  Males: $D = 1.1533 - 0.0643 \times (\log \Sigma)$
  Females: $D = 1.1369 - 0.0598 \times (\log \Sigma)$
e. Percentage body fat is calculated from D using the following formula[c]:
  Body Fat: $\% = [(4.95/D) - 4.5] \times 100$

[a]Adapted from ref. 21.
[b]Adapted from ref. 22.
[c]Adapted from ref. 54.

Table 54.4
Anthropometric Equations for Prediction of Percentage Fat from Two Skinfold Sites (8 to 18 years)[a]

White males	
Prepubescent:	1.21 (TSF + SUBSF) − 0.008 (TSF + SUBSF) − 1.7
Pubescent:	1.21 (TSF + SUBSF) − 0.008 (TSF + SUBSF) − 3.4
Postpubescent:	1.21 (TSF + SUBSF) − 0.008 (TSF + SUBSF) − 5.5
Black males	
Prepubescent:	1.21 (TSF + SUBSF) − 0.008 (TSF + SUBSF) − 3.2
Pubescent:	1.21 (TSF + SUBSF) − 0.008 (TSF + SUBSF) − 5.2
Postpubescent:	1.21 (TSF + SUBSF) − 0.008 (TSF + SUBSF) − 6.8
All females:	1.33 (TSF + SUBSF) − 0.013 (TSF + SUBSF) − 2.5
If (triceps + subscapular) greater than 35 mm	
Males:	0.783 (TSF + SUBSF) + 1.6
Females:	0.546 (TSF + SUBSF) + 9.7

From Slaughter M, Lohman T, Boileau R, et al. Hum Biol 1988;60:709–23, with permission.

[a]TSF, Triceps skinfold (mm); SUBSF, subscapular skinfold (mm); Prepubescent, Tanner stages 1 & 2; Pubescent, Tanner stage 3; Postpubescent, Tanner stage 4 & 5. See ref. 1 and Table 54.1.

nancy is important. Premature infant growth charts are available for both weight and length (28), which were developed from cross-sectional data of infants born between 24 and 42 weeks gestation. Though a sufficient number of infants were assessed, the sample from which the charts were derived has an undetermined bias because "premature birth itself is probably related to unphysiological states of either the mother or fetus" (29). These charts are often used until the infant reaches 40 weeks postconceptual age (full term), after which the NCHS growth charts (cited above) are used, and the child's age is adjusted for the degree of prematurity until the child is 2 years of age. However, the time at which catch-up growth is complete remains controversial (30, 31). For neonates in an intensive care unit, HC is the preferred assessment tool because clinical instability makes it difficult to measure weights and lengths accurately and reproducibly. Weights may vary daily due to fluctuations in fluid status and attached clinical equipment (e.g., intravenous catheters, endotracheal tubes, and chest tubes). HC should be measured 3 days postnatally to allow head edema and molding to resolve and then repeated for longitudinal assessment. HC data are commonly combined with MAC to provide information on the proportionality of body growth. MAC:HC reference data have been published for premature infants from 24 to 42 weeks postconceptual age (32).

ALTERNATIVE ASSESSMENT TOOLS FOR THE PHYSICALLY DISABLED CHILD

Body composition assessment of children with chronic diseases is essential in understanding their patterns of growth and development. Chronic disease is frequently associated with inadequate food intake, feeding problems, pica, drug-nutrient interactions, constipation, diarrhea, and/or altered energy needs resulting in poor nutritional status defined as decreased weight and/or height velocity accompanied by depletion of normal fat or fat-free mass stores (5, 33–34). Comparing the growth of children with moderate-to-severe physical and/or developmental disabilities with NCHS growth charts is inappropriate; special growth charts are available (Table 54.5).

Upper-Arm Length and Lower-Leg Length

Upper-arm length and lower-leg length are alternative measures of linear growth when length and stature measurements are not possible because of body habitus abnormalities such as scoliosis, spasticity, contractures, and/or poor cooperation due to cognitive or motor deficits. Both upper-arm length and lower-leg length are reliable and valid indexes of stature in children with developmental disabilities (36).

For young infants, sliding calipers (0–20 cm; Seritex Inc., NJ) are used; older infants and children require a Harpenden digital anthropometer (0–57 cm; Seritex Inc., NJ). These instruments are recommended for ease and accuracy of measurements. For infants and young children (0–24 months), upper-arm length is measured as shoulder-elbow length, and lower-leg length is measured as knee-heel length. A detailed description of the measurement technique is provided in Spender et al. (35), and revised reference percentiles for upper-arm length and lower-leg length are given for boys and girls aged 3 to 18 years (25, 36) (see Appendix Table III-A-14-f-1 and 2 and g-1 and 2). Percentiles and/or z-scores can be assigned and used as a proxy for length/height measurement. In nonambulatory children it is common for lower-

Table 54.5
Growth Charts Available for Specific Diseases/Syndromes in Children

Disease/ Syndrome	Growth Charts Available[a]	Reference
Achondroplasia	HT for age, HT velocity, HC	Horton et al., 1978 (55)
Down syndrome	HT for age, WT for age	Cronk et al., 1988 (56)
Fragile X syndrome	HT for age, WT for age, HC	Butler et al., 1992 (57)
Marfan syndrome	HT for age, WT for age	Pyeritz et al., 1985 (58)
Myelomeningocele	HT for age, WT for age	Ekvall, 1993 (63)
Noonan syndrome	HT for age	Ranke et al., 1988 (59)
Prader-Willi syndrome	HT for age	Holm, 1988 (60)
Turner syndrome	HT for age, HT velocity	Ranke et al., 1983 (61)
Willliams syndrome	HT for age, HC	Pankau et al. 1992 (62)

Adapted from refs. 6 and 64.

[a]HT: height, WT: weight, HC: head circumference.

leg length to be more severely affected than upper-arm length relative to reference standards (25).

OTHER METHODS OF BODY COMPOSITION ASSESSMENT

An extensive review of body composition assessment methods is found in Chapter 49. Total-body electric conductivity (TOBEC), bioelectric impedance, and isotope dilution are some of the safe and reliable methods for assessing body composition in infants and children, more often used for research purposes. A discussion of these methods is presented in Chapter 49, and reviews are available (37–41).

One method in particular, dual-energy x-ray absorptiometry (DXA) is being used increasingly to assess body composition in adults and more recently in children in both clinical and research settings. A thorough review is available (42). DXA exposes the child to low-level radiation, approximately 1/10th that of a chest x-ray. The ratio of low- to high-energy attenuation in soft tissue is used to distinguish between fat, FFM, and bone. DXA correlates well with densitometry, considered the gold standard for FFM measurement in adults (43). However, validation of new body composition methods in children is more problematic because of variation in FFM composition with age and change in the total-body water component (see Chapter 49); consequently, there is no accepted gold standard technique for infants and young children. DXA has been validated by carcass analysis of piglets (44) as well as by comparison with other frequently used methods of body composition in children (45). Body composition assessment by DXA has many advantages to densitometry; in particular, it was shown to be more precise in repeated measurement analysis (46). DXA can measure the body as a whole or in regions to obtain specific information about regional fat distribution and FFM. DXA has the potential to become the gold standard for body composition analysis in children because, in addition to the advantages listed above, it is less dependent on the assumption of biologic consistency than other methods.

USE OF RESTING ENERGY EXPENDITURE IN CLINICAL PEDIATRICS

The energy requirement for children, as stated by the World Health Organization (WHO), "includes the energy needs associated with the deposition of tissues (growth) . . . at rates consistent with good health" (47). For infants, children, and adolescents, the goal is to provide energy to achieve normal growth at the individual's genetic potential, achieve normal body composition, and maintain a normal pattern of activity. Chapter 5 provides a comprehensive review of the estimation and measurement of energy requirements. The focus here is on the estimation and measurement of energy expenditure in children, in both the inpatient and outpatient settings, with specific reference to indirect calorimetry.

Various sources in the literature provide tables of the predicted total daily energy needs for groups of healthy, normally grown children with the RDA being the standard for the United States (see Appendix Table II-A-2-a-1; for those of other countries see Tables A3–7). Yet in the practice of clinical medicine, the medical team needs to know the energy requirement of an individual patient who has a medically significant illness and possibly abnormal body composition, growth, and/or physical activity. The estimate of energy required is translated into a prescription for the appropriate number of calories from food, tube feeding, or intravenous nutritional support.

Estimating Resting Energy Expenditure

For many years, the only alternative to population-based recommendations for energy intake was using one of the various mathematical formulas to predict the basal metabolic rate or resting energy expenditure (REE), and then adjusting the REE with sets of physical activity and illness factors reflecting the patient's condition to predict the total daily energy needs of that patient. The most commonly used calculations were developed almost 80 years ago, mostly from adults, and therefore are not appropriate for the pediatric population (48). More recently, the WHO created new pediatric REE prediction equations ([47], Appendix Tables II-A-8-a-2-a and b). A more detailed evaluation of the WHO data resulted in the Schofield equations (Table 54.6), which use both weight and height, as well as age group and gender to predict REE (49). These equations assess the energy needs of normal healthy children quite well; however, the energy needs of hospitalized or chronically ill children are difficult to predict because of variations in metabolic demands of growth, body composition, and extra energy needs for the disease state. Many common pediatric gastrointestinal diseases (i.e., inflammatory bowel disease, cystic fibrosis, and liver disease) directly affect energy expenditure because of the associated malabsorption, inflammation, chronic infection, or changes in body composition. Thus, the energy needs of children with illnesses are difficult to pre-

Table 54.6
Schofield Equations for Predicting Resting Energy Expenditure in Children (0 to 18 Years)

Age Range (years)	Kcal/day[a,b]
Males	
0–3	0.167 W + 15.174 H − 617.6
3–10	19.59 W + 1.303 H + 414.9
10–18	16.25 W + 1.372 H + 515.5
Females	
0–3	16.252 W + 10.232 H − 413.5
3–10	16.969 W + 1.618 H + 371.2
10–18	8.365 W + 4.65 H + 200.0

Adapted from Schofield WN: Hum Nutr Clin Nutr 1985;39C(1s):5–42.

[a]Also see WHO equations for predicting basal metabolic rate from body weight, Appendix Table III-A-10-b.

[b]W, weight (kg); H, height (cm).

dict accurately from standard dietary recommendations designed from the requirements of healthy children. REE measurement is the best available method of accurately determining individual energy needs for use in clinical medicine to promote weight gain or loss or provide for weight maintenance.

Measuring Resting Energy Expenditure

The study of energy metabolism in clinical settings is now possible because of the availability of open-circuit ventilated-hood indirect calorimeters. The indirect calorimeter, or metabolic cart, measures oxygen consumption and carbon dioxide production by the patient, and these values are used to calculate the REE, expressed in absolute terms as kilocalories or kilojoules per day, or relative to body size as kilocalories or kilojoules per kilogram body weight. The instrument provides minute-by-minute values that are averaged over the testing interval to provide the final REE value. Clinical and research REE measurements are conducted under standardized conditions to ensure the accuracy of the data and thus that of the clinical interpretation. Detailed instructions on using indirect calorimetry to measure REE in children have been published (24, 25).

REE is measured to estimate the total caloric needs of an individual patient to achieve a specific clinical goal (weight maintenance, loss, or gain). To estimate the total daily energy requirements of a patient from measurement of the REE over a 1-h period requires further calculations and an understanding of the components of the total energy expenditure in health and disease. Children who are significantly ill and/or hospitalized have less spontaneous physical activity, and an activity factor of 1.3 to 1.5 times REE is usually an adequate estimate of the total energy needs. However, an additional correction factor for disease severity may be used to adjust the REE in some settings (i.e., burn patients, sepsis, significant protein losses). For example, the REE for children with cystic fibrosis is adjusted for the degree of pulmonary disease and/or fat malabsorption (51).

If indirect calorimetry is not available to measure REE, the WHO and/or Schofield equations are preferred and should be used to estimate the energy needs of the hospitalized child rather than the RDA values, which are based on population data. After calculations are made, recommendations may be adjusted for activity and disease factors, as stated above. Weight *must* be monitored routinely and caloric intake adjusted according to the nutritional goals for the child.

USE OF BONE MINERAL MEASURES IN CLINICAL PEDIATRICS

Bone mass accounts for up to 80% of the variance in skeletal strength and thus is the most important factor in preventing fracture. Since most bone mass accretion occurs during childhood and adolescence, increasing attention is focused on the components of bone health during the pediatric years. Bone mass is estimated from indirect, noninvasive measurements of bone mineral content (BMC) in grams or bone mineral density (BMD) in grams per square centimeter in selected skeletal regions or the whole body. Several methods were used previously; however, DXA is increasingly available in clinical settings and has several advantages for pediatric care (48). The precision of the measurement is excellent, 1 to 2%, and the radiation dose is small, less than 3 mrem (53). The most commonly performed scan for bone mineral determination is at the anterior-posterior (AP) lumbar spine site and can be completed within 3 minutes.

In most settings, data from the DXA scan of the AP view of the lumbar vertebrae (L1–4) is used for clinical interpretation and compared with results from healthy children of the same gender and chronologic age. The report includes information such as bone area (square centimeters), BMC, and BMD for each vertebral body and the mean of all four. The z-score for the patient is given, which allows comparison with the reference database. A z-score of zero is the mean (similar to the 50th percentile on a growth chart) for the reference data, with +1, +2, and −1 and −2 representing plus or minus one and two standard deviations of the reference mean. Since DXA measurements are new to clinical pediatrics, the approach to interpretation of the scans is evolving. In general, a DXA result that shows the patient with a z-score less than −2 (two standard deviations below the mean) for age and gender is clinically significant and treatment should be considered. In some high-risk settings, such as a child with significant malabsorption, steroid medications, poor oral intake, and/or decreased physical activity, intervention may be considered with a z-score below −1.

MANAGEMENT OF NUTRITIONAL PROBLEMS

Identification and treatment of nutritional and growth abnormalities are clearly standard pediatric practice. In general, dietary intake, food practices, and food beliefs are reviewed at each major well-child evaluation from infancy through adolescence. This information is the basis of individualized dietary and nutritional guidance provided by the primary care provider or dietitian. Therapeutic diets and vitamin or mineral supplements are prescribed on the basis of specific diagnoses and poor dietary patterns.

Monitoring incremental growth and development is also essential to the care of children and the detection of nutrition-related abnormalities. Care providers are concerned when a child's weight, height, or HC changes unexpectedly from the established growth channel on the standard NCHS growth charts or disease-specific charts. Crossing the chart percentile channel, either accelerating or faltering, requires careful review of the patient's general health, nutritional intake and needs, and psychosocial environment. This evaluation may again involve several members of the health care team. Management of undernutrition in otherwise healthy infants and premature infants is presented in Chapter 51, obesity in Chapter 63, and nutritional problems specific to disease in Chapters 59, 61, 62, and 64.

CONCLUSIONS

Assessment of growth, body composition, and energy requirements are essential components in the overall nutritional assessment and clinical care of children. Together with dietary and biochemical assessment, they reflect the current and previous nutritional status of the child and are essential for both monitoring changes in nutritional status that occur with normal growth and monitoring clinically indicated nutritional intervention.

ACKNOWLEDGMENTS

Special thanks to Babette Zemel, Ph.D., for significant contributions in preparing this manuscript.

REFERENCES

1. Tanner JM. Growth at adolescence. 2nd ed. Oxford: Blackwell Scientific Publications, 1962.
2. Morris NN, Udry JR. J Youth Adolesc 1980;9:271–80.
3. Gibson RS. Principles of nutritional assessment. New York: Oxford University Press, 1990.
4. McLaren DS. A colour atlas and text of diet related diseases. New ed. London: Wolfe Medical Publications, 1992.
5. American Dietetic Association. J Am Diet Assoc 1997;97: 189–93.
6. Zemel BS, Riley EM, Stallings VA. Annu Rev Nutr 1997;17: 211–35.
7. Johnston FE, Ouyang Z. Choosing appropriate reference data for the anthropometric assessment of nutritional status. In: Himes JH, ed. Anthropometric assessment of nutritional status. New York: Wiley-Liss, 1991;337–46.
8. Centers for Disease Control. CASP anthropometric software package. DHEW publ no. (PHS) 78-1650. Atlanta, GA: Division of Nutrition, CCDPHP, Centers for Disease Control.
9. Cameron N. The methods of auxological anthropology. In: Falkner F, Tanner JM, eds. Human growth: a comprehensive treatise, vol 3. 2nd ed. New York: Plenum Press, 1986;3–46.
10. Lohman TG, Roche AF, Martorell R, eds. Anthropometric standardization reference manual. Champaign, IL: Human Kinetics Books, 1988.
11. Hamill PW, Drizd TA, Johnson LL, et al. Am J Clin Nutr 1979;32:607–29.
12. Guo S, Roche AF, Fomon SF, et al. J Pediatr 1991;119:355–62.
13. Roche AF, Himes JH. Am J Clin Nutr 1980;33:2041–52.
14. Roche AF, Davila GH. Growth 1974;38:313–20.
15. Tanner JM, Davies PSW. J Pediatr 1985;107:317–29.
16. Himes J, Roche A, Thissen D, et al. Pediatrics 1985;75:304–13.
17. Roche AF, Mukherjee D, Guo S, et al. Pediatrics 1987;79: 706–12.
18. Frisancho AR. Am J Clin Nutr 1981;34:2540–5.
19. Cronk CE, Roche AF. Am J Clin Nutr 1982;35:347–54.
20. Frisancho AR. Anthropometric standard for assessment of growth and nutritional status. Ann Arbor, MI: University of Michigan Press, 1990.
21. Brook CGD. Arch Dis Child 1971;46:182–4.
22. Durnin JVGA, Rahaman MM. Br J Nutr 1967;21:681–9.
23. Slaughter M, Lohman T, Boileau R, et al. Hum Biol 1988;60: 709–23.
24. Tomezsko JL, Scanlin TF, Stallings VA. Am J Clin Nutr 1994;59:123–8.
25. Stallings VA, Cronk CE, Zemel BS, et al. J Pediatr 1995;126: 5:833–9.
26. Reilly JJ, Wilson J, Durnin JVGA. Arch Dis Child 1995; 73(4):305–10.
27. Pereira GR, Georgieff MK. Nutritional assessment. In: Polin RA, Fox WW, eds. Fetal and neonatal physiology. Philadelphia: WB Saunders, 1992;277–85.
28. Babson SG, Benda GI. J Pediatr 1976;89:814–20.
29. Lubchencho LO, Hansman C, Dressler M, et al. Pediatrics 1963;32:793–800.
30. Casey PH, Kraemer HC, Bernbaum J, et al. J Pediatr 1990;117: 298–307.
31. Ouden LD, Rijke M, Brand R, et al. J Pediatr 1991;118: 399–404.
32. Sasanow SR, Georgieff MK, Periera GR. J Pediatr 1986;109: 311–15.
33. Cronk C, Stallings V. Am J Hum Biol 1989;1:727–36.
34. Thommessen M, Kase BF, Riis G, et al. Eur J Clin Health 1991;45:479–87.
35. Spender QW, Cronk CE, Charney EB, et al. Dev Med Child Neurol 1989;31:206–14.
36. Stallings VA, Zemel BS. Nutritional assessment of the disabled child. In: Sullivan PB, Rosenbloom L, eds. Feeding the disabled child. London: Cambridge University Press, 1996;62–76.
37. Fiorotto ML, deBruin NC, Brans YW, et al. Pediatr Res 1995;37:94–100.
38. Schoeller DA, van Santen E, Peterson DW, et al. Am J Clin Nutr 1980;33:2686–93.
39. Goran JL, Kaskoun MC, Carpenter WH, et al. J Appl Physiol 1993;75:1776–80.
40. Houtkooper LB, Going SB, Lohman TG, et al. J Appl Physiol 1992;72:366–73.
41. deBruin NC, VanVelthoven KAM, Stijen T, et al. Am J Clin Nutr 1995;61:1195–205.
42. Mazess RB, Barden HS, Bisek JP, et al. Am J Clin Nutr 1990;51:1106–12.
43. VanLoan M, Mayclin P. Eur J Clin Nutr 1992;46:125–30.
44. Brunton J, Bayley H, Atkinson S. Am J Clin Nutr 1993;58: 839–45.
45. Gutin B, Litaker M, Islam S, et al. Am J Clin Nutr 1996;63:287–92.
46. Pritchard JE, Nowson CA, Strauss BJ, et al. Eur J Clin Nutr 1993;47:216–28.
47. WHO. Energy and protein requirements. Tech Rep Ser 724. Geneva: World Health Organization, 1985.
48. Harris JA, Benedict FG. A biometric study of basal metabolism in man. Publ no. 279. Washington, DC: Carnegie Institution, 1919.
49. Schofield WN. Hum Nutr Clin Nutr 1985;39C(1s):5–42.
50. Krick J, Murphy PE, Markham JFB, et al. Dev Med Child Neurol 1992;34:481–7.
51. Ramsey BM, Farell PM, Pencharz P, et al. Am J Clin Nutr 1992;55:108–16.
52. Ponder SW. Clin Pediatr 1995;34:237–40.
53. Lewis MK, Blake GM, Fogelman I. Osteoporosis Int 1994;4: 11–15.
54. Siri WE. Body volume measurements by gas dilution. In: Brozek J, Henschel A, eds. Techniques for measuring body composition. Washington, DC: National Academy of Sciences, 1961;108–17.

55. Horton WA, Rotter JI, Rimoln DL, et al. Pediatrics 1978;93: 435–8.
56. Cronk CE, Crocker AC, Pueschel SM, et al. Pediatrics 1988;81: 102–10.
57. Butler MG, Brunschwig A, Miller LK, Hagerman RJ. Pediatrics 1992;89:1059–62.
58. Pyeritz RE, Murphy EA, Lin SJ, Rosell EM. Growth and anthropometrics in the Marfan syndrome. In: Papadatos CJ, Bartsocas CS, eds. Endocrine genetics and the genetics of growth. New York: Alan R Liss, 1985:335–66.
59. Ranke MB, Heidemann P, Knupfer C, et al. Eur J Pediatr 1988;148:220–7.
60. Holm VA. Growth charts for Prader-Willi syndrome. In: Greensway LR, Alexander PC, eds. Management of Prader-Willi syndrome. New York: Springer-Verlag, 1988;appendix A.
61. Ranke MB, Pfluger H, Rosendahl W, et al. Eur J Pediatr 1983;141:81–8.
62. Pankau R, Tartsch CJ, Gosch A, et al. Eur J Pediatr 1992;151: 751–5.
63. Ekvall SW. Pediatric nutrition in chronic diseases and developmental disorders. New York: Oxford University Press, 1993;435–6.
64. Ranke MB. Horm Res 1996;45(Suppl 2):35–41.

SELECTED READINGS

Gibson RS. Principles of nutritional assessment. New York: Oxford University Press, 1990.

Lohman TG, Roche AF, Martorell R, eds. Anthropometric standardization reference manual. Champaign, IL: Human Kinetics Books, 1988.

Pereira GR, Georgieff MK. Nutritional assessment. In: Polin RA, Fox WW, eds. Fetal and neonatal physiology. 2nd ed. Philadelphia: WB Saunders, 1997.

Sullivan PB, Rosenbloom L, eds. Feeding the disabled child. London: MacKeith Press, 1996.

Walker WA, Watkins JB, eds. Nutrition in pediatrics. 2nd ed. Ontario: BC Decker, 1997.

55. Clinical and Functional Assessment of Adults

JEANETTE M. NEWTON and CHARLES H. HALSTED

Malnutrition, defined as an unintentional weight loss of more than 10% associated with a serum albumin level below 3.2 g/dL (1), is not infrequent in hospitalized patients in the modern era of medicine (2). Two different studies in the 1970s reported the prevalence of malnutrition in adult medical patients at 48% and in adult surgical patients at 50%, respectively (3, 4). Regardless of etiology, malnutrition is associated with a suboptimal surgical outcome (5), increased rate of infection (6), longer hospital stay (3), impaired wound healing (7, 8), frequent hospital readmission for the elderly (9), more frequent postoperative complications (10), and increased risk of death (5).

Determining the optimal approach to nutritional assessment in the clinical setting is difficult because nonnutritional factors alter many of the parameters used to determine nutritional status. For example, the serum albumin level can be affected by body fluid redistribution, sepsis, hepatic or renal disease, or the postoperative state (11, 12). Furthermore, the long half-life of serum albumin makes this measurement insensitive to rapid changes in nutritional status (12, 13). Urine and fecal nitrogen excretion and immune skin tests require up to 48 hours for results (14). Difficulty in obtaining complete 24-hour collections of urine and feces poses another potential clinical limitation on assessment of nitrogen balance (12). While there is no single irrefutable measure of nutritional status, proficiency in detecting malnutrition in its early stages is essential for effective treatment and prevention of adverse clinical outcomes, and interval assessments of nutritional status are required to evaluate the efficacy of any nutritional intervention (15, 16).

Malnutrition results from alterations in the intake, digestion and/or absorption, metabolism, excretion, and/or metabolic requirements of dietary energy, protein, and other nutrients. Understanding the pathophysiology of the patient's disease is essential to the likelihood of finding a component of malnutrition. Furthermore, the severity of clinical illness may be an independent variable of nutritional compromise (17, 18). Bedside nutritional assessment requires integration of the medical history, the physical examination, selected laboratory data, estimation of nutritional requirements, and approaches to nutritional intervention and its outcome. Accurate bedside assessment allows the physician to determine which patients may benefit from nutritional intervention, and careful patient selection is essential to the cost-benefit of nutritional support (19).

NUTRITIONAL HISTORY

The four main components of the nutritional history include the clinical, dietary, socioeconomic, and family histories. Unintentional loss of more than 10% of usual weight in the 3 months prior to evaluation may be associated with physiologic dysfunction, while loss of between 10 and 20% of usual weight is associated with impaired organ functions (5, 20), significantly higher in-hospital morbidity, and prolonged hospitalization of surgical patients (5).

The nutrition-oriented medical history should include the present illness, past medical and surgical history, family history, a medication list, and a review of systems. Special attention should be paid to the use of supplemental vitamins, hormone replacement therapy, mineral supplements, herbal remedies, and over-the-counter medications, which sometimes are not considered medications by patients. Chronic use of alcohol and medications such as glucocorticoids, immunosuppressive and cytotoxic agents, laxatives, appetite stimulants or suppressants, caffeine, and illicit drugs should be specifically noted. The history should assess changes in diet, including amounts and types of foods eaten and dental status, especially in the elderly. Chronic diseases such as gastric cancer or esophageal strictures may present with alterations in taste or dietary pattern. Table 55.1 lists the mechanisms by which malnutrition can result from many common diseases. Important nutrition-oriented questions for the review of systems are listed in Table 55.2.

Many socioeconomic factors contribute to malnutrition (21). Homeless patients, chronic alcoholics, and patients with low fixed incomes are examples of groups susceptible to poor dietary choices independent of the mechanisms listed in Table 55.1 (22). The absence of poverty does not ensure adequate nutrition. Factors that affect the patient's ability to participate in self-care include education level, physical or mental limitations that prevent access to food, and the ability to cook or store food. Self-prescribed or religious food preferences, food allergies, food intolerance, and the use of alcohol, illicit addictive drugs (e.g., methamphetamine), vitamins, various dietary supplements, and tobacco influence appetite and meal patterns (23). Alcohol abuse affects 5% of the population, with wide-ranging potential impact on health and increased risk of liver disease (24).

Table 55.1
Mechanisms of Malnutrition

Impaired dietary intake	Impaired food intake and/or delivery of energy and nutrients to the small intestine	AIDS Anorexia nervosa Aspiration Bulimia nervosa Cancer Cerebrovascular accident Chronic alcoholism Depression Dysmotility Gastroparesis Gingivitis Hyperemesis gravidarum Obstruction (esophageal, gastric, or intestinal) Poor dentition Poverty Senescence Social isolation Substance abuse
Maldigestion	Inability to digest macronutrients	Cholestasis from any cause Disaccharidase deficiency Intestinal bacterial stasis Pancreatic insufficiency Cystic fibrosis Radiation enteritis Short bowel syndrome
Malabsorption	Impaired transport of nutrients across the intestinal mucosa	AIDS Celiac disease Intestinal lymphoma Radiation enteritis Short bowel syndrome Tropical sprue Whipple's disease
Impaired metabolism	Altered metabolism of energy and nutrients	AIDS Cancer Chronic liver disease Chronic renal disease Corticosteroid use Inborn errors of metabolism
Nutrient excretion	Excessive loss of nutrient	Diarrhea (zinc, magnesium) Diabetes (glycosuria) Inflammatory bowel disease (Protein-losing enteropathy Occult GI bleeding (iron)
Increased requirements	Increased requirements for energy, protein, and other nutrients	Burns Chronic infection Chronic inflammatory diseases Chronic lung disease Hyperthyroidism Major surgery Sepsis Trauma

The family and dietary history are pertinent to both malnutrition and obesity (25–28). As described in the National Health and Nutrition Examination Survey (NHANES) III report, 33.4% of adults over the age of 20 are overweight, and obesity affects people of all socioeconomic strata (23). As described elsewhere (Chapter 87), obesity is associated with significant comorbidities of adult-onset diabetes, hypertension, hyperlipemia, and respiratory insufficiency. Diets high in saturated-fat calories and low in fiber are associated with increased risks for obesity (23) and colon cancer (29, 30), while diets low in vitamin B_{12} and vegetable sources of folate may predispose to hyperhomocysteinemia and cardiovascular disease (31) (see also Chapters 34 and 88).

Details of the dietary history are provided in Chapter 58. Health care providers should use the food guide pyramid to help their patients identify problem areas in food choices (32). In addition to features related to clinical illness and socioeconomic factors, the nutritional status of hospitalized patients may be affected adversely by factors unique to the inpatient setting, including withholding of meals for diagnostic testing, failure to recognize increased nutritional needs of injury or illness, major surgery, infection, and delay of nutritional support (33). If height and

Table 55.2
Nutritional Questions for the Review of Systems

General
Usual adult weight
Current weight
Prepubertal weight
Maximum, minimum weights
Weight 1 and 5 years prior
Recent changes in weight and time period
Recent changes in appetite or food tolerance
Presence of weakness, fatigue, fever, chills, night sweats
Recent changes in sleep habits, daytime sleepiness
Edema and/or abnormal swelling
Alimentary
Abdominal pain, nausea, vomiting
Changes in bowel pattern (normal or baseline)
Diarrhea (consistency, frequency, volume, color, presence of cramps, food particles, fat drops)
Difficulty swallowing (solids vs. liquids, intermittent vs. continuous)
Early satiety
Indigestion or heartburn
Food intolerance or preferences
Lesions in the mouth (aphthous ulcers, tooth decay)
Pain with swallowing
Sore tongue or gums
Neurologic
Confusion or memory loss
Difficulty with night vision
Gait disturbance
Loss of position sense
Numbness, paresthesias, and/or weakness
Skin
Appearance of a diagnostic rash
Breaking of nails
Dryness of skin
Hair loss, recent change in texture

weight are not recorded in the chart, a decline in nutritional status may not be detected until the patient is in a severe state of depletion. If a patient consumes 70% of a meal but has emesis, recording only the dietary intake is misleading. Communication between the physician, nurse, and dietitian improves the quality of nutritional care (33).

PHYSICAL EXAMINATION

The physical examination confirms the presence of under- or overnutrition suggested by the history. While undernutrition is often recognized, malnutrition in the presence of overnutrition may require a higher index of suspicion. Measurements of the severity of obesity and its complications are provided in Chapter 87. The multiple physical signs of malnutrition and their interpretations are listed in Table 55.3 according to different anatomic sites and organ systems.

INTEGRATED BEDSIDE ASSESSMENT

Since the early reports on malnutrition in hospitalized patients (3, 4, 15), there have been numerous attempts to define a series of parameters for accurate bedside assessment of nutritional status. Comprehensive assessment tools are too sophisticated for routine use by practitioners not trained in clinical nutrition (32, 35). The Likelihood of Malnutrition (LOM) score based upon eight defined measurements correlated with the length of hospitalization but included many parameters that are influenced by nonnutritional factors (3). The eight parameters used to define the LOM score in hospitalized medical patients included serum folate level, serum vitamin C level, triceps skinfold thickness, serum albumin level, absolute lymphocyte count, hematocrit, midarm muscle circumference, and body weight. While the LOM showed that 48% of patients were malnourished upon admission, 69% of patients hospitalized longer than 2 weeks demonstrated further decline in six nutritional parameters, and worsening of the LOM score was associated with prolonged hospitalization and increased mortality (3). Twelve years later, fewer medical patients were hospitalized with a high LOM score, and patients had shorter hospital stays, underscoring the importance of effective nutritional assessment and intervention in hospitalized patients (36).

The Prognostic Nutritional Index (PNI) that included serum albumin, serum transferrin, delayed hypersensitivity, and triceps skinfold measurements correlated with postoperative complications and mortality (37, 38). However, each of these measurements can be influenced by the severity of illness (38). The Instant Nutritional Index (INI) identifies available parameters that can alert the practitioner to a more thorough nutritional assessment. In the INI, the serum albumin level and the absolute lymphocyte count correlated with the incidence of hospital infection (39, 40), and a subsequent study added weight loss to the INI (41). However, like the PNI, the INI is limited by low sensitivity and specificity as well as the severity of the patient's illness. Another study of 216 patients assessed the significance of the seven parameters most frequently used in the various indices for nutritional assessment: weight for height, serum albumin level, serum total protein, midarm muscle area, triceps skinfold thickness, creatinine/height index, and hand grip strength. The best correlation with body cell mass was found for weight for height ($r = 0.82$), while the creatinine/height index had the worst correlation ($r = 0.37$). However, all parameters had wide 95% confidence intervals, and multiple linear regression predicted malnutrition in 22 of 69 normal subjects (32% false positives) and failed to predict malnutrition in 9 of 79 malnourished patients (11% false negatives) (42).

SUBJECTIVE GLOBAL ASSESSMENT

The Subjective Global Assessment (SGA) provides an integration of historical and physical data that allows a trained physician to make a bedside assessment of nutritional status (43). The SGA yields immediate results, which allow rapid intervention and avoidance of expensive tests with long turnaround times. Five features of the history and four features of the physical examination are

Table 55.3
Physical Signs of Abnormal Malnutrition

Site	Sign	Deficiency
General appearance	Loss of subcutaneous fat	Calories
	Sunken or hollow cheeks	Calories, fluid
Hair	Easily plucked hair, alopecia	Protein
	Dry, brittle hair	Protein, biotin
	Corkscrew hairs	Vitamin C
Nails	Spooning	Iron
	Transverse depigmentation	Protein
Skin	Dry and scaly flaky paint	Vitamin A, zinc
	Nasolabial seborrhea	Essential fatty acid deficiency
	Psoriasiform rash	Vitamin A, zinc
	Pallor	Iron, vitamin B_{12}, folate
	Follicular hyperkeratosis	Vitamin A
	Perifollicular hemorrhage	Vitamin C
	Easy bruising	Vitamin K or C
	Hyperpigmentation	Niacin
Eyes	Night blindness	Vitamin A, zinc
	Photophobia, xerosis	Vitamin A
	Conjunctival inflammation	Riboflavin, vitamin A
	Retinal field defect	Vitamin E
Mouth	Glossitis (smooth red tongue)	Riboflavin, pyridoxine, niacin, folic acid, vitamin B_{12}, iron
	Bleeding gums	Vitamin C, riboflavin
	Angular stomatitis	Riboflavin, pyridoxine, niacin
	Cheilosis	Riboflavin, pyridoxine, niacin
	Decreased taste or smell	Zinc
	Tongue fissuring	Niacin
	Tongue atrophy	Riboflavin, niacin, iron
	Loss of tooth enamel	Calcium
Neck	Goiter	Iodine
	Parotid enlargement	Protein
Heart	High output failure	Thiamin
Chest	Respiratory muscle weakness	Protein, phosphorus
Abdomen	Ascites	Protein
	Hepatomegaly	Protein, fat
Extremities	Edema	Protein
	Bone tenderness	Vitamin D
	Bone/joint pain	Vitamin A or C
	Muscle pain	Thiamin
	Joint swelling	Vitamin C
Muscles	Atrophic muscles	Protein
	Decreased grip strength	Protein
Neurological	Dementia	Thiamin, vitamin B_{12}, folate, niacin
	Acute disorientation	Phosphorus, niacin
	Nystagmus	Thiamin
	Ophthalmoplegia	Thiamin
	Wide-based gait	Thiamin
	Peripheral neuropathy	Thiamin, pyridoxine, vitamin E
	Loss of vibratory sense	Vitamin B_{12}
	Loss of position sense	Vitamin B_{12}
	Tetany	Calcium, magnesium
	Paresthesias	Thiamin, vitamin B_{12}
	Wrist or foot drop	Thiamin
	Diminished reflexes	Iodine

*Adapted from Halsted CH, Van Hoozen CM, Ahmed B. Preoperative nutritional assessment. In: Quigley EM, Sorrell MF, eds. The gastrointestinal surgical patient; preoperative and postoperative care. Baltimore: Williams & Wilkins 1994;27–49.

combined to assess nutritional status (Table 55.4). The historical features include *(a)* weight loss, *(b)* changes in dietary intake, *(c)* significant gastrointestinal symptoms, *(d)* the patient's functional status or energy level, and *(e)* the metabolic demand of the patient's underlying disease state. Weight loss is expressed as kilograms lost during the preceding 6 months and the 2 weeks prior to evaluation. Changes in the dietary pattern include the types of foods eaten, reduced intake, and duration of change. Assessment of abnormal food intake includes estimates of starvation, reliance on hypocaloric liquids, a complete liquid diet, or a suboptimal solid diet. Gastrointestinal symptoms are considered significant if they persist for more than 2 weeks and include anorexia, nausea, vomiting, and diarrhea. Energy level and functional capacity are graded from bedridden to full capacity. The severity of underlying

Table 55.4
Features of Subjective Global Assessment (SGA)

Select appropriate category with a checkmark, or enter numerical value where indicated by A "#".

A. History

1. Weight change and height
   Overall loss in past 6 months: Amt. = # ______kg; % loss = #______Height = #______cm
   Change in past 2 weeks:______ increase, ______ no change, ______ decrease.
2. Dietary intake change (relative to normal)
   ______ No change.
   ______ Change ______ duration = # ______ weeks.
   Type: ______ suboptimal solid diet, ______ full liquid diet,
   ______ hypocaloric liquids, ______ starvation.
   Supplement: (circle) nil, vitamin, minerals, # ______ frequency/week.
3. Gastrointestinal symptoms (that persisted for > 2 weeks)
   ______ none, ______ nausea, ______ vomiting, ______ diarrhea, ______ anorexia.
4. Functional capacity
   ______ No dysfunction (e.g., full capacity).
   ______ Dysfunction: duration # ______ weeks.
   type: ______ working suboptimally, ______ ambulatory, ______
   ______ bedridden.
5. Disease and its relation to nutritional requirements
   Primary diagnosis (specify) ______________________________
   Metabolic demand (stress): ______ no stress, ______ low stress, ______ moderate stress, ______ high stress.

B. Physical (for each trait specify: 0 = normal, 1+ = mild, 2+ = moderate, 3+ = severe)

# ______ Loss of subcutaneous fat (triceps, chest)	#______ Ascites
# ______ Muscle wasting (quadriceps, deltoids, temporalis)	#______ Mucosal lesions
#______ Ankle edema	#______ Cutaneous lesions
#______ Sacral edema	#______ Hair change

C. SGA rating (select one)
   ______ Well nourished.
   ______ Moderately (or suspected of being) malnourished.
   ______ Severely malnourished.

From Jeejeebhoy KN. Clinical and functional assessments. In: Shils ME, Olson JA, Shike M, eds. Modern nutrition in health and disease. 8th ed. Philadelphia: Lea & Febiger 1994;805–11.

disease is assessed according to its influence on the metabolic demand and hence nutritional requirement.

Physical findings are scored as normal (0), mild (1+), or severe (3+) and include depletion of subcutaneous fat, muscle wasting in the quadriceps and deltoid muscles, and the presence of edema and ascites. The triceps region and the midaxillary line at the level of the lower rib are assessed subjectively for subcutaneous tissue loss by pinching between thumb and forefinger. Palpation of the quadriceps and deltoid muscles assesses loss of tone and bulk. Ankle and sacral edema and ascites should be interpreted cautiously in the presence of comorbid disease states such as renal failure, congestive heart failure, or liver disease. Although not included in the original description of the SGA in Table 55.4, a careful neurologic examination should be included as part of the bedside nutritional evaluation. As indicated in Table 55.3, several micronutrient deficiencies can be identified by the bedside neurologic examination. For example, paresthesias of the face and hands may be the first sign of magnesium deficiency, more florid tetany is a sign of hypocalcemia, altered mental status may be a sign of hypophosphatemia, nystagmus or ataxic gait may be the only sign of thiamin deficiency, and loss peripheral of vibratory and position sense is a sensitive indicator of vitamin B_{12} deficiency.

Based on the history and physical examination findings, patients are ranked according to the following three categories: A, good nutrition; B, moderate or suspected malnutrition; and C, severe malnutrition. Weight loss, poor dietary intake, loss of subcutaneous tissue, and muscle wasting are considered the most significant factors. Conversely, the presence of ascites, edema, or a large tumor mass reduces the significance of body weight. Patients fall into rank B if there is at least a 5% weight loss in the 2 weeks prior to admission without stabilization or weight gain, together with reduction in dietary intake and mild loss of subcutaneous tissue. Patients assigned a C rank demonstrate obvious physical signs of malnutrition with ongoing weight loss, an overall decline of at least 10% of their normal weight, and change in the other parameters (43). These rankings are illustrated by the following cases.

CASE STUDIES

Case A. A 52-year-old previously healthy man was admitted for elective transverse colectomy. Over the prior 4 months, he had experienced alternating diarrhea and constipation with loss of 8% of his usual weight that had improved with use of oral supplements. The physical examination showed normal subcutaneous fat and muscle mass with no evidence of edema or ascites. In view of weight stabilization and absence of physical findings of malnutrition, the patient was classified as A.

Case B. A 47-year-old man with a history of alcohol abuse was transferred from another hospital for evaluation and management of a suspected pancreatic pseudocyst that followed a bout of acute pancreatitis 2 weeks previously. While in hospital he had lost 10% of his normal admission weight and continued to experience abdominal pain on eating. The physical examination was remarkable for moderate loss of subcutaneous fat over the triceps, a squared-off appearance of the shoulders, and pitting edema over the sacrum and ankles. The patient was classified as moderately malnourished, or B.

Case C. A 75-year-old previously healthy man had lost 20% of his usual weight in association with progressive dysphagia in the preceding 6 months. Physical examination showed obvious loss of subcutaneous fat and wasting of the deltoid and quadriceps muscles, with trace edema over the ankles. Following upper endoscopy, adenocarcinoma of the esophagus was diagnosed, and he was admitted for further evaluation and elective surgery. On the basis of marked and progressive weight loss and significant physical findings of fat and skeletal muscle loss, the patient was classified as C, or severely malnourished.

The SGA was used to evaluate 59 patients electively admitted to a general surgical ward. Two trained observers agreed on the SGA classification of 48 of the 59 patients (44). The incidence of infection, the use of antibiotics, and the length of hospital stay correlated with the clinical diagnosis of malnutrition including serum albumin, transferrin, actual weight/ideal weight, creatinine/height index, body fat/body weight, and delayed cutaneous hypersensitivity. The SGA correlated with other objective parameters but not with the total lymphocyte count (44). The sensitivity of SGA was 82% and the specificity was 72% (45, 46).

The SGA was also used to predict development of major postoperative nutrition-associated complications. Patients in SGA class C with a low serum albumin level were identified at greatest risk of complications among patients undergoing major gastrointestinal surgeries (47). Another study found no association between the SGA and the incidence of postoperative complications in surgical patients. However, the highest postoperative mortality was found in patients classified with the worst malnutrition according to the SGA; preoperative malnutrition was present in 43% of the survivors versus 100% of those who died (48). These findings are consistent with findings from the Veterans Affairs Total Parenteral Nutrition Cooperative Study Group, in which preoperative total parenteral nutrition support was significantly beneficial only to severely malnourished patients, but not to adequately nourished patients (10).

Another group applied the SGA to 59 chronic uremia patients, including 23 patients on continuous ambulatory peritoneal dialysis and 36 patients on intermittent hemodialysis, and found malnutrition in 30%. The SGA correlated with muscle wasting, loss of fat, or the presence of gastrointestinal symptoms, but not with weight loss or the presence of edema (49).

In general, the SGA is a widely available and low-cost technique for nutritional assessment with good reproducibility. Its quantitative scale can be successfully applied to different patient populations. However, the published applications of the SGA involved physicians who either were trained in clinical nutrition or had undergone instruction in nutritional assessment. It remains unclear whether the results of the SGA are reproducible when used by untrained physicians.

FUNCTIONAL ASSESSMENT

The physiologic impairment that accompanies significant weight loss may be the primary cause of increased morbidity and mortality (50); thus, bedside assessment of functional status may be an important component of clinical nutritional assessment (51). In a study of functional assessment, surgical patients were preoperatively categorized into three groups: 1, preoperative weight loss of less than 10%; 2, weight loss greater than 10% without physiologic dysfunction; and 3, weight loss greater than 10% with physiologic impairment of at least two systems. Physiologic function was assessed by overall activity, exercise tolerance, grip strength, respiratory function, wound healing, and plasma albumin concentration. Major complications were more frequent in group 3 than in group 2 (15 vs. 3%) and included sepsis (18 vs. 4%) and pneumonia (10 vs. 1%). Patients in group 3 had a longer hospital stay, increased incidence of wound infection, and a higher mortality (50).

In the alert and cooperative patient, impaired skeletal muscle function can be assessed by testing grip strength with a hand dynamometer (52, 53). Hand grip strength was found to be the most sensitive indicator of complications in 102 patients undergoing major abdominal surgery. Complications were predicted in 87% of patients whose preoperative hand grip strength was less than 85% of normal (54, 55). Specificity was improved when age- and sex-derived standards were used (56). Hill et al. described a bedside technique that requires a patient to squeeze the clinician's index and middle fingers for at least 10 seconds. The determination of impairment was then subjectively based upon the patient's age, sex, and body habitus (20).

Measuring the contraction of the adductor pollicis muscle in response to electrical stimulation of the ulnar nerve is an alternative technique that does not require patient cooperation but may be uncomfortable for an awake and alert patient (57). This technique assesses the relationship between the force of contraction and the frequency of the stimulus, as well as the rate of muscle relaxation. Starvation increases the force to frequency of contraction parameter while slowing the relaxation rate, and these changes are corrected by refeeding prior to improvement in body nitrogen retention (58). These measurements have been used to predict nutritional complications in preoperative surgical patients (59). Others noted that involuntary muscle function in this test can be normal (60) or even elevated (61) in the presence of significant protein depletion if the subject is receiving adequate energy. Difficulty has been experienced in applying this technique to patients requiring intensive care; when results were obtainable they did not reflect the extent of proteolysis but were indicative of the state of cellular energetics (61).

Exercise tolerance and the ability to perform the usual activities of daily living also reflect functional status. Bedside assessment of respiratory muscle function includes static compliance in the ventilated patient, while respiratory muscle strength can be assessed in the awake and cooperative patient by holding a strip of paper 10 cm from the mouth and observing its movement in response to respiration (20). The results must be interpreted with caution in the presence of comorbid disease like chronic obstructive pulmonary disease or congestive heart failure.

Measures of immunocompetence include delayed hypersensitivity skin testing and the absolute lymphocyte count. The absolute lymphocyte count (total white count × percentage lymphocytes; normal, >1200/mm^2) is available to the clinician within hours of admission. However, as an isolated value, the absolute lymphocyte count is a poor predictor of outcome, since it is also influenced by stress, injury, surgery, corticosteroids, immunosuppressive agents, and infection.

Skin testing is an uncertain means of assessing immune status because the immune response can be depressed in normal patients following major surgery (62). The clinical utility of skin testing is limited in critically ill patients by the 24- to 72-hour delay required for the test results. Anergy is associated with severe malnutrition, but lesser degrees of malnutrition do not cause anergy. The immunosuppressive effects of corticosteroids, stress, and infection; the low predictive value of the test; and the depressed response in many other disease states led to the conclusion that routine use of skin testing is not indicated in nutritional assessment of the sick patient (63).

Rapid identification of processes that increase metabolic stress and nutritional requirements is essential to risk assessment. The presence of metabolic stress is usually suggested by the history and physical examination. Sepsis, as evidenced by a temperature above 38°C, pulse faster than 100/min, respiratory rate above 30/min, white blood count below 3,000/L or above 12,000/L, a positive blood culture, active inflammatory bowel disease, or defined focus of infection, is a major cause of metabolic stress. Other causes of stress that can potentially increase nutrient requirements include major trauma or major surgery.

ACKNOWLEDGMENTS

The authors gratefully acknowledge the following people for their assistance with this manuscript: Kathleen Newman, R.D.; Thomas E. Taylor, computer resource specialist, Office of Curricular Support; and Diane Hardy, administrative assistant, Division of Clinical Nutrition and Metabolism.

REFERENCES

1. Swails WS, Samour PQ, Babineau TJ, et al. J Am Diet Assoc 1996;96:370–3.
2. McWhirter JP, Pennington CR. BMJ 1994;308:945–8.
3. Weinsier RL, Hunker EM, Krumdieck CL, et al. Am J Clin Nutr 1979;32:418–26.
4. Bistrian BR, Blackburn GL, Hallowell E, et al. JAMA 1974;230:858–60.
5. Studley HO. JAMA 1936;106:458–60.
6. Cannon PR, Wissler RW, Woolridge RL, et al. Ann Surg 1944;120:514–25.
7. Breslow RA, Hallfrisch J, Guy DG, et al. J Am Geriatr Soc 1993;41:357–62.
8. Pinchcofsky-Devin GD, Kaminski MV. J Am Geriatr Soc 1986;34:435–40.
9. Sullivan DH. J Am Geriatr Soc 1992;40:792–8.
10. Veterans Affairs Total Parenteral Nutrition Cooperative Group. N Engl J Med 1991;325:525–32.
11. Brackeen GL, Dover JS, Long CL. Nutr Clin Pract 1989;6: 203–5.
12. Phinney, SD. Clin Lab Med 1981;1:767–74.
13. Baker JP, Detsky AS, Wesson DE, et al. N Engl J Med 1982;306:969–72.
14. Linn BS. Am Surg 1987;53:628–31.
15. Bistrian BR, Blackburn GL, Vitale J, et al. JAMA 1976;235: 1567–70.
16. Phinney SD, Siepler J, Bach HT. West J Med 1996;164:130–6.
17. Charlson ME, Sax FL, Mackenzie CR, et al. J Chronic Dis 1986;39:439–52.
18. Dionigi R, Cremashi RE, Jemos V, et al. World J Surg 1986;10: 2–11.
19. Detsky AS, Jeebjeebhoy KN. JPEN J Parenter Enteral Nutr 1984;8:632–7.
20. Hill GL, Windsor JA. Nutrition 1995;11(2 Suppl):198–201.
21. Winkleby MA, Jatulis DE, Frank E, et al. Am J Public Health 1992;82:816–20.
22. Reicks M, Randall JL, Haynes BJ. J Am Diet Assoc 1994;94: 1309–11.
23. Kuczmarski RJ, Flegal KM, Campbell SM, et al. JAMA 1994;272: 205–11.
24. Halsted CH. Alcohol: medical and nutritional effects. In: Ziegler EE, Filer LJ, eds. Present knowledge in nutrition. 7th ed. Washington, DC: ILSI Press, 1996;547–56.
25. Jousilahti P, Puska P, Vartiainen E, et al. J Clin Epidemiol 1996;49:497–503.
26. Parent ME, Ghadirian P, Lacroix A. Genet Epidemiol 1996;13: 61–78.
27. Colditz GA, Willett WC, Rotnitzky A, et al. Ann Intern Med 1995;122:481–6.

28. Allen JK, Young DR, Blumenthal RS, et al. Arch Intern Med 1996;156:1654–60.
29. Statland BE. Clin Chem 1992; 38:1587–94.
30. Mettlin C. Surg Clin North Am 1986;66:917–29.
31. Selhub J, Rosenberg IH. Folic acid. In: Ziegler EE, Filer LJ, eds. Present knowledge in nutrition. 7th ed. Washington, DC: ILSI Press, 1996;206–19.
32. Achterberg C, McDonnell E, Bagby R. J Am Diet Assoc 1994;94:1030–5.
33. Council on Practice Quality Management Committee. J Am Diet Assoc 1994;94:838–9.
34. Blackburn GL, Bistrian BR, Maini BS, et al. JPEN J Parenter Enteral Nutr 1977;1:11–22.
35. Harvey KH, Moldawer LL, Bistrian BR, et al. Am J Clin Nutr 1981;34:2013–22.
36. Coats KG, Morgan SL, Bartolucci AA, et al. J Am Diet Assoc 1993;93:27–33.
37. Buzby GP, Mullen JL, Matthews DC, et al. Am J Surg 1980;139: 160–7.
38. Mullen JL, Buzby GP, Waldman MT, et al. Surg Forum 1979;30;80–2.
39. Seltzer MH, Bastidas JA, Cooper DM, et al. JPEN J Parenter Enteral Nutr 1979;3:157–9.
40. Seltzer MH, Fletcher HS, Slocum BA, et al. JPEN J Parenter Enteral Nutr 1981;5:70–2.
41. Seltzer MH, Slocum BA, Cataldi-Betcher E, et al. JPEN J Parenter Enteral Nutr 1982;6:218–21.
42. Forse RA, Shizgal HM. Surgery 1980;88:17–24.
43. Detsky AS, McLaughlin JR, Baker JP, et al. JPEN J Parenter Enteral Nutr 1987;11:8–13.
44. Baker JP, Detsky AS, Wesson DE, et al. N Engl J Med 1982;306:969–72.
45. Detsky AS, Baker JP, Mendelson RA, et al. JPEN J Parenter Enteral Nutr 1984;8:153–9.
46. Baker JP, Detsky AS, Whitwell J, et al. Clin Nutr 1982;36C: 233–41.
47. Detsky AS, Baker JP, O'Rourke K, et al. JPEN J Parenter Enteral Nutr 1987;11:440–6.
48. Hirsch S, de Obaldia N, Petermann M, et al. J Am Coll Nutr 1992;11:21–4.
49. Enia G, Sicuso C, Alati G, et al. Nephrol Dial Transplant 1993;8:1094–8.
50. Windsor J, Hill G. Ann Surg 1988;207:290–6.
51. Pettigrew RA, Hill GL. Br J Surg 1980;73:47–51.
52. Vaz M, Thangam S, Prabhu A, et al. Br J Nutr 1996;76:9–15.
53. Kalfaerntzos F, Spiliotis J, Velimezis G, et al. JPEN J Parenter Enteral Nutr 1989;13:34–6.
54. Klidjian AM, Archer TJ, Foster KJ, et al. JPEN J Parenter Enteral Nutr 1982;6:119–21.
55. Klidjian AM, Foster KJ, Kammerling RM, et al. Br Med J 1980;281:899–901.
56. Webb AR, Newman LA, Taylor M, et al. JPEN J Parenter Enteral Nutr 1989;13:30–3.
57. Lopes J, Russell DM, Whitwell J, et al. Am J Clin Nutr 1982;36:602–10.
58. Jeejeebhoy KN, Detsky AS, Baker JP. JPEN J Parenter Enteral Nutr 1990;14:193S.
59. Zeiderman MR, McMahon MJ. Clin Nutr 1989;8:164–6.
60. Christie PM, Hill GL. Gastroenterology 1990;99:730–6.
61. Finn PJ, Plank CD, Clark MA, et al. JPEN J Parenter Enteral Nutr 1996;20:332–7.
62. Slade MS, Simmons RL, Yunis E, et al. Surgery 1975;78:363–72.
63. Twomey P, Ziegler D, Rombeau J. JPEN J Parenter Enteral Nutr 1982;6:50–8.
64. Halsted CH, Van Hoozen CM, Ahmed B. Preoperative nutritional assessment. In: Quigley EM, Sorrell MF, eds. The gastrointestinal surgical patient; preoperative and postoperative care. Baltimore: Williams & Wilkins, 1994;27–49.
65. Jeejeebhoy KN. Clinical and functional assessments. In: Shils ME, Olson JA, Shike M, eds. Modern nutrition in health and disease, 8th ed. Philadelphia: Lea & Febiger, 1994; 805–11.

56. Nutritional Assessment of Malnutrition by Anthropometric Methods

STEVEN B. HEYMSFIELD, RICHARD N. BAUMGARTNER, and SHEAU-FANG PAN

Depletion of body nutrient stores and ultimate loss of specific cellular functions are common to many acute and chronic diseases. A hypothetical chronic illness of long duration is shown in Figure 56.1 (1). Progressive loss of fat-free body mass (FFM) is associated with the evolution of various complications, including loss of cell-mediated immunity, infections, bedsores, and, ultimately, death. A series of linkages implicit in Figure 56.1 is central to the nutritional assessment examination:

food intake < nutrient losses → negative protein balance → depletion of FFM → loss of protein-mediated cellular functions → clinical complications

With nutritional therapy, loss of nutrients can be prevented or reversed, thus minimizing or eliminating the risk of clinical complications. This chapter further explores these relations, specifically to give a general overview of the anthropometric component of the nutritional assessment examination, which can be used to evaluate acutely and chronically ill malnourished patients.

ASSESSMENT COMPONENTS

Maintaining optimum health requires adequate tissue levels of essential nutrients and a source of energy. More than 40 syndromes develop if tissue levels of these components are either too low or too high (2). The emphasis in this chapter is on protein and energy because the large majority of patients seen for clinical evaluation have a disorder of protein-energy nutriture (3, 4).

Steady-State Relations

The sequence of changes in progressive protein-energy malnutrition involves negative nutrient balance, loss of cellular functions, and finally clinical complications. This section gives an overview of the steady-state relationships that exist among energy exchange, body weight, and body composition in health and describes how they are altered in pathologic states that cause negative nutrient balance. Body weight is a fundamental component of nutritional assessment because it is an indirect marker of protein mass and energy stores. The relationships among body weight, protein mass, and body energy content are shown in Figure 56.2.

A major portion of tissue function can be attributed to proteins that are activated by energy derived from metabolism of organic fuels (5). Protein is also a metabolic fuel and under conditions of weight stability, oxidation of amino acids provides about 15% of daily energy requirements (6). The energy-producing reactions take the general form

$$\begin{aligned}\text{Fuel} + O_2 &\rightarrow \text{high energy intermediate}\\ &\rightarrow O_2 + H_2O + \text{heat} + \text{urea} \qquad (56.1)\end{aligned}$$

Urea is not metabolized further and is excreted unchanged in urine. During periods of nutritional deprivation, approximately half the total body protein mass can be used as metabolic fuel (7). A greater loss of protein is incompatible with survival. Therefore, when food intake is less than nutrient losses, amino acids from proteins are oxidized to provide energy, various tissue functions are altered, and, ultimately, protracted negative protein balance results in a rapid rate of lean tissue depletion and death (see Chapter 41 on starvation).

The main sources of nonprotein energy are glycogen and fat or triglyceride. Glycogen is distributed primarily in liver and skeletal muscle (8). Glycogen stores are small (~400 g), and carbohydrate oxidation on a usual diet in the United States accounts for about 50% of daily energy production (6). Fat is found almost entirely within adipocytes or fat cells (9). Fat stores vary widely in humans, with fatty acid oxidation representing about 35% of energy production in the average American diet (6). Both glycogen and fat are oxidized in reactions similar to that for protein (Eq. 56.1), except urea is produced only with amino acid oxidation.

The sum of protein, glycogen, and fat constitutes total body energy content (Fig. 56.2). These fuels account for over 90% of the nonaqueous portion of body weight (10). Generalizations can be made on how body weight, protein, glycogen, fat, and energy stores relate to each other. Glycogen and protein are both solubilized by water and electrolytes. About 2 to 4 g water binds to 1 g of either

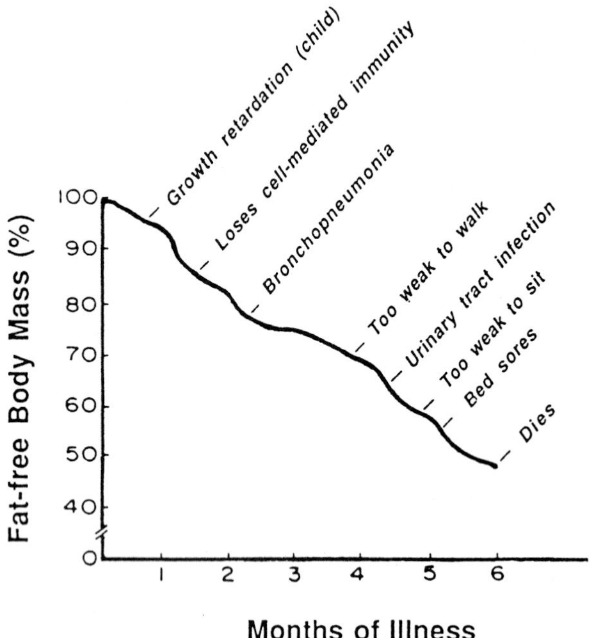

Figure 56.1. Natural history of protein-energy malnutrition in a patient with chronic wasting illness. (Modified from Heymsfield SB, Bethel RA, Ansley JD, et al. Ann Intern Med 1979;90:63–71.)

glycogen or protein (11). Changes in glycogen or protein balance are thus associated with greater changes in body weight than can be attributed to loss of the actual chemical component. For example, oxidation and loss of 100 g glycogen would result in approximately a 0.5-kg reduction in body weight.

The main remaining chemical components exclusive of fat are minerals, found primarily in the skeleton (9, 10). The total fat-free portion of body weight thus consists of protein, glycogen, water, and minerals. In healthy adults, the steady-state fractional contribution of three of these components to total FFM is reasonably constant: protein, 0.195; water, 0.725; and minerals, 0.08; respectively. Glycogen levels vary throughout the day and represent a fraction of FFM of 0.01 to 0.02. With long-term weight loss, the change in FFM is approximately the same as the relative reduction in protein (2). Sharp changes in body weight and FFM may also reflect alterations in glycogen and fluid balance.

Fat maintains a relatively constant, although more complex, relation to fat-free components. Figure 56.3 shows a plot of total body fat/height^2 (Ht) versus body weight/Ht^2 in 414 women. Fat was measured in the women using a four-component model (9). The ratio body weight:Ht^2, referred to as body mass index (BMI, kg/m^2), is discussed below in more detail. This figure illustrates two important points. First, the intercept for zero total body fat is a BMI of approximately 13. This extrapolated value represents a theoretical female subject without any fat, a condition incompatible with survival. Second, the slope of the regression line (i.e., the change in fat adjusted for stature/the change in body weight adjusted for stature) of approximately 0.74 indicates that body weight added above a BMI of about 13 is about three-fourths fat and one-fourth FFM. Webster et al. refer to the weight above a BMI of 13 as "excess weight" and suggest that weight gain or loss should approximate this composition (12). The composition of "excess weight" may differ between men and women and between young and old subjects. A more complex analysis of the relations among body weight, protein, and fat is presented by Forbes (13) (see also Chapter 49.)

These associations among body weight, total body protein mass, energy content, and fluid form an important concept: under most conditions, body weight is an indirect marker of protein mass and energy stores. A loss or gain in body weight is usually assumed to reflect changes in protein mass and/or energy content. Thus, body weight, total body protein mass and energy content, and chemical components are associated according to relatively simple rules. How these rules change in disease is important in anthropometric nutritional assessment, as described below.

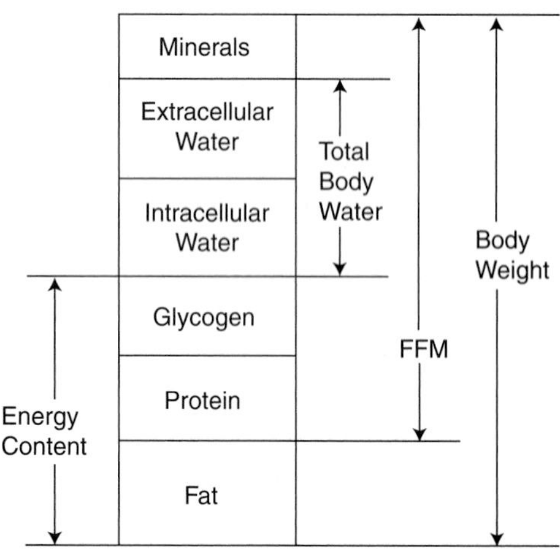

Figure 56.2. Major molecular body composition level components and how they relate to total body energy content.

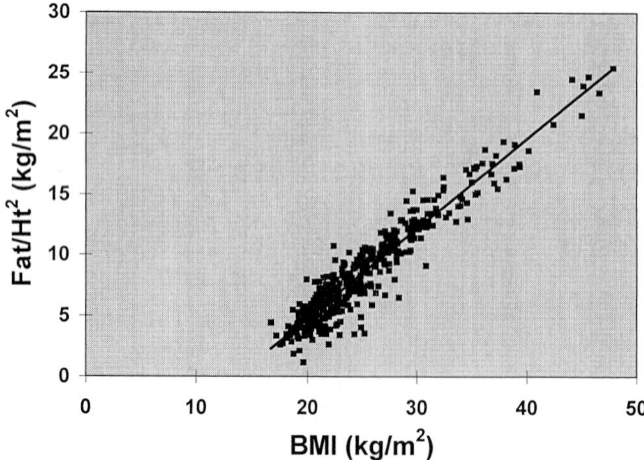

Figure 56.3. Relationship between total body fat (measured by four-component model [9]) adjusted for stature and body mass index (BMI) in 414 healthy women (R^2 = 0.91, P < .001).

Balance

Body composition is in a dynamic state throughout the day. Both total body protein mass and energy content decline between meals because of obligatory amino acid oxidation and metabolism of other fuels (8, 14). The result is negative protein and energy balance. With food intake, balance becomes positive, and total body protein and energy content increase. Over a typical day, net protein and energy balance are zero and body weight remains constant. These relationships are depicted in Figure 56.4 (2), which presents a hypothetical healthy subject at point *A*. Body weight is stable, and long-term balances of energy, protein, and water are zero. Figure 56.4 presents protein as nitrogen *(N)* as the two are related by a "constant" (protein = 16% N = 6.25 × N).

If the individual at point *A* develops an acute or chronic illness, food intake may be inadequate to replace nutrient losses; then net energy and nitrogen balance become negative, and body weight is lost. If the condition persists and balance remains negative, the subject approaches the point at which survival is no longer possible (B_u in Fig. 56.4). As mentioned above, the limits of survival with long-term underfeeding are a 50% loss in total body protein and a BMI of about 13. Loss of functional proteins and other essential nutrients results in the clinical complications described at the beginning of this chapter (Fig. 56.1) and shown in Figure 56.4 as C_u. Clinically significant abnormalities in physiologic function and loss of total body protein are seen in most hospitalized patients who lose more than 20% of their preillness body weight (15).

Overeating relative to nutrient losses results in positive balance; if sustained, the individual gains weight (Fig. 56.4). The maximum survivable body weight is approximately 500 kg or a body BMI of about 150. As with undernutrition, obesity is associated with complications (C_o in Fig. 56.4). The proposed mechanisms that lead to these complications are described in Chapter 87.

Thus, some hypothetic optimal state of health exists (point *A* in Fig. 56.4) in which long-term balance is zero and health risks are at a minimum. Weight loss or gain is secondary to a change in energy and nitrogen balance and increases the individual's risk of developing various medical complications.

Figure 56.4 embodies the main components of nutritional assessment: to define the patient's status between points *A*, *B*, and *C*. These aims can be formulated into four specific questions:

1. What is the patient's body weight and body composition status relative to an arbitrarily defined healthy range?
2. If the patient is under- or overnourished, what are the mechanisms leading to either negative or positive nutrient balance?
3. Is the patient at risk of developing a complication related to altered nutritional status?
4. With nutritional treatment is balance altered, and over time, is the patient's weight and body composition moving toward the healthy range?

Question 2 is examined in other chapters and is not discussed further here. This review focuses on undernutrition (Chapter 87 describes the evaluation of obese patients).

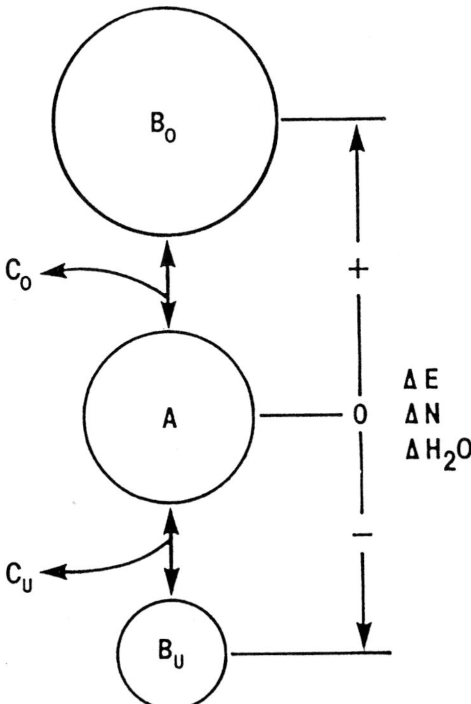

Figure 56.4. Model depicting changes in metabolic balance and body composition in protein-energy malnutrition and obesity. Point *A* is the range of body composition and tissue function found in health. Weight is stable, and balances of energy, nitrogen *(N)*, and water are zero. Disease causes negative metabolic balance, weight loss, and changes in body composition and tissue function. Point B_u is the minimal range of body composition and tissue function that is compatible with survival. The course of a patient moving between points *A* and B_u may be interrupted by a complication related to malnutrition, indicated by point C_u. Positive balance leads to obesity, and a similar set of endpoints, B_o and C_o, are designated.

Function

An important assumption of nutritional assessment is that body composition is an indirect measure of cellular function. Body composition estimates are usually highly correlated with specific functional tests. For example, anthropometric midarm muscle area is strongly correlated with forearm grip strength (16). However, body composition should not be assumed to be equivalent to tissue function; the two are different types of biologic measurements that serve different purposes but can, under certain conditions, replace one another. An example of mass and function dissociating is the patient with cardiomyopathy. Massive enlargement of the heart muscle is possible, yet the capacity of the myocardium to generate force and eject blood into the systemic circulation is severely impaired. The distinction between body composition estimates and cellular function indices should be kept in mind in interpreting the results of a patient's anthropometric and biochemical evaluations (15).

ANTHROPOMETRY

History

Anthropometry, developed in the late 19th century by anthropologists, uses simple measuring devices to quantify differences in human form. The potential of anthropometric methods in assessing nutritional status was first realized in the late 19th century by Richer, who used skinfold thickness as an index of fatness (17). The modern era of nutritional anthropometry began with the studies of Matiegka during World War I (18). Matiegka's interest in the physical efficiency of soldiers led him to develop methods of anthropometrically subdividing the human body into muscle, fat, and bone. Anthropometric techniques are now widely used in many areas of human biologic research, and three important multiauthor books on the subject appeared within the last decade (19–21).

Five-Level Model

The purpose of anthropometric measurements is to quantify the amount and distribution of major compositional determinants of body weight. A full appreciation of anthropometric measurements requires an understanding of human body composition and its organizational levels. The human body composition can be studied at five levels (9): I, atomic; II, molecular; III, cellular; IV, tissue-system; and V, whole body. The five levels and their major components are shown in Figure 56.5.

Atomic

The first level of body composition consists of major elements that make up body weight, such as oxygen, hydrogen, carbon, nitrogen, and calcium. Whole-body measurements at this level are usually made by research techniques such as in vivo neutron activation analysis (22–26) (see Chapter 57). Elemental measurements are important in the study of body composition as they are used either directly (e.g., nitrogen balance as a measure of protein change) or to estimate components at other levels (e.g., total body calcium to indicate total bone mineral) (23). Anthropometric methods are available for estimating total body nitrogen, calcium, and potassium at the atomic level (24).

Molecular

The second level of body composition consists of the major molecular components that constitute body weight, such as water, protein, glycogen, minerals (osseous and nonosseous), and fat (Fig. 56.5), which can now all be quantified in vivo except glycogen (22). It is possible to quantify hepatic and skeletal muscle glycogen stores (27). Total body protein can be estimated from total body nitrogen (an atomic-level component) (22, 25, 26) in a calculation that assumes that most total body nitrogen is incorporated into protein and that the nitrogen content of protein is 16% (28). Another component, total body fat, can be estimated by use of a two-component model in

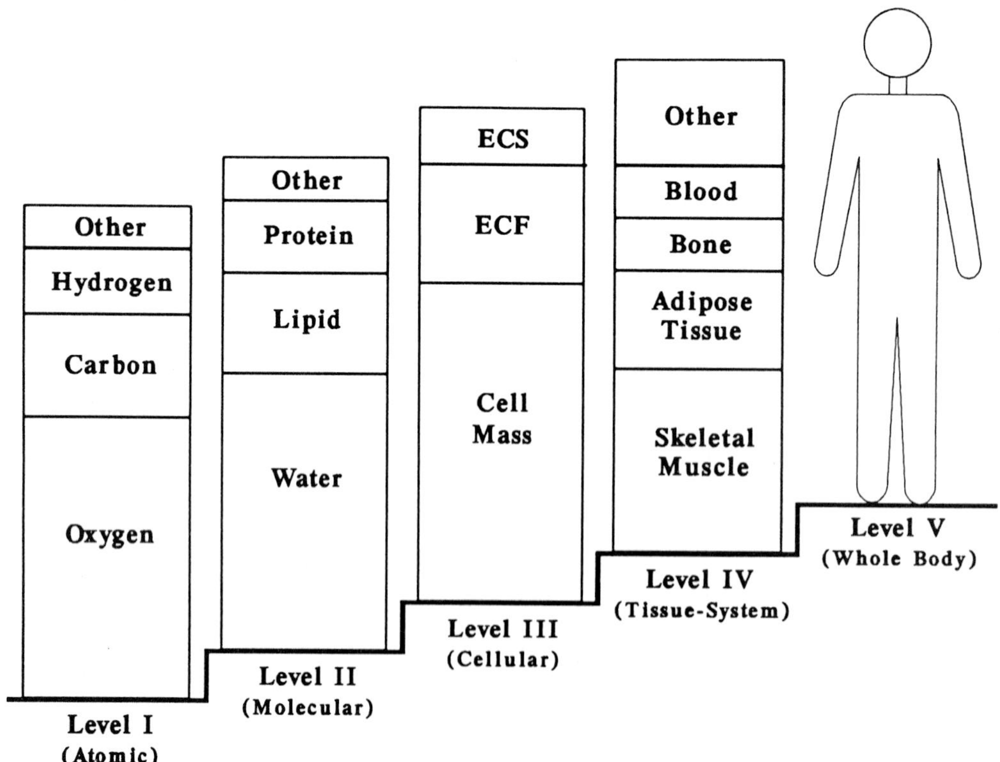

Figure 56.5. Five-level model of body composition. *ECF* and *ECS*, extracellular fluid and solids. (From Wang ZM, Pierson RN, Heymsfield SB. Am J Clin Nutr 1992;56:19–28, with permission.)

which the molecular level is simplified to body weight = fat + FFM (Fig. 56.5). Several two-component methods are used to estimate fat, such as underwater weighing, total body potassium, and total body water (TBW) (29). Each method relies on one or more assumptions that relate measurable body composition quantities to the unknown component of interest. For example, the TBW two-component method assumes that FFM has an average hydration of 73% (i.e., TBW/FFM = 0.73, or FFM = TBW/0.73). FFM and fat (i.e., body weight − FFM) can thus be estimated from TBW. Anthropometric methods of estimating total body fat are usually developed using one of these techniques as the reference standard for quantifying fat.

The second level of body composition is important in nutritional assessment because fat and FFM are the major components in which energy stores are distributed, and FFM contains all the functional components of body weight. Fat has an energy density of 9.4 kcal/g, and all but 1 to 2 kg is metabolically available during periods of protracted negative energy balance. Protein and glycogen have respective energy densities of 5.65 and 4.1 kcal/g. Assuming that the proportions of protein and glycogen are relatively normal in FFM, the metabolically available energy from FFM is 1.02 kcal/g (30, 31). Accordingly,

$$\text{Total body kcal} = [9.4 \times \text{total fat (g)}] + [1.02 \times \text{FFM (g)}] \quad (56.2)$$

Half of the energy contained in FFM is usually available as fuel during long-term semistarvation (31). Evaluation of fat and FFM thus allows the investigator or clinician to estimate total body energy content, available energy stores, and changes in energy balance over time.

FFM, the metabolically active component at the molecular level of body composition, is generally accepted as an index of protein nutriture. Changes in FFM over time are assumed to represent alterations in protein balance. Resting oxygen consumption, carbon dioxide production, and heat production (i.e., energy expenditure) are highly correlated with FFM, and FFM accounts for about 50 to 80% of the individual variation in energy expenditure (32). For example, Cunningham pooled data from seven studies to derive the resting metabolic rate (RMR, kcal/day) prediction equation (28):

$$\text{RMR (kcal/day)} = 370 + 21.6 \times \text{FFM (kg)} \quad (56.3)$$

where FFM is in kg. Anthropometric methods are available for estimating TBW, FFM, and fat at the molecular level (19, 20, 22, 24, 33, 34).

Cellular

The cellular level of body composition consists of three main components: cells, extracellular fluid, and extracellular solids (9). Measurement techniques are available for quantifying extracellular fluid and solids, although total cell weight or the weight of specific cell groups is difficult to quantify in vivo. A widely used model of body weight components at this level was suggested by Moore et al. (34). Cell mass was considered as two components: fat (a molecular-level component) and fat-free cell mass. They referred to fat-free cell mass as "body cell mass" (BCM), a component responsible for most of the body's metabolic processes. These investigators proposed that total body potassium (TBK) or exchangeable potassium (both atomic-level components, approximately equal in amount) could be used to estimate BCM because the potassium concentration of intracellular fluid is relatively constant at 150 mmol/L, and the ratio of intracellular fluid to solids is approximately 4:1 (i.e., intracellular fluid = BCM × 0.80). BCM could then be calculated using these relationships combined with an estimate of either total body or exchangeable potassium (i.e., BCM = [TBK/150] × [1/0.80], or 0.0083 TBK). Thus, according to Moore et al., body weight was equal to fat plus BCM plus extracellular fluids and solids.

Cells are the main functional components, and quantification of BCM enables investigators to explore important physiologic and functional relationships. At present, several anthropometric equations can be used to predict BCM at the cellular level (24, 34)

Tissue-System

The tissue-system level of body composition consists of the major tissues and organs. Body weight at this level is equal to adipose tissue plus skeletal muscle plus skeleton plus residual. Adipose tissue includes fat cells or adipocytes, blood vessels, and structural elements (9). It is the primary site of fat storage, and in healthy adults, the chemical composition of adipose tissue averages 80% fat, 18% water, and 2% protein (10).

Adipose tissue is distributed mainly into the subcutaneous and internal or visceral compartments. The proportions of total adipose tissue in the subcutaneous and visceral compartments are not constant. Distribution of adipose tissue is under hormonal and genetic control, and metabolic properties of adipose tissue vary in different anatomic locations (35). Men, the elderly, and obese subjects tend to have a higher percentage of total adipose tissue in the visceral compartment than women, young, and lean subjects, respectively (2, 35, 36). Weight gain or loss is associated with different relative rates of adipose tissue change in the subcutaneous and visceral compartments and from different subcutaneous sites (37). This differential loss of adipose tissue is important in interpreting anthropometric measurements. A strong positive correlation exists between the amount of visceral adipose tissue and the health risks of obesity (see Chapter 87).

Skeletal muscle is the largest component within the adipose tissue–free body mass (ATFM), accounting for approximately half of ATFM in healthy adults (9, 10). Skeletal muscle consists of muscle tissue, nerves, and tendons. Anatomic skeletal muscle also includes interstitial adipose tissue, which increases in amount in some diseases (e.g., Duchenne muscular dystrophy) and with aging. Approximately 20% of adipose tissue–free skeletal muscle is protein, and muscle is the largest tissue reservoir of amino acids (7). Depletion of up to 75% of skeletal muscle mass is possible during prolonged semistarvation (7).

The response of visceral organs to semistarvation varies. Organs decrease in weight at different rates during uncomplicated semistarvation. For example, liver mass decreases rapidly in rodents with underfeeding, whereas heart weight decreases at about the same rate as body weight (37). The pattern of visceral organ changes in protein-energy malnutrition associated with physiologic stress may differ from that of uncomplicated underfeeding. An example is the severe weight loss that often accompanies metastatic malignant disease. Cancer cachexia in both animals and humans is accompanied by preservation of some visceral organs despite loss of body weight and atrophy of skeletal muscles (38) (see Chapters 82 and 96). Preservation of visceral organs with physiologic stress may represent an adaptive response to injury or infection that is the anatomic counterpart to increased synthesis of serum acute-phase reactants.

Magnetic resonance imaging (MRI) and computed tomography are used by investigators to quantify total body and regional adipose tissue and skeletal muscle (22). Imaging and ultrasonic techniques can also be used to estimate visceral organ and skeletal weights. Skeletal muscle and adipose tissue are important components in nutritional assessment because they are readily estimated by anthropometric techniques. At present, many anthropometric equations can be used to predict total and visceral adipose tissues, skeletal muscle, and bone mass at the tissue-system level (9, 39, 40).

Whole Body

The whole body level of body composition includes the main anthropometric dimensions such as stature, circumferences, breadths, and skinfold thicknesses. Other whole-body measures include body weight, density, and volume (see also Chapter 49).

Features of the Model

The five-level model has several important features. First, the model is consistent as a whole and each component is distinct (9). Connections between components are important in relation to anthropometric methods, however; for example, a group of related components at atomic to tissue-system levels: calcium, bone mineral, extracellular solids, skeleton, and bone breadths. Each of these components is distinct, and yet all five are linked because they are different constituents or dimensions of the human skeleton (9).

Second, steady-state relationships exist between many components at the same or different levels (9). Steady state as used here means a stable relationship between components over a specified time interval, usually months or years. Some steady-state relations were described above (e.g., the hydration of FFM = 0.73, and intracellular potassium concentration = 150 mmol/L). These quantitative associations are important in developing body composition models that relate a known component to an unknown component of interest. For example, TBW can be measured and FFM then calculated as TBW/0.73 (9). Steady-state relationships are particularly important in anthropometry because although all anthropometric measurements are at the whole-body level, they are used primarily to infer information about the first four body-composition levels. Steady-state relationships allow us to establish connections between the whole-body level and other levels. Additionally, they are often altered across gender, age, and ethnic groups and with disease, thus changing the quantitative associations established between anthropometric dimensions and other body components.

Following is a summary of anthropometric methods in the context of the five-level model.

Measurements

The anthropometric measurements in general use for evaluation of malnutrition include body weight, stature, skinfold thicknesses, circumferences, and bone breadths. These whole-body measurements can be used in nutritional assessment, in indices, or in equations that estimate an absolute value component at one of the other levels (Table 56.1). The following discussion groups the various anthropometric measurements and techniques into three categories: *(a)* body weight and stature; *(b)* estimates of fat-

Table 56.1
Some Characteristic Components at Levels I to IV and Related Anthropometric Dimensions at Level V

Characteristic Compartments				Anthropometric Dimensions (Level V)				
Level I	Level II	Level III	Level IV	BW	Stature	Circumferences	Skinfolds	Breadths
TBC	fat	fat cells	adipose tissue	X		X	X	
TBO	TBW	BCM + ECF	ATFW	X		X	X	
TBCa, TBP	Mo	ECS	bone, skeleton	X	X			X
TBN, TBK	Pro, Ms	BCM	muscle + viscera	X	X	X	X	
TBNa, TBCl	Ms	ECF	blood + ISF	X	X			

ATFW, adipose tissue-free body weight; BCM, body cell mass; BW, body weight; ECF, extracellular fluid; ECS, extracellular solids; FFM, fat-free body mass; ISF, interestitial fluid; levels I to V: atomic, molecular, cellular, tissue-system, and whole-body levels of body composition, respectively; Mo, bone mineral; Ms, soft tissue mineral; Pro, protein; TBC, TBCa, TBCl, TBK, TBN, TBNa, TBO, TBP, total body carbon, calcium, chloride, potassium, nitrogen, sodium, oxygen, and phosphorus, respectively; TBW, total body water.

ness and energy stores; and *(c)* lean tissue indices, protein mass, and functional components.

Body Weight and Stature

Body weight is the sum of all components at each level of body composition. As described above, body weight is a rough measure of total body energy stores, and changes in weight parallel energy and protein balance. A significant correlation exists ($r = 0.6$, $P < 0.05$) between loss of body weight and change in total body protein in seriously ill adults (15).

Body weight usually varies less than ±0.1 kg/day in healthy adults (2). A weight loss of more than 0.5 kg/day either indicates negative energy or water balance or a combination of the two. Clinically significant weight loss is considered a relative decrease in weight of more than 10% over an interval of less than 6 months (2).

The severity of weight loss in an individual is determined by two factors: the rate of weight change over time and the total reduction in weight. The rate of weight loss in total starvation is approximately 0.4 kg/day, and survival is sustained to about 70% of desirable (i.e., ideal) body weight (2). Semistarvation, the more typical cause of negative energy balance in patients, results in a more gradual weight loss than total starvation. In patients with chronic disease, the weight change may occur over years or decades. The minimal survivable body weight in humans is between 48 and 55% of desirable body weight, or a BMI of about 13 (i.e., point B_u in Fig. 56.4). Body weight at this point consists of less than 5% metabolically available fat (2). Exhaustion of the remaining usable fat mass results in rapid depletion of lean tissue and death.

The absolute body weight and rate of change in weight have prognostic value, and two aspects are recognized. First, an absolute body weight below 55 to 60% of desirable places the subject at or near the survival limits of starvation (2); further negative balance could not be tolerated for long. Second, a significant weight loss from preillness weight (between 10 and 20%) over an interval of less than about 6 months places the patient at risk of developing functional impairment of multiple organ systems and an adverse clinical outcome.

Studley was among the first to associate weight loss with disease outcome (41). In 1936, this pioneering investigator made the classic observation that marked weight loss prior to surgical procedures for peptic ulcer resulted in a higher postoperative mortality rate than in weight-stable patients. Modern workers have identified weight loss as a major determinant of prognosis in many disease states and conditions, such as survival time in patients with carcinoma of the colon (42) and chronic obstructive lung disease (43). Seltzer et al. found a 19-fold increase in mortality in adult patients undergoing elective surgery who lost more than 10 lb body weight preoperatively, compared with patients with little or no weight loss (44). Hirsch et al. (45) observed a 21% preoperative weight loss in patients who died postoperatively, compared with a 12% preoperative weight loss in survivors.

An important study by Windsor and Hill refined Studley's classic observation by demonstrating that the postoperative patients with weight loss who are at the highest risk of complications are those who also have clinically obvious impairment in organ function (46). Postoperative patients with clinically apparent organ impairment in this study also had significant abnormalities of a variety of measured physiologic functions and a reduced weight of total body protein. Summarizing this and other studies from his laboratory, Hill concluded that a loss of less than 10% of preillness body weight is usually not associated with functional abnormalities; loss of between 10 and 20% of preillness body weight is accompanied by functional abnormalities in some patients; and a loss of >20% of preillness body weight is associated with protein-energy malnutrition and multiple functional abnormalities in almost all patients (15). Weight loss is thus an important indirect index of multiple physiologic functions and the underlying severity of disease and is a guide to a patient's prognosis. Body weight is measured longitudinally to establish the effectiveness of nutritional therapy. A change in weight reflects energy, protein, and water balance.

Measurement. In the hospital, body weight should be measured within ±0.1 kg on a calibrated physician's scale. Special scales should be used for bedridden or wheelchair-bound patients. Edema, if present, should be recorded with the weight. The general procedure is to obtain a morning weight following evacuation of the bladder. The weight of the hospital gown can be subtracted from the total weight to obtain nude weight. When comparing the patient's weight with standard values, the attire is usually presented in a footnote on the table. Serial weights should be measured on the same or a carefully calibrated scale. Intake and output records may be useful in interpreting the significance of weight changes.

Reference tables provide a standard weight for height, and in some cases, an adjustment is made for frame size (see Appendix Tables III-A-12 to 15). Height is usually measured by a sliding bar attached to the physician's scale, although more-accurate techniques are used for research purposes. Height can be estimated in bedridden patients using knee-height or arm-span prediction equations (47–50) (Table 56.2). Knee height is measured in the sitting position with an anthropometric caliper. The bottom of the foot is placed flat on the floor to form a right angle with the knee. The heel is raised, and the caliper blade is placed under the heel. The caliper's movable blade is then lowered to the top of the thigh at a minimum of 2 inches posterior to the kneecap. Methods for recumbent measurement of knee height are also available. Arm span is defined as the distance between the tips of the longest finger of each hand with subjects standing erect against the wall and both arms fully stretched horizontally (48, 50).

Table 56.2
Recommended Equations for Predicting Stature in Adults and Children

Group	Age Group	Equation[a]	Reference
White men	18–60	Stature = 1.88 (knee height) + 71.85	47
	17–67	Stature = 2.31 (knee height) + 51.1	48
	60–80	Stature = 2.08 (knee height) + 59.01	49
	17–67	Stature = 2.30 (knee height) − 0.063 (age) + 54.9	48
	17–67	Stature = 0.762 (arm span) + 40.7	48
Black men	18–60	Stature = 1.79 (knee height) + 73.42	47
	60–80	Stature = 1.37 (knee height) + 95.79	49
White women	18–60	Stature = 1.87 (knee height) − 0.06 (age) + 70.25	47
	22–71	Stature = 1.84 (knee height) + 70.2	48
	22–71	Stature = 1.91 (knee height) − 0.098 (age) + 71.3	48
	60–80	Stature = 1.91 (knee height) − 0.17 (age) + 75.00	49
	22–71	Stature = 0.693 (arm span) + 50.3	48
Black women	18–60	Stature = 1.86 (knee height) − 0.06 (age) + 68.10	47
	60–80	Stature = 1.96 (knee height) + 58.72	49
White boys	6–18	Stature = 2.22 (knee height) + 40.54	47
Black boys	6–18	Stature = 2.18 (knee height) + 39.60	47
Chinese boys	4–16	Statute = 1.75 (lower segment) + 26.56	50
	4–16	Stature = 0.92 (arm span) + 10.84	50
White girls	6–18	Stature = 2.15 (knee height) + 43.21	47
Black girls	6–18	Stature = 2.02 (knee height) + 46.59	47
Chinese girls	4–16	Stature = 1.81 (lower segment) + 22.75	50
	4–16	Stature = 0.93 (arm span) + 10.34	50

[a]Arm span, knee height, and stature are in cm; lower segment (subischial leg length) in cm = standing height minus sitting height; and age in years.

The body weight reference table usually specifies the technique used to estimate frame size.

Interpretation. Interpretation of body weight as an index of available energy supply must be done with caution in four conditions:

1. Edema and ascites cause a relative increase in extracellular fluid and may mask losses in chemical or cellular components.
2. Massive tumor growth or organomegaly can mask loss in fat or lean tissues such as skeletal muscle.
3. Lean tissue and cellular atrophy are partially masked by residual fat and connective tissue in obese patients undergoing rapid or severe weight loss. Patients may still be overweight and yet suffer severe protein-energy malnutrition and also be at increased risk of adverse health outcomes secondary to semistarvation.
4. Large changes in energy intake cause corresponding changes in glycogen mass and bound water over several days. Similarly, large changes in sodium intake are associated with brief periods of fluid readjustment and body weight change.

For these reasons, and also to characterize body composition more completely, anthropometric methods are used for further assessment of body weight. These methods are described under two general headings as they relate to nutritional assessment: measures of fat stores and measures of lean tissues.

Fat

Although fat refers specifically to a chemical component at the molecular level of body composition, this section as a whole relates to the following five-level sequence: atomic, carbon; molecular, fat; cellular, fat cells; tissue-system, adipose tissue; and whole-body, anthropometric dimensions (e.g., skinfolds/circumferences) (see Table 56.1). Although more accurate and reproducible methods of estimating fatness exist, anthropometric methods are the simplest, safest, most practical, and least costly of the available techniques because of easy access to subcutaneous adipose depots.

The amount of fat in healthy subjects varies greatly, with relatively small amounts in some highly trained athletes and relatively large amounts during the later stages of pregnancy. During protracted undernutrition, all but a small amount of total body fat can be used as metabolic fuel (2). Two factors determine the adequacy of fat: the amount of total body triglyceride present and energy balance. Very little fat is sufficient if the individual is healthy and in zero energy balance. In contrast, a small amount of fat in the presence of marked negative energy balance implies a limited survival time. The usual practice is to compare fat values from an individual patient with reference standards and also to follow trends over time. During nutritional therapy, the fat measurement provides an indirect guide to energy balance.

Measurement and Interpretation. Three methods of assessing fatness are available: *(a)* the single skinfold method; *(b)* the limb fat area method; and *(c)* total body fat (or adipose tissue) calculated from multiple anthropometric measurements. The measurements common to all three techniques are now briefly reviewed, and the interested reader should consult additional references for added details (19–21).

Measuring body fat requires two instruments: a skinfold caliper and a tape measure. The caliper should be a

Table 56.3
Skinfold Measurement Sites

1. **Biceps skinfold thickness.** Lift the skinfold on the anterior aspect of the upper arm, directly above the center of the cubital fossa, at the same level as the triceps skinfold and midarm circumference. The arm hangs relaxed at the patient's side, and the crest of the fold should run parallel to the long axis of the arm.
2. **Triceps skinfold thickness.** Grasp the skin and subcutaneous tissue 1 cm above the midpoint between the tip of the acromial process of the scapula and the olecranon process of the ulna. The fold runs parallel to the long axis of the arm. Care should be taken to ensure that the measurement is made in the midline posteriorly and that the arm hangs relaxed and vertical.
3. **Subscapular skinfold.** The skin is lifted 1 cm under the inferior angle of the scapula with the patient's shoulder and arm relaxed. The fold should run parallel to the natural cleavage lines of the skin; this is usually a line about 45° from the horizontal extending medially upward.
4. **Suprailiac skinfold.** Pick up this skinfold 2 cm above the iliac crest in the midaxillary line. The crest of this fold should run horizontally.
5. **Thigh skinfold.** The skin is picked up on the posterior aspect at the same level as the thigh circumference. The crest of the skinfold should run parallel to the leg.
6. **Calf skinfold.** This skinfold is picked up on the posterior aspect of the calf at the same level as the calf circumference. The crest of the skinfold should run parallel to the leg.

rugged and light instrument, and jaw pressure should be maintained at 10 g/mm^2 throughout the measurement range. The contact surface area of the jaws can vary between 30 and 100 mm^2, and the jaws on some calipers remain parallel as they are opened wider. A calibration block is usually supplied with the instrument.

The tape measure should be durable, resist stretching, and have an accuracy of ±0.1 cm. Plastic and fiberglass tapes meet these criteria, and calibration should be checked periodically against a meter stick.

Two types of measurement are usually made: skinfold thicknesses and limb or trunk circumferences. The location of six widely used skinfold sites and circumferences is described in Tables 56.3 and 56.4 (2). Skinfolds represent a double layer of subcutaneous tissue, including a small and relatively constant amount of skin and variable amounts of adipose tissue. Components at all five levels of body composition are thus represented by a skinfold measurement. For arm measurements, the most important aspect is to use the same arm for repeated measurements. Some workers recommend evaluating the nondominant arm; when comparing the patient's measurements with standard values, consult the arm selected in the reference table. Measuring techniques and methods of optimizing precision are presented in reference 19 and in Tables 56.5 and 56.6. Skinfold measurements are not accurate in massively obese patients.

Table 56.4
Circumferential Measurement Sites

1. **Midupper arm.** This circumference is taken at the midpoint between the acromial and olecranon processes of the scapula and the ulna, respectively. The arm should hang relaxed at the patient's side.
2. **Midthigh.** The subject stands with feet slightly apart and with weight evenly distributed on both feet. The tape is placed around the thigh horizontally at the midpoint between the lower extent of the gluteal fold and the crease immediately posterior to the patella.
3. **Midcalf.** With the subject standing in the same position as for the thigh circumference, the measurement is made with the tape horizontal at the maximal circumference of the calf.

The absolute skinfold thickness can be used directly for comparison with reference tables and for longitudinal follow-up (see Appendix Table III-A-14 and its subdivisions). The limitation of evaluating one skinfold thickness is that a single measurement is a relatively poor predictor of the absolute amount and rate of change in total body fat because *(a)* large interindividual differences exist in fat distribution, *(b)* as total body fat changes, each skinfold site responds differently, and *(c)* the relationship between skinfold thickness and total body fat is complex (e.g., an exponential relationship exists between subcutaneous skinfold thickness and total body fat and between subcutaneous fat and visceral fat) (39, 51). Other factors that limit a single skinfold thickness as a measure of fatness include changes in the composition of adipose tissue with age and nutritional status, variation in skinfold distribution and compressibility with age, and the inclusion of a small amount of nonadipose tissues (e.g., skin) in the measurement (2, 20, 39). The final consideration is that the day-to-day variability in measuring the same skinfold is large, even when the rigorous procedures outlined in Tables 56.5 and 56.6 are followed. Skinfold thickness should thus be considered a qualitative measure of the amount and rate of change in total body fat. The advantages are ease and rapidity of measurement, especially in bedridden patients.

Combining a limb skinfold thickness with a corresponding circumference allows calculation of limb fat areas (Table 56.7). Most of the problems related to a single skinfold measurement also occur with the limb fat area. The advantage generally ascribed to area calculations is that the result includes the contribution of limb

Table 56.5
Methods of Measuring Skinfolds and Circumferences

Skinfolds

1. Arrive at the anatomic site as described in Tables 56.3 and 56.4
2. Lift the skin and fat layer from the underlying tissue by grasping the tissue with the thumb and forefinger.
3. Apply calipers about 1 cm distal from the thumb and forefinger, midway between the apex and base of the skinfold.
4. Continue to support the skinfold with the thumb and forefinger for the duration of the measurement.
5. After 2 to 3 seconds of caliper application, read skinfold to the nearest 0.5 mm.
6. Measurements are then made in triplicate until readings agree within ± 1.0 mm; results are then averaged.

Circumferences

1. The tape should be maintained in a horizontal position touching the skin and following the contours of the limb, but not compressing underlying tissue.
2. Measurements should be made to the nearest millimeter, in triplicate, as previously described for skinfolds.

Table 56.6
Methods for Optimizing Precision

1. Train observers by skilled professionals.
2. Use one rather than multiple observers for the same subject over time.
3. Mark the anatomic site of the skinfold and circumferential measurement with indelible ink when repeatedly measuring the same patient over a short time span.
4. Learn the anatomic landmarks, how to grasp the skinfold, how long to compress the skinfold site, and how to properly read the caliper scale.
5. Periodically assess interobserver and between-day measurement differences of the staff.

circumference; two limbs with equal skinfolds but unequal circumferences have different amounts of fat.

Many prediction equations are available for calculating total body fat from measured skinfold thicknesses (see Appendix Tables III-A-17-a to c), circumferences, body weight, and stature. All methods presently in use are "descriptive" in that measured anthropometric dimensions are converted to total body fat or other components using statistically derived equations in the absence of an underlying theory of mechanism. In contrast, some body composition methods are based on theoretical or mechanistic models (e.g., BCM is calculated from exchangeable potassium by use of a model that assumes a constant intracellular potassium concentration). All descriptive methods, including anthropometry, share in common the following: development in a well-defined subject group, use of a criterion method for estimating total body fat, and a prediction model formulated by use of regression analysis. Some methods, for convenience and speed, are based only on gender, body weight, stature, and circumferences (52, 53). As all prediction formulas are population specific, they should be cross-validated in new subject groups prior to application. Ideally, the fat-prediction formula is used in a group similar to the population on whom it was developed.

A good example and the most widely applied total body fat–prediction formula was developed by Durnin and Womersley using underwater weighing as the criterion for fat estimation (54) (Table 56.8). The sample contained 209 Caucasian men and 272 women, less than 68 years of age, and on average normal or slightly overweight. Once total body fat is known, it can be subtracted from body weight to provide a value for FFM.

A literature search will turn up many fat-prediction formulas that are applicable in specific populations and that vary in measurement type (i.e., circumferences and skinfolds) and anatomic location. Some examples of methods in current use for females are presented in Table 56.9. In most of these formulas the dependent (i.e., predicted) variable is body density. These methods were developed using underwater weighing as a reference for body density estimation and setting anthropometric dimensions along with such other covariates as age in regression models as independent variables. The anthropometric "predicted" density cam be converted to percentage fat by use of traditional two-component body composition models as outlined in Table 56.8.

The advantages of calculating total body fat are *(a)* more than one skinfold site is usually included in the calculation and *(b)* the result (in kilograms) can be used directly to calculate energy reserves as fat. The latter values can then be integrated with estimates of energy balance calculations, thus providing a more physiologic description of the patient's nutritional state. A cautionary note, as with all prediction equations, results are most accurate on populations on which the equation was derived. The accuracy of the Durnin-Womersley equation (Table 56.8) and those presented in Table 56.9 is unknown in patients with severe weight loss, and the techniques should not be applied when a gross distortion in body habitus or obvious fluid accumulation is present (54). As emphasized by Damon and Goldman, skinfold thicknesses describe, but do not measure, total body fat (55). The error of prediction of total body fat from skinfolds may be considerable in some individuals, even when group means are accurate. More-accurate methods of measuring fat are therefore usually applied in research studies of body composition.

It is customary to express total body fat estimates as a percentage of body weight. However, as an individual gains or loses weight, both fat and FFM change, which leads to problems in interpretation. Additionally, the relationship between body fat and body weight has a nonzero intercept (Fig. 56.3), so that a curvilinear relationship exists between total body fat (12), expressed as a percent-

Table 56.7
Equations for Calculating Limb Fat Areas

Extremity	Equation	Comments
Upper arm	Arm fat area (cm^2) = $\left[\frac{MAC \times TSF}{2}\right] - \left[\frac{\pi \times (TSF)^2}{4}\right]$	This general equation assumes a circular limb and muscle compartment and a symmetrically distributed fat rim; the accuracy of this equation in predicting midupper arm fat area is unknown TSF, triceps skinfold (cm);MAC, midarm circumference (cm)
Thigh	Thigh fat area (cm^2) = $\left[\frac{MTC \times THSF}{2}\right] - \left[\frac{\pi \times (THSF)^2}{4}\right]$	THSF, thigh skinfold (cm); MTC, midthigh circumference (cm)
Calf	Calf fat area (cm^2) = $\left[\frac{MCC \times CSF}{2}\right] - \left[\frac{\pi \times (CSF)^2}{4}\right]$	CSF, calf skinfold (cm); MCC, midcalf circumference (cm)

Table 56.8
Calculation of Fat and Fat-Free Body Mass According to the Method of Durnin and Womersley

1. Determine the patient's age and weight (kg).
2. Measure the following skinfolds in mm; biceps, triceps, subscapular, and suprailiac (Tables 56–3 and 56–5).
3. Compute Σ by adding the four skinfolds.
4. Compute the logarithm of Σ.
5. Apply one of the following age- and sex-adjusted equations to compute body density (D, g/ml)

   Equations for men:

Age range	
17–19	$D = 1.1620 - 0.0630 \times (\log \Sigma)$
20–29	$D = 1.1631 - 0.0632 \times (\log \Sigma)$
30–39	$D = 1.1422 - 0.0544 \times (\log \Sigma)$
40–49	$D = 1.1620 - 0.0700 \times (\log \Sigma)$
50+	$D = 1.1715 - 0.0779 \times (\log \Sigma)$

   Equations for women:

Age range	
17–19	$D = 1.1549 - 0.0678 \times (\log \Sigma)$
20–29	$D = 1.1599 - 0.0717 \times (\log \Sigma)$
30–39	$D = 1.1423 - 0.0632 \times (\log \Sigma)$
40–49	$D = 1.1333 - 0.0612 \times (\log \Sigma)$
50+	$D = 1.1339 - 0.0645 \times (\log \Sigma)$

6. Fat mass is then calculated as fat mass (kg) = body weight (kg) $\times \left[\frac{4.95}{D} - 4.5\right]$
7. Fat-free body mass is then calculated as FFM (kg) = body weight (kg) − fat mass (kg)

Adapted from the data of Durnin JVGA, Womersley J. and reprinted from Wright RA, Heymsfield SB, eds. Nutritional assessment. Boston: Blackwell Scientific, 1984.

age of body weight, and body weight or BMI (Fig. 56.6). These complex relationships can result in some confusing situations, as when a severely obese patient loses a relatively large amount of weight with a relatively small change in the percentage of fat. A highly trained athlete and a severely malnourished patient might have an equivalent percentage of body weight as fat. They could also have a similar absolute fat weight. To overcome these difficulties, Van Itallie et al. suggest calculating a fat (or FFM)-stature index similar to BMI as fat/Ht^2 (56). A low or high "fat mass index" would then represent a reduced or increased actual fat mass relative to stature, respectively. For example, the fat mass index of a malnourished patient would be lower than that of a highly trained athlete, even though they had an equivalent percentage of body weight as fat. This is because the athlete with a similar percentage of body weight as fat would have a much larger absolute fat mass and also a much larger FFM and greater body weight than the malnourished patient.

Lean Tissues

Lean tissues refer in general to the following sequence of components at the five levels of body composition: atomic—nitrogen, potassium, and calcium; molecular—FFM, water, and protein; cellular—BCM; tissue-system—skeletal muscle, skeleton, and visceral organs; whole body—anthropometric measurements (e.g., skinfolds/circumferences) (see Table 56.1). These various components are associated with the major portion of whole-body metabolic activity and biologic functions.

Semistarvation. Semistarvation results in negative balances of energy, protein, water, and minerals, a reduction in FFM and BCM, and atrophy of tissues and organs (2, 57) (see Chapter 41). Not all lean components change at the same rate during periods of negative balance. At the molecular level, cellular proteins are depleted rapidly, and connective tissue proteins are lost at a slower rate (2). Similarly, at the cellular level, rapid changes can occur in BCM, whereas extracellular fluid is lost more slowly or may even increase in volume (57). Organs and tissues also differ in their rate of weight loss during semistarvation. Liver mass decreases rapidly and brain weight changes little if at all in uncomplicated semistarvation; liver and other visceral organs may be preserved in chronic catabolic conditions such as metastatic malignant diseases (37). Skeletal muscle is a major reservoir of amino acids for acute-phase protein synthesis and can decrease by up to 75% in weight

Table 56.9
Anthropometric Equations That Predict Body Density in the Female Population[a,b]

Authors (Date; ref.)	Equation	n	Mean or Range	*r*	SEE
Katch and McArdle (1973;84)	Density = 1.09246 − [0.00049 (scapula SF)] − [0.00075 (iliac SF)] + [0.00710 (ED)] − [0.00121 (thigh C)]	69	25.6 ± 6.4%	0.84	0.0086 (3.6%)
Jackson et al. (1980;85)	Density = 1.1470 − [0.0004293 (chest SF + midaxillary SF + triceps SF + subscapular SF + abd SF + suprailiac SF + thigh SF)] + [0.00000065 $(7SF)^2$] − [0.00009975 (A) 2 [0.000621415 (gluteal C)]	249	4–44%	0.87	0.0079 (3.6%)
Wright et al. (1980;86)	Density = [1.051 (biceps C)] − [1.522 (forearm C)] − [0.879 (neck C)] + [0.326 (abd_2 C)] + [0.597 (thigh C)] + 0.707	181	2–37%	0.73	(4.1%)
Hodgdon and Beckett (1984;52)	Density = −(0.35004 [$\log_{10}$ (waist C + hip C − neck C)] + (0.22100 [$\log_{10}$ (H)]) + 1.29579	214	10–47%	0.80	0.0080 (3.7%)
Vogel et al. (1988;87)	% Body fat = [0.173 (hip C)] + (105.328 [$\log_{10}$ (Wt)]) − 0.515 (H)] − [1.574 (forearm C)] − [0.533 (neck C)] − [0.200 (wrist C)] − 35.6	266	5–50%	0.77	(3.9%)
Tran and Weltman (1989;88)	Density = 1.168297 − [0.00284 (abd C)] + [0.0000122098 (abd^2)] − [0.000733128 (hip C)] + 0.000510477 (H)] − [0.00021616 (A)]	400	35.9 ± 7.7%	0.89	0.0095 (4.2%)

[a]A, age (years); abd, average waist and abdomen at navel (cm); C, circumference (cm); ED, elbow diameter (cm); H, height (cm); SF, skinfold (mm); and Wt = weight (kg). Correlations are shown, for test group samples unless otherwise specified. The interested reader should consult original sources for information regarding application of specific equations.

[b]Density in g/cc or kg/L.

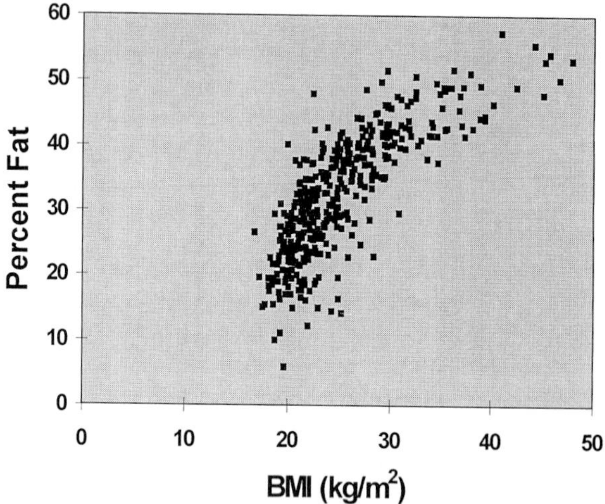

Figure 56.6. Percentage of body weight as fat in 413 healthy women versus body mass index (BMI). Fat was measured by the four-component model (9).

during protein-energy malnutrition (7, 37). The malnourished patient with a reduced body weight therefore differs in composition at each of the five levels from his or her normally nourished counterpart. This explains why anthropometric equations developed in normal subjects may not predict a specific component with equal accuracy in an undernourished seriously ill patient.

In anthropometrically assessing the severity of malnutrition, an important goal is defining the amount and rate of change in total body or skeletal muscle protein (7, 37). The main anthropometric indices used for this assessment are FFM (molecular level) and limb muscle areas (tissue-system level). As lower limits compatible with survival are known for both types of measurement (2), the severity of protein-energy malnutrition is usually judged as the patient's value relative to the normal range on the one hand and the minimal range on the other. In terms of prognostic value, these measurements provide some index of potential survival time; given the patient's anthropometric FFM or muscle index and nitrogen balance, progression toward or away from potentially lethal starvation can be established. During nutritional therapy and follow-up, the anthropometric FFM indices are used as measures of nitrogen balance; specific details regarding interpretation are presented in the following paragraphs.

Measurement and Interpretation. FFM is measured by anthropometric methods, such as those described above in the section on fat (Tables 56.8 and 56.9). The cautions in measurement technique and selection of patients noted in that earlier discussion also apply to FFM. With regard to interpretation, in theory, multiplying FFM (in grams) by 0.195 and 1.02 provides the amount of total body protein in grams and metabolizable energy in kilocalories. Of the metabolizable energy in the healthy subject, about half of that in FFM is available during prolonged periods of semi-starvation (2). Combined with balance data and information on total body fat, these bedside calculations often provide an interesting insight into a patient's course. Unfortunately, the information needed for accurate prediction of total body protein cannot be derived from anthropometric FFM because of the changes in body hydration and variability of skinfold measurements described above. A large tumor burden or organomegaly of any cause may also add metabolically unavailable mass (as water, protein, and mineral) to FFM. In patients without serious derangements in body composition, FFM can be used in equation 56.3 to calculate RMR (28). This FFM-based calculation of RMR is largely independent of sex and age (28, 32), although evidence is accumulating that ethnic RMR difference exist, even after controlling for body composition.

Calculating the amount of limb muscle tissue from anthropometric data requires only two measurements: the limb circumference and the corresponding skinfold thickness. The midportion of the upper limb is usually studied, and little additional information is gathered by also measuring thigh and calf muscle areas (37). Calf muscle measurement would, of course, be useful in subjects whose upper extremities are burned, amputated, edematous, or immobilized by casts or traction devices. The upper arm muscles tend to atrophy slightly more rapidly during semi-starvation than the muscles of the thigh or calf, but the differences are not large (37). The equations for calculating the limb muscle indices are provided in Table 56.10.

Limb muscle measurements are used primarily to obtain a measure of the amount and rate of change in skeletal muscle protein. The following three factors should therefore be considered (2):

1. The mass of a skeletal muscle represents a three-dimensional measurement (i.e., volume), whereas limb muscle area and circumference are two- and one-dimensional indices, respectively (2, 37). As the muscle volume changes, the corresponding proportional changes in muscle area and circumference are smaller. For example, a 50% decrease in muscle volume corresponds to theoretical decreases in muscle area and circumference of 37 and 21%, respectively. As a rule, the relative change in muscle area is larger than the change in muscle circumference.
2. The equations for calculating limb muscle indices are based upon simple theoretical assumptions regarding arm geometry (2, 37). Actually, the calculated arm muscle area overestimates the amount of skeletal muscle by 15 to 25% in relatively young, nonobese subjects. Half of this overestimate is due to the inclusion of bone in the calculated area, and the remainder is due to errors in the assumptions and the inclusion of nonmuscle tissue (e.g., neurovascular bundle) in the result (58). Two methods of correcting this overestimate of muscle area are available. The first is to express results as a percentage of standard, because the standard value also contains these "nonskeletal muscle" components. The second approach is to calculate a value for bone-free arm muscle area, as described in Table 56.10. Studies by Forbes et al. and Baumgartner et al. suggest that arm muscle area assumptions are also inaccurate in obese and elderly subjects, respectively (59, 60). Rolland-Cachera et al. recently proposed a new anthropometric approach for calculating upper midarm mus-

Table 56.10
Anthropometric Equations for Calculating Muscle Mass

Equation	Comment
(1) Calf muscle area $(cm)^2 = \frac{[MCC - \pi \times CSF]^2}{4\pi}$	Includes bone area; assumes circular limb and muscle compartment and symmetric fat rim; abbreviations as inTable 56.7 Table 56.7
(2) Thigh muscle area $(cm^2) = \frac{[MTC - \pi \times THSF]^2}{4\pi}$	Bone corrections area available
(3) Arm muscle circumference (cm) = $MAC - \pi \times TSF$	Same assumption as for equations 1 and 2; includes bone; note that as muscle loses mass or volume in protein-energy malnutrition, circumferential measurements will change proportionately less than area measurements; the latter therefore more realistically depict severity of muscle atrophy
(4) Arm muscle area $(cm^2) = \frac{[MAC - \pi \times TSF]^2}{4\pi}$	Same assumption as equations 1 and 2; includes bone; equation overestimates actual muscle area; by expressing absolute value as a percentage of standard, the error is partially corrected
(5) Arm muscle area $(cm^2) = \frac{[MAC - \pi \times TSF]^2}{4\pi} - 10$ (men) Arm muscle area $(cm^2) = \frac{[MAC - \pi \times TSF]^2}{4\pi} - 6.5$ (women)	Same assumptions as equations 1 and 2; the overestimate in equation 4 is corrected, and the average value for bone area is also subtracted; resulting value is therefore bone-free arm muscle area; as for all muscle derivatives on this table, the resulting value remains an approximation (±8%) of actual muscle area; arm muscle area estimates may be particularly inaccurate in obese and elderly subjects
(6) Total body skeletal muscle mass (g) = $STAT \times (0.0553 \times CTG^2 + 0.0987 \times FG^2 + 0.0331 \times CCG^2) - 2445$	Based on cadaver studies.[40] STAT, stature (cm); CTG, thigh circumference corrected for the front thigh skinfold thickness (cm); FG, uncorrected forearm circumference (cm); CCG, calf circumference corrected for the medial calf skinfold thickness (cm)

cle area (61). In this model, the unrolled fat rim is assumed to be a rectangle with length equal to upper arm circumference (C) and width equal to triceps skinfold thickness/2. Upper mid-arm fat area then equals C × (triceps skinfold thickness/2), and the remaining tissue, mainly muscle, is derived as total upper midarm area minus upper midarm fat area. Promising correlations were observed in normal-weight and obese children with MRI as the midarm cross-sectional component area reference method. This approach has not yet been examined in adult populations. Further studies are needed to improve our understanding of the relationship between anthropometric muscle estimates at the whole-body level and actual skeletal muscle mass at the tissue-system level.

3. Atrophic skeletal muscle differs in chemical composition from normal tissue. Per gram of muscle, the amounts of water, total lipid, and collagen are increased, whereas non-collagen protein is reduced (Fig. 56.7). Thus, the concentration of functional proteins per unit arm muscle area or circumference is relatively lower in atrophied muscle. Another chemical consideration is that muscle size can abruptly change by ±5 to 10% in response to rapid changes in muscle glycogen resulting from the water-binding properties of glycogen (37).

Thus, both anthropometric FFM and muscle indices are truly indirect markers of the active protein component of body weight. The two lean tissue indices should be considered approximate bedside guides to the amount of total body protein. Despite their approximate nature, anthropometric muscle estimates correlate with more complex methods of estimating skeletal muscle (e.g., total limb muscle area vs. total body skeletal muscle volume by MRI; Fig. 56.8) over the broad biologic range of muscle mass in humans.

Small changes in total body protein cannot be detected by anthropometry; nitrogen balance and other techniques must be used for this assessment. An example of the limi-

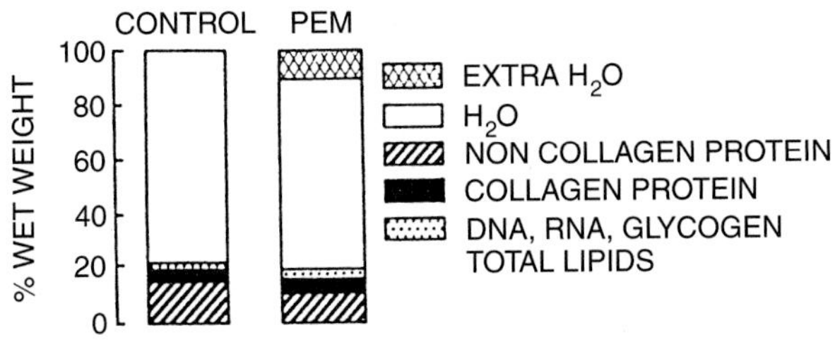

Figure 56.7. Muscle composition per gram of wet muscle weight in control subjects and in protein-energy malnourished *(PEM)* humans. Muscle specimens were collected at autopsy. Undernourished patients had more water (including extra water), collagen proteins, and total lipids than controls. The extra water was calculated by assuming that muscle dry weight is normally 21% of wet weight. (From Heymsfield SB, Stevens V, Noel R, et al. Am J Clin Nutr 1982; 36:131–142; with permission.)

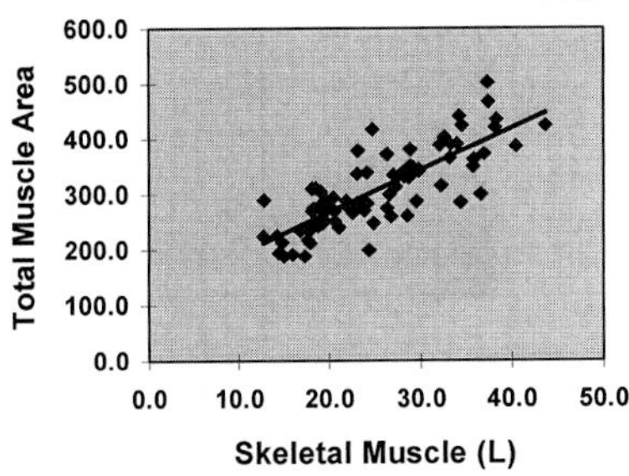

Figure 56.8. Correlation between total limb muscle area (sum of arm, calf, and thigh muscle areas in cm^2) and total body skeletal muscle volume in L by whole-body MRI in healthy subjects. (N = 79; total muscle area [cm^2] = 7.6 − skeletal muscle [L] + 115.4; $R^2 = 0.6423$, $P < 0.001$).

tation of anthropometry is shown in Figure 56.9, where short-term changes in anthropometric arm muscle area with nutritional support show no correlation with nitrogen balance. Martin et al. (40) developed an anthropometric prediction formula for total-body skeletal muscle mass, but the accuracy of this method in monitoring changes in muscle mass and associated protein content has not been reported.

Reference Values

Body Weight

The patient's body weight is evaluated using two reference sources. The first reference values are those of the patient, and these include a "usual weight" by history or previous measured weight. This is important because many obese patients who lose weight during an illness and are thus potentially malnourished are still overweight by conventional standards. The second reference source is the healthy population. In this approach, the individual's actual body weight is compared with that of a gender-, stature-, and age-appropriate reference or a desirable body weight (see Appendix Tables III-A-12 to 15 and their subtables). The subject's actual body weight is expressed as a percentage of the desirable weight. The normal range for desirable body weight varies among different sources, but it usually is set between 90 and 120%. A body weight below or above these levels is consistent with undernutrition and obesity, respectively. A historical review of the development of reference body weight tables is provided in Appendix Table III-A-12-a.

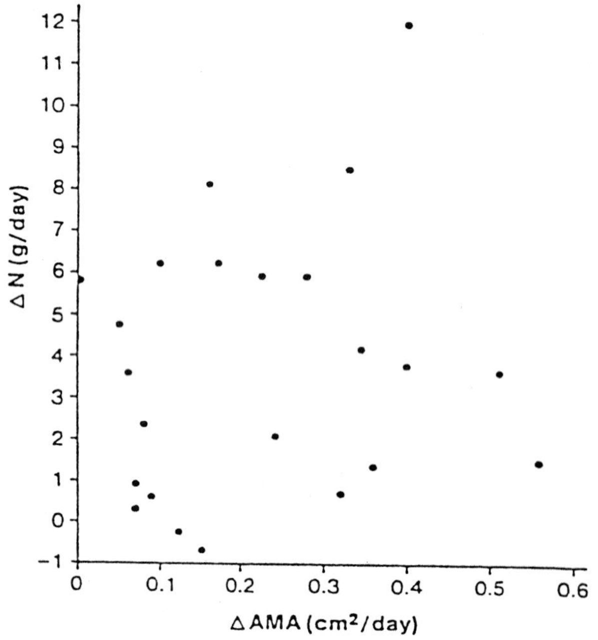

Figure 56.9. Nitrogen balance *(N)* measured on a metabolic ward versus change in arm muscle area *(AMA)* in subjects undergoing 1-week balance studies. (From Heymsfield SB, Casper K. JPEN J Parenter Enteral Nutr 1987;11:36S–41S.

Another method of comparing the patient's weight with that of a reference population is to calculate a body weight (BW)-stature (S) index (62). Most weight-stature indices in present use take the form W/S^P (59). The term P indicates how stature is to be scaled. The main assumptions of weight-stature indices are that they are independent of height, represent an indirect index of body composition, correlate with health outcomes, and can be generalized across different populations.

At present, BMI, calculated as BW/Ht^2, is gaining acceptance as a weight-stature index for use in diagnosing both protein-energy malnutrition and obesity (63–65). Most of the assumptions of weight-stature indices are fulfilled by BMI, although several limitations should be noted. First, although the correlation between BMI and total body fat is relatively strong ($r = 0.5–0.8$), individual variation is large, and some subjects can be misclassified as undernourished or obese (63). For example, some athletic subjects have a large skeletal muscle mass and a high BMI but are not obese. Another example, reported by Smalley et al., is that a man with a BMI of 27 can have total body fat ranging from 10 to 31% of body weight (66). Note that in studies such as these some of the observed error may be in the reference method for estimating body fat. BMI may also have a small stature dependence, because individuals with short legs for their height have higher BMI values independent of fatness (62, 64). Finally, Gallagher et al. recently used a four-component model as the criterion for body fat estimation (67) and found that BMI as a measure of fatness in their healthy cohort was age and sex dependent but independent of ethnicity in their black and white adults.

Although no consistent BMI ranges are accepted by all investigators, a useful set of guidelines is presented in Table 56.11. The table gives a normal range (18.5 to <25) and three grades of both chronic protein-energy malnutrition and obesity. The investigators proposing these guidelines based their criteria on extensive reviews of functional measurements and health outcomes at various levels of BMI (21, 64, 68). The BMI range considered nor-

Table 56.11
Body Mass Index and Grades of Chronic Protein-Energy Malnutrition and Obesity

Grade	Body Mass Index
Obesity	
III	>40
II	30–40
I	25–29.9
Normal	≥18.5–<25
Protein-energy malnutrition	
I	17.0–18.4
II	16.0–16.9
III	<16

Adapted from James WPT Ferro-Luzzi A, Waterlow JC. Eur J Clin Nutr 42:969–981, and McLaren DS. A fresh look at anthropometric classification schemes in protein-energy malnutrition. In: Himes JH, ed. Anthropometric assessment of nutritional status. New York: Wiley-Liss, 1991; 273–286.

mal is similar to the healthy weight range suggested in the "Dietary Guidelines for Americans" of 19 to 25 kg/m^2 (69). The diagnosis of protein-energy malnutrition or obesity and their associated risks is often multifactorial and may require additional estimates including body composition, energy expenditure, organ/tissue function, and biochemical markers.

Fat and Lean

Two methods are used to process anthropometric data other than body weight. The first expresses the individual's values relative to a healthy reference population. This method provides the anthropometric component used to assess whether and to what extent the patient is malnourished. Anthropometric reference tables present the results of large surveys and usually describe the general population. Appendix Tables III-13 to 18 include reference values for the United States population as a whole.

The reference tables usually present data in three forms: *(a)* as a mean ($\bar{x}$) value, *(b)* as $\bar{x}$ and standard deviation (SD), and *(c)* as percentiles. Describing a population in terms of $\bar{x}$ and SD assumes that the measurement under study is symmetrically (normally) distributed. If the data fit this model, then $\bar{x} \pm 2$ SD includes 95% of the population. An abnormal value is more than 2 SD units above or below $\bar{x}$. Some tables provide only $\bar{x}$; the patient's value is then expressed as a percentage of the standard or reference value. A weakness of this approach is that tables of this type do not provide a method of determining whether the result is within the normal range. The second type of table includes the SD, or 95% range of the healthy population, thus indicating whether and to what degree the patient is abnormal. The third mode of expression is in terms of percentiles (e.g., see various Appendix Tables III-A-16, 18). If results are expressed as a percentile rather than as a percentage of a standard, the reference population need not be symmetrically distributed. Often anthropometric surveys of populations produce "skewed" distributions, and thus the easiest option is to present results in percentiles (70). In this approach, the values of the subject exactly in the middle of the group define the 50th percentile. If the patient's value is between the 5th and 95th percentile, the result is considered normal; below or above these respective values is abnormal.

No simple method of judging the severity or potential morbidity of protein-energy malnutrition from anthropometric data is available. Studies in adults have not yet clearly defined the "risk" of a subnormal anthropometric index, especially for results falling just below the normal range. Combining anthropometric data with the results of other components of the nutritional assessment provides some measure of potential morbidity (71).

The second method of expressing anthropometric data is in terms of the individual's total-body energy content, fat, and FFM. Combining estimated energy and nitrogen balance with these body composition data permits a whole spectrum of potential calculations. Of course, these are approximations, but they are often useful in teaching and solving simple clinical questions.

CLINICAL APPLICATIONS

The following are suggested applications of anthropometry:

1. Weight and height should be recorded in the chart of every hospitalized patient. Weight indices, such as recent weight loss, should be added to the database for all patients who have a history of weight change. All patients undergoing short-term nutritional support should be weighed daily.
2. One skinfold measurement, limb fat area, and limb muscle area are helpful
   a. When body weight is an invalid index of energy reserves because of edema or massive tumor burden. The upper limb is usually not affected by dependent edema.
   b. When body weight is unmeasurable because of immobilizing devices such as a cast or respirator.
   c. When patients are seen for nutritional consultation or are seen at rounds removed from the bedside. Anthropometric estimates provide a quantitative description of what is usually visible at the bedside. Although weight alone is useful in this regard, two patients of the same height and weight may differ in body composition.
   d. During the initial evaluation of hospitalized patients prescribed short-term nutritional support. Although changes in fat and lean tissue will most likely not be detected over a 1- to 2-week period, the baseline anthropometric data become a permanent component of the nutritional database, and are thus available if a future reevaluation is needed.
3. Total body fat and FFM are useful indices
   a. In patients who are undergoing long-term nutritional follow-up over months or years. Limb muscle area measurements, preferably of the upper arm, should also be included in this group to complete the body composition database.
   b. In groups of subjects forming the basis of nutritional studies, when a more critical assessment of body composition is often useful and more-accurate techniques of evaluating body composition are not available.
   c. In estimating RMR based upon FFM.
   d. For teaching purposes, when the interrelation of metabolic balance, body composition, and nutritional therapy are being considered.

AGING AND ANTHROPOMETRIC INDICES

Body composition changes throughout the adult life span, which must be considered in evaluating anthropometric indices. Height declines and, assuming constant body weight, an elderly subject has more fat and less FFM than a younger individual of the same sex (48, 72–74). Most of the loss in FFM can be accounted for by a decrease in both skeletal muscle and visceral organs. A summary of how body composition changes with age and how anthropometric measures are affected is presented in Table 56.12. Because of these changes in body size, shape, and

Table 56.12
Effects of Aging on Body Composition and Anthropometric Measurements

Anthropometric Measurement	Comment
Weight	The average population value increases until the fifth decade and then plateaus or declines
Height	Height decreases by 1 to 3 cm/20 years after maturity; the rate of height decline is race and sex dependent
Fat	Fat increases as a percentage of body weight; redistribution occurs from subcutaneous to internal fat and between different subcutaneous sites
Skinfold	The compressibility of skinfolds changes with age; there is a loss in the elastic recoil of skin and an increase in viscoelastic recovery time; skinfolds in the elderly are often pendulous and difficult to measure
Fat-free body mass	Fat-free body mass decreases as a percentage of body weight mainly because of a loss in skeleton and skeletal muscle mass; the mass of visceral organs remains unchanged or decreases only slightly with age; skeletal muscle undergoes compositional changes, which include a relative increase in connective tissue and fat and relative loss in myofibrillar proteins

Based on refs. 41 and 70.

proportions, investigators now advocate geriatric-specific anthropometric body-composition prediction equations (75, 76).

Estimation of height is difficult in the elderly, especially in the wheelchair-bound, bedridden, or kyphotic subject. Specialized approaches such as recumbent anthropometry may be useful with hospitalized or nursing home patients (77). Another useful approach is measuring knee height or arm span (Table 56.2) to predict adult stature. Knee height and arm span undergo little change with age in adults and provide an estimate of stature that is difficult to obtain by conventional methods. The estimated value for height can then be used in calculating other assessment indices and comparing these results to height-adjusted reference values. Alternatively, knee height can be used in place of stature in such indices as fat/knee height (2, 78).

Anthropometric measurements may be useful in diagnosing malnutrition in hospitalized elderly subjects. Lansey et al. (79) examined 47 consecutive geriatric patients admitted to an acute care facility and found that approximately 45% of the patients had two anthropometric measures (i.e., midarm circumference and muscle area; subscapular and triceps skinfold) below the fifth percentile, indicating severe malnutrition. In contrast, only 28% of patients were below 90% of ideal body weight. Anthropometric measurements may therefore supplement, and be more sensitive than, body weight and stature in evaluating malnutrition in hospitalized elderly persons.

Anthropometric measures may also predict mortality in elderly populations. For 40 to 46 months, Campbell et al. (80) measured bone-corrected arm muscle area and triceps skinfold thickness in 758 subjects over age 70 years. In a logistic regression model, both low arm muscle area and triceps skinfold thickness were associated with significantly increased mortality risk.

Because of the ability of anthropometry to detect malnutrition and potentially predict mortality in elderly subjects, screening methods are being developed or have been reported for use in older cohorts. For example, in their "mini nutritional assessment," Guigoz et al. (81) include as screening measures, midarm circumference, calf circumference, and BMI. The usefulness of these anthropometric measurements beyond that of weight and height alone has not been established.

EVALUATING AND CONTROLLING ERROR SOURCES

Like all measurements, anthropometric evaluations include error. This section provides an introduction to anthropometric error sources; the interested reader is referred to comprehensive reviews for an advanced discussion of this important topic (19, 21, 82). Error can be considered in the context of the fundamental body composition methodology equation as shown in Figure 56.10. This equation indicates that error in the estimation of a body composition component (e.g., total body fat) from anthropometric measurements is a function of two main error sources, measurement of a quantity (Q) and mathematical function (i.e., descriptive or mechanistic). The figure also notes that errors of measurement may be either systematic (nonrandom) or random, or both. Errors due to misspecification of mathematical functions are always systematic. The following discussion first considers measurable quantity errors and then proceeds to an overview of mathematical function errors.

A subject's anthropometric dimensions can be evaluated at a single point in time or on repeated occasions over time. Measurement error is the main concern with a single evaluation, and measurement error combined with normal biologic variation must be considered with repeated measurements. Measurement error can be caused by instrument error and observer error. Methods of minimizing instrument error were reviewed above and mainly involve the correct choice of measurement instruments and accurate calibration. Observer error is related to three factors: precision, reliability, and accuracy.

Accuracy is the level of agreement between the measured value and the "true" dimension. Accuracy of an anthropometric dimension is usually established by comparison to a reference method. For example, subcutaneous adipose tissue thickness estimated using a skinfold caliper can be compared with corresponding estimates by computerized axial tomography or MRI. Of course any such analysis also includes instrument and observer errors. In clinical situations, measurements by an anthropometrist are usually compared with those of a designated "expert" (21).

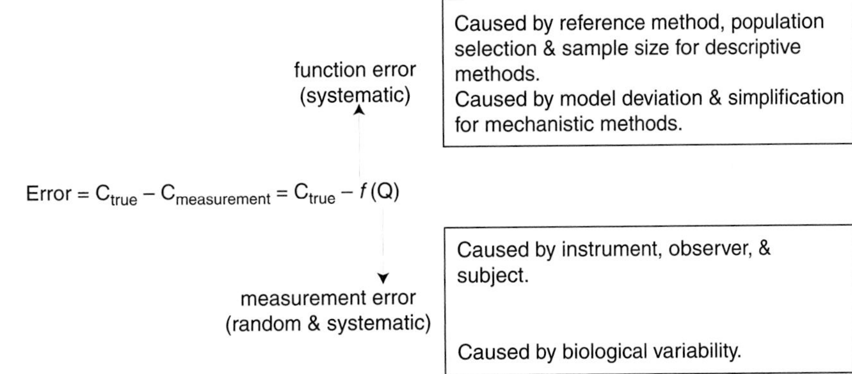

Figure 56.10. Sources of error in anthropometric methods (see text).

Precision, distinct from accuracy, defines the quality of a measurement in terms of being sharply defined or exact. In this sense, precision refers to the scale of measurement; for example, a skinfold measured to the nearest 1 mm is more precise than one measured to the nearest 0.5 cm. A highly precise measurement (e.g., body weight measured to the nearest gram) is not necessarily accurate if the weight scale used is improperly calibrated. The definition of precision overlaps to some extent with that of *reliability.* Reliability is the degree to which a measurement can be replicated by the same or a different observer using the same instrument. This is linked to precision because it is difficult for a measurement to be precise or exact if it is unreliable (83).

The precision of an anthropometric measurement can be quantified as the variability among repeated measurements over a short time in the same subject (21). Precision can be expressed as the *technical error of measurement,* which is the standard deviation of repeated measurements on the same subject by the same or different observers. The technical error of measurement, which is expressed in the same units as the measured quantity, can also be expressed as a percentage, a *coefficient of variation* (SD/mean × 100) (19, 21).

Reliability is also referred to as "reproducibility" or "repeatability." Reliability, as distinct from precision, is more commonly expressed in terms of the intraclass correlation among repeated measurements, sometimes called the "reliability coefficient." Measures of reliability often include both measurement error and physiologic variation.

The total variation in an anthropometric measurement monitored over time includes measurement variation and biologic variation. Biologic variation occurs even in the healthy individual, as weight and fluid balance fluctuate over time. This aspect of measurement variability is the difference between total anthropometric dimension variation over time and that due to measurement error. Some measures, such as stature, are extremely stable in adults; others, such as selected skinfold thicknesses, are moderately variable over time. In practice, this biologic component of variability is often included in estimates of the reliability of anthropometric measurements.

Anthropometric dimensions are often used directly, for example, triceps skinfold thickness as a measure of fatness. Mathematically transforming an anthropometric measurement to a component estimate involves error sources. The "validity" of an anthropometric method in this context is the degree to which it accurately measures or predicts a specific component. Descriptive or type I methods are population specific, and error may arise in applying a prediction formula to a new subject group or one outside the original subject range for age, weight, and stature. Mechanistic or type II methods include "model" error. For example, calculation of arm muscle area from triceps skinfold and midarm circumference is based on a simple geometric model (Table 56.10). Actual arm muscle area may deviate from the assumed model, which introduces error into the component estimate. Both types of error are nonrandom, or systematic.

Anthropometry is applied widely in evaluating a single subject or whole populations. Professionals who apply anthropometry in their clinical work or research should fully comprehend the anthropometric error sources and apply procedures to maximize the quality of their measurements. It is a good policy to set up an evaluation program for the anthropometrists as outlined in references 19, 21, and 82. An approach such as that suggested in these reports will help maintain a high-quality measurement standard.

CONCLUSION

Anthropometry is one of the oldest approaches to quantifying body composition, and it is the most practical for field and clinical settings. The severity, response to nutritional treatment, and aspects of subject malnutrition risk can be established using relatively simple and easily acquired anthropometric measurements. For these reasons, anthropometry is an indispensable tool for the practitioner of clinical nutrition.

REFERENCES

1. Heymsfield SB, Bethel RA, Ansley JD, et al. Ann Intern Med 1979;90:63–71.

2. Heymsfield SB, Tighe A, Wang ZM. Nutritional assessment by anthropometric and biochemical methods. In: Shils ME, Olson JA, Shike M, eds. Modern nutrition in health and disease. 8th ed. Philadelphia: Lea & Febiger, 1994;812–41.
3. Bistrian BR, Blackburn GL, Vitale J, et al. JAMA 1976;235: 1567–70.
4. Bistrian BR, Blackburn GL, Hallowell E. JAMA 1974;230:858.
5. Crim MC, Munro HN. The proteins and amino acids. In: Shils ME, Olson JA, Shike M, eds. Modern nutrition in health and disease. 8th ed. Philadelphia: Lea & Febiger, 1994;3–35.
6. Garrow JS. Obesity and related diseases. Edinburgh: Churchill Livingstone, 1988.
7. Heymsfield SB, Smith J. Am J Clin Nutr 1982;35:1192–9.
8. Stryer L. Biochemistry. 4th ed. New York: WH Freeman, 1995; 582.
9. Heymsfield SB, Baumgartner RN, Ross R. Evaluation of total and regional body composition. In: Bray GA, Bouchard C, James WPT, eds. Handbook of obesity. In press.
10. International Commission on Radiologic Protection. Report of the Task Group on Reference Man: adopted by the commission in October. New York: Pergamon, 1974.
11. Heymsfield SB, Stevens V, Noel R. Am J Clin Nutr 1982; 36:131–42.
12. Webster JD, Hesp R, Garrow JS. Hum Nutr Clin Nutr 1984;38: 299–306.
13. Forbes GB. Nutr Rev 1987;45:225–31.
14. Heymsfield SB, Casper K, Funfar J. Am J Cardiol 1987;60: 75G–81G.
15. Hill GJ. JPEN J Parenter Enteral Nutr 1992;16:197–218.
16. Klidjian AM, Foster KJ, Kammerling RM. Br Med J 1980;281: 899–901.
17. Richer P. Nouv Inconogr Salpetriere 1890;3:20–6.
18. Matiegka J. Am J Phys Anthropol 1921;3:223–30.
19. Lohman TG, Roche AF, Martorell R, eds. Anthropometric standardization reference manual. Champaign, IL: Human Kinetics Books, 1988.
20. Himes JH. Anthropometric assessment of nutritional status. New York: Wiley-Liss, 1991.
21. Norton K, Olds T, eds. Anthropometrica: a textbook of body measurement for sports and health courses. 1st ed. Sydney, Australia: UNSW Press, 1996.
22. Heymsfield SB, Wang Z, Baumgartner RN, et al. Human body composition: advances in models and methods. Annu Rev Nutr 1997;17:527–58.
23. Ellis KJ, Shypailo R, Schoknecht P, et al. J Radioanal Nucl Chem 1995;195:139–44.
24. Ellis KJ. Biol Trace Elem Res 1990;26–27:385–400.
25. Dilmanian FA, Weber DA, Yasumura S, et al. Performance of the neutron activation systems at Brookhaven National Laboratory. In: Yasumura S, McNeill KG, Woodhead AD, Dilmanian FA, eds. Advances in in vivo composition studies. New York: Plenum Press, 1990.
26. Ellis KJ. Whole-body counting and neutron activation analysis. In: Roche AF, Heymsfield SB, Lohman TG, eds. Human body composition. Champaign, IL: Human Kinetics, 1996; 45–62.
27. Jue T, Rothman DL, Shulman GI, et al. Proc Natl Acad Sci USA 1989;86:4489–91.
28. Cunningham JJ. Am J Clin Nutr 1991;54:963–9.
29. Heymsfield SB, Waki M. Nutr Rev 1991;49:97–108.
30. Merrill AL, Watt BK, eds. Energy value of foods. Washington, DC: United States Government Printing Office, 1973.
31. Heymsfield SB, Casper K. JPEN J Parenter Enteral Nutr 1987;11:36S–41S.
32. Ravussin E, Bogardus C. Am J Clin Nutr 1989;49:968–75.
33. Ellis KJ, Yasumura S, Vartsky D, et al. J Lab Clin Med 1982;99:917.
34. Moore FD, Olesen KH, McMurray JD, et al., eds. The body cell mass and its supporting environment. Philadelphia: WB Saunders, 1963.
35. Kissebah AH, Freedman DS, Peiris AN. Med Clin North Am 1989;73:111–38.
36. van der Kooy K, Seidell JC. Int J Obes Relat Metab Disord 1993;17:187–96.
37. Heymsfield SB, McManus CB III, Seitz SB, et al. Anthropometric assessment of adult protein-energy malnutrition. In: Wright RA, Heymsfield SB, eds. Nutritional assessment. Boston: Blackwell Scientific Publications, 1984;27–82.
38. Heymsfield SB, McManus CB. Cancer 1985;55:238–43.
39. Sjostrom L. Int J Obes Relat Metab Disord 1991;15:19–30.
40. Martin AD, Spenst LF, Drinkwater DT, et al. Med Sci Sports Exerc 1990;22:729–33.
41. Studley HO. JAMA 1936;106:458–60.
42. Nixon DW, Heymsfield SB, Cohen AB, et al. Am J Med 1980;68: 683–90.
43. Vandenbergh E, Van de Woestijne KP, Gyselen A. Am Rev Respir Dis 1967;195:556–66.
44. Seltzer MH, Slocum BA, Cataldi-Betcher ML. JPEN J Parenter Enteral Nutr 1982;6:218.
45. Hirsch S. de Obaldia N, Petermann M, et al. J Am Coll Nutr 1992;11:21–4.
46. Windsor JA, Hill G. Ann Surg 1988;207:290–6.
47. Chumlea WC, Guo S, Steinbaugh ML. J Am Diet Assoc 1994;94:1385–8, 1391.
48. Han TS, Lean ME. Int J Obes Relat Metab Disord 1996;20: 21–7.
49. Chumlea WC, Guo SS. J Gerontol 1992;47:M197–203.
50. Cheng JC, Leung SS, Lau J. Clin Orthop 1996;323:22–30.
51. Schreiner PJ, Terry JG, Evans GW, et al. Am J Epidemiol 1996;144:335–45.
52. Hodgdon JA, Beckett MB. Prediction of percent body fat for U.S. Navy men from body circumferences and height. Report no. 84-11. San Diego, CA: Naval Health Research Center, 1984.
53. Hodgdon JA, Beckett MB. Prediction of percent body fat for U.S. Navy women from body circumferences and height. Report no. 84-92. San Diego, CA: Naval Health Research Center, 1984.
54. Durnin JV, Womersley J. Br J Nutr 1974;32(1):77–9.
55. Damon A, Goldman RF. Hum Biol 1964;36:32–44.
56. Van Itallie TB, Yang MU, Heymsfield SB, et al. Am J Clin Nutr 1990;52:953–9.
57. Keys A, Brozek J, Henschel A, et al., eds. The biology of human starvation, vols I and II. Minneapolis: University of Minnesota Press, 1950.
58. Knapik JJ, Staab JS, Harman EA. Med Sci Sports Exerc 1996;28(12):1523–30.
59. Forbes GB, Brown MR, Griffiths HJL. Am J Clin Nutr 1988;47:929–31.
60. Baumgartner RN, Rhyne RL, Garry PJ, et al. J Nutr 1993;123(2 Suppl):444–8.
61. Rolland-Cachera M-F, Brambilla P, Manzoni P, et al. Am J Clin Nutr 1997;65:1709–13.
62. Cole TJ. Weight-stature indices to measure underweight, overweight, and obesity. In: Himes JH, ed. Anthropometric assessment of nutritional status. New York: Wiley-Liss, 1991.
63. Garn SM, Leonard WR, Hawthorne VM. Am J Clin Nutr 1986;44:996–7.
64. James WPT, Ferro-Luzzi A, Waterlow JC. Eur J Clin Nutr 1988;42:969–81.

65. Luke A, Durazo-Arvizu R, Rotimi C, et al. Am J Epidemiol 1997;145:620–8.
66. Smalley KJ, Knerr AK, Kendrick ZV, et al. Am J Clin Nutr 1990;52:405.
67. Gallagher D, Visser M, Sepúlveda D, et al. Am J Epidemiol 1996;143:228–39.
68. McLaren DS. A fresh look at anthropometric classification schemes in protein-energy malnutrition. In: Himes JH, ed. Anthropometric assessment of nutritional status. New York: Wiley-Liss, 1991.
69. United States Department of Agriculture, United States Department of Health and Human Services. Dietary guidelines for Americans. 1995.
70. Galen RS, Gambino SR. Beyond normality: the predictive value and efficiency of medical diagnoses. New York: John Wiley & Sons, 1975.
71. Jeejeebhoy KN, Detsky AS, Baker JP. JPEN J Parenter Enteral Nutr 1990;14:193S–6S.
72. Forbes G. Human body composition: growth, aging, nutrition and activity. New York: Springer-Verlag, 1987.
73. Baumgartner RN. Prog Food Nutr Sci 1993;17:223–60.
74. Baumgartner RN, Stauber PM, McHugh D, et al. J Gerontol A Biol Med Sci 1995;50(6):M307–16.
75. Visser M, van den Heuvel E, Deurenberg P. Br J Nutr 1994;71:823–33.
76. Reilly JJ, Murray LA, Wilson J, et al. Ann Hum Biol 1994;21: 613–6.
77. Chumlea WC, Guo SS, Vellas B, et al. J Gerontol A Biol Sci Med Sci 1995;50A(Spec. no.):45–51.
78. Roubenoff R, Wilson PW. Am J Clin Nutr 1993;57:609–13.
79. Lansey S, Waslien C, Mulvihill M, et al. Gerontology 1993; 39:346–53.
80. Campbell AJ, Spears GFS, Brown JS, et al. Age Ageing 1990;19: 131–5.
81. Guigoz Y, Vellas B, Garry PJ. Nutr Rev 1996;54(1 pt 2):S59–65.
82. WHO Expert Committee. Physical status: the use and interpretation of anthropometry. WHO tech. rep. series 854. Geneva: World Health Organization, 1995.
83. Last SM. A dictionary of epidemiology. New York: Oxford University Press, 1983.

SELECTED READING

Heymsfield SB, Wang Z, Baumgartner RN, et al. Human body composition: advances in models and methods. Annu Rev Nutr 1997;17:527–58.

Hines JH, ed. Anthropometric assessment of nutritional status. New York: Wiley-Liss, 1991.

Roche AF. Growth, maturation, and body composition. The Fels longitudinal study 1929–1991. New York: Cambridge University Press, 1992.

Roche AF, Heymsfield SB, Lohman TG, eds. Human body composition. Champaign, IL: Human Kinetics, 1996.

57. Laboratory Tests for Assessing Nutritional Status

NANCY W. ALCOCK

LABORATORY TESTS

Measurement of relevant individual analytes in body tissues, fluids, or excretions—feces, urine, sweat or expired air—provides specific, sensitive, and quantitative indices of a subject's nutritional status. Such measurements are often of value in supporting, modifying, or negating nutritional history and physical examination. Impaired absorption of dietary nutrients from the gut or renal tubule is a major cause of malnutrition and may be due to any one of a number of factors that have been reviewed in chapters related to specific nutrients and to clinical considerations, including Chapters 39 and 68–71. To the complexity of causes of malnutrition is added the number of nutrients that may be involved singly or in combination, endpoints that result from byproducts of intestinal tract activity and/or digestive and absorptive defects, and finally the varied methodologic and technical issues of analyses.

Caregivers must have sufficient knowledge of the value, availability, reliability, and interpretation of results of tests to use the laboratory to advantage. Chapter 65 discusses the clinical approach and use of various test procedures to detect and determine the cause of malabsorption. Types of tests for diagnosing the presence, severity, and possible site(s) of suspected malabsorption are listed in Table 57.1.

This chapter endeavors to provide the basis for laboratory involvement in investigating nutritional status. Standards that must be met for reliable results are discussed, tests useful in diagnosis and their methodology are reviewed, and a brief discussion is appended of instrumentation useful in physical methods of assessment.

Specimen Collection and Handling

A most important, often neglected, factor in obtaining accurate results for analysis of any nutrient or its product, is the appropriateness of the procedure used in collection and subsequent handling of the specimen. This requires organization and planning at the clinical, transport, storage, and laboratory phases of the investigation. This topic has been reviewed (1). Requirements may include *(a)* protection of the specimen from exposure to light, *(b)* temperature stability of components to be measured, and *(c)* possible contamination from vessels used for collection or storage of samples to be tested for trace metals and other components.

Detection Limit, Sensitivity, and Specificity of Tests

Evaluation of a biochemical or biophysical method and hence selection of the most appropriate method for a particular application requires the following considerations.

Detection Limit

The detection limit of a particular test is the smallest concentration or absolute quantity of the analyte that can be detected with reasonable certainty. The amplitude of the blank readings and the precision or reproducibility of the method on repeated performance are important considerations in establishing the detection limit (2).

Sensitivity

The sensitivity of a method is defined as a change in signal relative to a change in concentration, absolute quantity, or property of the analyte (2). A method with high sensitivity has a low limit of detection; for example, the limit of detection of copper in urine is 1.0 μg/L. This low level of detection makes the test highly sensitive.

Specificity

The specificity of a method defines the accuracy with which the method measures the true value of an analyte,

Table 57.1
Types of Tests for Determining Presence, Severity, and Possible Site(s) of Suspected Malabsorption[a]

Tests for possible malabsorbed macronutrients: fat, carbohydrates, proteins (nitrogen)
Direct measurement of the macronutrient in feces, urine, blood
Direct measurement of surrogate compounds (e.g., xylose)
Indirect measurements (e.g., breath tests)
Load test of suspect malabsorbed substance (e.g., lactose tolerance test)
Test for possible malabsorbed micronutrients
Direct measurements in feces, urine, blood
Indirect measurements of relevant enzymes and abnormal metabolites

[a]One of the issues in making a diagnosis is deciding which specific nutrient parameters to test in the early workup to provide relevant information about the extent and severity of suspected or known malabsorption and the nutritional status of the patient.

especially in the presence of other analytes with similar chemical properties or substances that may interfere with the particular analytical method (3).

Matrix to Be Analyzed

In assessing nutritional status, measurement of an analyte or a metabolite of a substrate is usually made in blood—whole blood, serum, plasma, or erythrocytes, depending upon its normal distribution—or in urine, but other sources are often valuable. Leukocyte fractions isolated from whole blood and platelets isolated from plasma have been analyzed for various nutrients to assess status. Fecal analysis is extremely important in assessing the balance of a nonmetabolizable nutrient or a component, for example, nitrogen, trace metals that are excreted in bile, and components of pancreatic secretions in protein-losing enteropathy, and α-antitrypsin clearance. Analysis of expired air for a radioactively labeled metabolite—usually CO_2 or H_2 generated by bacterial action in the gut—or a stable isotope ratio (e.g., $^{13}CO_2$:$^{14}CO_2$) enables the absorption of carbohydrates or fat to be determined. Labeled expired air is also analyzed for O_2 or CO_2 by indirect or direct calorimetry and more recently by isotope dilution methods using $^2H_2{}^{18}O$ to determine resting energy expenditure (see Chapter 5).

While depletion of a nutrient is often detected by its low concentrations, depletion may be indicated by increased concentration of a related metabolite occurring because of altered intermediary metabolism; for example, high homocysteine levels in the absence of the folate or vitamin B_{12} coenzyme required for its conversion to methionine.

An alternative to measuring the concentration of a specific mineral, trace element, or vitamin in blood or urine uses a test that indicates the function of a related component in the body; for example, enzymatic activities in erythrocytes for which thiamin pyrophosphate, pyridoxal-5-phosphate, or flavin adenine dinucleotide (FAD) are the coenzymes of the vitamins thiamin, pyridoxine, and riboflavin, respectively (4). If addition of the cofactor raises the respective in vitro enzyme activity more than 20% above its initial value, a deficiency of the vitamin in vivo is indicated.

IMPORTANT ANALYTICAL TECHNIQUES: PRINCIPLES AND PROCEDURES

Some analytical techniques frequently used are illustrated in Figures 57.1 to 57.4 and discussed in detail elsewhere (5).

Assays

Immunoassays

A competitive simultaneous radioimmunoassay uses a radiolabeled (usually with ^{125}I) form of the nutrient being analyzed (termed the *antigen*) that competes for binding to antibody when the level of unlabeled antigen in the sample is in the range of 30 to 80% of labeled antigen. The amount of bound labeled antigen is inversely proportional to the amount of unlabeled analyte. In the competitive sequential assay, bound labeled antigen is separated, and the radioactivity counted is directly proportional to the amount of bound unlabeled antigen. In noncompetitive assays, a solid phase such as plastic beads, the surface of a tube or well, or magnetic beads permits adherence of antibody-bound antigen and labeled complex. Radioactivity counts are directly proportional to the amount of unlabeled antigen. The various assays are illustrated in Figure 57.1.

Immunosorbent Assay

An enzyme-linked immunoabsorbent assay uses a solid phase on which analyte to be measured (antigen) is immobilized. Enzyme-labeled antibody and sample are added. Only those antibody-enzyme binding sites not occupied by the sample analyte will bind to the immobilized antigen. The solid-phase antigen:antibody-enzyme complex is washed with buffer prior to the addition of substrate for enzymatic reaction. The concentration of the reaction product is directly proportional to the amount of analyte in the specimen (Fig. 57.2). Alkaline phosphatase is the enzyme frequently used. An example of this assay is described below in the immunoassay for vitamin B_{12}.

High-Performance Liquid Chromatography

Figure 57.3 shows the components of a high-performance liquid chromatography (HPLC) system for chromatographic separation and quantitation of components of a solution. The procedure is highly specific and sensitive for components with similar properties, such as fat-soluble vitamins, retinol, α-tocopherol, and β-carotene, which are suitably extracted in an organic solvent before chromatography.

Atomic Absorption Spectrophotometry

Atomic absorption spectrophotometry is the most specific and sensitive technique for measuring minerals and

A. Competitive Simultaneous Radioimmunoassay

Ab + Ag + Ag* ⇄ Ab:Ag + Ab:Ag*
(free) (bound)

B. Competitive Sequential Radioimmunoassay

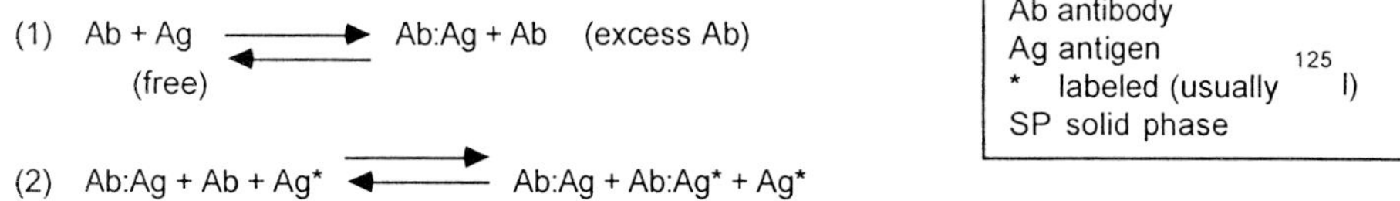

C. NonCompetitive Radioimmunoassay

SP + Ab → SP-Ab —Ag sample→ SP-Ab:Ag —Ab*→ SP-Ab:Ag:Ab*

Figure 57.1. Diagrammatic representation of reactions in radioimmunoassay (RIA) techniques. *A*, Competitive simultaneous assay; *B*, competitive sequential (two-step) assay; *C*, noncompetitive assay.

trace elements. The components of a typical instrument for flame atomic absorption spectrophotometry or the more sensitive graphite furnace atomic absorption spectrophotometry are shown in Figure 57.4. High specificity is obtained by the measurement of absorption by neutral atoms in the vapor state from a lamp that emits light of a wavelength characteristic of the element being measured.

TESTS FOR ASSESSING MALABSORPTION AND MALNUTRITION

Carbohydrate Absorption

D-Xylose Tests

D-Xylose Oral Test. Carbohydrate absorption may be assessed by the D-xylose absorption test. D-xylose, a nondietary pentose, is more poorly absorbed than glucose; it is not rapidly metabolized after absorption and hence appears in the urine. An oral dose of 25 g of D-xylose (Pfanstiehl Labs, Inc., Waukegan, IL) in 250 to 500 mL water is administered over 10 minutes to a fasting subject. Preferably, D-xylose is then measured both in blood (at hourly intervals up to 5 h), and in the 5-h urine (with its creatinine level measured to ensure complete collection). For pediatric patients a smaller dose, 2 g, and a single 1-h blood analysis is reported to give a reliable index of absorption.

The recommended analytical method for D-xylose is that of Roe and Rice (6), as described in detail (7). After a 25-g dose, blood or plasma D-xylose should rise to 30 to 35 mg/dL or above within 2 hours, and then decrease gradually; at least 25% of the dose should be excreted in the 5-h urine specimen. Variation in the dose and appropriate results are given in reference 7. The test also serves

Enzyme-linked immunosorbent assay

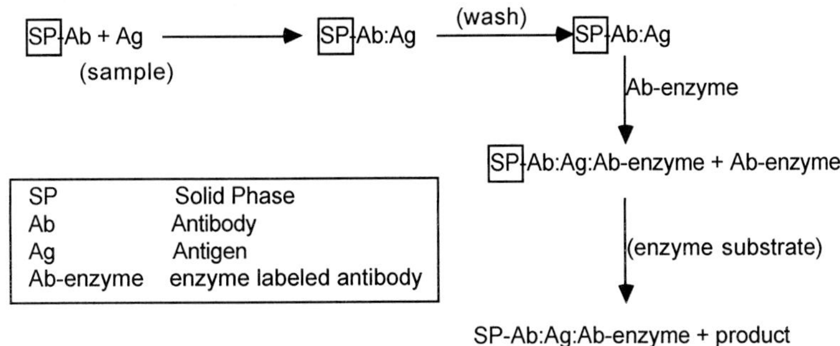

Product is measured and this value is directly proportional to the amount of Ag in the sample

Figure 57.2. Schematic diagram of steps involved in enzyme immunoassay techniques. *Ab*, antibody; *Ag*, antigen; *SP*, solid phase. The product measured is directly proportional to the amount of Ag in the specimen.

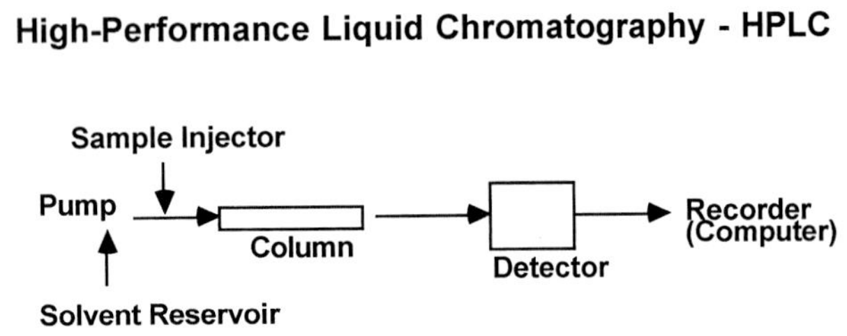

High-Performance Liquid Chromatography - HPLC

Sample Injector
Pump
Column
Detector
Recorder (Computer)
Solvent Reservoir

Figure 57.3. Components of a system for sequential flow of solvent sample for HPLC separation of components in solution. Detector may be UV-VIS, fluorometric, or electrochemical.

to measure intestinal mucosal and renal function. Interpretation of results must consider the renal clearance of D-xylose because of its dependence on glomerular filtration. Hence, measurement of urine or serum creatinine or of blood urea nitrogen is essential. Figure 57.5 presents the results of serial D-xylose absorption tests conducted over 15 months following major bowel resection in a patient and demonstrates progressive improvement in gastrointestinal function (8). Misleading results may occur when bacterial overgrowth of the jejunum is present. In this situation, a repeat of the oral test after a trial of antibiotics provides more accurate data on D-xylose absorption and confirms the effect of the bacteria.

^{14}C-Breath D-Xylose Test. Gases produced by colonic bacteria from unabsorbed carbohydrate or those resulting from bacterial overgrowth in the small intestine are absorbed into the circulation and excreted by the lungs. ^{14}C-D-Xylose showed 85 to 100% specificity of increased exhaled $^{14}CO_2$ within 60 minutes of ingestion of 1 g of unlabeled D-xylose and 10 mCi of ^{14}C-D-xylose (9) by subjects with bacterial overgrowth. Normally, most of the D-xylose is absorbed in the jejunum; the little that reaches the colon is subject to significant bacterial action as was shown when an oral dose of 25 g was given (Fig. 57.6). Delayed gastric emptying can complicate the interpretation of results from this test. Exhaled CO_2 collected in a vial containing 1 to 2 mmol/L hyamine hydroxide and phenolphthalein indicator is converted to carbonic acid and counted in a scintillation counter.

Atomic Absorption Spectrophotometry

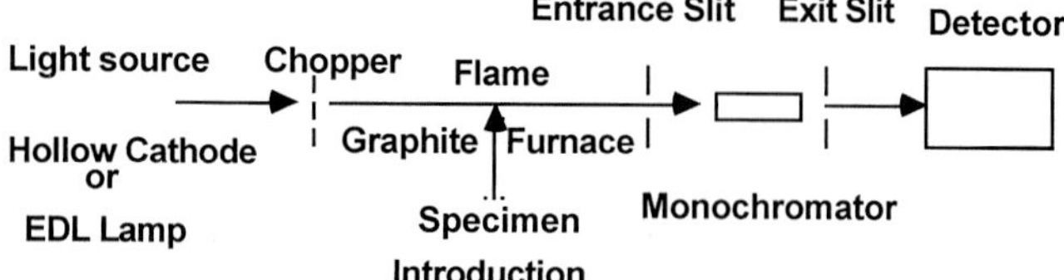

Figure 57.4. Components of an atomic absorption spectrophotometer for flame or graphite furnace analysis of minerals or trace metals. See text for comments on specificity and sensitivity.

Lactose Absorption

Oral Load Test with Glucose Determination. Lactose is hydrolyzed by the mucosal enzyme lactase to its component sugars, glucose and galactose. Plasma glucose levels are measured before administration of a 50-g oral dose of lactose, and 1 and 2 hours afterward. An increase of more than 20 mg/dL is considered a normal response, indicating absence of lactase deficiency. Delayed gastric emptying

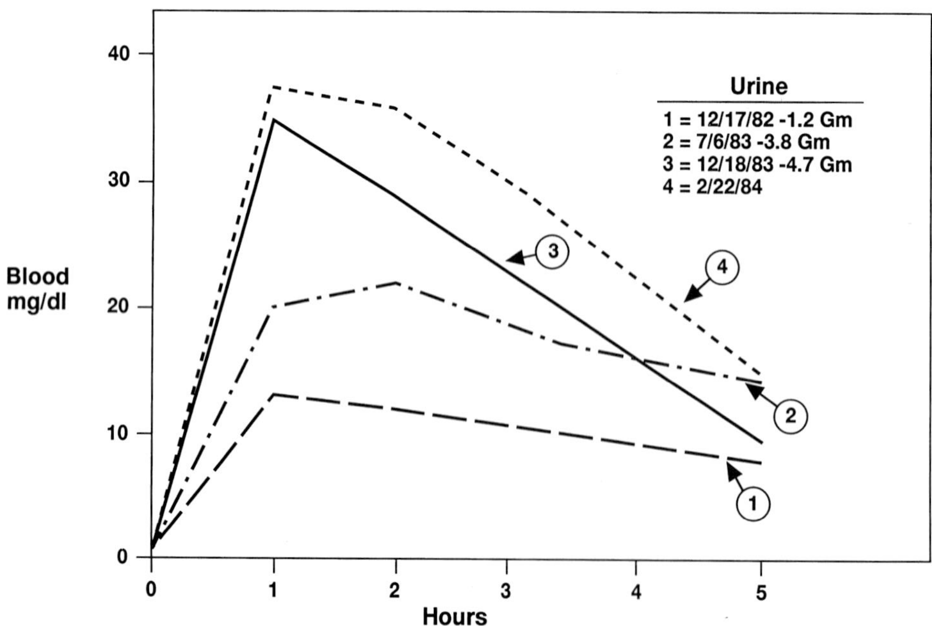

Figure 57.5. Changes in D-xylose levels with time following major bowel resection in a 30-year-old malnourished female patient. When first tested, she failed to achieve normal blood and urine levels from a standard 25-g D-xylose load. She was initially treated with parenteral nutrition and subsequently with tube feeding, followed by partial tube feeding with oral supplements. The data indicate progressive improvement into the normal range, presumably because of hyperplasia of the remaining jejunum in response to improved nutrition. (Shils ME, unpublished data).

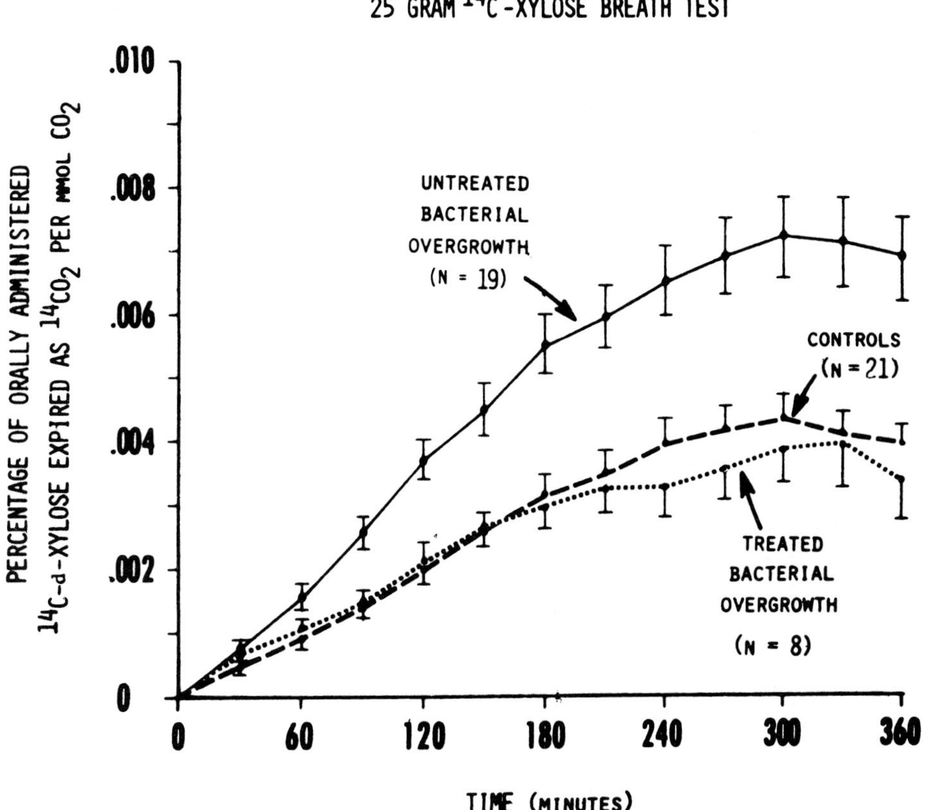

Figure 57.6. Concentration of $^{14}CO_2$ (percentage of administered dose expired as $^{14}CO_2$ per mmol CO_2) after oral administration of 25 g xylose and 10 μCi ^{14}C-xylose. Untreated patients with intestinal bacterial overgrowth exhaled significantly more $^{14}CO_2$ than controls ($P < .005$, 60–360 min) and treated patients ($P < 0.01$ after 60 min). (From King CE, Toskes PP, Spivey JC, et al. Gastroenterology 1979;77:75–82, with permission.)

may result in a negative response. Lactase deficiency may be confirmed by measuring glucose absorption from a glucose load.

Breath Hydrogen. General carbohydrate malabsorption may be assessed by measuring breath hydrogen 3 to 4 hours after a meal. Malabsorption of a specific carbohydrate is determined by a more rigidly controlled collection of hydrogen at hourly intervals up to 8 hours in a fasted subject who has been given a dose (usually <50 g) of the specific carbohydrate. Details of the procedure for performing the test and interpretation of results are given in reference 10. ^{2}H and methane (which is sometimes produced but does not interfere with the results) are determined by gas chromatography with a dedicated instrument (Fig. 57.7). The breath test is useful in discriminating between pancreatic insufficiency, small bowel disease, and diseases unlikely to affect carbohydrate absorption. Bacterial overgrowth in elderly hypochlorhydric subjects does not affect carbohydrate or fat absorption (11), but breath tests are not reliable in this condition.

Fat Absorption

Classical Fat Test. Fat absorption may be determined either by weighing the isolated lipids or by titrating free fatty acids after hydrolysis of dietary and fecal specimens and lipid extraction into organic solvent (12). A 72-hour equilibration period on the diet and fecal collection for 72 hours are required. Although hospitalization is preferable, current costs prohibit this. A well-motivated patient, given precise instructions and collection devices can complete

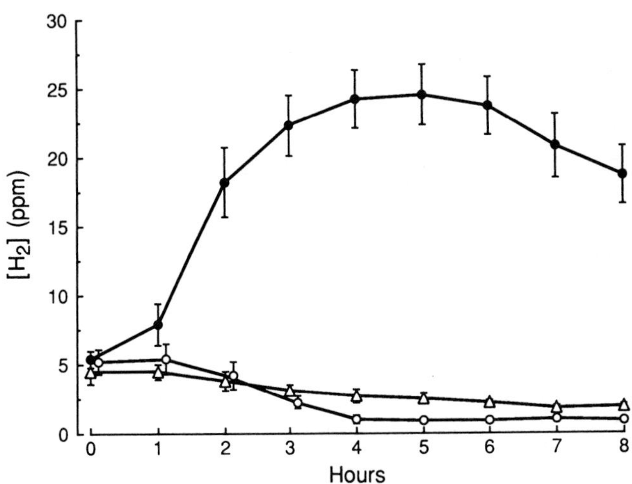

Figure 57.7. Breath H_2 response (mean ± SEM) to ingestion of 10 g of lactulose *(solid circle)*, 10 g of glucose *(open triangles)*, or Colyte *(open circle)*. (From Strocchi A, Corazza G, Ellis CJ, et al. Gastroenterology 1993;105:1404–10, with permission.)

the collections. Less than 7% of the fat in the diet should normally be excreted in the fecal specimen.

$^{14}CO_2$ Breath Test. A tracer dose of radioactive ^{14}C uniformly labeled triglyceride given with 20 to 30 g of nonlabeled triglyceride provides a test meal for the semiquantitative assessment of the metabolism of fat to CO_2 and H_2O. ^{14}C is collected and counted as described above. Experience with this test showed variability in results, compared with fecal fat analysis. However, it is a semiquantitative convenient method of assessing fat absorption (13). Alternatively, a stable isotope, ^{13}C-triglyceride, may be given, but a mass spectrometer is required to quantitate the stable isotope.

ASSESSMENT OF NITROGEN BALANCE

The ultimate assessment of nutritional status is a reliable determination of the balance (positive, negative, or zero) between dietary intake and total loss from the body of a particular nutrient that is unchanged in metabolism (e.g., a mineral) or a basic element that is a marker for a nutrient (e.g., nitrogen). The metabolic basis for an inclusive scheme for balance studies owes much to Reifenstein Albright and Wells (14). The diet and all excreta must be chemically analyzed. The patient's intake must be equilibrated on a standardized diet for varying times prior to complete collection of fecal, urinary, and any other losses from the body for 72 hours or longer. Appropriate losses in sweat, hair, and nails must be assumed for particular nutrients. The costly requirement for hospitalization in a metabolic or similarly equipped unit restricts such studies to research centers with a federally funded Clinical Research Center (CRC) or equivalent. However, with careful planning and provision of prepared meals, a well-motivated, supervised patient can make the necessary collections at home (15).

Intake of a particular nutrient by a patient maintained entirely on an enteral formula or on total parenteral nutrition can be accurately calculated from the amount of administered nutritional support. When nutrients are administered intravenously and nothing but water is being ingested, stool loss for most components of interest can be considered to be zero if stool output is insignificant.

Nitrogen Balance

Net change in total body protein may be assessed by estimating nitrogen balance. Approximately 16% of protein is nitrogen, and almost all total body nitrogen is in protein. In a stable, healthy adult, dietary intake equals nitrogen excreted in urine and feces together with losses due to hair and nail growth, sweat, and sloughing of cutaneous cells. The individual in this state is said to be in zero nitrogen balance, or equilibrium. Ideally, following a period of days for equilibration on the diet, the actual nitrogen balance is determined from analysis of complete dietary intake over 3 or more days and the collection and analysis of nitrogen in complete fecal (between markers) and urinary output over the period.

Serum levels of some specific proteins useful in monitoring changes in nutritional status are shown in Table 57.2. Since factors other than nutrition (e.g., infection, hepatic and renal functions, surgery, and thyroid status) influence these, the patient's clinical status must be evaluated carefully when interpreting results (17).

Methods of Analysis. Methods for estimation of total nitrogen include the classical Kjeldahl procedure or chemoluminescence for the measurement of nitrogen in urine or digests of fecal and dietary samples. A much simplified estimate of nitrogen balance can be obtained from assessment of nitrogen in the diet from published food composition tables for protein, estimation of urinary nitrogen from urea and ammonia excretion, and an assumed daily fecal nitrogen output (16). The nitrogen content of protein is assumed to be 16%, although for special formulae, this factor may be in error. Heymsfield et al. (17) consider that total daily urine nitrogen can be approximated as urea nitrogen plus 1.5 to 2.0 g for most hospitalized patients. Allowance for fecal loss varies, depending upon the composition of the oral intake or

Table 57.2
Nutritional Assessment: Serum Proteins, Reference Ranges, and Half-Lives

Metabolite(s)	Method	Reference Range				Half-Life[a]
		Age	Sex	Conv. unit	SI units	
Albumin	Dye binding					18–20 days
		21–44	male	33–61 g/L	500–920 μmol/L	
		20–44	female	28–57 g/L	440–920 μmol/L	
		45–54	male	29–61 g/L	420–860 μmol/L	
		45–54	female	25–54 g/L	380–820 μmol/L	
		55–93	male	32–55 g/L	490–830 μmol/L	
		55–81	female	32–53 g/L	490–800 μmol/L	
Transferrin	Rate nephelometry			2.6–4.3 g/L	28.6–47.3 μmol/L	8–9 days
Prealbumin	Rate nephelometry			0.2–0.4 g/L	3.64–7.27 μmol/L	2–3 days
Retinol-binding protein (RBP)	Rate nephelometry			30–60 mg/L	1.43–2.86 μmol/L	12 hours
Insulin-like growth factor–1				0.55–1.4 IU/mL		2–6 hours
Fibronectin[b]	Turbidometri			1.66–1.98 g/L	3.77–4.50 μmol/L	4–24 hours

[a]Based in part on data from reference (17).
[b]A glycoprotein found in many tissues. A soluble form in blood has opsonic properties. Considered a marker to monitor changes in nutritional status during depletion or repletion.

intravenous fluids, whether the patient has malabsorption, and other factors related to protein metabolism associated with the patient's condition (17).

TESTS FOR ASSESSING SOME INDIVIDUAL NUTRIENTS

Folic Acid

The most common causes of depletion of this vitamin are listed in Chapters 26 and 88. Experimental folate deficiency in man showed that the earliest biochemical change was a reduction in serum folate to less than 3 ng/mL, which was evident by day 22 of the deficiency (18). Red cell folate, which is a better indicator of tissue status, was reduced to less than 20 ng/mL by day 123. Impairment of histidine conversion to glutamate, which involves folate-dependent pathways, was evident at day 49; this may be detected by an increase in 8-h urinary excretion of formiminoglutamate (FIGLU) following an oral dose of 15 g of histidine. Normal excretion is approximately 17 mg FIGLU. In folate deficiency, levels of 185 to 2047 mg are common. The test is not specific for folate deficiency, as a percentage of vitamin B_{12}–deficient patients also have elevated FIGLU excretion.

Methods of Analysis. Serum or plasma folate is determined by competitive binding assay (Fig. 57.1). Various instrument manufacturers provide kits that usually permit simultaneous assay for folate and vitamin B_{12}. However, as pointed out by McNeely (19), kits must be carefully evaluated, as they frequently focus on the vitamin B_{12} assay at the expense of the folate requirements. These assays employ a specific folate-binding protein from milk. If a boiling step necessary to eliminate serum folate binding is not included, the accuracy and specificity of the procedure must be validated. Kits usually contain tritiated pteroylglutamate as a tracer, since tritiated methyltetrahydrofolate has very low specific activity and is unstable. Using liquid scintillation to count beta particles is inconvenient; kits with ^{125}I are becoming available for evaluation and offer more convenient counting capability. The simple procedures required for manual performance of the competitive binding assay are described in reference 19. Red cell folate determinations can be done on a hemolysate.

Table 57.3
Diagnosis of Vitamin B_{12} Deficiency with the Schilling Test

Cause of Deficiency	Free B_{12}	B_{12}-IF	Antibiotic	Pancreatic
Normal	Normal	—	—	—
Pernicious anemia (lack of intrinsic factor, IF)	Abnormal	Corrected	—	—
Bacterial overgrowth syndrome	Abnormal	Abnormal	Corrected	—
Pancreatic insufficiency	Abnormal	Abnormal	Abnormal	Corrected
Ileal disease or resection	Abnormal	Abnormal	Abnormal	Abnormal

Reproduced from Table 65.2, Chapter 65, with permission. See also reference 20.

Cobalamin (Vitamin B_{12})

Causes of depletion of vitamin B_{12} are given in chapters 37 and 88. The diagnosis of deficiency can be made with certainty by appropriate laboratory techniques, whose results are shown in Table 57.3 (20).

Methods of Analysis

The reference method for estimation of serum vitamin B_{12} is the microbiologic assay. This method requires specialized treatment of the sample and laboratory facilities and is no longer feasible for the large volume of requests in chemistry laboratories. A second problem is the possible presence in the serum sample of antibiotics to which the microorganisms may be sensitive.

Immunoassays. For routine purposes, microbiologic assay has been replaced by techniques that can be performed on various autoanalyzers. These use competitive binding proteins and either count a radioactive label or take a spectrophotometric reading of an immunochemistry product. Folic acid and vitamin B_{12} assays are frequently required on the same serum sample, and kits are available to perform the two assays simultaneously. ^{57}Co-labeled vitamin B_{12} and ^{125}I-labeled folate are used as tracers. The two radionuclides are counted simultaneously in pulse-height multichannel gamma scintillation counters without interference from the differences in energy.

For vitamin B_{12} determination, purified intrinsic factor, free from a rapidly migrating R protein, must be used to measure the true biologically active vitamin B_{12}. If intrinsic factor is contaminated with R protein, cobinimide, an analogue of vitamin B_{12}, must be present to block binding of endogenous B_{12} to the R protein. Most kits use purified porcine intrinsic factor and a folate-specific binder from milk, and require off-line denaturation of the endogenous serum binding proteins in a boiling-water bath with subsequent cooling. An alternative method using alkali denaturation (21) requires incubation and neutralization of the extract prior to the competitive binding reaction, and therefore is not considered to have an advantage over boiling.

An alternative competitive magnetic-separation immunoassay for vitamin B_{12} can be performed entirely automatically on the Technicon Immuno 1 system. Serum must be used in this assay. Vitamin B_{12} is released from serum binders and reacted with intrinsic factor. Alkaline phosphatase–labeled vitamin B_{12} is added, which competes with vitamin B_{12} in the serum for binding sites on the intrinsic factor. Addition of monoclonal immunomagnetic particles allows separation of bound and unbound enzyme-labeled B_{12}. Detection is by spectrophotometric measurement at 405 nm of the product *p*-nitrophenoxide from the substrate *p*-nitrophenyl phosphate.

Deoxyuridine Suppression Test. The deoxyuridine suppression test in a suspension of bone marrow cells was found highly sensitive for detection of early, subtle, or occult deficiency of vitamin B_{12} or folate (22).

Homocysteine. The association of high plasma homocysteine levels with neurologic and cardio- and cerebrovascular disease and the inverse relationship between plasma homocysteine and plasma folate and, to a lesser extent, vitamins B_6 and B_{12}, emphasizes the possible role of administration of the appropriate vitamins for amelioration or prevention of such diseases (23). The biochemical and clinical aspects of hyperhomocysteinemia are discussed in Chapters 26, 27, 34, 61, 75, and 95.

Methylmalonic Acid Excretion. Isomerization of methylmalonyl-COA to succinyl-COA is vitamin B_{12} dependent. Increased urinary excretion of methylmalonic acid results from vitamin B_{12} deficiency. The assay method of choice is isotope dilution involving gas chromatography–mass spectrometry (24, 25).

Schilling Test. The Schilling test is used to investigate absorption of vitamin B_{12} from the ileum as affected by various conditions in the alimentary tract. There are a number of variations in the time schedule for carrying out the procedure (26). An oral dose of ^{57}Co radioactively labeled B_{12} may be administered, followed 1 to 8 hours later (as specified) by a larger flushing dose of unlabeled vitamin. Urine is collected during the following 24 to 72 hours. From 8 to 15% of the radioactivity should be excreted normally if renal function is adequate. Since intrinsic factor is required for absorption, low excretion of radioactivity may be due to lack of secretion of this cofactor. The test should thus be repeated with intrinsic factor given at the same time as the labeled B_{12}. Bacterial overgrowth in the upper intestine results in loss of absorbable vitamin B_{12} and false results are obtained; in this situation, a trial antibiotic therapy helps in making the diagnosis. Hence, this test serves to monitor gastric, pancreatic, jejunal and ileal functions (Table 57.3).

Retinol (Vitamin A)

Fasting blood samples for retinol determination should be protected from exposure to light, centrifuged promptly (preferably at 4°C), and have the serum removed and stored at −20°C or below until analysis is performed. Exposure to UV light during analysis should be avoided.

Vitamin A status is most commonly assessed by its serum level. An elevated level usually indicates an excess of vitamin A. However, increased amounts are present when renal failure increases the level of retinol-binding protein (RBP). Similarly, low serum levels may not be associated with decreased stores of the vitamin when impaired protein synthesis results in low levels of serum RPB. In zinc deficiency, low RPB synthesis or release from the liver is also associated with low serum retinol when liver stores are not depleted.

Methods of Analysis

Chromatography. The recommended method of measuring retinol in a hexane extract of serum is HPLC. A variety of solvent systems, mainly methanol based, using reverse-phase, isocratic chromatography enable the separation of retinol, α-tocopherol, and β-carotene in a single run in less than 20 minutes (27). Following addition of an internal standard and serum deproteinization, the lipid-soluble vitamins are extracted, evaporated, and reconstituted in chloroform-ethanol-BHT (butylated hydroxytoluene) prior to chromatography. This method has a sensitivity of 0.1 mg/L. The between-day coefficient of variation at a level of 0.32 mg/L is 4.4%.

A fluorometric method (28) involves ethanol precipitation of serum proteins and extraction of retinol in hexane. A silicic acid column chromatographic step is required to remove an interfering substance, phytofluene. Retinol is determined in the eluate by measuring fluorescence at 490 nm after excitation at 340 nm.

A relative dose response (RDR) test is useful in estimating vitamin A status (29). A baseline fasting blood sample (A_o) is collected before oral administration of 1.6 to 3.5 μmol (450–1000 μg) vitamin A. A second blood sample (A_t) is taken at 5 hours. Response is expressed as the ratio of the increment in serum retinol over the 5-h period divided by the 5-h value expressed as a percentage.

RDR (%) = [(Serum retinol (5 h) − serum retinol (baseline) × 100]/serum retinol (5 h)

An RDR above 50% indicates severe deficiency; 20 to 50%, marginal deficiency; and less than 20%, adequate status.

Serum Retinol-Binding Protein

RPB binds one molecule of retinol and is the carrier protein for this vitamin. The complex is associated with one molecule of thyroxine-binding prealbumin. It has a half-life of only approximately 12 hours and has been shown to respond rapidly to protein and energy deprivation and to dietary treatment. Serum RPB is decreased in vitamin A deficiency and in zinc deficiency, since zinc is required for mobilization of RPB from the liver. Following vitamin A and or zinc supplementation, the serum level increases (30). A specific RPB antibody is available (Behring, San Jose, CA) for determination of the protein by rate nephelometry (Table 57.2). Radial immunodiffusion is also available, but its sensitivity is not good for the low levels of this protein normally present in serum.

Iron

Iron deficiency is a common problem in many populations, particularly in growing children. The ability to assess body iron stores in epidemiologic evaluations of nutritional status is important and has been reviewed (31). Biochemical measurements can differentiate between iron stores and those associated with depleted iron in the functional pool. Storage iron parameters for iron deficiency include the absence of hemosiderin in bone marrow smears, a total iron-binding capacity below 400 μg/dL and serum ferritin below 12 μg/L. Serum transferrin saturation below 16%, and hemoglobin below 130 g/L in men or 120 g/L in women are functional indicators of iron deficiency. A mean cell volume below 80 fL, and erythrocyte protoporphyrin below 70 μg/dL RBCs indicate low iron stores. In iron deficiency, low serum iron is associated with low serum ferritin and increased total iron-binding capacity of serum transferrin. Serum ferritin and serum iron increase and total iron-binding capacity decreases in iron overload. Normal total iron-binding capacity is associated with elevated serum iron and ferritin in megaloblastic anemia. Serum transfer receptor level is elevated in iron deficiency anemia (normal range 1.3–3.3 mg/L) but not in the anemia of chronic illness (31a).

Methods of Assay

Serum Ferritin. Serum ferritin can be determined by any one of a number of immunoassays. Either ferritin or antibody is labeled with ^{125}I. In immunoradiometric assays the radioactivity of the bound labeled antibody is determined and is directly related to the serum ferritin concentration. Radioimmunoassays use competition between serum ferritin and radiolabeled ferritin for antibody. The antibody-antigen complex is precipitated and counted. Radioactivity is inversely proportional to serum ferritin concentration. Enzyme immunoassays use enzyme activity as an endpoint. Antiferritin-coated solid phase is incubated with serum plus antiferritin conjugated to an enzyme (usually alkaline phosphatase or peroxidase). Serum ferritin binds to the immobilized antibody and in turn is bound by the conjugate. Enzyme reaction with the appropriate substrate yields a color for spectrophotometric endpoint. Details of the procedures and a list of the various types of assay kits and vendors who supply them are given elsewhere (32). Sensitivity varies from 1 to 4 ng/mL for most assays. Reported precision (CV) between runs ranged from 3.5 to 10.8%. The CV between laboratories ranged from 10.9 to 20.5%. Each laboratory must develop a reference range for serum ferritin for each method used.

Serum Iron. Spectrophotometric assays for serum iron involve release of ferric iron from transferrin, its reduction to the ferrous state, and reaction with one of a number of chromagens. Ferrene and ferrozine, which have absorption maxima at 600 and 560 nm, respectively, are most commonly used. Detailed procedures are described elsewhere (33). Kits for some assays are available (35).

An alternative method uses coulometry, based upon the electrochemical potential developed at the interface of the iron-containing serum and an electrode. The electrode is maintained at a constant potential that is determined from the electropositivity of the iron atom. The current required to maintain the electrode at this potential is measured. This current is a function of the electropositivity of iron and its concentration in the serum. Since the electropositivity is known, the concentration can be calculated. The technique requires a specialized instrument (36) such as that available from Environmental Sciences Associates (ESA).

A third method appropriate for research uses atomic absorption spectrophotometry (37). Iron is complexed with basophenanthroline, and the complex is extracted into methylisobutylketone. The concentrated iron can then be measured by flame atomic absorption spectrophotometry. Graphite furnace atomic absorption spectrophotometry can be applied for direct analysis of serum iron (38). It is mandatory that hemolysis of the blood specimen be avoided.

Total Iron-Binding Capacity. In addition to the total serum iron, the total amount of iron that transferrin can bind—total iron-binding capacity (TIBC)—must be determined to assess iron status. TIBC is determined by measuring excess iron in the supernatant from a known amount of iron added to serum to saturate transferrin, which is separated by protein precipitation (34). The same methods used for serum iron determination may be used to measure the unbound iron. The number of available iron-binding sites of transferrin (UIBC) is the difference between the concentration of added iron standard (e.g., 5000 μg/L) and the free iron measured in the supernatant.

$$\text{UIBC} + \text{serum Fe} = \text{TIBC}$$

Zinc

Results of analysis of zinc in serum or erythrocytes do not consistently reflect zinc status. Approximately 65% of serum zinc is bound to albumin, and most of the remainder to α_2-macroglobulin, hence a low serum zinc concentration may be associated with a low serum protein level. In severe zinc deficiency, serum zinc is low, but very low serum zinc levels may be attained in other conditions such as an acute phase response, in which the element is redistributed to other tissues. Erythrocyte zinc concentration is approximately ten times that in plasma, and changes that occur slowly because of the long half-life of the cell are not easily detected. Platelets, lymphocytes, and granulocytes are rich in zinc and are depleted in zinc deficiency of the host (39). Although isolation of these cells and platelets is tedious, it is easily accomplished with a little practice. Performing a zinc loading test and monitoring plasma levels with time is of limited value in assessing zinc status.

Recent application of stable isotopes of zinc (40) has provided promising results; however, the applicability of this technique for clinical use is limited because inductive plasma mass spectrometry is needed for measuring isotope ratios to monitor the disappearance from plasma following administration of an enriched isotope.

Using hair zinc levels to assess zinc status has the advantage of an easily accessible sample. Hair zinc was found to be low in preschool children whose zinc bioavailability was considered low (19a). Age- and sex-matched groups are necessary for comparison (19b). A change in the rate of hair growth was suggested in the interpretation of results of decreased zinc (μg/g hair) in children given zinc supplements (19c). In conditions of malnutrition, hair growth rate may be decreased; hence the zinc content per unit weight increases, introducing a source of error. Hair may be a useful tissue to monitor response to supplementation, provided that errors of bias are ruled out and that care in specimen preparation and analysis avoids environmental contamination, including some hair shampoos and dyes as sources of zinc.

Although many enzymes that require zinc as a cofactor (e.g., alkaline phosphatase, lactic dehydrogenase, erythrocyte carbonic anhydrase) have decreased activity and ribonuclease activity is increased in experimental zinc deficiency in animals, no consistent changes have been demonstrated in human zinc deficiency.

Methods of Analysis

Plasma, Serum, or Urinary Zinc. Zinc in plasma, serum, or urine is best measured by flame atomic absorption spectrophotometry (41). To compensate for viscosity differences, calibration standards for a five-fold dilution of plasma or serum with deionized water are prepared in 5% glycerin. Erythrocyte zinc is determined on the hemolysate from a 50-fold dilution of cells. The result may be expressed as μg/dL red cells or in terms of hemoglobin concentration. Leukocyte and platelet zinc determinations require graphite furnace analysis (39). Rigid adherence to a meticulous protocol is required at every stage of the procedure to prevent contamination.

Other Vitamins

Tests to assess the status of other vitamins and suggested analytical methods with normal reference ranges for adults are given in Table 57.4 and discussed in relevant chapters of this book. Detailed analytical procedures by individual authors are described (42) and discussed elsewhere (42, 43), with reference ranges listed (44).

Other Minerals and Trace Elements

Tests to assess the status of various minerals and trace elements are noted in the relevant chapters. Suggested analytical methods and reference ranges for serum con-

Table 57.4
Laboratory Tests for Assessment of Vitamin Status

Vitamin	Assay[a]	Method[b] (Reference)	Reference Conventional Units	Range SI Units
A	Retinol(S)	Reverse-phase HPLC	0.45–0.80 mg/L males 0.35–0.75 mg/L females	1.57–2.79 μmol/mL
D	25(OH) vitamin D (S)	RIA	4–60 ng/mL	10–150 nmol/L
D	1,25 $(OH)_2$ vitamin D	RIA	20–65 pg/mL	48–156 pmol/mL
E	α-tocopherol (S)	Reverse-phase HPLC	5.0–20.0 mg/L	11.6–46.4 μmol/mL
K	Prothrombin time (P)	Functional test	11–15 sec	
K_1	Phylloquinone	Reverse-phase HPLC	0.5–2.0 ng/mL	1.1–4.4 nmol/mL
Total β-carotene	Total β-carotene (S)	Reverse-phase HPLC	10–85 μg/dL	0.18–1.58 μmol/mL
B_1 (thiamin)	Transketolase activity coefficient (RBC)	Spectrophotometric	Stimulation by TPP <20%	
B_2 (riboflavin)	Glutathione reductase activity coefficient (RBC)	Spectrophotometric	Stimulation by FAD <20%	
B_6 (pyridoxal-5-phosphate)	Alanine aspartate aminotransferase activity coefficient (RBC)	Spectrophotometric	Stimulation by P-5-P <20%	
	Pyridoxal-5-phosphate (S)	Reverse-phase HPLC	7.41–8.64 μg/L	30–35 nmol/L
Folate	Folic acid (S)	Radioimmunoassay	1.9–14 ng/mL	4.3–31.7 nmol/L
B_{12}	Cobalamin(s) (S)	Radioimmunoassay	180–960 pg/mL	133–708 pmol/L
C	Ascorbic acid (P)	HPLC	6.0–20.0 mg/L	0.034–0.110 μmol/L
	Ascorbic acid, leukocytes	HPLC	20–53 μg/10^8 cells	

Prepared from data from references 42–44. Reference 42 is continually updated on CD ROM, Pesce & Kaplan, Publishers, Inc. Cincinnati, OH.

[a]S, serum; P, plasma; RBC, erythrocytes.

[b]HPLC, high-performance liquid chromatography; RIA, radioimmunoassay.

Table 57.5
Laboratory Tests Values: Serum Levels Electrolytes

Electrolyte	Analytical Method	Reference Conventional Units	Range SI Units
Sodium	Flame AA	135–145 mEq/L	135–145 mmol/L
Potassium	Flame AA	3.6–5.0 mEq/L	3.6–5.0 mmol/L
Calcium	Flame AA	80–105 mg/L	2.0–2.6 mmol/L
Magnesium	Flame AA	18.0–23.0 mg/L	0.75–0.95 mmol/L
Phosphate	Spectrophotometric	25–48 mg/L	0.81–1.55 mmol/L

Prepared from references 42–44. Reference 42 is continually updated on CD ROM, Pesce & Kaplan, Publishers, Inc. Cincinnati, OH.

centrations of electrolytes and trace elements are listed in Tables 57.5 and 57.6, respectively. Analytical procedures are described in detail by individual authors (42), with reference ranges listed (43, 44).

PHYSICAL AND INSTRUMENTAL ANALYTIC METHODS

Stable Isotopes

Nutritional Assessment and Metabolic Studies. Radioactive isotopes as tracers for nutritional assessment cannot be given to children or pregnant women. In contrast, stable isotopes, the naturally occurring isotopes of an element, are not radioactive. Their safety is a distinct advantage, as is the absence of decay. Disadvantages of the enriched stable isotopes are their greater expense and the required larger dose, which, unlike the radioactive tracer dose, may add significantly to the body pool of the element being studied. Sample pretreatment required for stable isotope measurements is usually more extensive than for radioactivity, and equipment is more expensive. In addition, whole-body counting is not possible with stable isotopes. Sandstrom et al. (45) have published a comprehensive discussion of various aspects of stable isotope application.

Minerals and Trace Metals

Stable isotopes of calcium, chromium, copper, iron, magnesium, manganese, selenium, and zinc have been used in nutritional studies. Ideally, the enrichment achieved should approach 100%, but this is sometimes difficult because of the cost and availability of the isotope. If a less abundant isotope is selected, a larger dose is required. Stable isotopes may be quantified by any one of a number of systems, and the advantages and disadvantages of each are discussed elsewhere (45), as are the doses of various available enriched isotopes, methods introducing the isotope, comparisons of the metabolism of intrinsically and extrinsically labeled foods for a number of elements (e.g., zinc, copper, calcium, magnesium, and selenium) (45). Numerous studies measuring absorption of zinc, copper, and iron from fecal monitoring of stable isotopes have been summarized (45). Most studies require fecal collections for up to 15 days, which emphasizes the high costs associated with these research tools. Instrumentation costs are also a major consideration.

Zinc status may be assessed from very short term observations of isotope ratios in plasma and urine following intravenous administration of stable isotope (40).

Table 57.6
Laboratory Values: for Serum Levels of Trace Elements and Associated Protein

Trace Element	Assay	Method	Reference Conventional Units	Range SI Units
Copper	Copper	Flame AA	0.7–1.4 mg/L (males) 0.8–1.55 mg/L (females)	11.0–22.0 μmol/L (males) 12.6–24.4 μmol/L (females)
	Ceruloplasmin	Rate nephelometry	150–600 mg/L	1.0–4.0 μmol/L
	Cytochrome c oxidase	Enzymatic		
Iron	Iron	Flame AA	400–1600 μg/L	7.16–28.6 μmol/L
	Transferrin	Rate nephelometry	1.87–3.12 g/L	21–35 μmol/L
	Iron-binding capacity	Flame AA	2.6–4.3 mg/L	46.0–77.0 μmol/L
	Ferritin	RIA or EIA	20–200 μg/L	45–450 pmol/L
Selenium	Glutathione peroxidase	Spectrophotometric	455–800 U/L	
	Selenium	Graphite furance AA	103–190 μg/L	1.3–2.4 μmol/L
Zinc	Zinc	Flame AA	654–1150 μg/L	10.0–17.6 μmol/L

Prepared from data from references 42–44. Reference 42 is continually updated on CD ROM, Pesce & Kaplan, Publishers, Inc. Cincinnati, OH.

Whole-Body Counting

Whole body [K] is an accurate index of the body cell mass and can be determined by ^{40}K measurement. Instruments can accommodate a wide range of body size, from low-birth-weight infants to obese adults (46). Of the naturally occurring isotopes of potassium, ^{40}K represents approximately 0.018% of the total. This isotope emits gamma rays, which are easily detected and quantitated.

In Vivo Neutron Activation Analysis (IVNAA)

IVNAA (47, 48) enables chemical analysis of body composition. When exposed to neutrons, elements of interest undergo a nuclear reaction. The resulting gamma emissions are characteristic of the tissue elements to be determined and can be easily counted. The technique has been applied to many elements, including calcium, sodium, chloride, phosphorus, nitrogen, zinc, and carbon. Partial-body IVNAA can be applied to individual organs that are target organs for a particular element. Counting statistics may be calculated either by delayed gamma-activation analysis or prompt gamma-activation analysis, described below.

Delayed Gamma-Activation Analysis. Delayed gamma-activation analysis involves neutron capture by an atom of the element (48), transformation of the atom to another nuclear state, and radioactive decay with gamma emission. The activation time, delay time between the end of activation and the beginning of counting, and the counting time are used to correct for decay of the radioactive element. This technique has been used mainly in research in laboratories and development of instrumentation has been innovative, so there is a lack of standardization for calculation of results.

Prompt Gamma-Activation Analysis. Capture of a neutron by a nucleus of an element results in an excited nuclear state because of the energy provided by the neutron. The excited nucleus promptly returns to its lower energy state, with emission of gamma rays. Since the excitation and gamma emission occur within a fraction of a nanosecond, the signal must be measured at the time of neutron exposure. The total activity is then directly proportional to the activation time. Prompt gamma-activation analysis is currently used to estimate total body protein, assuming that the nitrogen content of protein is 16%. The technique and instrument design, a detailed discussion of assumptions and their validity, equipment, aspects of measurement procedures, precision, accuracy of the techniques, and cost factors are presented elsewhere (48).

Bioelectrical Impedance

The water and electrolyte content of fat-free tissue permits greater conduction of an applied electrical signal than does fat. Thus, by placing electrodes dermally on the ankle and wrist and applying an electrical signal, one can determine various parameters of total body composition by applying Ohm's law. Electrical impedance measurements are used to determine total body water and subsequently to estimate fat-free mass and the percentage of body fat. The assumptions, exceptions to be considered for other than healthy subjects, and need for standardization in applying the technique are discussed elsewhere (49). (See also chapters 49 and 56.)

REFERENCES

1. Young DS, Bermes EW Jr. Specimen collection and processing: sources of biological variation. In: Burtis CA, Ashwood ER, eds. Tietz fundamentals of clinical chemistry. 4th ed. Philadelphia: WB Saunders, 1996;33–52.
2. Freiser H, Nancollas GH. Compendium of analytical nomenclature—definitive rules 1987. International Union of Pure and Applied Chemistry, Analytical Chemistry Division. Oxford: Blackwell, 1987;114–7.
3. Clinical Laboratory Improvement Act of 1988, final rule. Fed Regist 1992;57:7002–288.
4. Bayoumi RA, Rosalkie S. Clin Chem 1976;22:327–35.
5. Burtis CA, Ashwood ER, ed. Tietz fundamentals of clinical chemistry. 4th ed. Philadelphia: WB Saunders, 1996.
6. Roe JH, Rice EW. J Biol Chem 1948;173:507–12.
7. McNeely MMD. D-xylose. In: Pesce AJ, Kaplan LA, eds. Methods in clinical chemistry. St. Louis: CV Mosby, 1987;862–7.
8. Shils ME, unpublished data.
9. King CE, Toskes PP, Spivey JC, et al. Gastroenterology 1979;77:75–82.
10. Strocchi A, Corazza G, Ellis CJ, et al. Gastroenterology 1993;105:1404–10.
11. Saltzman JR, Kowdley KV, Pedrosa MC, et al. Gastroenterology 1994;106:615–23
12. Van de Kamer, JH. Total fatty acids in stool. In: Seligson D, ed. Standard methods of clinical chemistry. New York: Academic Press, 1958;II:34–9.
13. Shils ME, Alcock NW, unpublished data.
14. Reifenstein EC Jr, Albright F, Wells SL. J Clin Endocrinol 1945;5:367–95.
15. Powell DW. Approach to the patient with diarrhea. In: Yamada T, ed. Textbook of gastroenterology. 2nd ed. Philadelphia: JB Lippincott, 1995;813–63.
16. Mackenzie TA, Clark NG, Bistrian BR, et al. J Am Coll Nutr 1985;4:575–81.
17. Heymsfield SB, Tighe A, Wang ZM. Nutritional assessment by anthropometric and biochemical methods. In: Shils ME, Olsen RA, Shike M, eds. Modern nutrition in health and disease. 8th ed. Philadelphia: Lea & Febiger, 1994;812–41.
18. Herbert V. Am J Clin Nutr 1967;20:562–72.
19. McNeely MDD. Folic acid. In: Pesce SJ, Kaplan LA, eds. Methods in clinical chemistry, St. Louis: CV Mosby, 1987;539–42.

19a. Smit Vanderkooy PD, Gibson RS. Am J Clin Nutr 1987;45:609–16.

19b. Klevay LM. Am J Clin Nutr 1970;23:284–9.

19c. Alcock NW, Sandstead HH, Chen YJ, et al. FASEB J 1996;10:A785

20. Kelly DG. Small intestine and its disorders. In: Shearman D, Finlayson N, Carter D, Camilleri M, eds. Diseases of the gastrointestinal tract and liver. 3rd ed. Edinburgh: Churchill Livingstone, 1997;13.1–13.41.

21. Chen IW, Sperling MJ, Heminger LA, et al. Clin Chem 1983;29:1241.
22. Das KC, Herbert V. Am J Hematol 1989;31:11–20.
23. Cornwell PE, Morgan SL, Vaughn WH. J Chromatogr 1993;617:136–99.
24. Matchar DB, Feussner JR, Millington DS, et al. Ann Intern Med 1987;106:707–10.
25. Normon EJ, Martelo OJ, Denton MD. Blood 1982;59:1128–31.
26. Nickoloff E. Crit Rev Clin Lab Sci 1988; 26:263–76.
27. MacCrehan WA, Schonberger E. Clin Chem 1987;33:1585–92.
28. Thompson JN, Erdody P, Brien R. Biochem Med 1971;5:67–89.
29. Loerch JD, Underwood BA, Lewis KC. J Nutr 1979;109:778–86.
30. Jacob R, Sandstead HH, Solomons NW, et al. Am J Clin Nutr 1978;31:638–44.
31. Shreiber WE. Iron, porphyrin and bilirubin metabolism. In: Pesce AJ, Kaplan LA, eds. Clinical chemistry, theory, analysis and correlation. 3rd ed. St. Louis: CV Mosby, 1996;696–715.
31a. Suomineu P, Punnonen K, Rajamaki A et al. Clin Chem 1997;43:1641–46.
32. Franco RS. Ferritin. In: Pesce AJ, Kaplan LA, eds. Methods in clinical chemistry. St. Louis: CV Mosby, 1987;1240–2.
33. Peters T, Giovanniello T. J Lab Clin Med 1956;48:280–8.
34. Levy A, Vitacce P. Clin Chem 1961;7:241–8.
35. Perotta G. In: Pesce AJ, Kaplan LA, eds. Methods in clinical chemistry. St. Louis: CV Mosby, 1987;1259–61.
36. Ferro Chem Model 3050 Analyzer instruction manual. 2nd ed. Bedford, MA: Environmental Sciences Associates, revised February 1981.
37. Olsen AD, Hamlin WB. Clin Chem 1969;15:438–41.
38. Lewis SA, O'Haver TC, Harnley JM. Anal Chem 1984;56:1551–4.
39. Wang A, Prasad A, DuMouchelle EA. J Micronutr Anal 1989;5:181–90.
40. Yokoi K, Alcock NW, Sandstead HH. J Lab Clin Med 1994;124:852–61.
41. Smith JC Jr, Butrimovitz GP, Purdy WC. Clin Chem 1979;45:1487–91.
42. Pesce AJ, Kaplan LA. Methods in clinical chemistry; with 101 contributors. St. Louis: CV Mosby, 1987.
43. Morrow FD, Sahyoun N, Jacob RA, et al. Clinical assessment of the nutritional status of adults. In: Linder MC, ed. Nutritional biochemistry and metabolism with clinical applications. 2nd ed. Norwalk, CT: Appleton & Lange, 1991:391–424.
44. Anonymous. Reference values inside front and back covers. In: Kaplan LA, Pesce AJ, eds. Clinical Chemistry, theory, analysis, correlation. 3rd ed. St Louis, CV Mosby, 1996.
45. Sandstrom B, Fairweather-Tait S, Hurrell R, et al. Nutr Res 1993;6:71–95.
46. Ellis KJ, Shypailo RJ. Whole body potassium measurements independent of body size. In: Ellis KJ, Eastman JD, eds. Human body composition: in vivo methods and assessment. New York: Plenum Press, 1993;371–5.
47. Ellis KJ. Whole body-counting and neutron activation analysis. In: Roche AE, Heymsfield SB, Lohman TG, eds. Human body composition. New York: Plenum Press, 1996;45–60.
48. Russell DM, Pendergast PJ, Darby PL, et al. Am J Clin Nutr 1983;38:229–37.
49. NIH Technology Assessment Conference Statement. Biolectrical impedance analysis in body composition measurement. December 12–14, 1994;1–35.

58. Dietary Assessment

JOHANNA DWYER

Dietary assessment began in ancient times, but only when knowledge of food composition expanded in the 20th century was it linked to intakes of nutrients and other constituents that affect health (1, 2). Technologic advances now include biochemical measures for estimating intakes of some constituents to supplement or corroborate dietary intake data (3, 4). Microcomputers and computerized dietary analysis software now permit direct data entry using structured dietary recall interviews. Semi-quantitative food frequency questionnaires are available in computerized forms (5). Computerized nutrient analysis programs and automated data processing ease the burdens of calculating nutrient intakes and rapidly provide summaries of the analyses in databases and tables. These advances help standardize dietary assessment tools and extend their uses from the bedside to large surveys. Statistical techniques for analyzing dietary data have also been refined. The pressing challenges of the future include development of better methods for rapidly screening and assessing dietary intakes and incorporating results routinely into computerized databases and other communications to optimize patient care.

This chapter guides readers in selecting appropriate dietary assessment methods for their purposes and describes the nutritionist's role in carrying out these tasks.

BASIC QUESTIONS TO ANSWER WHEN SELECTING A DIETARY ASSESSMENT METHOD

All dietary assessment methods are imperfect. Their validity and reliability depend heavily on the skill of the interviewer; the instruction, training, and cooperation of the subject; and a valid, reliable nutrient database or other system of analysis. The "best" method depends on the purpose of the investigation. Incorrect inferences may be made about nutritional status if intake data are used alone. For estimating individual nutritional status and developing dietary treatments, a combination of dietary, biochemical, clinical, and anthropometric methods will continue to be the "gold standard." No indicator provides a definitive diagnosis of all forms of malnutrition and the information needed for shaping dietary interventions in individual cases (6, 7).

Why Is Dietary Intake Being Evaluated?

The answer to this question influences the type of data that must be collected, the number of observations necessary, and the best methods to use. One may collect dietary intakes to screen, assess, evaluate, plan interventions or monitor dietary intake or nutritional status of individuals, groups, or nations.

What Is Being Assessed?

Nutrients, other food constituents, foods, food groups, and dietary patterns may be assessed (Table 58.1). The methods required for each purpose differ. Information on the entire diet is usually needed if the focus is on intakes of several nutrients that are widely dispersed in the food supply (as is the case for most clinical purposes) and if nutrient-nutrient interactions exist, since the absorption, use, and health effects of one nutrient may be influenced by the presence of others (8). Collection of food frequencies or food groups is less time consuming and may suffice for screening purposes, but data are inaccurate for assessing absolute levels of nutrient intake. Special food-group-

Table 58.1
Types of Dietary Information of Interest

Entire diet	One or many nutrients or food constituents
	Interrelationships between these
Foods or meals	Intake frequency of a single food or foods
	Form of food (such as retentiveness of sugar-containing foods in studies of dental caries)
	Type of food (animal, plant)
	Cooking or preparation method
	Food diversity
	Source of foods (feeding or meal program)
Food groups	Intake frequency of food groups
	Conformity with a food guidance system (basic four food groups, food exchange lists, or some other system)
Dietary patterns and characteristics	Typical meals
	Meal frequency
	Temporal patterns (time of meal, snacking, drinking, breakfast eating)
	Location of eating (home or away from home)
	Use of vitamin-mineral supplements
	Other patterns (bingeing, spells of illness, fasting, dieting)
	Conformity to some recommended pattern (introduction of solids or weaning)
	Source of meals
	Associations of consumption with some other characteristics (such as mood or time in menstrual cycle)
	Type of feeding (breast, mixed, bottle)

ing systems such as food or diet exchange lists provided for those on modified diets furnish rough estimates of some nutrients. For descriptive purposes, additional information on food consumption patterns or dietary characteristics may also be helpful.

Who Is the Target of the Assessment?

The respondent's capabilities must be well matched to the assessment methods (9). Table 58.2 lists some respondent characteristics that limit the choice of methods. The generalizability of results also depends on who is targeted. Population sampling techniques must be used if individuals are to be representative of a larger population. The variability of the target's dietary intake will influence how many days of observation are necessary to get a true representation of usual intakes.

What Time Frame Is Important?

Typical intakes that span many weeks or months are usually the time frame of interest for nutritional purposes. Sometimes, as in investigations of food intoxication incidents, only a single day's intake is needed, greatly simplifying the task.

What Is the Focus of Analysis?

The appropriate target may be an individual or group. Intake alone may be of interest, or how it is associated with some other characteristic, such as morbidity or mortality. Methods differ in their validity and reliability for describing individual intakes (10). If the focus of analysis is to characterize the diets of individuals, more observations are usually needed than if the focus is on groups (11). For epidemiologic and educational purposes, stable relative rankings for groups of respondents rather than absolute levels of nutrient intakes may suffice. Statistical methods for analysis of dietary data have been well described (12, 13).

How Great Is Respondent Burden?

The respondent's time burden varies from a few minutes to several hours, depending on the method chosen. Psychologic burdens of respondents include the time, annoyance, and work involved in recording, remembering, and reporting minute details about food intake, especially when the reporter considers the information embarrassing or sensitive. Tradeoffs must often be made between the investigator's desire to collect information that could conceivably be of interest and respondents' willingness to give it.

What Are the Costs?

Objectives of data collection must be matched to resources. Some costs are immediately apparent: forms, food models, computers, interviewer time, and respondent honoraria. There are also hidden costs such as the time needed for protocol development, calibration, interview training, checking and coding of records, other quality assurance activities, calculating and interpreting intake data, and communicating findings. These are usually much greater than one imagines (14).

What Other Constraints Are Present?

Other limitations include the social and physical context and setting for the interview; the availability, skill, interest, and training of the interviewers; assessment techniques; and the time and facilities available for analyzing the resulting data. When patients are being assessed, their illness or the necessity for other treatments may limit the means available (15).

How Accurately Must the Characteristic Be Measured?

Accuracy depends on validity and reproducibility, and it varies from one method to another. Differences between actual and measured intakes in dietary assessment depend not only on how representative the data are but also on the many factors that affect measurement accuracy.

Misclassification can be corrected for by sampling sufficient and representative numbers of days of observation for individuals, by using sample size formulas that take misclassification into account, by increasing the number of respondents, and by using other formulas to adjust the

Table 58.2
Considerations in Choosing Dietary Assessment Methods for Particular Target Groups

Pregnant women	Intakes change over the course of pregnancy, so usual intakes must be assessed at specific points in time during pregnancy
	Distortion of intakes owing to fear of noncompliance may be an issue
	Intakes of certain substances such as alcohol and supplements may be of particular concern
Lactating women	Maternal intakes and breast-feeding practices vary over the course of lactation and by individual
	Maternal intakes are affected by extent to which infant is breast-feeding
	Infant intakes may be supplemented with nutrients or foods
	Composition of breast milk varies
Infants	Intakes of breast milk must be assessed using special techniques such as test weighing or indirect estimates from doubly labeled water studies
	Mixed feedings (breast and other food) complicate assessment
	Surrogate respondents must be used
	Eating patterns and intakes vary greatly from month to month, hampering retrospective reporting methods
	Special foods (formulas, baby and weaning foods) and portions commonly used must be included in food tables
Preschool children	Surrogate respondents must be used (often several, because no one person is aware of child's entire intakes)
	Intakes vary greatly from day to day
School children	Recall is limited; surrogate respondents or records may be needed to supplement recall
	Literacy may be limited
	Vocabulary and ability to describe foods may be limited
	Reports may be of what was served, or what parent believes should have been provided, not what was eaten
	Children have limited attention spans
	Intakes may differ greatly between school days and other days
Adolescents	Intakes change rapidly, especially during pubertal growth spurt, and may be more highly associated with physical maturation than age
	Usual patterns, including frequent meal skipping, snacks at unusual times of day, dieting, fasting, bulimia, self-induced vomiting, laxative abuse, and sports training regimens may be present and not immediately apparent
	Recall of childhood food habits of interest may be unknown (e.g., duration of breast-feeding, weaning patterns)
Elderly	Recall may be limited
	Disabilities in hearing, sight, or attention may complicate assessment
	Intakes may vary greatly from day to day if chronic illnesses affecting food intake are present
Illiterate persons	Methods using printed information, instructions, or records cannot be used
Acutely ill	Reporting may be biased because of fears that noncompliance will be punished
	Intakes may vary greatly from day to day with exacerbations in illness
	Recall may be distorted by disease or by recollection of "usual" diet when well
	Ability to pay attention, read, write, or hear may be affected by illness
	"Net" intake may be affected by such conditions as fasting, vomiting, and diarrhea
	Special dietary supplements or foods may be consumed in large amounts
Unusual lifestyles or patterns	"Usual" intakes may be difficult to describe; athletes and dancers may have special regimens while training or during competition or performance; shift workers may have different patterns of eating on and off duty

size of the confidence intervals (16, 17). These issues are discussed in depth elsewhere (18).

DIETARY SCREENING AND ASSESSMENT IN HEALTH CARE

Dietary evaluation is part of a continuum that begins by identifying individuals who have certain risk factors or characteristics of interest and ends with integrating the results of the assessment with other information to reach appropriate conclusions about dietary, nutritional, or general health status. Dietary data are collected in most health care settings to furnish a sound basis for developing and implementing nutritional care plans. The individual's condition and the health care delivery setting will dictate the specific focus. It may concentrate primarily on developing information for later health promotion, disease prevention and control, rehabilitation, or, if prevention or cure are not possible, guide interventions devoted to amelioration or palliation. At present, there is no consensus on the best method for assessing dietary or nutritional status in clinical settings (19).

Nutritional Screening in Acute and Chronic Care

It is no longer possible to rely solely on the goodwill and individual subjective judgments of health professionals in accurately screening for nutritional risk. Certainly, subjective impressions are useful in identifying some individuals who need further nutritional assessment, but selections based solely on such criteria tend to be idiosyncratic and vary in their validity from one practitioner to another. Moreover, those individuals who need services the most may be the very ones who are the least likely to come to the attention of health professionals, and they will be missed. Valid, objective screening criteria that are mutually agreed upon by all on the health team help to avoid these difficulties.

Screening is helpful in establishing priorities for the most efficient use of available time and money in health care settings. Standardized guidelines for nutritional screening are still in their infancy in clinical practice, but they are gradually coming into more widespread use. The Joint Commission on Accreditation of Hospitals and

Health Care Organizations (JCAHO) now recognizes the need for some method of identifying all patients at high nutritional risk and requires it within 24 hours of hospital admission, although standardized methods are not specified (20). Nutritional screening is included in the U.S. Preventive Services Task Force recommendations on nutritional counseling (21, 22). Screening has also been proposed as a factor for measuring the quality of managed care services as part of the HEDIS 3.0, a set of quality indicators widely used to evaluate managed care organizations (23). In the future, it is likely that dietary intake and nutritional status will be routinely screened in all patient assessments (24).

Changes in health care financing, constraints on economic and human resources, the advent of managed care, and the growth of comprehensive networks for care that span various delivery settings are revolutionizing medical, public health, and nutritional care delivery. In acute care settings, illness severity has increased, patient lengths of stay have decreased, and patients are often discharged while they are still very ill. Rapid patient turnover makes it essential to screen and assess quickly patients most likely to need nutritional care so that it can be provided in a timely fashion. Professionals working in outpatient, community, and public health settings are now encountering individuals with severe and complex nutritional problems who need evaluation. However, even very simple and straightforward questions about eating and diet are often omitted on standard clinical history forms and patient interviews in all of these settings (25). These trends have stimulated the need for standardized nutritional screening and assessment methods to identify those most in need of nutritional assistance, which can be performed quickly and communicated easily to all who need the findings for providing health care.

The most important attributes of risk factors for screening purposes in acute care settings are that they are already collected or are easily and rapidly abstracted from existing data, they are available on all patients, and they result in clinically meaningful categorizations of patients by risk status. Preferably, they should be available on computerized patient record summaries or other information systems that can be rapidly perused. Once risk is ascertained, it should be entered into the same system so that all providers have access to the information.

Presently, many health professionals are uncertain about what should be screened to detect malnutrition and whether screening is effective. Although many dietary and other characteristics are used for nutritional screening, few of them have been formally evaluated for specificity, sensitivity, and predictive value. This is an important area for future research.

Dietary Assessment in Health Settings

Further dietary assessment is necessary in health care practice settings because screening by any single measure is likely to identify both individuals who will respond to dietary measures and others who will not. Because the causes of malnutrition vary, dietary screening or assessment may indicate a deficit in nutritional status, but without additional information, one cannot assume that better alimentation will solve the problem. Dietary measures can only remedy forms of malnutrition that are primarily due to diet, such as inadequate, imbalanced, or excessive dietary intake. Much malnutrition secondary to physical ill health and psychosocial problems occurs even in the face of adequate food in the environment, and even if the individual is provided with an adequate diet. The presence of certain diseases or conditions provides clues that malnutrition secondary to disease may be involved. Even when it is, there is often a component that involves dietary deficiency, and this may be treated or prevented if dietary intakes are improved. Assessment aids in identifying forms of malnutrition that are likely to respond to nutritional measures and those that require other measures.

Changes in dietary intake are among the earliest signs of nutritional problems. Theoretically, dietary intakes should be ideal for screening and assessment. However, dietary screening and assessment measures also have major limitations. These include the heterogeneity of malnutrition itself, inability to completely describe why intake is poor or whether improved intake will correct the problem, and methodological limitations such as specificity and sensitivity. These limitations make it necessary to use other types of information in the assessment process as well (26).

Many forms of malnutrition exist, ranging from starvation and deficiencies of specific vitamins and minerals to imbalances and excesses of food energy or other nutrients. No single screening or assessment indicator signals the presence of all of them. All of these need to be evaluated, since they may be present and relevant to prognosis. The best indicator for each specific form of malnutrition may be dietary in some instances, clinical, biochemical, or anthropometric in others, depending on the validity, reliability, and specificity of the indicator in question. However, few indicators of nutritional status are definitive and unambiguous in themselves; usually several indicators are necessary to signal the presence of problems.

Early, less severe, and presumably more easily remediable forms of malnutrition may signal their presence only by decreased dietary intakes, but the errors in dietary intake assessment in the clinical setting may be so large that true decreases in dietary intake are indistinguishable from the error in the method itself. Thus, dietary assessment has methodological limitations. Dietary reporting is rarely entirely valid, and some individuals may not be able to provide estimates at all. Food intake varies considerably from day to day so that intraindividual variability is high. It is time consuming and difficult to obtain estimates of food intake over a long enough time for valid qualitative descriptions of intakes in individuals, particularly if respondents are sick. Finally, memory problems confuse results with retrospective methods, and changes in intake during recording may make intakes unrepresentative with prospective methods.

Further examination of the patient found to be at risk involves not only dietary assessment but also a review of available biochemical, anthropometric, clinical, functional, dietary, and medical history information. Such a review gives more insight into the causes of the malnutrition, and the most reasonable and fruitful interventions or therapies can be determined.

HOW METHODS FOR OBTAINING INFORMATION ABOUT FOOD INTAKE DIFFER

Degree of Detail Required

The degree of detail and range of information provided by screening measures is less complete than that furnished by assessment measures.

Screening

Screening is the process of identifying individuals who have characteristics (risk factors) that potentially place them at high risk for dietary or nutritional problems. To identify such individuals, screening criteria must be simple, inexpensive, relatively straightforward, and easy to administer, preferably by generalists or those with little special expertise, in a variety of settings. However, risk factors are probabilistic; they only signify increased risk, not the definitive presence of malnutrition. Thus, they are not definitive in individual cases.

Screening and assessment must be valid and reliable to be effective (27). They must identify those who truly are malnourished and those who are not. Screening must avoid producing large numbers of false positives (persons who have the risk factor but who are not malnourished on further assessment) and false negatives (persons who are judged on screening to be well nourished but who, after later testing with more definitive standards, are shown to be malnourished). The screening test must also detect malnutrition earlier than without screening and do so accurately (i.e., without large numbers of false positives and false negatives). Finally, early detection must be effective. Those judged to be malnourished who are detected and treated early should have better clinical outcomes than those detected without screening.

Dietary Risk Factors. Dietary risk factors are easily identified characteristics that are associated with an increased likelihood of poor diet or nutritional status. They include indices of poor diet such as perceived inadequate quantity or quality of food intake, presence of certain acute or chronic diseases or conditions, need for assistance with eating, and physiologic vulnerability, evidenced by medication use and dental problems, for example. Psychosocial factors such as social isolation, demographic characteristics known to be associated with poor nutritional status such as poverty, and membership in a nutritionally vulnerable group such as extreme youth or old age, pregnancy, or lactation are also useful indicators of dietary risk. Note that they identify risk of poor diet and not necessarily dietary factors per se.

Dietary Assessment

Dietary assessment is the measurement of indicators of dietary status to identify more definitively the possible occurrence, nature, and extent of poor diet or impaired nutritional status. Assessment should follow screening and give priority to those found to be at high risk. Individuals whose characteristics at screening suggest nutritional risk require further assessment. This consists of a more detailed investigation to identify diet, eating habits, food resources, disease-related issues, or other factors that may affect nutritional status adversely.

Short Dietary Assessment Tools

Short dietary assessment tools are brief methods that provide either qualitative or quantitative information on food groups, a food, or sometimes a specific nutrient. They include abbreviated food-frequency questionnaires, food checklists, questionnaires on specific eating or drinking behaviors (e.g., consumption of fruits and vegetables, alcoholic beverage intake), self-monitoring tools such as fat gram counters for keeping track of the intake of a nutrient, and counting the number of food groups consumed. The short dietary assessment tools fall between screening methods and the more detailed and comprehensive descriptions of diet (described below) in the time they take to administer and the information they provide. The detail they provide may suffice for some clinical purposes. Their advantages are that they are short and easy to administer by nonprofessionals and may be useful for nutritional education. Their disadvantages are that they do not provide the quantitative accuracy of the other assessment methods, nor do they provide quantitative estimates of more than a few nutrients or food groups. Specific tools for use in various settings are discussed below.

Reference Time Period

Methods differ in when the respondent is asked to provide information. Methods may focus on past intake (retrospective), on intake to be collected after the instruction (prospective), or combinations of the two. Table 58.3 summarizes the major methods. Examples of existing instruments are available (Dietary Assessment Resource Manual [28] and in greater detail elsewhere [29, 30]). For research purposes, a register that lists dietary assessment calibration and validation studies comparing dietary intake estimates from two or more assessment methods is available (31). Correlations between methods vary; usually those with a correlation coefficient, r, of 0.5 or higher are considered acceptable (32). Table 58.4 summarizes the advantages and disadvantages of the various methods;

Table 58.3
Dietary Assessment Methods

Method	Description
Retrospective methods	
24-Hour recall	Interviewer prompts a respondent to recall and describe all foods and beverages consumed over the past 24 hours, usually starting with the meal immediately preceding the interview; food models, measuring cups and spoons, and other tools are used to get rough estimate of portion sizes; may be face-to-face or by telephone
Food-frequency questionnaire	Respondent records or describes usual intakes of a list of different foods and the frequency of consumption per day, week, or month, over a period of several months or a year; the number and type of food items vary, depending on the purpose of the assessment; nutrient analyses are usually not possible
Semiquantitative food-frequency questionnaire	Similar to a food-frequency questionnaire; portion sizes are specified as standardized portion size or choice (of a range of sizes); foods are chosen to encompass the most frequently consumed foods as well as the most common source of nutrients; the major sources of nutrients for a given population should be included for questionnaire to be valid
Burke-type dietary history	Respondent orally reports all foods and beverages consumed on a usual day, then the interview progresses to questions about the frequency and amount of consumption of these foods; often, the respondent provides additional documentation of several days' intakes in the form of food diaries; food models, cross-checks on food consumption, careful probing, and other techniques are also used
Prospective methods	
Weighed food record	With a food record, the individual weighs on a small scale all food and drink consumed rather than simply estimating portion sizes; all is recorded as eaten; the individual records in his food diary everything eaten or drunk, including estimated portion sizes at the time of consumption for several days, or only at specified times
Telephone record	Instead of personal face-to-face interviews, telephones are used to report food intakes as soon as they have occurred
Photographic or videotape records	Individual photographs or videotapes all foods to be eaten, at standardized camera distance
Electronic records	Respondent records food intake on a specially programmed computer program or hand-held computer
Portable electronic set of recording scales	Respondent records intake on an electronic weighing scale recording device with a built-in memory; it operates by pressing a single button, weighing the foods to be eaten; weights are automatically recorded, then the description of the food is dictated on a microphone connected to the tape recorder and weighing scale
Duplicate portion analysis	A duplicate portion of the foods and beverages consumed by an individual is collected; foods are then chemically analyzed to obtain a direct nutrient analysis; applicable to confined individuals, usually in institutions; all foods entering and leaving the room are measured; the difference is assumed to be what the respondent ate
Direct observation by video recording	Video cameras are used to monitor the individual's food intakes over a certain period; videotapes may then be reviewed and intakes recorded accordingly
Direct observation by trained observers	In controlled or highly supervised environments intakes may be directly watched by trained observers who use any of the methods mentioned above; sometimes this observation is covert

these are discussed briefly below. The suitability of each method for estimating specific nutrients and additional details are discussed elsewhere (33, 34).

Retrospective Methods

Retrospective methods include the 24-hour recall, food-frequency recalls, semiquantitative food-frequency recalls, and dietary histories. All rely heavily on the individual's memory and motivation to recall diets eaten in the near or more distant past. Accuracy of recall is related to interview setting, characteristics of the interviewer, effects of instruction, respondent variables such as commitment, memory, sex, age, education, recent health status and diet, the stability of the respondent's diet over time, social desirability, and other factors (35, 36). With the proper incentives and training, most adults can recall what they ate over the past day or week well enough to place them reliably in tertiles or sextiles (37). Recalls of actual food consumption during the previous 24 to 48 hours are the most reliable, with the maximum period thought to be a month (38). Usual or customary habits and relative rankings of food intake patterns going back much farther in time are probably also recalled (39). Intakes collected retrospectively usually give lower estimates of intakes than those collected prospectively because of forgetting. However, intrusions or false memories (e.g., remembering the consumption of a food that was not eaten) may also occur; these may be important in studies of food intoxication. The accuracy of long-term recall data is poor for individuals (40, 41). The reliability of recall after 1 or 2 years is insufficient to classify individuals into tertiles or quantiles of nutrient intakes, although it may be possible to do so for groups (42). Long-term recall is also biased by current diet; these errors may affect patients differently than controls in epidemiologic studies (43). In case-control studies when individuals cannot be categorized reliably with respect to differences in timing, dose, frequency, or duration of intakes of the dietary factors of interest, the associations between diet and later disease or mortality are obscured.

24-Hour Recalls. Twenty-four-hour recalls can be obtained on single or multiple occasions. They provide the respondent with the opportunity, without suggesting responses, to describe all the food, drink, and dietary supplements that may have been consumed. Underreporting can be decreased by probing, but it is still considerable—usually at least 20% for calories and most nutrients. A sin-

Table 58.4
Advantages and Disadvantages of Different Dietary Assessment Methods

Methods and Advantages	Disadvantages
Retrospective	
24-Hour recall Easy to administer Time required to administer is short Inexpensive Respondent burden is low Useful in clinical settings More objective than diet history Serial 24-hour recalls can provide estimates of usual intakes on individuals Data obtained can be repeated with reasonable accuracy Good reliability between interviewers	Does not provide adequate quantitative data on nutrient intakes Individual diets vary daily, so that a single day's intake may not be representative An experienced interviewer is required Relies heavily on memory, making it unsuitable for certain groups, such as the elderly Selective forgetting of foods such as liquids, high-calorie snacks, alcohol, and fat occurs Reported intake may not be actual intake but rather what the interviewer wants to hear Does not reflect differences in intake for weekday vs. weekend, season to season, or shift to shift Data may not accurately reflect nutrient intakes for populations because of variations in food consumption from day to day May be a tendency to overreport intake at low levels and underreport intake at high levels of consumption, leading to "flat-slope syndrome" with reports of group intakes
Food-frequency questionnaire May be either self-administered or interviewer administered Inexpensive Quick to administer Good at describing food intake patterns for diet and meal planning No observer bias Can be used for large population studies Useful when purpose is to study association of a specific food or a small number of foods and disease such as alcohol and birth defects Specific information about nutrients can be obtained if food sources of nutrients are confined to a few sources Can be analyzed rapidly for nutrients or food groups using a computer Foods can be ranked in relation to intakes of certain food items or groups of foods	Response rates may be lower if questionnaire is self-administered Incomplete responses may be given Lists compiled for the general population are not useful for obtaining information on groups with different eating patterns (foods inappropriate) Total consumption is difficult to obtain because not all foods can be included in lists; underestimation can occur Respondent burden rises as the number of food items queried increases Analysis is difficult without use of computers and special programs Reliability is lower for individual foods than for food groups Foods differ in extent to which they are over- and underreported (errors are not random) Each questionnaire needs validation Translation of food groups to nutrient intakes requires many assumptions
Semiquantitative food-frequency questionnaires Inexpensive May be self-administered Rapid Usual diets are not altered Can rank or categorize individuals by rank of nutrient intakes rather than measuring group means Precoding and direct data entry to computer available to speed up analysis on some versions Correlations between this and other methods are satisfactory for food items and targeted nutrients when groups are the focus of the analysis Sufficiently simple to obtain dietary information in large epidemiologic studies that would not be possible with other methods Can provide useful information on intake of a wide variety of nutrients Validation studies are proceeding rapidly Respondent burden varies	Good only for the general population, but not necessarily for specific groups Culture specific—i.e., assessment of intake in a culturally distinct group requires creation and validation of another instrument Unvalidated for individual dietary assessments Needs to be constantly updated Questionnaires available for adults cannot be used for children Specific nutrients are measured, not all nutrients or food constituents Not yet validated for those who eat modified or unusual diets (frequency and amount of intake from food groups may differ) Ability to monitor short-term changes in food intake (weeks or months) is not known Correlations for individual nutrient intakes obtained with semiquantitative food-frequency questionnaires are poor compared with those obtained with diet histories and food records in household measures May be reliable but invalid in some cases Default codes with estimated variables may influence results unduly May only reflect "core diets" of a week's duration
Burke-type dietary history Produces a more complete and detailed description of both qualitative and quantitative aspects of food intake than do food records, 24-hour recalls, or food-frequency questionnaires Eliminates individual day-to-day variations Takes into consideration seasonal variations Good for longitudinal studies	Highly trained nutritionists required to administer dietary histories Difficult to standardize because of considerable variability among and within interviewers Depends on subject's memory Time-consuming (takes about 1–2 hours to administer) Diet histories overestimate intakes compared with food records collected over the same period because of bigger portion sizes and

continued

Methods and Advantages	Disadvantages
Provides good description of usual intake Provides some data on previous diet before beginning prospective studies	greater frequencies reported; also does not account for missed meals or sick days Time frame actually used by subject for reporting intake history is uncertain, probably no longer than a few weeks Costs of analysis are high because records must be checked, coded, and entered appropriately
Prospective methods	
Food diary	
What is eaten is recorded (or should be recorded at time of consumption) Recording error can be minimized if subjects are given proper directions Does not rely heavily on memory, and thus may be good for the elderly Can be obtrusive	Food intake may be altered Respondent burden is great Individual must be literate and physically able to write Respondent may not record intakes on assigned days Difficult to estimate portion sizes Food models or picture may help Underreporting is common Number of sampled days must be sufficient to provide usual intake Records must be checked and coded in standardized way Measured food intakes are more valid than records above Costs of coding and analysis are high Sex difference exists—i.e., women are more competent than men in recording Number of days surveyed depends on the nutrient being studied The very act of recording may change what is eaten
Weighed food diary	
Increased accuracy of portion sizes over food diaries (where errors are substantial—up to 40% for foods and 25% for nutrients)	Respondent burden great, and may increase dropout rates Consumption may be altered during recording days Expensive May restrict choice of food Subjects must be highly motivated Other disadvantages similar to those of food diary Not highly portable Obtrusive Time consuming Scales may break
Telephone interviews	
Some anonymity is maintained Validity is good Respondent burden is low Respondent acceptance is good Effect of forgetting minimum Outreach is greater May be easier to carry out after a face-to-face interview and instruction	Makes assumptions that portion sizes reported are actually eaten Validation studies are incomplete
Records for monitoring specific foods or nutrients	
Immediate feedback Easy, rapid way to monitor specific foods or nutrients for monitoring and adherence purposes in patients	Inaccurate for research All food sources of nutrients not included
Special records	
Can be correlated with other measures such as hunger, blood sugar, mood	Time consuming Difficult to analyze
Photographic records	
Validity is good	Problems result with estimating portion sizes and identifying some foods from photographs Food waste may not be taken into consideration, leading to overestimating Necessary details may be lacking Obtrusive Respondent burden is high
Duplicate portion collection and analysis	
Highly accurate in metabolic research Duplicate portion permits direct chemical analysis Helpful for validating other methods for constituents on which food composition data are incomplete Good for individuals consuming unusual foods	Intakes may be altered Differences between duplicate portions and weighed records are large (7% for energy, larger for other nutrients) Expensive Time consuming and messy
Electronic records	
Preliminary validations are good Decreased respondent burden Eliminates time for coding and data entry, as well as associated errors occurring at those stages	Requires considerable instructions and training Special food groups must be constructed for population to be studied Portion size estimates are often imprecise (147)

continued

Methods and Advantages	Disadvantages
Can be used for patients who cannot write	
Measured intakes and outputs	
Low respondent burden	Others in the room may have eaten the food
Assessment can be accomplished without individual knowing about it	Staff may forget to deliver or collect the food
Good for individuals incapable of writing or remembering	
Portable electronic set of tape recording	
Used for patients who cannot write	Expensive
Cumulative weight is automatically recorded	Does not take plate waste into consideration
Records cannot be altered once entered	
Measures actual and habitual food intake	
Has been initially validated	
Time saved for coding and data entry	
Eliminates errors occurring during coding and data entry	
Direct observation by video recording	
Low respondent burden	High initial cost
Measures usual and habitual food intake	Not good for large studies
Highly accurate	May have technical problems (e.g., angle of camera, low quality, picture detail)
Details may be observed	Intakes may be altered if individual is aware of observation
Individual may or may not know he or she is being observed	
Direct observation by trained observers	
Low respondent burden	Obtrusive
Overt to covert observation is possible	Expensive and time consuming for observer
Precise measurements may be obtained	Not ideal for large studies
	Intakes may be altered especially if person is aware of observation
	Details may be overlooked

gle 24-hour recall cannot precisely identify individuals whose intakes are likely to be high or low in the population. Group mean intakes from single 24-hour recalls may be reliable, since those who report very high intakes on a given day are balanced out by those reporting very low intakes. However, the individuals with high intakes will not necessarily maintain their rankings on a second occasion; even though group means may be constant, their values usually exhibit regression toward the mean (44). Thus, quantitative estimates of usual intakes from single 24-hour recall data are highly suspect for individuals. With several 24-hour recalls accuracy improves. Computerized dietary assessment interview schedules permitting direct data entry by either an interviewer or the respondent are now available in English, Spanish, and other languages. They make it possible to obtain several random 24-hour recalls; these provide estimates of usual intake that are as accurate as semiquantitative food-frequency questionnaires. They have the advantage of including foods that may not be assessed with the frequency questionnaire, and they avoid the prompting of a food list. Multiple unannounced 24-hour recalls offer advantages over food records and semiquantitative food-frequency questionnaires in monitoring dietary changes during intervention studies because they are less susceptible to recording bias and show recent dietary changes (45).

Single 24-hour recalls should not be used in surveys to report the number of individuals below some cutoff point for dietary adequacy. They will overestimate those whose intakes are truly low, compared with dietary assessment measures that better reflect typical or usual intakes and rely less on forgetting. Compared with longer observation periods, distributions of nutrient intake obtained from single 24-hour recalls are more spread out, with more very high and very low values. Simply adding respondents does not compensate for this. Because intraindividual variability is high, single 24-hour recalls are poorly correlated with biochemical parameters that reflect usual diet, even when a strong association actually exists; multiple recalls are more satisfactory. Errors of estimates of usual levels of absolute intake depend on how many days are included and vary from one nutrient to the next.

Food Frequency Recalls. The first food-frequency questionnaires were used chiefly in abbreviated versions based on food groups in clinical situations and for special studies. Food frequency recalls are good for describing groups but have serious limitations for making statements about the absolute magnitude of individual nutrient intakes of respondents. If only a single nutrient is of interest, lists are now available of about 100 foods that, by virtue of their composition, portion size, and the frequency with which they are eaten contribute the most to intakes of that nutrient in national surveys of representative samples of Americans (46, 47). Special lists are available to obtain detailed information on single nutrients such as calcium (48) and lactose (49). Various approaches can be used in selecting the most informative foods to use for estimating nutrient intakes in epidemiologic studies (50). Food frequency recalls tailored for ethnic groups such as Native Americans have also been developed (51).

Burke-Type Dietary History. The Burke-type dietary history method is used infrequently today because it takes so long, it requires a trained, highly skilled nutritionist, and the results are difficult to code and process. It is less directive than list-based methods, and for some purposes it may be appropriate, because it completely profiles an individual diet (52).

Semiquantitative Food-Frequency Questionnaires. Today, semiquantitative food-frequency questionnaires are available that are based on lists of the most common food and vitamin-mineral supplement sources of nutrients in a representative sample of the American population. These are useful for providing semiquantitative rankings to classify individuals into low, medium, and high intakes of a specific nutrient. The two semiquantitative food-frequency questionnaires presently in widespread use that have been tested most extensively are the instrument developed by Willett et al. at Harvard University (53, 54) and that developed by Block and coworkers at the National Cancer Institute (55–58). They differ from each other in their method of construction; the reference populations used to select foods; the extent to which they have been validated; the reference portion sizes used; the number of foods they contain; the nutrient intakes they are designed to assess; the proportion of target nutrients they account for; the questions they ask on vitamin, mineral, and other dietary constituents; the construction of the nutrient databases used for translating responses into nutrient intakes; and probably in other respects. Special questionnaires have also been developed to assess dietary fiber intake (59), and additional interview schedules may be included to increase the accuracy of assessment of energy and fat intake (60) or specific nutrients (61). Questionnaires for participants in the Women, Infants and Children Supplementary Food Program (WIC) (62) and for specific ethnic groups are also available (63, 64).

Recently questionnaires have been developed to assess other biologically active substances in foods, such as carotenoids (65). Questionnaires constructed from population-based surveys are good tools for estimating the usual nutrient intakes of groups. The questionnaires are now being widely and sometimes incorrectly used to provide quantitative assessments of absolute levels of intakes of individuals. The basic problem with this procedure is that the nutrient values for each food category on the questionnaire are derived from weighted averages or medians (based on group estimates) of frequency, portion size, and number of servings per occasion for each food in the category among the population used for validating the questionnaire. Thus, nutrient intakes for each food category are derived from weighted group estimates and reflect *population, not individual, values.* Individuals then provide their frequency of consumption of each food group category, with some estimate of portion and servings, and from these, individual intake profiles are derived. However, overall nutrient intakes for individuals do not reflect their own individual weighted averages of food consumption frequency within each category. Rather, they are rough estimates of intakes of food groups, whose nutrient contents are assumed to be similar to that of the reference population at a given point in time, introducing a strong group effect. Also, intraindividual variation is not measured. True differences between individuals may therefore be impossible to ascertain unless replicates are used. Finally, statistical adjustments for energy intakes may not reflect true energy intakes.

Single food-frequency, semiquantitative food-frequency, and dietary history questionnaires help minimize intraindividual variation by focusing on typical or usual intakes. However, their within-individual variation is often unknown, and threats to validity exist due to forgetting, unequal estimation errors, and the use of different periods as the interval for reporting. Correlation coefficients rarely exceed 0.5 to 0.6 from one administration to the next. Correlations of this magnitude present problems when data on usual intakes of individuals are required for correlation with biochemical or clinical parameters; unless very large numbers of subjects are available, significant correlations may be masked (66).

Prospective Methods

Table 58.3 describes the many prospective methods for obtaining food records at the time the food is eaten or shortly thereafter. These include collection of duplicate portions of all food eaten, records of weighed intakes using scales, food diaries, precoded lists for monitoring frequency of intake of foods with respect to how much of a specific nutrient it provides, other special records, telephone interviews on current intake, and photographic, videotaped, and electronic microcomputer records of consumption.

The prospective methods' strengths and limitations are presented in Tables 58.3 and 58.4 and are discussed in detail elsewhere (67–69). They are more reliable and precise for estimating mean intakes for individuals because they reduce the intraindividual variability attributable to day-to-day variations in diet (70, 71) and are less affected by forgetting than retrospective methods. However, the very act of recording food intake may inadvertently stimulate greater consciousness about intake or otherwise lead the respondent to alter intakes during recording periods. Before prospective studies are undertaken for epidemiologic purposes, it is important to do substudies of dietary intake measurements to correct relative risk estimates for biases due to measurement error and to account for statistical power losses when estimating the sample size requirements of the cohort (72). The results of calibration studies show that efficiency of instruments varies (73).

Combinations of Methods

Often dietary assessment studies for research purposes use several methods simultaneously to increase accuracy (74). For example, the United States Department of Agriculture (USDA) National Food Consumption Survey used a 24-hour recall combined with either 2- or 3-day written records, and the Department of Health and Human Service's National Health and Nutrition Examination

Survey (NHANES) used a 24-hour recall and food frequency information (75). The monumental yearlong diet study conducted by the USDA also used a variety of methods (76). Newer national surveys are using telephone recalls and interactive computer recalls in addition to food records (77).

Mode of Administration

Methods differ in other relevant attributes, such as the mode of administration and technologies used. Many methods are observer administered. They may use in-person interviews, telephone interviews, direct observation of food consumption, collection of duplicate food samples, information on food served and plate waste, and novel methods such as closed-circuit television cameras or collection of garbage. Others are completed by the respondent, including questionnaires, food records or self-monitoring tools, interactive computerized interview schedules, and electronic aids such as tape recorders or handheld computers for immediately recording intakes.

THE DIETITIAN'S ASSESSMENT

Standards of Nutritional Care

For optimal function, the nutritional care team today must include both clinicians and administrators who collaborate to ensure that nutritional information and tracking systems are in place and operate smoothly. The vital elements include nutritional standards for screening and assessment (with priorities for which patients will be seen and for what), care plans, and systems for monitoring and evaluating the quality, quantity, costs, and outcomes of the care provided. These fit well with the performance-based interdisciplinary delivery of nutritional services that is now mandated by the JCAHO (78).

Dietitian's Responsibilities

Dietitians have direct responsibilities in the nutritional care of patients on modified diets and special routes of alimentation and those on usual diets. In addition, dietitians have broader duties as members of the multidisciplinary health team in setting and implementing standards of care and as consultants on food and nutrition. Finally, they must serve as liaisons to ensure that patients have access to appropriate food or alimentation by other means.

Inpatient Settings

Inpatient and institutional settings are particularly challenging today. Health care restructuring has decreased the dietitian:patient ratio in most settings, so that priorities must be set in terms of which patients will be seen, by whom, and for what indications. Patients who might benefit the most from nutritional care are most likely to receive it when dietitians and others on the nutritional care team use systematic, standardized criteria to screen and identify those at nutritional risk and use standardized guidelines for subsequent nutritional care.

All patients in institutional settings must be fed; only some need pharmaceutical or other specialized medical care. It follows that dietitians working in these settings must ensure that all patients are fed appropriately for their health conditions. To do this requires patient screening, assessment, and nutritional care planning. The dietitian is responsible for ensuring that all patients receive the initial nutritional screening. Individuals found to be at nutritional risk must have their dietary and nutritional status further assessed, and relevant observations and recommendations for nutritional care or further consultation proposed. These may include modified diets, feeding assistance, or special feeding routes. The dietitian must also arrange for all patients, regardless of their risk status, to be provided with safe food in a form suitable for their condition and aesthetically acceptable. Dietitians are responsible for jointly establishing and implementing standards of nutritional care in collaboration with relevant medical, nursing, pharmacy, and food service staff to ensure that all patients receive these essential nutritional services. The standards must be implemented, monitored, and periodically evaluated to ensure that they are having the intended results. Dietitians must serve as liaisons between the clinical and food services to ensure not only that patients are fed appropriately, but that they receive appropriate guidance and education on dietary measures that may be necessary after discharge. Dietitians also provide referrals, information, and liaison with home care and extended care services if needed.

Initial Screening. In hospital settings, high patient turnover and the need for efficient screening within the first 24 hours of admission require that the initial screening method rapidly identifies patients in greatest need of help. Initial screening may be done by the dietitian or by some other individual, such as a diet technician or nurse (79). The content of dietary screening is the same no matter who actually does the task. Many risk factors may be used for screening; the critical issue is rapid and valid triage. Table 58.5 summarizes some commonly used risk factors for screening patients in acute and chronic care settings to find those at high risk of malnutrition who need further assessment. Diet-related risk factors for screening patients in these settings mostly involve signs of obviously inadequate intake or of difficulty in eating, since these require immediate action (80). Long-standing dietary imbalances, excesses, and obesity are less amenable to immediate remediation in acute care settings. The remaining items listed in Table 58.5 rely on proxies often associated with dietary inadequacy that are sometimes readily available on charts or computerized patient information systems, such as anthropometric indices; clinical observations and diagnoses likely to be associated with disrupted intake; abnormal absorption, metabolism, or output; or biochemical tests that are rou-

Table 58.5
Possible Risk Factors for Screening for Dietary Inadequacy in Acute and Chronic Healthcare Facilities

Characteristic	Examples
Signs of obviously inadequate intake or difficulty in eating	NPO status (patient is taking nothing by mouth)
	Scheduled for extensive tests which preclude food intake for more than a day
	Nausea, consistent food refusal
	Vomiting, diarrhea
	Fluid intake from all sources very low (e.g., less than 1 quart liquids per day)
	Unable to eat without assistance
	Frequent chart notes on patient's difficulty in eating or refusal to eat
	Comatose or rapidly altering states of consciousness limiting food intake
	Intake below estimated resting metabolism (or 800 kcal) for 5 or more days
	Not currently eating even if offered food, or eats less than two-thirds of food provided in institutional setting
	Dysphagia and swallowing problems, pica, rumination
	Chewing problems (edentulous, failure to use dentures, broken dentures, extensive oral and dental disease)
	Goes without food 1 or more days a month
	Eats less than 2 meals a day
	Failure to use vitamin mineral supplements (e.g., iron supplements, renal vitamins, etc.) or oral nutritional supplements when appropriately prescribed
	Frequent spells of illness or disability with no or very low intake prior to admission
	Physician orders for oral nutritional supplements, special enteral or parenteral feedings noted but not implemented
	Usually fails to eat one or more servings from each of the food groups on the USDA pyramid, basic four food groups, or some other simple food grouping system (i.e., milk and milk products, grains and cereals, fruits and vegetables, meat/poultry/fish/eggs and beans)
	High alcohol intake
	Following a physician-prescribed therapeutic diet
	Following an inappropriate, rigid therapeutic diet
	Following a self-imposed restrictive dietary regimen or other dietary practices
	Consuming a diet modified in consistency (pureed, liquid, etc.)
	Patient forgets to eat
	Special route of feeding (enteral, parenteral, mixed oral and special routes, or in process of being weaned from special routes to oral feedings)
Anthropometric indices of malnutrition	Body mass index (BMI) below 19 or above 30 in adults (148)
	Weight loss >2.5 kg since hospital admission
	Edema, dehydration
Clinical diagnosis	Fever, diarrhea, malabsorption
	Burn-fistula, draining abscess, or other condition increasing nutrient losses
	Major disease of the upper or lower gastrointestinal tract, obstruction, or surgery for these conditions
	Conditions requiring admission to medical, surgical, pediatric, or neonatal intensive care unit
	Advanced cancer, diabetic ketoacidosis
	Alcoholism, drug addiction
Biochemical indicators suggesting undernutrition	If available on computerized record; low serum albumin, hemoglobin, hematocrit
Functional indicators	Low activities of daily living (ADL) or instrumental activities of daily living (IADL)
Composite indicators	Composite prognostic index based on ADL deficits, number of comorbidities, clinical diagnosis of malnutrition, and low serum albumin predicted mortality and length of hospital stay satisfactorily; no single indicator is useful in critically ill patients (149)

tinely performed and available on all patients, which may be depressed in malnutrition.

Nutrition-related items that measure physical functional status (including the ability to feed oneself) are included in the widely used activities of daily living (ADL) instrument developed by Katz (81, 82) for institutionalized populations. Loss of the capacity to eat independently is associated with both morbidity and mortality in institutionalized populations (83). The instrumental activities of daily living (IADL) measures social function and the ability of individuals to continue to live independently in the community. It includes three food-related items: food preparation, shopping, and ability to use the telephone (84, 85). The ADL and IADL are useful in identifying both serious and moderate functional impairment that is missed in usual clinical assessments, but they are not sensitive enough to identify mild impairments (86, 87). A low ADL or IADL score does not necessarily suggest that the individual is malnourished, nor does it indicate that health status will improve with nutritional rehabilitation. Other measures of eating dependency have been developed for use in screening and assessing children with special developmental and health needs and patients with specific diseases.

The nonspecificity of existing scoring systems for identifying malnutrition has stimulated efforts to develop more specific nutritional screening tools over the past two decades. The earliest composite measures, such as the

Prognostic Nutrition Index (PNI), were made up of combinations of anthropometric, biochemical, and immunologic measures and were validated by examining later morbidity or mortality. Those who scored high on risk did have increased death rates, but high scores did not predict whether nutritional intervention would alter their prognosis. The PNI and similar scoring systems were not adopted for use in most clinical settings because they did not identify malnourished patients whose prognosis would benefit from nutrition interventions better than well-standardized clinical assessment by skilled professionals (88). Also some components of the indices were costly, difficult to collect, not obtained on many patients, or unavailable for several days after admission, and the scores were rarely included in hospital computerized clinical data systems.

Efforts have been devoted to developing simple screening tools based solely on questions to patients and other easy-to-obtain information to predict malnutrition, but none of these tools yet provide the specificity and sensitivity needed for a truly useful assessment battery (89). One effort is the Nutrition Screening Initiative. It initially focused on developing a consensus on nutritional risk and assessment factors for use among the elderly. However, most of the risk factors identified are also helpful in considering patients at nutritional risk at other ages.

To organize the information on characteristics predisposing to malnutrition in older Americans, the Nutrition Screening Initiative suggested the mnemonic DETERMINE, which represents the first letter in some of the most common risk factors for malnutrition and other types of ill health. These include *d*isease, *e*ating poorly, *t*ooth loss and swallowing difficulties, *e*conomic hardship, *r*educed social contact, *m*ultiple medications, *i*nvoluntary weight loss or gain, *n*eed for assistance in self care, and *e*lderly aged above 80. Recommendations are provided for subjective and objective risk factors and indicators for further assessment. The DETERMINE list (with the addition of another risk factor, *sedentary lifestyles and physical inactivity*) summarizes most of the major risk factors commonly associated with malnutrition and ill health in older Americans, and it may be useful for identifying such persons, particularly in community settings (90–92). Nutrition Screening Initiative manuals are available to assist those who wish to develop nutritional screening, assessment, and intervention programs. They provide specific recommendations for applications in acute and long-term care, outpatient medical office practices (93), and community settings (94).

Other simple screening batteries, such as the Mini Nutritional Assessment (MNA), are also available to assess the nutritional status of patients in acute care hospitals, nursing homes, and other institutional settings (95, 96).

At present, screening methods vary from one institution to the next; many may be used. For example, in the author's institution, patient height and weight (measured) are entered into the computerized medical record; body mass index (BMI) is calculated automatically and appears on the computer screen along with other patient information. In addition, such obvious risk factors as NPO (nothing by mouth) status, use of special enteral or parenteral feedings, and certain diagnoses or easily ascertainable characteristics that place the patient at risk are also used. On the basis of these criteria, patients are categorized as high, moderate, or low risk. Those at highest risk are given first priority for further assessment and attention. Any patient for whom an attending physician or a nurse requests assistance is also placed in the high-risk category.

Ongoing Nutritional Assessment. In acute care settings today, half or more of all patients require modified diets or special enteral and parenteral alimentation. Ongoing nutritional assessment is required by the JCAHO and is essential to ensure that nutritional interventions are linked to outcomes (97, 98). Clinical rounds with the health care team can be helpful in making initial assessments and in updating other providers about the admitted patient's status or progress.

The most appropriate dietary assessment method to use depends on the route of administration, patient diagnosis, health status, length of stay, dietary issues others on the health team may raise, and time available. For example, with acutely ill patients, little patient participation may be possible, and intakes and outputs may need to be relied upon; whereas, for chronically ill patients in skilled nursing facilities, the focus of assessment is on collecting data for nutritional care planning to achieve long-term quality of life and rehabilitation. Both retrospective methods (e.g., food frequencies or dietary recalls) and prospective methods (e.g., monitoring intakes and outputs or enteral and parenteral alimentation received) may be used under such circumstances. The initial chart note should concisely summarize the relevant aspects of the dietary assessment. It should clearly state any suggestions about the nutritional prescription and indicate that the dietitian is informed about the patient's status (99). Long handwritten notes are usually not read. The note should contain recommendations about changes in diet orders if these are called for, and it should be signed and dated. It is illegal to remove notes from the chart. Increasingly, summaries or reassessments of risk are included in computer databases to permit other professionals to scan relevant dietary issues easily.

After consultation with the physician and other members of the nutritional team, the dietitian is responsible for ensuring that a nutritional care plan is developed, implemented, and revised as needed. Such interventions must be cost-effective (100, 101).

Reassessment is in order whenever a patient's status or mode of alimentation changes and for any patient who remains in the hospital for more than a week or whose physician requests assistance. Follow-up notes should be concise and to the point; they may consist of no more than a single line stating that the patient is doing well and should continue on the same regimen.

Many patients leave the hospital on modified diets, on special routes of feeding, or before all of their diet-related problems are resolved. It is essential to provide a discharge dietary assessment and counseling. A timely warning system must be in place to allow the dietitian several hours before discharge to find an appropriate time to provide the needed counseling and instruction to the patient and family in an unhurried manner and to make appropriate arrangements for follow-up. It is unreasonable to assume that this can be done on a few minutes' notice as the patient is leaving. The dietitian and others on the health care team have the obligation to see that necessary dietary instructions are communicated to the patient, the referring health care provider, and any other organizations (such as home care companies, visiting nurse associations, community hospitals, or extended care facilities) that will be involved in aftercare. For patients who return to settings in which dietary assistance is unavailable, special attention must be paid to discharge planning.

It is especially important to document and communicate assessments and nutritional care plans for the many patients who require modified diets or special feeding routes after discharge. Written instructions to patients, their families, and the referring physician are helpful. Means of ensuring nutritional continuity of care, including electronic transmission of the results of nutritional assessment between acute care, outpatient, and community settings, are therefore essential.

Outpatient and Community Settings

In outpatient settings, dietitians usually do not have direct responsibility for providing appropriate diets. Rather, they counsel and educate patients and their families on how to implement necessary dietary modifications in their daily lives. They also provide consultation to other health care providers and serve as resources on nutritional care planning to optimize dietary and nutritional status. Traditionally, outpatient care mostly involved primary prevention and chronic disease control activities. In recent years, ambulatory practice has become increasingly more complex and demanding. It now includes the care of acutely and terminally ill persons and demands new skills.

In public health and community settings, the reasons for screening and assessment are more likely to involve primary prevention, health promotion, or education rather than developing nutritional care plans. Table 58.6 summarizes some recent measures used for these purposes. In community settings, self-reports and sociodemo-

Table 58.6
Risk Factors for Dietary Risk Used in Community Settings

Factor	Examples of Uses
Food insecurity	For homeless persons whose major sources of dietary intake are food obtained in shelters or soup kitchens, comparisons of the food groups provided by these sources vs. the USDA food pyramid guide and the number of meals eaten per day provided rough indicators of groups at risk for malnutrition (150); an indirect estimate of likely food insecurity at the community level to identify the characteristics of families at risk is the cost of the U.S. Department of Agriculture's Thrifty Food Plan market basket relative to food stamp allotments and costs and types of food available in area supermarkets (151); comparisons of costs of the Thrifty Food Plan to local food costs identify poor rural and urban communities possibly at risk for food insecurity (152)
Food insufficiency in household	Questionnaires to elderly receiving home-delivered meals in Great Britain (153); food sufficiency questions included in the National Center for Health Statistics' Third National Health and Nutrition Examination Survey (NHANES III) at the household level on perceived food sufficiency, the number of days per month on which there was no food or money to buy food, and reasons for such a lack of food; at the individual level seven specific questions about the frequency and reasons for going without food were asked along with a 24-hour dietary recall (154)
Composite score based on various factors associated with risk of mal- and undernutrition (DETERMINE checklist; see text)	Nutrition Screening Initiative DETERMINE checklist, an awareness tool to help identify older persons living in the community who are at risk for poor nutrition and health problems (155–157); evaluations to date using the checklist indicate that half of all elders score in the moderate to high ranges on the tool, suggesting it probably overidentifies potential nutritional and general health problems (158, 159); an unknown number of these individuals identified as at risk cannot be successfully treated with nutritional or other therapies, and the checklist has been criticized on these grounds (161); the checklist is sensitive, but not specific, so it reports too many false positives; also, many individuals do not understand the concept of risk, indicating the need for more educational efforts to accompany the checklist (162); intervention materials for remedying identified shortfalls in food intakes are available (163)
Dietary diversity and food variety	Omission of major food groups used as a measure of dietary quality found to be associated with poor dietary quality (164–166) and increased risk of various chronic degenerative diseases or mortality in large surveys (167, 168)
Dietary quality	The Diet Quality Index, a composite of eight food and nutrient-based recommendations for adequacy and moderation from the National Academy of Sciences was used to evaluate dietary trends in national surveys; over time, it has risen, indicating better dietary quality, but socioeconomic differences still exist (169); other diet-quality indices emphasize dietary adequacy based on intakes of food groups, nutrients, or both (170); they tend to be more highly associated with disease risk than are individual foods or nutrients
Fruit and vegetable consumption	Number of servings of fruits and vegetables is used as an index of dietary quality in this respect (171)

graphic factors must be relied on to a greater degree to infer malnutrition because the paraphernalia are lacking to carry out laboratory tests, anthropometric measurements, clinical examinations, or actual monitoring of intakes and outputs. Also, situational or general determinants of nutritional risk may be of greater interest. Rapid assessment procedures (RAPS) are early warning indices such as key infant feeding practices, anthropometric indicators, or deficiency diseases that are associated with poor nutritional status. These are already used in nutritional surveillance activities in developing countries (102). Similar indicators are now being developed in this country. Table 58.7 presents some new dietary assessment methods for different groups that are suitable for community settings.

DESIGNING DIETARY ASSESSMENT STUDIES

Dietary assessment is becoming increasingly important in clinical trials and epidemiologic studies. The reader is referred to the 8th edition of this textbook and to other texts that deal with these issues in greater detail.

Dietary assessment methods differ in the ease with which representative samples of intake can be obtained. Representativeness of the study population, the period under study, and the heterogeneity of food habits in the population are important considerations in drawing samples for study. Dietary methods also differ in their validity and reliability, and thus in their potential uses.

Validity. Validity is the degree to which a method measures what it claims to measure. Validity is affected the most by bias (systematic errors) and to a lesser extent by random response errors. Estimates of validity are needed so that suitable corrections in analysis can be made to account for errors, and comparisons can be made to other studies (103, 104).

Guidelines for validating methods for estimating habitual diets have been proposed (105). The most common validation technique used is "calibration," or estimation of concurrent validity; this involves evaluating the test dietary method against a "gold standard" reference method thought to be particularly accurate and precise (106). These are important to carry out since the relationships between methods differ from one population to another (107). It is difficult to assess the absolute validity of dietary methods because diet is constantly changing, the very act of observing often alters intakes, and the reference standard itself may be flawed. Neither the test method nor the reference method may reflect true intake levels. In actuality, because subjective response errors and bias are likely to be present in both methods, concurrent validity really only measures apparent validity; it does not tell whether the assessment method is producing the correct answer, only that it is producing the same answer.

Lately, efforts have been made to obtain better estimates of validity that eliminate this subjective element. One method is surreptitious weighing or observation of food intakes at the same time that the individual keeps records. Biochemical markers to validate intakes of some nutrients are now available, including doubly labeled water to estimate energy intake. In general, energy intakes are underestimated, and the bias is greatest in those reporting the lowest intakes (108, 109). Calculations of predicted versus actual energy intake, using estimates of resting metabolism and a coefficient for physical activity, show differential reporting bias by those who are heavier and less well educated, especially among women (110). Comparisons of energy intakes with weight changes may also be helpful. Urinary nitrogen appearance (UNA) is used as a proxy for protein intakes (111, 112). However, it cannot be considered a perfect reference standard since it is not accurate if urine collections are incomplete, if the individual is in a catabolic state, or if kidney function is poor and the kidney secretes nitrogen into the urine. There are also sex differences between UNA and recalls (113). The normalized protein catabolic rate (nPCR) is a similar biochemical index of protein catabolism that is

Table 58.7
Risk Factors for Dietary Risk Used in Community Settings

Group	Examples of questionnaires
Pregnant women	Quick assessment methods are available (172)
Lactating women	Various methods used in national evaluations (173, 174)
Infants	
Preschool children	
School children	Child reporting of 24-hour recalls by telephone and using tape recorders were satisfactory when compared to personal monitoring and documentation of food frequencies and nutrient intakes (175); serial 24-hour recalls have also been used (176); for groups, fruit and vegetable frequency questionnaires, 175-item food-frequency questionnaire (177) exhibited low correlation with dietary records; other food frequencies (178, 179) were higher compared with food records; 24-hour recalls used successfully in two large surveys of schoolchildren's diets (180, 181); unclear if concept of dietary pattern underlying food frequencies is understood at early school ages, although children are aware of what they eat (182)
Adolescents	Youth Adolescent Questionnaire (YAQ) (183, 184) is a reliable semiquantitative food-frequency questionnaire that compares well with three 24-hour recalls; 24-hour recalls used successfully to describe children's diets in grades 1–12 (185); food-frequency questionnaire for Norwegian adolescents correlated well with 7-day records and was reliable, ranking most nutrients (186)
Elderly	Semiquantitative food-frequency questionnaire for elderly correlated well with dietary histories (187)

obtained from kinetic modeling to provide estimates of protein intake in hemodialysis patients (114).

Reproducibility. Reproducibility is the degree to which the method gives the same results when it is used repeatedly in the same situation. It is affected most seriously by random response errors and within-person variation in food intake. Observer training and standardized techniques can reduce random response errors. Test-retest reliability is commonly used to measure reproducibility. Larger numbers of observations can improve accuracy (115).

Causes and Control of Variation between Actual and Measured Intake

Table 58.8 summarizes the major sources of error that account for the differences between actual and measured diets, and likely vulnerabilities of each dietary assessment method. These problems and some ways to control them are described in greater depth elsewhere.

Population Sampling Errors and Biases

Differences between actual and measured intakes that are caused by unrepresentative study population or days of intake sampled can be partially controlled with good study design. The population studied must be representative of the reference population and unbiased in physical, environmental, or other significant ways that threaten inference. Population sampling error is controlled by an appropriate sampling design that selects individuals who are representative of the larger population, with appropriate substitutions for those who fail to volunteer, who drop out, or who are uncooperative.

Choice of an atypical period of observation limits generalization of measured intakes to usual actual intakes. Systematic variability within individuals may be due to fluctuations from weekday to weekend, season to season, sick and well days, or "dieting" and nondieting days. In clinical trials (116), intakes on reporting days often differ in important ways from typical diets. To avoid sampling bias, typical fluctuations in intake patterns must be identified. Then, a suitable sampling design and weighting system can be developed so that each major source of illness, event, or time-related variability is represented appropriately.

Heterogeneity of food intakes is considerable from day to day in affluent Western countries, further complicating sampling of typical intakes. Variation within individuals in their food intake consists of day-to-day variations not accounted for in the design of the study, and other random measurement errors that cannot be disentangled from true individual biologic variation. Within-individual variation is usually much greater than the variation between individuals, and when it is high, reproducibility decreases (117). The size of the intraindividual variability in intake of a nutrient depends on the food patterns of the individual being studied, the food constituent being assessed, the time frame of interest, and the dietary assessment technique used. Within-individual variability is not constant; it varies depending on the population studied and the assessment method used. Intraindividual variability should be assessed directly when planning studies; rough estimates of its usual size among adults (118), young infants, and other special populations are available (118–120). The stability of estimates of usual intake can be enhanced by sampling greater numbers of days for nutrients or individuals exhibiting high within-person variability.

Between-person variation is that existing between people in their habitual food pattern. It varies for each nutri-

Table 58.8
Sources of Error in Dietary Assessment Methods

Method	Duplicate Portion	Weighed Records	Estimated Record	24-Hour Recall	Diet History	Food Frequency
Population sampling error and bias	+	+	+	+	+	+
Response bias	?	?	?	?	?	?
Response errors						
Omitting foods	–	?	?	+	+	+
Adding foods	–	–	–	+	+	+
Estimate of weight of foods	–	–	+	+	+	+
Estimate of servings	–	–	–	–	+	+
Estimate of food consumption frequency	–	–	–	–	+	+
Day-to-day variation	+	+	+	+	–	–
Changes in diet	+	+	?	–	–	–
Coding errors	–	+	+	+	+	+
Errors in conversion of foods to nutrients						
Food-sampling errors	+	–	–	–	–	–
Direct analysis	+	–	–	–	–	–
Food composition tables	–	+	+	+	+	+
Nutrient database values used for groups of foods	–	–	–	–	–	+
Dietary analysis computational errors	+	+	+	+	+	+

Adapted from Bingham SA. Dietary assessment of individuals: methods, accuracy, new techniques and recommendations. Nutr Abstr Rev 1987; 57:709, and Bingham SA, Nelson M, Paul AA, et al. Methods for data collection at the individual level. In: Manual on methodology for food consumption studies. Cameron ME, Van Staveren WA, eds. Oxford: Oxford University Press, 1988;98.

ent and increases with the heterogeneity of the population being studied. Within some populations, systematic but unrecognized alterations in food intake may be present in certain subgroups. These include dieting, bingeing, and periodic low intakes due to lack of money or illness. Large between-person variation in habitual food intake increases the difficulty of achieving representativeness in drawing samples from the population and increases the sample size needed. Between-person variation can be reduced by identifying causes of heterogeneity and controlling them by stratifying in sample selection or in later analysis.

Duration of Data Collection

When nutrients are of concern, intra- and interindividual variation in intakes of each nutrient determine the number of days needed to describe intakes. If these are known, the measurement periods necessary to achieve different levels of accuracy can be calculated. The number of individuals or groups to be studied also influences the number of days data must be collected to get satisfactory accuracy. Several days' worth of intakes are generally necessary to characterize usual nutrient intakes reliably. For example, to classify nutrient intakes of individuals reliably into tertiles, a week's worth of dietary records suffices for some nutrients, but for nutrients with very large intraindividual variations in intakes (e.g., vitamin A, riboflavin, iron, and cholesterol), a longer time is needed. For some nutrients, so many days of observation are needed and respondent burden is so great that the study is not feasible. Estimates of how long data must be collected that are gleaned from the literature may be helpful in preliminary planning. However, empirical evidence on the actual population to be measured is also necessary because within-individual variation is not fixed; it varies from one study to another (121).

Response Errors and Bias

Most people are only vaguely aware of what they eat. Without instruction, food records and recalls collected from people will lack sufficient detail to be useful for most research purposes. Random reporting errors include memory failures that lead to omissions and additions of foods. They arise from the type of diet eaten, assessment method used, ability and training of the respondent, and the skill of the interviewer. Simple and stereotypical intakes are probably recalled best. Frequency of consumption errors (times per day and servings per time) are common with all methods (122). Errors in estimating the portion size are also frequent (123). When foods are not actually weighed, these are very large—as high as 50% for foods and 20% for nutrients. The quality of reporting can be improved by training respondents and by the use of probes, memory aids, food models, and cross checks on reports of intakes, but retraining is needed after about a month (124).

Response biases constitute serious threats to validity. With prospective record keeping individuals may consciously or unconsciously eat differently on reporting days, either to make recording easier or to conform to what they perceive is an appropriate food intake. This bias is common in clinical trials among dietary intervention groups; individuals "eat to the study objectives" on recording days. Retrospective recalls of previous diet are also often inaccurate. Because current diet exerts a strong influence on recollection of past diet, faulty memory may be involved. Also, with both prospective and retrospective methods, respondents may wish to provide intakes they regard as "good" eating habits that will please the interviewer (127).

Coding Errors

Coding dietary records validly and reliably requires a record with enough detail to code and coder training. The best practice is to obtain adequate information to begin with by training both interviewers and respondents so that a complete record is obtained that provides sufficient detail on foods that are major sources of the target nutrients. Whenever possible, additional information needed on portion sizes, brands, and the like should be obtained directly from the respondent, the cook, or someone else who is familiar with the respondent's eating habits. Probing should concentrate especially on foods that are consumed frequently or very rich sources of the target nutrient. Information on composition from recipes (which vary greatly in ingredients), restaurants, or manufacturers may also be helpful for key items. Supplement and condiment intakes may also be important for some nutrients. Checking records and further probing the respondent prior to coding helps resolve some of the ambiguities (130, 131). When respondents describe foods vaguely or illegibly, many plausible food-coding alternatives exist, and errors are large, especially when each coder interprets the food description differently. Even when high-quality records have been received, well-standardized decision rules and coding methods for handling unknowns and ambiguous items are necessary. Allowing coders to use their own discretion introduces error.

Precoded interview schedules such as food frequency and semiquantitative food frequency questionnaires also need to be screened and checked since some respondents misunderstand instructions.

Disaggregating Foods into Nutrients

All dietary assessment methods involve conversion of foods into nutrients or other constituents. The process involves many problems and assumptions that can lead to substantial errors in estimating intakes (125, 126). Generally, a food composition table or computerized nutrient database is used that summarizes existing chemical analyses of the foods in question. Specialized databases with complete values and extensive detail on certain constituents are available for some purposes.

Errors in Sampling Foods

Food composition values are approximations, not absolute and immutable quantities with the accuracy of atomic weight determinations. Errors due to food composition include true random variability in composition of the individual food item and biased food composition data owing to inadequate sampling. However, some error is inevitable, since the nutrient composition of food is inherently variable. Samples of genetically similar foods differ in their composition because of inherent biologic variability. In addition, environmental factors such as the soil in which food plants are grown, the feed consumed by livestock, postharvest or postslaughter handling, time or circumstances of storage, and the effects of light, heat, humidity, and other conditions may alter nutrient composition. Food processing and inappropriate choices of ingredients in recipe or composite foods introduce additional variability. The effects of these factors vary from one food constituent to another. The best way to avoid these errors is to have an individual who is familiar with food preparation use a nutrient database or food table that is as representative of the food supply as possible and that provides complete data or reasonable imputed values when direct analyses are not available.

For calculations of nutrient intakes to be valid, they must be based on food samples that represent the food supply. The information in some food composition databases includes samples of convenience or lacks documentation for values provided, making the data of uncertain quality. Content and comprehensiveness also differ between databases. The USDA has the largest and most comprehensive program for collecting food composition data in the world and reports average values representing the nutrient composition of foods available in the United States (127). Information on food composition is best when it is based on samples drawn to be representative (as is done in the USDA program) rather than from samples of convenience. Errors may occur when nutrient values are compiled from several sources or laboratories to develop single representative values used in food tables.

Keeping food composition tables up to date is a continuing struggle. As the food supply, formulations, and processing techniques change, new analyses are required to update nutrient composition values. USDA strives constantly to upgrade the quality, quantity, and completeness of information and its documentation. The number of foods has quintupled in USDA tables of food composition over the past three decades, and the number of nutrients for which values are available has nearly doubled (128). Methods of determining many nutrients and other constituents in foods are still being developed, and data are still sparse for many items of interest, such as dietary fiber, specific fatty acids, and candidate nutrients such as glutamine, phytochemicals, and other biologic substances thought to be significant to health. Demand is currently outstripping the agency's economic resources and analytic capability; more research is needed in this important area.

Users need to be aware of the limitations of food tables. For example, recently vitamin D toxicity was discovered among a population obtaining milk from a dairy that was overfortifying its products with the vitamin; use of food composition tables did not reveal the cause, and direct analysis of the suspected food was required.

Errors in Direct Chemical Analysis

For research purposes, values are sometimes obtained from direct chemical analysis of duplicate food samples to achieve greater precision or to provide information on food constituents that is unavailable in standard tables. Representative samples of foods in the total diets of the American population as determined from dietary surveys are collected in conjunction with chemical analysis to determine dietary intakes of selected pesticides, industrial chemicals, and radionuclides in diets (129). Military rations have also been chemically analyzed (130). Potential errors include both sampling errors in assuming that the foods chosen for analysis are representative of the entire food supply, and laboratory errors in the chemical analyses or biologic assays themselves.

Calculated and chemically analyzed values for individual foods rarely agree perfectly. For most nutrients, comparisons between calculated and chemically analyzed values for total diets are closer than those for individual foods. In general, calculated and analyzed values for protein are closest. Values for total calories, carbohydrate, and fat are also fairly reliable, although the fat content of meat and cooking, serving, and eating practices vary a good deal and may increase errors. In contrast, the vitamin and mineral content of foods, especially that of the trace elements, is subject to much greater variation, some of which is environmentally determined or affected by food preparation. Therefore, the differences between calculated and analyzed values are likely to be much greater for these nutrients (131).

Food Composition Tables

Calculations of nutrient intakes must be based on foods as actually eaten to be accurate. Once the food is purchased, food preparation, trimming, and cooking techniques may further alter nutrient content. Food composition databases must therefore provide values for processed and prepared as well as raw foods, with as much detail as possible to be helpful for most purposes.

Many different food composition tables and databases are in use in the United States today. They vary in the timeliness, number, completeness, and specificity of the information they provide on food constituents. The major source of data on food composition in all of them is that compiled by the USDA and other government agencies. However, USDA data frequently do not identify a source or brand name for prepared foods, some proprietary food manufacturer data are not included, reports of additional research on food composition since publication of the tables may not be included, not all constituents of possible interest are necessarily covered, and data availability is limited to published tables of food composition or data tapes. For these reasons, other food tables that provide information on these issues have come into common use for many purposes (132).

Some databases are in the public domain (e.g., USDA databases). Others are proprietary and for sale commercially. Publications of the National Nutrient Database Conferences provide information on these newer systems. The advantages of the proprietary databases are that they often are produced in microcomputer-usable versions; are easy to use; provide additional values for special foods, brands of foods, and vitamin-mineral supplements, oral nutritional supplements and parenteral and enteral formulas (133); and include computer programs for manipulating and presenting the results of the analysis in a variety of ways. However, these databases differ in the criteria used to assess food quality, the composition data they accept, the number of items or nutrients included, timeliness of data updates, descriptions of the source of the data, timeliness of values, ease of use, and many other respects. Systems for reviewing databases are available (134).

Composition information on foods eaten in other countries is available from the International Network of Food and Data Systems (INFOODS), which has recently produced an international directory of food composition tables (126). Differences exist between values obtained from nutrient databases among industrialized countries and even within countries at different times (133). Some of these differences are real, and others are due to methodological and reporting conventions (136). Therefore, caution is indicated when information from various food tables is combined. Although the completeness of information on food composition leaves much to be desired in the United States and other highly industrialized countries, in developing countries, the information available on food composition is considerably more fragmentary and incomplete.

Missing Values. A major difficulty with food tables for diet assessment purposes is missing values, especially for certain nutrients, phytochemicals such as fiber or carotenoids, toxicants, environmental contaminants, and intentional food additives. New food products are being developed, and the number of food components of potential interest is immense. Few analyses are available for many components, and for others, food analytic methods are not yet developed. Thus, complete information on each component of each food consumed in this country is unlikely to ever be available.

When data are lacking, imputed values, or "best estimates," of nutrients in similar foods can be used. Botanic and zoologic taxonomy and knowledge of food processing techniques may also be helpful in establishing the presence of some constituents and possibly produce rough quantitative estimates. However, when chemical analyses are lacking, values are only approximations, and additional assumptions and errors are introduced. Good estimates can minimize errors. Pennington (137) has developed tables of imputed values for many nutrients. Estimation of values for other food constituents is more difficult. Consensus on standard protocols for imputation will facilitate comparisons between studies. Finally, the quality and quantity of the available food-composition data may be so inadequate for many of the less-studied food constituents (e.g., biotin, vitamin K, or the flavonoids) that accurate calculations of their intakes are impossible, and only rough estimates can be obtained (137).

Bioavailability. Intakes calculated from food composition databases do not necessarily represent those actually biologically available and absorbed from the gut. Most databases include adjustments to account for usual net absorption and utilization for energy-providing nutrients, so that biologically available nutrients can be calculated directly. However, if disease or other causes of malabsorption are present, these assumptions may need adjustment. For minerals and vitamins, estimates of net bioavailability are not incorporated in food tables because so many constituents of foods may promote or inhibit absorption; separate calculations may be necessary.

Errors in Nutrient Databases Used in Food-Frequency Questionnaires

The computerized nutrient databases used to analyze semiquantitative food-frequency questionnaires usually consist of average values for different categories or groups of foods derived from the intake of a U.S. reference population. Alternatively, foods contributing to variation among individuals are used to generate the lists. These food tables are vulnerable to errors due to differences (compared with the reference group) in frequency of consumption (which is especially important), changes in the nutrient composition of individual foods, and differences in portion size of various foods within the food groups or categories. Also, the use of closed-ended rather than open-ended questions on some food-frequency questionnaires introduces further errors (138). Because they are based on American foods and consumption patterns, these food tables are obviously inappropriate for use without adaptation in other countries. Because the food supply and consumption patterns are constantly changing, even within categories, errors arise if these questionnaires are not updated periodically. Before they are used in large-scale studies, validation is necessary. Finally, defaults and imputations may be incorrect or invalid.

Computational Errors Using Nutrient Analysis Systems

Computerized nutrient analysis systems greatly reduce inadvertent computational errors and minimize the otherwise onerous task of calculation (139). However, computerized dietary analysis systems are only computational aids, not panaceas. They cannot cope with or compensate for careless data collection, coding, or interpretation of results. Moreover, programming mistakes or assumptions in some programs introduce errors. Errors in some nutrient analysis systems are so large that they obscure the effects of treatments or changes in intakes. Differences in calculated intakes exist between systems, even when the same records are analyzed (140). Comparison across studies is facilitated by standardization. Not only the disparate nutrient databases but also assumptions in calculations give rise to these errors. Assumptions include differences in portion sizes and weight/portion equivalence, factors for conversion from raw to prepared foods, listings of ingredients in recipe foods, values provided for nutrient-fortified foods, estimates of bioavailability of nutrients, and the defaults or imputed values used. A systematic method for reviewing nutrient database capabilities has been devised (141, 142). It should be used to test programs before a dietary analysis system is chosen. It is important to know the strengths and limitations of the programs to avoid misinterpreting their outputs (143).

RESEARCH NEEDS

The growth of interest in assessing upper safe levels of nutrient intakes has implications for dietary assessment. Vitamin, mineral, botanic, herbal, and oral nutrient supplements provide highly concentrated sources of nutrients and other substances, and thus use of such substances must be an integral part of dietary assessment. Better methods for obtaining such information and tables of supplement composition are sorely needed.

Assessing intakes of nonnutrient substances in food such as flavonoids that have biologic activity that may be relevant to health is another challenge (144). Tables of food composition of these substances are just becoming available; the major limitation is the lack of resources to perform analyses (145). Adequate food intake data are also needed for more accurate estimations of potential exposures to environmental contaminants such as radionuclides or pesticide residues and intentional or unintentional food additives (146).

Most computerized nutrient analysis programs provide outputs expressed as total intakes of nutrients per meal or per day; outputs expressed by groups of foods, dietary patterns, or food grouping systems are needed as well.

Finally, brief nutritional screening and assessment methods are needed for specific clinical and educational purposes.

ACKNOWLEDGMENTS

Partial support for the preparation of this manuscript was furnished by a grant from the Gerber Foundation and through the following grants, which were subcontracts to New England Medical Center: 5R25-CA49612-02 from the National Cancer Institute and grant U01HL47098 from the National Heart, Lung, and Blood Institute, National Institutes of Health. This paper has also been funded at least in part from federal funds from the United States Department of Agriculture (USDA), Agricultural Research Service, under contract 533K065-10. The contents of this publication do not necessarily reflect the views or policies of USDA.

REFERENCES

1. Grivetti LE. Nutr Today 1991;26:13–24.
2. Medlin C, Skinner JD. J Am Diet Assoc 1988;88:1250–7.
3. Gibson RS. Principles of nutritional assessment. New York: Oxford University Press, 1990.
4. Looker AC, Gunter EW, Johnson CL. Nutr Rev 1995;53(9): 246–54.
5. Block G, Hartman AM, Dresser CM, et al. Am J Epidemiol 1986;124:453.
6. Tarasuk V. Nutritional epidemiology. In: Zeigler EE, Filer LJ, eds. Present knowledge in nutrition. 7th ed. Washington, DC: International Life Sciences Institute, 1996;508–16.
7. Anderson SA, ed. Guidelines for use of dietary intake data. Bethesda, MD: Life Sciences Research Office, Federation of American Societies for Experimental Biology, 1986.
8. Calvo MS, Park YK. J Nutr 1996;126 (4 Suppl):68S–80S.
9. Pao EM, Cypel YS. Estimation of dietary intake. In: Brown ML, ed. Present knowledge in nutrition. Washington, DC: International Life Sciences Institute, 1990;399–406.
10. Bingham S. Nutr Abstr Rev 1987;57:707–42.
11. Basiotis PP, Thomas RG, Kelsay JL, et al. Am J Clin Nutr 1989;50:448–53.
12. Borelli R, Cole TJ, DiBiase G, et al. Eur J Clin Nutr 1989;43: 453–63.
13. Willett W. Nutritional epidemiology. New York: Oxford University Press, 1990.
14. Black AE. Appl Nutr 1982;36A:85–94.
15. Burk MC, Pao EM. Home economics research report no. 40. Washington, DC: United States Department of Agriculture, 1976.
16. Liu K, Stamler J, Dyer A, et al. J Chronic Dis 1978;31:399–418.
17. Walker AM, Blettner M. Am J Epidemiol 1985;121:783–800.
18. Harlan L, Block G. Epidemiology 1990;1:224–31.
19. Charney P. Nutr Clin Pract 1995;10(4):131–9.
20. Joint Commission on Accreditation of Hospitals and Health Care Organizations. Accreditation manual for hospitals. Oakbrook Terrace, IL: Joint Commission on Accreditation of Health care Organizations, 1995.
21. Soltesz KS, Price JH, Johnson LW. Arch Fam Med 1995;4: 589–93.
22. U.S. Public Health Service. Put prevention into practice. Washington, DC: U.S. Government Printing Office, 1994.
23. Nutrition Screening Initiative. Managed Care Med 1995; S1–S18.
24. Field MJ, Lohr KN, eds. Institute of Medicine Committee on

Clinical Practice Guidelines. Guidelines for clinical practice: from development to use. Washington, DC: National Academy Press, 1992.
25. Glanz K, Tziraki C, Albright CL, et al. J Gen Int Med 1995;10(2):89–92.
26. Dwyer JT. Concept of nutritional status and its measurement. In: Himes JH, ed. Anthropometric assessment of nutritional status. New York: Wiley-Liss, 1991;5–28.
27. U.S. Preventive Services Task Force. Guide to clinical preventive services: an assessment of the effectiveness of 169 interventions. Report of the U.S. Preventive Services Task Force. Philadelphia: Williams & Wilkins, 1989;xxix–xxxii.
28. Thompson FE, Byers T, Kohlmeier L. J Nutr 1994;124(11S): 2245S–317S.
29. Pao EM, Cypel YS. Estimation of dietary intake. In: Zeigler EE, Filer LJ, eds. Present knowledge in nutrition. 7th ed. Washington, DC: International Life Sciences Institute Nutrition Foundation, 1996;498–505.
30. Sempos CT, Briefel RR, Johnson C, et al. Vital Health Stat 1992;4(27):85–90.
31. Thompson F, Moler JE, Freedman Clifford C, Willett WC. Dietary assessment calibration/validation studies register: a status report. Bethesda, MD: National Cancer Institute, 1994.
32. Jain M, Howe GR, Rohan T. Am J Epidemiol 1996;143(9): 953–60.
33. Cameron ME, Van Staveren WA, eds. Manual on methodology for food consumption studies. Oxford: Oxford University Press, 1988.
34. Block G, Hartman AM. Dietary methods. In: Moon TE, Micozzi M, eds. Nutrition and cancer prevention. New York: Marcel Dekker, 1989;159–81.
35. Dwyer JT, Krall EA, Coleman KA. Nutr Res 1988;8:829–41.
36. Krall EA, Dwyer JT. J Am Diet Assoc 1987;87:1374–7.
37. Wu ML, Whittemore AS, Jung DL. Am J Epidemiol 1986; 124:326–35.
38. Van Staveren WA, West CE, Hoffmans MD, et al. Am J Epidemiol 1986;123:884–93.
39. Mackerras E. Interpreting dietary data. Sydney: Sydney Department of Public Health, University of Sydney, 1990.
40. Block G. Am J Epidemiol 1982;115:492–505.
41. Willett WC, Reynolds RD, Cottrell-Hoehner S, et al. J Am Diet Assoc 1987;87:43–7.
42. Dwyer JT, Gardner J, Halvorsen K, et al. Am J Epidemiol 1989; 130:1033–46.
43. Bakkum A, Bloemberg B, Van Staveren WA, et al. Nutr Cancer 1988;11:41–53.
44. Food and Nutrition Board, National Research Council. Nutrient adequacy. Assessment using food consumption surveys. Washington, DC: National Academy Press, 1986.
45. Buzzard IM, Faucett CL, Jeffery RW, et al. J Am Diet Assoc 1996;96:574–9.
46. Block G, Dresser CM, Hartman AM, et al. Am J Epidemiol 1985;122:13–40.
47. Pao EM, Flemming KH, Guenther DM, et al. Human Nutrition Information Service, Home economics research report no. 49. Washington, DC: United States Department of Agriculture, 1982.
48. Wilson P, Horwath C. Eur J Clin Nutr 1996;50(4):220–8.
49. Cooper GS, Busby MG, Fairchild AP. Ann Epidemiol 1995;5(6):473–7.
50. Mark SD, Thomas DG, Decarli A. Am J Epidemiol 1996; 143(5):514–21.
51. Smith CJ, Nelson RG, Hardy SA, et al. J Am Diet Assoc 1996;96(8):778–84.
52. Jain M. J Am Diet Assoc 1989;89:1647–52.
53. Willett WC, Stampfer MJ, Underwood BA, et al. Am J Clin Nutr 1983;38:631–69.
54. Willett WC, Sampson L, Stampfer MJ, et al. Am J Epidemiol 1985;122:51–65.
55. Block G, Hartman AM, Dresser CM, et al. Am J Epidemiol 1986;124:453–69.
56. National Cancer Institute, Division of Cancer Prevention and Control. Health habits and history questionnaire. Bethesda, MD: National Institutes of Health, 1985.
57. Block G, Hartman AM, Naughton D. Epidemiology 1990;1: 58–64.
58. Block G, Woods M, Potosky A, et al. J Clin Epidemiol 1990;43:1327–35.
59. Rimm EB, Ascherio A, Giovannucci E, et al. JAMA 1996;275: 447–51.
60. Patterson RE, Kristal AR, Coates RJ, et al. J Am Diet Assoc 1996;96(7):670–9.
61. Enger SM, Longnecker MP, Shikany JM, et al. Cancer Epidemiol Biomarkers Prev 1995;4(3):201–5.
62. Suitor CJW, Gardner J, Willett WC. J Am Diet Assoc 1989;889: 1786–94.
63. Hankin JH. Am J Clin Nutr 1989;(5):1121–7.
64. Hankin JH, Kolonel LN, Hinds WW. J Natl Cancer Inst 1984;73:1417–22.
65. Kushi LH, Fee RM, Sellers TA, et al. Am J Epidemiol 1996;144: 165–74.
66. Potosky AL, Block G, Hartman AM. J Am Diet Assoc 1990;90: 810–3.
67. Black AE. Pitfalls in dietary assessment. In: Howard AN, Baird IM, eds. Recent advances in clinical nutrition. London: John Libbey, 1981.
68. Fehily AM. Hum Nutr Appl Nutr 1983;37:419–25.
69. Howat PM, Mohan R, Champagne C, et al. J Am Diet Assoc 1994;94:169–73.
70. Millen Posner BE, Martin-Munley SS, Smigelski C, et al. Epidemiology 1992;3(2):171–7.
71. Beaton GH, Milner J, Corey P, et al. Am J Clin Nutr 1979;32:2546–59.
72. Kaaks R, Riboli E, Van Staveren W. Am J Epidemiol 1995;142(5):548–56.
73. Carroll RJ, Freedman LS, Hartman AM. Am J Epidemiol 1996;143(4):392–404.
74. Gable CB. Am J Epidemiol 1990;121:381–94.
75. Harris T, Woteki C, Briefel RR, Kleinman JC. Am J Clin Nutr 1989;50:1145–9.
76. Mertz W, Tsui JC, Judd JT, et al. Am J Clin Nutr 1991;54: 291–5.
77. Andersson I, Rossner S. J Am Diet Assoc 1996;96(7):686–92.
78. Wesley JR. Nutr Clin Pract 1995;10(6):219–28.
79. Reilly H. Br J Nurs 1996;5(1):18, 20–4.
80. Dwyer JT, Roy J. Diet therapy. In: Wilson JD, Braunwald E, Isselbacher KJ, et al., eds. Harrison's principles of internal medicine. 12th ed. New York: McGraw Hill, 1990;420–7.
81. Katz S, Akpom CA. Int J Health Serv 1976;6:493–508.
82. Katz S, Ford AB, Moskowitz RW, et al. JAMA 1963;185:914–9.
83. Siebens H, Trupe E, Siebens A, et al. J Am Geriatr Soc 1986;34:192–8.
84. Katz S. J Am Geriatr Soc 1983;31:(12):721–7.
85. Katz S, Stroud MW. J Am Geriatr Soc 1989;37:267–71.
86. Pinholt EM, Kroenke K, Hanley JF, et al. Arch Intern Med 1987;147:484–8.
87. Miller DK, Morley JE, Rubenstein LZ, et al. J Am Geriatr Soc 1990;38:645–51.

88. Detsky AS, Baker JP, Mendelson RA, et al. JPEN J Parenter Enteral Nutr 1984;8:153–9.
89. Watson RR, Mohs ME. Adult protein-calorie malnutrition in developing countries. In: Watson RR, ed. CRC handbook of nutrition in the aged. Boca Raton, FL: CRC Press, 1985; 57–73.
90. Nutrition Screening Initiative. Nutrition screening manual for professionals caring for older Americans. Maple Grove, MN: Nutrition Screening Initiative, 1992.
91. Nutrition Screening Initiative. Nutrition interventions manual for professionals caring for older Americans. Washington, DC: Nutrition Screening Initiative, 1993.
92. Nutrition Screening Initiative Technical Review Committee: Barrocas A, Blackburn GL, Chernoff R, et al. J Am Diet Assoc 1995;95:647–8.
93. Nutrition Screening Initiative. Incorporating nutrition screening and interventions into medical practice: a monograph for physicians. Washington, DC: Nutrition Screening Initiative, 1994.
94. Gallagher Allred CR. Implementing nutrition screening and intervention strategies. Washington, DC: Nutrition Screening Initiative, 1993.
95. Guigoz Y, Vellas BJ, Garry PJ. Nutr Rev 1996;54:S59–S64.
96. Vellas BJ, Guigoz Y, Garry PJ, et al. Nutritional assessment as part of the geriatric evaluation: the Mini Nutritional Assessment. In: Vellas BJ, Garry PJ, Albanede JL, eds. The Mini Nutritional Assessment (MNA) facts and research in gerontology (supplement nutrition). New York: Serdi Publishing, 1994;11–32.
97. Morrison Health Care. MHC policies and procedures manual: cross-reference for Joint Commission 1996 standards. Atlanta, GA: Morrison Health Care, 1995.
98. Abbott Laboratories. Nutrition intervention and patient outcomes: a self-study manual. Columbus, OH: Ross Products Division, 1995.
99. Peterson AE, Maryniuk MD. Diabetes Educ 1996; 22(3):205–6, 209–10.
100. Splett PL. The practitioner's guide to cost-effectiveness analysis of nutrition interventions. Maternal and Child Health Interorganizational Nutrition Group (MCHING), U.S. Department of Health and Human Services, Public Health Service, Health Resources and Services Administration, 1996.
101. Disbrow DD. J Am Diet Assoc 1989;89(4 Suppl).
102. Scrimshaw NS, Gleason GR, eds. RAP: rapid assessment procedures: qualitative methodologies for planning and evaluation of health related programmes. Boston: International Nutrition Foundation for Developing Countries (INFDC), 1992.
103. Block G, Hartman AM. Am J Clin Nutr 1989;50:1133–8.
104. Bazzarre TL, Klwiner SM, Litchford MD. J Am Coll Nutr 1990;9:136–42.
105. Garrow JS. Eur J Clin Nutr 1995;49(4):231–2.
106. Lee HH, McGuire V, Boyd NF. J Clin Epidemiol 1989;42: 269–79.
107. Stram DO, Longnecker MP, Shames L, et al. Am J Epidemiol 1995;142(3):353–62.
108. Livingstone MB. Br J Biomed Sci 1995;52(1):58–67.
109. Schoeller DA. Nutr Rev 1990;48:373–9.
110. Klesges RC, Eck LH, Ray JQ. J Consult Clin Psychol 1995;63(3):438–44.
111. Bingham SA, Cummings JH. Am J Clin Nutr 1985;42:1276–89.
112. Hulten B, Bengtsson C, Isaksson B. Eur J Clin Nutr 1990;44:169–74.
113. Kahn HA, Whelton PK, Appel LJ, et al. Ann Epidemiol 1995;5(6):484–9.
114. Maroni BJ. Requirements for protein, calories, and fat in the predialysis patient. In: Mitch WE, Klahr S, eds. Nutrition and the kidney. 2nd ed. Boston: Little, Brown, 1993;185–212.
115. El Lozy M. J Chronic Dis 1983;36:237–49.
116. Ballard-Barbash R, Graubard I, Krebs-Smith SM, et al. Eur J Clin Nutr 1996;50(2):98–106.
117. Sempos CT, Johnson NE, Smith EL, et al. Am J Epidemiol 1985;12:120.
118. Black AE, Cole TJ, Wiles SJ, et al. Hum Nutr Appl Nutr 1983;37:448–58.
119. De Boer JP, Knuiman JT, West CE, et al. Hum Nutr Appl Nutr 1987;41:225–32.
120. Nelson M, Black AE, Morris JA, et al. Am J Clin Nutr 1989;5:155–67.
121. Liu K. Am J Epidemiol 1988;12:864–74.
122. Flegal KM, Larkin FA. Am J Epidemiol 1990;131:1046–58.
123. Cohen NL, Laus MJ. The contribution of portion data to estimates of nutrient intakes by food frequency. Res. bull. no. 73. Amherst, MA: Massachusetts Agricultural Experiment Station, College of Food and Natural Resources, University of Massachusetts, 1990.
124. Dwyer JT. Assessing and monitoring dietary behaviors. In: Snetselaar LG, ed. Nutrition counseling skills: assessment, treatment, and evaluation. Rockville, MD: Aspen Press, 1989;91–122.
125. Rand WM. J Am Diet Assoc 1985;85:1081–3.
126. Rand WM, Windham CT, Wyse BW, et al., eds. Food composition data: a user's perspective. Tokyo: United Nations University, 1987.
127. Consumer and Food Economics Institute, U.S. Department of Agriculture. Composition of foods: raw, processed, prepared. Agricultural handbook no. 8-1 to 8-15. Washington, DC: United States Department of Agriculture, 1989 to 1991.
128. Stewart KK. Food Nutr Bull 1983;5:54–65.
129. Gunderson EL. FDA J APAC Int 1995;78(6):1353–63.
130. Warber J, Haddad E, Hodgkin G, Lee J. Military Med 1995; 160(9):438–42.
131. Beecher GR, Khachik R. Analysis of micronutrients in foods. In: Moon TE, Micozzi MS, eds. Nutrition and cancer prevention. New York: Marcel Dekker, 1989;103–58.
132. Pennington JAT, Church HN. Bowes and Church's food values of portions commonly used. 14th ed. Philadelphia: JB Lippincott, 1985.
133. Bell SJ, Stack JA, Forse RA, et al. Nutr Clin Pract 1995;10(6): 237–41.
134. Hoover LW, Perloff BP. Model for review of nutrient database capabilities. Columbia, MO: University of Missouri, 1981.
135. Deleted in proof.
136. Rand WM. J Am Diet Assoc 1985;85:1081–3.
137. Pennington JAT. Dietary nutrient guide. Westport, CT: AVI Publishing, 1976.
138. Tylavsky FA, Sharp GB. Am J Epidemiol 1995;142(3):342–52.
139. Thompson JK, Dwyer JT. Clin Nutr 1987;6:185–91.
140. Adelman MO, Dwyer JT, Woods M, et al. J Am Diet Assoc 1983;83:422–8.
141. Hoover LW, Perloff BP. J Am Diet Assoc 1983;82:506–8.
142. Hoover LW, Dowdy RP, Hughes KV. J Am Diet Assoc 1985;85:297–304, 307.
143. Windham CT, Helm AA, Wyse BW. Crit Rev Food Sci Nutr 1990;29:149–6.
144. American Institute of Cancer Research. Dietary phytochemicals in cancer prevention and treatment. New York: Plenum Press, 1996.
145. Greenfield H, Southgate DAT. Food composition data: production, management and use. London: CEC Agro-Industrial Research, Elsevier Applied Science, 1992.

146. MacDonald I. Monitoring dietary intakes. Berlin: Springer-Verlag, 1991;259.
147. Young LR, Nestle MA. Nutr Rev 1995;53(6):149–58.
148. Bailey V, Ferro-Luzzi A. Bull WHO 1995;73(5):673–80.
149. Manning EM, Shenkin A. Crit Care Clin 1995;11(3):603–34.
150. Cohen BE, Chapman N, Burt MR. J Nutr Educ 1992;24: 45S–51S.
151. Morris PM, Neuhauser L, Campbell C. J Nutr Educ 1992;24: 52S–8S.
152. Crokett EG, Clancy KL, Bowering J. J Nutr Educ 1992;24: 72S–9S.
153. Gerontology Nutrition Unit. Catering and nutrition in residential homes: assessment kit. London: Queen Elizabeth College, 1981.
154. Briefel RR, Woteki CE. J Nutr Educ 1992;24:24S–8S.
155. Posner BM, Jette AM, Smith KW, et al. Am J Public Health 1993;83:972–8.
156. Melnik TA, Helferd SJ, Firmerly LA, Wales KR. J Am Diet Assoc 1994;12:1425–1427.
157. Wellman NS. Nutr Rev 1994;52(8):44–7.
158. Posner BM, Jette A, Smigelski C, et al. J Gerontol 1994;49: M123–92.
159. Wilson D, Benedict J. Nutr Rev 1996;54:S45–7.
160. Deleted in proof.
161. Rush D. Am J Public Health 1993;83:944–5.
162. Sahyoun NR, Jacques PF, Russell RM. J Am Diet Assoc 1994; 94:A13.
163. American Dietetic Association Foundation. Physician nutrition education. Chicago, IL: American Dietetic Association, 1995.
164. Krebs-Smith SM, Smicklas-Wright H, Guthrie HA, et al. J Am Diet Assoc 1987;87:897–903.
165. Kant AK, Schatzkin A, Block G, et al. J Am Diet Assoc 1991;91:1532–7.
166. Kant AK, Block G, Schatzkin A, et al. J Am Diet Assoc 1991;91:1526–31.
167. Kant AK, Schatzkin A, Ziegler RG. J Am Coll Nutr 1995;14: 233–8.
168. Kant AK, Schatzkin A, Harris TB, et al. Am J Clin Nutr 1993;57:434–40.
169. Popkin BM, Siega-Ris AM, Haines PS. N Engl J Med 1996;335:716–20.
170. Kant AK. J Am Diet Assoc 1996;96:785–91.
171. Krebs-Smith SM, Cook A, Subar AF, et al. Arch Pediatr Adolesc Med 1996;150(1):81–6.
172. Subcommittee on Nutritional Status and Weight Gain During Pregnancy. Dietary intake during pregnancy. In: Institute of Medicine, Subcommittee on Nutritional Status and Weight Gain During Pregnancy. Washington, DC: National Academy Press, 1990;258–71.
173. Rush D. In: The National WIC evaluation: an evaluation of the Special Supplemental Food Program for Women, Infants, and Children, vol III. Chapel Hill NC: Research Triangle Institute and New York State Research Foundation for Mental Hygiene, 1987, V:3–32, VI:4–45.
174. Subcommittee on Nutrition During Lactation. Nutrition during lactation. Washington, DC: National Academy Press, 1991.
175. Van Horn LV, Gernhofer N, Moag-Stahlberg A, et al. J Am Diet Assoc 1990;90:412–6.
176. Haraldsdottir J, Hermansen B. Eur J Clin Nutr 1995; 49(10):729–39.
177. Jenner DA, Neylon K, Croft S, et al. Eur J Clin Nutr 1989;43:663–73.
178. Blom L, Lundmark K, Dahlquist G, Persson LA. Acta Paediatr Scand 1989;78:858–64.
179. Frank GC, Nicklas TA, Webber LS, et al. J Am Diet Assoc 1992;92:313–8.
180. Osganian SK, Nicklas T, Stone E, et al. Am J Clin Nutr 1995;61(1 Suppl):241–4S.
181. Burghart JA, Devaney BL, Gordon AR. Am J Clin Nutr 1995;61(1 Suppl):252S–7S.
182. Baranowski T, Domel S. Am J Clin Nutr 1994;59:2125–75.
183. Rockett HRH, Breitenbach MA, Frazier AL, et al. Prev Med, in press.
184. Rockett HR, Wolf AM, Colditz GA. J Am Diet Assoc 1995;95:336–40.
185. Gordon AR, McKinney P. Am J Clin Nutr 1995;61(1 Suppl):232S–40S.
186. Andersen LF, Nes M, Lillegaard IT, et al. Eur J Clin Nutr 1995;49(8):543–54.
187. Grootenhuis PA, Westenbrink S, Sie CM, et al. J Clin Epidemiol 1995;48(7):859–68.

SELECTED READINGS

Bingham SA. The dietary assessment of individuals: methods, accuracy, new techniques and recommendations. Nutr Abstr Rev 1987;57:705–42.

Cameron ME, Van Staveren WA. Manual on methodology for food consumption studies. Oxford: Oxford University Press, 1988.

Gibson RS. Principles of nutritional assessment. New York: Oxford University Press, 1990.

Pao EM, Cypel YS. Estimation of dietary intake. In: Brown ML, ed. Present knowledge in nutrition. Washington, DC: International Life Sciences Institute, 1990;399–406.

Tarasuk V. Nutritional epidemiology. In: Zeigler EE, Filer LJ, eds. Present knowledge in nutrition. 7th ed. Washington, DC: International Life Sciences Institute, 1996;508–16.

Thompson FE, Byers T, Kohlmeier L. Dietary assessment resource manual. J Nutr 1994;124(11S):2245S–317S.

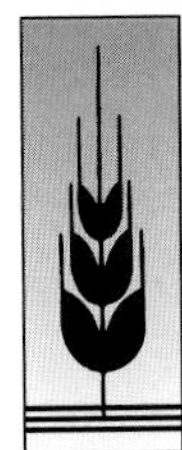

PART IV.

Prevention and Management of Disease

59. Protein-Energy Malnutrition

BENJAMIN TORUN and FRANCISCO CHEW

Protein-energy malnutrition (PEM) results when the body's needs for protein, energy fuels, or both cannot be satisfied by the diet. It includes a wide spectrum of clinical manifestations conditioned by the relative intensity of protein or energy deficit, the severity and duration of the deficiencies, the age of the host, the cause of the deficiency, and the association with other nutritional or infectious diseases. Its severity ranges from weight loss or growth retardation to distinct clinical syndromes, frequently associated with deficiencies of minerals and vitamins.

Dietary energy and protein deficiencies usually occur together, but sometimes one predominates and, if severe enough, may lead to the clinical syndrome of *kwashiorkor* (predominantly protein deficiency) or *marasmus* (mainly energy deficiency). *Marasmic kwashiorkor* is a combination of chronic energy deficiency and chronic or acute protein deficit. It is difficult to recognize which deficit predominates in milder forms of the disease.

The origin of PEM can be *primary,* when it is the result of inadequate food intake, or *secondary,* when it is the result of other diseases that lead to low food ingestion, inadequate nutrient absorption or use, increased nutritional requirements, and/or increased nutrient losses. Its onset can be relatively fast, as in starvation due to abrupt withholding of food, or gradual. This chapter discusses primary PEM of a relatively gradual onset, in which the metabolic alterations and clinical characteristics of protein and/or energy deficits predominate. PEM secondary to other diseases and the metabolic and clinical manifestations of starvation and of specific vitamin and mineral deficiencies are described in other chapters.

HISTORICAL BACKGROUND

It has long been recognized that inadequate food intake produces weight loss and growth retardation and, when severe and prolonged, leads to body wasting and emaciation. It took much longer to understand the nature of the edematous forms of PEM, probably because they could be found among children who were not starving and in families in good socioeconomic position. Descriptions of the disease in the early part of this century paid special attention to dermatologic signs and led to the belief that the disease was caused by tropical parasites or a vitamin deficiency (1–7). This was questioned by various authors in the late 1920s and 1930s. The real nature of the disease was studied more carefully after Cicely Williams' descriptions in the mid-1930s of "kwashiorkor" (8, 9). This term, used by the Ga tribe in the Gold Coast (now Ghana) for "the sickness the older child gets when the next baby is born," already suggested that the disease could be associated with an inadequate diet during the weaning period.

Other pediatricians who worked in tropical countries in the 1930s showed that the edematous disease could be cured by feeding milk or other high-protein foods (10, 11). In the 1940s, researchers showed that most patients had low concentrations of serum proteins, which could also be related to the quality of dietary proteins (12).

The nature and importance of this disease gained worldwide recognition in the 1950s, partly owing to publications such as those of Brock and Autret (13), Autret and Behar (10), and Trowell et al. (11). By then, more than 40 names had been given to this clinical syndrome (11). Some of them, such as "síndrome policarencial de la infancia" (infantile pluricarential syndrome), indicated that young children were mainly affected and that a deficit of various nutrients was involved. Others,

Abbreviations: **AP**—acute-phase reactant proteins; **BMI**—body mass index; **IL-1**—interleukin-1; **PEM**—protein-energy malnutrition; **TNF**—tumor necrosis factor.

such as "Mehlnahrschade" (damage by cereal flours), "starch edema," and "sugar babies," indicated that it was caused by the intake of foods with high carbohydrate and low protein content. Today, the more comprehensive term *protein-energy (or protein-calorie) malnutrition* is universally accepted (14), and its severe forms are most often called "marasmus," "kwashiorkor," and "marasmic kwashiorkor." The term *malnutrition* is usually used in lay language for PEM.

Studies done in the last 30 years showed that marasmus and kwashiorkor have distinct metabolic features, that some manifestations, such as anemia and reduced physical activity, are partly due to adaptive mechanisms, that the immune response of severely malnourished patients is impaired, and that physical and emotional stimulation is important in treating malnourished children. These findings are the basis of current therapeutic measures.

ETIOLOGY AND EPIDEMIOLOGY

Protein-energy malnutrition is the most important nutritional disease in developing countries because of its high prevalence and its relationship with child mortality rates, impaired physical growth, and inadequate social and economic development. An epidemiologic analysis from 53 developing countries indicated that 56% of deaths in children 6 to 59 months old were due to malnutrition's potentiating effects in infectious diseases and that mild and moderate malnutrition was involved in 83% of those deaths (15). Associated deleterious effects on mental growth and maturation have been demonstrated in experimental animals and seem to occur in humans, but environmental support and stimulation can improve the cognitive state of malnourished children (16). PEM occurs more frequently when infections impose additional demands, induce greater losses of nutrients, or produce metabolic alterations.

Magnitude of the Problem

There are about 800 million undernourished people in the world. Most live in developing countries, about 30% each in southern and eastern Asia, 25% in sub-Saharan Africa, and 8% in Latin America and the Caribbean. Consequently, 36% (193 million) of the children under the age of 5 in the developing world are underweight, 43% (230 million) are stunted, and 9% (50 million) are wasted, on the basis of a deficit of more than 2 standard deviations below the WHO/NCHS reference values (17, 18) for weight-for-age, height-for-age, and weight-for-height, respectively. This prevalence ranges from 12% underweight, 22% stunted, and 3% wasted in Latin America and the Middle East to 62% underweight, 61% stunted, and 17% wasted in southern Asia.

A long-term analysis shows a decade-by-decade gradual improvement in the prevalence of child malnutrition, if countries are not disturbed by natural and manmade disasters such as droughts, desertification, wars, and economic crisis. However, the total number of malnourished children has not decreased because of the rise in population in the countries where malnutrition is highly prevalent. In sub-Saharan Africa, current population growth rates of about 3.0%—the highest in the world—suggest that the number of malnourished children will continue growing unless the prevalence of PEM and/or the population growth rates are dramatically reduced (19). In industrialized countries, primary PEM is seen mainly among young children of the lower socioeconomic groups, the elderly who live alone, and adults addicted to alcohol and drugs.

Causes

Social, economic, biologic, and environmental factors may be underlying causes for the insufficient food intake or ingestion of foods with proteins of poor nutritional quality that lead to PEM.

Social and Economic Factors

Poverty that results in low food availability, overcrowded and unsanitary living conditions, and improper child care is a frequent cause of PEM. *Ignorance,* by itself or associated with poverty, leads to poor infant- and child-rearing practices, misconceptions about the use of certain foods, inadequate feeding during illnesses, and improper food distribution within the family. A decline in the practice and duration of breast-feeding, combined with *inadequate weaning practices* when breast milk is withdrawn or can no longer provide sufficient dietary energy and protein to the infant, is associated with growing rates of infantile PEM.

Social problems such as child abuse, maternal deprivation, abandonment of the elderly, alcoholism, and drug addiction can result in PEM. *Cultural and social practices* that impose food taboos, some food and diet fads particularly popular among adolescents and women, and the migration from traditional rural settings to urban slums can also contribute to, or precipitate, the appearance of PEM.

Biologic Factors

Maternal malnutrition prior to and/or during pregnancy is more likely to produce an underweight newborn baby (20). Intrauterine malnutrition can be compounded after birth by insufficient food to satisfy the infant's needs for catch-up growth, resulting in PEM.

Infectious diseases are major contributing and precipitating factors in PEM. Diarrheal disease, measles, acquired immunodeficiency syndrome (AIDS), tuberculosis, and other infections frequently result in negative protein and energy balance because of anorexia (reduced food intake), vomiting, decreased absorption (increased nutrient losses), and catabolic processes (increased requirements and metabolic losses). Intestinal parasites have little or no effect unless the infection is extensive and causes anemia or diarrhea (21).

Diets with low concentrations of proteins and energy, as occur with overdiluted milk formulas or bulky vegetable foods that have low nutrient densities, can lead to PEM in young children whose gastric capacity does not allow ingestion of large amounts of food and in elderly persons with anorexia or difficulty in eating without assistance. Diets poor in protein and rich in carbohydrates are particularly likely to produce kwashiorkor.

Environmental Factors

Overcrowded and/or unsanitary living conditions lead to frequent infections. This is an important cause of PEM, especially among weanlings who develop severe or frequent episodes of diarrhea. *Agricultural patterns, droughts, floods, wars, and forced migrations* lead to cyclic, sudden, or prolonged food scarcities and can cause PEM in whole populations. Postharvest losses of food because of bad storage conditions and inadequate food distribution systems contribute to PEM, even after periods of agricultural plenty.

Age of the Host

PEM can affect all age groups but it is more frequent among infants and young children whose growth increases nutritional requirements, who cannot obtain food by their own means, and who, when living under poor hygienic conditions, frequently become ill with diarrhea and other infections. Infants who are weaned prematurely from the breast or who are breast-fed for a prolonged time without adequate complementary feeding become malnourished for lack of adequate energy and protein intake.

The long-term intake of insufficient food can result in marasmus, the most common form of severe PEM before 1 year of age. Kwashiorkor, the edematous form of the disease, is more frequent after 18 months of age and typically occurs in children with diets consisting of starchy gruels, diluted cereal-based beverages, and vegetable foods rich in carbohydrates but almost devoid of proteins of good nutritional quality (i.e., lacking one or more essential amino acid). Most often, the severe protein deficit is associated with chronic dietary energy deficit and results in a combined form of marasmic kwashiorkor. The appearance of edema is frequently preceded or accompanied by acute diarrhea or other infectious disease.

Older children usually have milder forms of PEM because they can cope better with social and food availability constraints. Infections and other precipitating factors become less severe, and early survival may imply a natural selection of the more fit. Pregnant and lactating women can also have PEM because of their increased nutritional requirements; however, their dietary deficiencies affect mainly the growth, nutritional status, and survival rates of their fetuses, newborn babies, and infants. The elderly who are unable to care properly for themselves tend to suffer from PEM. Gastrointestinal alterations can be an important contributing factor. Adolescents, adult men, and nonpregnant, nonlactating women usually have the lowest prevalence and the mildest forms of the disease because of greater opportunities to obtain food and cultural practices that protect the productive members of the family.

Severe PEM occurs as a primary disorder in conditions of extreme privation and famine or of social or chemical dependency without adequate support, as may be the case with mental patients, prisoners, alcoholics, and drug addicts. It is more frequently secondary to other illnesses, such as chronic infections, cancer, AIDS, malabsorption, and liver and endocrine diseases. In such cases, both the malnutrition and the underlying cause must be treated.

PATHOPHYSIOLOGY AND ADAPTIVE RESPONSES

PEM develops gradually over weeks or months. This allows a series of metabolic and behavioral adjustments that result in decreased nutrient demands and a nutritional equilibrium compatible with a lower level of cellular nutrient availability. If the supply of nutrients becomes persistently lower, the patient can no longer adapt and may even die. Metabolic disruptions can be due to severe nutrient deficit, complications (such as infections), or inadequate treatment (such as abrupt administration of large amounts of dietary energy or protein). Patients whose PEM develops slowly—as is usually the case in marasmus—are better adapted to their current nutritional status and maintain a less fragile metabolic equilibrium than those with more acute PEM, as in kwashiorkor of rapid onset.

Energy Mobilization and Expenditure

A decrease in energy intake is quickly followed by a decrease in energy expenditure, accounting for shorter periods of play and physical activity in children (22) and for longer rest periods and less physical work in adults (23). When the decrease in energy expenditure cannot compensate for the insufficient intake, body fat is mobilized, with a decrease in adiposity and weight (24). Lean body mass diminishes at a slower rate, mainly as a consequence of muscle protein catabolism with increased efflux of amino acids, primarily alanine, that contribute to the energy sources. As the cumulative energy deficit becomes more severe, subcutaneous fat is markedly reduced, and protein catabolism leads to muscular wasting. Visceral protein is preserved longer, especially in the marasmic patients.

In marasmus, these alterations in body composition lead initially to increased basal oxygen consumption (i.e., basal metabolic rate) per unit of body weight, and it decreases in more severe stages (25). In kwashiorkor, the severe dietary protein deficit leads to an earlier visceral depletion of amino acids that affects visceral cell function and reduces oxygen consumption; therefore, basal energy expenditure decreases per unit of lean or total body mass.

Table 59.1
Selected Enzyme Activity Changes in Protein-Energy Malnutrition

Cells	Enzyme Activity[a]
Muscle and leukocytes	↓Aldolase
	↓Amino acid dehydrogenases
	↓Pyruvic kinase
	↑Aminotransferases
Liver	↓Phenylalanine hydroxylase
	↓Urea cycle enzymes
	↑Amino acid activating enzymes

Adapted from Viteri FE. Primary protein-energy malnutrition: clinical, biochemical, and metabolic changes. In: Suskind RM, ed. Textbook of pediatric nutrition. New York, Raven Press, 1981.

[a] ↓, ↑, decrease or increase in activity.

Blood glucose concentration remains normal, mainly at the expense of gluconeogenic amino acids and glycerol from fats, and it falls in severe PEM or when complicated by serious infections or fasting.

Protein Breakdown and Synthesis

The poor availability of dietary proteins reduces protein synthesis (26). Adaptations lead to the sparing of body protein and preservation of essential protein-dependent functions. The gradual and inevitable loss of body protein as a result of long-term dietary protein deficit is primarily from skeletal muscle. Table 59.1 illustrates some enzymatic changes that favor muscle protein breakdown and liver protein synthesis, as well as energy mobilization from fat depots. Some visceral protein is lost in the early development of PEM but then becomes stable until the nonessential tissue proteins are depleted; the loss of visceral protein then increases, and death may be imminent unless nutritional therapy is successfully instituted.

Under normal conditions about 75% of the free amino acids that enter the body pool from dietary and tissue proteins are recycled or reused for protein synthesis, and 25% are broken down for other metabolic purposes. When protein intake is reduced, there is not so much a decrease in total nitrogen or amino acid turnover but an adaptive increase to 90 to 95% in the proportion recycled for synthesis and a proportional decrease in amino acid catabolism (26, 27), which markedly reduces urea synthesis and urinary nitrogen excretion.

The half-lives of several proteins increase. The rate of albumin synthesis decreases initially, but after a lag of a few days, the rate of breakdown also falls and its half-life increases. In addition, a shift of albumin from the extravascular to the intravascular pool helps maintain adequate levels of circulating albumin in the face of reduced synthesis. When protein depletion becomes too severe, the adaptive mechanisms fail, and the concentration of serum proteins, and especially albumin, decreases. The ensuing reduction in intravascular oncotic pressure and outflow of water into the extravascular space contributes to development of the edema of kwashiorkor.

Endocrine Changes

Hormones are important in the adaptive metabolic processes. However, circulating levels of hormones do not always explain endocrine changes in PEM, because cellular responses to hormonal stimulation may also be altered. Table 59.2 summarizes the main changes in hormonal activity in patients with severe energy or protein deficiencies. They contribute to the maintenance of energy homeostasis through increased glycolysis and lipolysis; increased amino acid mobilization; preservation of visceral proteins through increased breakdown of muscle proteins; decreased storage of glycogen, fats, and proteins; and decreased energy metabolism. These effects can be summarized as follows (Fig. 59.1):

1. Decreased food intake tends to reduce plasma concentrations of glucose and free amino acids, which in turn reduce insulin secretion and increase glucagon and epinephrine release; the latter further reduces insulin secretion.
2. The low plasma amino acid levels, seen mainly in kwashiorkor, also stimulate secretion of human growth hormone and reduce somatomedin activity; this produces a further increase in growth hormone levels because of the absence of feedback inhibition; the increased levels of growth hormone and epinephrine influence the reduction in urea synthesis, thereby favoring amino acid recycling.
3. The stress induced by low food intake and further amplified by fever, dehydration, and other manifestations of the infections that frequently accompany PEM also stimulates epinephrine release and corticosteroid secretion; this occurs more in marasmus than in kwashiorkor, probably because of the greater energy deficit of marasmus. Resistance to the peripheral action of insulin increases, probably from the increased plasma free fatty acid concentration resulting from the lipolytic activity of growth hormone, glucocorticoids, and epinephrine.
4. The low levels of circulating insulin and high levels of circulating cortisol may further reduce secretion of somatomedins.
5. Decreased 5′-monodeiodinase activity reduces triiodothyronine production with a concomitant increase in the inactive reverse T_3; thyroxine levels are also reduced, possibly by a decrease in iodine uptake by the thyroid. The reduction in active thyroid hormone levels decreases thermogenesis and oxygen consumption, leading to energy conservation.

Secretion of hormones involved in nonvital growth-related functions such as gonadotropins decreases; the functional capacities of the hypothalamic-pituitary axis and adrenal medulla are preserved, thus allowing endocrine and metabolic responses to stress conditions. Some investigators have postulated that the evolution of PEM into either kwashiorkor or marasmus may be partly related to differences in adrenocortical response, whereby the better response will preserve visceral proteins more efficiently and lead to the better-adapted syndrome of marasmus.(29)

Hematology and Oxygen Transport

The reduction in hemoglobin concentration and red cell mass that almost always accompanies severe PEM is, at

Table 59.2
Summary of Selected Hormonal Changes Usually Seen in Severe PEM and Their Main Metabolic Effects

Hormone	Influenced in PEM By	Hormonal Activity in: Energy Deficit	Hormonal Activity in: Protein Deficit	Effects of Abnormality in PEM
Insulin	Low food intake (↓glucose) (↓amino acids)	Decreased	Decreased	↓Muscle protein synthesis ↓Lipogenesis ↓Growth
Growth hormone (GH)	Low protein intake (↓amino acids) Reduced somatomedin synthesis	Variable	Increased	↑Visceral protein synthesis ↓Urea synthesis ↑Lipolysis ↓Glucose uptake by tissues
Somatomedins (insulin-like growth factors)	Low protein intake Low circulating insulin High circulating cortisol	Variable	Decreased	↓Muscle and cartilage protein synthesis ↓Collagen synthesis ↓Lipolysis ↓Growth ↑Production of growth hormone
Epinephrine	Stress of food deficiency, infections (↓glucose)	Normal but can increase	Normal but can increase	↑Lipolysis ↑Glycogenolysis inhibits insulin secretion
Glucocorticoids	Stress of hunger Fever (↓glucose)	Increased	Normal or increased	↑Muscle protein catabolism ↑Visceral protein turnover ↑Lipolysis ↑Gluconeogenesis ↓Somatomedin-dependent actions of GH
Renin-aldosterone	↓Blood volume ↑Extracellular K? ↓Serum Na?	Normal	Increased	↑Sodium retention and ↑Water retention contributes to appearance of edema
Thyroid hormones	↓5′-deiodinase (↑reverse T_3) Defect in I uptake?	T_4 normal or decreased; T_3 decreased	T_4 usually decreased; T_3 decreased	↓Glucose oxidation ↓Basal energy expenditure ↑Reverse T_3
Gonadotropins	Low protein intake? Low energy intake?	Decreased	Decreased	Delayed menarche

↓, low or reduced; ↑, high or increased.

least in part, an adaptive phenomenon related to tissue oxygen needs (30). The reduced lean body mass and lower physical activity of malnourished patients also lower oxygen demands. The simultaneous decrease in dietary amino acids results in reduced hematopoietic activity, which spares amino acids for synthesis of other more necessary body proteins. As long as the tissues receive sufficient oxygen, this should be considered an adaptive response, not a "functional" anemia (i.e., with tissue hypoxia). When tissue synthesis, lean body mass, and physical activity begin

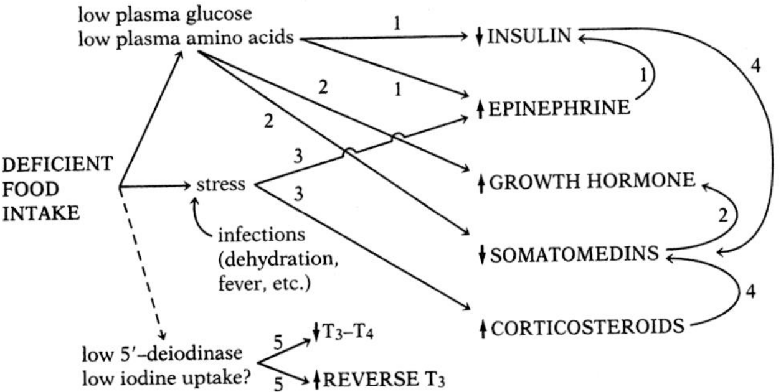

Figure 59.1. Endocrine adaptive functions in severe protein-energy malnutrition related to energy and protein metabolism. See text for an explanation of the numbered events.

improving with dietary treatment, oxygen demands rise, necessitating accelerated hematopoiesis. If sufficient iron, folic acid, and vitamin B_{12} are not available, functional anemia with tissue hypoxia will develop.

Figure 59.2 shows that administration of hematinics to a severely malnourished patient does not induce a hematopoietic response until dietary treatment produces an increase in lean body mass. Figure 59.3 shows that the reticulocyte response is related to protein intake when erythropoietic substances are not limiting (28).

The severely malnourished patient may have relatively high body iron stores (31) and retains the ability to produce erythropoietin and reticulocytes in response to acute hypoxia (32, 33). Nevertheless, these patients tend to develop functional, severe anemia if there is a superimposed dietary deficiency of iron or folic acid, or a chronic blood loss, as in hookworm infection.

Other Physiologic and Metabolic Changes

Not all pathophysiologic changes lead to advantageous adjustments. Certain functions are affected, and some nutrient reserves decrease, making the malnourished individuals more susceptible to injuries that a well-nourished individual can withstand with little repercussion.

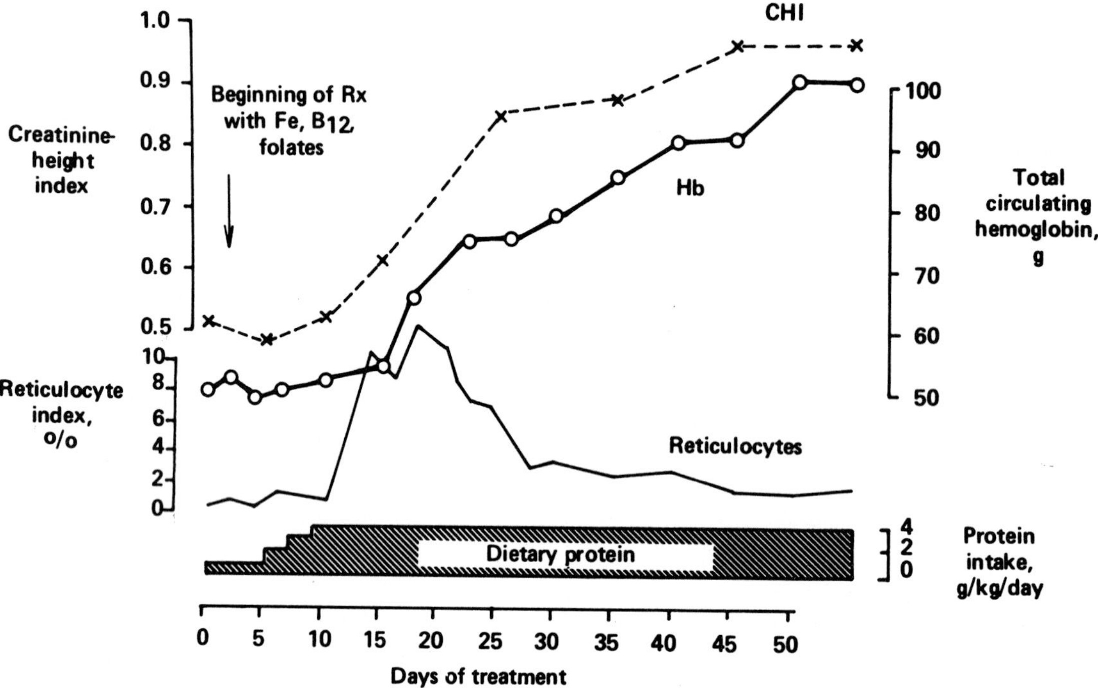

Figure 59.2. Hematologic response of a child with severe protein-energy malnutrition. Treatment with iron, folic acid, and vitamin B_{12} began on day 2; dietary energy and proteins were increased gradually to 150 kcal and 4 g protein/kg/day on day 9. No reticulocyte or hemoglobin response occurred until lean body mass, assessed by the creatinine-height index, began increasing.

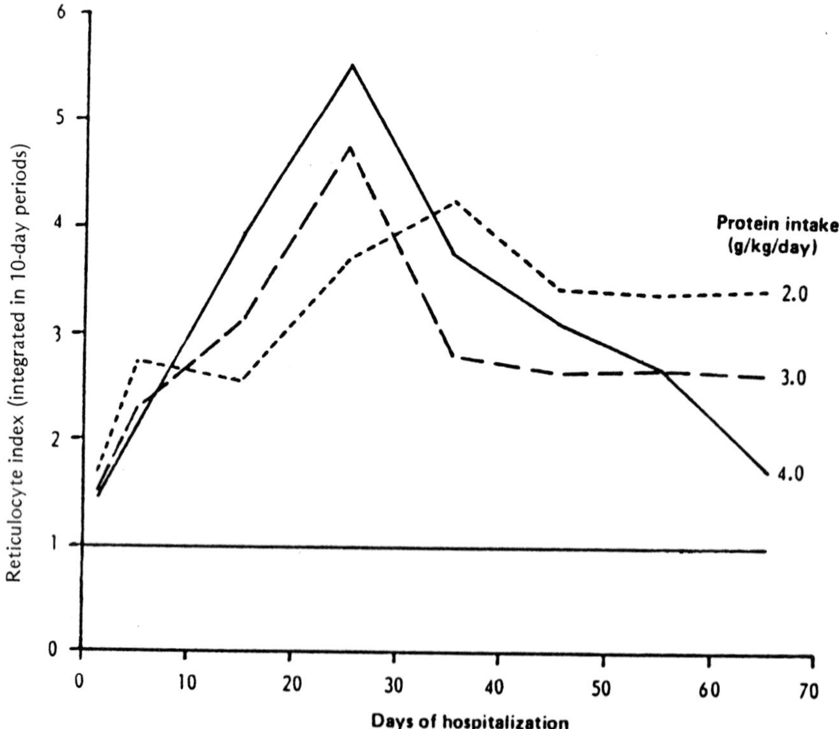

Figure 59.3. Reticulocyte response of children treated for severe protein-energy malnutrition with different amounts of dietary energy and hematinics. (From Viteri FE. Primary protein-energy malnutrition: clinical, biochemical, and metabolic changes. In: Suskind RM, ed. Textbook of pediatric nutrition. New York: Raven Press, 1981.)

Cardiovascular and Renal Functions

Cardiac output, heart rate, and blood pressure decrease, and central circulation takes precedence over peripheral circulation (34, 35). Cardiovascular reflexes are altered, leading to postural hypotension and diminished venous return. In severe PEM, peripheral circulatory failure comparable to hypovolemic shock may occur. Hemodynamic compensation occurs primarily from tachycardia rather than from increased stroke volume. Renal plasma flow and glomerular filtration rates may be reduced because of the decreased cardiac output, but water clearance and the ability to concentrate and acidify urine appear unimpaired (36–38).

Immune System

The major defects seen in severe PEM seem to involve T lymphocytes and the complement system (39). Lymphocytes from the thymus are depleted markedly and the gland atrophies. In addition, cells from the T-lymphocyte regions of the spleen and lymph nodes are depleted, probably owing to a decrease in thymic factors (40, 41). Alteration in monokine metabolism, particularly decreased interleukin-1 (IL-1) activity, may contribute to the low proliferation of T cells in severe malnutrition (42). Production of several complement components, the functional activity both the classic and alternative pathways of the complement system, and the opsonic activity of serum are depressed in severe PEM (43). These deficiencies may explain the high susceptibility of severely malnourished patients to gram-negative bacterial sepsis. Phagocytosis, chemotaxis, and intracellular killing are also impaired, partly because of the defects in opsonic and complement functional activities. The B-lymphocyte areas of spleen and lymph nodes and the circulating levels of B cells and immunoglobulin are relatively normal, but there may be defects in antibody production (e.g., secretory IgA) (39).

The overall consequences of all these alterations in severe PEM are a greater predisposition to infections and to severe complications of otherwise less important infectious diseases. The defects in immune functions disappear with nutritional rehabilitation, except perhaps those due to intrauterine malnutrition (40).

Monokines

Monokines or cytokines are peptide/glycoprotein mediators of the body's response to injury (see Chapters 44, 45, and 96). They are synthesized primarily by activated monocytic and phagocytic cells lining the liver and spleen. These peptides activate neighboring tissue in a paracrine fashion and also enter the circulation to exert more-distant effects. The most extensively characterized monokines are IL-1 and cachectin, or tumor necrosis factor (TNF).

Macrophages from children with severe edematous PEM have decreased IL-1 activity (42). In addition to the immunologic alterations mentioned above, this might contribute to the poor febrile response and low leukocyte count in infections (44). On the other hand, serum levels of TNF seem to be increased in severe malnutrition (45). This could be associated with the anorexia, muscle wasting, and lipid abnormalities of PEM.

Electrolytes

Total body potassium decreases in PEM because of the reduction in muscle proteins and loss of intracellular potassium. The low insulin action and diminished intracellular energy substrates reduce the availability of adenosine triphosphate (ATP) and phosphocreatine. This process probably alters the cellular exchange of sodium and potassium, leading to potassium loss and increased intracellular sodium levels (46). Water accompanies the sodium influx, and although total body intracellular water is decreased because of the loss in lean body mass, there may be intracellular overhydration. These alterations in cell electrolytes and energy sources may explain, at least in part, the increased fatigability and reduced strength of skeletal muscle (47).

Gastrointestinal Functions

Impaired intestinal absorption of lipids and disaccharides and a decreased rate of glucose absorption occur in severe protein deficiency. The greater the protein deficit, the greater the functional impairment. A decrease in gastric, pancreatic, and bile production is also observed, with normal to low enzyme and conjugated bile acid concentrations (48–50). These alterations further impair the absorptive functions. Nevertheless, ingestion of nutrients in high therapeutic amounts usually allows sufficient uptake for nutritional recovery (51). Malnourished persons, however, are prone to have diarrhea because of these alterations and possibly also because of irregular intestinal motility and gastrointestinal bacterial overgrowth. Diarrhea aggravates the malabsorption and can further impair nutritional status. Malabsorption disappears with nutritional recovery unless there is an underlying food or nutrient intolerance unrelated to primary PEM.

Central and Peripheral Nervous System

Individuals who suffer severe PEM at an early age may have decreased brain growth, nerve myelination, neurotransmitter production, and velocity of nervous conduction. The long-term functional implications of these alterations have not been clearly demonstrated, and they cannot be correlated with later behavior and level of intelligence (52). In the human, it is impossible to separate nutrition from other factors that can affect gross and fine motor skills, intelligence, and behavior. Factors that can determine developmental outcome include the severity, timing, and duration of nutritional deprivation, the quality of nutritional rehabilitation and psychosocial support, the degree of family stimulation, and a host of positive and negative environmental factors.

FACTORS LEADING TO KWASHIORKOR

The concept that marasmus or kwashiorkor is the end result of either severe energy or protein deficiency is too simplistic. Nevertheless, the classic theory of a dietary cause of kwashiorkor and marasmus, which states that a diet deficient in protein and with a low protein:energy ratio is an important (perhaps even principal) factor in the production of kwashiorkor, still is valid. The deficiency of vitamins and minerals associated with food sources of protein, and the variability in nutrient requirements between children, may explain why some children develop the edematous and others the nonedematous form of the disease. It also explains, at least in part, some epidemiologic features of PEM, such as the predominance of marasmus in infants under 1 year of age and the predominance of either marasmus, kwashiorkor, or marasmic kwashiorkor in different parts of the world and in urban or rural areas.

Other factors such as overloading a severely malnourished person with carbohydrates, or metabolic changes induced by infections, may cause or contribute to the appearance of kwashiorkor with its characteristic edema, hypoalbuminemia, and enlarged fatty liver. Some investigators have postulated that the evolution of PEM into either kwashiorkor or marasmus may be partly related to differences in adrenocortical response, so that a greater response preserves visceral proteins more efficiently and leads to the better-adapted syndrome of marasmus (29, 53). Others have proposed that kwashiorkor results from aflatoxin poisoning (54, 55), but there is no clear difference in the amounts of aflatoxin or its metabolites in the diet, urine, or tissues of children with kwashiorkor and marasmus.

Another theory is related to the production of toxic free radicals and their safe disposal (56–58). Among the factors that would increase free radicals are infections, toxins, sunlight, trauma, and catalysts such as iron. Formation of free radicals is decreased by the antioxidant function of vitamins A (or β-carotene), C, and E, by ceruloplasmin and transferrin that bind free iron and favor its oxidation, and by zinc-metallothionein, which acts as a free radical sink. Free radicals and the peroxides they generate are removed via reactions catalyzed by enzymes in which glutathione and trace minerals are important, such as Cu-Zn and Mn superoxide dismutase, and Se-containing glutathione peroxidase. The toxic effects of free radicals would be responsible for cell damage leading to the alterations seen in kwashiorkor, such as edema, fatty liver, and skin lesions. This theory has not been firmly established or subjected to the test of animal experiments; nevertheless, it has drawn attention to factors and processes in the pathogenesis of severe PEM that have previously been neglected, and it may have important implications for treatment (59).

When there is a severe lack of food, endocrine adjustments mobilize fatty acids from adipose tissue and amino acids from muscle tissue; plasma protein concentration remains normal, and hepatic gluconeogenesis is enhanced (60). An increase in carbohydrate intake when protein intake is very low can produce a breakdown of those adjustments, as follows:

1. Carbohydrate intake induces insulin release and reduced production of epinephrine and cortisol (61, 62).
2. Lipolysis decreases, which decreases the inhibitory effects of free fatty acids on the peripheral action of insulin, and insulin action is enhanced (63).
3. Muscle protein breakdown is reduced and the body pool of free amino acids decreases; the decreased supply of muscle amino acids to the other organs results in less visceral protein synthesis (64–66).
4. Decreased synthesis of plasma proteins in the liver, particularly albumin, reduces intravascular oncotic pressure. Plasma water decreases and accumulates in extravascular tissues, tissue pressure rises, and cardiac output diminishes. This contributes to the appearance or increase of edema, as discussed below.
5. Increased hepatic fatty acid synthesis from the excess carbohydrate, impaired lipolysis, and reduced production of apo-β-lipoproteins for lipid transport lead to fatty infiltration of the liver and hepatomegaly.

Infections in undernourished children also can precipitate the onset of kwashiorkor. How this occurs has not been satisfactorily explained, but the following mechanisms may be involved:

1. Infections might divert the meager amino acid pool to production of globulins and acute-phase reactant proteins (APs) instead of albumin and transport proteins.
2. The increase in APs that are proteinase inhibitors, such as α_1-antitrypsin and α_1-antichymotrypsin, may impair muscle protein breakdown (67).
3. Impaired production and use of ketone bodies for energy during infections might lead to the use of more amino acids for gluconeogenesis (68).
4. Protein catabolism and nitrogen losses are enhanced by many viral and febrile infections, probably through increased epinephrine and cortisol actions (69, 70). Regardless of the mechanisms involved, protein losses during severe infections can amount to as much as 2% of muscle protein per day (71).
5. Leukocytes stimulated by infectious organisms produce large quantities of superoxide and hydrogen peroxide (72), which are released into the surrounding medium and contribute to the production of kwashiorkor, according to the free-radical theory (56, 57).

The pathogenesis of edema in severe PEM has aroused much discussion because of its key role in the diagnosis of kwashiorkor and because it may give clues about the patient's dietary background and other precipitating factors of the disease. The edema of kwashiorkor has been classically linked to hypoalbuminemia through a reduction in colloid osmotic pressure of the plasma, which leads to outflow of fluid from the capillaries into the interstitial space. However, serum albumin levels between edematous and nonedematous PEM in children and adults overlap. Experimental studies on dogs fed a low-protein diet showed that many animals with plasma albumin levels below 20 g/L did not have edema, but almost all edematous dogs had albumin levels below that value (73). Furthermore, the edema of kwashiorkor is reduced by treatment with protein-free or low-protein diets that contain potassium and other minerals and moderate amounts of carbohydrates. All this suggests that hypoalbuminemia may be a necessary but not sufficient cause for edema, and that some other factors may be needed, at least in some cases (59). These factors include potassium deficiency, which promotes water and sodium retention (74), excessive administration of water and sodium, and extravasation of fluid because of increased capillary permeability in infection.

A theory for the production of edema in severe PEM involved a reduction in renal blood flow (RBF) and glomerular filtration rate (GFR) because of decreased plasma volume and decreased cardiac output as consequence of hypoalbuminemia. Decreased RBF and GFR would lead to sodium retention and production of renin and aldosterone, which in turn would increase the tubular reabsorption of sodium and water, leading to edema (75). However, there is conflicting evidence about the changes in plasma volume in kwashiorkor, and aldosterone activity may increase in children with marasmus as well as in children with edema (76, 77). Other theories include an increase in ferritin that stimulates production of antidiuretic hormone by the posterior pituitary (78, 79), energy deficiency that does not allow adequate function of the sodium pump and restoration of intracellular potassium (80), and, more recently, leakiness of cell membranes caused by the damaging effects of free radicals (56–58). None of these theories have been fully demonstrated, and some have conflicting evidence. Possibly the pathogenesis of edema in PEM is not a single entity and it differs, depending on the multiple nutritional deficiencies, patient age, and other concomitant conditions. However, except for iatrogenic water overload, hypoproteinemia—especially hypoalbuminemia—is an essential component.

DISRUPTION OF ADAPTATION

When the supply for tissue and cell energy can no longer be maintained by patients with severe energy deficiency, a serious decompensation occurs, causing hypoglycemia, hypothermia, impaired circulatory and renal functions, acidosis, coma, and death. These events can occur within a few hours. Metabolic decompensation because of severe protein deficiency, in addition to the changes discussed in the onset of kwashiorkor, may include hemorrhagic diathesis and jaundice because the liver fails to synthesize several clotting factors and transport proteins; various degrees of renal failure with acidosis and water and sodium retention; decreased cardiac work, pulmonary congestion, and increased susceptibility to pulmonary infections; coma; and death.

A high-carbohydrate, low-protein diet is not the only iatrogenic cause of serious metabolic disruption in patients who have, or are prone to develop, edematous PEM. Abrupt administration of too much protein to patients with edematous PEM can also have life-threatening consequences. When such patients have been eating minute amounts of protein or none at all and they are suddenly fed large amounts of protein or given large transfusions of plasma or blood, they may experience a rapid increase in intravascular protein concentration and entry of extracellular fluid into the vascular compartment leading to cardiovascular insufficiency and pulmonary edema. In fact, premature introduction of a high-energy or high-protein diet may be fatal to a severely malnourished patient (81, 82).

DIAGNOSIS

The clinical, biochemical, and physiologic characteristics of PEM vary according to the severity of disease, the patient's age, the presence of other nutritional deficits and infections, and the predominance of energy or protein deficiency.

Classification of PEM

The classification scheme shown in Table 59.3 is useful for the diagnosis and treatment of PEM and the application and evaluation of public health measures. *Severity* is determined mainly by anthropometry, because other clinical findings and biochemical indexes usually do not show changes unless the disease is well advanced. More-accurate measurements, such as assessment of body composition, are not practical or feasible in most of the settings in which primary PEM occurs, and they are usually used for research rather than for clinical purposes. The so-called functional indicators are not well standardized, can be influenced by deficits of more than one single nutrient, or may be too complex to measure routinely (83).

Classification of the *course* or *duration* of the disease as acute, chronic, or acute with a chronic background is also done by anthropometry to assess current nutritional status and degree of growth retardation in children. Dietary history is useful, especially in adults, as are dietary surveys in population groups. The relative contributions of dietary *protein and energy deficits* in the mild and moderate forms of PEM are assessed mainly by the individual's dietary history or the population's dietary habits and food availability.

Table 59.3
Classification of PEM According to Severity of Disease, Its Course or Duration, and Predominant Nutrient Deficiency

Severity	Course	Main Deficit
Mild	Acute	Energy
Moderate	Chronic	Protein
Severe	Both	Both

Clinical characteristics and biochemical data confirm the diagnosis in severe PEM.

Anthropometric Measurements

The choice of anthropometric measurements depends on their simplicity, accuracy, and sensitivity; on the availability of measuring instruments; and on the existence of reference standards for comparison.

To allow international comparisons, it is sensible to use the same standard of reference for various populations. International or universal standards based on reliable anthropometric data can be used because *(a)* most children have similar growth potentials, regardless of ethnic background (84, 85), *(b)* the relationship of various anthropometric measurements, especially weight and height, is relatively constant in normal, healthy individuals of all age groups, *(c)* the reference standards are merely for purposes of comparison and do not necessarily represent an ideal or target, and *(d)* the interpretation of the comparison (i.e., the values that separate "normal" from "deficient" and further divide the latter into "mild," "moderate," and "severe" forms) is a matter of judgment that comes into play when deciding whether the expected normal value for a given population should be 100%, 90%, or another proportion of the standard. Setting different cutoff points relative to a single standard is more practical than constructing local standards that, in a country with heterogeneous population groups, may pose the same problem as a "foreign" commonly used reference. At present, the World Health Organization recommends the data from the United States National Center for Health Statistics (NCHS) (86) as reference for weight and height (87).

The best anthropometric assessment of nutritional status and PEM is based on measurements of weight and height or length, and records of age, to calculate two indexes: *weight for height,* as an index of current nutritional status, and *height for age,* as an index of past nutritional history. Deficient height for age may represent a short period of growth failure at an early age or a longer period at a later age. Waterlow suggested the terms *wasting* for a deficit in weight for height and *stunting* for a deficit in height for age (88). Patients may then fall into four categories: *(a)* normal, *(b)* wasted but not stunted (suffering from acute PEM), *(c)* wasted and stunted (suffering from acute and chronic PEM), and *(d)* stunted but not wasted (past PEM with present adequate nutrition, or "nutritional dwarfs"). The intensity of wasting and stunting can be graded by calculating weight as a percentage of the reference median weight for height, and height as a percentage of the reference median height for age, as follows:

$$\text{\% weight-for-height (or height-for-age)} = \frac{\text{observed weight (or height)}}{\text{reference weight for patient's height (or reference height for patient's age)}} \times 100$$

The use of centiles or standard deviations from the mean, instead of percentage deviation from the median, is statistically more adequate. However, percentage deviation is easier for the general public to understand and for field workers to calculate. The grading shown in Table 59.4 is suggested for most countries, although some might find it convenient to use different cutoff points for specific groups. For example, the normal height for age in populations that are genetically short could be less than 95% of the reference. Color-coded charts and graphs have been devised to simplify the measurements and their interpretation (89, 90).

The *body mass index* (BMI, or Quetelet's index), weight in kg/height in meters^2, is recommended for adolescents and adults. Table 59.5 shows the criteria for classification of chronic energy deficiency in adults proposed by an international working party (91). We suggest using the same BMI criteria to classify current PEM in adults. There will be more body fat in women than in men at all three cutoff points, but this is an intrinsic biologic phenomenon. Therefore, the same cutoff points can be used for both sexes (91).

In adolescents, interpretation of BMI must take into account sexual maturation (92). We suggest that, in general, the diagnosis of PEM in adolescent boys and girls can be based on a BMI *below 15.0 at ages 11 to 13 years,* and *below 16.5 at ages 14 to 17 years.* The corresponding values for *severe* PEM would be *below 13.0* and *below 14.5,* respectively.

The use of deficit in weight for age does not differentiate between a truly underweight child (current PEM) and one who is short but well proportioned in weight (past PEM); furthermore, the information about chronologic age is not always reliable. However, the classification of PEM as grades I (75–90% of reference weight for age), II (60–74%), and III (less than 60%) is useful in public health and epidemiologic studies, because it indicates the proportion of children in a population group who at some time in their lives have had malnutrition (93).

Table 59.4
Classification of Severity of Current ("Wasting") and Past or Chronic ("Stunting") PEM in Infants and Children, Based on Weight for Height and on Height for Age[a,b]

	Normal	Mild	Moderate	Severe
Weight for height (deficit = wasting)	90–110 (±1 Z)[b]	80–89 (−1.1 to −2 Z)	75–79 (−2.1 to −3 Z)	<75, or with edema (<−3 Z)
Height for age (deficit = stunting)	95–105 (±1 Z)	90–94 (−1.1 to −2 Z)	85–89 (−2.1 to −3 Z)	<85 (<−3 Z)

[a]Expressed as percentage relative to the median NCHS standard (86, 87).
[b]In parentheses: standard deviations from the NCHS median, or "Z scores" (87).

Table 59.5
Classification of Intensity of Protein-Energy Malnutrition in Adult Men and Women

Body Mass Index (BMI)	PEM
≥18.5	Normal
17.0–18.4	Mild
16.0–16.9	Moderate
<16.0	Severe

Based on the classification proposed for chronic energy deficiency in James WPT, Ferro-Luzzi A, Waterlow JC. Eur J Clin Nutr 1988;42:969–81.

Use of the upper arm circumference has been advocated under field conditions without access to a weighing scale. It is not a sensitive index, but one can differentiate between a moderately to severely malnourished child and one with better nutritional condition.

Mild and Moderate PEM

The main clinical feature of mild and moderate PEM is weight loss. A decrease in subcutaneous adipose tissue may become apparent. When PEM is chronic, children show growth retardation in terms of height (stunting). Populations in which PEM is highly prevalent or "endemic" show slow weight gains, as illustrated in Figure 59.4.

Physical activity and energy expenditure of children decrease (24, 94–96). Other functional indicators of immunocompetence, gastrointestinal functions, and behavior may be altered, but their assessment is not yet practical for diagnostic purpose (28, 40, 97). Nonspecific manifestations include more-sedentary behavior, frequent episodes of diarrhea, and apathy, lack of liveliness, and short attention spans.

In adults, mild to moderate PEM results in leanness with reduction in subcutaneous tissue. The most common change in body composition is a reduction of adiposity below 12 and 20% in men and women, respectively. Capacity for prolonged physical work is reduced, but this change is usually apparent only in persons engaged in intense, energy-demanding occupations (23, 98). Malnourished women have a higher probability of giving birth to infants with low birth weights (99). As in children, there may be other functional alterations not yet well characterized.

Biochemical information is not consistent in mild and moderate PEM. Laboratory data related to low protein intakes may include low urinary excretion of creatinine, leading to a low creatinine-height index in children (100), low urinary urea nitrogen and hydroxyproline excretions, altered plasma patterns of free amino acids with a decrease in branched-chain essential amino acids, slight decreases in serum transferrin and albumin levels, and a reduced number of circulating lymphocytes.

Severe PEM

The diagnosis of severe PEM is principally based on dietary history and clinical features. Marasmus is usually associated with severe food shortage, prolonged semistarvation, early weaning, or infrequent feeding of infants, and kwashiorkor with late weaning and poor protein intakes. Chronic or recurrent diarrhea and infections are common features.

Marasmus

Generalized muscular wasting and absence of subcutaneous fat give the patient with severe nonedematous PEM a "skin and bones" appearance (Figs. 59.5 and 59.6). Marasmic patients frequently have 60% or less of the weight expected for their height, and children have marked retardation in longitudinal growth. The hair is sparse, thin, and dry, without normal sheen; it is easily

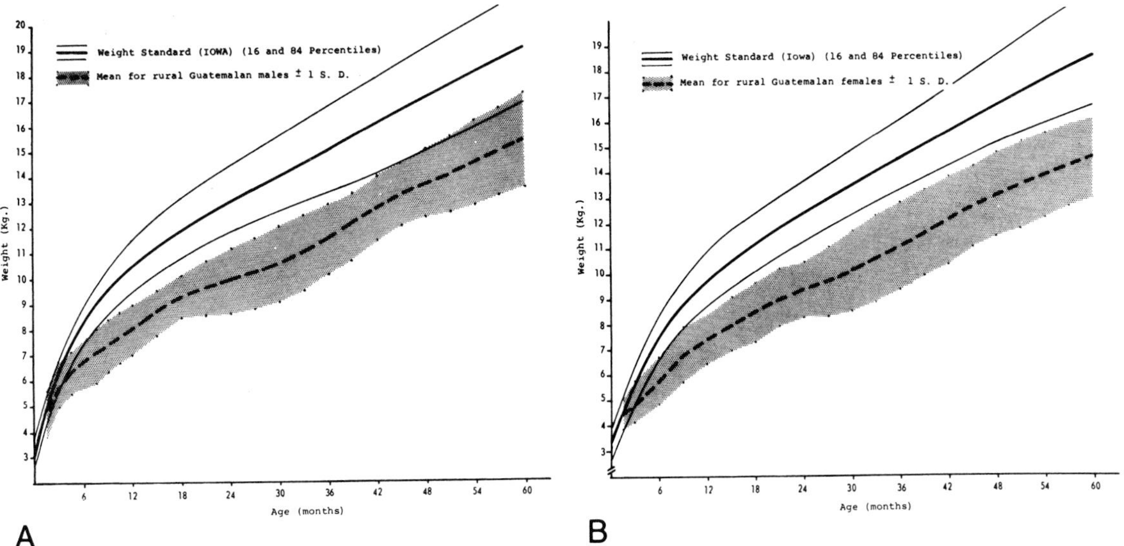

Figure 59.4. Pattern of weight gain, from birth to 5 years, in 431 boys (**A**) and 436 girls (**B**) from low-income families in rural Guatemala. (From INCAP. Evaluación nutricional de la población de Centro América y Panamá: Guatemala. Guatemala: Instituto de Nutrición de Centro América y Panamá, 1969.)

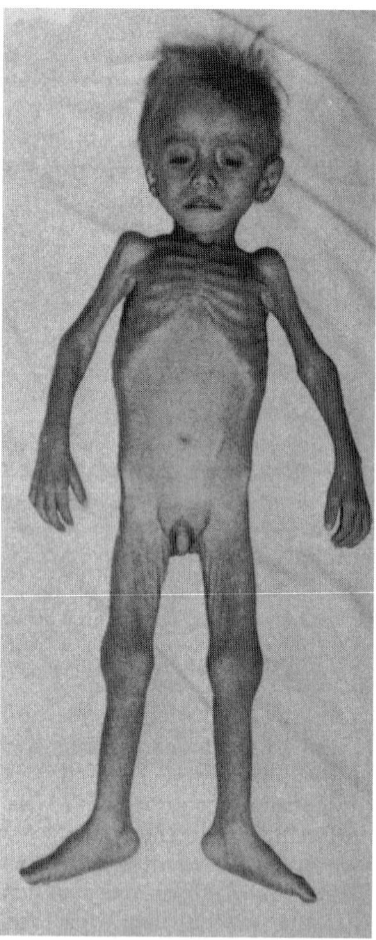

Figure 59.5. Marasmus in a 21-month-old child. (From Viteri FE. Primary protein-energy malnutrition: clinical, biochemical, and metabolic changes. In: Suskind RM, ed. Textbook of pediatric nutrition. New York, Raven Press, 1981.)

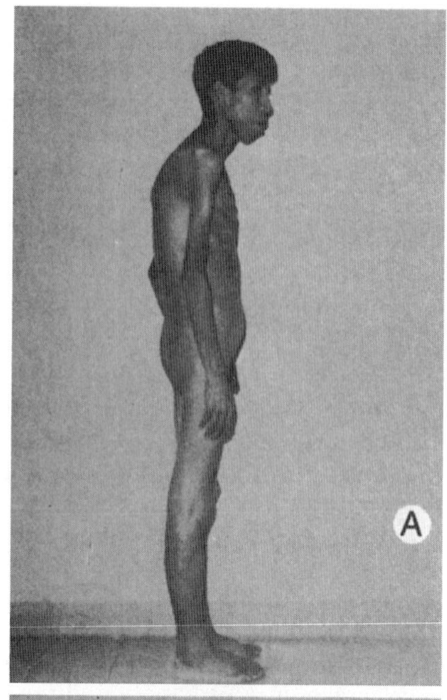

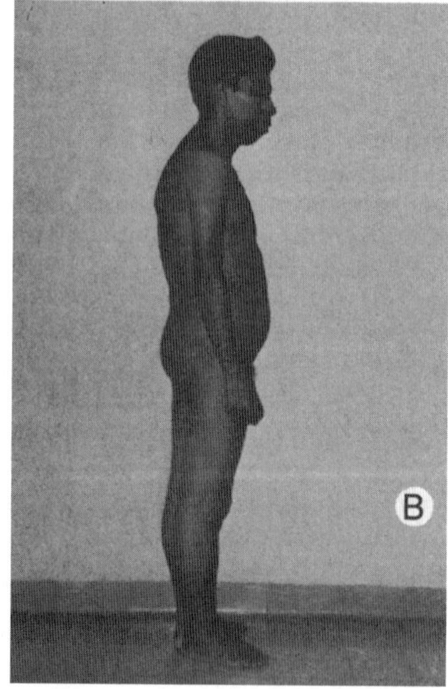

Figure 59.6. A. Marasmic protein-energy malnutrition in a 29-year-old man. **B.** The same patient after 3 months of treatment.

pulled out without causing pain. The skin is dry and thin, with little elasticity, and wrinkles easily. Patients are apathetic but usually aware and have an anxious look. These features and the sunken cheeks caused by disappearance of the Bichat fat pads, which are among the last subcutaneous adipose depots to disappear, give the marasmic child's face the appearance of a monkey's or an old person's face.

Some patients are anorectic, while others are ravenously hungry, but they seldom tolerate large amounts of food, and they vomit easily. Diarrhea may be present. There is marked weakness, and children frequently cannot stand without help. Heart rate, blood pressure, and body temperature may be low, but tachycardia may be present. Hypoglycemia can occur, especially after fasting for 6 or more hours, and is often accompanied by hypothermia of 35.5°C or less. The viscera are usually small. Abdominal distention may be present. The lymph nodes are easily palpable.

Differential diagnosis must be made from the secondary PEM of AIDS and other body-wasting diseases; dietary history plays an important role.

Common complicating features are acute gastroenteritis, dehydration, respiratory infections, and eye lesions due to hypovitaminosis A. Systemic infections lead to septic shock or intravascular clotting with high mortality rates.

Kwashiorkor

The predominant feature of kwashiorkor is soft, pitting, painless edema, usually in the feet and legs, but extending to the perineum, upper extremities, and face in severe cases (Fig. 59.7). Most patients have skin lesions, often confused with pellagra, in areas of edema, continuous pressure (e.g., the buttocks and back), or frequent irrita-

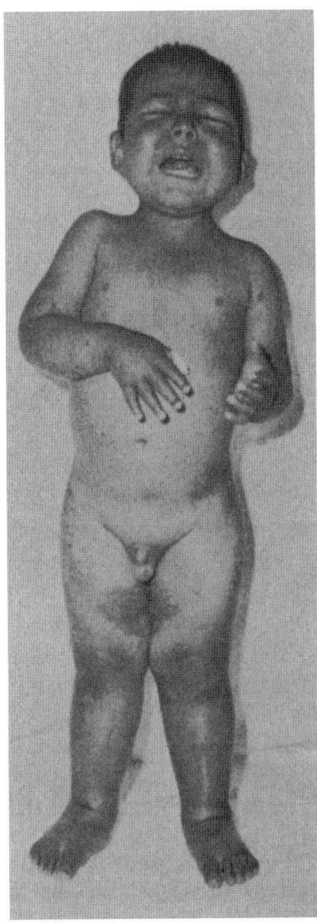

Figure 59.7. Kwashiorkor in a 36-month-old child. Note that subcutaneous tissues were preserved in the trunk and face.

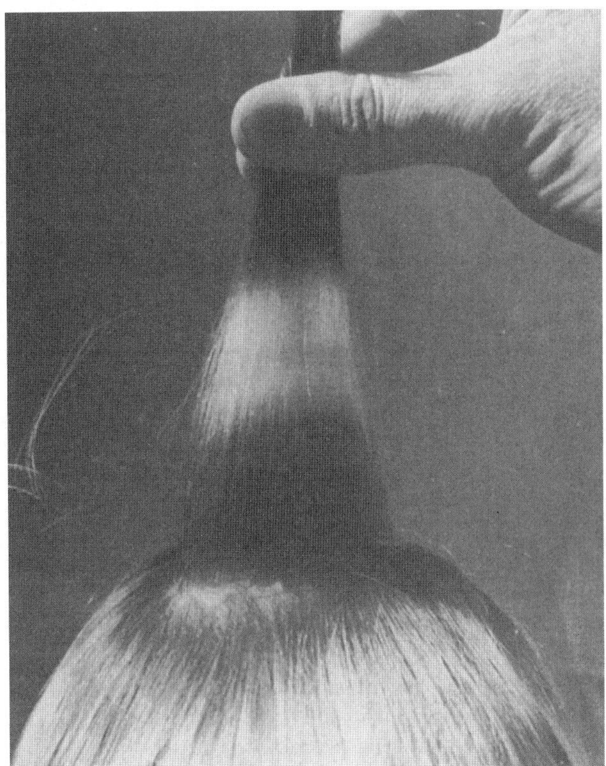

Figure 59.8. "Flag-sign": bands of depigmented and normal hair caused by alternating periods of poor and relatively good protein intake. (From Torun B, Viteri FE. Protein-energy malnutrition. In: Warren KS, Mahmoud AAF, eds. Tropical and geographical medicine. 2nd ed. New York, McGraw-Hill, 1990.)

tion (e.g., the perineum and thighs). The skin may be erythematous, and it glistens in the edematous regions with zones of dryness, hyperkeratosis, and hyperpigmentation, which tend to become confluent. The epidermis peels off in large scales, exposing underlying tissues that are easily infected. Subcutaneous fat is preserved, and there may be some muscle wasting. Weight deficit, after accounting for the weight of edema, is usually not as severe as in marasmus. Height may be normal or retarded, depending on the chronicity of the current episode and on past nutritional history.

The hair is dry, brittle, and without normal sheen, and it can be pulled out easily without pain. Curly hair becomes straight, and the pigmentation usually changes to dull brown, red, or even yellowish white. Alternating periods of poor and relatively good protein intake can produce alternating bands of depigmented and normal hair, termed the *flag sign* (Fig. 59.8).

Patients may be pale, with cold and cyanotic extremities. They are apathetic and irritable, cry easily, and have an expression of misery and sadness. Anorexia (sometimes necessitating nasogastric tube feeding), postprandial vomiting, and diarrhea are common. These conditions improve without specific gastrointestinal treatment as nutritional recovery progresses. Hepatomegaly with a soft round edge caused by severe fatty infiltration is usually present. The abdomen is frequently protruding because of distended stomach and intestinal loops. Peristalsis is irregular and frequently slow. Muscle tone and strength are greatly reduced. Tachycardia is common. Both hypothermia and hypoglycemia can occur after short periods of fasting.

Differential diagnosis must be made from other causes of edema and hypoproteinemia and from secondary PEM due to impairment in protein absorption or metabolism. The same complications occur as in marasmus, but diarrhea and respiratory and skin infections are more frequent and severe. Fatal infections may occur, frequently without fever, tachycardia, respiratory distress, or appropriate leukocytosis. The most common causes of death are pulmonary edema with bronchopneumonia, septicemia, gastroenteritis, and water and electrolyte imbalances.

Marasmic Kwashiorkor

The marasmic kwashiorkor form of edematous PEM combines clinical characteristics of kwashiorkor and marasmus. The main features are the edema of kwashiorkor, with or without its skin lesions, and the muscle wasting and decreased subcutaneous fat of marasmus (Figs. 59.9 and 59.10). When edema disappears during early treatment, the patient's appearance resembles that of marasmus. Biochemical features of both marasmus and kwashiorkor are seen, but the alterations of severe protein deficiency usually predominate.

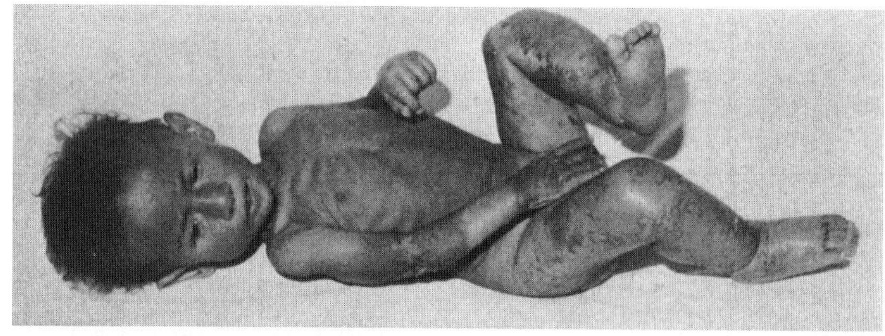

Figure 59.9. Marasmic kwashiorkor in a 22-month-old child. Note the edema in the lower part of the body, the emaciated upper part, and the skin lesions. (From Torun B, Viteri FE. Protein-energy malnutrition. In: Warren KS, Mahmoud AAF, eds. Tropical and geographical medicine. 2nd ed. New York, McGraw-Hill, 1990.)

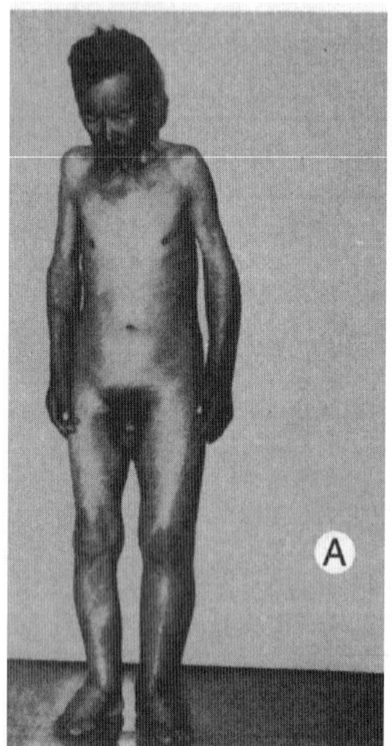

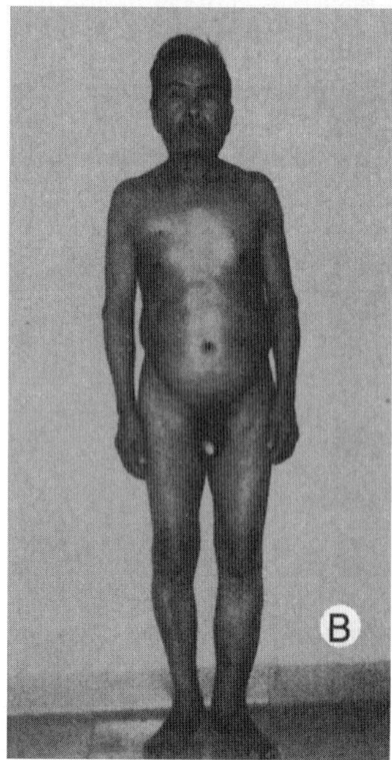

Figure 59.10. A. Edematous protein-energy malnutrition in a 46-year-old man. **B.** The same patient after 3 months of treatment.

Biochemical and Histopathologic Features of Severe PEM

The most common biochemical findings are the following:

1. Serum concentrations of total proteins, and especially albumin, are markedly reduced in edematous PEM, and normal or moderately low in marasmus.
2. Hemoglobin and hematocrit are usually low, more so in kwashiorkor than in marasmus.
3. The ratio of nonessential to essential amino acids in plasma is elevated in kwashiorkor and usually normal in marasmus.
4. Serum levels of free fatty acids are elevated, particularly in kwashiorkor.
5. Blood glucose level is normal or low after fasting 6 or more hours.
6. Urinary excretion of creatinine, hydroxyproline, 3-methylhistidine, and urea nitrogen is low. Edematous children have markedly reduced urinary creatinine excretion in relation to their height, leading to a low creatinine-height index (100), whereas marasmic children may have a normal or somewhat low index.

Plasma levels of other nutrients vary and tend to be moderately low. They do not necessarily reflect the body stores. For example, serum iron and retinol levels may be normal with almost depleted body stores, or in kwashiorkor they may be relatively low with adequate stores because of alterations in the transport proteins, transferrin and retinol-binding protein.

Many other biochemical changes have been described in severe PEM. Some are discussed in the section "Pathophysiology and Adaptive Responses"; others are listed in Table 59.6. Although they have little practical importance in diagnosing the disease, they allow better understanding of the pathophysiologic modifications.

Body protein is lost slowly, most of it from muscle, and the greater loss of adipose tissue results in a relative increase in total body water (i.e., per unit of body mass), mainly as intracellular water. In severe protein deficiency (kwashiorkor), extracellular water also increases. The intracellular concentrations of potassium and magnesium decrease and that of sodium increases, although the serum concentrations of electrolytes do not necessarily reflect these alterations (101).

Table 59.6
Additional Selected Biochemical Changes Observed in Severe PEM

	Marasmus	Edematous PEM
Body composition		
Total body water	High	High
Extracellular water	High	Higher
Total body potassium	Low	Lower
Total body protein	Low	Low
Serum or plasma		
Transport proteins[a]	Normal or low	Low
Branched-chain amino acids	Normal or low	Low
Tyrosine:phenylalanine ratio	Normal or low	Low
Enzymes (in general)[b]	Normal	Low
Transaminase	Normal or high	High
Liver		
Fatty infiltration	Absent	Severe
Glycogen	Normal or low	Normal or low
Urea cycle and other enzymes[c]	Low	Lower
Amino acid synthesizing enzymes	High	Not as high

From Torún B, Viteri FE. Protein-energy malnutrition. In: Warren KS, Mahmoud AAF, eds. Tropical and geographical medicine. 2nd ed. New York: McGraw-Hill, 1990.

[a]For example, transferrin, ceruloplasmin, retinol-, cortisol-, and thyroxine-binding proteins, α- and β-lipoproteins.

[b]For example, amylase, pseudocholinesterase, alkaline phosphatase.

[c]For example, xanthine oxidase, glycolic acid oxidase, cholinesterase.

Histopathologic studies show nonspecific atrophy, mainly in tissues with greater cell turnover rates such as intestinal mucosa, red bone marrow, and testicular epithelium; intestinal villi are flattened, and enterocytes lose their columnar appearance. In marasmus there is generalized atrophy of skeletal muscle. The skin changes consist of dermal atrophy, ecchymosis, ulcerations, and hyperkeratotic desquamation, seen primarily in areas subjected to irritation and not necessarily restricted to exposed areas, as in the case of pellagra. The liver in individuals with kwashiorkor is enlarged with fatty infiltration; periportal fat appears first and advances centripetally as severity increases. Other histologic analyses, special staining techniques, and electron microscopy reveal more alterations, not all of which result specifically from primary PEM. All do reflect generalized atrophy, however. Lesions due to superimposed infections and other nutrient deficiencies often are evident macroscopically and upon histopathologic examination. These changes usually revert to normal with nutritional recovery, although some residual lesions may persist for a long time.

PROGNOSIS AND RISK OF MORTALITY

Treatment of mild and moderate PEM corrects the acute signs of the disease, but children's catch-up growth in height may take a long time or might never be achieved. These children have been deprived not only of food but also of opportunities for development, and they may have missed critical periods for harmonic physical, mental, and social maturation. Weight for height can be restored easily, but the child may remain stunted, and a small body size may influence his or her maximal working capacity as an adult. Many severely malnourished children appear to have residual behavioral and mental problems in creativity and social interaction. However, the causal roles of malnutrition and a poor living environment are difficult to disassociate, and there is no irrefutable evidence that the damage cannot be corrected in a good, stimulating environment.

Mortality rates among children with severe PEM are associated with the quality of treatment. Worldwide, median case fatality has remained unchanged at 20 to 30% over the past 50 years, due to outmoded and faulty case management, with the highest levels (40–60%) among those with edematous PEM (102). Low mortality is attainable with adequate treatment, and in some centers it is as low as 4 to 6% for both edematous and nonedematous forms. Table 59.7 lists the characteristics that generally indicate a poor prognosis and demand close surveillance.

TREATMENT

Severe PEM

Patients with uncomplicated PEM should be treated outside the hospital whenever possible. Hospitalization increases the risk of cross-infections, and the unfamiliar setting may increase apathy and anorexia in children, making feeding more difficult. Severely malnourished children with signs of a poor prognosis (Table 59.7) or other life-threatening complications and those living under deplorable social conditions that do not permit adequate medical and nutritional treatment as outpatients must be hospitalized.

Treatment strategy can be divided into three stages: *(a)* resolving life-threatening conditions, *(b)* restoring nutritional status without disrupting homeostasis, and *(c)* ensuring nutritional rehabilitation.

Table 59.7
Characteristics That Indicate Poor Prognosis in Patients with PEM

- Age less than 6 months
- Deficit in weight for height greater than 30%, or in weight for age greater than 40%
- Signs of circulatory collapse: cold hands and feet, weak radial pulse, diminished consciousness
- Stupor, coma or other alterations in awareness
- Infections, particularly bronchopneumonia or measles
- Petechiae or hemorrhagic tendencies (purpura is usually associated with septicemia or a viral infection)
- Dehydration and electrolyte disturbances, particularly hypokalemia, and severe acidosis
- Persistent tachycardia, signs of heart failure or respiratory difficulty
- Total serum proteins below 30 g/L
- Severe anemia with clinical signs of hypoxia
- Clinical jaundice or elevated serum bilirubin level
- Extensive exudative or exfoliative cutaneous lesions, or deep decubitus ulcerations
- Hypoglycemia
- Hypothermia

Resolving Life-Threatening Conditions

On admission, the child with severe PEM is often a medical emergency. Restoration of nutrition should start as soon as possible, but it can be delayed until life-threatening conditions are resolved. The most frequent life-threatening conditions follow.

Fluid and Electrolyte Disturbances. The assessment of dehydration is not easy in severe PEM, because classic signs of dehydration, such as sunken eyeballs and decreased skin turgor, are frequently found in well-hydrated patients, whereas hypovolemia may coexist with subcutaneous edema, and irritability or apathy makes assessment of the mental state difficult. Useful signs are a history of watery diarrhea or vomiting, thirst, low urinary output, weak and rapid pulse, low blood pressure, cool and moist extremities, and a declining state of consciousness. The therapeutic approach differs from that in well-nourished patients because of water and electrolyte peculiarities of severe PEM: *(a)* hypoosmolality with moderate hyponatremia, *(b)* mild-to-moderate metabolic acidosis, which decreases or disappears when the patient receives dietary or parenteral energy and when electrolyte balance is reestablished, *(c)* high tolerance to hypocalcemia, partly because the acidosis produces a relative increment in ionized calcium and partly because hypoproteinemia makes less protein available to bind calcium ions, *(d)* decreased body potassium without hypokalemia, and *(e)* decreased body magnesium, with or without hypomagnesemia.

Fluid repletion should allow a diuresis of at least 200 mL in 24 hours in children and 500 mL in adults, or a micturition every 2 to 3 hours. Whenever possible, oral or nasogastric rehydration should be used. Many clinicians report good results with the use of the oral rehydration salt (ORS) solution promoted by the WHO for children who are not severely malnourished. But in keeping with recent WHO recommendations for the management of severe malnutrition, it is preferable to use solutions that provide more potassium, magnesium, and (especially for edematous PEM) less sodium (103). Opinions regarding the concentration of sodium vary between 30 and 60 mmol/L (104). A practical approach is preparation of a mineral mix to complement the diet, which can be combined with WHO's regular ORS and sucrose to prepare a *modified ORS* solution for patients with severe PEM. This solution will have magnesium to begin replenishing the body stores and help potassium retention as well as other minerals that usually are deficient in severely malnourished patients. Table 59.8 shows the composition of the mineral mix, and Table 59.9 shows the composition of the modified ORS prepared by diluting one standard WHO ORS packet, *two* 3.12-g packets of mineral mix (*or* 40 mL of concentrated mineral mix solution), and 50 g of sucrose in *2* L of water (103).

The ORS solution should be given *orally* in small quantities (a teaspoonful or sips from a cup) every few minutes to provide between 70 and 100 mL/kg body weight over a period of 12 hours, starting with about 10 mL/kg/h during the first 2 hours for children with mild-to-moderate dehydration and up to 30 mL/kg/h for severe dehydration. This is slower than is customary for less undernourished, dehydrated children (105). Additional ORS solution should be given to compensate for the losses of diarrhea and vomiting. As a general guide, give 50 to 100 mL after each loose stool to children under 2 years old and twice as much to older children. Breast-feeding should continue during the period of rehydration, approximately every half-hour. *Patients must be evaluated every hour.* As soon as the patient improves, usually 4 to 6 hours after beginning rehydration, small amounts of liquid dietary formula with potassium, calcium, magnesium, and other electrolytes should be offered every 2 to 3 hours. If signs of dehydration are still present after 12 hours but the condition is improving, another 70 to 100 mL ORS/kg can be given over the next 12 hours. When there are signs of overhydration, such as when the child's eyelids become puffy, edema increases, the jugular veins become full, or respiratory rate increases, only breast milk or liquid diet should be given instead of ORS.

Table 59.8
Mineral Mix for Preparation of Modified Oral Rehydration Salt (ORS) Solution and to Complement Liquid Foods[a]

Salt	Amount (g)	mmol in 1 g	mmol in 3.71 g
Potassium chloride	89.5	6.47 K	24 K
Tripotassium citrate	32.4	1.62 K	6 K
Magnesium chloride · $6H_2O$	30.5	0.81 Mg^{2+}	3 Mg
Zinc acetate · $2H_2O$	3.3	0.081 Zn^{2+}	0.300 Zn
Copper sulfate · $7H_2O$	0.56	0.011 Cu^{2+}	0.040 Cu
Total	156.26[b]		

[a] 1 mmol K = 39.1 mg; 1 mmol Mg = 24.3 mg; 1 mmol Zn = 65.4; 1 mmol Cu = 63.5 mg.

[b] Add water to make 1000 mL concentrated mineral mix solution that can be stored at room temperature, or prepare packets with 3.12 g of dry mineral mix. Add 20 mL of the concentrated solution or 1 packet to each liter of modified ORS solution or liquid food (based on WHO recommendations [103]).

Table 59.9
Composition of *Modified* Oral Rehydration Solution for Severely Malnourished Children[a,b]

Component	Concentration (mmol/L)[b]
Glucose	125
Sodium	45
Potassium	40
Chloride	70
Citrate	7
Magnesium	3 (6 mEq)
Zinc	0.3
Copper	0.04
Osmolarity	300

[a] Prepared by diluting *one* standard WHO ORS packet, *two* 3.12-g packets or 40 mL of concentrated mineral mix solution shown in Table 59.8, and 50 g sucrose in *two* liters of water (103).

[b] 1 mmol glucose = 180 mg; 1 mmol Na = 23.0 mg; 1 mmol K = 39.1 mg; 1 mmol Cl = 35.5 mg; 1 mmol citrate = 207.1 mg; 1 mmol Mg = 24.3 mg; 1 mmol Zn = 65.4; 1 mmol Cu = 63.5 mg.

Children who vomit constantly or who cannot be fed orally should be rehydrated by *nasogastric tube,* giving 3 to 4 mL of ORS solution/kg slowly or drop by drop every half-hour. In addition to what was described for oral rehydration, the following actions must be taken on the basis of frequent evaluations: if there is repeated vomiting or increasing abdominal distension, give the fluid more slowly and in smaller portions; if hydration is not improving after 4 hours, begin intravenous rehydration; when vomiting ceases and hydration improves, give modified ORS by mouth and, if the child tolerates oral solutions for the next 2 hours, remove the nasogastric tube.

Intravenous fluids must be used when there is repeated vomiting or persistent abdominal distension, and in severe dehydration with hypovolemia and impending shock. Hypoosmolar solutions (200–280 mOsm/L) must be used. Potassium (when urinating) and sodium should not exceed 6 and 3 mmol/kg per day, respectively, and glucose must provide at least 63 to 126 kJ (15–30 kcal)/kg/day. Solutions that have been successfully used include a 1:1 mixture of 10% dextrose in water (D/W) either with isotonic saline (i.e., 5% glucose in 0.5 N saline) or with Darrow's solution; a 1:2:3 mixture of 0.17 sodium lactate:isotonic saline:10% D/W; or Hartmann's solution (Ringer's lactated solution). One of these should be infused *during the first hour* at a rate of 10 to 30 mL/kg, depending on the patient's condition. After that, 5% glucose in 0.2 N saline (800 mL of 5% D/W, 20 mL of 50% D/W, and 200 mL of isotonic saline), or a 1:2:6 mixture of lactate:isotonic saline:5% glucose with 50 mL of 50% D/W added to each 500 mL, should be infused at a rate of 5 to 10 mL/kg/h, based on hourly evaluations of the patient, until oral therapy is initiated. When the patient is urinating, 2 g KCl (27 mmol K) is added to each liter of the infusion solution.

Increases in pulse and respiratory rate with weight gain after accounting for weight of excreta, pulmonary rales, and appearance or exacerbation of edema indicate overhydration. An increase in pulse and respiratory rate with weight loss, low urine output, and continuing losses from diarrhea and vomiting suggest insufficient fluid therapy.

Patients with severe hypoproteinemia (less than 30 g/L), anuria, and signs of hypovolemia or impending circulatory collapse should be given 10 mL plasma per kg in 1 to 2 hours, followed by 20 mL/kg/h of a mixture of two parts of 5% dextrose and one part of isotonic saline for 1 or 2 hours. This will increase plasma protein concentration by about 5 to 10 g/L and help prevent the rapid exit of water from the intravascular compartment. If diuresis does not improve, the dose of plasma can be repeated 2 hours later. Further treatment is similar to that of well-nourished patients. Unless the patient is at risk of imminent death, only plasma tested to be human immunodeficiency virus (HIV)-negative should be used.

Hypocalcemia may occur secondary to magnesium deficiency. When the patient has symptoms of hypocalcemia and serum magnesium determinations are not available, it is essential not only to give calcium infusion but also to give magnesium intravenously or intramuscularly. When the serum concentration of calcium rises to normal or, in the absence of laboratory data, when the symptoms of hypocalcemia disappear, calcium infusion may be discontinued. Intramuscular or oral magnesium supplementation should follow the initial parenteral magnesium until the patient is repleted with this ion as indicated by maintenance of serum and urine magnesium concentrations. When there are no laboratory facilities to monitor Mg concentrations, a general therapeutic guideline is to give magnesium intramuscularly as a 50% solution of magnesium sulfate in doses of 0.5, 1, and 1.5 mL for patients who weigh less than 7, between 7 and 10, and more than 10 kg, respectively. The dose can be repeated every 12 hours until there is no recurrence of the hypocalcemic symptoms and oral magnesium supplementation of 0.25 to 0.5 mmol Mg (0.5 to 1 mEq)/kg/day can be given, as described later. Certain antibiotics, such as amphotericin, can cause loss of magnesium and potassium into the urine, increasing the need for both ions.

Infections. Malnourished patients are particularly prone to infections, which are frequently the immediate cause of death in severe PEM. Paradoxically, clinical manifestations may be mild, and the classic signs of fever, tachycardia, and leukocytosis may be absent. Antigen-antibody reactions are often impaired, and skin tests such as tuberculin, often give falsely negative results.

When an infection is suspected, appropriate antibiotic therapy must be started immediately, even before obtaining the results of microbiologic cultures. The choice of drug will vary with the suspected etiologic agent, the severity of the disease, and the pattern of drug resistance in that area. Although antibiotics should not be used prophylactically, when patients cannot be monitored closely by experienced personnel for signs of infection, as is often the case in rural hospitals of developing countries, it is safer to assume that all ill and severely malnourished patients have a bacterial infection and to treat them with antibiotics to cover both gram-positive and gram-negative microorganisms; the latter are particularly common in PEM. When septicemia is suspected, a broad-spectrum antibiotic or a combination such as ampicillin and gentamicin (two inexpensive antibiotics generally available in developing countries) is usually given intravenously. Other supportive treatment may also be necessary, such as treatment for respiratory distress, hypothermia, and hypoglycemia.

However, clinicians should be aware that drug metabolism is likely to be altered and that detoxification mechanisms are likely to be compromised in severe PEM as a result of delayed absorption, abnormal intestinal permeability, reduced protein binding, changes in the volume of distribution, decreased conjugation or oxidation in the liver, and decreased renal clearance (106, 107). For example, in malnourished children the half-lives of chloramphenicol (108), sulfadiazine (109), and gentamicin (106) are increased, and their clearance is decreased. For this same reason, treatment for intestinal parasites, which is rarely urgent, should be deferred until nutritional rehabilitation is under way. This will decrease the risks of potential toxicity, including the possibility of absorbing drugs normally not absorbed by a healthy intestine.

Every child over 6 months old should be vaccinated against measles on admission, because of the high mortality rates associated with this disease in severe PEM. As seroconversion may be impaired at this early stage of treatment, a second dose of vaccine should be given before discharge.

Hemodynamic Alterations. Cardiac failure may develop when there is severe anemia, during or after administration of intravenous fluids, or shortly after the introduction of high-protein and high-energy feedings or of a diet with high sodium content, leading to pulmonary edema and frequent secondary pulmonary infection. These alterations may result from impaired cardiac function, sudden expansion of the intravascular fluid volume, severe hypoxia, or impaired membrane function. Diuretics such as furosemide (10 mg intravenously or intramuscularly, repeated as necessary) should be given, and other supportive measures should be taken. Many clinicians advocate the use of digoxin (0.03 mg/kg intravenously, every 6–8 hours). *The use of diuretics merely to accelerate the disappearance of edema in kwashiorkor is contraindicated.*

Severe Anemia. The routine use of blood transfusions endangers the patient; hemoglobin levels will improve with proper dietary treatment supplemented with hematinics. Therefore, blood transfusions should be given only to those with severe anemia with less than 40 g hemoglobin/L, less than 12% packed cell volume (hematocrit), clinical signs of hypoxia, or impending cardiac failure. In many developing countries with a high prevalence of infection with HIV and few or no resources for screening the blood supply, the risk of transmission of HIV is significant; the use of transfusion should be restricted except in life-threatening situations. Whole blood (10 mL/kg) can be used in marasmic patients, but it is better to use packed red blood cells (6 mL/kg) in edematous PEM. The transfusion should be given slowly, over 2 to 3 hours and repeated if necessary after 12 to 24 hours. If there are signs of heart failure, 2.5 mL blood/kg should be withdrawn before the transfusion is started and at hourly intervals so that the total volume of blood transfused equals the volume of anemic blood removed.

Hypothermia and Hypoglycemia

Body temperature below 35.5°C and plasma glucose concentration below 3.3 mmol/L (60 mg/dL) can be due to either impaired thermoregulatory mechanisms, reduced fuel substrate availability, or severe infection. Asymptomatic hypoglycemia can be treated (and prevented) by feeding small volumes of glucose- or sucrose-containing diets and solutions every 2 to 3 hours, day and night. Severe symptomatic hypoglycemia must be treated intravenously with 10 to 20 mL of 50% glucose solution followed by oral or nasogastric administration of 25 to 50 mL of 10% glucose solution at 2-hour intervals for 24 to 48 hours.

Body temperature usually rises in the hypothermic patient with frequent feedings of glucose-containing diets or solutions. Patients must be closely monitored when external heat sources such as heavy clothing, heat lamps, and radiators are used to reduce the loss of body heat, because they may rapidly become hyperthermic. It is best to keep the seminude patients in an ambient temperature of 30 to 33°C. Treatment must also be given as for hypoglycemia and systemic infection.

Severe Vitamin A Deficiency. Severe PEM is often associated with vitamin A deficiency. A large dose of vitamin A should be given on admission, because ocular lesions can result from increased demands for retinol when adequate protein and energy feeding begins. Water-miscible vitamin A as retinol should be given orally or intramuscularly on the first day at a dose of 52 to 105 μmol (15,000–30,000 μg, or 50,000–100,000 IU) for infants and preschool children, or 105 to 210 μmol (30,000–60,000 μg, or 100,000–200,000 IU) for older children and adults, followed by 5.2 μmol (1500 μg, or 5000 IU) orally each day for the duration of treatment. The initial dose should be repeated for 2 more days in symptomatic patients. Corneal ulcerations should be treated with ophthalmic drops of 1% atropine solution and antibiotic ointments or drops until the ulcerations heal.

Homeostatic Restoration of Nutritional Status

The next objective of therapy is to replace nutrient tissue deficits as rapidly and safely as possible. This should start as soon as the measures to manage the life-threatening conditions have been established. Based on the premise that the patient is adapted to the malnourished state, nutritional treatment must begin slowly to avoid deleterious metabolic disruptions. Various regimens provide a diet that meets daily maintenance requirements for a few days, followed by a gradual increase in nutrient delivery. It is best to begin with a liquid formula fed orally or by nasogastric tube, divided equally into 6 to 12 feedings per day, depending on the patient's age and general condition. This frequent feeding of small volumes, which must be given around the clock to avoid fasting for more than 4 hours, prevents vomiting and development of hypoglycemia and hypothermia. For older children and adults with good appetite, the liquid formula can be partly substituted with solid foods that have a high density of good-quality, easily digestible nutrients. The same diet can be used to treat marasmic and edematous patients. The only difference is that the marasmic patient may require larger amounts of dietary energy after 1 or 2 weeks of dietary treatment, which can be provided by adding vegetable oil to increase the diet's energy density. Diets that derive as much as 60 to 75% of their energy from fats are usually well tolerated; there may be some steatorrhea without profuse diarrhea, and 85 to 92% of the fat is absorbed (51). Intravenous alimentation is not justified in primary PEM and can increase mortality rates (110).

The protein source must be of high biologic value and easily digested. Cow's milk is frequently available, but some clinicians worry about the possibility of lactose malabsorption in severe PEM. However, cow's milk usually is well tolerated and assimilated by severely malnourished children and can be safely advocated (111, 112). Goat's, ewe's, buffalo's, and camel's milk can also be used. Human, mare's, and ass's milk, however, have very low protein concentrations. Cow's dried skimmed milk has very low energy density, which must be restored by adding sugar and/or vegetable oil. Eggs, meat, fish, soy isolates, and some vegetable protein mixtures are also sources of good protein. Most vegetable mixtures have protein digestibilities that are 10 to 20% lower than those of animal proteins, making it necessary to feed larger amounts. Their bulk might pose a problem in feeding small children, but energy density can be increased by adding sugar and/or vegetable oil. The latter will also provide the essential fatty acids needed.

The diet must be supplemented to provide daily about 5 to 8 mmol K and 0.5 to 1 mmol Mg (1–2 mEq) *per kg of body weight*, and 150 to 300 μmol Zn and 40 to 50 μmol Cu. Sodium content should be low, especially for patients with edematous PEM. This can be accomplished by adding to the diet appropriate amounts of a mineral mix, as indicated in Table 59.8. Additional supplements should include daily doses of 5.2 μmol (1.5 mg, or 5000 IU) vitamin A, 1.2 mmol (0.3 mg) folic acid, and other vitamins and trace elements in the doses provided by most commercial preparations, which should be higher than the daily recommended allowances for well-nourished persons. Supplemental calcium to provide about 15 mmol (600 mg) daily should be given when nondairy diets are used. Supplemental iron (1–2.1 mmol, or 60–120 mg daily) should be given beginning 1 week after starting dietary therapy. Earlier administration of iron will not elicit a hematologic response (Fig. 59.2); it might facilitate bacterial growth, and if the free-radical theory is true, it might produce metabolic disturbances, especially in patients who have or may develop edematous PEM.

To avoid the danger of initial excessive intakes of protein and energy by hungry patients, a relatively rigid regimen is recommended to deliver small amounts of nutrients initially and increase them gradually every 2 or 3 days. A practical way to do this, which can also be applied to extremely anorectic patients who must be fed by nasogastric tube, is based on the preparation of a *basic liquid food* with high protein concentration and high energy density; Table 59.10 gives several examples. Delivery of proteins and energy is gradually increased by use of different concentrations of the basic food, as shown in Table 59.11; the additional sugar compensates for the dilution of dietary energy. The liquid preparations must be fed at a dose of 100 mL/kg/day. *Additional water* must be given to provide at least 1 mL of total fluids per kilocalorie in the diet. After day 7, the patient can be allowed larger amounts of food (ad libitum). The intervals for the dietary increments in Table 59.11 can be lengthened to 3 to 5 days in severely malnourished children, especially those with less than 30 g/L plasma proteins or serious metabolic disturbances. The energy density of the diet of marasmic patients who are not gaining weight at an adequate rate by the second week (an average of at least 5 g/kg/day) should be increased at 5- to 7-day intervals by adding vegetable oil (Table 59.11).

Table 59.10
Formulations for High-Protein, High-Energy Liquid Foods (3–4 g protein and 565 to 605 kJ (135–145 kCal) per 100 mL

Food Used As Protein Source	Amount (g)	Sucrose (g)	Oil[a] (g)	Water (mL)
Cow's milk, full-cream powder	140	100[d]	40	900
Cow's milk, skimmed powder	110	100[d]	70	900
Cow's, goat's, or camel's milk, fresh	1000	100[d]	40	—
Buffalo's or ewe's (sheep's) milk, fresh	850	100[d]	15	150
Yogurt (cow's or goat's milk)	900	100[d]	40	—
ICSM[b]	170	100	40	900
Incaparina[c]	140	100	55	900

Adapted from Torún B, Viteri FE. Protein-energy malnutrition. In: Warren KS, Mahmoud AAF, eds. Tropical and geographical medicine. 2nd ed. New York, McGraw-Hill, 1990.
[a]Amount of vegetable oil can be substituted for up to one-half with isoenergetic amounts of sugar.
[b]Mixture of 63% cornmeal, 24% defatted soy flour, 5% skimmed milk powder, 5% soy oil, and 3% vitamin and mineral mix, distributed by U.S. AID and CARE.
[c]Mixture of 58% lime-treated corn flour, 38% cottonseed flour, and 4% vitamin, mineral, and lysine mix, developed by INCAP.
[d]50 g of sugar can be substituted by 50 g of cereal flour (rice, corn) to reduce osmolality.

Another option, which is particularly useful for relief and refugee camps, is advocated by WHO (103). It consists of giving during the initial phase of treatment a liquid diet based on a mixture of skim milk, cereal flour, sugar, oil, vitamins and minerals, which provides 1.2 g protein and 75 kcal (314 kJ) per 100 mL. The child is given at least 80, but not more than 100, kcal/kg/day. After the appetite has returned, another liquid diet is used, with higher concentrations of skim milk and vegetable oil, and without cereal flour, which provides 2.8 g protein and 100 kcal (418 kJ) per 100 mL. Intake is maintained at 100 kcal/kg/day until steady weight gain is established, and then the diet is fed to satiety. Additional water is offered between feedings. The diets can be purchased as a powder that is mixed with water, or they can be made from the basic ingredients, which include a mineral mix similar to that shown in Table 59.8 and a commercial multivitamin preparation.

Therapeutic diets for older children must be adjusted to their age. Initial treatment should provide average energy and protein requirements, followed by a gradual

Table 59.11
Example of a Dietary Therapeutic Regimen for Children, Based on Dilutions of the Basic High-Energy Foods Shown in Table 59.10[a]

Days from Beginning of Treatment	Proportions of Basic Food + Water	Additional Sugar (g/100 mL)	Additional Oil (mL/100 mL)	100 mL Will Provide Protein (g)	100 mL Will Provide Energy (kCAL)
1	1 + 2	10	—	1–1.3	85–90
3	1 + 1	10	—	1.5–2	110–115
5	3 + 1	5	—	2.3–3	120–130
7	Undiluted	—	—	3–4	135–145
Marasmus[b]					
12	Undiluted	—	3	3–4	160–170
17	Undiluted	—	6	3–4	185–195
22	Undiluted	—	9	3–4	210–220
etc.	Undiluted	—	†	3–4	b

From Torún B, Viteri FE. Protein-energy malnutrition. In: Warren KS, Mahmoud AAF, eds. Tropical and geographical medicine. 2nd ed. New York, McGraw-Hill, 1990.

[a]The formulas must be fed at 100 mL/kg/day. They must be supplemented with adequate amounts of vitamins, minerals, and electrolytes. Additional water must be given to provide at least 1 mL of total fluids per kcal in the diet.

[b]Marasmic patients may require more dietary energy; 2 to 3 mL (half a teaspoon) of vegetable oil per 100 mL of liquid diet should be added at 5-day intervals until the rate of weight gain becomes adequate.

increase to about 1.5 times the energy and 3 to 4 times the protein requirements by day 7. Dietary energy delivery to marasmic patients may have to be increased further.

The attitude of the person who feeds the patient is important to overcome the patient's lack of appetite. Patience and loving care are needed to coax the child gently to eat all the diet. The appearance, color, and flavor of the foods also affect appetite and food acceptance.

The initial response to the diet is either no change in weight or a decrease caused by loss of edema, accompanied by large diuresis (Fig. 59.11). After 5 to 15 days, there is a period of rapid weight gain or "catch-up." The catch-up is usually slower in marasmus than in kwashiorkor. In children, the rate of catch-up weight gain is generally 10 to 15 times the rate of weight gain of a normal child of the same age, and it can be as much as 20 to 25 times greater. Some patients only show a four- or fivefold increase in catch-up. Most often this is associated with insufficient energy intake (e.g., because of inadequately prepared formula, insufficient amounts of formula given at each feeding, too few feedings per day, anorexia, or lack of patience of the person who feeds the child) or with overt or asymptomatic infections; urinary infections and tuberculosis are the most commonly seen asymptomatic diseases.

Ensuring Nutritional Rehabilitation

The last stage of treatment usually begins 2 to 3 weeks after admission, when the child is without serious complications, eating satisfactorily, and gaining weight. It may start in the hospital and continue on an outpatient basis, preferably at a nutrition rehabilitation center or similar facility that gives daytime care by staff trained in the rehabilitation of malnourished children. When there is no such facility, the hospital must continue to provide care until the child is ready for discharge. The patient must continue to eat adequate amounts of protein, energy, and other nutrients, especially when traditional foods are introduced into the diet. Emotional and physical stimulation must be provided, and persistent diarrhea, intestinal parasites, and other minor complications must be treated. Children should be vaccinated during this period as well.

Introduction of Traditional Foods. Other foods, especially those available at home, are gradually introduced into the diet in combination with the high-energy, high-protein formula. This step should be taken when edema has disappeared, the skin lesions are notably improved, the patient is active and interacts with the environment, the appetite is restored, and adequate rates of catch-up growth have been achieved. For children, a daily minimum intake of 3 to 4 g of protein and 500 to 625 kJ (120 to 150 kcal)/kg of body weight (or more in marasmus) must be ensured. To achieve this, the energy density of solid foods must be increased with oil, and protein density and quality must be high, using animal proteins, soybean protein preparations, and good vegetable protein mixtures. Local traditional foods can be used in appropriate combinations (113–115) *in addition to the liquid formula,* as in the following examples: *(a)* one part of a dry pulse or its flour (e.g., black beans, soybeans, kidney beans, cowpeas) and three parts of a dry cereal or flour (e.g., corn, rice, wheat); fat or oil should be added to the mashed or strained pulse during or after cooking in amounts equal to the weight of the dry pulse or flour, and to the cereal preparations in amounts of 10 to 30 mL oil/100 g dry cereal product, depending on the type of preparation; and *(b)* four parts of a dry cereal (e.g., rice or wheat) and one part of fresh fish, fowl, or meat; fat or oil should be added in amounts equal to 20 to 40% of the dry weights. The food can be served as separate dishes or the parts can be mashed or blended and fed as paps to infants and young children.

Emotional and Physical Stimulation. The malnourished child needs affection and tender care from the beginning of treatment. This requires patience and understanding by

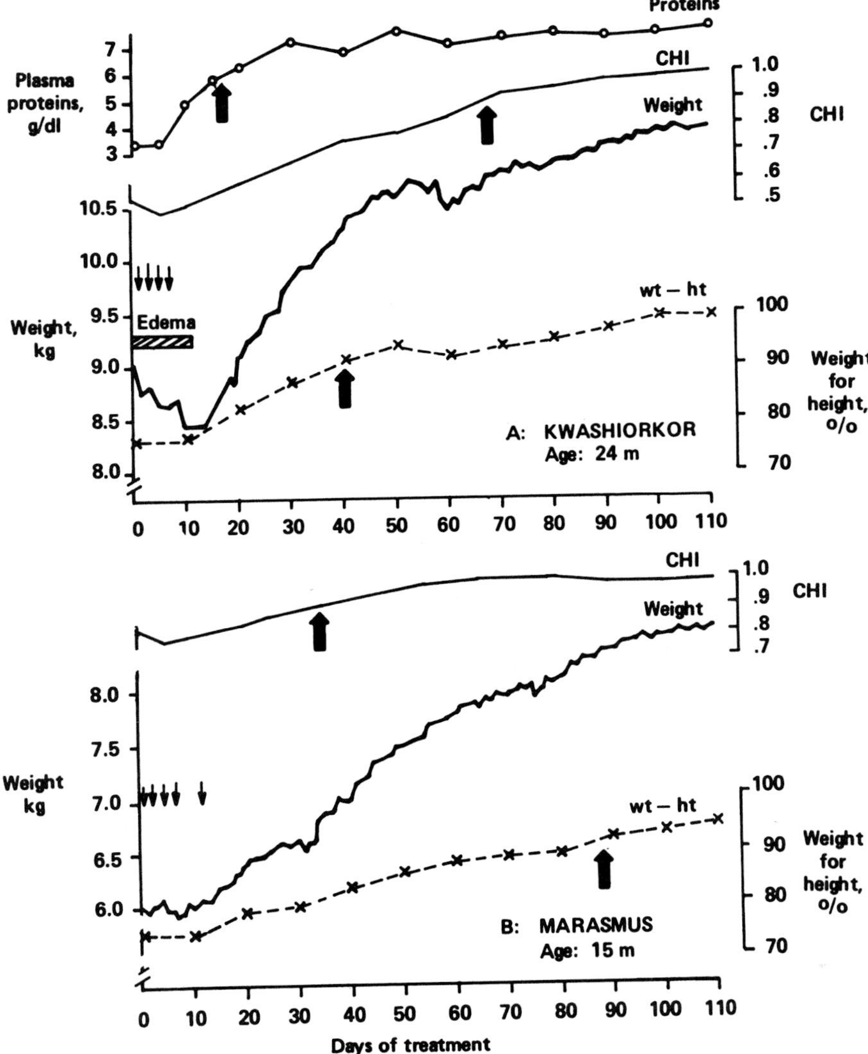

Figure 59.11. Weight gain and improvement in weight for height, creatinine-height index (CHI), and plasma protein concentration of two children treated at INCAP for kwashiorkor (child A) and marasmus (child B). The *thin, downward arrows* indicate gradual increments in dietary proteins and energy, as described in Table 59.11. The *thick, upward arrows* indicate the day when the lower limit of normal values was reached. The marasmic child had a normal plasma protein concentration on admission. Weight for height was calculated on child A on admission, after correcting for the weight of edema. Dietary energy was reduced on days 60 and 80 for child A and on day 100 for child B.

the hospital staff and relatives. Involvement of parents or relatives must be encouraged. Hospitals should be brightly colored and cheerful, with auditory stimulation such as music. As soon as the child can move without assistance and is willing to interact with the staff and other children, he or she must be encouraged to explore, to play, and to participate in activities that involve body movements. Relatively small increments in physical activity and energy expenditure during the course of nutritional rehabilitation result in faster longitudinal growth and accretion of lean body tissues (116, 116a). This can be achieved with games and activities that include walking uphill, running, tumbling, or climbing stairs. Parents should be encouraged to stimulate and teach their children by playing and talking. Toys and play materials can often be made from discarded local articles.

Adult patients should exercise regularly with gradual increments in cardiorespiratory workload.

Persistent or Recurrent Diarrhea and Other Health Problems. Mild diarrhea does not interfere with nutritional rehabilitation as long as fluid and electrolyte intakes maintain satisfactory hydration. This condition often disappears without specific treatment as nutritional status improves (117). However, persistent or recurrent diarrhea can contribute to development of a new episode of PEM and should be treated. Treatment is determined by the underlying cause of diarrhea, usually intestinal infections, excessive bacterial flora in the upper gut that ferment food substrates and deconjugate bile salts, intestinal parasites (particularly giardiasis, cryptosporidiosis, and trichuriasis), and intolerance to food components.

Lactose, milk protein, and gluten have commonly been held responsible for food intolerances. However, the apparent high prevalence of lactose malabsorption and intolerance in PEM is often based on inadequate diagnostic procedures (e.g., intolerance to 2 g lactose/kg in aqueous solution, rather than to the 7 to 15 g lactose contained in a milk meal) (49). When food intolerance is suspected, the diet should be modified, taking care to preserve its nutritional quality and density. Before branding a patient intolerant to a given food, the food should be reintroduced into the diet to confirm the diagnosis, and adequate diagnostic tests should be done.

Criteria for Recovery. Treatment until full recovery *should not* be in a hospital. Ideally, the patient should be referred to a nutrition clinic or rehabilitation center to continue treatment after all life-threatening conditions have been controlled, appetite is good, edema and skin lesions have disappeared, and the patient smiles, interacts with staff and other patients, and is gaining weight at a fast rate. The child's mother or caretaker must understand the importance of continuing the high-energy, high-protein diet until full recovery has taken place. If this can be done at home, the patient can continue treatment on an outpatient basis with regular follow-up in a nutrition clinic or its equivalent or by home visits by trained personnel.

An increase in plasma protein or albumin concentration indicates a good response but not full recovery (Fig. 59.11). The most practical criterion for recovery is weight gain, and almost all fully recovered patients should reach the weight expected for their height (see below). As shown in Figure 59.11, however, weight for height does not necessarily indicate protein repletion, and it is best to use it in conjunction with body composition indices. In children, if urine can be collected for 24 to 72 hours, the creatinine-height index (CHI) can be used as an indicator of body protein repletion. Premature termination of treatment increases the risk of a recurrence of malnutrition. As a general guideline, when body composition cannot be assessed, dietary therapy should continue for 1 month after the patient admitted with edematous PEM reaches an adequate weight for height without edema, and clinical and overall performances are adequate, or for 15 days after the marasmic patient reaches that weight. The minimum normal limits should be 92% of the weight expected for height (or 1 standard deviation below the reference median) and, especially in children, a CHI of 0.9. Some patients, however, do not reach those values because they are in the lower end of the normal distribution curve. If they continue growing at a normal rate and have no functional impairments, treatment can be terminated after 1 month of adequate dietary intake and weight for height and CHI stabilization. Specific treatment of other nutritional problems (e.g., iron deficiency) sometimes must be prolonged beyond discharge for PEM.

Before being discharged, patients or their parents must be taught about the causes of PEM, emphasizing rational and nutritious use of household foods, personal and environmental hygiene, appropriate immunizations, and early treatment—including dietary management—of diarrhea and other diseases.

Adolescents and Adults

The physiologic changes and principles of management of adolescents and adults with severe PEM are the same as those for children. Clinical and dietary history, as well as laboratory tests, are particularly important to identify underlying causes and to include them in the therapeutic program. Complications and life-threatening conditions must be treated as described for children.

Initial dietary treatment should provide average energy and protein requirements for the patient's age (45 kcal and 0.75 g protein/kg/day for adolescents, and 40 kcal and 0.6 g protein/kg/day for adults), followed by a gradual increase to about 1.5 times the energy and 3 to 4 times the protein requirements by day 7. Dietary energy delivery to marasmic patients may have to be increased further. Minerals and vitamins must be added in amounts at least twice the recommended daily allowances, following the same schedule as for children. Except for pregnant women, a single dose of 210 μmol (60 mg, or 200,000 IU) retinol should be given.

The liquid diets described for infants and young children can be given, especially to weak and anorectic patients. However, adults and adolescents are often reluctant to eat anything other than habitual foods, and liquid diets must be prescribed as a medicine, rather than as a food. When appetite improves, a diet should be given based on traditional foods but with added sugar and oil to increase energy density, plus vitamins and minerals. A wide variety of foods should be provided in amounts to satisfy appetite, taking into account the patient's inclinations and taboos. The liquid diet with vitamins and minerals should be given between meals and at night.

Adolescents and adults can be discharged when they are eating well and gaining weight, they have a reliable source of nutritious food outside the hospital, and other problems have been diagnosed and treatment begun. Supplementary feeding should continue on an outpatient basis until the BMI exceeds 15.0, 16.5, and 18.5, respectively, for adolescents 11 to 13 years old, adolescents 14 to 17 years old, and adults.

Mild and Moderate PEM

The less severe forms of PEM should be treated in an ambulatory setting, supplementing the home diet with easily digested foods that contain proteins of high biologic value, a high energy density, and adequate amounts of micronutrients. In some instances, therapy can be achieved merely by instructing the adult patient about adequate eating habits and a better use of food resources or by instructing mothers in improved child-feeding practices and more nutritious culinary habits. It is almost always necessary, however, to provide both nutritious food supplements and instructions for their use.

The quantity of food supplements will vary, depending on the degree of malnutrition and the relative deficit of proteins and energy. As a general guideline, the goal should be to provide a total intake, including the home diet, of *at least* twice the protein and 1.5 times the energy requirements. For preschool children, this would signify a daily intake of about 2 to 2.5 g of high-quality protein and 500 to 625 kJ (120 to 150 kcal)/kg of body weight, and for infants under 1 year, about 3.5 g protein and 625 kJ (150 kcal)/kg/day.

The ingestion of the food supplement by the malnourished person must be ensured. This is more likely to occur if it is appetizing to both child and mother, if it is ready-made or easy to prepare, if additional amounts are provided to feed other children living in the same household, and if it does not have an important commercial value outside the home that would make it easy and profitable for the family to sell the item for cash. A substitution effect on the home diet (i.e., a decrease in the usual food intake) is almost always unavoidable, but it can be reduced by using low-bulk supplements with high protein and energy concentrations. Special attention should be given to avoid a decrease in breast-feeding. The supplements for breast-fed infants should be paps or solid foods that will not quench the infant's thirst and thus not change the infant's demand or the mother's attitude toward lactation.

Adequate amounts of vitamins and minerals must be ensured, although mild deficiencies can be overcome by the micronutrients in the food or by use of fortified vehicles such as iron-enriched bread or sugar fortified with retinol.

PREVENTION AND CONTROL OF PEM

Poverty, ignorance, frequent infections, cultural customs, cyclic climatic conditions, and natural and man-made disasters are among the main causes of PEM. Therefore, its control and prevention require multisectoral approaches that include food production and distribution, preventive medicine, education, social development, and economic improvement. At a national or regional level, control and prevention can only be achieved through short- and long-term political commitments and effective actions to enforce the measure to eradicate the underlying causes of malnutrition.

Nevertheless, the physician, nutritionist, public health worker, and educator *can and must* play an active role in prevention of PEM, even though prevention is aimed at smaller population groups or individuals. If they have to attend only those at higher risk to develop PEM, because of limited resources, a profile of risk factors is useful. The most likely victims are children under 2 years of age from low socioeconomic strata whose parents have misconceptions concerning the use of foods, who come from broken or unstable families, whose families have a high prevalence of alcoholism, who live under poor sanitary conditions, in urban slums, or in rural areas frequently subject to droughts or floods, and whose societal beliefs prohibit the use of many nutritious foods. Special attention must be given to the availability and rational use of foods that optimize nutrient use, the control or reduction of infections, and health and nutrition education programs for the individual, the family, and the community.

Food Availability

Animal foods are the best protein sources, but they tend to be expensive, not always available, or prohibited by religious practices. Under such circumstances, the staple vegetable foods can be complemented with other vegetable foods combined in culturally acceptable ways to permit a good essential amino acid complementation and improve the biologic value of dietary protein. For example, corn and black bean combinations that provide proteins in a proportion of about 60:40, equivalent to about three parts of dry corn and one part of dry beans, have an excellent amino acid composition and permit adequate growth and function (118). The same is true of a series of other combinations of grains and pulses (113–115). The relatively low nitrogen digestibility of these vegetable sources must be considered in recommending the amounts to be eaten. Energy density can be increased by adding fats or carbohydrates.

It is often necessary to convince parents of the safety of using foods that, in some cultures, are fed only to adults and older children. This is especially true of foods used to complement mother's milk or to wean infants from the breast. Breast-fed infants from populations at risk of PEM should start receiving at 6 months of age—or earlier, if weight gain is not satisfactory—commercial preparations of cooked rice, oat, or wheat, or homemade paps prepared by mashing boiled rice, bread soaked in about 50% water, or cooked corn products (e.g., tamale, tortilla). After 6 months of age, fish, egg, or minced meat, or one part of a cooked pulse (e.g., kidney beans, soybeans, chick peas) should be added for every three parts of rice, corn, or bread to provide a better protein mixture. If the child is underweight, 1 teaspoon of vegetable oil or 2 teaspoons of sugar can be added to every 2 to 3 ounces of pap. Paps based on a pulse, such as black beans *(Phaseolus vulgaris)*, a cereal, and vegetable oil can be fed to babies as young as 3 months of age without intestinal discomfort and without decreasing breast milk intake. Examples of such paps are shown in Table 59.12.

Children who are fully weaned or only occasionally breast-fed must receive adequate amounts of energy- and protein-rich staples and, ideally, animal foods to satisfy their nutritional needs and allow adequate growth. It is also important to convince parents that food should not be withheld when a child has diarrhea, because in many developing countries children under 5 years of age have loose stools 15 to 20% of the time. Many local foods of vegetable origin that are rich in fiber can be safely used and may even shorten the duration of diarrhea (119).

Reducing Infections

The risk of infections must be reduced because of the interactions of nutrition with infection. High priority must

Table 59.12
Paps to Complement Breast Milk, Using Common Foods and Based on Combinations of a Legume with a Cereal or Potato, and Vegetable Oil

	A	B	C	D
Cooked beans (60% water)[a]	25 g	25 g	25 g	25 g
Corn dough (57% water)	75 g	—	—	—
White bread (50% water)	—	75 g	—	—
Boiled rice (55% water)	—	—	75 g	—
Boiled potatoes (33% water)	—	—	—	75 g
Water	25 mL	25 mL	25 mL	25 mL
Vegetable oil	10 mL	10 mL	10 mL	15 mL
Protein, g/100 g[b]	3.6	4.8	3.4	2.2
Energy, kcal/100 g[b]	176	176	183	147

Modified from unpublished observations by FE Viteri, B Garcia, and B Torún. Black beans (*Phaseolus vulgaris*) cooked, mashed, and strained. Corn dough cooked with limestone, according to Guatemalan customs. White bread soaked in equal weight of water.

[a] In parentheses: proportion of water added to prepare 100 g.

[b] Protein and energy content of 100 g of pap, ready to eat.

be given to immunizations, sanitary measures to reduce fecal contamination, and early oral rehydration and feeding of children with diarrhea (119).

Education

The presence of a malnourished child in a family indicates that something is wrong in that family and suggests that other members of the household might also be at risk of malnutrition. Therefore, nutritional and health education must not be restricted to rehabilitation of the index case but should include prevention of nutritional deterioration of other family members, especially siblings and pregnant and lactating women. Similarly, a high prevalence of children with malnutrition or growth retardation indicates that the entire community is at some risk of impaired nutrition. Consequently, education programs must be devised for community leaders, civic action groups, and the community as a whole. Such programs must emphasize promotion of breast-feeding, appropriate use of weaning foods, nutritional alternatives using traditional foods, personal and environmental hygiene, feeding practices during illness and convalescence, and early treatment of diarrhea and other diseases. Personal and communal involvement should be pursued through commitments to apply the recommendations. Toward this end, all educational programs *must* incorporate the community's own assessment of their nutritional problems and their feelings toward personal participation in solving these problems.

REFERENCES

1. Patron-Correa JP. Rev Med Yucatán (Mexico) 1908;3:89–96.
2. Normet L. Bull Soc Pathol Exot 1926;19:207–13.
3. Kerandel J. Bull Soc Pathol Exot 1926;19:302–11.
4. McConnell RE. Uganda Ann Med San Report (appendix 2). Entebbe: Government Printer, 1918.
5. Procter RAW. Kenya Med J 1927;3:264.
6. Mann WL, Helm JB, Brown CJ. JAMA 1920;75:1416–8.
7. Payne GC, Payne FK. Am J Hyg 1927;7:73–83.
8. Williams CD. Arch Dis Child 1932;8:423–33.
9. Williams CD. Lancet 1935;2:1151–2.
10. Autret M. Behar M. Síndrome policarencial infantil (kwashiorkor) and its prevention in Central America. FAO nutrition studies no. 113. Rome: Food and Agriculture Organization, 1954.
11. Trowell HC, Davies JNP, Dean RFA. Kwashiorkor. London: Edward Arnold, 1954.
12. Hegsted DM, Tsongas AG, Abbott DB, et al. J Lab Clin Med 1946;31:261–84.
13. Brock JF, Autret M. Kwashiorkor in Africa. FAO nutrition studies no. 8. Rome: Food and Agriculture Organization, 1952.
14. Jelliffe DB. J Pediatr 1959;54:227–56.
15. Pelletier DL, Frongillo EA, Schroeder DG, Habicht JP. Bull WHO 1995;73:443–8.
16. Kretchmer N, Beard JL, Carlson L. Am J Clin Nutr 1996;63: 997S–1001S.
17. De Onis M, Monteiro C, Akre J, Clugston G. Bull WHO 1993; 71:703–12.
18. UNICEF. The state of the world's children 1995. Oxford: Oxford University Press, 1996.
19. Garcia M. Malnutrition and food insecurity projections, 2020. Washington, DC: International Food Policy Research Institute, 1996.
20. Villar J, Rivera J. Pediatrics 1988;81:51–7.
21. Chagas C, Keusch GT, eds. The interaction of parasitic diseases and nutrition. Pontificiae academiae scientiarum scripta varia no. 61. Vatican: Pontifical Academy of Sciences, 1986.
22. Torun B. Short and long-term effects of low or restricted energy intakes on the activity of infants and children. In: Schurch B, Scrimshaw NS, eds. Activity, energy expenditure and energy requirements of infants and children. Lausanne: International Dietary Energy Consultancy Group, 1990;335–59.
23. Viteri FE, Torun B. Bol Of Sanit Panam 1975;78:58–74.
24. Torun B, Viteri FE. United Nations Univ Food Nutr Bull 1981;Suppl 5:229–41.
25. Viteri FE, Alvarado J. Rev Col Med Guatem 1970;21:175–230.
26. Waterlow JC, Garlick PJ, Millward JD. Protein turnover in mammalian tisues and in the whole body. Oxford: North Holland, 1978.
27. Tomkins AM, Garlick PJ, Schofield WN, Waterlow JC. Clin Sci 1983;65:313–24.
28. Viteri FE. Primary protein-energy malnutrition: clinical, biochemical, and metabolic changes. In: Suskind RM, ed. Textbook of pediatric nutrition. New York: Raven Press, 1981;189–215.
29. Reddy V. Protein-energy malnutrition: an overview. In: Harper AE, Davis GK, eds. Nutrition in health and disease and industrial development. New York: Alan R Liss, 1981;227–35.
30. Viteri FE, Alvarado J, Luthringer DG, et al. Vitam Horm 1968;26:573–615.
31. Caballero B, Solomons NW, Batres R, et al. J Pediatr Gastroenterol Nutr 1985;4:97–102.
32. MacDougall LG, Moodley G, Eyberg C, Quirk M. Am J Clin Nutr 1982;35:229–35.
33. Wickramasinghe SN, Mary-Cotes P, Gill DS, et al. Br J Haematol 1985;60:515–24.
34. Viart P. Am J Clin Nutr 1977;30:334–48.
35. Heymsfield SB, Bethel RA, Ansley JD, et al. Am Heart J 1978;95:584–94.

36. Alleyne GAO. Pediatrics 1967;39:400–11.
37. Paniagua R, Santos D, Mu§oz R, et al. Pediatr Res 1980;14: 1260–2.
38. Mahakur AC, Mishra AC, Panda SN, et al. J Assoc Physicians India 1983;31:79–81.
39. Keusch GT. Malnutrition, infection and immune function. In: Suskind RM, Lewinter-Suskind L, eds. The malnourished child. Nestlé Nutrition Workshop series vol. 19. New York: Raven Press, 1990;37–59.
40. Chandra RK. Am J Clin Nutr 1991;53:1087–101.
41. Olusi SO, Thurman GB, Goldstein AL. Clin Immunol Immunopathol 1980;15:687–91.
42. Bhaskaram R, Siwakumar B. Arch Dis Child 1986;61:182–5.
43. Keusch GT, Torun B, Johnson RB, et al. J Pediatr 1984;105: 434–6.
44. Kauffman CA, Jones RG, Kluger MJ. Am J Clin Nutr 1986;44: 449–52.
45. Cerami A, Ikeda Y, LeTrang N, et al. Immunol Lett 1985; 11:173–5.
46. Nichols BL, Alvarado J, Hazlewood CF, et al. J Pediatr 1972; 80:319–30.
47. Lopes J, Russell DM, Whitwell J, et al. Am J Clin Nutr 1982;36:602–10.
48. Viteri FE, Schneider R. Med Clin North Am 1974;58: 1487–505.
49. Torun B, Solomons NW, Viteri FE. Arch Latinoam Nutr 1979;29:445–94.
50. Lifshitz F, Teichber S, Wapnir RA. Malnutrition and the intestine. In: Tsang RC, Nichols BL, eds. Nutrition and child health: a perspective for the 1980's. New York: Alan R Liss, 1981.
51. Torun B. Nutrient absorption in malnutrition. In: Chagas C, Keusch GT, eds. The interactions of parasitic diseases and nutrition. Pontificiae academiae scientiarum scripta varia no. 61. Vatican: Pontifical Academy of Sciences, 1986;81–94.
52. Winick M. J Pediatr Gastroenterol Nutr 1987;6:833–5.
53. Jaya-Rao KS. Lancet 1974;1:709–11.
54. Hendrickse RG. Trans R Soc Trop Med Hyg 1984;78:427–35.
55. Coulter JBS, Suliman GI. Eur J Clin Nutr 1988;42:787–96.
56. Golden MHN. The consequences of protein deficiency in man and its relationship to the features of kwashiorkor. In: Blaxter KL, Waterlow JC, eds. Nutritional adaptation in man. London: John Libby, 1985;169–88.
57. Golden MHN, Ramdath D. Proc Nutr Soc 1987;46:53–68.
58. Golden MHN, Ramdath D, Golden BE. Free radicals and malnutrition. In: Dreosti IE, ed. Trace elements, micronutrients and free radicals. Clifton, NJ: Humana Press, 1990.
59. Waterlow JC. Protein energy malnutrition. London: Edward Arnold, 1992.
60. Olson RE. Am J Clin Nutr 1975;28:626–37.
61. Alleyne GAO, Trust PM, Flores H, et al. Br J Nutr 1972; 27:585–92.
62. Munro HN. General aspects of the regulation of protein metabolism by diet and by hormones. In: Munro HN, Allison JD, eds. Mammalian protein metabolism, vol 1. New York: Academic Press, 1964.
63. Felig P. N Engl J Med 1970;283:149–59.
64. Arroyave G, Wilson D, Funes C, et al. Am J Clin Nutr 1962; 11:517–24.
65. Holt LE, Snyderman SE, Norton PM, et al. Lancet 1963; 2:1343–8.
66. Vis HL. Aspects de mecanismes des hyperaminoaciduries de l'enfance. Paris: Editions Arsica, 1963.
67. Schelp FP, Migasena P, Pongpaew P, et al. Am J Clin Nutr 1978;31:451–6.
68. Neufeld HA, Pace JA, White FE. Metabolism 1976;25:877–84.
69. Beisel WR, Sawyer WD, Ryll ED, et al. Ann Intern Med 1967;67:744–79.
70. Beisel WR, Am J Clin Nutr 1977;30:1236–47.
71. Powanda MC. Am J Clin Nutr 1977;30:1254–68.
72. Gabig TG, Babior BM. Oxygen-dependent microbial killing by neutrophils. In: Oberly LW, ed. Superoxide dismutase, vol 2. Boca Raton, FL: CRC Press, 1982;1–15.
73. Weech AA. Bull NY Acad Med 1939;15:63–91.
74. Walter SJ, Shore AC. Clin Sci 1988;75:621–8.
75. Klahr S, Alleyne GAO. Kidney Int 1973;3:129–41.
76. Migeon CJ, Beitins IZ, Kowarski A, Graham GG. Plasma aldosterone concentration and aldosterone secretion rate in Peruvian infants with marasmus and kwashiorkor. In: Gardner LI, Amacher P, eds. Endocrine aspects of malnutrition. Santa Ynez, CA: Kroc Foundation, 1973;399–424.
77. Beitins IZ, Graham GG, Kowarski A, et al. J Pediatr 1974;84: 444–51.
78. Srikantia SG, Gopalan C. Am J Appl Physiol 1959;14:829–33.
79. Srikantia SG, Mohanham S. J Clin Endocrinol 1970;31: 312–14.
80. Golden MHN. Lancet 1982;1:1261–5.
81. Torun B, Viteri FE. Rev Col Med Guatem 1976;27:43–62.
82. Patrick J. Br Med J 1977;1:1051–4.
83. Benjamin DR. Pediatr Clin North Am 1989;36:139–61.
84. Habicht JP, Martorell R, Yarborough C, et al. Lancet 1974;1: 611–15.
85. Graitcer PL, Gentry EM. Lancet 1981;2:297–99.
86. United States Dept of Health, Education and Welfare (DHEW). NCHS growth curves for children from birth to 18 years. PHS publ 78-1650. Hyattsville, MD: DHEW, 1970.
87. WHO. Measuring change in nutritional status. Geneva: World Health Organization, 1983.
88. Waterlow JC. Classification and definition of protein-energy malnutrition. In: Beaton GH, Bengoa JM, eds. Nutrition in preventive medicine. Geneva: World Health Organization, 1976.
89. Nabarro D, McNab S. J Trop Med Hyg 1980;83:21–33.
90. Torun B, Samayoa C. Un sistema sencillo para evaluar el estado nutricional de niños, con participación comunitaria. In: Proceedings 9th Latin American Congress of Nutrition. San Juan, PR, 1991;159.
91. James WPT, Ferro-Luzzi A, Waterlow JC. Eur J Clin Nutr 1988;42:969–81.
92. WHO. Physical status: the use and interpretation of anthropometry. WHO Tech Rep Ser 1995, no. 854.
93. Gomez F, Ramos-Galvan R, Frenk S. Adv Pediatr 1955;7: 131–69.
94. Rutishauser IHE, Whitehead RG. Br J Nutr 1972;28:145–52.
95. Viteri FE, Torun B. Nutrition, physical activity and growth. In: Ritzen M, Aperia A, Hall K, et al., eds. The biology of normal human growth. New York: Raven Press, 1981;265–73.
96. Spurr GB, Reina JC. Eur J Clin Nutr 1988;42:819–34.
97. Allen LH. Clin Nutr 1984;3:169–75.
98. Viteri FE, Torun B, Immink MDC, et al. Marginal malnutrition and working capacity. In: Harper AE, Davis GK, eds. Nutrition in health and disease and international development. New York: Alan R Liss, 1981;277–83.
99. Habicht JP, Lechtig A, Yarborough C, et al. Maternal nutrition, birth weight and infant mortality. In: Elliott J, Knight J, eds. Size at birth. Ciba Found Symp 1974, no. 27.
100. Viteri FE, Alvarado J. Pediatrics 1970;46:696–706.
101. Parra A, Garza C, Garza Y, et al. J Pediatr 1973;82:133–42.
102. Schofield C, Ashworth A. Bull WHO 1996;74:223–9.
103. WHO. Management of the child with severe malnutrition: a

manual for physicians and other senior health workers. Geneva: World Health Organization, in press.

104. Briend A, Golden MHN. Eur J Clin Nutr 1993;47:750–4.
105. WHO. A manual for the treatment of diarrhea: programme for the control of diarrhea disease, WHO/CDD/SER/80.1 rev. 1 1990. Geneva: World Health Organization, 1990.
106. Krishnaswamy K. Clin Pharmacokinet 1989;17(Suppl 1): 68–88.
107. Mehta S. Drug metabolism in the malnourished child. In: Suskind RM, Lewinter-Suskind L, eds. The malnourished child. Nestlé Nutrition Workshop series, vol 19. New York: Raven Press, 1990;329–38.
108. Mehta S, Nain CK, Kalso HK, Mathur VS. Indian J Med Res 1981;74:244–50.
109. Mehta S, Naim CK, Sharma B, Mathur VS. Pharmacology 1980;21:369–74.
110. Janssen F, Bouton JM, Vuye A, et al. JPEN J Parenter Enteral Nutr 1983;7:26–36.
111. Solomons NW, Torun B, Caballero B, et al. Am J Clin Nutr 1984;40:591–600.
112. Torun B, Solomons NW, Caballero B, et al. Am J Clin Nutr 1984;40:601–10.
113. Cameron C, Hofvander Y. Manual on feeding infants and young children. 2nd ed. New York: United Nations Protein-Calorie Advisory Group, 1976.
114. Torun B, Young VR, Rand WM, eds. Protein-energy requirements of developing countries: evaluation of new data. Tokyo: United Nations Univ Food Nutr Bull (Suppl 5), 1981.
115. Rand WM, Uauy R, Scrimshaw NS, eds. Protein-energy requirement studies in developing countries: results of international research. Tokyo: United Nations Univ Food Nutr Bull (Suppl 10), 1984.
116. Torun B, Schutz Y, Bradfield RB, et al. Effect of physical activity upon growth of children recovering from protein-calorie malnutrition (PCM). In: Proceedings 10th International Congress Nutrition. Kyoto: Victory-sha Press, 1976; 247–9.
116a. Torun, Viteri FE. Eur J Clin Nutr 1994;48(Suppl 1):S186–90.
117. Torun B. Alimentación de niños con desnutrición proteínico-energética y diarrea, con énfasis en las experiencias del INCAP. In: Pan American Health Organization Meeting on Feeding of Children Ill with Diarrhea. Washington, DC: Pan American Health Organization, 1983.
118. Viteri FE, Torun B, Arroyave G, et al. Food Nutr Bull 1981;Suppl 5:202–9.
119. Torun B, Chew F. Trans R Soc Trop Med Hyg 1991;85:12–17.
120. INCAP. Evaluación nutricional de la población de Centro América y Panamá: Guatemala. Guatemala: Instituto de Nutrición de Centro América y Panamá, 1969.
121. Torun B, Viteri FE. Protein-energy malnutrition. In: Warren KS, Mahmoud AAS, eds. Tropical and geographical medicine. 2nd ed. New York: McGraw-Hill, 1990:1024–40.

60. Malnutrition among Children in the United States: The Impact of Poverty

ROBERT KARP

There are over 13 million children in the United States living in families with incomes below the poverty level (1, 2). Of these, approximately 10% have clinical malnutrition, mostly iron deficiency, but all poor children are at risk for the long-term consequences of malnutrition including continued poverty. It is the chronicity of poverty that leads to the consequences of malnutrition and learning failure, since the behavioral adjustments to chronic poverty may affect nutritional status adversely (3, 4). This chapter shows how poverty affects food intake, nutritional status, behavior, and intellectual performance. These consequences contribute to ongoing cycles of poverty (5–7).

Malnutrition among the poor in the United States is neither marked protein-energy malnutrition (marasmus or kwashiorkor) nor classic micronutrient deficiency (pellagra, beriberi, scurvy). Rather, both national surveys (3, 8) and those conducted in small communities (9, 10) show that growth retardation is an expression of malnutrition among poor children. Deficient intake and biochemical measures of micronutrient status, based solely on income, are found for folate (11–16), ascorbic acid (12–14, 16), vitamin A (12–14, 16), several of the B vitamin group (14), and continued iron deficiency (14, 17), even with a decade of decrease in response to successful food programs (17). These findings are striking in contrast to measures of nutrient intake and nutritional status in other industrial societies where poverty is uncommon (8, 17–20).

Mild protein-energy malnutrition associated with growth retardation (20, 21) and nutrition-related disorders including iron deficiency (5–7, 21–23) have contributed to observed learning failure, deprivation, and disease within poor families in the United States. Lead poisoning in childhood (24) has consequences similar to in utero exposure to drugs (25), alcohol (26), and products of tobacco smoking (25) because of its effect on diet, use of nutrients, and direct toxicity to metabolic pathways in the fetus. A covariance model is presented in which nutrition and environment operate synergistically in both cause and repair of developmental delay and associated consequences (5–7, 27).

An international survey, the Luxembourg Income Study of Families with Children, ranked 18 developed nations on the basis of both wealth and poverty (i.e., income at 10th and 90th percentile adjusted to U.S. dollars [28]). The United States ranked first in income of the wealthy and 16th in income of the poor; the rich:poor ratio of 6 was by far the highest. Moreover, unlike other industrial societies, in the United States having children reduces income substantially, and essential services such as medical care and support for children while their parents seek education or employment are not universally available (19, 28). The dimensions of this neglect "are spelled out in the growth of children" (8). The data presented in this chapter show that poverty has both direct effects on food intake and nutritional status and indirect affects through the use of drugs, alcohol, and tobacco.

UNDERNUTRITION AS AN INDICATOR OF POVERTY

Measures used to determine the nutritional status of individuals must be distinguished from those applicable to communities (29). Poverty is associated with poor growth and other clinical signs of malnutrition. For individuals, growth retardation may or may not be the result of undernutrition. However, when a disproportionate number of children in a community are growth retarded, fail to maintain linear growth, or are anemic, it is reasonable to assume that the community provides a suboptimal environment, with undernutrition as its most predictable outcome (29, 30).

Assessing Growth Retardation

Systems commonly used for assessing growth retardation are (a) weight adjusted for age (from Gomez) (29), (b) weight adjusted for height or, below 2 years of age, for length assessed simultaneously with height adjusted for age (from Waterlow) (30), (c) that from McLaren and Reed, commonly used in clinical practice, which considers actual weight as a percentage of ideal weight for actual height (31). Though effective in determining the degree of protein-energy malnutrition in individual children, this last method is rarely used to assess nutritional status in the community.

Under 5 years of age, weight for age combined with dietary surveys of the community and a careful diet and social history of the affected child provides the most sensitive indicators of deprivation (29). For example, in 1951, Widdowson (32) observed that a group of maltreated but well-fed German children living in an orphanage failed to grow as well as nurtured children with marginal diet in similar circumstances. Subsequently, Powell et al. (33) suggested impairment of the hypothalamic-pituitary axis as the cause. Recently, Skuse et al. (34) have documented growth hormone deficiency in growth-retarded children with excellent appetites living in stressful home situations.

Weight for age is an exquisitely sensitive indicator of disruptions in feeding and (unlike assessments that depend on measures of length or height) does not require extensive training to obtain accuracy. By contrast, as Gopalan writes, "Heights (or lengths) for age in children are more difficult to measure accurately, and height measurements are less sensitive to dietary deprivation" (29). Weight is the first parameter to change, and with longitudinal assessments, the age at which growth failure occurs tells investigators when disruption of nutrition or nurture occurs (3, 4, 29, 31). Data from the Pediatric National Nutrition Surveillance Survey (PedNSS), a poverty-weighted sample, show that 70% of low-birth-weight (LBW) babies are stunted at 3 months of age, and 30% at 1 to 2 years of age, compared with 10% of normal-weight infants at these later ages (4).

For older children, the Waterlow system considers height for age and weight for length (or height), first separately and then together as shown in Table 60.1 (30). "Wasting" (decreased weight for length or height) is associated with acute malnutrition and is distinguished from "stunting" (decreased length or height for age), seen with chronic malnutrition. This system is based on a standardized normal distribution using z-scores in which the 5th percentile is two standard deviation units below the mean. Stunted children at the 5th percentile have a height that is approximately 90% of the mean height for children of the same age and sex. Stunted growth with normalization of weight/height ratio has been misrepresented as an indicator of "nutritional adaptation" (29, 30), but children in developing countries who are either wasted or stunted are at greater risk from death from infection than children with neither wasting nor stunting (30). In the United States, growth retardation is associated with delayed neurodevelopment and school failure (3, 4, 35). Thus, of all measures of nutritional status for older children, none surpass "the great value of height measurements as an instrument for monitoring progress with respect to the state of health, nutrition and well being of communities" (29).

Table 60.1
The Waterlow System for Classification and Definition of Protein-Energy Malnutrition

		Length or height for age and sex	
		Normal range	<5th percentile
Weight for length or height and sex	Normal range	Normal	Stunting (chronic PEM)
	<5th %ile	Wasting (acute PEM)	Both acute and chronic PEM

Data from Martorell R. Child growth retardation: a discussion of its causes and its relationship to health. In: Blaxter K, Waterlow JC, eds. Nutritional adaptation in man. London: John Libby, 1985;13–30.

Short stature in early life may be accounted for by decreased birth length; and perhaps half of all LBW children with concomitant decreased length never completely achieve "catch-up" in linear growth (4, 36). The growth of small children is heavily influenced by multiple factors including the in utero environment, duration and quality of breast feeding, appropriate use of formula substitute, introduction of transitional food (beikost) at 4 to 6 months of age, and transitions to toddler and adult diets by 2 to 3 years of age (29).

In the United States, studies of children conducted in the 1960s showed consistent correlation among income and weight, height, and hemoglobin level (3, 4). Data for 1986 from the PedNSS showed a consistent decrease in weight for age as well as short stature for poor children under 5 years old of all racial and ethnic backgrounds (4). These data were supported by findings by Scholl and colleagues in Camden, NJ, where the white-poor (37) and abused children of any ethnicity (38) were most likely to demonstrate both wasting and stunting. Using data from the National Longitudinal Survey of Youth, Miller and Korenman showed that poverty affects the growth rate. Height for age was significantly lower among poor children than among average- and above-average-income children (4).

HOW POVERTY LEADS TO MALNUTRITION

Living in poverty means having economic resources below those needed to "obtain a minimally adequate standard of living" and/or essential goods and services (39). Simply stated, the poor cannot possibly enter the mainstream of American life and become self-supporting without an adequate income, capital, or other resources such as land inheritance or kinship networks available to them (39–42).

Defining Poverty

For over 40 years, the United States has used an absolute definition of poverty—"an income three times the value of a low cost diet for a family unit" (39). This definition originated with the need to provide economic support for the miner's widow or an incapacitated worker. It assumes economic dependency. Many in the United States have beliefs about the cause of poverty that tend to distinguish between people who deserve support and those who do not on the basis of how well they harbor their resources and how they behave (40–42a). This view fails to recognize that for the poor, behavior is shaped by the power of an environment they are unable to change (42a–44). Thus, the poor must prove their worth by higher rational and moral behavior than is required of people with higher incomes (42a, 43).

Recently, it was suggested that a relative definition of poverty should replace the absolute standard so that a recipient of support would have sufficient resources to escape dependency and enter the work force (39). The relativist model recognizes that financial resources are needed not simply to survive (food and housing) but also to work (cost of education, health care, clothing, day care, and transportation). With this model, the percentage of family income from employment or from unearned income is almost identical for poor and nonpoor alike so total income, with supports included, is the key difference (39).

Prevalence of Poverty

In the United States, almost 18 million (22.7%) of the 62.3 million children under 18 years of age live in poverty (2). Data from the 1993 U.S. Census reports show that the numerical majority of poor are white (9.75 million children; 9.4% of total for category); 5.12 million children (46.1%) of African American ancestry and 3.87 million (40.9%) of Hispanic ancestry are similarly affected.

Cipro and Michael recommended "that the poverty threshold concept apply to a reference family of two adults and two children" with threshold adjusted for families with special needs (39). The current poverty level income for this reference family is $14,306. They note, however, that the reference family is no longer predominant in the United States; one-adult households (25%) are most common, parents without children (22%) are second, and the two parent/two child reference (13%) is the third most common. As shown in Table 60.2, 9% of children in reference families live in poverty, with a rise from 25% to almost all children living in single-parent families of five or more; 48% of families with two children and one adult and 65% of three-children families with a single parent live in poverty (2).

Table 60.2
Children under 18 Years of Age in Families Living in Poverty[a]

Ratio = families living in poverty with children under 18 years
(All in 1000s)

	Number of Children						
	7	6	5	4	3	2	1
One adult	15	30	74	294	690	1220	1321
	15	32	78	350	1067	2538	3601
Percentage of these families in poverty	100	94	95	84	65	48	37
Two adults	47	25	101	253	581	825	578
	67	68	246	1017	3826	9589	8072
Percentage of these families in poverty	70	37	41	25	15	9	7

[a]For one adult/three child families, the poverty level is $14,705/year, compared with $11,602 for one adult/two child families, and $14,654 for reference families with two adults and two children (from Census data [2]).

The "New Approach" adjustment applied to single-parent two-child families would not shift them from poor to nonpoor if they were receiving aid-to-dependent families support (39). However, a parent who was working at a full-time job with the full range of deductions and had a need to pay for child care, work expenses, and out-of-pocket medical expenses would be recategorized as "poor" (39). Similarly, poverty status would not be changed for a similar family with a farm worker as head of household in the rural Midwest as opposed to a city-living family where the cost of living is thought to be higher. This may be an idealized view of the rural poor. In some areas, food costs are high, as is transportation for persons, goods, and services. Land is often unavailable, housing stock is expensive to rent and often deteriorated, and poor families lack the capital or credit rating to buy or rehabilitate a home.

Influence of Food Costs on Dietary Adequacy

An obvious need for poor and nonpoor alike is sufficient income to purchase food. Under pressure of rising food costs or decreasing income, food selection narrows to items containing the most energy at lowest cost (46, 47). Malnutrition ensues. This observation, called "Engels' Law" (46) from a description of eating patterns of English workers from the mid-19th century, is similar to one by Joseph Goldberger's in the rural American South at the turn of the 20th century (48). Goldberger "was well aware that pellagra was a problem of poverty and that only improvement in economic conditions would eradicate the disease" (48). More recently, evidence of iron deficiency anemia following a rise in food costs (47) and growth retardation associated with high housing costs (10) provide examples of Engels' law at work among innercity poor children.

Until recently, equal parts dairy products, meat, cereal grains, and fruits and vegetables—the "four food groups"—was the model for good nutrition, with a substantial contribution from fat to daily caloric intake (12). Recently, however, the model for good nutrition has been changed to a "food pyramid" that mimics the traditional low-income diet with its high cereal grain content but increases cost by recommending substantially more fruit (2–4 servings) and vegetables (3–5 servings) each day, with the hope of preventing the degenerative diseases of adult life. A poverty-weighted national sample of 3148 children 2 to 18 years old taken from the 1989–1991 Continuing Survey of Food Intakes by Individuals (CSFII) showed insufficient consumption of fruits and vegetables, with 25% of their intake of vegetables as french-fried potatoes.

Krebs-Smith et al. (12) compared the daily food intake of children from the poorest families (household incomes <$10,000/year) with that of children from the wealthiest families (>$50,000/year). They showed that 59.6% of the poorest children consumed less than one serving of fruit each day, compared with 46.5% of children from the wealthiest families. Moreover, the diet of poor children was less likely to contain the recommended five servings of fruits and vegetables (16.3 vs. 24.5%). Intake by the poor met the old standard from "four food groups" for fruits and vegetables but not the new standard. Of note, a minority of children in the United States meet the new standard, regardless of income (12).

Iron deficiency anemia affects the poor disproportionately because as incomes fall, food consumption narrows to those foods containing the most energy at the lowest cost (46). If this process continues long enough, essential nutrients disappear from the diet, and in the United States, iron deficiency occurs (47). As with growth retardation, this difference is documented in both national surveys and local studies. Using confirmatory biochemical markers to avoid overdiagnosing iron deficiency as the cause for anemia, the Second National Health and Nutrition Examination Survey (NHANES) of 1976–80 showed that 20.6% of children 1 to 2 years of age from families living below the poverty level had iron deficiency, compared with 6.7% for nonpoor children (49). For children 3 to 4 years of age, the difference is 9.7% compared with 2.5%. Older children take in more calories and thus more iron. These differences by economic status disappear until girls reach adolescence, when iron requirements increase. As shown in NHANES II, the values are 8.2% and 2.8% for poor and nonpoor teenage girls, respectively. All comparisons are highly significant (49).

Influence of Food Choices

Economics alone do not determine the nutritional status of individual children in a family or community. Parental beliefs and practices profoundly affect how much and what kind of food is brought into the family as well as the allocation to each member (29, 50) (see also Chapter 107). Gopalan writes, "differences in the nature of intrafamilial distribution of food, in particular in infant feeding and child-rearing practices, between the families and between communities can result in important differences with nutritional status (especially of children) between households, and between communities with nearly similar overall levels of dietary inadequacy" (29). Variables to be considered include the use of breast-feeding (how long and how well), use of appropriate formulas as a substitute, and the use and choice of beikost (29–31). Issues of parental competence, age, spacing and health of siblings, and the presence of drugs, alcohol, and tobacco affect a child's growth (51).

An important variable is the relationship that forms between the mother and the affected infant or child. Three studies in the United States (Pollitt [52], Karp et al. [53], and Casey et al. [54]) document that malnutrition is not an isolated occurrence in the families of undernourished children. In each of these studies, relationships between mothers and undernourished children were less effective than those in families with similar incomes and education and well-nourished children. In the study by Karp et al. (53), the families with an excessive use of low-nutritional-value foods ate predominantly convenience foods.

The use of convenience foods, characteristic of contemporary general food consumption patterns in the United States, illustrates how the Engels' phenomenon affects the poor. Cheaper convenience foods have lower nutrient density (high fat or sugar content) than the more expensive nutritious ones (46). A cereal grain, legume, plus a little meat diet, as recommended by the U.S. Department of Agriculture in its "Low Cost Food Plan" (LCFP), can be obtained within the allotment, but to achieve savings, families need an adult at home who can prepare food and a supermarket with low-cost staples (46). Some parents—the homeless or indigent, those living in motel rooms or in migrant labor camps—may have no alternative to convenience foods. They may be quite willing to purchase nutritious foods and prepare and distribute them to their children but are hampered by their circumstances. Their indigenous food preferences may be unique, and preferred nutritious food choices may be unavailable (46).

Thus, in the context of chronic poverty, what we see as "food choice" is a highly complex phenomenon influenced by the cost and availability of food and the dynamics of the family. These and related issues are discussed in greater detail in Chapter 107.

UNDERNUTRITION AND LEARNING FAILURE

In the United States, children from the poorest and least-educated families consistently perform poorly on measures of cognitive ability (5, 21, 23, 27). This section addresses links between nutrition and the environmental experience that underlies education. How children experience their environment predicts the effects of poverty better than family income or parental educational level alone (27). These standard measures of socioeconomic status are too broad to label the capability of individuals within any of these groups (27).

HISTORICAL PERSPECTIVE: HEREDITY, ENVIRONMENT, OR NUTRITION?

At the turn of the 20th century, examples of transgenerational mental retardation were widely represented by two socially dysfunctional families—the Jukes of New York State and the Kallikaks from central New Jersey (1, 55–58). The use to which their history (e.g., heredity) was put (1, 58) illustrates the failings of a main-effect model—heredity or environment or nutrition—as the cause for learning failure (27).

In 1877, Richard Dugdale recognized the interaction between heredity and environment among the Jukes. "In idiocy and insanity," notes Dugdale (56), "heredity is the preponderating factor in determining career; but it is, even then, capable of marked modification for better or worse by the character of the environment." Recognition that alcohol has toxic in utero effect is not new (26). The conceptual framework for a "fetal alcohol syndrome" (FAS) was stated by Elisha Harris in Dugdale's 1876 description of the Jukes (56), and Dugdale noted the possibility of in utero effects of alcohol affecting the future viability and function of exposed children (56). In 1899, two British police surgeons, Sullivan and Scholar (59) effectively separated the consequence of living in families of alcoholic mothers from that of in utero exposure in their classic study of incarcerated alcoholic women. The infants of alcoholic women imprisoned during pregnancy were less likely to have epilepsy than were siblings born to the same women living (and drinking) freely.

Fifteen years later, Henry H. Goddard, director of the Vineland Training School for Feeble-Minded Boys and Girls in New Jersey, failed to recognize the potential effect of alcohol. He believed that no amount of education or good environment could change a feeble-minded individual into a normal one (57). Pauline "Kallikak," a 19-year-old girl was photographed in 1911 as part of a series of studies of mentally retarded children conducted at Vineland (1, 57, 58). Goddard was fully aware of the alcoholism in this family. He found siblings of mentally retarded children of "drunkard" parents to be 63% more likely to be judged retarded than those of "nondrunkard" parents (57). Contemporary reanalysis of these data shows the difference to be statistically significant (58). While these findings might reflect the consequence of living in a family affected by alcoholism, Pauline's photograph reveals the characteristic features of FAS, a consequence of in utero alcohol exposure (26, 58) (Fig. 60.1).

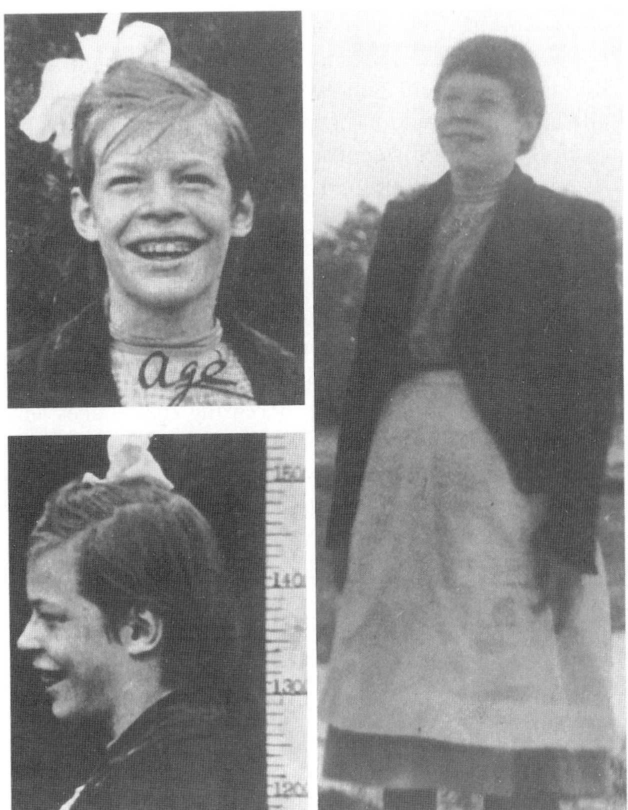

Figure 60.1. Characteristic appearance of child with fetal alcohol syndrome. (From Karp RJ. Introduction and overview of malnourished children in the United States. In: Karp RJ, ed. Malnourished children in the United States: caught in the cycle of poverty. New York: Springer, 1993;xix–2, with permission.)

SIMPLE CAUSES: BRAIN GROWTH AND CENTRAL NERVOUS SYSTEM EFFECTS

From 1920 to 1940, it was recognized that there are critical periods in a child's development during which malnutrition affects intellectual achievement (5–7, 60). By the 1960s, nutrition, separate from environment, was shown to affect cellular and metabolic changes in developing neural tissues, and attempts were made to use nutrition influences rather than multifactorial explanations for behavioral consequences (5–7, 61–63).

A "Brain Growth and/or C.N.S. Effects" model for assessing the consequences of malnutrition, shown as Figure 60.2, was developed by Winick and Rosso (61) from the work of Cravioto et al. (62) and his own studies of starved pregnant rats and newborn pups (61). This model was supported by observation of marked decreases in brain weight and DNA content in infants dying of protein-energy malnutrition with decreased head circumference and developmental delay in survivors (60, 61).

Thus, in the 1960s, it was suggested that retarded mental development was caused by permanent cellular

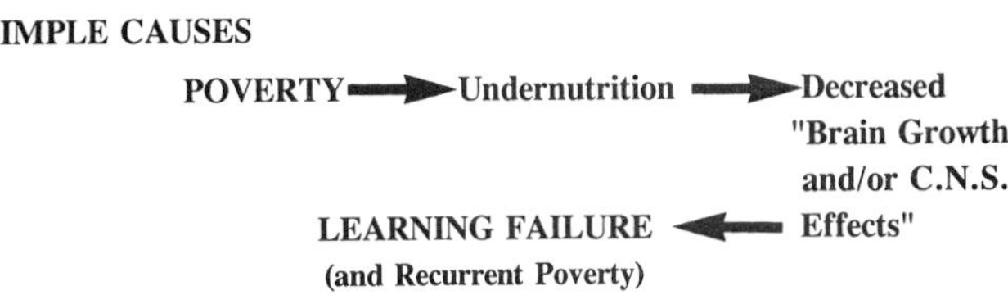

Figure 60.2. "Brain Growth and/or C.N.S. Effects" model for assessing the consequences of malnutrition.

changes induced by early undernutrition (60, 61). Oski was among the first to suggest that learning problems associated with iron deficiency were mediated by lack of iron availability for formation of specific structures and/or key enzyme systems in the central nervous system (CNS) (23). His case-controlled studies of children from impoverished northcentral Philadelphia found that intellectual performance was directly linked to iron status after controlling for other factors (23). In Oski's first study of 12- to 14-year-old junior high school students in northcentral Philadelphia, 92 iron-deficient children were compared with 101 nonanemic controls. A composite measure of intellectual accomplishment showed increasing differences with age between anemic and nonanemic children for both boys and girls. In Oski's second study, 38 anemic and nonanemic boys were matched. Significant differences were found for "Conduct Problems" for older anemic boys, whereas scales for "Personality Disturbances and Inadequacy-Immaturity" showed no significant differences. Oski postulated that behavior is affected by (a) deficiencies in iron-catalyzed CNS monoamine and cytochrome oxidase systems, (b) decreased iron stores in brainstem nuclei, and (c) effects on the γ-aminobutyric acid system in the CNS (22, 23, 63). This theory has been supported by the work of Brown and Pollitt, who writes "even at the very early stages of iron deficiency, a decrement in iron-dependent dopamine D2 receptors alters dopamine neurotransmission in the cortex, which in turn, impairs cognitive function" (6).

Neurotransmitter activity in the CNS is a direct function of the severity of iron deficiency, the decrease in hemoglobin levels (63). Studies in Latin America have shown minimal effects on learning with mild iron depletion (decreased ferritin level) and iron deficiency without anemia (decreased serum iron and percentage saturation). Learning failure occurs only in the last phase of iron deficiency in the presence of anemia. Inability to transport oxygen limits a child's ability to sustain motor activity (63), which is critical for learning by exploration and repetition (63–65). As appealing and elegant as the simple model seems, a contemporary conceptualization is that the interaction between nutrition and environment is more important than either taken alone (5–7, 27).

HOW NUTRITION AFFECTS LEARNING

Parallel to its direct CNS effects, malnutrition contributes to learning failure by affecting transitions, transactions, and the way children experience their environment. Because of the transitional nature of learning, cumulative learning failure results when critical phases in neurodevelopment are missed. Malnourished children are often developmentally unprepared to benefit from age-appropriate educational experiences (27, 64, 65). The transactions between malnourished children and their adult caregivers fail to satisfy the emotional needs of either the children or the adults. Malnourished infants' and children's lack of attention and responsiveness to social stimuli, along with their inability to elicit responses from others (27, 64, 65), undermine the enthusiasm of parents and teachers alike. These children are "temperamentally different from well nourished ones and will be treated so during the toddler and preschool years" (64). These consequences of malnutrition lead children to learn (i.e., to receive, process, comprehend, and transmit information and concepts) differently from well-nourished ones, and this is termed the experience of environment (27). Learning experiences throughout life and the likelihood of reward for success are affected (27, 64–66).

Unless parents living in poverty are taught how to respond to the special needs of malnourished children, the children's learning and nutrition will continue to cycle downward. Working with poor children in Providence, Rhode Island, Sameroff and Chandler (67) recognized that the variability in outcome of birth weight in medically compromised infants was a function of the "cluster effects" of multiple consequences of poverty. The transactional model for learning described below derives from their work.

Environment As a Cofactor

The effects of malnutrition must always be considered in the context of the particular social environment with or without evidence of direct toxic consequences of malnutrition (5–7, 21, 22, 27). Ineffective relationships within families and between parents and children affect the growth of poor children. Other family members are frequently undernourished (68). The pattern of single parenthood without a support system is common (1, 40–42). Medical, social, and educational resources are often inadequately available and used (1, 41). Delayed entry into school and poor attendance are likely (69). Often, the reduced somatic growth used to define malnutrition reflects the concomitant effects of iron and zinc deficiency (5–7), inadequate caloric intake (5, 6, 27), exposure to lead (24, 70), and to alcohol and drugs in utero (25, 26).

Life in Northcentral Philadelphia

Data collected in northcentral Philadelphia document the deteriorated social environment in which Oski worked. Northcentral Philadelphia is among the poorest urban sections in the United States (23). In 1975 and at present, over 70% of families with school children have incomes below the poverty level. In 1975, 17.2% of infants were of low birth weight or premature (vs. 15.6% in 1993); 64.4% of infants were born to unmarried mothers (85.6% in 1993); neonatal mortality (deaths under 1 month of age) was 23.8/1000 live births (9.5 in 1993); infant mortality (deaths under 1 year of age) was 36.6/1000 live births (18.1 in 1993). Though mortality figures have improved, these rates remain two to three times those for the United States.

Studies at the Pratt-Arnold school, a northcentral

Philadelphia elementary school, showed that malnourished children were more likely to live on numbered (long-running, heavy traffic, no trees, and deteriorated housing) rather than named (short-running, little traffic, and tree lined) streets. These differences in condition of housing stock and quality of life on the streets of north-central Philadelphia reflect the interaction between undernutrition and the environment that produces it.

At Pratt-Arnold, children with decreased height-for-age (stunting) were older than their classmates, reflecting delayed entry into school, another indicator of ineffective nurturing likely to diminish both school performance and nutritional status (5–7, 69). The undernourished children appeared to be of "normal" size and performance by grade (but not by age), compared with their younger classmates. Looking younger than their chronologic age, note Brown and Pollitt, would cause adults "to treat them as if they were younger than their actual age. Such a response would very likely slow cognitive development" (6). As in developing countries, these stunted children seem normal for their height/age because of the close parallel between height/age and social and intellectual development. Yet they are retarded compared with well-nourished children of the same age.

The growth-retarded children at Pratt-Arnold school had measures of perception and motor development that reflected height-age better than chronologic age (5, 21). Their height-age correlated with reading level when there was associated anemia or muscle wasting. With normal hemoglobin level and muscle mass, height and reading level were unrelated, suggesting the influence of undernutrition-associated short stature on learning (71). As Pollitt notes, the impact of various nutritional deprivations (linear growth, weight, anemia, muscle mass) occurring together is more important than an individual nutritional deprivation acting alone (72). The cluster effects of nutritional and nonnutritional influences (lead, drug, alcohol, and tobacco exposure) seem to have similar effects as cluster effects of poverty (67).

At Pratt-Arnold, nutritional status, cognitive function, and neurodevelopment were measured, along with a composite measure of school achievement. Using stepwise regression (age factored out), the data demonstrated that gradations in all anthropometric measures were significantly related to rising achievement scores, but anthropometric variables correlated better with academic achievement than with measures of cognitive ability or neurodevelopment (5, 21). This suggests common antecedents for undernutrition and learning failure—the cluster effects of poverty and consequences of failed mother/child interaction—affecting school achievement. Thus, for undernourished children, growth, nonverbal aspects of neurodevelopment, and learning seem to be on a "slow track."

Anthropometric variables were not significantly related to nonverbal measures of cognitive ability, suggesting that the protein-energy deprivation the children at the low end of the anthropometric scale was not significant enough to cause damage to basic cognitive processes (27). These findings explain in part why undernourished children who have been adopted into homes where they are well fed and well nurtured are better achievers in school, even when growth continues to be somewhat slow (73), and why early intervention aids the development of low- and normal-weight infants in families with limited parental education (74–76).

Effective Interventions

Following his studies of surviving, impoverished, and starved infants left to grow in deprivation, Winick examined formerly undernourished children from Korea adopted into middle-class and professional families in the United States. He found that children adopted before 3 years of age had subsequent I.Q. scores higher than the U.S. norm but lower than their nonadopted American siblings (73). Two large, multicenter studies that included disadvantaged innercity children of all races and ethnicities showed the effectiveness of concomitant nutritional and social intervention for LBW infants in multiple centers (74–76). In both studies, a substantial number of the children came from families with incomes below the poverty level.

According to Susser (77), proof of effectiveness requires temporal linearity, with undernutrition and learning failure followed by intervention, followed by recovery of normal nutritional status and learning ability. The intervention studies conducted in the United States fail Susser's stringent test, because linear growth is not universally recovered; perhaps one cannot expect LBW infants, especially those with simultaneous failure of linear growth to completely recover (36, 66, 66a). These studies do, however, quite effectively improve academic potential (66a). In 1990, the Infant Health and Development Program reported substantial increases in I.Q. for "socially disadvantaged" LBW premature children at a corrected age of 36 months, ranging from 6.5 points in the lightest infants to 13.2 in heavier ones (75). The intervention groups were all heavier and longer, but differences did not reach statistical significance. A contemporary review of children receiving nutritional supplements notes that infants with low birth weights are "likely to remain shorter and lighter throughout childhood, especially those who were intrauterine growth retarded rather than premature" (36, 76).

Consequences of Complacency

Iron deficiency, growth retardation, in utero exposure to alcohol or smoking, and lead poisoning cause downward shifts in the mean for any measure of behavior or learning (commonly assessed by I.Q.) of approximately 5 points (24). The effect of lead poisoning on intellectual development are shown in Figure 60.3.

Lead poisoning, a common occurrence in the "lead belt" neighborhoods of many innercities, mainly affects

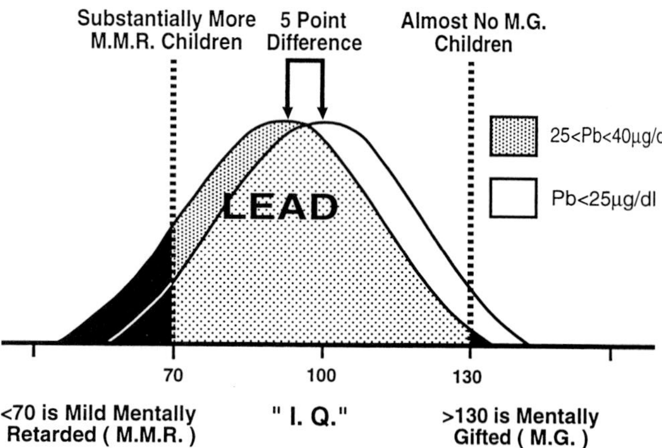

Figure 60.3. Effect of lead poisoning on intellectual development. (From Harris P, Clarke M, Karp RJ. The prevention of lead poisoning in disadvantaged children. In: Karp RJ, ed. Malnourished children in the United States: caught in the cycle of poverty. New York: Springer, 1993;91–100, with permission.)

African American children, many of whom are iron deficient and growth retarded (24, 70). Lead and nutrition interact in three ways: (a) iron and other divalent cation deficiencies enhance lead absorption, (b) markers for iron deficiency are affected by concomitant lead poisoning, and (c) lead's unique effects on CNS functions compound other effects of undernutrition. Lead and iron deficiency each contribute independently to learning failure among children (78). The phenomenon illustrated by the two curves in Figure 60.3 could represent iron deficiency alone; however, when these conditions coexist, children are four times more likely to show behavioral symptoms usually attributed to lead poisoning alone (70, 78).

This result may have little effect on the life of an individual child, but in communities, it disqualifies all children for programs designed for the mentally gifted while greatly expanding the need for services to children with mild mental retardation. In impoverished communities, classes for the mentally gifted (I.Q. two standard deviations above the mean [>130]) are almost empty, while classes for children who are mild mentally retarded (I.Q. two standard deviations below the mean [<70]) are filled to capacity (5). It may be comforting in a peculiar way to maintain discredited racial explanations for these findings (6, 7, 27) because they allow societal or personal inaction; however, the general success of interventions that are given time to work (73–76) provide the best challenge to their validity. Simply stated, there are no effects of race and social class on the inherent capabilities of children. Of note, as shown in NHANES III, an estimated 1.7 million (almost 9%) children between 1 and 5 years of age have blood lead levels above 10 μg/dL, the level at which lead effects are noted for small children (79, 79a).

An Ecology of Poverty, Malnutrition, and Learning Failure

Figure 60.4 shows an ecology of poverty, undernutrition, and learning failure (21) and suggests that learning failure is contingent on an interaction between social environment and nutrition. In developed countries, the prevalence and consequences of malnutrition in young children are related so closely to chronic poverty that one can only rarely distinguish the consequences of malnutrition from the consequences of living in the milieu in which it occurs. Giving food and micronutrients to nutritionally and socially deprived children without correcting their environment is unlikely, in the long run, to have any great effect on learning. Rather, combined social and nutritional intervention is more effective than either intervention alone (5, 6, 73–76).

NUTRITION-DRUG INTERACTIONS AND THEIR EFFECTS

Drug Abuse Increased by Poverty

Chronic poverty is associated with a sustained disproportionate use of both legal (tobacco and alcohol) (25, 80, 81) and illegal addictive mood-altering substances (marijuana, cocaine, and heroin) (25, 82). Alcohol, tobacco, and other drugs of abuse affect nutritional status in direct relation to duration of use (83, 84) (see Chapter 67). There are populations living in seemingly hopeless circumstances in which the prevalence and consequences of alcoholism are disproportionately high. These include Native Americans living on desolate reservations (an estimated 25% of infants are born with FAS), poor whites in decaying industrial cities (10% of school children with FAS in one town) (85), and inner-city, black families.

Particularly problematic is drug use during pregnancy. Among women of childbearing age, poverty engenders chronic depression (86) increasing the risk for drug abuse during pregnancy with concomitant increased risk for teratogenesis (87). As illustrated by studies of alcoholic mothers and children, there is a substantial variability in outcome for children exposed to drugs in utero (25, 87). To an extent that is not yet well determined, maternal nutrition and alcohol intake contribute to these differences. (83, 84, see Chapter 67) While there are severe consequences to the fetus from exposure to illicit drugs, the risks from alcohol consumption and smoking tobacco during pregnancy are better defined and more widespread (25, 26). Moreover, for people living in poverty, illicit drug use is unusual in a woman who neither smokes nor drinks alcohol. (The sum of research on in utero effects suggests that the order of biologic consequence is alcohol greater than tobacco greater than drugs, but punishments for sale and use of these substances are just the reverse.)

Prevalence and Consequences of Drug, Alcohol, and Tobacco Use

Alcohol

Alcohol produces a characteristic dysmorphism deriving from altered CNS growth and function. Children with FAS show midface hypoplasia, short palpebral fissures,

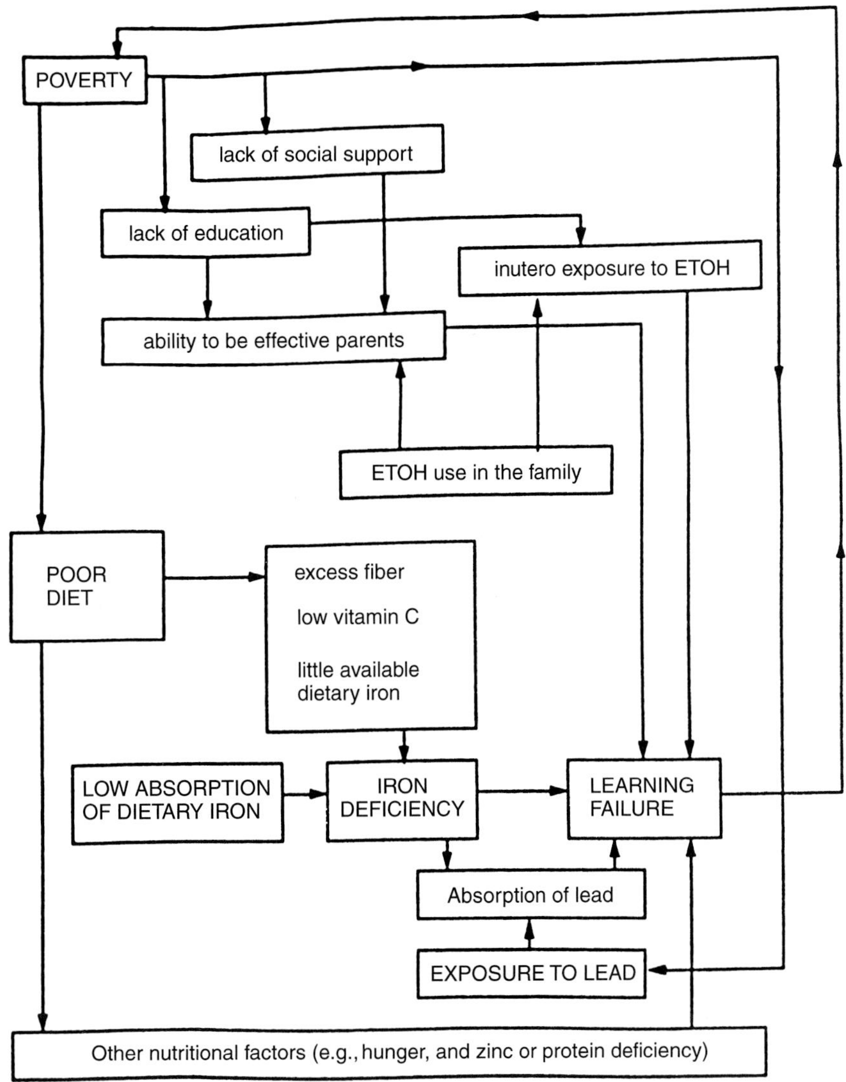

Figure 60.4. An ecology of poverty, undernutrition and learning failure. (From Sewell TE, Price VD, Karp RJ. The ecology of poverty undernutrition and learning failure. In: Karp RJ, ed. Malnourished children in the United States: caught in the cycle of poverty. New York: Springer, 1993;24–30, with permission, and derived from the work of Cravioto, DeLicardie, and Birch [62] and Hallberg [7].)

increased distance from the base of the nose to the upper lip, absent philtrum, and narrow vermilion border of the upper lip (26, 85) (Fig. 60.1). There is concomitant growth retardation at birth with failure to "catch-up" and persistent neurodevelopmental problems. Infants born to drinking mothers have CNS depression and withdrawal syndrome (85). Alcohol-related problems after birth are common, even without the full syndrome, because drinking severely hampers parental effectiveness. Recent data show that 4.4% of 21- to 30-year-old women have two or more drinks each day, and the percentage drops to 3.5% for ages 31 to 40 years (81). Chronic abuse, as opposed to binge drinking, is characteristic of older women. Abuse and dependency are less common among black women (2.88%) (81), but with respect to FAS, race along with age, parity, and length of alcohol use is an independent risk factor (82).

Specific alcohol/nutrition interactions likely to increase in utero effects include (a) decreased gastric alcohol dehydrogenase levels with age, allowing higher blood alcohol levels, (b) maternal loss of zinc and magnesium, (c) diminution of antioxidant nutrients, and (d) failure in hepatic degradation, allowing potentially toxic substances and metabolites to affect the fetus (83, 84) (see Chapter 67).

Hepatic dysfunction associated with chronic alcoholism alters the detoxification process for other drugs of abuse as well as for environmental pollutants, allowing toxic metabolites to reach the fetus. A contemporary view, from Lieber, is that "at cellular, biochemical and molecular levels, the nutritional and toxic effects of alcohol converge" (83). Thus, polydrug abuse concomitant to aging of mothers creates a nutrient-deprived in utero environment that increases the risk for teratogenic consequences of drug exposure on the growing fetus (81, 83, 84). A model for teratogen × malnutrition effects, derived from the work of Lieber (83), is shown in Figure 60.5.

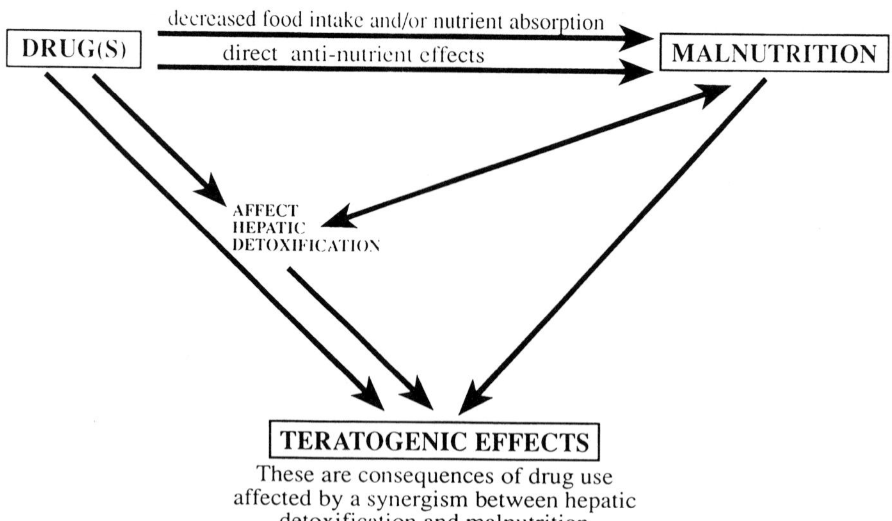

Figure 60.5. A model for teratogen [x] malnutrition effects. (From Leiber CS. Am J Clin Nutr 1993;58:430–42, with permission.)

Tobacco

The principal in utero consequence of smoking tobacco, growth retardation, is directly proportional to the number of cigarettes smoked per day (82). The decrease in mean birth weight for infants born to tobacco-smoking mothers is approximately 200 g, with a concomitant increase in infant morbidity and mortality above that expected from a simple shift to the left on birth weight–mortality curves (82, 87). The pattern of growth retardation tends to be symmetric, with all anthropometric measures—weight, length, and head circumference—affected equally. This pattern has been associated with failure to achieve catch-up growth and developmental delay (74). Specific smoking effects on the fetus or on the infant include (a) placental arterial spasm, (b) carbon monoxide binding of hemoglobin, (c) decreased maternal intake, and (d) reduced levels of ascorbic acid from the oxidative stress of both passive and active smoking (82, 87). Barker has provided epidemiologic data suggesting that much of the degenerative disease associated with smoking is caused by exposure in utero and during the first year of life (88). Lucas distinguishes between toxic effects of early nutritional deprivation and factors affecting perinatal health and infant nutritional status that reestablish themselves in childhood to influence the onset of cardiovascular disease (89). Recent studies show that smoking during pregnancy affects uterine artery spasm and blood pressures of infants, lasting through the first year (90), as well as older children exposed during the last trimester of pregnancy (91).

In the United States, tobacco use is more common among those with limited education and limited income (92); 35 to 40% of adults with a 12th grade education or less and income near or at the poverty level smoke, compared with approximately 20% of adults with more than 2 years of college education and an upper-middle income (93). Tobacco companies have been effective recently in reaching teenagers with special emphasis on recruiting African American and Hispanic adolescents, poorly educated boys of all races/ethnicities, and all girls (93).

Smoking and dietary inadequacies maintained into adult life are significant alterable contributors to the shortened life expectancies of the poor in this country (92). Data from Framingham show that 55% of attributable risk for coronary heart disease (CHD) before 55 years of age is from smoking. Data collected in the Multiple Risk Factor Intervention Trial (MRFIT) show a disproportional increase in CHD risk with smoking (94). At the highest quintile of serum total cholesterol in the MRFIT study (>240 mg/dL), concomitant hypertension (diastolic blood pressure > 90 mm Hg) with no smoking was associated with a 3.5-fold increase in CHD mortality, but for those in the third (200 mg/dL) and fourth (220 mg/dL) quintiles who smoked, CHD mortality increased approximately sixfold. Smoking transformed midlevel risk for CHD mortality to a risk greater than that for a hypercholesterolemic person who did not smoke (94). Data collected from 300 of Brooklyn's most disadvantaged children with truncated families and very young grandparents suggest a greater incidence of CHD at a young age likely to be caused by the concomitant harmful effects of smoking and untreated hypertension (94).

Like alcohol, smoking promotes malnutrition in two ways: first, the diets of smokers are of lower nutritional value than those of nonsmokers, and second, smoking has direct antinutrient effects such as reduced vitamin C levels with passive smoking (95). Steinberg has suggested that decreased intake and increased use of antioxidant nutrients (vitamins C and E and retinoids) accelerate oxidation of low-density-lipoprotein cholesterol and alter the balance between clotting and antithrombotic activity unfavorably (96). However, attempts to prevent degenerative diseases among smokers by providing antioxidant nutrients have had mixed results, as illustrated by one Scandinavian study in which the occurrence of lung cancer increased among carotenoid-supplemented subjects (96).

Illicit Drugs

Marijuana. Marijuana use is fairly widespread, with use by women of childbearing age ranging from 10 to 25% (97). Crack cocaine use is currently an inner-city, African American phenomenon associated with polydrug use as well as sexually transmitted diseases and lack of prenatal care. Bell and Lau give prevalence rates for cocaine use by high school seniors ranging from 2 to 17% (97). Socioeconomic differences in usage patterns for illicit drugs vary according to pressures from peers, law enforcement, educational efforts, and simple experimentation with new drugs. Data on prevalence for illegal drugs are highly suspect, and studies of effects must always be read cautiously.

Cocaine. Cocaine is a powerful sympathomimetic that affects both placental function and the fetus directly throughout pregnancy. Moreover, cocaine, like alcohol, marijuana, amphetamines, and heroin, produces a withdrawal syndrome in exposed children. Polydrug use affects the severity and duration of withdrawal in affected infants (87, 97). Though specific "fetal cocaine" and "fetal marijuana syndromes" have been hypothesized, clear documentation is lacking. Some infants exposed to marijuana show the stigmata of FAS which may reflect a heightened susceptibility to alcohol among marijuana or polydrug users. Infants born to cocaine using mothers have multiple perinatal complications including growth retardation and CNS bleeding. These children are often developmentally delayed and have seizure disorders. (82, 87, 97). Bell and Lau give prevalence rates for use by high school seniors ranging from 2 to 17% (97).

The principal effects on the fetus of cocaine use by the mother are symmetric growth retardation with reduced head circumference and premature delivery (87, 97, 98). In a recent study of 98 cocaine-exposed infants, Roizen et al. showed a significant developmental delay in these children compared with nonexposed controls, but this delay was predicted by the growth retardation concomitant to premature delivery and living in homes with drug-affected mothers or relatives rather than by cocaine exposure per se (98). Moreover, with respect to postnatal development (99) and growth (100), the social milieu in which cocaine use occurs (99) and concomitant alcohol and tobacco use during pregnancy (100) may be more important than the cocaine use. Again, these findings must be judged cautiously and in an environmental context.

IMPORTANCE OF PUBLIC POLICY: KEEPING NUTRITIOUS FOOD AVAILABLE TO THE POOR

Malnutrition as part of a "poverty syndrome" occurs in some poor families when society accepts the legitimacy of poverty and malnutrition (29). Chronic poverty involves more than lack of income, but mass poverty and malnutrition in society is caused by a nation's economic policy and the politics of entitlement (29, 43, 101). Policies that nurture and nourish children yield remarkable improvements in health and social stability. In the United States, the failure to implement policies supporting poor children and their families raises the question, "In what direction is our society going?"

The prevalence of malnutrition will depend on the depth of poverty to which society allows those with the least income and resources to sink (1). Failed or inadequate public policy predicts the prevalence of consequences of poverty, which include, of course, malnutrition. Which poor families are affected, however, depends on behavioral characteristics. Parents in affected families often lack the skills to nourish and nurture children. To resolve the problem of malnourished children in the United States, resources must be made available to provide nutritious food and to address the multiple interdependent problems faced by poor families. Support for the poorest in society begins with a broad base of support for everyone (29, 43, 101, 102). Otherwise, notes Chamberlin, "for every family whose functioning is improved by some kind of intensive intervention, several more medium-risk families will take their place as their life circumstances change" (102).

In the United States, provision of food stamps, school lunches and breakfasts, and the special program for Women, Infants and Children (WIC) has improved nutritional status both by providing nutritious food and by allowing the purchase of a higher quality diet with the same amount of money budgeted for food, thus effectively reversing Engels' law (46). These supports are often referred to as "welfare," implying an unearned benefit to the recipient. Actually, these supports benefit children, who in developed societies are not responsible for their own support, and they benefit everyone by creating a healthy population able to learn, work, and earn. They do not create "welfare dependence" since supplemental programs provide essential food to working families and their children. Contemporary food programs have never been shown to be a detriment to work. Rather, they are an alternative to the bread lines and soup kitchens of a post-Victorian era (101).

Childhood malnutrition in the context of poverty predicts various endpoints—learning failure, social dysfunction, increased risk for drug use, birth defects, and chronic illness later in life. While it is incorrect to maintain that any form of malnutrition is the solitary cause for recurrent poverty, ignorance, dysfunction, and disease, malnutrition in the context of poverty is a significant contributor to a self-sustaining system—an ecology of learning failure, poverty, and malnutrition (1, 28). These unfortunate outcomes are contingent on continued poverty and are concomitant to malnutrition. Yet, the poor in the United States live in social environments that are harsh and hostile rather than supportive, with substandard schools and an inadequate system for health care (1, 4, 5, 19, 27, 40–43, 102). The converging validity of data from various studies providing both nutritional supplementation and social support (36, 66, 66a, 75, 76) suggests that the rigor of Susser's criteria (77) should be tempered by the reality of effective interventions.

Eliminating poverty includes provision of food and structures of opportunity within which the poor can adapt and cope. Poor people must be treated as real individuals, not as caricatures of a defective culture. These calls for the investment of human and monetary resources may seem unrealistic, but the political unacceptability of effective policies should not cause us to "turn to politically acceptable formulas which provide no real solutions" (43).

ACKNOWLEDGMENTS

Appreciation is noted to William Bithoney, M.D., Annabelle Schaeffer, M.D., Ruth Sartisky, Ph.D., Theresa Scholl, Ph.D., Theodore Wachs, Ph.D., and Judy Wiley-Rosset, Ed.D., R.D.

REFERENCES

1. Karp RJ. Introduction and overview of malnourished children in the United States. In: Karp RJ, ed. Malnourished children in the United States: caught in the cycle of poverty. New York: Springer, 1993;xix–2.
2. Current Population Reports. Consumer income series P60-188. Income, poverty, and valuation of noncash benefits: 1993. U.S. Department of Commerce Economics and Statistics administration. Washington, DC: Bureau of the Census,
3. Miller J, Korenman S. Am J Epidemiol 1994;78:75–7.
4. Miller JE, Korenman S. Poverty, nutritional status, growth and cognitive development of children in the United States. Working paper no. 93-5. Princeton, NJ: Princeton University Office of Population Research, 1993.
5. Sewell TE, Price VD, Karp RJ. The ecology of poverty undernutrition and learning failure. In: Karp RJ, ed. Malnourished children in the United States: caught in the cycle of poverty. New York: Springer, 1993;24–30.
6. Brown L, Pollitt E. Sci Am 1996;274:38–43.
7. Hallberg L. Am J Clin Nutr 1989;50:598–606.
8. Garn SM, Clark DC. Pediatrics 1975;56:306–19.
9. Scholl TO, Karp RJ, Theophano J, et al. Public Health Rep 1987;102:278–83.
10. Meyers A, Frank DA, Roos N, et al. Arch Pediatr Adolesc Med 1995;149:1079–84.
11. United States Department of Agriculture, Human Nutrition Information Service. Nationwide food consumption survey: continuing survey of food intakes by individuals, low-income women 19–50 years and their children 1–5 years, 1 day, 1986, NFCS, CFSII report no. 86-2. Hyattsville, MD: USDA, 1987.
12. Krebs-Smith SM, Cook DA, Subar AF, et al. Arch Pediatr Adolesc Med 1996;150;81–6.
13. Alaimo K, McDowell MA, Breifel RR, et al. Dietary intake of vitamins and minerals, and fiber of persons age 2 months and over in the United States. Third National Health and Nutrition Examination Survey, phase I, 1989–91. Advance data from vital statistics; no. 258. Hyattsville, MD: National Center for Health Statistics, 1994.
14. Johnson RK, Guthrie H, Smicklas-Wright H, et al. Public Health Rep 1994;109:414–20.
15. Basch CE, Zybert P, Shea S. Am J Public Health 1994;84: 814–8.
16. Scholl TO, Hediger ML, Schall JI, et al. Am J Clin Nutr 1996: 63:520–5.
17. Yip R, Binken NJ, Fleshhood L, et al. JAMA 1987:258: 1619–23.
18. Bielicki T. Physical growth as a measure of the economic well-being of populations: the twentieth century. In: Falkner F, Tanner JM, eds. Human growth, vol 3. New York: Plenum, 1980;283–305
19. Karp RJ. J Am Coll Nutr 1995;14:561–2.
20. Floud R. Anthropometric measures of nutritional status in industrialized societies: Europe and North America since 1750. In: Osmani SR, ed. Nutrition and poverty. Oxford: Oxford University Press, 1992;218–42.
21. Wachs T. J Nutr 1995;125(Suppl):2245–54.
22. Pollit L. Annu Rev Nutr 1993;13:521–37.
23. Oski FA. Am J Dis Child 1979;133:315–22.
24. Needleman HL, Gatsonis CA. JAMA 1990;263:673–78.
25. Drews CD, Murphy CC, Yeargin-Allsop M, et al. Pediatrics 1996;97:547–53.
26. Streissguth AP, Aase JM, Clarren SK, et al. JAMA 1991;265, 1961–7.
27. Wachs TD. The nature of nurture. Newbury Park, CA: Sage Publications, 1993.
28. Rainwater L, Smeeding T. A comparative study of children's wealth. Luxembourg Income Study (LIS) working paper no. 127, Syracuse University, 1995.
29. Gopalan C. Undernutrition: measurement and implication. In: Osmani SR, ed. Nutrition and poverty. Oxford: Oxford University Press, 17-48
30. Martorell R. Child growth retardation: a discussion of its causes and its relationship to health. In: Blaxter K, Waterlow JC, eds. Nutritional adaptation in man. London: John Libbey, 1985;13–30.
31. Goldbloom RB. Pediatr Rev 1987;9:57–61.
32. Widdowson EM. Lancet 1951;1:1316–8.
33. Powell GF, Brasel JA, Raiti S, Blizzard RM. N Engl J Med 1967;276:1279–83.
34. Skuse D, Albanese A, Stanhope R, et al. Lancet 1996;353: 353–8.
35. Karp RJ, Martin R, Sewell T, et al. Clin Pediatr 1992:32: 336–40.
36. Blinken NJ, Yip R, Fleshhood L, et al. Pediatrics 1988;82: 828–34.
37. Scholl TO, Karp R. Theophano J, et al. Public Health Rep 1987;102:278–83.
38. Karp RJ, Scholl TO, Decker E, et al. Clin Pediatr 1984;28: 317–20.
39. Cipro CF, Michael RT, eds. Measuring poverty: a new approach. Washington, DC: National Academy Press, 1995.
40. Katz M. The undeserving poor. New York: Pantheon, 1989.
41. Wilson JW. The truly disadvantaged: the inner-city, the under class and public policy. Chicago: University of Chicago Press, 1987.
42. McLeod JD, Shanahan MJ. Am Sociol Rev 1993;58:351–66.
42a. Lampman R. Ends and means of reducing income poverty. Chicago: Markham Publishers, 1971.
43. Rosen D. Failure of response to poverty. In: Karp RJ, ed. Malnourished children in the United States: caught in the cycle of poverty. New York: Springer, 1993;250–2.
44. Bloom BS. Stability and social change in human characteristics. New York: Wiley, 1964;46.
45. Rural sociological task force. Persistent poverty in rural America. Boulder, CO: Westview Press, 1993.
46. Karp RJ, Greene GW. Bull NY Acad Med 1983;59:721.

47. Karp RJ, Fairorth JW, Kanofsky P, et al. Public Health Rep 1978;93:456–58.46.
48. Sebrell WH. J Nutr 1955;55:3–12.
49. Pilch SM, Senti FR. Assessment of the iron nutritional status of the U.S. population based on data collected in the Second National Health and Nutrition Examination Survey. Contract no. FDA 223-83-2384. Bethesda, MD: FASEB, 1984.
50. Engle PL, Zeitlin M, Medrano Y, et al. Growth consequences of low income Nicaraguan mothers' theories about feeding 1-year-olds. In: Harkness S, Super C, eds. Parents' cultural belief systems: their origins, expressions and consequences. New York: Guilford Press, 1996;428–6.
51. Bithony WG, Dubowitz HG. Organic concomittants of nonorganic failure to thrive: implications for research. In: Drotar D, ed. New directions in failure to thrive. New York: Plenum Press, 1986;47–56.
52. Politt E. Fed Proc 1975;34:1593.
53. Karp R, Snyder E, Fairorth, et al. J Fam Pract 1984;18:731.
54. Casey PH, Bradley R, Wortham B. Pediatrics 1984;73:348.
55. Degler C. In search of human nature. New York: Oxford University Press, 1991.
56. Dugdale R. "The Jukes": a study in crime, pauperism, disease, and heredity. 4th ed. New York: GP Putnam's Sons, 1895.
57. Goddard HC. Feeble-mindedness: its causes and consequences. New York: MacMillan, 1914.
58. Karp RJ, Qazi QH, Moller K, et al. Arch Pediatr Adolesc Med 1995;149:45–8.
59. Sullivan WC, Scholar S. J Ment Sci 1899;45:489–903.
60. Dobbing J. Introduction. In: Dobbing J, ed. Brain, behavior, iron in the infant diet. London: Springer Verlag, 1990.
61. Winick M, Rosso P. Pediatr Res 1969;3:181–4.
62. Cravioto J, DeLicardie ER, Birch HG. Pediatrics 1966; 38(Suppl):319–73.
63. Lozoff B. Has iron deficiency been shown to cause altered behavior in infants? In: Dobbing J, ed. Brain, behavior, iron in the infant diet. London: Springer Verlag, 1990.
64. Barret S. Nutr Rev 1986;44(Suppl):224–36.
65. Rutter M. Ciba Found Symp 1991;156:189–208.
66. Grantham-McGregor S, Powell C, Walker S, et al. Child Dev 1994;65:428–39.
66a. Grantham-McGregor SM, Walker SP, Chang SM, Powell CA. Am J Clin Nutr 1997;66:247–53.
67. Sameroff A, Seifer R, Barocas R, et al. Pediatrics 1987;79: 3453–50.
68. Karp RJ, Haaz W, Starko K, et al. Am J Dis Child 1972;1974: 128:18–20.
69. Karp RJ, Nuchpakdee M, Fairorth JW. Am J Clin Nutr 1976; 29:216–8.
70. Harris P, Clarke M, Karp RJ. The prevention of lead poisoning in disadvantaged children. In: Karp RJ, ed. Malnourished children in the United States: caught in the cycle of poverty. New York: Springer, 1993;91–100.
71. Karp R, Wadowski S. Arch Pediatr Adolesc Med 1995;149–51.
72. Pollitt E. Int Rev Res Ment Retardation 1988;15:33–80.
73. Winick M, Meyer KK, Harris RC. Science 1975;190:1173.
74. Casey PH, Kelleher KJ, Bradley RH, et al. Arch Pediatr Adolesc Med 1994;148:1071–7.
75. Gross RT, and the Infant Health and Development Program Staff. JAMA 1990;263:3035–42.
76. Casey PH, Kelleher KJ, Bradley RH, et al. Arch Pediatr Adolesc Med 1995;149:1041.
77. Susser M. Bull NY Acad Med 1989;65:1032–49.
78. Clark M, Royal J, Sealer R. Pediatrics 1988;81:247–54.
79. Anon. MMWR 1994;43:545–8.
79a. Anon. MMWR 1994;272:277–83.
80. Russell M. The epidemiology of alcohol. In: Estes NJ, Heinemann ME, eds. Alcoholism: development, consequences and interventions. St Louis, MO: CV Mosby, 1986;31–52.
81. Wilsnack SC, Wilsnack RW, Hiller-Sturmheofel S. Alcohol Health Res World 1994;18:173–80.
82. Jacobson JL, Sokol RJ, Martier SS, et al. J Pediatr 1994; 124:757–64.
83. Leiber CS. Am J Clin Nutr 1993;58:430–42.
84. Lieber CS. J Am Coll Nutr 1991;10:602–32.
85. Karp RJ, Qazi QH. Fetal alcohol syndrome. In: Karp RJ, ed. Malnourished children in the United States: caught in the cycle of poverty. New York: Springer, 1993;101–8.
86. Sidel R. Women and children last: the plight of poor women in affluent America. New York: Viking Penguin, 1986.
87. Berlin CM. Pediatr Rev 1991;12:232–7.
88. Barker DJP. Br Med J 1992;33–335.
89. Lucas A. Programming by early nutrition in man. CIBA Found Symp 1991;156:38–50.
90. Beratis NG, Panagoulias D, Varvarigou A. J Pediatr 1996;128: 806–12.
91. Morley R, Payne CL, Lucas A. Arch Dis Child 1995;72:120–4.
92. Winkelby MA, Ragland DR, Syme SL. Am J Epidemiol 1988; 128:1075–83.
93. Winkelby MA, Fortmann SP, Barrett DC. Prev Med 1990;19: 1–12.
94. Wadowski S, Karp, R Bachmann R, et al. Pediatrics 1994;93: 109–13.
95. Schwartz J, Weiss S. Am J Clin Nutr 1994;59:110–4.
96. Steinberg D. N Engl J Med 1995;346:36–8.
97. Bell GL, Lau K. Pediatr Clin North Am 1995;42:261–81.
98. Roizen NJ, Martinez S, Kime K, et al. (Abstract) Arch Pediatr Adolesc Med 1996;150:16.
99. Hurt H, Brodsky NC, Malmud E, et al. Arch Pediatric Adolesc Med 1997;151:1242–1246.
100. Frank DA, Cosal H. (Abstract) Pediatr Res 1996:39:264A.
101. Sen A. Poverty and famine. New York: Oxford University Press, 1981.
102. Chamberlin RW. Pediatr Rev 1992;13:64–71.

61. Nutritional Support of Inherited Metabolic Disease

LOUIS J. ELSAS II and PHYLLIS B. ACOSTA

GENETIC PERSPECTIVE

Geneticists approach the general subject of nutrition and the specific requirement for nutrients with the view that the recommended dietary allowance (RDA) for an essential nutrient is not optimum for all individuals. Rather, individuals in a population have genetically determined variations in their nutrient requirements that extend over a wide range. This concept arose historically from two older scientific disciplines: human biochemical genetics and nutrition science. The former discipline originated with Sir Archibald Garrod's Croonian lectures of 1908. Garrod defined four "inborn errors of metabolism" as blocks in the normal flow of metabolic processes. Biochemical and clinical expression of these metabolic blocks demonstrated patterns of inheritance consistent with Mendel's predictions for transmission of single genes with large effect on the phenotype. Thus arose the concept that genes controlled metabolism and that disease states were created by blocks in this metabolic flow, yielding accumulated precursors and deficient products.

Today, we recognize that "inborn errors" are discontinuous traits resulting from variation in the structure and function of enzymes or protein molecules. The amino acid sequences of enzymes and their quantity are dictated by genes. The control of enzyme function is predicated by molecular regulation through gene transcription, posttranscriptional processing of RNA, translation, posttranslational modification, and protein turnover. Over 8000 monogenic human disorders are cataloged and available. Of these, about 300 have a defined biochemical basis (1). The extent of normal variation in genes controlling enzyme activity suggests that about 30% of our population is heterozygous for common alleles (2). Within this continuous diversity, mutations produce discontinuous, relatively rare traits that are expressed as disease under normal environmental conditions.

Mutant gene frequencies vary in populations; for example, mitochondrial branched-chain α-ketoacid dehydrogenase (BCKAD) deficiency (maple syrup urine disease) occurs in 1 of approximately every 250,000 newborns worldwide, but occurs in 1 of 176 in an inbred Mennonite population (3). The mutation is one of few that are not private to individual families. The Mennonite mutation is in the E1α gene and changes a tyrosine at position 194 to asparagine (Y302N). In the homozygous state, it produces extreme toxicity due to accumulated branched-chain α-ketoacids (BCKAs) if affected newborns are fed the RDA during rapid growth. However, normal growth and development are expected if dietary isoleucine, leucine, and valine are restricted to 20 to 40% of the RDA during rapid growth in year 1 of life (4, 5).

Considerable human variation occurs in the structure and activity of enzymes involved in the catabolism of essential amino acids, but only a few are so impaired that ingestion of the RDA creates severe disease. Population-based newborn screening and dietary intervention are now applied through public health programs to at least five rare inborn errors for which newborn screening predicts genetic susceptibility to a normal diet (6). By contrast to these relatively rare inborn errors, all humans lack the enzyme that converts L-gulono-α-lactone to ascorbic acid, but scurvy does not occur if sufficient vitamin C is ingested and absorbed (7). Thus, the frequency of genetic susceptibility to a "normal" diet ranges from rare to common and extends to the metabolism of amino acids, carbohydrates, lipids, purines, pyrimidines, minerals, and vitamins.

GENETIC DISORDERS BENEFITED BY NUTRITIONAL SUPPORT

Over 300 genetic disorders have been reported in which toxic manifestations relate to accumulation, deficiency, or overproduction of normally occurring substrates and products of metabolic flow. In many of them, modifications of the dietary supply will alleviate the manifestations. In a large number, however, irreversible damage has already occurred by the time symptoms appear. Optimum management of these disorders depends on identifying affected subjects while they are presymptomatic or before irreversible disease has occurred. Because the disorders are genetic, markers are theoretically present from the moment of conception, and thus the genetic power of prediction and prevention is applicable. In practice, a number of disorders can be detected in the fetus in the 10th to 16th week of gestation by studies on chorionic villus or amniotic fluid cells. Prenatal diagnosis has been pushed forward to the 9th to 12th week of gestation through the use of chorionic villus biopsy (8). Some intrauterine sequelae of the inborn error, such as congenital cataracts in galactosemia, may be prevented by removing lactose from the mother's diet. Other inherited metabolic alterations are detected postnatally in the presymptomatic infant by analysis of blood, urine, erythrocytes, leukocytes, or cultured skin fibroblasts.

A selective search for presymptomatic genetic disease is often undertaken when there is a family history of inherited disease. Selective screening for inherited disease is also initiated for relatively common symptoms such as failure to thrive in childhood. Early treatment has proved effective for many diseases such as phenylketonuria (PKU), galactosemia, isovaleric acidemia, homocystinuria, maple syrup urine disease (MSUD), argininosuccinic aciduria, and citrullinemia. Irreversible brain damage occurs if treatment is not initiated in PKU before the 3rd week of life. In MSUD, galactosemia, isovaleric acidemia, and disorders of the urea cycle, irreversible damage to the brain may occur within the 1st week of life. To prevent this, population-wide nonselective screening of newborns has been instituted for PKU, MSUD, galactosemia, homocystinuria, and tyrosinemia. Thus, speed in diagnosis and treatment is of the utmost importance in preventing a poor outcome.

In the future, population-based presymptomatic detection will be extended to other disorders. However, before screening is initiated as a public health program, several principles should be fulfilled (Table 61.1). Knowledge of the pathogenesis, preventability, and availability of therapy must precede initiation of routine screening programs. Table 61.2 lists genetic disorders in which modification of nutrient intake has been employed. Effectiveness in preventing clinical sequelae is experimental in some of the therapies listed.

Although many patients with inherited disorders benefit from nutritional support, each would require a chapter for adequate discussion. Thus, this chapter emphasizes disorders for which population-based screening, retrieval, diagnosis, and nutritional support are available to prevent their irreversible, severe pathologic problems.

GENERAL PRINCIPLES OF GENETIC DISEASE MANAGEMENT

Specific enzymes produced under the direction of individual genes catalyze specific reactions as noted in the following genetic and metabolic sequences. A is converted to D through intermediates B and C using enzymes AB, BC, and CD:

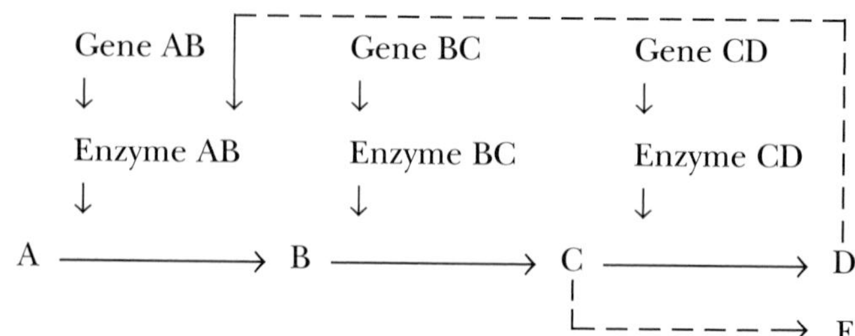

If enzyme CD were genetically impaired, at least six pathophysiologic consequences might occur:

1. Deficiency of product D. For example, in PKU, when phenylalanine is not hydroxylated to form tyrosine, not only is accumulated phenylalanine toxic, but tyrosine becomes an essential nutrient. Tyrosine must be supplemented to maintain proper growth in the dietary management of PKU.
2. Loss of feedback control. If product D normally functions in feedback control of enzyme AB, overproduction of an intermediate product may occur because D is not present in amounts necessary to regulate production of intermediates B and C. Exemplary of this phenomenon is acute intermittent porphyria, in which heme is deficient and does not exert feedback control on δ-aminolevulinic acid (δ-ALA) and porphobilinogen syntheses, with consequent excess accumulation and neuropathic sequelae.
3. Accumulation of C, the immediate precursor of the blocked reaction. In MSUD, toxic BCKAs accumulate because they cannot be decarboxylated and transacylated to their coenzyme A–acyl acid derivatives. The consequence in the neonate is severe central nervous system (CNS) depression and apnea, stupor, coma, and death. If the neonate survives, severe mental retardation ensues if the child is not treated by diet restriction within the 1st week of life.
4. Accumulation of A or B, remote precursors of the blocked reaction sequence, CD. If the preceding reactions are freely reversible, a precursor in addition to the one immediately before the block will accumulate. This process is illustrated in MSUD by increased leucine, isoleucine, and valine, which are

Table 61.1
Criteria for Nonselective Newborn Screening

1. The disorder produces a high burden to the affected individual yet is preventable
2. Methods for screening retrieval, diagnosis, and management must be practical and available to the population as a whole
3. Inheritance and pathogenesis of the disease should be understood
4. Benefit:cost ratio of the program should be greater than one
5. Patients' rights should be protected (including confidentiality and informed consent)
6. False-negative laboratory screening results should not occur
7. False-positive laboratory results should be minimized

Table 61.2
Nutritional Treatment of Genetic Disorders

Disorder	Therapy
Abetalipoproteinemia	Medium-chain triglycerides; vitamin A, D, E, and K parenterally or in excess orally
Acrodermatitis enteropathica	Zinc sulfate supplement
Adenine phosphoribosyltransferase deficiency	Purine restriction, allopurinol; avoid alkali
Alkaptonuria (ochronosis)	Ascorbic acid supplement; phenylalanine and tyrosine restriction
Anemia, hypochromic, sideroblastic	Pyridoxine supplement
Argininemia	Protein restriction; essential amino acids supplement; ornithine supplement
Argininosuccinic aciduria	Arginine, benzoic acid, and phenylbutyrate or phenylacetate supplements; protein restriction; essential amino acids supplement
β-Methylcrotonylglycinuria	Leucine restriction; L-carnitine supplements
β-Methylglutaconic aciduria	Leucine restriction; L-carnitine supplements
β-Sitosterolemia	Plant sterol restriction
Biotinidase deficiency	Biotin supplement
Carbamylphosphate synthetase deficiency	Arginine, benzoic acid, and phenylbutyrate or phenylacetate supplements; protein restriction; essential amino acids supplement; L-carnitine supplements
Chediak-Higashi syndrome	Ascorbic acid supplement
Chloride diarrhea	Sodium chloride supplement
Chylomicronemia	Restrict fat; medium-chain triglycerides
Citrullinemia	Protein restriction; supplemental essential amino acids, arginine, phenylbutyrate, or phenylacetate and benzoic acid; L-carnitine supplements
Combined hyperlipidemia	Energy, carbohydrate, saturated fatty acid restriction, nicotinic acid and mevinolin therapy, cholestyramine
Cystathioninuria	Pyridoxine supplements
Cystic fibrosis	Enteric enzyme supplements (trypsin, lipase, chymotrypsin)
Cystinosis	Alkali, phosphate, and vitamin D supplements; cysteamine to reduce cystine
Cystinuria	Alkali, hyperhydration, D-penicillamine
Diabetes insipidus	Water, low-solute diets; vasopressin
Diabetes mellitus	Insulin, controlled diet
Dibasic aminoaciduria	Arginine supplement; protein restriction
Ehlers-Danlos syndrome, lysyl hydroxylase defect	Ascorbic acid supplement
Fatty acid oxidation defects (mitochondrial)	Restrict fat; supplement; glycine, L-carnitine; avoid fasting
Folic acid reductase deficiency	N^5-Formyltetrahydrofolic acid supplement
Folic acid transport defect	Parenteral folate supplement
Fructose intolerance	Fructose-free diet
Fructose malabsorption	Fructose-free diet
Fructose-1,6-diphosphate deficiency	Frequent glucose, folate supplement, reduced fructose intake
Galactokinase deficiency	Galactose-restricted diet
Galactosemia	Galactose-restricted diet; aldose reductase inhibition
Gaucher's disease, type I	Intravenous β-glucocerebrosidase
Glucose-galactose malabsorption	Glucose, galactose restriction; fructose supplement
Glucose-6-phosphate dehydrogenase deficiency	Avoidance of fava beans and drugs that cause erythrocyte hemolysis
Glutaric acidemia type I	Restriction of lysine and tryptophan; supplement L-carnitine, riboflavin
Glutaric acidemia type II	Restriction of fat and protein; supplement L-carnitine, riboflavin
Glycogen storage	
Type I (glucose-6-phosphatase deficiency)	Frequent feeding, complex starch supplement (liver transplant)
Type III (amylo-1,6 glucosidase deficiency	Frequent feeding, high protein
Type VI (phosphorylase deficiency)	Frequent feeding
Type VIII (phosphorylase kinase deficiency)	Avoid fasting, high protein
Glutamate-aspartate transport defect	Glutamine supplement
Gout	Purine restriction; allopurinol
Growth hormone deficiency	Growth hormone (HGH) or releasing factor (GHRF)
Gyrate atrophy of choroid and retina	Arginine restriction; essential amino acids supplement; protein restriction
Hartnup disease	Nicotinamide supplement
Hereditary methemoglobinemia	Methylene blue, ascorbate, riboflavin supplements
Histidinemia	None
Homocystinuria:	
Cystathionine β-synthase deficiency	Methionine restriction; cysteine supplement; pyridoxine to augment block; folate and betaine to provide alternate routes
N^5, N^{10}-Methylenetetrahydrofolate reductase deficiency	Folic acid supplement
3-Hydroxy-3-methylglutaryl-CoA lyase deficiency	Leucine and fat restriction
Hydroxykynureninuria	Nicotinic acid supplement
Hyperbetaalaninemia	Pyridoxine supplement
Hypercholesterolemia	Restriction of saturated fatty acids and cholesterol; supplemental fiber; mevinolin, nicotinic acid, cholestyramine

continued

Disorder	Therapy
Hyperphenylalaninemia	
Dihydropteridine reductase deficiency	Phenylalanine restriction; carbidopa; 5-hydroxytryptophan; tetrahydrobiopterin
Biopterin biosynthetic blocks	Tetrahydrobiopterin, carbidopa; 5-OH-tryptophan
Hyperornithinemia—hyperammonemia—homocitrullinuria (HHH)	Protein restriction, essential amino acid supplement
Hypertriglyceridemia	Weight reduction; carbohydrate restriction
Hypophosphatemia	Vitamin D, phosphorus supplements
Isovaleric acidemia	Leucine restriction; L-carnitine, glycine supplements
Ketoacidosis of infancy	Alkali, glucose supplements
Lactic acidosis, intermittent	
Pyruvate decarboxylase deficiency	High-fat, low-carbohydrate diet, thiamin supplement; alkali
Pyruvate carboxylase deficiency	Frequent feeds, alkali, thiamin, and biotin supplements
Lactose intolerance	Lactose restriction
Lipoprotein lipase deficiency	Low fat diet, supplement with essential fatty acids and medium-chain triglycerides
Lysine intolerance (hyperlysinemia)	Protein restriction; citrulline supplements
Maple syrup urine disease (MSUD)	Restrict isoleucine, leucine, and valine; supplement thiamin
Methionine malabsorption	Methionine restriction; cysteine supplement
Methylmalonic aciduria	
Defective reduction or transport of cobalamin	B_{12} supplement, megadoses parenterally; betaine and OH-B_{12} orally
Impaired cobalamin methylation	Parenteral B_{12} megadoses; betaine and OH-B_{12} orally
Impaired synthesis of 5′-deoxyadenosylcobalamin	Parenteral B_{12} megadoses; betaine and OH-B_{12} orally
Methylmalonyl-CoA mutase/racemase deficiency	Isoleucine, methionine, threonine, valine restriction; L-carnitine supplementation
Multiple carboxylase deficiency	Biotin supplement
Niemann-Pick disease type C	Cholesterol restriction; mevinolin, cholestyramine
Nonketotic hyperglycinemia	Protein restriction, energy supplements; benzoic acid; dextromethorphan
Ornithine transcarbamylase deficiency	Arginine, benzoic acid and phenylacetate or phenylbutyrate supplements; protein restriction; essential amino acids; L-carnitine supplements
Orotic aciduria	Uridine supplements
Oxalosis	Pyridoxine magnesium orthophosphate, water supplements (liver and kidney transplant)
Periodic paralysis	
Hypokalemic	Carbohydrate restriction, potassium salts, sodium chloride
Hyperkalemic	Increased carbohydrates
Normokalemic	Sodium chloride
Peroxisome dysfunction	Supplement docosahexaenoic acid, bile acid, steroids, vitamin K
Phenylketonuria	Phenylalanine restriction, tyrosine supplement
Porphyria, acute intermittent	High glucose; hematin infusions for feedback control
Pseudohypoparathyroidism	Calcium and vitamin D supplement
Prolidase deficiency	L-Proline, $MgCl_2$, vitamin C
Propionic acidemia	Isoleucine, methionine, threonine, valine restriction; biotin and L-carnitine supplements
Pyridoxine dependency with seizures	Pyridoxine parenterally; oral pharmacologic B_6 supplements
Pyroglutamic aciduria	Alkali, protein restriction
Pyruvate dehydrogenase deficiency, partial	Thiamin supplement, carbohydrate restriction, energy supplements (lipids); ketogenic diet
Refsum's disease	Phytanic acid restriction (diet low in dairy and ruminant fats)
Sucrose-isomaltose malabsorption	Sucrose restriction, ingestion of sucrase-isomaltase containing *Streptomyces cerevesiae*
Tryptophanuria with dwarfism	Nicotinic acid
Tyrosinemia type I	Phenylalanine-tyrosine restriction, high-energy diet; NTBC, liver transplant
Tyrosinemia with keratosis and corneal dystrophy (type II)	Phenylalanine and tyrosine restriction
Tyrosinemia type III	Phenylalanine and tyrosine restriction
Valinemia	Valine restriction
Vitamin A defect (β-carotene 15, 15′-dioxygenase)	Vitamin A supplement
Vitamin B_{12} defect (conversion of B_{12} to precursor of 5′-deoxyadenosyl-B_{12} and methyl-B_{12})	Vitamin B_{12} supplement
Vitamin D–dependent rickets	1,25 dihydroxy D supplement
Vitamin K–dependent coagulation defects (factors VII, IX, and X; protein C, protein S deficiency)	Vitamin K supplement
Williams-Beuren syndrome	Calcium, vitamin D restriction
Wilson's disease	Copper restriction, D-penicillamine
Xanthinuria	Purine restriction; allopurinol, fluids, alkali supplements
Xanthurenic aciduria	Pyridoxine

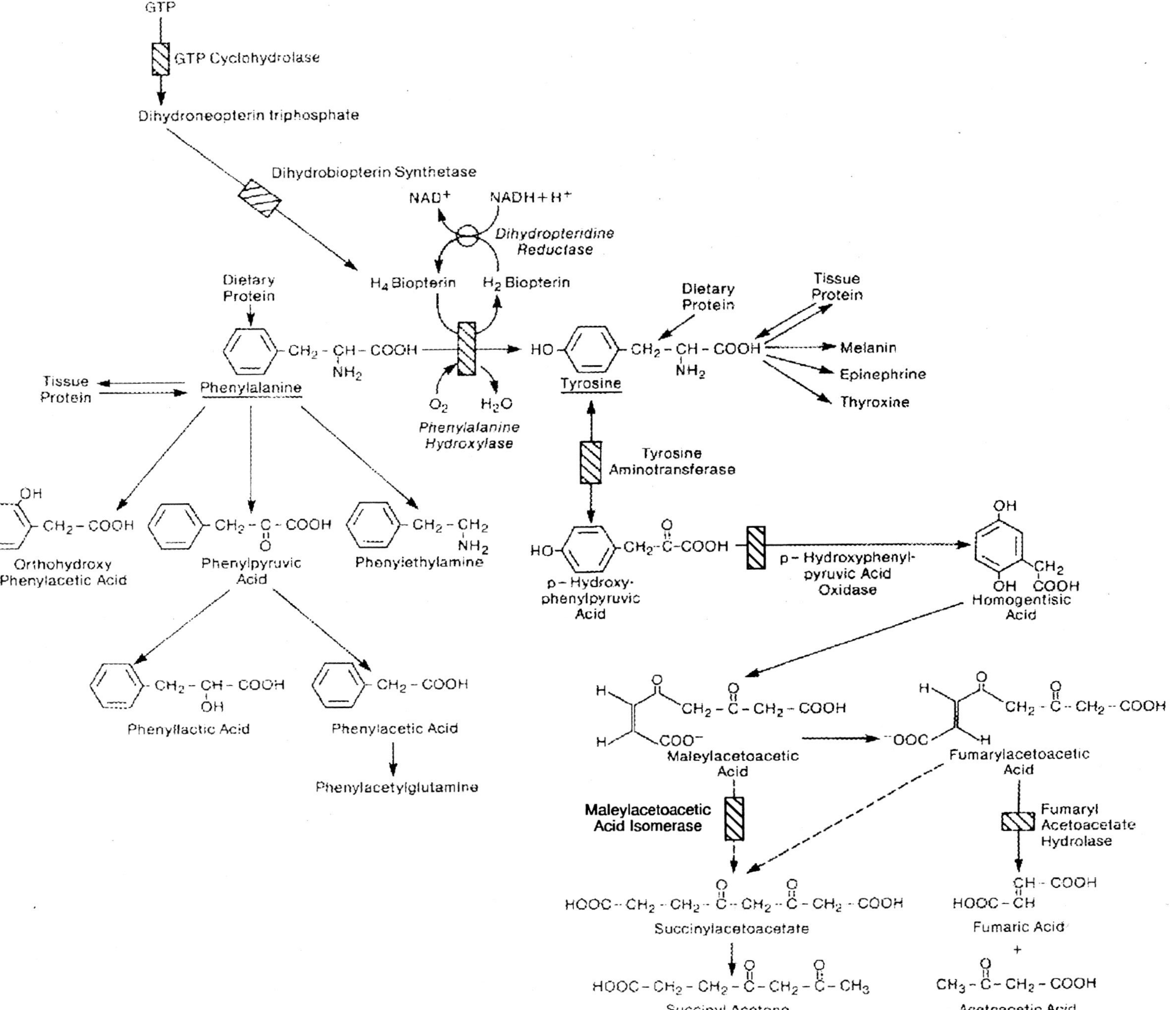

Figure 61.1. Metabolism of aromatic amino acids. The metabolic flow and nutrient interaction in disorders of phenylalanine and tyrosine are diagramed. *Crosshatched bars* represent impaired enzymes involved in biopterin biosynthesis, phenylketonuria, and tyrosinemia. See text for discussion.

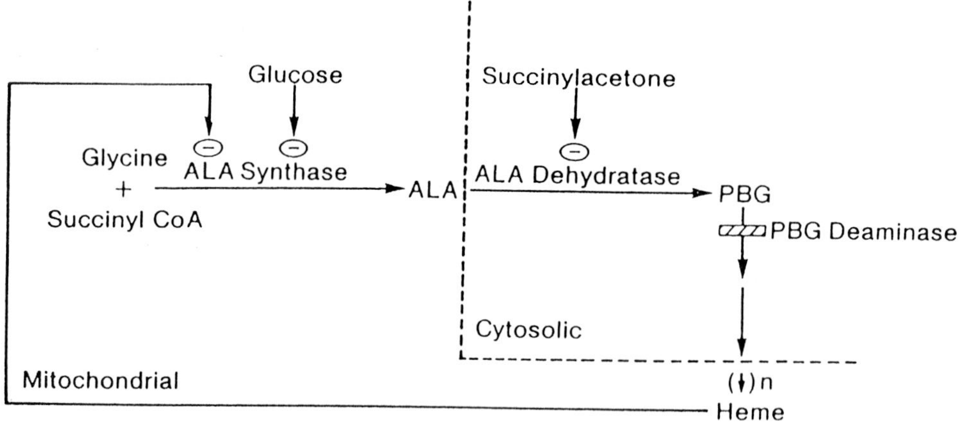

Figure 61.2. Inhibition site in heme biosynthesis of relevance to diagnosis and treatment of tyrosinemia type I. The *hatched bar* schematically represents the partial block in acute intermittent porphyria with resultant overproduction of δ-ALA (δ-aminolevulinic acid) and PBG (porphobilinogen) with decreased heme biosynthesis. In type I tyrosinemia, succinylacetone is produced and inhibits δ-ALA dehydratase with accumulation of δ-ALA alone, which is neurotoxic. δ-ALA accumulation can be reduced by addition of excess dietary glucose (calories) and by hematin infusions that negatively control δ-ALA synthase at levels of both enzyme and gene expression.

formed by reamination of the BCKAs α-ketoisocaproic, α-keto-β-methylvaleric, and α-ketoisovaleric acids, respectively.

5. Increased production of alternative products (E) through little-used metabolic pathways. As illustrated in Figure 61.1, when phenylalanine accumulates because of impaired phenylalanine hydroxylase (PAH), phenylpyruvic, phenylacetic, and phenyllactic acids are produced in larger than normal amounts through existing pathways that normally do not function at physiologic concentrations of cellular phenylalanine.
6. Inhibition of alternate pathways by accumulated substrate (i.e., C in CD impairment). For example, neurotransmitter synthesis may be depressed in PKU owing to increased blood phenylalanine that competitively inhibits tyrosine hydroxylase and tryptophan hydroxylase in the CNS. Another example is type I tyrosinemia. The accumulation of succinylacetone inhibits δ-ALA dehydratase (Fig. 61.2) and results in secondary accumulation of δ-ALA, attacks of acute porphyria with peripheral neuropathy, hypertension, and bizarre behavior.

Twelve approaches to therapy of inherited metabolic disease are discussed here. The choice of therapy depends on the mechanisms producing disease. Several therapeutic approaches may be tried sequentially or used simultaneously, depending on the acuteness of the disease process.

1. *Enhancing anabolism and depressing catabolism.* This involves the use of high-energy feeds, appropriate amino acid mixtures, and administration of insulin, if needed. Fasting should be prevented. This therapeutic maneuver should be common to all inborn errors involving catabolic pathways.
2. *Correcting the primary imbalance in metabolic relationships.* This correction involves a reduction through dietary restriction of accumulated substrate(s) that are toxic and provision of products that may be deficient. For example, in PAH deficiency, phenylalanine is restricted and tyrosine is supplemented.
3. *Enhancing excretion of accumulated substances that are overproduced.* Treatment of gout with uricosuric agents leads to lower blood uric acid levels by blocking renal reabsorption. The tissue deposits of uric acid salts are then mobilized. A more general use is hydration to enable renal clearance of toxic compounds.
4. *Providing alternative metabolic pathways to decrease accumulated toxic precursors in blocked reaction sequences.* For example, the accumulated ammonia in enzyme defects of the urea cycle is reduced by removing nitrogen through administration of therapeutic amounts of phenylbutyric or phenylacetic acid to form phenylacetylglutamine from glutamine. Similarly, in isovaleric acidemia, innocuous isovalerylglycine (IVG) is formed from accumulating isovaleric acid (IVA) if supplemental glycine is provided to drive glycine-*N*-transacylase. IVG is excreted in the urine.
5. *Using metabolic inhibitors to lower overproduced products.* For example: allopurinol inhibits xanthine oxidase and decreases overproduction of uric acid in gout, Lovastatin and Compactin suppress hydroxymethylglutaryl–coenzyme A (CoA) reductase and reduce excess cholesterol biosynthesis in familial hypercholesterolemia, and 2-(2-nitro-4-trifluoromethylbenzoyl)-1,3-cyclohexanedione) (NTBC) inhibits *p*-OH-phenylpyruvic acid dioxygenase (*p*-OHPPAD) and thus succinylacetone production in type I tyrosinemia.
6. *Supplying products of blocked secondary pathways.* In cystic fibrosis, the exocrine pancreas does not function in a normal manner to produce and secrete digestive enzymes. Administration of these pancreatic enzymes partially corrects this insufficiency.
7. *Stabilizing altered enzyme proteins.* The rate of biologic synthesis and degradation of holoenzymes depends on their structural conformation. In some holoenzymes, saturation by coenzyme increases their biologic half-life and thus overall enzyme activity at the equilibrium produced by mutant proteins. This therapeutic mechanism is exemplified in homocystinuria and MSUD. Pharmacologic intake of vitamin B_6 in homocystinuria or vitamin B_1 in MSUD increases intracellu-

lar pyridoxal phosphate or thiamin pyrophosphate and will increase the specific activity of cystathionine β-synthase (CBS) or BCKAD complex, respectively (8, 9).

8. *Replacing deficient coenzymes.* A variety of vitamin-dependent disorders are due to blocks in coenzyme production and are "cured" by lifetime pharmacologic intake of a specific vitamin precursor. This mechanism presumably involves overcoming a partially impaired enzyme reaction by mass action. If reactions are impaired that are required to produce methylcobalamin and/or adenosylcobalamin, homocystinuria or methylmalonic aciduria (or both) will result. Daily intake of milligram quantities of vitamin B_{12} may cure both disorders (10). In biotinidase deficiency, the coenzyme biotin is not released from its covalently bound state. Reviews of "vitamin-dependency syndromes" have been published (11, 12).
9. *Artificially inducing enzyme production.* If the structural gene or enzyme is intact, but suppressor, enhancer, or promoter elements are not functional, abnormal amounts of enzyme may be produced. It should be possible to "turn on" or "turn off" the structural gene and enable normal enzymatic production to occur. In the acute porphyria of type I tyrosinemia, excessive δ-ALA production may be reduced by suppressing transcription of the δ-ALA synthase gene with excess glucose and hematin (Fig. 61.2).
10. *Replacing enzymes.* Many attempts to replace deficient enzymes by plasma infusion and microencapsulation have been tried with limited success. Recently the use of polyethylene glycol coating of adenosine deaminase significantly prolonged the biologic half-life of this enzyme in treating severe combined immunodeficiency (13). The engineering of β-glucosidase with a high mannan receptor site enables intravenous use of Ceredase to treat type I Gaucher's disease.
11. *Transplanting organs.* Kidney transplant in Fabry's disease and liver transplant in type I glycogen storage disease benefit systemic metabolism with the return of organ function replacing deficient enzyme activity.
12. *Correcting the underlying defect in DNA so that the body can manufacture its own functionally normal enzymes.* This experimental approach has great possibility for the future. The DNA for many proteins such as adenosine deaminase, hypoxanthine-guanine phosphoribosyl transferase, ornithine transcarbamylase, and the LDL cholesterol receptor has been cloned, and retroviral constructs containing their cDNA transfected into dividing somatic cells from affected individuals. Human gene therapy is currently contemplated for these inborn errors, although several technical problems in gene stability and expression must be solved first. Other molecular approaches such as homologous recombination to correct mutant sequences on endogenous genes are also future possibilities (14).

Nutritional management remains a principal component in treating all of these inherited disorders, and some practical considerations for nutritional support should be considered. Foremost is the need to maintain normal growth, which cannot be achieved without adequate intake of energy and amino acids. Energy requirements are greater than normal when natural protein is restricted and L-amino acids supply protein equivalent (15). L-Amino acids administered in one daily dose are oxidized to a much greater extent than those in the same dose divided and administered throughout the day (16). Nitrogen balance was improved considerably when L-amino acids were ingested in several doses throughout the day with whole protein, rather than in one dose (17). If adequate energy and amino acids cannot be ingested to support normal growth through oral feeds, nasogastric, gastrostomy, or parenteral feeds should be used. Failure to adapt nutrient intake to the individual needs of each patient can result in mental retardation, metabolic crises, neurologic crises, growth failure, and, with some inherited metabolic diseases, death. When specific amino acids or nitrogen requires restriction, total deletion of the toxic nutrient for 1 to 3 days in the presence of excess energy intake is the best approach to initiating therapy. Longer deletion or overrestriction may precipitate deficiency of the amino acid(s) or nitrogen. Because the most limiting nutrient in the diet determines growth rate, overrestriction of an amino acid, nitrogen, or energy will result in further intolerance of the toxic nutrient(s).

Dietary restrictions to correct imbalances in metabolic relationships often require the use of chemically defined or elemental medical foods (18). These medical foods must be accompanied by small amounts of whole natural protein that supply the restricted amino acid(s). Natural foods seldom supply more than 50%, and often much less, of the protein requirements of patients. Nitrogen-free natural foods that provide energy are limited in their range of nutrients. Consequently, care must be taken to provide nutrients often considered to be contaminants because their essentiality has been demonstrated through long-term use of total parenteral nutrition (19). Thus, in addition to nutrients for which an RDA is established, other nutrients must be supplied in adequate amounts. These include the trace minerals chromium and molybdenum; the vitamins biotin and pantothenic acid; choline and inositol; and carnitine when excess acylcarnitines are produced and excreted, as in methylmalonic acidemia or propionic acidemia. Other possible conditionally essential nutrients for patients with PKU have been described (20).

Elemental medical foods consist of small molecules that often provide an osmolality that exceeds the physiologic tolerance of the patient. Abdominal cramping, diarrhea, distention, nausea, and vomiting result from hyperosmolar feeds. Aside from gastrointestinal distress, more-serious consequences can occur such as hypertonic dehydration, hypovolemia, hypernatremia, and death. Osmolalities of selected medical foods intended for inherited diseases of amino acid metabolism have been published (21).

AROMATIC AMINO ACIDS

Inborn errors of the aromatic amino acids were historically the first to respond to nutritional support. Phenylketonuria was discovered in 1933, and the prevention of its resultant mental retardation by dietary intervention is classic. Today, more than 200 different mutations at the PAH gene locus are described (22).

BIOCHEMISTRY

The essential amino acid phenylalanine is used for two major purposes: tissue protein synthesis and hydroxylation to form tyrosine. The hydroxylation reaction requires PAH, O_2, tetrahydrobiopterin, dihydropteridine reductase (DHPR), and NADH plus H^+ (Fig. 61.1). The normal adult uses only 10% of the RDA for phenylalanine for new protein synthesis, and approximately 90% is hydroxylated to form tyrosine. The growing child uses 60% of the required phenylalanine for new protein synthesis, and 40% is hydroxylated to form tyrosine. Mass spectrometry and stable isotope studies of patients with PKU provide information on other pathways available for phenylalanine metabolism. These alternative pathways, outlined in Figure 61.1, are minor in the metabolism of phenylalanine at 50 μmol concentration in the plasma of normal individuals. However, byproducts become apparent when phenylalanine is not hydroxylated to tyrosine and accumulates to over 500 μmol (22).

Tyrosine is the normal immediate product of phenylalanine and is essential to five pathways (Fig. 61.1), including synthesis of protein, catecholamines, melanin pigment, and thyroid hormones. Tyrosine also provides energy when catabolized through *p*-hydroxyphenylpyruvate to fumarate and acetoacetate. Enzymes required in this latter degradative pathway include tyrosine aminotransferase, *p*-hydroxyphenylpyruvic acid dioxygenase (*p*-OHPPAD), homogentisic acid oxidase, and fumarylacetoacetic acid hydrolase (FAH) (Fig. 61.1).

Phenylketonuria

Phenylketonuria is a group of inherited disorders of phenylalanine metabolism caused by impaired PAH activity. The disease is expressed at 3 to 6 months of age and is characterized by developmental delay, microcephaly, abnormal electroencephalogram, eczema, musty odor, and hyperactivity. If not treated before 3 weeks of age, the metabolic imbalance produces irreversible mental retardation. The defect in metabolism in classic PKU is associated with less than 2% of the activity of normal PAH, and these "classic" mutations are now defined (23). The enzyme is expressed primarily in liver but not in peripheral blood cells, bone marrow, or cultured cells. Five of the most frequent mutations in a U.S. clinic include I65T, R408W, Y414C, L348V, and IVS10nt546, which account for more than 50% of mutant PAH alleles. Genotypes with R408W and IVS10nt546 result in more severe PAH impairment while Y414C and I65T have relatively mild phenotypes (23). Heterozygous parents for "classic" PKU have 50% enzyme and can be identified by increased ratios of semifasting phenylalanine squared to tyrosine (P^2/T) in vivo (24).

The genetic bases for disorders of PAH followed localization of the PAH gene to chromosome 12q22-q24 and cloning of the gene, which has 90 kilobases (kb), 13 exons, and 12 introns (22). At least 200 different mutations have been identified that cause the "PKU phenotype," and these involve deletions in coding frames, missense mutations, and intron splice site mutations (22, 23). Ethnic variation occurs in the type and frequency of PAH mutations, a fact that provides clues to migration of populations in history (22). Cloning of this gene and identification of different mutations have assisted in genotyping probands, counseling families, and predicting the amount of dietary phenylalanine that will be required (23). Preventive newborn screening with immediate and lifelong avoidance of excess phenylalanine in the diet continues to be the principal paradigm of therapy despite these advances in molecular genetics.

Other forms of PKU may result from defects in other enzymes involved in the overall reaction. DHPR, an enzyme normally present in many tissues, reduces the quininoid form of dihydrobiopterin to tetrahydrobiopterin (Fig. 61.1). The gene for DHPR is located on chromosome 4p15.1-p16.1. Several other types of PKU result from defects in the synthesis of tetrahydrobiopterin (25) (Fig. 61.1). In addition to functioning as a coenzyme for PAH, tetrahydrobiopterin is also required by tyrosine hydroxylase and tryptophan hydroxylase (26, 27) (Fig. 61.1). Because these enzymes produce essential neurotransmitters, defects in biopterin synthesis are associated with progressive neurologic disease unless tetrahydrobiopterin, L-3,4-dihydroxyphenylalanine (L-DOPA), and serotonin are replaced (26).

Although the precise pathogenesis of mental retardation in classic PKU is not known, accumulation of phenylalanine or its catabolic byproducts, deficiency of tyrosine or its products, or all four circumstances will produce CNS damage if phenylalanine accumulates in plasma above normal concentrations during critical periods of brain development. The pathologic consequence varies with the time in brain development at which the chemical insult occurs. Deficient myelination and abnormalities in brain proteolipids and/or proteins occur in late gestation and during the first 6 to 9 months of life (28). During this period, oligodendroglia migration may also be impaired, resulting in irreversible brain damage later in childhood. Protein synthesis in the brain is also depressed, probably owing to competitive inhibition by high phenylalanine concentrations on blood-brain barrier transport, with consequent imbalance in intraneuronal amino acid concentrations (29). In the mature brain, neurodegeneration (30), behavioral difficulties, and prolonged performance times may result from depressed neurotransmitter synthesis (31, 32). Impairment of these neuropsychologic functions in the mature brain may be reversible when phenylalanine returns toward normal concentrations in cells and blood (31, 32).

Screening

The disorders of phenylalanine metabolism require identification, diagnosis, and appropriate therapy before clinical expression of the disease is apparent. Nutritional and possibly other therapy should be instituted before the 3rd week of life. Thus a tetrapartite public health program involving screening, retrieval, diagnosis, and treatment must be coordinated and efficient to prevent mental retardation. A screening test using the bacterial inhibition assay (33) detects potential cases in the newborn population. One laboratory can effectively screen 20,000 to 200,000 samples per year using these methods. Although other methods such as fluorometry are more quantitative, the Guthrie test is used worldwide because of its ease of application and low cost. Newborns with blood phenylalanine concentrations above 121 μmol/L (2 mg/dL) on the screening test are restudied. The actions taken in "retrieval" depend on the concentration of blood phenylalanine, days of age, and protein intake at the time of screening.

Protein ingestion may not be required for a positive PKU screen, but quantitative normal concentrations during the first 48 hours of life are needed for comparison (34). Almost all infants with PKU have blood phenylalanine concentrations above normal during the 1st day of life, even before the first feeding if they have "classic" PKU mutations (23, 24). Neonates with PAH gene mutations resulting in less severely impaired PAH may take longer to develop an elevated blood phenylalanine concentration. Some infants with relatively mild elevation of blood phenylalanine have serious neuropathology that is progressive due to a defect in synthesis of tetrahydrobiopterin. Therefore, diagnosis of "positive" newborn screenees should include measurement of urinary tetrahydrobiopterin (BH_4) and erythrocyte DHPR.

Newborn screening in most of the 50 states, in conjunction with aggressive approaches to retrieval and diagnosis, has led to early institution of diet therapy and prevention of mental retardation (34). To be successful, state-mandated screening programs must enable collection and rapid evaluation of specimens while providing an organized, efficient retrieval system of babies whose screening tests yield positive results (34, 35). With the present early infant discharge from the newborn nursery and the increase in breast feeding, lower phenylalanine concentrations of 121 to 242 μmol/L (2 to 4 mg/dL) are considered "positive," and follow-up is initiated (36). Approximately 1 in 10,000 Caucasian newborns in the United States is affected with PKU, whereas 1 in 132,000 newborns in the black population is affected (35). Data in Table 61.3 detail the number of cases of PKU diagnosed since the inception of an exemplary statewide screening program in Georgia. The mean frequency of PKU is based on a population of newborns that is 63% Caucasian.

Table 61.3
Incidence of Inherited Metabolic Diseases in Georgia's Newborn Population

Disease	Total	Incidence
PKU[a]		
Classic	70	1:24,649
Hyperphenylalaninemia	34	1:50,748
Total	104	1:16,591
Tyrosinemia[a]		
Type I (hepatorenal)	6	1:287,574
Type II (oculocutaneous)	3	1:575,147
Type III (transient neonatal)	1909	1:904
Total	1918	1:900
Maple syrup urine disease[a]	14	1:123,246
Homocystinuria[a]		
CBS deficiency	5	1:345,088
Hypermethioninemia	39	1:44,242
Total	45	1:38,343
Galactosemia[b]		
Classic	41	1:41,212
Variant	169	1:9,998
Total	214	1:7,896

[a]Based on 1,725,442 newborn screenees.
[b]Based on 1,689,692 newborn screenees.

Diagnosis

Patients with initial blood phenylalanine concentrations above 121 μmol/L (>2 mg/dL) should have the test repeated immediately. If the initial or follow-up screening test yields levels above 484 μmol/L (8 mg/dL), plasma amino acids should be quantitated by ion-exchange chromatography with the infant on a known phenylalanine intake from natural protein sources. A precise diagnosis is necessary to establish the mode of therapy.

Differential diagnosis requires several laboratory procedures. These include ion-exchange chromatography to determine plasma phenylalanine, tyrosine, and other amino acid concentrations; genotyping of parents and proband (37); and assays of biopterin and DHPR (26). DNA analysis using restriction fragment length polymorphisms (RFLP) and cDNA probes for the PAH gene help in classifying patients and determining the amount of dietary phenylalanine to prescribe (22, 23). For families with an affected child, prenatal diagnosis is available through direct mutational analysis of fetal cell DNA for known PAH genes, or indirect RFLP analysis of PAH in parents and proband for unknown fetal PAH genes (22, 38). Because PAH is not expressed in cultured amniotic fluid cells and because phenylalanine concentrations do not rise in amniotic fluid until the last trimester, prenatal monitoring was not possible before molecular techniques became available.

Treatment

Patients with plasma phenylalanine concentrations above 250 μmol, plasma tyrosine concentrations below 50 μmol, and normal BH_4 and DHPR require prompt treatment with a phenylalanine-restricted, tyrosine-supplemented diet. The objective of nutritional support of the child with classic PKU is to maintain blood phenylalanine concentrations that will allow optimum growth and brain development by supplying adequate energy, protein, and other nutrients while restricting phenylalanine and supplementing tyrosine intake.

Although the effects of moderately elevated plasma phenylalanine are not yet known, optimum blood levels should be as close to normal as possible. This objective is met through use of a combination of medical and natural foods. Some investigators have supplemented the phenylalanine-restricted diet with isoleucine, leucine, and valine and have found improvement in behavior and decreased plasma phenylalanine (39). This may be related to inhibition of phenylalanine transport by competition at either the intestinal or blood-brain barrier uptake steps (29). Gene replacement therapy using recombinant viruses containing the PAH gene requires more fundamental research before being of practical use. Recombinant retroviruses containing the cDNA for PAH can introduce a functioning PAH gene into dividing liver cells, but long-term PAH expression is limited (22, 40). These approaches are under study and require not only stable transformation and PAH expression, but also coordinating DHPR and biopterin synthesis to accomplish the overall reaction. Thus, gene therapy is not yet applicable to practical therapy of PKU.

Therapy of the child with biopterin-deficient forms of hyperphenylalaninemia requires administration of tetrahydrobiopterin and use of the phenylalanine-restricted, tyrosine-supplemented diet in combination with L-DOPA and carbidopa (26). Serotonin that is derived from tryptophan may also improve behavior, since tryptophan hydroxylase is also impaired by diminished tetrahydrobiopterin (26, 27, 41).

Initiation of Nutritional Support. Blood phenylalanine concentration at the time of diagnosis may be rapidly lowered by feeding the infant a 20-kcal/oz (67 kcal/dL) low-phenylalanine or phenylalanine-free formula (42). A minimum of 120 kcal/kg/day intake is necessary. Within a mean of 4 days (SD ± 3), blood phenylalanine concentration should drop to treatment range on a phenylalanine-free formula. Treatment should be initiated in hospitalized infants to enable adequate parental information transfer and to monitor blood amino acids daily. Laboratory results should be available promptly to prevent precipitation of phenylalanine deficiency and to enable rapid replacement of phenylalanine and tyrosine to optimum blood concentrations.

If the infant or child is not hospitalized for initiation of nutritional support or if only weekly blood phenylalanine concentrations are obtained, 48 hours of a phenylalanine-free formula followed by maintenance formula containing adequate phenylalanine from an appropriate source should be prescribed. Blood phenylalanine concentration will fall to treatment range within a mean of 10 days (SD ± 5) with this approach (42). Blood phenylalanine concentrations should be between 120 and 300 μmol as soon as possible, but no later than the 3rd week of life.

Chronic Care. Long-term care of the patient with classic PKU dictates that medical and natural foods provide all nutrients in required amounts.

Nutrient Requirements. Table 61.4 outlines the suggested ranges of phenylalanine, tyrosine, protein, energy, and fluid to offer. A formal prescription must be written that is individualized to the specific genotype (23, 43–45), growth rate, and consequent needs of each patient. Weekly adjustments in the diet prescription may be necessary, particularly during the first 6 months of life, based on hunger, growth, development, and laboratory analyses of plasma phenylalanine and tyrosine concentrations. The prescribed phenylalanine should maintain the 3- to 4-h postprandial blood phenylalanine concentration between 60 and 300 μmol (46). Phenylalanine is an essential amino

Table 61.4
Approximate Daily Requirements for Selected Nutrients by Infants, Children, and Young Adults with Selected Inherited Disorders of Amino Acid Metabolism

		Age						
Nutrient[a]	Unit	0 < 6 months	6 < 12 months	1 < 4 years	4 < 7 years	7 < 11 years	11 < 15 years	15 < 19 years
Energy	kcal/kg	145–95	135–80	—	—	—	—	—
	kcal/day (range)	—	—	1300 (900–800)	1700 (1300–2300)	2400 (1650–3300)	2200–2700 (1500–3700)	2100–1800 (1200–3900)
Fluid	mL/kg[b]	160–135	145–120	95	90	75	50–55	50–65
Protein	g/kg	3.5–3.0	3.0–2.5	—	—	—	—	—
	g/day	—	—	30	35	40	50–55	50–65
Carbohydrate	g/day	kcal × 0.35 to 0.30 ÷ 4				kcal × 0.50 to 0.60 ÷ 4		
Fat	g/day	kcal × 0.50 ÷ 9				kcal × 0.35 ÷ 9		
Isoleucine	mg/kg	90–30	90–30	85–20	80–20	30–20	30–20	30–10
Leucine	mg/kg	100–60	75–40	70–40	63–35	60–30	50–30	40–15
Methionine	mg/kg	35–20	35–15	30–10	20–10	20–10	20–10	10–5
Phenylalanine	mg/kg	70–20	50–15	40–15	35–15	30–15	30–15	30–10
Tyrosine, PKU	mg/kg	350–300	300–250	230	175	140	110–120	110–120
Tyrosinemias	mg/kg	80–60	60–40	60–30	50–25	40–20	30–15	30–10
Valine	mg/kg	95–40	60–30	85–30	50–30	30–25	30–20	30–15

[a]All known essential amino acids, essential fatty acids, minerals and vitamins must be provided in adequate amounts.
[b]At least 1 mL of fluid should be offered for each kcal of energy ingested by the infant.

Table 61.5
Formulation, Nutrient Composition, and Sources of Medical Foods for Selected Inborn Errors of Metabolism

Disorder and Medical Foods	Modified Nutrient(s) (mg/100 g)	Protein Equivalent (g/100 g), source	Fat (g/100 g), source	Carbohydrate (g/100 g), source	Energy (kcal/100 g)	Minerals Not Added
Aromatic amino acids						
PKU and hyperphenylalaninemia						
Lofenalac[a]	PHE-80, TYR-800, TRP-195; L-carnitine, taurine added	15 Enzymically hydrolyzed casein, L-amino acids	18 Corn oil	60 Corn syrup solids, modified tapioca starch	460	Chromium Molybdenum
Periflex[b]	PHE-0, TYR-1850, TRP-270; L-carnitine-20, added taurine	20 L-Amino acids	17 Canola oil, hybrid safflower oil, fractionated coconut oil	40.5 Corn syrup solids	395	None
Phenex-1[c]	PHE-0, TYR-1500, TRP-170; L-carnitine-20, added taurine	15 L-Amino acids	23.9 Palm oil, hydrogenated coconut oil, and soy oil	46.3 Hydrolyzed cornstarch	480	Chromium[d] molybdenum[d]
Phenex-2[c]	PHE-0, TYR-3000, TRP-340; L-carnitine-40, added taurine	30 L-Amino acids	15.5 Palm oil, hydrogenated coconut oil, and soy oil	30 Hydrolyzed cornstarch	410	Chromium[d] Molybdenum[d]
XP Analog[b]	PHE-0, TYR-1370, TRP-300; L-carnitine-10, added taurine	13 L-Amino acids	20.9 Peanut oil, refined lard, hydrogenated coconut oil	59 Corn syrup solids	475	None
XP Maxamaid[b]	PHE-0, TYR-2650, TRP-570; L-carnitine-20, added taurine	25 L-Amino acids	<1.0 None added	62 Sucrose, hydrolyzed corn-starch	350	None
XP Maxamum[b]	PHE-0, TYR-4030, TRP-890; L-carnitine-20, added taurine	39 L-Amino acids	<1.0 None added	45 Surcose, hydrolyzed corn-starch	301	None
Phenyl-Free[a]	PHE-0, TYR-2000, TRP-280; L-carnitine, taurine added	19.8 L-Amino acids	6.6 Corn and coconut oils	66 Sucrose, corn syrup solids, modified tapioca starch	410	Chromium Molybdenum
PKU 1[a]	PHE-0, TYR-3400, TRP-1000; no L-carnitine, taurine	50 L-Amino acids	0 None added	19 Sucrose	280	Chromium Selenium
PKU 2[a]	PHE-0, TYR-4500, TRP-1400; no L-carnitine, taurine	67 L-Amino acids	0 None added	7 Sucrose	300	Chromium Selenium
PKU 3[a]	PHE-0, TYR-6000, TRP-1400; no L-carnitine, taurine	68 L-Amino acids	0 None added	3 Sucrose	290	Chromium Selenium
Tyrosinemia type I						
Tyromex-1[c]	PHE-0, TYR-0, MET-0; L-carnitine-20, added taurine	15 L-Amino acids	23.9 Palm oil, hydrogenated coconut oil, soy oil	46.3 Hydrolyzed cornstarch	480	Chromium[d] Molybdenum[d]
Tyrex-2[c]	PHE-0, TYR-0; L-carnitine-40, added taurine	30 L-Amino acids	15.5 Peanut oil, refined lard, hydrogenated coconut oil	30 Hydrolyzed cornstarch	410	Chromium[d] Molybdenum[d]
XPHE, TYR, MET Analog[b]	PHE-0, TYR-0, MET-0; L-carnitine-10, added taurine	13 L-Amino acids	20.9 Peanut oil, refined lard, hydrogenated coconut oil	59 Corn syrup solids	475	None
XPHE, TYR Maxamaid[c]	PHE-0, TYR-0; L-carnitine-20, added taurine	25 L-Amino acids	<1.0 None added	62 Sucrose, hydrolyzed cornstarch	350	None
Tyrosinemia type II, type III						
Low PHE/TYR Diet Powder[a]	PHE-75, TYR<38; L-carnitine, taurine added	15 Enzymically hydrolyzed casein, L-Amino acids	18 Corn oil	60 Corn syrup solids, modified tapioca starch	460	Chromium Molybdenum

Disorder and Medical Foods	Modified Nutrient(s) (mg/100 g)	Protein Equivalent (g/100 g), source	Fat (g/100 g), source	Carbohydrate (kcal/100 g), source	Energy (g/100 g)	Minerals Not Added
TYR 1[a]	PHE-0, TYR-0 no-L-carnitine, taurine	47 L-Amino acids	0 None added	21 Sucrose	270	Chromium Selenium
TYR 2[a]	PHE-0, TYR-0 no L-carnitine, taurine	63 L-Amino acids	0 None added	12 Sucrose	300	Chromium Selenium
Tyrex-2[c]	PHE-0, TYR-0; L-carnitine-40, added taurine	30 L-Amino acids	15.5 Peanut oil, refined lard, hydrogenated coconut oil	30 Hydrolyzed cornstarch	410	Chromium[d] Molybdenum[d]
XPHEN, TYR Analog[b]	PHE-0, TYR-0; L-carnitine-10, added taurine	13 L-Amino acids	20.9 Peanut oil, refined lard, hydrogenated coconut oil	50 Corn syrup solids	475	None
XPHEN, TYR Maxamaid[b]	PHE-0, TYR-0; L-carnitine-20, added taurine	25 L-Amino acids	<1.0 None added	62 Sucrose, hydrolyzed cornstarch	350	None
Branched-chain amino acids						
Maple syrup urine disease						
Ketonex-1[c]	ILE-0, LEU-0, VAL-0; L-carnitine-100; added taurine	15 L-Amino acids	23.9 Palm oil, hydrogenated coconut oil, soy oil	46.3 Hydrolyzed cornstarch	480	Chromium[d] Molybdenum[d]
Ketonex-2[c]	ILE-0, LEU-0, VAL-0; L-carnitine-200; added taurine	30 L-Amino acids	15.5 Palm oil, hydrogenated coconut oil, soy oil	30 Hydrolyzed cornstarch	410	Chromium[d] Molybdenum[d]
MSUD 1[a]	ILE-0, LEU-0, VAL-0; L-carnitine-0, taurine-0	49 L-Amino acids	0 None added	29 Sucrose	280	Chromium Selenium
MSUD 2[a]	ILE-0, LEU-0, VAL-0; L-carnitine-0, taurine-0	54 L-Amino acids	0 None added	22 Sucrose	310	Chromium Selenium
MSUD Analog[b]	ILE-0, LEU-0, VAL-0; L-carnitine-10, added taurine	13 L-Amino acids	20.9 Peanut oil, refined lard, hydrogenated coconut oil	59 Corn syrup solids	475	None
MSUD Diet Powder[a]	ILE-0, LEU-0, VAL-0; added L-carnitine, taurine	8.8 L-Amino acids	20 Corn oil	63 Corn syrup solids, modified tapioca starch	470	Chromium Molybdenum
MSUD Maxamaid[b]	ILE-0, LEU-0, VAL-0; L-carnitine-10, added taurine	25 L-amino acids	<1.0 None added	62 Sucrose, hydrolyzed cornstarch	350	None
MSUD Maxamum[b]	ILE-0, LEU-0, VAL-0; L-carnitine-20, added taurine	39 L-Amino acids	<1.0 None added	45 Sucrose, hydrolyzed cornstarch	340	None
Isovaleric acidemia						
I-Valex-1[c]	ILE-430, LEU-0, TRP-170, VAL-480; L-carnitine-900; GLY-1000; added taurine	15 L-Amino acids	23.9 Palm oil, hydrogenated coconut oil, soy oil	46.3 Hydrolyzed cornstarch	480	Chromium[d] Molybdenum[d]
I-Valex-2[c]	ILE-860, LEU-0, TRP-340, VAL-960; L-carnitine-1800; GLY-3020; added taurine	30 L-Amino acids	15.5 Palm oil, hydrogenated coconut oil, soy oil	30 Hydrolyzed cornstarch	410	Chromium[d] Molybdenum[d]

Disorder and Medical Foods	Modified Nutrient(s) (mg/100 g)	Protein Equivalent (g/100 g), source	Fat (g/100 g), source	Carbohydrate (kcal/100 g), source	Energy (g/100 g)	Minerals Not Added
XLEU Analog[b]	ILE-400, LEU-0, TRP-260, VAL-450- GLY-2500; L-carnitine-10, added taurine	13 L-Amino acids	209 Peanut oil refined lard, coconut oil, soy oil	59 Corn syrup solids	475	None
XLEU Maxamaid[b]	ILE-780, LEU-0, TRP-500, VAL-870, GLY-3990; l-carnitine-20, added taurine	25 L-Amino acids	<1.0 None added	62 Sucrose, hydrolyzed cornstarch	350	None
Homocystinuria, pyridoxine-nonresponsive						
HOM 1[a]	MET-0; CYS-2500; L-carnitine-0, taurine-0	52 L-Amino acids	0 None added	18 Sucrose	280	Chromium Selenium
HOM 2[a]	MET-0; CYS-3400 L-carnitine-0, taurine-0	69 L-Amino acids	0 None added	5 Sucrose	300	Chromium Selenium
Hominex-1[c]	MET-0, CYS-450; L-carnitine-20, added taurine	15 L-Amino acids	23.9 Palm oil, hydrogenated coconut oil, soy oil	46.3 Hydrolyzed cornstarch	480	Chromium[d] Molybdenum[d]
Hominex-2[c]	MET-0, CYS-900; L-carnitine-40, added taurine	30 L-Amino acids	15.5 Palm oil, hydrogenated coconut oil, soy oil	30 Hydrolyzed cornstarch	410	Chromium[d] Molybdenum[d]
XMET Analog[b]	MET-0, CYS-390; L-carnitine-10, added taurine	13 L-Amino acids	20.9 Peanut oil, refined lard, hydrogenated coconut oil	59 Corn syrup solids	475	None
XMET Maxamaid[b]	MET-0, CYS-750; L-carnitine-20, added taurine	25 L-Amino acids	<1.0 None added	62 Sucrose, hydrolyzed cornstarch	350	None
XMET Maxamum[b]	MET-0, CYS-1180; L-carnitine-20, added taurine	39 L-Amino acids	<1.0 None added	45 Sucrose, hydrolyzed cornstarch	340	None
Urea cycle enzyme defects						
Cyclinex-1[c]	Nonessential amino acids-0; L-carnitine-190; added taurine	7.5 L-Amino acids	27 Palm oil, hydrogenated coconut oil, soy oil	52 Hydrolyzed cornstarch	515	Chromium[d] Molybdenum[d]
Cyclinex-2[c]	Non-essential amino acids-0; L-carnitine-370; added taurine	15 L-Amino acids	20.7 Palm oil, hydrogenated coconut oil, soy oil	40 Hydrolyzed cornstarch	480	Chromium[d] Molybdenum[d]
UCD 1[a]	Nonessential amino acids-0; no L-carnitine, taurine	67 L-Amino acids	0	8 Sucrose	260	Chromium Magnesium Selenium
UCD 2[a]	Nonessential amino acids-0; no L-carnitine, taurine	67 L-Amino acids	0	6 Sucrose	290	Chromium Magnesium Selenium
Pro-Phree[c]	Protein-0; L-carnitine-25; added taurine	0	31.0 Palm oil, hydrogenated coconut oil, soy oil	60.0 Hydrolyzed cornstarch	520	Chromium[d] Molybdenum[d]
Protein-Free Diet Powder[a]	Protein-0; L-carnitine, taurine added	0	23.0 Corn oil	72.0 Corn syrup solids, modified tapioca starch	500	Chromium Molybdenum

[a]Mead Johnson Nutritional Division, Evansville, IN; 1/800-457-3550.
[b]Scientific Hospital Supplies, North American Division, Gaithersburg, MD; 1/800-365-7354.
[c]Ross Products Division, Abbott Laboratories, Columbus, OH; 1/800-551-5838.
[d]*Note:* values listed, although accurate at time of publication, are subject to change. The most current information may be obtained by referring to product labels.

acid (47) and cannot be deleted from the diet without producing death (48). Excess restriction produces growth failure, rashes, bone changes, and mental retardation (48).

The infant with classic PKU requires 20 to 50 mg phenylalanine per kilogram body weight for growth, with younger infants requiring the larger amount (49). The phenylalanine requirement declines rapidly between 3 and 6 months of age as growth rates decline. Requirements for phenylalanine in the 6- to 12-month-old patient with classic PKU may fall to 15 mg/kg/day, but they vary considerably (Table 61.4). Frequent monitoring of blood phenylalanine concentration and intake is required to prevent excess intake when growth rate decelerates and to prevent inadequate intake when growth rate is at its peak, as in early infancy and during the prepubertal and pubertal growth spurts and during the later half of gestation.

Tyrosine is an essential amino acid for individuals with PKU. For this reason, plasma tyrosine concentrations must be monitored; if they are low, L-tyrosine supplements are given. Dietary proteins contain, by weight, 5.5% phenylalanine and 4.5% tyrosine, on average. The normal individual hydroxylates some 40 to 90% of phenylalanine to form tyrosine. To supply a normal tyrosine intake to patients with PKU, 10% of protein prescribed should be as tyrosine. Tyrosine supplements alone will not prevent mental retardation in classic PKU (50).

The protein content of the diet for patients with PKU has traditionally been higher than normal. Protein requirements are increased when either an L-amino acid mix or casein hydrolysate is the primary protein source rather than natural protein (51). Thus, recommendations for protein for nutritional support exceed the RDA (52, 53). Mean protein intake 24% above the 1989 RDA for age was associated with greater phenylalanine tolerance and growth in infants with PKU than was found when mean protein intake was 9% above RDA (54). Recommendations for energy and fluid intake (Table 61.4) are the same as those for normal individuals (52, 55).

Low-Phenylalanine and Phenylalanine-Free Medical Foods. Adequate protein cannot be obtained from natural foods without ingesting excess phenylalanine (natural proteins contain 2.4–9% phenylalanine by weight) (56–61). Thus, special medical foods are used to provide protein (62–64). Formulations, composition of major nutrients, and sources of these products are given in Table 61.5.

Natural Foods. Serving lists are available to simplify the phenylalanine-restricted diet for families and professional persons guiding them (Table 61.6). The lists are similar to diabetic exchange lists in that foods of similar phenylalanine content are grouped together and can be exchanged for one another within a list to vary the diet (63). Portion sizes of foods in each list may be found in reference 63.

Diet plans for children with PKU at different ages using different medical foods may be found in Tables 61.7 and 61.8. For instance, Lofenalac, Phenex-1, PKU 1, or XP Analog could be used to initiate a prescribed diet for a neonate at 55 mg phenylalanine/kg/day (Table 61.7). By 4 years of age, patients with some genotypes might require as much as 25 mg/kg/day. To allow as many natural foods as possible, Periflex, Phenex-2, Phenyl-Free, or XP Maxamaid are more likely to be the medical food of choice (Table 61.8), since they contain no phenylalanine (Table 61.5).

Management Problems. Management problems described for children with PKU occur in other children with inherited disorders of metabolism. Principles described here apply to children with other disorders as well but are not reiterated in other sections.

Maintenance of an adequate intake of protein and energy is important for the infant and child with PKU even though phenylalanine must be restricted. Nutritional support must be aggressive, and if intake fails to meet prescription, a nasogastric or gastrostomy tube should be placed to achieve anabolism. This is extremely important in disorders of branched-chain amino acids (BCAAs) and nitrogen metabolism. Protein is obtained from medical

Table 61.6
Average Nutrient Content of Servings Lists for Phenylalanine and/or Tyrosine and Protein-Restricted Diets

Food List	Phenylalanine (mg)	Tyrosine (mg)	Methionine (mg)	Protein (g)	Carbohydrate (g)	Fat (g)	Energy (kcal)
Breads/cereals	30	20	13	0.6	7	0	30
Fats	5	4	2	0.1	0.0	5	60
Fruits	15	10	8	0.5	15	0	60
Vegetables	15	10	6	0.5	2	0	10
Free foods[a]	5	4	2	0.1	18	0	65
Free foods B[a]	0	0	0	0	14	Varies	55
Enfamil with Iron[b], concentrate, 100 mL	116	134	58	3.0	13.9	7.6	135
Isomil[c] concentrate, 100 mL	18.8	126	80	3.3	13.9	7.4	135
ProSobee[b], concentrate, 100 mL	198	138	73	4.0	13.5	7.2	135
Similac[c] with Iron, concentrate 100 mL	129	113	73	2.8	14.6	7.3	135

[a]Low-protein pastas and breads not included.
[b]Mead Johnson Nutritional Division, Evansville, IN; 1/800-457-3550.
[c]Ross Products Division, Abbott Laboratories, Columbus, OH; 1/800-551-5838.

Table 61.7
Sample Diets for Phenylketonuria (2 weeks of age): Weight 3.25 kg

Prescription	Total	per kg			
Phenylalanine, mg	179	55			
Tyrosine, mg	980	302			
Protein, g	9.8	3.0			
Energy, kcal	390	120			
Medical Food #1	**Amount**	**PHE, mg**	**TYR[a], mg**	**Protein, g**	**Energy, kcal**
Lofenalac	40 g	30	316	5.9	182
Enfamil w/Iron, concentrate	127 mL	149	172	3.8	172
Table sugar	0.8 Tbsp	0	0	0	38
Volume, water to make	600 mL				
Totals		179	488	9.8	392
Medical Food #2					
Phenex-1	41 g	0	620	6.2	197
Similac with Iron, concentrate	139 mL	179	157	3.9	188
Table sugar	0.5 Tbsp	0	0	0	24
Volume, water to make	600 mL				
Totals		179	777	10.1	409
Medical Food #3					
PKU 1	10 g	0	349	5.2	28
Enfamil w/Iron, concentrate	153 mL	179	206	4.6	206
Vegetable oil	4 mL	0	0	0	32
Table sugar	2.6 Tbsp	0	0	0	124
Volume, water to make	600 mL				
Totals		179	555	9.8	390
Medical Food #4					
XP Analog	46 g	0	630	6.0	218
Similac With Iron, concentrate	139 mL	179	157	3.9	188
Volume, water to make	600 mL				
Totals		179	787	9.9	406

[a]Add L-tyrosine only if plasma tyrosine concentration is below the lower limit of the normal range.

foods; therefore, the amount of medical food offered must be varied to provide the protein needed. Nonprotein sources of energy such as corn syrup, Moducal and Protein-Free Diet Powder (Mead Johnson Nutritionals, Evansville, IN), Polycose Glucose Polymers, Pro-Phree (Ross Products Division, Abbott Laboratories, Columbus, OH), sugar, and pure fats can be added to maintain energy intake and to satisfy the child's hunger without affecting blood phenylalanine concentrations. Natural foods should be prescribed in numbers of servings and introduced at the appropriate ages and in the usual textures as for any child. Children should be given a variety of foods at the appropriate age so that these foods may be included in the diet later in life. In this way, increasing total phenylalanine requirements may be met.

A variety of factors may influence blood phenylalanine concentrations. Those that may elevate the blood phenylalanine concentration include acute infections with concomitant tissue catabolism, excessive or inadequate phenylalanine intake, and inadequate protein or energy intake. Infection affects plasma amino acid concentrations in normal adults (65). Similar increases in blood phenylalanine concentrations occur in febrile, treated patients with PKU. Because of this fact, any infection should be promptly diagnosed and appropriately treated. The best approach to nutritional support during short-term infections is to increase the intake of fluids and carbohydrates through the use of Pedialyte with added Polycose powder; fruit juices; high-carbohydrate, protein-free beverages; and soft drinks that do not contain caffeine.

Excess phenylalanine intake is the most common cause of elevated blood phenylalanine concentration in the older child with PKU. This condition may be due to overprescription, misunderstanding of the diet by the caretaker, or "snitching" of food by the child. Frequent evaluations of blood phenylalanine concentration with accompanying accurate diet records for calculation of intake are used to determine the dietary phenylalanine prescription. Diet records are also useful in determining parental understanding. Misunderstanding of diet requires additional education of parents. One of the most common "misunderstandings" in older children is the total number and size of servings allowed. In extended families living in close proximity, the child may receive three to four times the allowed amount of food from different well-intentioned but uninformed relatives. "Snitching" of food by the child is the most difficult problem to handle. The child should be given sound reasons

Table 61.8
Sample Diets for Phenylketonuria (4 years of age): Weight 17 kg

Prescription	Total	per kg			
Phenylalanine, mg	325	19			
Tyrosine, mg	3500	206			
Protein, g	35	2.0			
Energy, kcal	1700	100			
Medical Food #1	**Amount**	**PHE, mg**	**TYR, mg**	**Protein, g**	**Energy, kcal**
Phenex-2	91 g	0	2730	27.3	373
Table sugar	1.3 Tbsp	0	0	0	62
Volume, water to make	960 mL				
Foods			140		
Breads/cereals	7 svgs	210	20	4.2	210
Fats	5 svgs	25	40	0.5	300
Fruits	4 svgs	60	20	2.0	240
Vegetables	2 svgs	30	0	1.0	20
Free foods B	9 svgs	0		0	495
Totals		325	2950	35.0	1700
Medical Food #2					
Phenyl-Free	138 g	0	2760	27.3	566
Volume, water to make	960 mL				
Foods					
Breads/cereals	7 svgs	210	140	4.2	210
Fats	5 svgs	25	20	0.5	300
Fruits	4 svgs	60	40	2.0	240
Vegetables	2 svgs	30	20	1.0	20
Free foods B	7 svgs	0	0	0	385
Totals		325	2980	35.0	1721
Medical Food #3					
XP Maxamaid	109 g	0	2790	27.3	381
Polycose Powder	2.5 Tbsp	0	0	0	55
Volume, water to make	960 mL				
Foods					
Breads/cereals	7 svgs	210	140	4.2	210
Fats	5 svgs	25	20	0.5	300
Fruits	4 svgs	60	40	2.0	240
Vegetables	2 svgs	30	20	1.0	20
Free foods B	9 svgs	0	0	0	495
Totals		325	3010	35.0	1701

for avoiding foods not allowed on the diet, and this responsibility should be shifted to the child by 4 to 6 years of age. Appropriate disciplinary action by the parents should also be supported if the patient is unwilling to accept this responsibility. Lifetime nutritional support should be emphasized to the parents at the onset of therapy, and to both parents and child at recurring intervals.

Phenylalanine deficiency associated with inadequate phenylalanine intake has three specific stages of development (66). The first stage is characterized biochemically by decreased blood and urine phenylalanine. Clinically, the child may appear normal, lethargic, or anorectic and may fail to gain length or weight. In the older child, increases in blood alanine and β-hydroxybutyric and acetoacetic acidemia result from muscle alanine production and β-lipolysis. In the second stage, blood phenylalanine levels increase as a result of muscle protein degradation, but blood tyrosine may be low. BCAA concentrations may increase with decreases in other plasma amino acids. Aminoaciduria appears because of renal tubular malabsorption (67). In this stage, body protein stores are catabolized, energy sources are depleted, and "active" membrane transport functions are impaired (67). Eczema is common. In the third stage of phenylalanine deficiency, blood phenylalanine is below normal, as are other amino acids. Accompanying clinical manifestations include failure to gain weight, failure to gain height, osteopenia, anemia, sparse hair, and finally death if the deficiency is not corrected by supplemental dietary phenylalanine and tyrosine.

Insufficient protein intake results in an inadequate supply of essential amino acids and/or nitrogen for growth. When protein synthesis is decreased, phenylalanine is no longer used for growth and accumulates in the blood. If catabolism occurs because of prolonged lack of nitrogen and/or amino acid intake, blood phenylalanine concentration increases because tissue protein contains some 5.5% phenylalanine. In instances of protein insufficiency, medical food intake should be increased to supply the required nitrogen and/or essential amino acids.

Energy, the first requirement of the body, is necessary for growth. When energy is provided as carbohydrate and fat, and if adequate nitrogen is available, nonessential amino acids may be synthesized from their ketoacid precursors. Furthermore, carbohydrate ingestion leads to insulin secretion, and insulin promotes amino acid transport into the cell and consequent protein synthesis (68, 69). The mechanisms by which insulin regulates amino acid uptake in muscle change with increasing age (69). When energy intake is inadequate, tissue catabolism occurs to meet energy needs. Such catabolism releases phenylalanine, leading to elevated blood phenylalanine concentrations. Sufficient energy must be provided through generous use of nonprotein and low-protein foods to ensure a normal growth rate.

Low blood phenylalanine concentrations (<25 μmol) may lead to depressed appetite (70), decreased growth (71), and, if prolonged, mental retardation (46, 48). Low blood phenylalanine concentrations are often due to inadequate prescription of phenylalanine for the affected child during rapid growth phases. In such cases, the prescription for phenylalanine can be increased by addition of measured amounts of milk and/or solid foods. In some situations, medical food may be diluted to a volume that is too great for the child to consume in the allotted time. The volume must be decreased to the amount the child can ingest. Concentrated medical foods are frequently used without any untoward side effects. They may be mixed as a paste and spoon-fed, even to the young infant. The practice could begin at 3 to 4 months of age or when tongue thrust is no longer a problem for solid food intake. Extra fluid must then be offered between feedings to maintain appropriate water balance.

Assessment of Nutritional Support. Along with biweekly assessment of growth through measurement of height, weight, and head circumference and evaluation of development by appropriate developmental scales, the adequacy of phenylalanine and tyrosine intake is determined by twice-weekly quantitation of the blood phenylalanine and tyrosine concentrations. The 1st year is the period of most rapid growth and of greatest vulnerability to nutritional insult. Thus, twice-weekly blood tests are suggested during the first 3 months and weekly thereafter until the child is 1 year of age. After 1 year of age, weekly blood tests suffice for monitoring diet. If, however, blood phenylalanine concentrations exceed 300 μmol (5 mg/dL), more frequent determinations should be obtained. When indicated, the prescription for phenylalanine is decreased, and frequent blood tests are obtained until blood phenylalanine concentrations are between 60 and 300 μmol.

For blood tests to be of use in adjusting the prescription, laboratory analyses must be both accurate and prompt. Quantitative methods of phenylalanine determination using automated ion-exchange chromatography and liquid blood are preferable. This method allows evaluation of all amino acids. The microbiologic (Guthrie) method is acceptable for screening, but is nonquantitative and invalid if antibiotics are used. Fluorimetric methods are quantitative and preferred to the Guthrie test to monitor blood phenylalanine (72). If properly instructed, parents may be given responsibility for obtaining the specimens on filter paper or in microcapillary tubes and mailing them to a central laboratory.

A record of food ingested before and during blood sampling for blood phenylalanine measurement is essential and should be kept by the child's caregiver. The correlation between the child's intake of phenylalanine, tyrosine, protein, and energy; the child's clinical status; and the blood phenylalanine and tyrosine concentrations is considered when the diet is altered.

The success of early diet management rests with the parents and depends on their understanding of the disease and their ability to cope with the diet. Later, the child's understanding of the diet and ability to assume responsibility for it are critical. These factors in turn are related to the support the parents and patient receive from various professional members of the genetic team. Roles and functions of some team members have been described (73).

Results of Therapy. Early diagnosis and treatment of infants with PKU with a nutritionally adequate, phenylalanine-restricted, tyrosine-supplemented diet have promoted normal growth and prevented severe mental retardation. A study showed that mean height, weight, and head circumference of 111 children treated from before 120 days of age were the same as those of normal children at 4 years of age (74). Assessment of mental development in these same children at 4 years of age yielded a mean IQ score of 93 on the Stanford Binet Intelligence Scale (75). Delay in treatment and suboptimal control of blood phenylalanine concentration produced lower IQs than projected from parental IQs. More-recent programs with tighter control of plasma phenylalanine have improved overall outlook for normal IQs (46). Trefz et al. (37) reported that when blood phenylalanine concentration was kept below 360 μmol, there was no difference in mean IQ by genotype of 9-year-old children.

The semisynthetic nature of the phenylalanine-restricted diet has led to questions concerning its adequacy. Mean serum carnitine (total, free, and esters) of 16 treated patients was about one-third that of normal children of similar age (76). Low plasma tyrosine concentrations were found in both treated and untreated patients (77–79). Following an overnight fast, concentrations of all essential plasma amino acids were below the lower limit of normal and the concentration of plasma glycine was elevated in patients who ingested two different medical foods (80). The elevated concentration of plasma glycine occurred even in patients receiving a glycine-free medical food (PeriflexR, Scientific Hospital Supplies, Inc., Gaithersburg, MD). Treated patients with PKU often have below-normal concentrations of prealbumin (81, 82).

Depressed plasma concentrations of total cholesterol have been reported in treated children and untreated adults with PKU (83–85). Lower than normal plasma and erythrocyte docosahexaenoic acid concentrations and higher than normal *n*-6 series fatty acid concentrations have been found in patients undergoing therapy for PKU (86, 87). The significance of these differences is unclear, but they appear to be diet related.

Calculation indicates that intake of major nutrients is adequate (88), compared with the RDAs. Balance studies of calcium, phosphorus, magnesium, and iron in 8 girls, 6 to 8 years of age, on Lofenalac suggested that magnesium may be inadequate to provide for optimal nutrition (89). Studies of chromium, iron, ferritin, and selenium in children with PKU revealed low concentrations (90, 91). Iron deficiency has been reported in significant numbers of children undergoing therapy for PKU despite more than adequate iron intake (92, 93). Low activity of glutathione peroxidase and low plasma selenium have been found in treated children with PKU who were receiving medical foods without added selenium (94–96). Potentially life-threatening cardiac dysrhythmia was found in one selenium-deficient treated child with PKU (97). Significantly reduced mitogenesis to optimal concentrations of monoclonal antibody (OKT3) and plant lectin phytohemagglutinin was demonstrated in a group of patients with PKU with reduced serum selenium, compared with a normal group (98). Patients with PKU with low selenium concentrations had elevated concentrations of T4 and rT3, which decreased significantly with selenium supplementation (99). Inadequate intake may be responsible, since patients receiving medical food with adequate added selenium have normal plasma concentrations. Plasma retinol concentrations of infants and children with PKU undergoing treatment are often below those of normal subjects (82). When Lofenalac is the protein source, the intake of vitamin E suffices for normal plasma concentrations despite the high intake of polyunsaturated fatty acids (100). Adequacy of niacin status in children on Lofenalac is questionable because of limited intake of tryptophan and niacin and disturbances in tryptophan metabolism (101).

Bone changes noted radiographically were reported as early as 1956 in treated children with PKU. Bone mineral content of 11 treated children were more than 1 SD below the mean (102). Bone osteocalcin, a calcium-binding protein with a high content of δ-carboxyglutamic acid, was considerably below the normal range, and 80% of patients had serum calcium levels below 9.0 mg/dL. The mean of the three most recent serum phenylalanine concentrations correlated negatively with the bone mineral content and osteocalcin. Hillman et al. (102) suggested that bone abnormalities were related to lack of control of plasma phenylalanine. McMurry et al. (103) found normal bone mineralization in preschool children with PKU in good dietary control. As blood phenylalanine increased in older patients under poorer dietary control, values for bone mineral content, bone width, and bone density were always lower than control values. Trabecular bone mineral content was recently assessed in 11 young adults with PKU who had been treated from early childhood with a diet restricted in complete protein plus added amino acids, minerals, and vitamins. Bone mineral content was significantly lower in patients than in the normal population (104). Amino acid imbalances, inadequate protein intake, and the need for phosphorus to buffer organic acids made from excess dietary phenylalanine could have contributed to bone abnormalities. Mean plasma concentrations of IgA and IgM were significantly lower in patients with PKU undergoing therapy (105) than in normal children.

Diet Discontinuation. Certain clinicians have suggested that the diet might be discontinued at 4, 6, or 12 years of age with no adverse effects (106–108). Investigators have questioned this possibility because studies have shown significant differences in performance and intelligence in children (109, 110) and neurologic function in adults who discontinued the diet and those who remained on the diet (30, 111). Severe agoraphobia (112) reversible by a return to the phenylalanine-restricted diet also has been reported in adults. Vitamin B_{12} deficiency resulting in hematologic changes and neurologic disease occurs in off-diet patients who refuse foods of animal origin but fail to supplement with phenylalanine-free medical foods (113).

In studies using the patient as his or her own control, elevated plasma phenylalanine concentrations prolonged the performance time on neuropsychologic tests of higher integrative function, reduced the mean power frequency of the electroencephalogram (EEG), and decreased urinary dopamine excretion and plasma L-DOPA in older treated patients with PKU (114, 115). A correlation was found between high plasma phenylalanine concentrations, prolonged performance time on the neuropsychologic tests, and decreased urinary dopamine in 10 patients (114). In a study of eight additional patients, statistically significant decreases were found in the mean power frequency of the EEG and in plasma L-DOPA when plasma phenylalanine concentration increased (115). EEG slowing occurred in PKU heterozygotes at concentration changes of blood phenylalanine that are induced by aspartame ingestion (150 μmol) (31). These effects were reversible and correlated in the reverse direction when plasma phenylalanine was reduced. Severe neurologic deterioration occurred in several off-diet PKU patients (30, 111). Reversal of most of the symptoms was possible in a patient who returned to a phenylalanine-restricted, medical food–containing diet (30). Elevated plasma phenylalanine may be concentrated by the blood-brain barrier in neural cells and inhibit L-DOPA and serotonin synthesis by competing for tyrosine and tryptophan hydroxylases (115).

Maternal Phenylketonuria

Pregnant women with PKU who are untreated at conception and during gestation have offspring with intrauterine growth retardation, microcephaly and congenital anomalies, often severe and incompatible with life. Mental retardation is common in offspring of mothers whose plasma phenylalanine is above 150 μmol (116). The pathogenesis of the fetal damage is uncertain but is believed to be related to elevated maternal blood phenylalanine concentration (117) because phenylalanine is actively transported across the placenta to the fetus (118). Fetal blood phenylalanine concentrations are 1.5 to 2 times those of maternal blood (119). Such elevated fetal plasma phenylalanine concentrations are again concentrated 2- to 4-fold by the fetal blood-brain barrier (120, 121). Intraneuronal phenylalanine concentrations of 600 μmol interfere with brain development by one or more of the several previously described mechanisms, including abnormal oligodendroglial migration and/or myelin and other protein synthesis (122). Thus, it is extremely important to maintain normal plasma phenylalanine concentrations in the reproductive female with PKU before conception and throughout gestation. Offspring of untreated women who survive fail to grow and develop normally. In fact, Kirkman (123) predicted that if the fertility of these women is normal and they are not treated with dietary control of phenylalanine intake, the incidence of PKU-related mental retardation could return to the prescreening level after only one generation.

In 1984 the Collaborative Study of Maternal Phenylketonuria (MPKUCS) was initiated to answer questions related to diet and reproductive outcome in women with PKU (124). Interim results of the MPKUCS support the premise that a phenylalanine-restricted diet and the gestational age at which it is initiated affect reproductive outcome (125). Little is known of the effect of dietary phenylalanine in artificial sweeteners on newborn outcome in the general population.

Nutritional Support of MPKU. Adherence to a phenylalanine-restricted diet by pregnant women is a major problem. These women must adjust to the taste of the phenylalanine-free medical food and be able to withstand the social pressures to eat proscribed foods, such as animal protein. Therefore, the phenylalanine-restricted diet should be initiated at least 3 months before a planned pregnancy by women who have PKU, if they have previously discontinued diet.

The objectives of therapy for pregnant women with PKU are a healthy mother and a normal, healthy newborn. To obtain adequate protein and fat storage in early pregnancy to support last trimester fetal growth, careful attention must be paid to prescribing diet and evaluating nutritional status. Although the blood phenylalanine concentration most likely to yield the best reproductive outcome is unknown (124), one group of investigators suggests that these objectives may be achieved by a phenylalanine-restricted diet that maintains blood phenylalanine concentration between 60 and 180 μmol/L (126). Plasma phenylalanine concentrations below 60 μmol/L may lead to maternal muscle wasting and poor fetal growth. Recommended phenylalanine intake to prescribe for initiating therapy is given in Table 61.9 (127). Other indices of nutritional status should be in the normal range for pregnant women. After initiation of diet with the minimum recommended phenylalanine prescription (Table 61.9), plasma phenylalanine concentration and weight should be monitored twice weekly, if possible, to enhance weight gain and maintain targeted plasma phenylalanine concentration.

Table 61.9
Recommended Phenylalanine (PHE), Tyrosine (TYR), Protein and Energy Intakes for Pregnant Women with PKU

	Nutrients				
				Energy[d] (kcal/day)	
Trimester and age (years)	PHE[a,b] (mg/day)	TYR[c] (mg/day)	Protein[d] (g/day)	Mean	Range
Trimester 1: (0 < 14 weeks gestation)					
15 < 19	200 < 820	≥7600	≥76	2500	1600–3400
19 < 24	180 < 800	≥7400	≥74	2500	2100–3200
≥24	180 < 800	≥7400	≥74	2500	2100–3400
Trimester 2: (14 < 27 weeks gestation)					
15 < 19	200 < 1000	≥7600	≥76	2500	1600–3400
19 < 24	180 < 1000	≥7400	≥74	2500	2100–3200
≥24	180 < 1000	≥7400	≥74	2500	2100–3400
Trimester 3: (27 < 41 weeks gestation)					
15 > 19	330 < 1200	≥7600	≥76	2500	1600–3400
19 < 24	310 < 1200	≥7400	≥74	2500	2100–3200
≥24	310 < 1200	≥7400	≥74	2500	2100–3400

[a]Recommended range of PHE intake covered about 80% of MPKUCS women studied.

[b]Initiate diet with the lowest amount recommended for trimester and age. Frequent monitoring of plasma PHE is essential to prevent deficiency or excess. Modify prescription based on frequent plasma PHE and TYR concentrations; intakes of PHE, TYR, protein, and energy and maternal weight gain.

[c]L-TYR is very insoluble in water; consequently any supplemental L-TYR should be mixed with fruit purees, mashed potatoes, or soup for ingestion. Recommended intake is from MPKUCS data (128).

[d]Modified from Food and Nutrition Board, 1989 (52). Energy requirements for some women may be greater than the upper limit of the range given, to obtain appropriate weight gain.

Even after plasma phenylalanine concentration is stabilized in the treatment range, frequent changes in the individualized diet prescription are required as pregnancy progresses, based on concentrations of plasma phenylalanine, tyrosine, and other amino acids and on weight gain. Phenylalanine and tyrosine requirements of each pregnant woman depend on genotype, age, state of health, and trimester of pregnancy (127, 128). About midpregnancy, phenylalanine tolerance increases considerably (127, 128). Specific numbers of servings of low-protein cereals, fruits, fats, and vegetables (Table 61.6) are prescribed by the nutritionist to supply the individual amount of tolerated phenylalanine.

As noted for the child with PKU, the amount of protein prescribed (Table 61.9) exceeds the RDA because of the use of L-amino acids as the primary source of protein equivalent. A phenylalanine-free medical food (Table 61.5) is used to provide most of the protein prescribed and nitrogen-free foods (Free Foods B, Table 61.6), such as pure sugars and pure fats, are used to provide the remaining energy needs. A protocol is available that suggests a step-by-step approach to planning and evaluating nutritional support for the pregnant woman with PKU (63).

Birth measurements of neonates of women with PKU are negatively correlated with maternal plasma phenylalanine concentrations and positively correlated with maternal energy and protein intake and weight gain during pregnancy. The plasma phenylalanine concentration of the pregnant woman with PKU is negatively correlated with total protein intake (128), suggesting that total protein intake should minimally be at the amount recommended in Table 61.9 for better control of plasma phenylalanine.

Appropriate weight gain is related to height and prepregnancy weight and is greater for underweight than for normal-weight women (129). Data in Table 61.10 describe recommended pregnancy weight gain for underweight, normal-weight, and overweight women.

Two families of fatty acids, linoleic (C18:2, *n*-6) and α-linolenic (C18:3, *n*-3) are essential for humans (130). Linoleic acid should supply about 7% (52) and α-linolenic acid should supply 0.7 to 2.5% of energy in the diet (131), especially during pregnancy.

Women in the MPKUCS who had a good reproductive outcome had a greater fat intake throughout pregnancy than women with a poor outcome (128). Whether the poor outcome was due to inadequate essential fatty acids is not clear. Because most of the medical foods are devoid of, or contain very little, α-linolenic acid (Table 61.5), the fat used to supply 30 to 40% of energy in the diet should be obtained from cooking and salad oils, margarines, salad dressing, and shortenings with either unhydrogenated canola or soybean oil as the first ingredient in the ingredient list (132).

Table 61.10
Recommended Weight Gain during Pregnancy for Women with PKU

	Recommended Weight Gain (kg)	
Weight Status[a]	1st Trimester	Total
Normal weight	1.6	15.5–16.0
Underweight	2.3	12.5–18.0
Overweight	0.9	7.0–11.5

Data from the Subcommittee on Nutritional Status and Weight Gain During Pregnancy, 1990 (129).
[a]Weight status at conception.

Intakes of iron, zinc, and selenium require monitoring to prevent deficiency. Supplemental iron may be required if maternal plasma ferritin concentration decreases to less than 12 ng/mL. Women with PKU who are on a low-protein diet and do not ingest medical food daily before pregnancy may have many nutrient deficiencies, including protein, iron, selenium, and vitamin B_{12} (113). Because all of the vitamin B_{12} and most of the zinc in the diets of Americans are derived from animal protein, pregnant women with PKU are at risk for developing deficiencies of these nutrients if adequate medical food is not ingested.

Phenylalanine-free medical foods that provide prescribed protein for the pregnant woman with PKU also provide the required amounts of vitamins. Therefore, a prenatal vitamin capsule containing vitamins A and D should not be prescribed for women ingesting adequate amounts of phenylalanine-free medical food. In fact, supplementation may provide vitamin A at levels approaching those that are teratogenic (133).

Morning sickness and changes in food preferences that accompany pregnancy may make adherence to the diet difficult for some pregnant women. Healthcare professionals need to support these patients and work with metabolic nutritionists to improve the palatability and acceptance of the phenylalanine-free medical foods. One option might be to schedule the medical food at times when nausea is less likely to occur. Additional suggestions to help control nausea are available in the *Nutrition Support Protocols* (63).

Monitoring Nutritional Support. Ongoing monitoring of women with PKU involves more than measuring plasma concentrations of phenylalanine and tyrosine. Maternal weight gain, concentrations of plasma amino acids, albumin, ferritin, selenium, and zinc should be assessed on a regular basis. Because pregnant women with PKU are at risk for spontaneous abortion and premature delivery, they should be treated as high-risk patients, even if their blood phenylalanine concentration is in the targeted treatment range. Multiple ultrasound studies, beginning at 16 to 20 weeks' gestation, may be requested to monitor fetal head size and intrauterine growth patterns. Level II ultrasound to scan for heart defects and other malformations may also be ordered.

Tyrosinemias

Several known disorders of tyrosine metabolism (Table 61.11) may be amenable to nutritional support (see Fig.

Table 61.11
Inherited Disorders Producing Increased Plasma Tyrosine

Designation	Enzyme Defect	Clinical Features
Hepatorenal tyrosinemia (type Ia)	Fumarylacetoacetate hydrolyase	Cirrhosis, renal Fanconi syndrome, acute porphyria, (succinylacetone), hepatocellular carcinoma
Hepatorenal tyrosinemia (type Ib)	Maleylacetoacetate isomerase	Liver failure, Fanconi syndrome, psychomotor retardation (no succinylacetone)
Oculocutaneous tyrosinemia (type II)	Hepatic cytosol tyrosine aminotransferase	Eye and skin disorders with variable mental retardation
Primary *p*-OHPPAD deficiency (type IIIa)	*p*-OHPPAD	Neurologic abnormalities, mental retardation
Hawkinsinuria (type IIIb)	*p*-OHPPAD	Metabolic acidosis, microcephaly
Transient neonatal (IIIc)	*p*-OHPPAD	Prematuriy, possibly benign
Tyrosinosis (Medes)	Probably type II	Myasthenia (possibly acute porphyric attack)

[a]*p*-OHPPAD is *p*-OH-phenylpyruvic acid dioxygenase.

61.1). Precise biochemical diagnosis is important because disorders such as liver disease, scurvy, and prematurity may produce increases in blood tyrosine that are not due to permanent, specific enzyme defects in tyrosine metabolism.

Seven clinical forms of hereditary tyrosinemia have been reported (Table 61.11). Type Ia is caused by a primary defect of hepatic FAH with the production of an abnormal metabolite, succinylacetone (134). The gene for FAH has been localized to chromosome 15q23-25 (135). Succinylacetone is formed from the accumulated substrate fumarylacetoacetate (Fig. 61.1). If maleylacetoacetic acid isomerase is functional, succinylacetone is also formed from maleylacetoacetate. Succinylacetone is extremely toxic and is associated with impaired active transport function and disordered hepatic enzymes, including *p*-OHPPAD and δ-ALA dehydratase (136). Decreased activity of both hepatic and erythrocyte δ-ALA dehydratase has been reported in these patients and is postulated to be the mechanism for development of acute porphyric-like episodes (Fig. 61.2) (137–138). Using the drug NTBC to inhibit *p*-OHPPAD has prevented acute porphyric episodes and decreased rates of progression of cirrhosis and Fanconi syndrome (139).

Tyrosinemia type Ia is characterized by a generalized renal tubular impairment with hypophosphatemic rickets, progressive liver failure producing cirrhosis and hepatic cancer, hypertension, episodic behavioral and peripheral nerve deficiencies, and elevated concentrations of blood phenylalanine and tyrosine, with succinylacetone and δ-ALA excretion in urine (140). The most common mutant allele is a splice donor site gain in intron 12 (IVS12G → A+5). Many other missense and nonsense mutations are known. Reversion of the IVS12 mutation to normal in noncancerous hepatic nodules is described. FAH is expressed in amniotic and chorionic villus cells, and prenatal diagnosis is available by biochemical or molecular techniques (140).

Tyrosinemia type Ib, believed to be due to a deficiency of maleylacetoacetate isomerase, has been reported in one infant (140). Liver failure, renal tubular disease, and progressive psychomotor retardation occurred prior to death at 1 year of age. Succinylacetone did not accumulate. If this is confirmed, the pathophysiology of tyrosinemia type I will require reevaluation.

Tyrosinemia type II is characterized by greatly elevated concentrations of blood and urine tyrosine and increases in urinary phenolic acids, *N*-acetyltyrosine and tyramine. A deficiency of hepatic cytosolic tyrosine aminotransferase (TAT) has been demonstrated (140). Characteristic physical findings include stellate corneal erosions and plaques and bullous lesions of the soles and palms. Persistent keratitis and hyperkeratosis occur on the fingers and palms of the hands and on the soles of the feet. These skin abnormalities respond to restriction of dietary phenylalanine and tyrosine. Intracellular crystallization of tyrosine is thought to cause these inflammatory responses. Mental retardation may occur. The *TAT* gene is located on human chromosome 16q22. Missense, deletions, nonsense, and splice site mutations are known.

Three clinical subsets of type III tyrosinemia result from dysfunctions of *p*-OHPPAD (Fig. 61.1) (Table 61.10). The most severe is type IIIa with no hepatic *p*-OHPPAD. Neurologic abnormalities, including seizures, ataxia, and mental retardation have been reported in untreated patients with type IIIa. Hawkinsinuria (type IIIb) is named for the 2-L-cysteinyl 5-1,4-dihydroxycyclohexenyl-5,1-acetic acid that presumably is formed from an intermediate of impaired *p*-OHPPAD reaction. Metabolic acidosis and failure-to-thrive with "swimming pool"-like odor are described. Tyrosine restriction improves the critical condition.

Type IIIc is "benign" neonatal tyrosinemia, associated with increased plasma and urinary concentrations of tyrosine and its metabolites. It occurs in 0.2 to 10% of neonates (140). Short-term protein restriction to 1.5 to 2.0 g/kg body weight/day has lowered plasma tyrosine concentrations in most patients within 4 weeks of life. Whether added ascorbate will stabilize and increase the activity of *p*-OHPPAD in this disorder is not clear. Persistence of hypertyrosinemia in this disorder may lead to impaired mental function, and short-term dietary and ascorbate therapy are recommended (141).

Diagnosis

Differential diagnosis is imperative for institution of appropriate therapy. Quantitation of plasma amino acids by ion-exchange chromatography and mass spectrometry (GC/MS) is a necessary approach to diagnosis. The more severe tyrosinemia type I may not be detected by newborn screening using the bacterial inhibition assay because newborn blood tyrosine may not be above 8 mg/dL. Many newborn screening programs consider 440 μmol/L (8 mg/dL) within normal limits and do not retrieve these babies for further diagnosis. We routinely retest newborns with blood tyrosine levels above 220 μmol/L (4 mg/dL) if no other cause is clinically evident. If blood tyrosine is above 8 mg/dL at 14 days of age, we evaluate renal tubular and hepatic function as well as urine by organic acid analysis for the presence of *p*-hydroxyphenyl acids and succinylacetone. Prenatal diagnosis of type I hereditary tyrosinemia has been made by measurement of succinylacetone in amniotic fluid (142), by measurement of FAH activity in cultured amniotic fluid cells, and by molecular analyses. Type II tyrosinemia has a marked increase in urinary *p*-OH-phenylacids and blood tyrosine (143). It increases with increasing age of the infant, whereas type IIIc decreases. Hawkinsinuria is measured by its ninhydrin reaction using ion-exchange chromatography.

Treatment

The objective of nutritional support for the hereditary tyrosinemias is to provide a biochemical environment that allows normal growth and development of intellectual potential. It will prevent pathophysiologic changes only in types II and III. Plasma phenylalanine concentrations should be maintained between 40 and 80 μmol, and plasma tyrosine concentrations between 50 and 150 μmol. Plasma methionine may need to be regulated by dietary means in tyrosinemia type I. We follow plasma methionine as an index of *S*-adenosylmethionine (SAM) transferase deficiency produced by liver damage and restrict dietary methionine when plasma methionine is elevated.

Nutritional therapy of the hereditary tyrosinemias requires a firm diagnosis because the approaches to therapy between types are different. Phenylalanine and tyrosine restriction is less severe and prognosis is excellent for types II and III. In type I, however, progressive liver and renal failure may occur as well as acute episodes of porphyria. Renal impairment must also be treated in tyrosinemia type I. Generalized renal tubular failure may result in metabolic acidosis, hypophosphatemia, rickets, and hypokalemia unless replacement of bicarbonate, phosphate, 1,25-dihydroxycholecalciferol, and potassium is instituted. Rapid treatment of infections is required to prevent a "catastrophic" catabolic state with overproduction of succinylacetone.

Many of the "porphyric" symptoms are due to overproduction of δ-ALA secondary to the inhibitory effect of succinlyacetone on δ-ALA dehydratase and/or decreased heme biosynthesis (Fig. 61.2). Parenteral nutrition with 20 to 25% dextrose solutions may control these acute porphyric attacks (144). Continued or progressive loss of energy-requiring functions that involve loosely bound heme to heme-protein (plasma membrane transporters, cytochrome P-450) may be due to rapid turnover and insufficient heme biosynthesis (Fig. 61.2). Infusions of hematin have produced transient decreases in δ-ALA and have improved acute attacks of intermittent porphyria, but this invasive therapy is not recommended unless NTBC is not available (145, 147). Hepatocellular carcinoma, however, will *not* be prevented and will require liver transplant to prevent metastases (140, 145). The drug NTBC, which inhibits the activity of *p*-OHPPAD (148) in the treatment of tyrosinemia type I, may reduce the need for liver transplants and is an indicated adjunct to diet therapy (149). Patients should be on "protocol." There is an excellent mouse model (149).

Nutritional Requirements. When one is planning nutritional support for the infant or child with tyrosinemia, a formal prescription that recommends daily amounts of phenylalanine, tyrosine, protein, energy, and fluid should be written. The prescription for phenylalanine and tyrosine is based on blood analyses correlated with intake that indicate the child's requirement and/or tolerance for each amino acid. Data in Table 61.4 describe amounts of phenylalanine, tyrosine, protein, energy, and fluid to offer as beginning therapy.

Because a large portion of phenylalanine is normally hydroxylated to form tyrosine (150), phenylalanine must also be restricted in the diet of patients with tyrosinemia. Phenylalanine requirements appear to be greater for children with tyrosinemia than for children with PKU. In general, the more distal the block is in the catabolic pathway, the more normal the amino acid requirement is. Tyrosine needs of children with tyrosinemia have been inadequately described and will vary with the metabolic state of the child and the accumulation of succinylacetone. If plasma tyrosine is inadequately controlled in NTBC-treated patients, symptoms of tyrosinemia type II occur.

Some investigators suggest that patients with tyrosinemia type I have decreased ability to metabolize methionine, whereas others believe that the elevated plasma methionine concentrations are secondary to liver damage (140). Whatever the cause for hypermethioninemia, some have recommended methionine restriction when blood methionine concentrations are above 40 μmol in the absence of hepatocellular damage. Although the extent of methionine restriction to maintain normal blood methionine concentration is unknown, one recommendation is 50 mg/kg of body weight for a 15-month-old child (151). L-Cysteine supplementation is also recommended for children with tyrosinemia type I, particularly if methionine restriction is implemented (152).

Recommended protein intakes for infants and children with tyrosinemia are given in Table 61.4. Because the primary protein source used for the infant is either an L-amino acid mix or a casein hydrolysate, recommended intake is greater than for the normal infant (51, 52). For tyrosinemia type I, when NTBC is administered, energy needs are similar to those of normal infants (52).

Medical Foods Low in or Free of Phenylalanine and Tyrosine. Adequate protein cannot be obtained from natural foods without ingesting excess phenylalanine and tyrosine (proteins contain by mass 1.4 to 5.8% tyrosine). Thus, special medical foods are used that contain little or no phenylalanine or tyrosine. Several medical foods are available to provide protein (62–64). Formulations, composition of major nutrients, and sources of medical foods are given in Table 61.5.

The methionine content of Low Phe/Tyr Diet Powder; XPHEN, TYR Analog; XPHEN, TYR, Maxamaid; TYR 1, and TYR 2 (Table 61.5) is too great for use if dietary methionine must be restricted. In such a situation, Tyromex-1 Amino Acid Modified Medical Food with Iron; XPHEN, TYR, MET Analog and XPHEN, TYR, MET Maxamaid (Table 61.5), which contain no phenylalanine, tyrosine, or methionine, could be used.

Serving Lists. Serving lists are available for the phenylalanine-tyrosine-restricted diet (Table 61.6) (63). Methionine content is given for each list in the event that methionine restriction is required for type I. Portion sizes of individual foods in each list are given in reference 63.

Initiation of Nutritional Support. The most rapid decline of blood tyrosine concentration at the time of diagnosis may be obtained by feeding a 20 kcal/oz (67 kcal/dL) phenylalanine- and tyrosine-free formula with no added source of phenylalanine and tyrosine. Total energy intake above 120 kcal/kg/day is required to prevent a catabolic phase. Laboratory results of blood phenylalanine and tyrosine should be rapidly available or a deficiency of phenylalanine and tyrosine (153) could be precipitated. Catabolism, either due to inadequate energy intake and/or phenylalanine and tyrosine is particularly undesirable in treating tyrosinemia type I because a catabolic phase with overproduction of succinylacetone will worsen the clinical state. Protein sources containing 20 to 70 mg phenylalanine and 60 to 80 mg tyrosine/kg body weight/day are usually required after 3 to 4 days of total restriction in the newborn period.

Assessment of Nutritional Support. Frequency of assessment is dictated by the type of tyrosinemia and clinical course of the patient. In tyrosinemia type I, vital signs, height, weight, head circumference, neurologic examination, and development are documented weekly for the first 3 months, biweekly for the second 3 months, and monthly between 6 months and 1 year of life. Plasma amino acids are quantitated by ion-exchange chromatography and succinylacetone and *p*-hydroxyphenyl organic acids by GC/MS. Additional laboratory studies include urinary δ-ALA, blood and urine assessment of renal losses (HCO_3, K^+, Na^+), and liver status (α-fetoprotein and liver function tests). Clinical status, dietary intake, and laboratory data should be monitored and correlated in managing tyrosinemia type I at intervals indicated previously. Application for inclusion in NTBC trials and for eventual liver transplant should be initiated within the 1st year of life for patients with type I tyrosinemia.

Outcomes of Nutritional Support. Outcomes, to date, have been variable with tyrosinemia type I. Some of this "variation" is caused by the lack of clear diagnostic criteria in the past to delineate the various types of tyrosinemia. Early detection and diagnosis using GC/MS; low-phenylalanine and low-tyrosine, high-carbohydrate diets; hematin infusions; and early replacement of renal tubular losses bring success at early ages in treated tyrosinemia type I. Although NTBC may be the ultimate treatment for tyrosinemia type I, institution of the treatment immediately after birth may be necessary to prevent hepatocellular carcinomas, but there are few data to support outcome in this regard (139). The low-phenylalanine, low-tyrosine diet has been successful in several patients with tyrosinemia types II and III, with rapid resolution of clinical signs and symptoms (140). Neonatal tyrosinemia requires early but transient protein restriction. The efficacy of oral ascorbate at 50 mg/day is unclear. Controlled outcome data are not yet available.

BRANCHED-CHAIN AMINO ACIDS

Disorders of BCAA metabolism provide an interesting interface between clinical and basic sciences. Using the nutritional model of preventing mental retardation through screening, retrieval, diagnosis, and management of newborns, many rare experiments of nature have become available and have advanced our knowledge concerning nutrition needs and metabolic use of isoleucine, leucine, and valine (154).

Biochemistry

The BCAAs isoleucine, leucine, and valine are essential nutrients. In the newborn, 75% of the amounts ingested is used for protein synthesis. That present in excess of need for synthetic purposes is degraded through many steps to provide energy (Fig. 61.3). The initial step in catabolism is reversible transamination, requiring a specific transaminase and the coenzyme pyridoxal phosphate. The second step is irreversible oxidative decarboxylation, which uses the BCKAD complex. This complex is located in the inner mitochondrial membrane and requires the coenzymes thiamin pyrophosphate, lipoic acid, CoA, and NAD+ (154–159). Figure 61.3 diagrams this overall reaction, which is impaired in MSUD. At least six proteins are involved: E1α, E1β, E2, E3, a kinase, and phosphatase.

The loci for these genes are E1α at chromosome 19q13.1q13.2; E1β at 6p21-p22; E2 at 1p31; and E3 at 7q31-q32 (154). The BCKAD-specific kinase and phosphatase have not been cloned, nor have chaperonin proteins, which are involved in their mitochondrial assembly process. Almost all mutations in these proteins that pro-

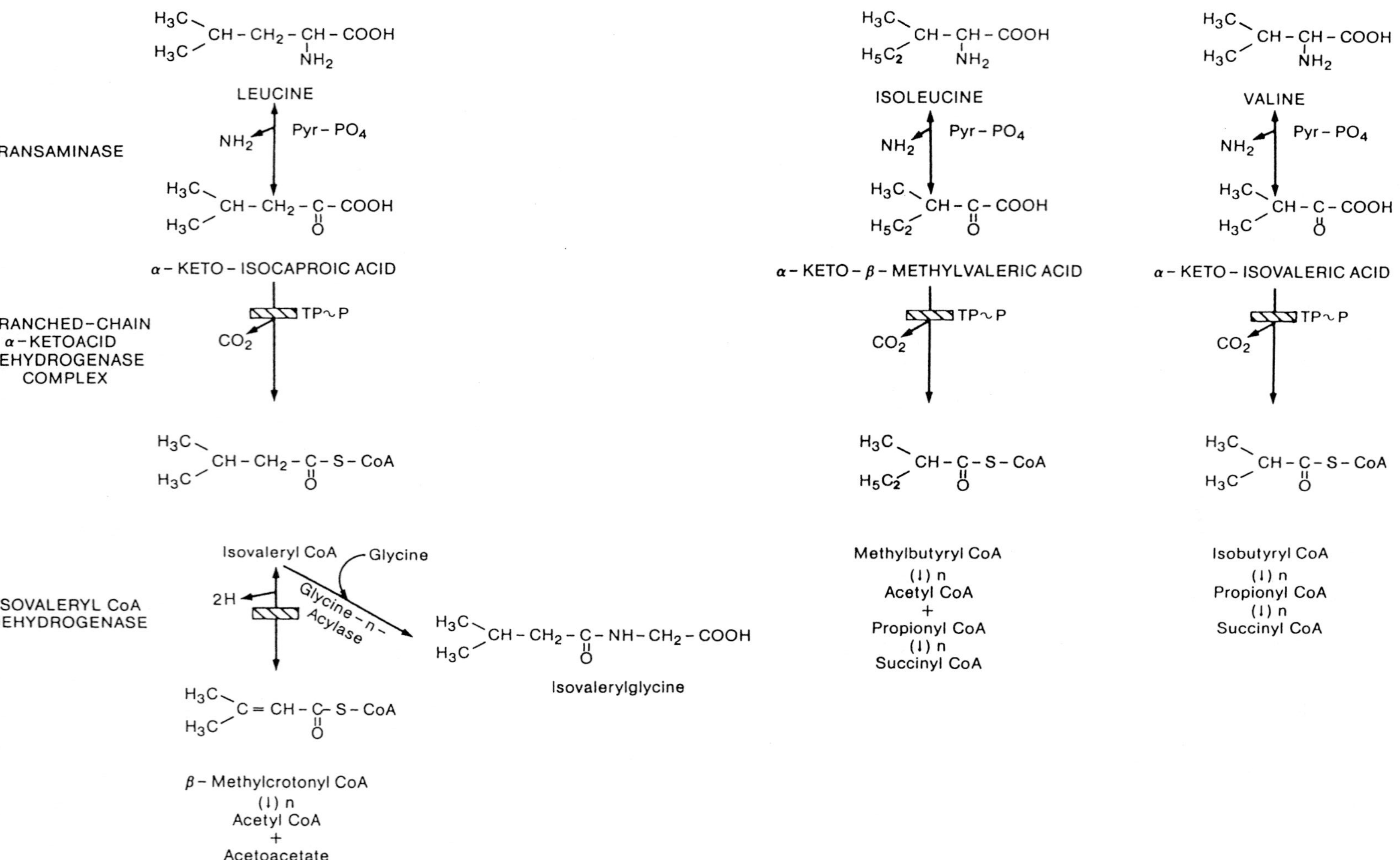

Figure 61.3. Catabolism of branched-chain amino acids. *Crosshatch bars* represent blocks in maple syrup urine disease (branched-chain α-ketoacid dehydrogenase complex) and in isovaleric acidemia (isovaleryl-CoA dehydrogenase). *TPP*, the cofactor thiamin pyrophosphate; *(n)*, several catalyzed intermediate steps.

duce MSUD are private. The only one common among Mennonites is in the E1α protein and is a conversion of tyrosine to asparagine at amino acid 393 (Y393N).

Relatively little help in managing MSUD has resulted from these advances except for the role of pharmacologic cofactors. When thiamin pyrophosphate saturates its site on E1α, the biologic turnover of BCKAD is decreased. Increasing thiamin ingestion increases intracellular thiamin pyrophosphate (TPP), and the TPP-binding sites on the decarboxylase (E1α) moiety of the BCKAD complex become saturated. When these TPP-binding sites are occupied, the multienzyme complex undergoes a conformational change that makes it more resistant to chymotrypsin and heat degradation. The biologic half-life of the enzyme and overall activity are increased when a new equilibrium of enzyme synthesis and degradation is reached. This model has been tested and is supported by clinical, functional, and structural studies (155–160) (Fig. 61.4).

Branched-Chain α-Ketoaciduria (Maple Syrup Urine Disease)

MSUD is a group of inherited disorders of isoleucine, leucine, and valine metabolism (154, 161). These disorders result from several different mutations that impair various components of the multienzyme BCKAD (Fig. 61.3). Although most mutant enzymes are immunologically present, one reported patient had absent branched-chain acyl transferase (E2) as a cause of thiamin-resistant MSUD (156, 162). An autosomal recessive mode of inheritance was found in all reported cases, supporting nuclear, rather than mitochondrial, origin of these proteins. The cellular mechanisms involved in assembling the products of these nuclear genes into a multienzyme complex in mitochondria are of considerable clinical and fundamental importance and are still unresolved.

Infants with MSUD appear normal at birth and are clinically well until after they eat a protein-containing feed. The most severely impaired enzymes may produce seizures, apnea, and death within 10 days of birth. The disorder is characterized by elevated blood, urine, and cerebrospinal fluid concentrations of the BCKAs, their amino acid precursors, and the pathognomonic alloisoleucine. Progressive neurologic dysfunction and production of fragrant urine with the odor of burnt sugar (caramel) or maple syrup follow. The sweet smell may only be evident in earwax, easily sensed after otoscopic examination. Neurologic impairment in the newborn is manifested by poor sucking, irregular respiration, rigidity alternating with periods of flaccidity, opisthotonos, progressive loss of Moro reflex, and seizures.

Several variants covering a spectrum of impaired mito-

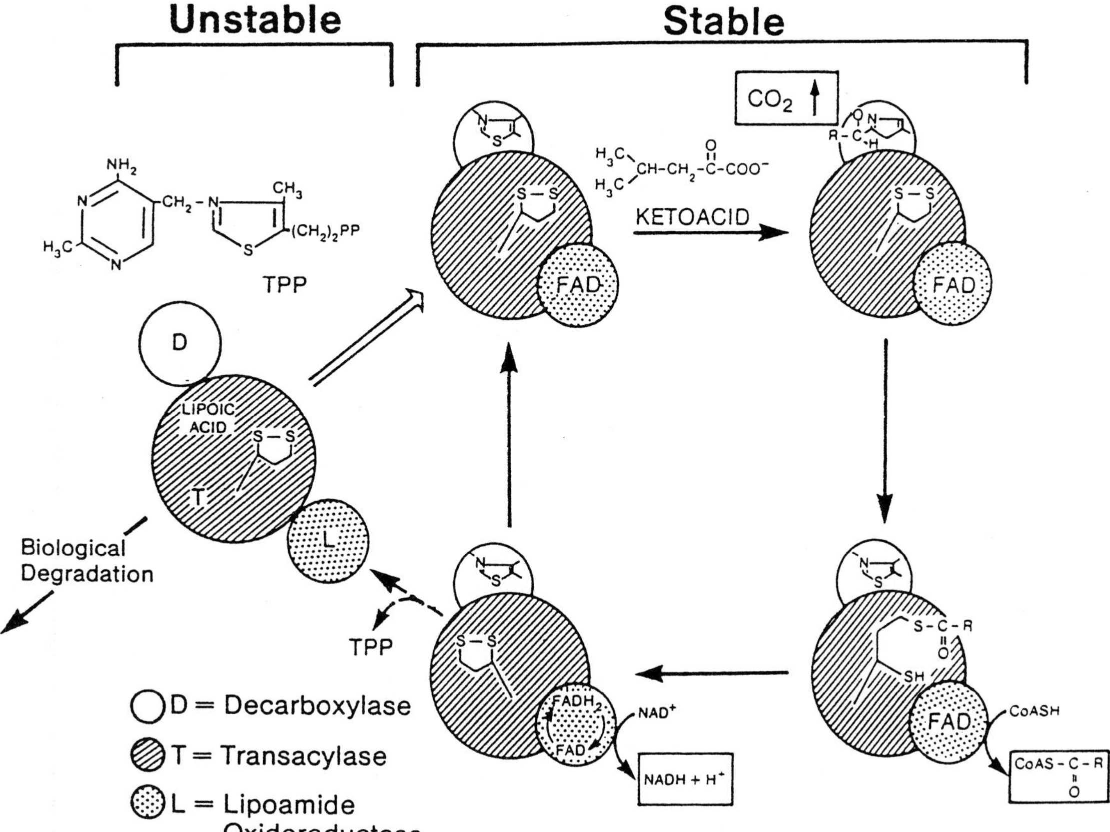

Figure 61.4. Model for stabilization of branched-chain α-ketoacid dehydrogenase by thiamin pyrophosphate. The multienzyme complex branched-chain α-ketoacid dehydrogenase has a configuration that is more stable to degradation when thiamin pyrophosphate (TPP) binding sites on its decarboxylase moiety are occupied. *FAD* and *NAD*, flavin and nicotinamide adenine dinucleotide.

chondrial BCKAD complexes have been reported. Clinical manifestations are expressed intermittently upon protein loading or with febrile illness in patients with partial enzyme activity between 5 and 20% of normal. Patients with 3 to 30% BCKAD complex activity express an intermediate form of the disease. A thiamin-responsive form with expression similar to the intermediate form has been described (154). Whole-body leucine-1-^{13}C oxidation to $^{13}CO_2$ may be the best method to ascertain total body needs, because peripheral cells may not reflect liver and renal BCKAD function (156, 158).

Untreated patients with classic MSUD (0–2% BCKAD complex activity) who survive beyond early infancy have retarded physical and mental development (4, 5). Early diagnosis and therapy lead to normal growth and development. If death occurs in the first few days of life, few unique abnormalities are seen in the brain. With prolonged survival, deficient myelination is thought to be due to enzymes involved in myelin formation, inhibition of amino acid transport, and inhibition by BCKAs of oxidative phosphorylation (4, 5).

Screening

Because apnea and death may be the first clinical manifestations of the classic disorder, newborn screening, retrieval, and initiation of therapy are urgent, and all four processes must be completed within the 1st week of life. Nonselected screening of the newborn population is currently in progress (in some states) using a bacterial-inhibition assay for blood leucine concentrations (3, 35). Bedside screening in selected children uses the urinary dinitrophenylhydrazine (DNPH) reaction for branched-chain α-ketoaciduria. This reaction can also be used to monitor dietary progress. International newborn screening indicates that the incidence of MSUD is about 1 in 216,000 (163). The incidence in Georgia, where 37% of newborns are black, is approximately 1 per 123,000 live births (Table 61.3). Little information comparing frequencies among ethnic groups is available, although some inbred communities have a high frequency (154).

Diagnosis

Any infant with a blood leucine concentration above 4 mg/dL (305 μmol/L) on the newborn screening test should be immediately evaluated. Most infants with the classic disease have more than 8 mg/dL (610 μmol/L) leucine at 72 hours of age. Diagnosis is confirmed using ion-exchange chromatography to quantitate plasma isoleucine, leucine, valine, and alloisoleucine and GC/MS to identify urinary BCKAs. The extent of enzyme impairment should be determined on cultured cells such as dermal fibroblasts to enable future prenatal diagnosis, since prenatal monitoring is available if the cellular phenotype is confirmed in fibroblasts cultured from the patient's skin (164). In some families with severely impaired enzyme function, heterozygotes can also be identified from enzymatic assays of cultured dermal fibroblasts (162). However, total-body leucine oxidation using stable isotopes and the $^{13}CO_2$ "breath test" is the most reliable diagnostic tool to establish dietary needs, including thiamin responsivity (156, 158). Except in Mennonites, molecular analysis is useful only for research purposes.

Treatment

Although hemodialysis with nitrogen-free dialysate (165, 166) or exchange transfusion (165) may be required when diagnosis is delayed, if screening, retrieval, and diagnosis are completed within 8 to 10 days of life, these actions are seldom necessary. Because hemodialysis superimposes iatrogenic risk and prolongs a catabolic phase, it is not recommended. BCAA-free orogastric feeding of protein and energy should begin as soon as the diagnosis is made. The objective is to produce anabolism in the infant and thereby prevent accumulation of neurotoxic BCKAs (167). If orogastric feeding is not acceptable, gastrostomy or a central line for hyperalimentation with dextrose and lipid should be initiated for initial care of classic MSUD during the neonatal period. Except during illness, restricting protein intake to 1.5 g/kg/day may be adequate therapy for those with 20% or more of enzyme activity.

Long-term therapy for MSUD is dietary. The objective of long-term nutritional support in the child with MSUD is to maintain plasma concentrations of BCAAs that will allow maximal development of intellect while supplying adequate energy, protein, and other nutrients for optimal growth. Plasma concentrations of BCAAs (3–4 hours after a meal) should be maintained within the following ranges: isoleucine, 40 to 90 μmol; leucine, 80 to 200 μmol; and valine, 200 to 425 μmol. Isoleucine deficiency results in skin lesions that resemble acrodermatitis enteropathica (168, 169). With a deficiency of isoleucine or valine, plasma concentration of leucine remains elevated. With deletion of the BCAAs, plasma isoleucine returns to normal first, followed by valine. If adequate dietary isoleucine and valine are then added to maintain normal plasma concentrations, plasma leucine concentration returns to normal in 5 to 10 days (170).

The objectives of nutritional support are met by using a combination of medical foods (Table 61.5) and natural foods (Table 61.12). Most patients with MSUD who have detectable BCKAD multienzyme complex by immunoassay respond to oral thiamin administration of 100 to 1000 mg daily (156, 158, 160, 171). In classic MSUD, thiamin is only an adjunct therapy, and dietary restriction of isoleucine, leucine, and valine is needed. Supraphysiologic amounts of oral thiamin should be added for at least a 3-month trial period because it stabilizes the enzyme complex (Fig. 61.4). Increased residual specific activity of mitochondrial membrane-bound enzymes may require this prolonged period because of the biologic half-life of this subcellular organelle. During this period, decreased sensitivity to dietary BCAAs is usually observed, and more can be added

Table 61.12
Average Nutrient Content of Equivalent Lists for Branched-Chain Amino Acid–Restricted Diets

Food List	Isoleucine (mg)	Leucine (mg)	Valine (mg)	Protein (g)	Fat (g)	Energy (kcal)
Breads/cereals	18	35	25	0.5	0	30
Fats	7	10	7	0.1	8	70
Fruits	17	25	22	0.6	0	75
Vegetables	22	30	24	0.6	0	15
Free foods A[a]	3	5	4	0.1	0	50
Free foods B	0	0	0	0	Varies	55
Enfamil with Iron[b], concentrate, 100 mL	181	310	184	3.0	7.6	135
Isomil[c] concentrate, 100 mL	162	286	160	3.3	7.4	135
ProSobee[b], concentrate, 100 mL	186	310	186	4.0	7.2	135
Similac[c] with Iron, concentrate, 100 mL	146	275	158	2.8	7.3	135

[a]Low-protein pastas and breads not included.
[b]Mead Johnson Nutritionals, Evansville, IN; 1/800-457-3550.
[c]Ross Products Division, Abbott Laboratories, Columbus, OH; 1/800-551-5838.

to the diet. Evaluation of total body leucine oxidation before and during thiamin administration gives direct evidence for responsivity (156, 158).

Nutrient Requirements. Data in Table 61.4 outline the suggested amounts of BCAAs, protein, energy, and fluid to offer the infant or child with MSUD. Because the BCAAs are essential, they cannot be deleted from the diet without producing growth failure and death. In planning nutritional support of the infant or child with MSUD, a formal prescription should be written that includes recommended daily amounts of BCAAs, protein, energy, and fluid. Frequent adjustments in the dietary prescription are necessary. Adjustments are needed daily during the first few weeks and biweekly during the first 6 months of life, based on appetite, growth, development, and laboratory analyses of plasma BCAAs and BCKAs. Because leucine residues are more prominent than isoleucine and valine in most proteins, supplemental L-isoleucine and L-valine as free amino acids may be necessary in the newborn period and beyond to prevent deficiency of these two essential amino acids. However, competition between the free BCAAs at the intestinal cell can cause imbalances in plasma amino acids (172).

Requirements for isoleucine, leucine, and valine vary considerably depending on age, type and extent of enzyme defect, growth rate, and state of health. Younger infants normally have greater requirements per unit body weight than older infants. A rapid decline occurs in requirements for BCAAs between 3 and 6 months of age. Careful monitoring of plasma concentrations and intake of BCAAs is required to prevent excess intake when growth rate declines and to provide adequate intake when growth is accelerated as in early infancy, during prepuberty and puberty, and during the last half of gestation. There has been one successful pregnancy in an adult with MSUD whose protein requirements were those of a normal adult but fell dramatically after delivery (154).

The recommended protein intake for infants with MSUD (Table 61.4) exceeds that for normal infants and children because the primary protein source consists of L-amino acids (51). Recommended energy intake after the initial acute period is the same as for normal infants and children, but may vary considerably (see Table 61.4) (52). During the neonatal acute period, up to 170 kcal/kg/day may be required (173).

Medical Foods Free of Branched-Chain Amino Acids. Adequate protein cannot be obtained from ordinary foods without ingesting more BCAAs than are required in classic MSUD. The BCAA content of foods as a percentage of protein ranges from approximately 3.5 to 8.5% (56–61). Because of the BCAA content of most proteins, medical foods are used that are formulated from L-amino acids free of BCAAs. In the United States, several products are available to provide protein (62–64). Formulations, major nutrient composition, and sources of these products are given in Table 61.4.

Equivalent Lists. Equivalent lists of foods are available to provide variety and needed natural protein in the diet (63). The lists are similar to diabetic exchange lists in that foods of similar leucine content are grouped together and may be exchanged for one another within the same list. Average isoleucine, leucine, valine, protein, and energy contents of these lists are given in Table 61.12.

Initiation of Nutritional Support. A rapid decline in plasma isoleucine and valine can be achieved at the time of diagnosis by feeding formula free of BCAAs. However, plasma leucine will continue to increase over the first 4 days of life, even if dietary BCAA restriction is implemented at birth (170). Most patients are not anticipated at birth, and infants whose screening results are positive are treated at 7 to 14 days of life. In our experience, branched-chain ketoacidosis can be averted by high-energy intake with no added BCAAs over a 72-h period if instituted between 8 and 11 days of age. There is an association among the degree of α-ketoisocaproic acid excretion, leucine elevation, and clinical outcome (174). Laboratory results of plasma BCAAs should be rapidly available to prevent the predicted deficiency in isoleucine and valine. When replacement is begun, these two amino acids may be added as free L-amino acids to increase their ratio to leucine in natural protein. High-energy intake of 140 to 170 kcal/kg of body weight during this period prevents catabolism of body protein. If the osmolality of formula permits, protein at 3.0 to 3.5 g/kg should be offered. This regimen will lower the concentrations of BCAAs to near normal ranges. If deficiency of either isoleucine or valine occurs, plasma leucine concentrations will remain elevated as a function of muscle catabolism or decreased protein synthesis.

Sample diets for management of children with MSUD are listed in Tables 61.13 and 61.14. The leucine required at birth may fall from 70 to 40 mg/kg/day at 2 years. Medical foods designed for MSUD should be used for therapy, but to prevent deficiency of the essential amino acids isoleucine and valine, solutions of these two BCAAs are added back to the formula. As described in these sample dietary guides, this need persists over this 2-year developmental period.

Assessment of Nutritional Support. Frequency of assessment is dictated by the clinical course and the response of plasma amino acids. Monitoring of therapy should use three combined approaches. Ion-exchange chromatography should be used daily to quantitate plasma amino acid concentrations for approximately 3 weeks after birth; these help determine requirements for the individual BCAAs. Urine can be evaluated at bedside for decline in the DNPH reaction much like Clinitest was used to monitor diabetic ketoacidosis. Quantitation of organic acids by GC/MS can detect decline in BCKAs and presence of β-lipolysis.

After requirements are established, plasma amino acid concentrations are determined approximately every 2 weeks to ensure that the child has not "outgrown" the prescription. Samples should be obtained at midday before the noon feeding. We have found organic acid analysis of urine to be helpful. BCKAs decrease under optimum dietary conditions. If energy or a specific amino acid is overrestricted, evidence of β-lipolysis (acetoacetic acid, β-OH-butyric acid) is found.

After hospital discharge, daily testing of urine with DNPH by a parent at home screens rapidly for ketoaciduria. As a rule, "preventive" clinical evaluation of the child for cryptogenic infections before overt ketoacidosis occurs is more effective than trying to treat the child after a catabolic phase has produced its attendant ketoacidosis. If the urine DNPH results are positive, a blood sample should be collected on filter paper for leucine assay and the urine should be further analyzed by GC/MS to differentiate "ketonuria" from branched-chain α-ketonuria.

Table 61.13
Sample Diets for Branched-Chain Ketoaciduria (2 weeks of age): Weight 3.25 kg

Prescription	Total	per kg				
Isoleucine, mg	163	50				
Leucine, mg	228	70				
Valine, m	195	60				
Protein, g	9.8	3.0				
Energy, kcal	390	120				
Medical Food #1	**Amount**	**ILE, mg**	**LEU, mg**	**VAL, mg**	**PRO, g**	**Energy, kcal**
Ketonex-1	50 g	0	0	0	7.5	240
Similac w/Iron, concentrate	83 mL	121	228	131	2.3	112
Table sugar	1 Tbsp	0	0	0	0	48
ILE, 10 mg/mL	4.6 mL	46	0	0	0	0
VAL, 10 mg/mL	6.4 mL	0	0	64	0	0
Volume, water to make	600 mL			0		
Totals		167	228	195	9.8	400
Medical Food #2						
MSUD Analog	55 g	0	0	0	7.2	261
Isomil concentrate	80 mL	129	228	128	2.6	108
Polycose liquid	1.25 mL	0	0	0	0	29
ILE, 10 mg/mL	3.4 mL	34	0	0	0	0
VAL, 10 mg/mL	6.6 mL	0	0	66	0	0
Volume, water to make	600 mL					
Totals		163	228	194	9.8	398
Medical Food #3						
MSUD Diet Powder	86 g	0	0	0	7.6	362
Enfamil w/Iron concentrate	73.3 mL	133	228	135	2.2	99
ILE, 10 mg/mL	3 mL	30	0	0	0	0
VAL, 10 mg/mL	6 mL	0	9	60	0	0
Volume, water to make	600 mL					
Totals		163	228	195	9.8	461[a]

[a]To supply adequate protein with, MSUD Diet Powder, energy prescription must be exceeded.

Table 61.14
Sample Diets for Branched-Chain Ketoaciduria (4 years of age): Weight 17 kg

Prescription	Total	per kg				
Isoleucine, mg	455	27				
Leucine, mg	520	30				
Valine, mg	481	28				
Protein, g	35.0	2.1				
Energy, kcal	1700	100				
Medical Food #1	**Amount**	**ILE, mg**	**LEU, mg**	**VAL, mg**	**PRO, g**	**Energy, kcal**
Ketonex-2	92 g	0	0	0	27.7	377
ILE, 10 mg/mL	15 mL	150	0	0	0	0
VAL, 10 mg/mL	9.3 mL	0	0	93	0	0
Volume, water to make	960 mL					
Foods						
Breads/cereals	9 svgs	162	315	225	3.6	225
Fats	7 svgs	49	70	49	0.7	490
Fruits	3 svgs	51	75	66	1.8	225
Vegetables	2 svgs	44	60	48	1.2	30
Free foods B	6.5 svgs	0	0	0	0	358
Totals		456	520	481	35.0	1705
Formula #2						
MSUD Diet Powder	315 g	0	0	0	27.7	1480
ILE, 10 mg/mL	15.7 mL	157	0	0	0	0
VAL, 10 mg/mL	9 mL	0	0	90	0	0
Volume, water to make	960 mL					
Foods						
Breads/cereals	11 svgs	198	385	275	4.4	275
Fruits	2 svgs	34	50	44	1.2	150
Vegetables	3 svgs	66	90	72	1.8	45
Totals		455	525	481	35.0	1950[a]
Formula #3						
MSUD Maxamaid	111 g	0	0	0	27.7	388
ILE, 10 mg/mL	15 mL	149	0	0	0	0
VAL, 10 mg/mL	9.3 mL	0	0	93	0	0
Volume, water to make	960 mL					
Foods						
Breads/cereals	9 svgs	162	315	225	3.6	225
Fats	7 svgs	49	70	49	0.7	490
Fruits	3 svgs	51	75	66	1.8	225
Vegetables	2 svgs	44	60	48	1.2	30
Free foods B	6 svgs	0	0	0	0	330
Totals		455	520	481	35.0	1688

[a]To supply adequate protein with MSUD Diet Powder, energy prescription must be exceeded.

A physician should evaluate the child for infection or other causes of ketoacidosis. With a dietary history, a physician's examination, and laboratory analyses, one can usually differentiate among overrestriction, intercurrent infection, or dietary underrestriction as a cause for branched-chain α-ketoaciduria. Weekly quantitation of leucine, isoleucine, and valine and dietary records are useful for chronic management. Every effort should be made to maintain plasma BCAAs in the normal range. Plasma leucine concentrations above 600 μmol are associated with clinically significant α-ketoacidemia and appearance of ataxia (4, 174). Changes suggesting dysmyelination were found in the white matter in the cerebral hemispheres, brainstem, mesencephalon, thalamus, and globus pallidus of patients with chronically elevated concentrations of BCAAs (175).

Episodes of infection can evoke catabolism of tissue protein and increase plasma concentrations of BCAAs. Clinical improvement is rapid if some BCAAs are administered along with an amino acid mix that provides 150 to 200 kcal/kg/day. Parenteral amino acid solutions free of BCAAs have also caused a rapid decline in plasma BCAAs during infection, with concomitant clinical improvement (176).

Outcome of Nutritional Support. Patients diagnosed at 5 days of age or less had IQs (97 ± 13 SD) above those of normal siblings or parents (177). Factors influencing IQ were age at the time of diagnosis, neonatal condition, and long-term metabolic control. Reproductive outcome of a woman with classic MSUD, whose blood BCAAs were controlled by diet, was excellent (178).

The first attempt to manage an 8-month old infant with MSUD used pure amino acids totaling approximately 50 g daily. Oil and sugar were used to yield 1500 kcal/day. Mineral and vitamin mixtures were also provided. Plasma concentrations of BCAAs decreased significantly, and the maple syrup odor disappeared from the urine. During the dietary trial, length and weight increased from the 3rd to the 50th percentile (179).

Nutritional support of a neonate with BCKA was subsequently described (180). Plasma amino acids were measured as a basis for dietary changes. Approximate protein intake ranged from 3.5 to 3.0 g/kg/day between 3 and 8 months of age, respectively. Energy intake was about 125 kcal/kg/day. At birth, the infant was at the 10th percentile for length and weight; during the 1st year of life, length increased toward the 50th percentile, but weight remained at about the 10th percentile. Anemia, with a hemoglobin of 8.5 g/dL, was present from 1 to 3 months of age. At 55 weeks of age, the patient had a developmental quotient of 97, which is in the normal range (180).

Experience with seven patients with MSUD, three of whom expired, was reported (181). The surviving patients received an L-amino acid mix free of BCAAs to which corn oil (43% of energy), dextrimaltose (45% of energy), minerals, and vitamins were added. Protein and energy intake was not reported. Linear growth of one patient by 1 year of age was considerably below the 10th percentile. Three of the four surviving patients had weights below the 10th percentile; length/height percentiles were not given.

A number of other investigators have reported poor growth in treated children with BCKA (181–187). Except for Henstenberg et al. (187), who indicated that mean protein and energy intakes were 78 and 86% of RDA, respectively, few authors reported protein or energy intake. However, intake of both protein and energy by children with MSUD has been reported to be below that of comparably aged normal children (188). Whether failure to thrive is due to the underlying disease or to iatrogenic dietary effects is unclear. Some investigators reported normal growth when adequate protein and energy were fed (156, 158, 179, 180).

Selenium deficiency has been found in treated patients with MSUD (189). B vitamin deficiencies resulting in anemia, angular stomatitis, and skin lesions occurred in one baby when the B vitamin mixture was not added to the diet for 6 weeks (180). Folic acid deficiency was reported in an infant after about 4 months on a synthetic diet (190). Acidosis occurred in an infant treated with an amino acid mix in which several amino acids were provided as the HCl salt (191).

Termination of Nutritional Support. Patients with classic MSUD are unable to terminate diet, even if they respond to thiamin. The occurrence of death in variants with intermittent MSUD suggests the need for some form of ongoing therapy in even these relatively stable patients (154). The BCKAs are relatively acute neurotoxins and probably interfere with oxygen consumption and adenosine triphosphate (ATP) production in the medullary reticular substance of the brain (154).

Isovaleric Acidemia

First described in 1967, isovaleric acidemia was identified by the urinary excretion of IVA (189). Subsequently, a deficiency of isovaleryl-CoA dehydrogenase (IVD) was defined in cultured skin fibroblasts (170). This enzyme is a mitochondrial flavoprotein that uses electron transfer factor (ETF). Although ETF deficiency is also reported, mutations in the apoenzyme are specific for isovaleryl-CoA as substrate. IVD deficiency blocks the catabolism of leucine at the next step after the BCKAD complex (Fig. 61.3). The IVD gene was assigned to chromosome 15q14-q15 (191), and molecular heterogeneity is defined and five classes proposed on the basis of the effects of various mutations on IVD (191, 192). Class I has normal-sized IVD and missense mutations. Classes II, III, and IV have smaller proteins, and class V has no immunologically detectable IVD (192a). IVA, 3-hydroxyisovaleric acid (3-OHIVA), and the adduct IVG accumulate in body fluids. Gas-liquid chromatography and mass spectrometry can identify these compounds in body fluids (161).

The phenotypic abnormalities result from the toxic accumulation of free IVA. An alternate pathway producing IVG using glycine-*N*-acylase reduces the accumulation of the toxic precursors. Thus, clinical differences in phenotype are due to the degree of impaired IVD and epigenetic phenomena such as the degree of alternate detoxification available to this alternative pathway (161, 193, 194). Carnityl adducts offer an additional alternate pathway to detoxify free IVA.

Despite molecular advances in understanding the mutations affecting IVD, two disease forms continue to be clinically useful classifications: the acute form and the chronic intermittent form (161). Patients with the acute form of isovaleric acidemia are generally normal full-term infants at birth. Within the first days of life, poor feeding, tachypnea, vomiting, and a characteristic "sweaty-feet" odor (due to IVA) of the blood and urine are frequently noted. Diarrhea, lethargy, hypotonia, and tremors (161) may also be found. In some cases, patients do not respond to treatment; they may become cyanotic or comatose, and death often results (161). The exact cause of death is frequently unknown. Severe metabolic acidosis, hyperammonemia, CNS hemorrhage, cardiac arrest, and sepsis are some probable causes. Infants who are detected early and respond to treatment survive the neonatal period and develop appropriately. If the acute neonatal disease is prevented, they progress into the chronic intermittent type of isovaleric acidemia (161).

In the chronic intermittent form, babies are normal at birth. During late infancy they may develop episodes of vomiting, acidosis, stupor, and coma. A sweaty-feet odor is usually present, and a transient alopecia is occasionally seen. These episodes may begin as early as 2 weeks of age, and the frequency of attacks seems to decrease with age. Urinary tract and upper respiratory infections frequently trigger these episodes, as do excessive intake of protein and aspirin. Many children affected by the intermittent form prefer fruits and vegetables over meat and milk. The degree of enzyme (IVD) impairment and capacity of the alternate IVG-producing pathway, as well as intake, probably produce these clinically different presentations.

Several patients with either the acute or the chronic form of isovaleric acidemia have had moderate-to-severe hematologic abnormalities, including leukopenia and thrombocytopenia, with pancytopenia being the most common. IVA inhibits granulopoietic progenitor cell proliferation in bone marrow cultures and may account for the neutropenia often seen in isovaleric acidemia (195). In one instance, transfusion of packed red cells and platelets prevented further complications. Depressed hemoglobin levels were also seen in several patients. Transient alopecia seems to be more common with the chronic intermittent form than with the acute form of the disease and may be nutritionally related (161). Hyperammonemia (up to 1200 μmol) has also been reported during neonatal crises (161).

Diagnosis

Because IVG is excreted during both remission and ketotic attacks, measurement of urinary IVG by GC/MS is the best method of diagnosis. Normal 3- to 5-year-old unaffected children have no detectable urinary IVG (<2 mg/day). Affected children of the same age excrete from 40 to 250 mg/day (161). During ketotic episodes, urinary 3-OHIVA, 4-OHIVA, and methylsuccinic acid are excreted in large quantities as well (161).

Diagnosis is confirmed by measuring the impaired ability of skin fibroblasts cultured from affected individuals to oxidize leucine-2-^{14}C to $^{14}CO_2$ (190, 196). A more complicated assay using mitochondria and 1-^{14}C-IVA has also been used (197). High-field proton nuclear magnetic resonance is a promising new technique for rapid diagnosis of isovaleric acidemia because it can readily detect IVG in a small sample of urine (198).

Prenatal diagnosis is available by combined organic acid analysis of amniotic fluid and enzyme assay of cultured amniotic fluid cells. A heterozygote for IVD has been detected prenatally (199).

Treatment

During acute ketotic attacks, parenteral fluid therapy and correction of the metabolic acidosis are indicated as adjuncts to high energy intake and L-carnitine and glycine therapy (161). Serum and urine IVA concentrations are monitored during ketotic attacks. GC/MS analysis is the most accurate means of determining serum and urinary IVA (161). A special method of GC/MS allows separate quantitation of the two isomers, IVA and 2-methylbutyric acid (161). Serum IVA ranges from 0.1 to 84 mg/dL (161) depending on the patient's clinical status. A simple and rapid method of determining 4-OHIVA concentrations in the plasma has recently been devised (200); however, elevations of this metabolite lag at least 36 hours behind the maximum plasma level of IVA (200), which limits its use clinically. Monitoring urinary IVG provides a good parameter of nutrition therapy. Titration of IVG with free glycine to a stable optimum is desirable. However, excess glycine over free substrate (IVA) may inhibit IVG production (Fig. 61.5). When leucine restriction is optimal and the patient is stable, about 90 mg/kg/day is optimal. During acute disease, a higher intake (300–600 mg/kg/day) of glycine may be necessary until infection or dietary leucine indiscretions are removed (202).

Nutrient Requirements. A low-protein diet of 1.2 to 1.5 g/kg/day in children under 1 year of age improves clinical symptoms, and many patients restrict protein by choice (161). This represents only 60% of the RDA. Protein restriction alone is therefore not the best mode of therapy because overrestriction of essential BCAA (ILE, VAL) is inevitable if leucine is adequately restricted in natural food.

Leucine restriction and the use of pharmacologic doses of glycine have been reported. In six patients with isovaleric acidemia, glycine therapy resulted in decreased IVA in plasma and urine (161). Urinary IVG simultaneously increased, often two- to threefold (Fig. 61.5). Clinical

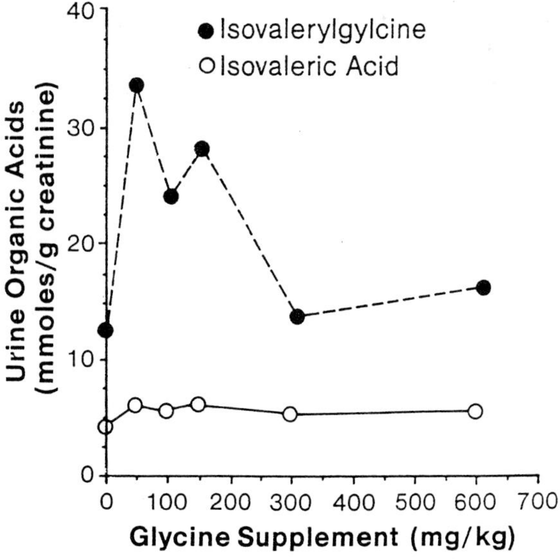

Figure 61.5. Effect of oral glycine supplement on isovalerylglycine production in stable isovaleric acidemia. Oral glycine supplements indicated on the *abscissa* were administered at weekly intervals to a patient with isovaleric acidemia while she was maintained on a constant leucine-restricted diet. Isovalerylglycine (IVG) and isovaleric acid were quantitated by gas chromatography. Symbols represent the mean of duplicate 24-h urine samples collected over the last 2 days of each interval. Note the increase in IVG production at 50–150 mg/kg/day with increased IVG production at 300 and 600 mg/kg/day of dietary glycine supplement. (Courtesy of Division of Medical Genetics, Emory University, Atlanta, GA).

improvement occurred that was characterized by increased growth, control of acidosis, and resolution of pancytopenia with glycine supplements and protein restriction over a 2-week period.

Glycine used to remove IVA through an alternative pathway is a prototype for nutritional detoxification of accumulated substrates in inborn errors of metabolism (Fig. 61.5) (201, 202). The ubiquitous enzyme glycine-*N*-acylase has a broad range of substrates (Table 61.15) that accumulate in other inborn errors of metabolism and might also be amenable to this approach. The relative amounts of glycine required to optimize removal of IVA (or other substrates for the glycine-*N*-acylase reaction) need careful evaluation and will change with the clinical condition of the patient (202).

Some evidence exists for substrate inhibition of the reaction when excess glycine is added under stable conditions (Fig. 61.5). The optimal dose of supplemental glycine was determined for a 9-year-old Caucasian girl with isovaleric acidemia who was well and maintained on a leucine intake of 54 ± 3.6 mg/kg/day. Supplementation with glycine below or above the range of 50 to 150 mg/kg resulted in a 50% decrease in IVG excretion. Urinary IVA excretion was consistent throughout the study. No β-hydroxy-IVA was detected in plasma or urine. The results of this study indicated that *(a)* the optimal dose of glycine for this patient under these stable clinical and nutritional conditions was 50 to 150 mg/kg, *(b)* an optimal dose of glycine should be quantitated for specific ages, clinical states, degree of enzyme activity, and leucine intake in the treatment of isovaleric acidemia, and *(c)* glycine supplements above 300 mg/kg/day increased plasma and urinary concentrations of glycine but resulted in decreased IVG excretion, as if this substrate inhibited glycine-*N*-acylase when concentrations of its cosubstrate, isovaleryl-CoA, were controlled (202).

Systemic carnitine deficiency was demonstrated in several patients with isovaleric acidemia (203). Although plasma levels of carnitine were low in these patients, the acylcarnitine ester—isovaleryl carnitine (IVC)—was increased, especially during illness (203, 204). Relative deficiency of muscle carnitine and use of carnitine as an adduct for IVA are two reasons for treating with extra L-carnitine. The relative therapeutic value of L-carnitine has been compared with that of glycine in the treatment of isovaleric acidemia in a 4.5-year-old black male (204). Administration of glycine plus leucine resulted in excretion of more IVA as IVG than when leucine was administered alone. Leucine plus L-carnitine increased IVC excretion from a pretreatment level of 7 μmol per 24 hours to a posttreatment level of 1470 μmol per 24 hours. Large doses of carnitine are needed, in the range of 100 to 200 mg/kg/day, to accomplish this therapeutic excretion, whereas 100 to 150 mg/kg/day of glycine will suffice. Smaller doses of carnitine supplements are recommended to prevent "deficiency."

Table 16.15
Kinetic Constants for Glycine-*N*-Acylase from Bovine Liver

Substrate	K_M (10^{-4} M)	V_{MAX} (μmol/min/mg protein)
Tiglyl-CoA	1.1	33.3
Isovaleryl-CoA	1.8	12.3
Benzoyl-CoA	0.09	10.4
2-Methylbutyryl-CoA	1.1	8.3
3-Methylcrotonyl-CoA	0.14	5.7
Propionyl-CoA	1.8	4.4
Acetyl-CoA	2.1	1.6

From Barlett K, Gompertz D. Biochem Med 1974;10:15, with permission.

Medical Foods Free of Leucine. Four medical foods free of leucine have been designed specifically for nutritional support of patients with isovaleric acidemia and other disorders of leucine catabolism. Formulations, major nutrient composition, and sources of these medical foods are given in Table 61.5.

Outcome of Nutritional Support. A male infant with isovaleric acidemia, treated from the neonatal period with a medical food designed for MSUD with added L-isoleucine and L-valine and whole protein to supply essential restricted leucine, had normal growth and development. Height and weight were between the 25th and 50th percentile. Head circumference was at the 50th percentile. On average, the diet supplied 2.5 to 3.0 g protein/kg/day and 100 mg leucine/kg/day. L-Carnitine and glycine were not a part of the dietary regimen (205).

Growth of a male infant diagnosed prenatally with isovaleric acidemia has been reported. At birth the infant was breast-fed ad libitum, and 250 mg glycine/kg/day was administered. In spite of the low protein intake from human milk and the glycine supplement, the patient became acidotic and began to vomit and hyperventilate at 3 days of age. Breast-feeding was discontinued, and a leucine-free diet providing 125 kcal/kg supplemented with 380 mg glycine/kg/day was begun. His clinical status improved rapidly. Dietary leucine at 45 mg/kg/day with glycine at 250 mg/kg/day and protein at 2.0 g/kg was introduced at 5 days of age. At 2 years of age, the patient was developmentally normal and above the 95th percentile for height and weight. Diet at 2 years of age supplied per kg: 46 mg leucine, 1.7 g protein, and 72 kcal. Only one hospitalization for vomiting and dehydration was required during the 2-year period (202).

Outcomes in nine patients with isovaleric acidemia managed by protein restriction (1.5–2.0 g/kg in infancy, 0.8–1.5 g/kg thereafter) and 250 mg glycine/kg/day have been reported (206). Since all patients had secondary carnitine deficiency (total serum carnitine 19 ± 3 μmol/L), four of the children were supplemented with 50 mg/kg/day L-carnitine, and in these, serum carnitine returned to normal (51 ± 5 μmol/L). Actual height, weight, and head circumference of patients were not reported, although growth velocities were stated to be normal after diet initiation. Developmental quotients or IQ scores of the five subjects in whom diet was initiated during the neonatal period ranged from 49 to 115 (206).

In a study by one of the authors (PBA), the patient failed to grow normally, most probably because of low energy intake; however, development was normal. Food refusal has been reported in a patient with isovaleric acidemia (207). Both physiologic and behavioral components to feeding problems were reported. The physiologic component involved altered serotonin metabolism. Any factor such as hyperammonemia or a high-carbohydrate, low-protein diet that stimulates the transport of tryptophan, a precursor of serotonin, into the brain, could lead to anorexia. A low-tryptophan diet was suggested as one alternative to the treatment of anorexia (208).

Of 11 reported French patients with isovaleric acidemia, 8 were alive after the neonatal period. Leucine restriction and glycine supplementation were used to manage patients. Six of the eight surviving patients have normal development (209).

SULFUR-CONTAINING AMINO ACIDS

The biochemistry and nutritional requirements for sulfur-containing amino acids have been largely elucidated in humans by studies of inherited blocks in their metabolic pathways.

Biochemistry

Natural protein contains approximately 0.3 to 5.0% methionine. Some dietary methionine is used by the body for tissue protein synthesis, but most is used in the transsulfuration pathway to form adenosylmethionine, adenosylhomocysteine, homocysteine, cystathionine, α-ketobutyrate, cysteine, and their derivatives (Fig. 61.6). The first step in the transsulfuration pathway is synthesis of SAM, a reaction catalyzed by methionine-*S*-adenosyltransferase (MAT). Impaired MAT results in hypermethioninemia and variable clinical expression from sulfurous breath odor to mental retardation. The hepatic isoform of MAT only is deficient (212). In this reaction, the adenosyl portion of ATP is transferred to methionine. Biologically important compounds that obtain their methyl group from SAM include creatine, choline and phosphatidylcholine, methylated DNA and RNA, and epinephrine. Decarboxylated SAM is the source of the three carbon moieties of spermidine and spermine. *S*-Adenosylhomocysteine is formed as an intermediary product in this pathway and is hydrolyzed to homocysteine.

Homocysteine then has four possible pathways open to it. Homocysteine reacts with serine in the presence of cystathionine β synthase (CBS), found in liver and brain, to form cystathionine (Fig. 61.6). CBS requires pyridoxal phosphate as a coenzyme. Homocysteine can also be remethylated to form methionine through two different enzymatic reactions. In one reaction, the methyl group is derived from betaine and is catalyzed by betaine-homocysteine methyltransferase. The second reaction requires N^5-methyltetrahydrofolate as a methyl donor and methylcobalamin (CH_3-B_{12}) as coenzyme (Fig. 61.6) and is catalyzed by 5-methyltetrahydrofolate-homocysteine methyltransferase. Finkelstein and Martin used an in vitro system that approximated in vivo conditions in rat liver to measure the simultaneous product formation by the three enzymes that use homocysteine (210). In this control system, 5-methyltetrahydrofolate-homocysteine methyltransferase, betaine homocysteine methyltransferase, and CBS accounted for 27, 27, and 46%, respectively, of the homocysteine consumed. The fourth pathway open to homocysteine is spontaneous oxidation to homocystine (Fig. 61.6). This reaction occurs only when homocysteine is present in tissue in abnormal amounts. It is essentially irreversible because the disulfide bond of homocystine is covalent. Homocystine is not further metabolized. CBS metabolizes most homocysteine with high affinity to cystathionine, using serine as cosubstrate and pyridoxal phosphate as coenzyme. Cystathionine is then hydrolyzed to cysteine and α-ketobutyrate. The enzyme cystathionase, which also uses pyridoxal phosphate as coenzyme, is required for this reaction (Fig. 61.6). A deficiency of cystathionase results in cystathioninuria, which has no pathologic consequence. α-Ketobutyrate is converted to propionyl-CoA, which is carboxylated to methylmalonyl-CoA and isomerized to succinyl-CoA, a Krebs cycle intermediate. L-Cysteine is catabolized to pyruvate, NH_3, and H_2S.

Homocystinuria

Defects in the function of CBS or 5-methyltetrahydrofolate-homocysteine methyltransferase result in classical homocystinuria. Impaired activity of the latter enzyme may be caused by failure to synthesize methylcobalamin from vitamin B_{12} or by a deficiency in 5,10-methylenetetrahydrofolate reductase, as well as by mutations in the apoenzyme, CBS (211). Several different defects impair the uptake, transfer, and conversion of dietary vitamin B_{12} to methylcobalamin (11, 212, 213).

The most common form of homocystinuria is caused by a deficiency of CBS. The human *CBS* locus has been mapped to chromosome 21q-22.3 (214). The gene has been cloned, and over 20 mutations are characterized in expression systems. Although phenotypes vary for the same genotype, some mutations respond to vitamin B_6 (I278T, P145L, A114V) and others do not (G307S) (215). Severely impaired enzyme function produces accumulation of plasma homocyst(e)ine and methionine and decreased cyst(e)ine in cells and physiologic fluids. If this biochemical circumstance is not treated early in life, skeletal changes, dislocated lenses, intravascular thromboses, osteoporosis, malar flushing, and, in some patients, mental retardation will occur.

The skeletal changes and dislocated lenses are presumably due to a structural defect in collagen formation produced by α-homocystine interaction with aldose groups on collagen (212). Intravascular thromboses may occur at any

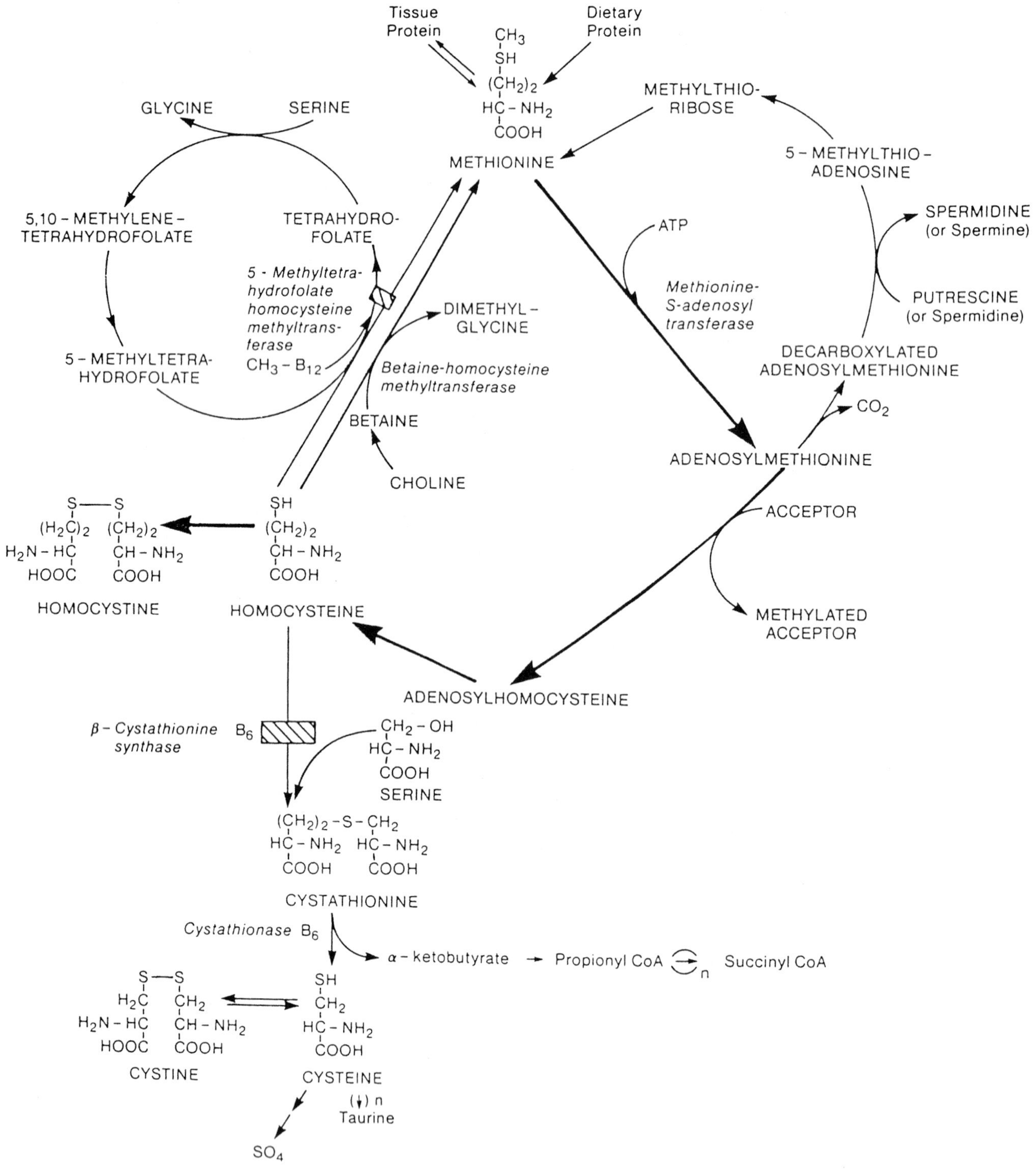

Figure 61.6. Metabolic pathways of sulfur amino acids. *Hatched bars* represent impaired reactions in three inherited metabolic disorders resulting in hyperhomocyst[e]inemia.

age and have been found in coronary, renal, carotid, and intracranial arteries. Some 50% of untreated patients die before 20 years of age, and 95% before 50 years of age (216). The natural history of homocystinuria due to CBS deficiency has been clarified in a large series of patients (217). Heterozygosity for some mutations in CBS (and/or in tetrahydrofolate reductase) may predispose patients to development of premature occlusive arterial disease (218). Further information on the relationship between total plasma homocyst(e)ine and premature coronary disease is given in Chapter 34.

It is not known to what degree the mental retardation seen in homocystinuria is due to a metabolic sequela, such as a deficiency of cystathionine in myelin formation, or results from multiple small cerebrovascular thromboses. In a series of 84 patients, half were of average intelligence, several were university graduates, and one held a Ph.D. (216). Mental deficiency may occur with severely impaired CBS as a consequence of multiple cerebral-arteriolar obstructions if homocystinemia is not controlled by diet.

Screening

CBS deficiency is inherited as an autosomal recessive disease. Accurate estimates of the incidence for homocystinuria are not available, but newborn screening in 13 countries found 1 in 344,000 infants screened (212). Screening for homocystinuria in Georgia yielded an incidence of approximately 1 per 345,088, with hypermethioninemia occurring in 1 per 44,242 live births (Table 61.3). Homocystinuria occurs in many ethnic groups, but has a higher frequency in persons of Irish extraction than in other ethnic groups, 1 in 58,000 (212). This finding may be a bias of ascertainment because of the original description of, and continued screening for, this disorder in the Irish population. Vitamin B_6–responsive mutations in CBS are probably not ascertained by neonatal screening for elevated blood methionine.

Selective screening uses the inexpensive urinary nitroprusside reaction. In this reaction, excessive amounts of reduced homocysteine and cysteine form a stable red color with nitroprusside. This selective screening test for sulfur amino acids should be included in the evaluation of any patient with an unknown cause for arterial thrombosis, dislocated lens, marfanoid habitus, or mental retardation. This test is also positive in cystinuria and should be included as a screen for patients with nephrolithiasis.

In a large survey of patients with homocystinuria due to CBS deficiency, only 13% responded to vitamin B_6 (217). Most of these patients were "leaky mutants" who had residual CBS activity and expressed their disease in adolescence or young adulthood rather than early childhood. Response to vitamin B_6 occurs in several mutations with some residual enzyme activity. The mechanism involves stabilizing CBS to biologic degradation (212). The more residual enzyme activity present, the more dramatic the response to vitamin B_6. Hypermethioninemia may not be present in the newborn if CBS activity exceeds 15% of normal. Some patients with CBS deficiency have no activity in the fibroblasts, yet appear to be B_6 responsive (215).

Diagnosis

Positive results in a newborn screen by bacterial inhibition assay for methionine must be followed by assay of plasma amino acids using ion-exchange chromatography because many environmental, as well as genetic, variations cause neonatal hypermethioninemia. With a CBS defect, homocystine, cysteine-homocysteine, and methionine are all elevated in plasma and increase with increased protein intake (Fig. 61.6). Demonstration of significantly decreased CBS, folate, CH_3-B_{12}, or homocysteine methyltransferases is necessary to confirm the diagnosis and implement appropriate therapy. Methionine may be elevated in the absence of homocystinemia in liver disease and in specific impairment of SAM. By contrast, in defects of homocysteine remethylation to methionine, methionine is low or normal, whereas homocysteine concentrations are elevated. Hyperhomocysteinemia due to disorders of cobalamin methylation to CH_3-B_{12} or the two homocysteine methyltransferases will not be detected by nonselective newborn screening for elevated blood methionine. Similarly, B_6-responsive "mild" CBS deficiency is missed by newborn screening. Thus, selective screening using urinary nitroprusside reaction or plasma amino acid analysis is indicated for all children or adults with ectopic lens, unexplained vascular occlusions, marfanoid habitus, and mental delay.

Management of CH_3-B_{12} deficiency or impaired methyl transfer with homocystinuria does not include methionine-restricted diets. Rather, pharmacologic amounts of vitamin B_{12}, folate, choline, or betaine are added, depending on the primary defect. Liver biopsy specimens, transformed lymphoblasts, or cultured skin fibroblasts express CBS and are used to confirm the most common cause of homocystinuria, and molecular screening and sequencing of the CBS gene are useful in predicting management. Prenatal diagnosis can be provided by direct enzyme assay of amniotic fluid cells or by DNA analysis if the mutations are known (212, 215, 217).

Treatment

Objectives of nutritional support in homocystinuria vary according to the age at which diagnosis is made and the specific cause. If homocystinuria is due to CBS deficiency expressed in the newborn, the clinical objectives are *(a)* to prevent the development of skeletal and ocular abnormalities, *(b)* to prevent intravascular thromboses, and *(c)* to ensure normal intellectual development.

Pharmacologic doses of pyridoxine should be tried in all patients with hypermethioninemia and homocystinemia (217–219). In newborns and early childhood, 25 to 100 mg/day should be tried for 4 weeks before methionine restriction. Older children and adults should be given oral pyridoxine (1 g/day). Pyridoxine's effect on plasma methionine and homocystine concentrations is monitored weekly on a "constant" protein intake. Because enzyme stabilization is the most common mechanism of vitamin responsivity, weeks may be required for a biochemical response to occur. If the plasma methionine and homocysteine concentrations are reduced, the amount of pyridoxine should be gradually lowered until the minimum dose required to maintain biochemical normality is reached. Doses of 25 to 750 mg/day have been required for some patients (219). Excess vitamin B_6 for prolonged periods may cause peripheral neuropathy (220) and liver injury (221); consequently, if vitamin B_6 is not helpful, it should be discontinued. Betaine supplements (6 g/day) will help maintain postprandial plasma homocysteine concentrations in the near-normal range in vitamin B_6-responsive individuals (222).

Patients who do not respond completely to pyridoxine require a methionine-restricted diet supplemented with L-cysteine. L-Cysteine becomes an essential amino acid in homocystinuria (Fig. 61.6). If plasma folate concentrations are below normal owing to excess use in remethylating homocysteine to methionine, folate should be added as a supplement.

Nutrient Requirements. In prescribing and implementing nutritional care plans for infants and children with homocystinuria due to CBS deficiency, one must consider energy, protein, methionine, cysteine, folate, vitamins B_6 and B_{12}, betaine, and fluid needs. Younger infants have a greater methionine requirement per kilogram of body weight than older infants. Suggested daily methionine intakes range from 35 mg/kg in the young infant to 5 mg/kg in the 15- to 19-year-old patient. Suggested beginning energy, protein, methionine, and fluid intakes for infants and children of different ages are given in Table 61.4. If the medical food mixture provides more than 24 kcal/oz, extra fluid should be offered between feedings to prevent dehydration.

Calcium cystinate, a soluble form of L-cysteine, should supplement the methionine-restricted diet at all ages. The young infant should be offered 300 mg/kg body weight. This amount may be decreased to 200 mg/kg at 6 months of age and 100 mg/kg at 3 years of age and thereafter. The calcium cystinate should be mixed with the chemically defined methionine-free medical food to provide even distribution throughout the day. Older children can sprinkle it in applesauce or other low-protein solids.

Methionine-Free Medical Foods. Several medical foods have been developed as protein sources for patients with homocystinuria (62–64). Formulations, composition of major nutrients, and sources of these products are given in Table 61.5.

Serving Lists. Methionine may be provided for the young infant by addition of specified amounts of proprietary infant formula to the methionine-free medical foods. As growth and development proceed, solid foods should be added at the usual ages. The methionine requirement is small, and most foods contain moderate amounts in relation to requirement (56–61). Because of this, the amount of solid food that can be ingested is small. To provide variety to the methionine-restricted diet, serving lists have been prepared (63). Average methionine, cystine, protein, and energy contents of these lists are given in Table 61.16.

Sample diets for children at 2 weeks and 4 years apply these principles in Tables 61.17 and 61.18. Prescription for methionine in a patient nonresponsive to vitamin B_6 will fall from about 35 mg/kg/day in the newborn period to about 10 mg/kg/day in the 2 year old.

Assessment of Nutritional Support. Following introduction of diet and stabilization, plasma methionine and cysteine concentrations should be monitored twice weekly until the patient is 3 months of age. Weekly monitoring is suggested until 6 months of age and twice monthly thereafter if blood methionine levels are stable. After a dietary change, plasma methionine and cysteine should be measured after 3 days have elapsed. A 3-day record prior to each blood sample is necessary to evaluate plasma methionine and cysteine. Plasma methionine should be maintained between 15 and 30 μM in fasting plasma. Little or no homocystine should be present in blood and urine. Growth and development as well as clinical evaluation of the pulses, skeletal growth and development, and ocular lenses are routinely assessed.

Results of Nutritional Support. In a retrospective study of 629 patients with CBS deficiency, methionine restriction initiated neonatally prevented mental retardation, decreased the frequency of lens dislocation, and reduced the incidence of seizures (217). Pyridoxine treatment of late-detected vitamin B_6–responsive patients decreased the rate of thromboembolic events (217). Weight and height in a girl with homocystinuria treated from the 9th day of life was at the 90th percentile (223). Hispanic male twins born at 38 weeks gestation with homocystinuria grew well during the entire 1st year of life while on nutrition support. Protein intake of these two patients averaged 3.7 g/kg/day during the first 6 months of life and 2.6 g/kg/day during the second 6 months. Energy intake averaged 131 kcal/kg during the first 6 months and 100 kcal/kg during the second 6 months (224).

Cysteine deficiency manifested as abnormally low plasma cysteine concentrations, elevated plasma methionine, and weight loss in a 3-year-old male with homocystinuria who received 32 mg/kg/day of L-cysteine was reported (225). The Hispanic twins referred to above received 58 to 118 mg cystine/kg/day, which resulted in

Table 61.16
Average Nutrient Content of Serving Lists for Methionine-Restricted Diets

Food List	Methionine (mg)	Cystine (mg)	Protein (g)	Fat (g)	Energy (kcal)
Breads/cereals	20	20	1.2	0	55
Fats	2	0	0.1	2	50
Fruits	5	5	0.5	0	60
Vegetables	10	8	1.0	0	20
Free foods A[a]	1	1	0.2	0	50
Free foods B	0	0	0	Varies	55
Enfamil with Iron[b], concentrate, 100 mL	58	35	3.0	7.6	135
Isomil[c], concentrate, 100 mL	80	48	3.3	7.4	135
ProSobee[b], concentrate, 100 mL	73	36	4.0	7.2	135
Similac[c] with Iron, concentrate, 100 mL	73	41	2.8	7.3	135

[a]Low-protein pastas and breads not included.
[b]Mead Johnson Nutritionals, Evansville, IN; 1/800-457-3550.
[c]Ross Products Division, Abbott Laboratories, Columbus, OH; 1/800-551-5838.

Table 61.17
Sample Diets for Homocystinuria (2 weeks of age): Weight 3.3 kg

Prescription	Total	per kg			
Methionine, mg	115	35			
Cystine, mg	975	300			
Protein, g	9.9	3.0			
Energy, kcal	390	120			
Medical Food #1	**Amount**	**MET, mg**	**CYS, mg**	**Protein, g**	**Energy, kcal**
Hominex-1	38 g	0	171	5.7	182
Similac w/Iron, concentrate	156 mL	114	64	4.4	211
L-CYS, 10 mg/mL	74 mL	0	740	0	0
Volume, water to make	600 mL				
Totals		114	975	10.1	393
Medical Food #2					
XMET Analog	42 g	0	164	5.5	200
Similac w/Iron, concentrate	156 mL	114	64	4.4	211
L-CYS, 10 mg/mL	75 mL	0	750	0	0
Volume, water to make	600 mL				
Totals		114	978	9.9	411

plasma cystine concentrations of 19 to 30 μmol/L (224). Up to 150 mg L-cysteine/kg/day may be required to maintain normal plasma cysteine concentrations (226).

Elevated plasma copper and ceruloplasmin concentrations were found in 15 patients with homocystinuria, compared with values found in age- and gender-matched normal controls. No relationship to plasma homocysteine could be found (227). The twins mentioned above had elevated serum copper concentrations of 151 and 144 μg/dL at about 13 months of age. Low plasma selenium concentration (about 15 μmol/L) and erythrocyte glutathione peroxidase activity (about 3 U/g Hgb) were found in a child with homocystinuria treated with a medical food free of selenium (228). Administration of 50 μg

Table 61.18
Diet Guide for Homocystinuria (4 years of age): Weight 17 kg

Prescription	Total	per kg			
Methionine, mg	139	8			
Cystine, mg	1950	115			
Protein, g	35.0	2.0			
Energy, kcal	1700	100			
Medical Food #1	**Amount**	**MET, mg**	**CYS, mg**	**Protein, g**	**Energy, kcal**
Hominex-2	84 g	0	756	25.2	344
L-CYS, 10 mg/mL	107 mL	0	1070	0	0
Table sugar	6 Tbsp	0	0	0	288
Volume, water to make	960 mL				
Foods					
Breads/cereals	4 svgs	80	80	4.8	220
Fats	5 svgs	10	0	0.5	125
Fruits	4 svgs	20	20	2.0	240
Vegetables	3 svgs	30	24	3.0	60
Free foods B	8 svgs	0	0	0	440
Totals		140	1950	35.5	1717
Medical Food #1					
XMET Maxamaid	103 g	0	772	25.8	370
L-CYS, 10 mg/mL	106 mL	0	1060	0	0
Sugar	6 Tbsp	0	0	0	228
Volume	960 mL				
Foods					
Breads/cereals	4 svgs	80	80	4.8	220
Fats	5 svgs	10	0	0.5	125
Fruits	4 svgs	20	20	2.0	240
Vegetables	3 svgs	30	24	3.0	60
Free foods B	8 svgs	0	0	0	440
Totals		140	1948	35.1	1733

selenium (in selenium-enriched yeast) every other day was required to maintain normal indices of selenium status. The twins mentioned above ingested, on average, 26 μg selenium (as sodium selenite) daily throughout the 1st year of life (224). Serum selenium concentrations ranged between 60 and 72 μg/L, very similar to values reported for normal human milk-fed babies (229).

Vitamin A absorption tests were carried out in eight untreated patients with homocystinuria by measuring the elevation in serum after administration of vitamin A alcohol (retinol). The explanation proposed for the resulting subnormal serum vitamin A elevation was that retinol was oxidized by -SH groups excreted into the gut (230). Of the eight plasma retinol values obtained on the twins studied, one was below 20 μg/dL and five were between 20 and 30 μg/dL. According to parental report, vitamin A intake was always more than adequate (1.20–5.58 times RDA for age). Serum transthyretin concentrations were all below 20 mg/dL (marginal), and two of the four values obtained were below 15 mg/dL (deficient) (224).

Fasting serum folate concentrations in eight untreated patients with homocystinuria were found to be abnormally low (4 ng/mL, compared with 8 ng/mL in control subjects). Two of these subjects were treated with 20 mg/day folate, which led to a decrease in urinary homocystine excretion (231). Severe folate deficiency was found in an untreated infant with homocystinuria who was receiving diluted boiled cow's milk for an episode of gastroenteritis. Excessive use of 5-methyltetrahydrofolate in the remethylation of homocysteine to form methionine is proposed as a reason for folate deficiency in untreated patients (232). The twins in our study had adequate hemoglobin concentrations after 4 months of age, and mean corpuscular volume was normal (224).

Termination of Nutritional Support. Most clinicians who treat individuals with homocystinuria believe that patients should be kept on the diet indefinitely. Termination of diet after growth is achieved may lead to thromboembolisms and ciliary muscle laxity with lens dislocation. When initiation or maintenance of nutritional support is not possible, acetylsalicylic acid (1 g/day) and dipyridamole (100 mg/day) increase platelet survival time and decrease thrombotic events (233). Vitamin B_6 in pharmacologic doses should be continued.

Reproductive Performance

Fewer conceptions are reported for both men and women who do not respond to vitamin B_6 than for those who do. Offspring of male patients do not suffer excess losses and are generally reported to be normal. A study showed that higher rates of fetal loss occurred in presumptive heterozygous fetuses carried by CBS-deficient mothers than occurred in normal women (217). Whether hypermethioninemia, homocysteinemia, or other metabolic variations in methionine metabolism are teratogenic is as yet unclear, but a teratogenic mechanism as defined for "maternal PKU" is possible. Also "folate"-responsive neural tube defects may involve hyperhomocyst(e)inemia as a pathophysiologic mechanism.

Carrier State. Heterozygotes for CBS deficiency may be at risk for premature vascular occlusion (222). The physician's duty to diagnose, inform, and treat extended family members of probands with CBS deficiency awaits further definition of this risk and outcomes of intervention (Chapter 34) (224).

AMMONIA

Nutritional management of disorders involving ammonia fixation and urea production uses traditional rules for treating inborn errors of metabolism. Three essential rules are restricting the toxic precursor, adding deficient product, and encouraging alternative pathways for nitrogen excretion. Furthermore, an anabolic state should be maintained to promote growth and prevent catabolism of lean body mass. Study of the biologic variation imparted on ammonia fixation and the urea cycle by heritable mutations in these biochemical reactions has greatly increased our understanding of the normal physiology, biochemistry, and molecular biology of human nitrogen metabolism (234).

Biochemistry

Central dogma holds that ammonia is converted to urea in the liver through the Krebs-Henseleit cycle (Fig. 61.7) and excreted in the urine. The first three enzymes of the cycle and *N*-acetylglutamate synthetase are mitochondrial. *N*-Acetylglutamate synthetase catalyzes the conversion of acetyl-CoA plus glutamate to *N*-acetylglutamate, an essential cofactor for carbamylphosphate synthesis. Carbamylphosphate synthetase I catalyzes the conversion of ammonia, ATP, and bicarbonate to carbamylphosphate. Ornithine transcarbamylase (OTC) uses carbamylphosphate and ornithine as cosubstrates to form citrulline, which is exported from mitochondria to the cytoplasm, where cytosolic reactions are linked to those three mitochondrial functions. Citrulline and aspartate form argininosuccinic acid, a reaction catalyzed by argininosuccinic acid synthetase. Fumarate is cleaved from argininosuccinic acid by argininosuccinic acid lyase, yielding arginine. Urea is then formed by the action of arginase, regenerating cytosolic ornithine, which is transported back into the mitochondria to react with OTC.

Urea Cycle Enzyme Deficiencies

Disorders of the urea cycle are a group of inherited defects in these six enzymes that produce urea (Fig. 61.7) (234). With the exception of OTC deficiency, all have an autosomal recessive mode of inheritance. OTC deficiency is inherited as an X-linked dominant trait that is usually lethal in males (234). Many of the genes for these enzymes have been localized to the human genome, cloned, and

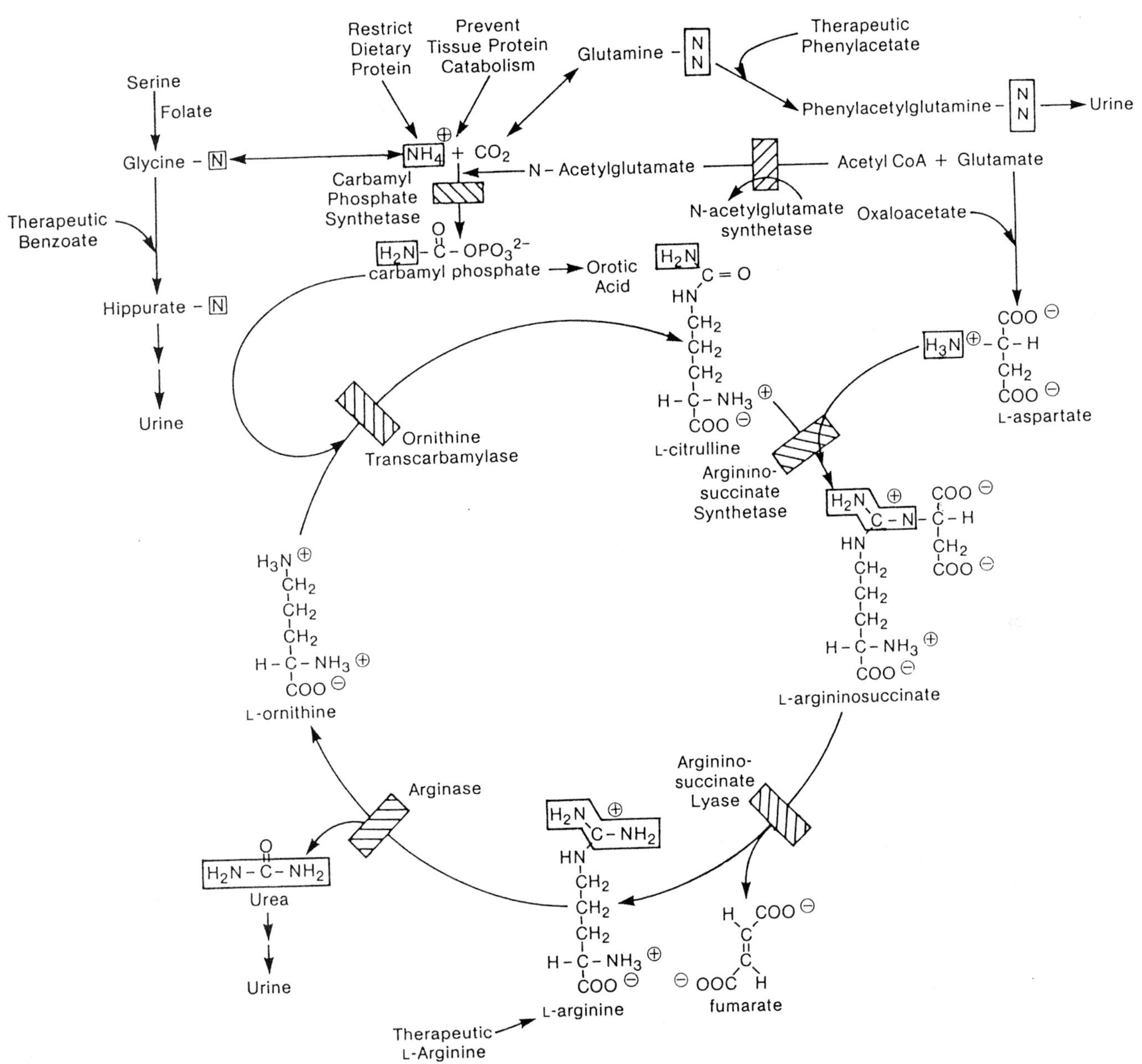

Figure 61.7. Inborn errors in the urea cycle and nutritional approaches to their management. Ammonia fixation and urea production are metabolically cycled with inherited blocks producing hyperammonemia indicated by *hatched bars*. Important nitrogen molecules and their biochemical origins are outlined in *boxes*. Mitochondrial enzymes in urea synthesis are carbamylphosphate synthetase, *N*-acetylglutamate synthetase, and ornithine transcarbamylase. Use of benzoate, phenylacetate, and phenylbutyrate is indicated to provide alternate pathways for nitrogen excretion. Dietary arginine is added to provide urea cycle substrate distal to genetically impaired reactions. Restriction of dietary protein and addition of dietary energy to prevent protein catabolism are also indicated.

had mutations defined. *OTC,* a 73-kb gene containing 10 exons, is located on Xp21.1. Over 20 mutations have been defined with some genotype/phenotype relationships. For example, the generation of stop codons from R109X and R109Q results in no residual liver enzyme and severe neonatal presentation. By contrast, the R129 to histidine mutation also present in the spf-ash mouse model of OTC deficiency has a milder phenotype and residual liver enzyme activity (235). Carbamylphosphate synthetase is located on 2p, argininosuccinic acid synthetase on 9q34, argininosuccinic acid lyase on 7q11, and arginase on 6q23. All are primarily expressed in liver, and all of these genes have defined mutations in their respective disorders (Table 61.19) (234–247). Argininosuccinic acid synthetase has several pseudogenes that confound DNA analysis (234, 243). In OTC deficiency, defects in the protein include disordered mitochondrial uptake and immunologically absent protein in this organelle (235). Arginase has two genes with differential expression in liver and erythrocytes. In addition to these defects in ureagenesis, a seventh cause of hyperammonemia is the HHH syndrome (hyperammonemia, homocitrullinemia, hyperornithinemia), which is caused by defective mitochondrial uptake of ornithine (247).

Table 61.19
Chromosomal Location, Gene Location, Gene Size, Number of Exons, and Tissue Distribution of Genes for Urea Cycle Enzymes

Enzyme	Chromosomal Location	cDNA/kb	Gene Size/No. Exons	Tissue Distribution
Mitochondria				
Carbamylphosphate synthetase	2p	5.2	Unknown	Liver, intestine, kidney (trace)
N-Acetylglutamate synthetase	Unknown	Unknown	Unknown	Liver, intestine, kidney (trace), spleen
Ornithine transcarbamylase	2q34-q35	1.06	73 kb/10	Liver, intestine, kidney (trace)
Cytosol				
Argininocuccinate synthetase	9q34, many pseudogenes	1.6	63 kb/14	Liver, kidney, fibroblasts, brain (trace)
Arginisosuccinate lyase	7cenq11.2	2.0	35 kb/16	Liver, kidney, brain, fibroblasts
Arginase	6q23	1.55	11.5 kb/8	Liver, erythrocytes, kidney, lens, brain (trace)

Hyperammonemia is a biochemical manifestation of all disorders of the urea cycle. Other biochemical characteristics of each defect follow: carbamylphosphate synthetase I defect causes decreased plasma citrulline; OTC deficiency results in orotic aciduria and X-linked patterns of transmission; argininosuccinate synthetase deficiency is associated with increased plasma citrulline accompanied by orotic aciduria; argininosuccinate lyase deficiency causes increased argininosuccinate in plasma and urine; and arginase deficiency has increased arginine in plasma and urine. Clinical features in the newborn suggesting urea cycle defects occur with protein ingestion. In increasing order of severity, these defects include poor feeding, vomiting, lethargy, hypotonia, stupor, bleeding diatheses, convulsions, coma, shock, and death. Mental retardation occurs in survivors of these disastrous newborn episodes, but successful control of hyperammonemia in the newborn may prevent this sequela.

Clinical Phenotypes

Hyperammonemia and its clinical sequelae of vomiting, lethargy, and coma relate to excessive protein intake or catabolism and are observed in all the defects. However, biochemical and phenotypic manifestations differ in the individual enzyme deficiencies. In argininosuccinate (ASA) lyase deficiency, a specific hair abnormality, trichorrhexis nodosa, is evident (Fig. 61.8). This condition is related to arginine deficiency and the relatively high arginine content of normal hair protein. Hair reverts to normal with arginine supplementation (Fig. 61.8). Adult siblings with ASA lyase deficiency may have little-to-no clinical manifestations despite identical mutations. In patients with defects of the first four enzymes, arginine deficiency has also been associated with progressive degeneration of the CNS, and a peculiar rash with control of hyperammonemia through protein restriction alone (236, 237).

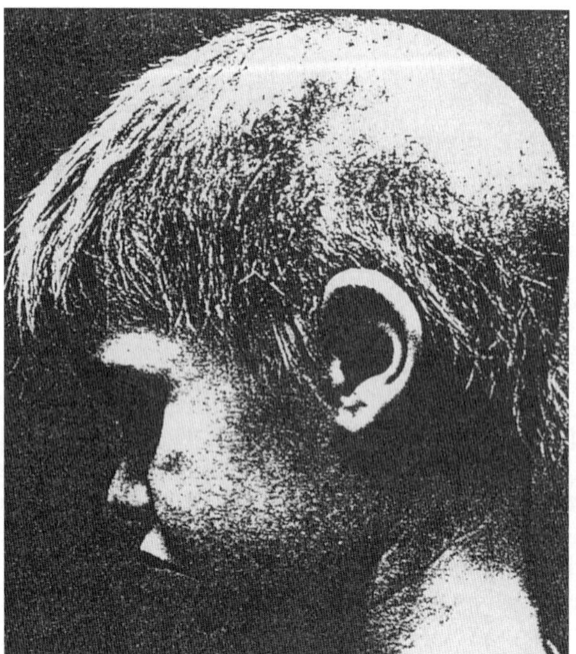

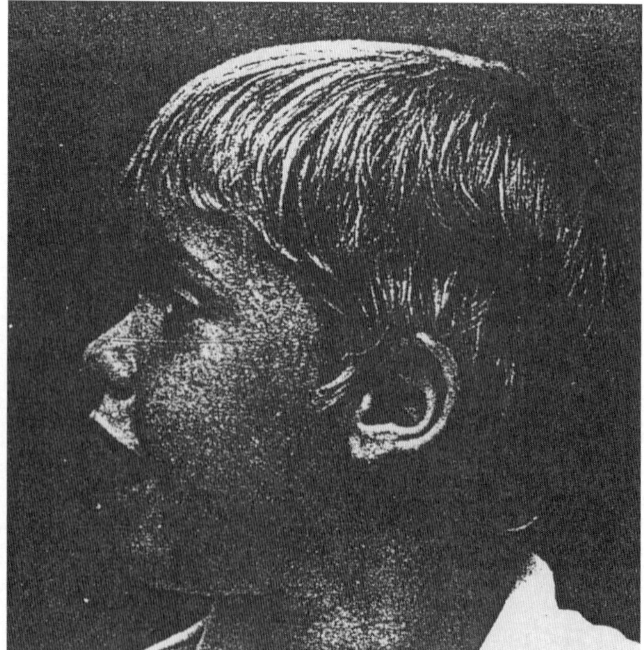

Figure 61.8. Effect of arginine on hair growth in argininosuccinic aciduria. A 6-year-old boy with hyperammonemia, trichorrhexis nodosa, and developmental delay was diagnosed with argininosuccinic aciduria. **A.** Before diet therapy he had diffuse, brittle hair. **B.** Six months later, while receiving 350 mg/kg/day arginine, he had luxuriant blond hair and his first haircut. (Courtesy of P. Fernhoff, Division of Medical Genetics, Emory University, Atlanta, GA).

Each enzyme defect has a spectrum of clinical manifestations ranging from death in the newborn period to cyclical vomiting and migraine in adolescence. For example, the typical male with OTC deficiency has less than 5% activity and dies in the neonatal period. A surviving male child with the "late-onset" form of OTC deficiency has immunologically present OTC with decreased affinity for ornithine, a shift of pH optimum, and 25% of normal activity under physiologic conditions (238). Mutational analyses of the *OTC* gene has differentiated "neonatal" from late-onset phenotypes (234, 235).

Enzymatic evidence for genetic heterogeneity comes from kinetic studies in fibroblasts of patients with argininosuccinic acid synthetase deficiency. Early biochemical studies showed that enzymes from patients with citrullinemia all exhibited decreased binding of citrulline and/or aspartate, but the residual argininosuccinic acid synthetase had a distinct and different curve of activity in each patient (239). Analyses of RNA in citrullinemic patients revealed heterogeneity, and over 20 different mutations are now defined (234, 240, 243).

Expression of the Heterozygous State for OTC Deficiency

The female heterozygote of OTC deficiency may have mild protein intolerance manifested clinically by migraine in adults and by cyclic vomiting with intermittent hyperammonemia in children (248). When protein or ammonium chloride loads were administered to 15 children with migraine and cyclic vomiting, 9 had abnormally high baseline plasma ammonium levels; the tests produced marked hyperammonemia in 8 and 6 developed migraine symptoms. Enzyme assay in seven girls with cyclical vomiting showed three with deficient OTC activity (248). Heterozygous females with OTC deficiency may be asymptomatic or as severely affected as hemizygous males (249).

Screening

Nonselected screening of all newborns for urea cycle disorders was routinely conducted in Massachusetts using a bacterial auxotroph that required arginine (250). Nine of 700,000 newborns were found to be homozygous-affected or heterozygous for ASA lyase deficiency (250). Selective screening tests for disorders of the urea cycle are available (251, 252). One method for selective screening for hyperammonemia in the newborn nursery requires drops of blood, can be performed at the bedside, and gives results in 15 minutes (253). This method can be readily adopted in offices and hospitals for selective screening. Its lack of use in this country is related to cost and demand.

The true incidence of urea cycle defects is not known because population-based screening has not been conducted, and many undiagnosed deaths may be caused by these disorders. The overall incidence is underestimated at 1 in 25,000 live births (254).

Diagnosis

Hyperammonemia in association with other characteristic biochemical and clinical findings is diagnostic of specific disorders in the urea cycle (234). The enzyme defect can be inferred from the metabolites (in addition to ammonia) that accumulate in blood and urine: orotic acid in the urine in OTC deficiency; and citrulline, argininosuccinic acid, and arginine in the plasma and urine in argininosuccinate synthetase, ASA lyase, and arginase deficiencies, respectively. Carbamylphosphate synthetase or the rare *N*-acetylglutamate synthetase deficiency is suggested by exclusion of these four enzymopathies and requires liver biopsy with enzyme analyses for diagnosis. Hyperammonemia can also be caused by acute or chronic liver diseases, galactosemia, neonatal Niemann-Pick type IC, tyrosinemia, hereditary fructose intolerance, Reye's syndrome, asparaginase treatment, propionic acidemia, hyperlysinemia, hyperornithinemia, isovaleric acidemia, methylmalonic aciduria, long-term use of parenteral amino acids, and a wide range of infectious agents in infancy. Definitive diagnosis depends on clinical acumen followed by appropriate laboratory studies. A suggested algorithm for differential diagnosis of urea cycle enzyme defects is given in Figure 61.9. A suspected urea cycle enzyme defect is a medical emergency and requires immediate intervention.

Treatment

The treatment of inherited urea cycle enzymopathies can be divided into short- and long-term therapy and depends on the specific diagnosis.

Short-Term Therapy. We prefer to begin orogastric perfusion with high energy intake (150 kcal/kg/day) but no protein. Pro-Phree or Protein-Free Diet Powder is useful for this approach (see Table 61.5). L-Arginine (350–500 mg/kg/day) should be added to this formulation. Sodium benzoate (300 mg/kg/day) can successfully reduce acute hyperammonemia in the neonatal period. Phenylbutyric acid or phenylacetic acid (500 mg/kg/day) is also given to form phenylacetylglutamine, which is excreted in the urine, eliminating from the body two nitrogen atoms per molecule (Fig. 61.7) (257). Addresses and telephone numbers of suppliers of these compounds are given in Table 61.20. Urinary potassium loss is enhanced by excretion of hippurate and phenylacetylglutamine. Consequently, plasma potassium concentrations should be monitored, and supplements given if needed.

Hemodialysis may be useful in the presence of coma in reducing plasma ammonium levels (255). Peritoneal dialysis for 7 days in a male neonate with OTC deficiency removed 50 times more ammonia than a single exchange transfusion did (256). However, peritoneal dialysis includes risks such as *Candida* peritonitis and continued catabolism. If dialysis is used, parenteral L-arginine and Ucephan (McGaw) should begin as well.

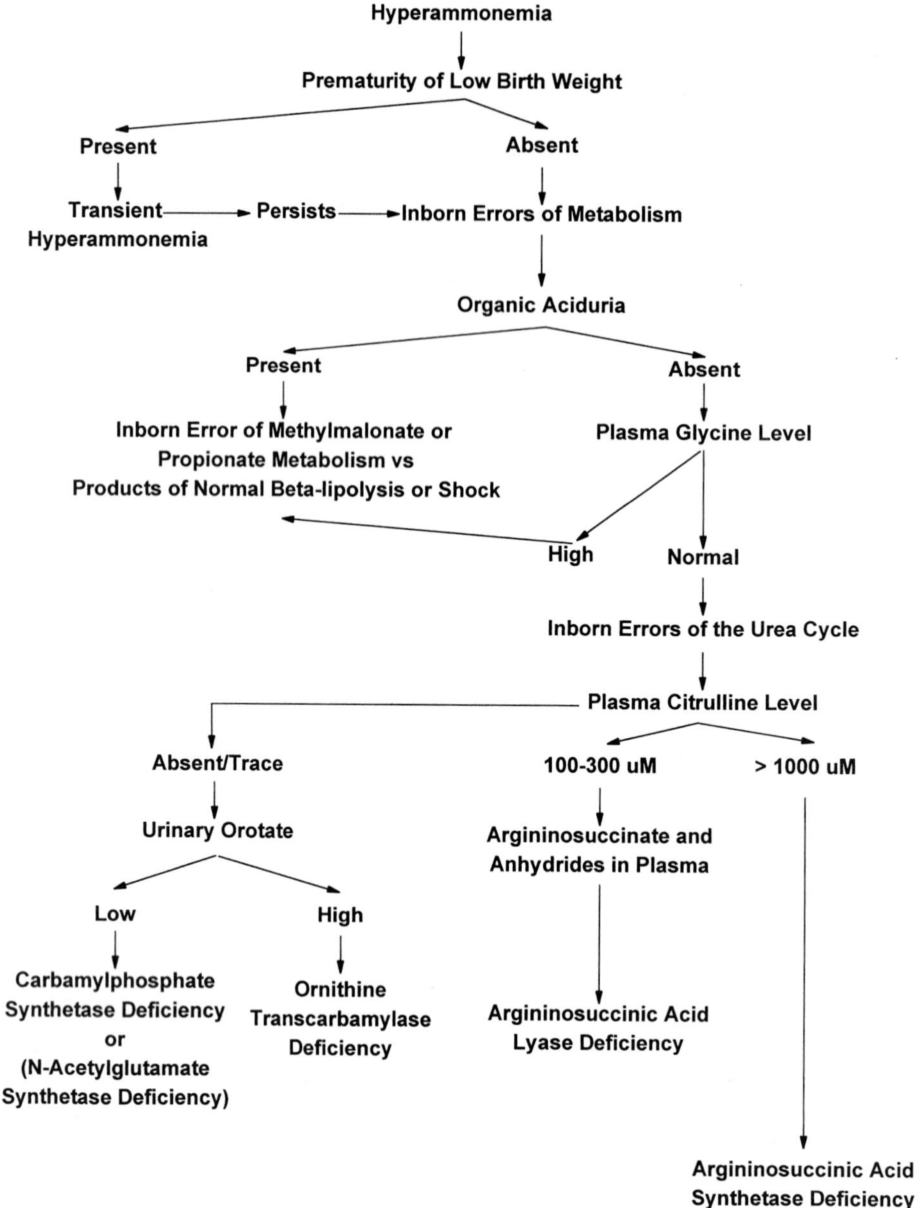

Figure 61.9. Algorithm for differential diagnosis of urea cycle disorders.

A priority of newborn therapy is to "force" the neonate into an anabolic phase with energy feedings. Peripheral venous hyperalimentation with 10 to 20% glucose and lipid (2–4 g/kg) may be necessary if gavage is not tolerated. As gavage feedings are increased, peripheral alimentation should be decreased. After 4 days of "no-protein," high-energy, arginine- and benzoate-supplemented feedings, blood ammonia levels should revert to near normal. Cautious addition of 1.0 to 1.5 g/kg/day of protein is then necessary.

Long-Term Therapy. The objectives of therapy in a child with a defect of the urea cycle are to maintain plasma concentrations of ammonia as near normal as possible, and to supply protein and other essential amino acids and nutrients that will allow maximal intellectual development and optimal growth. Four major approaches are used in treating individuals with urea cycle defects (Fig. 61.7): *(a)* reducing precursors of ammonia (protein intake), *(b)* correcting arginine deficiency, *(c)* enhancing alternate mechanisms of waste nitrogen loss, and *(d)* accelerating renal excretion of accumulated intermediates (234, 257).

Methods used to reduce ammonia precursors include protein restriction, prevention of body protein catabolism, and use of essential and "semiessential" amino acids. Any time intake of protein or essential amino acids is severely restricted, precursors for synthesis of carnitine (lysine, methionine), glutathione (cysteine, glutamate), and taurine (cysteine) may be limiting. Restricted methionine intake may result in a decrease in the available pool of labile methyl groups required for synthesis of important metabolic compounds.

Table 61.20
Suppliers of Medications and Nutritional Supplements Required for Treatment of Urea Cycle Disorders

Product	Supplier
Medications	
Sodium benzoate plus sodium phenylacetate (intravenous) (IND); Sodium phenylbutyrate powder and tablets (Buphenyl)	Ucyclyd Pharmacy, 10819 Gilroy Road, Hunt Valley, MD 21031, (410) 584-8188
Ucephan: a 10% solution of sodium benzoate plus 10% sodium phenylacetate (oral)	McGaw Laboratories, Inc., 2525 McGaw Avenue, Irvine, CA 92714, (800) 624-2963
Nutrition Supplements	
L-Arginine powder[a] (free base) L-Citrulline powder[a]	Ajinomoto USA, Inc., 500 Frank W. Burr Boulevard, Teaneck, NJ 07666-6894, (201) 488-1212; Tanabe USA, Inc., 7071 Convoy Court, San Diego, CA 93138, (619) 571-8410
L-Arginine powder[a] and capsules (free base)	Tyson and Associates, Inc., 12832 Chardron Avenue, Hawthorne, CA 90250-5525, (800) 367-7744
L-Arginine HCL[b] (10% pyrogen-free solution; 10% sterile solution for intravenous use)	KabiVitrum, Inc., 1311 Harbor Bay Parkway, Alameda, CA 94501, (800) 227-1518
L-Citrulline powder[a]	Seybridge Pharmacy, 37 New Haven Road, Seymour, CT 06483, (203) 888-0073, Ask for Peter Przybylski; Tyson and Associates, Inc., 1661 Lincoln Boulevard, Santa Monica, CA 90494, (800) 367-7744

[a]Amino acid powders have different densities. Consequently, they should be measured on a scale that reads in grams. A 1-week supply may be weighed and placed in a vial. The week's supply may then be mixed to a known volume in boiled water, capped, and stored in the refrigerator. The daily amount required may be measured in a disposable syringe or volumetric flask.

[b]Hyperchloremic acidosis may occur with high-dose L-arginine HCl. Consequently, plasma concentrations of chloride and bicarbonate should be monitored and bicarbonate administered if needed.

L-Arginine supplementation is required in all of the urea cycle enzyme defects except arginase deficiency. To maintain normal or slightly elevated plasma arginine concentrations, 100 to 500 mg/kg of body weight daily is used (258). L-Arginine can then produce ornithine for ammonia fixation and drive the cycle to citrulline and argininosuccinate (Fig. 61.7). These two amino acids are poorly absorbed by the kidney and allow nitrogen loss. Acceleration of renal excretion of accumulated intermediates in the impaired cycle is sought. Arginine supplementation increases citrulline and argininosuccinic acid excretion in argininosuccinic acid synthetase and ASA lyase deficiency, respectively (234, 258).

Waste nitrogen urinary loss can be enhanced by the use of sodium benzoate, phenylacetate, or phenylbutyrate (259) (Fig. 61.7). Glycine conjugates with benzoate via glycine-*N*-acylase, which leads to excretion of a nearly stoichiometric quantity of nitrogen as hippurate (Fig. 61.7). Toxicity is low on 200 to 500 mg/kg/day. Folate must be administered to provide a source of one-carbon fragments for synthesis of glycine from serine to prevent glycine depletion (260). Pyridoxine is necessary for transamination. Phenylbutyrate and phenylacetate increase urinary nitrogen excretion as phenylacetylglutamine (258, 259) (Fig. 61.7). The suggested dose is 500 mg/kg body weight. This efficient alternative pathway removes two molecules of nitrogen per molecule of phenylacetylglutamine and requires monitoring of protein intake to prevent deficiency. Excess use of these nitrogen-binding drugs can lead to nitrogen deficiency and poor growth.

Catabolism during a febrile illness or because of poor appetite may lead to life-threatening elevations in blood ammonia. In addition to prompt diagnosis and treatment of the infection, decreased protein intake (0 g for 1–2 days), increased energy intake, and peritoneal dialysis may all be required. Gastrostomy feedings may be required to ensure adequate intake and prevent inadequate growth or catabolism.

In planning nutritional support of the infant or child with a defect of a urea cycle enzyme, a formal prescription for the day should be written that includes recommended amounts of protein, energy, fluid, L-arginine, and drugs that enhance nitrogen loss. The prescription for protein should be based on the specific diagnosis, degree of impaired urea cycle, and blood ammonia concentrations and correlated with various parameters of growth, including rates of height and weight increase, and hair, nails, teeth, and skin changes.

Protein intakes suggested in Table 61.21 are based on amounts required to cover obligatory nitrogen losses and growth needs (261) of infants and children fed an excellent protein source such as egg or milk. Intakes may need to be increased if the child fails to grow adequately on the recommended intake or if sodium benzoate, phenylacetate, or phenylbutyrate is administered. Renal capacity to excrete excess acidity as NH_4^+ is modulated by the amount of protein ingested (262). Overrestriction of protein may lead to catabolism and impaired renal activity to excrete NH_4^+. Tryptophan intake should be at the minimal requirement for growth to prevent excess serotonin synthesis that suppresses appetite (207, 208).

Energy intakes recommended in Table 61.21 are somewhat higher than those for normal infants and children to provide ketoacid precursors from carbohydrate for synthesis of nonessential amino acids and to prevent protein degradation. Carbohydrate should not provide more than 50% of the energy because of frequently elevated plasma triacylglycerol concentrations.

In any situation in which protein-restricted diets are fed, L-carnitine supplements may be necessary. Recommended amounts of supplemental L-carnitine are 50 to 100 mg/kg/day. L-Carnitine supplements are reported to lower blood ammonium concentrations (263, 264).

Table 61.21
Recommended Daily Nutrient Intakes (Ranges) for Infants, Children, and Adults with Urea Cycle Disorders

	Nutrient			
Age	L-ARG[a] Free Base (g/kg)	Protein[b] (g/kg)	Energy (kcal/kg)	Fluid (mL/kg)
Infants				
0 to <3 months	500–100	2.20–1.25	150–125	160–130
3 to <6 months	400–100	2.00–1.15	140–120	160–130
6 to <9 months	300–100	1.80–1.05	130–115	150–125
9 to <12 months	300–100	1.60–1.00	120–110	130–120
	(g/day)	(g/day)	(kcal/day)	(mL/day)
Girls and boys				
1 to <4 years	1300–2600	8–12	945–1890	945–1890
4 to <7 years	2000–4000	12–15	1365–2415	1365–2445
7 to <11 years	2800–5600	14–17	1730–3465	1730–3465
Women				
11 to <15 years	4600–9200	20–23	1575–3150	1575–3150
15 to <19 years	5500–11000	20–23	1260–3150	1260–3150
≥19 years	5800–11600	22–25	1785–2625	1875–2625
Men				
11 to <15 years	4500–9000	20–23	2100–3885	2100–3885
15 to <19 years	6600–13200	21–24	2200–4095	2200–4095
≥19 years	7200–14400	23–32	2625–3465	2625–3465

[a]Not used with arginase deficiency.
[b]Protein intake may need to be increased if sodium benzoate, sodium phenylacetate, or sodium phenylbutyrate is prescribed.

Citrate deficiency has been reported in patients with ASA lyase deficiency, and supplementation was recommended (265, 266).

Medical Foods for Urea Cycle Disorders. Nutritional support of urea cycle disorders requires restricting nitrogen intake, which is best accomplished by providing about one-half to two-thirds the prescribed protein in the form of essential amino acids only. Formulation, composition, and sources of medical foods for urea cycle enzyme defects are given in Table 61.5. Cyclinex-1 and Cyclinex-2 contain 25 mg of L-carnitine per gram of protein (63).

Serving Lists. Serving lists of natural foods are available to simplify protein-restricted diets for professionals and for families (Table 61.6).

Assessment of Nutritional Support. Frequency of assessment is, in part, dictated by the clinical course of the patient. Blood ammonia concentrations should be monitored routinely and maintained below 50 μM. Plasma concentrations of amino acids should be monitored and maintained in the normal range. Plasma albumin and globulin concentrations are indices of protein status and should be evaluated frequently. Plasma transthyretin and retinol-binding protein have shorter half-lives than albumin and can provide information on protein status at an earlier stage in deficiency than albumin can. Caretakers should provide dietary diaries and records of health status in tandem with blood for ammonia and plasma amino acid determinations. Growth and development should be routinely assessed. If evidence of protein deficiency occurs or growth is not maintained, increased protein intake is necessary.

Results of Nutritional Support. Results of therapy in infants with complete or near-complete enzyme deficiencies have been less than optimal, with delayed death and below-normal development. If the serious brain swelling and coma are prevented in the neonatal period or if onset of disease expression is delayed, physical growth and mental development are more nearly normal with nutritional and pharmacologic support (234). If diagnosis is anticipated and treatment is begun during the neonatal period in affected siblings with citrullinemia or argininosuccinic acidemia, relatively normal outcome is observed even with severe enzyme defects (267).

GALACTOSE

Biochemistry

Because lactose is the principal carbohydrate and energy source for infants and young children, galactose maintains a central metabolic role in human nutrition. Lactose is hydrolyzed in the intestine by lactase to glucose and galactose, and 0.5 to 1.0 mg galactose/kg/min is produced (268). Galactose is converted to glucose-1-P and energy through the Leloir pathway. This occurs primarily in the liver, where galactose becomes glucose through three enzymatic steps (Fig. 61.10). First, galactose is phosphorylated to galactose-1-phosphate (Gal-1-P) by galactokinase. The rate-limiting and evolutionarily conserved step is the transfer of the uridyl moiety from uridine diphosphate (UDP)-glucose to UDP-galactose (UDP-Gal) with the consumption of Gal-1-P and release of free glucose-1-phosphate. This complex bimolecular, two-substrate catalytic reaction is catalyzed by Gal-1-P uridyltransferase (GALT) (Fig. 61.10). UPD-gal can be converted back to

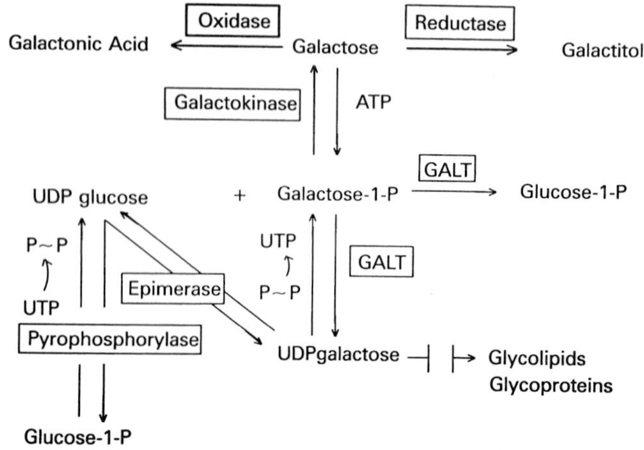

Figure 61.10. Metabolic blocks in galactose metabolism that lead to galactosemia. Genetic disorders of catalyzed reactions are indicated by *hatched bars*.

UDP-glucose through a reversible reaction to UDP-Gal-4-epimerase (Fig. 61.10). The glucose thus formed can be used for glycogen synthesis or phosphorylated to glucose-1-phosphate for further energy production. UPD-Gal is an important precursor for galactated membrane proteins and glycolipids.

Galactosemia

Galactosemia may occur because of deficient functioning of any of three enzymes: galactokinase, GALT, or UDP-Gal-4-epimerase (269) (Fig. 61.10). Patients with galactokinase deficiency have only cataracts, but also produce galactitol and galactonic acid through alternate pathways (Fig. 61.10). Galactokinase deficiency does not produce the acute hepatotoxic manifestations or the accumulation of Gal-1-P seen with GALT deficiency. Several variants with different degrees of function and structure have been described for mutant GALT (275). This gene locus is on chromosome 9p (270–272). The cDNA and gene for GALT have been accurately sequenced, and many different mutations identified (272–277).

Galactosemia due to deficiency of GALT leads to accumulation of Gal-1-P, which may act as a phosphate sink, reducing intracellular phosphate for high-energy phosphate bonds. Thus, ATP, GTP (guanosine triphosphate), and CTP (cytidine triphosphate) levels are reduced. Gal-1-P may also inhibit galactation of phospholipids and phosphoproteins by competitive inhibition. Several other hypotheses for the pathophysiology of GALT deficiency include UPD-gal deficiency, galactose excess with galactation of membrane proteins, and galactitol accumulation with deleterious effects on intracellular osmolality (278–280). Many or all of these postulated pathologic processes are probably involved.

Clinical symptoms of the GALT defect appear early in infancy. About 10% of infants with GALT deficiency are born with cataracts. Acute hepatotoxicity may appear with the start of milk feeding. Prolonged neonatal jaundice at 4 to 10 days of age is common. Hyperbilirubinemia and hyperammonemia may be exacerbated by toxic injury to liver cells by delayed maturation of glucuronyl transferase (281), mild hemolysis, and bleeding. Bleeding diatheses, *Escherichia coli* sepsis, and shock are catastrophic events that occur during the neonatal period. Therefore, rapid screening, retrieval, diagnosis, and treatment are essential for population-based newborn screening programs if the clinical sequelae of neonatal galactosemia are to be prevented. Other relatively minor symptoms occur. Anemia from various causes is present in about 40% of untreated patients. Lethargy, hypotonia, food refusal, vomiting, and diarrhea are also common symptoms in infancy.

Retarded mental and physical growth occur in most of the untreated patients who survive (282). The pathophysiology of galactosemia remains unclear, but early diet clearly prevents neonatal sepsis, shock, and bleeding. Whether intrauterine effects of accumulated galactose or deficiency of UDP-gal (286) causes the pathology remains for further study. Cataracts occur in about 45% of untreated children and are thought to result from formation and accumulation of galactitol in the lens of the eye, which is impermeable to efflux. Galactitol creates an osmotic gradient that allows glutathione to efflux and results in decreased concentrations of lens glutathione. When glutathione concentrations are decreased, glutathione peroxidase is inactivated, and hydrogen peroxide accumulates to toxic levels. Hydrogen peroxide denatures lens protein, producing lenticular cataracts (269, 281). Hepatomegaly occurs in nearly all cases of GALT deficiency, and cirrhosis develops in untreated patients. Liver damage results in decreased synthesis of liver coagulants and albumin, and a decrease in a wide range of liver functions. Because of decreased albumin synthesis and proteinuria, ascites and generalized edema occur in about 36% of untreated patients (281). The albumin synthesized by untreated patients with galactosemia contains large amounts of galactose, whereas albumin of normal individuals is free of galactose (287). Untreated or poorly controlled patients are extremely susceptible to infection with gram-negative organisms. Immunoincompetence is probably a direct result of inhibition by Gal-1-P of immune protein synthesis by lymphocytes and inactivation of leukocyte phagocytosis. Galactose and its accumulated metabolites are toxic to the glomeruli and tubules of the kidney. Additionally, active tubular transport is impaired because of deficient ATP, producing generalized aminoaciduria and loss of phosphate, potassium, and bicarbonate. On rare occasions, hypoglycemia occurs. Causes include defective hepatic gluconeogenesis, the inability to convert glycogen to glucose because of inhibition of phosphorylase kinase by Gal-1-P, and hyperinsulinemia that may result from galactose stimulation of pancreatic β cells and decreased hepatic extraction of insulin (281).

Despite early diagnosis and removal of galactose during the neonatal period, some patients with classic (G/G) galactosemia have long-term poor outcomes, including infertility in females, growth failure, dyspraxic speech, ataxia, and mental retardation (282, 283). This has been called the "enigma" of galactosemia (269, 278). This enigmatic outcome may be of intrauterine origin and has been associated with more-severe mutations in GALT. For example, the Q188R mutation in exon 6 is prevalent among Caucasians and more prevalent among classic galactosemia patients with two or more of the above chronic deficits (277, 278). By contrast, the S135L mutation in exon 5 of the GALT gene is associated with good outcomes in patients treated from birth, is prevalent in black patients, and has differential expression in different organs (284). Other variant mutations, such as the Duarte variant (N314D), when associated with G alleles such as E203K may return structural integrity and function to the dimeric GALT protein function and produce a "good" clinical outcome (273, 275, 276). Over 57 mutations have been defined to date in patients with galactosemia (Table 61.22).

Table 61.22
Sequence Changes in the Human GALT Gene found in Patients with Galactosemia

Amino Acid Changes	Exon	Nucleotide Change	Conserved
Del > 5KB (Δ GALT)	1–10		Yes
Asp 28 Tyr (D28Y)	1	GAC → TAC	No
Ile 32 Asn (I32N)	2	ATC → AAC	No
Gln 38 Pro (Q38P)	2	CAG → CCG	No
Val 44 Leu (V44L)	2	GTG → TTG	Yes
Val 44 Met (V44M)	2	GTG → ATG	Yes
Gln 54 Stop (Q54X)	2	CAG → T AG	Yes
Leu 62 Met (L62M)	2	CTG → ATG	No
Arg 67 Cys (R67C)	2	CGC → TGC	No
Leu 74 Pro (L74P)	2	CTG → CCG	Yes
Ala 81 Thr (A81T)	2	GCC → ACC	No
Del 38 (frameshift)	3	bp281 → 318	Yes
IVSC	4	bp956 A → C	Yes
Asp 113 Asn (D113N)	4	GAT → AAT	No
Phe 117 Ser (F117S)	4	TTC → TCC	No
Arg 123 Gly (R123G)	4	CGA → GGA	Yes
Lys 127 Glu (K127E)	5	AAG → GAG	No
Ser 135 Leu (S135L)	5	TCG → TTG	No
Thr 138 Met (T138M)	5	ACG → ATG	Yes
Leu 139 Pro (L139P)	5	CTG → CCG	No
Met 142 Lys (M142K)	5	ATG → AAG	No
Ser 143 Leu (S143L)	5	TCG → TTG	No
Arg 145 Gln (R148Q)	5	CGC → CAG	No
Arg 148 Trp (R148W)	5	CGG → TGG	No
Arg 151 Ala (V151A)	5	GTT → GCT	Yes
Trp 154 Gly (W154G)	5	TGG → GGG	Yes
Phe 171 Ser (F171S)	6	TTT → TCT	Yes
Gln 188 Arg (Q188R)	6	CAG → CGG	Yes
IVSF	7	bp1632 A → G	Yes
Ser 192 Asn (S192N)	7	AGC → AAC	No
Leu 195 Pro (L195P)	7	CTG → CCG	Yes
Ile 198 Met (II98M)	7	ATT → ATG	No
Arg 201 His (R201H)	7	CGT → CAT	No
Glu 203 Lys (E203K)	7	GAG → AAG	No
Tyr 209 Cys (Y209C)	7	TAT → TGT	Yes
Gln 212 Stop (Q212X)	7	CAG → TAG	No
Arg 231 His (R231H)	8	CGT → CAT	Yes
Arg 258 Cys (R258C)	8	CGT → TGT	No
Arg 259 Trp (R259W)	8	CGG → TGG	No
Lys 285 Asn (K285N)	9	AAG → AAT	No
Glu 291 Lys (E291K)	9	GAG → AAG	No
Glu 308 Lys (E308K)	10	GAG → AAG	No
Asn 314 Asp (N314D)	10	AAC → GAC	No
Trp 316 Stop (W316X)	10	TGG → TAG	Yes
His 319 Gln (H319Q)	10	CAC → CAA	Yes
Ala 320 Thr (A320T)	10	GCT → ACT	No
Tyr 323 Asp (Y323D)	10	TAC → GAC	Yes
Pro 324 Ser (P324S)	10	CCT → TCT	Yes
Ala 330 Val (A330V)	10	GCC → GTC	Yes
Arg 333 Trp (R333W)	10	CGG → TGG	Yes
Lys 334 Arg (K334R)	10	AAA → AGA	Yes
IVSJ	10	bp2919 C → T	Yes
Glu 340 Stop (E340X)	10	GAA → TAA	Yes
Thr 350 Ala (T350A)	10	ACC → GCC	No
Tyr 336 Stop (Y366X)	11	TAC → TAA	No
Gln 370 Stop (Q370X)	11	CAG → TAG	No

Screening

GALT deficiency of clinical importance to the neonate is found in approximately 1:8000 births (Table 61.3). Based on 1.7 million newborns screened in Georgia, about 1:40,000 have classic (G/G) galactosemia while about 1:10,000 have variant forms. The most common screening method used is the Beutler fluorescent test for galactosemia (288). This procedure consists of incubating dried blood on filter paper disks with a mixture of uridine diphosphoglucose (UDPG), galactose-1-P, and NADP. Erythrocytes from normal individuals containing GALT and phosphoglucomutase produce glucose-1-phosphate, glucose-6-phosphate, and fluorescent NADPH through the linked reaction of glucose-6-phosphate dehydrogenase. If heat has inactivated this reaction (e.g., in summer), glucose-1-phosphate is added to differentiate between heat inactivation of GALT and GALT deficiency (true galactosemia).

Galactose-1-P + UDP glucose
↓ galactose-1-P uridyl transferase
UDP galactose + Glucose-1-P
↓
Glucose-6-P + NADP
↓
6-P-gluconate + NADPH

Positive screening results occur with classic (G/G) GALT deficiency and with variants of GALT that are thermolabile such as the Duarte/galactosemia compound heterozygote. Confirmation of positive Beutler screening test results requires the use of erythrocyte hemolysates for quantitative enzyme activity determinations and quantitation of erythrocyte galactose and Gal-1-P content. A combined analysis of the GALT biochemical phenotype and molecular genotype is important for diagnosis, therapy, prognosis, and genetic counseling (275, 277).

Diagnosis

Patients with positive Beutler test results should have all lactose removed from their diets immediately while enzyme diagnosis and family workup proceed. Fresh, sterile heparinized blood should be sent to a central laboratory experienced in enzyme analyte and molecular analyses. Both patient and parents should be evaluated by the center for biochemical phenotype and molecular genotype. Diagnosis of galactosemia is accomplished through measurement of activity of GALT in erythrocytes, erythrocyte Gal-1-P content, and molecular analysis of the GALT gene for prevalent mutations. No activity occurs in individuals homozygous for the classic disease (G/G), whereas heterozygotes (G/N) have approximately one-half normal activity. Since the Q188R allele occurs in 70% of Caucasians with G/G galactosemia, it is easy to identify (277, 278). The Duarte allele (N314D) has a characteristic isozyme pattern when erythrocytes are studied by isoelectric focusing for the GALT enzyme. The need for therapy in patients with an activity of 25% or less of GALT, as in compound heterozygotes for Duarte/galactosemia alleles, has not been established. However, galactose should be restricted in early life for patients with any mutant genotype if erythrocyte Gal-1-P is more than 2 mg/dL or urinary galactitol exceeds 5 mmol/mol creatinine.

GALT is expressed in cultured amniotic fluid cells and chorionic villi. Thus, GALT deficiency can be detected prenatally by both direct enzyme assay and DNA analysis if the mutations are known. Amniotic fluid of a fetus with galactosemia has recently been found to have an elevated concentration of galactitol. Assessment of the galactitol content of amniotic fluid by GC/MS provides an ancillary method for prenatal diagnosis and may perhaps be related to enigmatic outcome (289).

Treatment

Objectives of therapy in galactosemia are to ameliorate or prevent symptoms while providing adequate energy and nutrients for normal growth and development. Treatment should begin as early in life as possible and consists of removal of all sources of lactose and galactose from the diet of patients with no enzyme activity. Patients with GALT activity above 5 to 10% of normal may tolerate small amounts of galactose found in muscle meats, fruits, and vegetables.

Nutrient Requirements. Energy and nutrient requirements of infants and children with well-controlled galactosemia are the same as those for normal individuals of the same age, gender, and physical activity level. Whether above-normal energy and protein intakes prevent the linear growth retardation seen in poorly controlled children is not known.

Formulas. Human milk contains 6 to 8% lactose; cow's milk, 3 to 4% lactose; and many proprietary infant formulas, 7% lactose. These milks must be replaced by a formula free of bioavailable galactose (Isomil Soy Formula with Iron, Ross Products Division, or Prosobee, Mead Johnson Nutritionals).

Formulas containing soy protein isolate have about 14 mg galactose/L in the form of raffinose and stachyose, oligosaccharides that contain galactose. At one time it was thought that these oligosaccharides yielded free galactose on hydrolysis in the intestine. It is now believed that the human intestine has no enzymes to hydrolyze these oligosaccharides (290). Thus, they may be safely used for feeding infants and children with galactosemia. RCF (Ross Products Division) and Next Step Soy Formula (Mead Johnson Nuritionals) may be used by children and adults who require a galactose-free formula. Casein hydrolysates such as Alimentum, Nutramigen, and Pregestimil (Mead Johnson Nutritionals) have been treated to remove lactose but may still contain small amounts of galactose. Data in Table 61.23 describe foods allowed in, and excluded from, the galactose-restricted diet.

Free Galactose in the Diet. Milk and milk products are well-known sources of lactose and casein. Less well known is that different forms of casein and cheeses contain galactose in various amounts (291–293). Based on studies by botanists and plant physiologists that began in the early 1950s, it is clear that cereals, fruits, legumes, nuts, seeds, tubers, and vegetables contain galactose. But many believe that the galactose in these foods is in linkages resistant to human digestive enzymes. Many fruits and vegetables, however, contain free (soluble) galactose in amounts ranging from less than 0.5 mg/100 g to 35.4 mg/100 g fresh weight (294). Ten of 12 baby foods had detectable amounts of free galactose, with applesauce and squash containing the largest amounts (295). Galactose has also been found in fermented cocoa beans (296).

Oral loads of raffinose and stachyose have been administered to one patient with GALT deficiency (290). No changes were observed in erythrocyte Gal-1-P, the analyte used to monitor dietary compliance. Soybean formula was fed to a 14 year old with GALT deficiency, and an insignificant change in Gal-1-P was found (297). These observations led clinicians to suggest that legumes could be used freely in the diets of patients with GALT deficiency, although explicit warning of the possible release of absorbable free galactose in the small intestine by bacteria when the patient had diarrhea had been given (290). Ingestion of legumes over a 5-year period led to a 21 to 100% increase in erythrocyte Gal-1-P in four patients with GALT deficiency, while of four patients who did not receive legumes, three had decreases in Gal-1-P of 17, 19, and 23%, and one patient had an increase of 37% (298). Chickpea flour contains 110 mg free galactose per 100 g flour (299). Free galactose in six types of cooked legumes ranged from 42 to 444 mg/100 g dry beans (300). Many legumes (dried beans and peas), cereals, fruits, nuts, seeds, and vegetables have not yet been analyzed for free galactose. Until such analyses are conducted, we will not know the extent of free galactose in foods.

Bound Galactose in Food and Drugs. Bound galactose is present in lactose, arabinogalactans I and II, feruloylated galactose, galactan, glycolipids, galactinol, galactopinitols, and rhamnogalacturonans I and II (300). Lactose is found in milk and dairy products and as an extender in many over-the-counter and prescription drugs (301). Hash-browned potatoes and some other prepared foods contain added lactose, and some chefs sprinkle meat with lactose before frying for faster and better browning (300, 302). Calcium lactobionate, the active ingredient in Neo-calglucon, a liquid calcium supplement, is a substrate of β-galactosidases (303) and yields free galactose.

Organ meats such as brain, kidney, liver, pancreas, and spleen contain galactosylcerebrosides, gangliosides, and lactosyl sulfatide. These compounds are constantly turned over in living organisms. In patients with GALT deficiency, the free galactose liberated is metabolized to Gal-1-P or other metabolites such as galactitol (304). Glycoproteins found in muscle meats contribute significant amounts of galactose to the diet (305).

Table 61.23
Galactose-Restricted Diet

Foods Allowed	Foods Excluded
Beverages	
Carbonated drinks; Isomil[a]; Next Step Soy Formula[b]; ProSobee[b]; RCF[a]; and other formulas made with soy protein isolate; fruit drinks free of apple, banana, papaya, pear, watermelon	Calcium caseinate– or sodium caseinate–containing beverages; some cocoas and instant coffees (read labels); hot chocolate; imitation or filled milks; malted milk; milk -all untreated of any species and all products containing milk, whether buttermilk, whole, skim, dried, evaporated, or condensed; milk treated with *Lactobacillus acidophilus* culture or lactase; Ovaltine; powdered soft drinks with lactose
Breads, cereals, and grains	
Breads, crackers, and rolls made without milk; Italian bread; some cooked and prepared creals (read labels), soda crackers, pasta; contact bakeries in each geographic area for milk-free breads; barley, buckwheat, oats, rye, rice, wheat	Prepared mixes, such as biscuits, muffins, pancakes, or waffles; some dry cereals (read labels carefully); instant Cream of Wheat; cereals, breads, crackers, French toast made with milk, zwieback
Cheeses	
None	All excluded
Desserts	
Water and fruit ices made with allowed fruit juices; gelatin, angel food cake; homemade cakes, pies, cookies made from allowed ingredients; puddings made with water, Isomil, ProSobee, or RCF; sorbets	Commercial cakes, cookies, and mixes; custard, ice cream, puddings, and sherbets made with milk; any containing milk chocolate; pie crust made with butter or margarine that contains milk or soy flour
Eggs	
All	Omelets and souffles containing milk
Fats	
Margarines and salad dressings that do not contain milk or milk products; bacon; lard; nut butters; oils; shortening; some nondairy creamers (read label)	Margarines and dressings containing milk or milk products or soy; butter, cream, cream cheese, peanut butter with milk solid fillers, salad dressings containing lactose or milk products; nondairy creamers containing sodium or calcium caseinate; sour cream; whipping cream
Fruits[c,d]	
Canned, fresh, or frozen fruits that do not contain galactose and are not processed with lactose; apricot; avocado; cantaloupe; fruit cocktail; grapefruit; grapes, green; nectarines; oranges; peaches	Any canned or frozen fruits processed with lactose; apples, applesauce; bananas; dates; figs; kiwi fruit; oranges; papayas; pears; persimmons, American; watermelon; and juices containing these fruits
Legumes, nuts, seeds	
Peanuts, peanut butter, nuts except hazel nuts	All legumes (dry beans and peas); hazel nuts; seed kernel or flour of pumpkin, safflower, sesame, sunflower
Meat, fish, poultry	
Plain beef, chicken, fish, ham, lamb, pork, veal, strained or junior meats that do not contain milk or milk products, kosher frankfurters	Creamed or breaded meat, fish, or fowl; sausage products such as cold cuts, liver sausage, wieners containing nonfat milk solids; brains, kidney, liver, pancreas, sweetbreads
Soups	
Clear consommes, cream soups, or soups made with nondairy creamers free of caseinate; vegetable soups made with allowed vegetables	Chowders; commercially prepared soups containing lactose; cream soups; vegetable soups unless made with allowed ingredients;
Vegetables[c,f]	
Canned, fresh, or frozen vegetables; artichokes; asparagus; bean sprouts, green; beets; cabbage; cauliflower; celery; chard; corn; cucumbers; eggplant; kale; lettuce; mushrooms, common; mustard greens; okra; parsley; parsnips; potatoes, white; radishes; rutabagas; spinach; turnips; squash, zucchini; all vegetables not containing galactose if prepared without lactose	Any vegetable to which lactose is added during processing; breaded, buttered, or creamed vegetables; instant potatoes, corn curls, and frozen French fries if processed with lactose; bell peppers; broccoli; brussels sprouts; carrots; onions; peas; pumpkin; sweet potatoes; tomatoes in any form; V-8 juice; yams
Miscellaneous	
Baker's cocoa; beet sugar; carob powder; corn syrup; gravy made with water; honey; jelly or marmalade; malt powder; molasses, olives; pickles; popcorn; pure monosodium glutamate; pure seasoning and spices; pure sugar candy; sugar	Artificial sweeteners containing lactose; Bean-O; butterscotch; caramels; dietetic preparations (read labels); certain drugs, such as estrogen and progestin, and vitamin and mineral preparations; some cocoas; chewing gum; milk chocolate; monosodium glutamate extender; Neocalglucon; peppermint; spice blends if they contain lactose; toffee

[a]Ross Products Division, Abbott Laboratories, Columbus, OH 43215.

[b]Mead Johnson Nutritional Division, Evansville, IN 47221.

[c]Gross KC, Acosta PB. J Inherited Metab Dis 1991;14:253–258.

[d]Matthews RH, Pehrsson R, Farhat-Sabet M. Sugar Content of Selected Foods; Individual and Total Sugars. USDA Home Economics research report No. 48. Washington, DC: U.S. Government Printing Office, 1987.

[e]Acosta PB, Gross KC. Eur J Pediatr 1995;154(Suppl 2):S87–S92.

[f]Gross KC, Sams CE. Phytochemistry 1984;23:2457–2461.

Enzymes That Degrade Compounds Containing Bound Galactose. α-Galactosidases, enzymes that digest carbohydrates with galactose in α-linkages, are found in human tissues and are probably responsible for the degradation of human galactosylcerebrosides, galactosylsulfatides, and gangliosides. α-Galactosidases also appear to be distributed in many plant tissues (306). Bean-O is an α-galactosidase isolated from *Aspergillus niger* and marketed by AkPharma, Inc., as a food enzyme that reduces gas formation from many vegetables. α-Galactosidases can hydrolyze the terminal galactose attached to digalactosyldiacylglycerol yielding galactose and monogalactosyldiacylglycerol (307).

β-Galactosidases are found in many foods, including apples and pears, peppers, tomatoes, and cocoa beans (308–312). The human intestine also contains β-galactosidases (313). The β-galactosidases in the human intestine digest lactose, but also have heterogenous activity on compounds with galactose in β-1,4 linkages (313). β-Galactosidase preparations from *E. coli* release galactose from ferulic acid and from monogalactosyldiacylglycerols (307, 314).

Results of Nutritional Support. Treatment of patients with GALT deficiency, although life saving, may not result in complete freedom from the sequelae of the disorder. Infants diagnosed and treated early who maintain excellent dietary control have better intellectual function than those who have poor control or are diagnosed late (282). Control is defined on the basis of erythrocyte Gal-1-P concentrations and is considered excellent if consistently below 2 mg/dL (315). However, even with deletion of all known galactose-containing foods, children frequently have a higher Gal-1-P and a lower IQ than their normal siblings (316). Patients may have difficulty with language, abstract thinking, visual perception, ovarian failure, and cataracts, despite good dietary control (315–319). These clinical deficits may be related to intrauterine damage from intrauterine accumulation of Gal-1-P or galactitol and/or maternal galactose transported into the vulnerable fetus. Embryonic membranes are constantly synthesized and degraded and require galactose and UPD-Gal. Galactose (i.e., milk) restriction in at-risk pregnant females is generally advised (320) although little change in outcome has been observed (282). This may be because many fruits, vegetables, and legumes contain free galactose, making restriction of all exogenous galactose impossible (300).

The recent observation that UDP-Gal is partially deficient in erythrocytes of patients with galactosemia offered another potential reason for poor outcome despite adequate lactose restriction (321). These findings have not been confirmed by others and uridine supplements have not been helpful in therapy (322, 324). Thus, other pathophysiological mechanisms or intrauterine development remain problematic.

Bone mineralization of both female and male patients with galactosemia was below that of normal age-, gender-, and ethnicity-matched subjects (325). Bone mineralization was positively correlated with calcium intake and in females was improved in those women who received estrogen (325).

A recently described mouse "knockout" for GALT has no acute hepatotoxicity or apparent ovarian failure. The mouse model differs from humans in having no aldose reductase and thus in not overproducing galactitol (Fig. 61.10). Thus, a pathological effect of polyol production and treatment using aldose reductase inhibitors is of considerable research interest for future therapeutic intervention (326, 327).

Assessment of Nutritional Support. Evaluation of growth, development, lens, liver function, erythrocyte Gal-1-P concentrations, and urinary galactitol excretion are necessary to determine adequacy of dietary intervention. Use of galactosylated hemoglobin A_1 as an index of dietary control has been suggested, but it is less sensitive and is an indirect test (328).

Diet Termination. Although some investigators have recommended liberalizing the galactose-restricted diet at 12 to 13 years of age, this is not warranted, because the potentially damaging effects of accumulated galactitol and Gal-1-P in the lens, liver, kidney, and brain remain. Females with galactosemia must continue treatment with galactose exclusion to reduce possible in utero damage to their future offspring (329). Diet termination is not recommended.

REFERENCES

1. McKusick VA. Mendelian inheritance in man: catalog of autosomal dominant, recessive, and X-linked phenotypes. 11th ed. Baltimore: Johns Hopkins University Press, 1994.
2. Harris H. The principles of human biochemical genetics. 3rd ed. Amsterdam: North Holland Publishing, 1980.
3. National Newborn Screening Reports. McLean, VA: National Maternal and Childhealth Clearinghouse, 1992, 1993.
4. Elsas LJ, Danner D, Lubitz D, et al. Metabolic consequences of inherited defects in branched-chain α-ketoacid dehydrogenase: mechanisms of thiamine action. In: Walser M, Williamson GR, eds. Metabolism and clinical implications of branched-chain amino acids and ketoacids. New York: Elsevier, 1981.
5. Snyderman E. Maple syrup urine disease. In: Wapnir LA, ed. Congenital metabolic disease: diagnosis and treatment. New York: Marcel Dekker, 1985.
6. Elsas LJ. Newborn screening. In: Rudolph AM, ed. Pediatrics. 20th ed. New York: Appleton-Century Crofts, 1994.
7. Burns JJ. Am J Med 1959;26:740.
8. Lipson MH, Kraus J, Rosenberg LE, et al. J Clin Invest 1980; 66:188.
9. Elsas LJ, Danner DJ. Ann NY Acad Sci 1982;378:404.
10. Baumgartner ER, Wick H, Linnel JC, et al. Helv Paediatr Acta 1979;34:483.
11. Elsas LJ, McCormick DB. Vitam Horm 1987;43:103.
12. Elsas L, McCormick D. Vitam Horm 1987;44:103–44.
13. Hershfield MS, Buckley RH, Greenberg ML, et al. N Engl J Med 1987;316:589.

14. Elsas LJ. Approach to the patient with metabolic disease. In: Bennett JC, Plum F, eds. Cecil's textbook of medicine. 20th ed. Philadelphia: WB Saunders, 1996;1078.
15. Pratt EL, Snyderman SE, Cheung MW, et al. J Nutr 1955;56: 231.
16. Hermann ME, Broesicke HG, Keller M, et al. Eur J Pediatr 1994;153:501.
17. Schoeffer A, Hermann ME, Brosicke HG, et al. J Nutr Med 1994;4:415.
18. Acosta PB. Construction of an amino acid-restricted diet. In: Kelly V, ed. Practice of pediatrics. Philadelphia: JB Lippincott, 1983:1–21.
19. Chipponi JX, Bleier JC, Santi MT, Rudman D. Am J Clin Nutr 1982;35:1112.
20. Acosta PB, Stepnick-Gropper S. J Inherited Metab Dis 1986; 9(Suppl 2):183.
21. Martin S, Acosta PB. J Am Diet Assoc 1987;87:48.
22. Scriver CR, Kaufman S, Woo SL, Eisensmith RC. The hyperphenylalaninemias. In: Scriver CR, Beaudet AL, Sly WS, Valle D, et al., eds. The metabolic and molecular bases of inherited disease. 7th ed. New York: McGraw-Hill, 1995.
23. Eisensmith RC, Martinez DR, Kuzmin AI, et al. Pediatrics 1996;97:512.
24. Griffin RF, Elsas LJ. J Pediatr 1975;86:572.
25. Niederwieser A, Ponzone A, Curtius HC, et al. J Inherited Metab Dis 1985;8(Suppl 1):34.
26. Kaufman S. J Inherited Metab Dis 1985;8(Suppl 1):20.
27. Curtius HC, Heintel D, Ghisla S, et al. J Inherited Metab Dis 1985;8(Suppl 1):28.
28. Dobbing J. The later development of the brain and its vulnerability. In: Davis JA, Dobbing J, eds. Scientific foundations of paediatrics. London: Heinemann, 1981.
29. Pardridge WM, Choi TB. Fed Proc 1986;45:2073.
30. Villasana D, Butler IJ, Williams JC, Roongta SM. J Inherited Metab Dis 1989;12:451.
31. Krause W, Halminski M, McDonald L, et al. J Clin Invest 1985;75:40.
32. Epstein CM, Trotter JF, Averbook A, et al. Electroencephalogr Clin Neurophysiol 1989;72:133.
33. Guthrie RA, Susi A. Pediatrics 1963;32:338.
34. Pass K, Levy H, eds. Impact of early discharge on screening for inborn errors of metabolism. Washington, DC: MCH CORN Clearinghouse, 1995.
35. Fernhoff PM, Fitzmaurice N, Milner J, et al. South Med J 1982;75:529.
36. Doherty LB, Rohr F, Levy HL. Pediatrics 1991;87:240.
37. Trefz F, Burgard P, Konig T, et al. Clin Chim Acta 1993;217:15.
38. Daiger SP, Lidsky AS, Chakraborty R, et al. Lancet 1986;1:229.
39. Jordan MK, Brunner RL, Hunt MM, Berry HK. Dev Med Child Neurol 1985;27:33.
40. Cournoyen D, Caskey CT. N Engl J Med 1990;323:601.
41. Reichle FA, Baldridge RC, Dobbs J, Trompetter M. JAMA 1961;178:939.
42. Acosta PB, Wenz E, Williamson M. J Am Diet Assoc 1978; 72:164.
43. Desviat LR, Pérez B, Ugarte M, et al. Hum Genet 1993;92:254.
44. Martinez-Pardo M, Colmenares AR, Garcia MJ, et al. J Inherited Metab Dis 1994;17:366.
45. Guttler F, Guldberg P. Acta Paediatr 1994;83(Suppl):407:49.
46. Smith I, Beasley, MG, Ades AE. Arch Dis Child 1990;65:472.
47. Rose WC. Nutr Abstr Rev 1957;27:631.
48. Hanley WB, Linsao L, Davidson W, et al. Pediatr Res 1970;4: 318.
49. Acosta PB. The contribution of therapy of inherited amino acid disorders to knowledge of amino acid requirements. In: Wapnir RA, ed. Congenital metabolic disease: diagnosis and treatment. New York: Marcel Dekker, 1985.
50. Batshaw ML, Valle D, Bessman SP. J Pediatr 1981;99:159.
51. Holt LE, Gyorgy P, Pratt EL, et al. Protein and amino acid requirements in early infancy. New York: New York University Press, 1960.
52. Food and Nutrition Board, National Research Council. Recommended dietary allowances. 10th ed. Washington, DC: National Academy Press, 1989.
53. Kindt E, Motzfeldt K, Halvorsen S, Lie S. Am J Clin Nutr 1983; 37:778.
54. Acosta PB, Yannicelli S. Acta Paediatr Scand Suppl 1994; 407:66.
55. Barness LA, Curran JS. Nutrition. In: Behrman RE, Kliegman RM, Arvin AM, eds. Nelson's textbook of pediatrics. 15th ed. Philadelphia: WB Saunders, 1996.
56. Douglass JS, Matthews RH, Hepburn FN. Composition of foods: breakfast cereals: raw, processed, prepared. Agricultural handbook 8-8. Washington, DC: US Government Printing Office, 1982.
57. Gebhardt JE, Cutrufelli R, Matthews RH. Composition of foods: fruits and juices: raw, processed, prepared. Agricultural handbook 8-9. Washington, DC: US Government Printing Office, 1982.
58. Haytowitz DB, Matthews RH. Composition of foods: vegetables and vegetable products: raw, processed, prepared. Agricultural handbook 8-11. Washington, DC: US Government Printing Office, 1984.
59. Pennington JAT, Church HN. Bowes and Church's food values of portions commonly used. 14th ed. New York: Harper & Row, 1985.
60. Posati LP. Composition of foods: poultry products: raw, processed, prepared. Agricultural handbook 8-5. Washington, DC: US Government Printing Office, 1979.
61. Posati LP, Orr ML. Composition of foods: dairy and egg products: raw, processed, prepared. Agricultural handbook 8-1. Washington, DC: US Government Printing Office, 1976.
62. Mead Johnson Nutritional Division. Products for dietary management of inborn errors of metabolism. Evansville, IN: Mead Johnson, 1994.
63. Acosta PB, Yannicelli S. Nutrition support protocols. Columbus, OH: Ross Laboratories, 1997.
64. Acosta PB. Nutrition support of inborn errors of metabolism. In: Queen P, Lang C, eds. Handbook of pediatric nutrition. Rockville, MD: Aspen Publishers, 1990.
65. Wannemacher RW. Am J Clin Nutr 1977;130:1269.
66. Umbarger B, Berry HK, Sutherland BS. JAMA 1965;193: 128.
67. Ingall GB, Sherman JD, Cockburn F, Klein R. J Pediatr 1964;65:1073A.
68. Elsas LJ, Albrecht I, Rosenberg LE. J Biol Chem 1968;243: 1846.
69. Elsas LJ, MacDonell RC, Rosenberg LE. J Biol Chem 1971; 246:6452.
70. Nakagawa I, Takahashi T, Suzuki T, Kobayashi K. J Nutr 1962; 77:61.
71. Sibinga MS, Friedman CJ, Steisel IM, Baker EC. Dev Med Child Neurol 1971;13:63.
72. McCaman RE, Robins AJ. J Lab Clin Med 1962;59:885.
73. Acosta PB, Wenz E, Koch R. PKU—a guide to management. Berkeley, CA: California State Department of Health, 1972.
74. Holm VA, Kronmal RA, Williamson M, Roche AF. Pediatrics 1979;63:700.
75. Dobson JC, Williamson ML, Azen C, Koch R. Pediatrics 1977;60:822.

76. Schulpis KH, Nounopoulos C, Scarpalerou A, et al. Acta Paediatr Scand 1990;79:920.
77. Brouwer M, De Bree PK, von Sprang FJ, et al. Lancet 1977;1:1162.
78. Francois B, Diel M, De La Brassinne M. J Inherited Metab Dis 1989;12(Suppl 2):332.
79. Nord AM, McCabe L, McCabe ERB. J Inherited Metab Dis 1988;11:431.
80. Buist NRM, Prince AP, Huntington KL, et al. Acta Paediatr Scand Suppl 1994;407:75.
81. Shenton A, Wells FE, Addison GM. J Inherited Metab Dis 1983;6(Suppl 2):109.
82. Acosta PB, Greene C, Yannicelli S, et al. Int Pediatr 1993;8:63.
83. Acosta PB, Alfin-Slater RB, Koch R. J Am Diet Assoc 1973; 63:631.
84. Galluzo CR, Ortisi MT, Castelli L, et al. J Inherited Metab Dis 1985;8(Suppl 2):129.
85. Schulpi KH, Scarpalezou A. Clin Pediatr 1985;28:466.
86. Galli C, Agostoni C, Mosconi C, et al. J Pediatr 1991;119:562.
87. Sanjurjo P, et al. J Inherited Metab Dis 1994;17:704.
88. Acosta PB, Wenz E, Williamson M. Am J Clin Nutr 1977; 30:198.
89. Wong R, Acosta PB, Jones D, Koch R. J Am Diet Assoc 1970;57:229.
90. Acosta PB, Fernhoff PM, Warshaw HS, et al. J Inherited Metab Dis 1982;5:107.
91. Acosta PB, Stepnick-Gropper S, Clarke-Sheehan N, et al. JPEN J Parenter Enteral Nutr 1987;11:287.
92. Bodley JL, Austin VJ, Hanley WB, et al. Eur J Pediatr 1993;152:140.
93. Gropper SS, Trahms C, Cloud HA, et al. Int Pediatr 1994;9: 237.
94. Lipson A, Masters H, O'Halloran M, et al. Aust Paediatr J 1988;24:128.
95. Lloyd B, Robson E, Smith I, Clayton BE. Arch Dis Child 1989;64:352.
96. Longhi R, Rotolli A, Vitorelli A, et al. Eur J Pediatr 1987;146(Suppl 1):A32.
97. Greeves LG, Carson DJ, Craig BG, McMaster D. Acta Paediatr Scand 1990;79:1259.
98. Collins RJ, Boyle AE, Clagne AE. Biol Trace Elem Res 1991;30:233.
99. Calomme M, Vanderpas J, Francois B, et al. Biol Trace Elem Res 1995;47:349.
100. Lewis JS, Pian AK, Baer MT, et al. Am J Clin Nutr 1973;26:136.
101. Lewis JS, Loskill S, Bunker ML, et al. Fed Proc 1974;33:666A.
102. Hillman LS, Schlotzhauer C, Lee D, et al. Eur J Pediatr 1996;155(Suppl 1):S148.
103. McMurry MP, Chan GM, Leonard CO, Ernst SL. Am J Clin Nutr 1992;55:997.
104. Carson DJ, Greeves LG, Sweeney LE, Crone MD. Pediatr Radiol 1990;20:598.
105. Gropper SS, Chaung HC, Bernstein LE, et al. J Am Col Nutr 1995;14:264.
106. Hudson FP. Arch Dis Child 1967;42:198.
107. Holtzman NA, Welcher DW, Mellits ED. N Engl J Med 1975;293:1121.
108. Horner FA, Streamer CW, Alejandrino LL, et al. N Engl J Med 266:79.1962;
109. Seashore MR, Friedman E, Novelly RA, Bapat V. Pediatrics 1985;75:226.
110. Holtzman NA, Kronmal RA, van Doorninck W, et al. N Engl J Med 1986;314:593.
111. Thompson JA, Smith I, Brenton D, et al. Lancet 1990; 336:602.
112. Waisbren SE, Levy HL. J Inherited Metab Dis 1991;14:755.
113. Hanley WB, Feigenbaum A, Clarke JT, et al. Lancet 1993; 342:997.
114. Krause W, Epstein C, Averbook A, et al. Pediatr Res 1986;20: 1112.
115. Elsas LJ, Trotter JF. Changes in physiological concentrations of blood phenylalanine produce changes in sensitive parameters of human brain function. In: Dietary phenylalanine and brain function. Boston: Birkhauser Publishing, 1987;187–95.
116. Lenke RR, Levy HL. N Engl J Med 1980;303:1202.
117. Levy HL. Enzyme 1987;38:312.
118. Kudo Y, Boyd CAR. J Inherited Metab Dis 1990;13:617.
119. Hanley WB, Clarke JT, Schoonheyt W. Clin Biol 1987;20: 149.
120. Fisch RO, Burke B, Bass J, et al. Pediatr Pathol 1986;5:449.
121. Kirby ML, Miyagawa ST. J Inherited Metab Dis 1990;13:634.
122. Okano Y, Chow IZ, Isshiki G, et al. J Inherited Metab Dis 1986;9:15.
123. Kirkman HN. Appl Res Mental Retard 1982;3:319.
124. Koch R, Friedman EG, Wenz E, et al. J Inherited Metab Dis 1986;9(Suppl 2):159.
125. Koch R, Levy H, Matalon R, et al. Acta Paediatr Suppl 1994; 407:111.
126. Smith I, Glossop J, Beasley M. J Inherited Metab Dis 1990; 13:651.
127. Acosta PB. Semin Perinatol 1995;19:182.
128. Acosta PB, Michals-Matalon K, Austin V, et al. Nutrition findings and requirements in pregnant women with phenylketonuria. In: Platt L, ed. Effects of genetic disorders on pregnancy outcome. London: Parthenon, 1996.
129. Subcommittee on Nutritional Status and Weight Gain during Pregnancy. Nutrition and pregnancy. Washington, DC: National Academy Press, 1990;430–1.
130. Innis SM. Prog Lipid Res 1991;30:39.
131. Neuringer M, Anderson GJ, Connor WE. Annu Rev Nutr 1988;8:517.
132. Hunter JE. Am J Clin Nutr 1990;51:809.
133. Rothman KJ, Moore LL, Singer MR, et al. N Engl J Med 1995;333:1369.
134. Lindblad B, Lindstedt S, Steen G. Proc Natl Acad Sci USA 1971;74:4641.
135. Phaneuf D, Labelle Y, Beruve D, et al. Am J Hum Genet 1991;48:525.
136. Sassa S, Kappas A. J Clin Invest 1983;71:625.
137. Christensen E, Brock-Jacobsen B, Gregersen N, et al. Clin Chim Acta 1981;116:331.
138. Kvittingen EA, Halvorsen S, Jellum E. Pediatr Res 1983;14: 541.
139. Lindstedt S, Holme E, Lock EA, et al. Lancet 1992;340:813.
140. Mitchell GA, Lambert M, Tanguay RM. Tyrosinemia and related disorders. In: Scriver CR, Beaudet AL, Sly WS, et al. The metabolic and molecular bases of inherited disease. 7th ed. New York: McGraw-Hill, 1995.
141. Mamunes P, Prince PE, Thornton NH, et al. Pediatrics 1976;57:675.
142. Gagne R, Lescault A, Grenier A, Laberge C. Prenat Diagn 1982;2:185.
143. Kvittingen EA, Steinmann B, Gitzelmann R, et al. Pediatr Res 1985;19:334.
144. Elsas LJ. Personal experience.
145. Sassa S, Granick S. Proc Natl Acad Sci USA 1970;67:517.
146. Goetsch CA, Bissell DM. N Engl J Med 1986;315:235.
147. Rank JM, Pascual-Leone A, Payne W, et al. J Pediatr 1991;118;136.
148. Kvittingen EA. J Inherited Metab Dis 1995;18:375.

149. Grompe M, Lindstedt S, Al-Dhalimy M, et al. Nat Genet 1995;10:453.
150. Tolbert BM, Watts DT. J Nutr 1963;80:111.
151. Michals K, Matalon R, Wang PWK, et al. J Am Diet Assoc 1978;73;507.
152. Soirdahl S, Lie SO, Jellum E, Stokke O. Pediatr Res 1979; 13:74.
153. Cohn RM, Yudkoff M, Yost B, et al. Am J Clin Nutr 1977; 30:209.
154. Chuang DT, Shih VE. Disorders of branched chain amino acid and ketoacid metabolism. In: Scriver CR, Beaudet AL, Sly WS, Valle D, eds. The metabolic and molecular bases of inherited disease. 7th ed. New York: McGraw-Hill, 1995.
155. Danner DJ, Armstrong N, Heffelfinger SC, et al. J Clin Invest 1985;75:858.
156. Ellerine NP, Herring WJ, Elsas LJ, et al. Biochem Med Metab Biol 1993;49:363.
157. Elsas LJ, Danner DJ. Ann NY Acad Sci 1982;378:404.
158. Elsas LJ, Ellerine NP, Klin PD. Pediatr Res 1993;33:445.
159. Heffelfinger S, Sewell ET, Elsas LJ, Danner DJ. Am J Hum Genet 1984;36:802.
160. Fernhoff PM, Lubitz D, Danner DJ, et al. Pediatr Res 1985; 19:1011.
161. Sweetman L, Williams JC. Branched-chain organic acidurias. In: Scriver CR, Beaudet AL, Sly WS, Valle D, eds. The metabolic and molecular bases of inherited disease. 7th ed. New York: McGraw-Hill, 1995.
162. Elsas LJ, Pask BA, Wheeler FB, et al. Metabolism 1972; 21:929.
163. Naylor EW, Guthrie R. Pediatrics 1978;61:262.
164. Elsas LJ, Priest JH, Wheeler, et al. Metabolism 1974;23:569.
165. Wendel LL, Langenbeck U, Lombeck I, et al. Eur J Pediatr 1982;138:293.
166. Clow CL, Reade TM, Scriver CR. Pediatrics 1981;68:856.
167. Thompson GN, Frances DEM, Halliday D. J Pediatr 1991;119:35.
168. Giacoia BP, Berry GT. Am J Dis Child 1993;147:954.
169. Koch SE, Packman S, Koch TK, Williams ML. J Am Acad Dermatol 1993;28:289.
170. DiGeorge AM, Rezvani I, Garibaldi LR, et al. N Engl J Med 1982;307:1492.
171. Duran M, Wadman SK. J Inherited Metab Dis 1985;8(Suppl 1):70.
172. Szmelcman S, Guggenheim K. Biochem J 1966;100:7.
173. Hammerson G, Wille L, Schmidt H, et al. Monogr Hum Genet 1978;9:84.
174. Snyderman SE, Goldstein F, Sansaricq C, Norton PM. Pediatr Res 1984;18:851.
175. Treacy E, Clow Cl, Reade TR, et al. J Inherited Metab Dis 1992;15:121.
176. Berry GT, Heidenreich R, Kaplan P, et al. N Engl J Med 1991;324:175.
177. Kaplan P, Mazur A, Field M, et al. J Pediatr 1991;119:46.
178. van Calcar S, Wolff J. Am J Med Genet 1992;44:641.
179. Dent CE, Westall RG. Arch Dis Child 1961;36:259.
180. Westall RG. Am J Dis Child 1967;113:58.
181. Snyderman SE, Norton PM, Roitman E, Holt LE. Pediatr 1964;34:454.
182. Scwartz JF, Kolendrianos ET. Dev Med Child Neurol 1969;11:460.
183. Dickinson JP, Holton JB, Lewis GM, et al. Acta Paediatr Scand 1969;58:341.
184. Gaull GE. Biochem Med 1969;3:130.
185. Committee for Improvement of Hereditary Disease Management. CMA J 1976;115:1005.
186. Parsons HG, Carter RJ, Unrath M, Snyder FF. J Inherited Metab Dis 1990;13:125.
187. Henstenberg JD, Mazur AR, Kaplan PB, et al. J Am Diet Assoc 1990;90(Suppl):A32.
188. Gropper SS, Naglak MC, Nardella M, et al. J Am Coll Nutr 1993;12:108.
189. Budd MA, Tanaka K, Holmes LB, et al. N Engl J Med 1967; 277:321.
190. Rhead WJ, Tanaka K. Proc Natl Acad Sci USA 1980;77:580.
191. Kraus JP, Matsubara Y, Barton D, et al. Genomics 1987;1;264.
192. Vockley J, Parimoo B, Tanaka K. Am J Hum Genet 1991; 49:147.
192a. Shigematsu Y, Sudo M, Momoi T, et al. Pediatr Res 1982;16:771.
193. Truscott RTW, Malegan D, McCairns E, et al. Clin Chim Acta 1981;110:187.
194. Lehnert W, Niederhoff H. Eur J Pediatr 1981;136:281.
195. Hutchinson RJ, Bunnell K, Thoene JG. J Pediatr 1985;106:62.
196. Dubiel B, Dabrowski C, Wetts R, Tanaka K. J Clin Invest 1983; 72:1543.
197. Ikeda T, Noda C, Tanaka K. Purification and characterization of isovaleryl-1-CoA dehydrogenases from a liver mitochondria. In: Walser M, Williamson GR, eds. Metabolism and clinical implications of branched-chain amino acids and ketoacids. New York: Elsevier, 1981.
198. Lehnert W, Hunkler D. Eur J Pediatr 1986;145:260.
199. Blascovics M, Donnell G. J Inherited Metab Dis 1978;1:9.
200. Shigematsu Y, Kikawa Y, Sudo M, et al. Clin Chim Acta 1984; 138:333.
201. Bartlett K, Gompertz D. Biochem Med 1974;10:15.
202. Naglak M, Salvo R, Madsen K, et al. Pediatr Res 1988;24:9.
203. Stanley CA, Hale DE, Whiteman DEH, et al. Pediatr Res 1983;17:296A.
204. Roe CR, Millington DS, Maltby DA, et al. J Clin Invest 1984;74:2290.
205. Lott IT, Erickson AM, Levy HL. Pediatr 1972;49:616.
206. Berry GT, Yudkoff M, Segal S. J Pediatr 1988;113:58.
207. Hyman SL, Porter CA, Page TJ, et al. J Pediatr 1987;111:558.
208. Hyman SL, Coyle JT, Parke JC, et al. J Pediatr 1986;108:705.
209. Rousson R, Guibaud P. J Inherited Metab Dis 1984;7(Suppl 1):10.
210. Finkelstein JD, Martin JJ. J Biol Chem 1984;259:9508.
211. Rosenblatt DS. Inherited disorders of folate transport and metabolism. In: Scriver CR, Beaudet AL, Sly WS, Valle D, eds. The metabolic and molecular bases of inherited disease. 7th ed. New York: McGraw-Hill, 1995.
212. Mudd SH, Levy HL, Skovby F. Disorders of transsulfuration. In: Scriver CR, Beaudet AL, Sly WS, Valle D, eds. The metabolic and molecular bases of inherited disease. 7th ed. New York: McGraw-Hill, 1995.
213. Fenton WA, Rosenberg LE. Inherited disorders of cobalamin transport and metabolism. In: Scriver CR, Beaudet AL, Sly WS, Valle D, eds. The metabolic and molecular bases of inherited disease. 7th ed. New York: McGraw-Hill, 1995.
214. Shih VE, Fringer JM, Mandell R, et al. Am J Hum Genet 1995;57:34.
215. Kraus JP. J Inherited Metab Dis 1994;17:383.
216. McCusick VA, Hall JH, Char F. The clinical and genetic characteristics of homocystinuria. In: Carson N, Raine N, eds. Inherited disorders of sulfur metabolism. London: Churchill Livingstone, 1971.
217. Mudd JH, Skovby F, Levy H, et al. Am J Hum Genet 1985;37:1.
218. Boers GHJ, Smals AG, Trijbels FJ, et al. N Engl J Med 1985;313:709.
219. Ferhoff PM, Danner DJ, Elsas LJ. Vitamin-responsive disor-

ders. In: Garry PJ, ed. Human nutrition: clinical and biochemical aspects. Washington, DC: American Association for Clinical Chemistry, 1980:219–38.
220. Schaumburg H, Kaplan J, Windebank A, et al. N Engl J Med 1983;309:445.
221. Yoshida I, Sakaguchi Y, Nakano M, et al. J Inherited Metab Dis 1985;8:91.
222. Wilcken DEL, Dudman NPB, Tyrrell PA. Metabolism 1985;34:1115.
223. Komrower GM, Sardharwalla IB. The dietary treatment of homocystinuria. In: Carson NAJ, Raine DN, eds. Inherited disorders of sulfur metabolism. London: Churchhill Livingstone, 1971.
224. Kang SS, Wong PW, Malinow MR. Annu Rev Nutr 1992;12:279.
225. Sansaricq C, Garg S, Norton PM, et al. Acta Paediatr Scand 1975;64:215.
226. Perry TL, Dunn HG, Hansen S, et al. Pediatrics 1966;37:502.
227. Dudman NPB, Wilcken DEL. Clin Chim Acta 1983;127:105.
228. Spooner NJ, Fell GS, Halls DJ, et al. Clin Nutr 1986;5:29.
229. Smith AM, Picciano MF, Milner JA. Am J Clin Nutr 1982;35:521.
230. Carey MC, Donovan DE, Fitzgerald O, et al. Am J Med 1968;45:7.
231. Carey MC, Fennelly JJ, Fitzgerald O. Am J Med 1968;45:26.
232. Wagstaff J, Korson M, Kraus JP, Levy HL. J Pediatr 1991;118:569.
233. Marcus AJ. N Engl J Med 1983;309:1515.
234. Brusilow S, Horwich A. Urea cycle enzymes. In: Scriver CR, ed. The metabolic and molecular bases of inherited disease. 7th ed. New York: McGraw-Hill, 1995.
235. Tuchman M. Hum Mutat 1993;2:174.
236. Kline JJ, Hug G, Schubert WK, Berry H. Am J Dis Child 1981;135:437.
237. Cederbaum S, Shaw KN, Valente M. J Pediatr 1977;90:5.
238. Levin B, Abraham JM, Obenholzer VG, Burgess EA. Arch Dis Child 1969;44:152.
239. Kennaway N, Harwood PJ, Ramberg DA, et al. Pediatr Res 1975;9:554.
240. Kobayashi K, Jackson MJ, Tick DB, et al. J Biol Chem 1990;256:1136.
241. Summar ML, Dasouki MJ, Schofield PJ, et al. Cytogenet Cell Genet 1995;71:266.
242. Beaudet A. Am J Hum Genet 1985;37:386.
243. Beaudet A, O'Brien WE, Bock HG, et al. Adv Hum Genet 1986;15:161.
244. Horwich AL, Fenton WA, Williams KR, et al. Science 1984;224:1068.
245. Kraus JP, Hodges PE, Williamson CL, et al. Nucleic Acids Res 1985;13:943.
246. Spector EB, Rice SCH, Cederbaum SD. Pediatr Res 1983;17:941.
247. Valle D, Simell O. The hyperornithinemias. In: Scriver CR, Beaudet AL, Sly WS, Valle D, eds. The metabolic and molecular bases of inherited disease. 7th ed. New York: McGraw-Hill, 1995.
248. Russell A. Mt Sinai J Med 1973;40:723.
249. Rowe PC, Newman SL, Brusilow SW. N Engl J Med 1986;314:541.
250. Levy H, Coulombe JT, Shih V. The New England experience. In: Bickel H, Guthrie R, Hammersen G, eds. Neonatal screening for inborn errors of metabolism. Berlin: Springer-Verlag, 1980.
251. Naylor EW. Pediatrics 1981;68:453.
252. Talbot HW, Sumlin AB, Naylor EW, Guthrie RS, et al. Pediatrics 1982;70:526.
253. Tada K, Okuda K, Watanabe K, et al. Eur J Pediatr 1979;130:105.
254. Brusilow SW. Hosp Pract 1985;20:65.
255. Batshaw ML, Brusilow SW, et al. Pediatr Res 1979;13:472.
256. Snyderman SE, Sansaricq C, Phansalkar SV, et al. Pediatrics 1975;56:65.
257. Bachmann C. Enzyme 1984;32:56.
258. Batshaw ML, Thomas GH, Brusilow SW, et al. Pediatrics 1981;68:290.
259. Brusilow SW. Pediatrics 1991;29:147.
260. Msall M, Batshaw ML, Suss R, et al. N Engl J Med 1984;310:1500.
261. Ad Hoc Expert Committee. Energy and protein requirements. Rome: Food and Agriculture Organization of the United Nations, 1973.
262. Remer T, Manz F. J Nutr Biochem 1995;6:431.
263. Ohtani Y, Ohyanagi K, Yamamoto S, Matsuda I. J Pediatr 1988;112:409.
264. Ohtsuka Y, Griffith OW. Biochem Pharmacol 1991;41:1957.
265. Iafolla AK, Gale DS, Roe CR. J Pediatr 1990;117:102.
266. Renner C, Sewell AC, Bervoets K, et al. Eur J Pediatr 1995;154:909.
267. Sanjurjo P, Rodriguez-Soriano J, Vallo A, et al. Eur J Pediatr 1991;150:730.
268. Wilson O, Schfert W, Ballatore A, Sparks WJ. Pediatr Res 1995;37:323A.
269. Segal S. Berry GT. Disorders of galactose metabolism. In: Scriver CR, Beaudet AL, Sly WS, Valle D, eds. The metabolic and molecular bases of inherited disease. 7th ed. New York: McGraw-Hill, 1995.
270. Sparkes RC, Sparkes MC, Funderburk SJ, et al. Ann Hum Genet (London) 1980;43:343.
271. Flach JE, Reichardt J, Elsas L. Mol Biol Med 1990;7:365.
272. Leslie ND, Immerman EB, Flach JE, et al. Genomics 1992;14:474.
273. Elsas LJ, Dembure PP, Langbein S, et al. Am J Hum Genet 1994;54:1030.
274. Gathof BS, Sommer M, Podskarbi T, et al. Hum Genet 1995;96:721.
275. Elsas LJ, Langley S, Steele E, et al. Am J Hum Genet 1995;56:630.
276. Fridovich-Keil JL, Langley SD, Mazur LA, et al. Am J Hum Genet 1995;56:640.
277. Elsas LJ, Langley S, Paulk EM, et al. Eur J Ped 154(Suppl 1995;2):20.
278. Elsas LJ, Fridovich-Keil J, Leslie ND. Int Pediatr 1993;8:101.
279. Kadhom N, Baptista J, Brinet M, et al. Biochem Med Metab Biol 1994;52:140.
280. Wolfrom C, Raynaud N, Kadhom N, et al. J Inherited Metab Dis 1993;16:78.
281. Sidbury JB Jr. Investigations and speculations on the pathogenesis of galactosemia. In: Hsia D, ed. Galactosemia. Springfield, IL: Charles C Thomas, 1969.
282. Waggoner DD, Buist NRM, Donnell GN. J Inherited Metab Dis 1990;13:802.
283. Schweitzer S, Shin Y, Jakobs C, Biodehl J. Eur J Pediatr 1993;152:36.
284. Lai K, Langley K, Singh R, et al. J Pediatr 1995;128:89.
285. Berry GT, Nissin I, Lin Z, et al. Lancet 1995;346:1073.
286. Xu YK, Kaufman FR, Donnell GN, et al. Clin Chim Acta 1995;240:21.
287. Urbanowski JC, Cohenford MA, Levy HL, et al. N Engl J Med 1982;306:84.
288. Beutler B. J Lab Clin Med 1966;68:137.

289. Jakobs C, Kleijer WJ, Allen J, Holton JB. Eur J Pediatr 1995; 154(Suppl 2):S33.
290. Gitzelman R, Auricchio S. Pediatrics 1965;36:231.
291. Harvey CD, Jeness R, Morris HA. J Dairy Sci 1981;64:1648.
292. Hettinga DH, Miah AH, Hammond EG, Reinbold GW. J Dairy Sci 1970;53:1377.
293. Reynolds LM, Henneberry BO, Baker BE. J Dairy Sci 1959;42:1463.
294. Gross KC, Acosta PB. J Inherited Metab Dis 1991;14:253.
295. Gropper SS, Gross KC, Olds SJ. J Am Diet Assoc 1993;93:328.
296. Cerbulis J. Arch Biochem Biophys 1954;49:442.
297. Koch R, Acosta P, Ragsdale N, Donnell GN. J Am Diet Assoc 1963;43:216.
298. Holton JB. Galactosemia. In: Schaub J, van Hoof F, Vis HL. Inborn errors of metabolism. New York: Raven Press, 1991.
299. Lineback DR, Ke CH. Cereal Chem 1975;52:334.
300. Acosta PB, Gross KC. Eur J Pediatr 1995;154(Suppl 2):S87.
301. Kumar A, Weatherly MR, Beaman DC. Pediatrics 1991;87:352.
302. Smith JS, Villalobos MC, Kottemann CM. J Food Sci 1986; 51:373.
303. Harju M. Milk Sci Int 45(1990;7):411.
304. Segal S. Int Pediatr 1992;7:75.
305. Weismann VN, Rosé-Butler B, Schluchter R. Eur J Pediatr 1995;154(Suppl 2):S93.
306. Pridham JB, Dey PM. The nature and function of higher plant alpha-galactosidases. In: Pridham JB, ed. Plant carbohydrate biochemistry. New York: Academic Press, 1974.
307. Carter HE, McCluer Rh, Slifer ED. J Am Chem Soc 1956;78: 3735.
308. Gross KC, Watada AE, Kang MS. Physiol Plant 1986;66:31.
309. Jarvis MC. Plant Cell Environ 1984;7:153.
310. Knee M, Bartley JM. Composition and metabolism of cell wall polysaccharides in ripening fruits. In: Friend J, Rhodes MJC, eds. Recent advances in the biochemistry of fruits and vegetables. New York: Academic Press, 1981.
311. Pressey R. Plant Physiol 1983;71:132.
312. Roelofsen PA. Adv Food Res 1958;8:225.
313. Asp NG. Biochem J 1971;191:229.
314. Fry SC. Biochem J 1982;203:493.
315. Donnell G, Bergran WR, Perry G, Koch R. Pediatrics 1963;31:802.
316. Gitzelman R, Steinmann B. Enzyme 1984;32:37.
317. Waisbren SE, Norman TR, Schnell RR, Levy HL. J Pediatr 1983;102:75.
318. Kaufman FR, Xu YK, Ng WG, Donnell GN. J Pediatr 1988;112:754.
319. Irons M, Levy HL, Puschel S, Castree K. J Pediatr 1985;107: 261.
320. Fenson AH, Benson PF, Blunt S. Br Med J 1974;4:386.
321. Ng WG, Xu YK, Kaufman FR, Donnell GN. J Inherited Metab Dis 1989;12:257.
322. Gibson JB, Reynolds RA, Palmieri MJ, et al. Metabolism 1995;44:597.
323. Kaufman FR, Xu YK, Ng WG, et al. Pediatr Res 1995;37:149A.
324. Manis FR, Cohn L, McBride-Chang C, et al. Pediatr Res 1995;37:150A.
325. Kaufman FR, Loro ML, Azen C, et al. J Pediatr 1993;123:365.
326. Berry GT. Eur J Pediatr 1995;154(Suppl 2):53.
327. Leslie N. Personal communication.
328. Howard NJ, Monaghan H, Martin JM. Acta Paediatr Scand 1981;70:695.
329. Komrower GM. J Inherited Metab Dis 1982;5(Suppl 2):96.

SELECTED READINGS

Desnick RJ, ed. Treatment of genetic diseases. New York: Churchill Livingstone, 1991;350.

Elsas LJ. In: Bennett JC, Plum F, eds. Cecil's textbook of medicine. 20th ed. Philadelphia: WB Saunders, 1996;142;1078, 1111.

Fernandes J, Saudubray JM, Tada K, eds. Inborn metabolic diseases. Diagnosis and treatment. New York: Springer-Verlag, 1990;730.

Scriver CR, Beaudet A, Sly W, Valle D, eds. The metabolic and molecular bases of inherited disease, vol 1. 7th ed. New York: McGraw-Hill, 1995;1650.

62. Inherited Metabolic Disease: Defects of β-Oxidation

JERRY VOCKLEY

β-Oxidation, which results in sequential cleavage of two-carbon units from fatty acids, is an important source of energy for the body during fasting and metabolic stress. Free fatty acids released into the blood via catabolism of fat stores or from dietary sources are metabolized in two intracellular compartments: the peroxisomes and the mitochondria. Peroxisomes (sometimes referred to as microbodies) are subcellular organelles bounded by a single lipid bilayer membrane (1). They are ubiquitously distributed in tissues but are particularly abundant in liver and kidney (2). Most peroxisomal proteins are synthesized in the cytosol in their final form, although several are made in a precursor form that requires posttranslational proteolytic processing. All peroxisomal proteins are encoded in the nuclear genome and transported to the organelle posttranslationally. This process involves at least three mechanisms (3, 4). The most common is the presence of a serine-lysine-leucine amino acid motif at the carboxy terminus of the protein, which serves as a targeting signal to direct the protein to peroxisomes. A second mechanism uses an amino terminus–targeting signal. The third entails an internal amino acid motif.

Mitochondria are more complex structures than peroxisomes and are bounded by two lipid bilayer membranes (the inner and outer mitochondrial membranes). The intermembrane space constitutes a distinct compartment within the mitochondrion, while the space bounded by the inner mitochondrial membrane is known as the matrix. Mitochondria are unique organelles in animals in that they contain their own genetic information. The mitochondrial genome is composed of a circular DNA molecule encoding several protein subunits that constitute part of the electron transfer chain complexes as well as genes for specific tRNA and ribosomal RNA molecules necessary for mitochondrial protein translation.

Human sperm cells are nearly devoid of mitochondria, while human oocytes contain numerous mitochondria. Genes on the mitochondrial chromosome therefore are inherited strictly from the mother by both sexes and can be passed on to subsequent generations only by females. This leads to the characteristic pattern of maternal inheritance seen in disorders associated with defects in the mitochondrial genome. Most proteins found in the mitochondria, however, are nuclear encoded and thus are inherited in a standard mendelian fashion. In general, they are synthesized in a larger precursor form containing information in an amino-terminal signal peptide necessary for targeting the proteins to the mitochondria (5–10). These signal sequences are usually removed after the protein is imported into the mitochondrion. More than one targeting signal may be necessary to direct the imported protein to the correct mitochondrial space or membrane. Peroxisomes and mitochondria arise by division of previously existing organelles and are randomly distributed to daughter cells upon cellular division.

Mitochondrial fatty acid oxidation is predominantly responsible for the oxidation of fatty acids of carbon length 20 or less, while the peroxisomal pathway is physiologically more relevant for longer-chain fats. Mitochondrial β-oxidation is a complex process involving transport of activated acyl-CoA moieties into the mitochondria and sequential removal of 2-carbon acetyl-CoA units (11) (Fig. 62.1). These in turn are used as fuel for the tricarboxylic acid cycle or production of ketone bodies (Fig. 62.2). The end result is generation of reducing equivalents that are funneled into the electron transport chain and ultimately lead to production of ATP. Ketones derived from hepatic fat metabolism can be used as an auxiliary fuel by most tissues, including the brain. At least 25 enzymes and specific transport proteins are responsible for carrying out the steps of mitochondrial fatty acid metabolism, some of which have only recently been recognized (Fig. 62.1 and Table 62.1). Of these, defects in at least 15 have been shown to cause disease in humans. The first of these disorders was identified only 20 years ago (12, 13), and most have been identified in the past 10 years.

Fatty acid oxidation in peroxisomes uses a different set of enzymes (14, 15) (Fig. 62.3) and Table 62.2. While this system functions optimally for fats of carbon chain lengths between 12 and 16, its role in oxidation of fats longer than

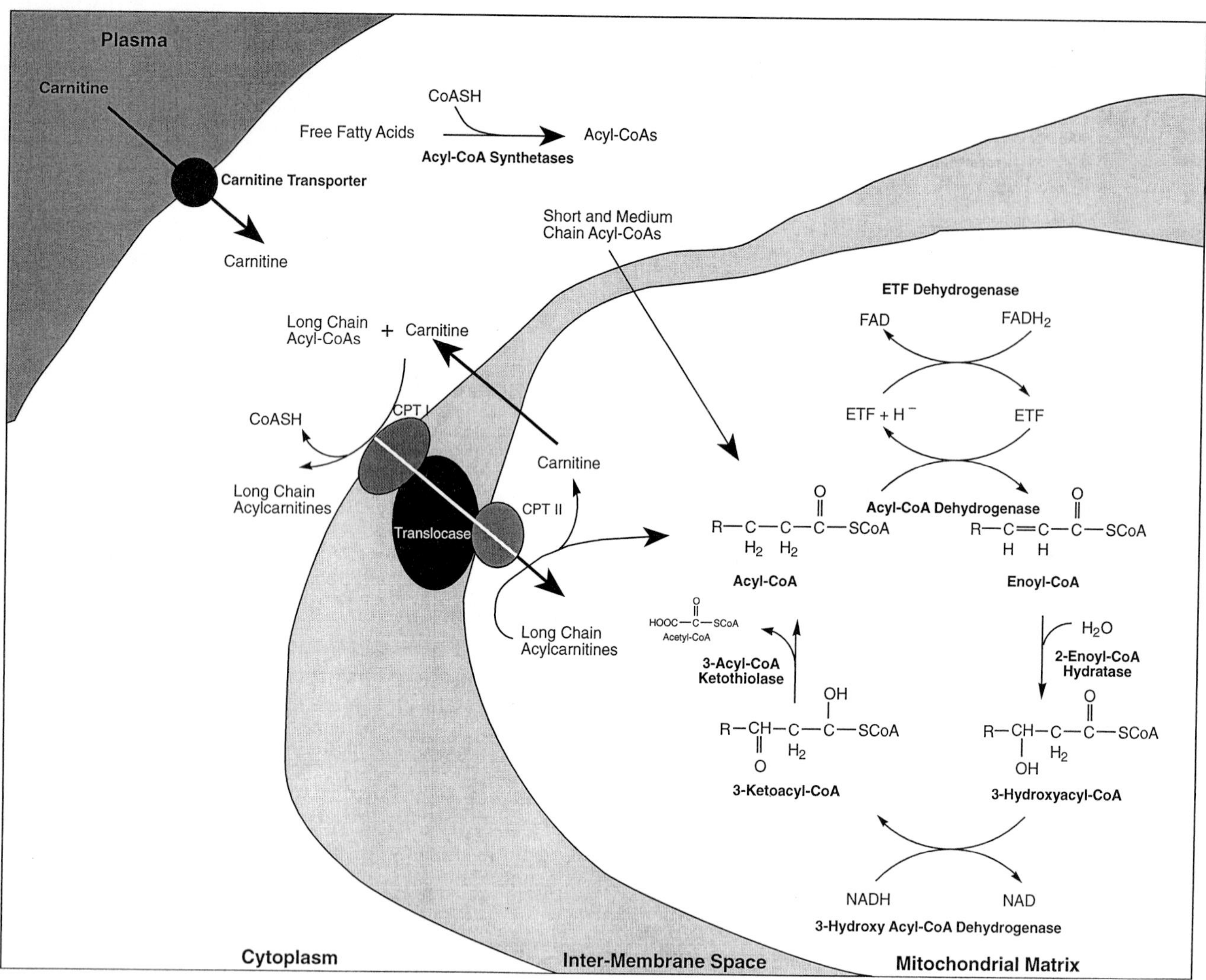

Figure 62.1. Pathway of enzyme and transporter proteins involved in mitochondrial β-oxidation. Abbreviations are as in the text. Modified and reprinted with permission of the Mayo Clinic and Foundation.

20 carbons may be physiologically more relevant, since these molecules are not good substrates for the mitochondrial enzymes of β-oxidation. Activation of fatty acids to fatty acyl-CoAs is probably coincident with transport into peroxisomes (16). Following a series of enzymatic steps that shorten the acyl-CoA moiety in 2-carbon-unit increments to a minimum of 6 carbons, reaction products can be exported from the peroxisome as acylcarnitines. They are also available for use in intraperoxisomal anabolic pathways such as cholesterol synthesis. β-oxidation in peroxisomes involves fewer enzymes than in mitochondria (perhaps as few as five), and defects in all of them have been identified as causes of human disease. However, abnormalities of peroxisomal biogenesis leading to multiple enzymatic deficiencies are much more common in humans.

ENZYMES OF β-OXIDATION

Mitochondria

Free fatty acids are transported through the blood after intestinal absorption or mobilization from endogenous stores by the use of albumin as a carrier protein or in the form of triacylglycerols in lipoprotein complexes (17). Transport of free fatty acids intracellularly and through the cytoplasm is probably accomplished by a specific transport process; however, the mechanism is not well characterized (18, 19). Before undergoing β-oxidation, free fatty acids must be activated to their corresponding acyl-CoA thioesters. Long-chain-specific acyl-CoA synthetases can be found in various subcellular locations but are thought to arise from a single gene product (20). Short- and medium-chain carboxylic acids directly enter the mitochondrial matrix, where they are activated. In contrast, long-chain fats are activated in the cytoplasm and require active transport into mitochondria. Transport of long-chain acyl-CoAs requires at least two enzymes, a transporter protein, and carnitine as an intermediate carrier molecule. Carnitine is itself transported intracellularly by a specific transporter protein (21, 22). Two carnitine transporters have been described, one specific to liver and a second with a more ubiquitous distribution, including kidney, muscle, and fibroblasts (23). Long-chain acyl-CoAs are conjugated to

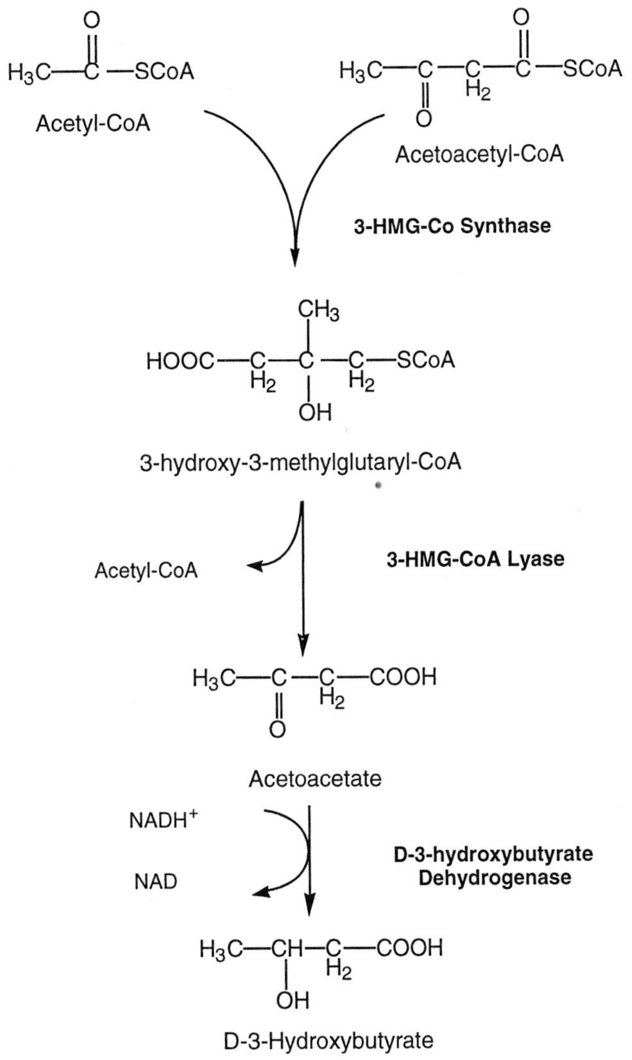

$$H_3C-C(=O)-SCoA \text{ (Acetyl-CoA)} + H_3C-C(=O)-CH_2-C(=O)-SCoA \text{ (Acetoacetyl-CoA)}$$

3-HMG-Co Synthase

$$HOOC-CH_2-C(CH_3)(OH)-CH_2-C(=O)-SCoA$$

3-hydroxy-3-methylglutaryl-CoA

Acetyl-CoA ← 3-HMG-CoA Lyase

$$H_3C-C(=O)-CH_2-COOH$$

Acetoacetate

NADH⁺ → NAD — D-3-hydroxybutyrate Dehydrogenase

$$H_3C-CH(OH)-CH_2-COOH$$

D-3-Hydroxybutyrate

Figure 62.2. Generation of ketone bodies from the products of β-oxidation.

carnitine by carnitine palmitoyl transferase I (CPT I) (17, 24). This enzyme is located on the inner aspect of the outer mitochondrial membrane. Tissue-specific isoforms of this enzyme probably exist. Long-chain acylcarnitines are then passed to carnitine palmitoyl transferase II (CPT II) in the inner mitochondrial membrane by a translocase (25).

Once present in the mitochondrial matrix, acyl-CoAs of all chain lengths undergo a series of enzymatic reactions which results in release of the 2-carbon-unit acetyl-CoA and a new acyl-CoA molecule that is two carbons shorter. The first step in this cycle is dehydrogenation of the acyl-CoA to 2-enoyl-CoA. This reaction is catalyzed by a family of related enzymes, the acyl-CoA dehydrogenases (ACDs) (26–29). Four different members of this family are active in β-oxidation: very long, long-, medium-, and short-chain acyl-CoA dehydrogenases (VLCAD, LCAD, MCAD, and SCAD, respectively), which differ in their chain-length specificity. The ACDs differ from most other dehydrogenases because they use electron-transfer flavoprotein (ETF) as a final electron acceptor and thus can channel electrons directly into the ubiquinone pool of the electron transport machinery by way of ETF dehydrogenase. The ACDs are homotetramers that are synthesized in a larger precursor form in the cytoplasm from nuclear-encoded transcripts and transported into mitochondria. Once inside the mitochondrial matrix, the leader peptide is removed by a specific protease, and the mature subunits assemble into the active homotetramer. One molecule of flavin adenine dinucleotide (FAD) is noncovalently attached to each ACD subunit. cDNAs for each of these proteins have been cloned, and sequence analysis shows that they are approximately 30 to 35% conserved, suggesting evolution from a common primordial gene (29–32).

2-Enoyl-CoAs produced by the ACDs are hydrated to 3-hydroxy-acyl-CoAs. These in turn undergo 2,3 dehydrogenation to 2-ketoacyl-CoAs, followed by cleavage of the thioester bond. This releases acetyl-CoA and completes one turn of the β-oxidation cycle. The exact mechanism of these steps varies for substrates of differing chain length. A trifunctional protein (TF) has recently been identified that has 2-enoyl-CoA hydratase, 3-hydroxy-acyl-CoA dehy-

Table 62.1
Enzymes Involved in Mitochondrial Fatty Acid Oxidation

Enzyme	Proven Clinical Disorder
Fatty acid activation	
Acyl-CoA synthetase	No
Carnitine cycle	
Plasma membrane carnitine transporter	Yes
CPT I	Yes
Carnitine/acylcarnitine translocase	Yes
CPT II	Yes
Mitochondrial β-oxidation spiral	
Very long chain acyl-CoA dehydrogenase (membrane)	Yes
LCAD (matrix)	No
MCAD	Yes
SCAD	Yes
Trifunctional protein	Yes
Long-chain 2-enoyl CoA hydratase	
Long-chain 3-hydroxyacyl-CoA dehydrogenase	Yes (isolated)
Long-chain 3-ketoacyl-CoA thiolase	
Crotonase (short-chain 2-enoyl-CoA hydratase)	No
SCHAD	Yes
Short-chain 3-ketoacyl-CoA thiolase	Possible
Enzymes of β-oxidation of unsaturated fats	
Long-chain δ^3, δ^2-enoyl-CoA isomerase	No
Short-chain δ^3, δ^2-enoyl-CoA isomerase	No
2,4-Dienoyl-CoA reductase	Possible
Enzymes of ketone body production	
HMG-CoA synthase	
HMG-CoA lyase	
D-3-hydroxybutyrate dehydrogenase	

drogenase, and 3-acyl-CoA ketothiolase activities for longer-chain acyl-CoA substrates (33–36). This complex is an octamer consisting of 4 α and 4 β subunits. LCHAD activity resides on the α subunit along with that of 3-enoyl-CoA hydratase, while the β subunit contains the 3-keto-acyl-CoA thiolase activity. In contrast, individual proteins that catalyze these reactions for shorter-chain substrates have been identified and purified, each with a single activity (37). There is, however, considerable overlap in the substrate specificity of these enzymes, and additional enzymes with yet different substrate optima have been postulated to exist for some of these steps (38). Enzymes catalyzing several additional sets of reactions are necessary for complete oxidation of unsaturated fatty acyl-CoA molecules.

Ketone bodies are produced exclusively in the liver from acetyl-CoA generated by β-oxidation (Fig. 62.2). HMG-CoA synthase forms 3-hydroxy-3-methylglutaryl-CoA (HMG-CoA) from acetoacetyl-CoA and acetyl-CoA. Acetyl-CoA and acetoacetate are then produced by cleavage of HMG-CoA by HMG-CoA lyase. Finally, acetoacetate is reduced to D-3-hydroxybutyrate by D-3-hydroxybutyrate dehydrogenase within mitochondria.

Several alternative metabolic pathways become important when mitochondrial β-oxidation is impaired. Peroxisomal β-oxidation allows continued metabolism of longer-chain fats, while ω-oxidation in the cytosol (which proceeds from the opposite end of the fatty acid) results in production of the characteristic dicarboxylic acids often present in these disorders. In addition, deacylation of acyl-CoA by cytosolic thioesters, and conjugation of acyl-CoAs to glycine and carnitine, become important mechanisms of CoA scavenging and detoxification, respectively.

Peroxisomes

Activation of fatty acids with chain lengths between 12 and 24 carbons and import into the peroxisomes is probably accomplished concomitantly by an acyl-CoA synthetase (16). A second enzyme with activities toward longer-chain substrates may exist (39, 40). The actual β-oxidation cycle in peroxisomes differs from that in mitochondria in a number of important ways (14, 41). The first step of the cycle in the peroxisomal matrix is oxidation by palmitoyl-CoA oxidase, leading to production of an enoyl-CoA (42). This enzyme transfers electrons directly to molecular oxygen, producing hydrogen peroxide, and may be, evolutionarily, distantly related to the mitochondrial acyl-CoA dehydrogenases. Additional oxidases can perform similar reactions using 2-methyl branched-chain acyl-CoAs and CoA intermediates of bile acids as substrates. The second and third steps of the β-oxidation cycle are carried out by a trifunctional protein complex containing enoyl-CoA hydrotase and 3-hydroxyacyl-CoA dehydrogenase activities associated with the inner aspect of the peroxisomal membrane (43, 44). A peroxisomal-specific 3-ketoacyl-CoA thiolase catalyzes the final step of the cycle, producing acetyl-CoA and regenerating an acyl-CoA (45). Carnitine acyltransferases likely facilitate removal of acetyl-CoA and acyl-CoAs from peroxisomes for subsequent metabolism in mitochondria or elsewhere (46–48). Additional enzymes involved in the metabolism of unsaturated long chain fats in peroxisomes include organelle-specific 2,4-dienoyl-CoA reductase, 3/2 enoyl-CoA isomerase, 2-enoyl-CoA hydratase, 2,5 enoyl-CoA reductase, and 3,5/2,4-dienoyl-CoA isomerase.

DEFECTS OF FATTY ACID METABOLISM

Mitochondria

Defects of Carnitine Biochemistry

Deficiencies of several steps of carnitine biochemistry and acylcarnitine transport into mitochondria have been described. These include defects of the specific plasma membrane carnitine-transporter proteins, CPT I and II, and the carnitine-acyl-carnitine translocase. Deficiency of the plasma membrane carnitine transporter represents a true primary carnitine deficiency (23). Carnitine is freely filtered by the kidney and must be reabsorbed from the proximal tubules to preserve plasma levels. Because the transporter for carnitine is deficient in kidney as well as other tissues in this defect, carnitine cannot be reabsorbed. This leads to a carnitine deficiency in end organs and impaired long-chain fatty acid metabolism.

Patients with carnitine-transporter deficiency can pre-

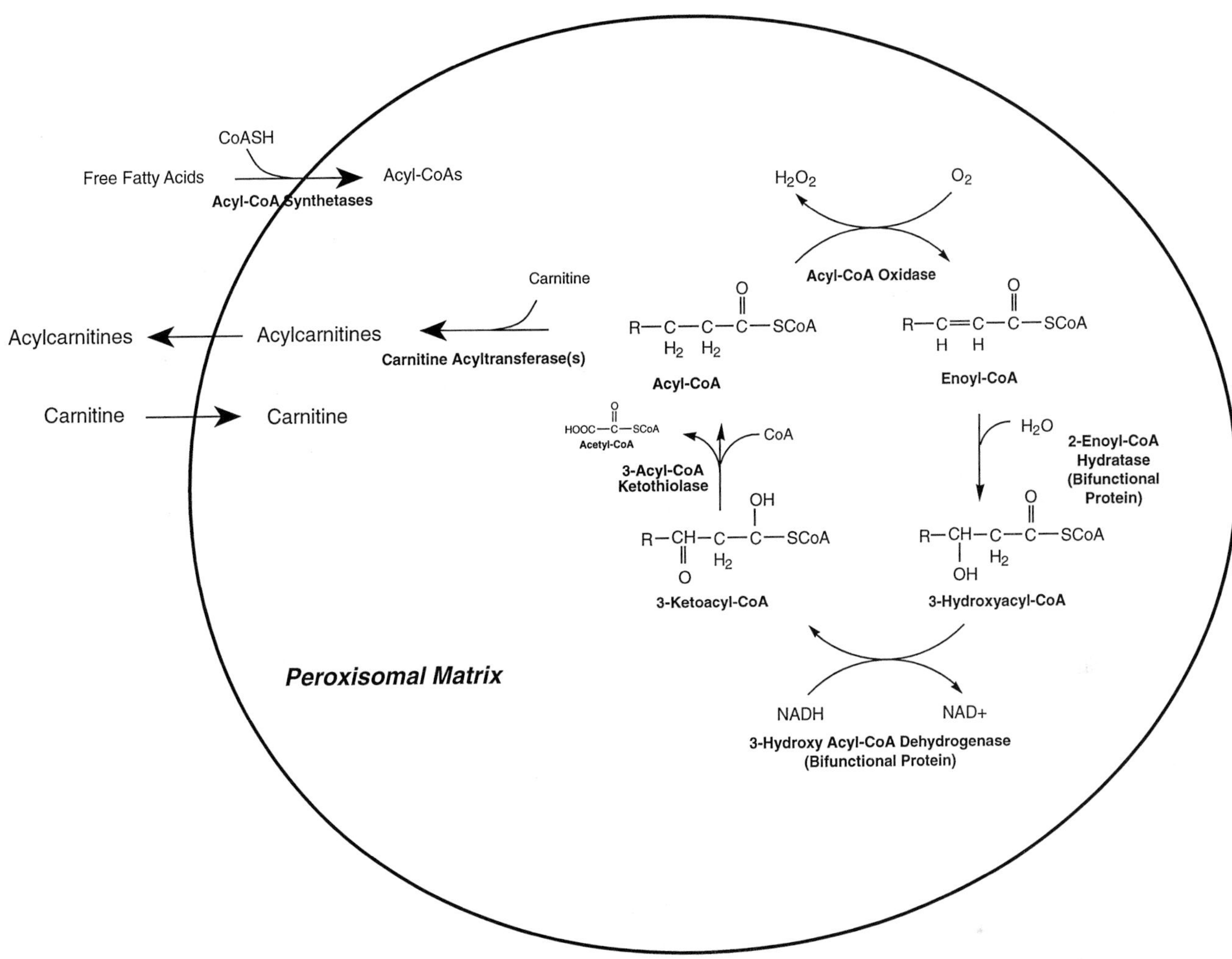

Figure 62.3. β-Oxidation of fatty acids in the peroxisome.

sent with severe hypoglycemia and dilated cardiomyopathy in infancy or childhood. Alternatively, they may show onset of hypertrophic cardiomyopathy, progressive muscle weakness, and muscle lipid storage in the first year of life. A mixed picture of these findings has also been seen. Fetal hydrops secondary to this disorder has been reported (49, 50). Plasma carnitine levels are extremely low or undetectable in these children, and a dramatic rise is seen upon

Table 62.2
Enzymes of Peroxisomal β-Oxidation

Acyl-CoA synthetase
Acyl-CoA oxidase
Bifunctional protein
2-Enoyl-CoA hydratase
3-Hydroxyacyl-CoA dehydrogenase
3-Ketoacyl-CoA thiolase
Carnitine acyltransferase
Enzymes of β-oxidation of unsaturated fats
2,4-Dienoyl-CoA reductase
3/2 Enoyl-CoA isomerase
2-Enoyl-CoA hydratase
2,5 Enoyl-CoA reductase
3, 5/2, 4-Dienoyl-CoA isomerase

supplementation with pharmacologic doses of carnitine (100 mg/kg body weight). Patients' symptoms also show dramatic resolution with therapy. Outcome for these children is likely to be good if diagnosis is prompt and therapy is instituted.

CPT I deficiency is a rare disorder characterized by the onset in infancy of episodic hypoketotic hypoglycemia and multiorgan system failure (51). Less than a dozen cases have been reported. Muscle symptoms are not present. In one case, an apparently healthy girl aged 2 years 9 months developed hepatomegaly and coma following a viral illness and died (52). Organic aciduria is not prominent in this disorder, but hyperammonemia may be present. Plasma carnitine levels are normal or elevated, with a high free fraction. Elevated levels of creatine kinase were seen in sibs from one family. Analysis of samples from patients with CPT I deficiency has revealed normal CPT I levels in muscle, but low activity in other tissues including liver (51, 53). Patients with an isolated deficiency of muscle CPT I have not been reported. Patients thus far have not responded well to therapy with carnitine.

Deficiency of the carnitine-acyl-carnitine translocase has recently been reported (54–56). Patients presented in the newborn period with severe hypoketotic hypoglycemia and cardiac arrhythmias and/or hypertrophy. All have had a grossly elevated acylcarnitine:free carnitine ratio, while dicarboxylic aciduria was reported in one. One child died at 36 months of age following a prolonged course of progressive muscle weakness (54). He had episodes of coma associated with intercurrent illness and fasting which left him profoundly weak for 2 to 3 weeks following recovery. Another patient died at 8 days of age of a pulmonary hemorrhage, probably secondary to liver failure (55). Mild hyperammonemia was present in both cases. Organic aciduria was not prominent. Two sibs died at age 2 months of liver failure, after presentation at age 2 days (56). Carnitine supplementation did not appear to improve clinical symptoms in either patient.

CPT II deficiency is the most common of this group of disorders. It classically presents in late childhood or early adulthood as episodes of recurrent exercise- or stress-induced myoglobinuria (57), which can be severe enough to occasionally lead to acute renal failure. Patients are typically well between episodes. There is no tendency to develop hypoglycemia. Weakness and muscle pain are common. The characteristic diagnostic finding in these patients is a low total plasma carnitine level with increased acylcarnitine fraction and no dicarboxylic aciduria. Long-chain acylcarnitines may in fact be elevated (58). A more severe variant of CPT II deficiency similar in symptoms to CPT I deficiency has recently been reported (58, 59). These patients presented with neonatal hypoglycemia, hepatomegaly, and cardiomyopathy. A severe reduction in CPT II activity was found in all tissues tested, including liver, heart, muscle, and fibroblasts, while CPT I activity was normal. This decrease in enzyme activity was in the same range as that seen with the later-onset form of the disease. Plasma carnitine was not increased. Mutations in the cDNA for CPT II have been described, and expression studies of mutant CPT II alleles suggest that the level of residual function of the mutant enzyme may determine the clinical phenotype (59–61). A common mutation has been reported to account for half of mutant alleles in the late-onset form of the disease. Carnitine supplementation has not been of benefit in the severe form of CPT II deficiency (62).

Defects of ACDs

Deficiencies of VLCAD, LCAD, and SCAD have been described in relatively few patients. VLCAD deficiency has only recently been recognized. The first patient presented with ventricular fibrillation and respiratory arrest at 2 days of age and exhibited massive dicarboxylic aciduria (63). Plasma glucose and ammonia levels were not reported. She was treated with a low-lipid diet and carnitine supplementation. Despite the dramatic neonatal presentation, she recovered and is reported well at 2 years of age, without muscle or cardiac abnormalities. The patient's older sib died suddenly at 2 days of age and showed hepatic steatosis at necropsy. It is now clear that VLCAD deficiency is commonly, but not invariably, associated with early-onset cardiac and skeletal myopathy (64). One patient with onset of recurrent exercise-induced myoglobinuria in adolescence has been described (65). Hypoketotic hypoglycemia, hyperammonemia, and hepatocellular failure have been reported, and 3-hydroxy-dicarboxylic acids or saturated dicarboxylic acids may be present in the urine (63, 66). Cloning of the gene for VLCAD has allowed identification of a variety of genetic defects, but no common mutations have been found (32, 67–70).

Putative LCAD deficiency has been reported, but all patients originally categorized as LCAD deficient subsequently were proven to have a deficiency of VLCAD instead (71–73). Thus, there are no known patients with bona fide LCAD deficiency.

A number of patients with SCAD deficiency have been described (74–78). Clinical findings have included episodes of intermittent metabolic acidosis, neonatal hyperammonemic coma, neonatal acidosis with hyperreflexia, and infantile-onset lipid-storage myopathy with failure to thrive and hypotonia. Hypoglycemia has not been reported in this disorder. The characteristic metabolites of ethylmalonic and methylsuccinic acids seen in SCAD deficiency have also been described in individuals who appear to have normal SCAD activity in fibroblasts. It has been suggested that a relatively common variant of SCAD may predispose to excess production of these metabolites, but the role of this in disease remains unclear (79).

In the past several years, MCAD deficiency has emerged as one of the most common inborn errors of metabolism in certain populations. The most frequent presentation is one of intermittent hypoketotic hypoglycemia with onset in the second year of life (clinical features reviewed in [11]). Mild hyperammonemia and coma may or may not be present. These findings often lead to inappropriate diagnosis of Reye syndrome. The patient is usually well between episodes. Dicarboxylic aciduria is extensive during times of illness, but can be undetectable by routine means when the patient is well. Similarly, micro- and macrovesicular steatosis present during acute illness may resolve between acute episodes. Most patients who have subsequently been shown to have died of MCAD deficiency have survived an initial episode. Thus, recurrent Reye syndrome–like episodes especially should trigger suspicion of this disorder. Sudden death in a previously healthy child has been described in numerous cases of MCAD deficiency. In the appropriate age range, such deaths are often misascribed to "sudden infant death syndrome" (SIDS). Autopsy usually reveals the characteristic micro- and macrovesicular steatosis and should suggest the diagnosis. Finally, completely asymptomatic individuals have been identified in the course of family studies of patients. The diagnosis of MCAD deficiency in asymptomatic individuals has been made possible in the past several years by dramatic advances in laboratory techniques based on identification of alternate metabolites that accumulate in various bodily fluids (80, 81).

Remarkable progress has been made in recent years in our understanding of the molecular mechanisms responsible for MCAD deficiency. Following cloning of the cDNA for MCAD, several groups simultaneously reported that a single common mutant allele was responsible for up to 90% of mutant alleles in patients with this disorder (82). Substitution of a G for an A residue at position 985 results in replacement of a lysine by a glutamic acid residue, leading to production of an unstable protein (83). Furthermore, screening of newborn blood samples has revealed that the carrier frequency for this disorder is quite high in some populations. Allele frequencies for the A to G^{985} mutation range from 1 in 40 in northern European populations to less than 1 in 100 in Asian and some southern European populations. In the United States, a carrier frequency for all mutations of 1 in 60 has been estimated for Caucasians (84). This translates into a predicted disease frequency of 1 in 15,000. MCAD deficiency has not yet been diagnosed in an African American. The public health issues surrounding a disease of potentially such high frequency have been vigorously debated. The predicted incidence of MCAD deficiency on the basis of these studies is similar to, or greater than, that for phenylketonuria (PKU), a disorder screened for in all 50 states in the United States. Thus, some groups feel strongly that newborn screening for MCAD deficiency is warranted.

Deficiency of Other β-Oxidation Enzymes

Patients with a deficiency of long-chain 3-hydroxy acyl-CoA dehydrogenase (LCHAD) have tended to fall into two clinical subclasses (85–90). One group presented primarily with symptoms of cardiomyopathy, myopathy, and hypoglycemia. Peripheral neuropathy with or without pigmentary retinopathy and recurrent myoglobinuria may be present (38, 91, 92). These patients are deficient in all three enzymatic activities of the trifunctional protein. The other group has shown a picture of severe hepatocellular disease. Considerable overlap in these groups has been described, however, and LCHAD deficiency has also been reported in patients with recurrent Reye syndrome–like symptoms and in sudden infant death. Defects in the α subunit appear to destabilize trifunctional protein, resulting in the multiple enzymatic deficiencies seen in some patients (93–95). A common G to C mutation at nucleotide position 1528 accounts for approximately 80% of mutant alleles thus far identified in this gene (94). Heterozygosity for trifunctional protein α subunit deficiency has recently been implicated as a potential risk factor in the development of fatty liver of pregnancy or "hemolysis, elevated liver enzymes, low platelet" (HELLP) syndrome (96, 97). Mutations in the β subunit of trifunctional protein have been less well characterized but can also destabilize trifunctional protein (95). The reason for the clinical heterogeneity in this disorder remains to be elucidated (98).

Three patients have been reported with a deficiency of short-chain 3-hydroxy acyl-CoA dehydrogenase (SCHAD) (99, 100). The first was a 16-year-old previously healthy girl who developed episodic myoglobinuria at age 13 years. At age 16 years she developed a flulike illness with generalized weakness, hypoketotic hypoglycemia, and lethargy. She subsequently died of a cardiac arrhythmia. Dicarboxylic and 3-hydroxydicarboxylic aciduria were present acutely. An older brother died at age 8 years of encephalopathy after a 6-year history of intermittent episodes of irritability, ataxia, and mild mental retardation. The 16-year-old girl had 35% of normal SCHAD activity in muscle, compared with controls, but activity for long-chain substrates was preserved. A second patient exhibited episodic vomiting, dehydration, and hyperammonemia beginning at age 13 months (100). Urine findings during acute episodes included elevated 3-hydroxybutyrate and acetoacetate levels along with dicarboxylic acids and 3-hydroxydicarboxylic acids of chain length C6 to C14. Urinary carnitine was increased and was mostly conjugated. A final patient displayed a complex clinical picture complicated by a concurrent chromosomal abnormality but with biochemical findings similar to those of the second patient. Only the last patient exhibited hypoglycemia. SCHAD activity in isolated mitochondria from the latter two patients was reduced to about 5% of normal (100).

Three patients have recently been described with developmental delay and muscle weakness; one of them, who died of a Reye-like illness, had urine metabolite findings suggesting a defect in 3-ketoacyl-CoA dehydrogenase (101). Definitive enzyme testing has not been performed. An isolated defect of 3-enoyl-CoA hydratase deficiency has not been reported.

One patient has been reported to have a potential defect in the enzyme 2,4-dienoyl-CoA reductase (102). This patient presented in the newborn period with persistent hypotonia. She was found to have elevated lysine and decreased carnitine levels in plasma. 2-*trans*,4-*cis*-Decadienenoylcarnitine was identified in plasma and urine, and reduced activity of 2,4-dienoyl-CoA reductase was found in liver and muscle. The patient died at 4 months of age of respiratory acidosis. Confirmation of the clinical significance of these biochemical abnormalities awaits identification of additional patients.

Multiple Acyl-CoA Dehydrogenation Disorder (MAD)

Abnormalities of ETF or ETF dehydrogenase deficiency lead to an in vivo deficiency of all dehydrogenases that use ETF as an electron acceptor (103). This includes the ACDs discussed above, as well as isovaleryl-CoA dehydrogenase, 2-methylbutyryl-CoA dehydrogenase, glutaryl-CoA dehydrogenase, dimethylglycine dehydrogenase, and sarcosine dehydrogenase, enzymes involved in the intermediate metabolism of branched-chain amino acids, tryptophan, lysine, and choline. Intermediate compounds accumulate related to blockages in all of these pathways. Because glutaric acid is present in the urine of some patients, this disorder is frequently referred to as glutaric aciduria type II (GA II) to distinguish it from a primary deficiency of glutaryl-CoA dehydrogenase (GA I).

Clinical manifestations of MAD are extremely heterogeneous. A neonatal form can be seen with severe hypotonia, dysmorphic features, and cystic kidneys. These infants also exhibit metabolic acidosis and hypoglycemia. Milder variants are common, with nonspecific neurologic signs, myopathy, fasting hypoketotic hypoglycemia, and/or intermittent acidosis. In some patients, only fasting hypoketotic hypoglycemia and/or intermittent acidosis is seen. In these patients, the organic acid profile in times of illness is usually dominated by ethylmalonic (EMA) and adipic acids, leading to the alternate name of EMA-adipic aciduria for this disorder.

Analysis of fibroblasts from patients with MAD has revealed defects in both protein subunits of ETF and in ETF dehydrogenase (104). Cell lines with and without immunologically cross-reactive material have been described. cDNAs for both subunits of ETF and ETF dehydrogenase have been cloned, and direct mutational analysis has revealed a variety of defects in patients. Thus far, correlation of the mutation with severity of clinical symptoms has not been possible.

Riboflavin-Responsive Defects of Fatty Acid Metabolism

Riboflavin is the precursor to FAD, an essential cofactor for the ACDs, ETF, and ETF dehydrogenase. Several sets of patients with biochemical abnormalities suggesting β-oxidation defects have responded with clinical improvement to pharmacologic doses of riboflavin (100–200 mg/kg/day). One group clinically resembles patients with multiple dehydrogenase deficiency and appears to represent a variant of ETF or ETF dehydrogenase with an as yet undefined defect in interaction with FAD. Increasing intramitochondrial concentrations of FAD by administration of riboflavin apparently allows enough cofactor binding to restore activity. A second set of patients shows a picture of late-onset lipid-storage myopathy and muscle weakness with some level of hepatic dysfunction. These patients also appear to respond to therapy with riboflavin, but their defect remains undefined. Marked clinical heterogeneity within each group has been documented.

Deficiencies of Ketone Body Production

HMG-CoA synthase deficiency has been reported in a child with fasting hypoketotic hypoglycemia. Deficiency of HMG-CoA lyase, which is also active in the metabolism of leucine, presents with hypoketotic hypoglycemia with hyperammonemia and acidosis (105). Identification of hydroxymethylglutaric acid in the urine is diagnostic.

Peroxisomes

Defects of Peroxisomal Biogenesis

Deficiencies of single peroxisomal enzymes exist for a number of the steps of peroxisomal β-oxidation (Table 62.2). Defects of peroxisomal biogenesis with a resulting failure to import all or a subset of matrix enzymes are far more common, however. Absence or significant reduction in the number of peroxisomes occurs in four disorders historically considered distinct: Zellweger syndrome, neonatal adrenoleukodystrophy, infantile Refsum disease, and pipecolic acidemia (1, 106). It is now clear that these are related disorders that form a spectrum of clinical severity from the early lethal phenotype seen in Zellweger syndrome to the later-onset symptoms of infantile Refsum disease and pipecolic acidemia.

Zellweger syndrome was the first disorder of peroxisomal biogenesis to be identified (107). Classic findings include characteristic dysmorphic facial features and other malformations accompanied by severe neurologic dysfunction with hypotonia, seizures, and ultimate deterioration. Liver function is abnormal, as is that of the gastrointestinal tract, leading to failure to thrive. Neuronal heterotopia and renal cortical cysts are seen pathologically. Proximal limb shortening may be present. Death usually occurs within the first few months of life. Peroxisomes are completely absent in all tissues examined, and the enzymatic functions associated with peroxisomes are similarly absent or mislocalized to the cytosolic compartment. This results in severe impairment of cholesterol synthesis, bile acid metabolism, β-oxidation of very long chain fats and branched-chain fats, ether phospholipid synthesis, and phytanic acid and pipecolic acid metabolism.

Neonatal adrenoleukodystrophy and infantile Refsum disease can manifest in the first 6 months of life with a presentation resembling that of Zellweger syndrome, but with slightly later onset of symptoms (108, 109). These disorders, along with pipecolic acidemia, can also appear in early childhood (less than 3 years of age) with findings of psychomotor retardation (108, 109), ophthalmologic abnormalities, and other neurologic deficits, including neurosensory impairment and nystagmus. Biochemical findings in patients with neonatal adrenoleukodystrophy, infantile Refsum disease, and pipecolic acidemia resemble those of Zellweger syndrome but may be more subtle.

Understanding of the molecular basis for deficient peroxisomal biogenesis in this group of disorders is evolving rapidly. Complementation analysis of fibroblasts from these patients reveals that at least 10 separate genes are affected (110). Three of these have been identified as a protein import receptor, a peroxisomal assembly factor, and a 70-kd peroxisomal membrane protein, with the latter defect found in the largest group of patients

(111–114). Some of the complementation groups are rare and so far identified only in patients with the Zellweger phenotype, but this is likely to be an ascertainment bias (110). Patients in the remaining complementation groups may exhibit any of the clinical phenotypes.

Disorders of Single Enzymes

X-linked adrenoleukodystrophy is the most common disorder involving peroxisomal β-oxidation, affecting 1/20,000 males (15). Biochemical studies originally characterized an impaired ability to activate fatty acids to their acyl-CoA esters and suggested that this was a disorder of an acyl-CoA synthetase. Recent molecular data, however, have identified defects in an ATP-binding transporter located in the peroxisomal membrane as responsible (115). Why this defect affects the activity of acyl-CoA synthetase remains to be elucidated. Regardless, patients show a severely impaired ability to metabolize very long chain fatty acids in the peroxisomes. Several clinical phenotypes have been associated with defects at this locus (115–120). Classical cerebral childhood adrenoleukodystrophy is the most common of these and accounts for 50% of cases. Boys are usually well until the second half of the first decade of life, when progressive quadriplegia, blindness, and dementia develop. Death generally occurs within 5 years of onset of symptoms. In 30% of individuals, a later-onset disorder designated adrenomyeloneuropathy is seen in which male patients experience progressive spastic paraparesis with peripheral neuropathy beginning in the second or third decade of life. Up to 30% of females who are carriers of X-linked adrenoleukodystrophy show a similar picture beginning at about age 30 years. Finally, some males with a defect in this gene show only adrenal insufficiency (which also accompanies almost 90% of adrenoleukodystrophy and adrenomyeloneuropathy). There may be great clinical heterogeneity within families.

The remaining defects in peroxisomal β-oxidation are relatively rare, with only a handful of reported cases each. Acyl-CoA oxidase deficiency is characterized by early-onset seizures, psychomotor retardation, and neurologic degeneration similar to neonatal adrenoleukodystrophy and is often referred to as "pseudo–neonatal adrenoleukodystrophy" (121). Dysmorphic features are not seen. Hepatic peroxisomes are present and an isolated elevation of very long chain fatty acids is found in blood and urine. Peroxisomal trifunctional protein deficiency also presents similarly to neonatal adrenal leukodystrophy, but with accumulation of trihydroxycoprostanoic acid in addition to very long chain fatty acids (122–125). Dysmorphic features may be present. Several patients with clinical and pathologic features identical to those of Zellweger syndrome have been described who have abundant hepatic peroxisomes and an isolated defect of the peroxisomal 3-ketoacyl-CoA thiolase (126, 127). This entity has been referred to as "pseudo-Zellweger syndrome." Very long chain fatty acids, pipecolic acid, and bile acid intermediates are all elevated in these patients.

Classic Refsum disease due to deficiency of phytanic acid oxidase is not a defect of peroxisomal β-oxidation per se but deserves mention because of the confusing nomenclature. Clinical findings include retinitis pigmentosa, cerebellar ataxia, and peripheral neuropathy, with onset of symptoms varying from childhood to the fifth decade of life (128). There is no mental retardation, dysmorphic features, or hepatomegaly. This disorder is characterized by accumulation of phytanic acid in blood and tissues, while measures of other peroxisomal enzyme functions are normal.

DIAGNOSIS OF DEFECTS OF FATTY ACID METABOLISM

Mitochondria

Diagnosis of defects of mitochondrial fatty acid metabolism requires a high level of suspicion in the appropriate clinical settings (Table 62.3). This is crucial because, in many instances, the biochemical abnormalities that might suggest a defect of β-oxidation often resolve along with clinical symptoms. Thus, individuals with unexplained hypoglycemia, acidosis, hyperammonemia, myopathy with or without recurrent myoglobinuria, or progressive neuropathy should be considered candidates for one of these disorders. All cases of Reye syndrome, patients with Reye syndrome–like symptoms, "SIDS," or unexplained sudden or near death in childhood should be evaluated for a defect in fat metabolism.

When an individual presents with such a clinical picture, it is critical to obtain blood and urine samples acutely for appropriate analysis, since biochemical findings may disappear when the patient is well. Because routine organic acid analysis is often normal when patients are not in an acute crisis, these patients should be more extensively evaluated if a diagnosis is not immediately obvious. This is best done in a referral center by a specialist trained in the evaluation of these patients. Plasma free and total carnitine levels can often suggest whether a deficiency is

Table 62.3
Findings Suggestive of a Defect in Mitochondrial β-Oxidation

Hypoketotic hypoglycemia with fasting or stress
Reye syndrome (especially recurrent)
Hypotonia and/or muscle weakness
Peripheral neuropathy
Coma
Sudden death in infancy or childhood
Cardiomyopathy
Unexplained metabolic acidosis ± hyperammonemia
Hyperuricemia
Recurrent myoglobinuria
Elevated serum creatine kinase
Dicarboxylic aciduria
Carnitine deficiency

Table 62.4
Plasma Carnitine Levels in Defects of β-Oxidation

Enzyme Defect	Total Carnitine	Free Carnitine	Free/Total Carnitine
Carnitine Transporter	Very Low	Low	Normal
CPT I	Normal or high	High	High
Translocase and CPT II	Low	Very low	Low
VLCAD, LCAD, MCAD, SCAD, LCHAD, SCHAD, ETF and ETFdehydrogenase and 2,4-dienoyl-CoA reductase	Low	Low	Normal or low

primary or secondary (Table 62.4). Laboratory clues to the diagnosis of one of these disorders include dicarboxylic or 3-hydroxydicarboxylic aciduria, hypoglycemia in the face of little or no ketosis, mild lactic acidosis, and mild hyperammonemia. Hyperuricacidemia is a useful sign if present but is nonspecific. Myoglobin in blood or urine and elevated plasma creatine kinase levels can be seen when muscle involvement is present. Highly sensitive techniques, using mass spectrometry, can detect minute quantities of intermediates specific for certain fatty acid oxidation disorders. These intermediates are often not detectable by routine organic acid analysis (80, 81). All patients with a suspected defect in fatty acid metabolism should receive an echocardiogram because of the high incidence of cardiomyopathy in many of these disorders. A fasting test with or without a subsequent challenge test with medium- or long-chain triglycerides may induce excretion of a diagnostic metabolite but should only be undertaken in a hospital setting by someone experienced in performing such tests. A medium-chain triglyceride loading test must only be performed *after* specifically excluding the diagnosis of MCAD deficiency, as catastrophic consequences can result in patients with MCAD deficiency. Direct DNA mutational analysis is readily available for the common A to G^{985} mutation responsible for MCAD deficiency (82). Specific enzyme analysis can be performed for many of these defects on cultured fibroblasts and/or liver or skeletal muscle. Newborn screening for MCAD deficiency has been suggested but remains controversial (129, 130).

Peroxisomes

Diagnosis of defects of peroxisomal β-oxidation is more straightforward than that of mitochondrial defects since clinical symptoms and biochemical abnormalities are not intermittent. Clinical findings suggesting a defect of peroxisomal biogenesis or an isolated defect in β-oxidation are summarized in Table 62.5. These diagnoses should be considered in the setting of unexplained seizures and/or developmental delay, especially if accompanied by hypotonia. Screening plasma and/or urine for very long chain fatty acids, pipecolic acid, phytanic acid, and prystanic acid will identify most patients. Additional investigations can include quantitation of bile acid and cholesterol synthesis intermediates, red blood cell membrane plasmalogen level, and presence or absence of peroxisomes in cultured skin fibroblasts. Finally, specific enzyme analysis on cultured skin fibroblasts as well as complementation analysis can be performed to identify the precise nature of the defect in a patient. Molecular mutational analysis remains largely a research tool.

Table 62.5
Findings Suggestive of a Defect in Peroxisomal β-Oxidation

- Seizures
- Hypotonia
- Dysmorphic features
  - Large fontanelle
  - High forehead
  - Epicanthal folds
  - Malformed ears
  - Inverted nipples
  - Rhizomelic chondrodysplasia
- Hepatomegaly and/or hepatic failure
- Renal cysts
- Neurologic and/or intellectual degeneration
- Ophthalmologic abnormalities
  - Peripheral neuropathy
  - Optic atrophy
  - Cataracts
  - Retinopathy
- Hearing impairment
- Failure to thrive

GENETICS OF DEFECTS OF FATTY ACID METABOLISM

All of the defects of mitochondrial fatty acid metabolism identified thus far and all of the peroxisomal disorders except X-linked adrenoleukodystrophy are inherited in an autosomal recessive fashion. The recurrence risk for subsequent sibs is therefore 25%. X-linked adrenoleukodystrophy is inherited as an X-linked trait. Affected males are hemizygous for one abnormal gene, while carrier women are heterozygous for one normal and one mutant allele. Thus, carrier women face a 50% risk of having an affected male or carrier female with each pregnancy. There may be great clinical heterogeneity within families, and individuals with the severe childhood onset and less severe myeloneuropathy forms may be present in the same family. To explain this, it has been proposed that one or more additional autosomal genes modulate the clinical severity of this disorder.

SUDDEN INFANT DEATH AND DEFECTS OF FATTY ACID METABOLISM

The role of mitochondrial β-oxidation defects in SIDS bears special mention. Precision is required when discussing SIDS. Since the definition of SIDS includes normal autopsy findings, many patients with defects of β-oxidation will be eliminated from this population by careful microscopic study of muscle, heart, and liver. Unfortunately, not all deaths reported as SIDS receive the same level of scrutiny, and thus cases of β-oxidation disorders may still be represented. In addition, some disorders of β-oxidation can clearly present with minimal or no tissue changes, making postmortem diagnosis far more difficult. An early claim that 15 to 17% of cases of SIDS are caused by defects of β-oxidation has been tempered by additional data, but it is likely that approximately 1 to 3% of unexplained sudden deaths in infancy and childhood are related to such disorders (131–133). Because of this high frequency and because of the lack of reliable autopsy findings, all children who die suddenly from unexplained causes (whether or not they are infants) should be evaluated for possible metabolic defects, including disorders of β-oxidation.

Postmortem examination should include analysis of blood, urine, or aqueous humor for organic acids and acylglycines and/or acylcarnitines. Tissue samples of liver, skeletal muscle, and heart should be rapidly frozen and stored at −70°C for future enzymatic analysis, and a skin fibroblast culture should be started when possible. Only such an intense effort to determine a diagnosis in these cases will permit accurate counseling for the family regarding recurrence risks and identification of asymptomatic siblings. It has been suggested that newborn screening for MCAD deficiency could reduce the incidence of SIDS, but this remains to be substantiated (129, 130).

TREATMENT OF DEFECTS OF FATTY ACID METABOLISM

Mitochondria

The mainstay for therapy of defects of mitochondrial β-oxidation is avoidance of fasting. By not allowing patients with these disorders to become dependent on β-oxidation for energy needs, accumulation of intermediate metabolites and development of symptoms can be minimized. Thus, during periods of wellness, fat consumption should ideally be restricted to the ADA minimum nutritional requirements for age. This may be difficult to achieve in practice, and a goal of 25% of calories by fat may be more realistic.

Increased caloric intake may be necessary during intercurrent illness because of increased metabolic demands on the body. This can be met via oral or nasogastric tube (NG) administration of an appropriate formula or by intravenous (IV) infusion of glucose (8–10 mg/kg/min) if oral intake is inadequate. Orally administered corn starch (1.5–2.0 g/kg/dose) has been used as an alternative glucose source in some patients with long-chain fat metabolism defects to reduce dependence on NG or IV calories.

Substitution of medium-chain triglycerides for complete dietary fats in patients with defects in long-chain fat metabolism has been reported to be of value, as fats in this preparation can bypass the metabolic block. Carnitine at a dose of 100 mg/kg can completely reverse the symptoms of carnitine-transporter deficiency and may be necessary to replete carnitine levels that are secondarily lowered in other patients.

The concept of carnitine as a completely benign therapy has been called into question for patients with β-oxidation defects (134, 135). Theoretically, promoting entry of long-chain fats into mitochondria, the physiologic role of carnitine, may be counterproductive in patients unable to subsequently metabolize those substances. Adverse effects of such therapy have been reported (134). In addition, few controlled studies are available regarding the efficacy of carnitine therapy in defects of fatty acid metabolism other than primary deficiencies. Finally, carnitine may interfere with production of acylglycines in some instances and actually decrease the total amount of excreted metabolites (80, 135).

Conjugation of acyl-CoAs with glycine occurs via a specific enzymatic reaction and represents a major route for excretion of excess acyl-CoAs as well as other organic acids. Glycine therapy (300 mg/kg/day) has been advocated for patients with multiple dehydrogenase deficiency and has been shown to increase metabolite excretion in these and other patients (136). Concern over toxicity has tempered its use, however. Riboflavin (200 mg/kg/day) may be useful in some patients with multiple acyl-CoA dehydrogenase deficiency and riboflavin metabolism defects.

Peroxisomes

Treatment of patients with defects in peroxisomal β-oxidation has been problematic and, in recent years, controversial. Therapy for X-linked adrenoleukodystrophy has received the most attention. Several inhibitors of very long chain fatty acid synthesis have been used in an attempt to control excess accumulation of very long chain fats in patients. These include oleic acid, glycerol trioleate, and glycerol trierucate. The most extensive therapeutic trial to date used a diet that provided 10% of calories as fat, with less than 10 to 15 mg of C26:0 fatty acid per day (137). In addition, 1.7 g/kg body weight/day of glycerol trioleate oil and 0.3 g/kg body weight/day were also given, along with 10 to 15 mL safflower oil and 2 g fish oil (to avoid a deficiency of essential fatty acids). Using this regimen, very long chain fatty acid levels were normalized in patients with either adrenoleukodystrophy or adrenomyeloneuropathy, but little or no clinical improvement could be documented (137). It is still not known whether presymptomatic treatment will prevent or delay appearance of symptoms, but this now seems the best possible alternative for patients with this deficiency. Liver transplant has been used in this disorder with mixed results. Therapy of the other single-enzyme defects of peroxisomal β-oxidation has not been reported.

Treatment of the disorders of peroxisomal biogenesis has been problematic because of the multisystemic disease and the numerous metabolic pathways affected in these individuals. In addition to reduction of very long chain fatty acid intake, patients may benefit from reduction of phytanic acid intake (10 mg/day) as in adult Refsum disease (128). Dairy products, ruminant fats, and ruminant meats are the prime dietary sources of phytanic acid. Green vegetables, originally excluded from the diet, are no longer believed to contribute significantly to the physiologic phytanic acid load. Unfortunately, limited information is available on many food items. Since it is difficult to reduce dietary intake below 10 to 20 mg/day, it may be necessary to supplement with an artificial liquid formula. Benefits in uncontrolled studies have been reported for supplementation of patients with oral formulations of ether lipids, cholic (100 mg/day) and deoxycholic acids (100 mg/day), and docosahexenoic acid (250 mg/day), but large-scale controlled studies are necessary for rigorous evaluation of the efficacy of these treatments (138–140). Regardless, based on experience with X-linked adrenoleukodystrophy, these therapies are likely to be helpful (if at all) only when begun presymptomatically, and perhaps only in the milder disorders of peroxisomal biogenesis.

REFERENCES

1. Lazarow PB, Moser HW. Disorders of peroxisome biogenesis. In: Scriver C, Beaudet AL, Sly W, et al., eds. The metabolic basis of inherited disease. 7th ed. New York: McGraw-Hill, 1995;2287–324.
2. Molzer B, Bernheimer H, Budka H, et al. J Neurol Sci 1981;51:301–10.
3. Purdue PE, Lazarow PB. J Biol Chem 1994;269:30065–8.
4. Subrammani S. Annu Rev Cell Biol 1993;9:445–78.
5. Hartl F-U, Pfanner N, Nicholson DW, et al. Biochim Biophys Acta 1989;988:1–45.
6. Glick B, Schatz G. Annu Rev Genet 1991;25:21–44.
7. Horwich AL, Kalousek F, Rosenberg LE. Proc Natl Acad Sci USA 1985;82:4920–33.
8. Horwich AL, Kalousek F, Mellman I, et al. EMBO J 1985;4:1129–35.
9. Horwich AL, Kalousek F, Fenton WA, et al. Cell 1986;44:451–9.
10. Rosenberg LE, Fenton WA, Horwich AL, et al. Ann NY Acad Sci 1987;488:99–108.
11. Roe CR, Coates PM. Mitochondrial fatty acid oxidation disorders. In: Scriver C, Beaudet AL, Sly W, et al., eds. The metabolic basis of inherited disease. 7th ed. New York: McGraw-Hill, 1995;1501–33.
12. Engel AG, Angelini C. Science 1973;899–902.
13. DiMauro S, DiMauro PMM. Science 1973;182:929–31.
14. Hashimoto T. Ann NY Acad Sci 1982;386:5–12.
15. Moser HW, Smith KD, Moser AB. X-linked adrenoleukodystrophy. In: Scriver C, Beaudet AL, Sly W, et al., eds. The metabolic basis of inherited disease. 7th ed. New York: McGraw-Hill, 1995;2325–49.
16. Krisans SK, Mortensen RM, Lazarow PB. J Biol Chem 1980;255:9599–607.
17. McGarry JD, Foster DW. Annu Rev Biochem 1980; 49:395–420.
18. Stremmel W, Strohmeyer G, Borchard F, et al. Proc Natl Acad Sci USA 1985;82:4–8.
19. Stremmel W, Strohmeyer G, Berk PD. Proc Natl Acad Sci USA 1986;83:3584–8.
20. Abe T, Fujino T, Fukuyama R, et al. J Biochem 1992;111: 123–8.
21. Bremer J. Physiol Rev 1983;63:1420–80.
22. Martinuzzi A, Vergani L, Rosa M, et al. Biochim Biophys Acta 1991;1095:217–22.
23. Treem WR, Stanley CA, Finegold DN, et al. N Engl J Med 1988;319:1331–6.
24. Murthy MSR, Pande SV. Proc Natl Acad Sci USA 1987;84:378–82.
25. Pande SV. Proc Natl Acad Sci USA 1975;72:883–7.
26. Iafolla AK, Thompson RJ, Roe CR. J Pediatr 1994;124:409–15.
27. Ikeda Y, Dabrowski C, Tanaka K. J Biol Chem 1983;258: 1066–76.
28. Ikeda Y, Tanaka K. J Biol Chem 1983;258:1077–85.
29. Matsubara Y, Indo Y, Naito E, et al. J Biol Chem 1989; 264:16321–31.
30. Matsubara Y, Ito M, Glassberg R, et al. J Clin Invest 1990;85:1058–64.
31. Kelly D, Kim J, Billadello J, et al. Proc Natl Acad Sci USA 1988;85:4068–72.
32. Aoyama T, Souri M, Ueno I, et al. Am J Hum Genet 1995;57:273–83.
33. Uchida Y, Izai K, Orii T, et al. J Biol Chem 1992;267:1034–41.
34. Carpenter K, Pollitt RJ, Middleton B, et al. Biochem Biophys Res Commun 1992;183:443–8.
35. Kamijo T, Aoyama T, Miyakaki J, et al. J Biol Chem 1993;268:26452–60.
36. Kamijo T, Aoyama T, Komiyama A, et al. Biochem Biophys Res Commun 1994;199:818–25.
37. Mori M, Amaya Y, Arakawa H, et al. Biosynthesis and mitochondrial import of fatty acid oxidation enzymes. In: Tanaka K, Coates PM, eds. Progress in clinical and biological research: fatty acid oxidation. Clinical, biochemical and molecular aspects. New York: Alan R Liss, 1990;23–36.
38. Jackson S, Kler RS, Bartlett K, et al. J Clin Invest 1992;90:1219–25.
39. Wanders RJ, van Roermund CW, van Wijiland MJ, et al. Clin Chim Acta 1987;166:255–63.
40. Wanders RJ, van Roermund CW, van Wijiland MJ, et al. Biochim Biophys Acta 1987;919:21–5.
41. Vandenbosch H, Schutgens RBH, Wanders RJA, et al. Annu Rev Biochem 1992;61:157–97.
42. Van Veldhoven PP, Vanhove G, Assselberghs S, et al. J Biol Chem 1992;267:20065–74.
43. Palosaari PM, Vihinen M, Mantsala PI, et al. J Biol Chem 1991;266:10750–3.
44. Palosaari PM, Hiltunen JK. J Biol Chem 1990;265:2446–9.
45. Hijikata M, Wen JK, Osumi T, et al. J Biol Chem 1990;265:4600–6.
46. Markwell MA, Tolbert NE, Bieber LL. Arch Biochem Biophys 1976;176:497–88.
47. Markwell MA, Bieber LL. Arch Biochem Biophys 1976;172:502–9.
48. Markwell MA, McGroarty EJ, Bieber LL, et al. J Biol Chem 1973;248:3426–32.
49. Steenhout P, Elmer C, Clercx A, et al. J Inherited Metab Dis 1990;13:69–75.
50. Shapira Y, Glick B, Harel S, et al. Pediatr Neurol 1993;9:35–8.
51. Demaugre F, Bonnefont J-P, Mitchell G, et al. Pediatr Res 1988;24:308–11.
52. Vianey-Saban C, Mousson B, Bertrand C, et al. Eur J Pediatr 1993;152:334–8.
53. Demaugre G, Bonnefont J-P, Cepanec C, et al. Pediatr Res 1990;27:497–500.
54. Stanley CA, Sunaryo F, Hale DE, et al. J Inherited Metab Dis 1992;15:785–9.
55. Pande SV, Brivet M, Slama A, et al. J Clin Invest 1993;91:1247–52.

56. Pande SV, Murthy M. Biochim Biophys Acta 1994;1226:269–76.
57. Angelini C, Trevisan C, Isaya G, et al. Clin Biochem 1987;20:1–27.
58. Hug G, Bove KE, Soukup S. N Engl J Med 1991;325:1862–4.
59. Taroni F, Verderio E, Fiorucci S, et al. Proc Natl Acad Sci USA 1992;89:8429–33.
60. Taroni F, Verderio E, Dworzak F, et al. Nature Genet 1993;4:314–20.
61. Bonnefont JP, Taroni F, Cavadini P, et al. Am J Hum Genet 1996;58:971–8.
62. Elpeleg ON, Joseph A, Gutman A. J Pediatr 1994;124:160–1.
63. Bertrand C, Largilliere C, Zabot MT, et al. Biochim Biophys Acta 1993;1180:327–9.
64. Aoyama T, Souri M, Ushikubo S, et al. J Clin Invest 1995;95:2465–73.
65. Ogilvie I, Pourfazam M, Jackson S, et al. Neurology 1994;44:467–73.
66. Aoyama T, Uchida Y, Kelley RI, et al. Biochem Biophys Res Commun 1993;191:1369–72.
67. Orii KO, Aoyama T, Souri M, et al. Biochem Biophys Res Commun 1995;217:987–92.
68. Andresen BS, Bross P, Vianeysaban C, et al. Hum Mol Genet 1996;5:461–72.
69. Strauss AW, Powell CK, Hale DE, et al. Proc Natl Acad Sci USA 1995;92:10496–500.
70. Andresen BS, Vianeysaban C, Bross P, et al. J Inherited Metab Dis 1996;19:169–72.
71. Hale DE, Batshaw ML, Coates PM, et al. Pediatr Res 1985;19:666–71.
72. Tream WR, Stanley CA, Hale DE, et al. Pediatrics 1991;87:328–33.
73. Yamaguchi S, Indo Y, Coates PM, et al. Pediatr Res 1993;34:111–3.
74. Amendt B, Green C, Sweetman L, et al. J Clin Invest 1987;79:1303–9.
75. Coates PM, Hale DE, Finocchiaro G, et al. J Clin Invest 1988;81:171–5.
76. Bhala A, Willi SM, Rinaldo P, et al. J Pediatr 1995;126:910–5.
77. Sewell AC, Herwig J, Bohles H, et al. Eur J Pediatr 1993;152:922–4.
78. Turnbull DM, Bartlett K, Stevens DL, et al. N Engl J Med 1984;311:1232–6.
79. Kristensen MJ, Kmoch S, Bross P, et al. Hum Mol Genet 1994;3:1711.
80. Rinaldo P, O'Shea JJ, Coates PM, et al. N Engl J Med 1988;319:1308–13.
81. Millington DS, Tereca N, Chace DH, et al. The role of tandem mass spectrometry in the diagnosis of fatty acid oxidation disorders. In: Coates PM, Tanaka K, eds. Oxidation. New York: Wiley-Liss, 1992;339–54.
82. Matsubara Y, Narisawa K, Shigeaki M, et al. Biochem Biophys Res Comm 1990;171:498–505.
83. Yokota I, Saijo T, Vockley J, et al. J Biol Chem 1992;267:26004–10.
84. Matsubara Y, Narisawa K, Tada K, et al. Lancet 1991;338:552–3.
85. Hale DE, Thorpe C, Braat K, et al. The L-3-hydroxyacyl-CoA dehydrogenase deficiency. In: Tanaka K, Coates PM, eds. Progress in clinical and biological research: fatty acid oxidation. Clinical, biochemical and molecular aspects. New York: Alan R Liss, 1990;503–10.
86. Pollitt RJ. Clinical and biochemical presentations in 20 cases of hydroxydicarbocylic aciduria. In: Tanaka K, Coates PM, eds. Progress in clinical and biological research: fatty acid oxidation. Clinical, biochemical and molecular aspects. New York: Alan R Liss, 1990;495–502.
87. Hagenfeldt L, van Dobein U, Holme E, et al. Pediatrics 1990;116:387–92.
88. Wanders RJA, Ijlst L, van Gennip AH, et al. J Inherited Metab Dis 1990;13:311–4.
89. Rocchiccioli F, Wanders RJA, Aybourg P, et al. Pediatr Res 1990;28:657–62.
90. Wanders RJA, Ijlst L, Duran M, et al. J Inherited Metab Dis 1991;14:325–8.
91. Vici CD, Burlina AB, Bertini E, et al. J Pediatr 1991;118:744–6.
92. Bertini E, Dionisivici C, Garavaglia B, et al. Eur J Pediatr 1992;151:121–6.
93. Brackett JC, Sims HF, Rinaldo P, et al. J Clin Invest 1995;95:2076–82.
94. Ijlst L, Wanders RJ, Ushikubo S, et al. Biochim Biophys Acta 1994;1215:347–50.
95. Ushikubo S, Aoyama T, Kamijo T, et al. Am J Hum Genet 1996;58:979–88.
96. Wilcken B, Leung KC, Hammond J, et al. Lancet 1993;341:407–8.
97. Sims HF, Brackett JC, Powell CK, et al. Proc Natl Acad Sci USA 1995;92:841–5.
98. Ijlst L, Uskikubo S, Kamijo T, et al. J Inherited Metab Dis 1995;18:241–4.
99. Tein I, Devivo DC, Hale DE, et al. Ann Neurol 1991;30:415–9.
100. Bennett MJ, Weinberger MJ, Kobori JA, et al. Pediatr Res 1996;39:185–8.
101. Bennet MJ, Sherwood WG. Clin Chem 1993;39:897–901.
102. Roe CR, Millington DS, Kodo NN, et al. J Clin Invest 1990;85:1703–7.
103. Frerman FE, Goodman SI. Glutaric acidemia type II and defects of the mitochondrial respiratory chain. In: Scriver C, Beaudet AL, Sly W, et al., eds. The metabolic basis of inherited disease. 6th ed. New York: McGraw-Hill, 1989;915–31.
104. Loehr JP, Goodman SI, Frurman FE. Pediatr Res 1990;27:311–5.
105. Sweetman L, Williams JD. Branched chain organic acidurias. In: Scriver C, Beaudet AL, Sly W, et al., eds. The metabolic and molecular basis of inherited disease. 6th ed. New York: McGraw-Hill, 1995;1387–422.
106. Wanders RJA, Schutgens RBH, Barth PG. J Neuropathol Exp Neurol 1995;54:726–39.
107. Zellweger H. Dev Med Child Neurol 1987;29:821–9.
108. Thomas GH, Haslam RH, Batshaw ML, et al. Clin Genet 1975;8:376–82.
109. Gatfield PD, Taller E, Hinton GG, et al. Can Med Assoc J 1968;99:1215–33.
110. Moser AB, Rasmussen M, Naidu S, et al. J Pediatr 1995;127:13–22.
111. Braverman N, Dodt G, Gould SJ, et al. Hum Mol Genet 1995;4:1791–8.
112. Slawecki ML, Dodt G, Steinberg S, et al. J Cell Sci 1995;108:1817–29.
113. Dodt G, Braverman N, Wong C, et al. Nature Genet 1995;9:115–25.
114. Shimozawa N, Tsukamota T, Suzuki Y, et al. Science 1992;255:1132–4.
115. Mosser J, Lutz Y, Stoeckel ME, et al. Hum Mol Genet 1994;3:265–71.
116. Scotto JM, Hadchouel M, Odievre M, et al. J Inherited Metab Dis 1982;5:83–90.
117. Ulrich J, Herschkowitz N, Heitz P, et al. Acta Neuropathol 1978;43:77–83.

118. Schaumburg HH, Powers JM, Raine CS, et al. Neurology 1977;27:1114–9.
119. Griffin JW, Goren E, Schaumburg H, et al. Neurology 1977;27:1107–13.
120. Budka H, Sluga E, Heiss WD. J Neurol 1976;213:237–50.
121. Poll-The BT, Roels F, Ogier H, et al. Am J Hum Genet 1988;42:422–34.
122. Wanders RJ, van Roermund CW, Schelen A, et al. J Inherited Metab Dis 1990;13:375–9.
123. Clayton PT, Lake BD, Hjelm M, et al. J Inherited Metab Dis 1988;11:165–8.
124. Watkins PA, Chen WW, Harris CJ, et al. J Clin Invest 1989;83:771–7.
125. Wanders RJ, van Roermund CW, Brul S, et al. J Inherited Metab Dis 1992;15:385–8.
126. Goldfischer S, Collins J, Rapin I, et al. J Pediatr 1986;108:25–32.
127. Schram AW, Goldfischer S, van Roermund CW, et al. Proc Natl Acad Sci USA 1987;84:2494–6.
128. Steinberg D. Refsum disease. In: Scriver C, Beaudet AL, Sly W, et al., eds. The metabolic basis of inherited disease. 7th ed. New York: McGraw-Hill, 1995;2351–69.
129. Ziadeh R, Hoffman EP, Finegold DN, et al. Pediatr Res 1995;37:675–8.
130. Lemieux B, Giguere R, Cyr D, et al. Pediatrics 1993;91:986–8.
131. Pollitt RJ. J Inherited Metab Dis 1989;12(Suppl 1):215–30.
132. Harpey J-P, Charpentier C, Paturneau-Jouas M. Biol Neonate 1990;58(Suppl 1):70–80.
133. Bennett MJ, Ragni MC, Hood I, et al. Ann Clin Biochem 1992;29:541–5.
134. Green A, Preece MA, deSousa C, et al. J Inherited Metab Dis 1991;14:691–7.
135. Rinaldo P, Schmidtsommerfeld E, Posca AP, et al. J Pediatr 1993;122:580–4.
136. Rinaldo P, Welch RD, Previs SF, et al. Pediatr Res 1991;30:216–21.
137. Aubourg P, Adamsbaum C, Lavallardrousseau MC, et al. N Engl J Med 1993;329:745–52.
138. Setchell KD, Bragetti P, Zimmer-Nechemias L, et al. Hepatology 1992;15:198–207.
139. Martinez M. Prog Clin Biol Res 1992;375:389–97.
140. Martinez M, Pineda M, Vidal R, et al. Neurology 1993; 43:1389–97.

SELECTED READINGS

Aubourg P, Adamsbaum C, Lavallardrousseau MC, et al. A 2-year trial of oleic and erucic acids (Lorenzo oil) as treatment for adrenomyeloneuropathy. N Engl J Med 1993:329:745–52.

Matsubara Y, Indo Y, Naito E, et al. Molecular cloning and nucleotide sequence of cDNAs encoding the precursors of rat long chain acyl-CoA, short chain acyl-CoA, and isovaleryl CoA dehydrogenases: sequence homology of four enzymes of the acyl-CoA dehydrogenase family. J Biol Chem 1989:264: 16321–31.

Moser AB, Rasmussen M, Naidu S, et al. Phenotype of patients with peroxisomal disorders subdivided into sixteen complementation groups. J Pediatr 1995:127:13–32.

Rinaldo P, Schmidtsommerfeld E, Posca AP, et al. Effect of treatment with glycine and L-carnitine in medium-chain acyl-coenzyme-A dehydrogenase deficiency. J Pediatr 1993:122:580–4.

Vockley J. The changing face of disorders of fatty acid oxidation. Mayo Clin Proc 1994:69:249–57.

63. Childhood Obesity

WILLIAM H. DIETZ

DEFINITION

Use of the Triceps Skinfold and Body Mass Index

Because weight and height change throughout childhood, the cutoff points of any measure used to define obesity must be age and gender dependent. The ideal anthropometric measure of fatness is one that correlates reasonably well with fat as a percentage of body weight. Among children and adolescents, weight for height, body mass index, and triceps skinfold demonstrate comparable correlation coefficients with fat as a percentage of body weight, measured by underwater weighing (1). Despite the similarity of the correlation coefficients, variants of weight for height and triceps skinfold thickness probably capture different aspects of body fat. Although the triceps skinfold thickness provides a direct measure of fat, it only does so at one location in the body. Furthermore, because body fat redistributes at adolescence to a more central distribution, the triceps skinfold thickness may decrease even as body fat increases. Weight and height measures do not measure fatness directly, but use of an index such as body mass index (BMI; wt/ht^2) may remove the covariance of weight and height and thereby provide a more direct measure of the effect of increased fat on weight.

In adolescents, a convenient algorithm (2) exists to screen patients for obesity (Fig. 63.1). The algorithm begins with a BMI in excess of the 95th percentile for age and gender, using tables derived from representative surveys of the U.S. population (3) (see also Appendix Tables III-A-18-b-1 and 2), or a BMI of 30.0 or above. If the BMI exceeds the 95th percentile for age or gender or if it is greater than 30 BMI units, an in-depth medical assessment is warranted. The details of the medical assessment are considered below. The same algorithm could reasonably be applied to screen younger children. In both adolescents and young children, selection of the 95th percentile as a screening tool reduces the sensitivity of the measure but increases its specificity (4). This approach therefore minimizes the likelihood that obesity will be overdiagnosed and thus lead to excessive concern about weight when no significant problem exists.

Changes in Body Fat and Fat Distribution with Age

The BMI and triceps skinfold do not change synchronously with age. In females after the first year of life, the triceps skinfold thickness remains stable, then begins to increase in early adolescence (5). Female adolescence is characterized by an increase in body fat from a mean of 17% of body weight to 25% of body weight. In males, changes in fatness are somewhat more complex. The triceps skinfold decreases at approximately 4 years of age, increases immediately before puberty, and subsequently decreases during the adolescent growth spurt. Male adolescence is characterized by a decline in body fat from a mean of 18% of body weight to 11% of body weight.

Changes in BMI with age are similar for both genders. BMI rises between birth and 9 months of age and subsequently declines to a nadir at approximately 4 to 5 years of age (6). Thereafter, BMI rises through adolescence. The point at which BMI begins to increase after the nadir is known as the period of adiposity rebound.

The pattern of fat distribution also changes with age and differs for males and females. In both genders during adolescence, body fat redistributes from peripheral to central sites (7, 8). In girls, more fat is deposited in the gluteal regions than in the abdomen. In males, fat tends to be deposited more centrally.

Changes in adipocyte numbers tend to parallel the changes in body fatness that occur from early childhood. Adipocyte replication occurs as body fat increases, regardless of whether the increase in body fat is normal or excessive (9, 10). Adipocyte size increases in early infancy. However, after early infancy, adipocyte size remains relatively constant until puberty, when another small increase occurs. The factors that control the regionalization of body fat and adipocyte replication throughout childhood remain unclear.

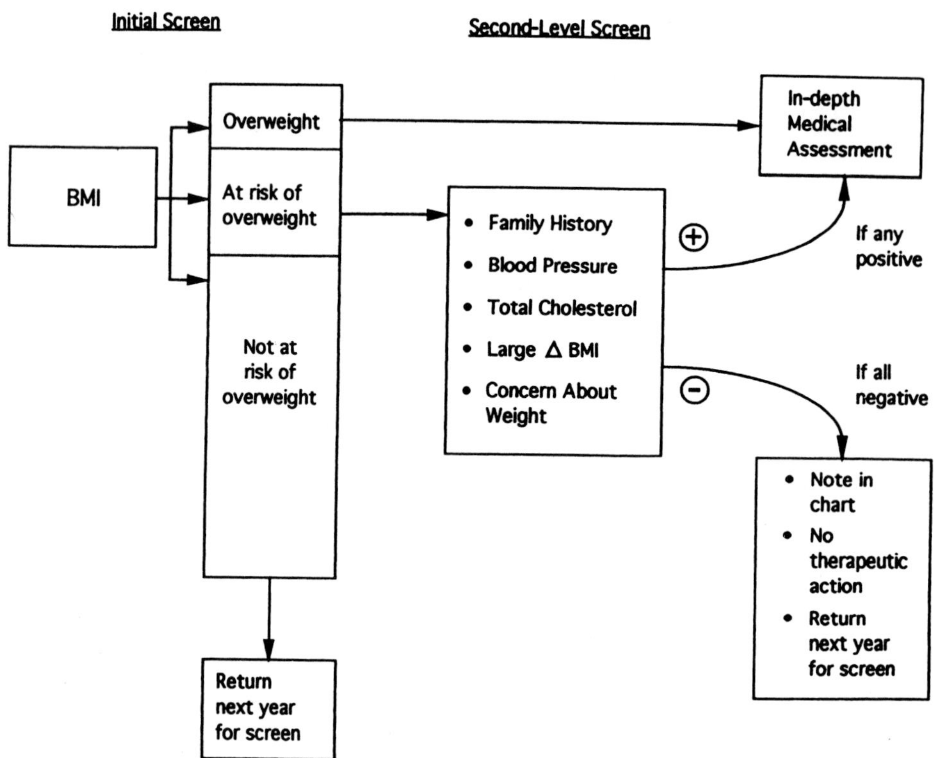

Figure 63.1. A convenient algorithm (2) exists to screen patients for obesity. The algorithm begins with a BMI in excess of the 95th percentile for age and gender, using tables derived from representative surveys of the U.S. population (3), or a BMI ≥ 30.0. If the BMI exceeds the 95th percentile for age or gender or if it is greater than 30 BMI units, an in-depth medical assessment is warranted.

EPIDEMIOLOGY

Prevalence

Both triceps skinfold and BMI data suggest that the prevalence of obesity among children and adolescents in the United States has increased rapidly over the last 30 years. Based on the use of a triceps skinfold greater than the 85th percentile among children and adolescents studied in the National Health Examination Surveys (NHES; 1963–1970), the prevalence of obesity appeared to increase by 54% in children aged 6 to 11 years by the time the second National Health and Nutrition Examination Survey (NHANES II) was conducted in 1980 (11). Over roughly the same time period, the prevalence of obesity among adolescents aged 12 to 17 years had increased by 30%. Increases in the prevalence of superobesity, defined as a triceps skinfold above the 95th percentile, increased even more rapidly over the same time period. More-recent data, collected between 1980 and 1990, when the NHANES II and NHANES III examinations were completed, and based on an age- and gender-specific BMI above the 85th percentile in the NHES (12), demonstrated that the prevalence of obesity increased by 12% in boys and 44% in girls aged 6 to 11 years. In male and female adolescents aged 12 to 17 years, the prevalence of overweight increased by 45 and 37%, respectively. Increases in more severe obesity, defined by the authors as a BMI above the 95th percentile, ranged from 37 to 137%. These estimates suggest that one in five children and adolescents in the United States is now overweight. Furthermore, both the triceps skinfold data, which provide direct measures of fat, and the BMI data indicate that the prevalence of severe obesity has increased more rapidly than more modest degrees of excess fatness.

The reasons for the changes in prevalence have not been carefully examined. Although dietary fat intake in the population has declined (13), increased quantities of food are consumed outside of the home. The fat and caloric content of foods consumed outside the home remains unclear and may contribute to caloric imbalance. Likewise, although Neilsen estimates of time spent viewing television by children have not changed substantially over the last 20 years (14), the Neilsen estimates may be biased because only half of those families invited to participate do so (14). More-recent data from the National Longitudinal Survey of Youth suggest that children and adolescents currently watch more than 1 hour more of television per day than they did before 1963–1970 (15). Approximately 30% of children watch 5 or more hours of television daily. Nonetheless, the relative contributions of diet and inactivity to the increases in prevalence of obesity remain unclear.

Critical Periods for Onset of Childhood Obesity

A critical period for development of obesity is defined as a developmental stage in which physiologic alterations increase the later prevalence of obesity (16). Fetal life, the period of adiposity rebound, and adolescence appear to be critical periods for onset of obesity in children and adolescents. Several groups appear at risk for development of obesity or its complications as a consequence of intrauterine developments. Low-birth-weight infants appear to have an increased risk of hypertension and cardiovascular disease as adults (17). However, it is not clear that adults born with low birth weights have an increased prevalence of obesity in adulthood, although visceral fat may be increased (18). The best evidence that fetal life constitutes a critical period for development of obesity derives from studies of infants of diabetic mothers. These infants are fatter at birth than infants whose mothers are not diabetic. By 1 year of age, the differences in fatness at birth are no longer present (19). However, by 5 to 6 years of age, children of mothers diabetic during pregnancy have an increased prevalence of obesity that persists through 18 years of age (20).

The second critical period in childhood is the period of adiposity rebound. Children with early adiposity rebound appear at increased risk for development of obesity that persists into adulthood (21, 22).

Adolescence, particularly in girls, represents a third critical period in childhood for development of obesity. Longitudinal data suggest that the risk of persistence of adolescent obesity into adulthood is threefold greater in adolescent girls than in boys (23). Furthermore, obesity in adolescence carries an increased risk of all-cause and cardiovascular mortality in adult males and cardiovascular morbidity in both male and female adults that appears independent of adult weight (24).

Regardless of the age of onset, fatness appears increasingly canalized with age (25, 26). Furthermore, estimates suggest that 30 to 80% of overweight children remain overweight as adults (27). Adults who were overweight during childhood may account for a disproportionate percentage of morbidly obese adults (28).

The mechanisms that act to entrain obesity and its complications at these periods remain unclear. The relationship between early fetal undernutrition and morbidity may be mediated by fetal adaptations to stress, such as hypercortisolism (29). Whether fetal undernutrition also leads to increased body fat or enhances the likelihood of comorbidities of obesity remains unclear. The increase in body fatness that occurs in infants of diabetic mothers may entrain either the number of fat cells, the central regulation of fatness by the hypothalamic-pituitary-adrenal axis, or adipocyte factors concerned with regulation of body fat. Factors that regulate body fatness during the period of adiposity rebound remain less certain. Adiposity rebound may represent the period when the genetic predisposition to obesity may be expressed. Conversely, the period of adiposity rebound may represent the first important period in life when social forces that affect activity and diet begin to operate. Entrainment of these behaviors could have a disproportionate effect on the onset and persistence of later obesity. As indicated above, adolescence represents a period when major changes in body fat and fat distribution occur in both genders. Excessive increases in body fat during female adolescence appear to increase the risk that increased body fat will persist. In males, the risks of adult disease that adolescent obesity entrains may reflect the central redistribution of fat that occurs in adolescence (7, 8).

Role of the Physical Environment

Childhood obesity has been associated with a variety of variables within the physical environment, including season, region, and population density (30). Obesity among children and adolescents is also more prevalent in winter and spring than in summer and fall. Childhood obesity is more prevalent in the northeastern United States, followed in descending order by the Midwest, South, and West. Within each region, obesity is more prevalent in densely settled urban areas than in areas with lower population densities.

The mechanisms that account for the variations induced by season, region, and population density remain unclear. However, regional and seasonal differences in diet and activity represent likely candidates. Other cultural factors such as differences in the amount of clothing worn and its consequent effect on the perception of body appearance represent reasonable hypotheses. In highly urbanized areas, reduced access to exercise facilities or heightened concern about safety may reduce the opportunity for activity.

Role of the Behavioral Environment

Family Environment

A variety of familial and behavioral variables have also been associated with childhood obesity. Children whose parents are obese have an increased risk of obesity (5). Obesity is most prevalent among single children and less prevalent among children from large families (31).

The role of socioeconomic class in the genesis of childhood obesity remains unclear. Although an early study demonstrated an inverse relationship of obesity to socioeconomic class (32), other studies have shown either a direct (33) or no significant relationship (34). Several sources of data suggest that obesity may represent a determinant rather than a consequence of socioeconomic class in young adults (35, 36). The effect of social class on the prevalence of obesity has not been examined in more recent representative surveys of the U.S. population.

Children who are the victims of parental neglect (37) and those who suffer from increased psychosocial problems (38, 39) also appear at increased risk for development of obesity.

Diet

Energy balance can be expressed as $TEE = RMR + TEF + ACT$, where TEE is total daily energy expenditure, RMR

is resting metabolic rate, *TEF* is the thermic effect of food, and *ACT* is the energy spent on activity. Obesity occurs when energy intake exceeds energy expenditure. The only two discretionary components of the energy balance relationship are food intake and energy spent on activity.

The absence of a clear relationship of dietary intake to development of obesity in children derives from the difficulties inherent in accurately measuring dietary intake. For example, overweight children rarely gain more than 5 extra kilograms per year. Assuming that all excess weight is fat, that the cost of synthesis of adipose tissue is minimal, and that a kilogram of adipose tissue contains 150 to 200 g of water (40, 41), the daily caloric excess necessary to produce a gain of 5 kg of adipose tissue annually approximates a caloric imbalance of 100 kcal/day (Table 63.1).

Comparisons of reported dietary intake with energy expenditure measured by the doubly labeled water method emphasize the difficulties inherent in accurate measurement of the minor caloric imbalances necessary to generate obesity. For example, careful dietary records collected from normal-weight and overweight adolescents underestimated measured energy expenditure by 20% and 40%, respectively (42). Although younger children may provide more-accurate estimates of food intake (43, 44), dietary records still cannot provide the valid caloric intakes necessary to establish the source of caloric imbalance that generates excess weight gain. However, dietary records may help identify foods that are the appropriate target of therapy or eating patterns that could be modified to reduce caloric intake for the individual patient.

Because dietary records to establish caloric intake are inaccurate, studies of patterns of eating or food consumption may be a more fruitful approach to the examination of the role of diet in the genesis of childhood obesity. Such studies have not been done. The increased caloric density of fat and the possibility that individual differences in fat oxidation account for a differential susceptibility to weight gain (45, 46) suggest that reduced dietary fat intake is an appropriate target for preventive efforts.

Activity

As indicated above, energy expenditure includes the energy spent on resting or basal metabolic rate, the thermic effect of a meal, and the energy spent on activity. Although an initial report demonstrated that maternal obesity appeared related to reduced energy expenditure in infants (47), subsequent studies have failed to reveal any significant differences in energy expenditure between infants born of normal and overweight mothers (48). Furthermore, total energy expenditure at 12 weeks of life failed to predict changes in body fat that had occurred by 9 months and 2 years of age (49).

Studies of resting metabolic rate conducted in obese and nonobese children (50) and adolescents (51) have consistently shown an elevated resting metabolic rate in the obese subjects, even after normalization for fat-free mass. Although the thermic effects of food were lower in obese than in nonobese children, no differences were observed after weight reduction (52). Furthermore, no significant differences have been observed between obese and nonobese adolescents (53).

Reduced energy spent on activity could also increase susceptibility to obesity in children and adolescents. For example, vigorous physical activity declines markedly in girls during adolescence and may increase the risk of obesity onset during this period (54, 55). As indicated in Table 63.2, doubly labeled water studies indicated that the energy spent on activity, calculated from TEE measured with doubly labeled water and resting metabolic rate, gradually increases throughout childhood (56–59). If reduced energy spent on physical activity represented a risk factor for development of obesity, the incidence of obesity should be inversely related to the energy spent on physical activity. However, the increases with age in the energy spent on activity suggest that alterations in activity do not adequately account for the increased risk of obesity that accompanies either the period of adiposity rebound or adolescence. Nonetheless, reductions in the energy spent on metabolic rate, the thermic effects of food, or activity could predispose individuals or subgroups to an increased risk for development of obesity.

Inactivity

The decreased activity in adolescents (54, 55) and adults (60) in the United States has focused attention on inactivity as a potential cause of obesity. Activity within populations, measured by time of participation in activities, may have an effect on the prevalence of obesity that is independent of the effect of inactivity, measured by television time (61). If inactivity was the reciprocal of activity, the effects of activity and inactivity on the prevalence of obesity would not be independent. These data also suggest that inactivity may be better understood as sedentary behavior rather than as function of energy expenditure.

Table 63.1
Caloric Excess Necessary to Gain 5 kg of Adipose Tissue per Year

Adipose tissue = 20% H_2O
1 g fat = 9 kcal/g
1 kg adipose = 800 g fat = 7200 kcal
5 kg adipose tissue = 36,000 kcal/365 days = 98 kcal/day

Table 63.2
Mean (SD) Energy Costs of Activity (TEE/RMR) in Humans of Different Ages (Determined by the Doubly Labeled Water Method)

Age Group	(reference)	Males	Females
5 years	(56)	1.36 (.13)	1.40 (.17)
9–12 years	(58)	1.61 (.23)	1.53 (.15)
12–18 years	(51)	1.79 (.20)	1.69 (.28)
Adults	(57)		1.70 (.23)

The principal sedentary behavior in the United States is television viewing. Current estimates suggest that approximately one-third of children in the United States view more than 5 hours of television per day (15). Television viewing occupies more time on an annual basis than any other behavior except sleep. Television viewing has been linked with a variety of adverse health outcomes (14), including obesity (15, 62). Furthermore, the relationship between television viewing and obesity may be causal (62). Television viewing is associated with reduced activity, although metabolic rate may not be lower than when children engage in other sedentary activities such as reading (63). Television viewing is also associated with increased food intake, and the foods consumed are those advertised on television (64).

Several sources of data are consistent with the view that the covariation of inactivity with other behaviors may contribute to the adverse effects of inactivity on obesity. For example, although television viewing is a sedentary activity, television viewing has been significantly associated with increased fat intake (63). Furthermore, recent studies in adolescents (65, 66) demonstrated significant relationships between inactivity and other adverse health practices, such as smoking, consumption of less healthy foods, or increased fat intake.

CLINICAL EFFECTS

Syndromes Associated with Childhood Obesity

Table 63.3 includes most of the clinical syndromes associated with childhood and adolescent obesity (67). Even in specialty clinics that deal with childhood obesity, syndromes associated with obesity are rare. Most syndromes associated with obesity are readily identified by physical examination because of short stature, dysmorphic features, or ocular anomalies.

Because childhood obesity is generally accompanied by an increase in linear growth (68), short stature in association with obesity should prompt a careful search for other characteristics associated with potential clinical syndromes. Additional features common to more than one syndrome include ocular (Alstrom-Hallgren syndrome [69], Bardet-Biedl syndrome [70], pseudohypoparathyroidism), hand (Carpenter syndrome, Cohen syndrome, Bardet-Biedl syndrome, Prader-Labhart-Willi syndrome [71, 72], pseudohypoparathyroidism), or menstrual abnormalities (Cushing's syndrome [73], hypothalamic dysfunction [74], Bardet-Biedl syndrome, polycystic ovary disease [75], Prader-Labhart-Willi syndrome, Turner's syndrome).

Table 63.3
Clinical Syndromes Associated with Childhood Obesity

Alstrom-Hallgren syndrome
Carpenter syndrome
Cohen syndrome
Cushing syndrome
Growth hormone deficiency
Hyperinsulinemia
Hypothalamic dysfunction or tumor
Hypothyroidism
Laurence-Moon-Biedl syndrome
Polycystic ovary disease
Prader-Labhart-Willi syndrome
Pseudohypoparathyroidism
Turner syndrome

Consequences of Obesity in Childhood

Although many of the consequences of childhood obesity resemble those in adults, they occur less frequently. Several are unique to childhood-onset obesity. Among the most prevalent consequences of obesity in children is the discrimination that overweight children suffer at the hands of their peers. Young children learn to associate obesity with other undesirable characteristics. For example, children as young as 6 years of age consistently rank obese children as less desirable candidates as friends than children with any other handicap (76). As children grow older, discrimination becomes more institutionalized. Among adolescents, college acceptance rates for obese girls are lower than those for nonobese girls with comparable academic credentials (77). As adults, girls overweight in late adolescence and early adulthood complete fewer years of education, marry significantly less frequently, and have lower family incomes and increased rates of poverty (35).

Orthopaedic problems unique to childhood occur more frequently among the obese. Slipped capital femoral epiphysis occurs among children with a prevalence of approximately 3/100,000 persons per year (78), but most children with this problem are obese (79). The disease probably reflects the susceptibility of the epiphysis of the femoral head to the increased stress of weight bearing. The disease may present only with hip pain or a limp. Blount's disease (80), or bowed tibia with a consequent deformity of the medial aspect of the proximal tibial metaphysis, occurs with increased frequency among obese children. Blount's disease reflects the effects of increased weight bearing on cartilaginous bone, with compensatory overgrowth of the tibia. Surgery may be necessary to correct the deformity. Minor injuries, such as ankle sprains, may resolve more slowly or become chronic in overweight children and adolescents and may account for persistent extremity pain.

Although the cardiovascular consequences of obesity occur less frequently than they do in adults, the precursors of adult disease are present in childhood. Acanthosis nigricans, an increased pigmentation of the skin of the neck and axillae, may be a consequence of the increased friction between skinfolds but may also indicate abnormal glucose tolerance and hyperinsulinemia (81). However, frank non-insulin-dependent diabetes mellitus is rare in children and adolescents in the absence of a strong family history of diabetes. Hyperlipidemia is frequent among obese children. Furthermore, the lipoprotein pattern is characterized by elevated levels of low-density lipoproteins and decreased levels of high-density lipoproteins (82, 83).

Hepatic abnormalities occur in a sizable fraction of overweight children. These abnormalities generally consist of modest elevations of liver enzymes and may reflect hepatic steatosis (84). In severely obese patients, hepatic steatosis may progress to cirrhosis. Weight loss can normalize the abnormal levels of liver enzymes. As in adults, obesity may also be associated with cholecystitis (85). A more common cause of abdominal pain is gastroesophageal reflux caused by the increased intra-abdominal pressure of visceral or subcutaneous abdominal fat.

The two most serious and urgent complications of childhood and adolescent obesity are sleep apnea (86) and pseudotumor cerebri. Severe sleep apnea invariably occurs in association with snoring, and parents may describe the apneic episodes. Long apneic episodes are associated with hypoxia and may trigger a fatal cardiac arrhythmia. Up to 50% of children with pseudotumor may be obese (87), although the role that obesity plays in the pathophysiology of pseudotumor remains unclear. Compression of the optic nerve may produce visual field cuts. Rapid weight reduction is essential for both problems.

Clinical Assessment

Few causes or consequences of obesity occur in the absence of signs or symptoms. Therefore, a careful history and physical examination are crucial to exclude underlying associated syndromes or to identify complications of obesity.

History

A careful history of the age of onset of obesity may help identify underlying risk factors that may predispose to the persistence of the disease. Such factors include gestational diabetes in the mother or onset of obesity at the time of adiposity rebound. Questions regarding discrimination in school represent a useful mechanism to engage the child's or adolescent's interest and participation in the therapeutic process. A family history of severe obesity or associated hypertension, diabetes, or cardiovascular morbidity heightens concern about future comorbidities in the pediatric patient and helps establish the level of family concern regarding the medical complications of obesity.

Although the dietary history cannot be used to establish the level of caloric intake, a 24-hour recall and a brief series of quantitative questions about the consumption of juice, milk, soft drinks, fast food, and high-caloric-density snacks such as candy bars, chips, cookies, ice cream, or frozen yogurt may identify specific foods that can be permanently altered or eliminated from the diet. Questions about time spent outdoors, participation in vigorous activities, and time spent viewing television are essential to establish the level of activity and identify potential approaches to reduce inactivity or increase vigorous activity.

The review of systems should include questions that address the principal morbidities outlined above. Headaches or visual changes may indicate the presence of pseudotumor cerebri or the rare hypothalamic tumor. Snoring in association with daytime somnolence suggests the possibility of sleep apnea. Dyspnea on exertion provides a functional measure of activity and the restriction on activity imposed by obesity. Abdominal pain may be functional and may result from school avoidance, but it may also indicate the presence of gastroesophageal reflux or cholecystitis. Irregular periods or amenorrhea may indicate polycystic ovary disease. Hip pain or a limp suggests imminent or acute slipped capital femoral epiphysis.

Physical Examination

The physical examination should begin with a careful plot of height and weight on a growth chart to establish the severity of obesity. Measurement of the triceps skinfold thickness will help establish whether the excess weight represents body fat or increased frame size. Measurement of the waist and hip circumferences provides a crude estimate of visceral fat distribution. Determination of blood pressure with an appropriate-size cuff and the use of age-appropriate standards is essential.

Short stature or dysmorphic features should prompt careful exclusion of one of the syndromes associated with childhood obesity. The presence of acanthosis nigricans or the violaceous striae that characterize Cushing's syndrome can be noted on inspection of the skin. A careful funduscopic examination should be performed to exclude papilledema suggestive of increased intracranial pressure. Enlarged tonsils may contribute to sleep apnea. If a tonsillectomy is warranted, careful postoperative care is essential, because obese children are at high risk for postoperative obstruction from the peripharyngeal swelling that follows a tonsillectomy. Abdominal tenderness may reflect cholecystitis or cholelithiasis. Limited range of motion of the legs at the hip may be the only indication of slipped capital femoral epiphysis. In younger children, bowed extremities require radiologic examination to exclude the possibility of early Blount disease.

Laboratory Assessment

Serum cholesterol levels to exclude the possibility of hyperlipidemia, liver enzyme levels to identify hepatic steatosis, and a urinalysis to exclude glucosuria should be done routinely. Abnormal liver function tests in a child with a history of abdominal pain or a family history of gall bladder disease require an ultrasound examination of the abdomen to exclude cholelithiasis. Fasting glucose and insulin levels may help clarify the risk of diabetes mellitus in a child or adolescent with acanthosis nigricans. A history consistent with sleep apnea warrants a sleep study to determine the frequency and severity of apneic episodes. Sex hormones, luteinizing hormone, and follicular stimulating hormone may be helpful adjunct measures in girls with signs or symptoms of polycystic ovary disease. Additional laboratory studies that are not suggested by concerns identified during the history or physical examination are rarely helpful.

TREATMENT

Family involvement in the treatment of childhood and adolescent obesity is crucial (88, 89) because the pediatric patient is rarely responsible for the purchase, preparation, or serving of food. Such involvement is implicit in the description of the therapeutic approaches that follow.

Regardless of the severity of obesity, the first consideration for any overweight individual is weight maintenance. For some children, such as those who are 120% of their ideal weight, weight maintenance for 1 year may be the only step necessary to achieve ideal weight for height. However, aggressive therapy must be considered from the outset for the morbidly obese adolescent who is 200% of ideal weight. Although dietary therapy is necessary to achieve weight reduction, increased levels of activity may be essential to achieve weight maintenance after weight loss has been accomplished.

Education

Education of the obese child or adolescent rarely proves successful as an isolated intervention in treatment of childhood obesity. However, several principles are useful in the treatment of children and families. Use of the Food Guide Pyramid to guide food choices may help to reduce dietary fat intake (90). Furthermore, use of labels to establish fat and caloric content will help families purchase lower fat and calorie options.

Dietary Modification

Reduced caloric intake must remain the cornerstone of weight reduction therapy, because it is easier to achieve a caloric deficit by reduced food intake than by increased activity. As indicated above, the most useful function of a dietary history is to identify foods that can be altered or eliminated.

Low-Fat Diets

Reductions in dietary fat represent the first step in modification of dietary intake. According to the current recommendation of the American Academy of Pediatrics, dietary fat intakes should approximate 30% of calories for children over the age of 2 years. Several caveats accompany this recommendation. First, although no comparable studies in children have been done, reductions in dietary fat in the absence of reduced caloric intake may only achieve modest weight reduction in adults (91). Although anecdotal reports suggest that excessive concerns about the effects of dietary fat have led to growth failure in young children (92), concerns about the effect of caloric restriction on the growth of the population become moot in obese children where the potential for minor adverse effects of diet are exceeded by the risks of persistent obesity.

A second alternative for children and young adolescents is the "Stop-light Diet" (93). This approach classifies foods as green, yellow, and red, according to whether the food can be consumed freely, with caution, or only on rare occasions. The stop-light diet has been used repeatedly and effectively in weight-reduction studies of 8- to 12-year-old children.

The manner in which dietary modifications are introduced may be as important as the dietary modification itself. For example, children appear to respond better when the emphasis is on foods that families *can* eat, rather than on foods that are restricted (89). This observation is consistent with the finding that children and adolescents for whom specific diets were recommended did poorly in comparison to children and adolescents for whom recommended diets were less specific (94). Both observations suggest that the results of therapy are likely better when more control of the choices remain in the hands of children and their families.

Use of Restrictive Diets

Severely obese adolescents whose weight is 180% or more in excess of ideal, or children or adolescents with a major complication of excess body weight, may require more aggressive dietary interventions such as the protein-modified fast. The protein-modified fast should be used cautiously in patients with renal or cardiac disease; however, it may be highly beneficial in patients with liver disease that results from hepatic steatosis. Before the diet is started, it is essential to determine whether the candidate for the diet is capable of weight maintenance. If weight maintenance is impossible before the diet is started, the patient is more likely to relapse after the diet is discontinued.

The protein-modified fast consists of a carbohydrate-free diet that contains 2.0 to 2.5 g protein/kg ideal body weight/day provided as meat or other high-quality protein, supplemented with 30 mEq KCl, 800 mg Ca, and a multivitamin with minerals daily (67, 95). Vegetables low in carbohydrate may be consumed ad libitum. Fluid intake should be maintained at a level of 48 oz of noncaloric fluids daily. Ketosis appears within 48 to 72 hours of the initiation of the diet and can be used to monitor dietary adherence. After the diet is started, it should be continued for several months. Weight losses are most rapid in the first 2 weeks of the diet and thereafter average 0.5 to 1.0 kg/week. Patients should be seen frequently during the diet to monitor adherence, identify potentially adverse effects of the diet, and provide ongoing family support. Blood counts, liver function tests, and amylase and albumin levels should be monitored monthly. At the termination of the diet, carbohydrates should be reintroduced gradually over several weeks.

Complications of the protein-modified fast include malaise during the transition to ketosis, orthostatic hypotension, and diarrhea or constipation. Although gall bladder disease may occur in association with fat-free diets, this complication is rare in children and adolescents following the protein-modified fast, probably because the fat contained in a meat-based diet may cause gall bladder contractions and thereby reduce biliary sludging. Nonetheless, if a patient develops abdominal pain with weight reduction, an ultrasound of the abdomen is essential to exclude cholelithiasis or pancreatitis.

Alterations in Activity

Increased Activity

Increased activity may have several benefits during weight reduction. In adults, increased activity may block the adaptive decrease in metabolic rate that occurs in response to a hypocaloric diet, perhaps by a reduction in the loss of fat-free mass (96, 97). Second, increased activity in association with a low-calorie diet may increase the rate of weight loss. Finally, increased levels of activity may increase the likelihood of weight maintenance after weight loss is achieved. Reasonable recommendations for activity are those proposed by the International Consensus Conference on Physical Activity Guidelines for Adolescents, which suggest that adolescents should participate in three or more sessions per week of moderate to vigorous activity that last 20 minutes or more (98). However, recommendations for vigorous activity are not appropriate for massively obese adolescents who may achieve maximal energy expenditure with walking. For this group, simple increases in activity should be the goal.

Increased activity among obese preadolescents increases total energy expenditure and is not apparently counterbalanced by reduced activity in other areas (99). As in adults (100), losses of fat are likely to depend on the individual's capacity for fat oxidation, the intensity of exercise, and the quantity of fat in the diet.

How increases in activity are accomplished may contribute to the long-term success of the intervention. For example, lifestyle activities chosen by the child may accomplish more sustained rates of weight reduction than structured exercise programs that provide fewer choices (101), perhaps because children are more likely to participate in an activity that they choose. Furthermore, when children make a choice, they may feel more responsible for the decision to change (102).

Reduced Inactivity

As indicated above, both increased activity and reduced inactivity may have beneficial effects on weight changes in the population. The long-term effects of increased activity and reduced inactivity on weight reduction have only recently been carefully examined (102). When the effect on weight of increased activity was compared with that of reduced activity, 4-month and 1-year weight losses were significantly greater for the group reinforced for reductions in inactivity than in the group that was reinforced for increased activity. Furthermore, attitudes toward high-intensity activity were more positive among children who were reinforced for decreased sedentary activity than among children reinforced for increased activity. These data suggest again that efforts to reduce inactivity under circumstances in which children choose the alternative activity are more effective than when children are reinforced for the activity itself. Further trials of the effects of reductions in inactivity are essential.

Behavior Modification

Behavior modification is not an additional therapeutic endeavor but rather the mechanism by which changes in diet and activity are effected. As indicated above and in repeated studies by Epstein and his colleagues (88), parental involvement in weight reduction programs aimed at children is essential.

The major components of behavior modification are contracting, self-monitoring, and social reinforcement and modeling (88). Contracting provides reinforcement to promote adherence to the weight reduction regimen or incentives for weight loss. Self-monitoring involves careful daily observation of diet and activity. Social reinforcement and modeling involves teaching children and parents how to model behaviors related to diet and activity for other family members. The capacity to make free choices between alternatives appears highly beneficial to adherence and should be central in the design of weight reduction programs for children and adolescents.

Other therapies aimed at the modification of family behaviors, such as family therapy, have not been studied as intensively. One reason is that interventions such as family therapy are not as readily quantified. Likewise, because studies of behavior modification have focused most intensively on children less than 12 years of age, the effectiveness of this intervention in other age groups has not been established.

Alternative Therapies

Therapies for morbid obesity in adolescents, as in adults, are associated with a high relapse rate. For example, virtually all patients studied as inpatients in a variety of studies of hypocaloric diets regained their weight after discharge from the study. Furthermore, substantial numbers of patients may not be able to initiate hypocaloric diets or may be so incapacitated by their weight that movement is impossible. For these patients, more aggressive therapies such as pharmacotherapy or gastric bypass surgery may be warranted. Unfortunately, experience with these therapies in adolescents is limited.

Pharmacotherapy

Few trials of pharmacotherapy in adolescents have been reported. Although combined trials of phenteramine and fenfluramine have been performed (103) or are under way in adults, few comparable data exist for adolescents. Therefore, at present, pharmacotherapy must be reserved for morbidly obese adolescents but only after other, more conservative, approaches, including the protein-modified fast, have been exhausted.

Only one report has considered the effects of *d,l*-fenfluramine on overweight children and adolescents. In a trial that compared 30 or 60 mg of *d,l*-fenfluramine in 11- to 17-year-old patients with a placebo-treated group (104), mean weight loss at 6 months was 3.3 BMI units, and at 12 months was 5.1 BMI units for the treated group. These losses approximate 8.25 and 12.75 kg, respectively. Although side effects appeared minor, use of pharmacotherapy should be reserved for morbidly obese adolescents in whom all more conservative therapies have failed, until trials involving larger numbers of patients are available. Furthermore, adolescents and their physicians must retain realistic expectations regarding the response to therapy. Pharmacotherapy will probably not achieve the massive weight reduction necessary for the morbidly obese patient to achieve ideal body weight.

Surgery

Gastric bypass surgery or vertically banded gastroplasty must be considered therapy of last resort for the morbidly obese adolescent who has failed all other conventional therapies. Only two reports have been published regarding the use of surgery to treat obesity in this age group (105, 106). These studies suggest that mean weight losses are in excess of 40 kg, depending on the type of operation and gender of the patient. These results may underestimate the effects of surgery, because weight gains in some of the operative patients would have continued unabated without intervention. Surgery is probably not warranted for patients with Prader-Labhart-Willi syndrome, many of whom promptly regain the weight that they lose. Acute complications of surgery include leaks at the anastomosis and wound infections. Long-term complications include anemia. Nonetheless, weight losses have been sustained in almost all patients for over 7 years.

Outcome

Childhood- and adolescent-onset obesity appears to account for approximately 30% of obesity present in adult women. Furthermore, in both males and females, obesity in adolescents appears associated with a risk of adult morbidity and mortality that seems independent of the effect of adolescent weight on adult weight. These observations suggest that effective treatment of obese children and adolescents may exert a substantial effect on the morbidity and mortality of adult obesity.

Children also appear more responsive to weight reduction therapies than adults. For example, Epstein et al. (88) have shown that the long-term effects of a family-based program of diet and activity promoted by behavior modification could still be demonstrated 10 years after the program was introduced. These results indicate that children should be targeted for an increased proportion of the resources and efforts aimed at weight control in the U.S. population.

REFERENCES

1. Roche AF, Siervogel RM, Chumlea WC, et al. Am J Clin Nutr 1981;34:2831–8.
2. Himes JH, Dietz WH. Am J Clin Nutr 1994;59:307–16.
3. Must A, Dallal GE, Dietz WH. Am J Clin Nutr 1991;54:773.
4. Himes JH, Bouchard C. Int J Obes 1989;13:183–93.
5. Garn SM, Clark DC. Pediatrics 1976;57:443–55.
6. Rolland-Cachera M-F, Deheeger M, Guilloud-Bataille M, et al. Ann Hum Biol 1987;14:219–29.
7. Goran MI, Kaskoun M, Shuman WP. Int J Obes 1995;19:279–83.
8. Mueller WH. Soc Sci Med 1982;16:191–6.
9. Malina RM, Bouchard C. Adipose tissue changes during growth. In: Malina RM, Bouchard C, eds. Growth, maturation, and physical activity. Champaign, IL: Human Kinetics Books, 1991;133–49.
10. Knittle JL, Timmers K, Ginsberg-Fellner F, et al. J Clin Invest 1979;63:239–46.
11. Gortmaker SL, Dietz WH, Sobol AM, et al. Am J Dis Child 1987;141:535–40.
12. Troiano RP, Flegal KM, Kuczmarski RJ, et al. Arch Pediatr Adolesc Med 1995;149:1085–91.
13. Life Sciences Research Office. Third Report on Nutrition Monitoring in the United States, vol 2. Washington, DC: US Government Printing Office, 1995.
14. Dietz WH, Strasburger VC. Curr Prob Pediatr 1991;21(1):8–31.
15. Gortmaker SL, Must A, Sobol AM, et al. Arch Pediatr Adolesc Med 1996;150:356–62.
16. Dietz WH. Am J Clin Nutr 1994;59:955–9.
17. Barker DJP, Hales CN, Fall CHD, et al. Diabetologia 1993;36:62–7.
18. Law CM, Barker DJP, Osmond C, et al. J Epidemiol Community Health 1992;46:184–6.
19. Vohr BR, Lipsitt LP, Oh W. J Pediatr 1980;97:196–9.
20. Pettit DJ, Baird HR, Aleck KA, et al. N Engl J Med 1983;308:242–5.
21. Rolland-Cachera M-F, Deheeger M, Bellisle F, et al. Am J Clin Nutr 1984;39:129–35.
22. Siervogel RM, Roche AF, Guo S, et al. Int J Obes 1991;15:479–85.
23. Braddon FEM, Rodgers B, Wadsworth MEJ, et al. Br Med J 1986;293:299–303.
24. Must A, Jacques PF, Dallal GE, et al. N Engl J Med 1992;327:1350–5.
25. Crisp AH, Douglas WB, Ross JM, et al. J Psychosom Res 1970;14:313–20.
26. Serdula MK, Ivery D, Coates RJ, et al. Prev Med 1993;22:167–77.
27. Lloyd JK, Wolff OH, Whelen WS. Br Med J 1961;2:145–8.
28. Rimm IJ, Rimm AA. Am J Public Health 1976;66:479–81.
29. Barker DJP. Br Med J 1995;311:171–4.
30. Dietz WH, Gortmaker SL. Am J Clin Nutr 1984;39:619–24.
31. Ravelli GP, Belmont L. Am J Epidemiol 1979;109:66–70.
32. Stunkard A, d'Aquili E, Fox S, et al. JAMA 1972;221:579–84.
33. Garn SM, Clark DC. Pediatrics 1975;56:306–19.

34. Lissau-Lind-Sorensen I, Sorensen TIA. Int J Obes 1992;16: 169–75.
35. Gortmaker SL, Must A, Perrin JM, et al. N Engl J Med 1993;329:1008–12.
36. Sargent JD, Blanchflower DG. Arch Pediatr Adolesc Med 1994;148:681–7.
37. Lissau I, Sorensen TIA. Lancet 1994;343:324–7.
38. Mellbin T, Vuille J-C. Acta Paediatr Scand 1989;78:568–75.
39. Mellbin T, Vuille J-C. Acta Paediatr Scand 1989;78:576–80.
40. Martinsson A. Acta Med Scand 1967;182:795–803.
41. Bjorntorp P, Hood B, Martinsson A. Acta Med Scand 1966;180:123–7.
42. Bandini LB, Schoeller DA, Dietz WH. Am J Clin Nutr 1990;52:421–5.
43. Bandini LG, Cyr H, Must A, et al. Am J Clin Nutr 1997;65:1138S–41S.
44. Livingstone MBE, Prentice AM, Coward WA, et al. Am J Clin Nutr 1992;56:29–35.
45. Flatt JP. Ann NY Acad Sci 1987;499:104–23.
46. Zurlo F, Lillioja S, Esposito-Del Puente A, et al. Am J Physiol 1990;259:E650–7.
47. Roberts SB, Savage J, Coward WA, et al. N Engl J Med 1988;318:461–6.
48. Davies PSW, Wells JCK, Fieldhouse CA, et al. Am J Clin Nutr 1995;61:1026–9.
49. Davies PSW, Day JME, Lucas A. Int J Obes 1991;15:727–31.
50. Maffeis C, Schutz Y, Micciolo R, et al. J Pediatr 1993;122:556–62.
51. Bandini LG, Schoeller DA, Dietz WH. Pediatr Res 1990;27:198–203.
52. Maffeis C, Schutz Y, Pinelli L. Eur J Clin Nutr 1992;46:577–83.
53. Bandini LG, Schoeller DA, Edwards J, et al. Am J Physiol 1989;256:E357–67.
54. Wolf AM, Gortmaker SL, Cheung L, et al. Am J Public Health 1993;83:1625–7.
55. Heath GW, Pratt M, Warren CW, et al. Arch Pediatr Adolesc Med 1994;148:1131–6.
56. Fontvieille AM, Harper IT, Ferraro RT. J Pediatr 1993;123: 200–7.
57. Schulz LO, Schoeller DA. Am J Clin Nutr 1994;60:676–81.
58. Livingstone MBE, Coward WA, Prentice AM, et al. Am J Clin Nutr 1992;56:343–52.
59. Black AE, Coward WA, Cole TJ, et al. Eur J Clin Nutr 1996;50:72–92.
60. Centers for Disease Control. MMWR 1993;42:576–9.
61. Ching PLYH, Willett WC, Rimm EB, et al. Am J Public Health 1996;86:25–30.
62. Dietz WH, Gortmaker SL. Pediatrics 1985;75:807–12.
63. Dietz WH, Bandini LG, Morelli JA, et al. Am J Clin Nutr 1994;59:556–63.
64. Robinson TN, Killen JD. J Health Educ 1995;26(Suppl):91–8.
65. Lytle LA, Kelder SH, Perry CL, et al. Health Ed Res 1995;10:133–46.
66. Raitakari OT, Porkka KVK, Taimela S, et al. Am J Epidemiol 1994;140:195–205.
67. Dietz WH, Robinson TN. Pediatr Rev 1993;14:337–44.
68. Forbes GB. J Pediatr 1977;91:40–2.
69. Alstrom-Hallgren, Goldstein JL, Fialkow PJ. Medicine 1973;52:53–71.
70. Green JS, Parfrey PS, Harnett JD, et al. N Engl J Med 1989;321:1002–9.
71. Holm VA, Sulzbacher SJ, Pipes PL. Prader-Willi syndrome. Baltimore: University Park Press, 1981.
72. Greenswag LR, Alexander RC. Management of Prader-Willi syndrome. New York: Springer-Verlag, 1988.
73. Magiakou MA, Mastorakos G, Oldfield EH, et al. N Engl J Med 1994;331:629–36.
74. Dunger DB, Wolff OH, Leonard JV, et al. Lancet 1980;1:1277–81.
75. McKenna TJ. N Engl J Med 1988;318:558–62.
76. Richardson SA, Hastorf AH, Goodman N, et al. Am Sociol Rev 1961;26:241–7.
77. Canning H, Mayer J. N Engl J Med 1966; 275:1172–4.
78. Kelsey JL, Keggi KJ, Southwick WO. J Bone Joint Surg 1970;52-A:1203–16.
79. Kelsey JL, Acheson RM, Keggi KJ. Am J Dis Child 1972;124:276–81.
80. Dietz WH, Gross WL, Kirkpatrick JA Jr. J Pediatr 1982;101:735–7.
81. Richards GE, Cavallo A, Meyer WJ III, et al. J Pediatr 1985;107:893–7.
82. Freedman DS, Burke GL, Harsha DW, et al. JAMA 1985;254:515–20.
83. Lauer RM, Lee J, Clarke WR. Pediatrics 1988;82:309–18.
84. Mallory GB Jr, Fiser DH, Jackson R. J Pediatr 1989;115:892–7.
85. Baldridge AD, Perez-Atayde AR, Graeme-Cook F, et al. J Pediatr 1995;127:700–4.
86. Crichlow RW, Seltzer MH, Jannetta PJ. Dig Dis 1972;17:68–72.
87. Weisberg LA, Chutorian AM. Arch Dis Child 1977;131: 1243–8.
88. Epstein LH, Valoski A, Wing RR, et al. JAMA 1990;264: 2519–23.
89. Epstein LH. Int J Obes 1996;20(Suppl 1):S14–21.
90. Kennedy E, Goldberg J. Nutr Rev 1995;53:111–26.
91. Sheppard L, Kristal AR, Kushi LH. Am J Clin Nutr 1991;54:821–8.
92. Pugliese MT, Weyman-Daum M, Moses N, et al. Pediatrics 1987;80:175–82.
93. Epstein LH, Squires S. The stop-light diet for children. Boston: Little Brown & Co, 1988.
94. Haddock CK, Shadish WR, Klesges RC, et al. Ann Behav Med 1994;16:235–44.
95. Dietz WH, Schoeller DA. J Pediatr 1982;100:638–44.
96. Prentice AM, Goldberg GR, Jebb SA, et al. Proc Nutr Soc 1991;50:441–58.
97. Ballor DL, Poehlman ET. Int J Obes 1994;18:35–40.
98. Sallis JF, Patrick K. Pediatr Exerc Sci 1994;6:302–14.
99. Blaak EE, Westerterp KR, Bar-Or O, et al. Am J Clin Nutr 1992;55:777–82.
100. Tremblay A, Almeras N. Int J Obes 1995;19(Suppl4):S97–101.
101. Epstein LH, Wing RR, Koeske R, et al. Behav Ther 1982;13:651–65.
102. Epstein LH, Valoski AM, Vara LS, et al. Health Psychol 1995;14:109–15.
103. Weintraub M. Clin Pharmacol Ther 1992;51:581–646.
104. Pedrinola F, Cavaliere H, Lima N, et al. Obes Res 1994;2:1–4.
105. Soper RT, Mason EE, Printen KJ, et al. J Pediatr Surg 1975;10:51–8.
106. Greenstein RJ, Rabner JG. Obes Surg 1995;5:138–44.

SELECTED READINGS

Dietz WH, Robinson TN. Assessment and treatment of childhood obesity. Pediatr Rev 1993;14:337–44.

Epstein LH, Valoski A, Wing RR, et al. Ten-year follow-up of behavioral, family based treatment for obese children. JAMA 1990;264:2519–23.

Himes JH, Dietz WH. Guidelines for overweight in adolescent preventive services: recommendations from an expert committee. The Expert Committee on Clinical Guidelines for Overweight in Adolescent Preventive Services. Am J Clin Nutr 1994;59:307–16.

64. Nutritional Management of Infants and Children with Specific Diseases and/or Conditions

WILLIAM C. HEIRD and ARTHUR COOPER

The generalized deficiency of all nutrients, i.e., protein-energy malnutrition, is by far the most common nutritional deficiency in the world today. Although this condition is rare in developed countries, it occurs in a number of infants and/or children with the underlying medical problems discussed below. Thus, it is helpful to consider the special nutrient needs and nutritional management of these children within the framework of protein-energy malnutrition as encountered in many underdeveloped parts of the world.

Protein-energy malnutrition results from a lack, in varying proportions, of protein and energy. It is seen most frequently in infants and young children and may occur in epidemic (famine-related) or endemic (disease-related) forms. Whether the cause is primary (e.g., insufficient food supply) or secondary (e.g., poor absorption, increased excretion, increased requirements), the physicochemical pattern of the tissues, defensive capacity to environmental aggressors, and efficiency and ability for work are affected adversely. Moreover, the condition is associated with a high mortality rate.

Protein-energy malnutrition includes two distinct syndromes, marasmus and kwashiorkor, as well as a mixed syndrome, often termed *marasmic kwashiorkor. Marasmus* refers to the state of chronic total undernutrition (i.e., a deficiency of both protein and energy). It results in growth failure as well as gradual emaciation and inanition. *Kwashiorkor,* derived from the Ga language of Ghana, was used initially to refer to the protein deficiency of weanling infants, i.e., "the disease that the first child gets when the second is on the way" (1). Clinically, it is characterized by signs of protein deficiency, including edema and ascites, as well as growth failure.

Both conditions occur in varying degrees in the groups of pediatric patients discussed below. Mild and moderate forms of both distinct syndromes are subclinical and characterized only by growth failure and possibly some retardation of mental development. Whether or not these latter consequences are permanent is a matter of debate; on balance, it appears that most can be ameliorated with appropriate treatment (2).

CYSTIC FIBROSIS AND OTHER CHRONIC PULMONARY DISEASES

Cystic fibrosis is characterized by progressive deterioration of pulmonary and pancreatic function. The former may increase nutrient requirements somewhat, but probably its greatest nutritional impact is an adverse effect on intake, particularly during acute exacerbations and in older children with severe pulmonary disease. Pancreatic insufficiency severely limits the absorption of fat, a major energy source of most diets. Thus, the cause of malnutrition in infants and children with this disease can be both primary (i.e., inadequate nutrient intake) and secondary (i.e., fecal losses of protein and, particularly, fat). The latter cause usually can be controlled with appropriate pancreatic enzyme replacement.

Traditionally, a high-protein, low-fat diet has been advocated for patients with cystic fibrosis. However, with appropriate pancreatic enzyme replacement, most patients can maintain a reasonable nutritional status with a "normal" diet. Younger patients usually have very good appetites, but with advanced pulmonary disease, appetite usually decreases. Many patients with advanced disease take in far less protein and especially energy than is recommended. From time to time, the theoretical possibility of essential fatty acid deficiency secondary to poor fat absorption is mentioned. However, unless the intake of essential fatty acids is quite low, this is rarely a significant problem.

There is some concern that malnutrition may hasten deterioration of pulmonary function, but there is no definitive proof that this is the case. Nonetheless, acute improvement of nutritional status improves muscle strength (3). Thus, attempts either to improve nutritional status or to prevent even minimal deterioration of nutritional status are warranted.

In recent years, high-fat formulas have been advocated for patients with chronic pulmonary disease. The rationale, supported adequately by fact, is that oxidation of fat produces less carbon dioxide than oxidation of carbohydrate and, hence, a high-fat intake imposes less stress on the already compromised pulmonary system. This obviously is an important consideration in patients who require mechanical ventilation or who have severely compromised pulmonary function. One product based on this principle (Pulmocare, Ross Laboratories) is available for patients with pulmonary disease. Although designed for adults, the product is used in pediatric patients; however, its sodium content is quite high.

CONGENITAL HEART DISEASE

Chronic protein-energy malnutrition, manifested chiefly by growth failure, is also a common finding in infants with congenital heart disease, particularly those with conditions associated with congestive heart failure. Although not studied extensively, the nutrient needs of patients with heart disease do not appear to be much greater, if at all, than those of infants or children without heart disease. Rather, in most patients, the cause of the accompanying malnutrition can be traced to inadequate intake. In some patients, this is a result simply of poor appetite; in others, it appears to be due to excessive tiring during feeding. In addition, fluid and sodium intakes frequently are restricted as a part of treatment and use of diuretics is common. Either practice, of course, may limit growth, even if intake of protein and energy is adequate.

The most common form of nutritional therapy for infants with congenital heart disease is use of a high-nutrient-density formula, which reduces the volume that must be ingested. Tube feeding via either a nasogastric or gastrostomy tube is frequently necessary, particularly in infants whose disease is sufficiently severe to cause excessive tiring during feeding. In general, if sufficient nutrients are delivered, most such patients will grow at a reasonably "normal" rate.

GASTROINTESTINAL DISORDERS

Malnutrition is endemic among infants and children with gastrointestinal disorders. The cause is usually loss of nutrients secondary to the specific derangement in gastrointestinal function, either diarrhea or vomiting. However, both diarrhea and vomiting are frequently "treated" by withholding all nutrients except water and electrolytes. This practice, of course, contributes to development of malnutrition.

Acute Diarrhea

Acute diarrhea caused by most common organisms rarely persists for more than 4 to 5 days. During this time, the major goal of therapy is to maintain a normal state of hydration. This can be accomplished with use of oral rehydration solutions and/or special formulas (Table 64.1). Hospitalization and intravenous fluid therapy may be necessary, particularly if fever and/or vomiting accompany the diarrhea.

What to feed and whether to feed the child with acute diarrhea have been subjects of considerable controversy for many years, and both remain unresolved. In general, stool output is greater in the patient who is fed, but this does not mean necessarily that feeding should be proscribed. Most patients can ingest at least some nutrients; however, the nature of this intake must be selected carefully, taking into account the probable etiology of the diarrhea. The approach followed by the authors is outlined below; other approaches, of course, may be equally successful.

In general, the etiology of most cases of acute diarrhea is either bacterial or viral. Thus, a stool culture to detect the specific pathogen is indicated. In most developed countries, the recognized enteropathogenic bacteria (*Salmonella, Shigella,* and enteropathogenic *Escherichia coli*) are infrequent causes of diarrhea. Rather, most acute bacterial diarrheas are caused by one of the many toxicogenic strains of most gram-negative organisms. Thus, a routine stool culture, unless it suggests a predominant organism, usually is not helpful. On the other hand, since the pathogenesis of toxicogenic bacterial diarrhea (i.e., a secretory diarrhea resulting from stimulation of the adenylate cyclase system, as occurs in cholera [4]) differs from that of viral diarrhea (i.e., an osmotic diarrhea secondary to inhibition of glucose transport as described for rotavirus [5]), testing the stool for pH and reducing substances can be very helpful. In general, a low pH (<6.0) and the presence of reducing substances suggest a viral etiology. The stool must be tested, of course, following a period of adequate intake of a reducing sugar (e.g., a 5% glucose solution or a rehydration solution); in addition, the water content of the stool rather than any solid matter should be tested.

If the etiology of the diarrhea appears to be viral, a carbohydrate-free formula (Table 64.1) is usually well tolerated. However, such formulas result in ketosis and sometimes hypoglycemia; thus, some carbohydrate intake is necessary. In the hospitalized child, this can be provided intravenously. Most who do not require hospitalization usually tolerate at least some sugar intake by the enteral route. In general, 0.5 g of glucose or sucrose per ounce of formula, provided intake is adequate but not excessive, is well tolerated and prevents ketosis and/or hypoglycemia. If this preparation is tolerated, the amount of carbohydrate can be increased daily or every other day as tolerance for carbohydrate increases. Once full carbohydrate content (i.e., approximately 2 g/oz) is tolerated, the patient usually can be switched to a carbohydrate-containing formula.

If the etiology of the diarrhea is a toxicogenic bacterium, feeding usually does not affect the volume of stool output. In many cases, in fact, a glucose-electrolyte solution appears to decrease the volume of stool output. In such patients, therefore, decisions concerning feeding must be based on clinical experience.

Table 64.1
Composition (amount/100 kcal) of Special Formulas for Infants with Deranged Intestinal Function

Component	RCF[a,c]	Pregestamil[b]	Nutramigen[b]	Portagen[b]	Alimentum[a]	Pediasure[a]
Protein (g)	4.95 (Soy protein isolate)	2.8 (Casein hydrolysate, cystine, tyrosine, and tryptophan)	2.8 (Casein hydrolysate, cystine, tyrosine, and tryptophan)	3.5 (Sodium caseinate)	2.75 (Casein hydrolysate, cystine, tyrosine, and tryptophan)	3.0 (Low-lactose whey protein and sodium caseinate)
Fat (g)	8.91 (Soy and coconut oils)	5.6 (MCT; corn, soy and high-oleic safflower oils)	3.9 (Corn and soy oils)	4.8 (MCT, corn oil)	5.54 (MCT; safflower and soy oils)	5.0 (MCT; soy and high-oleic safflower oils)
Carbohydrate (g)	0	10.3 (Corn syrup solids, modified corn-starch, dextrose)	13.4 (Corn syrup solids, modified cornstarch)	11.5 (Corn syrup solids, sucrose)	10.2 (Sucrose, modified tapioca starch)	11.0 (Hydrolyzed cornstarch; sucrose)
Calcium (mg)	173	94	94	94	105	97
Phosphorus (mg)	124	63	63	70	75	80
Magnesium (mg)	12.4	10.9	10.9	20	7.5	20
Iron (mg)	0.37	1.88	1.88	1.88	1.8	1.4
Zinc (mg)	1.2	0.94	0.78	0.94	0.75	1.2
Manganese (μg)	50	31	31	125	30	250
Copper (μg)	124	94	94	156	75	100
Iodine (μg)	25	7	7	7	15	9.7
Selenium (μg)	3.5	2.3	2.3	—	2.8	2.3
Sodium (mg)	73	39	47	55	44	38
Potassium (mg)	180	109	109	125	118	131
Chloride (mg)	103	86	86	86	80	101
Vitamin A (IU)	500	380	310	780	300	257
Vitamin D (IU)	100	75	63	78	45	51
Vitamin E (IU)	5.0	3.8	3.1	3.1	3.0	2.3
Vitamin K (IU)	25	18.8	15.6	15.6	15	3.8
Thiamine (mg)	100	78	78	156	60	270
Riboflavin B_2 (μg)	150	94	94	188	90	210
Vitamin B_6 (μg)	100	63	63	210	60	260
Vitamin B_{12} (μg)	0.75	0.31	0.31	0.62	0.45	0.6
Niacin (μg)	2230	1250	1250	2100	1350	1690
Folic acid (μg)	25	15.6	15.6	15.6	15	37
Pantothenic acid	1240	470	470	1050	750	1000
Vitamin C (mg)	13.6	11.7	8.1	8.1	9.0	10
Biotin (mg)	7.5	7.8	7.8	7.8	4.5	32
Choline (mg)	13	13.3	13.3	13.3	8	30
Inositol (mg)	8	4.7	4.7	4.7	5	8

[a]Ross Laboratories, Columbus, Ohio.
[b]Mead Johnson Nutritional Division, Evansville, Indiana.
[c]Note that formula contains no carbohydrate, which accounts for the markedly different nutrient content of it versus the others shown.

The tendency to avoid feeding lactose to infants with diarrhea, regardless of etiology, probably is unnecessary. If stool pH is normal when the child is first seen and reducing substances are not present, lactase deficiency is an unlikely contributor to the diarrhea.

If the acute episode of diarrhea does not resolve in the usual 4 to 5 days, as happens in a small number of patients, nutritional therapy management becomes a much more important consideration. While most infants can tolerate a 4- to 5-day period with little or no nutritional intake, few can tolerate more than 2 weeks without becoming malnourished and developing secondary intestinal changes due to both persistent diarrhea and malnutrition. Such infants are much more likely to develop secondary deficiencies of mucosal hydrolases (e.g., lactase deficiency and, less commonly, sucrase deficiency) and also monosaccharide intolerance. Managing these infants without hospitalization is much more difficult. Choice of formula, again, must be made on the basis of the suspected or culture-proven cause of the diarrhea; in addition, the much greater likelihood of secondary mucosal hydrolase deficiencies must be taken into account. If small volumes of a particular formula are reasonably well tolerated, it frequently is possible to deliver enough to meet nutritional needs by a continuous infusion technique (6). This usually requires hospitalization of small infants.

Many other congenital and/or acquired forms of chronic diarrhea (e.g., abetalipoproteinemia, celiac disease), if not managed appropriately, frequently result in the same secondary changes in mucosal function. Nutritional management, in general, is similar to that described above and must be coordinated with the usual medical management of these conditions. Although diet is a major aspect of the therapy of most chronic diarrheas, a detailed discussion of this aspect of therapy is beyond the scope of this chapter.

Vomiting

Most acute episodes of vomiting are of short duration and present few nutritional problems. However, chronic vomiting accompanies a number of conditions. The most common of these conditions intrinsic to the gastrointestinal tract is gastroesophageal reflux. To some extent, this condition is physiologic in infancy; however, it assumes pathologic significance if it results in failure to thrive and/or recurrent pulmonary aspiration.

In the early stages, nutritional management of this condition includes maintaining the patient in an upright position during and immediately following feeding and reassuring the parents that the persistent vomiting is causing no harm so long as the infant is gaining weight normally and is not having respiratory symptoms. If either growth failure or a decrease in weight-for-height develops despite optimal medical management, remedial nutritional therapy is indicated (i.e., feedings delivered continuously into the duodenum or jejunum to minimize the risk of further reflux). Many patients require corrective surgery.

Short Bowel Syndrome

Functionally, short bowel syndrome can be considered in the same way as chronic diarrhea. In this condition, alterations of gastrointestinal motility, secretion, digestion, and absorption are secondary to massive small intestinal loss rather than bacterial and/or viral invasion and the secondary effects of these organisms and malnutrition. In general, the severity of the short bowel syndrome is related inversely to the length of the remaining intestinal segment; however, loss of the ileocecal valve, which acts as a physiologic sphincter to slow transit time and prevent backwash ileitis, also increases severity (7). Specific symptoms also result from removal of specific segments of intestine. Since disaccharidase activity is greater in jejunal cells and since cholecystokinin and other intestinal hormones are secreted by jejunal sites, removal of the jejunum results in more-severe carbohydrate malabsorption and, perhaps, decreased biliary and pancreatic secretion as well as deranged motility. Ileal loss, on the other hand, results in loss of both bile salt uptake and absorption of vitamin B_{12}. In general, the ileum's potential for adaptation appears to be superior to that of the jejunum. Thus, loss of jejunum usually is better tolerated than loss of the ileum.

The early phase of the short bowel syndrome immediately after massive resection usually is associated with massive fluid and electrolyte losses, making effective enteral alimentation impossible. Thus, during both this phase and the early part of the intermediate phase, most nutrient requirements must be provided parenterally. As the remaining small bowel gradually adapts, enteral intake usually can be advanced, but this must proceed slowly. In general, continuous feeding via either an indwelling nasogastric or gastrostomy tube is better tolerated during this phase than bolus feeding. In addition, elemental formulas (Table 64.1) are generally better tolerated than nonelemental formulas.

Eventually, maximum adaptation is achieved, and more complex proteins and carbohydrates can be introduced. Even during this final phase, however, frequent small feedings may be necessary. During all phases, pharmacologic manipulations (e.g., cholestyramine to chelate bile acids; loperamide and/or paregoric to slow transit time; antibiotics to eradicate significant bacterial overgrowth) may provide symptomatic as well as physiologic improvement. (See Chapter 68.)

GENERAL APPROACH TO NUTRITIONAL THERAPY

Accurate determination of nutritional status obviously is the first step in all types of nutritional therapy. However, assessing the nutritional status of infants is difficult (8), in part because malnutrition is not precisely defined and in part because the earliest changes of malnutrition are subtle adaptations that tend to ameliorate the effects of malnutrition. Nonetheless, some objective evaluation of nutritional status should be applied to every child who is a potential candidate for nutritional therapy. If for no other reason, this evaluation provides a baseline for monitoring the results of therapy. Physical growth charts, height and weight velocity curves, and other anthropometric data are given in Appendix Tables III-A-14-b-1 to g-2.

Many anthropometric and biochemical assessment techniques are available (see Chapter 54); their specific advantages, disadvantages, and limitations have been discussed extensively (8). In general, no single test or combination of tests is ideal. Indeed, clinical judgment based upon knowledge of the disease process and the status of the body's nutritional reserves appears to be as reliable as any of the commonly used "objective" tests (9). In the authors' experience, assessment of weight in relation to height (length) is one of the most useful indices of nutritional status. A child who falls below the 10th percentile on this standard curve, regardless of either weight for age or height (length) for age, can be assumed to be malnourished and in need of nutritional therapy.

The situation of the child whose weight is appropriate for height (length) but whose weight and height are low for age (i.e., the stunted child) is more problematic (10). There is no convincing evidence that such a child is malnourished and in need of aggressive nutritional intervention. On the other hand, an attempt to permit the child to achieve his or her growth potential is warranted. This usually requires both a nutritional history and a more extensive medical evaluation, including evaluation of endocrinologic status (see also Chapter 59).

In general, the approach advocated for nutritional management of the low-birth-weight (LBW) infant (Chapter 51) is equally applicable to any malnourished infant or child—indeed, any infant or child with an underlying condition predisposing to malnutrition. Initially, particularly in less severely affected individuals, attempts should be made to increase nutrient intake by conventional means. If this approach is unsuccessful, one of several commercially available supplements can be used. However, these often replace usual food intake and thus may not result in the desired increased total intake. Moreover, most of the products currently available were designed for adults and are not optimal for pediatric patients. One exception is Pediasure (Table 64.1).

If conventional foods are not tolerated, use of special formulas or supplements and perhaps delivery by tube, either as a bolus or continuously, are the next steps (Chapter 100). The choice of both formula and method of delivery, of course, must be dictated by the patient's underlying condition. Tube feedings can be given throughout the day or only during part of the day (e.g., at night), depending upon the patient's age, condition, and nutritional status. If the patient's condition (e.g., pulmonary disease) makes an indwelling nasal tube inadvisable, a gastrostomy tube, inserted percutaneously or surgically, should be considered. If gastrointestinal tolerance of even elemental formulas is severely limited, parenteral nutrients can be used, either as the sole source of nutrition or as a supplement to tolerated enteral nutrient combinations.

PARENTERAL NUTRITION

The now widespread use of parenteral nutrition (see Chapter 101) is usually considered one of the major contributing factors to the current low mortality of infants born with surgically correctable lesions of the gastrointestinal tract (e.g., omphalocele, gastroschisis, intestinal atresias) as well as those with short bowel syndrome and intractable diarrhea (11). Although the role of parenteral nutrient delivery in decreasing the mortality and morbidity of other groups of pediatric patients (e.g., LBW infants) is less clear, the technique is used in a wide variety of pediatric patients. Moreover, despite the many hazards of the technique, most agree that the obvious anabolism that can be achieved with parenteral delivery of nutrients is preferable to the inevitable continuation of catabolism if delivery of adequate nutrients by other routes is impossible. This is particularly true if careful attention is paid to every aspect of the technique, thereby minimizing its hazards and maximizing its benefits.

Route of Administration

Parenteral nutrients can be infused by either central vein or peripheral vein. An energy intake of 70 to 80 kcal/kg/day can be provided consistently and safely by the peripheral venous route, but for obvious reasons, the duration of this type of delivery is limited. Much greater intakes (100 to 120 kcal/kg/day) can be delivered for a longer period by the central venous route. Acceptable intakes of all other nutrients are possible by either route.

Although the advantages and disadvantages of these two routes of delivery are frequently discussed, both are efficacious when used in the appropriate circumstances. In general, the time that parenteral nutrients are likely to be required and the nutrient needs of the patient should determine which route is chosen. If parenteral nutrients are likely to be required for more than approximately 10 days, central venous delivery usually is preferable.

In LBW infants, the infusate frequently is delivered by umbilical vessel catheters. Although this route of delivery is convenient, it cannot be recommended without reservation. The flow characteristics of the umbilical vessels do not permit sufficient dilution of a concentrated nutrient infusate to circumvent intimal damage. Also, the incidence of thrombosis with umbilical catheters is quite high, malposition of these catheters can result in severe consequences, and the incidence of sepsis appears to be greater when nutrients are delivered by umbilical vessels than when delivered by either central or peripheral vein.

The Nutrient Infusate

The nutrient infusate should include amino acids as well as sufficient energy (glucose and lipid), electrolytes, minerals, and vitamins. Suitable infusates for both central vein and peripheral vein delivery are shown in Table 64.2. While these are acceptable for most infants and children, modification may be required to reflect the specific needs of individual patients.

Several crystalline amino acid mixtures are available (Table 64.3); all contain most essential amino acids (exceptions are cystine and tyrosine, which are either unstable or insoluble in aqueous solution) and varying amounts of nonessential amino acids. An amino acid intake of 2.5 to 4.0 g/kg/day is recommended. Higher intakes, although tolerated by most infants, are more likely to result in elevated plasma amino acid concentra-

Table 64.2
Composition of Suitable Parenteral Nutrition Infusate(s)

Component	Amount/kg/day
Amino acids	2.5 g–4.0 g
Energy	60–120 kcal
Glucose[a]	15–30 g
Lipid[b]	0.5–3.0 g
Electrolytes and minerals	
Sodium (as chloride)	2–4 mEq
Potassium (as phosphate and chloride)[c]	2–4 mEq
Calcium (as gluconate)	1.5–2.0 mmol
Magnesium (as sulfate)	0.25 mEq
Phosphorus (as potassium phosphate)[c]	1.5 mmol
Trace minerals	See Table 64.4
Vitamins	See Table 64.5
Volume	100–150 mL

[a]For peripheral vein infusion, glucose concentration should not exceed 10–12.5%.
[b]Lipid must be infused separately (see text).
[c]Potassium, as phosphate, should be limited to 2.5 mEq/kg/day (approximately 1.7 mmol phosphate) unless chemical monitoring suggests need for more phosphate; if only additional potassium is required, it should be provided as the chloride salt.

Table 64.3
Amino Acid Content (mg/2.5 g) of Commercially Available Amino Acid Mixtures

Amino Acid	Aminosyn[a]	Aminosyn-Pf[a]	Travasol (B)[b]	Novamine[c]	FreAmine III[d]	TrophAmine[d]
Isoleucine	180	191	120	124	175	204
Leucine	235	297	155	174	228	350
Lysine	180	170	145	198	182	204
Methionine	100	45	145	124	132	83
Phenylalanine	110	107	155	174	140	121
Threonine	130	129	105	124	100	104
Tryptophan	40	45	45	41	38	50
Valine	200	161	115	162	165	196
Histidine	75	79	109	147	71	121
Cystine	0	0	0	<12	<6	<8
Tyrosine	11	16	10	9	0	58
Taurine	0	18	0	0	0	6
Alanine	320	175	518	353	178	133
Aspartic acid	0	132	0	74	0	79
Glutamic acid	0	206	0	124	0	125
Glycine	320	96	518	174	350	92
Proline	215	204	104	147	280	171
Serine	105	124	0	100	148	96
Arginine	245	308	258	247	238	304

[a]Abbott Laboratories, North Chicago, IL.
[b]Clintec, Deerfield, IL.
[c]Kabi-Vitrum, Inc, Franklin, OH.
[d]McGaw Laboratories, Irvine, CA.

tions and azotemia. Some advocate amino acid intakes below 2.5 g/kg/day for the LBW infant, particularly during the first few days of therapy when nonprotein energy intake is low (due to glucose and lipid intolerance). Recent studies suggest that there is no reason to advocate this practice, even if concomitant energy intake is quite low (12).

Glucose is the preferred nonlipid parenteral energy source; however, the ability of some infants to metabolize it is limited. Many infants, particularly during the early period of parenteral nutrition, develop hyperglycemia and osmotic diuresis with concomitant urinary loss of electrolytes when the amount of glucose infused exceeds tolerance. Careful, continuous administration of small doses of insulin appears to alleviate glucose intolerance in LBW infants, thereby permitting administration of much greater glucose intakes (13). Whether this practice is desirable remains to be determined.

Most LBW infants tolerate 5 to 7% solutions of dextrose (3.5–5.0 mg/kg/min, or 18–25 kcal/kg/day) if volume is limited to 100 mL/kg/day), even during the first few days of life; thus, in very small and/or unstable infants, it is wise to begin parenteral nutrition with these lower glucose intakes and increase the intake as the infant's tolerance for glucose improves. In older, more stable infants, an initial glucose intake of 15 g/kg/day (about 50 kcal/kg/day) is usually well tolerated and can be delivered easily by the peripheral route without exceeding a glucose concentration of 10%. With central venous delivery, much greater intakes (i.e., 25–30 g/kg/day, or 85–102 kcal/kg/day) are eventually tolerated. Even in the most stable patients, however, these higher intakes should be achieved gradually with daily increments of no more than 5 g/kg/day. In all patients, glucose tolerance should be closely monitored as glucose intake is being increased (see below). Once achieved, the higher intakes usually are well tolerated so long as the patient's condition remains stable.

Electrolyte requirements vary from patient to patient; thus, the amounts suggested in Table 64.2 should not be interpreted as absolute requirements. Adjustments are often necessary and should be made on the basis of close monitoring (see below).

The amounts of calcium and phosphorus required for optimal skeletal mineralization (i.e., 100–120 and 60–75 mg/kg/day, respectively) in the "normally growing" LBW infant often cannot be incorporated into the parenteral nutrition infusate because of the chemical incompatibility of calcium and phosphate. (See also Table 101.7 and text in Chapter 101 concerning avoidance of coprecipitation of these two ions.) In general, the amounts suggested in Table 64.2 are compatible and cause no problems over the short term. However, if parenteral nutrition is required for weeks to months, skeletal mineralization may be inadequate, particularly that of the LBW infant.

Addition of trace minerals to the infusate is recommended if exclusive parenteral nutrition is likely to exceed 7 to 10 days. Suggested intakes (14) are given in Table 64.4. Many advocate including zinc and copper from the outset. Issues related to the recommended doses of trace elements and commercially available multitrace element solutions for infants and children are discussed in Chapter 101.

Parenteral vitamin requirements are not known with certainty. Obviously, the usual recommended dietary allowances (RDAs) may not apply with parenteral administration. Recommended parenteral intakes are given in Table 64.5 (14). Currently, however, a multivitamin prepa-

Table 64.4
Recommended Parenteral Intakes (amount/kg/day) of Trace Minerals[a]

Trace Minerals[b]	Preterm Infants	Term Infants and Children[c]
Zinc (μg)	400	250 (5000)
Copper (μg)	20	20 (300)
Selenium(μg)	2.0	2.0 (30)
Chromium(μg)	0.2	0.2 (5)
Manganese (μg)	1.0	1.0 (50)
Molybdenum (μg)	0.25	0.25 (5)
Iodide (μg)	1.0	1.0 (1)
Iron[d]		

[a]The American Society for Clinical Nutrition Committee on Clinical Practice Issues (14).
[b]If parenteral nutrients are used as a supplement for tolerated enteral feeds or as sole source of nutrients for <4 weeks, only zinc and, perhaps, copper are needed.
[c]Maximum recommended intake per day is shown in parentheses.
[d]Iron dextran (1–2 mg/L) has been used safely in adults, but reported experience in children, particularly infants, is limited. Estimated requirements, based on the assumption that 10% of the recommended enteral intake is absorbed, are 100 and 200 μg/kg/day, respectively, for the term and preterm infant.

ration that provides the recommended intakes of all vitamins for underweight premature infants is not available. Intakes provided by the most commonly used U.S. pediatric multivitamin mixture, which is deemed suitable for children aged 1 to 11 years, are also shown in Table 64.5. (See also Tables 101.11 and 101.12 for European pediatric formulas.)

Use of Parenteral Lipid Emulsions

Infants who receive fat-free parenteral nutrition, particularly LBW infants and nutritionally depleted infants, develop classic essential fatty acid (EFA) deficiency (i.e., an elevated triene:tetraene ratio) very quickly (i.e., days) when growth and/or regrowth is initiated (15). Thus, it is desirable to use lipid emulsions to prevent this deficiency, which is detectable biochemically (eicosatrienoic acid:arachidonic acid > 0.25) before clinical signs appear. Parenteral lipid emulsions are also a useful source of energy. Emulsions of either soybean oil (Intralipid, Kabi-Vitrum; Travamulsion, Travenol Laboratories; Liposyn III, Abbott Laboratories) or a mixture of safflower and soybean oils (Liposyn II, Abbott Laboratories) are available in both 10 and 20% concentrations (see Table 101.5 for the composition of such formulations). A dose of only 0.5 g/kg/day of soybean oil emulsion prevents classic EFA deficiency; since the linoleic acid content of the emulsion of soy and safflower oils is even greater, a smaller dose may suffice. The linolenic acid content of the latter emulsion is somewhat lower but is probably adequate.

All infants, including LBW infants, usually tolerate the small dose of parenteral lipid emulsion necessary to prevent EFA deficiency. However, the ability of an individual infant to tolerate a larger dose is quite variable. In general, the ability to metabolize intravenous fat emulsions is related directly to maturity (16), but the stressed and/or malnourished patient (i.e., the small-for-gestational-age LBW infant and the nutritionally depleted older child) also may have difficulty metabolizing these preparations (17).

Doses of fat emulsion in excess of the infant's ability to metabolize it results in accumulation of triglyceride in the bloodstream. This in turn may decrease pulmonary diffusion capacity, presumably secondary to accumulation of small lipid droplets within the pulmonary capillaries (18). It also results in recruitment of the reticuloendothelial system for lipid clearance and, hence, lipid accumulation in these cells (19). This lipid accumulation is a likely explanation for the impaired host defense mechanisms reported in patients receiving lipid emulsions (20). Metabolism of the infused lipid increases serum concentrations of free fatty acids, which compete with bilirubin and other substances for binding to albumin (21). Thus, administration of large doses of lipid emulsion may be hazardous for infants with pulmonary disease, infection, and/or hyperbilirubinemia.

Considering the difficulties of monitoring serum concentrations of both triglyceride and free fatty acids, it probably is wise to limit the dose of lipid emulsion given to patients who are likely to be intolerant to 0.5 to 1.0 g/kg/day. Most other patients usually tolerate a dose of 3 g/kg/day or more, but even in these patients, it is wise to begin with a smaller dose (e.g., 1–1.5 g/kg/day) and increase the dose slowly. In LBW infants, administration of lipid emulsion should be initiated with a relatively low dose (0.5 g/kg/day) and increased gradually to a maximum of 3 g/kg/day. In all patients, the emulsion should be infused continuously throughout the day.

Table 64.5
Suggested Parenteral Intakes of Vitamins[a]

Vitamin	Preterm Infants[b] (Amount/kg/day)	Term Infants and Children[c] (Amount/day)
A (μg)	500	700
E (mg)	2.8	7
K (μg)	80	200
D(μg)	4 (160 IU)	10
Ascorbic acid (mg)	25	80
Thiamin (mg)	0.35	1.2
Riboflavin (mg)	0.15	1.4
Pyridoxine Cl (mg)	0.18	1.0
Niacin (mg)	6.8	17
Pantothenate (mg)	2.0	5
Biotin (μg)	6.0	20
Folate(μg)	56	140
B_{12} (μg)	0.3	1.0

[a]The American Society for Clinical Nutrition Committee on Clinical Practice Issues (14).
[b]Total daily dose should not exceed that recommended for term infants and children. A dose of 2 mL of reconstituted MVI-Pediatric (Armour Pharmaceutical Co., Chicago, IL) provides the following intakes (amount/kg/day): vitamin A, 280 mg; vitamin E, 2.8 μg; vitamin K, 80 μg; vitamin D, 4 μg (160 IU); ascorbic acid, 32 mg; thiamin, 0.48 mg; riboflavin, 0.56 mg; pyridoxine, 0.4 mg; niacin, 6.8 mg; pantothenate, 2.0 mg; biotin, 8.0 μg; folate, 56 μg; vitamin B_{12}, 0.4 μg.
[c]These amounts are provided by a vial of reconstituted MVI-Pediatric.

The 20% soybean oil emulsion appears to be cleared more rapidly than the 10% emulsion and thus is less likely to cause hypertriglyceridemia (22). Hyperphospholipidemia and hypercholesterolemia, both of which occur routinely in patients receiving the 10% soybean emulsion, do not occur with use of the 20% emulsion (22), presumably because of the lower phospholipid:triglyceride ratio of the 20% emulsion.

Since the size of the lipid particles of the emulsions (0.4–0.5 microns) exceeds the pore size of an effective filter (0.22 microns), filters cannot be used for infusion of fat emulsions. In the author's opinion, the emulsions should not be mixed directly with other components of the infusate. This practice, which appears to be relatively common, may not destroy the emulsion but it certainly inhibits detection of chemical incompatibilities within the complicated infusate (e.g., precipitation of calcium phosphate). The potential hazards of the latter possibility are compounded, of course, by the fact that filters cannot be used.

Complications of TPN

Despite its obvious nutritional efficacy, total parenteral nutrition (TPN) is associated with a number of complications, both catheter (or infusion) related and metabolic. At the time of central vein catheter insertion, pneumothorax, hemothorax, injury to an artery, and/or hematoma may occur. Thrombosis, dislodgment, perforation, infusion leaks (pericardial, pleural, mediastinal), and infections have been reported during use of central vein catheters. The most common infusion-related problem is infection. Phlebitis and soft tissue sloughing are the most frequent complications of peripheral vein infusions. All these complications can be controlled, but it is difficult to prevent them entirely. Careful attention to care of the central catheter, including frequent dressing changes, is particularly important for controlling infection. Careful frequent observation of the infusion site is necessary to prevent infiltration of infusates delivered by peripheral vein and to ensure proper long-term function of central vein catheters.

Metabolic complications result either from either the limited metabolic capacity of the patient for the various components of the nutrient infusate or from the infusate itself. The metabolic complications most commonly observed and their probable causes are listed in Table 64.6. One of the more troublesome of these is the occurrence of abnormal plasma amino acid patterns with use of many of the currently available amino acid mixtures (23). Cyst(e)ine and tyrosine, both thought to be essential amino acids for the newborn and perhaps for all patients receiving parenteral nutrients, are unstable and/or only sparingly soluble; hence, none of the currently marketed mixtures contains appreciable amounts of these amino acids (Table 64.3). Furthermore, all result in very low plasma cyst(e)ine and tyrosine concentrations (23). Many available mixtures also have large amounts of only a few nonessential amino acids (e.g., glycine) rather than a mixture of all nonessential amino acids (Table 64.3); thus, extremely high plasma concentrations of the amino acid(s) present in excess are commonly seen.

Table 64.6
Metabolic Complications of Total Parenteral Nutrition and Their Probable Etiology

Complication	Probable Etiology
Disorders related to metabolic capacity of patient	
Hyperglycemia	Excessive intake (either excessive concerntration or infusion rate); Change in metabolic state (e.g., infection; surgical stress)
Hypoglycemia	Sudden cessation of infusion
Azotemia	Excessive nitrogen intake
Electrolyte disorders	Excessive or inadequate intake
Mineral disorders	Excessive or inadequate intake
Vitamin disorders	Excessive or inadequate intake
Essential fatty acid deficiency	Failure to provide essential fatty acids
Hyperlipidemia	Excessive intake; change in metabolic state (e.g., stress; sepsis)
Disorders related to infusate components	
Metabolic acidosis	Use of hydrochloride salts of amino acids (e.g., cysteine)
Hyperammonemia	Inadequate arginine intake
Abnormal plasma aminograms	Amino acid pattern of nitrogen source
Hepatic disorders	Unknown; suggested etiologies include prematurity, malnutrition, sepsis, inadequate stimulation of bile flow, toxic effects of amino acids, specific amino acid deficiency, excessive amino acid and/or carbohydrate intake, nonspecific response to lack of feeding
Bone disease	Inadequate calcium and/or phosphorus intake and, perhaps, other unknown reasons

Whether these abnormal plasma amino acid patterns are hazardous, or even undesirable, is not known. However, considering the well-known relationship between abnormally high plasma amino acid concentrations and mental retardation in infants with inborn errors of metabolism (e.g., phenylketonuria) as well as the relationship between inadequate intake of a specific amino acid and a low plasma concentration of that amino acid, normalization of plasma amino acid patterns seems warranted. Some of the newer amino acid mixtures (e.g., TrophAmine, Kendall-McGaw Laboratories, Inc.) accomplish this to a large extent (24).

Although some metabolic complications are unavoidable, many can be controlled by careful monitoring and appropriate adjustment of the infusate. A suggested monitoring schedule is given in Table 64.7. The monitoring required to ensure safe and efficacious use of lipid emulsions is the most problematic. The most common practice, inspecting the plasma for turbidity, may not reliably detect elevated plasma triglyceride and free fatty acid concentrations (25), which requires chemical determinations that are usually not practical. A reasonable compromise is to observe the plasma frequently (at least 3 times a day) for

Table 64.7
Suggested Monitoring Schedule During Total Parenteral Nutrition

Variables to be Monitored	Suggested Frequency (per week)[a] Initial Period[a]	Later Period[a]
Growth variables		
Weight	7	7
Length	1	1
Head circumference	1	1
Metabolic variables		
Plasma electrolytes	3–4	2
Plasma calcium, magnesium, phosphorus	2	1
Blood acid base status	3–4	1
Blood urea nitrogen	2	1
Plasma albumin	1	1
Liver function studies	1	1
Serum lipids[b]		
Hemoglobin	2	2
Urinary glucose	2–6/day	2/day
Variables for detection of infection		
Clinical observations (activity, temperature, etc.)	Daily	Daily
WBC count	As indicated	As indicated
Cultures	As indicated	As indicated

[a]Initial period is the time during which the desired energy intake is being achieved or the time(s) of metabolic instability.
[b]See text.

evidence of lipid accumulation (primarily triglyceride) and measure triglyceride and free fatty acids less frequently. Careful monitoring is particularly important when the lipid dose is being increased, when the infant is unstable, and when a change in the infant's condition occurs. If the plasma becomes turbid, the rate of infusion should be decreased or the infusion stopped completely until the turbidity clears. Usually, infusion can then be resumed at a lower rate. Once the desired dose of intravenous fat is achieved, serum turbidity should be checked once a day (unless the patient becomes unstable) and actual determinations of serum triglyceride and free fatty acid concentrations should be made weekly. The development of cholelithiasis is discussed in Chapter 101.

Weaning Infants from TPN

In most infants, administration of parenteral nutrients need not interfere with introducing enteral feedings as soon as they are likely to be tolerated. Once started, the volume of enteral feedings can be advanced as tolerated by the infant, and the volume of the parenteral nutrition infusate decreased. During the period of combined enteral and parenteral nutrition, care should be taken to ensure that nutrient requirements are met as nearly as possible and that tolerance for both fluids and nutrients is not exceeded. This requires careful attention to the total (parenteral *plus* enteral) intake and frequent downward adjustment of the parenteral intake as enteral intake increases.

Home Parenteral Nutrition

Today, most patients who require parenteral nutrients for a long period of time leave the hospital and receive this therapy at home. Considering the many difficulties of in-hospital parenteral nutrition (see above), the potential problems of TPN at home seem formidable. Nonetheless, both patients who can tolerate some enteral intake and patients who can tolerate only parenteral nutrients have been treated successfully at home for several months to years. In many cases, sufficient nutrients can be administered during only a portion of the day, allowing the older patient to pursue reasonably normal daytime activities and the younger patient (and his or her parents) to sleep with little danger of accidental disconnection of the infusion system. Small portable infusion pumps are available such that the necessary apparatus can be enclosed in vests, backpacks, etc., allowing even the patient who requires constant infusion of parenteral nutrients to pursue a reasonably normal life. Obviously, home parenteral nutrition is more likely to be successful for the older child, adolescent, or adult. However, with careful patient selection, young infants can also be managed quite successfully at home.

The Broviac catheter, which can be used for several months, frequently years, is usually used for home parenteral nutrition. Standard nutrient infusates are obtained from the hospital pharmacy or from a number of commercial concerns and stored in a small home refrigerator. Catheter care is managed by the patient or by a family member after careful training prior to discharge.

All the usual metabolic and catheter-related complications of parenteral nutrition can occur at home as well as in the hospital. However, patients who can be managed successfully with home parenteral nutrition usually have reached the point at which requirements are reasonably stable. Thus, less frequent monitoring is sufficient. Nonetheless, successful home parenteral nutrition, particularly for the young pediatric patient, requires frequent outpatient visits as well as frequent telephone contact. Some commercial home parenteral nutrition services include frequent home visits by a nurse.

Overall, administration of parenteral nutrients at home has been much more successful than initially envisioned. Certainly, the practice improves the quality of life for patients who require long-term parenteral nutrition. However, the purpose of parenteral nutrition is to provide the necessary nutrients transiently while the compromised gastrointestinal function necessitating use of parenteral nutrition recovers. Some patients, of course, may never be able to survive without parenteral nutrition, but attempts to increase enteral intake must continue. In the authors' experience, this is not always the case; rather, discharge from the hospital often is viewed as the goal of therapy, and once achieved, attempts to increase tolerance of enteral intake slow or stop. This attitude should not become more common.

REFERENCES

1. Williams CD. Arch Dis Child 1933;8:423–33.
2. Grantham-McGregor SM, Powell CA, Walker SP, Himes JH. Lancet 1991;338:1–5.
3. Mansell AL, Andersen JC, Muttart CR, et al. J Pediatr 1984; 109:700–5.
4. Sack RB. Bacterial and parasitic agents of acute diarrhea. In: Bellanti JA, ed. Acute diarrhea: its nutritional consequences in infancy. New York: Raven Press, 1983;53–65.
5. Hamilton JR. Viral enteritis: a cause of disordered small intestinal epithelial renewal. In: Lebenthal E, ed. Chronic diarrhea in children. New York: Raven Press, 1984;269–76.
6. Parker P, Stroop BS, Greene H. J Pediatr 1981;99(3):360–4.
7. Wilmore DW. J Pediatr 1972;80:88–95.
8. Cooper A, Heird WC. Am J Clin Nutr 1982;35:1132–41.
9. Baker JP, Detsky AS, Wesson DE, et al. N Engl J Med 1982; 306:969–72.
10. Waterlow JC. Br Med J 1972;3:566–9.
11. Heird WC. Justification of total parenteral nutrition. In: Yu VYH, MacMahon RA, eds. Intravenous feeding of the neonate. London: Edward Arnold, 1992;166–75.
12. Kashyap S, Heird WC. Protein requirements of low birthweight, very low birthweight, and small for gestational age infants. In: Räihä NCR, ed. Protein metabolism during infancy. Nestlé Nutrition Workshop Series, vol 33, Nestlé Ltd. New York: Vevey/Raven Press, 1995;133–51.
13. Collins JN, Hoope M, Brown K, et al. J Pediatr 1991;118:921–7.
14. Greene HL, Hambidge KM, Schanler R, et al. Am J Clin Nutr 1988;48:1324–42.
15. Paulsrud JR, Pensler L, Whitten CF, et al. Am J Clin Nutr 1972;25:897–904.
16. Shennan AT, Bryan MD, Angel A. J Pediatr 1977;91:134–7.
17. Park W, Paust H, Brösicke H, et al. JPEN 1986;10:627–30.
18. Greene HL, Hazlett D, Demree R. Am J Clin Nutr 1976;29: 127–35.
19. Friedman Z, Marks MH, Maisels J, et al. Pediatrics 1978;61:694–8.
20. Loo LS, Tang JP, Kohl S. J Infect Dis 1982;146:64–70.
21. Odell GTB, Cukier JO, Ostrea EM Jr, et al. J Lab Clin Med 1977;89:295–307.
22. Haumont D, Deckelbaum RJ, Richelle M, et al. J Pediatr 1989; 115:787–93.
23. Winters RW, Heird WC, Dell RB, et al. Plasma amino acids in infants receiving parenteral nutrition. In: Green HL, Holliday MA, Munro HN, eds. Clinical nutrition update: amino acids. Chicago: American Medical Association, 1977;147–54.
24. Heird WC, Dell RB, Helms RA, et al. Pediatrics 1987;80:401–8.
25. Schreiner RL, Glick MR, Nordschow CW, et al. J Pediatr 1979; 94:197–200.

65. Assessment of Malabsorption: A Tutorial

DARLENE G. KELLY

HISTORY

The term *malabsorption* is frequently used broadly to include intraluminal processes that primarily involve maldigestion, dysfunction at the mucosal level, which alters transport or absorption per se, as well as postabsorptive handling of nutrients. From a nutritional point of view, the end result of malabsorption resulting from maldigestion tends to be more specific in that only one or a few nutrients may be affected, while mucosal disease usually involves generalized malabsorption.

Malabsorption may be implicated in the patient who presents with growth failure, delayed sexual maturation, weight loss, clinical evidence of specific nutrient deficiencies, or bloating and flatulence. Gastrointestinal symptoms may range from frequent passage of large volumes of watery diarrhea, usually associated with carbohydrate malabsorption, to steatorrhea consisting of less-frequent bulky, oily, foul-smelling stool, more commonly seen with fat malabsorption. However, it is not uncommon for gastrointestinal symptoms to be absent or minimal. Other signs and symptoms that can result from malabsorption include fatigue, malaise, anemia, edema, easy bruising, bleeding, muscle weakness, hyporeflexia, bone pain, pathologic fractures, altered taste sensation, poor wound healing, cramps, paresthesias, tetany, and numbness. Although these features are not specific to malabsorption and none is pathognomonic of gastrointestinal dysfunction, malabsorption should enter the differential diagnostic considerations when they are present. A careful history and physical examination should be used to guide an efficient laboratory evaluation of malabsorption (Table 65.1).

Medical

In an adult, a history of growth failure or childhood diarrhea may suggest a chronic or latent process, such as celiac sprue. Previous surgical procedures, especially gastric and intestinal resections, may be important in the etiology of malabsorption. Gastric operations often alter the ability to take in sufficient calories, to regulate stomach emptying and/or small bowel transit or to absorb specific nutrients, such as iron and calcium. Intestinal resection, even when restricted, can selectively alter nutrient absorption (i.e., vitamin B_{12} and bile salts with ileal resection) and when extensive can cause generalized malabsorption because of decreased mucosal surface area. Bacterial overgrowth of the small bowel may be the consequence of surgical resections as a result of decreased gastric acid production or of creation of a blind loop. Prior abdominal or pelvic radiation therapy can contribute to significant nutritional compromise as a result of radiation enteritis and dysmotility from desmoplastic reactions of the serosal surface of the bowel or fibrotic changes in the muscularis.

Recent onset of diarrhea in conjunction with weight loss may indicate the onset of malabsorption. Diarrhea, abdominal discomfort, and distention following a meal may indicate malabsorption-type diarrhea, and the association with the meal differentiates this diarrhea from secretory-type diarrhea.

Associated nongastrointestinal symptoms often help determine the diagnosis of malabsorption syndromes. Rheumatologic symptoms including Raynaud's phenomenon and arthralgias may suggest scleroderma, inflammatory bowel disease, or Whipple's disease. Evidence of extensive vascular disease frequently accompanies mesenteric ischemia. The presence of endocrine diseases, such as hyperthyroidism, diabetes mellitus, and hypoparathyroidism, can suggest that malabsorption may result from these disorders. Pulmonary disease in children with steatorrhea may point to a diagnosis of cystic fibrosis.

Medication history often explains malabsorption of certain nutrients. For example, cholestyramine binds bile salts, decreasing solubilization of fat and fat-soluble vitamins. Similarly, a history of alcohol abuse may contribute to chronic liver disease or pancreatic insufficiency, both of which may cause fat malabsorption. Other social factors, including homosexual practices and intravenous drug abuse, which predispose to HIV infection and *Giardia lamblia,* may provide clues to causes of malabsorption.

Diet

Diet histories, when accurate and comprehensive, may be helpful in detecting one of the common reasons for growth failure and weight loss, namely inadequate intake. This may result from anorexia related to the underlying disease or to psychosocial issues such as depression, stress, or eating disorders. Additionally, a variety of other factors lead to poor intake. Often, pain curtails food intake. Occasionally, one learns that health professionals and

Table 65.1
Symptoms and Laboratory Evaluation of Nutrient Malabsorption

Malabsorbed Nutrient	Clinical Manifestations	Laboratory Tests
Fat	Pale, bulky greasy malodorous stool; diarrhea without distention or gas	Fecal fat
Protein	Edema, muscle atrophy	Fecal nitrogen α-1 antitrypsin, and albumin
Carbohydrate	Watery diarrhea, flatus, borborygmi, abdominal distension	Breath H_2 excretion
Vitamin B_{12}	Macrocytic anemia, neurologic sequelae	MCV, Schilling test, serum B_{12}
Folic acid	Macrocytic anemia	MCV, serum and RBC folate
B-complex vitamins	Angular cheilosis, painless glossitis, acrodermatitis	
Iron	Microcytic anemia, painful glossitis koilonychia	MCV, serum ferritin, serum iron
Magnesium	Paresthesias, tetany	Serum magnesium
Calcium and vitamin D	Paresthesias, tetany, bone pain or fractures positive Chvostek's and Trousseau's signs, muscle cramps	Serum calcium and phosphate, plasma vitamin D, serum alkaline phosphatase
Vitamin A	Night blindness, follicular hyperkeratosis	Retinal esters
Vitamin E	Decreased deep tendon reflexes	Serum tocopherol
Vitamin K	Easy bruising, hemorrhage	Prothrombin time/INR
Fluid, electrolytes	Tachycardia, hyperpnea, dry mouth	Electrolyte panel, creatinine, BUN
Bile salts	Watery diarrhea	

Adapted from Earnest DL. Steatorrhea and disorders of intestinal mucosal absorption. In: Winawer SJ, eds Management of gastrointestinal diseases. New York: Gower Medical Publishing, 1992;14.1–14.41, with permission.

well-meaning acquaintances have instituted programs that unnecessarily restrict the diet. A careful history of diet that reveals a poor intake may prevent an uncomfortable, expensive, and time-consuming evaluation of presumed malabsorption.

Family

Several malabsorptive disorders are characterized by a positive family history. These include inflammatory bowel diseases, celiac sprue, and lactase deficiency. Lack of a positive family history, however, does not exclude these diagnoses. A history in family members of various non-gastrointestinal disease states often associated with malabsorption may be helpful in arriving at an ultimate diagnosis.

PHYSICAL EXAMINATION

In severe or prolonged malabsorption, wasting of muscle mass (particularly noticed in the temporal and gluteal regions) and of subcutaneous fat stores is common. When there is marked hypoalbuminemia, peripheral edema or even anasarca can be found. On abdominal examination, distention, visible peristalsis, and borborygmi are sometimes present. Abdominal tenderness is not usually present except in inflammatory conditions. Other stigmata of malnutrition that are discussed in elsewhere (Chapters 30, 54, and 55) may suggest specific nutrient deficiencies.

LABORATORY ASSESSMENT

Laboratory tests used to diagnose malabsorptive disorders can be broadly divided into categories. The initial tests are typically those considered screening tests, primarily general hematology and chemistry studies. This initial battery of tests may be helpful in directing subsequent assessment. A second group of tests is diagnostic or suggestive of generalized mucosal failure. The next series of studies is used to determine specific dysfunction of luminal digestion or specialized absorption mechanisms. Based on a knowledge of absorption (Chapter 39), it should be possible to do a systematic, direct, and economical laboratory workup. The choice and order of laboratory tests, however, is not universally agreed upon and may be modified by availability and expertise at any given institution. The rationale, general procedures, and interpretation of a number of biochemical and laboratory tests are presented in Chapter 57.

Initial Testing

The complete blood count, particularly hemoglobin or hematocrit, mean corpuscular volume, and RDW (red cell distribution width) (see Chapter 88) in conjunction with a peripheral blood smear may suggest iron deficiency (microcytosis and hypochromasia), macrocytosis related to vitamin B_{12} or folate deficiency, or possibly a combination of these suggested by an elevated RDW. Iron deficiency is most commonly encountered in blood loss but can occur from malabsorption, especially after gastric resection and occasionally as the sole manifestation of celiac sprue. Vitamin B_{12} malabsorption occurs after gastric resection, distal ileal resection, bacterial overgrowth, extensive ileal Crohn's disease, and in cases of prolonged pancreatic insufficiency. Folate deficiency is found in proximal mucosal disease, such as celiac sprue or tropical sprue. Based on the findings of the blood count and smear, follow-up tests including measurements of ferritin (1), red blood cell and serum folate or vitamin B_{12} levels may be indicated. A Schilling test can then be used to determine which of several abnormalities is responsible for vitamin B_{12} deficiency (Table 65.2).

Serum albumin is commonly regarded as helpful in assessing malabsorption and nutritional status, but albumin levels are also affected by sepsis, trauma, liver disease, and inflammation (2). Hypoalbuminemia in gastroin-

Table 65.2
Diagnosis of Vitamin B_{12} Deficiency with the Schilling Test

Cause of Deficiency	Free B_{12}	B_{12}-IF	Antibiotics	Pancreatic
Normal	Normal	—	—	—
Pernicious anemia (lack of intrisic factor)	Abnormal	Corrected	—	—
Bacterial overgrowth syndrome	Abnormal	Abnormal	Corrected	—
Pancreatic insufficiency	Abnormal	Abnormal	Abnormal	Corrected
Ileal disease or resection	Abnormal	Abnormal	Abnormal	Abnormal

Reprinted from Kelly DG. Small intestine and its disorders. In: Shearman D, Finlayson N, Carter D, Camillerí M, eds. Diseases of the gastrointestinal tract and liver. 3rd ed. Edinburgh: Churchill Livingstone 1997;13.1–13.41 with permission.

testinal disease commonly indicates protein-losing gastroenteropathies rather than malabsorption (3). Hypoproteinemia is unusual at the initial diagnosis of malabsorption on the basis of mucosal disease or pancreatic insufficiency. In pancreatic insufficiency, low lipase levels causing steatorrhea and wasting markedly antedate (by 5 years on average) clinically significant decreased protease production and resultant protein maldigestion (4). Albumin levels are useful, however, in interpreting levels of minerals, since many minerals are albumin bound, and low levels are to be expected in hypoalbuminemic patients.

While a common cause of a decreased serum calcium is a low albumin level, a clinically significant decrease in the calcium level may also result from decreased calcium absorption. (In most cases, bone resorption induced by parathyroid hormone (PTH) compensates for low calcium absorption and normalizes the serum calcium level. Still, hypocalcemia can be seen secondary to calcium malabsorption.) Calcium malabsorption may be the result of poor absorption of vitamin D or of binding of calcium with unabsorbed fats to form unabsorbable soaps. A serum 1,25-dihydroxycholecalciferol level is helpful in determining whether a low calcium level (in the presence of a normal albumin) is based on malabsorption of fat-soluble vitamins. Hypomagnesemia is commonly found in short bowel syndrome, as well as occasionally in Crohn's disease and celiac sprue (Chapter 9). Decreased serum zinc levels are most commonly observed in patients with enterocutaneous fistulae where losses of zinc are high (Chapter 11).

An increased prothrombin time resulting from vitamin K deficiency in conjunction with evidence of vitamin D deficiency suggests fat malabsorption, which is often accompanied by fat-soluble vitamin malabsorption. Decreased levels of vitamin A and E may be found in this setting as well.

Tests of Mucosal Dysfunction

Gut mucosal failure resulting in weight loss, diarrhea, and generalized nutritional deficiencies may occur in such disorders as celiac sprue, Crohn's disease, Whipple's disease, radiation enteritis, mesenteric ischemia, and intestinal resection. While various mechanisms are involved in these disorders, the overall result tends to be generalized nutritional deficiencies.

Serum carotene is frequently intended as a screening tool for mucosal failure. The test, however, is quite insensitive, and apart from mucosal disease and fat malabsorption, low concentrations can be found in patients with poor dietary intake of carotene and with liver disease. Normal levels of carotene may help to exclude mucosal disease as a cause of malabsorption.

The D-xylose test is also used to screen noninvasively for malabsorption and to distinguish mucosal from intraluminal disease. Urinary excretion of less than 4 g of D-xylose in 5 hours is found in more than 90% of patients with celiac sprue, while a small percentage of those with pancreatic dysfunction and no mucosal disease have decreased excretion (5). False-negative results can occur in mucosal disease limited to the distal small bowel or with mild proximal disease. False-positive results are found in myxedema, in vomiting, with ascites, following gastric surgery when rapid transit decreases absorption, in bacterial overgrowth syndrome, and during treatment with aspirin, neomycin, glipizide, and indomethacin. Incomplete urine collection and renal insufficiency also cause false-positive results. In this case, serum levels obtained 1 hour after the test dose or a 5-h breath test (6) can be measured to circumvent these problems (see Chapter 57 for methodology).

In general the "gold standard" diagnostic tests are structural studies for mucosal disorders. In the case of short bowel syndrome, the history of resection, details of residual small bowel length, and anatomy (proximal vs. distal) provide sufficient evidence to determine whether the malabsorption is consistent with the degree of resection (Chapter 68). When details of resection are unavailable, x-ray studies of the small intestine may help determine the length of remaining small bowel (Fig. 65.1). In cases of Crohn's disease or ischemia, the small bowel x-ray is helpful in determining the diagnosis, as well as the extent of disease. Enteroclysis (a specified barium study of the small bowel, which provides a detailed picture of the ischemia) may be preferred to standard x-ray, since it avoids or delays flocculation of barium, allows better distention of the lumen, and provides a better assessment of the folds of Kerkring to provide more accurate diagnosis (7). Specialized radiologic examinations, such as angiography or Doppler ultrasonography for the diagnosis of mesenteric insufficiency and lymphangiography for the identification of intestinal lymphangiectasia, are essential to establish some diagnoses.

Another structural test that is often helpful in diag-

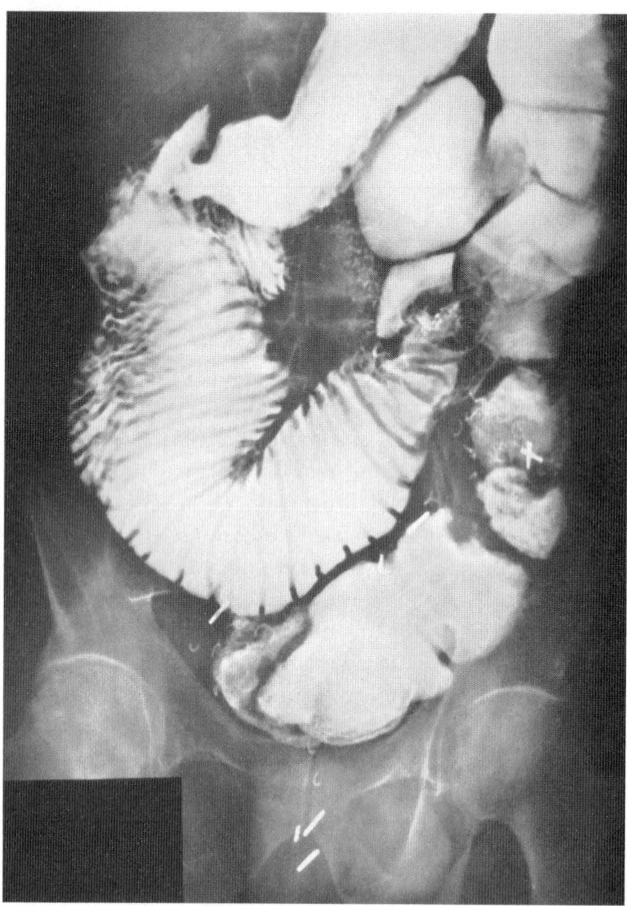

Figure 65.1. Short bowel syndrome. A small bowel follow-through x-ray demonstrates a short small bowel and a marked dilatation of the residual duodenum and jejunum. The jejunum is anastomosed to the distal colon.

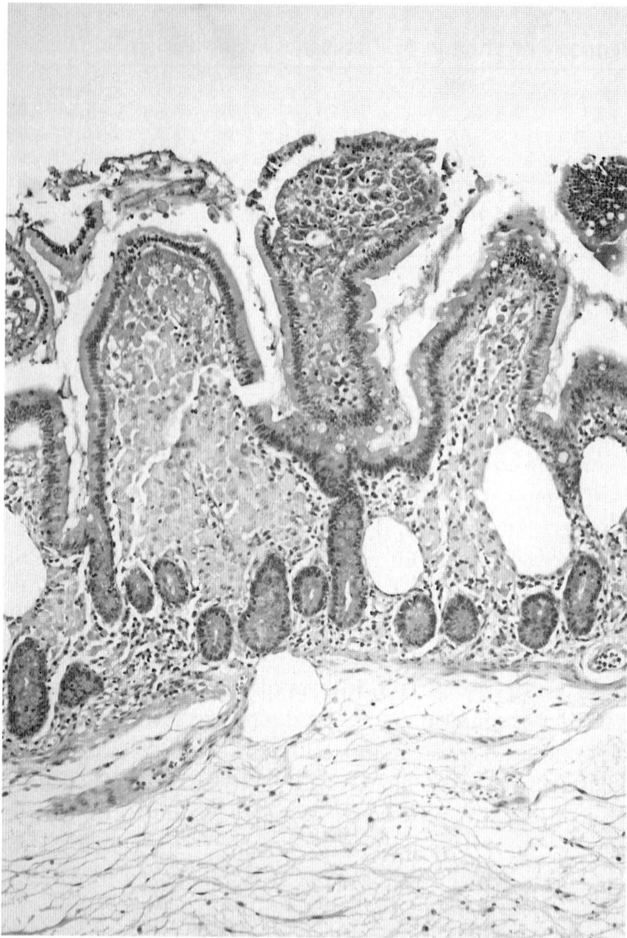

Figure 65.2. Whipple's disease, small bowel resection. The lamina propria contains numerous macrophages with abundant eosinophilic cytoplasm, resulting in thickened and mildly blunted villi. While *Mycobacterium avium-intracellulare* could show similar changes, special stains for mycobacteria were negative, and polymerase chain reaction (PCR) was positive for Whipple's bacilli *(Tropheryma whippelii)*. The dilated lymphatic spaces are also characteristic of Whipple's disease. (H&E, ×40). (Courtesy of KP Batts, MD.)

nosing suspected mucosal disease is the small bowel biopsy. The biopsy can be diagnostic in diseases such as amyloidosis, mastocytosis, or Whipple's disease (Fig. 65.2). In other diseases, including bacterial overgrowth, celiac sprue (Fig. 65.3), or radiation enteritis, the findings are suggestive but not diagnostic. For a diagnosis of celiac sprue based solely on biopsy results, the classic mucosal changes of absence of villi, elongation of crypts, and lymphocytic infiltration of the epithelium and lamina propria must be demonstrated, with subsequent resolution during 6 to 12 months of a strict gluten-free diet. The purist also insists on withholding the diagnosis until a biopsy following gluten rechallenge of the effectively treated patient again reveals villous damage. This is most important in children, in whom infectious gastroenteritis can mimic celiac sprue. The biopsy results can be supplemented with noninvasive antibody studies to confirm celiac sprue, particularly in adults and in those who are not IgA deficient. IgA endomysial antibody immunofluorescence in this setting has excellent sensitivity and specificity (approaching 100%), while IgA antigliadin is somewhat less sensitive and specific (82–83%) (8). An unequivocal response to a strict gluten-free diet also provides supporting evidence to confirm the diagnosis of celiac sprue.

While mechanisms of fat absorption involve both luminal and mucosal steps, tests indicating the presence of excess fat in stool can be extremely helpful in diagnosing mucosal dysfunction, since fat malabsorption is a feature of most mucosal diseases. Microscopic examination of a single sample of feces using Sudan red stain is favored by some as a key screening test (9). However, it is only reliable when there is moderate or severe steatorrhea. The "gold standard" test for fat malabsorption remains the 48- or 72-h quantitative fecal fat determination, which expresses results as the coefficient of fat absorption

$$[\text{Dietary fat intake} - \text{fecal fat excreted})/\text{Dietary fat intake}] \times 100$$

While normal fecal fat levels are quoted as up to 7% of intake, it has been shown recently that with diarrhea

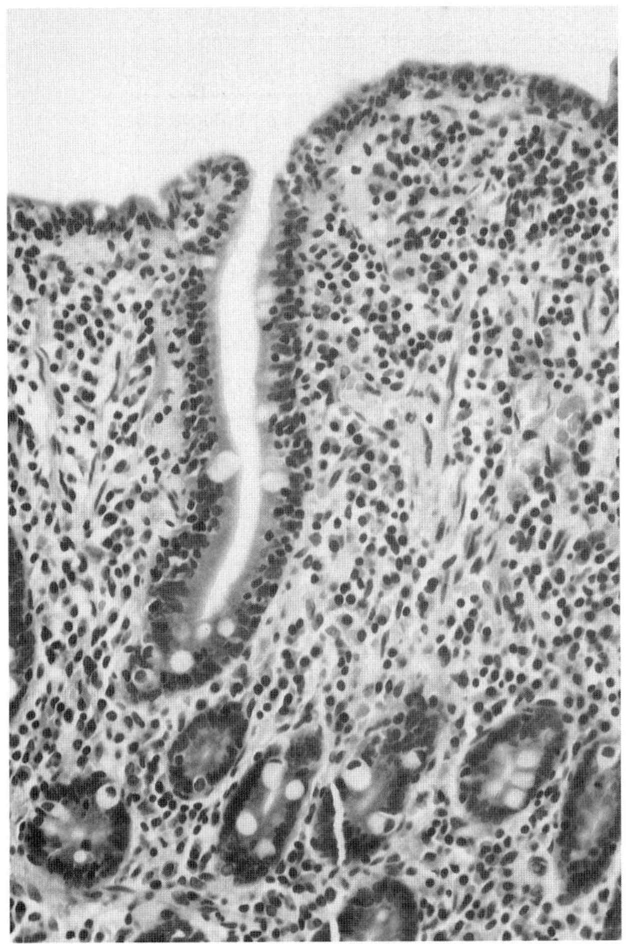

Figure 65.3. Celiac sprue, small bowel biopsy. The total villous atrophy, crypt hyperplasia, and relatively squat, cuboidal surface epithelium all indicate mucosal injury. The prominent intraepithelial lymphocytosis as well as similar inflammatory infiltrate in the lamina propria suggests celiac sprue. (H&E, ×140). (Courtesy of KP Batts, MD.)

induced in healthy subjects, up to 14% of intake can appear in stool subjected to rapid gut transit (10). Although fraught with problems of incomplete collection and unpopularity among patients and laboratory personnel, this test not only offers a coefficient of fat absorption but also gives data concerning the amount of stool excreted and the amount of water in the stool. These advantages of the fecal fat determination make it superior to triolein breath tests and Sudan staining (11).

Tests of Luminal Dysfunction

Bacterial overgrowth syndrome results from surgical creation of blind loops, achlorhydria from gastric atrophy, surgical intervention, or prolonged treatment with acid inhibitors. The effect of bacterial overgrowth on nutritional status is related to bacterial deconjugation of bile salts, utilization of vitamin B_{12} by the bacteria, and mucosal damage causing disaccharidase destruction, protein-losing enteropathy, altered intestinal transport, and secretion of water and electrolytes (Fig. 65.4). The results are malabsorption of fats, fat-soluble vitamins, vitamin B_{12}, and carbohydrates (12). The medical history, constellation of symptoms, and results of screening blood tests may be highly suggestive of this diagnosis, which should prompt one to order a small-bowel aspirate for quantitative aerobic and anaerobic cultures. Cultures of duodenal and jejunal aspirates yield bacterial numbers exceeding the normal level of 10^5 cfu/mL, but specific pathogenic organisms are usually not identified. Alternatively, noninvasive tests have been developed for bacterial overgrowth, with the ^{14}C-xylose breath test offering specificity and sensitivity similar to those of cultures, albeit at the expense of exposure to low doses of radionuclide (13). A subsequent barium x-ray study often identifies the etiology of bacterial overgrowth. Effective treatment with antibiotics, usually on a cyclic basis, confirms this diagnosis as the cause of malabsorption.

Giardia lamblia infestation results in weight loss in up to 65% of cases. If stool examinations for ova and parasites are negative, examination of a duodenal aspirate or a biopsy specimen can be helpful in making this diagnosis (14).

In AIDS, particularly, infectious causes for malabsorption are quite common. Stool and jejunal fluid cultures and examinations for ova and parasites, as well as jejunal and colonic mucosal cultures and histology, are helpful in identifying organisms involved (15).

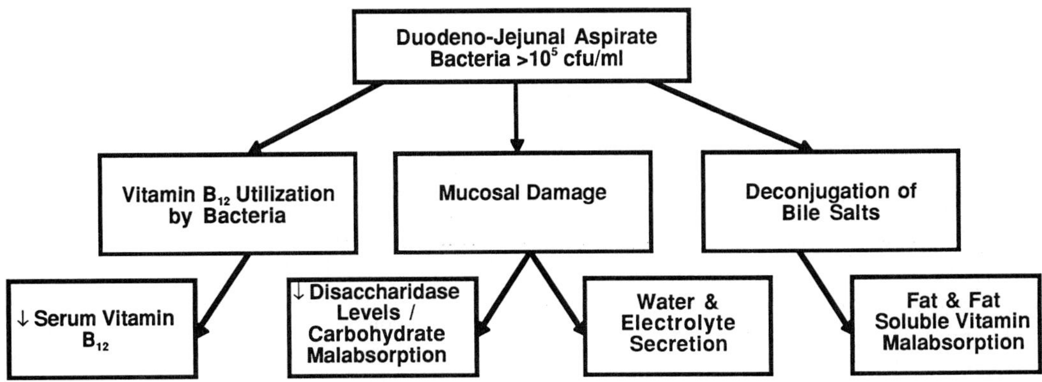

Figure 65.4. The pathogenesis of malabsorption in bacterial overgrowth syndrome.

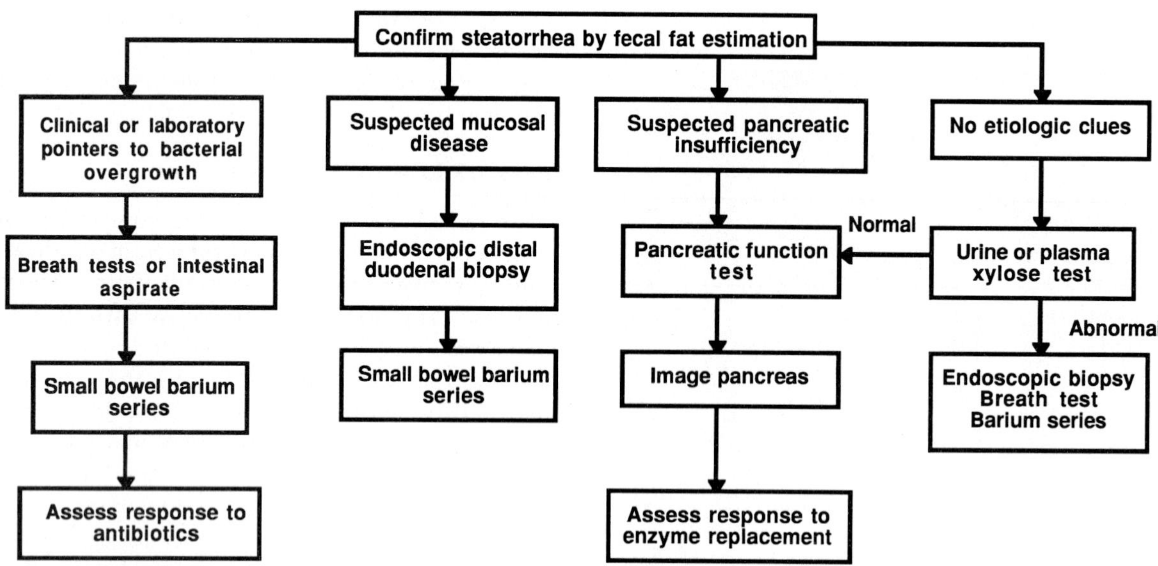

Figure 65.5. An algorithm for the evaluation of steatorrhea. (Modified from Riley SA, Turnberg LA. Maldigestion and malabsorption. In: Sleisenger MH, Fordtran JS, Scharschmidt BF, Feldman M, eds. Gastrointestinal disease pathophysiology/diagnosis/management. Philadelphia: WB Saunders, 1993;1009–27, with permission.)

Pancreatic insufficiency is manifest years after chronic pancreatitis occurs, owing to the large reserve of pancreatic enzymes. Steatorrhea does not occur until lipase levels are less than 10% of normal (16). The tests that are considered the "gold standard" for diagnosis are those that directly measure stimulated pancreatic exocrine function. These tests use intravenous cholecystokinin and/or secretin and a duodenal tube to collect pancreatic juice for measurement of lipase and trypsin and/or bicarbonate. This test is highly sensitive and specific (96 and 93%, respectively) but is invasive, costly (~$600) and of limited availability (16). Tubeless assays such as the fecal chymotrypsin, bentiromide, and pancreolauryl tests tend to be abnormal when intestinal malabsorption is present. In many patients, a very high level of fecal fat and the presence of pancreatic calcification detected on abdominal x-ray or by computerized axial tomography (CAT scan) are highly suggestive of pancreatic insufficiency, and a successful trial of adequate enzyme replacement may suffice for diagnosis in such cases (Fig. 65.5). However, pancreatic malignancy can also present with pancreatic insufficiency, so ultrasound, CAT scan, or ERCP may be necessary to exclude the diagnosis in some cases.

Isolated disaccharidase deficiency presents with watery diarrhea, distention, and flatulence. For patients who have symptoms clearly associated with milk ingestion, especially in those whose ethnic origin and family history are consistent with the diagnosis, a trial of lactose withdrawal with relapse on rechallenge may suffice for a diagnosis of lactase deficiency. In those whose symptoms are more subtle and less clearly associated with specific foods, hydrogen breath tests performed with various disaccharides often clarify the diagnosis of disaccharidase deficiency.

REFERENCES

1. Fairbanks VF. Hosp Pract 1991;26:15–24.
2. McMahon MM, Bistrian BR. Disease-a-month 1990;36:375–415.
3. Riley SA, Turnberg LA. Maldigestion and malabsorption. In: Sleisenger MH, Fordtran JS, Scharschmidt BF, Feldman M, eds. Gastrointestinal disease pathophysiology/diagnosis/management. Philadelphia: WB Saunders, 1993;1009–27.
4. DiMagno E, Malagelada J-R, Go V. Ann NY Acad Sci 1975;252:200–7.
5. Craig RM, Atkinson AJ. Gastroenterology 1988;106:615–23.
6. Casellas F, Malagelada J-R. Dig Dis Sci 1994;39:2320–6.
7. Herlinger H. Radiologe 1993;33:335–42.
8. Vogelsang H, Genser D, Wyatt J, et al. Am J Gastroenterol 1995;90:394–8.
9. Roberts IM. Compr Ther 1994;20:10–5.
10. Fine KD, Fordtran JS. Gastroenterology 1992;102:2163–4.
11. Newcomer AD. Physiologic and diagnostic approach to diarrheal diseases. In: Winawer SJ, Almy TP, eds. Management of gastrointestinal diseases. New York: Gower Medical Publishing, 1992;12.1–12.18.
12. Toskes PP. Adv Intern Med 1993;38:387–407.
13. Saltzman JR, Russell RM. Compr Ther 1994;20:523–30.
14. Hill DR. Giardia lamblia. In: Mandell GL, Douglas J, Bennett RG, Bennett JE, eds. Principles and practice of infectious disease. 3rd ed. New York: Churchill Livingstone, 1990;2110–5.
15. Friedman SL. Gastrointestinal manifestations of the acquired immunodeficiency syndrome. In: Sleisenger MH, Fordtran JS, Scharschmidt BF, Feldman M, eds. Gastrointestinal disease pathophysiology/diagnosis/management. Philadelphia: WB Saunders, 1993;239–67.
16. Raimondo M, DiMagno EP. Pract Gastroenterol 1996;20:54–9.
17. Earnest DL. Steatorrhea and disorders of intestinal mucosal absorption. In: Winawer SJ, Almy TP, eds. Management of gastrointestinal diseases. New York: Gower Medical Publishing, 1992;14.1–14.41.
18. Kelly DG. Small intestine and its disorders. In: Shearman D, Finlayson N, Carter D, Camilleri M, eds. Diseases of the gas-

trointestinal tract and liver. 3rd ed. Edinburgh: Churchill Livingstone, 1997;13.1–13.41.

SELECTED READINGS

Earnest DL. Steatorrhea and disorders of intestinal mucosal absorption. In: Winawer SJ, Almy TP, eds. Management of gastrointestinal diseases. New York: Gower Medical Publishing, 1992;14.1–14.41.

Kelly DG. Small intestine and its disorders. In: Shearman D, Finlayson N, Carter D, Camilleri M, eds. Diseases of the gastrointestinal tract and liver. 3rd ed. Edinburgh: Churchill Livingstone, 1997;13.1–13.41.

Newcomer AD. Physiologic and diagnostic approach to diarrheal diseases. In: Winawer SJ, Almy TP, eds. Management of gastrointestinal diseases. New York: Gower Medical Publishing, 1992;12.1–12.18.

Raimondo M, DiMagno EP. Chronic pancreatitis: selective use of diagnostic laboratory procedures. Pract Gastroenterol 1996;20:54–59.

Riley SA, Turnberg LA. Maldigestion and malabsorption. In: Sleisenger MH, Fordtran JS, Scharschmidt BF, Feldman M, eds. Gastrointestinal disease pathophysiology/diagnosis/management. Philadelphia: WB Saunders, 1993;1009–27.

66. Nutrition in Relation to Dental Medicine

DOMINICK P. DEPAOLA, MARY P. FAINE, and CAROLE A. PALMER

CELLULAR AND STRUCTURAL CHARACTERISTICS OF THE ORAL TISSUES

Distinctive characteristics of oral tissues may render them particularly sensitive to nutritional extremes. For example, the inability of enamel to remodel coupled with the high cellular turnover rate of oral mucosa and the rates of alveolar bone growth and saliva production make oral tissues a unique indicator of physiologic perturbations.

In the same vein, nutrition and oral health and disease transcend the relationship between fermentable carbohydrates and dental caries. The oral cavity is the site of chronic disease (e.g., caries, periodontal disease(s), AIDS, nutritional anemias, herpes, salivary gland disorders, osteoporosis, cancer), congenital anomalies (e.g., cleft lip and palate), and environmentally induced birth defects (e.g., fetal alcohol syndrome), which could relate to nutritional status. Nutrients interact with physiologic systems in the oral cavity, such as cell replication, cell repair, and immune response mechanisms, in such a manner as to increase or decrease the risk of disease. Thus, the oral tissues constitute a major site of interactions between nutritional factors and the physiologic systems, a relationship that makes oral health no less vulnerable to the effect of nutrition than general health. In this regard, the oral tissues and fluids mirror subtle changes in nutritional status and are often the first visible site to exhibit signs of nutritional disorders. Thus, nutritional disorders affect the oral tissues and fluids both directly and indirectly.

Most importantly, the linkages between oral disease and systemic health are frequently being clarified and scientifically validated, with some startling and profound observations. Within the last 5 years, clear linkages have been established between periodontal diseases and cardiovascular disease, diabetes, bronchitis, stroke, and low birth weight. The infectious nature of the oral diseases approximately doubles the risk of stroke (1) and cardiac disease (2), as well as increasing the risk for a low-birth-weight infant (3). Since the inherent nature of the infectious oral diseases dictates that the host have an adequate functional immune and cellular repair system and unequivocal data link nutrient intake and these host defense mechanisms, the relationships between oral health, systemic health, and nutrition require careful attention by physicians, dentists, dental hygienists, nurses, and virtually all healthcare providers.

To better appreciate these complex relationships, one must understand the structure and function of the craniofacial-oral-dental complex. Teeth, specialized structures vital for the initial processing of food, are composed of three mineralized tissues—enamel, dentin, and cementum—that encase the highly vascular dental pulp, or "nerve." These relationships can be seen in the schematic cross section of a tooth in Figure 66.1. The teeth are retained in their bony sockets by means of a fibrous structure termed the *periodontal membrane or ligament.* Influences that affect the integrity of this structure and bone surrounding the socket result in periodontal disease that may progress sufficiently to cause loosening and loss of the teeth (4).

Each tooth develops from a tooth bud or germ located in the jaws. The bud consists of an epithelial component that arises as an invagination from the surface and produces enamel. The mesenchymal component consists of the dental papilla, which produces the tooth pulp and

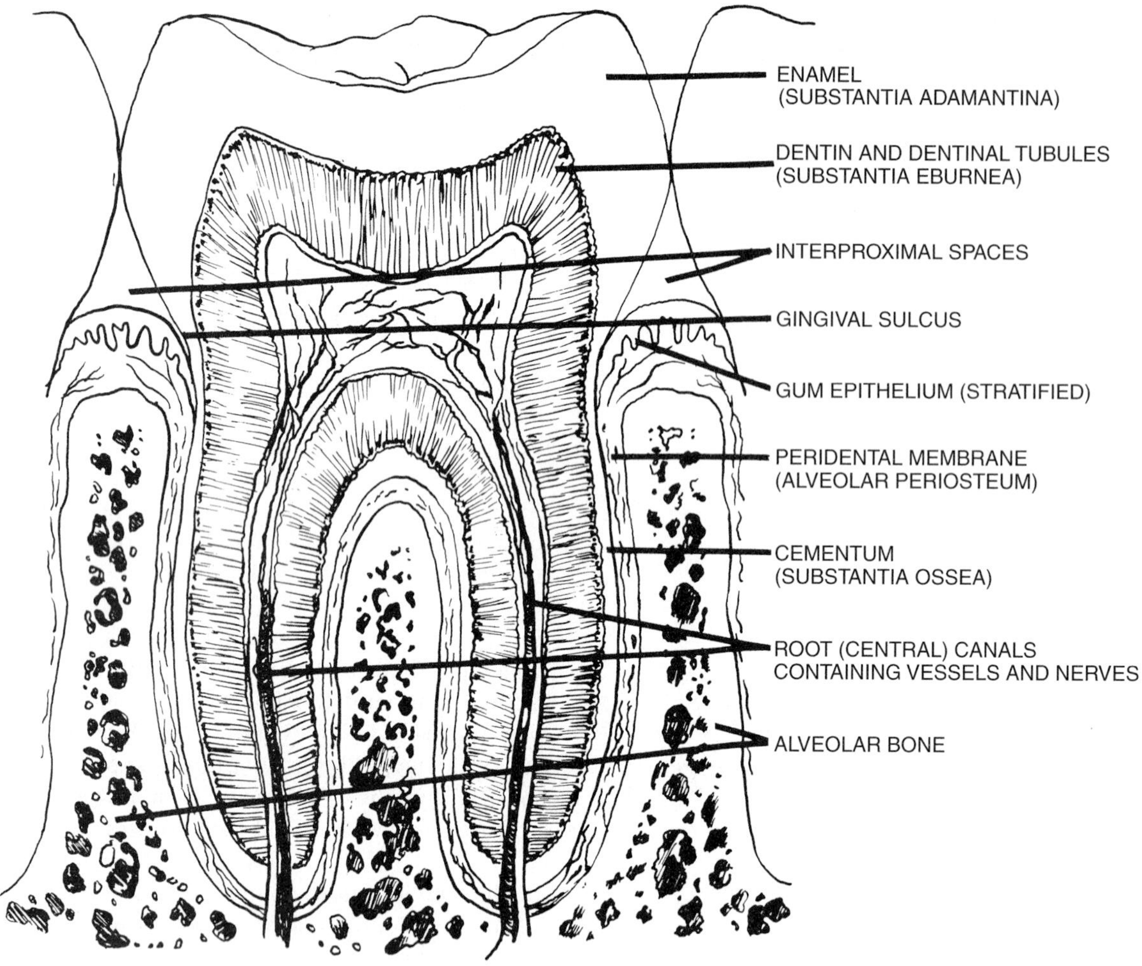

Figure 66.1. Schematic illustration of teeth in contact with the alveolar bone.

dentin, and the dental follicle, which produces the cementum and periodontal ligament once the tooth has formed. Table 66.1 details the chronology of the human dentition. Primary teeth begin forming about 6 weeks in utero, when cells in the primitive oral cavity differentiate to form the dental lamina, which is the site of tooth bud development. Formation of the crown of the tooth begins with secretion of a dentin matrix containing collagen fibrils. Mineral ions then enter the matrix to form small crystals on or between the collagen fibrils. Enamel formation begins as soon as the first dentin layer has been laid down. This mineralization process constitutes the maturation of enamel and continues after all the matrix is formed. As can be seen in Table 66.1, the mineralization process begins as early as 4 months in utero and continues into late adolescence. After the tooth erupts into the oral cavity, it continues to incorporate minerals (including fluoride) into its structure from saliva, food, and drinking fluids (5).

The life history of a tooth may be divided into three main eras: *(a)* the period when its crown is forming and mineralizing in the jaw, *(b)* the period of maturation when the tooth is erupting into the oral cavity and its root or roots are forming, and *(c)* the maintenance period while it is functioning in the oral cavity (4). During the preeruptive period, the developing enamel and dentin are subject to nutritional deficiencies or imbalances in the same manner as any other developing tissues. Indeed, nutrient deficiencies can affect either the secretory or the maturation stage of enamel formation. For example, hypoplastic lesions in the enamel reflect disturbances affecting the secretory process, whereas hypomineralized defects reflect interference with the maturation process. These are systemic effects of nutrient imbalances. Of course, both hypoplasia and hypocalcification can be induced by other environmental stresses, such as febrile episodes, genetic defects, and toxic chemicals. Following eruption into the oral cavity, the enamel is bathed in saliva and is exposed to oral microorganisms and their byproducts as well as food, so nutritional deficiencies or excesses and dietary habits may affect teeth in a totally different or more local manner (5).

At least three striking differences exist between the mineralized tissues of the teeth and the other tissues of the body. First, enamel contains no capillary or lymphatic vessels to act as transport systems; however, the intimate relationships between the organic and inorganic components of enamel suggest that pathways in the enamel exist for diffusion of ions and small molecules from saliva and pos-

Table 66.1
Chronology of Development of the Human Dentition

Tooth	Hard Tissue Formation Begins	Amount of Enamel Formed at Birth	Enamel Completed	Eruption	Root Completed
Primary dentition					
Maxillary					
Central incisor	4 months in utero	Five-sixths	1½ months	7½ months	1½ years
Lateral incisor	4½ months in utero	Two-thirds	2½ months	9 months	2 years
Cuspid	5 months in utero	One-third	9 months	18 months	3¼ years
First molar	5 months in utero	Cusps united	6 months	14 months	2½ years
Second molar	6 months in utero	Cusp tips still isolated	11 months	24 months	3 years
Mandibular					
Central incisor	4½ months in utero	Three-fifths	2½ months	6 months	1½ years
Lateral incisor	4½ months in utero	Three-fifths	3 months	7 months	1½ years
Cuspid	5 months in utero	One-third	9 months	16 months	3¼ years
First molar	5 months in utero	Cusps united	5½ months	12 months	2¼ years
Second molar	6 months in utero	Cusp tips still isolated	10 months	20 months	3 years
Permanent dentition					
Maxillary					
Central incisor	3–4 months	—	4–5 years	7–8 years	10 years
Lateral incisor	10–12 months	—	4–5 years	8–9 years	11 years
Cuspid	4–5 months	—	6–7 years	11–12 years	13–15 years
First bicuspid	1½–1¾ years	—	5–6 years	10–11 years	12–13 years
Second bicuspid	2–2¼ years	—	6–7 years	10–12 years	12–14 years
First molar	At birth	Sometimes a trace	2½–3 years	6–7 years	9–10 years
Second molar	2½–3 years	—	7–8 years	12–13 years	14–16 years
Mandibular					
Central incisor	3–4 months	—	4–5 years	6–7 years	9 years
Lateral incisor	3–4 months	—	4–5 years	7–8 years	10 years
Cuspid	4–5 months	—	6–7 years	9–10 years	12–14 years
First bicuspid	1¾–2 years	—	5–6 years	10–12 years	12–13 years
Second bicuspid	2¼–2½ years	—	6–7 years	11–12 years	13–14 years
First molar	At birth	Sometimes a trace	2½–3 years	6–7 years	9–10 years
Second molar	2½–3 years	—	7–8 years	11–13 years	14–15 years

Adapted from Logan WAG, Kronfeld R. J Am Dent Assoc 1933;20:420 (slightly modified by McCall, Shour) with permission of the American Dental Association.

sibly from blood. Although the dentin likewise contains no formed vascular elements, it is more readily permeable to extracellular fluids from the blood because dentinal tubules traverse the dentin. Interchange between elements in the enamel takes place through the bathing of its external surface with saliva. In contrast, interchange in the dentin occurs by reason of the ions present in the blood supply to the pulp or periodontal membrane (4).

Second, owing to the absence of cells, mineralized dental tissues do not have a microscopically or chemically detectable ability to repair improperly formed or mineralized areas, and the tooth cannot repair itself after a portion has been destroyed by tooth decay or mechanical injury. An exception is the remineralization of slightly demineralized, superficial areas of the enamel where the organic matrix and surface integrity are still intact, commonly referred to as "white spots." In addition, the odontoblasts, which persist throughout life on the pulpal surface of the dentin, form secondary dentin in response to chemical stimuli from an advancing carious lesion in an effort to wall off the noxious influence. Lack of ability to repair dental tissues is in direct contrast to bone, with its continual turnover and ability to remodel (4).

Third, unlike other tissues, the mineralized tissues of teeth have a partial change of environment midway in their life. When the tooth begins to emerge into the oral cavity, the vascular supply to the enamel organ is severed, and the enamel surface comes in contact with a complex mixture of saliva, microorganisms, food debris, and epithelial remnants. Thus, instead of a pure systemic environment, the erupted tooth has, in addition, an oral or external environment. As a consequence, the enamel and cementum surfaces on which carious lesions are initiated by microbial action are largely outside the influences of humoral immune systems, so immune relationships with the caries process are primarily limited to those in saliva (4).

The development and maintenance of the soft tissues and bone that support the teeth are also subject to nutritional defects. The periodontium, as seen in Figure 66.1, comprises the gingiva; the periodontal ligament (peridental membrane), which joins the root cementum to the alveolar bone; the root cementum, a specialized, mineralized tissue similar to bone, which covers the root of the tooth; and the alveolar bone, which forms and supports the tooth sockets. Alveolar bone grows in response to dental eruption, is modified by dental changes, and resorbs when teeth are lost. The finite space between the tooth and the gingiva, known as the gingival sulcus, is lined by a nonkeratinized epithelium. In addition, dental plaque, one of the primary agents responsible for initiating both dental caries and gingivitis, contains a high concentration of bacteria, which, in the gingival sulcus, are juxtaposed with a "naked" epithelium. Thus, bacteria and their byproducts or antigens can permeate the gingival epithelium and precipitate a classic inflammatory response that denotes periodontal disease(s). In fact, an intact immune system, which is highly dependent on nutritional status, is vital to maintain periodontal health. Another unique characteristic of the oral soft tissues is their rapid turnover rates; thus, continued optimum levels of nutrients are necessary to promote oral health and to prevent disease. Indeed, the diversity of hard and soft tissues that comprise the oral structures and the distinctive nutritional needs of each contribute to the uniqueness of the mouth as an external reflection of past and present nutritional problems (6).

ROLE OF NUTRITION IN CRANIOFACIAL AND ORAL TISSUE DEVELOPMENT

Many severe and even moderate nutritional deficits can result in defective tooth development. The most commonly studied nutrients and conditions that have affected tooth integrity, enamel solubility, and salivary flow and composition in animal models include protein/calorie malnutrition, ascorbic acid, vitamin A, vitamin D, calcium/phosphorus, iron, zinc, and fluoride. Only protein/calorie malnutrition, deficiencies of vitamin A, ascorbic acid, vitamin D, and iodine, and fluoride excess have been demonstrated to affect the human dentition (Table 66.2).

Characteristically, enamel hypoplastic defects and hypomineralization have been the hallmarks of under- or overnutrition during tooth development. For example, Sweeney et al. noted that 73% of Guatemalan children with third-degree malnutrition and 43% of children with second-degree malnutrition had hypoplasia of enamel formed prior to the diagnosis of malnutrition (7). Data on 45 malnourished children in a marginal population (8) supported Sweeney's findings.

Vitamin A deficiency has been implicated as a critical factor because it frequently accompanies protein/calorie malnutrition and is known to affect epithelial tissue development, tooth morphogenesis, and odontoblast differentiation (9). Protracted vitamin A deficiency during tooth development results in atrophy of the enamel organ, metaplasia of the ameloblasts, and defective apposition and calcification of dentin (6). The interference with calcification is expressed clinically by enamel hypoplasia (10). Additionally, vitamin A excess during the first trimester of pregnancy (as in individuals taking retinoic acid analogues to treat cystic acne) can result in severe craniofacial and oral clefts and limb defects (11).

Vitamin D, calcium, and phosphorus deficiencies all significantly affect tooth development and resistance to the caries challenge. Vitamin D deficiency appears to exert its metabolic effect through lowering plasma calcium levels; it has been difficult to localize vitamin D metabolites in target tooth and bone cells (12). Leaver demonstrated that extreme calcium and phosphorus deficiencies may result in hypomineralization of developing teeth (13). The deficit must be severe enough to reduce plasma levels of calcium and phosphorus, which suggests that this mechanism is unlikely to occur in humans because of the highly

Table 66.2
Effects of Nutrient Deficiencies on Tooth Development

Nutrient	Effect on Tissue	Effect on Caries	Human Data
Protein/calorie malnutrition	Tooth eruption delayed Tooth size Enamel solubility decreased Salivary gland dysfunction	Yes	Yes
Vitamin A	↓Epithelial tissue development Tooth morphogenesis dysfunction ↓Odontoblast differentiation ↑Enamel hypoplasia	Yes	Yes
VitaminD/calcium/phosphorus	Lowered plasma calcium Hypomineralization (hypoplastic defects) Tooth integrity compromised Delayed eruption patterns	Yes	Yes
Ascorbic acid	Dental pulpal alterations Odontoblastic degeneration Aberrant dentin	No	No
Fluoride	Stability of enamel crystal (enamel formation) Inhibits demineralization Stimulates remineralization Mottled enamel (excess) Inhibits bacterial growth	Yes	Yes
Iodine	Delayed tooth eruption Altered growth patterns Malocclusion?	No	Yes
Iron	Slow growth Tooth integrity? Salivary gland dysfunction	Yes	No

effective homeostatic mechanisms that mobilize calcium from the skeleton to maintain normal plasma calcium levels. Bawden postulates that vitamin D hypovitaminosis may be more important in considering hypomineralization due to inadequate calcium transport into developing dental tissues (14). Vitamin D deficiency also affects tooth structure and delays their eruption patterns (15).

In childhood vitamin D deficiency, the teeth are characterized microscopically by a widened layer of predentin, by the presence of interglobular dentin, and by interference with enamel formation (hypoplastic defects) (16). Young children with rickets have delayed eruption of the deciduous teeth, and the sequence of eruption is altered (6). The permanent incisors, cuspids, and first molars are usually affected because their development coincides with the age at which rickets is most common (6). Vitamin D–resistant rickets results in more frequent and severe tooth defects than with primary rickets, including large pulps with developmental "exposures" of the pulp.

Vitamin C deficiency also affects tooth development and eruption. Deciduous and permanent teeth of scorbutic infants contain minute pulpal hemorrhages attributable to vitamin C deficiency. In older vitamin C–deficient children, the dental pulp undergoes hyperemia, edema, necrosis, and aberrant calcification, and the dentin shows odontoblastic degeneration and irregular formation (17). The relationship of vitamin C deficiency to dental caries is poorly defined, however. Indeed, although it is likely that the primary mechanism of vitamin C deficiency–induced tooth, gingival, and bone disease involves disruption of collagen biosynthesis, no study has clearly demonstrated the relationship between scurvy and dental caries (18).

In areas where goiter is endemic, children born to mothers with severe iodine deficiency display marked mental and physical growth retardation. Eruption of both primary and secondary teeth is often greatly delayed and precluded. Malocclusion is relatively common because of the altered patterns of craniofacial growth and development (6).

Perhaps the most intriguing and important data on nutritional status during development and oral disease come from observations on malnutrition and dental caries. Several studies demonstrated delayed tooth eruption, compromised tooth integrity (especially enamel surface solubility), and increased dental caries in animals and in chronically malnourished children (19, 20). Studies in Lima, Peru, demonstrated significant delays in tooth eruption and exfoliation in three groups of malnourished children; such delays were associated with, and appeared to be the direct cause of, a significant temporal delay in caries development in the primary teeth (21). These data support previous studies on malnourished children in India and Guatemala (22, 23).

Clearly, the development of teeth and salivary glands is intimately associated with the nutrient supply. Teeth subjected to nutritional insult during critical stages of development show a diminished ability to withstand caries and thus are at a higher risk. In many studies, impaired salivary function accompanied the morphologic changes in teeth, which may be a primary factor in the subsequent increase in caries susceptibility (24). These data also explain the positive association between socioeconomic status and the prevalence of dental caries in deciduous but not permanent teeth (20). Nutritional injuries early in life may affect tooth formation and may result in increased caries susceptibility, whereas chronic malnutrition is associated with delayed tooth emergence and a shift in the curve for caries prevalence versus age (20). Thus, to understand any cross-sectional survey on caries prevalence, the nutritional history must be taken into account.

On a broader scale, 7% of babies born in the United States each year have some mental or physical defect evident at birth or later (25). Prominent among these defects are structural, functional, or biochemical abnormalities involving the craniofacial complex. The most common of these malformations are cleft lip and cleft palate, affecting 1 out of 600 white infants; the incidence is higher among Asians, Native Americans, and Eskimos and lower among blacks (25). One out of 1600 babies born alive suffers from craniofacial anomalies other than cleft lip or palate, including jaw deformities, defects in ossification, malformed or missing teeth, facial asymmetries, and defects that are a component of other syndromes, such as fetal alcohol syndrome (25). Fetal alcohol syndrome consists primarily of small size for gestational age, dysmorphism (especially of the face and eyes, heart, joints, and internal genitalia), and mental deficiency. Of particular interest are the facial aberrant growth patterns, which include a low nasal bridge, short palpebral fissures, indistinct philtrum of the lip, thin upper lip, short nose, small midface, epicanthic folds, and small head circumference (26).

In addition, certain other craniofacial orodental disorders such as craniosynostosis, hemifacial microsomia, anodontia, amelogenesis imperfecta, dentinogenesis imperfecta, osteogenesis imperfecta, chondrodystrophies, and juvenile periodontitis represent major challenges to human oral health (27). Neural tube defects, among the most common birth defects with a rate of occurrence of 1 to 2 per 1000 births, have been linked to folate deficiency, range in severity, and can result in incomplete formation of cranial bones (28). Many of these malformations and disorders have a genetic basis or an environmental cause. Certain nutrients given in excess, especially early in pregnancy (e.g., retinoic acid and other lipophilic molecules such as vitamins K and E), induce craniofacial orodental malformations. As stated above, therapeutic doses of 13-*cis* retinoic acid administered during the first trimester of pregnancy to treat cystic acne have resulted in significant craniofacial orodental malformations. The molecular mechanisms during these genetic-environmental interactions are not precisely known but are believed to interfere with developmental processes by reducing the number of cells required for normal morphogenesis of the head, face, jaws, skeleton, and neural tube, among others (28).

A small proportion of craniofacial malformities can be traced to specific genetic or chromosomal disorders, and others result from environmental factors, such as malnutrition, maternal disease, exposure to drugs, and obstetric problems. Most investigators believe, however, that craniofacial malformations have a multifactorial basis, in which particular genes alter the ability of the developing fetus to adapt to environmental factors (25). Indeed, evidence from studies of identical twins clearly establishes the role of environmental and genetic factors in cases of isolated cleft lip or cleft palate (25).

The regulatory genes and gene products functioning as transcriptional factors for the bronchial arches that give rise to the midface and lower face are being discovered, and their interactions with nutrients (e.g., retinoic acid via its specific receptors) are critical to craniofacial orodental morphogenesis (29). A superfamily of genes is now considered to interact with nutrients during instructive stages of craniofacial development in the mammalian embryo (i.e., about 19 to 26 days of gestation in the human). Endogenous retinoic acid appears to function as a developmental organizer during limb development and limb regeneration. Excess exogenous retinoic acid produces significant craniofacial malformations associated with clefting, dental development, hemifacial microsomia, spina bifida, eye defects, and limb morphogenesis (30). The function of endogenous retinoic acid in craniofacial development and how excess levels of retinoic acid might produce congenital malformations are central questions in this area (28, 31) (see also Chapters 17 and 18 on the roles of vitamins A and D on differentiation and morphogenesis). A striking illustration of the need to understand the effects of nutrition on birth defects is the recent demonstration that folate supplements provided near the time of conception significantly reduced the recurrence of neural tube defects among high-risk individuals in the United Kingdom (32). Similar data relate folic acid or multivitamins in congenital craniofacial malformations such as cleft lip and/or cleft palate (28, 33).

Dietary advice following thorough diagnostic endeavors can materially benefit expectant mothers, lactating women, and infants. Proper oral tissue development clearly depends on adequate nutrition. When dietary advice is provided during such critical development times, it is appropriate to consult with other professionals, including physicians, dietitians, and nutritionists, to ensure reasonable and substantive therapy. Most important, appropriate dietary counseling, particularly with reference to critical developmental times, and intake of essential nutrients, can ensure optimal oral health. Clearly, this knowledge base has profound implications for the continuing advancement of nutrition in the education of professionals and in integrating dentistry more closely with medicine. In this manner, dental/oral healthcare professionals can provide critical points of entry into the healthcare delivery system for at-risk patients.

NUTRITION AND DENTAL CARIES

Dental caries is a preventable infectious disease of the oral cavity and a major cause of tooth loss in children and adults in the United States. Caries has declined among children, however. A measure of the level of dental caries in a population is the decayed-missing-filled-surfaces (DMFS) rate, which is the number of permanent tooth surfaces (out of a possible 128 surfaces on 32 teeth) that are decayed, missing, or filled. An oral examination was included in the Third National Health and Nutrition Examination Survey (NHANES III) conducted between 1988 and 1991. Among U.S. children aged 5 to 17 examined, over half (54.7%) had a caries-free permanent dentition; however, the mean DMFS was 2.5 (34). In the 1979 to 1980 NIDR survey, 37% of school children examined had no caries in their permanent teeth, and the mean DMFS was 4.77. However, dental decay increases with age; by 15 years of age, about two-thirds of U.S. teens had experienced caries in their permanent dentition (Fig. 66.2). Cavitation occurs most frequently on the occlusal or chewing surface of the tooth. Decay on the smooth surfaces of teeth has declined since 1980, and interproximal caries (between the teeth) is nearly eradicated in the younger age groups.

Caries was also common in the primary teeth. Although more than 60% of those under 9 years of age had a caries-free deciduous dentition, an average of 3.1 primary tooth surfaces were decayed or filled (34). Mexican American children had the highest mean number of decayed-filled primary tooth surfaces (4.8). About 31% of children aged 6 to 8 years had untreated decay in their primary or per-

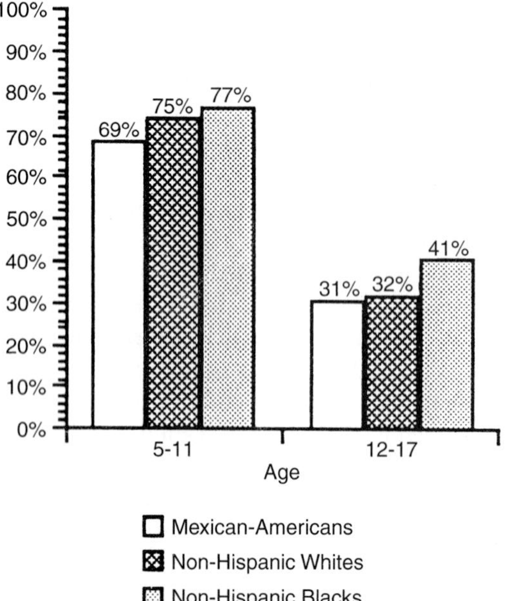

Figure 66.2. Percentage of U.S. children and adolescents caries free, by age and ethnicity. (From National Center for Health Statistics. Plan and operation of the third National Health and Nutrition Examination Survey, 1988–94. DHHS publ. no. (PHS) 94-1308, series 1, no. 322. Hyattsville, MD: National Center for Health Statistics, 1994.)

manent teeth (35). The prevalence of unfilled tooth surfaces was greater among low-income, Mexican American, and non-Hispanic black children and teens.

Based on data collected in the NHANES III survey, 93.8% of dentate adults have treated or untreated coronal caries. The average number of decayed and filled coronal tooth surfaces for adults aged 25 to 34 was 16.5 and climbed to 73.1 in adults 65 to 74.9 (36). The rate of edentulousness continues to decline. In the 1988 to 1991 survey, 26% of adults 65 to 69 years of age were edentulous, compared with 32% of adults in the 1985 to 1986 NIDR adult survey (37). Many adults have had fluoride exposure part of their lives; as a result, teeth are being retained longer.

The decline in caries prevalence does not imply that caries is no longer a public health problem; it is the most common disease of childhood and remains one of, if not the most, prevalent disease(s) in the world. Even the most optimistic data indicate that nearly 50% of children still have the disease. However, most of the caries in the permanent dentition are found in a small number of children; in those aged 5 to 17 years, 80% of the caries were seen in 25% of the children (34). Thus, the target group for intervention (including dietary intervention) has shifted to individuals at high risk, such as those of lower socioeconomic status, immigrants to the United States from developing countries, developmentally disabled individuals, persons undergoing head and neck radiation, and individuals with compromised host defenses because of complicating medical and pharmacy regimens that affect the oral tissues.

For many years, dental caries was thought to be irreversible. Recently it was determined that caries is a dynamic process with three phases: *(a)* demineralization, *(b)* equilibrium, and *(c)* remineralization of tooth enamel. With frequent fermentable carbohydrate exposure and poor oral hygiene, incipient lesions may develop rapidly. In the early stage of tooth decay, the process can be reversed. When no bacterial fermentation is occurring, calcium, phosphorus, and fluoride released from the tooth enamel can be redeposited to remineralize the tooth. A clinical cavity (caries) is the final stage in the disease process. The average time for progression of incipient caries to a carious lesion in children is about 18 ± 6 months.

Etiology of Dental Caries

The direct relationship between diet and dental caries is clearly established. Dental caries results from the interaction of four factors in the mouth: *(a)* cariogenic plaque bacteria, *(b)* fermentable substrate, *(c)* host and tooth factors including fluoride and other minerals, and *(d)* saliva (38) (Fig. 66.3). These factors must be present simultaneously in the oral cavity for a long enough time to interact.

Dental plaque is a sticky gelatinous mass composed of gram-positive bacteria, extracellular polysaccharides, proteins of salivary and dietary origins, and lipids. Without

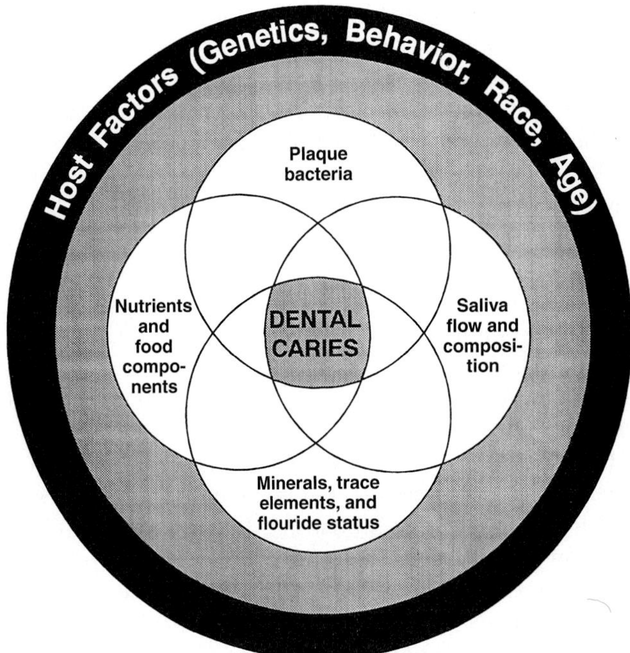

Figure 66.3. Major factors that interact in the dental caries process. (Adapted, with permission, from Navia JM. Am J Clin Nutr 1994;59:719S–27S.)

effective oral hygiene, plaque may cover all surfaces of the teeth. When foods are ingested, plaque bacteria metabolize the carbohydrate component, sugars and starches, to form organic acids—lactic, butyric, acetic, formic, and propionic—on the surfaces of the teeth. This fermentation begins within minutes and may continue for hours. These acids lower the pH of plaque and can dissolve tooth structure. Demineralization of enamel is thought to occur between pH 5.3 and 5.7. Stephan proposed using a pH of 5.5 as the "critical pH" in measuring the cariogenicity of a food (39). Frequent intake of carbohydrates that depress the plaque pH below 5.5 can cause repeated acid attacks. When substrate is exhausted, acid production stops and the plaque pH returns to a resting state. Changes in plaque pH have been used to estimate the cariogenicity of foods and snacks.

Dental caries is one of the most common bacterial diseases in humans. In 1960, Fitzgerald and Keyes demonstrated that dental caries was an infectious disease in animals (40). When germ-free animals were fed a high-sucrose diet, no caries developed. When sucrose-fed animals were inoculated with mutans streptococci or exposed to infected animals, they developed smooth-surface and fissure caries. The cariogenicity of *Streptococcus mutans* in humans has been established by monitoring the levels of the organism in the fissures of teeth until they become carious. The number of *S. mutans* increases at sites where caries is diagnosed; caries-free tooth surfaces have low levels of *S. mutans*. Elevated numbers of mutans streptococci are found in children, teens, and adults with high rates of dental caries. Six genetically distinct species of mutans streptococci are now recognized (41). *S. mutans* (serotype

C) has been identified as the principal organism responsible for the initial destruction of enamel and the underlying dentin in North American populations. The ability to survive and metabolize carbohydrate in the low-oxygen, acidic environment of dental plaque is a unique property of *S. mutans*. In addition to streptococci, species of actinomyces and lactobacilli are linked to dental caries.

Human clinical trials to measure the effect of dietary habits on the development of caries or to confirm the findings of epidemiologic studies are considered unethical and are prohibited today. Thus, rats, hamsters, and monkeys have been widely used in caries research and for testing foods for cariogenicity. Rats have been used most extensively because the etiologic agents are essentially the same as in man (42). Caries can be produced within a few weeks in rats, whereas it takes 6 to 18 months for caries to develop in monkeys or humans. Although tooth morphology and saliva composition differ, lesions develop in the pits, fissures, smooth surfaces, and roots of rodents' teeth. As in humans, *S. mutans* are the critical cariogenic microbes, but fermentable carbohydrate must be present for caries to occur. In animal studies, essential nutrition can be provided by gastric intubation to bypass the oral cavity or given orally as animal chow or a gelled nutrient supplement. Poor growth and high mortality have occurred in animals undergoing gastric intubation, however, so this technique is less common than provision of an oral noncariogenic diet.

A programed feeding machine is used so that the caloric intake, quantity, and frequency of intake of foods tested for cariogenicity can be monitored (43). A measured amount of food can be given to the animals up to 17 times during the day. At approximately 35 days, the animals are sacrificed and the teeth are scored for carious lesions. By using the feeding machine, researchers have shown that caries activity is linked to the quantity and frequency of fermentable carbohydrate intake (42). The results of animal trials cannot be extrapolated directly to humans, but they support a probable role of carbohydrates in human caries.

Role of Carbohydrates in Dental Caries

Epidemiologic surveys, extensive animal experiments, and early controlled human studies all link sugars to the development of dental caries. When refined sugar was introduced into the diets of primitive populations such as Eskimos, Tahitians, and Bushmen, their caries prevalence increased dramatically. As the per capita consumption of sucrose increased in England and the United States in the last 100 years, the prevalence of caries rose. Caries rates fell when sugar was rationed in Europe during World War II but increased again when sugar rationing ended (44). Sreebny showed that the average DMFT index in 12-year-old children in 47 countries was highly correlated with the amount of sugar available per capita daily (45). Populations with low sugar intakes had low caries scores; children who had high sugar consumption developed high rates of caries. In the United States today, total sugars minus lactose constitute 20% of children's total caloric intake (46). Most dietary sugars are added to manufactured foods rather than being added to foods by the consumer at home. The relationship between sugar intake and caries is stronger today in developing countries than in developed countries, where fluoride exposure, regular oral hygiene, and professional care have weakened this relationship (47).

In rodents, monkeys, and humans, the presence of sucrose in the mouth increases the volume and rate of plaque formation. Sucrose has a unique role in permitting bacteria to colonize on the teeth. When high concentrations of sucrose are present, *S. mutans* can produce extracellular polysaccharides, glucans, which form an organic matrix on the tooth. These insoluble, sticky polymers permit bacterial colonies to adhere to the tooth. In addition to glucans, *S. mutans* produces intracellular polysaccharides (primarily fructans) from sucrose, which are stored and used in glycolysis when dietary carbohydrates are unavailable. Figure 66.4 depicts the relationship of nutritive and nonnutritive sweeteners to the caries process and microbial metabolism. The critical concentration of carbohydrate in a food that will cause caries in man is unknown; however, foods with 15% sugars by weight are considered high-sugar foods. In animals, caries scores increase as the sugar content increases (48). The Hopewood House Study showed that children eating diets containing complex carbohydrates but few refined sugars had low caries increments (49). The relationship of sugar intake to caries increment was examined in a longitudinal study of school children in England where the fluoride level in drinking water was low; the highest significant correlation was between grams of sugar eaten daily and caries experience (50). The weak correlations found between food habits and caries increment can be attributed to several factors: a low level of caries in all children, a high intake of sugary foods by all children, and widespread use of topical fluorides.

The other mono- and disaccharides (glucose, fructose, maltose, and lactose) found in fruits, dairy products, and processed foods are also readily used by oral microorganisms. These sugars diffuse rapidly through dental plaque to become available for bacterial fermentation. Within a few minutes of ingestion, fructose and glucose cause falls in plaque pH similar to those with sucrose; thus, they are considered as cariogenic as sucrose.

When eaten with meals, fresh fruits have low cariogenic potential. This is attributed to the high water content and the presence of citric acid, which stimulates saliva secretion. Fresh fruits vary in sucrose content from 10 to 15% by weight in apples, bananas, and some grapes; 7 to 8% in citrus fruits; to 2% in berries, cherries, and pears. However, orchard workers who ate large quantities of apples and grapes daily showed a high caries rate (51). Highly acidic foods may prevent bacterial fermentation but cause enamel erosion.

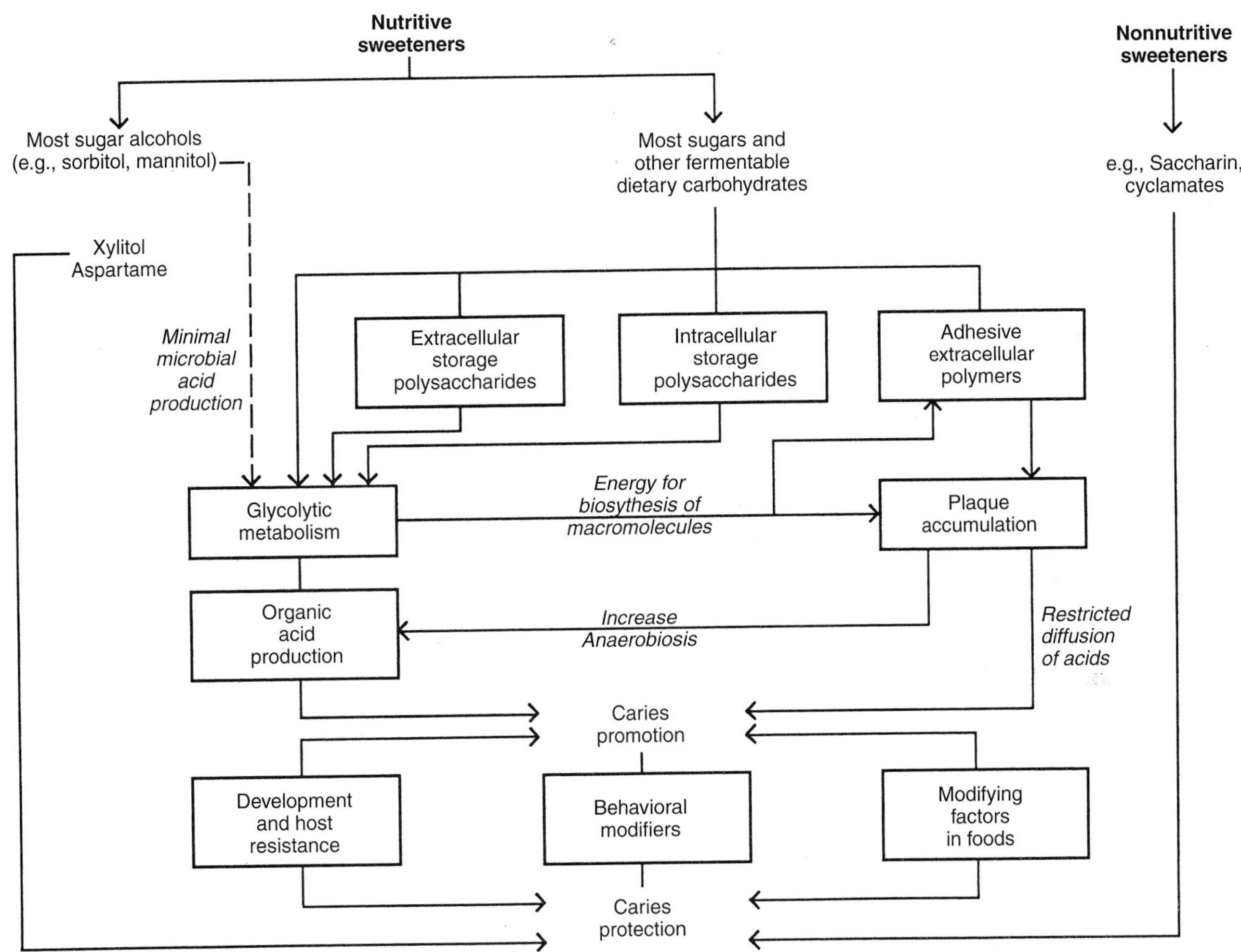

Figure 66.4. Relationship of nutritive and nonnutritive sweeteners to oral microbial metabolism and dental caries. (Adapted from Alfano MC. Food Technol 1980;34:70–4.)

Sugars in solution have been considered less harmful to teeth than solid sweets because beverages clear the mouth quickly. In the 1940s, however, Stephan showed that a 10% glucose rinse lowered the plaque pH below 5.5 (39). The total sugar content in carbonated beverages, fruit drinks, and fruit juices is about 10%, and sport drinks contain about 4.4% total sugars. Based on sugar content, acidity and changes in plaque pH after rinsing with these beverages, all of them appear to have similar cariogenic potential (52). Analysis of dental data from 1971 to 1974 (NHANES I study) showed that frequent between-meal intake of sweetened beverages was associated with increased caries (53). Teenagers and young adults who drank sugar-sweetened soft drinks three or more times between meals daily, increased their odds of having a high DMFT score by 179%. Since then, food manufacturers have replaced some of the sucrose in beverages with high-fructose corn syrup, saccharin, or aspartame. Whether beverages formulated with high-fructose corn syrup are less cariogenic is unknown. Substitution of sport drinks or ion drinks for carbonated beverages or fruit drinks was associated with decalcification of Japanese children's teeth (54). Most of these drinks have a pH below 4. Slowly drinking sugar-sweetened tea or coffee can also dissolve enamel. Use of sugar-based liquid oral medication may affect the oral health of chronically sick children. English children taking long-term liquid oral medicine had significantly more caries of deciduous anterior teeth than their siblings (55).

Extensive studies of the sugar alcohols show that they result in limited acid production by plaque bacteria. Plaque bacteria can ferment sorbitol and mannitol but too slowly to induce dental caries in most people. If sorbitol-sweetened products are used frequently, some evidence suggests that bacterial adaptation may occur (56). After several weeks of regular sorbitol mouth rinses, increased acid production was measured in adults given additional sorbitol. However, acid production may be clinically significant only in xerostomic patients who are at high risk of developing caries if they use sorbitol-mannitol-sweetened gums and candies regularly to relieve the symptoms of dry mouth. Xerostomic patients should be cautioned about the cariogenic potential of these products (57).

Xylitol, a five-carbon sugar alcohol, has been used in Canada and Europe to replace sucrose in candies, gum, and medicines. In the United States, it is approved by the

Food and Drug Administration (FDA) for use in special dietary products. Ingestion of solutions of xylitol does not lower plaque pH because oral bacteria lack the enzymes to ferment xylitol to organic acids. A 2-year clinical trial in Finland showed that young adults eating foods sweetened solely with xylitol developed no new caries, whereas groups ingesting fructose and sucrose developed caries (58). Later studies confirmed that xylitol was noncariogenic. Xylitol, however, is not widely used because it is costly to produce.

Saccharin, found in beverages, dietetic foods, and dentifrices and as a table sweetener for diabetics, inhibits tooth decay in rats. Low caries scores and low recoveries of *S. mutans* resulted when rats were challenged with a cariogenic diet supplemented with saccharin (59). The effects of saccharin on human oral bacteria have not been reported. Aspartame does not support the growth of *S. mutans*, acid production in the mouth, or plaque formation. Frequent rinsing with aspartame was no more cariogenic in rats than distilled water (60). Because soft drinks are a popular cariogenic snack, the use of aspartame in these beverages is safer for teeth.

Frequent use of chewing gum sweetened with xylitol or xylitol/sorbitol mixtures significantly reduces dental plaque as well as plaque and saliva levels of *S. mutans* (61). The Turku chewing gum study showed that those chewing four sticks of xylitol gum daily had 80% less dental decay than subjects chewing sucrose-sweetened gum (62). Gum chewing stimulates salivary flow and pushes saliva into the interproximal area where salivary buffers can neutralize bacterial acids. Chewing also removes food particles from plaque and soft tissues. The net result is that the stimulation of salivary flow caused by the physical act of chewing, coupled with the helpful effects of a noncaloric sweetener, can benefit dental health by "neutralizing" the plaque bacteria's acid response to fermentable carbohydrate–containing foods.

The effect of starch-containing foods on teeth depends on their form, whether the starch is raw or cooked, and whether sucrose is present. Raw starches found in vegetables have low cariogenicity in animals. Vegetables lacking sugars do not cause intraoral acid production or demineralization of enamel in man. Adults with hereditary fructose intolerance are a unique study group who consistently avoid fruits, table sugar, and refined starches containing sucrose because they cause nausea, but these persons eat wheat, rice, potatoes, and root vegetables. An examination of the caries status of these young adults showed that 15 of 27 adults examined were caries free, and the remainder had low DMFT scores. Siblings without the inborn error of metabolism had a higher caries prevalence, similar to that of the general population (63).

Because starch is a large molecule, it cannot diffuse through dental plaque. However, when cereal grains are refined in the production of breads or crackers and are cooked, they are more easily hydrolyzed by salivary and plaque amylases. Fermentation of the resulting sugar, maltose, yields acids that demineralize enamel rapidly. Mixtures of starches and sugars in ready-to-eat breakfast cereals, bread, pastries, and many convenience foods are often retained longer in the interproximal plaque than high-sugar foods. This may make heated sugar-starch combinations more cariogenic than sugar alone (64, 65). Foods previously thought to be of low cariogenicity—breads, muffins, crackers, chips—are no longer considered safe for teeth, especially when they are eaten between meals, because they are retained and can serve as substrate for plaque microbial fermentation.

Other Factors Affecting Cariogenicity

Sugar and starches are not the only factors that determine the cariogenic potential of a food. Frequency of intake, physical consistency, and position of a food in the meal are also important. In rats, the intervals between eating snacks or meals profoundly affect the number of *S. mutans* in plaque and the number of cavities formed. Few caries develop in rats fed a cariogenic diet two or three times a day. As the frequency of sugar and starch exposure increases, however, the caries risk increases. In the 1950s, the classic human intervention trial, the Vipeholm study, was conducted in Sweden (66). Institutionalized adults were fed an adequate diet and supplemented with either retentive sweets (chocolate, toffee, and caramels) between meals or nonsticky, sweet foods at meal time. Subjects provided up to ten times the sucrose at meals did not experience a significant increase in caries relative to the control subjects. However, the group receiving between-meal sweets developed more caries than subjects receiving sugar at mealtimes. Similarly, analysis of the NHANES I data obtained in a cross-sectional survey revealed that individuals with high DMFT scores consumed table sugars, syrups, sugary desserts, and snacks more frequently than persons with low DMFT scores (67). In a 3-year longitudinal study of 11- to 15-year-old Michigan children living in nonfluoridated areas, teens who developed two or more carious lesions derived more calories from snack carbohydrates and high-sugar foods than children with low caries increments (68). In rat experiments, granola cereal, french fries, bananas, cupcakes, and raisins had a cariogenic potential equal to or greater than that of sucrose (64).

The sequence of eating foods in a meal affects the magnitude of a drop in plaque pH. If a piece of aged cheese is eaten after an acidogenic food such as canned pears in syrup, the plaque pH rises above the danger zone immediately (69). Sugared coffee elicits a rapid drop in pH, but it will rise if followed by an unsweetened food. Sugared coffee at the end of a meal, however, will cause a prolonged drop in plaque pH. Placing acidogenic items between other foods lessens the risk of demineralization.

Saliva and protective components in foods modify the effect of fermentable carbohydrates on the teeth (70). The importance of saliva in caries prevention is perhaps best demonstrated by the rampant caries that develop in xerostomic patients. Saliva flow is stimulated by chewing, by citric acid in fruits, and by sugars. The composition of saliva is also influenced by dietary components.

Four protective mechanisms of saliva are important in caries prevention. First, saliva prevents bacterial aggregation on the tooth surface and speeds clearance of food particles and sugars from the mouth. Second, proteins, bicarbonates, and phosphates in saliva dilute and neutralize plaque acids. Third, immunoglobulins present in saliva protect the teeth by depressing bacterial activity. Finally, calcium, phosphate, and fluoride ions in saliva promote the remineralization of tooth enamel.

Food components can have two protective effects on tooth enamel. Some foods decrease the solubility of enamel (demineralization); others stimulate salivary secretion or remineralization of tooth enamel. Substances that make the enamel less soluble include fluoride in tea, an unidentified factor in cocoa, phytate, oxalate, and proteins in milk. Citric acid found in citrus fruits stimulates saliva production and thereby increases the amount of bicarbonate and phosphate buffers in the mouth.

Much research has been done on the effects of cheese on plaque pH. Over 21 aged cheeses have been identified that do not cause the plaque pH to fall (71). The protective properties of these cheeses are attributed to their texture (which increases the salivary secretion rate) and their protein, calcium, and phosphorus content (which neutralizes plaque acids). Cheese seems to prevent demineralization and promote remineralization (72). A "protective pH rise factor" has been hypothesized, but none has been identified.

Measuring the Cariogenic Potential of Human Food

Plaque acidogenicity is considered a valid indirect measure of the cariogenic potential of foods in humans. The results of three indirect types of tests (73), taken together, on a variety of commonly consumed foods reveal that the foods with high cariogenic potential are those with high fermentable carbohydrate content, eaten frequently, that adhere to the teeth. Tests also demonstrated that the following foods cause the pH at interproximal sites to fall below pH 5.5, implying that if they are ingested frequently, the risk of caries will substantially increase: dried fruits, breads, cereals, cookies, snack crackers, and potato chips (74). Generally, the more processing a food undergoes, the greater its cariogenicity. Foods that are noncariogenic (i.e., do not drop the plaque pH below 5.5) include some vegetables, meats, fish, aged cheeses, and nuts. These tests are useful predictors of cariogenicity, but additional factors determine if caries actually develop, including host susceptibility, virulence of the oral bacteria, how frequently a food is eaten, the sequence in which foods are eaten in a meal, and the interaction between foods eaten concurrently.

In addition to the continuing concern regarding food cariogenicity and caries prevalence and experience in the so-called normal population, two other specific groups have been targeted as high-risk groups, primarily because of eating and social behavioral patterns: the infant/toddler, at risk of early childhood caries, and the elderly, at risk of developing root surface caries.

Root Caries

Dietary factors are also important in the initiation and progression of root caries. When gingival tissues recede, the root surfaces of teeth are exposed to the oral environment. Because roots lack the protective enamel layer, they are highly susceptible to dental caries. Root caries lesions are primarily a disease of older adults. In the NHANES III survey, root surface lesions were found in 54% of males and 41% of females 65 to 74 years of age. The mean number of decayed and filled root surfaces for 65 to 74 year olds was 2.2 (75). About 60% of the lesions had been restored. Older adults at greatest risk of developing root caries include persons with coronal caries, gingival recession, low saliva flow, low fluoride exposure, and frequent intake of fermentable carbohydrates.

High levels of *S. mutans* are found in adults with root caries (76). Examination of ancient skulls and dentition of members of primitive societies revealed that root caries was more common than coronal caries. Because these groups consumed starches but not refined sugars, complex carbohydrates are implicated in the development of root caries. Adults who have periodontitis or have had periodontal surgery resulting in exposed root surfaces frequently develop root caries if their intake of fermentable carbohydrates is high (77). A high sugar intake is positively associated with root caries, and a high cheese intake is negatively associated with root caries (78, 79). In a cross-sectional study of healthy, free-living elderly persons, high daily intake of semisolid and sticky, slowly dissolving fermentable foods such as ice cream, gelatin, hard candies, and antacids was positively correlated with root caries (80).

In a 2-year longitudinal study of elderly Bostonians, subjects in the highest quintile for root caries had significantly higher intakes of sweetened liquids, solid fermentable carbohydrates, and starches than subjects who were free of root caries (81). Adults who were free of root caries ate 50% more cheese and 25% more milk than persons with caries. Because root caries develop more rapidly than coronal caries, preventive measures are critical. Nutritional counseling, home oral care, and fluoride therapy should be provided to older adults with gingival recession. Thus, the dietary etiology of root caries seems to be similar to that of coronal caries. Both the amount and frequency of fermentable carbohydrates are important.

Early Childhood Caries

Severe tooth decay in infants and toddlers is a preventable disease associated with inappropriate feeding practices. Early childhood caries, often referred to as nursing caries or baby bottle tooth decay, occurs between 1 and 3 years of age, develops rapidly, and can cause severe dental pain and infection. The prevalence of early childhood caries in the United States is estimated to be between 1 and 12%. However, much higher prevalence rates have been reported among Hispanic, Southeast Asian, innercity, and American Indian/Alaska Native children (>50%) (82).

Children with nursing caries are at greater risk of developing additional caries in the primary and permanent teeth than children who are caries free (83). Initially, the smooth surfaces of the four primary maxillary incisor teeth are involved; later, decalcification of the maxillary and mandibular molars and canines occurs (84). The tongue protects the lower anterior four incisors. First white spot lesions develop on the gingival third of the maxillary front teeth; this stage often goes undetected by parents. Within 6 months, these lesions may progress to a dull white band of demineralization rapidly developing along the gum line of the upper incisors. If the disease advances further, a brown or black collar encircles the necks of the teeth. The four maxillary incisors may be completely destroyed so that only brownish root stumps remain. When nursing caries progresses to the development of abscesses, the abscesses may affect the underlying developing permanent dentition. Restoration of severe caries is expensive and emotionally traumatic for parents and children. The young child must often be treated under general anesthesia. Loss of incisors alters the arch dimension, affects appearance and speech, and may have a psychologic impact on the child.

Nursing caries results from the interaction of pathogenic oral microorganisms, fermentable carbohydrates, and susceptible teeth. *S. mutans* is not part of the indigenous flora of the oral cavity at birth. When the deciduous teeth erupt at about 6 months of age, bacterial colonies begin to form in the mouth. *S. mutans* is believed to be transmitted to infants by caregivers. If mothers have high levels of *S. mutans,* their infants are at greater risk of having elevated levels of these cariogenic organisms in their plaque (85). As discussed above, early malnutrition may increase a tooth's susceptibility to caries.

Early decay of the primary dentition may result from use of a nursing bottle at naptime and/or bedtime that contains milk, fruit juice, or another sweetened solution. Sweetened liquids pool around the teeth of a child who habitually falls asleep with a bottle in the mouth, leading to demineralization of the enamel. The same pattern of dental decay may result from ad libitum breast-feeding (86). Breast-fed infants with rampant decay have reportedly been allowed to sleep with the mother and remain on the breast for long periods of time. During sleep, diminished flow rates greatly reduce the protective action of saliva. Severity of the disease is linked to the number of decay-causing bacteria present in the oral cavity, the number of feedings per day, and the duration of bottle or breast-feeding.

To prevent early childhood caries, education must occur before the child's primary teeth erupt. All caregivers—parents, grandparents, and daycare workers—must be counseled about the recommended feeding practices with the baby bottle. Nap or nighttime bottle feeding in bed should be discouraged. If a bedtime bottle is offered, the only safe liquid is water. Parents should be encouraged to offer juices from a cup after 6 months of age. Allowing breast-fed infants to sleep with the nipple in the mouth during the night should be avoided after the first primary tooth begins to erupt. Infants should be removed from the breast when they fall asleep. Children should be weaned from the bottle by 12 months of age. Information about nursing caries should be provided in dental offices, pediatric clinics, WIC (Women, Infants, and Children) clinics, birthing centers, and Head Start programs. One-on-one counseling with caretakers of infants and communitywide education programs have been successful in reducing BBTD among southwestern American Indian children (87). The American Academy of Pediatric Dentistry recommends that infants visit a dentist within 6 months after the first tooth erupts in the mouth.

FLUORIDE

The decline in coronal caries in industrialized countries in the past 30 years is attributed primarily to the widespread use of fluorides. This mineral is universally present in nature; trace amounts are found in soils, water, plants, and foodstuffs. Currently, the primary sources of fluoride for humans are community water supplies, foods, beverages, dentifrices, and other dental products. The ionic fluoride ingested in water has a systemic effect prior to tooth eruption and a topical effect after eruption. Dietary fluoride supplements are prescribed for children when fluoride is lacking in the water supply. Professionally applied topical applications of fluoride in higher concentrations are used to protect erupted teeth and are not swallowed. The preventive benefits of fluoride depend upon the concentration of fluoride used, whether it is given systemically or topically, and the type of agent used, whether in water, tablet, drops, a rinse, or a gel. The caries preventive properties of systemic and topical fluoride are additive. Fluoride is more effective in preventing smooth surface caries than occlusal caries.

Mechanisms of Action

Although the cariostatic properties of fluoride are widely recognized, the mechanisms of action of fluoride in the oral environment are not fully understood. At least three mechanisms of action are recognized (88). First, fluoride ions replace some of the hydroxyl groups of the hydroxyapatite in developing teeth to form fluoridated hydroxyapatite. This increases the stability of the enamel crystals because fluoridated hydroxyapatite is less soluble in organic acids than hydroxyapatite. Fluoride uptake by calcified tissues is extremely high (90%) in infancy but decreases with age. Second, low concentrations of fluoride in the saliva can decrease the rate of demineralization and enhance remineralization of early carious lesions. When enamel is partially demineralized by organic acids, calcium, phosphate, and fluoride from the tooth can diffuse back into the surface layers of enamel and accelerate recrystallization. Third, fluoride has direct effects on the acidogenic plaque bacteria. In higher concentrations, fluoride inhibits growth of *S. mutans* found in dental plaque, and in low concentrations, it inhibits bacterial enzymes, reducing acid production from catabolism of fermentable carbohydrates.

Water Fluoridation

Fluoridation of community water supplies is the most effective method of providing fluoride to large populations. Through extensive epidemiologic studies of naturally fluoridated communities in the United States in the 1930s, the protective properties of fluoride in the prevention of dental caries were fully recognized (89). In 21 U.S. cities, an inverse relationship was shown between caries prevalence in children and the fluoride content of the drinking at an optimal range (Fig. 66.5).

In 1945, Grand Rapids, Michigan, became the first city in the world to fluoridate its drinking water. Between 1950 and 1980, clinical studies conducted in 20 countries showed that adding fluoride to community water supplies reduced caries by 40 to 50% in primary teeth and by 50 to 60% in permanent teeth (90). Recent comparisons of caries in U.S. children who had always lived in optimally fluoridated communities with children never exposed to fluoridated drinking water revealed 25% lower DMFS scores in the fluoridated group (91). The decline in caries prevalence among children living in communities with nonfluoridated water is attributed to intake of foods and beverages processed with fluoridated water, use of fluoride-containing dentrifrices, and use of topical fluorides in the dental office and at home. Adults also benefit from consumption of fluoridated water. The prevalence of coronal and root caries seems to be 20 to 30% lower in adults living in optimally fluoridated communities than in adults residing in cities with lower levels of fluoride in the water supply (92).

According to the United States Public Health Service, the desirable fluoride concentration for dental caries prevention is about 1 part per million (0.7–1.2 ppm, based on climactic temperature). By 1990, 42 of the 50 largest cities in the United States had fluoridated their water supplies. In 1992, in the United States, approximately 144 million people, or 62% of the population on public water supplies, drink water with fluoride levels of 0.7 ppm or higher (93). This includes 9 million people who drink water with natural fluoride at optimal levels. Continuous exposure to fluoride is desirable. In communities where water fluoridation has been interrupted or eliminated, a significant increase in dental caries has been observed (92).

Water fluoridation is the most cost-effective method of preventing tooth decay in the United States. The current average cost for delivering fluoride in the drinking water is less than a dollar per person per year. Even though scientists, health professionals, and the courts generally agree that community water fluoridation is safe, effective, economical, and legally valid, some members of the public remain confused about fluoride's safety. Opponents to fluoridation have attempted to link it to AIDS, Alzheimer's disease, and cancer, but they have provided no scientific evidence to support their claims. Over 50 epidemiologic studies have demonstrated no association between water fluoride and the risk of cancer. In addition, animal studies have failed to establish a relationship between fluoride and cancer (88). Water fluoridation cannot be taken for granted. Health professionals—nutritionists, physicians, dentists, pharmacists, nurses, and public health specialists—have a responsibility to educate patients and the public about the health and economic benefits of fluoridation.

Dietary Supplementation

Children living in cities and rural areas with suboptimal water fluoridation can receive the caries-preventive benefits of fluoride by taking a prescribed fluoride supplement. Children given fluoride drops or tablets daily from 6

Number of cities studied	Number of children examined	Number of DMF teeth per 100 examinees (0 100 200 300 400 500 600 700)	Fluoride content of water (ppm)
11	3867		< 0.5
3	1140		0.5 - 0.9
4	1403		1.0 - 1.4
3	847		>1.4

Figure 66.5. Relationship between caries prevalence and fluoride content of drinking water in 21 cities. (With permission from Newbrun E. Fluorides and dental caries. 3rd ed. Springfield, IL: Charles C Thomas, 1986.)

Table 66.3
Supplemental Fluoride Dosage Schedule (mg/day[a]) According to Fluoride Concentration of Drinking Water

	Concentration of Fluoride in Drinking Water (ppm)		
Age	Less than 0.3	0.3 to 0.6	More than 0.6
6 months to 3 years	0.25 mg	0	0
3 to 6 years	0.50 mg	0.25 mg	0
6 to 16 years	1.00 mg	0.50 mg	0

From ADA Council on Access, Prevention & Interpersonal Relations. J Am Dent Assoc 1995;126:Special Supplement, 19S.
[a]ppm = parts per million; 2.2 mg sodium fluoride contains 1 mg fluoride.

months of age through the early teenage years show a low prevalence of caries. The level of dietary supplementation is determined by the age of the child and the concentration of fluoride in the water supply. Well water should be tested for fluoride concentration by the local water district or the county or state health department. Table 66.3 presents the levels of daily fluoride supplementation recommended by the American Dental Association (ADA) Council on Scientific Affairs and the American Academy of Pediatrics. No fluoride supplementation is recommended in areas where the drinking water contains 0.6 ppm fluoride or more. For those consuming water with less than 0.30 ppm fluoride, 1 mg of fluoride is not recommended until age 6. The upper limit of fluoride intake appears to be 0.05 mg/kg body weight. Future dosage schedules may be based on body weight rather than age.

Liquid fluoride supplements (drops) are recommended for infants and young children. Fluoride drops or tablets alone are as effective as fluoride-vitamin supplements. A list of accepted fluoride supplements is published regularly by the ADA Council on Scientific Affairs (94). Fluoride-vitamin supplements are not recommended by the ADA because when vitamins are discontinued, fluoride use may cease. Few healthy, full-term, formula-fed infants require a vitamin-mineral supplement. The fluoride present when commercial formula is diluted with fluoridated water is 95 to 100% available. If infant formula is prepared with nonfluoridated water, however, fluoride drops should be prescribed. The fluoride concentration of breast milk and cow's milk is very low (0.1 ppm).

For older children, fluoride tablets are available in the following doses: 0.25 mg F, 0.5 mg F, or 1 mg F. Tablets are formulated with neutral sodium fluoride or acidulated phosphate fluoride (APF). The caries preventive effects of neutral fluoride tablets is similar to that of APF tablets. Chewable fluoride tablets seem to have both topical and systemic benefits. Patients should be instructed to allow the tablet to dissolve by chewing before swallowing. Administering the appropriate dosage of fluoride preparations should be carefully explained to parents, because excess fluoride may lead to dental fluorosis.

Other countries have incorporated fluoride into the food supply by fluoridating salt, milk, flour, or sugar. If community water fluoridation is impractical, these foods appear to be possible vehicles for fluoride. Unfortunately, individual intake of these foods varies widely, so formulating a dosage regimen is difficult.

Primary tooth development begins before birth; therefore, the efficacy of prenatal fluoride supplementation is of interest. During pregnancy, fluoride diffuses across the placental barrier and is incorporated into fetal bones and teeth. Fluoride concentration in fetal blood appears to be about 25% of that in maternal blood (95). Although prenatal supplements are considered safe for mother and fetus, the benefits of supplementation in reducing caries are unproven. Dental caries rates of children whose mothers received fluoride supplements during pregnancy and children whose mothers did not, did not differ significantly at 3 and 5 years of age (96). Both groups lived in cities without fluoridation of the water supply.

Dental Fluorosis

Fluorosis is characterized by white opaque flecks, white or brown staining, or in severe cases, pitting of the tooth enamel. Because the crowns of all permanent teeth are forming between birth and 14 years of age, the effects of excess systemic fluoride are limited to this age group. The most critical time for developing fluorosis appears to be the first or second year of life when maturation of upper anterior permanent teeth enamel occurs and the daily fluoride ingestion exceeds 2 ppm (97). Fewer than 2% of school children in the 1986 to 1987 NIDR survey had moderate-to-severe fluorosis (98). An increase in the prevalence of mild/very mild dental fluorosis is observed more often in fluoridated than nonfluoridated communities (Fig. 66.6). This is primarily a cosmetic problem and does not increase the teeth's susceptibility to caries. Fluorosis is not considered a public health problem in North America today.

Exposure to multiple sources of fluoride increases a child's risk of developing fluorosis (99, 100). More than two-thirds of the fluorosis cases can be explained by inappropriate use of fluoride supplements and use of more than the recommended amount of toothpaste (99). If a child receiving optimal amounts of fluoride from dietary sources or fluoridated water swallows large amounts of dentifrice, fluorosis can occur. Nearly all U.S. toothpastes contain fluoride that is readily absorbed when ingested. Toothpaste is generally swallowed rather than expectorated by children under 6 years of age. Therefore, parents should dispense a pea-sized amount of toothpaste for young children to prevent excess fluoride intake.

Substantial amounts of fluoride can be introduced into the infant's diet through food processing. In the 1970s, it was discovered that infant formulas contained variable and often high levels of fluoride. To reduce the risk of infants receiving too much fluoride, beginning in 1979, infant formula manufacturers voluntarily reduced the amount of fluoride in formulas. Soy-based formulas

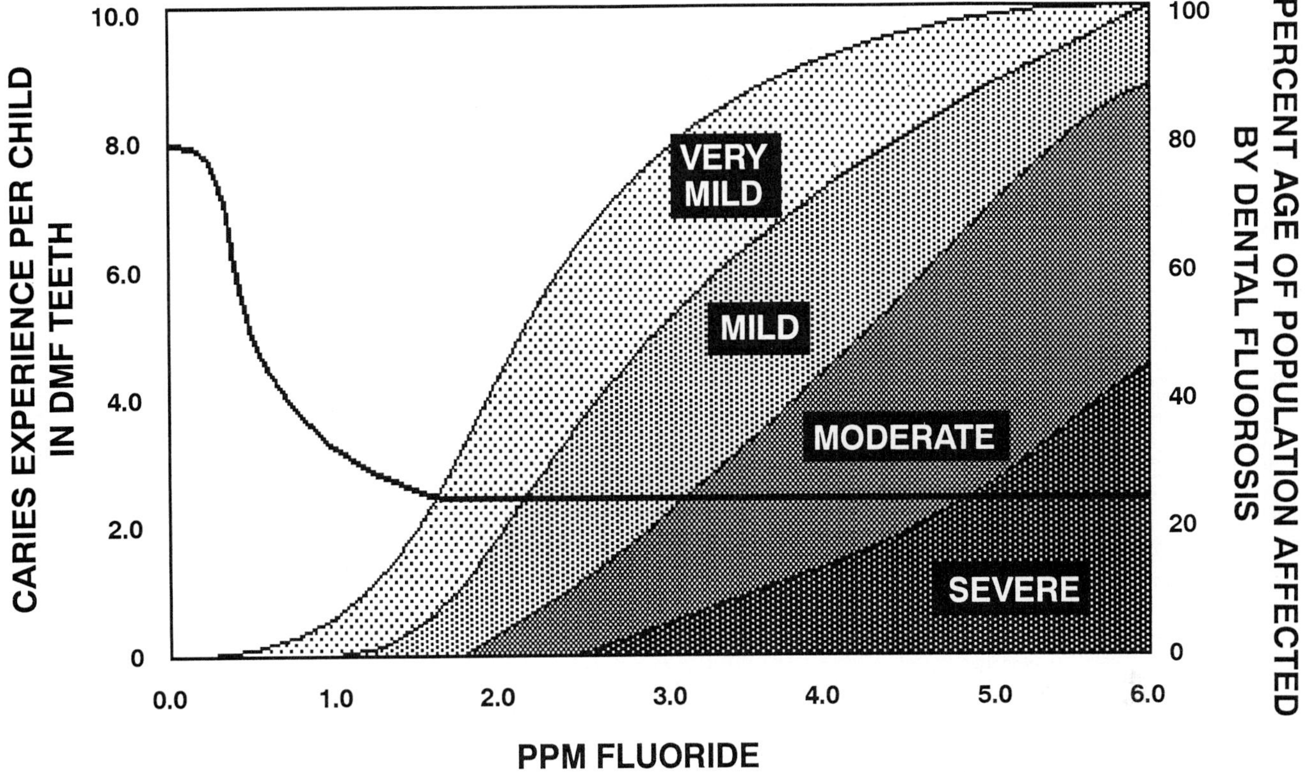

Figure 66.6. Prevalence of dental caries and dental fluorosis in relation to fluoride in drinking water. (From Department of Health and Human Services, Public Health Service Review of Fluoride Benefits and Risks. Report of the Ad Hoc Subcommittee on Fluoride of the Committee to Coordinate Environmental Health and Related Programs. Washington, DC: U.S. Government Printing Office, 1991.)

appear to have higher fluoride levels than milk-based formulas because the soy products contain components that bind fluoride. Ready-to-feed infant fruit juices, tea, fish, dried seafood products, and chicken products can contain high levels of fluoride. Continued monitoring of the fluoride content of a "market basket" of infant and toddler foods in the United States is needed to ensure that fluoride intake remains within safe limits. When the pathogenesis of enamel fluorosis is better understood, the appropriateness of the current fluoride supplementation schedule can be determined.

EFFECT OF NUTRITION ON ORAL SOFT TISSUES

Nutrient Deficiencies

The oral mucosa is particularly susceptible to physiologic or anatomic changes resulting from nutritional deficit or toxicity. Since the turnover rate of oral mucosal cells is relatively rapid (gingival sulcular epithelial cells have a turnover rate of 3 to 7 days), sufficient nutrients must be available at the appropriate times and in the correct concentration for DNA replication, protein synthesis, and cell and tissue maturation to occur. The oral epithelium acts as an effective barrier against invasion of toxic substances, particularly antigens derived from oral microbes, into the underlying collagenous connective tissue. Inadequate nutrition can cause the oral epithelia to either break down or be compromised, thus increasing the tissue's susceptibility to infectious disease.

For these reasons, the oral cavity is one of the first regions of the body to exhibit clinical signs of malnutrition. Virtually every classic nutritional deficiency or toxicity, including scurvy, beriberi, and pellagra, has signs and symptoms in the oral cavity and surrounding structures. The lips, tongue, oral mucosa, and gingiva may all reflect nutritional aberrations long before they are apparent elsewhere in the body. Table 66.4 summarizes the oral signs and symptoms of nutritional aberrations. Nutritionally induced oral changes may include anatomic lesions, color changes, functional changes (e.g., burning mouth and tongue), textural changes, and inflammation of the lips, oral mucosa, corners of the mouth, tongue, and gingiva (6).

For example, the dorsum of the tongue may undergo changes in size or color, and taste changes may result from atrophy or hypertrophy of tongue papillae. Longstanding nutrient deficiencies may lead to atrophy of the papillae and denudation of the dorsum. A bright red, painful tongue and swelling of the oral mucosa may be early symptoms of pernicious anemia due to a lack of vitamin B_{12}. Inflammation, a burning sensation, and tenderness of the tongue or palate may be caused by a deficiency of vitamin B complex, protein, or iron. Burning mouth syndrome

Table 66.4
Oral Signs and Symptoms of Nutritional Aberrations

Nutrient	Deficiency or (Excess)
Vitamins	
Vitamin C	**Deficiency** Mild: exaggerated tissue response to and increased risk of infection, blood vessel fragility, increased periodontal signs and symptoms, delayed wound healing Severe: (scurvy) red swollen gingiva, gingival friability and bleeding on provocation, interdental papillary infusions, petechiae, sore burning mouth, increased risk of candidiasis, subperiosteal hemorrhages, periodontal destruction, increased tooth mobility and exfoliation, soft tissue ulceration, teeth are malformed with normal enamel but inadequate dentin that can easily fracture (**Excess:** chronic overdosing can increase metabolism of vitamin C as an adaptation; rebound scurvy may occur after dose normalization)
Vitamin D	**Deficiency:** abnormal bone regeneration, osteoporosis, osteomalacia, incomplete calcification of teeth and alveolar bone, rickets (**Excess:** pulp calcification, enamel hypoplasia)
Vitamin K	**Deficiency:** increased risk of bleeding and candidiasis
Vitamin A	**Deficiency:** inadequate differentiation of cells leading to impaired healing and tissue regeneration; desquamation of oral mucosa; early keratinization of mucosa (keratosis); increased risk of candidiasis, gingival hypertrophy and inflammation; leukoplakia, decreased taste sensitivity, xerostomia, disturbed or arrested enamel development leading to poor or absent calcification and hypoplasia in mature teeth Severe: may lead to irregular tubular dentin formation and increased caries risk (**Excess:** also impairs cell differentiation and epithelialization resulting in delayed and impaired healing of oral tissues mimicking signs and symptoms of deficiency)
B-complex in general	**Deficiency:** angular cheilosis of lips, leukoplakia, burning tongue, papillary atrophy, magenta tongue, fissuring, glossitis
B_2 Riboflavin	**Deficiency:** angular cheilosis, atrophy of filiform papillae, enlarged fungiform papillae, shiny red lips, magenta tongue, sore tongue
B_3 Niacin	**Deficiency:** angular cheilosis, mucositis, stomatitis, oral pain, ulceration, denuded tongue, glossitis, glossodynia, (tongue: tips are red, swollen, beefy, dorsum is smooth and dry), ulcerative gingivitis
Folic acid	**Deficiency:** angular cheilosis, mucositis, stomatitis, sore or burning mouth, increased risk of candidiasis, inflamed gingiva glossitis (tongue: red, swollen tip or borders, slick bald pale dorsum), apthous-type ulcers
B_6 Pyridoxine	**Deficiency:** angular cheilosis, sore burning mouth, glossitis, and glossodynia
B_{12} Cynocobalamin	**Deficiency:** angular cheilosis, sore burning mouth, mucositis/stomatitis, hemorrhagic gingiva, halitosis, epithelial dysplasia of oral mucosa, oral paresthesia (numbness, tingling), detachment of periodontal fibers, loss or distortion of taste, glossitis, glossodynia (tongue: beefy red, smooth, glossy), delayed wound healing, xerostomia, bone loss, apthous-type ulcers
Minerals	
Fluoride	**Deficiency:** decreased resistance to dental caries (**Excess:** fluorosis leading to enamel hypoplasia: *mild* = mottled enamel (white spots)/high caries resistance; milder signs of toxicity are esthetically unpleasant but increase caries resistance; *moderate* = unsightly brown stain/high caries resistance; *severe* = hypoplasia of enamel, with decreased caries resistance; more severe toxicity results in interference with amelogenesis and decreased caries resistance)
Iron	**Deficiency:** angular cheilosis, pallor of lips and oral mucosa, sore, burning tongue, atrophy/denudation of filiform papillae, glossitis, increased risk of candidiasis
Calcium	**Deficiency:** incomplete calcification of teeth, rickets, osteomalacia, excessive bone resorption and bone fragility, osteoporosis, increased tendency to hemorrhage, and increased tooth mobility and premature loss
Copper	**Deficiency:** decreased trabeculae of alveolar bone, decreased tissue vascularity, increased tissue fragility
Zinc	**Deficiency:** loss or distortion of taste and smell acuity, loss of tongue sensation, delayed wound healing, impaired keratinization of epithelial cells, epithelial thickening, atrophic oral mucosa, increased susceptibility to periodontal disease and candidiasis, xerostomia, increased susceptibility to caries if present during tooth formation
Magnesium	**Deficiency:** alveolar bone fragility, gingival hypertrophy
Phosphorus	**Deficiency:** incomplete calcification of teeth, increased susceptibility to caries if present during tooth development, increased susceptibility to periodontal disease via effects on alveolar bone
Other nutrients	
Carbohydrates	**Deficiency:** caries rate generally decreases when carbohydrate intake decreases in populations and individuals (**Excess:** increased frequency of any carbohydrates (other than fiber) is a causative risk factor for dental caries; cariogenic characteristics include physical form of foods, constancy of intake, total oral contact time with caries-susceptible dentition)
Fats	**Deficiency:** no direct effect/difficult to get deficiency (**Excess:** no direct effect, but fats may coat teeth and protect them against cariogenic challenges)
Proteins	**Deficiency:** defects in composition, eruption pattern, and resistance to decay during periods of tooth development, increased susceptibility to infection in soft tissues, poor healing and tissue regeneration
Water	**Deficiency:** dehydration and fragility of epithelial tissue, decreased muscle strength for chewing, xerostomia, burning tongue

Data from Martin WE. In: Chernoff R, ed. Oral health in the elderly in geriatric nutrition, the health professional's handbook. Gaithersburg, MD: Aspen Publishers, 1991;107–81. McKinney RV. Oral and dental diseases. In: Feldman EB, ed. Essentials of clinical nutrition. Philadelphia: FA Davis, 1988.

has been associated with vitamin B-complex deficiencies (101), and vitamin B-complex supplementation resolved the symptoms in 85% of subjects. A bright red, inflamed mucosa from a vitamin B-complex deficiency may be seen in long-term alcoholics. The mucosa may become pale in anemias induced by deficiency of iron, folic acid, or vitamin B_{12}. Atrophy of the filiform papillae of the tongue (glossitis) is a sign of malnutrition usually resulting from multiple nutritional deficiencies. A highly significant positive correlation between papillary health and plasma vitamin E status provides some indication that vitamin E may be a marker nutrient for papillary health (102).

In ascorbic acid deficiency, the classic oral signs of scurvy are first seen in the oral cavity, including red, swollen interdental papillae that bleed readily and inflamed, swollen marginal and attached gingiva. Although no longer a public health problem, ascorbic acid deficiency still occurs in isolated cases, usually as a result of total elimination of vitamin C sources from the diet. Most epidemiologic studies have not supported a direct relationship between periodontal disease and ascorbic acid status. However, one study did show a weak association between periodontal disease and ascorbic acid deficiency in an elderly population (103). Consumption of ascorbic acid in excess of recommended allowances has not been shown to be associated with increased periodontal health (104).

No clinical sign is of significance by itself, however, because several etiologic factors usually contribute to a differential diagnosis. For example, inflammation or cracking of the lips may be due to allergies, licking of the lips, or drooling, as well as to nutritional aberrations. Angular cheilosis can result not only from vitamin deficiencies, but also when overclosure of the jaw by denture wearers allows the skin folds at the corners of the mouth to provide a moist area for bacterial or fungal infections to develop. The painful oral lesions that result from nutrient deficiency can alter a patient's food selection and oral hygiene behavior, thus increasing the risk of oral and systemic diseases.

Nutrient Excesses

Nutrient excesses can also affect the oral cavity. Vitamin A toxicity can impair proper development of the oral mucosal epithelium and result in a variety of oral changes including delayed wound healing (105). Clinical effects reported in a patient taking 200,000 IU/day of vitamin A for over 6 months included gingival erosions and ulcerations, bleeding, swelling, loss of keratinization, and color changes in the oral cavity along with desquamation of the lips and dry mouth. Two months after withdrawal of the supplementation, all clinical manifestations had disappeared (106).

Rebound scurvy is a condition in which scurvy develops as an adaptation result of fast withdrawal after chronic high intake levels of vitamin C in animals (107). Its existence in human populations has been questioned (108), but some supportive evidence (109) has been reported clinically in patients who abruptly terminated megadosing on vitamin C. The resulting scurvy is first manifested in the oral cavity and diagnosed by the dental professional.

Periodontal Disease

Periodontal disease is a general term describing bacterial infection of either the gingiva (that part of the oral mucosa that covers the root and the apical portion of the crown) or both the gingival and the attachment apparatus (ligamentous attachment of the tooth to the surrounding alveolar bone). If the infection is confined to the gingival unit, the resulting disease is called *gingivitis*. If the infection involves destruction of the tissue attaching tooth to bone, the disease is termed *periodontitis*. The two diseases are not a continuum of the same process, but are in fact two separate diseases, each associated with different plaque flora. The etiology of gingivitis is relatively simple, that of periodontitis is extremely complex. Though bacterial plaque is the major etiologic agent in both conditions, other local and systemic factors, many unidentified, play a large role as well.

Most forms of periodontitis result in a slow loss of attachment of the tooth from the surrounding alveolar bone. Although most individuals have some mild periodontal disease, severe periodontal destruction is confined to approximately 24% of the adult population (110).

The reaction of the periodontal tissues to microbial antigens and byproducts is a classic chronic inflammatory-immune response like that observed in infectious diseases in general. Optimal functioning of the host's cellular and humoral immune system and the phagocytic system, as well as the integrity of the oral mucosa (particularly the gingival sulcular epithelium), is important for maintenance of periodontal health and prevention of periodontal disease.

Evidence directly linking diet and nutritional factors to periodontitis is somewhat controversial (111). In both the animal model and man, numerous longitudinal studies have attempted to associate either nutritional deficiency or supplementation with gingivitis. The few well-controlled animal and human longitudinal studies demonstrated associations between deficiencies of ascorbate and folate and severity of gingivitis (112–114). However, an increase in gingivitis does not necessarily mean an increase in susceptibility to periodontitis, the destructive disease that compromises tooth support.

Epidemiologic studies have attempted to link periodontitis directly to nutrition by looking at the degree of periodontal destruction in societies where malnutrition is pervasive or by attempting to relate intake of specific nutrients to the degree of periodontal destruction in well-nourished societies (115, 116). In general, there was more periodontal destruction in malnourished populations than in well-nourished societies. The role of nutrition as a contributing factor is unclear, however, since these malnourished populations consistently demonstrate poor oral hygiene as well. Massive pathogenic plaque accumulation would lead to greater loss of attachment without the possible effects of malnutrition. When the periodontal destruction measured resulted from previous disease, an attempt to correlate this with present nutritional intake is problematic.

Although little evidence links nutritional aberrations directly to periodontal disease, nutritional status has been associated with level of immune response, phagocytic activity, and mucosal integrity, all of which affect the periodontal condition (117, 118).

Nutrition may thus contribute to the pathogenesis of destructive periodontal disease. Rational assumptions for testing can be made by extrapolating data about the importance of various aspects of the host's defense mechanism to the pathogenesis of the disease and further extrapolating known relationships between nutrition and these defense mechanisms. For example, patients with deficiencies of polymorphonuclear neutrophil leukocytes (PMNs) have increased susceptibility to destructive periodontal disease (119). Thus, although little direct evidence of the interrelationships of nutrition and PMN function and periodontitis exists, chronic deficiencies of ascorbate and iron are associated with impaired PMN function, and these deficiencies could contribute to an altered host response to plaque pathogens, making the affected individual more susceptible to periodontitis.

Likewise, several animal and human studies have demonstrated a positive correlation between deficits of ascorbic acid, iron, folate, and zinc and increased permeability or diminished integrity of the gingival sulcular epithelium (an important host defense mechanism) (112, 120). Zinc deficiency in rats resulted in parakeratotic and hyperplastic buccal epithelium due to decreased keratinolytic enzyme activity (121). Dietary vitamin E supplementation accelerated gingival wound healing in albino rats and decreased alveolar bone loss in rice rats (122, 123).

A study comparing fruit farmers and grain farmers showed that periodontal pockets 4 mm and deeper occurred less frequently in workers who ate large amounts of different fruits and were the least frequent in those consuming citrus fruits (124). Malnutrition almost always has a synergistic interaction with infection. Since periodontitis is an infection, one could hypothesize that malnutrition would render the host more susceptible to destructive periodontal disease. This susceptibility to infection may be even more pronounced in the periodontium because these tissues are constantly exposed to toxic and antigenic challenges from the omnipresent bacterial plaque and thus are in a state of continuous repair.

New evidence from human aging studies gives more credence to these hypotheses (125). Periodontal diseases increase with aging, and the immune response declines in old age in both humans and animals (although older persons are less homogeneous in immune responses than younger persons). As immune function declines, the incidence of infections, cancers, and immune complex diseases increases. Nutritional deficiencies result in impaired immune response. Even children and young adults consistently show an adverse impact of nutritional deficiencies on cell-mediated immunity, complement system, secretory IgA response, and phagocyte function (125, 126). In a group of elderly with no systemic disease, those with clinical, hematologic, and biochemical evidence of nutritional deficiency also showed reduced immune function. When given appropriate nutrition guidance and supplements, immune function improved. When elders (even those with adequate diets) were given physiologic doses of vitamins and trace elements, immune response increased, and the incidence of infections decreased. The nutrients significantly correlated with improved immune response were zinc, vitamin E, folic acid, vitamin B_6 and β-carotene (117, 118, 125).

Some evidence indicates that periodontal tissues may be susceptible to end-organ deficiencies (127). In other words, although systemic levels of a specific nutrient measured biochemically in serum may be within normal limits, increased challenges at a local site may be such that levels normally considered adequate are unable to maintain optimal health at the local site. Such end-organ deficiencies have been reported in other organ systems (128).

Alveolar Bone Health, Osteoporosis, and Dentate Status

One of the more dramatic clinical signs of severe periodontal disease is resorption of alveolar bone, which ultimately results in tooth loss. The literature has long speculated that calcium deficiency is a major etiologic factor in periodontitis and that periodontal disease may foreshadow systemic metabolic bone disorders (129, 130) that then lead to tooth loss. Well-designed studies to determine whether individuals with destructive periodontal disease have any greater disposition to metabolic bone disorders or whether calcium deficiency predisposes the periodontium to destructive disease are only now emerging (131).

The alveolar process (crest of the maxilla and mandible) is composed primarily of trabecular bone. Histologically, it is the same type of bone found in the distal radius, neck of the femur, and vertebrae. When negative calcium balance occurs in the body, calcium is more easily mobilized from skeletal sites consisting of trabecular than cortical bone. Thus, the alveolar bone provides a potential labile source of calcium to meet other tissue needs. Since the alveolar process is thought to undergo resorption prior to other bones; change in the alveolar process may be used for early diagnosis of osteoporosis.

In females, a high correlation has been shown between dental bone mass and total bone mass. Women with low bone density have fewer teeth. Women with severe residual ridge resorption have osteopenia on the iliac crest, and those with severe postmenopausal osteoporosis are three times more likely to be edentulous than normal controls (132).

Approximately 32% of U.S. women and men aged 65 to 69 are edentulous (110), and tooth loss may reflect osteoporotic loss of alveolar bone. A study of 329 healthy postmenopausal women (133) showed that systemic bone loss may be associated with tooth loss. An inverse relationship was shown between bone mineral density and number of existing teeth, with women who got dentures after the age of 40 having the lowest bone mineral density. In another study, mandibular bone density in edentulous subjects showed significant correlations with bone density elsewhere in the body, especially in the hip (134). In a study of 208 postmenopausal women, those with osteoporosis were more likely to have dentures by age 60 than those without osteoporosis (135). Conversely, postmenopausal estrogen use, which protects against osteoporosis, has been associated with decreased tooth loss (136).

In another study, both mandibular bone mass and the number of teeth were strong predictors of osteoporosis (although not predictors of other periodontal indicators such as mean pocket depth or recession) (137). This study is consistent with previous observations that severe alveolar resorption was related to low bone density of the radius of edentulous subjects (137).

Mandibular bone mass correlated with total body calcium and bone mass of the radius and vertebrae in dentate and edentulous postmenopausal women with osteoporosis (130), with the highest correlation between total body and mandibular bone mass. Thus, the mandible seems to reflect the mineral status of the entire skeleton. Calcium intake in postmenopausal osteoporotic women was also correlated with mandibular density, supporting the hypothesis that low calcium intake may contribute to reduced bone density (137). Thus, the oral healthcare professional must carefully assess an individual's mandibular bone density, which can result in early diagnosis or detection of osteoporosis.

Dentate Status

Resorption of the alveolar process is a widespread problem among patients with dentures. Remodeling of the alveolar bone occurs in response to occlusal forces associated with chewing. With the loss of teeth, the alveolar bone is no longer required for tooth support; as a consequence, bone resorption is accelerated, and bone height is diminished. Bone loss is greatest during the first 6 months following tooth extractions. The reduction in residual ridge height is more pronounced in women than in men; and resorption is greater in the mandible than in the maxilla. Severe mandibular resorption makes it difficult to construct a mandibular denture with good stability and retention. Low calcium intake may compound bone loss in denture wearers. In a small group of edentulous adults, those with the greatest loss of vertical height had lower calcium intakes (138). Calcium supplementation for new denture wearers may help maintain calcium balance and may slow the rate of alveolar resorption. Positive calcium balance may be especially important to help preserve the integrity of the residual ridges of edentulous postmenopausal women.

Although an intact dentition is not absolutely essential to maintain nutritional health, loss of teeth or of the supporting periodontium can affect food selection and subsequent nutritional status. Periodontal disease with its associated tissue soreness, tooth sensitivity, bone resorption, and tooth mobility can lead to a preference for soft foods of low nutritional value and avoidance of foods requiring chewing. The same may be true for those with severe dental caries and those with dentures.

The number of missing teeth can affect masticatory efficiency and consequent food selection (139). The biting force and the ability to chew food to a particle size that can be swallowed is reduced in partially edentulous (fewer than 10–13 teeth per side of the mouth) or fully edentulous individuals (140). The average denture wearer's chewing ability is thought to be only about 20% that of the dentate adult (141).

Dentate status has also been associated with quality of nutrient intake (142, 143). In one study, individuals with one or two complete (upper and lower) dentures had a 20% decline in the nutrient quality of their diets compared with individuals with partial dentures or their own teeth (144, 145). Another study showed that edentulous participants ate fewer vegetables, less fiber and carotene, and more cholesterol, saturated fat, and calories than did participants with 25 teeth or more (146). Edentulousness has also been associated with gastrointestinal disorders (147), and among the frail elderly, poor oral health is associated with the involuntary weight loss resulting from protein-calorie malnutrition (148). Totally edentulous individuals seem to increase caloric intake after dentures are inserted and they adjust to the new prosthesis (149). The condition of existing teeth can also affect diet. Large carious lesions and considerable loss of periodontal attachment resulting in mobile teeth leads to a preference for soft foods of lower nutrient density and avoidance of hard or fibrous foods that require chewing.

Dentures can also affect taste and swallowing ability, especially if they are maxillary (upper) dentures. The denture covers the upper palate where some taste buds are located and thus can blunt normal taste sensitivity. An upper denture can also impede swallowing. When the upper palate is covered, it is difficult for the tongue to determine the location of food in the mouth. As a result, dentures are said to be the major cause of choking in adults (150).

The dentally impaired can maintain good nutriture by continuing to choose nutritious foods of more chewable consistency, by eating more slowly, by chewing longer, and by cooking foods and/or cutting them into bite-sized pieces.

Food-Related Injury

Thermal or mechanical injury can result from drinking hot beverages, chewing ice cubes, or puncturing oral tissues and cause tooth or mouth pain. This, in turn, may alter an individual's food selection behavior. Fortunately, the oral tissues turn over more rapidly than other body tissues, possibly as an adaptation to just such insults. As a result, tissue repair is fairly rapid and should not cause long-term dietary problems. Tooth sensitivity is often associated with gingival recession, which is common in middle-aged and older adults. Other causes of sensitivity include toothbrush abrasion, caries, and the side effects of periodontal treatment. Tooth sensitivity sometimes can be corrected by use of over-the-counter desensitizing products.

Failure to Thrive in Children

Oral conditions are often overlooked as contributing factors to eating problems or failure to thrive (FTT) in children. Sore teeth and gums may lead a child to avoid chewing or eating. The foods they will or can eat may not provide adequate calories or nutritional value to meet their growth needs (151). If caregivers are not alerted to look for oral problems, or if the children are not receiving regular dental care, the oral implications may be missed.

Oral Surgery

In general oral surgical situations, food consumption is impaired for a relatively short period of time, and the risk of nutritional deficiency is low, except in those already at nutritional risk. A soft or liquid diet and multivitamin supplementation may be recommended. For the patient who has a wired jaw, however, eating may be totally impaired for long periods of time, and nutritional status can suffer unless appropriate dietary guidelines are provided. Often patients prefer purees of normal foods to commercial liquid supplements. Diet suggestions *must* be provided that allow these individuals to meet their caloric needs via liquid food sources alone (152).

Oral Infections and Immune Deficiency Diseases

Oral infections such as herpes simplex and oral candidiasis can result in painful oral lesions that impair the desire and ability to eat. Usually, palliative oral care and appropriate food choices (bland, easily masticated) effectively help maintain nutritional status. However, when these conditions are longstanding (e.g., in HIV-AIDS), nutritional status can be undermined, thus contributing to further virulence of the disease.

The oral cavity is a principal site of lesions associated with human immunodeficiency virus (HIV) infection, which are often painful and drastically limit the intake of nutrients at a time when nutrition is essential. These lesions include HIV-associated gingivitis and periodontitis, oral candidiasis, recurrent herpes simplex infection, xerostomia, and Kaposi's sarcoma. Curative or palliative therapy for these lesions is relatively successful in allowing normal ingestion of nutrients. Excellent reviews on the management of these lesions are available (153, 154). The occurrence of many of these lesions can be drastically curtailed or their severity reduced by the use of prophylactic regimens. Unfortunately, oral manifestations of HIV are often ignored until they reach crisis proportion and contribute to the anorexia-cachexia syndrome common to cancer patients.

Crohn's disease may have oral manifestations such as ulcers, lip fissures, angular cheilitis, polypoid lesions, perioral erythema, and gingival bleeding in addition to weight loss and diarrhea. Pyostomatitis vegetans is a rare eruption of the oral mucosa that is characterized by small yellow pustules and is considered a marker for inflammatory bowel disease. In one study, oral zinc supplementation caused regression of the pyostomatitis vegetans leading to the conclusion that this oral lesion may be caused by zinc deficiency secondary to malabsorption (155).

Oral and Pharyngeal Cancers

In 1996 it was estimated that 8260 Americans would die from oral cancers. Oral cancer was projected to comprise 2% (29,490) of all 1996 estimated new cancer cases in the United States (155a). The 5-year relative survival rate for persons with oral cancers is 52%, among the lowest survival rates of the major cancers. Most of these malignant neoplasms are squamous cell carcinomas. Tobacco use and heavy alcohol consumption are considered the primary causative agents of oral cancers (155b), and a variety of consumables such as charcoal-grilled and salt-preserved foods have been implicated as well (156).

Recent evidence is mounting that several foods and food factors protect against oral carcinomas. The protective effect of liberal fruit and vegetable consumption has been the most consistent finding (157). Antioxidant nutrients, β-carotene, and vitamin E have shown oral chemopreventive effects in animal models, epidemiologic surveys (158), intervention trials to reverse premalignancies (159–161), and prevention of malignancies in high-risk persons. In a case-controlled cohort study of 25,802 adults, serum levels of all individual carotenoids, especially β-carotene, were lower in subjects who developed oral and pharyngeal cancer, and the risks of malignancy decreased with increasing serum level of each carotenoid. Those in the highest tertile of total carotenoids had one-third lower cancer risk than those in the lowest tertile (158). In a study of cigarette smokers in the United States, β-carotene supplementation at 30 mg/day for 6 months resulted in complete or partial remission of precancerous lesions in 71% of participants (162). A study by Toma had a 44% response rate with 90 mg β-carotene daily for 6 months (159). A 60% response rate was reported in a group given 24 mg/day of β-carotene, 1000 mg/day of vitamin C, and 800 mg/day of vitamin E (163).

In laboratory and animal studies, both β-carotene and vitamin E can inhibit oral carcinogenesis and cause clinical regression of oral leukoplakia (160), which is a precursor to oral cancer. However, methodological difficulties have resulted in less definitive results in humans to date (164, 165).

Radiation therapy for head and neck cancers causes several conditions that can adversely affect systemic nutrition (166, 166a). If not treated prior to irradiation, chronic pulpal and periodontal infections can become acute because of radiation-associated changes and can lead to osteoradionecrosis. These lesions are extremely painful and difficult to treat and can impair systemic nutrition for months. Radiation therapy can also lead to oral mucositis with complications similar to those previously described for the chemotherapeutic patient. In addition, if the radiation beam passes through the major salivary glands, fibrosis of the gland occurs, with all the resultant problems associated with xerostomia. If the salivary glands are not the primary foci of irradiation, lead shields can be individually fabricated for the patient to protect the glands from unnecessary irradiation. If the radiation beam is aimed through the muscles of mastication, fibrosis of the musculature may occur. This fibrosis results in limitation of mandibular movement, called trismus, which usually becomes evident 3 to 6 months after irradiation. Trismus makes it difficult for patients to consume a normal diet. Though it will not stop fibrosis of the musculature, physiotherapy, such as range-of-motion and isometric exercises starting prior to the onset of the fibrosis, can decrease the extent of mandibular immobility (167).

Some of the same oral lesions associated with HIV infections are also seen in cancer patients undergoing chemotherapy. The antimetabolic activity of these drugs often induces a mucositis (see Chapter 82), rendering the tissues more susceptible to physical trauma from sharp tooth edges and hard bits of food. Ulceration, secondary infection, and painful stomatitis may result. Generally, the more intense the cytotoxic therapy, the more common the oral complications. Proper prophylactic therapy prior to chemotherapy can prevent or minimize many lesions and result in fewer problems in ingesting required nutrients (168).

Surveys show that between 60 and 64% of head and neck cancer patients are nutritionally compromised at the time of initial diagnosis (169). The amount of weight loss prior to surgery is a good predictor of the risk of developing postoperative complications. Depending on the procedure, food intake may be severely compromised after surgery, and it should be closely monitored throughout treatment. The least invasive method of providing essential nutrients to maintain weight should be used. Blended foods given by mouth are tolerated by some patients. If adequate calories cannot be obtained orally, tube or parenteral feeding must be provided (see Chapters 100 and 101); however, oral feeding should resume as soon as possible in oral cancer patients (170).

Since oral and pharyngeal cancers are very prevalent, carry extremely high morbidity and morality rates, and are highly detectable, all healthcare providers should work closely to identify early those patients with signs and symptoms of cancer. Appropriate and timely therapy is essential to increase survival from this very detectable and often visible cancer.

Effects of Saliva on Oral Health and Nutrition

Saliva is a primary factor in both the function and maintenance of the oral cavity. In addition to being important in speech and deglutition, certain antimicrobial and nonantimicrobial systems in saliva protect both the hard and soft tissues of the mouth. Cessation or severe decrease of salivary flow from such causes as surgical removal of salivary glands, radiation therapy, and Sjögren's syndrome can lead to microbial infection of the oral cavity, rampant caries, and loss of taste acuity, as well as inability to lubricate, masticate, and swallow food. All these conditions have a profound effect on food selection and thus on systemic nutrition. In fact, significant deficiencies of fiber, vitamin B_6, iron, calcium and zinc were found in xerostomic older adults (171). Comfort in wearing dentures depends on lubrication of the soft tissues by saliva. Patients with oral dryness retain their dentures poorly and may develop ulcerations at denture borders that make mastication difficult and painful.

It was once believed that the aging process brought with it a "natural" reduction of salivary flow, but in fact, salivary flow in healthy individuals does not decrease due to age (172). Nearly 50% of elderly subjects are taking medications that diminish salivary flow; however, though salivary flow is decreased in these individuals, it generally still does not interfere with either deglutition or maintenance of hard and soft tissues (173). Nonetheless, these patients often feel as if their mouths are dry and frequently use hard candies or gum to stimulate salivary flow throughout the day. Because most candies and gum contain fermentable carbohydrates, the constant exposure may promote root caries and altered food intake because of discomfort or loss of integrity of the dentition. Patients taking xerostomia-producing drugs should be counseled about side effects and should be advised to use candies and gums containing relatively nonfermentable sugar alcohols such as sorbitol, mannitol, or xylitol. Table 66.5 lists xerostomia-inducing drugs by class. The use of artificial saliva, though not a panacea, may benefit some of these patients. To prevent rampant caries in such individuals, aggressive home care emphasizing effective oral hygiene and daily fluoride application is usually recommended.

Acid Reflux Disorders (Gastroesophageal Reflux and Bulimia)

Both gastric reflux and self-induced vomiting observed in eating disorders (see Chapter 93) commonly irritate oral

Table 66.5
Xerostomia-Inducing Drugs by Class

Analgesics	Antiinflammatory agents
Anticholinergics	Antiparkinson agents
Antidepressants	Antipsychotic agents
Antihypertensive agents	Decongestants
Systemic antihistamines/decongestants	Diuretics
Systemic bronchodilators	Gastrointestinal agents

Adapted from Levy SM, Baker KA Semla TP, et al. Gerodontics 1988;4:121.

tissues and destroy dental enamel (174). The extent of oral tissue damage depends on the frequency of the purging and cariogenicity of the diet. Because they are often the first healthcare providers to see these patients, dentists may make an early diagnosis of eating disorders. Some symptoms that may cause these patients to seek dental treatment are sensitivity to hot and cold temperatures or air, dental pain, and concern about the appearance of their teeth.

The most obvious clinical symptom of bulimia nervosa is loss of tooth enamel and dentin on the lingual and incisal surfaces of anterior teeth and occlusal surfaces of posterior teeth. Enamel erosion is primarily caused by chronic regurgitation of the acidic contents of the stomach. Erosion may also result from frequent intake of fruit juices high in citric acid, sucking on chewable vitamin C tablets, disulfiram (Antabuse) therapy for alcoholism, or exposure to industrial acids. Contact and thermal hypersensitivity occurs when the dentin is exposed. The acidic oral environment irritates the oral mucosa, including the gingiva, palate, and pharynx. With repeated vomiting, esophageal tears may develop. The lips may become cracked, and fissures may develop at the corners of the mouth. Enlargement of the parotid glands, which are painful to palpation, may occur 2 to 6 days after vomiting. Patients with eating disorders have lower resting salivary flow rates than normal adults, which may result in xerostomia (175, 176).

Dental treatment must be coordinated with the primary healthcare provider. Definitive restorative treatment cannot occur until the vomiting behavior is under control. Temporary restorations are placed on eroded tooth surfaces to prevent further loss of enamel and to prevent hypersensitivity. The patient is encouraged to practice meticulous oral hygiene. Patients are cautioned against brushing immediately after vomiting, to prevent further erosion of dental enamel. Instead, a sodium bicarbonate or magnesium hydroxide rinse is recommended to neutralize acid in the mouth. Neutral pH sodium fluoride rinses (0.5%) or home application of stannous fluoride gels (0.4%) in custom trays will prevent dental erosion and enhance remineralization of teeth (177). Patients should be counseled to limit fruit juices with high citric acid content and to avoid sticky, sweet foods between meals. Foods of low cariogenicity—nuts, seeds, cheese and vegetables—are desirable snacks. If dry mouth is a problem, chewing paraffin wax, sugarless chewing gum, or sugar-free lemon drops may stimulate saliva flow.

The Aging Patient

In the past three decades, the population of individuals age 65 and up has increased by 85.8%, and the population over age 85 increased by 225% (178). The aging process involves a host of changes that can affect and be affected by the oral condition. Dental problems are considered a primary contributor to malnutrition in the elderly (148). Sore or missing teeth make it difficult to consume a normal diet. When an individual is edentulous or has ill-fitting dentures, diet quality often suffers (145), and the soft consistency of manageable foods can lead to constipation. With age, the sense of smell declines (179), often leading to increased use of cariogenic foods. It was formerly believed, on the basis of threshold studies, that advancing age produced taste loss as well, which could also contribute to decreased nutrient intake. However, these elevations in threshold are relatively small and have fewer clinical effects. The hypogeusia observed in some elderly individuals is possibly associated with specific disorders leading to taste loss, rather than being a normal component of the aging process (180). Xerostomia is common because of multiple drug use and often results in root caries. Nearly 50% of those aged 75 and older take two or more medications daily (181), and one-third to one-half of older adults may experience xerostomia (182). With between 68% of those 65 to 69 years old and 51% of those over 80 being at least partially dentate, dental caries remains a potential problem. Root caries affects over 60% of dentate individuals, and the caries rate increases with age (183). Periodontal disease is also a problem for older adults, with approximately one-third showing evidence of severe periodontitis (183). Oral cancer is also more common with age, almost tripling between the 55- to 64-year-old group and those aged 85 or older. Tooth loss, pain, malpositioning, loss of vertical dimension, joint dysfunction, and dental prostheses can all impair mastication. In addition, social interactions surrounding eating, and subsequent nutrition can be impaired by mobile or fractured teeth and the condition and/or retention of dental prostheses (181).

Since the elderly are at particular risk of nutritional and oral problems, all health professionals are encouraged to broaden the scope of their routine screening beyond their own discipline. To accomplish this, the Nutrition Screening Initiative (a collaborative project between the American Academy of Family Physicians, the American Dietetic Association, and the National Council on the Aging) has developed simple screening questionnaires based on the major contributors to nutritional risk for use by health professionals in screening the elderly (184). There are screening forms for medical problems, drug interactions, psychosocial factors, nutrition, and oral health. When used consistently, all healthcare providers, including nutritionists and dental professionals, will be able to screen for a variety of factors contributing to nutritional risk and refer to the appropriate provider for further care.

Diabetes and Oral Health

The diabetic condition increases the risk and severity of periodontal disease. In both type I and type II diabetes mellitus, physiologic changes result in a decrease in overall resistance. Increased oral infections and *Candida albicans* are common (181). Severe periodontal problems and tooth loss are often associated with poorly controlled diabetes. In one recent study, tooth loss was significantly associated with non-insulin-dependent diabetes and obesity in adults. Functionally edentulous subjects (<6 teeth) were found to be at significantly greater risk for NIDDM than those who were partially edentulous (7–25 teeth) or dentate. Since obesity was also significantly associated with greater risk for NIDDM, this appeared to confound the relationship between functional edentulism and NIDDM (185). When diabetes is poorly controlled, frequent use of hard candies may counteract bouts of hypoglycemia. This habit, combined with the xerostomia common to diabetes, can lead to rampant dental caries.

With proper management techniques, oral health can be maintained despite the diabetes. A regimen of controlled diet, conscientious and effective oral hygiene, and topical fluoride when indicated, can maintain oral health integrity throughout life (186, 187).

SUMMARY: IMPLICATIONS FOR THE FUTURE

Observations made in recent years suggest that diet and nutrition are intimately linked to general and oral tissue health promotion and disease prevention (188). The oral condition can have a major influence on diet and ultimate nutritional status. Conversely, food choices can affect oral tissues directly and indirectly. Research findings linking systemic nutritional factors and oral conditions in humans are expanding rapidly, complementing the traditional relationships between local dietary factors and dentition.

The discovery that people can change their eating behavior as a consequence of aggressive health promotion and disease prevention programs and that better, more sensitive measures of nutritional status exist, will have a major impact on our understanding of nutrient–oral tissue relationships and subsequent dietary intervention programs. The key role of the oral healthcare professional identifying patients at risk for systemic nutrition-related disease is essential in providing early entry into the healthcare system. In this regard, *Healthy People 2000* places nutrition and oral health in the appropriate context, articulating that lifestyle and systemic health are associated with oral health, and setting goals for achieving better oral health outcomes. The impact of nutrition on dental education and clinical practice will be profound, provided appropriate academic programs are implemented to train investigators and clinicians in nutrition and oral health science. The consequences will be nothing short of integrating dental medicine more closely into the healthcare delivery system and improving public health and welfare.

REFERENCES

1. Grau AJ, Buggle F, Hacke W. Nervenarzt 1996;67:639–49.
2. Beck J, Garcia R, Heiss G, et al. J Periodontol 1996;67(10 Suppl):1123–37.
3. Offenbacher S, Katz U, Fertik G, et al. J Periodontol 1996;67 (10 Suppl):1103–13.
4. Shaw JH, Sweeney EA. Nutrition in relation to dental medicine. In: Shils ME, Young VR. Modern nutrition in health and disease. 7th ed. Philadelphia: Lea & Febiger, 1988;1070–1.
5. Surgeon General's report on nutrition and health: dental diseases. U.S. Department of Health & Human Services, publ. no. 88-50210. Washington, DC: U.S. Government Printing Office, 1988;345–80.
6. Dreizen S. Pediatrician 1989;16:139–46.
7. Sweeney EA, Saffir AJ, deLeon R. Am J Clin Nutr 1971;4: 29–31.
8. Sawyer DR, Kwoku AL. J Dent Child 1985;54:141–5.
9. Punysingh JT, Hoffman S, Harris SS, et al. J Oral Pathol 1984;13:40–57.
10. Boyle PE. J Dent Res 1933;13:139–50.
11. Slavkin H. J Am Dent Assoc 1996;127:681–2.
12. Kim YS, Stumpf WA, Clark SA, et al. J Dent Res 1983;62:58–9.
13. Leaver AG. Clin Orthop 1971;8:90–107.
14. Bawden JW. Anat Rec 1989;24:226–33.
15. Mellanby M. Br Dent J 1923;44:1031–41.
16. Wolf JJ. Am J Dis Child 1935;49:905–11.
17. Boyle PE. J Dent Res 1934;14:172.
18. Schiltz JR, Rosenbloom J, Levinson GE. J Embryol Exp Morphol 1977;37:49–57.
19. Alvarez JO, Eguren JC, Caleda J, et al. J Dent Res 1990;69: 1564–6.
20. Alvarez JO, Navia JM. Am J Clin Nutr 1989;49:417–26.
21. Alvarez JO, Lewis CA, Saman C, et al. Am J Clin Nutr 1988; 48:368–72.
22. Rami-Reddy V, Vijayalakshmi PB, Chandrasekhar-Reddy BK. Odont Pediatr 1986;7:1–5.
23. Delgado H, Habicht JP, Yarbrough C, et al. Am J Clin Nutr 1975;38:216–24.
24. Menaker L, Navia JM. J Dent Res 1973;52:688–91.
25. National Institute of Dental Research. Mineralized tissues, craniofacial development, dentofacial malrelations and trauma. In: Broadening the scope: long-range research plan for the nineties. NIH publ. no. 90-1188. Washington, DC: U.S. Government Printing Office, 1990.
26. Iber FL. Nutr Today 1990;15:5.
27. Slavkin HC. Cleft Palate J 1990;27:101–9.
28. Slavkin HC. J Am Dent Assoc 1997;128:1308–13.
29. Akam M. Cell 1989;57:347–9.
30. Lammer EJ, Chen DT, Hoar RM, et al. N Engl J Med 1985;313:837–41.
31. Slavkin HC. Personal communication, 1992.
32. MRC Vitamin Study Research Group. Lancet 1991;338:131–7.
33. Tolarova M, Harris J. Teratology 1995;51:71–8.
34. Kaste LM, Selwitz RJ, Oldakowski JA, et al. J Dent Res 1996; 75(Spec Iss):631–41.
35. Gift HC, Drury TF, Nowjack-Raymer RE, J Public Health Dent 1996;56:84–91.
36. Winn DM, Brunelle JA, Selwitz RH, et al. J Dent Res 1996;75(Spec Iss):642–51.
37. Oral health of United States adults. The National Survey of Oral Health in U.S. Employed Adults and Seniors, 1985–1986. NIH publ. (PHS) 87-2868.
38. Navia JM. Am J Clin Nutr 1994;59:719S–27S.
39. Stephan RJ. J Am Dent Res 1940;27:718–23.
40. Fitzgerald RJ, Keyes PH. J Am Dent Assoc 1960;61:9–19.

41. Loesche W. Microbiol Rev 1986;50:353–80.
42. Tanzer JM. J Dent Res 1986;65(Spec Iss):1491–7.
43. Konig KG, Schmid P, Schmid R. Arch Oral Biol 1968;13: 13–26.
44. Eriksen HM, Grythen J, Holst D. Acta Odontol Scand 1991; 49:163–7.
45. Sreebny LM. World Rev Nutr Diet 1982;40:19–65.
46. Gibney M, Sigman-Grant M, Stanton JL, et al. Am J Clin Nutr 1995;62:178S–94S.
47. Konig KG, Navia JM. Am J Clin Nutr 1995;62:275S–83S.
48. Ishii T, Konig KG, Muhlemann HR. Helv Odontol Acta 1968;12:41–7.
49. Harris R. J Dent Res 1963;42:1387–99.
50. Rugg-Gunn AJ, Hackett AF, Appleton DR. Caries Res 1987;21:464–78.
51. Grobler SR, Blignaut JB. Clin Prev Dent 1989;11:8–12.
52. Birkhed D. Caries Res 1984;18:120–7.
53. Ismail Al, Burt BA, Eklund SA. J Am Dent Assoc 1984;109: 241–5.
54. Motokawa W, Braham R, Ishii K, et al. Quintessence Int 1990; 21:983–7.
55. Maguire A, Rugg-Gunn AJ, Butler TJ. Caries Res 1996;30: 16–21.
56. Makinen KK, Isokangas P. Prog Food Nutr Sci 1988;12: 73–109.
57. Kalfas S, Svansater D, Birkhed D, et al. J Dent Res 1990;69: 442–6.
58. Scheinen A, Makinen KK. Acta Odontol Scand 1975;34: 179–216.
59. Tanzer JM, Slee AM. J Am Dent Assoc 1983;106:331–3.
60. Lout RK, Messer LB, Soberay A, et al. Caries Res 1988; 22:237–41.
61. Soderling E, Makinen KK, Chen CY. Caries Res 1989;23: 378–84.
62. Scheinen A, Makinen KK, Larmas M. Acta Odontol Scand 1975;39:269–78.
63. Newbrun E, Hoover C, Mettrauz G, et al. J Am Dent Assoc 1980;101:619–26.
64. Mundorff SA, Featherstone JDB, Bibby BC, et al. Caries Res 1990;24:344–55.
65. Pollard MA, Imfeld T, Higham SM, et al. Caries Res 1996;30:132–7.
66. Gustaffsson B, Quensel SE, Svenander-Lanke L, et al. Acta Odontol Scand 1954;11:232–64.
67. Ismail Al. J Dent Res 1986;65:1435–40.
68. Burt BA, Eklund SA, Morgan KJ, et al. J Dent Res 1988;67: 1422–9.
69. Rugg-Gunn AJ, Edgar WM, Jenkins GN. J Dent Res 1981;60: 867–72.
70. Lagerlof F, Oliveby A. Adv Dent Res 1994;8:229–38.
71. Jensen ME, Harlander SK, Schachtele CF, et al. Evaluation of the acidogenic and antacid properties of cheeses by telemetric recording of dental plaque. In: Hefferen JJ, Koehler HM, Osborn JC, eds. Food, nutrition and dental health. Park Forest South, IL: Pathotox, 1984.
72. Silva MF, Jenkins GN, Burgess RC, et al. Caries Res 1986;20: 263–9.
73. DePaola DP. J Dent Res 1986;65(Spec Iss):1540–3.
74. Schachtele CF, Harlander SK. J Can Dent Assoc 1984;50:213–9.
75. Winn DV, Brunelle JH, Selwitz RH, et al. J Dent Res 1996;75(Spec Iss):642–51.
76. van Houte J, Jordan R, Laraway R, et al. J Dent Res 1990;69:1463–8.
77. Ravald N, Hemp SE, Birkhed D. J Clin Periodontol 1986;13: 758–67.
78. Papas AS, Joshi A, Belanger AJ, et al. Am J Clin Nutr 1995;61:417S–22S.
79. Papas AS, Joshi A, Palmer CA, et al. Am J Clin Nutr 1995;61:423S–9S.
80. Papas AS, Palmer CA, McGandy R, et al. Gerodontics 1987;3:30–7.
81. Papas AS, Palmer CA, Rounds MC, et al. Ann NY Acad Sci 1989;561:124– 42.
82. Billings RJ. J Public Health Dent 1996;56:37.
83. O'Sullivan DV, Tinanoff N. J Dent Res 1993;72:1577–8.
84. Ripa LW. Pediatr Dent 1988;10:28–82.
85. Berkowitz R. J Public Health Dent 1996;56:51–4.
86. Gardner DE, Norwood JR, Eisenson JE. J Dent Child 1977;44: 186–91.
87. Bruerd B, Jone C. Public Health Rep 1995;111:63–5.
88. Department of Health and Human Services, Public Health Service. Review of fluoride benefits and risks. Report of the Ad Hoc Subcommittee on Fluoride of the Committee to Coordinate Environmental Health & Related Programs. Washington, DC: U.S. Government Printing Office, 1991.
89. Dean HT. Epidemiological studies in the United States. In: Moulton FR, ed. Dental caries and fluoride. Washington, DC: American Association for Advancement of Science, 1946.
90. Murray JJ, Rugg-Gunn AJ. Fluorides and dental caries. 2nd ed. Briston, England: John Wright & Sons, 1982.
91. Brunelle JA, Carlos JP. J Dent Res 1990;69(Spec Iss):723–7.
92. Newbrun E. J Public Health Dent 1989;49:279–89.
93. Centers for Disease Control and Prevention. MMWR 1992;41:372–81.
94. Jakush J. ADA News May 16,1996.
95. Kula K, Wei SHY. Fluoride supplements and dietary sources of fluoride. In: Wei SHY, ed. Clinical uses of fluoride. Philadelphia: Lea & Febiger, 1985.
96. Leverett DH, Vaughn BW, Adair SM, et al. (Abstract) J Public Health Dent 1993;53:205.
97. Ismail Al, Messer JG. J Public Health Dent 1996;56:22–7.
98. Brunelle JA. J Dent Res 1989;68:995.
99. Levy SM, Kahout FJ, Firitsy MC, et al. J Am Dent Assoc 1995;126:1625–32.
100. Pendry DG. J Am Dent Assoc 1995;126:1617–24.
101. Lamey PJ, Allam BF. Br Dent J 1986;160:81–3.
102. Drinka P, Langer E, Voeks S, et al. J Am Coll Nutr 1993;12:1, 14–20.
103. Ismail Al, Burk BA, Eklund SA. J Am Dent Assoc 1984;109:241–5.
104. Woolfe SN, Hume WR, Kenney EP. J West Soc Periodontol-Perio Abstracts 1980;28(2):44–56.
105. Hathcock J, Hattan DC, Jenkins M, et al. Am J Clin Nutr 1990;52:183–202.
106. DeMenezes AC, Costa IM, El-Guindy MM. J Periodontol 1984;55:474–6.
107. Tsao CS, Leung PY. J Nutr 1988;118:895–900.
108. Gerster H, Moser V. Nutr Res 1988;8:1327–32.
109. Omaye ST, Skala JH, Jacob RA. Am J Clin Nutr 1988;48:379–81.
110. National Institute of Dental Research. Oral health of U.S. adults: the national survey of oral health in United States employed adults and seniors: 1985–86. NIH publ no. 87-2868. Washington, DC: U.S. Government Printing Office, 1987.
111. Alfano MC. Dent Clin North Am 1976;20:519–48.
112. Alvares O, Siegel I. J Oral Pathol 1981;10:40–8.
113. Alvares O, Altman LC, Springmeyer S, et al. J Periodont Res 1981;16:628–36.
114. Leggott, PJ, Robertson PB, Rothman DC, et al. J Periodontol 1986;57:480–5.

115. Russell AL. J Dent Res 1963;42:233–47.
116. Burt AA, Eklund SA, Landis JR, et al. A study of dietary intake food patterns and dental health. Analysis of data from the HANES I Survey. Ann Arbor, MI: University of Michigan, 1980.
117. Meydani SN, Barklund PM, Liu S, et al. Am J Clin Nutr 1990;52:557–63.
118. Meydani S. Nutr Rev 1995;53:4:S52–8.
119. Genco RJ, Wilson ME, DeNardin E. Periodontal complications and neutrophil abnormalities. In: Genco R, Goldman H, Cohen DW, eds. Contemporary periodontitis. St. Louis: CV Mosby, 1990.
120. Vogel RI, Lanster IB, Wechsler SA, et al. J Periodontol 1986:472–79.
121. Hsu DJ, Daniel JC, Gerson SJ. Arch Oral Biol 1991;36:759–63.
122. Kim JE, Shklar G. J Periodont 1983:54:305–58.
123. Cohen ME, Meyer DM. Arch Oral Biol 1993;38(7):601–6.
124. Blignaut JB, Grobler SR. Clin Prev Dent 1992;14:25–8.
125. Chandra R. Nutr Rev 1995;53:4(pt 2)S80–5.
126. Bendich A, Chandra RK. Micronutrients and immune functions. New York: New York Academy of Sciences, 1990.
127. Malleck HM. An investigation of the role of ascorbic acid and iron in the etiology of gingivitis in humans. Doctoral thesis. Cambridge, MA, Institute Archives, Massachusetts Institute of Technology, 1978.
128. Whitehead N, Ryner F, Lindenbaum J. JAMA 1973;226: 1421–4.
129. Whalen J, Krook L. (Editorial) Nutrition 1996;12:53–4.
130. Kribbs PJ. J Prosthet Dent 1990;63:86–9.
131. Proceedings of the workshop on osteoporosis and oral bone loss. Leesburg, VA. Aug 26–28, 1992. J Bone Miner Res Dec 1993;8(Suppl 2):S443–606.
132. Jeffcoat MK, Chesnut C. J Am Dent Assoc 1993;124:49–56.
133. Krall EA, Dawson-Hughes B, Papas A, Garcia RI. Osteoporosis Int 1994;4:104–9.
134. Houki K, DiMuzio MT, Fattore L. J Bone Miner Res 1994;9(Suppl 1):S211.
135. Daniel HW. Arch Intern Med 1983;143:1678–82.
136. Grodstein F, Colditz G, Stampfer M. J Am Dent Assoc 1996;127:370–7.
137. Kribbs PJ. J Prosthet Dent 1990;63:218–22.
138. Wical KE, Swoope CC. J Prosthet Dent 1974;32:13–22.
139. Chauncy HH, Muench ME, Kapur KK, et al. Int Dent J 1984;34:98–104.
140. Wayler AH, Muench ME, Kapur KK, et al. J Gerontol 1984;39:284–9.
141. Kapur KK, Soman KK. J Prosthet Dent 1964;14:1054–64.
142. Sebring NG, Guckes AD, Li S, McCarthy GR. J Prosthet Dent 1995;74:358–63.
143. Greksa LP, Parraga IM, Clark CA. J Prosthet Dent 1995;73:142–5.
144. McGandy RB, Russell RM, Hartz SC. Nutr Res 1986;6:785–98.
145. Papas A, Herman J, Palmer C, et al. Gerodontology 1984;3:147–55.
146. Joshipura K, Willett W, Douglass C. J Am Dent Assoc 1996;127:459–67.
147. Brodeur J, Laurin D, Vallee R, Lachapelle D. J Prosthet Dent 1993;70:468–73.
148. Sullivan DH, Martin W, Flaxman N, Hagen JE. J Am Geriatr Soc 1993;41:725–31.
149. Rimm EWB, Ascherio A, Giovannucci E, et al. Am J Epidemiol 1995;141:S17.
150. Anderson DA. Int Dent J 1977;27:349.
151. McKinney L, Palmer C, Dwyer JT, Garcia R. Top Clin Nutr 1991:6:70–5.
152. Patten JA. Compend Contin Educ Dent 1995;16:200–14.
153. Robertson PB, Greenspan JS. Perspectives on oral manifestations of AIDS: diagnosis and management of HIV-associated infections. Littleton, MA: PSG Publishing. 1988.
154. Winkler JR, Murray PA, Grassi M, et al. J Am Dent Assoc 1989;119(Suppl):25S–34S.
155. Ficarra G, Cicchi P, Armorosi A, Piluso S. Oral Surg Oral Med Oral Pathol 1993;75:220–4.
155a. Parker SL, TongT, Bolden S, et al. CA 1996;46:5–27.
155b. Winn DM. Am J Clin Nutr 1995;61(Suppl):437S–45S.
156. DeStefani E, Oreggia F, Ronco A, et al. Cancer Epidemiol Biomarkers Prev 1994;3:381–5.
157. Gridely G, McLaughlin JK, Block WJ, et al. Am J Epidemiol 1992;135:1083–92.
158. Zheng W, Blot W, Diamond E, et al. Cancer Res 1993;53: 795–8.
159. Toma S, Benso S, Albanese E, et al. Oncology 1992;49:77–81.
160. Benner S, Winn R, Lippman S, et al. J Natl Cancer Inst 1993;85:1:44–7.
161. Stich JH, Rosin MP, Hornby AO, et al. Int J Cancer 1988;42:195–9.
162. Garewal HS. Ann NY Acad Sci 1992;669:261–7.
163. Kaugers G, Brandt R. Carcaise-Edinboro P, et al. Oral Surg Oral Med Oral Pathol 1990;70:607–8.
164. Garewal H. Am J Clin Nutr 1995;62(Suppl):1410S–16S.
165. Garewal H, Meyskens F, Friedman S, et al. Prev Med 1993;22:701–11.
166. Nikoskelainen J. J Clin Periodont 1990;17:504–7.
166a. NIH Consensus Development Panel. NCI Monogr 1990;9.
167. Montgomery MT. Irradiation. In: Rose L, Kaye D, eds. Internal medicine for dentistry. St. Louis: CV Mosby, 1990;393–4.
168. Toth BB, Martin JW, Flemming RJ, Clin Periodontol 1990;17:508–15.
169. Bassett MR, Dobie RA. Otolaryngol Head Neck Surg 1983;91:119–25.
170. Dwyer J, Efstathion A, Palmer C, Papas A. Nutr Rev 1991;49:11:332–7.
171. Rhodus NL, Brown J. J Am Diet Assoc 1990;90:1688–92.
172. Heft MW, Baum BJ. J Dent Res 1984;63:1182–5.
173. Beck JD, Hunt RJ. J Dent Educ 1985;49:407–25.
174. Schroeder PL, Filler SJ, Ramirez B, et al. Ann Intern Med 1995;122:809–10.
175. Tylenda AA, Robert MW, Elin RJ. J Am Dent Assoc 1991;122:37–41.
176. Brown S, Bonifazi DZ. Compend Contin Educ Dent 1993;141:1596–1602.
177. Gross KBW, Brough KM, Randolph PM. J Dent Child 1986;53:378–81.
178. U.S. Bureau of the Census. Statistical abstract of the United States 1991. 111th ed. Washington, DC: U.S. Government Printing Office.
179. Schiffman SS. Taste and smell losses with age. Contemporary Nutrition, General Mills Nutrition Department 1991; 16(2):6–8.
180. Bartoshuk LM. Chemical sensation: taste. In: Pollack R, Kravitz R, eds. Nutrition in oral health and disease. Philadelphia: Lea & Febiger, 1985.
181. Berkey D, Berg R, Ettinger R, et al. JADA 1996;127:321–32.
182. Atkinson JC, Fox PC. Salivary gland dysfunction. In: Baum BJ, ed. Clinics in geriatric medicine. Oral and dental problems in the elderly. Philadelphia: WB Saunders, 1992;8:499–511.
183. U.S. Public Health Service, National Institute of Dental Research. Oral health of United States adults: national findings. NIH publ. no. (PHS) 88-1593, series 10, no. 165. Washington, DC: U.S. Government Printing Office, 1988.

184. Nutrition screening manual for professionals caring for older Americans. Nutrition screening initiative, 2626 Pennsylvania Avenue NW, Suite 301, Washington, DC 20037.
185. Cleary TJ, Hutton JE. Diabetes Care 1995;18:1007–9.
186. Holdren RS, Patton LL. Diabetes Spectrum 1993;6:11–7.
187. Touger-Decker R, Sirois D. Dental care of the person with diabetes. In: Powers MA, ed. Handbook of diabetes nutrition management. 2nd ed. Rockville, MD: Aspen, 1996.
188. Navia JM. Am J Clin Nutr 1995;61(Suppl):407S–9S.

SELECTED READINGS

Bowen WH, Tabak L. Cariology for the nineties. Rochester: University of Rochester Press, 1993.

Curzon MEJ, tenCate JM, eds. Diet, nutrition and dental caries. Proceedings of the Second European Congress on Diet, Nutrition and Dental Caries. Caries Res 1990;24(Suppl 1):1–79.

Enwonwu CO. Cellular and molecular effects of malnutrition and their relevance to periodontal diseases. J Clin Periodontol 1994;21:643–57.

National Research Council. Diet and health: implications for reducing chronic disease risk. Washington, DC: National Academy Press, 1989.

Nizel AE, Papas AS. Nutrition in clinical dentistry. 3rd ed. Philadelphia: WB Saunders, 1989.

Pollack RL, Kravitz E. Nutrition in oral health & disease. Philadelphia: Lea & Febiger, 1985.

67. The Esophagus and Stomach

WILLIAM F. STENSON

MOUTH, PHARYNX, AND ESOPHAGUS

The digestive process is initiated by placing food in the mouth. Chewing and salivary secretion result in formation of a food bolus, a rounded, lubricated mass suitable for swallowing (Fig. 67.1). Movement of the bolus from the mouth to the pharynx initiates the process of swallowing. The presence of the bolus in the pharynx activates glossopharyngeal and vagal fibers connected to the swallowing center in the brainstem (1). The swallowing center coordinates initiation of swallowing, opening the upper esophageal sphincter, peristalsis in the upper esophagus, and momentary cessation of breathing. The presence of food in the mouth also activates neural pathways that result in salivary secretion, gastric acid secretion, pancreatic secretion, contraction of the gallbladder, and relaxation of the sphincter of Oddi. Thus, although the mouth and pharynx have little direct role in digestion and absorption of nutrients, neurally mediated events initiated by the presence of food in the mouth and pharynx are important in coordinating the initial phases of the integrated response of the entire gastrointestinal (GI) tract to a meal.

Human saliva contains two digestive enzymes, salivary amylase and lingual lipase. Lingual lipase has a limited role in digestion of dietary triglycerides; however, salivary amylase plays an important role in digestion of dietary starches. Although salivary amylase is secreted with the saliva into the mouth, little starch digestion occurs in the mouth because of the limited time of interaction of food with saliva there. Most of the enzymatic activity of salivary amylase occurs in the stomach, where there is a much longer time for it to interact with dietary starch.

After leaving the pharynx, the food bolus passes through the upper esophageal sphincter to enter the esophagus (2, 3). In the resting state, both the upper and lower esophageal sphincters are closed. After initiation of a swallow there is increased pressure in the pharynx and relaxation of the upper esophageal sphincter. This combination of events pushes the food bolus from the pharynx into the upper esophagus. Then the upper sphincter closes, and a peristaltic wave pushes the bolus through the esophagus. The lower esophageal sphincter relaxes after initiation of the swallow and contracts again after the bolus passes through it.

GASTRIC MOTILITY

Gastric Motility after a Meal

After a meal, the stomach relaxes, and its volume increases to accommodate the ingested food. In addition to this reservoir function, the stomach also grinds food into smaller particles through the action of the antral musculature. Finally, the stomach releases the gastric contents into the duodenum in a regulated fashion. The net effects of the motor activity of the stomach are to prepare food for digestion and absorption in the intestine by reducing it to small particles and to present these particles to the intestine at a rate that facilitates digestion and absorption by allowing maximal mixing with pancreatic and biliary secretions and maximal contact time with the small-intestinal mucosa (4).

Motility is markedly different in the proximal and distal parts of the stomach (5). The proximal stomach, which includes the fundus and the upper part of the body, relaxes as it is filled with food. This relaxation increases gastric volume without increasing intragastric pressure. Relaxation of the proximal stomach in response to a meal includes both "receptive relaxation" and "gastric accommodation" (5, 6). Receptive relaxation is a reduction in proximal gastric tone in response to swallowing; it is mediated by neural pathways and occurs within 10 seconds of swallowing. In contrast, "gastric accommodation" is the reflex relaxation of the proximal stomach in response to gastric distention; this process is mediated by vagovagal reflexes. The vagal afferents are activated by the effects of gastric distention on pressure receptors in the gastric wall. The afferent messages are processed in the brain in the dorsal vagal complex of the medulla. This processing in turn initiates vagal efferent activity, which elicits effects in the stomach and other portions of the GI tract. In the

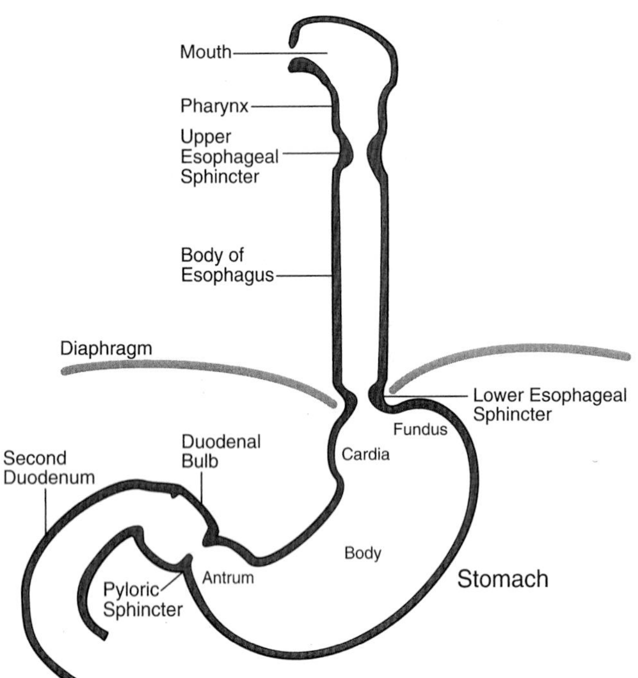

Figure 67.1. Anatomy of the upper gastrointestinal tract in man.

stomach, the vagal efferent activity causes muscle relaxation in the proximal stomach (gastric accommodation), and muscle contraction in the antrum; it also induces secretion of gastric acid, pepsinogen, and gastrin. Vagal efferent activity induced by gastric distention also causes increased enzyme secretion in the pancreas, contraction of the gallbladder, and relaxation of the sphincter of Oddi.

The period of relaxation in the proximal stomach after a meal is followed by a period of contraction, which increases intragastric pressure. The proximal stomach produces slow, sustained tonic contractions to push the contents of the meal into the distal stomach. The intragastric pressure created by the tonic contraction of the proximal stomach increases the rate of gastric emptying, especially the emptying of liquids. Contraction of the proximal stomach is regulated by neural and hormonal input; among the hormones that influence this process are cholecystokinin (CCK), motilin, and gastrin.

The distal stomach includes the lower part of the body and the antrum. In contrast to the tonic contractions of the proximal stomach, the contractions of the distal stomach are phasic. (In "tonic" contractions, the muscle contracts over a long period of time; in "phasic" contractions, there is a rhythmic contraction and relaxation.) Tonic contractions of the proximal stomach influence the rate of gastric emptying, whereas phasic contractions of the distal stomach grind food into small particles. Phasic motor activity in the distal stomach migrates as a ring contraction, increasing in amplitude as it approaches the pylorus; these contractions can generate intragastric pressures as high as 100 mm Hg. Phasic contractions originate in an area of spontaneously depolarizing muscle in the proximal body termed the *gastric pacemaker;* depolarization travels in a wavelike manner from the pacemaker through the distal body and the antrum. The pattern of phasic antral contractions seen in the fed state begins 5 to 10 minutes after the ingestion of a meal and persists as long as food remains in the stomach. Fluoroscopic studies demonstrate that antral contractions first propel ingested material distally toward the pylorus. The pylorus is closed tightly enough that larger food particles cannot pass. The ingested material is then directed back from the distal antrum into the more proximal stomach, and the process is repeated (7). This to-and-fro action mixes and grinds solid food.

The pylorus is a sphincter that sits at the junction of the antrum and the duodenal bulb. It regulates the flow of intraluminal contents from the stomach into the duodenum (8). The rate of gastric emptying is determined by the pressure generated in the proximal stomach and by the size of the pyloric opening; the higher the pressure and the larger the opening, the faster the rate of emptying. During feeding, the pylorus acts as a sieve that impairs the emptying of particles greater than 1 mm in diameter (9). If the stomach is presented with a meal that is a mixture of small (<1 mm) and large (>2 mm) particles, the pylorus passes the smaller ones and retains the larger ones. Antral grinding of the larger particles reduces them to a size that can pass through the pylorus.

Gastric Motility during Fasting

In addition to the motor activity seen in the stomach in response to a meal, there is also activity in the fasting state. The migrating motor complex (MMC) clears the stomach and small intestine of undigested food particles and other particulate debris (10). The MMC has three phases of activity that repeat at periods of 90 to 100 minutes. Phase I, which occupies 40 to 60% of the cycle, is a period of little phasic motor activity. Phase II, which lasts 20 to 30% of the cycle length, is a period of irregular contractions of various amplitudes. Phase III lasts 5 to 10 minutes and is marked by high-pressure, propagative waves accompanied by pyloric relaxation. These waves clear undigested food particles from the stomach. Phase III is mediated by cyclic release of motilin from duodenal mucosal cells.

GASTRIC EMPTYING

Nonnutritional liquids, nutritional liquids, and solids each empty from the stomach at different rates, and these rates are regulated by different mechanisms (5, 11). Nonnutritional liquids, such as water or isotonic saline, empty rapidly from the stomach. The volume emptied into the duodenum is a constant fraction of the volume of liquid in the stomach. Thus, the initial rate of emptying of a 400-mL bolus of water is twice that of a 200-mL bolus; half the volume of a bolus of water empties from the stomach in about 10 to 15 minutes (12). The rate of emptying of liquids from the stomach is determined by the tonic contractions of the proximal stomach but is also influenced by the degree of pyloric resistance and the capacity of the duodenum to receive a volume of fluid.

When nutrients such as glucose are present in a liquid meal, the rate of gastric emptying is slowed in response to feedback from the small intestine (13). Neural reflexes from the small intestine modulate contraction of the muscles of the proximal stomach and thus affect intragastric pressure and the rate of gastric emptying. The rate of emptying of a liquid from the stomach is influenced by its caloric concentration, osmolality, fat content, and pH. Liquids of high caloric density empty more slowly than those with fewer calories per unit volume. The emptying of nutrients occurs at a rate that delivers approximately 200 kcal/h into the intestine. Carbohydrates and amino acids modulate intestinal nutrient delivery through their effects on small intestine osmolality. Nutritional liquids of high osmolality empty more slowly than those of low osmolality. A bolus of 300 mL of 0.1 M glucose empties from the stomach three times as fast as a bolus of 300 mL of 0.3 M glucose (14). The effects of fats on gastric emptying are complex. Liquid fats empty from the stomach more slowly than aqueous liquids. Fats bind to solid food particles and float on the surface of aqueous gastric secretions, which slows their emptying from the stomach. The rate of liquid emptying from the stomach is also influenced by pH; acid solutions empty more slowly than neutral solutions. This reflex prevents acid solutions from entering the duodenum at a rate high enough to lower the pH of the duodenal contents and thus diminish the activity of pancreatic enzymes. Slowing the release of acid solutions from the stomach provides more time for neutralization by bicarbonate in biliary and pancreatic secretions.

Digestible solids empty from the stomach at a slower rate than liquids. Food particles need to be reduced in diameter to a maximum of 1 to 2 mm to allow passage through the pylorus (15). Small particles have a higher surface:volume ratio than large particles, which makes more of their contents accessible to the action of digestive enzymes in the intestine. Digestible solids empty after an initial lag phase that persists for up to an hour after the end of a meal. During the lag phase there is extensive mixing and grinding of solid food, but little or no solid material exits the stomach. The smaller the food particles, the shorter the lag phase. After this initial grinding period, the particles empty at a linear rate that is independent of the volume remaining in the stomach. Food particles larger than 2 mm in diameter that cannot be further reduced in size are emptied from the stomach by active contraction during phase III of the MMC. These strong contractions also clear foreign bodies from the stomach. In adults, coins as large as a quarter are cleared through the pylorus by the MMC.

DISORDERS OF GASTRIC EMPTYING

Most disturbances of gastric motor activity delay gastric emptying (16). Interference with production of normal gastric tone in the proximal stomach delays emptying of both liquids and solids, whereas disorders that interfere with grinding activity in the antrum result in delayed emptying of solids but normal emptying of liquids. The symptoms associated with delayed gastric emptying are nausea, vomiting, early satiety (feeling full after eating a small portion of a normal meal), weight loss, and abdominal distention. Delayed gastric emptying can result in vomiting of recognizable food particles many hours after ingestion of a meal. Delayed gastric emptying due to disorders of gastric motility may be difficult to distinguish from that due to gastric outlet obstruction by ulcer, scarring, or tumor; the two conditions cause the same set of symptoms.

Delayed gastric emptying is seen in a variety of conditions. Certain drugs can delay gastric emptying; among these are opiates, tricyclic antidepressants, phenothiazines, and calcium channel blockers. Alcohol, tobacco, and marijuana can also delay gastric emptying. Delayed gastric emptying is seen in anorexia nervosa. Malnutrition itself can delay gastric emptying; treatment of patients with anorexia nervosa with dietary supplements to induce weight gain improves gastric emptying.

The most common cause of clinically significant delayed gastric emptying is diabetic gastroparesis (17). This is especially common in insulin-dependent diabetes of long standing and is often associated with peripheral or autonomic neuropathy. At least 25% of insulin-requiring diabetics who have had their disease for 10 years, will have delayed emptying of liquids and/or solids (18). For some patients with long-standing insulin-dependent diabetes, gastroparesis is a major cause of morbidity; severe upper abdominal discomfort, frequent vomiting, and substantial weight loss are common. The pathogenesis of the delay in gastric emptying in diabetes is not well understood, but there is evidence that it results primarily from neuropathy of the autonomic nervous system, with vagal neuropathy being the dominant abnormality (19). Reduced vagal input to the distal stomach results in reduced antral contractions. Pyloric dysfunction also occurs in diabetes and results in increased pyloric resistance and impairment of emptying. Evaluation of diabetic gastroparesis is difficult, and most patients are treated on the basis of suggestive symptoms in an appropriate clinical setting. Delayed gastric emptying may be suspected from retained gastric contents after a fast for an upper GI examination or endoscopy.

A radionuclide gastric-emptying study is the most sensitive clinical test. Solid-phase radionuclide tracers are normally used, as patients with delayed emptying for either liquids or solids may be detected by this method. Radionuclide emptying studies have a broad range of normal, and the results need to be carefully standardized. The correlation between symptoms and radionuclide studies is not good; some asymptomatic patients have markedly abnormal radionuclide studies, and some patients with severe symptoms have relatively normal studies.

The first approach to symptomatic relief in diabetic

gastroparesis is better control of the blood sugar; hyperglycemia itself is thought to have adverse effects on gastric motor function. Other approaches include removing offending medications, increasing the liquid content of the diet, and reducing dietary fat. Over the past few years, a number of drugs that stimulate gastrointestinal motility have become available. Although some of these prokinetic agents are effective in diabetic gastroparesis, their efficacy is variable and tends to diminish over time. Metoclopramide has dopamine-antagonist and cholinergic-enhancing effects (20). The cholinergic effects increase the amplitude and frequency of antral contractions and relax the pylorus. Thus, metoclopramide produces an effect that mimics phase III of the MMC. The central dopamine antagonism of metoclopramide can cause side effects that mimic Parkinson's disease. The prokinetic effect of metoclopramide on the stomach is diminished after about 4 weeks of therapy. Cisapride accelerates emptying of both liquids and solids by enhancing the coordination of gastric and duodenal motor events (21). Like metoclopramide, cisapride produces a phase III–like effect through acetylcholine release. The prokinetic effects of cisapride are more sustained than those of metoclopramide but still diminish after 6 months. In contrast to metoclopramide, which activates motility primarily in the stomach and proximal small intestine, cisapride activates motility in the entire GI tract from esophagus to colon; as a consequence, diarrhea is its major side effect.

Accelerated gastric emptying occurs most commonly in patients who have had gastric surgery for peptic ulcer disease. This topic is discussed below in the section "Nutrition and Gastric Surgery."

GASTRIC SECRETION AND DIGESTION

The major organ for digestion and absorption of nutrients is the small intestine. The stomach primarily prepares ingested food for digestion and absorption in the small intestine by grinding it into smaller particles and regulating its flow into the small intestine for optimal digestion and absorption. Although the intestine is the major digestive organ, appreciable digestion of carbohydrates, protein, and fats occurs in the stomach (22). Moreover, the stomach is the source of intrinsic factor, a protein required for absorption of vitamin B_{12} in the ileum. Although the stomach facilitates digestion of macronutrients, its contribution to digestion is not absolutely required. Patients who have undergone total gastrectomy can maintain normal nutritional status on a regular diet despite the absence of the stomach. The only exception to this is the eventual requirement for administration of parenteral vitamin B_{12} to compensate for the malabsorption of dietary vitamin B_{12} due to the absence of intrinsic factor. In patients with gastrectomies, the major morbidity is not the absence of the stomach as a digestive organ but, rather, the absence of the stomach as a food reservoir and regulator of the flow of ingested food into the small intestine.

Digestive events in the stomach are tied to the functional capacity of the different populations of cells forming the gastric epithelial lining. The gastric lining consists of thick folds, each of which contains microscopic gastric pits (23). Four or five gastric glands drain into each of these pits. The mucosa of the body and fundus of the stomach contains oxyntic glands (Fig. 67.2). (The term *oxyntic gland* comes from the oxyntic, or parietal, cell, which is a prominent component of these glands.) Oxyntic glands are lined by parietal cells that secrete gastric acid (HCl) and intrinsic factor and by chief cells that secrete pepsinogen and gastric lipase. In contrast, the pyloric glands that form the mucosa of the antrum contain almost no parietal cells or chief cells but, rather, contain mucus-secreting cells and G cells, which produce the hormone gastrin.

Gastric Acid Secretion

The physiologic function most closely associated with the stomach is the production of gastric acid (22). The physiologic stimulus for gastric acid production is food;

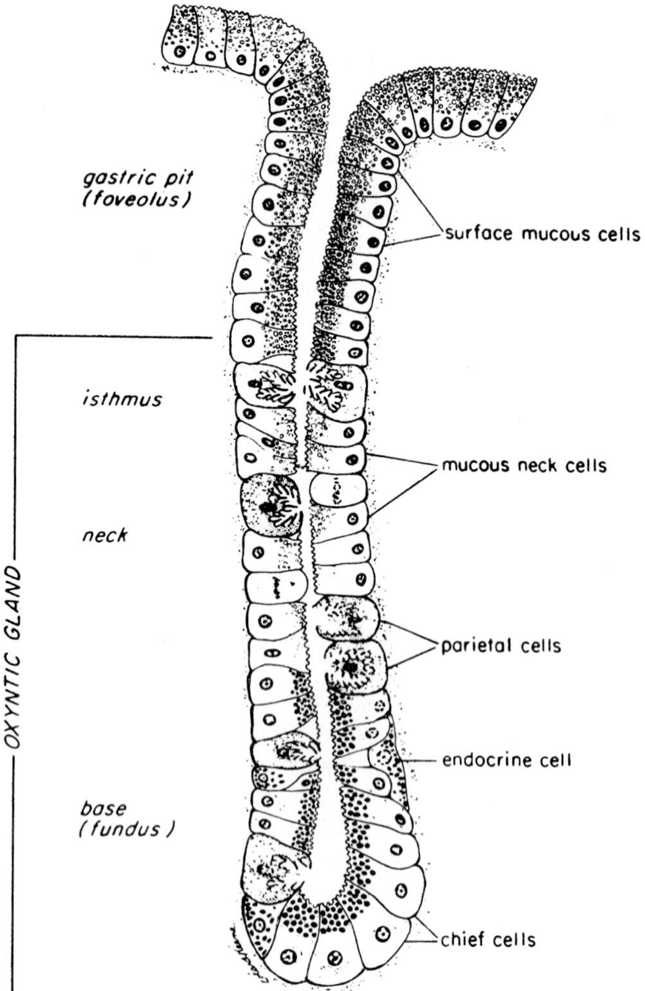

Figure 67.2. Gastric gland from the body of a mammalian stomach. (From Ito S, Winchester RJ. J Cell Biol 1963;16:541–78, with permission.)

although gastric acid is produced in response to a meal, it plays a relatively minor role in digestion. Patients treated with drugs that inhibit gastric acid secretion by blocking the parietal cell proton pump do not have clinically significant problems with maldigestion or malabsorption. Nonetheless, gastric acid does play some role in digestion. Conversion of pepsinogen to pepsin requires an acid pH that can only be achieved by gastric acid secretion. Moreover, pepsins, which break down proteins into peptides, have pH optima in the acid range. Gastric lipase cleaves triglycerides to yield free fatty acids. The pH optimum for gastric lipase is between 4 and 5.5; it is much less active at the neutral pH seen in the absence of gastric acid secretion. However, neither pepsins nor gastric lipase are required for digestion of food. The functional reserves of pancreatic peptidases and pancreatic lipase are large enough to make up for the loss of the contribution of pepsins and gastric lipase to digestion. Gastric acid secretion is important in the absorption of iron, particularly nonheme iron. Ferric salts are insoluble at neutral or slightly acid pH, whereas ferrous salts are much more soluble in this pH range (24). In acidic solutions (pH < 4), ferric salts dissolve and can be reduced to ferrous salts, which remain in solution at the neutral pH found in the duodenum where they are absorbed.

Gastric acid is secreted constantly, but the rate of secretion is increased with meals. During fasting, gastric acid is secreted at about 15% of its maximal rate. The food-stimulated increase in gastric acid secretion occurs in three phases: cephalic, gastric, and intestinal (22). The cephalic phase refers to the stimulation of gastric acid secretion by the smell, taste, or even thought of food. Gastric acid secretion induced by chewing or swallowing food is also part of the cephalic phase. The cephalic phase is mediated primarily by the vagus nerve; vagotomy abolishes this phase of gastric acid secretion. When food enters the stomach, gastric acid secretion is stimulated. One mechanism for the gastric phase of acid secretion is distention of the stomach by food, which activates stretch receptors in the gastric wall and thus initiates gastric acid secretion mediated by a vagovagal reflex. A second mechanism is activation of chemoreceptors by amino acids and peptides formed by partial digestion of dietary proteins by pepsins. The entry of partially digested food into the small intestine initiates the intestinal phase of acid secretion. This process is mediated by distention of the small intestine and by the presence of proteins and the products of protein digestion in the partially digested food. In contrast to the cephalic and gastric phases of gastric secretion, the intestinal phase is not mediated by vagal reflexes; the intestinal phase remains intact even after vagotomy.

Gastric acid secretion increases at the start of a meal; within 1 hour after the end of the meal, the rate of acid secretion reaches a peak that is near the maximal capacity of the stomach to secrete acid. Two to 3 hours after a meal, gastric acid production is reduced by the presence of acid and the products of digestion in the stomach and intestine. Although the rate of acid secretion peaks within the first hour after a meal, the total amount of acid in the stomach rises for an additional 1 to 2 hours.

The presence of acid in the gastric antrum shuts down gastrin release and thus reduces acid secretion. The presence of acid, fat, or hyperosmotic solutions in the duodenum inhibits gastric acid secretion. The inhibition of acid secretion by duodenal contents is at least partially humoral, because it persists after vagotomy. A number of hormones including somatostatin, secretin, and CCK have been suggested as possible mediators of the inhibition of gastric acid secretion by duodenal contents.

Gastric acid secretion by parietal cells is regulated by acetylcholine, gastrin, and histamine (25). Parietal cells have specific receptors for each of these ligands. Acetylcholine is a neurotransmitter produced by the vagus and other parasympathetic nerves. Gastrin is a peptide hormone produced by G cells in the gastric antrum. Gastrin secretion is stimulated by specific nutrients in the gastric lumen, which include amino acids and small peptides but not glucose or fat. Gastrin release is also stimulated by a high pH in the gastric lumen. Histamine is secreted by mucosal mast cells and enterochromaffin-like cells. Drugs that block the binding of histamine to its receptor on parietal cells (H2 receptor antagonists) are potent inhibitors of gastric acid secretion.

Gastric Protein and Fat Digestion

In the stomach, dietary proteins are cleaved into smaller peptides by the action of pepsins, proteases that are maximally active at low pH (pH 1.5–2.5) and are inactivated by neutral or alkaline conditions (26). Pepsinogens, the inactive precursors of pepsins, are secreted by chief cells and are autocatalytically cleaved to form pepsins under acidic conditions (pH < 6). Secretion of pepsinogens by chief cells, like secretion of gastric acid by parietal cells, occurs in response to the ingestion of food. Gastrin and acetylcholine are important mediators of pepsinogen secretion in response to a meal. Chief cells store pepsinogen in apical granules; stimulation by gastrin or acetylcholine results in the exocytosis of these granules. Parallel stimulation of parietal cells provides the acid environment required for cleavage of pepsinogens to form pepsins. Pepsins cleave dietary proteins into peptides but do not generate large amounts of free amino acids; they only cleave about 10 to 15% of the peptide bonds in food proteins. Peptides generated by pepsin digestion of dietary proteins act as signals for secretion of gastrin by G cells in the antral mucosa. These peptides are further hydrolyzed to amino acids by the action of pancreatic peptidases in the intestine.

The stomach contributes to fat digestion both by emulsifying dietary fats to prepare them for digestion by lipases in the intestine and by lipolysis of ingested fats by gastric lipase (27). Emulsification of dietary fats is initiated in the stomach by body heat, which liquifies most dietary fat, and by the grinding action of the antrum, which promotes the interaction of dietary lecithin with dietary triglyceride droplets. Gastric lipase, like pepsinogens, is secreted by chief cells in the oxyntic mucosa; its secretion is regulated by the same mechanisms that regulate secretion of pepsinogens. Gastric lipase differs from pancreatic lipase in several important respects. It has a pH optimum of 4 to 5.5, as opposed to the neutral pH optimum of pancreatic lipase. Moreover, gastric lipase acts preferentially on the 3-position long-chain fatty acid esterified on triglyceride. Thus, the major products of gastric lipase action on triglycerides are free fatty acids and diglycerides. Also, gastric lipase is activated by bile salts, whereas pancreatic lipase is not. Under normal circumstances, gastric lipase accounts for the digestion of 20 to 30% of total dietary fats, with pancreatic lipase accounting for most of the rest. When pancreatic lipase is present in decreased amounts, as in patients with pancreatitis or surgical resections of the pancreas, gastric lipase can account for a considerably larger percentage of lipid digestion. Gastric lipase is also important in lipid digestion in neonates, because pancreatic lipase secretion is quite limited during the first weeks of life.

Intrinsic Factor

Intrinsic factor is secreted from parietal cells in response to stimulation by gastrin and acetylcholine (28). Dietary vitamin B_{12} (cobalamin) can only be absorbed in the ileum when complexed with intrinsic factor. Other luminal proteins can also bind cobalamin; in the acidic environment of the stomach, cobalamin preferentially binds to R protein, a protein secreted in saliva, rather than intrinsic factor. In the duodenum and jejunum, salivary R protein is degraded by pancreatic proteases, and cobalamin is released. In the neutral pH of the small intestine, cobalamin preferentially binds to intrinsic factor. The intrinsic factor–cobalamin complex is then bound to a specific ileal receptor and absorbed. Even though the stomach secretes intrinsic factor in excess, a partial gastrectomy (especially one that involves resection of a significant portion of the body) may result in substantial loss of intrinsic factor secretory capacity, with clinically significant effects on cobalamin absorption. In the complete absence of intrinsic factor secretion (e.g., after total gastrectomy), dietary cobalamin is not absorbed. The very large stores of cobalamin in the liver prevent development of the clinical manifestations of cobalamin deficiency for 3 to 6 years after gastrectomy. In addition to total or partial gastrectomy, the other common cause of intrinsic factor deficiency is pernicious anemia, a disease that typically affects elderly Caucasians. It is characterized by atrophy of the oxyntic mucosa with resultant loss of gastric acid and intrinsic factor secretion. Over a period of years, the absence of intrinsic factor leads to clinical cobalamin deficiency. Patients with pernicious anemia and those with total gastrectomy should receive parenteral cobalamin once a month. In patients with partial gastrectomies, the risk of cobalamin deficiency is great enough that either the serum cobalamin level should be monitored carefully or the patient should be placed on prophylactic vitamin B_{12} therapy.

DIET IN GASTROESOPHAGEAL DISEASES

Diet in Gastroesophageal Reflux Disease (GERD)

GERD is irritation and inflammation of the esophagus in response to reflux of gastric acid into the esophagus (29). In normal individuals, reflux of gastric contents into the esophagus is largely blocked by the lower esophageal sphincter (LES) at the junction of the esophagus and stomach. The LES is normally closed except during swallowing. Despite the presence of the LES, some reflux of gastric contents into the esophagus occurs in normal individuals. This reflux elicits esophageal contractions that push the refluxed gastric contents back into the stomach. GERD occurs when reflux of gastric contents into the esophagus occurs with excessive frequency or in excessive volume or if the refluxed gastric contents fail to elicit esophageal contractions to push them back into the stomach. When too much gastric acid is in contact with the esophageal mucosa for too long a time, the individual may experience heartburn. In milder cases of GERD, the patient experiences heartburn but the esophageal mucosa remains endoscopically and histologically normal. In more severe cases, the refluxed gastric contents cause the esophageal mucosa to become ulcerated. Healing of these esophageal ulcers can result in stricturing of the esophagus and thus difficulty swallowing. Among the factors that contribute to GERD are an excessive volume of acidic contents in the stomach, looseness of the LES, and motility disorders in the esophagus that impair its ability to generate a coordinated contraction in response to reflux of gastric contents. The amount of acid refluxed, the severity of heartburn, and the damage to the epithelium do not always correlate. Sometimes, severe heartburn is seen in the absence of mucosal injury, or severe injury is seen in patients with minimal heartburn.

GERD is treated with drugs, physical measures, and diet. The drugs used to treat GERD are those that decrease gastric acid secretion (H2 receptor antagonists and proton pump inhibitors), those that neutralize gastric acid (antacids), and those that enhance gastric emptying (metoclopramide and cisapride). One physical measure used to treat GERD is elevation of the head of the bed to keep gastric acid in the stomach and out of the esophagus during sleep.

Diet affects GERD in several ways. If the esophageal mucosa is damaged and sensory pain fibers are exposed or sensitized, acidic foods such as orange juice or tomato juice may elicit pain on swallowing. The more important impact of diet on GERD involves the effects of food on LES pressure and gastric acid secretion, which depend on both the kinds of food consumed and the timing of their ingestion. The amount of gastric acid in the stomach reaches a maximum 2 to 3 hours after a meal. When an individual is in the upright position, gravity keeps gastric acid in the lower portions of the stomach; however, reclining allows gastric acid to enter the upper part of the stomach where it can more easily reflux into the esophagus. Patients with GERD frequently complain that their symptoms worsen if they lie down after eating. Thus, patients with GERD should be told not to eat within 3 hours before going to bed. Alcohol, chocolate, and fatty foods have been implicated in relaxing the LES. In normal individuals, coffee tightens the LES; however, in patients with GERD it does not. Moreover, coffee and alcohol both increase gastric acid secretion. Thus, a bad combination of events for a patient with GERD is a large fatty meal eaten late in the evening and accompanied by alcohol, coffee, and chocolate.

Diet in Peptic Ulcer Disease

Peptic ulcer disease includes both gastric and duodenal ulcers (30). For many years, gastric acid secretion was thought to play a major role in the pathogenesis of peptic ulcer disease; however, recent studies have identified *Helicobacter pylori* as a causal agent for many, if not most, cases of peptic ulcer disease. Aspirin and other nonsteroidal antiinflammatory drugs play a part in the causation of many other cases of peptic ulcer disease. Although gastric acid does not have a primary causal role in the vast majority of cases of peptic ulcer disease, it does play a causal role when secreted at extremely high rates, as is seen in Zollinger-Ellison syndrome.

Although gastric acid does not play a primary causal role in the development of most cases of peptic ulcer disease, inhibition of gastric acid secretion is therapeutic. Both H2 receptor antagonists, which inhibit gastric acid secretion by blocking the histamine receptor on parietal cells, and proton pump inhibitors, which inhibit the parietal cell pump that secretes hydrogen ions into the gastric lumen, are therapeutic in peptic ulcer disease. Although these drugs that profoundly inhibit gastric acid secretion are therapeutic in peptic ulcer disease, there is no evidence that dietary manipulations that modulate gastric acid secretion are therapeutic.

Many ulcer patients remark that certain foods, particularly spicy foods, cause them epigastric discomfort, but there is no evidence that these foods cause peptic ulcer disease. Moreover, no causal role in peptic ulcer disease has been demonstrated even for foods known to be potent inducers of gastric acid secretion, such as milk, alcohol, and coffee. Just as there is no evidence for a causal role for diet in peptic ulcer disease, there is no evidence that diet influences the rate of ulcer healing. Many ulcer patients have been told to avoid alcohol, coffee, and other potent secretagogues, yet there is no evidence that these dietary factors, at least when taken in moderate quantities, retard ulcer healing. There are theoretical reasons to limit the consumption of alcohol, in particular, in patients with peptic ulcer disease. Beer and wine, even in modest amounts, induce near-maximal gastric acid secretion without providing any significant buffering capacity. There has been some interest in the potential role of dietary fiber in peptic ulcer disease; some studies suggest that the incidence of recurrence of peptic ulcer disease is higher in patients on low-fiber diets than in those on high-fiber diets (31).

Earlier in this century, diet management played a prominent, if unsubstantiated, role in the management of peptic ulcer disease. Patients were placed on bland diets and encouraged to consume small amounts of food frequently throughout the day. Pureed food was recommended to avoid mechanical irritation of the healing ulcer. Milk was a major component of these ulcer diets. These diets were based on the clinical observation that eating relieved ulcer pain and the laboratory observation that food, especially high-protein food, buffered gastric acid. Although these regimens were widely used for several decades, there was no scientific evidence to support their use. Controlled trials in the 1950s demonstrated no benefit of these ulcer diets to either the rate of ulcer healing or relief of symptoms compared with regular diets (32).

NUTRITION AND GASTRIC SURGERY

Surgery and Gastric Emptying

Two commonly performed surgical procedures for peptic ulcer disease are truncal vagotomy and pyloroplasty, and truncal vagotomy and antrectomy (for discussion of gastric surgery for cancer, see Chapter 82). Truncal vagotomy is cutting the main trunks of the vagus nerve on each side of the distal esophagus. Vagotomy is part of the surgical treatment of peptic ulcer disease because it eliminates the neural components of the stimulation of gastric acid secretion. However, truncal vagotomy also eliminates neural input to the antral musculature and thus reduces antral contractions and delays emptying of solids from the stomach. Truncal vagotomy also impairs relaxation of the pylorus, which further impairs gastric emptying. To compensate for these effects, truncal vagotomy is often accompanied by pyloroplasty, which is a surgical revision of the pylorus that makes it incapable of acting as a barrier to the emptying of gastric contents. A vagotomy and pyloroplasty results in accelerated emptying of liquids, whereas the emptying of solids is frequently slowed (34).

Vagotomy and antrectomy is a more aggressive surgical procedure for peptic ulcer disease. Antrectomy is the resection of the antrum and pylorus; resection of the antrum removes the gastrin-secreting portion of the stomach and thus eliminates the gastrin-dependent component of the stimulation of gastric acid secretion. There are two operations for attaching the gastric remnant to the intestine after antrectomy. In the Billroth I, the gastric remnant is anastomosed to the duodenal bulb, and the flow of gastric contents is directly into the bulb. In the Billroth II, the gastric remnant is anastomosed to the jejenum; in this procedure, gastric contents bypass the duodenum and proximal jejunum. A vagotomy and antrectomy results in rapid and unregulated entry of gastric contents into the intestine; it also allows solid food particles to enter the intestine without having been reduced in size by antral grinding. With an antrectomy, the intestine sees the sudden entry of a large volume of liquids and unground solids after a meal rather than the slow regulated presentation of liquids and finely ground particles seen with an intact stomach. The larger the gastric resection, the more severe the problems with rapid entry into the intestine.

The highly selective vagotomy, or proximal gastric vagotomy, is a surgical procedure for peptic ulcer disease that is designed to reduce gastric acid secretion without interfering with antral motility. In a standard truncal vagotomy, the vagal input to gastric secretion and to antral contraction is lost. Truncal vagotomy also eliminates vagal innervation of the gallbladder, pancreas, and small intestine. In a highly selective vagotomy, the vagal branches going to the body of the stomach are cut, while the branches going to the antrum are not. This results in decreased acid secretion without impaired antral motility, thus eliminating the need for a pyloroplasty and the associated rapid gastric emptying (35). This procedure also spares the vagal innervation of the gallbladder, pancreas, and small intestine.

Dumping Syndrome

A vagotomy and pyloroplasty results in rapid entry of liquids into the intestine, whereas vagotomy plus antrectomy results in rapid entry of both solids and liquids. When nutrients empty from the stomach and enter the intestine in a rapid and unregulated fashion, the digestive and absorptive capacity of the intestine can be overwhelmed. The symptom complex induced by accelerated gastric emptying is termed the *dumping syndrome* (34). Diarrhea, abdominal pain, and the symptoms associated with hypoglycemia (diaphoresis, palpitations, weakness) are prominent components of the dumping syndrome. In response to rapid entry of a hypertonic meal into the intestine, water enters the intestinal lumen through the intestinal wall in an attempt to make the intestinal contents isosmotic. The sudden influx of the meal and water into the proximal intestine stretches the intestinal wall, causing abdominal distention and pain. Diarrhea results from the inability of the intestine to deal with the sudden load of volume and osmoles. This early phase of the dumping syndrome may also be marked by systemic symptoms, including weakness, tachycardia, and palpitations, thought to be due to the sudden fluid shifts from the intravascular space into the intestine with the release of vasoactive substances (bradykinin, serotonin, substance P). There is also a late phase of the dumping syndrome, which is related to hypoglycemia. Rapid gastric emptying results in rapid glucose absorption from the intestine and an abrupt increase in insulin secretion. Not infrequently, insulin is secreted in excess of the amounts required to handle the glucose load. When carbohydrate absorption abruptly ceases and insulin secretion remains high, there can be a transient episode of hypoglycemia. In the dumping syndrome, diarrhea and abdominal pain occur 30 to 60 minutes after the meal, and the symptoms of hypoglycemia occur later. Some of the symptoms (weakness and palpitations) associated with hypoglycemia in the late phase of the dumping syndrome are similar to those seen with fluid shifts in the early phase. Dietary management usually controls the symptoms of the dumping syndrome. The core of dietary management is to avoid the sudden entry of large volumes into the proximal intestine. This is achieved by eating frequent small meals and by avoiding the intake of liquids with meals. Meals should be low in osmolality; thus, simple sugars should be avoided.

Iron and Calcium

Absorption of iron and calcium is frequently impaired after gastric ulcer surgery. Iron deficiency anemia is common in patients with vagotomy and antrectomy. There are several contributing factors. Frequently, total food intake is slightly decreased, especially in patients with antrectomy. There is also decreased digestion of iron-containing foods, particularly meats. Diminished acid secretion results in a higher gastric pH, which impairs the solubility of ferric ions and diminishes their conversion to the more easily absorbed ferrous ions (24). Moreover, the duodenum is an important site for iron absorption, and gastric surgery either bypasses the duodenum (Billroth II) or causes ingested materials to pass through the duodenum rapidly (Billroth I). When all these factors are combined with the marginal iron intake prevalent in society, the result is iron deficiency anemia.

Osteomalacia is also common after surgery for peptic ulcer disease (36). Osteomalacia is marked by low serum calcium, low urinary calcium, elevated alkaline phosphatase, and elevated parathyroid hormone levels and widened osteoid seams in the bones. The clinical outcome of this process is a fracture rate that is two to three times that of the general population (37). The mechanism for osteomalacia after gastric ulcer surgery is not fully defined. In normal individuals, the duodenum is an important site for calcium absorption, and the rapid transit through the duodenum seen after gastric ulcer surgery may contribute to calcium malabsorption. However, it is not clear that calcium malabsorption per se is a major feature in the pathogenesis of osteomalacia (see Chapter 83).

REFERENCES

1. Diamant NE. Physiology of the esophagus. In: Sleisenger MH, Fordtran JS, eds. Gastrointestinal disease. 5th ed. Philadelphia: WB Saunders, 1993;319–30.
2. Biancani P, Behar JB. Motility: esophageal motor function. In:

Yamada T, ed. Textbook of gastroenterology. 2nd ed. Philadelphia: JB Lippincott, 1995;159–81.
3. Conklin JL, Christensen J. Motor functions of the pharynx and esophagus. In: Johnson, LR, ed. Physiology of the gastrointestinal tract. 3rd ed. New York: Raven Press, 1994;903–29.
4. Jansson G. Acta Physiol Scand 1969;(Suppl);326:1–42.
5. Mayer EA. The physiology of gastric storage and emptying. In: Johnson LR, ed. Physiology of the gastrointestinal tract. 3rd ed. New York: Raven Press, 1994;929–76.
6. Hasler WL. The physiology of gastric motility and gastric emptying. In: Yamada T, ed. Textbook of gastroenterology. 2nd ed. Philadelphia: JB Lippincott, 1995;181–206.
7. Cannon WB. Am J Physiol 1898;1:359–370.
8. Schulze-Delrieu K, Wall JP. Am J Physiol 1983;245:G257–64.
9. Meyer JH, Thompson JB, Cohen MB, et al. Gastroenterology 1979;76:804–13.
10. Rees WDW, Malagelada JR, Miller LJ, Go VLW. Dig Dis Sci 1982;27:321–9.
11. Read NW, Houghton LA. Gastoenterol Clin North Am 1989;18:359–73.
12. McHugh PR, Moran TH. Am J Physiol 1979;236:R254–G260.
13. Hunt JN, Stubbs DF. J Physiol 1975;245:209–25.
14. Lin HC, Doty JE, Reedy TJ, Meyer JH. Am J Physiol 1989;256:G404–11.
15. Mayer EA, Thompson JB, Jehn D. Gastroenterology 1984;87:1264–71.
16. Lin HC, Hasler WL. Disorders of gastric emptying. In: Yamada T, ed. Textbook of gastroenterology. 2nd ed. Philadelphia: JB Lippincott, 1995;1318–46.
17. Feldman M, Schiller LR. Ann Intern Med 1983;98:378–84.
18. Keshavarzian A, Iber FL, Vaetch J. Am J Gastroenterol 1987;82:29–35.
19. Feldman M, Corbett DB, Ramsey EJ. Gastroenterology 1979;77:12–7.
20. Schulze-Delrieu K. Gastroenterology 1979;77:768–79.
21. McCallum RW. Am J Gastroenterol 1991;86(2):135–49.
22. DelValle J, Lucey MR, Yamada T. Gastric secretion. In: Yamada T, ed. Textbook of gastroenterology. 2nd ed. Philadelphia: JB Lippincott, 1995;295–325.
23. Ito S, Winchester RJ. J Cell Biol 1963;16:541–78.
24. Conrad ME. Factors affecting iron absorption. New York: Academic Press, 1970;87–115.
25. Hersey SJ, Sachs G. Physiol Rev 1995;75:155–90.
26. Hersey SJ. Gastric secretion of pepsins. In: Johnson LR, ed. Physiology of the gastrointestinal tract. 3rd ed. New York: Raven Press, 1994;1227–38.
27. Hamosh M. Gastric and lingual lipases. In: Johnson LR, ed. Physiology of the gastrointestinal tract. 3rd ed. New York: Raven Press, 1994;1239–54.
28. Seetharam B. Gastrointestinal absorption and transport of cobalamin (vitamin B_{12}). 3rd ed. Raven Press, 1994:1997–2026.
29. Kahrilas PJ, Hogan WJ. Gastroesophageal reflux disease. In: Sleisenger MH, Fordtran JS, eds. Gastrointestinal disease. 5th ed. Philadelphia: WB Saunders, 1993;378–400.
30. Soll AH. Gastric, duodenal, and stress ulcer. In: Sleisenger MH, Fordtran JS, eds. Gastrointestinal disease. 5th ed. Philadelphia: WB Saunders, 1993;580–678.
31. Rydning A,, Berstad A. Scand J Gastroenterol 1986;21:1–5.
32. Doll R, Friedlander P, Pygott F. Lancet 1956;1:5–9.
33. Matthews JB, Silen W. Operations for peptic ulcer disease and early postoperative complications. In: Sleisenger MH, Fordtran JS, eds. Gastrointestinal disease. 5th ed. Philadelphia: WB Saunders, 1993;713–30.
34. Meyer JH. Chronic morbidity after ulcer surgery. In: Sleisenger MH, Fordtran JS, eds. Gastrointestinal disease. 5th ed. Philadelphia: WB Saunders, 1993;731–92.
35. Lavigne ME, Wiley ZD, Martin P. Am J Surg 1979;138:644–51.
36. Klein KB, Orwoll ES, Lieberman DA. Gastroenterology 1987;92:608–16.
37. Nilsson BE, Westlin NE. Acta Chir Scand 1971;137:533–4.

SELECTED READINGS

Conklin JL, Christensen J. Motor functions of the pharynx and esophagus. In: Johnson, LR, ed. Physiology of the gastrointestinal tract. 3rd ed. New York: Raven Press, 1994;903–29.

Hersey SJ, Sachs G. Physiol Rev 1995;75:155–90.

Lin HC, Hasler WL. Disorders of gastric emptying. In: Yamada T, ed. Textbook of gastroenterology. 2nd ed. Philadelphia: JB Lippincott, 1995;1318–46.

Mayer EA. The physiology of gastric storage and emptying. In: Johnson LR, ed. Physiology of the gastrointestinal tract. 3rd ed. New York: Raven Press, 1994;929–76.

Meyer JH. Chronic morbidity after ulcer surgery. In: Sleisenger MH, Fordtran JS, eds. Gastrointestinal disease. 5th ed. Philadelphia: WB Saunders, 1993;731–92.

68. Short Bowel Syndrome

JAMES S. SCOLAPIO and C. RICHARD FLEMING[†]

Short bowel syndrome (SBS) is a collection of signs and symptoms used to describe the nutritional and metabolic consequences of major resections of the small intestine. The syndrome is characterized by diarrhea, fluid and electrolyte abnormalities, malabsorption, and weight loss. Patients who have not had intestinal resections but who have marked reduction of small bowel absorptive surface area (e.g., diffuse inflammatory bowel disease, sprue, radiation enteritis) may have the same nutritional sequelae.

LENGTH OF SMALL INTESTINE

The length of the normal small intestine varies widely among individuals. Measurement of 260 autopsy specimens found a mean length of 620 cm, with a range of 300 to 850 cm (1, 2). The discrepancy in length is secondary to both the method of measurement and the tone of the intestine when measured. While most autopsy studies report pylorus to ileocecal valve as small bowel length, operative studies report small bowel length from the ligament of Treitz to ileocecal valve (3). Loss of intestinal tone at autopsy results in overestimation of actual small bowel length compared with intraoperative measurements. Measurements from barium x-rays appear to correlate well with surgical measurements (4). Classification of SBS by the length of intestine that has been resected is generally not accurate. The length of residual small intestine best determines prognosis. Resection of 75% or more of the small intestine usually leaves a patient with 70 to 100 cm (2–3 feet) of small bowel. Patients with less than 100 cm of small bowel who do not have a colon in continuity usually require parenteral nutrition support (5).

The proximal two-fifths of small bowel is referred to as jejunum, and the distal three-fifths as ileum (6). Adults have approximately 240 cm of jejunum, 360 cm of ileum, and 150 cm of colon. Patients with SBS, depending on the extent of surgical resection, can be classified as either those with an end-jejunostomy or end-ileostomy, or those with a small bowel in continuity with colon (7). Knowledge of this classification is important for management and prognosis.

ETIOLOGY OF SHORT BOWEL SYNDROME

Crohn's disease, mesenteric vascular disease, and malignancy are the most common causes of SBS in adults. Crohn's disease may involve many segments of the small bowel that require multiple resections over several years before the SBS is functionally significant. Venous and/or arterial occlusion secondary to primary vascular disease or an underlying coagulopathy may result in intestinal infarction and subsequent resection. The jejunoileal bypass procedure that was popular 20 years ago for treatment of morbid obesity remains a major cause of SBS. Necrotizing enterocolitis, midgut volvulus, and intestinal atresia are the major reasons for SBS in infants.

FACTORS INFLUENCING PROGNOSIS

Positive prognostic factors after intestinal resection include youth, larger length of residual bowel, proximal resection (vs. distal), presence of ileocecal valve and colon, healthy residual bowel, and small bowel adaptation (8). Children have a better prognosis after massive small bowel resection because of a usual lack of comorbid conditions and greater potential for adaptation of the remaining bowel. Distal or ileal resections result in more disability than proximal or jejunal resections because of the specialized transport mechanisms for bile salts and vitamin B_{12} in the ileum and a slower rate of peristalsis in the ileum than in the jejunum (9). Also, ileal resections result in the removal of the "ileal brake," with more rapid transit through the stomach and proximal small bowel.

The ileocecal valve is a physiologic sphincter that controls the rate of delivery of chyme from the small bowel to the colon and prevents bacterial overgrowth in the small bowel (10). Bacterial overgrowth can cause the deconjugation of bile salts with subsequent malabsorption of fat (11). The presence of a colon not only gives added bowel length but also slows intestinal transit. The colonic bacteria ferment unabsorbed complex carbohydrates to short-

[†]Deceased.

chain fatty acids that provide a source of calories and trophic stimuli to the intestine (12, 13).

The colon is also an important organ of fluid and electrolyte salvage, which is more critical in patients with short bowel (14). The status of the residual intestine is an obvious factor in determining long-term prognosis in patients with SBS and probably explains why patients with Crohn's disease and radiation enteritis generally do worse than comparably aged patients with a bowel infarction and healthy remaining small bowel.

Small Bowel Adaptation

Following intestinal resection the remaining bowel undergoes both structural and functional changes that increase nutrient and fluid absorption (15). Structural changes (villus cell hyperplasia and increased crypt depth) begin days after resection and result in increased mucosal surface area. Functional adaptation (increased brush border enzyme activity and decreased gastrointestinal motility) also promotes fluid and nutrient absorption following resection (16–18).

The controlling mechanism(s) of gut adaptation is not totally understood. Potential stimuli include luminal nutrients, intestinal hormones and pancreaticobiliary secretions (19). Intraluminal nutrients are essential in promoting intestinal adaptation and probably work by more than one mechanism. Support for the intraluminal theory includes finding mucosal atrophy within 5 days after proximal enterectomy in dogs receiving only parenteral nutrition (20). Surgical diversion studies have shown that small bowel not receiving direct nutrient flow develops mucosal atrophy (21). The contents of the diet are also important; trophic factors include dietary fiber (22), short-chain fatty acids (23), and glutamine (24). Intraluminal nutrients may promote adaptation by a direct "bathing" effect on the mucosa and/or a stimulation of pancreaticobiliary secretions and intestinal hormones. Pancreatic and biliary secretions (PBS) appear to be important in the adaptive process. Diversion studies by Altmann et al. in which PBS were diverted to the distal small intestine resulted in distal intestinal hyperplasia (25). PBS may also help explain the proximal-distal gradient of villus height found in health. Growth hormone, insulin-like growth factor-I (IGF-I), epidermal growth factor, and insulin are peptide hormones that appear to increase mucosal hyperplasia following intestinal resection in experimental animals (26, 27). The clinical role of other hormones such as enteroglucagon, prostaglandins, neurotensin, and testosterone are less well defined. Intestinal hormones may work by stimulating the production of polyamines (putrescine, spermidine, and spermine), trophic compounds whose production is regulated by the enzyme ornithine decarboxylase (28). Polyamines are known to stimulate cell proliferation, and blockage of ornithine decarboxylase inhibits the proliferative process (28).

COMPLICATIONS

Nutritional Deficiencies

After large resections of the small intestine there is impaired absorption of most nutrients, each with characteristic clinical or biochemical findings (29–42) (Table 68.1, see also specific chapters on each nutrient). Inadequate dietary intake and loss of micronutrients in the stool contribute to the development of vitamin and mineral deficiencies. Patients with end-jejunostomies or proximal ileostomies are the most difficult to manage because of recurrent dehydration and deficiencies in electrolytes and divalent cations (Ca^{2+}, Mg^{2+}, Zn^{2+}). Particularly problematic is Mg deficiency. While Ca and Zn can be administered orally when there is adequate absorptive surface, Mg should not be because it induces diarrhea. In some situations, Mg has to be provided parenterally. The malabsorption of macronutrients (carbohydrates, fat, protein) can result in severe weight loss and malnutrition.

Bile salts are required for micellar solubilization of dietary fat and fat-soluble vitamins. After ileal resections, bile salts are malabsorbed, the bile salt pool becomes depleted, and consequently, fat malabsorption occurs. In addition to the malabsorption of fat and fat-soluble vitamins, the unabsorbed fatty acids complex with divalent cations such as calcium and magnesium, decreasing their availability. When the colon is present, malabsorbed bile and fatty acids can stimulate water and sodium secretion

Table 68.1
Clinical Presentation of Nutrient Deficiencies

Nutrient	Disease	Reference
Copper	Neutropenia, anemia, scorbutic bone lesions, ↓ ceruloplasmin, kinky hair, impaired CNS development	29, 30
Zinc	Nasolabial and perineal acrodermatitis, alopecia, ↓ T cell function, ↓ alkaline phosphatase, dysgeusia	31
Chromium	Glucose intolerance, peripheral neuropathy	32, 33
Selenium	Myalgias, cardiomyopathy, ↓ glutathione peroxidase and serum selenium	34, 35
Molybdenum	AA intolerance, tachycardia, tachypnea, central scotomas, irritability, ↓ uric acid	36
Essential fatty acids	Eczymoid dermatitis, ↑ 20:3/20:4	37
Vitamin A	Night blindness, impaired dark-field adaptation	38
Vitamin E	In vitro platelet hyperaggregation and H_2O_2-induced RBC hemolysis; signs and symptoms suggesting subacute combined degeneration (posterolateral columns) in the presence of a normal serum B_{12} level.	39
Biotin	Scaly dermatitis, alopecia, hypotonia in one child	40
Thiamin	Wernicke's encephalopathy, refractory lactic acidosis,cardiac failure	41
Cobalamin (B_{12})	Weakness, paresthesia, diarrhea, dementia, megaloblastic anemia, subacute combined degeneration	42

from the colonic mucosa and induce diarrhea, thus aggravating the clinical situation.

Most water-soluble vitamins are absorbed in the proximal jejunum. With the exception of vitamin B_{12} and folate, deficiencies of water-soluble vitamins are rarely seen in SBS. Vitamin B_{12} is absorbed by the terminal ileum after binding with intrinsic factor. When more than 60 cm of ileum has been resected, monthly B_{12} injections are required indefinitely.

Deficiencies of trace elements such as zinc, copper, selenium, iron, chromium, and molybdenum can also occur in the short bowel patient (29–36) (Table 68.1). Oral vitamin and mineral supplements usually prevent or correct deficiencies. Zinc may be an exception, since zinc losses may be enormous in the stool, nasogastric aspirates, and fistulous drainage, and intravenous replacement is sometimes needed to restore positive zinc balance. Serum zinc levels may also be low because of low serum albumin, the major zinc-binding protein, and not necessarily reflect zinc deficiency. Patients with extensive small intestinal resections also have reduced disaccharidase enzymes, most commonly lactase. This may result in significant lactose intolerance.

Peptic Ulcerations

Gastric acid hypersecretion following small bowel resections may result in peptic ulcer disease, inactivation of pancreatic lipase, and deconjugation of bile salts (43). Increased gastric acid secretion is usually a transient phenomenon that subsides within 3 to 6 months. It may be treated with histamine-2 receptor antagonists or proton pump inhibitors (44). Surgery is seldom required, unless complications of peptic ulcers occur.

D-Lactic Acidosis

D-Lactic acid is produced by fermentation of malabsorbed carbohydrates in the colon (44). Humans lack the enzyme necessary to metabolize D-lactic acid. Increased serum levels of D-lactic acid are associated with marked metabolic acidosis with patients developing dysarthria, ataxia, and confusion (45). D-Lactate acidosis should be suspected when there is an unexplained metabolic acidosis and elevated anion gap in patients with short bowel and colonic continuity. Management is focused on carbohydrate-restricted diets and administration of nonabsorbable antibiotics that diminish D-lactate production by eliminating colonic bacteria.

Nephrolithiasis

Dietary oxalate normally binds to intraluminal calcium to form an insoluble complex that is excreted in stool. However, in SBS, calcium binds to unabsorbed fatty acids and leaves free oxalate to be absorbed from the colon (46). Malabsorbed bile salts that reach the colon increase oxalate absorption by increasing intestinal permeability (47). Hyperoxaluria and formation of oxalate stones can lead to significant renal impairment and formation of kidney stones. In addition to an increase in urinary oxalate, there are frequently very low urinary levels of stone inhibitors such as citrate and magnesium. Chronic dehydration in patients without SBS and colonic continuity usually results in the production of uric acid stones.

Cholelithiasis

Patients with short bowel have a two- to threefold increased risk of cholesterol gallstones (48). Precipitation of cholesterol occurs because of the decreased concentration of bile salts in bile secondary to ileal resections and bile salt malabsorption (49). Long-term parenteral nutrition also increases the risk of gallstones because of lack of oral intake and gallbladder stasis. The gallstones in short bowel patients receiving long-term total parenteral nutrition (TPN) are predominantly calcium bilirubinate, with cholesterol as a minor component. Bilirubin and ionized calcium levels are increased in bile in both man and the prairie dog receiving TPN (50).

TREATMENT

Optimal care for the patient with a short bowel begins in the operating room, where the surgeon, recognizing the inevitable result of extensive resection of the small intestine, conserves as much bowel as possible, with a special effort to maintain the ileocecal valve and colon. Thereafter, medical care falls into three stages.

Stages of Medical Treatment

Stage I, the immediate postoperative period, dominated by problems with fluid and electrolyte balance, typically lasts 1 to 2 weeks. Fluid losses can exceed 2 L/day or more, which makes it very important to assess daily fluid balance and electrolytes. All patients require intravenous fluids and electrolytes to replace losses. Fluids should be infused to match losses and to maintain urine output of at least 1 L/d. Hypersecretion of gastric acid can contribute to significant intestinal fluid loss and can also inactivate pancreatic lipase, resulting in further fat malabsorption. Intravenous histamine-2 receptor antagonists can control gastric acid hypersecretion. Ranitidine (Zantac) 150 mg, or famotidine (Pepsid) 20 mg, can be given intravenously every 12 hours. Initially, diarrhea is managed by avoiding oral intake, to reduce any osmotic effects. If diarrhea exceeds 2 L/day, antidiarrheal agents can be used. Codeine in doses of 60 mg intramuscularly every 4 to 6 hours can be given. In some patients, octreotide, a somatostatin analogue, can reduce stool volume by 50% when given in a dose of 100 μg three times a day (51). Octreotide is usually reserved for patients with end-jejunostomies (<100 cm) who have more than 3 L of diarrhea per day (51). When the patient tolerates liquids by mouth, oral antidiarrheal agents can be used. Loperamide (Imodium), 16 to 20 mg/day in divided doses, or tincture of opium, 10 to 30 drops every 4 to 6 hours, can be used. Patients are usually started on clear oral liquids (small-volume isotonic feedings) when bowel sounds have returned postoperatively and stool losses are less than 2 L/day. Glucose-electrolyte solutions can be used for oral hydration. They should contain 3.4% glucose with at least 90 mmol/L of sodium (7). Oral hydration solutions are available commercially. They work by avoiding osmotic stimulation and promoting fluid and electrolyte absorption.

Stage II represents the transitional feeding period. The oral diet should be advanced slowly, using small, frequent feedings of solid food. The parenteral solution is reduced gradually as oral intake is increased. When oral caloric intake begins to exceed 1000 cal/day without worsening diarrhea, intravenous support can be reduced. There is no evidence that elemental or defined formula diets (DFDs) are more efficient than normal food in stimulating adaptation of the small bowel, and experimental evidence suggests that they may be less efficient (52, 53). It may take several weeks before the patient can completely discontinue TPN support.

Stage III begins when the patient is off parenteral nutrition, and attention to details of a permanent nutrition program becomes increasingly important.

Nutritional/Pharmacologic Treatment

Reduction of dietary fat from 90 to 100 g/day to 20 to 40 g/day was reported in early papers to decrease the number of stools, stool weight, and steatorrhea while increasing body cell mass (54). More-recent studies challenged the wisdom of low-fat diets in all patients with SBS (55). High-fat (60% of calories as fat) and low-fat (20% of calories as fat) diets were compared in crossover fashion in patients with the SBS. There were no differences in stool volumes between patients on the two diets (55). Hence, dietary restriction of fat may be detrimental by restricting the nutrient of greatest caloric density (9 kcal/g). There is no reason to restrict fat in short bowel patients without a colon in continuity. Patients with colonic continuity may occasionally have worsening diarrhea from a high-fat diet secondary to colonic mucosal irritation from free fatty acids, which stimulate water and sodium secretion, and should then be fed a diet high in complex carbohydrates (50% of calories) and lower in fat (30% of calories).

Patients with hyperoxaluria and calcium oxalate renal stones should be treated with a low-oxalate, low-fat diet and high fluid intake. If these measures do not normalize urinary oxalate and reduce stone formation, other helpful measures include cholestyramine to bind intraluminal oxalate; calcium supplements, which increase calcium oxalate insoluble complexes; citrate (polycitra) to correct low urinary citrate levels; and parenteral magnesium to normalize urinary magnesium levels.

Fat-soluble vitamins also need to be evaluated and replaced as needed. Because of the high incidence (36%) of osteomalacia in short bowel patients (56), vitamin D therapy is often required. Serum 25-OH vitamin D levels can usually be normalized by giving oral vitamin D (i.e., Drisdol) 50,000 IU every other day as maintenance until plasma levels normalize, and then once or twice per week may suffice. Vitamin A can be replaced by an aqueous preparation (Aquasol A) and vitamin E by Liquid E. Vitamin K can be replaced by giving 5.0 mg/day orally and titrating to the frequency required to maintain a normal prothrombin time.

Of the water-soluble vitamins, vitamin B_{12} is the one that may need to be replaced in patients with more than 60 cm of ileal resection. Since the enterohepatic circulation accounts for 10 μg/day, total malabsorption would require 300 μg/month for replacement. A monthly injection of 100 μg of vitamin B_{12} is usually adequate. Other water-soluble vitamins can usually be maintained with a daily oral multivitamin.

Control of diarrhea is also very important in the treatment of SBS. Antidiarrheal agents should be used to decrease diarrhea and electrolyte losses. Loperamide (Imodium), 16 to 20 mg/day in divided doses, or tincture of opium, 10 to 30 drops every 4 to 6 hours, can be used. Oral histamine-2 receptor antagonists or proton pump inhibitors, such as omeprazole, can also be helpful in reducing gastrointestinal secretions and fluid losses. Sorbitol-containing elixirs should be avoided.

INTRACTABLE SHORT BOWEL SYNDROME

Home Parenteral Nutrition

In patients with intractable gut failure, home parenteral nutrition (HPN) can be life saving, and in many patients it provides the time bridge necessary for maximal adaptation to occur. HPN is designed to improve daily function of patients with gut failure by providing most or all of the daily nutrient needs through a central venous catheter. Parenteral nutrition is infused during an 8- to 12-hour overnight period, which frees the patient during the day for regular activities. Venous access is usually gained by either implantable subcutaneous ports or silastic catheters that are placed in the subclavian vein and tunneled subcutaneously to exit low on the anterior chest wall.

The distribution of calories provided in parenteral nutrition varies, depending on what the patients eat and absorb. For patients who have to rely exclusively on HPN, 20 to 30% of total calories should be given as intravenous fat, which supplies 9 kcal/g fat and serves to prevent essential fatty acid deficiency. Patients are usually given 1.0 to 1.5 g protein/kg/day. The remaining calories are given as carbohydrate. Vitamins, minerals, and trace elements are given in TPN solutions in amounts adequate to maintain normal blood concentrations (Chapter 101).

Nutritional repletion by parenteral nutrition is dramatic. Ideal body weight is achieved in almost all patients. Measurements of visceral protein and skeletal muscle mass as well as body composition studies have confirmed nitrogen repletion. Many of these patients are also rehabilitated and return to gainful employment.

A rough estimate of the total U.S. home parenteral nutrition population in 1992 was 40,000 patients, with a major trend toward larger use in cancer patients (57). Active cancer is now the most common diagnosis, accounting for more than 40% of all new patients reported to the National HPN Registry (57).

Mortality from HPN complications has been approximately 5% (57). Outcome data have shown that HPN is safe, that the primary disease has the most impact on survival and rehabilitation, and that age is not a reason to deny HPEN (57). Crohn's disease tends to have the best, and AIDS or active cancer the worst, prognosis in patients on HPN. HPN-related complications requiring hospitalization are infrequent. In the 1970s, most of the reported complications were micronutrient deficiencies and complications of carbohydrate overfeeding (e.g., hepatic steatosis). The last decade brought complications that might have been expected with increasing duration of HPN use such as venous thrombosis, chronic liver disease, cholelithiasis, and metabolic bone disease (57). Catheter-related septicemia has been the most common major complication, with coagulase-negative staphylococci, *Staphylococcus aureus,* and *Candida* being the most common organisms isolated.

Hepatobiliary dysfunction is frequent in patients receiving parenteral nutrition support and occurs more often in children. Most vulnerable are premature infants. Patients on short-term parenteral nutrition usually have mild-to-moderate elevations in transaminases and alkaline phosphatase levels. Patients on long-term HPN may develop persistent elevations in liver tests and steatohepatitis, with progressive fibrotic liver disease (58). The pathogenesis of parenteral nutrition–induced liver disease is not well understood. Theories include a high fat:carbohydrate ratio, amino acids or metabolites acting as hepatic toxins, portal endotoxemia, lithocholic acid toxicity, and carnitine deficiency. Although several attempts at preventing TPN-associated steatohepatitis have been tried, none have proven totally successful. In patients with certain HPN-related complications such as liver dysfunction and lack of venous access, small bowel transplantation may be an option.

Recently Byrne and colleagues reported that the combination of human recumbent growth hormone, glutamine, and a high-carbohydrate, low-fat diet significantly increased nutrient absorption in an uncontrolled study of eight patients with SBS (58). Three weeks of this combination therapy resulted in a significant increase in protein, carbohydrate, sodium, and fluid absorption. In a subsequent uncontrolled study of 47 short bowel patients, the same investigators showed that 40% of treated patients remained off all parenteral support at 1-year follow-up (59). This form of therapy is thought to work by its ability to increase small bowel intestinal surface, i.e., increased villus height and crypt depth. However, it has not been shown in clinical trials that surface area is increased. Gastrointestinal motility may also be slowed with this therapy and allow increased contact time for nutrient absorption; however, this has never been documented with formal gastrointestinal transit studies. Most patients studied by Byrne et al. had colonic continuity, and since the colon can salvage calories by fermentation of carbohydrates to short-chain fatty acids, a high-carbohydrate diet may be the most important part of this regimen in those with colonic continuity. In fact, many patients can reduce their parenteral nutrition to three to four nights per week with appropriate use of diet and antidiarrheal agents alone. It remains to be determined whether such therapy as that proposed by Byrne and colleagues has long-term clinical benefit.

Surgical Treatment

The primary emphasis of surgery as it relates to SBS is to prevent intestinal resection by early diagnosis and conservative resections when possible. The two main goals of surgical treatment of SBS are to slow intestinal transit and increase intestinal surface area (60, 61).

Operations used to slow transit include construction of intestinal valves, antiperistaltic segments, colonic interposition, recirculating loops, and intestinal pacing. Clinical experience with intestinal valves is limited; complete intestinal obstruction and intussusception are concerns (61). Slowing intestinal transit by reversing segments of small intestine has been investigated. This procedure places a segment of bowel in the opposite direction of normal flow or peristalsis, which creates an antiperistaltic segment and hence slows transit, allowing added contact time for nutrient and fluid absorption. More than 30 patients have been reported in the literature, and 70% appear to have had good results. Other reports have not been so promising; these may be related to the length of the reversed small bowel segment used. Patients with short intestinal remnants are usually not able to sacrifice a 10-cm segment for reversal. Colonic interposition, both isoperistaltic and antiperistaltic, has been performed. Since colonic transit is slower than small bowel transit, this procedure slows transit and allows added contact time for nutrient absorption. Results with antiperistaltic colonic segments have been inconsistent (61). Recirculating loops are done by looping part of the small bowel, which theoretically allows luminal nutrients to be exposed to the absorptive mucosa several times before leaving the intestinal tract. However, recirculating loops are associated with high morbidity and mortality (61). Retrograde electrical pacing has been used in attempts to slow intestinal transit in dogs but has not been successful in man (62).

Operations used to increase the area of absorption include intestinal tapering and lengthening, intestinal transplantation, and growing neomucosa. Intestinal tapering and lengthening have been reported to have good results in children (61). This procedure is done by dissecting longitudinally along the mesenteric border of the small intestine. Once transected longitudinally, the two parallel intestinal segments that result can be anastomosed end to end so that the initial dilated segment becomes a tapered segment of twice the length. More than 40 cases of intestinal lengthening procedures have been reported in children, and 10-year follow-up suggests long-term benefit. Intestinal transplantation is promising, but until improved immunosuppression is developed, graft rejection remains the obstacle. More than 100 intestinal transplants have been performed in humans over the last decade (61). Individuals with TPN-induced complications such as liver failure and poor venous access may be appropriate candidates. At this time, no operative procedure for SBS is safe and effective enough to recommend for routine use.

REFERENCES

1. Bryant J. Am J Clin Nutr 1994;167:499–520.
2. Underhill BML. Br Med J 1995;2:1243–6.
3. Backman L, Hallberg D. Acta Chir Scand 1974;40:57–63.
4. Nightingale JMD, Bartram CI, Lennared-Jones JE. Gastrointest Radiol 1991;16:305–6.
5. Nightingale JMD, Lennard-Jones JE. Dig Dis 1993;11:12–31.
6. Scott JR. The small intestine—anatomy and physiology. In: Sabiston DC, ed. Textbook of surgery. 13th ed. London: WB Saunders, 1986;897–905.
7. Lennard-Jones JE. Aliment Pharmacol Ther 1994;8:563–77.
8. Guyton AC. Digestion and absorption in the gastrointestinal tract. In: Guyton AC, ed. Textbook of medical physiology. 7th ed. Philadelphia: WB Saunders, 1986:787–97.
9. Summers RW, Kent TH, Osborne JW. Gastroenterology 1970;59:731–9.
10. Phillips SF, Quigley EMM, Kumar D, et al. Gut 1988;29:390–406.
11. Gorbach SL, Plaut AG, Nahas L, et al. Gastroenterology 1967; 53:856–7.
12. Moran BJ, Jackson AA. Br J Surg 1992;79:1132–7.
13. Bond JH, Currier BE, Buchwald H, et al. Gastroenterology 1980;78:444–7.
14. Debongnie JC, Phillips SF. Gastroenterology 1978;74:698–703.
15. Williamson RCN. N Engl J Med 1978;298:1393–1402.
16. McCarthy DM, Kim YS. J Clin Invest 1973;52:942–51.
17. Remington M, Malagelada J-R, Zinsmeister A, et al. Gastroenterology 1983;85:629–36.
18. Quigley EMM, Thompson JS. Gastroenterology 1993;105: 791–8.
19. Dowling RH. Scand J Gastroenterol 1982;74:53–74.
20. Feldman EJ, Dowling RH, McNaughton J, et al. Gastroenterology 1976;70:712–9.
21. Bury KD. Surg Gynecol Obstet 1972;135:177–87.
22. Koruda MJ, Rolandelli RH, Settle RG, et al. JPEN J Parenter Enteral Nutr 1986;10:342–50.
23. Koruda MJ, Rolandelli RH, Bliss DZ, et al. Gastroenterology 1988;95:715–20.
24. Tamada H, Nezur R, Matsuo Y, et al. JPEN J Parenter Enteral Nutr 1993;17:236–42.
25. Altmann GG. Am J Anat 1971;132:167–78.
26. Shulman DI, Hu CS, Duckett G, et al. J Pediatr Gastroenterol Nutr 1992;14:3–11.
27. Chen K, Okuma T, Okamura K, et al. JPEN J Parenter Enteral Nutr 1995;19:119–24.
28. Dowling RH. Digestion 1990;46:331–8.
29. Shike M, Roulet M, Kurian R, et al. Gastroenterology 1981; 81:290–7.
30. Shike M. Bull NY Acad Med 1984;60:132–43.
31. Solomon NW. Trace elements. In: Rombeau JL, Caldwell MD, eds. Parenteral nutrition. 2nd ed. Philadelphia: WB Saunders, 1993;150.
32. Jeejeebhoy KN, Chu RC, Marliss EB, et al. Am J Clin Nutr 1977;30:531–8.
33. Freund H, Atamian S, Fischer JE. JAMA 1979;241:496–508.
34. Lane HW, Barroso AO, Englert D, et al. JPEN J Parenter Enteral Nutr 1982;6:426–31.
35. Brown MR, Cohen HJ, Lyons JM, et al. Am J Clin Nutr 1986;43:549–54.
36. Abumrad NN. Bull NY Acad Med 1984;60:163–71.
37. Press M, Hartop PJ, Prottery C. Lancet 1974;1:597–8.
38. Anderson CE. Vitamins. In: Schneider HA, Anderson CE, Coursin DB, eds. Nutritional support of medical practice. 2nd ed. Philadelphia: Harper & Row, 1983;23.
39. Farrell PM. Vitamin E. In: Shils ME, Young VR, eds. Modern nutrition in health and disease. 7th ed. Philadelphia: Lea & Febiger;1988:340.
40. Mock DM, de Lorimer AA, Liebman WM, et al. N Engl J Med 1981;304:820–3.
41. Kishi H, Nishii S, Ono T, et al. Am J Clin Nutr 1979;32:332–8.
42. Hoffbrand AV. Vitamin B-12 and folic acid. In: Krikler DM, ed. Post-gastrectomy nutrition. London: Lloyd-Luke, 1967;1–15.
43. Murphy JP, King DR, Dubois A. N Engl J Med 1979;300:80–1.
44. Satoh T, Narisawa K, Konno T, et al. Eur J Pediatr 1982; 138:324–6.
45. Stolberg L, Rolfe R, Gitlin N, et al. N Engl J Med 1982;306:1344–8.
46. Dobbins JW, Binder HJ. N Engl J Med 1977;296:298–301.
47. Chadwick VS, Gaginella TS, Carlson GL, et al. J Lab Clin Med 1979;94:661–74.
48. Manji N, Bistrian BR, Macioli EA, et al. JPEN J Parenter Enteral Nutr 1989;13:461–4.
49. Farkkila MA. Surgery 1988;104:18–25.
50. Broughton G, Fitzgibbon RJ, Geiss RW, et al. JPEN J Parenter Enteral Nutr 1996;20:187–193.
51. Farthing MJG. Digestion 1993;54:47–52.
52. Levy E, Frileux P, Sandrucci S, et al. Br J Surg 1988;75:549–53.
53. McIntyre PB, Fitchew M, Lennard-Jones JE. Gastroenterology 1986;91:25–33.
54. Andersson H, Isaksson B, Sjogren B. Gut 1974;15:351–9.
55. Woolf GM, Miller C, Kurian R, et al. Gastroenterology 1983;84:823–8.
56. Koo W. JPEN J Parenter Enteral Nutr 1992;16:386–94.
57. Howard L, Ament M, Fleming CR, et al. Gastroenterology 1995;109:355–65.
58. Fleming CR. Dig Dis 1994;12:191–8.
59. Byrne T, Morrissey T, Nattaksom T, et al. JPEN J Parenter Enteral Nutr 1995;19:296–302.
60. Byrne T, Persinger R, Young L, et al. Ann Surg 1995;222: 243–55.
61. Devine RM, Kelly KA. Gastroenterol Clin North Am 1989;18: 603–18.
62. Thompson JS, Langnas AN, Pinch LW, et al. Ann Surg 1995; 222:600–7.
63. Collin J, Kelly KA, Phillips SF. Gastroenterology 1979;76: 1422–8.

69. Inflammatory Bowel Disease

ANNE M. GRIFFITHS

Inflammatory bowel disease (IBD) encompasses at least two forms of chronic intestinal inflammation: Crohn's disease (CD) and ulcerative colitis (UC) (1). The two conditions are currently defined empirically on the basis of clinical, radiologic, endoscopic, and histologic features. Debate continues as to whether these two major forms of IBD represent different manifestations of the same disease or distinct disorders with some pathogenetic and clinical similarities. The latter contention is favored by genetic and immunologic data. The natural history of IBD is variable. The observed spectrum of disease severity and nutritional impact is wide, in part related to the site, nature, and extent of intestinal involvement.

CD is a panenteric inflammatory process with focal microscopic inflammation identifiable throughout the gastrointestinal tract. The anatomic distribution of macroscopic disease varies but includes the terminal ileum more frequently than any other site. Initial patterns of localization include terminal ileal disease only (25–35% of patients), involvement of the terminal ileum and colon (35–45%), isolated colonic disease (15–25%), and, least commonly, proximal or diffuse small intestinal inflammation (5–10%). Following intestinal resection, CD almost invariably recrudesces in a new site, most commonly proximal to the anastomosis. Wherever it occurs, macroscopic disease is characteristically segmental with spared areas ("skip lesions").

The inflammation in UC is always confined to the colonic mucosa and hence is curable by colectomy. Inflammation universally includes the rectum but extends proximally to varying degrees in a continuous fashion. Patients are typically classified as having proctitis, rectosigmoiditis, left-sided colitis, or extensive or pancolitis, depending on the length of diseased colon.

Many nutritional issues are important in the care of patients with IBD. Many patients feel that their problem is caused by, or is in need of, a special diet. This chapter reviews the question of the role of diet in the pathogenesis of IBD, discusses the problems of malnutrition and specific nutritional deficiencies and their management, and examines the use of nutritional therapies in the primary modulation of intestinal inflammation. Separate consideration of CD and UC is warranted, because of differences in the impact of disease on nutritional state and in the responsiveness of acute disease to nutritional therapies.

DIET AND THE PATHOGENESIS OF IBD

Pathogenesis of IBD: Current Concepts

Understanding the pathogenesis of UC and CD is a major challenge of gastroenterologic research (1). To date, a positive family history in a first-degree relative is the major known risk factor for IBD. Efforts to identify susceptibility genes through linkage studies among families with multiply affected members are under way. Environmental factors must also play a role, however, as evidenced by the increasing incidence of CD in recent decades and changing incidences of IBD in migrant populations (e.g., increased UC in Asians following emigration to England) (2).

The fundamental question regarding the pathogenesis of IBD has been framed as follows: does the chronic, recurring inflammatory activity reflect an appropriate response to a persistently abnormal stimulus (e.g., a persistent causative agent in the intestinal lumen) or an abnormally prolonged response to a normal stimulus (i.e., aberrant regulation of the immune response) (1). Although the search for a specific pathogen, in CD particularly, continues, the most widely accepted working hypothesis is that IBD represents a dysregulated immune response to intraluminal antigens, conceivably dietary, but more likely common enteric bacterial (1). An enormous antigenic load is regularly presented through the lumen of the gastrointestinal tract, but regulatory mechanisms normally prevent the immune and inflammatory responses from proceeding to cause tissue injury. The intestinal inflammation of IBD may be viewed as an exaggeration of the "physiologic" inflammatory response always present in the normal lamina propria of the intestine and colon. Candidate genes contributing susceptibility to IBD, therefore, include genes involved in determining the specificity of the immune system (class II genes of the HLA region, immunoglobulin genes, T-cell receptor genes) or the level of the immune response (cytokines, adhesion molecules) as well as mucin genes and genes responsible for the structures defining intestinal permeability (1). Such predisposing genes must interact with exogenous or endogenous triggers and modifying factors to result in a chronic inflammatory process in which tissue injury is mediated by the immune system (1).

Role of Diet

No specific dietary toxin or antigen has been incriminated. The rarity of IBD has limited traditional epidemiologic methods of determining causation to case-control studies, which have failed to provide a meaningful lead to the pathogenesis of CD and UC. Persson et al. reviewed studies comparing the reported preillness intake of refined sugar, cereals, fiber, and milk products by patients with CD or UC and controls (3). Increased intake of refined sugar before development of symptomatic CD has been fairly consistently reported, suggesting perhaps a modulating role, but the methodologic weaknesses of study design must be recognized (3). The association may represent a behavioral adaptation to, rather than a cause of, disease. Many IBD patients have circulating antibodies to milk protein, but this is also likely to be a secondary phenomenon; the inflamed intestine is abnormally permeable, permitting entry of intact dietary proteins to which an appropriate immune response is then mounted (4).

Recently, nutritional factors modulating the risk of IBD development have been examined. Breast feeding in infancy may reduce the risk of developing CD (2). Although not truly dietary, a clear dichotomy between UC and CD is indicated by the opposing effect of cigarette smoking on the two disorders (2). Smoking decreases and cessation of smoking increases the risk of developing UC, whereas smokers are at increased risk of developing CD. Some authors suggest that smoking may be a determinant of the type of IBD that develops in predisposed subjects. Finally, in a correlation study from Japan, the increasing incidence of CD in the racially homogeneous population was shown to parallel increasing daily intake of animal protein, total fat, and animal fat, especially n-6 polyunsaturated fatty acids (PUFAs) relative to n-3 PUFAs (5). These trends indicating "Westernization" of diet in Japan were determined from sequential population surveys of dietary habits. n-3 PUFAs found in marine oils have an antiinflammatory effect through modulation of proinflammatory cytokine synthesis (6). A recent placebo-controlled study using enteric-coated fish oil capsules designed for ileal release demonstrated a substantial reduction in clinical relapse rate among patients with CD in clinical but not biochemical remission at baseline (7). Confirmation from other studies is awaited. Prior studies with pharmacologic amounts of eicosapentanoic acid in UC and CD (but without such a coating to facilitate release in the distal intestine) have shown little or no clinical benefit.

INTESTINAL EFFECTS OF IBD

The impact of IBD on the gastrointestinal tract and its digestive and absorptive functions varies depending on the site(s), nature, and extent of intestinal inflammation.

Fat Absorption

Digestion and absorption of fat is unaffected by UC. In CD involving the ileum, fat digestion and absorption may be altered either by loss of gut surface area due to inflammation or by depletion of the circulating bile salt pool due to bile acid malabsorption in the diseased ileum or deconjugation by bacteria. However, studies years ago confirmed that significant impairment of fat absorption occurs only when the extent of inflammatory involvement is massive, when the absorptive surface has been reduced by extensive small intestinal resection, or conceivably when there is bacterial overgrowth secondary to luminal stenosis and incomplete bowel obstruction (8, 9). Filipsson et al. studied fecal excretion in CD patients prior to intestinal resection and found predominantly mild steatorrhea in 24% of patients with ileal disease, 26% of those with ileocolonic involvement, and 17% of those with Crohn's colitis. Following resection of the ileum and ileocecal valve, fecal fat excretion was elevated in 48% of patients (8). The frequency and severity of the steatorrhea correlated with the extent of ileal resection, and it was infrequent and mild with resections of less than 30 cm.

Enteric Losses

More prevalent and significant than fat malabsorption is enteric leakage of protein, blood, minerals, electrolytes, and trace elements from the bowel during periods of active inflammation in both UC and CD. Patients with CD, even when clinically asymptomatic, frequently have laboratory evidence of protein-losing enteropathy and consequent hypoalbuminemia (10).

Digestion and Absorption of Specific Nutrients

Specific digestive or absorptive defects may occur in CD, but these also are not universal (8, 9). Vitamin B_{12} malabsorption is the most common, because its site of absorption corresponds to the area most often inflamed. The prevalence of B_{12} malabsorption correlates with extent of ileal disease and, among operated patients, with the length of ileum resected. Vitamin B_{12} malabsorption has been reported in 21% of patients with less than 30 cm of terminal ileum involved, in 48% of those with 30 to 60 cm affected, and in 71% of patients with 60 to 90 cm resected (8). Other digestive or absorptive defects are uncommon, presumably reflecting the reserve of the gut and the large surface area that is usually relatively uninflamed. Lactase deficiency and lactose intolerance may coexist with IBD but are in general no more common than would be expected in an age- and ethnically matched control population (11).

Drug-Nutrient Interactions

Certain drugs used in the management of IBD contribute to selected nutrient malabsorption (12). For example, sulfasalazine reduces folate absorption, but supplementation to prevent anemia does not seem routinely necessary. Calcium metabolism is disturbed by corticosteroid treatment, which causes decreased absorption and increased urinary excretion.

NUTRITIONAL CONSEQUENCES OF IBD

Malnutrition

Weight loss and emaciation are the most prevalent nutritional disturbances in IBD (13, 14). Some 20 to 75% of adult patients experience weight loss with exacerbations, the incidence and magnitude of the loss varying with disease severity. At the time of first diagnosis, approximately 85% of pediatric CD and 65% of pediatric UC patients have lost weight.

Etiology of Malnutrition

As summarized in Table 69.1 multiple factors contribute to malnutrition. However, reduced intake, rather than excessive losses or increased needs, is the major cause of the caloric insufficiency. Abdominal cramps and diarrhea are aggravated by eating; thus the patient consumes less. Disease-related anorexia may be profound in CD, particularly; cytokines produced by the inflamed bowel are likely responsible. Tumor necrosis factor α has been shown to produce anorexia in rats (15).

Intestinal malabsorption may factor in the equation leading to energy imbalance, but it is seldom the major cause as discussed above. Increased energy expenditure associated with active inflammation has been suggested as a further mechanism accounting for the frequency of malnutrition. In general, resting energy expenditure (REE) does not differ from normal in patients with inactive disease but can exceed predicted rates in the presence of fever and sepsis (16). Furthermore, in comparison to comparably malnourished patients with anorexia nervosa a lack of compensatory reduction in REE has recently been described (17). Reduction in REE is a normal biologic response to conserve energy. Production of inflammatory mediators may explain the lack of REE adaptation in Crohn's patients and further augment the ongoing malnutrition.

Table 69.1
Factors Causing Malnutrition in Inflammatory Bowel Disease

Decreased nutrient intake
Disease-related anorexia
Iatrogenic (unjustified dietary restrictions)
Malabsorption
Diminished absorptive surface (disease, fistulae, resection)
Bacterial overgrowth
Bile salt deficiency
Increased gut losses
Protein-losing enteropathy
Electrolytes, minerals, trace metals (diarrhea and fistulae)
Bleeding
Increased requirements
Sepsis, fever
Increased cell turnover

Growth Impairment

Chronic malnutrition translates into impairment of linear growth and pubertal development in pediatric IBD (18). Inflammatory disease occurring during early adolescence is likely to have a major impact on nutritional status and growth because of the very rapid accumulation of lean body mass that normally occurs at this time. Furthermore, boys are more vulnerable to disturbances in growth than girls because their growth spurt comes at a later stage of normal pubertal development and is ultimately longer and greater. Growth impairment is much less common in UC than in CD, at least in part because the more subtle intestinal symptoms in CD often go unrecognized and the inflammatory disease therefore untreated for longer (18).

Prevalence of Growth Impairment in CD

Several recent studies have characterized the growth of children with CD as treated in the 1980s and into the 1990s (19–22). They show that impaired linear growth is common prior to disease recognition as well as during the subsequent years and that height at maturity is often compromised. The percentage of patients with CD whose growth is affected varies with the definition of growth impairment and with the nature of the population under study (tertiary referral center vs. population based). Height velocity is the most sensitive parameter for diagnosing impaired growth and following the effects of therapy on growth. Kanof et al. reported a decrease in height velocity prior to onset of intestinal symptoms in 46% of newly diagnosed children and after development of symptoms in an additional 42%, implying that linear growth was unimpaired in only 12% at the time of diagnosis (23). It is important to obtain preillness heights, so that the impact of the inflammatory bowel disease can be fully appreciated. The greater the height deficit at diagnosis, the greater the demands for catch-up growth.

Children already significantly stunted at the time of diagnosis are a particular concern. In a Toronto study of 100 children with CD diagnosed prior to or at an early stage of puberty, 17 were below the Tanner and Whitehouse third centile for height at the time of disease recognition. Despite gains in growth following disease treatment at least comparable to those of other patients,

10 of these failed to reach the third centile for adult height when followed to maturity (19). This emphasizes the need for early recognition of CD in young patients and also for new approaches to optimizing the catch-up growth of those diagnosed late.

Mechanisms of Growth Impairment in Crohn's Disease

Several interrelated factors contribute to growth impairment in children with CD. Most emphasis has been placed on the importance of chronic undernutrition as the primary cause of growth retardation (24). The multifactorial etiology of the caloric insufficiency has been discussed. Serum levels of insulin growth factor–1 (IGF-1) are low in most patients with growth abnormalities and likely reflect a poor nutritional state (25). However, the growth-retarding effect of chronic inflammation per se is still poorly defined. A recent study has shown that interleukin-6 (IL-6) secreted from the inflamed gut may act to suppress growth (26). Daily corticosteroid use may inhibit growth, but it is often difficult to separate the relative contributions of disease activity from corticosteroid usage in the pathogenesis of slow linear growth in pediatric CD (13, 19, 22). From the above discussion, it follows that optimization of treatment of intestinal inflammation and provision of adequate nutrition are of paramount importance in preventing or remedying growth impairment (27, 28).

Specific Nutrient Deficiencies

As with protein-calorie malnutrition, deficiencies of vitamins, minerals, and trace elements may result from either inadequate intake or increased losses. Most studies of micronutrition have focused on adults; reported frequencies pertain predominantly to CD (29). Observations based on small numbers of patients may not be generalizable. It is difficult to obtain an accurate and meaningful representation of the prevalence of specific deficiencies, but an appreciation of their relative frequencies is useful.

Water-Soluble Vitamins

Of the water-soluble vitamins, folic acid and vitamin B_{12} deficiencies are relatively commonly encountered; others are extremely rare.

Fat-Soluble Vitamins

Vitamin D deficiency is the most commonly reported fat-soluble vitamin deficiency (30). However, although osteomalacia may be encountered in CD, especially following ileal resection, a more prevalent problem appears to be osteoporosis related to a direct effect of inflammatory disease on bone deposition or resorption (31). Identification and attempts at prevention or correction of this metabolic bone complication will undoubtedly receive increasing attention in the years ahead.

Minerals and Trace Elements

Iron deficiency is common, related to gut losses and inadequate intake (32). The ability to absorb iron is usually preserved. Low serum ferritin is the most reliable indicator of reduced iron stores. Anemia in IBD is frequently due to chronic disease rather than to iron deficiency. Of other minerals and trace elements, zinc has received considerable attention (33). Nevertheless, the true frequency of deficiency and its role in growth retardation are highly controversial because of inaccuracies in the measurement of total body zinc. Low serum levels of zinc reflect more the degree of hypoproteinemia than depletion of body stores. Avoidance of milk products and the effects of corticosteroids on calcium absorption and excretion predispose to calcium deficiency; documented hypocalcemia, however, is usually due to hypoalbuminemia.

NUTRITION IN THE MANAGEMENT OF IBD

Nutritional support is a vital component of the management of patients with IBD. The frequently encountered macronutrient deficiency can lead to altered cellular immunity with increased risk of infection, prolonged cellular renewal of inflamed tissues, delayed wound healing, diminished skeletal muscle function, and, in children, growth retardation (13, 14). Undernutrition and its associated complications may hence become as debilitating as the underlying IBD. Management goals must include correction and prevention of nutritional deficits as well as control of symptoms. Nutritional assessment techniques are discussed in Chapters 54 to 57. Table 69.2 correlates with the above discussion of nutritional problems encountered in IBD and summarizes the evaluation that should be considered an essential minimum for proper patient care.

Table 69.2
Recommended Nutritional Assessment of Patients with IBD

Subject assessment
Detailed history
Complete physical examination, pubertal staging[a]
Dietetic evaluation (3-day diary)
Anthropometry
Height, weight
Growth velocity[a]
Height for age %[a], weight for height %
Midarm circumference
Triceps skinfold thickness
Laboratory data
Complete blood count, red-cell morphology
Serum albumin
Folic acid, vitamin B_{12}
Serum Fe, total iron-binding capacity, ferritin
Calcium, magnesium, alkaline phosphatase
Bone age[a]
Additional tests if growth failure or significant malnutrition is present
Vitamins A, D, E
Prothrombin time, partial prothrombin time
Zinc
Phosphorus

[a]In pediatric populations.

General Dietary Measures

For most ambulatory patients, the most important advice is to consume a diet liberal in protein, with sufficient calories to maintain or restore weight or to support growth in children and adolescents. A caloric input of 35 to 40 kcal/kilogram ideal body weight (IBW) per day and 1 to 1.5 g/kg IBW protein per day will meet the protein and energy requirements of most adult patients with active inflammatory bowel disease. For children, recommendations should be made according to their height, age, and need for catch-up growth. Liquid dietary supplements may help motivated patients to achieve these goals, although in young patients these will often simply displace ingested calories from regular food without increasing total caloric intake (34).

The merits and necessity of dietary restrictions need to be critically examined. Controlled studies have not supported a role for a low-residue diet nor for a high-fiber, low-refined-sugar diet in the maintenance of remission in IBD (35, 36). Recent studies have suggested that exclusion of specific foods on the basis of individual clinical intolerance improves the clinical course of CD (37).

A major problem with dietary modifications is that they frequently result in a less appetizing diet, which discourages optimal caloric intake. Imposition of dietary restrictions can result in a major source of conflict between children with IBD and their parents. Except in specific circumstances (e.g., a low-residue diet to reduce obstructive symptoms in the setting of small intestinal stricture) a full diet for age is most appropriate.

INTENSIVE NUTRITIONAL SUPPORT IN IBD

There are three broad indications for undertaking intensive nutritional support in patients with IBD. The first is adjunctive therapy to correct or avoid malnutrition and to facilitate growth. The second is primary therapy of active intestinal inflammation in CD but not in UC. The third includes the small proportion of CD patients who may require long-term nutritional support because of short bowel syndrome or extensive active disease. Nutritional therapy in these contexts may be provided by enteral nutrition using formulated food or via parenteral nutrition using a centrally placed intravenous catheter. Enteral nutrition has become the preferred and more frequent approach because of its lower complication rates and easier and less costly administration. Circumstances favoring long-term total parenteral nutrition (TPN) are limited to the patient with a very short gut or near-complete obstruction.

Adjunctive Nutritional Therapy

Adjunct to Drug Treatment

Intensive nutritional support will improve the nutritional status of the anorectic or malnourished patient with CD or UC. In the setting of acute severe colitis, which is often unresponsive to drug therapy, provision of TPN will prevent further loss of body protein and improve respiratory and peripheral muscle function (38). Postoperative respiratory complications were reduced among patients who ultimately required colectomy. These data argue for early use of parenteral nutrition in conjunction with corticosteroid therapy but do not justify delaying colectomy to improve nutritional state in the malnourished patient with fulminant disease who is clearly failing medical therapy.

Preoperative Nutritional Support

Adjunctive nutritional therapy has frequently been advocated prior to planned surgery in CD and UC to decrease postoperative morbidity on the basis of observations that protein-calorie malnutrition impairs wound healing and diminishes immunocompetence, thereby increasing the risk of infection. Collins et al. found that provision of calories with amino acids resulted in a lower complication rate postoperatively than either provision of amino acids alone or standard intravenous solutions (39). Clinically important benefits are observed only among patients with severe malnutrition (40).

Nutritional Treatment of Growth Impairment

Among children and adolescents prior to completion of puberty, consistent provision of adequate nutrition, either enterally or parenterally, effectively restores normal growth (13, 24, 41–43). The most common approach involves nocturnal nasogastric infusion of formulated food (41–43). Such intensive nutritional support rather than simple dietary counseling to increase caloric intake is required when growth is retarded (13).

Primary Nutritional Therapy of Active Disease

Enteral Nutrition

The potential role of exclusive enteral nutrition as primary therapy of active CD was discovered fortuitously. Patients given elemental formulas preoperatively experienced improvement not only in their nutritional status as intended, but also in the inflammatory activity of their disease.

Efficacy: Controlled Trial Data. The controversy surrounding seemingly divergent outcomes in early small controlled trials of exclusive enteral nutrition and subsequent larger multicenter studies has fueled several meta-analyses (44). As summarized in Table 69.3, in all but two small trials, more patients achieved clinical remission with steroids than with enteral nutrition. The pooled odds ratio for likelihood of clinical response to enteral nutrition using elemental, semielemental, or polymeric formulas versus corticosteroids was 0.35 (95% CI, 0.23–0.53) (44). Thus, treatment with corticosteroids has greater benefit than treatment with enteral feeding. Furthermore, sec-

Table 69.3
Results of Trials Included in Metaanalyses: Enteral Nutrition (EN) versus Corticosteroids

Study (ref.)	Number of Patients in Each Treatment Group: EN	Steroids	Formula Type	Percentage Achieving Remission: EN	Steroids	Difference in Remission Rate (EN − Steroids
Lochs 1991 (46)	55	52	Semielemental	53	85	−32
Malchow 1990 (47)	51	44	Semielemental	41	73	−32
Gonzalez-Huix 1993 (57)	15	17	Polymeric	80	67	−8
Lindor 1992 (58)	9	10	Semielemental	22	50	−28
Gorard 1993 (59)	22	20	Elemental	45	85	−40
O'Morain 1984 (60)	11	10	Elemental	82	80	+2
Seidman 1991 (61)	10	9	Elemental	80	67	+13
Seidman 1993 (62)	40	38	Elemental	75	90	−15

ondary metaanalysis excluding dropouts for apparent intolerance showed that poor compliance, although a factor, is not the major reason for the lower response rates to enteral nutrition (44).

No controlled trials have compared enteral nutrition with placebo or less effective drugs in active CD. Comparison of observed response rates to exclusive liquid diet therapy (53–82%) with usual placebo response rates in the controlled clinical trial setting suggests that enteral nutrition is of therapeutic benefit, even if efficacy does not equal that of corticosteroid treatment (44). Moreover, reduced gastrointestinal protein loss, decreased intestinal permeability, and reduced fecal excretion of indium-labeled leukocytes have all been demonstrated, suggesting a direct effect on intestinal inflammation (45).

There are situations in which risk/benefit considerations may justify a preference for exclusive enteral nutrition, even if steroids induce clinical remission in more patients. Children with CD need special approaches to therapy (13, 27, 28). Enteral nutrition can provide optimal macro- and micronutrients and appears to ameliorate intestinal inflammation, all of which should facilitate growth. Enteral nutrition does seem to be more feasible, if not inherently more efficacious, in pediatric populations. The formula can be infused nocturnally in the home setting and not interfere with normal activities.

Site-Specific Efficacy. The site of intestinal inflammation has been postulated to influence the likelihood of response to nutritional therapy. Specifically, it has been suggested on the basis of retrospective data that Crohn's colitis responds less well to enteral feeding than ileocolitis or isolated small bowel disease. The large European Collaborative Crohn's Disease Study could not relate outcome to the site of intestinal inflammation, but the numbers of patients with isolated colonic disease were small, even in these trials (46, 47). The lack of site-specific data concerning rates of induction of clinical remission in other trials precludes prospective appraisal of the relationship between anatomic localization of CD and responsiveness to exclusive enteral nutrition. In one trial comparing two types of enteral nutrition, two-thirds of patients had disease confined to the colon, but excellent clinical response rates of 67 and 73% to elemental and polymeric formulas, respectively, were nevertheless observed (48).

Mode of Action. The mode of action of enteral nutrition as primary treatment of active CD remains conjectural. Hypotheses have included alteration in intestinal microbial flora, elimination of dietary antigen uptake, diminution of intestinal synthesis of inflammatory mediators via reduction of dietary fat, overall nutritional repletion, or provision of important micronutrients to the diseased intestine (49).

Importance of Formula Composition. The importance of formula composition to efficacy can be addressed by sensitivity analyses of trials versus corticosteroids, grouped according to type of liquid diet, or by metaanalysis of data from trials comparing an elemental with a nonelemental formula (see Chapter 101 for formula content). Trials versus corticosteroids, employing a low-fat elemental diet, included too few patients for any definitive conclusion. Results from directly comparative trials as summarized in Table 69.4 do not support a benefit for elemental formulas. The pooled odds ratio for likelihood of attainment of remission using an elemental versus nonelemental formula was 0.87 (95% CI 0.41–1.83) (44). However, the number of patients in the total sample would preclude detection of a difference in response rate even as large as 30%. Furthermore, the elemental and "nonelemental" formulas used in these studies were not consistently disparate. All elemental formulas contained amino acids as their protein source, but the "nonelemental" formulas contained either oligopeptides (also of low antigenicity) or intact proteins. Similarly, the percentage of total calories derived from fat varied greatly. Both a low total fat content and a low ratio of n-6:n-3 PUFAs have been hypothesized as necessary for reduction of intestinal inflammation (5, 6, 49). Data from randomized controlled trials are at present insufficient to establish definitively whether either decreased antigenicity related to the protein content or an immunomodulatory or antiinflammatory effect related to low-fat content is important in reduc-

Table 69.4
Formula Composition and Outcome in Trials of Elemental versus Nonelemental Liquid Diet Therapy

	Elemental Diet				Nonelemental			
Study (ref.)	Number of Patients Treated	Percentage Achieving Remission	Protein Source	% Total Calories As Fat	Number of Patients Treated	Percentage Achieving Remission	Protein Source	%Total Calories As Fat
Raouf 1991 (63)	13	69	Amino acids	16.4	11	73	Intact milk	Not stated
Rigaud 1991 (48)	15	67	Amino acids	0.8	15	73	Intact milk protein and egg or milk protein	27 36
Park 1991 (64)	7	29	Amino acids	11	7	71	Whole whey	27
Royall 1994 (65)	19	84	Amino acids	3	21	71	Oligopeptides	33 (10 LCT +23 MCT)
Middleton 1991 (66)	11	73	Amino acids	16.4	15	73	Oligopeptides	24

ing intestinal inflammation. These possibilities should both be further explored.

Importance of "Bowel Rest." When used in the treatment of active CD, enteral nutrition is generally combined with "bowel rest." However, in a randomized trial of adjunctive nutritional treatments, Greenberg et al. observed that partial parenteral nutrition plus an ad libitum oral diet was as effective in inducing clinical remission as either elemental liquid diets administered by nasogastric tube or TPN and complete bowel rest among patients hospitalized because of continuing activity of their disease despite high-dose steroid therapy (50).

Maintenance of Remission. One of the limitations of liquid diet therapy has been the observed tendency for symptoms to recur promptly following its cessation. In most studies, 60 to 70% of patients experience a relapse within 12 months of stopping enteral nutrition and resuming a normal diet (42, 44, 48). Nutritional strategies have been used in pediatric studies to keep children well and growing for a longer time after attaining remission through use of exclusive enteral nutrition. In a Canadian Pediatric Collaborative Trial, patients attaining remission through exclusive enteral nutrition or prednisone treatment were rerandomized to receive for 18 months either cyclical exclusive semielemental liquid diet therapy for 4 weeks out of every 16 or low-dose alternate-day prednisone. As recently reported, linear growth was better and rate of clinical relapse lower with the nutritional treatment (27). This confirms an earlier retrospective report of the beneficial effects of cyclical exclusive enteral nutrition on disease activity and growth (43). Continuation of nocturnal nasogastric feeding four to five times weekly as supplement to an unrestricted ad libitum daytime diet was also associated with prolonged disease quiescence and improved growth in a historical cohort study (42). In the long term, allowing normal food at times when family and friends are eating is particularly important in achieving compliance. The observation that supplementary enteral nutrition is associated with prolonged clinical remission despite resumption of regular food is most consistent with a micro- or macronutritional effect (42).

Mode of Administration. Children become adept at passing a nasogastric silastic feeding catheter each night. However, if long-term therapy either in a cyclical exclusive or continuous supplementary fashion is contemplated, insertion of a gastrostomy tube may make administration easier. This procedure appears to be uncomplicated in CD patients, but experience is limited. One patient in a pediatric series had a persistent gastrocutaneous fistula when the gastrostomy tube was removed, but surgical closure was successful (51).

Parenteral Nutrition

Efficacy. Studies of TPN as primary treatment of active CD have been summarized in detail by Greenberg (14). In contrast to studies of enteral nutrition in active disease, there are numerous retrospective reports but few prospective, randomized, controlled trials of TPN. From retrospective series among CD patients, one can expect an in-hospital remission rate of 64% after 14 to 21 days of treatment, with isolated colonic CD responding less often than disease involving the small intestine alone or small intestine plus colon (14). Two small prospective controlled trials suggest that TPN combined with bowel rest is of no primary therapeutic efficacy in the management of patients with acute UC or of those with acute Crohn's colitis, although it will improve their nutritional status (52, 53). Only two randomized studies have compared TPN with exclusive enteral nutrition in the treatment of active disease; remission rates with either modality were comparable (50, 54). There is no evidence to suggest that TPN is superior to enteral nutrition in the treatment of acute inflammation. Indeed, enteral provision of nutrients may optimize the repair of inflamed mucosa. In animals, TPN administration is associated with subtotal villous atrophy of the intestine, and this physical alteration of the mucosal barrier promotes translocation of bacteria normally confined to the gastrointestinal tract (55). Permeability, in contrast, normalizes with enteral nutrition, so that access to factors that putatively may perpetuate intestinal inflammation is reduced (47).

Long-Term Nutritional Support

Fortunately, only a small minority of patients with CD have inadequate gastrointestinal reserve for maintaining a normal nutritional state on standard oral or enteral diets. Nevertheless, patients with CD often comprise the largest single group of adults on home TPN programs (56). The usual clinical setting involves persistent active inflammation after multiple small bowel resections. Either the remaining small bowel is incapable of sufficient nutrient absorption to sustain nutritional homeostasis (short bowel syndrome) or resection of the colon and ileum results in substantial losses of isotonic fluid, electrolytes, minerals, and trace elements, but with relatively normal macronutrient absorption (end-jejunostomy syndrome). Both of these circumstances may require permanent home parenteral nutrition for provision of complete nutritional support or alternatively to facilitate fluid and electrolyte balance. It is hoped that these situations will become less common with the more conservative approaches to surgery: operation for complications of disease only, limited resections of only the most severely diseased bowel, and use of stricturoplasty to preserve absorptive surface area (See also Chapter 101).

REFERENCES

1. Podolsky DK. N Engl J Med 1991;325:928–35, 1008–14.
2. Calkins BM, Mendeloff AI. Epidemiol Rev 1986;8:60–91.
3. Persson P-G, Alhbom A, Hellers G. Scand J Gastroenterol 1987; 22:385–9.
4. Lochs H, Genser D, Bühner S. Role of nutrition in IBD. In: Tytgat GNJ, Bartelsman JFWM, van Deventer SJH, eds. Inflammatory bowel diseases 1995. Hingham, MA: Kluwer Academic Publishers, 1995.
5. Shoda R, Matsueda K, Yamato S, et al. Am J Clin Nutr 1996;63: 741–5.
6. Blok WL, Katan MB, van der Meer JWM. J Nutr 1996;126: 1515–33.
7. Belluzzi A, Brignola C, Campieri M, et al. N Engl J Med 1996;334:1557–60.
8. Filipsson S, Hulten L, Lindstedt G. Scand J Gastroenterol 1978;13:529–36.
9. Dyer NH, Dawson AM. Br J Surg 1973;60:134–40.
10. Griffiths AM, Drobnies A, Soldin SJ, et al. J Pediatr Gastroenterol Nutr 1986;5:907.
11. Kirschner BS, Defavaro MV, Jensen W. Gastroenterology 1981;81:829–32.
12. Griffiths AM. Pharmacologic treatment of IBD. In: Durie P, Hamilton JR, Walker JA, Walker-Smith JA, eds. Pediatric gastrointestinal disease. 2nd ed. St. Louis: Mosby Year Book, 1996.
13. Seidman E, LeLeiko N, Ament M, et al. J Pediatr Gastroenterol Nutr 1991;12:424–38.
14. Greenberg GR. Semin Gastrointest Dis 1993;4:69–86.
15. Murch SH. Inflammatory mediators and suppression of growth in paediatric chronic IBD. In: Tytgat GNJ, Bartelsman JFWM, van Deventer SJH, eds. Inflammatory bowel diseases 1995. Kluwer Academic Publishers, 1995.
16. Chan ATH, Fleming CR, O'Fallon WM, et al. Gastroenterology 1986;91:75–8.
17. Ascue M, Rashid M, Griffiths A, et al. Gut 1997;41:203–8.
18. Kirschner BS. Acta Paediatr Scand 1990;(Suppl 366):98–104.
19. Griffiths AM, Nguyen P, Smith C, et al. Gut 1993;34:939–43.
20. Hildebrand H, Karlberg J, Kristiansson B. J Pediatr Gastroenterol Nutr 1994;18:165–73.
21. Markowitz J, Grancher K, Rosa J, et al. J Pediatr Gastroenterol Nutr 1993;16:373–80.
22. Motil KJ, Grand RJ, Davis-Kraft L, et al. Gastroenterology 1993; 105:681–91.
23. Kanof ME, Lake AM, Bayless TM. Gastroenterology 1988;95: 1423–7.
24. Kelts DG, Grand RJ, Shen G, et al. Gastroenterology 1979;76: 720–7.
25. Thomas AG, Holly JMP, Taylor E, et al. Gut 1993;34:944–7.
26. DeBenedetti F, Alonzi T, Moretta A, et al. J Clin Invest 1997;99: 643–50.
27. Griffiths AM. Medical management of Crohn's disease in a pediatric population. In: McLeod RS, Martin F, Sutherland LR, et al., eds. Trends in IBD therapy. Kluwer Academic Publishers, 1997.
28. Walker-Smith JA. Arch Dis Child 1996;75:351–4.
29. Harries AD, Heatley RV. Postgrad Med J 1983;59:690–7.
30. Driscoll RH, Meredith SC, et al. Gastroenterology 1982;83: 1252–8.
31. Bjarnson I, Macpherson A, Mackintosh C, et al. Gut 1997;40: 228–33.
32. Bartels U, Strandberg Pedersen N, Jarnum S. Scand J Gastroenterol 1978;13:649–56.
33. Hendricks KM, Walker WA. Nutr Rev 1988;46:40–6.
34. Harries AD, Danis V, Heatley RV, et al. Lancet 1983;1:887–90.
35. Levenstein S, Prantera C, Luzi C, et al. Gut 1985;26:989–93.
36. Ritchie JK, Wadsworth J, Lennard-Jones JE, Rogers E. Br Med J 1987;295:517–20.
37. Riordan AM, Hunter JO, Cowan RE. Lancet 1993;343:1131–4.
38. Christie PM, Hill GL. Gastroenterology 1990;99:730–6.
39. Collins JP, Oxby CB, Hill GL. Lancet 1978;1:788–91.
40. Veterans Affairs TPN Cooperative Study Group. N Engl J Med 1991;325:525–32.
41. Aiges H, Markowitz J, Rosa J, et al. Gastroenterology 1999;97: 905–10.
42. Wilschanski M, Sherman P, Pencharz P, et al. Gut 1996; 38:543–8.
43. Belli DC, Seidman E, Bouthillier L, et al. Gastroenterology 1988;94:603–10.
44. Griffiths AM, Ohlsson A, Sherman P, et al. Gastroenterology 1995;108:1056–67.
45. Teahon K, Smethurst P, Pearson M, et al. Gastroenterology 1991;101:84–7.
46. Lochs H, Steinhardt HJ, Klaus-Ventz B, et al. Gastroenterology 1991;101:881–8.
47. Malchow H, Steinhardt HJ, Lorenz-Meyer H, et al. Scand J Gastroenterol 1990;25:235–44.
48. Rigaud D, Cosnes J, Le Quintrec Y, et al. Gut 1991;32:1492–7.
49. Fernandez-Banares F, Cabre E, Gonzalez-Huix F, et al. Gut 1994;35:S55–9.
50. Greenberg GR, Fleming CR, Jeejeebhoy KN, et al. Gut 1988;29:1309–15.
51. Israel DM, Hassall E. Am J Gastroenterol 1995;90:1084–8.
52. Dickinson RJ, Ashton RM, Axon ATR. Gastroenterology 1980; 79:1199–204.
53. McIntyre PB, Powell-Tuck J, Wood SR, et al. Gut 1986;27: 481–4.
54. Alun Jones V. Dig Dis Sci 1987;32:1009–75.

55. Feldman FJ, Dowling RH, McNaughton J, et al. Gastroenterology 1976;5:712–9.
56. Richards DM, Irving MH. Gut 1997;40:218–22.
57. Gonzalez-Huix F, de Leon R, Fernandez-Banares F, et al. Gut 1993;34:778–82.
58. Lindor KD, Fleming R, Burnes JU, et al. Mayo Clin Proc 1992;67:328–33.
59. Gorard DA, Hunt JB, Payne-James JJ, et al. Gut 1993;34:1198–202.
60. O'Morain C, Segal AW, Levi AJ. Br Med J 1984;288:1859–62.
61. Seidman EG, Lohoues MJ, Turgeon J, et al. Gastroenterology 1986;90:1625A.
62. Seidman E, Griffiths AM, Jones A, et al. Gastroenterology 1993;104:778A.
63. Raouf AH, Hildrey V, Daniel J, et al. Gut 1991;32:702–7.
64. Park HR, Galloway A, Danesh JZD, Russell RI. Eur J Gastroenterol Hepatol 1991;3:483–90.
65. Royall D, Jeejeebhoy KN, Baker JP, et al. Gut 1994;35:783–7.
66. Middleton SJ, Riordan AM, Hunter JO. Ital J Gastroenterol 1991;23:609A

SELECTED READINGS

Greenberg GR. Nutritional management of inflammatory bowel disease. Semin Gastrointest Dis 1993:4:69–86.

Grimble RF. Nutrition and cytokine action. Nutr Res Rev 1990;3:193–210.

Heller AD. Nutrition in patients with inflammatory bowel disease. In: Korelitz B, Sohne N, eds. Management of inflammatory bowel disease. St. Louis: Mosby-Year Book, 1992.

Lochs H, Genser D, Buhner S. Role of nutrition in IBD. In: Tytgat GNJ, Bartelsman JFWM, van Deventer SJH, eds. Inflammatory bowel diseases 1995. Kluwer Academic Publishers, 1995.

Seidman E, Leleiko N, Ament M, et al. Nutritional issues in pediatric inflammatory bowel disease. Symposium report. J Pediatr Gastroenterol Nutr 1991;12:424–38.

70. Diseases of the Small Bowel

PENNY S. TURTEL and MOSHE SHIKE

Inflammatory bowel diseases (Chapter 69), the short bowel syndrome (Chapter 68), celiac disease (Chapter 71), and various intestinal parasite infections are the most common diseases of the intestinal tract that result in malabsorption and nutritional problems. This chapter addresses other, less common diseases that may also cause severe intestinal dysfunction, malabsorption, and malnutrition.

RADIATION ENTERITIS

Abdominal and pelvic radiation, commonly used in the treatment and palliation of various tumors can cause major gastrointestinal morbidity. With the development of supervoltage techniques, high doses can be administered to the tumor without skin toxicity, making gastrointestinal tolerance the main dose-limiting factor. The ileum and jejunum are felt to be the most susceptible, followed by the transverse colon, sigmoid, and rectum. During the time of radiation, most patients experience acute radiation toxicity, manifested by nausea, vomiting, abdominal cramps, and diarrhea. This form of toxicity is self limited and usually subsides within weeks of ending radiation therapy (RT). Chronic, late gastrointestinal complications occur less frequently and can cause major morbidity and mortality.

Risk factors predisposing to radiation injury of the small and large intestine include previous abdominal surgery, thin physique, hypertension, diabetes mellitus, and pelvic inflammatory disease (1). Concomitant chemotherapy, especially with actinomycin D, seems to compound the damage (2). Total dose administered and volume of bowel irradiated are major determinants of late radiation damage. Significant injury generally occurs when more than 5000 rads are administered.

Prevention

Besides limiting the amount of radiation and appropriately fractionating the total dose schedule, prevention efforts are aimed at minimizing bowel exposure during RT. Several surgical techniques have been described that displace small bowel from the pelvic radiation field. These include intraoperative placement of a polyglycolic, absorbable intestinal sling that suspends the small bowel above the pelvic radiation field and resorbs several months postoperatively (3, 4); the "pedicled omentoplasty," which uses the omentum as a sling to exclude the small bowel from the pelvis (5); and peritoneal reconstruction, used in patients with rectal carcinoma, in which the posterior rectus sheath and peritoneum are used to partition the abdominal cavity at the level of the umbilicus to the sacral promontory (6).

Medications have not generally been useful in prevention of radiation enteritis (RE). A randomized, placebo-controlled trial of 5-ASA, the active component of Azulfidine, did not demonstrate any protective effect and appeared to worsen diarrhea (7). An aminothiol drug, given intravenously prior to RT in one trial protected against radiation injury, presumably acting as a free radical scavenger (8). Sucralfate reduced acute diarrhea and prevented late bowel disturbances in one trial (9).

Pathology

Acute Phase

Acute radiation changes are manifested primarily in the mucosal layer. Mitotic activity in the segment of irradiated intestinal epithelium decreases within 12 hours of the first treatment, continues to drop during the first week and persists at low levels throughout treatment (10). Mucosal injury occurs with shortening of villi, decrease in mucosal thickness, edema, erosions, inflammation, and ulcerations. Within 2 weeks after completion of therapy, the histologic picture returns to normal in most patients (10).

Subacute Phase

Vascular and connective tissue damage becomes evident in the subacute period, from 2 to 12 months after radiation treatment. Large "foam cells" beneath the intima, abnormal fibroblasts, and submucosal fibrosis are characteristic. As a result, there is obliteration of venules and arterioles and progressive ischemia, which can then insidiously lead to clinically apparent chronic RE.

Chronic Phase

All layers of the gut wall and mesentery are involved in chronic radiation injury; submucosal fibrosis, edema, lymphatic ectasia, and obliterative endarteritis are characteristic (Fig. 70.1). These pathologic changes can result in ulcerations, perforations, strictures, and fistulas.

Clinical Manifestations

Acute Phase

Acute gastroenterologic symptoms from abdominal RT are common. Most patients experience anorexia, nausea, and vomiting early in treatment, which seem to be mediated through the central nervous system. After 2 to 3 weeks of RT, abdominal cramping and watery diarrhea may occur. Slight-to-moderate weight loss is common, occurring more frequently with abdominal than with pelvic RT, and is attributed mainly to decreased food intake. Malabsorption of water, fats, bile salts, carbohydrates, calcium, magnesium, iron, and vitamin B_{12} occurs commonly during RT. It is generally most pronounced at midtreatment and persists to the end of treatment.

Malabsorbed bile salts and carbohydrates play a major role in acute radiation-induced diarrhea. Bile salts that normally are absorbed in the terminal ileum reach the colon, where they induce secretion of fluids and minerals, inhibit absorption, and stimulate peristalsis ("cholerheic diarrhea"). Malabsorbed carbohydrates, presumably resulting from secondary brush border enzyme deficiencies, exert strong osmotic effects in the intestinal lumen, compounding the fluid losses.

In most patients, acute radiation symptoms resolve within several weeks after cessation of therapy (11). In a small percentage, symptoms persist and merge with those of chronic RE.

Chronic Phase

The relationship between acute and chronic RE is unclear. Absence of early symptoms does not guarantee protection from delayed morbidity. An estimated 5 to 15% of patients suffer late sequelae of radiation, with latency periods ranging from 1 year to over 20 years, commencing in most studies at 1 to 2 years (12, 13). These percentages represent reported series of patients with severe disease and probably underestimate the incidence of chronic overall morbidity (14). In one study of 17 women with previous pelvic radiation, none of whom sought attention for gastroenterologic complaints, 12 reported a permanent change in bowel habits, 16 had abnormal cholylglycine breath tests, and 8 had abnormal small bowel radiologic studies (15).

Colicky abdominal pain, diarrhea, steatorrhea, and weight loss are the most common clinical manifestations. Small bowel obstruction, fistula and abscess formation, bleeding, and perforation are less frequent, but graver complications, often requiring operation, with its attendant high postoperative morbidity and mortality (16). Gallstones and hyperoxaluria may develop as a consequence of ileal dysfunction.

Several factors contribute to the malabsorption that occurs in late radiation damage: *(a)* bacterial overgrowth

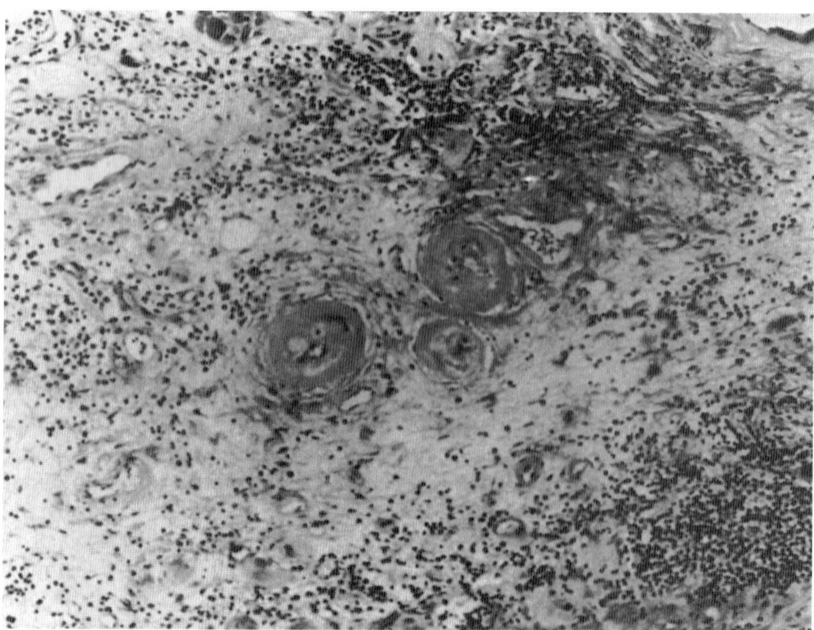

Figure 70.1. Chronic radiation enteritis. Small bowel biopsy demonstrating *(in the center)* three blood vessels partially occluded by fibrosis and inflammation in the walls.

secondary to strictures, fistulas, and stasis; *(b)* decreased available absorptive surface area because of radiation damage and resection; *(c)* chronic lymphatic obstruction causing steatorrhea and protein loss; *(d)* secondary disaccharidase deficiency and subsequent osmotic catharsis; *(e)* bile salt malabsorption leading to cholerheic diarrhea; and *(f)* rapid intestinal transit.

Management

Specific therapeutic modalities are used to treat gastrointestinal pathology when the mechanism can be identified, including antibiotics for bacterial overgrowth; cholestyramine for bile acid malabsorption; antidiarrheal medications for rapid transit; and anticholinergic and antispasmodic preparations for pain and cramps. Most treatments are largely empiric, with few controlled trials. Sucralfate decreased acute symptoms in one trial (9). Azulfidine, in some cases with corticosteroids, was helpful in managing diarrhea of RE in a small number of reports (17). Loperamide-*N*-oxide, a peripheral opiate agonist precursor, decreased stool frequency and volume, slowed small bowel and whole gut transit, and improved bile acid absorption in a double-blind, randomized controlled trial (18). In a recent case report, hyperbaric oxygen was dramatically effective in a woman with severe chronic RE. Therapy consisted of 20 sessions of 100% oxygen inhalation, at 3 bar in a hyperbaric chamber. During treatment, nausea, vomiting and diarrhea abated, and weight gain occurred. Four and one-half months later, clinical improvement persisted, and the D-xylose test, previously severely abnormal, normalized (19).

Nutritional Management

Nutrition is optimized by identifying the factors contributing to malabsorption and correcting those that are treatable. Dietary therapy can play a major role in both controlling symptoms and ensuring adequate nutrition. Enteral and parenteral nutrition should be used only in severe cases.

Acute Radiation Enteritis

During RT, control of diarrhea and prevention of weight loss constitute important goals. A diet low in lactose and fat is recommended, as transient ileal dysfunction and brush border enzyme deficiencies are highly prevalent, causing diarrhea and malabsorption. Experimental evidence suggests that intraluminal contents, especially pancreatic secretions and bile acids, potentiate acute small intestinal radiation damage (20). This finding has led to trials of enteral feeding with solutions containing amino acids or partially digested protein and very low fat content. These solutions are absorbed proximally in the small intestine and are thought to stimulate less pancreatic, biliary, and salivary secretion than normal diets. Studies in which patients received only such enteral feeding during RT indeed demonstrated less diarrhea and weight loss and less frequent interruption of the radiation schedule because of toxicity (21, 22). Enteral nutrition solutions used as dietary supplements provide no clinical benefit (23).

Despite data supporting the use of enteral feeding with partially or fully digested protein during RT, the transient nature of the acute injury, the inconvenience of limiting intake to these formulas, and their unpalatability requiring their administration through a tube make them impractical for general use. Such enteral feeding should be used only in patients who develop severe acute toxicity or who have preexisting malnutrition.

Several studies have evaluated the role of total parenteral nutrition (TPN) during pelvic and abdominal RT. TPN clearly prevents weight loss, and in some cases, lessens gastrointestinal toxicity, while enhancing the ability of the patient to tolerate RT on schedule. Survival is not affected. Two randomized prospective trials concluded that TPN should be reserved for patients malnourished before starting a course of curative RT (24, 25). This conclusion is reasonable considering the complexity of TPN and the fact that acute RE is a transient disorder.

Chronic Radiation Enteritis

Assessment of the functional outcome of chronic RE should be the first step in management of this disorder. The nutritional status of the patient should be evaluated, and a complete investigation for malabsorption and specific nutrient deficiencies should be performed (Chapters 57 and 65). These may include radiographic studies of the intestinal tract, absorption studies (D-xylose, stool fat, and Schilling test), and assessment of blood levels of selected nutrients.

Dietary management is effective in treating both the diarrhea and the nutritional deficiencies of chronic RE. Sequential restrictions of fat, fiber, lactose, and gluten may establish an optimal diet that provides symptomatic relief and improves nutrition. In addition, such an approach may clarify which pathophysiologic mechanisms are salient in an individual patient. The histologic similarity between RE and other malabsorptive diseases, such as sprue, has led to trials using specific dietary therapy as the major form of treatment for RE. A diet free of gluten, cow's milk protein, and lactose, with low fat and fiber content was given to five children with severe, delayed injury manifested by small bowel obstruction after whole abdominal irradiation (2). In all patients, clinical symptoms improved, and radiographic studies and histologic pictures normalized. After 1 to 2 years, the gradual addition of fiber, gluten, milk, and fat was well tolerated by all. In another trial, dietary fat was restricted to 40 g/day in nine women with diarrhea after pelvic irradiation (26). Three to 6 months later, fecal excretion of bile salts decreased, and diarrhea abated in eight of the nine patients.

A trial of low-fat, partially digested protein liquid formula given through a tube may benefit patients who fail to improve with oral dietary therapy. Significant reductions in fecal fluid, fat, and nitrogen with the use of enteral feedings (27) were reported, while other authors found no such benefit (13). Patients with limited absorptive capacity can benefit from enteral feedings given in a pump-controlled, slow infusion through a gastrostomy tube. This technique avoids overwhelming the intestine's limited absorptive capacity, which can occur with bolus feedings or oral feeding. Using this mode of nutrition, some patients can be maintained in good nutritional state without the use of TPN.

In patients with severe RE who are unable to maintain their weight with oral or enteral diets, TPN is lifesaving. It achieves weight gain, improves overall nutrition, and may help in decreasing fistula drainage (28). Some evidence also suggests a direct therapeutic role for TPN. In a report on 31 patients (29) with severe RE treated with TPN, significant improvement in intestinal function, nutritional status, and weight gain was observed. Oral feeding was resumed in 11 of 31 (36%) patients after a mean of 3.6 months, and 8 of these patients had a sustained benefit. Factors predicting a poor response were age above 60 years, hypertension, diabetes mellitus, vascular occlusive disease, and intestinal fistula or perforation. TPN was well tolerated and was associated with few complications. However, TPN does not affect morbidity, overall survival rate, or clinical recurrence of severe RE (34% at 1 year, 47% at 2 years). Although these results are encouraging, most data indicate that the role of TPN is supportive, not therapeutic, and that TPN should be reserved for patients with nutritional failure refractory to dietary therapy and enteral feeding.

Surgical Treatment

High postoperative morbidity and mortality have been reported for surgical management of chronic RE due to extensive adhesions, fibrosis, and poor tissue healing. Surgery is generally reserved for patients whose symptoms are not relieved by conservative measures, usually those with small bowel obstruction. In one recent series of 20 patients over a 22-year period who underwent surgery for chronic radiation injury, postoperative morbidity was 55%, consisting of diarrhea, fistula formation, ostomy complications, obstruction, and wound infection. The authors concluded that although intestinal resection and primary anastomosis are possible, judicious creation of stomas can avoid major morbidity and mortality (30).

EOSINOPHILIC GASTROENTERITIS

Eosinophilic gastroenteritis (EGE) is a spectrum of disorders characterized by food-related gastrointestinal symptoms, peripheral eosinophilia, and eosinophilic infiltration of the gastrointestinal tract (Chapter 92). Peak age of onset is in the third decade, and children constitute approximately 20% of reported cases (31). The disease shows a slight male predominance (32).

The cause of EGE remains unknown. An allergic basis is believed most likely, supported by frequent association with atopic disorders such as asthma, dermatitis, eczema, allergic rhinitis, and bronchitis and by the frequent finding of elevated serum IgE. The role of tissue eosinophilia remains unclear. Whether the eosinophils are mediating the injury or are responding to and modulating the inflammation is not known.

Parasitic infection can cause diffuse eosinophilic infiltration in the gut, with similar symptoms of abdominal complaints and weight loss. By definition, no infestation is found in idiopathic EGE, and in all cases, parasitic infection must be excluded with stool studies and careful inspection of biopsy specimens. Serologic testing and duodenal aspirate should be considered as well, particularly in patients from endemic areas.

Drug or toxin exposure can also produce a clinical picture of eosinophilic gastroenteritis, in particular, gold salts (33) and L-tryptophan ingestion (34).

Pathology and Clinical Manifestations

Three clinicopathologic patterns of EGE have been described (35).

Mucosal Layer–Predominant

Mucosal layer–predominant EGE is the most common pattern, generally involving the stomach alone or both the stomach and small intestine. Recent reports extend the spectrum of gastrointestinal tract involvement to include isolated eosinophilic esophagitis, paninvolvement of the gastrointestinal tract (36, 37), and cholangitis associated with colitis (38).

Presenting complaints include eating-related nausea, vomiting, and abdominal pain, occasionally with diarrhea. Approximately 50% of patients have a history of allergic disorders. Edema, pallor, occult fecal blood, and frequently, signs of allergic disease are present on physical examination. In children, growth retardation is prominent. Further evaluation typically reveals iron-deficiency anemia, peripheral eosinophilia (up to 55%), hypoproteinemia, and evidence of malabsorption and protein-losing enteropathy. The D-xylose test typically is abnormal, reflecting small intestinal mucosal dysfunction, whereas the Schilling test for vitamin B_{12} absorption and the fecal fat test are variably abnormal. Radiographic and endoscopic studies reveal edematous, distorted, and sometimes nodular folds, irritability, and increased secretion (39). Occasionally, ulcers are present, involving primarily the gastric antrum and proximal small intestine. The pathologic hallmark of the disease is eosinophilic infiltration and tissue edema without vasculitis (35). Villous architecture varies from normal to complete flattening as seen in sprue. Involvement is patchy, and several biopsies may be required to confirm the diagnosis.

Muscle Layer–Predominant

Obstructive symptoms are more prominent. Radiographic studies reveal thickening and rigidity of the gut. Full-thickness biopsy is often needed to demonstrate eosinophilic infiltration through the muscularis propria.

Subserosa-Predominant

The subserosa-predominant pattern is the least common. Patients typically present with ascites, which contains high numbers of eosinophils. The subserosa is thickened and infiltrated with eosinophils. Mucosal and muscle layers are variably involved.

Relationship to Food Allergy

EGE is distinguished from "food allergy" by the inability in EGE to identify a specific offending dietary agent. Many patients with EGE report intolerance to specific foods, most commonly beef, eggs, milk, and pork (35). Blind food challenges, using nasogastric tube delivery, demonstrate development of symptoms and an increase in white blood cells, IgE, and peripheral and tissue eosinophils in response to specific foods (35, 40–42). Yet, dietary manipulation is generally ineffective, and patients with EGE are thus distinguished by their requirement for steroids to induce remission and by their chronicity.

Management

Given the high prevalence of food intolerance in EGE, the first step in treatment should be a trial of eliminating the suspected offending agent. In the absence of a suspect agent, sequential elimination of milk, eggs, pork, beef, and gluten has been recommended (43). Although some patients respond transiently to such measures, sustained response is rare.

Corticosteroids are the mainstay of therapy. Although efficacy has not been documented in controlled clinical trials, anecdotally, they are highly effective, produce quick resolution of symptoms, and allow weight gain in most patients (35, 44). Many patients require small maintenance doses; others need dietary restriction and short courses of steroids for exacerbations only.

Cromolyn, a mast cell stabilizer useful in treating food allergies, has been used in small trials in EGE, with benefit in some (45, 46). A related drug, ketotifen, with antihistamine and mast cell stabilizing properties produced clinical improvement and weight gain and cleared tissue infiltration in a small open trial of six patients (47). Although these drugs do not appear to be as effective as steroids, they are worth a therapeutic trial because of their low toxicity. When patients fail to improve while receiving steroids and have exacerbation of symptoms with any oral intake (a rare occurrence), TPN and bowel rest may be necessary to provide nutrition and induce remission. In one such patient, TPN and intravenous administration of steroids led to a decrease in eosinophilia and in symptoms. When oral feeding was resumed, the disease worsened, and the patient died (48).

AMYLOIDOSIS

Amyloidosis is a multisystem pathologic complex characterized by extracellular deposition of amyloid. Amyloid consists of aggregated, linear glycoprotein fibrils arranged in a β-pleated sheet. Amyloid is classified to two major groups: primary amyloidosis is associated with no preceding or coexisting disease except in cases of multiple myeloma; secondary amyloidosis is associated with underlying conditions, mainly chronic infections (osteomyelitis, tuberculosis) and chronic inflammatory disorders (rheumatoid arthritis, inflammatory bowel disease). Other forms include localized, heredofamilial, senile, and β_2-microglobulin-derived amyloidosis.

The biochemical classification is based on the structure of the fibrils: immunoglobulin light chains in primary and in multiple myeloma–related amyloidosis (AL amyloid); protein A in secondary forms and in familial Mediterranean fever (AA amyloid); prealbumin in other familial forms (AF amyloid), and β_2-microglobulin (AH) in long-term hemodialysis–associated amyloid. Typically, AL affects the gastrointestinal tract (GIT), nerves, skin, heart, and tongue; AA more heavily involves liver, spleen, and kidneys; and AH the osteoarticular system, heart, GIT, and lungs. Actually, overlap exists, and the GIT is frequently involved in both primary and secondary forms.

Pathology

In the GIT, blood vessels are the earliest and most common site involved by amyloid deposition, usually at the submucosal level. Progression of vessel and wall thickening and luminal narrowing may cause bowel ischemia and infarction (49). Gastrointestinal smooth muscle is heavily infiltrated, leading to pressure atrophy and impaired motility. Only with massive deposition is mucosa invaded. Villous architecture in the small intestine most often is normal. Mucosal atrophy and ulceration may result from vascular insufficiency. Neurons in the myenteric plexus and visceral nerve trunks may be damaged by direct pressure from deposition (49).

Endoscopic features of small bowel amyloid vary according to the chemical type of amyloid protein. A fine granular appearance, mucosal erosions, friability, and shallow ulcers are more common in AA cases, reflecting the histologic pattern of wide granular deposition in the lamina propria, whereas multiple polypoid protrusions and thickening of the mucosal folds is found only in AA cases, relating to the massive AL amyloid deposits in the muscularis mucosa, submucosa, and muscularis propria (50).

On routine hematoxylin and eosin staining, amyloid appears pink and amorphous. Congo red staining viewed under polarized light reveals its unique apple-green birefringence. Electron microscopy demonstrates its fibrillar structure.

Clinical Manifestations

Gastrointestinal symptoms may predominate in all forms of systemic amyloidosis and are particularly prominent in the familial forms (51, 52). Constipation or diarrhea typically occurs early in the course. Progression to severe, disabling diarrhea, often with incontinence, may occur subsequently (52). Autonomic neuropathy of the gut nerves and direct muscle layer infiltration underlie these abnormalities, causing dysmotility, stasis, and often bacterial overgrowth.

Abdominal pain, infarction, perforation and bleeding are less common manifestations and reflect vascular insufficiency or direct invasion (49). Occult gastrointestinal bleeding is common. Mechanical obstructions may occur, usually from massive localized amyloid deposition or from ischemia-induced strictures, and must be differentiated from pseudoobstructions, which result from severe motility abnormalities, stasis, and dilatation.

Malabsorption may occur in all forms of amyloidosis, but it is particularly prominent in the familial forms, in which it is an important cause of cachexia and death (51, 52). Multiple factors are involved, including bacterial overgrowth, direct mucosal and submucosal destruction, vascular insufficiency, pancreatic insufficiency, and autonomic neuropathy. In familial amyloidosis with polyneuropathy, the degree of steatorrhea and evolution of gastrointestinal symptoms has been correlated with severity of electromyographic changes in peripheral nerves (52), implicating the neuropathy as a major factor in producing these symptoms. While direct amyloid infiltration of GIT nerves obviously impairs intestinal motility, a reduction in intestinal endocrine cell is reported in familial amyloid-associated polyneuropathy (FAP), suggesting that local hormonal abnormalities may contribute to the dysmotility of GI amyloid (53). In addition, bile acid malabsorption has been demonstrated in most patients with FAP (54). The degree of bile acid malabsorption correlated more closely with gastric retention than with amyloid deposition in small bowel biopsy specimens, supporting dysmotility as the major factor causing malabsorption.

Fecal weight and fat content are elevated in most patients with significant gastrointestinal involvement (49, 51), whereas D-xylose absorption and results of Schilling and bile acid breath tests are variably abnormal. Orocecal transit time, as measured by lactulose hydrogen breath tests, is significantly delayed in both symptomatic and asymptomatic amyloidosis patients (55). Prothrombin time may be elevated, and carotene levels often are depressed (49). Hypocalcemia and hypokalemia occur occasionally. Anemia, when present, may reflect iron or vitamin B_{12} deficiency or the underlying chronic disease. Hypoalbuminemia and edema are common (49), usually reflecting nephrotic syndrome (secondary to amyloid in the kidneys), hepatic dysfunction, malabsorption, and, rarely, protein-losing enteropathy (56).

The most common radiographic appearance is diffuse thickening of the small bowel valvulae conniventes and polypoid appearance (57). Other radiographic features include pseudonodularity, atypical large nodules, pseudoobstruction, ischemic manifestations, dilation without thickening, and blunting of plical folds (58).

The definitive diagnosis of amyloidosis is made by demonstrating amyloid on Congo red staining of a biopsy specimen. High-yield sites for biopsy include rectum, small bowel, and abdominal fat pad. Several biopsies should be performed because amyloid deposition may be patchy.

Management

The use of broad-spectrum antibiotics for enteric bacterial overgrowth often alleviates diarrhea, steatorrhea, and bile acid deconjugation (51); however, the effect is temporary, and repeated courses may be needed. A norepinephrine precursor, L-threo-3,4-dihydroxyphenylserine (L-threo-DOPS) has had efficacy in managing the diarrhea and orthostatic hypotension in amyloidosis (59), presumably acting on sympathetic nerve function. A recent study demonstrated significant short-term reduction in diarrhea and increased serum norephinephrine in patients with familial amyloid neuropathy using intranasal administration of this drug, whereas no significant effect was seen after oral administration, most likely because of drug malabsorption (59). Cisapride, a prokinetic agent, produced marked symptomatic resolution, with normalized bowel movements, decreased abdominal distention and peripheral edema, and increased serum albumin levels in a patient with intestinal pseudoobstruction due to amyloidosis (60).

In managing the nutritional state, special attention should be paid to supplement fat-soluble vitamins, which can be severely malabsorbed in the presence of steatorrhea. Sodium restriction is helpful in patients with edema, and dietary fat restriction is advisable for patients with significant steatorrhea. Pancreatic enzymes are useful when massive pancreatic acinar destruction contributes to the maldigestion. Both TPN and enteral feedings are useful in nutritional support of the cachectic patient with severe wasting and malabsorption related to gastrointestinal amyloidosis.

Combination chemotherapy with prednisone, melphalan, and colchicine may halt progression of nephropathy in some patients with AL amyloid (61). Treatment of the underlying inflammatory condition and adjunctive use of colchicine has been advocated in secondary amyloidosis (62–64). Enterostomy may benefit patients with intractable diarrhea with incontinence.

INTESTINAL LYMPHANGIECTASIA

Intestinal lymphangiectasia (IL) is a protein-losing enteropathy characterized by dilated small bowel lymphatic channels (Fig. 70.2), obstruction to lymph flow, and

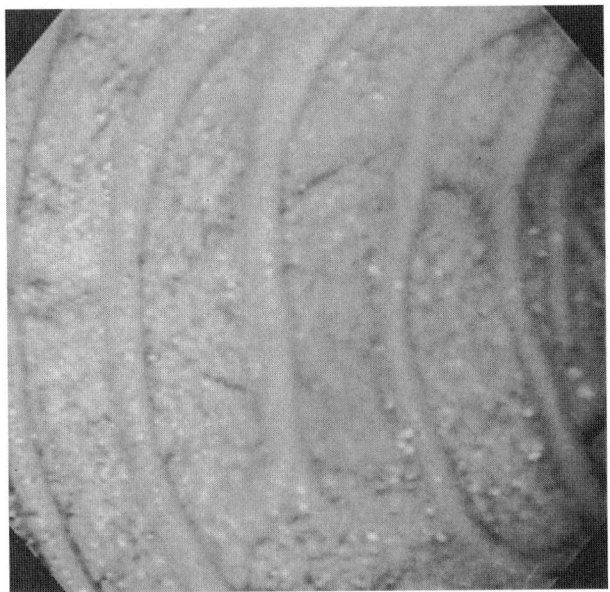

Figure 70.2. Endoscopic picture of the small bowel mucosa of a patient with lymphangiectasis. Dilated lymphatic channels can be seen in the form of many nodules carpeting the mucosal surface

leakage of protein and lymphocyte-rich chyle into the intestinal lumen. The primary form probably represents a congenital malformation of lymphatics and generally presents in early childhood. Family history is often positive in these cases, and lymphatic abnormalities outside the gastrointestinal tract are common. Lymphatic blockage may occur in several locations—lamina propria, submucosa, serosa, and mesentery. A transient acquired type of primary IL has also been described. Secondary IL develops in a variety of disease states in which lymph flow is obstructed. These diseases include constrictive pericarditis, chronic congestive heart failure, left subclavian venous obstruction, retroperitoneal fibrosis or neoplasms, Crohn's disease, mesenteric diseases, tuberculosis, sarcoid, mesenteric panniculitis, RE, and chronic pancreatitis and after abdominal surgical procedures. IL has been reported rarely in systemic sclerosis (65), systemic lupus erythematosus (66), and autoimmune polyglandular disease type I (67). Celiac disease and IL are rarely associated (68), and in some cases IL may masquerade as celiac disease (69).

Endoscopic changes of IL are occasionally seen incidentally, and despite biopsy demonstration of dilated lymphatics, laboratory studies are normal, and no clinical evidence of malabsorption is present, suggesting the presence of a "functional" degree of IL (70).

Pathology

The histologic hallmark is dilatation of mucosal and submucosal lymph vessels (Fig. 70.3). Foamy macrophages containing neutral lipids are found in the lymphatic channels, nodules, and lymph nodes. Mesenteric lymphatics are thickened by medial muscular hypertrophy, fibrosis, and elastosis.

Grossly affected small bowel is edematous and slightly dilated with thickened folds. The serosal surface appears congested. Serosal lymphatics are dilated and may contain yellow nodules. Mesenteric lymph nodes are variably enlarged and yellow. "Enlarged, bleblike tips" give the villous surface a pebbly, papillary appearance.

Clinical Manifestations

Edema, the typical presenting feature, may be generalized or localized. Diarrhea with variable steatorrhea, nau-

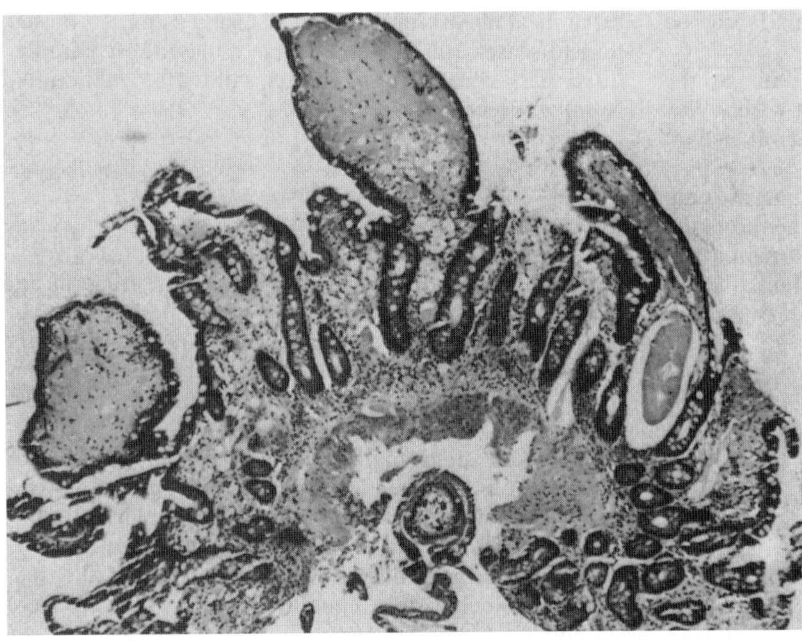

Figure 70.3. Intestinal lymphangiectasia. Small bowel biopsy demonstrating dilated lymphatic channels with widened distorted villi.

sea, and vomiting occurs at some time in most patients. Chylous effusions and abdominal distension with ascites are common, but significant abdominal pain is unusual. Growth retardation may be prominent in children. Bacterial infections, related to lymphopenia and hypogammaglobulinemia, and hypocalcemic tetany secondary to vitamin D malabsorption, may occur in severely affected patients.

Hypoproteinemia and lymphopenia are the salient laboratory features. Serum albumin and globulin levels are markedly reduced, whereas those of other proteins are moderately reduced. Coagulation studies usually are normal, as is the hemoglobulin concentration, although iron deficiency may occur. The cholesterol level is low to normal; deficiencies of fat-soluble vitamins occur to a variable extent. Hypocalcemia, hypomagnesemia, and alkalosis may develop. Results of fecal fat studies range from upper normal to significant steatorrhea. D-Xylose absorption typically is normal. ^{99m}Tc-Scintigraphy using labeled albumin is useful in demonstrating gastrointestinal protein loss, as well as in localizing the region involved (71). Endoscopic features include well-circumscribed xanthomatous plaques, white-tipped villi, multiple submucosal nodules, and, rarely, cystic masses that exude chylous material on biopsy (72). The typical radiographic feature is diffuse, symmetric thickening of folds with increased secretion. Less common findings include dilatation, spiculation, disorganization, punctuate lucencies, and jejunization of ileum. Double-contrast technique is more sensitive in demonstrating the characteristic smooth nodular protrusions (73). Lymphangiography, generally not needed for diagnosis, may be helpful in identifying discrete abnormalities amenable to surgical therapy.

Definitive diagnosis requires small bowel biopsy. The abnormally dilated submucosal lymphatics may be patchy; therefore, several biopsy samples should be obtained.

Management

Diet clearly plays a crucial role in the management of IL. Intestinal lymph production is stimulated by long-chain fatty acids in the intestinal lumen. Decreased production may diminish local lymphatic pressure, resulting in less enteral chyle leakage. Indeed, restricting fat to less than 5 g/day increases serum albumin and albumin half-life and decreases diarrhea and steatorrhea (74). A high-protein, fat-free diet with medium-chain triglyceride (MCT) supplements produced partial to complete remission in most of 15 patients (75).

The MCTs, containing C8-C10 fatty acids, are absorbed directly into the portal system and do not significantly increase lymph flow. When added to the fat-free diet of patients with IL, they enhance its palatability, while providing a good source of calories. In one report, all six children placed on a fat-free, MCT diet showed rapid and sustained long-term clinical improvement (76). Relapse occurred with introduction of long-chain triglycerides and responded to resumption of the previous diet. Despite clinical improvement, persistence of the underlying chyle leak was suggested by refractory lymphopenia and hypoglobulinemia. In several other reports, however, lymphocyte and globulin levels tended to parallel the disease course (75, 77). Short periods of fasting and TPN have been advocated to allow distended lymphatics to collapse and edema to resolve, maximizing conditions for treatment with a fat-free, MCT diet. This plan may be particularly useful for malnourished patients and those with severe diarrhea.

Low-sodium diets, diuretics, and intravenous albumin infusions provide symptomatic relief. Oral vitamin supplements are routinely prescribed. For the rare, highly localized lesion, segmental intestinal resection may be beneficial. Less often, lymphatic-mesenteric venous anastomosis and peritoneal LeVeen shunts are used (78).

Octreotide therapy resulted in a rise in serum albumin, normalization of sedimentation rate, and improvement in fecal albumin loss in a patient with IL associated with an inflammatory disorder that had been refractory to several other therapies (79). Antiplasmin therapy (*trans*-4-aminomethyl cyclohexane carboxylic acid) was dramatically helpful in one patient, with resolution of symptoms and of endoscopic lesions and normalization of protein levels (80), although in several other cases, no benefit was seen (81, 82). Corticosteroids, gluten-free diets, and γ-globulin injections have repeatedly been ineffective (76).

In most patients, the disease is permanent, and its course is marked by spontaneously fluctuating symptoms. Dietary management is successful, for the most part, in maintaining remission. Occasionally, the defect is transient and is completely reversible (75–77).

ABETALIPOPROTEINEMIA

Abetalipoproteinemia (AβL) is a rare, autosomal recessive disorder characterized by *(a)* abnormal lipid metabolism, *(b)* acanthocytosis (spiny or thorny red blood cells), *(c)* retinitis pigmentosa, and *(d)* progressive neurologic dysfunction. Failure of the intestinal mucosa to synthesize apoprotein B (apoB) is the basic defect. This results from mutations in the gene encoding for microsomal triglyceride protein (mtp), a lipid transfer protein within the endoplasmic reticulum of hepatocytes and enterocytes, required for assembly and secretion of apoB lipoproteins (83, 84). ApoB is essential for synthesis and structural integrity of chylomicrons (CMs) and very low density and low-density lipoproteins (VLDLs, LDLs). All of these lipoproteins are therefore absent in AβL. Defective CM formation leads to impaired transportation of fat out of enterocytes and malabsorption of fat-soluble vitamins. Acanthocytosis and lipid abnormalities are present from birth; neurologic and retinal findings generally develop in the second decade, perhaps reflecting deficiency states (vitamins E and A) rather than the underlying disease.

Pathology

Grossly, the mucosa has a diffuse yellow hue. Histologic appearance is unique. Enterocytes appear distended and vacuolated because of engorgement with lipid droplets, even in the fasting state. Nuclei are pressed to the base of cells (85). Villous structure is normal. In contrast to the enterocytes, the lacteals, submucosa, lamina propria, and lymphatics contain no fat. Immunofluorescence studies reveal absence of apoB in jejunal mucosa in the fasting state and lack of apoB synthesis after fat feeding (86).

Clinical Manifestations

Gastrointestinal symptoms of diarrhea, steatorrhea, anorexia, vomiting, and growth retardation manifest in the first year of life. In many cases, celiac sprue is diagnosed, and a gluten-free diet is administered without relief. When the appropriate diagnosis is made and a low-fat diet is prescribed, clinical improvement ensues. Symptoms of fat intolerance tend to diminish with age (86, 87), perhaps as a result of increased use of the portal route of fat absorption.

Neurologic problems begin toward the end of the first decade, years after the onset of gastrointestinal symptoms. These include ataxia, intention tremors, clumsiness, and muscle weakness. Examination reveals abnormalities of the posterior columns, peripheral nerves, cerebellum, and muscles similar to those in Friedreich's ataxia, which often is erroneously diagnosed. Visual complaints, scotomata, and decreased acuity are the last to develop. Ophthalmoscopic examination demonstrates fine mottling of the retina consistent with atypical retinitis pigmentosa. Decreased photoreceptor response in both light and dark conditions may be demonstrated on physiologic testing (electroretinography). Untreated, the neurologic and retinal features progress relentlessly and cause severe impairment (88).

The biochemical hallmark of AβL is complete absence of apoB and undetectable or small amounts of β-lipoproteins—LDLs, VLDLs, and CMs—on plasma lipid electrophoresis (88, 89). Serum cholesterol and triglyceride levels are low, 0.78 to 2.07 mmol/L (30–80 mg/dL) and less than 0.11 mmol/L (10 mg/dL), respectively, and the triglyceride level fails to rise after fat ingestion (89). Although linoleic acid levels are reduced in blood and in tissue, essential fatty acid (EFA) deficiency does not contribute significantly to the clinical picture (89, 90).

Fecal fat content is mildly to moderately increased. D-Xylose and Schilling absorption tests typically are normal, as are measurements of serum electrolytes and complete blood count. Examination of the blood smear preparations reveals spiny or thorn erythrocytes—acanthocytes. The lipid composition of the membranes of these red blood cells is abnormal with a unique phospholipid distribution: decreased lecithin and increased sphingomyelin (85). These changes may contribute to the abnormal configuration. Although acanthocytes function normally, increased autohemolysis and increased sensitivity to peroxide hemolysis, the latter of which is correctable with dietary vitamin E supplementation, are demonstrable (85).

A combination of impaired vitamin E absorption and defective transport (because of the absence of apoB, its normal carrier) results in severe vitamin E deficiency (88). Serum levels are undetectable; tissue levels are low (91). Vitamin E deficiency likely contributes significantly, if not entirely, to the neurologic and perhaps retinal manifestations of AβL (87, 88). Vitamin A is moderately to severely malabsorbed, and night blindness may compound the visual symptoms. Carotene levels are low. Coagulopathy from vitamin K deficiency is mild or nonexistent (85), whereas vitamin D deficiency has not been a clinical problem. The clinical features of fat malabsorption, growth retardation, and neurologic and visual abnormalities with acanthocytes on the blood smear and the absence of apoB strongly suggest the diagnosis. The histologic abnormality is diffuse, and small bowel biopsy is diagnostic. A normal biopsy rules out AβL (92).

Treatment

Oral supplementation with fat-soluble vitamins is the cornerstone of treatment. With high-dose oral supplementation (2.40–4.80 μmol of retinol [2286–4572 IU]/kg/day), vitamin A levels can be normalized (88, 93). Abnormalities in dark adaptation response and in electroretinography generally improve with supplementation, although retinal degeneration is not prevented (93). Massive oral doses of vitamin E (200–300 IU/kg/day) can produce detectable serum levels and correct in vitro red blood cell hemolysis (88, 91). Normal serum levels are rarely, if ever, attained (85, 88). Administration of vitamin E in the first few years of life may prevent retinopathy (93). Given later in the course of the disease, vitamin E may halt or retard neurologic and retinal deterioration and may even lead to improvement in some patients (88, 93). A water-soluble form of vitamin E has been used successfully in the treatment of serum vitamin E deficiency associated with fat malabsorption in chronic childhood cholestasis (94) and the short bowel syndrome (95). It is conceivable that this treatment may also be useful in patients with IL. Oral vitamin K, 5 mg twice a month, has corrected the coagulopathy that seldom occurs.

Moderate fat restriction, initially to approximately 10% of ingested calories, ameliorates the gastrointestinal symptoms of diarrhea and steatorrhea and allows resumption of normal growth and even "catch-up" growth (88, 93). With age, the capacity to absorb fat increases, and patients should be encouraged to increase fat intake as tolerated (85, 90). Additional polyunsaturated fat as corn oil is sometimes recommended to correct the associated biochemical EFA deficiency (90). MCTs are useful as a source of extra calories and clearly aid in weight gain; however, their potential to worsen long-chain fat malabsorption and to cause hepatic steatosis makes their use controversial (88). Gluten-free diets, steroids and ß-lipoprotein-rich plasma infusions have been administered without benefit (85, 89).

REFERENCES

1. Potish RA. Am J Clin Oncol 1982;5:189–94.
2. Donaldson SS, Jundt S, Ricour JC, et al. Cancer 1975;35: 1167–78.
3. Rodier JF, Janser JC, Rodier DL, et al. Cancer 1991;68:2545–9.
4. Meric F, Hirschl RB, Mahboubi S, et al. J Pediatr Surg 1994;29:917–21.
5. Logmans A, Trimbos JB, van Lent M. Eur J Obstet Gynecol Reprod Biol 1995;58:167–71.
6. Chen JS, Chang Chien CR, Wang JY, et al. Dis Colon Rectum 1992;35:897–901.
7. Baughan CA, Canney PA, Buchanan RB, et al. Clin Oncol 1993;5:19–24.
8. Liu T, Liu Y, He S, et al. Cancer 1992;69:2820–5.
9. Henriksson R, Franzen L, Littbrand B. J Clin Oncol 1992;10: 969–75.
10. Trier JS, Browning TH. J Clin Invest 1966;45:194–204.
11. Yeoh EK, Horowitz M. Surg Gynecol Obstet 1987;165:373–9.
12. Kinsella TJ, Bloomer WD. Surg Gynecol Obstet 1980;151: 273–84.
13. Loiudice TA, Lang JA. Am J Gastroenterol 1983;78:481–7.
14. Yeoh E, Horowitz M. Br J Hosp Med 1988;39:498–504.
15. Newman A, Katsaris J, Blendis LM, et al. Lancet 1973;2: 1471–3.
16. Galland RB, Spencer J. Lancet 1985;1:1257–8.
17. Goldstein F, Khoury J, Thornton J. Am J Gastroenterol 1976; 65:201–8.
18. Yeoh EK, Horowitz M, Russo A, et al. Gut 1993;34:476–82.
19. Neurath MF, Branbrink A, Meyer zum Buschenfelde K-H, et al. Lancet 1996;347:1302.
20. Mulholland MW, Levitt SH, Song CW, et al. Cancer 1984; 54:2396–402.
21. Bounous G, Lebel E, Shuster J. Strahlenther Onkol 1975;149: 476–83.
22. McArdle AH, Reid EC, Laplante MP, et al. Arch Surg 1986;121:879–85.
23. Brown MS, Buchanan RB, Karran SJ. Clin Radiol 1980;31: 19–20.
24. Kinsella TJ, Malcolm AW, Bothe A Jr, et al. Int J Radiol 1980;31:19–20.
25. Donaldson SS, Welsey MN, Ghavimi F, et al. Med Pediatr Oncol 1982;10:129–39.
26. Bosaeus I, Andersson H, Nystrom C. Acta Radiol Oncol 1979; 18:460–4.
27. Beer WH, Fan A, Halsted CH. Am J Clin Nutr 1985;41:85–91.
28. Howard L, Ament R, Fleming CR. Gastroenterology 1995;109: 355.
29. Silvain C, Besson I, Ingrand P, et al. Dig Dis Sci 1992;37: 1065–71.
30. Cross MJ, Frazee RC. Am Surg 1992;58:132–5.
31. Talley NJ. Eosinophilic gastroenteritis. In: Sleisinger MH, Fortran JS, eds. Gastrointestinal disease. 5th ed. Philadelphia: WB Saunders, 1993;1224–32.
32. Talley NJ, Shorter RG, Phillips SF, et al. Gut 1990;31:54–8.
33. Martin DM, Goldman JA, Gilliam J, et al. Gastroenterology 1981;80:1567–70.
34. Stein HB, Urowitz MB. J Rheumatol 1976;3(1):21–6.
35. Klein NC, Hargrove L, Sleisinger MH, et al. Medicine 1970; 49:299–319.
36. Vitellas KM, Bennett WF, Bova JG, et al. Radiology 1993; 186(3):789–93.
37. Matsushita M, Hajiro K, Morita Y, et al. Am J Gastroenterol 1995;90:1868–70.
38. Schoonbroodt D, Horsmans Y, Laka A, et al. Dig Dis Sci 1995;40(2):308–14.
39. Marshak RH, Lindner A, Maklansky D, et al. JAMA 1981; 245:1677–80.
41. Scudamore HH, Phillip SF, Swedlund HA, et al. J Allergy Clin Immunol 1982;70:129–38.
42. Greenberger NJ, Tannenbaum JI, Ruppert RD. Am J Med 1967;43:777–84.
43. Cello JP. Am J Med 1979;67:1097–104.
44. Katz AJ, Twarog FJ, Zeiger RS, et al. J Allergy Clin Immunol 1984;74:72–8.
45. Di Gioacchino M, Pizzicannella G, Fini N, et al. Allergy 1990;45:161–6.
46. Moots RJ, Prouse P, Gumpel JM. Gut 1988;29:1282–5.
46a. Caldwell JH, Tennenbaum JI, Bronstein HA. N Engl J Med 1975;292:1388–90.
46b. O'Connor CR, O'Dorisio TM. Ann Intern Med 1989;110: 665–6.
47. Melamed I, Feanny SJ, Sherman PM, et al. Am J Med 1991;90:310–4.
48. Tytgat GN, Grimj R, Dekker W, et al. Gastroenterology 1976;71:479–83.
49. Gilat T, Spiro HM. Dig Dis Sci 1968;13:619–33.
50. Tada S, Iida M, Yao T, et al. Gastrointest Endosc 1994;40: 45–50.
51. Feurle GE. Digestion 1987;36:13–7.
52. Steen LE, Ek BO. Scand J Gastroenterol 1984;19:480–6.
53. el Salhy M, Suhr O, Stenling R, et al. Gut 1994;35(10):1413–8.
54. Suhr O, Danielsson A, Steen L. Scand J Gastroenterol 1992; 27:201–7.
55. Matsumoto T, Iida M, Hirakawa M, et al. Dig Dis Sci 1991; 36:1756–60.
56. Hunter AM, Borsey DQ, Campbell IW, et al. Postgrad Med J 1979;55:822–3.
57. Gozzi G, Ballerdini G, Colombi R, et al. Acta Radiol 1990; 3:355–8.
58. Smith TR, Cho KC. Am J Gastroenterol 1986;81:477–9.
59. Ando Y, Gotoh T, Kawaguchi Y, et al. Pharmacology 1995; 15:345–9.
60. Fraser AG, Arthur JF, Hamilton I. Dig Dis Sci 1991;36:532–5.
61. Benson MD. Arthritis Rheum 1986;29:683–7.
62. Becker SA, Bass D, Nissim F. J Clin Gastroenterol 1985;7: 296–300.
63. Meyers S, Janowitz HD, Gumaste VK, et al. Gastroenterology 1988;94:1503–7.
64. Edwards P, Cooper DA, Turner J, et al. Gastroenterology 1988;95:810–5.
65. van Tilburg AJ, van Blankenstein M, Verschoor L. Am J Gastroenterol 1988;83:1418–9.
66. Edworthy SM, Fritzler MJ, Kelly JK, et al. Am J Gastroenterol 1990;85(10):1398–402.
67. Bereket A, Lowenheim M, Blethen SL, et al. J Clin Endocrinol Metab 1995;80(3):933–5.
68. Perisic VN, Kohai G. Arch Dis Child 1992;67:134–6.
69. Nazer HM, Abutalib H, Hugosson C, et al. Ann Trop Paediatr 1991;11:349–55.
70. Barnes RE, DeRidder PH. Am J Gastroenterol 1993;88:887–90.
71. Takeda H, Takahashi T, Ajitsu S, et al. Am J Gastroenterol 1991;86:450–3.
72. Salomons HA, Kramer P, Nikulasson S, et al. Gastroenterol Endosc 1995;41:516–8.

73. Aoyagi K, Iida M, Yao T, et al. Clin Radiol 1994;49(11):814–9.
74. Jeffries GH, Chapman A, Sleisinger MH. N Engl J Med 1964;270:761–7.
75. Vardy PA, Lebenthal E, Shwachman H. Pediatrics 1975;55: 842–51.
76. Tift WL, Lloyd JK. Arch Dis Child 1975;50:269–76.
77. Orbeck H, Larsen TE, Hovig T. Acta Paediatr Scand 1978;67: 677–82.
78. Fox U, Lucani G. Lymphology 1993;26:61–6.
79. Bac DJ, van Hagen PM, Postema PTE, et al. Lancet 1995;345:1639.
80. Mine K, Matsubayashi S, Nakai Y, et al. Gastroenterology 1989;96(6):1596–9.
81. Heresbach D, Raoul JL, Bretagne JF, et al. Gastroenterology 1991;100:1152–64.
82. Cohen SA, Diuguid D, Whitlock R, et al. Gastroenterology 1992;102(6):2193.
83. Narcisi TME, Shoulders CC, Chester SA, et al. Am J Hum Genet 1995;57:1298–310.
84. Ricci B, Sharp D, O'Rourke E, et al. J Biol Chem 1995; 270(24):14281–5.
85. Kayden HJ. Annu Rev Med 1972;23:285–96.
86. Glickman RM, Green PH, Lees JRS, et al. Gastroenterology 1979;76:288–92.
87. Muller JDPR. Clin Gastroenterol 1982;11:119–40.
88. Illingworth DR, Connor WE, Miller RG. Arch Neurol 1980;37:659–62.
89. Isselbacher KJ, Scheig R, Plotkin CR, et al. Medicine 1964;43:347–61.
90. Kayden HJ. Nutr Rev 1980;38:244–6.
91. Muller DPR, Harries JT, Lloyd JK. Gut 1974;15:966–71.
92. Trier JS. Hosp Pract 1988;23:195–211.
93. Muller DPR, Lloyd JK, Bird AC. Arch Dis Child 1977;52:209–14.
94. Sokol RJ, Herbi JE, Butler-Simon N, et al. Gastroenterology 1987;93:975–8.
95. Traber MG, Schiano TD, Steephen AC. Am J Clin Nutr 1994;59:1270–4.

71. Celiac Disease

J. JOSEPH CONNON

HISTORICAL BACKGROUND

An illness resembling celiac disease was described as early as the 1st century AD by Aretaeus of Cappadocia (1). In the 19th century, Dr. Samuel Gee provided an excellent clinical description and recommended dietary treatment of a diarrheal illness that he termed "the celiac affection" (2). However, determination of the cause and dietary therapy of celiac disease awaited the observations of W. R. Dicke, a Dutch pediatrician, who noted improvement followed by deterioration of his celiac patients as bread was first withdrawn and then reintroduced into their diets during and after the Second World War (3). Further progress in understanding the disease was facilitated by development of peroral intestinal biopsy devices by Shiner (4) and Crosby and Kugler (5) that confirmed Paulley's observation of intestinal mucosal flattening in surgically obtained specimens (6).

PATHOLOGY

The normal small bowel mucosa is thrown up in a series of concertina-like folds called the valvulae conniventes. Microscopically, the absorptive surface of the mucosa is configured as millions of villi covered by columnar epithelial cells, while the secretory mucosa primarily consists of the crypts of Lieberkuhn. In advanced celiac disease, the valvulae are thinner and more widely spaced than normal, and scalloping of their free margins has been described at endoscopy (7, 8). The microscopic changes are usually diffuse rather than focal and diminish in severity caudally. Changes range in severity from intraepithelial lymphocytic infiltration to complete loss of villi, crypt hyperplasia, and infiltration of the lamina propria by plasma cells, lymphocytes, neutrophils, eosinophils, and mast cells (9). The remaining absorptive cells are cuboidal and vacuolated. Occasionally, changes are patchy (10).

The effects of gluten extend beyond the small intestine. A lymphoplasmacytoid reaction responsive to gluten has been demonstrated in the rectal mucosa of patients with celiac disease (11). Changes similar to those of celiac disease have been described in other local and systemic disorders that affect the intestinal mucosa. These include lymphoma, giardiasis, tropical sprue, bacterial overgrowth, viral gastroenteritis, cow's milk protein intolerance, and graft-versus-host disease (12).

Dietary exclusion of gluten usually results in restoration of a more normal mucosal appearance within 2 to 3 months. In children, complete recovery may occur, but some residual villous blunting and lymphocytic infiltration is the rule (13). If rechallenge with gluten is felt necessary to confirm the diagnosis, 10 g gluten per day should be added to the diet for up to 2 months, followed by rebiopsy. Some patients are unable to tolerate gluten for more than a few days because of nausea, bloating, and diarrhea. Occasionally, gluten challenge fails to cause typical histologic changes in patients who relapse years later (14). The presence of a normal mucosa, even on a normal diet, does not preclude eventual development of celiac disease (latent celiac disease) (15).

Since some gluten-sensitized people may have a normal mucosa, even in the presence of antigluten antibodies, and others with advanced jejunal mucosal atrophy may be asymptomatic, Marsh has emphasized the need to reconsider traditional definitions of celiac disease (16). He proposed that gluten sensitivity be regarded as a state of heightened T- and B-cell–based immunologic responsiveness to gluten proteins in DQW2 individuals (see below.)

PREVALENCE

Celiac disease has worldwide distribution, but there are significant variations in prevalence, ranging from 1:300 in Ireland (17) to 1:3500 in Finland (18). It is extremely rare in blacks, Chinese, and Japanese but has been described in India (19). Celiac disease is more common in women especially during the reproductive years, but this may be an artifact related to increased case finding. The prevalence of celiac disease is higher in adults than in children, and most such adults have no history of childhood symptoms. Peak prevalence in women occurs between 35 and 44 years of age (20). In Scotland, the incidence of childhood celiac disease appears to have fallen since 1976, perhaps because of changes in weaning practice, with later introduction of cereal products to the infant diet. However, the incidence of celiac disease in Sweden has not declined, despite similar infant feeding practices (21). An increased prevalence in diabetic patients has been reported from Sweden and Italy (22, 23). Celiac disease is also more common in cryptogenic cirrhosis (24).

GENETICS

There is strong evidence for an inherited predisposition to celiac disease (25). It occurs up to 100 times more frequently in first-degree relatives of patients with the disease than in the general population. About half of these relatives are asymptomatic. Identical twin studies have shown a disease concordance of 70% (26). This inherited susceptibility is closely associated with HLAB8, HLA-DR3, and HLA-DQ alleles. The alleles encoding B8 are in linkage disequilibrium with DQW2 and DR3. More than 90% of celiac patients possess the HLA-DQW2 allele (27), but the nature of the pathogenetic connections between the HLA type and gluten sensitivity remains unclear. Some 70% of unaffected siblings have the same HLA-DR phenotype as their affected sibling (28), so some additional genetic or environmental factors appear necessary for gluten sensitivity to be manifest.

PATHOGENESIS

Gluten is a protein component of wheats, oats, barley, and rye, all of which belong to the genus *Triticum.* Gliadin is the toxic agent in gluten. It is rich in proline and glutamine, hence the term *prolamins* for alcoholic extracts of gluten. There are several subfractions of gliadin, the best studied being α, β, γ, and ω. These have in turn been subfractionated, and all the gliadin moieties appear harmful to the intestinal mucosa (29).

The causal relationship between dietary gluten and mucosal changes in susceptible patients is unquestioned. However, many questions remain regarding the mechanism by which gluten exerts its harmful effects. Initially, it was suggested that incomplete brush border hydrolysis of gluten as a consequence of enzyme deficiency led to formation of toxic products (30), but inability to demonstrate abnormally low mucosal peptidase or carbohydrase activity following treatment with a gluten-free diet rendered this hypothesis untenable (31).

There is widespread agreement that interaction between CD4 cells and prolamin peptides bound to a celiac-associated HLA-DQ molecule is important in bringing about the pathologic changes associated with celiac disease. Class II HLA molecules bind peptide fragments and present them after further intracellular processing on the cell surface, where they may interact with immunologically competent cells, causing crypt cell hyperplasia and villous atrophy (32). Translocation of gliadin has been shown in intraenterocyte vacuoles positive for HLA-DR antigens in patients with untreated celiac disease (33).

Kagnoff et al. noted significant structural amino acid homology between a gliadin fragment and a nonstructural component, E1B, of type 12 adenovirus and suggested that adenovirus infection of susceptible subjects brings about gluten sensitization through the process of molecular mimicry (34). Although his and other groups (35) found a significant increase in the prevalence of antiadenovirus 12 antibodies in patients with untreated celiac disease, others have failed to confirm this (36, 37).

A variety of antibodies directed against both dietary and self antigens have been found in serum and intestinal secretions of celiac patients (38–40). Antigliadin IgA antibodies are found in up to 90% of untreated celiac patients and their titer gradually diminishes on gluten withdrawal (41). Other food-related antibodies such as antiovalbumin and anticasein have been described. It appears likely that antibody production is related to increased paracellular intestinal permeability found in celiac disease. Although pathogenic mechanisms involving disordered humoral immunity have been proposed, such as antibody-dependent cell-mediated cytotoxic effects and immune complex formation, the role of antibodies in causing villous damage remains conjectural.

IgA antibodies directed against specific tissue components have also been identified. These include antireticulin (42), antijejunal (43), and antiendomysial (44) antibodies, which can be detected by immunofluorescence technique in both human and animal tissues. Antijejunal and antiendomysial antibodies likely recognize a common antigen (45). The endomysium is a delicate connective tissue layer surrounding intestinal smooth muscle, and antiendomysial antibodies have been found in more than 95% of patients with celiac disease (46, 47). The specificity of both antiendomysial and antigliadin antibodies is 90%. Antiendomysial antibody titers decrease after institution of a gluten-free diet. Measurement of antibody titers has been suggested as a screening test for celiac disease and a means of evaluating dietary compliance in nonresponsive patients (48, 49).

CLINICAL MANIFESTATIONS

The presentation of celiac disease is highly variable, ranging from mild, nonspecific features through monodeficiency states to a full-blown classic panmalabsorption syndrome (50). In adults, the classic form of the disease is now the least common presentation, and several authors have emphasized the need to consider celiac disease in patients with irritable bowel–like features occurring in association with another trigger finding such as anemia, weight loss, or a monodeficiency state (51, 52).

Diarrhea

Diarrhea is found in 70% of patients (53). It is usually intermittent, occurs three to four times daily, and is of mushy consistency. Celiac patients often have crampy abdominal pain that, in association with diarrhea and bloating secondary to fermentation of lactose and other maldigested compounds, may simulate the irritable bowel syndrome. In a few patients, the diarrhea is more severe, and stools have the classic malabsorptive features of large volume, frothiness, offensive odor, greasy appearance, and a tendency to float. This latter quality results from their increased gaseous content rather than their fat concentration.

Weight Loss

Some weight loss is usual, but the amount is highly variable, depending as much on associated anorexia as on malabsorption. Patients with villous atrophy confined to the proximal small intestine may lose no weight.

Malaise

A loss of general well-being is found in 80% of patients but is often so insidious in onset that it is only recognized retrospectively, after institution of a gluten-free diet.

Monodeficiency Syndromes

Isolated monomalabsorption of substances absorbed from the duodenum and proximal and midjejunum is well recognized (54). These include iron, vitamins D and K, calcium, magnesium, albumin, and folic acid (12, 55). A combination of iron and folate deficiency is not unusual. Bone mineral density is reduced in association with increased bone turnover and increased secretion of parathormone. The abnormal bone density may respond only partially to treatment with a gluten-free diet (56, 57). The increased metabolic demands of pregnancy may unmask marginal absorption, especially of iron and folate.

Associated Diseases

The clinical features of celiac disease may sometimes be overshadowed by the more dramatic manifestations of associated diseases, thus delaying diagnosis. Many of these diseases have an autoimmune basis. They include dermatitis herpetiformis (58), intestinal lymphoma (59), diabetes (60), thyroid disease (61), IgA deficiency (62), cerebellar atrophy (63), inflammatory bowel disease (64), and sclerosing cholangitis (65). Other diseases linked with celiac disease in addition to those listed above include psychiatric disorders, farmer's lung, autoimmune thrombocytopenia, anemia, and Berger's disease, but the evidence for these associations is not conclusive (75).

Dermatitis Herpetiformis

Dermatitis herpetiformis causes pruritic, vesicular, and papular lesions with an erythematous background, primarily on the extensor surfaces of the limbs. The lesions demonstrate granular or linear deposition of IgA at the junction of dermis and epidermis (66). Although intestinal symptoms are uncommon, virtually all patients with the granular pattern of IgA deposition show patchy mucosal changes identical to those of celiac disease. Linear deposition of IgA is not associated with celiac disease. Both the cutaneous and mucosal abnormalities respond to a gluten-free diet, and in some patients, dapsone therapy can be withdrawn (67, 68).

Malignancy

A number of malignant disorders have been associated with celiac disease, notably small intestinal lymphoma. Celiac-associated lymphoma is generally agreed to be of T-cell origin, though it has been variously described as a B-cell tumor and as a malignant histiocytosis (69). Although it has been suggested that the mucosal atrophy associated with this lymphoma is secondary to the lymphoma rather than vice versa (70), there is a reluctance to accept that the malignant features of lymphoma may be delayed for many years and that gluten exclusion would restore a normal mucosal appearance in intestinal lymphoma. Moreover, antigliadin antibodies have been noted in patients who develop lymphoma in the course of celiac disease, whereas these antibodies are absent in patients who present with a lymphoma without a prior history of celiac disease (71).

A variety of presentations have been noted including diarrhea, intestinal obstruction, intestinal perforation, weight loss, abdominal pain, intestinal bleeding, fever, and finger clubbing. IgA levels may increase. Enteropathy-associated T-cell lymphoma (EATL) may be very difficult to diagnose (72). If routine investigations, including small bowel enema and abdominal computed tomography (CT) scanning, are negative and the clinical picture is suspicious, a laparotomy with full-thickness biopsies should be done. Local resection is rarely possible, and response to systemic chemotherapy is poor.

Other cancers also occur with increased frequency in celiac disease, including esophageal and pharyngeal cancer as well as small intestinal adenocarcinoma (73). A reduced incidence of small bowel lymphoma has been reported in patients adhering to a gluten-free diet (74).

INVESTIGATIONS

Hematology

Anemia is present in 40 to 80% of patients (76, 77). Unexplained iron or folate deficiency anemia rather than florid malabsorption is increasingly responsible for raising the suspicion of celiac disease (78). The simultaneous deficiency of both iron and folate produces a dimorphic blood picture, giving rise to an increased red cell distribution width (RDW). Hyposplenism is common in celiac disease and produces Howell-Jolly bodies (79). Folate deficiency may cause a slightly low serum B_{12} level that responds to folate replacement. Rarely, mucosal atrophy extending to the terminal ileum or bacterial overgrowth secondary to celiac-associated intestinal stasis, may produce B_{12} deficiency.

Biochemistry

Biochemical abnormalities in celiac disease essentially reflect both the extent and duration of malabsorption and range from none to multiple changes involving fluids, minerals, proteins, fat, and gut hormones. The stool fat content is usually increased in celiac patients with diarrhea but may be normal in those presenting in a monosymptomatic fashion with iron, folate, or vitamin D deficiency (80). Steatorrhea tends to be less marked in celiac disease than in chronic pancreatitis, and stool fat concentration is also relatively lower because of greater fluid losses in the celiac stool. The importance of stool fat measurement has diminished with increasing use of endoscopic small bowel biopsy.

D-Xylose is an inert sugar absorbed in the upper small intestine. Serum or urinary levels following oral administration provide a measure of jejunal absorptive capacity, but test reliability is influenced by variations in gastric emptying, age, and renal function (82) (see Chapter 65). Selective mucosal absorption has been tested with probes of different molecular size for both diagnosis and follow-up of celiac disease. These molecules include mannitol, lactulose, and lactobiose. In celiac patients, larger molecules are selectively absorbed, probably via paracellular routes, and transcellular absorption of smaller molecules diminishes as a result of villous atrophy (83). Although a high sensitivity and negative predictive value have been claimed for tests of differential urinary excretion, they have not yet gained wide acceptance. Transaminase levels are frequently elevated in adult patients and normalize following treatment with a gluten-free diet (84, 85).

Radiology

The primary role of radiology of the small bowel is exclusion of other diseases such as Crohn's disease, jejunal diverticulosis, strictures, or lymphoma and barium studies are not routinely required. In celiac disease, the radiologic appearance is often normal but there may be dilatation of the lumen and thickening of mucosal folds.

Antigliadin and Antiendomysial Antibodies

Increasing recognition of the subtle and atypical modes of presentation of celiac disease has underlined the importance of noninvasive screening tests. Both IgG and IgA antigliadin antibodies are present in untreated celiac disease, but they lack sufficient diagnostic sensitivity and specificity, especially in the case of IgG antibodies. Antiendomysial antibodies, which are detected by binding to a variety of smooth muscle basement membranes including monkey esophagus and human umbilical cord (86), have a sensitivity and specificity of 100%. This results in a predictive accuracy of 100%, even with prevalence rates as low as 0.2% (87–89). Titers of both antigliadin and antiendomysial antibodies fall rapidly in patients on a gluten-free diet.

The role of serologic testing remains controversial. It will likely become a valuable screening test but will not supplant intestinal biopsy as a diagnostic test. The positive predictive value of antiendomysial antibody testing is sufficiently high for use as a population screening tool, which has been suggested.

Intestinal Biopsy

Endoscopic biopsy of the second or third portion of the duodenum has largely replaced use of the Crosby or Watson capsule. Although these latter devices provide larger biopsy specimens, frustration with the technical difficulties associated with them compared with the ease of obtaining multiple, albeit smaller, endoscopic samples has led to a marked decline in their use. An immediate diagnosis of villous atrophy can be made by dissecting-microscopic examination of the biopsy material. Gastric antral histologic changes have been reported in celiac patients.

Endoscopy may reveal macroscopic changes in some patients. These include thinning, wider separation and scalloping of the margins of the valvulae conniventes (7, 8). En face, the mucosa may have a mosaic appearance that is enhanced when it is partially covered with blood following biopsy. Diagnostic sensitivity and specificity of about 90% have been reported.

The appearance of celiac disease on biopsy specimens is nonspecific, and definitive diagnosis requires repeat biopsy to demonstrate histologic improvement on a gluten-free diet and reversion to abnormality after gluten challenge. In adults, the last step is frequently omitted.

TREATMENT

Dietary avoidance of gluten is central to management of celiac disease. Most patients notice a significant symptomatic improvement within days. Changes in mucosal histology take longer. A reduction in intraepithelial lymphocyte infiltration occurs within a few weeks (90), but recovery of the normal villous appearance usually takes 2 to 3 months. Some patients never fully recover, even though they feel well. The diet of patients with demonstrated deficiencies should be supplemented initially with appropriate vitamins and minerals, but long-term supplementation is unnecessary.

Wheat, barley, rye, and oats are the main sources of gluten, and foodstuffs derived from these products have been traditionally excluded. Oats contain less gluten than other cereals, and a recent Finnish study showed no adverse nutritional or mucosal effects from a daily intake of 50 g of oats (91). Adherence to a strict gluten-free diet may be difficult because cereal products are present in a variety of prepared foods, but deliberate noncompliance is a much larger problem. Dietary surveys show that 30% of patients admit to taking gluten and remaining asymptomatic (92, 93). However, in some patients, ingestion of even small amounts of gluten results in bloating and diarrhea. Attainment of expected adult stature may be compromised by gluten intake during childhood and adolescence (94). The desirability of adhering to a gluten-free diet is heightened by a study demonstrating a reduction in the malignancy rates of compliant patients (74). See Appendix Table V-A-36 for details of a gluten-free diet and associated precautions.

Significant differences exist internationally in the constituents of a gluten-free diet. In Canada, the diet must not contain any wheat, barley, rye, oats, or triticale, whereas in many European countries, levels ranging from 5 to 50 μg gliadin per day are acceptable. The Celiac Sprue Association U.S.A., in addition to recommending complete exclusion of gluten-containing cereals, also advises avoiding buckwheat and any foods using cereal mash in their manufacture. These include distilled alcoholic beverages and white vinegar, which contain no detectable gliadins. Beer contains 3 μg/L prolamin and probably should be avoided. In vitro studies have shown that gliadin-deficient wheat is less toxic to enterocytes, thus revealing potential approaches to dietary treatment (95).

TREATMENT FAILURE

If a patient fails to respond to treatment, deliberate or inadvertent intake of gluten must be considered as well as diagnostic error. If there is any doubt about the adequacy of the original intestinal biopsies, further tissue should be obtained. Consideration must be given to other disorders associated with mucosal flattening, especially ulcerative jejunoileitis and lymphoma.

True failure to respond to dietary treatment is rare, and its pathogenesis uncertain. Some patients respond successfully to corticosteroid treatment (96). Rapidly metabolized "first-pass" steroids have been used to treat celiac disease instead of dietary therapy, and such compounds may become the drugs of choice in nonresponsive patients (97). Cyclosporine has been used successfully in a few patients with resistant disease (98).

REFERENCES

1. Hude C. Aretaeus: Corpus Medicorum Graecorum II. 2nd ed. Berlin: Academy of Sciences, 1958.
2. Gee SJ. On the celiac affection. St. Bartholomew's Hosp Rep 1888;24:17–20.
3. Dicke WK. Coeliakie. PhD thesis. University of Utrecht, Utrecht, the Netherlands, 1950.
4. Shiner M. Lancet 1956;i:85.
5. Crosby WH, Kugler HW. Am J Dig Dis 1957;2:236–41.
6. Paulley JW. Proc R Soc Med 1949;42:241.
7. Jabbari M, Wild G, Goresky CA, et al. Gastroenterology 1988;95:1518–22.
8. Brocchi E, Corazza G, Treggiari EA, et al. N Engl J Med 1988;319:741–4.
9. Rubin CE, Brandborg LL, Phelps PC, et al. Gastroenterology 1960;38:28–49.
10. Scott BB, Losowsky MS. Gut 1976;17:984–92.
11. Ensarim A, Marsh MN, Loft DE, et al. Gut 1993;34:1225–9.
12. Cooke WT, Holmes GKT. Celiac disease. New York: Churchill Livingstone, 1984.
13. Rubin CE, Eidelman S, Weinstein WM. Gastroenterology 1970;58:409–13.
14. Kuitunen P, Savilahti E, Verkasalo M. Acta Paediatr Scand 1986;75:340–2.
15. Mäki M, Holm K, Koskimies S, et al. Arch Dis Child 1990;65:1137–41.
16. Marsh MN. Q J Med 1995;85:913.
17. Mylotte M, Egan-Mitchell B, McCarthy CF, et al. Br Med J 1973;1:703–5.
18. Simila S, Kokkonen J, Voulukka P, et al. Lancet 1981;i:494–5.
19. Misra RC, Kasthuri D, Chuttani HK. Br Med J 1966;2:1230–2.
20. Logan RAF, Rifkind EA, Busuttil A, et al. Gastroenterology 1986;90:334–42.
21. Ascher H, Krantz I, Kristiansson, B. Arch Dis Child 1991;66: 608–11.
22. Sigurs N, Johansson C, Elfstrand PO, et al. Acta Paediatr 1993;82:748–51.
23. Sategna-Guidetti C, Grosso S, Pulitano R, et al. Dig Dis Sci 1994;39:1633–7.
24. Lindgren S, Sjoberg K, Eriksson S. Scand J Gastroenterol 1994;29:661–4.
25. Mylotte M, Egan-Mitchell B, Fottrell PF, et al. Q J Med 1974;43:359–69.
26. Polanco I, Biemond I, van Leeuwen A, et al. In: McConnell RD, ed. Genetics of celiac disease: proceedings of international symposium. Lancaster, England: MTP Press, 1981.
27. Tosi R, Vismara D, Tanigaki N, et al. Clin Immunol Immunopathol 1983;28:395–404.
28. Kagnoff MF, Harwood JI, Bugawan TL, et al. Proc Natl Acad Sci USA 1989;86:6274–8.
29. Ciclitira PJ, Evans DJ, Fagg NLK, et al. Clin Sci 1984;66:357–64.
30. Frazer AC, Fletcher RF, Ross CA. Lancet 1959;2:252–5.
31. Davidson AGF, Bridges MA. Clin Chim Acta 1987;163:1–40.
32. Lundin KEA, Sollid LM, Qvigstad E, et al. J Immunol 1990;145:136–9.
33. Ciclitira PJ, Harms E. Gut 1995;36:703–9.
34. Kagnoff MF, Austin RK, Hubert JJ, et al. J Exp Med 1984;160:1544–57.
35. Lahdaaho ML, Parkkonen P, Reunala T, et al. Clin Immunol Immunopathol 1993;69:300–5.
36. Howdle PD, Blair Zajdel ME, Smart CJ, et al. Scand J Gastroenterol 1989;24:282–6.
37. Mahon J, Blair GE, Wood GM. Gut 1991;32:1114–6.
38. Kenrick KG, Walker-Smith JA. Gut 1970;11:635–40.
39. Ferguson A, Carswell F. Br Med J (Clin Res) 1972;1:75–7.
40. O'Mahony S, Arranz E, Barton JR, et al. Gut 1991;32:29–35.
41. Kelly CP, Feighery CF, Weir DG. Gastroenterology 1988;94: A221.
42. Mäki M, Hallstrom O, Vesikari T, et al. J Pediatr 1984;105: 901–5.
43. Kárpáti S, Török E, Kosnaii J. Invest Dermatol 1986;87:703–6.
44. Volta U, Molinaro N, Fusconi M, et al. Dig Dis Sci 1991;36: 752–6.
45. Karpati S, Meurer M, Burgin-Wolff A, et al. Gut 1992;33:191–3.
46. Chorzelski TP, Suley J, Tchorzewska H, et al. Ann NY Acad Sci 1983;420:325–34.
47. Kumar V, Lerner A, Valeski JE, et al. Immunol Invest 1989;18:533–44.
48. Cacciari E, Volta U, Lazzari R, et al. Lancet 1985;1:1469–71.
49. Mearin ML, Peña AS. Neth J Med 1987;31:279–85.
50. Mann JG, Brown WR, Kern F. Am J Med 1970;48:375–6.
51. Rifkind EA, Busuttil A, Ferguson A. Br Med J 1980;281:1637.
52. Swinson CM, Levi AJ. Br Med J 1980;281:1258–60.

53. Dawson AM. Neth J Med 1987;31:256–62.
54. Rossi E. Eur J Pediatr 1982;138:4–5.
55. Weir DG, Hourihane DOB. Gut 1974;15:450–7.
56. Gonzalez D, Mazure R, Mautalen C, et al. Bone 1995;16:231–4.
57. Cecchetti L, Tarozzi C, Corra O, et al. Gastroenterology 1995; 109:122–8.
58. Marks J, Shuster S, Watson AJ. Lancet 1966;2:1280–2.
59. Holmes GKT, Stokes PL, Sorahan TM, et al. Gut 1976;17: 612–9.
60. Walker-Smith JA. Arch Dis Child 1975;50:668.
61. Midhagen G, Jarnerot G, Kraaz W. Scand J Gastroenterol 1988;23:1000–4.
62. Mawhinney H, Tomkin GH. Lancet 1971;2:121–4.
63. Finelli PF, McEntee WJ, Ambler M, et al. Neurology 1980;30:245–9.
64. Shah A, Mayberry JF, Williams G, et al. Q J Med 1990;74:283–8.
65. Hay JE, Wiesner RH, Shorter RG, et al. Ann Intern Med 1988;109:713–7.
66. Lawley TJ, Strober W, Yaoita H, et al. J Invest Dermatol 1980;74:9.
67. Weinstein WM, Brow JR, Parker F, et al. Gastroenterology 1971;60:362–9.
68. Fry L, Seah PP, Riches DJ, et al. Lancet 1973;1:288–91.
69. Isaacson PG, O'Connor NT, Spencer J, et al. Lancet 1985;2:688–91.
70. Wright DH, Jones DB Clark H, et al. Lancet 1991;337(8754): 1373–4.
71. O'Farrelly C, Feighery C, O'Briain DS, et al. Br Med J (Clin Res) 1986;293:908–10.
72. Isaacson PG. Celiac disease: malignant lymphoma. In: Jewell DP, Ireland A, eds. Topics in gastroenterology, vol 14. Boston: Blackwell Scientific Publications, 1986.
73. Swinson CM, Slavin G, Coles EC, et al. Lancet 1983;1:111–5.
74. Holmes GKT, Prior P, Lane MR, et al. Gut 1989;30:333–8.
75. Mulder CJ, Tytgat GN. Neth J Med 1987;31:286–9.
76. Hoffbrand AV. Clin Gastroenterol 1974;3:71–89.
77. Corazza GR, Valentini RA, Andreani ML. Scand J Gastroenterol 1995;30:153–6.
78. Logan RAF, Tucker G, Rifkind EA. Br Med J 1983;286:95–7.
79. Ferguson A, Hutton MM, Maxwell JD, et al. Lancet 1970;1:163–4.
80. McGuigan JE, Volwiler W. Gastroenterology 1964;47:636–41.
81. Bow-Linn GW, Fordtran JS. Gastroenterology 1984;87:31—22.
82. Craig RM, Atkinson AJ Jr. Gastroenterology 1988;95:223–31.
83. Juby LD, Rothwell J, Axon AT. Gastroenterology 1989;96: 79–85.
84. Dickey W, McMillan SA, Collins JS, et al. J Clin Gastroenterol 1995;20:290–2.
85. Bardella MT, Fraquelli M, Quatrini M, et al. Hepatology 1995;22:833–6.
86. Ladinser B, Rossipal E, Bittschieler K. Gut 1994;35:776–8.
87. Hallström O. Gut 1989;30:1225–32.
88. Ferenci P, Granditsch G, Penner E. Am J Gastroenterol 1995;90:394–8.
89. Corrao G, Corazza GR, Andreani ML. Gut 1994;35:771–5.
90. Yardley JH, Bayless TM, Norton JH, et al. N Engl J Med 1962;267:1173–9.
91. Janatuinen EK, Pikkarainen PH, Kemppainen TA. N Engl J Med 1995;333:1033–7.
92. Kumar PJ, Clark ML, Dawson AM. Q J Med 1985;57:803.
93. Bardella MT, Molteni N, Prampolini L. Arch Dis Child 1994;70:211–3.
94. Colaco J, Egan-Mitchell B, Stevens FM, et al. Arch Dis Child 1987;62:706–8.
95. Frisoni M, Corazza GR, Lafiandra D. Gut 1995;36:375–8.
96. Taylor AB, Wollaeger EE, Comfort MW. Gastroenterology 1952;20:203–8.
97. Mitchison HC, al Mardini H, Gillespie S, et al. Gut 1991;32(3): 260–5.
98. Longstreth GF. Ann Intern Med 1993;119:1014–6.

72. Nutrition in Pancreatic Disorders

MASSIMO RAIMONDO and EUGENE P. DIMAGNO

Each disorder of the exocrine pancreas requires special attention to nutritional aspects of treatment. In acute pancreatitis, nutrition is important in moderate-to-severe disease because the disease process often is complicated and prolonged, precluding eating. In chronic pancreatitis and pancreatic cancer, there is reduced secretion of pancreatic enzymes leading to malabsorption. In the former, the disease primarily affects acinar cells that manufacture enzymes, and in the latter, the tumor obstructs the pancreatic ducts, blocking pancreatic enzymes from entering the duodenum. In this chapter, we briefly discuss important clinical aspects of these diseases, particularly the assessments that should lead to treatment of the nutritional deficits of the diseases, parenteral or enteral nutrition in acute pancreatitis, and pancreatic enzymes in chronic pancreatitis and pancreatic cancer.

ACUTE PANCREATITIS

Depending on the population, alcohol abuse and biliary tract disease cause acute pancreatitis in 75 to 85% of patients. In addition to these common causes of acute pancreatitis, other factors have been implicated in the pathogenesis of acute pancreatitis, such as metabolic, traumatic, operative, infectious, and pharmacologic etiologies (Table 72.1). Patients with acute pancreatitis typically present with acute abdominal pain and elevation of pancreatic enzymes in the serum; amylase is the enzyme most commonly measured.

Acute pancreatitis ranges in severity from a slight edematous inflammation (interstitial pancreatitis) that usually resolves spontaneously and completely in a few days to a fulminate process that can progress to necrotizing pancreatitis because of inflammation and tissue necrosis following intra- and extrapancreatic spreading of active pancreatic enzymes. In acute pancreatitis, toxicity and complications are caused by extravasation of enzymes into the pararenal spaces, lesser sac, and peritoneal cavity and into the circulation by absorption through retroperitoneal venous and lymphatic vessels. Extravasation of enzymes into the abdominal cavities produces a "burn," resulting in loss of protein and fluid. This third-space loss and escape of enzymes into the circulation causes hypovolemia and hypotension. In addition to circulatory collapse, this process also leads to other systemic complications such as renal insufficiency, respiratory distress syndrome, and findings akin to those of sepsis (leukocytosis, fever). Furthermore, escape of pancreatic enzymes and other pancreatic secretions into the pancreas and peripancreatic areas causes pancreatic and peripancreatic necrosis. Lipase most likely is the enzyme responsible for initiation of necrosis by digesting pancreatic and peripancreatic fat.

Clinical Assessment and Prediction of Need for Specialized Nutritional Treatment

Mild acute interstitial pancreatitis is characterized by abdominal pain, nausea, vomiting, anorexia, and low or no mortality (<2%). Although local complications such as third-space losses leading to hypovolemia and systemic complications such as respiratory or renal failure may occur in interstitial pancreatitis, they are uncommon, and resolution of symptoms and recovery occurs in several days. In these patients, simple supportive medical treatment suffices, and parenteral nutrition is rarely needed. However, in severe necrotizing pancreatitis, characterized by end-organ failure, the mortality rate may approximate 30% if the necrotic tissue is infected (1). These patients need parenteral nutrition instituted as soon as their severe pancreatitis is recognized, because a prolonged, complicated clinical course is extremely likely.

Clinical Predictors of Severity

Severity of acute pancreatitis is the major predictor of the outcome of an attack of pancreatitis and predicates the type of treatment patients will receive. Therefore, one *must* be able to predict the severity of the disease at presentation. A number of predictors of severity have been proposed, many carrying the name of the principal investigator who devised them. Among them are the criteria of Ranson (2), the first criteria proposed. In addition, Bank (3), Agarwal and Pitchumoni (4), and Imrie (5) have suggested criteria. All these criteria have the disadvantage of requiring 48 hours to measure at least some of their components. Ranson's criteria (Table 72.2) use age and laboratory measurements at admission and further clinical and laboratory measurements at 48 hours: 2 signs or less predict 0 mortality; 3 to 5 signs predict a mortality of 10 to 20%; and with 6 or more signs, mortality exceeds 50%. Patients with three signs or more have a high risk of devel-

Table 72.1
Etiology of Acute Pancreatitis

Biliary tract disease	Postoperative
Alcohol	Endoscopic retrograde pancreatogram
Idiopathic	Hypercalcemia
Anatomic causes	Infectious agents
Choledochocele	Pregnancy (usually biliary tract)
Pancreas divisum?	Hereditary
Duodenal diverticulum?	Pancreatic duct obstruction (worms, ampullary tumor)
Drugs	Hyperlipidemia (types I, IV, and V)
Cancer of the pancreas	Metastatic cancer to the pancreas
Vasculitis	Renal transplantation
Abdominal trauma	

oping pancreatic necrosis and systemic complications. The other named criteria are simpler and in general rely on development of cardiac, pulmonary, renal, metabolic, hematologic and neurologic complications within the first 48 hours; presence of one complication or more identifies patients with a high risk of complications and death.

At present, the most commonly used severity index is the APACHE-II score (*A*cute *P*hysiology and *C*hronic *H*ealth *E*valuation), with scoring on the basis of laboratory testing and vital signs. In contrast to other scoring systems, the APACHE score can be used repeatedly and at any time during the course of an attack. Scores of 9 or below predict survival, but scores of 13 or more have a high probability of death (6–10, 11). On the basis of these data, we recommend that scores of 10 or more, particularly during the first 48 hours, should trigger a move to the intensive care unit and consideration of initiating parenteral nutrition, among other supportive measures.

Imaging and Serum Tests

Of the imaging and laboratory tests, computed tomography (CT) is currently considered the best to assess the severity of acute pancreatitis. Originally, the scoring system of Balthazar and Ranson (12, 13) was used (grades A to E: A, normal pancreas; B, focal or diffuse enlargement; C–E, pancreatic enlargement; C with mild peripancreatic inflammation, D with fluid in the anterior pararenal space, and E with fluid collections in more than one area). The prognosis for grades A and B is excellent. For grade C, pancreatic necrosis and infection approximates 10%. For grades D and E, infection is 50%, and mortality may reach 15%. Currently, however, the state of the art is to do a bolus contrast-enhanced CT when severe pancreatitis is suspected. This technique clearly differentiates interstitial from necrotizing pancreatitis.

Other methods of detecting severe pancreatitis such as peritoneal tap (recovery of dark fluid or recovery of >20 mL of free peritoneal fluid of any color) or serum tests such as C-reactive protein, α_2-macroglobulin, phospholipase A_2 activity, and urinary trypsinogen activating peptide (TAP) are not popular because they are invasive or they lack proven diagnostic accuracy.

Table 72.2.
Ranson's Criteria of Severity

At admission
Age > 55 years
WBC > 16,000/mm^3
Glucose > 200 mg/dL
LDH > 350 IU/L
AST > 250 U/L
During initial 48 hours
Hct decrease of >10
BUN increase of >5 mg/dL
Ca^{2+} < 8 mg/dL
PaO_2 < 60 mm Hg
Base deficit > 4 mEq/L
Fluid sequestration > 6 L

From Banks PA. Medical management of acute pancreatitis and complications. In: Go VLW, et al., eds. The pancreas: biology, pathobiology, and disease. New York: Raven Press, 1993;593–611, with permission.

Treatment

Food and drink are withheld from all patients with acute pancreatitis. In addition, in moderate-to-severe attacks of pancreatitis, gastric contents are aspirated from the stomach through a nasogastric tube. Most patients have mild pancreatitis and are treated for several days with supportive care including pain control, intravenous fluids, and nothing by mouth. Most patients eat within 5 to 7 days and do not require parenteral nutrition. In contrast, patients with moderate-to-severe pancreatitis require nutritional support as a routine part of medical management (14), to prevent inanition because they rapidly become nutritionally depleted. However, total parenteral nutrition (TPN) does not affect the outcome of attacks (15).

Although resting energy expenditure in patients with uncomplicated acute pancreatitis (measured by indirect calorimetry) is no greater than predicted, 82% of patients with sepsis are hypermetabolic (120 ± 12% of predicted value) (16). Indeed, patients with pancreatitis exhibit some of the same metabolic, cardiovascular, and hemodynamic features observed in sepsis. In addition, if pseudocysts, abscesses, or fistulas develop, a protracted course with increased metabolic needs should be anticipated; nutritional complications are most likely to arise in this setting.

In moderate-to-severe acute pancreatitis, parenteral nutrition is initiated as soon as the cardiorespiratory systems are stable. Nutritional support should include *(a)* hypertonic dextrose; *(b)* solution of crystalline amino acids; *(c)* fat emulsion to prevent fatty acid deficiency (except in patients with hyperlipidemia-induced pancreatitis); *(d)* daily requirements of electrolytes, vitamins, and trace elements; *(e)* insulin to control hyperglycemia; and *(f)* proton pump inhibitors (omeprazole) or H_2 blockers to reduce gastric acid secretion. After paralytic ileus has subsided and in patients requiring surgery, oral low-fat feedings should be used instead of the parenteral route.

The oral route, rather than TPN, should be used whenever possible, to eliminate the potential complications of TPN (see Chapter 101).

TPN has the advantage of maintaining "pancreatic rest" better than enteral nutrition. However, enteral feedings have a number of advantages over TPN: maintenance of intestinal integrity and the gut mucosal barrier, which may decrease the risk of bacterial translocation and subsequent septic complications of acute pancreatitis, lower cost, and elimination of complications related to parenteral nutrition. The farther down the upper gastrointestinal tract an elemental diet is infused, the less stimulation of pancreatic exocrine secretion, because the normal cephalic, gastric, and intestinal (more potent) phases of pancreatic stimulation are bypassed. Unfortunately, to date no prospective randomized trials have assessed the effect of early enteral nutrition on the course and outcome of acute pancreatitis.

Refeeding

When to begin oral feeding, what to feed, and how often to feed are questions that occur with every patient with acute pancreatitis. The answers to these questions are not based on scientific data from studies in patients with acute pancreatitis. Instead, they are based on physiologic studies in normal humans to determine the effects of nutrients on pancreatic enzyme secretion and on personal anecdotal experience. The criteria we use to initiate oral feedings are *(a)* absence of abdominal pain and tenderness, *(b)* reduction of amylase levels to near-normal levels, and *(c)* absence of complications.

We begin feeding patients by giving 100 to 300 mL of liquids containing no calories every 4 hours for the first 24 hours. If this diet is tolerated, oral feeding is advanced to giving the same volume of liquids containing nutrients. Subsequently, if patients continue to do well, feedings are changed gradually over 3 to 4 days to soft, and finally solid, foods. All diets contain more than 50% carbohydrate calories, and the total caloric content is gradually increased from 160 to 640 kcal per meal.

These recommendations are based on our studies in healthy humans in which we found that the rate of pancreatic enzyme secretion was related to the nutrient composition of meals (18) and the rate of delivery of kilocalories to the duodenum (19). Secretion of pancreatic enzymes decreased as more carbohydrate was ingested, particularly when carbohydrates were 50% or more of the total caloric content of the diet (Fig. 72.1). In another study, we found that when nutrients were infused into the duodenum, pancreatic enzyme secretion was directly related to the rate of caloric infusion, i.e., there was less secretion at infusions of 40 kcal/h than at 90 or 160 kcal/h (Fig. 72.2) (19).

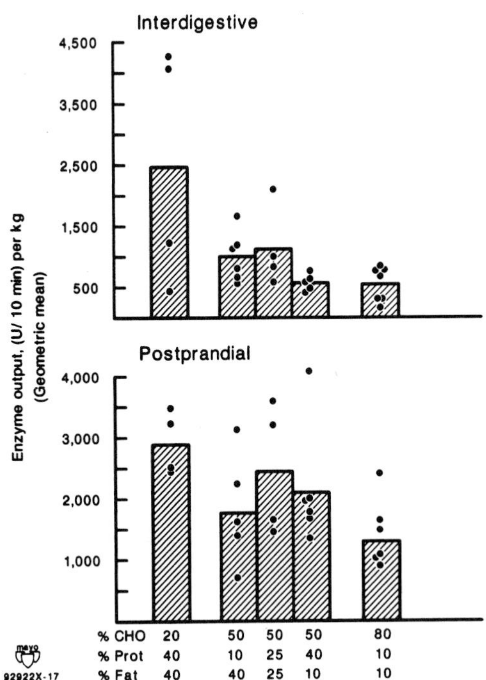

Figure 72.1. Interdigestive *(top panel)* and postprandial *(bottom panel)* geometric mean total enzyme output (combined outputs of amylase, lipase, and trypsin) after following one of the five diets for 2 weeks. The interdigestive and postprandial enzyme outputs were significantly different among the five diets (one-way ANOVA, $P < 0.05$). (From Boivin M, Lanspa SJ, Zinsmeister AR, et al. Gastroenterology 1990;99:1763–71, with permission.)

CHRONIC PANCREATITIS

Most patients who develop chronic pancreatitis are alcoholics, who may have nutritional deficiencies secondary to alcoholism (Chapter 96). However, about 20% of patients with chronic pancreatitis in our population have idiopathic chronic pancreatitis. Other causes of chronic pancreatitis are much less common (Table 72.3). Some conditions give rise to exocrine insufficiency and malabsorption and malnutrition without causing chronic

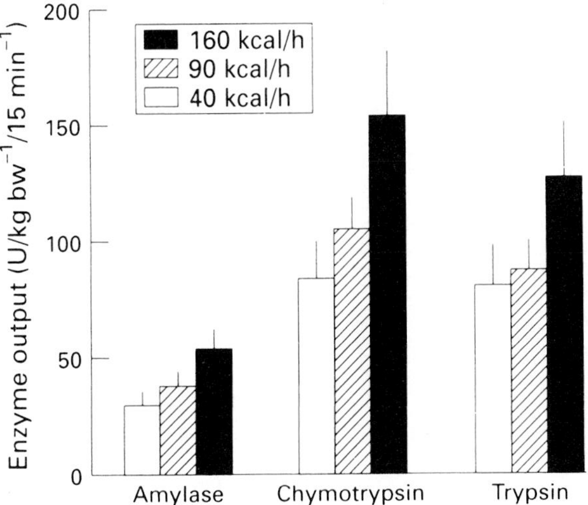

Figure 72.2. Mean (SEM) total enzyme outputs for the 300 minutes of the study. Outputs of amylase, chymotrypsin, and trypsin were significantly associated with 40, 90, and 160 kcal/h infused ($r = 0.44$, $P < 0.02$; $r = 0.44$, $P < 0.03$; and $r = 0.32$, $P < 0.05$; respectively. (From Holtmann G, Kelly DG, DiMagno EP. Gut 1996;38:920–4, with permission.)

Table 72.3
Etiology of Chronic Pancreatitis and Exocrine Insufficiency

Alcohol	Idiopathic
Nonalcoholic tropical chronic pancreatitis	
Hereditary	Hypercalcemia
Stricture of the duct of Wirsung	Cystic fibrosis
Carcinoma of the pancreas	Pancreatic fistula
Schwachman's syndrome	Trypsinogen-enterokinase deficiency
α_1-Antitrypsin deficiency	Isolated enzyme deficiency (e.g., lipase, colipase)

pancreatitis, such as trypsinogen or enterokinase deficiency or colipase or lipase deficiency, but these conditions are rare.

During early chronic pancreatitis in patients with abdominal pain but no steatorrhea, a low-fat, low-protein, high-carbohydrate diet is indicated. In dogs with profound exocrine pancreatic insufficiency, a diet containing a high proportion of fat (43 and 47%) along with sufficient lipolytic activity (bacterial or porcine lipase) decreases steatorrhea by increasing the coefficient of fat absorption (20).

Natural History and Clinical Aspects

Chronic pancreatitis causes both exocrine and endocrine insufficiency. What is not widely recognized is that the rate of progression to exocrine and endocrine insufficiency depends upon the underlying type of chronic pancreatitis. In our experience (21), about 60% of patients have chronic pancreatitis due to alcohol (defined as an average daily consumption of 50 g of alcohol or more), about 16% have idiopathic chronic pancreatitis, and the remainder ingest an unknown amount of less than 50 g of alcohol daily. The natural history of the latter group is not defined but is under study. However, patients with chronic pancreatitis due to alcohol develop exocrine (Fig. 72.3) and endocrine (Fig. 72.4) insufficiency a median of 13 and 20 years, respectively, from onset of disease. According to our studies, there are two forms of idiopathic chronic pancreatitis with quite different courses for development of pancreatic insufficiency. Patients with early-onset chronic pancreatitis (age 35 or younger) develop exocrine and endocrine pancreatic insufficiency at much slower rates (26 and 28 years from onset of disease vs. 17 and 12 years for late-onset disease).

The onset and severity of pain are important differences among the groups of patients with chronic pancreatitis. All patients with early-onset chronic pancreatitis have pain, mostly severe. In contrast, at onset of the disease, about 75% of patients with alcoholic pancreatitis have pain (50% severe), and only 50% of patients with late-onset idiopathic chronic pancreatitis have pain (mostly mild). Patients with late-onset chronic pancreatitis who do not have pain usually present with symptoms of malabsorption and later are found to have chronic pancreatitis; uncommonly, they may present with diabetes.

Clinically, recurrent attacks of abdominal and back pain characterize chronic pancreatitis of patients with alcoholic or early-onset idiopathic pancreatitis. Persistent abdominal pain usually indicates a complication, an inflammatory mass, pseudocyst, or obstruction of the bile duct or duodenum. Anorexia, nausea, and vomiting may accompany these complications. Eating may aggravate these symptoms as well as induce diarrhea. The clinical spectrum of chronic pancreatitis ranges from a benign chronic course to unremitting progressive weight loss and inanition complicated by narcotic abuse, addiction, and significant psychologic problems. Abdominal pain, malabsorption, and diabetes mellitus are complications of chronic pancreatitis that affect nutritional status and have

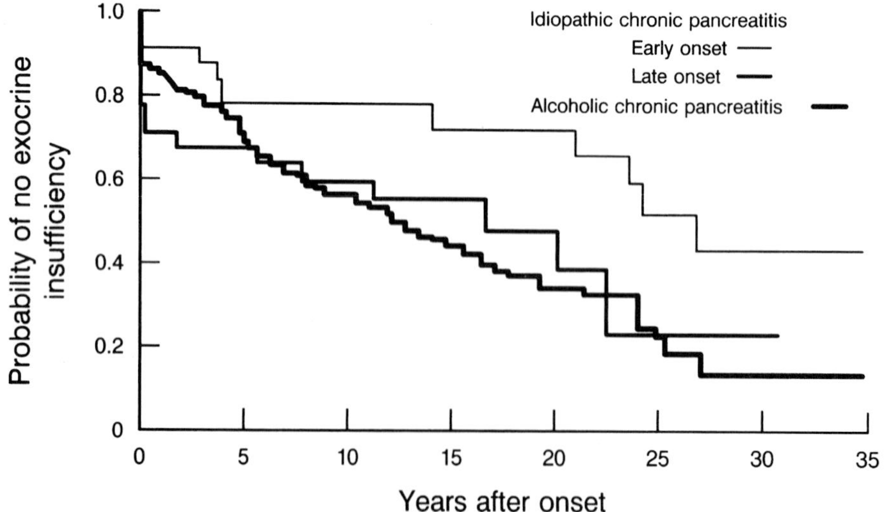

Figure 72.3. Probability of remaining free of exocrine insufficiency for patients with early-onset or late-onset idiopathic chronic pancreatitis and alcoholic pancreatitis. Differences were significant between early-onset idiopathic chronic pancreatitis and late-onset idiopathic chronic pancreatitis ($P = 0.024$) and between early-onset idiopathic chronic pancreatitis and alcoholic chronic pancreatitis ($P = 0.0008$). (From Layer P, Yamamoto H, Kalthoff L, et al. Gastroenterology 1994;107:1481–7, with permission.)

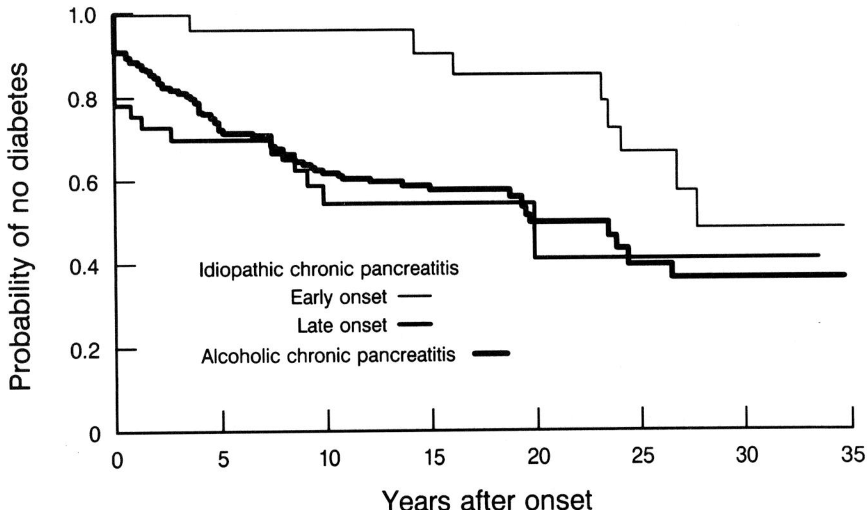

Figure 72.4. Probability of remaining free of diabetes mellitus for patients with early-onset or late-onset idiopathic chronic pancreatitis and alcoholic pancreatitis. Differences were significant between early-onset idiopathic chronic pancreatitis and late-onset idiopathic chronic pancreatitis ($P = 0.01$) and between early-onset idiopathic chronic pancreatitis and alcoholic chronic pancreatitis ($P = 0.0025$). (From Layer P, Yamamoto H, Kalthoff L, et al. Gastroenterology 1994;107:1481–7, with permission.)

important implications for nutritional treatment of chronic pancreatitis.

Some 33% of patients with chronic pancreatitis were reported to have a resting energy expenditure above the value predicted by the standard Harris and Benedict formula (16). In another series of stable outpatients with alcoholic chronic pancreatitis, hypermetabolism was observed in 48.5%, and this percentage rose to 65% in the subgroup of undernourished chronic pancreatitis patients (22). However, most patients with pancreatic insufficiency can maintain their weight and strength with a good appetite, high caloric intake, and ingestion of pancreatic enzymes. In our experience, more extensive measures are rarely needed to achieve or maintain an acceptable nutritional state. Usually, patients who become severely debilitated and malnourished do so in response to an acute complication such as an exacerbation of chronic pancreatitis, pancreatic ascites, or symptomatic pseudocysts. In these patients, enteral feeding or TPN may be necessary for extended periods of time. Similarly, enteral or parenteral nutritional support may be advisable to prepare a patient for surgery or to maintain the patient following an operation (23).

Assessment of Exocrine Insufficiency

Most patients with chronic pancreatitis who require long-term attention to nutritional status have malabsorption. Therefore, it is important to detect malabsorption promptly when suspected. The "gold standard" test for malabsorption is quantitative fecal fat excretion measurement (see Chapter 65). However, a qualitative fecal fat test may have more than 90% sensitivity (23). Other fecal tests devised to assess exocrine function (fecal chymotrypsin and elastase) as well as noninvasive tests of exocrine pancreatic function (bentiromide or pancreolauryl tests) are generally highly sensitive (>85%) only when malabsorption is present. Therefore, they can generally be used to detect malabsorption in chronic pancreatitis. The most accurate tests of pancreatic function are invasive tests that require duodenal intubation and stimulation of the pancreas by hormones (24) (we use CCK-OP; others use secretin or a combination of CCK and secretin). These tests measure the entire range of pancreatic function and are very useful to establish the diagnosis of chronic pancreatitis when mild or moderate exocrine dysfunction is present, but they are not necessary when malabsorption is present.

Relationship between Pancreatic Enzyme Secretion and Nutrition

As noted above, in chronic pancreatitis, it may take one to three decades for severe pancreatic chronic insufficiency with malabsorption to develop. Major reasons for the slow development of malabsorption are the slowly progressive destruction of the acinar cell mass and the large reserve capacity for enzyme secretion. There is a 10-fold reserve for exocrine pancreatic enzyme secretion; steatorrhea or azotorrhea occurs only after maximal lipase or trypsin secretion is reduced by more than 90% in patients with chronic pancreatitis or pancreatic cancer (25–28). In addition, in studies in normal humans we found that reducing intraluminal amylase activity to 10% of normal by use of an amylase inhibitor causes carbohydrate (starch) malabsorption (29, 30). Lipase secretion into the duodenum decreases more rapidly than secretion of proteolytic enzymes (26). Hence, steatorrhea often occurs earlier and is more severe than azotorrhea. This may be due to decreased pancreatic secretion of lipase relative to proteolytic enzymes, but lipase is much more fragile than proteolytic enzymes and amylase (31); it is more easily inactivated by acidic pH and is digested by proteolytic enzymes (chymotrypsin > trypsin) (32).

Effect of Pancreatic Enzyme Replacement on Absorption

Standard pancreatin treatment (a large amount of enzymes taken at doses of eight tablets with meals consisting of 25 g of fat) abolishes azotorrhea and reduces, but does not totally correct, steatorrhea (33) (Fig. 72.5). Most patients on this regimen achieve satisfactory nutritional status and become relatively asymptomatic. In many remaining symptomatic patients, simply reducing the amount of dietary fat alleviates diarrhea. For the occasional symptomatic patient, addition of cimetidine (34) or omeprazole (35) to standard pancreatin treatment usually abolishes steatorrhea and alleviates troublesome diarrhea. Similar results have been achieved with bicarbonate (36).

When gastric pH exceeds 4 for approximately 2 hours postprandially, altering the dose schedule from 8 tablets with meals to 2 tablets hourly may alleviate steatorrhea. By contrast, when gastric pH does not exceed 5 and duodenal pH is maintained relatively acidic (below 4) for long periods of time postprandially, microencapsulated preparations may be effective (37).

If symptoms and steatorrhea continue, special intraluminal studies may be necessary to determine whether intraluminal conditions permit certain dose schedules to be effective or if the intraluminal conditions have been altered by adjunctive therapy. For example, if administration of 300 mg of cimetidine does not keep the gastric pH above 4, gastric secretion was not reduced enough. Either more cimetidine should be given or, if intraluminal conditions are constantly acidic, Pancrease may be the best preparation to use. Although microencapsulated preparations containing a high dose of lipase may correct steatorrhea in some patients (38), these preparations have been withdrawn from the U.S. market because of the association of colonic strictures in children with cystic fibrosis who were ingesting large numbers of these capsules (39, 40).

Effect of Nutrients (Diet) on Normal Pancreas Secretion

Single nutrients have different effects on exocrine pancreatic secretion when infused into the gut (41). Essential amino acids (41) and poorly absorbed carbohydrates (mannitol) (42) cause 50% maximal enzyme secretion, but calcium (43), triglycerides, and long-chain (C18) fatty acids (44) induce maximal enzyme secretion.

Similarly, in normal persons, diets containing carbohydrate as 50 to 80% of the caloric content cause the least postprandial and interdigestive pancreatic enzyme secretion (18), and high-fat diets (40% of the calories) stimulate maximal postprandial and interdigestive secretion. Postprandial effects occur immediately, whereas the carbohydrate effect on interdigestive secretion occurs within 24 hours, and that for fat after 24 hours. Thus, in patients with pancreatitis, high-carbohydrate, low-fat, low-protein diets may be useful to minimally stimulate exocrine pancreatic secretion.

Effect of Unabsorbed Nutrients on Pancreatic Secretion

In normal humans, ileal infusions of carbohydrate (starch plus glucose) proportionally decrease trypsin and

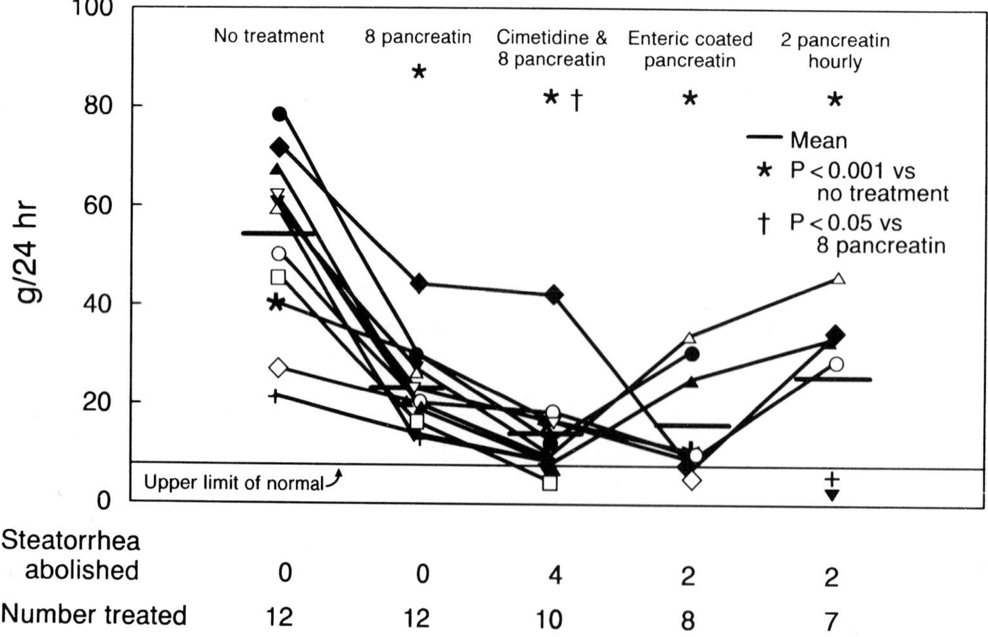

Figure 72.5. Results of various treatments on fecal fat excretions (g/24 h) in patients with chronic pancreatitis. Pancreatin used in these studies was Viokase. (From DiMagno EP, Layer P, Clain JE. Chronic pancreatitis. In: Go VLW, et al., eds. The pancreas: biology, pathobiology, and disease. New York: Raven Press, 1993;665–706, with permission.)

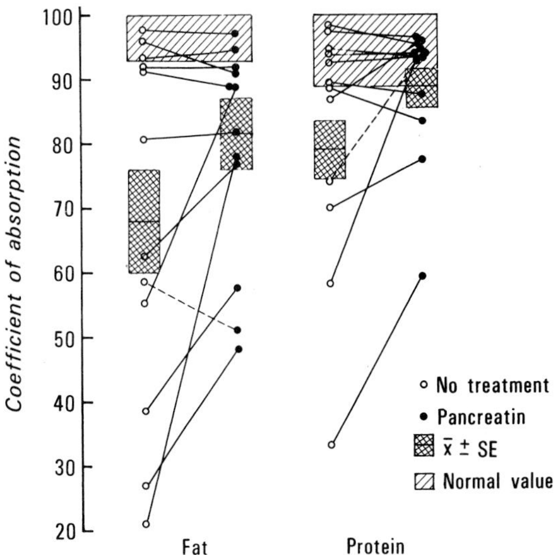

Figure 72.6. Coefficients of fat and protein absorption in pancreatic cancer patients with no treatment and when receiving pancreatic extract. The single patient who had severe steatorrhea and did not improve with pancreatin developed a biliary cutaneous fistula between no treatment and administration of pancreatin *(dotted line)*. (From Perez MM, Newcomer AD, Moertel CG, et al. Cancer 1983;52:346–52, with permission.)

bile acid secretion into the duodenum, slow gastric emptying (45), but increase amylase secretion relative to trypsin (46). These changes should increase digestion and absorption of carbohydrate by slowing gastric emptying of carbohydrate into the duodenum and increasing pancreatic amylase secretion. It is not known whether these changes in exocrine pancreatic secretion occur with other nutrients in the ileum or in diseases causing malabsorption.

PANCREATIC INSUFFICIENCY IN PANCREATIC CANCER

A common error in patients with pancreatic cancer is not recognizing that malabsorption is an important cause of weight loss (47). About 75 to 80% of pancreatic adenocarcinomas (the type of 90% of pancreatic cancers) arise in the head of the pancreas and are associated with obstruction of the pancreatic duct and severe exocrine pancreatic insufficiency (Fig. 72.6). In addition, patients who undergo the standard radical pancreaticoduodenectomy are frequently not given appropriate enzyme replacement therapy. These patients should receive pancreatin as described for treatment of chronic pancreatitis. In our experience, steatorrhea and creatorrhea can be appreciably improved (Fig. 72.6). (Also see Chapter 82.)

REFERENCES

1. Roscher R, Beger HG. Bacterial infection of pancreatic necrosis. In: Beger HG, Buchler M, eds. Acute pancreatitis. Heidelberg: Springer-Verlag, 1987:314–7.
2. Ranson JHC, Rifkind KM, Roses, et al. Surg Gynecol Obstet 1974;139:69–81.
3. Bank S, Wise L, Gersten M. Am J Gastroenterol 1983;78:637–40.
4. Agarwal N, Pitchumoni CS. Pancreas 1986;1:69–73.
5. Corfield AP, Williamson RCN, McMahon MJ, et al. Lancet 1985;24:403–7.
6. Demmy TL, Burch JM, Feliciano DV, et al. Am J Surg 1988;156:492–6.
7. Larvin M, McMahon MJ. Lancet 1989;2:201–4.
8. Wilson C, Heath DI, Imrie CW. Br J Surg 1990;77:1260–4.
9. Stanten R, Frey CF. Arch Surg 1990;125:1269–75.
10. Larvin M, Chalmers AG, Robinson PJ, et al. Br J Surg 1989;76:465–71.
11. Karimgani I, Porter KA, Langevin RE, et al. Gastroenterology 1992;103:1636–40.
12. Balthazar EJ, Ranson JHC, Naidich DP, et al. Radiology 1985;156:767–72.
13. Balthazar EJ, Robinson DL, Megibow AJ, et al. Radiology 1990;174:331–6.
14. Pisters PW, Ranson JH. Surg Gynecol Obstet 1992;175:275–84.
15. Goodgame JT, Fisher JE. Ann Surg 1977;186–651–8.
16. Dickerson RN, Vehe KL, Mullen JL, et al. Crit Care Med 1991;19:484–90.
17. Grant JP, James S, Grabowski V, et al. Ann Surg 1984;200:627–31.
18. Boivin M, Lanspa SJ, Zinsmeister AR, et al. Gastroenterology 1990;99:1763–71.
19. Holtmann G, Kelly DG, DiMagno EP. Gut 1996;38:920–4.
20. Suzuki A, Mizumoto A, Sarr MG, et al. Gastroenterology 1997;112:2048–55.
21. Layer P, Yamamoto H, Kalthoff L, et al. Gastroenterology 1994;107:1481–7.
22. Hebuterne X, Hastier P, Peroux J-L, et al. Dig Dis Sci 1996;41:533–9.
23. Newcomer AD, Hofmann AF, DiMagno EP, et al. Gastroenterology 1979;54:157–62.
24. Maringhini A, Nelson DK, Jones JD, et al. Gastroenterology 1994;107:231–5.
25. DiMagno EP, Go VLW, Summerskill WHJ. N Engl J Med 1973;288:813–5.
26. DiMagno EP, Malagelada J-R, Go VLW. Ann NY Acad Sci 1975;252:200–7.
27. DiMagno EP. Malagelada J-R, Go VLW. Mayo Clin Proc 1979;54:157–62.
28. Lankisch PG, Creutzfeld W. Therapy of exocrine and endocrine pancreatic insufficiency. In: Creutzfeld W, ed. Clinics in gastroenterology. Philadelphia: WB Saunders, 1984;985–99.
29. Layer P, Zinsmeister AR, DiMagno EP. Gastroenterology 1986;91:41–8.
30. Boivin M, Flourie B, Rizza R, et al. Gastroenterology 1988;94:387–94.
31. Layer P, Go VLW, DiMagno EP. Am J Physiol 1986;251: G475–80.
32. Thiruvengadam R, Sandberg R, Bentley K, et al. Gastroenterology 1986;90:1663.
33. DiMagno EP, Malagelada J-R, Go VLW, et al. N Engl J Med 1977;296:1318–22.
34. Regan PT, Malagelada J-R, DiMagno EP, et al. N Engl J Med 1977;297:854–8.
35. Heijrman HG, Lamers CB, Bakker W. Ann Intern Med 1991;114:200–1.
36. Graham DY. Dig Dis Sci 1982;27:485–90.
37. DiMagno EP. Mayo Clin Proc 1979;54:435–42.
38. Malesci A, Maiani A, Mezzi G, et al. J Clin Gastroenterol 1994;18:32–5.

39. Smyth RL, van Velzen D, Smyth AR, et al. Lancet 1994;343:85–6.
40. Taylor CJ. Lancet 1994;343:615–6.
41. Go VLW, Hofmann AF, Summerskill WHJ. J Clin Invest 1970;49:1558–64.
42. Owyang C, Miller LJ, DiMagno EP, et al. Gut 1982;23:357–61.
43. Holtermueller KH, Malagelada JR, McCall JT, et al. Gastroenterology 1976;70:693–6.
44. Malagelada J-R, DiMagno EP, Summerskill WHJ, et al. J Clin Invest 1976;58:493–9.
45. Jain NK, Boivin M, Zinsmeister AR, et al. Gastroenterology 1989;96:377–87.
46. Jain NK, Boivin M, Zinsmeister AR, et al. Pancreas 1991;6:495–505.
47. Perez MM, Newcomer AD, Moertel CG, et al. Cancer 1983;52:346–52.

73. Nutrition in Liver Disorders

C. S. LIEBER

The functional integrity of the liver is essential for use of nutrients. Disorders of this organ have far-reaching effects on nutritional status. This chapter first delineates the liver's role in normal processes. Then nutritional complications of liver dysfunction and approaches for correcting these nutritional deficiencies are assessed. Finally, nutritional factors that may themselves result in liver injury are discussed.

LIVER IN NORMAL NUTRITION

The liver influences nutritional status through its elaboration of bile salts and its role in intermediary metabolism of protein (amino acids), carbohydrate, fat, and vitamins.

Bile Salts

Bile salts are synthesized in the liver from cholesterol, secreted in bile, and mixed with intestinal contents in response to a meal. In the intestine, bile salts are active in the intraluminal phase of fat assimilation, their principal action being that of a detergent. Triglycerides enter the duodenum as an emulsion whose surface is covered by a relatively polar layer of phospholipids and proteins that must be removed by bile salts before lipolysis via pancreatic lipase can proceed. However, clearance of these polar substances from the emulsion also separates glyceride in the emulsion from lipase in the water phase; as a result, lipolysis becomes dependent on another enzyme, colipase, which is secreted with lipase in the pancreatic juice. By binding to lipase and altering its molecular conformation, colipase overcomes the inhibitory actions of bile salts on lipolysis (1, 2).

The products of lipolysis, such as fatty acids, monoglycerides, and small amounts of lysophospholipids form mixed micelles with bile salts. Intestinal uptake of long-chain fatty acids depends on these mixed micelles. In contrast, absorption of short- and medium-chain fatty acids proceeds in the absence of bile (3). Following uptake of fatty acids, bile salts are conserved by being recycled through an enterohepatic circulation. Bile salts, especially conjugates of the trihydroxy bile acid, cholic acid, are reabsorbed from the distal small bowel by an active, sodium-dependent process. Dihydroxy bile salts are absorbed by passive diffusion from the proximal small bowel (4). The liver extracts these reabsorbed bile salts from the portal vein blood and returns them to the biliary tree. Hepatic synthesis of bile salts replenishes the fraction of the bile salt pool that escapes reabsorption and is excreted in the feces (5).

Intermediary Metabolism

The liver plays a fundamental role in intermediary metabolism. This is a highly complex topic and is not covered here in an exhaustive manner. Instead, the highlights are reviewed to provide an overall view for understanding of the nutritional complications of liver injury.

Carbohydrates

The liver regulates carbohydrate metabolism by the synthesis, storage, and breakdown of glycogen. A polymeric form of glucose, large amounts of glycogen can be stored within the hepatocyte without major effects on the intracellular osmotic pressure. Glycogen is formed when the intake of glucose (or other gluconeogenic fuels) exceeds energy requirements; glycogen is broken down when intake lags behind energy needs. The principal enzymes controlling glycogenesis and glycogenolysis are glycogen synthase and phosphorylase, respectively. There is a reciprocal relationship between these two enzymes. Stimulation of glycogen synthetase is usually accompanied by inhibition of phosphorylase; conversely, agents that stimulate phosphorylase inhibit glycogen synthetase. Factors that control these enzymes include intracellular levels of glucose-6-phosphate and hormones such as epinephrine, glucagon, and insulin. Epinephrine and glucagon raise blood glucose levels by activating phosphorylase, whereas insulin lowers blood glucose, in part by stimulating glycogen synthetase.

Hepatocytes also possess enzymes that enable them to synthesize glucose from various precursors such as amino acids, pyruvate, and lactate (gluconeogenesis). Hypoglycemia promotes this process. The link between hypoglycemia and gluconeogenesis is probably mediated by secretion of cortisol from the adrenal medulla. Cortisol secretion is under pituitary control (adrenocorticotropic hormone, or ACTH) and is known to mobilize glycogenic amino acids from various tissues.

Fat

The liver is a major site of fatty acid breakdown and triglyceride synthesis. The breakdown of fatty acids provides an alternative source of energy when glucose is unavailable, as during fasting or starvation. Triglyceride in adipose tissue is hydrolyzed to release fatty acids. Bound to albumin in the blood, the released fatty acids are rapidly removed by the hepatocyte and transported into mitochondria by a carnitine-mediated process. Within the mitochondria, a number of enzymes degrade the fatty acid molecule to acetyl-CoA fragments, a sequence known as β-oxidation. In turn, acetyl-CoA can enter the citric acid cycle and generate adenosine triphosphate (ATP) by oxidative phosphorylation. Triglyceride synthesis occurs when carbohydrate intake exceeds energy requirements; under such conditions, glucose may overwhelm the glycogen reservoir, and the acetyl-CoA generated by glycolysis is not needed for oxidative phosphorylation. During such times of nutrient abundance, the energy charge inherent in acetyl-CoA is conserved by its conversion to fatty acids and, ultimately, triglycerides. Synthesis of fatty acids involves repetitive additions of two-carbon fragments (derived from acetyl-CoA) to malonyl-CoA. After reaction with α-glycerophosphate, the resulting triglycerides are transported to the adipose tissues as part of lipoproteins, specifically, the very low density lipoproteins (VLDL).

Proteins

The liver plays a central role in synthesis and degradation of protein. Thus it contains the enzymes necessary for transamination and oxidative deamination of amino acids as well as those required for urea synthesis. As noted above, amino acids can also participate in gluconeogenesis. Gluconeogenesis proceeds after conversion of deaminated amino acids to pyruvate or intermediates of the citric acid cycle. Plasma proteins, including albumin, coagulation factors, transferrin, and ceruloplasmin, constitute about one-half of the protein synthesized in the liver. These export proteins are synthesized on the rough endoplasmic reticulum and pass through intracellular pathways. Protein synthesis by the liver is influenced by the nutritional state, as well as by hormones, particularly insulin, glucagon, and glucocorticoids. Insulin and steroids stimulate synthesis of hepatic proteins, whereas glucagon inhibits their synthesis and promotes their degradation.

NUTRITIONAL CONSEQUENCES OF LIVER INJURY

Acute Liver Injury

Regardless of cause, acute liver injury is often associated with anorexia, nausea, and vomiting. When the liver injury is due to alcohol, these symptoms may be exacerbated by concomitant alcoholic gastritis. Thus, acute liver injury is likely to decrease the oral intake of food, but if the illness is short-lived and self-limited, nutritional consequences are minimal. Both alcoholic and nonalcoholic acute liver injury may cause fasting hypoglycemia. This has been attributed to depleted liver glycogen reserves and a block in gluconeogenesis from amino acids.

Chronic Liver Injury

Nutritional complications are frequent when hepatic function becomes impaired in chronic liver injury, particularly cirrhosis. Regardless of etiology, cirrhosis is likely to cause patients to have abnormal anthropometric measurements (i.e., muscle wasting) and to be anergic to common antigens on skin testing (6). Circulating levels of both fat- and water-soluble vitamins are low in a high percentage of patients with alcoholic cirrhosis. Low serum levels of fat-soluble vitamins (rather than the water-soluble variety) are more characteristic of nonalcoholic cirrhosis (7). These nutritional deficiencies arise as a result of one or more of the following factors: inadequate dietary intake, maldigestion, malabsorption, and defective metabolism.

Dietary Intake

Inadequate intake of protein is common, especially among alcoholics with cirrhosis. Indeed, if the alcoholic patient continues to drink despite cirrhosis, protein intake may be low, and the bulk of dietary calories may be derived from carbohydrates and alcohol per se. Calories derived from alcohol are, in a sense, "empty" because alcoholic beverages are devoid of proteins, minerals, vitamins, and significant amounts of carbohydrate. Furthermore, their actual caloric contribution is less than that of an equivalent amount of carbohydrates (see Chapter 94). Changes in mental status that result from hepatic encephalopathy may also contribute to the poor intake of patients with advanced liver disease. Hepatic coma in turn is likely to result in hospitalization, which may itself exacerbate nutritional deficiencies in these patients. Malnutrition in hospitalized patients results from both diagnostic (radiologic or endoscopic procedures) and therapeutic (e.g., variceal sclerotherapy) interventions.

Maldigestion and Malabsorption

Decreased bile salt secretion and pool size have been demonstrated in patients with cirrhosis (8). In light of the role of bile salts in fat digestion (see "Bile Salts" above), contraction of the bile salt pool would be expected to impair micelle formation and lead to abnormalities of fat assimilation, especially in patients with underlying pancreatic insufficiency. Steatorrhea in turn causes deficiencies in fat-soluble vitamins, with clinical manifestations such as night blindness, osteoporosis, and easy bruisability or hemorrhage.

Metabolic Changes

A number of defects in protein metabolism have been noted in patients with chronic liver failure. These include decreased hepatic synthesis of export proteins (albumin, coagulation factors), decreased urea synthesis (9), and decreased metabolism of aromatic amino acids. The effect of advanced liver disease on protein catabolism is controversial. Using stable isotopes such as ^{13}C leucine, turnover studies indicate that protein degradation is normal in fasted cirrhotic patients (10). However, after feeding, protein flux appears to increase (11). These alterations have important clinical consequences. Decreased synthesis of plasma proteins may lead to hypoalbuminemia and exacerbate the formation of ascites in patients with portal hypertension. Depressed levels of coagulation factors may predispose these patients to the risk of gastrointestinal (GI) hemorrhage. Failure to detoxify ammonia and the abnormal amino acid profile of patients with cirrhosis may in part increase the likelihood of hepatic encephalopathy. Despite these abnormalities in intermediary metabolism, overall nitrogen balance can be maintained at positive levels by amounts of dietary protein similar to that in the noncirrhotic individual (35 to 50 g/day) (12).

Glucose tolerance is frequently abnormal in the cirrhotic patient and has been linked to insulin resistance. The high fasting and postprandial insulin levels in these patients may be related to such factors as portosystemic shunting, increased levels of growth hormone, and depleted body stores of potassium (13, 14). Also, because glycogen stores are often depleted in the cirrhotic liver, fatty acid oxidation appears to supplant glucose as a source of fuel during fasting (10, 14–17). This is apparent when indirect calorimetry is performed, because stable cirrhotic patients have a significantly lower respiratory quotient (RQ) than normal controls. Energy expenditure in chronic liver injury is comparable to that in controls (15, 16, 18), making hypermetabolism per se an unlikely explanation for weight loss in these patients. A number of investigators have reported higher-than-predicted energy production rates in cirrhotic patients, but only when energy expenditure was related to urinary creatinine excretion (17, 19). However, as pointed out by Merli et al. (16) and Heymsfield et al. (20), the use of urinary creatinine excretion as a measure of active cell mass is invalid in patients with cirrhosis because their hepatic production of creatine is depressed. Isotopic methods involving labeled water and potassium have been recommended for estimating the metabolically active body cell mass in patients with decompensated cirrhosis (20).

Abnormalities of water- and fat-soluble vitamins are common in patients with cirrhosis. In the nonalcoholic with cirrhosis, deficiencies of fat-soluble vitamins are likely to arise from malabsorption. In part, abnormal bile salt metabolism and defective micelle formation limit the uptake of such vitamins in these patients. In the alcoholic, inadequate intake of vitamins, especially those that are water soluble (thiamin and folic acid), is important (see Chapter 94).

In addition to inadequate intake and decreased uptake, vitamin metabolism per se may be deranged in chronic liver injury. Defects have been described in phosphorylation of thiamin by alcoholic cirrhotic patients (21), in synthesis of retinol-binding protein (22), in degradation of pyridoxal-5′-phosphate (23), and in conversion of vitamin D to its active form (24). Hepatic vitamin A levels are depressed by both heavy alcohol consumption and drug use (25, 26). Part of the hepatic depletion may be due to mobilization, since hepatic lipoprotein secretion is increased by chronic alcohol consumption (27). "Induced" hepatic microsomes may enhance degradation of both retinol and retinoic acid (28–30). As a result of these derangements, vitamin repletion strategies require modification in patients with liver failure, as discussed below.

NUTRITIONAL THERAPY IN LIVER DISORDERS

Protein and Amino Acids

To the extent that patients with liver injury, either acute or chronic, are in negative nitrogen balance, it has been assumed that liver regeneration will be delayed and that muscle wasting will be accelerated. However, when feeding protein or administering amino acids, one must be aware of the precarious balance between the need to restore protein intake and the potential risk of precipitating hepatic encephalopathy. There is often only a small margin of safety in this respect. The amount of dietary protein that can be tolerated varies considerably. At times, only minimal amounts of protein can be ingested without altering the mental state. Under such circumstances, breakdown of remaining protein stores can be minimized by provision of calories in the form of fats and carbohydrates.

In acute liver injury, much work has focused on the role of protein or amino acid supplementation on the outcome of alcoholic hepatitis. Both enteral and parenteral routes have been used in these investigations. In general, studies in patients with acute hepatitis have demonstrated that hepatic encephalopathy can usually be avoided by judicious titration of dietary protein, that relatively little dietary protein can be associated with positive nitrogen balance, and that both symptomatic and biochemical improvement (if not prognosis) can be expected (31–37). Positive nitrogen balance can be attained in patients with chronic liver injury (cirrhosis) with daily amounts of dietary protein (0.74 g/kg) similar to that required by normal individuals (12). Conflicting results have been obtained regarding the extent to which the source of the dietary protein (animal or vegetable) affects overall nitrogen balance (38, 39).

Attempts have been made to normalize the plasma amino acid pattern found in patients with cirrhosis. The ratio of branched-chain amino acids (BCAAs; isoleucine, leucine, valine, and lysine) to aromatic amino acids (phenylalanine, tryptophan, and tyrosine) is abnormally low in these patients, especially those who are malnourished. However, compared with standard mixtures of amino acids, administration of BCAAs has shown no significant advantage in terms of nitrogen balance (40–43).

There was hope that correction of the abnormal amino acid profile in patients with cirrhosis would be beneficial in the treatment of hepatic encephalopathy. To this end, mixtures with high BCAA:aromatic amino acids ratios have been administered, and the source of protein (vegetable-derived protein is relatively low in aromatic amino acids) has been varied. A potential benefit seemed plausible in light of the false neurotransmitter hypothesis of Fischer and Baldersarini (44). In this scheme, entry of aromatic amino acids into the brain is favored by low plasma levels of BCAA. In the brain, sympathomimetic amines are generated from these aromatic amino acids (especially phenylalanine) and hinder neuronal transmission by competitive interactions with bona fide neurotransmitters at the receptor level. Initial studies in humans involving infusion of BCAA-enriched mixtures were encouraging, but these early clinical trials were not fully controlled or randomized (45). Using tighter designs, most subsequent studies failed to confirm the efficacy of intravenous or orally administered enriched mixtures in treating acute hepatic encephalopathy (6). Despite a recent metaanalysis that detected a trend favoring this therapy (46), the evidence does not support routine clinical use of these amino acid mixtures in acute encephalopathy (47). However, a subset of protein-intolerant patients with chronic encephalopathy (and better liver function) might benefit from BCAA (48).

Some success has been achieved in treating hepatic encephalopathy with protein derived from vegetable sources (38, 49). However, improvement in encephalopathy does not correlate with changes in the plasma amino acid profile. As a result, it has been suggested that the beneficial effects of vegetable protein are due to its fiber content rather than its amino acid composition per se (50). Fiber may increase elimination of nitrogenous waste, but the high fiber content of these diets is poorly tolerated.

Dietary restrictions of amino acids or protein are important in a number of inherited liver abnormalities, including disorders of the urea cycle and hypertyrosinemia (see Chapter 61). Specifically, reduced nitrogen intake is the cornerstone of therapy in hyperammonemia syndromes. In these disorders, activity of the urea cycle enzymes is diminished, ammonia accumulates in the blood, and central nervous system toxicity (lethargy, coma) develops. Depending on the specific location of the defect in the cycle, certain amino acids must also be supplemented. For example, in citrullinemia there is diminished conversion of citrulline to arginine as a result of a deficiency of argininosuccinic acid synthetase. Supplemental arginine bypasses this block and permits the urea cycle to proceed (51). In hypertyrosinemia, there is a defect in the final step in the breakdown of tyrosine and phenylalanine (52). This leads to high levels of tyrosine in the blood and urine, renal tubular dysfunction, and eventually death from liver failure. Dietary restriction of tyrosine and phenylalanine may be helpful.

Choline, Methionine, and *S*-Adenosyl-L-Methionine

For several decades, protein, methionine, and choline deficiencies have been implicated in the pathogenesis of liver injury. In growing rats, deficiencies in dietary protein and lipotropic factors (choline and methionine) can produce a fatty liver (53), and it has been reported that ethanol increases choline requirements in the rat (54), possibly by enhancing choline oxidation (55). Primates, however, are far less susceptible to protein and lipotropic deficiency than are rodents (56). Clinically, choline treatment of patients suffering from alcoholic liver injury has been ineffective in the face of continued alcohol abuse (57–60). Human liver contains very little choline oxidase activity, which may explain the species differences with regard to choline deficiency. In humans, choline deficiency (and thus a need for choline supplementation) has been documented in only very limited circumstances of extremely restricted diets (61). Moreover, in baboons fed ethanol, fatty liver as well as fibrosis (including cirrhosis) developed (62, 63) (Fig. 73.1), with striking ultrastructural changes (64), despite choline given at twice the dose recommended for the baboon (65).

Nevertheless, since the possibility existed that massive choline supplementation might have a favorable effect on the process, this was the subject of an experimental study in baboons (66). They were given either normal or choline-supplemented diets, each with or without ethanol. For 3 to 4 years, they were pair-fed liquid diets with 50% of total energy as ethanol or isocaloric carbohydrate. Ten animals were given the regular diets, and in eight, the choline content was increased fivefold. Choline supplementation failed to prevent alcohol-induced steatosis and fibrosis. All parameters remained normal in the eight baboons fed the regular control diet. However, in the choline-supplemented controls, serum bilirubin, and aspartate amino transferase (AST) and glutamate dehydrogenase (GDH) activities increased moderately, and serum albumin levels decreased. Occasional fat droplets appeared in hepatocytes with mitochondrial changes (enlargement and alterations of the cristae) and an abundance of "myelin" figures in the cytoplasm, indicating that choline supplementation had exerted moderate hepatotoxicity (66). It was concluded that massive choline supplementation does not prevent alcoholic liver injury but may, in fact, be hepatotoxic.

Liberal supplementation with methionine (62) also failed to prevent alcohol-induced liver injury, including cirrhosis, from developing in baboons. In man as well,

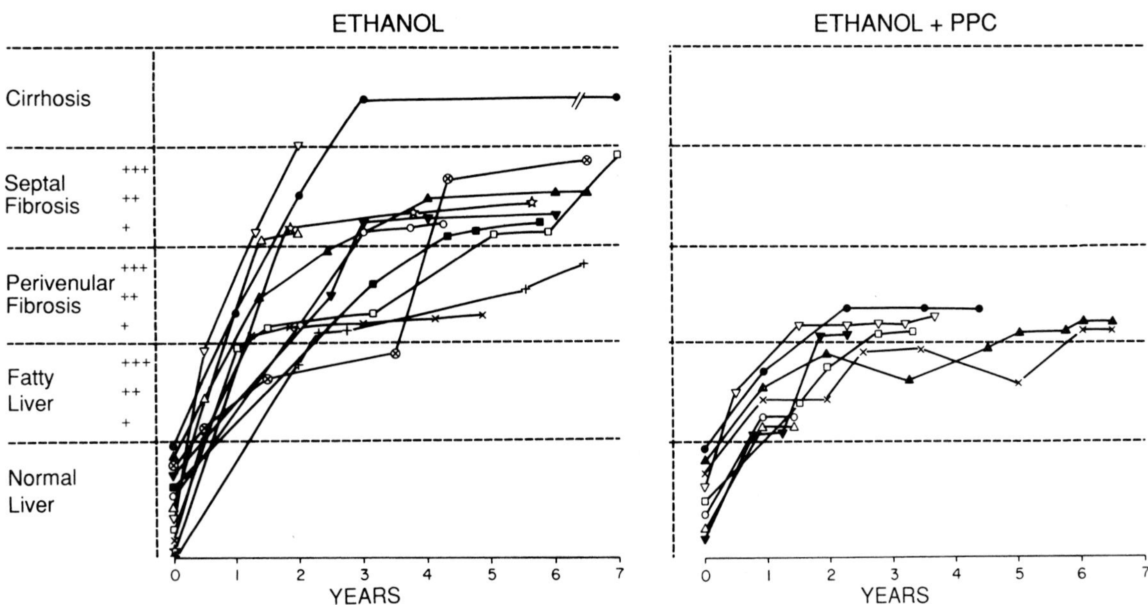

Figure 73.1. Sequential development of alcoholic liver injury in baboons fed ethanol with an adequate diet *(left panel)* and prevention of septal fibrosis and cirrhosis by supplementation with polyunsaturated phosphatidylcholine *(PPC) (right panel)*. Liver morphology in animals pair-fed control diets (with or without PPC) remained normal (not shown) (data form 117). Whereas no cirrhosis or septal fibrosis developed in the animals fed alcohol with PPC, in the aggregate 67 baboons fed ethanol with adequate diets (usually for 5 years) in this (117), as well as other (121, 169, 170) studies, cirrhosis was observed in 14, and septal fibrosis developed in an additional 14 animals, an incidence comparable to that observed in alcoholics.

methionine supplementation was considered for the treatment of liver diseases, especially the alcoholic variety, but some difficulties were encountered. Indeed, excess methionine has some adverse effects (67, 68). Furthermore, whereas in some patients with alcoholic liver disease, circulating methionine levels are normal (69), elevated levels have been reported in others (45, 70, 71). Kinsell et al. (72) observed a delay in clearance of plasma methionine after its systemic administration to patients with liver damage. Similarly, Horowitz et al. (73) reported that the blood clearance of methionine after an oral load was slowed in such subjects. Since about half of the methionine is metabolized by the liver, the above observations suggest impaired hepatic metabolism of this amino acid in patients with alcoholic liver disease. Indeed, Duce et al. (74) reported decreased *S*-adenosyl-L-methionine (SAMe) synthetase activity in cirrhotic livers. Chronic alcohol consumption was associated with enhanced methionine use and depletion (75). As a consequence, one can anticipate SAMe depletion as well as decreased availability. The baboon model of alcohol-induced liver injury was used to verify the latter hypothesis and to explore the possibility that SAMe repletion might oppose some of the adverse effects of alcohol on the liver (76). This study revealed that in the baboon, chronic ethanol consumption is associated with significant depletion of hepatic SAMe and that SAMe supplementation attenuates ethanol-induced liver injury.

Studies in rodents also showed prevention of fat accumulation in the liver by SAMe (77). The significant hepatic SAMe depletion in primates after long-term ethanol consumption (76) is due in part to increased use of reduced glutathione (GSH) secondary to enhanced free radical and acetaldehyde generation by the induced microsomal ethanol-oxidizing system (MEOS) (Fig. 73.2) as well as GSH leakage (78). Under these conditions, increased GSH turnover may ensue, as evidenced by a rise in α-amino-*n*-butyric acid (79, 80) (Figs. 73.2 and 73.3). However, synthesis of SAMe may become rate limiting, especially since it is decreased in cirrhosis (74). As a consequence of this enzymic defect, SAMe is depleted and methionine supplementation may be ineffective in alcoholic liver disease, whereas SAMe can correct the defect.

Potentially, SAMe depletion may have a number of adverse effects. SAMe is the principal methylating agent in various vital transmethylation reactions that are important to nucleic acid and protein synthesis. Methylation is important to cell membrane function (81, 82), with phospholipid methylation active in membrane fluidity and transport of metabolites and transmission of signals across membranes. Thus, by being detrimental for methyltransferase activity, decreased SAMe may thereby promote the membrane injury found in alcohol-induced liver damage (83). Not only is SAMe the methyl donor in almost all transmethylation reactions, but it also plays a key role in synthesis of polyamines and provides one source of the cysteine needed for glutathione production. Alcohol-induced depletion of glutathione is particularly striking in primates (76, 84).

In rats, chronic alcohol feeding results in decreased methionine formation via the *n*-5 tetrahydrofolate pathway, an effect compensated for through an adaptive

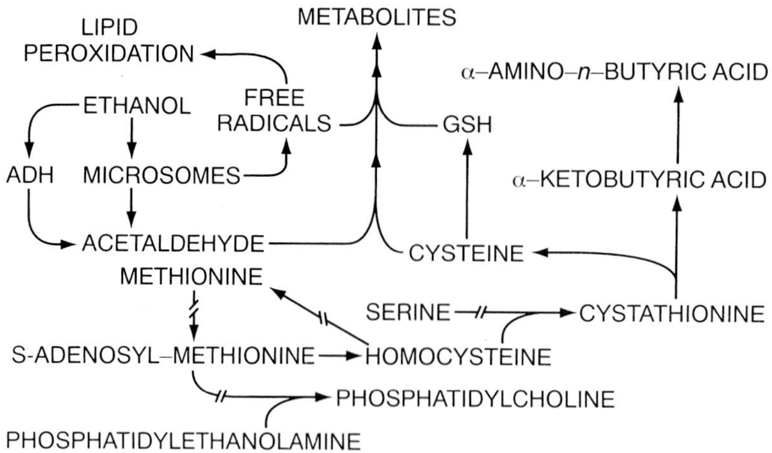

Figure 73.2. Link between accelerated acetaldehyde production and increased free radical generation by induced microsomes, resulting in enhanced lipid peroxidation with metabolic blocks due to alcohol, folate deficiency, and/or alcoholic liver disease, illustrating possible beneficial effects of GSH, its precursors (including *S*-adenosylmethionine [SAMe]) and phosphatidylcholine (166).

increase in betaine-homocysteine methyltransferase activity, which maintains hepatic SAMe levels (85). This adaptive process may be particularly operative in the rodents and much less so in primates. Indeed, as mentioned above, rodents contain higher levels of choline oxidase than primates and therefore can produce significantly greater amounts of betaine, which may be one reason why rodents are less susceptible to alcohol-induced liver injury than primates (56) (see above). Thus, replenishment of methionine (in its activated form, SAMe) may be particularly indicated in the primate subjected to an alcoholic insult.

Compared with methionine, administration of SAMe has the advantage of bypassing the deficit in SAMe synthesis from methionine, referred to above. Indeed, this deficit is due to decreased enzyme activity, not substrate, and hence it cannot simply be corrected by excess methionine. The hepatocyte can be replenished with SAMe via ingestion of the compound; blood levels of SAMe increase after oral administration in rodents (86) and in man (87). Although it has been claimed that the liver does not take up SAMe from the bloodstream (88), other results indicate uptake of SAMe by isolated hepatocytes at either pharmacologic (89) or physiologic (90, 91) extracellular levels. The liver SAMe transport system appears to be saturable (90, 92). Results in baboons (76) also clearly indicate hepatic uptake of exogenous SAMe. Furthermore, in these baboons, the ethanol-induced hepatic SAMe depletion was partially corrected by oral SAMe administration. In addition to uptake of extracellular SAMe, extracellular methionine appears to play a major role in the synthesis of newly acquired intracellular SAMe (91). Thus, orally administered SAMe may play a precursor role for intracellular SAMe, both as unchanged SAMe and also by the

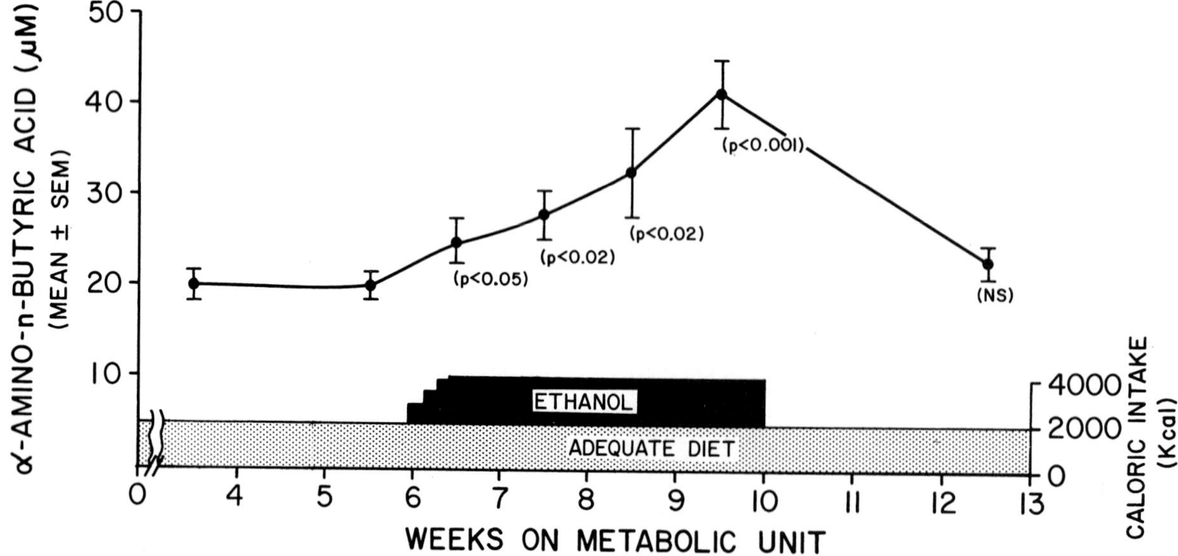

Figure 73.3. Effect of ethanol consumption on plasma α-amino-*n*-butyric acid (mean ± SEM); consumption of ethanol (4 g/kg/day) in addition to an adequate diet in three human volunteers resulted in doubling of plasma α-amino-*n*-butyric acid after 2 to 4 weeks, which was reversed after cessation of drinking (80).

methionine it provides. Since the SAMe transport system does not appear to be saturated under physiologic conditions, it is likely that SAMe levels in biologic compartments regulate, at least in part, the rate of transport across membranes. Indeed, hepatic levels of SAMe increase with increasing extracellular levels (91), and the intracellular concentrations reached are above or close to the K_m for SAMe of both phospholipid methyltransferase (92, 93) and catechol-*o*-methyltransferase (94). Furthermore, effective use of SAMe for both transmethylation and transsulfuration has been demonstrated in vivo (95).

Thus, the therapeutic use of SAMe is a good example of a beneficial result from replenishment of a naturally occurring molecule that has been depleted by liver disease. The exact role of SAMe in the treatment of liver disorders has been partly clarified by studies showing that this molecule is beneficial in intrahepatic cholestasis (reviewed in detail by Osman et al. [96].) Treatment with a stable salt of SAMe resulted in both improvement of standard liver function tests and reduction in symptoms such as itch. It has also been successfully used in severe cholestasis of pregnancy, where it has the advantage of few, if any, untoward effects. Treatment with SAMe also appears to be helpful in recurrent intrahepatic cholestasis and severe jaundice caused by androgens or estrogens, perhaps because of changes in membrane phospholipid composition. Experimentally, SAMe prevented total parenteral nutrition–induced cholestasis in the rat (97).

Potentially beneficial clinical effects of SAMe include enhanced bile salt conjugation with taurine in patients with liver cirrhosis (98). Other observations indicate that administration of exogenous SAMe prevents the hepatic glutathione depletion observed in patients with liver disease (99). Loguercio et al. (100) measured glutathione and cysteine concentrations in erythrocytes of alcoholics with and without liver cirrhosis. Glutathione levels decreased and cysteine levels increased in all patients. Parenteral treatment with SAMe corrected the erythrocyte thiol alterations. Furthermore, in patients given SAMe, long-term treatment doubled the plasma concentrations of the secondary sulfur-containing amino acids cystine and taurine (on average, low normal at baseline), without any change in the concentrations of methionine, neutral amino acids, and polyamines. No changes in plasma amino acids were observed in the control group (101). In experimental animals, SAMe prevented and reversed erythrocyte membrane alterations in cirrhosis (102). It also protected against liver damage induced by biliary obstruction in rats (103), prevented carbon tetrachloride–induced SAMe synthetase inactivation and associated liver injury (104), and improved the hepatic histologic picture in rats treated with CCl_4 and ethanol for 1 month (105). Betaine administration was reported to elevate hepatic SAMe levels and to prevent ethanol-induced fatty liver in rats (106).

Lack of methionine may also result from a deficit in methylation of homocysteine to methionine, mainly by the folate- and vitamin B_{12}–dependent enzyme methionine synthetase. Since most alcoholics have disturbed folate metabolism (attributable to multiple mechanisms, including an inadequate diet), elevated plasma homocysteine levels in alcoholics could have been anticipated and have now indeed been noted (107). Since hyperhomocysteinemia has been associated with premature vascular disease (108), the increased plasma homocysteine levels in alcoholics could contribute to the increased incidence of stroke in these patients. Furthermore, SAMe-dependent methylation of specific DNA cytosine bases to form 5-methylcytosine may block gene expression, and abnormalities in DNA methylation contribute to the loss of normal controls on protooncogene expression (109–111). Indeed, a methyl-deficient diet has been linked to early stages of colorectal neoplasia (112). These observations illustrate the need to correct underlying malnutrition in the alcoholic, which may exist irrespective of the social and medical situation of the patient (113). Nutritional support successfully decreased nutrition-associated complications in patients with alcoholic liver disease (114). The rationale for the various modalities of nutritional intervention has also been reviewed (115). It is now clear, however, that mere nutritional repletion may not suffice and that "supernutrients" may be needed, such as SAMe and possibly polyunsaturated phospholipids (see below).

Carbohydrates

Cirrhotic patients are prone to develop diabetes. As noted above, insulin resistance appears to account for this abnormality of glucose homeostasis. In patients with portal hypertension complicated by portosystemic shunting, an alteration in insulin metabolism may contribute to this resistance. Depleted body stores of potassium and elevated levels of growth hormone are probably also significant. As in other patients with diabetes, nutritional management plays an important role in therapy. Specifically, providing calories as complex carbohydrates effectively reduces insulin requirements. Increasing intake of complex carbohydrate may also be of benefit in hepatic encephalopathy because the nonabsorbable fiber found in such foods decreases colonic transit time and lowers colonic pH. Indeed, the efficacy of lactulose, one of the mainstays in treatment of hepatic encephalopathy, has been related to these same effects.

Inherited disorders of hepatic carbohydrate metabolism may also benefit from dietary manipulation. This heterogenous group of disorders, which includes galactosemia (see Chapter 61), glycogen storage disease, and fructose intolerance, can be traced to specific enzymatic deficiencies. These defects impair the orderly flow of substrates along pathways involved in anaerobic glycolysis. Accumulation of these substrates in various organs, especially the liver and muscle, results in organ injury and, frequently, hypoglycemia. Galactosemia can be successfully controlled by strict dietary exclusion of milk products containing galactose. Likewise, fruit, vegetables, and sucrose must be eliminated from the diets of children who are fructose intolerant. At least in type I glycogen storage disease (von Gierke's disease), biochemical improvement can be expected when hypoglycemia is prevented by frequent intake of glucose-rich formulas (116)

Lipids

Fat accumulation in the liver is strikingly affected by the amount and type of dietary triglycerides (see Chapter 94). With alcohol, the more triglycerides in the diet, the more fat accumulates in the liver (Fig. 73.4), at least down to a level of 10% of total energy. Below that, fat accumulates even when dietary fat is extremely low (2%), probably because of stimulation of lipogenesis.

Dietary phospholipids also have striking effects on liver structure and function. Indeed, in primates, chronic ethanol consumption results in a decrease in liver phospholipids and phosphatidylcholine (PC) levels; both can be corrected by PC supplementation (117). The total phospholipid content of the mitochondrial membranes is decreased, with significant reduction in the levels of PC (64); associated striking morphologic changes have a functional counterpart—diminished mitochondrial oxidation mainly due to decreased cytochrome oxidase activity (64, 118). The latter appears to result from alterations in the phospholipid composition of the mitochondrial membranes. Indeed, in vitro cytochrome oxidase activity could be restored with phospholipids extracted from normal mitochondria or synthetic ones, with PC being the most active (64).

The mechanism whereby chronic ethanol consumption alters phospholipids in unknown but may be related, at least in part, to decreased phosphotidylethanolamine/

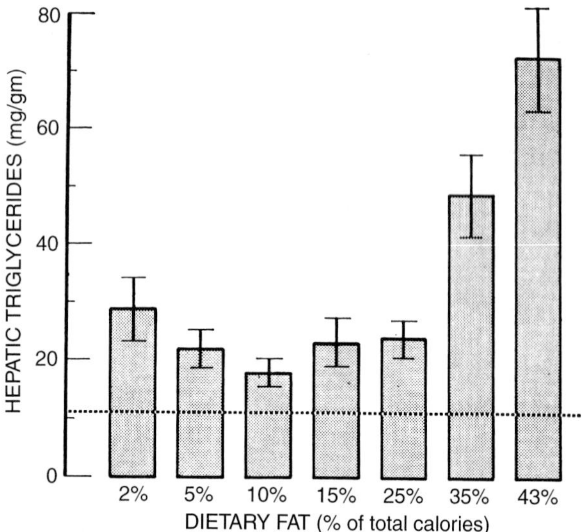

Figure 73.4. Effect of varying amounts of dietary fat. Hepatic triglycerides in seven groups of rats given ethanol (36% of calories) with a diet of normal protein (18% of calories). Average hepatic triglyceride concentration in the control animals is indicated by a *dotted line* (167).

methyltransferase activity described in cirrhotic livers (74) (Fig. 73.2). That this is not simply secondary to the cirrhosis but may in fact be a primary defect related to alcohol is suggested by the observation that the enzyme activity is decreased before development of cirrhosis (117). Ethanol may also affect phospholipids via formation of phosphatidylethanol, with possible impact on signal transduction, as shown in isolated rat hepatocytes (119). A third mechanism involves increased lipid peroxidation, as reflected by increased F_2 isoprostanes and 4-hydroxynonenal (120), which could explain the associated decrease of arachidonic acid in phospholipids (118).

In alcoholic patients, reduced phospholipid methyltransferase activity together with the decreased activity of SAMe synthetase (see above) may promote the membrane injury see experimentally in alcohol-induced liver damage (83). The question then is whether such deficiency could be attenuated, at least in part, by bypassing the enzyme defects via phospholipid supplementation. This was tested by feeding baboons alcohol in a diet supplemented with polyunsaturated lecithin. Administration of phospholipid preparations rich in polyunsaturated phosphatidylcholine (PPC) (121) or virtually pure PPC (63) (Fig. 73.1) was found to fully prevent alcohol-induced fibrosis and cirrhosis in the nonhuman primate. PPC contains choline, but, as discussed above, choline in the amounts present in PPC has no protective action against the fibrogenic effects of ethanol in the baboon (66). PPC is rich in linoleic acid, but this fatty acid per se is probably not responsible for the protective effect because the basic diet was supplemented with linoleate and contained large amounts of corn oil, which is rich in linoleic acid. Furthermore, this fatty acid has been incriminated as a permissive, rather than a protective, factor in alcoholic liver injury (122). Thus, the polyunsaturated phospholipids themselves appear to be responsible for protection, perhaps because of their high bioavailability and selective incorporation into liver membranes (123). Furthermore, PPC directly affects collagen metabolism and opposes the oxidative stress (120).

While there is still some discussion about the relative contributions of hepatocytes and stellate cells in the production of collagen in the liver, stellate cells are "activated" after chronic alcohol consumption and appear to play a major role (124, 125). When normal stellate cells are isolated and cultured on plastic surfaces, they undergo spontaneous transformation into myofibroblast-like cells, thus mimicking in vitro the "activation" that prevails in vivo after chronic alcohol consumption (126). These cells produce collagen in culture (126). When acetaldehyde is added to these cells, collagen accumulation increases further (126), with enhanced mRNA for collagen (127). Other aldehydes (such as malonaldehyde) are produced from lipid peroxidation, and they may also stimulate collagen production. Acetaldehyde stimulates collagen synthesis in cultured myofibroblasts as well (128), and a similar effect was observed with lactate. These cells were shown to proliferate in the perivenular zones of the liver after chronic alcohol consumption (129); they are similar to "activated" stellate cells, although they can be differentiated by ultrastructural and cytochemical characteristics (130). The normal liver contains a negligible number of "activated" stellate cells, whereas after chronic alcohol consumption, most stellate cells (more than 80%) are transformed. The protection afforded by PC against fibrosis (Fig. 73.1) was associated with a lesser transformation of stellate cells to transitional cells in vivo (48 vs. 81%). Thus, to the extent that transformation of stellate cells in alcohol-fed animals was responsible for the fibrosis, the lesser transformation after PC may be one reason for the decreased fibrosis.

Fibrosis and the associated collagen accumulation does not result simply from enhanced collagen production but from an imbalance between collagen production and breakdown. Breakdown was assessed in cultured rat stellate cells by measuring collagenase activity with different phospholipids, including various species of PC. It had been reported that a mixture of PCs affected the breakdown, but not the synthesis, of collagen under these conditions (131). The PC preparation used contained 18:2-18:2 PC (DLPC), 16:0-18:2 PC (PLPC) and other minor PC species. We found that pure DLPC stimulates collagenase activity in vitro. Increased collagenase activity can be expected to oppose collagen accumulation and development of fibrosis by promoting the breakdown of collagen. Increased collagenase activity was observed both in the absence and the presence of acetaldehyde, the metabolite of ethanol that has been incriminated in many of its effects (132). The specificity of the DLPC effect was illustrated by the fact that the other main component of the administered PC, namely PLPC, or other unsaturated or saturated PCs such as dioleoyl-PC, diarachidonoyl-PC, distearoyl-PC, dilauroyl-PC, or another polyunsaturated phospholipid (dilinoleoylphosphatidylethanolamine) or polyunsaturated free fatty acids (linoleic, arachidonic) had no effect on collagenase activity. A similar lack of effect had been shown earlier with dilauroyl-PC (131). Choline was inactive in vitro and found to be ineffective in vivo (see above). Taken together, these findings suggest that DLPC is responsible, at least in part, for the protection afforded by PPC against development of fibrosis and its ultimate stage of cirrhosis, most likely because of stimulation of collagen breakdown. Collagenase activity generally increases during the early stage of liver injury (133). Our previous studies revealed that fibrosis coincides with the stage at which collagen breakdown slackens and stops keeping pace with increased production (134). Thus these findings suggest that studies on collagenase activity associated with hepatic injury may be relevant to elucidation of the pathogenesis of liver fibrosis and its treatment and prevention.

PPC could of course also act in other ways. Phospholipids rich in essential fatty acids have a high bioavailability. More than 50% of orally administered PC is made biologically available either by intact absorption (lesser extent) or by reacylation of absorbed lysophosphatidylcholine (greater extent) (135). Pharmacokinetic studies in man, using $^3H/^{14}C$-labeled phosphatidylcholine, showed the absorption to exceed 90% (136). Similar observations were made in animals (137–139). Indeed, although much of the PC in the diet is degraded by pancreatic phospholipase A2 (140), the products (*l*-acyl-lysophosphatidylcholine and fatty acids) are absorbed in the jejunum (141). Animal studies show that PCs recovered in intestinal lymph after feeding fat enriched with single fatty acids are highly enriched in both *sn*-1 and *sn*-2 positions with the same acyl groups that were fed (142). Thus, it can be anticipated that during absorption of a diet enriched with 18:2 fatty acids, new PCs will be formed from dietary 18:2-lysoPC that will have an 18:2-18:2 composition. Various authors (123, 143, 144) reported PC accumulation in the liver during the first 24 to 48 h after administration. Furthermore, all 18:2 PCs were present in the liver in significantly increased amounts in baboons fed 18:2-18:2PC (117).

PC has been used before empirically in nonalcoholic liver diseases; beneficial histologic effects were reported in recovery from kwashiorkor (145), in HBsAG-positive patients with cirrhosis (146), and in inflammatory parameters in patients with chronic active hepatitis (147). PC was also used for treatment of alcoholic hepatitis (147) and alcoholic fatty liver (148), but not as yet for prevention or treatment of hepatic fibrosis or cirrhosis. In view of the lack of toxicity of PC (demonstrated in its use for these other indications) and its effectiveness in prevention of alcoholic fibrosis and cirrhosis in the baboon (demonstrated with a virtually pure PC preparation [63] and a less pure extract before [121]), PC or, if possible DLPC, both natural compounds, should now be tried for the control of alcoholic fibrosis and cirrhosis in humans. Since DLPC promotes breakdown of collagen, there is a reasonable hope that this treatment may not only affect the progression of the disease but may also reverse preexisting fibrosis, as demonstrated for CCl_4-induced cirrhosis in the rat (149). For the same reason, it may be useful for the management of fibrosis of nonalcoholic etiologies as well. Indeed, fibrosis is a common end stage for most chronic liver diseases.

Vitamins

Fat-Soluble Vitamins

Poor dietary intake, together with changes in bile salt metabolism and pancreatic function, increases the likelihood of fat-soluble vitamin deficiency in patients with both alcoholic and nonalcoholic cirrhosis.

Vitamin A. It is recommended that the diet of the nonalcoholic with cirrhosis be supplemented with 5000 to 15,000 IU vitamin A. In patients with alcoholic cirrhosis, caution must be exercised in this respect because microsomal induction may increase the toxicity of this vitamin (150, 151) (see Chapter 94), and ethanol can potentiate liver damage caused by excessive vitamin A (152). Although β-carotene, the precursor of vitamin A, is less toxic, studies in primates have shown that its toxic effects are also enhanced by alcohol (153). Furthermore, β-carotene increases the risk of pulmonary cancer in smokers (154), an effect related to a concomitant consumption of alcohol (155, 156). Thus, vitamin A or β-carotene supplementation must be used cautiously in alcoholics.

Vitamin D. Supplementation of the diet with vitamin D may fail to halt the progression of osteoporosis and osteopenia. However, there appears to be no hazard in recommending ingestion of additional 25-OH D_3 (100 to 300 nmol [40–120 μg]/day) when patients complain of bone pain or demonstrate pathologic fractures (157).

Vitamin E. In children with biliary atresia and cholestasis, vitamin E deficiency may be associated with a number of neurologic alterations. Although such infants and children may benefit from supplementation, repletion of vitamin E stores in adults with liver injury has no proven clinical benefit. Actually, in patients with liver disease of various etiologies, hepatic vitamin E concentrations were rather normal except in the presence of cirrhosis, alcoholic and nonalcoholic (Fig 73.5).

Vitamin K. Deficiency of vitamin K leads to easy bruisability and, at times, to overt bleeding from esophageal varices or hemorrhoids. When the prothrombin time is lengthened, parenteral supplementation of vitamin K (10 mg/day for 3 days) will serve to discriminate between vitamin K deficiency and failure of the liver to synthesize normal coagulation factors; after vitamin K, an abnormal prothrombin time is corrected in the former setting but not in the latter.

Water-Soluble Vitamins and Trace Minerals

Deficiencies of water-soluble vitamins (folic acid, thiamin, and pyridoxine) are most likely to occur in the malnourished alcoholic with advanced liver injury. Patients with Wilson's disease and those with chronic cholestasis (e.g., primary biliary cirrhosis) have excessive copper accumulation in the liver (158). Although chelation of copper by penicillamine is highly effective, it is also advantageous to reduce the intake of foods rich in this mineral. Foods rich in copper include chocolate, shellfish, and liver. Zinc deficiency occurs in alcoholics with liver injury and is discussed in Chapter 74.

EFFECT OF NUTRITION ON THE LIVER

At least in children, protein deficiency (kwashiorkor) is associated with development of fatty liver (159, 160). Studies performed during and after World War II indicated that severe malnutrition could also lead to liver injury in adults (161). These studies did not convincingly prove that malnutrition per se caused liver injury. Indeed, a number of other factors, including hepatotoxins (e.g., aflatoxin) and parasites (schistosomiasis) prevalent in war-ravaged or underdeveloped countries may have mediated

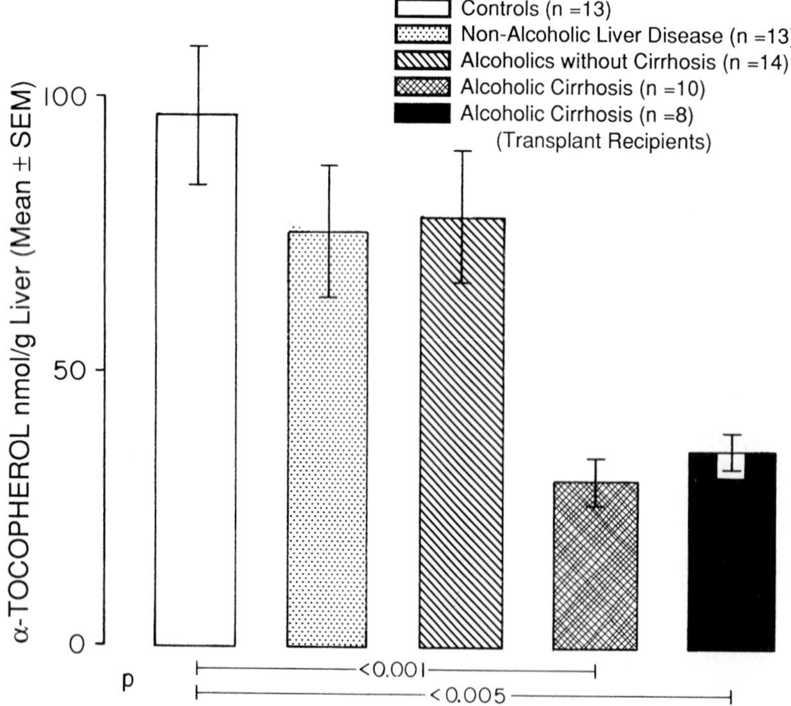

Figure 73.5. Effects of various liver diseases on total hepatic tocopherol levels. Only the cirrhotic groups had significantly lower α-tocopherol levels (168).

the relationship between liver injury and poor nutrition (162).

Because malnutrition is also common in alcoholics, these early findings were used to bolster the argument that malnutrition, rather than alcohol per se, could explain the pathogenesis of alcohol-induced liver injury. Over the past three decades, however, a more balanced view has evolved. Studies in humans, subhuman primates, and rodents have established that alcohol can cause liver damage in the absence of dietary deficits. Epidemiologic data also support this revised concept. In both France and Germany, a close correlation exists between per capita alcohol consumption and the likelihood of cirrhosis (163, 164). Moreover, no relationship has been documented between nutritional status and the severity of alcohol-induced liver injury as defined histologically (165). The above notwithstanding, it is now becoming clear that nutrition and the toxic effects of alcohol are often intertwined at the biochemical level. For example, by inducing microsomal cytochromes, chronic ethanol consumption results in energy wastage and promotes breakdown of nutrients, including retinol (28, 30, 152).

REFERENCES

1. Borgström B, Erlanson C. Gastroenterology 1978;75:382–6.
2. Borgström B, Erlanson-Albertsson C, Wielock F. J Lipid Res 1979;20:805–16.
3. Westergaard H, Dietschy JM. J Clin Invest 1976;58:97–108.
4. Lock L, Weiner IM. Fed Proc 1963;22:1334–8.
5. Carey MC. The enterohepatic circulation. In: Arias IM, Popper H, Schacter D, Shafritz DA, eds. The liver: biology and pathobiology. New York: Raven Press, 1982;429–65.
6. McCullogh AJ, Mullen KD, Smanik EJ, et al. Gastroenterol Clin North Am 1989;18:619–43.
7. Mezey E. Liver and biliary system. In: Paige DM, ed. Clinical nutrition. 2nd ed. St. Louis: CV Mosby, 1988;186–97.
8. Vhlachevic ZR, Buhac I, Farrar JJ, et al. Gastroenterology 1971;60:491–8.
9. Rudman D, DiFulco TJ, Galambos JT, et al. J Clin Invest 1973;52:2242–9.
10. Mullen KD, Denne SC, McCullough AJ, et al. Hepatology 1986;6:622–30.
11. Swart GR, Van DenBerg JWO, Wahimena JLD, et al. Clin Sci 1988;75:101–7.
12. Gabuzda GJ, Shear L. Am J Clin Nutr 1970;23:479–84.
13. Collins JR, et al. Arch Intern Med 1970;126:608–14.
14. Conn HO. Am J Med 1970;299:394–404.
15. Owen OE, Trapp VE, Reichard GA. J Clin Invest 1983;72: 1821–32.
16. Merli M, Riggio O, Romiti A, et al. Hepatology 1990;12:106–12.
17. Schneeweiss B, Graninger W, Ferenci P, et al. Hepatology 1990;11:387–93.
18. Jhongiani SS, Nanakram A, Holmes R, et al. Am J Clin Nutr 1986;44:323–9.
19. Shanbhogue RLK, Bistrian BR, Jenkins RL, et al. JPEN J Parenter Enteral Nutr1987;11:305–8.
20. Heymsfield SB, Waki M, Reinus J. Hepatology 1990;11:502–4.
21. Fennelly J, Frank O, Baker H, et al. Am J Clin Nutr 1967;20: 946–9.
22. Russell RM, Morrison SA, Smith FR, et al. Ann Intern Med 1978;88:622–6.
23. Mitchell D, Wagner C, Stone WJ, et al. Gastroenterology 1976; 71:1043–9.
24. Skinner RK, Sherlock S, Long RG, et al. Lancet 1977;1:720–1.
25. Leo MA, Lieber CS. N Engl J Med 1982;307:597–601.
26. Leo MA, Kim CI, Lowe N. Am J Clin Nutr 1984;40:1131–6.
27. Borowsky SA, Perlow W, Baraona E, et al. Dig Dis Sci 1980;25:22–7.
28. Sato M, Lieber CS. Arch Biochem Biophys 1982;213:557–64.
29. Leo MA, Lieber CS. J Biol Chem 1985;260:5228–31.
30. Leo MA, Lieber CS. J Nutr 1987;117:70–6.
31. Nasrallah SM, Galambos JT. Lancet 1980;2:1276–7.
32. Smith J, Horowitz J, Henderson JM, et al. Am J Clin Nutr 1982;35:56–72.
33. Calvey J, Davis M, Williams RJ. Hepatology 1985;1:141–51.
34. Diehl AM, Boitnott JK, Herlong HF, et al. Hepatology 1985;5:57–63.
35. Naveau S, Pelletier G, Poynard T, et al. Hepatology 1986;6:270–4.
36. Achord JL. Am J Gastroenterol 1987;82:871–5.
37. Simon D, Galambos JT. J Hepatol 1988;7:200–7.
38. Greenberger NJ, Carley J, Schenker S, et al. Dig Dis Sci 1977;22:845–55.
39. Shaw S, Worner TM, Lieber CS. Am J Clin Nutr 1983;38: 59–63.
40. Rocchi E. Casaanelli M, Gilbertini P, et al. JPEN J Parenter Enteral Nutr 1981;9:447–51.
41. Okundo M, Nagayama M, Takai T. J Surg Res 1985;39:93–102.
42. Mendenhall C, Bongiovanni G, Goldberg S, et al. JPEN J Parenter Enteral Nutr 1985;9:590–6.
43. Kaneinatsu T, Koyanagi N, Matsumata T, et al. Surgery 1988; 104:482–8.
44. Fischer JE, Baldersarini RJ. Lancet 1971;2:75–80.
45. Fischer JE, Yoshimura N, Aguirre A, et al. Am J Surg 1974; 127:40–7.
46. Naylor CD, O'Rourke K, Detsky AS, et al. Gastroenterology 1989;97:1033–42.
47. Vilstrup H, Gluud C, Hardt F, et al. J Hepatol 1990;10:291–6.
48. Horst D, Grace ND, Conn HO, et al. Hepatology 1984;4: 279–87.
49. Uribe M, Marquez MA, Ramos GG, et al. Dig Dis Sci 1982; 27:1109–16.
50. Weber FL, Minco D, Fresard KM, et al. Gastroenterology 1985:89:538–44.
51. Brusilow SW. J Clin Invest 1984;74:2144–8.
52. Lindblad B. Proc Natl Acad Sci USA 1977;74:4641–5.
53. Best CH, Hartroft WS, Lucas CC, et al. Br Med J 1949;2: 1001–6.
54. Klatskin G, Hrehl WA, Conn HO. J Exp Med 1954;100: 605–14.
55. Thompson JA, Reitz RC. Ann NY Acad Sci 1976;273:194–204.
56. Hoffbauer FW, Zaki FG. Arch Pathol 1965;79:364–9.
57. Lieber CS, Teschke R, Hasumura Y, DeCarli LM. Fed Proc 1975;34:2060–74.
58. Phillips GB, Davidson CS. Arch Intern Med 1954;94:585–603.
59. Post JJ, Benton B, Breakstone R, Hoffman J. Gastroenterology 1952;20:403–10.
60. Volwiler W, Jones CM, Mallory TB. Gastroenterology 1948;11: 164–82.
61. Chawla RK, Wolf DC, Kutner MH, et al. Gastroenterology 1989;97:1514–20.
62. Lieber CS, DeCarli LM. J Med Primatol 1974;3:153–63.
63. Lieber CS, Robins SJ, Leo MA. Alcoholism Clin Exp Res 1994; 18:592–5.
64. Arai M, Leo MA, Nakano M, et al. Hepatology 1984; 4:165–74.
65. Foy H, Kondi A, Mbaya V. Br J Nutr 1964;18:307–18.

66. Lieber CS, Leo MA, Mak KM, et al. Hepatology 1985;5:561–72.
67. Finkelstein JD, Martin JJ. J Biol Chem 1986;261:1582–7.
68. Hardwick DF, Applegarth DA, Cockcroft DM, et al. Metabolism 1970;19:381–91.
69. Iob V, Coon WW, Sloan M. J Surg Res 1967;7:41–3.
70. Iber FL, Rosen H, Stanley MA, et al. J Lab Clin Med 1957;50:417–25.
71. Montanari A, Simoni I, Vallisa D, et al. Hepatology 1988;8:1034–9.
72. Kinsell L, Harper HA, Barton HC, et al. Science 1947;106:589–94.
73. Horowitz JH, Rypins EB, Henderson JM, et al. Gastroenterology 1981;81:668–75.
74. Duce AM, Ortiz P, Cabrero C, et al. Hepatology 1988;8:65–8.
75. Finkelstein JD, Cello JP, Kyle WE. Biochim Biophy Res Commun 1974;61:475–81.
76. Lieber CS, Casini A, DeCarli LM, et al. Hepatology 1990;11:165–72.
77. Feo F, Pascale R, Garcea R, et al. Toxicol Appl Pharmacol 1986;83:331–41.
78. Speisky H, MacDonald A, Giles G, et al. Biochem J 1985;225:565.
79. Lieber CS. Pharmacol Biochem Behav 1980;13:17–30.
80. Shaw S, Lieber CS. Gastroenterology 1978;74:677–82.
81. Hirata F, Viveros OH, Diliberto EJ Jr, et al. Proc Natl Acad Sci USA 1978;75:1718–21.
82. Hirata F, Axelrod J. Science 1980;209:1082–90.
83. Yamada S, Mak KM, Lieber CS. Gastroenterology 1985;88:1799–1806.
84. Shaw S, Jayatilleke E, Ross WA, et al. J Lab Clin Med 1981;98:417–25.
85. Barak AJ, Beckenhauer HC, Tuma DJ, et al. IRCS Med Sci Biochem 1984;12:866–7.
86. Stramentinoli G, Gualano M, Galli-Kienle M. J Pharmacol Exp Ther 1979;209:323–6.
87. Bombardieri G, Pappalardo G, Bernardi L, et al. Int J Clin Pharmacol Ther Toxicol 1983;21:186–8.
88. Hoffman DR, Marion DW, Cornatzer WE, et al. J Biol Chem 1980;10:822–7.
89. Travers J, Varela I, Mato JM. Biochem Pharmacol 1984;33:1562–4.
90. Pezzoli C, Stramentinoli G, Galli-Kienele M, et al. Biochem Biophys Res Commun 1978;85:1031–8.
91. Engstrom MA, Benevenga NJ. J Nutr 1987;117:1820–6.
92. Zappia V, Galletti P, Porcelli M. FEBS Lett 1978;90:331–5.
93. Audubert F, Vance D. J Biol Chem 1983;258:10695–701.
94. Quiram DR, Weinshilboum RM. J Neurochem 1976;27:1197–203.
95. Giulidori P, Stramentinoli G. Anal Biochem 1984;137:217–20.
96. Osman E, Owen JS, Burroughs AK. Aliment Pharmacol Ther 1993;7:21–8.
97. Belli DC, Fournier LA, Lepage G, et al. J Hepatol 1994;21;18–23.
98. Angelico M, Gandin C, Nistri A, et al. Scand J Clin Invest 1994;54:459–64
99. Vendemiale G, Altomare E, Trizio T, et al. Scand J Gastroenterol 1989;24:407–15.
100. Loguercio C, Nardi G, Argenzio F, et al. Alcohol Alcohol 1994;29:597–604.
101. Marchesini G, Bugianesi E, Bianchi G, et al. Clin Nutr 1992;11:303–8.
102. Muriel P. J Appl Toxicol 1993;13:179–82.
103. Muriel P, Suarez OR, Gonzalez P, et al. J Hepatol 1994;21:95–102.
104. Corrales F, Giménez A, Alvarez L, et al. Hepatology 1992;16:1022–7.
105. Cutrin C, Meniño MJ, Otero X, et al. Life Sci 1992;51:113–8.
106. Barak A, Beckenhauer HC, Junnila M, et al. Alcohol Clin Exp Res 1993;17:552–5.
107. Hultberg B, Berglund M, Andersson A, et al. Alcohol Clin Exp Res 1993;17:687–9.
108. Stampfer MJ, Malinow MR, Willett WC. JAMA 1992;268:877–81.
109. Holliday R. Science 1987;283:163–70.
110. Nyce J, Weinhouse S, Magee PN. Br J Cancer 1983;48:463–75.
111. Hoffman RM. Biochim Biophys Acta 1984;738:49–87.
112. Giovannucci E, Stampfer MJ, Colditz GA, et al. J Natl Cancer Inst 1993;85:875–84.
113. Koehn V, Burnand B, Niquille M. JPEN J Parenter Enteral Nutr 1993;17:35–40.
114. Hirsch S, Bunout D, de la Maza P, et al. JPEN J Parenter Enteral Nutr 1993;17:119–24.
115. Lieber CS. Am J Clin Nutr 1993;58:430–442.
116. Greene HL, Slonim AF, O'Neill JA, et al. N Engl J Med 1976;294:423–5.
117. Lieber CS, Robins S, Li J, et al. Gastroenterology 1994;106:152–159.
118. Arai M, Gordon ER, Lieber CS. Biochim Biophys Acta 1984;797:320–7.
119. Hoek JB, Thomas AP, Rooney TA, et al. FASEB J 1992;6:2386–96.
120. Lieber CS, Leo MA, Aleynik SI, et al. Alcoholism Clin Exp Res 1997;21:375–379.
121. Lieber CS, DeCarli LM, Mak KM, et al. Hepatology 1990;12:1390–98.
122. Nanji AA, French SW. Life Sci 1989;44:223–27.
123. Lekim D, Graf E. Arzneimittelforschung 1976;26:1772–82.
124. Mak KM, Lieber CS. Hepatology 1988;8:1027–33.
125. Mak KM, Leo MA, Lieber CS. Gastroenterology 1984;87:188–200.
126. Moshage H, Casini A, Lieber CS. Hepatology 1990;12:511–18.
127. Casini A, Cunningham M, Rojkind M, et al. Hepatology 1991;13:758–65.
128. Savolainen E-R, Leo MA, Timple R, Lieber CS. Gastroenterology 1984;87:777–87.
129. Nakano M, Lieber CS. Am J Pathol 1982;106:145–55.
130. Takase S, Leo MA, Nouchi T, et al. J Hepatol 1988;6:267–76.
131. Li J-J, Kim C-I, Leo MA, et al. Hepatology 1992;15:373–81.
132. Lieber CS. Medical and nutritional complications of alcoholism: mechanisms and management, New York: Plenum Press, 1992;579.
133. Maruyama K, Feinman L, Okazaki I, et al. Biochim Biophys Acta 1981;658:124–31.
134. Maruyama K, Feinman L, Fainako M, et al. Life Sci 1982;30:1379–84.
135. Fox JM. Polyene phosphatidylcholine: pharmacokinetics after oral administration—a review. In: Avogaro P, Macini M, Ricci G, Paoletti R, eds. Phospholipids and atherosclerosis. New York: Raven Press, 1983.
136. Zierenberg O, Grundy SM. J Lipid Res 1982;23:1136–42.
137. Parthasarathy S, Subbaiah PV, Ganguly J. Biochem J 1974;140:503–8.
138. Rodgers JB, O'Brien RJ, Balint JA. Am J Dig Dis 1975;20:208–11.
139. Lekim D, Betzing H. Drug Res 1974;24:1217–21.
140. Arnesjö B, Nilsson Å, Barrowman J. Scand J Gastroenterol 1969;4:653–65.
141. Nilsson AKE. Biochim Biophys Acta 1968;152:379–90.
142. Patton GM, Clark SB, Fasulo JM, et al. J Clin Invest 1984;73:231–40.

143. Holz J, Wagner H. Z Naturforsch 1971;26:1151–8.
144. Lekim D, Betzing H, Stoffel W. Hoppe-Seyler's Z Physiol Chem 1972;353S:929–46.
145. Alliet J, Comlan G, Gourdier D. Ouest Med 1976;29:85–104.
146. Fassati P, Horejsi J, Fassati M, et al. Cas Lek Cesk 1981;120: 56–60.
147. Bird GLA, Panos MZ, Polson R, et al. Z Gastroenterol 1991;(Suppl 2)29:21–4.
148. Schüller-Pérez A, González-San Martin F. Med Welt 1985;36:517–21.
149. Ma X, Zhao J, Lieber CS. J Hepatol 1996;24:604–13.
150. Leo MA, Arai M, Sato M, et al. Gastroenterology 1982;82: 194–205.
151. Leo MA, Sato M, Lieber CS. Gastroenterology 1983;84: 562–72.
152. Leo MA, Lieber CS. Hepatology 1988;8:412–7.
153. Leo MA, Kim CI, Lowe N, et al. Hepatology 1992;15:883–91.
154. The Alpha Tocopherol–Beta Carotene Cancer Prevention Study Group. N Engl J Med 1994;330:1029–35.
155. Albanese D, Heinonen OP, Taylor PR, et al. J Natl Cancer Inst, 1996;88:1560–71.
156. Omenn GS, Goodman GE, Thornquist MD, et al. J Natl Cancer Inst, 1996;88:1550–9.
157. Long RG, Meinhard E, Skinner RK, et al. Gut 1978;19:85–90.
158. Gibbs K, Walshe JM. Clin Sci 1971;41:189–202.
159. Cook GC, Hutt MS. Br Med J 1967;3:454–7.
160. Ramalingswami V. Nature 1964;201:546–51.
161. Snapper I. Chinese lessons to western medicine. 2nd ed. New York: Grune & Stratton, 1965.
162. Conn HO, Atterbury CE. Cirrhosis. In: Schiff L, Schiff ER, eds. Diseases of the liver. Philadelphia: JB Lippincott, 1987;725–864.
163. Pequignot G, Chabert C, Eydowx H, et al. Rev Alcohol 1974;20:191–202.
164. Lelbach WK. Ann NY Acad Sci 1975;252:85–105.
165. Mills PR, Shankin A, Anthony RS, et al. Am J Clin Nutr 1983;38:849–59.
166. Lieber CS. Dig Dis 1997;15:42–66.
167. Lieber CS, DeCarli LM. Am J Clin Nutr 1970;4:474–8.
168. Leo MA, Rosman AS, Lieber CS. Hepatology 1993;6:977–86.
169. Lieber CS, DeCarli LM, Rubin E. Proc Natl Acad Sci USA 1975;72:437–41.
170. Popper H, Lieber CS. Am J Pathol 1980;98:695–716.

74. Nutrient and Genetic Regulation of Lipoprotein Metabolism

CLAY F. SEMENKOVICH

Lipoproteins are important in the pathogenesis of vascular disease. Production and removal of circulating lipoproteins are dynamic processes affected by many variables, two of which are nutrient intake and the genetic composition of an individual.

Nutrients transported into the cell can have direct effects by altering expression of a protein such as apolipoprotein B (apo B) critical for lipoprotein assembly. Effects can also be indirect, as when nutrients increase expression of other factors (e.g., insulin) not intrinsic to lipoproteins but critical for their metabolism. Genetic effects can also be complicated. Mutations (changes in the DNA sequence encoding a protein that alter expression of that protein) can result in a loss of function, a gain of function, or a dominant negative effect. The latter occurs when a protein has more than one subunit and a mutation in a single subunit dominantly interferes with the function of other nonmutated subunits. Inherited diseases may not be due to mutations in the gene for the protein affecting the phenotype; instead, the defect can reside in other genes controlling expression of the protein of interest (see abetalipoproteinemia below).

Regulated expression of genes involved in lipoprotein metabolism is necessary for survival. This regulation can occur at many levels (Fig. 74.1). However, for a particular gene and its protein product, there are one or two predominant levels of regulation. Typically, regulation can be classified as transcriptional, posttranscriptional, translational, or posttranslational. Figure 74.1 illustrates that genes, consisting of DNA, are transcribed to produce nuclear RNA that is processed to new messenger RNA (mRNA). Transcription can be affected by nutrients. For example, cholesterol decreases expression of the low-density lipoprotein receptor by suppressing transcription of its gene (see below), and transcription of the fatty acid synthase gene is blocked by essential amino acid deficiency (1) and polyunsaturated fatty acids (2). Regulation of gene expression can be posttranscriptional. One such mechanism is the regulation of mRNA stability; a stable message will be translated more times, forming more protein, than an unstable one. Nutrients can alter message stability. The nutrient iron regulates transferrin receptor expression by altering the stability of the transferrin receptor message; glucose increases fatty acid synthesis in part by stabilizing the fatty acid synthase mRNA (3).

Gene expression can be regulated at the level of translation. In this process, preexisting cytoplasmic mRNA becomes associated with ribosomes that synthesize the protein encoded by the mRNA. For example, iron regulates ferritin gene expression by a translational mechanism. Finally, genes can be regulated posttranslationally. The stability of preexisting proteins can be altered by nutrients. For example, cholesterol regulates HMG-CoA reductase expression by controlling the stability of the HMG-CoA reductase protein; dietary fats stabilize the apo B protein (see below). Posttranslational mechanisms are not limited to protein stability. Some proteins require posttranslational modifications for normal function. These modifications include glycosylation, the addition of sugars to peptides (see lipoprotein lipase below), and fatty acid acylation (see Chapter 25).

This chapter focuses on nutrient and genetic regulation of the expression of genes involved in lipoprotein synthesis and catabolism. The discussion illustrates several mechanisms of regulation, some of which are applicable to the regulation of numerous genes, and others, such as apo B editing, that are relatively unique.

APOLIPOPROTEIN B (APOB)

Apo B Expression

Apo B is the major protein of chylomicrons, chylomicron remnants, very low density lipoproteins (VLDL),

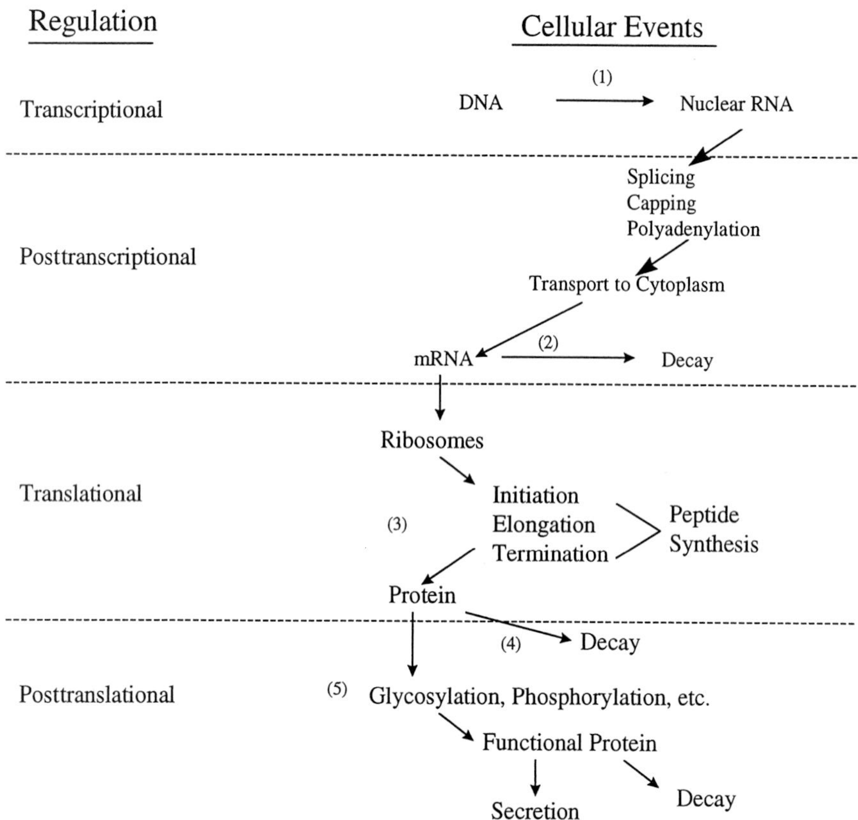

Figure 74.1. Regulation of gene expression. Major levels of regulation of gene expression are shown on the *left,* and corresponding cellular events are schematically depicted on the *right.* Transcriptional regulation is associated with recruitment of transcription factors to specific elements in the promoters of genes in response to nutrients, etc. These transcription factors affect production of new nuclear RNA by the enzyme RNA polymerase II at step 1. Expression of the LDL receptor is regulated at the transcriptional level. Posttranscriptional regulation can occur through changes in the processing (splicing, capping, and polyadenylation) of nuclear RNA and its transport to the cytoplasm as mRNA. Once in the cytoplasm, factors can affect mRNA stability; alteration of mRNA stability is another form of posttranscriptional regulation. Expression of the enzyme fatty acid synthase is regulated in part by controlling the rate of decay of its mRNA in the cytoplasm (step 2). Translational regulation involves the efficiency with which mRNA is translated into a peptide. Ferritin expression is regulated at this level (step 3) by the nutrient iron. Posttranslational regulation involves events following peptide synthesis. Such regulation can include control of the rate at which a newly synthesized peptide decays (step 4). Apo B expression is regulated at this level (Fig. 74.2). Posttranslational events can also include modifications to proteins, such as glycosylation (step 5). Lipoprotein lipase expression is regulated in part at posttranslational levels by nutrients.

intermediate-density lipoproteins (IDL), and low-density lipoproteins (LDL). In general, apo B–containing lipoproteins are associated with increased atherosclerotic risk. Therefore, lowering apo B levels is desirable. The protein exists in two forms, apo B100 (4536 amino acids) and apo B48 (2152 amino acids), so named because it is 48% of the size of apo B100. The two forms are derived from the same gene through editing of the apo B mRNA (see below). In humans, apo B100 is made only in the liver and apo B48 only in the small intestine. Human VLDL, IDL, and LDL contain B100, while human chylomicrons and their remnants contain B48. In other species, including rodents and dogs, both B100 and B48 are made in the liver (4).

Regulation of apo B expression occurs posttranslationally, i.e., after the protein is made (Fig. 74.2). Apo B gene transcription and mRNA translation appear to be constitutive; apo B protein is made continuously. If sufficient lipid associates with apo B at the appropriate intracellular location, the protein is stabilized, and VLDL particles (in the liver) or chylomicrons (in the intestine) are assembled around the scaffolding provided by apo B and secreted. Without sufficient lipid, the apo B protein is degraded. The exact lipid required to stabilize apo B and promote the maturation of nascent lipoproteins is uncertain; experimental evidence supports the role of both triglycerides (5) and cholesteryl esters (6). Excessive secretion of apo B–containing lipoproteins mediated by this mechanism likely contributes to human hyperlipidemia associated with excessive intake of dietary fat and cholesterol. These nutrients also affect LDL receptor expression (see below).

Apo B Editing

Apo B editing is a posttranscriptional event. As noted above, a single gene encodes apo B100 and apo B48. The apo B gene is transcribed into a single mRNA. In humans, this mRNA is modified only in the intestine, and the specificity of this modification is remarkable. Of the more than 14,000 nucleotide bases in the apo B mRNA sequence, only the cytidine at position 6666 is edited to uridine,

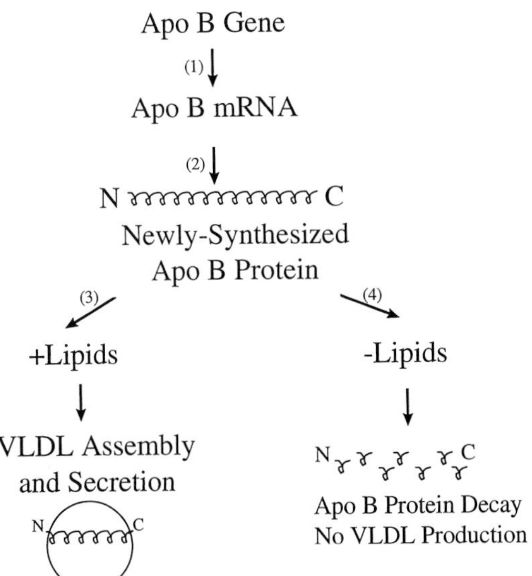

Figure 74.2. Posttranslational regulation of apo B gene expression in the liver. Apo B is a critical component of several lipoproteins. Its regulation is predominantly posttranslational. Transcription (step 1) and translation (step 2) for apo B are thought to be constitutive. These processes yield newly synthesized apo B protein with its amino terminus (indicated by "N") and carboxyl terminus ("C") connected by a *twisted line* representing the complex secondary structure of the protein. Dietary lipids are catabolized for absorption and eventually reach the hepatocyte. Triglycerides and cholesteryl ester are then resynthesized in the liver cell. When these lipids are available (step 3), they are transferred to apo B by microsomal transfer protein (MTP). The association of lipids with the apo B protein stabilizes the protein so it can be used for the assembly of VLDL, which is eventually secreted into the circulation. Absence of MTP produces the clinical disorder abetalipoproteinemia. Without new lipid (step 4), apo B protein is degraded, which prevents VLDL production.

resulting in the conversion of the glutamine codon CAA to the stop codon UAA (7). When this message associates with ribosomes, instead of placing a glutamine residue at this position and continuing with translation (as for apo B100), the translational complex stops synthesizing protein, yielding apo B48, 48% the size of apo B100.

A multisubunit enzyme edits apo B mRNA. The catalytic subunit is a zinc-dependent cytidine deaminase called apobec-1 (8). Inactivation of this subunit by genetic techniques in mice abolishes apo B mRNA editing (9). Editing is regulated by fasting and refeeding a high-carbohydrate diet in rats (10). Zinc is known to affect lipid metabolism, and apobec-1 is zinc-dependent, but zinc deficiency in rodents does not affect apo B editing (11).

Apo B100 is essentially the only protein in LDL, a critical lipoprotein in the development of atherosclerosis. Theoretically, it should be possible to decrease apo B100 levels (through metabolism to apo B48) in humans by supplying the liver with the editing enzyme via gene therapy. However, one group has reported that transgenic mice and rabbits expressing apobec-1 in liver develop hepatocellular carcinoma, perhaps because of editing of other messages involved in cell growth (12).

Abetalipoproteinemia and Microsomal Transfer Protein

Abetalipoproteinemia is a rare, autosomal recessive disorder characterized by absence of apo B in the plasma (see Chapter 70). Triglyceride and cholesterol levels are extremely low, even after ingestion of dietary fat. Chylomicrons, VLDL, and LDL are absent (see Chapter 75). Patients usually present with symptoms of fat malabsorption and, if untreated, develop debilitating neurologic dysfunction leading to death. Other complications include retinopathy, which progresses to blindness, and hematologic problems including anemia and coagulation defects. Clinical features of the disease are related to the inability to secrete apo B–containing lipoproteins. Because of this defect, patients are probably unable to deliver essential fatty acids to critical tissues and definitely unable to transport certain fat-soluble vitamins. Of the fat-soluble vitamins A, D, E, and K, vitamin E is the most severely affected in abetalipoproteinemia; high-dose supplementation with vitamin E may prevent clinical sequelae (13).

Surprisingly, defects in the apo B gene are not responsible for abetalipoproteinemia. Instead, the defect is probably exclusively associated with mutations in a protein essential for secretion of apo B–containing proteins, microsomal transfer protein (MTP) (14). The active MTP complex consists of two subunits, MTP itself and protein disulfide isomerase (PDI), an endoplasmic reticulum protein with several catalytic activities. This complex transfers triglycerides and cholesteryl esters from their site of synthesis to apo B, thereby preventing apo B degradation and facilitating lipoprotein assembly. Several MTP mutations have been described, and their characterization suggests that the carboxyl terminus of MTP is essential for lipid transfer activity (15).

Within 24 hours of high-fat feeding, MTP gene expression is stimulated in the intestine but not in the liver. Expression in the liver increases with longer-term dietary interventions (20). There is considerable interest in development of pharmacologic inhibitors of MTP activity; such agents would be expected to lower circulating lipids by interfering with the assembly of VLDL (in liver) and chylomicrons (in the intestine).

Hypobetalipoproteinemia

Unlike abetalipoproteinemia, hypobetalipoproteinemia is not usually associated with clinical manifestations. Patients have low LDL cholesterol levels (<90 mg/dL [2.33 mmol/L], roughly the fifth percentile for Western populations) but not absent concentrations of apo B lipoproteins. Although not well studied, these individuals may be at lower risk for cardiovascular disease. The causes of most cases of hypobetalipoproteinemia are unknown, but some are familial and inherited in an autosomal dominant fashion (17). A significant proportion of these families carry mutations encoding truncated forms of apo B.

Several apo B truncations have been described, ranging

from apo B2 (2% of the size of apo B100) to apo B89. The molecular bases for these truncations are diverse and include nonsense mutations (producing premature stop codons), frameshift mutations, and deletions. The production rate of these truncations is related to their size (i.e., very short apo B proteins are produced at very low rates). Most subjects are heterozygotes; they carry a truncated allele as well as a normal apo B100 allele. For unknown reasons, the rate of apo B100 production is much lower than expected in these heterozygotes.

Individuals with heterozygous familial hypobetalipoproteinemia do not malabsorb fat and are clinically normal. Patients carrying two alleles for apo B truncations can resemble those with abetalipoproteinemia.

Familial Defective Apo B and Other Variants

Apo B100 on LDL particles is a ligand for the LDL receptor. Substitution of glutamine for arginine at amino acid residue 3500 of the apo B100 protein interferes with the normal interaction of apo B with the LDL receptor, resulting in reduced clearance and hypercholesterolemia. This mutation, called familial defective apo B, is fairly common, with a frequency of 1:500 to 1:700 in the general population. These patients appear to respond appropriately (18) to dietary and pharmacologic therapies for hyperlipidemia (see Chapter 75).

There are several additional variants of the apo B gene, some of which appear to predict serum lipid responses to a high-fat diet (19). However, the exact regions of the gene responsible for these effects are unknown.

LIPOPROTEIN LIPASE (LPL)

Lipid Metabolism

The enzyme LPL is bound to proteoglycans on the capillary endothelium of essentially all adult tissues except the liver. This binding is disrupted by heparin, an agent commonly used to release LPL into the circulation to assess whole body stores of LPL enzyme activity. The greatest mass of LPL is found in adipose tissue, cardiac muscle, and skeletal muscle (20), and in the mammary glands during lactation. Free fatty acids produced after hydrolysis of triglycerides by LPL are taken up by adipose tissue for storage or by muscle for oxidation.

LPL hydrolyzes triglycerides in VLDL and chylomicrons, yielding the smaller, denser IDL and chylomicron remnants, respectively. During this process, excess lipoprotein surface components are released to form HDL particles. Thus, LPL is thought to be crucial for normal lipoprotein physiology. The recent inactivation of the LPL gene in mice (21) supports this concept; in the absence of LPL, triglyceride-rich lipoproteins accumulate in high concentrations since they cannot be metabolized, and HDL particles are not generated.

LPL Expression

High-fat intake increases heparin-releasable LPL activity in humans (22), but diet has complex, tissue-specific effects on LPL expression. In general, eating a mixed meal induces adipose tissue and suppresses skeletal muscle LPL activity. The differential response between muscle and fat may be due to meal-associated stimulation of insulin. Insulin infusion in humans increases adipose tissue and decreases skeletal muscle LPL (23). LPL is important for partitioning energy stores. It may play a role in certain types of obesity by preferentially directing triglyceride-rich particles to fat instead of muscle (24).

In adipose tissue, regulation of LPL expression by both macronutrients and insulin is predominantly posttranslational (25–27). Stores of inactive LPL protein probably exist intracellularly and are activated by insulin or nutrients. Normal LPL is glycosylated (28); glycosylation may be responsible for the posttranslational regulation of LPL activity. LPL regulation may be pretranslational in muscle. Exercise increases human muscle LPL pretranslationally (20), and insulin suppresses LPL mRNA in human muscle (29).

LPL Mutations

Rare individuals homozygous for mutations in the LPL gene can present with the chylomicronemia syndrome (30). Triglyceride concentrations commonly exceed 2000 mg/dL (22.6 μmol/L) in fasting plasma and can be considerably higher. Affected subjects have abdominal pain, recurrent episodes of pancreatitis, eruptive xanthomas (caused by uptake of chylomicrons by macrophages in the skin), hepatomegaly, and neurologic dysfunction, including memory loss and the carpal tunnel syndrome. Patients usually present in early childhood with failure to thrive. Treatment includes a diet that restricts fat to 15% or less of daily caloric intake.

While homozygous LPL deficiency is rare, heterozygous LPL deficiency is fairly common in the general population (~1:35). Heterozygotes (carrying one normal and one mutant LPL allele) may have normal fasting lipid levels. However, considerable evidence links lipid levels in the postprandial state with development of atherosclerosis, and individuals with heterozygous LPL deficiency have higher concentrations of atherogenic lipoproteins after intake of a fatty meal (31). More than 40 different mutations have been described in the LPL gene; the frequency of just one, a serine for asparagine substitution at amino acid residue 291, was recently reported to be 5.2% in patients with premature atherosclerosis (32). These data suggest that heterozygous LPL deficiency may interact with a high-fat diet to increase the risk for cardiovascular disease.

LOW-DENSITY LIPOPROTEIN (LDL) RECEPTOR

Lipid Metabolism

The LDL receptor binds LDL, an atherogenic lipoprotein carrying cholesterol. When low levels of the receptor are present because of nutrient or genetic effects on its expression, LDL accumulates in plasma, and the risk for cardiac disease increases. The LDL receptor is not thought to be directly involved in the pathogenesis of atherosclerosis. Normal LDL particles do not induce the cellular changes of early atherosclerosis. Such changes require modified (e.g., by oxidation) LDL. Modified LDL binds to scavenger receptors but not to the LDL receptor. The LDL receptor is found on essentially all cells, but the most important tissue for its expression is the liver, where the vast majority of LDL-cholesterol metabolism takes place (33). Humans cannot degrade cholesterol. However, free cholesterol in the liver can be converted to bile acids, and the major route for cholesterol excretion is through bile.

Both dietary cholesterol and saturated fatty acids increase LDL cholesterol levels by decreasing LDL receptor activity. When dietary cholesterol is high, cholesterol stores in the liver increase. This sterol pool has numerous effects on cell physiology. ACAT (acyl-CoA:cholesterol acyltransferase), the enzyme that esterifies cholesterol for intracellular storage, is induced. HMG-CoA reductase, the rate-limiting enzyme for cholesterol synthesis, is suppressed. Most importantly, increased cholesterol signals the hepatocyte to suppress transcription of the LDL receptor gene. Fewer receptors are synthesized, less LDL is removed from the plasma, and circulating LDL levels increase. Dietary fatty acids may also suppress transcription of the LDL receptor gene (34).

LDL Receptor Expression

The LDL receptor is a glycosylated protein that, after translation, is directed to the cell membrane where it binds apo B–containing lipoproteins such as LDL. Upon binding, receptors migrate to specialized regions of the cell surface known as coated pits. Bound lipoproteins then undergo endocytosis and are transported to lysosomes where the cholesteryl esters of LDL are hydrolyzed to yield free cholesterol. The level of free cholesterol in this sterol pool regulates transcription of the LDL receptor gene.

Promoters are regions of genes usually closely associated with the DNA encoding the protein of interest. Within promoters are response elements, comprising DNA sequences that bind to specific proteins known as transcription factors. The levels of these factors can be influenced by nutrients, their metabolites, and by intracellular signals sent by hormones. Transcription factors bind to response elements, causing genes to be transcribed, ultimately producing new mRNA.

For the LDL receptor, the critical transcription factors are two structurally similar sterol regulatory element–binding proteins (SREBPs) called SREBP-1 and SREBP-2 (35, 36). These proteins reside in an inactive form in the cytoplasm, attached to the endoplasmic reticulum. When free cholesterol levels are low, a sterol-sensitive protease cleaves an SREBP, releasing a large fragment of the protein. This amino-terminal fragment (the active transcription factor) migrates to the cell nucleus, binds to sterol regulatory elements in the LDL receptor promoter, and stimulates transcription of the LDL receptor gene. When intracellular free cholesterol levels increase, cleavage of the SREBP ceases, and the nuclear SREBP fragment is rapidly degraded. In hamsters, SREBP-2 appears to be more important than SREBP-1 in responding to changes in cellular cholesterol levels (37).

Familial Hypercholesterolemia

Familial hypercholesterolemia (FH) is an autosomal dominant disorder caused by mutations in the gene for the LDL receptor. More than 150 different mutations responsible for the disease have been described (38), including promoter mutations preventing normal transcription of the gene.

Homozygous FH (characterized by two defective LDL receptor alleles) is rare but clinically striking. Patients have extreme elevations of fasting cholesterol, with total cholesterol levels of ~700 mg/dL (18.1 μmol/L) and mean LDL cholesterol levels of ~625 mg/dL (16.1 μmol/L). They also have xanthomas (caused by deposition of lipid in skin and tendons) and severe premature atherosclerosis. Myocardial infarction (MI) has been described at age 18 months in this disorder. The frequency of heterozygous FH ranges from 1:200 to 1:500 in most populations. About 5% of all individuals who have suffered a premature MI (defined as before age 55 in males and 65 in females) are FH heterozygotes. These individuals have one normal allele, which allows them to respond to pharmacologic and dietary interventions aimed at lowering LDL cholesterol by increasing LDL receptor expression. Such treatments are discussed in Chapter 75.

APOLIPOPROTEIN E (APO E)

Lipid Metabolism

Apo E, like apo B100, is a ligand for the LDL receptor. It is a prominent component of triglyceride-rich lipoproteins such as VLDL and chylomicrons, as well as HDL. Apo E is necessary for normal clearance of triglyceride-rich lipoproteins from the circulation through its interaction with both the LDL receptor and another receptor, the LDL receptor–related protein (commonly known as the LRP). Genetic inactivation of apo E in mice results in massive hyperlipidemia and spontaneous atherosclerosis on a low-fat, low-cholesterol diet (39), compelling evidence that apo E is important in mediating cardiovascular risk.

Three common alleles at the apo E gene locus ($\epsilon 2$, $\epsilon 3$, and ϵ4) encode the three major isoforms of the apo E protein in plasma, E2, E3, and E4. E3 is considered normal and carries a cysteine at residue 112 and an arginine at residue 158. An arginine for cysteine substitution at residue 112 produces E4, and a cysteine for arginine substitution at residue 158 produces E2. Since humans have two copies of each chromosome and both alleles are expressed, the six phenotypes (with frequencies in parentheses) are E3/E3 (~60%), E3/E2 (~15%), E3/E4 (~20%), E4/E2 (~2%), E4/E4 (~2%), and E2/E2 (~1%). Individuals with E4 isoforms are at increased risk for cardiovascular disease and, surprisingly, Alzheimer's disease (40). The explanation for the latter is incomplete, but apo E is found in the senile plaques in the brain that characterize Alzheimer's disease. E2/E2 individuals are at risk for dysbetalipoproteinemia (see below).

Apo E and Diet

Apo E isoforms can predict responses to dietary interventions aimed at lowering serum lipoproteins. Subjects with the fairly common E3/E4 phenotype show greater decreases in LDL cholesterol than those with the E3/E3 or E3/E2 phenotypes when consuming a low-fat, low-cholesterol diet (41–43). In population studies, individuals with E2 isoforms have lower levels of LDL-cholesterol, E3 subjects have intermediate levels, and those with E4 have higher levels. E4 subjects may also have an impaired ability to clear atherogenic, postprandial triglyceride-rich lipoproteins (44).

Dysbetalipoproteinemia

Dysbetalipoproteinemia is rare but important to recognize because it can be effectively treated. Also called type III hyperlipoproteinemia, dysbetalipoproteinemia occurs in subjects with the E2/E2 phenotype. Although the frequency of this phenotype is 1:100, the rate for dysbetalipoproteinemia is from 1:5,000 to 1:10,000. Thus, the E2/E2 phenotype is necessary but not sufficient for development of the disorder. The clinical manifestations of the disease are usually not apparent until the middle decades of life. Additional factors postulated to be required for clinical manifestation of dysbetalipoproteinemia include alcohol intake, high intake of dietary fat, hypothyroidism, and inheritance of genes associated with obesity and diabetes.

Affected individuals classically have elevations of serum triglycerides and cholesterol, severe peripheral vascular disease, coronary artery disease, and xanthomas (30). While the latter can develop at several sites, xanthomas occurring in the palms of the hands are relatively specific for dysbetalipoproteinemia (see Chapter 75). Dietary and pharmacologic treatment of affected individuals is thought to decrease the risk of adverse clinical outcomes such as myocardial infarction and limb loss due to peripheral vascular disease.

HIGH-DENSITY LIPOPROTEIN (HDL)

Lipid Metabolism

There is a strong inverse relationship between HDL-cholesterol levels and the risk of cardiovascular disease. The exact basis for this epidemiologic observation is still unresolved. One possibility is that HDL is critical for reverse cholesterol transport, the process by which excess cholesterol in tissues (including the arterial wall, the site of atherosclerosis) is transported back to the liver for excretion from the body. Forward cholesterol transport is mediated by apo B100–containing lipoproteins, which are known to be atherogenic. By the former mechanism, elevated levels of HDL cholesterol reflect an efficient ability to excrete excess cholesterol.

Another possibility is that HDL serves as marker for the efficiency of metabolism of postprandial, triglyceride-rich lipoproteins. These lipoproteins are atherogenic, and their concentration is inversely related to HDL cholesterol levels: when triglycerides are elevated, HDL cholesterol levels are low. Thus, a low HDL cholesterol level may increase cardiac risk indirectly through its association with elevated concentrations of atherogenic, triglyceride-rich lipoproteins. There is also experimental evidence supporting other mechanisms. HDL carries paraoxonase, an enzyme that can protect LDL from oxidation in vitro. LDL modifications such as oxidation may be critical in the pathogenesis of atherosclerosis (see above). In a mouse model of diet-induced atherosclerosis, an atherogenic diet decreases both HDL and expression of the paraoxonase gene (45).

Not all HDL particles are necessarily associated with protection against atherosclerosis. Apo AI and apo AII are the major protein components of HDL particles. There are at least two populations of HDL particles: those containing apo AI only and those containing both apo AI and apo AII. Apo AI is clearly antiatherogenic. Overexpression of apo AI decreases atherosclerosis in mice with spontaneous atherosclerosis caused by genetic inactivation of the apo E gene (46). However, overexpression of apo AII in mice appears to be proatherogenic (47, 48).

Several factors are associated with lower HDL cholesterol levels, including central obesity, androgens such as testosterone, medications that block β-adrenergic receptors, smoking, and reduced intake of dietary fat. Aerobic exercise, estrogens, alcohol, and the vitamin niacin (in pharmacologic doses) increase HDL cholesterol levels.

Genetic Regulation of HDL Levels

Several familial disorders are associated with inherited changes in HDL levels. As noted above, LPL is involved in HDL synthesis, and defects in the LPL gene are associated with HDL deficiency. Normal clearance of HDL particles depends on cholesteryl ester transfer protein (CETP), and defects in the CETP gene are associated with elevated HDL levels (49). Hepatic lipase also participates in HDL clearance, and genetic defects in hepatic lipase are associated with elevated HDL levels. However, for each of these inherited defects, the level of HDL does not necessarily predict cardiovascular risk as it does in the general population. For example, despite very low levels of HDL in LPL deficiency, these patients do not appear to be at greatly increased risk for atherosclerosis.

Genetic absence of apo AI in humans results in HDL deficiency and increased susceptibility to cardiovascular disease (50). However, another human genetic variant of apo AI produces HDL deficiency but apparently protects from heart disease. This variant, apo AI_{Milano}, is caused by a cysteine for arginine substitution at amino acid residue 173 of the apo AI protein. This human variant diminishes vascular damage without affecting cholesterol levels in rabbits (51), suggesting that apo AI has a direct protective effect on the vascular wall.

In populations, genetics appears to play a major role in determining HDL levels, but the exact loci responsible for these effects are unknown. Kindreds with very low and very high HDL levels are fairly common and identified as having familial hypoalphalipoproteinemia and familial hyperalphalipoproteinemia, respectively. Until the use of genetic markers for determining vascular risk becomes widespread, family history is the most powerful way to determine the clinical significance of inherited levels of HDL cholesterol. For example, a very low HDL cholesterol in an asymptomatic patient with several first-degree relatives with low HDL cholesterol and premature cardiovascular disease indicates an increased risk of heart disease in that patient.

REFERENCES

1. Dudek SM, Semenkovich CF. J Biol Chem 1995;270:29323–9.
2. Clarke SD, Armstrong MK, Jump DB. J Nutr 1990;120:225–31.
3. Semenkovich CF, Coleman T, Goforth R. J Biol Chem 1993;268:6961–70.
4. Greeve J, Altkemper I, Dieterich J-H, et al. J Lipid Res 1993;34:1367–83.
5. Ginsberg HN. Curr Opin Lipidol 1995;6:275–80.
6. Thompson GR, Naoumova RP, Watts GF. J Lipid Res 1996;37:439–47.
7. Chen S-H, Habib G, Yang C-Y, et al. Science 1987;238:363–6.
8. Teng B, Burant CF, Davidson NO. Science 1993;260:1816–9.
9. Hirano K-I, Young SG, Farese RV Jr, et al. J Biol Chem 1996;271:9887–90.
10. Baum CL, Teng BB, Davidson NO. J Biol Chem 1990;265: 19263–70.
11. Nassir F, Blanchard RK, Mazur A, et al. J Nutr 1996;126:860–4.
12. Yamanaka S, Balestra ME, Ferrell LD, et al. Proc Natl Acad Sci USA 1995;92:8483–7.
13. Rader DJ, Brewer HB Jr. JAMA 1993;270:865–9.
14. Wetterau JR, Aggerbeck LP, Bouma ME, et al. Science 1992;258:999–1001.
15. Narcisi TME, Shoulders CC, Chester SA, et al. Am J Hum Genet 1995;57:1298–310.
16. Lin MCM, Arbeeny C, Bergquist K, et al. J Biol Chem 1994;269:29138–45.
17. Schonfeld G. Annu Rev Nutr 1995;15:23–34.
18. Myant NB. Atherosclerosis 1993;104:1–18.
19. Humphries SE, Talmud PJ. Curr Opin Lipidol 1995;6:215–22.
20. Seip RL, Angelopoulos TJ, Semenkovich CF. Am J Physiol 1995;268:E229–36.
21. Coleman T, Seip RL, Gimble JM, et al. J Biol Chem 1995;270:12518–25.
22. Campos H, Dreon DM, Krauss RM. J Lipid Res 1995;36:462–72.
23. Farese RV Jr, Yost T, Eckel RH. Metabolism 1991;40:214–6.
24. Pagliassotti MJ, Knobel SM, Shahrokhi KA, et al. Am J Physiol 1994;267:R659–64.
25. Semenkovich CF, Wims M, Noe L, et al. J Biol Chem 1989;264:9030–8.
26. Doolittle MH, Ben-Zeev O, Elovson J, et al. J Biol Chem 1990;265:44570–7.
27. Erskine JM, Jensen DR, Eckel RH. J Nutr 1994;124:500–7.
28. Semenkovich CF, Luo C-C, Nakanishi MK, et al. J Biol Chem 1990;265:5429–33.
29. Laville M, Auboeuf D, Khalfallah Y, et al. J Clin Invest 1996;98:43–9.
30. Semenkovich CF. Hypertriglyceridemia and combined hyperlipidemia. In: Vascular surgery: theory and practice. Stamford, CT: Appleton & Lange, 1995;105–17.
31. Miesenbock G, Holzl B, Foger B, et al. J Clin Invest 1993;91:448–55.
32. Reymer PWA, Gagne E, Groenemeyer BE, et al. Nature Genet 1995;10:28–34.
33. Spady DK. Semin Liver Dis 1992;12:373–85.
34. Horton JD, Cuthbert JA, Spady DK. J Clin Invest 1993;92: 743–9.
35. Yokoyama C, Wang X, Briggs MR, et al. Cell 1993;75:187–97.
36. Hua X, Yokoyama C, Wu J, et al. Proc Natl Acad Sci USA 1994;90:11603–7.
37. Sheng Z, Otani H, Brown MS, et al. Proc Natl Acad Sci USA 1995;92:935–8.
38. Hobbs HH, Brown MS, Goldstein JL. Hum Mutat 1992;1:445–66.
39. Plump AS, Smith JD, Hayek T, et al. Cell 1992;71:343–53.
40. Strittmatter WJ, Saunders AM, Schmechel D, et al. Proc Natl Acad Sci USA 1993;90:1977–81.
41. Cobb MM, Teitlebaum H, Risch N, et al. Circulation 1992;86:849–57.
42. Lopez-Miranda J, Ordovas JM, Mata P, et al. J Lipid Res 1994;35:1965–75.
43. Dreon DM, Fernstrom HA, Miller B, et al. Arterioscl Thromb Vasc Biol 1995;15:105–11.
44. Bergeron N, Havel RJ. J Clin Invest 1996;97:65–72.
45. Shih DM, Gu L, Hama S, et al. J Clin Invest 1996;97:1630–9.
46. Paszty C, Maeda N, Verstuyft J, et al. J Clin Invest 1994;94:899–903.
47. Warden CH, Hedrick CC, Qiao J-H, et al. Science 1993;261: 269–72.
48. Marzal-Casacuberta A, Blanco-Vaca F, Ishida BY, et al. J Biol Chem 1996;271:6720–8.
49. Tall A. Annu Rev Biochem 1995;64:235–57.
50. Breslow JL. Annu Rev Med 1991;42:357–71.
51. Ameli S, Hultgardh-Nilsson A, Cercek B, et al. Circulation 1994;90:1935–41.

SELECTED READINGS

Breslow JL. Mouse models of atherosclerosis. Science 1996;272: 685–8.

Dammerman M, Breslow JL. Genetic basis of lipoprotein disorders. Circulation 1995;91:505–12.

Gregg RE, Wetterau JR. The molecular basis of abetalipoproteinemia. Curr Opin Lipidol 1994;5:81–6.

Vance DE, Vance L, eds. Biochemistry of lipids, lipoproteins and membranes. Amsterdam: Elsevier, 1991;1–596.

75. Nutrition and Diet in the Management of Hyperlipidemia and Atherosclerosis

SCOTT M. GRUNDY

The last decade has witnessed growing acceptance of the concept that a high serum cholesterol level and related disorders of serum lipoproteins critically influence development of coronary heart disease (CHD) and other atherosclerotic diseases. Support for this concept comes from studies in animal models, surveys of different populations, findings of premature CHD in persons with genetic forms of hyperlipidemia, investigations in laboratory animals, and clinical trials (1, 2). Recent clinical trials (3–7) provide irrefutable evidence that high serum cholesterol levels predispose to CHD; these trials moreover demonstrate conclusively that reducing serum cholesterol levels decreases the incidence of CHD. Dramatic results from recent clinical trials (3–7) have greatly heightened interest in cholesterol as a risk factor for CHD.

This chapter outlines the major abnormalities of serum cholesterol and other disorders of serum lipids and lipoproteins. It also links these abnormalities to disease endpoints, notably, coronary atherosclerosis and CHD. Serum lipids (cholesterol and triglycerides) do not circulate as independent molecules but are solubilized by specific apolipoproteins to form macromolecular complexes called lipoproteins. The serum contains several distinct species of lipoproteins. Among these, low-density lipoprotein (LDL) is the major cholesterol-carrying lipoprotein. Strong evidence indicates that high serum levels of LDL, called hypercholesterolemia, accelerate coronary atherogenesis and predispose to CHD. An elevated serum LDL cholesterol has been identified as the predominant atherogenic lipoprotein by the U.S. National Cholesterol Education Program (NCEP) (1, 2). Although cholesterol has received more attention, another important lipid carried in serum lipoproteins is triglyceride. There are several species of triglyceride-rich lipoproteins (TGRLPs). Those made by the intestine are called chylomicrons; TGRLPs produced by the liver are named very low density lipoproteins (VLDLs). Although chylomicrons generally are not considered atherogenic lipoproteins, there is growing evidence that VLDL can have atherogenic potential. Another species of lipoprotein is high-density lipoprotein (HDL). This lipoprotein also contains cholesterol, but HDL does not promote atherosclerosis; in fact, high serum levels of HDL seemingly protect against CHD.

The lipoprotein disorders can be conveniently divided into three categories: hypercholesterolemia, chylomicronemia, and atherogenic dyslipidemia. Hypercholesterolemia occurs in varying degrees from mild to severe and is characterized by high serum levels of LDL cholesterol. Chylomicronemia consists of marked elevation of chylomicrons, with or without high VLDL levels. Finally, atherogenic dyslipidemia is a disorder characterized by multiple lipoprotein abnormalities occurring simultaneously in a single person; this disorder is described in more detail below. Each category of lipoprotein abnormality is considered separately.

HYPERCHOLESTEROLEMIA

Hypercholesterolemia denotes an isolated elevation of serum LDL cholesterol. Several lines of evidence indicate that elevated serum concentrations of LDL promote atherogenesis and increase the risk for CHD (1, 2). The increment in risk for CHD is proportional to the elevation of the serum LDL level (2). In fact, risk is compounded by progressively increasing serum LDL concentrations. Conversely, in populations in which serum LDL concen-

Abbreviations: **ACAT**—acyl-CoA cholesterol acyltransferase; **BMI**—body mass index; **CETP**—cholesteryl ester transfer protein; **CHD**—coronary heart disease; **FFA**—free (unesterified) fatty acid(s); **FDB**—familial defective apolipoprotein B; **FH**—familial hypercholesterolemia; **HDL**—high-density lipoprotein; **LDL**—low-density lipoprotein; **LPL**—lipoprotein lipase; **MTP**—microsomal lipid-transfer protein; **NCEP**—National Cholesterol Education Program; **NIDDM**—non-insulin-dependent diabetes mellitus; **SREBP**—sterol regulatory element–binding proteins; **TGRLP**—triglyceride-rich lipoproteins; VLDL, very low density lipoproteins.

Table 75.1
Classification of Total and LDL-Cholesterol

Classification	Total Cholesterol mg/dL (mmol/L)	LDL-Cholesterol mg/dL (mmol/L)
"Optimal"	<150 (<3.88)	<100 (<2.59)
Desirable	150–199 (3.88–5.15)	100–129 (2.59–3.34)
Borderline-high	200–239 (5.17–6.19)	130–159[a] (3.36–4.11)
High	≥240 (≥6.21)	≥160[b] (≥4.14)

[a]For LDL-cholesterol 130–159, the term *borderline-high risk* is used.
[b]For LDL-cholesterol ≥160, the term *high-risk* is used.

trations are very low, CHD is rare (8); this is true even when other CHD risk factors—cigarette smoking, hypertension, and diabetes mellitus—are relatively common. This latter observation (8) strongly suggests that LDL is an essential atherogenic agent. For populations, although not necessarily for all individuals, there is a high correlation between serum LDL-cholesterol levels and total cholesterol levels. This is because about two-thirds of the serum total cholesterol is normally transported as cholesteryl esters in LDL. However, this generalization does not necessarily hold for all persons; thus, for individuals, laboratory measurements of LDL cholesterol are required to accurately define the level.

The NCEP (1, 2) classifies total serum cholesterol according to the degree of severity as shown in Table 75.1; corresponding values for LDL cholesterol are also listed in Table 75.1. In the current review, this classification is modified slightly and expressed in terms of "hypercholesterolemia" (Table 75.2). According to this latter classification, hypercholesterolemia can be divided into mild, moderate, and severe categories. Lower ranges of serum cholesterol can be separated into "optimal" and "desirable." Optimal levels of cholesterol are those associated with minimal risk for CHD. Desirable levels can be somewhat higher than optimal but are usually associated with relatively low rates of CHD.

Optimal Cholesterol Levels

Total cholesterol levels below 150 mg/dL (LDL-cholesterol < 100 mg/dL) are considered "optimal" (2). Within this range, atherosclerosis develops at a very slow rate; consequently CHD is rare. Optimal serum cholesterol levels typically occur in children and young adults but also are present in middle-aged and older persons in various populations around the world (e.g., rural Asia). In these latter populations, intakes of saturated fatty acids and cholesterol typically are very low, daily physical activity is high, and body fat content is low; this combination of dietary and life habits apparently keeps serum cholesterol levels in the optimal range throughout life. The very low rates of atherosclerotic disease in these populations demonstrate the benefit of keeping serum cholesterol levels low (8). It has been suggested that very low serum cholesterol levels in these populations can be explained by genetic factors; however, changes in eating and exercise habits have caused cholesterol levels to rise, even in populations that historically have exhibited very low cholesterol levels (9).

Table 75.2
Classification of Hypercholesterolemia

Degree of Hypercholesterolemia	Total Cholesterol mg/dL (mmol/L)	LDL-Cholesterol mg/dL (mmol/L)
Mild	200–239 (5.18–6.19)	130–159 (3.36–4.11)
Moderate	240–299 (6.21–7.76)	160–219 (4.14–5.67)
Severe	≥300 (≥7.76)	≥220 (≥5.69)

Not only does an elevated serum cholesterol level promote atherogenesis, but restoration of serum cholesterol to optimal levels markedly reduces the risk for CHD, even in persons who already have advanced atherosclerotic disease. For example, in patients who have established CHD, reducing serum cholesterol levels to near the optimal range decreases their risk of recurrent myocardial infarction (3, 4). Similar risk reduction follows therapeutic lowering of serum cholesterol levels in hypercholesterolemic patients who have not yet developed CHD (5). Several other clinical trials (7, 10), in which coronary arteries were visualized directly by angiography, revealed that reducing serum cholesterol levels retards progression of coronary atherosclerosis. Thus, an elevation in serum cholesterol contributes to initiation and progression of coronary atherosclerosis; but of equal importance, it plays a critical role later in the course of atherosclerotic disease by predisposing to acute coronary events, e.g., myocardial infarction. Thus, there is a growing recognition that optimal cholesterol levels convey substantial protection against development of CHD.

Desirable Cholesterol Levels

The NCEP (1, 2) defines total cholesterol levels in the range of 150 to 199 mg/dL (LDL-cholesterol 100 to 129 mg/dL) as "desirable." Although "desirable" cholesterol levels may still promote atherogenesis, compared with optimal levels, premature CHD (i.e., onset of CHD before age 65) is relatively rare in the absence of other CHD risk factors (11). For most adult Americans living in an urbanized setting and other populations in similar circumstances, it is unrealistic to expect cholesterol levels to remain at optimal levels throughout life (e.g., LDL-cholesterol below 100 mg/dL). Serum levels in the somewhat higher but still desirable range are mainly the product of small increments in dietary saturated fatty acids and cholesterol, modest excesses in body fat, and failure to maintain vigorous physical activity (12). Premature CHD nonetheless is uncommon in people who have desirable cholesterol levels, provided they avoid cigarette smoking and maintain a normal blood pressure (11). It is a major goal of the NCEP to bring about a change in serum cholesterol levels in the American public so that a greater proportion of the population achieves and sustains cholesterol concentrations in the desirable zone (13). At present, almost half of all American adults have total cholesterol levels below 200 mg/dL (2, 14). Fortunately, serum cholesterol levels in the general public have been declining over the past three decades (14); as a result, a larger fraction of the population now has desirable cholesterol levels than it did in the past.

An important public health goal for adults of the general population thus is to maintain serum cholesterol levels in the desirable range. Reduction in intakes of saturated fatty acids and cholesterol over the past 3 decades in the United States has increased the proportion of the U.S. general population with desirable cholesterol levels. Table 75.3 compares current macronutrient intakes in the U.S. public (15) with intakes recommended by the NCEP (13) and the American Heart Association (AHA) (16). If population-mean intakes of saturated fatty acids and cholesterol could be reduced to recommended levels, a greater proportion of the population would achieve serum cholesterol levels in the desirable range.

Overweight is another factor responsible for the rise of serum cholesterol levels to above the desirable range. It has been estimated that the weight gain that typically occurs with aging accounts for a rise in serum cholesterol of approximately 25 mg/dL (12). The average American adult gains about 10 kg between ages 20 and 50 years. A significant increase in serum cholesterol levels is one consequence of this weight gain (18, 19). Thus, weight control, particularly a reduction in the amount of weight gained with aging, is an important public health goal. Weight gain with aging is due to two factors: *(a)* a decline in basal metabolic rate with aging (see Chapter 87) and *(b)* a reduction in physical activity. The metabolic rate decline results largely from a decrease in muscle mass (20), which likewise is due in part to reduced physical activity. Although increased physical activity that does not produce weight loss will not significantly lower cholesterol levels, maintaining a high enough level of exercise to prevent weight gain will contribute to lower serum cholesterol levels. In most persons, however, maintaining a moderate level of physical activity will not be enough to prevent an increase in body weight with aging; therefore, some reduction in caloric intake also will be required.

Table 75.3
Current Macronutrient Intakes in the American Public

	Recommended Intake[a] (% of total calories)	Current American Intake[b] (% of total calories)
Total fat	≤30	35
Cholesterol-raising fatty acids	<10	
Saturated		12
Trans		3
Monounsaturated fatty acids	10–15	14
Polyunsaturated fatty acids	<10	6
Carbohydrate	55	50
Protein	15	15
Cholesterol (mg/day)	<300	300–400

[a]Recommended macronutrient intakes (13, 16).
[b]Values approximated from existing data (15).

Table 75.4
Distribution of Body Mass Indexes in the American Public

Body Mass Index (kg/m^2)	Adult Men (%)	Adult Women (%)
21–24.9	37	55
25–26.9	25	15
27–29.9	25	10
≥30	13	20

Distribution of body mass indexes estimated from the data of Shah et al. (21).

In spite of the success in reducing serum cholesterol levels among Americans through decreased intakes of saturated fatty acids and cholesterol, the public has not been successful in weight control. Indeed, obesity in the United States has progressively increased (see Chapter 87). Table 75.4 shows the proportion of the U.S. population within each category of body mass index (BMI) (21). A desirable BMI ranges from 21 to 25 kg/m^2. In this category, cholesterol levels are at their lowest (18, 19). BMIs in the ranges of 25 to 26.9 kg/m^2, 27 to 29.9 kg/m^2, and more than 30 kg/m^2 can be called mild, moderate, and severe overweight, respectively. As noted in Table 75.4, approximately half of Americans fall into the overweight range. This high prevalence of overweight stands in the way of achieving desirable serum cholesterol levels for many persons.

Mild Hypercholesterolemia

About 25% of American adults have mild hypercholesterolemia (total cholesterol 200 to 239 mg/dL; LDL-cholesterol 130 to 159 mg/dL) (2). These levels are called "borderline high" by the NCEP. In middle-aged adults with mild hypercholesterolemia, the risk for CHD in the short term (5–10 years) is about 1.5 times that accompanying serum cholesterol levels in the desirable range (11). Recent analyses suggest that the risk differential over a lifetime is even greater, i.e., in the presence of mild hypercholesterolemia, long-term (30–40 years) risk is three to four times that associated with a desirable cholesterol level (22, 23).

In most persons, several causative factors underlie mild hypercholesterolemia (12): *(a)* diets high in cholesterol, *(b)* diets high in cholesterol-raising fatty acids (saturated fatty acids and *trans* fatty acids), *(c)* increasing body weight with aging, *(d)* aging per se, *(e)* genetic factors, and *(f)* estrogen loss in postmenopausal women. Each of these factors deserves some attention. If a greater portion of the public is going to achieve desirable cholesterol levels, it will be necessary to modify some of these factors. The effects of two factors—genetics and aging per se—cannot be mitigated short of treatment with cholesterol-lowering drugs; however, the other factors listed above can be changed by modifying life habits.

Causes of Mild Hypercholesterolemia

Genetic Causes. Some people appear to be unusually susceptible to higher serum cholesterol levels. In addition, the broad range of serum cholesterol concentrations in the general population suggests variability in genetic susceptibility. Genetic epidemiologists (24) have calculated that about 50% of the variation in cholesterol levels in the general population can be explained by polymorphism in the genes influencing serum total cholesterol and LDL-cholesterol.

Genetic factors potentially regulate LDL-cholesterol levels at multiple control points. A discussion of these sites of control requires examining the origins and fates of serum LDL. LDL is derived from catabolism of TGRLPs produced by the liver. Hepatic TGRLPs, called VLDLs, contain mainly triglycerides in their lipoprotein core and three apolipoproteins in their surface coat: apo-B-100 (apo-B), apo-Cs, and apo-E. VLDL-triglycerides are hydrolyzed by lipoprotein lipase (LPL) (see "Chylomicronemia," below), degrading VLDLs to smaller TGRLPs called VLDL remnants; most apo-Cs are lost from VLDL particles during this process (see Chapter 4). VLDL remnants can either be taken up by the liver (via LDL receptors) or converted to LDL. Hepatic triglyceride lipase (HTGL) probably hydrolyzes the remaining triglycerides in remnants, causing their conversion to LDL. The only apolipoprotein remaining on LDL is apo-B-100; it is apo-B-100 on LDL that is recognized by LDL receptors (25). Most LDL particles are removed via LDL receptors on liver parenchymal cells (25). Synthesis of each of the proteins that influence LDL levels is under genetic control and is subject to modification by genetic aberrations.

One factor influencing LDL levels is the rate of formation of lipoproteins by the liver. Most lipoproteins made by the liver are rich in triglycerides and hence are secreted as VLDLs. The amount of hepatic triglyceride available for incorporation into VLDL may influence the rate of VLDL secretion. In cultured hepatocytes, supplying more fatty acids for triglyceride synthesis increases the number of VLDL particles secreted by these liver cells (26). Transfer of triglycerides into newly forming VLDL particles is mediated by microsomal lipid-transfer protein (MTP) (27, 28). This protein shuttles both triglyceride and phospholipid into VLDL particles. In patients with a genetic absence of MTP, VLDL particles do not mature; affected individuals consequently lack apo-B-containing lipoproteins in the circulation (abetalipoproteinemia) (27). The rate of formation of apo-B-100 itself could affect the rate of VLDL secretion. At the other extreme, high serum levels of both cholesterol and triglycerides (combined hyperlipidemia) could be due to excessive synthesis of apo-B-100 by the liver (28); this possibility, however, has not been proved through definitive studies (29). Whether the availability of cholesterol in the liver influences the rate of secretion of VLDL also remains to be determined. In laboratory animals, high doses of drugs that inhibit cholesterol synthesis reduce VLDL secretion; whether usual doses of these drugs have this same effect in humans is uncertain. In sum, multiple factors under genetic control undoubtedly affect the assembly and secretion of hepatic VLDLs; and because LDL particles are derived from VLDL, VLDL secretion rates can influence LDL-cholesterol levels (28). Consequently, genetic aberrations leading to overproduction of apo-B-containing lipoproteins by the liver may be one of the causes of hypercholesterolemia.

The rate of removal of LDLs from the circulation also influences serum LDL levels. The clearance of LDLs has been studied extensively. Most circulating LDL particles are removed via LDL receptors located on liver cells (25). As noted above, LDL receptors specifically bind apo-B-100. Variation in the number of LDL receptors expressed on liver cells is a major determinant of serum LDL-cholesterol levels. A critical factor controlling expression of hepatic LDL receptors is the amount of cholesterol in the liver cell (25). When the cholesterol content of the liver rises, synthesis of LDL receptors is reduced.

The mechanisms whereby this occurs have recently been elucidated. Specialized proteins, called sterol regulatory element–binding proteins (SREBP), span the microsomal (endoplasmic reticulum) membranes (30). When the cholesterol content of membranes falls, an enzyme is activated that clips SREBP in two so that a fragment of SREBP is freed to move into the cell nucleus. This protein binds to the promoter region of the gene for the LDL receptor and stimulates its transcription (see Chapter 74). Increased availability of cholesterol in the liver has the opposite effect; namely, it suppresses LDL-receptor activity.

Steady-state amounts of cholesterol in the liver cells depend on the rate of synthesis of cholesterol, the rate of secretion of cholesterol into bile, and the rate of conversion of cholesterol into bile acids (12). All of these metabolic pathways are under genetic regulation; thus, genetic polymorphism of multiple proteins regulating these pathways could enhance the availability of intracellular cholesterol. This event, in turn, can raise LDL-cholesterol levels through the SREBP mechanism. Moreover, genetic variation in SREBPs, or the gene encoding LDL receptors, may affect the expression of LDL receptors. Future research may uncover a variety of genetic polymorphisms in the complex system of LDL-receptor regulation that lead to higher LDL-cholesterol levels. Genetic polymorphisms likely account for much of the variability in LDL cholesterol levels in the U.S. population, and some polymorphisms undoubtedly contribute to the development of mild hypercholesterolemia.

Rise of Cholesterol Levels with Age. *Decline in LDL Receptor Activity with Aging.* In the United States, the average serum total cholesterol level rises by about 40 to 50 mg/dL between ages 20 and 50 (2, 12). About half of this rise apparently results from increased body weight; but another portion seems to be linked to aging per se (31, 32). The aging process is accompanied by delayed clearance of LDL from the circulation; presumably, the complex mechanisms regulating LDL-receptor function become less efficient with aging. For example, hepatic disposal of cholesterol may be slightly retarded with aging, leading to increased hepatic cholesterol content. Alternatively, synthetic mechanisms for LDL receptors may become sluggish, causing decreased receptor expression and LDL catabolism. There is, however, a curious observation: serum cholesterol levels do not rise progressively from middle age into older age (2). Most of the increase occurs between the ages of 20 and 50 years; thereafter, LDL-cholesterol levels reach a plateau or even decline somewhat. This suggests that external, controllable factors, such as weight gain, play critical roles in the age-related increase in cholesterol levels.

Obesity and the Rise of Cholesterol with Aging. There is a strong correlation between changes in serum cholesterol concentrations and changes in body weight from young adulthood into middle age (18, 19). Most weight gain in adults occurs between ages 20 and 50 years; during this same period, serum cholesterol concentrations rise. Although epidemiologic studies have indicated that serum cholesterol levels rise with aging, even in persons who show little weight gain (18, 19), those who gain more weight manifest greater increments in serum cholesterol. The increase of serum cholesterol with aging occurs in both VLDL and LDL fractions (18, 19). This combined change further suggests an effect of obesity on serum cholesterol. The major influence of obesity on lipoprotein metabolism is upon the input pathway (33, 34), and isotope kinetic studies suggest that obesity induces overproduction of hepatic VLDLs (33, 34). Consequently, the rise in LDL-cholesterol levels with increasing body weight is likely to be secondary to an increased rate of input of VLDLs, followed by an increased rate of conversion of VLDLs to LDLs. Thus, it is not surprising that both VLDL and LDL levels rise concomitantly with increasing obesity.

Cholesterol-Raising Fatty Acids. Two classes of dietary fatty acids can raise serum cholesterol levels: saturated fatty acids (35) and *trans* monounsaturated fatty acids (36, 37). These fatty acids induce increments in total cholesterol levels that occur largely in the LDL fraction. Specifically, these fatty acids elevate LDL-cholesterol concentrations relative to the effects of other nutrients: polyunsaturated fatty acids, *cis* monounsaturated fatty acids, and carbohydrates (35). Since the latter nutrients do not raise LDL-cholesterol levels, they are called "neutral." Although saturated fatty acids as a class raise serum LDL levels, compared with "neutral" nutrients, even the different types of saturated fatty acids differ in their influence on LDL-cholesterol levels. The saturated fatty acid present in the largest quantities in the U.S. diet is palmitic acid (C16:0); a review of the literature shows palmitic acid to be a potent cholesterol-raising fatty acid (35). Another saturated acid, myristic acid (C14:0), occurs in lesser amounts in the diet, but it appears to be even more potent than palmitic acid in elevating the serum LDL-cholesterol concentration (38). Recent investigations reveal that shorter-chain saturates—lauric acid (C12:0) (36) and medium-chain fatty acids (C10:0 and C8:0) (40)—also raise serum LDL levels, although somewhat less than does palmitic acid. Still another saturated fatty acid, stearic acid (C18:0) (41, 42), *does not* increase LDL-cholesterol levels relative to unsaturated fatty acids. Hence, stearic acid is a "neutral" fatty acid. This apparently is because stearic acid is rapidly converted into oleic acid (C18:1) once it enters the body (43).

Although the saturated fatty acids make up the lion's share of cholesterol-raising fatty acids in the diet, recent studies have indicated that *trans* monounsaturated fatty acids also increase LDL levels (36, 37, 44). *Trans* fatty acids are produced by hydrogenation of vegetable oils. The *trans* configuration of these fatty acids gives them structural properties similar to those of saturated fatty acids, which may explain their action in raising serum LDL concentrations. In the typical American diet, *trans* fatty acids account for only about one-fourth as much energy intake as do saturated fatty acids; however, their role as a contributor to mild hypercholesterolemia is nonetheless significant and should not be discounted.

The mechanisms by which cholesterol-raising fatty acids elevate the serum LDL cholesterol concentration remain to be fully elucidated. Investigations carried out in animal models point to suppression of LDL-receptor activity as the primary site of the action of fatty acids (45). One hypothesis holds that these fatty acids interfere with esterification of cholesterol in the liver (46). Saturated fatty acids seemingly interfere with the cholesterol-esterifying enzyme acyl-CoA cholesterol acyl transferase (ACAT). If saturated fatty acids retard formation of cholesteryl esters in the liver, more unesterified cholesterol is available for action on SREBPs and hence, secondarily, for suppression of LDL-receptor activity, so that LDL accumulates in plasma. Other mechanisms have been proposed to explain the action of saturated fatty acids in raising cholesterol levels, but most data support the concept that, by one means or another, they suppress the activity of LDL receptors.

Dietary Cholesterol. In many animal models, high intakes of cholesterol exert a powerful hypercholesterolemic action (47, 48). The mechanism of this response seems to be straightforward. When the diet is enriched with cholesterol, hepatic cholesterol content rises. This suppresses SREBPs cleavage and thus downregulates LDL-receptor synthesis. The same mechanism presumably obtains in man. Humans, however, are less susceptible to the hypercholesterolemic action of dietary cholesterol than many experimental animals (49). Increasing dietary cholesterol apparently fails to induce such marked rises in unesterified cholesterol concentrations in the liver of humans. There could be several reasons. First, in humans, less than half of dietary cholesterol is absorbed, which limits its availability to the liver. Also, humans may be more efficient in esterifying cholesterol in hepatocytes or secreting it into bile; both mechanisms will reduce unesterified cholesterol in liver cells. In spite of these protective mechanisms, an increased amount of cholesterol in the diet definitely raises LDL-cholesterol in many people. A relatively high level of cholesterol in the American diet is one of several factors contributing to a high frequency of mild hypercholesterolemia in the general population.

Rise of Cholesterol after Menopause. Loss of estrogen after menopause leads to increased serum cholesterol in many women (2, 12). Estrogens stimulate LDL-receptor synthesis in several animal models (50), and the same response presumably occurs in humans. After menopause and with a loss of estrogens, LDL-receptor activity falls. This decline in receptor function and consequent rise in LDL-cholesterol levels can be reversed by estrogen replacement therapy after menopause (51).

Management of Mild Hypercholesterolemia

Detection and Classification. The first step in the management of mild hypercholesterolemia is measuring concentrations of serum lipids and lipoproteins. Initial measurements should include total cholesterol (C), triglycerides (TG), and HDL-cholesterol (HDL-C) (1, 2). When triglycerides are below 300 mg/dL, serum LDL-cholesterol (LDL-C) can be estimated as follows:

$$LDL\text{-}C = C - HDL\text{-}C - TG/5$$

The term *TG/5* represents the concentration of very low density lipoprotein (VLDL) cholesterol. When triglycerides exceed 300 mg/dL, measurement of LDL cholesterol requires removing VLDL by ultracentrifugation. After removal of VLDL, the LDL cholesterol is calculated as

$$LDL\text{-}C = (C - VLDL\text{-}C) - HDL\text{-}C$$

Sometimes the LDL-cholesterol level is in the desirable range even when total cholesterol falls into the elevated range; this occurs when HDL-cholesterol levels are relatively high. Alternatively, when the HDL-cholesterol level is low, the LDL-cholesterol level can be high, even when the total cholesterol concentration is in the desirable range. For purposes of clinical management, *mild hypercholesterolemia* can be defined as a serum LDL-cholesterol level of 130 to 159 mg/dL.

Modification of Diet Composition. For most people without established CHD, treatment of mild hypercholesterolemia consists of dietary modification. The major factors responsible for mild hypercholesterolemia are *(a)* relatively high intakes of cholesterol, *(b)* high intakes of cholesterol-raising fatty acids, and *(c)* overweight. Modifying the dietary composition by reducing offending nutrients and weight reduction thus will reduce LDL-cholesterol levels into the desirable range for many persons.

Modifying dietary composition requires adopting the step I diet of the American Heart Association (1, 2) (Table 75.5) or a similar diet plan. The essential features of the step I diet are reducing intake of cholesterol-raising fatty acids to less than 10% of total calories, dietary cholesterol to less than 300 mg/dL, and total fat to 30% of total calories or less. Most persons with mild hypercholesterolemia in the United States exceed these recommendations in all categories. Reductions designed to achieve the goals of the step I diet can be expected to decrease serum LDL-cholesterol levels by about 10% (52).

Cholesterol-raising fatty acids can be calculated as the sum of cholesterol-raising saturated fatty acids plus *trans* fatty acids. About two-thirds of saturated fatty acids in the American diet comes from animal fat. Sources of animal fat include milk fat and meat fat. Milk fat is more hypercholesterolemic than meat fat because of its higher content of cholesterol-raising fatty acids. The remainder of saturated fatty acids in the diet comes from vegetable fats. The tropical oils (i.e., palm oil, coconut oil, and palm kernel oil) have a very high content of saturated fatty acids. Other vegetable oils have a lower content but still contribute some saturated fatty acids to the diet. In recent years in the United States, use of tropical oils by the food industry has decreased. A further reduction in saturated fatty acids in the American diet must come through decreasing the consumption of animal fats. Replacing fatty meats, including fatty cuts of steak, hamburger, and processed meats, with leaner products is one important way to decrease saturated fatty acids. Also, replacing traditional milk-based products (whole milk, butter, cream, ice cream, and cheese) with low-fat or fat-free milk products likewise will reduce the consumption of saturated fatty acids. The goal for the general population is to decrease dietary saturated fatty acids by at least one-third.

Since *trans* fatty acids are now known to belong to the category of cholesterol-raising fatty acids, intake of these must also be reduced to achieve the goals of the step I diet. Estimates of the intake of *trans* fatty acids in the United States vary, ranging from 2 to 5% of total calories; the aver-

Table 75.5
Step I Diet

Nutrient	Percentage of Total Calories
Total fat	≤30
Cholesterol-raising fatty acids[a]	<10
Monounsaturated fatty acids	10–15
Polyunsaturated fatty acids	<10
Carbohydrates	≥55
Protein	15
Cholesterol	<300 mg/day

[a]Includes saturated fatty acids (C8–C16) and *trans* fatty acids.

age intake is about 3% of total calories. This percentage of *trans* fatty acids in the diet can be cut in half by avoiding hard (hydrogenated) margarine as a spread and baked products containing hydrogenated shortenings. At present, commercially produced bakery goods and snack foods tend to be rich in *trans* fatty acids. Thus, to promote lowering of cholesterol, the food industry should make an effort to decrease the *trans* fatty acid content of food products by modifying the types of fats used in food manufacture.

Reduced consumption of animal fats will also decrease cholesterol intake. This reduction will further lower serum LDL-cholesterol levels. Intakes of cholesterol typically are divided about equally among eggs, milk-based products, and meats. Keeping the intake of foods containing egg yolks low, using low-fat or fat-free milk products, and decreasing meat fats can cut the current cholesterol intake by one-third to one-half.

Weight Control. The rise of body weight with aging contributes importantly to mild hypercholesterolemia (12, 18, 19). Consequently, weight reduction also is required for many overweight people to restore serum cholesterol to the desirable range. For a large number of persons, reducing intake of cholesterol and cholesterol-raising fatty acids will not suffice to obtain the desirable range for serum cholesterol unless weight reduction is carried out concurrently. Effective weight reduction usually requires a combination of calorie control and increased exercise. Most people with mild hypercholesterolemia are moderately overweight and consume an excess of 300 to 500 calories/day (18, 19). Most overweight persons are only moderately overweight, i.e., they have a BMI ranging from 25 to 30 kg/m^2 (21). Restoring the caloric balance required to achieve and maintain desirable body weight thus should not be difficult, but it requires continuous attention to body weight, moderate reduction of food intake, increased exercise, and both mental and physical discipline.

Certain foods should be targeted for caloric restriction to achieve a desirable body weight. Highest on the list for elimination are animal fats (milk fat and meat fat); their removal will not only decrease caloric intake but also reduce the intake of saturated fatty acid and thereby lower serum cholesterol levels. To achieve weight loss, the animal fats removed from the diet must *not* be replaced by calories of other types. Second on the priority list for reduction are high-sugar foods, such as soft drinks, desserts, candies, and cookies. High-sugar products, advertised as low-fat, have become popular in the United States. The increased use of these foods has offset much of the benefit derived from reduction of high-fat foods. Thus, to achieve weight reduction, high-sugar foods must be controlled as well. Third on the list are high-starch foods such as breads, potatoes, rice, and pasta. When less-desirable sources of calories of the first and second type are removed, care must be taken not to replace them with excessive intakes of high-starch foods. The same holds for replacement with vegetable oils. Although oils such as olive oil, canola oil, and soy bean oil produce a favorable lipoprotein pattern compared with saturated fatty acids, too much of these oils can provide excess calories and prevent weight reduction.

A second approach to weight reduction is to increase physical activity. The caloric balance required to achieve and maintain desirable weight can be restored in part by increased use of calories in physical exercise. Suitable exercises include regular walking, swimming, biking, and competitive sports (2, 53). For purposes of caloric expenditure, aerobic exercise is preferable to weight training. The latter, however, is also useful in older persons to maintain muscle mass and improve musculoskeletal function, which may prevent falls (53). Thus, instituting an appropriate regimen of regular exercise that expends excess calories is an integral element in the management of mild hypercholesterolemia.

A third recommendation incorporated in the step I diet is to reduce the intake of total fat to 30% or less of total calories. Most of the fat calories in this diet should come from vegetable oils. Currently, the most desirable percentage of calories from fat in the diet is disputed. Some investigators favor a higher fat content (e.g., 30–35% fat [54]), and others a lower intake (e.g., 15–25% fat [55]). The argument favoring a lower percentage of fat is that it may promote weight reduction. Certainly, reducing animal fat intake without replacement of fat will decrease total calories and promote weight reduction. Whether vegetable oils should be listed as a high priority for reduced intake is problematic. Maintaining a moderate intake of vegetable oils will help to sustain a relatively low level of triglycerides and a high level of HDL cholesterol. Assigning a higher priority to reduction of high-sugar foods seems preferable to decreasing the intake of vegetable oils. The current recommendation of about 30% of total calories from fat, mostly in the form of vegetable oils, seems reasonable (16, 17).

The one category of foods that can be safely increased includes fruits and colored vegetables (56). These products are relatively low in calories and rich in other nutrients. The latter include antioxidants along with fiber, phytoestrogens, phytosterols, polyphenols, carotenoids, indoles, quinones, and organosulfur compounds. Epidemiologic studies and investigations in laboratory animals suggest that some of these substances may protect against CHD, stroke, or cancer (57). There also is interest in the possibility that supplemental antioxidants, especially vitamins E and C, will give added protection against CHD or cancer (58). Although studies of several types support this possibility, a benefit of antioxidant supplements has not been proved through controlled clinical trials. In many persons with hypercholesterolemia, elevated blood pressure is a concomitant risk factor; thus, reduced salt intake combined with increased consumption of potassium from fruits and vegetables may reduce the risk for CHD and stroke by decreasing blood pressure (59).

Estrogen Replacement Therapy. In postmenopausal women with elevated serum LDL-cholesterol, consideration can be given to estrogen replacement therapy (ERT). Estrogens partially restore LDL-receptor activity that normally declines after menopause (51). ERT thus reduces serum LDL-cholesterol levels by 10 to 15%. In addition, prospective studies suggest that postmenopausal ERT reduces the risks for both CHD and osteoporotic fractures (2). The major concern about ERT is the possibility of an increased risk for breast cancer. Expert opinion based on available data is divided about this risk. Moreover, the fear of breast cancer dissuades many women from starting ERT. Most investigators believe that the reduction in deaths from CHD and osteoporosis will exceed the increase in deaths from breast cancer, but the precise balance between positive and negative aspects of ERT must await a controlled clinical trial.

Maximal Nondrug Therapy. The combination of changes in eating habits and other life habits that reduce risk for CHD can be termed *maximal nondrug therapy*. The concept of maximal nondrug therapy is useful because it incorporates all of the changes, short of drugs, that can be used to achieve risk reduction. Table 75.6 lists the components of maximal nondrug therapy. In addition to the factors discussed above, avoiding smoking or smoking cessation must top the list. Adoption of this list of habits throughout life should lead to a low incidence of CHD into old age. What can be achieved by the combination of all of these beneficial life habits is illustrated by populations in many countries where CHD rates are low (60). Unfortunately, urbanization and industrialization occurring in many previously low-risk populations are changing eating patterns and life habits and are markedly increasing the risk for cardiovascular disease in these populations.

Cholesterol-Lowering Drugs. For patients with established CHD, it has been recommended that LDL-cholesterol levels be reduced to the optimal range (i.e., ≤100 mg/dL) (1, 2). Many patients with mild hypercholesterolemia cannot achieve this goal by dietary change alone. Cholesterol-lowering drug therapy is required in addition to dietary change. The drugs in this category and their characteristics are considered below.

Table 75.6
Maximal Nondrug Therapy

Smoking avoidance or cessation
Reduced dietary cholesterol-raising fatty acids
Reduced dietary cholesterol
Achieve and maintain desirable body weight
Regular physical activity
Reduced dietary salt
Increased fruits and colored vegetables
Antioxidant vitamins

Moderate Hypercholesterolemia

Total cholesterol levels in the range of 240 to 300 mg/dL constitute moderate hypercholesterolemia, defined more specifically as serum LDL-cholesterol levels in the range from 160 to 219 mg/dL (1, 2). These higher cholesterol levels produce a still greater increment in CHD risk. Approximately 20% of American adults have moderate hypercholesterolemia (2). The causes of moderate elevations of LDL-cholesterol are similar to those for mild hypercholesterolemia, except that genetic factors play an increasingly dominant role. For most people with moderate hypercholesterolemia, diet modification alone will not reduce their serum cholesterol levels to the desirable range. Instead, responsible genetic factors will maintain some LDL elevation. Our studies have identified several different patterns of LDL metabolism that underlie a rise in LDL-cholesterol from the mild to the moderate range (12, 61). These patterns include *(a)* higher rate of formation of LDL, *(b)* lower fractional clearance rate for LDL, and (c) enrichment of LDL particles with esterified cholesterol. The mechanisms underlying each of these factors are examined briefly below.

Causes of Moderate Hypercholesterolemia

Overproduction of LDL. In patients with moderate hypercholesterolemia, two potential mechanisms underlie the overproduction of LDL: *(a)* increased input of VLDL particles and *(b)* reduced uptake of VLDL remnants by the liver (12, 61). Both changes should increase total amounts of VLDL converted to LDL. Isotope kinetic studies (61) suggest that either mechanism can occur in persons with moderate hypercholesterolemia. These mechanisms seemingly can be distinguished by differences in the fractional catabolic rate (FCR) for LDL. In persons who overproduce VLDL particles, input rates for LDL are high and FCRs for LDL are relatively low; low FCRs for LDL occur because LDL receptors are relatively overloaded with an excess of lipoprotein particles, reducing the fractional clearance of LDL. On the other hand, in persons who have a decreased uptake of VLDL remnants, high rates of LDL input are combined with increased FCRs for LDL. High inputs of LDL are due to increased fractional conversion of VLDL to LDL; high FCRs for LDL can be explained by increased availability of LDL receptors because of reduced uptake of VLDL remnants by LDL receptors. Our studies (61) suggest that the first pattern (overproduction of lipoprotein particles) probably occurs because of heightened genetic sensitivity to the effects of mild obesity. The mechanism for the second pattern (reduced remnant uptake and increased conversion of VLDL to LDL) has not yet been determined.

Reduced Clearance of LDL. Another pattern of LDL metabolism responsible for moderate hypercholesterolemia is reduced fractional clearance of LDL. This abnormality presumably reflects decreased availability of

LDL receptors (12, 61). Some of the dietary or acquired factors listed above can suppress synthesis of LDL receptors. In patients with moderate hypercholesterolemia, however, genetic factors presumably become increasingly important. Since regulation of LDL-receptor expression is complex, the genetic aberrations underlying a moderately reduced synthesis of LDL receptors have not been fully elucidated. A few individuals may have mutations in the gene encoding LDL receptors (62), although such mutations usually produce severe hypercholesterolemia. Polymorphisms in other genes that indirectly influence LDL receptor synthesis are more likely candidates to explain moderate hypercholesterolemia. To date, few of these genetic polymorphisms have been discovered.

Cholesterol-Enriched LDL. Some individuals have moderately elevated serum LDL-cholesterol concentrations because their LDL particles contain excessive amounts of cholesteryl ester (12, 60–62). The reasons for this compositional change are not known. Cholesteryl ester–enriched LDL particles are more likely to occur in persons who have relatively low FCRs for LDL; in such persons, the slow clearance of LDL may allow more time for cholesteryl esters to enter LDL particles through the action of the plasma cholesteryl ester transfer protein (CETP) (64, 65). In patients without a reduced clearance rate for LDL, an increased plasma concentration of CETP may account for cholesterol-enriched LDL particles (65).

Management of Moderate Hypercholesterolemia

According to the NCEP (1, 2), the intensity of cholesterol-lowering therapy in patients with moderate hypercholesterolemia depends on their absolute risk status. Patients can be classified as being at either *moderate risk* or *high risk,* according to the number of other coronary risk factors present. The risk factors used in this classification are listed in Table 75.7. Patients with moderate hypercholesterolemia who have zero or one other risk factor are designated at moderate risk; those who have two or more additional risk factors are considered at high risk. All patients in these categories must be devoid of clinical CHD.

Table 75.8 outlines the general therapeutic approach to patients with moderate hypercholesterolemia, as recommended by NCEP (1, 2). Treatment decisions are based on LDL-cholesterol levels. Moderate-risk patients can be separated into those with moderately elevated LDL-cholesterol levels of 160 to 189 mg/dL and those with higher levels, from 190 to 219 mg/dL. The goal of therapy in both subgroups is to reduce the serum LDL-cholesterol level below 160 mg/dL. Most patients with LDL-cholesterol levels of 160 to 189 mg/dL should reach their treatment goal by maximal nondrug therapy (Table 75.6). However, some patients may require low doses of drugs to achieve their LDL-cholesterol target. Most patients with still higher LDL-cholesterol levels (190–219 mg/dL) will require cholesterol-lowering drugs at standard doses to lower LDL-cholesterol below 160 mg/dL. The major cholesterol-lowering drugs currently available are listed in Table 75.9. They include bile acid sequestrants and HMG-CoA reductase inhibitors (statins). The daily doses of sequestrants and statins required to produce approximately 15 and 30% lowering of LDL-cholesterol levels, respectively, are shown.

The major drugs currently in use in the United States are statins. These drugs inhibit cholesterol synthesis in the liver and raise the activity of LDL receptors (66, 68). All statins are identical in mechanism, but they differ in dose responsiveness. Side effects appear to be mechanism related; it is doubtful that any of the statins carry unique advantages. Bile acid sequestrants also can be effective cholesterol-lowering drugs. Sequestrants interfere with the reabsorption of bile acids by the intestine; this action

Table 75.7
Coronary Heart Disease Risk Factors

Cigarette smoking
Hypertension
Diabetes mellitus
Low HDL cholesterol (<35 mg/dL)
Advancing age
Men >45 years
Women >55 years or postmenopausal

Table 75.8
Treatment Decisions Based on LDL-Cholesterol

Dietary (nondrug) therapy		
	Initiation level	LDL goal
Without CHD and with fewer than 2 risk factors	≥160 mg/dL	<160 mg/dL
Without CHD and with 2 or more risk factors	≥130 mg/dL	<130 mg/dL
Drug treatment		
	Consideration level	LDL goal
Without CHD and with fewer than 2 risk factors	≥190 mg/dL[a]	<160 mg/dL
Without CHD and with 2 or more risk factors	≥160 mg/dL	<130 mg/dL

[a]In men under 35 years old and premenopausal women with LDL-cholesterol levels 190–219 mg/dL, drug therapy should be delayed except in high-risk patients such as those with diabetes.

Table 75.9
Cholesterol-Lowering Drugs

Drugs	Dose
Bile acid sequestrants	
Cholestyramine	8–12 g/day[a]
Colestipol	10–15 g/day[a]
HMG-CoA reductase inhibitors	
Lovastatin	40 mg[b]
Pravastatin	40 mg[b]
Simvastatin	20 mg[b]
Fluvastatin	80 mg[b]
Atorvastatin	10 mg[b]

[a]Dose required to produce an approximate 15% reduction in LDL-cholesterol.
[b]Dose required to produce an approximate 30% reduction in LDL-cholesterol.

enhances conversion of cholesterol into bile acids in the liver, reducing hepatic cholesterol content and enhancing the activity of LDL receptors (68).

Physicians may be tempted to use cholesterol-lowering drugs and ignore dietary modification in hypercholesterolemic patients who are at moderate risk for CHD. There are two reasons to resist this temptation. First, effective dietary modification alone may achieve the LDL-cholesterol target without the need for drugs; moreover, when drugs are required, the dose of drug may be lessened by use of maximal nondrug therapy (Table 75.6). Second, implementation of a maximal nondrug regimen addresses multiple factors involved in CHD risk and should reduce the risk for CHD beyond that achievable by lowering LDL-cholesterol per se.

The NCEP recommends that cholesterol-lowering drugs generally be avoided in men below age 35 and in premenopausal women who are at only moderate risk of CHD (2). The very long term consequences of cholesterol-lowering drugs are unknown; side effects possibly could develop after prolonged drug usage. In addition, the cost:benefit ratio for long-term therapy will be high. However, some authorities believe that bile acid sequestrants are indicated for young adult men who have LDL-cholesterol levels in the range of 190 to 219 mg/dL (2). Some authorities also contend that hypercholesterolemic, diabetic patients deserve intensive cholesterol-lowering therapy, even in the absence of other risk factors.

Maximal nondrug therapy for patients with moderate hypercholesterolemia includes the step II diet (Table 75.10). This diet calls for reducing dietary cholesterol to less than 200 mg/day and cholesterol-raising fatty acids to less than 7% of total calories (2). The step II diet should be supplemented by weight control, increased exercise, and other modifications noted in Table 75.6.

For patients classified as high risk because of multiple (two or more) risk factors, the goal of therapy is to reduce LDL-cholesterol to less than 130 mg/dL (2). Most high-risk patients will require cholesterol-lowering drugs to achieve this LDL-cholesterol target. Again, *maximal dietary therapy will facilitate obtaining this LDL target and will provide additional benefits to further reduce risk.*

Frequently, however, it is not possible to reach an LDL-cholesterol below 130 mg/dL without the use of cholesterol-lowering drugs. In patients with LDL-cholesterol levels in the higher ranges, appropriately higher doses of statins may be required. Alternatively, a lower dose of statin can be combined with a bile acid sequestrant to obtain an enhanced LDL-lowering response.

Table 75.10
Step II Diet

Nutrient	Percentage of Total Calories
Total fat	≤30
Cholesterol-raising fatty acids[a]	<7
Monounsaturated fatty acids	10–15
Polyunsaturated fatty acids	<10
Carbohydrate	≥55
Protein	15
Cholesterol	<200 mg/day

[a]Includes saturated fatty acids (C8-C16) and *trans* fatty acids.

The benefits of cholesterol-lowering drugs in high-risk patients with moderate hypercholesterolemia were demonstrated in the West of Scotland Coronary Prevention Study (WOSCOPS) (5). In this study, 6595 middle-aged men were randomized between placebo and the statin pravastatin (40 mg/day). After 5 years, pravastatin therapy produced a 31% reduction in recurrent coronary morbidity, a 33% reduction in CHD mortality, and a 22% reduction in total mortality.

In very high risk patients with moderate hypercholesterolemia (i.e., those with established CHD or other forms of clinical atherosclerotic disease), the target for LDL-cholesterol reduction is still lower, namely, 100 mg/dL or less (2). Most hypercholesterolemic patients with CHD require aggressive therapy with cholesterol-lowering drugs. The benefit of statin therapy in patients in this category was documented by the Scandinavian Simvastatin Survival Study (3). This study randomized 4444 hypercholesterolemic patients with established CHD to placebo or simvastatin (20–40 mg/day) for 5 years. At the end of this period, the group that received simvastatin therapy experienced a 34% reduction in myocardial infarction, a 42% reduction in CHD mortality, and a 30% reduction in total mortality, compared with the group receiving placebo.

Severe Hypercholesterolemia

Causes of Severe Hypercholesterolemia

A small portion of the population has *severe hypercholesterolemia,* i.e., serum LDL-cholesterol levels of 220 mg/dL or higher. Most patients with severe hypercholesterolemia have reduced LDL receptor activity, although the elevated LDL-cholesterol concentrations may be accentuated in some persons by overproduction of lipoproteins by the liver or by enrichment of LDL particles with cholesteryl ester (12, 61). Almost certainly, genetic factors play the predominant role in development of severe hypercholesterolemia; in most patients of this type, however, the precise genetic defect(s) has not been elucidated.

A small portion of severely hypercholesterolemic patients have mutations in the gene encoding the LDL receptor. This genetic abnormality produces the hereditary condition called familial hypercholesterolemia (FH) (25). Affected patients can have either heterozygous FH or homozygous FH, depending on whether one or both alleles for the LDL-receptor gene are defective. Heterozygous FH occurs once in 500 people, whereas homozygous FH is present once in 1,000,000 people. LDL-cholesterol concentrations are approximately doubled in heterozygous FH and are elevated fourfold in homozygous FH. A related disorder is called familial defective apolipoprotein B-100 (FDB) (69, 70). This form of hypercholesterolemia is characterized by a defect in the structure of the apo-B-100 protein such that it fails to bind normally to LDL receptors; consequently, clearance of LDL from the circulation is retarded. Patients with FDB can have either moderate or severe hypercholesterolemia.

Management of Severe Hypercholesterolemia

Patients with severe hypercholesterolemia must be considered at high risk, and most will require cholesterol-lowering drugs. However, the choice of drugs and timing of their institution requires clinical judgment. Drug therapy can be delayed in most children with heterozygous FH until adolescence (71). Exceptions are those with very severe hypercholesterolemia. Before adulthood, FH patients generally should avoid statins but can be treated with bile acid sequestrants. Later, statins can be introduced. In adults with heterozygous FH, use of statins and bile acid sequestrants in combination may be required to achieve an acceptably low level of LDL-cholesterol (72, 73). Even when drugs are used to treat heterozygous FH, maximal nondrug therapy should be used to maximize risk reduction. Patients with oligogenic (or polygenic) forms of severe hypercholesterolemia should be treated similarly to patients with monogenic, heterozygous FH.

The very rare patients with homozygous FH must undergo lipid-lowering therapy from early life. Some patients have defective but mildly functioning LDL receptors; these patients show some response to statin therapy. When serum cholesterol levels remain severely elevated, which is usually the case, a procedure to remove LDL directly from the circulation will be required. The procedure currently used, called LDL pheresis, filters plasma through a resin that binds LDL, reducing the plasma LDL concentration (74).

CHYLOMICRONEMIA

Chylomicrons are lipoproteins that carry newly absorbed dietary fat into the circulation. These lipoproteins derive their triglycerides from dietary fat (also see Chapter 4). When fat enters the intestinal tract, it is hydrolyzed by pancreatic lipase into fatty acids and monoglycerides. Uptake of these lipids into intestinal mucosal cells is facilitated by biliary products—the bile salts and phospholipids. Following uptake by enterocytes, fatty acids and monoglycerides are resynthesized into triglycerides. These triglycerides are transferred into newly formed chylomicron particles by MTP (27, 28).

The core of chylomicron particles is composed almost exclusively of triglycerides, but a small amount of cholesteryl ester, derived from newly absorbed cholesterol, also is present. The major apolipoprotein of chylomicrons is apo-B-48. In addition, apo-Cs (CII and CIII), and apo-As (AI and AIV) are present on the surface of chylomicrons. Chylomicrons are secreted into the lymphatic circulation where they pass via the thoracic duct into the systemic circulation. When chylomicrons distribute into the peripheral microcirculation, they come into contact with LPL located on the surface of capillary endothelial cells. LPL hydrolyzes the triglycerides of chylomicrons and releases their free (unesterified) fatty acids (FFAs) into the circulation. Much LPL is located in the capillary beds of adipose tissue and, consequently, much of the newly released FFA is taken up directly by adipocytes where FFAs are reesterified to form triglycerides for storage. FFA released during lipolysis of chylomicron triglyceride also can be taken up by liver or muscle. In fact, muscle cells also express LPL, which facilitates FFA uptake by muscle. When lipolysis of triglycerides is almost complete, a residual lipoprotein, called a chylomicron remnant, reenters the circulation and is removed rapidly by the liver. Chylomicron remnants are cholesterol-enriched lipoproteins, and some investigators believe that they have atherogenic potential.

Type I Hyperlipoproteinemia

Lipoprotein Lipase Deficiency

A lipoprotein pattern of increased chylomicrons with relatively normal VLDL concentrations is called *type I hyperlipoproteinemia* (75). Mutations in the gene for LPL can lead to deficient enzyme activity that results in type I hyperlipoproteinemia (75). The severity of the resulting chylomicronemia depends on the nature of the mutations. A few patients are homozygous for severe defects; they develop severe chylomicronemia when the diet contains appreciable amounts of fat. A sizable number of defects in the LPL gene responsible for this form of hyperlipidemia have been discovered (76). The severity of the resulting hypertriglyceridemia depends on whether the LPL gene is functionally absent or has some, but diminished, function.

Patients who completely lack LPL activity develop severe chylomicronemia shortly after birth (77). Depending on the level of fat intake, triglyceride levels can vary from 1,000 to 10,000 mg/dL. When triglycerides exceed 2000 mg/dL, the risk for acute pancreatitis increases greatly. Pancreatitis can occur even in infancy when chylomicronemia is severe. In LPL-deficient patients, increases in plasma triglycerides are predominantly in chylomicrons; serum VLDL triglycerides generally are not strikingly elevated. This lack of severely raised VLDL triglycerides probably reflects a relatively low hepatic output of VLDL particles by the liver. An increase in serum chylomicrons alone probably does not promote development of atherosclerosis, because chylomicrons are large lipoproteins and seemingly do not penetrate into the arterial wall.

Apolipoprotein CII Deficiency

Apo-CII is an apolipoprotein that activates LPL. Rare patients have a genetic deficiency of apo-CII (77, 78); as a result, LPL remains nonfunctional, and chylomicron triglycerides cannot be hydrolyzed. Affected patients have severe chylomicronemia similar to those with LPL deficiency. They, too, have the pattern of type I hyperlipoproteinemia.

Type V Hyperlipoproteinemia

Type V hyperlipoproteinemia is characterized by high serum levels of both chylomicrons and VLDL (75, 79). In contrast to genetic deficiencies of LPL and apo-CII, type V hyperlipoproteinemia typically appears later in life (79). Two defects in triglyceride metabolism appear to underlie this disorder (80): overproduction of VLDL particles by the liver and a delay in lipolysis of TGRLPs. An excess of circulating VLDL particles caused by overproduction will accentuate any defect in lipolysis for TGRLP, because lipolytic mechanisms become saturated with excess TGRLP, causing their retention in plasma (81). Elevations of chylomicrons in type V hyperlipoproteinemia can be explained in part by saturation of lipolysis with excess VLDL. In addition, the inherent activity of LPL may be reduced in some patients with type V hyperlipoproteinemia (77). This added defect exacerbates the serum accumulation of both VLDL and chylomicrons.

Overproduction of VLDL triglycerides in type V hyperlipoproteinemia usually results from hepatic overload of lipids secondary to excessive release of FFA by adipose tissue. High serum FFA levels most often result from obesity and other disorders of adipose tissue (82, 83). In obese patients, the rate of lipolysis of adipocyte triglyceride is abnormally high, leading to increased release of FFAs; increased hepatic uptake of FFAs; oversynthesis of hepatic triglycerides; and overproduction of VLDL triglycerides (84, 85). When obese patients have predominantly truncal obesity, the release of FFAs from adipose is further accentuated and hypertriglyceridemia is more severe (86, 87). The same is true in patients with non-insulin-dependent diabetes mellitus (NIDDM) in whom insulin levels are not raised enough to dampen FFA release from adipose tissue. Rare patients with partial lipodystrophy, in whom regions of adipose tissue are absent, are prone to hepatic lipid accumulation and type V hyperlipoproteinemia (88). An even more-severe accumulation of hepatic lipid occurs in patients who completely lack adipose tissue (generalized lipodystrophy) (89). Because of high serum FFA levels, patients with generalized obesity and other disorders of adipose tissue usually have lipid overloading in liver and skeletal muscle. These excess accumulations of tissue lipids interfere with the normal cellular metabolism of glucose, producing a condition called insulin resistance (90, 91). Insulin resistance in skeletal muscle interferes with glucose uptake by this tissue. Most patients with type V hyperlipoproteinemia also have insulin resistance in liver that appears to be intimately related to overproduction of VLDL triglycerides (92, 93).

As mentioned above, another defect in type V hyperlipoproteinemia is defective lipolysis of TGRLPs (80). Many patients appear to have an inherent defect in lipolytic capacity in addition to having the lipolytic system saturated by excess TGRLP. Some probably have polymorphisms in LPL that reduce lipase function. However, insulin resistance in the liver again is involved because it raises hepatic production of apo-CIII (94), an apolipoprotein that interferes with LPL activity (95). Thus, not only do lipid overload and insulin resistance in the liver lead to overproduction of VLDL triglyceride, but they also cause a lipolytic defect for TGRLP by inducing excessive synthesis of apo-CIII.

Management of Chylomicronemias

Type I Hyperlipoproteinemia

Patients with type I hyperlipoproteinemia lack LPL activity because of mutations in the LPL gene or the apo-CII gene. No triglyceride-lowering drugs are available to overcome these defects. The only effective means of preventing severe chylomicronemia is to reduce dietary fat. Fat intake should be reduced below 10% of total calories. Triglycerides containing medium-chain fatty acids can be substituted in part for long-chain fatty acids because medium-chain fatty acids are not incorporated into chylomicrons, and thus, their ingestion does not induce chylomicronemia. The purpose of treatment of severe chylomicronemia is to lessen the danger of acute pancreatitis—not to decrease the risk of CHD.

Type V Hyperlipoproteinemia

In type V hyperlipoproteinemia, very low fat diets also are necessary to reduce the severity of chylomicronemia. Moreover, weight reduction in obese patients, combined with increased physical activity, will lessen overproduction of VLDL by reducing hepatic lipid overload. However, in many patients with type V hyperlipoproteinemia, changes in eating and exercise habits alone do not effectively control their severe hypertriglyceridemia. Such patients require triglyceride-lowering drugs.

The fibric acids are one class of effective drugs (96). Available fibric acids include clofibrate, gemfibrozil, fenofibrate, and bezafibrate. Gemfibrozil is the agent currently used in the United States, whereas the latter two are more commonly used in Europe. All the fibric acids have a similar mechanism of action. Recent studies show that they act mainly by binding to the class of nuclear receptors called perioxisomal proliferation-activating receptors–α (PPAR-α) (97) (see also Chapter 36). Activation of these receptors initiates a cascade of reactions that elicits changes in apo-CIII and LPL: synthesis of apo-CIII in liver is reduced, and synthesis of LPL in peripheral tissues is increased. In addition, fibrates may increase oxidation of fatty acids in the liver. All of these changes act to lower serum concentrations of TGRLP. Most patients with type V hyperlipoproteinemia require fibric acids for effective control of hypertriglyceridemia. Reduction of chylomicronemia lessens the risk for acute pancreatitis; decreasing VLDL levels may also reduce the risk for developing CHD, although this latter benefit has not been proven.

Another agent for treatment of type V hyperlipoproteinemia is nicotinic acid. At low intakes, nicotinic acid acts as a vitamin (see Chapter 23); in high doses, it becomes a triglyceride-lowering drug. Its precise mechanism of action is not known, although it appears to act in the liver to reduce formation of VLDL (98). This action often controls severe hypertriglyceridemia. Although nicotinic acid is highly effective as a triglyceride-lowering drug, side effects are not uncommon. Typical side effects include gastrointestinal irritation, hepatotoxicity, flushing and itching of the skin, and hyperuricemia. In diabetic patients, nicotinic acid can worsen insulin resistance and raise glucose levels (99). For these reasons, this drug is used less frequently in the treatment of type V hyperlipoproteinemia than are the fibric acids.

ATHEROGENIC DYSLIPIDEMIA

Causes of Atherogenic Dyslipidemia

A third major category of lipoprotein abnormalities can be called *atherogenic dyslipidemia* (100). This form of dyslipidemia is characterized by a constellation of lipoprotein abnormalities occurring together. Four components typically make up atherogenic dyslipidemia: *(a)* mild hypercholesterolemia, *(b)* mild-to-moderate hypertriglyceridemia, *(c)* small, dense LDL particles, and *(d)* low HDL-cholesterol. Atherogenic dyslipidemia generally does not result from a single metabolic defect but from the coexistence of several defects. Five causes for atherogenic dyslipidemia are recognized: *(a)* obesity, *(b)* diets high in cholesterol-raising fatty acids, *(c)* physical inactivity, *(d)* aging, and *(e)* genetics (100). These causes resemble the categories of factors underlying hypercholesterolemia; however, among them, obesity and physical inactivity tend to predominate in atherogenic dyslipidemia, whereas a diet high in cholesterol-raising fatty acids and aging more commonly cause hypercholesterolemia. Patterns of genetic aberration also tend to differ in patients with atherogenic dyslipidemia and those with predominant hypercholesterolemia.

Atherogenic Dyslipidemia and the Metabolic Syndrome

The major causes of atherogenic dyslipidemia may, simultaneously, be responsible for other nonlipid risk factors, notably hypertension, NIDDM, and a prothrombotic state. The coexistence of these several risk factors can be called the syndrome of multiple metabolic risk factors, or simply the "metabolic syndrome" (100). This syndrome is extremely common in patients with atherogenic dyslipidemia. Obesity usually is present in patients with the metabolic syndrome and is often the predominant cause. As indicated above, obesity produces high levels of FFA that overload the liver with lipid, and excess hepatic lipid predisposes to atherogenic dyslipidemia. This sequence also causes insulin resistance, which may cause NIDDM; it also can raise blood pressure; and it may induce a prothrombotic state (101). These multiple actions of obesity that initiate the metabolic syndrome are commonly augmented by lack of exercise, aging, diet, and genetic factors. Because of the concurrence of several metabolic risk factors in the metabolic syndrome, it is difficult to dissect the relative contributions of each risk factor to atherogenesis. Nonetheless, evidence exists that each of them are independently atherogenic, and when the impact of all of the risk factors is summed, together they substantially raise the risk for CHD.

Some investigators postulate that the underlying abnormality responsible for the metabolic syndrome is a state of insulin resistance (102). The metabolic basis of insulin resistance is exceedingly complex and may arise from a host of different biochemical defects. These defects produce a generalized metabolic disorder. A common feature of this disorder is one in which fatty acids displace glucose as the predominant energy source (91, 92). For example, one cause of insulin resistance is tissue uptake of excess fatty acids derived from adipose tissue. The metabolic consequence of this overloading of tissues with lipids is inhibition of insulin action at the cellular level, which leads secondarily to hyperinsulinemia. Thus, a state of disordered metabolism, which has been called insulin resistance, is commonly present in patients exhibiting multiple metabolic risk factors, including atherogenic dyslipidemia (102). The following discussion briefly reviews the causes and features of each component of atherogenic dyslipidemia.

Components of Atherogenic Dyslipidemia

Mild Hypercholesteroemia

Most persons in the United States having the other components of atherogenic dyslipidemia also manifest mild hypercholesterolemia, i.e., a serum LDL-cholesterol concentration ranging from 130 to 159 mg/dL (borderline high, see Table 75.1). Since some LDL elevation is prerequisite for atherogenesis, LDL concentrations are usually in the mildly elevated range when patients with atherogenic dyslipidemia develop premature CHD. The causes of mild hypercholesterolemia are described above. In patients with atherogenic dyslipidemia, obesity often is a major contributing cause of elevated serum LDL, but the other factors considered above can play a role as well.

Mild-to-Moderate Hypertriglyceridemia

Most people with atherogenic dyslipidemia have some elevation in plasma triglycerides. Two categories of triglyceride elevation are mild hypertriglyceridemia (triglycerides 150–199 mg/dL) and moderate hypertriglyceridemia (200—500 mg/dL). Elevations of serum triglycerides occur mostly in the VLDL fraction. The usual cause of mild-to-moderate hypertriglyceridemia is increased hepatic production of VLDL secondary to obesity (84, 85). Production rates of VLDL triglycerides can be further enhanced by decreased physical inactivity or by high-carbohydrate intakes (103). Overproduction of VLDL triglycerides often unmasks mild defects in lipolysis; this combination of abnormalities frequently raises serum triglycerides into the hypertriglyceridemic range (85, 104). Mild lipolytic defects may be of genetic origin, possibly due to mild abnormalities in the expression of LPL. As already noted (69), insulin resistance, common in patients with atherogenic dyslipidemia, is accompanied by overproduction of apo-CIII (94), an apolipoprotein that inhibits the activity of LPL (95) and induces a lipolytic defect.

An important question is whether an elevation of VLDL particles directly promotes development of atherosclerosis. To address this question, it must be recognized that VLDL particles are not homogenous in size or composition. At least two varieties of VLDL should be distinguished: *(a)* newly secreted VLDL and *(b)* VLDL remnants. Although they are similar in density, the lipid compositions of newly secreted VLDL and VLDL remnants differ. VLDL remnants consist of partially catabolized VLDL; some of their triglycerides have been hydrolyzed, and they have acquired more cholesteryl esters. In fact, in fasting serum, most VLDL particles are remnants. There is growing evidence that VLDL remnants have an atherogenic potential comparable to that of LDL. In contrast, newly secreted VLDLs probably are not atherogenic. The atherogenicity of VLDL remnants is most striking in type III hyperlipoproteinemia (75, 105). In this condition, catabolism of VLDL remnants is curtailed because of a genetic defect in the structure of apo-E that impairs binding of VLDL remnants to hepatic LDL receptors (105). Because of their slow removal from the circulation, remnants in type III hyperlipoproteinemia accumulate excessive amounts of cholesteryl esters; apparently, this excess cholesterol makes them highly atherogenic.

Small Dense LDL Particles

Another feature of atherogenic dyslipidemia is an abnormality in LDL particle size, specifically, the abnormally small LDL particles (100, 106). Small LDL particles frequently occur in patients with premature CHD (106–108). They may have greater atherogenic potential than normal-sized LDL. The unusually high atherogenicity of small LDLs could have several reasons. For example, they could enter the arterial wall more readily than larger LDLs. Moreover, they appear to be more sensitive to oxidation than larger LDLs (109); this too could enhance their atherogenicity. In spite of these possibilities, it is difficult to quantify the increased risk that accompanies having small LDL particles, mainly because of confounding associations between small LDLs and other components of atherogenic dyslipidemia and/or other risk factors of the metabolic syndrome (100).

One cause of small LDL particles is an elevation of serum triglycerides. High triglyceride levels partially deplete LDLs of cholesteryl esters because cholesteryl esters in LDLs are exchanged for excess triglycerides in VLDLs. As hydrolysis of LDL triglycerides by LPL continues, small relatively cholesterol-depleted LDLs are formed. Another cause of small LDLs may be an increased activity of HTGL. This enzyme degrades both triglycerides and phospholipids in LDLs, thereby reducing LDL size and increasing LDL density. The link between small LDL and elevated HTGL also may result from elevated HTGL activity. High HTGL activity may accelerate catabolism of VLDL remnants to LDLs, which will result in fewer VLDL remnants being removed directly by the liver. Consequently, more LDL receptors are available to remove LDLs, and the fractional clearance rate for LDL increases. The amount of cholesteryl ester that accumulates in LDL is a function of the half-life of LDL. If the half-life of LDL is shortened by increased HTGL activity, LDL particles should be smaller and deficient in cholesteryl esters.

Low HDL-Cholesterol

The fourth component of atherogenic dyslipidemia is a low concentration of HDL-cholesterol. In particular, there is a tight link between elevated triglycerides, small LDL particles, and low HDL-cholesterol (106). Prospective epidemiological studies reveal a strong inverse relation between low HDL-cholesterol levels and risk of CHD (110–113). This inverse correlation may have several explanations. First, HDL may directly retard atherogenesis by blocking the atherogenic action of LDL; second, a low HDL level can be a marker for the presence of other components of atherogenic dyslipidemia; and third, a low HDL commonly denotes the presence of the nonlipid risk factors in the metabolic syndrome (114). These several links may explain why low HDL levels have been reported to be such a strong predictor of CHD (110–113).

The underlying causes of low HDL-cholesterol are the same as those for other causes of atherogenic dyslipidemia: obesity, lack of exercise, aging, diet, and genetics. Increasing obesity causes a progressive fall in HDL-cholesterol concentration (18, 19). Sedentary life habits lower HDL levels; these low levels can be reversed by regular and vigorous exercise (115). Both obesity and lack of exercise increase insulin resistance, and insulin resistance is reported to be common in patients with low HDL-cholesterol levels (116). One dietary pattern resulting in low HDL levels is a low-fat, high-carbohydrate diet (117, 118). Cigarette smoking also reduces serum HDL levels (119). Finally, genetic polymorphism accounts for about 50% of the variation in serum HDL-cholesterol levels in the general population (120, 121); therefore, genetic factors probably contribute to many cases of low serum HDL levels.

There is genetic control over a large number of key

metabolic pathways affecting the level of HDL-cholesterol. For instance, multiple genetic factors contribute to higher serum triglyceride levels. Higher serum triglycerides, in turn, are accompanied by lower HDL-cholesterol concentrations (122). Triglycerides in TGRLP exchange for cholesteryl esters in HDL, thereby lowering HDL-cholesterol levels. One factor under genetic control that affects both triglyceride and HDL-cholesterol levels is LPL; patients with low HDL levels often have reduced LPL activity (123, 124). Another determinant of HDL levels is HTGL activity. Increased HTGL activity commonly accompanies reduced serum HDL-cholesterol levels (114, 124). Recent studies (121, 125) indicate that polymorphism in the HTGL gene accounts for about half of the genetic contribution to variation in HDL-cholesterol concentrations. Current evidence suggests that increased HTGL activity facilitates degradation of HDL particles and promotes HDL catabolism (126). Enhanced catabolism of HDL also may occur because of high CETP activity (127); this protein promotes transfer of cholesteryl ester from HDL to TGRLP (64). Genetic polymorphism of the CETP gene accounts for about 20% of the variability of CETP levels in plasma (128). Studies of apolipoprotein kinetics (129, 130) reveal that increased HDL catabolism is responsible for most cases of low serum HDL-cholesterol levels. Accelerated HDL catabolism may be secondary to increased serum triglycerides, reduced LPL activity, increased HTGL activity, and increased CETP activity. All of these changes can be influenced by genetic polymorphism, although acquired factors (e.g., insulin resistance) also may contribute (116). Finally, reduced production of apo-AI may be another cause of low HDL-cholesterol levels (130); production rates of apo-AI likewise appear to be under genetic control (121) (see Chapter 74). Thus, low HDL-cholesterol concentrations, which often are part of the syndrome of atherogenic dyslipidemia, appear to be determined in part by polymorphism in a few key genes that regulate HDL metabolism and in part by external influences on these genes. When patients become insulin resistant, the genetic influences on HDL metabolism are magnified.

Management of Atherogenic Dyslipidemia

The strategy for management of atherogenic dyslipidemia is based on its twofold origin. First, a generalized metabolic disorder—a state of insulin resistance—commonly is present in dyslipidemic patients. But since the severities of particular components of atherogenic dyslipidemia are modified by genetic factors, treatment must be directed toward *(a)* lessening insulin resistance and, when necessary, *(b)* direct therapeutic modification of individual components of the dyslipidemic pattern.

Treatment of Insulin Resistance

Insulin resistance is best reduced by caloric restriction and increased physical activity. Both changes in life habits will lower serum insulin levels and dampen the lipid abnormalities characteristic of atherogenic dyslipidemia. Therefore, weight control and increased physical activity are the foundation of management of atherogenic dyslipidemia.

In recent years, there has been a growing interest in the use of drugs designed specifically to reduce insulin resistance. One drug of this type is metformin. Its primary site of action appears to be the liver. The precise biochemical target of metformin action is not known. However, one consequence of its action is reduced hepatic glucose production, which leads to a decrease in peripheral insulin resistance (131). Associated with this change can be a reduction in plasma triglyceride levels (132). Unfortunately, metformin does not fully correct the metabolic abnormalities characteristic of the insulin-resistant state, and hence, dyslipidemia is only partially improved.

The thiazoladinediones are another class of drugs that can modify cellular metabolism and lessen insulin resistance. Among these, troglitazone is the one currently in clinical use. The thiazoladinediones appear to act by binding to the nuclear receptor, PPAR-γ(133). The biochemical consequences of this action are not fully understood. One response, however, appears to be an inhibition of FFA release from adipose tissue. This action alone should reduce the availability of FFAs for accumulation as lipids in liver and skeletal muscle. Troglitazone also may act directly on liver and skeletal muscle to modify metabolism favorably. These actions result in decreased plasma insulin levels, indicating reduced insulin resistance (134). There are reports that treatment of patients with troglitazone improves atherogenic dyslipidemia (135). However, insulin resistance is only partially corrected by thiazoladinediones, and serum lipid patterns, although improved, usually remain abnormal.

Available data indicate that effective weight reduction and increased physical exercise correct insulin resistance as effectively as drugs (136, 137). In some patients, insulin "sensitizers" may be a useful adjunct, but current agents are too weak to normalize the serum lipid pattern in most patients. The foundation of treatment of atherogenic dyslipidemia, therefore, is weight reduction and physical activity. Unfortunately, in many patients, changes in life habits do not suffice to normalize serum lipids, and lipid-lowering drugs are necessary to normalize the lipoprotein profile.

Treatment of Lipoprotein Disorders of Atherogenic Dyslipidemia. The primary therapeutic target for lipid modification in atherogenic dyslipidemia is elevated serum LDL-cholesterol (100). Reducing the intake of fats containing cholesterol-raising fatty acids and cholesterol will produce some decrease in plasma LDL-cholesterol concentrations. The goals of LDL-lowering therapies depend on a patient's absolute risk for CHD (outlined above in the section "Management of Hypercholesterolemia"). Patients with a high or very high risk of

CHD often require LDL-lowering drugs. The statins are the first line of therapy in higher-risk patients with atherogenic dyslipidemia. Many patients in the CARE study (4) had a lipoprotein pattern characteristic of atherogenic dyslipidemia; the marked reduction in acute coronary events in CARE patients who received pravastatin therapy reveals the benefit of aggressively lowering LDL-cholesterol levels.

The second abnormality of atherogenic dyslipidemia is a high level of VLDL. Reduction in LDL-cholesterol concentrations with statin therapy typically is accompanied by a concomitant decrease in VLDL levels (138, 139), best reflected by decreased VLDL-cholesterol levels. Statin therapy causes similar percentage reductions in both LDL-cholesterol and VLDL-cholesterol levels (138, 139). Much of the reduction in VLDL levels during statin therapy reflects a fall in VLDL remnants. Thus, some of the CHD risk reduction accompanying treatment with statins in patients with atherogenic dyslipidemia probably is due to a decreased level of atherogenic VLDL remnants.

Nonetheless, even with statin therapy, many patients with mild-to-moderate hypertriglyceridemia maintain some elevation of VLDL levels. The question thus arises whether addition of a triglyceride-lowering drug, combined with statins, will provide further benefit. Available drugs to use in combination with statins are fibric acids and nicotinic acid. Their use is attractive because of reports that these drug combinations can normalize lipoprotein patterns (140). However, the incremental benefit of combined drug therapy over statins alone has never been documented in clinical trials designed to quantify CHD risk reduction. Until such trials are carried out, it remains uncertain whether combined-drug therapy, in spite of its theoretical benefits, is advantageous in patients with mild-to-moderate hypertriglyceridemia. Unfortunately, combined-drug therapy carries an increased risk for side effects; combining a fibric acid with a statin raises the likelihood for severe myopathy, whereas use of nicotinic acid in combination therapy increases the chances of hepatotoxicity.

The third component of atherogenic dyslipidemia consists of small dense LDL particles, discussed above. Treatment with statins certainly reduces the concentration of small LDL particles in the circulation, which itself should reduce atherogenic risk. Adding a triglyceride-lowering drug to statin therapy helps convert smaller dense LDL particles into larger particles with lower atherogenic potential (141). This is one theoretical benefit of combined drug therapy. Should future clinical trials show combined-drug therapy to be advantageous, one mechanism of benefit may involve a change in the particle size of LDLs.

The fourth component of atherogenic dyslipidemia is a low HDL-cholesterol level. Statins and fibric acids can elicit modest elevations in HDL-cholesterol levels, in combination they produce moderate increases in HDL-cholesterol (138, 141). However, the best available agent for raising HDL-cholesterol levels is nicotinic acid (142, 143). The combination of a statin and nicotinic acid leads to a particularly striking increase in HDL-cholesterol. In spite of this beneficial response, many patients cannot tolerate nicotinic acid because of its side effects (see above). Certainly, in very high risk patients, an effort can be made to lower LDL-cholesterol concentrations maximally and to raise HDL-cholesterol levels by combined drug therapy. Alternatively, if combining a triglyceride-lowering drug with a statin is unacceptable, the prudent approach may be to lower the LDL-cholesterol level more effectively with a higher dose of statin, thus partially offsetting the risk of a low HDL-cholesterol level.

REFERENCES

1. Expert Panel on Detection, Evaluation, and Treatment of High Blood Cholesterol in Adults. JAMA 1993;269:3015–23.
2. Expert Panel on Detection, Evaluation,and Treatment of High Blood Cholesterol in Adults. Circulation 1994;89:1329–445.
3. Scandinavian Simvastatin Survival Study Group. Lancet 1994;344:1383–9.
4. Sacks FM, Pfeffer MA, Moye LA, et al. N Engl J Med 1996;335:1001–9.
5. Shepherd J, Cobbe SM, Ford I, et al. N Engl J Med 1995; 333:1301–7.
6. Byington RP, Jukema JW, Salonen JT, et al. Circulation 1995;92:2419–25.
7. Brown BG, Zhao X-Q, Sacco DE, Albers JJ. Circulation 1993;87:1781–91.
8. Grundy SM, Wilhelmsen L, Rose R, et al. Eur Heart J 1990; 11:462–71.
9. Anderson TJ, Meredith IT, Yeung AC, et al. N Engl J Med 1995;332:488–93.
10. Brown BG, Zhao X-Q, Bardsley J, Albers JJ. J Intern Med 1997;241:283–94.
11. Stamler J, Wentworth D, Neaton JD. JAMA 1986;256:2823–8.
12. Grundy SM. Arterioscler Thromb 1991;11:1619–35.
13. National Cholesterol Education Program. Circulation 1991; 83:2154–232.
14. Johnson CL, Rifkind BM, Sempos CT, et al. JAMA 1993;269: 3002–8.
15. Federation of American Societies for Experimental Biology, Life Sciences Research Office. Prepared for the Interagency Board for Nutrition Monitoring and Related Research. Third report on nutrition monitoring in the United States, vol 1. Washington, DC: US Government Printing Office, 1995.
16. National Cholesterol Education Program. Circulation 1991; 83:2154–232.
17. Krauss RM, Deckelbaum RJ, Ernst N, et al. Circulation 1996;94:1795–800.
18. Denke MA, Sempos CT, Grundy SM. Arch Intern Med 1993; 153:1093–103.
19. Denke MA, Sempos CT, Grundy SM. Arch Intern Med 1994; 154:401–10.
20. Tzankoff SP, Norris AH. J Appl Physiol 1978;45:536–9.
21. Shah M, Hannan PJ, Jeffery RW. Int J Obes 1991;15:499–503.
22. Law MR, Wald NJ, Wu T, et al. Br Med J 1994;308:363–6.
23. Law MR, Wald NJ, Thompson SM. Br Med J 1994;308:367–73.
24. Perusse L, Despres J, Tremblay A, et al. Arteriosclerosis 1989; 9:308–18.
25. Goldstein JL, Hobbs HH, Brown MS. Familial hypercholesterolemia. In: Scriver CR, Beaudet AL, Sly WS, et al., eds. The

metabolic and molecular bases of inherited disease. New York: McGraw Hill, 1995;1981–2030.
26. Dixon JL, Furukawa S, Ginsberg HN. J Biol Chem 1991;266:5080–6.
27. Wetterau JR, Aggerbeck LP, Bouma M-E, et al. Science 1992; 258:999–1001.
28. Grundy SM. J Lipid Res 1984;25:1611–8.
29. Grundy SM, Vega GL. What is meant by overproduction of apo B-containing lipoproteins? In: Malmendier CL, Alaupovic P, Brewer HB Jr, eds. Hypercholesterolemia, hypocholesterolemia, hypertriglyceridemia. New York: Plenum Press, 1992;213–22.
30. Yokoyama C, Wang X, Briggs MR, et al. Cell 1993;75:187–97.
31. Grundy SM, Vega GL, Bilheimer DW. Arteriosclerosis 1985; 5:623–30.
32. Ericsson S, Eriksson M, Vitols S, et al. J Clin Invest 1991;87:591–6.
33. Kesaniemi YA, Beltz WF, Grundy SM. J Clin Invest 1985; 76:586–95.
34. Egusa G, Beltz WF, Grundy SM, et al. J Clin Invest 1985; 76:596–603.
35. Grundy SM, Denke MA. J Lipid Res 1990;31:1149–72.
36. Mensink RP, Katan MB. N Engl J Med 1990;323:439–45.
37. Judd JT, Clevidence BA, Muesing RA, et al. Am J Clin Nutr 1994;59:861–8.
38. Zock PL, de Vries JHM, Katan MB. Arterioscler Thromb 1994;14:567–75.
39. Denke MA, Grundy SM. Am J Clin Nutr 1992;56:895–8.
40. Cater NB, Heller HJ, Denke MA. Am J Clin Nutr 1997; 65:41–5.
41. Bonanome A, Grundy SM. N Engl J Med 1988;318:1244–8.
42. Denke MA, Grundy SM. Am J Clin Nutr 1991;54:1036–40.
43. Bonanome A, Bennett M, Grundy SM. Atherosclerosis 1992; 94:119–27.
44. Zock PL, Katan MB. J Lipid Res 1992;33:399–410.
45. Dietschy JM, Turley SD, Spady DK. J Lipid Res 1993; 34:1637–59.
46. Daumeri CM, Woollett LA, Dietary JM. Proc Natl Acad Sci USA 1992;89:10797–801.
47. McGill HC Jr, McMahan CA, Kruski AW, Mott GE. Arteriosclerosis 1981;1:3–12.
48. Rudel LL, Parks JS, Bond MG. Ann NY Acad Sci 1985;454:248–53.
49. Grundy SM, Barrett-Connor E, Rudel LL. Arteriosclerosis 1988;8:95–101.
50. Ma PT, Yamamoto T, Goldstein JL, Brown MS. Proc Natl Acad Sci USA 1986;83:792–6.
51. Denke MA. Am J Med 1995;99:29–35.
52. Denke MA, Grundy SM. Arch Intern Med 1994;154:317–25.
53. U.S. Department of Health and Human Services. Physical activity and health: a report of the surgeon general. Atlanta, GA: U.S. Department of Health and Human Services, Centers for Disease Control and Prevention, National Center for Chronic Disease Prevention and Health Promotion, 1966.
54. Katan MB, Grundy SM, Willett WC. N Engl J Med 1997, in press.
55. Connor WE, Connor SL. N Engl J Med 1997, in press.
56. U.S. Department of Agriculture/Department of Health and Human Services. Nutrition and your health: dietary guidelines for Americans, ed 232. Home and garden bull., 1990.
57. Committee on Comparative Toxicity of Naturally Occurring Carcinogens, National Research Council. Carcinogens and anticarcinogens in the human diet: a comparison of naturally occurring and synthetic substances. Washington, DC: National Academy Press, 1996.
58. Jialal I, Devaraj S. J Nutr 1996;126:1053S–7S.
59. Appel LJ, Moore TJ, Obarzanek E, et al. N Engl J Med 1997; 336:1117–24.
60. Keys A. Seven countries: a multivariate analysis on death and coronary heart disease. Cambridge, MA: Harvard University Press, 1980;132.
61. Vega GL, Denke MA, Grundy SM. Circulation 1991;84:118–28.
62. Arca M, Vega GL, Grundy SM. JAMA 1994;271:453–9.
63. Vega GL, Grundy SM. Arterioscler Thromb Vasc Biol 1996; 16:517–22.
64. Tall AR. J Lipid Res 1993;34:1255–74.
65. Tato F, Vega GL, Tall AR, Grundy SM. Arterioscler Thromb Vasc Biol 1995;15:112–20.
66. Endo A. J Lipid Res 1992;33:1569–82.
67. Grundy SM. N Engl J Med 1988;319:24–33.
68. Grundy SM. Bile acid resins. Mechanisms of action. In: Pharmacological control of hyperlipidemia. S.A., J.R. Prous Science Publishers, 1986;3–19.
69. Vega GL, Denke MA, Grundy SM. J Clin Invest 1986;78: 1410–4.
70. Innerarity TL, Mahley RW, Weisgraber KH, et al. J Lipid Res 1990;31:1337–49.
71. National Cholesterol Education Program. Pediatrics 1992; 89(3 Pt 2):525–84.
72. Bilheimer DW, Grundy SM, Brown MS, Goldstein SL. Proc Natl Acad Sci USA 1983;80:4124–8.
73. Bilheimer DW, Eisenberg S, Levy RI. Biochim Biophys Acta 1972;260:212–21.
74. Thompson GR, Maher VM, Matthews S, et al. Lancet 1995;345:811–6.
75. Fredrickson DS, Levy RI, Lees RS. N Engl J Med 1967; 276:34–42, 94–103, 148–56, 215–25, 273–81.
76. Santamarina-Fojo S, Dugi KA. Curr Opin Lipidol 1994; 5:117–25.
77. Brunzell JD. Familial lipoprotein lipase deficiency and other causes of the chylomicronemia syndrome. In: Scriver CR, Beaudet AL, Sly WS, et al., eds. Metabolic and molecular bases of inherited disease. New York: McGraw-Hill, 1989;1116–250.
78. Breckenridge WC, Little JA, Steiner G, et al. N Engl J Med 1978;298:1265–73.
79. Nikkila E: Familial lipoprotein lipase deficiency and related disorders of chylomicron metabolism. In: Stanbury JB, Wyngaarden JB, Fredrickson DS, et al., eds. The metabolic basis of inherited disease. New York: McGraw Hill, 1983;622–42.
80. Kesaniemi YA, Grundy SM. JAMA 1984;251:2542–7.
81. Brunzell JD, Hazzard WR, Porte D Jr, et al. J Clin Invest 1973;52:1578–85.
82. Bjorntorp P, Bergman H, Varnauskas E. Acta Med Scand 1969;185:351–6.
83. Lillioja S, Bogardus C, Mott DM, et al. J Clin Invest 1985;75:1106–15.
84. Grundy SM, Mok HY, Zech L, et al. J Clin Invest 1979;63: 1274–83.
85. Grundy SM. Metabolism of very low density lipoprotein-triglycerides in man. In: Gotto AM, Smith LC, Allen B, eds. Atherosclerosis V. New York: Springer Verlag, 1980;586–90.
86. Freedman DS, Jacobsen SJ, Barboriak JJ, et al. Circulation 1990;81:1498–506.
87. Cigolini M, Seidell JC, Charzewska J, et al. Metabolism 1991;40:781–7.
88. Chait A, Janus E, Mason AS, Lewis B. Clin Endocrinol 1979;10:173–8.
89. Stacpoole PW, Alig J, Kilgore LL, et al. Metabolism 1988;37:944–51.

90. Randle PJ, Garland PB, Hales CN, et al. Lancet 1963;I:785–9.
91. Randle PJ, Priestman DA, Mistry S, Newsholme EA. Diabetologia 1994;37:S155–61.
92. Steiner G, Vranic M. Int J Obes 1982;6(Suppl 1):117–24.
93. Kissebah AH, Alfarsi S, Adams PW, et al. Diabetologia 1976; 12:563–71.
94. Damerman M, Sandkuijl LA, Halaas JL, et al. Proc Natl Acad Sci USA 1993;90:4562–6.
95. Aalto-Setala K, Fisher EA, Chen X, et al. J Clin Invest 1992; 90:1889–900.
96. Grundy SM, Vega GL. Am J Med 1987;83:9–20.
97. Staels B, Vu-Dac N, Kosykh VA, et al. J Clin Invest 1995;95:705–12.
98. Grundy SM, Mok HYI, Zech L, Berman M. J Lipid Res 1981;22:24–36.
99. Garg A, Grundy SM. JAMA 1990;264:723–6.
100. Grundy SM. Circulation 1997;95:1–4.
101. Beck-Nielsen H, Hother-Nielsen O. Obesity in non-insulin-dependent diabetes mellitus. In: Le Roith D, Taylor SI, Olefsky JO, eds. Diabetes mellitus. Philadelphia: Lippincott-Raven, 1996;475–84.
102. Reaven GM. Am Heart J 1991;121:1283–8.
103. Knittle JL, Ahrens EH Jr. J Clin Invest 1964;43:485–95.
104. Grundy SM, Vega GL. Are plasma triglyceride concentrations explained by saturation kinetics? In: Berman M, Grundy SM, Howard BV, eds. Lipoprotein kinetics and modeling. New York: Academic Press, 1982;271–86.
105. Mahley RW, Rall SC Jr. Type III hyperlipoprotein (dysbetalipoproteinemia): the role of apolipoprotein E in normal and abnormal lipoprotein metabolism. In: Scriver CR, Beaudet AL, Sly WS, et al., eds. The metabolic and molecular bases of inherited disease. New York: McGraw-Hill, 1995;1953–80.
106. Austin MA, King M-C, Vranizan KM, Krauss RM. Circulation 1990;82:495–506.
107. Austin MA, Breslow JL, Hennekens CH, et al. JAMA 1988; 260:1917–21.
108. Austin MA, Hokanson JE, Brunzell JD. Curr Opin Lipidol 1994;5:395–403.
109. de Graaf J, Hak-Lemmers HLM, Hectors MPC, et al. Arterioscler Thromb 1991;11:298–306.
110. Miller NE, Thelle DS, Forde OH, Mjos OD. Lancet 1977; 1:965–8.
111. Gordon T, Castelli WP, Hjortland MC, et al. Am J Med 1977; 62:707–14.
112. Assman G, Schulte H, Oberwittler W, et al. New aspects in the prediction of coronary artery disease: the Prospective Cardiovascular Munster Study. In: Fidge NH, Nestel PJ, eds. Atherosclerosis VII. Amsterdam: Elsevier Science Publishers, 1986;19–24.
113. Gordon DJ, Probstfeld JL, Garrison RJ, et al. Circulation 1989;79:8–15.
114. Vega GL, Grundy SM. Curr Opin Lipidol 1996;7:209–16.
115. Durstine JL, Haskell WL. Exerc Sport Sci Rev 1994; 22:477–521.
116. Karhapaa P, Malkki M, Laakso M. Diabetes 1994;43:411–7.
117. Ettinger WH. Med Clin North Am 1989;73:1525–30.
118. Mensink RP, Katan MB. Lancet 1987;1:122–5.
119. Craig WY, Palomaki GE, Haddow JE. Br Med J 1989; 298:784–8.
120. Heller DA, de Faire U, Petersen NL, et al. N Engl J Med 1993;328:1150–66.
121. Cohen JC, Wang Z-F, Grundy SM, et al. J Clin Invest 1994;94:2377–84.
122. Schaefer EJ, Levy RI, Anderson DW, et al. Lancet 1978; 2:391–3.
123. Nikkila EA, Taskinen M-R, Rehunen S, Harkonen M. Metabolism 1978;27:1661–71.
124. Blades B, Vega GL, Grundy SM. Arterioscler Thromb 1993; 13:1227–35.
125. Guerra R, Wang JP, Grundy SM, Cohen JC. Proc Natl Acad Sci USA 1997;94:4532–7.
126. Groot PHE, Scheek LM, Jensen H. Biochim Biophys Acta 1983;751:393–400.
127. Tato F, Vega GL, Grundy S. Arterioscler Thromb Vasc Biol 1995;15:446–51.
128. McPherson R, Grundy SM, Guerra R, et al. J Lipid Res 1996;37:1743–8.
129. Brinton EA, Eisenberg S, Breslow JL. J Clin Invest 1991; 87:536–44.
130. Gylling H, Vega GL, Grundy SM. J Lipid Res 1992;33:1527–39.
131. Widen EI, Eriksson JG, Groop LC. Diabetes 1992;41:354–8.
132. DeFronzo RA, Goodman AM, and the Multicenter Metformin Study Group. N Engl J Med 1995;333:541–9.
133. Forman BM, Chen J, Evans RM. Proc Natl Acad Sci USA 1997;94:4312–7.
134. Nolan JJ, Lukvik B, Beerdsen P, et al. N Engl J Med 1994;331:1188–93.
135. Iwamoto Y, Kosaka K, Kuzuya T, et al. Diabetes Care 1996;19:151–6.
136. Niskanen I, Uusitupa M, Sarlund H, et al. Int J Obes 1996; 20:154–60.
137. Perseghin G, Price TB, Petersen KF, et al. N Engl J Med 1996;335:1357–62.
138. Vega GL, Grundy SM. Arch Intern Med 1990;150:1313–9.
139. Garg A, Grundy SM. N Engl J Med 1988;318:81–6.
140. East C, Bilheimer DW, Grundy SM. Ann Intern Med 1988; 109:25–32.
141. Vega GL, Grundy SM. JAMA 1985;253:2398–403.
142. Vega GL, Grundy SM. Arch Intern Med 1994;154:73–82.
143. Martin-Jadraque R, Tato F, Mostaza JM, et al. Arch Intern Med 1996;156:1081–8.

SELECTED READINGS

Brown BG, Zhao X-Q, Bardsley J, Albers JJ. Secondary prevention of heart disease amongst patients with lipid abnormalities: practice and trends in the United States. J Intern Med 1997;241:283–94.

Denke MA, Sempos CT, Grundy SM. Excess body weight: an underrecognized contributor to dyslipidemia in white American women. Arch Intern Med 1994;154:401–10.

Expert Panel on Detection, Evaluation, and Treatment of High Blood Cholesterol in Adults (Grundy SM, chairman). National Cholesterol Education Program: second report of the Expert Panel on Detection, Evaluation, and Treatment of High Blood Cholesterol (Adult Treatment Panel II). Circulation 1994;89:1329–445.

Grundy SM, Denke MA. Dietary influences on serum lipids and lipoproteins. J Lipid Res 1990;31:1149–72.

Grundy SM. Small LDL, atherogenic dyslipidemia and the metabolic syndrome. Circulation 1997;95:1–4.

76. Nutrition, Diet, and Hypertension

THEODORE A. KOTCHEN and JANE MORLEY KOTCHEN

Between 1971 and 1991, national health examination surveys document a downward trend of blood pressure levels and the prevalence of hypertension in the US (1). Adoption of healthier lifestyles may have contributed to this favorable trend. Nevertheless, hypertension continues to be a major risk factor for cardiovascular disease (1a). As many as 50 million people in the United States have elevated blood pressure (systolic blood pressure >140 mm Hg and/or diastolic blood pressure >90 mm Hg) or are taking antihypertensive medications (2). Blood pressure–associated risks ensue incrementally and progressively over a wide range of blood pressure levels, and a critical value of blood pressure above which individuals are classified as "hypertensive" is arbitrary. Furthermore, even among normotensive individuals, blood pressure level is predictive of morbidity and mortality from stroke, heart disease, and renal impairment (3). Although categorization of individuals as hypertensive or normotensive provides pragmatic guidelines for medical intervention, it insufficiently addresses blood pressure–related risks. Indeed, between 30 and 40% of all blood pressure–related cardiovascular disease events occur in individuals with average blood pressures below currently defined hypertensive levels but above 120/80 mm Hg. A recent consensus report recommended that the goal of treating hypertensive patients is to maintain blood pressure levels below 140/90 mm Hg, and possibly to levels of 130/85 mm Hg, while concurrently controlling other modifiable risk factors (2).

This chapter reviews evidence that specific nutrients and interactions among nutrients influence blood pressure. Figure 76.1 presents a schematized, incomplete compilation of highly interrelated physiologic factors that contribute to regulation of arterial pressure. As discussed below, many of these factors have been implicated as potential mechanisms by which specific nutrients affect blood pressure. An understanding of the relationship between diet and blood pressure has important implications not only for the treatment of hypertension but also for developing population-based strategies to decrease the long-term risk of cardiovascular disease.

SODIUM CHLORIDE

A high sodium chloride (NaCl) intake convincingly contributes to elevated arterial pressure in a number of genetic and acquired models of experimental hypertension. The chimpanzee is phylogenetically close to the human, and in a carefully controlled study, it was recently demonstrated that addition of NaCl to the usual diet of the chimpanzee (a fruit and vegetable diet that is low in sodium and high in potassium) over 20 months results in a significant elevation of blood pressure (4). Blood pressure did not increase in control animals maintained on their usual diets. Despite individual variation, blood pressures increased progressively with progressive increases in dietary NaCl, and at the highest NaCl intake studied, systolic and diastolic pressures increased by 33 mm Hg and 10 mm Hg, respectively. These increases were completely reversed within 6 months of cessation of the high NaCl intake. Animal studies (as well as limited epidemiologic and clinical observations) also suggest that diets high in NaCl may have deleterious cardiovascular consequences independent of blood pressure, e.g., cerebral arterial disease and stroke, left ventricular hypertrophy, renal vascular disease, and glomerular injury (5).

In the human, evidence for an association between NaCl intake and blood pressure is provided by both observational and intervention studies (6–10). The effect of NaCl on blood pressure increases with age, with the height of the blood pressure, and, in normotensive individuals, with a family history of hypertension (11). There may also be a modest association between higher NaCl intake and higher blood pressure in children and adolescents (11a), and results of a recently published randomized trial suggest that a high NaCl intake during the first 5 weeks of life is associated with higher blood pressures during adolescence (11b).

Among populations, the prevalence of hypertension is related to NaCl intake. The Intersalt study describes the relationship between blood pressure and 24-h urine

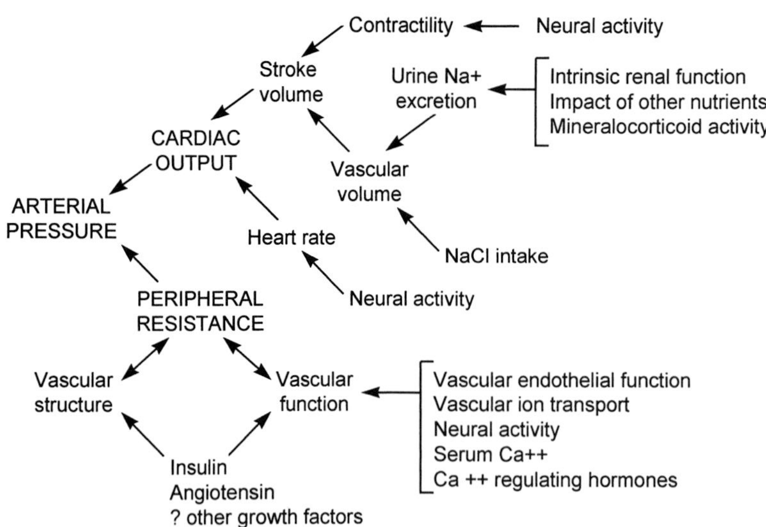

Figure 76.1. Interrelated physiologic factors that contribute to the regulation of arterial pressure. Arterial pressure is determined by cardiac output and peripheral vascular resistance, and cardiac output is determined by stroke volume and heart rate. Cardiac contractility and vascular volume determine stroke volume. Structural and functional changes in the vasculature affect vascular resistance, and increased vascular resistance induces structural and functional changes in the vasculature. Factors that contribute to the regulation of myocardial contractility, vascular volume, and vascular structure and function are also noted.

sodium excretion in over 10,000 individuals at 52 centers around the world (12, 13). Two principal findings of this study are *(a)* a difference of 100 mEq/day in sodium intake is associated with a 3 to 6 mm Hg difference in systolic blood pressure, and *(b)* lowering the sodium intake by 100 mEq/day attenuates the rise of systolic blood pressure in those between the ages of 25 and 55 years by 10 mm Hg.

NaCl Sensitivity

Based on results of acute NaCl depletion or acute NaCl loading protocols (depending on criteria for the definition of NaCl sensitivity), approximately 30 to 50% of hypertensives and a smaller percentage of normotensives are estimated to be NaCl sensitive, i.e., arterial pressure is decreased by NaCl depletion and/or increased by NaCl loading (14, 15). In short-term intervention trials of the effects of moderate NaCl restriction on blood pressure, the overall reduction of blood pressure is relatively small. As reviewed in two recent metaanalyses, reduction of blood pressure by NaCl restriction is more prominent in hypertensive (4.9/2.9–3.7/0.9 mm Hg) than in normotensive (1.7/1.0–1.0/0.1 mm Hg) individuals (16, 17). These modest reductions of blood pressure in normotensives has led some to question recommendations for reducing NaCl intake in the general population (18). However, many of the trials included in the metaanalyses were of short duration (<2 weeks), and the full impact of NaCl reduction on blood pressure may increase over time. It has been estimated that these small reductions of blood pressure in the population would reduce risks of stroke by 15% and coronary heart disease by 6% (19).

The anion accompanying sodium is important in determining the magnitude of the blood pressure increase in response to high dietary intake of NaCl. The full expression of NaCl-sensitive hypertension depends on concomitant administration of both sodium and chloride (20). In both experimental models of NaCl-sensitive hypertension and in the human, blood pressure is not increased by high dietary sodium intake with anions other than chloride, and a high chloride intake without sodium has less effect on blood pressure than NaCl. The failure of nonchloride sodium salts to produce hypertension may be related to their failure to expand plasma volume. In usual diets, however, sodium is generally consumed as NaCl.

Blood pressure responses to sodium may be modified by other components of the diet. Both epidemiologic and clinical evidence suggest that dietary intake of potassium or calcium below the recommended daily allowances (RDA) potentiate NaCl sensitivity of blood pressure (21, 22). Conversely, high dietary intake of potassium or calcium prevents or attenuates development of NaCl-induced hypertension in several animal models. Increasing evidence, primarily in the rat, suggests that high intakes of sucrose potentiate NaCl sensitivity of blood pressure (23); this may be related to an antinatriuretic effect of sucrose.

Within a population, overall blood pressure responses to NaCl restriction may mask individual variability. Experimental models of hypertension and increasing information in the human provide convincing evidence for a genetic susceptibility and a genetic resistance to the effects of dietary NaCl on arterial pressure. A familial resemblance in the change of blood pressure in response to salt restriction has been described, and a phenotype of haptoglobin may be a marker of NaCl sensitivity (24, 25). In the United States, compared with Caucasians, a larger proportion of both normotensive and hypertensive African Americans are NaCl sensitive. Reasons for this are not entirely clear but may in part be genetic. Clinically, there is evidence for heritability of sodium excretion, levels of hormones that regulate sodium excretion, and salt sensitivity of blood pressure in both Caucasians and African Americans. African Americans excrete sodium less efficiently than whites; plasma renin activity tends to be suppressed in African Americans, and low plasma renin may be a surrogate marker for salt sensitivity of blood pressure (26). It has been estimated that more than 50% of African American hypertensives in the U.S. are salt sensitive; the prevalence of diuretic-sensitive (and presumably salt-sensitive) blood pressures approaches 75% (27).

Physiologic Mechanisms of NaCl Sensitivity

Several interrelated blood-pressure control mechanisms may contribute to blood pressure elevations induced by NaCl (Fig. 76.1). Experimental and clinical evidence suggests that a genetically determined decreased capacity to excrete sodium contributes to NaCl-induced elevations of arterial pressure in the susceptible host (28). The Dahl salt-sensitive (Dahl-S) rat is a well-characterized genetic model of low-renin, NaCl-sensitive hypertension associated with insulin resistance (29). In this model, the pressure natriuresis curve (inflow pressure vs. sodium excretion) from the isolated kidney is shifted to the right, i.e., the kidney of the NaCl-sensitive animal requires a greater pressure to excrete sodium than the kidney from the salt-resistant (Dahl-R) rat. Similarly, in the human, several, but not all, investigators reported that NaCl-sensitive hypertensives retain more sodium in response to a NaCl load than NaCl-resistant patients (30).

Nitric oxide is a vascular endothelium–derived vasodilator. In the normal rat, nitric oxide activity increases in response to a high NaCl intake, perhaps facilitating natriuresis and blood pressure homeostasis, and impaired nitric oxide synthase activity may contribute to NaCl sensitivity of blood pressure (31). Pharmacologic inhibition of nitric oxide synthesis shifts the pressure/natriuresis relationship to higher levels of arterial pressure and produces hypertension (28); conversely, long-term treatment with arginine shifts the pressure/natriuresis relationship to lower pressures and prevents development of hypertension in the Dahl-S rat and the spontaneously hypertensive rat (SHR).

Increased sympathetic nervous system activity and impaired baroreflex function may also contribute to NaCl-sensitive hypertension in the experimental animal and in man (32–34). In the Dahl-S rat, dietary NaCl loading potentiates the increment of vascular resistance in response to neural stimulation and increases the rate of basal firing of the splanchnic nerve (32, 35). A high NaCl intake increases vascular reactivity to norepinephrine in the prehypertensive Dahl-S rat. A high NaCl diet also exacerbates impairment of baroreceptor reflex control of heart rate in the Dahl-S rat, whereas in the Dahl-R rat, a high NaCl diet enhances afferent discharge of aortic baroreceptors and augments sympathoinhibitory responses to volume expansion. In the normotensive rat, dog, and rabbit, impaired baroreflex function renders the animal susceptible to NaCl-induced blood pressure elevations.

NaCl sensitivity of blood pressure is also associated with alterations of ion transport in vascular smooth muscle that favor vasoconstriction (36). Based primarily on studies in circulating blood cells, most evidence suggests that active membrane Na+ transport is suppressed by high NaCl intake and that suppression of sodium transport by a high NaCl diet may be less prominent in circulating cells of hypertensives than of normotensives. Hypertension is also associated with increased red blood cell Li^+Na^+ countertransport and decreased $Na^+K^+/2\ Cl^-$ cotransport; increased red cell Li^+Na^+ countertransport may be a marker for NaCl sensitivity of blood pressure. Dietary NaCl loading has been reported to increase intracellular calcium in lymphocytes of NaCl-sensitive humans. Based on nuclear magnetic resonance spectroscopy studies of the intracellular ionic consequences of NaCl loading, patients with salt-sensitive hypertension have an exaggerated increase in intracellular sodium and, in contrast to non-salt-sensitive individuals, elevation of cytosolic free calcium, and suppression of intracellular pH and magnesium levels (37). These ionic alterations may contribute to increased peripheral resistance.

OBESITY

An association between obesity and hypertension has been amply documented. Data from cross-sectional studies indicate a direct linear correlation between body weight (or body mass index) and blood pressure (38–43). Centrally located body fat is a more important determinant of blood pressure elevation than peripherally located body fat in both women and men. In longitudinal studies, there is a direct correlation between change in weight and change in blood pressure over time, even when dietary salt intake is held constant (43). The proportion of the prevalence of hypertension attributable to obesity is an important public health question. It has been estimated that 60% of hypertensives are more than 20% overweight. The high prevalence of overweight combined with the corresponding increase in risk of developing high blood pressure has led to estimates that 20 to 30% of hypertension can be attributed to this exposure (44).

A reduction of blood pressure by weight loss has been clearly documented in short-term trials in both hypertensive and normotensive individuals. Based on pooling results of controlled dietary intervention trials, it has been estimated that a mean change in body weight of 9.2 kg is associated with a 6.3 mm Hg change in systolic blood pressure and 3.1 mm Hg change in diastolic blood pressure (43).

Obesity-related hypertension has been variously ascribed to hypervolemia and an increased cardiac output without an appropriate reduction of peripheral resistance, to increased sympathetic nervous system activity, and to insulin resistance (45, 46).

INSULIN RESISTANCE

Obesity is associated with resistance to insulin-stimulated glucose uptake and hyperinsulinemia, and weight loss increases insulin sensitivity (47). Depending on the populations studied and methodologies for defining insulin resistance, approximately 25 to 40% of nonobese, nondiabetic hypertensives are also insulin resistant (48). The constellation of insulin resistance, reactive hyperinsulinemia, increased serum triglyceride concentrations, decreased HDL cholesterol, and hypertension has been designated "syndrome X." Independent of obesity, centripetal distribution of body fat is also associated with insulin resistance and elevated blood pressure. Insulin resistance is also associated with alterations in the blood clotting cascade that accentuate thrombosis by increasing coagulation and inhibiting fibrinolysis. In both women and men, centripital obesity is predictive of coronary heart disease, independent of body mass index, and waist:hip ratio may be a better predictor of cardiovascular risk than body mass index (48).

Increasing evidence suggests that insulin resistance is associated with salt sensitivity of blood pressure in both normotensive and hypertensive individuals (47–49). Like patients with salt-sensitive hypertension, even in the absence of hypertension, obese individuals and/or individuals with type II diabetes mellitus reportedly also have elevated intracellular calcium and suppressed intracellular magnesium levels, and these ionic alterations may contribute to insulin resistance.

Syndrome X may in part be heritable; however, in the rat, simple carbohydrate feeding (sucrose, glucose, or fructose) also results in insulin resistance, dyslipidemia, and increased blood pressure (47). Sucrose feeding also potentiates development of hypertension in the SHR, in a rat model of adrenal regeneration hypertension, and in normotensive rats fed high NaCl. Although a number of putative mechanisms have been proposed, it is unclear whether insulin resistance and/or hyperinsulinemia actually cause hypertension. Putative mechanisms include antinatriuretic effect of insulin, increased sympathetic nervous system activity, augmented vasoconstriction in response to norepinephrine and angiotensin, impaired endothelium-dependent vasodilatation, and stimulation of vascular smooth muscle growth by insulin.

POTASSIUM

Potassium loading prevents or ameliorates development of hypertension in several animal models of genetic and NaCl-induced hypertension (21). Conversely, in both Dahl-S and Dahl-R rats on a high NaCl diet, a low potassium intake results in blood pressure elevation and renal vascular remodeling (increased wall:lumen ratio), indicating increased renal vascular resistance (50).

In societies with high potassium intakes, both mean blood pressure and the prevalence of hypertension tend to be lower than in societies with low potassium intakes (21, 51). Several large surveys have demonstrated a significant inverse correlation between potassium intake and blood pressure among individuals within a population; this inverse association is more prominent on a high NaCl diet (12, 21). However, in some studies, after adjusting for other variables (e.g., age, weight, consumption of alcohol, fiber, magnesium), dietary potassium was not found to be independently associated with blood pressure (52), and not all surveys have documented an association between potassium intake and either level of blood pressure or prevalence of hypertension. Failure to observe this association may be related to insufficient sample sizes. The urine sodium:potassium ratio appears to be a stronger correlate of blood pressure than either sodium or potassium alone (12, 21, 51, 53); in children, the rise of blood pressure with age is directly related to the urine sodium:potassium ratio (54).

Almost 70 years ago, Addison reported that a high potassium intake has an antihypertensive effect in humans (55). More recently, results of two metaanalyses of clinical trials concluded that oral potassium supplements significantly lower both systolic and diastolic blood pressures (56, 56a). The magnitude of the blood pressure lowering effect is greater in hypertensive, than in normotensive, individuals and is more pronounced with a longer duration of supplementation. The effect of a high potassium intake on blood pressure is also more pronounced in blacks than in whites and in individuals consuming a high NaCl diet (21). Increased intake of potassium has been reported not to affect blood pressure in hypertensive men on a low NaCl diet (57); however, reduced sodium and increased potassium and magnesium intake lowered blood pressure in men and women with mild-to-moderate hypertension (58). Conversely, potassium depletion induced either by a low-potassium diet or by diuretics is associated with blood pressure elevation (59, 60).

Proposed mechanisms by which a high dietary intake of potassium may lower blood pressure include a natriuretic effect of potassium, inhibition of renin release, antagonism of the pressor response to angiotensin II, direct vasodilatation, augmentation of endothelium-dependent vasodilatation, decreased production of the vasoconstrictor thromboxane, and increased production of the vasodilator kallidin (21).

Dietary potassium may affect morbidity and mortality, independent of an effect on blood pressure. Unrelated to changes of blood pressure, a high potassium diet was reported to decrease stroke mortality in the stroke-prone SHR and to decrease renal damage in several rat models of hypertension (61–63). Similarly, in a prospective clinical study, the 12-year risk of stroke death was negatively associated with potassium intake, independent of blood pressure (54). In a prefecture in Japan, introducing a diet with a low sodium:potassium ratio was associated with a reduced 10-year stroke mortality rate (64).

CALCIUM

As recently reviewed, more than 80 studies have reported that blood pressure is lowered by increasing dietary calcium in experimental models of hypertension (65). This effect of calcium on blood pressure may be more pronounced in models of salt-sensitive hypertension (66).

Within and among human populations, like potassium, there is an inverse association between dietary calcium intake and blood pressure, and low calcium intake is associated with an increased prevalence of hypertension (22, 67). Data from both epidemiologic reports and animal studies suggest a threshold for calcium intake below which arterial pressure increases (68), and a low calcium intake may amplify the effects of a high NaCl diet on blood pressure. In the human, diets with less than 600 mg calcium per day are most clearly associated with hypertension (65). Based on results of two published metaanalyses including 23 and 66 populations, weak but statistically significant inverse correlations were observed for association of dietary calcium with both systolic and diastolic blood pressures (69, 70). However, because of the size of the estimate, the heterogeneity among studies, the difficulty of assessing calcium intake, and the possibility of confounding and publication bias, the authors conclude that increasing calcium intake above the RDA is not recommended for the prevention or treatment of high blood pressure. Dietary calcium is also inversely related to systolic blood pressure in young children (71).

Most clinical trials evaluating the effect of increased dietary calcium on blood pressure have supplemented diets with 1000 to 1500 mg of elemental calcium per day. Reductions of blood pressure have been modest and inconsistent, and no gradient of calcium effect or threshold intake level has been identified. Two recently published metaanalyses of randomized clinical trials have shown a small, statistically significant reduction of systolic, but not diastolic, blood pressure (72, 73). Like the data in the observational studies, results of these clinical trials do not justify recommending calcium supplementation to the general population for prevention or treatment of hypertension.

Within a population, it may be possible to identify subgroups who are more likely to be responsive to calcium. For example, calcium supplementation may preferentially lower blood pressure in patients with NaCl-sensitive hypertension and low-renin hypertension, whereas calcium may actually increase blood pressure in patients with high-renin or renin-dependent hypertension (22). During pregnancy, calcium supplementation has been reported to reduce both systolic and diastolic blood pressure (74). Despite earlier evidence to the contrary (75), results of a recent, randomized, multicenter trial indicate that calcium supplementation during pregnancy does not prevent preeclampsia or pregnancy-associated hypertension (75a). Calcium supplementation more convincingly lowers blood pressure in individuals consuming low-calcium diets (68, 76).

There is considerable speculation about mechanisms by which dietary calcium may affect blood pressure (77). Calcium has a natriuretic effect, which may explain the apparent greater sensitivity of patients with NaCl-sensitive hypertension to the blood pressure–lowering effect of calcium. Conversely, in both the human and the intact rat, NaCl loading increases urinary calcium excretion and serum parathyroid hormone (PTH) and 1,25-dihydroxyvitamin D concentrations. Hypercalcuria, decreased plasma ionized calcium concentrations, and increased plasma concentrations of PTH and 1,25-dihydroxyvitamin D have been observed in experimental models of NaCl-sensitive hypertension and in patients with low-renin hypertension (78, 79). It has been hypothesized that PTH results in vasoconstriction by influencing neural activity and/or vasoactive hormones either directly or indirectly via changes in serum calcium (77–79). Other studies have emphasized a role for vitamin D, especially in NaCl-related hypertension.

Conceivably, NaCl-sensitive hypertension may be a calcium-losing state, resulting in secondary hyperparathyroidism (65, 77–79). Calcium supplementation may reduce blood pressure by correcting this calcium deficiency and the associated hyperparathyroidism. Alternatively, alterations of calcium metabolism and calcium-regulating hormones may be epiphenomena of NaCl loading that are not causally related to development of hypertension.

Other putative mechanisms by which high dietary calcium intake may lower blood pressure include decreased calcium influx into vascular smooth muscle cells and increased capacity of these cells to extrude calcium, potential vasoactive effects of calcium-regulating hormones (PTH, 1,25-dihydroxyvitamin D, calcitonin-gene-related peptide), and modulation of sympathetic nervous system activity.

MAGNESIUM

Relatively little information is available concerning dietary magnesium and blood pressure. Although magnesium is found in a variety of foods, it is not easily identified and quantified. High magnesium intakes lower blood pressure in rat models of hypertension, and in the rat, blood pressure increases in response to magnesium deprivation (80, 81).

In the human, as with calcium, there is suggestive evidence for an association between lower magnesium in the diet and higher blood pressures (22). Over the past century, the availability of magnesium-rich foods has declined, and consumption of processed foods that have lost magnesium has increased. It has been proposed that subclinical magnesium deficiency has developed in industrialized countries, and that this has paralleled the increased prevalence of hypertension (82). Conversely, persons consuming vegetarian diets, which are usually high in magnesium and fiber content, tend to have lower blood pressures than nonvegetarians, raising the possibility that dietary magnesium is inversely related to blood pressure. However, in one cross-sectional study of 9- to 10-year-old girls, after adjusting for dietary fiber, a significant inverse association between magnesium intake and blood pressure was no longer discerned (83). In older persons, diets high in both magnesium and potassium are associated with lower blood pressures (58). Limited evidence suggests that dietary intake of magnesium is lower in hypertensives than in normotensives; in one prospective study, lower calcium (<400 mg/day vs. >800 mg/day) and lower magnesium (<200 mg/day vs. >300 mg/day) intake predicted risk of subsequent hypertension (84). In another prospective study, dietary magnesium, potassium, and fiber were each significantly associated with lower risk of hypertension when considered separately; however, when these nutrients were considered simultaneously, only dietary fiber had an inverse association with hypertension (85).

Limited information is available about the effects of magnesium supplementation on blood pressure in hypertensives, and the results are inconsistent (see also Chapter 9). At best, the overall hypotensive response to magnesium supplementation is small and may become more apparent in trials of more than 6 months duration (86, 87). The capacity of magnesium to lower blood pressure appears to be greater in hypertensives who are hypomagnesemic and/or are taking diuretics (88, 89).

There is a plausible physiologic rationale for an effect of magnesium on blood pressure. Magnesium decreases vascular tone and contractility, possibly by decreasing cellular uptake of calcium and thereby decreasing cytosolic calcium (22). In addition, magnesium administration in endothelial cells and in humans stimulates production of prostaglandin I_2, a vasodilator, when serum magnesium is raised acutely (90). Conversely, magnesium deficiency is associated with resistance to insulin-stimulated glucose uptake and enhanced vascular contractility.

ALCOHOL

Observational studies suggest a J-shaped relationship between alcohol consumption and blood pressure (91–94). Light drinkers (one to two drinks per day) have lower blood pressures than teetotalers (95), whereas in comparison to nondrinkers, there is a small but significant elevation of blood pressure in individuals consuming three or more drinks per day (a standard drink contains approximately 14 g of ethanol and is defined as a 12-ounce glass of beer, a 6-ounce glass of table wine, or 1.5 ounces of distilled spirits). These higher blood pressures are not related to potentially confounding variables such as age and body mass. The assumption is that alcohol is a vasodilator at low doses but a vasoconstrictor at higher doses.

The contribution to the prevalence of hypertension attributed to consuming more than two drinks of alcohol per day has been estimated to be 5 to 7%; the contribution in men is greater than in women, although in women the risk of hypertension increases progressively with alcohol intake in excess of 20 g/day. Several short-term studies suggest that decreasing alcohol consumption has therapeutic benefit to hypertensives (96). In controlled studies, reduction of alcohol consumption has been associated with a reduction of 4 to 8 mm Hg in systolic blood pressure and a lesser reduction of diastolic pressure. Blood pressure of normotensives may also decrease in response to a reduction of alcohol consumption.

The mechanism(s) by which alcohol may affect blood pressure has not been established. In both the rat and the human, alcohol ingestion augments sympathetic nervous system activity (95). Alcohol also stimulates corticotropin-releasing hormone (CRH) and cortisol secretion, and CRH appears to stimulate sympathetic neural activity. In normal subjects, it has recently been reported that dexamethasone inhibits both the augmented neural discharge and blood pressure increment in response to alcohol infusion (97). This observation suggests that the alcohol-induced elevation of blood pressure is related to CRH-mediated sympathetic activation. Additionally, short-term administration of alcohol results in an early rise in serum magnesium level followed by a transient decrease in PTH, associated with a transient hypocalcemia and hypercalciuria and followed by a late rise in PTH. What relation, if any, this may have to alcohol-induced increases of blood pressure is not clear.

LIPIDS

Both animal and human data suggest that polyunsaturated n-3 and n-6 fatty acids play a role in blood pressure regulation (99). In experimental models of hypertension, both linoleic acid (a long-chain n-6 polyunsaturated fatty acid) and fish oil (rich in eicosapentaenoic and docosahexaenoic acids, both n-3 fatty acids) attenuate development of renin-dependent hypertension (100). Limited epidemiologic evidence suggests a direct association between diets high in saturated fats and blood pressure, and many populations that have low mean blood pressure levels consume diets low in total fat and saturated fatty acids (101). Conversely, diets high in n-3 fatty acids may be associated with lower blood pressures (102). Several trials have failed to show a significant blood pressure effect by varying the dietary content of fat or by exchanging polyunsaturated fatty acids for saturated fatty acids, and there is ongoing debate as to whether reducing saturated fat and/or increasing polyunsaturated fat in the diet lowers blood pressure (103). Limited evidence suggests that linoleic acid–enriched diets reduce blood pressure in normotensive and hypertensive humans.

Results of a recent metaanalysis of 31 controlled trials showed a small, statistically significant reduction of blood pressure by fish oil (3.0/1.5 mm Hg) at an overall mean dose of 4.8 g of n-3 fatty acids (or approximately 10 capsules) per day (104). In these trials, there was little or no effect among healthy normotensive individuals; however, hypertensive patients showed a dose-response hypotensive effect of fish oil. Fish oil also had a moderate effect on blood pressure in hypercholesterolemic patients and patients with athersclerotic cardiovascular disease. The authors concluded that fish oil is unlikely to benefit healthy subjects for the prevention or treatment of hypertension, given the uncertainty of response and the large dose required to elicit small changes in blood pressure. Despite some earlier evidence to the contrary, a recent randomized, controlled trial concluded that fish oil in doses that reduce blood pressure in hypertensive persons does not adversely affect insulin sensitivity or glucose metabolism (105).

In contrast to n-3 polyunsaturated fatty acids, results of clinical trials show little or no evidence that saturated fats and n-6 polyunsaturated fats have an independent effect on blood pressure beyond changing body weight (106, 107). The blood pressure reductions attributed to n-3 fatty acids may be related to alterations of prostaglandin metabolism, alterations of vascular endothelial function, increased vascular responsiveness to pressor agents, and inhibition of vascular smooth muscle proliferation.

PROTEIN

Several recent observational studies, including the Intersalt study, suggest that blood pressure level is inversely associated with dietary protein consumption (12, 108). However, limited clinical intervention trials show no evidence that amount or type of protein in the diet affects blood pressure (95, 96). Conceivably, specific amino acids could affect neurotransmitters or humoral substances that control blood pressure. For example, acute administration of tryptophan or tyrosine (either peripherally or directly into the central nervous system) reduces blood pressure in experimental animals, possibly via effects on neuronal pathways involved in blood pressure control (108).

CARBOHYDRATE

As discussed above, simple carbohydrate feeding induces insulin resistance. In the rat, high dietary intake of glucose, sucrose, or fructose may increase arterial pressure in the normotensive animal, may augment NaCl sensitivity of blood pressure, and may potentiate development of hypertension in several experimental models (23, 47). However, in the human, there is no evidence that manipulating the carbohydrate content of the diet affects blood pressure.

VEGETARIAN DIET

In general, results of both observational and intervention studies demonstrate that lacto-ovo vegetarian diets consumed by acculturated individuals are associated with a decreased prevalence of hypertension and lower blood pressure levels than omnivorous diets (109–112). A strict lacto-ovo vegetarian diet consists of a relatively low intake of saturated fat, a high polyunsaturated:saturated fat ratio, and a high intake of fruits, vegetables, and other fiber. Dietary intakes of carbohydrate, potassium, magnesium, and calcium tend to be increased, and dietary protein is lower than that in omnivores.

The DASH Trial is a randomized multicenter study that evaluated the effects of three dietary patterns over 8 weeks on blood pressure in 459 adults with high-normal blood pressure or mild hypertension (112a). The dietary interventions were *(a)* control diet, with potassium, calcium, and magnesium levels close to the 25th percentile of U.S. consumption; *(b)* a diet rich in fruits and vegetables; and *(c)* a "combination" diet rich in fruits, vegetables, and low-fat dairy products. Sodium chloride content was equivalent in all three diets (8 g/day). Systolic and diastolic blood pressures were significantly reduced by the fruit and vegetable diet (−2.8 and −1 mm Hg, respectively) and, compared with controls, were reduced even more by the combination diet (−5.5 and −3.0 mm Hg, respectively).

The specific nutrients responsible for the blood pressure reduction associated with vegetarian diets have not been defined. Although vegetarians tend to be slimmer, the lower blood pressure appears not to be totally accounted for by body weight. Results of randomized controlled dietary trials suggest that the hypotensive effect of a vegetarian diet is also not due to the absence of meat protein per se (111). Substituting animal fat with starch and sugar appears not to lower blood pressure, whereas blood pressure is lowered by replacing fat with vegetable products, including vegetable oils (109). The effect of dietary fiber on blood pressure remains an unresolved issue (113); carefully controlled studies with different types of fiber are needed. Additionally, vegetables are a primary source of vitamin C, and several observational studies suggest an inverse correlation between plasma vitamin C levels and blood pressure; however, the limited available clinical trial data do not demonstrate a convincing blood pressure reduction with increased consumption of vitamin C (114).

PRIMARY PREVENTION AND TREATMENT OF HYPERTENSION

In children, there is a strong correlation between obesity and blood pressure, and a direct association between changes in body weight and change in blood pressure (115). In addition, blood pressures in the young tend to track over time, and a large proportion of obese children become obese adults. Prevention of obesity, beginning in childhood, would seem important for the primary prevention of hypertension and cardiovascular disease.

Several recent trials have tested the efficacy of preventing hypertension in adults through altered dietary intake. In one trial, approximately 200 subjects with diastolic blood pressures in the high-normal ranges (80–89 mm Hg) were assigned to either a control group or a combined intervention consisting of weight loss, sodium restriction, moderate alcohol restriction, and moderate isotonic physical activity (116). Subjects were followed over a 5-year period. Nine percent of intervention subjects developed hypertension, compared with 19% of control subjects ($P < 0.027$). In a second prevention trial, 841 men and women between the ages of 25 and 49 years with diastolic blood pressures between 78 and 89 mm Hg were assigned to one of five groups: *(a)* control, *(b)* reduced calories, *(c)* reduced sodium, *(d)* reduced calories and sodium, and *(e)* reduced sodium and increased potassium (117). Calorie counseling reduced mean diastolic and systolic blood pressures at 6 months (2.8 and 5.1 mm Hg, respectively) and 3 years (1.8 and 2.4 mm Hg). Somewhat unexpectedly, the combination of calorie and sodium counseling was less effective than calorie counseling alone. The other interventions did not significantly affect blood pressure.

The Trial of Hypertension Prevention (TOPH) was designed to evaluate nonpharmacologic interventions in the primary prevention of hypertension in men and women with diastolic blood pressures ranging from 80 to 89 mm Hg. Different groups of subjects were exposed to different interventions. In phase I (which included 2182 subjects), stress management or dietary supplementation for 6 months with calcium, magnesium, potassium, or fish oil did not significantly reduce systolic or diastolic blood pressure, compared with controls; however, blood pressure was reduced by weight reduction and to a lesser extent by modest salt restriction over an 18-month period (118–120). Phase II was designed to test the effects of weight loss and sodium restriction, alone and in combination, on blood pressure over 3 to 4 years in overweight adults with high normal blood pressures (120). Both weight loss and reduction of sodium intake, individually and in combination, lowered systolic and diastolic blood pressures in the short term (6 months), although the effects of the two interventions were not additive. Beyond 6 months, the interventions were less effective in maintaining both weight loss and sodium restriction, and although their impact on blood pressure (although still significant) lessened, hypertension incidence was reduced. Additional studies evaluating the impact of diet modification and the interaction of nutrients on blood pressure in adults with "high normal" blood pressures are in progress.

The impact of dietary intervention on blood pressure is most pronounced in individuals with hypertension. With appropriate dietary modifications, it may be possible to treat hypertensive patients with fewer drugs and with lower doses; in a significant percentage of hypertensives, particularly patients with mild hypertension, dietary modifications may totally obviate the need for drug therapy (121–124). In hypertensives whose blood pressures have been controlled with medications, weight loss or NaCl restriction more than doubles the likelihood of maintaining normal blood pressure after withdrawal of drug therapy. The following lifestyle modifications have been recommended as adjunctive or definitive therapy for hypertension: weight reduction if overweight; aerobic exercise; limited NaCl and alcohol intake; maintenance of adequate dietary potassium, calcium, and magnesium intake; smoking cessation and reduced dietary saturated fat and cholesterol intake for overall cardiovascular health (2).

PUBLIC HEALTH IMPLICATIONS

Observational and interventional studies in humans, supported by findings from animal studies, provide a clear rationale for the following population-based recommendations to optimize the effect of diet on blood pressure: reduce NaCl intake; control body weight; consume adequate amounts of potassium, calcium, and magnesium; and moderate alcoholic beverage intake. Blood pressure–lowering interventions applied to the entire community would result in a small downward shift in the blood pressure distribution, which would have a substantial impact on preventing hypertension and reducing the burden of blood pressure–related cardiovascular disease (44, 112, 125). There is strong rationale for a population-based educational approach to blood pressure control through diet. A population-based approach reaches children during years when lifestyles and dietary preferences are established. It also reinforces recommended dietary changes for hypertensive individuals. We found that educational efforts directed to an entire community significantly decreased blood pressure levels and improved control of high blood pressure (126).

It is estimated that 20 to 30% of hypertension can be attributed to overweight (43, 44). The strength of the association between body weight and blood pressure and between change in weight and change in blood pressure over time indicates that weight reduction in overweight individuals and avoidance of obesity should be key strategies for both prevention and treatment of hypertension.

Opinion is divided concerning a recommendation on NaCl restriction for the entire population (44, 127). Arguments for this recommendation include the following: current NaCl intake exceeds the physiologic need; the tendency for blood pressure to increase with high NaCl intake occurs over the entire population; although relatively large differences in dietary NaCl have a relatively small impact on blood pressure within and across populations, these blood pressure differences may significantly affect the overall incidence of cardiovascular disease; within a population, a certain percentage of individuals may be particularly susceptible to the effect of dietary NaCl on blood pressure; and identification of NaCl-sensitive individuals is not practical. Arguments against the recommendation for reduction of NaCl consumption for the entire population include the following: limited or no proven blood pressure reduction for a large segment of the population; little evidence that reduction of NaCl intake affects cardiovascular disease endpoints (e.g., stroke, heart attack, and kidney disease); and potential adverse health consequences of NaCl restriction.

Despite these reservations, it is generally recommended that excessively high intake of dietary NaCl be avoided. Current estimates of NaCl intake in the U.S. are in the range of 8 to 10 g/day. As an example of a specific guideline, the U.S. Dietary Guidelines Advisory Committee and the American Heart Association recommended that dietary NaCl be restricted to no more than 6.0 g/day, and more rigorous NaCl restriction may be recommended for hypertensive individuals. In the absence of blatant salt-losing disorders, there is no convincing evidence that this modest reduction in salt intake has any long-term, adverse health consequences; nevertheless, this concern has been raised. Alderman et al. reported increased incidence of myocardial infarction over an average 3.8-year follow-up in drug-treated hypertensive men with the lowest levels of sodium excretion (<4 g NaCl per day) at entry (18). The design of this observational study makes it impossible to exclude the influence of such potentially confounding variables as severity of underlying disease, presence of other cardiovascular disease risk factors, and usual long-term NaCl consumption.

Recommendations about other nutrients should also be considered. Because of the strong association of alcohol intake with blood pressure, a recommendation to restrict alcohol intake to two drinks per day would seem reasonable, particularly in individuals with hypertension. Low intake of potassium, calcium, or magnesium has been associated with higher levels of blood pressure, and the effects of a high NaCl intake on blood pressure may be amplified by diets low in both potassium and calcium. Furthermore, dietary deficiencies of these ions may be associated with other disorders such as calcium deficiency and osteoporosis. Recent National Academy of Science recommendations for calcium consumption are 1300 mg/day for adolescents (ages 9–18 years), 1000 mg/day for adults under 50 years of age, and 1200 mg/day for those over age 50 (see Chapter 7 and Appendix Table II-A-2-b-1). Although serum cholesterol and hence cardiovascular disease risk may be modified by dietary fat intake, there is currently insufficient information to make recommendations about dietary intake of lipids or carbohydrates for the prevention or treatment of hypertension.

Strategies for the prevention and treatment of hypertension should address overall cardiovascular disease risk, not simply elevated blood pressure. Dietary recommendations should be incorporated into a comprehensive program that also addresses other cardiovascular disease risk factors such as elevated serum cholesterol concentrations, cigarette smoking, and a sedentary lifestyle. In developing recommendations, the potential impact of changing the intake of a single nutrient on the dietary content and/or bioavailability of a wide range of nutrients should also be considered.

Several population-based dietary education initiatives have recently been introduced in the U.S. The U.S. Department of Agriculture has released revised recommendations for dietary intake for Americans. Dietary intake recommendations are communicated by the "food pyramid," which emphasizes a diet based on increased intake of complex carbohydrates and limited intake of calorically dense foods. In addition, the National Cancer Institute and others have promoted "Five a Day for Better Health," the recommendation that Americans consume five fruits and vegetables a day as a tangible way to improve dietary intake. Through federally published dietary guidelines, revised recommendations for sodium intake are being promoted. The U.S. Department of Agriculture has made major changes in nutritional standards for reimbursable school breakfasts and lunches (128). These changes require decreased salt and fat in the foods provided in schools. In addition, there is federal support for nutritional education programs in schools for children and for food service employees. Finally, federally mandated food labeling permits individuals to assess their nutritional intake accurately and modify it more readily.

REFERENCES

1. Burt VL, Cutler JA, Higgins M, et al. Hypertension 1995;26: 60–69.
1a. Kannel WB. JAMA 1996;275:1571–6.
2. National High Blood Pressure Education Program/National Institutes of Health. The fifth report of the Joint National Committee on Detection, Evaluation, and Treatment of High Blood Pressure. NIH publ. no. 93-1088, 1993.
3. Stamler J, Stamler R, Neaton JD. Arch Intern Med 1993;153: 598–615.
4. Denton D, Weisinger R, Mundy N, et al. Nature Med 1995;1:1009–16.
5. Antonios TF, MacGregor GA. Clin Exp Pharmacol Physiol 1995;22:180–4.
6. Law MR, Frost CD, Wald NJ. Br Med J 1991;302:811–5.
7. Frost CD, Law MR, Wald NJ. Br Med J 1991;302:815–8.
8. Law MR, Frost CD, Wald NJ. Br Med J 1991;302:819–24.
9. Weinberger MH. The effects of sodium on blood pressure in humans. In: Laragh JH, Brenner BM, eds. Hypertension: pathophysiology, diagnosis, and management. 2nd ed. New York: Raven Press, 1995;2703–14.
10. Simpson FO. Blood pressure and sodium intake. In: Laragh JH, Brenner BM, eds. Hypertension: pathophysiology, diagnosis, and management. 2nd ed. New York: Raven Press, 1995;273–81.
11. Overlack A, Ruppert M, Kolloch R, et al. Hypertension 1993;22:331–8.
11a. Simons-Morton DG, Obarzanek E. Pediatr Nephrol 1997; 11:244–9.
11b. Geleijnse JM, Hutman A, Witteman JCN, et al. Hypertension 1997;29:913–7.

12. Intersalt Cooperative Research Group. Br Med J 1988; 297:319–28.
13. Elliott P, Stamler J, Nichols R, et al. Br Med J 1996;312: 1249–53.
14. Weinberger MH, Miller JH, Luft FC, et al. Hypertension 1986;8(Suppl II):127–34.
15. Sullivan JM, Prewitt RL, Ratts TE. Am J Med Sci 1988;295: 370–7.
16. Cutler JA, Follmann D, Elliott P, et al. Hypertension 1991; 17(Suppl I):27–33.
17. Midgley JP, Matthew AG, Greenwood CM, et al. JAMA 1996;275:1590–7.
18. Alderman MH, Madhavan S, Cohen H, et al. Hypertension 1995;25:1144–52.
19. Cook NR, Cohen J, Hebert P, et al. Arch Intern Med 1995; 155:701–9.
20. Boegehold M, Kotchen TA. Hypertension 1991;17(Suppl I):158–61.
21. Morris RC, Sebastian A. Potassium responsive hypertension. In: Laragh JH, Brenner BM, eds. Hypertension: pathophysiology, diagnosis, and management. 2nd ed. New York: Raven Press, 1995;2715–26.
22. Harlan WR, Harlan LC. Blood pressure and calcium and magnesium intake. In: Laragh JH, Brenner BM, eds. Hypertension: pathophysiology, diagnosis, and management. 2nd ed. New York: Raven Press, 1995;1143–54.
23. Johnson MD, Zhang HY, Kotchen TA. Hypertension 1993;21:779–85.
24. Miller JZ, Weinberger MH, Christian JC, et al. Am J Epidemiol 1987;126:822–30.
25. Weinberger MH, Miller JZ, Fineberg NS, et al. Hypertension 1987;10:443–6.
26. Grim CE, Luft FC, Weinberger MH, et al. Aust NZ J Med 1984;14:453–7.
27. Freis ED, Reda DJ, Materson BJ. Hypertension 1988;12: 244–50.
28. Cowley AW, Roman RJ. JAMA 1996;275:1581–9.
29. Kotchen TA, Zhang HY, Covelli M, et al. Am J Physiol 1991;261:E692–7.
30. Gill JR, Gullner HG, Lake CR, et al. Hypertension 1988;11: 312–9.
31. Tolins JP, Shultz PJ. Kidney Int 1994;46:230–6.
32. Reddy RS, Baylis C, Kotchen TA. Am J Physiol 1990;260: R32–8.
33. Sullivan JM. Hypertension 1991;17(Suppl I):61–8.
34. Shimamoto H, Shimamoto Y. J Hypertens 1992;10:855–61.
35. Reddy SR, Kotchen TA. J Lab Clin Med 1992;120:476–82.
36. Rusch NJ, Kotchen TA. Vascular smooth muscle regulation by calcium, magnesium and potassium in hypertension. In: Swales JD, ed. Textbook of hypertension. London: Blackwell Scientific Publications, 1994;188–99.
37. Resnick LM, Gupta RK, DiFabio B, et al. J Clin Invest 1994; 94:1269–76.
38. Kannell W, Brand N, Skinner J, et al. Ann Intern Med 1967;67:48–59.
39. Chiang BN, Perlman LV, Epstein RH. Circulation 1969;39: 403–21.
40. Epstein FH. Am J Epidemiol 1965;81:307–22.
41. Stamler R, Stamler J, Riedlinger WE, et al. JAMA 1978;240:1607–10.
42. National Institutes of Health Consensus Development Panel on the Health Implications of Obesity. Ann Intern Med 1985;103:1073–7.
43. MacMahon SW, Cutler J, Brittan E, et al. Eur Heart J 1987; 8(Suppl B):57–70.
44. National High Blood Pressure Education Program Working Group. Arch Intern Med 1993;153:186–208.
45. Dustan HP. Diabetes Care 1991;14:488–504.
46. Krieger DR, Landsberg L. Obesity and hypertension. In: Laragh JH, Brenner BM, eds. Hypertension: pathophysiology, diagnosis, and management. 2nd ed. New York: Raven Press, 1995;2367–88.
47. O'Shaughnessy IM, Kotchen TA. Curr Opin Cardiol 1993;8:757–64.
48. Kotchen TA, Kotchen JM, O'Shaughnessy IM. Curr Opin Cardiol 1996;11:483–9.
49. Zavaroni I, Coruzzi P, Bonini L, et al. Am J Hypertens 1995;8:855–88.
50. Resnick LM, Gupta R, Bhargava KK, et al. Hypertension 1991;17:951–7.
51. Khaw KT, Barrett-Conner E. Circulation 1985;77:653–61.
52. Ascherio A, Rimm EB, Giovannucci EL, et al. Circulation 1992;86:1475–84.
53. McCarron D, Morris C, Henry H, et al. Science 1984;224: 1392–8.
54. Khaw KT, Barrett-Conner E. N Engl J Med 1987;316:235–40.
55. Addison W. Can Med Assoc J 1928;18:281–5.
56. Cappuccio FP, MacGregor GA. J Hypertens 1991;9:465–73.
56a. Whelton PK, He J, Cutler JA, et al. JAMA 1997;277:1624–32.
57. Grimm RH, Neaton JD, Elmer PJ, et al. N Engl J Med 1990;322:569–74.
58. Geleijnse JM, Witteman JC, den Breeijen JH. J Hypertens 1996;14:737–41.
59. Lawton WJ, Fita AE, Anderson EA, et al. Circulation 1990;81:173–84.
60. Krishna GC, Kapoor SC. Ann Intern Med 1991;115:77–83.
61. Tobian L, Lange JM, Ulm KM, et al. Hypertension 1984;6(Suppl 3):363–6.
62. Tobian L, MacNeill D, Johnson MA, et al. Hypertension 1984;6(Suppl 1):170–6.
63. Liu DT, Wang MX, Kincaid-Smith P, et al. Clin Exp Hypertens 1994;16:391–414.
64. Yamori Y, Horie R. Health Rep 1994;6:181–8.
65. Hatton DC, McCarron DA. Hypertension 1994;23:513–30.
66. Butler TV, Cameron J, Kirchner KA. Am J Hypertens 1995;8:615–21.
67. Cutler JA, Brittain E. Am J Hypertens 1990;3:137s–46s.
68. McCarron DA, Hatton D. JAMA 1996;275:1128–9.
69. Cappuccio FP, Elliott P, Allender PS. Am J Epidemiol 1995;9:935–45.
70. Pryer J, Cappuccio FP, Elliott P. J Hum Hypertens 1995;9: 597–604.
71. Gillman MW, Oliveria SA, Moore LL, et al. JAMA 1992;267:2340–3.
72. Bucher HC, Cook RJ, Guyatt GH, et al. JAMA 1996;275: 1016–22.
73. Allender PS, Cutler JA, Follmann D, et al. Ann Intern Med 1996;124:825–31.
74. Bucher HC, Guyatt GH, Cook RJ, et al. JAMA 1996;275: 1113–7.
75. Belizan JM, Villar J, Gonzalez L, et al. N Engl J Med 1991; 325:1399–405.
75a. Levine RJ, Hauth JC, Curet LB, et al. N Engl J Med 1997;337:69–76.
76. Gillman MW, Hood MY, Moore LL, et al. J Pediatr 1995;127:186–92.
77. McCarron DA, Hatton D, Roullet JB, et al. Can J Physiol Pharmacol 1994;72:937–44.
78. Resnick LM. Ionic disturbances of calcium and magnesium metabolism in essential hypertension. In: Laragh JH, Brenner

BM, eds. Hypertension: pathophysiology, diagnosis, and management. 2nd ed. New York: Raven Press, 1995;1169–91.
79. Kotchen TA, Ott CE, Whitescarver SA, et al. Am J Hypertens 1989;2:749–53.
80. Rayssiguier Y, Mbega JD, Durlach V, et al. Magnesium Res 1992;5:139–46.
81. Summanen JU, Vuorela HJ, Hiltunen RK. J Pharm Sci 1994;83:249–51.
82. Durlach J, Bara M, Guiet-Bara A. Magnesium 1985;4:5–15.
83. Simon JA, Obarzanek E, Daniels SR, et al. Am J Epidemiol 1994;139:130–40.
84. Witteman JCM, Willett WC, Stampfer MJ, et al. Circulation 1989;80:1320–7.
85. Ascherio A, Rimm EB, Giovannucci EL, et al. Circulation 1992;86:1475–84.
86. Whelton P, Klag M. Am J Cardiol 1989;63:26G–30G.
87. Witteman JCM, Grobbee DE, Derkx FHM, et al. Am J Clin Nutr 1994;60:129–235.
88. Lind L, Lithell H, Pollare T, et al. Am J Hypertens 1991;4:674–9.
89. Zemel PC, Zemel MB, Urberg M, et al. Am J Clin Nutr 1990;5:665–9.
90. Nadler JL, Rude RK. Endocrinol Metab Clin N Am 1995;24: 623–41.
91. MacMahon S. Hypertension 1987;9:111–21.
92. Witteman JCM, Willett WC, Stampfer MJ, et al. Am J Cardiol 1990;65:633–7.
93. Klatsky AL. Blood pressure and alcohol intake. In: Laragh JH, Brenner BM, eds. Hypertension: pathophysiology, diagnosis, and management. 2nd ed. New York: Raven Press, 1995;2649–68.
94. Klag MJ, He J, Whelton PK, et al. Hypertension 1993;22: 365–70.
95. Victor RG, Hansen J. N Engl J Med 1995;332:1782–3.
96. Puddey IB, Parker M, Bellin LJ, et al. Hypertension 1992;20:533–41.
97. Randin D, Vollenweider P, Tappy L, et al. N Engl J Med 1995;332:1733–7.
98. Laitinen K, Lamberg-Allardt L, Tunninen R. N Engl J Med 1991;327:721–7.
99. Pietinen P. Ann Med 1994;26:465–8.
100. Reddy SR, Kotchen TA. J Am Coll Nutr 1996;15:92–6.
101. Sacks FM. Nutr Rev 1989;47:291–300.
102. Knapp HR. Nutr Rev 1989;47:301–13.
103. Iacono JM, Dougherty RM. Blood pressure and fat intake. In: Laragh JH, Brenner BM, eds. Hypertension: pathophysiology, diagnosis, and management. New York: Raven Press, 1990;257–76.
104. Morris M, Sacks F, Rosner B. Circulation 1993;88:523–33.
105. Toft I, Bonaa KH, Ingebretsen OC, et al. Ann Intern Med 1995;123:911–8.
106. Beilin LJ. Ann NY Acad Sci 1993;683:35–45.
107. Morris MC. J Cardiovasc Risk 1994;1:21–30.
108. Obarzanek E, Velletri PA, Cutler JA. JAMA 1996; 275:1598–603.
109. Moore TJ, McKnight JA. Endo Metab Clin N Am 1995;24: 643–55.
110. Rouse IL, Beilin LJ. Hypertensive disease and kidney structure. In: Laragh JH, Brenner BM, eds. Hypertension: pathophysiology, diagnosis, and management. New York: Raven Press, 1990;241–56.
111. Beilin LJ, Burke V. Clin Exp Pharmacol Physiol 1995;22: 195–8.
112. Melby CL, Toohey ML, Cebrick J. Am J Clin Nutr 1994;59: 103–9.
112a. Appel LJ, Moore TJ, Obarzanek E, et al. N Engl J Med 1997;336:1117–24.
113. Swain JF, Rouse IL, Curley CB. N Engl J Med 1990;322:147–52.
114. Ness AR, Khaw KT, Bingham S, Day NE. J Hypertens 1996;14:503–8.
115. Kotchen JM, Holley J, Kotchen TA. Semin Nephrol 1989;9:296–303.
116. Stamler R, Stamler J, Gosch FC, et al. JAMA 1989;262:1801–7.
117. Hypertension Prevention Trial Research Group. Arch Intern Med 1990;150:153–62.
118. Trials of Hypertension Prevention Collaborative Research Group. JAMA 1992;267:1213–20.
119. Yamamoto ME, Applegate WB, Klag MJ, et al. Ann Epidemiol 1995;5:96–107.
120. Trials of Hypertension Prevention (Phase II) Cooperative Research Group. (Abstract) J Hyperten 1996;14(Suppl 1):pS–210.
121. Langford HG, Davis BR, Blaufox D, et al. Hypertension 1991;17:210–7.
122. Treatment of Mild Hypertension Research Group. Arch Intern Med 1991;151:1413–23.
123. Ramsay LE, Yeo WW, Chadwick IG, et al. Br Med Bull 1994;50:494–508.
124. Beilin LJ. J Hypertens 1994;12:S71–81.
125. Cook NR, Cohen J, Hebert P, et al. Arch Intern Med 1995;155:701–9.
126. Kotchen JM, McKean HE, Thayer St, et al. JAMA 1986;255:2177–82.
127. Swales JD. Blood pressure 1992;1:201–4.
128. Dairy Council Digest 1996;67:19–24.

77. Chronic Congestive Heart Failure

CHARLES HUGHES and PATRICIA KOSTKA

Over the last 50 years, attempts to define heart failure have remained difficult. Paul Wood offered the classic definition in 1950 as "a state in which the heart fails to maintain an adequate circulation for the needs of the body." This description does not provide clinically useful diagnostic criteria and ignores the fact that cardiac output may be maintained. Cohn has offered an operational definition. He describes heart failure as a syndrome in which cardiac dysfunction is associated with impaired left ventricular function, reduced exercise tolerance, a high incidence of ventricular arrhythmia, and a shortened life expectancy (1). Although this definition is operational, it is not absolute. First, symptoms may be present without demonstrable systolic dysfunction, and secondly, exercise tolerance may be normal with severe systolic impairment.

EPIDEMIOLOGY

Advances in treatment of cardiac disease has led to a significant decline in myocardial infarction and strokes in the United States. Paradoxically, the incidence and prevalence of congestive heart failure has increased.

ETIOLOGY

In the United States, two million patients have congestive heart failure, and 400,000 new cases occur each year (2). The age-adjusted death rate for heart failure increased from 3.8/1000 in 1968 to about 7.7 in 1984. The incidence of death increases exponentially with age in both sexes. Hospitalization rates for heart failure have increased sharply among people older than 55 in the United States and Western Europe (3). Given a mortality that varies from 15 to 50% per year and the high cost of hospitalization, congestive heart failure is a costly public health issue.

PATHOPHYSIOLOGY

Heart

Recent models suggest that heart failure results from the combined effect of positive feedback mechanisms. These mechanisms include aortic impedance, ventricular preload, myocardial hypertrophy, myocardial ischemia, and neurohormonal activation (sympathetic nervous system, renin-angiotensin system, antidiuretic system, and natriuretic peptide).

Neurohormones

Following myocardial injury, ventricular performance is impaired. As a result of the diminished ventricular function, neurohormonal activation occurs to support the declining cardiac output. The major response is an increase in norepinephrine, which induces vasoconstriction. This initial response of the sympathetic nervous system activation is beneficial, enhancing contractility and promoting diastolic relaxation. However, this may be countered by redistribution of blood and increased afterload on the left ventricle because of vasoconstriction, both of which are factors in the progression of heart failure (4).

The second major neuroendocrine response is activation of the renin-angiotensin-alderosterone system. Many stimuli exist for activation of the renin-angiotensin aldosterone system in heart failure. In addition to decreased renal perfusion, circulating norepinephrine increases renin activity. The elevated activity of the renin-angiotensin-alderosterone system leads to increased angiotensin and alderosterone production, intensifying vasoconstriction and fluid retention, respectively. The subsequent increase in ventricular afterload and fluid retention promotes ventricular dilatation. This combination leads to further impairment of ventricular function (5).

Although the neurohormonal activation associated with congestive heart failure has major hemodynamic effects, specifically vasoconstriction with a consequent reduction in ejection fraction, the cellular effects of the neurohormones must be considered as well. Neurohormones, especially norepinephrine and angiotensin II, have definite effects on cellular growth. Myocyte hypertrophy occurs in response to nonspecific loading conditions. Mechanical stretching causes an increase in messenger RNA (mRNA), leading to protein synthesis associated with cell growth (6). Studies of neonatal myocytes show that norepinephrine promotes myocardial cell growth independent of loading conditions (7).

Remodeling

Angiotensin II induces hypertrophy of the myocytes independent of elevated peripheral vascular resistance and altered afterload. Secondly, angiotensin II has mitogenic properties. Increased levels of angiotensin II induces fibroblast proliferation and collagen synthesis leading to increased myocardial collagen content. The fibroblast stimulation may be more important than the hemodynamic effect of angiotensin II on myocytes because the myocardium contains more fibrocytes than myocytes (8). The excess collagen alters the filling characteristics of the left ventricle and impairs contractile function. The increase in chamber radius produces increased wall stress and accentuates myocardial oxygen requirements (9). The combined effect of neurohormones on both hemodynamics and cellular structure leads to remodeling of the heart.

Remodeling is an alteration in the geometry (volume and shape) of the ventricular cavity independent of alteration in distending pressures (10). Initially, it is a compensatory mechanism that preserves stroke volume. Although incompletely understood, it is apparent that remodeling results from the interaction between the infarcted and noninfarcted myocardium. Infarct expansion involves acute dilatation and thinning of the infarcted area. Several tissue changes are involved, including myocyte slippage and loss of intracellular space. Echocardiographically, the process is associated with lengthening of noncontractile elements in the noninfarcted area. Studies indicate progressive increase in end-diastolic length in the noninfarcted myocardium, with ventricular enlargement as early as 2 weeks after myocardial injury. The extent of wall motion abnormality correlates closely with the degree of ventricular cavity enlargement. As a result of the ventricular dilatation and inadequate hypertrophy, increased wall stress leads to self-perpetuating dysfunction of the noninfarcted ventricle. Remodeling is progressive and increases mortality by a factor of 3 (11, 12).

CLINICAL RECOGNITION

Hemodynamic changes associated with remodeling include a progressive increase in end-diastolic volume and a decrease in the ejection fraction of the ventricle. Left ventricular end-diastolic pressure rises initially and is transmitted to the left atrium, pulmonary wedge pressure, pulmonary artery, right ventricular pressure, and finally right atrial pressure. Over time, the decreased ejection fraction leads to diminished cardiac output.

The increased left atrial pressure produces exudation of fluid from the intravascular space to the pulmonary interstitium, leading to decreased pulmonary compliance or stiff lungs. When fluid exudes into the alveoli, there is a reduction in air space volume as well as decreased oxygen exchange. These changes are manifested clinically by dyspnea and orthopnea in the heart failure patient.

The reduced cardiac output is manifested clinically by fatigue and weakness. This effect results not only from absolute reduction of cardiac output but also from redistribution of flow, favoring the vital organs. The reduced blood flow to the kidneys leads to renin release, elaboration of angiotensin II, and finally elevated aldosterone levels. The increase in aldosterone levels produces significant fluid retention, manifested clinically by jugular venous distention, pulmonary rales or pleural fluid, S3 gallop, enlarged tender liver, hepatojugular reflux, ascites, and peripheral edema.

The routine laboratory procedures useful in evaluating heart failure include complete blood count, urinalysis, serum electrolytes, BUN, creatinine, liver function test, arterial blood gases, and drug levels such as digoxin levels. The chest x-ray (cardiac size and shape) and electrocardiogram can be extremely useful in defining the cause of the cardiac problem. The echocardiogram defines chamber size and volume, valvular integrity, wall motion abnormalities, and presence or absence of pericardial fluid.

Exercise testing quantifies the degree of functional impairment, and prognostic and therapeutic information may also be obtained. It has become a standard method for evaluating the response to chronic drug therapy as well as detecting ST abnormalities associated with ischemic heart disease. It is inexpensive, repeatable, and safe (13).

As heart failure progresses, symptoms of dyspnea and fatigue increase. Weakness develops, and weight loss may occur in advanced cases. Development of weakness associated with loss of lean body mass in patients with heart failure constitutes a well-recognized syndrome known as cardiac cachexia. Cachexia involves primarily the depletion of metabolically active lean body mass, with subsequent declines in strength, performance status, and immune competence (14–16). Nutritional surveys of hospitalized patients have revealed that between 50 and 68% of patients with CHF are significantly malnourished, based on anthropometric measurements, total body weight, and plasma protein status (16). Although Hippocrates was the first to observe the association of heart failure (dropsy) with cachexia, the mechanisms of this syndrome remain obscure (14). Multiple mechanisms include decreased caloric intake, increased metabolic needs, hypermetabolism, decreased energy and nutrient assimilation, and increased cytokine production (14).

Decreased caloric intake may be secondary to anorexia, directly related to the nausea, dyspnea, or fatigue of heart failure. Some investigators have reported inadequate intake of both calories and vitamins in heart failure. Others have shown that negative nitrogen and calorie balance could be reversed with voluntary improvement in food intake (15–17). Although the exact mechanism of anorexia is unknown, visceral congestion, unpalatable diets (salt free), and severe depression may contribute to this problem. Drugs often prescribed to treat heart failure may inadvertently contribute to development of cardiac cachexia. Diuretics may deplete potassium and zinc stores, leading to hypomotility of the gastrointestinal tract and decreased taste acuity, respectively. Likewise, digitalis intoxication may cause nausea, vomiting, and anorexia. Quinidine may also decrease gastrointestinal tolerance to food (18). The loss of lean body mass, however, exceeds that expected from anorexia alone (15).

Steatorrhea is recognized clinically, and fat balance studies have demonstrated a rough correlation between fat malabsorption and the severity of CHF (19). Iodine-labeled triolein studies have confirmed steatorrhea in 30% of heart failure patients, compared with 2% of normal controls (20). Defective absorption of amino acids and protein-losing enteropathy have been reported, but the mechanism of protein loss has not been fully explained (21).

Hypermetabolism is an established state in chronic congestive heart failure. It may be divided into increased metabolic needs of specific tissues or a generalized calorigenic effect. Of the increased metabolic demands, dyspnea due to the increased work of breathing has been documented. Generalized factors involved in hypermetabolism include low-grade fever and enhanced sympathetic nervous system (SNS) activity. Investigators reviewing records of 200 hospitalized heart failure patients found only 4 entirely free of fever. At autopsy of the 50 patients who expired, pulmonary infarction was found in half, and pneumonia was present in 40% of the patients (22).

Poehlman has compared 20 men with advanced heart failure and reduced ejection fractions with 40 age-matched healthy males (see Chapter 5). The patients had a lower fat-free mass than the controls. The two groups did not differ in fat mass. The measured metabolic mass had a higher resting metabolic rate (18%) in heart failure patients than in healthy volunteers. The difference was clinically significant and was felt to contribute to weight loss and musculoskeletal wasting. These investigators could not confirm that caloric expenditure associated with meals, deconditioned state, or voluntary reduction in caloric intake adequately explained the weight loss. A more likely explanation is the increase in SNS activity (23). Elevated SNS activity is established in heart failure and accounts for many other adverse aspects including tachycardia, sweating, and vasoconstriction.

Recently, there has been interest in tumor necrosis factor in heart failure and cardiac cachexia (23). Tumor necrosis factor-α (TNF-α) is a proinflammatory cytokine. It is a low-molecular-weight protein that acts at shorter distances than classic endocrine hormones. Classically, cytokines are released by monocytes and macrophages in response to viral and bacterial infection. In heart failure, TNF-α activity appears to respond to cardiac tissue injury and is produced by impaired myocytes and not the white cells of the immune system (24).

TNF-α has a moderate negative inotropic effect in humans. Prolonged infusion of TNF-α leads to irreversible cardiomyopathy. It may activate remodeling by activating a collagenase gene, leading to breakdown of the collagen framework of the heart (25). In addition, TNF-α produces fever and cachexia in experimental cardiac failure. Elevated circulating TNF-α levels have been noted in severe heart failure. Other studies comparing measured body weights reveal an inverse correlation between circulating TNF level and body weight. This continued loss of muscle tissue contributes to morbidity and mortality.

The clinical manifestations of cardiac cachexia are well described. Subclavicular and temporal wasting generally is evident, and the skin texture is like parchment. Measurements of triceps skin fold and midarm muscle circumference may be reduced to 60% of normal. Generally a 10% loss of lean body mass is recorded, which is more significant than loss of total body weight (14).

Several biochemical parameters are significant to the nutritional assessment of the patient with congestive heart failure: reduced serum albumin and transferrin levels, depressed total lymphocyte counts, elevated BUN and creatinine, and reduced potassium and magnesium levels. Creatinine-height index is generally a reliable indicator of protein stores in patients with cardiac failure. The ratio of blood urea nitrogen to blood creatinine may also be used as an accurate measure in stable patients. It is important to note that commonly used visceral protein markers such as serum albumin and transferrin may be artificially low because of dilutional effects of excessive extracellular fluid rather than malnutrition per se (15). Cell-mediated immunity as assessed by delayed hypersensitivity has been observed to be reduced. Electrolyte imbalances may also result from diuretic medications and excess fluid restriction.

TREATMENT

Surgical

Once the cause of the heart failure has been established, the clinician must select the appropriate therapy. Medical therapy consists of elimination of precipitating causes such as pulmonary emboli, infection, anemia, dietary indiscretion, and medication noncompliance. Surgical therapy is a reasonable choice in selected cases. Revascularization may be helpful in patients with viable but hibernating myocardia. Current intervention includes coronary artery bypass or coronary angioplasty (13). Certain congenital and acquired valvular problems respond nicely to valve replacements. In view of the poor outlook (50% mortality/year), eligible patients with the most advanced congestive heart failure should be considered for cardiac transplantation. In the modern era of immunosuppression, survival rates for transplants exceed 80% at 1 year and 70% at 3 years. Quality of life is markedly improved by successful cardiac transplantation. At present, however, organ donation is low relative to the demand, and the cost is high.

Medical

Basic drug therapy in the current era includes the appropriate application of diuretics and the use of inotropics, specifically digoxin and vasodilators. More recently, angiotensin-converting enzyme (ACE) inhibition has been shown effective in increasing survival in patients with severe heart failure (26, 27). More controversial medical therapy includes the cautious use of β-blockers, which may have a role in selected cases. Calcium-channel blockers have not yet been shown beneficial in this syndrome. Current data suggest that the use of first-generation calcium-channel blockers is harmful in dilated cardiomyopathy.

Diuretics are used in heart failure to alleviate symptoms and prevent accumulation of fluid in both the central and peripheral circulations, preventing associated breathlessness and swelling. The major benefit of this therapy is reduction of edema. To date, no trials have demonstrated that diuretics improve prognosis in heart failure. They are, however, generally safe, although electrolyte abnormalities and metabolic disturbances may be noted. The most severe adverse effects include electrolyte abnormalities with abnormalities that are associated with cardiac arrhythmias, glucose intolerance, elevation of LDL cholesterol level, and hyperuricemia.

Digitalis is a mainstay in the treatment of chronic congestive heart failure. Digoxin is a mildly positive inotrope that increases ejection fraction as well as exercise tolerance in heart failure. It is apparently most effective in dilated forms of cardiomyopathy and usually is not indicated in patients with sinus rhythm and preserved systolic function. It may, however, be useful in this group when atrial arrhythmias become a problem. Digitalis toxicity may occur in 10 to 12% of patients but rarely causes death. The interaction of digoxin compounds with other drugs such as quinidine, verapamil, and amiodarone must be carefully weighed, as these agents reduce digoxin binding and may enhance digoxin toxicity. Several studies are pending to clarify the effects of digoxin on survival.

In 1986, Cohn showed that the combination of digoxin, diuretics, and the vasodilators hydralazine and isordil was beneficial in prolonging the survival of patients with chronic congestive heart failure (26). In the V-HeFT I studies, there was a reduction of 34% in mortality over a 2-year period, compared with placebo. In 1991, the V-HeFT II and SOLVD groups assessed the efficacy of the ACE inhibitor enalapril in chronic congestive heart failure. Both groups showed a significant beneficial effect on survival when these agents were added to a fixed regimen of digoxin and diuretics. However, isordil and hydralazine induced greater hemodynamic improvements, e.g., increased both ejection fraction and exercise capacity, compared with the ACE inhibitors (27, 28).

Fatigue interferes with the activities of daily living in heart failure. The potential mechanisms include impaired arteriolar compliance, increased neurohormonal vasoconstriction, and endothelial dysfunction. Most studies have demonstrated a decline in the biochemical and ultrastructural indicators of oxidative capacity. Exercise training regimens are safe in compensated heart failure and improve both the endurance and strength of trained muscles (16, 29).

Nutritional Management

The basic objectives in nutritional management of congestive heart failure are *(a)* to reduce the workload of the heart as much as possible, *(b)* to maintain appropriate dry weight, and *(c)* to achieve and maintain overall optimal nutritional status. Nutritional management encompasses a threefold process of assessment, intervention, and education.

Nutritional Assessment

Accurate assessment of a wide spectrum of dietary, anthropometric, biochemical, and clinical indices provide the data upon which the clinician can implement appropriate therapy. Physical examination, medical history, and individual interview are all essential components of the nutritional assessment of the patient with congestive heart failure (see Chapter 55). Indications of nutrient deficiencies and imbalances may be identified by general examination, patient interview, and medical history. It is especially important to include the patient's family or caregivers in the interview process. Evaluation of the patient's usual weight, rate of weight change, reported dietary intake, and medication compliance as well as the rate of weight change will help not only in determining the presence and degree of malnutrition and fluid retention but also in assessing the patient's level of comprehension and compliance with therapeutic recommendations. Also, concomitant diseases such as diabetes, atherosclerotic coronary artery disease, and chronic renal failure may necessitate monitoring pertinent indices and integrating additional appropriate diet and clinical therapy. The diet should not be overly restricted, especially since many of these patients are immunocompromised.

Nutrition Intervention

The goal of achieving and maintaining the patient at or slightly below dry weight while protecting and even improving overall nutritional status forms the basis for determination of the specific therapeutic diet prescription. Diet modification centers on sodium restriction and management of fluid intake. Although individual response to sodium restriction varies, most patients who have congestive heart failure with edema respond to a diet restricted to 1.5 to 2.0 g sodium per day (30, 31). A reasonable determination for effective sodium restriction should be based on individual assessment. A brief oral interview can delineate estimated sodium intake as well as medication compliance.

Ordinarily, fluid intake for patients with congestive

heart failure need not be restricted. In fact, fluid intake up to 2500 to 3000 mL daily may enhance diuresis (31). However, with the progressive pump failure associated with cardiac cachexia, fluid restriction to about half the normal daily requirement, or 1500 mL, is advisable (32).

In advanced heart failure, especially when the patient's general and cardiac condition has deteriorated, significant edema—both pulmonary and peripheral—may appear to be refractory to treatment. Even with administration of potent diuretics, unusual retention of fluid can develop on a low-sodium diet and unrestricted fluid intake. This leads to dilutional hyponatremia in which there is a dilutional lowering of extracellular sodium concentration, although the total body sodium content is usually excessive. Administration of salt is useless and often dangerous. Since there is a refractoriness to diuretics, fluid restriction is urgently indicated along with appropriate treatment for the underlying causes of the aggravated circulatory failure. Restoration of serum sodium concentration after spontaneous water diuresis may then occur, with improvement in the patient's general status (31, 33).

In an acute CHF event, it is often difficult to ascertain the cause and best treatment approach. Asking patient and family about recent diet and medication compliance often provides the clinician the key to the appropriate treatment plan. Weight monitoring is fundamental in management of congestive heart failure. Laboratory indicators to monitor include serum urea nitrogen and serum creatinine levels. Elevated serum urea nitrogen and elevated creatinine usually reflect decreased renal flow due to pump failure or dehydration (34). If the patient presents with increased weight with elevated urea nitrogen and creatinine levels, sodium restriction should be intensified, fluid should be restricted, and diuretic therapy may require adjustment. Conversely, weight loss with elevated urea nitrogen and elevated creatinine levels indicates volume depletion, and thus treatment should consist of increased oral or intravenous fluids, suspension of diuretic therapy, and maintenance of moderate dietary sodium intake.

The clinician should be cautioned to maintain close observation of patients adhering to a low-sodium diet. Very low sodium diets can result in depletion of body sodium stores, particularly in those with chronic renal insufficiency. Excretion of urinary sodium exceeding intake accompanied by weight loss and decreased renal function indicates that more sodium is needed. Too little sodium in the diet can produce muscle cramps, convulsions, hypovolemia, hypotension, and further deterioration of renal function (33). Elderly patients may be more vulnerable to abrupt sodium withdrawal than younger persons.

In addition to sodium and fluid considerations, other diet management factors should be integrated into the diet prescription and nutrition counseling. Total caloric needs may require adjustment to achieve and maintain the patient at a healthful weight. Emphasis in counseling should be placed on achieving the most nutrient-dense composition possible.

Protein needs of the well-nourished adult range between 0.75 and 1.0 g per kg body weight (35). However, patients with cardiac cachexia and those with loss of protein in the urine as a result of increased glomerular permeability or in the feces because of impaired digestion and absorption may have increased protein needs (18, 19, 32).

Dietary supplements of magnesium, potassium, folate, and thiamin are indicated to offset losses of water-soluble vitamins and electrolytes associated with high diuretic doses (36). Broad-range vitamin and mineral supplementation also may be indicated, depending on the patient's dietary intake and nutritional status. Also, problems with gastrointestinal absorption may interfere with adequate absorption of fat-soluble vitamins and minerals, especially calcium and magnesium. In addition, small frequent feedings are often better tolerated by these patients and may better help them meet their caloric requirements.

Education

The central objective of education of the patient with congestive heart failure is to increase long-term compliance to reduce episodes of acute congestive heart failure requiring hospitalization and to improve and maintain optimal overall nutritional status. Patients often fail to comply with prescribed treatment because *(a)* they do not understand what they are supposed to do and the rationale behind the recommendations; *(b)* they forget to follow the advised regimen or are not convinced that the treatment is beneficial; or *(c)* they cannot consistently adhere to the regimen because of financial, psychosocial, or other constraints. Therefore, the educational process must be designed to provide an interdisciplinary, patient- and family-centered, threefold approach encompassing needs assessment, instruction, and long-term support.

Needs assessment should address the critical self-management issues that affect the patient's ability to comply with recommendations. These include age, financial limitations, visual and physical impairments, dentition, literacy and language differences, other medical conditions, and family or social support. In addition, long-term psychologic and motivational factors related to depression and isolation, often seen in this population, have significant influence on long-term compliance.

Education should be individualized and reinforced by all members of the health care team. Patients and caregivers need to understand the rationale for each recommendation. Nutritional education should include instruction regarding basic nutrition, sodium content of basic foods, nutrition labeling of packaged foods, and food preparation modifications.

Patients should be encouraged to keep a diet and medication diary plus a daily weight chart and to review them with health care providers on a regular basis. Involving the patient as an active member of his or her health care team fosters self-responsibility and communication, both of which are critical to achieving and maintaining long-term compliance. Group educational and support programs have proven to be cost-effective measures resulting in improved compliance and fewer hospitalizations (29).

SUMMARY

In summary, until the precise mechanism of cardiac cachexia is defined, one can only intensify therapy for the underlying heart failure and provide supportive therapy. Long-term compliance is significantly improved when the treatment is individualized and not only meets the patient's clinical needs, but also encompasses his or her capabilities and psychosocial influences. In clinical practice, it appears that patient-centered, interdisciplinary education of the patient and family or caregivers is the single most important factor in long-term compliance and management of the patient with congestive heart failure.

REFERENCES

1. Cohn J. Circulation 1988;78:1099–110.
2. Kannel WB. Cardiol Clin 1989;1–9.
3. Ghali JK, Cooper R, Ford E. Arch Intern Med 1990;150:769–73.
4. Barnett DB. The sympathetic nervous system and myocardial adrenoreceptor function and regulation of cardiac failure. In: Barnett DB, Pouleur H, Francis G, eds. Congestive cardiac failure. New York: Marcel Dekker, 1993;29–45.
5. McDonald K, Francis GS. Pathophysiology of heart failure. In: Barnett DB, Pouleur H, Francis G, eds. Congestive cardiac failure. New York: Marcel Dekker, 1993;46–61.
6. Komuro I, Kaida T, Shibazuki G, et al. J Biol Chem 1990;265:3595.
7. Fuller SJ, Gaitanaki CJ, Sugden PH. Biochem J 1990;727–36.
8. Ganten D, Scheling P, Flugel RM, et al. Int Res Common Med Sci 1975;3:327.
9. Cohn J. Clin Cardiol 1995;18:4–12.
10. Baughn DE, Lamas A, Pfeffer M. Left ventricular remodeling. In: Barnett DB, Pouleur H, Francis G, eds. Congestive cardiac failure. New York: Marcel Dekker, 1993;71–4.
11. Hammermesiter KE, DeRoven TA, Dodge HT. Circulation 1979;59:42–50.
12. Pfeffer MA, Lamas GA, Vaughan DE, et al. N Engl J Med 1988;319:80–6.
13. Hosenpud JD, Greenberg BH. Congestive heart failure. New York: Springer-Velag, 1994;594–613.
14. Ansari A. Prog Cardiovasc Dis 1987;30:45–60.
15. Pittman JG, Cohen P. N Engl J Med 1964;271:403–8.
16. Freeman L, Roubenoff R. Nutr Rev 1994;52:340–7.
17. Heymsfield SB, Smith J, Redd S. Surg Clin North Am 1981;61:635–50.
18. Kris-Etherton P. Cardiovascular disease: nutrition for prevention and treatment. Chicago: American Dietetic Association 1990;151–3.
19. Pittman JG, Cohen P. Pathogenesis of cardiac cachexia. N Engl J Med 1964;271:453–60.
20. Hakkula J, Mahila TE, Halonen PI. Am J Cardiol 1960;5:295–9.
21. Davidson JD, Waldman TA, Goodman DS, et al. Lancet 1961;1:899–902.
22. Kinsey D, White PD. Arch Intern Med 1990;65:163–70.
23. Poehlman ET, Schiffers J, Gottlieb SS, et al. Ann Intern Med 1994;121:860–2.
24. Levine B, Mayer L, et al. N Engl J Med 1990;223:236–41.
25. Oral H, Kapsadia S, Nakumo M, et al. Clin Cardiol 1995;18:20–7.
26. Cohn J, Archibald D, Ziesche S. N Engl J Med 1986;314:1547–52.
27. Cohn J, Johnson G, Ziesche S, et al. N Engl J Med 1991;325:303–10.
28. SOLVD Investigators. N Engl J Med 1991;325:294–8.
29. Dracup K, Baker D, Dunbar S, et al. JAMA 1994;272:1442–6.
30. American Dietetic Association. Handbook of clinical dietietics. Hanover, MA: Yale University Press 1981;G5–6.
31. Goodhart R, Shils M. Modern nutrition in health and disease. 5th ed. Philadelphia: Lea & Febiger, 1978;888–91.
32. Gottschlich M, Matarese L, Shronts E. Nutrition support dietetics—core curriculum. 2nd ed. Silver Spring, MD: American Society for Parenteral and Enteral Nutrition 1993;243–9.
33. Schneider H, Anderson C, Coursin D. Nutritional support of medical practice. Hagerstown, MD: Harper & Row, 1977;250–1.
34. Loeb S. Illustrated guide to diagnostic tests. Springhouse, PA: Springhouse Corp, 1993;419–32.
35. National Research Council. Recommended dietary allowances. 10th ed. Washington, DC: National Academy Press, 1989;59–60.
36. Pronsky Z. Food-medication interactions. 8th ed. Pottstown, PA: Food-Medication Interactions, 1993;88,118,205.

78. Molecular Basis of Human Neoplasia: A Tutorial

PAUL D. SAVAGE

Current dogma in molecular oncology is built on the premise that cancer is the end result of an accumulation of genetic alterations, some that may be acquired, some that may be inherited. The genes that are altered are those involved in fundamental, normal cellular processes such as cell cycle regulation, signaling, and differentiation, many of which are discussed elsewhere in this book. Many environmental agents are felt to cause such genetic abnormalities. These include viruses, chemicals, dietary factors, and radiation; however, when focusing on a specific gene, specific abnormality, or a specific type of cancer, the list shortens considerably. This dogma—that cancer results from the accumulation of genetic abnormalities—unifies the current hypotheses of physical carcinogenesis (chemicals and radiation), viral carcinogenesis, and genetics, in that all of these can cause changes in a cell's DNA.

This tutorial describes the crucial classes, or families, of genes and genetic systems that are altered as part of the basic processes of carcinogenesis in which a normal cell is transformed into a malignant one. The promise for the future is that by better understanding the molecular basis of carcinogenesis, specific treatments or preventive measures can be undertaken that will be nontoxic to the normal cells and tissues of the patient, thus providing more effective cancer therapy.

ONCOGENES AND TUMOR SUPPRESSOR GENES (ANTIONCOGENES)

The homeostatic state of most cells results from a balance between opposing processes, akin to a car that is moving at constant speed on level ground with both the accelerator and brake pedals partially "on." When a cell needs to adjust to a stimulus or new conditions, the "action" is often the result of a relative change in balance between opposing forces; using the model of the car, as it climbs a hill, it must either increase the accelerator, decrease the brake, or both to maintain a constant speed; once on level ground, the previous ratio is restored to again maintain the constant speed. Similarly, if there is a need to change the speed (e.g., to go slower), the accelerator:brake ratio must change (decrease, favoring the braking mechanism).

Analogously, regulation of the cell cycle (which determines the replication rate of cells) is a balance between gene products that induce a cell to replicate and gene products that deter cells from replicating; in many cancers, defects in these regulatory systems have occurred, causing the cells to be driven into uncontrolled replication. Genes that can cause resting cells to divide are in a class of genes referred to as protooncogenes (i.e., the "accelerator" on the car model), whereas the genes that can prevent a cell from dividing are members of the family of tumor suppressor genes (i.e., the "brakes") (Table 78.1). Cancer often results in part from a "lack of brakes" (absence of tumor suppressor activity), "too much accelerator" (overactivity of oncogenes), or both. Understanding how "the brakes fail" or "the accelerator gets stuck on the floor" forms the basis for understanding molecular oncogenesis.

Oncogenes

As early as 1911 it was established that particular tumors (avian sarcomas) could be induced in healthy birds by an extract derived from established avian sarcomas (1); this was not the case for sarcomas in other species nor other tumors (at that time). Although neither viruses nor DNA were recognized, considerable information was gleaned from these initial observations, such as species specificity (only birds) and tumor reproducibility (always sarcomas). Not until many years later was a viral agent proven as causative, and not until the mid-1970s was the viral genome analyzed, and it was realized that the particular virus described in the 1911 paper (which bears the author's name—the Rous Sarcoma virus) contained extra genetic material and that this material alone could induce a malignant sarcoma in healthy birds. Intense studies on this "cancer gene," or oncogene, yielded the following, unexpected revelations unprecedented for genetics theory and models at that time (2, 3):

- This oncogene was closely related to sequences found in normal, healthy cells from *all* mammalian species (the normal counterpart gene is formally referred to as a protooncogene)
- The degree of similarity (homology) between species was quite high—higher than for any other genetic system studied
- Only a single copy of the (abnormal) oncogene was needed to transform a normal, healthy cell to a full-blown malignant one

Not until 1982, after a number of viral oncogenes had been isolated from virus-induced tumors in nonhuman

Table 78.1
Examples of Oncogenes and Tumor Suppressor Genes

Oncogenes	
Growth factors	
c-fps	Colony-stimulating factor-1 (CSF-1, or M-CSF [monocyte colony-stimulating factor])
c-sis[a]	α-chain of PDGF (platelet-derived growth factor)
Growth factor receptor	
c-fms	CSF-1 receptor
c-erb-A	Thyroid hormone receptor
Protein kinases	
c-abl	Exact function unknown; overexpression seen in chronic myelogenous leukemia
Mediators of signal transduction	
ras	Nucleoside phosphatase (GTP → GDP)
Nuclear factors/DNA-binding proteins	
c-jun	Heterodimerizes with *c-fos* to form AP-1 transcription complex
c-fos	Heterodimerizes with *c-jun* to form AP-1 transcription complex
ets family (*ets*-1, *ets*-2, *erg*-1, . . .)	A family of proteins that bind to genomic DNA and regulate gene expression; possibly interacts with the AP-1 complex in the cases of some genes
c-myc	Binds to DNA (via MAX protein), causing transcription of genes that initiate S-phase; overexpression seen in both solid tumors and hematologic neoplasms; "hallmark" neoplasms are B-cell lymphomas, most notably Burkitt's lymphoma
c-myb	Hallmark neoplasm when overexpressed—acute nonlymphocytic leukemias
Antiapoptosis	
bcl-2	Expression blocks apoptosis; originally characterized as a result of its role in low-grade non-Hodgkin's lymphoma (it is overexpressed, and leading to prolonged life span of the neoplastic B lymphocytes)
Tumor Suppressor Genes	
p53	Termed the "guardian of the genome," one of the major functions attributable to *p53* is its regulation of apoptosis; when sufficient "genomic damage" has occurred, apoptosis is induced, leading to the death of the cell; inactivity is associated with many solid tumor types; hereditary deficiency is associated with the Li-Fraumeni syndrome, leading to increased incidences of breast cancers, sarcomas, brain tumors, and possibly colorectal and prostate carcinomas
rb-1	Codes for a nuclear phosphoprotein that acts as a major checkpoint in cell cycle; progression through the G_1/S transition of the cell cycle is controlled by the phosphorylation status of *rb-1;* control of differentiation in certain cell lines in vitro is also associated with changes in phosphorylation status of *rb-1;* inactivity of *rb-1* is associated with development of retinoblastoma, osteosarcoma, and breast carcinomas

[a]The names of genes are in lower case italics; their derived proteins are in capitals (see text).

mammals, was the first evidence obtained that oncogenes were involved in human malignancy. In this setting, the *c-myc protooncogene, originally isolated as the* cellular homolog to the avian leukemia *v*irus oncogene VMYC (the avian *my*elo*c*ytosis virus, hence the name *myc*), was shown to be structurally altered in virtually all cases of a lymphoid tumor called Burkitt's lymphoma; furthermore, chromosomal abnormalities that were routinely and consistently seen on cytogenetic analysis of Burkitt's lymphoma (and felt to be "hallmark findings" unique to Burkitt's lymphoma) were found to have their molecular basis in rearrangement of the c-*myc* oncogene (4). It was soon determined that the consequence of c-*myc* rearrangement was constitutive (i.e., constant, unregulated) overproduction of the CMYC protein to hundreds of times normal levels, regardless of the cell-cycle phase the lymphoma cell was in. It was later established that *(a)* exposure of a normal resting cell to a mitogenic stimulus resulted in a "burst" of CMYC oncoprotein expression (lasting only 5–10 minutes), followed by subsequent decrease in CMYC protein levels to basal resting levels as a result of normal degradative processes and *(b)* the high levels of CMYC protein associated with the "burst" were associated with that cell's entry into the S-phase of the cell cycle and subsequently by cell division and the formation of two daughter cells. Thus, the evolving picture of Burkitt's lymphomagenesis is that of a B cell whose DNA is altered so that the cell is always producing an endogenous protein that drives it into S phase and cell division (Fig. 78.1). Clearly, uncontrolled replication alone does not explain all facets of Burkitt's lymphoma (or any other malignancy), but it does explain why these (lymphoid) cells replicate in the absence of exogenous growth factors, something not seen in normal lymphocytes.

Today there are approximately 65 genes that are considered oncogenes or candidate oncogenes. Alteration of these protooncogenes to activated forms capable of inducing neoplastic transformation can occur via a variety of mechanisms, outlined below. One common feature of (activated) oncogenes is their *dominance,* in that only one of the two copies needs to be altered to induce neoplastic transformation. Furthermore, the biochemical activity of the oncoprotein is usually (but not always) more active than the normal gene product; referring to the car model, oncogene activity can, therefore, be viewed as having the gas pedal stuck to the floor in the "full open" position, accelerating the car out of control, beyond the capacity of the brakes to slow it down. It is important to realize that the abnormal oncoprotein activity (and the activated oncogene itself) are found only in tumor tissue—the remaining normal cells of the patient contain the normal protooncogene and normal gene product.

Protooncogenes can be activated to oncogenes by a

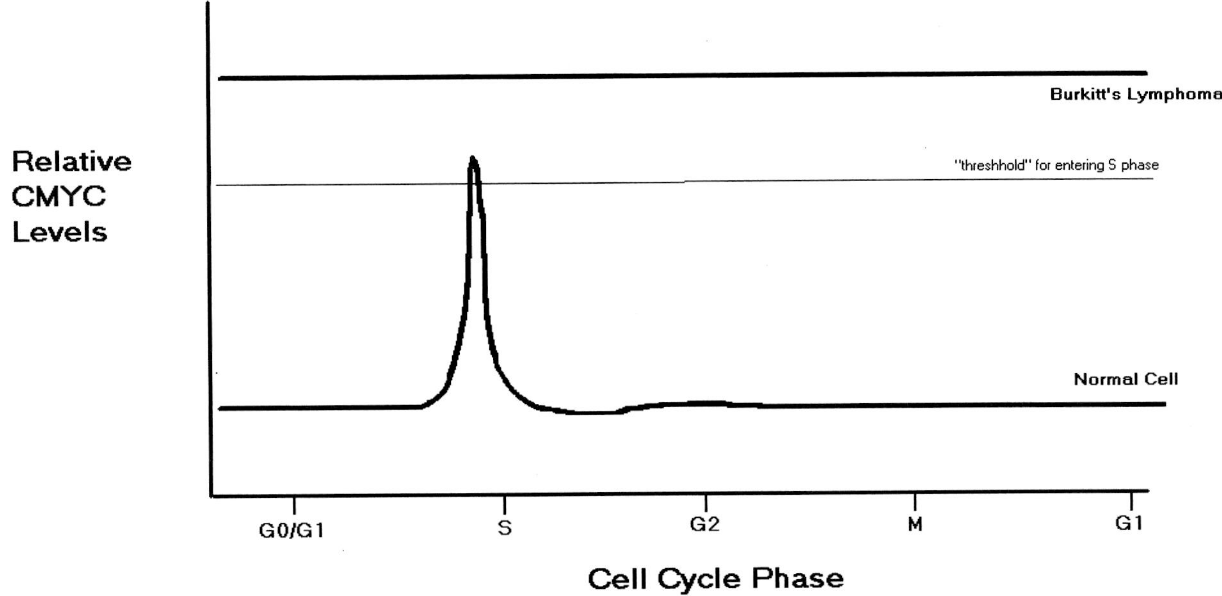

Figure 78.1. Schematic demonstrating CMYC oncoprotein levels in a normal cell and a neoplastic Burkitt's lymphoma cell. In normal cells, the level of CMYC oncoprotein is tightly regulated and linked to the cell cycle; in Burkitt's lymphoma, because of the chromosomal translocation involving the c-*myc* protooncogene, the CMYC oncoprotein is constitutively overexpressed, regardless of the phase of the cell cycle.

variety of mechanisms; the common end result is aberrant activity of a protein that the cell cannot properly control and that ultimately drives the cell into replication. The commonly observed mechanisms are best highlighted by the following examples, in which a "normal DNA sequence" (presented as 3-letter words, akin to the triplet anticodon sequence that codes for the specific amino acid sequences of a protein) is altered in a pattern analogous to the alteration in protooncogenes:

–THE RED CAT ATE THE OLD RAT —

Point Mutations/Transversions

Point mutations/transversions frequently result from exposure to chemical carcinogens and radiation. There are two types of point mutations—sense mutations, in which the altered triplet codon is a legitimate codon (i.e., is "readable"), and nonsense mutations, in which the new codon does not code for anything. Activating sense mutations usually result in amino acid substitutions (a different amino acid replacing the correct one), although the codon can code for a "stop" signal, which would result in a shortened, truncated protein; activating nonsense mutations always result in a prematurely truncated product.

The following is an example of a sense mutation (i.e., the altered sequence can still be "read," although its meaning is altered):

— THE RED CA*R* ATE THE OLD RAT —

below is an example of a nonsense mutation (i.e., the altered sequence cannot be "read"):

— THE RED CA*X* ATE THE OLD RAT —

Protooncogenes whose activation occurs as the result of premature truncation are usually overactive, as the missing sequences are frequently the regulatory sequences that control the protein's activity. When the normal gene codes for a receptor, the deleted portion is often the ligand-binding portion, with the truncated product being the catalytic activity portion that performs the biochemical process. This truncated protein can now carry out its activity in the absence of the ligand, *as if the ligand were always present*; the presence or absence of the ligand now becomes irrelevant, and the protein activity is uncontrollable.

Frameshift Mutations

Frameshift mutations result from insertions or deletions; these alterations can involve a single nucleotide or large quantities of DNA. Such mutations can easily result in an unreadable sequence (such as deletion of the "D" of "red" illustrated below), which frequently results in premature truncation of the protein:

— THE REC ATA TET HEO LDR AT? —
(? denotes the next base in the DNA sequence)

Amplification

Amplification is a process whereby a protooncogene, instead of being present in two copies within a cell, is found in increased numbers—anywhere from 10 copies to hundreds of copies per cell. In this scenario, the cellular compensatory mechanisms simply are not strong enough to overcome a signal of such magnitude. This would be akin to a well-matched pair of arm wrestlers in which one player suddenly became hundreds of times stronger; the weaker of the two players would now lose consistently. In neuroblastomas and breast cancer, the copy number of the N*myc* and c-*erb-B2/HER2/neu* oncogenes, respectively, is of independent prognostic importance for survival. The mechanisms that cause amplification are not yet established, although some data suggest that errors in mismatch-repair may play a role. In the following example the sequence is amplified three times, in tandem:

—THE RED CAT ATE THE OLD RAT THE RED CAT ATE THE OLD RAT THE RED CAT ATE THE OLD RAT —

Translocations

Translocations result in the fusion of two genes—a protooncogene and another cellular gene—forming the transforming oncogene. The fusion gene often codes for a novel protein not found under any other circumstances. Alternatively, translocations can bring the intact protooncogene coding sequences under the regulatory control of a strong(er) promoter, resulting in overexpression of a normal protooncogene product (this end result would be biologically indistinguishable from amplification). This latter case is the situation for Burkitt's lymphoma, in which the coding sequences of c-*myc* are translocated to the immunoglobulin genes in such a way that the *c-myc* coding sequences are under the control of the immunoglobulin gene regulatory sequences.

chromosome A: — THE RED CAT ATE THE OLD RAT —
chromosome B: — THE DOG SAW THE NEW FLY—
becomes
chromosome A*: — THE RED CAT SAW THE NEW FLY—
chromosome B*: — THE DOG ATE THE OLD RAT —

With rare exceptions, there is nothing specific about a given oncogene abnormality and the type of tumor caused by that abnormality; rather, a normal cell can undergo transformation to a neoplastic (malignant) cell if a particular protooncogene within that cell becomes altered in a fashion that results in activation. For example, the *ras* protooncogene family has three members—H-*ras,* N-*ras,* and Ki-*ras,* which have unique locations within the genome. Each *ras* member can become activated by a point mutation at any of three particular codons (12, 13, or 61), which results in an amino acid substitution. As shown in Table 78.2, the same abnormality of H-*ras* (i.e., Glu → Leu transversion of codon 61), for instance, has been identified in lung cancers and melanomas, while lung cancer has been reported to have abnormalities of either H-*ras,* N-*ras,* or Ki-*ras,* albeit not to equal extents. Thus, there is not a specific lung cancer abnormality within the *ras* system, nor does a specific *ras* abnormality cause a particular cancer. A notable exception is a specific abnormality of Ki-*ras* that is seen in over 95% of human pancreatic carcinomas; the high frequency of this association suggests that this alteration may be causative for this malignancy.

A second example involves the *c-erb-B2/HER2/neu* oncogene (this gene has three names, reflecting the three different means by which it was independently studied and named prior to the realization that it was in fact one gene). In human breast cancers this oncogene is amplified, with copy number having prognostic importance. This contrasts with this gene's first isolation from rat *neu*ro- and glioblastomas, in which it is activated by point mutations.

Table 78.2
Alterations Associated with *ras* Activation and Tumor Types

	Amino Acid Residue			
Oncogene Allele	12	13	61	Tumor Type
c*-H-*ras*[a]	Gly	Gly	Glu	(Normal)
			Leu	Melanoma
			Leu	Lung cancer
	Val			Bladder cancer
	Asp			Breast
c-Ki-*ras*	Gly	Gly	Glu	(Normal)
	Val			Colon
	Cys			Lung
c-N-*ras*	Gly	Gly	Glu	(Normal)
			Lys	Neuroblastoma
			Arg	Lung
		Val or Asp		Acute myeloid leukemia

[a]c, denotes cellular homologue.

Tumor Suppressor Genes

As alluded to above, tumor suppressor genes serve as "braking mechanisms," preventing cells from undergoing uncontrolled growth; tumors may result, therefore, when such gene activity is *absent.* Since these genes are autosomal (i.e., cells contain two copies—one maternally derived and one paternally derived), tumor formation requires that *both* genes become defective (within a cell) to lose genetic (tumor suppressor) activity. Using our automobile analogy, this situation would arise when the brakes are suddenly lost, with the result being that the car accelerates uncontrollably, since the gas pedal is "on" (remember, "normal" is a balance in which the gas and brakes are both (partially) "on"). As with oncogenes, particular abnormalities of a tumor suppressor gene are not specific for tumor type, nor are particular tumor types associated with specific tumor suppressor abnormalities, although there are exceptions (much like the association of Ki-*ras* abnormalities with >95% of human pancreatic carcinomas). For example, alteration of codon 132 of *p53* has been reported for cancers of the ovary, breast, lung, and colon; ovarian cancers, on the other hand, have been associated with abnormalities of codons 132, 139, 151, 172, 237, and 242, to name only a few. A striking association exists between abnormalities involving codon 249 and hepatocellular carcinomas from individuals in high-risk regions (5). Most abnormalities of *p53* that have been associated with malignancies involve those regions of the gene with highly conserved sequences between the human and other mammals.

The tumor suppressor genes are the class of genes that are responsible for many, if not all, of the inherited cancer syndromes (6). These syndromes have variable penetrance (i.e., virtually all members of one family may develop cancer, while only a few members of another family may become victim to the disease). Such patterns of presentation would be predicted, since abnormalities of one allele would not be expected to give rise to malignancy, but such patients would be more susceptible to cancer development when exposed to other factors. This predisposition arises since all cells in these patients already have one of the two abnormalities (of a given suppressor gene) necessary for tumor development; furthermore, such predisposition would lead to earlier and more frequent tumor development than seen in the sporadic cases, since the sporadic cases require two abnormalities to be acquired within the same cell (against a normal background). Indeed, this is the situation a) in patients with hereditary retinoblastoma (who have a defect in *rb-1*) versus those with sporadic retinoblastoma, b) for development of neurofibrosarcomas in patients with hereditary neurofibromatosis (who have a defect in *nf-1*) versus those with sporadic neurofibrosarcoma, and c) for development of sarcomas and breast cancers in patients with the Li-Fraumeni syndrome (who have a defect in *p53*) versus the general population. These are a few of many cases. Although the responsible genes have not been definitively identified, the identification and inheritance pattern of approximately 20 to 30 familial cancer syndromes is consistent with their molecular etiology being an inherited defective tumor suppressor gene.

As with the oncogenes, many mechanisms can alter tumor suppressor genes. The most intuitive (to eliminate a gene's activity)—that of deleting or eliminating the gene itself—occurs frequently among these genes. The first indication of this was at the cytogenetic level, when a small percentage of retinoblastomas demonstrated a shortened chromosome 13, specifically a shortened long arm; a very rare patient's tumor demonstrated abnormalities of both chromosome 13s. As loss of function can occur with deletion or substitution of just a single critical base, the biologic significance of deletions of larger amounts of genetic material (sometimes the entire chromosome) is not clear. Base substitution (point mutation) is the other abnormality frequently seen in defective tumor suppressor genes. For unclear reasons, most tumors that have been analyzed have demonstrated a consistent pattern: one allele is completely deleted, while the other one contains small, intragenic deletions or point mutations. Which came first, or why both alleles are not altered by the same means to the same extent, is unclear.

The concept of cancer being a multistep process, likely involving multiple genetic defects, is best exemplified in the hereditary cancer syndromes, since these represent situations in which every cell in the body contains the identical (single) allelic defect. Were a tumor to arise from whatever cell acquired the second necessary defect (in the normal allele), then all types of cancers would be seen in affected families. Yet specific syndromes are identifiable because of the limited spectrum of tumor type(s) seen for a particular syndrome. For example, patients with hereditary retinoblastoma are predisposed to becoming homozygous with respect to *rb-1* (the retinoblastoma suppressor gene); to date, this gene has been implicated as having a central role in the cell cycle, which all living cells use. Yet patients with hereditary retinoblastoma only demonstrate increased incidences of retinoblastomas, osteosarcomas, and breast cancers; notably "absent" from this list are tumors from tissues that are very active and are always dividing and cycling—primarily skin and gastrointestinal tract but also the respiratory tract. Hence, as with the oncogenes, a given gene defect likely is necessary but not sufficient.

Some of the most intriguing experiments being conducted that hold promise for future treatments involve reintroduction of missing tumor suppressor genes into tumor cells. Such genetic manipulation in vitro has resulted in reversal of some (if not all) of the properties of malignant cells, with return of growth control (cessation of growth, inability to form a tumor mass), loss of metastatic capabilities (inability to spread), and even tumor cell death (7, 8). Such manipulations are still limited to in vitro conditions in which the missing gene, part of the chromosome containing the missing gene, or the entire chromosome on which the missing gene lies, is directly introduced into the cell by nuclear microinjection or by exposing cells in culture to nonphysiologic conditions (such as extremes in acidity, salt concentrations, or electrical fields) (9). Despite the inapplicability of such manipulations to the intact organism, these experiments form the basis and rationale for developing gene therapy as a treatment modality because they demonstrate that restoration of absent genetic function can arrest the natural progression of an established malignancy. Additionally, such experiments may ultimately lead to a better understanding of the exact function(s) of the missing gene(s), which could suggest an alternative means of compensating for the genetic deficiency, possibly by providing the protein itself or its product or by manipulating the affected pathway farther downstream through conventional pharmacologic means.

Oncogenes, Growth Factors, Hormones, and Their Receptors

Recent studies have elucidated a system of growth factors, receptors, and transporters related to insulin and its receptors—the insulin-like growth factor superfamily. This system of ligands (insulin-like growth factors, or IGFs), receptors (insulin-like growth factor receptors [IGFRs]), and binding proteins (insulin-like growth factor–binding proteins [IGFBPs]) is abnormally expressed or regulated in malignant cells and may serve an autocrine or paracrine function in tumor cell proliferation.

Breast cancer is one of only a few malignancies that express estrogen and progesterone receptors (ER and PR, respectively) on the surface of the tumor cells. When these receptors are present, there is an (approximately) 80% likelihood the tumors will respond to hormonal blockade with antiestrogenic agents such as tamoxifen; interestingly, about one-third of patients whose tumors do not express hormone receptors also respond to hormonal manipulation, for previously unclear reasons.

Studies on breast cancer that have examined the IGFs have not only demonstrated abnormal expression of these growth factors, their receptors, and binding proteins but also suggested that an interaction may exist between the "classic" hormone/receptor system (i.e., estrogen, progesterone, and their receptors) and the IGF system of growth factors and receptors. Specifically, tissues from both receptor-positive and receptor-negative breast tumors express increased levels of IGFBPs (10), and tamoxifen decreases circulating levels of IGF-1 (11, 12); this lowering of circulating IGF-1 may explain why tamoxifen works in some breast cancer patients whose tumors are receptor negative. Analogously, all-*trans* retinoic acid, which induces differentiation of certain tumors in vivo and in vitro (see Chapter 17), inhibits breast cancer cells in vivo by altering expression and release of IGFBPs (13).

MISMATCH REPAIR

DNA replication is an imperfect system; it is estimated that one of every 100,000 bases (i.e., 10^{-5}) that is replicated is initially replicated erroneously. As the genome of each human cell contains approximately 1 billion (10^9) bases, 10,000 errors would be acquired within every cell with each division were there no mechanisms to correct these mistakes. Many mechanisms have been demonstrated in organisms as simple as bacteria and yeast that "proofread" the DNA as it is being replicated and correct these errors, so that the error rate in bacteria is estimated to be on the order of $1/10^{10}$ bases (10^{-10}). Although there are no estimates for mammalian (and particularly, human) cells, the rates are probably of the same order of magnitude. One of the most important mechanisms and the one with strong implications for human cancer is the mismatch-repair system, or the human homologue to the bacterial MutS system. This system reads the double helix as it is being replicated, and if an incorrect base has been inserted (creating a mismatch), this system excises the incorrect base, allowing insertion of another base (statistically, the correct one).

This system was first established as being important in human cancer when it was shown that the vast majority of patients with hereditary nonpolyposis colon cancer (HNPCC) had defective mismatch repair and that this defect was likely the heritable lesion (14); soon thereafter it was shown that (colon) tumors from most patients with sporadic colon cancer were also deficient in mismatch repair, whereas normal tissues from these patients were not.

Cancer cells have been noted to have a higher spontaneous mutation rate than their normal counterparts in vitro and in vivo. This is almost certainly requisite for solid tumor development if the current model, which predicts that tumors arise as the result of the accumulation of *multiple* genetic defects, is correct (see Fig. 78.2, for the model of colorectal carcinogenesis). Such a hypothesis is supported by recent observations that defects in mismatch repair result in higher mutation rates. Thus, errors in mismatch repair are likely early events in tumorigenesis; these errors then predispose the cells (deficient in mismatch repair) to even more errors and mutations, probably within critical oncogenes and tumor suppressors, leading to a growth advantage over the normal cells. The increased growth rate contributes to further errors in DNA replication, ultimately leading into a "vicious cycle" that would continue until either sufficient damage is acquired to be lethal or the "right combination" of errors occurs in critical genes to allow autonomous uncontrolled growth.

TELOMERES AND TELOMERASE

One of the latest discoveries in molecular oncology involves the regulation of telomeres—the "capping" sequences found at the ends of chromosomes. Structurally, telomeres are tandem repeat sequences whose length and integrity are maintained by the enzyme telomerase. Every time a cell divides, the telomeres of the daughter cells are slightly shorter because of the way that DNA replication is initiated; furthermore, as a resting cell ages (chronologically), telomerase activity within that cell steadily decreases. The end result of these processes is progressively shorter telomeres, both as a result of endogenous, normal enzymatic degradation of the ends of the chromosomal DNA and by imperfect DNA replication.

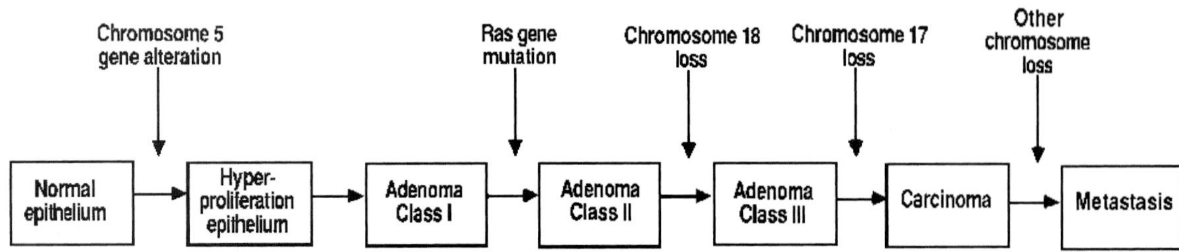

Figure 78.2. Schema of colorectal tumorigenesis, demonstrating accumulation of multiple genetic abnormalities required to achieve a malignant neoplastic cell. Note that the ability to metastasize requires acquisition of additional abnormalities that remain to be elucidated. (Adapted from Stanbridge EJ, et al., Science 1990;247:12–13.)

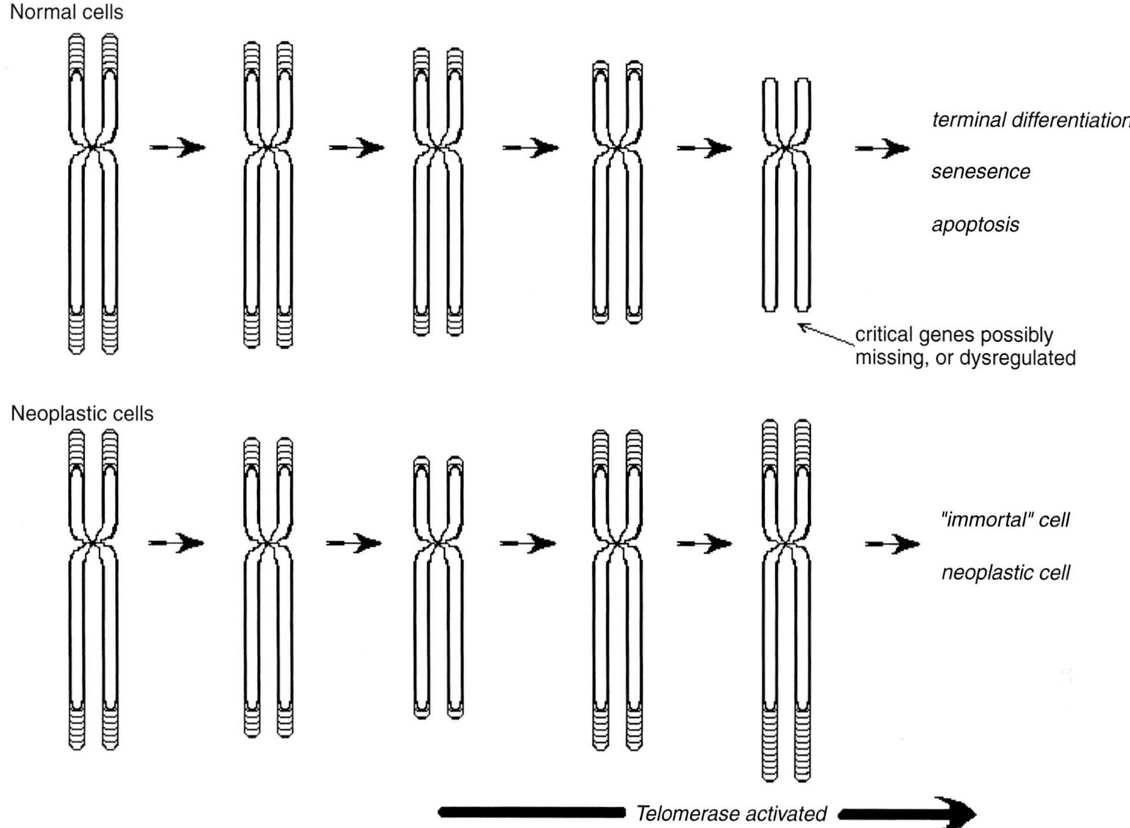

Figure 78.3. Effect of telomete length in normal and (some) neoplastic cells. In normal cells, the telomeres become progressively shorter with each replication of the cell or as part of normal turnover and DNA repair in some nondividing resting cells. In neoplastic cells, telomerase activity, normally absent in somatic cells, is present, often above the levels found in germ cells and fetal tissues. The telomeres do not shorten over time or with replication; thus the cells can potentially live "indefinitely."

At some critical point, the telomeres become so short that the genes at the ends of the somatic portion of the chromosomes become inactive, because of either altered regulation or actual structural degradation, and the cell undergoes apoptosis (programed cell death). In vitro, immortal cells (cells that can be passaged and propagated "indefinitely") have constant, and sometimes increased, levels of telomerase, and their telomeres are often longer than those in the parental nonimmortalized cells (Fig. 78.3).

Analysis of tumor cells from certain malignancies in humans and other species revealed increased telomerase activity and telomere length in the tumor cells relative to the normal surrounding tissue. This "phenotype" (increased telomerase activity and long telomeres) is present in some human renal cell carcinoma cell lines. In renal cell carcinoma, the short arm of chromosome 3 is frequently lost, and occasionally the entire chromosome is lost. Cell lines derived from these tumors have longer telomeres than those found in normal renal cells and higher telomerase levels than normal renal cells; these cell lines are immortal. Reintroduction of a normal chromosome 3 into the nuclei of cells from these cell lines (by nuclear microinjection) results in decreased telomerase levels, progressive shortening of the telomeres, and eventual senescence of the cells that were microinjected (15). How widespread this phenomenon is among human tumors has not yet been determined, but potential differences in telomere biology between normal and cancer tissue clearly provides a new avenue for investigation and intervention. To date, no hereditary disease or condition (other than cancer) is attributable to abnormal telomerase, although some premature aging syndromes (e.g., progeria) are candidates for investigation into this area.

REFERENCES

1. Rous P. J Exp Med 1911;13:397–411.
2. Spector DH, Varmus HE, Bishop JM. Proc Natl Acad Sci USA 1978;75:4102–6.
3. Stehelin D, Varmus HE, Bishop JM, et al. Nature 1976;260: 170–3.
4. Taub R, Kirsch I, Morton C, et al. Proc Natl Acad Sci USA 1982;79:7837–41.
5. Hollstein M, Sidransky D, Vogelstein B, et al. Science 1991; 253:49–53.
6. Knudson AG. Proc Natl Acad Sci USA 1993;90:10914–21.
7. Trent JM, Stanbridge EJ, McBride HL, et al. Science 1990; 247(4942):568–71.
8. Leone A, Flatow U, King CR, et al. Cell 1991;65(1):25–35.
9. Vigneron JP, Oudrhiri N, Fauquet M, et al. Proc Natl Acad Sci USA 1996;93:9682–6.

10. LeRoith D, Baserga R, Helman L, et al. Ann Intern Med 1995;122:54–9.
11. Pollak MN, Huynh HT, Lefebvre SP. Breast Cancer Res Treat 1992;22:91–100.
12. Colletti RB, Roberts JD, Devlin JT, et al. Cancer Res 1989; 49:1882–4.
13. Adamo ML, Shao ZM, Lanau F, et al. Endocrinology 1992; 131:1858–66.
14. Fishel R, Lescoe MK, Rao MRS, et al. Cell 1994;75(5):1027–38.
15. Ohmura H, Tahara H, Suzuki M, et al. Jpn J Cancer Res 1995;86:899–904.

SELECTED READING

Cooper GM, ed. Oncogenes. 2nd ed. Sudbury: Jones and Bartlett, 1995:1–400.

79. Diet, Nutrition, and the Prevention of Cancer

WALTER C. WILLETT

CANCER AS A PUBLIC HEALTH PROBLEM

Following cardiovascular disease, cancer is the second leading cause of death in most affluent countries and also contributes importantly to mortality rates among adults in developing countries (1, 2). In the U.S., about one in three persons will be diagnosed with cancer during their lifetime, and about 60% of those diagnosed will die of cancer (3). Because rates of cardiovascular death have been declining rapidly and overall cancer mortality has not substantially changed, it is likely that cancer will become the most important cause of death in the U.S. (2, 4). Although overall cancer rates among adults vary only modestly around the world, the types of cancers are dramatically different (1, 2). In affluent countries cancers of the lung, colon, breast, and prostate contribute most to incidence and mortality (Fig. 79.1*A* and *B*). In poorer regions and the Far East, cancers of the stomach, liver, oral cavity, esophagus, and uterine cervix are most important. In Japan, for example, rates of breast cancer have until recently been only about one-fifth those of the U.S., and the differences in rates of colon and prostate cancers have been even greater (5). However, cancer incidence rates are very dynamic; many areas of the world are experiencing a transition from the cancer incidence patterns of poorer to those of affluent areas (1). In almost all countries, rates of breast cancer have been increasing.

Although development of cancer is characterized by alterations in DNA and some of these changes can be inherited, inherited mutations cannot account for the dramatic differences in cancer rates seen around the world. Populations that move from countries with low rates of cancer to areas with high rates, or the reverse, almost invariably achieve the rates characteristic of the new homeland (6–8). The rate of change can vary, though, from several decades in the case of colon cancer, to about three generations for breast cancer (8–11). The dramatic changes in cancer rates within countries provide further evidence for the importance of noninherited factors. For example, in Japan, rates of colon cancer mortality increased about 2.5-fold between 1950 and 1985 (5).

The dramatic variations in cancer rates around the world and changes over time imply that these malignancies are potentially avoidable if we knew and could alter the causal factors. For a few cancers, such as lung cancer, the primary causes are well known, in this case smoking, but for most others, the etiologic factors are less well established. However, there are strong reasons to suspect that dietary and nutritional factors may account for many of these variations in cancer rates. First, a role of diet has been suggested by observations that national rates of specific cancers are strongly correlated with aspects of diet such as per capita consumption of fat (12). Also, numerous studies in animals, including a series of detailed experiments conducted during the 1930s (13), clearly demonstrated that dietary manipulations could dramatically influence tumorigenesis.

Also, a multitude of steps in the pathogenesis of cancer have been identified in which dietary factors could plausibly act either to increase or decrease the probability that clinical cancer will develop. For example, carcinogens in specific foods that can directly damage DNA are discussed in Chapter 80, and other dietary factors may block endogenous synthesis of carcinogens or induce enzymes involved in the activation or deactivation of exogenous carcinogenic substances (14). Oxidative damage to DNA is likely to be an important cause of mutations and can potentially be enhanced by some dietary factors, such as polyunsaturated fats, or reduced by dietary antioxidants or nutrients that are cofactors for antioxidant enzymes, such as selenium or copper (15). Inadequate intake of dietary factors needed for DNA synthesis, such as folic acid, could also influence the risk of mutation. The rate of cell division influences whether DNA lesions are replicated and is thus likely to influence the probability of cancer developing (15). Thus, energy balance and growth rates, which can be influenced by a variety of essential nutrients, could affect cancer rates. Dietary factors can influence endogenous hormone levels, including estrogens and various growth factors, which can influence cell cycling and thus, potentially, cancer incidence. Estrogenic substances found in some plant foods can also interact with estrogen receptors and thus could either mimic or block the effects of endogenous estrogens (14). Many other aspects of diet can alter cell proliferation or differentiation, either by direct hormonal effects, such as by vitamins A or D, or indirectly by influencing inflammatory or irritative

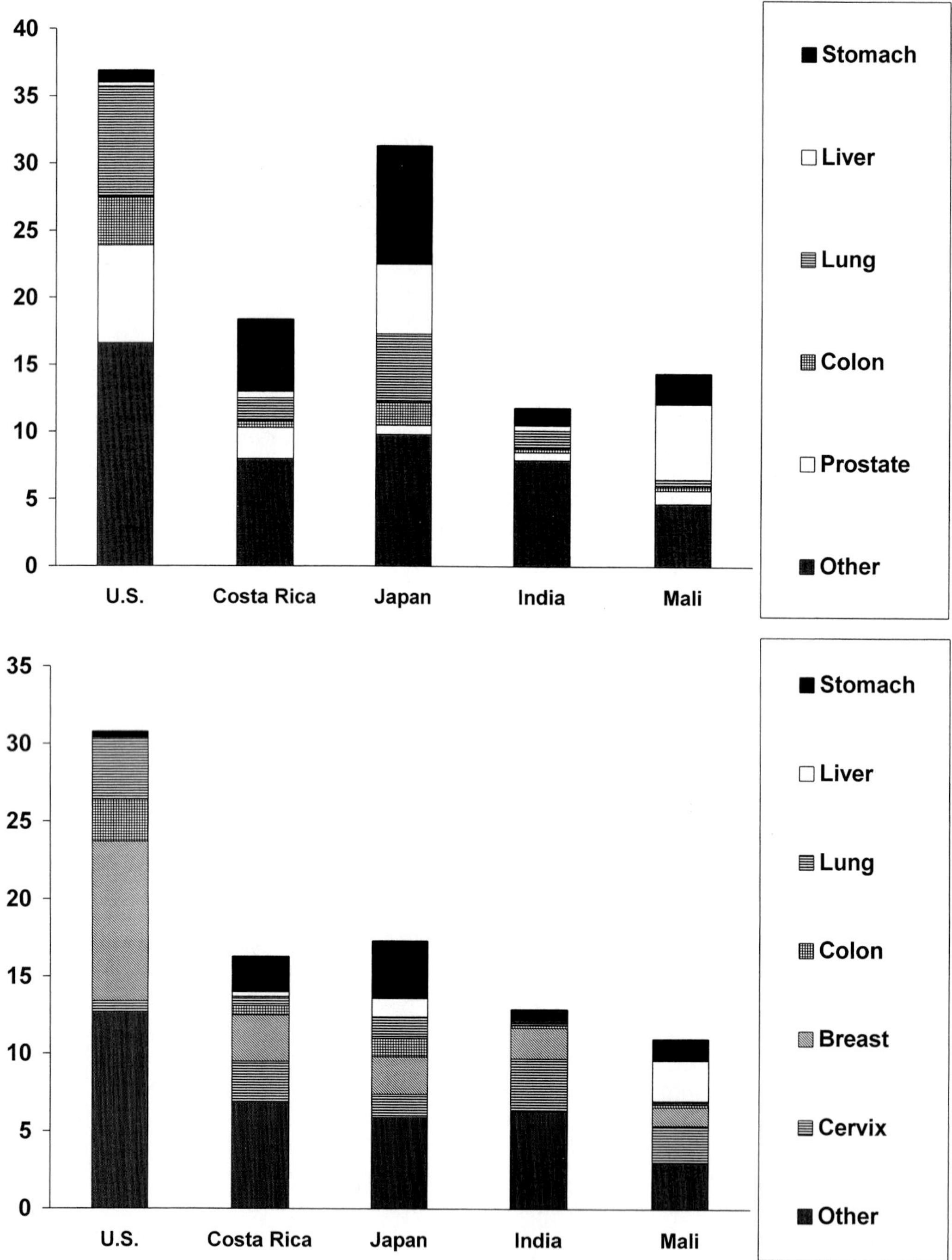

Figure 79.1. A. Cancer incidence rates for men in several countries. Cumulative incidence 0–74 years (per 100,000 population). (U.S.-SEER-nationwide, Costa Rica-nationwide, Japan-Osaka, India-Bangladore, Mali-Bamako) (skin cancers not included) (2, 170) **B.** Cancer incidence rates for women in several countries. Cumulative incidence 0–74 years (per 100,000 population). (U.S.-SEER-nationwide, Costa Rica-nationwide, Japan-Osaka, India-Bangladore, Mali-Bamako) (skin cancers not included) (2, 170).

processes, such as specific fatty acids that are precursors of prostaglandins or that inhibit their synthesis. Many other examples can be given of how dietary factors could plausibly influence the development of cancer (14, 15).

EPIDEMIOLOGIC INVESTIGATION OF DIET AND CANCER RELATIONSHIPS

The strong suggestion from international comparisons, animal studies, and mechanistic investigations that various aspects of diet might importantly influence risk of cancer raises two critical sets of questions: Which dietary factors are actually important determinants of human cancer? and What is the nature of the dose-response relationships? The nature of the dose-response relationships is particularly important because a substance could be carcinogenic to humans, but there could be no important risk within the range of intakes actually consumed by humans. Alternatively, another factor could be critical for protection against cancer, but all persons in a population may already be consuming sufficient amounts to receive the maximal benefit. In either case, there is no potential for reduction in cancer rates by altering current intakes. The important factors to identify are those of which at least some part of the population is either consuming a toxic level or is not eating a sufficient amount for optimal health.

A variety of epidemiologic approaches can be used to investigate diet and human cancer relationships (Table 79.1). Relationships between diet, nutrition, and cancer incidence in epidemiologic studies can be evaluated by collecting data on dietary intake, by using biochemical indicators of dietary factors, or by measuring body size and composition. Food frequency questionnaires have been used to assess diet in most epidemiologic studies because they provide information on usual diet over an extended period of time and are sufficiently efficient to be used in large populations. Food frequency questionnaires have been shown to be sufficiently valid to detect important diet-disease relationships in comparisons with more detailed assessments of diet and biochemical indicators (16). Biochemical indicators of diet can be useful in some situations, but for many dietary factors of interest, such as total fat, fiber, and sodium, no useful indicators exist. DNA specimens collected from participants in many studies allow examination of gene-diet interactions. Until now, most information on diet and cancer has been obtained from case-control studies. However, a number of large prospective cohort studies of diet and cancer in various countries are now ongoing and will be producing reliable data at an exponentially increasing rate as their populations age.

Epidemiologic investigations should be viewed as complementary to animal studies, in vitro investigations, metabolic studies of diet in relation to intermediate endpoints, such as hormone levels, and randomized controlled studies. Although conditions can be controlled to a much greater degree in laboratory studies than in free-living human populations, the relevance of findings to humans will always be uncertain, particularly in regard to dose-response relationships. Ultimately, our knowledge is best based on a synthesis of epidemiologic, metabolic, animal, and mechanistic studies.

SPECIFIC ASPECTS OF DIET

Diet is a complex composite of various nutrients and nonnutritive food constituents, and there are many types of human cancer, each with its own pathogenetic mechanisms; thus, the combinations of specific dietary factors and cancer are almost limitless. This brief overview focuses primarily on the major cancers of affluent populations and aspects of diet for which there are strong hypotheses and substantial epidemiologic data. Several dietary factors that are thought to have preventive roles are discussed in detail in Chapter 81.

Energy Balance, Growth Rate, and Body Size

Studies by Tannenbaum and colleagues (13, 17) during the first half of the 20th century indicated that energy restriction could profoundly reduce development of mammary tumors in animals. This finding has been consistently replicated in a wide variety of mammary tumor models and has also been observed for a wide variety of other tumors (18–22). For example, restricting energy intake by approximately 30% can reduce mammary tumors by as much as 90% (23). The possibility that this relationship, which is the most consistent and strong effect of diet in animal studies, might also apply to humans has received relatively little attention until recently.

In evaluating the effect of energy restriction on cancer rates in humans, it may be tempting to examine the association between energy intake and incidence of cancer. However, such an approach is likely to be completely misleading because in free-living populations, variation in energy intake is determined largely by energy expenditure in the form of physical activity (24). Thus, for example, energy intake is inversely associated with risk of coronary heart disease. This is attributed to the fact that increased exercise is actually the driving force for the increased food intake (16). The most sensitive indicators of the balance between energy intake and expenditure are growth rates and body size, which can be well measured in epidemiologic investigations, although they also reflect genetic and other nonnutritional factors. Adult height can provide an indirect indicator of preadult nutrition, and adult weight gain and obesity reflect positive energy balance later in life.

Internationally, the average national height of adult women is strongly associated with risk of breast cancer (25). Also, in case-control and cohort studies, greater height has generally been associated with an increased risk of breast cancer (26). For example, in a representative U.S. sample, taller women had nearly twice the risk of

Table 79.1
Types of Studies That Address Effect of Diet on Human Cancer

Study	Methods	Potential Limitations
Descriptive	Comparison of cancer rates in populations having different diets by assessing average intake of specific nutrients and determining cancer incidence or mortality	Diet is only one of many variables that distinguish different populations; gathering even crude data on average nutrient intake is difficult; these studies are probably best used to generate hypotheses
Case-control	Comparison of earlier diets reported by patients with a particular type of cancer with diets reported by matched controls without cancer	Selection bias can occur if controls do not accurately represent the population from which cases arose; recall bias results when patients systematically differ from controls in ability to recall diets; memory of dietary habits can be faulty among patients with controls[a]; in studies of rapidly fatal cancers, researchers must often rely on recall of proxy respondents such as spouses
Cohort (prospective or follow-up)	Comparison of incidence of cancer in people whose diets and other potentially relevant traits are determined before follow-up begins	Selection bias and recall bias should not occur, but cohort studies must enroll thousands or even tens of thousands of people and monitor their health for many years before statistical power can be achieved
Interventional	Comparison of incidence of cancer in two groups randomized to specific interventions or sometimes to no interventions	Compliance with substantial dietary changes is difficult for many people; subjects cannot be easily blinded to their status. Optimal dosages (e.g., of supplemental nutrients) and dose-response relationships can be difficult to ascertain; duration of intervention required is generally unknown but may be decades

From Willett WC. Adv Oncol 1995;11:3–8.
[a]In case-control and cohort studies of the effect of vitamins, measurements of vitamins in blood are sometimes substituted for dietary recall questionnaires; however, this strategy is not universally applicable. For example, retinol levels in blood do not accurately reflect intake of vitamin A, for example, whereas β-carotene blood levels are a good index of dietary intake. Blood levels must be interpreted with caution in case-control studies because cancer can change the level of a vitamin in plasma.

breast cancer of the shortest (27). Taller height has also been associated with risk of colon and other cancers (28, 29). In populations who were traditionally short, such as the Japanese, rapid gains in height during the last several decades (30) have corresponded to increases in breast cancer rates. Further support for an important role of growth rates comes from epidemiologic studies of age at menarche. Early menarche is a well-established risk factor for breast cancer. The difference in the late age in China, approximately 17 years (31), compared with 12 and 13 years of age in the U.S. (32), contributes importantly to differences in breast cancer rates between these populations. Body mass index, height, and weight have consistently been strong determinants of age at menstruation (33–35), but the composition of diet appears to have little if any effect. Collectively, these studies provide strong evidence, consistent with animal experiments, that rapid growth rates prior to puberty play an important role in determining future risk of breast and probably other cancers. Whether the epidemiologic findings are due only to restriction of energy intake in relation to requirements for maximal growth or whether the limitation of other nutrients, such as essential amino acids, may also play a role cannot be determined from available data.

A positive energy balance during adult life and the resultant accumulation of body fat also contributes importantly to several human cancers. The best-established relationships are with cancers of the endometrium and gall bladder (36–40). Greater adiposity also increases the risk of colon cancer in both women (41) and men, particularly when assessed as abdominal circumference (42). The relationship between body fatness and breast cancer is more complex. Prior to menopause, women with greater body fat have reduced risks of breast cancer (43, 44), and after menopause a positive, but weak, association with adiposity is seen. These findings are probably the result of anovulatory menstrual cycles in fatter women prior to menopause (45), which should reduce risk, and the synthesis of endogenous estrogen by adipose tissue in postmenopausal women (46), which is presumed to increase risk of breast cancer.

Dietary Fat and Meat Intake

In the landmark 1982 National Academy of Sciences review of diet, nutrition, and cancer (47), reduction in fat intake to 30% of calories was the primary recommendation; this objective has been echoed in subsequent dietary recommendations as well (48, 49).

Interest in dietary fat as a cause of cancer began in the first half of the 20th century when studies by Tannenbaum and colleagues (13, 17) indicated that diets high in fat could promote tumor growth in animal models. In this early work, energy (caloric) restriction also profoundly reduced the incidence of tumors. A vast literature on dietary fat and cancer in animals has subsequently accumulated (reviewed elsewhere [22, 47, 50–52]).

Dietary fat has a clear effect on tumor incidence in many models, although not in all (53, 54); however, a central issue has been whether this is independent of the effect of energy intake. An independent effect of fat has been seen in some animal models (22, 50, 51), but this has been either weak (55) or nonexistent (23) in some studies designed specifically to address this issue. A possible relationship of dietary fat intake to cancer incidence has also been hypothesized because the large international differences in rates of cancers of the breast, colon, prostate, and endometrium are strongly correlated with apparent per capita fat consumption (12, 56, 57). These correlations are limited to animal (not vegetable) fat (58)

Fat and Breast Cancer

Although a major rationale for the dietary fat hypothesis has been the international correlation between fat consumption and national breast cancer mortality (12), in a study of 65 Chinese counties (59) in which per capita fat intake varied from 6 to 25% of energy only a weak positive association was seen between fat intake and breast cancer mortality. Notably, five counties consumed approximately 25% of energy from fat, yet experienced rates of breast cancer far below those of U.S. women with similar fat intake (60), thus providing strong evidence that factors other than fat intake account for the large international differences. Breast cancer incidence rates have increased substantially in the United States during this century, as have the estimates of per capita fat consumption based on food disappearance data. However, surveys based on reports of individual actual intake, rather than food disappearance, indicate that consumption of energy from fat, either as absolute intake or as a percentage of energy, has actually declined in the last several decades (61, 62), a time during which breast cancer incidence has increased (63).

A number of case-control studies have investigated the effect of dietary fat on breast cancer risk. In the largest study so far (64), animal fat and total fat intake were not associated with breast cancer. The results from twelve smaller case-control studies have been summarized in a metaanalysis by Howe et al. (65), which included 4312 cases and 5978 controls. The pooled relative risk was 1.35 ($P < .0001$) for a 100-g increase in daily total fat intake, and the risk was somewhat stronger for postmenopausal women (relative risk, 1.48; $P < .001$). This magnitude of association, however, could potentially be compatible with biases due to recall of diet or the selection of controls (66).

A substantial body of data from cohort studies is now available to assess the relationship between dietary fat intake and breast cancer in developed countries. In a pooled analysis of the prospective studies, which included nearly 5000 cases of breast cancer (67), no overall association was seen for overall fat intake ranging from below 20% to more than 45% of energy from fat (Fig. 79.2). A similar lack of association was seen among postmenopausal women only and for specific types of fat. Only among the small number of women consuming less than 15% of energy from fat was a significant association seen; breast cancer risk was twofold higher in this group. These cohort findings therefore do not support the results of the case-control studies cited above.

Although empirical evidence is limited, endogenous estrogen levels are thought to be related to risk of breast cancer. Thus, the effects of fat and other dietary factors on estrogen levels are of potential interest. Vegetarian women, who consume higher amounts of fiber and lower amounts of fat, have lower blood levels and reduced urinary excretion of estrogens, apparently due to increased fecal excretion (68). In studies without concurrent controls, estrone sulfate, but not other estrogens, decreased among women fed diets high in fiber and low in fat (69); among postmenopausal women, estradiol but not estrone sulfate decreased on a low-fat diet (70). These studies are difficult to interpret because of a lack of a concurrent control group.

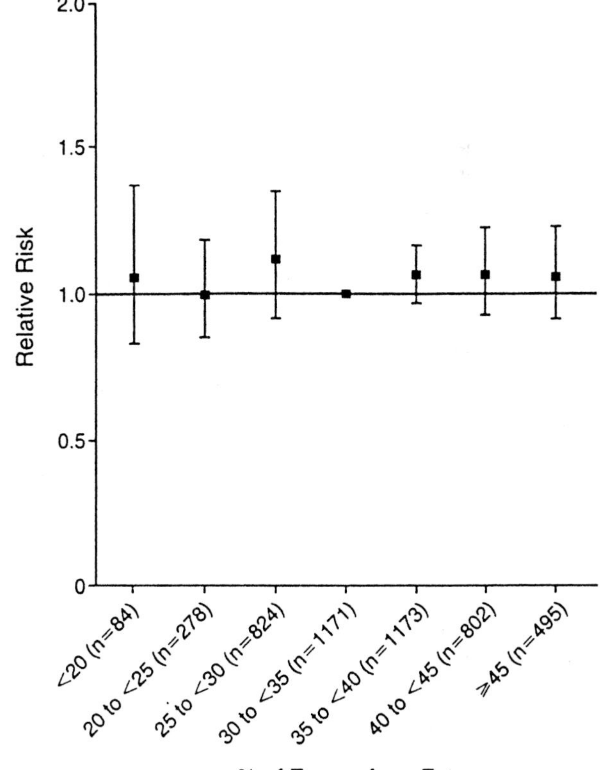

Figure 79.2. Pooled relative risks and 95% confidence intervals for various levels of energy from fat. A level of 30 to less than 35% of total energy from fat was designated as the reference category. *N*, number of cases in each category. (From Hunter DJ, Spiegelman D, Adami H-O, et al. N Engl J Med 1996;334:356, with permission.)

Although total fat intake has been unrelated to breast cancer risk in prospective epidemiologic studies, some evidence suggests that the type of fat may be important. In animal mammary tumor models, the tumor-promoting effect of fat intake has been observed primarily for polyunsaturated fats fed in diets containing approximately 45% of energy from total fat (71, 72). However, in a metaanalysis of case-control studies (65), increased risk of breast cancer was somewhat greater for saturated (relative risk, 1.46) and monounsaturated fats (relative risk, 1.41) than for polyunsaturated fats (relative risk, 1.25). Data based on the detailed food frequency questionnaire administered in 1984 in the Nurses' Health Study, showed an inverse association between monounsaturated fat and breast cancer (60). This is an intriguing observation given the relatively low rates of breast cancer in Southern European countries that have high average intakes of monounsaturated fats because olive oil is the primary fat. In case-control studies in Spain and Greece, women who used more olive oil had reduced risks of breast cancer (73, 74). Furthermore, olive oil has been protective relative to other sources of fats in some animal studies (50).

Fat and Colon Cancer

In comparisons among countries, rates of colon cancer are strongly correlated with national per capita disappearance of animal fat and meat, with correlation coefficients ranging between 0.8 and 0.9 (12, 58). Based on these epidemiologic investigations and animal studies, a hypothesis has developed that dietary fat increases excretion of bile acids, which can be converted to carcinogens or promoters (75). However, recent evidence from many studies that higher levels of physical activity reduce risk of colon cancer means that at least part of the high rates in affluent countries previously attributed to fat intake are probably due to sedentary lifestyle.

With some exceptions (76–79), case-control studies have generally shown an association between risk of colon cancer and intake of fat (80–87) or red meat (88–93). However, in many of these studies, a positive association between total energy intake and risk of colon cancer has also been observed (80–84, 86, 87), raising the question of whether it is general overconsumption of food or the fat composition of the diet that is etiologically important. A recent metaanalysis by Howe and colleagues of 13 case-control studies found a significant association between total energy and colon cancer, but saturated, monounsaturated, and polyunsaturated fat were not associated with colon cancer independently of total energy (94).

The relation between diet and colon cancer has been examined in several large prospective studies. These have not confirmed the positive association with total energy intake in case-control studies (95–99), suggesting that the case-control studies were distorted by reporting bias. The Nurses' Health Study showed that women in the highest quintile of animal fat intake had about a 2-fold higher risk of colon cancer than those in the lowest quintile (95). In a multivariate analysis of these data, which included red meat and animal fat intakes in the same model, red meat intake remained significantly predictive of risk of colon cancer, whereas the association with animal fat was eliminated. A cohort study from the Netherlands showed a significant direct association between intake of processed meats and risk of colon cancer, but no relationship was observed for fresh meats or overall fat intake (96). A cohort study in Iowa women also found a direct association with processed meats, although this was not statistically significant (97). Among a large cohort study of men, a direct association between red meat consumption and risk of colon cancer was seen, but no association was observed with other sources of fat (98). In this study, no overall relationship existed between total or saturated fat and colon cancer despite a substantial range in fat intake. A similar association was noted for colorectal adenomas in the same cohort of men. (75) In the large American Cancer Society Cohort (99), little relation was seen between either meat or fat intake and mortality due to colon cancer, but the dietary questionnaire was brief and of uncertain validity. The apparently stronger association with red meat than with fat in several recent cohort studies needs further confirmation but could result if the fatty acids or nonfat components of meat (e.g., the heme iron or carcinogens created by cooking) were the primary etiologic factors. This issue does have major practical implications, as current dietary recommendations (100) support daily consumption of red meat as long as it is lean.

Fat and Prostate Cancer

An association between fat intake and risk of prostate cancer has been seen in many case-control studies (101–111), but sometimes only in subgroups. In a recent large case-control study among various ethnic groups within the U.S. (112), consistent associations with prostate cancer risk were seen for saturated fat, but not with other types of fat.

The association between fat intake and prostate cancer risk has been assessed in only a few cohort studies. In a cohort of 8000 Japanese men living in Hawaii, no association was seen with intake of total or unsaturated fat (113); however, diet was assessed with a single 24-h recall, so the lack of association may not be informative. In a study of 14,000 Seventh-Day Adventist men living in California, a positive association was seen between the percentage of calories from animal fat and prostate cancer risk was seen, but it was not statistically significant (114). More recently, two large prospective studies have been published. In the Health Professionals Follow-up Study of 51,000 men, a positive association seen with intake of red meat and total and animal fat was largely limited to aggressive prostate cancers (115). No association was seen with vegetable fats. In another cohort from Hawaii, increased risks of prostate cancer were seen with consumption of beef and animal fat (116).

Although further data are desirable, the evidence from international correlations, case-control, and cohort studies is reasonably consistent in supporting an association between consumption of fat-containing animal products and prostate cancer incidence. This evidence does not generally support a relation with intake of vegetable fat, which suggests that either the type of fat or other components of these animal products are responsible. Evidence also suggests that animal fat consumption may be most strongly associated with aggressive prostate cancer, which suggests an influence on the transition from the widespread indolent form to the more lethal form of this malignancy.

Other Cancers

Rates of other cancers that are common in affluent countries, including those of the endometrium and ovary, are also correlated with fat intake internationally. Although these have been studied in a small number of case-control investigations, consistent associations with fat intake have not been seen (117–126). In a prospective study among Iowa women (127), no evidence of relation between fat intake and risk of endometrial cancer was observed. Positive associations have been hypothesized between fat intake and risks of skin cancer (128) and lung cancer, but relevant data in humans are limited.

Assessment of Fat and Cancer

As the findings from large prospective studies have become available, support for a major relationship between fat intake and breast cancer risk has weakened considerably. For colon cancer, the associations seen with animal fat internationally have been supported in numerous case-control and cohort studies. However, more-recent evidence suggests that this might be explained by factors in red meat other than simply its fat content. Further, the importance of physical activity as a protective factor against colon cancer indicates that international correlations probably overstate the contribution of diet to differences in colon cancer incidence. The available evidence most strongly supports an association between animal fat consumption and risk of prostate cancer, particularly the aggressive form of this disease. As with colon cancer, however, the possibility remains that other factors in foods containing animal fat contribute to risk.

Fruits and Vegetables

A massive body of epidemiologic data indicates that higher consumption of fruits and vegetables is associated with a reduced risk of cancers at many sites. Inverse relationships with intake of these foods have been observed in over 200 case-control and prospective cohort studies (129, 130), and additional support comes from studies in which biochemical indicators of fruit and vegetable consumption, such as serum carotenoid levels, are also associated with reduced risks. The studies are particularly numerous and consistent for cancers of the lung (131) and stomach (132); inverse associations have also been observed in many case-control studies of colon cancer but prospective data are still limited. Somewhat fewer studies have also indicated inverse associations with cancers of the oral cavity, larynx, esophagus, endometrium, cervix, bladder, kidney, and breast (133). Although inverse associations have not been seen between fruit and vegetable consumption in general and risk of prostate cancer, inverse associations with tomato products, the primary source of the carotenoid lycopene, have been seen in several case-control and prospective studies (105, 114, 134).

Although the evidence that high consumption of fruits and vegetables can reduce the risk of many cancers is strong, which constituents of these foods are responsible for these reduced risks is less clear. These foods contain a myriad of biologically active chemicals, including both recognized nutrients and many more nonnutritive constituents that could potentially play a role in protection against cancer (14). Among the potentially protective factors are various carotenoids, folic acid, vitamin C, phytoestrogens (see Chapter 81) and fiber (discussed below). Identification of the specific protective constituents, or combination thereof, is a daunting task and may never be completely possible. Further details on the types and amounts of fruits and vegetables that appear to be particularly protective could provide additional practical guidance for those wanting to select an optimally healthy diet.

Dietary Fiber

Interest in dietary fiber is largely the result of Dr. Denis Burkitt's observation of low rates of colon cancer in areas of Africa where fiber consumption and stool bulk were high (135). Fiber was originally seen simply as providing bulk to dilute potential carcinogens and speed their transit through the colon. Other hypotheses have suggested that fiber may act by binding carcinogenic substances (136), altering the colonic flora (137–140), reducing the pH (141), or serving as the substrate for the generation of short-chain fatty acids that are the preferred substrate for colonic epithelial cells (142).

As epidemiologic evidence has accrued, the importance of dietary fiber in reducing risk of colon cancer has become less clear. First, the populations with high fiber consumption and low rates of colon cancer are also typically those of poorer countries where meat consumption and obesity are low and physical activity is high. Evidence has become clearer that each of these factors reduces risk and thus is likely to explain at least part of the geographic associations between low intake of dietary fiber and colon cancer rates. Also, in case-control studies, intake of cereal products or fiber from grains has not usually been associated with reduced risks of colon cancer, in contrast to the abundant evidence for a protective effect of fruits and vegetables (143, 144). Indeed, in some studies higher consumption of grains has been associated with greater risks of colon cancer (76, 89, 145, 146). Also, in several large prospective studies, even overall fiber intake has not been clearly associated with lower risk of colon cancer after adjustment for other risk factors (95–98). Thus, fiber intake does not appear to account for the reduced risk of colon cancer associated with consumption of fruits and vegetables, and evidence supporting higher consumption of grain fiber to reduce risk of colon cancer is weak.

Higher intake of fiber has also been hypothesized to reduce risk of breast cancer by interrupting the enterohepatic circulation of estrogens (147). However, in prospective studies, little or no relationship has been observed between fiber intake and risk of breast cancer (60, 148, 149).

Alcoholic and Caffeinated Beverages

High consumption of alcohol, particularly in combination with cigarette smoking, is a well-established cause of cancer of the oral cavity, larynx, esophagus, and liver (150). More recently, substantial evidence from case-control and cohort studies indicates that amounts as low as one or two drinks per day increase risk of breast cancer (151, 152). Moderate alcohol consumption appears to increase endogenous estrogen levels, which may account for this effect (46, 153, 154). Moderate alcohol consumption also appears to be associated with risk of cancers of the colon and rectum (144). Alcohol interferes with the availability of folic acid, which may account for its relationship with large bowel cancers (155–157).

Coffee contains multiple mutagenic substances (15), and concern has thus existed that it might be an important cause of cancer in humans. Although early evidence suggested a possible positive association with pancreatic cancer, this has not been supported in most subsequent studies (158–160). Similarly, for breast cancer, coffee consumption has been unassociated (161) or even weakly inversely associated with risk (162). Green tea contains polyphenolic compounds that inhibit tumors in experimental animals (163) and inverse associations between green tea consumption and risk of gastric cancer have been seen in case-control studies from Japan (164) and China (165). Notably, however, rates of gastric cancer in the U.S., where tea consumption is low, are among the lowest in the world; this has been attributed in part to relatively low salt intake (132).

Vitamin Supplements

Relatively few data are available on vitamin supplement use and cancer incidence. High-dose supplements of vitamins C and E have not been associated with reductions in breast cancer incidence (148, 166). In the study by Hunter, there was a suggestion that vitamin A supplements at the RDA level might be associated with reductions in breast cancer risk among women whose dietary intakes were relatively low, but higher intakes did not confer additional reductions in risk. Limited data suggest that folic acid contained in multiple vitamins might reduce risk of large bowel cancer (155, 156), but this needs confirmation. In a single case-control study, vitamin E supplements were associated with a reduced risk of oral cancer (167). In a randomized trial conducted in a region of China with low consumption of fruits and vegetables, a supplement containing β-carotene, vitamin E, and selenium reduced incidence of stomach cancer (168). Although further research is needed, on the basis of available evidence, the prevention of cancer does not provide justification for the use of vitamin supplements by most persons with a reasonable diet.

CONCLUSIONS

Evidence from both animal and epidemiologic studies indicate that throughout life, excessive energy intake in relation to requirements increases risk of human cancer. Rapid growth rates in childhood lead to earlier age at menarche, which in turn increases risk of breast cancer, and accumulation of body fat in adulthood is related to cancers of the colon, kidney, and endometrium as well as postmenopausal breast cancer. Higher intake of vegetables and fruits has been associated with lower risks of many cancers. The constituents responsible for these apparent protective effects remain uncertain, although evidence supports a contribution of folic acid. Recent evidence suggests that the percentage of energy from fat in the diet is not a major cause of cancers of the breast or colon. Higher intake of meat and dairy products has been associated with greater risk of prostate cancer, which may be related to their saturated fat content. Also, red meat consumption has been associated with risk of colon cancer in numerous studies, but this appears to be unrelated to its fat content. Excessive consumption of alcohol increases risks of upper gastrointestinal tract cancer, and even moderate intake appears to increase cancers of the breast and large bowel. Although many details remain to be learned, evidence is strong that remaining physically active and lean throughout life, consuming an abundance of fruits and vegetables, and avoiding high intakes of red meat, foods high in animal fat, and excessive alcohol will substantially reduce risk of human cancer.

REFERENCES

1. Parkin DM. Cancer Surveys 1994;19-20:519–61.
2. International Agency for Research on Cancer. Cancer incidence in five continents, vol VI. Parkin DM, Muir CS, Whelan SL, et al., eds. IARC scientific publ. no. 120. Lyon: International Agency for Research on Cancer and International Association of Cancer Registries, World Health Organization, 1992.
3. American Cancer Society. Cancer facts and figures. Atlanta, GA: American Cancer Society, 1996.
4. Devesa SS, Blot WJ, Stone BJ, et al. J Natl Cancer Inst 1995;87: 175–82.
5. Aoki K, Hayakawa N, Kurihara M, et al. Death rates for malignant neoplasms for selected sites by sex and five-year age

group in 33 countries, 1953–57 to 1983–87. International Union against Cancer. Nagoya, Japan: University of Nagoya Coop Press, 1992.
6. Haenszel W, Kurihara M. J Natl Cancer Inst 1968;40:43–68.
7. Buell P. J Natl Cancer Inst 1973;51:1479–83.
8. Shimizu H, Ross RK, Bernstein L, et al. Br J Cancer 1991;63:963–6.
9. Thomas DB, Karagas MR. Cancer Res 1987;47:5771–6.
10. Kolonel LN, Hankin JH, Lee J, et al. Br J Cancer 1981;44: 332–9.
11. Ziegler RG, Hoover RN, Pike MC, et al. J Natl Cancer Inst 1993;85:1819–27.
12. Armstrong B, Doll R. Int J Cancer 1975;15:617–31.
13. Tannenbaum A, Silverstone H. Adv Cancer Res 1953;1: 451–501.
14. Steinmetz KA, Potter JD. Cancer Causes Control 1991;2: 427–42.
15. Ames BN, Gold LS, Willett WC. Proc Natl Acad Sci USA 1995;92:5258–65.
16. Willett WC. Nutritional epidemiology. New York: Oxford University Press, 1990.
17. Tannenbaum A. Cancer Res 1942;2:468–75.
18. Ross MH, Bras G. J Natl Cancer Inst 1971;47:1095–113.
19. Weindruch R, Walford RL. Science 1982;215:1415–8.
20. Birt DF. J Nutr 1995;125(Suppl):1673S–6S.
21. Birt DF, Kris ES, Choe M, et al. Cancer Res 1992; 52(Suppl):2035s–9s.
22. Birt DF. Adv Exp Med Biol 1986;206:69–84.
23. Boissonneault GA, Elson CE, Pariza MW. J Natl Cancer Inst 1986;76:335–8.
24. Willett WC, Stampfer MJ. Am J Epidemiol 1986;124:17–27.
25. Micozzi MS. Yearb Phys Anthropol 1985;28:175–206.
26. Hunter DJ, Willett W. Epidemiol Rev 1993;15:110–32.
27. Swanson CA, Jones DY, Schatzkin A, et al. Cancer Res 1988;48:5363–7.
28. Swanson CA, Potischman N, Wilbanks GD, et al. Cancer Epidemiol Biomarkers Prev 1993;2:321–7.
29. Chute CG, Willett WC, Colditz GA, et al. Cancer Causes Control 1991;2:117–224.
30. Micozzi MS. Horm Res 1993;39(Suppl 3):49–58.
31. Chen J, Campbell TC, Tunyao L, et al. Diet, lifestyle and mortality in China: a study of the characteristics of 65 Chinese counties. Oxford: Oxford University Press, 1990.
32. Wyshak G, Frisch RE. N Engl J Med 1982;306:1033–5.
33. Moisan J, Meyer F, Gingras S. Cancer Causes Control 1990;1:149–54.
34. Maclure M, Travis LB, Willett WC, et al. Am J Clin Nutr 1991;54:649–56.
35. Merzenich H, Boeing H, Wahrendorf J. Am J Epidemiol 1993;138:217–24.
36. Austin H, Austin JM Jr, Partridge EE, et al. Cancer Res 1991;51:568–72.
37. Goodman MT, Nomura AMY, Kolonel LN, et al. Case-control study of the effect of diet and body size on the risk of endometrial cancer. In: Rao RS, Deo MA, Sanghvi LD, eds. Proceedings of the International Cancer Congress New Delhi, India. Bologna, Italy: Monduzzi Editore, 1994;2325–8.
38. Parazzini F, La Vecchia C, Bocciolone L, et al. Gynecol Oncol 1991;41:1–16.
39. Tornberg SA, Carstensen JM. Br J Cancer 1994;69:358–61.
40. Garfinkel L. Cancer 1986;58(Suppl):1826–9.
41. Martinez ME, Giovannucci E, Spiegelman D, et al. Am J Epidemiol 1996;143:S73.
42. Giovannucci E, Ascherio A, Rimm EB, et al. Ann Intern Med 1995;122:327–34.
43. Tretli S. Int J Cancer 1989;44:23–30.
44. London SJ, Colditz GA, Stampfer MJ, et al. JAMA 1989;262:2853–8.
45. Rich-Edwards JW, Goldman MB, Willett WC, et al. Am J Obstet Gynecol 1994;171:171–7.
46. Hankinson SE, Willett WC, Manson JE, et al. J Natl Cancer Inst 1995;87:1297–302.
47. Committee on Diet, Nutrition and Cancer, Assembly of Life Sciences, National Research Council. Diet, nutrition, and cancer. Washington, DC: National Academy Press, 1982.
48. Committee on Diet and Health, National Research Council. Diet and health: implications for reducing chronic disease risk. Washington, DC: National Academy Press, 1989.
49. Food and Nutrition Board. Recommended dietary allowances. 10th rev. ed. Washington, DC: National Academy of Sciences, 1989.
50. Welsch CW. Cancer Res 1992;52(Suppl 7):2040S–8S.
51. Freedman LS, Clifford C, Messina M. Cancer Res 1990;50: 5710–9.
52. Albanes D. Cancer Res 1987;47:1987–2.
53. Sonnenschein E, Glickman L, Goldschmidt M, et al. Am J Epidemiol 1991;133:694–703.
54. Appleton BS, Landers RE. Adv Exp Med Biol 1986;206:99–104.
55. Ip C. Quantitative assessment of fat and calorie as risk factors in mammary carcinogenesis in an experimental model. In: Mettlin CJ, Aoki K, eds. Recent progress in research on nutrition and cancer: proceedings of a workshop sponsored by the International Union against Cancer, Nagoya, Japan, November 1–3, 1989. New York: Wiley-Liss, 1990;107–17.
56. Carroll MD, Abraham S, Dresser CM. Dietary intake source data: United States, 1976–1980, series 11. Washington, DC: National Center for Health Statistics, 1983.
57. Prentice RL, Sheppard L. Cancer Causes Control 1990;1: 81–97.
58. Rose DP, Boyar AP, Wynder EL. Cancer 1986;58:2263–71.
59. Marshall JR, Yinsheng Q, Chen J, et al. Eur J Cancer 1992;28A:1720–7.
60. Willett WC, Hunter DJ, Stampfer MJ, et al. JAMA 1992;268: 2037–44.
61. Stephan AM, Wald NJ. Am J Clin Nutr 1990;52:457–69.
62. McDowell MA, Briefel RR, Alaimo K, et al. Energy and macronutrient intakes of persons ages 2 months and over in the United States: third national health and nutrition examination survey, phase I, 1988–1991. National Center for Health Statistics, Centers for Disease Control, Public Health Service, U.S. Department of Health and Human Services, 1994.
63. American Cancer Society. Cancer facts and figures. Atlanta, GA: American Cancer Society, 1994.
64. Graham S, Marshall J, Mettlin C, et al. Am J Epidemiol 1982;116:68–75.
65. Howe GR, Hirohata T, Hislop TG, et al. J Natl Cancer Inst 1990;82:561–9.
66. Giovannucci E, Stampfer MJ, Colditz GA, et al. Am J Epidemiol 1993;137:502–11.
67. Hunter DJ, Spiegelman D, Adami H-O, et al. N Engl J Med 1996;334:356–61.
68. Goldin BR, Aldercreutz H, Gorbach SL, et al. N Engl J Med 1982;307:1542–7.
69. Woods MN, Gorbach SL, Longcope C, et al. Am J Clin Nutr 1989;49:1179–93.
70. Prentice R, Thompson D, Clifford C, et al. J Natl Cancer Inst 1990;82:129–34.
71. Hopkins GJ, Carroll KK. J Natl Cancer Inst 1979;62:1009–12.
72. Hopkins GJ, Kennendy TG, Carroll KK. J Natl Cancer Inst 1981;66:517–22.

73. Martin-Moreno JM, Willett WC, Gorgojo L, et al. Int J Cancer 1994;58:774–80.
74. Trichopoulou A, Katsouyanni K, Stuver S, et al. J Natl Cancer Inst 1995;87:110–6.
75. Giovannucci E, Stampfer MJ, Colditz GA, et al. J Natl Cancer Inst 1992;84:91–8.
76. Macquart-Moulin G, Riboli E, Cornee J, et al. Int J Cancer 1986;38:183–91.
77. Berta JL, Coste T, Rautureau J, et al. Gastroenterol Clin Biol 1985;9:348–53.
78. Tuyns AJ, Haelterman M, Kaaks R. Nutr Cancer 1987;10: 181–96.
79. Meyer F, White E. Am J Epidemiol 1993;138:225–36.
80. Jain M, Cook GM, Davis FG, et al. Int J Cancer 1980;26: 757–68.
81. Potter JD, McMichael AJ. J Natl Cancer Inst 1986;76:557–69.
82. Lyon JL, Mahoney AW, West DW, et al. J Natl Cancer Inst 1987;78:853–61.
83. Graham S, Marshall J, Haughey B, et al. Am J Epidemiol 1988;128:490–503.
84. Bristol JB, Emmett PM, Heaton KW, et al. Br Med J Clin Res Ed 1985;291:1467–70.
85. Kune GA, Kune S, Watson LF. Nutr Cancer 1987;9:5–56.
86. West DW, Slattery ML, Robison LM, et al. Am J Epidemiol 1989;130:883–94.
87. Peters RK, Pike MC, Garabrandt D, et al. Cancer Causes Control 1992;3:457–73.
88. Manousos O, Day NE, Trichopoulos D, et al. Int J Cancer 1983;32:1–5.
89. La Vecchia C, Negri E, Decarli A, et al. Int J Cancer 1988;41: 492–8.
90. Miller AB, Howe GR, Jain M, et al. Int J Cancer 1983;32: 155–61.
91. Young TB, Wolf TB. Int J Cancer 1988;42:167–75.
92. Benito E, Obrador A, Stiggelbout A, et al. Int J Cancer 1990;45:69–76.
93. Lee HP, Gourley L, Duffy SW, et al. Int J Cancer 1989;43: 1007–16.
94. Howe GR, Aronson KJ, Benito E, et al. Cancer Causes Control 1997;8:215–28.
95. Willett WC, Stampfer MJ, Colditz GA, et al. N Engl J Med 1990;323:1664–72.
96. Goldbohm RA, van den Brandt PA, van't Veer P, et al. Cancer Res 1994;54:718–23.
97. Bostick RM, Potter JD, Kushi LH, et al. Cancer Causes Control 1994;5:38–52.
98. Giovannucci E, Rimm EB, Stampfer MJ, et al. Cancer Res 1994;54:2390–7.
99. Thun MJ, Calle EE, Namboodiri MM, et al. J Natl Cancer Inst 1992;84:1491–500.
100. U.S. Department of Agriculture. The food guide pyramid. Home and Garden Bulletin no. 252. Washington DC: Government Printing Office, 1992.
101. Talamini R, La Vecchia C, Decarli A, et al. Br J Cancer 1986;53:817–21.
102. Rotkin ID. Cancer Treat Rep 1977;61:173–80.
103. Mishina T, Watanabe H, Araki H, et al. Prostate 1985;6:423–36.
104. Talamini R, Franceschi S, La Vecchia C, et al. Nutr Cancer 1992;18:277–86.
105. Schuman LM, Mandel JS, Radke A, et al. Some selected features of the epidemiology of prostatic cancer: Minneapolis-St. Paul, Minnesota case-control study, 1976–1979. In: Magnus K, ed. Trends in cancer incidence: causes and practical implications. Washington, DC: Hemisphere Publishing Corp, 1982:345–54.
106. Graham S, Haughey B, Marshall J, et al. J Natl Cancer Inst 1983;70:687–92.
107. Ross RK, Shimizu H, Paganini-Hill A, et al. J Natl Cancer Inst 1987;78:869–74.
108. West DW, Slattery MI, Robison LM, et al. Cancer Causes Control 1991;2:85–94.
109. Kolonel LN, Yoshizawa CN, Hankin JH. Am J Epidemiol 1988;127:999–1012.
110. Heshmat MY, Kaul L, Kovi J, et al. Prostate 1985;6:7–17.
111. Kolonel LN. Cancer Causes Control 1996;7:83–94.
112. Whittemore AS, Kolonel LN, Wu AH, et al. J Natl Cancer Inst 1995;87:652–61.
113. Severson PK, Nomura AMY, Grove JS, et al. Cancer Res 1989;49:1857–60.
114. Mills PK, Beeson WL, Phillips RL, et al. Cancer 1989;64:598–604.
115. Giovannucci E, Rimm EB, Colditz GA, et al. J Natl Cancer Inst 1993;85:1571–79.
116. Le Marchand L, Kolonel LN, Wilkens LR, et al. Epidemiology 1994;5:276–82.
117. Cramer DW, Welch WR, Hutchison GB, et al. Obstet Gynecol 1984;63:833–8.
118. La Vecchia C, Decarli A, Negri E, et al. J Natl Cancer Inst 1987;79:663–9.
119. Shu XO, Gao YT, Yuan JM, et al. Br J Cancer 1989;59:92–6.
120. Byers T, Marshall J, Graham S, et al. J Natl Cancer Inst 1983;71:681–6.
121. Slattery ML, Schuman KL, West DW, et al. Am J Epidemiol 1989;130:497–502.
122. Risch HA, Jain M, Marrett LD, et al. J Natl Cancer Inst 1994;86:1409–15.
123. Levi F, Franceschi S, Negri E, et al. Cancer 1993;71:3575–81.
124. Barbone F, Austin H, Partridge EE. Am J Epidemiol 1993;137:393–403.
125. Potischman N, Swanson CA, Brinton LA, et al. Cancer Causes Control 1993;4:239–50.
126. Shu XO, Zheng W, Potischamn N, et al. Am J Epidemiol 1993;137:155–65.
127. Zheng W, Kushi LH, Potter JD, et al. Am J Epidemiol 1995;142:388–94.
128. Black HS, Herd JA, Goldberg LH, et al. N Engl J Med 1994;330:1272–5.
129. Steinmetz KA, Potter JD. Cancer Causes Control 1991;2:325–57.
130. Block G, Patterson B, Subar A. Nutr Cancer 1992;18:1–29.
131. Ziegler RG, Mayne ST, Swanson CA. Cancer Causes Control 1996;7:157–77.
132. Kono S, Hirohata T. Cancer Causes Control 1996;7:41–55.
133. Willett WC, Trichopoulos D. Cancer Causes Control 1996;7:178–80.
134. Giovannucci E, Ascherio A, Rimm EB, et al. J Natl Cancer Inst 1995;87:1767–76.
135. Burkitt DP. Cancer 1971;28:3–13.
136. Story JA, Kritchevsky D. Am J Clin Nutr 1978; 31(Suppl):S199–202.
137. Reddy BS, Mastromarino A, Wynder EL. Cancer Res 1975;35:3403–6.
138. Reddy BS. Fed Proc 1971;30:1772.
139. Reddy BS, Weisburger JH, Wynder EL. J Nutr 1975; 105:878–84.
140. Klurfeld DM. Cancer Res 1992;52(Suppl):2055s–9s.
141. Cummings JH. Lancet 1983;1:1206–9.
142. Stephen AM, Cummings JH. Nature 1980;284:283–4.

143. Willett W. Nature 1989;338:389–94.
144. Potter JD. Cancer Causes Control 1996;7:127–46.
145. Wynder EL, Kajitani T, Ishikawa S, et al. Cancer 1969;23: 1210–20.
146. Bidoli E, Franceschi S, Talamini R, et al. Int J Cancer 1992;50: 223–9.
147. Gorbach SL, Goldin BR. Prev Med 1987;16:525–31.
148. Rohan TE, Howe GR, Friedenreich CM, et al. Cancer Causes Control 1993;4:29–37.
149. Verhoeven DTH, Assen N, Goldbohm RA, et al. Am J Epidemiol 1996;143(Suppl):S37.
150. International Agency for Research on Cancer. IARC Mongr Eval Carcinog Risk Hum 1988;44:194–207.
151. Longnecker MP, Newcomb PA, Mittendorf R, et al. J Natl Cancer Inst 1995;87:923–9.
152. Longnecker MP. Cancer Causes Control 1994;5:73–82.
153. Reichman ME, Judd JT, Longcope C, et al. J Natl Cancer Inst 1993;85:722–7.
154. Ginsburg ES, Walsh BW, Gao XP, et al. J Soc Gynecol Invest 1995;2:26–9.
155. Giovannucci E, Stampfer MJ, Colditz GA, et al. J Natl Cancer Inst 1993;85:875–84.
156. Giovannucci E, Rimm EB, Ascherio A, et al. J Natl Cancer Inst 1995;87:265–73.
157. Freudenheim JL, Graham S, Marshall JR. Int J Epidemiol 1991;20:368–74.
158. International Agency for Research on Cancer. IARC Monogr Eval Carcinog Risk Hum 1991;51.
159. Gold EB. Surg Clin North Am 1995;75:819–43.
160. Gordis L. Cancer Lett 1990;52:1–12.
161. Folsom AR, McKenzie DR, Bisgard KM, et al. Am J Epidemiol 1993;138:380–3.
162. Hunter DJ, Manson JE, Stampfer MJ, et al. (Abstract) Am J Epidemiol 1992;136:1000–1.
163. Yang CS, Wang ZY. J Natl Cancer Inst 1993;85:1038–49.
164. Kono S, Ikeda M, Tokudome S, et al. Jpn J Cancer Res 1988;79:1067–74.
165. Yu GP, Hsieh CC, Wang LY, et al. Cancer Causes Control 1995;6:532–8.
166. Hunter DJ, Manson JE, Colditz GA, et al. N Engl J Med 1993;329:234–40.
167. Gridley G, McLaughlin JK, Block G, et al. Am J Epidemiol 1992;135:1083–92.
168. Blot WJ, Li JY, Taylor PR, et al. J Natl Cancer Inst 1993;85:1483–92.
169. Willett WC. Adv Oncol 1995;11:3–8.
170. Miller BA, Ries LAG, Hankey BF, et al. In: SEER Cancer Statistics Review: 1973–1990. National Cancer Institute, Bethesda, MD, 1993.

80. Carcinogens in Foods

TAKASHI SUGIMURA and KEIJI WAKABAYASHI

It is widely accepted that dietary factors are deeply involved in human neoplasia. Cancer is a disease of DNA, and genetic alterations are essential for its development. Individual cancers are caused by multiple factors, including both genotoxic substances and nongenotoxic tumor promoters. 12-*O*-Tetradecanoylphorbol-13-acetate (TPA), teleocidines, and aplysiatoxins are well known as typical tumor promoters (1, 2). However, human exposure to these typical tumor promoters is very limited. In contrast, major dietary components, salt and fat, may have a sizeable influence on cancer development as tumor promoters in our actual environment. Many reports indicate the presence in foodstuffs of various types of genotoxic carcinogens (i.e., mutagens/carcinogens), which can be divided into several groups. The first group comprises the naturally occurring mycotoxins and plant-origin mutagenic and carcinogenic compounds. The second includes the compounds produced during cooking, food storage, and food processing. The third group, which consists of food additives and pesticide residue contaminants, is the subject of rigorous control by regulatory agencies; thus this chapter is mainly concerned with the genotoxic carcinogens, mutagens/carcinogens classified into the first and second groups. Additionally, as examples of factors responsible for tumor promotion and progression, the effects of salt and fat are discussed.

AFLATOXINS AND OTHER MYCOTOXINS

Mycotoxins are toxic substances produced by fungi. A number of mycotoxins have been reported, and some of these have proven to be carcinogenic. In 1960, numerous turkeys died of a disease syndrome called the "turkey X disease" in the United Kingdom. The etiologic factor appeared to be the diet, which was contaminated with a potent carcinogen subsequently identified as aflatoxin. Aflatoxins are very toxic metabolites produced by *Aspergillus flavus.* Among many derivatives, aflatoxin B_1 exerts the strongest carcinogenicity (3). Its structure is shown in Figure 80.1. Aflatoxin B_1 induces hepatocarcinomas in many species of experimental animals such as rodents, monkeys, birds, and fishes. Male Fischer rats are the most sensitive among rodents, with a TD_{50} of 1.3 μg/kg body weight/day (1). Aflatoxin B_1 has been classified as a group 1 human carcinogen by the International Agency for Research on Cancer (IARC) (4) and is found as a contaminant of foodstuffs consumed by inhabitants in several areas, mainly in Asia and Africa. Levels of aflatoxin B_1 as low as micrograms per kilogram of food may increase the incidence of liver cancer in man. The carcinogenicity of other derivatives of aflatoxins are much weaker, but aflatoxin M_1, a hydroxy derivative often found in milk, does produce hepatocellular carcinomas in rats (5). Aflatoxins G_1 and B_2 can also induce tumors in experimental animals.

Induced Mutations

Aflatoxin B_1 induces gene mutations in mammalian cells as well as bacteria. In addition, it causes unscheduled DNA synthesis and cell transformation in mammalian cell lines including human fibroblasts in vitro and micronucleus formation in rats in vivo (6, 7). Aflatoxin B_1 is metabolically activated to its 8,9-epoxide, the ultimate carcinogen, by cytochrome P-450s including CYP1A2 and 3A4. This epoxide modifies DNA to form an adduct, 8,9-dihydro-8-(N^7-guanyl)-9-hydroxyaflatoxin B_1 (8). The level of aflatoxin binding to hepatic DNA is correlated with hepatocarcinogenicity among different species (9). Several studies concerned with mutation spectra indicate that aflatoxin B_1 preferentially induces GC to TA transversions (10, 11). In addition, it has been associated with a G to T transversion in codon 249 of the *p53* tumor suppressor gene in human hepatocytes (12). This mutation has been recognized as a mutational hotspot in human hepatocellular carcinomas (13). The frequency is more than 50% in Qidong, China, where the inhabitants are exposed to high levels of aflatoxins, but less than 5% in most developed countries (14–17). These findings suggest that aflatoxin B_1 ingested with contaminated foods is directly involved in hepatocarcinogenesis in humans by inducing G to T mutations in codon 249 of the *p53* gene.

Urine specimens have been used to estimate human

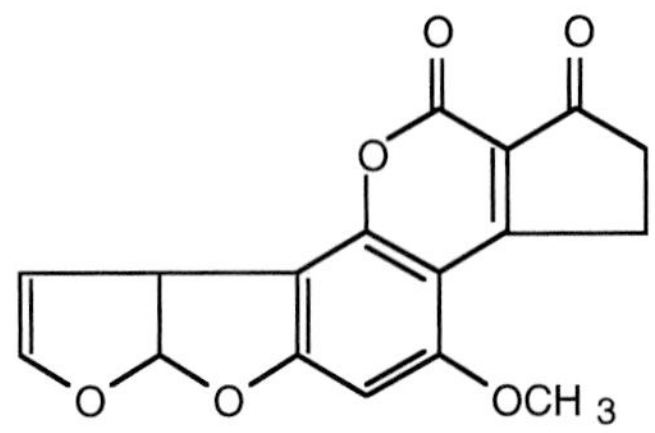

Figure 80.1. Structure of aflatoxin B_1.

exposure to aflatoxins, and a number of biomarkers including aflatoxin-DNA adducts and metabolites have been identified in human urine. The dose of aflatoxin B_1 correlates with the level of aflatoxin B–N^7-guanine in rat urine (18). Moreover, a follow-up study in China suggested that persons demonstrating detectable amounts of aflatoxin-DNA adduct or other aflatoxin biomarkers in their urine have a significantly elevated risk of developing primary liver cancer (19). Aflatoxin-protein adducts in serum albumin can also used as a biomarker of aflatoxin exposure, since the aflatoxin B_1 form binds to lysine residues in this protein (20).

Other Mycotoxins

Fumonisin, produced by the corn pathogen *Fusarium moniliforme,* is carcinogenic in rats (21, 22). It consists of fumonisin B_1, B_2, and other forms, which are all closely related structural analogues. Sterigmatocystin, generated by *Penicillium, Aspergillus,* and *Biopolaris,* also induces hepatocellular carcinomas in rats (23). Ochratoxin A, produced by *Aspergillus ochraceus* and other fungi, causes tubular cell carcinomas of the kidney in female rats (24).

PLANT-ORIGIN CARCINOGENS

Pyrrolizidine Alkaloids

Pyrrolizidine alkaloids are esters of amino alcohols derived from pyrrolizidine, which exist in a wide range of Asteraceae and other plant species, often at more than 1% by weight. Some of the alkaloids are known to cause serious hepatic damage in humans and animals. Petasitenine, which has an otonecine moiety, is present in a kind of coltsfoot, *Petasites japonicus* Maxim, and induces hemangioendothelial sarcomas in rats (25). The young flower stalk of the plant has been used as a food and an herbal remedy in Japan. Senkirkine, which also has an otonecine moiety, is a main alkaloid component in another coltsfoot, *Tussilago farfara* L. The dried buds of coltsfoot are taken as an herbal remedy for coughs in China and Japan. Feeding *Tussilago farfara* L also induces hemangioendothelial sarcomas in rats (26). Heliotrine, whose necine base is heliotridine, occurs in *Heliotropium* species and was the cause of an outbreak of venoocclusive disease in Afghanistan. Heliotrine and another alkaloid containing the same necine base, lasiocarpine, induce islet cell tumors and hepatocellular carcinomas, respectively, in rats (27, 28). Monocrotaline, which has a retronecine moiety, is also carcinogenic in the rat (29). The mutagenicity of some pyrrolizidine alkaloids has been shown in *Salmonella typhimurium* strain TA100 with S9 mix by the preincubation method.

Aquilide A/Ptaquiloside

Bracken fern, *Pteridium aguilinum,* is grown in many areas of the world and is eaten by residents of some countries, including Japan (Fig. 80.2). Cows allowed to graze in fields where bracken fern grows often develop hematuria with tumors of the urinary bladder. Moreover, feeding bracken fern induces adenocarcinomas and urinary bladder carcinomas in rats. (30, 31) The active principle of bracken fern was isolated as a mutagenic compound and termed aquilide *A* by van der Hoeven et al. (32). Aquilide A, a norsesquiterpene glucoside of the illudane type, itself is not mutagenic to *Salmonella,* but becomes so after alkaline treatment. Thus, an aglycone of aquilide A has been suggested as the mutagenic component. Hirono et al. isolated the same compound by monitoring the carcinogenicity of various fractions from bracken fern and named it ptaquiloside (33). Ptaquiloside was also found to induce multiple ileal adenocarcinomas and mammary cancers in rats (34). Thus aquilide A/ptaquiloside was concluded to be the carcinogenic component in bracken fern. Its structure is shown in Figure 80.2. Since the carcinogenic activity of bracken fern is essentially lost after boiling, exposure of humans to aquilide A/ptaquiloside in cooked bracken fern is probably small.

Mushroom Hydrazines

The commonly cultivated edible mushroom, *Agaricus bisporus,* contains a hydrazine, *β*-*N*-[*γ*-*S*(+)-glutamyl-4-hydroxymethylphenylhydrazine (agaritine) as well as derivatives that in some cases have been shown to be carcinogenic to experimental animals. Toth et al. demonstrated that the *N′*-acetyl derivative of 4-hydroxymethylphenylhydrazine induces adenocarcinomas of the lung and angiosarcomas of the blood vessels in mice (35). Subcutaneous injection and intragastric instillation of

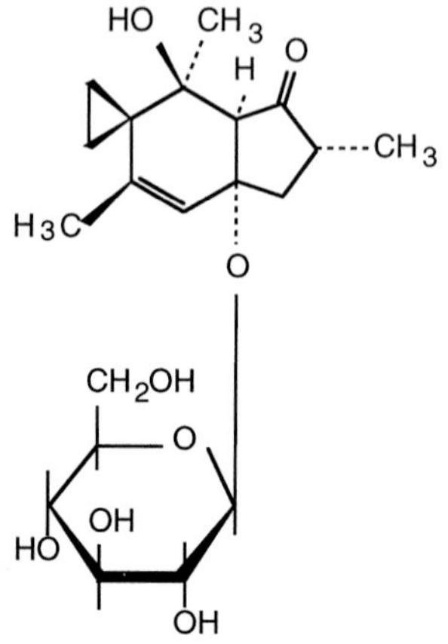

Figure 80.2. Structure of aquilide A/ptaquiloside.

4-(hydroxymethyl)benzenediazonium ion, stabilized as the tetrafluoroborate salt, causes subcutis and skin cancers, and glandular stomach cancers, respectively (36, 37). These results suggest that the edible mushroom may have carcinogenic potential in animals. In fact, uncooked cultivated *Agaricus bisporus* itself is carcinogenic in mice (38). The shiitake *(Lentinus edodes),* which is a popular edible mushroom in Japan, also contains agaritine. Another edible mushroom, false morel *(Gyromitra esculenta),* contains several hydrazine derivatives, including acetaldehyde methylformylhydrazone (gyromitrin), *N*-methyl-*N*-formylhydrazine, and methylhydrazine. *N*-Methyl-*N*-formylhydrazine induces malignant histiocytomas and liver cell carcinomas in hamsters (39).

Cycasin

Cycad is a plant classified as a gymnosperm that grows in tropical areas. Its nuts have been used as a source of starch for food by the inhabitants in some tropical areas including Guam and the Amami Oshima islands. Carcinogenicity of cycad nuts was first reported by Laqueur et al. (40). The β-D-glucoside of methylazoxymethanol, cycasin, is responsible for the carcinogenicity of cycad nuts. Cycasin itself is not an ultimate carcinogen; its hydrolysis is required to produce the aglycon methylazoxymethanol by intestinal microflora. Methylazoxymethanol acts as an methylating agent and is carcinogenic for the rat colon (41).

Alkenylbenzenes

1-Allyl-3,4-methylenedioxybenzene, safrole, is a major constituent of the oil of the sassafras tree and has been used as a fragrance in soft drinks and soaps. Estragole is present in tarragon and sweet basil and is used as an essence. Miller et al. showed that these two alkenylbenzenes induce hepatomas and angiosarcomas in mice, both apparently being metabolically activated to 1′-hydroxy derivatives (42). In addition, isosafrole (3,4-methylenedioxy-1-propenylbenzene) and methyleugenol (1-allyl-3,4-dimethoxybenzene) were reported to induce hepatocarcinomas in rats and mice, respectively (42, 43). The related β-asanone (*cis*-1-propenyl-2,4,5-trimethoxybenzene) causes highly malignant mesenchymal tumors of the small intestine in rats (44).

NITROSAMINES

N-Nitrosamines are both mutagenic and carcinogenic compounds. One example of their toxicity was provided by the severe liver disease observed in sheep fed a diet containing fishmeal preserved with nitrite (45). The toxic principle was subsequently identified as *N*-nitrosodimethylamine (46), which led to estimation of nitrosamine contamination of human foodstuffs. *N*-Nitrosamines are formed by the reaction of secondary amines with nitrite under acidic conditions, both in vitro and in vivo (47). Nitrite exists in various foods and is also produced endogenously from nitrate contained mainly in vegetables. In addition, highly reactive nitric oxide formed from L-arginine by nitric oxide synthase in inflammatory processes is involved in generation of *N*-nitroso compounds (48). Nitrosation of *N*-nitrosamines can occur not only with nitrous acid but also with the oxides of nitrogen formed by combustion in open fires. *N*-Nitrosodimethylamine was found in cooked bacon, cheese, and some nitrite-preserved foods in microgram amounts per kilogram, and *N*-nitrosopyrrolidine was also identified in cooked bacon (49). Beer has been known to contain *N*-nitrosodimethylamine. This nitroso compound is produced during direct-fire drying of barley malt by the reaction of oxides of nitrogen with the barley malt alkaloids, gramine and hordenine, which possess a dimethylamine moiety as a common structure (49). Discovery of this problem led to adoption of an improved method for drying malt to reduce the level of *N*-nitrosodimethylamine.

CARCINOGENS IN HEATED MATERIALS

Polycyclic Aromatic Hydrocarbons

Polycyclic aromatic hydrocarbons produced by heating crude materials are widely distributed in our environment, being present in cigarette smoke, exhaust gas, and cooked food. Charred parts of biscuits have been found to contain benzo[*a*]pyrene (50), and broiled steak is reported to be contaminated by various polycyclic aromatic hydrocarbons (51). Among these, benzo[*a*]pyrene is present at an average of 8 ng per gram of steak. Benzo[*a*]pyrene requires metabolic activation to the ultimate diol epoxide form, which binds to DNA and predominantly forms adducts at the N2 position of guanine (52). A high frequency of G to T transversions in the *p53* gene has been observed in benzo[*a*]pyrene-induced mouse skin tumors (53).

Heterocyclic Amines

As was the case with cigarette smoke condensate, the smoke particles collected on a glass-fiber filter by broiling fish over a naked gas flame were found to be mutagenic in Ames's *Salmonella* assay in the presence of the metabolic activation system, S9 mix (54, 55). The charred parts of broiled fish and meat also proved to be mutagenic. *S. typhimurium* TA98, a detector of frameshift mutations, was more sensitive to the mutagenicity of these agents than TA100, a detector of base-pair change mutations. Although the polycyclic aromatic hydrocarbons were reported earlier in samples of smoke condensate and charred material, their levels could not account for most of the mutagenicity. Actually, the mutagenic activity was mainly associated with the basic fraction of charred materials obtained from broiled fish and meat. In addition to broiled fish and meat, formation of mutagens in cooked ground beef and beef extract was also the subject of an early report (56).

By monitoring the mutagenicity at each purification step with *S. typhimurium* TA98 or TA1538 with S9 mix, a series of new mutagenic substances were purified, and their structures determined. One approach was to isolate mutagenic substances from pyrolysates of amino acids and proteins that are constituents of foods. For example, Trp-P-1 and Trp-P-2 were isolated from a pyrolysate of D,L-tryptophan, Glu-P-1 and Glu-P-2 from that of L-glutamic acid. AαC and MeAαC were isolated from a pyrolysate of a protein, soybean globulin. Some of these mutagenic heterocyclic amines (HCAs) were also found in cooked foods.

The second approach was to isolate mutagens directly from cooked fish and meat. IQ and MeIQx were isolated from broiled sardines and MeIQx from fried beef. PhIP was also isolated from fried ground beef. This class of HCAs have a 2-aminoimidazole moiety as a common structure and are formed by heating mixtures of creatine, sugars, and amino acids, which are present in raw meat and fish. So far, 19 HCAs have been isolated as mutagens and their structures determined (2, 57–60). Their chemical structures, chemical names, and abbreviations are shown in Figure 80.3.

All HCAs show higher mutagenicity in *S. typhimurium* TA98 than in TA100 with S9 mix made with S9 that was prepared from livers of rats treated with polychlorinated biphenyls. The mutagenicity of 19 HCAs varies, depending on the chemical structure, ranging from 2 to 661,000 revertants/μg. Some HCAs show higher mutagenicity than typical mutagens/carcinogens such as aflatoxin B_1, 4-nitroquinoline 1-oxide, and benzo[*a*]pyrene.

These HCAs are also mutagenic to cultured mammalian cells including Chinese hamster lung cells with diphtheria toxin resistance (61) and repair-deficient Chinese hamster ovary cells with 6-thioguanine resistance (62). Further, HCAs induce sister-chromatid exchanges and chromosomal aberrations in cultured mammalian cells (63–66).

Ten HCAs (Trp-P-1, Trp-P-2, Glu-P-1, Glu-P-2, AαC, MeAαC, IQ, MeIQ, MeIQx, and PhIP) were chemically synthesized in large scale to test long-term carcinogenicity in CDF_1 mice and F344 rats of both sexes. These HCAs were mixed with diet at concentrations of 100 to 800 ppm and given to animals continuously throughout the experiments. All HCAs tested were carcinogenic (2, 57, 58, 67–70). All these compounds, except PhIP, induced tumors in the liver. Other tumors were also found in the small and large intestines, Zymbal glands, clitoral gland, skin, oral cavity, urinary bladder, prostate, and mammary glands of rats, and in the forestomach, lung, hematopoietic system, lymphoid tissue, and blood vessels of mice.

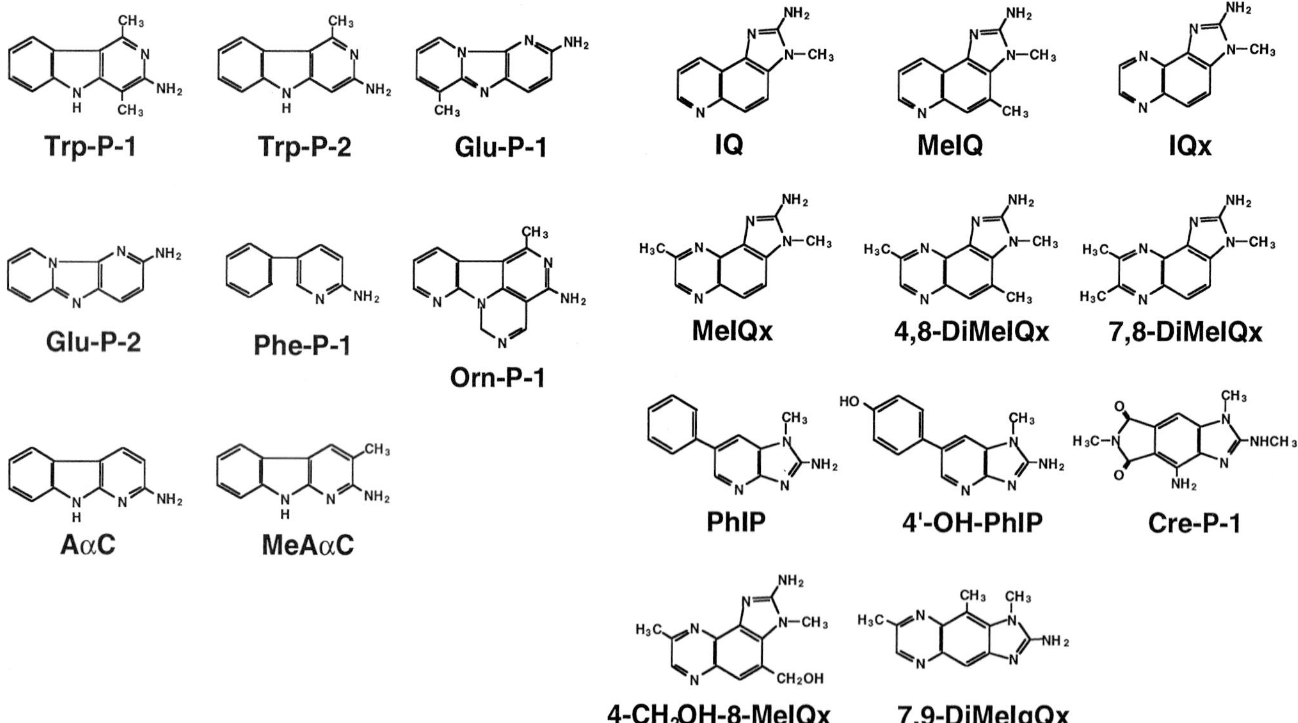

Figure 80.3. Structures of heterocyclic amines. Trp-P-1, 2-Amino-1,4-dimethyl-5*H*-pyrido[4,3-b]indole; Trp-P-2, 3-Amino-1-methyl-5*H*-pyrido[4,3-*b*]indole; Glu-P-1, 2-Amino-6-methyldipyrido[1,2-*a*: 3′,2′-*d*]imidazole; Glu-P-2, 2-Aminodipyrido[1,2-*a*: 3′,2′-*d*]imidazole; Phe-P-1, 2-Amino-5-phenylpyridine; Orn-P-1, 4-Amino-6-methyl-1*H*-2,5,10,10*b*-tetraazafluoranthene; AαC, 2-Amino-9*H*-pyrido[2,3-*b*]indole; MeAαC, 2-Amino-3-methyl-9*H*-pyrido[2,3-*b*]indole; IQ, 2-Amino-3-methylimidazo[4,5-*f*]quinoline; MeIQ, 2-Amino-3,4-dimethylimidazo[4,5-*f*]quinoline; IQX, 2-Amino-3-methylimidazo[4,5-*f*]quinoxaline; MeIQx, 2-Amino-3,8-dimethylimidazo[4,5-*f*]quinoxaline; 4,8-DiMeIQx, 2-Amino-3,4,8-trimethylimidazo[4,5-*f*]quinoxaline; 7,8-DiMeIQx, 2-Amino-3,7,8-trimethylimidazo[4,5-*f*]quinoxaline; PhIP, 2-Amino-1-methyl-6-phenylimidazo[4,5-*b*]pyridine; 4′-OH-PhIP, 2-Amino-1-methyl-6-(4-hydroxyphenyl)imidazo[4,5-*b*]pyridine; Cre-P-1, 4-Amino-1,6-dimethyl-2-methylamino-1*H*,6*H*-pyrrolo-[3,4-*f*]benzimidazole-5,7[dione; 4-CH_2OH-8-MeIQx, 2-Amino-4-hydroxymethyl-3,8-dimethylimidazo[4,5-*f*]quinoxaline; 7,9-DiMeIgQx, 2-Amino-1,7,9-trimethylimidazo[4,5-*g*]quinoxaline.

PhIP induced lymphoma in mice (68) and colon, mammary gland, and prostate cancers in rats (69, 70). IQ was also carcinogenic in monkeys (71).

Cultured mammalian cells infected with vaccinia virus bearing cloned cDNA of a single molecular species of cytochrome P-450 were used to identify the particular molecular species of P-450 responsible for metabolic activation of HCAs. All HCAs tested were most effectively oxidized to their *N*-hydroxyamino derivatives by CYP1A2 (72). These results are consistent with the observation that S9 obtained from the liver of rats treated with polychlorinated biphenyls and 3-methylcholanthrene is more active than that treated with phenobarbital (73). The *N*-hydroxyamino derivatives of HCAs are further activated to final forms by esterification with acetic acid and sulfuric acid, and these final metabolites react with guanine bases in DNA. HCAs such as Trp-P-2, Glu-P-1, IQ, MeIQx, and PhIP form DNA adducts, primarily at the C-8 position of guanine residues, N^2-(deoxyguanosin-8-yl)-HCA in vitro and in vivo (58, 74, 75). In the case of IQ, 5-(deoxyguanosin-N^2-yl)IQ (dG-N^2-IQ) was also identified as a minor adduct in vitro and in vivo (76). Removal of dG-N^2-IQ was much slower than that of dG-C8-IQ in the liver and kidney of rats.

Formation of adduct of the guanine base in DNA with HCAs is involved in induction of mutations in cancer-related genes. Mutations of H-*ras*, K-*ras*, and *p53* were observed in Zymbal gland, mammary, forestomach, and liver cancers induced by HCAs (77–79). In the case of colon cancer induced by PhIP, IQ, and Glu-P-1, mutations of K-*ras* and *p53* were very rare (79). Instead, a specific mutation of the *Apc* gene, deletion of a guanine base at a 5′-GGGA-3′ site, was frequently detected in rat colon cancers induced by PhIP (80). Moreover, microsatellite mutation is more frequent in colon and mammary cancers induced by PhIP than in those induced by IQ and 7,12-dimethylbenz[*a*]anthracene, respectively (81, 82).

Quantification of HCA levels in cooked foods and human urine samples indicates that humans are continuously exposed to low levels of HCAs derived from their daily diet (83). For example, daily exposure to MeIQx of 10 healthy volunteers living in Tokyo was estimated to be 0.3 to 3.9 μg per person (84). A linear relationship was observed between the dose of MeIQx and the MeIQx-DNA adduct level in the livers of rats and mice by ^{32}P-postlabeling and accelerator mass spectrometry analyses (85, 86). This suggests that MeIQx could form DNA adducts in human organs, even at doses as low as human exposure levels. Actually, MeIQx-DNA adducts were found in human tissues, colon, rectum, and kidney at levels of 14, 18, and 1.8/10^{10} nucleotides, respectively (87).

There are now several epidemiologic studies indicating a positive association between cooked meat consumption and development of colorectal, pancreatic, and urothelial cancers (88–91). Moreover, rapid metabolic phenotypes for acetyltransferase and CYP1A2 significantly increase the risk of colorectal neoplasia associated with cooked meat intake in man (92, 93). Thus, these findings suggest that HCAs are involved in human cancer development.

MAJOR COMPONENTS IN FOOD FOR PROMOTING CARCINOGENESIS

Sodium Chloride

Epidemiologic studies have linked sodium chloride intake and development of human gastric cancer (94). Administration of a high concentration of dietary sodium chloride after treatment with a gastric carcinogen, *N*-methyl-*N*′-nitro-*N*-nitrosoguanidine (MNNG) also significantly enhanced development of adenomas and adenocarcinomas in the glandular stomach of rats (95). Excess sodium chloride results in formation of malondialdehyde in the mucosa of the glandular stomach and increases its excretion into the urine (96). Thus, lipid peroxidation occurs in the glandular stomach damaged by sodium chloride.

Fat

Epidemiologic studies have generally associated high-fat diets with a high risk of colon and breast cancer (97). Consistent with these epidemiologic data, experiments with rodents demonstrated that elevated levels of dietary fat can enhance mammary and colon carcinogenesis in rats (98, 99). In these experiments, vegetable oils containing large amounts of ω6 polyunsaturated fatty acids were found to enhance the carcinogenicity more effectively than saturated fat. Although the mechanism of the effect of fat is not yet fully elucidated, it probably acts at the tumor-promotion stage. High fat intake could yield a tumor-promoting condition for colon cancer development through increased bile acid formation (100) and for breast cancer development through increased estrogen production by aromatase in adipose tissues (101).

PUBLIC HEALTH SIGNIFICANCE

Cancer development in man can be viewed as a multistage process involving multiple genetic alterations. The multiple genetic alterations are caused by various kinds of environmental xenobiotics including the food-derived carcinogens detailed above as well as autobiotics, such as endogenously generated oxygen radicals, which can also induce DNA damage. Chronic inflammation may be involved in cancer development by causing continuous cell turnover and creating a favorable environment for carcinogenesis. For example, infection with *Helicobacter pylori* resulting in gastritis is a risk factor for gastric cancer in man. On the other hand, a number of foods appear protective because they contain a variety of cancer preventive substances such as fiber, fish oil, polyphenols and vitamins. Although single carcinogenic factors are not in themselves sufficient to induce cancers, their genotoxic effects accumulate. Moreover, carcinogenic factors interact with each other and thus could play some role in carcinogenesis. Thus, it is desirable to avoid exposure to carcinogens in food as much as possible and adapt all feasible measures to reduce their adverse effects.

REFERENCES

1. Hecker E. Naturwissenschaften 1967;54:282–4.
2. Sugimura T. Science 1986;233:312–8.
3. Wogan GN. Cancer Res 1992;52(Suppl):2114s–8s.
4. IARC Monogr Eval Carcinog Risk Chem Hum 1987; 7(Suppl):83–7.
5. Hsieh DPH, Cullen JM, Ruebner BH. Food Chem Toxicol 1984;22:1027–8.
6. Milo GE Jr, DiPaolo JA. Nature 1978;275:130–2.
7. Trzos RJ, Petzold GL, Brunden MN, Swenberg JA. Mutat Res 1978;58:79–86.
8. Croy RG, Essigmann JM, Reinhold VN, Wogan GN. Proc Natl Acad Sci USA 1978;75:1745–9.
9. Lutz WK. Mutat Res 1979;65:289–356.
10. Foster PL, Eisenstadt E, Miller JH. Proc Natl Acad Sci USA 1983;80:2695–8.
11. Antrup H, Jorgensen ECB, Jensen O. Mutagenesis 1996; 11:69–73.
12. Aguilar F, Hussain SP, Cerutti P. Proc Natl Acad Sci USA 1993; 90:8586–90.
13. Hsu IC, Metcalf RA, Sun T, et al. Nature 1991;350:427–8.
14. Bressac B, Kew M, Wands J, et al. Nature 1991;350:429–31.
15. Ozturk M, Bressac B, Puisieux A, et al. Lancet 1991; 338:1356–59.
16. Murakami Y, Hayashi K, Hirohashi S, Sekiya T. Cancer Res 1991;51:5520–5.
17. Scorsone KA, Zhou Y-Z, Butel JS, Slagle BL. Cancer Res 1992; 52:1635–8.
18. Groopman JD, Hasler JA, Trudel LJ, et al. Cancer Res 1992;52:267–74.
19. Ross RK, Yuan J-M, Yu MC, et al. Lancet 1992;339:943–46.
20. Sabbioni G, Skipper P, Buchi G, Tannenbaum SR. Carcinogenesis 1987;8:819–24.
21. Jaskiewicz K, van Rensburg SJ, Marasas WFO, Gelderbloom WCA. J Natl Cancer Inst 1987;78:321–5.
22. Gelderbloom WCA, Kriek NPJ, Marasas WFO, Theil PG. Carcinogenesis 1991;12:1247–51.
23. Terao K. J Toxicol Toxin Rev 1983;2:77–110.
24. National Toxicology Program. NTP technical report on the toxicology and carcinogenesis studies of ochratoxin A in F344/N rats, NTP TR 358, NIH publ. no. 88–2813. Research Triangle Park, NC: National Toxicology Program, 1988.
25. Hirono I, Mori H, Yamada K, et al. J Natl Cancer Inst 1977; 58:1155–7.
26. Hirono I, Mori H, Culvenor CCJ. Gann 1976;67:125–9.
27. Shoental R. Cancer Res 1975;35:2020–4.
28. Svoboda DJ, Reddy JK. Cancer Res 1972;32:908–12.
29. IARC Monogr Eval Carcinog Risk Chem Man 1976;10:291–302.
30. Evans IA, Mason J. Nature 1965;208:913–4.
31. Hirono I, Shibuya C, Fushimi K, Haga M. J Natl Cancer Inst 1970;45:179–88.
32. Van der Hoeven JCM, Lagerweij WJ, Posthumus MA, et al. Carcinogenesis 1983;4:1587–90.
33. Hirono I, Yamada K, Niwa H, et al. Cancer Lett 1984;21: 239–46.
34. Hirono I, Aiso S, Yamaji T, et al. Gann 1984;75:833–6.
35. Toth B, Nagel D, Patil K, et al. Cancer Res 1978;38:177–80.
36. Toth B, Patil K, Jae H-S. Cancer Res 1981;41:2444–9.
37. Toth B, Nagel D, Ross A. Br J Cancer 1982;46:417–22.
38. Toth B, Erickson J. Cancer Res 1986;46:4007–11.
39. Toth B, Patil K. J Cancer Res Clin Oncol 1979;93:109–21.
40. Laqueur GL, Mickelsen O, Whiting MG, Kurland LT. J Natl Cancer Inst 1963;31:919–51.
41. Laqueur GL, Matsumoto H. J Natl Cancer Inst 1966;37: 217–32.
42. Miller EC, Swanson AB, Phillips DH, et al. Cancer Res 1983;43:1124–34.
43. IARC Monogr Eval Carcinog Risk Chem Man 1976;10:231–44.
44. Gross MA, Jones WI, Cook EL, Boone CC. Proc Am Assoc Cancer Res 1967;8:24.
45. Koppang N, Slagsvold P, Hansen MA, et al. Nord Vet Med 1964;16:343–62.
46. Sakshaug J, Sögnen E, Hansen MA, Koppang N. Nature 1965;206:1261–2.
47. Mirvish SS. Toxicol Appl Pharmacol 1975;31:325–51.
48. Leaf C, Wishnok JS, Tannenbaum SR. Carcinogenesis 1991; 12:537–9.
49. Scanlan RA. Cancer Res 1983;43(Suppl):2435s–40s.
50. Kuratsune M. J Natl Cancer Inst 1956;16:1485–96.
51. Lijinsky W, Shubik P. Science 1964;145:53–5.
52. Jeffrey AM, Weinstein IB, Jennette KW, et al. Nature 1977; 269:348–50.
53. Ruggeri B, DiRado M, Zhang SY, et al. Proc Natl Acad Sci USA 1993;90:1013–7.
54. Sugimura T, Nagao M, Kawachi T, et al. Mutagen-carcinogens in food, with special reference to highly mutagenic pyrolytic products in broiled foods. In: Hiatt HH, Watson JD, Winsten JA, eds. Origins of human cancer. Cold Spring Harbor, NY: Cold Spring Harbor Laboratory, 1977;1561–77.
55. Nagao M, Honda M, Seino Y, et al. Cancer Lett 1977;2: 221–6.
56. Commoner B, Vithayathil AJ, Dolara P, et al. Science 1978; 201:913–6.
57. Sugimura T. Science 1992;258:603–7.
58. Wakabayashi K, Nagao M, Esumi H, Sugimura T. Cancer Res 1992;52:2092s–8s.
59. Felton JS, Knize MG, Shen NH, et al. Carcinogenesis 1986;7:1081–6.
60. Becher G, Knize MG, Nes IF, Felton JS. Carcinogenesis 1988; 9:247–53.
61. Nakayasu M, Nakasato F, Sakamoto H, et al. Mutat Res 1983; 118:91–102.
62. Thompson LH, Tucker JD, Stewart SA, et al. Mutagenesis 1987;2:483–7.
63. Ishidate M Jr, Sofuni T, Yoshikawa K. GANN Monogr Cancer Res 1981;27:95–108.
64. Tohda H, Oikawa A, Kawachi T, Sugimura T. Mutat Res 1980; 77:65–9.
65. Holme JA, Wallin H, Brunborg G, et al. Carcinogenesis 1989; 10:1389–96.
66. Aeschbacher HU, Ruch E. Carcinogenesis 1989;10:429–33.
67. Ohgaki H, Takayama S, Sugimura T. Mutat Res 1991;259: 399–410.
68. Esumi H, Ohgaki H, Kohzen E, et al. Jpn J Cancer Res 1989;80:1176–8.
69. Ito N, Hasegawa R, Sano M, et al. Carcinogenesis 1991;12: 1503–6.
70. Shirai T, Sano M, Tamano S, et al. Cancer Res 1997;57:195–8.
71. Adamson RH, Thorgeirsson UP, Snyderwine EG, et al. Jpn J Cancer Res 1990;81:10–14.
72. Aoyama T, Gonzalez FJ, Gelboin HV. Mol Carcinog 1989;1: 253–9.

73. Kato R, Yamozoe Y. Gann 1987;78:297–311.
74. Lin D, Kaderlik KR, Turesky RJ, et al. Chem Res Toxicol 1992; 5:691–7.
75. Fukutome K, Ochiai M, Wakabayashi K, et al. Jpn J Cancer Res 1994;85:113–7.
76. Turesky RJ, Markovic J, Aeschlimann JM. Chem Res Toxicol 1996;9:397–402.
77. Kudo M, Ogura T, Esumi H, Sugimura T. Mol Carcinog 1991; 4:36–42.
78. Ushijima T, Kakiuchi H, Makino H, et al. Mol Carcinog 1994; 10:38–44.
79. Ushijima T, Makino H, Kakiuchi H, et al. Genetic alterations in HCA-induced tumors. In: Adamson RH, Gustafsson J, Ito N, et al., eds. Heterocyclic amines in cooked foods: possible human carcinogens. Princeton, NJ: Princeton Scientific Publishing, 1995;281–91.
80. Kakiuchi H, Watanabe M, Ushijima T, et al. Proc Natl Acad Sci USA 1995;92:910–4.
81. Canzian F, Ushijima T, Serikawa T, et al. Cancer Res 1994; 54:6315–7.
82. Toyota M, Ushijima T, Weisburger JH, et al. Mol Carcinog 1996;15:176–82.
83. Wakabayashi K, Ushiyama H, Takahashi M, et al. Environ Health Perspect 1993, 99:129–33.
84. Ushiyama H, Wakabayashi K, Hirose M, et al. Carcinogenesis 1991;12:1417–22.
85. Yamashita K, Adachi M, Kato S, et al. Jpn J Cancer Res 1990;81:470–6.
86. Turteltaub KW, Felton JS, Gledhill BL, et al. Proc Natl Acad Sci USA 1990;87:5288–92.
87. Totsuka Y, Fukutome K, Takahashi M, et al. Carcinogenesis 1996;17:1029–34.
88. Norell SE, Ahlbom A, Erwald R, et al. Am J Epidemiol 1986; 124:894–902.
89. Steineck G, Hagman U, Gerhardsson M, Norell SE. Int J Cancer 1990;45:1006–11.
90. Schiffman MH, Felton JS. Am J Epidemiol 1990;131: 376–8.
91. Gerhardsson de Verdier M, Hagman U, Peters RK, et al. Int J Cancer 1991;49:520–5.
92. Lang NP, Butler MA, Massengill J, et al. Cancer Epidemiol Biomarkers Prev 1994;3:675–82.
93. Roberts-Thomson IC, Ryan P, Khoo KK, et al. Lancet 1996;347:1372–4.
94. Hirayama T. Gann Monogr 1971;11:3–19.
95. Takahashi M, Nishikawa A, Furukawa F, et al. Carcinogenesis 1994;15:1429–32.
96. Takahashi M, Hasegawa T, Furukawa F, et al. Carcinogenesis 1991;12:2201–4.
97. Caroll KK, Khor HT. Progr Biochem Pharmacol 1975;10: 308–53.
98. Caroll KK, Khor HT. Lipids 1971;6:415–20.
99. Reddy BS. Cancer 1975;36:2401–6.
100. Reddy BS, Cohen LA, McCoy GD, et al. Adv Cancer Res 1980;32:238–345.
101. O'Neill JS, Elton RA, Miller WR. Br Med J 1988;296:741–3.

81. Chemoprevention of Cancer

DIANE F. BIRT, JAMES D. SHULL, and ANN L. YAKTINE

This chapter reviews recent information on cancer prevention by diet. The role of macronutrients such as dietary fat and properties of macronutrients, such as calorie contribution, are covered to emphasize their importance. Since macronutrient effects on cancer epidemiology are covered in Chapter 79, this chapter is limited to a consideration of the animal and mechanistic studies. Micronutrient effects on cancer prevention emphasize nutrient interactions and specific micronutrients that have been extensively studied or for which recent provocative observations have been reported. The discussion of the role of nonnutrient components of diet in cancer prevention emphasizes agents and classes of agents that have received considerable recent attention. These compounds are grouped according to the major potential mechanism for cancer prevention.

MACRONUTRIENTS AND PROPERTIES OF MACRONUTRIENTS

Dietary Energy

Laboratory Studies

Dietary energy restriction is one of the most potent and reproducible inhibitors of carcinogenesis in rodent tumor models (1). Restriction of energy from carbohydrate or carbohydrate and fat inhibited mammary (2), colon (3), liver (4), and skin (5) carcinogenesis in recent studies. The rodent energy restriction paradigm is not a starvation protocol. The dietary energy–restricted rodents do eat their diet over a shortened time frame (meal eaters), and they do gain less weight than the fully fed rodent, but they live considerably longer than their fully fed controls (1). The fully fed rodents can reasonably be considered overfed. Epidemiologic studies that suggest obesity as a risk factor for cancers of the colon, endometrium, prostate, and breast and indicate the role of physical activity in prevention of cancers of the colon and breast provide strong support for a role of dietary energy and energy balance in cancer.

Energy restriction appeared somewhat more effective in prevention of late events in carcinogenesis studies with breast (6) and skin (7), but this may simply be due to the carcinogenesis protocols, which attempt to divide cancer into initiation and promotional events. Research in breast (6) and skin (7) cancer suggested that energy restriction must be of long duration for effective cancer prevention. However, peripubertal dietary restriction inhibited virus-induced mammary carcinogenesis later in life in mice (8).

Mechanism of Action

Oxidative Processes. Numerous mechanisms have been explored for prevention of cancer by dietary energy restriction. Energy and/or diet restriction of rodents and humans reduces oxidative damage (9, 10). Restriction changes numerous metabolic processes, including reduced oxidative metabolism, improved elimination of carcinogens, and slowing of the age-related decline in various repair processes (11).

Hormonal Modulation. Hormonal adaptation to dietary energy restriction may be an important mediator of energy-restriction prevention of cancer. Glucocorticoid hormones increase in response to dietary energy restriction in mice (12) and in anorexia nervosa patients (cortisol) (13). Glucocorticoid hormones and glucocorticoid drugs have long been known to inhibit skin tumor promotion in mouse skin, and more recent studies demonstrated the importance of an intact adrenal gland in prevention of cancer by energy restriction. When mice were adrenalectomized and fed restricted diets, skin tumor promotion was not inhibited. However, parallel groups with intact adrenal glands demonstrated striking inhibition of skin tumor promotion in the energy-restricted mouse (12) (Fig. 81.1). Recent studies demonstrated the importance of an intact adrenal gland in prevention of lung carcino-

Abbreviations: **DMBA**—7,12-dimethylbenz[*a*]anthracene; **MNU**—methylnitrosourea.

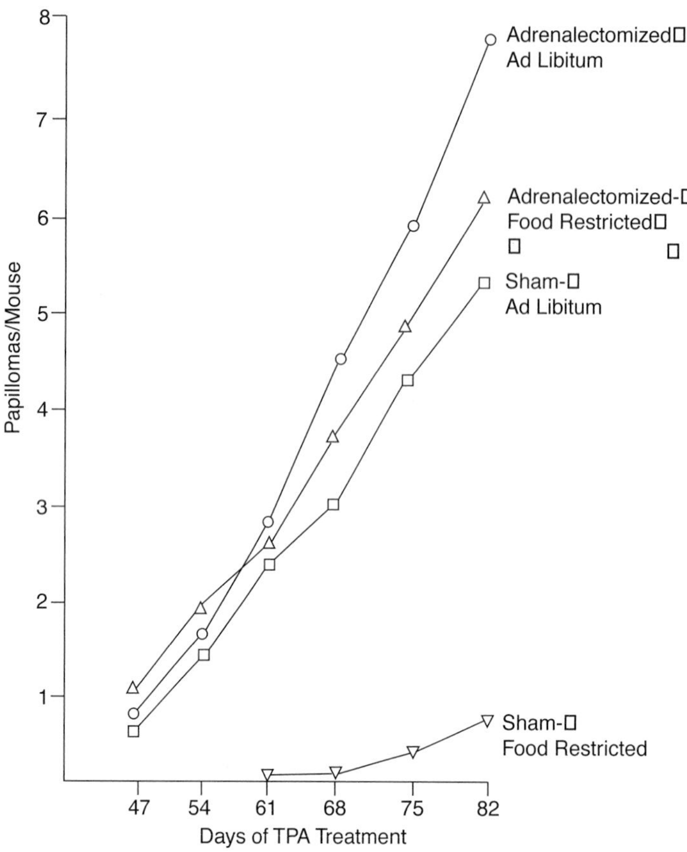

Figure 81.1. Inhibition of papilloma development by food restriction and its reversal by adrenalectomy. (From Pashko LL, Schwartz AG. Carcinogenesis 1992;13:1925–8, with permission.)

genesis by dietary restriction (14). These studies do not indicate which adrenal hormones were necessary for energy-restriction prevention of skin and lung carcinogenesis because of the number of hormones produced by the adrenal gland. However, the fact that energy restriction increased glucocorticoid hormone secretion and that glucocorticoid hormones are potent inhibitors of skin carcinogenesis (15) supports the hypothesis that energy–restriction inhibition of lung and skin carcinogenesis may require glucocorticoid hormone.

Studies are currently testing the hypothesis that the elevated glucocorticoid hormone secretion may mediate downstream events that are necessary for energy–restriction inhibition of carcinogenesis. Birt et al. previously demonstrated inhibition of epidermal protein kinase C (PKC) α and ζ (two of the four isoforms of the enzyme) in the skin of the energy–restricted mouse (16). This reduction may be relevant to energy–restriction inhibition of cancer, since the phorbol ester tumor promoter 12-*O*-tetradecanoylphorbol-13-acetate (TPA) binds to specific PKC isoenzymes with phorbol ester binding domains. This interaction is believed to be important for skin tumor promotion by TPA (17). Indeed, epidermal cells from energy–restricted mice had reduced phorbol ester–binding sites (16). It is possible that the reduction in PKC isoforms is mediated, at least in part, by the elevated glucocorticoid hormone. A number of studies have suggested that PKC may play a role in downstream signaling from the glucocorticoid receptor (18) (see also Chapter 37). Furthermore, our preliminary studies suggest that glucocorticoid treatment of adrenalectomized mice reduces PKC ζ expression (Birt et al., unpublished).

Cellular Proliferation and Apoptosis. Observations from other laboratories demonstrate the importance of inhibition of cellular proliferation and enhanced programed cell death (apoptosis) in tissues from energy–restricted rodents. In particular, James and Muskhelishvili (19) demonstrated inhibition of hepatic cell proliferation and accelerated hepatic apoptosis in the liver of energy–restricted mice (Fig. 81.2). In parallel studies, energy restriction inhibited spontaneous hepatoma development (19). Earlier studies focusing on regression of nafenopin, a peroxisome proliferator that induces hepatocellular carcinomas and adenomas in diet-restricted rats, suggested that enhanced apoptosis of preneoplastic cells, in addition to reduced cell replication, was responsible for the protective effect of diet restriction (20). The evolving role for PKC in the process of apoptosis suggests the possibility that changes induced in PKC by dietary-energy restriction may play a role in induction of apoptosis in the restricted animal (21).

Immunologic Modulation. Dietary restriction is certainly important in modulation of immunologic responses (22,

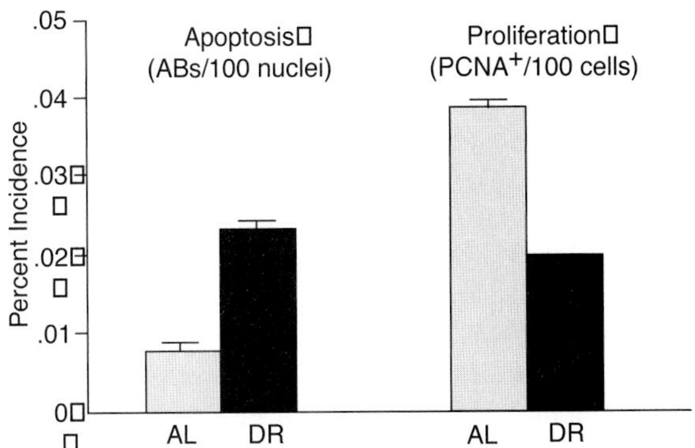

Figure 81.2. Rates of apoptosis (apoptosis bodies/100 nuclei) and proliferation (proliferating cell nuclear antigen+/100 hepatocytes) within livers of 12-month-old ad libitum and 40% diet-restricted B6C3F$_1$ mice. Comparison of indices between the two dietary groups demonstrates the relative increase in incidence of apoptotic bodies and decrease in incidence of proliferating cell nuclear antigen+ cells in livers of diet-restricted mice compared with ad libitum mice. (From James SJ, Muskhelishvili L. Cancer Res 1994;54:5508–10, with permission.)

23). How alterations in immune function in underfed animals relate to reduced rates of cancer development is unclear, but this is a fertile area for further research.

Gene Expression. Dietary food restriction causes significant alterations in gene expression that may be important in cancer development. For example, heat-shock proteins, which are important for normal cell growth and homeostasis as well as in protecting cells from the toxic effects of extreme temperatures, were induced to a greater extent in aged diet-restricted rats than in aged control-fed rats (24).

Dietary Fat

Laboratory Studies

The level and type of dietary fat have been extensively studied in animal models for cancer modulation. In general, diets rich in polyunsaturated fatty acids have enhanced development of mammary (25), colon (26), pancreas, (27), and prostate (28) cancer. Investigations on dietary fat and skin cancer promotion provide different results, depending upon experimental design (5). It has been suggested that the influence of diets rich in polyunsaturated fatty acids (PUFAs) on carcinogenesis in the mammary gland and colon may be caused by the content of linoleic acid in such diets. A threshold of linoleic acid was demonstrated to be necessary for cancer enhancement in mammary gland (29) (Fig. 81.3).

In a number of studies, oils rich in oleic acid, such as olive oil, were found to result in lower cancer rates than diets rich in PUFAs such as corn oil (30). This observation may relate more to the removal of high levels of dietary linoleic acid in corn oil than to addition of olive oil (30).

Diets rich in ω-3 fatty acids have also been investigated for their influence on cancer at a number of sites. Studies in the breast and colon have provided some evidence for cancer prevention, but in general, fish oil does not appear to prevent cancer induction; it simply lacks cancer-enhancing properties (30).

Mechanism of Action

There are probably more mechanisms for dietary fat modulation of cancer than there are convincing data that dietary fat is an important risk factor for human cancer. The major problem may be the complexity of lipids in the human diet and the possibility that only specific fatty acids are really important in cancer cause and prevention.

Eicosanoid Metabolism. A favorite hypothesis for involvement of dietary fat in carcinogenesis is that different lipids provide alternative substrates for eicosanoid synthesis. Furthermore, experimental studies provide the most compelling evidence for a promotional role for linoleic acid, and linoleic acid is the dietary precursor to arachidonic acid. Arachidonic acid clearly plays a central role in cellular regulation as the precursor of eicosanoid synthesis. Our poor understanding of the role of eicosanoids in human cancer cause and development makes it difficult to assess the importance of dietary modulation of eicosanoid synthesis in cancer. Another problem with trying to relate diet to prostaglandin production is that radical changes in dietary fat intake are required, such as an essential fatty acid deficiency or a linoleate:saturated fatty acid ratio greater than 5 (31). Some of the

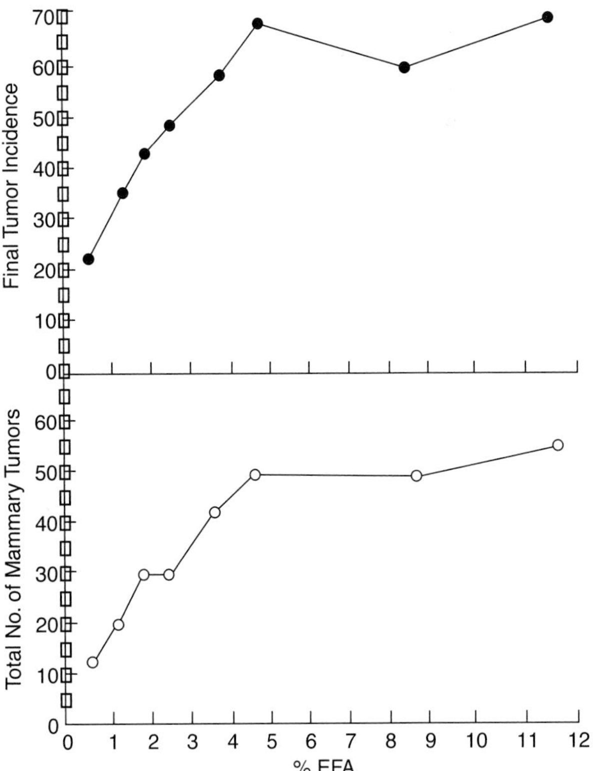

Figure 81.3. Autopsy data of tumor incidence and tumor yield of rats fed diets containing different levels of EFA. There were 30 rats/group. (From Ip C, Carter CA, Ip MM. Cancer Res 1985;45:1997–2001, with permission.)

influence of ω-3 fatty acids on cancer prevention may possibly be related to reduced basal prostaglandin levels.

However, compelling data on the importance of prostaglandin synthesis in cancer has been obtained from studies using inhibitors of prostaglandin synthesis as inhibitors of cancer. A number of inhibitors have been very effective, especially in inhibition of colon carcinogenesis (32). However, these drugs inhibit many other enzymes as well as prostaglandin synthesis, and it is impossible to know which effects are the most important.

Cellular Proliferation. Dietary fat may also influence cellular proliferation. Studies in colon (33) and breast (34) suggest that high-fat diets result in greater cellular proliferation than low-fat diets. Since this is also influenced by dietary energy, it is important to know if the animals fed high-fat diets had an equivalent intake of dietary energy. In general, dietary fat influences a number of processes, which may account for the observed enhancement of cell proliferation. High-fat diets were shown to increase colonic ornithine decarboxylase (ODC) activity (35). ODC is the rate-limiting enzyme in polyamine synthesis, and polyamines are needed for DNA replication. Thus, a number of agents that increase cell proliferation induce ODC activity. Induction of ODC appears necessary, but not sufficient, for tumor promotion in the skin (36), and overexpression of ODC in transgenic mice increased the incidence of spontaneous skin tumors (37). Tyrosine kinase activity was also increased in association with accelerated cellular proliferation, and studies determined increased tyrosine kinase activity in the colon of rats fed a high-fat diet (35). Since oxidative products of fatty acids appear to induce ODC and tyrosine kinase activity, lipid oxidation may possibly be necessary for these observations (38).

Protein Kinase C (PKC). Recent studies have assessed the role of dietary fat in modulation of PKC. PKC, as mentioned above, is important in cellular proliferation and differentiation. Our understanding of the specific tissue and isoenzyme selectivity in modulating cellular proliferation and differentiation is in its infancy (39). A series of studies focused on mouse epidermis suggested that high dietary fat (24.6%) increased the activity of PKC in comparison with diets low in fat (5%) (40). This increased PKC activity was associated with a 36% increase in 1,2-*sn*-diacylglycerol (DAG), an activator of PKC (40). Further investigations to assess if this increase was due to changes in the expression of specific isoforms indicated that dietary fat did not influence the expression of PKC α, ϵ, δ, and ζ (16). These results suggest that dietary fat effects on PKC in the epidermis must have been due to changes in the activation of the epidermal enzyme. This is certainly possible, since PKC is known to respond to cellular lipid composition and metabolism (41).

Recent studies in in vitro systems and in rodents fed diets containing different levels and types of fat have explored the relationship of dietary fat to colonic PKC activity and isoenzyme expression. Weinstein and collaborators (42) explored the hypothesis that dietary fat in the colonic mucosa results in generation of DAG, which is then available to activate colonic PKC (Fig. 81.4). This activation is hypothesized to result in a proliferative environment in the colonic epithelium. Assessment of colonic DAG in rats fed diets differing in fat (corn oil and fish oil) and fiber (cellulose and pectin) indicated approximately 2.5-fold more DAG excretion in animals fed cellulose than in those fed pectin and somewhat higher DAG excretion in rats fed corn oil than in those fed fish oil (43). These results demonstrate that diet can alter fecal DAG concentration and excretion. Lafave et al. (44) compared a diet containing 15% beef tallow and 5% corn oil with a diet containing 5% corn oil and reported that the high-fat diet caused a translocation of PKC activity from soluble to particulate fractions, which is consistent with increased PKC in the plasma membrane, believed to be the more active state. Davidson et al. (45) compared colonic PKC isoform

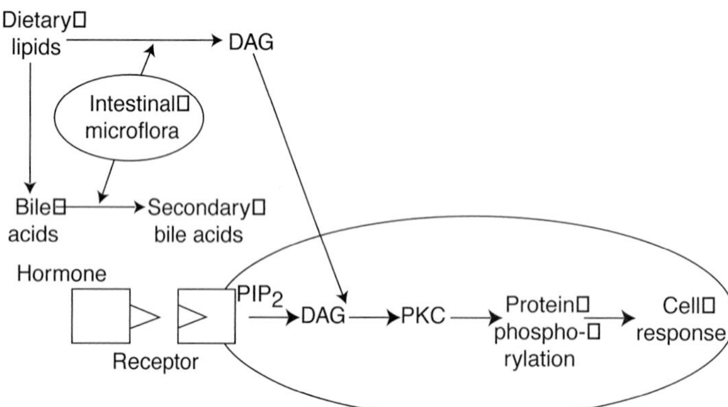

Figure 81.4. Hypothesis relating production of diacylglycerol *(DAG)* by the intestinal microflora to colon cancer. Conversion by intestinal bacteria of dietary phospholipids to DAG would be enhanced by a high-fat diet and by secondary bile acids. Intestinal bacteria also play a role in conversion of bile acids to secondary bile acids. It was proposed that the DAG thus produced enters colonic epithelial cells and stimulates protein kinase C directly. This mechanism would bypass the usual pathway in mammalian cells in which hormones and other agonists occupy membrane-associated receptors leading to activation of cellular phospholipase C. (From Weinstein IB. Cancer Res 1991;51(Suppl):5080s–5s, with permission.)

expression in rats fed diets differing in fiber and fat. Their results provided little evidence that the type of dietary fat affected colonic PKC isoform expression.

Modulation of Gene Expression. Another potential role of dietary fat in cancer is alteration of gene expression. Studies of transcription of mouse mammary tumor virus (MMTV) proviral DNA at the MTV-1 locus in mammary glands from C3H Heston mice fed 23.5% or 5% corn oil diets demonstrated accelerated transcription in the mice fed the high-fat diet (46). Mice fed the high-fat diet had accelerated mammary tumor development with shorter tumor latency and development of tumors after fewer litters (46). High dietary fat may also preferentially promote mammary tumor development in methylnitrosourea-induced tumors that contain the wild-type *ras* gene, suggesting differential patterns of signal transduction and gene expression (47).

Conjugated Linoleic Acid

Occurrence

In contrast to linoleic acid, with double bonds at carbons 9 and 12, which has been studied as a potential factor in cancer promotion in animal and human studies, conjugated linoleic acid (CLA), which has conjugated double bonds at carbons 10 and 12 or at carbons 9 and 11, has antimutagenic and anticarcinogenic activity (48). CLA was first isolated from a fraction of cooked meat that had antimutagenic activity (49). It is now apparent that CLA is present in human diets, and the primary sources appear to be dairy and meat products. For example, cooked beef was reported to contain 6.6 to 8.2 mg/g fat (50). The most prevalent form of CLA in foods is the *cis* 9,11 isomer of CLA.

Laboratory Studies

CLA was effective in inhibiting carcinogenesis of skin (49) and forestomach (51). Studies in the laboratory of Dr. Clement Ip demonstrated inhibition of mammary and breast carcinogenesis (52). Triglyceride-CLA is as effective as free fatty acid–CLA in preventing mammary carcinogenesis (53). This is important, because dietary CLA is in the form of triglyceride-CLA, and previous carcinogenesis studies were done with fatty acid–CLA.

MICRONUTRIENT INTERACTIONS

Vitamin D, Calcium, and Phosphorus

Epidemiologic and Clinical Studies

The hypothesis that dietary calcium and vitamin D protect against colon cancer, and that dietary phosphorus may block this protection, has received considerable attention in recent years. The biochemical basis for this hypothesis comes from the ability of calcium to chemically interact with bile acids and fatty acids and potentially reduce their toxicity. The proposed antagonism by phosphorus is based on the ability of phosphorus to interfere with calcium absorption and use. Data supporting the hypothesis that dietary vitamin D and/or calcium could prevent cancer came from the observation of a gradient of increasing colon cancer mortality rates with increasing latitude north (55). Such an association could be due to the impact of ultraviolet light on synthesis of vitamin D in the skin and, subsequently, on absorption of dietary calcium. A 19-year prospective study in Chicago demonstrated a 50% reduction in colon cancer risk in men with a daily intake of 3.75 μg vitamin D and a 75% reduction in men with a daily intake above 1200 mg calcium (55). Levels of circulating 25-hydroxy-vitamin D were higher in controls than in patients (55). A prospective study on women in Iowa further supported the hypothesis that vitamin D and/or calcium protect against colon cancer (56).

Further investigation into the relationship of calcium intake and colon cancer has not generally supported this hypothesis. Studies in the Netherlands focused on the relationship between consumption of fermented dairy products or dietary intake of calcium and the risk of colon cancer in a case-control study (57). Consumption of fermented dairy products, hard cheese, and unfermented dairy products was not associated with the risk of colon cancer. Furthermore, consumption of total dietary calcium was positively (significant in men but not in women) associated with colon cancer risk. In a prospective study on the relationship between serum levels of vitamin D metabolites and colon cancer in Washington County, Maryland, no relationship was observed between 25-hydroxy-vitamin D or 1,25-hydroxy-vitamin D levels and the subsequent risk of colon cancer in 20,305 subjects (58).

Recently, prostate cancer risk was similarly reported to be inversely associated with exposure to ultraviolet light and hypothesized to be another cancer related to vitamin D intake (59). This hypothesis is supported by the presence of vitamin D receptors in the normal prostate (60) and by evidence of vitamin D involvement in regulation of differentiation and gene expression (61).

Studies on the influence of calcium supplementation on colon cancer prevention have also been inconclusive (62, 63). Early investigations in subjects at high risk for colon cancer suggested that calcium supplements were effective in reducing cell proliferation, a potential biomarker for colon cancer risk (64). However, these studies were neither blinded nor placebo controlled, and they generally had short follow-ups. More-comprehensive placebo-controlled studies with longer follow-up have not shown appreciable reduction in colonic cell proliferation in calcium-supplemented subjects. In spite of these inconclusive results, the hypothesis continues to find support in human investigations. In a study of intestinal bypass patients, calcium supplementation (2.4 or 3.6 g/day) for 3 months reduced rectal hyperproliferation and decreased fecal DAG output. DAG is a second messenger for PKC, a key enzyme in cellular growth regulation. The authors hypothesized that the reduction in fecal DAG in calcium-supplemented patients was, at least in part, responsible for the reduced rectal cell proliferation (65).

Laboratory Studies and Mechanism of Action

The importance of dietary phosphorus in antagonizing protective effects of calcium was studied in rats supplemented with calcium from calcium carbonate, calcium phosphate, and milk mineral (66). This study was designed to determine whether the phosphorus in calcium phosphate or in milk mineral would block bile acid excretion and decrease cytolytic activity of fecal water, which was associated with calcium supplementation. The influence of these supplements on epithelial cell damage and proliferation and on serum gastrin was also measured. All three calcium sources decreased soluble bile acids and fatty acids and decreased the cytolytic activity of fecal water. Only minor differences between groups were observed, demonstrating that the hypothesized interference by phosphorus did not occur in this experimental paradigm.

Newmark and Lipkin (67) conducted an extensive series of experiments in rodents to assess a diet designed to mimic four of the suggested dietary risk factors for colon cancer: high fat and phosphate, and low calcium and vitamin D. They first demonstrated that feeding this "stress diet" for 12 weeks resulted in hyperproliferation in the sigmoid colon (67). Subsequent experiments demonstrated that increasing the level of dietary calcium in the "stress diet" could return colonic proliferation to normal values (68). Parallel studies assessed the influence of a "western-style stress diet" on mammary ductal epithelial cell hyperproliferation and hyperplasia (69). Following 20 weeks of consumption of the diet high in phosphorus and fat and low in calcium and vitamin D, the authors observed more mammary ducts and more proliferating cells in the small terminal ducts, a cancer-prone region of the mammary gland, in the experimental animals than in controls. Studies with cultured cells revealed induction of apoptosis in breast cancer cell lines treated with vitamin D or antiestrogens (70). The growth inhibitory properties of 1,25-dihydroxy-vitamin D_3 against cultured mouse keratinocytes were associated with induction of vitamin D receptor in an experiment comparing cells resistant to vitamin D growth inhibition with wild-type cells in which vitamin D receptor was induced (71).

Studies with rats treated with the colonic carcinogen 1,2-dimethylhydrazine (DMH) and fed graded levels of calcium and vitamin D showed that both of these nutrients reduced colonic carcinogenesis and altered colonic cell kinetics (72). Comparable studies on mammary carcinogenesis by 7,12-dimethylbenz[*a*]anthracene (DMBA) suggested that high dietary calcium and vitamin D protected against mammary carcinogenesis, while high dietary phosphate increased susceptibility (73).

Methyl Deficiency; Folic Acid, Vitamin B_{12}, Choline, and Methionine Interactions

Laboratory Studies

Observations on methyl group deficiency (folic acid, choline, and methionine) and increased cancer were originally made in animal models. In the early studies, combined deficiencies of choline and methionine were induced using diets contaminated with aflatoxin (74). The induced liver cancers were attributed to the aflatoxin. However, it was apparent that methyl deficiency was a potent facilitator of carcinogenesis. Further investigations demonstrated that methyl deficiency alone, using a deficiency of choline and methionine (75), or folic acid, vitamin B_{12}, choline, and/or methionine (76), induced preneoplastic or neoplastic lesions in animal livers. These observations led to the hypothesis that DNA methylation by methyl donors is important in cancer prevention.

Epidemiologic and Clinical Studies

Although it was not clear if imbalanced methyl-deficient conditions were present in human diets, the prevalence of inadequate folate intake had been documented (77). A role for folic acid in cancer prevention was suspected because folic acid is abundant in vegetables and fruits, and consumption of such foods has been associated with reduced cancer rates. Furthermore, the importance of adequate dietary folic acid for regulation of normal gene expression suggests a potential role in cancer prevention. However, a case-control study of colon and rectal cancer did not show any association with dietary folate intake (78). Studies of women in the Nurses' Health Study and men in the Health Professionals Follow-up Study showed that dietary folate was inversely associated with risk of adenoma in women and men, alcohol intake above 30 g/day was positively associated with adenoma risk, and dietary methionine was inversely associated with risk of an adenoma 1 cm or larger (79). Combined intakes of high alcohol and low folate and methionine significantly increased the risk for adenomas 1 cm or larger (Table 81.1). These results support the importance of methyl group availability in preventing human colorectal cancer.

Mechanism of Action

Recent studies in laboratory animals demonstrated that deficiencies of choline, methionine, or folic acid in rats fed semipurified diets could result in imbalances in deoxynucleotide pools, which are known to produce mutagenic events (80). In particular, folic acid–derived, one-carbon groups are required for synthesis of purines and the pyrimidine thymidylate. Deficiencies of folate and methionine in cultured rat splenic T-cells resulted in increased deoxythymidine pools and depleted deoxyguanosine triphosphate pools (81). These changes were associated with a decreased proportion of cells in the S phase of the cell cycle and an increase in cells in the

Table 81.1
Relative Risk (95% CIS) of Adenoma ≥1 cm of the Left Colon or Rectum by Combination of Alcohol, Methionine, and Folate Intake

	High-Alcohol[a] Low-Folate vs. Low-Alcohol High-Folate	High-Alcohol Low-Methionine vs. Low-Alcohol High-Methionine	Low-Folate-Low-Methionine vs. High-Folate High-Methionine
Total	1.99[b]	2.21[c]	2.39[c]
	(1.12–3.53)	(1.32–3.69)	(1.25–4.60)
Women	2.57[d]	2.17[b]	2.09[b]
	(1.31–5.06)	(1.18–3.98)	(1.04–4.18)
Men	1.16	2.50	5.72
	(0.39–3.43)	(0.93–6.71)	(0.85–38.3)

Data from Giovannucci E, Stampfer MJ, Colditz GA, et al. J Natl Cancer Inst 1993;85:875–84.
[a]High alcohol is defined as more than 20 g/day and low alcohol as less than 5 g/day; high and low folate are defined by high and low quintiles of intake. For women, median values are 0.9 g/day for low alcohol and 26.1 g/day for high alcohol; for men, 38.6 g/day for high alcohol and 1.8 g/day for low alcohol. Daily median energy-adjusted folate levels for women are 166 μg for the low category and 711 μg for the high category; for men, they are 241 μg and 847 μg. Daily median energy-adjusted methionine levels for women are 1.4 g for the low category and 2.5 g for the high category; for men, they are 1.6 g and 2.7 g.
[b]$0.01 < P \leq 0.05$.
[c]$0.001 < P \leq 0.05$.
[d]$0.0001 < P \leq 0.001$.

G_2/M phase (81). Studies in Chinese hamster ovary cells demonstrated similar imbalances that, under conditions of long-term culture, resulted in massive cell death and apoptosis (82). However, minor subpopulations in these cells adapted to the folate-deficient conditions and exhibited phenotypic, biochemical, and genetic abnormalities that gave them a growth advantage (82).

Studies with severe methyl deficiency in animal models (diet lacking choline, methionine, folic acid, and vitamin B_{12}) demonstrated hypomethylation of CCGG sites in genes involved in cell proliferation and cancer, such as c-*myc*, c-*fos*, and c-Ha-*ras* (83). Similarly, rats fed a diet deficient in methionine, choline, and folic acid for 9 weeks exhibited genomewide strand breaks, hypomethylation, and increased DNA methyltransferase activity (84). In exon 5 of the *p53* gene, strand breaks were associated with significant hypomethylation. Folate deficiency also potentiates the genetic damage by carcinogens, possibly by limiting DNA repair (85).

Choline deficiency appears to play a role beyond contributing methyl groups in the combined lipotrope deficiency (86). In particular, when a single nutrient deficiency is imposed, choline is the only lipotrope that induces cancer (76). Choline-deficiency cancer induction has been associated with induction of free radicals leading to necrosis and cancer (86). Furthermore, choline is required for a major membrane phospholipid, phosphatidylcholine (PC), and PC plays a role in cellular signaling as well as being a component of the membrane (87). Choline deficiency in rats was accompanied by a three- to five-fold increase in hepatic DAG in as short as 6 weeks of feeding (88). DAG is important in cellular signaling, as part of the activation of PKC (41). Rats fed choline-deficient diets had activated PKC, supporting the hypothesis that increases in hepatic DAG in choline deficiency activate PKC and contribute to increases in cell proliferation and hepatocellular carcinoma (89).

MICRONUTRIENTS

Dietary Iron and Neoplasia

Iron Overload As a Risk Factor for Cancer

Dietary iron is implicated in the pathogenesis of neoplasia in liver, lung, and colorectal tissues when cellular levels are excessively elevated. Iron overload, resulting from either excessive dietary intake or idiopathic hemochromatosis, is associated with increased risk for hepatocellular, gastric, and colorectal cancer (90). Site-specific associations between high iron stores and cancer risk have also been made for lung, esophageal, and bladder cancers (91, 92).

Southern Africa has the highest incidence of hepatocellular carcinoma in the world, with a reported incidence of 0.1% of the total population of Mozambique (93). By comparison, the incidence in the United States is approximately 0.004% (94). Although the high risk for hepatocellular cancer has been commonly linked to the high incidence of hepatitis B infection, Gangaidzo and Gordeuk (95) proposed that the similarity in pathology between dietary iron overload and idiopathic hemochromatosis suggests a strong correlation between excessive iron intake and hepatocellular cancer in the southern African population. They identified the source of dietary iron overload as consumption of a traditional home-brewed beer. However, beer consumption alone is not likely to result in toxic iron overload. Apparently, beer drinkers who also are genetically predisposed to iron overloading are at greatest risk (96).

Iron overload is also a factor in development of cirrhosis and may therefore be an indirect risk factor for hepatocellular cancer. Hepatocellular carcinoma is more likely to develop when cirrhosis is present, independent of iron status (97).

Iron and Cellular Proliferation

The role of iron in cellular proliferation and differentiation has been studied in normal and transformed lymphomyeloid cells and hepatocytes (98). In normal cells, iron uptake is stimulated by growth factors specific to the cell type. Iron is presented to cells in transferrin, the plasma transport protein, binds to cell-surface receptors, and is incorporated through endocytosis (see Chapter 10). Iron-free transferrin acts to inhibit proliferation. However, as transferrin becomes saturated with iron, proliferation increases (98). Transferrin saturation levels over 60% have been associated with significantly elevated risk for cancer (99).

In cell-cycle studies, cancer cells have been shown to require iron to maintain a proliferative state (100). Although they have greater numbers of transferrin receptors than normal cells, cancer cells have a lower iron content and do not accumulate iron in the presence of iron overload (101).

In vivo, iron also has a mitostimulatory effect. However, the role of iron in initiation and/or promotion in vivo is not known (105). An important step in the progress of hepatocytes from normal to neoplastic is development of cirrhosis. Whether iron is a singular factor in that process or enhances other hepatocarcinogens is not clear (102).

Iron accumulation in cells has been proposed to be genotoxic because of free radical damage to DNA and to be mitogenic, stimulating proliferation of preneoplastic cells (102). Iron removed from ferritin by ascorbate and other reducing agents forms a small pool of non-protein-bound iron that can move freely between transferrin, cytoplasm, mitochondria, and ferritin (103). This small pool of free iron is subject to reaction with H_2O_2 to produce hydroxyl radicals in the Fenton reaction (104). Hydroxyl radicals attack DNA and yield single-strand breaks or 8-hydroxyguanine mutations that give rise to base substitutions (102).

Although iron is required for cellular proliferation, its role as a mitogenic agent remains unclear. Experiments in human hepatoma cell systems have demonstrated that iron deprivation results in cell cycle arrest at G_2. However, whether these reactions also take place in vivo is not known.

Prevention and Therapy

Preventing iron overload in susceptible individuals is an important component of risk reduction for hepatic and other iron-associated cancers. Inclusion of dietary fiber that contains phytic acid suppresses iron absorption in rats and in humans (105). Phytic acid chelates polyvalent metals. Phytic acid included in the drinking water significantly reduced the incidence of intestinal tumors in rats treated with the chemical carcinogen azoxymethane (105).

Another method of depriving neoplastic cells of iron is to expose them to an antibody to the transferrin receptor. As the primary iron-transport protein, transferrin has a significant role in regulating iron availability to normal and neoplastic cells. In hematopoietic tumors, the combined effect of anti–transferrin receptor antibody and an iron chelating agent, such as deferoxamine, was even more efficacious in suppressing tumor growth in cultured lymphoid tumor cells (106).

Antioxidant Vitamins (A, E, and C) and Cancer

Vitamin Status Is Inversely Related to Risk for Cancer

An abundance of epidemiologic evidence exists to support or refute the antitumorigenic effects of retinol and related compounds. Most studies that support the antitumorigenicity of retinoids have found a correlation between low intake of vitamin A from fruits and vegetables or low levels of retinoids in serum or plasma and increased risk for certain cancers (107). On the other hand, studies that have tested the hypothesis that elevated levels of blood retinol decrease cancer risk have not been conclusive, in part because blood levels of retinol remain stable despite variations in intake, making it difficult to draw conclusions about possible protective effects of vitamin A based on such data. For example, studies of oral contraceptive (OCA) users, whose blood retinol levels were significantly higher than those of non-OCA users, failed to find convincing evidence for a reduced cancer risk due to the increased blood retinol levels (108). Studies of retinol intake may be further confounded by the fact that foods high in preformed vitamin A are also sources of animal fats, which may be a factor in tumor promotion (91). Additionally, food sources of carotenoids are also sources of other antioxidants, such as α-tocopherol and ascorbate, which have been shown to act cooperatively as inhibitors of tumorigenesis.

Epidemiologic evidence in support of an inhibitory role in tumorigenesis for α-tocopherol and ascorbate shows an inverse relationship between serum levels of ascorbate and α-tocopherol and risk for cancer (109). Byers et al. (110) examined a number of epidemiologic studies by cancer site and intake of vitamins E and C from dietary sources and found that the highest vitamin C intake from fruits and vegetables was correlated with the lowest risk for cancers of the gastrointestinal tract and lung. Studies of subjects taking vitamins E and C from oral supplements failed to show consistent correlations with decreased cancer risk from all sites. Furthermore, blood levels of these nutrients were not associated with cancer risk.

An inverse relationship between vitamin C intake and gastric cancer was found in the Seven Countries Study (111), in which 16 cohorts from seven different countries were compared for mortality from lung, stomach, and colorectal cancer and intake of antioxidant (pro)vitamins from dietary sources. However, this study failed to find a significant inverse relationship between vitamin C intake and lung or colorectal cancer.

Site specificity is an important consideration in determining whether a specific nutrient is an effective chemopreventive agent. In a review of epidemiologic studies on such chemopreventive agents, Bertram et al. (112) cited studies identifying associations between cancer site and specific nutrient. This review reported inverse associations between vitamin A and risk for oral, esophageal, bladder, reproductive, lung, and stomach cancers; vitamin C and risk for colon, esophageal, stomach, lung, and oral cancers; and vitamin E with risk for lung and breast cancers. However, many of the epidemiologic studies reviewed by Bertram et al. (112) assessed intake of the antioxidant vitamins from food sources. This type of evaluation does not consider potential interactions between the many nutritive and nonnutritive components of foods and thus cannot determine specific chemopreventive effects of these vitamins.

Experimental and Clinical Trials

Evidence supporting a role for vitamin A or carotene deficiency in enhancing carcinogenesis is more convincing than evidence supporting prevention by supplementation. Peto et al. (108) reported that low intake of β-carotene from fruits and vegetables predicted increased risk for lung cancer. The same conclusion was reached in another study involving male smokers who also regularly consumed alcohol (113). Individuals in this study who had lower than average intakes of β-carotene, vitamin C, and fiber had higher incidences of oral cancers than those whose intakes were above the mean.

More recently, a study was carried out in the Chinese county of Linxian, where consumption of β-carotene, α-tocopherol, and ascorbic acid in foods was low and the incidence of esophageal and gastric cardia cancer was high (114). Although blood levels of retinol, β-carotene, and other nutrients were low in this population, signs of deficiency were not present. Subjects in this study who were given supplements of β-carotene, vitamin E, and selenium, up to twice the recommended dietary allowance (RDA), had significantly lower mortality rates due to cancer than subjects who did not receive supplements; subjects given ascorbic acid and molybdenum had the same incidence of cancer as the controls.

In contrast to the large body of evidence supporting a chemopreventive role for β-carotene, the Alpha-tocopherol, Beta Carotene Cancer Prevention Study (ATBC) (115) conducted on male subjects in Finland suggested that β-carotene was ineffective or might even enhance risk for lung cancer in male smokers. The study provided β-carotene (and vitamin E) as supplements for 5 to 8 years. The subjects in this study differed, however, in being male smokers at increased risk for lung cancer. The results of the study in part supported the finding of the Linxian study, in that subjects with the lowest baseline levels of serum β-carotene had a greater incidence of cancer than those with higher levels. However, this study found that subjects who took β-carotene supplements had an 18% greater incidence of lung cancer than those who did not. Subjects supplemented with α-tocopherol showed no difference in incidence of lung cancer from unsupplemented controls (Fig. 81.5). The level of β-carotene supplementation in the ATBC study was more than three times the level in the Linxian study. However, finding an association between increased incidence of cancer and increased intake of β-carotene does not necessarily suggest a role for this nutrient in development of lung cancer, because of the long latency period (10–30 years) from initiation to diagnosis of cancer.

In a similar study, CARET, subjects received a daily supplement of 30 mg β-carotene and 25,000 IU retinyl palmitate. Initial results of the trial showed a 28% increased incidence of lung cancer in patients receiving supplements compared with controls. The increase in lung cancer and an increase in mortality among the supplemented subjects resulted in termination of the trial before the scheduled completion date in 1997. The similarity in results from the ATBC and the CARET trials exemplify the need for further evaluation of the role of carotenoids in lung cancer in populations at risk, i.e., smokers and individuals exposed to carcinogenic agents such as asbestos.

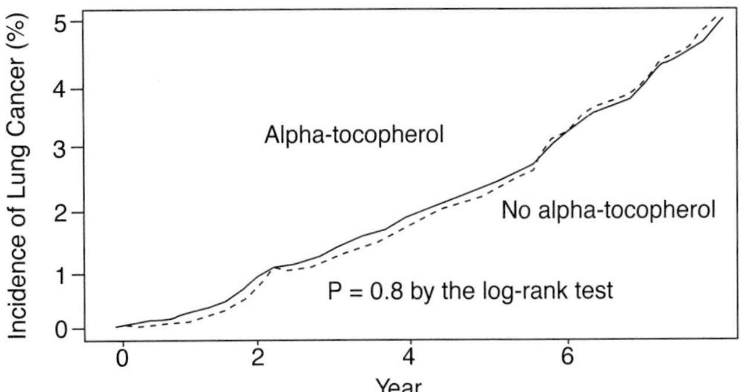

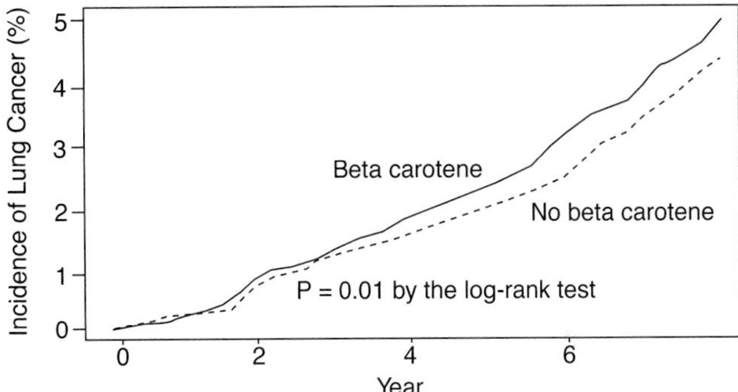

Figure 81.5. Kaplan-Meier curves for the cumulative incidence of lung cancer among participants who received α-tocopherol supplements and those who did not *(upper panel)* and among participants who received β-carotene supplements and those who did not *(lower panel)*. Data are shown only through 7½ years of follow-up because of the small numbers of participants beyond that time. Reprinted by permission of The New England Journal of Medicine. (From The Alpha-Tocopheral, Beta Carotene Cancer Prevention Study Group. N Engl J Med 1994;330(15):1029–1035, with permission.)

Other carotenoids, in particular α-carotene, may be more effective chemopreventive agents than β-carotene. Murakoshi et al. (117) studied the inhibitory effect of α- and β-carotene alone and mixed carotenoids in palm oil on both spontaneous and induced tumorigenesis. These experiments were carried out in mice that consumed the carotenoids through their drinking water. The fewest tumors in liver, lung, and skin occurred in the mice who received mixed carotenoids, followed by the α- and β-carotenoid groups, respectively. A similar study (118) also determined that mixed carotenoids were the most effective in inhibiting induced skin, lung, and liver tumorigenesis and that α-carotene was more effective than β-carotene in inhibiting tumorigenesis. Taken together, these studies suggest that dietary sources of carotenoids are more effective than supplementation with individual carotenoids and that there may be a cooperative or synergistic effect between carotenoids to achieve tumor inhibition.

The mechanism(s) through which vitamin A derivatives, particularly the carotenoids, vitamin C, and vitamin E inhibit tumorigenesis has not been elucidated. Wattenberg (119) proposed three levels at which chemopreventive agents could act: *(a)* as inhibitors of carcinogenic precursors, *(b)* as blocking agents preventing carcinogens from acting at a target site, and *(c)* as suppressing agents that diminish the effect of a carcinogen already present (Fig. 81.6).

A number of in vitro studies support the hypothesis that retinoids and carotenoids function as antioxidants in the promotional phase of carcinogenesis (120, 121). The antioxidant activity of carotenoids has been demonstrated in vivo by inhibition of lipid peroxidation (122).

The findings of a human study appear to support the inhibition of lipid peroxidation by carotenoids (123). In this study, volunteers were initially depleted of β-carotene, which significantly decreased their serum carotene levels. After 2 weeks, lipid peroxide measures were significantly decreased after supplementation, compared with peroxide levels in depleted subjects before supplementation. Serum β-carotene levels in the supplemented groups were twice the baseline levels. However, since the subjects were depleted of β-carotene prior to supplementation, it is difficult to determine if the response was due to the increased serum concentration of β-carotene or to repletion from a deficient state.

As with the carotenoids, vitamin C status has been found to be inversely related to risk for certain cancers, and experiments testing inhibition of tumorigenesis with supplementary vitamin C have shown mixed results (124). In clinical trials testing tumor recurrence in the presence and absence of supplemental vitamin C, no change in the incidence of tumor recurrence was found between the

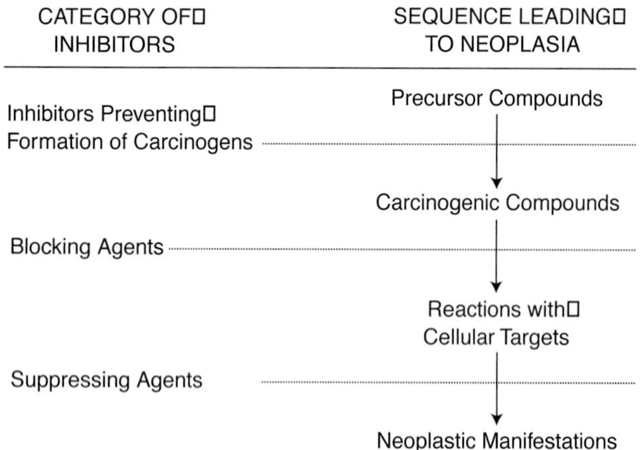

Figure 81.6. Classification of chemopreventive agents on the basis of the time at which they exert their protective effects. (From Wattenberg LW, Cancer Res 1985;45:1–8, with permission.)

supplemented group and controls. However, when cellular proliferation assays were done with tissue samples, the vitamin C–supplemented subjects had significantly less proliferation in colonic crypts (125). A similar study, in which subjects received a combination of retinol and vitamins E and C, also found significantly less proliferation in the supplemented group than in controls (126).

The role of ascorbic acid and α-tocopherol as inhibitors of tumorigenesis is similar to that of retinoids and carotenoids in that they share antioxidant properties (127). Additionally, in vitro, both ascorbic acid and α-tocopherol act as inhibitors at initiation by scavenging mutagens such as free radicals and by preventing formation of nitroso compounds (128). Nitrosamines are strongly implicated in the pathogenesis of gastric cancer, and thus ascorbic acid may be an important chemopreventive agent in this disease process (112). These and other studies further suggest that antioxidant vitamins are most effective in combination rather than as isolated supplements (115).

Prevention and Therapy

An important aspect of retinol as a chemopreventive agent is its toxicity in humans. Although a number of in vitro studies using retinol have shown inhibition of oncogene expression and decreased damage to DNA (97, 129), preformed vitamin A cannot be considered a supplemental chemopreventive vitamin at therapeutic doses. Supplementation may, however, be a factor in preventing esophageal-gastric carcinomas in a population that is deficient in vitamin A (130).

As an alternative to vitamin A supplementation, retinoid analogues have been studied as potential chemopreventive agents. Hong et al. (131) showed that the analogue 13-*cis*-retinoic acid effectively suppressed further development of premalignant lesions of the oral cavity and also reduced the incidence of second primary tumors in patients with squamous-cell carcinomas of the head and neck. However, primary tumor recurrence was not suppressed by the retinoid analogue (132).

Selenium and Cancer

Epidemiology of Selenium and Cancer Risk

Associations between selenium and cancer have been studied for more than 25 years. However, the findings of these studies remain controversial and contradictory. Correlations between selenium status and tumorigenesis are derived from studies demonstrating an increase in cancer risk with decreased blood, tissue, or intake levels of this micronutrient (133).

Early studies examined correlations between geographic regions with high forage plant–selenium levels and incidences of cancer. Clark (reviewed in [137]) reported from studies by Shamberger et al. and Kuboto that areas of high forage selenium were inversely related to incidences of lung, colon, rectal, bladder, esophageal, and pancreatic cancer and positively related to liver and stomach cancer, Hodgkin's lymphoma, and leukemia. In a subsequent study, Clark et al. (134) assessed the association of cancer mortality incidence and forage selenium in smaller geographic segments, by county rather than by state or nation. This study also found an inverse correlation between forage selenium level and cancer mortality. More recently, however, the work of Nakadaira et al. (135) on soil selenium concentrations and cancer mortality failed to find any correlation. Vinceti et al. (136) also failed to find a correlation between levels of naturally occurring selenium in the drinking water and mortality from various cancers, except that a positive correlation was found in females between selenium and cancers of lymphatic and hematopoietic tissues, including non-Hodgkin's lymphoma.

Although forage selenium reflects exposure to this micronutrient within a geographic region, intake levels of selenium may vary because of consumption of foods transported from other geographic areas. Alternatively, tissue indicators of selenium status have been used, including urine, blood, or serum measures and selenium levels in hair and nails. However, blood selenium level may not be an accurate measure of selenium status as the plasma pool shifts with short-term changes in intake. Furthermore, selenium status changes in individuals with cancer, because of such factors as chemotherapy, radiotherapy, and stage of disease (133).

Clark et al. (137) examined plasma selenium levels in subjects with basal cell and squamous cell carcinomas. These skin cancers were chosen for study because of the low ratio of tumor mass to normal tissue and the decreased likelihood of influencing metabolic parameters, such as selenium level.

Another important consideration in determination of biologic/anticarcinogenic activity of selenium is its chemical form. Although the predominant form of selenium in the human diet is selenomethionine ([Se]Met), other forms, particularly selenite, have greater anticarcinogenic activity (142).

Selenite or [Se]Met enter the selenium metabolic pathway, where the initial compound is converted to methylated products or incorporated into selenoamino acids (see Chapter 14) (143). The methylated selenium products, particularly the monomethylated species, are proposed to have the greatest anticarcinogenic potential (149). Furthermore, the form of selenium, i.e., selenite, initially entering the metabolic pathway appears to determine the anticarcinogenic efficacy (145).

To be activated for anticarcinogenic potential, selenium compounds first go through the methylation pathway (146). Hydrogen selenide, an important intermediate in the pathway, can enter the assimilatory pathway and generate selenoproteins, such as glutathione peroxidase, or it can enter the detoxification pathway and undergo methylation.

In addition to the forms of selenium mentioned, other analogues, such as selenobetaine and se-methylselenocysteine, have been tested for anticarcinogenic potential (143). Both of these forms of selenium are metabolized to monomethylated selenide. However, the yield is much greater than from selenomethionine or selenite (143). Animal studies have shown that the partially methylated species have greater efficacy as antitumorigenic agents than the fully methylated species (143).

Aside from a role in inhibiting free radical formation, selenium compounds also induce programed cell death, or apoptosis, in cultured cells (147). The ability of cells to program their own death provides a mechanism to control mutations.

Clinical Trials of the Efficacy of Selenium in Cancer Inhibition

Clinical trials testing the anticarcinogenic effects of selenium obtained from foods or supplements have been carried out in areas of the world where nutrient deprivation is common, as in parts of China and India. Linxian, China, has been studied because it is part of a large region of high cancer mortality as well as micronutrient deficiency (130). Blot et al. (114) conducted supplementation trials that included combinations of micronutrients. Although neither of these studies evaluated the chemopreventive activity of selenium alone, both studies did find that selenium in combination with other nutrients, particularly vitamins A and E, had an inhibitory effect on esophageal and stomach cancers (reviewed in [118, 134]).

Prasad et al. (148) studied the inhibitory effects of a micronutrient cocktail of vitamin A, riboflavin, zinc, and selenium on tumorigenesis in tobacco chewers and smokers in India. The population chosen has a high incidence of both oral and upper airway cancers and of micronutrient deficiencies (149). Dietary assessment of study participants revealed that blood levels of micronutrients were similar, low-normal or deficient in all subjects (150). At the completion of the 1-year study, significantly fewer in the supplemented group developed oral lesions or ulcers than in the placebo group. Furthermore, of those subjects who had lesions initially, significantly fewer receiving the supplements regressed to more serious cancers. Biochemical assessment of study participants showed that formation of DNA adducts, an indicator of carcinogenicity, was significantly lower in the supplemented subjects than in those receiving placebo (150).

These trials among population groups at risk for micronutrient deficiencies suggest that supplementation with selenium (and other micronutrients) reduces the carcinogenic potential of other cancer-causing factors. Among a nutritionally healthy population, however, such a chemopreventive effect is not as clearly seen.

Inhibition of Carcinogenesis by Selenium in Animal Models

Inorganic selenium compounds, such as sodium selenite, inhibit tumorigenesis in laboratory animal models.

These models have been used to demonstrate selenium inhibition of many types of cancer, including liver, skin, pancreas, mammary gland, and colon (151). Experiments in rats demonstrated that dietary selenium, in the form of sodium selenite in drinking water, inhibited formation of DMBA-DNA adducts and decreased the incidence of mammary tumors (152). In hamsters, sodium selenite inhibited *N*-nitrosobis(2-oxopropyl)amine (BOP)-induced pancreatic cancer, in a dose-dependent fashion (153). Decreased carcinogen-induced damage to DNA supports a role for selenium inhibition of cancer at the stage of initiation, and increased latency to tumor development suggests inhibition of tumor promotion. However, earlier studies by Birt et al. (152) found that dietary supplementation with sodium selenite and D,L-selenomethionine (153) had no inhibitory effect on pancreatic tumors in BOP-treated male hamsters or enhanced pancreatic carcinogenesis in BOP-treated male hamsters fed high-fat diets (153).

Recently developed compounds, such as 1,4-phenylene-bis(methylene)selenocyante or xylene selenocyanate (p-XSC), have been found to be more efficacious inhibitors of mammary and colon carcinogenesis (154). This modified form of selenium has an LD_{50} greater than 1 g/kg body weight, compared with an LD_{50} of 35 mg/kg for sodium selenite and 125 mg/kg for benzyl selenocyanate (BSC) (155). Furthermore, when administered during initiation, p-XSC inhibited tumor formation by 80% (155). Although the inorganic selenocyante compounds have been shown to be effective inhibitors of tumorigenesis in animal models, they are not yet applicable to humans.

Selenium in Chemoprevention and Therapy

Selenium enrichment of foods has shown promise as a means of increasing selenium intake and decreasing tumor incidence in animal models (156). The similarity between sulfur and selenium metabolism in plants has been exploited to increase the selenium content of foods rich in sulfur compounds (157). Garlic, an ideal candidate for selenium enrichment, demonstrated inhibition of mammary tumorigenesis in rat experiments. Ip et al. (158) fed freeze-dried powdered garlic, grown in normal soil or grown in selenium-enriched soil, to rats during DMBA initiation or through initiation and postinitiation until the end of the experiment. The total number of mammary tumors that developed were compared among rats fed regular garlic, selenium-enriched garlic, and supplemented with inorganic selenium compounds. Tumor inhibition was achieved in all three groups, but the rats fed selenium-enriched garlic had 69% inhibition compared with controls whereas the group fed regular garlic had 40% inhibition.

The advantage of dietary intake of selenium-enriched garlic, in addition to the increased tumor inhibition, was that tissue selenium levels were not elevated to the near-toxic levels seen with inorganic selenium compounds. Also, glutathione peroxidase activity was not perturbed by selenium-enriched foods (157). While selenium enrichment of garlic and other foods may be a practical means of providing this chemopreventive agent at nontoxic levels, further research is needed to determine efficacy and feasibility in humans.

NONNUTRIENT DIETARY COMPONENTS

Flavonoids

Occurrence and Intake

Flavonoids are widely distributed in fruits and vegetables. They are composed of a number of related compounds with the general structure shown in Figure 81.7. It is estimated that we consume approximately 1 g of flavonoids daily, and the bulk of these compounds are in our diets as glycosides (159). Recent studies assessed the intake of particular flavonoids in the Netherlands, and an estimated daily consumption of 16 mg/day was made for quercetin (160, 161). However, the analysis of foods for these compounds is problematic, and estimates should be considered tentative. As indicated below, many of the biologic effects are associated more with the free aglycone that is released in the intestine than with the compound bound in the glycoside.

Mutagenicity Studies

Quercetin is the most extensively studied dietary flavonoid. Quercetin is a widely distributed flavonol that was initially studied for potential carcinogenicity because it functions as a frame-shift mutagen (162). Mutagenicity in a number of Ames strains was shown to require the 3′ and 4′ hydroxyls of quercetin and rhamnetin (163). Parallel studies with quercetin, rhamnetin, isohamnetin, apigenin, and luteolin isolated from medicinal herbs provided no evidence of mutagenicity for apigenin and luteolin (163). A number of studies reported inhibition of mutagenicity by a variety of flavonoids. In a study of 64 flavonoids for mutagenicity against the heterocyclic amines, Edenharder et al. (164) found that a carbonyl function at C-4 of the flavone nucleus was essential for antimutagenicity. Furthermore, increasing polarity by

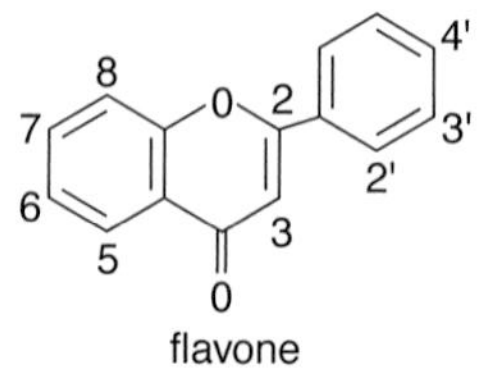

Common Name	Substituents 3	4	5	7	3′	5′
Acacetin	H	H	OH	OH	H	OCH_3
Apigenin	H	H	OH	OH	H	OH
Chrysin	H	H	OH	OH	H	H
Kaempferol	OH	H	OH	OH	H	OH
Quercetin	OH	H	OH	OH	OH	OH

Figure 81.7.

addition of hydroxyl groups reduced antimutagenicity, and 6-hydroxy- and 2′-hydroxy-substituted flavonoids were considerably less potent antimutagens. Apigenin treatment resulted in potent antimutagenesis compared with other phytochemicals when tested against nitropyrenes in *Salmonella* strains and in Chinese hamster ovary cells (165). In addition, apigenin inhibited mutagenicity induced by benzo[*a*]pyrene and 2-aminoanthracene induced in the Ames assay with TA98 bacteria (166).

Laboratory Studies

More-recent studies have focused on the ability of quercetin to prevent carcinogenesis (162). Quercetin was effective in prevention of skin carcinogenesis in the two-stage model of DMBA-initiated and TPA-promoted cancer (167). In addition, quercetin inhibited azooxymethanol (AOM)-induced aberrant crypt foci (ACF) (168, 169). Similar observations were reported for liquritin, a glucosylated flavonoid (170). Quercetin and rutin, a common dietary source of quercetin, were not equally effective in prevention of colon carcinogenesis (168). Incorporation of 2% dietary quercetin decreased the incidence of colon cancer in AOM-treated rats from 25 to 6% ($P < 0.003$), while 4% dietary rutin (roughly equivalent to the amount of quercetin in the 2% diet) decreased colon cancer incidence to 10% (not significant) in the same study. Later studies from the same laboratory demonstrated inhibition of AOM-induced ACF in mice fed high-fat diets with quercetin but not with rutin (169). Furthermore, rutin was not effective in another laboratory in inhibition of ACF (171).

Four citrus flavonoids (quercetin, taxifolin, nobiletin, and tangeretin) were studied in the in vitro growth of human squamous cell carcinoma cells, HTB43 (172). Nobiletin and tangeretin, hydroxymethylated flavonoids, markedly inhibited the growth of cells at doses from 2 to 8 μg/mL; quercetin and taxifolin were ineffective.

Studies have explored skin cancer prevention by flavonoids. Research in the Birt laboratory has focused on apigenin (4′,5,7,-trihydroxyflavone), a widely distributed flavone. Apigenin inhibited both ultraviolet light–induced and DMBA- and TPA-induced skin carcinogenesis (166, 173, 174) (Fig. 81.8). In initial studies, apigenin inhibited ornithine decarboxylase activity induced by the tumor promoter TPA or by the complete carcinogen UV light in a dose-responsive manner (166, 174).

Flavonoids have recently been demonstrated to be effective in prevention of cellular proliferation and carcinogenesis in a number of other models. For example, bioflavonoids inhibited lymphocyte proliferation induced by con A or LPS in studies by Lee et al. (175).

Mechanism of Action

Protein Phosphorylation. Numerous mechanisms have been suggested for flavonoid inhibition of carcinogenesis. Some of these may relate to the inhibition of cell cycle as discussed below, while others may be independent effects that interact with inhibition of cell cycle in the prevention of cancer. Several laboratories have associated changes in protein phosphorylation of cancer cell lines with growth inhibition by flavonoids. For example, apigenin, kampherol, and genistein (25 μM) reversed the transformed phenotype of v-H-*ras*-transformed NIH3T3 cells (176). Twelve other flavonoids were not effective. The observed reversion was associated with reduced phosphotyrosine content in the cells (176), and recent work from this group suggested that apigenin could inhibit mitogen-activated protein kinase (MAPK) (177). This inhibition was associated with reductions in c-*jun* and c-*fos* expression, but mRNA expression and protein level of *ras* were not influenced.

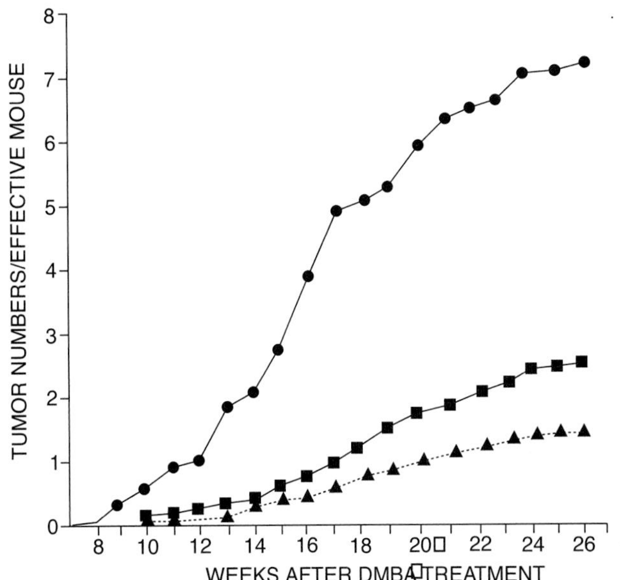

Figure 81.8. Skin papilloma multiplicity in apigenin-treated and control groups. *(circles)*, 7,12-Dimethylbenz[*a*]anthracene (DMBA)/dimethylsulfoxide (DMSO)/12-0-tetradecanoylphorbol-13-acetate(TPA); *(squares)*, DMBA/5 μmol apigenin/TPA; *(triangles)*, DMBA/20 μmol apigenin/TPA. Average papilloma number of DMBA/DMSO/TPA is significantly higher than that of two apigenin-treated groups ($P < 0.001$), while there is no significant difference between two apigenin-treated groups by Student's *t* test. (From Wei H, Tye L, Bresnick E, et al. Cancer Res 1990;50:499–502, with permission.)

Topoisomerase Inhibition. A number of flavonoids are topoisomerase antagonists; myricetin, quercetin, fisetin, and morin inhibited both Topo I and Topo II, while phoretin, kaempherol, and 4′,6,7-trihydroxyisoflavone inhibited only Topo I. Apigenin, prunetin, quercetin, and kaempferol stabilized the Topo II DNA complex (178). In addition, apigenin and tangeretin enhanced gap junctional intracellular communication in rat liver epithelial cells. Increased dye transfer was associated with increases in connexin 43 protein (179).

Antioxidant and Antiinflammation Activity. Flavonoids have also demonstrated antioxidant and antiinflammation properties. Thirty-five phenolic compounds, primarily flavonoids, were studied for their ability to prevent carbon tetrachloride lipid peroxidation of rat liver microsomes (180), and a number of flavones, flavonols, and related compounds were active. Furthermore, apigenin-7-glucoside was effective in prevention of skin inflammation induced by a number of generators of reactive oxygen species (181). In studies of 24 flavonoids, Tordera et al. (182) found a number of compounds to be effective in inhibiting β-glucuronidase activity, lysosome release, and arachidonic acid release from membranes.

Cell Cycle Arrest. Matsukawa et al. reported that a number of flavonoids, flavone, quercetin, and luteolin, arrested cells at G_2/M or G_1 (183). Flow-cytometric analysis showed that the flavonoids and daidzen induced cell cycle arrest at G_1, but genistein almost completely arrested the cell cycle progression at G_2/M. Cell cycle arrest by genistein was reversed in HGC-27 gastric cancer cells when genistein was removed from the culture medium. Quercetin inhibited the cell cycle at late G_1 in human leukemic T cells (184). Human colon cancer cells were also arrested in late G_1 (COLO320) (185), and the arrest was associated with inhibition of a cell cycle–related 17-kDa protein (1985). Another laboratory reported that apigenin induces G_2/M arrest in rat neuronal cells (186). Lepley et al. (187) demonstrated that apigenin arrests human promylocytic leukemia cells and murine keratinocytes at G_2/M and that this effect is reversible. In the apigenin-treated keratinocytes, inhibition of $P34^{cdc2}$ kinase and reduction in the cyclin B protein, the cyclin associated with $P34^{cdc2}$ kinase, was noted. In studies with immunoprecipitated $P34^{cdc2}$ kinase, quercetin and genistein were reported to inhibit this kinase (188).

Wei et al. recently reported induction of apoptosis by quercetin in several tumor cell lines (K562, Molt-4, Raji, and MCAS), resulting in nuclear fragmentation, condensation of nuclear chromatin, and a subdiploid peak by DNA flow cytometry (189).

Absorption and Metabolism of Flavonoids

The literature has little information on the absorption and metabolism of flavonoids. Recent reports demonstrated good absorption of quercetin in female ileostomy patients (190). Absorption was estimated from oral intake minus ileostomy excretion, with correction for 14% degradation in the ileostomy bag. Estimated quercetin absorption from quercetin glycosides in onions was 52 ± 15%, absorption from quercetin rutinoside (the common form in tea) was 17 ± 15%, and absorption from quercetin aglycone was 24 ± 9% (190). Regarding the importance of flavonoid metabolism in cancer prevention, apigenin inhibition of skin carcinogenesis and cell cycle arrest do not appear to require apigenin metabolism (191). No evidence was found of apigenin metabolism in mouse skin, tissue culture systems, or cultured epidermal (C50) cells under conditions in which apigenin has been demonstrated to inhibit skin carcinogenesis in the intact animal or to cause cell cycle arrest in cultured cells (187, 191).

Isoflavonoids

Epidemiologic and Clinical Studies

Several epidemiologic studies indirectly suggest that consumption of dietary isoflavones may lend protection against certain cancers. Although these epidemiologic studies alone are not conclusive, they are supported by numerous laboratory studies indicating that isoflavones exhibit a large number of diverse biologic effects, both in vivo and in vitro, that may be associated with anticancer activities. Consequently, isoflavones receive much attention as possible cancer prevention agents.

Breast Cancer. Perhaps the strongest evidence suggesting that isoflavones possess anticancer activities in humans stems from studies demonstrating an inverse correlation between consumption of soy-derived products, known to contain substantial amounts of isoflavones, and risk of developing breast cancer (reviewed in [192, 193]). Nomura et al. (194) evaluated the association between the dietary practices of 6860 Hawaiian men of Japanese ancestry, who were participants in the Honolulu Heart Study, and breast cancer in their spouses, under the assumption that husbands and wives consume similar diets. The husbands of women with breast cancer consumed significantly less Japanese miso (fermented soybean paste) soup than husbands of women without breast cancer. Although the breast cancer group also consumed 22% less tofu (soy bean curd) than the control group, the difference was not statistically significant. Interpretation of these data was confounded by the observation that the husbands of women with breast cancer consumed significantly more beef and wieners than the control group. In a prospective study of 142,857 Japanese women, Hirayama (195) demonstrated a significant inverse correlation between consumption of soybean paste soup and breast cancer risk. An inverse correlation between breast cancer risk and consumption of soy protein as well as total soy products was observed by Lee et al. (196) in a study of premenopausal Singapore Chinese women.

Prostate Cancer. The incidence of prostate cancers in North America and western Europe is much greater than in Asian populations. Because of this, it is often suggested that consumption of a diet high in soy provides protection against prostate cancer. However, two large prospective studies failed to reveal such an effect (197, 198).

Laboratory Studies

Several animal studies suggest that isoflavones possess anticarcinogenic properties. Some of these studies evaluated the effects of dietary soy on experimental carcinogenesis (192), whereas others evaluated specific isoflavones for their anticarcinogenic activities.

Experimental Mammary Cancer. Barnes et al. (199) demonstrated that consumption of diets containing either powdered soybean chips or isolated soy protein inhibited development of mammary tumors in female Sprague-Dawley rats treated with either *N*-methyl-*N'*-nitrosourea (MNU) or DMBA (Fig. 81.9). In this study, inhibition of mammary tumorigenesis was revealed by both a decreased tumor burden and an increased latency. Cooking the soybean chips did not eliminate their antitumorigenic activity, suggesting that isoflavones or other heat-stable components, not heat-labile proteinase inhibitors, may have been the active soy constituent. In a subsequent study, these investigators demonstrated that consumption of soy protein isolate, but not an alcohol-extracted soy protein isolate, inhibited DMBA-induced mammary carcinogenesis in the female Sprague-Dawley rat (200). These data again suggest that isoflavones, which are alcohol-soluble and therefore extracted from the protein isolate, contain the antitumorigenic activity in the soy diet.

An antitumorigenic effect of soy protein isolate was also observed by Hawrylewicz et al. (201), who initiated mammary tumorigenesis with MNU and began feeding the soy diet 5 weeks thereafter. Their data indicate that soy protein isolate exerts its inhibitory effect during the promotion and/or progression phases of mammary tumorigenesis. Baggott et al. (202) demonstrated that miso consumption protected against DMBA-induced mammary adenocarcinomas in the Sprague-Dawley rat. Although cancer incidence was reduced and latency was increased by miso consumption, this protective effect was not attributed to consumption of soy-derived isoflavones. In contrast to the studies of Barnes and Hawrylewicz, Carroll (203) reported similar mammary tumor yields following DMBA treatment of female Sprague-Dawley rats fed diets in which the protein was derived from either casein or soy. The reason for these disparate observations is not clear. In summary, several studies suggest soy-containing diets may suppress chemically induced mammary cancers in the female rat. However, without additional evidence, the antitumorigenic activity in the different soy-containing diets cannot be attributed to isoflavones.

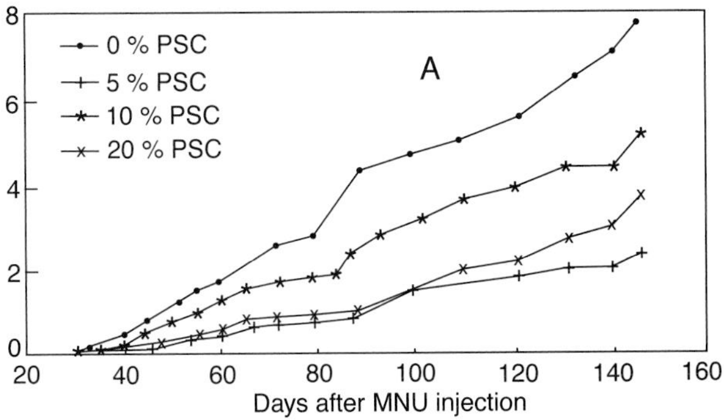

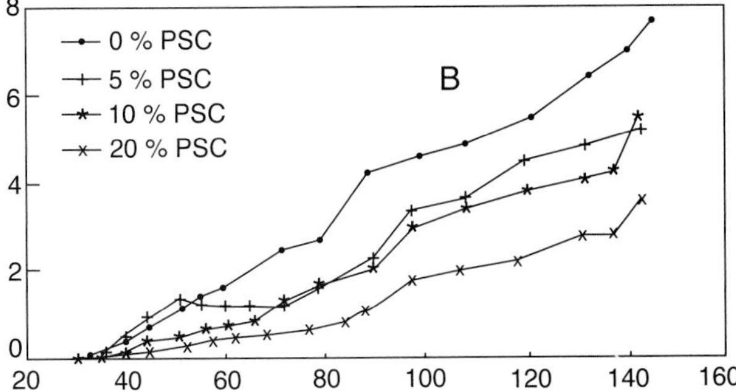

Figure 81.9. Inhibition of mammary tumors induced by MNU in rats by addition of nonautoclaved (**A**) and autoclaved (**B**) powdered soybean chips (PSC) to AIN-76A diet. (From Barnes S, Grubbs C, Setchell KDR, et al. Prog Clin Biol Res 1990;347:239–53, with permission.)

Genistein administered by subcutaneous injection to neonatal female Sprague-Dawley rats inhibited development of mammary tumors following subsequent treatment with DMBA at 50 days of age (204). Genistein treatment also altered the course of mammary gland development, leading to increased lobuloalveolar structures and decreased terminal end buds at the time of DMBA treatment. Because terminal end buds are highly susceptible to chemically induced tumorigenesis (205), it was suggested that induction of differentiation of end buds to lobules is the probable mechanism of genistein inhibition of mammary tumorigenesis in the DMBA-treated rat.

Formononetin was shown to stimulate mammary cell proliferation in ovariectomized mice (206). In this study, formononetin, administered for 5 days by subcutaneous injection at a dose of 40 mg/kg, stimulated mammary cell proliferation 3.3-fold, increased the level of estrogen receptor in the mammary tissues 2-fold, and increased the level of circulating prolactin 1.7-fold. Although these data strongly suggest that formononetin exerts weak estrogenic activity in the mouse mammary and anterior pituitary tissues, the relevance of this estrogenic activity to mammary cancer development and chemoprevention remains to be assessed.

Isoflavones inhibit proliferation of a number of human breast cancer cell lines. Peterson and Barnes (207) demonstrated that genistein, daidzein, and biochanin A each inhibit proliferation of the breast cancer cell lines MCF-7 and MDA-468, with IC_{50} values of 39, 74, and 110 μM, respectively. Because similar IC_{50} values for each of these isoflavones were observed in MCF-7 cells, which are estrogen-receptor positive, and MDA-468 cells, which do not express estrogen receptor, it was concluded that the inhibitory effects of these isoflavones on cell proliferation, at least in MDA-468 cells, are not mediated through the estrogen receptor. When treated with genistein at a concentration of 10 μM, MCF-7 cells were reversibly arrested at the G_2/M cell cycle boundary; at concentrations of 50 μM, G_2/M arrest was not reversible, and cells underwent apoptosis (208). Kievitone, an isoflavonoid from red kidney beans, is a potent inhibitor of basal and growth factor–stimulated proliferation of the estrogen receptor–positive MCF-7 and T47D breast cancer cell lines, and the estrogen receptor–negative SKBR3 breast cancer cell line (209). At this time, the molecular mechanism of isoflavone inhibition of breast cancer cell proliferation in culture is not fully elucidated. Also not clear is whether isoflavones can exert selective inhibitory effects on breast cancer cell proliferation in vivo.

Other studies have revealed stimulatory effects of isoflavones on breast cancer cell proliferation. Welshons et al. (210) established and validated a highly sensitive assay for evaluating the phytoestrogen content of animal feeds. Using this assay, it was demonstrated that the isoflavones genistein, biochanin A, daidzein, and formononetin stimulate MCF-7 cell proliferation with potencies ranging from 3 to 5 orders of magnitude less than that of 17β-estradiol. The ability of each of these isoflavones to stimulate MCF-7 cell proliferation was correlated with their binding affinities for the estrogen receptor. Moreover, the antiestrogens tamoxifen or LY156758 blocked induction of MCF-7 cell proliferation by each of these isoflavones, indicating that their effects on proliferation were mediated through the estrogen receptor. Stimulatory effects of genistein and biochanin A on MCF-7 cell proliferation have recently been reported by a second group (211), but no antiestrogenic activities of isoflavones were observed in this study. Sathyamoorthy et al. (212) observed that equol and daidzein added to estrogen-depleted culture media to a concentration of 1 μM stimulate MCF-7 cell proliferation. From these studies, it would appear that at physiologically relevant concentrations, isoflavones display estrogenic, not antiestrogenic, activities in cultured breast cancer cell lines.

Experimental Prostate Cancer. Genistein has been demonstrated to inhibit, in a concentration-dependent manner, proliferation of both human (PC-3) and rat (Dunning R-3327-MAT-LyLu) prostate cancer cell lines. However, when administered by either addition to the drinking water or intraperitoneal injection, genistein failed to inhibit growth of MAT-LyLu rat prostate cancer cells maintained as subcutaneous transplants in male Copenhagen rats (213). A probable explanation for the observed inability of genistein to inhibit prostate cancer cell proliferation in vivo is that the micromolar concentrations of the isoflavone required for inhibition of proliferation were not achieved within the transplanted tumor cells.

Mechanisms of Action

Estrogenic and Antiestrogenic Activities. *Interaction of Isoflavones with the Estrogen Receptor.* Probably the first indication that isoflavones interact with the estrogen receptor was the observation that genistein inhibited, in a dose-dependent manner, the uptake of 17β-estradiol by the uterus and vagina of the immature mouse (214). Shutt and Cox (215) demonstrated that genistein, equol, daidzein, *O*-desmethylangolensin, biochanin A, and formononetin each inhibit binding of 17β-estradiol to estrogen receptor in cytosol prepared from sheep uterus. Experiments in which a plasmid encoding the human estrogen receptor and a plasmid containing an estrogen-regulated promoter/reporter gene construct (pERE/TK/CAT) are transfected into HeLa cells indicate that genistein, biochanin A, daidzein, and formononetin each act through the estrogen receptor to enhance expression of the reporter gene (216). Genistein and biochanin A behaved as full agonists in this experimental system, whereas daidzein and formononetin behaved as partial agonists. Together, these data strongly suggest that several isoflavones bind to the estrogen receptor and display agonistic activity.

Estrogen-Related Biologic Activities in Humans. It has recently been demonstrated that consumption of a diet containing soy protein and associated isoflavones modulates the menstrual cycle in young women (217). In a dietary intervention study, six young women were monitored over several consecutive menstrual cycles, initially while consuming a control diet and subsequently while consuming a diet that incorporated 60 g/day soy protein containing 45 mg of isoflavones. Consumption of the soy diet resulted in a 1000-fold increase in urinary excretion of isoflavones, primarily daidzein, genistein, and equol, and a significant lengthening of the menstrual cycles due to an extended follicular phase. The midcycle surges of luteinizing hormone and follicle-stimulating hormone were significantly diminished by the soy diet, but no effect on circulating sex hormone–binding globulin (SHBG) levels was observed. These data strongly suggest that dietary isoflavones exert physiologic effects in premenopausal women, possibly because of actions mediated through the estrogen receptor. Because the highest level of mammary epithelial cell proliferation occurs during the luteal phase of the menstrual cycle, it has often been suggested that prolongation of the follicular phase of the cycle would reduce the number of total cycles a woman would display in her lifetime and might thereby provide protection against development of breast cancer.

Incorporation of soy flour into the diets of 23 postmenopausal women markedly increased urinary excretion of the isoflavones daidzein and equol and significantly lessened menopause-associated symptoms, including hot flushes, when these symptoms were evaluated 6 and 12 weeks after initiation of the dietary intervention (218). No effects of soy flour consumption on vaginal cytology or circulating follicle-stimulating hormone (both regulated by estrogens) were observed in that study. Consequently, it is not clear that the reported relief of menopause symptoms was due to estrogenic activities of the soy-derived isoflavones. Another recently published dietary intervention study failed to demonstrate that consumption of a diet high in soy modulated any of four estrogen-regulated parameters in postmenopausal women (219). In this study, 91 postmenopausal women consumed for 4 weeks either a "normal" omnivorous diet (25 women) or a diet in which soy products accounted for approximately one-third of caloric intake (66 women). Although the women consuming the soy-based diet ingested substantially more isoflavones, as evidenced by a greater than 100-fold increase in urinary excretion of the isoflavones daidzein, genistein, and equol, no statistically significant changes in the levels of circulating luteinizing hormone, follicle-stimulating hormone, or SHBG or in vaginal cytology were observed.

Estrogen-Related Biologic Activities in Experimental Animals. A number of laboratory studies suggest that isoflavones may modulate estrogen-regulated functions. Six-week-old rats that had been treated as neonates with genistein administered by subcutaneous injection exhibited an altered pituitary gonadotroph response to administered gonadotropin-releasing hormone, suggesting neonatal exposure to this isoflavone may influence development of the hypothalamic-pituitary axis (220). In contrast, pituitary gonadotroph responsiveness to gonadotropin-releasing hormone was not altered by prenatal exposure to genistein, although female rats exposed to this isoflavone in utero did display delayed onset of puberty (221).

Other Estrogen-Related Biologic Activities. Isoflavones modulate several biologic activities that could potentially affect production or action of endogenous estrogens. The physiologic relevance of these modulatory effects remains to be assessed, however. SHBG, present in the systemic circulation, binds estrogens and androgens with high affinity and thereby modulates the availability of these hormones for binding to their respective intracellular receptors. Genistein has been reported to increase production of SHBG by Hep-G_2 cells, a human hepatoma cell line, cultured under estrogen-depleted conditions (222). Induction of SHBG production occurred at genistein concentrations of 20 μM or greater, which are greater than that observed in the circulation of humans consuming large amounts of dietary soy (223, 224). Although a positive correlation between isoflavone consumption, as indicated by urinary excretion, and the level of circulating SHBG has been reported (225), two dietary intervention studies failed to reveal significant effects of increased consumption of soy-derived isoflavones on circulating SHBG in women (217, 219). Thus, it is not clear that dietary isoflavones modulate SHBG levels in vivo.

Aromatase is a cytochrome P450 that catalyzes the conversion of androgens to estrogens. Numerous studies indicate the potential of certain isoflavones to competitively inhibit aromatase and thereby inhibit estrogen production (226–228), but it has yet to be demonstrated that diet-derived isoflavones can modulate aromatase activity in vivo.

17β-Hydroxysteroid oxidoreductase type I (17β-HSOR) catalyzes the interconversion of estrone and 17β-estradiol. It has recently been reported that genistein, but not biochanin A, inhibits 17β-HSOR, both enzyme purified from human placenta and endogenous enzyme in T47D human breast cancer cells (225). In T47D_{21} cells, which overexpress 17β-HSOR activity because of a stably transfected cDNA, reduction of estrone to 17β-estradiol was observed to predominate over oxidation of 17β-estradiol to estrone. Interestingly, estrone reduction was inhibited by genistein, whereas oxidation of 17β-estradiol was unaffected. At concentrations required to inhibit 17β-HSOR activity in T47D cells, genistein displayed significant inherent estrogenic activity.

Inhibition of Protein Tyrosine Kinases. Tyrosine-specific protein kinases are a family of related enzymes that catalyze the addition of phosphate derived from ATP to the hydroxyl group of specific tyrosine residues in proteins. The membrane-associated receptors for a variety of cellular growth factors, such as insulin, insulin-like growth factor I (IGF-I), and epidermal growth factor (EGF), possess intrinsic tyrosine kinase activity. Mutations in the genes encoding these and other protein tyrosine kinases that result in unregulated kinase activity are often associated with the transformed phenotype displayed by cancer cells.

Akiyama et al. (230) were the first to demonstrate that the isoflavone genistein is a specific inhibitor of protein tyrosine kinases. Inhibition of kinase activity was competitive with respect to ATP binding. Although genistein was a potent inhibitor of the EGF receptor and the protein products of the v-*src* and v-*fes* viral oncogenes, each of which possesses tyrosine kinase activity, no inhibition of kinases that phosphorylate serine and threonine residues, cyclic AMP-dependent protein kinase, and protein kinase C, was observed.

Genistein inhibits proliferation of a wide variety of cell lines (231). For example, genistein inhibits, in a concentration-dependent manner (IC_{50} = 12 μM), proliferation of NIH-3T3 fibroblasts that are growth stimulated by EGF (232). Interestingly, genistein, at concentrations ($\leq$40 μM) that effectively inhibited cellular proliferation, did not inhibit the ability of EGF to induce expression of the c-*myc* gene, a cellular response that is well known to require the protein tyrosine kinase activity of the EGF receptor. From these data it would appear that inhibition of cellular proliferation by genistein is independent of inhibition of EGF receptor protein tyrosine kinase activity (232). Similar results were observed by Peterson and Barnes in studies of genistein action in DU-145 prostate cancer stimulated with EGF (233). Abler et al. (234) demonstrated that the ability of genistein to inhibit certain insulin-regulated responses in isolated rat adipocytes did not correlate with its ability to inhibit insulin receptor tyrosine kinase activity. Together, these data indicate that it should not be assumed that the protein tyrosine kinases are the cellular targets through which genistein exerts it cytostatic and cytotoxic properties.

Inhibition of Topoisomerases. Topoisomerases are enzymes that relieve torsional stress in DNA generated during replication and transcription. A number of widely used chemotherapeutic drugs, such as etoposide (VP-16), mitoxantrone, and adriamycin, act through inhibition of topoisomerase activity. Genistein inhibits the activities of purified preparations of both topoisomerase I and topoisomerase II (235) and appears to promote accumulation of topoisomerase-DNA intermediates, which may lead to single-strand and double-strand breaks in the DNA

(235–237). The isoflavone orobol (5,7,3′,4′-tetrahydroxyisoflavone) displays a similar inhibitory effect on topoisomerase II activity (237), whereas biochanin A and daidzein do not (236, 237). Markovits et al. (236) demonstrated that different variants of the DC-3F Chinese hamster lung cell line display differing degrees of growth inhibition in response to genistein and that the variant cell line (DC-3F/9-OH-E) most resistant to genistein appears to express an altered form of topoisomerase II. These data were interpreted to suggest that the cytotoxic effects of genistein on cell proliferation may be mediated through inhibition of topoisomerase II activity. It has yet to be established whether topoisomerases are suitable in vivo targets for isoflavone-based chemoprevention or chemotherapeutic strategies.

Regulation of Cell Cycle Progression, Differentiation, and Apoptosis. The replicative cycle of cells can be divided into four major stages: G_1 (gap_1); S (synthesis), the stage of the cycle where cellular DNA is replicated; G_2 (gap_2); and M (mitosis), the stage during which the replicated chromosomes segregate. Terminally differentiated and other nonreplicating cells represent a quiescent stage often referred to as G_0. Apoptosis is an active process in which cells undergo genetically programed death. An understanding of the molecular events regulating cell cycle progression (238) and apoptosis (238–241) is rapidly emerging.

Genistein inhibits proliferation of HL-60 human promyelocytic leukemia cells and MOLT-4 human lymphocytic cells at IC_{50} concentrations of 31 and 48 μM, respectively (142). Genistein at higher concentrations (185 μM) promoted apoptosis within the treated HL-60 and MOLT-4 cell populations, whereas normal proliferating lymphocytes were unaffected by genistein at concentrations up to 739 μM. HL-60 and MOLT-4 cells treated with genistein were arrested at the S/G_2 boundary. In a subsequent study, genistein, at concentrations of 200 to 400 μM, was demonstrated to arrest progression of HL-60 cells in G_2 and to promote apoptosis independent of cell-cycle stage (243). Matsukawa et al. (183) demonstrated that genistein inhibited, in a concentration-dependent and reversible manner, progression of HGC-27 human gastric cancer cells in G_2/M. Interestingly, daidzein inhibited progression of this cell line in G_1. Therefore, it cannot be assumed that closely related isoflavones act through the same mechanisms to inhibit cell proliferation.

A number of reports indicate that isoflavones can induce differentiation of a variety of cell lines (reviewed in [244]). Genistein (37 μM) promotes differentiation of HL-60 human promyelocytic leukemia cells and K-562 human erythroid leukemia cells (245). Honma et al. (246) demonstrated that genistein and a second inhibitor of protein tyrosine kinase activity, herbimycin A, promote differentiation of K-562 cells and suggested this might occur either through inhibition of the tyrosine kinase encoded by the *c-abl* gene or the chimeric protein encoded by the *bcr/abl* oncogene, which results from a genetic translocation involving chromosomes 9 and 22. Genistein, at a concentration of 40 to 55 μM, effectively induced differentiation of mouse F9 embryonal carcinoma cells to cells displaying phenotypic features of parietal endoderm (247). Daidzein (37 μM) promotes differentiation of HL-60 cells while arresting cell cycle progression in G_1 (248). Although it has been suggested that induction of differentiation in these various cell systems results from inhibition of protein tyrosine kinases or topoisomerases, this has yet to be demonstrated conclusively.

Inhibition of Angiogenesis. Formation of new vasculature is required for a cancer to grow and metastasize. Consequently, much effort has been focused on identifying antiangiogenic agents that inhibit development and dissemination of tumors. Isoflavones, in particular genistein, have been identified as antiangiogenic factors contained in urine of healthy women consuming a diet high in fruits and vegetables (248). Genistein inhibits proliferation of bovine brain capillary endothelial cells in culture, whereas equol, daidzein, and *O*-desmethylangolensin are significantly less active in this regard. Genistein also displayed an inhibitory effect in an in vitro angiogenesis assay in which the ability of bovine microvascular endothelial cells to invade a collagen matrix serves as the surrogate indicator (249). Whether isoflavones, either consumed in the diet or administered by other means, are capable of modulating angiogenesis in vivo remains to be determined.

Modulation of Metabolism. Discussed above were data indicating that specific isoflavones can inhibit enzymes involved in estrogen metabolism. Effects of isoflavones on other metabolic processes are summarized in this section.

Isoflavones as Antioxidants. Much information suggests that reactive oxygen species play an important role in aging and cancer. Soy-derived isoflavones possess antioxidant activity (250). Genistein and, to a lesser extent, daidzein inhibit induction of H_2O_2 production by HL-60 cells treated with the tumor promoter TPA (251). In contrast, biochanin A had no effect on TPA-induced H_2O_2 production by HL-60 cells. Genistein, prunectin, and daidzein inhibit production of superoxide anion by xanthine oxidase, whereas biochanin A is ineffective in this regard (251). The investigators hypothesized that the antioxidant properties of genistein provide the mechanism for the antitumorigenic activity of this isoflavone in mouse skin during DMBA/TPA-mediated tumorigenesis.

Isoflavones as Inhibitors of Carcinogen Metabolism. In a search for natural products that inhibit metabolic activation of known carcinogens, Cassady et al. (252) identified biochanin A as the active component of an alcohol extract of red clover. Purified biochanin A was demonstrated to inhibit metabolic activation of benzo[*a*]pyrene (B[*a*]P) by approximately 50%. In a subsequent study, these investigators further defined the inhibitory effects of biochanin

A on B[*a*]P metabolism and demonstrated that it significantly diminished the mutagenicity of B[*a*]P in a V79 cell–based assay (253). Biochanin A also inhibits the mutagenic effects of the direct-acting carcinogen *N*-methyl-*N'*-nitro-*N*-nitrosoguanidine in a TA100 bacterial assay (254). More recently, it has been demonstrated that treatment of mice with genistein and daidzein inhibits DMBA-induced sister chromatid exchange in bone marrow cells, suggesting that these isoflavones may reduce the amount of DNA damage resulting from DMBA treatment (255). Although the mechanisms through which isoflavones inhibit metabolic activation and mutagenesis have not been elucidated, each of these studies provides evidence of potential anticancer activity of isoflavones.

Occurrence

Isoflavones are broadly distributed within the plant and bacterial worlds. Leguminous plants such as soybean and clover contain large amounts of specific isoflavones. In plants, isoflavones exist primarily as conjugated glycosides. The isoflavone conjugates are hydrolyzed by glucosidases produced by the bacterial flora of the gut. The unconjugated isoflavones appear to be more readily absorbed from the gut than the conjugated forms. The structures of several biologically active isoflavones are illustrated in Figure 81.10.

Phytoestrogens

Several classes of plant-derived chemicals possess estrogenic activity in mammalian species. Among these phytoestrogens, the isoflavones discussed above, have been most widely studied. Other phytoestrogens include lignans such as enterolactone and enterodiol, coumestans (e.g., coumestrol), and resorcyclic acid lactones (e.g., the fungal compounds zearalenone and zearalenol).

Epidemiologic and Clinical Studies

Several epidemiologic studies suggest that consumption of diets high in whole grains, fruits, and vegetables are associated with a relatively low risk of developing cancers at a variety of sites. Because individuals who consume diets high in whole grains, fruits, and vegetables consume large amounts of phytoestrogens, it has been hypothesized that the low risk of developing cancer is due in part to anticancer activities of various phytoestrogens (256). Studies focused on dietary isoflavones are discussed above. Summarized here are studies investigating other classes of phytoestrogens.

Enterolactone and enterodiol are present in human urine (257, 258). Although originally thought to be of gonadal origin, these compounds are now recognized to be derived from dietary sources (256, 259). Urinary excretion of the lignans enterodiol and enterolactone correlates with fiber consumption (225, 260). Moreover, Adlercreutz et al. (225, 260) demonstrated that urinary lignan excretion among various groups of women was lowest in the group with breast cancer, prompting the hypothesis that formation and adsorption of antiestrogenic lignans may protect against breast cancer. Although this hypothesis is supported by correlative data, it has yet to be directly verified.

Little information exists concerning the levels of lignans in the systemic circulation and tissues of humans. Dehennin et al. (261) reported plasma enterolactone concentrations (total) of 37 to 127 nM in a group of 6 men. Most of this lignan was conjugated. Adlercreutz et al. (224) reported plasma enterolactone concentrations (total) of 10.4 to 74.1 nM (mean, 33.3 nM) in a group of 14 omnivorous women and 17.9 to 1078.2 nM (mean, 252.6 nM) in a group of 14 vegetarian women. Approximately 20 to 30% of total plasma enterolactone was either in the free or sulfated forms. Much lower levels of plasma enterodiol were observed in this study. Bioavailability of the various circulating lignans to peripheral tissues has not been assessed. Consumption of a diet supplemented with soy flour, red clover sprouts, and linseed, all of which contain substantial amounts of several phytoestrogens, promoted maturation of vaginal epithelial cells in a group of 23 postmenopausal women (262). Although the quantities and identities of the phytoestrogens consumed were not determined, these data nonetheless suggest that dietary phytoestrogens exert detectable estrogenic activity in the reproductive tract of the human female.

isoflavone

Common Name	Substituents 5	7	4′	5′
Daidzein	H	OH	OH	H
Genistein	OH	OH	OH	H
Formonetin	H	OH	CH_3	H
Biochanin A	OH	OH	OCH_3	H
Genistin	OH	O glucose	OH	H
Prunectin	OH	OCH_3	OCH_3	H
Prunetin	OH	OCH_3	OH	H
Orobol	OH	OH	OH	OH
Tectorigenin	OH	OH	OH	H

Figure 81.10.

Laboratory Studies Using Animal Models

Enterolactone, administered subcutaneously, was unable to elicit an estrogenic response (stimulation of RNA synthesis) in the uterus of the immature rat (263). When administered concurrently with, or 12 hours before, 17*β*-estradiol, enterolactone did not inhibit the ability of the estrogen to stimulate uterine RNA synthesis. When administered 22 hours prior to 17*β*-estradiol, enterolactone partially inhibited induction of uterine RNA synthesis by 17*β*-estradiol. The mechanism for this inhibition was not established, and Waters and Knowler did not conclude that the classic antiestrogenic mechanism involving competition for binding to the estrogen receptor was responsible for the observed partial inhibition (263). Based upon our present knowledge of the relative affinities of enterolactone and 17β-estradiol for the estrogen receptor, it would appear that the dose of enterolactone administered by Waters and Knowler was inadequate to allow effective competition with 17β-estradiol for binding to the receptor.

Coumestrol, incorporated into a semipurified diet at levels approximating those consumed by humans and fed for 4 days, elicited a significant trophic effect in the uterus of the immature female rat (264). In addition to stimulating uterine growth, coumestrol consumption increased the number of progesterone receptors in the uterus, anterior pituitary, and hypothalamus (264, 265). Coumestrol, either consumed in the diet or injected subcutaneously, did not antagonize the ability of 17β-estradiol to increase uterine growth (266). Together, these data indicate that coumestrol displays estrogenic, as opposed to antiestrogenic, activities in the female rat.

Verdeal et al. (267) observed binding of coumestrol, zearalenone, and zearalenol to estrogen receptor (ER) in rat uterine cytosol. These investigators demonstrated that coumestrol, administered orally at doses of 0.1, 2, and 5 mg/day, was unable to support the growth of estrogen-dependent, DMBA-induced mammary cancers in Sprague-Dawley rats, suggesting that at this dose and route of administration, coumestrol was devoid of estrogenic activity. Interestingly, the orally administered coumestrol was similarly devoid of antiestrogenic activity. However, when administered by subcutaneous injection at a dose of 1.5 mg/day, coumestrol stimulated growth of these mammary tumors, indicating that this phytoestrogen exerts estrogenic activity in the rat mammary gland.

Mechanisms of Action

Regulation of Estrogen Receptor–Dependent Parameters in Cultured Cells. The abilities of various phytoestrogens to bind to the estrogen receptor (ER) have been well documented. A common method for examining binding of a potential ligand to the ER is to demonstrate that it effectively competes with 17β-estradiol for the binding site on the receptor. It is often wrongly assumed or stated that an ability of a compound to compete with an endogenous estrogen such as 17β-estradiol for binding to the ER is synonymous with that compound possessing antiestrogenic activity. For a ligand to be classified as an antiestrogen, the compound must bind to the ER yet lack estrogenic activity. We now review known biologic effects of phytoestrogen interactions with the ER.

Shutt and Cox (215) noted that coumestrol can bind to the ER and noted a correlation between the relative abilities of coumestrol, the synthetic estrogen diethylstilbestrol, and a variety of isoflavone phytoestrogens to bind to the ER and their uterotrophic potencies in vivo. A similar correlation was noted by Shemesh et al. (268).

Martin et al. (269) demonstrated that coumestrol, zearalenone, and zearalenol each bind to the ER in MCF-7 breast cancer cells, albeit with an affinity significantly less than that of 17β-estradiol. Each of these compounds displayed estrogenic activity in MCF-7 cells, as evidenced by their abilities to stimulate proliferation of this cell line (269). Enterolactone also stimulates MCF-7 cell proliferation (212, 270). Welshons et al. (210) (Fig. 81.11) further demonstrated that zearalenol, zearalenone, coumestrol, and β-zearalenol behave as full agonists with respect to their ability to stimulate proliferation of MCF-7 cells cultured under estrogen-depleted conditions. Similar observations were reported by Mäkelä et al. (211). The latter study is noteworthy in that none of the phytoestrogens examined displayed antiestrogenic activity in the presence of 17β-estradiol.

In contrast to studies discussed above (212, 270) that demonstrated a proliferative response of MCF-7 breast cancer cells to enterolactone, Mousavi and Adlercreutz (271) reported that enterolactone and 17β-estradiol each

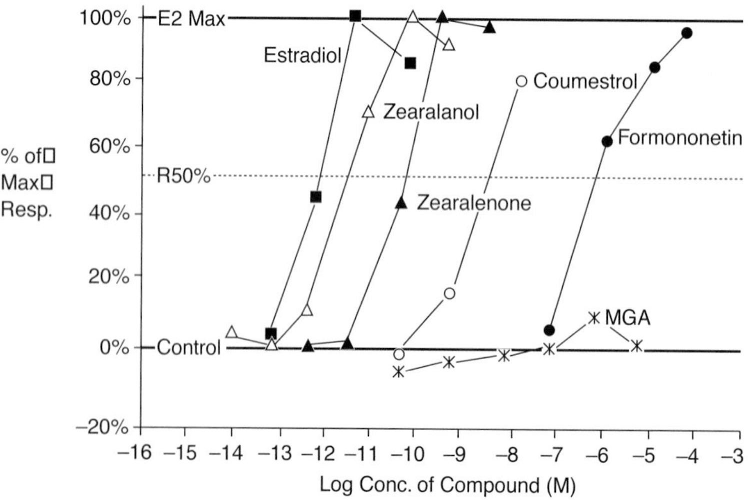

Figure 81.11. Dose-response curves for several of the estrogens. *MGA,* melengestrolacetate. (From Welshons WV, Rottinghaus GE, Nonneman DJ, et al. J Vet Diagn. Invest 1990;2:268–73, with permission.)

inhibit the other's ability to stimulate proliferation of this cell line. In that study, 17β-estradiol itself either failed to stimulate MCF-7 cell proliferation or simulated proliferation only weakly. The proliferative response to enterolactone was also small. Therefore, the validity of the stated conclusion must be questioned. Enterolactone and enterodiol have been demonstrated by Hirano et al. (272) to inhibit proliferation of ZR-75-1 human breast cancer cells. These investigators suggested that inhibition of proliferation may be due to inhibition of membrane-associated N^+,K^+-ATPase activity.

Coumestrol, zearalenone, β-zearalenol, and phloretin were demonstrated to enhance expression of an estrogen-responsive reporter plasmid (pERE/TK/CAT) in HeLa cells (216). This stimulation was inhibited by the anti-estrogens ICI164384 and 4-hydroxytamoxifen. Moreover, no stimulation of expression was observed in the absence of cotransfected expression plasmid encoding the human ER. Together these data clearly indicate that these phytoestrogens exert their estrogenic activities by binding to and activating the ER. Although these phytoestrogens were less potent than 17β-estradiol in this model system, coumestrol, zearalenone, and β-zearalenol were each more potent than the isoflavone phytoestrogens genistein, daidzein, and biochanin A. Mäkelä et al. (211), using a similar transfection assay, demonstrated that coumestrol and zearalenone exert estrogenic activities that are mediated through the ER.

Modulation of Estrogen Metabolism. Enterolactone and, to a lesser extent, enterodiol inhibit aromatase activity in microsomes prepared from human placenta (226). Inhibition by enterolactone is competitive. These lignans also inhibit aromatase activity in cultured preadipocytes (228) and JEG-3 human choriocarcinoma cells (226). These data suggest that certain lignans at micromolar concentrations may inhibit production of estrogens.

Another study (211) indicates that different phytoestrogens may inhibit 17β-HSOR in an isoform-specific manner and thereby inhibit conversion of estrone to 17β-estradiol.

Occurrence

The lignans enterolactone and enterodiol have been identified in human urine. They are formed from plant lignans matairesinol and secoisolariciresinol by intestinal flora (256, 259). Lignans are contained in whole grains, beans, and peas (269). Although not widely consumed by humans, flax seed contains the highest amount of lignan of any plant source examined (273). Coumestrol is contained in a variety of legumes. Zearalenone and zearalenol are produced by the fungus *Fusarium graminearum*. Structures of some of these common phytoestrogens are shown in Figure 81.12.

Isothiocyanates

Occurrence

Isothiocyanates are common constituents of cruciferous vegetables (274). Volatile isothiocyanates are released from thioglucosides in vegetables and contribute to the distinctive odor and flavor of cruciferous vegetables. Allyl isothiocyanate was identified nearly 50 years ago as particularly prevalent in cabbage (274). Widely used by the food industry, it is the component that gives the horseradish bite to brown mustard (275). Sulphoraphane was recently isolated from broccoli by following its potent induction of phase 2 detoxication enzymes in cultured mouse hepatoma cells (276). Phenetyl isothiocyanate is abundant in water cress (277).

Laboratory Studies

More than 20 natural and synthetic isothiocyanates have been studied for their ability to prevent carcinogenesis, as was comprehensively reviewed (278).

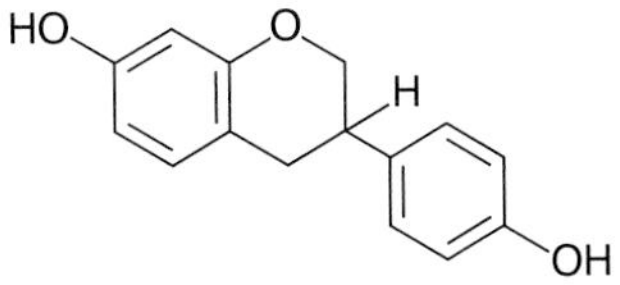

equol
(metabolite of diadzein,
formmonetin, and genistein)

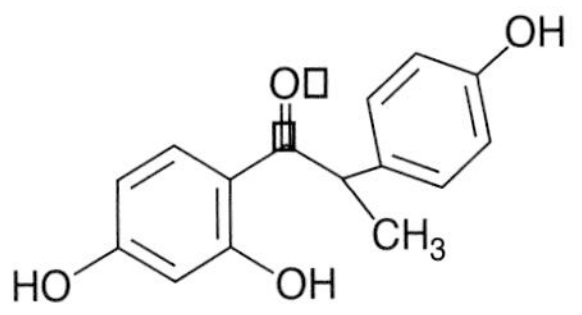

O-desmethoxylangoleinsin
(metabolite of daidzein)

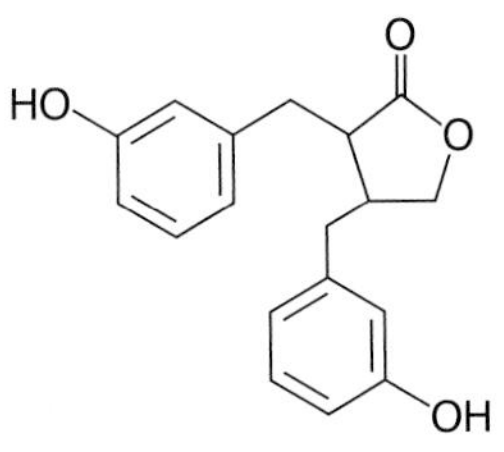

enterolactone

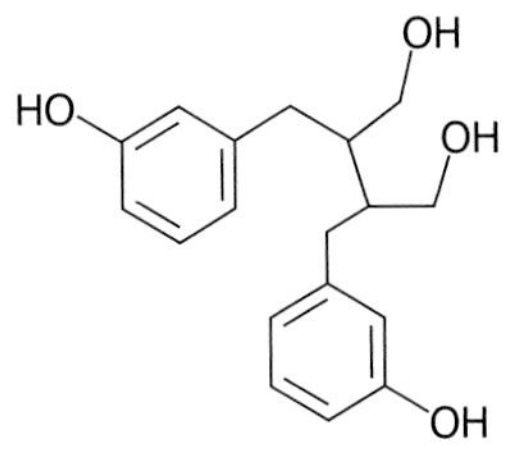

enterodiol

Figure 81.12. Some common phytoestrogens and metabolites.

Isothiocyanates are generally effective in cancer prevention when administered near the time of carcinogen treatment, suggesting that their main mode of action is to enhance detoxication and inhibit activation pathways. Early investigations of the anticarcinogenicity of isothiocyanates demonstrated inhibition of liver cancer in animals treated with α-naphthyl and β-naphthyl iosthiocyanate prior to, or with, 3-methyl-4-dimethylaminoazobenzene (DAB) (279).

In recent years, laboratories have focused on intervention in lung and nasal cavity carcinogenesis in rats and mice by a variety of isothiocyanates (280). The naturally occurring phenethyl isothiocyanate and benzyl isothiocyanate have been extensively studied as inhibitors of tobacco-specific nitrosamine (4-(methylnitrosamino)-1-3-pyridyl)-1-butanone; NNK) and polycyclic hydrocarbon (benzo[*a*]pyrene; BaP) carcinogenesis (278). Phenethyl isothiocyanate was effective in the inhibition of lung tumorigenesis by NNK, and butyl isothiocyanate was effective against BaP-induced cancer (278).

Prevention of mammary carcinogenesis was reported for sulphoraphane and related norbornyl isothiocyanates (281, 282). Oral intubation of these compounds near the time of treatment with 9,10-dimethyl-1,2-benzanthracene inhibited development of mammary tumors. Earlier studies demonstrated inhibition of DMBA-induced mammary tumors in rats pretreated with benzyl isothiocyanate, phenethyl isothiocyanate, and phenyl isothiocyanate (283). Mixed results were observed in prevention studies of esophageal carcinogenesis (284, 285). In contrast to studies at other sites, studies of colon cancer using the azoxymethane-rat model reported no inhibition of foci of aberrant crypts in rats treated with phenyl isothiocyanate, and an enhancement of small intestinal and colon carcinomas was observed in rats fed 6-phenylhexyl isothiocyanate (286). The latter study suggested that 6-phenethyl isothiocyanate promotion of colon carcinogenesis may be due to elevated eicosanoid synthesis. Because of the extensive consumption of allyl isothiocyanate, the National Toxicology Program conducted a bioassay of this compound at maximally tolerated doses in rats and mice (275). No evidence of carcinogenicity was observed in mice or in female rats. In male rats, a small but statistically significant rate of transitional cell papilloma of the urinary bladder was observed (275). Since excessive doses of the compound were used in the bioassay, it is improbable that allyl isothiocyanate presents any risk to humans at normal dietary levels.

Mechanisms of Action

Cancer prevention by isothiocyanates generally requires that the isothiocyanate treatment be administered at or near the time of treatment with carcinogen (278). This observation predicted that isothiocyanates would modify metabolic pathways for carcinogen activation and/or detoxication and elimination. Indeed, both inhibition of cytochrome P450–mediated activation and enhancement of glutathione sulfatransferase–mediated detoxication have been demonstrated for a wide variety of isothiocyanates. However, data showing a block in cell cycle progression in cells treated with isothiocyanates (287) suggests that isothiocyanates may be able to prevent cell proliferation and thus inhibit later events in cancer.

An extensive series of investigations demonstrated that isothiocyanates inhibit oxidative metabolism of a number of carcinogens and result in reduced DNA damage. Studies focused on liver metabolism indicated that phenyl isothiocyanate and phenethyl isothiocyanate inhibited α-hydroxylation of *N*-nitrosodimethylamine and of the tobacco-specific nitrosamine NNK. This result was associated with reduced DNA methylation (288). In addition, benzyl isothiocyanate and benzyl thiocyanate suppressed DNA synthesis and cell proliferation induced by several carcinogens in the liver (289). Esophageal tumorigenesis by *N*-nitrosomethylbenzylamine and DNA methylation were inhibited by phenethyl isothiocyanate in parallel studies (284). Inhibition of DNA methylation is shown in Figure 81.13. Studies have assessed isothiocyanate effects on tobacco carcinogenesis in the oral cavity and lung. A variety of isothiocyanates inhibited metabolic activation of NNK in the lung and oral cavity (290). Structure activity studies suggested that 4-phenylbutyl isothiocyanate and 6-phenylhexyl isothiocyanate were the most effective inhibitors of NNK activation and that they were more

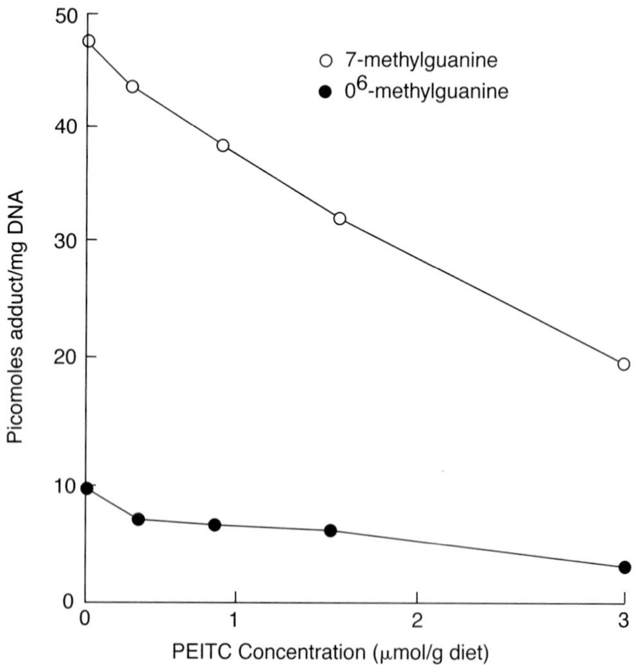

Figure 81.13. Effect of dietary phenethylisothiocyanate *(PEITC)* on nitrosomethylbenzylamine (NMBA)-induced DNA methylation. Groups of 20 rats were administered control or experimental diets for 14 days before administration of [^{3}H-methyl]NMBA. Animals were killed 24 h later. Esophageal 7-methylguanine and O^6-methylguanine were isolated and analyzed. (Reprinted from Morse MA, Zu H, Galati AJ, et al. Cancer Lett 1993;72, 1–2, 103–110, with permission.)

effective than phenethyl isothiocyanate. These observations may be useful in designing increasingly effective inhibitors of tobacco-induced cancer.

Isothiocyanate inactivates and inhibits the enzymes necessary for NNK activation (291). Phenyl isothiocyanate was particularly effective in the inhibition of hepatic demethylase (cytochrome P450-2E1 dependent) (292) and was a potent inhibitor of cytochrome P450-1A1, which is involved in formation of oxidative metabolites of NNK (298). Recent studies with the broccoli constituent sulphoraphane demonstrated its ability to inhibit cytochrome P450-2E1 (294). Human studies assessing debrisoquine metabolism as an indicator of cytochrome P450-2D6 activity indicated inhibition by phenethyl isothiocyanate in vitro with human liver microsomes, but no evidence of inhibition was observed in the in vivo study (295).

Several lines of evidence support a role of isothiocyanates in induction of phase II metabolism, which results in reduced toxicity and accelerated elimination of many toxic and carcinogenic substances. For example, early studies reported an increase in glutathione sulfatransferase, the enzyme responsible for conjugation of a wide variety of electrophiles with the sulfhydryl group of glutathione, in the mouse forestomach following dietary administration of benzyl isothiocyanate (296). More-recent studies demonstrated that compounds that induce glutathione transferase also induce NAD(P)H:(quinone-acceptor)oxidoreductase (297), another important enzyme defense against toxicity and carcinogenicity of chemicals. Furthermore, isothiocyanates including sulphoraphane, benzyl isothiocyanate, allyl isothiocyanate, and phenethyl isothiocyanate are substrates and inducers of human glutathione transferase (298).

Recent investigations demonstrated the induction of c-Jun N-terminal kinase by isothiocyanates in ovarian HeLa cells and in fibrosarcoma cells (HT1080) (299). Phenethyl isothiocyanate treatment resulted in the most-sustained induction, while 3-phenylpropyl and 4-phenylbutyl isothiocyanate stimulated transient activation. The authors speculate that c-Jun N-terminal kinase induction may be involved in induction of phase II detoxication enzymes. However, it is not clear if the cellular concentrations of the isothiocyanates in this investigation were comparable to concentrations achieved in vivo.

Diallylsulfide

Epidemiology of Allium Foods and Cancer

Allium vegetables are members of the lily family and include garlic, onions, leeks, scallions, and chives (300). These foods share the common property of generating organic molecules that incorporate sulfur atoms when the plant is cut or cooked. Many different organosulfur compounds are present in allium foods. For example, garlic contains diallyl sulfide, allyl methyl disulfide, allyl methyl trisulfide, *S*-allyl cysteine, diallyl trisulfide, and others (301). Allium foods have been used for centuries for their antibiotic and antithrombotic activity. They have also been shown, in animal models, to have anticarcinogenic properties (302).

Studies in human populations have evaluated the incidence of certain cancers in subjects relative to their consumption of allium vegetables. As with the micronutrients that have been studied for their chemopreventive effect, allium vegetables yield mixed results in epidemiologic cancer research. Two retrospective studies, conducted in the province of Shandong, China, which has an exceptionally high rate of stomach cancer mortality, showed that subjects who consumed garlic had a tenfold lower risk for gastric cancer than those who did not (303).

Haenszel et al. (304) compared stomach cancer risk in Hawaiian Japanese populations consuming native foods and Western foods. This study found an increased cancer risk among subjects who consumed dried and salted fish and pickled vegetables and a decreased risk among those who consumed Western vegetables, including onions. In addition to the overall lower relative risk for stomach cancer in onion consumers, the investigators found that risk declined further as the frequency of onion consumption increased.

Another investigation, in which consumption of garlic and onions together was studied, found that relative risk for gastric cancer declined as frequency of intake increased (305). This study also found that the reduced risk associated with consumption of raw onions did not exist for cooked onions, although risk was significantly decreased for consumption of cooked garlic.

In contrast to epidemiologic studies demonstrating decreased gastric cancer risk with garlic and onion consumption, a case-control study of a Japanese cohort (306) found that consumption of certain vegetables, including onion, was associated with a significantly elevated relative risk for stomach and colorectal cancers. The increased cancer risk associated with onion consumption remained even when variables for education, smoking, alcohol, and high-salt food consumption were taken into account (306). Although most epidemiologic evidence supports a role for allium vegetables in decreasing risk for gastric and colorectal cancers, studies that show either no change or an increased cancer risk suggest the need for further investigation, particularly into possible mechanisms of action for this compound as a chemopreventive agent.

Chemoprevention by Allium Compounds in Animal Models

Administration of high doses of garlic compounds to rodents has demonstrated significant inhibition of chemically induced mammary, colon, esophageal, and other cancers in these animal models. The first study to show that dietary garlic increased latency and decreased mammary tumor incidence in rats provided organosulfur compounds (OGCs) as garlic powder added at levels of 2 and 4% to semipurified diet (307). Although specific organosulfur compounds were not identified, a dose-responsive inhibition of tumorigenesis was demonstrated following consumption of the garlic in the rat diet. Furthermore, inhibition was seen in both the initiation and promotional phases of tumor development. Similar results were obtained in subsequent studies by Amagase et al. using 20 g/kg garlic powder in semipurified diets (308, 309). These studies also established an inhibition of DMBA-DNA adduct formation in mammary tissue in animals fed the garlic-supplemented diets.

In contrast to the findings of Amagase and Milner (308), Pereira and Khoury (310) found no significant inhibition of cancer foci in the colons of mice fed 0.1% diallyl sulfide in semipurified diets. The diallyl sulfide treatment was begun 1 week prior to administration of carcinogen. Tumor inhibition by the OGCs in garlic may be the result of interaction between other compounds in the garlic powder that were not present in the diallyl sulfide–supplemented diet. Also, the level of diallyl sulfide in the diet (0.1%) may have been too low to achieve an inhibitory effect.

In studies by other investigators, garlic extracts have been administered by intragastric gavage. Sumiyoshi and Wargovich (311) and Wargovich et al. (312) administered diallyl sulfide and other OGCs in doses of 50 400 mg/kg body weight to rats in serial gavages prior to injection with carcinogen. This experimental protocol resulted in a significant decrease in chemically induced colon tumor incidence in the rats when diallyl sulfide and other lipophilic OGCs were used.

Gastric gavage delivers the OGC in a concentrated form directly to the absorptive surface of the gut. Whether this method of delivery is more effective than dietary administration has not been established. Also, dosage and timing in intragastric OGC administration can affect the outcome of chemically induced tumorigenesis. Takada et al. found that high doses (up to 150 mg/kg) of DAS and related OGCs administered intragastrically during the promotional stage increased rather than decreased the number of tumor foci and nodules in hepatic tissue of mice (313). Such varied outcomes in chemopreventive effects of OGCs suggests that these compounds function quite differently as food components than as purified compounds administered in supraphysiologic doses.

Mechanisms of Inhibition of Tumorigenesis by Organosulfur Compounds

Organosulfur compounds may mediate tumor inhibition through various pathways. Two notable mechanisms that have been studied are the induction of cytochrome p450 enzymes and induction of glutathione *S*-transferase. Cytochromes p450 are a group of microsomal enzymes found in most tissues but predominantly in the liver (314). They are involved in hydroxylation reactions that result in increased solubility in metabolism and excretion of toxic compounds. However, some compounds (e.g., carcinogens) enter the p450 pathway and become activated rather than detoxified (314).

In the case of agents such as benz[*a*]pyrene that form DNA adducts, inhibition of certain p450 enzymes results in decreased tumorigenicity (91). However, not all organosulfur compounds are effective p450 inhibitors. Furthermore, specific OGCs inactivate certain p450 species following induction by specific carcinogens. For example, diallyl sulfoxide, diallyl sulfone, and diallyl sulfide inactivate the p450 isoform 2E1 induced by NNK and DMH, although at different rates (91).

Previous research using carbon disulfide established that p450 inactivation is due to the sulfur compound (329). This mechanism may in part account for the decreased tumor inhibitory properties of onion, which contains saturated (*n*-propyl) substituents, compared with garlic with unsaturated alkyl groups (330).

The glutathione *S*-transferases (GSTs) catalyze the conjugation of glutathione to electrophilic species produced from cytochrome p450 activity. These transformed metabolites are rendered less toxic and more soluble for excretion (317). GST activity has been measured following administration of chemical carcinogens. In the presence of OGCs such as diallyl sulfide, diallyl trisulfide, and others, GST activity is increased and tumor incidence is decreased (311). Glutathione may exert its inhibitory effect by conjugating carcinogenic compounds and rendering them unavailable to bind to DNA and initiate damage. However, GST activity is clearly only one of many components of the cancer inhibitory effect of diallyl sulfide and other OGCs.

Chemoprevention with Garlic Extract

Concentrated extract of fresh garlic has been used in rodent models to demonstrate inhibition of tumor growth from injected transplantable tumors and inhibition of chemically initiated and promoted tumors. Garlic was administered to mice either orally or peritoneally concomitantly with injection of tumor cells or chemical initiation and promotion (318), and survival time and tumor incidence in the mice were determined. Interestingly, garlic extract was only effective in increasing survival and decreasing tumor incidence in the group that received orally administered extract. In another study, garlic extract was injected intraperitoneally simultaneously with the cytotoxin cyclophosphamide, followed by injection of tumor cells 14 days later (319). This group was compared with mice that received only the tumor cells. The animals that received injected garlic extract, cyclophosphamide, and tumor cells survived longer than those receiving injected garlic extract and tumor cells only. The results of the study suggest that the garlic extract could protect normal cells from the cytotoxic agent but had little or no effect on inhibiting tumor growth.

Tea and Tea Polyphenols

Epidemiologic and Clinical Studies

Epidemiologic studies on the relationship between tea consumption and human cancers have not provided clear evidence for cancer prevention by tea. However, as discussed below, studies in experimental animals and cultured cells provide strong evidence for cancer prevention by tea and its constituent polyphenols (reviewed in [320]). A number of the human studies focused on esophageal cancer because early reports indicated a causal role for tea consumption. In general, consumption of tea at high temperature, near boiling, was associated with esophageal cancer in some studies, while consumption at more moderate temperatures was protective or had no effect (320). Tea consumption was suggested to increase, decrease, or have no effect on stomach, lung, breast, colon and rectum, and kidney cancer in epidemiologic investigations (320). Urinary bladder and nasopharynx cancer were not associated with tea intake.

In a recent prospective study conducted with the Netherlands Cohort Study on Diet and Cancer, black tea consumption was not associated with rates of colorectal cancer, was positively associated with breast cancer, and was inversely associated with stomach and lung cancers. However, tea drinkers tended to smoke less and consume more fruits and vegetables. When the data were corrected for these covariants, the protective association disappeared, indicating that tea itself was not related to these cancers (321). Since green tea contains higher concentrations of many of the compounds suspected to protect against cancer, it is possible that human study designs must clearly distinguish the influences of green and black teas. Furthermore, some of the studies indicating that tea consumption was protective were conducted in areas of the world where green tea is more frequently consumed (322). It is possible that these populations are also more prone to micronutrient deficiencies, and thus tea (green or black) may be more effective in cancer prevention in populations that are deficient in micronutrients. In summary, there is no conclusive evidence that consumption of tea at normal temperature protects against cancer, and consumption at excessively high temperature may be a risk factor for esophageal cancer.

Laboratory Studies

Investigations with experimental animals provide strong evidence of cancer prevention properties for tea (320). Green or black tea, polyphenol-rich extracts from tea, or specific tea polyphenolic compounds have been shown to inhibit both chemically and ultraviolet light–induced skin cancer and chemically induced cancer of the esophagus, lung, forestomach, liver, colon, small intestine, breast, pancreas, and prostate (reviewed in [320]). Inhibition of skin carcinogenesis by tea and tea constituents has been extensively studied. Both topical and oral application of green tea or black tea extracts were effective in preventing carcinogenesis by DMBA and TPA or by UV light (320). Inhibition of UV light–induced skin tumors by black tea is shown in Figure 81.14. Furthermore, all stages of chemical carcinogenesis, initiation, promotion, and conversion of papillomas to carcinomas were inhibited by tea.

Oral administration of tea also reduced the number of spontaneous lung metastases from mouse Lewis lung carcinoma cells (323). Parallel in vitro studies demonstrated inhibition of Matrigel invasion, a proxy assay for tissue invasion, in the presence of green tea infusion or in the presence of gallate-containing catechins (323).

Most studies on tea inhibition of experimental carcinogenesis have focused on green tea and green tea constituents, probably because many of the chemicals suspected to be important in cancer prevention by tea are present in higher concentration in green tea. For example, catechins such as epigallocatechin and epigallocatechin-3-gallate have been shown to have cancer preventive properties similar to those of tea or phenolic-rich extracts from tea (320). Green tea extract is 30 to 42% catechins, while black tea is only 3 to 10% catechins (320) (Table 81.2). However, some studies found similar potency in cancer prevention by green and black tea (324) and others found that cancer prevention by tea did not appear to be consistently related to the presence of the major catechin, (-)-epigallocatechin-3-gallate (325). These results

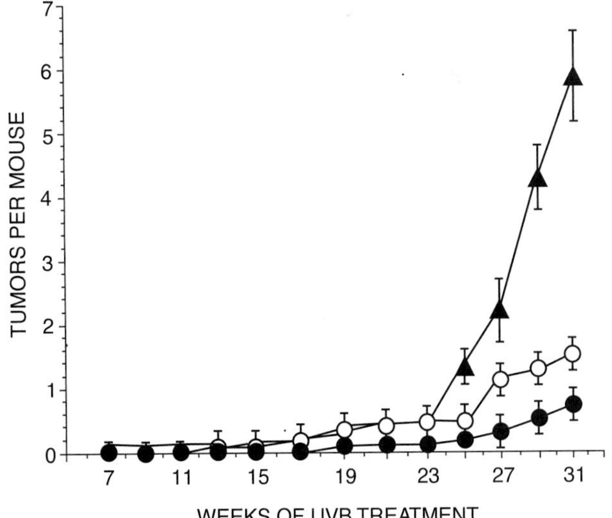

Figure 81.14. Inhibitory effect of oral administration of two doses of black tea, 0.63% *(open circles)* and 1.25% *(closed circles)*, in the drinking water on the formation of UVB-induced skin tumors in mice previously initiated with DMBA; controls *(triangles)*. Female SKH-1 mice were initiated with 200 nmol of DMBA. One week later, the mice were given gradually escalating doses of tea in the drinking water for 1 week, followed by full-strength tea for 1 week before and during treatment with UVB (30 mJ/cm^2) twice weekly for 31 weeks. Each value is the mean from 29–30 mice; bars, SE. (From Wang ZY, Huang M-T, Con Y-R, et al. Cancer Res 1994;54:3428–35. Br J Cancer 1994;69:879–82, with permission.)

Table 81.2
Principal Polyphenolic Components Present in Green and Black Tea (measured in weight % of extract solids)

Components	Green Tea	Black Tea
Catechins	30–42	3–10
Flavonols	5–10	6–8
Other flavanoids	2–4	—
Theogallin	2–3	—
Gallic acid	0.5	—
Quinic acid	2.0	—
Theanine	4–6	—
Methylxanthines	7–9	8–11
Theaflavins	—	3–6
Thearubigens	—	12–18

From Katiyar SK, Mulchtar H. Int J Oncol 1996;8:221–38. Carcinogenesis 1989;10: 781–3, with permission.

suggest that many components of green and black tea may have cancer prevention properties.

Mechanisms of Action

A major barrier to understanding the mechanisms of cancer prevention by tea and its constituents is that the particular compounds that contribute to cancer prevention by tea and tea extracts are not well identified. Although several components have been isolated and their activities have been studied, it appears that many compounds contribute to cancer prevention by tea. Irrespective of this barrier, a wide range of activities have been identified for tea and its constituents. Augmentation of the antioxidant defense system and phase II metabolism was reported by Khan et al. (326). Dietary administration of a 0.2% phenol-rich fraction from green tea for 30 days increased the activities of glutathione peroxidase, catalase, and quinone reductase in the small bowel, liver, and lungs. In addition, glutathione *S*-transferase activity was elevated in the small bowel and liver. In studies designed to assess the inhibition of colon cancer by green tea and green tea catechins, Pingzhang et al. (327) observed increased expression of colonic superoxide dismutase by immunohistochemistry. Oxidative metabolism of the tobacco-specific nitrosamine NNK and DNA methylation by lung microsomes was inhibited by tea extracts (328). The catechin (-)-epigallocatechin-3-gallate was the most effective component of the tea extracts. This compound also inhibited the catalytic activity of several p450 enzymes (328). However, in vivo studies did not provide evidence for the importance of the inhibition by tea of metabolism and DNA alkylation in vivo.

Pretreatment of mouse skin with polyphenolic-rich tea extracts inhibited epidermal inflammation induced by the phorbol ester tumor promoter TPA (329). TPA-induced edema, hyperplasia, and neutrophil infiltration were all inhibited by green tea polyphenols (329). Further research by the same laboratory demonstrated that induction of the inflammatory cytokine interleukin-1α by a number of agents that induce epidermal inflammation was inhibited by several green tea polyphenols (330).

Monoterpenes

Laboratory Studies

Experimental Mammary Tumorigenesis. Consumption of orange peel oil (5%), of which the monoterpene limonene is the predominant component, inhibited development of mammary tumors in Sprague-Dawley rats treated with DMBA (331). In that experiment, orange peel oil was fed to the rats beginning 1 week after treatment with DMBA. D-Limonene, fed to female Sprague-Dawley rats at levels of 0.1 and 1.0% (w/w) beginning 1 week before, and continuing for 27 weeks after, administration of DMBA, inhibited development of mammary tumors in a dose-dependent manner, as evidenced by an increased latency (332) (Fig. 81.15). When consumed for a 1-week period bracketing DMBA treatment, limonene (5%) increased latency and reduced the number of tumors per animal (333). Limonene consumption, beginning 1 week before initiation with DMBA and continuing for the duration of a 25-week promotion/progression phase, reduced the number of tumors per animal but had no effect on latency. These data indicate that limonene exerts anticarcinogenic effects during both the initiation and promotion/progression phases of DMBA-induced mammary tumorigenesis. Also, limonene inhibits development of mammary tumors during the promotion/progression phase in female Wistar-Furth rats treated with the direct-acting carcinogen nitrosomethylurea (NMU) (334).

Consumption of a diet containing limonene (10% of diet by weight) promotes regression of DMBA-induced mammary cancers in female F2 progeny resulting from a cross between F344 and Wistar-Furth rats (335). This observation has been confirmed and extended by Jirtle et al. (336). These data suggest that limonene may have therapeutic potential. Regressing tumors displayed increased levels of immunoreactive transforming growth factor–β1 (TGF-β1) and mannose 6-phosphate/insulin-like growth factor II receptor (M6P/IGF-II receptor). Regressing tumors in limonene-treated animals showed approximately twice as much mRNA encoding the M6P/IGF-II receptor as nonregressing tumors from control animals or nonregressing tumors in limonene-treated animals. No effect of limonene on TGF-β1 mRNA was observed. These investigators proposed that the observed increase in M6P/IGF-II receptor expression might enhance conversion of latent TGF-β1 to its active form. Because TGF-β1 exerts an inhibitory effect on mammary cell proliferation (337), Jirtle et al. suggested (336) that the increase in TGF-β1 observed in association with regressing tumors might be the mechanism through which regression occurs. More recently, limonene (5–10% w/w) was shown to promote regression of NMU-induced mammary cancers in female Ludwig/Wistar/Olac rats (338).

Other monocyclic monoterpenes also display anticancer activities in the rat mammary gland. Russin et al. (339) demonstrated that dietary (-)-menthol (1% w/w) during the initiation phase significantly inhibits DMBA-

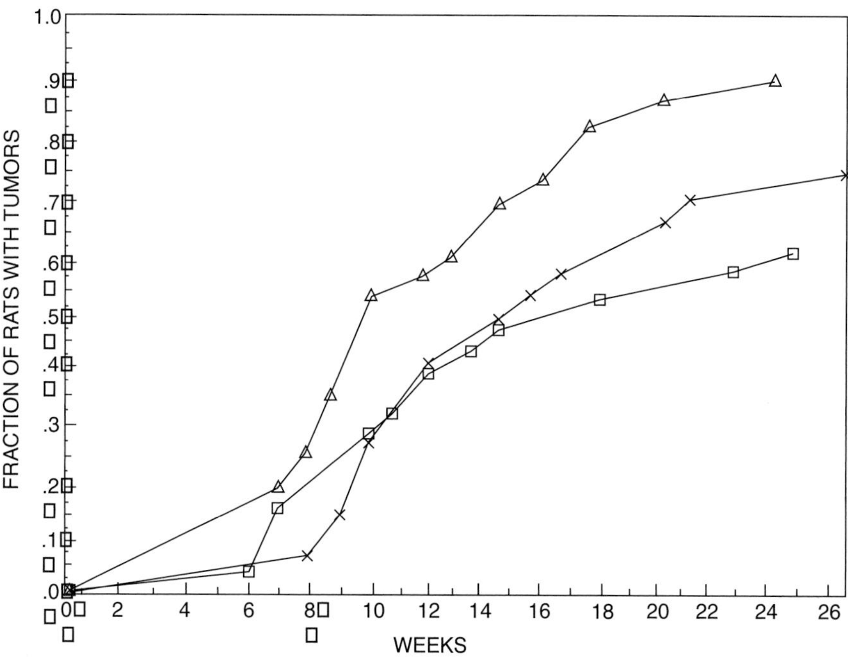

Figure 81.15. Appearance of first tumor (1 × 1 mm) in rats treated with DMBA (week 0) and fed diets containing 0 ppm *(triangles)*, 1000 ppm *(X)*, or 10,000 ppm *(squares)* d-limonene. The diets were fed for 1 week prior to and 27 weeks after DMBA. (From Elegbede JA, Elson CE, Qureshi A, et al. Carcinogenesis 1984;5:661–4. J Natl Cancer Inst 1976;56:1237–42, with permission.)

induced mammary tumorigenesis in female Sprague-Dawley rats. Carveol and uroterpenol, two hydroxylated derivatives of limonene identified in urine of rats and humans, and sobrerol, a derivative of α-pinene, inhibit DMBA-induced mammary tumorigenesis during the initiation phase (340). When fed to female Wistar-Furth rats at a level of 1% beginning 2 weeks before, and continuing for 1 week after, treatment with DMBA, uroterpenol, and sobrerol significantly increased latency, whereas all three monoterpenes significantly decreased tumor multiplicity. Of these compounds, sobrerol appeared most active in inhibiting mammary cancer development in DMBA-treated animals. Perillyl alcohol, a hydroxylated analogue of limonene, has recently been shown to be more potent than limonene in promoting regression of DMBA-induced mammary cancers (341). Relative to limonene, perillyl alcohol produced higher circulating levels of perillic acid and dihydroperillic acid, suggesting that the differing potencies of limonene and perillyl alcohol may result from pharmacokinetic factors.

Experimental Gastric Tumorigenesis. When administered by oral intubation 1 hour prior to *N*-nitrosodiethylamine (NDEA), D-limonene and D-carvone markedly inhibited development of forestomach papillomas and carcinomas in female A/J mice (342).

Experimental Lung Tumorigenesis. Limonene, administered by weekly intravenous injections, inhibited spontaneous development of lung adenomas in A/J mice, whereas both limonene and orange oil inhibited dibenzpyrene (DBP)-induced lung tumorigenesis (343). Wattenberg (342) demonstrated that limonene and carvone, administered by oral intubation 1 hour prior to NDEA, inhibited development of pulmonary adenomas in A/J mice. Together, these data suggest that monoterpenes may inhibit lung tumorigenesis at both the initiation and promotion/progression stages.

Experimental Skin Tumorigenesis. Orange oil, as well as other citrus oils, promotes development of skin papillomas in strain 101 mice treated topically with DMBA (344). In this experiment, mice were treated weekly by topical application of the citrus oils at the site of carcinogen treatment. Skin tumors did not develop in response to treatment with orange oil in mice that were not pretreated with DMBA, indicating that the orange oil itself was devoid of carcinogenic activity. A terpene-containing fraction of orange oil was shown to contain the active skin tumor–promoting agent. Elegbede et al. (345) demonstrated that orange peel oil and limonene, when applied topically, are each capable of weakly promoting development of skin tumors in CD-1 mice following initiation with DMBA. In contrast, neither orange peel oil nor limonene promoted DMBA-induced skin tumors when consumed in the diet.

Van Duuren and Goldschmidt (346) observed a slight inhibitory effect of limonene on DMBA-induced skin tumorigenesis in ICR/Ha Swiss mice when the two compounds were administered together. Similar results were reported by Gould et al. (347) who observed a slight, but not statistically significant, inhibitory effect of limonene on DMBA-induced skin tumorigenesis in CD-1 mice when limonene was administered for a total of 6 days flanking DMBA treatment. From these data it would appear that limonene, depending upon when and how it is administered, can either promote or inhibit DMBA-induced skin tumorigenesis.

Experimental Hepatocarcinogenesis. Mills et al. (348) recently demonstrated that consumption of perillyl alcohol (1–2% w/w) inhibits development of diethylnitrosoamine (DEN)-induced liver tumors in the male F344 rat. Tumor mass was markedly smaller in animals consuming perillyl alcohol than in animals fed the control diet. Although consumption of perillyl alcohol had no effect on proliferation of normal and neoplastic liver cell populations, the number of apoptotic cells within the tumors was significantly increased in the animals fed perillyl alcohol, suggesting that this monoterpene may inhibit hepatocarcinogenesis by promoting apoptosis within the tumor cell population.

Experimental Pancreatic Tumorigenesis. It was recently demonstrated that consumption of perillyl alcohol (3% w/w) markedly inhibits growth of a pancreatic cancer cell line (PC-1) maintained subcutaneously in male Syrian hamsters (349). Perillyl alcohol also inhibited proliferation of PC-1 (hamster pancreatic ductal carcinoma cells harboring activating mutation in the K-*ras* gene) and MIA PaCa-2 cells (human pancreatic carcinoma cell line harboring mutations in the K-*ras* and *p53* genes) maintained in culture.

Other Experimental Cancers. Orange oil administered to C57BL/6 mice by subcutaneous injection at the same site 24 hours following the carcinogen dibenzpyrene markedly inhibited development of subcutaneous fibrosarcomas (343). Limonene and a mixture of limonene and limonene hydroperoxide also inhibited DBP-induced tumor development in this animal model.

Mutations in the *p53* tumor suppressor gene are common in human malignancies. Mice in which both alleles of the *p53* gene have been inactivated by insertional mutagenesis rapidly and spontaneously develop a variety of tumors, including lymphomas. Hursting et al. (350) recently examined the effect of limonene consumption (7.5% w/w) on tumorigenesis in *p53*-knockout mice. Although limonene consumption slightly inhibited development of lymphoma, other nonhematopoietic tumors developed, and survival was not prolonged.

Clinical Studies

Although phase I clinical studies are in progress, information about the effectiveness of monoterpenes as therapeutic or chemopreventive agents in humans is not available. Crowell et al. (351) performed a study to assess toxicity and metabolism of limonene in human subjects. Consumption of limonene (100 mg/kg body weight) did not result in detectable toxicity. The ingested limonene was extensively metabolized within 4 hours, with the major circulating metabolites being perillic acid, dihydroperillic acid, and limonene-1,2-diol. Lesser metabolites included the methyl esters of perillic acid and dihydroperillic acid.

Mechanisms of Action

Chemically induced mammary cancers in rats are often associated with activating mutations in the c-Ha-*ras* gene (352). Moreover, the ability of p21*ras* to transform NIH3T3 cells requires that this protein be farnesylated (353). Limonene has been demonstrated to inhibit, in cultured NIH3T3 cells, isoprenylation of several proteins of 21 to 26 kDa, including $p21^{ras}$, the product of the c-Ha-*ras* protooncogene (354). Perillic acid and dihydroperillic acid, both major circulating metabolites of limonene in the rat and human (351, 355), also inhibit protein isoprenylation in NIH3T3 cells (354). Crowell et al. (356) evaluated the abilities of a number of monoterpenes to inhibit protein isoprenylation in NIH3T3 cells. The following structure-activity relationship was observed in that study: monohydroxyl = ester = aldehyde > thiol > acid = diol = epoxide > triol = unsubstituted. Moreover, the monoterpenes displayed the same structure-activity relationship when their abilities to inhibit proliferation of HT-29 human colon carcinoma cells was examined. More recently, Gelb et al. (357) demonstrated that limonene, perillyl alcohol, and perillic acid weakly inhibit protein farnesyl transferase and protein geranylgeranyl transferase, whereas a minor metabolite, perillic acid methyl ester, markedly inhibits these enzymes. Based on these data, Gould and colleagues suggested that limonene and/or its circulating metabolites might exert their anticancer activities by inhibiting farnesylation of $p21^{ras}$, thereby modulating the intracellular localization and activity of this protein. Ruch and Sigler (358) demonstrated that limonene, perillyl alcohol, perillic acid, menthol, and pinene each inhibit proliferation of a v-Ha-*ras*-transformed rat liver epithelial cell line (WB-ras). However, inhibition of cellular proliferation by these monoterpenes could not be attributed to inhibition of *ras* farnesylation.

In the rat, limonene consumption has been shown to inhibit formation of DMBA-DNA adducts in the liver, spleen, kidney, and lung; increase urinary excretion of DMBA and DMBA-derived metabolites; and induce the levels and activities of hepatic cytochrome P450s of the CYP2B and CYP2C families as well as the activity of epoxide hydratase (EH) (340, 359). Urinary excretion of DMBA and its metabolites is also increased by consumption of sobrerol (340). Paradoxically, limonene and sobrerol increased formation of DMBA 3,4-dihydrodiol, which is considered by many to represent the proximate carcinogen of DMBA (359). Although these data indicate that limonene modulates the activities of phase I metabolizing enzymes, the relationship between these enzymes and the anticancer effects of this monoterpene are not clear.

Consumption of diets containing limonene and sobrerol resulted in increased activities of the phase II enzymes GST and uridine diphosphoglucuronsyl transferase (UDPGT) in the liver (360). Consequently, the investigators suggested that induction of phase II enzymes may be responsible for much of the anticancer actions of these monoterpenes during initiation of mammary tumorigenesis by DMBA.

ACKNOWLEDGMENTS

The authors appreciate the excellent secretarial and word processing support provided by Ms. Mary Doty, the editing assistance of Ms. Robin Amerine, and generation of structures for figures by Dr. Barry Gold.

REFERENCES

1. Weindruch R, Albanes D, Kritchevsky D. Hematol Oncol Clin North Am 1991;5:79–89.
2. Klurfeld DM, Welch CB, Davis MJ, et al. J Nutr 1989; 119:286–91.
3. Kritchevsky D. Mutat Res Fundam Mol Mech Mutagen 1993;290:63–70.
4. Fu PP, Dooley KL, Von Tungeln LS, et al. Carcinogenesis 1994;15:159–61.
5. Birt DF, Kris ES, Luthra R. Modification of murine skin tumor promotion by dietary energy and fat. In: Mukhtar H, ed. Skin cancer: mechanisms and human relevance. Boca Raton, FL: CRC Press, 1995;371–81.
6. Kritchevsky D, Welch CB, Klurfeld DM. Nutr Cancer 1989;12:259.
7. Birt DF, Pelling JC, Anderson J, et al. Carcinogenesis 1994;15:2341–5.
8. Engelman RW, Day NK, Good RA. Cancer Res 1994;54: 5724–30.
9. Wachsman JT. Mutat Res Fundam Mol Mech Mutagen 1996;350:25–34.
10. Loft S, Velthuis-te Wierik EJM, Van den Berg H, et al. Cancer Epidemiol Biomarkers Prev 1995;4:515–29.
11. Manjgaladze M, Chen S, Frame LT, et al. Mutat Res 1993; 295:201–22.
12. Pashko LL, Schwartz AG. Carcinogenesis 1992;13:1925–8.
13. Kennedy SH, Brown GM, McVey G, et al. Biol Psychiatry 1991;30:216–24.
14. Pashko LL, Schwartz AG. Carcinogenesis 1996;17:209–12.
15. Slaga TJ, Lichti U, Hennings H, et al. J Natl Cancer Inst 1978;60:425–31.
16. Birt DF, Copenhaver J, Pelling JC, et al. Carcinogenesis 1994; 15:2727–32.
17. Blumberg PM, Acs G, Areces LB, et al. Prog Clin Biol Res 1994;387:3–19.
18. Robertson NM, Bodine PVN, Hsu T-C, et al. Cancer Res 1995;55:548–56.
19. James SJ, Muskhelishvili L. Cancer Res 1994;54:5508–10.
20. Grasl-Kraupp B, Bursch W, Ruttkay-Nedecky B, et al. Proc Natl Acad Sci USA 1994;91:9995–9.
21. Lee S, Christakos S, Small MB. Curr Biol 1993;5:286–91.
22. Moriguchi S, Toba M, Kishino Y. J Nutr Sci Vitaminol 1989;35: 49–59.
23. Mizutani H, Engelman RW, Kurata Y, et al. J Nutr 1994;124: 2016–23.
24. Heydari AR, Conrad CC, Richardson A. J Nutr 1995;125: 410–8.
25. Rose DP. Adv Exp Med Biol 1994;364:1–10.
26. Reddy BS. Lipids 1992;27:807–13.
27. Birt DF, Roebuck BD. In: Ip C, Birt DF, Mettlin C, et al, eds. Dietary fat and cancer. New York: Alan R Liss, 1986;331–55.
28. Rose DP, Connolly JM. Lipids 1992;27:798–803.
29. Ip C, Carter CA, Ip MM. Cancer Res 1985;45:1997–2001.
30. Ip C. Prev Med 1993;22:728–37.
31. Mathias MM, Dupont J. Lipids 1979;14:247–52.
32. Reddy BS. Cancer Metastasis Rev 1994;13:285–302.
33. Newmark HL, Lipkin M, Maheshwari N. J Natl Cancer Inst 1990;82:491–6.
34. Lok E, Ratnayake WMN, Scott FW, et al. Carcinogenesis 1992; 13:1735–41.
35. Rao CV, Reddy BS. Carcinogenesis 1993;14:1327–33.
36. Russell DH. Drug Metab Rev 1985;16:1–88.
37. Megosh L, Gilmour SK, Rosson D, et al. Cancer Res 1995;55: 4205–9.
38. Ames BN, Gold LS. Proc Natl Acad Sci USA 1990;87:7772–6.
39. Nishizuka Y. Cancer 1989;63:1892–903.
40. Choe M, Kris ES, Luthra R, et al. J Nutr 1992;122:2322–9.
41. Nishizuka Y. FASEB J 1995;9:484–96.
42. Weinstein IB. Cancer Res 1991;51(Suppl):5080s–5s.
43. Pickering JS, Lupton JR, Chapkin RS. Cancer Res 1995; 55:2293–8.
44. Lafave LMZ, Kumarathasan P, Bird RP. Lipids 1994;29: 693–700.
45. Davidson LA, Lupton JR, Jiang Y-H, et al. J Nutr 1995; 125:49–56.
46. Etkind PR, Qiu L, Lumb K. Nutr Cancer 1995;24:13–21.
47. Lu J, Jiang C, Fontaine S, et al. Nutr Cancer 1995;23:283–90.
48. Pariza MW, Ha YL, Benjamin H, et al. Adv Exp Med Biol 1991;289:269–72.
49. Ha YL, Grimm NK, Pariza MW. Carcinogenesis 1987;8: 1881–7.
50. Shantha NC, Crum AD, Decker EA. J Agric Food Chem 1994;42:1757–60.
51. Ha YL, Storkson J, Pariza MW. Cancer Res 1990;50:1097–101.
52. Ip C, Chin SF, Scimeca JA, et al. Cancer Res 1991;51:6118–24.
53. Ip C, Scimeca JA, Thompson H. Nutr Cancer 1995;24:241–7.
54. Garland CF, Garland FC. Int J Epidemiol 1980;9:227–31.
55. Garland CF, Garland FC, Gorham ED. Am J Clin Nutr 1991; 54(Suppl):193S–201S.
56. Bostick RM, Potter JD, Sellers TA, et al. Am J Epidemiol 1993; 137:1302–17.
57. Kampman E, Van't Veer P, Hiddink GJ, et al. Int J Cancer 1994;59:170–6.
58. Braun MM, Helzlsouer KJ, Hollis BW, et al. Am J Epidemiol 1995;142:608–11.
59. Hanchette CL, Schwartz GG. Cancer 1992;70:2861–9.
60. Berger U, Wilson P, McClelland RA, et al. J Clin Endocrinol Metab 1988;67:607–13.
61. Minghetti PP, Norman AW. FASEB J 1988;2:3043–53.
62. Kleibeuker JH, Cats A, Van der Meer R, et al. Dig Dis 1994; 12:85–97.
63. Kleibeuker JH, Van der Meer R, De Vries EGE. Eur J Cancer [A] 1995;31A:1081–4.
64. Lipkin M, Newmark H. N Engl J Med 1985;313:1381–4.
65. Steinbach G, Morotomi M, Nomoto K, et al. Cancer Res 1994; 54:1216–9.
66. Govers MJAP, Termont DSML, Van der Meer R. Cancer Res 1994;54:95–100.
67. Newmark HL, Lipkin M. Cancer Res 1992;52(Suppl): 2067s–70s.
68. Richter F, Newmark HL, Richter A, et al. Carcinogenesis 1995;16:2685–9.
69. Khan N, Yang K, Newmark H, et al. Carcinogenesis 1994; 15:2645–8.
70. Welsh J. Biochem Cell Biol 1994;72:537–45.
71. Park K, Bae H, Heydemann A, et al. Cancer Res 1994;54: 6087–9.

72. Beaty MM, Lee EY, Glauert HP. J Nutr 1993;123:144–52.
73. Carroll KK, Jacobson EA, Eckel LA, et al. Am J Clin Nutr 1991;54(Suppl):206S–8S.
74. Copeland DH, Salmon WD. Am J Pathol 1946;22:1059–79.
75. Ghoshal AK, Farber E. Carcinogenesis 1984;5:1367–70.
76. Zeisel SH. Adv Exp Med Biol 1995;369:175–84.
77. Committee on Diet and Health. Nutrient assessment. In: Food and Nutrition Board, ed. Diet and health: implications for reducing chronic disease risk. Washington, DC: National Academy of Sciences Press, 1989;41–84.
78. Freudenheim JL, Graham S, Marshall JR, et al. Int J Epidemiol 1991;20:368–74.
79. Giovannucci E, Stampfer MJ, Colditz GA, et al. J Natl Cancer Inst 1993;85:875–84.
80. James SJ, Cross DR, Miller BJ. Carcinogenesis 1992;13: 2471–4.
81. James SJ, Miller BJ, McGarrity LJ, et al. Cell Prolif 1994; 27:395–406.
82. James SJ, Basnakian AG, Miller BJ. Cancer Res 1994;54: 5075–80.
83. Christman JK, Sheikhnejad G, Dizik M, et al. Carcinogenesis 1993;14:551–7.
84. Pogribny IP, Basnakian AG, Miller BJ, et al. Cancer Res 1995;55:1894–901.
85. Branda RF, Blickensderfer DB. Cancer Res 1993;53:5401–8.
86. Ghoshal AK, Farber E. Lab Invest 1993;68:255–60.
87. Zeisel SH. FASEB J 1993;7:551–7.
88. Blusztajn JK, Zeisel SH. FEBS Lett 1989;243:267–70.
89. Da Costa K-A, Garner SC, Chang J, et al. Carcinogenesis 1995;16:327–34.
90. Nelson RL, Davis FG, Sutter E, et al. J Natl Cancer Inst 1994; 86:455–60.
91. Creasey WA. Diet and cancer. Philadelphia: Lea & Febiger, 1985.
92. Selby JV, Friedman GD. Int J Cancer 1988;41:677–82.
93. Van der Merwe. Gastroenterol Forum 1990;1:7–16.
94. Rustgi VK. Gastroenterol Clin North Am 1987;16:545–51.
95. Gangaidzo IT, Gordeuk VR. Gut 1995;37:727–30.
96. Bacon BR. N Engl J Med 1992;326:126–7.
97. Stal P, Hultcrantz R, Moller L, et al. Hepatology 1995; 21:521–8.
98. Brock JH. The biology of iron. In: de Sousa M, Brock JH, eds. Iron in immunity, cancer and inflammation. 3rd ed. New York: John Wiley & Sons, 1989;35–53.
99. Knekt P, Reunanen A, Takkunen H, et al. Int J Cancer 1994;56:379–82.
100. Reddel RR, Hedley DW, Sutherland RL. Exp Cell Res 1985; 161:277–84.
101. Eriksson LC, Torndal UB, Andersson GN. Carcinogenesis 1986;7:1467–74.
102. Stal P. Dig Dis 1995;13:205–22.
103. Halliwell B, Gutteridge JM. Biochem J 1984;219:1–14.
104. Halliwell B, Gutteridge JMC, Cross CE. J Lab Clin Med 1992; 119:598–620.
105. Ullah A, Shamsuddin AM. Carcinogenesis 1990;11:2219–22.
106. Sussman HH. Pathobiology 1992;60:2–9.
107. Block G, Patterson B, Subar A. Nutr Cancer 1992;18:1–29.
108. Peto R, Doll R, Buckley JD, et al. Nature 1981;290:201–8.
109. Zheng W, Blot WJ, Diamond EL, et al. Cancer Res 1993; 53:795–8.
110. Byers T, Guerrero N. Am J Clin Nutr 1995;62:1385S–92S.
111. Ocke MC, Kromhout D, Menotti A, et al. Int J Cancer 1995;61:480–4.
112. Bertram JS, Kolonel LN, Meyskens FL. Cancer Res 1987;47:3012–31.
113. Kune GA, Kune S, Field B, et al. Nutr Cancer 1993;20:61–70.
114. Blot WJ, Li JY, Taylor PR, et al. J Natl Cancer Inst 1993;85:1483–92.
115. Heinonen OP, Albanes D. N Engl J Med 1994;330:1029–35.
116. Omenn GS, Goodman GE, Thornquist MD, et al. N Engl J Med 1996;334:1150–5.
117. Murakoshi M, Nishino H, Satomi Y, et al. Cancer Res 1992;52:6583–7.
118. Nishino H. J Cell Biochem [Suppl] 1995;22:231–5.
119. Wattenberg LW. Chemoprevention of cancer. Cancer Res 1985;45:1–8.
120. Palozza P, Luberto C, Ricci P, et al. Arch Biochem Biophys 1996;325:145–51.
121. Palozza P, Krinsky NI. Methods Enzymol 1992;213:401–84.
122. Krinsky NI. Annu Rev Nutr 1993;13:561–87.
123. Mobarhan S, Bowen P, Andersen B, et al. Nutr Cancer 1990; 14:195–206.
124. Burr ML, Samloff IM, Bates CJ, et al. Br J Cancer 1987;56: 163–7.
125. Cahill RJ, O'Sullivan KR, Mathias PM, et al. Gut 1993;34:963–7.
126. Paganelli GM, Biasco G, Brandi G, et al. J Natl Cancer Inst 1992;84:47–51.
127. Wang W, Higuchi CM. Cancer Lett 1995;98:63–9.
128. Mirvish SS. J Natl Cancer Inst 1983;71:629–47.
129. Prasad KN, Edwards-Prasad J. J Am Coll Nutr 1990;9:28–34.
130. Mobarhan S. Nutr Rev 1994;52:102–5.
131. Hong WK, Endicott J, Itri LM, et al. N Engl J Med 1986;315: 1501–5.
132. Hong WK, Lippman SM, Itri LM, et al. N Engl J Med 1990; 323:795–801.
133. Clark LC. Fed Proc 1985;44:2584–9.
134. Clark LC, Cantor KP, Allaway WH. Arch Environ Health 1991;46:37–42.
135. Nakadaira H, Endoh K, Yamamoto M, et al. Arch Environ Health 1995;50:374–80.
136. Vinceti M, Rovesti S, Gabrielli C, et al. J Clin Epidemiol 1995;48:1091–7.
137. Clark LC, Graham GF, Crounse RG, et al. Nutr Cancer 1984; 6:13–21.
138. Clark LC, Combs GF Jr, Turnbull BW, et al. JAMA 1996;276:1957–63.
139. Colditz GA. JAMA 1996;276:1984–5.
140. Guo WD, Hsing AW, Li JY, et al. Int J Epidemiol 1994;23:1127–32.
141. van Noord PAH, Maas MJ, Van der Tweel I, et al. Breast Cancer Res Treat 1993;25:11–9.
142. Buell DN. Semin Oncol 1983;10:311–21.
143. Reddy BS, Upadhyaya P, Simi B, et al. Anticancer Res 1994; 14:2509–14.
144. Sunde RA. Annu Rev Nutr 1990;10:451–74.
145. Ip C, Hayes C, Budnick RM, et al. Cancer Res 1991;51:595–600.
146. Ip C, Ganther HE. Relationship between the chemical form of selenium and anticarcinogenic activity. In: Wattenberg L, Lipkin M, Boone CW, et al., eds. Cancer chemoprevention. Boca Raton, FL: CRC Press, 1992;479–88.
147. Krishnaswamy K, Prasad MPR, Krishna TP, et al. Oral Oncol Eur J Cancer 1995;31B:41–8.
148. Prasad MPR, Mukundan MA, Krishnaswamy K. Oral Oncol Eur J Cancer 1995;31B:155–9.
149. Szarka CE, Grana G, Engstrom PF. Curr Probl Cancer 1994;18:6–79.
150. Liu JZ, Gilbert K, Parker HM, et al. Cancer Res 1991;51: 4613–7.
151. Kise Y, Yamamura M, Kogata M, et al. Int J Cancer 1990;46:95–100.

152. Birt DF, Julius AD, Runice CE, et al. J Natl Cancer Inst 1986; 77:1281–6.
153. Birt DF, Julius AD, Runice CE, et al. Nutr Cancer 1988;11: 21–33.
154. Ip C, el Bayoumy K, Upadhyaya P, et al. Carcinogenesis 1994;15:187–92.
155. el Bayoumy K, Chae YH, Upadhyaya P, et al. Cancer Res 1992;52:2402–7.
156. Ip C, Lisk DJ, Scimeca JA. Cancer Res 1994;54:1957s–9s.
157. Ip C, Lisk DJ. Carcinogenesis 1994;15:1881–5.
158. Ip C, Lisk DJ, Stoewsand GS. Nutr Cancer 1992;17:279–86.
159. Middleton E. Trends Pharmacol Sci 1984;5:335–8.
160. Hertog MGL, Hollman PCH, van de Putte B. J Agric Food Chem 1993;41:1242–8.
161. Hertog MGL, Hollman PCH, Katan MB. J Agric Food Chem 1992;40:2379–83.
162. Stavric B. Clin Biochem 1994;27:245–8.
163. Czeczot H, Tudek B, Kusztelak J, et al. Mutat Res 1990; 240:209–16.
164. Edenharder R, von Petersdorff I, Rauscher R. Mutat Res 1993;287:261–74.
165. Kuo ML, Lee KC, Lin JK. Mutat Res 1992;270:87–95.
166. Birt DF, Walker B, Tibbels MG, et al. Carcinogenesis 1986; 7:959–63.
167. Kato R, Nakadate T, Yamamoto S, et al. Carcinogenesis 1983; 4:1301–5.
168. Deschner EE, Ruperto J, Wong G, et al. Carcinogenesis 1991;12:1193–6.
169. Deschner EE, Ruperto JF, Wong GY, et al. Nutr Cancer 1993;20:199–204.
170. Kawamori T, Tanaka T, Hara A, et al. Cancer Res 1995;55:1277–82.
171. Pereira MA, Barnes LH, Rassman VL, et al. Carcinogenesis 1994;15:1049–54.
172. Kandaswami C, Perkins E, Soloniuk DS, et al. Cancer Lett 1991;56:147–52.
173. Wei H, Tye L, Bresnick E, et al. Cancer Res 1990;50:499–502.
174. Birt DF, Mitchell D, Gold B, et al. Anticancer Res 1997;17:85–92.
175. Lee SJ, Choi JH, Son KH, et al. Life Sci 1995;57:551–8.
176. Kuo M-L, Lin J-K, Huang T-S, et al. Cancer Lett 1994;87:91–7.
177. Kuo ML, Yang NC. Biochem Biophys Res Commun 1995;212: 767–5.
178. Constantiou A, Mehta R, Runyan C, et al. Surg Oncol 1994;1: 2–3.
179. Chaumontet C, Bex V, Gaillard-Sanchez I, et al. Carcinogenesis 1994;15:2325–30.
180. Cholbi MR, Paya M, Alcaraz MJ. Experientia 1991;47:195–9.
181. Fuchs J, Milbradt R. Arzneimittelforschung 1993;43:370–2.
182. Tordera M, Ferrandiz ML, Alcaraz MJ. Z Naturforsch C 1994; 49:235–40.
183. Matsukawa Y, Marui N, Sakai T, et al. Cancer Res 1993; 53:1328–31.
184. Yoshida M, Yamamoto M, Nikaido T. Cancer Res 1992;52: 6676–81.
185. Hosokawa N, Hosokawa Y, Sakai T, et al. Int J Cancer 1990;45:1119–24.
186. Sato F, Matsukawa Y, Matsumoto K, et al. Biochem Biophys Res Commun 1994;204:578–84.
187. Lepley DM, Li BY, Birt DF, et al. Carcinogenesis 1996;17: 2367–75.
188. Losiewicz M, Carlson B, Kaur G, et al. Biochem Biophys Res Commun 1995;201:589–95.
189. Wei Y-Q, Kariya Y, Fukata H, et al. Cancer Res 1994;54: 4952–7.
190. Hollman PCH, De Vries JHM, Van Leeuwen SD, et al. Am J Clin Nutr 1995;62:1276–82.
191. Li B, Birt DF. Pharmaceutical Res 1996;13:1710–5.
192. Messina MJ, Persky V, Setchell KDR, et al. Nutr Cancer 1994;21:113–31.
193. Cassidy A, Bingham S, Setchell K. Br J Nutr 1995;74:587–601.
194. Nomura A, Henderson BE, Lee J. Am J Clin Nutr 1978;31: 2020–5.
195. Hirayama T. A large scale cohort study on cancer risks by diet—with special reference to the risk of reducing effects of green-yellow vegetable consumption. In: Hayashi Y, et al. eds. Diet, nutrition and cancer. Tokyo: VNU Scientific Press, 1986;41–53.
196. Lee HP, Gourley L, Duffy SW, et al. Lancet 1991;337:1197–200.
197. Hirayama T. Natl Cancer Inst Monogr 1979;53:149–55.
198. Severson RK, Nomura AMY, Grove JS, et al. Cancer Res 1989;49:1857–60.
199. Barnes S, Grubbs C, Setchell KDR, et al. Prog Clin Biol Res 1990;347:239–53.
200. Barnes S, Peterson G, Grubbs C, et al. Adv Exp Med Biol 1994;354:135–47.
201. Hawrylewicz EJ, Huang HH, Blair WH. J Nutr 1991;121: 1693–8.
202. Baggott JE, Ha T, Vaughn WH, et al. Nutr Cancer 1990;14: 103–9.
203. Carroll KK. Cancer Res 1975;35:3374–83.
204. Lamartiniere CA, Moore J, Holland M, et al. Proc Soc Exp Biol Med 1995;208:120–3.
205. Russo J, Russo IH. Role of differentiation of transformation of human breast epithelial cells. In: Medina D, Kidwell W, Heppner G, et al, eds. Cellular and molecular biology of mammary cancer. New York: Plenum Press, 1987;399–417.
206. Wang W, Tanaka Y, Han Z, et al. Nutr Cancer 1995;23:131–40.
207. Peterson G, Barnes S. Biochem Biophys Res Comm 1991;179: 661–7.
208. Pagliacci MC, Smacchia M, Migliorati G, et al. Eur J Cancer 1994;30A:1675–82.
209. Hoffman R. Biochem Biophys Res Comm 1995;211:600–6.
210. Welshons WV, Rottinghaus GE, Nonneman DJ, et al. J Vet Diagn Invest 1990;2:268–73.
211. Mäkelä S, Davis VL, Tally WC, et al. Environ Health Perspect 1994;102:572–8.
212. Sathyamoorthy N, Wang TTY, Phang JM. Cancer Res 1994; 54:957–61.
213. Naik HR, Lehr JE, Pienta KJ. Anticancer Res 1994;14: 2617–20.
214. Folman Y, Pope GS. J Endocr 1969;44:213–8.
215. Shutt DA, Cox RI. J Endocrinol 1972;52:299–310.
216. Miksicek RJ. J Steroid Biochem Mol Biol 1994;49:153–60.
217. Cassidy A, Bingham S, Setchell KDR. Am J Clin Nutr 1994; 60:333–40.
218. Murkies AL, Lombard C, Strauss BJG, et al. Maturitas 1995;21:189–95.
219. Baird DD, Umbach DM, Lansdell L, et al. J Clin Endocrinol Metab 1995;80:1685–90.
220. Faber KA, Hughes CL Jr. Biol Reprod 1991;45:649–53.
221. Levy JR, Faber KA, Ayyash L, et al. Proc Soc Exp Biol Med 1995;208:60–6.
222. Mousavi Y, Adlercreutz H. Steroids 1993;58:301–4.
223. Adlercreutz CHT, Goldin BR, Gorbach SL, et al. J Nutr 1995;125(Suppl):757S–70S.
224. Adlercreutz H, Fotsis T, Lampe J, et al. Scand J Clin Lab Invest 1993;53(Suppl 215):5–18.
225. Adlercreutz H, Höckerstedt K, Bannwart C, et al. J Steroid Biochem 1987;27:1135–44.

226. Adlercreutz H, Bannwart C, Wähälä K, et al. J Steroid Biochem Mol Biol 1993;44:147–53.
227. Campbell DR, Kurzer MS. J Steroid Biochem Mol Biol 1993;46:381–8.
228. Wang C, Mäkelä T, Hase T, et al. J Steroid Biochem Mol Biol 1994;50:205–12.
229. Mäkelä S, Poutanen M, Lehtimäki J, et al. Proc Soc Exp Biol Med 1995;208:51–9.
230. Akiyama T, Ishida J, Nakagawa S, et al. J Biol Chem 1987; 262:5592–5.
231. Barnes S, Peterson TG. Proc Soc Exp Biol Med 1995;208: 103–8.
232. Linassier C, Pierre M, Le Pecq J-B, et al. Biochem Pharmacol 1990;39:187–93.
233. Peterson TG, Barnes S. Prostate 1993;22:335–45.
234. Abler A, Smith JA, Randazzo PA, et al. J Biol Chem 1992; 267:3946–51.
235. Okura A, Arakawa H, Oka H, et al. Biochem Biophys Res Comm 1988;157:183–9.
236. Markovits J, Linassier C, Fossé P, et al. Cancer Res 1989;49: 5111–7.
237. Yamashita Y, Kawada S-Z, Nakano H. Biochem Pharmacol 1990;39:737–44.
238. Kroemer G, Petit P, Zamzami N, et al. FASEB J 1995;9: 1277–87.
239. Vaux DL. Proc Natl Acad Sci USA 1993;90:786–9.
240. King KL, Cidlowski JA. J Cell Biochem 1995;58:175–80.
241. Osborne BA, Schwartz LM. Trends Cell Biol 1994;4:394–9.
242. Traganos F, Ardelt B, Halko N, et al. Cancer Res 1992; 52:6200–8.
243. Gorczyca W, Gong J, Ardelt B, et al. Cancer Res 1993;53: 3186–92.
244. Constantinou A, Huberman E. Proc Soc Exp Biol Med 1995;208:109–15.
245. Constantinou A, Kiguchi K, Huberman E. Cancer Res 1990;50:2618–24.
246. Honma Y, Okabe-Kado J, Kasukabe T, et al. Jpn J Cancer Res 1990;81:1132–6.
247. Kondo K, Tsuneizumi K, Watanabe T, et al. Cancer Res 1991;51:5398–404.
248. Jing Y, Nakaya K, Han R. Anticancer Res 1993;13:1049–54.
249. Fotsis T, Pepper M, Adlercreutz H, et al. Proc Natl Acad Sci USA 1993;90:2690–4.
250. Hammerschmidt PA, Pratt DE. J Food Sci 1978;43:556–9.
251. Wei H, Bowen R, Cai Q, et al. Proc Soc Exp Biol Med 1995; 208:124–30.
252. Cassady JM, Zennie TM, Chae Y-H, et al. Cancer Res 1988;48:6257–61.
253. Chae Y-H, Coffing SL, Cook VM, et al. Carcinogenesis 1991;12:2001–6.
254. Francis AR, Shetty TK, Bhattacharya RK. Carcinogenesis 1989;10:1953–5.
255. Giri AK, Lu L-JW. Cancer Lett 1995;95:125–33.
256. Adlercreutz H. Scand J Clin Lab Invest 1990;50(Suppl 201):3–23.
257. Stitch SR, Toumba JK, Groen MB, et al. Nature 1980;287:740–2.
259. Setchell KDR, Borriello SP, Gordon H, et al. Lancet 1981;2:4–7.
260. Adlercreutz H, Fotsis T, Heikkinen R, et al. Lancet 1982; 2:1295–9.
261. Dehennin L, Reiffsteck A, Jondet M, et al. J Reprod Fertil 1982;66:305–9.
262. Wilcox G, Wahlqvist ML, Burger HG, et al. Br Med J 1990;301:905–6.
263. Waters AP, Knowler JT. J Reprod Fertil 1982;66:379–81.
264. Whitten PL, Russell E, Naftolin F. Steroids 1992;57:98–106.
265. Whitten PL, Naftolin F. Steroids 1992;57:56–61.
266. Whitten PL, Russell E, Naftolin F. Steroids 1994;59:443–9.
267. Verdeal C, Brown RR, Richardson T, et al. J Natl Cancer Inst 1980;64:285–90.
268. Shemesh M, Lindner HR, Ayalon N. J Reprod Fertil 1972; 29:1–9.
269. Martin PM, Horwitz KB, Ryan DS, et al. Endocrinology 1978;103:1860–7.
270. Welshons WV, Murphy CS, Koch R, et al. Breast Cancer Res Treat 1987;10:169–75.
271. Mousavi Y, Adlercreutz H. J Steroid Biochem Mol Biol 1992;41:615–9.
272. Hirano T, Fukuoka K, Oka K, et al. Cancer Invest 1990; 8:595–602.
273. Thompson LU, Robb P, Serraino M, et al. Nutr Cancer 1991;16:43–52.
274. Clapp RC, Long L Jr, Dateo GP, et al. J Am Chem Soc 1959;81:6278–81.
275. Dunnick JK, Prejean JD, Jaseman J, et al. Fundam Appl Toxicol 1982;2:114–20.
276. Zhang Y, Talalay P, Cho C, et al. Proc Natl Acad Sci USA 1992;89:2399–403.
277. Chung FL, Morse MA, Eklind KI, et al. Cancer Epidemiol Biomarkers Prev 1992;1:383–8.
278. Hecht SS. J Cell Biochem Suppl 1995;22:195–209.
279. Lacassagne A, Hurst L, Xuong MD. C R Soc Biol 1970; 164:230–3.
280. Chung FL, Morse MA, Eklind KI. Cancer Res 1992;52: 2719s–22s.
281. Zhang Y, Talalay P. Cancer Res 1994;54(Suppl):1976s–81s.
282. Zhang Y, Kensler TW, Cho C, et al. Proc Natl Acad Sci USA 1994;91:3147–50.
283. Wattenberg LW. J Natl Cancer Inst 1977;58:395–8.
284. Morse MA, Zu H, Galati AJ, et al. Cancer Lett 1993;72:103–10.
285. Stoner GD, Siglin JC, Morse MA, et al. Carcinogenesis 1995;16:2473–6.
286. Rao CV, Rivenson A, Simi B, et al. Cancer Res 1995;55:4311–8.
287. Hasegawa T, Nishino H, Iwashima A. Anticancer Drugs 1993;4:273–9.
288. Chung F-L, Wang M, Hecht SS. Carcinogenesis 1985;6: 539–43.
289. Sugie S, Yoshimi N, Okumara A, et al. Carcinogenesis 1993; 14:281–3.
290. Guo Z, Smith TJ, Thomas PE, et al. Cancer Res 1991;51: 4798–803.
291. Smith TJ, Guo Z, Li C, et al. Cancer Res 1993;53:3276–82.
292. Guo Z, Smith TJ, Wang E, et al. Carcinogenesis 1992;13: 2205–10.
293. Smith TJ, Guo ZY, Guengerich FP, et al. Carcinogenesis 1996;17:809–13.
294. Barcelo S, Gardiner JM, Gescher A, et al. Carcinogenesis 1996;17:277–82.
295. Caporaso N, Whitehouse J, Monkman S, et al. Pharmacogenetics 1994;4:275–80.
296. Sparnins VL, Wattenberg LW. J Natl Cancer Inst 1981;66: 769–71.
297. Spencer SR, Xue L, Klenz EM, et al. Biochem J 1991;273:711–7.
298. Kolm RH, Danielson UH, Zhang Y, et al. Biochem J 1995; 311:453–9.
299. Yu R, Jiao JJ, Duh JL, et al. Cancer Res 1996;56:2954–9.
300. Block E. Sci Am 1985;252:114–9.
301. Fenwick GR, Hanley AB. Crit Rev Food Sci Nutr 1985;22: 199–271.

302. Weisberger AS, Pensky J. Cancer Res 1958;18:1301–8.
303. Han J. Prev Med 1993;22:712–22.
304. Haenszel W, Kurihara M, Segi M, et al. J Natl Cancer Inst 1972;49:969–88.
305. Buiatti E, Palli D, Decarli A, et al. Int J Cancer 1989;44:611–6.
306. Tajima K, Tominaga S. Jpn J Cancer Res 1985;76:705–16.
307. Liu J, Lin RI, Milner JA. Carcinogenesis 1992;13:1847–51.
308. Amagase H, Milner JA. Carcinogenesis 1993;14:1627–31.
309. Amagase H, Schaffer EM, Milner JA. J Nutr 1996;126:817–24.
310. Pereira MA, Khoury MD. Cancer Lett 1991;61:27–33.
311. Sumiyoshi H, Wargovich MJ. Cancer Res 1990;50:5084–7.
312. Wargovich MJ, Imada O, Stephens LC. Cancer Lett 1992; 64:39–42.
313. Takada N, Matsuda T, Otoshi T, et al. [Published erratum appears in Cancer Res 1995;55(11):2484.] Cancer Res 1994;54:2895–9.
314. Guengerich FP. Cancer Res 1988;48:2946–54.
315. Chengelis CP, Neal RA. Biochem Pharmacol 1987;36:363–8.
316. Sparnins VL, Barany G, Wattenberg LW. Carcinogenesis 1988;9:131–4.
317. Chasseaud LF. Adv Cancer Res 1979;29:175–274.
318. Unnikrishnan MC, Kuttan R. Cancer Lett 1990;51:85–9.
319. Unnikrishnan MC, Soudamini KK, Kuttan R. Nutr Cancer 1990;13:201–7.
320. Katiyar SK, Mukhtar H. Int J Oncol 1996;8:221–38.
321. Goldbohm RA, Hertog MGL, Brants HAM, et al. J Natl Cancer Inst 1996;88:93–100.
322. Gao YT, McLaughlin JK, Blot WJ, et al. J Natl Cancer Inst 1994;86:855–8.
323. Sazuka M, Murakami S, Isemura M, et al. Cancer Lett 1995; 98:27–31.
324. Wang ZY, Huang M-T, Lou Y-R, et al. Cancer Res 1994;54: 3428–35.
325. Cao J, Xu Y, Chen JS, et al. Fundam Appl Toxicol 1996;29: 244–50.
326. Khan SG, Katiyar SK, Agarwal R, et al. Cancer Res 1992; 52:4050–2.
327. Pingzhang Y, Jinying Z, Shujun C, et al. Cancer Lett 1994;79:33–8.
328. Shi ST, Wang Z-Y, Smith TJ, et al. Cancer Res 1994;54:4641–7.
329. Katiyar SK, Agarwal R, Ekker S, et al. Carcinogenesis 1993; 14:361–5.
330. Katiyar SK, Rupp CO, Korman NJ, et al. J Invest Dermatol 1995;105:394–8.
331. Wattenberg LW. Cancer Res 1983;43(Suppl):2448s–53s.
332. Elegbede JA, Elson CE, Qureshi A, et al. Carcinogenesis 1984; 5:661–4.
333. Elson CE, Maltzman TH, Boston JL, et al. Carcinogenesis 1988;9:331–2.
334. Maltzman TH, Hurt LM, Elson CE, et al. Carcinogenesis 1989;10:781–3.
335. Elegbede JA, Elson CE, Tanner MA, et al. J Natl Cancer Inst 1986;76:323–5.
336. Jirtle RL, Haag JD, Ariazi EA, et al. Cancer Res 1993;53: 3849–52.
337. Knabbe C, Lippman ME, Wakefield LM, et al. Cell 1987;48: 417–28.
338. Chander SK, Lansdown AGB, Luqmani YA, et al. Br J Cancer 1994;69:879–82.
339. Russin WA, Hoesly JD, Elson CE, et al. Carcinogenesis 1989; 10:2161–4.
340. Crowell PL, Kennan WS, Haag JD, et al. Carcinogenesis 1992;13:1261–4.
341. Haag JD, Gould MN. Cancer Chemother Pharmacol 1994; 34:477–83.
342. Wattenberg LW, Sparnins VL, Barany G. Cancer Res 1989;49:2689–92.
343. Homburger F, Treger A, Boger E. Oncology 1971;25:1–10.
344. Roe FJC, Peirce WEH. J Natl Cancer Inst 1960;24:1389–403.
345. Elegbede JA, Maltzman TH, Verma AK, et al. Carcinogenesis 1986;7:2047–9.
346. Van Duuren BL, Goldschmidt BM. J Natl Cancer Inst 1976;56:1237–42.
347. Gould MN, Wacker WD, Maltzman TH. Chemoprevention and chemotherapy of mammary tumors by monoterpenoids. In: Anonymous ed. Mutagens and carcinogens in the diet. Wiley-Liss, 1990;255–68.
348. Mills JJ, Chari RS, Boyer IJ, et al. Cancer Res 1995;55:979–83.
349. Stark MJ, Burke YD, McKinzie JH, et al. Cancer Lett 1995;96:15–21.
350. Hursting SD, Perkins SN, Haines DC, et al. Cancer Res 1995;55:3949–53.
351. Crowell PL, Elson CE, Bailey HH, et al. Cancer Chemother Pharmacol 1994;35:31–7.
352. Zarbl H, Sukumar S, Arthur AV, et al. Nature 1985;315:382–5.
353. Jackson JH, Cochrane CG, Bourne JR, et al. Proc Natl Acad Sci USA 1990;87:3042–6.
354. Crowell PL, Chang RR, Ren Z, et al. J Biol Chem 1991;266: 17679–85.
355. Crowell PL, Lin S, Vedejs E, et al. Cancer Chemother Pharmacol 1992;31:205–12.
356. Crowell PL, Ren Z, Lin S, et al. Biochem Pharmacol 1994; 47:1405–15.
357. Gelb MH, Tamanoi F, Yokoyama K, et al. Cancer Lett 1995;91:169–75.
358. Ruch RJ, Sigler K. Carcinogenesis 1994;15:787–9.
359. Maltzman TH, Christou M, Gould MN, et al. Carcinogenesis 1991;12:2081–7.
360. Elegbede JA, Maltzman TH, Elson CE, et al. Carcinogenesis 1993;14:1221–3.

SELECTED READINGS

Hecht SS. Chemoprevention by isothiocyanates. J Cell Biochem Suppl 1995;22:195–209.

Katiyar SK, Mukhtar H. Tea in chemoprevention of cancer: epidemiologic and experimental studies (review). Int J Oncol 1996;8:221–38.

Kleibeuker JH, Cats A, Van der Meer R, et al. Calcium supplementation as prophylaxis against colon cancer. Dig Dis 1994;12:85–97.

Knekt P, Reunanen A, Takkunen H, et al. Body iron stores and risk of cancer. Int J Cancer 1994;56:379–82.

Krinsky NI. Actions of carotenoids in biological systems. Annu Rev Nutr 1993;13:561–87.

Mason JB. Folate and colonic carcinogenesis: searching for a mechanistic understanding. J Nutr Biochem 1994;5:170–5.

Messina MJ, Persky V, Setchell KDR, et al. Soy intake and cancer risk: a review of the in vitro and in vivo data. Nutr Cancer 1994;21:113–31.

82. Nutritional Support of the Cancer Patient

MAURICE E. SHILS and MOSHE SHIKE

The designation cancer includes many disease conditions characterized by growth of cells that have lost their usual growth regulation and thus multiply and spread. The localized and/or distant spread interferes with the function of adjacent organs and often has detrimental systemic effects. Potent factors produced by tumor cells or by other body cells in reaction to the cancer may also have profound local and systemic effects.

HEALTH BURDEN OF CANCER

This chapter reviews the many effects of malignant diseases on the nutritional state of the patient and the roles of diet and nutrition in the management of such patients. The genetic basis of cancer is reviewed in Chapter 78 and the contributions of diet to cancer development and its prevention are reviewed in Chapter 79; chemoprevention of cancer is considered in Chapter 81.

Mortality from Cancer

The estimated number of deaths from cancer in 1996 in the United States was 554,740, up from 331,000 in 1970 and 514,000 in 1991 (1). The total number of deaths from cancer was second only to that from cardiovascular disease (2), but this gap has been narrowing for both men and women in the United States (3) (Table 82.1). This trend is attributable to the continuing decline in deaths from ischemic heart disease and stroke. Mortality rates from cancer in the United States in persons below the age of 45 and especially below 20 years decreased markedly for men and women (4) but were more than made up by mortality in older groups prior to 1990. In 1992, cancer accounted for 23.9% of all deaths, compared with 33% of deaths from heart disease (2).

Death rates from cancer at common anatomic sites at intervals from 1930 to 1992 are presented in Figure 82.1 for females and males. The striking changes over the 7 decades have been the dramatic rise in death from lung cancer and the marked decline in mortality from gastric and uterine (predominantly cervical) malignancies. The rise in lung cancer deaths has been caused primarily by cigarette smoking, while the decline in uterine cancer mortality is attributed to early detection by widespread screening with the Papanicolaou (Pap) smear. The reasons for the decrease in gastric cancer mortality, seen throughout the world, are not completely clear. Improvements in food refrigeration and decline in use of salt, nitrates, and nitrites for food preservation are thought to have played an important role.

After decades of steady increase, the age-adjusted mortality due to cancer has recently declined, as shown by recent data based on the Surveillance, Epidemiology and End Results Program (SEER) of the National Cancer Institute. This program collects incidence and survival data on cancer from five states (Connecticut, Hawaii, Iowa, New Mexico, and Utah) and four metropolitan areas (Detroit, Atlanta, San Francisco-Oakland, and Seattle-Puget Sound).

The American Cancer Society applies incidence rates from SEER for 1979–93 to the estimated total U.S. pop-

Table 82.1
Comparative Mortality in the United States from Cancer, Ischemic Heart Disease (IHD), and Stroke in 1955 and 1986

		Men		Women	
Cause	Year	Percentage of All Deaths	Probability of Dying from Cause (%)	Percentage of All Deaths	Probability of Dying from Cause (%)
Cancer	1955	14.5	14.6	17.5	15.5
	1986	22.7	22.5	21.9	19.5
IHD	1955	33.1	35.8	27.9	32.3
	1986	24.8	26.4	24.6	26.5
Stroke	1955	9.6	11.1	13.7	15.7
	1986	5.4	6.0	9.0	9.9

Data from Lopez AD. Ann NY Acad Sci 1990;609:70, 72 (Tables 1 and 2).

ulation (e.g., for 1996) to give current incidence rates. These rates indicate that cancer mortality declined by 3.1% between 1990 and 1995 (5), mainly because of a decrease of 3.9% in lung cancer deaths and 2% in other smoking-related cancers. The overall decrease of 3.1% has been credited to cancer prevention activities (e.g., decreased cigarette smoking, earlier detection) and improved therapies. The changes have been greatest among children and adults under 55 years of age (6). Using data from other sources, it has been estimated that cancer mortality on an age-related basis decreased by 1.0% between 1991 and 1994 (6).

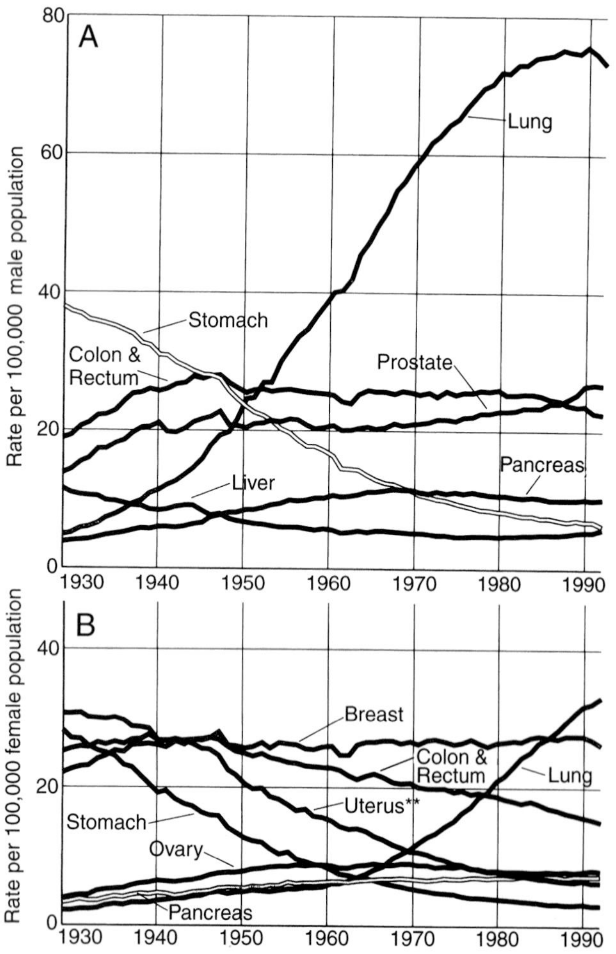

Figure 82.1. Changes in cancer mortality in the United States in males (**A**) and females (**B**) between 1930 and 1992. (From Anon. Cancer facts and figures, 1996. Atlanta, GA: American Cancer Society, 1996, with permission.)

Table 82.2
1996 Incidence, 5-Year Survival and Death Rates of Specific Cancers in the United States

Cancer Site	Incidence	5-Year Survival (%)	Annual Death (1996)
Lung	177,000	13.4	158,700
Colorectal	133,500	61	54,100
Breast	185,700	83.2	44,560
Prostate	317,000	85.8	41,400
Pancreatic	26,300	3.6	27,800
Non-Hodgkin's Lymphoma	52,700	51	23,300
Leukemia	27,600	Variable[a]	21,000
Ovarian	26,700	44.1	14,800

Data compiled from Anon. Cancer facts and figures, 1996. Atlanta, GA: American Cancer Society, 1996.

[a]Varies from 68.6% for chronic lymphatic leukemia and 11.4% for acute myelocytic leukemia.

The incidence, 5-year survival, and annual 1996 estimated death rates for the eight major cancers are listed in Table 82.2. Treatment of some neoplasms including testicular cancer and some forms of leukemia and lymphoma has been very successful; however, in most common cancers (lung, breast, colorectal), treatments have had moderate or no success. Primary prevention measures such as avoidance of smoking and sun exposure, diet modification, control of infection, and moderation in alcohol use have decreased cancer incidence and mortality (7, 8). Significant progress in secondary prevention by detecting and removing premalignant or early cancerous lesions can improve cure and survival rates and decrease mortality. Thus, Pap smears for detection of in situ cervical cancer and mammography for detection of breast cancer are effective early measures for reducing mortality from female cancers. Fecal occult blood testing and sigmoidoscopy can detect polyps and early cancers in the colon, and their removal reduces colon cancer mortality.

PREVALENCE AND SIGNIFICANCE OF MALNUTRITION

An involuntary weight loss of more than 10% in the cancer patient—especially when rapid—is generally agreed to be cause for concern and is frequently an independent risk factor for survival (9). In quantitative terms, the degree of undernutrition at which survival is minimal is associated with a corrected muscle area of 9 to 11 cm^2 in cancer patients (10). The degree and prevalence of malnutrition, if any, in cancer patients depend on tumor type and stage, the organs involved, the types of anticancer therapy used, and patient response. Concurrent nonmalignant conditions such as diabetes and intestinal diseases can be important contributing factors.

Determining the true prevalence of malnutrition can

be difficult because it depends on the sensitivity and specificity of the parameters used for nutritional assessment (Chapters 54–56) and because of the lack of universal agreement on the validity of these parameters. Most studies in cancer patients used weight loss as the primary nutritional assessment criterion and found that between 40 and 80% of patients suffer from malnutrition (11).

The prevalence of weight loss during the 6 months preceding the diagnosis of cancer was reported from a multicenter cooperative study of patients with 12 types of cancer (9). The lowest frequency (31–40%) and severity of weight loss were found in patients with breast cancer, hematologic cancers, and sarcomas. Intermediate frequency (54–64%) of weight loss was found in patients with colon, prostate, and lung cancers. Patients with gastrointestinal (GI) cancers (pancreas and stomach) had the highest frequency (over 80%) and severity of weight loss, with more than one-quarter of the patients presenting with weight loss exceeding 10% of body weight. The study did not report on patients with esophageal or head and neck cancers, in whom weight loss is also very frequent and severe because of dysphagia (12). Other studies revealed that over 40% of patients undergoing medical treatment for cancer were malnourished (11, 13).

Breast cancer is usually associated with relatively little or no weight loss when it is confined or metastatic to the bones only (9). In a study of 923 women newly diagnosed with breast cancer and without metastases, 13% were undernourished, 42.4% were at their desired weight, 22.1% were overweight, and 22.4% were obese. Obesity at time of diagnosis was associated with an increased risk for recurrence (14).

Among surgical patients in VA hospitals, 39% of those undergoing a major operation for cancer were malnourished, as judged by either a nutritional risk index or a combination of weight loss and low serum proteins (15). In patients with early pancreatic cancer deemed suitable for curative resection, malnutrition was common, with weight loss up to 22% of body weight and an average of 6.3% (16). As noted above, patients with more-advanced pancreatic cancer present with more-severe malnutrition and weight loss (9). The degree of malnutrition among children admitted to the hospital with malignant diseases was similar to that seen in children with benign diseases (17, 18). In a prospective study, children with newly diagnosed cancer were commonly malnourished with a significantly reduced food intake (19).

Malnutrition may have a major clinical impact on the cancer patient and is associated with increased morbidity and mortality, first pointed out in a report by Warren in 1932 (20). Studying data from autopsies, Warren concluded that cachexia was the leading cause of death among patients with various cancers. More-recent studies have confirmed the association of malnutrition with poor prognosis and quality-of-life of the cancer patient. In the aforementioned multicenter cooperative study of patients receiving chemotherapy (9), those who had experienced weight loss prior to diagnosis had decreased performance status and survival compared with those without weight loss. In a study of patients with limited, inoperable lung cancer, weight loss was a major predictor of survival (13).

The negative impact of malnutrition was also demonstrated in surgical patients with malignant diseases. Malnourished patients undergoing a major operation were at greater risk for postoperative infectious and noninfectious morbidity and mortality than well-nourished patients (15). In patients with cancer of the esophagus, significant weight loss was associated with increased postoperative morbidity including higher rates of anastomotic leak and infection (21). Analysis of prognostic factors for survival in patients with cancer of the head and neck (stages 3 and 4) undergoing chemotherapy revealed that pretreatment weight loss was the strongest predictor of survival (18). Patients with no weight loss had a median survival of 44.3 months, compared with 10.6 months for patients with more than 10% weight loss. The extent of weight loss in these patients was also a significant negative predictor of decreased performance status.

These studies do not establish a clear causal relationship between malnutrition and poor outcome. It is reasonable to suppose that a poor nutritional state is an independent prognostic factor for a poor outcome, but malnutrition may merely indicate a more serious type and stage of illness rather than causing a poor outcome. A few studies have attempted to isolate the effect of malnutrition from the direct effects of the disease (9, 22). Without a clear demonstration that reversal of malnutrition independently improves the outcome, it is hard to establish it as an independent factor in the course of the disease. However, one *must* appreciate that in a particular patient, various ill effects result from malnutrition and will respond to nutritional support.

EFFECTS OF CANCER ON NUTRITIONAL STATUS

Malignancies can induce a number of adverse changes in nutritional status (Table 82.3). An understanding of these changes provides the basis for evaluating their causes and for planning and providing support when indicated. Malignant tumors can produce signs and symptoms at the site of the original tumor or distally, by metastasis. In addition, humoral factors produced by cells of the immune or neuroendocrine system exert local or distant effects termed *paraneoplastic syndromes*.

Anorexia, Wasting, and Other Paraneoplastic Effects

Loss of appetite (anorexia) in patients with various cancers occurs as a manifestation of a systemic effect but also as a consequence of infection, surgery, radiation, chemotherapy, or other medications. It is often intensified by fear and depression. Although anorexia is not unique

Table 82.3
Nutritional Problems Associated with the Presence of Neoplastic Disease

Anorexia with progressive weight loss and undernutrition
Taste changes causing depressed or altered food intake
Alterations in protein, carbohydrate, and fat metabolism
Increased energy expenditure despite weight loss
Impaired food intake and malnutrition secondary to
  Mechanical bowel obstruction at any level
  Intestinal dysmotility induced by various tumors, particularly lung cancer
Malabsorption associated with
  Deficiency or inactivation of pancreatic enzymes
  Deficiency or inactivation of bile salts
  Failure of food to mix with digestive enzymes (e.g., enzyme dilution, pancreaticocibal asynchrony)
  Fistulous bypass of small bowel
  Infiltration of small bowel wall or lymphatics and mesentery by malignant cells
  Blind loop syndrome with depressed gastric secretion or partial upper small bowel obstruction leading to bacterial overgrowth
  Malnutrition-induced villous hypoplasia in the small intestine
Protein-losing enteropathy
Metabolic abnormalities induced by tumor-derived eutopic hormones
  Hypercalcemia induced by parathyroid hormone–like polypeptides, osteolytic processes, increased calcitriol
  Osteomalacia with hypophosphatemia often associated with depressed serum calcitriol
  Hypoglycemia induced by insulin-secreting tumors
  Hyperglycemia, e.g., with islet glucagonoma or somatostatinoma
Anemia of chronic blood loss and bone marrow suppression
Electrolyte and fluid problems with
  Persistent vomiting with intestinal obstruction or intracranial tumors
  Intestinal fluid losses through fistulas or diarrhea
  Intestinal secretory abnormalities with hormone-secreting tumors (e.g., carcinoid syndrome, Zollinger-Ellison syndrome [gastrinoma], Verner-Morrison syndrome [VIPoma], increased calcitonin, villous adenoma)
  Inappropriate antidiuretic hormone secretion associated with certain tumors (e.g., lung carcinomas)
  Hyperadrenalism with tumors producing corticotropin or corticosteroids
Miscellaneous organ dysfunction with nutritional implications (e.g., intractable gastric ulcers with gastrinomas, Fanconi's syndrome with light-chain disease, coma with brain tumors)
Tumor products stimulating monocyte production of various interleukins (see text)

to cancer, its high incidence and severity in certain types of malignancies can contribute to significant weight loss.

Onset of anorexia and weight loss may be insidious and may not be accompanied by specific disease manifestations. A dictum of medicine states that the patient with an unexplained weight loss should be examined for an occult neoplasm. Detailed initial medical evaluation usually reveals the cause (23).

Cancer-induced anorexia appears to be a general phenomenon exhibited by humans and other tumor-bearing species. Anorexia in these species, as in humans, is not necessarily induced by all tumor types. A comparison of the reactions of rats to transplanted tumors of different types is instructive (24). A Leydig's cell–derived tumor (LTW) caused early anorexia and growth failure when transplanted in young rats. A breast carcinosarcoma, however, was not associated with significant anorexia; tumor and host grew almost until death. Parabiotic studies were performed in which two rats were subcutaneously attached so that a small persistent blood exchange occurred. In each pair, one rat had either the LTW or the breast tumor type and the other had no tumor. Attached cancer-free rats served as controls. Over time, none of the rats with breast cancer lost weight (as expected), and neither did their parabiotic non-tumor-bearing partners. In contrast, the rats with the LTW tumor lost weight (as expected), and their parabiotic non-tumor-bearing partners also lost significant weight. Such general results have been observed by others (25).

Such studies suggest that one or more mediators from anorexia-inducing tumors can (directly or indirectly) act on the neuroendocrine system to affect food intake adversely and to induce metabolic changes characterized as paraneoplastic syndromes. Data derived from laboratory animals with a variety of transplanted human tumor cells and from cancer patients indicate that the mediators differ among tumors and that tumor burden is not necessarily correlated with degree of wasting and other effects. The nature of the mediators and their mechanisms of action are the focus of much current research as indicated below in the section on mediators of metabolic changes affecting nutritional status.

Energy Expenditure

Because patients with cancer tend to lose weight, some at a relatively early stage, many measurements of resting energy expenditure (REE) have been performed to determine whether increased REE is a possible causative factor. One type of study compared the daily REE of cancer patients as measured by indirect calorimetry with values predicted by the Harris-Benedict equation. Some investigators noted a hypermetabolic rate (i.e., 10% above the predicted value) in varying degrees (26, 27). Others found that the daily REEs of patients with GI cancer were variable, with some patients hypometabolic, some normometabolic, and some hypermetabolic (28, 29). Still others found no difference in the REEs of patients with colon and rectal cancer (30).

More-relevant data have been obtained by making direct comparisons between cancer patients with different degrees of weight loss and those with nonmalignant diseases having similar weight changes.

Alimentary Tract Tumors. The data on REE are contradictory. Investigators reported a small absolute increase in REE in patients with GI cancer who were losing weight, compared with patients without malignant disease ($P < .05$) (31); the presence of liver metastases or more extensive disease increased the REE (31). Other studies found no increase (30, 32, 33). Patients with similar cancers and weight loss (average, 17%) had a significantly higher daily REE than patients with benign disease who had lost a similar percentage of weight. This relationship held true when REE was expressed per kilogram per day or per millimole of total body potassium (34). Regardless of the presence of weight loss, the cancer patients had similar daily REEs and REEs per kilogram, but the REE in relation to total body potassium was higher in those who had lost weight (34).

Other studies have found no significant differences in REE between patients with gastric or colorectal cancer and an average loss of 18% body weight and those with benign gastric diseases and an average loss of 16% body weight, whether the loss was expressed in $kg^{0.75}$/day, kg/day, or kg lean body mass (LBM)/day (32). When a relatively large group of patients with colon and non-small-cell lung cancer with some weight loss were compared with malnourished patients without cancer and with healthy volunteers, no difference appeared in their daily REE/kg LBM (34). No significant difference existed among weight-losing or weight-stable patients with gastric or colon cancer or among weight-losing patients with benign GI diseases in their REE per day, per kilogram body weight, or per kilogram fat-free mass (FFM) (36). Patients who were in a semistarving condition with localized resectable esophageal cancer had an REE/kg body weight similar to that of better-nourished controls admitted for minor surgery (37). In contrast, cachectic patients with pancreatic cancer had an increased REE (38). Weight-stable patients with cancer and healthy volunteers had a significantly higher ($P < .001$) total daily REE than weight-losing patients with cancer or GI diseases, but no difference in REE existed among any groups in relation to body weight or FFM (33).

Sarcomas. In patients with bony and soft tissue sarcoma, those with localized tumor and a 7.2% average weight loss had a total daily REE similar to that of age- and sex-matched controls; also, the REE/$kg^{0.75}$/day was not different (39). Four of these patients had diffuse disease and a 15.4% mean weight loss; their total daily REE was the same as that of the other two groups, but their REE/kg/day and REE/$kg^{0.75}$/day were increased. Tumor resection led to a postoperative fall in REE (39).

Several groups noted that the Harris-Benedict equation tended to underestimate the REE/day for weight-losing cancer patients (32, 34). On the other hand, Fredrix et al. concluded that this equation overestimated energy expenditure in all groups studied, with or without cancer and weight losing or weight stable (33). They found that the current FAO/WHO/UNU prediction equation reduced the predicted number of "hypermetabolic" patients (40).

Although some controlled studies indicated increased REE in patients with cancer, especially those with weight loss, the differences among patients with and without cancer were not marked, and some studies indicated no differences. Furthermore, expressing data in terms of weight or LBM tends to eliminate or decrease differences. However, some weight-losing cancer patients maintain their preweight-loss level of energy expenditure in contrast to otherwise healthy, semistarving, weight-losing individuals, who decrease their energy expenditure (41).

Further insight into the question of energy expenditure is provided by examining cancer patients for evidence of an inflammatory response to their cancer. Cachectic pancreatic cancer patients had appreciably higher REE per kilogram body cell mass than age-matched healthy controls; REE was even greater in patients with an acute-phase response (APR) (38). Similarly, among 87 patients with primary non-small-cell lung cancer, 67 had increased REE. This response was positively correlated with increased APR and with other evidence of a systemic inflammatory response, including elevated levels of IL-6 and soluble tumor necrosis factor (TNF) receptors as well as weight loss (42).

Carbohydrate Metabolism

Glucose intolerance has been noted frequently in patients with cancer (43); it may be mild in early stages, and it increases with tumor burden (Table 82.4). This glucose intolerance results from increased insulin resistance to both exogenous and endogenous insulin and perhaps from inadequate insulin release. This may be nonspecific in part, because such nontumor factors as weight loss, bed rest, and sepsis cause similar changes in other diseases (44).

Gluconeogenesis and Glucose Turnover and Disappearance

The reports of an increased rate of endogenous glucose production in cancer patients are numerous. Tumor type, stage, and histology influence the rate. This increased production, combined with other changes in carbohydrate metabolism, is associated with weight loss (41, 43–45). In contrast, weight loss caused by uncomplicated starvation is associated with reduced glucose turnover (46). Rates of glucose and urea turnover and glucose oxidation have been determined in normal volunteers, in a group of patients with early GI (colon) cancer, and in those with advanced GI (esophagus, stomach, pancreas) cancer (47). Basal rates of glucose turnover were similar in the normal and early cancer groups but were significantly higher in the advanced cancer group. The glucose oxidation rate increased progressively in proportion to tumor burden (23.9% for controls, 32.8% for early tumors, and 43.0% for advanced tumors). After curative resection in the early tumor groups, glucose use decreased significantly.

Table 82.4
Carbohydrate Metabolism Abnormalities Associated with Advanced Cancer

Glucose intolerance
Insulin resistance
Abnormal insulin secretion
Delayed glucose clearance
Increased glucose production
Increased glucose turnover
Variably increased Cori cycle activity

In those with early and advanced GI cancer, glucose production was suppressed with glucose infusion by 76 and 69%, respectively, whereas in normal volunteers, glucose production was almost completely suppressed (94%) (47). Glucose infusion significantly suppressed urea turnover in the healthy control group but did not induce a significant decrease in the high-urea-turnover advanced-tumor group (47). Glucose turnover rates in patients with sarcoma and leukemia have been 2 to 3 times those of normal volunteers; on the other hand, no difference from the normal rate was observed in patients with lymphoma (48). Glucose infusion into patients with sarcoma and leukemia suppressed hepatic glucose production by less than one-third (48).

Cori Cycling. In the Cori cycle, glucose released by peripheral tissues is metabolized to lactate, which is then resynthesized to glucose in the liver (46, 49–51). An increased rate of Cori cycling has been reported in cancer patients. The process consumes energy because six adenosine triphosphate molecules (ATP) are required for glucose resynthesis, whereas only two are produced in the glycolytic cycle; hence, the term *futile cycle.* If anaerobic glycolysis by tumor cells with release of lactate is substantial, a considerable amount of energy would be consumed by Cori cycling of lactate in the liver. Hence, increased Cori cycling could theoretically be a significant factor in the development of weight loss from diminished energy production. Increased cycle activity has been noted in patients with metastatic disease and progressive weight loss but not in patients with cancer and stable weight (49). Cycling was significantly higher in patients with cancer—fasting or fed—than in patients without cancer but with a similar degree of weight loss (50).

The source of recycled lactate that accompanies accelerated Cori cycling in human cancer cachexia has not been completely elucidated (44). Earlier work focused on glucose consumption by the tumor with lactate formation because glucose use by the tumor can be substantial. A massive tumor, however, would be required to consume the amount of glucose reportedly used; such a size is unusual for most human tumors of the type often associated with cancer cachexia (45). More-recent reports have emphasized release of lactate from glucose recycling in peripheral tissues (45). The quantitative significance of Cori cycling to cancer wasting is uncertain (50, 51).

Information on the relation of lactate production to weight loss is gained from comparison of two experimental colonic tumors. When transplanted into the animal host (52), tumor Mac 13 consumed much more glucose than Mac 16 did; however, both tumors were the largest glucose consumers after the brain. Although Mac 13 used glucose at a greater rate than Mac 16, Mac 13 did not induce cachexia whereas Mac 16 did. In this model, at least, increased glucose oxidation and lactate production by the tumor were divorced from cachexia and from glucose use by normal tissues.

Lipid Metabolism

Many reports have stated that the major portion of weight loss in many cancer patients is attributable to fat depletion (43, 53, 54). Fat metabolism abnormalities in cancer patients are listed in Table 82.5.

Fat Mobilization

Fat from adipose tissue is mobilized in the fasting state by the action of specific lipases that eventually complete the lipolytic conversion of triglycerides to free fatty acids and glycerol. The lipase that releases the first fatty acid, triglyceride lipase, is regulated by various circulating hormones, some of which, especially catecholamines, are stimulatory, whereas insulin is antilipolytic. In the nonfasting state, fatty acids are derived from chylomicrons and very low density lipoprotein (VLDL) under the influence of lipoprotein lipase (LPL).

Klein and Wolfe (55) have reviewed mechanisms that may increase lipolytic rates in cancer patients: decreased food intake, weight loss, stress response to illness with adrenal medullary stimulation and increased circulating catecholamine levels, insulin resistance, and release of lipolytic factors produced by the tumor itself or by myeloid tissue cells. Hence, these mechanisms must be controlled insofar as possible to delineate the role of the tumor per se (55). The evidence for an increased lipolytic rate is contradictory. Weight loss per se in the absence of cancer has been associated with increased lipolytic rate. Other reports concerning whole-body lipolytic rates in patients with cancer vary; rates were normal in some and increased in others (55).

Body fat is lost when both lipolysis and fatty acid oxidation are increased. Increased lipolysis without a corresponding increase in fatty acid oxidation increases triglyceride–fatty acid cycling; that is, released fatty acids are subsequently reesterified to triglyceride. Although this cycle does not increase net flux of reactants, the reaction requires energy. β-Adrenergic activity stimulates both lipolysis and triglyceride–fatty acid recycling in burn patients (56); serious undernutrition may be such a stimulus as well (55).

In laboratory animal models with transplanted tumors, including those in the genetically abnormal nude mouse, carcass lipid depletion occurs with varying degrees of tumor burden (57). Assays showed that urine and plasma from mice and human subjects with cancer cachexia had higher lipid-metabolizing activity than urine and plasma from either normal controls or volunteers after a period of acute starvation (58).

Table 82.5
Fat Metabolism Abnormalities Associated with Advanced Cancer

Excess body fat depletion relative to protein loss
Increased lipolysis, free fatty acids, and glycerol turnover
Decreased lipogenesis
Hyperlipidemia

Hyperlipidemia

Elevated lipid levels usually are not marked in cancer patients but do occur in association with certain tumors. One mechanism for this elevation is decreased LPL activity, which has been noted in rodents bearing transplanted tumors and in patients with lung cancer. The lowest levels of LPL activity in lung cancer patients were associated with the greatest weight loss. Patients with breast cancer had normal LPL and minimal weight loss (59).

Fat Oxidation

The considerable literature reporting that fat is oxidized at an increased rate in patients with cancer has been summarized (43). Fat oxidation rates were higher and carbohydrate oxidation rates were lower in those patients with cancer (colorectal and gastric) who had lost significant weight than in patients with cancer who had not lost weight or in patients with benign disease who had lost weight (32).

Protein Metabolism (Table 82.6)

The rates of whole-body protein turnover and the synthetic and catabolic rates of muscle protein increase with advancing stage of disease and its clinical expression of weight loss (60–62). Whole-body protein turnover increased 50% or more in patients with small-cell sarcoma (62) and 50 to 70% in those with lung and colorectal cancer (35). On the other hand, subpopulations of patients exist with turnover rates varying from increased to normal. In malnourished cancer patients, providing nutrition by the intravenous route did not reverse the increased turnover rate (63). Whole-body protein turnover was 32 and 35% greater in a group of malnourished untreated cancer patients without liver metastasis than in malnourished patients with benign disease and in healthy subjects starved for 10 days, respectively (64). Thus, patients with cancer and weight loss usually have increased protein turnover, synthesis, and proteolysis in contrast to the reduced rates that are the normal adaptive response to acute malnutrition in benign disease states.

By the use of labeled leucine during intraoperative periods, no significant differences were noted in whole-body protein synthesis, whole-body protein catabolism, net protein catabolism, or albumin fractional synthesis rates between groups of patients with benign disease who had maintained weight and those with cancer who had also maintained weight (65). In contrast, patients with cancer cachexia (e.g., 15% weight loss) had significantly elevated whole-body protein catabolism, somewhat elevated whole-body protein synthesis, and an increased net protein catabolic rate. They also had significantly higher fractional synthetic rates in skeletal muscle, liver, and albumin. It was concluded that patients with cancer cachexia were actively losing protein as a result of increased whole-body protein catabolism that was only partially compensated for by increased whole-body protein synthesis. Protein fractional synthetic rates did not significantly differ in the primary tumors of those patients, with or without weight loss.

Table 82.6
Abnormalities in Protein Metabolism Associated with Advanced Cancer

Increased whole-body protein turnover
Increased protein fractional synthetic rates in liver
Reduced fractional synthetic rates in muscle
Increased hepatic protein synthesis
Persistent muscle protein breakdown
Decreased plasma branched-chain amino acids

A key question is the nature of the catabolic pathway(s) involved in such proteolysis in muscle. One pathway is lysosomal energy-dependent proteolysis, another involves calcium-dependent proteases, and a third is the ubiquitin-proteasome-dependent pathway (66). Skeletal muscle from rats with hepatoma had a higher proteolytic rate during in vitro incubation than muscle from non-tumor-bearing control animals. The first two pathways mentioned were not affected, but ATP-dependent proteases were involved, and ubiquitin conjugates were increased in skeletal muscle of tumor-bearing rats. Thus, the ubiquitin-protease-dependent pathway seems to play a role in cancer-related muscle wasting (67).

Cancer patients who have lost significant weight often have protein kinetics similar to those of traumatized or infected individuals, including mobilization of skeletal muscle protein with an efflux of amino acids from peripheral stores to liver and increased urinary nitrogen excretion (68, 69) (see also Chapter 96). The same changes are noted in animal tumor models (68).

Organ imaging in a small sample of patients with cancer cachexia indicated that liver size has been spared, presumably as the result of transfer of nitrogen to the liver (70). Patients with cancer and serious weight loss had significantly decreased percentage of lean body mass, while the percentage of nonmuscle lean body mass (i.e, visceral protein) rose markedly (54). The patients had an average total weight loss of 15.2 kg over a 6-month period, which represented loss of 7.4 kg of body water, 6.2 kg of fat, and 1.6 kg of protein (71).

Taste and Appetite Changes

Many patients ascribe diminished appetite and food intake to unpleasant and unacceptable alterations in the taste of foods. Anatomic, physiologic, and other factors affecting taste and smell are complex (see Chapter 42), as are those regulating food intake (reviewed in [72] and Chapter 40). Earlier studies of altered taste in patients with cancer used the method of detecting the lowest perceptible solution concentration of sodium chloride (salt), hydrochloric or citric acid (sour), urea (bitter), and sucrose (sweet). This method has been criticized, and forced-choice methods, although more time consuming, have been recommended to eliminate some response biases (73).

An early paper in this field (74) noted that 25 of 50 patients with metastatic carcinoma of various primary sites stated that food didn't taste as good. This change was associated with an elevated taste threshold for sweetness (i.e., food tasted less sweet) and a lowered taste threshold for bitterness (74). Subsequent papers have challenged the concept of a consistent pattern of altered taste (75, 76); others have found no abnormalities (77, 78). While such findings on taste are inconsistent with respect to pattern, altered responses to the taste of foods are frequent. When such responses cause rejection of nutritious foods, they contribute to anorexia and decreased intake. Physicians and dietitians should ascertain the food preferences and dislikes of their individual patients and develop appropriate menus based on their responses.

Learned Food Aversions

The impact on appetite of fear and uncertainty engendered by the diagnosis of cancer and the stress of diagnostic procedures is exacerbated by the physiologic and metabolic effects of various antitumor interventions. One aspect of these stresses is so-called learned or conditioned food aversion, which stems from unconscious or conscious association (by person or laboratory animal) of consumption of a particular food with a concurrent or subsequent unpleasant reaction, such as nausea or vomiting. The result is avoidance of that food. In cancer patients, unpleasant reactions may be associated with antitumor therapy, such as a chemotherapeutic drug or ionizing radiation. Children who were to be given anticancer drugs that induced nausea or vomiting were tested for learned food aversion: the test group was offered an unusual flavor of ice cream shortly before drug administration, while controls were given ice cream, but not of this flavor. When tested later for aversion to the unusually flavored ice cream, controls chose it three times more frequently than did the experimental groups (79). Such studies were extended to include adult patients.

The possible role of learned food aversions in tumor-bearing animals was based on the hypothesis that tumor-bearing rats would avoid foods associated with aversive physiologic effects of the tumor itself without any relation to treatment. The results have been variable and have depended, in part, on the tumor and diets tested (80, 81).

Conditioned food preferences and aversions are discussed in Chapter 40, with reference to neural pathways. The conditioned aversion associated with cancer chemotherapy depends on a serotonergic mechanism, because 5-HT_3 antagonists abolish it (82). The neural pathways that mediate learned aversions depend on both forebrain and hindbrain interactions (83, 84).

MEDIATORS OF METABOLIC CHANGES AFFECTING NUTRITIONAL STATUS

The deleterious effects on nutritional status that occur when malignancy reaches a certain critical stage are summarized above. This section summarizes current information on specific factors that may cause such paraneoplastic changes: various hormones, cytokines (also called interleukins and, in the Japanese literature, toxohormones), and related growth factors. A later section considers the effectiveness of nutritional intervention in reversing these paranoeplastic changes in tumor growth and in host response.

Cytokines and Growth Factors

Laboratory Animal Research

Efforts to delineate a specific role for certain hormones known to reduce appetite (e.g., cholecystokinin [85] or serotonin [86]) in tumor-induced anorexia and weight loss have been unsuccessful. More recently, attention has been directed to polypeptides (cytokines and growth factors) derived from mononuclear blood cells (lymphocytes and macrophages) under the influence of tumor-derived substances. These factors provide communication between cells that influences their proliferation, differentiation, and metabolism. Individual cytokines can influence other cytokines in activated blood cells. Their production and activation is also influenced by neuroendocrine secretions (e.g., glucocorticoids and catecholamines). Certain cytokines are produced also in response to infection or trauma; these "proinflammatory" cytokines include TNF-α), interleukin-6 (IL-6), and interferon-α (INF-α). Their regulation involves antiinflammatory cytokines (e.g., IL-10) that decrease secretion of proinflammatory cytokines and suppress macrophage and T-cell functions.

Much attention was directed to studies of TNF-α as a factor in wasting following the initial studies of Cerami and associates, who noted wasting of body proteins and fat in association with anorexia and suppression of LPL in rabbits infected with *Trypanosoma brucei* (reviewed in ref. 87).

More-recent animal studies have revealed a more complex situation, namely, other mediators may be present in larger amounts than TNF-α, and the presence and levels of such mediators vary with specific tumors. In addition to TNF-α, IL-6, INF-α and leukemia-inhibitory factor (LIF) are produced by some cachexia-inducing human cancer cell lines, which may act indirectly by inhibiting LPL (88). In nude mice transplanted with any single one of eight human cancer cell lines from widely divergent tissues, all of which induced cachexia, two had elevated IL-6, two had elevated LIF, and one had elevated LIF, IL-6, and IL-11; the three others had no increase in measured cytokines. mRNA for the *ob* gene was not expressed in any of these cell lines that induced wasting (89). Normal mice injected with leptin or rats with continuously high leptin levels had severe depletion of fat stores (90). IL-6 injected into mice with a cachexia-inducing subclone of an adenocarcinoma and into normal controls induced anemia, thrombocytosis, and visceral organ hypertrophy but not anorexia, body weight loss, or lymphocytopenia (91). These latter signs are characteristically observed in the cachexia-inducing subclone that enhances tumor growth and elevates IL-6 (91).

Investigation of murine adenocarcinoma MAC 16 led to isolation of a 24K proteoglycan from the host mouse splenocytes; this agent produced cachexia in vivo by inducing catabolism of skeletal muscle. It was also present in the urine of cachectic cancer patients but not in urine from patients with weight loss due to trauma and cancer patients with little or no weight loss (92).

Cachexia-inducing transplanted tumors may exert their effects through hypothalamic neuroendocrines, namely, neuropeptide Y (NPY) and corticotropin-releasing factor (CRF), which are, respectively, a stimulant and an inhibitor of feeding behavior. These neuropeptides are discussed in Chapter 40 and reference 72. In Yoshida sarcoma–bearing rats, NPY activity is impaired and CRF activity is not suppressed (93).

Clinical Studies

No significant elevations of serum TNF were found in patients with solid tumors who were without sepsis or acute parasitic infections (38, 42, 94, 95). Similarly, TNF-α and IL-1β levels were not elevated in patients with renal cell carcinoma, regardless of weight loss or fever. In contrast, IL-6 concentrations were higher in the cancer patients than in healthy individuals, and higher in those with fever or weight loss and lymph node or metastatic spread. The higher IL-6 concentrations correlated with C-reactive protein blood values (94). Elevated serum IL-6 has been related to weight loss in lung cancer patients (42) and correlated with the degree of weight loss, tumor size, tumor invasion, noncurative resectability, serum albumin and C-reactive protein levels in patients with esophageal or pancreatic cancer (96). The rise in IL-6 levels, however, was not always related to the acute-phase response (38).

Continuous infusion of low doses of recombinant human TNF into normal subjects for 4 weeks did not modify REE, body weight, serum TNF, or the level of common laboratory nutritional markers (97). Infusion of this cytokine into cancer patients for 5 days was associated with negative nitrogen balance attributed to TNF-induced anorexia rather than to a specific effect on protein metabolism (98).

Failure to observe elevated TNF levels does not necessarily signify that TNF is not involved in the wasting and other metabolic changes observed in advanced cancer. Increased production of TNF and IL-6 by peripheral mononuclear blood cells was found in patients with pancreatic cancer who had an acute-phase response, although serum TNF was not present (38). Increased soluble TNF in hypermetabolic lung cancer patients (42) suggests that local activity at the production site, without first circulating through the blood, is important in development of the hypercatabolic state.

Data from laboratory animals support the concept of local effects. A liver tumor (LIV) weighing approximately 1% of total body weight produced anorexia, weight loss, acute-phase response, and systemic cytokine responses similar to those associated with the subcutaneous (SQ) tumor weighing approximately 10% of body weight. Neither tumor-bearing group had abnormal liver function tests or evidence of obstructive biliary pathology. TNF was detected in both tumors as well as in histologically normal liver tissue remote from the tumor of the LIV group but not in livers of animals in control and SQ groups. The proximity of the tumor to the competent tissue macrophage populations, such as hepatic Kupffer cells, may suffice to induce cachexia (99).

In contrast, TNF-α levels can be very high in the serum of children with leukemias, lower in those with pediatric solid tumors (Wilms, osteosarcoma, etc.) than in healthy controls (100, 101), and decline to undetectable levels in those with complete remission (101). In adult B-cell chronic lymphocytic leukemia, TNF-α levels were high in serum, circulating monocytes, and leukemic cells (102).

Hormone- and Cytokine-Induced Paraneoplastic Syndromes

Secretion of various polypeptide hormones by a number of malignant tumors has been known for many decades to cause distinct paraneoplastic syndromes (103–105). Multiple endocrine neoplasia syndromes also occur, e.g., MEN I, II, and IIA (104a). In addition to these classic endocrine disturbances, various cytokines and growth factors are also expressed by tumors and can interact with each other.

Every known naturally occurring hormone has been reported to be produced by one or more human tumor types. Unlike the firmly regulated feedback controls of the normal endocrine system, such hormone production is more autonomous. Hence, unregulated production can have a powerful influence on adjacent and distant organs. Table 82.7 lists a number of clinical syndromes that induce hormone formation, and others are discussed below. These tumor-produced hormones were believed earlier to be abnormal with respect to source. However, many normal cells not previously considered hormone producers are now known to be capable of making small amounts of hormones (103). For example, chorionic gonadotropin made by colonic adenocarcinoma can also be produced in normal colonic mucosa; ACTH and calcitonin made "ectopically" by bronchiogenic cancer can be produced in small amounts by normal bronchial epithelial cells. Hence, tumor-derived peptide production is more appro-

Table 82.7
Clinical Syndromes That Induce Hormone Formation

Clinical Syndromes	Hormones[a]
Flushing/diarrhea	Serotonin, substance P, NKA, TCT, PP
Ulcer disease	Gastrin
Hypoglycemia	Insulin, TNF, IGF-II
Dermatosis, dementia, diabetes, deep vein thrombosis	Glucagon
Diabetes, steatorrhea, cholelithiasis	Somatostatin
Acromegaly	GHRH
Cushing's disease	ACTH/CRH
Hypercalcemia	HHM (PTHrP), PTH, VIP
Inappropriate antidiuretic hormone	Vasopressin, atrial natriuretic peptide
Pigmentation	Melanocyte-stimulating hormone
Silent vascular liver metastases	PP

Modified from Perry RR, Vinick AI. Annu Rev Med 1996;47:57–68.
[a]NKA, neurokinin A; TCT, calcitonin; PP, pancreatic polypeptide; TNF, tumor necrosis factor; IGF-II, insulin-like growth factor II; GHRH, growth hormone–releasing hormone; ACTH, adrenocorticortropic hormone; CRH, corticotrophin-releasing hormone; VIP, vasoactive intestinal polypeptide; HHM, humoral hypercalcemic factor of malignancy; PTHrP, parathyroid hormone–related protein; PTH, parathyroid hormone.

priately designated as "eutopic", that is, production is abnormal with respect to quantity but not with respect to source. Metabolic, nutritional, electrolytic, and other clinical problems can result from increased production of eutopic hormones.

Gastrointestinal Syndromes

Approximately 50% of the tumors inducing such syndromes are carcinoids, 25% are gastrinomas, 15% are insulinomas, 6% are VIPomas, 2 to 5% are glucagonomas, and less than 2.5% are a variety of rare types (104). In addition to the GI hormones listed in Table 82.7, somatostatins, enkephalins, and neurotensin may be produced. More than one can be secreted by a given tumor type, and the symptoms elicited may be intermittent and vary in severity.

The classic carcinoid syndrome (flushing and diarrhea) with elevated levels of serotonin and various peptides is associated with tumors most commonly found in the appendix and terminal ileum but can be found throughout the GI tract as well as in the pancreas and lungs. Loss of parietal cells in pernicious anemia can be associated with development of gastric carcinoid tumors (106). Secretory diarrhea occurs with *(a)* carcinoids; *(b)* VIPomas that induce the Verner-Morrison syndrome with watery diarrhea, hypokalemia, hypochlorhydria, and acidosis (107); *(c)* gastrinomas that occur in the pancreas, duodenum, and porta hepatitis and cause the Zollinger-Ellison syndrome, which is also associated with severe ulcers and steatorrhea [108]); *(d)* medullary carcinoma of the thyroid; *(e)* one type of somatostatinoma; and *(f)* secreting villous adenoma of the rectum.

Hypoglycemia from islet cell insulinomas is associated with an elevated insulin:glucose ratio and proinsulin and C-peptide levels (103). In contrast, the nonislet tumors that also induce hypoglycemia usually lack insulin. Insulin-like growth factor (IGF) II, often present in elevated amounts in this tumor and in the blood, is postulated to bind to and activate insulin receptors (105).

Some polypeptide hormones produced by tumors may have activities of other hormones because of common peptide sequences in their molecules. Many hormones produced by neuroendocrine tumors contain opioid peptide sequences. Secretion of opioid peptides has been postulated to contribute to psychiatric disturbances such as depression, mood swings, and psychosis (109).

Several drugs have proved useful in the management of some of these gut-derived endocrine tumors when resection is not feasible. Omeprazole and H_2-blocking drugs that inhibit acid secretion by the gastric mucosa can eliminate or greatly reduce the gastrin effects in the Zollinger-Ellison syndrome. When administered in several daily subcutaneous injections, the analogue of somatostatin, octreotide, has proved beneficial in suppressing endocrine secretions associated with the Verner-Morrison syndrome (VIPomas) and the carcinoid syndrome. Octreotide has also been reported of benefit with insulinomas and glucagonomas (110).

Hypercalcemia

Hypercalcemia, one of the most common metabolic complications of cancer, is probably the most common paraneoplastic syndrome. Approximately 20 to 40% of patients with breast, squamous, bladder, and renal carcinomas, multiple myeloma, and lymphomas develop hypercalcemia at some point. The total incidence of these cancer-related effects is about one-half that seen with primary hyperparathyroidism. It is steadily progressive unless treated and may be symptomatic at calcium concentrations lower than those found in hyperparathyroidism. The more common symptoms are nausea, muscle weakness, excess urinary secretion, elevated blood pressure, anorexia, lethargy, confusion, and stupor progressing to coma. The etiologies of tumor-related hypercalcemia include the following (111, 112):

1. Local osteolytic hypercalcemia. This syndrome is involved in 20 to 40% of malignancy-associated cases of hypercalcemia, primarily in breast cancer, multiple myeloma, lymphomas, and leukemias. The primary cause is tumor cell secretion of paracrine factors that stimulate nearby osteoclasts to reabsorb bone. IL-1α, IL-1β TNF-α, TNF-β and TGF-α stimulate osteoclastic bone resorption in vitro and cause hypercalcemia when infused into mice; which of these polypeptides are involved in this syndrome is not yet established (112). While serum calcium levels are elevated, serum phosphorus is normal, and PTH and calcitriol are reduced secondary to the hypercalcemia (111, 112). The herpesvirus that is associated with Kaposi's sarcoma, when present in the bone marrow dendritic cells of multiple myeloma patients, has been found to transcribe IL-6; the human homologue of IL-6 is a growth factor for multiple myeloma (113).

2. Osteoclastic bone resorption. This hypercalcemia results from discrete lytic lesions caused by bone-metastasizing solid tumors (breast, lung, and pancreatic).
3. Humeral hypercalcemia of malignancy (HHM). HHM is the dominant form of cancer-related hypercalcemia in 75–80% of such cases, mainly in squamous, renal, and urothelial malignancies (112). This syndrome of diffuse osteoclastic bone resorption is normally caused by a tumor distant from the skeleton. Although there may be tumor metastases to the bone, the generalized loss of calcium from bone results from secretion of a hormone designated PTH-related protein (PTHrP), which is related genetically to PTH but whose gene is much more complex than that of PTH (112). Its biochemical effects result from its interaction with PTH receptors in skeleton and kidneys; hence, the elevated serum calcium is associated with both a low serum phosphate and a high nephrogenous cyclic AMP; PTH and calcitriol are low, and bone formation is suppressed. Patients with HHM are typically severely hypercalcemic and in marked negative calcium balance.
4. Excessive calcitriol associated with lymphomas. Although hypercalcemia in this condition is uncommon, about 50% of hypercalciuric patients with lymphomas have elevated serum calcitriol levels (114).

There have been several cases of true ectopic PTH production in patients with lung, ovarian, and neuroectodermal cancer (112).

Syndrome of Inappropriate Antidiuretic Hormone Secretion (SIADH)

SIADH is probably the second most common endocrine-related complication in malignant conditions. It is associated primarily with the presence of small-cell carcinoma of the lung, but it may occur with intestinal and urothelial cancers. Originally, it was associated with ADH (vasopressin) excess, hence the name. Because it is now known to be associated also with production of atrial natriuretic peptide and perhaps other hormones, it might be better described as the humoral hyponatremia of malignancy (115). This syndrome with hyponatremia induced by excessive and inappropriate retention of water is discussed in Chapter 6, where it is noted that other factors also induce this syndrome, including pulmonary lesions and a variety of medications.

Osteomalacia

Certain tumors are associated with reduced plasma concentrations of calcitriol, PTH, and calcium in conjunction with hypophosphatemia, renal phosphate wasting, and normal calcidiol, thereby inducing an oncogenic osteomalacia. Approximately 50 such cases were reported as of 1986. Most reported cases have involved benign nonendocrine tumors of mesenchymal origin (e.g., hemangiopericytoma) or giant cell tumors of epithelial origin (116). In addition, hypophosphatemic osteomalacia has been noted with prostatic carcinoma (117). Muscle weakness of varying degree and variable back pain have been frequent complaints. GI malabsorption of calcium and phosphate has been observed. When resection of the tumor has been possible, serum calcitriol and phosphate levels rose within 36 hours, with subsequent correction of the bone disease (117).

LOCALIZED TUMOR EFFECTS

In addition to the systemic effects of cancer, more-localized effects of various neoplasms may lead to nutritional problems (Table 82.3).

Intestinal Obstruction

The most common direct effect of alimentary tract neoplasms on nutritional status relates to partial or complete obstruction at one or more sites. Approximately 20% of surgical hospital admissions for acute abdominal conditions are associated with intestinal obstruction; the second most common cause of obstruction in adults is neoplasm of the alimentary tract (118). Esophageal, gastric, and colorectal carcinomas are important etiologic factors in older persons. Obstructive symptoms can result from peritoneal tumor seeding and intestinal dysfunction without mechanical obstruction and may develop secondary to abdominal metastases. Acute obstruction almost always leads to immediate medical attention. Most neoplasms, however, obstruct slowly and progressively; consequently, a significant number of patients wait until one or more of their symptoms and signs (anorexia, dysphagia, weight loss, weakness, nausea, vomiting, pain, diarrhea, or anemia from chronic blood loss) cause them to seek medical care.

Malabsorption

Malabsorption occurs for numerous reasons.

Intestinal Villous Changes

Creamer (119) suggested that malignant tumors external to the gastrointestinal tract induced an abnormal intestinal mucosa with resultant malabsorption and weight loss characteristic of malignant disease. In a more definitive study, Barry (120) showed that malnourished patients with extra-alimentary-tract malignant tumors often displayed abnormal mucosal cell structure, epithelial cell loss, and decreased xylose absorption. Because he found similar changes in seriously malnourished patients without cancer, he suggested that the mucosal changes result from malnutrition rather than being a direct effect of non-GI malignant tumors (120). Once present, impaired mucosal function contributes further to malnutrition.

Blind Loop Syndrome

Blind loop syndrome occurs with partial obstruction in the small bowel, the presence of jejunal diverticula, or lack of motility in an intestinal loop. The associated overgrowth of bacteria in the small bowel may result in steatorrhea and vitamin B_{12} deficiency. Not only is there direct interaction of bacteria with certain nutrients, but resulting abnormalities of the intestinal epithelium also cause malabsorption (121). (See also Chapter 65.)

Fistula

Bypass of a significant portion of the bowel can result from fistula formation between widely separated portions of the GI tract. The degree of malabsorption depends on the site, completeness, and extent of the bypass. Severe malabsorption occurs with fistulas between stomach and large bowel (gastrocolic type), between small bowel and large bowel (enterocolic type), between small bowel and small bowel (enteroentero fistula), or from small bowel to skin (enterocutaneous fistula).

Malignancies of the Small Bowel

Malignancies of the small bowel, uncommon in the duodenum and small intestine, account for only about 1% of all malignancies of the GI tract. They may be associated with pain and bleeding (often occult, resulting in microcytic anemia), weight loss, partial obstruction, and diarrhea or steatorrhea, especially with lymphomas of the upper intestine. Celiac disease is associated with increased incidence of intestinal lymphoma and carcinoma (122, 123) (Chapter 71). A type of intestinal lymphoma in individuals in the Middle East involves the mesenteric lymph nodes, with resultant malabsorption (124).

Protein-Losing Enteropathy

Infiltration of the lamina propria and draining lymph nodes by tumor cells can lead to obstruction and dilation of the lymphatics within the intestinal villi; this, in turn, can lead to development of protein-losing enteropathy with hypoalbuminemia, hypoglobulinemia, and lymphocytopenia (125). This condition was described originally with intestinal lymphoma and gastric carcinoma but now is known to occur with tumors arising outside the alimentary tract (e.g., malignant melanoma, ovarian carcinoma, and metastatic lung carcinoma).

Anemia

Anemia occurs in cancer patients for a number of reasons. Nutritional deficiencies occur secondary to chronic blood loss (iron deficiency) and malabsorption (folic acid deficiency). However, in those with solid tumors, most anemias are normocytic and normochromic and are secondary to hemolysis, bone marrow failure, infection, or a paraneoplastic effect of a distant tumor (126).

NUTRITIONAL MANAGEMENT OF PATIENTS WITH SPECIFIC CANCERS

Reversal of the undesirable clinical, metabolic, and nutritional changes secondary to progressive systemic and localized effects of cancer depends primarily on its complete eradication or major palliation. As with all chronic wasting diseases, one cannot and should not expect to induce significant improvement in the nutritional state in a short period of time. Urgent antineoplastic treatment cannot and should not be postponed until nutritional rehabilitation is achieved. In such a situation, acute or chronic vitamin and mineral deficiencies, blood loss, and electrolyte and fluid imbalances can usually be corrected rapidly. When malnutrition is present or is a risk factor, nutritional therapy should be incorporated in the overall treatment program as early as possible.

When surgery, radiation, and/or chemotherapy are indicated for a debilitated patient who faces a further significant period of little or no voluntary oral intake, efforts to improve nutritional and metabolic status by adequate enteral (Chapter 100) or parenteral feeding (Chapter 101) may help decrease morbidity, thereby shortening the period of convalescence. The efficacy of such support is reviewed below.

Significant nutritional problems may arise not only from the local and systemic effects of the malignant condition but also from treatments undertaken to control the neoplastic process. The nutritional impact of such therapies is summarized in Table 82.8 and in the following sections.

Head and Neck Cancer

Patients with cancer of the head and neck often present with significant weight loss and malnutrition because the obstructing tumor impairs food intake. In addition, patients often have a history of chronic heavy alcohol intake and smoking; many may be nutritionally depleted prior to therapy. Treatment often involves combined surgery and radiation, with chemotherapy also used in some cases.

The overall 5-year survival rate is 52%. Radiation can induce mucositis, loss of taste ("mouth blindness"), xerostomia (dry mouth) as the result of salivary gland damage, trismus (spasm of jaw muscles) and some nerve damage, depending on the site irradiated. Injury to teeth may also occur, but this outcome can be minimized by adequate dental care. Some of these effects subside within 3 months after completion of radiotherapy, but they may persist for prolonged periods in some patients. Of 13 such patients studied 1 to 7 years after radiotherapy, 9 had measurable taste losses (especially for salt and bitter), 12 had reduced salivary flow and secretion rates, 9 complained of dry mouth, and 7 had no saliva (127).

Surgery may include partial or total glossectomy and mandibulectomy, and resection of portions of the hard or soft palate and of soft tissues of the lower face and neck. These procedures add to the difficulties in chewing and swallowing. The likelihood of chronic aspiration during swallowing may be serious enough to require tube feeding. Chemotherapy may produce serious systemic effects that can severely impair the patient's ability to ingest, digest, and absorb food (Table 82.9).

Nutritional Support

For the patient who is seriously malnourished on presentation, early nutritional intervention with appropriate

Table 82.8
Consequences of Cancer Treatment Predisposing to Nutrition Problems

Radiation treatment
- Oropharyngeal area: destruction of sense of taste; xerostomia and odynophagia; loss of teeth
- Lower neck and mediastinum: esophagitis with dysphagia; fibrosis with esophageal stricture
- Abdomen and pelvis: bowel damage (acute and chronic), with diarrhea, malabsorption, stenosis, and obstruction; fistulization

Surgical treatment
- Radical resection of oropharyngeal area
  - Chewing and swallowing difficulties
- Esophagectomy
  - Gastric stasis and hypochlorhydria secondary to vagotomy
  - Steatorrhea secondary to vagotomy
  - Diarrhea secondary to vagotomy
  - Early satiety
  - Regurgitation
- Gastrectomy (high subtotal or total)
  - Loss of reservoir and early satiety
  - Malabsorption
  - Vitamin B_{12} deficiency
  - Hypoglycemia
  - Dumping syndrome
- Intestinal resection
  - Jejunum
    - Decreased efficiency of absorption of many nutrients
  - Ileum
    - Vitamin B_{12} deficiency (terminal ileum resection)
    - Bile salt losses with diarrhea or steatorrhea
    - Hyperoxaluria and renal stone
    - Calcium and magnesium depletion
    - Fat and fat-soluble vitamin malabsorption
  - Massive bowel resection
    - Life-threatening malabsorption
    - Malnutrition
    - Metabolic acidosis
    - Dehydration
  - Ileostomy and colostomy
    - Complications of salt and water balance
- Blind loop syndrome
  - Vitamin B_{12} malabsorption
- Pancreatectomy
  - Malabsorption
  - Diabetes mellitus

Drug treatment
- Corticosteroids
  - Fluid and electrolyte problems
  - Nitrogen and calcium losses
  - Hyperglycemia
- Sex hormone analogues
  - Fluid retention
  - Nausea
  - Megesterol acetate (glucocorticoid effects)
- Immunotherapy
  - Tumor necrosis factor (TNF)
    - Fluid retention
    - Hypotension
    - Nausea, vomiting
    - Diarrhea
  - Interleukin-2
    - Hypotension
    - Fluid retention
    - Azotemia
  - Interferons
    - Anorexia
    - Nausea/vomiting
    - Diarrhea
    - Azotemia
- Cytotoxic chemotherapy (see Table 82.9)

diet, nutritional supplements, or enteral feeding may be desirable. Patients receiving nutritional supplements throughout radiation therapy maintained good body weight and completed radiation therapy without interruption (128). The widespread use of percutaneous endoscopic gastrostomy allows tube feeding patients with cancer of the head and neck despite severe dysphagia and obstructing tumors (see Chapter 100). Enteral feeding given prior to and during radiation therapy can prevent weight loss, dehydration, and interruption in therapy as well as minimizing admissions to the hospital. In the malnourished patient scheduled for surgery or chemotherapy, pretreatment enteral feeding can improve the nutritional state and may decrease morbidity (129). In a randomized study, malnourished patients with head and neck cancer who received enteral nutrition prior to surgery had decreased postoperative complications and hospitalization (130). In the immediate postoperative period, most patients require a short course of enteral feeding, mostly provided through a tube placed during the operation with the tip in the esophagus. Such feedings are usually required for a few days to allow healing of the operative wounds or improvement in the ability to swallow improves. In patients who continue to experience mild to moderate dysphagia postoperatively, nutritional treatment is directed to providing attractive foods with pleasant aroma, which are lubricated by gravies and salad dressings and have high caloric content. Nutritious liquid formulas that can be administered by mouth are also helpful.

For patients with significant nonresolving dysphagia, endoscopic gastrostomy tubes greatly facilitate provision of nutrition by feedings administered 3 to 4 times a day (131). For patients who are at serious risk of aspiration of regurgitated food (tendency to vomit, absent gag reflex, significant pulmonary disease), bolus feeding through a tube with its tip in the stomach increases the risk. This danger is reduced by placing the tip of the tube in the small bowel and using a pump to infuse the formula by slow drip over several hours.

Patients who require long-term enteral feedings at home should be trained in enteral feeding techniques, including recognition of safety problems, information about nutritious formulas, and issues of cost. Regular medical follow-up is important to ensure the adequacy of the patient's regimen and allow appropriate adjustments as required (e.g., with diabetes, heart and kidney failure). These issues are reviewed further in Chapter 100.

Esophageal Cancer

Malnutrition is highly prevalent in patients with carcinoma of the esophagus, primarily because of the severe dysphagia. This symptom, most commonly found on initial presentation, is seen in about 90% of all patients. In a report on 110 patients, average weight loss at presentation totaled 9 kg (132). A review of 83,783 patients from 122

Table 82.9
Potential Adverse Nutritional Effects of Cytotoxic Chemotherapeutic Agents

	N/V[a]	D[b]	Cons[c]	Mucositis	Wt. Gain	Anorexia	Abnormal Electrolytes	Other
Alkylating agents								
Busulfan	–	+	–	–	–	+	–	
Carboplatin	+++	–	–	–	–	+	+	Renal toxicity
Chlorambucil	+	–	–	–	–	–	–	
Cisplatin	++++	–	–	–	–	+	++	Renal toxicity
Cyclophosphamide	++++	–	–	–	–	++	++	
Nitrogen mustard	++++	++++	++	–	–	–	+	Metallic taste
Antibiotics								
Doxorubicin	+++	+	–	++	–	+	–	
Daunorubicin	++	+	–	++	–	+	–	
Mitomycin	++	–	–	++	–	++	–	
Antimetabolites								
Cytarabine	++	+	–	++	–	++	–	GI hemorrhage
5-Fluorouracil	++	+		++++	–	++++		Proctitis
Gemcytabine	+++	–	–	–	–	++	–	Flulike syndrome
Methotrexate	+	+	–	++++	–	++++	–	Gingivitis, pharyngitis
Hormonal agents								
Tamoxifen	+	–	–	–	++	–	–	
Megestrol acetate	+	–	–	–	++	–	–	Increased appetite
Anastrozole	+	+	+	–	+	+	–	
Plant alkaloids								
Vincristine	+	–	+++	–	–	++	–	Paralytic ileus
Vinblastine	+	–	++	+	–	+	–	Abdominal pain
Vinorelbine	+	+	–	–	–	+	–	
Taxoids								
Paclitaxel	++	+	–	+++	–	+	–	
Docetaxel	++	+	–	+++	–	+	–	
Topoisomerase inhibitors								
Irinotecan	++	++++	–	++		–	+	Weight loss
Topotecan	++	++	+	+	+	–	++	
Miscellaneous								
Etoposide	+	+	–	–	–	+	–	Pancreatitis
Bleomycin	+	–	–	–	–	–	–	Pheumonitis or lung changes

[a]N/V, nausea, vomiting.
[b]D, diarrhea.
[c]Cons, constipation.

studies revealed a mean weight loss of 10 kg on initial presentation (12).

Surgery is the primary treatment modality of patients with carcinoma of the esophagus, with radiation and chemotherapy often given preoperatively. The outcome is still poor, with an overall 5-year survival rate of only 11%. Surgical treatment usually involves total or distal esophagectomy requiring bilateral vagotomy, proximal gastrectomy, and anastomosis of the retained portion of the esophagus to the remaining stomach, which is placed in the chest. Frequent regurgitation, rapid satiety, decreased rate of gastric emptying of solid food (despite pyloroplasty), diarrhea, and steatorrhea (mild to moderate) are common complications of this surgery (Table 82.8). The causes of diarrhea and steatorrhea are not easily identified. If troublesome, their cause should be identified; vagotomy should be suspect (133).

Esophagectomy is often associated with short- and long-term complications that can severely limit the patient's ability to consume adequate amounts of food. Such complications include anastomotic leak, stricture, dysmotility of the stomach, early satiety, regurgitation, and vomiting. Of 46,692 patients enrolled in different studies, serious postoperative complications occurred in 36% (134). When strictures occur postoperatively, dilatation can help increase the diameter of the esophageal lumen; however, strictures often recur.

Radiation to the esophagus can induce esophagitis. Although this complication usually subsides following cessation of therapy, some patients may develop fibrosis with resultant esophageal stricture. Fistulas (particularly esophagotracheal) and hemorrhage are commonly related to regrowth of the cancer. Chemotherapy may induce nausea, anorexia, sore mouth, and odynophagia, thus further inhibiting food intake and decreasing the acceptance of tube feeding. In a series of patients receiving radiation plus chemotherapy or radiation alone, severe or life-threatening upper digestive tract complication with accompanying nutrition problems occurred in 33 and 18%, respectively (135). These complications included mucositis, ulcerations, dysphagia, necrosis, fistulas, and perforations.

In the patient presenting with advanced, nonresectable esophageal cancer, dysphagia is usually a major problem.

Dilatation and laser therapy often temporarily improve the patient's ability to swallow, but dysphagia usually recurs, requiring repeated treatments. In these patients, placement of a gastrostomy tube can be very helpful in providing nutrition.

Nutritional Support

Many patients present with significant weight loss secondary to progressive dysphagia. Weight loss and malnutrition are negative prognostic factors (136). When obstruction is mild and regurgitation is not a problem, ingestion of an adequate amount of well-planned meals and liquid formulas often prevents or ameliorates malnutrition. Dietary management of various stages of dysphagia is reviewed in Appendix Tables V-A-34-a to e. When dysphagia is moderate or severe, special oral and/or enteral feeding should be initiated. It can be administered through an endoscopically or surgically placed gastrostomy or jejunostomy tube. Because patients with esophageal cancer have functional GI tracts distally, enteral nutrition should be used rather than TPN when there is no contraindication (i.e., severe nausea, vomiting, and/or diarrhea).

Following resumption of oral intake by the patient who has undergone esophagectomy, the nutritional plan should provide for frequent small meals (to overcome easy satiety and the tendency to regurgitate). The diet should be high in carbohydrates and adequate in protein and fat.

If postoperative strictures occur, the patient may temporarily require special diets or oral or tube-fed liquid formulas to ensure adequate intake until the stricture is overcome.

Carcinoma of the esophagogastric junction creates pre- and postoperative physiologic and nutritional problems similar to those described above. Because an appreciably larger portion of the proximal stomach may be resected, early satiety may be more marked and production of gastric juice may be reduced, thereby resulting in decreased vitamin B_{12} absorption.

Gastric Cancer

Patients with gastric cancer frequently present with weight loss, abdominal pain, anorexia, and weakness. Surgical treatment for gastric cancer involves either a radical subtotal gastrectomy (80–85%) with a gastrojejunal anastomosis or a total gastrectomy with an esophagojejunal anastomosis with or without some type of reservoir in the upper jejunum. The 5-year survival of gastric cancer patients in the United States varies from 43% for stage 1 to 20% for stage 4 (136). Long-term survival following curative surgery is better in Japan (where gastric cancer is highly prevalent) than in the United States (137).

Radiation and/or chemotherapy are used for the treatment of patients with resected but residual localized disease. Patients who present with metastatic disease usually receive only palliative therapy; surgery is performed only to relieve gastric obstruction or to manage severe bleeding.

Removal of most or all of the stomach reduces or eliminates its reservoir, digestive, secretory, diluting, and metering functions. These modifications have both physiologic and nutritional consequences that may vary from mild to severe, depending on the extent of resection, the individual patient response, and the postoperative care (Table 82.8). The most common nutritional problems in patients postgastrectomy are early satiety and the inability to ingest adequate amounts of food during a meal. Consequently, they often exhibit weight loss and nutrient deficiencies.

Depending on the types and amounts of foods ingested postoperatively and on the response of the patient, various signs and symptoms, termed the *dumping syndrome,* can occur (138). Usually the signs and symptoms occur within 15 to 30 minutes following ingestion of a meal, termed *early dumping* (139). Vasomotor manifestations include diaphoresis, palpitations, weakness, and faintness; in addition, GI signs and symptoms include abdominal bloating, cramping, and diarrhea, which may become pronounced shortly after the meal. Another set of symptoms, which often occur in conjunction with those just mentioned but usually $1^1/_2$ to 2 hours after eating *(late dumping)* (139), is characterized also by sweating, tachycardia, and faintness; confusion may also occur. This set of symptoms and signs is related to catecholamine discharge mediated by hypoglycemia induced by a heightened insulin response to rapid entry of the meal into the upper small bowel. This syndrome may be intense enough to discourage food consumption. A diagnostic provocation test consists of measuring the heart rate after oral ingestion of 50 g of glucose. The sensitivity and specificity of a positive response (i.e., a heart rate increase $\geq$ 10 beats/min in the first hour) were 100 and 94%, respectively. An early rise in breath hydrogen in the same protocol had an 84 and 94% sensitivity and specificity, respectively (139).

Fat malabsorption occurs especially in patients who have undergone total or near-total gastrectomy (138). Deficiencies of iron, calcium, and fat-soluble vitamins may also develop. Lack of gastric acidity, intrinsic factor, and R protein inhibits both cobalamin availability and absorption from food and its absorption from a vitamin supplement unless accompanied by intrinsic factor equivalent (Chapter 27).

Numerous reports have described the benefits of somatostatin and especially of its analogue octreotide, both short and long term, in the treatment of the dumping syndrome. In dumping provocation tests induced by diet, the drug reduced or abolished the early and late signs and symptoms associated with hypovolemia and hypoglycemia, respectively (140, 141). Some patients benefited from long-term use, but many could not tolerate the drug because of diarrhea (140). The use of octreotide has provided important information on the possible cause of the dumping syndrome; the plasma levels of pancreatic polypeptide, neurotensin, and glucagon were markedly elevated during the "dump" in patients treated with placebo but were suppressed in those pretreated with octreotide. It has been postulated that neurotensin is most likely the mediator peptide (141).

Patients with gastric cancer who do not undergo curative resection may have very severe nutritional problems because of obstruction, abdominal pain, recurrent nausea and vomiting, and bloating. In such patients, enteral feeding through a jejunostomy may play an important supporting role in providing adequate hydration and nutrition for an interim period.

Nutritional Support

Attention to dietary treatment and appropriate education of the patient and family may alleviate many of the nutritional problems that arise postgastrectomy, especially when there has been a major resection. The dumping syndrome can be greatly minimized or prevented by adherence to an antidumping diet (see Appendix Table V-A-35). Small meals should be taken five to six times per day. In general, such a diet is high in protein, adequate in fat, quite low in simple carbohydrates, and restricted in fluids at mealtime. The foods should be calorically dense and relatively low in insoluble fiber, since high fiber content both increases satiety and decreases transit time; thus, high-fiber diets can diminish food intake and increase the risk of diarrhea. Those who continue to be symptomatic should recline for a period immediately after eating. Use of a pectin derivative has been reported to prolong gastric emptying, thus decreasing dumping with its blood volume changes, to exert better control on the early serum insulin rise, and to minimize the later fall in blood sugar (see also Chapter 43) (142).

Deficiencies of vitamins and minerals can be prevented or treated by adequate oral administration of iron with ascorbic acid and by supplements containing both water-soluble and fat-soluble vitamins (high-potency vitamin formulations are usually not necessary). Monthly injections of 100 μ2g of vitamin B_{12} are necessary because of the inability to extract bound B_{12} from food secondary to loss of gastric juice and an inability to absorb ordinary amounts of oral B_{12} because of the absence of intrinsic factor.

Symptoms of milk (lactose) intolerance, which are common in these patients, can be prevented by lactase-treated milk or yogurt. If these approaches are unsatisfactory, the more soluble calcium salts should be taken in divided doses over the day to provide at least 1 g of this nutrient.

The weight loss seen so often in patients postgastrectomy is only partly due to malabsorption; it is primarily attributable to poor food intake. In addition to food antipathy related to early satiety and the unpleasant dumping syndrome with meals, discomfort associated with eating may result from obstructive symptoms, the afferent loop syndrome, esophagitis secondary to bile regurgitation, anorexia, depression, or the side effects of drugs and/or radiation. Hence, a careful diet history, adequate explanation of the basis for dietary modifications, and periodic review to manage new problems as they arise are important.

When the most careful dietary advice and adherence to an antidumping diet do not prevent weight loss and dumping, nocturnal enteral feeding given via a pump that controls continuous drip into the jejunum can provide up to 1800 calories/night and provide a substantial portion of the required nutrients and fluids. Such feeding requires placing a jejunal feeding tube, which can be done endoscopically.

Pancreatic Cancer

Pancreatic ductal adenocarcinoma is an aggressive disease, and by the time of diagnosis, most patients have significant weight loss and are at a stage at which curative treatment is not feasible. Although histologically similar, adenocarcinoma of the distal bile ducts and of the ampulla of Vater usually have a better prognosis because of a higher rate of resectability (143).

The adverse impacts on nutritional status of this type of tumor and its treatments are listed in Table 82.8. Pancreatic carcinoma is often associated with presenting complaints of abdominal pain, anorexia, nausea, and vomiting or of weight loss; some nausea and vomiting is associated with duodenal obstruction. Eating may aggravate pain. Carcinoma of the pancreas may cause digestive enzyme deficiency when the pancreatic duct is obstructed, and the resulting malabsorption, combined with anorexia, contributes to progressive weight loss. Bile insufficiency may result from tumor obstruction of the ampulla of Vater or the common bile duct behind the pancreatic head or at the porta hepatis. Bile insufficiency may reduce absorption of fat and fat-soluble vitamins.

Surgical resection offers the only chance of cure at present, but less than 20% of patients are resectable (143a). Pancreaticoduodenectomy was described by Whipple et al. in 1935 for the surgical treatment of carcinoma of the ampulla of Vater; this procedure is now used for surgical management of cancer of the ampulla of Vater, head of the pancreas, distal common bile duct, and duodenum. In the standard operative procedure, the distal half of the stomach is removed, the pancreas is transected (usually at its neck, but varying amounts or even the entire organ may be removed), and the entire duodenum and a few inches of jejunum distal to the ligament of Treitz are resected. Ligation of the pancreatic duct with oversewing of the transected end of the pancreas (a procedure that is occasionally done) leads to complete exocrine pancreatic insufficiency (144). Even when the remainder of the duct in the pancreatic stump is anastomosed into the small bowel in an effort to use exocrine secretions, fat malabsorption occurred in 27% (144) and 50% (145, 146) of patients. Total pancreatectomy is still performed in a small minority of patients.

The evolution, current status of modifications, and morbidity and mortality of this procedure in cancer patients have been summarized recently (147). Over the past 35 years, the perioperative mortality rate has declined from about 20% to less than 5% or even 2% or less. Early postoperative delay in gastric emptying (up to 6 weeks) is still a problem, as is leakage at the pancreatic anastomosis. The standard procedure is associated with the morbidities attributable to hemigastrectomy: dumping, marginal ulceration (minimized with use of H_2 blockers), and bile reflux gastritis. A pylorus-preserving modification reduces bile reflux and dumping, but its use in patients with pancreatic cancer is problematic. The 5-year survival rate following the standard procedure for adenocarcinoma of the head of the pancreas has been poor (about 4%) in the 50 years up to 1986; more-recent large-scale studies report survivals of about 20%, but the data require confirmation (147).

Approximately 10 to 12% of patients with carcinoma of the pancreas are overtly diabetic, and depending on the site of the tumor, 10 to 35% have asymptomatic glycosuria or hyperglycemia (145). Decreased glucose tolerance has been noted in postpancreaticoduodenectomy patients with normal fasting blood sugar but an insufficient insulin response to a glucose load (148).

Patients with an unresectable tumor undergo a "double bypass," which is performed to alleviate an actual or impending obstruction of the duodenum and bile duct. The operation consists of a gastrojejunostomy and choledochojejunostomy. Despite this procedure, patients often continue to suffer from early satiety, abdominal pain following a meal, distention, and lack of appetite. The GI tract dysfunction is due to compression of the stomach and small bowel by the tumor. Usually these patients have severe weight loss, weakness, pain, and anorexia.

Nutritional Support

Pancreaticoduodenectomy results in early satiety, rapid transit, diarrhea, and generalized feeling of anorexia. The end result is a substantial decrease in food intake and weight loss. Malabsorption and glucose intolerance can further aggravate the nutritional state. When the tumor recurs in the abdomen (usually within a year or two), generalized dysmotility of the GI tract (due to mesenteric carcinomatosis), intestinal obstruction, ascites, and liver involvement may further aggravate the nutritional state. Exocrine pancreatic secretions may be deficient following pancreaticoduodenectomy. This requires adequate amounts of pancreatic enzyme preparations, which should be administered with all meals and snacks, particularly when moderate-to-severe fat malabsorption exists (145). Dietary therapy should aim at providing sufficient amounts of calories and nutrients to compensate for the malabsorption. Because glucose oligosaccharides do not require pancreatic enzymes for their hydrolysis, their use may provide better glucose absorption than use of long-chain carbohydrates. Concern for glucose intolerance requires appropriate testing. Frequent small meals may help the patient increase intake because early satiety secondary to the partial gastric resection may limit the ability to consume large meals. In patients with or without a curative resection, nocturnal enteral feeding through an endoscopically placed jejunostomy tube can supplement the oral intake and provide significant amounts of calories and nutrients.

Colorectal Cancer

Patients with colorectal cancer usually present with little or no weight loss. Surgical therapy involves removal of the segment of the colon containing the tumor. The overall 5-year survival rate of patients is 61% (1). In patients with familial polyposis or with ulcerative colitis, the whole colon is removed. Resection of part or all of the colon does not result in significant nutritional problems. Although patients may experience transient diarrhea postoperatively, this usually subsides and does not cause significant fluid or mineral depletion. Patients with Duke's stage B and C routinely receive a 5-fluorouracil-based adjuvant chemotherapy postoperatively, which can result in transient diarrhea that usually does not create nutritional or hydration problems.

Resection of the right colon with the ileocecal valve and a portion of the distal ileum may be associated with watery diarrhea, in large part caused by entry of increased amounts of bile salts into the colon as well as by functional loss of the valve (149). Cholestyramine binds bile salts and may markedly attenuate the diarrhea. Only a small segment of distal ileum usually is sacrificed; thus, vitamin B_{12} deficiency is not likely.

When a significant segment of the large bowel is taken out of continuity by a diverting procedure that leaves the distal colon in place but without the stream of stool, an inflammatory process, termed *diversion colitis,* can develop in this residual area. Diversion colitis occurs at variable times after the operation and is characterized by persistent histologic features resembling those of ulcerative colitis: absent or variably symptomatic abdominal cramping with mucoid or bloody diarrhea. Resolution occurs only with reanastomosis (150). Infusion of a salt solution containing short-chain fatty acids (SCFAs) into the rectal remnant appears to have a healing effect (151). Butyric acid, one of the SCFAs, is the primary energy source for colonocytes. SCFAs are active factors in colonic cell differentiation, which may explain their role in healing the colonic mucosa.

Ileal Resection

Major resection of the small bowel because of primary GI malignant tumors is relatively uncommon, as is resection of only the jejunum. The ileum may be damaged, bypassed, or removed to varying extents in cancer patients because of involvement with metastatic disease, fistula development, or radiation enteritis. Resection of the ileum leads to significant physiologic and nutritional problems that are reviewed in Chapters 65 and 68 and listed in Table 82.8.

NUTRITIONAL IMPACT OF CANCER THERAPIES

The nutritional impact of surgery is discussed above for specific cancer sites. The effects of radiation therapy are reviewed in Chapter 70.

Chemotherapy

Combinations of chemotherapy drugs are administered cyclically in maximum tolerated dosages either as the only antitumor therapy or in combination with surgery or radiation. The therapeutic effectiveness of available agents against certain malignant tumors is significant. High percentages of cures, particularly of childhood malignancies, have been reported for acute leukemias, lymphomas, testicular tumors, Wilms' tumor, osteogenic sarcoma, and rhabdomyosarcoma. Adjuvant therapy (chemotherapy given following curative resection) is highly effective in increasing survival of patients with breast and colon tumors. On the other hand, other cancers (e.g., those of the lung, stomach, pancreas and liver) respond poorly to chemotherapy and adjuvant chemotherapy. Major efforts continue to develop and test new agents and to vary the combinations of drugs and their dosages to obtain better responses.

Nutrition-Related Side Effects

Because the activities of chemotherapy drugs are not specific to cancer cells, side effects on host cells are common. The severity and manifestation of these side effects are related to the specific agent, dosage, duration of treatment, accompanying drugs, and individual susceptibility. Because the epithelial cells of the alimentary tract have a relatively rapid turnover, many of the drugs affecting cell division have adverse effects on this tissue, with severe nutritionally related consequences. Chemotherapeutic agents may also have pronounced damaging effects on bone marrow and renal tubules as well as on hepatic, cardiac, pulmonary, and nerve cells. Nausea and vomiting are among the most common side effects of chemotherapy, but development of effective drugs to counteract chemotherapy-induced emesis (CIE) has helped ease these problems (see below).

Table 82.9 lists some of the more commonly used chemotherapeutic agents and summarizes their biochemical actions and potential side effects that influence nutritional status. Severe nausea and vomiting tend to result from usual dosages of cisplatin, cyclophosphamide, nitrogen mustard, doxorubicin, and gencytabine. Mucositis and stomatitis may be severe with 5-fluorouracil, methotrexate, paclitaxel, and docetaxel. Diarrhea may be marked with nitrogen mustard, 5-fluorouracil, and methotrexate. Vincristine may cause neurologic damage leading to severe ileus and constipation. Abdominal pain occurs with dactinomycin, cyclophosphamide, methotrexate, and vincristine. Hepatotoxicity occurs with busulfan in high doses, pentostatin, and asparaginase. Nephrotoxicity is frequent with asparaginase, cisplatin, gallium nitrate, pentostatin, and methotrexate. Cisplatin leads to renal wasting of magnesium, with resultant hypokalemia and hypocalcemia if the hypomagnesia is not corrected (152). Doxorubicin is cardiotoxic. Bleomycin and busulfan may induce pulmonary toxicity. Some hormonal agents (e.g., diethylstilbestrol and tamoxifen) may induce nausea and vomiting. Corticosteroids cause sodium and water retention and nitrogen and calcium loss. The dose-limiting toxicity of many chemotherapeutic agents is leukopenia and thrombocytopenia.

Another common effect on the nutritional status is negative nitrogen balance despite continuing nutrient supply. This was illustrated by a study of protein kinetics during parenteral nutritional support before and during multiple chemotherapy in patients with advanced testicular carcinoma. Nitrogen equilibrium before starting vinblastine, cisplatin, and bleomycin changed to negative balance; protein turnover, synthesis, and catabolism decreased by 23, 34, and 30%, respectively (153).

Chemotherapy-Induced Emesis (CIE) and Antiemetics. Distinct types of CIE occur, including acute, delayed, and anticipatory emesis (154). *Acute emesis* has its onset within 24 hours of administration of emetogenic chemotherapy. *Delayed emesis* is a syndrome of nausea and/or vomiting that begins approximately 24 hours after administration of chemotherapy, most commonly described following high-dose cisplatin. *Anticipatory emesis* is a learned behavior that develops over time, most commonly in patients who experience acute or delayed emesis.

Certain patient-related factors are highly predictive of severe vomiting following chemotherapy (154). Female patients, young adults (40 years old or younger), and patients with no history of heavy alcohol consumption tend to vomit heavily following chemotherapy. Of greatest importance in predicting the incidence of CIE is the emetogenic potential of the chemotherapy agent or combination of agents being administered.

The discovery that serotonin receptors play a pivotal role in CIE led to development of specific serotonin-receptor antagonists (155). Ondansetron (Zofran) and granisetron (Kytril), the two serotonin antagonists licensed for use in the United States, are now routinely used as effective first-line agents for prevention of CIE. These drugs should be given just before administration of the emetogenic chemotherapy rather than after symptoms begin. Previously available agents, such as high-dose metoclopramide, are associated with disturbing side effects (dystonic reactions, agitation, and restlessness). In contrast, the side effects of serotonin antagonists are less severe, and include headache, constipation or diarrhea, and transient elevations of liver enzymes. When used in combination with dexamethasone (which improved the efficacy of serotonin antagonists by 10–15%), complete control of emesis, defined as complete absence of nausea and vomiting, has been demonstrated in 45 to 55% of patients receiving highly emetogenic chemotherapy (156, 157). The remaining patients generally experience fewer than two vomiting episodes and only mild nausea. Ondansetron and granisetron are therapeutically equivalent, and the decision to use one agent over another often depends on dosage, schedule, and cost.

Blood Cell–Stimulating Factors

Bone marrow injury with high-dose chemotherapy leads to neutropenia and thrombocytopenia, with the risk of life-threatening infections and bleeding. This can be overcome in most patients by the use of autologous bone marrow transplant or peripheral stem cell rescue. The production by recombinant DNA technology of hematopoietic colony-stimulating factors for granulocytes (G-CSF) and for granulocytes and macrophages (GM-CSF) has allowed clinical studies of their effectiveness in overcoming neutropenia induced by chemotherapy. Despite their widespread use in cancer patients and despite the fact that G-CSF does shorten the duration of neutropenia, evidence to date suggests that use of G-CSF had no clinical benefit over standard practice with antibiotics in adults (158) and children (159). GM-CSF and G-CSF may have value for patients undergoing peripheral blood stem cell transplantation after chemotherapy (160). GM-CSF has been associated with development of hypomagnesemia, hypocalcemia, hypokalemia, and hypoalbuminemia (161, 162).

Dietary Influences on Toxicity and Efficacy

Protein and Amino Acids. Numerous laboratory animal studies have addressed the effects of the nutritional state and different types of diets on toxicity of certain chemotherapeutic compounds. Protein-caloric malnutrition in rats is associated with increased methotrexate toxicity because of reduced drug clearance (163). When protein-depleted rats were repleted with protein-enriched diets, tumor response to methotrexate administration was enhanced (164). Casein-based diets enhanced the gastrointestinal toxicity and weight loss of methotrexate, while soy concentrates or peptide-based diets offered significant protection (165). The inhibitory effect of soy-based diets on growth of various tumors in rats has been reviewed (166); part of the effect appears to be secondary to methionine deficiency (167). When methotrexate was administered to rats with transplanted mammary tumors 2 hours after initiating various nutritional regimens, tumor volumes were significantly lower in those given either adequate parenteral or oral diets or amino acid supplements than in those given a protein-depleted diet (168–170).

Conditionally Essential Nutrients: Arginine, N-3 Fatty Acids and RNA. In a randomized study, the effects of a standard feeding formula were compared with a formula enriched with ω-3 fatty acids, arginine, and RNA (Impact), which was designed to enhance the immune response (171). The group receiving the supplemented formula had fewer wound complications and infections and a shorter hospitalization; however, the results of this study have been criticized on several grounds (172). A subsequent study comparing Impact with routine intravenous fluids in postsurgery cancer patients showed no clinical benefits from routine postoperative enteral feeding with the immunity-enhancing formula (173).

Conditionally Essential Nutrients: Glutamine. The metabolic roles and clinical significance of glutamine and its precursors are discussed in detail in Chapters 35, 96, 98, 101. The evidence of its value as a supplement in affecting survival and hospital stay was considered at a recent meeting (174). Hospital stays of bone-marrow transplant patients (175, 176) and of patients resected for colorectal cancer (177) were reduced by supplementation of the parenteral solutions. Oral supplementation of glutamine to cancer patients, however, did not reduce manifestations of stomatitis (178) and intestinal and hematologic toxicity induced by chemotherapy (179, 180).

Biologic Therapies

Immunotherapy

The term *immunotherapy* has been given to various biologic strategies designed to destroy cancer cells by use of cells and cell products of the natural defense mechanisms of the immune system (181). They are mentioned here because they may either influence nutritional state or be influenced by some dietary modification.

Monoclonal Antibodies. Tumor cells often bear surface molecules that are immunogenic in the natural host or in other animal species. By immunizing animals with tumor cell preparations, antisera can be prepared that recognize the various antigens found on the surface of the tumor cell. Each clone of cells produces a single type of antibody, termed a *monoclonal antibody,* that has a single type of antigen-binding site. These cells can be grown in large numbers, and the monoclonal antibody can be highly purified in essentially unlimited amounts. Monoclonal antibodies can be used to radiolocalize tumors and as carriers of cytotoxic substances for cancer therapy. They can also be used to purge bone marrow in vitro of either T lymphocytes (to prevent graft-versus-host disease) or tumor cells before autologous transplantation in conjunction with high-dose systemic chemotherapy (182). Monoclonal antibodies have been used in the treatment of melanoma and colorectal, breast, and ovarian cancers (183). This type of therapy is evolving, and new generations of antibodies are being evaluated.

Cytotoxic Effects of Cytokines (Interleukins). It was noted approximately 18 years ago that lymphocytes exposed to IL-2 developed the ability to kill fresh tumor cells but not normal cells (181). IL-2 was shown to be effective in the treatment of renal cell carcinoma and, to a lesser degree, melanoma. However, toxicity may be severe, resulting in hypotension; renal, hepatic, and central nervous dysfunction; nausea; vomiting; diarrhea; and, in extreme cases, death (184). A nutritional complication of both IL-2 and interferon is their induction of the enzymes that degrade tryptophan to kynurenine, with resultant decline in the concentration of this essential amino acid (185).

Interferons have also been used as therapeutic agents against a variety of tumors and viruses (particularly hepatitis B and C viruses). They are effective against chronic leukemias (particularly hairy cell and myeloid types), lymphomas, and a variety of solid tumors including melanoma, Kaposi's sarcoma, and ovarian and basal cell carcinoma. Side effects include a flulike syndrome, significant weight loss, nausea, vomiting, and neurologic disturbances (186). Other cytokines given singly or in combination with chemotherapy or interferon are currently being assessed for activity against a variety of cancers.

Differentiation Therapy

The strategy of differentiation therapy is to use chemical compounds to induce differentiation of human cancer cells rather than to destroy them.

Retinoid Analogues. Some success has been achieved with the retinoids 13-*cis*-retinoic acid (isotretinoin) (see Chapter 17) and all-*trans*-retinoic acid (ATRA). Isotretinoin caused regression of premalignant leukoplakia of the buccal mucosa and has prevented secondary primary tumors in patients with squamous cell carcinoma of the head and neck. Objective responses have been observed in patients with squamous cell carcinoma of the skin and cervix treated with isotretinoin and interferon (187).

ATRA has induced an aggregate rate of complete remission of approximately 80% in acute promyelocytic leukemia (APL); however, remissions solely by ATRA are brief, so consolidation chemotherapy must follow (188). This retinoid induces differentiation of immature neoplastic cells into mature granulocytes. ATRA has side effects similar to those of other retinoids given in high doses (see Chapter 17). In addition, APL patients are very susceptible to reactions termed the *retinoic acid syndrome*, which consists of fever, respiratory distress, edema, pleural or pericardial effusions, and episodic hypotension. Early treatment with high-dose dexamethasone resulted in prompt improvement and recovery (188).

Synthetic Vitamin D Analogues. Vitamin D analogues—including new ones that are much less likely to induce hypercalcemia—have nuclear receptors and induce tumor cells to differentiate (189, 190). (See also Chapter 18.)

Gene Therapy

Gene therapy involves transfer of DNA into cells to correct pathologic processes that result from abnormalities in the genetic makeup of the cell. There are two major categories of gene therapy: *(a)* in vitro therapy, in which the gene is inserted into the target cells in vitro and then the cells are returned to the animal or patient, and *(b)* in vivo therapy, in which the gene is transferred into the target cell by introducing the gene directly into the body (191). Systems used to transfer the genes are mostly viruses, but nonviral systems are also used. Gene replacement has been useful in slowing growth of malignant cells in vitro and occasionally in vivo. However, major obstacles in the use of gene therapy against cancer include the presence of numerous genetic aberrations in tumors (requiring transfer of many genes) and the potential need to introduce genes into all the malignant cells to achieve effective therapy. A more promising use of gene therapy is the application of gene transfer–mediated antitumor immunotherapy. Current laboratory studies and planned clinical trials will address these issues.

EFFICACY OF NUTRITIONAL SUPPORT

Two major and apparently contradictory themes are apparent in considering the relationship of advanced cancer and nutritional support. One is the need to prevent to minimize the severe undernutrition frequently accompanying advanced cancer. The other is the altered metabolism induced by tumor-mediated cytokines in many of these patients, which renders current nutritional therapies ineffective unless the underlying malignant condition can be eradicated or significantly palliated by antitumor treatments.

In contradistinction to patients with active malignancies that require immediate therapy, a group of patients have primary nutritional support needs. Included in this category are those whose effective antitumor therapies—curative or significantly palliative—have resulted in significant short- or long-term nutritional problems (e.g., alimentary tract dysfunction of various kinds). Nutritional support of some kind is usually effective for such patients.

Evaluation of Total Parenteral Nutrition

Total parenteral nutrition (TPN) has been a primary method of ensuring continued administration of nutrients to seriously ill patients undergoing antitumor treatments. Early retrospective and uncontrolled reports suggested that with such nutritional support, undernourished cancer patients had improved nutritional status, were more responsive to radiation therapy and/or chemotherapy, and had fewer side effects from treatment (192, 193). Better-controlled studies followed, but they differed with respect to patient numbers, ages, and gender; the types and stages of malignant disease; the nature and duration of accompanying antitumor treatments; and the types, duration, and frequency of administration of TPN formulations. This variability often makes it difficult to compare findings of individual studies. This section summarizes this complex field.

Chemotherapy with or without Radiation and Total Parenteral Nutrition

TPN can improve some nutritional parameters in patients receiving chemotherapy; it can yield better hydration, increase body fat and weight, and correct specific nutrient depletion (27, 194). In patients with advanced cancer, TPN does not suppress the cancer-induced increased glucose oxidation and turnover (47, 48), muscle proteolysis and protein turnover (64, 65), or redistribution of body protein and increased lipolysis (54). Although some specific nutritional parameters can be improved, the more relevant issue is whether TPN can improve morbidity rates, quality of life, and survival when given in conjunction with chemotherapy. These clinical issues have been examined in a number of randomized studies using a variety of chemotherapy drugs, with different cancer sites: lung (195, 196), colon (197), testes (198), lymphoma (199), and others (200, 201).

Patients enrolled in many of these studies were not malnourished, and some had adequate oral intake and GI function, making elucidation of a potentially favorable effect of TPN difficult. The results of such studies, judged individually or in combination, indicated that routine nondiscriminatory use of TPN in patients treated with chemotherapy offered no treatment outcome advantage and no decrease in chemotherapy-induced complications.

A metaanalysis evaluated a pool of 12 randomized studies of cancer patients receiving chemotherapy and given TPN (202). The American College of Physicians report based on this analysis concluded that TPN did not result in any improvement in overall survival or response to chemotherapy (203). This analysis supported the conclusions of an earlier analysis of 28 clinical trials indicating that TPN had little or no effect on decreasing chemotherapy toxicity (204). TPN was associated with a significant increase in risk of infection, and the data revealed no conditions for which TPN could be shown to be beneficial (203).

Eighteen trials were reviewed in which adults were given only chemotherapy and five trials in which children were treated with chemotherapy alone or with additional radiation (205). The author concluded that although weight gain or decreased weight loss can often be achieved with nutritional support, "early weight gain with nutritional support usually results from accumulation of water and fat" and that "this is of questionable benefit. Consistent improvement in other nutritional parameters has not been found in the trials. This reviewer would argue that changes in nutritional parameters without concomitant improvement in clinical outcome are of no clinical utility. . . . Based upon prospective, randomized, controlled clinical trials *with the exception of bone marrow transplantation* [author's emphasis], there appears to be little support for the routine aggressive nutritional support in the nonsurgical oncology patient." Nevertheless, the author recognized circumstances in which aggressive nutrition by any route should be provided. These circumstances include prolonged inability to eat (especially when malnutrition is secondary to poor intake), a nutritional support team to decrease complications, and the presence of a tumor deemed likely to respond to treatment (205).

Patients treated with bone marrow transplantation (BMT) can benefit from TPN because the cytoreductive chemotherapy and radiation often cause prolonged severe GI dysfunction with mucosal injury, nausea, vomiting, diarrhea, and abdominal pain. These symptoms can severely limit oral intake for weeks. In a randomized study, BMT recipients received either TPN starting 6 days prior to cytoreductive therapy or, alternatively, intravenous fluids with minerals and vitamins until metabolic dysfunction occurred, at which point TPN was given. In the TPN group, the incidence of malignant relapse was lower and survival was longer (206). In children receiving BMT for acute nonlymphocytic leukemia, TPN improved body mass and bone marrow function (207).

In a prospective randomized study comparing TPN with ad libitum food and fluid intake in children given chemotherapy plus high-dose abdominal and/or pelvic radiation, TPN was found safe and maintained nutritional status; one-third of controls became malnourished and required TPN. However, there was no clinical benefit of "bowel at rest" or decreased toxicity. Most patients lost the weight gained on TPN when TPN was discontinued and chemotherapy was continued (208). These studies suggest that patients receiving BMT and others who cannot eat for a prolonged time (particularly if they are severely malnourished) may benefit from TPN or, if the GI tract is functioning, from enteral feeding.

Surgery and Total Parenteral Nutrition

Numerous randomized studies in surgical cancer patients examined whether TPN decreased postoperative complications and improved survival (15, 16, 209, 210). Ten days of preoperative TPN was associated with nutritional improvement and significant reduction in major postoperative complications and mortality in patients with GI cancer (209). However, these positive results could not be confirmed in other studies. In a multiinstitution Veterans Administration prospective randomized study, of whom two-thirds were cancer patients, TPN was not associated with a reduction in postoperative morbidity or in 90-day mortality (15). The authors concluded that perioperative TPN should be given only to severely malnourished patients.

Patients in one hospital undergoing curative resection for pancreatic cancer (n = 117) were randomized to receive TPN or intravenous fluids and electrolytes in the postoperative period (16). No benefit from routine postoperative TPN was noted. However, routine perioperative TPN in patients (n = 144) undergoing hepatectomy for hepatocellular carcinoma exerted a clear benefit (210). The TPN group in this randomized study had a lower overall postoperative morbidity mostly because of fewer septic complications. There was also less deterioration in liver function postoperatively.

Two early metaanalyses found that pooled results from studies in which patients received perioperative TPN showed that postoperative complications and mortality were significantly reduced in the TPN groups (202, 211). A more recent analysis concluded that routine TPN did not improve the complication rate and mortality following surgery in cancer patients (212).

It appears from various randomized studies that indiscriminate use of TPN in the surgical cancer patient offers no benefit. Severely malnourished patients may benefit from preoperative TPN because of improved nutritional status prior to possible interference with nutrient use as a result of the surgical injury. In specific operations (e.g., hepatectomy), routine perioperative TPN may offer benefits, but more studies are required to clarify this issue.

The role of TPN in patients with severe, prolonged, postoperative complications (abdominal abscess, anastomotic leak, prolapsed ileus) has not been examined specifically. Such patients are usually given TPN 7 to 10 days after the operation if gastrointestinal dysfunction persists. This practice seems warranted at the present time.

Total Parenteral Nutrition and Infection

Infection is a particularly serious matter in patients on chemotherapy because of the frequency of associated leukopenia and depressed immunity, especially in malnourished patients. The metaanalysis summary of the American College of Physicians indicated a fourfold risk of infection in patients given chemotherapy and TPN, compare with those not receiving TPN (203). However, in only four of seven studies analyzed by Koretz was there a statistically significant difference in infection rates associated with TPN in nonsurgical patients on chemotherapy with or without radiation (212). In the VA perioperative study, the increased infection rate in the TPN group (compared with controls) occurred only in borderline or mildly malnourished patients (15). In contrast, the severely malnourished group on TPN had rates of infectious complications comparable to those in the control group (15). Infection rates were not greater with TPN, chemotherapy, or undernutrition in another study (201). There is evidence in neonates that the use of Intralipid is associated with increased infection rates (213). This possible relationship with parenteral lipids has not been reported in appropriately designed studies in cancer patients nor has there been such a comparison among newer lipid formulations.

Critique of the Analyses of Standard TPN. The preceding section provides good evidence that indiscriminate use of TPN in cancer patients undergoing antitumor therapies has generally shown no statistically significant benefit. Nevertheless, the reader should be aware of specific issues that were not always adequately considered or discussed in various reviews.

One issue involves the adequacy of the TPN solutions given during the trials. Because several clinical trials were published in 1981 or earlier, most of the subjects in these studies were given TPN solutions that were not nutritionally adequate. Prior to 1981, complete vitamin formulations were not commercially available, and prior to 1983, a number of essential trace elements were not added to TPN solutions. Unless these missing nutrients were obtained or prepared separately by the pharmacist or physician, their provision to the patients was very problematic. Because common use of Intralipid in the United States began in the late 1970s, glucose-based TPN solutions were generally used in that period. Secondly, in most of the studies with cyclical chemotherapy continued at home, TPN was given for relatively short periods of 2 to 4 weeks. Thus, a number of patients were not appreciably malnourished at the outset. Furthermore, such patients were usually discharged home without receiving TPN in the intervals. Thirdly, most of the surveys did not include survival data. Failure of chemotherapy to have a significant effect on the downhill course of most advanced adult solid tumors guaranteed progressive debility and death.

Some of the studies implied that provision of TPN significantly shortened survival. An analysis of one trial is instructive. This study involved patients with advanced colorectal cancer treated with chemotherapy, randomized to receive either an ad libitum diet or TPN. One of its conclusions was that "overall median survival was significantly decreased in TPN patients (79 vs. 305 days, P= .03)" (197). Analyses of the protocol and results reveal that TPN was given for 14 days prior to chemotherapy and continued during the first course only, which lasted an average of 12 days. TPN was discontinued thereafter, although chemotherapy was continued every 4 weeks with oral intake. While shortened survival was attributed to TPN, there were significant other reasons for earlier demise, including major group differences in sex distribution and maldistribution of patients with liver metastases.

Another major problem lies in evaluating the significance of the findings of trial summaries and metaanalyses. The variability between and among studies in terms of patient diagnoses, disease severity, complications, medications, and outcome assessment makes statistical comparison difficult. The uncertainty has led to calls for prospective randomized intervention studies (214, 215).

Evaluation of Enteral Nutrition

Chemotherapy

A few randomized studies evaluated the efficacy of enteral nutrition in patients receiving chemotherapy. They included patients with lung (216, 217), GI (217,

218), breast (219), hematologic (220), and metastatic cancer (221). These studies did not demonstrate a clear benefit from enteral nutrition with regard to treatment toxicity, tumor response, or survival. However, the small number of patients in each study and the poor designs weaken the validity of their conclusions.

Surgical Patients

Little information is available for assessing the role of standard enteral nutrition in the perioperative period. Randomized studies in patients who had surgery for GI cancers included small numbers of patients and encountered major difficulties in providing the planned nutritional regimens because of nausea, vomiting, distention, and dysfunction of the needle jejunostomy tubes (222–225). No evidence exists currently to justify routine enteral feeding postoperatively in cancer patients. However, provision of enteral nutrition to seriously malnourished patients should be considered.

Home Nutritional Support

Long-term TPN in the home can be lifesaving and life sustaining for prolonged periods for appropriately selected cancer patients (see also Chapters 100, 101). These include individuals with massive intestinal resection, those with severe radiation enteritis, and those suffering from major radiation-induced unresectable stenosis but who show good evidence that malignancy has been cured. Survival rates and TPN-related complications in such patients are comparable to those seen in patients with diseases such as the short bowel syndrome and Crohn's disease who require home TPN. However, among patients with widely metastatic disease who have failed all therapy, home TPN offers limited benefit, with only 15% of such patients surviving longer than 1 year (226). Recently developed techniques for placing feeding tubes, even in the presence of upper GI obstruction, make it possible to feed such patients enterally and thus obviate the need for TPN. Ethical issues related to administration of fluids and nutritional supplements to the terminally ill patient or to those in a persistent vegetative state are discussed in Chapter 102.

PHARMACOLOGIC AGENTS

With the limited success of total parenteral or enteral nutrition in reversing the wasting of advanced cancer, there has been renewed interest in anabolic agents such as hormones, appetite stimulants, and, more recently, cytokine inhibitors.

Hormones

The effects of insulin, IGF, anabolic steroids, growth hormone (GH), and related agonists have been tested in laboratory animals and in patients with cancer and other hypercatabolic states. This literature is reviewed in Chapters 44, 96, and 98 and by Herrington et al. (227) regarding clinical trial results in cancer and HIV patients.

Laboratory Animal Studies. In sarcoma-bearing rats treated with doxorubicin, growth hormone (GH) significantly attenuated weight loss and preserved host body composition without stimulating tumor growth (228). Rats bearing mammary adenocarcinoma given GH also had greater carcass weight, muscle weight, and protein content than did controls; deprivation of protein and provision of GH inhibited tumor growth (229).

Because IGF-I mediates many of the anabolic growth properties of GH, the influence of IGF-I has been assessed in tumor-bearing rats. In three reports using different tumor transplants, there were variable effects when rats that had the hormone (or an analogue) infused subcutaneously over many hours on a daily basis were compared with tumor-bearing controls. With a transplanted methylcholanthrene-induced sarcoma, Fischer rats receiving IGF-I had significantly better host weight and attenuated loss of host muscle protein and lean tissue without tumor growth stimulation, compared with saline-treated controls (230). Wistar-Furth rats with a dimethylhydrazone-induced colon cancer transplant were randomly assigned to IGF-I, insulin, or control solutions, with paired feeding (230a). Neither IGF-I nor insulin had any significant effect on rate of tumor growth, but IGF-I very significantly ameliorated the loss of host body mass, compared with insulin or control infusion, with no changes in circulating glucose or insulin. In contrast, in a study using a transplanted mammary adenocarcinoma, IGF-I was associated with decreased food intake and circulating insulin and glucose, failure to promote muscle protein accretion, and increased tumor growth, compared with controls (231). Insulin infusion alone increased food consumption, decreased tumor growth, and increased carcass protein and fat. LR^3-IGF-I, a potent analogue of IGF-I, had no positive effect when given alone; however, when insulin and LR^3-IGF-I were infused together, there was a synergistic effect on host weight. It was postulated that IGF-I may exacerbate an insulin insufficiency with resulting decreased metabolic substrates available to the host. As noted above, experimental animal tumors may differ in their production of cytokines and growth factors, which may be of importance in accounting for the variable effects of IGF-I. In another study, insulin maintained the normal ratio of inorganic phosphorus to ATP in the liver of tumor-bearing rats, compared with non-insulin-treated controls; this was associated with better food intake and weight maintenance without increased tumor growth (232). In earlier long-term studies, insulin was not considered effective because it did not extend survival.

When the anabolic β_2 agonist cimaterol was administered, tumor-bearing and control rats exhibited large increases in muscle protein and weight resulting from increased protein synthesis and decreased degradation (233). Tumor-bearing adult mice given a similar drug, clenbuterol, had no significant change in food intake or body composition (234). When the anabolic steroid norandrolone propionate was given to tumor-bearing mice, their weight increased, but 85% of the gain was water (235).

Clinical Studies. Growth hormone and IGF-I in their recombinant human forms have been given to patients with the wasting syndrome of HIV infection, as reviewed recently (227). While there was some weight gain, most patients did not have any improvement in quality of life.

Corticosteroids of various potencies have been tested in cancer patients undergoing antitumor therapies. In most studies, the effects on nutritional indices and appetite have been either minimum or short-lived; long-term use has been associated with negative nitrogen and calcium balances, glucose intolerance, and immunosuppression (227). The anabolic steroid nandrolone did not prevent weight loss in lung cancer patients undergoing chemotherapy (236).

Inhibitors of Cytokine-Related Paraneoplastic Syndromes

Studies in Laboratory Animals. Monoclonal antibody against TNF has had variable effects when injected into animals with various transplanted or induced tumors. It decreased anorexia and loss of body protein or fat in mice but did not reverse anemia, hypoalbuminemia, or acute-phase responses in one study (237). Both anti-TNF and antibody to IL-1 decreased anorexia and tumor growth in mice, but the effects were not additive; neither changed the acute-phase responses or decreased the elevated serum IL-6 (238). Anti-TNF lowered to varying extents the rates of proteolysis of various organs in tumor-bearing rats (239). Antibody against IL-6 significantly (but only partially) suppressed cachexia in mice (240). Similarly, antibody against IFN-γ prevented severe cachexia induced in nude mice bearing hamster ovary tumor cells genetically engineered to produce this cytokine (241).

Clinical Studies. Pentoxyifilline was reported to decrease TNF messenger RNA. However, a randomized double-blind, placebo-controlled trial did not demonstrate any benefit in treating cancer-associated anorexia or cachexia (242). A preliminary study with melatonin reported lower serum TNF levels and less weight loss in the treated group (243).

Summation. Agents that effectively slow or inhibit wasting in cancer patients could be very useful if their actions on tumors and paraneoplastic syndromes could be separated from the deleterious effects on normal cell growth and normal cell differentiation. This would allow *(a)* significant improvement in the state of well-being and function of patients primarily at home during intensive antitumor treatment and *(b)* increased survival by decreasing mortality from infection and improving response to therapies. This approach is still in its early stages and will require clinical application with randomized studies and adequate follow-up studies.

Appetite Stimulants

Megesterol Acetate

Megesterol acetate, a synthetic progestational agent used to treat metastatic endometrial and breast cancers, has also shown some promise in improving appetite and weight. A recent review summarized results of nine trials of this drug used as an anticachectic agent in adult cancer patients with either hormone-sensitive or hormone-insensitive tumors; daily dosages varied from 160 mg/day to 1600 mg/day. Some were randomized, double-blind placebo-controlled trials; others were randomized tests of different dosages (227). In general, the results were positive for increased appetite and weight. In some studies, edema was apparent in a minority of the patients. While the actual changes in body composition have not been studied in detail, fat accumulation was indicated. This review (227) did not mention any possible survival benefit of megesterol acetate.

This agent in daily doses as low as 60 mg has been given in conjunction with cytokines INF-α and IL-2 to a variety of patients who failed standard antitumor therapy; decreased anorexia and weight loss were reported (244). Increased appetite, weight gain, and quality of life were reported when this agent was given between chemotherapy cycles to patients with head and neck cancer; however, performance status (Karnofsky) did not improve (245). It is available (Megace) on prescription as an oral suspension at 800 mg (20 mL) once daily for treatment of anorexia and cachexia in patients with HIV infection. The manufacturer notes that cases of adrenal suppression have been observed. It may exacerbate preexisting diabetes and is contraindicated in pregnancy.

Medroxyprogesterone acetate, which was tested some years ago as an appetite stimulant, has apparently not been used further for this purpose. Similarly, cyproheptadine has failed to prevent weight loss in patients with advanced cancer (227).

Cannabinoids

Marijuana and its derivative dronabinol were claimed to enhance appetite and induce weight gain in cancer patients in two studies that were not properly randomized and controlled (227). Dronabinol has Food and Drug Administration approval for the treatment of nausea and vomiting associated with chemotherapy and for anorexia with weight loss in HIV patients. Randomized studies are needed to evaluate the effects of these agents. Despite lack of such information, several states have decriminalized the use of such agents for cancer patients.

GUIDELINES FOR NUTRITIONAL SUPPORT

While recognizing the uncertainties of a positive response of patients to nutritional support, nevertheless, the physician frequently has to make a decision concerning its initiation and withdrawal. Individual responses to such support vary, and there are no simple objective tests that will enable the physician to predict who will and who will not benefit. The following guidelines are offered to assist in decision making:

1. Early nutritional assessment and serial follow-up are indicated for patients who have developed or are at risk of developing significant and persistent nutritional deficits as a consequence of the tumor or therapy. This evaluation should be followed where indicated by appropriate nutritional intervention and periodic evaluation to ensure adequate therapy.
2. For the patient with mild-to-moderate anorexia and taste changes who may require prolonged treatment, careful evaluation of food preferences and provision of attractive solid and liquid foods and supplements, properly timed, may make the difference between weight maintenance and loss.
3. An important criterion for instituting nutritional support is progressive and serious weight loss or the likelihood of significant weight loss in a patient deemed likely to respond to therapy. The specific period of active support depends on the nature and duration of the antitumor therapy or therapies and on patient responsiveness. For example, enteral feeding may greatly benefit the patient with cancer of the head and neck with severe dysphagia who is undergoing radiation and chemotherapy.
4. Factors influencing the choice of enteral versus parenteral route are reviewed in Chapters 100 and 101. In general, the seriously ill leukopenic and thrombocytopenic patient with seriously impaired GI function is a candidate for parenteral nutrition through a central vein. Patients undergoing BMT are in this category. If the GI route can be safely used without significant distress to the patient, oral and tube feeding are advised. In general, if the gut works, use it. Enteral and parenteral nutritional formulations for the cancer patient are basically the same as those for the mildly to moderately ill patient without cancer. Due consideration must be given, however, to special problems related to organ failure and the effects of the various antitumor or other therapies being used.
5. For the patient requiring major surgery who has lost little (<5%) or no weight, routine fluid and electrolyte support in the postoperative period is indicated unless serious complications postpone enteral intake for at least 7 to 10 postoperative days. In this instance, TPN is indicated unless gastrostomy or jejunostomy tube feedings are appropriate and feasible.
6. A patient requiring major surgery who has severe weight loss (15–20% body weight loss) should be considered for 12 to 14 days of preoperative nutritional therapy, usually through a gastrostomy or jejunostomy tube. Patients with carcinoma of the esophagus, stomach, or pancreas may fall in this category.
7. Enteral feeding should be used for the seriously anorectic patient who is no longer a candidate for antitumor therapy, who has a functioning alimentary tract, and whose quality of life is reasonably acceptable and likely to be maintained or improved by enteral supplementary feeding at home.
8. The patient with an aggressive malignancy and persistent intestinal obstruction or other severe intestinal dysfunction who has failed all therapy and cannot be sustained on some type of enteral feeding will experience a rapid downhill course as an inpatient or outpatient without intravenous feeding. This situation presents difficult emotional problems, especially for the family, when the patient is to be discharged home without TPN, particularly if prior use of parenteral nutrition had improved strength and weight. The physician frequently is pressured to continue this method at home despite clear indication that TPN will not benefit the patient and may induce serious complications. The physician, preferably with the assistance of other health professionals, should present to the patient and/or family members the options and drawbacks of home parenteral nutrition (including financial costs). The mentally competent patient or the family or surrogate of the incompetent patient must then make the decision. Our personal experience and recent data (230) indicate a poor outcome (mean survival ≤3 months) for most of these patients.
9. The cancer patient with a chronic severely dysfunctional alimentary tract (the result of radiation, surgery, chemotherapy, or a combination thereof) who is free of residual malignant disease has an entirely different prognosis from that of the cancer patient in item 8. Proper management of such patients by oral, enteral, and/or parenteral feedings can lead to prolonged survival of good quality. (See Chapters 68, 70, 100, and 101.)

UNPROVEN DIETARY AND NUTRITIONAL CLAIMS

Historically, diseases with major morbidity and mortality and a relatively poor response rate to conventional medical practice of the time have attracted therapeutic "innovations" that have little or no evidence of proof of efficacy. Cancer is no exception because *(a)* it ranks second in terms of mortality, *(b)* major cancers of solid organs at the disseminated stage currently have relatively low "cure" rates by the best medical practice, and *(c)* expensive conventional therapies for cancer often have unpleasant, but usually transient, side effects with no certainty of "cure."

How many cancer patients in the United States and elsewhere are being given treatments that are not accepted by the medical profession is unknown. Although probably a minority of all cancer patients, they are a very "visible minority" (246). Such treatments are called "fraud," "quackery," "unproven," or disproved" (e.g., laetrile) by those mainly in scientific medicine, "unconventional" or "unorthodox" by those less oriented to scientific method, and "alternative" or "complementary" by those favorable to unproven methods. The "alternative" movement embraces the postmodernist doctrine that science is not necessarily more valid than pseudoscience (247).

The nature of some of these "alternative" nutrition treatments, their claims for efficacy, and the characteristics of their practitioners are reviewed in Chapter 110 with the relevant literature. Many of these unconventional treatment programs have special dietary and nutritional components and regimens and use herbal and gland extracts, purgatives, enemas, laetrile, special "immunizing" agents, and spiritual guidance, often combined to form a particular "system" of management. Some of the agents and procedures appear innocuous; others raise a concern for safety. Of special concern is the patient who decides to forgo accepted medical therapy for an "alternative" program. Physicians, dietitians, and nurses who care for cancer patients should be aware of the extent of this problem, know the details and costs of some of the more common components of unproven systems of care, and be willing to discuss this area frankly with patients who ask about such methods (245, 248–251).

The need for an informed and understanding approach to patients on this issue is underscored by data collected on cancer patients by Cassileth et al. (251). Interviews were conducted with 304 inpatients at a cancer center and with 356 cancer patients (primarily outpatients) under the care of "unorthodox" practitioners; 31% were treated with conventional (i.e., medically accepted) therapy only, 49% were treated with both conventional and unorthodox therapy, and 8% were treated with unorthodox therapy only. In addition to the 171 patients treated with both types of therapies who received chemotherapy and/or radiation and/or surgery, 10% of the remaining patients had refused recommended chemotherapy, 9% had refused recommended radiation therapy, and 2% had refused recommended surgery. Of the patients treated with unorthodox therapy only, 28% had refused recommended chemotherapy, 26% had refused recommended radiation therapy, and 28% had refused recommended surgery. Of the 325 patients treated with both types of therapies, 64% had sought conventional treatment first and then added alternative treatment an average of 24 months later; although 60% continued both systems of treatment, 40% had discontinued conventional care entirely after an average of 8 months.

This study revealed that physicians constituted 60% of unorthodox practitioners; they played an active role in prescribing unorthodox treatments for the 378 patients receiving such therapies, particularly "metabolic," megavitamin, and "immune" treatments. Of patients treated with dual systems, 75% had informed their regular physicians of their adoption of alternative care; 39% of these physicians reacted with disapproval to this information, 30% were supportive, and 12% were neutral. Disapproval resulted in 4% of patients being denied further treatment by their physicians. No data were provided on the nature of the unorthodox treatments that led to rejection, disapproval, or approval by physicians (251).

Two major claims made by proponents of "alternative" therapies are *(a)* superior patient support is offered by the therapists and *(b)* their remedies are effective against cancer. Both aspects were examined in a prospective randomized study of patients with advanced malignant disease and an expected median survival time of not more than 1 year. One group received care at an academic cancer center and the other at a cancer clinic that provided its "autogenous immune enhancing vaccine" plus the conventional care of the academic center (253). Survival times were the same in these two settings, but the quality-of-life scores were consistently better among those treated at the academic center beginning from the time of enrollment.

Summation. As indicated above, conventional medical treatments for cancer, while prolonging or saving life, may induce significant adverse side effects. Most patients who have chosen to explore alternative remedies first started with conventional therapy. Presumably because of dissatisfaction with the effectiveness of that therapy, because of painful side effects, or for other reasons, they initiated alternative treatment described by practitioners, friends, or the media as effective, less painful alternatives. Randomized, well-controlled studies have not been performed by their proponents to demonstrate benefit. Nonetheless, new, more effective, and less stressful modalities in the treatment of cancer are clearly needed. One hopes that their development will render ineffective alternatives less attractive.

REFERENCES

1. Anon. Cancer facts and figures, 1996. Atlanta, GA: American Cancer Society, 1996.
2. Parkes S, Tong T, Bolden S, et al. Cancer statistics. CA 1996; 65:5–27.
3. Lopez AD. Ann NY Acad Sci 1990;609:58–74.
4. Doll R. Am J Epidemiol 1991;134:675–88.
5. Cole P, Rody B. Cancer 1996;78:2045–8.
6. Bailar JC III, Gornik HL. N Engl J Med 1997;336:1569–74.
7. Sporn MB. Lancet 1996;347:1377–81.
8. Ames BN, Gold LS, Willet WE. Proc Natl Acad Sci USA 1995; 92:5258–65.
9. DeWys WD, Begg D, Lavin PT, et al. Am J Med 1980;69:491–7.
10. Heymsfield SB, McManus C, Smith J, et al. Am J Clin Nutr 1982;36:680–90.
11. Ollenschlager G, Viell B, Thomas W, et al. Cancer Res 1991; 121:249–59.
12. Goodwin WJ, Byers PM. Med Clin North Am 1993;77: 597–610.
13. Lanzotti VJ, Thomas DR, Boyle LE. Cancer 1977;39:303–13.
14. Serrie R, Rosen PP, Rhodes P, et al. Ann Intern Med 1992; 116:26–32.
15. Veterans Affairs Total Parenteral Nutrition Cooperative Study Group. N Engl J Med 1991;325:525–32.
16. Brennan MF, Pisters PW, Posner M, et al. Ann Surg 1994; 220:436–41.
17. Donaldson SS, Wesley MN, DeWys WD, et al. Am J Dis Child 1981;135:1107–12.
18. Carter P, Carr D, Van Eys J, et al. J Am Diet Assoc 1983; 82:616–22.
19. Smith DE, Stevens ME, Booth IW. Eur J Pediatr 1991; 150:318–22.
20. Warren S. Am J Med Sci 1932;184:610–5.
21. Patil PK, Patel SG, Mistry RC, et al. J Surg Oncol 1992; 49:163–7.
22. Mick R, Vokes EE, Weichselbann RR, et al. Otolaryngol Head Neck Surg 1991;105:62–73
23. Morton KI, Sox HC, Krupfs JR. Ann Intern Med 1981; 95:568–74.
24. Mordes JP, Rossini AA. Science 1981;213:565–7.
25. Norton JA, Moley JF, Green MV, et al. Cancer Res 1985;45: 5547–52.
26. Bozzetti F, Pagnoni A, Del Vecchio M. Surg Gynecol Obstet 1980;150:229–34.
27. Russell DM, Shike M, Marliss B, et al. Cancer 1984;44: 1706–11.
28. Knox CS, Crosby CO, Feuer IB, et al. Ann Surg 1983;197: 152–62.

29. Dempsey DT, Feuer ID, Knox CS, et al. Cancer 1984;53: 1265–73.
30. Merrick HW, Long CL, Grecos GP, et al. JPEN J Parenter Enteral Nutr 1988;12:8–14.
31. MacFie J, Burkenshaw L, Oxby C, et al. Br J Surg 1982; 69:443–6.
32. Hansell DT, Davies JWL, Born HJG. Ann Surg 1986;203: 240–5.
33. Fredrix EWHM, Soeters PB, Rouflart MJJ, et al. Am J Clin Nutr 1991;53:1318–22.
34. Lindmark L, Bennegard K, Eden E, et al. Gastroenterology 1984;87:402–8.
35. Nixon DW, Kutner M, Heymsfield S, et al. Metabolism 1988;37:1059–64.
36. Fearon KCH, Hansell DT, Preston T, et al. Cancer Res 1988;48:2590–5.
37. Thomson SR, Hirschberg A, Haffaje AA, et al. JPEN J Parenter Enteral Nutr 1990;14:119–21.
38. Falconer JS, Fearon KCH, Plester CE, et al. Ann Surg 1994;219:325–31.
39. Arbeit JM, Lees DE, Corsey R, et al. Ann Surg 1984;199: 292–8.
40. FAO/WHO/UNU. Energy and protein requirements. WHO Tech Rep Ser no. 724. Geneva: World Health Organization, 1985.
41. Douglas RG, Shaw JHF. Br J Surg 1990;77:246–54.
42. Staal-van den Brekel J, Denteuer MA, Schals AM, et al. J Clin Oncol 1995:13:2600–5.
43. Kern KA, Norton JA. JPEN J Parenter Enteral Nutr 1988; 12:286–98.
44. Chlebowski FR, Heber D. Surg Clin North Am 1986;66: 957–68.
45. Cerosimo E, Pisters PWT, Persola G, et al. Surgery 1991; 109:459–67.
46. Holyroyde CP, Reichard GA. Cancer Treat Rep 1981;65(Suppl 5):55–9.
47. Shaw JHF, Wolfe RR. Surgery 1987;101:181–91.
48. Shaw JHF, Humberstone DM, Wolfe RR. Ann Surg 1988;207:283–9.
49. Holyrode CP, Gabuzda TG, Putnam RC, et al. Cancer Res 1975;35:3710–4.
50. Eden E, Edstrom S, Bennegard K, et al. Cancer Res 1984; 1717–24.
51. Young VR. Cancer Res 1977;37:2336–47.
52. Mulligan HD, Tisdale MJ. Biochem J 1991;277:321–6.
53. Lundholm K. Surg Clin North Am 1986;66:1013–24.
54. Cohn S, Gartenhaus W, Sawitsky A, et al. Metabolism 1980; 30:222–9.
55. Klein S, Wolfe RR. J Clin Invest 1990;86:1403–8.
56. Wolfe RR, Herndon DN, Jahoor F, et al. N Engl J Med 1987; 317:403–8.
57. Hollander DM, Ebert EC, Robert AI, et al. Surgery 1986; 100:292–7.
58. Beck, SA, Tisdale MJ. Br J Cancer 1991;63:846–50.
59. Vlassara H, Spiegel RJ, Doval DS, et al. Horm Metab Res 1986;18:698–703.
60. Kokal WA, McCullough A, Wright PO, et al. Ann Surg 1983;198:146–50.
61. Eden E, Ekman L, Lindmark L, et al. Metabolism 1984;33: 1020–7.
62. Heber D, Chlebowski RT, Ishibashi DE, et al. Cancer Res 1982;42:4815–9.
63. Norton JA, Stein TP, Brennan MF. Ann Surg 1981;194:123–8.
64. Jeevandaman M, Horowitz GD, Lowry SF, et al. Lancet 1984;1:1423–6.
65. Shaw, JHF, Humberstone DA, Douglas RG, et al. Surgery 1991;109:37–50.
66. Tiao G, Fagan JM, Samuels N, et al. J Clin Invest 1994;94: 2255–64.
67. Llovera M, Garcia-Martinez C, Agell N, et al. Int J Cancer 1995;61:138–41.
68. Warren RS, Jeevanadam M, Brennan MF. J Surg Res 1987; 42:43–50.
69. Lundholm K, Edstrom S, Ekman LA. Cancer 1978;42:453–61.
70. Heymsfield SB, McManus CB. Cancer 1985;55:238–49.
71. Cohn SH, Gartenhaus W, Vartsky D, et al. Am J Clin Nutr 1981;34:1997–2004.
72. Schwartz MW, Seeley RJ. N Engl J Med 1997;336:1802–11.
73. Bartoshuk LM. Am J Clin Nutr 1978;31:1068–77.
74. DeWys WD, Walters K. Cancer 1975;36:1888–96.
75. Williams LA, Cohen MH. Am J Clin Nutr 1978;31:122–5.
76. Carson JAS, Gormican A. J Am Diet Assoc 1977;70:361–5.
77. Kamath S, Booth P, Lad TE, et al. Cancer 1983;52:386–9.
78. Trant AS, Serin J, Douglass HO. Am J Clin Nutr 1982;36: 46–58.
79. Bernstein IL. Cancer Res 1982;42(Suppl):715S–20S.
80. Bernstein IL, Fenner DP. Appetite J Intake Res 1983;74: 79–86.
81. Levine SA, Emering PW. Br J Cancer 1987;56:73–8.
82. Costall B, Naylor J, Tyers MB. Rev Neurosci 1988;2:41–65.
83. Houpt TA, Philopena JM, Joh TH, et al. Learn Memory 1996; 3:25–30.
84. Bernstein IL. Neurosci Behav Rev 1996;20:177–81.
85. Van Lammeren FM, Chance WT, Fischer JE. Peptides 1984; 5:97–101.
86. Chance WT, von Myenfeldt M, Fischer JE. Pharmacol Biochem Behav 1983;18:115–21.
87. Moldower LL, Lowry SF, Cerami A. Annu Rev Nutr 1988;8: 585–609.
88. Tisdale MJ. Anticancer Drugs 1993;4:115–25.
89. Kajimara N, Isehi H, Tanaka R, et al. Cancer Chemother Pharmacol 1996;38(Suppl)S48–52.
90. Flier JS. Proc Natl Acad Sci USA 1997;94:4242–5.
91. Soda K, Kawakami M, Kashii A, et al. Int J Cancer 1995;62: 332–6.
92. Todorov P, Carick P, McDevitt T, et al. Nature 1996; 379:739–42.
93. McCarthy HD, McKibbin PE, Perkins AV, et al. Am J Physiol 1993;264:E638–43.
94. Dosquet C, Schaetz A, Faucher C, et al. Eur J Cancer 1994; 30A:162–7.
95. Maltoni M, Fabbri L, Nauno O, et al. Support Care Cancer 1997;5:130–5.
96. Oka M, Yamamoto K, Takahashi M, et al. Cancer Res 1996; 56:2776–80.
97. Hardin TC, Koeller JM, Kuhn JG, et al. JPEN J Parenter Enteral Nutr 1993;17:541–55.
98. Michie HR, Sherman ML, Spriggs DR, et al. Ann Surg 1989;209:19–24.
99. Fong Y, Moldawer LL, Marano M, et al. Surg Oncol 1992;1:65–71.
100. Abrahamson J, Carlsson B, Mellander C. Am J Pediatr Hematol Oncol 1993;15:364–9.
101. Saarunun UM, Koseko EK, Teppo AM. Cancer Res 1990;50: 592–5.
102. Adami F, Guarini A, Pini M, et al. Eur J Cancer 1994;30A: 1259–63.
103. Odell WD, Wolfsen AR. Annu Rev Med 1978;29:379–406.
104. Perry RR, Vinick AI. Annu Rev Med 1996;47:57–68.
104a. Gardner DG. Adv Intern Med 1997;42:597–627

105. LeRoith D, seminar moderator. In LeRoith D, Baserga R, Helman L, Robert CI Jr. Ann Intern Med 1995;122:54–9.
106. Case records of the Massachusetts General Hospital, case 9-1997. N Engl J Med 1997;336:861–7.
107. Fahrenkrug J. J Clin Gastroenterol 1980;9:633–43.
108. Shimoda SS, Saunders DR, Rubin CE. Gastroenterology 1968; 705–23.
109. Bostwick DG, Null WE, Holmes D, et al. N Engl J Med 1987; 317:1439–43.
110. O'Donnell LDJ, Farthing MGJ. Gut 1989;30:1165–72.
111. Mundy GR. J Clin Invest 1988;82:1–6.
112. Wysolmerski JJ, Broadus AE. Annu Rev Med 1994;45:189–200.
113. Rettig MB, Ma HJ, Vescio RA, et al. Science 1997;276:1851–4.
114. Adams JS, Fernandes M, Gacad MA, et al. Blood 1989;73: 235–9.
115. Shapiro J, Richardson GE. Crit Rev Oncol Hematol 1995;18: 129–35.
116. Siris ES, Clemens TL, Dempster DW, et al. Am J Med 1987; 82:307–12.
117. Case records of the Massachusetts General Hospital, case 52-1989. N Engl J Med 1989;321:1812–21.
118. Schwartz SI, Storer EH. Manifestations of gastrointestinal disease. In: Schwartz SI, Shires GT, Spencer FC, eds. Principles of surgery. 5th ed. New York: McGraw Hill, 1989;980.
119. Creamer B. Br Med J 1964;2:1435–6.
120. Barry RE. Gut 1974;15:562–5.
121. Mathias JR, Clench MH. Am J Med Sci 1985;289:243–8.
122. Herbsman H, Wetstein L, Rosen Y, et al. Curr Probl Surg 1980;17:121–84.
123. Case records of the Massachusetts General Hospital, case 15-1996. N Engl J Med 1996;334:1316–22.
124. Novis BH, Banks S, Marks SW, et al. Q J Med 1971;40:521–40.
125. Waldman TA, Broder S, Strober W. Ann NY Acad Sci 1974;230:306–17.
126. Spivak JL. Semin Oncol 1994;21(2 Suppl 3):3–8.
127. Mossman K, Schatzman A, Chencharick J. Int J Radiat Oncol Biol Phys 1982;8:991–7.
128. Nagel H, Choniemy E, El Haddad S. J Surg Oncol 1994;55: 33–6.
129. Fietkau R, Iro H, Sailer D, et al. Cancer Res 1991;121: 269–82.
130. Flynn MB, Leighty FF. Am J Surg 1987;157:359–62.
131. Shike M, Berner YN, Gerdes H, et al. Otolaryngol Head Neck Surg 1989;101:549–54.
132. Gelfand GA, Finley RJ, Nelems B, et al. Arch Surg 1992;127: 1164–8.
133. Shils ME. Surg Gynecol Obstet 1971;132:709–15.
134. Muller JM, Erasmi H, Stelzner M, et al. Br J Surg 1990;77: 845–57.
135. Herskovic A, Martz K, Al-Sassaf M, et al. N Engl J Med 1992;326:1592–8.
136. Lawrence W, Menck HR, Steele GD, et al. Cancer 1995;75:1734–44.
137. Bandoli T, Isoyama T, Toyoshima H. Surgery 1991;109: 136–42.
138. Lawrence W. Cancer Res 1977;37:2379–88.
139. Vander Kleij FGH, Vecht J, Lamers CB, et al. Scand J Gastroenterol 1996;31:1162–6.
140. O'Donnell LDJ, Farthing MGJ. Gut 1989;30:1165–72.
141. Geer RJ, Richards WO, O'Dorisio TM, et al. Ann Surg 1990; 212:678–87.
142. Leeds AR, Ralphs DNC, Ebeid F, et al. Lancet 1981;1:1075–8.
143. Rosewicz S, Wiedenmann B. Lancet 1997;349:485–9.
143a. Conlon KC, Klimstra DS, Brennan MF. Ann Surg 1996;223:273–9.
144. Goldsmith HS, Ghosh BG, Huvos AG. Surg Gynecol Obstet 1971;132:87–92.
145. Wallaeger EE, Comfort MW, Clagett OT, et al. JAMA 1948;137:838–48.
146. Brooks JR, Culebras JM. Am J Surg 1976;131:516–20.
147. Strasberg SM, Drebin JA, Soper NJ. Gastroenterology 1997; 983–4.
148. Miyata, M, Takao T, Uozumi T, et al. Ann Surg 1974;179: 494–8.
149. Weser E, Fletcher JT, Urban E. Gastroenterology 1979;77: 575–9.
150. Glotzer OJ, Glick ME, Goldman W. Gastroenterology 1981; 80:438–42.
151. Haing JM, Soergel KN, Komorowski, RA, et al. N Engl J Med 1987;320:23–8.
152. Schilsky RL, Anderson T. Ann Intern Med 1979;90:929–31.
153. Hermann VM, Garnick MB, Moore FD, et al. Surgery 1984;90:381–7.
154. Kris MG, Pizzo B. Chemotherapy-induced nausea and vomiting. In: Holland GF, ed. Cancer medicine. 4th ed. Baltimore: Williams & Wilkins, 1997;3111–6.
155. Miner WD, Sanger GJ. Br J Pharmacol 1986;88:497–9.
156. Italian Study Group for Antiemetic Research. N Engl J Med 1995;332:1–5.
157. Hesketh PJ, Harvey WW, Hasker HG, et al. J Clin Oncol 1994;12:596–600.
158. Hartmann LC, Tschetter LK, Habermann TM, et al. N Engl J Med 1997;1776–80.
159. Pui CH, Boyett JM, Hughes WT, et al. N Engl J Med 1997; 336:1781–6.
160. Hoelzer D. (Editorial) N Engl J Med 1997;336:1822–4.
161. Potter MN, Mott MG, Oakill A. Ann Intern Med 1990;112: 715.
162. Kaczmarski, RS, Mufti GJ. Br Med J 1990;301:1312–3.
163. Charland SL, Bartlett D, Torosian MH. JPEN J Parenter Enteral Nutr 1994;18:45–9.
164. Reynolds HM, Daly JM, Rowlands BJ, et al. Cancer 1980;45: 3069–74.
165. Chaurean N, Funk-Archuleta M. Nutr Cancer 1995;23: 185–204.
166. Hawrylewicz EJ, Zapata JJ, Blair WH. J Nutr 1995;125(3 Suppl):698S–708S.
167. Goseki N, Yamazaki S, Endo M, et al. Cancer 1992;69:1865–9.
168. Torosian MH, Mullen JL, Miller EE, et al. Surgery 1983;94:291–9.
169. Torosian MH, Mullen JL, Stein TP, et al. J Surg Res 1988;39:103–13.
170. Torosian MH, Mullen JL, Miller EE, et al. JPEN J Parenter Enteral Nutr 1983;7:337–45.
171. Daly JM, Lieberman MD, Goldfine J, et al. Surgery 1992;112: 56–67.
172. Koretz RL. Gastroenterology 1993;104:936–8.
173. Heslin MJ, Latkany L, Leung D, et al. Ann Surg 1997; 226:567–80.
174. Powell-Tuck J, Williamson DH, Hardy G, eds. Third Oxford glutamine workshop. Nutrition 1997;13:725–61.
175. Ziegler TR, Young LS, Benfell K, et al. Ann Intern Med 1992;116:821–8.
176. Schloerb P, Amare M. JPEN J Parenter Entereral Nutr 1993; 17:407–13.
177. Morlion BJ, Sjedhoff HP, Furst P, et al. (Abstract) Clin Nutr 1996;15(Suppl):48.
178. Jebb SA, Osborne FJ, Maughar TS. Br J Cancer 1995;70: 732–5.
179. Jebb SA, Marcus R, Elia M. Clin Nutr 1995;14:143–6.

180. Bozetti F. Nutrition 1997;13:748–51.
181. Rosenberg SA. Cancer Res 1991;51(Suppl):5074S–9S.
182. Dillman RO. Ann Intern Med 1989;111:592–603.
183. Bast RC, Zalutksy MR, Frankel AE. Monocolonal serotherapy. In: Holland GF, ed. Cancer medicine. 4th ed. Baltimore: Williams & Wilkins 1997;1245–62.
184. Siegal JP, Pusi RK. J Clin Oncol 1991;9:694–704.
185. Brown RR, Lee CM, Kobler PC, et al. Cancer Res 1989;49: 4941–4.
186. Quesada JR, Talpaz M, Ris W. J Clin Oncol 1986;4:234–8.
187. Parkinson DR, Smith MA. (Editorial) Ann Intern Med 1992;117:338–40.
188. Warrell RP. Annu Rev Med 1996;47:555–65.
189. Colston KW, Chander SK, Mackay AG, et al. Biochem Pharmacol 1992;44:693–720.
190. Wali RK, Bissonette M, Khare S, et al. Gastroenterology 1996;111:118–26.
191. Fine HA, Kufe DW. Cancer gene therapy. In: Holland GF, ed. Cancer medicine. 4th ed. Baltimore: Williams & Wilkins, 1997;1265–78.
192. Copeland EM, MacFayden BV, Lanzotti VJ, et al. Am J Surg 1975;129:167–73.
193. Copeland EM, Souchon EA, MacFayden BV, et al. Cancer 1977;36:609–16.
194. Shike M. Russel DM, Detsky A, et al. Ann Intern Med 1984;101:303–9.
195. Serrou B, Cupissol D, Plagne R, et al. Cancer Treat Rep 1981;65 (Suppl):151–5.
196. Valdivieso M, Bodner GP, Benjamin RS, et al. Cancer Treat Rep 1981;65(Suppl 5):145–50.
197. Nixon DW, Moffitt S, Lawson DH, et al. Cancer Treat Rep 1981;65(Suppl 5):121–8.
198. Samuels ML, Selig DE, Ogden S, et al. Cancer Treat Rep 1981;65:615–27.
199. Daly JM, Reynold J, Thom A, et al. Ann Surg 1988;208:512–23.
200. Fletcher JP, Little JM. Surgery 1986;100:21–4.
201. DeCicco M, Panarello G, Fantin D, et al. JPEN J Parenter Enteral Nutr 1993;17:513–8.
202. McGeer AJ, Detsky AS, O'Rourke K. Nutrition 1990;6:478–83.
203. American College of Physicians. Position paper. Parenteral nutrition in patients receiving cancer chemotherapy. Ann Intern Med 1989;110:734–6.
204. Klein SM, Simes J, Blackburn GL. Cancer 1986;58:1378–86.
205. Lipman TO. Hemotol Oncol Clin North Am 1991;5:91–102.
206. Weisdorf SA, Lysne J, Wind D, et al. Transplantation 1987; 43:833–8.
207. Hays DM, Merritt RF, White L, et al. Med Pediatr Oncol 1983;11:137–9.
208. Ghavimi F, Shils ME, Scott BF, et al. J Pediatr 1982;4:530–7.
209. Muller JM, Brenner U, Dienst C, et al. Lancet 1982;1:68–71.
210. Fan St, Lo M, Lai ECS, et al. N Engl J Med 1994;331:1547–2.
211. Detsky AS, Baker JP, O'Rourke K, et al. Ann Intern Med 1987;107:195–203
212. Koretz RZ. J Clin Oncol 1984;2:534–8.
213. Freeman J, Goldmann DA, Smith NE, et al. N Engl J Med 1990;323:301–8.
214. Souba WW. N Engl J Med 1997;336:41–8.
215. Wolfe BM, Mathiesen KA, JPEN J Parenter Enteral Nutr 1997;21:1–6.
216. Lipschitz DA, Mitchell CO. JPEN J Parenter Enteral Nutr 1980;4:593–217.
217. Evans WK, Nixon DW, Dalyn JM, et al. J Clin Oncol 1987;5: 113–24.
218. Tandon SP, Gupta SC, Sinha SN, et al. Indian J Med Res 1984;80:180–8.
219. Elkort RJ, Baker FL, Vitale JJ, et al. JPEN J Parenter Enteral Nutr 1981;5:385–90.
220. Cousineau L, Bounous G, Rochon M, et al. Clin Res 1973;21:1067 (Abstract).
221. Bounous G, Gentile JM, Hugon J. Can J Surg 1971;14:312–24.
222. Ryan JA, Page CP, Babcock L. Ann Surg 1981;47:392–4.
223. Shukla HS, Rao RR, Banu N, et al. Indian J Med Res 1984; 80:339–46.
224. Smith RC, Haremink FJ, Hollinshead JW, et al. Br J Surg 1985;72:458–61.
225. Flynn MB, Leightty FF. Am J Surg 1987;154:359–62.
226. Howard L, Ament R, Fleming R, et al. Gastroenterology 1995; 109:355–65.
227. Herrington AM, Herrington JD, Church CA. Nutr Clin Pract 1997;12:101–13.
228. Ng B, Wolf RE, Weksler B, et al. Cancer Res 1993;53:5483–4.
229. Bartlett DC, Stein TP, Torosian MH. Surgery 1995;117:260–7.
230. Ng EH, Rock CS, Lazarus DD, et al. Am J Physiol 1992; 262:R426–31.
230a. Dong Y-L, Fleming RY, Huang KF, et al. J Surg Oncol 1993;53:121–7.
231. Tomas FM, Chandler CS, Coyle P, et al. Biochem J 1994;301:769–75.
232. Brauer M, Inculet RI, Bhatnagar G, et al. Cancer Res 1994;54:6383–6.
233. Stallion A, Foley-Nelsae T, Chance WT, et al. J Surg Res 1995;59:387–92.
234. Hyltander A, Svaninger G, Lundholm K. Biosci Rep 1993;13:325–31.
235. Lyden E, Cvetkovska E, Westin T, et al. Metabolism 1995; 44:445–51.
236. Chlebowski RT, Herrold J, Ali I, et al. Cancer 1986;58:183–6.
237. Sherry BA, Gelin J, Fang Y, et al. FASEB J 1989;3:1956–9.
238. Gelin J, Moldawer LL, Lonnroth C, et al. Cancer Res 1991; 51:415–21.
239. Castelli P, Carbo N, Tessitore L, et al. J Clin Invest 1993;9: 2783–6.
240. Fujimoto-Ouchi K, Tamura S, Mori K, et al. Int J Cancer 1995;61:522–8.
241. Mattys P, Dijkmans R, Proost P, et al. Int J Cancer 1991;49:77–82.
242. Goldberg RM, Loprinzi CL, Mailliard JA, et al. J Clin Oncol 1995;13:2856–9.
243. Lissoni P, Paolorossi F, Tancini G, et al. Eur J Cancer 1996; 32A:1340–3.
244. Ackermann M, Kirchner H, Atzpodien J. Anticancer Drugs 1993;4:585–7.
245. Montovani G, Maccio A, Bianchi A, et al. Int J Clin Lab Res 1995;25:135–41.
246. U.S. Congress, Office of Technology Assessment. Unconventional cancer treatments. OTA-H-405. Washington, DC; Government Printing Office, 1990.
247. Sampson W. Antiscience trends in the rise of the "alternative medicine" movement. In: Gross PR, Levitt N, Lewis MW, eds. The flight from science and reason. NY Acad Sci 1996;775:188–97.
248. Cassileth BR, Lusk EJ, Guerrey Du P, et al. N Engl J Med 1991;324:1180–5.
249. American Society for Clinical Oncology. Ineffective cancer therapy: a guide for the lay person. J Clin Oncol 1983;1: 154–63.
250. Anon. Questionable methods of cancer management. New York: American Cancer Society, 1992.
251. Cassileth BR, Lusk EJ, Strouse TB, et al. Ann Intern Med 1984;101:105–12.

83. Bone Biology in Health and Disease: A Tutorial

ROBERT P. HEANEY

BONE COMPOSITION AND STRUCTURE

Bone is a tissue in which cells make up only 2 to 5% of the volume, and nonliving material, 95 to 98%. It is the nonliving material that gives the bone its mechanical properties of hardness, stiffness, and resiliency. This nonliving material consists of a mineral-encrusted protein matrix (also called *osteoid*), with the mineral comprising about half the volume and the matrix the other half. Unlike other connective tissues, there is virtually no free water in the bony material itself. Embedded in this solid material are cells, called *osteocytes,* residing in lacunae in the matrix, and communicating with one another through an extensive network of long cellular processes lying in channels called *canaliculi* that ramify throughout the bone. As a consequence of this arrangement, virtually no volume of normal bone is more than a few micrometers distant from a living cell. Furthermore, even in the dense bone of the shafts of long bones, there is an extensive network of vascular channels, so that the most remote osteocyte is typically no more than 90 μm away from a capillary.

Bone Mineral

The mineral of bone is a carbonate-rich, imperfect hydroxyapatite with variable stoichiometry. Calcium comprises 37 to 40%, phosphate 50 to 58%, and carbonate 2 to 8% of this mineral. These values vary somewhat from species to species, and the carbonate component is particularly sensitive to systemic acid-base status (decreasing in acidosis and rising in alkalosis). In addition, bone mineral contains small amounts of sodium, potassium, magnesium, citrate, and other ions present in the extracellular fluid at the time the mineral was deposited, adsorbed onto the crystal surfaces and trapped there as the water in the recently deposited matrix is displaced by the growing mineral crystals.

Protein Matrix

The protein matrix of bone, as for tendons, ligaments, and dermis, consists predominantly of collagen, which comprises about 90% of the organic matrix. For bone, the collagen is type I. Collagen is a long fibrous protein, coiled as a triple helix. For the molecules of the protein to coil tightly, there can be no side chains projecting off the peptide backbone on the side facing inward; hence every third amino acid in the body of the collagen molecule is glycine. Projecting outward, however, are the side chains of various amino acids, such as lysine, which allow posttranslational formation of tight covalent bonds between collagen fibers. This cross-linking helps prevent fibers from sliding along one another when bone is stressed along the axis of the fibers.

Noncollagenous Matrix Proteins (1)

Noncollagenous proteins make up about 10% of the organic matrix of bone. They include a family of proteins in which glutamic acid residues are carboxylated in the γ position, called *gla-proteins,* the best studied of which is osteocalcin (or bone gla-protein, BGP), which comprises about 1.5% of the matrix. Other proteins include osteonectin, fibronectin, matrix gla-protein, osteopontin, and bone sialoprotein. The functions of these many constituents are unclear. Some doubtless serve as chemoattractants for osteoclasts, while others stimulate osteoblasts to lay down new bone. Because of these properties of the matrix proteins, bone seems to contain the chemical signals for its own remodeling (see below).

The shape and three-dimensional structure of bone is determined by its protein matrix. A bone that has been completely demineralized in the laboratory (by soaking in acid or EDTA) looks entirely normal, and when sectioned, stained, and examined under a microscope, reveals all the fine structure of bone. In fact, prior demineralization has been the traditional first step in studying bone histologically (since mineralized bone tends to damage the microtome knives used by histologists to make their sections).

BONE CELLS AND THEIR FUNCTIONS

There are four principal bone cells: lining cells, osteoblasts, osteoclasts, and osteocytes. They are responsible both for maintaining the mechanical properties of bone and for mediating the calcium homeostatic function of bone.

Lining cells are flat, fibrocyte-like cells covering free surfaces of bone. They are probably derived from, or closely related to, the osteoblast cell line. They form a membrane that completely covers free bone surfaces and insulates them from the cells and hormones in the general circulation.

Osteoblasts, derived from marrow stromal cells, are the cells that lay down bone, first synthesizing, depositing, and orienting the fibrous proteins of the matrix, then initiating changes that render the matrix capable of mineralization. Osteoblasts lay down this matrix between and beneath themselves on a preexisting bone surface, thereby pushing themselves backward as they add new bone.

Bone matrix, when freshly deposited, consists of about half protein and half water and is not immediately mineralizable, just as the similar collagen-based structures, tendon and ligament, do not normally calcify. So the osteoblast still has more work to do after forming and depositing the matrix. The details of the process are not completely clear, but they involve secretion of proteins by the osteoblast into the matrix that it had previously laid down. These somehow help create a three-dimensional configuration that attracts calcium and phosphate ions and arranges them in the apatite crystal habitus. Osteoblasts also secrete an enzyme called *alkaline phosphatase* that hydrolyzes organic phosphate compounds in the vicinity, which would otherwise inhibit mineralization. Finally, as mineral is deposited, it displaces the water of the original matrix. The apatitic crystals that form are spindle shaped and are oriented parallel with, and lie between, the collagen fibers.

Osteoclasts are derived from the monocyte-macrophage line of cells, are usually multinucleated, and are the cells that resorb bone. They do this by attaching firmly to a microscopic bony surface, walling off a small region of that surface, and then secreting acid and proteolytic enzymes into this confined space. These dissolve the mineral and digest the matrix. The osteoclasts then release the breakdown products into the extracellular fluid around the resorption site, from whence they are carried away by the circulating blood. The calcium and phosphorus released into the bloodstream are usually used to mineralize other bone-forming sites elsewhere in the skeleton, while the protein fragments are metabolized or excreted. After working for a short time (a few days), the osteoclasts undergo programed cell death (apoptosis), leaving their excavation to be refilled by osteoblasts.

Osteocytes are osteoblasts that have stopped matrix synthesis and have become embedded in bone as other bone-forming cells around them continue to add new layers of matrix. Osteocytes are responsible for monitoring the amount of strain (bending) occurring in their domains when bone is mechanically loaded and for reporting that information to lining cells on nearby anatomic bone surfaces, which may then initiate local bone remodeling projects.

The activity of these bone cells is influenced by a large number of both systemic and local hormonal agents. Additionally, the cells influence the activity of one another. Table 83.1 lists a few of the many agents influencing osteoblasts and osteoclasts. This is a rapidly developing field of investigation with much still to be learned. Osteoblasts or cells of the osteoblast lineage occupy a central position, not just in forming bone, but in processing systemic signals to the bone-remodeling apparatus (see below, "Revision of Bony Material"). Thus, although parathyroid hormone (PTH) is responsible for stimulating bone resorption, there are no PTH receptors on the osteoclast. Rather they are found on osteoblasts (and related cells) which, in response to PTH-binding, release agents that stimulate osteoclast activity. By contrast, the osteoclasts do possess calcitonin (CT) receptors and are thus able to respond very rapidly to the antiresorptive stimulus provided by CT.

BONE ARCHITECTURE

Bone consists of a dense outer shell, or cortex, and an internal, chambered system of interconnected plates,

Table 83.1
Humoral Factors Acting on Bone Cells

Osteoblasts	Osteoclasts
Parathyroid hormone	Calcitonin
$1,25(OH)_2D$	Bisphosphonate drugs
Glucocorticoids	Interleukin-1
Insulin-like growth factors (IGFs)	Colony stimulating factor (CSF-1)
Transforming growth factor-β (TGF-β)	TGF-α
Interleukin-6	TGF-β
Parathyroid hormone–related peptide (PTHrP)	Gallium nitrate

rods, and spicules called *cancellous, or trabecular bone* (Fig. 83.1). In the shafts of the long bones the cortical component predominates, creating a hollow tube, while nearer the joints the cortex becomes thinner, and the interior is made up of an extensive latticework of cancellous bone. Bones such as the vertebrae, pelvis, sternum, and shoulder blades possess a thin outer rind of cortex and a more or less even distribution of cancellous bone on the inside.

The proportions both of mineral and matrix and of calcium and phosphorus are essentially identical in cortical and cancellous bone. The issue has been sometimes confused in the literature because of the difficulty of removing adherent marrow elements from cancellous bone samples prior to analysis. Fundamentally, however, bone is bone. Cancellous bone, however, turns over (remodels) much more rapidly than cortical bone. This is partly because of the much greater surface area of cancellous bone. (Remodeling always proceeds from a microanatomic bone surface into the bony material. See below, "Revision of Bony Material.") It is also partly due to the generally greater contact with hemopoietic marrow in cancellous bone. In fact, the partition between bone with and without red marrow is probably more important than the partition between cortical and trabecular bone.

The end segments of bones are called *epiphyses* (Fig. 83.2). The shafts of long bones are called *diaphyses,* and the flared portion of the shaft merging with the region of the growth plate is called a *metaphysis.* The lining cells on the outside of the bone form a tough sheet or membrane, called the *periosteum,* while the cells on the inside surfaces of both cortical and trabecular bone are called the *endosteum.*

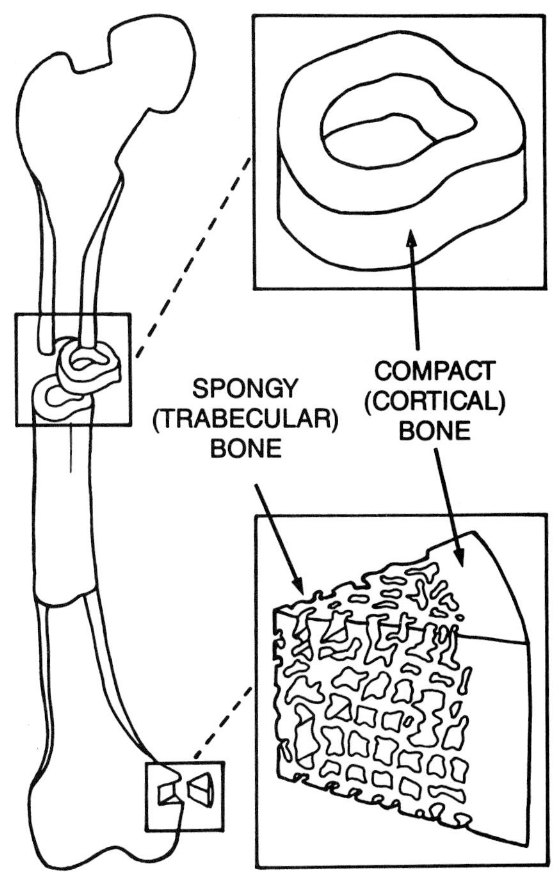

Figure 83.1. Gross and microarchitecture of a typical long bone. (Copyright Robert P. Heaney, 1996; used with permission.)

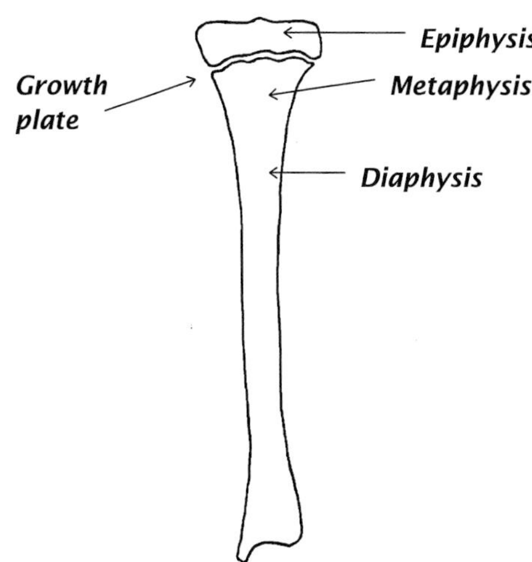

Figure 83.2. Principal regions of a growing long bone. (Copyright Robert P. Heaney, 1996; used with permission.)

The spaces between the trabecular plates and spicules are filled with bone marrow. Early in life much of that marrow is hemopoietic, but later the blood-producing marrow is confined to the bones of the trunk, and the peripheral skeletal marrow spaces are filled mostly with fat.

In dense cortical bone, remodeling over the years produces a series of internal structures called *osteons* or Haversian systems, in which concentric cylindrical layers of bone are laid down along the course of a capillary. These are produced by the usual remodeling process (see below, "Revision of Bony Material"). First a tubular hole is created in the bone by osteoclastic resorption; then it is filled in by successive waves of osteoblasts moving from the outside inward.

At their ends, where bones meet one another, is a joint; the bony surface is covered with a layer of cartilage, rather than with periosteum. In health, this cartilage is highly hydrated and is lubricated by synovial fluid held there by a tough connective tissue sac called the *joint capsule.* This arrangement ensures that the bones move on one another smoothly.

BONE DEVELOPMENT

In utero, most bones are formed first as cartilage models that are gradually replaced by bone. In this process, blood vessels invade the cartilage, calcification ensues, and the calcified cartilage is then removed by osteoclasts and replaced by bone laid down by osteoblasts. In infancy and childhood, bone development is somewhat similar. However, to accommodate growth, most bones possess one or more plates of cartilage perpendicular to the main axis of growth, separating, for example, the bone at the ends of a long bone from the bone of the shaft. This structure, called a *growth plate* (Fig. 83.2), consists of rapidly proliferating cartilage cells that, as they multiply, push the ends of the bones away from the shafts. Blood vessels invade these columns of proliferating cartilage cells from the shaft side and initiate calcification of the cartilage and bone replacement in a process similar to that occurring in utero. Meanwhile, the ends of the bone are being pushed still farther away, so that there continues to be an anatomic and temporal sequence consisting of growth plate, proliferating cartilage, calcifying cartilage, and bony replacement, progressing down the metaphysis from the epiphyses toward the diaphysis.

Growth stops when the ossification process catches up with the formation of new cartilage and bony bridges develop across the growth plate, firmly anchoring the ends to the shaft of the bone. This closure process is initiated by the high levels of estrogen produced at puberty in both girls and boys. During the time when growth in length is occurring, the process of modeling (see below) shapes the outsides of the bones to keep them in proper proportion with the growth in length. At midshaft this typically involves periosteal new bone formation and endosteal resorption.

REVISION OF BONY MATERIAL

Although the intercellular bony material, which makes up 95 to 98% of the volume of bone, is nonliving, nevertheless it is capable of being revised and replaced, just as are soft tissues, whose cellular constituents are constantly and invisibly turning over. With bone, the revision process occurs at discrete locations and can be readily visualized microscopically. The process normally follows a stereotyped sequence of activation first, then resorption, then reversal, and finally formation. This sequence is shown diagrammatically in Figure 83.3.

In the activation step, lining cells on a bone surface retract, exposing the bony substance directly to the circulating blood. Mineralized bone serves as a chemoattractant for osteoclast precursors, which migrate to the exposed site, coalesce, attach to bone as osteoclasts, and begin to erode into the bone. After removing a suitable volume of bone, osteoclasts undergo apoptosis and disappear from the scene. A reversal phase follows. Then osteoblasts move in and begin to replace the bone removed from the cavity. They orient the collagen fibers in parallel arrays, layer by layer, often alternating direction of the fibers every few micrometers. In this way they build what is termed *lamellar bone,* which is similar in a sense to plywood (in which the grain of the wood runs in different directions in different layers). In the adult, osteoblasts advance at a rate of about 0.5 μm/day, and mineralization lags about 10 days behind the advancing matrix deposition. Some of the osteoblasts, as noted above, stay behind in cavities within the bone and become osteocytes.

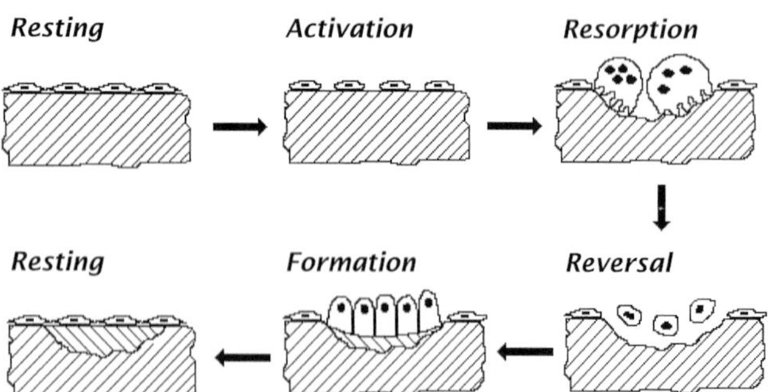

Figure 83.3. Schematic diagram of some of the major bone cells, indicating their role in the bone remodeling sequence. In the resting state, the bone surface is covered by lining cells. These retract at activated sites. Multinucleated osteoclasts move in and excavate a cavity. Then, after reversal, columnar osteoblasts deposit new bone matrix. Finally, the resting state is reestablished. (Copyright Robert P. Heaney, 1996; used with permission.)

When this revision process is finished at a particular site, the remaining surface osteoblasts become quiescent, flatten out, and turn into lining cells, effectively sealing the new bone surface until, at some later time, a new remodeling project is initiated locally. In healthy adults, this sequence, from start to finish, takes about 3 months at any given site. The resorptive phase takes about 2 to 3 weeks and formation, 2 to 3 months. The process is more rapid in infants and small children and slower in the elderly.

The process just described is technically called *remodeling.* One of its principal purposes is to replace damaged bone with fresh new material. But during growth, and indeed at any time when the shape of the bone is being revised, the resorptive and formative processes occur, not at the same site, but in different parts of the bone. For example, the small shafts of the long bones of a child enlarge to adult size by osteoblastic formation on the periosteal surface and corresponding osteoclastic resorption on the endosteal surface. This process is technically called *modeling,* and is similar to remodeling in most respects except that the new bone is laid down at a location different from the site of resorption.

One of the ways this revision process can be readily visualized is by administration of carefully timed doses of a fluorescent compound such as one of the tetracycline antibiotics. The molecules of these markers bind to mineralizing bone sites and are trapped as the site is buried by layers of new bone. The markers become readily visible when, on undecalcified bone biopsy, specimens are viewed microscopically under ultraviolet illumination (Fig. 83.4.).

BONE FUNCTIONS

Bone serves two distinct functions: provision of mechanical rigidity and stiffness to our bodies, and provision of a homeostatic buffer, particularly to help our bodies maintain a constant level of calcium in the circulating body fluids and to provide a reserve supply of phosphorus. The mechanical function is necessary so that we can resist gravity and move about on dry land. (Strictly speaking a

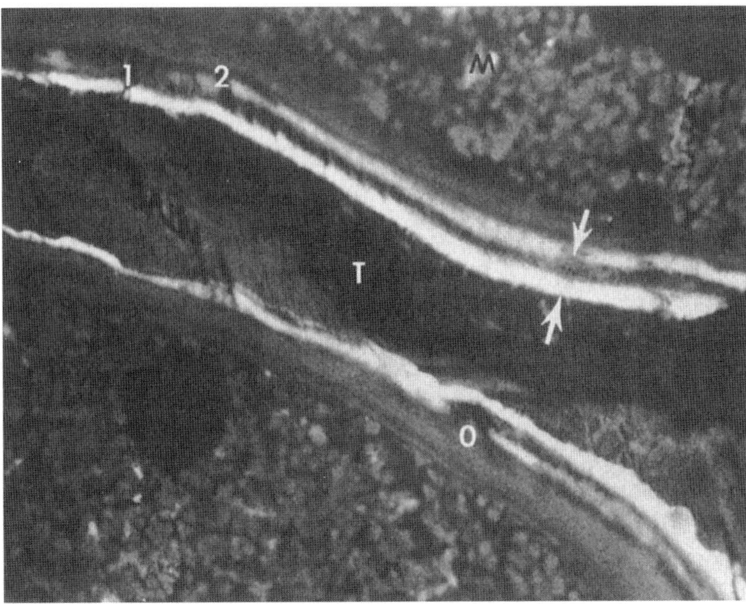

Figure 83.4. Section through trabecular bone obtained from the iliac crest. *M,* marrow; *O,* osteoid; *T,* trabecular bone; *1* and *2,* first and second tetracycline labels. The *distance between the arrows* represents the amount of bone deposited during the time between administration of the two tetracycline labels. (From Fallon MD. Morphology and dynamics of bone nutritional interactions. In: Shils ME, Olson JA, Shike M, eds. Modern nutrition in health and disease. 8th ed. 1994;889.)

rigid skeleton would not be necessary in a fully buoyant medium such as water. For example, some originally bony fish, such as the sturgeon, have lost nearly all of their skeleton over the millennia of evolution. Still they function mechanically perfectly well.) The homeostatic function is the older of the two from the standpoint of evolution and is, in a sense, the more fundamental, since the body will sacrifice the structural function before it will risk losing the homeostatic one. In other words, the body will weaken the bone structurally to maintain the calcium levels of the blood and extracellular fluid.

Mechanical

In the mechanical function of bone, nature strikes a balance between a skeleton so massive that it would resist most forces but be too heavy to carry around and one so flimsy that while adequate to meet calcium homeostatic needs would be too fragile to sustain the mechanical forces of exertion or of minor injuries. Bone finds the middle ground by adjusting its mass, using a classic negative-feedback loop so that it bends under routine use by about 0.1–0.15% in all dimensions (Fig. 83.5). This bend-

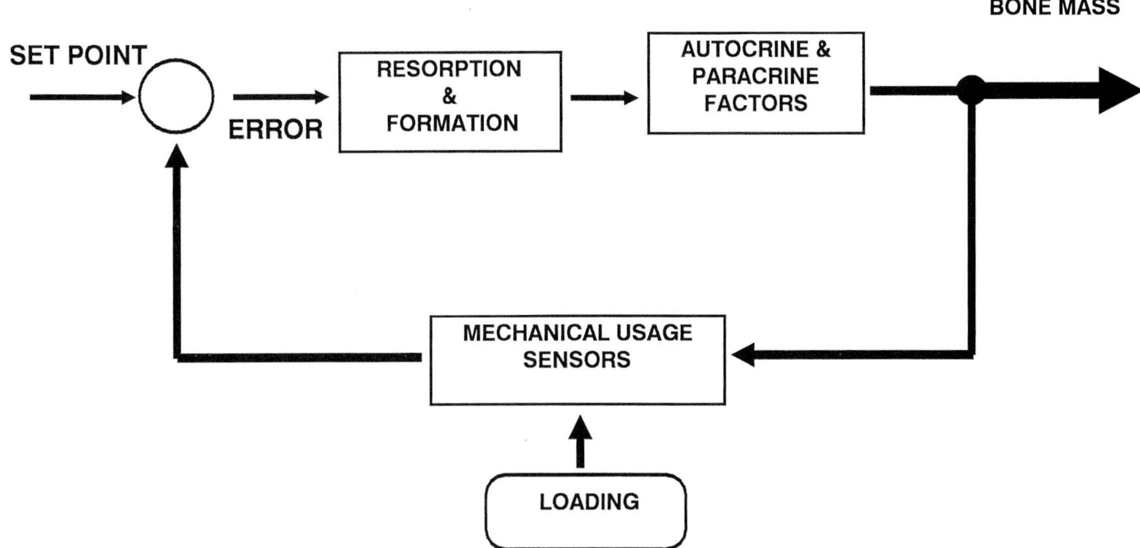

Figure 83.5. Feedback loop regulating bone mass. Mechanical sensors detect the amount of bending occurring under loading, compare that with the reference level, or setpoint, and if the two differ, send signals to the remodeling apparatus, either to initiate remodeling or to adjust the balance between resorption and formation. (Copyright Robert P. Heaney, 1990. Reproduced with permission.)

ing setpoint is a major determinant of bone *size* during growth and bone *density* during adult remodeling.

In the operation of this control loop, the osteocytes detect the amount of bending (or strain) in a local region of bone and send signals to nearby cells of the remodeling apparatus, which mediate the balance between resorption and formation. The result is that when bone is loaded locally so heavily that its strain is greater than the reference amount (as with an increase in strenuous exercise), the processes of modeling and remodeling work to increase local bone density. And when bone is loaded less heavily, so that its strains are less than this reference amount, remodeling removes more bone than it replaces, thereby lightening the structure and making it less stiff. For example, the bones in the dominant arm tend to be denser than those on the nondominant side, and the bones of athletes denser than those of nonathletes. This effect on bone mass is illustrated in Figure 83.6, which shows how this difference in bone mass between the dominant and nondominant arms is exaggerated in world-class tennis players relative to nonathletes.

The strength of a bony structure is proportional to approximately the square of the bony density. This relationship makes bone strength sensitive to relatively small changes in density and helps explain why fracture risk doubles at bone density values only 10 to 15% lower than normal.

It is important to grasp the meaning of this doubling of fracture risk. If an average individual's risk of fracture is, for example, one chance in 100 in any given year, doubling the risk means simply two chances in 100. The average individual will not perceive any difference, since the typical individual will not actually experience fracture (i.e., 98 of 100 will be fracture free). Nevertheless, at a population level, the group of all individuals experiencing this decline in bone mass will have twice as many fractures,

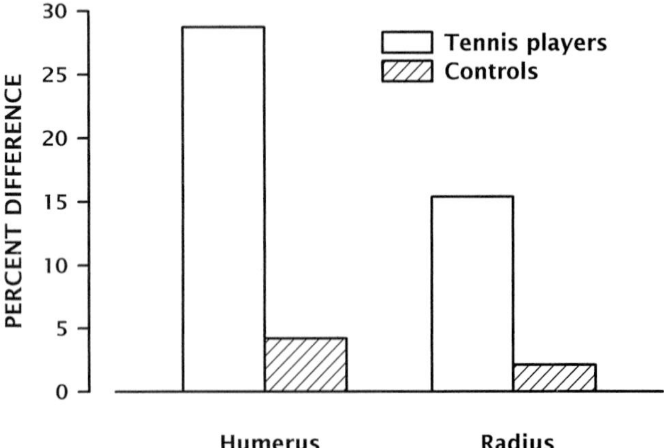

Figure 83.6. Difference in humeral and radial bone mass between dominant and nondominant arms of world class tennis players and nonathletic controls. Note that, even in the controls, the greater use of the dominant arm results in more bone on that side. This difference is greatly amplified in the tennis players. (Adapted from Kannus P, Haapasalo H, Sievanen H, et al. Bone 1994;15:279–84; copyright Robert P. Heaney, 1996; used with permission.)

and health care costs or demands on the health care system will rise accordingly.

Homeostatic

The bone remodeling process also mediates the homeostatic function of bone. While the pattern of strain under loading is the major determinant of *where* bone remodeling occurs, parathyroid hormone (PTH) is the principal determinant of *how much* remodeling is occurring and how readily bone cells in any given locus respond to local stimuli to initiate a remodeling project. PTH secretion is directly responsive to the body's need for calcium. It is important to note that calcium is never simply removed from bone. Instead whole volumes of bone are removed and their calcium then scavenged to meet body needs.

As noted above, resorption precedes formation. This produces local asynchrony of mineral movement: remodeling at any given site first makes its calcium and phosphorus available to the body (as mineral is removed during resorption). The same site later creates a demand for calcium and phosphorus as the mineralizing site extracts mineral from the blood flowing past. Averaged over the whole skeleton, these processes are about equal at any given time: new remodeling sites are releasing as much calcium as the older sites are depositing. However, this local asynchrony also means that when remodeling activity is increased, resorption changes first and more calcium is released from bone than previously initiated remodeling sites need. Thus, an additional supply of calcium is made temporarily available to the body. Conversely, when remodeling is acutely suppressed, resorption drops immediately, while previously initiated formation continues, and thus the skeleton can soak up a temporary excess of calcium from the blood (Fig. 83.7). Modulation of remodeling in this way by the hormones PTH and calcitonin (CT) is a major part of the basis of the regulation of blood calcium levels by the skeleton.

Two examples with nutritional relevance illustrate how this system operates. During the absorption of large quantities of calcium from milk in infant feeding, CT is secreted to suppress osteoclastic resorptive activity, thereby reducing release of calcium from bone. This allows the demands of rapidly mineralizing bone to be met by absorbed calcium from the milk, and at the same time prevents the absorbed calcium from causing a dangerous increase in blood [Ca^{2+}]. Later, during the postabsorptive phase, CT levels drop, and PTH levels rise to stimulate resorption again. This action sustains the blood [Ca^{2+}] at normal levels despite the ongoing mineral demands of bone formation and wide swings in calcium input from the intestine. Another example is found during antler formation in deer. Each spring the demands of the growing antler exceed the calcium available from the late-winter foliage that makes up the deer's diet. So a burst of PTH-mediated remodeling occurs throughout the skeleton at the time antler mineralization begins. This creates a tem-

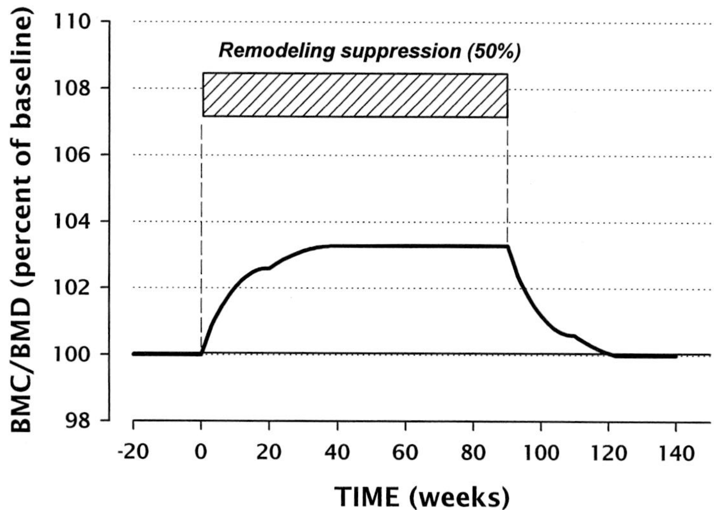

Figure 83.7. Positive bone remodeling transient in a healthy individual who is not calcium deficient, in response first to a large increase in calcium intake (sufficient to suppress remodeling by 50%) and then to its later withdrawal. The vertical axis is bone mass (i.e., either bone mineral content, *BMC*, or bone mineral density, *BMD*), expressed as percentage of the baseline value. Note that the initial rise in bone mass does not continue past one remodeling cycle (40 weeks in this illustration), and that the bone gained by remodeling suppression is lost once again when remodeling returns to its previous level. (Copyright Robert P. Heaney, 1996. Reproduced with permission.)

porary surplus of calcium from skeletal remodeling, which is used to mineralize the bone of the rapidly forming antler. Later, when the new bony remodeling sites throughout the skeleton enter their own formation phase, they are filled in with calcium made available from the calcium-rich summer grasses and foliage.

NUTRIENTS IMPORTANT TO SKELETAL INTEGRITY

Total nutritional status influences bone cell function just as it does the function of other tissues. However, cellular malnutrition affects mainly bone currently being remodeled, while the strength of bony structures at any given time depends not so much on current cell function as on the mass of bony material accumulated by bone cellular activity over many years. For that reason, acute nutritional stresses or deficiencies rarely produce overt skeletal symptoms in adults, even when they severely compromise bone cell function. Children and growing animals show effects more promptly, both because they have less skeletal capital in their bone banks and because they are revising it much more rapidly. Nevertheless, a few nutrients are more likely than others to produce skeletal manifestations when deficient: calcium, phosphorus, vitamin D, vitamin K, and certain of the trace minerals.

Calcium and Phosphorus

In addition to buffering absorptive oscillations in blood calcium levels, bone serves as a nutrient reserve for both calcium and phosphorus. This reserve is to the calcium (and phosphorus) functions of the body as body fat is to energy metabolism. But unlike most nutrient reserves, this one (bone) has acquired a distinct function in its own right, i.e., mechanical/structural support. In other words, we walk around on our calcium reserve. It follows that any influence, nutritional or otherwise, that alters the size of the calcium reserve will alter bone strength.

Bone is a very rich source of calcium. Total skeletal calcium averages 1100 to 1500 g, and each cubic centimeter of bone contains more calcium than the entire circulating blood in an adult. Thus, in comparison with other nutrients, the calcium reserve is huge. While low-calcium diets usually deplete the bony reserves, they do so slowly. Thus, while *population-level* risk of fracture rises immediately, it will take many years for bone strength to be sufficiently reduced to lead to a detectable increase in an *individual's* risk of fracture (see above). The slow expression of the effect of calcium deficiency has led many nutritional scientists in the past to the erroneous conclusion that calcium was not important for adult bone strength. Nevertheless, a nutritional deficiency that develops over 30 years is just as much a deficiency as one that develops over 30 days.

Low intakes of calcium and phosphorus can both limit bone acquisition during growth and cause bone loss after maturity. Calcium intake operates most directly through modulation of remodeling, as described above. In the antler example previously cited, if summer foliage were not calcium rich, each cycle of antler formation would deplete the skeleton, bony replacement would fail to occur, and bone mass would fall progressively over the animal's adult life. Because human calcium requirement rises with age (3) and because calcium intakes tend to fall in the elderly, precisely such depletion occurs in most human populations as they age.

Inadequate phosphorus availability also affects bone, but in a different way. The osteoblast environment is one of continuous mineralization, with the matrix extracting phosphate (as well as calcium) from the fluid bathing the bone-forming cells. While calcium makes up about 40% of the bone mineral, phosphate accounts for nearly 60%. Thus, phosphorus is fully as important for bone building as is calcium. Rapid growth is not possible without a high blood phosphate level, which explains the substantially higher blood phosphate values in children. When phosphate levels in the blood entering bone are low, mineralization extracts as much phosphate as it can from the fluid around the osteoblast. In so doing, it creates a local environment severely depleted of phosphate. But osteoblasts, like all cells, need phosphate for their own metabolism. The result is serious interference with osteoblast function; matrix deposition is slowed and osteoblast initiation of mineralization is reduced even more. These abnormalities produce the typical histologic pattern in bone of rickets and osteomalacia (see below).

Vitamin D

Vitamin D has many bony effects, such as facilitating development of osteoclast precursors at an activated remodeling locus and augmenting osteoclast response to resorptive stimuli. The vitamin also stimulates synthesis and release of osteocalcin by osteoblasts (see above). But its major importance for bone is to facilitate absorption of calcium (and to some extent phosphorus) from the diet. Severe vitamin D deficiency causes rickets and osteomalacia (see below). Milder shortages of the vitamin reduce calcium availability to the body and produce a situation of calcium deficiency. Because of the traditional (if simplistic) identification of vitamin D *deficiency* with rickets and osteomalacia, it is customary to refer to less extreme degrees of vitamin D shortage as *insufficiency*.

Vitamin K

Vitamin K functions in the γ-carboxylation of the glutamic acid residues of three bone gla-proteins, the best studied of which is osteocalcin. Vitamin K deficiency results both in undercarboxylation of osteocalcin and in reduced osteocalcin synthesis. The net effect of these changes on bone strength or integrity is not certain.

Micronutrients

Vitamin C and certain trace minerals (notably copper, zinc, and manganese) are important cofactors for synthesis or cross-linking of matrix proteins. Copper and vitamin C are perhaps the best studied in this regard. Copper is the cofactor for lysyl oxidase, the enzyme responsible for cross-linking collagen fibrils. Interference with cross-linking results in structurally weak bone. Ascorbic acid is also a required cofactor for the cross-linking of collagen fibrils, and in its absence bone strength is impaired. In the face of deficiencies of these micronutrients during growth, severe bone abnormalities can result. These abnormalities include stunting of growth, deformity of bones, and epiphyseal dysplasia. Whether adults can develop sufficient deficiencies of these nutrients to interfere significantly with bone integrity remains unknown.

SKELETAL DISORDERS AND THEIR NUTRITIONAL CORRELATES

Osteoporosis

Osteoporosis is a multifactorial condition of the skeleton in which skeletal strength is reduced to such an extent that fractures occur on minor trauma (see also Chapter 85). Generally, osteoporosis exhibits reduced bone mass (i.e., both matrix and mineral) as well as various microstructural disturbances of bony architecture (4). A simple decrease in quantity of bone is sometimes called "osteopenia" (literally, "shortage of bone"). By current World Health Organization standards, osteopenia is a bone mass value between −1 and −2.5 standard deviations below young-adult normal values. Bone mass or density values more than 2.5 standard deviations below young-adult normal are now called osteoporosis, whether or not a fracture is present.

Lack of exercise, alcohol abuse, smoking, gonadal hormone deficiency, and inadequate intakes of calcium and vitamin D can all contribute to development of this disorder. Given diets typical of the elderly in Europe and North America, it can be estimated that inadequate calcium intake accounts for one-third to two-thirds of osteoporotic fractures. (This is why the U.S. Food and Drug Administration allows an osteoporosis health claim on labels of certain calcium-rich foods.)

Rickets and Osteomalacia (5)

Rickets is a disorder of the growth apparatus of bone (see above) in which the growth cartilage fails to mature and mineralize normally. Growth is stunted, and various deformities about the growth plates occur. Osteomalacia is the corresponding disorder of adults, in which the newly deposited bone matrix fails to mineralize adequately. New matrix formation is slowed in both conditions, but mineralization is retarded even more; thus unmineralized matrix accumulates on microscopic bone surfaces. For this reason, the proportion of mineral to matrix drops. In severe cases, unmineralized bone may constitute so large a proportion of the skeleton that individual bones lose their stiffness and become severely deformed.

The stereotypical forms of rickets and osteomalacia are those associated with vitamin D deficiency. The principal pathogenesis of these common forms follows from insufficient intestinal absorption of calcium and phosphorus from the diet. In attempting to keep blood calcium levels close to normal levels, the body raises PTH secretion. Because one of the effects of PTH is to increase renal clearance of phosphate, this adaptive response drives the already reduced blood phosphate concentrations down to levels such that severe phosphate deficiency develops—first locally in the vicinity of the osteoblasts and chondrocytes, and then in other tissues as well (producing, e.g., muscle weakness, tenderness, and pain).

Rickets and osteomalacia develop for other reasons beside vitamin D deficiency, including fluoride toxicity and cadmium poisoning, as well as in association with certain rare vascular malignancies. Presumably the toxins or some product of tumor metabolism interferes with normal osteoblast function. More important is a group of heritable abnormalities of renal phosphate transport, the most common of which is X-linked hypophosphatemia (6). These share the inability to maintain the blood phosphate levels required for growth. Such forms of rickets produce their bony effects solely because of severe hypophosphatemia. This group of disorders in the past has been called vitamin D–resistant rickets. They do not respond to usual doses of vitamin D (hence their name). Therapy is directed at elevating serum phosphate levels.

Paget's Disease of Bone

Paget's disease is a local, but often multifocal, disorder of the bone remodeling process of uncertain etiology. Resorption proceeds erratically, with formation filling in with new bone behind it. Architecture and even external bone shape is disordered. During the early resorptive phase, the bone is excessively fragile and may fracture readily. The high level of bone remodeling is usually accompanied by high levels of remodeling markers (see below), particularly serum alkaline phosphatase. When the process involves the skull, bony growths may constrict the cranial nerve passages and lead to, for example, deafness. There are no known nutritional correlates of this disorder.

Parathyroid Dysfunction

Since PTH is the principal determinant of the amount of remodeling activity in the skeleton, one might expect significant skeletal manifestations of parathyroid functional disorders. The reality, however, is complicated. Patients with hypoparathyroidism have reduced remodeling, slightly greater than average bone mass, and probably fewer fractures. By contrast, patients with severe, long-standing hyperparathyroidism may have reduced bone mass, subperiosteal bone loss, widespread, very active bone remodeling, and even cysts in bone filled with osteoclast-like cells. Such cases are extremely rare today, and generally patients with primary hyperparathyroidism have no abnormalities of the skeleton detectable by ordinary x-rays. In fact, when PTH hypersecretion is pulsatile and the peaks are short-lived, PTH is actually trophic for bone and can produce quite large increases in spine bone density. For that reason, PTH is now an investigational therapy for osteoporosis.

Osteogenesis Imperfecta

Osteogenesis imperfecta (OI) is a group of heritable disorders in which there may be one of several mutations in the genes encoding for the collagen molecules that comprise the bulk of bone matrix (7). Patients with OI have fragile skeletons with reduced bone mass. In one of the common forms of OI, long bones typically have narrow shafts as well as reduced mass. Patients with OI commonly suffer many fractures throughout life, often starting in utero. When some other amino acid replaces glycine in the collagen molecule, the triple helix will not coil properly, collagen synthesis is reduced, and the matrix is abnormal. The severity of the defect depends upon the position of the substitution in the collagen molecule chain. Fractures heal normally. Other collagen-based connective tissues are also affected in certain forms of the disease, including dentin, ligaments and tendons, and the sclerae. Despite the manifest abnormality of the bone matrix, the reason for the reduced bone mass is unclear.

Bony Manifestations of Diseases of Nonskeletal Systems

Patients with chronic liver disease, especially biliary cirrhosis, commonly have a bone disease that is basically osteoporosis (8). Patients coming for liver transplant often have severe osteoporosis, attributable to a combination of the underlying disease, the immobilization that inevitably accompanies the severe disability of these very sick patients, and the treatments they have received.

Patients with end-stage renal disease often have a complex bone disease consisting of a varying mixture of osteosclerosis, osteomalacia, and hyperparathyroid bone disease (9). Exact expression of these varied abnormalities depends upon the medical regimens the patients have received, specifically on how these regimens have managed calcium, phosphorus, and vitamin D metabolism for the patient.

Patients with a variety of disorders of the small intestine, but especially those with gluten-sensitive enteropathy, malabsorb fat-soluble vitamins and hypersecrete calcium and magnesium into the digestive juices. As a result, they are commonly deficient in vitamin D, calcium, and magnesium. They often have severe osteoporosis and may have osteomalacia as well.

Patients who have had organ transplants commonly have osteoporosis (10), in part because they come to transplant with already reduced bone mass, and in part because the immunosuppressive therapy used to sustain the transplant itself causes bone loss.

Aluminum and Bone

Aluminum (Al) is not strictly speaking a nutrient, but it is extremely common in the environment, is a major component of antacids, and is widely used as cookware. Only a small portion of ingested Al is absorbed, and in healthy individuals, absorbed Al is promptly excreted in the urine. However, in patients with severely compromised renal function, particularly in those treated with large doses of Al-containing antacids to block phosphorus absorption, Al accumulates at the mineralizing sites of the bone remodeling process. It was thought at one time to be responsible for the unique bony pathology of end-stage renal disease, but Al is now considered to be at most only a minor contributor to renal osteopathy. Experimentally, Al has shown an ability to increase trabecular bone density in animals, particularly in combination with fluoride. The ultimate significance of this finding remains uncertain.

SKELETAL MANIFESTATIONS OF SYSTEMIC NUTRIENT DEFICIENCIES

Protein-Calorie Malnutrition

As noted above, the cells of bone are as dependent upon total nutrition as are other cells, and bone suffers in starvation just as do other tissues. However, bone strength is not immediately affected in acute malnutrition, especially in adults. There are two situations in which the bony effects of protein-calorie malnutrition are most obvious. One is during growth, when both growth rates and bone mass accumulation are retarded by malnutrition. The other is in repair of fractures, especially in the elderly. Protein-calorie malnutrition is common among the old elderly, and when they break a bone, such as the hip, serious complications and even death may develop. Protein supplementation reduces these complications substantially and is an important and necessary component of the treatment of most patients with hip fractures (11).

Magnesium Deficiency

Magnesium deficiency occurs with severe intestinal malabsorption (such as gluten-sensitive enteropathy, fistulas, or ileal resection, especially with high-fat diets) or with urinary losses from renal tubular defects. Initially, magnesium deficiency impairs bony responsiveness to PTH and thus leads to hypocalcemia despite a rising PTH level. As deficiency progresses, parathyroid response falters, and PTH secretion falls. The hypocalcemia of magnesium deficiency is thus due to impairment of the calcium regulatory system and is unresponsive to calcium supplementation (12) (see also Chapter 9). Less severe degrees of magnesium deficiency in these same syndromes are associated with reduced bone mass, also unresponsive to calcium supplementation. In addition to other needed treatments (such as calcium), magnesium supplements may be helpful in these patients.

INVESTIGATION OF NUTRIENT EFFECTS ON THE SKELETON

As noted above, the effects of nutrient deficiencies on the skeleton are expressed slowly in the adult. For this same reason, nutrient effects on the skeleton of any kind are difficult to detect and easy to misinterpret.

Change in Bone Mass

As noted above, bone is a composite of mineral and matrix, and "bone mass" refers, technically, to the quantity of such bone present in the whole organism (or in a body region). Technically, changes in bone mass itself cannot be measured in vivo, since there are no ways of detecting the organic component of the composite. However, in conditions of health, and in fact in most bone diseases, the proportion of mineral and matrix is about the same (50:50, by volume), and there are quite good methods for measuring bone mineral. Mineral content can be measured either for the whole skeleton or for various regions of interest by absorptiometric methods (see below). Change in bone mass is measured either by classic metabolic balance methods or by serial absorptiometry.

The classic nutritional approach to nutrient status is measurement of a metabolic balance, in this case, calcium (or phosphorus) balance. Since better than 99% of body calcium is in the skeleton, total body calcium balance reflects predominantly bone. And, since calcium is essentially never removed from or added to preformed bone tissue (rather units of tissue itself are removed or added), it follows that body calcium balance is a direct measure of bone tissue balance. The balance method is theoretically the ideal way of assessing change in bone mass, but it is expensive, and balance studies are difficult to perform accurately. The principal source of this difficulty, for poorly absorbed nutrients such as calcium, is that net absorption is low, and most of the ingested calcium ends up in the feces. Accurate timing of fecal excretion is nearly impossible. Moreover, lag time between ingestion and fecal excretion averages several days in healthy adults, and failure to take that lag into account leads to serious misinterpretation of calcium balance results (13). Colored dye markers demarcating treatment periods are not adequate safeguards. Rather, continuous intake markers (such as PEG 4000) are required, and fecal output must be adjusted both for its PEG content and for the time lag.

A newer approach, ideally suited to measurement of the quantity of bone present, is the direct measurement of bone mineral (13), either in a specific region or in the skeleton as a whole, by the technique of dual-energy x-ray absorptiometry (DEXA). A tightly collimated beam of x-rays is passed back and forth across the body (or one of its regions), and absorption of its photons is measured by a detector on the side opposite the x-ray source. Absorption is a function of the amount of mineral present in the path of the beam. This method measures, for example, spine mineral content in as little as 2 to 5 minutes and has a reproducibility on the order of 1 to 2%.

Because total body calcium in an adult is in the range of 900 to 1500 g, and because change in bone mass (in other words, positive or negative calcium balance) is rarely more than ±100 mg/day (and usually much less), it follows that closely spaced, repeat measurements by DEXA will produce results within the reproducibility error of the method. For that reason, measurements in individuals must usually be separated by 12 to 24 months (less time will not allow measurable change to occur). Thus, while DEXA permits rapid and accurate measurement of bone *mass*, it is not very sensitive to the sorts of *change in mass* that have physiologic or nutritional significance.

The Remodeling Transient

Any intervention, nutritional or otherwise, that alters bone remodeling activity will produce a transient change (15) in calcium balance (or bone mass) which is due to the asynchrony of the remodeling cycle (see above). Because of the temporal separation of resorption and formation at each remodeling site, suppression of remodeling will produce a prompt but temporary increase in bone mass (Fig. 83.7). If this follows, for example, administration of supplemental calcium, phosphorus, or vitamin D, the retention of bone mineral should not be interpreted to indicate a preexisting deficiency. (There may be such a deficiency, of course, but positive balance will occur whether or not deficiency is present, simply because, initially, the resorptive component of remodeling is reduced more than the formative component.) Since the remodeling cycle lasts at least 3 months in healthy young adults, bone mass (and calcium balance) continues to change under the influence of this asynchronous remodeling for at least that long. It may actually take a year or more in the elderly for formation and resorption once again to come into equilibrium. Response to nutritional interventions can only be interpreted *after* the transient is complete. If, at that time, balance is more positive (or bone mass by DEXA is still increasing), only then can one safely conclude that the subjects needed more of the nutrient than they had previously been receiving.

Bone Histomorphometry

The term *histomorphometry* means the measurement of shapes on histologic specimens of bone (16). As noted above, many substances attach to bone crystals as they are forming and then become trapped as more bone is laid down on top of them. Some of those substances, like the tetracycline antibiotics, fluoresce brilliantly when illuminated by ultraviolet light. Histomorphometry takes advantage of that property by giving patients paired, timed doses of tetracycline several days before obtaining a bone biopsy (typically from the iliac crest). Specimens are sectioned on special microtomes without first removing the mineral and then examined with an ultraviolet microscope. Figure 83.4 presents a typical photomicrograph from such a labeled biopsy. Since the distance between fluorescent lines can be measured with a calibrated eyepiece and since the times of administration are known, one can derive a reasonably precise estimate of the rate at which the remodeling cells are working and how active the remodeling process may be. Among other histologic features, measurements are made not only of the distance between labels but of the extent of bone surface covered with a label. This method is very useful for studying bone biology and disease but has limited applicability to the study of nutritional problems affecting bone.

Biochemical Markers of Bone Remodeling

In the synthesis of bone collagen, the ends of the collagen molecules are clipped off as the triple helix is assembled, the proline molecules in the peptide chain are converted to hydroxyproline, and cross-links are developed between collagen molecules. Additionally, both alkaline phosphatase and the noncollagenous proteins are secreted into the matrix; in this process, some of these substances leak into the bloodstream. Later, when bone is broken down, the hydroxyproline residues and the cross-links, since they cannot be recycled, are metabolized or excreted. All these activities leave residues or produce effects that can be measured in serum or urine. Collectively, these circulating or excreted substances are called biochemical biomarkers of bone remodeling (17). They reflect in a general way the level of bone remodeling activity. Table 83.2 summarizes the principal markers currently in use, together with the component of remodeling they are thought to reflect most directly. It is important to note, in this connection, that, when remodeling activity changes, *both* resorption and formation generally change, almost always in the same direction, and often to nearly the same extent. So, for most situations, a marker for either formation or resorption may be used as an index of remodeling activity.

While measurements of bone biomarkers can be a relatively inexpensive way of assessing bone remodeling activity under differing nutritional conditions, they are at best only semiquantitative. In other words, a 50% drop in a resorption marker does not mean a 50% reduction in the amount of bone resorbed. Also, the markers exhibit important discrepancies among themselves. For example, serum alkaline phosphatase is high in nutritional rickets despite a generally low level of new bone apposition, and $1,25(OH)_2$ vitamin D elevates serum osteocalcin without, apparently, altering actual bone-forming activity (18).

The effects of nutritional deficiencies on the relationship between marker level and the process it reflects have not been studied. Nevertheless, to the extent that a nutritional deficiency alters bone remodeling, one can expect to find corresponding changes in remodeling marker levels. Thus, the accelerated bone loss of the aged, which is due to calcium deficiency, is associated with elevated excretion of deoxypyridinoline and hydroxyproline. Calcium supplementation both stops or

Table 83.2
Biochemical Markers of Bone Remodeling

Formation	Resorption
Serum alkaline phosphatase	Urine hydroxyproline
Bone specific	Urine pyridinium cross-links
Total	Pyridinoline
Serum osteocalcin	Deoxypyridinoline
Serum procollagen type I propeptide	Urine peptide cross-links
Carboxyterminal (P1CP)	Amino terminal (NTx)
Amino terminal (P1NP)	Carboxyterminal (crosslaps)

slows the bone loss and reduces urinary excretion of deoxypyridinoline

REFERENCES

1. Robey PG, Boskey AL. The biochemistry of bone. In: Marcus R, Feldman D, Kelsey J, eds. Osteoporosis. San Diego: Academic Press, 1996;95–183.
2. Kannus P, Haapasalo H, Sievanen H, et al. Bone 1994; 15:279–84.
3. NIH Consensus Conference. JAMA 1994;272:1942–8.
4. Marcus R. The nature of osteoporosis. In: Marcus R, Feldman D, Kelsey J, eds. Osteoporosis. San Diego: Academic Press, 1996;647–59.
5. Klein GL. Nutritional rickets and osteomalacia. In: Favus MJ, ed. Primer on the metabolic bone diseases and disorders of mineral metabolism. 8th ed. New York: Raven Press, 1993;264–8.
6. Glorieux FH. Hypophosphatemic vitamin D resistant rickets. In: Favus MJ, ed. Primer on the metabolic bone diseases and disorders of mineral metabolism. 8th ed. New York: Raven Press, 1993;279–82.
7. Shapiro JR. Osteogenesis imperfecta and other defects of bone development as occasional causes of adult osteoporosis. In: Marcus R, Feldman D, Kelsey J, eds. Osteoporosis. San Diego: Academic Press, 1996;899–924.
8. Herlong HF, Recker RR, Maddrey WC. Gastroenterology 1982; 83:103–8.
9. Goodman WG, Coburn JW, Ramirez JA, et al. Renal osteodystrophy in adults and children. In: Favus MJ, ed. Primer on the metabolic bone diseases and disorders of mineral metabolism. 8th ed. New York: Raven Press, 1993;304–23.
10. Epstein S. J Bone Miner Res 1996;11:1–7.
11. Delmi M, Rapin C-H, Bengoa J-M, et al. Lancet 1990;335: 1013–6.
12. Rude RK. Hypocalcemia due to magnesium deficiency. In: Favus MJ, ed. Primer on the metabolic bone diseases and disorders of mineral metabolism. 8th ed. New York: Raven Press, 1993;200–2.
13. Heaney RP. Bone Miner 1986;1:99–114.
14. Wahner HW. Use of densitometry in management of osteoporosis. In: Marcus R, Feldman D, Kelsey J, eds. Osteoporosis. San Diego: Academic Press, 1996;1055–74.
15. Heaney RP. J Bone Miner Res 1994;9:1515–23.
16. Chavassieux P, Arlot M, Meunier PJ. Clinical use of bone biopsy. In: Marcus R, Feldman D, Kelsey J, eds. Osteoporosis. San Diego: Academic Press, 1996;1113–21.
17. Delmas PD, Garnero P. Utility of biochemical markers of bone turnover in osteoporosis. In: Marcus R, Feldman D, Kelsey J, eds. Osteoporosis. San Diego: Academic Press, 1996;1075–88.
18. Feldman D, Malloy PJ, Gross C. Vitamin D: metabolism and action. In: Marcus R, Feldman D, Kelsey J, eds. Osteoporosis. San Diego: Academic Press, 1996;205–35.

84. Nutrition and Diet in Rheumatic Diseases

CLAUDIO GALPERIN, BRUCE J. GERMAN, and M. ERIC GERSHWIN

The nutritional requirements of healthy humans are relatively well described and are the basis of nutrient intake recommendations of several governmental and health agencies. However, rheumatic diseases represent an important deviation from the norm, and vital issues relevant to nutrient intakes need to be resolved. Are the nutrient requirements recommended for normal healthy children and adults sufficient to minimize the progression and destructive effects during development of these various pathologic conditions? Does the rheumatic disease condition represent a significantly altered physiologic state in which the spectrum and balance of nutrients recommended for normal healthy children and adults are no longer adequate? Rheumatic diseases represent a serious health hazard to a large minority of the adult population, and relatively little attention has been paid to the role of diet in the progression of this family of diseases, the severity once established, or the effect of the diseases on nutrient requirements. Nevertheless, the role of particular foods in mitigating disease severity has been widely speculated in folk medicine, and many individuals alter their diets in the hopes of beneficial effects. Rheumatic and inflammatory conditions are now known to increase demand on proteins because of increased turnover, on minerals because of increased mobilization, on antioxidant vitamins because of free radical scavenging, and on particular vitamins because of altered metabolism and bioavailability.

NUTRITIONAL IMBALANCE

Protein-Energy Malnutrition

Malnutrition in variable degrees is a common finding in patients with rheumatic diseases, including rheumatoid arthritis (RA), rheumatoid spondylitis, systemic necrotizing vasculitis, systemic sclerosis (SSc), and systemic lupus erythematosus (SLE) (1–3). Such data have profound implications for patients with chronic disease and may be a predisposing factor for infection and morbidity. For instance, results of a 2-year prospective study of hospitalized adult patients with RA found that malnutrition was associated with a poor prognosis, as assessed by rehospitalization and/or mortality rate (4).

Cytokine-Mediated Catabolism

Lean body mass, consisting of the body cell mass and connective tissue, accounts for nearly all metabolic activity of the body (5). Loss of body cell mass in chronic disease is associated with deficient immune competence (6) and has been shown to be a major predictor of outcome in certain critical illnesses. The mechanism of these effects is not clear, but inflammatory cytokines, such as interleukin-1β (IL-1β) and tumor necrosis factor-α (TNF-α), are associated with hypermetabolism and loss of body cell mass in animals (7). Similar effects have been shown following cytokine infusion studies in humans.

Adults with RA have significantly reduced body cell mass (8), and high levels of TNF-α and IL-1β have been demonstrated in synovial fluid and in the circulation of these patients (9, 10). A decrease of approximately one-third of the body cell mass was noted in patients with RA (11), which was associated with elevated levels of circulating IL-1β and TNF-α; the latter were associated with elevated energy expenditure (hypermetabolism). Significantly, this association was noticed even in a group with low disease activity, suggesting that hypermetabolism, a feature of chronic inflammation, lingers even when good clinical control of RA is achieved.

Anorexia

Poor appetite, a common finding among different chronic diseases, including SLE (12), and RA (11), appears to be more prevalent during periods of active disease. Although the contribution of drugs used in the treatment of these disorders should not be ignored, inflammatory cytokines appear to play a critical role. The proinflammatory cytokines IL-1 and TNF cause profound anorexia in experimental animals and humans (13) and, as discussed above, are present in elevated levels in patients with RA (14). Further support of this view comes from the recent report that documents an inverse association between IL-1β production and dietary intake in patients with RA (11). Perhaps, the anorexia induced by IL-1β aggravates the loss of body cell mass that occurs in the hypermetabolic state by preventing these patients from increasing their intake to meet their higher energy needs.

Gastrointestinal Involvement

Oral Cavity Abnormalities. Involvement of the oral cavity in rheumatic disease represents an additional impairment to adequate nutritional intake. Reduction of the oral aperture in SSc and arthritis of the temporomandibular joint and hypoplasia of the mandible in juvenile RA limit mouth opening, cause pain with chewing, and difficulty in swallowing. For these reasons, foods requiring extensive mastication should be avoided. Patients with Sjögren's syndrome exhibit several dietary problems. Inadequate amounts of saliva to properly masticate and mix food makes swallowing solid aliments difficult. Many patients tend to reduce dietary variety and rely on the few foods that do not cause discomfort to eat, a practice that is invariably detrimental for adequate nutrition. Maintenance of proper hydration by drinking plenty of fluids, avoidance of caffeine and other beverages that exert a diuretic effect, sucking on noncaloric "candies," and preparation of food with a consistency agreeable to these patients are among possible nutritional strategies (15). Artificial saliva is currently available, and its use has been helpful in selected cases. Oral ulcerations, a common manifestation of systemic vasculitis and SLE, may decrease the palatability of foodstuffs and thus contribute to impaired food intake. Moreover, many fruits, juices, and some vegetables of higher acidic content are not well tolerated.

Esophageal Dysfunction. Abnormal esophageal motility is observed in nearly 90% of patients with SSc and has also been observed in a subset of patients with mixed connective tissue disease (MCTD). Uncoordinated peristalsis of the lower two-thirds of the esophagus often causes dysphagia and odynophagia for solid foods. The potential complications arising from gastroesophageal reflux include *Candida* esophagitis, erosive esophagitis, Barrett's metaplasia (with its accompanying potential for adenocarcinoma), strictures, and aspiration (16).

Malabsorption. Malabsorption has been described as a manifestation of many rheumatic syndromes, including RA, Behçet syndrome (17), and polyarteritis nodosa (18). In advanced SSc, in which nutrition is usually a major management problem, malabsorption can be the immediate cause of death (19). In SSc, malabsorption may result from bacterial overgrowth of the small intestine, abnormalities of the intestinal absorptive surface, and pancreatobiliary insufficiency (20). There is no predictably effective therapy other than treatment of bacterial overgrowth and nutritional support. Antibiotics and nutritional supplementation with fat-soluble vitamins, vitamin C, low-residue and elemental diets, and medium-chain triglycerides, are the foundation of therapy (16). In extreme circumstances, when oral intake is not adequate to sustain normal nutrition, tube feeding or total parenteral nutrition might be indicated (21).

Protein-Losing Enterophathy. Increased protein loss from the bowel is a rare manifestation of SLE (22, 23). This diagnosis should be suspected when diarrhea and severe hypoalbuminemia without proteinuria are found. Although infrequent, identification of this condition is important because of its deleterious nutritional implications and because many patients improve with corticosteroid therapy (23).

Nephrotic Syndrome

The kidney is one of the organs most commonly affected in SLE (24). In many instances, glomerulonephritis may be associated with the nephrotic syndrome (NS), a condition characterized by increased glomerular permeability to protein, often resulting in loss of more than 3 g of albumin per day in the urine. An important feature of NS is hyperlipidemia, characterized by increased plasma levels of potentially atherogenic lipids such as very low density (VLDLs), intermediate-density, and low-density lipoproteins (LDLs) and, as the disorder progresses, also by hypertriglyceridemia and decreased concentrations of high-density lipoproteins (HDLs) (25, 26). These abnormalities are associated with an increased risk of coronary heart disease and may predispose to more rapid progression of renal disease. Moreover, uncontrolled NS can be complicated by increased susceptibility to infection, renal vein thrombosis, and protein-energy malnutrition (27).

In the past, high-protein diets were often prescribed for NS patients in an attempt to compensate for urinary protein losses and to restore normal serum albumin levels. More recently, however, it has become clear that increased dietary protein does not correct low serum albumin levels satisfactorily but does increase urinary protein excretion and may accelerate renal damage (28). The current general approach is to offer a diet with moderate protein restriction (containing no less than 0.6 g/kg body weight per day of protein of high biologic value), supplemented with an amount of protein equal to urinary loss. This strategy delays the progression of further loss of renal function (28–30). The energy intake, nevertheless, should be closely monitored to avoid overt nutritional deficiency and be adjusted upward if concurrent infection or another condition increases energy output.

The effect of a vegetarian soy diet on hyperlipidemia was studied in 20 patients with longstanding NS (31). After a baseline control period of 8 weeks on their usual diets, patients were given a vegetarian soy diet (low fat, cholesterol free, and rich in monounsaturated and polyunsaturated fatty acids and fiber) for 8 weeks. After the diet period, patients resumed their usual diet for another 8 weeks (washout period). During the soy-diet period there were significant decreases in serum cholesterol (total, VLDL, HDL) and urinary protein excretion.

Obesity

Osteoarthritis

Several earlier studies have suggested that obesity is associated with osteoarthritis (OA), particularly knee OA (32–35). Obesity also aggravates joint dysfunction in patients with rheumatic diseases whose joint function has been compromised by articular damage. Diseases of weight-bearing joints are particularly affected by obesity, which further compromises already impaired ambulation.

Intestinal Bypass Arthritis

In the past, patients with morbid obesity were subjected to jejunocolic or jejunoileal bypass to limit intestinal surface for absorption. Follow-up of these patients revealed that up to 54% of them developed arthritis (36), presumably related to chronic bacterial overgrowth, immune complex formation and deposition on the synovial tissue, and complement activation (37–39). The arthritis in these patients had a predilection for small joints of the upper and lower extremities (39). Oral antibiotics given intermittently or continuously reduce symptoms by reducing bacterial overgrowth (40). Surgical reversal of the intestinal bypass is usually associated with prompt and invariable remission of the arthritis (36) and, in some instances, correlates with a decline of circulating levels of immune complexes (37).

METABOLIC DISORDERS AFFECTING CONNECTIVE TISSUE

Gout

Diet and alcohol are among the common and important environmental factors that contribute to hyperuricemia. Studies of patients with gout have not revealed any significant difference in dietary intake from control groups, with the exception of a greater intake of beer by patients with gout (41). Prolonged consumption of alcohol increases urate synthesis, presumably by enhancing the turnover of adenine nucleotides (42), while acute intoxication produces transient lacticacidemia and ketosis, which might lead to inhibition of renal secretion and consequent hyperuricemia (43). A diet rich in purines is well known to raise serum uric acid level. Nevertheless, when compared with dietary sources as the origin, more than 80% of the urate formed each day comes as an end product of tissue nucleic acid turnover.

A purine-free diet is unpleasant, difficult to follow, and largely unnecessary because of the effectiveness of drug therapy. The only consideration currently given to diet is avoidance of purine-rich foods such as liver, kidney, sardines, fish roe, anchovies, and sweetbreads, particularly by patients with massive tophaceous deposits (44). Control of obesity, reduction in alcohol intake, and, when necessary, control of hyperlipidemia, remain important aspects of the nutritional management of gout. However, abrupt loss of weight induced by severe dietary restriction for control of obesity can lead to ketosis accompanied by a fall in urate excretion and thus should be avoided (45).

Hyperlipidemia

Since the first description of a series of patients with an apparently distinct hyperlipidemic arthropathy (46), the true existence of such an entity has been controversial. Support from epidemiologic studies is largely lacking (47–49), and if any agreement emerges from them, it is that features of inflammatory arthropathy are uncommon in patients with primary hyperlipidemia. In a clinical study, 18 patients homozygous for type II hyperlipidemia were identified among 14 families (46); 10 (56%) of them experienced a transient migratory polyarthritis with a pattern similar to that observed in rheumatic fever. Large joints were most frequently involved, and no relationship could be established between the joint affected and concomitant presence of xanthomas. Subsequent studies, although occasionally describing some of these features, contrasted with others, particularly the high incidence of rheumatic complaints reported. For heterozygotes, the evidence for an association is even scantier. Indeed, studies that support an association between type II hyperlipidemia and arthropathy show considerable diversity in the rheumatic syndrome reported. Of all possible associations with type II hyperlipidemia, the evidence for periarthritis, particularly Achilles tendinitis, is strongest (50–52). The predilection of xanthomas for the Achilles tendon suggests a possible causal relationship (53).

An oligoarthropathy with or without symptoms suggesting inflammation has been reported in some patients with type IV hyperlipidemia (54, 55). There is an accepted association between gout and type IV hyperlipidemia (familial hypertriglyceridemia), although the basis of the association is not entirely delineated. In contrast to the controversy regarding the existence of a unique arthropathy resulting from primary hyperlipidemic conditions, the occurrence of rheumatic syndromes secondary to lipid-lowering drugs is well established. The most frequently implicated drugs are the fibric acid derivatives (e.g., clofibrate) and hydroxymethylglutaryl–coenzyme A (HMG-CoA) reductase inhibitors (e.g., lovastatin, simvastatin) (56, 57). The myopathy may manifest simply as asymptomatic increases in muscle enzyme levels, such as creatine phosphokinase (CPK) and aldolase, or alternatively as pain and predominantly proximal muscle weakness. Less commonly, this process can be so severe as to result in renal failure secondary to rhabdomyolysis.

Alkaptonuria (Ochronosis)

Alkaptonuria is a rare autosomal recessive disorder characterized by complete deficiency of the enzyme homogentisic acid oxidase (58), which causes accumulation of homogentisic acid in various tissues, leading to major sequelae. Because such pigment is preferentially deposited in cartilage, a degenerative arthropathy is an inevitable complication. Clinical manifestations are generally apparent in the fourth decade, when severe disability usually occurs secondary to articular and cardiovascular complications.

SPECIFIC NUTRIENTS IN RELATION TO RHEUMATIC DISEASES

Trace Minerals

Iron

Anemia is a frequent finding in patients with chronic inflammatory rheumatic diseases and may arise from different mechanisms. Most commonly, it is the anemia of chronic disease (ACD). A cytokine-mediated failure of the bone marrow to increase red blood cell production in response to erythropoietin and an impaired release of iron from the reticuloendothelial system are the most likely underlying mechanisms (60). Less commonly, true iron deficiency anemia due to poor dietary intake or gastrointestinal blood loss secondary to medication might occur in RA patients.

Numerous investigators have observed deposition of large amounts of iron in the synovial tissue of patients with RA (61–63) and associated them with the occurrence of persistent joint inflammation (60). It has been hypothesized that excessive iron deposits may catalyze the formation of reactive oxygen species and thus contribute to inflammation and tissue injury in RA (64, 65). Intravenous infusion of iron produces synovitis in murine models (66) and precipitates flares of joint inflammation, with evidence of oxygen-free radical reaction products in serum and synovial fluid, in patients with RA (67, 68). Degradation of hyaluronate in RA synovial tissue was completely inhibited by iron chelators (69). Ferric nitrilotriacetate increased the production of collagenase and prostaglandin (PG) E_2, as well as the number of rabbit synovial fibroblasts in vitro (70). Iron stimulated the DNA synthesis by synovial cells in vitro and exerted an additive effect on the activity of human cytokines (IL-1β, IL-7, TNF-α, IFN-γ) for RA synovial cell proliferation (71).

Zinc

Plasma zinc levels are reduced in patients with many chronic inflammatory diseases including RA (72). The modifications in zinc status produced by inflammatory processes, however, appear to differ from that observed in subjects depleted of zinc by diseases such as alcoholic cirrhosis, diabetes, or renal insufficiency. With inflammation there is a redistribution of this element within the body compartments, characterized by decreased plasma zinc concentrations and increased zinc concentrations in mononuclear leukocytes, urine, and synovial fluid (73–76). These modifications significantly correlate with the degree of inflammation.

The clinical effects of zinc supplementation in RA were first examined by Simkin in 1976, who reported clinical improvement in patients suffering from chronic refractory RA by using 660 mg/day of zinc sulfate (77). These results could not be confirmed by several subsequent trials. The fad of zinc supplementation is not exempt from side effects (78). Significant impairment of lymphocyte and neutrophil functions (79) and a potentially harmful increased LDL:HDL ratio (80) have been described in healthy adults with excessive intake of zinc (≥150 mg/day, a 10-fold excess of the recommended dietary allowance [81]).

Copper

Copper, along with zinc, is a constituent in cytoplasmic superoxide dismutase (SOD). Both ceruloplasmin and SOD possess antioxidant properties and have an essential protective role against free radical–mediated tissue damage observed in inflammatory states (82, 83). Copper bracelets were used by the ancient Greeks to relieve aches and pains (84) and presently are used as a folk remedy for RA. Open trials using copper salts to treat RA and OA have been reported (85, 86). Although uncontrolled observations account for mild improvement in some of these patients, many side effects have been reported, and it is unlikely that copper compounds will play any relevant role in RA or OA therapy (87). Elevated copper levels have been observed in both serum and synovial fluid of patients with RA (88–91), with most studies showing a positive correlation with disease activity (89). Normalization of levels along with acute-phase reactants has been reported following pharmacologic control of disease (89).

Selenium

The antiinflammatory and immunomodulatory properties of selenium prompted studies of its role in RA, juvenile RA (JRA), OA, psoriatic arthritis, and SLE. In most of the studies of RA (92–96) and JRA patients (97, 98), plasma levels of selenium were significantly lower than those of healthy controls. In one study, selenium levels in the serum of patients with psoriatic arthritis were significantly lower than those of healthy controls (99). In another study, plasma selenium levels were within the normal range in patients with SLE, although a trend to lower values was observed in active disease (100). However, most selenium supplementation trials, (usually using organic selenium compounds) failed to demonstrate any significant improvement in any of these diseases, even when the deficient selenium status was corrected (101–103). While selenium supplementation (250 mg/day) significantly increases selenium concentration in serum and red blood cells of both RA and control subjects (101, 102), it does not increase selenium levels in PMN leukocytes from patients with RA as it does in PMNs from control subjects (104). Moreover, while selenium supplementation substantially increased glutathione reductase (GSH-Px) activity in serum, red blood cells, and platelets from RA patients, activity did not reach control levels in PMN leukocytes of these same patients. Given the important role of PMN leukocytes in the inflammatory process in RA, these findings agree with the lack of a benefit from selenium supplementation in controlled studies of RA patients. Altogether, these observations suggest that altered selenium metabolism rather than dietary deficiency underlies the observed levels.

Vitamins

Vitamin A and Retinoids

Both isotretinoin and etretinate have been associated with development of hyperostosis, especially in the cervical spine, and extraspinal calcifications of tendons and ligaments (105). These spinal changes at times resemble those seen in diffuse idiopathic skeletal hyperostosis (DISH), often developing in individuals younger than those usually afflicted with spontaneous DISH. Growth retardation and premature epiphyseal plate closure have been described in children under chronic therapy with large doses of vitamin A and, in a few instances, after administration of isotretinoin or etretinate (106).

Vitamin C (Ascorbic Acid)

Ascorbic acid is essential for the synthesis of collagen, the main extracellular protein of connective tissue. Its deficiency, such as seen in patients with scurvy, accounts for inadequate synthesis of collagen and consequent impaired wound healing and capillary fragility. An accurate differential diagnosis is needed because scurvy lesions in the skin can, at times, mimic those seen in cutaneous vasculitis (107). Decreased synthesis of collagen, however, is not a key feature in any of the rheumatic diseases. Low levels of ascorbic acid, in plasma, blood cells, and synovial fluid have been described in RA patients, irrespective of drug therapy. In the 1940s, vitamin C was used to treat RA. Nevertheless, large vitamin C supplements given to normalize serum levels had no effect on the clinical course of RA or laboratory parameters of inflammation (108).

Vitamin B_6 (Pyridoxine)

Low vitamin B_6 levels in the circulation is a well-described metabolic abnormality in patients with RA (11, 109). Low plasma levels of pyridoxal-5′-phosphate (PLP), the metabolically active form of B_6, also occur in these patients (110) and appear to be related to the degree of inflammation and the levels of inflammatory cytokines such as TNF-α (109). Given its role as a cofactor in numerous enzymatic reactions involving aminoacids and proteins, including nucleotide and protein synthesis and cellular proliferation (111), altered bioavailability of B_6 has been hypothesized to affect the balance between protein synthesis and degradation (109). Vitamin B_6 administration to patients with RA, including those with low serum levels of PLP, failed to show any clinical improvement in disease activity (110).

Vitamin E

While peroxidative damage has been associated with the loss of certain T-cell receptor activities (112), human lymphocytes have been shown to be protected from lipid peroxidation when cultured with vitamin E (113). Data from studies assessing the plasma levels of vitamin E in patients with RA conflict; some studies found a normal baseline (114, 115), while others reported significantly lower levels (116) than those in normal individuals. Concentrations of α-tocopherol in the synovial fluid significantly lower than those of paired serum samples have been observed in patients with RA (115). In one study, multiple regression analysis indicated that depletion of α-tocopherol was largely independent of the concomitant lower concentrations of cholesterol, triacylglycerol, and LDL in the inflamed joint (117). At least in vitro, the antioxidant activity of vitamin E is regenerated by electron donation from vitamin C (118, 119). Because vitamin C levels are low in RA joint fluid, it has been hypothesized that this is caused by local consumption of α-tocopherol (117). Nonetheless, whether low levels of α-tocopherol in the synovium contribute to oxidative damage of the joint or are an indirect marker of the local oxidative stress remains to be properly addressed. Fish oil preparations used in clinical trials of RA (discussed below) are enriched in α-tocopherol, which prevents peroxidation of its polyunsaturated fatty acids (PUFAs). Since the degree of unsaturation of the cell membrane increases the risk for lipid peroxidation and generation of toxic-free radicals, the α-tocopherol requirement depends on the amount of PUFA consumed. Data from several studies, however, show that despite a substantial increase in consumption of fish oil PUFAs, the amount of α-tocopherol added to fish oil capsules usually suffices to prevent deficiencies in cellular and plasma levels of vitamin E (114, 118–120). The clinical benefit of dietary fish oil supplementation in RA does not depend on the antioxidizing properties of the low dose of α-tocopherol (10.3–12.9 mg/day) in fish oil capsules (114, 121). In fact, aside from subjective parameters, no significant clinical improvement was observed even when patients with RA were supplemented with 1200 mg/day of α-tocopherol (122).

Histidine

Several studies have demonstrated a selective low level of serum histidine in patients with RA, compared with normal subjects including family members (123). The extent of reduction of histidine levels correlates with the degree of disease activity as assessed by clinical and laboratory parameters (124). Available in health food stores, L-histidine has been used empirically to treat patients with RA; however, a placebo-controlled trial, failed to demonstrate any convincing benefit of a dietary supplement of L-histidine in RA (125).

FOOD AND RHEUMATIC DISEASES

Diet has been hypothesized to affect rheumatic diseases by two possible mechanisms that are not mutually exclusive. First, food-related antigens might induce hypersensitivity responses leading to rheumatic symptoms. Second, nutritional factors might alter inflammatory and immune responses and consequently modify manifestations of rheumatic diseases.

Food Hypersensitivity

The belief that food-related antigens might provoke hypersensitivity responses leading to rheumatic symptoms is not a recent one (126, 127). This thesis has gained some support from sporadic but convincing case reports of the reproducible onset of a selected rheumatic syndrome shortly after ingestion of certain aliments. For a response to food to be linked plausibly to a hypersensitivity reaction resulting in a rheumatic symptom, food antigens would have to cross the gastrointestinal barrier and circulate in an antigenic form until recognized by effector or intermediary cells in the immune system. Although large molecules with antigenic proprieties are known to have very limited access to the circulation, some food antigens do cross the gastrointestinal barrier and circulate not only as food antigens but also as immune complexes (128, 129). The M cell, a specialized epithelial cell that covers the intestinal lymphoid tissue, being free from glycocalyx, is in direct contact with the intestinal contents. These cells, by active pinocytosis, randomly pick up foreign antigenic material from the intestinal lumen and present it to the underlying macrophages and lymphocytes (130). Antigenic molecules may also pass through the intestinal mucosa, in a less controlled manner, through gaps in the epithelium caused by allergic, infectious, or toxic processes (130). Nonsteroidal antiinflammatory drugs (NSAIDs), largely used for symptomatic management of pain, might lead to a loss of intestinal integrity, thus facilitating food antigen absorption (131). Because no reliable laboratory test is available, the diagnosis of food hypersensitivity still rests mostly on clinical grounds (see Chapter 92).

Food Hypersensitivity Associated with Inflammatory Arthritis

A relationship between food intake and inflammatory (rheumatoid or rheumatoid-like) arthritis has been suggested by a number of clinical observations (132–137). It is possible that cases are underreported, because patients may not necessarily be aware of possible sensitivities to commonly ingested foods in the diet. The small number of documented cases in the literature, however, suggests that the syndrome is probably rare.

Food Hypersensitivity Associated with Systemic Lupus Erythematosus

In the late 1970s, alfalfa meal was shown to reduce plasma cholesterol levels significantly and induce regression of atherosclerotic lesions in cholesterol-fed monkeys (138) and rabbits (139). Subsequent studies indicated that ingestion of alfalfa seeds was also associated with reduced plasma cholesterol levels in humans (140). In one study, however, after prolonged ingestion of alfalfa seeds, one human volunteer developed clinical and serologic features of SLE (141). Upon cessation of the dietary supplement of alfalfa seeds, these abnormalities reverted to normal. Because alfalfa sprouts had become an increasingly popular diet constituent in humans, further studies were undertaken to investigate potential side effects of their ingestion, in particular the induction of autoimmunity. These studies confirmed that alfalfa triggered an SLE-like syndrome in normal monkeys fed with alfalfa seeds and reactivated disease in susceptible animals (142). Isolated reports also suggest a similar role of alfalfa in inducing or reactivating human SLE (143). A nonprotein amino acid, L-canavanine, has been proposed to be the alfalfa component responsible for triggering an SLE-like syndrome (142). Canavanine is the principal free amino acid of a number of legumes such as clover and alfalfa, and it has also been reported to be a constituent of several food crops, including onions and soybeans (144). Interestingly, most of the toxic proprieties of L-canavanine appear to be destroyed by heating or cooking (145), which might explain why humans have not been affected more adversely by its toxicity (144). Altered synthesis of messenger RNA with resultant altered transcription has been hypothesized as the mechanism by which L-canavanine induces the generation of autoantibodies (144). Also, antibodies to alfalfa seeds appear to cross-react with DNA (146).

Food Hypersensitivity Associated with Other Systemic Rheumatic Diseases

Walnut extract has been reported to exacerbate Behçet's syndrome within 48 hours of its ingestion (147). In ex vivo studies, lymphocytes from these patients exhibited significantly decreased reactivity to both walnut extract and *Candida* antigens, which was associated with an increase in frequency and severity of their symptoms. Although it has been suggested that this transient suppression of lymphocyte reactivity may be responsible for the deleterious effects on the course of the disease, the mechanism by which English walnuts exacerbate Behçet's syndrome remains unknown.

Hypersensitivity to different foods has been hypothesized to be the cause of at least some cases of palindromic rheumatism and, in one instance, occurred secondary to sodium nitrate in food preservatives (148). Rarely and mostly in anecdotal reports, food hypersensitivity has been implicated as a cause of vasculitis. In 1929, Alexander et al. reported six patients with Henoch-Shöenlein purpura that improved when certain foods were excluded and recurred when those foods were reintroduced (149). Twenty-three patients with allergic purpura related to ingestion of certain foods were reported by Akroyd in 1953 (150). Azo dyes, particularly tetrazine, has also been occasionally implicated as a cause of purpura in a few patients (151, 152).

Eosinophilia-Myalgia Syndrome (EMS)

L-Tryptophan (LT) is an essential amino acid found in meats, dairy products, and some vegetable protein sources. Dietary supplementation with LT is associated with a unique rheumatic disease (EMS). Marketed as an over-the-counter food supplement in the United States since 1974 (153), LT became popular among health professionals and nutrition enthusiasts as a natural remedy for depression, insomnia, and premenstrual symptoms (154). The rationale for use was based partly on evidence that serotonergic activity is decreased in patients with depression. However, the clinical data that support its use are scant and at times conflicting (155, 156). In fall 1989, an outbreak of eosinophilia and severe myalgia was associated with ingestion of tryptophan (157, 158); this syndrome became known as eosinophilia-myalgia syndrome. Within 6 months after the initial description, 1511 cases (including 38 fatal cases) were reported to the Centers for Disease Control and Prevention (CDC) (159). Intensive epidemiologic investigation has established that all traceable EMS cases were linked to ingestion of LT produced by a single manufacturer (160) and that most likely identified contaminants such as 1,1′-ethylidenebis[tryptophan] play a role in the pathogenesis of EMS, although the mechanism remains unclear (161, 162).

Dietary Therapy

Dietary therapy for rheumatic diseases can be divided into two modalities: *(a) elimination therapy,* which includes both removal of selected foods from the diet and fasting, and *(b) supplementation therapy,* in which foods are added to the diet.

Elimination Therapy

The use of different diets to treat RA has been the subject of numerous studies and endless speculation. In 1983, Panush et al. (163) studied the effect of a commercially popular diet (the Dong diet [164]) in a 10-week placebo-controlled blinded study of 26 patients with active RA. This diet consists of simple Chinese foods, free of additives, preservatives, fruit, red meat, herbs, dairy products, and alcohol. The authors found no significant differences between patients on the Dong and placebo diets. However, two patients on the Dong diet experienced considerable clinical improvement and had recurrences of symptoms when they deviated from it. In 1986, Darlington et al. published the results of a nonblinded, placebo-controlled study of 6 weeks of dietary elimination therapy in 53 patients with RA (134). After a washout period during which no treatment was prescribed, the patients randomly received either the trial diet, which excluded cereal, or a placebo diet. No significant objective differences were observed between the two groups.

The role of diet in the treatment of RA remains controversial, partially because existing trials do not provide clear-cut results. Such trials have difficulty in ensuring compliance and in the ever-greater problem of blinding the trial and placebo diets. Moreover, the trial design might be inappropriate if the study population is heterogeneous and only a small number of patients are capable of being improved (165). In this context, studies with individual patients who have their symptoms exacerbated on a sufficient number of occasions by exposure to the alleged offending food provide more compelling evidence that in fact selective patients might benefit from exclusion of the offending food. In general, however, especially until methodologic impediments can be overcome, patients should be encouraged to follow balanced healthy diets and avoid elimination diets and fad nutritional practices that can lead to, or increase, preexisting nutritional deficiencies (166).

In 1979, Sköldstam et al. (167) reported that fasting for 7 to 10 days resulted in objective improvement of disease in 5 of 15 patients with classic RA, whereas only 1 of 10 control subjects improved. Equivalent results were subsequently presented by other investigators (168–171). The mechanism by which fasting improves RA symptoms is not fully understood. In a controlled trial conducted by Kjeldsen-Kragh et al. (168), 7 to 10 days of fasting, followed by an individualized vegetarian diet for a year, resulted in sustained advantage for the diet group. Nonetheless, in the vast majority of studies, the antirheumatic effects of fasting disappear shortly after eating is reinstated, whether the patients return to an ordinary Western diet (170), lactovegetarian diet (167), or strict vegetarian diet (vegan) (172). Complete fasting for periods beyond 1 week is considered unsafe (even for patients with no complicating disorders), with potential risk for protein-energy malnutrition (PEM) and renal and cardiac complications (172, 173).

Supplementation Therapy

Among dietary supplements, the most extensively investigated in rheumatic diseases are the ω-3 and ω-6 polyunsaturated fatty acids. Increasing experimental and clinical data supports the use of oral-feeding antigens in an attempt to treat RA. The use of vitamins and trace elements in treatment of rheumatic disorders was discussed above in this chapter.

ω-Fatty Acids. Fatty acids in the cellular membranes are substrates for the production of prostaglandin (PG) and leukotriene (LT) species fundamental for many biologic activities, including modulation of the inflammatory and immune responses; ω-3 (w-3) and ω-6 (w-6) fatty acids can only originate from diet and are considered essential because their deficiency can result in growth retardation and death. The composition of phospholipids in cellular membranes is determined by nutritional intake, and alterations in dietary lipids can cause major changes in the synthesis of lipid-derived mediators of inflammation. By far the most common polyunsaturated fatty acid constituents in the Western diet are the ω-6 fatty acids, predominantly from terrestrial sources. This represents a great departure from the nutritional habits throughout most of human evolution, which were characterized by consumption of a higher percentage of polyunsaturated fat, more ω-3 fatty acids, more fiber, and less total fat than the present Western diet. This relatively recent change in dietary patterns may have affected the development of some major chronic diseases in industrialized society. Epidemiologic studies, for example, have shown a lower incidence of myocardial infarction, asthma, diabetes mellitus, and psoriasis in Greenland Eskimos than in European controls (174). A study from the Faroe Islands reported that RA takes a milder course in this population than in other Nordic countries (175). Such evidence suggests that these findings are, at least in part, attributable to a high dietary intake of marine oils containing ω-3 polyunsaturated fatty acids.

In Western societies, arachidonic acid (AA) (20:4, ω-6) is predominantly present in cellular membranes and leads to the formation of the most potent PGs ("2" series), via the action of cyclooxygenase, and LTs ("4" series), via the action of 5-lipoxygenase. Marine polyunsaturated ω-3 fatty acids, such as eicosapentanoic acid (EPA) (20:5, ω-3) and docosahexanoic acid (DHEA) (22:6, ω-3), competitively inhibit the use of AA and become a substrate for the production of alternative biologically active products through the cyclooxygenase and 5-lipoxygenase cellular metabolic pathways. As a result, generation of PGs of the "3" series and LTs of the "5" series increases, both of which have considerably less proinflammatory effects than the corresponding AA metabolites. LTB_5, for instance, which is usually undetectable in humans consuming a Western diet, has only approximately 10% the potency of LTB_4 (176). Platelet-activating factor–acether (PAF-acether) generation of stimulated monocytes is also significantly diminished after fish oil ingestion (177). This is of considerable interest in the context of inflammation because PAF can stimulate endothelial cell generation of TNF and is 1000 times more potent than histamine in inducing vascular permeability. Alteration of the cell membrane composition by PUFAs may also result in changes in the signaling pathways critical for regulation of immune responses and cell adhesion. Of particular interest, eicosanoids modulate the immune system either directly by stimulating target cells or indirectly by modulating the production of other soluble regulatory factors such as cytokines. Normal individuals given a diet enriched with fish oil exhibit significantly reduced monocyte production of IL-1 and to some extent TNF (177).

The benefit of dietary supplementation with marine ω-3 fatty acids has been demonstrated in some, but not all, models of chronic inflammatory disease (178–180). The most striking results were observed in New Zealand Black × New Zealand White F1 hybrid mice (NZB/W), which spontaneously develop SLE-like features such as hemolytic anemia, antinuclear autoantibodies, and glomerulonephritis. NZB/W mice fed a diet rich in EPA experience notably lower levels of proteinuria, significantly lower levels of antibodies binding native DNA, and a greatly improved survival rate. The beneficial effect on glomerulonephritis is observed even if dietary supplements are withheld until after the kidney disease is established. Importantly, fish oil reduction of autoimmune disease severity in NZB/W mice does reduce immune competence, at least not in terms of susceptibility to bacterial, yeast, or viral attack.

Because this strain provides a good model in several respects, the use of marine lipids has been postulated to be of therapeutic value for human SLE. Unfortunately, this assumption has been to date only seldom, and inadequately, tested. A placebo-controlled study of 39 patients with SLE failed to show significant improvement in disease activity after 12 months of fish oil administration (181). However, the heterogeneous population enrolled in this study makes interpretation difficult. In another study, Westberg and Tarkowski (182), using a double-blind, crossover design, evaluated for a period of 6 months the effect of EPA in 17 patients with moderately active SLE. Significant improvement of clinical and serologic parameters was observed in the treated group after 3 months, but at 6 months no differences could be observed between this and the group control, suggesting a short-lived effect of EPA on SLE.

Kremer et al. pioneered the systematic study of essential polyunsaturated fatty acid supplementation (EPA and DHA) in patients with RA, and showed a significant improvement in the number of tender joints and morning stiffness in the treated group (183). Since then, several other studies have been carried out (184–187), most of which reported findings similar to those of Kremer's original study. Taken together, they indicate that ω-3 fatty acid supplementation exerts significant but modest antiinflammatory effects in patients with RA. These benefits appear to be dose dependent, more consistently observed after 18 to 24 weeks of fish oil administration, and in some instances accompanied by a decrease of LTB_4 and/or IL-1, and elevation of LTB_5. A modest sparing effect was observed in the studies that used reduction or discontinuation of NSAID therapy as the measure of outcome.

Raynaud's phenomenon, a condition marked by increased vascular reactivity to cold exposure, can be a primary disorder or part of the constellation of symptoms in SSc. Episodes of blanching or cyanosis of the fingers are the most characteristic clinical features. Infarction of tissue at the fingertip, however, may also lead to digital pitting scars or frank gangrene. DiGiacomo et al. observed that some of the biologic effects of ω-3 fatty acids in cardiovascular disease could potentially benefit such patients (188). These effects include decreased plasma viscosity, a more favorable vascular response to ischemia, a reduced vasospastic response to catecholamines and angiotensin, an increase in the levels of tissue plasminogen activator, and an increase in the endothelium-dependent relaxation of arteries in response to bradykinin, serotonin, adenosine diphosphate, and thrombin. A single prospective, double-blind controlled study of the effect of dietary supplementation with 3.96 g of EPA and 2.64 g of DHA was conducted for 3 weeks in 32 patients with primary or secondary Raynaud's phenomenon (188). Patients with primary, but not secondary, Raynaud's phenomenon who ingested fish oil showed significant improvement in the time-to-onset of Raynaud's phenomenon triggered by hand immersion in cold-water baths.

ω-6 Fatty Acids. Other fatty acids also exhibit antiinflammatory and immunomodulatory effects in experimental models and preliminary clinical trials. γ-Linolenic acid (GLA) (18:3, ω-6), a fatty acid found in seeds from the evening primrose (EPO) and borage, has been the focus of substantial investigation. GLA is a precursor of other ω-6 fatty acids, including AA, and may be converted by an elongase enzyme to dihomogamma-linolenic acid (DGLA) (20:3, ω-6). In humans, the delta 5 desaturase that converts DGLA to AA is inefficient. Since GLA is rapidly converted to DGLA, concentrations of AA do not increase appreciably. Hence, DGLA competes with AA for cyclooxygenase, reducing the generation of prostanoids derived from arachidonate (see Chapter 4). While AA leads to the formation of PGs of the "2" series, DGLA, as a substrate for cycloxygenase, generates prostaglandins of the "1" series, for which it has been shown to hold beneficial antiinflammatory and antithrombotic properties. Although the biologic activities of corresponding members of the monoenoic ("1" series) and dienoic ("2" series) are qualitatively similar in many instances, in some respects they differ considerably. For example, PGE_1 inhibits aggregation of human platelets in vitro, whereas PGE_2 does not influence this activity. Also, PGE_1 is much more effective than PGE_2 in increasing levels of cAMP in human synovial cells in culture and in suppressing synovial cell proliferation.

Along with its influence on the generation of PGs, it is of considerable importance that DGLA cannot be converted to inflammatory leukotrienes by 5-lipoxygenase (189). Instead, DGLA is converted to hydroperoxyl DGLA, which has additional aptitude to inhibit 5-lipoxygenase activity (190). Independent of its role as a prostaglandin precursor, DGLA may have an important role in regulating immune responses by suppressing IL-2 production by human PBMC and proliferation of IL-2-dependent T lymphocytes. GLA dietary supplementation suppresses acute and chronic inflammation, as well as joint tissue injury, in several experimental animal models (191). In ex vivo studies, addition of DGLA to human synovial cells grown in tissue culture inhibits IL-1β–stimulated growth fivefold, compared with cell growth in medium supplemented with AA (192). Compared with cells in control medium, those incubated with DGLA displayed a 14-fold increase in PGE_1 and a 70% decrease in PGE_2 levels.

Studies of dietary supplementation with GLA in humans have yielded somewhat mixed results. EPO used in short-term studies (12 weeks), with a small number of patients ($n = 20$) with RA has shown no apparent clinical benefit (193). GLA (in the form of EPO) was also used in a 12-month placebo-controlled, double-blinded study (193) in which 49 patients with active RA were randomly allocated in three groups receiving *(a)* 540 mg/day GLA, *(b)* 240 mg/day EPA and 450 mg/day GLA, or *(c)* an inert oil as placebo. In both treated groups, reduction of pain, together with a reduction or even termination of NSAIDs therapy, was reported. Nevertheless, no significant objective changes in clinical or laboratory parameters were demonstrated. Pullman-Moore et al. (194) used a higher dose of GLA (1.1 g/day), in the form of borage seed oil, to treat seven patients with active RA for 12 weeks. The authors reported significant clinical improvement in morning stiffness and in the number of swollen and tender joints. Although the larger dose of GLA used might explain the apparent favorable results, the lack of a placebo control in this study makes this assumption impossible to assess. More recently, two prospective double-blinded, placebo-controlled studies observed significant clinical improvement in RA patients taking GLA (195, 196). Although the initial study design was well conceived, the study included a limited number of patients, limited follow-up duration, possible interference by concomitant use of other medications, and a high number of dropouts, making further controlled studies necessary.

Because phosphatidylinositol (PI), a critical source of AA, is remarkably insensitive to dietary modification by ω-3 PUFAs, it has been hypothesized that alternative strategies to replace PI could displace a more significant amount of cell membrane AA and therefore exert a more potent antiinflammatory and immunomodulatory effect (196). Dietary *Platycladus orientalis* seed oil, which is rich in 5,11,14-eicosatrienoic acid and 5,11,14,17-eicosatetranoic acid, alters the fatty acid composition of PI in the cell membrane (197), displacing a significant amount of AA (198). Moreover, *P. orientalis* seed oil suppresses anti-erythrocyte autoantibodies, and significantly prolongs the survival of NZB mice, suggesting that the use of unique exotic oils might have a place in the nutritional therapy of autoimmune-mediated diseases. No clinical studies with such derivatives have been reported to date.

In summary, convincing clinical evidence supporting

the therapeutic use of ω-6 fatty acids in rheumatic diseases has yet to be demonstrated. The choice of an appropriate placebo for clinical studies on both EPO and fish oil has been the focus of evolving dispute. Because some fatty acids, such as olive oil, are thought to have potentially significant immunologic effects, it has been hypothesized that some of the so-called placebo fatty acids used in different studies could produce beneficial effects. The controversial issue of the ideal placebo dietary intervention to compare with EPO or fish oil remains to be settled.

NUTRITIONAL ASPECTS OF PEDIATRIC RHEUMATIC DISEASES

Pediatric rheumatic diseases are a heterogeneous group of illnesses that cause inflammation in a variety of tissues, including joints, muscles, skin, and visceral organs. Juvenile rheumatoid arthritis (JRA) is the most common pediatric rheumatic disease and one of the more prevalent chronic diseases of childhood (199). Other relatively less common disorders include SLE and juvenile dermatomyositis (JDM). In spite of the fact that growth retardation was noted over 90 years ago in the original description of JRA (200), not until recently have studies addressed the nutritional status of pediatric populations suffering from rheumatic diseases and the possible association between nutrition and growth in these patients (201). The developmental abnormalities observed in this group include generalized short stature in JRA, SLE, and JDM; diffuse muscle atrophy in JDM and JRA; and localized asymmetric growth abnormalities in JRA and JDM (202).

Protein-energy malnutrition has been identified in up to 50% of patients with JRA (202, 206). Multiple factors contribute to increase nutritional risk in children with JRA. Intermittent or persistent anorexia, at least in part mediated by overproduction of IL-1 and TNF, occurs most commonly in periods of increased disease activity. In one study, dietary analysis revealed that the mean caloric and selected nutrient intakes (calcium, iron) of patients with JRA ranged from 50 to 80% of those of healthy children of comparable age and sex, as reflected in the U.S. recommended allowances (203). As in adult patients with RA, decreased serum levels of selenium, vitamin C, iron, and zinc have been reported in JRA. Additional risk for malnourishment arises from mechanical feeding difficulties. Up to 30% of JRA patients develop arthritis of the temporomandibular joint and hypoplasia of the mandible, which limit mouth opening and can cause pain with chewing. Nearly 30% of these patients develop hypoplasia of the mandible, resulting in malalignment of the teeth and difficulty swallowing (204).

Children with rheumatic diseases are also at high risk for developing osteoporosis (205). This increased risk is due to multiple factors including limited physical activity, immobility, limited sunlight exposure (especially for those suffering from SLE in which sunlight is known to trigger relapse of disease), inadequate dietary intake of calcium and vitamin D, low body weight, and use of corticosteroids. In a preliminary crossover study with 10 corticosteroid-treated children with rheumatic disease and osteoporosis, the use of calcium and vitamin D supplementation significantly improved spinal bone density (205). Corticosteroid therapy also intensifies the preexisting risk for growth retardation of JRA patients during childhood and into adulthood.

When planning nutritional intervention in pediatric patients with rheumatic diseases, potential changes in nutrient requirements for children with a great degree of persistent inflammation should be considered; patients with active disease often require increased dietary energy and protein. Although PEM and growth abnormalities ameliorate as the underlying inflammatory process is controlled through medication, most rheumatic disorders are chronic, and they may remain active for several years or for a lifetime. National statistics reveal that the pediatric rheumatology patient population is nutritionally largely underserved; only 8% of these patients are seen by a dietitian. In fact, this is probably an overestimation, since these studies were conducted on university-based pediatric rheumatology centers where there is more likely to be a dietitian. Pediatric dietitians must be included in the interdisciplinary team involved in the care of these patients, to ensure prompt and effective management of nutritional problems (206).

REFERENCES

1. Lom-Orta H, Diaz-Jouanen E, Alarcon-Segovia D. J Rheumatol 1980;7:178–83.
2. Helliwell M, Coombes EJ, Moody BJ, et al. Ann Rheum Dis 1984;43:386–9.
3. Lundberg A-C, Åkesson A, Åkesson B. Ann Rheum Dis 1992; 51:1143–8.
4. Weinsier RL, Hunker EM, Krumdieck CL, et al. Am J Clin Nutr 1979;32:418–26.
5. Moore FD. JPEN J Parenter Enteral Nutr 1980;4:228–60.
6. Chandra S, Chandra RK. Prog Food Nutr Sci 1986;10:1–65.
7. Tocco-Bradley R, Georgieff M, Jones CT, et al. Eur J Clin Invest 1987;17:504–10.
8. Roubenoff R, Roubenoff RA, Ward LM, et al. J Rheumatol 1992;19:1505–10.
9. Eastgate JA, Wood NC, DiGiovine FS, et al. Lancet 1988; ii:706–9.
10. Saxne T, Paladino D, Heinegard N, et al. Arthritis Rheum 1988;31:1041–4.
11. Roubenoff R, Roubenoff RA, Cannon JG, et al. J Clin Invest 1994;93:2379–86.
12. Harvey AM, Schulman LE, Tumulty A, et al. Medicine 1954; 33:291–303.
13. Tracey KJ, Wei H, Manogue KR, et al. J Exp Med 1988; 167:1211–27.
14. Roubenoff R, Holland SM, Stevens MB. Arthritis Rheum 1989;32:S154–7.
15. Ferris AM, Reece EA. Am J Clin Nutr 1994;59(Suppl): 465S–73S.
16. Sjogren RW. Arthritis Rheum 1994;9:1265–82.
17. Shimizu T, Ehrlich GE, Hayashi K. Semin Arthritis Rheum 1979;8:223–60.

18. Carron DB, Douglas AP. Q J Med 1965;34:333–40.
19. Piper WN, Helwig EB. Arch Dermatol Cytol 1955;72:535–46.
20. Kaye SA, Lim SG, Taylor M, et al. Br J Rheumatol 1995; 34:265–9.
21. Grabowski G, Grant JP. JPEN J Parenter Enteral Nutr 1989; 13:147–51.
22. Castañeda S, Moldenhauer F, Herrero-Beaumont G, et al. J Rheumatol 1985;12:1210–2.
23. Alarcón-Segovia D, Cardiel MA. Baillière's Clin Rheumatol 1989;3:371–92.
24. Boumpas DT, Austin HA III, Fessler BJ, et al. Ann Intern Med 1995;122:940–50.
25. Appel GB, Blum CB, Chien S, et al. N Engl J Med 1985;312:1544–8.
26. Keane WF, Kaiske BL. N Engl J Med 1990;323:603–4.
27. Dwyer J. Nutr Rev 1993;51:44–56.
28. Ihle BU, Becker GJ, Whitworth JA, et al. N Engl J Med 1989;321:1773–7.
29. Rosman JB, ter Wee PM, Maijer S, et al. Lancet 1984;2:1291–6.
30. AcchiardoSR, Moore LW, Cockrel S. Clin Nephrol 1986; 25:289–94.
31. D'Amico GD, Gentile MG, Manna G, et al. Lancet 1992;339: 1131–4.
32. Acheson RM. Ann Rheu Dis 1982;41:325–34.
33. Hartz AJ, Ficher ME, Bril G, et al. J Chronic Dis 1986;39: 311–9.
34. Anderson JJ, Felson DT. Am J Epidemiol 1988;128:179–89.
35. Van Saase JLCM, Vandenbroucke JP, van Romunde LKJ, et al. J Rheumatol 1988;15:1252–8.
36. Delamere JP, Buddeley RM, Walton KW. Ann Rheum Dis 1983;42:553–8.
37. Clegg DO, Zone JJ, Samuelson CO, et al. Ann Rheum Dis 1985;44:239–43.
38. Inman RD. Rheum Dis Clin North Am 1991;17:309–21.
39. Rose E, Espinoza LR, Osterland CK. J Rheumatol 1977;4: 129–34.
40. Stein HB. Schlappner OL, Boyko W, et al. Arthritis Rheum 1981;24:684–90.
41. Gibson T, Highton J, Potter C. Ann Rheum Dis 1980;39: 417–23.
42. Faller J, Fox IH. N Engl J Med 1982;307:1598–602.
43. MacLachlan MJ, Rodnan GP. Am J Med 1967;42:38–57.
44. Scott JT. Baillière's Clin Rheumatol 1987;1:525–46.
45. Fam AG. Baillière's Clin Rheumatol 1990;4:177–92.
46. Khachadurian AK. Arthritis Rheum 1968;11:385–93.
47. Welin L, Larsson B, Svardsudd K, et al. Scand J Rheumatol 1978;7:7–12.
48. Wysenbeck AJ, Shani E, Beijel Y, et al. J Rheumatol 1989;16:643–5.
49. Struthers GR, Scott DL, Bacon PA, et al. Ann Rheum Dis 1983;42:519–23.
50. Mathon G, Gagne C, Brun D, et al. Ann Rheum Dis 1985; 44:599–602.
51. Glueck CJ, Levy RI, Friedrickson DS. JAMA 1968;206:2895–9.
52. Shapiro JR, Fallat RW, Tsang RC, et al. Am J Dis Child 1974; 128:486–90.
53. Careless DJ, Cohen MG. Semin Arthritis Rheum 1993;23: 90–8.
54. Goldman JA, Glueck CJ, Abrams NR, et al. Lancet 1972;2: 449–52.
55. Buckingham RB, Bole GG, Basset DR. Arch Intern Med 1975; 135:286–90.
56. Le Quintrec J-S, Le Quintrec J-L. Baillière's Clin Rheumatol 1991;5:91–8.
57. Zuckner J. Semin Arthritis Rheum 1990;19:259–68.
58. Schumacher HR, Holdsmith DE. Semin Arthritis Rheum 1977;6:207–46.
59. O'Brien WM, La Du BN, Bunimm JJ. Am J Med 1963; 34:813–38.
60. Means RT, Krantz SB. Blood 1992;80:1639–47.
61. Muirden KD, Senator GB. Ann Rheum Dis 1968;27:38–48.
62. Giordano N, Vaccai D, Cintorino M, et al. Clin Exp Rheumatol 1991;9:463–7.
63. Morris CJ, Blake DR, Wainwright AC, et al. Ann Rheum Dis 1986;45:21–6.
64. Blake DR, Gallagher PJ, Potter AR, et al. Arthritis Rheum 1984;27:495–501.
65. Blake DR, Hall ND, Bacon PA, et al. Lancet 1981;2:1142–4.
66. DeSousa M, Dynesius-Trentham R, Mota-Garcia, et al. Arthritis Rheum 1988;31:653–61.
67. Wyniard PG, Blake DR, Chirico S, et al. Lancet 1987;1:69–70.
68. Blake DR, Lunec J, Ahern M, et al. Ann Rheum Dis 1985; 44:183–7.
69. Schenk P, Schneider S, Miehlke R, et al. J Rheumatol 1995; 22:400–5.
70. Okazaki I, Brinckerhoff CE, Sinclair JF, et al. J Lab Clin Med 1981;97:396–402.
71. Nishiya K. J Rheum 1994;21:1802–7.
72. Job C, Menkes CJ, Delbarre F. Nouv Presse Med 1978;7:760–7.
73. Mattingly PC, Mowat AG. Ann Rheum Dis 1982;41:405–6.
74. Peretz A, Nève J, Jeghers O, et al. Am J Nutr 1993;57:690–4.
75. Sorenson RJ. Inorg Perspect Biol Med 1978;2:1–16.
76. Peretz A, Nève J, Jeghers O, et al. Clin Chem Acta 1991; 203:35–46.
77. Simkin PA. Lancet 1976;ii:539–42.
78. Chandra RK. Lancet 1983;i:688–9.
79. Chandra RK. JAMA 1984;252:1443–7.
80. Hooper PL, Visconti L, Gary PJ, et al. JAMA 1980;244:1960–1.
81. Food and Nutrition Board, National Research Council. Recommended dietary allowances. 9th ed. Washington, DC: National Academy of Sciences, 1980.
82. McCord JM, Fridovich J. J Biol Chem 1969;250:6049–54.
83. Gutteridge JMC. Ann Clin Biochem 1978;15:293–6.
84. Sorenson JRJ. Prog Med Chem 1978;15:211–60.
85. Sorenson JRJ, Hangarter W. Inflammation 1977;217–38.
86. Sorenson JRJ. Agents Actions 1981;(Suppl) 8:305–25.
87. Panush RS. Bull Rheum Dis 1985;34:1–10.
88. Scudder PR, Al-Timini D, McMurray W, et al. Ann Rheum Dis 1978;37:67–70.
89. Brown DH, Buchanan WE, El-Ghobarey A, et al. Ann Rheum Dis 1979;38:174–82 .
90. Youssef AAR, Wood B, Baron DN. J Clin Pathol 1983;36:14–9.
91. Scudder PR, McMurray W, White AG, et al. Ann Rheum Dis 1978;37:71–82.
92. Munthe E, Aaseth J, Jellun E, et al. Acta Pharmacol Toxicol 1986;59:365–73.
93. Peretz AM, Nève JD, Vertongen F, et al. J Rheumatol 1987;14:1104–7.
94. Tarp U, Graudau H, Overvad K, et al. J Trace Elem Health Dis 1989;3:93–6.
95. Tarp U, Overvad K, Hansen JC, et al. Scand J Rheum 1985; 14:97–101.
96. Sullivan JF, Blotcky AJ, Jetton MM, at al. J Nutr 1989; 109:1432–7.
97. Mäkela AL, Hiörä H, Vuorinen K, et al. Scand J Rheumatol 1984;53:94–103.
98. Honkanen V, Pelkonen P, Mussalo-Rauhamaa H, et al. J Rheumatol 1989;8:64–70.
99. Azzini M, Girelli D, Olivieri O, et al. J Rheumatol 1995;22: 103–8.

100. Almroth G, Westberg NG, Sandstrom BM. J Rheumatol 1985; 12:633–4.
101. Tarp U, Hansen JC, Overvad K, et al. Arthritis Rheum 1987;30:1162–6.
102. Tarp U, Overvad K, Thorling E, et al. Scand J Rheumatol 1985;4:364–8.
103. Hill J, Bird HA. Br J Rheumatol 1990;29:211–3.
104. Tarp U, Stengaard-Pedersen K, Hansen JC, et al. Ann Rheum Dis 1992;51:1044–9.
105. Pittsley RA, Yoder FW. N Engl J Med 1983;308:1012–4.
106. Pease CN. JAMA 1962;182:980–5.
107. Adelman HM, Wallach PM, Gutierrez F, et al. Cutis 1994; 54:111–4.
108. Hall MG, Darling RC, Taylor FHC. Ann Intern Med 1939; 13:415–23.
109. Roubenoff R, Roubenoff RA, Selhub J, et al. Arthritis Rheum 1995;1:105–9.
110. Schumacher HR, Bernhard FW, Gyorgy P. Am J Clin Nutr 1975;28:1200–3.
111. Rall LCR, Meydani SN. Nutr Rev 1993;51:217–25.
112. Grever MR, Thompson VN, Balcerzac SP, et al. Blood 1980; 56:284.
113. Topinka J, Binkova B, Sram RJ, et al. Mutat Res 1989;225: 131–7.
114. Tulleken JE, Limburg PC, Muskiet AJ, et al. Arthritis Rheum 1990;33:1416–9.
115. Wasil M, Hutchinson DCS, Cheesman P, et al. Biochem Soc Trans 1992;20:277S–80S.
116. Honkanen V, Kontinnen YT, Mussalo-Rauhamaa H. Clin Exp Rheum 1990;7:465–9.
117. Fairburn K, Grootveld M, Ward RJ, et al. Clin Sci 1992;83: 657–64.
118. Packer JE, Slater TF, Wilson RL. Nature (London) 1979; 278:737–8.
119. Doba T, Burton GW, Ingold KU. Biochem Byophis Acta 1985; 835:298–303.
120. Knapp HR, Reilly IAG, Alessandrini P, et al. N Engl J Med 1986;314:937–42.
121. Scherak O, Kolarz G. Arthritis Rheum 1991;34:1205–6.
122. Kolarz G. Scherak O, Shohoumi M, et al. Aktuel Rheumatol 1990;15:223–37.
123. Gerber DA. J Clin Invest 1975;55:1164–72.
124. Gerber DA, Tanembaum L, Ahrens M. Metabolism 1976;25: 655–62.
125. Pinals RS, Harris ED, Burnett JB, et al. J Rheumatol 1977; 4:414–22.
126. Panush RS. Rheum Dis Clin North Am 1991;17:259–72.
127. Zeller M. Ann Allergy 1947;7:200.
128. Walker WA, Bloch KJ. Ann Allergy 1983;51:240–5.
129. Paganelli R, Levinsky RJ, Brostoff J, et al. Lancet 1979;1: 1270–2.
130. Darlington LG, Ramsey NW. Br J Rheumatol 1993;32:507–14.
131. Bjarnason I, Williams P, So A, et al. Lancet 1984;11:1171–3.
132. Parke AL, Hughes GRV. Br Med J 1981;282:2027–9.
133. Ratner P, Schneeyour A, Eshel E, et al. Isr J Med Sci 1985; 21:532–4.
134. Darlington LG, Ramsey NW, Mansfield JR. Lancet 1986;i: 238–76.
135. Mandel M, Conte A. Ann Allergy 1980;44:51–7.
136. Turnbull JA. Boston Med Surg J 1924;438–40.
137. Panush RS. J Rheumatol 1990;17:291–4.
138. Malinow MR, McLaughlin P, Naito HK, et al. Atherosclerosis 1978;30:27–35.
139. Malinow MR, McLaughlin P, Stafford C, et al. Atherosclerosis 1980;37:433–8.
140. Malinow MR, McLaughlin P, Stafford C, et al. Experientia 1980;36:562–4.
141. Malinow MR, Bardana EJ, Goodnight SH. Lancet 1981;1: 615–7.
142. Malinow MR, Bardana EJ, Pirofsky B, et al. Science 1982; 216:415–7.
143. Robert JL, Hayashi JA. N Engl J Med 1983;308:1361–4.
144. Montanaro A, Bardana Jr EJ. Rheum Dis Clin N Am 1991; 17:323–32.
145. Malinow MR, McLaughlin P, Bardana EJ, et al. Food Chem Toxicol 1984;22:583–7.
146. Bardana EJ, Malinow MK, Craig S, et al. J Allergy Clin Immunol 1983;71:102–8.
147. Marquardt JC, Snyderman R, Oppenheim JJ. Cell Immunol 1973;9:263–72.
148. Epstein S. Ann Allergy 1969;27:343–50.
149. Alexander HL, Eyermann CH. JAMA 1929;92:2092–4.
150. Akroyd JF. Am J Med 1953;14:605–32.
151. Kubba R, Champion RH. Br J Dermatol 1975;93(Suppl 11): 61–2.
152. Michaelsson G, Pettersson L, Juhlin L. Arch Dermatol 1974;109:49–52.
153. Medsger TA. N Engl J Med 1990;322:926–8.
154. Belongia EA, Hedberg CW, Gleich GJ, et al. N Engl J Med 1990;323:357–65.
155. Boman B. Aust NZ J Psychiatry 1988;22:83–97.
156. Byerley WF, Judd LL, Reimherr FW, et al. J Clin Psycopharmacol 1987;7:127–37.
157. Centers for Disease Control. MMWR 1989;38:765–7.
158. Hertzman PA, Blevins WL, Mayer J, et al. N Engl J Med 1990;322:869–973.
159. Information update on the outbreak of the eosinophilia-myalgia syndrome associated with the ingestion of L-tryptophan. Atlanta, Ga: Centers for Diseases Control Press Office; May 1, 1992.
160. Jaffe RM. Int J Biosocial Med Res 1989;11:181–4.
161. Mayeno AN, Lin F, Foote CS, et al. Science 1990;250:1707–8.
162. Taylor R, McNeil JJ. Med J Aust 1993;158:51–5.
163. Panush RS, Carter RL, Katz P, et al. Arthritis Rheum 1983;26:462–71
164. Dong CH, Banks J. New York: Ballantine, 1975.
165. Buchanan HM, Preston SJ, Brooks PM, et al. Br J Rheumatol 1991;30:125–34.
166. Panush RS. Rheum Dis Clin North Am 1991;17:443–4.
167. Sköldstam L, Larsson L, Lindström FD. Scand J Rheumatol 1979;8:249–57.
168. Kjeldsen-Kragh J, Haugen M, Borchgrevink C, et al. Lancet 1991;ii:899–902.
169. Lithell H, Bruce A, Gustafsson IB, et al. Acta Dermatovererol (Stockh) 1983;63:397–403.
170. Halfströn I, Ringertz B, Gyllenhammar H, et al. Arthritis Rheum 1988;31:585–92.
171. Trang EL, Lövgren O, Bendz R, et al. Scand J Rheumatol 1980;9:229–38.
172. Sköldstam L. Scand J Rheumatol 1986;15:219–26.
173. Palmblad J, Halfströn I, Ringertz B. Rheum Dis Clin North Am 1991;17:351–62.
174. Kromann N, Green A. Acta Med Scand 1980;208:401–6.
175. Recht L, Helin P, Rasmussen JO, et al. J Intern Med 1990; 227:49–55.
176. Prescott SM. J Biol Chem 1984;259:7615–21.
177. Endres S, Ghorbani R, Kelley VE, et al. N Engl J Med 1989;320:265–9.
178. Prickett JD, Robinson DR, Steinberg AD. J Clin Invest 1981;68:556–62.

179. Robinson DR, Prickett JD, Makaoul GT, et al. Arthritis Rheum 1986;29:539–46.
180. Prickett JD, Trentham DE, Robinson DR. J Immunol 1984; 132:725–9.
181. Moore GF, Yarboro C, Sebring NG, et al. Arthritis Rheum 1987;30:S33.
182. Westberg C, Tarkowski A. Scand J Rheumatol 1990;19:137–43.
183. Kremer JM, Bigauotte J, Michalek A, et al. Lancet 1985; 1:184–7.
184. Kremer JM, Lawrence DA, Jubiz W, et al. Arthritis Rheum 1990;33:810–20.
185. Lau CS, Morley KD, Belch JJF. Br J Rheumatol 1993;32:982–9.
186. Van der Tempel H, Tulleken JE, Limburg PC, et al. Ann Rheum Dis 1990;49:76–80.
187. McCarthy GM, Kenny D. Semin Arthritis Rheum 1992;21: 368–75.
188. DiGiacomo RA, Kremer JM, Shah DM. Am J Med 1989;86:158–64.
189. Callegari PE, Zurier RB. Rheum Dis Clin N Am 1991;17: 415–25.
190. Hammarström S. J Biol Chem 1981;256:7712–4.
191. Tate G, Mandell FB, Laposata M, et al. J Rheumatol 1989;16: 1729–36.
192. Baker DG, Krakauer KA, Tate G, et al. Arthritis Rheum 1989;32:1273–8.
193. Belch JJF, Ansell D, Madho KR, et al. Ann Rheum Dis 1988;47:96–104.
194. Pullman-Moore S, Laposata M, Lem D, et al. Arthritis Rheum 1990;33:1526–30.
195. Leventhal LJ, Boyce EG, Zurier RB. Ann Intern Med 1993; 119:867–73.
196. Brzeski M, Madhok R, Capell HA. Br J Rheumatol 1991; 30:370–2.
197. Berger A, Fenz R, German JB. J Nutr Biochem 1993;4:409–20.
198. Lai LTY, Naiki M, Yoshida SH, et al. Clin Immunol Immunopathol 1994;71:293–302.
199. Cassidy JT, Nelson AM. Arthritis Rheum 1988;15:525–6.
200. Still GF. Trans R Med Chir Soc 1897;62:47–50.
201. Bacon MC, White PH, Raiten DJ, et al. Semin Arthritis Rheum 1990;20:97–106.
202. Johansson V, Portinsson S, Akesson A, et al. Hum Nutr Clin Nutr 1986;40:57–67.
203. Miller ML, Chacko JA, Young EA. Arthritis Care Res 1989;2:22–4.
204. Larheim TA, Hoyeraal HM, Stalbrun AE, et al. Scand J Rheumatol 1982;11:5–12.
205. Warady BD, Lindsley CB, Robinson RG, et al. J Rheumatol 1994;21:530–5.
206. Henderson CJ, Lovell D. Rheum Dis Clin North Am 1991;17: 403–13.

85. Osteoporosis

ELIZABETH A. KRALL and BESS DAWSON-HUGHES

One and a half million osteoporotic fractures of the spine, hip, wrist, and other sites occur each year, primarily in postmenopausal white women. The number of osteoporosis cases among men and nonwhite individuals, however, is expected to rise substantially in the next several decades as life expectancy increases and the world population expands. In the United States, direct medical costs of fractures among the population aged 45 and older totaled nearly 14 billion dollars in 1995 (1). Treatment of men accounted for approximately 3 billion dollars, or 20% of the total amount. In addition, fractures of the hip and spine often contribute to disability, dependence, and increased risk of death.

Osteoporosis is typically defined as a reduction in bone mineral mass that results in decreased bone strength and increased susceptibility to fracture with only mild-or-moderate trauma. For a discussion of normal bone development, metabolism, and composition and the roles of various nutrients in bone health and disease, see Chapter 83. Osteoporotic bone tissue is characterized by demineralized, disconnected trabeculae and thinning of the outer cortical surfaces (Fig. 85.1). The etiology and symptoms of osteoporosis and its link to the menopause were first described by Albright et al. more than 50 years ago (2). Several causes were known or suspected at that time, including immobilization, diet, and metabolic diseases. In subsequent years, the list of risk factors has grown, and it is now recognized that bone mass throughout the life span and the risk of osteoporotic fracture are determined by heredity and a large number of environmental factors. Diet remains of critical interest in this multifactorial disease because it is one of the few determinants that can be safely modified.

BONE DENSITY ASSESSMENT

Much of our knowledge of the influence of nutrition and other factors on bone status and fracture risk has been gained since the introduction of precise, noninvasive methods to measure bone mineral density (BMD). Widely used methods for both clinical diagnosis and research purposes include single photon or single x-ray absorptiometry, which is appropriate for measuring sites without much overlying fat and muscle tissue (e.g., wrist and heel), and dual photon or dual x-ray absorptiometry for sites such as the hip, spine, and whole body, where thicker layers of soft tissue surround the bone. Bone density is proportional to the amount of energy that is absorbed as it passes from an energy source located on one side of the bone to a detector on the opposite side. Low-radiation x-ray absorptiometry has largely replaced the older technologies that used a photon energy source. A bone density scan of the hip is shown in Figure 85.2.

Quantitative computed tomography (QCT) and quantitative ultrasound are two alternative research techniques for assessing bone status. QCT is primarily used to selectively assess trabecular bone, which is metabolically more active than cortical bone. Quantitative ultrasound measures the attenuation and velocity of sound waves as they pass through bone and other tissues. These measures are thought to assess qualitative factors such as bone architecture and elasticity in addition to bone mineral mass. Advantages of ultrasound are the lack of radiation exposure and the compact size of ultrasound units, which allows bone status measurements in field settings.

EPIDEMIOLOGY OF OSTEOPOROSIS

The descriptive epidemiology of osteoporosis depends to some extent on the method used to define the disorder. Fractures resulting from moderate trauma (e.g., a fall from

Abbreviations: **BMD**—bone mineral density; **25(OH)D**—25-hydroxyvitamin D; **$1,25(OH)_2D$**—1,25-dihydroxyvitamin D.

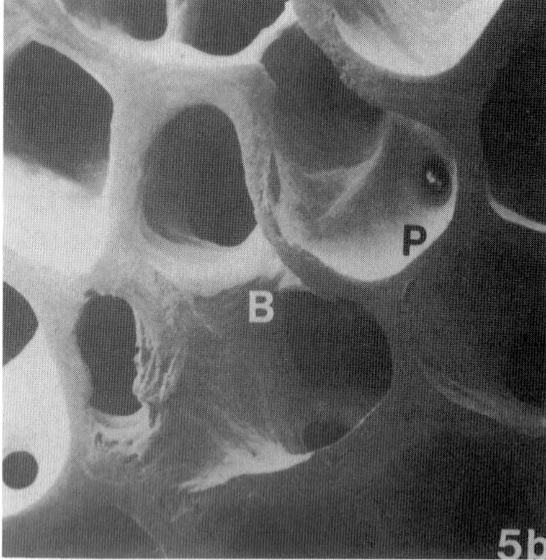

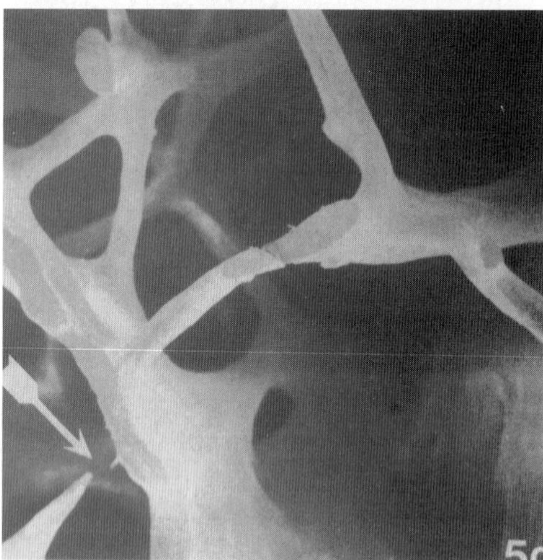

Figure 85.1. Electron micrographs of iliac crest biopsies illustrating normal bone *(upper panel)* and osteoporotic bone *(lower panel)*. Normal bone consists of a series of plates *(P)* interconnected by thick rods *(B)*. The osteoporotic bone has few plates, and several rods are fractured or disconnected *(arrow)*. (From Dempster DW, Shane E, Horbert W, et al. J Bone Miner Res 1986;1:15, with permission.)

standing height or less) are the most important clinical outcome of osteoporosis. The incidence of fractures rises sharply in the fourth decade of life and, at the hip and spine, continues to rise exponentially with age in men and women. At age 50, a white woman has a 30% chance of suffering a nonvertebral fracture sometime during her remaining life, and a man has about a 13% chance of fracture. Osteoporosis in women can also be defined solely in terms of BMD, regardless of whether an individual has suffered a fracture. There is a continuous inverse relationship between BMD and risk of fracture (3), as shown in Figure 85.3. The fracture rate for a given decrease in BMD is greater in older than in younger individuals *(left panel)*, which indicates that qualitative properties of bone that are not measured by BMD are important in determining fracture risk.

Overall, the likelihood of fracture increases 1.5- to 3-fold for each standard deviation decrease in bone density. The WHO Consensus Development Conference criteria for the definition of osteoporosis are based on this relationship: BMD that is not more than 1 standard deviation below a young female reference value is considered normal; osteopenia (low BMD) is defined as BMD more than 1 but less than 2.5 standard deviations below the reference value; and osteoporosis is present when BMD is more than 2.5 standard deviations below the reference value. Using these criteria, it is estimated that 7 to 9.4 million women in the U.S. have osteoporosis, and at least 13 million are osteopenic (4). Less than 15% of white women aged 50 have BMD in the osteoporotic range, but the prevalence rises to 70% among women aged 80 and older. Accepted definitions of osteopenia and osteoporosis based on BMD need to be developed for men.

Patterns of Peak Bone Density and Bone Loss

BMD in the older adult has been influenced by the peak bone mass achieved in young adulthood as well as

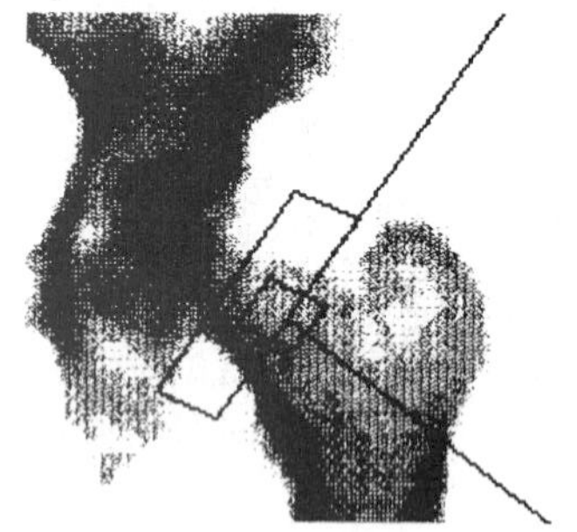

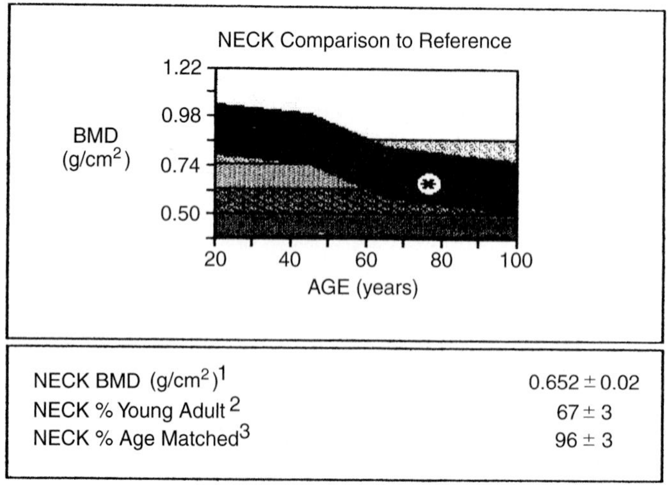

NECK BMD (g/cm^2)[1]	0.652 ± 0.02
NECK % Young Adult[2]	67 ± 3
NECK % Age Matched[3]	96 ± 3

Figure 85.2. Dual-energy absorptiometry of the femur site of a 78-year-old woman. The femoral neck is the area outlined by the *large box* in the picture on the *left*. The graph and percentages on the *right* compare the subject's bone mineral density *(BMD)* with the mean value of 20-year-old women *(% young reference)* and the mean value for women the same age as the subject *(% age-matched)*. The total width of the *dark band* in the center of the graph encompasses 1 standard deviation (SD) above and 1 SD below the mean BMD at various ages.

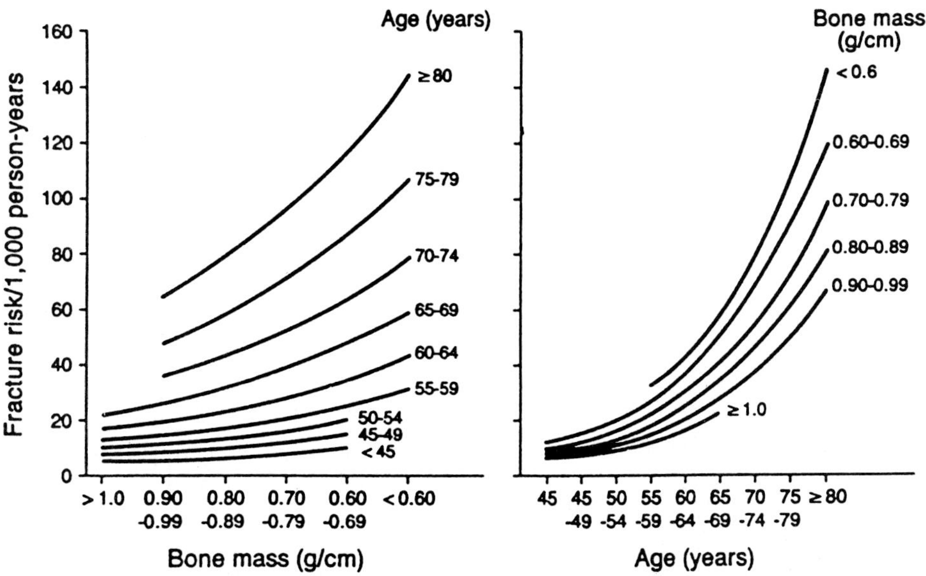

Figure 85.3. Relationships between bone mass of the radius, age, and rate of all nonvertebral fractures in women. For a given age, the risk of fracture increases with progressively decreasing bone mass *(left panel)*. The relationship between fracture risk and age is stronger, however, as seen by the steeper rise in risk with advancing age at a given level of bone mass *(right panel)*. (From Hui SL, Slemenda CW, Johnston CC Jr. J Clin Invest 1988;81:1804–9, with permission.)

the rate of bone loss in later years. The patterns of peak BMD, rates of bone loss, and fracture incidence vary with sex, age, ethnic group, and possibly skeletal site. Women, on average, have lower BMDs than men. This sex difference becomes evident in adolescence and is enhanced in later adulthood by several years of rapid bone loss surrounding the menopause. Blacks tend to have higher BMDs than whites and Asians, and this difference is first apparent in early childhood (5).

Growth in childhood is accompanied by an increase in bone mass. Bone mass accumulates rapidly during the growth spurt that normally occurs between the ages of 11 and 14 years in girls and 13 to 17 years in boys. After the growth spurt, bone continues to increase in density but at a slower rate until peak bone mass is achieved sometime in young adulthood, about the same time that the bones cease to grow in length and the epiphyses close (6). Small increments in bone mass may continue until the late 20s or 30s.

Bone loss in young adults is believed to be minimal, and the age of onset may vary by skeletal site (7). Longitudinal studies of women indicate that bone loss at the spine and radius occurs before menopause, but the rate is not greater than 1%/year. Within the first 1 to 5 years after the onset of menopause, the rate of bone loss is two to six times premenopausal levels, but it gradually returns to about 1% annually about the 10th year after menopause. In older women, bone loss continues at a rate of approximately 1% annually into advanced ages (8, 9), although the rate may accelerate again after age 75 (8). An apparent increase in lumbar spine density with age has been reported in elderly women and men, but this is attributed to coexisting osteoarthritis or calcification of soft tissue in the region of the spine, such as the aorta, which interferes with bone density measurement.

Until recently, men were frequently excluded from studies of osteoporosis and bone loss. The higher average bone mass seen in men beginning at puberty is maintained throughout the life span, and it is not clear at what age bone loss begins in men. Cross-sectional studies indicate that decreases in bone density at various skeletal sites among men over 50 are similar in magnitude to the declines seen in women more than 10 years postmenopause (10, 11). These findings have been confirmed in several longitudinal studies in men in which rates of bone loss from the hip (9) and radius (12) were approximately 1%/year.

Epidemiology of Fractures

The incidence of fractures peaks in childhood and then declines until age 40, when rates begin to rise again. Most fractures among children and young adults result from severe trauma and are not highly dependent on bone density, but after age 40, an increasing proportion of fractures result from mild or moderate trauma. Patterns of fracture incidence in older adults generally reflect the variations in bone mass and rates of loss by age and race, although there are distinct patterns of incidence at different skeletal sites.

Radius

The incidence of fractures of the forearm or distal radius (Colles' fracture) rises after age 40 and tends to level off by age 55 in men or age 65 in women. The incidence of Colles' fractures among women in Rochester, Minnesota, increased from 107/100,000 person-years between the ages of 35 and 39 to a maximum of 640/100,000 person-years at ages 60 to 64 (13). Among men, the rate increased from 44/100,000 person-years at ages 35 to 39 to a maximum of 118/100,000 person-years at ages 50 to 54. The ratio of forearm fracture in females and males varies from 2:1 at age 35 to more than 8:1 after age 80.

Femur

Beginning at age 40, the rate of hip fracture doubles about every 6 or 7 years in men and women in the United States, and this exponential rise continues among the very old (14). Among white individuals aged 85 years, the annual incidence rate of femoral fracture is approximately 2300/100,000 in women and 1200/100,000 in men. By age 95, the rates rise to 3600/100,000 in women and 2500/100,000 in men. The risk in black women is 50% higher than in black men at age 85 (900 and 600/100,000, respectively). Men and women of Asian descent living in the United States also have a reduced risk of hip fracture, comparable to that in blacks. International comparisons indicate that incidence rates of hip fracture in black and Asian men and women are approximately one-quarter to one-half those of white women in northern Europe and the United States. On average, an Asian women has half the risk of hip fracture of a white male living in the United States or northern Europe. Among white women aged 80 years and older, 20% of all fractures are hip fractures, which are nearly four times more common than fractures of the extremities. Of all osteoporotic fractures, those at the hip are associated with the highest risk of death and disability.

Spine

A vertebral compression fracture is typically diagnosed when the height of the vertebra decreases by 20% or more. As a result, the normally cube-shaped vertebra frequently becomes concave or wedge shaped. A severe consequence of vertebral fractures is kyphosis, or the curved spine known as "dowager's hump." Vertebral fractures arising from mild or moderate trauma occur more than three times more frequently in women than in men in the United States, 137 versus 44 fractures per 100,000 population per year, respectively (15). There is considerable geographic variation in the prevalence of this type of fracture. Estimates of the prevalence of vertebral fractures in the population over age 65 years vary from less than 3% in Finland to more than 20% in the United States (16). Because vertebral fractures can be asymptomatic or easily misdiagnosed, rates of vertebral compression fracture estimated by radiographic evaluations are much higher than those obtained from hospital admissions and clinical presentation.

Other Sites

Osteoporotic fractures at sites other than the radius, spine, or hip account for approximately half of all fractures among women aged 65 and above. Pelvic fracture resulting from moderate trauma in women in Rochester, Minnesota, rose from 17/100,000 person-years at ages 35 to 54 to 446/100,000 over age 85 (17). In men, the rate reached 64/100,000 by age 85. Fractures of the humerus display a similar gender-specific pattern, rising from 120/100,000 at ages 50 to 69 to 317/100,000 above age 70 in women, and from 27 to 51/100,000 in men (18). In contrast, fractures such as those of the ankle, ribs, patella, and hands do not appear to follow the age- or sex-specific incidence patterns of other osteoporotic fractures (14).

Falls

More than 90% of fractures among the elderly are caused by falls. Factors associated with an elevated risk of falling include use of sedatives, diminished muscle strength, gait and balance difficulties, arthritis, poor vision, Parkinson's disease, and disabilities of the lower extremities (19, 20). The chance of falling increases as more risk factors are present. In addition to bone density, biomechanical and individual characteristics influence the likelihood of fracture due to a fall. Hip fractures occur more frequently after a fall to the side (21), while Colles' fractures are more often associated with forward falls. The height of the fall is directly related to the force of impact and risk of fracture, but individuals with a high body mass index are less likely to sustain a fracture (21). Most falls occur after tripping or slipping on environmental hazards (19), which implies that nonmedical interventions can significantly reduce the number of falls and fractures.

NUTRITIONAL DETERMINANTS OF BONE DENSITY AND FRACTURE RISK

Many nutritional factors have been examined for associations with osteoporosis and bone mass. Calcium, phosphorus, trace minerals, and protein are components of bone tissue. Vitamin D regulates calcium balance, and various other nutrients interact with calcium absorption and excretion. Thus, dietary intakes of these nutrients may affect bone mass, although the strength of associations may be expected to vary according to developmental phase, menopausal status, and habitual intake by the subjects studied.

Calcium

Calcium Intake and Bone Mass in Childhood

Bone mass during childhood and adolescence can be increased by raising calcium intake to the level of the 1989 RDA or above (1200 mg or 30 mmol per day for ages 11–24 years) or to the 1997 Food and Nutrition Board adequate intake (AI) values of 1300 mg (32.5 mmol) per day for ages 9 through 18 years and 1000 mg (25 mmol) ages 19 through 50 years for both males and females (see Appendix Tables II-A-2-a-2 and A-2-b-1). A 3-year randomized, double-blind, placebo-controlled trial was conducted in twins aged 6 to 14 years, during which the usual daily calcium intake (22.5 mmol, or 900 mg) of one of each pair was supplemented with 17.5 mmol (700 mg) daily (22). In prepubertal twins, the child taking the calcium supplement gained a total of 3 to 5% more bone mass at the radius and spine than his or her sibling, but there was no clear benefit of supplementation among older children. In another randomized study, calcium supplementation in girls, mean age 11.9 years, a daily calcium intake of 32.8 mmol (1314 mg) was associated with 2.6% higher bone densities at the spine and whole body bone density at the end of 2 years (23). A daily calcium intake of 30 mmol achieved with dairy foods instead of supplements was associated with larger gains in BMD at the spine and whole body in 9- to 13-year-old girls than in a control group (24). Intakes of phosphorus, vitamin D, and protein were also increased, and it is not certain if calcium or a combination of nutrients was responsible for the gains in bone mass. The benefit to bone mass of 18 months of added calcium in prepubertal children disappeared when supplementation was halted (25), suggesting that adequate calcium intake may need to be maintained throughout childhood and adolescence to have a meaningful impact on peak bone mass. Gains in peak bone mass may afford some protection against fracture in later life.

Calcium Intake and Bone Loss in Adult Women

Increased calcium intake causes a short-term reduction in bone turnover in adult women, but whether initial beneficial effects on the rate of bone loss can be maintained for an extended period of time is questionable. The bone remodeling rate generally returns to a steady state within a year after the introduction of calcium. In addition, early and sustained effects may differ in trabecular and cortical bone.

Premenopausal. Prospective studies indicate that increasing calcium intake may reduce the rate of bone loss in premenopausal women. Spinal bone loss was significantly lower in a group of women who used dairy foods to raise calcium intake from 22.5 to 37.5 mmol (900 to 1500 mg) daily (26). A similar level of calcium intake (37 mmol) attained through supplementation slowed bone loss from the humerus but not the radius or ulna (27). The effect of calcium on bone density at other skeletal sites such as the hip in young women is unknown.

Postmenopausal. The responsiveness of bone to nutritional intervention is blunted in the first few years of menopause, as falling endogenous estrogen levels create a new "set point" of bone metabolism. Thus, results of calcium supplement trials in older women vary according to the menopausal status of the participants. Findings of recent randomized, placebo-controlled trials in early and late postmenopausal women (28–31a) are summarized in Table 85.1. A 3-year study of early menopausal women found that the effect of supplementation on the femoral neck was sustained during the 2nd and 3rd years (28). Calcium supplementation also slowed the loss of total body calcium in that study. A 2-year controlled study of women aged 46 to 55 years found that daily supplements of 25 or 50 mmol (1 or 2 g) retarded spinal bone loss only within the 1st year (32). In the 2nd year, rates of loss in all groups were similar. Nevertheless, BMD in both supplemented groups remained higher than in the control group throughout the study, because of the benefits accrued in the 1st year. Calcium had no benefit on metacarpal bone mineral. Limited responses to added calcium were also observed in early menopausal women with low usual calcium intakes, under 16.2 mmol, or 650 mg (33).

The recent controlled trials of calcium supplementation in later postmenopausal women (29–31a) shown in Table 85.1 confirm earlier studies that demonstrated a reduction in bone loss (33, 34). Several also suggest that the benefits can be maintained over an extended period of time. In a 4-year study in which total calcium intake was raised to 42.5 mmol/day (1700 mg), a reduction in whole-body bone loss became apparent after the 1st year but continued at a slower rate throughout all remaining years of the study (29). Other factors have emerged in addition to menopausal age that may modify the effect of calcium intake on bone loss. The level of usual calcium intake affected the degree to which a supplement containing 500 mg (12.5 mmol) elemental calcium retarded bone loss among late menopausal women participating in a randomized, placebo-controlled study (33). The largest reductions in bone loss from the spine, hip, and radius were observed in women with usual daily calcium intakes below 10 mmol (400 mg). And, the benefit of increased calcium intake on weight-bearing sites such as the hip appears to be enhanced in women who also have high levels of physical activity (30, 34).

Calcium Intake and Bone Loss in Men

Daily milk consumption as a teenager, recalled several decades later, was associated with higher hip BMD among men aged 50 to 88 years (10). To date, there are few longitudinal studies of calcium supplementation among men to confirm the association (31a). A placebo-controlled study in men aged 30 to 87 found that added calcium did not reduce bone loss at the spine over 3 years (12). These men habitually consumed a high level of calcium, over 27.4 mmol (1100 mg) per day, and the treatment group received an additional 25 mmol/day. It is possible that there is a threshold of calcium intake above which more calcium has no measurable effect. Calcium supplementation benefited older men with lower usual dietary levels at multiple skeletal sites (31a).

Calcium Intake and Fracture Rates

Previous epidemiologic associations of increased calcium intake and reduced fracture rates are supported by placebo-controlled trials (29, 31, 35). The incidence of hip fractures and of all nonvertebral fractures in over 3000

Table 85.1
Summary of Recent Randomized Trials of Calcium Supplementation

Investigators (ref. no.)	Description of Subjects	Study Length	Mean Dietary Calcium (mg/day)	Intervention[a]	Effect on Bone Loss
Aloia et al. 1994 (28)	101 women, age 49–53 years, 6 months–6 years postmenopausal	3 years	<500	1000 mg/day Ca 400 IU vitamin D[c]	Total body calcium ↓ Femoral neck ↓ Spine n.s. Radius n.s.
Reid et al. 1995 (29)	78 women, mean age 58 years, mean 9.5 years since menopause	4 years	760	1000 mg/day Ca	Spine ↓ Whole body ↓ Hip ↓
Prince et al. 1995 (30)	168 women, age 50–70 years, at least 10 years postmenopausal	2 years	800	1000 mg/day Ca as supplement or milk products	Intertrochanteric hip ↓ Ankle ↓
Chevalley et al. 1994 (31)	79 women and men, age 62–87, prevalent spine fractures, no previous hip fractures	18 months	<700	800 mg/day Ca[d]	Hip ↓ Spine n.s.
Dawson-Hughes et al. 1997 (31a)	389 healthy men and women, age 65 years or older	3 years	<800	500 mg/day Ca 700 IU vitamin D	Hip ↓ Whole body ↓ Spine ↓

Abbreviations: Ca, calcium.
[a]1 mg calcium = 0.025 mmol; 1 IU vitamin D = 0.025 μg.
[b]↓ indicates calcium significantly reduced the rate of bone loss compared to placebo; n.s. indicates the treatment was not significantly different from placebo.
[c]Subjects in placebo group also received 400 IU vitamin D daily.
[d]Each subject in treatment and placebo groups was given 300,000 IU intramuscularly at baseline.

elderly French women was reduced by 26% in a group supplemented with 30 mmol (1200 mg) of calcium and 20 mg (800 IU) of vitamin D (35). The control group received placebos of both calcium and vitamin D, so it is not certain which agent contributed more to the reduction in fractures. The results of supplement trials of calcium only and the known function of vitamin D in promoting intestinal calcium absorption suggest calcium had a critical role. Three smaller studies are consistent with the French study (29, 31, 31a). Calcium supplementation reduced the rate of all fractures in a 4-year study of postmenopausal women, but the total number of fractures was small (29). Three years of calcium and vitamin D supplementation was associated with a reduction in nonvertebral fractures in elderly men and women (31a). In an 18-month trial, the rate of vertebral compression fractures was about 32% lower in the treatment group than in a placebo group, but again the number of fractures was small, and the difference was not statistically significant (31). The reduction in risk may have continued over a longer follow-up time.

Summary of Calcium Intake and Bone Mass

Observational studies and controlled trials with children, young adults, and the elderly all support the important and measurable role of calcium intake in building and maintaining bone mass and reducing bone loss. Studies in children demonstrate that increasing calcium intake to the RDA or above augments bone density. Dietary or supplemental calcium reduces bone loss, although it may not eliminate it, in premenopausal and postmenopausal women and reduces the risk of fracture. Our knowledge of the effect of calcium intake on rates of bone loss in older men is limited. Variations in the response to calcium at different skeletal sites may be related to the proportions of trabecular and cortical tissue in bone, usual calcium intake level, and the interaction of calcium with other dietary and lifestyle characteristics.

Vitamin D

Vitamin D is obtained from the diet in the forms of ergocalciferol and cholecalciferol as well as from cutaneous synthesis after exposure to sunlight. It is hydroxylated to 25-hydroxyvitamin D (25(OH)D, or calcidiol) in the liver and then to the active metabolite, 1,25-dihydroxyvitamin D (1,25$(OH)_2$D, or calcitriol), in the kidney. 1,25$(OH)_2$D stimulates calcium absorption across the intestine and is necessary for maintenance of healthy bone. Plasma level of 25(OH)D is a widely used clinical indicator of vitamin D status. Although it reflects both dietary and endogenous contributions, sunlight exposure appears to have a stronger influence on 25(OH)D level than diet at vitamin D intake levels typically consumed in the United States and Europe. However, diet takes on increased importance in wintertime at high latitudes in healthy adults and throughout the year in individuals who have limited sun exposure or a diminished ability to synthesize the vitamin. In the United States and Europe, the elderly ingest an average of 2.5 μg (100 IU) per day, which is only half the RDA in the United States.

The concentrations of parathyroid hormone (PTH),

25(OH)D, and 1,25(OH)$_2$D vary with season. In the northern hemisphere, PTH is higher and levels of 25(OH)D and 1,25(OH)$_2$D are lower in winter than in summer. The most striking seasonal variability is seen in individuals with dietary vitamin D intake below 5 μg, or 200 IU (36). Rates of bone loss have also been reported to vary by season, with more rapid loss during the period in which PTH is elevated and vitamin D levels are low (37).

The role of vitamin D insufficiency in osteoporosis is increasingly recognized. The lower intestinal calcium absorption and blood levels of 25(OH)D and 1,25(OH)$_2$D seen in many osteoporotic patients compared with healthy age-matched controls may result from inadequate dietary vitamin D or impaired 1,25(OH)$_2$ action. Plasma 1,25(OH)$_2$D and calcium absorption can be corrected by administration of calcitriol, but previous studies with small numbers of subjects did not agree on the impact on bone density and fracture rates. Spine BMD and total-body calcium were maintained by elderly osteoporotic women after treatment with calcitriol (despite the fact that dietary vitamin D was replete), but there was no effect on the rate of vertebral fracture (38). A large multicenter trial found that treatment with 0.5 μg/day of calcitriol reduced vertebral fractures in osteoporotic women, compared with treatment with 25 mmol (1000 mg) calcium (39). The benefit was greatest in women with mild-to-moderate preexisting spinal fractures.

Vitamin D supplementation appears to be effective in preventing fracture in the frail elderly. Annual intramuscular injections of ergocalciferol to institutionalized and free-living elderly persons in Finland reduced the number of upper body fractures (e.g., radius, humerus, ribs) but surprisingly had no apparent effect on lower limb fractures (40). Injections overcame the problems of poor intestinal absorption and noncompliance. The large controlled trial of 20 μg cholecalciferol and calcium supplementation in elderly French women showed a substantial reduction in risk of fracture (35). Compared with the placebo group, there was a 26% reduction in the number of hip fractures and other nonvertebral fractures with vitamin D treatment. There was also a significant 6% difference between treatment and placebo groups in bone density of the hip in a subset of women measured over the 18-month interval. In contrast, rates of hip and other types of fracture were similar in a placebo group and a group supplemented with a lower dose of vitamin D (10 μg) without calcium in a large study in the Netherlands (41). Major differences in the population characteristics and treatments in these two trials that could have contributed to the contradictory findings are condensed in Table 85.2. The overall risk of fracture may have been lower in the Dutch study because of the inclusion of men, noninstitutionalized persons, and individuals with high usual calcium intake. The French study suggests that a large segment of the population with low calcium intakes would possibly benefit from increased vitamin D intake.

The 1997 FNB adequate intake (AI) values for vitamin D were doubled to 10 μg/day for women aged 51 and above, compared with the 5 μg (as cholecalciferol) in the 1989 RDA (see Appendix Tables II-A-2-a-2 and A-2-b-4).

Table 85.2
Summary of Differences in Two Large Intervention Trials of Dietary Vitamin D on Fracture Rates in Elderly Subjects

	France (35)	The Netherlands (41)
Subjects	3270 women	1916 women 662 men
Residence type	All institutionalized	60% institutionalized 40% free living
Daily supplement[a,b,c]	20 μg vitamin D with 1200 mg calcium and 600 mg phosphorus	10 μg vitamin D
Usual dietary calcium[b]	511 mg/day	868 mg/day
Duration of trial	18 months	3.5 years
Effect of intervention on fracture rate	26% reduction in hip fractures and all nonvertebral fractures	None

[a]1 μg vitamin D = 40 IU.
[b]1 mg calcium = 0.025 mmol.
[c]1 mg phosphorus = 0.032 mmol.

Phosphorus

An increase in serum phosphorus concentration arising from high dietary phosphorus intake stimulates PTH secretion, which in turn suppresses 1,25-(OH)$_2$D production and intestinal calcium absorption. As a consequence, excess phosphorus intake may be a concern. Increased phosphorus has an opposing effect on calcium balance, however, by reducing the amount of calcium lost through the urine, and this action may adequately offset the adverse effects on calcium absorption and bone metabolism in healthy adults. The phosphorus:calcium ratio may be more important than the level of phosphorus alone. A diet high in phosphorus (55 mmol or 1700 mg/day) and low in calcium (10 mmol/day) produced an increase in PTH secretion (42). If extended over a long period of time, it is suspected that this common dietary pattern could lead to unfavorable bone balance, but this has not been demonstrated.

Prolonged dietary phosphorus deficiency can deplete the serum level and result in enhanced resorption of this mineral from the bones. For a portion of the elderly population, phosphorus deficiency is a concern. Low serum phosphorus levels can result from malnutrition, excessive use of phosphorus-binding antacids, and intestinal malabsorption. The phosphorus content of calcium triphosphate supplements may have contributed to some degree to the reduction in fracture rate in the French study of vitamin D and calcium intervention (35). The 1997 FNB RDA for phosphorus in men and women above 19 years (700 mg/day) is lower than the 1989 RDA of 1200 mg at 19 to 24 years and 800 mg thereafter (see Appendix Tables II-A-2-a-2 and A-2-b-2).

Protein

The average protein intake in many industrialized countries is at least 50% above recommended levels. Excess protein intake has been proposed as a reason for the high incidence of osteoporosis in such populations despite moderate-to-high average calcium intakes. The proposed mechanism is the calciuric effect of protein. Over a wide range of protein intake, an average increase in dietary protein of 1 g results in the loss of an additional 1 mg of calcium in the urine. The effect of protein is rapid and is not balanced by a change in calcium absorption. Calcium losses of this magnitude could be very important in individuals with a low usual calcium intake or impaired calcium absorption. The importance of the protein effect in healthy adults is less clear. The interactions of protein, calcium, and phosphorus at various intake levels of these nutrients require further study.

Although reducing protein intake conserves calcium, intakes below the RDA can have serious adverse effects in the elderly. Patients with hip fracture are frequently protein and calorie malnourished. Protein-rich dietary supplements administered to hip fracture patients reduced the rates of complications and death immediately after surgery, and the rates remained lower than those of nonsupplemented patients for a period of 6 months (43).

Sodium

Sodium causes an increase in renal calcium excretion. At the high levels of sodium intake typical in the United States, over 90% of ingested sodium is excreted, and urinary sodium is a valid estimate of dietary intake. For each 500-mg increment in sodium excretion (or sodium intake) there is approximately a 10-mg increase in the amount of calcium lost in urine. Because, on average, only 25% of ingested calcium is absorbed, this means calcium intake must be raised 40 mg to compensate for a 500-mg increment in sodium intake. The impact of sodium intake on the rate of bone loss at the hip was evaluated in postmenopausal women (44). Over a wide range of sodium excretion (1–6 g/day), there was an increasingly negative change in hip bone density with higher levels of urinary sodium. In that population, optimal intakes to minimize bone loss were estimated at approximately 25 mmol (1000 mg) of calcium and no more than 87 mmol (2000 mg) of sodium daily.

Caffeine

Caffeine ingestion causes a short-term (within 1–3 h) increase in urinary calcium loss, but controlled studies have failed to document sustained effects of caffeine on urinary or fecal calcium excretion (45, 46). Such a temporary increase may be expected to have a minor effect on net calcium balance. However, among older individuals with low calcium intakes, the effect may possibly take on relatively greater importance as the body fails to adequately compensate for the additional calcium loss. A study of postmenopausal women found that coffee intake of two or more cups per day was associated with lower BMD in those who did not drink milk on a daily basis (47). Bone loss was more rapid in a subgroup of women with calcium intake below the RDA of 800 mg/day and caffeine intake of more than two to three cups of brewed coffee per day (46). Coffee consumption has also been associated with greater risk of hip fracture (48) in elderly women.

Alcohol

Chronic alcoholism and osteoporosis commonly co-occur in men (49). Ethanol directly affects bone tissue by suppressing bone formation. Its use is also associated with multiple nutritional deficiencies, hepatic damage, and hypogonadism, all of which have deleterious effects on bone metabolism. Moderate or social use, on the other hand, appears to have the opposite effect on BMD and bone loss. Several population studies have reported that moderate alcohol use is associated with higher mean bone density levels (50) and reduced rates of bone loss (51). Alcohol stimulates the conversion of androstenedione to estrone, an estrogenic compound with bone-preserving properties. A potential reduction in fracture risk among alcohol users arising from a modest increase in bone density may be offset by an increased likelihood of falling, however.

Fluoride

Fluoride stimulates osteoblast activity and can replace hydroxyl ions in the hydroxyapatite structure of bone. This substitution results in bone with increased crystalline size but decreased elasticity and quality. Thus, although the compression strength of fluoride-enriched bone is greater, the tensile quality may decline. An association between increased bone density on radiographs and naturally occurring high fluoride in drinking water, at concentrations between 0.21 and 0.30 mmol (4–5.8 mg) per liter, was observed in an early study (52). In contrast, fluoridated drinking water that supplies 0.05 to 0.16 mmol (1–3 mg) per day has neither beneficial nor deleterious effects on bone density (53) or hip fracture rates (54).

When used in high doses as a therapeutic agent for osteoporosis, fluoride increases spinal bone density, but the effect on fracture incidence is less clear. No protection against vertebral fractures was found in two trials of 3.9 mmol (75 mg) fluoride, and there was a suggestion that nonvertebral fractures might have increased on fluoride therapy (55, 56). More recently, a lower dose of slow-release sodium fluoride (1.3 mmol or 25 mg/day) administered cyclically increased bone density of the spine and hip and decreased the rate of vertebral fracture (57).

Trace Minerals

Increasing boron intake may result in a drop in urinary excretion of calcium, phosphorus, and magnesium and a simultaneous increase in serum estradiol level (58). Such findings suggest that boron may play a role in maintaining calcium balance. Although the mechanism is unknown, it is postulated that boron is necessary for formation of certain steroid hormones or hydroxylation of 25(OH)D. More information is needed on usual dietary intakes and boron requirements before its importance in the development of osteoporosis can be fully understood.

Bone tissue contains approximately half of the body stores of magnesium. In animals, dietary magnesium restriction is associated with increased bone resorption and decreased formation. When magnesium depletion is induced in humans, decreased PTH secretion, hypocalcemia, hypocalciuria, and a positive calcium balance result. Reports of altered levels of magnesium in bone of osteoporotic and control subjects have not been substantiated.

Manganese, zinc, and copper are cofactors for enzymes essential to bone tissue. The effect of these three trace minerals on bone loss at the spine, alone or in combination with calcium, was evaluated in a 2-year trial of postmenopausal women (59). Spine BMD in the group supplemented with a combination of 25 mol (1 g) calcium, 0.09 (5 mg) mmol manganese, 0.04 mmol (2.5 mg) copper, and 0.23 mmol (15 mg) zinc showed no decline compared with that in the control group, which lost an average of 3.5% of bone mass. The role of these trace minerals in maintaining bone mass has not yet been established.

OTHER RISK FACTORS FOR OSTEOPOROTIC FRACTURE

Body Weight and Body Composition

Bone loss that occurs during prolonged immobilization and weightlessness in space flight demonstrates the importance of gravitational force in preserving bone density. Body weight is directly correlated with bone density, and higher weight protects against fracture (60). Apart from the contribution of total weight on bone mass, the two major components of body weight, fat-free mass (primarily muscle) and fat tissue, may influence bone through other mechanisms. Fat tissue is a source of endogenous estrogen. In postmenopausal women, this source takes on increased importance as gonadal hormone production declines. Muscle size is influenced by some of the same factors that stimulate bone formation, such as physical activity, insulin, growth hormone, and androgens. There is no agreement on whether the fat (61) or fat-free (62) component of body weight is more important in building and preserving bone density. However, excess body fat is strongly associated with increased risk of numerous chronic diseases.

Smoking

Cigarette smokers often possess characteristics associated with low bone density independently of their exposure to tobacco. These include lower body weight, greater consumption of caffeine and alcohol, and, in women, earlier menopause. Controlling for some or all of these factors, women who smoke have lower bone density and more rapid rates of bone loss than nonsmokers (63, 64). The effect of smoking is thought to be related, in part, to alterations in estrogen metabolism. Smoking increases the hepatic conversion of estradiol into biologically inactive metabolites at the expense of active hormones estrone and estriol (65). Although one population study of hip fracture in elderly women reported that smoking reduced the benefit of hormone replacement therapy (66), another found no difference in bone loss rates between smokers who did use supplemental estrogen and those who did not (64). Smoking is associated with lower BMD, increased rate of bone loss, and higher fracture risk in men, as well (67). It is not known if smoking affects circulating androgen levels or has other direct effects on bone tissue.

Physical Activity

Part of the decrease in bone density that accompanies aging may be due to declining physical activity levels in later life. Vigorous, high-impact activity in young men and premenopausal women results in modest increases bone mass. Evidence suggests that initiating an exercise regime in older, previously sedentary individuals will increase bone density or slow bone loss. It is not known if any one type of activity is best for maintaining bone health. Vigorous aerobic activity and muscle-strengthening exercises have each been associated with increased or maintenance of bone density, particularly at skeletal sites that are directly stressed by the activity (68, 69). In postmenopausal women, aerobic exercise for 20 minutes, three times a week in conjunction with muscle-strengthening exercise is recommended to help stabilize bone density. Physical activity also improves muscle function and may play a role in reducing fall-related fractures.

Heredity

Like many anthropometric traits, bone density displays a family resemblance. The similarities arise from the influences of genetic factors and shared environment on peak bone mass, rates of bone loss, or both. Family and twin studies have reported moderate-to-strong correlations of bone density among relatives over a wide age range (70–72), indicating a substantial genetic component to peak bone mass and possibly rates of bone loss.

A genetic marker, the vitamin D receptor (VDR), has been associated with bone density and rates of bone loss in several different populations (73, 74) but not in others (75, 76). Interactions of VDR alleles with calcium intake have been reported (77, 78). Women with the low-bone-density genotype exhibit more-rapid bone loss when their usual calcium intake is very low (77) and lack a compensatory increase in calcium absorption in response to a reduction in dietary calcium (78). These relationships have yet to be confirmed. Other hormone receptors such as the estrogen (79) and PTH receptors are also potential markers of bone density.

Glucocorticoid Medications

Glucocorticoids are a class of drugs used to treat a range of chronic inflammatory diseases such as rheumatoid arthritis, inflammatory bowel diseases, asthma and other respiratory disorders, and systemic lupus, and to suppress the rejection of transplanted organs. Adverse effects associated with their use include decreased intestinal absorption and increased urinary excretion of calcium, reduced gonadal hormone levels, inhibition of osteoblast function, and increased bone resorption; each of these mechanisms can result in accelerated bone loss and increased risk of fracture. Osteoporosis occurs in more than half of patients who receive long-term glucocorticoid treatment. It is estimated that 4 million cases of osteoporosis in the United States, or 20% of the total number, are attributable to corticosteroid use (80).

THERAPIES FOR OSTEOPOROSIS

Diet modification alone is not sufficient treatment for established osteoporosis, although adequate dietary calcium and vitamin D intakes are necessary components of therapy. For patients with osteoporosis, the most promising treatments are estrogen replacement, calcitonin, and bisphosphonates. These commonly prescribed medications are described briefly below.

Estrogen

Estrogen receptors have been identified in normal human osteoblast-like bone cells in vitro, providing a means by which estrogen can directly influence bone turnover (81). Estrogen enhances calcium absorption through its trophic effect on $1,25(OH)_2D$ and perhaps also directly.

Conjugated equine estrogens are the most commonly prescribed hormone replacement for postmenopausal women in the United States. A dosage of 0.625 mg of conjugated estrogens, alone or in combination with progestins, prevented bone loss at the hip and spine in early postmenopausal women and increased BMD in older women participating in a 3-year randomized, double-blinded, placebo-controlled trial (65). Most of the increase in BMD occurred within the 1st year, but smaller increments were observed in the 2nd and 3rd years as well. Another estrogen, ethinyl estradiol, at doses ranging from 3.7 to 37 nmol (1–10 μg) reduced bone loss in early postmenopausal women (82). Hormone therapy also reduces fracture rates at the hip (83). Estrogen replacement must be maintained to prevent the onset of rapid bone loss; when therapy is discontinued, bone loss similar to that seen immediately after menopause ensues. Estrogen has widespread effects on other body tissues, including the cardiovascular system, serum lipids, the uterus, and breast.

Calcitonin

Calcitonin, a small peptide hormone produced by the C cells of the thyroid gland, is secreted in response to increased serum calcium concentration. Its primary function is to inhibit bone resorption. Women with osteoporosis have an attenuated calcitonin response to a calcium challenge.

Salmon calcitonin is a more potent inhibitor of bone resorption than is human calcitonin and is more effective therapeutically. Treatment with calcitonin prevented bone loss from the proximal radius and reduced the rate of loss at the distal radius by 65% in osteoporotic patients (84). A similar trend was seen at the spine. Calcitonin does not appear to be effective at the hip. It is commonly administered as a nasal spray.

Bisphosphonates

Bisphosphonates are structural analogues of pyrophosphate. Their metabolic actions include inhibition of hydroxyapatite formation, inhibition of bone resorption through a direct dose-related effect on osteoclasts, and alteration of serum phosphorus levels. The bisphosphonates were developed to treat disorders such as Paget's disease, ectopic calcification, and metastatic disease of the skeleton. They have recently been approved for treatment of osteoporosis. Therapy involving intermittent cyclic administration of etidronate and phosphorus (as a bone "activator") and continuous calcium increased spinal bone density by about 4% and femoral bone density by 2% over controls and decreased the rate of new vertebral deformities among women with previous spine fractures (85). The treatment effect was even greater in a subgroup of women with low spinal bone density and a history of multiple vertebral fractures.

An aminobisphosphonate, alendronate, is more potent than etidronate, selectively inhibits bone resorption without accompanying detrimental effects on bone matrix mineralization, and does not require intermittent administration. Alendronate given to postmenopausal women with osteoporosis produced gains in bone density of the whole body, hip, and spine over a 24-month period and a 48% reduction in new vertebral fractures (86).

REFERENCES

1. Ray NF, Chan JK, Thamer M, Melton LJ III. J Bone Miner Res 1997;12:24–35.
2. Albright F, Smith PH, Richardson AM. JAMA 1941;116: 2465–74.
3. Hui SL, Slemenda CW, Johnston CC Jr. J Clin Invest 1988; 81:1804–9.
4. Looker AC, Johnston CC Jr, Wahner HW, et al. J Bone Miner Res 1995;10:796–802.
5. Bell NH, Shary J, Stevens J, et al. J Bone Miner Res 1991; 6:719–23.

6. Theintz G, Buchs B, Rissoli R, et al. J Clin Endocrinol Metab 1992;75:1060–5.
7. Sowers MR, Galuska DA. Epidemiol Rev 1993;15:374–98.
8. Ensrud KE, Palermo L, Black DM, et al. J Bone Miner Res 1995;10:1778–87.
9. Jones G, Nguyen T, Sambrook P, et al. Br Med J 1994;309: 691–5.
10. Glynn NW, Meilahn EN, Charron M, et al. J Bone Miner Res 1995;10:1769–77.
11. Hannan MT, Felson DT, Anderson JJ. J Bone Miner Res 1992;7:547–53.
12. Orwoll ES, Oviatt SK, McClung MR, et al. Ann Intern Med 1990;112:29–34.
13. Owen RA, Melton LJ, Johnson KA, et al. Am J Public Health 1982;72:605–7.
14. Nevitt MC. Rheum Dis Clin North Am 1994;20:535–59.
15. Cooper C, Atkinson EJ, O'Fallon WM, et al. J Bone Miner Res 1992;7:221–7.
16. Kanis JA, McCloskey EV. Bone 1992;13(Suppl 1):S1–10.
17. Melton LJ III, Sampson JM, Morrey BF, et al. Clin Orthop 1981;155:43–7.
18. Rose SH, Melton LJ, Morrey BF, et al. Clin Orthop 1982;168:24–30.
19. Tinetti ME, Speechley M, Ginter SF. N Engl J Med 1988; 319:1701–7.
20. Grisso JA, Kelsey JL, Strom BL, et al. N Engl J Med 1991;324:1326–31.
21. Greenspan SL, Myers ER, Maitland LA, et al. JAMA 1994; 271:128–33.
22. Johnston CC Jr, Miller JZ, Slemenda CW, et al. N Engl J Med 1992;327:82–7.
23. Lloyd T, Andon MB, Rollings N, et al. JAMA 1993;270:841–4.
24. Chan GM, Hoffman K, McMurray M. J Pediatr 1995;126:551–6.
25. Lee WTK, Leung SSF, Leung DMY, et al. Am J Clin Nutr 1996;64:71–7.
26. Baran D, Sorensen A, Grimes J, et al. J Clin Endocrinol Metab 1989;70:264–70.
27. Smith EL, Gilligan C, Smith PE, et al. Am J Clin Nutr 1989; 50:833–42.
28. Aloia JF, Vaswani A, Yeh JK, et al. Ann Intern Med 1994; 120:97–103.
29. Reid IR, Ames RW, Evans MC, et al. Am J Med 1995;98:331–5.
30. Prince R, Devine A, Dick I, et al. J Bone Miner Res 1995;10: 1068–75.
31. Chevalley T, Rizzoli R, Nydegger V, et al. Osteoporosis Int 1994;4:245–52.
31a. Dawson-Hughes B, Harris SS, Krall EA, et al. N Engl J Med 1997;337;670–6.
32. Elders PJM, Netelenbos JC, Lips P, et al. J Clin Endocrinol Metab 1991;73:533–40.
33. Dawson-Hughes B, Dallal GE, Krall EA, et al. N Engl J Med 1990;323:878–83.
34. Lau EM, Woo J, Leung PC, et al. Osteoporosis Int 1992;2: 168–73.
35. Chapuy MC, Arlot ME, Duboeuf F, et al. N Engl J Med 1992; 327:1637–42.
36. Krall EA, Sahyoun N, Tannenbaum S, et al. N Engl J Med 1989; 321:1777–83.
37. Dawson-Hughes B, Dallal GE, Krall EA, et al. Ann Intern Med 1991;115:505–12.
38. Gallagher JC, Goldgar D. Ann Intern Med 1990;113:649–55.
39. Tilyard MW, Spears GF, Thomson J, et al. N Engl J Med 1992; 326:357–62.
40. Heikinheimo RJ, Inkovaara JA, Harju EJ, et al. Calcif Tissue Int 1992;51:105–10.
41. Lips P, Graafmans WC, Ooms ME, et al. Ann Intern Med 1996; 124:400–6.
42. Calvo MS, Kumar R, Heath A III. J Clin Endocrinol Metab 1990;70:1334–7.
43. Delmi M, Rapin CH, Bengoa JM, et al. Lancet 1990;335: 1013–6.
44. Devine A, Criddle RA, Dick IM, et al. Am J Clin Nutr 1995; 62:740–5.
45. Barger-Lux MJ, Heaney RP, Stegman MR. Am J Clin Nutr 1990;52:722–5.
46. Harris SS, Dawson-Hughes B. Am J Clin Nutr 1994;60:573–8.
47. Barrett-Connor E, Chang JC, Edelstein SL. JAMA 1994;271: 280–3.
48. Kiel DP, Hannan MT, Anderson JJ, et al. Am J Epidemiol 1990;132:675–84.
49. Kelepouris N, Harper KD, Gannon F, et al. Ann Intern Med 1995;123:452–60.
50. Felson DT, Zhang Y, Hannan MT, et al. Am J Epidemiol 1995;142:485–92.
51. Hansen MA, Overgaard K, Riis BJ, et al. Osteoporosis Int 1991;1:95–102.
52. Bernstein DS, Sadowsky N, Hegsted DM, et al. JAMA 1966;198:499–504.
53. Cauley JA, Murphy PA, Riley TJ, et al. J Bone Miner Res 1995;10:1076–86.
54. Suarez-Almazor ME, Flowerdew G, Saunders LD, et al. Am J Public Health 1993;83:689–93.
55. Riggs BL, Hodgson SF, O'Fallon WM, et al. N Engl J Med 1990;322:802–9.
56. Kleerekoper M, Peterson EL, Nelson DA, et al. Osteoporosis Int 1991;1:155–61.
57. Pak CY, Sakhee K, Adams-Huet B, et al. Ann Intern Med 1995;123:401–8.
58. Nielsen FH, Hunt CD, Mullen LM, et al. FASEB J 1987;1:394–7.
59. Strause L, Saltman P, Smith KT, et al. J Nutr 1994;124:1060–4.
60. Cummings SR, Nevitt MC, Browner WS, et al. N Engl J Med 1995;332:767–73.
61. Reid IR, Legge M, Stapleton JP, et al. J Clin Endocrinol Metab 1995;80:1764–8.
62. Aloia JF, Vaswani A, Ma R, et al. Am J Clin Nutr 1995; 61:1110–4.
63. Krall EA, Dawson-Hughes B. J Bone Miner Res 1991;6: 331–8.
64. The Postmenopausal Estrogen/Progestin Interventions (PEPI) Trial Investigators. JAMA 1996;276:1389–96.
65. Michnovicz JJ, Hershcopf RJ, Naganuma H, et al. N Engl J Med 1986;315:1305–9.
66. Kiel DP, Baron JA, Anderson JJ, et al. Ann Intern Med 1992;116:716–21.
67. Slemenda CW, Christian JC, Reed T, et al. Ann Intern Med 1992;117:286–91.
68. Nelson ME, Fiatarone MA, Morganti CM, et al. JAMA 1994;272:1909–14.
69. Forwood MR, Burr DB. Bone Miner 1993;21:89–112.
70. Matkovic V, Fontana D, Tominac C, et al. Am J Clin Nutr 1990;52:878–88.
71. Pocock NA, Eisman JA, Hopper JL, et al. J Clin Invest 1987;80:706–10.
72. Kelly PJ, Nguyen T, Hopper J, et al. J Bone Miner Res 1993; 8:11–7.
73. Morrison NA, Qi JC, Tokita A, et al. Nature 1994;367:284–7.
74. Riggs BL, Nguygen TV, Melton LJ III, et al. J Bone Miner Res 1995;10:991–6.
75. Hustmyer F, Peacock M, Hui S, et al. J Clin Invest 1994;94: 2130–4.

76. Garnero P, Borel O, Sornay-Rendu E, et al. J Bone Miner Res 1995;10:1283–8.
77. Krall EA, Parry P, Lichter JB, et al. J Bone Miner Res 1995; 10:978–84.
78. Dawson-Hughes B, Harris SS, Finneran S. J Clin Endocrinol Metab 1995;80:3657–61.
79. Kobayashi S, Inoue S, Hosoi T, et al. J Bone Miner Res 1996; 11:306–11.
80. American College of Rheumatology Task Force on Osteoporosis Guidelines. Arthritis Rheum 1996;39:1791–1801.
81. Eriksen EF, Colvard DS, Berg NJ, et al. Science 1988;241:84–6.
82. Speroff L, Rowan J, Symons J, et al. JAMA 1996;276:1397–1403.
83. Cauley JA, Seeley DG, Ensrud K, et al. Ann Intern Med 1995;122:9–16.
84. Overgaard K, Riis BJ, Christiansen C, et al. Clin Endocrinol 1989;30:435–42.
85. Harris ST, Watts NB, Jackson RD, et al. Ann Intern Med 1993;95:557–67.
86. Liberman UA, Weiss SR, Bröll J, et al. N Engl J Med 1995; 333:1437–43.

SELECTED READINGS

Anonymous. Optimal calcium intake. NIH Consensus Statement. 1994;12:1–31.

Orwoll ES, Klein RF. Osteoporosis in men. Endocr Rev 1995;16:87–116.

Welten DC, Kemper HC, Post GB, van Staveren WA. A meta analysis of the effect of calcium intake on bone mass in young and middle aged females and males. J Nutr 1995;125: 2802–13.

86. Nutritional Management of Diabetes Mellitus

JAMES W. ANDERSON

Diabetes mellitus afflicts 18 million persons in the United States and is emerging as a major health problem throughout the world. In the U.S., it is the fourth leading cause of death by disease and a major cause of blindness and kidney disease. The estimated costs of diabetes in the U.S. exceed $100 billion and are increasing (1). Medical nutritional management is the cornerstone in management of all persons with diabetes, since appropriate dietary practices decrease all the risks and complications associated with diabetes and can potentially restore normal life expectancy. Central to management of diabetes and lipid risk factors is a high-carbohydrate, high-fiber, low-fat diet. Exercise is second in importance in diabetes management. Self-monitoring of blood glucose levels and appropriate adjustment of food intake, exercise, and medications lead to good glycemic control with a minimum of hypoglycemic episodes. Because of the high risk for atherosclerotic cardiovascular disease, persons with diabetes should develop a preventive program to normalize serum lipid levels and consider regular use of aspirin and antioxidant vitamins. Healthcare team members counsel diabetic individuals to enable them to manage their diabetes and lifestyle to maintain optimal health.

HISTORICAL OVERVIEW

Ancient civilizations in Egypt, Greece, Rome, and India recognized diabetes and the effect of dietary intervention. The Roman Aretaeus, AD 70, noted polydipsia and polyuria and named the condition *diabetes,* meaning "to flow through." Thomas Willis, a London physician, later introduced the term *mellitus* or "honeylike" after noting the sweet taste of urine. Early dietary recommendations were based on theory rather than on scientific fact. As today, debate raged on the amount of carbohydrate allowed. Champions of low-carbohydrate, high-fat diets argued that excess sugar present in blood and urine required restriction of carbohydrate. Proponents of high-carbohydrate diets argued that dietary carbohydrate was needed to replace that lost in urine. Universally agreed, and still relevant today, was that diabetes is best treated by energy-restricted diets (2).

Frederick M. Allen (3) of New York developed the famous "Allen starvation treatment" of diabetes in 1912. Using 1000-kcal diets containing 10 g carbohydrate, he sustained the lives of a few young men until insulin became available. Thus, just prior to the discovery of insulin, diabetes was treated with low-carbohydrate, semi-starvation regimens (2). Over the years, many sources of carbohydrate were identified as therapeutic including milk, vegetables, rice, potatoes, and oatmeal. Even after insulin was discovered in 1921, most Western diabetes specialists used low-carbohydrate, high-fat diets to treat lean diabetic individuals. The few clinicians to report that high-carbohydrate, low-fat diets benefited diabetic individuals included Geyelin et al. (4) in 1935, Sansum et al. (5) in 1926, and Kempner et al. (6) in 1958.

Table 86.1
Nutritional Recommendations[a] for Persons with Diabetes: 1930–1997

Nutrient	1930	1955	1970	1990	1997
Carbohydrates, total, g/day	70	176	225	290	280
% Energy	14	35	45	58	56
Simple, g/day	40	71	112	130	90
Complex, g/day	30	105	113	160	190
Fat, total, g/day	153	99	82	60	67
% of Energy	69	45	37	27	30
Saturated, g/day	87	46	35	14	18
Monounsaturated, g/day	50	37	31	26	31
Polyunsaturated, g/day	9	11	13	17	18
Cholesterol, mg/day	1060	690	550	150	150
Protein, g/day	85	101	90	75	70
% of Energy	17	20	18	15	14
Dietary fiber, g/day	8	15	20	40	35

[a]Values for a 2000 kcal diet.

Recent scientific data analyzed by the British (7), Canadian (8), and American Diabetes Associations (9) support recommendations of a generous carbohydrate, fat-restricted diet. Table 86.1 lists major changes in nutritional recommendations in America over 50 years. Recommended carbohydrate intake increased steadily since 1930 and recently reached a plateau. Total fat intake steadily declined, and protein intake has remained about the same. Recommended fiber intake has increased dramatically (2).

CLASSIFICATION

Diabetes mellitus can result from a variety of genetic, metabolic, and acquired conditions eventuating in hyperglycemia. Metabolic derangements in glucose metabolism and profound abnormalities in metabolism of fat, protein, and other substances characterize the pathology of diabetes. Current research recognizes that diabetes mellitus has several antecedents, though each type has a similar outcome once established. A heterogeneous disorder both genetically and clinically, all classifications of diabetes have in common, hyperglycemia, due to either insulin insufficiency or insulin resistance. The traditional classification segregates hyperglycemic conditions into the following groups: insulin-dependent diabetes mellitus (IDDM or type I); non-insulin-dependent diabetes mellitus (NIDDM or type II); impaired glucose tolerance (IGT), and gestational diabetes mellitus (Table 86.2). Other conditions leading to diabetes mellitus are malnutrition-related diabetes mellitus, and a variety of other genetic, drug-induced, and acquired conditions (10).

Type I diabetes accounts for approximately 5% of diabetes and is manifested in insulin deficiency caused by destruction of the pancreatic β cells. Type II diabetes accounts for about 90% diabetes and is characterized by two primary defects: insulin resistance (diminished tissue sensitivity to insulin) and impaired β-cell function (delayed or inadequate insulin release). Other causes account for the remaining 5% of diabetes in the U.S.

Impaired glucose tolerance affects more people than have type I and type II diabetes combined. It is a serious public health problem because affected persons often progress to overt diabetes and frequently have other cardiovascular disease risk factors, such as hypertension, dyslipidemia, and obesity. The onset of gestational diabetes typically occurs between the 24th and 28th weeks of pregnancy, when the body's demand for insulin is dramatically

Table 86.2
Classification of Diabetes Mellitus and Glucose Intolerance

Clinical Classes	Subclasses	Comments
Diabetes mellitus		
Type I (insulin-dependent diabetes mellitus, IDDM)	1A Classical	
	1B Autoimmune	
Type II (non-insulin-dependent diabetes mellitus, NIDDM)	Nonobese NIDDM	May be insulin-treated or non-insulin-treated
	Obese-NIDDM	
	Maturity-onset diabetes of the young (MODY)	
Malnutrition-related diabetes mellitus (MRDM)	Fibrocalculous pancreatic diabetes	
	Protein-deficient pancreatic diabetes	
Other types	Pancreatic disease	
	Hormonal etiology	
	Drug- or chemical-induced	
	Certain genetic syndromes	
	Insulin receptor antibodies	
	Other conditions	
Impaired glucose tolerance (IGT)	IGT in nonobese	
	IGT in obese	
	IGT in MODY	
	IGT in other conditions	
Gestational diabetes (GDM)		

Modified from Fajans SS. Definition and classification of diabetes including maturity-onset diabetes of the young. In: LeRoith D, Taylor SI, Olefsky JM, eds. Diabetes mellitus. Philadelphia: Lippencott-Raven, 1996;27:251–60.

increased. It affects about 2 to 4% of all pregnancies. Nutritional intake and glycemic control influence the outcome of pregnancy. Other forms of diabetes are detailed elsewhere (10).

EPIDEMIOLOGY

An estimated 18 million persons in the United States have diabetes. Over 600,000 persons are newly diagnosed with diabetes each year. Only 750,000 (about 5%) have type I diabetes; the remainder have type II. Of those with type II diabetes, approximately half, or 7 million, are undiagnosed (1). Type I diabetes is much more common in northern Europeans (Caucasians) and is uncommon among African Americans and Native Americans (11). While the prevalence of diabetes has increased dramatically over this century in the U.S., it has stabilized since 1980 and remains fairly constant (1). In the U.S., the prevalence of diabetes is highest among Native Americans; adult Pima Indians have a prevalence of about 50%. African Americans and Hispanics have substantially higher rates of diabetes than do U.S. white individuals (12).

The prevalence of diabetes varies widely around the world; certain Chinese populations have very low rates, and Micronesian populations have very high rates. The prevalence of diabetes is increasing steadily in emerging or developing countries and parallels the increase in obesity; both diabetes and obesity increase progressively as the percentage of energy from fat increases. By the year 2000, an estimated 100 million persons in the world will have diabetes (13).

Genetic and environmental factors contribute to development of type II diabetes (14). A genetic predisposition to diabetes is usually present but not required. Environmental factors contributing to development of type II diabetes are obesity, lack of physical exercise, and high-fat, low-fiber diets (13, 15, 16). Obesity, clearly the overriding risk factor, may be responsible for more than 75% of the emergence of type II diabetes (13).

DIAGNOSIS

Classic symptoms such as polydipsia, polyuria, and rapid weight loss associated with gross and unequivocal elevation of blood glucose (over 11.1 mmol/L, or 200 mg/dL) make the diagnosis of diabetes mellitus. A fasting plasma glucose level above 7.0 mmol/L (126 mg/dL) on two occasions is diagnostic. An oral glucose tolerance test (OGTT) can be performed for impaired fasting plasma glucose (6.1–7.0 mmol/L, 110–126 mg/dL), when 2-hour postprandial plasma glucose exceeds 7.8 mmol/L (140 mg/dL) or for individuals at high risk of diabetes (10, 10a).

The OGTT identifies individuals with diabetes, impaired glucose tolerance, and gestational diabetes. For proper interpretation, the individual must be ambulatory, otherwise healthy, and taking no medications that impair glucose tolerance (10). For at least 3 days before the test, individuals use a weight-maintaining diet providing at least 150 g of carbohydrate daily. After an overnight fast of 10 to 16 hours, an oral glucose load of 75 g (or 40 g/m^2) is given. The subject remains seated during the test. Water is permitted, but smoking is not. Blood is taken before glucose administration and 0.5, 1, 1.5, and 2 hours later for plasma glucose determination (17).

Nondiabetic adults have fasting plasma glucose levels below 7.0 mmol/L (126 mg/dL) and values during the OGTT below 7.8 mmol/L (140 mg/dL) at 2 hours and below 11.0 mmol/L (200 mg/dL) at 0.5, 1, and 2 hours. Diabetes mellitus is present in nonpregnant adults when two OGTT results are abnormal, with plasma glucose levels exceeding 11.0 mmol/L (200 mg/dL) at 2 hours and one other time (0.5, 1, 1.5 hours). The diagnosis of gestational diabetes is established when two or more of the following criteria are met or exceeded after the glucose tolerance test: fasting, 105 mg/dL; 1 hour, 190 mg/dL; 2 hours, 165 mg/dL; and 3 hours, 145 mg/dL (10).

Glycosylated hemoglobin levels are convenient screening tests for diabetes. A glycosylated hemoglobin level more than three standard deviations above the "normal" mean indicates diabetes, but this test is much less sensitive than the OGTT (17) (Table 86.3).

BODY FUEL REGULATION

Role of Hormones

Cleavage of proinsulin results in the C-peptide (31 amino acids) and insulin (51 amino acids). Insulin is the hormone primarily responsible for the metabolism and storage of ingested body fuels. The body secretes insulin in response to increased blood glucose after a meal. This postprandial secretion of insulin promotes glucose, amino acid, and fat uptake by tissues (primarily liver, adipose, and muscle tissue) where the glucose is used or stored. Insulin production drops as the blood glucose level decreases (18).

Amylin, the most recently discovered pancreatic hormone, affects the rate of gastric emptying. This 37-amino-acid peptide is stored in pancreatic β cells with insulin, is

Table 86.3
Diagnosis of Diabetes and Related Conditions

Fasting or Hour after Glucose	Normal	Impaired (IGT)	Diabetes[a]	Gestational Diabetes[b]
Fasting	<110	<126	≥126	≥105
0.5 and/or 1 and/or 1.5	<200	≥200	≥200	≥190
2	<140	140–199	≥200	≥165
3				≥145

Modified from Fajans SS. Definition and classification of diabetes including maturity-onset diabetes of the young. In: LeRoith D, Taylor SI, Olefsky JM, eds. Diabetes mellitus. Philadelphia: Lippencott-Raven, 1996;27:251–60.

[a]From the Expert Committee on the Diagnosis and Classification of Diabetes Mellitus. Diabetes Care 1997;20:1183–97.

[b]If 2 or more of 4 values meet criteria.

cosecreted with insulin, and acts to affect the rate of intestinal absorption of nutrients (18).

Genuth (19) calculated insulin secretion rates in nondiabetic and diabetic subjects, Healthy lean adults secrete approximately 31 U insulin daily. Because of peripheral insulin resistance, obese nondiabetic adults secrete about 114 U daily. Type I diabetic individuals release only up to 4 U insulin daily, on average, whereas lean type II diabetic individuals with diabetes for more than 10 years produce only about 14 U daily. These estimates support other evidence that diabetes usually results from an absolute or relative deficiency of insulin.

Insulin is the main signal to the body for the "fed" or "fasting" states. After a large meal, high serum insulin levels stimulate fuel and energy storage. After an overnight fast, low serum insulin levels permit mobilization of fuel and energy from storage depots. Glucagon, the pancreatic α cell hormone, facilitates fuel and energy release with low blood insulin levels (Fig. 86.1). Under stressful circumstances, hypoglycemia, or trauma, glucagon and other "counterregulatory" hormones that oppose or counter insulin action are released. These hormones—glucagon, catecholamines, glucocorticoids, and growth hormone—act specifically to decrease glucose use, promote glucose production, and mobilize fatty acids. During fasting, exercise, and stress, fatty acids are a major source of energy (17, 18).

Energy Stores

A healthy 70-kg man stores approximately 70 g of liver glycogen, 200 g of muscle glycogen, and 30 g of glucose in body fluids, totaling 5023 kJ (1200 kcal). Available glucose stores can meet energy needs for only 12 to 18 hours. However, adipose tissue triglycerides typically represent energy deposits of 502,320 kJ (120,000 kcal), 100 times the glucose energy reserves. During starvation or stress, fatty acids are released for energy. Body proteins, skeletal and visceral structures, and other vital components are unavailable for energy except under conditions of prolonged starvation or severe stress (17).

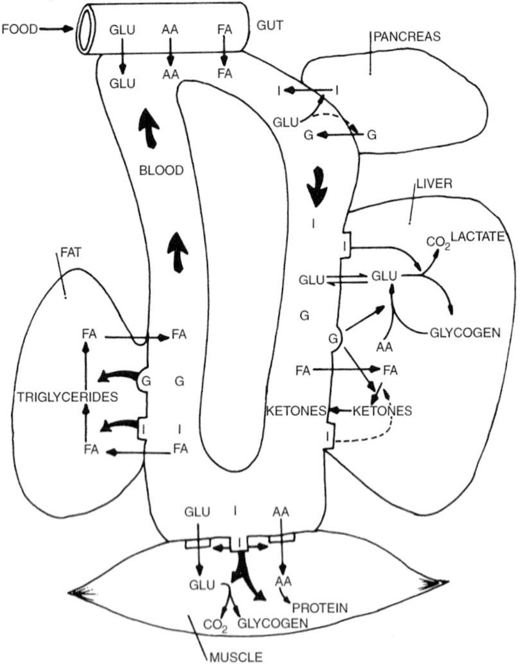

Figure 86.1. Action of insulin and glucagon shown schematically. *GLU*, glucose; *AA*, amino acids; *FA*, fatty acids; *I*, insulin; *G*, glucagon.

Fed State

A multifaceted system of hormones, nervous tissue, and digestive tissue is necessary to sustain the fed individual. This state begins as food travels down the digestive tract and is enzymatically broken down into smaller units, such as amino acids, sugars, glycerol, and fatty acids. These smaller particles are absorbed by the small intestine and then transported further. The portal blood carries amino acids and sugars to the liver. Lymph carries lipids as chylomicrons from the small intestine to the circulatory system where they are transported to numerous tissues (17).

Pancreatic β cells release insulin in response to perfusion by blood enriched with glucose, amino acids, pancreatic hormones, and other secretogogues. The same action of glucose decreases production of glucagon by pancreatic α cells. Various processes that occur in response to insulin release ensure that nutrients are taken up and stored in cells and tissues (18). Insulin stimulates glycogen synthesis, aerobic and anaerobic glycolysis, protein synthesis, and fatty acid synthesis in liver. Insulin inhibits glycogenolytic, gluconeogenic, proteolytic, and lipolytic processes. After activation by phosphorylation, glucose enters glycogen depots, generates energy in glycolytic and Krebs cycle pathways, and yields precursors for fatty acid and protein synthesis. Other simple sugars enter the glycogen pool, generate energy, or become precursors for synthetic processes. Amino acids enter precursor pools for protein synthesis (17).

Muscles and adipose tissue receive a large percentage of glucose and amino acids released after large meals. High serum insulin concentrations specifically stimulate transport of glucose and amino acids into muscle cells and glucose into adipose tissue. In muscle cells, under the influence of insulin, glucose enters glycogen depots and generates energy, while amino acids serve as precursors for protein synthesis. Insulin also facilitates conversion of glucose products to fatty acids for storage as triglycerides in fat cells. Most other tissues are freely permeable to glucose as well as amino acids and use the nutrients for glycogen formation, energy, and protein synthesis (17, 18).

Gut, liver, and other tissues handle ingested fat differently from glucose and amino acids. Gut hydrolyzes fats to fatty acids, glycerol, cholesterol, phospholipids, and other constituents. Short- and medium-chain fatty acids are absorbed and enter the portal vein for use in the liver. Long-chain fatty acids, cholesterol, and phospholipids are repackaged by gut mucosa and enter lymphatics as chylomicrons, which enter the superior vena cava through the thoracic duct. In the systemic circulation, chylomicrons release fatty acids for use by liver, muscle, fat, and other cells (17).

High serum insulin levels affect lipid metabolism in several ways. Insulin stimulates synthesis of lipoprotein lipases, which are secreted onto capillary membranes. These lipases extract fatty acids from triglyceride-rich circulating lipoproteins and facilitate entry of fatty acids into various tissues. In the fed state, a large proportion of these fatty acids are extracted by adipose tissue and incorporated into triglyceride storage. Liver cells exposed to generous amounts of insulin extract fatty acids from chylomicrons and repackage them as very low density lipoprotein (VLDL) particles, which are secreted into the systemic circulation. VLDLs also deliver fatty acids to adipose tissue for deposition (17, 18).

Fasting State

When the level of nutrients in the blood is decreased, as in a 12-hour fast, the individual is said to be in the postabsorptive, or fasting, state. This phase commences as nutrients cease to move from the intestines to the liver (17), accompanied by a gradual fall in serum insulin concentrations and a rise in serum glucagon levels. When the insulin:glucagon ratio decreases, the liver switches its enzyme machinery from glucose use to glucose production through gluconeogenesis and glycogenolysis. After 12 or more hours of fasting, half the liver glycogen is depleted. During longer starvation, hepatic glycolytic rates and activities of key glycolytic enzymes decline over 48 to 96 hours and then stabilize; hepatic gluconeogenesis rates and key gluconeogenic enzyme activity increase. After 72 hours of fasting, the liver has low glycolytic rates and has retooled for maximal gluconeogenesis (17).

Brain, other nervous tissues, red blood cells, and renal medulla have ongoing requirements for glucose for energy, whereas other tissues begin using fatty acids and ketones for energy. Low serum insulin levels stimulate lipolysis in adipose tissue; fatty acids are released at rates required for energy by various tissues. Lipolysis is further stimulated by high serum concentrations of glucagon and catecholamines. Liver burns fatty acids to meet energy needs and to fuel gluconeogenesis. Ketones are hepatic byproducts of fatty acid oxidation. Glucogenic amino acids released by muscles and other tissues are major substrates for active gluconeogenesis. When glycogen reserves of liver and muscle are exhausted, most tissues depend on fatty acids and ketones to meet their energy needs (17).

High levels of free fatty acids decrease the number of insulin receptors on various tissues and act in other ways to block insulin action. Because of low serum insulin and high serum free fatty acids, glucose and other amino acids are not transported into muscle cells. Protein synthesis stops, and proteolysis is activated, with amino acids released into circulation. Glucocorticoids also foster release of amino acids to support gluconeogenesis in liver (17).

During a short-term fast, serum insulin and glucagon orchestrate changes in fuel homeostasis resulting in a steady supply of glucose to brain and other glucose-dependent tissues while mobilizing free fatty acids to meet energy needs of other tissues. After a 7- to 10-day fast, brain develops the capacity to use ketones for fuel and the need to convert amino acids to glucose abates, allowing adjustment to long-term fasting with sparing of skeletal and visceral proteins (17).

METABOLIC DERANGEMENTS

Diabetes resembles fasting, especially in the responses of liver, muscle cells, and adipose tissues. With low serum ratios of insulin to glucagon and high levels of fatty acids, liver produces glucose while other tissues use fatty acids and ketones instead of glucose. Muscle cells and adipose tissue respond by using ketones and fatty acids. Although the resemblance between fasting is diabetes are striking, pathologically low serum insulin levels disrupt the efficiency seen during fasting (17).

With low insulin, key glycolytic enzyme activities decrease. Glucose use falls far below levels seen during fasting. Concurrently, hepatic gluconeogenic enzyme activities increase and gluconeogenic rates rise. Bombarded with free fatty acids, the liver increases gluconeogenesis, secreting large amounts of VLDLs, and accumulates fatty acids in droplet form. A long-term toxic effect of diabetes is accumulation of 25% more lipid than normal. In the diabetic state, the liver oxidizes these fatty acids and produces acetone, acetoacetate, and β-hydroxybutyrate (17).

Muscle cells and adipose tissue also show major metabolic changes in diabetes. Muscle glycogen almost disappears, and muscle protein is broken down to support gluconeogenesis. Cardiac and skeletal muscles meet their energy needs from ketones and fatty acids. Fat cells actively release fatty acids under the lipolytic stimuli of glucagon, catecholamines, and insulin deficiency (17).

Non-insulin-dependent tissues respond to diabetes totally differently. Hexokinase, the key stimulus of glucose use, is increased in jejunal mucosa, renal cortex, and peripheral nerves of diabetic animals. In hyperglycemia, glucose use increases, and sugars accumulate. Excess glucose accumulation leads to tissue damage. Diabetic rats have 30% more total body glycogen than nondiabetic rats. Glycogen accumulates in renal tubules to values 50 times those in nondiabetic rats. Glycogen accumulation may contribute to tubular dysfunction and susceptibility to damage from x-ray dyes. Unimpeded entry of glucose into many tissues increases cellular glucose, producing linkage of glucose to tissue proteins (glycosylation). The diabetic state damages non-insulin-dependent tissues, including glomeruli, retinal vessels, nerves, and circulating blood cells (17).

DIABETIC COMPLICATIONS

Acute Problems

Diabetes can first manifest with either symptomatic hyperglycemia or a medical emergency caused by severe hyperglycemia, ketoacidosis, or severe hyperlipidemia. Most symptoms of diabetes are related to hyperglycemia or accumulation of glucose in various tissues. As hyperglycemia develops, individuals have increased polyuria, thirst, lack of energy, irritability, blurred vision, and weight loss. Adults usually develop these symptoms over weeks to months, whereas children may develop them in hours or days. If hyperglycemia goes undetected or if stress or illness intervenes, the individual develops stupor or coma (Table 86.4).

The most frequent complication for diabetic individuals treated with insulin is hypoglycemia. Below-normal levels of blood glucose characterize this complication. Insulin administration may decrease the blood glucose concentration, which necessitates replenishing circulating glucose; otherwise, brain function will be permanently altered. Hypoglycemia may be triggered by missed or late meals, consumption of insufficient quantities of food, consumption of alcohol without food, or physical work. The symptoms of a hypoglycemic reaction differ for each patient; however, an individual's incidents resemble one another. Some symptoms of hypoglycemia are confusion, headaches, deficient coordination, irritability, shakiness, anger, sweating, and even coma or death. Desired treatment for hypoglycemia is 15 g of carbohydrate administered to raise the blood glucose level between about 50 or 100 mg/dL; this rise usually takes about 15 minutes (20).

Individuals with type I diabetes are vulnerable to diabetic ketoacidosis (DKA) characterized by hyperglycemia and ketonemia, which results from either insulin deficiency or stress. Either hyperglycemic nonketotic state or ketoacidosis can be fatal. DKA is most frequently caused by lack of patient education or inadequate compliance with instructions. Symptoms of DKA include nausea and confusion. Therapy for DKA includes administration of electrolytes, fluid, and insulin, because untreated DKA could result in coma or death (21, 22).

Adults with type II diabetes are likely to develop the hyperglycemic nonketotic state characterized by plasma glucose values above 750 mg/dL without significant ketonemia. These individuals may be protected from ketoacidosis by circulating insulin in spite of low-normal or low levels. The hyperglycemic nonketotic condition can be precipitated by excessive sugar intake, dehydration, heat exposure, illness, or drug therapy. Impaired renal function, hyperosmolarity, lack of ketosis, and/or central nervous system problems may occur with this condition. Usually, the hyperglycemic nonketotic state is seen in individuals with type II diabetes. In addition, these individuals have decreased, but not completely deficient, insulin levels released from the pancreas. The hyperglycemic nonketotic state is often caused by dehydration or by diabetes associated with a coexisting illness. Symptoms of this con-

Table 86.4
Diabetic Complications and Pathophysiologic Considerations

Complication	Pathophysiologic Consideration
	Acute
Hypoglycemia	Excess insulin
Moderate hyperglycemia	Polydipsia, polyuria, weight loss, fatigue, blurred vision
Severe hyperglycemia	Hyperglycemic nonketotic state
Severe ketosis	Diabetic ketoacidosis
Hypertriglyceridemia	Chylomicronemia syndrome with neurologic, skin, or pancreatic manifestations
	Short-term
Protein glycosylation	Premature aging of collagen, lens, and other tissue proteins; functional abnormalities of hormones, lipoproteins, and membranes
Susceptibility to oxidation	Contributes to atherosclerosis, premature aging, and susceptibility to cancer
Polyol accumulation	Nerve, lens, and kidney dysfunction
Mucopolysaccharide abnormalities	Alterations in arterial walls
Glycogen accumulation	Renal tubular and hepatic lesions
Dyslipidemia	Accelerated atherosclerosis
Vascular permeability abnormalities	Protein leakage from capillaries
Microcirculation defects	Abnormal renal, muscle, and eye blood flow
White blood cell abnormalities	Altered response to infection and immune challenges
Platelet abnormalities	Contribution to micro- and macrovascular complications and thrombosis
Erythrocyte abnormalities	Stiffness and altered oxygen transport
Nerve dysfunction	Decreased nerve conduction velocity
Kidney dysfunction	Hyperfiltration leading to nephropathy
	Long-term
Renal glomeruli	Nodular or diffuse thickening
Retinal vessels	Hemorrhage, ischemia, new vessel formation
Neurologic disorders	Numerous defects affecting central, peripheral, and autonomic nervous systems
Capillary disorders	Basement membrane thickening and microcirculation abnormalities
Arterial disorders	Generalized and accelerated atherosclerosis affecting coronary arteries, cerebral vessels, and peripheral vessels

dition include dehydration, hypotension, decreased mental ability, confusion, seizures, and coma. Therapy for the hyperglycemic nonketotic state includes insulin therapy and electrolyte and fluid replacement as well as treating basic causes (21).

Severe hypertriglyceridemia can be a serious medical emergency. Serum triglycerides exceed 22.6 mmol/L (2000 mg/dL) and may be accompanied by neurologic symptoms, skin lesions, or abdominal symptoms from pancreatitis. Treatment includes intravenous fluids or a clear liquid diet to lower serum triglycerides, insulin to control hyperglycemia, and appropriate therapy for other medical problems (23).

Short-Term Complications

Sustained hyperglycemia alters glucose metabolism in virtually every tissue. Cells that are non-insulin-dependent are particularly vulnerable because sugar alcohols (polyols) accumulate and proteins are glycosylated. Most tissues gradually convert glucose to polyols, which are used slowly. Hyperglycemia causes high intracellular glucose concentrations, leading to rapid formation of polyols (Fig. 86.2) that accumulate rapidly but are degraded slowly. Sorbitol and fructose, the major polyols, accumulate and cause cell distention and toxicity. Blurred vision, for example, is caused by distention of the lens. Polyol accumulation can alter the function of peripheral nerves (18, 24).

Excess glucose affects production of glycoproteins, proteins containing sugar side chains (Fig. 86.3). The condensation reaction between glucose and an amino acid component of protein has two stages: *(a)* the aldehyde group of glucose links to the amino group of an amino acid forming an aldimine (Schiff base) and *(b)* the unstable aldimine releases glucose or undergoes an Amadori rearrangement to form the stable ketoamine linkage. This process occurs spontaneously without enzyme action and is termed *nonenzymatic glycosylation*. Hemoglobin, serum albumin, and many other proteins are glycosylated. In diabetes, glycosylation is related to the magnitude and duration of hyperglycemia (18).

The sugar content of hemoglobin, the best-characterized glycoprotein, is normally less than 6%. In diabetes, the percentage of glycosylated hemoglobin can exceed 25% of total hemoglobin. When erythrocytes are incubated with glucose, glycohemoglobin doubles within hours. Most glucose is attached by the unstable aldimine linkage, which can be dissociated if erythrocytes are incubated in low glucose solutions. Long-term exposure to high glucose levels causes formation of irreversible

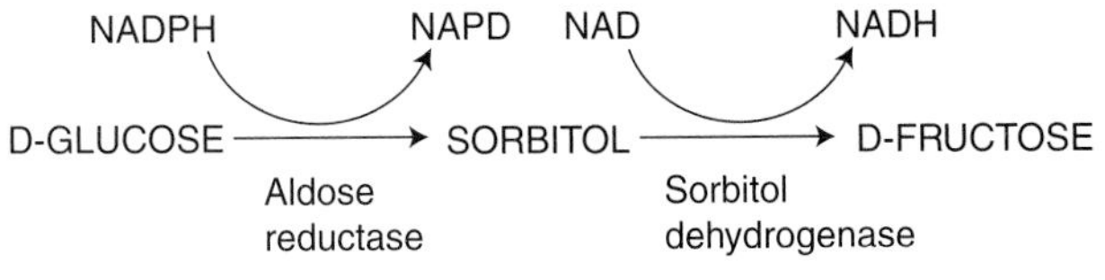

Figure 86.2. Polyol pathway.

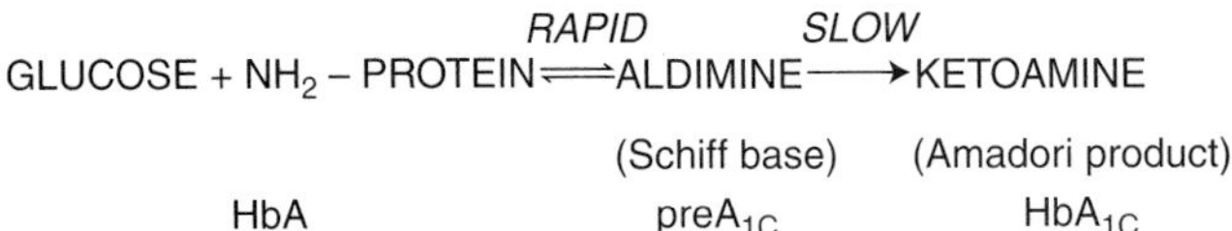

Figure 86.3. Pathway for nonenzymatic glycosylation.

ketoamine linkages that persist until the cell is degraded. Thus, glycohemoglobin measurements reflect glycemic control over the previous 6 to 8 weeks. In patients with excellent glycemic control, glycohemoglobin concentrations are normal. Poor diabetic control yields glycohemoglobin values exceeding 9%. The degree of glycosylation of circulating proteins, hormones, lipoproteins, plasma membranes of cells, basement membranes, and other proteins in diabetes has not been determined. This may contribute to basement membrane thickening, vascular permeability, microcirculation defects, and functional abnormalities of erythrocytes, leukocytes, and platelets (18, 25).

Hyperglycemia induces a host of other metabolic derangements. Glycogen accumulates in non-insulin-dependent tissues. Increased flux of glucose through insulin-insensitive pathways such as mucopolysaccharide synthesis leads to abnormalities of mucopolysaccharides, possibly contributing to atherosclerosis. Hyperglycemia alters the orderly formation of glycoproteins in the kidney and other tissues, contributing to diabetic glomerulosclerosis. Many short-term problems of hyperglycemia can be avoided by maintaining satisfactory plasma glucose concentrations, and in some cases, derangements can be reversed by good glycemic control (18).

Long-Term Complications

The pathogenesis of the long-term manifestations (Table 86.4) of diabetes is still under intense study and remains poorly understood. Metabolic, genetic, and other factors affect major diabetic complications: retinopathy, nephropathy, and neuropathy (24, 26). Most authorities believe that chronic hyperglycemia accelerates development of these complications. Long-term complications cannot be prevented, but risks can be lowered with good diabetic control. The Diabetes Control and Complication Trial (DCCT) was a landmark study of type I diabetes documenting that improved control decreases development of diabetic retinopathy, nephropathy, and neuropathy (27, 28).

Pirart (29) carefully documented the prevalence of diabetic complications among 4400 diabetic patients (Fig. 86.4). After 25 years, most patients had complications of some type; however, complications were less frequent in patients who maintained fairly good glycemic control than in those who had maintained poor diabetic control. Individual genetic tendencies toward complications also affect their frequency. Some diabetic individuals develop complications at an accelerated rate despite reasonable glycemic control, whereas others show little tendency toward these complications.

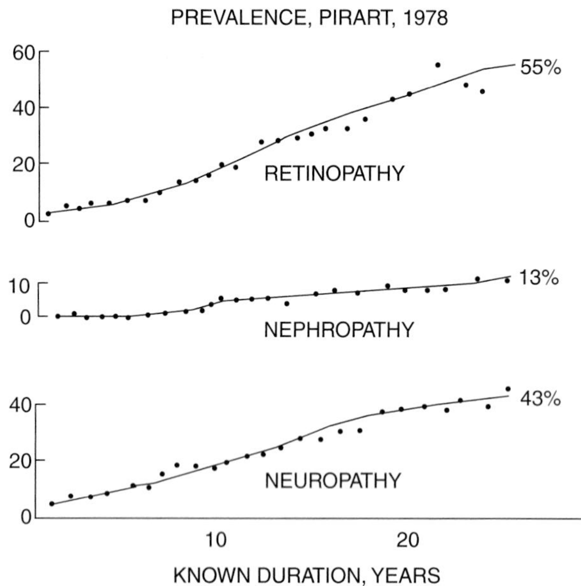

Figure 86.4. Prevalence of diabetic complications over time. (Redrawn from Pirart J. Diabetes Metab 1977;3:97–107).

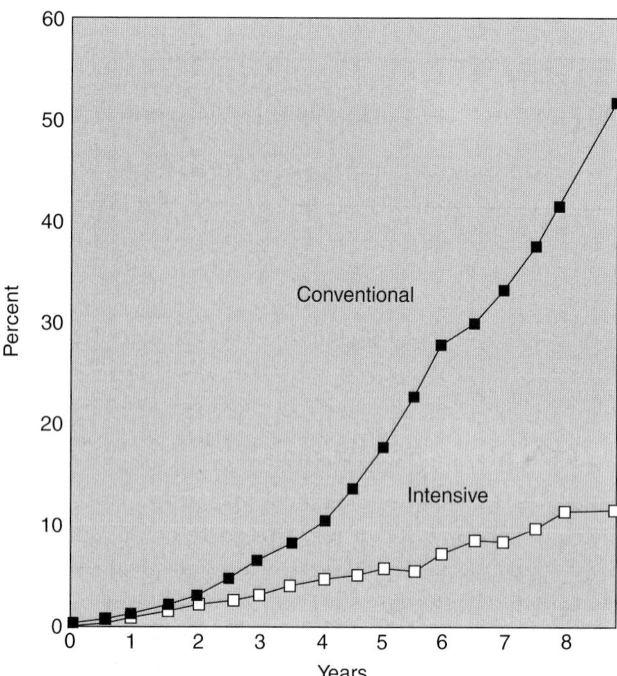

Figure 86.5. Effect of glycemic control on development of diabetic retinopathy in the Diabetes Control and Complication Trial (DCCT). Subjects had no evidence of retinopathy at entry and developed retinopathy at the indicated rate. Intensive therapy was associated with a 76% reduction in risk compared with conventional therapy.

The DCCT was a carefully controlled clinical study conducted by the National Institute of Digestive and Kidney Disease in the U.S. The study shows that keeping blood glucose levels as close to normal as possible slows the onset and progression of eye, kidney, and nerve diseases caused by diabetes. This was the largest and most comprehensive diabetes study ever conducted and included 1441 type I diabetic subjects at 29 medical centers in the U.S. and Canada. Over a 7-year period, the study compared the effects of a standard treatment regimen with an intensive treatment regimen. The study showed that lowering blood glucose concentrations reduced risk for diabetic retinopathy by 76%, for diabetic nephropathy by 50%, and for diabetic neuropathy by 60%. Figure 86.5 compares the effects of standard therapy and intensive control on development of diabetic retinopathy (27, 30).

Atherosclerosis

Atherosclerosis is the most common complication of diabetes. Diabetic men have a two- to threefold higher risk of coronary heart disease, stroke, and peripheral vascular disease, whereas diabetic women have a three- to fourfold higher risk than matched nondiabetic individuals. Mechanisms responsible for accelerated atherosclerosis are not understood, and many interacting factors contribute. Figure 86.6 illustrates major risk factors for atherosclerosis in diabetes and indicates the influence of nutrition. Reducing risk of vascular disease requires improved glycemic control, avoidance of cigarette smoking, normal blood pressure, and desirable serum lipoprotein levels. Hypertension is the major risk factor for coronary heart disease in type I diabetes. Diabetic individuals, particularly women, develop hypertension more frequently than the general population. Hypertension-related factors may act synergistically with arterial wall abnormalities, cellular dysfunction, lipoprotein abnormalities, and platelet derangements to accelerate atherosclerosis (25).

Lipoprotein abnormalities play a major role in atherosclerosis. Serum low-density lipoprotein (LDL) abnormalities, decreased serum high-density lipoproteins (HDL), and increased serum triglycerides contribute to accelerated atherosclerosis in diabetes. LDL may be glycosylated or altered in other ways to enhance atherogenicity in diabetes. Many lipoprotein alterations in diabetes increase the risk of atherosclerosis (25).

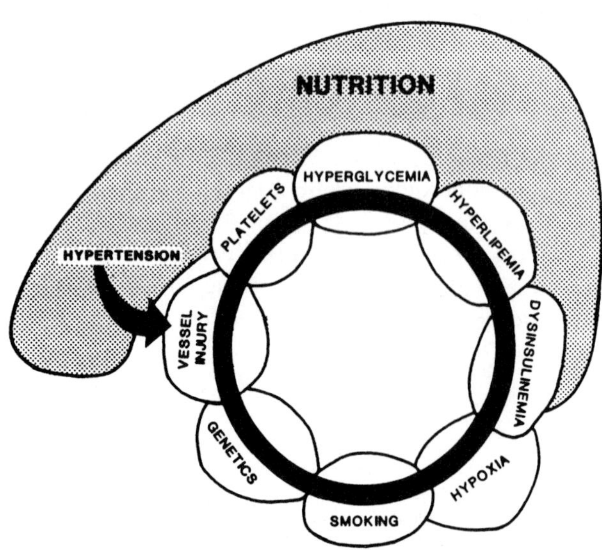

Figure 86.6. Relationship of diabetes, nutrition, and atherosclerosis.

Table 86.5
Risk Factors for Atherosclerotic Cardiovascular Disease in Diabetes

Nonmodifiable Risk Factors	Modifiable Nonlipid Risk Factors	Modifiable Lipid Risk Factors	Risk Factors Unique to Diabetes
Male gender	Obesity[a]	High LDL-cholesterol	Platelet aggregation[a]
Age	Hypertension[a]	Low HDL-cholesterol[a]	Increased coagulation[a]
Atherosclerotic disease[a]	Cigarette smoking	High triglycerides[a]	Protein glycosylation[a]
			Leukocyte dysfunction[a]
			Macrophage dysfunction[a]
			Susceptibility to oxidation[a]
			HDL dysfunction[a]

[a]Risk factors more likely present in diabetes.

In addition to hypertension and lipoprotein derangements, diabetic individuals have increased prevalence of other cardiovascular risk factors (Table 86.5): elevated serum insulin (31), elevated fibrinogen and von Willebrand factor (32), platelet function abnormalities (33), glycosylation of proteins throughout the body, leukocyte abnormalities contributing to vascular endothelial dysfunction and coagulation, macrophage dysfunction leading to foam cell formation, increased susceptibility to oxidation of LDL, and HDL dysfunction. The nutritional plan focuses on reducing the risk of atherosclerosis by reducing saturated fat intake, achieving desirable serum lipoproteins, and reducing other cardiovascular risk factors (17).

GOALS FOR MEDICAL NUTRITIONAL THERAPY

Medical nutritional therapy is pivotal in the management and care of diabetes. The objective is to provide diabetic individuals with an approach to diet that enables them to maintain a near-normal metabolic state. Glycemic control goals are outlined in Table 86.6. Nutritional intervention provides a cost-effective strategy for reducing the complications, hence the morbidity and mortality, of diabetes. Recent results from the DCCT (34) indicate the following: persons who reported following their prescribed meal plan more than 90% of the time had average glycohemoglobin levels 0.9% lower than those who followed their meal plan less than 45% of the time; overconsumption of food to treat hypoglycemia was associated with significantly higher glycohemoglobin values, emphasizing the importance of appropriate treatment of hypoglycemia; glycohemoglobin values were also lower in persons who said they responded to high blood glucose levels and changes in planned meals by adjusting their insulin dose according to meal size and content; and eating extra nighttime snacks was associated with higher glycohemoglobin levels than eating the prescribed evening snack more consistently.

The DCCT model establishes the following mandates for medical nutritional therapy (34):

1. Nutritional self-management education begins with a nutritional assessment. For persons taking insulin by injection, insulin can be integrated into usual eating and exercise habits. Goals, not rules and regulations, should be emphasized. Recommendations must be practical, achievable, and acceptable for the person with diabetes.
2. A variety of meal-planning approaches and educational tools were used in the DCCT. Educational tools that persons with diabetes can easily understand and use should be selected. Consistent follow-up for evaluation and continued self-management education is essential.
3. A team approach is necessary to promote positive nutritional behaviors. Optimal glycemic control was achieved only when patients applied nutritional principles learned through diabetes-nutrition self-management education.

The American Diabetes Association (ADA), in 1994, revised its nutritional recommendations and principles for persons with diabetes (9, 35). Table 86.7 lists specific and general targets of nutritional therapy. Specific guidelines apply to the diabetic individual, while general guidelines apply to all individuals. The first and preeminent goal is

Table 86.6
Glycemic Control for Persons with Diabetes

Measurement	Nondiabetic[a]	Goal (diabetes)	Action Suggested[b]
Preprandial glucose, mmol/L (mg/dL)	<6.4 (115)	4.4–6.7 (80–120)	<4.4 (80) >7.8 (140)
Bedtime glucose, mmol/L (mg/dL)	<6.7 (120)	5.6–7.8 (100–140)	<5.6 (100) >8.9 (160)
Glycohemoglobin, %	<6.0	<7[a]	>8

Modified from American Diabetes Association. Standards of reduced care for patients with diabetes mellitus. Diabetes Care 1995;18(Suppl 1):8–15.
[a]<15% above normal limit for laboratory; these values are for nonpregnant adults.
[b]"Action suggested" is tailored to the individual.

Table 86.7
Goals for Nutritional Therapy for Diabetes

Specific
- Achieve physiologic blood glucose levels
- Maintain desirable plasma lipids
- Reduce likelihood of specific diabetic complications
- Retard development of atherosclerosis

General
- Provide optimal selection of nutrients
- Attain and maintain desirable body weight
- Meet energy needs in a timely manner
- Address special requirements (such as pregnancy)
- Tailor for therapeutic needs (such as renal disease)

achieving and maintaining blood glucose levels as near normal as possible by balancing food intake with insulin (either endogenous or exogenous) or antidiabetes agents. Optimizing glucose use, normalizing glucose production, and enhancing insulin sensitivity will also regulate safe levels of fatty acids, ketones, and amino acids. Immoderate hyperglycemia, as well as ensuing hypoglycemia, is hazardous and should be minimized by diet. Second in priority is achieving and maintaining optimal serum lipid levels. Cardiovascular disease is the most common complication of diabetes. Lipoprotein abnormalities play a major role in atherosclerosis. Except for enhancing glycemic control, we do not know how to tailor the diet to reduce specific complications of diabetes; emerging research suggests that a diet moderate in protein (10–12% of energy) or one substituting vegetable protein for animal protein may decrease risk for diabetic nephropathy (36). Measures to retard development of atherosclerosis include maintaining desirable body weight and sustaining a diet high in dietary fiber, soy protein, and antioxidants and low in fat, saturated fat, and cholesterol (37). Regardless of the type of diabetes present, utmost consideration must be given to individual preferences, cultural or social mores, and ability to understand and follow the prescribed diet. All the nutritional planning in the world will do no good if it is not implemented.

General goals consider the provision of variety, balance, and moderation. *Dietary Guidelines for Americans* (38) and the *Food Guide Pyramid* (39) summarize and illustrate nutritional guidelines and nutrient needs for all healthy Americans and can be used by people with diabetes and their family members (35). Optimal selection of nutrients is addressed through food-value exchanges, allowing individual preferences to reign yet including foods from each of the food groups. Energy needs are met by distributing meals throughout the day, with allowances for snacks when indicated. Meal distribution and close monitoring of blood glucose levels limit the frequency of hyper- or hypoglycemic episodes. Eliminating excessive calories and fats is indicated to attain and maintain a reasonable weight for adults, especially non-insulin-dependent diabetics. However, provision of adequate calories is crucial for normal growth and development of children and adolescents, increased metabolic needs during pregnancy and lactation, or recovery from catabolic illnesses. Medical nutritional therapy aims at reducing and preventing complications of diabetes during short-term illnesses, exercise-related problems, and long-term complications such as renal disease, hypertension, and atherosclerotic cardiovascular disease. Special tailoring is needed for existing complications such as renal failure.

The DCCT (27) substantiated that goal achievement results from a coordinated team effort by the physician, nurse, dietitian, and diabetic individual. Effective self-management training requires an individualized approach, appropriate for the personal lifestyle and management goals of the diabetic individual. To facilitate compliance, sensitivity to cultural, ethnic, and financial considerations is of prime importance. Monitoring blood glucose and glycohemoglobin levels, serum lipids, blood pressure, and renal status is essential to evaluate nutrition-related outcomes (35). If goals are not met, changes must be made in the overall diabetes care and management plan. Nutritional assessment is used to determine what the individual with diabetes is able and willing to do. A major consideration is the likelihood of compliance with nutritional recommendations.

Methods of Diet Prescription

Nutritional Therapy and Type I Diabetes

Usual food intake and pattern preference should be determined and used as the basis for insulin requirement prescriptions (34). Eating at consistent times is vital for appropriate use of insulin. Intensified therapy may be considered for those willing and able to comply and can provide considerably more flexibility in meal planning. Individuals can be taught to adjust premeal insulin to compensate for changes in their meal plans, to delay premeal insulin for meals that are late, and to administer insulin for snacks that are not part of their meal plan. Insulin can also be adjusted for changes in physical activity. Intensified therapy may include carbohydrate counting with adjusted multiple injections or use of an insulin pump. The individual's skill and educational level must be considered.

Nutritional Therapy for Type II Diabetes

Emphasis should be placed on maintenance of desired weight and glucose, lipid, and blood pressure goals. Loss of 10% of current weight was shown to improve diabetes control (18). Strategies may be aimed at improving food selection (e.g., reducing dietary fats and saturated fats), spreading meals throughout the day, and incorporating regular exercise habits. If dietary and behavioral intervention is not successful, an antidiabetes agent may be needed. Stopping or changing oral agents is preferable to dietary manipulation for type 2 diabetic patients who are experiencing hypoglycemia. Insulin therapy should be a last resort after all combinations of oral medications have been exhausted, as it may exacerbate concomitant hyperinsulinemia and promote weight gain.

NUTRITIONAL PLAN

Consensus recommendations, though still somewhat controversial, have evolved considerably over the past few years. Areas of debate remain, and dogmatic or narrow recommendations would be inappropriate (7). Probably, there is more than one suitable diet composition. Wolever et al. (40) reported results in a randomized, controlled study, consistent with the recent move away from universal recommendation of high-carbohydrate diets toward individualizing the nature and amount of dietary carbohy-

Table 86.8
Nutritional Recommendations for Persons with Diabetes

Nutrient	ADA[a]	HCF Nutrition Fdn[b,c]
Carbohydrate, % of kcal	about 50%[d]	50–60%
Protein, %	10–20%	10–15% (0.8 g/kg)
Fat, total, %	≤30%[d]	≤30%[e]
Saturated, %	<10%	<10%
Monosaturated, %	10–20%	10–15%
Polyunsaturated, %	<10%	<10%
Cholesterol, mg/day	<300 mg/day	<200 mg/day
Fiber, g/day	20–35 g/day	about 35 g/day (15–25 g/1000 kcal)
Sodium, mg/day	<2400 mg if hypertensive	<1000 mg/1000 kcal
Alcohol	≤2 drinks/day	Men ≤2 drinks/day Women ≤1 drink/day
Vitamin supplements	Not recommended	Multivitamin-mineral daily Antioxidant supplements

[a]American Diabetes Association. Nutrition recommendations and principles for people with diabetes mellitus. JADA 1994;94–504.

[b]Anderson JW, Geil PB. Nutrition management of diabetes mellitus. In Shils M. Modern nutrition in health and disease, 8th Edition. Philadelphia: Lea & Febiger, 1994;1259–86.

[c]Anderson JW. Professional guide to high fiber fitness plan. Lexington, KY: HCF Nutrition Research Fdn. 1995;10.1–10.22.

[d]Individualization recommended. More fat permitted and less carbohydrate acceptable.

[e]Up to 35% of energy from fat can be used for nonobese individuals with acceptable serum triglyceride values if the additional fat comes from monounsaturated sources and saturated and polyunsaturated fats remain under 10% each.

drates. Associations between diet and glucose control varied in different groups of subjects with type II diabetes; higher carbohydrate or higher dietary fiber intakes were associated with improved blood glucose control in those treated by diet alone, insulin, or metformin, but not in subjects on sulfonylureas. Low glycemic index was associated with improved glucose control only in subjects treated by diet alone. Nutritional recommendations are outlined in Table 86.8.

Carbohydrates

Carbohydrates should provide 50 to 60% of energy intake. Greater amounts, up to 70%, are tolerated in research studies and by highly committed individuals but are not generally recommended for most persons with diabetes. Simple carbohydrates (not as severely restricted in the past) should make up less than 1/3 of total carbohydrate intake. Unrefined carbohydrates, with natural fiber intact, have distinct advantages over highly refined versions because of their other benefits such as a lower glycemic index, greater satiety, and cholesterol-lowering properties.

Amount

About 1980, the American and the British Diabetes Associations finally relinquished the antiquated strategy of carbohydrate-restricted diets for diabetic individuals, aiming instead for a diet restricted in fat but higher in complex carbohydrate and dietary fiber (2). While considered radical by some, many other countries introduced essentially identical policies. The enthusiasm for high-carbohydrate, high-fiber diets has waned somewhat, but these diets still have the strongest scientific basis for recommendation. Under certain circumstances, especially with low fiber intake, high-carbohydrate, low-fat diets can worsen blood glucose control, increase serum triglyceride concentrations, and lower HDL-cholesterol concentrations (41, 42). The fiber content of the diet appears critical in preventing these problems (17, 43). (See Appendix Table IV-A-20 for fiber contents of many foods.) The popularity of the "Mediterranean diet" has led some to recommend lower-carbohydrate, higher monounsaturated fat intake to alter serum lipid concentrations favorably and reduce risk for oxidation of LDL. However, only a few controlled studies support this recommendation, and the effect of higher fat intake on obesity in type II diabetes is a major concern (17, 44).

Glycemic Response

Carbohydrates in foods have traditionally been classified as either "simple" (sugars) or "complex" (starches). Simple carbohydrates from commonly used foods raise blood glucose concentrations more than complex carbohydrates from starchy foods. The glycemic response to 50 g glucose is much greater than the response to a variety of foods providing 50 g starch. Whereas glucose, maltose, and sucrose produce large increases in the blood glucose level, fructose does not (Fig. 86.7). Fructose, metabolized without insulin, evokes little increase in serum insulin in nondiabetic individuals; it produces only minimal increases in blood glucose levels in nondiabetic and diabetic persons with reasonable glycemic control. Fructose may play a role as a sweetener for selected individuals with diabetes (17). Although simple carbohydrate worsens glycemic control and promotes weight gain, the ADA has suggested that "modest amounts of sucrose and other refined sugars may be acceptable, contingent on metabolic control and body weight" (45).

Complex carbohydrates in different forms also evoke different glycemic responses. Bread and potatoes raise blood glucose levels much more than beans (Fig. 86.7). Many investigators have compared the glycemic response of foods rich in complex carbohydrates (46, 47). Jenkins et al. introduced the term *glycemic index* to describe these responses, comparing test foods to the glycemic response from a reference food such as bread or glucose (46). Table 86.9 compares the glycemic responses to selected foods (see Appendix Table V-A-26-a for more quantitative data).

Many factors influence the glycemic response to foods (Table 86.10). Sipping 50 g of glucose slowly over several hours produces a much smaller increase in blood glucose than rapid intake of the same amount. Eating three apples

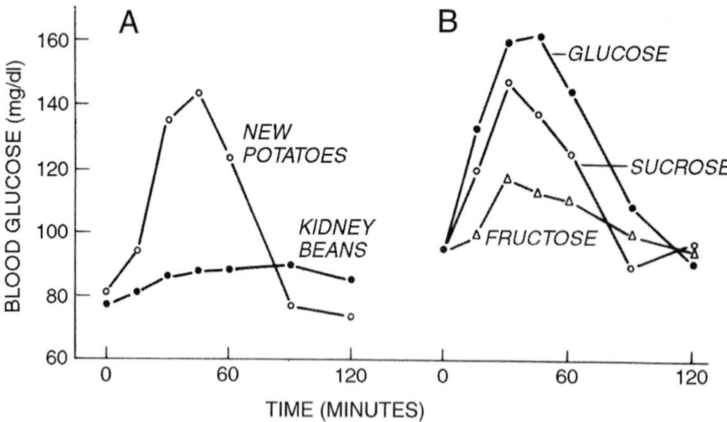

Figure 86.7. *A.* Glycemic response of nondiabetic individuals to 50 g carbohydrate from new potatoes or kidney beans. *B.* Glycemic response of healthy individuals to 50 g of glucose, sucrose, or fructose.

takes 15 minutes, whereas their juice can be consumed in 1.5 minutes. Differences in fiber content and ingestion time influence the resultant glycemic response. Fat, protein, water-soluble fiber, and other factors influence gastric emptying time. Food form has a major impact on digestion time; bread can be digested more rapidly than pasta. Methods of processing and cooking foods (and in the case of fruit, degree of ripeness) influence glycemic response. Foods with higher ratios of amylopectin to the amylose form of starch are digested more rapidly than those with low ratios (17).

Fiber is only one of many components of food that influence the glycemic response. Beans have lower glycemic indices than any other group of carbohydrate-rich foods. The low glycemic response to beans is probably related to their high soluble fiber content, food form (usually eaten as cooked rather than in bakery products), and naturally occurring starch blockers (inhibitors of digestive enzymes responsible for hydrolysis of starch). Finally, fiber fermentation products such as short-chain fatty acids are absorbed from the colon into the portal vein; in the liver, they may directly affect glucose metabolism (48). Factors influencing the glycemic response to foods require more investigation. The complexities of teaching and applying the glycemic index concept to individual patients make practical application difficult at this time. However, when using carbohydrate counting, more insulin is required for higher glycemic foods than for lower glycemic foods.

Proteins

The adult recommended dietary intake (RDI) of 0.8 g protein/kg body weight meets metabolic and nutritional needs. Though current ADA recommendations allow 10 to 20% of energy intake as protein, we recommend a more conservative 10 to 15% of total energy needs as protein. Diabetic individuals, on average, consume more protein than nondiabetic individuals, (49) and excessive protein intake has been linked to diabetic nephropathy (36, 50). According to current guidelines, in the presence of diabetic nephropathy, protein should not exceed 0.8 g/kg or 10% of total calories (9, 35).

At present, there is insufficient evidence to support protein allowances higher or lower than that for the general population. Protein of high biologic value should be given consideration, though protein should be included from both animal and vegetable sources. With the onset of

Table 86.9
Glycemic Index (GI) Ranking of Selected Starchy Foods

Class I (Higher: GI >90)	Class II (Intermediate: GI = 70–90	Class III (Lower: GI <70)
Most breads	All bran	Pumpernickle bread
Plain crackers	Oatmeal	Most pasta
Most breakfast cereals	Most cookies or biscuits	Parboiled rice
Most potatoes	Polished rice	Most dried legumes
Millet	Buckwheat	Nuts
Corn chips	Sweet corn	Barley
	Boiled new potatoes	Bulgar (cracked wheat)
	Yams	
	Sweet potatoes	

Adapted from Wolever TMS, Jenkins DJA. Diet and diabetes. In: Carroll KK, ed. Diet, nutrition and health. Montreal: McGill-Queen, 1995.

Table 86.10
Factors Affecting the Glycemic Response to Food

- Rate of ingestion
- Food form
- Food components
  - Fat content
  - Fiber content
  - Protein content
  - Starch characteristics
  - Food ingredients
- Methods of cooking and processing
- Physiologic effects
  - Pregastric hydrolysis
  - Gastric hydrolysis
  - Gastric emptying rate
  - Intestinal response
  - Intestinal hydrolysis and absorption
  - Pancreatic and gut hormone responses
  - Colonic effects

nephropathy, protein intake should be no greater than the recommended dietary allowance (RDA) of 0.8 g/kg. Ten percent of daily calories should be sufficiently restrictive and is recommended for individuals with evidence of nephropathy (9). Higher amounts (over 12%) are likely in diets with greater emphasis on vegetable sources of protein, particularly the cereals and legumes, which are recommended for diabetes from other considerations. Further work is required to establish whether a higher protein intake is acceptable from the renal point of view if it comes mainly from vegetable sources (36). Current research indicates that soy protein diets reduce hyperfiltration in diabetic individuals, and substituting soy protein for animal protein should be considered as a preventive measure for diabetic individuals (36).

Fat

Fat intake generally should not exceed 30% of energy. Most importantly, saturated fats, because of their atherogenic potential, should be held at a maximum of 10% of energy needs. Polyunsaturates, with their tendency to lower HDL-cholesterol values and their susceptibility to oxidation, should also be held under 10%. However, up to 35% of energy from fat can be used for nonobese individuals with acceptable serum triglyceride values if the additional fat comes from monounsaturated sources such as canola or olive oils. Cholesterol intake, though less influential than saturated fats on serum lipid values, should be held under 300 mg/day; we recommend less than 200 mg/day. These recommendations are consistent with those of the American Heart Association and other groups (17, 44).

Amount

In 1928, Dr. Elliott P. Joslin (51) stated that "with an excess of fat diabetes begins and from an excess of fat diabetics die." The weight of scientific evidence still supports this prescient observation. Excessive fat intake contributes to obesity, insulin resistance, hypertension, and atherosclerotic cardiovascular disease. Maintaining serum lipid levels is one of the most important goals in diabetes management. Hyperlipidemia, common in type II diabetics, is a major risk factor for cardiovascular disease. Epidemiologic evidence indicates that high-fat diets contribute to atherosclerosis. In fact, almost all risk factors for cardiovascular disease occur more frequently in diabetics. Hyperlipidemia, glycosylated lipoproteins, platelet dysfunction, arterial wall changes, hyperinsulinemia, hypertension, and obesity are correlated with atherosclerosis in diabetics. High-fat diets cause insulin resistance and impaired intracellular glucose metabolism. High-fat diets decrease the number of insulin receptors in several tissues, decreasing glucose transport into muscle and adipose tissue and decreasing activities of insulin-stimulated processes. Glycogen synthesis rates, glycogen accumulation, and glucose oxidation are also lower with high-fat diets (17).

Fat reduction has been identified as the most difficult dietary recommendation for diabetic patients to follow. Reducing fat intake may be relatively more important in type II diabetes, whereas limitation in protein intake may be more important in type I diabetes.

Type

The long-term effects of altering the type of fat in the diabetic diet are not well documented. One long-term (30-week) study compared diets rich in polyunsaturated fat with diets rich in saturated fat in patients with non-insulin-dependent diabetes. Compared with the saturated-fat diet, the polyunsaturated-fat diet significantly lowered cholesterol and LDL cholesterol without affecting triglycerides, HDL cholesterol, or apoproteins (52). A high-carbohydrate diet was compared with a diet high in monounsaturated fat in patients with non-insulin-dependent diabetes; after 4 weeks, the monounsaturated-fat diet significantly decreased insulin dose, glucose, triglycerides, and VLDL cholesterol while significantly increasing HDL cholesterol and apolipoprotein A-I (42). Although increased intake of fat usually leads to decreased insulin sensitivity, this preliminary short-term study suggests that this may not occur with monounsaturated fat intake.

Monounsaturated Fats. There is a growing consensus that diets for diabetic individuals should include only modest amounts of saturated fat but could include moderate-to-high levels of monounsaturates. Partial replacement of complex carbohydrates with monounsaturates in NIDDM patients does not increase the level of LDL cholesterol and may improve glycemic control and triglyceride and HDL-cholesterol levels (42, 53). If triglycerides and VLDLs are elevated, a moderate increase in monounsaturated fat intake may be liberalized to include up to 20% of calories with a more moderate intake of carbohydrate (9). However, increased monounsaturated fat intake may enhance insulin resistance and, in obese individuals, may perpetuate or aggravate the obesity.

Polyunsaturated Fats. Some increase in polyunsaturates and the polyunsaturated/saturated ratio can be expected as saturated fatty acids are reduced (7). Artificially high intakes and supplemental polyunsaturates are not advised, and the ADA recommends restriction to below 8% of energy. The World Health Organization (WHO) recommendation for the general population is 3 to 7% of energy from polyunsaturates. High intakes of polyunsaturates have been suggested to be potentially damaging, relating to increased production of lipid peroxides (43).

ω-3 Fatty Acids. Certain essential fatty acids of the ω-3 class lower serum cholesterol moderately and serum triglyceride levels markedly (54). These ω-3 fatty acids, popularly known as fish oils, may also decrease platelet aggregation, which may potentially reduce the cardiovascular disease risk in diabetes. Initially, fish oil supplementation in individuals with non-insulin-dependent diabetes appeared to improve their insulin sensitivity. The most potentially beneficial effects of ω-3 fatty acids are on plasma triglycerides, commonly elevated in type II diabetic patients. In pharmacologic quantities, ω-3 fatty acids reduce elevated plasma cholesterol and triglyceride concentrations and blood pressure. Diabetic patients may experience disadvantages associated with higher doses of ω-3 fatty acid supplements. Intake of more than 4 g/day may aggravate hyperglycemia and elevate serum LDL-cholesterol concentrations. Dietary supplementation with 10 g/day of fish-oil capsules in a prospective double-blind placebo-controlled study improved hypertriglyceridemia but with deleterious effects in factor VII and blood glucose levels in NIDDM subjects (55). Recent research indicates that the benefits of fish-oil supplements outweigh the disadvantages and that these supplements can benefit carefully monitored subjects (54). More studies are needed to be conclusive. Increased intake of oily fish is reasonable as an alternative to foods such as meat and cheese products with high saturated fat content. Higher intake of total fat, mostly from olive oil, occurs in Mediterranean countries and is associated with lower risk of heart disease (7).

Fat Substitutes. Olestra, a sucrose polyester, is a fat substitute recently approved by the Food and Drug Administration (FDA). While release of this food ingredient generated considerable attention, it seems well tolerated by most consumers; gastrointestinal side effects probably will limit overuse by persons who do not tolerate it well. Olestra is a nondigestible fat made from sucrose bonded with eight long-chain fatty acids into a molecule too large to be hydrolyzed in the small intestine. It currently is available in potato chips and similar snack foods.

Another product, Simplesse, is made from the protein of egg white and milk. Manufactured by a microparticulation process, it imparts a creamy smooth sensation much like that of fat. Since this product is a protein, it contains only 3.8 kcal/g instead of the 9 kcal/g in actual fats. Oattrim, is a product produced from oat bran. Clinical tests indicate that this product in useful in decreasing glycemic responses and in lowering serum cholesterol concentrations in nondiabetic subjects.

Controlled studies using these fat substitutes in the diabetic diet are needed to establish their potential usefulness. If results are positive, fat substitutes may foster improved dietary fat compliance in the diabetic population (35).

Fiber

Fiber has emerged as a major dietary component in the management of diabetes. It has therapeutic value and may reduce the prevalence of diabetes. The ADA currently recommends 20 to 35 g/day. We recommend approximately 35 g/day or 15 to 25 g/1000 kcal for our patients (44). In 1960, Trowell reported that diabetes was rare in African hospital patients (56). Walker then postulated that increased cereal fiber intake might prevent development of diabetes (57). Walker et al. documented that healthy Bantu school children in South Africa had lower glycemic responses than urban children and that these differences were related to dietary fiber intake (58). Trowell speculated that prolonged intake of fiber-depleted starch promoted development of diabetes and formulated the dietary fiber hypothesis of the etiology of diabetes (59). Epidemiologic data indicate that low fiber intake correlates with a higher prevalence of diabetes (15, 16, 57).

The therapeutic value of fiber in diabetes emerged in 1976 when the Oxford group reported that fiber supplements reduced postprandial glycemic responses (60), and we (61) reported that high-fiber diets decreased the insulin requirements of lean diabetic individuals. Many others confirmed that either fiber-supplemented diets or high-fiber diets benefit diabetic individuals (7, 62–64).

O'Dea et al. (64) compared the impact of different diets for 2 weeks on blood glucose and lipid values in type II diabetic individuals (Table 86.11) and showed the detrimental effects of high fat intake on blood glucose and lipid values and the beneficial effects of a high-carbohydrate, high-fiber, low-fat diet. Although a low-carbohydrate, low-fat, high-protein intake providing 221 g of protein daily was used to test the effects of low carbohydrate and low fat intake, this diet is impractical and contraindicated in diabetic individuals at risk of diabetic nephropa-

Table 86.11
Effect of Diets on Glycemic Control and Serum Lipids

Parameter	High Carbohydrate, High Fiber	High Carbohydrate, Low Fiber	Low Carbohydrate, High Fat	Low Carbohydrate, Low Fat
Carbohydrate, % energy	65	63	27	23
Protein, % energy	24	25	18	62
Fat, % energy	10	12	55	15
Fiber, g/day	45	20	14	13
Fasting glucose, % change	−17[a]	1	27[a]	−30
Oral glucose test change, mmol/L	−2.6	−0.9	2.5	−1.8
Serum cholesterol, % change	−16[a]	−2	6	−9
LDL cholesterol, % change	−22	1	7	−14
Serum triglycerides, % change	−17	−11	4	−30

Adapted from O'Dea K. J Am Diet Assoc 1989;89:1016.
[a] $P < .05$ vs. initial values.

Table 86.12
High Fiber Intakes: Advantages and Disadvantages

Advantages
- Slow nutrient digestion and absorption
- Decrease postprandial plasma glucose
- Increase tissue insulin sensitivity
- Increase insulin receptor number
- Stimulate glucose use
- Attenuate hepatic glucose output
- Decrease counterregulatory hormone release (e.g., glucagon)
- Lower serum cholesterol
- Lower fasting and postprandial serum triglycerides
- May attenuate hepatic cholesterol synthesis
- May increase satiety between meals

Disadvantages
- Increase intestinal gas
- Temporarily may cause abdominal discomfort or gastrointestinal distress
- May alter pharmocokinetics of certain drugs

thy. This study demonstrates the clear superiority of a high-carbohydrate, high-fiber diet to either a high-carbohydrate, low-fiber diet or a low-carbohydrate, high-fat diet.

Table 86.12 lists the pros and cons of recommending increased dietary fiber intake in diabetic individuals. For many individuals, the advantages outweigh the disadvantages. In addition to its effects on the gastrointestinal tract, fiber enhances peripheral sensitivity to insulin (65). Increasing dietary fiber intake offers these major advantages: improved glucose control with decreased swings in blood glucose resulting in less hyperglycemia and less hypoglycemia; decreased requirements for insulin or sulfonylureas; lower atherogenic lipoproteins; and other health benefits such as lower blood pressure (64), reduced risk of coronary heart disease (66), enhanced weight management (67), and reduced risk of colorectal cancer (68). Generous intake of dietary fiber from fruits, vegetables, legumes, whole-grain cereals, and breads also fosters intake of many nutrients such as vitamins and minerals.

Different types of fiber are distinguished by their physiologic properties and systemic effects. Water-insoluble fiber, found primarily in wheat, vegetables, and most grain products, alters gastrointestinal function by decreasing intestinal transit time and increasing fecal bulk. Insoluble fiber generally does not lower blood glucose or cholesterol levels. Soluble fiber becomes viscous or gummy when mixed with water, increasing intestinal transit time, delaying gastric emptying, and slowing glucose absorption. These actions lower postprandial blood glucose concentrations and decrease blood cholesterol, both important goals for individuals with diabetes. Food sources of soluble fiber include fruits, oats, barley, and legumes. Research into fiber supplements such as pectin, guar, and psyllium has documented the beneficial effects of these substances in diabetes control (69), but fiber supplements are not commonly used in clinical practice. Newly developed, safe, and palatable fiber supplements may help patients to reach recommended levels of fiber intake and improve metabolic control.

The major disadvantages of increased fiber intake relate to gastrointestinal symptoms. Theoretical concerns about detrimental effects on vitamin or mineral availability have not been documented (70, 71). The mild abdominal discomfort experienced by some individuals can usually be avoided by gradually increasing fiber intake, and it usually disappears after a few days. Most individuals have more flatulence with increased fiber intake; this usually persists but is better tolerated in time. Increased fiber intake increases fecal bulk and usually increases frequency of bowel movements. Individuals with irritable bowel syndrome often do not tolerate an abrupt increase in fiber intake well and should increase fiber intake slowly to avoid gastrointestinal symptoms. Individuals with autonomic neuropathy of the gastrointestinal tract need special consideration. Increased soluble fiber may aggravate delayed gastric emptying. Increased fiber intake may benefit diabetic diarrhea and also promote laxation for individuals with constipation. In our experience, dietary fiber has a beneficial effect in most diabetic individuals with autonomic neuropathy. Most diabetic individuals who gradually increase fiber consumption have net beneficial effects.

Many national health organizations recommend that healthy adults increase their dietary fiber intake by 50 to 100%. Because the average fiber intake of American adults is approximately 13 g/day for women and 18 g/day for men, this recommendation suggests that an intake of 20 to 35 g/day would be healthy and desirable (72). In 1987 the ADA recommended that diabetic adults consume approximately 40 g/day of dietary fiber or 15 to 25 g/4186 kJ (1000 kcal) (45). These recommendations are appropriate for diabetic individuals because of such fiber-related benefits as increased insulin sensitivity, better glycemic control, and lower atherogenic serum lipids. This level of fiber intake can easily be achieved using high-carbohydrate, high-fiber (HCF) exchanges (Table 86.13) or ADA exchanges (Table 86.14), with an emphasis on higher-fiber choices such as whole-grain breads, high-fiber cereals, generous intake of fruits and vegetables, and regular use of legumes (73). While foods rich in dietary fiber have many health benefits for diabetic individuals, the ADA recently decreased the amount it recommends and now recommends 20 to 35 g/day, the recommended level for the general population (9).

Table 86.13
Nutrient Values per Serving: 1987 High-Carbohydrate, High-Fiber (HCF) Exchange List

Food Group	Energy (kcal)	Carbohydrate (g)	Protein (g)	Fat (g)	Fiber (g)
Starches	70	15	2	—	2
Cereals	90	20	3	—	4
Proteins	50	—	8	2	—
Beans	95	17	7	—	5
Vegetables	25	5	1	—	2
Fruits	60	15	—	—	2.5
Skim milk	85	12	8		
Fats	45	—	—	5	—

Table 86.14
Nutrient Values per Serving: 1986 American Diabetes Association (ADA) Exchange List[a]

Food Group	Energy (kcal)	Carbohydrate (g)	Protein (g)	Fat (g)
Starch/bread	80	15	3	trace
Meat and substitutes				
Lean	55	—	7	3
Medium-fat	75	—	7	5
High-fat	100	—	7	8
Vegetables	25	5	2	—
Fruit	60	15	—	—
Milk				
Skim	90	12	8	trace
Low-fat	120	12	8	5
Whole	150	12	8	8
Fat	45	—	—	5

[a]Multiplying the grams of carbohydrate and protein by 4 in the starch/bread and skim milk lists will not yield the total number of calories given for these two lists. These exchanges contain less than a gram of fat per serving and the term *trace* is used to make teaching easier. Dietitians may wish to use 1 g of fat in their calculations to achieve the total caloric value for the exchange group.

Sweeteners

Traditionally, diabetic individuals have been advised to curtail intake of foods that aggravate hyperglycemia, increase serum triglyceride concentrations, and foster additional weight gain. Often, these same foods contain excessive amounts of fat and calories contributing to poor metabolic control. Much of the focus has been on limiting refined sweets and processed foods. Recently, the ADA and others have eased their restrictions on the use of sweets in the diet. However, this should not be construed as a recommendation to increase the amount of sweets consumed in the total diet. It merely illustrates that a variety of foods may be included as they fit into a well-balanced meal plan. It is still wise to limit the consumption of sugar in patients with diabetes to that recommended for the general population (35). This represents a major change in eating habits for many people. Up to 25 g of added sucrose may be allowed, provided it is part of a low-fat, high-fiber diet and that it substitutes for an isocaloric amount of fat or high-glycemic-index food or other nutritive sweeteners. There is no strong reason to recommend fructose in preference to sucrose within this limit.

There are two basic categories of sweeteners: nutritive (calorie containing) and nonnutritive (noncaloric). Nutritive sweeteners, such as fructose found in fruits, and common sugar alcohols, the polyols (sorbitol, mannitol, or xylitol), are acceptable in modest amounts in the diabetic meal plan.

Fructose as a natural component of foods is sweeter than other sugars and is metabolized without the use of insulin, thus producing less hyperglycemia. Though fructose may increase an already high blood glucose level in poorly controlled diabetics, its effect is minimal in those with adequate control. Substituting fructose for sucrose or glucose lowers average blood glucose levels, producing a glycemic response of 20% and 33%, respectively. When we incorporated 50 to 60 g of fructose/day in a prudent diet for 14 diabetic men for 24 weeks, no adverse effects were noted in plasma glucose, glycohemoglobin, cholesterol, triglycerides, lactate, or uric acid concentrations. Inclusion of fruits containing fructose in accordance with the dietary guidelines for Americans, 2 to 4 servings per day according to calorie and activity level, should provide balance and variety in the diabetic individual's diet.

The polyols are formed by partial hydrolysis and hydrogenation of edible starches. Polyols also produce a lower glycemic response than sucrose and other carbohydrates. There appear to be no significant advantages of the polyols over other nutritive sweeteners. Excessive amounts of polyols may, however, have a laxative effect (35).

Alternative sweeteners, noncaloric, are an acceptable means of checking the amounts of excess refined sugars in the diet. Though adequately safe, to avoid excesses of any one type, a multiple-type approach is recommended. Each sweetener has its distinctive taste, advantages, and risks. Saccharin, aspartame, and acesulfame K are approved by the FDA for use in the United States. The FDA also determines an acceptable daily intake for approved additives, including nonnutritive sweeteners. Nonnutritive sweeteners approved by the FDA are safe to consume by all people with diabetes (35).

Saccharin, one of the first artificial sweeteners, is a petroleum derivative with potential association with bladder cancer when ingested in excessive quantities. Though the typical diet certainly would not exceed a moderate amount, pregnant women are advised to avoid saccharin, and children should not exceed two cans of saccharin-sweetened soft drinks daily. Aspartame, a dipeptide containing aspartic acid and phenylalanine, is present in a large variety of foods and is contraindicated only for individuals with phenylketonuria. Its use is limited to foods that do not rely on heat exposure in processing or for baking (35). Acesulfame potassium, a derivative of acetoacetic acid, is approved for broad product applications. Intake of artificial sweeteners should be limited to established safe levels. Practical resources are available to assist in counseling patients with diabetes in regard to sweeteners (35).

Diabetic Foods

So-called diabetic specialty foods are not recommended for people with diabetes or for anyone else. There is no evidence that the foods or drinks offer any advantage to people with diabetes, compared with conventional products. They often contain large amounts of sorbitol or fructose and similar energy to the conventional equivalent. The term *diabetic* attached to a food for promotional purposes has been interpreted by patients and relatives as meaning freely available and even therapeutically beneficial. The main arguments for their use relate to risks of dental caries and of becoming overweight. Reduced-sugar products labeled "diabetic" are usually more expensive; ordinary reduced-sugar products should be used. There also is a risk of hypoglycemia if reduced-sugar foods are taken inadvertently by insulin-treated patients (35).

Alcohol

Because of its potential hypoglycemic effects, heavy alcohol use is not recommended in the diabetic population. However, if alcohol is included in the diet, it should be limited to no more than 2 drinks per day for men and no more than 1 drink per day for women. One drink consists of a 1.5-oz shot of distilled spirits (i.e., whiskey, scotch, vodka, gin, rum), a 4-oz glass of wine, or 12 oz of beer (see Appendix Table IV-A-19). Alcohol does not require insulin to be metabolized; it is directly absorbed from the stomach, duodenum, and jejunum. The liver is the site of alcohol metabolism and oxidation. Excessive alcohol enters the general circulation and exerts its effects on the central nervous system.

In diabetics, alcohol induces fasting hypoglycemia by inhibiting gluconeogenesis. If consumed, it should be ingested with a meal. Alcohol also provokes hypertriglyceridemia and interacts with concurrent medications (particularly the disulfiram reaction of flushing, nausea, and dizziness that may occur when alcohol and chlorpropamide are used). Impaired judgment from alcohol intake may disrupt otherwise stable eating patterns and insulin dosage.

Alcoholic beverages provide 7 kcal/g, similar to fat and metabolized much the same. This may result in excessive energy intake without corresponding nutritive value. For insulin-dependent diabetes, the caloric value should be counted in the meal plan. In the non-insulin-dependent diabetic diet, alcohol is best substituted as a fat exchange (one alcoholic beverage equals two fat exchanges). Additional calories from mixers must be included (44).

A thorough assessment of a diabetic should include inquiry about alcohol use. Individuals may not be aware of the effects of alcohol and should be provided with at least the following guidelines: *(a)* potential or current intake should be discussed with the physician and nutrition counselor; *(b)* alcohol should be consumed slowly and with food to lessen hypoglycemic episodes; *(c)* identification should be worn indicating diabetic diagnosis since the symptoms of insulin reaction and intoxication are similar; *(d)* drinking to the extent of impaired judgment or operating a motor vehicle should be avoided; *(e)* poorly controlled diabetics should abstain from alcohol use, and of course pregnant women, diabetic or not, should not use alcohol (35).

Micronutrients

Two minerals commonly mentioned in relation to diabetes are chromium and magnesium. Animal studies have also examined vanadium, but only one clinical study (74) is available for humans. Chromium deficiency has been related, hypothetically, to development of diabetes in humans for many years, but persuasive studies in Western people are not available for recommendation of chromium supplementation for diabetic individuals. The only clear-cut circumstance in which chromium replacement has any beneficial effect on glycemic control is for people who are chromium deficient as a result of long-term chromium-deficient parenteral nutrition (35). However, it appears that most people with diabetes are not chromium deficient, and thus chromium supplementation cannot be routinely recommended. Similarly, although magnesium deficiency may play a role in insulin resistance, carbohydrate intolerance, and hypertension, the available data suggest routine evaluation of serum magnesium levels only in patients at high risk for magnesium deficiency. Magnesium should be repleted only if hypomagnesemia is demonstrated. The magnesium question is controversial, and the ADA held a consensus conference in 1992 and recommended measuring serum magnesium in persons at risk for magnesium deficiency (75) (see also Chapter 9). Potassium loss may be sufficient to warrant dietary supplementation in patients taking diuretics. Hyperkalemia sufficient to warrant dietary potassium restriction may occur in patients with renal insufficiency or hyporeninemic hypoaldosteronism or in those taking angiotensin-converting enzyme inhibitors.

ADDITIONAL CONSIDERATIONS

Children

Diabetic children have unique needs. It is important to address their fears, their level of understanding, and family support. Each stage of childhood requires revision of the diabetic management plan. Both child and parent should participate in the learning process. As therapy progresses, the child should be allowed to assume increased responsibility for the management goals. Restoring the sense of wellness, of "feeling good," is the primary goal. Eliminating the hallmark signs of diabetes such as polydipsia, polyuria, and polyphagia; preventing ketoacidosis, hypoglycemia, and hyperglycemia are specific preliminary objectives to be covered with the child and caregiver.

Growth should be monitored and can be plotted on standardized charts appropriate for the child's age and gender several times yearly, especially during the initial learning phase. An individualized plan including adequate nutrition with consideration for preferences and eating habits and normal-for-age levels of physical activity are the cornerstone of child diabetes management.

A generous carbohydrate and fiber intake coupled with limited fat provides the same advantages for children as for adults with diabetes (35, 76). During periods of rapid growth or increased energy requirements, more carbohydrates may be added. Consistent levels of food intake are more important than carbohydrate distribution for the insulin-dependent diabetic child. Three meals, each providing approximately 20 to 25% (65% total) of energy needs, and an additional three snacks using the remaining 35% of energy needs are appropriate. The dietitian may develop a meal plan based on the child's food preferences and daily schedule, and then insulin doses are tailored to achieve good glycemic control.

Simple guidelines should be provided about appropriate glycemic range and increasing snack intake for increased physical activities. Self-monitoring of blood glucose is extremely important in preventing hypoglycemic or hyperglycemic episodes experienced with physical activity, changes in meal intake, and sedentary or sick days. By trial and error, the child and caregiver will learn which variables require adjustment or closer monitoring. Autonomy and acceptance are necessary in development of a healthy well-adjusted adult without physical or psychosocial limitations. Periodic nutritional reassessment is needed to adjust requirements for growth and physical activity. Changes in insulin dosage and meal planning should evolve as the child matures (35, 76).

Elderly Patients

Diabetes is a major chronic problem for a growing elderly population. The prevalence of diabetes is almost 10% for Americans over age 60 and approximately 20% for those over 80 years old. Diabetic individuals over age 65 have a relative risk of mortality approximately 1.5 times that of nondiabetic individuals. Factors that contribute to glucose intolerance and development of diabetes in the elderly include decreased physical activity, intake of less complex carbohydrate and a higher percentage of energy from fat, and increased adiposity with decreased lean body mass. Other illnesses or medications may contribute to development of diabetes in the elderly (35).

Because the elderly have multiple defects, including impaired insulin secretion, decreased action of insulin to suppress hepatic glucose output, and peripheral insulin resistance, treatment should first focus on increasing sensitivity to insulin through nutrition and physical activity. For consideration, an α-glucosidase inhibitor may be tried as the first antidiabetes agent in older individuals, since these agents do not cause hypoglycemia and may enable sluggish insulin secretion to keep pace with slowed absorption of carbohydrates. When required, second-generation sulfonylureas should be given. If insulin is necessary, a single injection of NPH or a premixture of NPH and regular (e.g., 70/30 insulin) often supplements endogenous insulin secretion adequately. Commonly, the sulfonylurea agent is continued after insulin is instituted to minimize the amount of insulin required. The goals for blood glucose control are tailored to each individual's circumstances.

Eating a nutritious diet providing adequate energy from a variety of foods is extremely important. Fat intake should be less than 30% of energy, with limited saturated fat and cholesterol. The generous carbohydrate intake can include simple and complex carbohydrates rich in dietary fiber. Fruits, juices, and sweeteners usually do not need to be limited if fat guidelines are followed. The antidiabetes agent or insulin regimen can usually be adjusted to allow individuals to follow meal plans that suit their preferences or circumstances. Special teaching skills and patient involvement are required to optimize learning for elderly diabetic individuals. Nutritional counselors need a positive attitude, patience, and use of praise to enable elderly individuals to change lifelong dietary and exercise habits successfully.

Pregnancy

Pregnancy changes eating habits, exercise patterns, emotional state, insulin sensitivity, and hormone secretions. These changes alter glucose control and insulin requirements. In the nondiabetic woman, as placental and ovarian hormones decrease insulin sensitivity, more insulin is secreted to maintain satisfactory glucose levels. Two to 4% of women lack the pancreatic reserve to meet this challenge and develop gestational diabetes. This condition usually abates after delivery, but these women are much more likely to develop diabetes during subsequent pregnancies or later in life, particularly if they are obese. For all diabetic women, reduction of maternal, fetal, and perinatal risks requires excellent glucose control (17).

Insulin requirements change dramatically during pregnancy. To sustain a healthy fetus, the diabetic woman must adjust her nutrient intake and insulin dose to control glucose levels and avoid ketosis. During the first half of pregnancy, insulin requirements drop by 20 to 30% because of decreased food intake and increased glucose uptake by the fetus and placenta. During the second half of pregnancy, insulin requirements rise by 60 to 100% above prepregnancy levels because of placental hormone production and insulin resistance related to other factors. After delivery and removal of the placenta, insulin requirements drop precipitously; much smaller doses are required the week after delivery, but insulin requirements gradually increase to prepregnancy levels by 6 weeks after delivery. Proper adjustment of insulin therapy during pregnancy and the postpartum period requires careful blood glucose monitoring (17).

Pregnant women have lower fasting glucose levels than nonpregnant women; normal fasting blood glucose is 55 to 65 mg/dL. This level normally peaks at 140 mg/dL 1 hour after a meal; the 24-hour average is 80 to 85 mg/dL. To ensure the best possible outcome, normal glucose levels are the goal for diabetic pregnant women. Goals during pregnancy include meeting the nutritional needs of both mother and fetus while maintaining excellent blood glucose control. Specifically, these goals are to achieve glucose control before gestation and during the early weeks of pregnancy to reduce the risks of congenital malformations; to provide energy intake for appropriate weight gain (a range of 6.8 to 18.1 kg [15 to 40 lb], based on prepregnancy body mass index [BMI]), to meet increased protein needs; to provide carbohydrate to minimize ketosis, meeting the needs of the fetus and placenta; to optimize tissue sensitivity to insulin; and, during the critical 3 to 4 weeks prior to delivery, to maintain excellent glucose control to reduce neonatal risk and fetal macrosomia (17, 35).

Requirements for most nutrients increase with pregnancy and are similar for diabetic and nondiabetic women. During the first trimester, most women should gain 0.9 to 1.8 kg (2–4 lb); this can be achieved by increasing energy intake by 419 kJ (100 kcal) per day. During the second and third trimesters, a gain of about 1 lb/week depending on prepregnancy BMI is the goal. This is achieved by increasing energy intake by 15%, or 1256 kJ (300 kcal) per day. To meet increased needs, intake of high-quality protein is increased by 30 g/day to at least 1.3 g protein/kg body weight. Carbohydrate should provide at least 50% of the energy intake; some individuals benefit from higher intakes of complex carbohydrate and fiber. Fat provides the remaining energy intake. Most women require supplemental iron and folic acid; a multiple vitamin and mineral supplement including these is usually prescribed if evidence indicates that usual intake is low enough to produce adverse effects on maternal or fetal health or on the outcome of the pregnancy (17).

Gestational Diabetes (GDM)

Onset of GDM and duration during pregnancy occur in about 2 to 4% of all pregnant women, or approximately 90,000 American women each year (1). This makes it the most common medical disorder affecting pregnancy. It appears to occur only rarely in women under 20 years of age. Although the vast majority of these women return to normal glucose tolerance after delivery, 40 to 60% of them may develop NIDDM in 15 to 20 years. Those who maintain a reasonable body weight and exercise regularly have a decreased incidence of developing NIDDM. From the 24th to the 28th week of pregnancy, the body's need for insulin increases dramatically. Risks for GDM include occurrence of GDM during an earlier pregnancy, delivery of a previous macrocosmic infant (>9 lb birth weight), a family history of diabetes, and maternal obesity (>120% of ideal body weight) (17).

Pregnancy in Overt Diabetes

A successful diabetic pregnancy requires planning and commitment of time and money. Because poorly controlled diabetes threatens the health of the mother and safety of the fetus and newborn, most women make these commitments. To reduce the risks of congenital malformations, excellent glycemic control prior to conception and during early pregnancy is necessary. Maintaining excellent glycemic control throughout pregnancy demands careful attention to diet, exercise, and insulin adjustments. Health professionals educate women about special needs during pregnancy, with the patient, physician, dietitian, and nurse educator working as a team to accomplish goals.

Nutritional management plans for pregnant and nonpregnant women with overt diabetes are similar, but pregnancy necessitates greater attention to the day-to-day nutritional plan. Guidance during early pregnancy includes special consideration of food cravings or nausea. An individualized nutritional plan that evolves throughout pregnancy is essential to meet changing nutritional needs and insulin requirements. Three meals and three snacks supply energy requirements in the timely fashion necessary to prevent hypoglycemia.

The pregnant diabetic woman requires intensive management to achieve a successful outcome. Frequent office visits and vigorous nutritional therapy are important. Using frequent home blood glucose measurements, the individual strives to maintain normal fasting and postprandial glucose values while avoiding frequent or severe hypoglycemic reactions. The healthcare team monitors the fetus and assesses fetal maturity to select the optimal time for, and mode of, delivery. Hospitalization may be necessary to reestablish blood glucose control; early hospitalization for glycemic control prior to delivery is advisable. Finally, intensive neonatal management is essential. Use of these principles can reduce maternal risk to near that of nondiabetic women and their offspring.

Diabetic women should be encouraged to breast-feed their infants, while paying special attention to changing insulin and food requirements. A caloric intake of 31 kcal/kg maternal body weight is associated with the ability of mothers with insulin-dependent diabetes to sustain lactation (35).

Renal Disease

Renal disease is a major complication that affects 30 to 50% of type I and over 20% of type II diabetic individuals. Diabetic nephropathy is accompanied by proteinuria, decreased glomerular filtration rate, and hypertension. Development of *microalbuminuria,* urine protein of 40 to 300 mg/24 hours, is the forerunner of overt nephropathy. Hypertension accelerates development and progression of renal disease, whereas poor glycemic control and high protein intake may contribute to development and progression of nephropathy (36).

Protein restriction in management of chronic renal failure is discussed elsewhere (see Chapter 89). High protein intake is thought to lead to renal damage in diabetic individuals by various mechanisms. Extensive protein feeding increases glomerular filtration rate, renal blood flow, single-nephron glomerular filtration rate, and transcapillary hydraulic pressure in laboratory animals (36).

Unlimited protein intake is inappropriate in patients with diabetic nephropathy. Protein restriction decreases the progression of chronic renal failure in nondiabetic individuals and perhaps in diabetic nephropathy. At present, it appears prudent to restrict protein intake to 0.6 g/kg body weight for individuals with established diabetic nephropathy, with appropriate adjustments for proteinuria and careful clinical monitoring. Carbohydrate should provide at least 50% of energy intake, and saturated fat and cholesterol intake should be restricted. Recent research indicates that substitution of soy protein for animal protein may decrease risk for developing diabetic nephropathy (36). Furthermore, substituting soy protein for animal protein may reduce proteinuria and slow progression of nephropathy. Further research is required to rigorously test this "soy protein for diabetic nephropathy" hypothesis (36).

Hyperlipidemia

Most diabetic individuals have lipoprotein abnormalities. There are multiple abnormalities of VLDL, LDL, and HDL composition and metabolism. Hypertriglyceridemia and low HDL-cholesterol values are seen more commonly in diabetic than nondiabetic individuals. Hypertriglyceridemia appears to confer a higher risk of atherosclerotic cardiovascular disease on diabetic than on nondiabetic individuals; low HDL-cholesterol values are another major risk factor (25, 77).

Serum lipid and lipoprotein goals for diabetic individuals are still being actively discussed. To minimize the risk of atherosclerotic cardiovascular disease, the following desirable or goal fasting values for diabetic individuals are recommended: total cholesterol, <200 mg/dL (<5.2 mmol/L); LDL cholesterol, <100 mg/dL (<2.6 mmol/L); triglycerides, <150 mg/dL (<1.7 mmol/L); and HDL cholesterol for males, >45 mg/dL (>1.2 mmol/L) and for females, >55 mg/dL (>1.4 mmol/L). Because abnormally low HDL-cholesterol levels are difficult to increase by dietary or pharmacologic measures, LDL cholesterol should be decreased to achieve ratios of LDL:HDL cholesterol below 2.2 for males and below 1.8 for females (44, 78).

The diabetes nutritional plan outlined in this chapter and elsewhere is the basic approach for most hyperlipidemic individuals (44). Good glycemic control, attaining and maintaining a desirable body weight, regular exercise, and moderation in alcohol intake—practices recommended for all diabetic individuals—reduce hyperlipidemia. Approach to hyperlipidemia can focus on management of elevated LDL cholesterol, elevated triglycerides, decreased HDL cholesterol, or combinations of these disorders.

Elevated LDL-cholesterol levels occur with the same frequency in diabetic and nondiabetic individuals; treatment is similar. A high-carbohydrate (55–60% of energy), high-fiber (25 g/4186 kJ [1000 kcal]), low-fat (about 25% of energy with less than 10% saturated), low-cholesterol (<200 mg/day) diabetes diet is the first step. This diet should include generous amounts of soluble dietary fiber from oat and bean products. Increasing soluble fiber intake by 6 g/day without other changes in diet can decrease LDL cholesterol by 10 to 20% (44, 79, 80). The second step is daily inclusion of 4 to 12 g of psyllium, a well-tolerated concentrated source of soluble fiber (80, 81). When desirable LDL-cholesterol levels are not achieved, a bile acid sequestrant is added. Bile acid sequestrants and psyllium can be mixed together in 8 to 12 oz of fluid and taken two or three times daily. Hydroxymethylglutaryl coenzyme-A (HMG-CoA) reductase inhibitors are the second pharmacologic agent of choice (44).

Because of the accelerated risk for atherosclerotic disease in diabetic individuals, some authorities recommend LDL-cholesterol goals below 2.6 mmol/L (100 mg/dL) for diabetic adults. These authorities also recommend low-dose HMG-CoA reductase inhibitor therapy for adults with LDL-cholesterol values above 2.6 mmol/L (100 mg/dL). Further study is required to justify this aggressive therapy.

Hypertriglyceridemia is more common in diabetic individuals, especially in type II diabetes, than in nondiabetic individuals and carries a greater risk of atherosclerosis. Almost all individuals can be managed effectively with a high-fiber, high-carbohydrate diet if they decrease their fat intake to a low enough level (44, 82). Figure 86.8 illustrates the responses of serum triglyceride values to intensive high-carbohydrate, high-fiber, low-fat diets for diabetic individuals at our medical center. Persistently elevated triglyceride levels usually are due to excessive dietary fat intake, because triglyceride levels plummet when individuals are hospitalized and receive a low-fat diet. Sometimes excessive alcohol or simple sugar intake aggravates hypertriglyceridemia. Fibric acid derivatives, nicotinic acid, or a combination of HMG-CoA reductase inhibitors with nicotinic acid are pharmacologic choices for those not responding to diet.

Type II diabetic individuals commonly have decreased HDL-cholesterol levels. Regular physical exercise such as

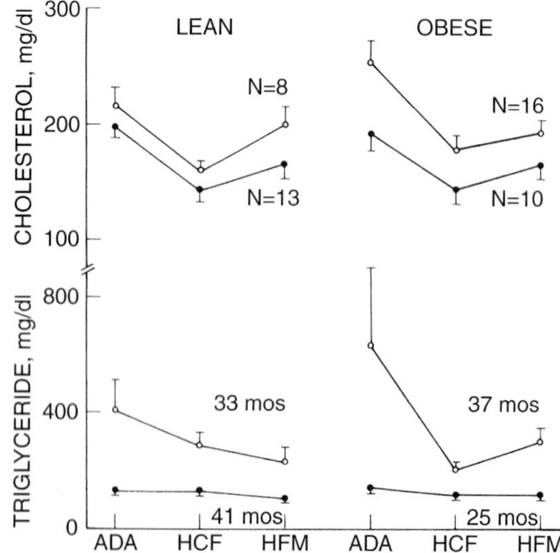

Figure 86.8. Response of serum cholesterol and triglyceride concentration to high-carbohydrate, high-fiber *(HCF)* and high-fiber-maintenance *(HFM)* diets in lean and obese diabetic individuals. *Open circles* represent individuals with elevated fasting serum triglyceride values on an American Diabetes Association *(ADA)* diet. Duration of follow-up is indicated in months.

walking 2 to 3 miles daily and not smoking are important lifestyle practices to increase HDL cholesterol. Dietary measures to decrease serum triglycerides and the regular use of oat products may increase HDL cholesterol by 10 to 20% (83). HDL cholesterol usually decreases when intensive nutritional measures are used. Decreases in HDL cholesterol may parallel decreases in LDL-cholesterol levels for several months before HDL cholesterol levels begin to increase. The increase in HDL cholesterol with exercise and diet occurs slowly over 3 to 6 months. However, most individuals cannot increase HDL-cholesterol levels by more than 0.13 to 0.26 mmol/L (5–10 mg/dL) by these lifestyle measures. Often, LDL-cholesterol levels must be decreased to below goal levels to achieve desirable LDL:HDL ratios below 2.2 for males or 1.8 for females. Pharmacologic agents that increase HDL cholesterol somewhat are fibric acid derivatives and HMG-CoA reductase inhibitors. These agents are introduced when LDL-cholesterol or triglyceride concentrations do not reach goal levels with dietary measures.

The hyperlipidemia of most diabetic individuals responds well to nutritional measures. Most individuals with LDL-cholesterol levels of 4.13 mmol/L (<160 mg/dL) can be managed effectively with high-fiber diets including generous amounts of soluble fiber. Most hypertriglyceridemic individuals respond to a high-fiber diet moderately or severely restricted in saturated and total fat. New nutritional considerations include use of soy protein to decrease LDL-cholesterol and triglyceride concentrations (84) and antioxidant supplements (85). Regular exercise (e.g., walking 2 to 3 miles daily) and achieving and maintaining a desirable body weight also enhance the lipoprotein response to nutritional measures.

Obesity

About 75% of type II diabetic individuals in the United States are obese; obesity is a major contributor to development and maintenance of the diabetic state. Achieving and maintaining a desirable body weight through diet and exercise is the treatment of choice. Antidiabetes drugs and insulin are important adjunctive measures, but they cannot be substituted for exercise and a diet appropriate in energy, fat, and complex carbohydrate.

Weight-Loss Programs

The healthcare team sets the stage for effective weight loss by being empathetic and supportive while continuing to emphasize the detrimental effects of overeating on diabetes and health. However, the obese individual must be committed to losing weight before nutrition counseling is effective. Our team offers a variety of weight-loss programs, including instruction in a hypocaloric diet; referral to a community program; an intensive high-fiber, weight-reduction diet with frequent medical and dietetic follow-up; and medically supervised low-calorie or very low calorie diet programs. Diabetic individuals with a BMI above 30 kg/m^2 or who need to lose more than 22.7 kg (50 lb) should have medical supervision during the weight-loss phase and should not enroll in medically unsupervised programs (44).

Weight Maintenance

Weight loss is not the cure for obesity. This chronic condition requires a long-term maintenance program and access to lifelong counseling about lifestyle changes important in weight maintenance. After nonsurgical weight-loss programs, long-term weight maintenance as a percentage of initial weight loss is reported to be about 36% at 2 years and about 5% at 5 years. Most obese individuals who complete community weight-loss programs, behavioral modification programs, and very low calorie programs regain all the weight they lost within 2 to 5 years. Newer very low calorie diet programs that stress physical activity, use the best available behavioral techniques, and facilitate achievement of desirable body weights are obtaining better long-term weight maintenance. Obese individuals completing the HMR Fasting Program at the University of Kentucky (UK) are maintaining about 63% of their initial weight loss 2 years after completing the weight-loss phase (86). Recent data indicate that "graduates" of the UK program are maintaining about 20% of their weight loss at 7 years; approximately 25% are maintaining a loss of at least 10% of their initial weight (i.e., maintaining more than 10 kg of weight loss) (Anderson JW, unpublished observations). The best predictors of good weight maintenance are low fat intake and good levels of physical activity such as walking 20 miles/week. Much further development is required to enable formerly obese individuals to maintain desirable weights for long periods.

High-Fiber Weight-Loss Programs

High-carbohydrate, high-fiber, weight-reducing diets are excellent choices for diabetic individuals with BMIs ranging from 28 to 35 kg/m^2 (62). The diet is individualized to provide 5 to 7 kcal/lb actual weight, so many women receive 4186- to 5023-kJ (1000- to 1200-kcal) diets and many men receive 5023- to 6698-kJ (1200- to 1600-kcal) diets. These diets provide 55 to 60% of energy from carbohydrate, 50 to 70 g protein, the remainder of energy from fat, and about 15 to 25 g fiber per 4186 kJ (1000 kcal). Patients also are encouraged to walk 2 to 3 miles/day and keep records of food intake, exercise, and blood glucose values. Initially, patients are seen every 2 weeks, then every 3 to 6 weeks during the weight-loss phase, and then every 4 to 8 weeks during the 1st year after completing the weight-loss phase (44, 68).

Low-Calorie and Very Low Calorie Weight-Loss Programs

Intensive low-calorie or very low calorie diet programs are the treatment of choice for obese diabetic individuals with BMIs exceeding 35 kg/m^2. Responsible very low calorie diets programs provide careful medical evaluation and ongoing medical supervision by trained physicians; a high-quality supplement adequate in protein, carbohydrate, vitamins, and minerals; a weekly program providing the most current behavioral and lifestyle education; an emphasis on physical activity that enables average participants to achieve and maintain the expenditure of 8372 kJ (2000 kcal) per week in physical activity such as walking; and a maintenance program of 18 or more months (87, 88).

Medication Adjustment with Low-Calorie Diets

Because high energy intakes sustain hyperglycemia and requirements for insulin or sulfonylureas, energy-restricted diets reduce requirements for these medications. Figure 86.7 shows insulin-dose reductions over 12 weeks when 20 insulin-treated type II diabetic individuals were given low-calorie or very low calorie diets providing 2093 to 3349 kJ (500–800 kcal) per day. Insulin doses decreased about 50% during the 1st week. We routinely decrease insulin doses by 50% when we initiate low-calorie or very low calorie diets. With less severe energy restriction, we reduce insulin doses by 10 to 30%, based on prior glycemic control and extent of energy restriction. Subsequent doses are decreased as required on the basis of home glucose monitoring. Similarly, sulfonylurea doses must be reduced when diabetic individuals initiate energy-restricted diets. Usually, we reduce sulfonylurea doses by 50% when initiating low-calorie or very low calorie diets. Individuals treated with either insulin or sulfonylureas must monitor their glucose when initiating energy-restricted diets, to avoid serious hypoglycemia (87) (Fig. 86.9).

EXERCISE

A routine exercise program is important for all people. Exercise is excellent for weight control, enhanced physical and psychologic fitness, better capacity to work, improved body composition, and increased HDL concentration

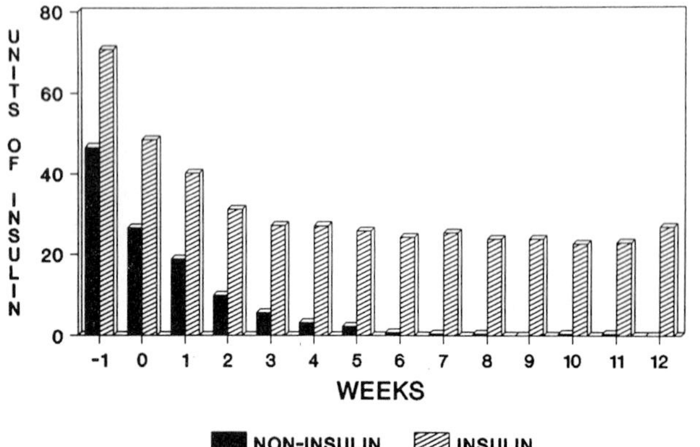

Figure 86.9. Reduction in insulin dose for type II individuals treated for 12 weeks with low-calorie diets. Subjects designated *non-insulin* were able to discontinue insulin during the 12-week study.

Table 86.15
Various Exercises That Are Equivalent to Walking One Mile

Exercise	Time or Distance Equivalent to Walking One Mile
Jogging or running	1 mile
Outdoor bicycling	3 miles
Stair climbing	25 flights
Stair machine (fast pace)	8 min
Cross-country skiing machine	8 min
Swimming	10 min
Sitting rowing machine (E-Force)	10 min
Rowing machine (20 strokes/min)	10 min
Stationary bicycle	12 min
Aerobic dancing	12 min
Basketball (noncompetitive)	12 min
Golf (not riding a cart)	20 min

Adapted from Anderson JW, Breecher MM. Dr. Anderson's antioxidant, antiaging health program. New York: Carroll & Graf. 1996;1(1):1–270.

[a]Amount of aerobic activity achieved (or activity equivalent to walking 1 mile) depends on the intensity of the exercise for most activities.

(44). Diabetics prosper in additional ways, including better glucose tolerance, raised insulin sensitivity, reduced atherosclerosis risk factors, decreased blood pressure (44), and improved cardiovascular fitness.

The most beneficial exercise program differs for each person, but walking is best for obese individuals. A good way to ease into an exercise regimen is to start walking 10 to 20 minutes once or twice each day, increasing this gradually over a few weeks to 30 minutes twice a day. On average, most diabetics should walk 12 to 14 miles/week.

Other exercises such as bicycling, stair climbing, swimming, and aerobic dancing are good alternatives to walking, but more time should be spent on these machines to equal desired walking time (Table 86.15). It is beneficial to use the upper body during exercise. A Cardioglide or E-Force machine is an excellent choice for persons who are limited in the exercises they can perform with their lower extremities. These machines allow cardiovascular exercise without working the legs. With the vast selection of exercise equipment available, all individuals can find something appropriate for their needs and physical condition. After patients have set an exercise goal and selected an appropriate program, they should keep a written reminder of the goal. In addition, a personal exercise journal keeps patients focused and helps them remember what they have done (43).

While exercise has definite benefits, there are also hazards to vigorous exercise, such as irritation of poorly regulated hyperglycemia, hypoglycemia or ketonemia, or unexpected death during exercise. Therefore, exercise safety for diabetics is of the utmost importance. Diabetics should monitor their blood glucose levels so food intake or insulin adjustment can be determined. Packing a snack while exercising outside prepares patients for times when they feel poorly. Also, an exercise partner who is educated on the patient's condition or having the patient wear identification can be useful in cases of hypoglycemia or an insulin reaction (89).

INSULIN THERAPY

Although insulin replacement therapy has been used for about 70 years, physiologic replacement of insulin for diabetic individuals remains an elusive goal. In lean, nondiabetic adults, insulin is secreted into the portal system in the basal state at a rate of approximately 1 U/h. After food intake, the rise in blood glucose and gastrointestinal hormones triggers a five- to tenfold increase in insulin secretion rates. Basal plus food-related insulin secretion totals approximately 40 U/day for lean, nondiabetic adults. Even though human insulin is available, this physiologic response cannot be mimicked (18).

Both diet and exercise have major effects on insulin sensitivity in type I and type II diabetic individuals. High-carbohydrate, high-fiber diets increase insulin sensitivity and decrease insulin requirements, whereas high-fat diets have opposite effects (65, 66). For example, a slender 38-year-old farmer required 57 U of insulin daily for good glycemic control on a conventional high-fat (37% of energy), low-carbohydrate (43% of energy), low-fiber diet in 1974 (44). After 16 years of good adherence to a high-carbohydrate (about 60% of energy), high-fiber (about 45 g/day), low-fat (less than 25% of energy) diet, he takes 36 U of insulin daily to maintain fairly good control as an outpatient. Regular physical activity appears to act similarly by increasing skeletal muscle sensitivity to insulin. For example, when a family-practice physician trains for marathons by running over 60 miles/week, he requires only 20 U of insulin daily, but when not in training, he requires about 50 U daily. Physiologic considerations, risks, and benefits of exercise are reviewed elsewhere (44).

These two case studies indicate that algorithms based on body weight have limited accuracy. The farmer had a 37% reduction in insulin dose related to diet without change in body weight or physical activity. While in his busy practice, the physician required 250% of the insulin dose needed when in training for marathons, without significant changes in body weight. Likewise, algorithms for premeal insulin doses used for carbohydrate counting are better based on total insulin dose of the individual than on body weight. For example, if someone takes 50 U of insulin daily, about 40%, or 20 U, is related to basal insulin needs and should be provided as intermediate (e.g., NPH) or long-acting (e.g., Ultralente). Thus, 30 U is assigned to premeal and presnack doses. If the person consumes 2400 kcal/day and 300 g of carbohydrate, one can "guestimate" a carbohydrate:insulin ratio of 10:1 and initiate carbohydrate counting and premeal insulin on this basis.

The insulin regimen is usually tailored to the nutritional plan and the physical activity of the individual. Some nutritional guidelines for insulin-treated type II diabetic individuals, type I diabetic individuals receiving conventional insulin therapy, and type I diabetic individuals receiving intensive insulin therapy are presented. Table 86.16 compares insulin preparations widely used in the United States.

Table 86.16
Usual Timing and Action of Human Insulins

Type	Onset (h)	Peak (h)	Maximum Duration (h)
Lyspro	0.25–0.5	1–1.5	2–3
Regular	0.5–1	2–3	4–6
70/30[a]	0.5–1	2–3,4–10	14–18
NPH	2–4	4–10	14–18
Lente	3–4	4–12	16–20
Ultralente	6–10	"peakless"	20–30

[a]Mixture of 70% NPH and 30% Regular.

More than 2 million type II diabetic individuals receive insulin therapy in the United States. Many receive sulfonylurea therapy as well as insulin because this combination decreases the amount of insulin required (44, 90). About 75% of these insulin-treated type II individuals are obese. When diabetes and obesity occur together, termed *diabesity,* overeating is the major cause of hyperglycemia. Any reduction in energy intake promptly reduces insulin requirements. When starting any weight-reduction diet, reduced insulin need should be anticipated.

Insulin therapy in type II diabetes usually supplements endogenous insulin and often is given as a single injection before breakfast or at bedtime. When doses exceed 50 U/day, injections are usually given twice daily, before breakfast and the evening meal. Some patients mix NPH insulin and regular insulin for these injections or use premixed combinations of 70% NPH insulin and 30% regular insulin (70/30 insulin). Most insulin-treated type II diabetic individuals can be managed with three meals and a bedtime snack. The major adverse effects of insulin therapy in type II diabetes are hypoglycemic attacks and weight gain. Because overeating is the major contributor to hyperglycemia, undereating predictably produces hypoglycemia in the insulin-treated, obese type II diabetic individual. Avoiding hypoglycemia and weight gain in these individuals challenges both the physician who counsels the patient on insulin dosage and the dietitian who counsels on diet.

Conventional insulin management in type I diabetes usually involves two daily injections of a mixture of NPH and regular insulin and a meal plan including three meals and two to three snacks. Many individuals can achieve fairly good glycemic control if they self-monitor the blood glucose (SMBG) and make appropriate adjustments in food intake, physical activity, and insulin doses on the basis of their blood glucose level. Because most type I diabetic individuals do not adjust their own insulin doses based on twice-daily SMBG, energy intake at meals and snacks must be consistent from day to day. Most of these individuals benefit from a meal plan based on exchanges (91).

Intensive insulin therapy is now used more widely by type I diabetic individuals and is the treatment of choice for most. An intensive therapy program includes multiple daily injections of insulin or use of an insulin infusion pump; multiple SMBG daily; careful balance of food intake, physical activity, and insulin dose through self-monitoring and self-adjustment of these parameters; and careful and frequent coaching and support by the health care team. The diet plan for these individuals is highly tailored to their needs, and patients must be able to make daily adjustments in food intake in response to blood glucose values and physical activity.

Carbohydrate counting is a popular adjunct to intensive insulin therapy (92–94). While the time-honored method of intensive insulin therapy relates to eating a standardized diet from day to day and adjusting insulin on the basis of blood glucose deviations from target values, carbohydrate counting provides more flexibility. However, this does complicate the insulin regimen, since premeal insulin doses must be adjusted for anticipated carbohydrate intake as well as current blood glucose level. For highly motivated, highly trainable type I individuals, this regimen brings flexibility to the treatment plan.

ANTIDIABETES DRUG THERAPY

The 1990s ushered in several new antidiabetes agents that allow better tailoring of therapy to the presumed pathologic defect. Table 86.17 outlines current thinking about the pathogenesis of type II diabetes and how the various antidiabetes agents approach these defects. As previously outlined (95), three organs—the liver, pancreas, and skeletal muscle—play a major role in the pathophysiology of diabetes. Recently added on the basis of emerging evidence related to amylin, is the gut. Currently, these four organs are considered to play major roles in the pathobiology of diabetes. Briefly, the liver exhibits excessive and uncontrolled gluconeogenesis and the skeletal muscles are resistant to the action of insulin. Because of hypertrophy related to hyperphagia and hyperglycemia, the intestines absorb glucose more rapidly than normal. The pancreas, of course, has defective secretion of insulin. As newer antidiabetes agents become available, we will be better able to tailor the agent to the presumed major pathophysiologic defect of the individual.

Within recent years, several new hypoglycemic agents have become available and a few are still in the research stage, awaiting approval. However, for years, sulfonylureas were the only oral hypoglycemic agents available in the United States. The sulfonylureas lower blood glucose principally by stimulating insulin secretion from the pancreatic β cells. These agents may also enhance peripheral sensitivity to insulin by unknown mechanisms. Persons of normal weight and obese individuals who develop diabetes after age 40, those who have had diabetes for less than 5 years, or those whose diabetes is well controlled on 20 U of insulin for lean persons or 40 U for obese persons are likely to respond well to sulfonylurea agents.

Nearly 40% of type II diabetic individuals take sulfonylureas; chlorpropamide, glipizide, and glyburide account for 75% of the market. (1). The two second-generation sulfonylureas are the preferred agents for initiating therapy. All sulfonylureas have the same mechanism of action, but they differ in potency, duration of action, and metabolic fate. The second-generation agents, glipizide and glyburide, are more potent than the first-generation agents, have fewer side effects, and may have other advantages (91). A significant disadvantage of sulfonylureas is the tendency for individuals to gain weight as they achieve good glycemic control. An overview of antidiabetes agents available or available shortly in the U.S. is presented in Table 86.18.

The combination of insulin and sulfonylureas is widely used for type II diabetes because it lowers insulin requirements and frequently improves glycemic control. Theoretically, the sulfonylureas increase peripheral sensitivity to insulin and reduce hyperinsulinemia. When insulin doses exceed 70 to 100 U/day for obese type II diabetic individuals, we incorporate sulfonylureas into the regimen (91).

Diet and exercise retain central importance in the management of type II diabetes. Our experience indicates that approximately three-fourths of type II individuals treated with insulin, sulfonylureas, or the combination can be managed with diet and exercise alone. Whether insulin or sulfonylureas are used or not, overeating is the major cause of hyperglycemia in type II diabetes; a mildly energy-restricted diet generous in complex carbohydrate and fiber and restricted in fat almost universally improves glycemic control as it facilitates weight loss (44, 91).

Metformin, another new oral hypoglycemic agent, is effective for the control of hyperglycemia without causing weight gain or hypoglycemia. Metformin is used to treat NIDDM when control of glucose levels cannot be achieved solely by diet. It is also used in combination with sulfonylureas when either drug alone is ineffective. There are

Table 86.17
Pathophysiologic Derangements in Type II Diabetes and Proposed Mechanisms of Action of Antidiabetes Agents

Organ	Basic Defect	Sulfonylurea Action	Metformin Action	Acarbose Action
Pancreas	Decreased insulin secretion	Increases insulin release in response to glucose	No action	(Allows slowly released insulin to work better)
Liver	Increased gluconeogenis	Decreases gluconeogenesis	Decreases gluconeogensis	No action
Muscle	Decreased insulin sensitivity	Increases sensitivity	Increases sensitivity	No action
Gut	Accelerated glucose absorption	No action	Decreases glucose absorption	Slows glucose absorption

Table 86.18
Antidiabetes Drugs

Agent	Class	Usual Starting Dose	Maximum Dose	Mechanism of Action
Glyburide	Sulfonylurea	2.5 mg/day	10 mg b.i.d.	Enhances insulin secretion and increases muscle sensitivity to insulin
Glynase	Sulfonylurea	3 mg/day	12 mg/day	Enhances insulin secretion and increases muscle sensitivity to insulin
Glipizide	Sulfonylurea	5 mg/day	20 mg b.i.d.	Enhances insulin secretion and increases muscle sensitivity to insulin
Glipizide GITS	Sulfonylurea	5 mg/day	20 mg/day	Enhances insulin secretion and increases muscle sensitivity to insulin
Glimiperide	Sulfonylurea	1–2 mg/day	8 mg/day	Enhances insulin secretion and increases muscle sensitivity to insulin
Metformin	Biguanide	500 mg t.i.d.	850 mg t.i.d.	Decreases hepatic output of glucose, decreases intestinal glucose absorption, and increases muscle sensitivity to insulin
Acarbose	α-Glucosidase inhibitor	25 mg b.i.d.	100 mg t.i.d.	Delays digestion of ingested carbohydrates
Troglitazone	Thiazolidinediones	200 mg/day	600 mg/day	Enhances peripheral sensitivity to insulin
Bromocriptine	Dopamine agonist	not available	not available	Enhances peripheral sensitivity to insulin

several advantages to using metformin. It does not exhaust the pancreas. Instead of stimulating the pancreas to make more insulin (and later causing the pancreatic cells to become depleted) as sulfonylureas do, metformin makes insulin receptors more sensitive. Metformin reduces insulin resistance in the cells so the body can use the insulin it has already produced. Other benefits of metformin are its appetite suppressant effect, as well as its ability to decrease the concentrations of blood lipids, especially triglycerides. Nausea, gastrointestinal discomfort, diarrhea, metallic taste, and anorexia are common side effects of metformin use. Side effects tend to lessen with decreased dosage. One important precaution is that metformin should not be used by individuals with kidney disease, since they are at higher risk for lactic acidosis (96–99).

Acarbose, a new antidiabetes agent available in the U.S. since early 1996, inhibits hydrolysis of complex carbohydrates and dietary disaccharides. In addition, it reduces the normal increase of insulin and blood glucose seen after a meal by impeding glucose release from disaccharides and complex carbohydrates. The recommended dosage of 25 to 50 mg should be taken at the beginning of each meal, totaling three doses daily. Side effects of acarbose include cramps, flatulence, borborygmus, abdominal distention, and diarrhea. However, these adverse effects lessen with time. This medication may also cause anemia and lower absorption of iron, but decreased weight is not an adverse effect of this medication. Administration of acarbose with metformin is *not* recommended, (100, 101).

Combining use of metformin and sulfonylureas is effective. Sulfonylureas cause the pancreas to make more insulin as metformin causes cells to better use the insulin produced. Also, addition of metformin to existing sulfonylurea therapy improves lipid levels and glucose metabolism (97, 98).

Troglitazone is another oral hypoglycemic agent recently approved for use in the U.S., specifically for type II individuals treated with insulin. This agent increases peripheral sensitivity to insulin. When troglitazone is administered to patients with type II diabetes, hyperglycemia and resistance to insulin are reduced (102, 103).

EDUCATION AND COUNSELING

The social and cultural importance of eating behavior has often been neglected, and the difficulty in making permanent changes to entrenched eating habits is still greatly underestimated. Many diabetic patients consider diet to be the most traumatic aspect of their treatment. Compliance with diabetic diets is notoriously poor, as is probably the case with any therapeutic diet where the short-term penalties for noncompliance are not always apparent and the reward for keeping to the diet is a negative one (absence of complications) in the distant future.

Full goals are probably attained by rather few patients. The degree to which dietary advice can be implemented varies between individuals. All patients should, with guidance, be able to improve their diets significantly, but not all will be willing or able to achieve the full goals, and certainly not overnight. Finding the right balance where nutritional goals are desirable, beneficial, and attainable is key. Dietary goals should continue to be presented, consistently, by all members of the diabetes care team.

About 64% of diabetics in the 1989 NHIS reported following a diet for their diabetes, but 87% believed that diet is important in control of their diabetes (1). A variety of situations were problematic in maintaining the diet, most notably the desire to eat foods that are not on the diabetes diet. Of importance, two situations were not issues: lack of support from family and friends and being unsure about what foods they should eat. In general, difficulties with following a diet for diabetes were expressed less frequently as age increased. Patient education can translate into increased self-management skills, but only 35% of people with diabetes in the 1989 NHIS had ever attended a diabetes educational class or course.

It is important to identify the types of situations that make nutritional adherence difficult for a particular person. Clinically, the idea of adherence barriers allows us to improve patient education and intervention efforts—teaching beyond generalized information.

1. Ensure that the healthcare team realizes that nutritional intervention is an important component of intensive therapy; many physicians and nurses are unaware that diet is vital in optimizing glycemic control.
2. Individualize the diet to include lifestyle and food preferences and expand counseling beyond nutritional requirements. Social and environmental influences greatly affect choices; the patient needs to have options to address these situations. "Ideal" meal plans that are generic for all patients are often never implemented.
3. Teach IDDM patients how to estimate food intake. Patients adjusting insulin doses to match intake must be able to identify portions and/or grams of carbohydrate.
4. During the initial stages of intervention, have the patient keep food records that can be correlated with glycemic control and adjusted accordingly.
5. Remind patients able to implement intensive therapy that though they may "cover" any food with insulin, weight gain carries considerable risk if it causes increased caloric consumption (101).

Simplified systems of nutritional education are again coming of age and should be considered for certain individuals. Some nutritional experts no longer use formal carbohydrate exchange lists. The British Diabetic Association notes that although these lists have some reference value and give confidence to some patients, such as the newly diagnosed, they are probably unnecessary for most routine management and are not essential in the initial stages (7). Recommendations may instead involve general nutritional goals such as quenching thirst with water or other drinks without sugar; having regular meals, avoiding fried and very sugary foods; eating plenty of vegetables with cereal, bread, pasta, potato, or rice as the main part of each meal; having meat, egg, or cheese as a small part of each meal; and remembering fish and legumes as alternatives (34).

One attractive approach is the "plate model" advocated by the Swedish Diabetic Association and the Community Nutrition Group of the British Dietetic Association (7). A simple system of fat exchanges might be useful for limiting fat intake. Identifying or naming a nutrient in a dietary prescription always carries the connotation of restriction. Since fat is the nutrient principally restricted and complex carbohydrate intake is generally encouraged, identifying the fat components of the diet might be preferable to the current system of defining the diet in terms of carbohydrate content.

Education and management of diabetes have become oriented more toward prevention and less toward crisis

Table 86.19
Diabetes Nutritional Education Topics

Survival Skills
Relation of food to insulin and activity
Importance of good nutrition in the control of blood glucose and lipid levels
Necessity of maintaining normal weight
Types and amounts of food in meal plan
Modification of food intake during brief illnesses
In-depth counseling
Meal planning
Types of nutrients, their functions, relation to insulin, and effect on blood glucose and lipid levels
Caloric level of meal plan and percentages of carbohydrate, protein, and fat
Food sources of fiber
Importance of reducing total fat, saturated fat, and cholesterol in the diet
Relation of sodium to hypertension
Proper serving sizes
Changes in food intake based on activity level
Eating out and special occasions
Label reading and grocery shopping
Use of sweeteners, alcohol, and "dietetic" foods
Food modifications for other disorders
Incorporation of favorite recipes

Adapted from Franz M, Krosnick A, Maschak-Carey BJ, et al. Goals for diabetes education. Chicago: American Diabetes Association, 1986.

intervention. Whichever educational approach is deemed appropriate, dietary guidelines for the diabetic remain similar to nutritional principles of the general American population. Reduction in saturated fat and total fat and increased fiber intake are among the most important of these recommendations (Table 86.19).

INDIVIDUALIZATION

To be effective in the long term, the nutritional plan must be individually tailored. Readily available, preprinted diet sheets provide clues to changes in eating habits, but they allow no flexibility and are doomed to eventual failure. Although the effects of dietary components such as carbohydrate and fat have been extensively studied, diet implementation has received much less attention. The best nutritional plans will not work if they are not followed.

Initially, team members must realistically assess the motivation and capability of the patient and family or support group. An optimistic approach is imperative; previous failures do not necessarily predict failure with a nutritional plan at this point. An individual unable to learn an exchange system should be taught a "no-added-sugar" plan. Shortly after the diagnosis of diabetes, some individuals are best taught a simplified "survival" diet, with more-detailed nutritional education provided when they are better able to cope with their condition.

After initial evaluation, the dietitian assesses exercise habits, work schedule, socioeconomic level, living situation, and past eating habits. Diet recalls, food records, or food-frequency checklists provide useful information. A history of food eaten in the past 24 hours is a practical way to estimate energy intake and the percentage contributions of carbohydrate, protein, and fat. A 7-day food-frequency survey offers a better overview of food intake. To obtain accurate information, the interviewer should ask nonjudgmental questions. Finally, food preferences are elicited. Information about prior food habits forms the foundation for building a solid nutritional plan.

Desirable body weight estimations are made during the initial nutritional assessment. After obtaining a weight history (lightest and heaviest adult weights, recent weight changes, prior use of weight-reducing regimens), we often ask individuals how much they would like to weigh. Ideally, the individuals identify "good" weight goals, and we avoid designating a weight they consider unrealistic. Desirable body weight estimations from tables or formulas provide guidance in setting weight goals. The diabetic individual and dietitian work together to develop targets for short- and long-term weight. The simple process of establishing an estimate of desirable body weight signals diabetic individuals that management of their condition is a partnership venture.

Developing the specific nutritional plan is the next step. Based on the available information, the dietitian and physician decide which nutritional strategy best suits the individual. For some, a plan avoiding sucrose and foods rich in sugars works best. Simplified educational materials have been developed for this purpose. For others, a plan using food exchanges is more appropriate. Some individuals are good candidates for high-fiber diets. Once the team establishes a basic plan, it must be modified for other conditions such as hyperlipidemia, congestive heart failure, or weight loss.

Tailoring the diet to the specific individual is probably the most difficult task in the management of nutrition in diabetes. In doing so, the dietitian considers the treatment regimen (frequency and type of insulin injections or use of oral hypoglycemic agents) as well as other factors. The individualized nutritional plan should be as compatible as possible with the food habits and lifestyle of the patient, but an effective nutritional plan usually requires change. The dietitian's goal is to develop the most therapeutically effective plan and to train the diabetic individual and support group to put this plan into practice.

FOOD EXCHANGES

Flexibility has slowly become an integral part of the diabetes nutritional plan. The American Diabetes Association and American Dietetic Association Exchange Lists for Meal Planning, first released in 1950, have remained the most acceptable, universal method of meal planning. To better reflect current nutritional recommendations for people with diabetes, these exchanges were revised in 1986 (17). Other specialized exchange plans have been developed based upon the same principles (44).

Table 86.20
Worksheet for Developing 2000-kcal Exchange Meal Plan

Exchange	Servings	Energy (kcal)	Carbohydrate (g)	Protein (g)	Fat (g)
Starch/bread	8	640	120	24	trace
Meat and substitutes	3	165	—	21	9
Vegetables	7	175	35	14	—
Fruit	7	420	10	—	—
Milk	2	180	24	16	trace
Fat	10	450	—	—	50
Total	—	2030	284	75	59
Target	—	2000	290	75	60

Exchange-based nutritional plans provide flexibility and choice while maintaining consistency from day to day.

Exchange groups include foods of similar nutrient composition; all serving sizes or portions in one exchange provide similar amounts of energy, carbohydrate, protein, and fat. Using an exchange diet, an individual chooses a certain number of items from each food group daily. Because each exchange group includes many different foods, the diet can be quite varied (Table 86.20) (see Appendix Table V-A-25-a to k). Although several methods of dietary instruction are available, exchange nutritional plans are widely used by health professionals. When individuals change healthcare providers, use of a universally understood nutritional plan facilitates communication and continuity of care.

Step-by-Step Guide to Exchange Diet Calculations

1. Estimate energy requirements. The Harris-Benedict equation may be used or an allowance of kilocalories per pound of current body weight. For middle-aged persons, the following approximations apply: sedentary individuals, 10 to 12 kcal/lb is adequate; for moderately active adults, 13 to 15 kcal/lb; and for very active adults, 16 to 20 kcal/lb. For weight reduction, subtract 500 kcal/day for a weight loss of 1 lb/week.
2. Calculate desired energy intake for each macronutrient based on caloric level. If following suggested guidelines, carbohydrate is calculated at 50 to 60% of energy needs, protein at 12 to 15%, and fat at about 30%. For example, with an energy requirement of 1500 kcal: 1500 × 0.55 CHO = 825 kcal from carbohydrate.
3. Convert kilocalories to grams, dividing by the appropriate conversion factors: protein and carbohydrate each have 4 kcal/g; fat has 9 kcal/g. Using the above example: 825 kcal of carbohydrate ÷ 4 kcal/g = 206 g of carbohydrate
4. Exchange lists are readily available for all caloric levels and include variations for individual preferences. However, it is a good idea to tailor each exchange on the basis of individual preferences and eating habits. Compliance is much greater if the diet is based on cultural, ethnic, and personal eating habits. Begin by estimating servings of starch/bread, vegetables, fruit, and milk to meet the carbohydrate goal. Add the meat and meat substitute required to meet the protein goal. Finally, add the fat exchanges. In tailoring personal exchange plans, vegetarian, nondairy, or other dietary preferences can be accounted for.

5. Assign exchanges to the meal/snack plan. Our meal plans routinely include three meals and an evening snack. Most persons taking insulin need midmorning and midafternoon snacks. Distribute energy intake according to the following guidelines. The three main meals should provide at least 65% of energy and snacks up to 35%. Breakfast has 20 to 30%, the noon meal 20 to 35%, and the evening meal 25 to 40% of energy intake. Snacks provide 0 to 15% each at midmorning, midafternoon, and evening. Insulin-treated individuals should be taught how to increase their food intake in response to exercise or hypoglycemia.
6. Finally, calculate the fiber content of the diet. The exchange worksheet diet provides 18 g of fiber from starches/breads, 12 g from vegetables, and 15 g from fruits, for a total of 45 g fiber. These values are based on fiber values developed for the high-carbohydrate, high-fiber (HCF) exchange list (104). This is a generous-fiber meal plan, a goal of approximately 35 g of fiber/day is currently recommended.

Carbohydrate Counting

Carbohydrate counting is an effective method of allowing diabetic patients to obtain needed nutrition while attaining the desired blood glucose values. This approach focuses on carbohydrate intake because carbohydrates have the most significant effect on blood glucose levels (93, 94, 105). Patients with an insulin pump or daily injections of insulin or individuals who desire more choices in food selection are good candidates for this method (94).

There are several methods of carbohydrate counting, each with advantages and disadvantages that would be considered for each individual. The patient should feel comfortable with the math involved and satisfied with the blood glucose levels that result. Carbohydrate counting can involve difficult or simple math; more-complex math allows greater freedom in choosing a food plan (93).

ACKNOWLEDGMENTS

I deeply appreciate the assistance of Kathy Johnson, RD, Meredith Crisp, and Kamara Gray.

REFERENCES

1. Anonymous. Diabetes facts. Alexandria, VA: American Diabetes Association, 1996;1.
2. Anderson JW. Adv Intern Med 1981;26:67–95.
3. Allen FM. JAMA 1914;63:639–43.
4. Geyelin HR. JAMA 1935;104:1203–8.
5. Sansum WD, Blatherwick NR, Bowden R. JAMA 1926;86: 178–81.
6. Kempner W, Peschel RL, Schlayer C. Postgrad Med 1958;24: 359–71.
7. Nutrition Subcommittee of the Professional Advisory Committee of the British Diabetic Association. Diabetic Med 1992;9:189–202.
8. Expert Committee of the Canadian Diabetes Advisory Board. Can Med Assoc J 1992;147:697–712.
9. Anonymous. Diabetes Care 1994;17:519–22.
10. Fajans SS. Definition and classification of diabetes including maturity-onset diabetes of the young. In: LeRoith D, Taylor SI, Olefsky JM, eds. Diabetes mellitus. Philadelphia: Lippincott-Raven, 1996;27:251–60.

10a. 'The Expert Committee on the Diagnosis and Classification of Diabetes Mellitus. Diabetes Care 1997;20:1183–97.

11. Atkinson MA, Maclaren NK. N Engl J Med 1994;331:1428–36.
12. Carter JS, Pugh JA, Monterrosa A. Ann Intern Med 1996; 125:221–32.
13. Bennett PH. Epidemiology of non-insulin-dependent diabetes. In: LeRoith D, Taylor SI, Olefsky JM, eds. Diabetes mellitus. Philadelphia: Lippincott-Raven, 1996;49:455–9.
14. Polonsky KS, Sturis J, Bell GI. N Engl J Med 1996;334:777–83.
15. Salmeron J, Manson JE, Stampfer MJ, et al. JAMA 1997;277: 472–7.
16. Marshall JA, Hamman RF, Baxter J. Am J Epidemiol 1991; 134:590–603.
17. Anderson JW, Geil PB. Nutritional management of diabetes mellitus. In: Shils MW, Olson JA, Shike M, eds. Modern nutrition in health and disease. 8th ed. Philadelphia: Lea & Febiger, 1994;1259–86.
18. LeRoith D, Taylor SI, Olefsky JM. Diabetes mellitus. A fundamental and clinical text. Philadelphia: Lippincott-Raven, 1996.
19. Genuth SM. Diabetes mellitus In: Cahill GF, Jr. ed. Harrison's principles of internal medicine. 9th ed. New York: McGraw-Hill, 1980;873–89.
20. Brodows RG, Williams C, Amatruda JM. JAMA 1984;252: 3378–81.
21. Kitabchi AE, Wall BM. Med Clin North Am 1995;79:9–35.
22. DeFronzo RA, Matsuda M, Barrett EJ. Diabetes Rev 1994;2:209–38.
23. Chait A, Brunzell JD. Adv Intern Med 1991;37:249–73.
24. Nathan DM. N Engl J Med 1993;328:1676–85.
25. Bierman EL. Arteriosc Thromb 1992;12:647–56.
26. Clark CM, Lee DA. N Engl J Med 1995;332:1210–7.
27. The Diabetes Control and Complications Trial Research Group. N Engl J Med 1993;329:977–86.
28. The Diabetes Control and Complications Trial Research Group. Ann Intern Med 1995;122:561–8.
29. Pirart J. Diabetes Metab 1977;3:97–107.
30. Colwell JA. Diabetes Rev 1994;2:277–91.
31. Stout RW. Diabetes Care 1990;13:631–4.
32. Colwell JA, Winocour PD, Lopez-Virella M. Am J Med 1993;75:67–79.
33. Colwell JA, Winocour PD, Holushka PV. Diabetes 1983;35:14–9.
34. Franz M, Kulkarni K, Leontos C, et al. Maximizing the role of nutrition in diabetes management. Alexandria, VA: American Diabetes Association 1994;1.
35. Franz M, Horton ES, Bantle JP, et al. Diabetes Care 1994;17:490–518.
36. Anderson JW, Sim JE, Turner J, Smith BM. Am J Clin Nutr 1998, in press.
37. Anderson JW, Breecher MM. Dr. Anderson's antioxidant, antiaging health program. New York: Carroll & Graf 1996;1.
38. U.S. Department of Agriculture. Nutrition and your health: dietary guidelines for Americans. 3rd ed. Hyattsville, MD: USDA Human Nutrition Information Service 1990;11.
39. U.S. Department of Agriculture. The food guide pyramid. Hyattsville, MD: USDA Human Nutrition Information Service, 1992;1.
40. Wolever TMS, Nguyen P, Chaisson J, et al. Nutr Res 1995;15:843–57.
41. Garg A, Bantle JP, Henry RR, et al. JAMA 1994;271:1421–8.

42. Garg A, Bonanome A, Grundy SM, et al. N Engl J Med 1988;319:829–34.
43. Anderson JW, Gustafson NJ. Dr. Anderson's high fiber fitness plan. Lexington, KY: University Press of Kentucky 1994;1.
44. Anderson JW. Professional guide to high fiber fitness plan. Lexington, KY: HCF Nutrition Fdn 1995;1.
45. American Diabetes Association. Diabetes Care 1987;10: 126–32.
46. Jenkins DJA, Wolever TMS, Taylor RH, et al. Am J Clin Nutr 1981;34:362–6.
47. Foster-Powell K, Miller JB. Am J Clin Nutr 1995;62:871S–93S.
48. Anderson JW, Spencer DO, Riddell-Mason S, et al. Metabolism 1995;44:848–54.
49. Anderson JW. Med Exerc Nutr Health 1993;2:65–8.
50. Zeller K, Whittaker E, Sullivan L, et al. N Engl J Med 1991;324:78–84.
51. Joslin EP. The treatment of diabetes mellitus. 4th ed. Philadephia: Lea & Febiger 1928.
52. Heine RJ, Mulder C, Popp-Snijders C. Am J Clin Nutr 1989;49:448–56.
53. Parillo M, Rivellese AA, Ciardullo AV, et al. Metabolism 1992;41:1373–8.
54. Connor WE. Ann Intern Med 1995;123:950–2.
55. Hendra TJ, Britton ME, Roper DR, et al. Diabetes Care 1990;13:821–9.
56. Trowell HC. Non-infective disease. London: Edward Arnold, 1960.
57. Walker ARP. S Afr Med J 1961;35:114–5.
58. Walker ARP, Walker BF, Richardson BD. Lancet 1970;2:51–2.
59. Trowell HC. Diabetes 1975;24:762–6.
60. Jenkins DJA, Leeds AR, Gassull MA. Lancet 1976;2:172–4.
61. Chapman MJ. J Lipid Res 1980;21:789–853.
62. Anderson JW, Bryant CA. Am J Gastroenterol 1986;81:898–906.
63. Vinik AI, Jenkins DJA. Diabetes Care 1988;11:160–73.
64. O'Dea K, Traianedes K, Ireland P. J Am Diet Assoc 1989;89: 1076–86.
65. Fukagawa NK, Anderson JW, Hageman G, et al. Am J Clin Nutr 1990;52:524–8.
66. Anderson JW, Zeigler JA, Deakins DA, et al. Am J Clin Nutr 1991;54:936–43.
67. DeCosse JJ, Miller H, Lesser ML. J Natl Cancer Inst 1989;81: 1290–7.
68. Anderson JW, Akanji AO. Diabetes Care 1991;14:1126–31.
69. Colwell JA, Bingham SF, Abraira C, et al. J Diabetic Complic 1989;3:191–7.
70. Behall KM, Scholfield DJ, McIvor ME. Diabetes Care 1989;12:357–64.
71. Anderson JW, Gustafson NJ. Diabetes Educ 1989;15:429–34.
72. Anderson JW, Deakins DA, Floore TL, et al. Crit Rev Food Sci Nutr 1990;29:95–147.
73. Anderson JW, Story L, Zettwoch N, et al. Diabetes Care 1989;12:337–44.
74. Cohen N, Halberstam M, Shlimovich P, et al. J Clin Invest 1995;95:2501–9.
75. Anonymous. Diabetes Care 1995;18:83–5.
76. Connell JE, Thomas-Dobersen D. J Am Diet Assoc 1991; 91:1556–64.
77. Ginsberg HN. Diabetes Care 1991;14:839–55.
78. Anonymous. Diabetes Care 1995;18:86–93.
79. Anderson JW, Gustafson NJ. Am J Clin Nutr 1988;48:749–53.
80. Anderson JW, Floore TL, Geil PB, et al. Arch Intern Med 1991;151:1597–602.
81. Anderson JW, Zettwoch N, Feldman T, et al. Arch Intern Med 1988;148:292–6.
82. Anderson JW. Can Med Assoc J 1980;123:975–9.
83. Anderson JW, Story L, Sieling B, Chen WJL. J Can Diet Assoc 1984;45:140–9.
84. Anderson JW, Johnstone BM, Cook-Newell ME. N Engl J Med 1995;333:276–82.
85. Anderson JW, Gowri MS, Turner J, et al. Antioxidant supplementation effects on low-density lipoprotein oxidation for individuals with non-insulin-dependent diabetes mellitus. Submitted for publication.
86. Anderson JW, Hamilton CC, Brinkman-Kaplan V. Am J Gastroenterol 1992;87:6–15.
87. Anderson JW, Brinkman-Kaplan VL, Hamilton CC, et al. Diabetes Care 1994;17:602–4.
88. Henry RR, Gumbiner B. Diabetes Care 1991;24:802–23.
89. Horton ES. Exercise in patients with non-insulin-dependent diabetes mellitus. In: LeRoith D, Taylor SI, Olefsky JM, eds. Diabetes mellitus. 1st ed. Philadelphia: Lippincott-Raven, 1996;71:638–43.
90. Yki-Jarvinen H, et al. N Engl J Med 1992;327:14–26.
91. Anderson JW, Angulo MO. Diabetes mellitus in adults. In: Rakel R, ed. Conn's current therapy. New York: Lea & Febiger, 1994;519–27.
92. Gregory RP, Davis DD. Diabetes Educ 1994;20:406–9.
93. Daly A, Barry B, Gillespie S, et al. Carbohydrate counting: level 1- getting started; level 2-moving on; level 3-using carbohydrate/insulin ratios. Alexandria, VA: American Diabetes Association 1995;11–3.
94. Brackenridge BP, Fredrickson L, Reed C. Counting carbohydrates: how to zero in on good control. Sylmar, CA: MiniMed Technologies 1995;1.
95. DeFronzo RA. Diabetes 1988;37:667–87.
96. Bailey CJ, Turner RC. N Engl J Med 1996;334:574–9.
97. Anderson JW, Siesel AE. Hypocholesterolemic effects of oat products. In: Furda I, Brine CJ, eds. New developments in dietary fiber, physiologic, physicochemical, and analytical aspects. New York: Plenum Press, 1990;17–36.
98. Reaven GM, Johnstone P, Hollenbeck CB, et al. J Clin Endocrinol Metab 1992;74:1020–6.
99. DeFronzo RA, Goodman AM, and Multicenter Metformin Study Group. N Engl J Med 1995;333:541–9.
100. Chaisson J, Josse R, Hunt JA, et al. Ann Intern Med 1994; 121:928–35.
101. Coniff RF, Shapiro JA, Seaton TB. Arch Intern Med 1994;154:2442–8.
102. Nolan JJ, Ludvik B, Beerdsen P, et al. N Engl J Med 1994;331:1188–93.
103. Iwamoto Y, Akanuma Y, Kosaka K, et al. Diabetes Care 1996;19:151–6.
104. Leake DS, Rankin SM. Biochem J 1990;270:741–8.
105. Grunewald KK. J Food Sci 1982;47:2078–9.

SELECTED READING

American Diabetes Association. Nutrition recommendations and principles for people with diabetes mellitus. Diabetes Care 1994;17:519–22.

Anderson JW. Dietary fibre, complex carbohydrate and coronary heart disease. Can J Cardiol 1995;11:55G–62G.

Bierman EL. Atherogenesis in diabetes. Arterioscl Thromb 1992;12:647–56.

Clark CM, Lee DA. Prevention and treatment of complications of diabetes mellitus. N Engl J Med 1995;332:1210–7.

Connell JE, Thomas-Dobersen D. Nutritional management of children and adolescents with insulin-dependent diabetes mellitus:

a review by the Diabetes Care and Education Dietetic Practice Group. J Am Diet Assoc 1991;91:1556–64.

Diabetes Control and Complications Trial Research Group. The effect of intensive treatment of diabetes on the development and progression of long-term complications in insulin-dependent diabetes mellitus. N Engl J Med 1993;329:977–86.

Franz M, Kulkarni K, Leontos C, et al. Maximizing the role on nutrition in diabetes management. 1. Alexandria, VA: American Diabetes Association, 1994;164.

LeRoith D, Taylor SI, Olefsky JM. Diabetes mellitus. A fundamental and clinical text. Philadelphia: Lippencott-Raven, 1996; 1:1–876.

Nathan DM. Long-term complications of diabetes mellitus. N Engl J Med 1993;328:1676–85.

Zeller K, Whittaker E, Sullivan L, et al. Effect of restricting dietary protein on the progression of renal failure in patients with insulin-dependent diabetes mellitus. N Engl J Med 1991;324:78–84.

87. Obesity

F. XAVIER PI-SUNYER

DEFINITION AND CLASSIFICATION

Obesity, characterized by an excess accumulation of fat, is a detriment to good health and well-being. It is easy for individuals to take on excess fat as soon as enough food and leisure are available in a society, because of an imbalance between energy intake and energy expenditure. Although there continues to be disagreement as to which side of this energy equation is more important in the epidemic of obesity, both sides certainly play a role.

Criteria for Weight Normality

A population cannot be precisely divided into normal and obese, because with gradually increasing fat accumulation, there is not a biphasic distribution with a "normal" and an "abnormal" group, nor is there a normal bell-shaped curve of weights in Western industrialized societies. Rather, the curve is skewed to the right, with excess weights trailing out.

Even in a genetically homogenous population, weight is variable. In the modern world, with the great intermixing of ethnic and racial groups, wide genetic heterogeneity exists. The heterogeneity is manifested by differing heights, body circumferences (chest, waist, hips), and heaviness of frame. It is undesirable to focus on a single number of kilograms for height in centimeters as the "normal" weight, particularly because it is not clear what the criterion for "normal" weight should be. Should it be low mortality, low morbidity, a combination of the two, or the longest extended "optimal health" or "well-being" of the individual?

For lack of a better database, life insurance industry statistics have been used widely to develop tables of normality. These tables give weight ranges for height and frame size and are associated with the greatest longevity in individuals who were healthy at the time of initial examination when their height and weight were measured. (See Appendix Table III-A-12-a-1 to 4 for a history of their development and Tables IIIA12b-l for actual tables.)

Although these (Appendix Tables III-A-12-a and b) are some of the best data available, they are inadequate in several ways. They predominantly reflect data from upper-middle-class white groups. They are sex and height specific but not age specific. As such, they provide data on the basis of the predictive longevity of relatively young persons generally weighed in their 20s and 30s and followed to their death. These tables have been used on the assumption that whatever weight is desirable at age 21 years is also desirable at age 45 or 65. Yet, in Western society, weight changes with age in a normal population, gradually increasing in women from 20 to 60 years and more gradually increasing for men from 20 to 50 years, with a fall after that (1). In addition, body composition changes with age, with gradual accretion of fat and loss of lean body mass even if weight remains stable (see Appendix Tables III-A-12-c-1 and 2 and A-15-a–c). It is unclear whether the "normal" weight should be the same as age advances or whether it can rise somewhat as the proportion of body fat increases, so that lean body mass remains as constant as possible.

A classification that is useful clinically is based on two simple measurements: height without shoes and weight with minimal clothing. The weight/height^2 (W/H^2), called the body mass index (BMI), is then calculated, with weight expressed in kilograms and height in meters. The population, whether male or female, can be divided by extent of obesity as follows:

Normal weight	W/H^2	20–24.9
Overweight	W/H^2	25–29.9
Grade I: obesity	W/H^2	30–34.9
Grade II: obesity	W/H^2	35–40
Grade III: severe obesity	W/H^2	>40

The major weakness of the use of W/H^2 (originally proposed by Quetelet in 1871) (2) is that some muscular individuals may be classified as obese when they are not (3). The number of such persons will be small, however. BMI is a relative weight index that shows a reasonable correlation with independent measures of body fat (4). The BMI range of 20 to 24.9, classified as normal, coincides well with the lowest level of mortality derived from life insurance tables. The mortality ratio increases at BMI levels above 25 and more steeply above 27, and it is at this level that health professionals must be concerned (5).

Although the increase in mortality with overweight ($W/H^2 = 25–29.9$) is not great, it is important because it is transitional to obesity grades I to III, which truly create health risks for the individual (5). Data on BMI by percentiles in U.S. males and females aged 1–74 years and a nomograph for estimating BMI are given in Appendix Tables III-A-13-a and b, respectively.

Other Relative Weight Measures

Skinfolds

Over half the fat in the body is deposited under the skin, and the percentage increases with increasing weight. The thickness of this subcutaneous fat can be measured at various sites by using standardized skin calipers. The distribution and amount of subcutaneous fat change with age and are also quite different by sex. One difficulty with skinfold measurement is that there is no agreement on the number and sites that best reflect actual body fat content. Also, an inexperienced or careless observer can easily make large errors, particularly if the patient is too obese.

Data on skinfolds for children have been obtained in cross-sectional population studies and are less reliable than those for adults. Arbitrary definitions of obesity (e.g., 85th percentile and above of weight) have been set (see Appendix Table III-A-18-b-1 to 3). Sex differences in percentage total body fat occur early in life, so that by 5 years of age, different standards are necessary for males and females. In adults, sex differences are marked. Subcutaneous fat is about 11% of body weight in lean men and 18% in women (6). Tables are available for triceps and subscapular percentile distributions for ages 1–74 years (see Appendix Tables III-A-16-a and b and references 7a and 7b).

Because the amount of fat distributed from place to place in the body varies, some investigators have suggested that the sum of skinfolds from different areas better reflects total body fat. For example, Durnin and Womersley (8) derived tables relating the sum of four skinfolds (biceps, triceps, subscapular, and suprailiac) to the fat content of the body. Other sets of skinfold thicknesses have been used to estimate body fat stores (see Appendix Table III-A-17-a to d and Chapters 49 and 56).

Other measurements to estimate body fat and other body compartments are more difficult, expensive, and time consuming and have generally been used for research purposes. These include indirect estimates of body fat by measuring the weight of the fat-free compartment and subtracting this amount from total body weight to derive the weight of fat.

Density

The density of the whole body is derived from the density of the various body components (bone, water, fat, protein), which are all slightly different. It is easier to think of the body as divided into fat and fat-free masses, with fat having a density of 0.900 g/mL and the fat-free mass a density of 1.100 g/mL. Therefore, as the proportion of fat in the body increases, the density decreases. The amount of fat in the body can be determined by measuring the density of the entire body. This requires total submersion of an individual and accurate correction for lung and abdominal air (9).

Tritiated or Deuterated Water

Total body water can be measured by dilution of tritiated (^3H_2O) or deuterated (D_2O) water. Both deuterium and tritium oxides rapidly equilibrate in body water, so the test can be done in 2 to 3 hours. Deuterium is nonradioactive and thus is preferentially used in children and women of childbearing age. Water is then assumed to be a fixed proportion of fat-free mass (FFM); that is, FFM = water mass/0.73. The calculated FFM is subtracted from total body weight to obtain total body fat (10). Alternatively, the naturally occurring ^{40}K in the body can be counted in a whole body counter. Total body ^{40}K can be measured as an index of lean body mass because potassium is present only in the fat-free compartments of the body. ^{40}K makes up 0.012% of the total potassium, and since it is naturally radioactive, it can be detected by a sensitive counter. Using an estimated value for the meq of K in lean body, one can calculate the lean body mass and once again derive total body fat (11) (see also Chapter 49).

Bioelectrical Impedance

Bioelectrical impedance is based on the passage of an electrical current through the body (see Chapter 49). Differing proportions of fat to lean tissue cause differing speeds of transmission of the signal. By appropriate calibration, the transmission can be converted to the proportion of fat and lean tissue in the body (12). This method is not as accurate as hydrodensitometry, total body water, or ^{40}K, but it is cheaper and more convenient and can be used in doctors' offices and for epidemiologic studies.

Inert Gases

The most tedious method for estimating fat uses an inert gas, such as krypton or xenon, which is soluble in fat but poorly soluble in water. The gas must be breathed for several

Table 87.1
Age-Adjusted Percentages of Overweight Persons Aged 20 to 74 Years from the National Health and Nutrition Examination Survey (NHANES) II and the NHANES by Ethnicity and Sex

	Male Overweight (%)	Female Overweight (%)
White	32.0	33.5
Black	31.5	49.6
Mexican	39.5	47.9

From Kuczmarski RJ, Flegal KM, Campbell SM, Johnson CL. JAMA 1994;272:205–11.

hours to allow equilibration with tissues. The proportion of gas retained reflects the amount of fat in the body (13).

PREVALENCE

Standards of Normality

Efforts to produce standards of obesity for the population, against which individuals can be compared, have generally concentrated on weight and have taken two forms. The first is the use of "desirable" weight, that is, weight (stratified for sex, height, and frame size) correlated with the greatest longevity. These weights come from life insurance data. The 1983 tables of the Metropolitan Life Insurance Company (14) are presented in Appendix Tables III-A-12-a-2 and 4. The second is the use of average weights of subsamples of a general population stratified by sex, age, and height. Examples are the Health and Nutrition Examination Survey (NHANES) tables produced by the National Center for Health Statistics in 1960 to 1962 (15), 1971 to 1974 (16), 1976 to 1980 (17), and 1988 to 1991 (18). The data are presented in Appendix Tables III-A-14 (graphs) for infants, children, and adolescents (Appendix Tables III-A-14), youths and adults. The data are given as means and as percentiles.

In these tables, it is necessary to designate a percentile level at which values are considered abnormal. The National Center for Health Statistics defines overweight as a BMI at or above the 85th percentile for the 20- to 30-year-old groups measured in 1960 to 1962 and severe overweight as at or equal to the 95th percentile (17). Appendix Tables III-A-18-a and b provide such graphic and tabular data for ages 1–74 years. Age-adjusted percentages of overweight persons by ethnicity and sex in the United States are shown in Table 87.1.

Two facts are evident from the Metropolitan Life tables and the NHANES tables. First, as a rule, the desirable weights on the insurance tables are lower than the average weights describing the U.S. population, although this is less true of the 1983 Metropolitan Life tables, which were set considerably higher than the 1959 tables (Appendix Table III-A-13-f). Second, the NHANES data show weight increasing by age from 18 years to 54 years, then a plateau, followed by a fall. Thus, in the U.S. population, weight is not static with age once maturity is reached but is actually a function of age.

The insurance companies used the terms *ideal weight* or *desirable weight* to describe weights that actuarially were associated with the least mortality. In subsequent use of these tables, overweight has been defined as 10% above an ideal or desirable weight and obesity as 20% or more above this point. Using such criteria, researchers found a high incidence of overweight in the NHANES survey of 1960 to 1962 (15). Data from the NHANES surveys of 1971 to 1974 and of 1976–1980 show that U.S. adults measured at that time were comparably obese (16, 17). The latest survey available (1988 to 1991), however, found a continuing obesity trend (18). These latest data are shown in Table 87.2 and Figure 87.1.

Figure 87.1 makes clear that an alarming percentage of Americans are overweight. As shown in Table 87.3, this percentage increases with age, particularly among women. What constitutes "healthy weight" at various ages is controversial. It has been suggested that as a person ages, some increase in weight is acceptable and not harmful (19). The NIH geriatrics tables allowed for such an increase (20) (Appendix Table III-A-12-b). The 1990 weight guidelines of the U.S. Departments of Agriculture and Health and Human Services also reflected this point of view (21). However, these more liberal tables have been vigorously attacked as unjustifiably lenient (22). The most recently released recommended dietary allowances from the U.S. Department of Agriculture make no allowance for weight gain with age, and acceptable weight for height is set as a constant for adult life (23).

Obesity in Children

The prevalence of obesity in the Western world begins in infancy. Available studies, though imperfect, suggest that one-third or more infants in the Western industrialized world are too heavy (24–26). Data for schoolchildren are less available, and estimates vary between 6 and 15% (24, 27, 28). Adolescent obesity rates have been calculated

Table 87.2
Age-Adjusted Percentages of Overweight Persons Aged 20 to 74 Years by Race and Sex in the United States

NHANES Survey Years	White				Black			
	'60–'62	'71–'74	'76–'80	'88–'91	'60–'62	'71–'74	'76–'80	'88–'91
Male	23.0	23.8	24.2	32.0	22.1	23.9	26.2	31.8
Female	23.6	24.0	24.4	33.5	41.6	43.1	44.5	49.2

From Kuczmarski RJ, Flegal KM, Campbell SM, Johnson CL. JAMA 1994;272:205–11.

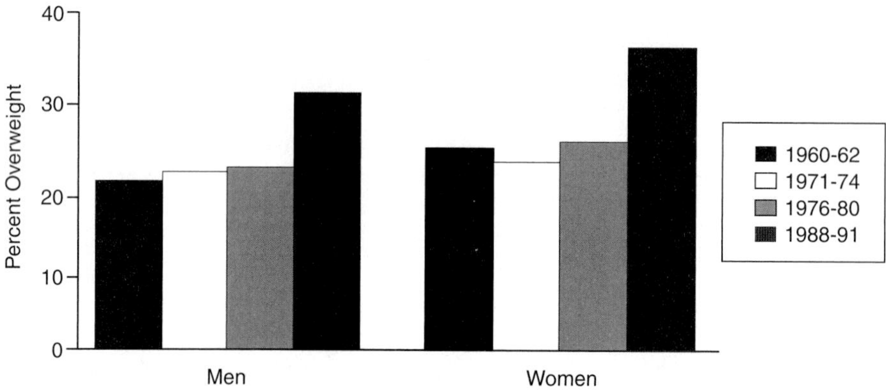

Figure 87.1. Age-adjusted percentages of overweight persons aged 20 to 74 years by sex in the United States. (From Kuczmarski RJ, Flegal KM, Campbell SM, Johnson CL. JAMA 1994;272:205–11.)

at 20 to 30% (26, 28–30). Studies suggest that young women are more likely to be obese than are young men. The most recent national data are shown in Figure 87.2, with comparisons of previous surveys. As in adults, overweight prevalence is increasing in children and adolescents (31) (see also Chapter 63).

Whether childhood obesity leads to obesity in the adult has been widely debated. Some retrospective studies have suggested a direct progression from a fat child to a fat adult (32). Rimm and Rimm report that 50% of adult women in every age group weighing more than 18% of ideal body weight were obese adolescents (33). In addition, it has been stated that 30% of obese adults become obese during childhood. About 80% of obese adolescents become obese adults (34), and they have been reported to be fatter than those who become obese as adults (33). Of obese infants and children, 26.5% were still obese two decades later, compared with the 15% expected by chance (35). The more severe the obesity in childhood, the greater the likelihood of persistence to adulthood (36).

Table 87.3
Unadjusted Age-Specific Prevalence of Overweight and Mean Body Mass Index (BMI), U.S. Population 20 Years of Age or Older, 1988 to 1991[a]

Age (years)	Sample Size	Prevalence of Overweight (SE) %	Mean BMI (SE)
		Men	
20–29	858	20.2 (2.25)	24.9 (0.21)
30–39	759	27.4 (2.28)	26.1 (0.29)
40–49	643	37.0 (2.73)	27.3 (0.36)
50–59	493	42.1 (2.05)	27.6 (0.16)
60–69	588	42.2 (2.84)	26.9 (0.22)
70–79	495	35.9 (3.06)	26.5 (0.29)
≥80	373	18.0 (2.24)	24.7 (0.24)
		Women	
20–29	755	20.2 (2.17)	24.1 (0.29)
30–39	771	34.3 (2.46)	26.4 (0.39)
40–49	624	37.6 (2.70)	26.7 (0.29)
50–59	464	52.0 (2.53)	28.5 (0.41)
60–69	595	42.5 (2.43)	27.3 (0.27)
70–79	446	37.2 (2.57)	26.7 (0.29)
≥80	396	26.2 (2.11)	24.6 (0.23)

From Kuczmarski RJ, Flegal KM, Campbell SM, Johnson CL. JAMA 1994;272:205–11.
[a]Pregnant women excluded.

Socioeconomic Influence

Epidemiologic studies have shown a strong association between socioeconomic status and the prevalence of obesity. This relationship is much stronger in women. The effect of social environment on obesity was investigated many years ago in the "Midtown Manhattan Study," which in 1965 studied a population with both high- and low-income groups. Socioeconomic status and the prevalence of obesity were found to be inversely related (37). As many as 30% of women of lower socioeconomic class were obese, 16% of middle-status women, and 5% of upper status. Men showed similar but less exaggerated trends. Similar socioeconomic trends have been found in other countries (38, 39). In the Manhattan study, obesity was also related to ethnicity (40), with Eastern Europeans being particularly heavy. Others have also found ethnicity to be an important variable (41). Religious affiliation was also important (42).

In the NHANES data, persons below the poverty line have a significantly greater prevalence of obesity (43). Although a relationship exists in the United States between increasing prevalence of obesity and socioeconomic status, it is not all clear-cut. For example, an English study showed a low prevalence of overweight in males of lower socioeconomic status engaged in heavy manual labor (44).

Race also affects obesity. The prevalence of overweight in whites, blacks, and Mexican Americans in the United States is shown in Figure 87.3. Mexican American men and both black and Mexican American women have higher prevalences of overweight (17). The reason for these findings is not presently evident, though it is thought to be partly socioeconomic, partly cultural, and possibly partly genetic.

MORTALITY AND MORBIDITY

Overweight has been associated with excess mortality in many studies (45–49). Table 87.4 summarizes mortality data

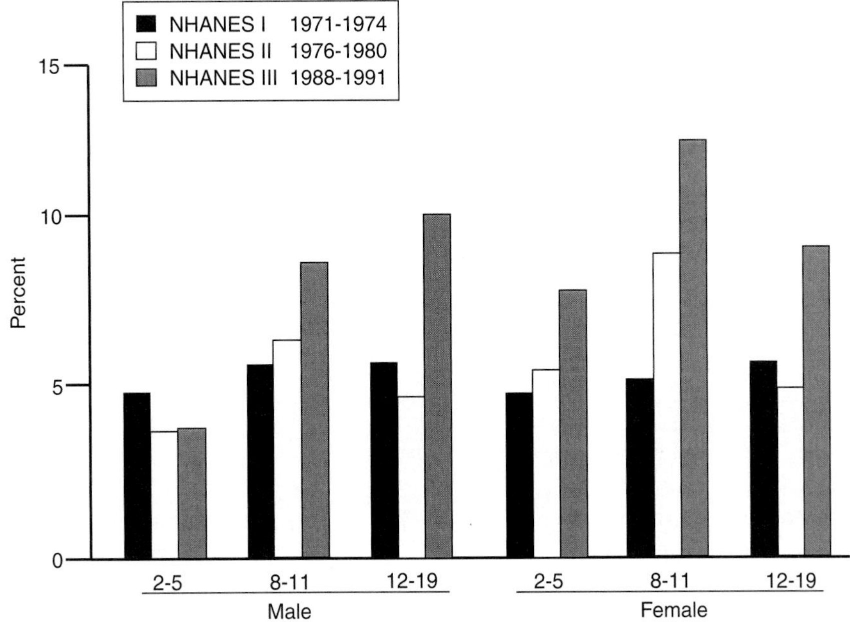

Figure 87.2. Overweight prevalence in American children and adolescents over time. (From MMWR 1997;46:198–202.)

for three such studies: the Build and Blood Pressure Study of 1959 (47), the Build and Blood Pressure Study of 1979 (48), and the American Cancer Society study (49). All three studies show increasing mortality with increasing overweight, with higher mortality risks in men than in women.

The American Cancer Society study, which was not an insurance study, counteracts the objection that it is not valid to relate weight at insurance to death some 35 years afterward because insured lives are not typical of the general population, as insured individuals tend to be richer and predominantly white. The American Cancer Society data are similar to the insured data, and they help validate the use of actuarial data of insured lives. Because insurance companies relate only to healthy persons, their data generally exclude ill people. On the other hand, the American Cancer Society study in all likelihood overstated the mortality of underweight persons, because it only lasted 12 years, and the general population it studied no doubt included some persons with illness and unintentional weight loss that could have caused early death.

The mortality rate increase is not linear with increasing weight. Accelerated mortality occurs as people get heavier, particularly males (50). In addition, in the insurance data, the relative mortality is higher in males who are overweight than in females, whereas this is not so in the general population, as reflected by the American Cancer Society study. Many studies do not show increased risk of mortality at relative weights up to 20% above desirable

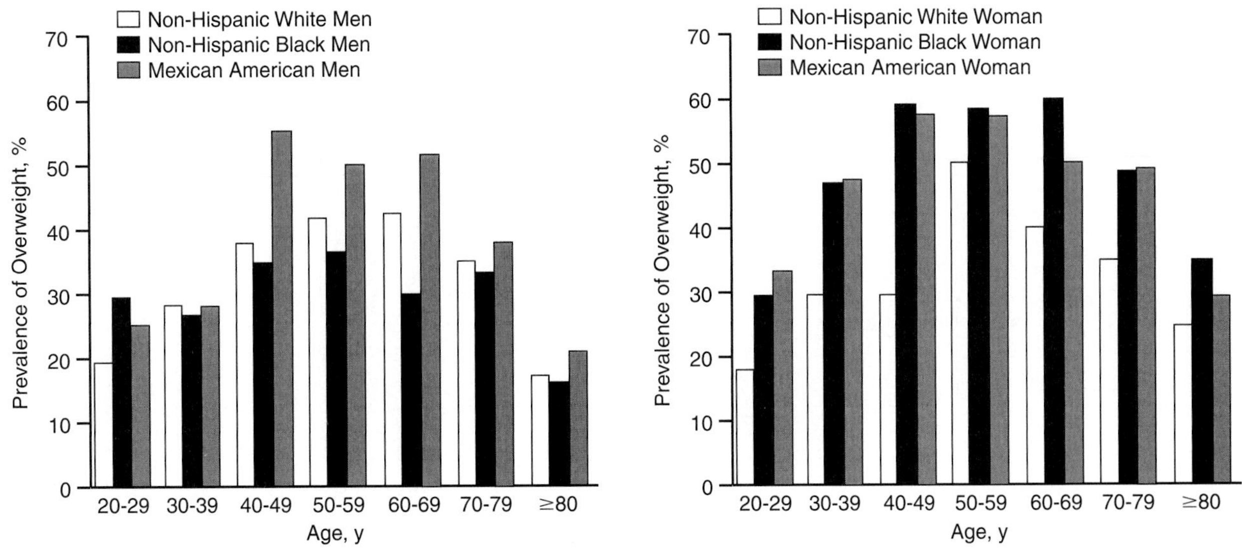

Figure 87.3. Prevalence of overweight by age and race/ethnicity for men and women, U.S. population 20 years of age and older, 1988–1991. (From Kuczmarski RJ, Flegal KM, Campbell SM, Johnson CL. JAMA 1994;272:205–11.)

Table 87.4
Mortality Ratios According to Variations in Weight[a]

	Build and Blood Pressure Study 1959		American Cancer Society Study		Build and Blood Pressure 1979	
Weight Group	Male	Female	Male	Female	Male	Female
20% Underweight	95	87	110	110	105	110
10% Underweight	90	89	100	95	94	97
10% Overweight	113	109	107	108	111	107
20% Overweight	125	121	121	123	120	110
30% Overweight	142	130	137	138	135	125
40% Overweight	167		162	163	153	136
50% Overweight	200		210		177	149
60% Overweight	250				210	167

From Van Itallie TB. Am J Clin Nutr 1979;32:2723–33, with permission of the American Society for Clinical Nutrition.
[a]Each study measured departures from its own set of average weights, where mortality would be 100.

level (50–54). In the extensive Norwegian study, which took weights and heights in a large proportion of the population between 1963 and 1975, relative mortality increased as the BMI increased above 27 (55). The so-called J-curve of mortality in relation to BMI is shown in Figure 87.4 (56).

Evidence exists that the relationship between weight and mortality differs at different times of life. The Whitehall study of 18,000 English civil servants showed that the relationship between weight quintile and mortality changes with age; for the youngest men, coronary heart disease (CHD) mortality increases linearly from lowest weight quintile to highest, whereas no relationship is evident for the oldest men (57). Other studies have investigated the relationship of weight and mortality in the elderly. All seem to agree on a protective effect of moderately increased weight in old age (58–60).

The relationship of obesity and mortality may be obscured by the fact that fatness may relate to the type of death as well as to overall mortality. That is, with increasing obesity, individuals are at greater risk of death from cardiovascular disease and diabetes but not from cancer (61). Thus, it may not be possible to assign a single optimum weight or an optimum level of fatness. There may be "different optima for different causes of death at different time periods and . . . no single value of weight or fatness is optimal for all" (62).

Causes of Death and Morbidity

The causes of death in men 20 and 40% above average weight as derived from the data of the American Cancer Society study (49) and the Build Study of 1979 (48) are shown in Table 87.5.

Cardiovascular Disease

Prospective studies of cardiovascular morbidity and mortality have shown an association with obesity. Studies that control for smoking show lowest mortality in the leanest weight category (63–66). The effect of obesity on cardiovascular disease has not always been independent but has generally involved exacerbation of other risk (64) such as hypertension, diabetes, and dyslipidemia (65). This finding is not surprising because blood pressure, blood

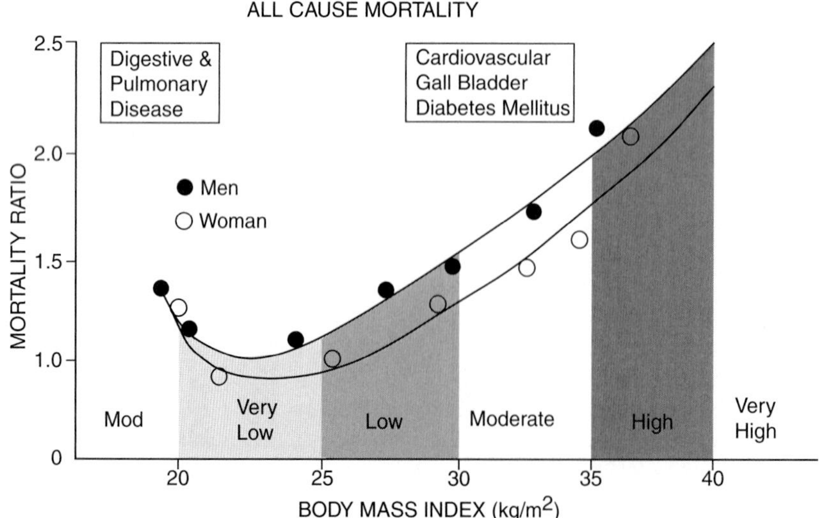

Figure 87.4. J-Curve of mortality.

Table 87.5
Mortality Ratios (Factor of Increased Risk)[a]

	Men 20% above Average Weight		Men 40% above Average Weight	
Cause of Death	Build Study 1979	American Cancer Society	Build Study 1979	American Cancer Society
Coronary heart disease	118	128	169	175
Cerebral "hemorrhage" (stroke)	110	116	164	191
Cancer	100	105	105	124
Diabetes	250	210	500	300
Digestive diseases	125	168	220	340
All causes	120	121	150	162

From Van Itallie TB. Am J Clin Nutr 1979;32:2723–33, with permission of the American Society for Clinical Nutrition.

[a]Each study measured departures from its own set of average weights, where mortality would be 100.

lipids, and glucose values increase when individuals gain substantial amounts of weight (67). The predictable increase in cardiovascular risk factors by increasing weight was well quantified in the Framingham study. For every 10% rise in relative weight, systolic blood pressure rises 6.5 mm, plasma cholesterol rises 12 mg/dL, and fasting blood glucose rises 2 mg/dL (68). Although the association of these cardiovascular risk factors is not as strong in women as in men, the association of obesity to cardiovascular disease is as strong in women as in men. The Nurses Health Study (66) showed this clearly.

Evidence indicates that obesity that occurs at an earlier age (20–40 years) has a greater influence on cardiovascular disease than later-onset obesity (69). The Manitoba Study, which compared the 26-year incidence of CHD and had a young average entry age of 30.8 years, found that BMI was significantly related to CHD (70). Myocardial infarction, sudden death, and coronary insufficiency were all associated with a high BMI. This association was not evident until the 10th year of follow-up. This was also true in the Framingham study, in which the effect of obesity on cardiovascular mortality increased with time of follow-up (71). Thus, short-term studies or studies concentrating on older individuals may not show an independent effect of obesity because they are too short or have not focused on the correct age group.

Finding a relationship between obesity and increased mortality at a young age (<40 years of age) and no such relationship at an older age implies that it is continuous obesity over many years that affects health and can lead to death. Moreover, as people grow older, other risk factors for death take on increased importance.

Studies by Chapman et al. using ponderal index ($W^{0.33}/H$) as a measure of obesity found a higher rate of myocardial infarction in men under age 40 and not in those older (72). In the Whitehall study, 10-year CHD mortality increased from the lowest- to the highest-weight quintiles for younger men but showed no effect of weight in older men (57). In addition, the effect of weight is small when blood pressure, cholesterol, and smoking are accounted for. For older men, the highest mortality is in the lowest weight quintile.

Numerous studies now show that the pattern of body fat distribution affects morbidity and mortality from cardiovascular diseases (73–76). In fact, this risk factor is as important as smoking, hypertension, and hypercholesterolemia (77). The effect is more important at younger ages and tends to lose importance after the seventh decade (77).

Blood Lipids

Triglycerides. Although hypertriglyceridemia has been associated with obesity (78), the association is not strong. Triglycerides are transported predominantly as very low density lipoproteins (VLDLs) (79). Hypertriglyceridemia may be related to the insulin resistance and consequent hyperinsulinemia of obesity (80), which increases hepatic triglyceride synthesis and secretion (79, 81). In addition, because free fatty acid (FFA) levels are raised in obesity, the increased hepatic uptake of FFA may increase the rate of triglyceride secretion (82). Enhanced triglyceride production may also come from more glucose precursors extracted by the liver (82). Despite this increased triglyceride production, the triglyceride level in obese persons is often normal or only slightly elevated. Because lipoprotein lipase activity is elevated in obesity (83) and rises higher after weight loss (84, 85), it is possible that this activity enhances VLDL clearance at the periphery. After weight reduction, plasma triglycerides that were high tend to fall (79). This change is associated with decreased VLDL-triglyceride production and decreased insulinemia (79). In families carrying the combined hyperlipidemia trait, obese relatives tend to manifest high levels of VLDL, whereas nonobese relatives show elevated low-density lipoproteins (LDLs) (86).

Cholesterol. Much less evidence exists of cholesterol elevation in obesity. Only marginally significant correlations have been shown (87, 88). High-density lipoprotein (HDL) cholesterol is usually low in obesity, and because of this, the LDL:HDL ratio is elevated, which enhances the risk of CHD. Low HDL-cholesterol concentrations are a risk factor for CHD, independent of the concentration of LDL-cholesterol (89, 90).

While LDL-cholesterol levels may be normal, the quality of the particles is different. Persons with insulin resistance tend to have small dense LDL particles (91, 92), which are considerably more atherogenic than larger particles, enhancing CHD risk (93, 94).

Diabetes Mellitus

A strong association exists between obesity and diabetes mellitus. In fact, obesity can be considered the most important "environmental" determinant in the manifestation of diabetes. In epidemiologic studies including many geographic areas, races, and cultures, West and Kalbfkeisch noted a marked correlation between prevalence of diabetes and overweight (95). This has also been shown in other, more recent studies (96). Even moderate obesity can raise the risk of diabetes tenfold (96). In the Framingham study, women in the upper quintile of weight were four times as likely to develop glucose intolerance as women in the lower quintile (97). In the Nurses Study (98), in which the nurses have been followed for 16 years, there is a gradually increasing risk with increasing BMI as shown in Figure 87.5. Also, the gain from baseline is important, with increased risk for the same amount of weight gain as baseline BMI increases (98).

Body fat distribution has been implicated as a predictor of glucose intolerance and hyperinsulinemia (99–103). It is also a predictor of frank diabetes (104, 105). Why the abdominal area is related to metabolic disturbance while the thigh area is not is unclear. This increased risk with abdominal fat suggests that a "male" pattern of fat distribution poses a greater risk for diabetes than a "female" pattern. The important factor is intraabdominal or visceral obesity (106). Possibly, visceral fat is more lipolytic, delivering more FFAs to the liver in a setting of high glycerol and insulin levels which make for enhanced VLDL production, small dense LDL particles, decreased HDL production, and enhanced gluconeogenesis (107, 108).

Hyperinsulinemia and Insulin Resistance. Obesity is associated with hyperinsulinemia (109); in general, the fatter an individual, the higher the basal or fasting insulin level (80). In addition, in nondiabetics, the height of the insulin response to glucose or other stimuli is related to basal insulin and therefore is closely correlated with the degree of obesity (80). In obese subjects with abnormal glucose tolerance, however, the percentage increase of insulin over basal values is actually lower than that of lean subjects. Thus, the impairment of glucose disposal can often be explained by an accompanying impairment of insulin secretion. This impairment is first observed in the early phase of insulin response, but as carbohydrate tolerance deteriorates, the entire time course of the insulin response is affected.

The phenomenon of excessive blood insulin levels in obesity, both basal and after stimuli, demonstrates that insulin resistance or insensitivity is present. This is manifested by tissue resistance at the muscle and liver level, decreasing glucose uptake at the periphery and increasing hepatic glucose output (110, 111); adipose tissue sensitivity remains high, and possibly nutrients are thus shunted to this tissue for storage (111).

Insulin Receptor and Postreceptor Defects. The first step in the action of insulin on the cell is the binding of the hormone to a specific receptor on the outer plasma membrane (see also Chapters 37 and 44). This process then initiates a series of "postreceptor" biochemical events such as glucose and amino acid transport, stimulation of protein synthesis, activation of certain enzymes, inhibition of others, stimulation of certain gene transcription, and inhibition of others (112). Generally, when high levels of insulin prevail in the blood, low levels of insulin receptors are present. This self-regulation of the membrane insulin receptor, so that high insulin levels cause a lowering of insulin receptor number, is called downregulation (113). It now seems clear that cells of insulin-sensitive tissues (e.g., fat and muscle) from obese humans present a decreased number of insulin receptors at the surface cell

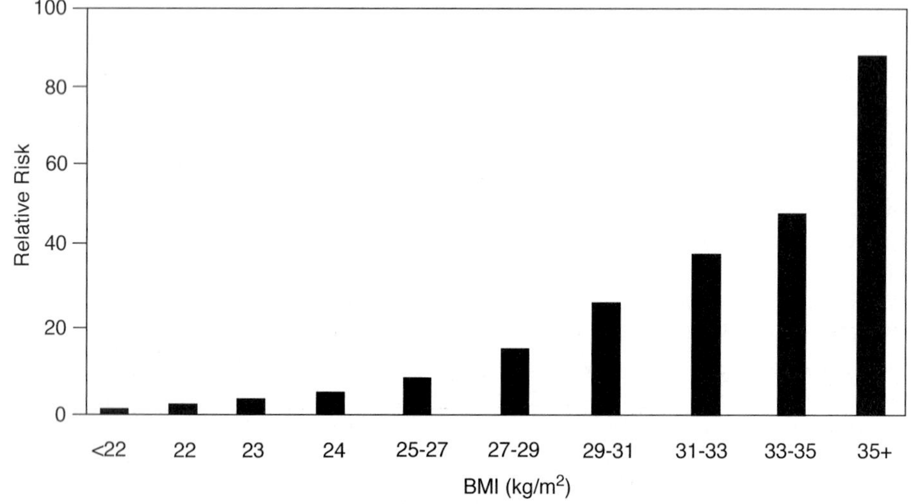

Figure 87.5. Risk of NIDDM using BMI (Nurses Study). (From Colditz GA, Willett WC, Rotnitzky A, et al. Ann Intern Med 1995;122:481–6, with permission.)

membrane (114, 115). Although part of the insulin resistance in obesity can be attributed to changes in insulin receptor number and/or receptor affinity for insulin, the tissues of obese animal models show intracellular postreceptor defects in glucose metabolism that account for the major part of insulin resistance.

In obese humans, the degree of insulin resistance is much greater than that predicted from the magnitude of the decrease of insulin receptors. Using the euglycemic glucose clamp technique, researchers can study in vivo insulin dose-response curves. The least hyperinsulinemic, least insulin-resistant patients show only a receptor defect, whereas the most hyperinsulinemic show the largest postreceptor defect. The nature of the postreceptor defect is being actively investigated. The β subunit of the receptor, which faces inward, when stimulated by insulin, expresses kinase activity toward its tyrosine residues (116, 117). This tyrosine phosphorylation is faulty, causing defective signaling within the cell. The postreceptor defect could also be due to an abnormality in the glucose transporter system within the affected cells. Because levels of glucose transporter protein and mRNA are normal in skeletal muscle cells of insulin-resistant persons, the defect may rest in the functional activity or insulin-mediated translocation of the transporters (118), although thus far this has not been satisfactorily documented (see also Chapter 37).

Significance of Hyperinsulinemia. Production of excessive quantities of insulin for a prolonged period may lead to pancreatic exhaustion in those who are genetically predisposed (119). Eventually, insulin response can decrease to the point of metabolic decompensation (120). Support for this position comes from data suggesting that the duration of obesity rather than the degree is best correlated with carbohydrate intolerance in obese adults.

Hypertension

Blood pressure elevation is a common concomitant of obesity (121–123). The causes of the association of obesity and hypertension are not clear. A relationship between weight gain and increased blood pressure is well documented (124, 125). In hypertensive patients, weight reduction reduces blood pressure (126–128), and weight regain raises pressure. The fall in blood pressure with weight reduction is associated with decreased blood volume, cardiac output, and sympathetic activity (129).

The cardiac output and the peripheral vascular resistance are the most important determinants of the blood pressure. These, in turn, are affected by the total body sodium content and by neurohumoral factors. Data of Dahl et al. incriminated sodium loss rather than weight loss as the cause of lowered blood pressure with caloric restriction (130). Others, however, have reported that it is weight reduction that is important (131).

Insulin may play a role in the hypertension of obesity (132), because changes in the plasma insulin concentration can affect sodium transport in the human kidney (133). Insulin reduces sodium excretion independent of changes in plasma glucose. This effect can be noted without concurrent changes in filtered load of glucose, glomerular filtration rate, renal blood flow, and plasma aldosterone levels (134). Natriuresis occurs during fasting or hypocaloric diets, when insulin levels fall, and antinatriuresis occurs with refeeding, when insulin levels rise again (135). The hyperinsulinemia of obesity may raise the blood pressure by increasing renal sodium absorption, which in turn expands the extracellular fluid volume, raising cardiac output, peripheral resistance, and blood pressure (132). Whether catecholamines play a role in the hypertension of obesity is unclear, although Landsberg and Young reported decreased sympathetic nervous system activity during weight loss diets and an increase during refeeding (136).

The distribution of fat in the body may have an important effect on blood pressure risk, as it does in diabetes, with central fat or upper body fat being more likely to raise blood pressure than the lower body fat of the gluteal and thigh region (103, 137, 138). The reasons for this tendency are not clear, although it is now known that insulin resistance is associated with hypertension (139) and may actually be important in the etiology (140).

Respiratory Problems

As an individual becomes more obese, the muscular work required for ventilation increases. If movement of the chest wall is limited enough, CO_2 retention occurs, which can lead to lethargy and somnolence. CO_2 narcosis can also lead to periods of apnea that usually occur during sleep and exacerbate the problem of CO_2 retention (141). In addition, polycythemia may occur, which can enhance thrombosis. In severe cases of respiratory disease, pulmonary hypertension, cardiac enlargement, and congestive heart failure may develop.

Gallbladder Disease

The risk for gallbladder disease rises as obesity in creases and is greater for women than for men (142–146). An increased body fat reservoir is associated with certain conditions that predispose individuals to gallstone formation. There is a supersaturation of the cholesterol in bile (147, 148) and increased biliary cholesterol excretion (149). Hypomotility of the gallbladder also occurs, allowing pooling and nucleation of stones (150). As a result, cholesterol stone formation is enhanced (151).

Arthritis

The clinical impression is that the incidence of osteoarthritis of the weight-bearing joints is higher in obese than in lean persons and that this condition tends to become worse with higher weight (152). No good prevalence studies are available, however.

Gout

The cause for the rise in uric acid levels with increasing weight is unclear. The effect is more common in men than women; thus, body fat distribution may play a role. Usually, this uric acid elevation is asymptomatic, but the occurrence of gouty attacks is higher in obese than in lean individuals, particularly when overweight reaches 30% above ideal.

Cancer

Obesity has been implicated as a risk factor in development of certain cancers. In a large prospective study, mortality ratios for cancer in persons who were more than 40% overweight were 1.33 for men and 1.55 for women (153). In men, the higher mortality was for colorectal and prostate cancer, and in women, for endometrial, gallbladder, cervical, ovarian, and breast cancers (153). Cancer of the endometrium has been particularly implicated (154–156). Cancer of the gall bladder also increases with increasing obesity. It is possible that this association is related to endocrine abnormalities, and increased conversion of estrone to androstenedione in adipose tissue has been implicated. In addition, obesity is correlated with increasing estrogenicity of cervical smears (157). Although such increased estrogen activity could cause the increased risk of breast cancer reported in postmenopausal women (158–161), no proof of this effect is available. The increased cancer risk may be related to a dietary component rather than the obesity per se.

GENETICS AND ENVIRONMENT

Genetics

In the last few years, a great deal has been learned about the genetics of animal models of obesity, and this has lent strength to the proposition that human obesity is to a large extent genetically determined. The *ob/ob* mouse was the first rodent model of obesity whose genetic defect was clarified, and the gene for the *ob* protein, leptin, was cloned (162). Two different mutations were identified in the *ob* gene of the *ob/ob* mouse, either of which produced a deficient, truncated, inactive leptin or no leptin at all. If *ob/ob* animals are injected with normal leptin, food intake drops, thermogenesis increases, and weight decreases (163–165). The leptin gene is primarily expressed in fat cells. As fat cells enlarge, they secrete more leptin. Thus, this hormone appears to be a signal of fat surfeit that communicates with the central nervous system to decrease food intake and enhance thermogenesis. The receptor for leptin has also been cloned (166).

The *db/db* mouse has a defective leptin receptor (167). This mouse has high circulating levels of leptin (168) and does not respond to injections of leptin (164). The *fa/fa* rat, like the *db/db* mouse, has a defective receptor that does not respond to high levels of normal leptin (169).

The yellow agouti mouse, which develops obesity, has a defective gene that produces an abnormal 108–amino acid protein, which in turn antagonizes the melanocortin-4 receptor (MC4-R) in the hypothalamus (170). One possible effect of losing MC4-R activity is a disturbance of hypothalamic signaling. This could, for instance, stimulate release of either neuropeptide Y or galanin, both of which stimulate food intake.

Other models of obesity are the *tub/tub* mouse, which has a defective phosphodiesterase, and the *fat/fat* mouse, which has a defective carboxypeptidase E, preventing appropriate conversion of a large number of prohormones to the active hormones. The exact mechanisms by which these defects cause obesity require further investigation. These animal models and their genetic defects are shown in Table 87.6.

Identification and cloning of the genes for these animal models have generated great interest in the genetics of human obesity. The relationship of these one-gene defects in animal models of obesity to human obesity is not clear. However, very recently, two obese persons, an adult and a child, have been found to be leptin deficient (171). These are the first descriptions of one-gene defects in humans. In general, obese humans demonstrate high circulating levels of leptin (172, 173) and normal leptin receptors (174). Thus, if a defect is present in obese persons with regard to leptin, it must be beyond the leptin receptor in a postreceptor signaling process. Neuropeptide Y has been suggested as the possible substance not adequately suppressed by leptin (175) (see also Chapters 37 and 40). Whether this will be borne out requires further investigation. Clinical trials of leptin in humans are under way but have not yet been completed, so the effect of leptin injection on body weight is not yet known.

Environmental Influences

The role of inherited factors in the origin of obesity is not well defined. Whereas clear genetic effects exist, they are modified by environmental and behavioral factors. Twin studies have been pursued to try to determine the relative importance of genetic inheritance and environmental influences in obesity. The weights of identical twins

Table 87.6
Molecular Genetics–Molecular Biologic Techniques

Rodent Obesity Mutations[a]	Gene	Inheritance	Chromosome Location	Human Syntenic Region
Mouse				
yellow	A^y	AD	2	20q11
diabetes	*db*	AR	4	1p31
fat	*fat*	AR	8	?16p
obese	*ob*	AR	6	7q31
tubby	*tub*	AR	7	11p15
Rat				
fatty	*fa*	AR	5	1p31
	fa^{cp}			

[a]Mouse and rat obesity mutations are indicated as well as their mode of inheritance (AR, autosomal recessive; AD, autosomal dominant), chromosome location, and corresponding syntenic chromosomal regions in the human genome.

raised in separate homes have been reported to be similar (176), suggesting that heredity contributes significantly to weight. Although Newman et al. showed a greater difference in twins raised apart than in twins raised together (implicating environment), they also found that fraternal twins raised apart showed a greater weight difference than did identical twins, suggesting a strong genetic component (177). Studies of twins by Stunkard et al. reinforce the importance of heredity (178, 179). Using a model of path analysis, Bouchard studied BMI and reported a total transmissible variance across generations of about 35% but a genetic effect of only 5% (180). The response to overfeeding in a group of pairs of identical twins has been studied. The intrapair resemblance was high, and the resemblance between pairs varied much more (181). Thus, the genotype seems important with regard to weight gain during overfeeding. The heritability of body fat distribution, particularly of central or visceral fat, has also been studied (166). The abdominal depot is also determined partly by genotype (182).

The Ten-State Nutrition Study suggests that environmental factors may be most important in the obesity found in families. Skinfold thicknesses were compared in 429 adoptive parent-child pairs and in 198 genetically unrelated siblings. In addition, 6372 pairs of biologic parent-child pairs and 3713 biologic pairs of siblings were measured. No difference was found between the correlations for biologic sibling pairs and those of genetically unrelated siblings (183). In addition, the correlations in skinfolds between parents and children were high (184). When parents were classified as lean, medium, or obese and various mother-father combinations (lean-lean, lean-obese, obese-lean, obese-obese) were examined, the children were fatter as the parents increased in fatness. This latter finding, however, does not prove a genetic risk; food may be more plentiful in households with fatter parents and result in fatter children.

Studying adoptive parent-child pairs, Withers could find no evidence that the correlation of fatness between a parent and an adopted child differed from that between a parent and a biologic child (185). However, Biron et al. (186) studied 374 families with one or more adopted children and found no correlation in weight between adopted children and their adoptive parents and siblings. Common environment seems to have less influence as children grow older. Rao et al., studying 1068 families in Brazil, found that the influence of shared family environment on weight could account for only 18% of the variance (187). Thus, the relative importance of genetics and environment on weight remains unclear.

PATHOGENESIS

Endocrinopathy in Obesity

Although obesity is popularly ascribed to glandular troubles, endocrinopathy is actually a rare cause of obesity. Overactivity of the adrenal gland, leading to Cushing's syndrome, causes central obesity. Why adipocytes located at the center of the body are stimulated to multiply and fill in this condition while those at the extremities are not is unclear. The central obesity is associated with hypertension and diabetes.

In severe hypothyroidism, some increased adipose mass may occur, but most of the increased weight is water. Few obese patients suffer from hypothyroidism.

Hypogonadism is sometimes associated with mild obesity, although the reason is not clear. Women with polycystic ovarian syndrome (PCOS) are generally overweight. Although the origin of this syndrome is unclear, investigators have documented that the ovaries are the major source of androgens in PCOS (188). Not only are excess androgens produced, but in obesity, sex hormone–binding globulin is decreased (189), so less androgen is bound. These women have significant insulin resistance (188). The relationship between increased androgens and insulin resistance is not clear.

A hypothalamic lesion caused by tumor, infection, or, rarely, trauma may lead to obesity (190). This is secondary to damage to nerve fibers coursing through the ventromedial area that are important in food intake regulation.

In children, obesity may be seen with certain congenital syndromes, but its cause is unknown. The syndromes include Prader-Willi syndrome, Laurence-Moon-Biedl syndrome, adiposogenital dystrophy (Fröhlich's syndrome), Bongiovanni-Eisenmenger syndrome, and pseudohypoparathyroidism.

Whereas the cause of obesity is seldom a hormonal abnormality, obesity may lead to abnormal hormone levels (191). Owing to the development of insulin resistance, insulin levels in the blood rise, as discussed above. Triiodothyronine (T_3) rises in conditions of high caloric intake with adequate carbohydrate (though not to abnormal levels). Thyroxine levels are normal. Urinary excretion of free cortisol and hydroxycorticoids, sometimes elevated in obesity, is probably related to increased cortisol turnover. These changes are related to the higher lean body mass in the obese. Blood cortisol levels are usually in the normal range in obesity, and diurnal patterns are generally normal. Growth hormone levels are in the low-normal range. Stimulatory tests with arginine, insulin hypoglycemia, or L-dopa demonstrate a poor growth hormone response, which reverts toward normal with weight loss.

Food Intake

Food intake regulation, while investigated for many years, is still very incompletely understood. There are clear internal and external controllers, which interrelate in a very complex manner. It has long been postulated that signals from the periphery are monitored by hypothalamic centers and create a feedback loop for body weight regulation (192, 193). Whether these signals relate to weight, fat, lean body mass, or some other marker has been the object of much debate. After food intake, satiety signals have been divided into preabsorptive and postabsorptive. Preabsorptive signals are probably responsible for cessation of eating after a single meal. Many preabsorptive signals of satiety have been proposed, and highest in rank are the gut peptides (194). The most documented of these is cholecystokinin (195). Others are bombesin, glucagon, and glucagon-like peptide 1. These hormones are released from the gut and pancreas after eating. How they signal the brain is not clear, but some may do so through the afferent branch of the vagus nerve.

Longer-range signals of satiety may be related to fat burden. Leptin is an example of such a signal. While its exact mechanism of action is unclear, secretion of this hormone from fat cells increases as fat cell size increases, and the leptin in some fashion signals the brain to decrease food intake and increase thermogenesis. Other long-range signals may monitor other aspects of body composition.

The central nervous system network that turns food intake on and off is very complicated (see Chapter 40). Neuropeptide Y is a powerful stimulator of eating, galanin also stimulates but is more macronutrient specific, while corticotropin-releasing factor and cholecystokinin inhibit (196–200). Dopaminergic, noradrenergic, and serotoninergic neurotransmission is also involved. How all these substances and others work in concert to create a coherent regulatory pattern is unknown.

Thermogenesis

Obese individuals have been described as using energy calories more "efficiently" than lean subjects. They have been characterized as requiring fewer calories per unit of lean body mass. If they take in the same number of calories as a lean subject, more of the calories are available as extra energy to be deposited as fat. Whether this phenomenon is important is unsettled. The expenditure of energy takes three forms: basal metabolic rate (BMR), activity, and the thermic effect of food.

Basal Metabolic Rate

The BMR is that energy required for the basic maintenance of the cells of the body and body temperature. In most sedentary adults, the BMR makes up about 60 to 70% of total energy expenditure (201). Fat-free mass, fat mass, sex, and age explain about 80% of the variance in BMR (202). Because the metabolic rate is defined primarily by the cell mass of the body, it is reasonable to express it in terms of the lean body mass (LBM). The contribution of the LBM to the BMR is much greater per kilogram than that of body fat (203, 204). The correlation of BMR with LBM explains why men with a higher LBM have higher metabolic rates than women and why metabolic rates decrease with age. The high metabolic rate of children can be ascribed to the energy cost of growth (205, 206).

However, metabolic rates differ in individuals matched for age, sex, and LBM (207). These differences can be as high as 30%. As a result, at a given fixed intake per kilogram of LBM, one individual may gain weight while another does not. Thus, different people maintain weight on different caloric intakes.

The BMR of obese persons is higher than that of lean individuals (208, 209). Since obese people have a higher LBM than lean people, this finding is not surprising. The obese often have a lower BMR than lean individuals if it is expressed per kilogram of body weight. This finding is reasonable because per unit of weight, they have relatively less metabolizing cell mass. If one expresses BMR as total energy expended per unit time, the obese expend more calories than lean people. Individuals with a low relative metabolic rate are at risk for gaining weight and becoming obese (210–212). Further studies are necessary to confirm this interesting phenomenon that suggests one mechanism by which individuals may be gaining weight. Moreover, a high 24-hour respiratory quotient (an index of carbohydrate/fat oxidation) has been shown to predict weight gain (213), and insulin resistance has predicted a low rate of weight gain (214).

Thermic Effect of Food

The rise of metabolic rate above basal level after eating has been called the thermic effect of food (TEF). About 10% of absorbed nutrients are lost as heat, which is created in intermediary metabolism of substrates, in the use of ATP, and in formation of ATP from reduced coenzymes by oxidative phosphorylation.

Although some studies suggest that obese people have a lower TEF than lean people (215–217), others report no difference (218–220). Insulin may be required for a full TEF effect (221). Insulin deficiency and/or resistance leads to defective glucose oxidation and impaired thermogenesis (222). Thus, whether obese individuals show impaired or delayed TEF depends on their insulin sensitivity or insulin response (223). The TEF seems to be diminished in the obese as a function of insulin resistance (222–223). Although an independent effect of obesity has also been described (224), the decreased TEF in obese subjects seems to be secondary to obesity rather than primary (225). Thus, an impaired TEF is unlikely to play a role in the development of obesity. In addition, even in those studies showing a decreased TEF, if TEF is added to the elevated BMR all obese persons manifest, the total energy expenditure (BMR plus TEF) is higher than that of lean persons.

Thermogenesis and Overfeeding

Neumann suggested 90 years ago that when a lean individual overate, the excess calories were dissipated as heat (luxus consumption) and normal weight was maintained (226). Garrow, investigating further, summarized the results of 15 studies in which lean and obese subjects were overfed (227). Most show fairly conclusive evidence that significant overfeeding (>2000 extra calories per day) of lean subjects for at least 10 days leads to some energy wastage. However, the four studies that evaluated obese subjects showed no evidence of luxus consumption. Thus, it is possible that the lean people are more adept at burning off excess ingested energy than are the obese. Even in lean people, however, caloric wastage has only been documented with caloric intake that is much higher than usual.

The suggestion of a deficient ability to increase thermogenesis with overingestion in obese humans is attractive because it has been documented in genetically obese rodents (228). Increased thermogenesis results from activation of an uncoupling protein (UCP-1), which allows ATP to be converted to ADP with the release of energy. UCP-1 is present in brown adipose tissue, but it is doubtful whether enough brown fat is available in adult humans to produce such excess heat. The extrapolation of small animal data to man is not valid at this time. However, recently, two uncoupling proteins (UCP-2 and UCP-3) have been discovered. UCP-2 is expressed in many tissues (228a, 228b), while UCP-3 is expressed preferentially in skeletal muscle and brown and white human adipose tissue (228c, 228d). The significance of UCP-2 in human obesity remains to be determined.

Does exercise potentiate TEF? Again, the data are contradictory. Some studies support this theory (229, 230), others do not (231, 232). Overfeeding did not potentiate the effect of exercise in two studies (233, 234), and even in studies that suggest a potentiating effect of exercise on TEF, the effect is small (235, 236). If a difference exists between lean and obese individuals, it is smaller still.

In summary, experimental evidence at present does not suggest that lean and obese individuals differ in wasteful energy production to any stimulant. There are two exceptions. First, it is probable that with great overfeeding (2000 kcal or more above the usual intake) for a long period of time (10 days or more), some wasteful energy production occurs, which may be greater in the lean than the obese person. Second, it is possible that obese patients with insulin resistance or insulin deficiency, having a defective glucose disposal system, have a depressed TEF.

FAT CELLS

Fat Cell Size and Number

Fat cells, or adipocytes, are distributed throughout the body. They form an elastic energy reservoir that can expand and contract to accommodate the energy balance of the organism. The depot can expand in two ways: by increasing the size of the fat cells or by increasing their number. Although fat cell size is generally tightly regulated between 0.3 and 0.9 μg, the number is more expandable, averaging from as low as 2×10^{10} to as high as 16×10^{10} (237). Thus, enormous flexibility exists for expansion of the adipose reservoir.

Fat cells develop from fat cell precursors called preadipocytes. It is unclear what stimulatory signal activates the preadipocyte to differentiate into an adipocyte and begin to accumulate lipid, although insulin and cortisol are required. Adipocytes gradually increase in size if energy balance continues to be positive, until a cell size of about 1.0 μg is reached. At this point, adipocytes appear unable to enlarge further. If positive energy balance persists, adipocyte proliferation is triggered, and cell number begins to rise. Because the cell number is virtually unlimited, the adipose reservoir can reach huge dimensions if caloric intake remains high.

Key time periods of adipose cell proliferation have been a controversial subject. It was initially reported that rat fat cell numbers increased in the preweaning phase (238) and not in the postweaning phase (239). However, others have since shown that rat fat cells can proliferate in the postweaning period (240–242). Although data in humans are more sparse, evidence indicates an increase in fat cell size in the initial year of life, with a subsequent rise in fat cell number (243) such that fat cell number increases fivefold between 1 and 22 years of age.

In humans, fat cell number may continue to increase as long as nutritional excess occurs; thus, excess storage energy is accommodated. Once fat cells are formed, however, it seems to be difficult to dedifferentiate them. The number seems to remain fixed even if weight is lost (244), although some decrease in number with weight loss has been reported. The net effect of weight loss is then to bring fat cell size down toward normal and eventually, if enough weight is lost, to below normal.

If infants attain maximum fat cell size at 1 year of age and then create additional fat reserves by increasing fat cell number, the child overfed on a long-term basis will develop an excess number of fat cells (hyperplasia). This condition is well documented. However, the hyperplastic child is not destined inevitably to become a hyperplastic adult. Obesity at age 2 or 3 does not necessarily predict obesity at age 21. Even though hyperplastic children have more fat cells than their lean contemporaries, they have fewer than lean adults. Thus, they may "outgrow" their obesity by maintaining their greater number of fat cells, which, if kept constant, may gradually approach normality. (See also Chapter 63.)

Obesity can thus be classified as either hypertrophic or both hypertrophic and hyperplastic. Obese patients are not hyperplastic without being hypertrophic unless they have lost weight by dieting or illness. This classification may have prognostic importance in treatment. Hypertrophic obese patients have been reported to maintain weight loss better than hyperplastic ones (245). This possibility requires further investigation.

Fat Cells As Endocrine Organs

It has become clear in recent years that the adipocyte is not the passive receptacle of lipid that was once thought. It secretes a number of active substances that have an impact on physiologic function elsewhere in the body (246). Fat cells increase leptin secretion when they enlarge and decrease it when they are depleted. Leptin levels increase with satiation and plummet with fasting and starvation. How this secretory process is controlled is presently unknown and the preoccupation of many laboratories.

Another substance secreted by the adipocyte is tumor necrosis factor alpha (TNF-α) TNF-α has been postulated to decrease insulin sensitivity and may be important in the insulin resistance associated with obesity (247, 248). Adipocytes from obese animals and humans have greatly increased TNF-α expression (248). Also secreted from the adipocyte are angiotensin-1 and adipsin, a serine protease that is on the alternative complement pathway (249). Prothrombin activator inhibitor-1 (PAI-1) has also been described as being released by fat cells (250, 251).

Thus, the adipocyte possesses the machinery to communicate with other cells in the body and influence physiology at distant sites. For example, recent information suggests that leptin may be involved in sexual maturation and reproductive function (252).

Lipoprotein Lipase

Adipose tissue lipoprotein lipase (LPL) is an enzyme that determines the rate of uptake by fat cells of circulating plasma triglyceride. It originates in adipocytes and muscle cells and is secreted to the capillary endothelium where it acts on circulating VLDL triglyceride. Activated LPL enhances breakdown of triglycerides to glycerol phosphate and FFAs; the smaller molecular weight substances can enter adipose cells, be reesterified, and be stored as triglyceride (see also Chapter 74).

Adipose tissue LPL activity is elevated in human obesity (83, 253). When adipose LPL is expressed per cell, it correlates significantly with fat cell size and with percentage of desirable weight (83, 253, 254). This correlation is not true of postheparin LPL, muscle LPL, or hepatic lipase (253). Racial differences also seem to exist in LPL. For example, Pima Indians, a group renowned for their high prevalence of obesity, have lower levels than obese Caucasians (254).

Obese individuals could have elevated LPL as a primary defect that enhances their ability to "pull" triglyceride into cells, or obesity could develop from some other cause and the enhanced LPL activity could be secondary to the enlarged fat cells. LPL activity rises further with weight loss and returns to lower (though elevated) values with weight regain (255, 256). The further elevation of LPL with any weight drop tends to enhance lipid clearance, to raise stored triglyceride levels, and to restore the obese state (84, 85).

After stabilized significant weight reduction, the elevated adipose tissue LPL activity drops (253, 257), whereas other tissues lipases are not affected (253). In addition, with refeeding, LPL activity rapidly rises above previous baseline levels (257). Thus, this change may enhance the capacity to store the circulating triglycerides that result from increased food intake, thus contributing to efficient weight regain by a refeeding obese patient who was previously on a hypocaloric regimen.

Weight Regain

Some 80 to 85% of patients who lose significant amounts of weight regain it (258). This dismal record is not readily explained, but a few hypotheses bear mentioning.

The first is that a reducing obese patient has decreased energy requirements. Patients on a reducing diet experience a 15 to 20% drop in metabolic rate (259, 260). As a result, it is more difficult for them to lose weight on the same hypocaloric diet in the second month than in the first, and in the third than the second (259). This reduced metabolic rate also may make it easier to regain weight on returning to a more normal diet. After a fast or a hypocaloric diet, refeeding is associated with a supranormal tissue response to nutrients. This response is characterized by a "repletion reaction" that includes generalized increased substrate utilization with adaptive hyperlipogenesis in adipose tissue and liver. In adipose tissue, this hyperlipogenesis is characterized by marked production of triglyceride and CO_2 from glucose (261, 262). The rapid transfer of glucose into the tissues, enhanced by increased insulin levels plus greater tissue insulin sensitivity, may increase lipogenesis and lower blood glucose levels, which may enhance hunger and stimulate greater food intake (262).

Rats demonstrate increased efficiency after fasting. Animals fasted for 4 days and then refed could maintain their new lower weight (90% of baseline) on 60% of the original daily calories (263). In addition, fasted rats refed their original daily caloric intake could regain their lost weight without overeating. These reports suggest that during the refeeding period, animals can use the same number of calories more efficiently (264).

Evidence suggesting a similar phenomenon is beginning to emerge from human studies. In morbidly obese patients whose weight was significantly reduced (from an average 152 to 100 kg), 7-day energy intake requirements to maintain weight dropped from 1432 to 1021 kcal/m^2/day (265). The figure of 1021 kcal/m^2/day was significantly lower than the 1341 kcal/m^2/day found in normal lean individuals weighing a mean of 63 kg. Because this weight loss was recent, a second metabolic study was executed with reduced obese patients who had maintained their weight loss for 4 to 6 years. These women also showed requirements averaging 1031 kcal/m^2/day to maintain their weight.

More recently, obese subjects were studied whose weight fell 10% from baseline and was maintained there for some weeks. Total energy expenditure was reduced by a mean of 6 kcal/kg fat-free mass and 8 kcal/kg weight/day. It is interesting that the reduction in resting energy expenditure was appropriate for the loss of lean body mass. The primary cause of reduced caloric expenditure was reduced nonresting energy expenditure; that is, individuals required fewer calories to carry out similar activity patterns (266). Others have reported similar data.

This finding suggests that at least some reduced obese individuals have lowered caloric requirements that may persist for years and that if caloric intake is increased above 1000 kcal/m^2/day, weight regain will occur. This theory may help to explain the poor record in maintaining weight loss after dieting.

Adipose tissue mass may be regulated by an ability of the organism to sense the filling of adipose cells with triglyceride. That is, weight regain in a refeeding animal seems to continue until fat cells have returned to their original size. Some investigators have suggested that in this way adipose tissue exerts a regulatory function on energy intake and energy balance (257). It is clear that Leptin works in this way (163–165). This process could explain why reduced obese patients have such difficulty staying on hypocaloric diets after they have dropped to a certain weight. At that point, their fat cells are at the lower limits of normal size. To drop weight further, these cells would need to become abnormally small. If hyperplastic obese persons do succeed in lowering their weight to the extent that fat cell size is below normal, they will be unable to remain at that weight, regain will occur, and fat cells will be filled to at least a "normal" size (268). The role of the fat cell in energy regulation is intriguing, and more investigative studies in this area are necessary.

THERAPY FOR OBESITY

Dietary Management

Many strategies for losing weight have been tried over the years because, as a rule, losing weight and keeping it off are extremely difficult. This is particularly true for individuals who are 25% or more overweight.

Impaired Absorption

Impairment of intestinal absorption of ingested calories is one suggested strategy. Fiber has been particularly touted in this regard, although little evidence exists that fiber significantly affects total intestinal absorption (269). Nondigestible fat substitutes have been developed. For example, sucrose polyester can be used in the diet as a replacement for fat. Whether the gastrointestinal side effects of fat malabsorption will be acceptable is presently unclear, as is the effectiveness of the substance.

Unbalanced Low-Calorie Diets

All unbalanced low-calorie diets have a marked imbalance of macronutrients that can also cause an imbalance of micronutrients. They emphasize particular food groups (carbohydrate, protein, or fat) and prohibit or deemphasize others. Their focused nature makes them easier for individuals to follow, which makes them popular.

They can be divided into different types. The ketogenic diets are high-protein, high-fat, low-carbohydrate diets. Carbohydrate generally makes up less than 20% of the calories. Proponents suggest that ketosis causes appetite suppression, but the effectiveness of ketone in inhibiting food intake has not been effectively demonstrated. Such diets tend to be low in vitamin C, and calcium loss can be enhanced. The high uric acid production may be dangerous for those predisposed to gout. These diets have a high cholesterol content, dangerous for people with hypercholesterolemia (270). They often cause nausea, hypotension, and fatigue (270).

The aforementioned diets have been modified to be high protein (40–45%), low fat (30–35%), and low carbohydrate (20–25%). These diets tend to be lower in calories because of limitation of fat, a high-calorie item. They are still ketogenic, with the same side effects of nausea, hypotension, and fatigue. They tend to be high in saturated fats and cholesterol and low in vitamins A, C, and thiamin and iron. The amount of cholesterol may be triple that in a regular diet (271).

A radically different type of diet is high in carbohydrate, low in protein (35 g/day), and low in fat (as low as 10%) (272). The emphasis is on fruits, vegetables, breads, and cereals. No table fats, oil, or dairy products except skim milk are allowed. Often these diets prohibit sugar. If taken faithfully, such diets may be low in salt, iron, essential fatty acids, and fat-soluble vitamins. Most commonly used today are diets relatively low in fat (20–30% of calories) that are also hypocaloric and have adequate protein. Such diets have successfully induced weight loss (273–275).

Some physicians have proposed total fasting as a way of losing weight (276, 277). Advocates have used it intermittently in treating obese type 2 diabetics. The problem with a total fast is that not only fat, but also much lean body mass, is lost (278). Lean body mass is difficult to regain, particularly in older individuals. In addition, the induced diuresis can result in significant mineral losses.

Protein-Supplemented Modified Fasts (PSMF)

Because of the deficiencies of total fasting, regimens called protein-supplemented modified fasts (PSMFs) have become popular (279). These severely limited diets of 400 to 700 calories generate rapid weight loss. The protein is given in the form of either formula or natural foods such as lean meat, fowl, or fish. These diets have been given for extensive periods of time, although the consensus is that it is dangerous to use them for longer than 16 weeks (280). Patients lose 1.5 to 2.3 kg/week on these diets. The protein that the patients take needs to be of high biologic quality to help prevent the loss of body protein that occurs during a standard fast (279).

Nitrogen Loss. In a fasting subject, nitrogen excretion is initially high (11–23 g/day) (281). Nitrogen loss decreases steeply in the first few days to a nadir of obligate nitrogen excretion (282). With total fasting, a cumulative nitrogen loss of 154 g of nitrogen or 963 g of protein occurs after

15 days (283). Simply adding 100 g of carbohydrate daily decreases nitrogen loss by 40% (284). Administering 55 g of high-quality protein daily causes negative nitrogen balance for the first 10 days, but many patients achieve balance at about 20 days (285). These low-caloric diets were given large-scale trials by three groups (286–288). All required vitamin and mineral supplements daily as well as essential fatty acids (287). They reported little morbidity. Vertes et al., with 1200 outpatient years of experience, had four deaths, which they describe as fewer than expected for the population treated (289).

It has been hypothesized that these diets spare protein by decreasing the insulin level and enhancing ketonemia (290). The ketonemia in turn inhibits release of amino acids from muscle (291). Little experimental evidence supports this hypothesis, because insulin levels are not absolute determinants of protein sparing (292, 293).

Morbidity and Mortality with PSMF. With the popularization of these PSMF diets, numerous commercial preparations of liquid protein have become available for over-the-counter purchase. Fifty-eight deaths were associated with the use of these formulas in the 1970s (294). Although the reason for these deaths is unclear, 17 of them were investigated (295, 296). Patients seemed to develop refractory ventricular arrhythmias. Whether this condition was secondary to myocardial protein atrophy, myocarditis, potassium deficiency, or other mineral losses is unclear (295, 297, 298). These deaths have been attributed to poor-quality protein in the commercial-formula diets. The proteins eaten in a regular diet, such as dairy products, meat, fish, poultry, and grain and cereal products, provide about 87% of the calcium, 80% of the phosphorus, 60% of the magnesium, 74% of the iron, 80% of the zinc, 57% of the copper, 80% of the manganese, and 100% of the selenium in a usual diet. Many of the poor-quality hydrolyzed protein diets did not adequately replace these minerals and others. The more recent formula preparations have used high-quality protein (casein or soy protein), have replaced micronutrients adequately, and have not led to untoward events (299).

Morbidity also occurs with these diets. Orthostatic hypotension may result from the sodium diuresis and volume depletion that occur (300). This condition is probably secondary to the natriuretic effect of hyperketonemia (301) and the impaired norepinephrine secretion associated with it (300). Other symptoms and signs include dehydration, cold intolerance, fatigue, dry skin, hair loss, and menstrual irregularities. Cholecystitis, pancreatitis, and peroneal nerve palsy have occasionally been reported.

Although nitrogen balance is better with PSMF than with starvation, there is little evidence that PSMF is better than a mixed diet. Comparison of an 800-kcal mixed diet, an 800-kcal all-protein ketogenic diet, and starvation in obese subjects showed that starvation gives the most negative nitrogen balance, while the mixed and the all-protein diet are not much different and result in less nitrogen loss (302). Over a 10-day period, 2.8 kg of weight is lost with a mixed diet and 4.7 kg with the ketogenic diet, but all the extra weight lost with the ketogenic diet is water. Longer 60-day studies show no difference in nitrogen balance between a mixed diet and a ketogenic diet (303).

Balanced Hypocaloric Diets

In view of the aforementioned risks and problems of unbalanced diets and the prolonged periods of time that restricted diets must be followed, a well-balanced mixed diet seems a sensible approach. Diets in the 1100- to 1200-kcal range can include appropriate macro- and microelements, vitamins, and protein (304). They can be followed for months without specific supplements. The nutrients most likely to be deficient are iron, folacin, vitamin B_6, and zinc (304). In such a diet, the percentage of protein is raised, so at least 240 calories or about 60 g/day are from protein. The protein should be of high quality and should make up about 25% of calories. At least 20% of the rest of the dietary calories should be carbohydrate and at least 20% fat. In this way, fat-soluble vitamins and essential fatty acids will be available from fat, and fiber and antiketogenic effect from carbohydrate. Diets of 800 to 1100 kcal must be supplemented with vitamins and minerals. In general, the caloric deficit should not exceed 500 to 1000 kcal/day, and total calories should not be below 800 kcal unless the individual is under tight medical surveillance.

A balanced diet for micronutrients and vitamins should contain food items from the following foods: *(a)* meat, fish, poultry, and meat substitutes; *(b)* milk and milk products; *(c)* cereals and cereal products; and *(d)* vegetables and fruits. The nutrients obtained are *(a)* protein, fat, niacin, iron, and thiamin; *(b)* vitamins A and D, calcium, magnesium, and zinc; *(c)* carbohydrates, fat, phosphorus, magnesium, zinc, and copper; and *(d)* carbohydrate, vitamins A and C, iron, and magnesium (304).

Because obese individuals need to be on a diet for a long time, the diet *must* be acceptable. It must fit the individual's tastes and habits and be flexible enough to allow eating both inside and outside the home.

Exercise

The therapeutic use of exercise to reverse obesity has been widely hailed. As mentioned above, body weight is determined by a balance between energy intake and energy expenditure. If energy expenditure can be increased by incremental physical activity and energy intake is kept constant, weight will drop. A number of points must be emphasized. First, a significant amount of physical effort is required to expend a significant number of calories. Calorie charts for expenditure usually list the total caloric expenditure for a given period of time. However, an individual who is not doing the activity does not expend zero calories but something above basal levels (sitting, standing). For example, an obese woman exercising on a treadmill at 4 mph expends about 7.0 kcal/min, or 210 calories if she continues this exercise for 30 min. Sitting in a chair, such a woman expends about 1.3

kcal/min, or 39 kcal over 30 min. Thus, her exercise-induced expenditure would not be 210 kcal but 210 minus 39, or 171 kcal. Therefore, in looking at expenditure tables, one must always subtract between 1 and 1.5 kcal/min for the resting or sitting metabolic expenditure that would occur anyway.

The second point that must be clarified is the purported prolonged elevation of oxygen consumption for long periods after exercise. Such a sustained effect of exercise lasting for 7 to 48 hours has been described, but two reviews of the literature concluded that no sustained increase could be demonstrated after exercise (305, 306). Studies support a lack of a sustained effect using exercise levels that are realistic for individuals on weight-control programs (307–310). Because little appreciable caloric loss occurs beyond that generated by the exercise period itself, claims for sustained effects of exercise on resting metabolic rate in weight control programs are unwarranted.

The third point relates to the effect of exercise on food intake. Although it has been generally suggested that exercise inhibits food intake, this phenomenon has not been documented. In lean individuals, exercise generally leads to increased energy intake and maintenance of body weight (311). This tendency is true with both mild (~400 kcal/day) and moderate (~775 kcal/day) exercise (312). Obese individuals may respond to exercise by defending weight to the same extent as lean persons.

Most studies of the effect of exercise on obese subjects only measured weight or body fat; they did not measure food intake. As mentioned above, if expenditure is increased and food intake remains stable, weight loss will be commensurate with the increased expenditure. Such a result has been described (313). Other studies, however, have documented amounts of weight loss that suggest curtailed food intake (314, 315). Some studies show no effect of exercise on weight at all (316). Two metabolic ward studies over long periods of time, 19-day (307) or 57-day (308) intervals, suggest that obese women tend to fix on an intake and remain at that intake even if the amount of activity is changed. Intake changes seemed more related to dietary characteristics than to level of exercise (316). Prospective epidemiologic studies show a lower risk for overweight in more physically active persons (317). With regard to weight loss, one review describes a modestly greater effect of diet and exercise over diet alone (318). A beneficial effect of exercise is best documented in the weight maintenance phase, predicting greater success (319).

Although exercise does not magically sustain an enhanced metabolic rate or inhibit food intake, every calorie expended can help in the battle to use significantly more calories than are ingested. Moreover, exercise helps to maintain weight loss while allowing less stringent diets—a more acceptable regimen to many patients.

Pharmacologic Treatment

The most widely used drugs for weight control are appetite suppressants; others attack food intake and metabolism at other sites, such as digestion, absorption, lipid synthesis, or thermogenesis. The anorectic agents, which suppress appetite, are considered first.

The first was amphetamine. Amphetamine, a β-phenethylamine, seems to induce anorexia via brain catecholamines, specifically norepinephrine and dopamine, although the relative importance of each in man is not yet clear. It causes not only anorexia, but also many other effects including central stimulation, mood enhancement, cardiovascular excitation, and a selective effect on certain neural transmitters, especially catecholamines. Some of these effects can lead to abuse (320). In addition, in a few patients, discontinuing the drug seems to be associated with onset of depression. Six anorectic agents that been shown to induce dependence have been most commonly used: diethylpropion, mazindol, *d,l* -fenfluramine, *d*-fenfluramine, phentermine, and phenylpropanolamine.

Diethylpropion seems to have little effect on sleep, and addiction has not been a problem. It is closest in structure to amphetamine, being modified by addition of a keto group on the β carbon and of ethyl groups on the amine terminal. Mazindol is thought to prolong the action of norepinephrine and also stimulates the central nervous system (321). It is a tricyclic compound with a long plasma half-life (33–55 hours). Fenfluramine has an ethyl group on the amine terminal and a CF_3 on the phenyl ring. Its action is mediated through a central serotonergic system. It has no central stimulant effect (322). Phentermine resin has methyl groups substituted on the carbon. It seems to be as effective as amphetamine, with lower stimulatory properties; however, dry mouth, tachycardia, and increased blood pressure often occur. Phenylpropanolamine, a derivative of amphetamine, has an extra hydroxyl group. It is available over the counter and as a result is widely used. Its effect is generally modest (323, 324).

Although we cannot yet classify obesity in terms of etiology, it probably has differing causes. The drugs available also differ. Thus, it is not surprising that the response differs from person to person. These drugs may be a useful adjunct for the treatment of obesity in some patients. The widespread belief in some medical circles that all appetite-suppressant drugs are useless and that tolerance quickly develops is not necessarily true. In addition, although side effects are common with excess dosage, they do not necessarily occur at recommended dosages. An anorectic agent can be helpful in some people. However, the drug can only be effective if appropriate dosage is given and blood levels are adequate. It is also wise to individualize use to a patient's dietary habits. One would not administer a relatively short-acting drug in the morning if a patient eats no breakfast and is an evening and night eater. Recently, the suggestion has been put forward that long-term drug therapy for obesity should be considered (325). Certain experimental studies have reported moderate success with long-term therapy using *d,l*-fenfluramine (326), sibutramine (327), and a combination of phentermine and fenfluramine (328).

Recently, the drugs *d,l*-fenfluramine and fenfluramine

have been withdrawn from the market by their manufacturer. The reason for this was development of heart valve lesions with the use of these agents (328a). The lesions, primarily in the aortic and mitral valve, consist of thickening of the valve, similar to what occurs with carcinoid syndrome. The result is development of aortic and mitral regurgitation. Twenty-seven persons required valve replacement, with three deaths reported (328b). The incidence of this side effect is not clear, but the Food and Drug Administration (FDA) has suggested that it may be as high as 30% (328b). On the basis of these side effects as well as the already known increased incidence of pulmonary hypertension (328c, 328d), these two drugs have been withdrawn from the market.

In 1998, a new drug, sibutramine, was approved by the FDA for long-term use. It is a norpinephrine and serotonin reuptake inhibitor. In clinical trials, it produces about the same degree of weight loss as the fenfluramines (327). A side effect of this drug is possible elevation of heart rate and blood pressure, so patients need to be monitored carefully (327a).

Another pharmacologic agent, orlistat, inhibits dietary lipid absorption by decreasing intestinal lipase activity. Clinical trials suggest an effect on weight loss comparable to that of the drugs described above (329). The safety profile of this drug seems high, although some fat-soluble vitamin levels may drop slightly.

There is an effort to develop thermogenic agents, but no satisfactory drug is available to date. Thyroid preparations, digitalis, or human chorionic gonadotrophin have no place in the treatment of obesity. Diuretics are rarely necessary and certainly should never be used in combination with low-calorie diets. Bulking agents such as methylcellulose and other fibers have been touted as aids in weight loss, but no evidence of this is available. They do not cause malabsorption and have not been shown to decrease food intake (330).

In summary, though drugs may be helpful in some individuals at some periods in weight loss and weight maintenance, they do not hold first rank in any therapeutic program.

Psychotherapy

The psychologic treatment of obesity has not enjoyed much success. Although a few optimistic reports have stated the effect of psychoanalysis in producing weight loss (331, 332), particularly in adolescents (331), therapeutic failure is the common result. Many obese patients may have emotional problems, but these vary. Some have anxiety, some are depressed, but some have no evident psychiatric problems at all, except for overeating and/or underactivity (333). No particular personality type is obese.

Although some investigators have suggested that obesity may be protective for underlying neurotic behavior, this possibility has not been confirmed by patients undergoing surgical treatment of obesity. Some psychiatrists predicted that morbidly obese individuals would develop other addictive tendencies or overt neurotic or psychotic traits as weight loss occurred. This has not happened. Patients either have had no psychiatric change or have improved; few have deteriorated (334).

A distortion of body image does seem to exist in a minority of obese patients, with overestimation of body size (333). In a study of morbidly obese subjects whose weight was reduced enough to have significant changes in body size, the distortion of body image persisted, particularly in those obese from childhood (335). Some psychiatrists have even reported evidence of low anxiety and depression in obese individuals (336), and epidemiologic evidence suggests that they have a lower incidence of suicide than the general population. Because no evidence indicates that all or even most obese subjects are neurotic, health professionals must individually evaluate each patient.

Some persons who wish to lose weight are binge eaters. If they have true bulimia nervosa with vomiting, laxative use, and electrolyte changes, this condition should be addressed by a psychiatrically trained professional. If an obese person engages in binge eating without purging, it seems wise to direct therapy to the binge eating before attempting weight loss (337).

Behavior Modification

Because of the poor record in the treatment of obesity by classic psychoanalysis and psychotherapy, behavior modification has gained favor. Behavior modification programs grew out of the hypothesis that the obese overeat because they are stimulus bound and environmental food-relevant cues control eating rather than any psychogenic neurotic states (338). This "externality theory" suggested that external environmental stimuli overrode whatever internal hunger or satiety cues generally caused lean individuals to initiate or stop eating (339). This theory differentiating obese from lean is now questioned because others have not been able to duplicate these differences in the two groups (340). Nevertheless, the theory won wide recognition and stimulated interest in behavior modification programs to control food intake by diminishing the number of external cues that led to overeating (341).

The first step in a behavior modification program is identifying the eating and activity patterns of an individual. Careful diaries are kept in which patients record not only when and what was eaten, but where, with whom, how (sitting, standing, walking), as well as their feelings and hunger. In addition to the diary of food-related behavior, a diary of all activity-related behavior is kept, including when, with whom, where, and feelings at the time. Food management behavior must also be itemized, including buying, storing, preparing, serving, and cleaning up food. These diaries are analyzed so that possible environmental (e.g., television) or emotional (e.g., depression) clues to overeating may be recognized and controlled. Once these cues have been identified, then techniques are invoked to try to control or evade them. Environmental stimuli to eating are controlled. Food shopping habits, visual cues, food preparation habits, and food storage habits are changed.

Techniques to control the act of eating are also imposed. These include always eating in the dining room, sitting, concentrating on eating (no reading or watching television), eating more slowly, taking more and smaller bites, putting utensils down between bites, not skipping meals, not taking snacks, changing high-calorie foods for low-calorie ones, and eating at prescribed times only. Besides these efforts to diminish environmental cues, new discriminative stimuli are introduced to develop new eating patterns. These include distinctive sites for eating, new and smaller plates, and eating with others as often as possible. Finally, behavior modification programs try to change the consequences of eating. A reward system is introduced for changing behavior. The rewards are generally immediate and may be monetary or social feedback. Family, friends, group members, and group leaders can all contribute.

Mahoney outlined the assumptions of the behavior modification movement (342):

1. Obesity is a learning disorder created by, and amenable to, principles of conditioning
2. Obesity is a simple disorder resulting from excess calorie intake
3. The obese individual is an overeater
4. Obese persons are more sensitive to food stimuli than are nonobese individuals
5. Important differences exist in the "eating style" of obese and nonobese persons
6. Training an obese person to behave like a nonobese one will result in weight loss

Many, if not all, of these assumptions are now considered untrue; thus many of the strategies for weight loss in behavioral modification programs were founded on false assumptions. Though the theoretical background may be incorrect, the strategy developed is effective. This argument is probably valid. Stunkard reviewed 30 controlled trials and found that behavioral treatment was more successful in producing weight loss than a variety of other treatments (343). Behavior modification programs seemed to be more successful than group psychotherapy, nutritional education, and relaxation training. That success is not universal, however; some patients do well and others poorly. To date, it has not been possible to identify the characteristics that determine success.

Although some weight has been lost, it has not been impressive. Jeffrey et al. reviewed 21 studies and found a mean weight loss of 11.5 lb (344). This amount, although a loss, is not clinically of much importance. In addition, not many persons have lost weight after termination of the program (345), and maintenance of weight loss in the long term has been poor (346).

In summary, it is difficult to be certain at this point whether behavioral treatment is better, and if so, how much better, than other forms of treatment. Well-controlled follow-up studies suggest that the same problem of failure to maintain weight loss that is true of other weight-control programs is true of behavior modification programs.

Surgical Treatment

The refractoriness of many patients with morbid obesity to diet, psychotherapy, behavior modification, drugs, and exercise programs has led to physician pessimism about the likelihood of long-term therapeutic success. As a result, surgical treatment has been attempted, based on one of two principles: *(a)* a short bowel is created to produce malabsorption of ingested calories and *(b)* a small stomach is created to prevent much caloric intake at any one time.

Short Bowel Procedure

Many variations of the jejunoileal bypass procedure existed (347), depending on how much jejunum and how much ileum was bypassed. The earliest procedure connected 12 to 15 in. of jejunum to 4 to 8 in. of ileum. Connections were end to end or end to side. The bypass loop was either left to drain in situ (end to side) or was reconnected to drain into the ascending or transverse colon (end to end). Various-sized segments were left in continuity (14–4 in., 10–10 in., 14–8 in.). Weight loss did generally occur, although it was variable, and few patients lost only a small amount of weight. The bypass procedure created malabsorption of both exogenous nutrients and endogenous gastrointestinal secretions. Complications made this procedure unacceptable (347), including hypokalemia, hypocalcemia, vitamin B deficiency, hepatic toxicity, renal calculi, and polyarthritis. There were also operative risks, including pulmonary embolus, pneumonia, wound infections, wound dehiscence, and phlebitis. Because of all these problems, the procedure was discontinued.

Gastric Surgery. The gastric bypass operation was first described by Mason and Ito in 1967 (348). In this operation, the stomach was transected (or stapled) to create a small upper pouch (30–50 mL) that was anastomosed to a loop of jejunum. The opening between pouch and jejunum was 9 to 11 mm in diameter. This operation made a blind loop of much of the stomach, the duodenum, and the proximal jejunum.

More commonly now, a modification of this operation, the gastroplasty, is done. The stomach is stapled across, creating a small 50- to 60-mL reservoir on top and a small 1-cm outlet to the rest of the stomach on the lesser, middle, or greater curvature. Another recent procedure is the vertical banded gastroplasty (349). In this procedure, a 20- to 30-mL stomach pouch is made by two longitudinal staple lines. In addition, the pouch can be wrapped with Teflon mesh to prevent pouch distention and stoma widening.

These operations have been associated with considerably less morbidity than the intestinal operations (350, 350a). The problems are generally postoperative and include anastomotic leaks, transient gastrojejunostomy obstruction, and intraabdominal abscess. Wound infection, dehiscence, pulmonary embolism, and atelectasis can also occur. Subsequent to these early problems, late morbidity depends greatly on patient education and compliance. Vomiting is frequent if the speed or amount of eating is too great. Late complications consist primarily of revisions caused by suture-line disruption or channel size problems. If chronic vomiting persists, esophagitis, hypokalemia, and malnutrition with dehydration can occur. The success rate with gastroplasty has been variable, depending greatly on the surgeon. It is difficult to construct a stoma small enough to inhibit too-rapid transit from the small reservoir to the large, yet not small enough to cause obstructive symptoms. Mason and Ito reported a 36-kg average weight loss in 3 years, but others have not done as well (348). In addition, patients can ensure failure by consuming high-caloric-density liquid or semisolid food that can easily pass through the small stoma.

Lipectomy. Lipectomy is not a treatment for obesity. It is surgical removal of adipose tissue for cosmetic purposes. Not enough fat can be removed to make a real impact on obesity, and it should not be performed for this reason. Lipectomy may be used to treat localized unsightly adiposity. A recent modification of this procedure is suction lipectomy. Long-term results of this procedure are unavailable.

WEIGHT CYCLING

In recent years, data have suggested that weight cycling (i.e., gaining and losing weight several times) may be detrimental. Although some studies have suggested increased morbidity and mortality (351, 352), others have not borne this out (353, 354).

REFERENCES

1. Kuczmarski RJ. Am J Clin Nutr 1992;55:495S–502S.
2. Quetelet LA. J. Anthropomètrie pour mesure des différentes facultés de l'homme. Brussels: C. Muquardt, 1981;479.
3. Simopolous AP, VanItallie TB. Ann Intern Med 1984;100: 285–95.
4. Gallagher D, Visser M, Sepulveda D, et al. Am J Epidemiol 1996;143:228–39.
5. Pi-Sunyer FX. Ann Intern Med 1993;119:655–60.
6. Wilmer HA. Proc Soc Exp Biol Med 1940;43:386–8.
7. National Center for Health Statistics. DHHS publ. no. (PHS) 81-1669. Vital Health Stat (11) no. 219. 1981.

7a. Bishop EW, Bowen PE, Ritchey SJ. Am J Clin Nutr 1981; 34:2530–9.

7b. Frisancho AR. Anthropometric standards for the assessment of growth and nutritional status. Ann Arbor: University of Michigan Press, 1990.

8. Durnin JVGA, Womersley J. Br J Nutr 1974;32:77–9.
9. Behnke AR, Wilmore JH. Evaluation of body build and composition. Englewood Cliffs, NJ: Prentice Hall, 1974.
10. Pace N, Rathbun E. J Biol Chem 1945;158:685–91.
11. Smith T, Hesp R, Mackenzie J. Phys Med Biol 1979;24:171–5.
12. Lukaski HC, Bolonchuk WW, Hall CB, et al. J Appl Physiol 1986;60:1327–32.
13. Lesser GT, Deutsch S, Markofsy J. Metabolism 1971;20:792–804.
14. 1983 Metropolitan Height and Weight Tables. Stat Bull Metrop Insur Co 1984;64:2–9.
15. National Center for Health Statistics, Roberts J. PHS publ. no. 1000. Vital Health Stat (14) 1966.
16. National Center for Health Statistics, Abraham S, Johnson CL, Najjar MF. DHEW publ. no. (PHS) 79-1656. Vital Health Stat (11) no. 208, 1979.
17. Najjar MF, Rowland M. Vital Health Stat (11) no. 238. 1987.
18. Kuczmarski RJ, Flegal KM, Campbell SM, Johnson CL. JAMA 1994;272:205–11.
19. Andres R, Elahi D, Tobin JD, et al. Ann Intern Med 1985; 103:1030–3.
20. Andres R. Mortality and obesity: the rationale for age specific height-weight tables. In: Bierman EL, Hazzard WR, eds. Principles of geriatric medicine. New York: McGraw-Hill, 1985;311–8.
21. U.S. Departments of Agriculture and Health and Human Services. Nutrition and your health: dietary guidelines for Americans. 3rd ed. Publ. no. 273-930. Washington, DC: U.S. Government Printing Office, 1990;1–27.
22. Willet WC, Stampfer M, Manson J, et al. Am J Clin Nutr 1991;53:1102–3.
23. U.S. Department of Agriculture. Dietary guidelines for Americans. 4th ed. Washington, DC: U.S. Government Printing Office. Home and Garden Bull no. 232, 1996.
24. Taitz LS. Br Med J 1971;1:315–6.
25. Shukla A, Forsyth HA, Anderson CM, et al. Br Med J 1972;4:507–15.
26. Jelliffe DB, Jelliffe EF. Environ Child Health Monogr 1975;41:124–238.
27. Johnson ML, Burke BS, Mayer J. Am J Clin Nutr 1975;4:231–8.
28. Hathaway ML, Sargent DW. J Am Diet Assoc 1962;40:511–5.
29. Garn SM, Clark DC. Pediatrics 1976;57:443–56.
30. Colley JRT. Br J Prev Soc Med 1976;28:221–5.
31. NHANES 1988–91. MMWR 1994;43:818–21.
32. Mossberg H. Acta Paediatr Scand 35 1948;11(Suppl):1–122.
33. Rimm IJ, Rimm AA. Am J Public Health 1976;66:479–81.
34. Abraham S, Nordseick M. Public Health Rep 1960;75: 263–273.
35. Garn SM, LaVelle M. Am J Dis Child 1985;139:181–5.
36. Borjeson M. Acta Paediatr 1962;51(Suppl 132):1–76.
37. Goldblatt PB, Moore ME, Stunkard AJ. JAMA 1965;192: 1039–44.
38. Baird IM, Silverstone JT, Grimshaw JJ, et al. Practitioner 1974;212:706–14.
39. Noppa H, Bengston C. J Epidemiol Community Health 1978;34:134–42.
40. Stunkard AJ. Fed Proc 1968;27:1367–73.
41. Ross CE, Mirowsky J. J Health Soc Behav 1983;24:288–96.
42. Moore ME, Stunkard AJ, Srole L. JAMA 1962;181:962–6.
43. Height and Weight of Adults Ages 18–74 Years by Socioeconomic Status and Geographic Variables, United States. DHHS publ. no (PHS) 81-1674. Hyattsville, MD: National Center for Health Statistics, 1981.
44. Silverstone JT, Gordon RP, Stunkard AJ. Practitioner 1969; 202:682–8.
45. Armstrong DB, Dublin LI, Wheatley GM, et al. JAMA 1951; 147:1007–14.

46. Lew EA. J Am Diet Assoc 1961;39:323–7.
47. Build and Blood Pressure Study 1959, vol 1. Chicago: Chicago Society of Actuaries, 1960.
48. Build and Study 1979. Chicago: Chicago Society of Actuaries and Association of Life Insurance Medical Directors, 1980.
49. Lew EA, Garfinkel LL. J Chronic Dis 1979;32:563–76.
50. Belloc NB. Prev Med 1973;2:67–81.
51. Andres R, Elahi D, Tobin JD, et al. Int J Obes 1980;4:381–6.
52. Dyer AR, Stamler J, Berkson DM, et al. J Chronic Dis 1975; 28:109–23.
53. Keys A, Aravanis C, Blackburn G, et al. Ann Intern Med 1972; 77:15–27.
54. Keys A. Nutr Rev 1980;38:297–307.
55. Waaler HT. Acta Med Scand 1984;679(Suppl):1–56.
56. Gray DS. Med Clin North Am 1989;73:1–13.
57. Jarrett JJ, Shipley MJ, Rose G. Br Med J 1982;285:535–7.
58. Libow LS. Geriatrics 1974;29:75–88.
59. Milne JS, Lauder IJ. Age Ageing 1978;7:129–37.
60. Burr MI, Lennings CI, Milbank JE. Age Ageing 1982;11:249–55.
61. Rissanen A, Heliovaara M, Knekt P, et al. J Clin Epidemiol 1988;42:781–9.
62. Garn SM, Hawthorne VM, Pilkington JJ, et al. Am J Clin Nutr 1983;38:313–9.
63. Linsted K, Tonstad S, Kuzma JW. Int J Obes 1990;15:397–406.
64. Sidney S, Friedman GD, Siegelaub AB. Am J Public Health 1987;77:317–22.
65. Keys A. Overweight and the risk of heart attack and sudden death. In: Bray GA, ed. Obesity in perspective. NIH publ. no. 75. Washington, DC: Dept of Health Education and Welfare, 1976;708:215–23.
66. Manson JE, Colditz GA, Stampfer MJ, et al. N Engl J Med 1990;372:882–9.
67. Kannel WB, LeBauer EJ, Dawber TR, et al. Circulation 1967;35:734–44.
68. Kannel WB, Gordon T. Physiological and medical concomitants of obesity: the Framingham study. In: Bray GA, ed. Obesity in America. NIH publ. no. 79. Washington, DC: Dept of Health Education and Welfare, 1979;359:125–63.
69. Ostfeld AM, Gibson DC. Epidemiology of aging. NIH publ. no. 75. Washington, DC: Dept of Health Education and Welfare, 1975;711:217–9.
70. Rabkin SW, Mathewson FAL, Hsu PH. Am J Cardiol 1977;39:452–8.
71. Feinlieb M. Ann Intern Med 1985;103:1019–24.
72. Chapman JM, Coulson AH, Clark VA, et al. J Chronic Dis 1971;23:631–45.
73. Bouchard C, Bray G, Hubbard VS. Am J Clin Nutr 1990; 52:946–50.
74. Donahue RP, Abbott RD, Bloom E, et al. Lancet 1987;1:821–4.
75. Ducimetiere P, Richard JL. Int J Obes 1989;13:111–22.
76. Lapidus L, Bengtsson C, Larsson B, et al. Br Med J 1984;289: 1257–61.
77. Larsson B, Svardsudd K, Welin L, et al. Br Med J 1984; 288:1401–4.
78. Albrink MH, Meigs JW. Am J Clin Invest 1974;53:64–76.
79. Olefsky J, Reaven GM, Farquhar JW. J Clin Invest 1974;53: 64–76.
80. Bagdade JD, Bierman EL, Porte D Jr. J Clin Invest 1967; 46:1549–57
81. Olefsky J, Farquhar JW, Reaven GM. Am J Med 1974;57: 551–60.
82. Havel RJ, Kane JP, Balasse EO, et al. J Clin Invest 1970;49: 2017–35.
83. Pykalisto OJ, Smith P H, Brunzell JD. J Clin Invest 1975; 56:1108–17.
84. Eckel RH, Yost TJ. J Clin Invest 1987;80:992–7.
85. Kern PA, Ong JM, Saffari B, et al. N Engl J Med 1990; 322:1053–9.
86. Brunzell JD, Hazzard WR, Motulsky AG, et al. Clin Res 1974; 22:462a.
87. Rifkind BM, Begg T. Br Med J 1966;2:208–10.
88. Montoye HJ, Epstein FH, Kjelsberg MO. Am J Clin Nutr 1966;18:397–406.
89. Kannel WB, Castelli WP, Gordon T. Ann Intern Med 1979; 90:85–91.
90. Yaari S, Doldbourt U, Even-Zohar S, et al. Lancet 1971; 1:1011–5.
91. Austin MA, Breslow JL, Hennekens CH, et al. JAMA 1988;200:1917–21.
92. Després JP, Moorjani SJ, Lupien PJ, et al. Arteriosclerosis 1990;10:497–511.
93. Lamarche B, Moorjani S, Lupien PJ, et al. Circulation 1996; 94:273–8.
94. Steinberg D, Parthasarathy S, Carew TE, et al. N Engl J Med 1989;320:915–24.
95. West KM, Kalbfkeisch JM. Diabetes 1971;20:99–108.
96. Hartz AJ, Rupley DC, Kalkhoff RD, et al. Prev Med 1983; 12:351–7.
97. Kannel WB. Health and obesity: an overview. In: Conn HL Jr, DeFelice EA, Kuo P, eds. Health and obesity. New York: Raven Press, 1983.
98. Colditz GA, Willett WC, Rotnitzky A, et al. Ann Intern Med 1995;122:481–6.
99. Haffner SM, Stern MP, Hazuda HP, et al. Diabetes Care 1986;9:153–61.
100. Feldman R, Sender AJ, Siegelaub AB. Diabetes 1969;18: 478–86.
101. Hartz AJ, Rupley DC, Kalkhoff RD, et al. Prev Med 1983;2: 351–7.
102. Kissebah AH, Vydelingum N, Murray R. J Clin Endocrinol Metab 1982;54:254–260.
103. Krotkiewski M, Bjorntorp P, Sjostrom L, et al. J Clin Invest 1983;72:1150–62.
104. Dowling HJ, Pi-Sunyer FX. Diabetes 1993;42:537–43.
105. Ohlson LO, Larsson B, Svardsudd K, et al. Diabetes 1985;34: 1055–8.
106. Haffner SM, Stern MP, Hazuda HP, et al. JAMA 1990; 263:2893–8.
107. Bjorntorp P. Obesity Res 1993;1:206–22.
108. Després JP. Nutrition 1993;9:452–9.
109. Karam JH, Grodsky GM, Forsham PH. Diabetes 1963;12: 197–204.
110. DeFronzo RA. Diabetes 1988;37:667–87.
111. Caro JF, Dohm LG, Pories WJ, et al. Diabetes Metab Rev 1989;5:665–89.
112. Granner DK, O'Brien RM. Diabetes Care 1992;15:369–95.
113. Kahn CR, Neville DM Jr, Roth J. J Biol Chem 1973;248: 244–50.
114. Archer JA, Gorden P, Roth J. J Clin Invest 1975;55:166–74.
115. Olefsky JM. J Clin Invest 1976;57:1165–72.
116. Kahn CR, White MD. J Clin Invest 1988;82:1151–4.
117. Rosen O. Diabetes 1989;38:1508–14.
118. Garvey WT. Diabetes Care 1992;15:396–417.
119. Pfeifer MA, Halter JB, Porte D Jr. Am J Med 1981;70:579–88.
120. DeFronzo RA, Bonadonna RC, Ferrannini E. Diabetes Care 1992;15:318–68.
121. Berchtold P, Sims EA, Horton ES, et al. Biomed Pharmacother 1983;37:251–8.
122. Stamler J, Stamler R, Romberg A, et al. J Chronic Dis 1975; 28:499–525.

123. Tobian L. N Engl J Med 1978;298:46–8.
124. Johnson BC, Karunas TM, Epstein FH. Clin Sci Mol Med 1973;45(Suppl 1):355–455.
125. Kannel WB, Brand N, Skinner JJ. Ann Intern Med 1967;67:48–59.
126. Oberman A, Lane NE, Harlan WR, et al. Circulation 1967; 36:812–22.
127. Tyroler HA, Heyden S, Harnes CG. Weight and hypertension: Evans County studies of blacks and whites. In: Paul O, ed. Epidemiology and control of hypertension. New York: Stratton Intercontinental Medical Book, 1975;177–201.
128. Reisin E, Abel R, Modan M, et al. N Engl J Med 1978;298:1–6.
129. Reisen E, Frolich ED, Messerli FH, et al. Ann Intern Med 1983;98:315–9.
130. Dahl LK, Silver L, Christie RW. N Engl J Med 1958;258: 1186–92.
131. Salzano JV, Gunning RV, Mastopaulo TN, et al. J Am Diet Assoc 1958;34:1309–12.
132. DeFronzo RA. Insulin and renal sodium handling: clinical implications. In: Björntörp P, Cairella M, Howard AN, eds. Recent advances in obesity research III. London: John Libbey, 1980;32–41.
133. DeFronzo RA, Goldberg M, Agus Z. J Clin Invest 1976;58: 83–9.
134. DeFronzo RA, Cooke CR, Andres R, et al. J Clin Invest 1975;55:845–55.
135. Kolanowski J, Godson A, Desmecht P, et al. Eur J Clin Invest 1978;8:277–82.
136. Landsberg L, Young JB. N Engl J Med 1978;298:1295–301.
137. Weinsier RL, Norris DJ, Birch R, et al. Hypertension 1985;7:578–85.
138. Björntörp P. Ann Intern Med 1985;103:994–5.
139. Ferranninni E. The phenomenon of insulin resistance: its possible relevance to hypertensive disease. In: Laragh JH, Brener BM, eds. Hypertension: physiology, diagnosis and management. 2nd ed. New York: Raven 1995;2281–300.
140. Resnick LM. Am J Hypertens 1993;6:123S–34S.
141. Kopelman PG, Apps MC, Cope T, et al. Int J Obes 1986;10:211–7.
142. Rimm AA, White PL. Obesity: its risks and hazards. In: Bray GA, ed. Obesity in America. NIH publ. no. 79. Washington, DC: Dept of Health, Education and Welfare, 1979;359: 103–24.
143. GREPCO. The Rome Group for Epidemiology and Prevention of Cholelithiasis. Hepatology 1988;129:587–95.
144. Jorgensen T. Gut 1989;30:528–34.
145. Maclure KM, Hayes KC, Colditz GA, et al. N Engl J Med 1989;321:563–9.
146. Stampfer MJ, Maclure KM, Colditz GA, et al. Am J Clin Nutr 1991;55:652–8.
147. Bennion LJ, Grundy SM. J Clin Invest 1975;56:996–1011.
148. Reuben A, Qureshi Y, Murphy GM, et al. Eur J Clin Invest 1985;16:133–42.
149. Miettinen TA. Horm Metab Res 1974;14:35–44.
150. Marzio L, Capone F, Neri M, et al. Dig Dis Sci 1988;33:4–9.
151. Grundy SM, Metzger AL, Adler RD. J Clin Invest 1972;51: 3026–43.
152. Leach RE, Baumgard S, Broom J. Clin Orthop 1973;93:272–3.
153. Garfinkel L. Ann Intern Med 1985;103:1034–6.
154. Blitzer PH, Blitzer EC, Rimm AA. Prev Med 1976;5:20–31.
155. McMahon B. Gynecol Oncol 1974;2:122–9.
156. Dunn LJ, Bradbury JT. Am J Obstet Gynecol 1967;97:465–71.
157. Garfinkel L. Cancer 1986;58:1820–9.
158. DeWaard F, Baanders-Van Halewijn EA. Acta Cytol 1969;13:675–8.
159. DeWaard F. Cancer Res 1975;35:3351–6.
160. Wynder EL, Bross IJ, Hirayama T. Cancer 1960;13:559–601.
161. Beer AE, Billingham RE. Lancet 1978;1:296.
162. Zhang Y, Proenca R, Maffei M, et al. Nature (London) 1994;372:425–32.
163. Halaas J, Gajiwala K, Maffei M, et al. Science 1995;269:543–6.
164. Campfield L, Smith F, Guisez Y, et al. Science 1995;269:546–8.
165. Pellymounter M, Cullen M, Baker M, et al. Science 1995;269: 540–3.
166. Tartaglia LA, Dembski M, Weng X, et al. Cell 1995;83: 1263–71.
167. Chen H, Charlat O, Tartaglia LA, et al. Cell 1996;84:491–5.
168. Lee GH, Proença R, Montez JM, et al. Nature 1996;379:632–5.
169. Chua SC Jr, Chung WK, Wu-Peng XS, et al. Science 1996;271: 994–6.
170. Michaud EJ, Bultman SJ, Klebig ML, et al. Proc Natl Acad Sci USA 1994;91:2562–6.
171. Montague CT, Farooqi IS, Whitehead JP, et al. Nature 1997; 387:903–8.
172. Maffei M, Halaas J, Ravussin E, et al. Nature Med 1995;1: 1155–61.
173. Considine RV, Sinha M, Heiman M, et al. N Engl J Med 1995; 334:292–5.
174. Considine RV, Considine EL, Williams CJ, et al. Diabetes 1996;45:992–4.
175. Schwartz MW, Figlewitz DP, Woods SC, et al. Ann NY Acad Sci 1993;692:60–71.
176. Shields J. Monozygotic twins brought up apart and brought up together. London: Oxford University Press, 1962.
177. Newman HH, Freeman FN, Holzinger KJ. Twins: a study of heredity and environment. Chicago: University of Chicago Press, 1937.
178. Stunkard AJ, Foch TT, Hrubec Z. JAMA 1986;256:51–4.
179. Stunkard AJ, Harris JR, Pedersen NL, et al. N Engl J Med 1990;322:1438–87.
180. Bouchard C. Inheritance of human fat distribution. In: Bouchard C, Johnson FE, eds. Fat distribution during growth and later health outcomes. New York: Alan R Liss, 1988.
181. Bouchard C. Acta Med Scand 1988;723(Suppl):135–41.
182. Bouchard C, Tremblay A, Despres JP, et al. N Engl J Med 1990;322:1477–82.
183. Garn SM, Bailey SM. Am J Clin Nutr 1976;29:1067–8.
184. Garn SM, Clark DC. Pediatrics 1976;57:443–55.
185. Withers RFJ. Eugen Rev 1964;56:81–90.
186. Biron P, Mongeau JG, Bertrand D. J Pediatr 1977;91:555–8.
187. Rao DC, MacLean CJ, Morton NE, et al. Am J Hum Genet 1975;27:509–20.
188. Dunaif A, Givens JR, Haseltine F, et al. The polycystic ovary syndrome. Cambridge, MA: Blackwell Scientific, 1991.
189. Plymate SR, Fariss BL, Bassett ML, et al. J Clin Endocrinol Metab 1981;52:1246–8.
190. Bray GA. Pediatr Ann 1984;13:525–36.
191. Sims EAH, Danforth E Jr, Horton EJ, et al. Recent Prog Horm Res 1973;29:457–76.
192. Kennedy GC. Proc R Soc Lond (B) 1953;140:578–92.
193. Mrosovsky N. Physiol Behav 1986;38:407–14.
194. Smith GP, Gibbs J. Fed Proc 1984;43:2889–92.
195. Kissileff HR, Pi-Sunyer FX, Thornton J, et al. Am J Clin Nutr 1981;34:154–60.
196. Hoebel BG, Hernandez L. Basic neural mechanisms of feeding and weight regulation. In: Stunkard AJ, Wadden TA, eds. Obesity. Theory and therapy. 2nd ed. New York: Raven Press, 1993;43–62.
197. Leibowitz SF. Brain Res Bull 1991;27:333–7.
198. Sahu A, Kolra SP. Trends Endocrinol Metab 1993;4:217–24.

199. Kyrkouli SE, Stanley BG, Hutchinson R, et al. Brain Res 1990;521:185–91.
200. Smith GP, Gibbs J. Ann NY Acad Sci 1994;713:236–41.
201. Ravussin E, Lilioja S, Anderson TE, et al. J Clin Invest 1986;78:1568–78.
202. Bogardus C, Lillioja S, Ravussin E, et al. N Engl J Med 1986;315:96–100.
203. Bernstein RS, Thornton JC, Yang MU, et al. Am J Clin Nutr 1983;37:595–602.
204. Zurlo F, Larson K, Bogardus C, et al. J Clin Invest 1990; 86:1423–7.
205. Millward DJ, Garlick PJ. Proc Nutr Soc 1976;35:229–349.
206. Spady BW, Payne PR, Picou D, et al. Am J Clin Nutr 1976;29: 1073–88.
207. Boothby WM, Berkson J, Dunn HL, et al. Am J Physiol 1936; 116:468–84.
208. James WPT, Trayhurn P. Br Med Bull 1981;37:43–8.
209. Ravussin E, Burnand B, Schutz Y, et al. Am J Clin Nutr 1982;35:566–73.
210. Roberts SB, Savage J, Coward WA, et al. N Engl J Med 1988;318:461–6.
211. Griffiths M, Payne PR, Stunkard AJ, et al. Lancet 1990; 336:76–7.
212. Ravussin E, Lillioja S, Knowler WC, et al. N Engl J Med 1988;318:467–72.
213. Zurlo F, Lillioja S, Esposito-Del Puente A, et al. Am J Physiol 1990;259:E650–7.
214. Swinburn BA, Nyomba BL, Saad MF. J Clin Invest 1991;88: 168–73.
215. Shetty PS, Jung RT, James WPT, et al. Clin Sci 1981;60:519–25.
216. Pittet P, Chappuis P, Acheson K, et al. Br J Nutr 1976; 35:281–8.
217. Ravussin E, Bogardus C, Schwartz RS, et al. J Clin Invest 1983;72:893–902.
218. Strang JM, McClugage HB. Am J Med Sci 1931;182:79–81.
219. Clough DP, Durnin JVGA. J Physiol 1970;207:89P.
220. Felig P, Cunningham J, Levitt M, et al. Am J Physiol 1983;244:E45–51.
221. Rothwell NJ, Stock MJ. Metabolism 1981;30:673–8.
222. Golay A, Schutz Y, Meyer HU, et al. Diabetes 1982;31:1023–8.
223. Segal KR, Lacayanga I, Dunaif A, et al. Am J Physiol 1988;256:E573–9.
224. Segal KR, Albu J, Chun A, et al. J Appl Physiol 1991;71: 2402–11.
225. Thorne A. Acta Chir Scand 1990;559(Suppl):6–59.
226. Neumann RO. Arch Hyg 1902;45:1–87.
227. Garrow JS. The regulation of energy expenditure in men. In: Bray GA, ed. Recent advances in obesity research, vol 2. London: Newman, 1978;200–10.
228. James WPT, Trayhurn P. Obesity in mice and men. In: Beers RF, Barrett EG, eds. Nutritional factors: modulating effects on metabolic processes. New York: Raven Press, 1981;123–38.
229. Bradfield RB, Curtis DE, Margen S. Am J Clin Nutr 1968;21: 1208–10.
230. Segal KR, Gutin B. Metabolism 1983;32:581–9.
231. Swindells YE. Br J Nutr 1972;27:65–73.
232. Hansen JJ. J Appl Physiol 1973;35:587–91.
233. Warnold I, Lenner RA. Am J Clin Nutr 1977;30:304–15.
234. Strong JA, Shirling D, Passmore R. Br J Nutr 1967;21:909–19.
235. Sims EAH, Goldman RD, Gluck CM, et al. Trans Assoc Am Physicians 1968;81:153–70.
236. Segal KR, Pi-Sunyer FX. Med Clin North Am 1989;73:217–36.
237. Sjöström L. Fat cells and body weight. In: Stunkard AJ, ed. Obesity. Philadelphia: WB Saunders, 1980.
238. Knittle JL, Hirsch J. J Clin Invest 1968;47:2091–8.
239. Hirsch J, Han PW. J Lipid Res 1969;10:77–82.
240. Braun T, Kazdova L, Fabry P, et al. Metab Clin Exp 1968;17:825–32.
241. DiGirolamo M, Mendlinger S. Am J Physiol 1971;221:859–64.
242. Lemmonier D. J Clin Invest 1972;51:2907–15.
243. Hager A, Sjöström L, Arvidsson B, et al. Metabolism 1977;26:607–14.
244. Hager A, Sjöström L, Arvidsson B, et al. Am J Clin Nutr 1978;31:68–75.
245. Krotkiewski M, Sjöström L, Björntorp P, et al. Int J Obes 1977;1:395–416.
246. Flier JS. Cell 1995;80:15–8.
247. Hotamisligil GS, Shargill NS, Spiegelman BM. Science 1993;259:87–91.
248. Hotamisligil GS, Murray DL, Choy LN, et al. Proc Natl Acad Sci USA 1994;91:4854–8.
249. Rosen BS, Cook KS, Yaglom J, et al. Science 1989;224:1483–7.
250. Shimomura I, Funahashi T, Takahashi M, et al. Nature Med 1996;2:800–3.
251. Frederich R Jr, Kahn BB, Peach MJ, et al. Hypertension 1992;19:339–44.
252. Chehab FF, Lim ME, Lu R. Nature Genet 1996;2:318–20.
253. Lithel H, Boberg J, Hellsing K, et al. Ups J Med Sci 1978;83:45–52.
254. Reitman JS, Kosmakos FC, Howard BV, et al. J Clin Invest 1982;70:791–7.
255. Schwartz R, Brunzell J. Lancet 1978;1:1230–1.
256. Schwartz R, Brunzell J. J Clin Invest 1981;67:1425–30.
257. Rebuffe-Scrive M, Basdevant A, Guy-Grand B. Am J Clin Nutr 1983;37:974–80.
258. Wadden TA. Ann Intern Med 1993;119:688–93.
259. Apfelbaum M, Bostsarron J, Lacatis D. Am J Clin Nutr 1971;24:1405–9.
260. Grande F, Anderson JT, Keys A. J Appl Physiol 1958;12:230–8.
261. Owens JL, Thompson D, Shah N. J Nutr 1979;109:1584–91.
262. Björntörp P, Enzi G, Karlsson M, et al. Int J Obes 1980;4:11–9.
263. DiGirolamo M, Smith U, Bjorntorp P. Refeeding effects on adipocyte metabolism. In: Bjorntorp P, Cairella M, Howard AN, eds. Recent advances in obesity research III. London: John Libbey, 1980;99–105.
264. Björntörp P, Yang MU. Am J Clin Nutr 1982;36:444–9.
265. Leibel RL, Hirsch J. Metabolism 1984;33:164–70.
266. Leibel RL, Hirsch J. N Engl J Med 1995;332:621–8.
267. Faust JM, Johnson PR, Hirsch J. Science 1977;197:393–6.
268. Krotkiewski M, Sjöström L, Björntörp P. Int J Obes 1977; 1:395–416.
269. VanItallie TB. Am J Clin Nutr 1978;31:543–52.
270. Council on Foods and Nutrition. JAMA 1973;224:1415–9.
271. Rickman F, Mitchell N, Dingman J, et al. JAMA 1974;22S: 54–8.
272. Pritikin N. Live longer now: the first one hundred years of your life. New York: Grosset and Dunlap, 1974.
273. Lissner L, Levitsky DA, Strupp BJ, et al. Am J Clin Nutr 1987;46:886–92.
274. Kendall A, Levitsky DA, Strupp BJ, et al. Am J Clin Nutr 1991;53:1124–9.
275. Weinsier RL, Johnston MH, Doleys DM, et al. Br J Nutr 1982;47:367–79.
276. Thompson TJ, Runcie J, Miller V. Lancet 1966;2:992–6.
277. Drenick JJ, Swendseid ME, Blahd WH, et al. JAMA 1964;187:100–5.
278. Yang MU, VanItallie TB. Effect of energy restriction on body composition and nitrogen balance in obese individuals. In: Wadden TA, VanItallie TB, eds. Treatment of the seriously obese patient. New York: Guilford Press, 1992;83–106.

279. Lindner PG, Blackburn GL. Obes Bariatr Med 1976;5: 198–216.
280. Wadden TA, Stunkard AJ, Brownell KD. Ann Intern Med 1983;99:675–84.
281. Owen OE, Felig P, Morgan AP, et al. J Clin Invest 1969;48: 574–83.
282. Calloway DH, Odell ACF, Margen S. J Nutr 1971;101:775–86.
283. Felig P, Owen OE, Wahren J, et al. J Clin Invest 1969;48: 458–594.
284. Consolazio CF, Matoush LO, Johnson HL, et al. Am J Clin Nutr 1968;21:803–12.
285. Apfelbaum M, Bostarron J, Brigant L, et al. Gastroenterologia 1967;108:121–34.
286. Bistrian BR, Winterer J, Blackburn G, et al. J Lab Clin Med 1977;89:1030–5.
287. Baird IM, Parsons RL, Howard AN. Metabolism 1974;23: 645–57.
288. Genuth SM, Castro JH, Vertes V. JAMA 1974;230:987–991.
289. Vertes V, Genuth SM, Hazelton IM. JAMA 1977;238:2151–3.
290. Flatt JP, Blackburn FL. Am J Clin Nutr 1974;27:175–87.
291. Sherwin RS, Hendler RG, Felig P. J Clin Invest 1975;44: 1382–90.
292. Marliss EB, Murray FT, Nakhooda AFF. J Clin Invest 1978; 62:468–79.
293. Landau RL, Rochman H, Blix-Gruber P, et al. Am J Clin Nutr 1981;34:1300–4.
294. Frattali VP. FDA By-Lines 1979;9:179.
295. Sours HE, Frattali VP, Brand CD, et al. Am J Clin Nutr 1981;34:453–61.
296. Singh BN, Gaarder TD, Kanegae T, et al. JAMA 1978;240:115–9.
297. VanItallie TB. JAMA 1978;240:144–5.
298. Jones AOL, Jacobs RM, Fry BE, et al. Am J Clin Nutr 1980;33:2545–50.
299. Pi-Sunyer FX. Am J Clin Nutr 1992;56:240S–3S.
300. DeHaven J, Sherwin R, Hendler R, et al. N Engl J Med 1980;302:477–82.
301. Sigler MH. J Clin Invest 1975;55:377–87.
302. Yang MU, VanItallie TB. J Clin Invest 1976;58:722–30.
303. Yang M, Barbosa SJL, Pi-Sunyer FX, et al. Int J Obes 1981;5:231–6.
304. Pi-Sunyer FX. Obesity. In: Rackel RE, ed. Conn's current therapy. Philadelphia: WB Saunders, 1998;574–9.
305. Steinhaus AH. Physiol Rev 1983;13:103–47.
306. Karpovitch PV. Res Q 1941;12:423–31.
307. Woo R, Garrow JS, Pi-Sunyer FX. Am J Clin Nutr 1982; 36:470–7.
308. Woo R, Garrow JS, Pi-Sunyer FX. Am J Clin Nutr 1982;36: 478–84.
309. Freedman-Akabas S, Colt E, Kissileff HR, et al. Am J Clin Nutr 1985;4:545–9.
310. Adams RP, Welch HG. J Appl Physiol 1980;49:863–8.
311. Passmore R, Thomson JG, Warnock GM. Br J Nutr 1952;6:253–64.
312. Woo R, Pi-Sunyer FX. Metabolism 1985;34:836–41.
313. Dempsey JA. Res Q 1964;35:275–87.
314. Williams BT. J Am Geriatr Soc 1968;16:794–7.
315. Boileau RA, Buskirk ER, Horstman DH, et al. Med Sci Sports 1971;3:183–9.
316. Pi-Sunyer FX, Woo R. Am J Clin Nutr 1985;42:983–90.
317. Rissanen A, Heliovara M, Knekt P, et al. Eur J Clin Invest 1991;45:419–30.
318. King AC, Tribble DL. Sports Med 1991;11:331–49.
319. Pavlou KN, Krey S, Steffee WP. Am J Clin Nutr 1989;49: 1115–23.
320. Craddock D. Obesity and its management. 3rd ed. Edinburgh: Churchill Livingstone, 1978;92–109.
321. Evans RR, Wallace MG. Curr Med Res Opin 1975;4:132–7.
322. Sullivan AC, Cheng L. Appetite regulation and its modulation by drugs. In: Hathcock JN, Coon J, eds. Nutrition and drug interrelations. New York: Academic Press, 1978.
323. Griboff SL, Berman R, Silverman H. Curr Ther Res Clin Exp 1975;17:535–43.
324. Hoebel BG, Krauss I, Cooper J, et al. Obes Bariatr Med 1975;4:200–6.
325. Bray GA. Ann Intern Med 1991;115:152–3.
326. Guy-Grand B, Crepaldi G, Lefebvre P, et al. Lancet 1989;ii:1142–5.
327. Bray GA, Ryan DH, Gordon D, et al. Obes Res 1996;4:263–70.
327a. Eckel R. Circulation 1997;96:3248–50.
328. Weintraub M, Sundaresan PR, Madan M, et al. Clin Pharmacol Ther 1992;51:581–642.
328a. Connoly HM, Crary JL, McGoon MD, et al. N Engl J Med 1997;337:581–8.
328b. Anon. MMWR 1997;46:1061–2.
328c. Brenot F, Herve P, Petitprez P, et al. Br Heart J 1993;70:537–41.
328d. Abenhaim L, Moride Y, Brenot F, et al. N Engl J Med 1996;335:609–16.
329. James WPT, Avenell A, Broom J, et al. J Int Obes 1997; 1S24–S30.
330. VanItallie TB. Am J Clin Nutr 1979;32:2723–33.
331. Bruch H. Eating disorders: obesity anorexia nervosa and the person within. New York: Basic Books, 1973.
332. Rand CS, Stunkard AJ. J Am Acad Psychoanal 1977;5:459–97.
333. Powers PS. Obesity: the regulation of body weight. Baltimore: Williams & Wilkins, 1980.
334. Halmi KA, Stunkard JA, Mason EE. Am J Nutr 1980;33: 446–51.
335. Glucksman JL, Hirsch J. Psychosom Med 1969;31:1–7.
336. Crisp AH, McGuiness B. Br Med J 1975;1:7–9.
337. Telch CF, Agras WS, Rossiter E, et al. J Consult Clin Psychol 1990;58:629–35.
338. Schachter S. Am Psychol 1971;26:129–44.
339. Schachter S. Emotion, obesity and crime. New York: Academic Press, 1971.
340. Rodin J. The externality theory today. In: Stunkard AJ, ed. Obesity. Philadelphia: WB Saunders, 1980;226–39.
341. Stuart RB. Behav Res Ther 1967;5:357–65.
342. Mahoney MJ. Psychiatr Clin North Am 1978;1:651–60.
343. Stunkard AJ. Int J Obes 1978;2:237–49.
344. Jeffrey RW, Thompson PD, Wing RR. Behav Res Ther 1978;16:363–70.
345. Stalonas PM, Johnson WG, Christ M. J Consult Clin Psychol 1978;46:463–9.
346. Wadden TA, Sternberg JA, Letizia KA, et al. Int J Obes 1989;13:39–46.
347. Pi-Sunyer FX. Am J Clin Nutr 1976;29:409–16.
348. Mason EE, Ito C. Surg Clin North Am 1967;47:1345–51.
349. Tretbar LL, Sigers EC. Int J Obes 1981;5:538.
350. Kral J. Surgical treatment of obesity. In: Björntörp P, Brodoff BM, eds. Obesity. Philadelphia: JB Lippincott, 1992.
350a. Consensus Development Conference Panel. Ann Intern Med 1991;115:956–61.
351. Lissner L, Odell PM, D'Agostino RB. N Engl J Med 1991;324: 1839–44.
352. Hamm P, Shekele RB, Stamler J. Am J Epidemiol 1989; 129:312–8.
353. Wing RR. Ann Behav Med 1992;14:113–9.
354. Jebb SA, Goldberg GR, Coward WA, et al. Int J Obes 1991;15:367–74.

88. Nutritional Aspects of Hematologic Disorders

ISRAEL CHANARIN

The formation of blood cells (hematopoiesis) is sited in the bone marrow cavity (medulla) of virtually all bones in the newborn, but in adults, active blood formation is confined to the central skeleton (skull, vertebral column, ribs, and pelvis) and upper ends of the humerus and femur. All hematopoietic cells arise from a very small population of self-renewing stem cells, and no more than 5% of these are dividing at any one time (1). Stem cells are too few in number to be seen or, indeed, recognized in marrow aspirates but react with a monoclonal antibody designated CD 34. Stem cells, under the influence of a range of growth factors, give rise to red blood cells, white blood cells including neutrophil, eosinophil, and basophil polymorphonuclear leukocytes, monocytes, lymphocytes, and platelets.

The nutritional requirements for hematopoiesis are no different from those of any other tissue. However, turnover of blood cells is normally greater than that of other tissues in the body, and availability of three nutrients can become limiting: iron, cobalamin (cbl, vitamin B_{12}), and pteroylglutamic acid, (folic acid, or folate). Iron is required as the oxygen carrier in the hemoglobin molecule in erythrocytes, and cbl and folate are essential in the synthesis of three of the four nucleotides of DNA required for the doubling of the DNA content of the cell before mitosis. Lack of other nutrients only rarely causes anemia; these include vitamin A, vitamin B_6, riboflavin, ascorbic acid, vitamin E, and copper.

A vegetarian diet usually supplies adequate amounts of iron, but its availability is low unless food of animal origin or ascorbate are also present. Furthermore, a vegetarian diet contains no cbl other than that arising from bacterial contamination. However, such diets usually have adequate amounts of folate (see Chapter 106).

ANEMIA AND ITS CLINICAL CONSEQUENCES

Impairment of normal red cell production results in a fall in the hemoglobin concentration, red cell count, and packed cell volume below the levels shown in Table 88.1. Those living at an altitude of 4000 feet or more have higher blood values. There are no racial differences. The fall in blood values in turn leads to a reduction in the oxygen-carrying capacity of the blood and impairment of oxygen delivery to tissues. The effects of anemia are due not only to impaired oxygen delivery but also to the compensatory mechanisms that develop.

The compensatory mechanisms are of three kinds. There is an increase in the level of 2,3-diphosphoglycerate in anemic red blood cells, which leads to increased binding of this compound to deoxyhemoglobin and so reduces its affinity for oxygen. As a result, a greater proportion of the oxygen on hemoglobin can be released to tissues. A second adjustment to anemia is speeding circulation of blood by increasing cardiac output; this becomes clinically obvious when the hemoglobin concentration falls below 7 g/dL. Finally, the decline in oxygenation of the kidneys results in increased production of the erythropoietic hormone, erythropoietin, which leads to increased blood production and extension of hematopoiesis into fatty bone

Conversion factors to SI units: iron, 1 mg = 0.18 mmol, 1 μg = 0.18 μmol; ferritin, 1 ng = 3.51 nmol; hemoglobin, 1 g = 0.62 mmol; cobalamin, 1 ng = 7.4 pmol, 1 μg = 0.75 nmol; folate, 1 ng = 2.27 nmol, 1 μg = 2.27 μmol, 1 mg = 2.27 mmol.

Table 88.1
Values in a Blood Count below Which Anemia Is Present

	Females	Males
Red cell count ($10^6/mm^3$)	4.0	4.5
Hemoglobin (g/dL)	12.5	13.5
Packed cell volume (%)	37	40

marrow. In chronic anemia, these compensatory mechanisms allow the patient to continue relatively normal activity, so that the severity of anemia often appears out of keeping with the paucity of symptoms.

Most patients with significant anemia are tired and tire easily after exertion. They are pale, most evident on inspection of mucous membranes. Palpitations (awareness of the heart beat), tinnitus (ringing or whistling noise in the ears or head), headache, irritability, dizziness, and weakness may be present. Patients are short of breath and have a rapid heart beat and pulse and visible arterial pulsation. There are often systolic heart murmurs on cardiac auscultation that disappear when the anemia has been corrected. In older people, cardiac pain (angina) and cardiac failure may develop, the latter characterized by swelling of the feet, enlarged liver, and pulmonary edema.

A sore mouth and tongue is often present in iron, cbl, or folate deficiencies. In the latter two deficiencies, impaired squamous cell renewal in mouth and tongue can be blamed, and a high iron requirement may also explain these findings in iron deficiency. There may be cracks at the angles of the mouth termed *angular stomatitis* (Fig. 88.1). Other findings in particular deficiencies are dealt with below in this chapter.

IRON

Basic aspects are dealt with in detail in Chapter 10. Since most of the iron in the body is in red blood cells, blood loss is the major cause of iron deficiency. Major sites of blood loss are the gastrointestinal tract in both sexes and menstrual blood loss in women. Intestinal malabsorption of iron and increased iron requirements for growth or that are not met from the diet in pregnancy are other causes of iron deficiency. This account is concerned with nutritional factors involved in producing a negative iron balance and iron deficiency. Frequently nutritional factors and blood loss coexist; most importantly, poor iron availability from a vegetarian diet in large numbers of people may coexist with hookworm infestation of the small gut, which produces considerable blood loss.

Physiologic Considerations

In addition to hemoglobin iron (1600–2400 mg in an adult), iron is present in myoglobin (300 mg) and various heme and many nonheme enzymes (150 mg) including cytochromes concerned with oxidative reactions producing energy. Reserve (storage) iron linked to ferritin and hemosiderin is present in liver, spleen, and marrow. An adult man has some 500 to 1000 mg of storage iron, and older men even more. Iron stores in women seldom reach 500 mg. Indeed, when iron requirements are high, as in growing children, menstruating women and in pregnancy, iron stores are more usually absent or low. Disappearance of iron stores precedes development of overt anemia, but by itself, absence of iron stores does not produce symptoms. Iron stores are assessed by the serum ferritin level (the higher the level, the greater the iron store) and by the amount of stainable iron in aspirated bone marrow fragments or liver biopsy specimens.

Adult iron turnover is some 22 mg of iron each day: 20 to 21 mg coming from recycled iron recovered from effete red blood cells and only about 1 mg in men and 2 mg in women from absorption of dietary iron. The latter constitute iron requirements and arise from iron loss as a result of desquamation of epithelial cells and by iron lost in menstruation. Children require additional iron for growth, and pregnancy increases iron requirements substantially. Iron losses have been assessed as follows.

In adult males, iron losses have been measured at 0.9 mg/24 h or 14 μg/kg/24 h (2). Extrapolation of data from males indicates a basal iron loss of 0.8 mg/24 h for a 55-kg woman. Median menstrual blood loss in healthy women is between 25 and 30 mL per cycle. Averaged over the entire menstrual cycle, the daily iron loss is 0.5 mg/24 h. A quarter of women lose more than 0.8 mg/24 h, 10% more than 1.3 mg/24 h, and 5% more than 1.6 mg/24 h. When basal iron losses are added, the daily iron requirement in 5% of women exceeds 2.4 mg/24 h. Oral contraceptives reduce menstrual loss by about half, whereas intrauterine devices double the loss.

Pregnant women require iron to replace basal iron losses (220 mg iron during pregnancy going to term), to expand their red cell mass (500 mg), and to provide for the placenta and fetus. The full-term fetus has about 290 mg of iron, and placenta about 25 mg. Thus the total additional iron requirement in pregnancy is about 1000 mg. The increased requirement starts in the second trimester; the daily iron requirement increases from 0.8 mg in the first trimester to 4.4 mg in the second and to 6.3 mg daily in the third. In the latter two-thirds of pregnancy, iron needs cannot be satisfied from dietary iron alone. Unless one believes that at least 500 mg of iron is available as iron stores present before pregnancy, iron supplements need to be given. There is further iron loss due to bleeding during delivery. During pregnancy, iron loss from menstruation ceases, and during the puerperium, reduction of the red cell mass makes the iron in these surplus red cells available. Following delivery, several months elapse before menstruation is restored in a lactating woman. There is, however, a daily loss of 0.3 mg in breast milk. The mean iron requirement during 6 months of lactation is 1.1 mg daily.

Table 88.2
Iron Requirements for Infants and Children

Age (Years)	Mean Body Weight (kg)	Growth Requirement (mg/24 h)	Basal Losses (mg/24 h)	Total Requirement (mg/24 h)
0.25–1	3	0.56	0.21	0.77
1–2	11	0.24	0.25	0.49
2–6	16	0.22	0.34	0.55
6–12	29	0.38	0.55	0.94
12–16M	53	0.66	0.80	1.45
12–16F	51	0.35	0.79	1.62[a]

From FAO/WHO. Requirements of vitamin A, iron, folate, and vitamin B_{12}. FAO Food and Nutrition series no. 23. Rome, Italy: Food and Agriculture Organization, 1988:1–107.

[a]Allowing for menstrual loss of 0.47 mg/24h.

A normal newborn has about 75 mg of iron per kilogram, of which two-thirds is in hemoglobin. The physiologic decrease in red cell mass in the first 2 months of life returns some iron to stores. Absorption of dietary iron becomes significant only at 4 to 6 months of life, when initial iron stores have become considerably depleted. Premature (low-birth-weight) infants have much reduced iron stores and need dietary iron at a much earlier age than full-term infants. In childhood, additional iron is required for the expanding red cell mass and for growth. (See Table 88.2 for FAO-WHO recommendations and Table 88.3 for U.S. RDA.)

Absorption and Availability of Dietary Iron

There are two forms of dietary iron, heme iron and nonheme iron.

Heme Iron

Heme provides 10 to 15% of food iron taken in a mixed diet. The heme is present in hemoglobin and myoglobin of animal foods. Between 20 and 30% of heme iron is absorbed, and its absorption is largely independent of the overall composition of the diet. Heme iron may meet about one-quarter of iron requirements in those eating a diet of high meat content. In the enterocyte, the iron is split from the tetrapyrrol portion of the heme.

Table 88.3
Recommended Daily Dietary Allowances (U.S. 1989)

Age (Years)	Iron (mg)	Cobalamin (μg)	Folate (μg)
0–0.5	6	0.3	25
0.5–1.0	10	0.5	35
1–3	10	0.7	50
4–6	10	1.0	75
7–10	10	1.4	100
11–14 Males	12	2.0	150
15–18	12	2.0	200
19–51+	10	2.0	200
11–14 Females	15	2.0	150
15–50	15	2.0	180
51+	10	2.0	180
Pregnant	30	2.2	400
Lactating 1st 6 months	15	2.6	280
2nd 6 months	15	2.6	260

Nonheme Iron

Nonheme iron is present in cereals, pulses (seeds of leguminous plants), fruits, vegetables, and dairy produce. It provides 85 to 90% of dietary iron in a mixed diet and is the only source of iron in a largely vegetarian diet. The mixture of foods in a diet contains factors that either promote or inhibit iron absorption, and thus, the amount of iron absorbed may vary considerably.

Absorption of food iron is inhibited by phytates, polyphenols (3) including tannins present in tea, certain proteins, and certain dietary fibers. Inhibitors act by strongly binding ionic iron. Phytates are salts of inositol hexaphosphates, and about 90% arise from dietary cereals. Even small amounts of phytates have a strong inhibitory effect on iron absorption. Bran has a high phytate content as does high-extraction-rate flour. Fiber-rich foods have abundant phytates. A high dietary iron content does not counteract the inhibitory effect of fiber. Polyphenols are widely present in plants and some bind iron, particularly those in tea, coffee, and cocoa. They are also present in vegetables such as spinach and in some herbs and spices. Calcium as a salt or in milk and cheese interferes with both heme and nonheme iron absorption (4).

Absorption of food iron is enhanced by the presence of meat, poultry, seafood, and ascorbic acid. Ascorbic acid, as such or derived from fruit and vegetables, is a potent enhancer of iron absorption, probably by reducing ferric to ferrous iron. Iron can probably only be absorbed in its ferrous form. Apart from their effect as a reducing agent, iron-ascorbate complexes are absorbed as such. Other weak organic acids such as citric acid may also enhance absorption of nonheme iron. Why meat, fish, and other seafood enhance absorption of nonheme iron is not clear.

Apart from the composition of the diet, the amount of iron absorbed is affected by the subject's iron status. Substantial iron stores decrease iron absorption, particularly of nonheme iron, and conversely, iron deficiency is accompanied by an increase in iron absorption to a maximum of 4 mg/24 h. This, however, is still short of the daily iron requirement in the latter months of pregnancy.

Total Dietary Iron Intake

Daily iron intake per capita in 137 countries ranged from 14.4 to 20.2 mg (2). Animal produce was a major contributor of iron in only 23 of these countries. This iron intake should be enough to meet a requirement of 1 to 2 mg daily, but it often does not do so because of the low availability of the iron in these diets. A comparison of the diet and iron status of 50 vegetarians and 50 matched subjects on mixed diets showed that the vegetarians consumed 16.8 mg iron daily compared with 14.6 mg from the mixed diet, but those on a mixed diet had larger iron stores. Serum ferritin levels in vegetarians were 36.6 ng/mL, compared with 105.4 ng/mL in those on a mixed diet (6).

Diets provide iron of low, intermediate, or high bioavailability (2). The data refer to iron absorption by individuals with no iron stores but with normal iron transport. A low-iron-bioavailibilty diet (iron absorption about 5%) is a monotonous diet of cereals, roots, and/or tubers and negligible amounts of meat, fish, or foods likely to contain ascorbate. These foods often contain inhibitors to iron absorption present in maize, beans, whole wheat flour, and sorghum and are largely consumed in lower socioeconomic groups in developing countries. Diets consisting largely of cereals may allow only 1 to 2% of the iron to be absorbed. This diet does not meet the needs of menstruating or pregnant women but may suffice under other circumstances.

Intermediate-iron-bioavailability diets (iron absorption about 10%) consist mainly of cereals, roots and/or tubers, some food supplying ascorbate, and minimal food of animal origin. A low bioavailability diet can be changed into one of intermediate bioavailability by increased intake of meat, fish, or ascorbate. A high bioavailability diet can be changed to one of intermediate iron availibility by simultaneous consumption of tea or coffee, which contain inhibitors to iron absorption. This diet may meet the needs of some menstruating women but not the needs of pregnant women.

A high-iron-bioavailability diet (iron absorption about 15%) is a mixed diet with good quantities of meat, poultry, fish, and foods of high ascorbate content. It is typical of the diet in industrialized countries. It is adequate for menstruating women but without substantial iron stores will not meet the needs in many pregnancies.

Human breast milk contains about 0.5 mg iron per liter. The bioavailability is high; 50% of this iron is absorbed. This contrasts with cow's milk formulas or unfortified cow's milk, in which only 10 to 20% of the iron is available for absorption. Cow's milk formulas are usually fortified with iron to supply 6 to 12 mg/L. Breast milk supplies sufficient iron to full-term infants to meet their needs for the first 4 to 5 months of life. Weaning foods often consist of cereals with iron of low bioavailability. Thus many have iron and ascorbate added, and they are a major source of iron in the first year or two of life. The 1989 U.S. RDA for iron is shown in Table 88.3. See also Appendix Table II-A-2 for the U.S. and Tables II A 3–8 for other national and international standards.

Prevalence of Iron Deficiency

Conservative estimates indicate that at least 700 million individuals worldwide have overt iron deficiency anemia. Major factors contributing to widespread iron deficiency include diets low in available iron, intestinal blood loss where hookworm infestation is prevalent, and demands for iron that cannot be met during pregnancy and growth. In African countries, millet, sorghum, or maize is the staple food, and in many parts of Asia, it is rice. Anemia is present in 36% of the population in developing countries and in about 8% of the population of developed countries. It is the most prevalent nutritional deficiency in the world. The frequency of iron deficiency in the U.S. is shown in Table 88.4.

Table 88.4
Incidence of Iron Deficiency (%) in the United States Assessed by the National Health and Nutrition Examination Study

Age (Years)	Males	Females
1–2	9.2	9.2
3–10	6.1	6.1
11–14	3.5–12.1	6.1
15–44	About 2.0	2.5–14.2
45–74	About 2.0	6.1

In clinical practice, iron deficiency is equated with blood loss, except in pregnancy and early childhood, when unmet demands for iron are the main factors. This is the proper clinical approach, since bleeding lesions in the gut, benign or malignant, and menorrhagia in women are generally amenable to intervention. A mixed diet is expected to supply enough iron when there is a normal iron requirement.

Clinical practice in communities that are largely vegetarian brings home the fact that purely nutritional factors are of great importance. A study of megaloblastic anemia in an affluent Hindu community of strict lifelong vegetarians generally taking only cow's milk as the only form of animal food, showed that two-thirds of 138 patients had overt iron deficiency, 53 women and 38 men. Stainable iron stores in bone marrow were absent in 70%. There was no abnormal blood loss (14).

Signs and Symptoms in Iron Deficiency Anemia

There may be no clinical complaints, and evidence of iron deficiency may come to light as the result of a blood count. Most patients, however, have symptoms of anemia (described above). In addition, they may have complaints attributable to iron deficiency directly. These include difficulty in swallowing and a sensation of a lump in the throat. They may have a sensation of pins and needles (paresthesia) in hands and feet. Some have a sore mouth and tongue, which may be aggravated by hot drinks or spicy food. There may be angular stomatitis (Fig. 88.1) and possibly reversible gastric atrophy. Pica (eating of materials such as ice, clay, paper, dirt, etc.) occurs, particularly in children. Obsessive eating of ice (pagophagia) may be specific to iron deficiency and disappears within 1 to 2 weeks of iron treatment. Eating of ice was noted in 8.1% of 553 African American women with iron deficiency in pregnancy (5).

Examination reveals pallor, pale blue sclera, and nails that break easily and may be misshapen and even spoon shaped (koilonychia). Heart and pulse rate may be rapid, and in severely anemic patients of longstanding, the spleen may be enlarged, and the edge palpable under the left costal margin. Radiography may show a web in the oesophagus (postcricoid web) and atrophic gastritis. Less well established are observations indicating impaired work performance and muscle function, possibly due to an effect of iron lack on enzymes.

There is impairment of both cell-mediated (T-lymphocyte) immunity and neutrophil killing of phagocytosed bacteria by white blood cells from iron-deficient patients. Ingested organisms are killed by production of active oxygen species, including free hydroxyl radicals; this is termed the *respiratory burst.* Iron-containing enzymes including NADPH oxidase and cytochrome B are involved in generation of the active oxygen. Iron treatment, particularly with parenteral iron, can precipitate latent infection such as pyelonephritis and activate latent malaria. Indeed, patients from areas where malaria is endemic should be given iron therapy with antimalarial prophylaxis.

Impaired mental development was found when hemoglobin levels were below 10 g/dL at 5 years of age (7), manifested in lower scores in mental and motor function, although results became normal when tests were repeated after iron therapy. The children showed reduced attention and poor learning performance. The iron content of parts of the brain is comparable to that of liver and continues to increase until the third decade of life. Iron uptake in the central nervous system (CNS) is effected by a transferrin system comparable to that in the bone marrow.

In pregnancy, iron deficiency is accompanied by increased maternal morbidity including premature labor and low-birth-weight infants (8).

Diagnosis of Iron Deficiency

A blood count shows a reduced hemoglobin level and hematocrit (Table 88.1) and a fall in the size of the red blood cells to below 80 fL (femtoliters). Smaller red cells contain less hemoglobin, so that the mean corpuscular hemoglobin (MCH) is below 27 pg (picograms). In early anemia, the stained blood film often shows the smaller red cells to be fully hemoglobinized, but as the hemoglobin falls, hypochromia is visible. In severe anemia, the red cell appears as a thin pink ring (Fig. 88.2). The nuclei of the neutrophil polymorphs tend to have an increased number of lobes.

The serum iron level falls below the normal range of 11 to 28 μmol/L, and the serum iron-binding capacity rises above the normal range of 47 to 70 μmol/L. Transferrin saturation falls below the normal range of 16 to 60%. At these low iron levels, there is poor release of iron to normoblasts. Serum ferritin is below 11 μg/L, and stainable iron is largely absent from bone marrow particles.

Differential Diagnosis

Apart from iron deficiency, small red blood cells are found in only a few situations, and these must be differentiated from iron deficiency. The newborn has larger red blood cells than adults, but they are soon replaced by cells that are substantially smaller than adult red blood cells. Not until the midteens does the mean MCV reach adult levels. Diagnosis of iron deficiency in children requires confirmation by serum iron and serum ferritin levels.

Thalassemia syndromes are accompanied by small red cells. Suspicion that the diagnosis is thalassemia trait rather iron deficiency is suggested by a relatively high red cell count exceeding 5.5 to 6 million/μL. In uncomplicated thalassemia trait, serum iron and ferritin levels are normal, and the Hb A_2 level in red cells is raised in β-thalassemia trait.

Anemia of chronic disorders may resemble iron deficiency, both having small red blood cells and a low serum iron level, but the serum iron-binding capacity is normal or low in the anemia of chronic disorders, whereas in iron deficiency it is raised. However, serum ferritin levels are normal in the anemia of chronic disorders even when there is accompanying iron deficiency. Similarly serum ferritin levels remain normal when iron deficiency is accompanied by liver disease.

Copper deficiency may be accompanied by a microcytic anemia that is unresponsive to iron therapy.

Nutritional deficiency, as a factor in producing iron deficiency, may be suspected from a careful assessment of the diet. A diet likely to be deficient in available iron is a strictly vegetarian one from which foods of animal origin are excluded. At the same time, exclusion of blood loss is essential. A good clinical history often provides a clue to gastric or gut problems, medication with aspirin or nonsteroidal analgesics, and menstrual blood loss. Fecal blood loss is often intermittent, and repeated tests for occult blood loss are needed. Where hookworm is endemic, hookworm ova will be present in fecal samples.

Iron Deficiency in Pregnancy

Pregnancy is accompanied by important changes in plasma and red cell volume that affect the hemoglobin concentration. The plasma volume expands by about 1000 mL, and the red cell volume by about 300 mL. The greater expansion of plasma volume results in dilution of red cells. The mean hemoglobin falls from 13.5 g/dL in nonpregnant women to 12.5 and 12.0 g/dL at 15 and 30 weeks of pregnancy, respectively. Thereafter there is some hemoconcentration, with a rise in hemoglobin to a mean of 12.8 g/dL at 38 weeks. At 30 weeks gestation, hemoglobin in iron-replete women ranges from 10.0 to 14.5 g/dL. At the same time, there are physiologic changes in the size of the red cells. These increase in size from a mean of 85 fL to 89 fL, but in some women the increase can reach 20 fL, so that the MCV is 105 fL. This is not influenced by folate supplements but is diminished or absent if the subject also has iron deficiency and/or β-thalassemia trait.

An extra 1000 mg of iron must be found in the second and third trimester to meet the needs of a normal singleton pregnancy. This has to be set against the total body iron present in an adult woman of 2500 mg with a normal iron absorption of 1 to 2 mg/day, increasing to 4 mg/day in the third trimester. It is unusual for sufficient iron stores to be present to meet such demands, and this amount is more than can be absorbed from a good diet. Serum iron and ferritin levels both fall steadily throughout pregnancy. In a study of over 2000 women not given any iron during pregnancy, not only did the hemoglobin level remain low to term, but even 1 year after childbirth, the mean hemoglobin of the group was still below the level present in the first blood sample taken in early pregnancy (9). Iron deficiency in pregnancy is due to increased demands for iron that cannot be met from stores and diet. It is coupled with poor nutrition insofar as a poor iron intake prevents formation of adequate iron stores and fails to provide sufficient iron to meet immediate needs.

The diagnosis of iron deficiency in pregnancy is the same as in other situations. It is found in about one-third or more of pregnant women who do not receive an iron supplement from early pregnancy. A hemoglobin level below 10 g/dL is low. During the last 30 years, a combined iron and folic acid tablet has been given in pregnancy in most developed countries and proved so successful in removing anemia as a significant problem in pregnancy that a generation of midwives and obstetricians are in practice in affluent societies who see little anemia in their antenatal practice, and many advocate treatment only when anemia is diagnosed. It may be that better diet and widespread use of a contraceptive pill have improved the iron status of women, but it is unlikely to have changed the balance so greatly that women now have sufficient iron in pregnancy. A recent study comparing iron and placebo in pregnancy in Dublin showed the expected fall in hemoglobin in the placebo group; the mean hemoglobin level at term in the supplemented group was 13.6 g/dL, compared with 11.9 in the placebo group (10).

There is also some resistance to iron medication in pregnancy due to side effects experienced by some, including abdominal cramps and constipation. Much of the blame for this can be laid on the drug companies who want their pills to have at least as much iron as is supplied by their competitors, and this amount is 200 to 300 mg/day ferrous sulfate or its equivalent. The more iron, the greater are the side effects. As little as 30 mg ferrous sulfate once daily is fully adequate (11). Doses under 30 mg have not been tested but may well be enough.

Infants, Children, and Adolescents

In utero iron stores are built up in the fetus in the last few weeks of pregnancy. Premature birth curtails transfer of iron from mother to child, and premature infants need iron supplements at an earlier age than normal infants. Thereafter, rapid growth with expansion of the red cell mass increases iron needs, and if diet fails to supply enough iron, iron deficiency appears.

Fortification and Treatment

Fortification of food such as flour to improve intake of iron has not been successful. Addition of metallic iron was not beneficial because the iron remained insoluble and unavailable. Addition of soluble iron made the bread unpalatable. Addition of iron to individual foods such as cereals has been more successful, and iron is widely added to prepared infant foods. At present in the U.S., 4.4 mg iron is added per 100 g flour.

Iron deficiency is treated by soluble iron salts, of which ferrous sulfate, generally as a 200-mg tablet three times a day, is the most widely used. Many other preparations are available. They should be taken apart from meals, and ascorbate as in orange juice enhances iron absorption. Response to the iron is shown by clinical benefit and a rise in hemoglobin level of about 1 g/week. To build up iron stores, treatment should continue for about 6 months. Side effects include abdominal discomfort and constipation and are dealt with by reducing the dose. Symptoms usually disappear after about 10 days.

COBALAMIN

Cbl is a pink, water-soluble vitamin. The main part of the molecule is similar in structure to heme but with cobalt replacing iron in the center of the pyrrole ring. Cbl is required for the integrity of blood formation, maintenance of the nervous system, and normal function of folate. The source of cbl is bacterial synthesis. Cbl is present in all diets containing food of animal origin and is totally absent in strictly vegetarian diets except as a result of bacterial activity or contamination from animal sources. Fruit bats obtain cbl by inadvertent consumption of insects on fruit. Bats on a diet of washed clean fruit die of cbl neuropathy in 9 months. In man, nutritional cbl deficiency occurs only in strict vegetarians.

Physiologic Considerations

A full account of the basic aspects of cbl is set out in Chapter 27. Cbl is present in meat, poultry, fish and other seafood, and dairy products. In the U.S., meat, poultry, and fish supply 74.8% of dietary cbl, dairy products 19.7%, eggs 3.7%, and other foods 1.8% (12). Liver is a rich source (see Appendix Table IV-A-23-a). Cbl is stable, resists cooking, and is only destroyed in very alkaline conditions when the pH exceeds 12. In food, cbl is present as a coenzyme linked to protein in methionine synthase and in methylmalonyl-CoA mutase. Small amounts are present on transport proteins termed *transcobalamins.* There is no free dietary cbl.

Availability and Absorption of Cobalamin

Most cbl present in food is available for absorption, although there are reports of cbl in egg being less well absorbed. That from meat or liver is as well absorbed as aqueous cbl (13b). It has been proposed but not proven that failure to separate cbl from binding proteins in the gut is a cause of cbl malabsorption. If so, it is not a known cause of cbl deficiency producing anemia in man (13a).

There is a limit to the amount of cbl that is absorbed from a single dose or meal, probably because of saturation of cbl-intrinsic factor–binding sites in the small gut. This amount is about 1.0 to 1.5 μg (13). A second dose of cbl given 4 to 6 hours after the first is absorbed normally, so if three adequate meals are taken daily in a mixed diet, at least 4.5 μg of cbl can be absorbed. Daily food intake in men taking a mixed diet containing 70 g protein and 2400 kcal supplied 5.2 μg cbl, and one with 53 g protein and 1400 kcal in women had 5.6 μg cbl. The daily intake ranged from 0.4 to 85.5 μg, being heavily influenced by consumption of liver or other rich sources (13b). A vegetarian diet supplies between 0.25 and 0.5 μg cbl daily, derived from bacterial activity in the food, from water, and from animal products such as milk.

Cobalamin Requirement

Diets supplying 0.5 μg cbl or less daily are associated with a high proportion of subjects having abnormally low serum cbl levels. Among Hindu vegetarians, more than half the population have low serum cbl levels (14). Patients with megaloblastic anemia due to nutritional cbl deficiency have similar cbl intakes. Such a cbl intake is clearly not adequate; an adequate cbl intake is one that maintains the serum cbl at the level found in those on mixed diets. This intake is probably nearer 1 to 2 μg/day cbl, the usual RDA in most countries (Table 88.3). Cbl is one of the nutrients for which the dietary sources in a mixed diet exceed the requirement. The total body pool of cbl in adults taking a mixed diet ranges from 2.5 to 5 mg. With a daily requirement of 1.0 μg, such cbl stores should suffice for 2500 days or more.

Cobalamin-Folate Metabolism: The Formate-Starvation Hypothesis

The biochemical pathways requiring cbl are discussed in Chapter 27. The methyl-folate trap was proposed to explain how cbl interacted with folate, but the few studies that tested this hypothesis failed to support it (15). More recently, considerable evidence has pointed to a failure in the supply of formate needed for folate-mediated carbon unit transfers in cbl deficiency. This has been termed the *formate starvation hypothesis.*

The role of folate in transferring single carbon units including formate (-CHO) in the synthesis of a variety of compounds was noted 50 years ago. Some forms of formate could be used by cbl-deficient preparations, but others could not. Formate that was available to cbl-deficient tissue was termed *active formate.* Twenty-five years ago, two studies found increased formate in the urine of cbl-deficient rats.

The observation that the anesthetic gas nitrous oxide (N_2O) destroyed reduced cbl provided an easy way to produce experimental cbl deficiency. Continuous N_2O administration in man leads to fatal megaloblastic anemia, and intermittent inhalation, to cbl neuropathy. The cbl-requiring enzyme regenerating methionine from homocysteine, methionine synthase, was inactivated in all species and in all tissues by N_2O. All folate-mediated pathways were impaired including those in which cbl had no direct role.

Folate given to cbl-deficient animals was not converted into the active coenzyme unless the folate had a formate group as part of the molecule. This and many similar studies suggested that cbl was concerned with formation of "active formate" needed to convert folate (actually tetrahydrofolate) into N10-formyltetrahydrofolate. The enzyme producing formylfolate was induced in cbl deficiency, indicating a lack of formylfolate. With impaired formate utilization in cbl deficiency, formate accumulated in tissues including blood, liver, and brain, and hence was lost into the urine. Two compounds bypassed the effect of cbl deficiency in a large variety of systems including synthesis of thymidine and cbl deficiency in man; these were N5-formylfolate (folic acid or citrovorum factor)and methionine. Formyltetrahydrofolate simply provided active formate; methionine did as well.

The pathway by which methionine bypassed cbl deficiency was via *S*-adenosyl-methionine and its utilization in polyamine synthesis when the methionine gave up three of its carbons. The methionine residue, methylthioribose, is regenerated into a new molecule of methionine using carbons from ribose to replace the missing carbons used for the synthesis of polyamine. This reaction leaves behind a surplus carbon as formate (71). Using ^{14}C-methylthioribose incubated with bone marrow cells, it was shown that the residual labeled formate was used as a single carbon unit to provide carbons 2 and 8 of the purine nucleus and did so equally well in both normal and cbl-deficient bone marrow cells (72). Thus a major role for cbl and methionine is to make active formate available to the folate coenzyme (16).

The same defect likely underlies cbl neuropathy despite the wide variety of problems that have been described in relation to products of methionine metabolism (Chapters 26, 27, and 34). The reason for this view is that the fruit bat with fatal and histologically proven cbl neuropathy does not manifest any of these abnormalities of methionine metabolism, other than loss of methionine synthase activity, in the nervous system (17). However, the brain does accumulate formate in cbl deficiency, implying a defect of formate metabolism.

Prevalence of Nutritional Cobalamin Deficiency

As cbl is absent from the plant kingdom, cbl deficiency can occur with time in any strict vegetarian. This is the case with millions of subjects such as Hindu Indians. The mean serum cbl level among vegetarian Indian medical students was 121 pg/mL, compared with a mean level of 366 pg/mL in those taking a mixed diet. In London, 1000 consecutive samples from Indians who were largely vegetarian showed a mean serum cbl level of 198 pg/mL, compared with 334 pg/mL in an age-matched Caucasian group taking a mixed diet (18). The cbl level was low in 54% of the Indian subjects. A lower incidence of low cbl levels is encountered in Western subjects adopting a vegetarian diet. In Australia, an analysis of 3846 samples sent for cbl and red cell folate assay found 335 (8.7%) to be abnormal, and 20 of these patients appeared to have nutritional cbl deficiency (19).

Signs and Symptoms in Cobalamin Deficiency

Vast numbers of subjects who have nutritional cbl deficiency and a low serum cbl level as a result are well and appear to have no clinical problems. Thus among a community of 15,000 Hindu Indians, largely vegetarian, of whom 54% had low serum cbl levels, only 10 patients per year with cbl-deficient megaloblastic anemia were seen in one local hospital (14). Most are just in balance, with low cbl stores and a low cbl intake. Not infrequently, patients come to notice because macrocytosis has been found in a blood count, and such patients may have few complaints, though almost invariably, they feel better after cbl therapy. Most patients present with tiredness, lack of energy, shortness of breath, tingling in hands and feet, and a sore mouth and tongue.

A series of 95 patients with nutritional megaloblastic anemia, all Indian vegetarians, were seen over 14 years. There were 52 women and 43 men, and their ages ranged from 13 to 80 years (14). They complained of tiredness (33%), shortness of breath (25%), loss of appetite (23%), weight loss (22%), generalized aches (19%) generally due to calcium and vitamin D deficiency, vomiting (19%), paresthesia (11%), change in skin pigmentation (8%), sore mouth (7%), diarrhea (6%), headache (5%), and infertility (5%). In 6%, macrocytosis in a blood count was the first indication of clinical cbl deficiency. All these patients had a megaloblastic bone marrow, and all had low serum cbl levels.

Examination showed pallor, a smooth tongue in some (Figs. 88.3 and 88.4), and yellowish sclera in 13%. Indian patients may show increased pigmentation about the nails, and one patient with severe anemia showed splenomegaly. This 19-year-old male also had lost hair pigmentation and had gray hair; hair grown after the start of oral cbl therapy was jet black (Fig. 88.5).

Neuropathy, if present, may manifest as symmetric tingling sensations in fingers and/or toes. There may be spastic movements, stiffness, and weakness. Difficulty with micturition includes hesitancy, a poor urinary stream, and even retention. Constipation and postural hypotension may be due to an effect on the autonomic nervous system. Irritability, memory disturbance, mild depression, and even hallucinations may occur. Visual impairment is uncommon. Loss of vibration sense, appreciation of passive movement, and a positive Romberg's sign may be present. There may be exaggerated reflexes and an extensor plantar, but others have a flaccid paralysis. Muscles may be wasted. Abnormal nerve conduction is found on electrophysiologic testing in 25% of patients.

In severe anemia, there is a fast pulse rate and low blood pressure. A soft systolic murmur may be present. Patients with severe anemia may be in cardiac failure with distended neck veins, swollen ankles, and cardiac enlargement.

Laboratory Findings

The diagnosis of cbl deficiency cannot be made on clinical grounds alone; it must be established by appropriate tests in the laboratory. Of these tests, a blood count and serum cbl level are the most helpful.

Blood Count. It is extremely rare to have clinically significant cbl deficiency without changes in the blood, and the vast majority of patients have large red cells shown by a raised MCV. Some patients may have a second blood disorder that produces small red cells; this is either α- or β-thalassemia trait or iron deficiency. In such a case the two diseases cancel each other out in so far as red cell size is concerned, and the MCV is usually normal; despite the normal MCV, the blood film is very abnormal, with bizarre red cell fragments. Cbl therapy restores the smaller red cells that characterize thalassemia trait. Thalassemia trait is present in 5% or more of those of African or Asian stock.

Macrocytosis is the earliest change in the blood in cbl deficiency (Fig. 88.6) and, as the anemia becomes more severe, is followed by neutropenia and thrombocytopenia. The nucleus of the neutrophilic polymorphonuclear leukocyte tends to become hypersegmented (Fig. 88.7). With more severe anemia, variation in red cell size and shape appears. There are many causes of a raised MCV other than cbl deficiency; these include folate deficiency, alcoholism, hypothyroidism, young red blood cells, and medicinal drugs.

Bone Marrow. The blood changes are caused by abnormal blood formation in the marrow, and these changes, termed *megaloblastic,* are easily recognized with properly fixed and stained marrow preparations, even if the hemoglobin level is still 16 g/dL (Fig. 88.8). There is nothing particularly subtle about this as some have claimed. It has become very unfashionable to carry out marrow examination merely to establish megaloblastosis, and as a result, undue weight is being placed on other accompanying and newer laboratory tests that have not been well explored. When the blood count, blood film, and clinical picture all strongly suggest a megaloblastic anemia, marrow examination can be omitted, and one can await the results of serum cbl and red cell folate estimations.

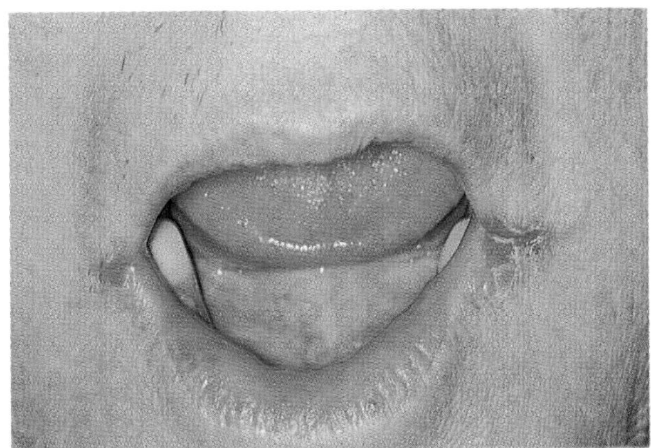

Figure 88.1. Angular stomatitis and a smooth shiny tongue in iron deficiency anemia.

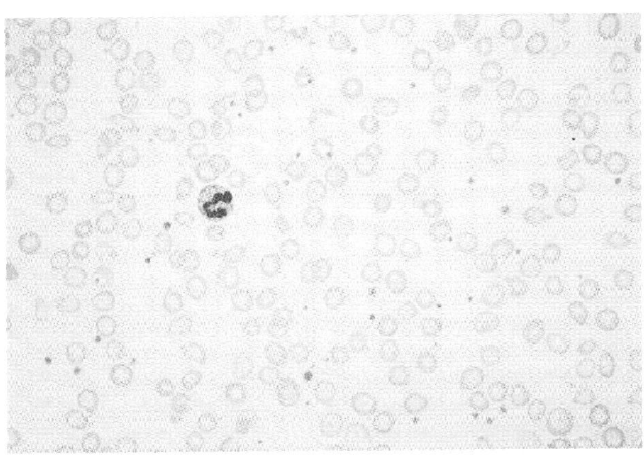

Figure 88.2. Peripheral blood film from a patient with severe iron deficiency anemia.

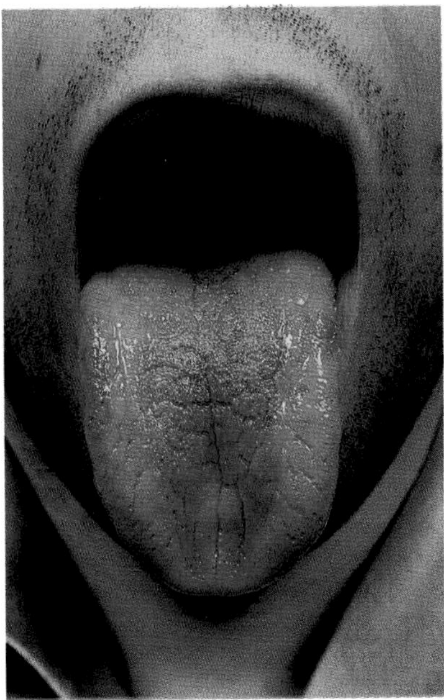

Figure 88.3. Red "beefy" tongue in a 23-year-old male with cobalamin deficiency. For 1 year he complained that spicy food and, in particular, whiskey, produced a painful mouth and tongue.

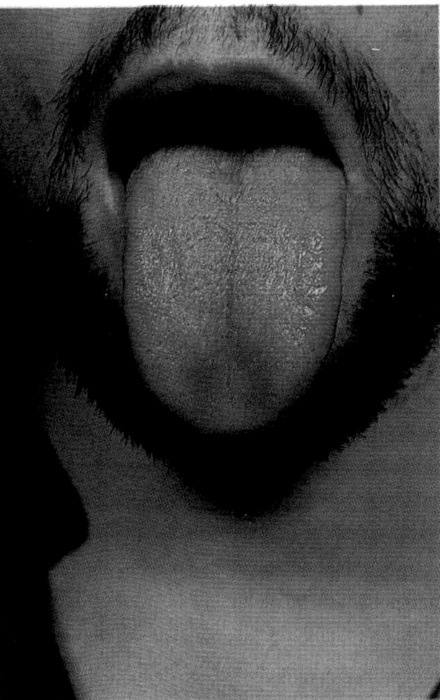

Figure 88.4. Same patient as in Figure 88.3 about 2 weeks after the start of cobalamin treatment. The tongue is normal in appearance, and the unpleasant symptoms after whiskey had disappeared.

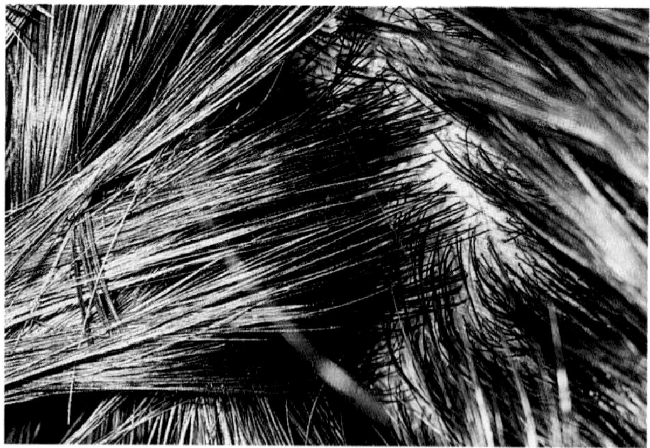

Figure 88.5. Scalp hair of a 19-year-old Indian with nutritional cobalamin deficiency and a severe megaloblastic anemia. On presentation his hair was a dingy grey color. This picture was taken about 2 months after the start of oral cobalamin, 5 μg/day. Cobalamin restored the normal pigment to the hair, which now grew jet black.

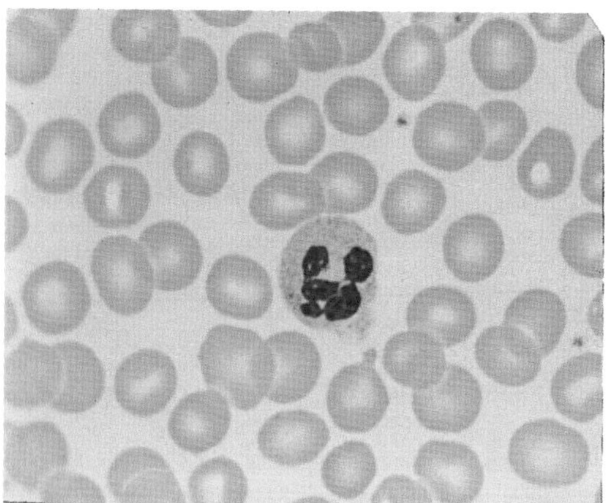

Figure 88.6. Early macrocytic anemia. The red blood cells are large compared with those in the strip on the *right,* which is a normal blood film.

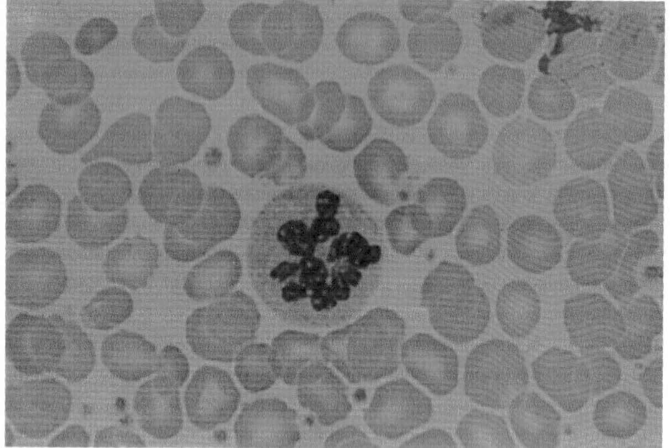

Figure 88.7. A blood film from a patient with cobalamin deficiency showing a strikingly hypersegmented neutrophil polymorphonuclear leukocyte. The red blood cells show variation in size (anisocytosis) and are generally larger than normal (macrocytosis).

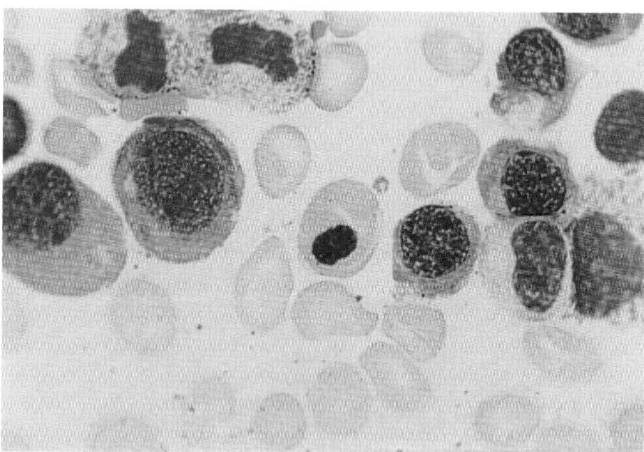

Figure 88.8. Bone marrow film from a patient with severe megaloblastic anemia. The cells with finely stippled nuclei and gray cytoplasm are red cell precursors called megaloblasts.

Serum Cobalamin Level. The serum cobalamin level is the most important single test needed for the diagnosis of cbl deficiency because it is always low, provided the patient has normal cbl-binding proteins. There are no exceptions to this rule! Nevertheless, recently it has been claimed that cbl deficiency, particularly with neuropathy, occurs in elderly patients with a normal blood count and a normal serum cbl level. These patients have an elevated level of methylmalonic (MMA) in serum and are said to respond to cbl therapy. A raised level of MMA is present in a large majority of patients with cbl-deficient megaloblastic anemia but also in subjects with normal cbl levels who do not have megaloblastic anemia (13a). The test, as currently performed, lacks specificity. It is far more likely that the correct diagnosis in the patients with neuropathy and a normal serum cbl level is something other than cbl deficiency, such as osteoarthritis, and such patients have osteophytes pressing on nerve fibers. As the nerve stretches to accommodate the pressure of the osteophyte, the neuropathy is relieved, and the cure is attributed to cbl therapy. A normal serum cbl level excludes a diagnosis of cbl deficiency. The normal level of serum cbl is 170 to 800 pg/mL, and levels below 170 are low. But there are other causes of low serum cbl that must always be considered.

Cbl assays are difficult to do well consistently, and at one time or another, most laboratories run into problems. It is not unusual for an assay to give too low a result and, less often, one that is too high. Rigid quality control procedures are essential to detect any problems in the test. These apply to isotope dilution methods with purified intrinsic factor as well as microbiologic assay methods. If there is any doubt a repeat assay in another laboratory is desirable. It is also wise to withhold treatment with cbl until such matters have been settled.

Some 30% of subjects with simple atrophic gastritis have a low serum cbl level and may even have cbl malabsorption, but the blood is and remains normal. At least 10% of the elderly have severe atrophic gastritis. Large numbers of strict vegetarians have low serum cbl levels but are hematologically normal. In these groups the low serum cbl level probably mirrors low cbl stores, with intake just balancing requirement. It is from these groups that patients with cbl-deficient megaloblastic anemia arise. About 5% of normal pregnant women have low serum cbl levels and are not cbl deficient. This is due to preferential transfer of absorbed cbl to the placenta and fetus in late pregnancy at the expense of maintaining the plasma level. About one-third of patients who have a megaloblastic anemia that is due to folate deficiency (and not to cbl deficiency) also have a low serum cbl level. The reason is not understood, and the serum cbl rises (often quite dramatically) into the normal range within a few days of folic acid treatment.

Not uncommonly, no explanation can be found for a low serum cbl level in a person who is otherwise normal. One report concerned 196 consecutive serum samples with cbl levels all below 170 pg/mL; 55% had a raised level of MMA and/or homocysteine and were accepted as being from patients with true cbl or folate deficiency, but 45% had no other abnormality. In a few such patients, liver biopsy has confirmed normal stores of cbl. Thus a low cbl level in the absence of the appropriate blood and bone marrow changes and in the absence of appropriate neuropathy is not likely to indicate clinically significant cbl deficiency (20). Such patients do not require treatment.

Methylmalonic Acid (MMA). MMA is formed from propionic acid and amino acids such as valine and isoleucine. MMA is converted to succinic acid by methylmalonyl-CoA mutase, which requires cbl as a coenzyme. MMA accumulates in cbl deficiency. Urinary excretion of MMA after an oral dose of 10 g valine was found to be abnormal in 74% of patients with proven cbl deficiency and a megaloblastic anemia; there were no abnormal results in 22 patients with folate-deficient megaloblastic anemia. The excretion of MMA returned to normal 3 to 5 days after cbl treatment. False-positive results were obtained when the assay was conducted by colorimetric methods (21). Although urinary excretion of MMA after stressing the pathway with a precursor such as valine is not applied widely, it may reflect the activity of this pathway more accurately than the newer serum MMA assay.

Recently, MMA has been assayed in serum. An increased MMA level in serum is found in a high proportion of patients with cbl deficiency, generally upward of 86% (22). More than 10% of subjects with normal serum cbl levels, such as elderly subjects in the Framingham population (23), 51 elderly European subjects (24), children on macrobiotic diets (25), alcoholics with folate deficiency (26), and patients with thyroid disease (27) have a raised serum MMA. One-third of sera from pregnant women had raised levels of MMA irrespective of the serum cbl level (60). The normal serum cbl level in these groups makes it unlikely that the raised MMA is due to significant cbl deficiency (13a).

The raised MMA levels with normal cbl levels were used to imply, generally with no additional evidence, that the serum cbl level was misleading and insensitive as a marker of cbl deficiency. This overlooks a half century of experience with the serum cbl level that has stood the test of time. It ignores enormous efforts made to detect cbl deficiency in the elderly and other possibly susceptible groups such as those with psychiatric and neurologic problems; these have failed to find missed examples of cbl deficiency. The largest discrepancy occurs in the elderly.

Data from claims to Medicare in the U.S. in 1991 indicate that in a 5% sample comprising 1.8 million persons, 18,068 made a claim relating to cbl deficiency. This is 1% of this population largely over 65 years of age. On the other hand, measurement of MMA levels in 548 elderly subjects in Framingham showed raised levels in 82 (15%) (23). The MMA level suggests a frequency of cbl deficiency 15-fold higher than the probably true incidence of pernicious anemia, the usual cause of cbl deficiency in the elderly.

It seems that more study is needed in relation to the precise significance of raised MMA serum levels. Megaloblastic anemia and cbl neuropathy are due to impaired methionine synthase; a raised MMA level is due to change in function of methylmalonyl-CoA mutase. Changes in activity of these two enzymes do not run in parallel; hence the different set of results when tests for these enzymes are used to assess cbl deficiency.

Serum Homocysteine (Hcy). Hcy is usually raised in most patients with megaloblastic anemia due to either cbl or folate deficiency and thus does not help differentiate between these two situations. There are other reasons for a raised Hcy level (see Chapters 34 and 61), so the test is of limited usefulness (19).

Deoxyuridine Suppression Test. The deoxyuridine suppression test is carried out with a suspension of bone marrow cells and measures the synthesis of thymidine, which is impaired in both cbl and folate deficiency. In the test, deoxyuridine, the precursor of thymidine, is added to bone marrow cells. Most of the thymidine needed by the bone marrow cells will be met by synthesis from deoxyuridine (the synthetic pathway). Thereafter tritium-labeled thymidine is added and any requirement not met by synthesis from deoxyuridine is met by uptake of thymidine (salvage pathway). DNA is extracted, and thymidine uptake is measured. Normally less than 10% of thymidine is taken up. A 100% value is obtained by incubating bone marrow cells with thymidine alone. In cbl- or folate-deficient marrows, more than 10% of the thymidine is taken up. The deoxuridine is held to have suppressed thymidine uptake.

In cbl deficiency, the defect is partially corrected by adding cbl to the system. Folate (as such or as 5-formyltetrahydrofolate) produces complete correction in both cbl and folate deficiency. This is a specific way of diagnosing these deficiencies, and results confirm the great value of serum cbl assays. The test becomes abnormal within a few hours of inactivating cbl by inhaling N_2O and returns to normal within a few hours of reversing the effect of cbl deficiency with folinic acid (16). However, some technicians have difficulty in carrying out this test properly. This may be indicated by failure to get a result of less than 10% uptake of labeled thymidine with normal marrow and, secondly, by a failure to get complete correction when folinic acid is added to the system.

A recent report found that among 50 patients with low serum cbl levels but normal or "limited megaloblastic" marrow change, 19 had a deoxyuridine suppression test result suggesting cbl deficiency, but only 10 had a raised MMA level (70). One-quarter of elderly patients selected on the basis of a low serum cbl level or a low red cell folate level had an abnormal deoxyuridine suppression test result, suggesting that the test may provide early evidence of transition to megaloblastic hematopoiesis (68).

The Hematologic Response. The response to treatment provides further evidence for the diagnosis of cbl deficiency, provided the response is optimal. In cbl deficiency, an injection of cbl is followed by a most gratifying clinical response with a remarkable feeling of well-being within 1 to 2 days and a dramatic return of appetite, etc.

There is a rise in reticulocytes (young red blood cells), which reach a peak 5 to 7 days after the start of treatment, and there is a rise in hemoglobin and red cells, which exceed 3 million/μl by the third week. Minor responses do not provide evidence of deficiency, since they are not uncommon after a host of interventions, including administration of substances given as part of diagnostic tests such as histidine and others such as glycine, choline, thymidine, pyrimidine, and even antibiotics and DNA (22, 28).

In the case of nutritional cbl deficiency, it is often desirable to treat with oral cbl; the response is far more subdued but in time restores a normal blood picture. Response to 5 μg cbl daily by mouth is proof of nutritional cbl deficiency.

Folate Estimations. If the patient has megaloblastic anemia, the usual alternate diagnosis to cbl deficiency is folate deficiency. Serum folate has little diagnostic value but can be marginally raised in a small proportion of patients with cbl deficiency. The red cell folate level is more useful. A normal value (145 to 450 ng/mL packed red cells) generally excludes folate deficiency other than in pregnancy, but a reduced value is almost always present in folate deficiency and is also present in about half of patients with cbl deficiency .

Cobalamin Absorption Tests. Other than nutritional cbl deficiency, all the conditions producing cbl deficiency share a failure in the intestinal absorption of cbl. The usual cbl absorption test, such as the Schilling test, involves giving the patient an injection of 1000 μg of cbl. This constitutes complete treatment and means that the chance of obtaining positive evidence for the diagnosis of nutritional cbl deficiency by demonstrating a response to 5 μg cbl once daily by mouth, is lost. If the absorption of cbl is normal and the patient responds hematologically following the injection of cbl, then the likely diagnosis remains nutritional cbl deficiency, provided that the patient is a strict longstanding vegetarian. If there is malabsorption of cbl, the most likely diagnosis is pernicious anemia or another disorder producing cbl deficiency. Such disorders include gastric surgery, abnormal small gut flora due to blind intestinal loops, strictures, diverticula, gut resections, and Crohn's disease. Disorders of the wall of the small gut producing cbl malabsorption include gluten sensitivity, tropical sprue, ileal bypass or resection, radiation damage, and drugs including alcohol. Five of 95 patients with nutritional cbl deficiency were found to have transient cbl malabsorption that disappeared after a few months of cbl therapy (14), and one-third had steatorrhea and xylose malabsorption. These latter findings also disappeared with cbl therapy.

Diagnosis

Diagnosis of nutritional cbl deficiency depends on establishing cbl deficiency in a person whose diet largely lacks all sources of cbl and in excluding cbl deficiency due to cbl malabsorption as in pernicious anemia, small intestinal bacterial overgrowth, and intestinal resection. Consumption of milk and occasional eggs and cheese will not supply enough cbl. Finding antibodies to intrinsic factor makes it likely that the diagnosis is pernicious anemia. In the study of Indian vegetarians, 95 patients had nutritional cbl deficiency, but another 20 had pernicious anemia, and only 4 had folate-deficient megaloblastic anemia, associated with excess alcohol in 2 and pregnancy in the other 2 (14). Restoration of a normal blood picture with 5 μg/day cbl by mouth prove that the diagnosis is nutritional cbl deficiency, since those with cbl malabsorption will not absorb sufficient cbl from this dose to restore normal hematopoiesis.

Cobalamin and Infection

Recurrent infections were found in a 6-year-old boy with an inherited abnormality of cbl transport (transcobalamin II deficiency) and consequent severe cbl deficiency. They were caused largely by the inability of this patient to produce antibodies; he could not generate a lymphoid response following contact with a foreign antigen until he was given regular cbl therapy (29).

Cbl-deficient neutrophils have an impaired respiratory burst, which prevents normal killing of phagocytosed bacteria. All patients with cbl deficiency and a red cell count below 2.0 million/μL gave an abnormal result when tested for neutrophil killing of phagocytosed bacteria, including several with nutritional cbl deficiency. Patients with folate deficiency were normal, other than those who were alcoholics. Phagocytosis was normal. The abnormal tests returned to normal 10 to 17 days after cbl treatment. This is the time required to produce a new post-cbl population of neutrophils in the bone marrow and have them reach the blood and tissues (30).

There is a high incidence of tuberculosis in the Indian community in the U.K. A survey of tuberculosis notification in the U.K. showed that if the incidence of tuberculosis in Caucasians was given a value of 1, in Asiatic Indians it was 38, in Africans from the Caribbean it was 3, and in Africans it was 13. Tuberculosis is known to be more common in new immigrant communities, but the Indian community in the U.K. is relatively prosperous. It was wondered whether the impaired neutrophil and presumably impaired macrophage killing of ingested bacteria in cbl deficiency could have a role in increasing susceptibility to tuberculosis. Furthermore, one of the components of the cell wall of *Mycobacterium tuberculosis* is mycocerosic acid, and MMA is an obligatory substrate for its synthesis. MMA accumulates in cbl-deficient tissues. To test whether cbl deficiency had a role in producing the high susceptibility to tuberculosis a dietary questionnaire was sent to over 2400 Indian subjects whose names were obtained from lists of patients registered with doctors in the Harrow area of London. At the same time, permission was sought to look at the clinical records of the patients for history of tuberculosis. A positive response was obtained from 1187 subjects. Tuberculosis had been diagnosed in 13.3% of vegetarians and 4.8% of those on mixed diets. This difference was highly significant (18).

Nutritional Cobalamin Deficiency in Infancy

Cbl stores are tranferred to the fetus in the last 2 months of pregnancy. Cbl levels in cord blood (373 pg/mL) are significantly higher than those in maternal blood at term (240 pg/mL). Low cbl stores in the mother, whether due to a longstanding vegetarian diet or to undetected pernicious anemia, is accompanied by inadequate cbl transfer in utero. Furthermore, the cbl level in breast milk is the same as that in maternal serum, and if this is low, the infant will not receive enough cbl. Most severely cbl-deficient women are infertile, but some do conceive and may have a relatively uncomplicated pregnancy. A significant number of infants with megaloblastic anemia and even neuropathy due to nutritional cbl deficiency have been reported, and even irreversible mental impairment has ensued.

Almost all such infants develop normally for the first 4 months of life. Thereafter they decline and are usually seen clinically between 6 to 14 months of age. The infants become irritable and lethargic, decline solid food, and are weak. They stop smiling, do not support their heads, and do not turn over. They have marked hypotonia and some choreoathetoid movements of upper limbs or constant wringing of hands. Their eyes do not fix or follow objects. They may even be in coma. Some have abnormal pigment on the back of their hands and about the nails. There is developmental delay, anemia (sometimes very severe), and usually enlarged liver and spleen. The blood is macrocytic, and marrow is megaloblastic. The serum cbl level is low, as is that of the mother. Response to cbl is excellent, and provided the delay in diagnosis has not been too long, recovery is complete and rapid (31, 32).

Treatment of Cobalamin Deficiency

With the exception of nutritional cbl deficiency, all patients with cbl deficiency have cbl malabsorption. Thus treatment must be given by intramuscular injection of large doses of cbl, usually 1000 μg every 2 months. Large doses of cbl can be given by mouth when, even in PA, about 1% is absorbed by passive diffusion. This must be taken daily to achieve an adequate intake of at least 1 μg/day. It is not recommended.

Patients who have nutritional cbl deficiency can absorb cbl normally and should be treated with oral cbl taken once daily. The preparation often has up to 50 μg cbl per tablet. This has to continue as long as they maintain a largely cbl-free vegetarian diet. Addition of cbl to cereals is widely practiced and is an important source of cbl in a vegetarian diet.

FOLATE

Folates are a group of labile compounds required for transfer of single-carbon units in a variety of biochemical pathways including synthesis of three of the four nucleotides of DNA. They are discussed in Chapter 26.

Physiologic Considerations

All foods contain folates. They are all reduced (i.e., they are tetrahydrofolates); most have five to six glutamic acids (i.e., they are folatepolyglutamates), two-thirds carry a methyl group, a quarter a formyl group, and 9% are without an additional single-carbon unit. Endogenous enzymes called conjugases, present in foods and tissues, remove all glutamate residues but one, and the reduced state of the pteridine moiety renders the folate very susceptible to oxidation, even by atmospheric oxygen. This is aided by exposure to UV light and by warmth. The oxidized molecule tends to be split into separate pteridine and *p*-aminobenzoate portions, so the folate is destroyed.

Intestinal Absorption

Folates are absorbed in the upper gut. Enzymes on the brush border as well as in the lysosome of the intestinal cell remove all glutamate residues but one, and in the enterocyte, the folate monoglutamate is converted into 5-methyltetrahydrofolate, which enters the portal circulation. Studies with tritium-labeled folates and a fecal excretion method in which the tritium of the unabsorbed folate was converted to tritium-labeled water showed almost complete absorption of reduced folate monoglutamates and some 79% absorption of oxidized pharmacologic pteroylglutamic acid. Precise data on the absorption of reduced folate polyglutamates are not available, but most believe some 70% are absorbed.

Folate Intake

Data on dietary folate are relatively imprecise because of the instability of natural folates, the large number of folate analogues present, and the difficulties in carrying out reliable microbiologic folate assays in complex material. A tired lettuce purchased days ago may have half the folate shown in food tables; one just collected from the vegetable patch may have twice the content. The folate content of foods is given in Appendix Table II-A-23. Assays of duplicate food collections are probably better than data derived from food tables. A Swedish study using duplicate food collection among the elderly, found a 24-h folate intake for men of 361 μg and for women, 129 μg (33). A Canadian diet supplied 205 μg/24 h for men and 149 μg for women (34). In the U.S., 24-h folate intakes have been reported from 152 to 250 μg, and in the U.K., the daily intake assessed over 3 years was between 210 and 213 μg. The recommended daily allowance is generally agreed to be 3.1 μg folate per kg body weight per day (Table 88.3). This is about 200 μg folate daily for a 65-kg male and 170 μg for a 55-kg female. Total body content of folate in man is about 10 to 15 mg.

Both mixed and vegetarian diets supply ample folate, but poor cooking practices can reduce the folate content considerably. Reducing substances such as ascorbate protect natural folates from oxidation and degradation. Much of the folate is lost by boiling in large volumes of water, but steaming has an equal effect. The loss is between 80 and 95%. Frying foods in an open pan results in loss of 50 to 95%. Dietary intake has been assessed on cooked foods.

Prevalence of Nutritional Folate Deficiency

Surveys of red cell folate levels in populations taking apparently adequate amounts of folate show low levels in 8% of the population. The frequency of low red cell folates in the NHANES II study in the U.S. is shown in Table 88.5. (See also Appendix Tables II-A-2 to A-8 for various national and international standards.) The frequency of low results is 8% in adult males, but 13% in women between the ages of 20 and 44 years. Surveys among the elderly based on 14 reports found a frequency of low red cell folate of 8.7% in persons living at home and 18% in those living in institutions (35). However, liver folate concentrations measured in samples collected at autopsy in Canada found only two low folate values among 560 samples (34). Perhaps the liver samples should have the last word, as clinical nutritional folate deficiency in adults without other complications is rare in Western society. More commonly, inadequate folate intake accompanies other problems such as alcoholism, pregnancy, chronic hemolytic states, or medication with anticonvulsant drugs. Nutritional folate deficiency, however, remains common in Third World countries, although documentation is poor. In Africa, between one-quarter and one-third of adults have low red cell folate levels (36).

The frequency of megaloblastic anemia in pregnancy is an excellent guide to the folate status of women in the population. The additional amount of folate required in a singleton pregnancy is approximately the same everywhere, and the ability to meet the additional requirement

Table 88.5
Frequency of Red Cell Folate Levels below 140 ng/mL in the U.S. Assessed by the National Health and Nutrition Examination Study (1988)

	Males		Females	
Age (Years)	Number Examined	% Low	Number Examined	% Low
0.5–9	243	2	201	2
10–19	178	5	173	8
20–44	299	8	389	13
45–74	503	8	439	4

Table 88.6
Frequency of Megaloblastic Marrow Changes in Pregnancy Near Term

Area	Bone Marrows Showing Megaloblastic Hematopoiesis As % of Total Performed
U.S., Houston	24
U.K., London	25
Canada, Montreal	25
South Africa, Johannesburg	25
Ireland, Dublin	30
Nigeria	30
India, Vellore	54 and 60

From Chanarin I. The megaloblastic anemias. 2nd ed. Oxford: Blackwell, 1979.

depends on folate stores on entering pregnancy and on the dietary folate intake. The best test is the presence of megaloblastic changes in the marrow, since concurrent iron deficiency makes it difficult to assess changes in peripheral blood. Such data are available from around the world and are shown in Table 88.6 (37). One-quarter of women in Western countries show changes of folate deficiency that largely disappear when a folate supplement is given during pregnancy, and this frequency rises to 60% in south India. Thus dietary folate intake in the West does not meet the requirements of pregnancy, and this is demonstrable hematologically in a quarter of such women and well over half the women in Third World countries.

Red cell folate levels underestimate the frequency of folate deficiency in pregnancy because folate is put into the red cell in the marrow at the time of formation of the red blood cell and remains locked there for about 110 days, which is the life span of the red blood cell. Lowering red cell folate levels requires replacing existing red blood cells by new cells of lower folate content. Maximum folate requirement corresponds to the time of greatest fetal growth in late pregnancy; at this time there is a markedly negative folate balance with a falling red cell level, but in about a third of women with megaloblastic marrows, the level has not yet fallen below the conventional normal range when full term is reached. Birth of the baby restores more normal folate needs. In Nigeria, 85% of all primigravidae have low red cell folate levels (38).

Apart from pregnancy, folate deficiency can be a problem among premature infants and among the elderly.

Signs and Symptoms in Folate Deficiency

The signs and symptoms in folate deficiency are the same as those described under cbl deficiency, since the ultimate defect is a failure of folate function in both cbl and folate deficiency. The exception is that neuropathy is extremely rare in folate deficiency.

Laboratory Findings

Blood and Bone Marrow. The changes that characterize megaloblastic hematopoiesis are identical in either cbl or folate deficiency and are described above under cbl.

Serum Cobalamin. A normal serum cbl level, for all practical purposes, in a patient with normal cbl serum binders (assessed by the uptake of labeled cbl by an aliquot of serum) and a megaloblastic blood film and/or marrow excludes a diagnosis of cbl deficiency and indicates that the deficiency is of folate. However, one-third of patients with folate-deficient megaloblastic anemia have a low serum cbl level that rises to normal within days of treatment with folic acid alone (39). The clinical circumstances may help in deciding which is the more likely diagnosis. Pregnancy, alcoholism, anticonvulsant drugs, and bulky stools may favor folate deficiency; neuropathy, a vegetarian diet, and other autoimmune disorders such as thyroid disease may favor cbl deficiency. Diagnosis thus depends on the final clinical and laboratory situation. If in doubt, it is best to start treatment with cbl and if there is no response switch to folate. Folate-deficient patients do not respond to cbl, but both deficiencies can respond to folate.

Serum Folate. Serum folate levels are of little diagnostic help as they are often low in ill patients with no folate problem.

Red Cell Folate. As indicated, red cell folate level is the best test for folate deficiency. The normal range is 145 to 450 ng/mL packed red cells. Unfortunately, commercial kits used in folate assays are designed for serum assays, and poor results for red cell assays are common.

Methylmalonic Acid and Homocysteine. Some 12% of folate-deficient patients, mostly alcoholics, have a raised serum MMA level (26) as do many other apparently healthy subjects (13a). This is not the case with MMA excretion in the urine after oral valine, which remains normal. A normal serum MMA in a patient with megaloblasic anemia favors a diagnosis of folate deficiency but by no means excludes cbl deficiency. As the serum homocysteine level can be elevated in both folate and cbl deficiency, the result is of no help.

Deoxyuridine Suppression Test. The deoxyuridine suppression test is abnormal in virtually all patients with megaloblastic anemia, and full correction of the defect in thymidine synthesis by addition of N5-formyltetrahydrofolate (folinic acid) but no correction with cbl confirms a diagnosis of folate deficiency.

Hematologic Response. A hematologic response to 200 μg/day of folate generally confirms a diagnosis of folate deficiency. This can only be done in patients who are sufficiently anemic to show a suitable response. Failure to respond to cbl providing that there are no interfering factors such as an intercurrent disorder or infection, favors a diagnosis of folate deficiency, confirmed by a response to folate.

Diagnosis of Folate Deficiency

In the absence of blood changes, subclinical folate deficiency is diagnosed by a low red cell folate level. When blood changes indicating a megaloblastic form of hematopoiesis are present, folate deficiency is diagnosed by excluding cbl deficiency by a normal serum cbl level and a normal serum MMA level, bearing in mind the limitations in the interpretation of these test results. Positive evidence is a low red cell folate level and a raised serum homocysteine level. No hematologic response to cbl, given orally if nutritional cbl deficiency is suspected or by injection if cbl malabsorption is more likely, favors folate deficiency and is confirmed by a full response to folate therapy.

Clinical Situations

Prematurity

Folate is actively transferred to the fetus in the last weeks of pregnancy. Assay of paired maternal and cord blood samples for serum and red cell folate showed values of 3.2 and 149 ng/mL for the mother and 17.1 and 325 for the fetus (40). Premature birth reduces fetal folate stores, with reduction of red cell folate levels averaging 270 ng/mL in samples from infants of 25 to 37 weeks gestation, compared with 340 ng/mL in infants at term. Red cell folate levels reach their nadir at 7 to 10 weeks postnatally in premature infants and at 11 to 12 weeks in full-term infants. After this time, the infant depends on dietary sources for folate.

Stored or frozen human milk shows a fall in folate content from about 45 μg/L to 30 μg/L at 4 weeks, to 25 μg at 8 weeks, and 19 μg at 12 weeks. Pasteurization of milk destroys the ascorbate, and reheating such a sample causes a fall of folate from 54 to 10 μg/L. Powdered milk is usually supplemented with folate.

Clinically the neonate fails to gain weight, and the anemia, if due to folate deficiency, does not respond to oral iron, which is the more usual cause. It does respond to oral folate.

Growth

Poor dietary folate intake, particularly when the folate requirement is increased (e.g., in children with sickle cell anemia and with the increased requirement for normal growth), can delay growth and the onset of menstruation in girls. This was shown dramatically in Nigeria, where folate therapy in women over the age of 20 was followed by growth spurts and the onset of normal menses (41).

Goat's Milk Anemia

Goat's milk has very low levels of both folate and cbl: 6 μg/L of folate in goat's milk (vs. 52 in human milk) and 0.1 μg/L cbl in goat's milk (vs. 4 μg in human milk). The kid grazes within days of birth and does not depend on maternal sources for either folate or cbl. Human infants reared on goat's milk develop a folate-deficient megaloblastic anemia at 3 to 5 months of age. If goat's milk must be used, a folate supplement is necessary (13b).

Neural Tube Defects (NTD)

NTDs arise from a failure of the neural tube to close completely at about the fourth week of embryonic life. The disorders include anencephaly (in which most of the brain and skull are absent), encephalocele (in which brain protrudes through a defect in the skull), and spina bifida (in which the spinal canal is not closed). The more severe defects are not compatible with life, and severer forms of spina bifida lead to very severe handicaps with paralysis of legs and bladder. The prevalence is about 4 per 1000 births, and most of these are diagnosed by raised α-fetoprotein levels in maternal blood and amniotic fluid and an ultrasound scan. Most such pregnancies are terminated, and defects present at birth now number about 0.3/1000 births.

In 1991, randomized, double-blind trials confirmed earlier evidence that supplemental folate given at conception and in the early weeks of pregnancy, reduced the frequency of NTDs by about 70% (42–45). The daily folate supplement given varied from 0.36 to 5.0 mg. On the whole, the data did not suggest that affected women had conventional folate deficiency, although there were indications of an association with poor diet. Study of women who had two episodes of NTD showed no evidence of a reduced folate intake (46), and usually red cell folate levels were normal. Thus the reason for a localized folate deficiency that led to a failure to close the neural tube is not clear. Possibly, in some women, vascularization of the placental site is inadequate in the early weeks and prevents folate access; raising the blood folate level significantly by increasing oral folate intake facilitates diffusion or active transfer of folate to the embryo. Other factors that produce NTDs include chromosomal abnormalities and maternal obesity (46a) and are not likely to be influenced by folate. A suggestion of a defective enzyme, methylenetetrahydrofolate reductase, was not confirmed because the frequency of the defect was similar in controls and in mothers who had a pregnancy complicated by NTD (46b).

Whatever the explanation for the beneficial effect of folate, it is now imperative to increase dietary folate in very early pregnancy, indeed, at a time when many women will not know that they are pregnant. As there is a risk of a second NTD in a subsequent pregnancy, women who have already had a pregnancy complicated by an NTD can be advised to take supplemental folate if they plan a further pregnancy. But half of all pregnancies are unplanned. Many authorities have issued advice on taking folate-rich food and on getting folate supplements, which has been largely unheeded by most women (47). It seems inescapable that the only way to increase dietary folate in very early pregnancy to all at risk is folate fortification of food such as flour. This will increase the folate intake of the population at large from about 0.2 mg/day to somewhere in the region of 0.5 to 1.0 mg/day. What are possible disadvantages of such a policy?

When folate became available after 1947, it was used by some to treat all megaloblastic anemias, including those that involved primarily cbl deficiency. It soon became clear that a high proportion of patients who needed cbl responded well initially to folate but, after several months, relapsed with damage to the nervous system and, ultimately, return of megaloblastic anemia. Generally the picture was restored by treatment with cbl, but some retained permanent neurologic damage (48). The plot thickened when it was realized that folates present in multivitamin preparations purchased without medical prescription could also produce a response in the blood in undiagnosed cbl deficiency but allow cbl neuropathy to develop. Although in the U.S. the amount of folate in the multivitamin preparation was not permitted to exceed 0.4 mg/day, many persons took the view that if one pill was good for you, up to six a day was even better. Folate restored normality to the blood pictures of those with undiagnosed cbl deficiency, which made it difficult for the clinician to suspect that the symptoms and signs were due to cbl deficiency with normal blood. Those at risk are usually patients with, as yet, undiagnosed pernicious anemia, which has a frequency of about 1.0% above the age of 60.

In the early 1950s, assays for serum cbl became widely available. A low serum cbl level was always present in cbl deficiency, and the test became mandatory when faced with a neuropathy that could be due to cbl deficiency. Since the early 1960s, reports of cbl deficiency concealed by folate therapy have been few, and it must be concluded that cbl deficiency is being properly diagnosed, despite the fact that 40% of North American adults take regular multivitamin supplements that include folate, sometimes in amounts that should prevent NTDs. It has been estimated that about one-third of American women take enough folate to prevent NTDs (49).

Proposals have been made to fortify flour so that the total folate intake should not exceed 1.0 mg/day. Such proposals are now being implemented in the U.S.

Pregnancy

The increased folate requirement in pregnancy arises from its role in increasing the mother's red cell mass, formation of the placenta, growth of the uterus and the fetus, and, finally, providing folate to be transferred to the fetus in the last few weeks before term (40). An increased folate requirement is evidenced at the 20th week of pregnancy by the more rapid clearance from the blood to tissues of a small injected dose of folate (50). Folate requirement increases throughout pregnancy and is maximal near term.

At the same time there is increased urinary loss of folate in pregnancy because of a lower renal threshold. Folate in the urine in pregnancy averages 14 μg/day, versus 4.2 μg/day in nonpregnant women and 3.5 μg in the puerperium. In some women, the urinary loss in pregnancy exceeds 50 μg/day (51). Claims of excessive folate catabolism in pregnancy await confirmation (52). The increased folate requirement, which has been assessed at 100 μg/day (53, 54), has to be met from the diet and from whatever folate stores are available.

In the U.S., 13% of women of childbearing age have a low red cell folate level (Table 88.5), and thus it is not surprising that 16% of women in New York had low red cell folate levels at their first visit to an antenatal clinic (55). Similar figures have been noted elsewhere, and in Nigeria, the frequency of a reduced red cell folate level at the first visit was 31%.

The red cell folate level generally falls throughout pregnancy, and in a London study, mean red cell folate levels at 12, 24, and 36 weeks and in the puerperium were 317, 302, 288, and 252 ng/mL packed red cells (54). This indicates a negative folate balance in pregnancy, but in Denmark and Australia, folate levels were maintained during pregnancy, implying a more adequate folate intake. Generally one-quarter to one-third of women have abnormally low folate blood levels at term, which corresponds to the frequency with which megaloblastic marrow changes have been found at term (Table 88.6). The serum folate level also falls during pregnancy, and at presentation, 30 weeks, 35 weeks, and puerperium, mean serum folate levels were 6.6, 5.2, 4.5, and 3.7 ng/mL. In part this is due to expansion of the plasma volume. Low levels are found in 15 to 54% of women.

Iron deficiency is the major cause of anemia in pregnancy, and folate deficiency comes next. The frequency of significant folate deficiency is related to the efforts made in its detection. Overt megaloblastic anemia is easily recognized, but more often it is concealed by accompanying iron deficiency; if there is no response to iron, marrow examination is the only certain way to make the diagnosis. Short of that, it can be suspected in a stained blood film by the presence of macrocytes in a microcytic red cell population, although responding iron deficiency can be similar, and hypersegmented neutrophils can be common to both deficiencies. The high frequency of megaloblastic anemia seen on bone marrow examination is shown in Table 88.6. Examination of the blood film will raise suspicion of megaloblastic anemia in only about 2% of women in late pregnancy.

Diagnosis is usually made in the last few weeks of pregnancy, and in about half of patients, in the puerperium. Megaloblastic anemia is 10 times more frequent in twin pregnancies, is more common in multigravidae, and has a seasonal incidence, with the highest frequency following the time of year when fresh vegetables are least available. In pregnancy, it is always due to folate deficiency. Women who get a megaloblastic anemia in pregnancy enter pregnancy with the lowest folate stores as assessed by the red cell folate level at presentation (54). Iron deficiency occurs in the same women who become folate deficient and implies a dietary deficiency of both nutrients (11).

Although a variety of consequences have been attributed to folate deficiency in pregnancy, only one has been established beyond doubt: prematurity and low-birth-weight infants. Pregnancy outcome in South Africa was compared in groups of well-nourished women taking a mixed diet and groups whose staple diet was boiled maize (corn). There were three supplements to each of 50 to 60 women, iron alone, iron and folate, or iron, cbl, and folate, and these were taken once daily. The supplements did not affect either birth weights or duration of gestation in the well-nourished group. In the group with maize as the main dietary item 19 of 63 women taking only iron had low-birth-weight babies weighing less than 2270 g, which fell to 4 of 65 in women taking iron and folate. The mean birth weight increased from 2466 g to 2798 g in those given iron and folate. Addition of cbl made no difference (56). Folate increased gestation by 1 week and increased placental weight from 456 g to 517 g (57). These findings have been widely confirmed, and only in well-nourished, affluent societies did folate supplements make no difference.

A folate supplement of 100 μg/day throughout pregnancy caused a rise in red cell folate levels during the first half of pregnancy, and thereafter the red cell folate did not change (54). There was a marked fall in the number of patients with megaloblastic marrows in the folate-supplemented group, but it was not abolished because not all the volunteers took their tablets. Since dietary folate intake in pregnancy can vary from less than 60 to over 200 μg/day, the daily folate supplement given in a single tablet with 30 mg ferrous sulfate needs to be no less than 200 μg folate to meet the needs of all pregnant women. The RDA for folate in pregnancy in the U.S. is 400 μg/day. Treatment of megaloblastic anemia in pregnancy is 5 mg folic acid given once or twice daily and continued for 4 weeks after delivery.

Lactation

Most patients with megaloblastic anemia in pregnancy are diagnosed in the puerperium. With delivery, folate requirements decline, and undiagnosed megaloblastosis will remit with dietary folate. This must be the case with most of the 25% of women who have a megaloblastic marrow at this time and who never come to clinical notice in the usual course of events. But in some, dietary folate is insufficient, and lactation poses a persistent increase in folate requirement. Human milk after the 2nd month of lactation contains 25 μg/L of folate; with secretion of 700 mL, this involves a loss of about 20 μg/day of folate. Milk contains an avid folate-binding protein, and small doses of folate given to the mother appear in the milk without any measurable rise in the maternal serum level (58). In Third World countries, megaloblastic anemia is more often diagnosed 2 to 18 months after birth than during pregnancy (59). The RDA during the first 6 months of lactation is 280 μg/day of folate, and in the second 6 months, 260 μg (Table 88.3). Treatment of megaloblastic anemia found during lactation is 5 mg of oral folic acid once daily.

The Elderly

The elderly are another group reported to be vulnerable to nutritional folate deficiency. In Western society, poverty and a very poor diet has been associated with clinical folate deficiency. Institutionalized elderly persons are more vulnerable than those living in their own homes. A survey of 17 studies on red cell folate levels in the elderly found that the incidence of low levels ranged from zero to 42.9% of subjects (69). The variation probably represents variation in assay technique rather than real differences in the samples tested. Very few of these subjects had anemia, and there was no obvious benefit from folate treatment. Diagnosis of significant folate deficiency must be based on a blood count and the additional tests set out above, but it is not common today except where there is general malnutrition.

Folate and Alcohol

There is a strong association between excessive alcohol consumption, folate deficiency, and megaloblastic anemia, and not infrequently, alcohol abuse turns out to be the explanation for an otherwise puzzling anemia. Alcohol has a direct toxic effect on hematopoietic cells in the bone marrow and perhaps on cells in the peripheral blood as well; it promotes excessive iron absorption, and patients who substitute alcohol for food can develop nutritional folate deficiency. The direct toxic effect is most obvious in those on a high alcohol intake and is best seen in the bone marrow, where there is megaloblastosis, vacuolation of red and white cell precursors, and ringed sideroblasts, that is, red cell precursors with iron granules forming a ring around the nucleus. These changes disappear within 10 days of alcohol withdrawal.

The peripheral blood in alcoholics may show a mixture of hypochromic and normochromic red cells, called a dimorphic blood picture, or just macrocytosis present in over 80% of alcoholics taking more than 80 g ethanol daily. The first diagnosis in a patient with a normal hemoglobin level and large red blood cells is alcohol abuse. Indeed, routine health screens carried out on the employees of a large U.S. insurance company showed that almost all the employees with large red blood cells and a normal hemoglobin level were taking excessive amounts of alcohol. The changes in the peripheral blood, although resulting from a direct toxic effect of alcohol on the marrow, take up to 100 days to disappear, related more to the survival of red cells in the circulation than to events in the marrow.

Folate deficiency occurs in those who substitute alcohol for food; they show low serum, red cell, and liver folate levels (61). It is seen in spirit drinkers rather than beer drinkers, since beer is a good source of folate. It occurs in one-third of alcoholics. They give a history of not taking an adequate meal during the day.

There is no good evidence that alcohol has a direct effect on folate metabolic pathways. Evidence does indicate that alcohol produces transient malabsorption of a variety of nutrients, including cbl and folate, but there is enhanced absorption of iron, leading to iron overload. This situation has been reproduced in alcoholic, folate-deficient rabbits but not in rabbits just given alcohol (62).

Diagnosis of folate deficiency in alcoholics, which is nutritional folate deficiency, is the same as that described above in this section.

Fortification and Treatment

The addition of folate to food is of importance in the prevention of NTDs. Furthermore, raised plasma levels of homocysteine may predispose for blood vessel damage and heart disease, and the homocysteine level is reduced by folate (73). New regulations in the U.S. indicate that flour must be enriched with 0.15 mg folate per 100 g flour, milled rice by 0.154 mg folate per 100 g, alimentary paste should contain 0.198 to 0.265 mg folate per 100 g, and enriched bread, 0.96 mg folate per 100 g bread.

Treatment of folate deficiency is by oral folate; tablets containing 5 mg are the usual dose given once or twice daily for 4 to 6 weeks. In sickle cell anemia and in chronic myelofibrosis there is a high folate requirement, and one 5-mg folate tablet is given daily for life. In pregnancy, a combined iron and folate supplement is strongly recommended.

LESS COMMON NUTRITIONAL DEFICIENCIES AFFECTING THE BLOOD

Ascorbic Acid (Vitamin C)

A full account of ascorbic acid is given in Chapter 29. Ascorbic acid and folate are both heat-labile water-soluble vitamins, and they occur in the same kind of foods. A diet deficient in one is likely to be deficient in the other. Ascorbate in food protects folate from oxidative destruction. A large proportion of patients with clinical scurvy have megaloblastic hematopoiesis or even frank megaloblastic anemia. Most of these patients respond only to ascorbate, but some may respond to folate (63). The relationship is likely to be a nutritional deficiency of both these substances in the same individual. There is no good evidence for a biochemical relationship other than the protective effect of ascorbate as a reducing agent preventing oxidation of labile tetrahydrofolate analogues, which occurs in an in vitro situation.

A cow's milk diet in monkeys led to development of severe ascorbate deficiency followed by a severely megaloblastic bone marrow about 2 weeks later (64). The liver had very low levels of both ascorbate and folate. As little as 1 mg ascorbate daily produced a response in both the scurvy and in the megaloblastic anemia, with accumulation of folate in the liver. Addition of folate alone to the diet precipitated clinical scurvy. The authors concluded that there was an increased folate requirement in scurvy, but they did not find a role for ascorbate in normal folate metabolism.

Pyridoxine

Pyridoxine metabolism is dealt with in Chapter 24. Pyridoxine-responsive anemias are not uncommon and are associated with pyridoxine antagonists such as cycloserine and pyrazinamide used to treat tuberculosis and with a group of anemias called sideroblastic anemias in which iron accumulates in erythroblasts as a ring around the nucleus. The accumulation of iron granules linked to mitochondria accompanies a failure of hemoglobin formation so that the cytoplasm of the erythroblast is pale and, if this cell matures, will give rise to an iron-deficient red cell. Apart from pyridoxine antagonists, sideroblastic anemia occurs as a preleukemic refractory anemia in older people or as sex-linked hereditary anemia in males. Folate deficiency is common, so there is a megaloblastic overlay.

All these disorders are suspected by examination of the stained blood film, which shows a mixture of iron-deficient (hypochromic) and normochromic red blood cells, also called a dimorphic blood picture. A dimorphic blood film is also present after a blood transfusion to an iron-deficient patient or after iron treatment in iron deficiency. The pyridoxine responsiveness is not due to nutritional deficiency but to a biochemical problem with pyridoxine metabolism, and high doses of pyridoxine in excess of 100 mg/day are needed for a response. Folate-deficient patients respond to folate in small doses (65).

Protein-Energy Deficiency (Kwashiorkor)

Children with protein malnutrition as recorded in Third World countries almost invariably have other problems, including infection and lack of other nutrients. Anemia is common and may be normocytic and normochromic. Hemoglobin levels may be below 8 g/dL, and the blood film may show anisocytosis. Some show evidence of scurvy, and slow hematologic responses follow repletion with protein. Marrows are often megaloblastic, and low blood folate levels are not infrequent. In some, megaloblastosis due to folate deficiency becomes evident only after protein repletion has been started. Blood changes have been reviewed (66).

Vitamin E Deficiency

Vitamin E deficiency is discussed in Chapter 19. α-Tocopherol serves as an antioxidant. Deficiency of vitamin E is rare but does occur in premature infants at about 4 to 6 weeks of age. There is anemia not responding to iron and recognizable from the appearance of the blood film, which shows contracted red blood cells and polychromasia. Polychromatic red cells are new red cells or reticulocytes; when increased under these circumstances, they indicate a response to increased red cell destruction (a hemolytic anemia), presumably due to loss of the protective effect of vitamin E. The hemolytic anemia is accompanied by a raised platelet count and edema of the dorsum of the feet and pretibial area. These symptoms and signs disappear with vitamin E treatment. It has been suggested that the anemia may be related to a diet rich in polyunsaturated fatty acids. A mild hemolytic anemia responding to vitamin E may also occur in cystic fibrosis.

Riboflavin

Riboflavin is discussed in Chapter 22. Experimental deficiency in volunteers was accompanied by anemia only affecting the red blood cells. Clinically, anemia due to riboflavin deficiency is rare, and is said to accompany alcohol abuse when a smooth, cherry-red tongue is a feature. The author encountered anemia responding well to riboflavin in a young woman with anorexia nervosa, with a hemoglobin level of 6 g/dL and a cherry-red tongue.

Copper

Copper deficiency has been described in malnourished children and in patients on parenteral nutrition. It is dealt with in Chapter 12. Copper is required in a number of enzymes; it is carried in plasma bound to a protein termed *ceruloplasmin*. The level is low in copper deficiency. Anemia and neutropenia rarely occur in copper deficiency and are said to be similar to those in iron deficiency but unresponsive to iron. An undoubted example of a macrocytic anemia responding to copper has been documented (67).

REFERENCES

1. Lajtha LG, Possi LV, Schofield R, et al. Cell Tissue Kinet 1969;2:39–49.
2. FAO/WHO. Requirements of vitamin A, iron, folate and vitamin B_{12}. FAO Food and Nutrition series no. 23. Rome, Italy: Food and Agriculture Organization, 1988;1–107.
3. Gillooly M, Bothwell TH, Torrance JD, et al. Br J Nutr 1983; 49:331–42.
4. Hallberg L, Rossander-Hulten L, Brune M, et al. Eur J Clin Nutr 1992;46:317–27.
5. Edwards CH, Johnson AA, Knight EM, et al. J Nutr 1994; 124(Suppl):954S–62S.
6. Alexander D, Ball MJ, Mann J, et al. Eur J Clin Nutr 1994; 48:538–46.
7. Lozoff B, Jimenez E, Wolf AW. N Engl J Med 1991;325:687–94.
8. Lieberman E, Ryan KJ, Momsen RR, et al. Am J Obstet Gynecol 1988;159:107–14.
9. Magee HE, Milligan EHM. Br Med J 1951;ii:1307–10.
10. Barton PP, Joy MT, Lappin TR, et al. Am J Obstet Gynecol 1994;170:896–901.
11. Chanarin I, Rothman D. Br Med J 1971;ii:81–4.
12. Life Sciences Research Office, FASEB. Third report on nutrition monitoring in the United States. Washington, DC: U.S. Government Printing Office, 1995;2:VA-33.
13. Chanarin I. The megaloblastic anaemias. 3rd ed. Oxford: Blackwell, 1990;30.
13a. Chanarin I, Metz J. Br J Haematol 1997;97:695–700.
13b. Chanarin I. The megaloblastic anaemias. 2nd ed. Oxford: Blackwell, 1979;55.
14. Chanarin I, Malkowska V, O'Hea LA-M, et al. Lancet 1985;ii:1168–72.
15. Deacon R, Perry J, Lumb M, et al. Br J Haematol 1990;74: 354–9.
16. Chanarin I, Deacon R, Lumb, et al. J Cin Path 1992;45: 277–83.
17. Vieira-Makings E, Metz J, Van der Westhuyzen, et al. Biochem J 1990;266:707–11.
18. Chanarin I, Stephenson E. J Clin Path 1988;41:759–62.
19. Curtis D, Sparrow R, Brennan L, et al. Eur J Haematol 1994;52: 227–32.
20. Green R, Gatautis V, Jacobsen DW. Blood 1990;76(Suppl):33a.
21. Ref. 13b, pp. 230–3.
22. Stabler SP, Allen RH, Savage DG, et al. Blood 1990;76:871–81.
23. Lindenbaum J, Rosenberg IH, Wilson PW, et al. Am J Clin Nutr 1994;60:2–11.
24. Joosten E, Van den Berg A, Riezle R, et al. Am J Clin Nutr 1993;58:468–76.
25. Schneede J, Dagnelie PC, Van Staveren WA, et al. Pediatr Res 1994;36:194–201.
26. Savage DG, Lindenbaum J, Stabler SP, et al. Am J Med 1994;96:239–46.
27. Chong Y-Y, Gupta MK, Jacobsen DW, et al. Blood 1993; 82(Suppl):94a.
28. Chanarin I. The megaloblastic anaemias. 2nd ed. Oxford: Blackwell 1979;296–8.
29. Hitzig WH, Kenny AB. Clin Exp Immunol 1975;20:105–11.
30. Skacel PO, Chanarin I. Br J Haematol 1983;55:203–15.
31. Chanarin I. The megaloblastic anaemias. 3rd ed. Oxford: Blackwell, 1990;99–100.
32. Graham SM, Arvela OM, Wise GA. J Pediatr 1992;121:710–4.
33. Borgstrom B, Norden A, Akkesson B, et al. Nutrition and old age. Oslo: Universitets Forleget, 1979;236–64.
34. Department of Health and Welfare. Canada food consumption pattern report. 1977. Ottawa.
35. Rosenberg IH, Bowman BB, Cooper BA, et al. Am J Clin Nutr 1982;36:1060–6.
36. Ref. 13b, pp. 135–9.
37. Ref. 13b, p. 475.
38. Fleming AF, Hendriks JDdeV, Allan NC. J Obstet Gynaecol Br Commonw 1968;75:425–32.
39. Mollin DL, Waters AH, Harriss E. Clinical aspects of the metabolic interrelationships between folic acid and vitamin B_{12}. In: Heinrich HC, ed. Vitamin B_{12} und intrinsic factor. Stuttgart: Enke, 1961;735–55.
40. Ek J. Acta Obstet Gynaecol Scand 1982;61:17–20.
41. Watson-Williams EJ. East Afr Med J 1962;39:213–20.
42. Laurence KM, James N, Miller MH, et al. Br Med J 1981; 282:1509–11.
43. Smithells RW, Sheppard S, Schorah CJ, et al. Arch Dis Child 1981;56:911–8.
44. MRC Vitamin Study Research Group. Lancet 1991;338:131–7.
45. Czeizel AE, Dudas I. N Engl J Med 1992;327:1832–5.
46. Wild J, Seller M, Schorah CJ, et al. Br J Obstet Gynaecol 1994;101:197–202.
46a. Werler MM, Louik C, Shapiro S, et al. JAMA 1996;275:1089–92.
46b. Wilcken DEL, Wang XL. Lancet 1996;347:340.
47. Clark NA, Fisk NM. Br J Obstet Gynaecol 1994;101:709–10.
48. Chanarin I. Clin Invest Med 1994;17:271–9.
49. Romano PS, Waitzman NJ, Scheffler RM, et al. Am J Public Health 1995;84:667–76.
50. Chanarin I, MacGibbon BM, O'Sullivan WJ, et al. Lancet 1959;ii:634–9.
51. Landon MJ, Hytten FE. J Obstet Gynaecol 1971;78:769–75.
52. McPartlin J, Halligan A, Scott JM, et al. Lancet 1993; 341:148–9.
53. Hansen H, Rybo G. Acta Obstet Gynaecol Scand 1967; 46(Suppl 7):107–12.
54. Chanarin I, Rothman D, Ward A, et al. Br Med J 1968;ii:390–4.
55. Herbert V, Colman N, Spivack M, et al. J Obstet Gynecol 1976;123:175–9.
56. Baumslag N, Edelstein T, Metz J. Br Med J 1970;i:16–7.
57. Iyengar L, Rajalakshmi K. J Obstet Gynecol 1975;122:332–6.
58. Metz J. Am J Clin Nutr 1970;23:843–7.
59. Izak G, Rachmilewitz M, Zan S, et al. Am J Clin Nutr 1963;13: 3669–77.
60. Metz J, McGrath K, Bennett M, et al. Am J Hematol 1995; 48:251–5.

61. Wu A, Chanarin I, Levi AJ. Lancet 1974;i:829–31.
62. Celada A, Rudolf H, Donath A. Blood 1979;54:906–15.
63. Ref. 13b, pp. 537–40.
64. May CD, Hamilton A, Stewart CT. Blood 1952;7:972–91.
65. Ref. 13b, pp. 535–7.
66. Ref. 13b, pp. 451–3.
67. Oppenheimer SM, Hoffbrand BI, Dormandy TL, et al. Postgrad Med J 1987;63:205–7.
68. Blundell EL, Matthews JH, Allen SM, et al. J Clin Pathol 1985; 38:1179–84.
69. Matthews JH. Megaloblastic anaemia. In: Wickramasinghe SN, ed. Clinical Haematology. London: Balliere Tindall 1995;3: 679–97.
70. Carmel R, Rasmussen K, Jacobsen DW, et al. Br J Haematol 1996;93:311–8.
71. Trackman PC, Abeles RH. Biochem Biophys Res Commun 1981;103:1238–44.
72. Deacon R, Bottiglieri T, Chanarin I, et al. Biochim Biophys Acta 1990;1034:342–6.
73. Brattstrom LE, Israelsson B, Jeppsson JO, et al. Scand J Clin Lab Invest 1988;48:215–21.

SELECTED READING

Chanarin I. The megaloblastic anaemias. 2nd ed. Oxford: Blackwell, 1979;1-783.

Chanarin I. The megaloblastic anaemias. 3rd ed. Oxford: Blackwell, 1990;1–209.

Craig WJ. Iron status of vegetarians. Am J Clin Nutr 1994; 59(Suppl):1233S–7S.

Dwyer JT. Vegetarian eating patterns: science, values, and food choices—where do we go from here? Am J Clin Nutr 1994; 59(Suppl):1255S–62S.

89. Renal Disorders and Nutrition

JOEL D. KOPPLE

KIDNEY FUNCTION

The kidney has three primary functions: excretory, endocrine, and metabolic. All three functions may be impaired in renal disease and may affect the patient's nutritional status and management. When injury, necrosis, and scarring of the renal parenchyma cause a loss of renal function, the amount of substances filtered by the kidney falls. However, many aspects of renal function undergo changes that preserve homeostasis and minimize the derangements in plasma and tissue concentrations of substances normally excreted by the kidney. Prominent among these adaptations is nephron hypertrophy and an increase in blood flow and glomerular filtration rate in those nephrons that are still functional.

Many organic compounds accumulate in renal failure (1); most are products of amino acid and protein metabolism. Quantitatively, the most prominent are urea, creatinine, other guanidine compounds, and uric acid (Fig. 89.1). Some of these compounds are considered toxic in high concentrations. Low protein intake reduces accumulation of many of these substances. Eventually, renal failure may become so severe that the aforementioned adaptive mechanisms can no longer maintain homeostasis, even with special dietary therapy that restricts intake of fluid, electrolytes, and protein. Accumulation of these compounds, the endocrine and metabolic disturbances, and the clinical signs and symptoms that result from renal failure are referred to as uremia. If this condition is not treated by hemodialysis, peritoneal dialysis, or renal transplantation, death will supervene.

Excretion and regulation of body water, minerals, and organic compounds are clearly the most important functions of the kidney. Without renal excretory function, patients rarely live longer than 4 to 5 weeks and often less than 10 days, particularly if they are hypercatabolic. In contrast, anephric patients can be kept alive for years with intermittent hemodialysis or peritoneal dialysis, even though endocrine and metabolic functions of the kidney are not replaced.

The kidney elaborates hormones with diverse metabolic effects, including 1,25-dihydroxycholecalciferol, erythropoietin, renin, and kallikreins. These effects have been the subject of many excellent and comprehensive reviews (2–5). The kidney plays an essential role in vitamin D metabolism (4) (see Chapter 18). Vitamin D_3 (cholecalciferol) is hydroxylated in the liver to form 25-hydroxycholecalciferol. This compound is then converted in the kidney to 1,25-dihydroxycholecalciferol (1,25-dihydroxyvitamin D). The actions of 1,25-dihydroxyvitamin D are discussed in Chapter 18. In renal failure, impaired synthesis of 1,25-dihydroxyvitamin D contributes to a vitamin D–deficient state associated with impaired intestinal calcium absorption, hyperparathyroidism, resistance to the actions of parathyroid hormone on bone, and development of renal osteodystrophy.

Erythropoietin is a glycoprotein that stimulates erythropoiesis in bone marrow (5, 6). The anemia of chronic renal failure is primarily caused by impaired erythropoiesis. Decreased red cell formation is mainly due to reduced erythropoietin production in the diseased kidneys, although compounds that accumulate in renal failure may also suppress erythropoiesis. A mild hemolysis often contributes to the anemia. Certain kidney diseases such as kidney cysts or tumors occasionally increase erythropoietin synthesis, which enhances erythropoiesis and

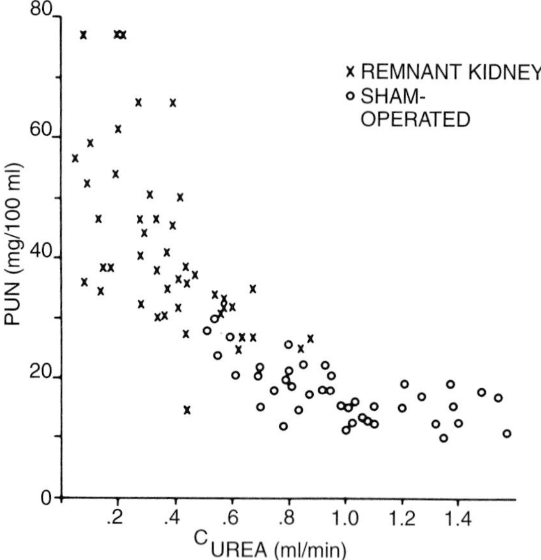

Figure 89.1. Relationship between the plasma urea nitrogen *(PUN)* and GFR as indicated by urea clearance in Sprague-Dawley rats with chronic renal insufficiency and sham-operated controls. Chronic renal failure was produced by ligation of two-thirds to three-fourths of the arterial supply to the left kidney and contralateral nephrectomy. (From Kopple JD. Nutrition and the kidney. In: Alfin-Slater RB, Kritchevsky D, eds. Human nutrition: a comprehensive treatise, vol 4. New York: Plenum Publishing, 1979;409–57, with permission.)

leads to elevated hemoglobin and hematocrit levels. Recombinant DNA–synthesized human erythropoietin is commonly used to increase blood hemoglobin levels in nondialyzed patients with advanced renal failure and those undergoing maintenance dialysis (7).

Renin stimulates conversion of angiotensin I to angiotensin II, a potent vasoconstrictive agent that raises blood pressure and also may stimulate collagen formation and cell proliferation in the kidney and probably other tissues. Renal renin secretion is stimulated by renal ischemia (e.g., in renal artery stenosis) and sometimes other renal diseases; increased plasma renin levels can cause hypertension. Renal disease and particularly renal failure also may engender hypertension by other mechanisms, including retention of sodium chloride and water.

INTERRELATIONSHIPS BETWEEN NUTRIENTS AND KIDNEY FUNCTION

Kidney function both regulates, and is influenced by, the body's pools and concentrations of water, minerals, and many other nutrients and their metabolites. The reader is referred elsewhere in this text for a discussion of water, sodium, potassium, and acid-base physiology (Chapter 6) and calcium and phosphorus (Chapter 8), magnesium (Chapter 9) and trace element (Chapters 10–15) metabolism.

Effects of Malnutrition on the Kidney

Malnutrition can have important, but usually reversible, effects on renal function. In humans, malnutrition decreases the glomerular filtration rate (GFR) (8, 9) as well as the capacity to concentrate and acidify urine (9–11). If nutritional intake improves, these functions may normalize. GFR falls reversibly in obese subjects placed on weight-reduction diets that contain no protein or calories but provide water, vitamins, and small quantities of minerals. This phenomenon is at least partly due to a reduction in extracellular body water, circulating blood volume, and renal blood flow. Increased salt and water intake rapidly reverses this condition. The low or absent protein intake also contributes to the lower renal blood flow and GFR (8, 9).

Ichikawa et al. investigated the mechanisms responsible for the reduction in GFR with protein malnutrition (12). They found that in rats pair-fed a low-protein (6%) diet as compared with an isocaloric high-protein (40%) diet, the GFR was almost 35% lower. Increased resistance was evident in the arterioles leading into (afferent) and out of (efferent) the glomerulus. The glomerular capillary plasma flow rate was about 25% lower, and the glomerular capillary ultrafiltration coefficient was almost 50% lower. Glomerular transcapillary hydraulic pressure differences were similar in the two groups. A reduction in insulin-like growth factor–I (IGF-I) levels may contribute to these changes (13, 14).

Malnourished individuals often have lower specific gravity in random urine specimens and increased daily urine volumes. Impaired concentrating ability probably contributes to the nocturia that may occur in malnutrition. The inability of the malnourished patient to concentrate urine normally appears to be due to low protein intake and consequent low rate of urea synthesis (10). Urea is critical for normal urinary concentration. Some urea filtered by the glomerulus is reabsorbed in the renal tubule and accumulates in the interstitium of the renal medulla where it attracts water from the collecting duct by osmotic pressure. Loss of water from the collecting duct lumen concentrates the urine. When protein intake is low, urea synthesis falls, and serum urea nitrogen (SUN) decreases; less urea is filtered by the glomerulus and reabsorbed into the renal medulla. Thus, medullary hypertonicity falls, and there is less tendency for water to move from the distal tubule and collecting duct to the medulla; hence maximum renal concentrating ability is reduced. Ingestion of urea or more protein by malnourished subjects or those who eat low protein diets improves renal concentrating ability (10). The capacity to dilute urine is normal in malnutrition.

Malnourished subjects are more likely to develop acidosis after an acid load (11). Urinary phosphate and ammonia are primary carriers of acid in the urine. Hydrogen ion secretion into the lumen of the distal nephron lowers the pH of tubular fluid and converts HPO_4^{2-} to $H_2PO_4^-$ and ammonia to NH_4^+. In individuals who have a low phosphorus intake, phosphate filtered in the kidney is largely reabsorbed, which conserves body phosphate pools; less phosphorus is excreted in the urine, however, which reduces the capacity of the kidney to excrete acid. Infusion of phosphate improves urinary excretion of titratable acid in malnourished patients (11). In malnutrition, renal production and excretion of ammonium are also reduced, both under basal conditions and after an acid load (11).

During prolonged starvation, the kidney may account for up to 45% of endogenous glucose production, although part of this percent increase in glucose synthesis is due to a fall in total body glucose production (15). In extended starvation, net renal extraction of lactate, pyruvate, amino acids, and glycerol also occurs (15). The carbon skeleton in these compounds is almost completely converted into glucose. During prolonged starvation, free fatty acids and β-hydroxybutyrate are also extracted by the kidney, and acetoacetate is released (15).

Acute starvation and other conditions associated with increased catabolism of nucleic acids, purines, and amino acids, such as may occur with chemotherapy of leukemias and certain other tumors, can markedly increase uric acid production. Hyperuricemia can lead to deposition of uric acid sludge in the kidney and lower urinary tract and may cause acute renal failure. Treatment consists of allopurinol (which inhibits synthesis of uric acid), maintaining good hydration and large urine flow, and alkalinizing the urine to increase the solubility of uric acid (16).

Effects of Protein and Amino Acid Intake on Renal Function

Protein intake appears to engender both an immediate and a longer-term increase in renal blood flow and GFR in humans. A transient increase in renal blood flow and GFR of about 20 to 28% occurs following ingestion of a protein or amino acid load (17, 18). The rise occurs about 2 hours after the meal and generally lasts about 1 hour. Renal blood flow and GFR increase more quickly and also transiently following an intravenous infusion of a mixture of essential and nonessential amino acids (19) or a 30-minute infusion of arginine hydrochloride (20).

The mechanisms responsible for the rise in renal blood flow and GFR following intake of protein or amino acids are not well delineated. Data concerning potential hormonal causes are either negative, inconclusive, or conflicting (21). Cytokines, paracrines, and other intrinsic renal processes, such as enhanced renal tubular amino acid and sodium reabsorption and altered tubuloglomerular feedback, have been proposed (21). Infusion of somatostatin blocks the rise induced by an amino acid infusion, indicating that peptide hormones may mediate the amino acid and protein enhancement of renal blood flow and GFR (19).

An infusion of glucagon that raises blood glucagon levels to those observed after an amino acid load is reported to increase renal blood flow and GFR (22). Hence glucagon may play a role in the amino acid– or protein-induced increase in renal blood flow and GFR. However, in some studies, the amount of glucagon necessary to increase renal blood flow and GFR exceeded that which occurs after a meat meal (23) or after ingestion or infusion of amino acids (18, 24). Moreover, infusing glucagon directly into the renal artery in dogs (25) and humans (24) does not increase renal blood flow or GFR, although infusion into the portal vein does. Acromegalic patients have an abnormally high GFR (26). An injection of growth hormone into normal humans increases renal blood flow and GFR after several hours (27). IGF-I appears to mediate the growth hormone–induced rise in renal hemodynamics (13, 28).

Most patients with renal insufficiency also demonstrate a protein- or amino acid–induced rise in renal blood flow and GFR (17, 21). This increase has been called the *renal functional reserve.* Some investigators have suggested that the maximum renal blood flow and GFR after a protein or amino acid load in patients with renal disease (compared with normal subjects) better estimates the magnitude of renal damage and scarring than the basal levels of these hemodynamic parameters. This has not been confirmed, because the maximum renal blood flow and GFR following a protein load appear to vary, depending on the individual's previous daily protein intake. The changes in renal blood flow and GFR in patients with diabetes mellitus given protein or amino acids are quite variable in different studies (22).

EFFECT OF NUTRITIONAL INTAKE ON THE RATE OF PROGRESSION OF RENAL FAILURE

Mechanisms of Progression

Physicians have known for many decades that patients with chronic renal disease who have sustained a substantial loss of GFR often continue to lose renal function inexorably until they develop terminal renal failure (29–31). Although the rate of progression of renal failure varies greatly among patients, in many individuals, the decline in kidney function is linear (29–31). The percentage of patients with renal insufficiency who progress to renal failure is not known, but it seems likely that renal failure will continue to progress in most patients who lose 50% or more of GFR. Renal failure may progress because of the underlying renal disease or because of superimposition of other diseases that may contribute to renal injury such as hypertension, adverse effects of nephrotoxic medicines (e.g., antibiotics or radiocontrast material), obstruction, kidney infection, hypercalcemia, or hyperuricemia. However, continued progression is not rare even after the initial cause of the renal disease seems to have disappeared and when no superimposed illnesses are present (32–35). For example, renal failure may progress in patients after relief of urinary tract obstruction, control of hypertension, discontinuance of nephrotoxic medications, or partial recovery from acute renal failure.

Studies of animal and in vitro models of chronic renal disease or renal failure have led to the following observations. There is a rather common physiologic and biochemical response to chronic loss of renal function that is largely independent of the underlying type of kidney disease. When enough functioning nephrons are lost to cause renal insufficiency, the remaining individual functioning nephrons show a rise in glomerular plasma flow and GFR, and both glomeruli and tubules increase in size (i.e., nephron hypertrophy) (36, 37). The capillary blood flow of the remaining glomeruli increases as does the blood pressure gradient across the capillary wall (37, 38). In addition, the chemical, electrical, and pore-size barriers to movement of plasma proteins across the glomerulus and into the renal tubule are impaired (39, 40). Migration of leukocytes and monocytes, platelet aggregation, collagen deposition, cellular proliferation, and other inflammatory and scarifying changes may occur to a greater or lesser degree and may cause progressive renal damage. Many of these changes, some of which could be considered adaptive physiologic responses, are believed to promote further renal injury and lead to progressive renal failure.

Current thinking regarding potential causes of progressive renal failure is summarized in Table 89.1. Most of these processes have been investigated only in animal models, and a role in human renal disease is inferred. Many of these mechanisms appear susceptible to amelioration or reversal by nutritional therapy (Table 89.1); for example, protein-restricted diets reduce renal blood flow, GFR, and proteinuria in humans with renal disease (21).

Table 89.1
Potential Causes and Mechanisms of Progressive Renal Failure[a]

Continued activity of the underlying renal disease
Systemic hypertension[b]
High-protein diet[b]
High-phosphorus diet[b]
High-total-fat or -cholesterol diet[b]
High calcium-phosphorus product in serum[b]
Vitamin D overdose (causing hypercalcemia)[b]
High serum oxalate levels (can be enhanced by high ascorbic acid intake)[b]
Hyperuricemia
Acidemia
Nephrotoxic medicines (e.g., radiocontrast material, aminoglycoside antibiotics
Intraglomerular capillary pressure and capillary blood flow
Intraglomerular transcapillary hydraulic pressure
Glomerular and tubular hypertrophy
Lipoprotein and lipid deposition in glomerulus
Deposition of other proteins in glomerulus
Inflammatory response in kidney with release of cytokines and monokines
Platelet aggregation in kidney
Calcium phosphate or calcium oxalate deposition in the kidney
Release of growth factors in kidney
Increased mesangial matrix production
Enhanced renal tubular generation of ammonia leading to complement activation
Increased generation of reactive oxygen metabolites in remaining functional nephrons
Lead, cadmium toxicity

[a]Evidence that many of these factors may cause progressive renal failure is derived from animal models or in vitro systems.
[b]These causes of progressive renal failure may act through one or more of the mechanisms listed in the lower half of this table.

Experimental Evidence for Effects of Nutritional Intake on Progression of Chronic Renal Failure

Dietary protein restriction has been used for many decades to minimize uremic toxicity (41). In the first half of the 20th century, research in rats also indicated that protein restriction could retard progression of renal failure (42–44). The experimental design of these studies as well as observations in humans concerning the effects of dietary protein restriction on progression of renal disease were not well controlled, and the results were inconsistent.

In the 1970s and 1980s, studies in both rats and humans indicated that dietary control can retard progression of renal failure in a variety of renal diseases. In rats, several models of renal insufficiency were studied. These included surgical removal of the upper and lower poles of one kidney or ligation of about two-thirds to three-quarters of the arteries to one kidney; in both models, contralateral nephrectomy was performed. In some cases, experimental glomerulonephritis was created (45–49). In these animal models, diets low in protein and/or phosphorus retarded or prevented progression of renal failure (45–49). In addition, a diet low or high in certain fats may retard progressive renal damage (50–53). Moreover, administration of prostaglandins may affect the progression of chronic renal disease in animals (54–56).

Proteins

In experimental animals with renal disease, a high-protein diet stimulates an increase in GFR, glomerular capillary blood flow, blood pressure gradients across the glomerular capillary wall, and enlargement of individual nephrons, whereas a low-protein diet blunts or prevents this response (37). Moreover, normal rats with renal injury who are fed a high-protein diet develop renal failure, and when such animals are fed a low-protein diet, the progression of renal failure is retarded or arrested (43, 44, 48). A current theory postulates that a high-protein intake, by increasing both glomerular capillary blood flow and transcapillary glomerular hydraulic pressure, causes progressive renal injury to the basement membrane (filtering wall) of the glomerulus. These alterations, in turn, increase capillary permeability, enhance movement of large molecules across the glomerular basement membrane, and cause deposition of these compounds in the mesangium, mesangial expansion, an inflammatory response in the glomerulus, scarring, and glomerulosclerosis (38, 57, 58).

High-protein diets may also promote renal insufficiency by other mechanisms: *(a)* induction of nephron hypertrophy with activation of growth factors that stimulate cell hypertrophy, proliferation, and scarring in the glomerulus; *(b)* enhanced oxidation rates in the nephron with increased generation of reactive oxygen species (59); *(c)* an acid load that stimulates renal ammonium production and activation of complement C (60); *(d)* increased generation of urea, which itself may cause hypertrophy of segments of the renal tubule (61); and *(e)* generation of angiotensin II and other hormones (61a, 61b). A low-protein diet retards or stops progressive renal damage by preventing or reducing these phenomena. Diets providing soya protein, a vegetable protein, rather than casein, an animal protein, may be more effective in retarding progression of kidney failure in rats with remnant kidneys (62).

Diabetic rats with moderate hyperglycemia develop renal hypertrophy and increased hemodynamics (63), and similar abnormalities appear to occur in the intact kidney of humans with diabetes mellitus. Early in the course of diabetes mellitus, patients develop increased renal blood flow, increased GFR, and large kidneys (64). Ultimately, in a large proportion of these individuals, glomerulosclerosis occurs and renal failure supervenes (65, 66). In the early stages of diabetes, strict blood glucose control may reverse these phenomena.

Phosphorus and Calcium

As previously indicated, a low phosphorus intake independent of protein intake seems to retard progression of renal failure (45, 67, 68). The mechanism of action of the low phosphorus intake is unclear. One theory is that a low phosphorus intake decreases deposition of calcium phosphate in kidney tissue, which may cause further renal damage (67, 68). Indeed, in renal tissue obtained by biopsy or autopsy, a direct correlation exists between the calcium content and the serum creatinine concentration (69). Moreover, in rats with chronic renal insufficiency, administration of the calcium-channel blocker verapamil retards the rate of progression of renal failure, compared with treatment with an antihypertensive agent that does not impede intracellular movement of calcium (70). In general, the calcium concentration of renal tissue is higher in those parts of the kidney with more severe renal histopathologic changes.

Lipids and Lipoproteins

Many animal studies suggest a pathogenic role of dietary fat intake and hyperlipoproteinemia. Rats, rabbits, and guinea pigs fed a high-cholesterol diet developed hypercholesterolemia and progressive glomerulosclerosis and renal failure (50, 71, 72). The lipid composition of renal cortical tissue is altered, and both mesangial cellularity and matrix formation increase (71). Glomerular capillary pressure rises, even though systemic blood pressure is not very elevated, which suggests a role for glomerular hypertension in the loss of renal function in the dietary cholesterol or hypercholesterolemia model of renal insufficiency. Cholesterol-induced renal injury is much greater when cholesterol-supplemented rats have other underlying renal diseases. Drugs that lower serum lipoprotein levels may also ameliorate glomerular injury in rats (73).

Mesangial cells and monocytes have receptors for certain lipoproteins (74). Monocytes may ingest low-density lipoprotein (LDL) cholesterol and other lipoproteins. These compounds, once incorporated, may initiate a series of biochemical and physiologic processes that are pathologic. For example, monocytes from hypercholesterolemic animals have greater adherence to endothelial cells and migrate to the subendothelial spaces more effectively than normal monocytes (75). Activated macrophages produce more reactive oxygen species. Moreover, rats made hypercholesterolemic by high-cholesterol diets show evidence of increased glomerular arteriole contractility, probably by oxidized lipoprotein activation of thromboxane (76). Hypercholesterolemia may also alter the metabolism of certain fatty acids, including arachidonic and linoleic acid.

In addition to a number of growth factors (see above), many other compounds may affect renal physiology and progression of renal failure (5), including angiotensin and various eicosanoids. Angiotensin not only causes vasoconstriction but also alters glomerular permeability and may stimulate mesangial cell proliferation. The essential fatty acid linoleic acid can be metabolized in the kidney to several families of eicosanoids, including prostaglandins. Prostaglandins have far-reaching effects on blood flow and blood pressure inside the glomerulus, the propensity for platelets to clot in the glomerulus, and the inflammatory process. Certain eicosanoids have antagonistic effects; some increase glomerular blood flow and pressure and may impair platelet clotting, whereas others do the opposite and may also stimulate an inflammatory response. In renal insufficiency, elaboration of certain eicosanoids and other cytokines increases in the kidney (53, 77), and they appear important in the complex adaptive processes the nephron exhibits as kidney function deteriorates (78, 79). In various animal models of chronic renal disease, feeding or infusions of linoleic acid, vasodilatory prostaglandins, or injections of thromboxane or leukotriene B4 may retard progression of renal failure in rats (54–56, 80, 81). In rats with Heymann nephritis, dietary protein itself reduces eicosanoid synthesis (82). Hence the beneficial effects of dietary protein restriction may be partly due to its effects on eicosanoid production.

Medicines

Although results of the above studies in animals indicate an important role for dietary restriction of protein and phosphorus and reduction or increase of certain fats in controlling progressive renal failure, evidence indicates that certain medicines may be able to substitute for or add to these benefits. Angiotensin-converting enzyme inhibitors (which decrease blood pressure by inhibiting the enzyme that catalyzes conversion of angiotensin I to angiotensin II) also lower glomerular capillary blood flow and blood pressure gradients across the glomerular capillary wall in rats with renal insufficiency (83). They also appear to retard progressive renal failure in these animals (83, 84) and reduce urinary protein excretion in patients with kidney disease (85). These medicines also reduce or abolish microalbuminuria in diabetic patients and retard the rate of progression of renal failure in patients with type I and type II diabetes mellitus and nephropathy and in nondiabetic patients with renal disease (86, 87). Another class of antihypertensive medicines, calcium-channel blockers, may also inhibit progressive renal failure in animals (88, 89). Evidence also strongly suggests that blood pressure control, by itself, retards progressive renal failure (88, 90).

Medicines that bind phosphorus in the intestinal tract enhance the effectiveness of dietary phosphorus restriction in reducing progression of renal failure in animals (45, 68). These drugs are of particular value as an adjunct to dietary phosphorus restriction, because it is difficult to lower dietary phosphorus intake to necessary levels without making diets highly restrictive and unpalatable, which limits adherence.

Human Studies on the Effect of Dietary Therapy on Progression of Chronic Renal Failure

To what extent do the animal data apply to patients? From the mid-1970s to the present, virtually all dietary studies in humans with renal insufficiency have indicated that low intake of dietary protein and phosphorus is effective in retarding the rate of progression of renal failure (91–102). Some evidence indicates that low protein and phosphorus intakes may act separately to slow progressive renal failure (67).

Earlier studies of this question in humans generally suffered from one or more major defects in experimental design, including small sample size, inadequate or absent control groups, poor documentation of the patients' actual intake, and imprecise methods of measuring renal function. More-recent clinical trials have used more effective research protocols. These latter studies have generally compared a low-protein, low-phosphorus diet providing either about 0.40 to 0.60 g protein/kg body weight per day or about 0.28 g protein/kg/day supplemented with essential amino acids or ketoacids with either a more liberal diet containing approximately 1.0 g protein/kg/day and more phosphorus or an ad libitum diet.

The very low protein diet providing about 0.28 g/kg/day (e.g., about 16–25 g protein/day) is supplemented with 10 to 20 g per day of the nine essential amino acids or of mixtures of several essential amino acids, several nonessential amino acids, and ketoacid or hydroxyacid analogues of other essential amino acids (91, 93–96, 98, 101). The ketoacid or hydroxyacid analogue is structurally identical to its corresponding essential amino acid, except that the amino (NH_2) group attached to the second (α) carbon of the amino acid is replaced by a keto group or hydroxy group, respectively.

The ketoacid and hydroxyacid analogues can be transaminated in the body to the respective amino acids, although a proportion of the analogues are degraded rather than transaminated. Because the ketoacids and hydroxyacids lack the nitrogen-containing amino group on the α carbon, these compounds provide the patient with a lower nitrogen load. As they are degraded in the body, they should generate fewer waste products to accumulate in renal failure. Ketoacid analogues of the branched chain amino acids, especially of leucine, may be particularly likely to promote protein anabolism, possibly by decreasing protein degradation (103, 104). Hence it is possible, but not yet demonstrated, that these ketoacids may play a beneficial role in maintaining protein mass in patients with renal failure.

The largest and most intensive examination of whether dietary control will retard the rate of progression of renal disease was the Modification of Diet in Renal Disease (MDRD) Study funded by the National Institutes of Health (101, 102). This project investigated, in an intention-to-treat analysis, the effects of three levels of dietary protein and phosphorus intakes and two blood pressure management goals on the progression of chronic renal disease. A total of 840 adults with various types of renal disease (excluding insulin-dependent diabetes mellitus) were divided into two study groups according to their GFRs.

In study A, 585 patients with a GFR, measured by ^{131}I-iothalamate clearances, of 25 to 55 mL/1.73 m^2/min were examined. Patients were randomly assigned to either a usual-protein, usual-phosphorus diet (protein, 1.3 g/kg standard body weight per day; phosphorus, 16 to 20 mg/kg/day) or a low-protein, low-phosphorus diet (protein, 0.58 g/kg/day; phosphorus, 5–10 mg/kg/day) and also to either a moderate or strict blood pressure goal (mean arterial blood pressure, 107 mm Hg [113 mm Hg for those 61 years of age or older] or 92 mm Hg (98 mm Hg for those 61 years of age or older]). Study B included 255 patients with a baseline GFR of 13 to 24 mL/1.73m^2/min. Patients were randomly assigned to the low-protein, low-phosphorus diet or to a very low protein, very low phosphorus diet (protein, 0.28 g/kg/day; phosphorus, 4–9 mg/kg/day) with a ketoacid–amino acid supplement (0.28 g/kg/day). They were also randomly assigned to either the moderate or strict blood pressure control groups, as in study A. Adherence to the dietary protein prescription in the different diet groups was good.

In study A, those prescribed the low-protein diet had significantly faster declines in GFR during the first 4 months than those assigned to the usual protein diet. Thereafter, the rate of decline of the GFR in the low-protein, low-phosphorus group was significantly slower than that in the group fed the usual-protein, usual-phosphorus diet. Over the entire treatment period, the overall rate of progression of renal failure in the two diet groups did not differ. However, the initial greater fall in GFR in the patients prescribed the low-protein diet probably reflects a hemodynamic response to the reduced protein intake rather than more rapid progression of the parenchymal renal disease. This might in fact be beneficial, reflecting reduced intrarenal hyperfiltration and intrarenal hypertension. If this explanation is correct—and it is not proven that it is correct—the slower rate of disease progression after the first 4 months of dietary treatment is consistent with a beneficial effect of this intervention in renal disease. In study B, the very low protein group had a marginally slower decline of GFR than the low-protein group; the average rate of decline did not differ significantly between the two groups ($P = .07$).

In a secondary analysis of study B in which the decrease in GFR was correlated with the actual quantity of protein ingested, progression of renal failure was the same with ingestion of the low protein diet as with the very low protein diet supplemented with ketoacids and amino acids (102). However, if the two diet groups were analyzed together and the protein intake of the latter diet was considered to be the sum of the protein and ketoacid–amino acid supplement ingested, a significantly lower rate of decline in GFR was found in the patients who actually ingested the lower-protein diets (102). These findings suggest that a lower total protein intake, but not the ketoacid–amino acid preparation itself, retarded the rate of progression of renal failure.

The MDRD study did not compare the very low protein ketoacid/amino acid supplemented diet with the usual protein intake. Moreover, the lack of significant effect of the low-protein diet on progression of renal failure might possibly reflect the rather short mean duration of treatment in the MDRD study, 2.2 years. Indeed, if the trend toward slower progression of renal failure in the low-protein-diet groups that was present at the termination of the MDRD study had persisted during a longer follow-up period, statistically significant slower progression would have been observed with the 0.60 g/kg protein diet in study A and the very low protein, ketoacid–amino acid supplemented diet in study B. The response to low-protein diets may possibly be similar to the experience with the Diabetes Control and Complications Trial (DCCT) comparing intensive and more-conventional serum glucose control (105). After 2 years of study, there was no trend toward less microalbuminuria in the more rigorously controlled glucose group; however, when the study was terminated after a mean of 6.5 years, a much lower incidence of microalbuminuria was found in these latter patients.

Two other factors may have reduced the differences in the rate of progression between the diet groups. Many patients assigned to each diet in the MDRD study showed no progression of kidney disease. Also, a disproportionately large number of patients had adult polycystic kidney disease, which may be less responsive to dietary therapy.

Two recent meta-analyses each evaluated several clinical trials of the effects of low-protein and (in some studies) low-phosphorus diets on the rate of progression of kidney failure (106, 107). The two metaanalyses evaluated a somewhat different series of clinical trials, and only one included the MDRD trial (107). Both metaanalyses concluded that low-protein diets retard the rate of progression of renal failure. One of these studies also analyzed the results of five prospective clinical trials of the effects of such diets on progression of renal failure in patients with insulin-dependent diabetes mellitus (107). This metaanalysis indicated that low-protein diets also retard progression in these individuals. However, the results were much less definitive because many fewer patients were analyzed; two of the trials had no randomized, concurrent control group; and the key endpoints were less definitive.

Vegetarian diets providing soy protein may retard progression of chronic renal failure more effectively than diets of similar protein content that contain animal protein (62, 108, 109). The mechanism of such an effect is not known, but it may be related to the total content and different composition of fats in the vegetarian diet. The latter diet is reported to improve the serum lipid profile in patients with chronic renal disease and the nephrotic syndrome (109, 110).

An interesting ancillary question concerning these studies of the effects of diet on progression of renal failure is whether diet may promote or retard development of renal failure in individuals with no underlying renal disease. As indicated above, very high cholesterol diets may cause renal failure in animals. Rats without renal disease or with only one kidney that are allowed to eat ad libitum or are fed high-protein diets throughout life have a higher incidence of renal disease in old age (111–114). In normal humans, after about the fourth decade of life, renal function falls progressively with age (115); possibly high-protein diets play a role in this phenomenon. As indicated above, in healthy young men and women, high-protein intake increases renal blood flow and GFR (21). Moreover, similarities exist between the type of scarring that occurs in normal aging human kidneys as compared with kidneys of rats fed high-protein diets. Adults with congenital absence, developmental failure, or surgical removal of one kidney during childhood have a slightly higher incidence of spontaneous glomerular scarring in the remaining kidney (116). The cause of this phenomenon is not known. It is possible, but by no means established, that the typical protein intake of Americans, which is considerably higher than the recommended dietary allowances (RDAs) for dietary protein (117), may increase glomerular capillary blood flow and hydraulic pressure and cause progressive renal injury.

NUTRITIONAL ALTERATIONS IN THE NEPHROTIC SYNDROME

The nephrotic syndrome is a kidney disorder characterized by loss of large quantities of protein in the urine (≥3.0 g/day), low serum albumin concentrations, high serum levels of cholesterol and other fats, and accumulation of excess body water to form edema (118). This condition is caused by diseases that affect the glomerulus and increase glomerular permeability to protein. Because they have large urinary protein losses and their appetite is frequently poor, patients with the nephrotic syndrome often develop protein malnutrition and debility. Certain vitamins and most trace elements are protein bound in plasma, and these patients are therefore also at risk for developing deficiencies of these nutrients. Vitamin D deficiency has been reported in patients with the nephrotic syndrome (118, 119). Malnutrition may occur in nephrotic patients even when they do not have advanced kidney failure. For a given type of renal disease, heavy proteinuria is associated with more-rapid progression of renal failure, possibly because of incorporation of proteins into the glomerular mesangium, which may cause sclerosis or inflammatory responses (120). Many growth factors and other bioactive substances are also bound to proteins filtered by the leaky glomerulus in patients with the nephrotic syndrome. It is postulated that some of these bioactive compounds may promote progressive renal damage (121).

Studies indicate that both protein-restricted diets and angiotensin-converting enzyme inhibitors reduce proteinuria in nephrotic patients without decreasing serum albumin levels or albumin pools (122–125). Treating nephrotic syndrome patients with both an angiotensin-converting enzyme inhibitor, which may decrease proteinuria, and a higher-protein diet, to increase protein synthesis, has been suggested as the most effective way to maintain a more normal albumin mass in these individuals (122–125). This has been demonstrated in one study in nephrotic rats but has not yet been well tested in nephrotic patients (125).

NUTRITIONAL AND METABOLIC CONSEQUENCES OF CHRONIC RENAL FAILURE

Chronic renal failure causes pervasive nutritional and metabolic disorders that may affect virtually every organ system. These abnormalities are reviewed briefly below.

Clinical, Nutritional, and Metabolic Disorders

Patients with chronic renal failure develop azotemia and uremia. Azotemia refers to accumulation of nitrogenous metabolites in the blood. Uremia is the combination of azotemia with the clinical signs and symptoms of advanced renal failure. Chronic advanced renal failure is a complex disorder caused by marked reduction in the excretory, endocrine, and metabolic functions of the kidney.

The many symptoms of uremia include weakness, a feeling of ill health, insomnia, fatigue, loss of appetite, nausea, vomiting, diarrhea, itching, muscle cramps, hiccups, twitching or jerking of the extremities, fasciculations, tremors, emotional irritability, and decreased mental concentration and comprehension. A characteristic fetid breath is often present. The sodium and water disturbances associated with renal failure include retention leading to congestive heart failure and hypertension or, if excessive sodium depletion occurs, reduction in extracellular fluid volume and a fall in blood pressure.

Altered serum concentrations of other electrolytes and acidosis can occur and can have profound and life-threatening effects on the physiologic processes and metabolism of the body (Fig. 89.1). Abnormalities in water and electrolyte balance and acidosis are caused by impaired ability of the failing kidney to regulate the content of water, salts, and acids in the body. Most of these clinical and metabolic disorders can be controlled or prevented with dietary therapy or dialysis. Untreated uremia can lead to lethargy, loss of consciousness, coma, convulsions, and death.

Chronic advanced renal failure causes pervasive alterations in the absorption, excretion, and metabolism of many nutrients. These disorders include accumulation of chemical products of protein metabolism (1); decreased ability of the kidney either to excrete a large sodium load or to conserve sodium rigorously when dietary sodium is restricted (126); impaired renal ability to excrete water, potassium, calcium, magnesium, phosphorus, trace elements, acids, and other compounds; a tendency to retain phosphorus (126a, 127, 128); decreased intestinal absorption of calcium (127) and possibly iron (128); and a high risk for developing certain vitamin deficiencies, particularly of vitamin B_6, vitamin C, folic acid, and the most potent known form of vitamin D, 1,25-dihydroxycholecalciferol (127, 129). The patient with chronic renal failure is also likely to accumulate certain potentially toxic chemicals such as aluminum that normally are ingested in small amounts and excreted in the urine (128).

Uremia is also a polyendocrinopathy, and many of its metabolic and clinical manifestations are caused by the endocrine disorders. A number of hormone concentrations are elevated in renal failure, particularly those of the peptide hormones, because of the impaired ability of the kidney to degrade peptides. These substances include parathyroid hormone, glucagon, insulin, growth hormone, prolactin, luteinizing hormone, often follicle-stimulating hormone (FSH), and gastrin (127, 130–138). Increased secretion of some hormones, such as parathyroid hormone and insulin, may contribute to elevated plasma levels. Chronically uremic patients have altered thyroid hormone levels that are similar to those in the euthyroid sick syndrome, but hypothyroidism is not common (139). Of the hormones elaborated by the kidney, plasma erythropoietin and 1,25-dihydroxycholecalciferol are reduced (4–7, 127), and plasma renin activity may be increased, normal, or decreased. Serum IGF-I (somatomedin C) levels, measured by radioreceptor assay or radioimmunoassay, are usually reported to be normal in renal failure, but there is resistance to the activity of IGF-I (140, 141). Sensitivity to the actions of glucagon increases; this is reversed by hemodialysis, but hyperglucagonemia persists (131). Resistance to the peripheral action of insulin occurs (142). These effects on insulin and glucagon contribute to the mild glucose intolerance usually present in chronic renal failure (132). Impaired actions of hormones in uremia may be due to circulating inhibitors in serum, downregulation of receptor number, or postreceptor defects in the signal transduction system. Cytosolic calcium participates in certain cell signaling systems. Elevated basal cytosolic calcium, induced by hyperparathyroidism, appears to be one of the postreceptor signal transduction disorders induced by chronic renal failure (143).

The ability of the failing kidney to synthesize or to metabolize many compounds, including amino acids, is impaired. In chronic renal insufficiency, the kidney displays reduced catabolism of glutamine, impaired synthesis of alanine, and decreased conversion of glycine to serine (144, 145). Many products of metabolism accumulate in renal failure; the majority are derived from amino acids and proteins (146). Most of these compounds accumulate because of decreased excretion, although in some instances enhanced synthesis or impaired degradation by the diseased kidney or other organs plays a role. Abnormal metabolism in the gastrointestinal tract and probably the liver also contributes to increased levels of certain metabolites in renal failure (147).

Quantitatively, the most important end product of nitrogen metabolism is urea (146). In a clinically stable patient with chronic renal failure who eats at least 40 g of protein daily, the net quantity of urea produced each day contains an amount of nitrogen equal to about 80 to 90% of the daily nitrogen intake. Guanidines are the next most abundant end product of nitrogen metabolism; these compounds include creatinine, creatine, and guanidinosuccinic acid (1, 146). The "middle molecules" are a class of compounds midway in size between the small, readily dialyzable substances that accumulate in renal failure and small proteins. Most middle molecules are considered to have molecular weights of approximately 300 to 2500 and contain amino acids. Levels of some middle-molecule compounds increase in uremic sera (1, 146). Despite decades of study, the compounds that cause uremic toxicity are not well defined; probably, many compounds contribute to this toxicity. Prime suspects as uremic toxins include urea, guanidine compounds, phenolic acids, middle molecules, and some of the hormones elevated in uremic plasma, especially parathyroid hormone and possibly glucagon (1, 131, 143, 146, 148, 149).

Altered gastrointestinal function may affect nitrogen metabolism in uremic patients. The gastrointestinal tract metabolizes urea, uric acid, creatinine, and choline and synthesizes (or releases from larger molecules) dimethylamine, trimethylamine, ammonia, sarcosine, methylamine, and methylguanidine (146). Gut metabolism or synthesis of many of these compounds increases in chronic renal failure, possibly because of increased numbers of intestinal bacteria (147).

Some of the metabolic alterations in uremia are adaptive homeostatic responses that both benefit and harm the patient (148). Hyperparathyroidism is an example. As the kidneys fail, impaired excretion of phosphorus leads to phosphorus retention. Concomitantly, the diseased and scarred renal parenchyma is less able to convert 25-hydroxycholecalciferol to 1,25-dihydroxycholecalciferol (127). Low plasma concentrations of 1,25-dihydroxycholecalciferol lead to an increase in parathyroid hormone secretion. In addition, deficiency of 1,25-dihydroxycholecalciferol both impairs intestinal calcium absorption and causes resistance to the actions of parathyroid hormone in bone. These alterations also promote hypocalcemia, low serum levels of both calcium and 1,25-dihydroxycholecalciferol, and lead to development of hyperparathyroidism. Elevated serum parathyroid hormone reduces renal tubular reabsorption of phosphorus (enhancing urine phosphorus excretion), lowers serum phosphorus, promotes renal synthesis of 1,25-dihydroxycholecalciferol, mobilizes calcium from bone, and increases intestinal calcium absorption (although intestinal calcium absorption usually remains low or, in mild renal insufficiency, normal). The benefits derived from these homeostatic actions are that more normal concentrations of plasma phosphorus and calcium are maintained. The "trade-off" is development of hyperparathyroidism (148, 149). Parathyroid hormone has been implicated as a pervasive uremic toxin that adversely affects many organs and tissues and contributes to the uremic syndrome (149).

With the institution of dietary therapy or treatment with hemodialysis or peritoneal dialysis, blood levels of many metabolic products that accumulate in uremic plasma decrease, and the patient may experience clinical improvement. Maintenance hemodialysis or peritoneal dialysis enables patients to live for many years with essentially no renal function. Despite such improvement, however, many clinical and metabolic disorders may persist or even progress. These include *(a)* a type IV hyperlipidemia and other disorders of lipid metabolism, (150, 151); *(b)* a high incidence of cardiovascular disease (152); *(c)* osteodystrophy with disordered bone architecture, osteoporosis, or osteomalacia (aluminum toxicity often contributes to the osteomalacia) (127, 153); *(d)* anemia (5–7); *(e)* impaired immune function and decreased resistance to infection; *(f)* mildly impaired peripheral and central nervous system function; *(g)* muscle weakness and atrophy; *(h)* frequent occurrence of viral hepatitis (154); *(i)* sexual impotence and infertility; *(j)* generalized wasting and malnutrition (155–163); *(k)* a general feeling of ill health or emotional depression; and *(l)* poor rehabilitation (164). Most of these complications can be aggravated by poor nutritional intake or improved with good nutrition.

Anemia, usually primarily due to impaired erythropoiesis caused by erythropoietin deficiency, can be treated effectively with this hormone (7). To reduce the risks and cost of therapy, usually enough erythropoietin is given to raise the hematocrit to only 33 to 36%. When kidney failure is a complication of an underlying systemic disease, such as diabetes mellitus, hypertension, or lupus erythematosus, other manifestations of the underlying disease may also adversely affect the patient and may progress. All the above problems do not seriously affect every patient, and many patients with chronic uremia or who undergo dialysis lead full and productive lives.

The above considerations indicate that intestinal absorption, excretion, and/or metabolism of virtually every nutrient may be altered in chronic renal failure. In addition, decreased intake of food and excessive intake of certain minerals (e.g., aluminum from ingestion of aluminum phosphate binders) may alter nutritional status. Medicinal therapy may also adversely affect nutrient metabolism in renal failure. For example, anticonvulsant medicines may cause deficiencies of vitamin D and folic acid; hydralazine, isoniazid, and other medicines may cause vitamin B_6 deficiency (165). The many altered nutritional requirements and tolerances that occur in chronic renal failure are a challenge for the dietary therapy of such patients.

Wasting Syndrome

The patient with chronic renal failure frequently shows evidence of wasting or protein-energy malnutrition (Table 89.2) (155–163, 166). Evidence includes decreased relative body weight (i.e., the patient's body weight divided by the median weight of normal people of the same age, height, sex, and skeletal frame size), skinfold thickness (an estimate of total body fat), arm muscle mass, and total body nitrogen and potassium; low growth rates in children; decreased serum concentrations of many proteins including albumin, transferrin, and certain complement proteins; and low muscle alkali-soluble protein. The plasma amino acid pattern, which is pathognomonic for renal failure, also resembles that found in malnutrition. The findings of malnutrition are sometimes observed in nondialyzed patients with chronic renal failure but are more prevalent in patients undergoing maintenance hemodialysis or chronic peritoneal dialysis. Not every dialysis patient shows evidence of these disorders; however, virtually every survey of maintenance dialysis patients indicates that as a group, these patients show evidence of malnutrition (155–163, 166). Malnutrition is mild to moderate in most malnourished chronic dialysis patients; about 6 to 8% of dialysis patients have evidence of severe wasting. In addition to protein-energy malnutrition, patients with chronic renal failure are at higher risk for malnutrition of iron, zinc, and certain vitamins, including vitamin B_6, vitamin C, folic acid, 1,25-dihydroxycholecalciferol and possibly carnitine (167–172).

Table 89.2
Evidence for Protein-Energy Malnutrition in Patients with Advanced Chronic Renal Failure

Anthropometry, Body Composition, and Isotope Dilution Studies[a]	Biochemistry[a]
Decreased	**Decreased**
Body weight	Serum
Height (children)	Total protein
Growth (children)	Albumin
Body fat (skinfold thickness)	Transferrin
Fat-free solids	Prealbumin
Intracellular water	C3
Muscle mass (midarm muscle circumference)	C3 Activator
	Cholinesterase
Total body potassium (nondialyzed patients)	Plasma
	Leucine
Total body nitrogen (CPD patients)	Isoleucine
	Total tryptophan
Total albumin mass, synthesis, and catabolism	Valine
	Tyrosine
Valine pools (nondialyzed patients)	Valine:glycine ratio
	Essential:nonessential ratio
	Muscle
	Alkali-soluble protein
	RNA:DNA ratio
	Valine
	Tyrosine
	Normal to increased
	Plasma glycine

[a]Patients with chronic renal failure may have normal values for these parameters, but statistical comparisons indicate that the levels are often abnormal in these individuals.

There are many causes of protein-energy malnutrition in chronic renal failure (158). First, dietary intake is often inadequate, particularly for energy requirements (156, 157, 173–177). The low dietary intake is mainly due to anorexia, caused by uremic toxicity, the debilitating effects of acute or chronic illness, and depression. The effects of acute superimposed illness on the patient's ability to eat or to accept tube feeding also reduce nutrient intake. In addition, the dietary prescription in renal failure, which is low in protein and other nutrients and may be difficult to prepare or unpalatable, can lead to low nutrient intake.

Second, patients with renal failure have a high incidence of superimposed catabolic illnesses (178–180). Third, the dialysis procedure itself may induce wasting. Hemodialysis and peritoneal dialysis remove free amino acids, peptides or bound amino acids (181–184), water-soluble vitamins (129), proteins (with peritoneal dialysis and, rarely, with hemodialysis) (182, 185), glucose (during hemodialysis with glucose-free dialysate) (186), and probably other bioactive compounds. Hemodialysis also increases net protein breakdown, especially by activating the complement cascade system and inducing release of catabolic cytokines (187, 188). This catabolic stress is particularly likely when bioincompatible dialyzer membranes are used (187, 188) and can be mitigated with use of dialyzers made from more biocompatible materials (188, 188a). Fourth, patients with renal failure sustain blood loss. Because blood is a rich source of protein, this loss might contribute to protein depletion. Blood loss results from frequent sampling for laboratory testing, occult gastrointestinal bleeding (common in renal failure), and sequestration of blood in the hemodialyzer and blood tubing (189).

Other possible but unestablished causes of wasting include *(a)* altered endocrine activity, particularly resistance to insulin (142) and IGF-I (140, 141), hyperglucagonemia (131), hyperparathyroidism (127, 143, 148,

149), and deficiency of 1,25-dihydroxycholecalciferol (127); *(b)* endogenous uremic toxins *(c)*; exogenous uremic toxins, such as aluminum; and *(d)* loss of metabolic functions of the kidney. Because the kidney synthesizes or degrades many biologically valuable compounds, including amino acids (144, 145), loss of these activities in kidney failure could possibly disrupt the body's metabolism and promote wasting.

Several investigators have shown an inverse relationship between dietary protein consumption (as determined by the patient's urea nitrogen appearance [UNA] or average SUN level) and morbidity and mortality (166, 190–192). Moreover, a striking inverse relationship exists between the serum albumin level and the mortality rate in these patients (166). These studies were not prospective with randomized assignment to different nutritional intakes, and it is likely that the patients' underlying illnesses contributed to both their high mortality and the low protein intake or serum albumin. Nonetheless, the data are consistent with the thesis that poor nutrient intake and malnutrition adversely affect prognosis in patients receiving maintenance hemodialysis or peritoneal dialysis.

DIETARY MANAGEMENT OF CHRONIC RENAL DISEASE AND CHRONIC RENAL FAILURE

A recommended plan for nutrient intake is given in Table 89.3 for patients with chronic renal failure who are not undergoing dialysis therapy as well as for patients undergoing maintenance hemodialysis or chronic peritoneal dialysis. This approach to dietary management of these patients is explained below.

General Principles of Dietary Therapy

The widespread metabolic and nutritional disorders, frequent occurrence of protein-energy malnutrition, and evidence that diet may retard the progression of renal failure indicate that nutritional management is critical to the treatment of chronic renal failure. The three goals of dietary therapy are *(a)* to maintain good nutritional status, *(b)* to prevent or to minimize uremic toxicity and the metabolic derangements of renal failure, and *(c)* to retard or to stop the rate of progression of renal failure.

Adherence to specialized diets is difficult and stressful for most patients and their families. Generally, patients must make a major change in their behavior patterns and forsake many of their traditional sources of daily pleasure. They must procure special foods, prepare special recipes, usually forgo or severely limit intake of many favorite foods, and often eat foods that are not desirable. Demands are made on the time, effort, and emotional support of family or close associates. Thus, it is incumbent on the physician not to prescribe radical changes in dietary intake without a clear indication that they may benefit the patient. To ensure successful dietary therapy, patients with renal failure must undergo extensive training in the principles of nutritional therapy and the design and preparation of diets and receive continuous encouragement regarding dietary adherence. They must receive repeated retraining with regard to their nutritional therapy. When nutritional intake is not carefully monitored, patients tend to adhere poorly to dietary prescriptions and may eat too little of certain nutrients rather than too much.

A team approach to dietary management may improve adherence to the special diet. The team should include the physician, dietitian, close family members, nursing staff, and (where available) psychiatrists or social workers. A problem-oriented approach to dietary compliance can be very effective (193). Diet plans should be tailored to the patient's tastes, and at each visit, the physician should monitor dietary intake and discuss the results with the patient.

The physician must strongly support the dietitian's efforts to train and counsel the patient and to obtain dietary compliance. Generally, the patient's spouse or other close relatives or friends should work closely with the patient to provide moral support and assist with acquisition and preparation of food. To promote adherence to the diet, the entire medical team should assume an energetic, positive, and sympathetic approach. Research indicates that these techniques enable many patients to attain acceptable dietary compliance (193).

Patients with advanced renal failure are at particular risk for inadequate energy intake. Because the prescribed diets are often marginally low in some nutrients (e.g., protein) and high in others (e.g., calcium) and malnutrition is frequent, the adequacy of the diet and the patient's nutritional status must be monitored periodically. Dietary intake should be assessed by interviews, dietary diaries, and measurement of UNA and nutritional status evaluated by anthropometry, biochemical measurements, bone radiography, and other parameters (194) (see Table 89.2). The dietitian is often best qualified to perform nutritional evaluation. In general, to maintain good dietary compliance and to monitor fluid and electrolyte disorders and clinical and nutritional status, patients with advanced renal failure should be seen monthly by the physician and the dietitian. Patients with slowly progressive mild-or-moderate renal insufficiency, under some circumstances may see the physician less frequently but may still need to see the dietitian monthly to promote adherence to the diet.

Evidence suggests that chronically uremic patients are at greatest risk for protein energy malnutrition when the GFR falls below 5 mL/min and when the patient is beginning maintenance dialysis therapy (158, 175, 195, 196). Moreover, the nutritional status of patients at the onset of chronic dialysis treatment appears to be a good predictor of nutritional status 1 to 2 years later (158, 197). Hence, particular effort should be made to prevent malnutrition as the patient approaches the time when dialysis should be instituted and during the first few weeks of chronic dialysis therapy. This effort should be directed toward maintaining good nutritional intake, rapidly instituting therapy

Table 89.3
Recommended Nutrient Intake for Nondialyzed Patients with Chronic Renal Failure and Patients Undergoing Maintenance Hemodialysis or Peritoneal Dialysis

	Chronic Renal Failure[a]	Maintenance Hemodialysis or Chronic Peritoneal Dialysis (CPD)[b]
Protein	Low-protein diet 0.55–0.60 g/kg/day ≥0.35 g/kg/day of high-biologic-value protein	Hemodialysis[b] 1.0–1.2 g/kg/day ≥50% high-biologic-value protein CPD 1.2–1.3 g/kg/day, ≥50% high-biologic-value protein; malnourished CPD patients may be given up to 1.5 g/kg/day
Energy[c]	≥35 kcal/kg/day unless the patient's relative body weight is >120% or the patient gains unwanted weight	
Fat (% of total energy intake)[d,e]	30–40	30–40
Polyunsaturated: saturated fatty acid ratio[g,e]	1.0:1.0	1.0:1.0
Carbohydrate[f]	Rest of nonprotein calories	
Total fiber intake[g,e]	20–25 g	20–25 g
Minerals	Range of intake	
Sodium	1000–3000 mg/day[g]	750–1000 mg/day[g]
Potassium	40–70 mEq/day	40–70 mEq/day
Phosphorus	5–10 mg/kg/day[h,i]	8–17 mg/kg/day[h]
Calcium	1400 to 1600 mg per day[i]	1400 to 1600 mg per day[i]
Magnesium	200 to 300 mg per day	200 to 300 mg per day
Iron	≥10 to 18 mg per day[j]	≥10 to 18 mg per day[j]
Zinc	15 mg per day	15 mg per day
Water	up to 3000 mL per day as tolerated[g]	usually 750–1500 mL/day[g]
Vitamins	Diets to be supplemented with these quantities	
Thiamin	1.5 mg/day	1.5 mg/day
Riboflavin	1.8 mg/day	1.8mg/day
Pantothenic acid	5 mg/day	5 mg/day
Niacin	20 mg/day	20 mg/day
Pyridoxine HCl	5 mg/day	5 mg/day
Vitamin B_{12}	3 μg/day	3 μg/day
Vitamin C	60 mg/day	60 mg/day
Folic acid	1 mg/day	1 mg/day
Vitamin A	No addition	No addition
Vitamin D	See text	See text
Vitamin E	15 IU/day	15 IU/day
Vitamin K	None[k]	None[k]

[a]GFR above 5–5 mL/1.73 m²/min and below about 70 mL/1.73 m² (see text).
[b]Protein intake for hemodialysis patients generally should be at or near 1.2 g/kg/day; for CPD patients who are not malnourished, it should be about 1.2–1.3 g/kg/day.
[c]This includes energy intake from dialysate in the CPD patients.
[d]Refers to percentage of total energy intake (diet plus dialysate); if triglyceride levels are markedly elevated, the percentage of fat in the diet may be increased to about 40% of total calories; otherwise, 30% of total calories is preferable. (These recommendations are based upon evidence indicating that triglyceride synthesis and serum triglyceride concentration may be stimulated by sugar intake [238, 239].)
[e]These dietary recommendations are considered less crucial than the others, unless hyperlipidemia is present (see text).
[f]Should be primarily complex carbohydrates, if tolerated by the patient.
[g]Can be higher in CPD patients or in nondialyzed patients with chronic renal failure and hemodialysis patients who have greater urinary losses.
[h]Phosphate binders (calcium carbonate, acetate, or citrate or aluminum carbonate or hydroxide) are often needed as well.
[i]Dietary intake usually must be supplemented to provide these levels.
[j]10 mg/day for males and nonmenstruating females; ≥18 mg/day serum for menstruating females.
[k]Vitamin K supplements may be needed for patients who are not eating and who are receiving antibiotics.

for supervening illnesses, and maintaining good nutritional intake during such illnesses.

Urea Nitrogen Appearance and the Serum Urea Nitrogen:Serum Creatinine Ratio

Control of protein intake is pivotal to nutritional management of patients with acute or chronic renal failure. Hence one must accurately monitor nitrogen intake. Fortunately, this is possible for most patients. Those who are in nitrogen balance should have a total nitrogen output equal to nitrogen intake minus about 0.5 g nitrogen per day for unmeasured losses from growth of skin, hair, and nails and from sweat, respiration, flatus, and blood drawing (198). For clinical purposes, a slightly positive or negative balance does not substantially alter the use of the nitrogen output to estimate intake. If patients are in very positive or negative balance (e.g., from pregnancy or severe infection), nitrogen output may not reflect intake. However, it is usually readily apparent to the clinician whether the patient is in very positive or negative balance and whether the nitrogen output will reflect intake.

Measurement of total nitrogen output is too laborious and expensive to be widely applied for clinical uses. However, because urea is the major nitrogenous product of protein and amino acid degradation, the UNA can be used to estimate total nitrogen output and hence nitrogen intake (199–201). UNA refers to the amount of urea that appears or accumulates in body fluids and all output, such as urine, dialysate, and fistula drainage. The term *urea nitrogen appearance* (UNA) is used rather than urea production or generation because some urea is degraded in the gastrointestinal tract; the ammonia released from urea is largely transported to the liver and converted back to urea (202, 203). Thus, the enterohepatic urea cycle has little effect on urea or total nitrogen economy, and this cycle can be ignored without compromising the ability of the UNA to estimate total nitrogen output or intake accurately. Moreover, urea recycling cannot be measured without costly and time-consuming isotope studies.

UNA is calculated as follows:

Equation 1:

$$\begin{aligned}\text{UNA} = {} & \text{urinary urea nitrogen} \\ & + \text{dialysate urea nitrogen} \\ & + \text{change in body urea nitrogen}\end{aligned}$$

where all values are in grams per day.

Equation 2:

$$\begin{aligned}&\text{Change in body urea nitrogen (g/day)} = \\ &\quad (\text{SUN}_f - \text{SUN}_i,\ \text{g/L/ day}) \times \text{BW}_i\ (\text{kg}) \times (0.60\ \text{L/kg}) \\ &\quad + (\text{BW}_f - \text{BW}_i,\ \text{kg/day}) \times \mathit{SUN}_f(\text{g/L}) \times (1.0\ \text{L/kg})\end{aligned}$$

where *i* and *f* are the initial and final values for the period of measurement, SUN is serum urea nitrogen (grams per liter), BW is body weight (kilograms), 0.60 is an estimate of the fraction of body weight that is water, and 1.0 is the fractional distribution of urea in the weight that is gained or lost (i.e., 100%).

The estimated proportion of body weight that is water may be higher in patients who are edematous or lean and lower in individuals who are obese or very young. Changes in body weight during the 1- to 3-day period of UNA measurement are assumed to be due entirely to changes in body water. In patients undergoing hemodialysis, the urea concentration in dialysate is low and difficult to measure accurately, and UNA can be calculated during the interdialytic interval and then normalized to 24 hours. Because many patients undergoing dialysis have little or no urinary excretion, the equation for calculating their UNA during the interdialytic interval often can be simplified to Equation 2.

In our metabolic studies, the relationship between UNA and total nitrogen appearance (output) in chronically uremic patients not undergoing dialysis is as follows (201):

Equation 3:

$$\text{Total nitrogen appearance} = 1.19\ \text{UNA} + 1.27$$

where all values are in grams per day. If the individual is more or less in neutral nitrogen balance, the UNA also correlates closely with nitrogen intake. Equation 4 describes our observed relationships between UNA and dietary nitrogen intake in clinically stable, nondialyzed, chronically uremic patients in neutral protein balance.

Equation 4:

$$\text{Dietary nitrogen intake} = 1.20\ \text{UNA} + 1.74$$

where all values are in grams per day. Multiplying Equation 3 by 6.25 converts total nitrogen output to net protein degradation (grams per day), that is, the difference between the absolute rates of protein degradation and protein synthesis in the study. Multiplying Equation 4 by 6.25 converts dietary nitrogen intake to dietary protein intake (grams per day). When both nitrogen intake and UNA are known, nitrogen balance can be estimated from the difference between nitrogen intake and nitrogen output estimated from the UNA.

If the patient is markedly anabolic (e.g., as in pregnancy, particularly in its later stages), Equation 4 will underestimate nitrogen intake. For patients who have large protein losses, such as from nephrotic syndrome or peritoneal dialysis, or who are acidemic and have sufficient kidney function to excrete large quantities of ammonia, equations 3 and 4 will underestimate both nitrogen output and nitrogen intake. In most circumstances, however, these conditions are not present, and the UNA provides a powerful tool for monitoring nitrogen output and intake or estimating balance. Maroni et al. and other researchers have described similar techniques for monitoring these parameters (199, 200).

The relationships between the UNA, total nitrogen output, and dietary nitrogen intake in patients undergoing continuous ambulatory peritoneal dialysis are shown in Equations 5 and 6 (201). Other researchers have described similar equations (204). Since protein losses in peritoneal dialysate are variable, some equations have an independent term for the daily protein losses in peritoneal dialysate. As indicated above, multiplying these terms by 6.25 converts the equations to net protein output (grams per day) or, in clinically stable patients who are in approximately neutral protein balance, to dietary protein intake (grams per day).

Equation 5:

$$\text{Total nitrogen output (g/day)} = 0.94\ \text{UNA} + 5.54$$

Equation 6:

$$\text{Dietary nitrogen intake (g/day)} = 0.97\ \text{UNA} + 6.80$$

The UNA (also called Gu) in hemodialysis patients can be calculated by urea kinetic modeling (199, 205). This technique essentially involves pre- and postdialysis SUNs and body weights, the urea clearance characteristics of the dialysis, and the blood flow, dialysate flow, and duration of dialysis therapy. The relationships between UNA, net protein degradation, and dietary nitrogen intake in maintenance hemodialysis patients have been described in other studies. A critique of the precision and reproducibility of these calculations is presented elsewhere (201, 205).

The SUN:serum creatinine ratio also correlates closely with dietary protein or amino acid intake in chronically uremic patients who are not undergoing dialysis treatment (206). This relationship can be used to estimate the recent daily intake of such patients. Although this ratio is not as precise as the UNA and is influenced by certain clinical factors, it is easy and inexpensive to measure.

Dietary Prescription

For purposes of nutritional prescription, the body weights in this chapter refer to the standard (normal) body weights from the NHANES data (207). An exception is individuals who are obese (e.g., more than 115% of standard body weight) or very underweight (e.g., less than 90% of standard body weight). For these patients, the adjusted actual body weight (aBW) may be used for the body weight term (207a). The adjusted aBW appears to be gaining in popularity but has not yet been validated by experimental data. The aBW, modified from the American Dietetic Association report (207a), is calculated as follows:

Adjusted aBW = standard (normal) BW
+ ([edema-free aBW − standard (normal) BW] × 0.25)

Protein, Amino Acid, and Ketoacid Intake

GFR above 70 mL/1.73 m²/min. Virtually no data exist concerning the optimal dietary protein and phosphorus intakes for patients with chronic renal disease and mildly impaired renal function. As more information becomes available, dietary guidelines doubtless will change. At present, we do not routinely restrict protein for patients with a GFR above 70 mL/1.73 m^2/min, except perhaps to 0.80 to 1.0 g/L/day, unless renal function is continuing to decline. In the latter case, the patient is treated as indicated in the next paragraph.

GFR of 25 to 70 mL/1.73 m²/min. The studies, including the metaanalyses (see above), indicating that low-protein, low-phosphorus diets may retard progression of renal failure are sufficiently convincing to warrant offering patients dietary therapy. Currently, our policy is to discuss with the patient the evidence that such diets retard progression and to indicate that the data justify restricting dietary protein. If the patient agrees to dietary therapy, a diet is offered providing 0.55 to 0.60 g protein/kg/day, of which at least 35 g/kg/day is high-biologic-value protein to ensure sufficient intake of the essential amino acids. This quantity of protein should maintain neutral or positive nitrogen balance, and for many patients, it should not be excessively burdensome.

GFR below 25 mL/1.73 m²/min without Dialysis. When GFR falls below 25 mL/1.73 m^2, the potential advantages of a low-protein, low-phosphorus diet become more compelling. First, at this degree of renal insufficiency, potentially toxic products of nitrogen metabolism begin to accumulate in larger quantities. The low-protein diet will generate fewer potentially toxic nitrogenous metabolites. Second, because the low-protein diet generally contains less phosphorus and potassium, intake of these minerals can be reduced more readily with this diet (see later sections on recommended phosphorus and potassium intakes). Third, some patients with chronic renal insufficiency eat too little protein rather than too much. Specific training and encouragement to follow a prescribed diet may increase the likelihood that the patient will not ingest too little protein. The dietary prescription should include 0.60 g of protein/kg/day with at least 0.35 g/kg/day of high-biologic-value protein (Table 89.3). This diet will generally maintain neutral or positive nitrogen balance as long as energy intake is not deficient and should generate a low UNA (200, 201, 208, 209). The protein content of this diet should be increased by 1.0 g of high-biologic-value protein daily for each gram of protein excreted in the urine each day.

Because of the lack of definitive evidence in large-scale clinical trials that the ketoacid–amino acid supplemented, very low protein diets retard progression of renal failure, these supplements are not currently available in the United States. Some researchers consider this unfortunate because smaller-scale studies suggest that these compounds are very effective in slowing progression (98, 210). There is insufficient research experience to evaluate the potential for essential amino acid–supplemented, very low protein diets to retard progression, and these diets are therefore not currently recommended for this purpose.

When the GFR falls below 5 mL/1.73 m^2/min, there is inconclusive evidence that patients fare as well with low-nitrogen diets as with regular dialysis and higher protein intake. Because patients with these low GFR levels may be at high risk for malnutrition (158, 175, 195), it is recommended that maintenance dialysis treatment or renal transplantation be inaugurated at this time.

Nephrotic Syndrome. Formerly, it was recommended that patients with the nephrotic syndrome be prescribed high-protein diets to prevent protein malnutrition (211). Current evidence that a high-protein intake may accelerate progression of renal failure has caused a rethinking of the dietary protein prescription for nephrotic patients. Moreover, low-protein diets (e.g., 0.80 g/kg/day) may decrease urinary protein excretion and may maintain or actually slightly increase serum albumin levels (123, 124, 212). A vegetarian, soy-based, low-protein diet may decrease proteinuria and serum lipid levels in nephrotic patients (108–110). Until more information is available, it is recommended that patients with the nephrotic syndrome be prescribed a diet containing about 0.70 g protein/kg/day and an additional 1.0 g/day of high-biologic-value protein for each gram of urinary protein lost each day above 5.0 g/day. The angiotensin-converting enzyme inhibitors may reduce proteinuria (122) and thus should be given preference in treating hypertension in these patients. Patients with the nephrotic syndrome should be given multivitamins, including vitamin D supplements, and must be monitored closely for depletion of protein and protein-bound nutrients, including vitamin D analogues and trace elements.

Maintenance Dialysis Therapy. Although few studies of dietary protein requirements have been conducted in patients undergoing maintenance hemodialysis (213–215), it seems clear that these patients have greater protein needs because of the removal of amino acids and peptides by dialysis procedures (181–183) and possibly because of other metabolic disorders that occur with end-stage renal disease, such as catabolic stimulus of hemodialysis (188, 188a, 214). On the basis of available evidence from nitrogen balance studies and clinical monitoring of outpatients, it is recommended that patients undergoing maintenance hemodialysis receive 1.0 to 1.2 g protein/kg/day (Table 89.3). Because many maintenance hemodialysis patients have evidence of protein malnutrition, a protein intake of 1.2 g/kg/day is preferable for most individuals. Patients undergoing chronic daily peritoneal dialysis (CPD) lose about 9 g of protein per day into dialysate as well as a small amount of peptides and about 2.5 to 4.0 g/day of amino acids (184, 185). Nitrogen balance studies suggest that CPD patients should, in general, be prescribed 1.2 to 1.3 g protein/kg/day (216). Protein-depleted patients undergoing CPD may be prescribed up to 1.5 g protein/kg/day (216).

At least 50% of the daily protein intake of all patients undergoing maintenance dialysis should be of high biologic value. Some physicians suggest that maintenance hemodialysis or CPD patients may maintain their body protein mass with lower dietary protein intake (e.g., about 0.9 g/kg/day). The above recommendations, although based upon relatively small numbers of studies, are designed to maintain good protein nutrition for the great majority of maintenance dialysis patients. Hence, although some patients may maintain good protein nutrition with lower daily protein intake, there is no demonstrated method for identifying these individuals. Because there is a high incidence of protein malnutrition in these patients (154–163, 166, 191, 192), we suggest that the higher protein intakes recommended in this chapter should be prescribed.

Energy

Studies in nondialyzed chronically uremic patients and in those undergoing maintenance hemodialysis indicate that energy expenditure is normal or nearly normal when patients are lying in bed or sitting, following ingestion of a standard meal, and during defined exercise (217–220). Nitrogen balance studies in nondialyzed chronically uremic patients ingesting diets providing 0.55 to 0.60 g protein/kg/day and 15, 25, 35, or 45 kcal/kg/day indicate that the energy intake necessary to ensure neutral or positive nitrogen balance is approximately 35 kcal/kg/ (217). Similar findings were obtained in nitrogen balance studies of maintenance hemodialysis patients who were ingesting 1.1 g protein/kg/day and 25, 35, or 45 kcal/kg/day (221). However, virtually every survey of energy intake in nondialyzed chronically uremic patients and in patients undergoing maintenance hemodialysis or CPD indicates that on average, the dietary intake is below this level and usually substantially below 30 kcal/kg/day (157, 177, 222–224). In nondialyzed patients with advanced renal failure and in patients undergoing hemodialysis, decreased body fat is one of the more prominent alterations in nutritional status, which supports the contention that these patients require more energy than they usually ingest (157, 160, 163, 224). In contrast, CPD patients not uncommonly gain fat, probably because of additional energy intake from peritoneal absorption of glucose from dialysate.

We currently recommend that nondialyzed chronically uremic patients and patients undergoing maintenance hemodialysis or CPD ingest at least 35 kcal/kg/day. Obese patients with an edema-free body weight more than 120% of desirable body weight may be treated with lower calorie intakes. Some patients, particularly those with mild renal insufficiency and young or middle-aged women, may become obese on this energy intake or may refuse to ingest the recommended calories out of fear of obesity. These individuals may require a lower energy prescription.

Many commercially available high-calorie foodstuffs are low in protein, phosphorus, sodium, and potassium. A nephrology dietitian can recommend these foodstuffs as well as other low-protein, high-calorie foods that can be prepared easily at home.

Lipids and Obesity

Nondialyzed chronically uremic patients and patients undergoing maintenance hemodialysis and CPD have a high incidence of type IV hyperlipoproteinemia with increased serum triglyceride levels, elevated serum LDL and very LDL (VLDL) levels, and a low serum high-density-lipoprotein (HDL) cholesterol level (150, 225–229). Serum lipoprotein (a) [Lp(a)] is frequently elevated (228, 229), and serum VLDL cholesterol and total cholesterol may also be increased in CPD patients. In chronic renal failure, a number of serum apolipoproteins and apolipoprotein fragments are increased and the composition of apolipoproteins may be altered (229).

One cause of hypertriglyceridemia is impaired clearance of triglyceride-rich LDL and VLDL from blood. In addition, because diets for patients with renal failure are usually restricted in protein, sodium, potassium, and water, it may be difficult to provide sufficient energy without resorting to a large intake of purified sugars, which may increase triglyceride production. Activities of plasma and hepatic lipoprotein lipase and lecithin cholesterol acyltransferase (LCAT) are decreased (230). Moreover, carnitine actions may sometimes be impaired (231, 232).

Patients with the nephrotic syndrome have hypercholesterolemia. Elevated serum cholesterol is caused by increased hepatic synthesis of lipoproteins and cholesterol and reduced LDL-receptor activity, which plays an important role in clearance of intermediate-density lipoproteins (IDL). These changes are stimulated by hypoalbuminemia. Decreased activity of lipoprotein lipase contributes to the elevated serum triglyceride levels. Serum triglycerides, phospholipids, and apoproteins B, C-II, C-III, and E are increased, whereas apoproteins A-I and A-II are normal (233). Plasma lipoprotein(a) [Lp(2)] is elevated (234). Both serum LDL and VLDL may be increased. There is elevated plasma cholesterol ester transfer protein (CETP) and decreased catabolism of LDL apolipoprotein, at least by the more typical receptor pathway.

Renal transplant recipients may have type IIb hyperlipidemia with high serum total cholesterol. Types II-a and IV hyperlipidemia also often occur after kidney transplantation, particularly if renal failure persists (235–237). Medicinal therapy (glucocorticoids, cyclosporine A, diuretics, antihypertensives), renal failure, fasting hyperinsulinemia, and obesity, which occurs frequently after renal transplantation, all may add to the high incidence of serum lipid disorders in renal transplant patients. Because these abnormalities may contribute to the high incidence of atherosclerosis and cardiovascular disease in patients with chronic renal failure, those undergoing maintenance dialysis, and those receiving renal transplants, attention has been directed toward reducing serum cholesterol and triglycerides and increasing HDL cholesterol.

Serum triglycerides may be lowered by a diet in which the carbohydrate content is reduced to about 35% of total calories, the fat content is increased to about 55% of total calories, and the polyunsaturated:saturated fatty acid ratio is raised to about 1.5:1.0 (Table 89.3) (238, 239). However, evidence suggesting that high cholesterol and fat intakes increase the risk of atherosclerotic vascular disease argues against using such diets, particularly because hypertriglyceridemia is not a strong risk factor for atherosclerotic vascular disease. Several investigators have reported that serum triglycerides may be decreased if dialysis patients take L-carnitine, which is often low in their plasma and possibly muscle (see below) (231, 232); other investigators have not confirmed this effect (240, 241). Fibric acids (e.g., gemfibrozil) also lower serum triglyceride levels in uremic patients, but owing to the altered pharmacokinetics of this drug in renal failure, the risk of developing myopathy or other toxicities is high (242). ω-3 Fatty acids, such as eicosapentanoic acid and docosahexanoic acid, which are found in fish oil, lower serum triglyceride and total cholesterol levels as well as phospholipids and may be tried (243). Fish oil also decreases platelet aggregation and exerts antiinflammatory effects (243). Some evidence suggests that ω-3 fatty acids or fish oil may retard progression of chronic renal failure, particularly when it is caused by IgA nephropathy (244). Ingestion of activated charcoal may lower serum cholesterol and triglycerides in chronically uremic rats (245).

At present, we recommend a dietary plan based upon the National Cholesterol Education Program (NCEP) for patients with chronic renal failure, patients with the nephrotic syndrome, and renal transplant recipients (see Chapter 75). This diet provides (246) no more than 30% of total calories from fat: up to 10% of total calories from polyunsaturated fatty acids, 10–15% of calories from monounsaturated fatty acids, less than 10% of calories from unsaturated fatty acids, and a cholesterol content of 300 mg/day or less. We treat hypertriglyceridemia by dietary modification when serum triglyceride levels are approximately 400 mg/dL or above. Dietary fat intake is not increased above 40% of total calories and as much as possible of the carbohydrate should be complex carbohydrates. The patient's energy intake should be monitored with this diet to ensure that it does not fall.

If serum triglyceride levels are substantially elevated, serum carnitine should be measured. If serum carnitine is low, 0.5 to 1.0 g/day orally may be given to nondialyzed patients with chronic renal failure and to patients undergoing maintenance dialysis. Alternatively, patients undergoing hemodialysis may be given L-carnitine, 1.5 g orally or intravenously, at the end of each dialysis. Fish oil supplements may be tried for severe hypertriglyceridemia (247). Hypercholesterolemia is most effectively treated by giving hydroxymethylglutaryl coenzyme A (HMG-CoA) reductase inhibitors (248) (see Chapter 75).

No established treatment exists for low serum concentrations of HDL in uremic patients, although a small amount of alcohol (e.g., one glass of red wine per day) and exercise may increase levels (249). As indicated above, while hemodialysis patients rarely gain substantial amounts of body fat, patients undergoing CPD commonly gain excessive body fat, probably because of the additional 400 to 700 kcal they receive from glucose absorbed from dialysate.

There are virtually no long-term data on the effects of dietary fat and carbohydrate intake, obesity, or changing serum lipid levels on the clinical course of patients with specific renal diseases, the nephrotic syndrome, renal failure, or renal transplantation. The recommendations given here are largely derived from data obtained from populations without renal disease, recognizing that patients with renal disease or renal failure have a high incidence of abnormal serum lipid and lipoprotein levels and atherosclerotic vascular disease, and from studies in animals with renal disease that indicate that high lipid intake or elevated lipoprotein levels may accelerate progression of renal failure, as discussed above.

Carnitine

Carnitine is an essential nutrient that is both synthesized in the body and ingested. Carnitine facilitates transfer of long-chain (>10 carbon) fatty acids into mitochondria and probably other cellular structures (250). Since fatty acids are the major fuel source for skeletal and myocardial muscle at rest and during mild-to-moderate exercise, this process is considered necessary for normal skeletal muscle and myocardial function. (See Chapter 31.)

Patients with chronic renal failure have low free carnitine and increased acylcarnitines (fatty acid/carnitine compounds) in serum (240, 241). In skeletal muscle, some but not all studies describe low free carnitine and increased acylcarnitines (251, 252). As a result of these observations, it was postulated that patients with chronic renal failure had carnitine deficiency, presumably caused by decreased synthesis and intake and increased losses from dialysis (240, 241). More recently, it has been suggested that carnitine actions may be impaired in chronic renal failure, possibly because of interference by the increased concentration of acylcarnitines.

Clinical studies in patients with chronic renal failure suggest that carnitine may improve physical exercise capacity, reduce dialysis-related symptoms of skeletal muscle cramps and hypotension, improve overall sense of well-being, increase blood hemoglobin levels, reduce cardiac arrhythmias, and improve cardiac function (253–257). Some studies indicate that carnitine will lower serum triglyceride levels; other studies have not confirmed this (240, 241). Many nephrologists are unconvinced by this research, in part because of the suboptimal experimental design of many of these studies and also because many of the reported benefits are not easy to quantify. New clinical trials of carnitine therapy should help determine more definitively the therapeutic potential of carnitine for patients with chronic renal failure. L-Carnitine appears to be a safe drug.

Until more-definitive information is available, we consider using L-carnitine for patients who satisfy both of the following criteria: *(a)* disabling or very bothersome skeletal muscle weakness or cardiomyopathy, skeletal muscle cramps or hypotension during hemodialysis treatment, severe malaise, or anemia refractory to erythropoietin therapy for no apparent reason and *(b)* these disorders do not respond to standard treatments. The patient is given a 3- to 6-month trial of L-carnitine (9 months for refractory anemia). If the symptoms do not improve by the end of the treatment period, carnitine therapy is discontinued. L-Carnitine may be administered orally, intravenously, or in dialysate. Oral L-carnitine is less expensive, but intestinal absorption is somewhat unpredictable in nonuremic individuals and has not been examined well in patients with chronic renal failure. The optimal dose of carnitine is not defined. Carnitine may be infused intravenously, 10 to 20 mg/kg, at the end of each hemodialysis, three times weekly, or given orally, about 0.50 g/day (253, 256).

Carbohydrates

The patient should be encouraged to eat complex rather than purified carbohydrates to reduce triglyceride synthesis and (where pertinent) to improve glucose tolerance.

Fiber

Studies in the normal population suggest that high dietary fiber intake may reduce the incidence of constipation, irritable bowel syndrome, diverticulitis, and neoplasia of the colon (258). Fiber may improve glucose tolerance in diabetic patients including those with chronic renal failure (259). Soluble fiber, which is soluble in the intestinal lumen but is not absorbed, includes pectins, certain gums, and psyllium. Supplemental soluble dietary fiber may also reduce plasma total cholesterol and LDL cholesterol levels in hypercholesterolemic men (260) and may decrease serum fasting triglyceride levels in hypertriglyceridemic patients with diabetes mellitus (261). A high dietary fiber intake also may reduce the SUN by decreasing colonic bacterial ammonia generation and enhancing fecal nitrogen excretion (262). High-fiber intake may promote fecal losses of trace elements. Foods high in fiber are often high in potassium, phosphorus, and low-quality protein. Thus, caution must be exercised when prescribing high-fiber diets to patients with renal failure. Because patients with renal failure may benefit from fiber intake, we currently encourage them to eat 20 to 25 g of total fiber daily.

Phosphorus

In patients with chronic renal failure, a high dietary phosphorus intake can lead to a high plasma phosphorus and calcium phosphorus product, with increased risk of calcium phosphate deposition in soft tissues (127). Moreover, hyperphosphatemia, by lowering serum calcium levels, provides a strong stimulus to development of hyperparathyroidism. As discussed above, both animal and human studies suggest that low phosphorus intake may reduce progression of chronic renal failure (45, 67, 69).

The optimal dietary phosphorus intake for patients with renal insufficiency has not been established. For the nondialyzed patient, one approach is to attempt to maintain normal renal tubular reabsorption of phosphorus to prevent elevated serum parathyroid hormone levels. This approach would require an extremely low phosphorus intake, lower than can usually be obtained with the combination of a low-phosphorus diet and phosphate binders, unless ketoacid- or essential amino acid–supplemented very low protein diets are used and the GFR is above 15 mL/min (Table 89.3). At least, in both nondialyzed and dialyzed patients, the morning fasting serum phosphorus concentrations should always be maintained at normal or possibly slightly elevated levels (e.g., about 5.0 mg/dL). Because a rough correlation exists between the protein and phosphorus content of the diet, it is easier to restrict phosphorus if protein intake is reduced.

For nondialyzed patients with a GFR below 25 mL/1.73 m^2/min who are prescribed 0.55 to 0.60 g/day of protein, phosphorus intake generally is decreased to about 5 to 10 mg/kg/day. This may make the diet more burdensome, particularly at lower phosphorus intakes. This level of dietary phosphorus restriction usually does not maintain serum phosphorus levels within normal limits in patients with a GFR below about 15 mL/min, even with reduced renal tubular reabsorption of phosphorus. Hence phosphate binders are also used. Traditionally, the two most commonly used phosphate binders have been aluminum carbonate and aluminum hydroxide. Usually, two to four 500-mg capsules taken three to four times daily are needed. Higher doses may be used if necessary. Evidence that aluminum-induced osteomalacia, anemia, and possibly dementia could result from intake of aluminum phosphate binders has made many nephrologists reluctant to use them (262a, 263).

Several alkaline calcium salts are often used to bind phosphate: calcium carbonate, calcium acetate, and calcium citrate. Calcium acetate may be slightly more potent than calcium carbonate at binding phosphate in the intestinal tract, whereas calcium citrate appears to be the least effective binder (264–267). Calcium acetate may be more likely to induce gastrointestinal discomfort (267). Patients should not ingest calcium citrate if they are also taking aluminum, because the citrate anion may complex with aluminum and enhance its intestinal absorption (264). The calcium salts are taken in divided doses with meals and should not be given unless the serum phosphorus level is normal or nearly normal, to avoid precipitation of calcium phosphate in soft tissues. Thus, hyperphosphatemic patients may be treated with an aluminum binder of phosphate until serum phosphorus falls to normal and then be placed on calcium carbonate or calcium acetate. Concern exists that calcium binder doses providing more than about 2.0 g of elemental calcium daily may cause excessive accumulation of calcium in soft tissues.

For patients with a GFR between 25 and 70 mL/1.73 m^2/min or with a higher GFR and progressive loss of renal function, 7 to 12 mg of phosphorus/kg/day may be prescribed with the 0.55 to 0.60 g of protein/kg/day diet. Even this level of reduction in phosphorus intake is difficult for many patients to accept, and lower phosphorus intakes make the diet too restrictive for virtually all patients. These individuals generally are not given phosphate binders unless serum phosphorus levels are above normal. The recommended phosphorus intake for patients undergoing maintenance hemodialysis or CPD is about 17 mg/kg/day or less. This higher upper limit was chosen because dialysis patients, with their greater protein intakes, cannot readily ingest less phosphorus without making the diet too restrictive. Patients undergoing maintenance dialysis usually require phosphate binders as well as this dietary phosphorus restriction to prevent hyperphosphatemia.

At present, no lower safe limit for the serum phosphorus level in renal failure has been defined. Experience suggests that if fasting serum phosphorus is maintained above the lower limit of normal, patients will not develop manifestations of phosphate depletion. More work is necessary to test the validity of this perception.

Calcium

Patients with chronic renal failure, including those undergoing maintenance dialysis therapy, usually have an increased dietary calcium requirement because they have both vitamin D deficiency and resistance to the actions of vitamin D. These disorders, which lead to impaired intestinal calcium absorption, are compounded by the low calcium content of diets for uremic patients. A 40-g protein, low-phosphorus diet, for example, generally provides only about 300 to 400 mg of calcium daily. Dietary calcium intake is low because many foods high in calcium are high in phosphorus (e.g., dairy products) and are thus restricted for uremic patients.

Nondialyzed chronically uremic patients usually require 1200 to 1600 mg of calcium daily for neutral or positive calcium balance (268). The current recommendation is to provide a total daily calcium intake (diet plus supplement) of 1400 to 1600 mg. Thus, low-protein diets need to be supplemented with 1000 to 1400 mg of elemental calcium daily. Supplemental calcium should not be given unless the serum phosphorus concentration is normal or only slightly elevated (e.g., 2.5 to about 5.5 mg/dL), to prevent calcium phosphate deposition in soft tissues. In addition, frequent monitoring of serum calcium is important because hypercalcemia may develop, particularly if serum phosphorus should fall to low-normal or low levels. This is especially likely to occur if the patient also has hyperparathyroidism, a common complication of chronic renal failure (127). Patients undergoing maintenance hemodialysis or peritoneal dialysis may require 1.0 g/day of supplemental oral calcium even though there is net calcium uptake from dialysate. The supplemental calcium should be taken in two or three divided doses each day.

Calcium comprises 40% of calcium carbonate, 25% of calcium acetate, 21% of calcium citrate, and 9% of calcium gluconate. Treatment with vitamin D analogues may decrease the daily calcium requirement by enhancing intestinal calcium absorption. To reduce the total daily calcium load to the dialysis patient who is taking calcium binders of phosphate, the calcium content of dialysate is often reduced. Currently, this is easier to arrange with chronic peritoneal dialysis than with maintenance hemodialysis.

As indicated above, the use of calcium binders of phosphate often results in a daily calcium intake that exceeds these levels. It is not known whether these large intakes of calcium cause hazardous calcium deposits in skeletal or soft tissues. A syndrome called aplastic or hypoplastic bone disease has been described in chronic dialysis patients (127, 269–271). It is characterized by relatively low serum parathyroid hormone concentrations, decreased bone osteoblasts, and marked reduction in bone turnover. The syndrome can be caused by aluminum toxicity but also occurs in the absence of such toxicity (127, 269, 270). Treatment with large doses of calcium binders of phosphate with consequent suppression of parathyroid hormone has been postulated to cause this disorder (127, 269, 271).

Magnesium

In chronic renal failure, there is net absorption of approximately 50% of ingested magnesium from the intestinal tract (net absorption is the difference between dietary intake and fecal excretion) (268). The absorbed magnesium is excreted primarily by the kidney. Hence, in renal failure, hypermagnesemia may occur (272). Because the restricted diets of uremic patients are low in magnesium (usually about 100 to 300 mg/day for a 40-g protein diet), their serum magnesium levels are usually normal or only slightly elevated unless the patient ingests substances with high magnesium content, such as magnesium-containing antacids and laxatives (268, 272). Nondialyzed chronically uremic patients require about 200 mg/day of magnesium to maintain neutral balance (268). The optimal dietary magnesium allowance for the chronic dialysis patient is not well defined and is influenced by the level of magnesium in the dialysate; at current dialysate magnesium concentrations, the optimal magnesium allowance is probably about 200–250 mg/day.

Sodium and Water

Sodium is freely filterable by the glomerulus. In the normal kidney, the renal tubules reabsorb well over 99% of the filtered sodium. As renal insufficiency progresses, both glomerular filtration and fractional reabsorption of sodium fall progressively. Thus, many patients with renal failure can maintain sodium balance with a normal salt intake. Normally, only about 1 to 3 meq/day of sodium are excreted in the feces, and in the nonsweating individual, only a few milliequivalents of sodium are lost daily through the skin. Despite an adaptive reduction in renal tubular reabsorption of sodium when end-stage renal disease supervenes, patients may be unable to excrete the quantity of sodium ingested, and they may develop edema, hypertension, or congestive heart failure. This syndrome is particularly likely to occur when the GFR is below 4 to 10 mL/min. When renal insufficiency is complicated by congestive heart failure, the nephrotic syndrome, or advanced liver disease, the propensity for sodium retention is increased. With decreased ability to excrete sodium, restriction of sodium and water intake and the use of diuretic medications may be necessary. In renal failure, hypertension often is more easily controlled with sodium restriction and may be accentuated with increased sodium intake, possibly because of expansion of the extracellular fluid volume (273).

In addition, nondialyzed patients with chronic renal failure are often unable to conserve sodium normally (126, 126a). A low sodium intake may not be sufficient to replace urinary and extrarenal sodium losses, and the patient may develop sodium depletion, decreased extracellular fluid volume, blood volume, and renal blood flow, and a further reduction in GFR. Volume depletion may be difficult to recognize. An unexplained weight loss or decrease in blood pressure may signal this condition. Nondialyzed patients with chronic renal failure who do not have evidence for fluid overload, hypertension, or heart failure may be cautiously given a greater sodium intake to determine whether their GFR can be improved slightly by extracellular volume expansion.

In general, when sodium balance is well controlled, thirst will regulate water balance adequately. However, when the GFR falls below 2 to 5 mL/min, there is a particular risk of overhydration. In diabetics, hyperglycemia may also increase thirst and enhance positive water balance. For patients with far-advanced renal failure whose total body water is at the desired level (as indicated by normal or near-normal blood pressure, absence of edema, and normal serum sodium), urine volume may be a good guide to water intake. The daily water intake should equal the urine output plus approximately 500 mL to replace insensible losses.

In most nondialyzed patients with advanced renal failure, a daily intake of 1000 to 3000 mg (40–130 meq) of sodium and 1500 to 3000 mL of fluid will maintain sodium and water balance. The requirement for sodium and water varies markedly, and each patient must be managed individually. Patients undergoing maintenance hemodialysis or peritoneal dialysis usually become oliguric or anuric after several weeks to 1 or 2 years of treatment. For hemodialysis patients, sodium and total fluid intake generally should be restricted to 1000 to 1500 mg/day and 700 to 1500 mL/day, respectively. Patients undergoing CPD usually tolerate a greater sodium and water intake because salt and water can be easily removed each day by using hypertonic dialysate, which increases the flow of water from the body into the peritoneal cavity where it can be drained. Maintaining a large dietary sodium and water intake allows the quantity of fluid removed from the CPD patient and, hence, the daily dialysate volume to be increased. This increase may be advantageous because the daily clearance of small molecules with CPD is directly related to the volume of dialysate outflow. In nondialyzed chronically uremic patients or in those undergoing maintenance dialysis who are not anuric and who gain excessive sodium or water despite attempts at dietary restriction, a potent loop diuretic, such as furosemide or bumetanide, may be tried to increase urinary sodium and water excretion.

Potassium

Normally, the kidney provides the major route for potassium excretion. In renal failure, potassium retention may occur and may lead quickly to fatal hyperkalemia. Two factors act to mitigate this process in renal failure. First, as long as urine output remains at approximately 1000 mL/day or above, tubular secretion of potassium in the remaining functioning nephrons tends to be increased, and thus renal potassium clearance does not fall as markedly as the GFR. Second, fecal excretion of potassium is increased owing to enhanced intestinal secretion (208). Thus, patients with chronic renal failure usually do not become hyperkalemic unless there is *(a)* excessive intake of potassium; *(b)* acidosis, oliguria, or hypoaldosteronism (e.g., secondary to decreased renin secretion by the diseased kidney or renal tubular resistance to the actions of aldosterone); or *(c)* catabolic stress. Patients with chronic renal failure and those undergoing maintenance hemodialysis, in general, should receive no more than 70 meq of potassium daily. Some patients, particularly those with less-advanced chronic renal failure, may tolerate higher potassium intakes; they may be identified by liberalizing their dietary potassium and carefully monitoring serum potassium levels.

Trace Elements

Several factors tend to either increase or decrease the body burden of certain trace elements in renal failure patients (274–276). Many trace elements are excreted primarily in the urine and may accumulate with renal failure (275, 277). Elements such as iron, zinc, and copper, which are protein bound, may be lost in excessive quantities when there are large urinary protein losses, as in the nephrotic syndrome (277). The effect of the altered dietary intake of the uremic patient on body pools of trace elements is unknown (276). Since many trace elements bind avidly to serum proteins, when present even in small quantities in dialysate, they may be taken up into blood and cause toxicity. Therefore, dialysate should be routinely purified of trace elements prior to use. In certain circumstances, therapeutic doses of trace elements might be administered through dialysis, as has been done for zinc (278). Assessing the trace element pools in renal failure patients is difficult because the serum binding-protein concentrations or affinities for trace elements may be altered, and red cell levels of trace elements may not reflect concentrations in other tissues.

Dietary requirements for trace elements have not been well defined in uremic patients (Table 89.3). Trace element supplementation should be undertaken cautiously, because impaired urinary excretion of trace elements increases the risk of overdosage. Oral iron supplements are often given to patients who are iron deficient or patients who have a propensity to develop iron deficiency (e.g., individuals who frequently have marginal or low serum iron, reduced percentage saturation of the iron-binding capacity, or decreased ferritin levels). Iron requirements increase when erythropoietin therapy is started and hemoglobin synthesis rises. Ferrous sulfate, 300 mg up to three times per day, one-half hour after meals, may be used. Some patients develop anorexia, nausea, constipation, or abdominal pain with ferrous sulfate and may tolerate other iron compounds better, such as ferrous fumarate, gluconate, or lactate. Patients who are intolerant of oral iron supplements or who have iron deficiency that does not respond to oral iron therapy may be treated with intramuscular or intravenous iron. Recent data indicate that higher serum iron concentrations may reduce the dose of erythropoietin necessary to maintain a given blood hemoglobin level.

The zinc content of most tissues is normal in renal failure (276), although serum and hair zinc may be low and red cell zinc is increased (275, 278–280). In nondialyzed chronically uremic patients, the fractional urinary excretion of zinc is increased; however, since the GFR is reduced, total urinary excretion of zinc may be normal or reduced (274). Fecal zinc is increased (279), and a dietary zinc intake above the RDA (117) may be necessary to maintain normal body zinc pools. Further studies are needed to confirm this. Some reports indicate that dysgeusia, poor food intake, and impaired sexual function, which are common problems of uremic patients, may be improved by giving patients zinc supplements (278, 279, 281, 282); however, other studies have not confirmed this (283).

As indicated above, in nondialyzed chronically uremic patients and in those receiving maintenance dialysis, an increased body burden of aluminum has been implicated as a cause of a progressive dementia syndrome (particularly in hemodialysis patients), osteomalacia, weakness of the muscles of the proximal limbs, and anemia (127, 262a, 263, 269, 270). Although contamination of dialysate with aluminum previously was the major source of aluminum toxicity in many dialysis centers, current methods of water treatment have removed virtually all aluminum from dialysate. At present, ingestion of aluminum binders of phosphate is probably the major cause of the excess body burden of aluminum (262a, 263). Consequently, many nephrologists now use aluminum binders more sparingly and rely more upon low-phosphorus diets and nonaluminum phosphate binders, particularly calcium carbonate or acetate, to control serum phosphorus levels (264–267). Aluminum toxicity may be treated by reducing aluminum intake and by intravenous infusions of desferrioxamine, a chelator of aluminum (284). This chelator can be removed from the body by hemodialysis or peritoneal dialysis. Since desferrioxamine may predispose to serious infections, nephrologists tend to use this medicine infrequently.

Vitamins

Chronically uremic patients are prone to deficiencies of water-soluble vitamins unless supplements are given (129). Vitamin deficiencies occur for the following reasons. First, vitamin intake is often low because of anorexia and poor food intake and also because many foods that are high in water-soluble vitamins are often restricted owing to the elevated potassium content. The typical diet for nondialyzed chronic renal failure and maintenance dialysis patients is frequently below the RDAs for certain water-soluble vitamins (117). Second, the metabolism of certain water-soluble vitamins tends to be altered in chronic renal failure (285, 286). Third, many medicines interfere with intestinal absorption, metabolism, or actions of vitamins (165, 187). Vitamin B_6, vitamin C, and folic acid are the water-soluble vitamins most likely to be deficient in nondialyzed patients with chronic renal failure and in maintenance dialysis patients. Vitamin B_{12} deficiency is uncommon in uremia because the daily requirement is small (2 μg/day for normal nonpregnant, nonlactating adults) (117), the body can store relatively large quantities of this vitamin, and vitamin B_{12} is protein bound in plasma and, hence, is poorly dialyzed.

Many of the studies that indicated a need for routine multivitamin supplementation in nondialyzed patients with chronic renal failure or those undergoing maintenance dialysis were carried out in the 1960s and early 1970s, when the incidence of poor nutritional intake of these patients may have been greater than it is today (288). Indeed, some more-recent studies suggest that many maintenance hemodialysis patients may subsist for months with no vitamin supplementation without developing deficiencies of water-soluble vitamins (289). However, these studies have not demonstrated that without vitamin supplements, a small but substantial proportion of patients will not develop water-soluble vitamin deficiencies, particularly after one or more years of dialysis treatment. Because water-soluble vitamin deficiencies are caused by several different mechanisms in these patients and because the water-soluble vitamin supplements are safe, it would seem prudent to continue to use them routinely until these issues are more completely resolved.

Daily supplements for most vitamins are not well defined in renal failure (129). Evidence indicates that in addition to vitamin intake from foods, the following daily supplements of vitamins will prevent or correct vitamin deficiency (Table 89.3): pyridoxine hydrochloride, 5 mg in nondialyzed patients and 10 mg in maintenance hemodialysis or peritoneal dialysis patients (290); folic acid, 1 mg; and the RDA for normal individuals for the other water-soluble vitamins (117). Patients with renal failure probably require less than 1.0 mg of folic acid daily; however, since this vitamin is safe and some evidence suggests that there may be competitive interference with its actions (285, 288), it may be advisable to prescribe this dose of folic acid until more definitive studies of the requirements are carried out. A supplement of only 60 mg/day of vitamin C is advised because ascorbic acid can be metabolized to oxalate. Large doses of ascorbic acid have been associated with increased plasma oxalate levels in renal failure patients (291, 292). Oxalate is highly insoluble, and there is concern that high plasma oxalate concentrations may lead to precipitation in soft tissues. Moreover, in the nondialyzed patient with chronic renal insufficiency, oxalate deposition in the kidney might further impair renal function.

Because serum retinol-binding protein and vitamin A are elevated in uremia (293), routine use of supplemental vitamin A is not recommended, particularly since even relatively small doses of vitamin A (i.e., 7500–15000 IU/day) may cause bone toxicity (294). Additional vitamin E and K are probably not necessary. However, patients who receive antibiotics for extended periods and who do not ingest foods containing vitamin K may need vitamin K supplements (295).

Although in renal failure many of the beneficial effects of 1,25-dihydroxycholecalciferol can be reproduced by administration of other vitamin D analogues such as dihydrotachysterol, cholecalciferol, or 25-hydroxycholecalciferol, 1,25-dihydroxycholecalciferol is the most potent agent (127). Because it is given in smaller doses and has a shorter half-life, there is little storage of this compound. Hence, it may be a safer agent to use. The high potency of 1,25-dihydroxycholecalciferol, however, increases the risk of hypercalcemia and hyperphosphatemia (127).

Treatment with oral 1,25-dihydroxycholecalciferol increases intestinal calcium and phosphorus absorption, raises serum calcium, lowers serum parathyroid hormone, decreases serum alkaline phosphatase activity, reduces bone resorption, decreases endosteal fibrosis, and often improves osteomalacia (127). Therapy with 1,25-dihydroxycholecalciferol or other active vitamin D analogues is indicated for hyperparathyroidism, osteitis fibrosa, mixed osteomalacia, and severe hypocalcemia. Some chronically uremic patients with vitamin D deficiency develop a myopathy, primarily of the proximal limb muscles, and may present with severe weakness. Strength may improve with vitamin D therapy. 1,25-Dihydroxycholecalciferol has many immunologic effects in vitro (296, 296a); whether treatment of patients with renal failure with this substance improves their immune function is not known. Uremic children require vitamin D analogues to promote growth.

It has been argued that because of the high incidence of vitamin D deficiency in patients with advanced chronic renal failure and patients undergoing maintenance hemodialysis and the pervasive benefits of vitamin D, 1,25-dihydroxycholecalciferol or other active vitamin D analogues should be used rather routinely in these patients unless there are specific contraindications to its use (e.g., hypercalcemia, severe hyperphosphatemia).

Treatment with 1,25-dihydroxycholecalciferol usually is started at 0.25 to 0.50 μg/day. The serum calcium concentration must be monitored carefully, and if it is low and does not rise by more than 0.5 mg/dL with any particular dosage, the dose may be increased by 0.25 to 0.50 μg/day every 4 to 6 weeks. Hypercalcemia is treated by temporary withdrawal of 1,25-dihydroxycholecalciferol. Ultimately, the best criterion for effective treatment with 1,25-dihydroxycholecalciferol is improved bone anatomy as determined by bone histology, radiographs, and densitometry. Improved muscle function or abolition of severe hypocalcemia also may indicate appropriate dosage of 1,25-dihydroxycholecalciferol. With time, the requirement for 1,25-dihydroxycholecalciferol and tolerance for this vitamin may decrease, and the maintenance dosage may have to be reduced. This change may occur after there has been sufficient bone healing so that the skeleton no longer serves as a sink for calcium and phosphorus. 1,25-Dihydroxycholecalciferol should not be started unless serum calcium is not elevated, serum phosphorus is not more than slightly increased, and the calcium-phosphorus product is below 45. Serum calcium and phosphorus should be monitored during therapy to ensure that the concentrations are normal.

In patients receiving maintenance hemodialysis or CPD, intravenous or oral boluses of 1,25-dihydroxycholecalciferol, given about 3 times weekly, are more effective than routine daily doses of the oral preparation in suppressing secretion and serum levels of parathyroid hormone and ameliorating osteitis fibrosa (297, 298). Intravenous or oral 1,25-dihydroxycholecalciferol boluses may exert a greater effect because less of the dose may be taken up by the small intestine, where it promotes calcium absorption and hypercalcemia. Thus, greater amounts of 1,25-dihydroxycholecalciferol can be administered safely. Hence, with this treatment, higher blood concentrations of the vitamin can be obtained, and the parathyroid glands may be suppressed more readily.

Acidosis

Metabolic acidosis occurs frequently in nondialyzed patients with chronic renal failure because the ability of the kidney to excrete acidic metabolites is impaired. In earlier stages of chronic renal failure, metabolic acidosis can also be caused by excessive renal loss of bicarbonate. The rate of acid production is probably normal or below normal in stable chronically uremic patients. Acidosis is reported to cause bone reabsorption, net protein degradation (299, 300), and symptoms of lethargy and weakness.

Ingestion of low-nitrogen diets may prevent or reduce the severity of acidosis by decreasing the endogenous generation of acidic products of protein metabolism. Alkali supplements are usually effective in preventing or treating the acidosis of chronic renal failure. Calcium carbonate, 5 g/day, may correct mild acidosis, provide needed calcium, and reduce intestinal phosphate absorption. For more severe acidosis, sodium bicarbonate or citrate may be administered orally or intravenously. If the nondialyzed chronically uremic patient is not oliguric and is not likely to develop edema, sodium is usually readily excreted when administered as sodium bicarbonate or citrate.

Alkali therapy should probably be initiated if the arterial pH is below 7.35 or the serum bicarbonate is less than 20–22 meq/L. Before alkali therapy is implemented, it must be ascertained that the low serum bicarbonate is not a compensatory response to chronic respiratory alkalosis. If acidosis is severe and not controlled by the foregoing measures, hemodialysis or peritoneal dialysis may be used.

Prioritizing Dietary Goals

The number and magnitude of dietary modifications for chronically uremic patients are so great that if they are all presented to the patient at one time, demoralization and noncompliance are likely. Hence, we often list goals for dietary treatment according to priority. Control of protein, phosphorus, sodium, energy, potassium, calcium, and magnesium intake generally is emphasized. Unless the patient has a lipid disorder that carries a high risk of atherosclerotic disease, recommendations concerning the types and amounts of carbohydrates and fats ingested are usually given lower priorities. Also, a high dietary fiber intake is given lower priority.

NUTRITIONAL THERAPY IN ACUTE RENAL FAILURE

Metabolic Derangements

Acute renal failure is characterized by sudden reduction or cessation in GFR. The most common causes of acute renal failure include shock, severe infection, trauma, medicines, obstruction, and certain types of glomerulonephritis. In most instances, patients who survive the underlying diseases recover from the acute renal failure. Patients who sustain acute renal failure are likely to develop fluid and electrolyte disorders, uremic toxicity, and wasting. These disorders are particularly likely when the patient is both oliguric and hypercatabolic, which are common complications of acute renal failure.

Patients with acute renal failure, particularly those with underlying catabolic illnesses, frequently undergo metabolic changes that promote degradation of protein and amino acids and consumption of fuel substrates. Energy expenditure is often increased (301). In vitro studies with rat muscle tissue indicate that protein degradation is enhanced and protein synthesis is reduced (302, 303). In addition, hepatic gluconeogenesis increases. If livers from these animals are perfused or incubated with amino acids, the elevated hepatic glucose and urea production is further enhanced (304). The metabolic changes promoting catabolism are not uncommonly severe in patients with acute renal failure, and these individuals may be among the sickest and most metabolically deranged patients in the hospital. As a result of these metabolic derangements, these patients often cannot use protein, amino acids, and energy substrates efficiently. Hence, it may be difficult to maintain and improve the nutritional status of these patients by enteral or parenteral nutrition (305–307).

General Nutritional Principles

Because available data concerning optimal nutritional therapy for patients with acute renal failure are both limited and conflicting, it is not possible to strongly justify any treatment plan for such patients. The following therapeutic approach is based upon our analysis of the literature and personal experience.

Fluid and mineral balance should be carefully monitored in patients with acute renal failure to prevent overhydration or electrolyte disorders. Water intake, in general, should equal output from urine and all other measured sources (e.g., nasogastric aspirate, fistula drainage) plus 400 mL/day. This regimen takes into account the contributions of endogenous water production from metabolism and the insensible water losses (primarily respiration and skin losses) to water balance. In general, if the patient is catabolic, weight should be allowed to decrease by 0.2 to 0.5 kg/day to avoid excessive fluid accumulation. Sodium, potassium, phosphorus, and magnesium intake should be restricted to prevent accumulation of these minerals. Energy and, if feasible, protein intake should satisfy the patient's nutritional requirements, which may exceed normal. By controlling the water and electrolyte intake and lowering the UNA, one may be able to reduce the need for dialysis treatments.

The patient's desirable nutrient intake depends upon the nutritional status, catabolic rate, residual GFR, and clinical indications for initiating dialysis therapy. For example, if a patient is wasted, one might be more inclined to give a surfeit of nutrients and to provide dialysis as needed. A patient with acute renal failure who has a high residual GFR also may receive larger quantities of nutrients, because there is less risk of developing fluid and electrolyte disorders or accumulating potentially toxic metabolites. On the other hand, for a patient who has little or no urine flow and who is not very catabolic or uremic, intake of small quantities of water, minerals, and amino acids may reduce the need for dialysis; this approach may be particularly beneficial if it is anticipated that the patient will not tolerate dialysis well. Similarly, a patient who is starting to recover from acute renal failure may be given this latter treatment to avoid dialysis for a few days until renal function becomes adequate. In these latter patients, high-calorie diets providing small amounts of essential amino acids or ketoacids with little or no protein may be used for short periods.

Whenever feasible, patients with acute renal failure should receive oral nutrition. If the patient will not eat adequately, use of liquid formula diets, elemental diets, and tube or enterostomy feeding should be considered. Often parenteral nutrition is the only technique that will provide adequate nutrient intake (Table 89.4).

Specific Nutrient Intakes

Protein and Amino Acid Intake

The quantity of nitrogen and the composition of the amino acid formulations that are administered enterally or parenterally to patients with acute renal failure are the subject of controversy. Abel and associates carried out a series of studies suggesting that parenteral nutrition benefitted patients with acute renal failure (308–310). The patients were infused with solutions containing hypertonic D-glucose and 12 to 30 g/day of essential amino acids but no nonessential amino acids. The authors reported that the SUN and serum potassium, phosphorus, and magnesium often stabilized or decreased, and dialysis therapy sometimes could be postponed or avoided. In a prospective, randomized, double-blind study, these investigators compared infusion of hypertonic glucose and essential amino acids with an isocaloric infusion of hypertonic glucose that contained no amino acids (310). Patients receiving glucose and essential amino acids had significantly greater survival until renal function recovered; hospital survival was slightly but not significantly increased. In retrospective studies with nonconcurrent controls, parenteral nutrition that provided essential and nonessential amino acids appeared to improve morbidity and mortality, particularly in patients who had more complicated clinical courses (311, 312).

Leonard et al. reported that parenteral nutrition with hypertonic glucose and about 21 g/day of essential amino acids had no advantages over isocaloric infusions with glucose alone with regard to SUN levels, nitrogen balance, or survival in patients with acute renal failure (313). Feinstein et al. carried out a randomized, prospective, double-blind study of individuals with acute renal failure who could not eat adequately (305). Thirty patients were treated with one of three isocaloric parenteral nutrition formulations: hypertonic glucose with no amino acids, hypertonic glucose with 21 g/day of essential amino acids, or hypertonic glucose with 21 g/day each of essential and nonessential amino acids. The mean duration of study was 9.2 days per patient. The metabolic balance data indicated that many of these patients were severely catabolic with net rates of protein degradation as high as 240 g/day (determined by the difference between nitrogen intake and UNA). UNA tended to be lower with the essential amino acid regimen. Neither nitrogen balance nor mortality rates were significantly different with any of the three infusion regimens, but each tended to be less adverse with the essential amino acid intake.

It has been argued that more than 40 g/day of a mixture of essential and nonessential amino acids may be more effective at improving nitrogen balance. Feinstein et al. tested this hypothesis in a randomized prospective trial (306). Patients received total parenteral nutrition (TPN) providing 21 g/day of essential amino acids or TPN with essential and nonessential amino acids provided in a 1.0:1.0 ratio. With the latter treatment, attempts were made to infuse a quantity of nitrogen equal to the UNA. Thirteen patients with acute renal failure were randomly assigned to one of the two treatments. The results indicated that although the nitrogen intake was five times greater with the latter regimen, nitrogen balance, determined from the difference between intake and UNA, was not different. The UNA fell significantly only in the patients receiving essential amino acids, and it tended to rise in the other group.

These data suggest that high-calorie solutions providing about 21 g/day of essential amino acids may be used more effectively than isocaloric preparations containing larger quantities of essential and nonessential amino acids (e.g., 40–70 g/day) provided in an essential: nonessential ratio of 1.0:1.0 (307). Essential amino acid solutions seem to reduce the UNA and total nitrogen output more than those solutions with essential and nonessential amino acids. Consequently, nitrogen balance seems to be no more negative with the former preparations, but accumulation of nitrogenous metabolites is lower. Studies in clinically stable patients with chronic renal failure also indicate that diets providing small amounts of essential amino acids as the sole nitrogen source maintain nitrogen balance more effectively than diets providing similar quantities of protein (314). It would be of interest to examine the response to a TPN regimen that provides greater quantities of essential and nonessential amino acids but with a larger proportion of essential amino acids.

The data from rat studies are also inconclusive. Toback and associates induced acute renal failure in rats by injecting mercuric chloride (315, 316). The rats infused with glucose and a mixture of essential and nonessential amino acids had greater regeneration of renal cortical cells, as determined by ^{14}C-choline incorporation into phospholipids, than rats that were infused with glucose alone. Amino acids promoted intracellular protein synthesis as determined by ^{14}C-leucine uptake (317). The maximum serum creatinine concentration also was lower in the rats infused with glucose and amino acids, suggesting that these nutrients enhanced recovery of renal function. However, Oken et al. were unable to show a consistent benefit of glucose and essential amino acids or glucose and essential and nonessential amino acids over glucose alone on the rate or incidence of recovery of renal function or survival in rats with acute renal failure (318).

These conflicting observations probably result from the following factors: *(a)* the clinical course of patients with acute renal failure is so complex and variable that it would be necessary to study large numbers of patients to show statistically significant benefits of nutritional therapy if such benefits exist; *(b)* many of these studies were retrospective or not randomly controlled and thus may contain unintentional biases; *(c)* the optimal composition of nutrients in the TPN solutions has not been defined, and the use of suboptimal formulations may reduce the clinical benefits of nutritional therapy; and *(d)* catabolic patients or rats with acute renal failure may need both good nutrition and metabolic intervention to suppress catabolic processes and to promote anabolism, and providing nutrients without metabolic intervention may not benefit nutritional status or clinical outcome, particularly in the first days after onset of acute renal failure.

It is pertinent that the prospective studies of parenteral nutrition in patients with acute renal failure compared different regimens of nutritional therapy; that is, infusion of high-calorie solutions containing amino acids versus isocaloric infusions without amino acids and administration of isocaloric solutions with essential amino acids versus those with essential and nonessential amino acids (305, 306, 310, 313). No prospective, randomized study has compared the clinical course of patients receiving nutritional therapy with that of patients receiving no nutritional support.

Our current policy for amino acid or protein intake in patients with acute renal failure is as follows (Table 89.4): Patients may be prescribed a low enteral or intravenous nitrogen intake if there is a low UNA (i.e., 4–5 g N/day), if they have no evidence of severe protein malnutrition, if they are anticipated to recover renal function within the next 1 or 2 weeks, and if there is an indication to avoid dialysis therapy (307). Under these conditions, we may prescribe 0.3 to 0.5 g/kg/day of primarily high-quality protein or essential amino acids, preferably with arginine. We do not give more than 0.4 g/kg/day of essential amino acids as the sole nitrogen source because larger quantities of the nine essential amino acids may cause serious amino acid imbalances (307, 319). Diets providing 0.10 to 0.30 g/kg/day of miscellaneous protein and 10 to 20 g/day of essential amino acids or ketoacids may also be used in patients who can eat. These regimens should minimize the rate of accumulation of nitrogenous metabolites and, unless the patient is severely catabolic, will usually maintain neutral or only mildly negative nitrogen balance. Hence, the need for dialysis therapy may be minimized or avoided. Patients with substantial residual renal function (e.g., GFR of 5–10 mL/min) who are not very catabolic may be treated as nondialyzed patients with chronic renal failure. They would receive 0.55 to 0.60 g protein or amino acids/kg body weight daily.

For patients who are more catabolic and have a higher UNA (>5 g N/day), are severely wasted, or are undergoing regular dialysis therapy and either have or are anticipated to have acute renal failure for more than 2 weeks, we are inclined to prescribe a higher protein or amino acid intake, up to 1.0 to 1.2 g/kg/day. If tolerated, 1.2 g protein or amino acids/kg/day is preferable. In comparison to small quantities of essential amino acids, these larger nitrogen intakes may improve nitrogen balance, particularly after the first 1 or 2 weeks of dialysis treatments. However, the UNA almost invariably rises, and the increased azotemia and, in those patients receiving TPN, the larger volumes of fluid necessary to provide this amount of amino acids may increase the need for dialysis.

If acute renal failure persists for more than 2 to 3 weeks, patients undergoing regular dialysis treatment are treated as maintenance dialysis patients, with about 1.0 to 1.2 g/kg/day of protein or amino acids for hemodialysis patients or 1.2 to 1.3 g/kg/day for peritoneal dialysis patients.

Table 89.4
Typical Composition of Solutions for Total Parenteral Nutrition in Patients with Acute Renal Failure[a]

	Daily Quantity or Concentration to be Infused	
Volume	liters	1.0
Essential and nonessential free crystalline amino acids (4.25–5.0%)[b] or	g/L	42.5–50
Essential amino acids (5%)[b]	g/L	12.5–25
Dextrose (D-glucose)[c]	g/L	350
Lipid emulsion[c]	10 or 20%	50 or 100 g/500 mL
Energy (approx)[c]	kcal/L	1140
Electrolytes[d]		
Sodium[e]	mmol/L	40–50
Chloride[e]	mmol/L	25–35
Potassium	mmol/day	≤35
Acetate	mmol/day	35–40
Calcium	mmol/day	5
Phosphorus	mmol/day	8
Magnesium	mmol/day	4
Iron	mmol/day	2
Trace elements		see text
Vitamins		
Vitamin A[f]		see text
Vitamin D		see text
Vitamin K[g]	mg/week	7.5
Vitamin E[h]	IU/day	10
Niacin	mg/day	20
Thiamin HCl (B_1)	mg/day	2
Riboflavin (B_2)	mg/day	2
Pantothenic acid (B_3)	mg/day	10
Pyridoxine HCl (B_6)	mg/day	10
Ascorbic acid (C)	mg/day	60
Biotin	μg/day	100
Folic acid	mg/day	2
Vitamin B_{12}	μg/day	3

[a]These nutrients are present in each bottle containing 500 mL of 8.5–10% crystalline amino acids or 250–500 mL of 5% essential amino acids and 500 mL of 70% dextrose. The vitamins and trace elements are an exception because they are added to only one bottle per day. The patient's fluid status and serum electrolytes and glucose must be monitored closely. Composition and volume of the infusate may need to be changed if the patient is very uremic, acidotic, or volume overloaded; if the serum electrolyte concentrations are not normal or are changing; or if dialysis therapy is not readily available or is particularly hazardous to the patient (see text).

[b]For patients who are more catabolic (e.g., UNA ≥5 g/day), are undergoing regular dialysis treatments (particularly for 2 or more weeks), or who are wasted, essential and nonessential amino acids may be infused: about 1.0–1.2 g/kg/day for hemodialysis patients and 1.2–1.3 g/kg/day for intermittent or CPD patients (see text). For patients who are less wasted, are less catabolic, are not undergoing regular dialysis therapy, and will not be receiving TPN for more than 2 or 3 weeks, 0.30–0.50 g/kg/day of the nine essential amino acids (preferably with arginine) may be infused. Patients undergoing CCVH or CVVHD may be given up to 1.5–2.5 g/kg/day of essential and nonessential amino acids, depending upon their clinical and metabolic status. See text for discussion of the formulations of amino acids. Only solutions of crystalline amino acids should be used.

[c]To attain an energy intake of 30–40 kcal/kg/day, 70% dextrose is added as necessary (see text). Lower energy intakes may be used in very obese patients. For the higher levels of energy intake (i.e., 35–40 kcal/kg/day), additional 70% dextrose may be added to the solutions. To balance the sources of calories and to prevent essential fatty acid deficiency, lipid emulsions may be used. For patients who are septic or at high risk for sepsis, about 10–20% of calories or less may be given as lipids. Lipid emulsions probably should be infused over at least 12 hours, if not 24 hours, to reduce the hyperlipidemia that occurs with intravenous infusion of lipid emulsions (see text). Lipid emulsions may be infused in a separate line or mixed with the amino acid and dextrose solutions and infused soon after mixing (see text). A 20% lipid emulsion may be used to reduce the water load. The approximate caloric values are dextrose monohydrate, 3.4 kcal/g; amino acids, 3.5 kcal/g; lipid emulsions 10%, 1.1 kcal/mL; 20%, 2.0 kcal/mL.

[d]When adding electrolytes, the amounts intrinsically present in the amino acid solution should be taken into account.

[e]Refers to the final concentrations of electrolytes after any additional 70% dextrose or other solutions have been added.

[f]Vitamin A probably should be avoided unless total parenteral nutrition is continued for more than several days (see text).

[g]Should be given orally or parenterally and not in the total parenteral nutrition solution because of antagonisms.

[h]May need to be increased with use of lipid emulsions.

Other Maneuvers to Improve Protein Balance and Clinical Outcome

Continuous arteriovenous hemofiltration (CAVH), CAVH with concurrent hemodialysis (CAVHD), continuous venovenous hemofiltration (CVVH), and CVVH with concurrent hemodialysis using low dialysate flow rates (CVVHD) are used increasingly for management of very ill patients with acute renal failure or other causes of fluid or nitrogen intolerance (e.g., severe liver or congestive heart failure). With CAVH, catheters are placed into a large artery and vein, such as the femoral artery and vein (320). The blood flows through a small filtering apparatus where some of the plasma water is filtered; the remaining blood is returned to the vein. CVVH/CVVHD are often preferred to CAVH or CAVHD because these procedures reduce the risks of complications caused by arterial catheter placement.

The following are among the advantages to this treatment (for simplicity, CVVH or CVVHD also refers to continuous arteriovenous hemofiltration with or without dialysis): *(a)* Large quantities of water, electrolytes, and metabolic products may be removed each day; *(b)* because the rate of removal of water and electrolytes is slow, CVVH/CVVHD is less likely to cause or worsen hypotension or induce other adverse physiologic changes (e.g., cardiac arrhythmias); *(c)* the high daily clearances of water and small molecules, including metabolic waste products, allow safer administration of large amounts of amino acids and other nutrients to the patient. Physicians frequently combine parenteral nutrition therapy with CVVH/CVVHD to provide intravenous nutrition while simultaneously controlling the water and salt balance and removing the metabolic products that accumulate in renal failure.

When CVVH/CVVHD is not used, patients with acute renal failure who receive parenteral nutrition may require treatment with a hemodialyzer as often as every day rather than three times weekly—the usual treatment for clinically stable patients receiving maintenance hemodialysis. With CVVH, and particularly CVVHD, standard hemodialysis treatments are usually needed less frequently and often can be avoided altogether. Indeed, CVVH/CVVHD often allows patients with acute renal failure to receive the amount of infused nutrients normally given to hypercatabolic, critically ill patients who do not have fluid, electrolyte, or nitrogen intolerance (i.e., patients who do not have renal, liver or heart failure). For patients receiving CVVHD, we often prescribe 1.5 to 2.5 g/kg/day of mixtures of essential and nonessential amino acids intravenously or similar amounts of protein given enterally. Amino acid losses with CVVH/CVVHD are generally about 4 to 7 g/day and are slightly higher when patients are receiving amino acid infusions than when they are not (321, 322).

Some investigators have proposed adding amino acids and additional glucose to the dialysate of patients undergoing CAPD or maintenance hemodialysis (323, 324). The nutrients diffuse into the body during dialysis. At present, these techniques may provide supplemental nutrition but cannot be used for total nutritional support.

Because the metabolic status of patients with acute renal failure often facilitates catabolism of protein, amino acids, and other energy substrates (302–307, 313), there may be advantages to administering agents that promote anabolic processes or reduce catabolic pathways. As mentioned above, nitrogen intake appears to be used more efficiently if a greater proportion of the administered amino acids is essential amino acids (305, 307, 314). This hypothesis has not yet been tested clinically. In addition, studies in catabolic patients without renal failure suggest that intravenous infusions in which a large proportion of the amino acids are branched-chain amino acids (i.e., isoleucine, leucine, and valine) may have a specific anabolic effect (325, 326). Not all studies confirm these findings. Ketoacid analogues of the branched-chain amino acids also promote anabolism, both when studied in in vitro preparations and when given to nonuremic individuals who are not hypercatabolic (103, 104). Intravenous infusion of the salt complex of α-ketoglutarate and ornithine in postoperative patients receiving TPN is reported to reduce UNA and to increase nitrogen balance (327). Severely stressed patients without renal failure display a rapid fall in intracellular muscle glutamine (328), and administration of glutamine improves protein balance in these patients (328, 329). Arginine has also been reported to increase nitrogen balance (330).

Anabolic steroidal compounds, many of which are androgenic and resemble testosterone, have been used in patients with acute renal failure (331, 332). These agents can reduce UNA and improve nitrogen balance and are reported to decrease the need for dialysis treatments. In vitro studies of skeletal muscle from rats with acute renal failure indicate that insulin may increase synthesis and reduce degradation of protein (303). Studies in catabolic patients who do not have renal failure indicate that insulin may decrease the UNA (333, 334). Recombinant DNA–synthesized human growth hormone has been used to improve nitrogen balance in postoperative, acutely stressed patients without renal failure, and the results are encouraging (335, 336). This hormone has also improved nitrogen balance in stable, malnourished patients undergoing maintenance hemodialysis (337). However, individuals acutely stressed from infection or physical trauma or who receive low quantities of nutrients sometimes become refractory to growth hormone, possibly because of downregulation of growth hormone receptors with reduced ability to express IGF-I (338).

These findings suggest that recombinant human IGF-I (rhIGF-I) therapy may be more beneficial than growth hormone treatment for hypercatabolic patients with acute renal failure. Indeed, studies in rats with ischemic- or toxin-induced acute renal failure indicate that rhIGF-I may enhance recovery of renal function (339, 340). However, a recent study suggests that rhIGF-I therapy does not enhance the rate of recovery of renal function, reduce the need for dialysis treatment, or improve survival in sick intensive care unit patients with acute renal failure (341). Because IGF-I appears to stimulate growth of dedifferentiated cells, neither growth hormone nor rhIGF-I should be given to patients with active malignancy.

Several other growth factors (epidermal growth factor [342], hepatocyte growth factor [343]), hormones (thyroxin [344], atrial natriuretic peptide [345]), or adenine nucleotides (346) are reported to enhance recovery of renal function in experimental animals or in preliminary studies in humans. None of these agents has yet been shown to improve renal function in well-controlled clinical trials in humans with acute renal failure.

Energy

Several lines of evidence suggest that patients with acute renal failure may benefit from a high energy intake. Because patients with acute renal failure are frequently in negative energy and nitrogen balance (301, 305, 306, 313), some investigators contend that greater energy intake may reduce protein wasting. Moreover, unlike nonuremic acutely ill patients who may receive large quantities of amino acids, patients with acute renal failure are usually given relatively small amounts of amino acids because of their excretory impairment. It is possible, although not proven, that higher energy intake may improve the utilization of low nitrogen intake. In two studies of patients with acute renal failure who were not randomized for energy intake, those who died were found to have a higher energy expenditure and more-negative energy balance (301) or lower energy intake (301, 305) than those who survived. As a result of these findings, we usually administer about 30 to 40 kcal/kg standard (normal) weight/day (Table 89.4) (207, 347), except in patients who are obese (e.g., above about 125% standard body weight) or very underweight (207a).

The higher intakes (40 kcal/kg/day) are used for patients who have a higher UNA, who are severely ill, and who are less obese. For example, if nitrogen balance, estimated from the difference between the patient's nitrogen intake and the nitrogen output calculated from the UNA, is negative, we try to provide an energy intake close to 40 kcal/kg/day. Alternatively, the patient's energy needs may be estimated by multiplying the Harris-Benedict equation (348) or the newer World Health Organization equations (349) for calculating the daily energy requirements of normal individuals by a stress factor to adjust for the patient's illness (350, 351) and by 1.25. The 1.25 is included to provide a surfeit of energy to promote anabolism or to diminish the rate of catabolism of the patient; the benefit of using this term has not been clearly demonstrated. Energy expenditure, measured by indirect calorimetry, can also be multiplied by 1.25 to estimate the daily energy requirement.

These energy intakes exceed those currently recommended for severely stressed patients without renal failure. However, because nitrogen intolerance limits the amount of amino acids or protein that can be given to the patient with renal failure and higher energy intake tends to reduce protein and amino acid degradation, the patient with renal failure may benefit from a larger energy load. Unfortunately, prospective studies to test this hypothesis are not available.

Larger energy intakes are not used because there appears to be little nutritional advantage to administering more calories to catabolic patients. Indeed, because high energy intakes generate more carbon dioxide from infused carbohydrate and fat, they can promote hypercapnia if pulmonary function is impaired (352). Carbon dioxide retention is particularly likely to occur with very high carbohydrate loads. In addition, high energy intakes may cause obesity and fatty liver (353), and they may increase the water load to the patient.

Because most patients with acute renal failure do not tolerate large water intakes, glucose is usually administered in a 70% solution. The glucose and amino acid solutions are mixed, so that amino acids and energy are provided simultaneously (Table 89.4). Patients receiving TPN for more than 5 days should receive lipid emulsions. Patients require about 25 g/day of a lipid emulsion to prevent essential fatty acid deficiency. Some investigators have recommended giving up 30 to 40% of calories as lipid emulsions to provide sufficient fatty acids to organs that normally use lipids as their main energy source and to approximate the normal American dietary intake more closely. However, some researchers have reported that infusions of large amounts of fat emulsions (e.g., 50 g over 8 to 12 hours) may impair the function of the reticuloendothelial system (354) and have questioned whether infusion of lipid emulsions might lower host resistance. A prudent approach may be to infuse lipid emulsions over at least 12 hours, if not 24 hours, to prevent marked increases in plasma lipids. For patients who are septic or at high risk of severe sepsis, probably no more than 10 to 20% of total calories should be provided from fat. For patients who are not septic and not at high risk of infection, about 20 to 30% of calories may be given as lipid emulsions.

Intravenous lipid emulsions are available in 10% (1.1 kcal/mL) and 20% (2.0 kcal/mL) solutions. Traditionally, lipid emulsions have been infused separately from the glucose and amino acid mixtures. With careful attention to aseptic control, the lipid emulsions may be mixed with glucose and amino acids; the mixtures should be infused shortly after preparation (355).

Minerals

A mineral prescription for parenteral nutrition in acute renal failure is shown in Table 89.4. Any recommended intake of minerals is tentative and must be adjusted according to the clinical status of the patient. If the serum concentration of an electrolyte is increased, it may be advisable to reduce the quantity infused or not administer it at the onset of parenteral nutrition. The patient must be monitored closely, because the hormonal and metabolic changes that often occur with initiation of parenteral nutrition may cause a rapid drop in serum electrolytes, particularly in potassium and phosphorus. On the other hand, a low concentration of a mineral may indicate a need for greater than usual intake of that element. Again, metabolic changes and the impaired GFR can lead to a rapid rise in the serum concentrations during repletion.

Except for iron and zinc, trace elements are probably not necessary in parenteral nutrition solutions given to catabolic patients with acute renal failure unless this is the sole source of nutritional support for at least 2 to 3 weeks. Nutritional requirements for trace elements have not been established for uremic patients receiving TPN.

Vitamins

The vitamin requirements have not been well defined for patients with acute renal failure. Tentative recommendations for vitamin intake for patients receiving parenteral nutrition are shown in Table 89.4. Much of the recommended intake is based on information obtained from studies in chronically uremic patients, normal individuals, or nonuremic acutely ill patients. Vitamin A is probably best avoided for the first several days of nutritional support, because serum vitamin A levels are elevated in chronic renal failure, and small doses of vitamin A have been reported to cause toxicity to chronically uremic patients (293, 294). After the first several days of nutritional therapy, a dose of vitamin A that is between one-half and the complete RDA (117) for normal individuals may be given daily.

Vitamin D is fat soluble, and vitamin stores should not become depleted during the few days to weeks that most patients with acute renal failure receive parenteral nutrition. However, turnover of its active analogue, 1,25-dihydroxycholecalciferol, is much faster. Hence, this analogue may be needed in patients with acute renal failure (297).

Although vitamin K is fat soluble, vitamin K deficiency has been reported in nonuremic patients who are not eating and are receiving antibiotics (295). Vitamin K therefore should be given routinely to patients receiving parenteral nutrition (Table 89.4). Ten milligrams per day of pyridoxine hydrochloride (8.2 mg/day of pyridoxine) is recommended because studies in clinically stable or sick patients undergoing maintenance hemodialysis indicate that this quantity may be necessary to prevent or correct vitamin B_6 deficiency (290). Patients should probably not receive more than 60 mg of ascorbic acid daily because of the risk of increased oxalate production (291, 292).

The nutrient intake of patients with acute renal failure must be carefully reevaluated each day and sometimes more frequently. This reevaluation is particularly important because these patients may undergo rapid changes in their clinical and metabolic condition.

Peripheral Parenteral Nutrition

Parenteral nutrition through a peripheral vein avoids the risks of inserting a catheter into the inferior vena cava. Because the osmolality of the infusate must be restricted to reduce the risk of thrombophlebitis, it is necessary to use a larger volume of fluid and/or a lower intake of nutrients. Both approaches may have undesirable consequences for patients with acute renal failure. It has been argued that the financial cost of TPN administered through a peripheral vein is about the same as, or greater than, the cost of administration through a central vein because of the large quantities of isotonic lipid emulsions used to provide the energy needs when peripheral veins are used.

Peripheral partial parenteral nutrition may be advantageous for patients with acute renal failure who can ingest or be tube fed only part of their daily nutritional requirements. Peripheral infusions may enable these patients to receive adequate nutrition without resorting to TPN through a large-flow vein. In these patients, it is often most practical to infuse an 8.5 to 10% amino acid solution or a 20% lipid emulsion into a peripheral vein and to administer as much as possible of the other essential nutrients, including carbohydrates, through the enteral tract. This treatment is used uncommonly.

The peripheral vascular access used for hemodialysis can also be used for parenteral nutrition. Because there is high blood flow through the vascular access used for hemodialysis, hypertonic solutions can be used, and the water load to the patient can be reduced. This technique probably increases the risk of infection or thrombosis in the vascular access, however, and it should not be used except in an emergency or in patients who will need a hemodialysis access for extended periods.

Supplemental Intradialytic Parenteral Nutrition

Amino acids, glucose, and/or lipids may be infused as a nutritional supplement to patients with acute or chronic renal failure who eat poorly. Supplemental amino acids, glucose, and/or lipids can be infused conveniently during the hemodialysis procedure. Because most patients in need of nutritional supplements have decreased intake of both amino acids and energy, I infuse 40 to 42 g of essential and nonessential amino acids and 200 g of D-glucose (150 g of D-glucose if the hemodialysate contains glucose). This preparation is infused throughout the hemodialysis procedure at a constant rate into the blood leaving the dialyzer. This technique minimizes the normal fall in amino acid and glucose pools that results from dialysis of these nutrients. Most of the infused glucose and amino acids are retained; amino acid losses into dialysate increase by only about 4 to 5 g (181). Lipid infusions have been substituted for some of the infused glucose, but they are more expensive and possibly pose some risk of reducing host resistance to infection (354). Patients who have low serum phosphorus or potassium concentrations at the onset of dialysis treatment may require supplements of these electrolytes during the amino acid and glucose supplementation. To prevent reactive hypoglycemia, the infusion should not be stopped until the end of hemodialysis, and the patient should eat a carbohydrate source 20 to 30 minutes before the end of the infusion.

Whether intravenous supplements with amino acids, glucose, and/or lipids thrice weekly for about 3–4 hours during hemodialysis benefit maintenance hemodialysis patients who eat poorly is controversial. Two recent retrospective analyses suggest that intradialytic parenteral nutrition may reduce the mortality rate in malnourished patients undergoing maintenance hemodialysis (356, 357). One study indicated that this benefit was only observed when the serum albumin was 3.3 g/dL or lower (357). Intradialytic parenteral nutrition should only be used in patients who cannot increase their intake of foods or take oral supplements. Intravenous supplements should be continued only if nutritional or clinical assessment indicates that they are beneficial.

Amino Acids That May Predispose to Acute Renal Failure

Several studies in rats suggest that amino acid or protein intake may increase the susceptibility to acute renal failure caused by ischemia or aminoglycoside nephrotoxicity (358–361). The nutrients seem to increase both the incidence and the severity of acute renal failure induced by these agents. Although some studies have demonstrated this effect with large doses of intravenous amino acids or dietary protein (358, 361), the quantities of amino acids and protein that might be prescribed for patients can also predispose to renal failure in animal studies (359, 360). D-Serine, DL-ethionine, and L-lysine appear to be particularly nephrotoxic (359, 361). It is not known whether amino acid or protein intake will predispose to renal failure in humans. If either one does, then patients who receive nephrotoxic medicines or who are at high risk for renal ischemia might benefit from low amino acid or protein intake for transient periods. On the other hand, in vitro studies also indicate that some amino acids, particularly L-glycine and L-alanine, may protect renal tubular cells from ischemic or nephrotoxic injury (362). Clearly, more research is needed in this area.

Future Direction for Nutritional Support

Several new techniques for improving nitrogen balance and host resistance could lead to major changes in nutritional support if the reported benefits are confirmed. The potential use of growth factors for patients with renal failure has been described previously (339, 340, 342, 343, 345). Arginine and glutamine supplements are reported to have specific effects on enhancing nitrogen balance (328–330). In addition, evidence indicates that supplemental arginine (330, 363), nucleotides (364), and ω-3 fatty acids (364) may improve parameters of immunologic function and host resistance. Peptides have been added to TPN solutions to increase the delivery of less soluble or less stable amino acids (e.g., tyrosine and glutamine) (329).

REFERENCES

1. Bergström J. Uremic toxicity. In: Kopple JD, Massry SG, eds. Nutritional management of renal disease. Baltimore: Williams & Wilkins, 1997;97–190.
2. Schoolwerth AC, Drewnowska K. Renal cell metabolism. In: Massry SG, Glassock RJ, eds. Massry & Glassock's textbook of nephrology, vol 1. 3rd ed. Baltimore: Williams & Wilkins, 1995;123–37.
3. Rabkin R, Dahl DC. Role of kidney in hormone metabolism. In: Massry SG, Glassock RJ, eds. Massry & Glassock's textbook of nephrology, vol 1. 3rd ed. Baltimore: Williams & Wilkins, 1995;161–71.
4. Kurokawa K, Taniguchi S. Effects of hormones on renal function. In: Massry SG, Glassock RJ, eds. Massry & Glassock's textbook of nephrology, vol 1. 3rd ed. Baltimore: Williams & Wilkins, 1995;172–81.
5. Kidney and endocrine system. In: Massry SG, Glassock RJ, eds. Massry & Glassock's textbook of nephrology, vol 1. 3rd ed. Baltimore: Williams & Wilkins, 1995;182–226.
6. Lakkis FG, Nassar GM, Badr KF. Hormones and the kidney. In: Schrier RW, Gottschalk CW, eds. Diseases of the kidney, vol 1. 6th ed. Boston: Little, Brown, 1997;251–92.
7. Eschbach JW, Kelly MR, Haley R, et al. N Engl J Med 1989;321:158–62.
8. Klahr S. Effect of malnutrition and of changes in protein intake on renal function. In: Kopple JD, Massry SG, eds. Nutritional management of renal disease. Baltimore: Williams & Wilkins, 1997;229–44.
9. Klahr S, Tripathy K. Arch Intern Med 1966;118:322–5.
10. Klahr S, Tripathy K, Garcia FT, et al. Am J Med 1967;43:84–96.
11. Klahr S, Tripathy K, Lotero H. Am J Med 1970;48:325–31.
12. Ichikawa I, Purkerson ML, Klahr S, et al. J Clin Invest 1980;65:982–8.
13. Hirschberg R, Kopple JD, Blantz RC, et al. J Clin Invest 1991;87:1200–6.
14. Hirschberg R, Kopple JD. J Am Soc Nephrol 1991;1:1034–40.
15. Owen OE, Felig P, Morgan AP. J Clin Invest 1969;48:574–83.
16. Gutman AB, Yu, T.-F. Am J Med 1968;45:756–79.
17. Bosch JP, Lew S, Glabman S, et al. Am J Med 1986;81:809–15.
18. Smoyer WE, Brouhard BH, Rassin DK, et al. J Lab Clin Med 1991;118:166–75.
19. Castellino P, Hunt W, DeFronzo RA. Kidney Int 1987;32 (Suppl 22):S15–20.
20. Hirschberg R, Kopple JD. Kidney Int 1987;32:382–7.
21. Woods LL. Kidney Int 1993;44:659–75.
22. Hirschberg R, Zipser RD, Slomowitz LA, et al. Kidney Int 1988;33:1147–55.
23. Premen AJ, Hall JE, Smith MJ Jr. Am J Physiol 1985; 248:F656–62.
24. Friedlander G, Blanchet-Benqué F, Nitenberg A, et al. Nephrol Dial Transplant 1990;5:110–7.
25. Premen AJ. Am J Physiol 1985;249:F319–22.
26. Christiansen JS, Gammelgaard J, Orskov H. Eur J Clin Invest 1981;11:487–90.
27. Hirschberg R, Rabb H, Bergamo R, et al. Kidney Int 1989; 35:865–70.
28. Hirschberg R, Kopple JD. J Clin Invest 1989;83:326–36.
29. Mitch WE, Walser M, Buffington GA, et al. Lancet 1976;2:1326–8.
30. Rutherford WE, Blondin J, Miller JP, et al. Kidney Int 1977;11:62–70.
31. Barsotti G, Guiducci A, Ciardella F, et al. Nephron 1981;27:113–7.
32. McCormack LJ, Beland JE, Schnekloth RE, et al. Am J Pathol 1958;34:1011–22.
33. Kleinknecht C, Grunfeld, J-P., Gomez PC, et al. Kidney Int 1973;4:390–400.
34. Rodriguez-Iturbe B, Garcia R, Rubio L, et al. Clin Nephrol 1976;5:198–206.
35. Torres VE, Velosa JA, Holley KE, et al. Ann Intern Med 1980;92:776–84.
36. Deen WM, Maddox DA, Robertson CR, et al. Am J Physiol 1974;227:556–62.
37. Hostetter TH, Olson JL, Rennke HG, et al. Am J Physiol 1981;241:F85–93.
38. Hostetter TH, Troy JL, Brenner BM. Kidney Int 1981;19: 410–5.
39. Olson JL, Hostetter TH, Rennke HG, et al. Proc Am Soc Nephrol Thorofare, NJ: Charles B Slack, 1979;87A.
40. Olson JL, Hostetter TH, Rennke HG, et al. Kidney Int 1982;22:112–26.
41. Kopple JD, Shinaberger JH, Coburn JW, et al. Am J Clin Nutr 1968;21:508–15.
42. Blatherwick NR, Medlar EM. Arch Intern Med 1937;59: 572–96.
43. Farr LE, Smadel JE. J Exp Med 1939;70:615–27.
44. Addis T. Glomerular nephritis, diagnosis and treatment. New York: Macmillan, 1948.
45. Ibels LS, Alfrey AC, Haut L, et al. N Engl J Med 1978;298: 122–6.
46. Karlinsky ML, Haut LL, Buddington B, et al. Kidney Int 1980;17:293–302.
47. Haut LL, Alfrey AC, Guggenheim S, et al. Kidney Int 1980;17:722–31.
48. Kirsch R, Frith L, Black E, Hoffenberg R. Nature 1968;217: 578–9.
49. Kenner CH, Evan AP, Blomgren P, et al. Kidney Int 1985;27: 739–50.
50. French SW, Yamanaka W, Ostwald R. Arch Pathol 1967;83: 204–10.
51. Hurd ER, Johnston JM, Okita JR, et al. J Clin Invest 1981;67:476–85.
52. Rothschild MA, Oratz M, Evans CD, et al. Albumin synthesis. In: Rosemoer M, Oratz M, Rothschild A, eds. Albumin structure, function and uses. New York: Pergamon Press, 1977;227–55.
53. Barcelli UO, Weiss M, Pollack VE. J Lab Clin Med 1982;100:786–97.
54. Zurier RB, Damjanov O, Sayadoff DM, et al. Arthritis Rheum 1977;20:1449–56.

55. Kelley VE, Winkelstein A, Izui S. Lab Invest 1979;41:531–7.
56. McLeish KR, Gohara AF, Cunning WT III. J Lab Clin Med 1980;96:470–9.
57. Brenner BM, Meyer TW, Hostetter TH. N Engl J Med 1982;307:652–9.
58. Meyer TW, Lawrence WE, Brenner BM. Kidney Int 1983;24 (Suppl 16):S243–7.
59. Schrier RW, Harris DCH, Chan L, et al. Am J Kidney Dis 1988;12:243–9.
60. Nath KA, Hostetter MK, Hostetter TH. J Clin Invest 1985;76:667–75.
61. Bouby N, Bachmann S, Bichet D, et al. Am J Physiol 1990;258:F973–9.
61a. Paller MS, Hostetter TH. Am J Physiol 1986;251:F34–9.
61b. Williams M, Young JB, Rosa RM, et al. J Clin Invest 1986;78:1687–93.
62. Walls J, Williams SJ. Contrib Nephrol 1988;60:179–87.
63. Mauer SM, Steffes MW, Azar S, et al. Kidney Int 1989;35: 48–59.
64. Mogensen CE. Diabetes 1976;25:872–9.
65. Mogensen CE, Steffes MW, Deckert T, et al. Diabetologia 1981;21:89–93.
66. Mogensen CE, Christensen CK, Vittinghus E. Diabetes 1983;32(Suppl 2):64–78.
67. Barsotti G, Giannoni A, Morelli E, et al. Clin Nephrol 1984;21:54–9.
68. Lumlertgul D, Burke TJ, Gillum OM, et al. Kidney Int 1986;29:658–66.
69. Gimenez LF, Solez K, Walker GW. Kidney Int 1987;31:93–9.
70. Harris DCH, Hammond WS, Burke TJ, et al. Kidney Int 1987;31:41–6.
71. Kasiske BL, O'Donnell MP, Schmitz PG, et al. Kidney Int 1990;37:880–91.
72. Wellmann K, Wolk BW. Lab Invest 1970;22:144–5.
73. Kasiske BL, O'Donnell MP, Cleary MP, et al. Kidney Int 1988;33:667–72.
74. Keane WF, O'Donnell MP, Kasiske BL, et al. J Am Soc Nephrol 1990;1:S69–74.
75. Alderson LM, Endemann G, Lindsay I, et al. Am J Pathol 1986;123:334–42.
76. Kaplan R, Aynedjian HS, Schlondorff D, et al. J Clin Invest 1990;86:1707–14.
77. Susuki S, Shapiro R, Mulrow PJ, et al. Prostaglandins Med 1980;4:377–82.
78. Knecht A, Fine LG, Kleinman KS, et al. Am J Physiol 1991;261:F292–9.
79. Anderson S, Meyer TW. Pathophysiology and nephron adaptation in chronic renal failure. In: Schrier RW, Gottschalk CW, eds. Diseases of the kidney, vol 1. 6th ed. Boston: Little, Brown, 1997;2555–80.
80. Rahman MA, Nakazawa M, Emancipator SN, et al. (Abstract). Kidney Int 1986;29:343.
81. Badr KF, Brenner BM, Wasserman M, et al. (Abstract). Kidney Int 1986;29:328.
82. Don BR, Blake S, Hutchison FN, et al. Am J Physiol 1989; 256:F711–8.
83. Anderson S, Meyer TW, Rennke HG, et al. J Clin Invest 1985;76:612–9.
84. Tolins JP, Raij L. Hypertension 1990;16:452–61.
85. Hostetter TH, Rosenberg ME. J Am Soc Nephrol 1990;1: S55–8.
86. Lewis EJ, Hunsicker LG, Bain RP, et al. N Engl J Med 1993;329:1456–62.
87. Viberti G, Mogensen CE, Groop LC, et al. JAMA 1994; 271:275–9.
88. Bauer JH, Reams GP. J Am Soc Nephrol 1990;1:S80–1.
89. Dworkin LD. J Am Soc Nephrol 1990;1:S21–7.
90. Anderson S. J Am Soc Nephrol 1990;1:S51–4.
91. Walser M. Clin Nephrol 1975;3:180–6.
92. Maschio G, Oldrizzi L, Tessitore N, et al. Kidney Int 1982;22: 371–6.
93. Alvestrand A, Ahlberg M, Bergstrom J. Kidney Int 1983;24 (Suppl 16):S268–72.
94. Barsotti G, Morelli E, Giannoni A, et al. Kidney Int 1983;24(Suppl 16):S278–84.
95. Gretz N, Korb E, Strauch M. Kidney Int 1983;24(Suppl 16):S263–7.
96. Mitch WE, Walser M, Steinman TI, et al. N Engl J Med 1984;311:623–9.
97. Rosman JB, Meijer S, Sluiter WJ, et al. Lancet 1984;2: 1291–5.
98. Walser J, LaFrance ND, Ward L, et al. Kidney Int 1987;32:123–8.
99. Ihle BU, Becker GJ, Whitworth JA, et al. N Engl J Med 1989;321:1773–7.
100. Zeller J, Whittaker E, Sullivan L, et al. N Engl J Med 1991;324:78–84.
101. Klahr S, Levey AS, Beck GJ, et al. N Engl J Med 1994;330: 877–84.
102. Levey AS, Adler S, Caggiula AW, et al. Am J Kidney Dis 1996;27:652–63.
103. Mitch WE, Walser M, Sapir DG. J Clin Invest 1981;67:553–62.
104. Tischler ME, Desautels M, Goldberg AL. J Biol Chem 1982; 257:1613–21.
105. The Diabetes Control and Complications Trial Research Group. N Engl J Med 1993;329:977.
106. Fouque D, Laville M, Boissel JP, et al. Br Med J 1992;304: 216–20.
107. Pedrini MT, Levey AS, Lau J, et al. Ann Intern Med 1996; 124:627–32.
108. Williams AJ, Baker F, Walls J. Nephron 1987;46:83–90.
109. D'Amico G, Gentile MG, Manna G, et al. Lancet 1992; 339:1131–4.
110. D'Amico G, Remuzzi G, Maschio G, et al. Clin Nephrol 1991;35:237–42.
111. Striker GE, Nagle RB, Kohnen PW, et al. Arch Pathol 1969;87:439–42.
112. Lalich JJ, Faith GC, Harding GE. Arch Pathol 1970;89:548–59.
113. Everitt AV, Porter BD, Wyndham JR. Gerontology 1982;28: 168–75.
114. Zucchelli P, Cagnoli L, Casanova S, et al. Kidney Int 1983;24:649–55.
115. Rowe JW, Anres R, Robin JD, et al. Ann Intern Med 1976;84:567–9.
116. Kiprov DD, Colvin RB, McCluskey RT. Lab Invest 1982;46: 275–81.
117. Food and Nutrition Board, National Research Council. Recommended dietary allowances. 10th ed. Washington, DC: National Academy Press, 1989.
118. Schnaper HW, Robson AM. Nephrotic syndrome: minimal change disease, focal glomerulosclerosis, and related disorders. In: Schrier RW, Gottschalk CW, eds. Diseases of the kidney, vol 1. 6th ed. Boston: Little, Brown, 1997;1725–80.
119. Kaysen GA. Nutritional management of nephrotic syndrome. In: Kopple JD, Massry SG, eds. Nutritional management of renal disease. Baltimore: Williams & Wilkins, 1997;533–61.
120. Ibels LS, Gyory AZ. Medicine 1994;73:79.
121. Hirschberg R. J Clin Invest 1996;98:116–24.
122. Taguma Y, Kitamoto Y, Futaki G, et al. N Engl J Med 1985; 313:1617–20.

123. Kaysen GA, Gambertoglio J, Jimenez I, et al. Kidney Int 1986;29:572–7.
124. Zeller KR, Raskin P, Rosenstock J, et al. Kidney Int 1986;29: 209.
125. Kaysen GA, Davies RW. J Am Soc Nephrol 1990;1:S75–9.
126. Gonick HC, Maxwell MH, Rubini ME, et al. Nephron 1966;3:137–52.
126a. Falkenhain M, Hartman J, Hebert LA. Nutritional management of water, sodium, potassium, chloride and magnesium in renal disease and renal failure. In: Kopple JD, Massry SG, eds. Nutritional management of renal disease. Baltimore: Williams & Wilkins, 1997;371–94.
127. Morton AR, Hercz G. Calcium, phosphorus, and vitamin D metabolism in renal disease and chronic renal failure. In: Kopple JD, Massry SG, eds. Nutritional management of renal disease. Baltimore: Williams & Wilkins, 1997;341–70.
128. Vanholder R, Cornelis R, Dhondt A, et al. Trace element metabolism in renal disease and renal failure. In: Kopple JD, Massry SG, eds. Nutritional management of renal disease. Baltimore: Williams & Wilkins, 1997;395–414.
129. Chazot C, Kopple JD. Vitamin metabolism and requirements in renal disease and renal failure. In: Kopple JD, Massry SG, eds. Nutritional management of renal disease. Baltimore: Williams & Wilkins, 1997;415–78.
130. Rabkin R, Simon NM, Steiner S, et al. N Engl J Med 1970;282:182–7.
131. Sherwin RS, Bastl C, Finkelstein FO, et al. J Clin Invest 1976;57:722–31.
132. Vajda FJE, Martin TJ, Melick RA. Endocrinology 1969;84:162–4.
133. Cuttelod S, Lemarchand-Beraud T, Magnenat P, et al. Metabolism 1974;23:101–13.
134. Davidson WD, Moore TC, Shippey W, et al. Gastroenterology 1974;66:522–5.
135. Samaan N, Freeman RM. Metabolism 1970;19:102–13.
136. Nagel TC, Frenkel N, Bell RH, et al. J Clin Endocrinol Metab 1973;36:428–32.
137. Lim VS, Fang VS. Am J Med 1975;58:655–62.
138. Tourkantonis A, Spiliopoulos A, Pharmakioltis A, et al. Nephron 1981;27:271–2.
139. Hershman JM, Krugman LG, Kopple JD, et al. Metabolism 1979;27:755–9.
140. Fouque D, Peng SC, Kopple JD. Kidney Int 1995;47:876–83.
141. Ding H, Gao X-L, Hirschberg R, et al. J Clin Invest 1996;97:1064–75.
142. McCaleb ML, Wish JB, Lockwood DH. Endocrinol Res 1985;11:113–25.
143. Fadda GZ, Hajjar SM, Perna AF, et al. J Clin Invest 1991;87:255–61.
144. Kopple JD, Fukuda S. Am J Clin Nutr 1980;33:1363–72.
145. Tizianello A, De Ferrari G, Garibotto B, et al. J Clin Invest 1980;65:1162–73.
146. Kopple JD. Products of nitrogen metabolism and their toxicity. In: Massry SG, Glassock RJ, eds. Massry & Glassock's textbook of nephrology, vol 1. 3rd ed. Baltimore: Williams & Wilkins, 1995;1317–24.
147. Simenoff ML, Burke JF, Saukkonen JJ, et al. Lancet 1976;2:818–21.
148. Bricker NS. N Engl J Med 1972;286:1093–9.
149. Massry SG, Smogorzewski M. Semin Nephrol 1994;14:219–31.
150. Krol E, Rutkowski B, Wroblewska M, et al. Miner Electrolyte Metab 1996;22:13–5.
151. Attmann PO, Alaupovic P. Nephron 1991;57:401–10.
152. Lindner A, Charra B, Sherrard D, et al. N Engl J Med 1974;290:697–701.
153. Malluche HH, Faugere MC. Kidney Int 1990;38:193–211.
154. Briggs WA, Lazarus JM, Birtch AG, et al. Arch Intern Med 1973;132:21–8.
155. Schoenfeld PY, Henry RR, Laird NM, et al. Kidney Int 1983;23(Suppl 13):S80–8.
156. Salusky IB, Fine RN, Nelson P, et al. Am J Clin Nutr 1983;38:599–611.
157. Wolfson M, Strong CJ, Minturn D, et al. Am J Clin Nutr 1984;39:547–55.
158. Kopple JD. Nutrition in renal failure: causes of catabolism and wasting in acute or chronic renal failure. In: Robinson RR, ed. Nephrology, vol 2. Proceedings of the IXth International Congress of Nephrology. New York: Springer-Verlag, 1984;1498–515.
159. Cano N, Fernandez JP, Lacombe P, et al. Kidney Int 1987;32:S178–80.
160. Marckmann P. Clin Nephrol 1988;29:75–8.
161. Bilbrey GI, Cohen TL. Dial Transplant 1989;18:669.
162. Young GA, Kopple JD, Lindholm B, et al. Am J Kidney Dis 1991;17:462–71.
163. Cianciaruso B, Brunori G, Kopple JD, et al. Am J Kidney Dis 1995;26:475–86.
164. Carlson DM, Duncan DA, Naessens JM, et al. Mayo Clin Proc 1984;59:769–75.
165. Hirschberg R. Drug-nutrient interactions in renal failure. In: Kopple JD, Massry SG, eds. Nutritional management of renal disease. Baltimore: Williams & Wilkins, 1997;799–815.
166. Lowrie EG, Lew NL. Am J Kidney Dis 1990;15:458.
167. Delano BG, Manis JG, Manis T. Nephron 1977;19:26.
168. Lawson DH, Boddy K, King PC, et al. Clin Sci 1971;41:345–51.
169. Mahajan SK, Prasad AS, Lambujon J, et al. Am J Clin Nutr 1980;33:1517–21.
170. Kopple JD, Mercurio K, Blumenkrantz MJ, et al. Kidney Int 1981;19:694–704.
171. Sprenger KBG, Bundschu D, Lewis K, et al. Kidney Int 1983;24(Suppl 16):S315–8.
172. Bellinghieri G, Savica V, Mallamace A, et al. Am J Clin Nutr 1983;38:523–31.
173. Kopple JD. Kidney Int 1978;14:340–8.
174. Kluthe R, Lüttgen FM, Capetianu T, et al. Am J Clin Nutr 1978;31:1812–20.
175. Kopple JD, Berg R, Houser H, et al. Kidney Int 1989;36(Suppl 27):S184–94.
176. Kopple JD, et al. Kidney Int, in press.
177. Dwyer JT, et al. (submitted).
178. Grodstein GP, Blumenkrantz MJ, Kopple JD. Am J Clin Nutr 1980;33:1411–6.
179. Keane WF, Collins AJ. Am J Kidney Dis 1994;24:1010–8.
180. United States Renal Data System. 1995 annual data report. United States Department of Health and Human Services. Health Care Financing Administration. Bethesda, MD: July 1995.
181. Wolfson M, Jones MR, Kopple JD. Kidney Int 1982;21:500–6.
182. Ikizler TA, Flakoll PJ, Parker RA, et al. Kidney Int 1994;46: 830–7.
183. Chazot C, Shahmir E, Matias B, et al. (Abstract). J Am Soc Nephrol 1995;6:574.
184. Kopple JD, Blumenkrantz MJ, Jones MR, et al. Am J Clin Nutr 1982;36:395–402.
185. Blumenkrantz MJ, Gahl GM, Kopple JD, et al. Kidney Int 1981;19:593–602.
186. Wathen RL, et al. Am J Clin Nutr 1978;31:1870.
187. Gutierrez A, Alvestrand A, Wahren J, et al. Kidney Int 1990;38:487–94.
188. Gutierrez A, Bergström J, Alvestrand A. Clin Nephrol 1992;38:20.

188a. Lindsay RM, Bergström J. Nephrol Dial Transplant 1994;9(Suppl 2):150.
189. Linton AL, Clark WF, Driedger AA, et al. Nephron 1977;19:95–8.
190. Acchiardo SR, Moore LW, Latour PA. Kidney Int 1983;24(Suppl 16):S199–203.
191. Churchill DN, Taylor DW, Cook RJ, et al. Am J Kidney Dis 1992;19:214–34.
192. Teehan BP, Schleifer CR, Brown JM, et al. Adv Perit Dial 1990;6:181–5.
193. Caggiula AW, Milas NC. Achieving patient adherence to diet therapy. In: Kopple JD, Massry SG, eds. Nutritional management of renal disease. Baltimore: Williams & Wilkins, 1997;843–56.
194. Kopple JD. ASAIO J 1997;43:246–50.
195. Kopple JD, Chumlea WC, Gassman JJ, et al. (Abstract). J Am Soc Nephrol 1994;5:335.
196. Ikizler TA, Greene JH, Wingard RL, et al. J Am Soc Nephrol 1994;6:1386–91.
197. Salusky IB, Fine RN, Nelson P, et al. (Abstract). American Society of Nephrology 15th Annual Meeting, December 1982;66A.
198. Calloway DH, Odell ACF, Margen S. J Nutr 1971;101:775–86.
199. Sargent JA, Gotch FA. J Am Diet Assoc 1979;75:547–51.
200. Maroni BJ, Steinman TI, Mitch WE. Kidney Int 1985;27: 58–65.
201. Kopple JD, Gao X-L, Qing DP-Y. Kidney Int 1997;52:486–94.
202. Varcoe R, Halliday D, Carson ER, et al. Clin Sci Mol Med 1975;43:379–90.
203. Walser M. J Clin Invest 1974;53:1385–92.
204. Bergström J, Fürst P, Alvestrand A, et al. Kidney Int 1993; 44:1048–57.
205. Blake P, Daugirdas J. Quantification and prescription: General principles. In: Jacobs C, Kjellstrand CM, Koch KM, Winchester JF, eds. Replacement of renal function by dialysis. 4th rev. ed. Dordrecht: Kluwer Academic Publishers, 1996; 619–56.
206. Kopple JD, Coburn JW. JAMA 1974;227:41–4.
207. Frisancho AR. Am J Clin Nutr 1984;40:808.
207a. American Dietetic Association. Manual of clinical dietetics. Chicago: American Dietetic Association, 1988;(appendix 48):623.
208. Kopple JD, Coburn JW. Medicine 1973;52:583–95.
209. Kopple JD. Treatment with low protein and amino acid diets in chronic renal failure. In: Barcelo R, Bergeron M, Carriere S, et al., eds. Proceedings of the VIIIth International Congress of Nephrology. Basel: S Karger, 1978;497–507.
210. Walser M, Hill SB, Ward L, et al. Kidney Int 1993;43: 933–9.
211. Blainey JD. Clin Sci 1954;13:567–81.
212. Kaysen GA, Al-Bander H. Am J Nephrol 1990;10:36.
213. Ginn HE, Frost A, Lacy W. Am J Clin Nutr 1968;21:385–93.
214. Borah MF, Schoenfeld PY, Gotch FA, et al. Kidney Int 1978; 14:491–500.
215. Kopple JD, Shinaberger JH, Coburn JW, et al. Trans Am Soc Artif Intern Organs 1969;15:302–8.
216. Blumenkrantz MJ, Kopple JD, Moran JK, et al. Kidney Int 1982;21:849–61.
217. Kopple JD, Monteon FJ, Shaib JK. Kidney Int 1986;29:734–42.
218. Monteon FJ, Laidlaw SA, Shaib JK, et al. Kidney Int 1986;30: 741–7.
219. Schneeweiss B, Graninger W, Stockenhuber F, et al. Am J Clin Nutr 1990;52:596–601.
220. Schwickardi M, Lange H. Resting metabolic rate in patients with different stages of pre-terminal renal disease. (Abstract) In: Abstracts of the 7th International Congress on Nutrition and Metabolism in Renal Disease, Stockholm, Sweden, May 29–June 1, 1994;51.
221. Slomowitz LA, Monteon FJ, Grosvenor M, et al. Kidney Int 1989;35:704–11.
222. Kopple JD. Kidney Int 1978;14:340–8.
223. Kluthe R, Luttgen FM, Capetianu T, et al. Am J Clin Nutr 1978;31:1812–20.
224. Blumenkrantz MJ, Kopple JD, Gutman RA, et al. Am J Clin Nutr 1980;33:1567–85.
225. Appel G. Kidney Int 1991;39:169–83.
226. Attman PO. Nephrol Dial Transplant 1993;8:294.
227. Cocchi R, Viglino G, Cancarini G, et al. Miner Electrolyte Metab 1996;22:22–5.
228. Wanner C, Bartens W, Nauck M, et al. Miner Electrolyte Metab 1996;22:26–30.
229. Wanner C. Lipid metabolism in renal disease and renal failure. In: Kopple JD, Massry SG, eds. Nutritional management of renal disease. Baltimore: Williams & Wilkins, 1997;35–62.
230. Chan MK, Varghese Z, Moorhead JF. Kidney Int 1981;19: 625–37.
231. Ciman M, Rizzoli V, Moracchiello M, et al. Am J Clin Nutr 1980;33:1489–92.
232. Bellinghieri G, Savica V, Mallamace A, et al. Am J Clin Nutr 1983;38:523–31.
233. Joven J, Villabona C, Vilella E, et al. N Engl J Med 1990;323: 579–84.
234. Wanner C, Rader D, Bartens W, et al. Ann Intern Med 1993; 119:263–9.
235. Ibels LS, Alfrey AC, Weil R III. Am J Med 1978;64:634.
236. Nelson J, Beauregard H, Gélinas M, et al. Transplant Proc 1988;20:1264–70.
237. Diměny E, Fellström B, Larsson E, et al. Transplant Proc 1992;24:366.
238. Sanfelippo ML, Swenson RS, Reaven GM. Kidney Int 1977;14: 54–61.
239. Sanfelippo ML, Swenson RS, Reaven GM. Kidney Int 1978;14:180–6.
240. Guarnieri G, Toigo G, Crapesi L, et al. Kidney Int 1987;32 (Suppl 22):S116–27.
241. Wanner C, Horl WH. Nephron 1988;50:89.
242. Pierides AM, Alvarez-Ude F, Kerr DNS, et al. Lancet 1979;2:1279–82.
243. Leaf A, Weber PC. N Engl J Med 1988;318:549.
244. Donadio JV Jr, Bergstralh EJ, Offord KP, et al. N Engl J Med 1994;331:1194–9.
245. Manis T, Deutsch J, Feinstein EI, et al. Am J Clin Nutr 1980; 33:1485–8.
246. Expert Panel on Detection, Evaluation, and Treatment of High Blood Cholesterol in Adults. JAMA 1993;269:3015.
247. Hamazaki T, Nakazawa R, Tateno S, et al. Kidney Int 1984;26:81–4.
248. Thomas ME, Harris KPG, Ramaswamy C, et al. Kidney Int 1993;44:1124–9.
249. Goldberg AP, Geltman EM, Hagberg JM, et al. Kidney Int 1983;24(Suppl 16):S303–9.
250. Bremer J. Physiol Rev 1983;63:1420.
251. Vacha GM, Corsi M, Giorcelli G, et al. Curr Ther Res 1985;37:505–15.
252. Hiatt WR, Koziol BJ, Shapiro JI, et al. Kidney Int 1992;41: 1613–9.
253. Golper TA, Wolfson M, Ahmad S, et al. Kidney Int 1990; 38:904–11.
254. Ahmad S, Robertson HT, Gloper TA, et al. Kidney Int 1990;38:912–8.

255. van Es A, Henny FC, Kooistra MP, et al. Contrib Nephrol 1992;98:28–35.
256. Golper TA, Ahmad S. Semin Dial 1992;5:94–8.
257. Labonia WD. Am J Kidney Dis 1995;26:757–64.
258. Symposium on Role Dietary Fiber in Health. Am J Clin Nutr 1978;31:S1–291.
259. Parillo M, Riccardi G, Pacioni D, et al. Diabetes Care 1985;8: 620.
260. Anderson JW, Zettwoch N, Feldman T, et al. Arch Intern Med 1988;148:292.
261. Anderson JW, Chen WL. Am J Clin Nutr 1979;32:346.
262. Rampton DS, Cohen SL, Crammond V De B, et al. Clin Nephrol 1984;21:159–63.
262a. Cannata JB, Briggs JD, Junor BJR. Br Med J 1983;286: 1937–8.
263. Sedman AB, Miller NL, Warady BA, et al. Kidney Int 1984; 26:201–4.
264. Nolan CR, Califano JR, Butzin CA. Kidney Int 1990;38: 937–41.
265. Schaefer K, Scheer J, Asmus G, et al. Nephrol Dial Transplant 1991;6:170–5.
266. Mai ML, Emmett M, Sheikh MS, et al. Kidney Int 1989;36: 690–5.
267. Pflanz S, Henderson IS, McElduff N, et al. Nephrol Dial Transplant 1994;9:1121.
268. Kopple JD, Coburn JW. Medicine 1973;52:597–607.
269. Sherrard DJ, Hercz G, Pei Y, et al. Kidney Int 1993;43:436–42.
270. Faugere MC, Malluche HH. Kidney Int 1986;30:717–22.
271. Hercz G, Pei Y, Greenwood C, et al. Kidney Int 1993;44:860–6.
272. Randall RE Jr, Cohen MD, Spray CC Jr, et al. Ann Intern Med 1964;61:73–8.
273. Koomans HA, Roos JC, Boer P, et al. Hypertension 1982; 4:190–7.
274. Lawson DH, Boddy K, King PC, et al. Clin Sci 1971;41:345–51.
275. Chen SM. J Formosan Med Assoc 1990;89:220.
276. Rudolph H, Alfrey AC, Smythe WR. Trans Am Soc Artif Intern Organs 1973;19:456–65.
277. Cartwright GE, Gubler CJ, Wintrobe MM. J Clin Invest 1954; 33:685.
278. Sprenger KBG, Bundschu D, Lewis K, et al. Kidney Int 1983; 24(Suppl 16):S315–8.
279. Mahajan SK, Bowersox EM, Rye DL, et al. Kidney Int 1989;27:S269–73.
280. Mansouri K, Halsted JA, Gombos EA. Arch Intern Med 1970;125:88–93.
281. Mahajan SK, Abraham J, Hessburg T, et al. Kidney Int 1983;24(Suppl 16):S310–4.
282. Antoniou LD, Shalhoub RJ, Sudhakar T, et al. Lancet 1977;2:895–8.
283. Rodger RS, Sheldon WL, Watson MJ, et al. Nephrol Dial Transplant 1989;4:888.
284. Navarro JA, Granadillo VA, Rodriguez-Iturbe B, et al. Clin Nephrol 1991;35:213–7.
285. Jennette JC, Goldman ID. J Lab Clin Med 1975;86:834–43.
286. Spannuth CL Jr, Warnock LG, Wagner C, et al. J Lab Clin Med 1977;90:632–7.
287. Shigetomi S, Kuchel O. Am J Hypertens 1993;6:33–40.
288. Kopple JD, Swendseid ME. Kidney Int 1975;7(Suppl 2):S79–84.
289. Sharman VL, Cunningham J, Goodwin FJ, et al. Br Med J 1982;285:96–7.
290. Kopple JD, Mercurio K, Blumenkrantz MJ, et al. Kidney Int 1981;19:694–704.
291. Balcke P, Schmidt P, Zazgornik J, et al. Ann Intern Med 1984;101:344–5.
292. Pru C, Eaton J, Kjellstrand C. Nephron 1985;39:112–6.
293. Smith FR, Goodman DS. J Clin Invest 1971;50:2426–36.
294. Yatzidis H, Digenis P, Fountas P, et al. Br Med J 1975;3:352–3.
295. Udall JA. JAMA 1965;194:127.
296. Kopple JD, Massry SG. Am J Nephrol 1988;8:437–48.
296a. Reichel H, Koeffler HP, Norman AW. N Engl J Med 1989; 320:980–91.
297. Slatopolsky E, Weerts C, Thielan J, et al. J Clin Invest 1984;74:2136–43.
298. Andress DL, Norris KC. N Engl J Med 1989;321:274–9.
299. May RC, Kelly RA, Mitch WE. J Clin Invest 1987;79:1099–103.
300. Reaich D, Channon SM, Scrimgeour CM, et al. Am J Physiol 1992;263:E735–9.
301. Mault JR, Bartlett RH, Dechert RE, et al. Trans Am Soc Artif Intern Organs 1983;29:390–4.
302. Flugel-Link RM, Salusky IB, Jones MR, et al. Am J Physiol 1983;244:E615–23.
303. Clark AS, Mitch WE. J Clin Invest 1983;72:836–45.
304. Frohlich J, Scholmerich J, Hoppe-Seyler G, et al. Eur J Clin Invest 1974;4:453–8.
305. Feinstein EI, Blumenkrantz MJ, Healy H, et al. Medicine 1981;60:124–37.
306. Feinstein EI, Kopple JD, Silberman H. Kidney Int 1983;26(Suppl 16):S319–23.
307. Kopple JD. JPEN J Parenter Enteral Nutr 1996;20:3–12.
308. Abel RM, Abbott WM, Beck CH Jr, et al. Am J Surg 1974;128:317–23.
309. Abel RM, Shih VE, Abbott WM, et al. Ann Surg 1974;180:350–5.
310. Abel RM, Beck CH Jr, Abbott WM, et al. N Engl J Med 1973;288:695–9.
311. Baek SM, Makabali GG, Bryan-Brown CW, et al. Surg Gynecol Obstet 1975;141:405–8.
312. McMurray SD, Luft FC, Maxwell DR, et al. Arch Intern Med 1978;138:950–5.
313. Leonard CD, Luke RG, Siegel RR. Urology 1975;6:154–7.
314. Kopple JD, Swendseid ME. Am J Clin Nutr 1974;27:806–12.
315. Toback FG. Kidney Int 1977;12:193–8.
316. Toback FG, Teegarden DE, Havener LJ. Kidney Int 1979;15:542–7.
317. Toback FG, Dodd RC, Maier ER, et al. (Abstract). Clin Res 1979;27:432A.
318. Oken DE, Sprinkel FM, Kirschbaum BB, et al. Kidney Int 1980;17:14–23.
319. Nakasaki H, Katayama T, Yokoyama S, et al. JPEN J Parenter Enteral Nutr 1993;17:86–90.
320. Mehta RL. Semin Nephrol 1994;14:64–82.
321. Davenport A, Roberts NB. Crit Care Med 1989;17:1010.
322. Davies SP, Reaveley DA, Brown EA, et al. Crit Care Med 1991;19:1510–5.
323. Feinstein EI, Collins JF, Blumenkrantz MJ, et al. Prog Artif Organs 1984;1:421–6.
324. Kopple JD, Bernard D, Messana J, et al. Kidney Int 1995;47:1148–57.
325. Cerra FB, Upson D, Angelico R, et al. Surgery 1982; 92:192–200.
326. Daly M, Mihranian MH, Kehoe JI, et al. Surgery 1983;94:151–9.
327. Leander U, Fürst P, Vesterberg K, et al. Clin Nutr 1985;4:43–51.
328. Hammarqvist F, Wernerman J, Ruston A, et al. Ann Surg 1989;209:455–61.
329. Stehle P, Zander J, Mertes N, et al. Lancet 1989;1:231–3.
330. Daly JM, Reynolds J, Thom A, et al. Ann Surg 1988; 208:512–23.

331. McCracken BH, Parsons FM. Lancet 1958;2:885–6.
332. Gjorup S, Thaysen JH. Acta Med Scand 1960;167:227–38.
333. Hinton P, Allison SP, Littlejohn S, et al. Lancet 1971;1:767–9.
334. Woolfson AMJ, Healtley RV, Allison SP. N Engl J Med 1979;300:14–7.
335. Ponting GA, Halliday D, Teale JD, et al. Lancet 1988;1:438–40.
336. Wilmore DW. N Engl J Med 1991;325:695.
337. Kopple JD. Miner Electrolyte Metab 1992;18:269–75.
338. Dahn MS, Lange P, Jacobs LA. Arch Surg 1988;123:1409.
339. Miller SB, Martin DB, Kissane J, et al. Proc Natl Acad Sci USA 1992;89:11876–80.
340. Ding H, Kopple JD, Cohen A, et al. J Clin Invest 1993;91:2281–7.
341. Kopple JD, Hirschberg R, Guler H-P, et al. (Abstract). J Am Soc Nephrol 1996;7:1375.
342. Humes HD, Cieslinski DA, Coimbra TM, et al. J Clin Invest 1989;84:1757–61.
343. Miller SB, Martin DR, Kissane J, et al. Am J Physiol 1994;266:F129–34.
344. Siegel NJ, Gaudio KM, Katz LA, et al. Kidney Int 1984;25:906–11.
345. Rahman SN, Kim GE, Mathew AS, et al. Kidney Int 1994;45:1731–8.
346. Siegel NJ, Glazier WB, Chaudry IH, et al. Kidney Int 1980;17:338–49.
347. Kopple JD, Jones MR, Keshaviah PR, et al. Am J Kidney Dis 1995;26:963–81.
348. Harris JA, Benedict FG. A biometric study of basal metabolism. Man. Publ. no. 279. Washington, DC: Carnegie Institute, 1919.
349. Garrel DR, Jobin N, de Jonge LHM. Nutr Clin Pract 1996;11:99–103.
350. Wilmore DW. The metabolic management of the critically ill. New York: Plenum, 1977;314.
351. Kopple JD. Nutritional management of acute renal failure. In: Kopple JD, Massry SG, eds. Nutritional management of renal disease. Baltimore: Williams & Wilkins, 1997;713–53.
352. Askanazi J, Elwyn DH, Silverberg BS, et al. Surgery 1980; 87:596–8.
353. Jeejeebhoy KN, Langer B, Tsallas G, et al. Gastroenterology 1976;71:943–53.
354. Seidner DL, Mascioli EA, Istfan NW, et al. JPEN J Parenter Enteral Nutr 1989;13:614–9.
355. Driscoll DF, Baptista BJ, Bistrian BR, et al. Am J Hosp Pharm 1986;43:416–9.
356. Capelli JP, Kushner H, Camiscioli TC, et al. Am J Kidney Dis 1994;23:808–16.
357. Chertow GM, Ling J, Lew NL, et al. Am J Kidney Dis 1994;24:912–20.
358. Zager RA, Johannes G, Tuttle SE, et al. J Lab Clin Med 1983;101:130–40.
359. Zager RA, Venkatachalam MA. Kidney Int 1983;24:620–5.
360. Malis CD, Racusen C, Solez K, et al. J Lab Clin Med 1984;103:660–76.
361. Andrews PM, Bates SB. Kidney Int 1987;32(Suppl 22):S76–80.
362. Weinberg JM. Semin Nephrol 1990;10:491–500.
363. Daly JM, Reynolds J, Sigal RK, et al. Crit Care Med 1990;18:S86–93.
364. VanBuren CT, Rudolph FB, Kulkarni A, et al. Crit Care Med 1990;18:S114–7.

90. Nutrition, Respiratory Function, and Disease

MARGARET M. JOHNSON, ROBERT CHIN, JR., and EDWARD F. HAPONIK

There has been increasing, although somewhat belated, appreciation of the important relationship between nutritional status and respiratory disease. During the past decade, a number of clinical investigations have appeared to support longstanding anecdotal impressions that nutritional compromise adversely affects the course of patients with diverse respiratory problems and that in some instances, improving nutritional support may complement other beneficial aspects of therapy. Progressively, basic science and clinical investigations are addressing the roles of nutrients in the genesis and modifications of pulmonary disease.

Cellular respiration is essential for normal function of all tissues. Food substrate is converted into usable energy by formation of high-energy phosphate bonds. Oxygen is required for efficient use of nutrients, and carbon dioxide is produced as a byproduct. The respiratory system is responsible for the uptake of oxygen and the elimination of carbon dioxide for the whole organism and can rapidly adjust these gas-exchange functions as necessary in response to dynamically changing metabolic needs. Such immediate adjustments are integrally related to overall substrate use. Moreover, compromise of nutritional status imposes major limits upon respiratory function in health and disease. This chapter provides an overview of the components of the respiratory system, their relationships to nutritional status, and how these interactions are altered by acute and chronic illnesses. In addition, we discuss the impact of nutrition on the epidemiology and pathogenesis of diverse pulmonary diseases and the challenges and potential benefits of nutritional modification in patients with these conditions.

THE RESPIRATORY SYSTEM

The respiratory system consists of *(a)* the lungs, including alveoli and blood vessels (where gas exchange occurs), the supporting structure, and the conducting airways; *(b)* the thoracic cage housing the lungs; *(c)* the respiratory muscles (the pump); *(d)* the central and peripheral nervous systems; and *(e)* the cellular constituents involved in host defense and the metabolic activity of the lungs (Table 90.1). Defects in any of these individual components can lead to clinical disease. The impact of nutritional state on development and progression of disease has only recently been investigated. Selected components of the respiratory system (central control of breathing, respiratory muscles, and the lung itself) are particularly affected by nutritional deficiency.

Control of Breathing

Rhythmic automatic respiration arises from neural input originating in the pontomedullary portion of the brainstem and sets the resting breathing pattern. Abnormal respiratory patterns can reflect a specific anatomic problem at one of the brainstem loci of respiratory neurons. Input from the higher voluntary center, the cerebral cortex, can modify the rate, rhythm, and depth of respiration or interrupt the automaticity to permit voluntary patterns of respiration (e.g., breath holding, cough, tachypnea, bradypnea). Rapid adjustments in the pattern of breathing are required to adapt to the changing metabolic demands of the organism. Feedback from the periphery allows integration of peripheral needs of the organism with the central output. Such adjustments maintain the acid/base and respirable gas (oxygen and carbon dioxide) balance within a narrow range. Thus, while higher centers set the automaticity of the respiratory system, peripheral receptors modify this pattern to accommodate metabolic needs. These intricate relationships enable the respiratory system to appropriately adjust bulk gas exchange.

The peripheral chemoreceptors (carotid and aortic bodies) respond to changes in the arterial partial pressure of oxygen (Pao_2), arterial partial pressure of carbon dioxide ($Paco_2$) and arterial pH. Reduced Pao_2 and pH and elevated $Paco_2$ result in increased chemoreceptor activity and respiratory stimulation. In humans, the carotid bodies are the dominant chemoreceptors (1). Central chemoreceptors located in the medulla respond to changes in cerebral spinal fluid pH (which reflects changes in the $Paco_2$,) but not to changes in Pao_2. Like the peripheral chemoreceptors, central chemoreceptors stimulate an increase in minute ventilation (the volume of gas inspired in a

Table 90.1
The Respiratory System

Central and peripheral nervous system
Control of breathing
Respiratory muscles
The "pump"
Thoracic Cage
Lungs
Conducting airways
Terminal respiratory unit and alveoli
Pulmonary vasculature
Supporting structures
Trafficking cells
Host defense cells

minute, V_e) (Table 90.2) in the presence of acidemia or hypercapnia but are slower to react to changes in the arterial blood.

Other sensors are located in the lungs, upper airways, and respiratory muscles and influence breathing in diverse ways. For the most part, receptors in the lungs and upper airways respond to focal conformational changes and irritant stimuli. They are important in originating the cough reflex, coordinating the upper and lower airway caliber, controlling inspiration and expiration, and producing and secreting mucus. The role of the sensors in respiratory muscle is unclear, but they may contribute to the balance between agonist and antagonist muscle groups, posture, and the sensation of dyspnea. Final integration of afferent and efferent information takes place in the spinal cord, from which segmental motoneurons destined for the respiratory muscles carry the fully integrated message.

Respiratory Muscles

Normally, at rest, inspiration is active and expiration occurs passively with relaxation of the inspiratory muscles.

Table 90.2
Definitions of Respiratory Physiology Terms and Abbreviations

Tidal volume (V_t): volume of gas moved during a single inspiration
Minute ventilation (V_E): total amount of air moved in and out of the lungs in one minute: V_E = Vt × respiratory rate (RR) in breaths per minute
Dead-space ventilation: inspired gas that does not participate in gas exchange because it does not reach alveoli that are perfused
V_d/V_t: fraction of each tidal volume that is dead space
Alveolar minute ventilation (V_A): amount of inspired air able to participate in gas exchange; alveolar ventilation is the difference between total minute ventilation and dead-space ventilation. $V_A = RR \times V_t - RR \times V_d = RR \times Vt\,(1 - V_d/V_t)$
Forced vital capacity (FVC): the volume of gas that can be forcibly exhaled after a maximal inhalation
Forced expiratory volume in one second (FEV_1): the volume of air expired within the first second of a forced expiration
Cardiac output (CO): the volume of blood pumped by the heart in one minute; the product of stroke volume and heart rate
Pao_2: partial pressure of oxygen in the arterial blood
$Paco_2$: partial pressure of carbon dioxide in the arterial blood
Vo_2: oxygen consumption (mL/min)
Vco_2: carbon dioxide production (mL/min)

With increased ventilatory demands, however, expiration may become an active process. Contraction of the inspiratory muscles leads to expansion of the thoracic cage, resulting in negative intrathoracic pressure (Boyle's law)

$$PV = K$$

where P is the pressure of a gas, V is volume, and K is a constant). Airflow is initiated when a pressure gradient develops between the opening of the respiratory system, the mouth, which is at atmospheric pressure and the alveoli, in which pressures become subatmospheric with inspiration. Inspiratory flow ceases when these pressures attain equilibrium. Return of the thoracic cage to its resting position by relaxation of the inspiratory muscles reverses the pressure gradient and leads to exhalation.

The muscles of the respiratory "pump" are the diaphragm, the intercostal and accessory muscles, and the abdominal muscles. The diaphragm is the major inspiratory muscle and anatomically separates the thoracic cavity from the abdominal cavity. It is composed of striated skeletal muscle with a rich vascular supply and a central tendon. At rest, it is dome shaped. With each contraction, the diaphragm flattens and descends, raising the lower ribs in the zone of apposition. This increases both the vertical and anterior-posterior dimensions of the thoracic cage and causes a decrease in intrathoracic pressure (Fig. 90.1). Although this muscle contracts rhythmically during the lifetime, it does not have intrinsic automaticity like the smooth muscle of the heart. The chest wall and abdominal muscles may also assist with inspiration and forced exhalation.

Like other skeletal muscle groups, the respiratory muscles are subject to fatigue from an imbalance between supply and demand. Roussos and Macklem defined muscle fatigue as a reversible inability of a muscle to continue to generate prior attainable force (2), whereas respiratory muscle weakness is the chronic inability of the muscle to attain adequate force. Both respiratory muscle fatigue and weakness can result in failure of the muscles to produce sufficient force to support continuous gas exchange in and out of the lung. Clinically, hypercapnic respiratory failure and, subsequently, hypercapnic and hypoxemic respiratory failure result from the respiratory system's incapacity to meet metabolic demands. Respiratory muscle fatigue may be central (resulting from loss of appropriate central neural drive), transmissional (resulting from reversible impairment of neural impulses through the nerves or across the neuromuscular junction), or peripheral (due to primary failure of muscle performance). Nutritional deficiencies affect primarily central and peripheral muscle fatigue.

Both fatigue and weakness have obvious, important relationships to nutritional status. The diaphragm and other respiratory muscles are composed of type I and type II muscle fibers. Type I fibers are slow-twitch fibers that require a longer period of time after stimulation to reach peak tension, have high levels of oxidative enzymatic capacity which makes them more resistant to fatigue, and

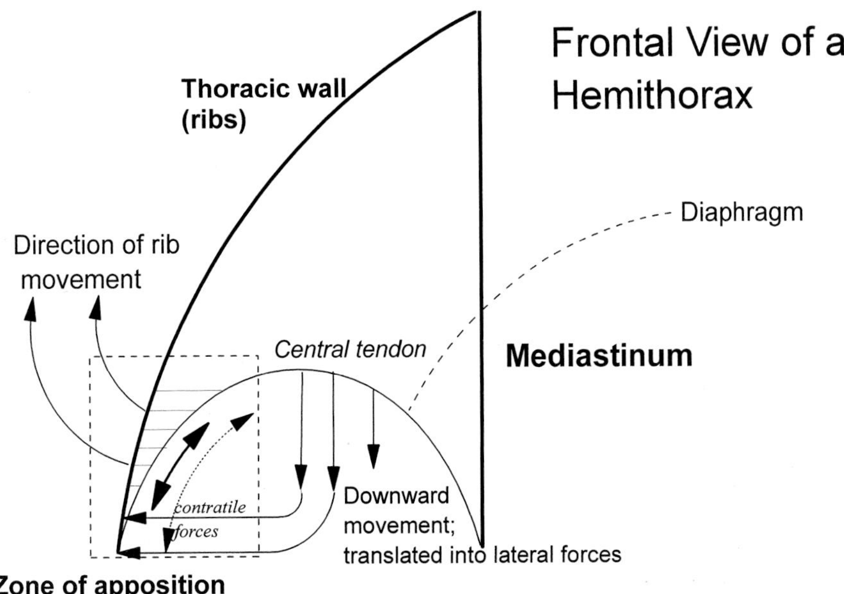

Figure 90.1. The diaphragm. Contraction of the diaphragm causes downward descent of the dome of the diaphragm. Contraction of the fibers that insert on the ribs, causes the ribs to lift and rotate outward. Additionally, the descent of the diaphragm increases the intraabdominal pressure leading to lateral outward movement of the lower thoracic cage. The net result is expansion of the thoracic cavity in both the vertical and horizontal dimensions.

are recruited earlier than type II, fast-twitch fibers. Type II fibers have relatively higher levels of glycolytic enzymes and less oxidative enzymatic capacity. Type II muscle fibers can generate a greater peak force than the type I fibers but are more easily fatigued.

The differential effects of malnutrition upon these two fiber types has been well studied. Lewis et al. studied rats subjected to 6 weeks of undernutrition (reduction of body weight to 50% of expected body weight) and found a significant reduction in the cross-sectional area of both types of fibers in the animal's diaphragm, but the fast-twitch fibers were quantitatively more affected (3). Goldspink and Ward (4) and Oldfors et al. (5) reported greater atrophy of fast-twitch fibers than of slow-twitch fibers in animal skeletal muscle preparations with malnutrition and protein-deficient nutrition, respectively. The fast-twitch fibers containing less oxidative enzymatic capacity were more affected than those fast twitch fibers with greater amounts of oxidative enzymes. Sieck et al. found that fatigue resistance was actually improved in an in vitro nerve-muscle-strip preparation from diaphragms of nutritionally deprived rats (daily food access restricted to one-third of estimated daily consumption until body weight was approximately 50% of the controls), despite a significant reduction in the cross-sectional area of both fibers (6). Type II fibers were selectively more affected than type I fibers (6). No change was noted in the oxidative capacity of the muscle fibers (6). These authors felt that the increase in fatigue resistance was most likely related to selective atrophy of the more fatiguable type II fibers (6). These observations suggest that malnutrition would result clinically in diminished peak-pressure generation by the respiratory muscles, with little or no effect on endurance.

However, in physiologic terms, inspiratory muscle fatigue can be predicted by the length of time in each respiratory cycle that the muscles are in active contraction and the ratio of tension developed to peak tension. Bellemare and Grassino defined the product of the ratio of inspiratory time to the total respiratory cycle (T_i/T_{tot}) and the ratio of diaphragmatic pressure generation to peak pressure (Pdi/Pdi_{max}) as the tension time index (7)

$$TTdi = Pdi/Pdi_{max} \times Ti/T_{tot}$$

In both normal subjects and patients with chronic airflow obstruction, a TTdi above 0.15 is associated with electromyographic evidence of diaphragmatic fatigue (7, 8). Therefore, any mechanism that increases Pdi/Pdi_{max}, Ti/T_{tot}, or both can lead to respiratory muscle fatigue. If the peak pressure that can be generated is reduced, any given pressure produced during the inspiratory cycle represents a greater percentage of the reduced peak pressure than of a normal peak pressure. Thus, if malnutrition contributes to a decline in peak pressure, the pressure required for a normal tidal breath represents a larger proportion of the "lower" peak pressure and can result in inspiratory muscle fatigue. Even if adaptation then leads to a lower inspiratory pressure per breath, the tidal volume (V_t, resting inspiratory volume) would have to fall, assuming lung mechanics remain the same. Therefore, to maintain the same minute ventilation

$$V_e = V_t \times RR$$

where *RR* is the respiratory rate in breaths per minute, the respiratory rate would have to increase, which would shorten each respiratory cycle and, given a static inspiratory time, increase T_i/T_{tot}. Again, this could lead to respiratory muscle fatigue.

Although diseases that primarily affect the respiratory muscles are much less common than those affecting the lung itself, the respiratory muscles are important as a compensating mechanism. Despite major alterations in the lung parenchyma or communicating airways, adequate gas exchange at the alveolar capillary membrane may still occur as long as an increase in bulk air exchange can offset the deficiencies. In fibrotic lung diseases, the elastic load to respiratory muscles is increased, whereas in obstructive airways diseases, the resistive load is increased. If the respiratory muscles can overcome such increased loads without fatigue, even though the work of breathing is markedly increased, function may be preserved. Unfortunately, with advancing disease or increased demand (e.g., in exercise), the imposed loads exceed the compensatory limits of the respiratory muscles, ultimately compromising the patient's functional status.

Lungs

The lungs comprise the conducting airways, the gas-exchange organ (alveoli and pulmonary capillary bed), the supporting structural elements, the pulmonary and bronchial vasculature, and trafficking immune effector cells.

Tracheobronchial Tree

The conducting airways are a series of dichotomously branching structures extending from the proximal main airway (the trachea) to the periphery (alveoli). There are two major types; the bronchi or cartilaginous airways and the bronchioles, noncartilaginous or membranous airways. As the bronchioles further divide toward the periphery, they are subdivided into nonrespiratory and respiratory bronchioles. The latter contain alveoli and participate in gas exchange as well as conduct the gas stream to more distal gas-exchange units (alveolar ducts and alveoli).

The airways not only conduct the gas to the alveoli but also further condition it (humidifying, warming, and filtering) through specialized bronchial epithelial cells and bronchial submucosal glands. The bronchial epithelium consists of ciliated columnar cells that sweep inhaled particles, by coordinated beating of the cilia, proximally for removal ("mucociliary elevator"). Other cell types include mucous and serous cells partially responsible for producing mucus that helps entrap particles for the ciliary elevator; basal and intermediate cells that migrate toward the surface to replace the luminal epithelial cells; argyrophil cells, which may have endocrine properties; and Clara cells found in the distal respiratory bronchioles, which may contribute to the luminal liquid lining (1). The submucosal bronchial glands contribute to the bronchial mucous layer and are most frequent in the medium-sized bronchi (1). In response to chronic irritation (e.g., chronic bronchitis), they can increase their output and size, thus narrowing the airway lumen.

Smooth muscle is found throughout the walls of the tracheobronchial tree. Muscle contraction imparts rigidity to the airways (1) and reduces the caliber of the airway lumen. Innervation is primarily through the parasympathetic and the nonadrenergic, noncholinengic nervous pathways, but receptors are present for other neurotransmitters. Gas flows through the tracheobronchial tree down a pressure gradient. Airflow is inversely related to the airway resistance, which in turn is inversely related to the fourth power of the radius of the tracheobronchial tube.

Terminal Respiratory Unit

The terminal respiratory unit consists of respiratory bronchioles, alveolar ducts, and alveoli. The total surface area of the alveoli in a normal human adult is estimated to be 140 m^2 (1). Gas exchange occurs at the alveolar-capillary membrane, which consists of the alveolar epithelium and capillary endothelium and their basement membranes, the tissue and cellular components of the contiguous interstitial space, and the surfactant lining (1). Surfactant, a complex phospholipid and protein mixture produced by the alveolar epithelium (type II pneumocyte), lines the alveolar airspace. Surfactant reduces the surface tension of the alveolus at the air interface, which decreases the tendency of the airway to collapse and thus maintains alveolar stability at low lung volumes.

Pulmonary Physiology

The ultimate purpose of the respiratory system is to facilitate transfer of O_2 from inspired gas to the bloodstream and CO_2 from blood to expirable gases. This exchange occurs at the alveolar-capillary interface. O_2-poor blood returns from the peripheral circulation to the right side of the heart where it is pumped through the pulmonary vasculature to the pulmonary capillaries. At the alveolar-capillary level, oxygen diffuses down a concentration gradient from the alveoli to the capillary blood. Most of the O_2 binds to and fully saturates hemoglobin in red blood cells; a small amount dissolves in the plasma. Simultaneously, CO_2 leaves the blood and enters the alveoli across a concentration gradient in the opposite direction. Inspired air, at sea level, has a partial pressure of O_2 of 160 torr (1 torr = 1 mm Hg) and a partial pressure of CO_2 of 0 torr. After hydration and mixing with the resident gas in the alveoli the normal partial pressures of O_2 and CO_2 in the terminal respiratory units and alveoli are approximately 100 and 40 torr, respectively. The partial pressures of O_2 and CO_2 in the capillary blood entering the gas exchange area are 40 and 46 torr, respectively; therefore, the driving pressure for O_2 is normally 60 torr, and for CO_2, 6 torr. Equilibrium between alveolar gas and entering capillary blood is achieved within the first 0.25 seconds of the total capillary transit time of 0.75 seconds at rest (1).

Implied in this system is rapid replenishment of fresh gas to alveoli to match the arrival of desaturated, CO_2-loaded blood to the alveolar-capillary unit. As described above, inspired gas enters the lungs when negative intrathoracic pressure is generated by respiratory muscle contraction. However, not all of an inspired breath can participate in gas exchange. About 30% of each breath remains in the conducting airways, which conduct gas to the lung parenchyma but do not participate in gas exchange. These large non-gas-exchanging airways are collectively termed *the anatomic dead space.* Some inspired gas also reaches alveoli that are not perfused and hence cannot participate in gas exchange. This volume is the physiologic dead space. Together, the anatomic and physiologic dead space make up the total dead space. Minute alveolar ventilation (V_A) is the difference between total minute ventilation and total dead space ventilation, that is, the portion of the tidal volume that participates in gas exchange times the respiratory rate (Table 90.2). This can be regarded as the "effective" minute ventilation.

Impairment of the fresh supply of gas to match perfusion of alveoli limits efficient gas exchange. The gas supply can be impaired by obstructed airflow (increased airway resistance) or limited expansion of the lungs (decreased compliance). These obstacles lead to ventilation and perfusion mismatch. When perfused alveoli are not ventilated, deoxygenated blood from these areas mixes with oxygen-saturated blood, reducing total oxygen content. This results in arterial hypoxemia and represents shunt physiology. Ventilation/perfusion mismatches ranging between the extremes of shunt and dead space ventilation have variable impact on overall gas exchange. Mechanical alterations increase the work of breathing, not only from the need to overcome increased airway resistance or decreased lung compliance, but also from the compensatory mechanisms (usually increased V_e) required to meet the continuing metabolic demands of the individual. Eventually, when metabolic demand exceeds respiratory reserve, gas exchange abnormalities appear.

In addition to its gas-exchange functions, the lung acts as a "filter" for blood and has extensive metabolic functions, including synthesis of surfactant, various proteins (both structural and enzymatic), and humoral substances (arachidonic acid metabolites, histamine, substance P, and vasoactive intestinal protein) and transformation of biochemical substances (1). Relatively little is known about the effects of altered nutrition is these areas.

In a broad sense, pulmonary diseases can be categorized on the basis of their primary physiologic abnormalities as obstructive airflow diseases or restrictive diseases, and either can be acute or chronic (Fig. 90.2). With

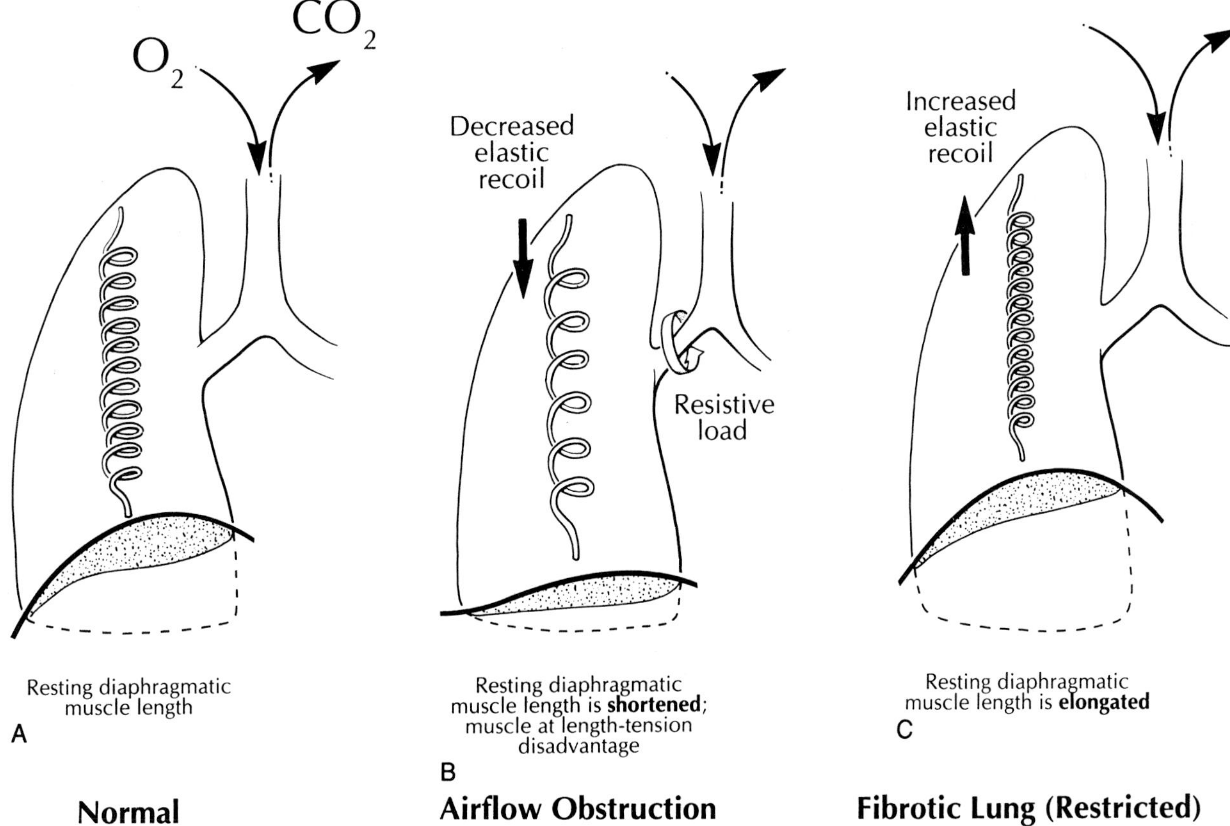

Figure 90.2. Normal (**A**), obstructive (**B**) and fibrotic (**C**) lungs. *Obstructive (B):* Airflow obstruction leads to an increased resistive load for the respiratory muscles to overcome. In emphysema, elastic recoil is lost because of destruction of multiple alveolar-capillary units. As expiratory flow is limited, the lungs become hyperinflated and flatten the normal curvature of the diaphragm. This places the diaphragm at a mechanical disadvantage by the shortened resting length of the diaphragm. The work of breathing is increased because of the increased resistive load and relative inefficiency of the respiratory muscles because of the shortened resting length. *Fibrotic (C):* Increased elastic recoil (decreased compliance of the lung) places an elastic load on the respiratory muscles and thus increases the work of breathing.

obstructive airflow disease, the primary problem is maintaining adequate V_A to match perfusion and allow adequate gas exchange in the setting of increased airflow resistance. The resulting ventilation/perfusion mismatch causes hypoxemia. CO_2 excretion is maintained initially by increased V_A; but if the V_A cannot increase or decreases, CO_2 excretion falls and the $Paco_2$ rises. In disease processes marked by decreased lung compliance (e.g., pulmonary fibrosis or air-space filling diseases such as pneumonia and pulmonary edema), loss of functioning alveolar-capillary units with varying degrees of ventilation/perfusion mismatch leads to hypoxemia. Compensation again occurs, usually with an increased respiratory rate to replenish alveolar oxygen stores, but the V_t may fall because of the increased work to inflate stiffer lungs; a greater pressure must be generated to achieve a given change of lung volume. If the process progresses or the respiratory reserve is diminished (e.g., respiratory muscle fatigue), CO_2 elimination decreases and $Paco_2$ rises, leading to hypercapnic, hypoxemic respiratory failure.

Arterial blood gas determinations at rest or with exertion can provide a guide to the efficiency of gas exchange. Pulmonary function tests that measure exhaled gas volumes and flow rates can identify abnormal lung compliance and airflow obstruction. The forced vital capacity (FVC), the volume of gas that can be forcibly exhaled after a maximal inhalation, reflects total lung volume. The forced expiratory volume in 1 second (FEV_1), the volume of gas that is forcefully exhaled in 1 second, can be reduced in both obstructive and restrictive lung diseases. This value allows quantitative information about both total lung volume and airflow resistance, since it is a timed maneuver. In restrictive lung diseases, the FEV_1 and the FVC are proportionally reduced, resulting in a normal FEV_1:FVC ratio; in obstructive diseases, the FEV_1 is reduced, but the FVC remains normal, resulting in a decrease in the FEV_1:FVC ratio, the hallmark of clinically important airflow obstruction.

Pulmonary function testing objectively reveals the presence and severity of respiratory diseases and has important implications for nutritional research investigations. Objective changes in lung volumes, flow rates, and respiratory muscle strength are commonly assessed endpoints when examining the effects of dietary modifications. The relevance of respiratory muscle function and exercise performance status to dyspnea and limitations in daily function have made measures of maximal inspiratory pressure (MIP), maximal expiratory pressure (MEP), walking distance (12-min walk), or more-comprehensive exercise testing valuable in assessing effects of nutritional supplementation. Terms used in these common physiologic indicators of lung and respiratory muscle function are defined in Table 90.2.

EFFECTS OF MALNUTRITION ON RESPIRATORY SYSTEM DEVELOPMENT, STRUCTURE, AND FUNCTION

Both laboratory investigations and clinical studies suggest that the major adverse effects of malnutrition upon the respiratory system are in respiratory muscle structure and function, ventilatory drive, and host immune defenses (Table 90.3). Appropriate nutritional support may reverse these effects. Malnutrition may affect adversely lung architecture, surfactant production, and reparative ability.

Developmental Effects

Both animal and human studies suggest that undernutrition during development can profoundly alter the structure and function of various organs. Fetal malnutrition in rats and guinea pigs can result in pulmonary hypoplasia (9, 10). Protein deprivation in developing rats can diminish collagen and elastin synthesis and simulate a defect pathologically similar to emphysema (11). Manifestations of developmental nutritional insults depend upon when they occur. Investigations in animal models showed that early undernutrition leads to small but normally proportioned animals, whereas later insults result in lungs that are disproportionately small for body size (12). In humans, airway division to the level of the terminal bronchiole is completed by gestational week 16; between weeks 17 and 20, a tremendous growth of lung cells occurs (12). Various authors have described associations between low birth weight and subsequent decreases in pulmonary function (13, 14). FEV_1 (adjusted for age and height) is directly related to birth weight, and mortality rates from chronic airflow obstruction are inversely related to birth weight (14). Rona et al. examined relationships between birth weight, gestational age, respiratory symptoms, and lung function in an attempt to define the independent effects of prematurity and intrauterine growth retardation (15). They found that birth weight corrected for gestational age correlated with measures of lung function whereas prematurity did not. Symptoms of wheezing and cough, however, correlated with prematurity (15).

Table 90.3
Respiratory Complications of Malnutrition

Established
Decreased respiratory muscle structure and function
Decreased ventilatory drive
Decreased pulmonary host immune defenses
Proposed
Altered lung architecture, especially in immature animals
Decreased ability to repair after injury
Decreased surfactant production

Effects on Respiratory Muscles

Studies based on animal models showed a linear correlation between diaphragm weight and body weight (16, 17). One investigation of the effects of a short-term fast in young rats leading to a 28% loss of body weight demonstrated a proportional loss in diaphragmatic weight (18). Similar correlation exists between body weight and diaphragm weight in normal humans (19) and persons with emphysema (20). Poorly nourished patients (body weights of 71 ± 6% of ideal body weight–based height and sex from Metropolitan Life Insurance tables) had diminished respiratory muscle strength, manifested by reductions in both MIP and MEP (21). The extent of muscle mass loss could not fully account for the disproportionately severe decline in respiratory muscle strength, and it was suggested that poor nutritional status could also result in possible myopathy of the remaining muscles (21). Although the effects of underlying disease (such as malignancy) cannot be excluded as contributing factors in this study, these observations suggest a clinical correlate to the anatomic findings.

Effect on Ventilatory Drive

Normal human subjects limited to a 500-kcal carbohydrate diet exhibit a decrease in both hypoxic ventilatory drive and metabolic rate (22), with significant correlation between the two (22). With refeeding, the hypoxic ventilatory response normalized (22). Normal male volunteers given only a daily infusion of 3 L of a 5% amino acid solution (550 kcal/day) for 10 days to maintain nitrogen balance had a lower hypoxic ventilatory drive than controls given a daily infusion of 3 L of 5% amino acid solution supplemented with 500 mL of 10% safflower oil emulsion (1100 kcal/day) (23). This suggests that a minimum caloric intake is necessary to preserve the normal ventilatory drive in semistarvation (23). However, neither study demonstrated significant alteration in the hypercapnic response in semistarvation. Conversely, in normal volunteers, after an overnight fast, enteral protein feeding (1000 kcal of egg albumin) caused the normal ventilatory response slope to CO_2 to rise, but the CO_2 response was unaffected by a carbohydrate meal (1000 kcal of a glucose solution); both feedings increased both resting metabolism and the hypoxic ventilatory response (24).

Both low V_e and low mouth occlusion pressure occurred in response to hypercapnea in a patient with severe anorexia nervosa who weighed 46% of ideal body weight (25). Mouth occlusion pressure correlates with the intensity of phrenic nerve stimulation and reflects the output of the respiratory center. Taken together, these data suggest that both abnormalities of central control of breathing and muscle weakness contributed to the abnormal response to hypercapnea (25). Refeeding can completely reverse the abnormalities seen with anorexia nervosa (25, 26).

Effect on Host Defenses

Along with a general susceptibility to infections, malnourished (both protein- and calorie-deficient) individuals are likely to develop alterations in pulmonary defense mechanisms. In infant rats, protein-calorie malnutrition reduced T lymphocyte–dependent alveolar macrophage function, although neutrophil-dependent alveolar macrophage function was preserved (27). In adult rats, effects of malnutrition on alveolar macrophage function are conflicting. One study recovered a reduced number of alveolar macrophages by bronchoalveolar lavage but showed normal phagocytic function in protein-restricted adult rats (28). In another investigation, more-severe starvation resulted in reduction in both alveolar macrophage phagocytosis and microbial killing (29). Protein-calorie malnutrition did not inhibit macrophage adherence or bacterial killing but did change the profile of inflammatory mediators produced by alveolar macrophages (30). Gram-negative bacterial adherence and colonization of the lower respiratory mucosa correlates inversely with nutritional status in tracheostomized patients (31). In malnourished patients with chronic obstructive pulmonary disease (COPD), absolute lymphocyte counts and reactivity to common skin test antigens improved with refeeding and weight gain, suggesting a link between these parameters (32). Malnourished subjects exhibit decreased tidal volumes and number of sighs leading to alveolar collapse (atelectasis) and inadequate clearance of secretions, which in turn may predispose to pulmonary infection (33). Studies in animals also suggest that adequate nutrition may be important in maintaining normal lung repair and structure (34) and surfactant production, but the clinical relevance of these observations is unclear.

PROTOTYPIC DISEASES OF THE LUNGS: RELATIONSHIPS TO NUTRITIONAL STATUS

Diseases of the pulmonary system can be grouped into those that cause acute alterations in normal function and those that cause chronic changes. The potential benefits, hazards, and clinical priorities of nutritional care differ in these settings. In acute lung injury, the general goal of nutritional support is to meet the expanded requirements of a hypercatabolic state to prevent protein breakdown. In chronic obstructive lung disease, emphasis is placed on maintaining respiratory muscle strength, mass, and function in an effort to optimize the patient's overall performance status and meet the demands of daily activities. In this section, we review acute respiratory failure and COPD as examples of the complex interactions of nutritional status and commonly encountered respiratory diseases.

Acute Lung Injury

Acute lung injury can result from a simple localized lung infection (pneumonia) or from a systemic process that leads to diffuse alveolar damage as seen with the acute respiratory distress syndrome (ARDS). Most acute respiratory illnesses are associated with the systemic symptoms of anorexia, fatigue, and malaise. When these are combined with cough and/or dyspnea, oral intake is generally poor. Patients with severe lung injury may require endotracheal intubation and mechanically assisted ventilation that precludes adequate oral intake. Acute lung injury often occurs in the setting of multisystem organ failure (MSOF) due to sepsis or trauma, conditions associated with a hypercatabolic state. The combination of decreased oral intake and increased metabolic demand can lead to negative nitrogen balance with decreased respiratory muscle strength because of protein catabolism, diminished ventilatory drive, and altered immune function (35). Nutritional support can potentially alleviate this imbalance between metabolic supply and demand.

Giner et al. prospectively evaluated the impact of malnutrition on outcome in an ICU population and found that patients who were malnourished at admission (defined by serum albumin levels and height:weight ratios) had a significantly higher incidence of complications and were less likely to be discharged from the hospital (36). Bartlett et al. showed that negative caloric balance postoperatively (measured by indirect calorimetry) correlated significantly with MSOF in 57 surgical patients (37). However, despite these correlations, optimal strategies for nutritional support have not been established.

Metabolic Requirements

The metabolic responses and requirements imposed by severe lung injury (e.g., ARDS) are similar to those associated with sepsis, trauma, major injury, or burns and differ from the normal fasting state. In ARDS, the degree of metabolic alteration depends more on the underlying insult than on the extent of lung injury because ARDS represents only the pulmonary response to an underlying local or distant injury. In the phase characterized by hypercatabolism, negative nitrogen balance generally occurs. Carbohydrate metabolism is altered; hyperglycemia results from increased glucose turnover because of relative insulin "resistance" with expanded hepatic gluconeogenesis and an excess of counterregulatory hormones (glucagon, epinephrine, and cortisol) (38). Fat oxidation appears to be preferred and may be the main caloric source in the stressed patient (39). However in shock states and MSOF, fat may be poorly used and may accumulate (38). Muscle proteolysis develops to maintain a steady glucose supply to the brain, leading to negative nitrogen balance (40). (See Chapter 96.)

The best method of determining energy requirements in the critically ill patient is not yet established. Energy requirements can be measured at bedside by indirect calorimetry or estimated using the Harris-Benedict equation (Table 90.4). Oxygen consumption (Vo_2) can be used

Table 90.4
Estimates of Energy Requirements

1. $EE = Vo_2 \times 4.7$ kcal/l $\times$ 1440 min/day
   or
   $EE = (3.9 \times VO_2 + 1.1 \times Vco_2) \times 1.44$
2. Harris-Benedict equation
   Females:
   $BEE = 655 + (4.3 \times wt\ (lb)] + [4.3 \times ht(in) - [4.7 \times age]$
   Males:
   $BEE = 65 + [6.2 \times wt(lb) + [12.7 \times ht(in) - [6.8 \times age)$

as an estimate of caloric use and can be calculated using the Fick equation

$$Vo_2 = CO \times (CaO_2 - CvO_2)$$

where CO is the cardiac output, CaO_2 is oxygen content of arterial blood and CvO_2 is the mixed venous content of blood. The disadvantages of this approach are the requirement for a pulmonary artery catheter to sample mixed venous blood, the need for a relatively stable patient, the inherent inaccuracies of using multiple measurements with their own standards of error to calculate a final product, and the intermittent timing of measurements. Despite these limitations, Liggett et al. found an excellent correlation (r = 0.90) between the calculated resting energy expenditure

$$REE = Vo_2 \times 4.86 \text{ kcal/L}$$

using the Fick method and the results of the gas-exchange method of calorimetry in 19 stable patients (41).

Alternatively, Vo_2 can be assessed by means of a metabolic cart (the gas-exchange method). This approach requires the technical ability to measure exhaled gases directly and is not universally available. Problems related to its use include availability, the need for skilled technicians trained to operate the analyzer, a leak-free system, a stable F_IO_2 (fraction of inspired oxygen), and expensive instrumentation. In addition, at the high F_IO_2 ($\geq$0.80) often required in patients with severe hypoxemic respiratory failure, the assumptions made in the derivation of the Vo_2 by this method begin to fail (42). Nevertheless, if it can be performed accurately, this approach can be used continuously and represents a more "direct" measurement. The Vo_2 (mL/min) obtained by either method is converted to kilocalories per day by simply using the caloric value of oxygen (4.69–5.05 kcal/L of O_2 consumed) based on a nonprotein respiratory quotient (RQ) (27) or by using the modified Weir equation if the Vco_2 (CO_2 production) is also known (42) (Table 90.4)

$$\text{Energy expenditure } (EE) = (3.9\ Vo_2 + 1.1\ Vco_2) \times 1.44$$

Another estimate of the resting energy requirement can be derived from standard regression formulas based on various population studies. The most common formula used is the Harris-Benedict equation (Table 90.4) (43). The regression equation was derived from studies on normal subjects at rest (43) and was not designed to address the stress and hypercatabolism seen in many disease states, especially those encountered in the critical care setting. Therefore, "stress factors" have been developed for certain commonly seen clinical scenarios. These range from 1.2 times the calculated REE for elective surgery (42) to 1.5 or more times the REE for burn patients (44). However, the correlation between the measured REE by indirect calorimetry and that predicted from the Harris-Benedict equation has been found to be only moderate in postoperative, hemodynamically stable, noncomatose but critically ill patients requiring mechanical ventilation (Fig. 90.3) (45). More recently, Ligget and Renfro have shown that in nonseptic mechanically ventilated medical ICU patients, the Harris-Benedict equation satisfactorily predicted the energy expenditure (EE) using the Fick method of determining Vo_2 without modification or stress factors (46). In patients with sepsis, the energy requirements were approximately 20% more than those predicted from the Harris-Benedict equation (46).

Because there are potential inherent complications of both underfeeding and overfeeding, proper estimation of caloric requirements is particularly important in patients with acute lung injury. Overfeeding can lead to fluid overload, glucose intolerance, fatty infiltration of the liver (with either parenteral or enteral feedings), diarrhea (with enteral feedings), net lipogenesis increasing the V_e demand secondary to increases in the net VCO_2 (CO_2 production), and an increase in the baseline REE due to diet-induced thermogenesis (DIT). Underestimation of caloric needs can lead to underfeeding and negative nitrogen balance with muscle proteolysis. Clinical evidence suggests that malnutrition has detrimental effects on pulmonary mechanics by impairing ventilatory drive, respiratory muscle function, and normal lung defense mechanisms (35), thereby increasing the need for mechanical assistance. Nutritional supplementation may aid in weaning patients with respiratory failure from mechanical ventilation (47, 48).

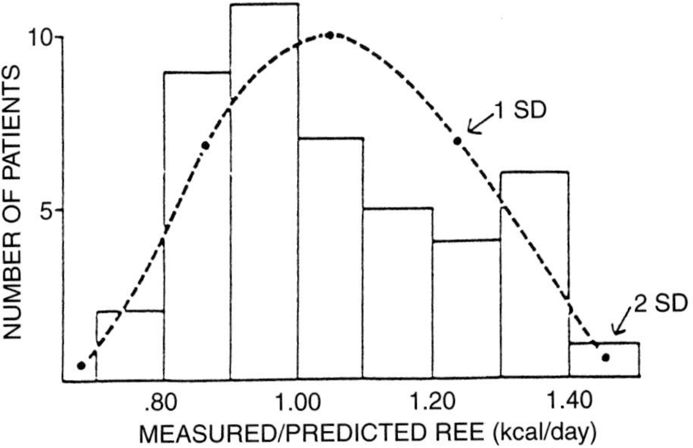

Figure 90.3. Distribution of the ratio of measured resting energy expenditure (REE) by indirect calorimetry to the predicted energy requirement using the Harris-Benedict equation in mechanically ventilated, postoperative, critically ill patients who were hemodynamically stable and noncomatose. Perfect correlation would have a value of 1.00. (From Weissman C, Kemper M, Askanazi J, et al. Anesthesiology 1986;64:673–9.)

Substrate Supplementation: Implications for Ventilatory Requirements

Nutritional supplementation can be in the form of protein, carbohydrate, or fat. The nutritional characteristics of these substrates are detailed in Chapters 2, 3, and 4. This chapter discusses the relative merits of these substrates as they relate to pulmonary diseases.

Most patients with acute respiratory failure who require mechanical ventilation are in a hypercatabolic state and will break down their protein stores to meet immediate metabolic needs. In addition, glucose-dependent tissue (brain, red blood cells, and healing wounds) requirements are met through gluconeogenesis from amino acids if glucose supplies are limited (49). Inhibition of glucose neosynthesis with protein sparing can be accomplished in normal fasting patients by administration of 100 g of glucose/day. By contrast, injured or septic patients may require up to 600 g or more (50). Intravenous fat emulsions can also spare protein if administered with at least 500 kcal/day of carbohydrate calories (either glycerol or glucose) (51). Exogenous protein administration can also replace endogenous protein stores as a substrate for gluconeogenesis and limit proteolysis (51). Protein supplementation may increase oxygen consumption (thermic effect of protein) (52), V_e (52), and the ventilatory response to hypercarbia and hypoxemia (24). Clinically, a high-protein diet could result in increased dyspnea in patients with an already augmented respiratory drive and/or those with borderline respiratory reserve. Because of the integral role of protein in normal physiologic and cellular function (e.g., structural support, enzyme activity, transport, receptor activity, and messenger activity), protein sparing is essential to recovery from any insult.

The appropriate mix of substrate (protein, carbohydrate, or fat) delivered depends on the clinical state and the desired goals. In acute or chronic respiratory failure where respiratory reserve is limited, carbohydrates impose a greater demand on the respiratory system than the other substrates because more CO_2 is produced during its oxidation. For every molecule of glucose completely oxidized, six molecules of CO_2 are produced, giving a respiratory quotient (RQ = molecule of O_2 used/molecule of CO_2 produced) of 1. On the other hand, the RQ of fat is 0.7 (less CO_2 produced for every molecule of O_2 consumed) and the RQ of protein is 0.8 (see Chapter 5). Therefore, more CO_2 is produced for the lung to eliminate in oxidizing carbohydrate than fat or protein (Fig. 90.4) (53). The partial pressure of arterial CO_2 is determined by the relationship

$$Paco_2 = K(Vco_2/V_A)$$

where K is a constant, Vco_2 is CO_2 production, and V_A is alveolar minute ventilation

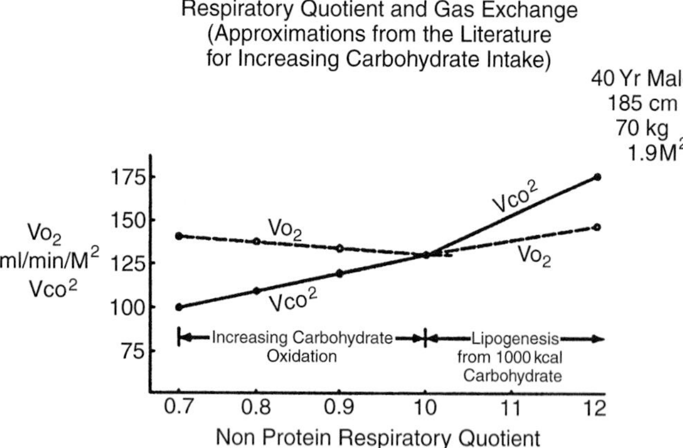

Figure 90.4. Effects of increased carbohydrate intake on CO_2 production, O_2 consumption, and RQ in a normal subject. As the carbohydrate intake increases, CO_2 production and eventually O_2 consumption increase. (From Elwyn DH, Askanazi J, Kinney JM. Acta Chir Scand 1981;507(Suppl):209–19.)

$$V_A = RR \times V_t(1 - Vd/V_t)$$

where *RR* is the respiratory rate, V_t is the tidal volume, and V_d/V_t is the fraction of wasted or dead space ventilation. Thus, if VCO_2 increases, V_A must also increase to keep the $Paco_2$ normal. Alveolar ventilation can be increased by increasing the respiratory rate or tidal volume, which in turn, increases the work of breathing. Reducing the physiologic dead space (that which is ventilated but not perfused) will also improve V_A, but such a reduction usually is not easily accomplished, because many patients with respiratory failure have an elevated dead space fraction because of their underlying pulmonary disease. If the patient has little or no respiratory reserve to meet the augmented ventilatory demand of increased CO_2 production, respiratory failure may be further exacerbated and complicate weaning from artificial ventilatory support.

Respiratory failure precipitated or aggravated by administration of high glucose loads to patients with compromised respiratory function has been reported (54–56). In chronically nutritionally depleted patients and acutely ill patients with injury or infection, Askanazi et al. studied the effect of total parental nutrition (TPN) supplementation at 1.5 times their REEs, with up to 50% of the nonprotein calories as either glucose or fat emulsions (54). No one in the two groups required assisted ventilation or was noted to have respiratory impairment. In the chronically nutritionally depleted group, however, VCO_2 rose by 20% and V_A (mostly due to an increase in V_t) rose by 26% after conversion from a high fat to a high glucose source (54). In the acutely ill individuals, VCO_2 also rose significantly by 21% (54). Changes in V_e in the acutely ill were not characterized in this report, but in an earlier investigation of high glucose TPN (1.2–2.25 × REE), V_e increased by 71% in the hypermetabolic patients and by 121% in those with mild or moderate injury (56). Respiratory deterioration was not reported in either study. Heymsfield et al. showed that the VCO_2 difference between a high-fat and a high-carbohydrate infusion in stable medical patients with chronic illness was exaggerated once supplementation was increased from a maintenance rate to a replenishment rate (57). This may be explained by the amount of CO_2 liberated in production of triglyceride from glucose, which is 30 times the amount of CO_2 produced in converting dietary fat into triglyceride (57).

Micronutrients may also be important in maintaining normal hemostasis. In rats, deficiency of selenium, an essential cofactor of the antioxidant enzyme glutathione peroxidase, increases susceptibility to lung injury induced by exposure to high oxygen concentrations (58, 59). Production of oxygen free radicals in excess of antioxidants is thought to contribute to acute lung injury (see Chapter 14). The clinical role of selenium and other trace elements in preventing lung injury is currently being investigated. Most enteral formulas contain sufficient levels of micronutrients, and it is unclear whether supplementation above these levels is beneficial.

Timing and Route of Nutritional Support

The relationships between malnutrition and worse outcomes support use of nutritional support in the critically ill. Despite these data and the hypothetical benefits of nutritional support, at present there are no prospective, randomized, controlled investigations that clearly demonstrate the efficacy of nutritional supplementation in this population (60) (see also Chapter 98). The optimal timing, composition of substrate, and route of administration of nutritional supplementation have not yet been unequivocally established either in the critically ill, but they are probably patient specific and greatly influenced by baseline nutritional status and type of imposed stress. The route of supplemental feeding may be either parental or enteral. The indications, techniques, formulations, goals, and complications are presented in detail in Chapters 51 and 64 (infants and children) and Chapters 98, 100, and 101.

Enteral Feeding and Pulmonary Issues

Enteral feeding is most commonly accomplished through a nasogastric feeding tube or a small-caliber (10-Fr) nasoduodenal tube. Potential mechanical risks are associated with enteric feeding tubes, including misplacement in the tracheobronchial tree beyond cuffed endotracheal tubes, occasionally with perforation into the pleural space (61), underscoring the need to confirm proper placement before use. In addition, epistaxis, sinusitis, esophagitis, tracheoesophageal fistula, and ruptured esophageal varices can complicate the use of nasoenteral tubes (62). Substituting oroenteral tubes for nasoenteral tubes can limit development of some upper airway complications. Theoretically, enteral feeding into the duodenum should reduce the likelihood of aspiration by bypassing the problem of delayed emptying secondary to gastric paresis and adding the pylorus as a barrier to regurgitation. Zaloga found a 30% incidence of aspiration when feeding tubes were placed in the stomach, compared with no occurrences when tubes were confirmed to be in the duodenum (63). On the other hand, Strong et al. demonstrated that the site of tube placement did not affect the incidence of aspiration (64). Various duodenal feeding tubes designed to be inserted either through the nose or through the abdominal wall (via surgery or endoscopy) have been developed (see Chapter 100). Unfortunately, the diagnosis of aspiration pneumonia cannot always be made with certainty, nor is it clear what degree of aspiration is clinically important. Maintaining patients in a semirecumbent rather than supine position can significantly decrease pulmonary aspiration of gastric contents in patients receiving nasogastric feeding (65).

Parenteral Nutrition and Pulmonary Issues

Parenteral nutrition (PN) can be accomplished through a central vein (allowing more concentrated and hypertonic solutions) or peripherally, unless a large amount of lipids is infused. Peripheral parenteral nutrition requires a greater obligate fluid load to meet similar caloric needs compared to the central route (see Chapter 101). Because impaired fluid handling is common in patients with acute lung injury, limited fluid intake is generally preferred and may be associated with improved outcomes (66).

Access is obtained through percutaneous catheterization of one of the central veins, most commonly the subclavian and jugular veins. Technical difficulties with insertion can lead to ipsilateral pneumothorax, arterial puncture, thoracic duct disruption, catheter misdirection, catheter fracture, thrombosis, catheter or air embolism, infection at the local site with subsequent bloodstream seeding, and local bleeding and hematoma formation. Complications associated with insertion occur more frequently when such catheters are placed by less experienced individuals (67). Catheter-related thrombosis can be diminished by adding 6000 U of heparin per day in the PN solution (68). Since PN solutions are also good media for microorganisms, strict aseptic technique *must* be used, and line disruptions minimized. Restricting catheter use to alimentation decreases infectious complications (69). Prolonged PN generally requires multiple catheter replacements (with their attendant risk) or surgical placement of a more permanent catheter (usually Silastic) tunneled in the subcutaneous tissues into a central vein.

Special formulations are available for different clinical circumstances often associated with acute lung injury. As noted above, if ventilatory reserve is limited, the formula that produces the least CO_2 during metabolism imposes the lowest demand on the ventilatory system and may facilitate weaning. Clearly, the net effects of multiple organ failure impose complex nutritional stresses (see Chapter 96 and 98); other problems arise in managing renal failure (see Chapter 89) and liver failure (see Chapter 94).

Studies from several centers have shown altered lung function (decreased oxygen saturation and diffusing capacity of carbon dioxide) in both humans and animal models given lipid emulsions (70). These changes appear to be caused principally by an increase in ventilation/perfusion inequalities induced by lipid infusions (70), but their clinical relevance even in the severely compromised is unknown. The choice of lipid may affect which inflammatory eicosanoids are produced. Linoleic acid, an ω-6 essential fatty acid, is converted to arachidonic acid (AA), the precursor of many proinflammatory eicosanoids (both prostaglandins and leukotrienes) (71). On the other hand, linolenic acid, an ω-3 fatty acid, is converted into eicosapentanoic acid (EPA), which produces different eicosanoids with markedly different actions (71). The eicosanoids (prostaglandins and leukotrienes) produced from AA are thought to perpetuate the inflammation associated with acute lung injury much more than those derived from EPA do (see Chapter 45.)

The quantity or composition of surfactant can be altered in acute lung injury. Some investigators have examined dietary fat supplementation as a way to enhance surfactant production. Baybutt et al. demonstrated that dietary supplementation with EPA, an ω-3 fatty acid, could increase the amount of whole-lung surfactant in a rat model but did not alter the amount of surfactant found in the alveolus (72). This study also demonstrated decreased AA content in the type II pneumocyte. Palombo et al. also demonstrated increased EPA in membrane phospholipids of lung tissue, alveolar macrophages, and surfactant after dietary supplementation with ω-3 fatty acids. (73). Although these data are intriguing, much still needs to be elucidated before a dietary fatty acid modification can be recommended to modulate inflammation in acute lung injury.

Chronic Lung Disease

Chronic lung disease is typically classified as either obstructive or restrictive, based upon the primary physiologic mechanism of ventilatory dysfunction. Obstructive pulmonary disease is a generic term encompassing asthma, emphysema, and chronic bronchitis. The hallmark of these diseases is airflow obstruction principally during expiration. Each of these diseases has unique characerisitics, but there is overlap in the pathophysiologic and clinical manifestations. Asthma is defined as airflow obstruction that is at least partially reversible, which is caused by airway smooth muscle contraction, bronchial inflammation and edema, and bronchial gland hypertrophy with mucous plugging. Chronic bronchitis is a clinical syndrome manifested as cough, mucus hypersecretion, sputum production, and bronchial gland hypertrophy. Emphysema is a pathologic finding in which there is destruction of lung tissue, loss of the "tethering effect" (elastic recoil) of lung, and resultant dynamic collapse of unsupported airways. In most patients, emphysema and chronic bronchitis are caused by tobacco smoking and are collectively labeled chronic obstructive pulmonary disease (COPD). Obstructive lung disease can result in hyperinflation and air trapping. Air trapping elevates the residual volume and causes flattening of the diaphragm (Fig. 90.1). The diaphragms are therefore placed at a mechanical disadvantage by being shortened in length prior to inspiratory contraction (the longer the precontractile fibers, the greater the tension that can be generated), and patients become limited during inspiration as well as expiration.

Restrictive lung diseases include infiltrative, fibrotic lung diseases and extrapulmonary conditions (e.g., musculoskeletal disease, obesity, neurologic disease) and are manifested by decreased total lung capacity, generally with preservation of expiratory flow rates. Restrictive lung disease causes decreased compliance of the lung, which increases the elastic load on the muscles and the work of breathing.

Most investigations of the interrelationships between nutrition and chronic pulmonary disease have focused on COPD, asthma, and cystic fibrosis. However, since most of these conditions also impose an inspiratory load on ventilatory mechanics, the management principles and interventions designed to improve respiratory muscle function in COPD are likely to prove helpful in these diseases as well. The other benefits of improved nutrition on lung function should also be advantageous in other specific lung diseases.

Role of Nutrition and Lifestyle in Development of Chronic Obstructive Pulmonary Disease

In 1984, COPD was the fifth leading cause of death in the United States (74). In the Tecumseh Community Health Study, the prevalence rate for obstructive airways disease, chronic bronchitis, or both was approximately 14% of adult men and 8% of the adult women (75).

Emphysema is thought to be due to an excess of proteases, causing destruction of the elastin and collagen matrix supporting the lung architecture. Tobacco smoking, overwhelmingly the most common cause of emphysema, causes an influx of neutrophils into the lung and a subsequent release of elastase and other proteases. Oxidants inhaled from tobacco smoke and released from activated inflammatory cells also play a role in the development of emphysema by impairing endogenous antiproteases.

There are several naturally occurring antioxidants (e.g., the enzymes superoxide dismutase and catalase and the peptide glutathione) present in lower respiratory tract to counteract inhaled oxidants. Ceruloplasmin, copper, methionine sulfoxide, retinols, and vitamins E and C may also protect against oxidant-induced destruction. The extent to which dietary supplementation with antioxidants might protect against environmentally encountered oxidants causing pulmonary disease is unknown. There are concerns about the use of the antioxidant β-carotene because of adverse findings. (See section on nutrition and lung cancers, below.) Interestingly, Massaro and Massaro reported reversal of elastase-induced emphysematous-like histologic changes in rats treated with all-*trans*-retinoic acid (75a).

Because only about 15 to 20% of cigarette smokers develop clinical evidence of COPD, several groups have evaluated the role diet may play in predisposing smokers to developing this disease. Several investigators have demonstrated an inverse relationship between dietary antioxidant intake and level of pulmonary function (76–80). It is, therefore, hypothesized that dietary antioxidants such as vitamin C and retinols may limit the destruction of lung tissue by proteases and protect against development of COPD. Recently, an analysis of a cohort of asbestos workers with a high rate of current or former cigarette smoking participating in the Carotene and Retinol Efficacy Trial (CARET), showed that β-carotene and retinol, based on serum levels, protect against the loss of ventilatory function in this group (81). These findings agreed with those from an earlier study (80) but differed from the baseline data in the Atherosclerosis Risk in Communities (ARIC) study (82).

Airway obstruction and wheezing have also been positively associated with dietary sodium:potassium ratios and negatively associated with serum niacin and zinc:copper ratios, independent of cigarette smoking (79, 83, 84). The clinical implications of these observations are not yet established.

Prostanoids from EPA have less inflammatory capabilities than those released from AA. The ARIC study investigators examined the relationships between dietary intake of ω-3 fatty acids and development of COPD in 8960 current or former smokers and found a quantity-dependent inverse relationship between the two after controlling for confounding variables including tobacco use (85). Sharp et al. and Schwartz and Weiss demonstrated similar results in 6346 and 2526 subjects, respectively (86, 87). Prostanoids released from AA are also thought to contribute greatly to the pathophysiologic changes seen in asthma. Epidemiologic studies from the 1960s and 1970s demonstrated a low incidence of asthma in populations whose diets were rich in EPA (88). Various investigators have, therefore, hypothesized that dietary supplementation with EPA could potentially attenuate manifestations of asthma. Although in vitro changes in inflammatory cells were demonstrated after dietary supplementation, the effects upon clinical markers of disease varied (89, 90).

It has been hypothesized that vitamin C may be beneficial in treating atopic asthma, although the mechanism by which this may occur has not been fully elucidated. A metaanalysis of this subject by Bielory and Gandhi was inconclusive (91). Adding intravenous magnesium to inhaled β-agonist therapy during an acute asthma exacerbation improves pulmonary function acutely better than β-agonist therapy alone in children (92), but its efficacy in adults with asthma has not been clearly demonstrated (93).

Malnutrition in COPD. Nutritional depletion is exceedingly common in persons with COPD; various authors have shown an incidence of malnutrition from 20 to 60% (94–101). Furthermore, many series demonstrate that nutritional depletion is an indicator of poor prognosis in patients with COPD (94, 102–106). A retrospective analysis of patients enrolled in the Intermittent Positive Pressure Breathing Trial found that individuals who were less than 90% of ideal body weight upon entry into the study had a greater overall 5-year mortality after normalization for the severity of their lung dysfunction (94) (Fig. 90.5). Low body mass index (BMI) has been identified as an independent predictor of mortality (105, 106), and BMI correlates with FEV_1, FEV_1:FVC ratio, and diffusion capacity (100). It is especially important to recognize malnutrition as an independent risk factor because it may potentially be modified.

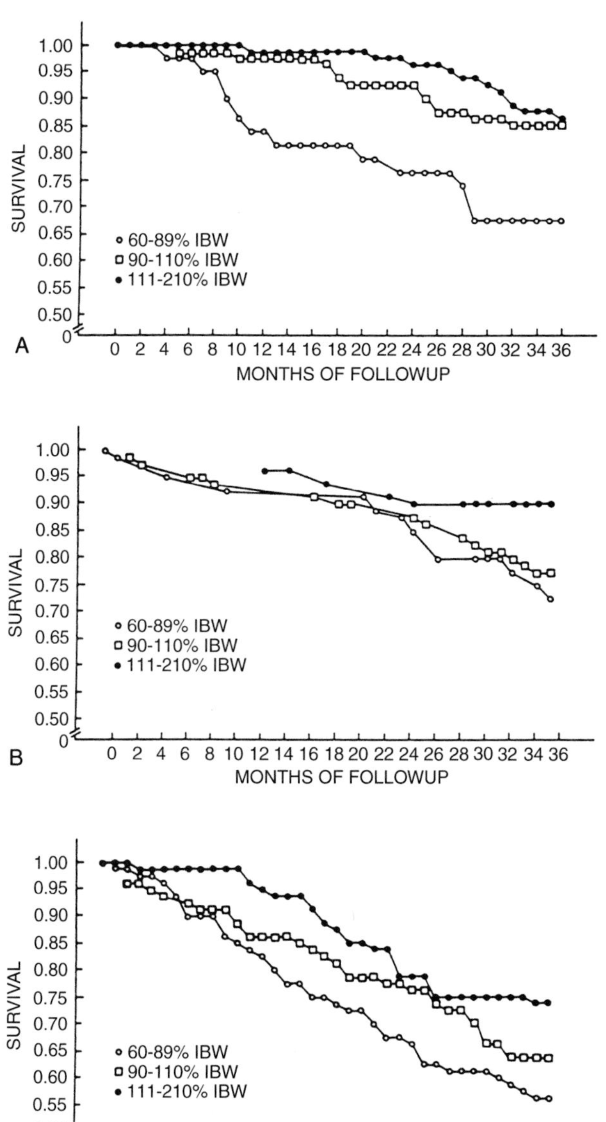

Figure 90.5. Survival curves for patients with COPD enrolled in the National Institutes of Health Intermittent Positive-Pressure Breathing Trial. **A.** Survival of patients with FEV_1 > 47% predicted by %IBW category; **B.** Survival of patients with FEV_1 = 35–47% predicted by %IBW category; **C.** Survival of patients with FEV_1 < 35% predicted by %IBW. (From Wilson DO, Rogers RM, Wright RC, et al. Am Rev Respir Dis 1989;139:1435–8.)

Mechanisms for this weight loss in patients with chronic lung disease have been summarized by Wilson et al. (34). Impaired gastrointestinal function, inadequate dietary intake (a potential adaptive mechanism to lower oxygen consumption to theoretically lower the work of breathing), altered pulmonary and cardiovascular hemodynamics limiting nutrient supply to other tissues, and a hypermetabolic state might all contribute to the malnutrition in these patients (34). Several investigators have shown that the measured REE in a large portion of stable patients with COPD, with and without weight loss, exceeds the REE calculated from the Harris-Benedict equation (95, 107, 108), although they do not seem to be hypercatabolic with preferential fat oxidation (107); some of these patients though may have been taking theophylline preparations that increase the REE in normal subjects (109). Donahoe et al. measured the oxygen cost of augmented ventilation with dead-space stimulation of ventilation in normal subjects and well-nourished and malnourished patients with COPD (108). Both groups of COPD patients had a higher oxygen cost of ventilation than the normal subjects, but the increase was greater in the malnourished group than in the well-nourished COPD patients (108). Patients with COPD had significantly increased energy expenditure for respiratory muscle activity (108). Although not quite analogous to ambulatory patients, Jounieaux and Mayeaux found a higher cost of breathing and lower somatic stores (arm muscle circumference and tricep skin fold) in emphysematous patients intubated for acute respiratory failure (110). Presumably, this elevation in energy requirements of the respiratory muscles for an increase in V_e can be extrapolated to the increases seen in daily activities of normal life.

Higher energy consumption by the respiratory muscles to meet the demands of daily life could produce a hypermetabolic state (compared with normal subjects) and lead to progressive weight loss when output exceeded caloric intake. Wilson et al. concluded that increased daily energy expenditure led to weight loss in patients with chronic lung disease related to increased resistive load and decreased respiratory muscle efficiency (34). Most studies show that caloric intake is adequate or better than that predicted for REE or measured at rest (95, 97, 111, 112) in COPD patients. However, these studies do not satisfactorily address the caloric expenditure necessary for activity (95) or intercurrent illness and also tend to use nutritional inventory (i.e., patient recall) to assess caloric intake rather than direct measurement (111). Conversely, Schols et al. found that although COPD patients with and without weight loss had similar REEs, those with weight loss had an inadequate dietary intake in relation to their energy expenditure and failed to adapt to undernutrition (112a). Baaraends et al. noted that the total free-living energy expenditure as measured by doubly labeled water was significantly higher in eight patients with stable COPD admitted to a pulmonary rehabilitation center than in eight matched controls. The REEs in the two groups were not significantly different. This supports the belief that there is a higher metabolic demand for physical activity in COPD patients than in matched healthy subjects (112b).

Tumor necrosis factor-α, a cytokine that can induce cachexia in laboratory animals, is elevated in weight-losing patients with COPD without acute infections (113). Although no causal relationship has been demonstrated, it is hypothesized that this could contribute to malnutrition in these patients.

Nutritional Supplementation in COPD. Despite the theoretical and proven benefits of improved nutritional status, realizing these goals is challenging. Attempts to augment caloric intake over baseline may be difficult because of respiratory and gastrointestinal symptoms (e.g., anorexia, early satiety, dyspnea, fatigue, bloating, constipation, and dental problems) (114). Some of these symptoms (bloating, satiety, anorexia) may be related to flattening of the diaphragm with impingement on the abdominal cavity. In hypoxemic COPD patients, arterial oxygen desaturation during eating may increase baseline dyspnea, further limiting intake (115). This change has been related to altered ventilation-perfusion relationships caused by diminished lung volume accompanying abdominal distention and, less often, increased splanchnic blood flow. Smaller, more frequent meals may alleviate some of these problems.

Most studies addressing nutritional supplementation in COPD have used less than ideal body weight as an index of poor nutritional status and changes in respiratory muscle function as the outcome assessed. Other pulmonary function tests (spirometry, lung volumes) should not be expected to improve and do not; they are related to the underlying cause of airflow obstruction, which nutritional support would not be anticipated to change directly. There are inherent limitations in this approach. Less than ideal body weight is only one manifestation of malnourishment, but it is related to prognosis (94). Changes in respiratory muscle strength may not be a good surrogate marker for prognosis, may lack clinical or functional significance, and/or may not only reflect nutritional deprivation or intervention.

The results of six efforts to improve the nutritional status of malnourished but clinically stable COPD patients are summarized in Table 90.5. Four studies (112, 116–118) noted significant weight gain that correlated with demonstrable improvement in respiratory muscle function. The other two studies showed an insignificant trend toward weight gain, but no improvement in respiratory muscle function, which might have been related to the shorter duration of nutritional supplementation (119, 120). The likelihood of improved respiratory muscle function may thus be linked to the amount of weight gain and, possibly, the severity of initial deficits. Further information is needed in this area.

Table 90.5
Nutritional Intervention in Malnourished COPD Patients

Author (ref)	No. Fed	Study Type	RMS[a]	Weight Gain
Wilson et al. (112)	6	Inpatient 3 weeks	MIP improved Mean: 143%	Yes
Whittaker et al. (117)	6	Inpatient 2.3 weeks	MIP improved Mean: 119%	Yes
Lewis et al. (119)	10	Outpatient 8 weeks	MIP no change Mean: 89%	No
Knowles et al. (120)	25	Outpatient 8 weeks	MIP no change[b] Mean: 105–115%	No
Efthimiou et al (116)	7	Outpatient 12 weeks	MIP improved Mean: 116%	Yes
Rogers et al. (118)	15	Inpatient 4 weeks	MIP improved Mean: 134%	Yes

[a]RMS, respiratory muscle strength; MIP, maximal inspiratory pressure; Mean, mean percentage of baseline after supplementation.
[b]No significant change in MIP between fed and control patients.

Both Lewis et al. (119) and Knowles et al. (120) noted the difficulty these COPD patients experience in ingesting and maintaining sufficient caloric intake to gain weight. It has been hypothesized that diet-induced thermogenesis (DIT) and/or the increased energy expenditure required while eating may compromise the value of ingested nutrients and contribute to inadequate nutrition. In a cohort of 11 stable COPD patients with REEs 10% above those predicted, DIT did not differ significantly from that of controls (121). These investigators also found no significant difference in 24-h energy expenditure by 16 patients with stable COPD and 12 normal controls, despite an increased basal metabolic rate in those with COPD (121). However, COPD patients compensated for the increased basal metabolic rate by decreasing their spontaneous physical activity (121). Dore also found no difference in DIT between undernourished patients with COPD and normally nourished patients with COPD, although the REE was approximately 120% of the predicted BMR in both groups (121a). In contrast, Goldstein et al. demonstrated that malnourished COPD patients had a greater increase in resting oxygen consumption after a meal than malnourished patients without COPD (122).

Recently, investigators have supplemented the diets of patients during hospitalization for an acute exacerbation of COPD (122a). Supplemented patients were able to consume significantly more calories per kilogram than the control groups without increased breathlessness. The FVC increased significantly more during treatment in the supplemented group than in the control group (122a). However, 6-min walking distance and overall feeling of well-being were the same, and both groups demonstrated negative nitrogen balance of similar magnitude, suggesting muscle wasting. All subjects, though, received systemic glucocorticoids, which may have contributed to the muscle wasting.

It is clear that low body weight is associated with a poorer prognosis in patients with COPD. It is much less clear that nutritional supplementation changes the outcome of these patients in a meaningful way. This is especially important in view of the difficulty in obtaining and maintaining weight gain and the cost of this intervention.

Roles of Hormone Administration. In a preliminary study, Suchner et al. found that administration of 60 μg/kg/day of growth hormone promoted positive nitrogen balance (123). Growth hormone supplmentation has also been associated with weight gain and increased MIP (124). Rudman et al. gave biosynthetic growth hormone (30 μg/kg/day) to a group of healthy elderly males and noted a significant increase in lean body mass and a decrease in adipose tissue compared with a control group with similar caloric intake (25–30 kcal/kg) (125). Schols et al. compared the effects of nutritional supplementation, with or without anabolic steroids, with placebo in 217 patients with COPD enrolled in a rehabilitation program and found that nutritional support in combination with anabolic steroids increased fat-free body mass and MIP in subjects who were depleted at baseline (126). The use of trophic agents in malnourished patients is also discussed in Chapters 96, 98, 101.

If body weight is an independent predictor of survival and nutritional support can improve and maintain body weight, one could hypothesize that optimizing nutritional support should improve survival. However, no long-term studies are available to substantiate that hypothesis.

Nutrient Composition and Administration. Since COPD patients have a limited ventilatory reserve, a high-carbohydrate diet that produces more CO_2 per mole of O_2 consumed for energy requirements might be expected to stress the respiratory system, whereas a high-fat diet would be expected to produce less CO_2 per mole of oxygen consumed and perhaps be beneficial. Angelillo et al. performed a randomized, double-blinded study of COPD patients with hypercarbia and found that a 5-day low-carbohydrate diet (28% carbohydrate calories, 55% fat calories) resulted in lower CO_2 production and arterial Paco2 than a 5-day high-carbohydrate diet (74% carbohydrate calories, 9.4% fat calories) (127). Kwan and Mir also noted that a low-carbohydrate diet benefited (reduced $Paco_2$) COPD patients with hypercapnia (128). In addition, Pao_2 and mouth pressure at 100 msec (a measure of respiratory center output) increased with carbohydrate restriction (128). A large carbohydrate load also reduced the 12-min walking distance in patients with COPD (129). Alternatively, Sue et al. found that altering dietary fat and carbohydrate proportions in normal subjects did not alter exercise gas exchange response or mean V_e during exercise (130).

Although the clinical significance is unclear, protein supplementation can increase oxygen consumption (from its thermic effect) (52), increase V_e (52), and increase the ventilatory response to hypoxemia and hypercarbia (24) that may potentially result in dyspnea in respiratory limited patients.

Electrolyte deficiencies such as hypophosphatemia, hypokalemia, and hypocalcemia can also adversely affect respiratory muscle function (see Chapters 6, 8, and 9). Aubier et al. showed that phosphorus replacement improved diaphragmatic contractility in hypophosphatemic patients with acute respiratory failure (131). This observation is particularly relevant to patients with COPD who are placed on mechanical ventilation; intracellular shifts commonly occur in these individuals after correction of respiratory acidosis (132). Serum phosphorus levels may drop acutely in asthmatics after intensive bronchodilator therapy, which is probably related to intracellular shifts and parallels improvement in the arterial pH and Paco2 (133, 134), but the clinical consequences of acute hypophosphatemia were not clear in these reports. Aubier et al. reported that lowering the serum calcium level acutely with a chelating agent (EDTA) can also reduce diaphragmatic maximal contraction (135). Restoring normal intracellular concentrations of these ions may account for acute improvements of respiratory muscle strength.

Cystic Fibrosis. Cystic fibrosis, physiologically resembles COPD, although a restrictive defect may also be present. In addition to lung involvement, the underlying defect in ion transport affects multiple organs. Pancreatic deficiency and resulting in malabsorption, glucose intolerance, intestinal obstruction, salt depletion, fatty liver, and gallbladder disease are common nonpulmonary complications of cystic fibrosis that increase the difficulty of maintaining an adequate nutritional status (see Chapter 69). Like patients with COPD, patients with cystic fibrosis have an REE about 20% higher than matched normals (136). However, as opposed to COPD, in which the oxygen cost of breathing is responsible for most, if not all, of the increase in baseline REE, only about 50% of the increase in REE is attributable to the oxygen cost of ventilation (136). Chronic infection and inflammation, increased sympathetic nervous activity, and (perhaps) increased energy expenditure at the cellular level as a consequence of the abnormal cystic fibrosis transmembrane conductance regulator (CFTR) may account for the other half of the increase in REE (136). Weight gain or loss correlates with the overall general health of the patient and is an important monitor and predictor of prognosis.

Although considerable advances have been made recently in delineating the genetic defect of cystic fibrosis, treatment is still largely supportive. A high-calorie, high-protein diet with supplemental pancreatic enzymes and multivitamin fortification is generally recommended to maintain weight. In a retrospective comparison between a traditional diet of low fat, high calorie, and an unrestricted diet of high fat and high energy with aggressive enzyme supplementation, there was improved survival from 21 years to 30 years in the latter group (137). Other studies have also shown that an aggressive approach to nutrition, even using enteral feedings, improves body weight and may even improve lung function (138). Caution is advised in providing dosages of pancreatic enzymes above 10,000 U/kg/day because of the reported association of higher dosages with fibrosing colonopathy in young patients (138a).

Role of Nutrition in Lung Cancer

Lung cancer is the leading cause of cancer deaths in both men and women. It is second in incidence only to prostate cancer in men and breast cancer in women. Over 80% of lung cancer cases can be attributed to tobacco abuse, principally cigarette smoking, with a direct relationship between the dose and duration of smoking and the incidence of this lethal disease. However, only approximately 10 to 20% of heavy smokers develop lung cancers. This has led to speculation that there may be a genetic predisposition to developing lung cancer and/or that other environmental factors may be involved. Studies with experimental cancers (both in vivo and in vitro) in animal models and case-control studies as well as cohort studies of dietary intake and serum levels have implicated dietary micronutrients (chemopreventive agents) in the development of malignancies (see Chapter 81).

Observations from epidemiologic studies have associated reduced intake and serum levels of carotenoids or retinoids with increased incidence of lung cancer and have led to several prospective studies. The first clinical randomized trial using retinoids in the prevention of secondary tumors in lung cancer patients began in 1985, at the National Cancer Institute in Milan (139). Patients with stage I (localized) disease were randomized to retinyl palmitate treatment (oral 300,000 IU daily for 12–24 months) or to a control group without treatment. There was significant improvement in the disease-free interval and the number of new malignancies related to tobacco use in the treatment group, but no improvement in overall survival. Subsequently, the Alpha-Tocopherol, Beta Carotene Cancer Prevention Group (ATBC), based in Finland, published results of a randomized, double-blind, placebo-controlled primary prevention trial consisting of 29,133 male smokers between the ages of 50 and 69 (140). Participants were randomized to one of four regimens: α-tocopherol (50 mg/day), β-carotene (20 mg/day), both α-tocopherol and β-carotene, or placebo. There was no significant reduction in the incidence of lung cancer among this group after 5 to 8 years of dietary supplementation with α-tocopherol or β-carotene. However, total mortality was 8% higher in participants who received β-carotene than in those who did not, primarily from increased mortality from lung cancer and ischemic heart disease. Two more-recent studies corroborate these findings. In a trial of β-carotene (30 mg) and vitamin A (25,000 IU) versus placebo in high-risk asbestos workers who were current or former smokers, the interventional group had a significantly higher relative risk (1.28) for lung cancer (141). A study of 22,000 male physicians taking β-carotene (50 mg) or placebo every other day for an average of 12 years found no difference in the rates of malignancy in general or in any specific type of malignancy (142). At this time, recommending dietary β-carotene supplementation for lung cancer chemoprevention does not appear warranted.

Other Clinical Considerations

In many commonly encountered clinical circumstances, compromised nutritional status may exacerbate or be worsened by respiratory illness. For example, protein malnutrition causing hypoalbuminemia alters the threshold for transudation of fluid into the lung and pleural space and results in pulmonary edema and pleural effusion formation. Both of these can cause a restrictive ventilatory defect and increase the work of breathing.

Occasionally, a respiratory disease may impose particular nutritional demands. Patients who have a malignancy metastatic to the pleura may leak large amounts of protein into the pleural space. Repeated drainage of this fluid may lead to severe protein wasting. In patients who develop chylothorax, disruption of the thoracic duct (generally due to trauma, cancer, or surgical complication) may lead to massive loss of protein, fat, electrolytes, and lymphocytes in the pleural space. While it may be necessary to use parenteral alimentation to maintain nutrition, administration of oral medium-chain triglycerides has been effective because they are directly absorbed from the portal vein rather than transported through the thoracic duct (143).

The medications administered to patients with respiratory disease have their own implications for nutritional supplementation. Systemic corticosteroids, commonly used in the treatment of respiratory diseases, have many untoward effects including glucose intolerance, sodium retention, nitrogen loss, hyperphagia, and weight gain with resultant increased load imposed on respiratory muscles (see Chapters 44, 84, 99). Improper administration of inhaled corticosteroids may lead to oropharyngeal fungal overgrowth and local pain, resulting in reduced oral dietary intake. Theophylline, commonly administered to patients with obstructive lung disease, and a variety of antibiotics for superimposed infections (e.g., bronchitis, pneumonia) may induce nausea or diarrhea, with obvious implications for nutritional status. Patients receiving anticoagulants for deep vein thrombosis and pulmonary embolic disease require particular attention to factors interfering with vitamin K metabolism. Dietary suppressants including aminorex and fenfluramine (Redux) have been associated with development of primary pulmonary hypertension (144).

Although particular emphasis has been placed on the adverse effects of malnutrition and low body weight on respiratory function, obesity also has imposing and potentially lethal respiratory sequelae. A restrictive ventilatory defect may be caused not only by the direct effects of increased weight on the chest and elevation of the hemidiaphragm due to increased abdominal pressure but also by structural and functional impairments of the respiratory muscles. In extreme clinical manifestations of this problem, these mechanical changes interact with abnormalities of the respiratory center (decreased sensitivity to hypoxemia and hypercarbia) and culminate in the "obesity-hypoventilation syndrome." Moreover, increased body weight is a major risk factor and clinical predictor for obstructive sleep apnea, a common and frequently unrecognized health hazard in the United States, associated with profound cardiovascular and functional sequelae. In patients with the spectrum of respiratory dysfunction related to obesity, weight loss is the primary measure for effectively improving the respiratory disease and its systemic consequences.

REFERENCES

1. Murray JF. The normal lung. 2nd ed. Philadelphia: WB Saunders, 1986;233–60.
2. Roussos C, Macklem PT. N Engl J Med 1982;307:786–97.
3. Lewis MI, Sieck HC, Founier M, Belman MJ. J Appl Physiol 1986;60:596–603.
4. Goldspink G, Ward PS. J Physiol (Lond) 1979;296:453–69.
5. Oldfors A, Mairk WGP, Sourander P. Neurol Sci 1983;59: 291–302.
6. Sieck GC, Lewis MI, Blanco CE. J Appl Physiol 1989;66 (5):2196–205.
7. Bellemare F, Grassino A. J Appl Physiol 1982;53:1190–5.
8. Bellemare F, Grassino A. J Appl Physiol 1983;55:8–13.
9. Lechner AJ, Winston DC, Bauman JE. J Appl Physiol 1986;60: 1610–4.
10. Faridy EE. J Appl Physiol 1975;39:535–40.
11. Kalenga M, Eeckhout Y. Pediatr Res 1989;26:125–7.
12. Shaheen SO, Barker DJ. Thorax 1994;49:533–6.
13. Chan KN, Noble-Jamieson CM, Elliman A, et al. Arch Dis Child 1989;64:1284–93.
14. Barker DJP, Godfrey KM, Fall C, et al. Br Med J 1991;303: 671–5.
15. Rona RJ, Gulliford MC, Chinn S. Br Med J 1993;306:817–20.
16. Davidson MB. Growth 1968;32:221–3.
17. Rochester DF, Pradel-Guena M. J Appl Physiol 1973;34: 68–74.
18. Goldberg AL, Odessey R. Am J Physiol 1972;223:1384–91.
19. Thurlbeck WM. Thorax 1978;33:483–7.
20. Arora NS, Rochester DF. J Appl Physiol 1982;56:64–70.
21. Arora NS, Rochester DF. Am Rev Respir Dis 1982;126:5–8.
22. Doekel RC, Zwillich AV, Scoggins CH, et al. N Engl J Med 1976;295:358–61.
23. Baier H, Somani P. Chest 1984;85:222–5.
24. Zwillich CW, Sahn SA, Weill JA. J Clin Invest 1977;60:900–6.
25. Ryan CF, Whittaker JS, Road JD. Chest 1992;102:1286–8.
26. Murciano D, Rigaud D, Pingleton S, et al. Am J Respir Crit Care Med 1994;150:1569–74.
27. Martin TR, Altman LC, Alvares OF. Am Rev Respir Dis 1983; 128:1013–9.
28. Moriguchi S, Sine S, Kishina Y. J Nutr 1983;113:40–6.
29. Shennib H, Chin RC, Mulder DS, Lough JO. Surg Gynecol Obstet 1984;158:535–40.
30. Skerrett S, Henderson W, Martin T. J Immunol 1990;144: 1052–61.
31. Niederman MS, Merrill WW, Feranti RD, et al. Ann Intern Med 1984;100:795–800.
32. Fuenzalida CE, Petty TL, Jones ML, et al. Am Rev Respir Dis 1990;142:49–56.
33. Rosenbaum SH, Askanazi J, Hyman AI, et al. Anesthesiology 1979;51:366S.
34. Wilson DO, Rogers RM, Hoffman RM. Am Rev Respir Dis 1985;132:1347–67.
35. Pingleton SK. Am Rev Resp Dis 1988;137:1463–93.
36. Giner M, Laviano A, Meguid MM, et al. Nutrition 1996; 12:23–9.
37. Bartlett RH, Dechert RE, Mault JR, et al. Surgery 1982; 92:771–8.
38. Kinney JM. Crit Care Clin 1987;3:1–10.
39. Wiener M, Rothkopf MM, Rothkopf G, et al. Crit Care Clin 1987;3:25–56.
40. Elwyn DH. Crit Care Clin 1987;3:57–69.
41. Liggett SB, St John RE, Lefrak SS. Chest 1987;91:562–6.
42. Damask MC, Schwarz Y, Weissman C. Crit Care Clin 1987; 3:71–96.
43. Harris JA, Benedict FG. Standard basal metabolism constants for physiologists and clinicians; a biometric study of basal metabolism in man. Philadelphia: JB Lippincott, 1919;223.
44. Saffle JR, Medina E, Raymond J, et al. J Trauma 1985;25:32–9.
45. Weissman C, Kemper M, Askanazai J, et al. J Anesth 1986; 64:673–9.
46. Liggett SB, Renfro AD. Chest 1990;98:682–6.
47. Bassili HR, Deital M. JPEN J Parenter Enteral Nutr 1981;5: 161–3.
48. Laaban JP, Lemaire F, Baron JF, et al. Chest 1985;87:67–72.
49. Wilmore DW. J Am Coll Nutr 1983;2:3–13.
50. Elwyn DH, Kinney JM, Jeevanandam M, et al. Ann Surg 1979;190:117.
51. Edens NK, Gil KM, Elywyn DH. Clin Chest Med 1986;7:3–17.
52. Weissman C, Askanazi J, Rosenbaum SH, et al. Ann Intern Med 1983;98:41–4.
53. Elwyn DH, Askanzi J, Kinney JM. Acta Chir Scand (Suppl) 1981;507:209–19.
54. Askanazi J, Elwyn DH, Silverbery PA, et al. Surgery 1980;8: 596–9.
55. Al-Saady NM, Blackmore CM, Bennett ED. Intensive Care Med 1989;15:290–5.
56. Herve L, Simonneau-Girard P, Cerrina J, et al. Crit Care Med 1988;13:537–40.
57. Heymsfield SB, Erbland M, Casper K, et al. Clin Chest Med 1986;7:41–67.
58. Kim HY, Picciano MF, Walig MA. J Nutr 1992;122:1760–7.
59. Coursin DB, Cihla HP. Thorax 1996;51:479–83.
60. Koretz RL. Chest 1990;98:524–6.
61. Miller KS, Tomlinson JR, Sahn SA. Chest 1985;88:230–3.
62. Berger R, Adams L. Chest 1989;96:372–8.
63. Zaloga GP. Chest 1991;100:1643–6.
64. Strong RM, Condon SC, Solinger MR, et al. JPEN J Parenter Enteral Nutr 1992;16:59–63.
65. Torres A, Serra-Batlles J, Ros E. Ann Intern Med 1992;116: 540–3.
66. Humphrey H, Hall J, Sznajder I, et al. Chest 1990;97:1176–80.
67. Bo-Linn GW, Anderson DJ, Anderson KC, et al. Cathet Cardiovasc Diagn 1982;8:23–7.
68. Imperial J, Bistrian BR, Bothe A, et al. J Am Coll Nutr 1983; 2:63–9.
69. Kruse JA, Shah NJ. Nutr Clin Pract 1993;8:163–70.
70. Hageman JR, Hunt CE. Clin Chest Med 1986;7:69–72.
71. Zaloga GP. Nutrition and prevention of systemic infection. In: Taylor RW, Shoemaker WC, eds. Critical care state of the art. Fullerton, CA: Society of Critical Care Medicine 1991;31–80.
72. Baybutt RC, Smith JE, Gillespie TG, et al. Lipids 1994; 29:535–9.
73. Palombo JD, Lydon EE, Chen PL, et al. Lipids 1994;29:643–9.
74. Higgins MW, Thom T. Curr Pulmonol 1988;9:1–24.
75. Higgins MW, Keller JB, Bedar M, et al. Am Rev Respir Dis 1982;125:144–51.

75a. Massaro GDC, Massaro D. Nature Med 1997;3:765–7.

76. Britton JR, Pavord ID, Richands KA, et al. Am J Respir Crit Care 1995;151:1383–7.
77. Strachnan DP, Cox BD, Erzinclioglu SW, et al. Thorax 1991; 46:624–9.
78. Schwartz J, Weiss ST. Am J Clin Nutr 1994;59:110–4.
79. Schwartz J, Weiss ST. Am J Epidemiol 1990;130:67–76.
80. Morabia A, Menkes MJS, Comstock GW, et al. Am J Epidemiol 1990;132:77–82.
81. Chuwers P, Barnhart S, Blanc P, et al. Am J Respir Crit Care Med 1997;155:1066–71.
82. Shahar E, Folsom SL, Melnik MS. Am J Respir Crit Care Med 1994;150:978–82.
83. Lieberman D, Heimer D. Thorax 1992;47:360–2.
84. Pistelli R, Forastiere F, Corbo GM, et al. Eur Res J 1993;6: 517–22.
85. Shahar E, Folsom AR, Melnick SL. N Engl J Med 1994; 331:228–33.
86. Sharp DS, Rodriguez L, Shahar E, et al. Am J Respir Crit Care Med 1994;150:983–7.
87. Schwartz J, Weiss ST. Am J Clin Nutr 1994;59:110–4.
88. Horrobin DF. Med Hypotheses 1987;22:421–8.
89. Arm JP, Horton CE, Spur BW, et al. Am Rev Respir Dis 1989;139:1395–400.
90. Thien FCK, Mencia-Huerta JM, Lee TL. Am Rev Respir Dis 1993;147:1138–43.
91. Bielory L, Gandhi R. Ann Allergy 1994;73:89–96.
92. Ciarrallo L, Sauer AH, Shannon MW. J Pediatr 1996;129: 809–14.
93. McLean RM. Am J Med 1994;96:63–76.
94. Wilson DO, Rogers RM, Wright RC, et al. Am Rev Resp Dis 1989;139:1435–8.
95. Braun SR, Keim NL, Dixon RM, et al. Chest 1984;86:558–63.
96. Schols A, Moslert R, Soetters P, et al. Chest 1989;96:247–9.
97. Hunter AMB, Carey MA, Larsh HW. Am Rev Respir Dis 1981;124:376–81.
98. Fiaccadori E, Canale SF, Coffrini E, et al. Am J Clin Nutr 1988;48:680–5.
99. Gray-Donald K, Gibbons L, Shupin SH, Martin JG. Am Rev Respir Dis 1989;140:1544–8.
100. Sahebjami H, Doers JT, Render ML, et al. Am J Med 1993; 94:469–74.
101. Schols AMWJ, Soeters PB, Dingemans AMC, et al. Am Rev Respir Dis 1993;147:1151–6.
102. Vandenbergh E, Van de Woestijne KP, Gyselen A. Am Rev Respir Dis 1967;95:556–66.
103. Boushy SF, Adhikari PK, Sakamoto A, Lewis BM. Dis Chest 1964;45:402–10.
104. Renzetti AD, McClement JH, Litt BD. Am J Med 1996; 41:115–29.
105. Chailleux E, Fauroux B, Binet F, et al. Chest 1996;109:741–9.
106. Gray-Donaldson K, Gibbons L, Shapiro SH, et al. Am J Respir Crit Care Med 1996;153:961–6.
107. Goldstein SA. Thomashaw BM, Kvetan V, et al. Am Rev Respir Dis 1988;138:636–44.
108. Donahoe M, Rogers RM, Wilson DO, Pennock BE. Am Rev Respir Dis 1989;140:385–91.
109. Sherman MS, Lang DM, Matityahu A, et al. Chest 1996; 110:1437–42.
110. Jounieaux V, Mayeux I. Am J Respir Crit Care Med 1995;152: 2181–4.
111. Ryan CF, Road JD, Buckley PA, et al. Chest 1993;103:1038–44.
112. Wilson DO, Rogers RM, Sanders MH, et al. Am Rev Respir Dis 1986;134:672–7.
112a. Schols AMWJ, Soeters PB, Mostert R, et al. Am Rev Respir Dis 1991;143:1248–52.
112b. Baarends EM, Shols AMNJ, Pannemans DLE, et al. Am J Respir Crit Care Med 1997;155;549–54.
113. DiFrancia M, Barbier D, Mege JL, et al. Am J Respir Crit Care Med 1994;150:1453–5.
114. Browning RJ, Olsen AM. Mayo Clin Proc 1961;36:537–43.
115. Schols AM, Mostert R, Cobben N. Chest 1991;100:1287–92.
116. Efthimiou J, Fleming J, Gomes C, Spiro SG. Am Rev Respir 1988;137:1075–82.
117. Whittaker JS, Ryan CF, Buckley PA, Road JD. Am Rev Respir Dis 1990;142:283–8.
118. Rogers RM, Donahoe M, Costantino J. Am Rev Respir Dis 1992;146:1511–7.
119. Lewis MI, Belman MJ, Dorr-Uyemura L. Am Rev Respir Dis 1987;135:1062–8.
120. Knowles JB, Fairburn MS, Wiggs BJ, et al. Chest 1988;93: 977–83.
121. Hugli O, Schutz Y, Fitting JW. Am J Rspir Crit Care Med 1996;153:294–300
121a. Dore MF, Labban JP, Orvoen-Frija E, et al. Am J Respir Crit Care Med 1997;155:1535–40.
122. Goldstein SA, Askanazi J, Weismann, et al. Chest 1987;91: 222–4.
122a. Saudny-Unterberger H, Martin JG, Gray-Donald K. Am J Respir Crit Care Med 1997;156:794–9.
123. Suchner U, Rothkopf MM, Stanilaus G, et al. Arch Intern Med 1990;150:1225–30.
124. Pape GS, Friedman M, Underwood LE, CLemmons DR. Chest 1991;99:1495–9.
125. Rudman D, Fellor AG, Nagraj HS. N Engl J Med 1991;323:1–6.
126. Schols AMWJ, Soeters PB, Mostert R, et al. Am J Respir Crit Care Med 1995;152:1268–74.
127. Angelillo VA, Sukhdarshan B, Durfee D, et al. Ann Intern Med 1985;103:883–5.
128. Kwan R, Mir MA. Am J Med 1987;82:751–8.
129. Brown SE, Nagendran RC, McHugh JW, et al. Am Rev Respir Dis 1985;132:960–2.
130. Sue DY, Chung MM, Grosvenor M, Wasserman K. Am Rev Respir Dis 1989;139:1430–4.
131. Aubier M, Murcianeo D, Lecocquic Y, et al. N Engl J Med 1985;313:420–4.
132. Laaban JP, Grateau G, Psychoyos I, et al. Crit Care Med 1989;17:1115–20.
133. Laaban JP, Waked M, Laromiguiere M, et al. Ann Intern Med 1990;112:68–9.
134. Brady HR, Ryan F, Cunningham J, et al. Arch Intern Med 1989;149:2367–8.
135. Aubier M, Viires N, Piquet J, et al. J Appl Physiol 1985; 58:2054.
136. Bell SC, Saunders MJ, Elborn JS. Thorax 1996;51:126–31.
137. Corey M, McLaughlin FJ, Williams M, et al. J Clin Epidemiol 1988;41:583–91.
138. Steinhamp G, von der Hardt H. J Pediatr 1994;124:244–9.
138a. Fitz Simmons SC. N Engl J Med 1997;336:1283–9.
139. Pastorino U, Infante I, Maioli M, et al. Am J Clin Oncol 1993; 11:1216–22.
140. The Alpha-Tocopherol, Beta-carotene Cancer Prevention Study Group. N Engl J Med 1994;330:1029–35.
141. Ommen GS, Goodman GE, Thornquist MD, et al. N Engl J Med 1996;334:1150–5.
142. Hennekens CH, Buring JE, Manson JE, et al. N Engl J Med 1996;334:1145–9.
143. Hashim SA, Roholt HB, Babayan VK, et al. N Engl J Med 1964;270:755–61.
144. Abenhaim L, Moride Y, Brenot F, et al. N Engl J Med 1996;335:609–16.

91. Nutrition and Retinal Degenerations

ELIOT L. BERSON

Degenerative diseases of the retina represent a significant cause of visual loss to people from all over the world. For the most part, these conditions result in visual loss due to compromise of the rod and cone photoreceptor cells in the outer retina. The role of adequate nutrition (especially vitamins A and E) in maintaining normal photoreceptor cell function and viability is well known. It is now apparent that some patients with photoreceptor cell degeneration can benefit from nutritional intervention. This chapter focuses on diseases involving the photoreceptor cells that have yielded to treatment with nutritional supplementation and/or dietary modification.

RETINITIS PIGMENTOSA

Background

Night blindness was first recognized in Egypt more than 3400 years ago as described in a papyrus called *The Book of the Eyes* found during archeologic excavations in Thebes. The Egyptians recommended a nutritional treatment for night blindness, namely, eating liver, which is now recognized as a rich source of vitamin A. In 1851 the ophthalmoscope was invented, and it became possible to visualize the living retina and underlying retinal pigment epithelium for the first time. Ophthalmoscopic examination of some night-blind individuals revealed a distinctive pattern of pigment around the peripheral retina, which led to the designation of their condition as retinitis pigmentosa (1).

Retinitis pigmentosa affects 50,000 to 100,000 people in the United States and an estimated 1.5 million people worldwide. Affected patients usually report impaired dark adaptation, night blindness, and loss of midperipheral visual field in adolescence. As the condition progresses, they lose far peripheral visual field and eventually lose central vision as well. Some patients become blind as early as age 30, and most are legally blind by age 60, with a central visual field diameter less than 20°. In addition to the characteristic intraretinal pigment seen around the midperiphery, findings on ophthalmoscopy include attenuation of the retinal vessels and, in some cases, waxy pallor of the optic discs. Histopathologic examination of autopsy eyes with advanced-stage disease show that loss of vision is due to degeneration of both rod and cone photoreceptor cells (2).

Retinitis pigmentosa can be detected in early life by electroretinographic testing. Electroretinograms (ERGs) are recorded in response to flashes of light with a contact lens electrode placed on the topically anesthetized cornea; responses are amplified and displayed on an oscilloscope. Patients with the early stages of retinitis pigmentosa have ERGs that are reduced in amplitude and delayed in their temporal aspects (Fig. 91.1). ERG amplitudes become smaller as the disease progresses; patients are usually legally blind when their cone ERG amplitudes fall below 0.05 microvolts (μV) (normal, 50–100 μV). Abnormal ERGs have been detected in asymptomatic children in some cases a decade before diagnostic changes are seen on a routine ophthalmoscopic examination. Individuals, age 6 and older, with normal ERGs and a family history of retinitis pigmentosa have not been observed to develop a widespread form of retinitis pigmentosa at a later time (2).

Retinitis pigmentosa can be inherited by an autosomal dominant, autosomal recessive, X-linked, digenic, or mitochondrial mode (2–4). Substantial genetic heterogeneity has been observed in this condition, with over 20 chromosomal loci mapped (5, 6). Mutations have been identified in eight genes (4, 7–14) and undoubtedly more abnormal genes will be discovered. Four of these genes encode proteins in the rod phototransduction cascade—rhodopsin, the α- and β-subunits of rod cGMP phosphodiesterase, and the rod cGMP cation-gated channel protein α-subunit. Two of these genes encode proteins involved in maintaining photoreceptor outer segment disc structure—peripherin/RDS and rod outer segment membrane protein 1 (ROM1). Mutations in the gene encoding myosin VIIa have been found in a form of autosomal recessive retinitis pigmentosa with associated profound congenital deafness

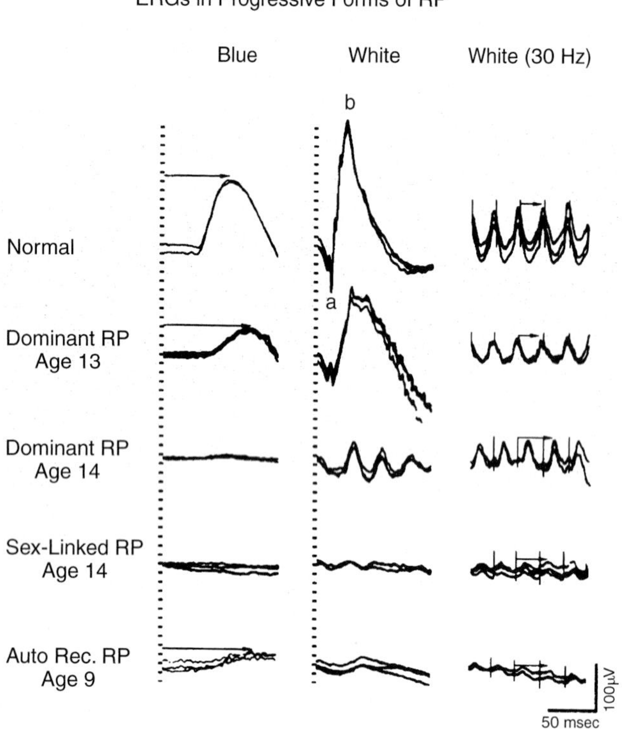

Figure 91.1. ERG responses for a normal subject and four patients (ages 13, 14, 14, and 9) with retinitis pigmentosa. Stimulus onset is *vertical hatched lines* for columns 1 and 2 and *vertical shock artifacts* for column 3. Rod b-wave implicit times in column 1 and cone implicit times in column 3 are designated with *arrows*. Calibration symbol *(lower right corner)* signifies 50 msec horizontally and 100 μvolts (μV) vertically for all tracings. Under these test conditions, normal amplitudes are ≥100 μV *(left column)*, ≥350 μV *(middle column)*, and ≥50 μV *(right column)*. Normal rod implicit time is ≤108 msec and normal cone implicit time is ≤32 msec. (From Berson EL. Invest Ophthalmol Vis Sci 1993;34:1659–76, with permission.)

(Usher syndrome, type I). Mutations have also been found in a GTPase regulator gene in a form of X-linked retinitis pigmentosa. Mutations in these eight genes account for about 20 to 25% of cases of retinitis pigmentosa in the United States. In the case of rhodopsin gene defects, patients with the same mutation display considerable variability in clinical expression at a given age, suggesting that some factor(s) other than the gene defect can affect the course of this condition (15, 16).

Treatment

While studying the course of the common forms of retinitis pigmentosa with the ERG from 1979 to 1983, it was observed that patients self-treating with a separate capsule of vitamin A or vitamin E appeared to be losing less ERG amplitude annually than those not taking these supplements. The relationship between vitamin A intake and ERG amplitude suggested that a total (i.e., diet plus supplement) intake of more than 15,000 IU of vitamin A or more than 200 IU of vitamin E or the combination was potentially therapeutic (17). These preliminary findings, as well as the known biologic roles of vitamin A and vitamin E in maintaining normal photoreceptor cell function and structure (18–21), prompted a randomized, controlled, double-masked trial with a 2 × 2 factorial design to determine whether vitamin A or vitamin E, alone or in combination, would halt or slow the progression of retinitis pigmentosa as monitored by the ERG. The main outcome variable was the 30-Hz cone-flicker ERG.

In broad outline, patients were evaluated twice over a 6-week interval prior to institution of vitamin supplementation. The screening visit was used to determine eligibility and the baseline visit to determine intervisit variability. The average of screening and baseline was used to provide pretreatment values. Patients were randomly assigned to one of four treatment groups: vitamin A, 15,000 IU/day, plus vitamin E, 3 IU/day (group A); vitamin A, 75 IU/day, plus vitamin E, 3 IU/day (group trace); vitamin A, 15,000 IU/day, plus vitamin E, 400 IU/day (group A+E); and vitamin A, 75 IU/day, plus vitamin E, 400 IU/day (group E). The procedure for randomization took into account the estimated dietary intake of vitamins A and E as well as the genetic type recorded at the screening examination. ERGs were monitored annually. Visual field areas and visual acuities were also followed as additional measures of visual function.

Mean annual rates of decline of remaining ERG amplitude were slowest for the group taking 15,000 IU/day of vitamin A and fastest for the group taking 400 IU/day of vitamin E. These rates were observed among all randomized patients as well as among a subgroup of 354 patients with slightly higher initial ERG amplitudes who could be followed more reliably; this subgroup was designated the higher-amplitude cohort. Mean annual rates of decline of the remaining 30-Hz ERG amplitude among this cohort were as follows: group A, 8.3%; group trace, 10%; group A+E, 8.8%; and group E, 11.8%. Rates of decline for visual field area showed similar trends, although the differences were not statistically significant. No significant differences were observed among groups with respect to rates of decline of visual acuity. These results are summarized in Table 91.1.

The mean declines in 30-Hz cone ERG from baseline for the higher-amplitude cohort by year are plotted in Figure 91.2. The greatest separation among treatment

Table 91.1
Mean Rates of Decline in Visual Function by Treatment Group

	All Randomized Patients				Higher-Amplitude Cohort			
Test	A	Trace	A+E	E	A	Trace	A+E	E
30 Hz[a]	6.1	7.1	6.3	7.9	8.3	10.0	8.8	11.8
0.5 Hz[a]	8.7	9.6	9.1	10.6	8.1	9.4	8.4	10.9
Field area[a]	5.6	5.9	6.2	6.3	6.3	7.2	7.3	7.8
Visual acuity[b]	1.1	0.9	0.7	0.9	0.8	0.8	0.7	0.7

Modified from Berson EL, Rosner B, Sandberg MA, et al. Arch Ophthalmol 1993;111:761–72, with permission of the American Medical Association, Chicago; copyright 1993, American Medical Association.

[a]Percentage decline in remaining function per year.

[b]Letters lost per year.

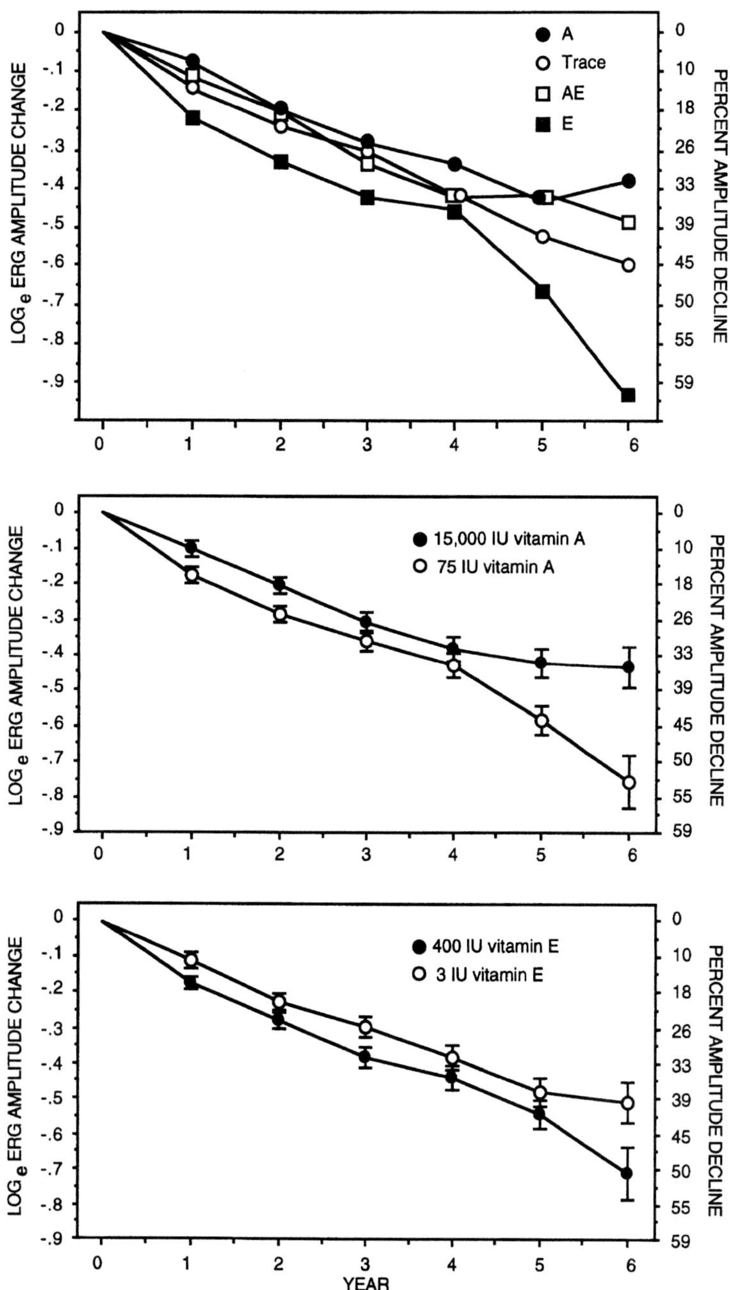

Figure 91.2. Mean change from baseline over 6 years in 30-Hz ERG amplitude in the higher-amplitude cohort by treatment group *(top),* by vitamin A main effect *(center);* and by vitamin E main effect *(bottom).* Sample sizes for years 1 through 6 respectively were n = 171, 167, 168, 164, 123, and 59 for patients receiving vitamin A, 15,000 IU/day, and n = 178, 182, 172, 171, 125, and 64 for patients receiving vitamin A, 75 IU/day. Sample sizes for years 1 through 6 respectively were n = 178, 177, 173, 168, 122, and 61 for the patients on vitamin E, 400 IU/day and n = 171, 172, 167, 167, 126, and 62 for patients receiving vitamin E, 3 IU/day. (From Berson EL, Rosner B, Sandberg MA, et al. Arch Ophthalmol 1993;111:761–72, with permission of the American Medical Association, Chicago; copyright 1993, American Medical Association.)

groups occurred at years 5 and 6. Mean change analyses revealed that the two groups receiving 15,000 IU/day of vitamin A had, on average, significantly smaller declines from baseline than those not receiving this dose at years 1, 2, 5, and 6 ($P < .01$ in each of these years), while the two groups receiving vitamin E at 400 IU/day had, on average, significantly greater declines in retinal function than those not on this dose at years 1, 3, and 6 ($P < .03$ in each of these years).

The mean declines from baseline in 30-Hz cone ERG amplitude were related to the total vitamin A intake (i.e., diet plus supplement) irrespective of randomization assignment. The average decline in amplitude in the higher-amplitude cohort was greatest for those with a daily vitamin A intake below 2,428 IU, intermediate for those between 2,428 and 16,946, and least for those with an intake of 16,947 IU or more (Fig. 91.3); a significant difference was found among these subgroups. These data show that the optimal total intake of vitamin A was approximately 18,000 IU per day; that is, a supplement of 15,000 IU plus a regu-

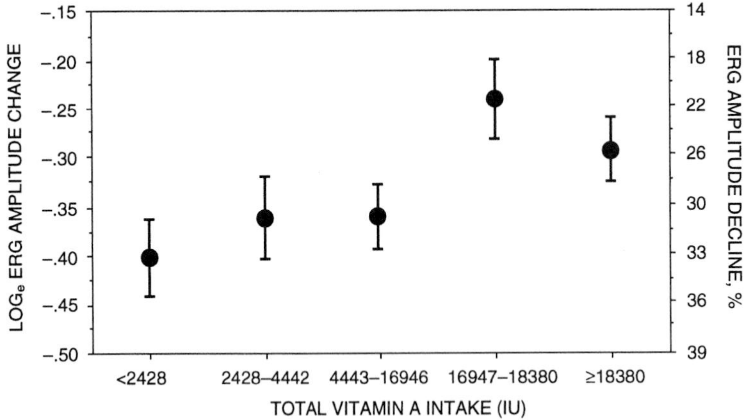

Figure 91.3. Mean ± SE decline from baseline in 30-Hz ERG amplitude by total vitamin A intake (diet plus capsules) irrespective of randomization assignment for all patients with retinitis pigmentosa in the higher-amplitude cohort. The mean decline was calculated as the mean of screening and baseline minus the mean of all follow-up visits by quintile of total vitamin A intake averaged over all visits. Sample sizes were 69, 72, 74, 65, and 74 for the lowest to highest quintiles of total vitamin A intake. *Vertical bars* indicate SEs. (From Berson EL, Rosner B, Sandberg MA, et al. Arch Ophthalmol 1993;111:761–72, with permission of the American Medical Association, Chicago; copyright 1993, American Medical Association.)

lar diet of about 3,500 IU of vitamin A daily resulted in the smallest ERG decline. Intake above 18,380 IU provided no greater benefit. Doses of 25,000 IU or more over the long term are considered potentially toxic (22–24).

These data support the hypothesis that a 15,000-IU supplement of vitamin A taken daily will slow the progression of the common forms of retinitis pigmentosa as monitored by ERG testing. The findings also suggest that a 400-IU supplement of vitamin E taken daily may adversely affect the course of the common forms of this disease. With respect to rates of decline of remaining 30-Hz cone ERG amplitude, the beneficial effect of vitamin A was shown for all randomized patients at the $P = .01$ level and for the higher-amplitude cohort at the $P < .001$ level. The possible adverse effect of vitamin E was shown for the higher-amplitude cohort ($P = .04$) but not for all randomized patients (17).

Based on these ERG results, it is recommended that most adults with the common forms of retinitis pigmentosa take 15,000 IU of vitamin A daily under medical supervision and avoid high-dose supplements of vitamin E such as the 400 IU/day used in the trial. It is also recommended that patients continue on a regular diet without specifically selecting foods containing high levels of preformed vitamin A. As a precaution, patients should have a pretreatment assessment of fasting serum vitamin A and liver function and annual evaluations thereafter. Because of the potential for birth defects, women who are pregnant or planning to become pregnant should not take this dose of vitamin A. Since patients under age 18 were not included in this study, no formal recommendation can be made for such patients.

No toxic side effects attributable to this vitamin A supplement were observed over 4 to 6 years. Furthermore, no reported case of toxicity in adults in good general health on this dose has been reported. The palmitate form of vitamin A used in the trial is recommended for therapeutic use; other forms might be suitable, but some are probably not, for example β-carotene which is not predictably converted to vitamin A from one patient to another.

The precise mechanism by which vitamin A preserves retinal function in retinitis pigmentosa is not known. Vitamin A may provide some of its benefit through the rescue of remaining cones, thereby explaining how one supplement may help a group of patients with a variety of different rod-specific gene defects. Vitamin E may adversely affect this condition by reducing the amount of vitamin A reaching the eye; serum vitamin A levels were observed to be significantly lower in patients on vitamin E (17, 25).

In this study, the rate of decline for the group taking 15,000 units of vitamin A daily was about 20% slower than the rate of decline for the trace group. Assuming that the rates of decline observed in this study are sustained over the long term, the estimated time to reach 0.05 μV (i.e., legal blindness) for an average patient with 1.3 μV who starts supplementation at age 32 would be age 70 for group A, 63 for group trace, 67 for group A+E, and 58 for group E. Thus, vitamin A supplementation would be expected to provide 7 additional years of useful vision for the average patient in this trial (17). A patient with twice the amplitude, or 2.6 μV, to 30-Hz white light who starts vitamin A at age 32 would reach 0.05 μV at age 78. Although not a cure, for some patients with retinitis pigmentosa and larger pretreatment ERGs, vitamin A supplementation may make the difference that allows them to retain some vision for their entire lives (17, 26).

BASSEN-KORNZWEIG SYNDROME

Background

In 1950, Bassen and Kornzweig described an 18-year-old girl, born of first cousins, who had a malabsorption syndrome, generalized retinal degeneration, a diffuse neuromuscular disease similar to Friedreich's ataxia, and a peculiar crenation of the red blood cells, now called acanthocytosis (27–29). In 1958, low serum cholesterol was observed (30). Soon thereafter, an absence of low-density plasma lipoproteins or so-called β-lipoproteins was found, and the term *abetalipoproteinemia* was assigned to this recessively inherited disorder (31–33) (see also Chapter 70). Other classes of lipoproteins have also been found to be abnormal (34).

Patients with the Bassen-Kornzweig syndrome can assimilate fat into the intestinal mucosa, but a defect exists in its removal from this site because of the lack of chylomicra. Intestinal biopsies have revealed normal-sized villi filled with lipid droplets that are essentially triglycerides. Mutations in the gene encoding a microsomal triglyceride-transfer protein have been found in patients with this condition (35). It appears that the liver and then the retina become depleted of vitamin A. Abnormal ERGs have been reported in a 15-month-old child (36) and a 6-year-old patient (37) in whom the fundi were still normal. The original patient described by Bassen and Kornzweig showed multiple white dots in the early stages, but by age 31, she developed multiple areas of pigment epithelial cell atrophy. In other patients, the typical intraretinal pigment associated with retinitis pigmentosa has been noted in the retinal periphery.

Treatment

Patients with this condition are treated with a low-fat diet and supplements of the fat-soluble vitamins A, E, and K. Vitamin A supplementation has been shown to restore elevated dark adaptation thresholds and reduced ERG responses to normal in two patients with the early stages (Fig. 91.4) (38–39). More-advanced patients have not responded, but in one instance, examination of the retina after the death of the patient revealed widespread loss of photoreceptor cells (40). Vitamin A therapy may not maintain retinal function over the long term, as patients have been reported whose vitamin A levels were restored to normal without halting progression of retinal degeneration (41, 42). Since these patients have low serum vitamin E levels, supplementation with vitamin E in addition to vitamin A has been advocated with reported stabilization of retinal function (43–45).

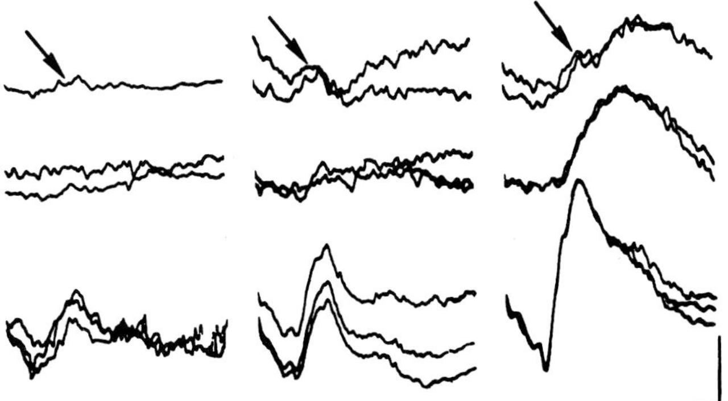

Figure 91.4. Full-field ERGs to a red *(top)* and a blue *(middle)* light, equal for rod vision, and a brighter white stimulus *(bottom)* from a patient with hereditary abetalipoproteinemia (dark adapted). Responses in the *left column* were obtained before vitamin A therapy, those in the *middle column* at 6 hours, and those on the *right,* 24 hours after vitamin A therapy. Two to three responses to the same stimulus are superimposed. *Arrows* indicate an exclusively cone response. The light stimulus begins with each trace. The calibration *(lower right)* signifies 0.06 mV vertically and 60 msec horizontally. (From Gouras P, Carr RE, Gunkel RD. Invest Ophthalmol Vis Sci 1971;10:784–93, with permission.)

Vitamin E supplementation has also been reported to be beneficial for patients with another rare recessively inherited form of ataxia associated with retinitis pigmentosa. These patients present with Friedreich-like ataxia, dysarthria, hyporeflexia, and decreased proprioceptive and vibratory sensation as well as markedly decreased serum vitamin E levels. They later can develop fundus changes of retinitis pigmentosa with abnormal ERGs. Molecular genetic analysis revealed a mutation in the α-tocopherol-transfer protein (α-TTP) gene (see also Chapter 19). Oral administration of vitamin E restored serum vitamin E levels to normal and appeared to halt or slow progression of the neurologic abnormalities and retinitis pigmentosa in three patients followed for 1, 4, and 10 years, respectively (46, 47).

REFSUM DISEASE

Background

Refsum disease is an inborn error of metabolism in which the patient accumulates exogenous phytanic acid. Findings include a peripheral neuropathy, ataxia, an increase in cerebrospinal fluid protein with a normal cell count, and retinitis pigmentosa. Anosmia, neurogenic impairment of hearing, and cardiac abnormalities can be present. Additional signs include pupillary abnormalities, lens opacities, skeletal malformations, and skin changes sometimes resembling ichthyosis. The fundus can be granular around the periphery, with a subnormal ERG in early stages or show more typical retinitis pigmentosa, with a nondetectable ERG in more advanced stages.

In 1946, Refsum recognized the clinical association of seemingly unrelated findings (48). Klenk and Kahlke (49) demonstrated the biochemical abnormality in 1963, namely, storage in many tissues of 3,5,7,11-tetramethylhexadecanoic acid or phytanic acid. In 1966, affected patients were found to have a defect in the first step in phytanic acid oxidation—introduction of a hydroxyl group on the α-carbon of phytanic acid (Fig. 91.5) (50, 51). This loss of activity of phytanic acid α-hydroxylase has been detected in cultured skin fibroblasts of affected patients; carriers of this autosomal recessive disorder have a partial deficiency (52). The relationship between elevated serum phytanic acid and the manifestations of Refsum disease is still unclear. One proposal is that phytanic acid can replace long-chain fatty acids in phospholipids and triglycerides with consequent malfunction. Another hypothesis is that phytanic acid accumulates in

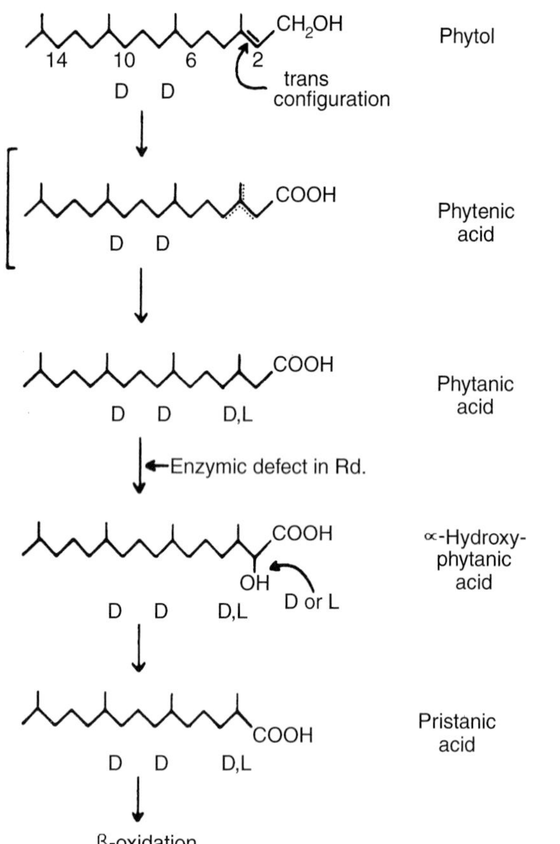

Figure 91.5. Phytanic acid, its immediate precursors and metabolites and site of enzyme defect in Refsum disease *(Rd)*. (From Eldjarn L, Stokke O, Try K. Biochemical aspects of Refsum's disease and principles for the dietary treatment. In: Vinken PJ, Bruyn GW, eds. Handbook of clinical neurology. Amsterdam: North-Holland, 1976;27: 528, with permission.)

the myelin lipid bilayer and disrupts the packing of myelin because of its branched methyl groups. In one autopsy specimen a large amount of fat-staining substance could be seen in the retinal pigment epithelium, which could presumably compromise the retinal pigment epithelial cells and eventually the photoreceptors (53).

Treatment

Phytanic acid is present primarily in dairy products, meat, and green leafy vegetables (54). Experiments in normal animals and man have shown that free phytol can be converted to phytanic acid in the body, but it is not clear whether the phytol bound to chlorophyll in green leafy vegetables is absorbed in the intestine. Therefore, until more is known, patients are advised to restrict not only milk products and animal fats (i.e., phytanic acid) but also green leafy vegetables containing phytol (55). Success in dietary treatment of Refsum disease depends on the patient receiving sufficient calories; if not, body weight becomes reduced and phytanic acid is released from tissue stores, resulting in increased serum phytanic acid levels that can exacerbate symptoms.

Refsum reported two patients whose serum phytanic acid levels were lowered to normal with subsequent improvement in motor nerve conduction velocity, some relief of ataxia, and return of the cerebrospinal fluid protein to normal (56). The retinitis pigmentosa and hearing impairment did not progress. One patient was followed for over 10 years and the other for many years. Other researchers have documented improvement in nerve conduction times and cerebrospinal fluid protein (57–59) as well as the histologic appearance of peripheral nerve (60). The long-term effects of dietary modification on retinal function in Refsum disease continue to be studied. Plasma exchange complementing the dietary regimen has been reported to be helpful in the treatment of this disease (61–63). Although the mechanism that links phytanic acid to the disease process remains to be defined, successful reversal of at least some of the abnormalities after dietary treatment supports the idea that the phytanic acid itself is responsible for some, if not all, of the clinical manifestations.

GYRATE ATROPHY OF THE CHOROID AND RETINA

Background

Gyrate atrophy of the choroid and retina is a chorioretinal degeneration with an autosomal recessive mode of inheritance (64, 65). Patients usually report night blindness and loss of peripheral vision between the ages of 10 and 20 years. Ocular findings include myopia, constricted visual fields, elevated dark adaptation thresholds, very small or nondetectable ERG responses, and chorioretinal atrophy distributed circumferentially around the peripheral fundus and sometimes near the optic disc. In addition to the ocular findings, abnormalities in electroencephalograms, muscle and hair morphology, and mitochondrial structure in the liver have been reported (66–69). Enlargement, coalescence, and posterior extension of areas of atrophy have been observed in young patients within 2 years (70). Patients develop cataracts and, if untreated, usually become virtually blind between the ages of 40 and 55 because of extensive chorioretinal atrophy (71).

Patients with gyrate atrophy have plasma ornithine concentrations 10 to 20 times normal (72, 73) due to a deficiency in ornithine-ketoacid-aminotransferase (OAT) activity (Fig. 91.6) (74–76). Patients cannot convert ornithine to pyrroline-5-carboxylic acid (PCA), and this deficiency can be detected in extracts of cultured skin fibroblasts. Patients have virtually no OAT activity in contrast to normal subjects, while carrier parents have a partial deficiency. Cultured cells from some patients have shown increased OAT activity when increasing concentrations of the cofactor for OAT, pyridoxal phosphate or vitamin B_6, are added to the media. Plasma lysine (77), glutamate, and glutamine (78), as well as serum and urine creatine (79) levels are reduced. More than 60 mutations have been discovered in the OAT gene on chromosome 10 in affected patients (80–83).

Intravitreal injections of ornithine in the normal

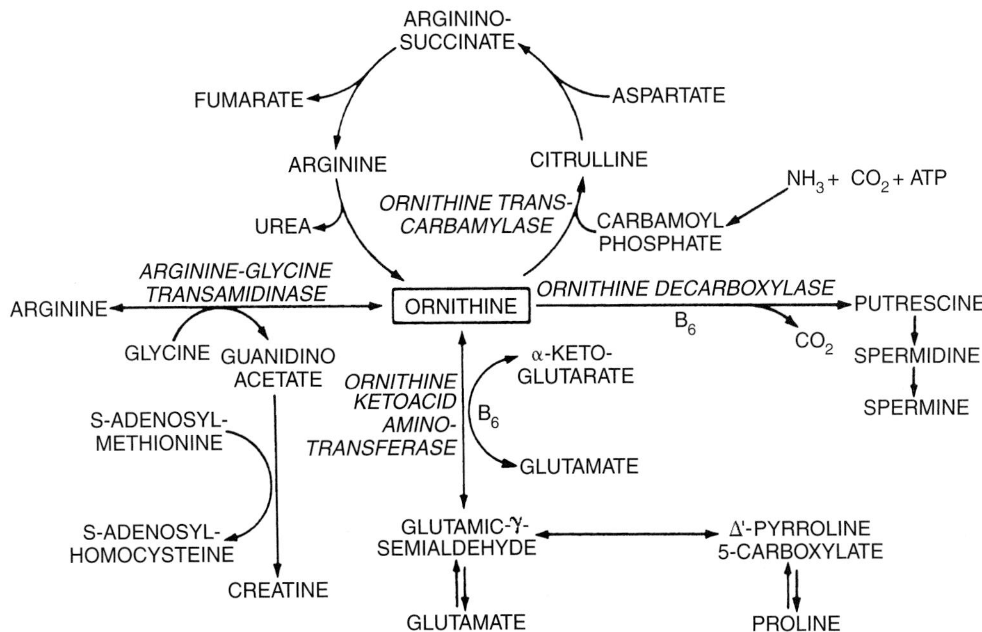

Figure 91.6. Pathways of ornithine metabolism. (From Weleber RG, Kennaway GN, Buist NR. Int Ophthalmol 1981;4:23–32, with permission.)

primate led to swelling and death of retinal pigment epithelial cells, with subsequent death of overlying photoreceptors (84). Moreover, the enzyme OAT is found in the normal pigment epithelium (85, 86), leading to the proposal that death of the pigment epithelial cells and then the photoreceptor cells results from elevated levels of ornithine combined with absence of OAT activity. Since arginine is a precursor of ornithine and since arginine (but not ornithine) is a constituent of food protein, it has been suggested that dietary restriction of protein and arginine would reduce plasma ornithine levels in these patients (87). OAT-deficient mice produced by gene targeting develop a retinal degeneration over several months that is amenable to treatment postweaning with an arginine-restricted diet (88, 89).

Treatment

The hyperornithinemia associated with gyrate atrophy has been lowered toward normal with low-protein, low-arginine diets in all patients so far studied (87, 90–93) and with vitamin B_6 (300–500 mg/day) in some cases (70, 94, 95). However, extreme protein restriction (10–15 g/day) with substantial lowering of plasma ornithine, accomplished under supervision in the hospital, has been difficult to achieve at home; thus many patients have followed modified (20–35 g/day) protein restriction with slight rises in their plasma ornithine levels. Some investigators have reported improvements in visual acuity, visual fields, dark adaptation thresholds, and/or ERGs in patients with gyrate atrophy after initiating either the diet or vitamin B_6 (91, 93, 96–98); others have not documented any significant improvement in visual function despite substantial reductions in plasma ornithine concentrations (92, 99). Improvement in muscle morphology following creatine supplementation was reported in several patients (100).

Kaiser-Kupfer and coworkers (101) reported results of severe arginine restriction of two pairs of siblings under 10 years of age who were followed for 5 to 7 years. Plasma ornithine levels were reduced to approximately the normal range (106 and 121 μmol/L) in one pair of siblings and reached twice the upper limit of normal (251 and 313 μmol/L) in the other pair. These younger siblings had significantly less atrophy than their elder siblings when they reached or approached the age at which their elders began the diet. Thus, there is evidence that a low-protein, low-arginine diet can slow progression of the chorioretinal degeneration, but only a small number of patients have been studied.

The goal of treatment is to maintain serum ornithine levels as close to normal as possible. Since some patients may respond to supplementation with pyridoxine (vitamin B_6), all patients are initially given a trial of this vitamin to determine to what extent, if any, it will lower plasma ornithine levels. Both pyridoxine-responsive and nonresponsive patients are then placed on a low-protein, low-arginine diet. Biochemical control is classified as good to excellent (≤200 μmol/L), fair (200–400 μmol/L), and poor (>400 μmol/L). In the management of children, expertise is required to be certain that growth and development remain normal while ornithine levels are lowered with a low-protein diet. An arginine-free essential amino acid mixture (e.g., Cyclinex-1 or -2 [Ross Laboratories], depending on the patient's age) is used to provide sufficient nitrogen and meet essential amino acid requirements. In adults, a low-protein diet is also likely to result in amino acid deficiency. Thus, adults should also be placed on an arginine-free essential amino acid mixture. Lysine supplementation may be necessary, depending on plasma levels. As a precaution, all patients are placed on a multivitamin preparation with minerals. In addition to a regular ocular examination, all patients on this treatment regimen should have their amino acid and protein levels monitored periodically (102).

SORSBY FUNDUS DYSTROPHY

Background

Sorsby fundus dystrophy is a rare autosomal dominant retinal degeneration in which patients report night blindness in young adulthood and then experience progressive loss of central vision in association with subretinal neovascularization and hemorrhage; in later stages, patients lose peripheral vision as well (103–106). The condition is caused by mutations in the tissue inhibitor of metalloproteinase-3 (TIMP3) gene on chromosome 22 (107). The exact pathogenesis of this condition remains to be defined, but it has been speculated that mutations lead to an abnormal lipid-containing deposit interposed between the photoreceptors and their blood supply in the choroid. This subretinal deposit, located within Bruch's membrane and present beneath the entire retina, appears to create a barrier to diffusion of nutrients to the photoreceptors.

Treatment

In a family with Sorsby fundus dystrophy, orally administered vitamin A in a dose of 50,000 IU/day reversed nightblindness within 1 week in early stages of the disease. Recovery of rod sensitivity in the macula followed recovery of rod sensitivity in the retinal periphery by several days, but once achieved, could not be maintained on a dose of 5,000 IU/day. Cone sensitivity in the central macula remained normal during the period of the study, while rod function varied (108).

The mechanism leading to a local deficiency of vitamin A in the retina in Sorsby fundus dystrophy is unknown. It has been suggested that the disturbance in the extracellular matrix caused by TIMP3 mutations may over decades impair storage of vitamin A in the retinal pigment epithelium and/or its transport to the photoreceptors. Photoreceptors deprived of vitamin A lose sensitivity to light and cannot regenerate functional visual pigment (i.e., opsin plus vitamin A) at a normal rate after exposure to light, resulting in slowed dark adaptation (108). Although supplementation with vitamin A has had short-term benefit for some patients with early stages of this condition, it remains to be determined whether vitamin A supplementation in doses considered safe for chronic administration (i.e., <25,000 IU/day) can be used to modify the course of this disease over the long term.

AGE-RELATED MACULAR DEGENERATION

Background

Age-related macular degeneration (AMD) is the leading cause of irreversible blindness in the United States among persons over age 50 (109, 110). The condition affects 1.7 million people in the United States and many millions worldwide (109). Patients develop moderate- to large-sized drusen (yellowish white spots) and a disturbance of the retinal pigment epithelium (RPE). Visual loss is related to atrophy of the RPE (dry form) or to a choroidal neovascular membrane (CNVM) that leads to hemorrhage, exudation, elevation of the macular retina, and scarring (wet form). There is no proven way to halt or slow progression in eyes with the dry form; and, despite the availability of laser photocoagulation, more than half of the eyes with a CNVM decline to a visual acuity below 20/200. Most patients who are legally blind as a result of AMD have the neovascular form of the disease (111).

Treatment

A high dietary intake of carotenoids has been associated with a lower risk for developing neovascular AMD. Those in the highest quintile of carotenoid intake had a 43% lower risk for developing an advanced stage of AMD than those in the lowest quintile. Lutein and zeaxanthin, primarily obtained from dark green leafy vegetables, were the carotenoids most strongly associated with a reduced risk for AMD. Several foods with a high content of carotenoids were inversely associated with AMD. Specifically, higher frequency intake of spinach or collard greens was associated with a substantially lower risk for AMD (P for trend $<.001$). Intake of preformed vitamin A (retinol) was not appreciably related to AMD. Moreover, neither vitamin E nor total vitamin C intake was associated with a statistically significant reduced risk for AMD. Based on these results, Seddon et al. have recommended that patients with AMD increase their consumption of vegetables, particularly, dark green leafy vegetables rich in lutein and zeaxanthin (112). VandenLangenberg et al. reported that higher intake of fruits and vegetables and certain carotenoids may be associated with decreased risk of developing the early fundus changes of AMD (113). Sanders et al. found no consistent differences in plasma concentrations of vitamin E, retinol, or carotenoids or in the erythrocyte phospholipid composition in patients with AMD compared with concentrations in a control population matched with respect to age and sex (114). These observational studies are helpful in generating hypotheses but should not be interpreted as conclusive for showing cause and effect.

Some preliminary evidence suggests that supplementation with zinc may slow the course of AMD (115). It has also been hypothesized that antioxidants—β-carotene, vitamin C, and vitamin E—might have a protective effect on the membranes of photoreceptors that are rich in polyunsaturated fatty acids (116–118). A randomized, controlled trial is in progress to determine whether β-carotene, vitamin C, and vitamin E as well as trace minerals (particularly zinc) will modify the course of this condition.

SUMMARY

Considerable progress has been made in the understanding and management of degenerative diseases of the retina involving photoreceptors. Nutritional approaches to treatment have proved successful in the case of the common forms of retinitis pigmentosa (supplementation with vitamin A), Bassen-Kornzweig disease (supplementation with vitamins A, E, and K), gyrate atrophy (low-protein, low-arginine diet and/or supplementation with vitamin B_6), and Refsum disease (low-phytol, low–phytanic acid diet). The night blindness associated with Sorsby fundus dystrophy can be reversed over the short term with vitamin A. A significant trend for decreased risk for advanced or exudative age-related macular degeneration has been reported among those whose diets contain a higher content of carotenoids, such as spinach and collard greens. A randomized trial is in progress to determine if β-carotene, vitamin C, and vitamin E as well as trace minerals, particularly zinc, will modify the course of age-related macular degeneration.

The difficulties that patients with retinal degenerations face as a result of their diminishing vision, sometimes over decades, cannot be underestimated. Nutritional therapy has proved effective in modifying the course of a number of these conditions; the therapeutic benefit of nutritional modification in diseases that have a genetic basis is of particular interest. Further research is warranted to determine the mechanisms by which these treatments provide their benefit, as well as to identify other conditions that may yield to nutritional intervention. Risk-factor analyses of well-defined populations followed over time with food-frequency questionnaires in conjunction with careful assessments of visual function may reveal other dietary constituents that can modify the course of degenerative diseases of the retina.

ACKNOWLEDGMENTS

Supported in part by grant EY00169 from the National Eye Institute, Bethesda, MD, and a center grant from the Foundation Fighting Blindness, Baltimore, MD.

REFERENCES

1. Bell J, ed. Retinitis pigmentosa and allied diseases. In: Pearson K, ed. The treasury of human inheritance. London: Cambridge University Press, 1922;3.
2. Berson EL. Invest Ophthalmol Vis Sci 1993;34:1659–76.
3. Dryja TP, Berson EL. Invest Ophthalmol Vis Sci 1995;36: 1197–200.
4. Kajiwara K, Berson EL, Dryja, TP. Science 1994;264:1604–8.
5. Dryja TP, Li T. Hum Mol Genet 1995;4:1739–43.
6. Daiger SP, Sullivan LS, Rodriguez JA. Behav Brain Sci 1995; 18:452–67.
7. Dryja TP, McGee TL, Reichel E, et al. Nature (London) 1990;343:364–6.
8. Farrar GJ, Kenna P, Jordan SA, et al. Nature (London) 1991; 354:478–80.
9. Kajiwara K, Hahn LB, Mukai S, et al. Nature (London) 1991;354:480–3.
10. McLaughlin ME, Sandberg MA, Berson EL, et al. Nature Genet 1993;4:130–3.
11. Dryja TP, Finn JT, Peng YW, et al. Proc Natl Acad Sci USA 1995;92:10177–81.
12. Huang SH, Pittler SJ, Huang X, et al. Nature Genet 1995; 11:468–71.
13. Weil D, Blanchard S, Kaplan J, et al. Nature (London) 1995; 374:60–1.
14. Meindl A, Dry K, Herrmann K. Nature Genet 1996;13:35–42.
15. Berson EL, Rosner B, Sandberg MA, et al. Arch Ophthalmol 1991;109:92–101.
16. Berson EL, Rosner B, Sandberg MA, et al. Am J Ophthalmol 1991;111:614–23.
17. Berson EL, Rosner B, Sandberg MA, et al. Arch Ophthalmol 1993;111:761–72.
18. Dowling JE, Wald G. Proc Natl Acad Sci USA 1960;46:587–608.
19. Dowling JE, Gibbons IR. The effect of vitamin A deficiency on the fine structure of the retina. In: Smelser G, ed. The structure of the eye. Orlando, FL: Academic Press, 1961;85–99.
20. Berson EL. Retina 1982;2:236–55.
21. Robison WG, Kuwabara T, Bieri JG. Retina 1982;2:263–81.
22. Bauernfeind JC. The safe use of vitamin A: a report of the International Vitamin A Consultative Group (IVACG). Washington, DC: The Nutrition Foundation, 1980.
23. Hathcock JN, Hattan DG, Jenkins MY, et al. Am J Clin Nutr 1990;52:183–202.
24. Geubel AP, De Galocsy C, Alves N, et al. Gastroenterology 1991;100:1701–9.
25. Berson EL, Rosner B, Sandberg, et al. Arch Ophthalmol 1993;111:1456–7.
26. Berson EL. Treatment trial for retinitis pigmentosa. In: Lakshminarayanan V, ed. Basic and clinical applications of vision science. Documenta ophthalmologica proceeding series 60. Dordrecht: Kluwer Academic Publishers, 1997;193–7.
27. Bassen FA, Kornzweig AL. Blood 1950;5:381.
28. Singer K, Fisher B, Perlstein MA. Blood 1952;7:577.
29. Druez G. Rev Hematol 1959;14:3–11.
30. Jampel RS, Falls HF. Arch Ophthalmol 1958;59:818–20.
31. Salt HB, Wolff OH, Lloyd JK, et al. Lancet 1960;2:325.
32. Druez G, Lamy M, Frézal J, et al. Presse Med 1961;69:1546–8.
33. DiFeorge AM, Mabry CC, Auerbach VH. Am J Dis Child 1961;102:580.
34. Scanu AM, Aggerbeck LP, Kruski AW. J Clin Invest 1974; 53:440–6.
35. Narcisi TME, Shoulders CC, Chester SA, et al. Am J Hum Genet 1995;57:1298–310.
36. Bach C, Polonovski J, Polonovski C, et al. Arch Fr Pediatr 1967;25:1093–111.
37. Lamy M, Frézal J, Polonovski J, et al. Pediatrics 1963:31: 277–89.
38. Carr RE. Birth Defects 1976;12:385–408.
39. Gouras P, Carr RE, Gunkel RD. Invest Ophthalmol Vis Sci 1971;10:784–93.
40. von Sallmann L, Gelderman AH, Laster L. Doc Ophthalmol 1969;26:451–60.
41. Wolff OH, Lloyd JK, Tonks E. Exp Eye Res 1964;3:439–42.
42. Bohlmann HG, Thiede H, Rosenstiel K, et al. Dtsch Med Wochenschr 1972;97:892–6.
43. Muller DP, Harries JT, Lloyd JK. Arch Dis Child 1970;45: 715.
44. Runge P, Muller DP, McAllister J, et al. Br J Ophthalmol 1986;70:166–73.
45. Rader DJ, Brewer HB Jr. JAMA 1993;270:865–9.
46. Yokota T, Shiojiri T, Gotoda T, et al. N Engl J Med 1996;335: 1770–1.

47. Yokota T, Shiojiri T, Gotoda T, et al. Ann Neurol 1997;41: 826–32.
48. Refsum S. Acta Psychiatr Neurol Scand 1946;38(Suppl):1.
49. Klenk E, Kahlke W. Hoppe-Seyler's Z Physiol Chem 1963;333: 133.
50. Avigan J, Steinberg D, Gutman A, et al. Biochem Biophys Res Commun 1966;24:838–44.
51. Eldjarn L, Stokke O, Try K. Scand J Clin Lab Invest 1966; 18:694.
52. Herndon JH, Steinberg D, Uhlendorf BW. N Engl J Med 1969;281:1034–8.
53. Toussaint D, Danis P. Am J Ophthalmol 1971;72:342.
54. Masters-Thomas A, Bailes J, Billimoria JD, et al. J Hum Nutr 1980;34:251–4.
55. Eldjarn L, Stokke O, Try K. Biochemical aspects of Refsum's disease and principles for the dietary treatment. In: Vinken PJ, Bruyn GW, eds. Handbook of clinical neurology. Amsterdam: North-Holland, 1976;27:528.
56. Refsum S. Arch Neurol 1981;38:605–6.
57. Steinberg D, Mize CE, Herndon JH Jr, et al. Arch Intern Med 1970;125:75–87.
58. Laudat P. Biochimie 1972;54:735–40.
59. Steinberg D. Phytanic acid storage disease (Refsum's syndrome). In: Stanbury JB, Wyngaarden JB, Frederickson DS, eds. The metabolic basis of inherited disease. 4th ed. New York: McGraw-Hill, 1978;688–706.
60. Lenz H, Sluga E, Bernheimer H, et al. Nervenarzt 1979;50: 52–60.
61. Dickson N, Mortimer JG, Faed JM, et al. Dev Med Child Neurol 1989;31:92–7.
62. Harari D, Gibberd FB, Dick JP, et al. J Neurol Neurosurg Psychiatry 1991;54:614–7.
63. Leppert D, Schanz U, Burger J, et al. Eur Arch Clin Neurosci 1991;241:82–4.
64. Fuchs E. Arch Augenheilkd 1896;32:111.
65. Takki K, Simell O. Br J Ophthalmol 1974;58:907–16.
66. McCullough C, Marliss EB. Am J Ophthalmol 1975;80: 1045–57.
67. Sipila I, Simell O, Rapola J, et al. Neurology 1979;29: 996–1005.
68. Kennaway NG, Weleber RG, Buist NRM. Am J Hum Genet 1980;32:529–41.
69. Kaiser-Kupfer MI, Kuwabara T, Askanas V, et al. Ophthalmology 1981;88:302–6.
70. Berson EL, Schmidt SY, Shih VE. Ophthalmology 1978;85: 1018–27.
71. Takki KK, Milton RC. Ophthalmology 1981;88:292–301.
72. Simmel O, Takki K. Lancet 1973;2:1030–3.
73. Takki K. Br J Ophthalmol 1974;58:3–23.
74. Valle D, Kaiser-Kupfer M, Del Valle LA. Proc Natl Acad Sci USA 1977;74:5159–61.
75. Kennaway NG, Weleber RG, Buist NRM. N Engl J Med 1977; 297:1180.
76. Trijbels JMF, Sengers RCA, Bakkeren JAJM, et al. Clin Chem Acta 1977;79:371.
77. Berson EL, Schmidt SY, Rabin AR. Br J Ophthalmol 1976;60:142–7.
78. Arshinoff SA, McCulloch JC, Matuk Y, et al. Metabolism 1979;28:979–88.
79. Sipila I. Biochim Biophys Acta 1980;613:79–84.
80. Valle D, Simell O. The hyperornithinaemias. In: Scriver C, Beaudet A, Sly W, et al., eds. The metabolic and molecular bases of inherited disease. New York: McGraw-Hill, 1995;1147–85.
81. Mitchell G, Brody LC, Loone J, et al. J Clin Invest 1988;81: 630–3.
82. Michaud J, Brody LC, Steel G, et al. Genomics 1992;13: 389–94.
83. Brody LC, Mitchell GA, Obie C, et al. J Biol Chem 1992; 267:3302–7.
84. Kuwabara T, Ishikawa Y, Kaiser-Kupfer MI. Ophthalmology 1981;88:331–4.
85. Baich A, Ratzlaff KO. Invest Ophthalmol Vis Sci 1980;19: 411–4.
86. Hayasaka S, Shiono T, Mizuno K, et al. Invest Ophthalmol Vis Sci 1980;21(Suppl):185.
87. Valle D, Walser M, Brusilow SW, et al. J Clin Invest 1980; 65:371–8.
88. Wang T, Lawler AM, Steel G, et al. Nature Genet 1995;11: 185–90.
89. Wang T, Milam AH, Valle D. Am J Hum Genet 1996;59 (Suppl):A15(70).
90. Stoppolini G, Prisco F, Santinelli R, et al. Helv Paediatr Acta 1978;33:429–33.
91. Kaiser-Kupfer MI, deMonasterio FM, Valle D, et al. Science 1980;210:1128–31.
92. Berson EL, Shih VE, Sullivan PL. Ophthalmology 1981;88: 311–5.
93. McInness RR, Arshinoff SA, Bell L, et al. Lancet 1981;1:513–7.
94. Weleber RG, Kennaway NG, Buist NRM. Lancet 1978;2:1213.
95. Kaiser-Kupfer MI, Valle D, Bron AJ. Am J Ophthalmol 1980;89:219–22.
96. Kaiser-Kupfer MI, deMonasterio FM, Valle D, et al. Ophthalmology 1981;88:307–10.
97. Weleber RG, Kennaway NG. Ophthalmology 1981;88:316–24.
98. Weleber RG, Kennaway GN, Buist NR. Int Ophthalmol 1981;4:23–32.
99. Berson EL, Hanson AH, Rosner B, et al. A two-year trial of low-protein, low-arginine diets of vitamin B_6 for patients with gyrate atrophy. In: Cotlier E, Maumenee I, Berman E, eds. Birth defects: original article series. New York: Alan R Liss, 1982;209–18.
100. Sipila I, Rapola J, Simell O, et al. N Engl J Med 1981;304: 867.
101. Kaiser-Kupfer MI, Caruso RC, Valle D. Arch Ophthalmol 1991;109:1539–48.
102. Acosta PB, Yannicelli S. Protocol 16—Gyrate atrophy of the choroid and retina. Nutrition support of infants, children, and adults with Cyclinex-1 and Cyclinex-2 amino acid-modified medical foods. In: The Ross metabolic formula system. Nutrition support protocols. Columbus: Ross Laboratories, 1993;359–92.
103. Sorsby A, Mason MEJ, Gardener N. Br J Ophthalmol 1949; 33:67–97.
104. Fraser HB, Wallace DC. Am J Ophthalmol 1971;71:1216–20.
105. Carr RE, Noble KG, Nasaduke I. Am J Ophthalmol 1978;85: 318–28.
106. Carr RE, Noble KG, Nasaduke I. Trans Am Ophthalmol Soc 1977;75:255–71.
107. Weber BHF, Vogt G, Pruett RC, et al. Nature Genet 1994;8:352–6.
108. Jacobson SG, Cideciyan AV, Regunath G, et al. Nature Genet 1995;11:27–32.
109. National Advisory Eye Council. Vision research, a national plan, 1994–1998. National Institutes of Health publ. no. 93-3186. Washington, DC: U.S. Government Printing Office, 1993.
110. Klein R, Klein B, Linton KLP. Ophthalmology 1992;99: 933–43.
111. Egan KM, Seddon JM. Age-related macular degeneration: epidemiology. In: Jakobiec FA, Albert DM, eds. Principles and

practice of ophthalmology, basic sciences. Philadelphia: WB Saunders, 1994;1266–74.
112. Seddon JM, Ajani UA, Sperduto RD, et al. JAMA 1994; 272:1413–20.
113. VandenLangenberg GM, Mares-Perlman JA, Klein R, et al. FASEB J 1997;11:A353(Abstract 2047).
114. Sanders TAB, Haines AP, Wormald R, et al. Am J Clin Nutr 1993;57:428–33.
115. Newsome DA, Swartz M, Leone NC, et al. Arch Ophthalmol 1988;106:192–8.
116. Organisciak DT, Wang HM, Li Z, et al. Invest Ophthalmol Vis Sci 1985;26:1580–8.
117. Morris DL, Kritchevsky SB, Davis CE. JAMA 1994;272: 1439–41.
118. Sperduto RD, Ferris FL, Kurinij N. Arch Ophthalmol 1990; 108:1403–5.

SELECTED READINGS

Bauernfeind JC. The safe use of vitamin A: a report of the International Vitamin A Consultative Group (IVACG). Washington, DC: The Nutrition Foundation, 1980.

Berman EL. Clues in the eye: ocular signs of metabolic and nutritional disorders. Geriatrics 1995;50:34–44.

Berson EL. Retinitis pigmentosa and allied diseases. In: Albert DM, Jakobiec FA, eds. Principles and practice of ophthalmology: clinical practice, vol 2. Philadelphia: WB Saunders, 1994; 1214–37.

Berson EL, Rosner B, Sandberg MA, et al. A randomized trial of vitamin A and vitamin E supplementation for retinitis pigmentosa. Arch Ophthalmol 1993;111:761–72.

Dowling JE, Proenza LM, Atwell CW, et al. Proceedings of a symposium on nutrition, pharmacology, and vision. National Research Council, National Academy of Sciences. Retina 1982;2:193–375.

Hathcock JN, Hattan DG, Jenkins MY, et al. Evaluation of vitamin A toxicity. Am J Clin Nutr 1990;52:183–202.

Saari JC. Retinoids in photosensitive systems. In: Sporn MB, Roberts AB, Goodman DS, eds. The retinoids: biology, chemistry, and medicine. 2nd ed. New York: Raven Press, 1994;351–85.

Sperduto RD, Ferris FL, Kurinij N. Do we have a nutritional treatment for age-related cataract or macular degeneration? Arch Ophthalmol 1990;108:1403–5.

Valle D, Simell O. The hyperornithinaemias. In: Scriver C, Beaudet A, Sly W, et al., eds. The metabolic and molecular bases of inherited disease. New York: McGraw-Hill, 1995;1147–85.

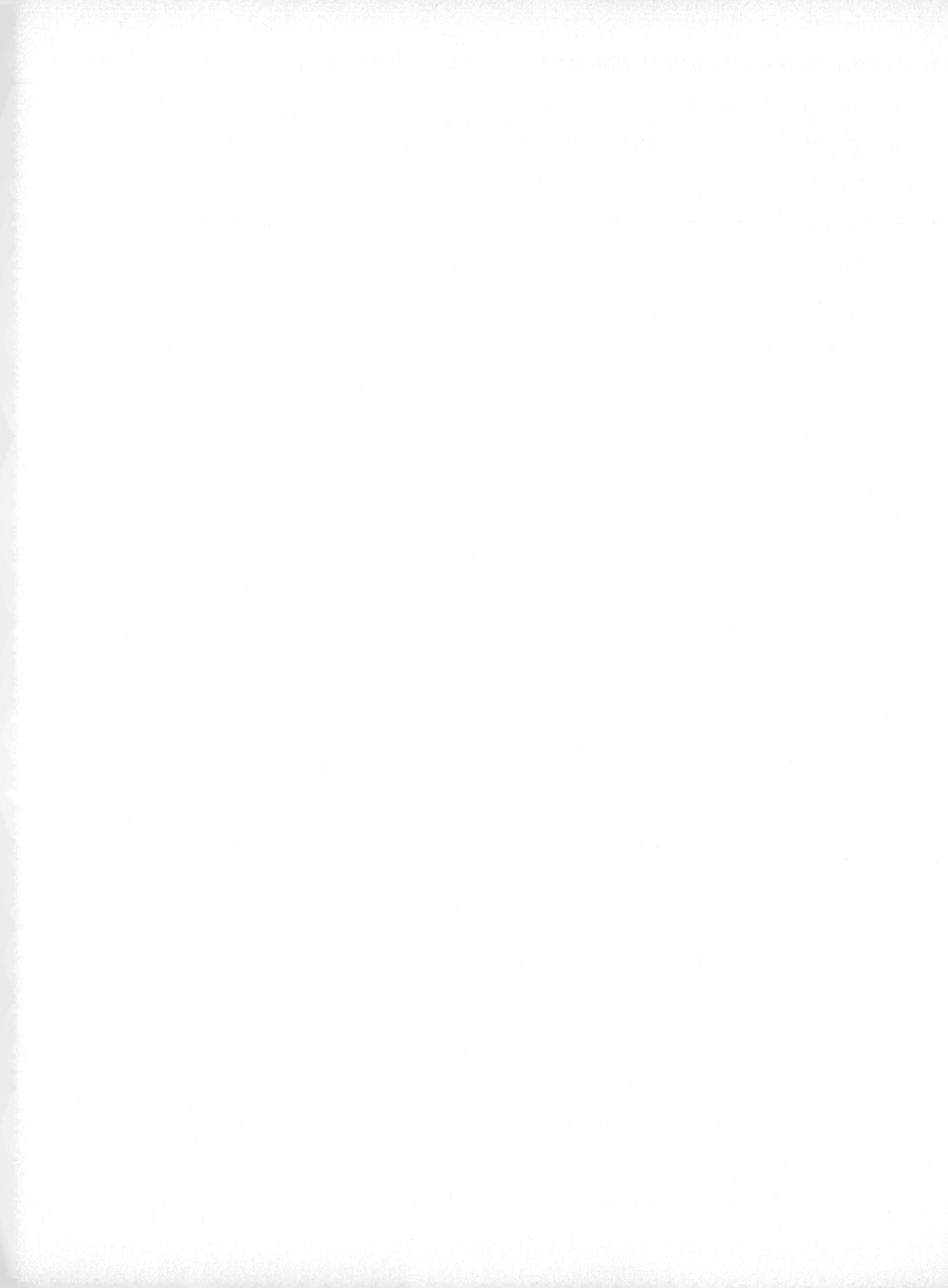

92. Diagnosis and Management of Food Allergies

HUGH A. SAMPSON

BACKGROUND AND DEFINITIONS

Hippocrates was among the first to record an adverse reaction to food over 2000 years ago. However, not until the turn of the century did scattered reports of food allergic reactions appear in the medical literature. Most accounts of food allergic reactions were based simply on histories provided by the patient, until 1950, when Loveless reported the first blinded, placebo-controlled food challenges; one study involving 8 patients for milk allergy (1) and one involving 25 patients for cornstarch sensitivity (2). Subsequently, Goldman et al. published a series of articles describing their studies in 89 children suspected of milk allergy (3, 4). The diagnosis of food allergy was considered established only when the patient had resolution of symptoms after withdrawal of milk from the diet and duplication of presenting symptoms on three successive challenges with milk. Although the "Goldman criteria" firmly established the diagnosis of food allergy, most investigators were reluctant to subject highly allergic patients to three challenges. In 1976, May introduced the use of double-blind, placebo-controlled oral food challenges (DBPCFC) to diagnose food allergy, ushering in the recent era of scientific investigation into food allergic disorders (5).

To facilitate investigation of adverse food reactions, the European Academy of Allergy and Clinical Immunology recently adopted standardized definitions for food reactions based solely on mechanism (6). An *adverse food reaction* is defined as any aberrant reaction following the ingestion of a food or food additive. Adverse food reactions are divided into *toxic* and *nontoxic* food reactions. Toxic reactions occur in anyone, provided a sufficient dose is ingested. Nontoxic reactions depend on individual susceptibility and may be the result of immune mechanisms *(allergy or hypersensitivity)* or nonimmune mechanisms *(intolerances)*. Type I, IgE-mediated food allergies have been most clearly delineated, but non-IgE-mediated immune reactions are clearly responsible for a variety of food allergic disorders, especially in the gastrointestinal tract. Food intolerances may be due to *pharmacologic* properties of the food (e.g., tyramine in aged cheeses, theobromine in chocolate), traits of the host such as *metabolic* disorders (e.g., lactase deficiency), or *idiosyncratic* responses. *Psychogenic* reactions can be reproduced only when patients are aware that they are ingesting a specific food.

PREVALENCE

The public "perceives" adverse reactions to foods and food additives as a common health problem. An American survey found that at least one family member was believed to have a food allergy in one-third of households (7). Similarly, approximately 20% of 7500 households surveyed in the United Kingdom reported a food intolerance (8). However, using DBPCFC to confirm patients' reports, the British study found the overall prevalence of adverse food reactions in adults to be 1.4 to 1.8%, while a comparable study in the Netherlands concluded that about 2% of the adult Dutch population is affected by adverse food reactions (9). A second large population survey in the United Kingdom evaluated the prevalence of adverse reactions to food additives in adults and following appropriate challenges, found a prevalence between 0.01 and 0.23% (10).

Adverse reactions to foods are more common in young children, which in part may relate to the feeding practices of the population evaluated. In a prospective study of 480 newborns followed in an American general pediatric practice for 3 years, parents reported adverse food reactions in 28% of the infants, but reactions were confirmed by oral challenge in only about one-third of suspected cases, or 8% of the total group (11). Reactions to fruits and fruit juices were analyzed separately. Overall, 56 (12%) infants experienced 60 positive challenges consisting of rashes and/or diarrhea following the ingestion of orange juice (14 children [3%]), tomato juice (14 children [3%]), apple juice (7 children [2.5%]), grape juice (4 children [1%]), and other fruit juices (21 children [4%]). Cow milk allergy has been studied extensively in young infants. Large prospective studies with appropriately performed milk challenges from four different countries revealed that 2.2 to 2.8% of infants experience cow milk allergy in the first 1 to 2 years of life (11–14). However, cow milk allergy is generally short-lived, with nearly 85% of sensitive infants losing their reactivity by 3 years of age (15). Adverse reactions to food additives also may be more common in children. In a study of 4274 Dutch school children, results of DBPCFC suggested a prevalence of about 1% (16).

Atopic individuals (i.e., atopic dermatitis [eczema], allergic rhinitis [hay fever], and/or asthma) appear to have a higher prevalence of food allergy. In children with moderate-to-severe atopic dermatitis, about one-third have skin symptoms provoked by food hypersensitivity (17). The more severe the atopic eczema in young children, the more likely they are to have food allergy (18). Studies of asthmatic children attending general pulmonary clinics indicated that 6 to 8% of children have food-induced wheezing (19, 20). Interestingly, infants with evidence of IgE antibodies to egg protein have a markedly higher risk of developing asthma than infants with no evidence of IgE sensitization (21, 22). Infants with non-IgE-mediated gastrointestinal allergy are not at increased risk for atopic disease.

PATHOPHYSIOLOGY

Foods and beverages ingested in everyday life constitute the largest exogenous antigenic load to which human beings are subjected, estimated by some to be in excess of several tons over a lifetime. The gastrointestinal tract uses a variety of immunologic and nonimmunologic mechanisms to prevent foreign proteins from entering the body. Nonimmunologic barriers include gastric acid secretion, proteolysis by various intestinal and pancreatic enzymes, peristalsis, the mucous coat, and the microvillous membrane. The gut enterocyte selectively absorbs small peptides and amino acids, and lysosomal activity further breaks down small peptides into nonantigenic fragments. The main immunologic barrier to foreign proteins is the secretion of secretory-IgA molecules into the gut lumen, which complex with foreign proteins and block their absorption. In addition, immune complexes promote both mucus release from goblet cells and mucosal surface proteolysis. Serum IgG and IgA antibodies may bind foreign proteins that gain access to the circulation, which leads to their clearing by the reticuloendothelial system (23).

Despite the intricate barrier network evolved to prevent the entry of foreign protein into the body, Walzer and colleagues established unequivocally that food proteins readily gain access to the circulation and are transported to distal target organs. In a series of experiments using Prausnitz-Kustner (P-K) tests with serum from highly food allergic individuals, Walzer demonstrated that food antigens gain access to the body at all levels of the gastrointestinal tract (24). In addition, other investigators have presented evidence to suggest that antigen permeability is increased after gastroenteritis and in young infants. The increased susceptibility of young infants to develop hypersensitivity reactions appears to result from immature "gut-associated lymphoid tissue," which is less proficient at developing normal oral tolerance, and immature, submaximal nonimmunologic mechanisms that allow increased antigenic penetration.

Food allergy results from an abnormal interaction between food allergens and the immune system and/or the gastrointestinal tract. The glycoprotein fractions of foods are implicated in allergic responses. The predominant allergenic glycoproteins are water soluble, largely heat resistant, acid stable, and commonly in the range of 10 to 60 kDa. Relatively few foods cause most allergic reactions: milk, eggs, peanuts, soy, and wheat in children and fish, shellfish, peanuts, and tree nuts in adults.

Normal individuals generate IgA, IgM, and IgG antibodies to the minute quantities of food antigens that pass the intestinal barrier or are selectively absorbed by M cells that overlie intestinal Peyer's patches and present antigens to resident lymphocytes. After a meal, circulating food antigen-antibody complexes often are found in normal individuals (25). In subjects developing food allergic reactions, food antigen–specific IgE antibodies and/or abnormal T cell responses develop.

IgE-Mediated Reactions

Food allergic reactions involving IgE antibodies are the best characterized. IgE antibodies bind to high-affinity Fc_E receptors on mast cells and basophils. Perivascular mast cells are prominent in all surfaces that confront the environment, such as the skin, respiratory tract, and gastrointestinal tract. When allergens react with IgE antibodies bound to mast cells, mediators such as histamine, prostaglandins, and leukotrienes are released. These mediators cause vasodilatation, smooth muscle contraction, and secretion of mucus, resulting in symptoms of immediate hypersensitivity. The activated mast cells also release a variety of cytokines, including interleukins (e.g., IL-4, IL-5, IL-6, and TNF_α), platelet-activating factor, and other mediators that promote the IgE-mediated late-phase response. Eosinophils and, to a lesser extent, basophils, lymphocytes, and monocytes infiltrate the area during the first 6 to 8 hours. These cells are activated and release a variety of mediators including platelet-activating factor, peroxidases, eosinophil major basic protein, eosinophil cationic protein, and cytokines. These mediators attract lymphocytes and monocytes in the subsequent 24 to 48 hours, which perpetuate the chronic inflammation. With repeated ingestion of a food allergen, mononuclear cells are stimulated to secrete "histamine-releasing factor" (HRF), a cytokine that interacts with IgE molecules bound to the surface of mast cells and basophils and increases their releasability (26). HRF production has been associated with bronchial hyperreactivity in patients with asthma (27) and cutaneous irritability in children with atopic dermatitis (28). IgE-mediated allergic reactions may provoke urticaria/angioedema, eczematous rashes, rhinoconjunctivitis, asthma, vomiting, and diarrhea.

Non-IgE-Mediated Reactions

Non-IgE-mediated reactions may consist of antibody-mediated (type II) hypersensitivity, immune complex reactions (type III), or cell-mediated (type IV) hypersensitivity, although few data are available to establish any of these mechanisms in food hypersensitivity disorders. In contrast to the IgE- mediated reactions, the non-IgE reactions may involve IgA, IgM, and IgG antibodies. The complexes formed by the interaction of non-IgE antibodies with antigen may or may not result in adverse reactions, but to date, support is minimal for type III, food antigen–immune complex–mediated disease (25). Studies in animal models reveal that cell-mediated (type IV) reactions can cause intestinal damage, including villus atrophy. Abnormal cell-mediated immune responses are responsible for some of the allergic gastrointestinal syndromes in humans, but data to delineate the exact mechanisms in man are absent. In both food allergic and nonallergic individuals, stimulation of peripheral blood lymphocytes with food antigens in vitro may result in cell proliferation, interleukin 2 (IL-2) production, and/or leukocyte inhibitory factor (LIF) production.

CLINICAL SIGNS AND SYMPTOMS

Symptoms attributed to food allergy are legion. However, relatively few specific symptoms have been documented as related to food hypersensitivity reactions. The most clearly delineated are the result of IgE-mediated reactions, but most reactions are probably the result of non-IgE-mediated mechanisms (Table 92.1).

Table 92.1
Food Allergy Reactions Substantiated by Blinded Challenges and Appropriate Laboratory Studies

IgE-mediated
- Skin
  - Urticaria/angioedema[a]
  - Atopic dermatitis
- Respiratory
  - Rhinoconjunctivitis
  - Laryngeal edema
  - Asthma
- Gastrointestinal
  - Nausea and abdominal cramps
  - Vomiting and diarrhea
  - Oral allergy syndrome
  - Infantile colic (rare)
- General
  - Anaphylactic shock[a]

Non-IgE-mediated
- Skin
  - Dermatitis herpetiformis
  - Contact dermatitis
- Respiratory
  - Heiner's syndrome
- Gastrointestinal
  - Food-induced enterocolitis
  - Food-induced eosinophilic proctocolitis
  - Food-induced enteropathy
    - celiac disease
  - Allergic eosinophilic gastroenteritis
  - Gastroesophageal reflux
  - Infantile colic (rare)
- Other
  - Migraine headaches
  - Iron deficiency anemia associated with gastrointestinal blood loss
  - Arthritis (two cases)

[a]Symptoms also may be provoked by ingesting specific food(s) in conjunction with exercising but not by ingestion of the food alone or exercise alone.

IgE-Mediated Reactions

IgE-mediated reactions typically develop within minutes to hours of the ingestion of a food allergen. However, frequent ingestion of a food allergen can lead to a "blunting" of immediate symptoms, and the chronic inflammatory reaction initiated by the immediate symptoms may last for several days. Skin symptoms are thought to be one of the most common manifestations of food allergic reactions. Acute urticaria/angioedema following ingestion or contact with a food is relatively common, although the actual prevalence is unknown. Most individuals with this disorder are aware of the association between ingestion of a specific food and development of symptoms and therefore simply avoid the food. Chronic urticaria/angioedema related to food allergy is rare (29, 30). The development of atopic dermatitis has been associated with food allergy in children. During blinded food challenges, a pruritic, erythematous morbilliform rash develops within 10 to 90 minutes of allergen ingestion (31). Repeated ingestion of the offending allergen leads to activation of cutaneous mast cells and infiltration of lymphocytes, both of which result in pruritus, consequent scratching, and development of eczematous lesions (32).

Both upper and lower respiratory symptoms have been demonstrated as a result of food allergy by DBPCFC (33, 34). Recently it was established that ingestion of food by food allergic patients with asthma could provoke increased airway hyperreactivity (asthma) (35), and two studies evaluating children attending pulmonary clinics demonstrated food-induced wheezing in 6 to 8% of unselected asthmatic patients (19, 20).

Symptoms involving the oropharynx and gastrointestinal tract may occur within minutes of ingesting a food allergen. Pruritus and swelling of the lips, tongue, and soft palate, as well as nausea, abdominal pain, vomiting, and diarrhea have all been demonstrated secondary to food allergy. The oral allergy syndrome consists of symptoms confined exclusively to the oropharynx and is most commonly reported in patients with seasonal allergic rhinitis following ingestion of one of a variety of fresh fruits and vegetables (36, 37). For example, patients with respiratory allergy to birch pollen may develop oral symptoms after ingestion of potatoes, carrots, celery, hazelnuts, and apples, whereas patients allergic to ragweed may develop oral symptoms after eating melons and bananas. Gastrointestinal anaphylaxis frequently accompanies symptoms in the skin or respiratory tract and presents as nausea, abdominal cramping, vomiting, and diarrhea. Repeated ingestion of food allergens in young children may induce partial "desensitization," resulting in less obvious symptoms, e.g., gastroesophageal reflux instead of projectile vomiting (38). A minority of patients with allergic eosinophilic gastroenteritis (discussed below) (39) and infantile colic (40) (inconsolable "agonized" crying, drawing up of the legs, abdominal distention, and excessive gas associated with feeding during the first several months of life) have symptoms attributed to IgE-mediated food hypersensitivity.

Food-induced systemic anaphylaxis was reported to be the leading cause of anaphylaxis seen in the Mayo Clinic Emergency Department (41). In two reports of fatal anaphylactic reactions (42, 43), the authors noted that all subjects had asthma, had unknowingly ingested the responsible food allergen, and had tended to minimize the symptoms initially and that initiation of emergency medical management was delayed. Anaphylactic shock in association with exercise 2 to 4 hours after ingestion of certain foods is being recognized increasingly, especially in young women (44, 45).

Non-IgE-Mediated Reactions

Non-IgE-mediated allergic reactions are believed to take several hours to days to develop, and a variety of disorders have been delineated. Although specific cell-mediated mechanisms often are implied, insufficient information is available to determine the exact immunopathogenic process involved.

A variety of gastrointestinal disorders believed to have an immunologic basis have been described. Food-induced enterocolitis syndrome is seen most frequently in young infants ingesting cow's milk– or soy-based formulas. It generally presents between 1 week and 3 months of age, with protracted diarrhea and projectile vomiting, often severe enough to produce dehydration (46), and about one-third of infants develop acidosis and transient methemoglobinemia (47). Stools generally contain occult blood, polymorphonuclear neutrophils (PMN), and eosinophils and are generally positive for carbohydrate (reducing substances) (48). The syndrome is also seen in exclusively breast-fed infants (secondary to the passage of food proteins in maternal milk) and occasionally in older children, associated with ingestion of egg, wheat, rice, peanut, nuts, chicken, turkey, and shellfish.

Benign eosinophilic proctocolitis also presents in the first few weeks to months of life and is often secondary to cow's milk or soy, although about half the infants are being exclusively breast fed (49, 50). Patients appear clinically well and present only with bloody stools (gross or occult) or hematochezia. Lesions are confined to the distal bowel and vary from mucosal edema to ulceration and linear erosions. Both enterocolitis and proctocolitis show dramatic clinical resolution within 72 hours of allergen elimination.

Food protein-induced enteropathy includes a spectrum of malabsorption disorders that generally present with protracted diarrhea, vomiting in up to two-thirds of patients, failure to thrive, and carbohydrate malabsorption. Increased fecal fat and abnormal *d*-xylose absorption generally are present. Cow's milk sensitivity is the most frequent cause of this syndrome, but it also has been associated with soy, egg, wheat, rice, chicken, and fish hypersensitivity. Patchy villous atrophy with cellular infiltrate on biopsy is characteristic of this disorder (51, 52). A more extensive enteropathy with total villous atrophy and extensive cellular infiltrate is associated with sensitivity to gliadin, a component of gluten (celiac disease). These patients often present with diarrhea or frank steatorrhea, abdominal distention and flatulence, weight loss, and occasionally nausea and vomiting (see Chapters 69 and 71). Dermatitis herpetiformis is a highly pruritic rash (sometimes mistaken for atopic dermatitis) associated with gluten-sensitive enteropathy (53). Biopsy of the rash reveals an infiltration of PMN and deposits of IgA at the dermal-epidermal junction. Administration of dapsone or other sulfones often relieves the skin itching within 24 hours. Like celiac disease, elimination of all gluten for 3 to 4 months may be required to normalize intestinal biopsy findings.

Allergic eosinophilic gastroenteritis (AEG) often presents as postprandial nausea with vomiting, abdominal pain, diarrhea, occasionally steatorrhea, and weight loss in the adult or failure to thrive in the infant (54). In the mucosal form, patients often have atopic disease, elevated serum IgE levels, positive immediate skin tests to a variety of foods and aeroallergens, peripheral eosinophilia, iron deficiency anemia, and hypoalbuminemia. Protein-losing enteropathy or pyloric obstruction may be the main feature in some infants with AEG (55, 56). A recent study of 10 patients with AEG and severe gastroesophageal reflux (GER) found that non-IgE-mediated food allergy may be a much more common cause of AEG than previously appreciated (57). Food hypersensitivity is a frequent cause of gastroesophageal reflux in young infants. Milk allergy was shown to be the cause of GER in 85 of 204 (42%) of infants less than 1 year of age (38). Removal of the suspect allergen for up to 12 weeks may be required to resolve symptoms and intestinal histologic changes.

Few non-IgE-mediated respiratory syndromes have been identified. Heiner's syndrome (a form of pulmonary hemosiderosis) is a chronic or recurrent pulmonary disease characterized by chronic rhinitis, pulmonary infiltrates and hemosiderosis, gastrointestinal blood loss, iron deficiency anemia, and failure to thrive. It is associated most often with a hypersensitivity to cow's milk, but reactivity to egg and pork have also been reported (58). Although peripheral blood eosinophilia and multiple serum precipitins to cow's milk are relatively constant features, the immunologic mechanisms responsible for this disorder are not known. Avoidance of the precipitating allergen leads to resolution of symptoms.

Given the presence of food antigen-immune complexes in many individuals after meals, several claims have been made for the use of fasting or hypoallergenic diets in the treatment of rheumatoid arthritis. However, only two patients have had exacerbation of arthritis associated with ingestion of a specific food established by DBPCFC (59).

Mechanism Unknown

In several clinical disorders, symptoms have been associated with reactivity to ingested foods, but an associated immune response is unclear. Reports since the turn of the century have suggested that oligoantigenic diets may be useful in the treatment of certain neurologic disorders. In one study, 15% of 104 adult patients with frequent migraine headaches had their headache cleared on a specific food elimination diet and their symptoms exacerbated during double-blind challenge with a single food (60). Two recent studies have raised the possibility that food allergic reactions may be responsible for some cases of sudden infant death syndrome (61, 62). Feeding pasteurized whole cow's milk to infants, especially those under 6 months of age, frequently leads to occult gastrointestinal blood loss and occasionally to iron deficiency anemia (63). Substitution of infant formula (including cow's milk–derived formulas that have been subjected to more extensive heating) for whole cow's milk generally normalizes fecal blood loss within 3 days. Considerable interest has resurfaced on the possible role of food allergy in inflammatory bowel disease (Crohn's disease and ulcerative colitis). Although considerable circumstantial evidence makes such hypotheses attractive, convincing proof is lacking.

Table 92.2 lists a variety of other symptoms reported to be related to food allergy. Convincing proof that any of these disorders manifest as isolated findings in association with food allergy is lacking. However, subjects experiencing a typical allergic reaction to a food may become irritable or lethargic following a reaction, and whether this response is due to the discomfort of the allergic symptoms or the release of various cytokines, such as IL-1, IL-6, and/or TNF_{α}, remains to be established.

Table 92.2
Unsubstantiated Symptoms and Disorders Ascribed to Food Allergy

- General
  - Fatigue (tension-fatigue syndrome)
  - Nervousness
  - Weakness
  - Sleep disturbances (other than infantile colic)
  - Learning disorders
  - Hyperactivity
  - Schizophrenia
  - Neuroses
  - Depression
  - Obesity
- Gastrointestinal
  - Crohn's disease
  - Ulcerative colitis
  - Irritable bowel syndrome
- Genitourinary
  - Enuresis
  - Dysmenorrhea
- Cardiovascular
  - Vasculitis
  - Recurrent phlebitis
  - Cardiac arrhythmias

DIAGNOSTIC TESTS

Much of the confusion surrounding food allergy has resulted from the lack of sensitive, specific laboratory tests to confirm the diagnosis. Confirmation of the diagnosis usually depends on a clinical test, the DBPCFC, which is the current "gold standard" for diagnosing food allergy (64, 65). Initial evaluation of a patient with suspected food allergy should focus on a careful history and physical examination. The history should emphasize the following points: food suspected and the approximate quantity ingested, time between ingestion and development of symptoms, description of the symptoms, frequency and reproducibility of symptoms, the most recent occurrence, and whether other factors (i.e., exercise) are necessary for the reaction to occur. The physical examination should note any atopic features, which frequently are present in individuals with IgE-mediated food allergy.

Several laboratory tests have evolved for use in the diagnosis of IgE-mediated food hypersensitivity reactions and may be used in the initial screening of food allergy complaints. Skin tests with food extracts are used to demonstrate the presence of food antigen–specific IgE antibodies on the surface of cutaneous mast cells, which are presumed to reflect the IgE present on mast cells in the gastrointestinal and respiratory tracts. Compared with DBPCFC, the negative puncture or prick skin test is extremely useful for excluding IgE-mediated food allergy but inadequate for predicting clinical reactivity (i.e., low positive predictive accuracy) (66). Intradermal skin tests are even less specific than prick skin tests and therefore are not recommended in evaluation of IgE-mediated food allergy. Standard radioallergosorbent tests (RASTs) or similar in vitro tests measure food antigen–specific IgE antibodies in the blood. RASTs performed in a reliable laboratory provide predictive information that is not significantly different from prick skin tests. Once suspected foods are identified by history and skin testing (or RAST), they are eliminated from the diet for 1 to 2 weeks. Because DBPCFC are so time-consuming, often single-blind challenges are performed to eliminate foods considered unlikely to provoke an allergic reaction. DBPCFC is then used to establish a diagnosis of food allergy (65). All challenges suspected to provoke an IgE-mediated response must be conducted in a physician's office or a hospital setting because of the risk of a generalized anaphylactic reaction. Although a DBPCFC is rarely equivocal when investigating typical IgE-mediated symptoms, a variety of laboratory measurements may be used to quantitate the response: plasma histamine level, spirometry, and/or nasal lavage histamine concentration.

No satisfactory laboratory tests have emerged to assist in the diagnosis of non-IgE-mediated food allergic disorders. For ailments in which cell-mediated reactions are considered important, peripheral blood mononuclear cells stimulated in vitro with specific food antigens have been tested for ^{3}H-thymidine uptake, leukocyte inhibitory factor production, and IL-2 generation. Although many patients with presumed food allergy have higher activity than normal controls, these tests are not discriminatory. In addition, no evidence exists that measurement of food antigen–specific IgG or IgG subclass antibodies or of food antigen-antibody complexes is of any diagnostic value. Other tests (e.g., cytotoxic tests, sublingual and intradermal provocation tests) have been suggested for use in diagnosing food allergy, but their diagnostic efficacies have never been validated.

Many gastrointestinal food hypersensitivities may be diagnosed with a single-blinded or open food challenge. In food-induced enterocolitis, up to 0.6 g of the implicated protein per kilogram of body weight is administered to the patient in a physician's office or hospital setting, because of the risk of protracted vomiting and hypotension (about 15% of cases). A positive challenge generally provokes vomiting and diarrhea, with occult or grossly apparent blood in the stools, an increase in stool PMN and eosinophils over baseline, and an increase in the total peripheral blood PMN count of 3500 cells/mm^3 over baseline at 6 to 8 hours postchallenge (48). Food-induced eosinophilic proctocolitis often has a characteristic appearance on sigmoidoscopy. The bowel wall is edematous, erythematous, and friable with scattered ulcerations. Biopsy reveals an inflammatory infiltrate and prominent eosinophilia (67). Examination of the stools reveals significant numbers of leukocytes, and examination of the blood may reveal a mild elevation in the number of peripheral blood eosinophils. Exclusion of the responsible allergen generally leads to resolution of symptoms within 72 hours, and refeeding provokes a recurrence of hematochezia within 24 to 48 hours.

Both food-induced enteropathy and allergic eosinophilic gastroenteritis require endoscopy and intestinal biopsy while the patient is ingesting the suspected allergen, after being on an allergen-exclusion diet for up to 3 months and after reinstituting the food allergen into the diet. Endoscopy and biopsy before challenge should reveal normal intestinal mucosa. Reintroducing the responsible allergen to patients with the malabsorption syndromes leads to villous atrophy, which may be partial or complete and is often patchy. In AEG, multiple food sensitivities are generally responsible for symptoms, so a 6- to 8-week trial on an elemental diet is often necessary for resolution of clinical symptoms. The characteristic eosinophilic infiltrate in AEG is frequently patchy, so multiple biopsies are required to exclude this diagnosis, especially in young children. Breath hydrogen and *d*-xylose absorption may be abnormal because of secondary disaccharidase deficiency. In celiac disease and dermatitis herpetiformis, both forms of malabsorption syndrome, IgA antigliadin and antiendomysial antibodies are present in over 90% of patients with untreated disease. In addition, IgA deposits in the dermal-epidermal junction is characteristic of patients with dermatitis herpetiformis.

Table 92.3
Disorders That Must Be Differentiated from Food Hypersensitivities

Food intolerances	
Postinfectious malabsorption (secondary disaccharidase deficiency, villous atrophy, bile salt deconjugation)	
Viral	Rotavirus
Bacterial	*Shigella, Clostridium difficile*
Parasitic	*Giardia, Cryptosporidium*
Bacterial enterotoxins	
Vibrio cholera, toxigenic *Escherichia coli, C. difficile*	
Metabolic disorders	
Transient fructose and/or sorbitol malabsorption	
Primary carbohydrate malabsorption—lactase deficiency, sucrase deficiency	
Hypo- or abetalipoproteinemia	
Acrodermatitis enteropathica	
Anatomic abnormalities	
Intestinal lymphangiectasia	
Short bowel syndrome	
Hirschsprung's disease (especially with enterocolitis)	
Ileal stenosis	
Other disorders	
Cystic fibrosis	
Chronic inflammatory bowel disease	
"Chronic nonspecific diarrhea of infancy"	
Tumors—Zollinger-Ellison syndrome (gastrin)	
Neuroblastoma (catecholamines or vasoactive inhibitory peptide)	

Confirmation of infantile colic resulting from food allergy requires at least two double-blind, placebo-controlled crossover trials of the suspected food allergen. For a positive result, symptoms should be prominent during the allergen challenges and absent during the placebo challenges.

As depicted in Table 92.3, many structural and enzymatic abnormalities in both children and adults can result in gastrointestinal symptoms that closely mimic food allergy reactions. The differential must be considered carefully in all patients undergoing evaluation, because many of these other disorders can also be life threatening (68). Foods may contain a variety of preservatives, dyes, and other chemicals that occasionally have been implicated in adverse reactions to foods. Many foods also have endogenous pharmacologic agents that can trigger symptoms in highly susceptible individuals. Occasionally, improper handling of food (scombroid poisoning) or ingestion of a toxin by an animal (ciguatera poisoning) results in symptoms that mimic an allergic reaction.

THERAPY

Once the diagnosis of food allergy has been established, the only proven form of therapy is strict elimination of the offending food. This action requires considerable time and effort (ideally with the help of a knowledgeable dietitian) to educate the patient (or parent). Teaching patients to read food labels is necessary to guarantee exclusion of many "hidden forms" of common foods (69). For example, most individuals are unaware that casein (milk protein) is found in some canned tuna fish; egg rolls often contain peanut butter; most nondairy creamers contain caseinate, etc. In addition, the importance of a nutritionally sound diet must be stressed. Many excellent educational materials can be obtained from the Food Allergy Network, a nonprofit organization (Fairfax, VA; phone: 800-929-4040).

In food-induced enterocolitis, a short course of corticosteroids may be lifesaving in the initial acute stages. However, long-term management involves identification and removal of the responsible food. Young infants diagnosed with cow's milk–induced enterocolitis should be placed on a "hypoallergenic" formula (e.g., Alimentum, Nutramigen), since up to 50% will develop soy-induced enterocolitis if placed on a soy formula (70). Allergic eosinophilic gastroenterocolitis often requires treatment with corticosteroids, especially when no food is clearly implicated. Although several other methods have been suggested for the treatment of food allergies (e.g., oral sodium cromolyn, ketotofin, desensitization), they have not been effective in controlled trials in which the diagnosis of food allergy has been established unequivocally.

NATURAL HISTORY

Results of follow-up studies on food allergic individuals indicate that food allergies may resolve after several years. Although children under 3 years of age appear more likely to lose ("outgrow") their food allergy (71, 72), loss of symptomatic, IgE-mediated food allergy occurred in approximately 40% of children and adults adhering to an allergen-exclusion diet for 1 to 3 years, even though results of skin tests and RAST did not change (i.e., food allergen–specific IgE was still present) (73, 74). The probability of symptomatic resolution appears to depend on compliance with the exclusion diet and the specific food provoking the symptoms; allergies to peanuts, tree nuts, fish, and other seafood are longer lasting, perhaps lifelong. In a cohort of cow's milk–allergic infants, 85% "outgrew" their milk allergy by their third birthday (15). Consequently, it is recommended that allergic children be rechallenged to most foods every 1 to 2 years and to peanuts, tree nuts, and seafood every 4 to 8 years to determine whether their clinical allergy persists. No evidence exists that individuals who lose a food allergy will redevelop symptomatic reactivity after reintroducing the food into the diet. In addition to the longevity of clinical allergy to peanuts, tree nuts, fish, and shellfish, patients with these allergies must be warned that these foods carry a greater risk of a generalized anaphylactic reaction.

Most infants with milk- or soy-induced enterocolitis and colitis syndromes "outgrow" their sensitivity in 1 to 2 years. However, infants developing both cow's milk– and soy-induced enterocolitis appear to have more persistent sensitivity, especially to soy protein. A similar presumption is that most infants with cow's milk–induced enteropathy "outgrow" their sensitivity. However, no studies have addressed this issue. Most clinicians agree that patients with celiac disease must exclude gluten-containing grains for life. Some patients with celiac disease can tolerate gluten-containing products with little gastrointestinal discomfort, especially after avoiding it for a time. However, the risk of malignancy of the mouth, pharynx, and esophagus and of non-Hodgkin's lymphoma is significantly increased in patients with celiac disease ingesting gluten, regardless of the presence of clinical symptoms (75). No information is available on the natural history of allergic eosinophilic gastroenteritis.

PROPHYLAXIS

The role of breast feeding and food allergen avoidance in prevention of atopic disease and food allergy remains highly controversial. Some studies suggest that breast feeding (especially with maternal avoidance of such major allergens as milk, egg, peanut, and fish during lactation) can prevent atopic dermatitis and food allergies in some high-risk infants. An infant is considered at "high risk" when both parents have atopic disease (i.e., atopic dermatitis, asthma, and/or allergic rhinitis), one parent and one sibling have atopic disease, or one parent or one sibling has atopic disease and the infant has an elevated cord blood IgE level (>0.9 IU/mL). In a large controlled trial, maternal and infant avoidance of allergenic foods (egg, milk, peanut, and fish) lowered the prevalence of atopic dermatitis, urticaria, and/or gastrointestinal disorders at 12 and 24 months but had no effect on the prevalence of asthma, allergic rhinitis, or positive skin tests to inhalant allergens (22, 76). Because of the difficulty in maintaining a prophylactic regimen, many investigators recommend prophylactic measures only in "high-risk" infants with highly motivated families until our understanding of immunologic sensitization to food allergens is more complete. This plan includes exclusive breast feeding, maternal avoidance of major food allergens, and supplementation with hypoallergenic formula (Alimentum, Nutramigen), if necessary, for the first 6 months of life. However, it may be prudent for lactating mothers to exclude peanuts and nuts from their diet, since these proteins may pass in the breast milk and sensitize the infant with a potentially lifelong allergy. Highly allergenic foods (i.e., peanuts, nuts, and fish) should also be excluded from the child's diet for the first 3 years.

SUMMARY

Food allergy affects 6 to 8% of young infants and 1.5 to 2% of the adult population. It has been implicated in all forms of atopic diseases, including anaphylactic shock and death, and a variety of gastrointestinal disorders. IgE-mediated food allergy reactions have been best characterized, but several other immunologic mechanisms are believed responsible for many adverse food reactions. Appropriate diagnosis of these disorders requires a provocative food challenge, preferably blinded, and in several gastrointestinal syndromes, endoscopy and intestinal biopsy. Rechallenges should be done at set intervals to determine whether clinical sensitivity has been lost, because most food allergies are not lifelong. At present, strict allergen avoidance remains the only documented form of therapy that is universally successful.

REFERENCES

1. Loveless MH. J Allergy 1950;21:489–99.
2. Loveless MH. J Allergy 1950;21:500–9.
3. Goldman AS, Anderson DW, Sellers WA, et al. Pediatrics 1963;32:425–43.
4. Goldman AS, Sellers WA, Halpern SR, et al. Pediatrics 1963; 32:572–9.
5. May CD. J Allergy Clin Immunol 1976;58:500–5.
6. Bruijnzeel-Koomen C, Ortolani C, Aas K, et al. Allergy 1995; 50:623–35.
7. Sloan AE, Powers ME. J Allergy Clin Immunol 1986;78:127–33.
8. Young E, Stoneham MD, Petruckevitch A, et al. Lancet 1994; 343:1127–30.
9. Niestijl Jansen JJ, Kardinaal AFM, Huijbers GH, et al. J Allergy Clin Immunol 1994;93:446–56.
10. Young E, Patel S, Stoneham MD, et al. J R Coll Physicians Lond 1987;21:241–71.
11. Bock SA. Pediatrics 1987;79:683–8.
12. Host A, Halken S. Allergy 1990;45:587–96.
13. Schrander JJP, van den Bogart JPH, Forget PP, et al. Eur J Pediatr 1993;152:640–4.
14. Hide DW, Guyer BM. Br J Clin Pract 1983;37:285–7.
15. Host A. Pediatr Allergy Immunol 1994;5:5–36.
16. Fuglsang G, Madsen C, Saval P, Osterballe O. Pediatr Allergy Immunol 1993;4:123–9.
17. Burks AW, Mallory SB, Williams LW, Shirrell MA. J Pediatr 1988;113:447–51.
18. Guillet G, Guillet MH. Arch Dermatol 1992;128:187–92.
19. Novembre E, de Martino M, Vierucci A. J Allergy Clin Immunol 1988;81:1059–65.
20. Oehling A, Cagnani CEB. Allergol Immunopathol 1980;8: 7–14.
21. Hattevig G, Kjellman B, Bjorksten B. Clin Allergy 1987;17: 571–8.
22. Zeiger R, Heller S. J Allergy Clin Immunol 1995;95:1179–90.
23. Walker W. In: Reinhardt D, Schmidt E, eds. Food allergy. New York: Raven Press, 1988;15–34.
24. Walzer M. J Lab Clin Med 1941;26:1867–77.
25. Paganelli R, Quinti I, D'Offizi G, et al. Ann Allergy 1987; 59:157–61.
26. Sampson HA, MacDonald SM. Springer Semin Immunopathol 1993;15:89–98.
27. Alam R, Kuna P, Rozniecki J, et al. J Allergy Clin Immunol 1987;79:103–8.
28. Sampson HA, Broadbent KR, Bernhisel-Broadbent J. N Engl J Med 1989;321:228–32.
29. Champion R, Roberts S, Carpenter R, Roger J. Br J Dermatol 1969;81:588–97.
30. Volonakis M, Katsarou-Katsari A, Stratigos J. Ann Allergy 1992; 69:61–5.
31. Sampson HA, McCaskill CC. J Pediatr 1985;107:669–75.
32. Sampson HA. Acta Derm Veneorol (Stockh) Suppl 1992;176: 34–7.
33. Bock SA. Pediatr Allergy Immunol 1992;3:188–94.
34. James JM, Bernhisel-Broadbent J, Sampson HA. Am J Respir Crit Care Med 1994;149:59–64.
35. James JM, Eigenmann PA, Eggleston PA, Sampson HA. Am J Respir Crit Care Med 1996;153:597–603.
36. Ortolani C, Ispano M, Pastorello E, et al. Ann Allergy 1988;61: 47–52.
37. Pastorello E, Ortolani C, Farioli L, et al. J Allergy Clin Immunol 1994;94:699–707.
38. Iacono G, Carroccio A, Cavataio F, et al. J Allergy Clin Immunol 1996;97:822–7.
39. Min K, Metcalfe D. Immunol Allergy Clin North Am 1991; 11:799–813.
40. Sampson HA. J Pediatr 1989;583–4.
41. Yocum MW, Khan DA. Mayo Clin Proc 1994;69:16–23.
42. Yunginger JW, Sweeney KG, Sturner WQ, et al. JAMA 1988;260:1450–2.
43. Sampson HA, Mendelson LM, Rosen JP. N Engl J Med 1992;327:380–4.
44. Horan R. Sheffer A. (Abstract) Immunol Allergy Clin North Am 1991;11:757.
45. Romano A, Fonso M, Giuffreda F, et al. Allergy 1995;50: 817–24.
46. Powell GK. J Pediatr 1978;93:553–60.
47. Murray K, Christie D. J Pediatr 1993;122:90–2.
48. Powell G. Compr Ther 1986;12:28–37.
49. Machida H, Smith A, Gall D, et al. J Pediatr Gastroenterol Nutr 1994;19:22–6.
50. Odze R, Wershil B, Leichtner A. J Pediatr 1995;126:163–70.
51. Kuitunen P, Visakorpi J, Savilahti E, Pelkonen P. Arch Dis Child 1975;50:351–6.
52. Nagata S, Yamashiro Y, Ohtsuka Y, et al. J Pediatr Gastroenterol Nutr 1995;20:44–8.
53. Hall RP. J Am Acad Dermatol 1987;16:1129–44.
54. Lee C, Changchien C, Chen P, et al. Am J Gastroenterol 1993; 88:70–4.
55. Waldman T, Wochner R, Laster R, et al. N Engl J Med 1967; 276:761–9.
56. Snyder JD, Rosenblum N, Wershil B, et al. J Pediatr Gastroenterol 1987;6:543–7.
57. Kelly KJ, Lazenby AJ, Rowe PC, et al. Gastroenterol 1995; 109:1503–12.
58. Lee SK, Kniker WT, Cook CD, Heiner DC. Adv Pediatr 1978; 25:39–57.
59. Panush RS. J Rheumatol 1990;17:291–4.
60. Weber RW, Vaughan TR. Immunol Allergy Clin North Am 1991;11:831–41.
61. Platt M, Yunginger J, Sekula-Perlman A, et al. J Allergy Clin Immunol 1994;94:250–6.
62. Holgate ST, Walters C, Walls A, et al. Clin Exp Allergy 1994;24:1115–22.
63. Wilson JF, Heiner DC, Lahey ME. JAMA 1964;189:568–72.
64. Sampson HA. Ann Allergy 1988;60:262–9.
65. Bock SA, Sampson HA, Atkins FM, et al. J Allergy Clin Immunol 1988;82:986–97.
66. Sampson HA, Albergo R. J Allergy Clin Immunol 1984; 74:26–33.
67. Goldman H, Proujanksy R. Am J Surg Pathol 1986;10:75–86.
68. Sampson HA. Curr Opin Immunol 1989;2:542–7.

69. Barnes Koerner C, Sampson HA. In: Metcalfe DD, Sampson HA, Simon RA, eds. Food allergy: adverse reactions to foods and food additives. Boston: Blackwell Scientific Publications, 1991;332–54.
70. Burks AW, Casteel HB, Fiedorek SC, et al. Pediatr Allergy Immunol 1994;5:40–5.
71. Bock SA. J Allergy Clin Immunol 1982;69:173–7.
72. Hill DJ, Firer MA, Ball G, Hosking CS. J Pediatr 1989;114:761–6.
73. Sampson HA. Scanlon SM. J Pediatr 1989;115:23–7.
74. Pastorello E, Stocchi L, Pravetonni V, et al. J Allergy Clin Immunol 1989;84:475–83.
75. Holmes G, Prior P, Lane M, et al. Gut 1989;30:333–8.
76. Zeiger R, Heller S, Mellon M, Pediatr Allergy Immunol 1992; 3:110–27.

93. Behavioral Disorders Affecting Food Intake: Anorexia Nervosa, Bulimia Nervosa, and Other Psychiatric Conditions

DIANE M. HUSE and ALEXANDER R. LUCAS

Eating disorders are deviations in eating behavior that lead to disease or disability. Mild deviations from the "norm" are extremely common and occur with great variation at any age. The eating disorders are classified on the basis of their visible end result (extreme thinness or fatness) or on the basis of variations in eating patterns (fasting, food restriction, binge eating). The most common eating disorder, obesity, is discussed elsewhere (see Chapter 87). This chapter deals with the eating disorders anorexia nervosa and bulimia nervosa, usually classified among psychiatric disorders. It also discusses disordered eating in other psychiatric conditions in children and in adults.

ANOREXIA NERVOSA AND BULIMIA NERVOSA

Anorexia nervosa is characterized by self-imposed weight loss, endocrine dysfunction, and a distorted psychopathologic attitude toward eating and weight. The illness typically occurs in females shortly after puberty or later in adolescence, but onset can be premenarchal or later in life. Rarely, the illness occurs in males.

Bulimia nervosa is a severe disorder characterized by frequent binge eating and purging associated with loss of control over eating and a persistent overconcern about body shape and weight. The disorder occurs predominantly in young adult women. Milder forms of binge eating and purging are common in normal-weight women.

Historical Note

Medical descriptions of anorexia nervosa exist from many centuries ago. The disease was formally identified simultaneously by Sir William Gull in England and Charles Lasègue in France (1). These authors recognized a psychologic cause, but for many years, no effective treatments existed. Bruch, in the 1960s, elucidated psychologic manifestations of the disorder and developed effective psychotherapeutic techniques (1). Recent research has focused on physiologic concomitants of the disorder and on the development of multifaceted treatment approaches (1).

The historical meaning of bulimia is ravenous appetite manifested by voracious eating. It was described in conditions of hypothalamic dyscontrol. In 1979, Russell (2) described bulimia nervosa as a distinct syndrome and serious variant of anorexia nervosa. Since then, much attention has been given to the many variants of eating disorders manifested by binge eating, self-induced vomiting, and other forms of purging.

Pathophysiology

The pathophysiologic changes in anorexia nervosa are similar to those in other states of semistarvation. For the most part, they are adaptive responses that allow the individual to survive a decreased dietary intake of sources of energy. Such adaptations, however, are not without their "cost": functional impairment in other systems that limits the capacity of an individual to perform normal physical and mental activities. Many of the symptoms and signs of anorexia nervosa can be understood within the context of "normal" adaptations to semistarvation (3). (See also Chapter 41.)

Starvation is associated with energy conservation, adaptations that spare glucose and protein while favoring use of fat, often dramatic shifts in fluid and electrolyte balances, and alterations in hypothalamic-pituitary function that result especially in amenorrhea and infertility. These adaptive changes may not account for all the decreased energy use. Diminished protein synthesis and turnover probably also contribute substantially. However, known alterations in insulin, thyroid, and catecholamine metabolism provide a framework for understanding some of the signs and symptoms experienced by semistarved patients, including reductions in pulse rate, respiratory rate, blood pressure, oxygen consumption, carbon dioxide production, cardiac output, gut motility, and other autonomic nervous system responses.

The alterations in thyroid hormone and catecholamine metabolism may also contribute to cold intolerance, dry skin, dry hair, hypercarotenemia, hypercholesterolemia, prolongation of ankle reflexes, constipation, and other symptoms of semistarvation. A more detailed discussion of fasting diuresis and refeeding edema, energy conservation, and endocrine adaptations in fasting and semistarvation, delineated in the classic studies by Benedict and Keys et al., is published elsewhere (3) (see Chapter 41).

The hypothalamic responses to energy deprivation are also adaptive, allowing the organism to survive better than it would if without such adaptations. The most obvious example is the altered control of secretion of pituitary gonadotropins, resulting in disruption of normal cyclic patterns and producing anovulation, amenorrhea, infertility, and reduced libido. Such adaptations decrease the likelihood of becoming pregnant and also preserve the iron and protein stores that normally would be lost during menstrual flow.

To the extent that semistarvation is a feature in bulimic syndromes, changes similar to those in anorexia nervosa occur. The diversity of eating patterns among patients with bulimic syndromes, however, makes it impossible to generalize regarding their physiologic changes. Like anorexia nervosa, the bulimic syndromes have multiple determinants. A depressive diathesis has been suggested because some patients respond favorably to antidepressant medication. One study showed impaired cholecystokinin metabolism and reduced postprandial satiety (4). Studies of normal-weight bulimic women indicate that they are in a state of semistarvation because they had once maintained a higher weight and being in the statistically "normal" weight range was suboptimal for them. They tended to have had greater maximum weights than control subjects and to have had weight fluctuations with periods of low weight. Resting metabolic rate was lower in this group of women than in controls, but much individual variation was noted (5).

Etiology and Pathogenesis

The prevailing view is that eating disorders have multiple interacting causes. Biopsychosocial conceptualization identifies roots in three spheres—biologic, psychologic, and social. This model suggests a unique interaction of variables for each individual. An unexplained physiologic predisposition with possible genetic determinants leads to a variable degree of biologic vulnerability in persons at risk for development of eating disorders. Specific early experiences and family influences may create intrapsychic conflicts that determine the psychologic predisposition (1). Despite some studies delineating certain "psychosomatic" family patterns (6), accumulated evidence indicates a considerable variety of psychodynamic patterns in the families of patients with anorexia nervosa (7, 8).

Social influences and expectations that exert special pressures on modern women play an important role in the development of eating disorders (9). The biologic factors that initiate anorexia nervosa are mediated by pubertal endocrine changes. Psychologic conflicts lead to personality and behavioral changes that promote and support dieting. The social climate, such as the cultural obsession with thinness, tends to reinforce the psychologic motivation. Each of the three factors has greater or lesser importance for particular individuals in whom the disease develops. Thus, some appear to have a strong, innate tendency toward development of the disorder despite a supportive family environment; others react particularly to conflicted family experiences; and still others are strongly influenced by societal pressures (1).

Most commonly, dieting begins at puberty, shortly after menarche. Sensitive about her developing figure and rapid weight gain associated with puberty, a girl in whom anorexia nervosa develops typically restricts her food intake by eliminating sweets, snacks, and calorically dense foods. This effort may at first seem like the innocent dieting so common among her peers. However, her efforts persist and become increasingly intense. Weight loss prompts further efforts at food restriction and setting lower and lower weight goals. Excessive exercise becomes ritualized. She becomes more and more compulsive, secretive, and idiosyncratic about her diet habits. Physical and mental signs of starvation begin to develop. The latter are often ignored or actively denied. She withdraws increasingly from social interaction, becomes quiet and seclusive, immerses herself in achievement-oriented activities, persists in dieting, and becomes increasingly active. Eventually, she becomes irritable and angry toward her family. School performance usually is maintained at a high level, but eventually it may decline, despite excessive hours of studying, as she becomes distractible, preoccupied and, ultimately, depressed and apathetic.

Overwhelming hunger may supervene as a reaction to chronic semistarvation. This urge may be suppressed for months or even years, or it may result in binge eating and rapid weight gain. If the bulimic individual with eating binges clings tenaciously to her pursuit of thinness, she will resort to vomiting or purging through laxative and diuretic abuse to maintain low body weight. This practice leads to chronic anorexia nervosa and bulimia nervosa.

Binge eating and purging also occur in normal-weight persons who have never had anorexia nervosa. Some may be overweight or may desire a much slimmer figure. A pattern characterized by meal skipping and choosing calorically restricted meals often starts the process.

Epidemiology

Anorexia nervosa most commonly begins in the second decade of life. Fewer than 10% of patients have premenarchal onset. Among females, more than one-half begin before age 20 years and about three-fourths before age 25 years (Fig. 93.1). The disorder occurs 8 to 12 times more frequently in females than in males. The prevalence in Rochester, Minnesota, in 1985 was 0.3% for females and 0.02% for males (10). Among 15- to 19-year-old girls, the prevalence was 0.5%. Among 15-year-old girls in Göteborg, Sweden, the prevalence was 0.84% (11).

Estimates of the annual incidence in Western countries based on hospitalized patients and psychiatric case registers have shown an apparent increase from 0.5/100,000 population in 1950 to 5.0/100,000 in the 1980s (12). In a population-based study from 1935 to 1984, a higher average incidence rate of 8.2/100,000 (14.6 for females, 1.8 for males) was found. No change occurred over time in the rates for females age 20 years and older or for males. For females 15 through 24 years old, the most susceptible group, a linear increase was noted, with rates rising from 13.4/100,000 during 1935 to 1939 to 76.1/100,000 during 1980 to 1984 (10).

The severe form of the disorder is still relatively rare. The population-based study suggests that the occurrence of this form of the disorder has not varied over time. Anorexia nervosa is thought to be more frequent in higher socioeconomic classes, but data from population-based studies do not bear this out. Confirmed cases are not reported from underdeveloped nations, but they would be difficult to identify among other forms of malnutrition. The disorder is rare in black persons, perhaps because of biologic protective factors affecting vulnerability.

Studies of the epidemiology of bulimic syndromes have focused on the prevalence of the disorders. The reliability and validity of many of the studies are questionable because of great variation in the diagnostic criteria used and because many of the studies are based on questionnaires and self-reports. Nonetheless, evidence is accumulating that when strict criteria for bulimia nervosa are used, with interviews, the prevalence rate among adolescent and young adult women is 1 to 2%. It is rare among males. When broader criteria for bulimia are used and data are based on self-reports, the prevalence rates are higher, from 3 to 9%. With broader criteria for binge eating, more males are included (13). The community-based incidence of bulimia nervosa rose sharply from 1980 to 1983, after the description of the syndrome, and then remained relatively constant through 1990. The incidence rates for residents of Rochester, Minnesota, during the 1980s were 26.5/100,000 population for females and 0.8/100,000 population for males. The mean age for females at diagnosis was 23 years. Among 15- through 24-year-old adolescent and young adult females, bulimia nervosa had become at least twice as common as anorexia nervosa (14).

Clinical Aspects and Complications

The signs and symptoms, as well as laboratory findings, in anorexia nervosa and in bulimic syndromes are understood most easily in the context of the stage of the illness and the diet pattern that has been followed. At the onset of the illness and for a considerable time thereafter, the patient may have no observable signs other than depletion of adipose tissue and no abnormalities on laboratory tests. The negative findings are simply confirmation that in a previously healthy individual, even starvation is compensated for by the homeostatic mechanisms of the body. The absence of abnormal findings tends to reinforce the patient's conviction that nothing is wrong. Bulimia (ravenous appetite) may lead to obesity. Occasional binge eating may be seen in normal-weight persons without complications. Bulimia alternating with prolonged fasting, vomiting, or purging leads to serious complications. Bulimia also occurs in certain forms of morbid obesity, notably Prader-Willi syndrome (15).

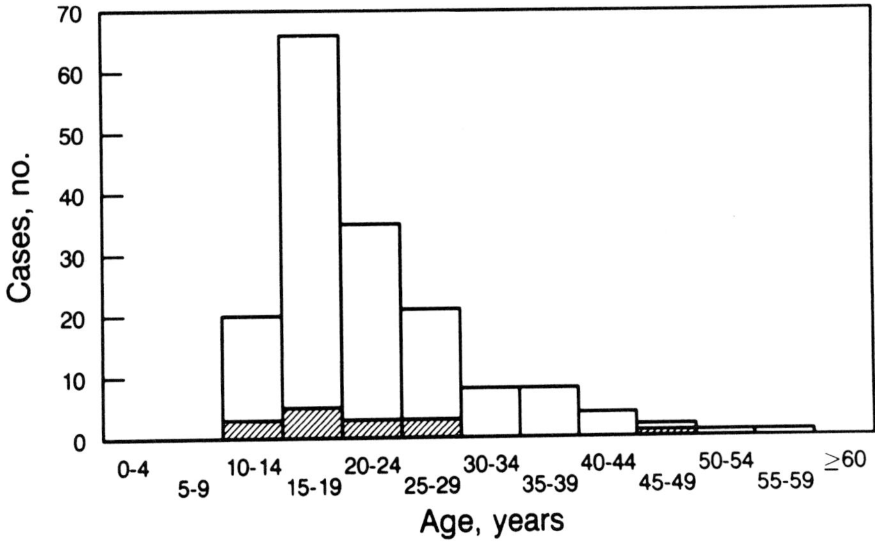

Figure 93.1. Distribution of age at diagnosis of anorexia nervosa in Rochester, Minnesota, from 1935 to 1984. *Open bars,* females (N = 166); *hatched bars,* males (N = 15). (From Lucas AR, Beard CM, O'Fallon WM, et al. Am J Psychiatry 1991;148:917–22, with permission of the American Psychiatric Association.)

Anorexia Nervosa

Many clinicians thought that patients with anorexia nervosa have similar diet patterns characterized by specific carbohydrate avoidance, but a study of diet patterns in 96 patients indicated much diversity (16). All restricted their calorie intake, but 38% maintained satisfactory quality in the selection of their diets. Of the 62% whose diets were unsatisfactory in quality, most had irregular meal patterns, and many indulged in binge eating, vomiting, or fasting. The great variability in diet preferences among anorectic patients has implications for planning individualized treatment.

Physical signs in anorexia nervosa include dry thin skin, sallow complexion, and loss of body fat. Bradycardia, hypotension, hypothermia, and cold intolerance occur. Often, patients experience abdominal pain and a sensation of fullness. Constipation is common. Amenorrhea is a constant feature in females; males experience an analogous loss of sexual interest. Excessive loss of scalp hair may occur, and eventually fine downy hair (lanugo) may appear on the body and face.

Premorbid personality features include model behavior, compliance, perfectionism, and high academic achievement. The patient usually presents a rigid, unspontaneous demeanor and is unusually serious and polite but inhibited and brief in responses. Others may be inappropriately cheerful and energetic, insisting that they are perfectly fine. Excessive activity occurs but may be concealed. Sleep disturbance is common. Eventually, manifestations of depression appear.

Bulimia Nervosa

Among normal-weight persons with bulimia, binge eating generally occurs frequently, at least several times a week. Usually, the episodes tend to last less than 2 hours, although they may last for many hours at a time. High-calorie, easily ingested foods, such as ice cream, bread products, and candy, tend to be eaten during binges. Vomiting is often a part of the syndrome, and patients with the disorder may also abuse laxatives and diuretics. Personality features differ from those in patients with anorexia nervosa who restrict intake. Depressive symptoms are common, and suicide attempts are frequent among bulimic patients. Many have impulse-control problems in other areas of their lives. Shoplifting (frequently of food) and other forms of stealing are reported. The positive association among substance abuse, alcoholism, and bulimia is being recognized more frequently.

A person with bulimia may demonstrate no physical signs of it until vomiting or other damaging behaviors have appeared. Nonpainful swelling of salivary glands suggests extreme variability in quantity of food intake. Erosion of dental enamel occurs with frequent vomiting, and calluses of the knuckles proclaim self-induced vomiting.

Laboratory Studies

Laboratory studies are of help chiefly in documenting the degree of physiologic adaptation to undernourishment, documenting complications of anorexia nervosa and bulimia, and identifying other illnesses resembling eating disorders. No laboratory profile is diagnostic. When a patient has physical signs and laboratory findings not usually associated with anorexia nervosa, such as increased heart rate, erythrocyte sedimentation rate, or leukocyte count, the physician should be alert to a possible medical complication or another disorder (17).

The laboratory profile varies considerably from normal to severely deranged and gives only a picture of these variables at the time of the test. In an illness that may last for many years, its stage is an important consideration in evaluating the laboratory findings. Abnormalities may not be observed until the illness is in an advanced stage. Serum electrolyte values usually are in the normal range, except when vomiting or laxative or diuretic abuse is a feature. The reported values may be high because of dehydration. The hematologic picture is variable because of changes in hydration. Anemia is a frequent finding in moderately severe cases, but it may be masked by hemoconcentration. Vomiting and laxative and diuretic abuse may be accompanied by serious electrolyte imbalances, notably hypokalemia, leading to cardiac arrhythmias, muscular weakness, renal impairment, and even death.

Dietary deficiencies lead to nutritional anemia in some patients. A peculiar morphologic change of erythrocytes resembling acanthocytosis is frequently present. The erythrocyte sedimentation rate usually is low. Leukopenia with relative lymphocytosis is common. Overt vitamin deficiencies are rare (18). Serum protein values tend to remain normal until the patient achieves advanced stages of starvation. The serum cholesterol level is increased in about one-third of patients, and the serum carotene value may be high.

Little documentation of the long-term complications exists in the literature, although various cardiovascular and renal complications can ensue. Demineralization of bone (osteoporosis) can be a long-term consequence (19). Kidney stones can occur. During the acute or subacute phases, gastrointestinal complications including decreased motility and atonic gut resembling paralytic ileus may occur. Pancreatitis has been reported, but its mechanism, like that of sialadenosis, is not known (20, 21).

Mortality Rates

Although mortality rates of up to 21.5% were reported in long-term follow-up of hospitalized patients, rates were less than 5% in over one-half of outcome studies (22). Preliminary findings suggest that the mortality rate in a community sample of subjects with anorexia nervosa will be lower (Lucas AR, unpublished data, 1997). Death from inanition is rare. It most often occurs from electrolyte disturbance or by suicide in persons with longstanding bulimia nervosa, but it also has been attributed to overwhelming infection and to cardiopulmonary complications. Death has also been attributed to overzealous refeeding, specifically, aspiration during tube feeding, and to fluid and electrolyte imbalance during intravenous therapy (23).

Diagnosis and Differential Diagnosis

Anorexia Nervosa

Diagnosis of anorexia nervosa is not difficult. It should be suspected when significant weight loss cannot be explained by physical illness. The physician then should inquire about whether weight loss was intentional. Psychologic characteristics, including the fear of becoming fat and misperception of body image, often are features of the illness. Three major features are required to make the diagnosis: *(a)* self-inflicted severe loss of weight by avoiding foods considered to be fattening, by self-induced vomiting or abuse of purgatives, or by excessive exercise; *(b)* a secondary endocrine disorder of the hypothalamus–anterior pituitary–gonad axis manifested in the female by amenorrhea and in the male by a diminution of sexual interest and activity; and *(c)* a psychologic disorder that has as its central theme a morbid fear of being unable to control eating and becoming too fat, either specified or implied by the eating behavior. Loss of appetite is not a usual feature of anorexia nervosa; rather, there is an aversion to eating and to gaining weight.

Patients with anorexia nervosa often insist that everything is all right, and they resent the implication that they are eating inadequately. Once a nonjudgmental atmosphere is established, however, they usually become more forthcoming about their true eating habits. An experienced dietitian familiar with disordered eating behaviors is best able to obtain an accurate diet history. If patients persist in denying the facts, their general attitude and physical appearance will make it obvious that modifications in eating behavior are necessary.

Other disorders associated with weight loss must be differentiated from anorexia nervosa. The chief physical diseases to be differentiated are gastrointestinal diseases involving malabsorption. Among psychiatric disorders, depression often manifests with true loss of appetite and weight loss. In schizophrenia, bizarre eating habits and delusions about food can lead to a clinical picture resembling anorexia nervosa.

Bulimia Nervosa

Diagnostic criteria for bulimia nervosa include the essential features of episodic binge eating; fear of not being able to stop eating voluntarily; self-induced vomiting; use of laxatives, diuretics, fasting, or vigorous exercise to prevent weight gain; and persistent overconcern with body shape and weight. Patients seeking help are more likely to reveal their true eating habits; others tend to be deceptive. Bulimia nervosa is a frequent sequel to anorexia nervosa. It also occurs in individuals who have always been normal in weight and occasionally in overweight individuals. It is associated with frequent weight fluctuations. Conditions to be differentiated include rumination syndrome in adolescence and involuntary vomiting.

Treatment

Although many cases of anorexia nervosa and bulimic syndromes can be managed by the family physician, internist, or pediatrician, they take time and sincere interest on the part of the physician. Patients mildly affected often respond to concerned counseling about adolescent growth, normal nutrition, and the consequences of starvation, binging, and purging. It has become customary to refer most patients to psychiatrists familiar with the treatment of eating disorders. Severe disorders are best managed by someone particularly experienced in treating the disorder. These patients need to be followed for a long time with various combinations of support, psychologic counseling, and diet counseling. When these symptoms are so severe that precipitous weight loss, binging, or purging continues despite outpatient treatment efforts, intensive hospital treatment is required.

Whether the patient remains at home or is hospitalized, the general principles of treatment involve education about the physiologic and psychologic consequences of starvation, encouragement to begin eating a healthy diet and control fasting, binging, and purging behaviors, and emotional support for the patient and the family.

Dietary Treatment

Treatment of anorexia nervosa and bulimic syndromes involves the joint efforts of a physician and a dietitian; they meet separately with the patient periodically, usually once a week, after the comprehensive evaluation. To achieve a working therapeutic relationship, the dietitian must first listen carefully to the patient, recognizing both the differences and the similarities among patients. It is helpful to know to what extent the evolution of the eating disorder was motivated by the patient's desire to be fit and healthy and how these goals can be supported but redirected by education. Patient education must begin early in the treatment and continue throughout. Included is a discussion of the effects of starvation and the extent to which disordered eating is not unique to eating disorders but rather occurs in starving people, whatever the cause. For many patients, understanding these issues as well as specific energy and nutrient needs (including growth needs) and the specifics of moderating practices in food choice leads to the realization that the dietitian and she have similar goals. This helps the patient to begin following the diet recommendations and then to experience a sense of relief and subsequently of greater well-being.

Both anorexia nervosa and bulimia nervosa patients benefit from these sessions. The goal for patients with anorexia nervosa is restoration of a normal weight. The goal for patients with bulimia nervosa is weight stabilization until eating behaviors are well regulated; additional emphasis is placed on education about, and control of, binging and purging.

Anorexia Nervosa. As in restoration of weight in other conditions involving starvation, a valid physiologic approach to treatment in anorexia nervosa is first to encourage the cessation of weight loss, to improve the nutritional state while low weight is maintained for a time, and then to encourage a gradual weight increase through normal self-feeding. Supplemental food products or parenteral feeding is usually unnecessary. Contrary to the ideas espoused by some authors, clinicians do not need to encourage anorectic patients to consume above-average quantities of food. Instead, because of the low body weight and hypometabolic state, unusually small quantities are necessary at first (see Appendix Table III-A-11-F). Estimated basal calorie requirements should be adjusted on the basis of the measured basal metabolic rate. The initial use of small quantities meets the psychologic needs of the patient, who fears gaining weight rapidly and becoming fat. Because some anorectic patients are realistically guarding against overeating, encouraging them to eat large quantities and high-calorie snacks is countertherapeutic. As the patient becomes less fearful of weight gain, physiologically acceptable weight goals can be set on the basis of the patient's height, body build, and weight history.

Management involves several phases: obtaining a detailed diet history, determining the caloric content of the initial diet, designing an appropriate diet plan, planning gradual progression in the diet, considering weight gain expectations, and, finally, designing a diet plan for weight maintenance. Specifics of this approach have been described in more detail elsewhere (24).

Bulimia Nervosa. The initial goals of dietary guidelines in bulimic syndromes are to encourage regularity in eating habits so that the patient can gain control of eating binges, to minimize the likelihood of the eating binges, and to avoid periods of fasting that may contribute to the binging, purging, and fasting cycle. Emphasis during the initial stages usually is on stabilizing weight while more acceptable eating patterns are being established.

For weight stabilization, the kilocalorie level of the initial diet can be defined by determining the patient's basal caloric needs for present weight (see Appendix Table III-A-11-f). A diet planned at this caloric level usually results in weight stabilization. If the patient is more active, a kilocalorie allowance for activity should be added to prevent weight loss. During the last phases of treatment, when the patient has regulated the dietary intake and is feeling more confident about controlling eating behaviors while keeping weight relatively stable, the need for a gradual weight loss program can be reassessed.

Treatment phases used in anorexia nervosa can be adapted for use with bulimia nervosa. Treatment should begin with a thorough discussion of the health consequences of bulimia nervosa, making certain that the patient can see how her specific symptoms fit. The patient must understand how erratic food patterns and purging lead to malnutrition and all its consequences despite maintenance of normal or even increased body weight. True understanding usually does not come until later in treatment. Concrete guidelines for altering eating behavior are often accepted when the patient begins to trust the dietitian. Many patients appreciate the structure provided.

Additional information needed to use anorexia nervosa treatment phases for bulimia nervosa includes identification of factors that trigger binging, vomiting, and fasting as well as the frequency of these behaviors. Knowing the types of foods eaten for a binge and what the patient identifies as a binge also helps in planning treatment strategies. This discussion usually allows the dietitian to understand the power food misconceptions and beliefs have in the patient's food choices and eating behaviors. The good-bad dichotomy about eating behaviors and exercise must be identified and explored for each patient before she is ready to risk modifying her behaviors to those recommended. Follow-up support and nutritional counseling need to continue even after weight has been stabilized and eating behaviors are regulated.

Psychotherapy

In addition to the dietary aspects of treatment aimed at normalizing eating patterns and weight, outpatient treatment deals with all aspects of the patient's functioning. Fears and misconceptions surrounding eating are addressed. Psychotherapy focuses on personal, family, and social conflicts that exist. With younger patients who are still living in their parental home, parents must be involved in the treatment, either with supportive counseling or in family therapy. A variety of individual and family treatment techniques have been developed, but the superiority of any one technique has not been established. These techniques have been described in detail (25, 26). Qualities in the therapist as well as characteristics of the illness and the patient are important in determining response to treatment. The individual needs of the patient are the most important considerations in planning a treatment program. Outcome studies are needed. Diet counseling alone can be effective in some cases, but data comparing it with psychotherapy are not available.

Hospital Treatment

The decision to hospitalize is based on the severity and rapidity of weight loss; the degree of malnutrition; the inability to control vomiting, laxative abuse, and other self-destructive behaviors; electrolyte disturbance or other hazardous complications; serious depression; suicidality; destructive family conflicts unresponsive to outpatient treatment; and the patient's lack of motivation for change. Hospital treatment requires a well-coordinated effort by the physician and hospital personnel on a unit that is geared to meeting the special needs of patients with eating disorders, not necessarily an "eating disorders unit." This may be a pediatric ward, an adolescent unit, a general medical ward, or a psychiatric unit for adolescents or adults. Essential considerations are that the staff have experience in treating patients with eating disorders and that patients be grouped by age. School-age children and adolescents need the opportunity to continue their education in the hospital (27).

Enteral nutrition and total parenteral nutrition have been used in severely undernourished patients with anorexia nervosa, particularly those who have failed to respond to treatment encouraging oral food intake. This group includes both patients who have steadfastly refused to eat and those who are so severely undernourished that it is difficult for them to take more than very small feedings. Although we encourage eating food orally, these alternative means of nutritional support may be necessary to sustain life and help the patient restore adequate nutritional uptake. These procedures can effectively improve the patient's nutritional state and, consequently, mental state. Nasogastric feeding no longer has all the negative implications of former times, because small-diameter tubes are available that can be inserted with minimal discomfort. Enteral nutrition is preferable to parenteral nutrition because the intestinal tract is kept active. When enteral nutrition and, especially, parenteral nutrition are used, some oral food intake should continue to prevent intestinal mucosal atrophy.

Parenteral nutritional support requires special precautions because of its associated risks. Complications developed in almost half of reported patients with anorexia nervosa undergoing parenteral nutrition. Infection is one of the most frequent. Technical complications associated with central venous catheterization, including vascular perforations, hemothorax, and pneumothorax, may occur. "Refeeding syndrome," caused by excessively rapid refeeding, leads to respiratory failure and cardiac decompensation (28). To minimize complications, an experienced parenteral nutritional support team should manage this phase of refeeding. Close monitoring of caloric intake, electrolyte changes, and fluid retention is essential.

The use of legal constraints (i.e., committing patients to a hospital and their forcing feedings) is usually more harmful than helpful; it creates an adversarial situation and compromises patient trust. In our experience, the necessary nutritional support can almost always be instituted without legal recourse. When a trusting relationship and open communications are established, severely undernourished patients almost always, albeit reluctantly, submit to enteral or parenteral nutritional support. When patients are so severely undernourished that they cannot competently make decisions about their basic needs, however, those decisions must come from their treating professionals and families. In the U.S., a competent adult may choose to forgo treatment for any medical condition, but allowing a patient to die from a treatable illness, as exemplified in a case report of a 24-year-old woman with anorexia nervosa who chose to go to a hospice to die, raises profound ethical questions (29). Ethical implications of forced feeding have been discussed by Hebert and Weingarten (30).

Medication

No evidence exists that neuroleptic or antidepressant medications either shorten the course of anorexia nervosa or improve the chance of recovery. Trials of medication have focused on their effect on short-term weight gain, but rapid weight gain bears no relationship to long-term outcome. On the other hand, antidepressant medications can reduce the frequency of binging and purging in bulimia nervosa over the short term, apparently independent of an antidepressant effect (26).

Outcome

Anorexia Nervosa

The course and outcome of anorexia nervosa are extremely variable. Meaningful conclusions about outcome require follow-up for at least 4 years. In reviewing such studies, Hsu (26) found that between 50 and 60% of patients were at normal weight, and about one-half had normal menses. Between 11 and 20% of patients were still underweight. The mortality rate was 0 to 5%. Findings from the longest-term studies, in which investigators have observed patients for several decades, underscore the conclusion that even after 6 years, some patients recover and others have recurrences. After 6 years of illness, about 50% of patients had recovered. As the observation time extended, more patients had recovered, but also more died. Twelve years after the onset of illness, 75% had recovered. The others had chronic illness, some with bulimic forms. Death from complications of starvation or from suicide continued to occur. Recovery after more than 12 years of illness was uncommon. After 33 years, 6% had poor outcomes and 18% had died (31).

Bulimia Nervosa

Outcome studies of bulimia nervosa are still rare, and few have more than 1 year of follow-up. Hsu (26) was encouraged about the short-term outcome in these studies. Two-thirds of patients no longer had symptoms of the disorder. Cautious optimism is justified until longer follow-up becomes available. Outcome is likely to vary greatly, with many patients recovering fully and others experiencing severe chronicity and complications.

DISORDERED EATING IN OTHER PSYCHIATRIC CONDITIONS

Attention-Deficit Hyperactivity Disorder

Estimates of the prevalence of attention-deficit hyperactivity disorder suggest that it affects between 3 and 9% of children (32). This disorder accounts for one-third to one-half of all referrals for child mental health services (33). The core clinical features of attention-deficit hyperactivity disorder are developmentally inappropriate activity levels, low frustration tolerance, impulsivity, poor organization of behavior, distractibility, and inability to sustain attention and concentration.

Multimodal treatment strategies that combine several forms of intervention have been considered the ideal. Sound clinical practice is necessary, including tailoring stimulant medication or psychosocial interventions (or both) to the particular needs of the individual children with attention-deficit hyperactivity disorder and their families.

Stimulant medications have been the major psychotropic agents used in the management of childhood behavior problems. The most commonly prescribed stimulants are methylphenidate (Ritalin), dextroamphetamine (Dexedrine), and pemoline (Cylert). Of these three, methylphenidate is by far the most widely used. The widespread clinical use of stimulant drugs stems from their demonstrated efficacy in dramatically treating a range of core attention-deficit symptoms. The most commonly reported side effects of stimulant medications are insomnia, anorexia, stomach pains, and weight loss. The anorexia and weight loss should not be surprising because these drugs are used as "diet pills" and were prescribed as appetite suppressors in the treatment of obesity in the past.

In 1972, Safer and Allen (34) suggested that growth-suppressant effects are present at all doses of dextroamphetamine and are dose dependent for methylphenidate. Subsequent studies of the influence of these medications on growth have conflicting findings. Results of a 1990 study suggest that methylphenidate use does not noticeably impair early adolescent growth velocities during 6 to 12 months of treatment. This finding contrasts with reports of at least temporary growth suppression in children and may indicate that early adolescent growth is relatively insensitive to methylphenidate (35).

Periodic monitoring of growth is standard practice when children receive stimulant medication. Many children are treated with these medications during their elementary school years and, frequently, into adolescence. Reducing the dosage, when practical, is indicated if growth suppression occurs. Parents of children receiving stimulants need to be taught to observe their child's appetite and changes in interest in meals and snacks and to report these changes to the child's physician. Closer monitoring of growth is needed in this population. If slowing weight gain or growth is noted, a 7-day food record of the child's intake should be kept by the parents and evaluated by a dietitian. The dietitian can use these records to recommend ways of increasing calories: using more calorically dense foods, encouraging regular meals and snacks, or supplementing intake with commercial products, if acceptable to the child. Encouraging the child to eat meals and snacks even when not hungry usually helps to avoid compromising growth. Children can be engaged in these efforts if they are provided with age-appropriate descriptions of the relationship between food intake and growth. Having the parents and child work with a dietitian to address nutritional needs and identify ways of meeting them within the family eating patterns and the child's preferences is effective for most children experiencing slowed growth with medication use.

Mood Disorders

Mood disorders are classified as unipolar or bipolar. Patients with unipolar disorder have episodes of depression only, whereas those with bipolar disorder have alternating episodes of mania and depression. The prevalence of unipolar depression is about 10% in women and 5% in men. Bipolar disorder is less frequent, about 0.5 to 1.0% in the population. These illnesses usually begin during the 20s, although they may occur earlier in life. Unipolar depression is more common in midlife and later (36).

Typically in major depression, loss of appetite occurs as well as loss of interest in the patient's surroundings and social relationships. Anorexia is manifested by loss of interest in eating and its associated pleasure. Depressed patients tend to ignore mealtime and to say that they do not feel hungry. Weight loss occurs frequently, is unintentional, and generally amounts to less than 15% of body weight. This can easily be differentiated from anorexia nervosa, in which the weight loss is intentional. If depression is unrecognized or untreated, however, weight loss may be substantial, and differentiation from chronic anorexia nervosa may be difficult. A minority of depressed patients have increased appetite and weight gain. Patients during a manic episode have pressured speech, hyperactivity, and sleeplessness, often associated with weight loss.

Treatment with antidepressant medication usually alleviates anorexia as other symptoms of depression are relieved. If weight loss was slight and there are no nutritional deficiencies, no other intervention is necessary. If there are significant nutritional deficiencies, as determined by a diet history, the assistance of a dietitian may be necessary to educate the patient about appropriate meal choices.

Treatment of depression with monoamine oxidase inhibitors such as tranylcypromine (Parnate), phenelzine (Nardil), and isocarboxazid (Marplan), requires that the patient follow a tyramine-controlled diet because of the risk of increased blood pressure with as little as 6 mg of tyramine; 25 mg of tyramine may induce a life-threatening hypertensive crisis. Thus, intake should be kept below 5 mg/day (37). With the availability of other antidepressants, these medications are now rarely used except in treatment-resistant patients.

Manic episodes are treated with lithium and antipsychotic medications. Almost half of patients receiving lithium gain weight. Lithium impairs glucose tolerance and may increase sensitivity to insulin. It also inhibits the effects of antidiuretic hormone, resulting in polyuria and polydipsia. If dietary sodium is restricted, lithium excretion decreases, and lithium toxicity may occur. Caffeine increases lithium excretion and may cause a decrease in plasma lithium levels. Dietitians should be aware of these metabolic effects in patients treated with lithium (36).

Schizophrenia

Schizophrenia is a chronic disorder characterized by hallucinations, delusions, illogical thinking, and bizarre behavior. Prevalence is 0.5 to 1.0%, with females and males about equally affected (36).

The patient with schizophrenia may have delusions about food and its effects on the body or command hallucinations (hearing a voice telling the patient not to eat) that lead to idiosyncratic or bizarre eating habits. Typically, patients believe that their food is poisoned or will harm their body. Those in an agitated state of psychosis may neglect eating. Others, such as those in a catatonic stupor, may be volitionally unable to eat. Untreated schizophrenic patients may lose a substantial amount of weight or acquire nutritional deficiencies because of prolonged fasting or idiosyncratic eating habits. Other patients with schizophrenia may eat ravenously (bulimia) and gain excessive weight. Effective treatment with antipsychotic medications restores rational thinking and eliminates the delusions. Eating habits usually normalize without specific nutritional intervention. When dietary irregularities of long duration have led to nutritional deficiencies, education by a dietitian may be necessary once the irrational thinking has resolved. Poorly functioning, chronically schizophrenic patients may need close monitoring of meals in hospitals or day treatment programs. Fluid retention and weight gain are common during long-term treatment with antipsychotic medications.

REFERENCES

1. Lucas AR. Mayo Clin Proc 1981;56:254–64.
2. Russell G. Psychol Med 1979;9:429–48.
3. Lucas AR, McAlpine DE. Eating disorders: anorexia nervosa, bulimia nervosa, pica, and rumination. In: Haubrich WS, Schaffner F, Berk JE, eds. Bockus gastroenterology, vol 4. 5th ed. Philadelphia: WB Saunders, 1995;3254–70.
4. Geracioti TD Jr, Liddle RA. N Engl J Med 1988;319:683–8.
5. Devlin MJ, Walsh BT, Kral JG, et al. Arch Gen Psychiatry 1990; 47:144–8.
6. Minucin S, Rosman BL, Baker L. Psychosomatic families: anorexia nervosa in context. Cambridge, MA: Harvard University Press, 1978.
7. Garfinkel PE, Garner DM. Anorexia nervosa: a multidimensional perspective. New York: Brunner/Mazel, 1982.
8. Strober M. An empirically derived typology of anorexia nervosa. In: Darby PL, Garfinkel PE, Garner DM, et al., eds. Anorexia nervosa: recent developments in research. New York: Alan R Liss, 1983;185–96.
9. Bruch B. Eating disorders: obesity, anorexia nervosa, and the person within. New York: Basic Books, 1973.
10. Lucas AR, Beard CM, O'Fallon WM, et al. Am J Psychiatry 1991;148:917–22.
11. Råstam M, Gillberg C, Garton M. Br J Psychiatry 1989;155: 642–6.
12. Lucas AR, Beard CM, O'Fallon WM, et al. Mayo Clin Proc 1988;63:433–42.
13. Fairburn CG, Beglin SJ. Am J Psychiatry 1990;147:401–8.
14. Soundy TJ, Lucas AR, Suman VJ, et al. Psychol Med 1995;25: 1065–71.
15. Holm VA, Sulzbacher S, Pipes PL, eds. The Prader-Willi syndrome. Baltimore: University Park Press, 1981.
16. Huse DM, Lucas AR. Am J Clin Nutr 1984;40:251–4.
17. Lucas AR. Mayo Clin Proc 1977;52:748–50.
18. Casper RC, Kirschner B, Sandstead HH, et al. Am J Clin Nutr 1980;33:1801–8.
19. Rigotti NA, Nussbaum SR, Herzog DB, et al. N Engl J Med 1984;311:1601–6.
20. Nordgren L, von Scheele C. Biol Psychiatry 1977;12:681–6.
21. Schoettle UC. J Am Acad Child Psychiatry 1979;18:384–90.
22. Hsu LK. Arch Gen Psychiatry 1980;37:1041–6.
23. Drossman DA, Ontjes DA, Heizer WD. Gastroenterology 1979; 77:1115–31.
24. Huse DM, Lucas AR. J Am Diet Assoc 1983;83:687–90.
25. Bruch H. The golden cage: the enigma of anorexia nervosa. Cambridge, MA: Harvard University Press, 1978.
26. Hsu LKG. Eating disorders. New York: Guilford Press, 1990.
27. Lucas AR, Duncan JW, Piens V. Am J Psychiatry 1976;133: 1034–8.
28. Mehler PS, Weiner KA. Nutr Clin Pract 1995;10:183–7.
29. O'Neill J, Crowther T, Sampson G. Am J Hosp Palliat Care 1994;11:36–8.
30. Hebert PC, Weingarten MA. Can Med Assoc J 1991;144:141–4.
31. Theander S. J Psychiatr Res 1985;19:493–508.
32. Richters JE, Arnold LE, Jensen PS, et al. J Am Acad Child Adolesc Psychiatry 1995;34:987–1000.
33. Popper CW. Disorders usually first evident in infancy, childhood, or adolescence. In: Talbott JA, Hales RE, Yudofsky SC, eds. The American Psychiatric Press textbook of psychiatry. Washington, DC: American Psychiatric Press, 1988;649–735.
34. Safer DJ, Allen RP. Pediatrics 1973;51:660–7.
35. Vincent J, Varley CK, Leger P. Am J Psychiatry 1990;147:501–2.
36. Gray GE, Gray LK. J Am Diet Assoc 1989;89:1492–8.
37. Nelson JK, Moxness KE, Jensen MD, et al. Mayo Clinic diet manual: a handbook of nutrition practices. 7th ed. St. Louis: CV Mosby, 1994;311–3.

SELECTED READINGS

Cahill GF Jr, Aoki TT, Rossini AA. Metabolism in obesity and anorexia nervosa. Nutr Brain 1979;3:1–70.

Garfinkel PE, Garner DM. Anorexia nervosa: a multidimensional perspective. New York: Brunner/Mazel, 1982.

Gray GE, Gray LK. Nutritional aspects of psychiatric disorders. J Am Diet Assoc 1989;89:1492–8.

Hsu LKG. Eating disorders. New York: Guilford Press, 1990.

Keys A, Brožek J, Henschel A, et al. The biology of human starvation, vols 1 and 2. Minneapolis: University of Minnesota Press, 1950.

Stunkard AJ, Stellar E. Eating and its disorders. Res Publ Assoc Res Nerv Ment Dis 1984;62:1–273.

94. Nutrition and Diet in Alcoholism

LAWRENCE FEINMAN and CHARLES S. LIEBER

The interactions between nutrition and alcoholism occur at many levels and are complex. Alcoholic beverages contain calories but almost no other useful constituents (1). Ethanol-containing beverages alter appetite and affect food intake and use. They displace required nutrients from the diet. Ethanol and nutrients have multiple interactions at almost every level of the gastrointestinal tract. Ethanol alters the storage, mobilization, activation, and metabolism of nutrients.

Ethanol is directly toxic to many body tissues. Its interplay with malnutrition in causing damage, particularly with respect to the liver, the predominant site of its metabolism, still needs clarification. Alcoholism remains one of the major causes of nutritional deficiency in the United States; alcohol-related illness poses an enormous medical burden and often entails complex nutritional therapy. Nutritional therapy is frequently a balance between maximizing recovery while avoiding iatrogenic complications.

NUTRITIONAL VALUE OF ALCOHOLIC BEVERAGES

Alcoholic beverages contain water, ethanol, variable amounts of carbohydrate, and little else of nutritive value (see Appendix Table IV-A-19). The carbohydrate content varies greatly: whiskey, cognac, and vodka have none, red and dry white wines have 2 to 10 g/L, beer and dry sherry 30 g/L, and sweetened white and port wines have as much as 120 g/L (2). Protein and vitamin content of these beverages is extremely low except for beer. Even if one used beer as a nutrient source, a liter would be necessary daily for nicotinic acid requirement, 15 to 20 L for protein, and 25 L for thiamin. Iron content may be appreciable, especially in wine (2). The amounts of iron, lead, or cobalt may reach harmful levels. The significance of congener content is mostly obscure (1).

Americans probably consume 4.5% of total calories as ethanol (3), and adult drinkers over 10%. Heavy drinkers may derive more than half their daily calories from ethanol. Combustion of ethanol in a bomb calorimeter yields 7.1 kcal/g; however, its biologic value is probably less than that of carbohydrates on a calorie basis. Lower body weight in alcohol drinkers than in nondrinkers is especially clear in women (4). Subjects given additional calories as alcohol under metabolic ward conditions did not gain weight (Fig. 94.1) (5, 6).

Hospitalized alcoholics on an open ward also gained no additional weight when 1800 calories from ethanol were added to their 2600-calorie diet (7). Isocaloric substitution of ethanol for carbohydrate, as 50% of total calories in a balanced diet, conducted under metabolic ward conditions, resulted in a decline in body weight (6); and when given as additional calories, ethanol resulted in less weight gain than equivalent carbohydrate or fat (1, 6). Others have found variable responses in weight to additional calories as ethanol (8). Body composition measurements were not reported. The ability of ethanol to support body weight may vary according to the quality of carbohydrate fed with it (9).

There is evidence that ethanol increases metabolic rate, which would at least partly explain its reduced biologic energy value. Ethanol increases oxygen consumption in normal subjects and does so to a greater degree in alcoholics (10). Substitution of ethanol for carbohydrates increases metabolic rate in humans and rodents (11, 12). Thermogenesis increased by 15% in rats fed ethanol for only 10 days in one study. Resting energy expenditure (REE) (13) and diet-induced thermogenesis (DIT) also increase in humans (11). Only a small portion of the energy waste in rats could be attributed to brown fat thermogenesis (14). It is theorized that energy waste during ethanol consumption may occur via oxidation (without phosphorylation) by the microsomal ethanol-oxidizing system (MEOS) (6). The MEOS is induced by chronic ethanol consumption, which aggravates energy waste (15,

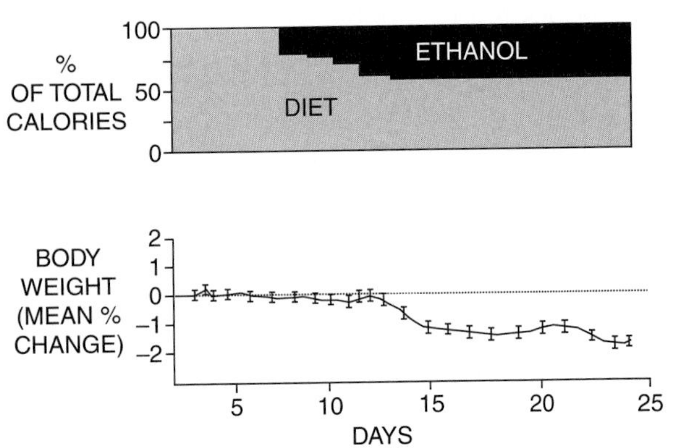

Figure 94.1. Effect of the isocaloric substitution of ethanol for carbohydrate calories on body weight. Substitution of ethanol as 50% of total calories results in body weight loss. (From Pirola RC, Lieber CS. Pharmacology 1972;7:185, with permission.)

16). The MEOS is unlikely to be solely responsible for energy wastage from ethanol metabolism. Oxidation of ethanol to acetaldehyde, catalyzed by the MEOS or alcohol dehydrogenase (ADH), represents only the first step in the metabolism of ethanol to carbon dioxide and water. Even when the MEOS is induced, much of the ethanol is metabolized by ADH to acetaldehyde, and most of the energy from ethanol is produced by oxidation of acetaldehyde to carbon dioxide and water. Acetaldehyde may contribute to energy wastage by promoting catecholamine release and by impairing various mitochondrial shuttles and mitochondrial oxidative phosphorylation. The appearance and metabolism of acetate, the next product in the oxidation of ethanol, is also associated with several energy-consuming features. Acetate increases myocardial contractility, coronary blood flow, and cardiac output. Hepatic damage itself, secondary to ethanol, decreases energy use, particularly from fat. A more detailed discussion of the energetics of ethanol metabolism is available (17). Some (18) have implicated uncoupling of mitochondrial NADH (the reduced form of nicotinamide adenine dinucleotide) reoxidation, perhaps abetted by a hyperthyroid state or catecholamine release (see above) to explain energy waste (18). The hyperthyroid state has been questioned (19).

NUTRITIONAL STATUS OF ALCOHOLICS

Alcoholism can undermine nutritional status. It was estimated that 20,000 alcoholics were suffering major illnesses due to malnutrition in the United States each year, accounting for 7.5 million days of hospitalization (20). Alcoholics hospitalized for medical complications of alcoholism have the most severe malnutrition. These alcoholics have inadequate dietary protein (21), signs of protein malnutrition (20, 22), and anthropomorphic measurements indicating impaired nutrition: their height: weight ratio is lower (23), muscle mass estimated by the creatinine-height index is reduced (22, 23), and triceps skin folds are thinner (22–24). Continued drinking results in weight loss and abstinence results in weight gain (25, 26) in patients with and without liver disease (24).

Many patients who drink to excess are either not malnourished or are less malnourished than the group hospitalized for medical problems. Women drinking one or more drinks per day weighed on average 2.3 kg less than nondrinkers, and they and their male counterparts maintained a more stable weight over the next 10 years than nondrinkers, whose weight rose (27). Other surveys, however, found that alcohol intake, especially when accompanied by high fat intake and sedentary behavior (28) favors truncal obesity, particularly in women (29). Those with moderate alcohol intake (30), even those admitted to hospital for alcohol rehabilitation rather than for medical problems (31), often hardly differ nutritionally from controls (matched for socioeconomic status and health history), except that females have a lower level of thiamin excretion than control patients following a thiamin load test (31).

The wide range in nutritional status of the alcoholic population surely reflects, in part, differences in what they eat. Moderate alcohol intake, alcohol accounting for 16% of total calories (alcohol included), is associated with slightly increased total energy intake (32). Perhaps because of the energy considerations already discussed, this group with higher total caloric intake has no weight gain despite physical activity levels comparable to those of the non-alcohol-consuming population. This level of alcohol intake and even slightly higher levels (23%) (33) are associated with substitution of alcohol for carbohydrate in the diet. In those consuming more than 30% of total calories as alcohol, significant decreases in protein and fat intake occur too, and their intake of vitamins A, C, and thiamin may fall below the recommended daily allowances (32). Calcium, iron, and fiber intake are also lowered (33).

The mechanisms underlying the altered pattern of food intake are not exactly known. Suppression of appetite has been postulated (34) but not been studied much. Depressed consciousness during inebriation, hangover, and gastroduodenitis due to ethanol partly explain the decreased food intake. The contribution of subtle nutritional alterations produced by ethanol to the pathogenesis of ethanol-induced or other disease states is largely undetermined. Nutritional therapy per se for alcoholism has not been successful (35).

EFFECTS OF ETHANOL ON DIGESTION AND ABSORPTION

Alcohol consumption is associated with motility changes in the gastrointestinal tract and affects the digestion and absorption of nutrients. Diarrhea and weight loss frequently occur in alcoholics. Ethanol effects may be direct or indirect, acute or chronic. One of the most intense changes, intestinal malabsorption secondary to folic acid deficiency, is not a direct effect of ethanol, but rather comes from diminished folic acid intake and abnormal metabolism accompanying alcoholism.

Gastrointestinal Tract

Patients with cirrhosis of the liver due to alcohol have edema, interstromal fat infiltration and fibrosis of the parotid glands, decreased basal- and citric acid–stimulated salivary flow, and lower salivary concentrations of sodium, bicarbonate, and proteins (36). Changes in esophageal peristalsis and lower esophageal sphincter pressure follow no consistent patterns (37–39) and usually do not lead to clinically significant dysphagia. However, the changes in saliva and esophageal motility and the direct effect of ethanol may be important in causing esophagitis and stricture, which are common in alcoholics and interfere dramatically with food intake.

Alcohol ingestion is a cause of acute gastritis and duodenitis (40). These areas of the gut are exposed to the highest concentrations of ethanol for the longest times. Damage to the gastric mucosal "barrier"' is important in making the mucosa more susceptible to acid and hyperosmolarity. Damage probably results from a combination of diminished gastric mucus production, altered mucosal blood flow, inhibition of active transport, increased permeability because of mast cell release of histamine and leukotriene C_4, cell membrane disruption, hyperosmolarity, changes in prostaglandin and cyclic adenosine monophosphate (cAMP) content of mucosa, and lipoperoxidative mechanisms. Erosive gastritis occurs, as does nonerosive hemorrhagic gastritis consisting of subepithelial hemorrhage of the foveolar region with surrounding edema (41). The effects of ethanol on gastric emptying of meals are concentration dependent; higher concentrations cause more consistent delay of passage of solid contents (42) and even enhance movement of liquids (43).

Alcoholics frequently suffer from diarrhea (44) and malabsorption. Acute effects of ethanol on motility and acute and chronic effects on the mucosa are responsible. Concomitant nutrient deficiencies can contribute significantly to mucosal changes, particularly folate deficiency. In the jejunum, ethanol decreases type I (impeding) waves, while in the ileum it increases type III (propulsive) waves. Decreases in villus height (45) and disaccharidase activity (46, 47) in mucosal biopsy specimens have been found in alcoholics with associated lactose intolerance, especially in black cirrhotics (47) (Fig. 94.2). The possibility of lactase deficiency must be considered in dietary treatment. Monosaccharide absorption is variably affected by ethanol; glucose is absorbed less well in rabbits after acute ethanol exposure (48), but chronic ethanol exposure enhances galactose absorption in rats (49) and glucose absorption in humans (50).

Acute depression of amino acid absorption can be readily demonstrated using high concentrations of ethanol (0.5 to 3.0%) in experimental models of ethanol exposure, using short segments of gut perfused in vivo or gut

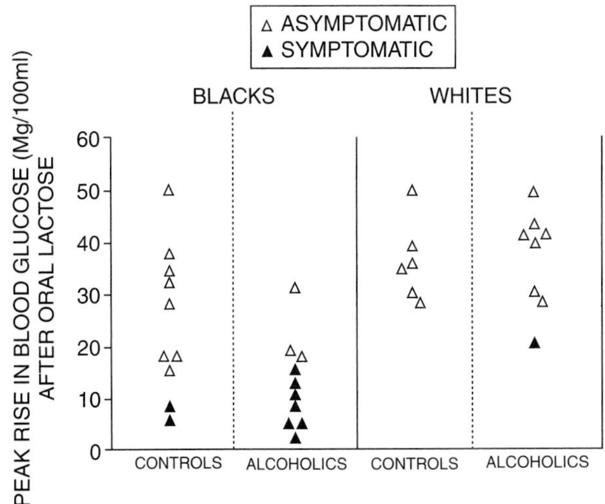

Figure 94.2. Effect of lactase deficiency on rise in serum glucose after oral lactase administration. Blood glucose rose the least in subjects with the most severe lactase deficiency. There was good correlation between symptoms and the lack of rise in glucose. (From Perlow W, Baraona E, Lieber CS. Gastroenterology 1977;72:680–4, with permission.)

sacs bathed in vitro. It has not been easy to demonstrate depressed absorption acutely using smaller concentrations of ethanol in whole intestines of living animals or in experimental models fed ethanol chronically. Several relevant topics are virtually unstudied: the effect of ethanol on amino acid absorption from complex mixtures (including peptides) and the possible effect of local changes in amino acid absorption on body nitrogen use.

Bile Salts

Steatorrhea, when it occurs in alcoholics, is mostly due to folic acid deficiency (see below) but luminal bile salt deficiency may contribute. Intraluminal bile salt levels are decreased by acute ethanol administration (51). In rodents, long-term ethanol administration delays the halftime excretion of cholic and chenodeoxycholic acids by decreasing the daily excretion and expanding the pool size slightly (52). Alcoholic cirrhotic patients may have bile low in deoxycholic acid, possibly because of impaired conversion of cholate to deoxycholate by bacteria (53). Thus, decreased cholic acid synthesis, decreased bile acid pool size (54), low concentrations of bile salts in intestinal juice, and bacterial deconjugation of bile salts by altered intestinal flora all promote steatorrhea in cirrhotics. Pigmented gallstones are more frequent in cirrhotics (55).

Pancreatitis and Pancreatic Insufficiency

Pancreatic function must be intact for optimal digestion and absorption of nutrients. The nutritional requirements of patients with acute pancreatitis or pancreatic insufficiency have to be met under conditions of handicap. Acute pancreatitis, with its associated hypermetabolic, hypercatabolic state, may increase energy expenditure by a sixth, in mild cases, and by half in severe ones. In many patients, oral food intake is limited by abdominal pain, nausea, and vomiting. Patients with chronic pancreatitis are often nutritionally depleted by inadequate food intake due to abdominal pain and by years of maldigestion secondary to insufficient exocrine secretion of digestive enzymes. Characteristically, patients have suffered weight loss. Initially, fat stores are diminished; eventually muscle mass is lost. Deficiencies of fat-soluble vitamins (A, D, and K) and minerals are frequently encountered. Nutritional repletion may be complicated by both abdominal pain, often exacerbated by oral intake, and maldigestion.

Acute alcoholic pancreatitis may be managed by oral feeding when the patient does not have ileus, nausea, or vomiting and when oral intake is not accompanied by increased abdominal pain. These conditions are often met in mild cases. Enteral feeding of elemental diets delivered via jejunostomy tube is theoretically attractive because the duodenal area is bypassed and release of pancreatic secretagogues is minimized, especially when low-fat mixtures are used; the requirement for digestion prior to absorption is small. However, the parenteral route is usual, since ileus is common. Standard total parenteral nutrition (TPN) formulations are used, which have glucose and lipid as energy sources. Usually the insulin requirement is reasonable, but if it exceeds 80 U/day, lipid substitution may be considered. Lipid has not been shown to be deleterious. Although nitrogen loss is diminished, improved survival has not been documented.

The nutritional approach to chronic pancreatic insufficiency requires alleviating abdominal pain to permit adequate oral food intake; replacing pancreatic exocrine secretion to prevent maldigestion, diarrhea, and energy wastage; and managing diabetes mellitus. Pancreatic enzyme replacement is effective given in adequate doses with meals. Lipase deficiency is usually responsible for symptoms such as steatorrhea and should be given in amounts up to 30,000 units as active enzyme. Sometimes antiacids such as H_2 blockers are needed to protect the enzymes from acid-mediated destruction, since the neutralizing action of bicarbonate secretion is lacking due to pancreatic damage. Diabetes mellitus due to pancreatic insufficiency may exhibit insulin sensitivity and hypoglycemia, perhaps because of concomitant glucagon deficiency. Insulin therapy has to be given with caution.

Alterations of Nutrient Metabolism

Water-Soluble Vitamins

Alcoholics tend to have clinical or laboratory signs of soluble vitamin insufficiency correlated with the increasing amount of alcohol they drink and a corresponding decrease in vitamin intake. This is true for thiamin, riboflavin, pyridoxine, folic acid, and ascorbic acid but has not been demonstrated for vitamin B_{12}. Alcohol effects on absorption, activation, and storage must also be considered. Alcohol clearly impairs thiamin absorption in rodents; human thiamin absorption may not be susceptible to alcohol. Alcohol interferes with riboflavin absorption in rodents, but this has not been studied in humans. Alcohol impairs folic acid absorption in malnourished humans, but the mechanism is unclear. Some experimental animals, even without malnutrition, have folic acid absorption impaired by alcohol; others do not. Hepatic retention of folic acid is inhibited by alcohol, which also interferes with hematologic use of folic acid and promotes its urinary and fecal loss. Whether alcohol interferes with the activation and storage of thiamin is controversial. Riboflavin and pyridoxine storage in the liver is adversely affected by alcohol, at least in experimental animals.

Thiamin. Thiamin deficiency is usually present in alcoholics in Western society and causes Wernicke-Korsakoff syndrome and beriberi heart disease and probably contributes to polyneuropathy. Neuroanatomic lesions comparable to the human syndrome can be produced in rhesus monkeys by prolonged thiamin deficiency without the need for alcohol intake (55, 56). There has been no confirmation of an inborn error of transketolase affinity for coenzyme in Wernicke-Korsakoff syndrome as was once claimed (57). Thiamin intake will be insufficient for those relying on alcoholic beverages for their energy needs. When obvious deficiency is not present, measuring the decrease in blood transketolase activity and its increase upon in vitro addition of cofactor thiamin pyrophosphate (TPP) is considered useful for diagnosis by some (58, 59) but not all (60). It is postulated that profound thiamin deficiency, alcohol intake (61), or liver disease (62) may affect levels of apoenzyme transketolase or its binding to cofactor and thus prevent the TPP effect. Others have found that decreased erythrocyte transketolase activity alone correlates best with thiamin deficiency in patients with Wernicke's encephalopathy (63). In any case, in experimental animals (64) and in well-nourished alcoholics who ingest normal amounts of thiamin or more, levels in the organs are maintained (65), and there is no abnormality in the relative amounts of phosphorylated species of thiamin (66).

Hospitalized alcoholics were reported to have poorer thiamin absorption than control patients when tested by radioactive thiamin excretion (67), a test also affected by steps not related to absorption. However, folic acid deficiency was not adequately excluded as a cause of thiamin malabsorption in these studies. Refined testing reveals reduced thiamin absorption due to alcohol in a minority of subjects (68). Jejunal perfusion studies showed no effect of 5% alcohol on thiamin absorption in man (69). Interestingly, thiamin absorption is lower in middle-aged subjects (alcoholics and controls) than in younger individuals. Studies in rats have progressed farther, but they may not be relevant to human disease (discussed above). In rodents, thiamin absorption is accomplished by an active system with a low K_m and a passive system with a higher K_m. Alcohol interferes with thiamin absorption via the low-concentration active pathway, and presumably (if humans are similarly constituted) is an important factor for alcoholics with marginal or low thiamin intake. The effects of alcohol on thiamin activation and storage in the liver are controversial (65).

Thiamin is well absorbed from sorghum beer despite its 3% alcohol content (69). Therefore, it is feasible to add thiamin to alcoholic beverages, but this is prohibited by the current laws against "adulteration" of alcoholic beverages. Thiamin should be provided to all alcoholics for a number of reasons: thiamin deficiency is common in alcoholics, assessing any but the most glaring thiamin deficiency syndromes is difficult, it is important to reverse early neurologic disease, and thiamin replacement is easy and safe. Thiamin should be given parenterally, 50 mg/day, until oral intake can be established, then orally, 50 mg/day, for weeks or longer if neurologic problems persist.

Riboflavin. When there is a general lack of B vitamin intake, riboflavin deficiency may be encountered (70). In one study, deficiency was found in 50% of a small group of patients with medical complications severe enough to warrant hospital admission (71). Although none of the patients exhibited classic signs of riboflavin deficiency, they had an abnormal activity coefficient (AC) that returned to normal 2 to 7 days after intramuscular replacement with 5 mg riboflavin daily. The AC is measured as the ratio of erythrocyte glutathione reductase activity upon addition of flavin adenine dinucleotide (FAD) to the activity with no additions. A study showed that riboflavin deficiency could be induced readily by feeding alcohol to the Syrian hamster; the most severe deficiency was seen in animals also restricted in riboflavin intake (72). Ethanol also impaired hepatic accumulation of riboflavin in rats given vitamins and alcohol by acute gavage, with evidence that ethanol markedly inhibited the enzymes that hydrolyze the vitamin forms–flavin mononucleotide (FMN), phosphatase, FAD, pyrophosphatase–and may decrease vitamin absorption.

Riboflavin replacement is easy because absorption occurs readily, excess is excreted in the urine, and there is no known toxicity. It is usually given to alcoholic patients as part of a multivitamin preparation.

Pyridoxine. Neurologic, hematologic, and dermatologic disorders can be caused in part by pyridoxine deficiency. Pyridoxine deficiency, as measured by low plasma pyridoxal-5′-phosphate (PLP) levels, was reported in over 50% of alcoholics without hematologic findings or abnormal liver function tests (73, 74). Inadequate intake may partly explain low PLP levels, but increased destruction and reduced formation may also obtain. PLP is more rapidly destroyed in erythrocytes in the presence of acetaldehyde, the first product of ethanol oxidation, perhaps by displacement of PLP from protein and consequent exposure to phosphatase (73, 75). Fairly high levels of acetaldehyde were used in the studies cited, so the significance of the proposed mechanism is uncertain. Previous studies showed that chronic ethanol feeding lowered hepatic content of PLP by decreasing net synthesis from pyridoxine (76–78), which depended on alcohol oxidation in some studies. The acetaldehyde produced was thought to enhance hydrolysis of PLP by cellular phosphatases (73). Actual displacement of PLP from its binding protein by acetaldehyde has been shown in rat hepatocytes (79). In later studies of mice (79) and rats (80), ethanol actually increased total hepatic levels of vitamin B_6 (PLP and pyridoxamine-5′-phosphate, or PMP), primarily because of an increase in PMP. However, plasma PLP may be lowered by plasma phosphatase activity (74).

Clinical management generally involves providing pyridoxine in the usual multivitamin dosage unless neuropathy or pyridoxine-responsive anemia has been diagnosed. Because of ataxia due to sensory neuropathy, which has been ascribed to toxicity from as little as 200 mg/day pyridoxine, indiscriminate use of large doses of vitamin must be avoided (81, 82).

Folic Acid. Alcoholics tend to have low folic acid status when they are drinking heavily and their folic acid intake is reduced. For example, a group of unselected alcoholics showed a 37.5% incidence of low serum folate levels and a 17.6% incidence of low red blood cell folate levels (83). More-recent studies correlated low serum and red cell folate levels to increased serum homocysteine levels in alcoholics, implying impaired disposition of the amino acid by transmethylation or transsulfuration (84). In monkeys, folate deficiency can be created by ethanol feeding (50% of total calories) for over 2 years, despite an otherwise adequate diet: hepatic folate is low and there is evidence for decreased folate absorption (85). In pigs fed ethanol for 11 months, folic acid absorption is normal, but jejunal folate hydrolase, an early enzyme of folate polyglutamate breakdown, is decreased (86, 87). In vitro preparations of rat intestine absorb folate less well when exposed to a variety of alcohols (88). Malnourished alcoholics without liver disease also absorb folic acid less well than their better-nourished counterparts (89). Folic acid absorption, usually increased by partial starvation, is increased less in rats when alcohol is ingested (90). It has not been clearly shown, however, that either protein deficiency or alcohol (89, 91) decreases folate absorption in vivo. Thus, it is still unclear what aspects of malnutrition adversely affect folate absorption and under what clinical circumstances alcohol may interfere with folate absorption.

Alcohol accelerates production of megaloblastic anemia in patients with depleted folate stores (92) and suppresses the hematologic response to folic acid in folic acid–depleted patients (93). Alcohol also has other effects on folate metabolism, but their significance is not clear: alcohol given acutely decreases serum folate, which is partly explained by increased urinary excretion (94); alcohol administered chronically to monkeys decreases hepatic folate levels, partly because the liver cannot retain folate (95) and perhaps because of increased urinary and fecal loss (96).

The clinical approach to folate deficiency without anemia is straightforward. A diet providing adequate folate, perhaps with additional folate, repletes stores in a matter of weeks. If malabsorption persists after this period, causes other than folate deficiency should be sought. When the patient is anemic, diagnostic evaluation is more complex (92). In addition to folate deficiency, the direct effect of alcohol on the bone marrow, liver disease, hypersplenism, bleeding, iron deficiency, infection, and use of anticonvulsants are all commonly encountered and will exert separate and combined influences on the hematologic picture. Remember, first, in well-nourished alcoholics folic acid deficiency is a rare cause of anemia (97), and second, a search for folic acid deficiency (serum or red cell folate levels) to explain anemia is unwarranted unless some or all of the morphologic features of the deficiency are present (macroovalocytes, hypersegmentation of polymorphonuclear leukocytes, megaloblastosis of the bone marrow).

The following sequence has been proposed for development of folic acid deficiency: negative folate balance (serum folate < 3 ng/mL); folate depletion (red blood cell folate < 160 ng/mL, serum folate < 120 ng/mL, neutrophil lobe average > 3.5, liver folate < 1.2 μg/g); folate-deficient anemia (low hemoglobin, elevated mean corpuscular volume, macroovalocytosis) (98). When there is combined iron and folate deficiency, the expression of macrocytosis is modified or a dimorphic red blood cell population may occur. Hypersegmentation of leukocyte nuclei and macroovalocytosis may persist for several weeks after folate replacement is started (92).

Some have proposed adding folate to alcoholic beverages because the taste of the beverage is not altered and vitamin absorption is adequate (99), but this is impermissible "adulteration" of alcoholic beverages under current law.

Vitamin B_{12}. Alcoholics do not commonly get vitamin B_{12} deficiency. Their serum levels are usually normal even when they are deficient in folate, whether they have cirrhosis (100, 101) or not (89, 90). This is probably due to large body stores of vitamin B_{12} and reserve capacity for absorption, since several factors in alcoholism would promote vitamin depletion. Pancreatic insufficiency, for example, results in decreased vitamin B_{12} absorption as measured by the Schilling test, because there is insufficient luminal protease activity and alkalinity, which normally serve to release vitamin B_{12} from the "R" protein secreted by salivary glands, intestines, and possibly the stomach (102). Alcohol ingestion also decreases vitamin B_{12} absorption in volunteers after several weeks of intake (103). The alcohol effect may be in the ileum, because coadministration of intrinsic factor or pancreatin does not correct the Schilling test results. Whether the binding of intrinsic factor–vitamin B_{12} complex to ileal sites is abnormal is controversial (104, 105).

Vitamin C. The vitamin C status of alcoholic patients admitted to a hospital is lower than that of nonalcoholics as measured by serum ascorbic acid, peripheral leukocyte ascorbic acid, or urinary ascorbic acid levels after an oral challenge (106). In addition to a lower mean ascorbic acid level, some 25% of patients with cirrhosis in one study had serum ascorbic acid levels below the range of healthy controls (106). Ascorbic acid status is low in alcoholic patients with and without liver disease. When alcohol intake exceeds 30% of total calories, vitamin C generally falls below recommended dietary allowances (RDAs) (107). Inadequate vitamin C intake provides only a partial explanation for low ascorbic acid status. The clinical significance is unknown for patients who have low ascorbic acid levels but who are not clearly scorbutic. Daily supplementation with 175 to 500 mg of ascorbic acid may be necessary for weeks or months to restore plasma and urinary ascorbate to normal levels (106).

Fat-Soluble Vitamins

Vitamin A. The interaction of alcoholism and vitamin A involves the intake, possibly the absorption of the vitamin, and its metabolism; there is evidence that alcohol may modulate the role of vitamin A in hepatotoxicity and carcinogenesis.

Vitamin A ingestion is not significantly below normal for Americans taking up to 400 kcal/day as alcohol (or less than 20% of total calories) (107), probably because the vitamin A density of the nonalcoholic portion of the diet is similar to that ingested by nonalcoholic populations. Americans taking 24% of total calories as alcohol ingest only 75% of the RDA for vitamin A (108). Probably those with intense alcoholism (i.e., individuals ingesting 50% or more of daily calories as alcohol) eat even less vitamin A. Chilean wine drinkers, for example, eat only 25% of the RDA for vitamin A when they ingest 150 g (1050 kcal) of alcohol per day (109). Elderly American men who consume alcohol regularly have a lower vitamin A intake (110); the mean intake of carotenes for men of all ages consuming over 50 g/day ethanol is lower than that of those drinking less (111). In a single study, vitamin A absorption was diminished 17% by 120 mL of wine (112).

Alcohol consumption is associated with raised blood β-carotene levels in both men (113) and women (114). Population studies showing lower blood β-carotene levels in drinkers may be explained by the lowering effect of concomitant smoking (111). Chronic alcoholic pancreatic insufficiency may substantially reduce vitamin A absorption, and the mean plasma vitamin A content is lower for these patients than for normal controls, correlating with the severity of steatorrhea (115). Low blood β-carotene levels were found in 98% of chronic alcoholics (150 g/day alcohol for 5–25 years) admitted to a hospital despite the lack of clinical signs of vitamin A deficiency (112).

The effect of short-term ingestion of alcohol on vitamin A blood levels has been variously reported as unchanged in man (116), increased in dogs (117), or increased as lipoprotein-bound retinol in rats (118). Experimental feeding of baboons with alcohol raises their blood β-carotene (119). Serum and liver levels of carotenoids and retinoids were recently measured in patients with liver diseases of alcoholic and nonalcoholic etiology, normal livers of transplant donors, and sera of normal control subjects (120). Total retinoids were decreased in the livers of alcoholics and nonalcoholics with liver disease, and decreases were more profound as alcoholic liver disease progressed to cirrhosis. Serum and liver concentrations of α- and β-carotenes were compared, and a substantial number of subjects with low hepatic levels had normal serum levels, suggesting that liver disease impairs the hepatic uptake, excretion, and/or metabolism of these compounds. Impaired conversion of ingested carotenes to hepatic retinoids during alcohol consumption may partially explain the decreased liver retinoid content, especially at advanced stages of alcoholic liver disease when plasma β-carotene is not raised much by carotene feeding (113, 119).

The experimental effect of long-term alcohol consumption on hepatic vitamin A in experimental animals is profound and is consistent with observations in humans: hepatic vitamin A stores are diminished whether dietary vitamin A is low, normal, or high. Rodents fed alcohol repeatedly in one study had lower hepatic vitamin A (121); 5 g/kg/day yielded a 20% decrease in the liver in another study (122). Higher intakes of alcohol—36% of calories or about 14 g/kg/day—decreased hepatic vitamin A by 60% in 4 to 6 weeks and by 72% in 7 to 9 weeks, without changes in serum vitamin A or retinol-binding protein (RBP) in another study (118). Five times the usual amount of vitamin A did not prevent hepatic depletion by alcohol. When baboons were fed 50% of calories as alcohol, a 60% decrease in hepatic vitamin A occurred after 4 months, and a 95% decrease after 24 to 84 months (118). Hepatic vitamin A levels decrease progressively with increasing severity of lesions to include cirrhosis in humans (Fig. 94.3) (123). Enhancement of hepatic vitamin A degradation due to alcohol consumption is one likely explanation for the drop in vitamin content. Vitamin A degradation by metabolism of retinoic acid to 4-hydroxy and 4-oxoretinoic acids and other polar metabolites is catalyzed by microsomal enzymes induced by ethanol consumption (123), but these enzymes are not active enough to deplete vitamin A stores. A more likely candidate for depleting hepatic vitamin A is a newly discovered microsomal pathway for oxidation of retinol to polar metabolites (124), also inducible by alcohol consumption (125). In addition, alcohol promotes vitamin A mobilization from the liver (125).

An important clinical consequence of low tissue vitamin A status is night blindness. A study showed that abnormal dark adaption occurred in 15% of alcoholics without cirrhosis and in 50% with cirrhosis (126). One can exclude retinal dysfunction with 95% confidence when the serum vitamin A level is 1.4 μmol/L (42.9 IU) or higher (127). The correlation of serum vitamin A with tissue stores is complicated by liver disease and protein deficiency.

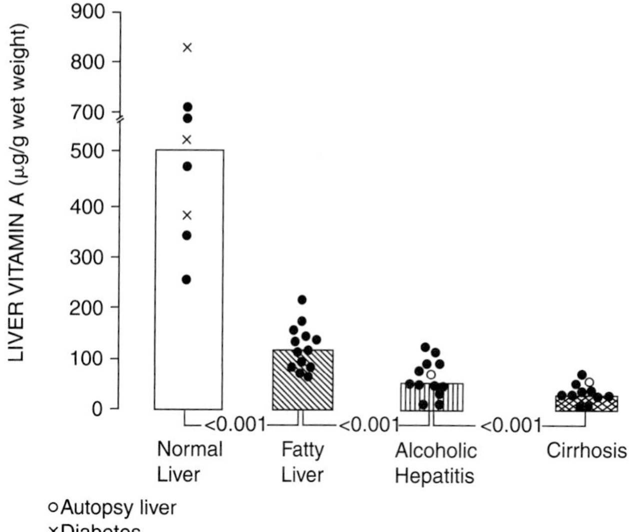

Figure 94.3. Hepatic vitamin A levels in subjects with normal livers, chronic persistent hepatitis, and various stages of alcoholic injury. (From Leo MA, Lieber CS. N Engl J Med 1982;37:597–601, with permission.)

The effects of vitamin A status and its related disease are widespread throughout the body and are in turn affected by ethanol consumption. Hepatotoxicity from diminished vitamin A includes the presence of multivesicular lysosomes and is potentiated by concomitant alcohol intake (128). Hepatotoxicity from increased vitamin A includes fibrosis (129, 130), which is potentiated by concomitant alcohol (131). The squamous metaplasia of rodent trachea due to vitamin A depletion is also enhanced by ethanol (132). Ethanol increases vitamin A in lung and esophagus (133). The role of alcohol in increasing vitamin A content of some tissues while having the opposite effect in others, speeding or altering the conversion of vitamin A to metabolites, probably has important consequences for the hepatotoxicity, fibrosis, and squamous metaplasia described above. Alcohol-mediated alterations of vitamin A status could be relevant to the association of low vitamin A or carotene levels with malignant diseases (133, 134); in a case-control study, mean levels of serum β-carotene and vitamin A were lower in both smokers and drinkers with oropharyngeal squamous cancer than in control patients hospitalized for minor surgical procedures, and protection was noted with increased intake of vitamin C, β-carotene, fruit, vegetables, and fiber (135).

Several factors make vitamin A therapy a complicated affair in the setting of alcoholism: assessment of tissue stores of vitamin A is difficult, vitamin A in high doses is toxic, even usual doses of vitamin A are potentially toxic with continued intake of alcohol (or other microsome-inducing drugs), and monitoring vitamin A hepatotoxicity is difficult in the presence of continued alcohol intake. Replacement with β-carotene was considered less hazardous, but in association with continued alcohol intake, it too shows evidence of hepatotoxicity (119, 136). Vitamin A replacement must therefore be modest for patients who cannot be ensured an alcohol- and drug-free environment. Replacement of vitamin A should be considered for patients who are confirmed to be vitamin deficient and who can be ensured abstinence from alcohol. Night blindness (or abnormal dark adaptation) with low serum vitamin A (<30 μg/dL or <1 μmol/L) may be considered evidence of deficiency. Vitamin A given at 2000 μg/day for several weeks should provide an adequate trial. Especially in the presence of night blindness, a low serum zinc level (<80 μg/dL) should be treated with 600 mg/day $ZnSO_4$. Considering the interrelationship of vitamin A and zinc metabolism, zinc therapy might also be tried when vitamin A therapy fails to correct night blindness. Documented fat malabsorption should prompt parenteral replacement of vitamin A. These recommendations appear reasonable but are not based on extensive clinical trials.

Vitamin D. Alcoholics have illness related to abnormalities of calcium, phosphorus, and vitamin D homeostasis. They have decreased bone density (137) and bone mass (138), increased susceptibility to fractures (139), and increased osteonecrosis (140). Low blood calcium, phosphorus, and magnesium levels, and low, normal, or high vitamin D_3 levels have been reported, indicating disturbed calcium metabolism (138).

In patients with alcoholic liver disease, vitamin D deficiency probably derives from too little vitamin D substrate, which results from poor dietary intake, malabsorption due to cholestasis or pancreatic insufficiency, and insufficient sunlight. (Vitamin D metabolism is discussed in Chapter 18.) The status of 25-hydroxylation appears adequate, even in advanced liver disease (138, 141, 142), although some disagree (143). The concentration of vitamin D–binding globulin, a protein synthesized in the liver, decreases in alcoholic liver disease (141), but because of its excess binding sites, its decrease is unlikely to cause 25-OH vitamin D_3 deficiency. Gascon-Barré says that although blood levels of 25-OH vitamin D_3 and 1,25-OH vitamin D_3 may be normal or even elevated in alcoholics, their stores of vitamin D_3 are often depleted, severely so in nutritionally depleted alcoholics (138). Insufficient intake of calcium and phosphorus or decreased calcium absorption in the presence of normal or increased 1,25-OH vitamin D_3 (and parathormone) might accelerate bone loss in alcoholics.

The diagnosis of osteopenia in liver disease may require bone densitometry because other clinical parameters of liver disease correlate poorly with osteopenia (144). Moreover, levels of free 25-OH vitamin D_3 may be normal in liver disease when total levels are low (145). Bone disease in patients with liver disease should be treated by increasing vitamin D_3 intake, ultraviolet light therapy, and correction of fat malabsorption to keep plasma calcium and phosphorus levels normal. Of course abstinence from alcohol is very important.

Vitamin K. Vitamin K deficiency in alcoholism may arise when fat absorption is interrupted by pancreatic insufficiency, biliary obstruction, or intestinal mucosal abnormality secondary to folic acid deficiency. Dietary vitamin K inadequacy is not a likely cause of clinical deficiency unless there is concomitant sterilization of the large gut, a reliable source of the vitamin. Alcohol-induced hepatocyte injury interferes with use of available vitamin K, with a consequent drop in blood levels of clotting factors II, VII, IX, and X, whose syntheses depend on this vitamin. Vitamin K is a cofactor for the microsomal carboxylase that effects posttranslational modification of these proteins, the conversion of glutamic acid (Glu) residues to δ-carboxyglutamic acid (Gla) residues, which is necessary for function. Abnormally high levels of inactive factor II (prothrombin) are found in the plasma in the presence of cirrhosis or vitamin K deficiency (146). Vitamin K may be given intramuscularly to test whether hepatocellular dysfunction or lack of availability of vitamin K to the liver is responsible for low levels of vitamin K–dependent clotting factors in the blood (147).

Vitamin E and Selenium. Vitamin E and selenium serve protective roles as antioxidants and interact physiologically (148–151). Vitamin E is a powerful antioxidant that prevents peroxidation of cellular and subcellular membrane phospholipids. Selenium is also involved in antioxidant functions and is a component of red blood cell glutathione peroxidase. Vitamin E and selenium function synergistically: vitamin E reduces the selenium requirement, prevents its loss from the body, and maintains it in an active form; selenium spares vitamin E and reduces the requirement for the vitamin (150).

Vitamin E deficiency is not a recognized complication of alcoholism, although patients with chronic alcoholic pancreatitis have a lower vitamin E:total plasma lipid ratio (115). Vitamin E deficiency has occurred in adults with diverse causes of fat malabsorption (148) and primary biliary cirrhosis (152) with clinical manifestations including decreased erythrocyte survival and neurologic disturbances (areflexia, gait disturbance, decreased proprioception and vibratory sensation, and ophthalmoplegia).

When rodents were fed ethanol repeatedly in one study their hepatic vitamin E levels (measured as α-tocopherol) were low (153); this was accompanied by increased hepatic lipid peroxidation when alcohol was combined with a low-vitamin E diet (154). The mechanism of hepatic vitamin E depletion by ethanol is probably enhanced oxidation of α-tocopherol (α-Toc) to α-tocopherol quinone (α-TQ) in liver microsomes (154). Alcohol-induced liver injury may be mediated, in part, by stress on cellular antioxidant mechanisms interrelated with vitamin E and selenium. Considering the findings in humans with fat malabsorption or severe cholestasis and the evidence of vitamin E depletion by chronic alcohol feeding of experimental animals, there would seem to be great potential for vitamin E deficiency in chronic alcoholics who may combine low vitamin E intake with steatorrhea from chronic pancreatitis or prolonged cholestasis. Indeed, low serum vitamin E levels have been reported in alcoholic patients with pancreatic insufficiency and fat malabsorption (115, 155). Vitamin E supplementation for 1 year to patients with chronic decompensated alcoholic cirrhosis significantly elevated serum vitamin E levels (156).

Selenium metabolism is of great theoretical interest to hepatologists in view of the proposed lipoperoxidative mechanism of drug- and alcohol-induced liver injury (133). Interestingly, serum selenium levels have been recorded as low in the alcoholic, especially in the presence of liver disease, but this may be a consequence of liver injury (133), because other nonalcoholic patients with liver disease also have low levels. Alcohol intake was not found to influence selenium excretion in the urine (157). No recommendation for dietary modifications of vitamin E or selenium intake in alcoholism can yet be made.

Water, Minerals, Electrolytes

Salt and Water Retention of Cirrhosis

Alcoholics with chronic liver disease often have disorders of water and electrolyte balance. Sodium and water retention are clinically apparent as weight gain, peripheral edema, ascites, and pleural effusions. Patients may have respiratory difficulties or umbilical herniation as further complications. Not only is sodium retained avidly, but a water load cannot be excreted normally (158). Low body potassium may result from vomiting, diarrhea, hyperaldosteronism, muscle wasting, renal tubular acidosis, or diuretic therapy. Potassium depletion may contribute to the appearance of renal vein ammonia and may worsen hepatic encephalopathy (159).

The pathogenesis of fluid retention and ascites is complex. At the hepatic level, portal hypertension, hypoalbuminemia, and alteration of lymph flow are important factors for ascites formation (160). Endocrine accompaniments and other phenomena suggest that the body is reacting to a diminished "effective circulating volume" (total blood volume is normal or elevated, but a disproportionately large fraction is sequestered in the splanchnic region) (161). Hyperreninemia, hyperaldosteronemia, and increased blood norepinephrine suggest diminished effective circulating volume. Reversal of salt and water retention by restoration of nonsplanchnic volume via head-out body immersion in water or via peritoneal venous (LeVeen) shunting of ascites suggests sequestration of blood volume in the splachnic area. Additionally, there may be a relative insufficiency of factors (or insensitivity to such factors) that promote salt loss by the kidneys, such as atrial natriuretic factor (ANF) (162), because the ANF level is raised (163, 164) and there is an abnormality of renal hemodynamics based in part on alterations in renal prostaglandins (162).

Patients with cirrhosis and fluid overload may require urgent relief, as when ascites and pleural effusion are causing respiratory difficulties or when imminent rupture of an umbilical hernia may result in lethal peritonitis. Thoracentesis, paracentesis, or both should be performed promptly. Usually, diuresis may be unhurried once a diagnostic tap has shown the fluid to be noninfected transudate. Treatment is aimed at preventing recurrence of fluid retention. Dietary management combines sodium and water restriction in selected cases of deficient water excretion. It is difficult to provide a palatable diet on a long-term basis with less than 0.5 to 1 g of sodium and 1500 to 2000 mL of total fluid daily. These amounts are recommended with addition of spironolactone, followed, if necessary, by small doses of diuretics (hydrochlorothiazide or furosemide), to achieve an initial daily weight loss of no more than 0.5 kg (165). More-rapid weight loss is probably safe when the patient has mobilizable peripheral edema and can be observed carefully (165). Accelerated diuresis risks renal failure. Use of prostaglandin inhibitors such as nonsteroidal antiinflammatory drugs (NSAIDs) carries the potential risk of altering renal hemodynamics and precipitating renal failure. Careful monitoring for development of hypokalemia (or hyperkalemia), hyponatremia, and renal failure is necessary. Recently, periodic large-volume paracenteses have again been used with intravenous fluid and albumin and seem to be as safe as diuretics (166). For patients in whom a reasonable program of salt and water restriction and diuretic therapy is not successful or for whom periodic paracentesis is cumbersome, a peritoneovenous (LaVeen) shunt may be useful (167–169). Best results have been obtained for patients without encephalopathy, coagulopathy, or severe jaundice.

Magnesium

Neuromuscular excitability in acute alcohol withdrawal resembles that seen in magnesium deficiency; thus the status of magnesium in alcoholism has been investigated for some time. Acute doses of ethanol cause magnesium loss in the urine (170), although chronic ethanol feeding does not change urinary magnesium levels (171). Flink summarized much work in the field to show that alcoholism is associated with magnesium deficiency (172): alcoholics have low blood magnesium and low body-exchangeable magnesium levels; symptoms in alcoholics resemble those in patients with magnesium deficiency of other causes; alcohol ingestion causes magnesium excretion; upon withdrawal from alcohol, magnesium balance is positive; and hypocalcemia in alcoholics in the setting of magnesium deficiency has been ascribed in part to impaired parathyroid hormone (PTH) secretion as well as renal and skeletal resistance to PTH (173), and the hypocalcemia may only respond to magnesium repletion. The correlation of magnesium content of blood with that of other tissues and with the severity of clinical symptoms in individual cases is imperfect, although it is statistically obvious among groups. Recently, a group of hospitalized alcoholics with normal serum total magnesium (tMg) levels were found to have significantly lower serum ionized magnesium (iMg) levels (174). Magnesium replacement should be seriously considered for symptomatic patients with measurably low serum magnesium, for anorectic patients with low serum magnesium, and for hypocalcemic alcoholics who do not respond to calcium replacement. Most alcoholics replete body stores of magnesium readily from normal dietary sources.

Iron

Iron metabolism is important in alcoholism in that there may be deficiency or there may be excess of iron in the body. The status of transferrin may provide a marker for chronic alcohol consumption. Alcoholics may be iron deficient as a result of the several gastrointestinal lesions to which they are prone that may bleed (esophagitis, esophageal varices, gastritis, and duodenitis). The usual laboratory indicators, red blood cell morphology (with alertness to altered morphology in the presence of folate deficiency), serum iron, and serum iron-binding capacity, are helpful. Iron therapy should be restricted to clearly diagnosed cases of deficiency.

Hepatic iron content is increased in autopsy studies of most patients with early alcoholic cirrhosis (175). Iron overload of the liver was described in Bantus who consumed alcoholic beverages prepared in iron containers that contributed a large amount of elemental iron to their diet. In most alcoholics, the iron content of the liver is normal or only modestly elevated, although there may be stainable iron in reticuloendothelial cells, possibly because of bouts of hemolysis. It is unclear whether increased intestinal absorption of iron because of alcohol (176) or hepatic uptake of iron from serum in established alcoholic liver disease (177) contributes significantly to increased hepatic iron levels. There should be little difficulty in distinguishing the hepatic iron increases of alcoholic liver disease from the much higher amounts characteristic of genetic hemochromatosis, by measuring absolute iron content per gram of liver with upward adjustments for age (178, 179). The contribution hepatic iron may make to liver damage via its role in lipid peroxidation (180) (perhaps in conjunction with the effects of alcohol) and its possible role in promoting fibrogenesis (181) are of great potential significance.

Alcoholism has been reported to result in qualitative changes in transferrin, the serum transport protein for iron: a higher fraction of molecules bear a reduced sialic acid content (182, 183). This provides a useful test for chronic alcohol consumption (184, 185). Synthesis of transferrin is decreased at the stage of alcoholic cirrhosis, as is serum transferrin concentration (186). At the stage of alcoholic fatty liver, the serum transferrin concentration is normal, although catabolic rate and presumably synthesis are both increased (186). The significance of these changes in transferrin is not apparent.

Zinc

Alcoholic cirrhosis is associated with abnormalities of zinc homeostasis, although the clinical implications are uncertain (for discussion of zinc metabolism, see Chapter 11). Patients have low plasma zinc (187), low liver zinc (188), and increased urinary zinc levels (188, 189). Acute ethanol ingestion, however, does not cause zincuria (190). The low zinc content of chronic alcoholics with cirrhosis is attributed to decreased intake and decreased absorption as well as increased urinary excretion. Many Americans have a diet marginal in zinc (191). Alcoholics fall into several of those groups with marginal intake. Interestingly, zinc absorption is low in alcoholic cirrhotics but not in patients with cirrhosis of other causes (192), although cirrhosis of varied etiologies is characterized by low serum zinc levels (193). Some instances of night blindness not fully responsive to vitamin A replacement (see vitamin A discussion) respond to zinc replacement. It is possible that human hypogonadism of alcoholism may involve perturbations of vitamin A and zinc interactions, but this is largely unstudied. Currently, the therapeutic use of zinc in alcoholism is restricted to treatment of night blindness not responsive to vitamin A. Sullivan and his colleagues could not raise serum zinc levels in patients with alcoholic cirrhosis; zinc was increased in the urine (194, 195).

Copper

Hepatic copper content is increased in advanced alcoholic cirrhosis (175). Elevated serum copper content has been reported in alcoholics independent of the stage of liver disease (196), but others report normal levels (195). These findings have no known clinical significance.

Trace Metals

Nickel levels are consistently high in alcoholic liver disease; manganese and chromium are unchanged (175). Intracellular shifts in trace metals have been described upon acute administration of alcohol (197). These shifts, with possible effects on organelle function, may be important but are not revealed in measurement of whole organ content. Versieck et al. reported high serum molybdenum levels in patients with acute liver disease (198); increased levels were not seen in those with cirrhosis. The clinical significance of trace metal changes is obscure, except for the cardiotoxicity ascribed long ago to alcoholic beverages with high cobalt content.

EFFECT OF ETHANOL ON METABOLISM OF CARBOHYDRATES, URIC ACID, LIPIDS, AND PROTEINS

Carbohydrates

The clinical problems of carbohydrate metabolism include hyperglycemia (frequent, but rarely severe or life threatening), hypoglycemia (infrequent, mostly occurring

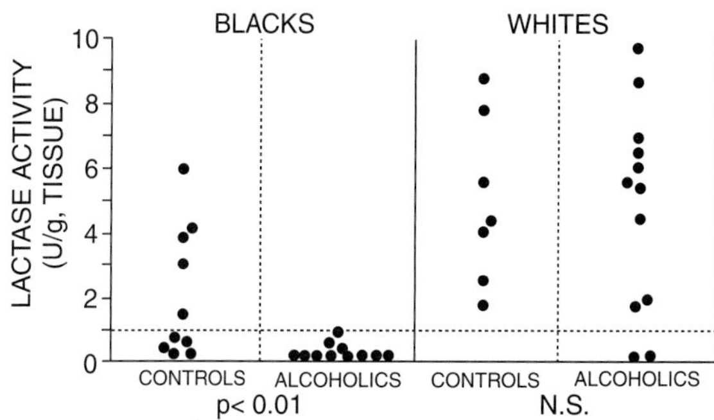

Figure 94.4. The effects of chronic alcohol consumption on lowering intestinal lactase activity. Black alcoholics were found to be especially sensitive. (From Perlow W, Baraona E, Lieber CS. Gastroenterology 1977;72:680–4, with permission.)

in conjunction with fasting or prolonged poor food intake except in children, but which can be lethal), and disaccharide (mostly lactose) malabsorption.

In large population studies, alcohol intake correlates with hyperglycemia (198). Except in patients with chronic pancreatitis and endocrine (insulin) insufficiency, there was no ready explanation for this until recently. The suspicion was that ethanol per se impairs glucose tolerance (199, 200), but this was difficult to prove because the elevated insulin levels that accompanied alcohol intake could have reflected insulin resistance due to alcohol or to the augmentation of insulin release that alcohol itself causes (201–203). Insulin resistance caused by alcohol has now been demonstrated in healthy subjects and in elderly men (204) by use of the insulin clamp technique in which glucose use is measured during glucose infusions at steady blood glucose and insulin levels (205).

In the fed state, when liver glycogen is abundant, glycogenolysis supports blood glucose levels. In the fasting state, concomitant metabolism of alcohol interferes with glycogenesis from amino acids and formation of glucose from glycerol, lactate, and galactose, pathways that can support blood glucose (206, 207). An increased NADH:NAD ratio from hepatic metabolism of alcohol is partly responsible for these metabolic changes. Changes in enzyme activities relevant to various metabolic steps of gluconeogenesis (208, 209) and lipogenesis (9) have also been described. Clinically, hypoglycemia must be suspected when an alcohol imbiber exhibits altered mental status (even in the fed state and especially children). Provision of glucose, usually intravenously, is simple and effective.

Monosaccharide malabsorption due to alcohol can be demonstrated experimentally, but as a clinical problem in alcoholics, malabsorption is probably restricted to those with folic acid deficiency. Malabsorption in alcoholics with folic acid deficiency can be documented by the xylose tolerance test (210, 211). Long-term ethanol ingestion depresses intestinal disaccharidase activities (sucrase, maltase, and lactase) (212) and is associated with lactose intolerance (Figs. 94.2 and 94.4) (47).

Uric Acid

It is an old observation that drinking alcoholic beverages is associated with precipitation of acute gouty attacks. Hyperuricemia accompanying bouts of intense alcohol intake has occurred in patients without known disorders of uric acid metabolism or renal function (212). An important mechanism of alcoholic hyperuricemia is decreased urinary excretion of uric acid secondary to elevated serum lactate. This is illustrated in data from one patient in Figure 94.5 (213). Lactate is produced in the liver from pyruvate by the action of NADH generated in the metabolism of ethanol by alcohol dehydrogenase. Depending on the metabolic state of the liver, NADH generation either enhances hepatic lactate production or prevents the liver from completing the Cori cycle and using lactate originating in peripheral tissues, especially lactate produced from muscle activity during alcohol withdrawal (214). Alcohol-associated ketosis or starvation may also provoke hyperuricemia. The renal mechanism neither depends on urinary pH (212) nor is abolished by probenecid (215): it remains unexplained.

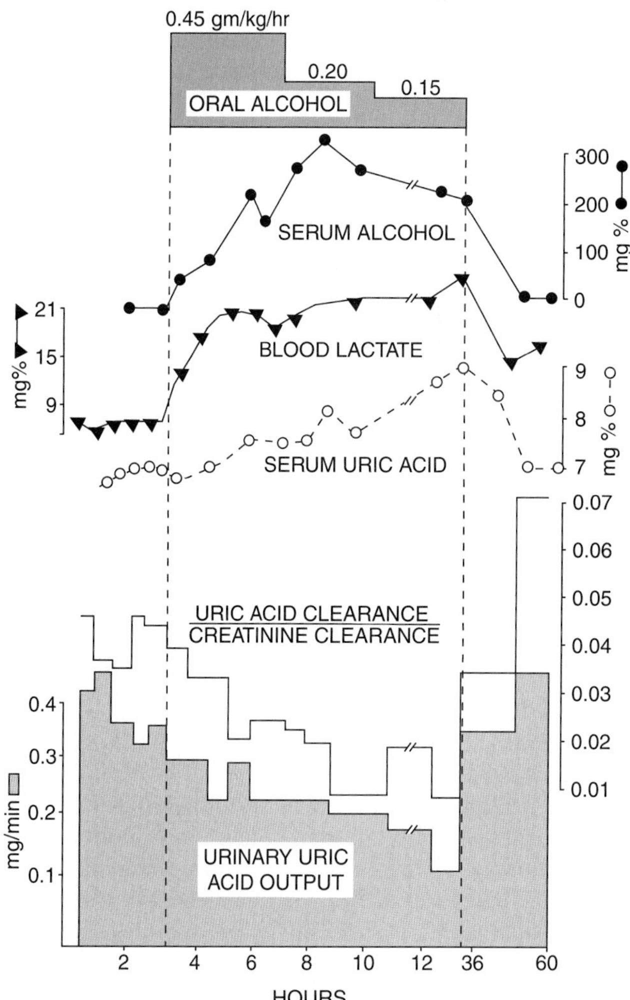

Figure 94.5. Effect of oral ethanol on blood and urine uric acid and lactate. (From Lieber CS, Jones DP, Losowsky MS, et al. J Clin Invest 1962;41:1863, with permission.)

Increased urate production partly due to increased adenosine nucleotide turnover has caused hyperuricemia in gouty volunteers (95). Urinary urate clearance was increased and urinary urate and oxypurines were higher in the study. This mechanism was demonstrated at lower blood alcohol levels than those in the lactate-related renal mechanism study, and blood alcohol levels were also lower than those usually seen in patients with alcoholic hyperuricemia.

The purine content (guanosine) of some beers may contribute to hyperuricemia and gout in alcoholic subjects (216). Patients with gout should refrain from significant alcohol intake, especially of purine-containing beers. The hyperuricemia encountered in the recent drinker should be observed during several days to a week of abstinence to allow alcoholic hyperuricemia to recede; a costly workup for other causes of hyperuricemia may thus be avoided.

Lipids, Fatty Liver, Hyperlipidemia, Ketoacidosis

Alcohol ingestion is associated with fatty infiltration of the liver, hyperlipidemia, and ketosis, each of which is largely explained by the effects that alcohol has on lipid metabolism (217). Fatty liver contains triglycerides with fatty acids derived from dietary sources, when available, but endogenously synthesized ones when dietary fatty acids are not available. High-fat diets increase the amount of fat that accumulates. Low-fat diets, high-protein diets, and even hypocaloric diets lessen the amount of fat that accumulates because of alcohol but do not completely prevent fatty liver. Dietary fat composed of medium-chain-length triglycerides causes less hepatic fat accumulation than fat containing triglycerides of long-chain fatty acids. The increased NADH:NAD ratio resulting from oxidation of alcohol to acetaldehyde by ADH reduces NAD availability for fatty acid oxidation via the citric acid cycle and thus depresses fatty acid oxidation. Structural damage to mitochondria inhibits oxidation of 2-carbon fragments from all sources. The major pathway of fatty acid synthesis in the cytosol is not increased. Fatty acid elongation by mitochondria is stimulated, probably by the increased NADH:NAD ratio. Glycerolipid synthesis increases because of the greater availability of fatty acids (as described above), the conversion of dihydroxyacetone phosphate to glycerol-3-phosphate favored by the increased NADH:NAD ratio, and possibly the increased capacity of lipid-synthesizing mechanisms. Activity of the rate-limiting enzyme, phosphatidate phosphohydrolase, which removes phosphorus from phosphatidic acid to form diacylglycerol, and of diacylglycerol acyl transferase, which catalyzes the formation of triglycerides increases. These enzymes are present in both endoplasmic reticulum and cytosol.

Administration of ethanol to man consistently results in hyperlipidemia; the extent is modified by associated dietary and pathologic conditions. The major increase occurs in serum triglycerides, with some cholesterol elevation; the involved lipoproteins are very low density lipoproteins (VLDLs) and chylomicrons, dietary particles formed by the intestines (Fig. 94.6). High-density lipoproteins (HDLs) are also increased by ethanol. Alcoholic hyperlipemia is usually classified as type IV according to the International Classification of Hyperlipidemias and Hyperlipoproteinemias because it is composed mostly of VLDLs, but it may be classified as type V when chylomicrons are also present. About 6% of alcoholics have type II hyperlipidemia, hypercholesterolemia due to an increase in low-density lipoproteins (LDLs). Alcohol-induced hyperlipemia may change rapidly in composition when clearing, because triglycerides are cleared more rapidly than cholesterol and phospholipids. The postprandial hyperlipidemia is greatly exaggerated by fat-containing meals (118). When alcohol is administered for several weeks at a dosage of 300 g/day, the initial several fold increase in triglycerides gradually returns to normal (219). This may be due to liver damage or increased lipoprotein lipase activity. Hyperlipemia is usually absent with severe liver injury (e.g., cirrhosis), and hypolipemia may be present (220–222).

Some patients may have marked hyperlipemia during alcohol ingestion. This most likely represents an underlying genetic defect in lipid metabolism, in addition to the effects of alcohol, such as hyperchylomicronemia (type I) due to decreased postheparin lipoprotein lipase activity

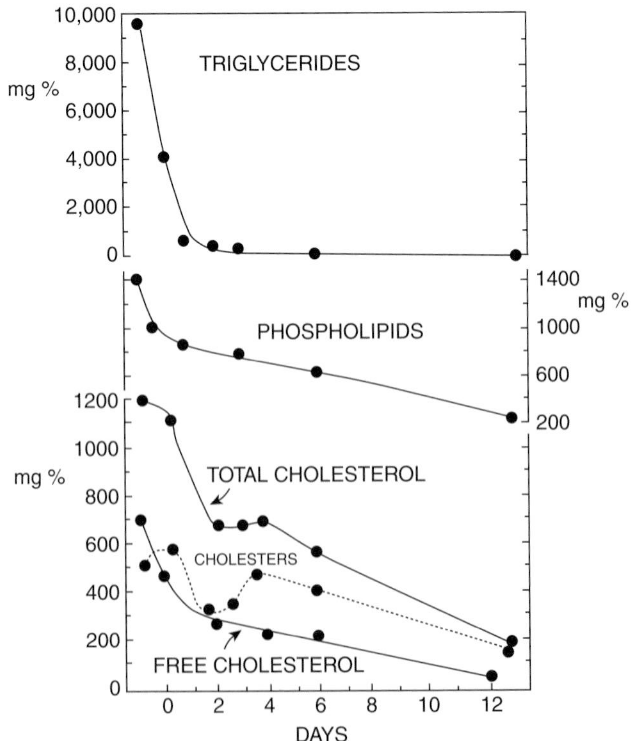

Figure 94.6. Serum lipids in the alcoholic and the effect of withdrawal from ethanol. Lipid fractions decrease at varying rates. (From Losowsky MS, Jones DP, Davidson CS, et al. Am J Med 1963;35:794, with permission.)

(213), carbohydrate-sensitive hyperlipidemia (223), diabetes, obesity, or pancreatitis.

Treatment of alcohol-induced hyperlipidemia consists of abstinence from alcohol and provision of a normal diet. A low-fat diet is unpalatable, may lead to inadequate energy intake (224), and is not usually necessary. The lipemia should rapidly disappear. Associated factors such as obesity and diabetes should be appropriately treated. Persistent hyperlipemia requires investigation for genetic or other causes not related to alcohol.

Moderate alcohol intake is associated with an increase in the fasting levels of a species of HDL-cholesterol (HDL_3) whose significance regarding risk for heart disease, unlike that for HDL_2, has not been fully established. Male red wine drinkers (46 g/kg/day of ethanol) tended to have elevated serum apolipoprotein A1 (225). Alcohol withdrawal led to a rapid decrease in both apo A1 and HDL_3 (226). Therefore, it is not clear whether any decreased risk for coronary heart disease associated with moderate alcohol intake can be explained by increased levels of HDL due to alcohol. HDL_2 increases with more substantial alcohol intake, but this level of intake is not cardioprotective and may even be deleterious (227). There are other possible mechanisms for a coronary protective effect of ethanol, in addition to its effect on HDL_3. Modest ethanol intake is associated with enhanced fibrinolysis via its effect on plasma concentration of plasminogen activator (228). Platelet aggregation is decreased by an acetaldehyde-mediated increase in prostacyclins (229) and by congeners in wine (230). However, there may be factors other than the alcoholic beverages which are responsible for the coronary-protective effect observed in modest drinkers, since apparent protection has been noted in people taking only one drink per day (231) or per month (232).

Alcohol intake is often accompanied by ketosis with minimal or absent acidosis. The blood glucose level is usually normal (233). The extent of ketosis will be underestimated unless care is taken to measure β-hydroxybutyrate in addition to acetoacetate, more common with diabetic ketosis. Abstinence from alcohol and a return to normal diet is usually the only required treatment. Fluid and electrolytes may be given. Insulin is usually not required.

Protein

Ethanol per se, measured as nitrogen balance, is nitrogen sparing when given as additional calories but increases urinary urea when given as an isocaloric substitute for carbohydrate (234, 235). Ethanol interferes with amino acid absorption in the gut in many experimental paradigms (see above), but the ultimate nutritional consequences are unknown because gross malabsorption of protein has not been demonstrated. An increase in urea nitrogen could represent protein that has escaped small bowel absorption, has been converted to ammonia in the colon, and subsequently has been converted to urea by the liver (235). Other explanations include protein catabolism in the heart (233), gastrointestinal tract (232), and other organs. As reviewed elsewhere (133), ethanol given in single doses impairs hepatic amino acid uptake, decreases gluconeogenesis, decreases leucine oxidation (234), increases serum branched-chain amino acids, and impairs synthesis of lipoproteins (236), albumin (237–240), and fibrinogen (234). Given over time, ethanol causes impaired protein secretion from the liver, probably related to alterations in microtubules and retention of proteins in enlarged hepatocytes (241). The importance of these effects on the hepatotoxicity of ethanol is being studied. Manipulation of dietary protein is not suggested during active alcoholism. The alterations in intermediary metabolism, including amino acids and nitrogen, in established cirrhosis and the implications for diet therapy are dealt with in Chapter 74.

EFFECTS OF DIETARY FACTORS ON ETHANOL METABOLISM

Alcohol is metabolized to acetaldehyde predominantly by ADH, a cytosolic enzyme, and also by the MEOS found in the endoplasmic reticulum. ADH is considered by some to be rate limiting for oxidation of ethanol (242). Low-protein diets reduce hepatic ADH in rats (243) and lower ethanol oxidation rates in rats (243) and in man (244). Prolonged fasting also decreases ethanol oxidation rates, as shown in isolated rat liver cells. A mechanism for lowered metabolism of ethanol during fasting is the lack of available metabolites to shuttle reducing equivalents from ethanol oxidation into mitochondria (245). For a given alcohol intake, malnourished alcoholics may develop higher blood alcohol levels and sustain them longer than normally nourished individuals (246), with possible deleterious consequences. An additional isozyme of ADH, σ ADH, exists in the stomach and contributes to the metabolism of ethanol before it reaches the portal circulation and the liver (247, 248). Gastric ADH is lower in women (249), allowing higher blood alcohol levels for similar alcohol ingestion occurring in men. Gastric ADH is also inhibited by the histamine H_2–receptor antagonist cimetidine taken orally.

A study showed that MEOS activity in the liver showed greater induction with a normal diet than with a low-fat diet in rats, although induction of the P4502E1 specific for ethanol metabolism was the same (250).

ALCOHOL, NUTRITION, AND ORGAN DAMAGE IN THE ALCOHOLIC

Liver

The role of nutrition in the pathogenesis of alcoholic liver injury (fatty liver, hepatitis, and cirrhosis) has been investigated from the perspectives of epidemiology, clinical therapeutic trials, and animal experimentation: the direct toxic effect of ethanol in each case was considered.

Malnutrition was previously thought to be important for development of alcoholic fatty liver: fatty liver is present in protein deficiency, particularly in children with kwashiorkor; a highly visible subset of alcoholics with fatty liver is malnourished (the "skid row" denizens); and rodents could readily be given fatty livers when subjected to diets deficient in lipotropes (see Chapter 73). Our current understanding is that alcohol per se, given in sufficient quantities, can cause fatty liver in man (and lower animals) despite an otherwise adequate diet (251–255). The lipid and protein composition of the diet modulates the amount and types of fat that accumulate in the liver. Reduction of dietary fat to 10% of total calories (but not lower) greatly lessens, but does not completely eliminate, hepatic fat accumulation. Fatty acids of the dietary chain length accumulate in the liver when available; otherwise, endogenously synthesized fatty acids deposit. Long-chain fatty acids in the diet have a greater tendency than medium-chain fatty acids to promote fatty liver in the presence of ethanol. However, providing more dietary protein than is usually recommended (25% of total calories) does not eliminate hepatic fat accumulation. The amount of fat accumulating in the ethanol-induced fatty liver is only one parameter of damage, and it must be considered along with organelle dysfunction and metabolic imbalances.

Lipotrope deficiency (choline and methionine) can cause fatty liver in rats (256), so attention was first directed toward the possible relevance of such deficiency for human alcoholic liver disease. However, there is no evidence that dietary choline deficiency causes human liver disease or is a part of ethanol-induced liver disease (see Chapter 73). Additionally, choline therapy is not effective when alcohol intake is continued (252–256). The difference in susceptibility to choline deficiency between rats and man is not surprising in view of the low choline oxidase activity in human liver.

The inappropriateness of extrapolating choline deficiency data in experimental animals to human alcoholic liver disease is also manifested by the differences between choline deficiency and ethanol-induced liver injury. The lesions differ ultrastructurally (257), in the levels of hepatic carnitine with which they are associated (increased with ethanol [258] and decreased with choline deficiency [259]), in their response to orotic acid supplementation (260), and in the decreased lipoprotein production and serum lipoproteins in choline deficiency (261, 262) and the opposite changes with alcohol (263). Even in rats, choline supplementation failed to fully prevent ethanol-induced lesions (264, 265). Dietary supplementation with choline, at times to extraordinary levels, did not prevent ethanol-induced fatty liver, fibrosis, and ultrastructural lesions (266) in nonhuman primates and was associated with hepatotoxicity of its own at high levels. Side effects such as nausea, vomiting, salivation, sweating, and anorexia have been noted with choline supplementation (267).

The role of nutrition in the pathogenesis of alcoholic hepatitis has been studied in much less detail. It is considered too severe to be induced in volunteers.

Alcoholic cirrhosis was directly linked to the intensity of ethanol consumption by its drop in the United States during the Prohibition Era and during World War II when alcoholic beverages were rationed (268, 269). The studies of Lelbach also show the direct influence of intensity of alcohol consumption (g/kg/day × years) on the incidence of chronic liver disease in patients admitted to alcohol rehabilitation spas in Europe (270). Neither the beverage source of ethanol nor concomitant malnutrition was noted to be an influence. These findings have been confirmed (271). The implied direct effect of ethanol in causing hepatic fibrosis and cirrhosis has been demonstrated in the baboon model of hepatic injury (272–274).

The direct hepatotoxic effect of ethanol has been shown histologically (by light and electron microscopy) and biochemically in both alcoholics and nonalcoholics, regardless of dietary variation in fat, protein, vitamins, and lipotropes (275–279). The mechanisms of ethanol-related cell injury includes alteration of the NADH:NAD ratio (a consequence of ethanol oxidation), alterations of calcium flux, and lipid peroxidation. Ethanol intake may influence lipid peroxidation via its induction of enzyme activities in the endoplasmic reticulum. Interactions of ethanol with selenium, iron, and copper, each of which is related to cellular control of peroxidation, are under study and have been reviewed (280). Dietary imbalances are not inferred, and dietary manipulations are not warranted from these very preliminary studies, except for such special circumstances as iron overload.

The role of nutrition in recovery from alcoholic liver injury was studied by clinicians before the pathogenesis of the injury was understood. Patek et al. (281, 282) and Morrison (283) demonstrated the efficacy of a normal-protein, normal-fat, vitamin-enriched diet in treatment of cirrhosis, as measured by clinical response and longevity. Erenoglu et al., extending previous work, treated cirrhotic patients with 198 mL of absolute ethanol daily and an adequate diet; they found no adverse effects and a possible benefit from higher dietary protein (284). This alcohol intake is much below the amount many alcoholics ingest spontaneously. In view of the current appreciation of the direct toxicity of ethanol and inability of most alcoholics to limit their alcohol intake, strict abstinence from alcohol is recommended.

The significance of congeners (285), moderate dosages of alcohol, genetic factors, and marginal nutritional deficiencies in alcohol-related tissue injury and in the recovery phase is under study. There is no established prophylactic regimen except abstinence. As discussed above, our best evidence indicates that acute liver damage consistently occurs if sufficient alcohol is ingested and cannot be prevented by a nutritious diet. There probably are safe levels of intake, although they have not been carefully established clinically. In any case, alcoholics are not usually able to confine their drinking to lower levels. Chronic liver injury from alcohol also appears to be dose and time related, with no indication that dietary manipulation will afford prevention. Patients with precursor lesions, such as perivenular fibrosis (280), require special attention, but the treatment approach is still mainly abstinence. Efforts to define populations with varying degrees of susceptibility to ethanol-induced liver disease on the basis of genetics or viral exposure have not been convincing; however, females are more susceptible than males (286, 287). We cannot advise a different approach for any group. Nutritional treatment of cirrhosis and its complications is described in Chapter 74.

Stroke

The incidence of stroke is strongly associated with advancing age, black race, obesity, and hypertension. Moderate-to-heavy alcohol consumption, over 45 g/day, was identified as an independent predictor of stroke after the increased risk due to hypertension and cigarette smoking were accounted for (288). A review of most of the English language literature concludes that moderate alcohol intake (<60 g/day) has a complex association with ischemic stroke in white populations (very low levels are possibly protective and higher levels are definitely deleterious) but little, if any, association in Japanese populations; by contrast, moderate drinking increases hemorrhagic stroke (intracerebral and subarachnoid hemorrhage) in diverse populations (289). Alcohol consumption may contribute to stroke by raising blood pressure to hypertensive levels as shown by most (32, 290–292), but not all (293), studies. Sodium intake and phosphorus intake were also positively identified as nutrient predictors of hypertension (32). Some authors have detected an immediacy of alcohol intake just prior to stroke (294) (although others have not [290]), which points to acute alcohol-induced changes that might precipitate stroke (295). If true, this finding is encouraging in that abstinence might yield early benefits.

Heart

Acute and chronic alcohol consumption affects the heart in some ways that are understood and in others that are obscure. The acute effects of even small amounts of hard liquor (several ounces) include measurable myocardial depression (296), a dose-dependent impairment of left ventricular emptying at rest (297), and such electrophysiologic effects as slight delay in atrial conduction and shortening of both the atrioventricular conduction time and the effective ventricular myocardial refractory period (298). These usually are not clinically apparent in people with normal hearts, especially because the impaired left ventricular emptying disappears with exercise (297). Patients with angina pectoris, even with congestive failure, have responses in left ventricular performance similar to those seen in controls at blood alcohol levels of 100 mg/dL (309). Patients with myocardial ischemia may experience an unfavorable distribution of coronary blood flow away from ischemic areas (299). The result of alcohol intake is thus not always predictable because it depends on the relative influence of alcohol on peripheral vasodilatation, coronary blood flow, direct myocardial depression, electrophysiologic changes, and the underlying cardiac reserve (300). Patients with chronic alcoholism or heart disease (300) and even normal nonalcoholic patients may develop atrial arrhythmias after substantial acute alcohol ingestion (301, 302).

Chronic alcohol consumption may result in heart disease by its association with hypertension, as discussed above in relation to stroke, or by its association with severe thiamin deficiency in the beriberi heart syndrome. Alcohol intake is associated with elevated serum homocysteine levels, as discussed in the sections on folic acid and the metabolism of one-carbon fragments. Elevated serum homocysteine levels have been linked to premature vascular disease (see Chapters 34 and 74). The relevance of alcohol-induced changes in serum HDL-cholesterol to the appearance of heart disease is not established (see above discussion of lipemia). Most epidemiologic studies of alcohol intake and either coronary artery disease or, more usually, total cardiac death rate, show a U-shaped relationship, with increased disease in abstainers, the lowest incidence in moderate drinkers (1 to 2 ounces of hard liquor or the equivalent per day), and the greatest incidence in those who consume larger amounts of alcohol. These results were found in the Hawaiian study (303), the Milwaukee study (304), and a study of the elderly in Massachusetts (305), but not clearly in the Albany experience (306). A prospective cohort study of 85,000 women demonstrated a similarly decreased mortality associated with very low alcohol intake compared with either abstainers or those using alcohol more heavily (307). Very low alcohol intake, 1.5 to 4.9 g/day or 1 to 3 drinks per week, was associated with the lowest mortality, but the "protective" effect was sustained up to 29 g or 2 drinks per day. Decreased mortality associated with alcohol intake reflected diminished fatal cardiovascular disease and occurred in those over 50 years of age and at risk for cardiovascular disease; younger women drinking similar amounts experienced increased mortality from external injury.

A fairly characteristic syndrome known as alcoholic cardiomyopathy has been described in a subset of these individuals with alcoholism and heart disease. It is a congestive cardiomyopathy seen typically in men aged 30 to 55 years who have been drinking 30 to 50% of calories as alcohol for 10 to 15 years (300). Arrhythmias are frequent. Coronary artery disease, hypertension, valvular abnormalities, and congenital heart disease must be excluded before the diagnosis of this disorder is made. Treatment with rest, diuretics, and abstention from alcohol may yield dramatic improvement (308, 309) but many times does not.

Blood and Bone Marrow

In addition to the anemias due to blood loss and folic acid deficiency discussed above, alcohol has direct or at least unexplained effects on the blood elements. Alcohol ingestion is associated with vacuolization of erythroid precursors, which is not prevented by adequate diet and pharmacologic doses of folic acid (310). Alcohol ingestion also causes granulocytopenia (probably mediated by nutritional inadequacy [310]), thrombocytopenia, and impaired platelet function (311, 312), which are partly attributed to direct effects because they are not mediated by folic acid or other identifiable nutritional deficiencies.

NUTRITIONAL THERAPY IN ALCOHOLISM

Nutritional therapy in alcoholism is directed at preventing illness due to alcoholism, treating documented or presumed deficiencies, and managing complications of alcoholism. As discussed above, individuals consuming over 30% of total calories as alcohol have a high probability of ingesting less than the recommended daily amounts of carbohydrate, protein, fat, vitamins A, C, and B (especially thiamin), and minerals such as calcium and iron. It is sensible to recommend a complete diet comparable to that of nonalcoholics to forestall deficiency syndromes, although this will not prevent some organ damage due to direct toxicity of alcohol (e.g., alcoholic liver disease). The feasibility and desirability of adding thiamin and perhaps folic acid to alcoholic beverages has been discussed previously but has not been done.

Management of observed deficiencies of protein and calories is straightforward in the absence of organ damage. The treatment of gross malnutrition of proteins and calories in the context of severe acute and chronic liver disease is discussed in chapter 74. Nervous system damage due to thiamin lack is serious and treatable with a great margin of safety; therefore thiamin deficiency should be presumed if not definitely disproved. Parenteral therapy with 50 mg of thiamin per day should be given until similar doses can be taken by mouth. Riboflavin and pyridoxine should be routinely given at the dosages usually contained in standard multivitamin preparations. Adequate folic acid replacement can be accomplished with the usual hospital diet. Additional replacement is optional unless deficiency is severe. Vitamin A replacement should only be given for well-documented deficiency and to patients whose abstinence from alcohol is ensured (see the above discussion on hepatotoxicity of hypervitaminosis A with alcohol). Vitamin A at doses of 2000 to 3000 μg/day may then be given. Zinc replacement should be given for night blindness unresponsive to vitamin A replacement. Magnesium replacement is recommended for symptomatic patients with low serum magnesium levels. Iron deficiency that has been clearly diagnosed may be corrected in the usual manner orally. Wernicke-Korsakoff syndrome requires at least 50 mg of thiamin daily (parenterally if necessary) for prolonged periods. Beriberi heart failure responds quickly to thiamin. Peripheral nerve damage necessitates months or years of vitamin B therapy. Acute pancreatitis may require withholding oral feeding for prolonged periods, during which time central venous alimentation must be given. Chronic pancreatic exocrine insufficiency is treated by dietary manipulation (often decreases in fat) with oral pancreatic enzymes at mealtime. The nutritional management of acute and chronic liver disease due to alcoholism aims to define feeding programs to reverse malnutrition, ameliorate liver disease, and decrease mortality, without promoting hepatic encephalopathy (see Chapter 74).

REFERENCES

1. Feinman L, Lieber CS. Alcohol Clin Exp Res 1988;12:2–6.
2. Pekkanen L, Forsander O. Nutr Bull 1977;4:91.
3. Scheig R. Am J Clin Nutr 1970;23:467.
4. Williamson DF, Forman MR, Binkin NJ, et al. Am J Public Health 1987;77:1324–30.
5. Lieber CS, Jones DP, DeCarli LM. J Clin Invest 1965;44:1009.
6. Pirola RC, Lieber CS. Pharmacology 1972;7:185.
7. Mezey E, Faillance LA. J Nerv Ment Dis 1971;153:445.
8. Crouse JR, Grundy SM. J Lipid Res 1984;25:486.
9. Guthrie GD, Myers KJ, Gesser EJ, et al. Clin Exp Res 1990; 14:17–22.
10. Tremolieres J, Carre L. Rev Alcoolisme 1961;7:202.
11. Stock MJ, Stuart JA. Nutr Metab 1974;17:297.
12. Stock AL, Stock MJ, Stuart JA. Proc Nutr Soc 1973;32:40A.
13. Klesges RC, Mealer CZ, Kesges LM. Am J Clin Nutr 1994; 59:805–9.
14. Rothwell NJ, Stock MJ. Metabolism 1984;33:768.
15. Pirola RC, Lieber CS. J Nutr 1975;105:1544.
16. Lieber CS. Am J Clin Nutr 1991;54:976–82.
17. Pirola RC, Lieber CS. Am J Clin Nutr 1976;29:90.
18. Israel Y, Videla L, Bernstein L. Fed Proc 1975;34:2052.
19. Teschke R, Moreno F, Heinen E, et al. Alcohol Alcohol 1983;18:151.
20. Iber FL. Nutr Today 1971;6:2–9.
21. Patek AJ, Toth EG, Saunder ME, et al. Arch Intern Med 1975;135:1053–7.
22. Mendenhall C, Bongiovanni G, Goldberg S, et al. JPEN J Parenter Enteral Nutr 1985;9:590–6.
23. Morgan MY. Acta Chir Scand 1981;507(Suppl):81–90.
24. Simko V, Connell AM, Banks B. Am J Clin Nutr 1982;35: 197–203.
25. World MJ, Ryle PR, Jones D, et al. Alcohol Alcohol 1984; 19:281–90.
26. World MJ, Ryle PR, Pratt OE, Thompson AD. Alcohol Alcohol 1984;19:1–6.
27. Liu S, Serdula MK, Williamson DF, et al. Am J Epidemiol 1994;140:912–20.
28. Armellini F, Zamboni M, Mandragona R, et al. Eur J Clin Nutr 1993;47:52–60.
29. Tremblay A, Buenmann B, Theriault G, et al. Eur J Clin Nutr 1995;49:824–31.
30. Bebb HT, Houser HB, Witschi JC, et al. Am J Clin Nutr 1971;24:1042–52.
31. Neville JN, Eagles JA, Samson G, et al. Am J Clin Nutr 1968; 21:1329–40.
32. Gruchow HW, Sobociaski KA, Barboriak JJ. JAMA 1985;253: 1567.
33. Hillers VN, Massey LK. Am J Clin Nutr 1985;41:356–62.
34. Westerfeld WW, Schulman MP. JAMA 1959;170:197–203.

35. Hillman RW. Alcoholism and malnutrition. In: Kissin B, Begleiter H, eds. Biology of alcoholism, vol III. New York: Plenum Press, 1974;513–60.
36. Dutta SK, Dukehart M, Narang A, et al. Gastroenterology 1989;96:510–8.
37. Winship DH, Carlton RC, Zaboralskie, et al. Gastroenterology 1968;55:173–8.
38. Silver LS, Worner TM, Korsten MA. Am J Gastroenterol 1986; 81:423–7.
39. Keshavarzian A, Iber F, Ferguson, Y. Gastroenterology 1987; 92:621–7.
40. Gottfried EB, Korsten MA, Lieber CS. Am J Gastroenterol 1978;70:587–92.
41. Laine L, Weinstein WM. Gastroenterology 1988;94:1254–62.
42. Barboriak JJ, Meade RC. Am J Clin Nutr 1970;23:1151–3.
43. Jian R, Cortot A, Ducrot F, et al. Dig Dis Sci 1986;31:604–14.
44. Keshavarzian A, Dangleis M, Wobbleton J, et al. Gastroenterology 1985;88:1444.
45. Hermos JA, Adams WH, Liu YK, et al. Ann Intern Med 1972;76:957–65.
46. Madzarovova-Nonejlova J. J Biol Gastroenterol 1971;4:325.
47. Perlow W, Baraona E, Lieber CS. Gastroenterology 1977;72: 680–4.
48. Thomson ABR. Dig Dis Sci 1984;29:267–74.
49. Mazzanti R, Debhaw ES, Jenkins WJ. Gut 1987;28:56–60.
50. Green PHR. Am J Med 1979;67:1066–76.
51. Marin GA, Ward NL, Fischer R. Dig Dis 1973;18:825–33.
52. Lefèvre A, DeCarli LM, Lieber CS. J Lipid Res 1972;13:48–55.
53. Knodell RG, Kinsey D, Boedeker EC, et al. Gastroenterology 1976;71:196–201.
54. Vlahcevic SR, Juttijudata P, Bell CC, et al. Gastroenterology 1972;62:1174–83.
55. Nicholas P, Rinaudo PA, Conn HD. Gastroenterology 1972; 63:112–8.
56. Witt ED, Goldman-Rakic PS. Ann Neurol 1983;13:396–401.
57. Blass JP, Gibson GE. N Engl J Med 1977;297:136–70.
58. Somogyi JC. Bibl Nutr Diets 1976;23:78–85.
59. Herve C, Beyne P, Letteron P, et al., Clin Chim Acta 1995; 234:91–100.
60. Camilo ME, Morgan MY, Sherlock S. Scand J Gastroenterol 1981;16:273–9.
61. Bitsch R, Hansen J, Hotzel D. Int J Vitam Nutr Res 1982; 52:126–33.
62. Fennelly J, Frank O, Baker H, et al. Am J Clin Nutr 1967; 20:946–9.
63. Wood B, Breen KJ, Penington DG. Aust NZ J Med 1977;7: 475–84.
64. Shaw S, Gorkin J, Lieber CS. Am J Clin Nutr 1981;34:856–60.
65. Hoyumpa AM. Alcohol Clin Exp Res 1983;7:11–4.
66. Dancy M, Evans G, Gaitonde MK, et al. Br Med J 1984; 289:79–82.
67. Thompson AD, Majumdar SK. Clin Gastroenterol 1981;10: 263–93.
68. Breen LJ, Buttigieg R, Iossifidis S, et al. Am J Clin Nutr 1985;42:121–6.
69. Katz D, Metz J, van der Westhuyzen J. Am J Clin Nutr 1985;42:666–70.
70. Van der Beek EJ, Lowik MR, Hulsof KF, et al. J Am Coll Nutr 1994;13:383–91.
71. Rosenthal WS, Adam MF, Lopez R, et al. Am J Clin Nutr 1973;26:858–60.
72. Kim C-I, Roe DA. Drug Nutr Interact 1985;3:99–107.
73. Lumeng L, Li T-K. J Clin Invest 1974;53:693–704.
74. Fonda ML, Brown SG, Pendleton MW. Alcohol Clin Exp Res 1989;3:804–9.
75. Lumeng L. J Clin Invest 1978;62:286–93.
76. Veitch RL, Lumeng L, Li TK. J Clin Invest 1975;55:1056–32.
77. Parker TH, Marshall JP, Roberts RK, et al. Am J Clin Nutr 1979;32:1246–52.
78. Lumeng L, Schenker S, Li T-K, et al. J Lab Clin Med 1984;103: 59–64.
79. Shane B. J Nutr 1982;112:610–8.
80. Liebman D, Furth-Walker D, Smolen TN, et al. Alcohol 1989;7:61–8.
81. Schaumberg H, Kaplan L, Windebank A, et al. N Engl J Med 1983;309:445–8.
82. Perry G, Bredesen DE. Neurology 1985;35:1466–8.
83. World MJ, Ryle PR, Jones D, et al. Alcohol Alcohol 1984; 19:281–90.
84. Cravo ML, Gloria LM, Selhub J, et al. Am J Clin Nutr 1996; 63:220–4.
85. Romero JJ, Tamura T, Halsted CH. Gastroenterology 1981;80: 99–102.
86. Reisenauer AM, Buffington CAT, Villanueva JA, et al. Am J Clin Nutr 1989;50:1429–35.
87. Naughton CA, Chandler CJ, Duplantier RB, et al. Am J Clin Nutr 1989;50:1436–41.
88. Said HM, Strum WB. Digestion 1986;35:129–35.
89. Halsted CH, Robles EZ, Mezey E. N Engl J Med 1971;285: 701–6.
90. Racusen LC, Krawitt EL. Am J Dig Dis 1977;22:915–20.
91. Lindenbaum J, Lieber CS. Effects of ethanol on the blood, bone marrow and small intestine of man. In: Roach MK, McIsaac WM, Cleaven PJ, eds. Biological aspects of alcohol, vol III. Austin: University of Texas Press, 1971;27–45.
92. Lindenbaum J, Lieber CS. Alcohol and the hematologic system. In: Lieber CS, ed. Medical disorders of alcoholism. Pathogenesis and treatment, vol 22. Philadelphia: WB Saunders, 1982;313–62.
93. Sullivan LW, Herbert V. J Clin Invest 1964;43:2048–62.
94. Russell RM, Rosenberg IH, Wilson PD, et al. Am J Clin Nutr 1983;38:64–70.
95. Tamura T, Romero JJ, Watson JE, et al. J Lab Clin Med 1981; 97:654–61.
96. Tamura T, Halsted CH. J Lab Clin Med 1983;101:623–8.
97. Eichner ER, Buchanan B, Smith JW, et al. Am J Med Sci 1972;273:35–42.
98. Herbert V. Am J Clin Nutr 1987;46:387–402.
99. Kaunitz JD, Lindenbaum J. Ann Intern Med 1977;87:542–5.
100. Herbert V, Zalusky R, Davidson CS. Ann Intern Med 1963; 58:977–88.
101. Klipstein FA, Lindenbaum J. Blood 1965;25:443–56.
102. Herzlich B, Herbert V. Am J Gastroenterol 1986;81:678–80.
103. Lindenbaum J, Lieber CS. Ann NY Acad Sci 1975;252:228–34.
104. Findlay J, Sellers E, Forstner G. Can J Physiol Pharmacol 1976; 54:469–76.
105. Lindenbaum J, Saha JR, Shea N, Lieber CS. Gastroenterology 1973;64:762.
106. Bonjour JP. Int J Vitam Nutr 1979;49:434–41.
107. Gruchow HW, Sobovinski KA, Barboriak JJ, et al. Am J Clin Nutr 1985;42:289–95.
108. Hillers VN, Massey LK. Am J Clin Nutr 1985;41:356–62.
109. Bunout D, Gattas V, Iturriaga H, et al. Am J Clin Nutr 1983; 38:469–73.
110. Barboriak JJ, Rooney CB, Leitschuh TH, et al. J Am Diet Assoc 1978;72:493–5.
111. Rimm E, Colditz G. Ann NY Acad Sci 1993;686:323–34.
112. Althausen TL, Uyeyama K, Loran K. Gastroenterology 1960; 38:942–5.
113. Ahmed S, Leo MA, Lieber CS. Am J Clin Nutr 1994;60:430–6.

114. Forman MR, Beecher GR, Lanza E, et al. Am J Clin Nutr 1995;62:131–5.
115. Marotta F, Labadarios D, Frazer L, et al. Dig Dis Sci 1994; 39:993–8.
116. Russell RM, Giovetti A, Garrett M, et al. Gastroenterology 1979;77:A36.
117. Lee M, Lucia SP. J Stud Alcohol 1965;26:1–8.
118. Sato M, Lieber CS. Gastroenterology 1980;79:1123.
119. Leo MA, Kim C-I, Lowe N, et al., Hepatology 1992;15:883–91.
120. Leo MA, Rosman AS, Lieber CS. Hepatology 1993;17:977–86.
121. Blomstrand R, Lof A, Osterling H. Nutr Metab 1977;21(Suppl 1):148–51.
122. Nadkarni GD, Deshpande UR, Pahuja DN. Experientia 1979;35:1059–60.
123. Leo MA, Lieber CS. N Engl J Med 1982;37:597–601.
124. Leo MA, Lieber CS. J Biol Chem 1985;260:5228–31.
125. Leo MA, Kim C, Lieber CS. Alcohol Clin Exp Res 1986; 10:487–92.
126. Bonjour JP. Int J Vitam Nutr Res 1981;51:166–77.
127. Carney EA, Russel RM. J Nutr 1980;110:552–7.
128. Leo MA, Sato M, Lieber CS. Gastroenterology 1983;84:562–72.
129. Leo MA, Lieber CS. Alcohol Clin Exp Res 1983;7:15–21.
130. Leo MA, Lieber CS. Hepatology 1983;3:1–11.
131. Leo MA, Arai M, Sato M, et al. Gastroenterology 1982; 82:194–205.
132. Mak KM, Leo MA, Lieber CS. Trans Assoc Am Physicians 1984;98:210–21.
133. Lieber CS. Alcohol and the liver. In: Arias IM, Frenkel MS, Wilson JHP, eds. Liver annual VI. Amsterdam: Excerpta Medica, 1987;163–240.
134. Anonymous. Lancet 1985;2:325–6.
135. Kune GA, Kune S, Field B, et al. Nutr Cancer 1993;20:61–70.
136. Leo MA, Lieber CS. N Engl J Med 1994;331:612.
137. Saville PD. J Bone Joint Surg (Am) 1965;47:492–9.
138. Gascon-Barré M. J Am Coll Nutr 1985;4:565–74.
139. Nilsson BE. Acta Chir Scand 1970;136:383–4.
140. Solomon L. J Bone Joint Surg (Br) 1973;55:246–61.
141. Long RG. Vitamin D in chronic liver disease. In: Bianchi L, Gerok W, Landmann L, et al., eds. Liver in metabolic diseases. Boston: MTP Press, 1983;421–7.
142. Posner DB, Russell RM, Absood S, Gastroenterology 1978;74: 866–70.
143. Jung RT, Davie M, Hunter JO, et al. Gut 1978;19:290–3.
144. Bonkovsky HL, Hawkins M, Steinberg K, et al. Hepatology 1990;12:273–80.
145. Bikle DD, Halloran BP, Gee E, et al. J Clin Invest 1986; 78:748–52.
146. Blanchard R, Furie BC, Jorgensen M, et al. N Engl J Med 1981;305:242–8.
147. Roberts HR, Cederbaum AI. Gastroenterology 1972;63: 297–320.
148. Bieri JG, Corash L, Hubbard VS. N Engl J Med 1983;308: 1063–71.
149. Scott ML. Fed Proc 1980;39:2736–9.
150. Martin DW Jr. Fat-soluble vitamins. In: Martin DW Jr, Mayes PA, Rodwell VW, Granner DK, eds. Harper's review of biochemistry. 20th ed. Los Altos, CA: Lange Medical Publications, 1985;118–27.
151. Levander OA, Burk RF. JPEN J Parenter Enteral Nutr 1986;10:545–9.
152. Knight RE, Bourne AJ, Newton M, et al. Gastroenterology 1986;91:209–11.
153. Bjorneboe G-E, Bjorneboe A, Hagen BF, et al. Biochim Biophys Acta 1987;918:236–41.
154. Kawase T, Kato S, Lieber CS. Hepatology 1989;10:815–21.
155. Kalvaria I, Labadarios D, Shephard GS, et al. Int J Pancreatol 1986;1:119–28.
156. de la Maza MP, Petermann M, Bunout D, et al., J Am Coll Nutr 1995;14:192–6.
157. Rodriguez EM, Sanz Alaejob MT, Diaz Romero C. Eur J Clin Chem Clin Biochem 1995;33:127–33.
158. Gabuzda GJ. Med Clin North Am 1970;54:1455–72.
159. Shear L, Gabuzda GJ, Shear L, et al. Am J Clin Nutr 1970;23: 614–8.
160. Summerskill WHJ, Barnardo DE, Baldus WP. Am J Clin Nutr 1990;23:499–507.
161. Epstein FH. N Engl J Med 1982;307:1577–8.
162. Epstein FH. Hepatology 1986;6:312–5.
163. Warner LC, Campbell PJ, Morali GA, et al. Hepatology 1990; 12:460–6.
164. Rector WG. Jr, Adair O, Hossack KF, et al. Gastroenterology 1990;99:766–70.
165. Boyer TD. Gastroenterology 1986;90:2022–3.
166. Kellerman PS. Ann Intern Med 1990;112:889–91.
167. LeVeen HH. Annu Rev Med 1985;453–69.
168. Smajda C, Franco D. Ann Surg 1985;201:488–93.
169. Wapnic S, Grossberg SJ, Evans MI. Br J Surg 1979;66:667–70.
170. McColister R, Prasad AS, Doe RP, et al. J Lab Clin Med 1958;52:928–32.
171. McDonald JT, Morgen S. Am J Clin Nutr 1979;32:823–33.
172. Flink EB. Alcohol Clin Exp Res 1986;10:590–4.
173. Abbott L, Nadler J, Rude RK, Alcohol Clin Exp Res 1994; 18:1076–82.
174. Wu C, Kenny MA. Clin Chem 1996;42:625–9.
175. Volini F, de la Huerga J, Kent G, et al. Trace metal studies in liver disease using atomic absorption spectroscopy. In: Sunderman FW, Sunderman FW Jr, eds. Laboratory diagnosis of liver disease. St. Louis: WH Green, 1968;199–206.
176. Chapman RW, Morgan MY, Bell R, et al. Gastroenterology 1983;84:143–7.
177. Chapman RW, Morgan MY, Boss AM, et al. Dig Dis Sci 1983;28:321–7.
178. Bassett ML, Halliday JW, Powell LW. Hepatology 1986;6: 24–9.
179. Olynk J, Hall P, Sallie R, et al. Hepatology 1990;12:26–30.
180. Bacon BR, Britton S. Hepatology 1990;11:127–37.
181. Chojkier M, Houglum K, Solis-Herruzo J, et al. J Biol Chem 1989;264:16957–62.
182. Stibler H, Allgulander C, Borg S, et al. Acta Med Scand 1978;204:49–56.
183. Stibler H, Sydow O, Borg S. Pharmacol Biochem Behav 1990; 13(Suppl):47–51.
184. Behrens UJ, Worner TM, Braly LF, et al. Clin Exp Res 1988; 12:427–37.
185. Behrens UJ, Worner TM, Lieber CS. Alcohol Clin Exp Res 1988;12:539–44.
186. Potter GJ, Chapman RWG, Nunes RM, et al. Hepatology 1985;5:714–21.
187. Vallee BL, Wacker WEC, Bartholomay AF, et al. N Engl J Med 1956;225:403–8.
188. Vallee BL, Wacker EC, Bartholomay AF, et al. N Engl J Med 1957;257:1055–65.
189. Sullivan JF. Gastroenterology 1962;42:439–42.
190. Sullivan JF. Q J Stud Alcohol 1962;23:216–20.
191. Sandstead HH. Am J Clin Nutr 1973;26:1251–60.
192. Valberg LS, Flanagan PR, Ghent CN, et al. Dig Dis Sci 1985; 30:329–39.
193. Poo JL, Rosas-Romero R, Rodriguez F, et al. Dig Dis 1995; 13:136–42.
194. Sullivan JE, Lankford HG. Am J Clin Nutr 1962;10:153–7.

195. Sullivan JF, Williams RV, Burch RE. Alcohol Clin Exp Res 1979;3:235–9.
196. Hartoma TR, Sontaniemi RA, Pelkonen O, et al. Eur J Clin Pharmacol 1977;12:147–51.
197. Szutowski MM, Lipsaka M, Bandolet JP. Pol J Pharmacol Pharm 1974;28:397–401.
198. Versieck J, Hoste J, Vanballenberghe L, et al. J Lab Clin Med 1981;97:535–44.
199. Phillips GB, Safrit HF. JAMA 1971;217:1513.
200. Rehfeld JF, Juhl E, Hilden M. Gastroenterology 1973;64: 445–51.
201. Dornhorst A, Ouyang A. Lancet 1971;2:957.
202. Metz R, Berger S, Mako M. Diabetes 1969;18:517.
203. Nikkilä EA, Taskin MR. Diabetes 1975;24:933.
204. Boden G, Chen X, Desantis R, et al. Diabetes 1993;42:28–34.
205. Yki-Järvinen H, Nikkilä EA. Metabolism 1985;61:941.
206. Krebs HA, Freedland RA, Hems R, et al. Biochem J 1969; 112:117.
207. Madison LL, Lochner A, Wulff J. Diabetes 1967;16:252.
208. Duruibe V, Tejwani GA. Mol Pharmacol 1981;20:621.
209. Stiffel FB, Green HL, Lufkin EG, et al. Biochim Biophys Acta 1976;428:633.
210. Dinda PK, Beck IT. Dig Dis Sci 1984;29:46.
211. Halsted CH, Robles EA, Mezey E. Gastroenterology 1973;64: 526–32.
212. Lieber CS, Jones DP, Losowsky MS, et al. J Clin Invest 1962;41:1863.
213. Losowsky MS, Jones DP, Davidson CS, et al. Am J Med 1963;35:794.
214. Newcomb DS. Metabolism 1972;21:1193.
215. MacLachlan MJ, Rodman GP. Am J Med 1967;42:38.
216. Gibson T, Rodgers AV, Simmonds HA, et al. Br J Rheumatol 1984;23:203.
217. Maddrey WC, Weber FL, Coutler AW, et al. Gastroenterology 1976;71:190–5.
218. Wilson DA, Schreibman PH, Brewster AC, et al. J Lab Clin Med 1970;75:264.
219. Lieber CS, Jones DP, Mendelson J, et al. Trans Assoc Am Physicians 1963;76:289.
220. Borowsky SA, Perlow W, Baraona E, et al. Dig Dis Sci 1980; 25:22.
221. Guisard D, Gonard JP, Laurent J, et al. Nutr Metab 1971;13: 222–9.
222. Marzo A, Ghiradi P, Sardini P, et al. Klin Wochenschr 1970;48: 949–50.
223. Ginsberg H, Olefsky J, Farquhar JW, et al. Ann Intern Med 1974;80:143–9.
224. Crews RH, Faloon WW. JAMA 1982;181:754.
225. Simonetti P, Brusamolino A, Pellegrini N, et al. Alcohol Clin Exp Res 1995;19:517–22.
226. Lamisse F, Schellenberg F, Bouyou E, et al. Alcohol Alcohol 1994;29:25–30.
227. Lieber CS. N Engl J Med 1984;311:846–8.
228. Ridker PM, Vaughan DE, Stampfer MJ, et al. JAMA 1994;272:929–33.
229. Guivernau M, Baraona E, Lieber CS. J Pharmacol Exp Ther 1987;240:59–64.
230. Renaud S, De Lrgeril M. Lancet 1992;339:1523–6.
231. Boffetta P, Garfinkel L. Epidemiology 1990;1:342–8.
232. Gronbaek M, Deis A, Sorsensen TIA. Br Med J 1995;310: 1165–9.
233. McGhee A, Henderson M, Milikan WJ, et al. Ann Surg 1983;197:288.
234. Klatskin G. Yale J Biol Med 1961;34:124.
235. Rodrigo C, Antezana C, Baraona E. J Nutr 1971;101:1307–10.
236. Schapiro RH, Drummer GD, Shimuzu Y, et al. J Clin Invest 1964;43:1338–47.
237. Rothschild MA, Oratz M, Mongelli J, et al. J Clin Invest 1971;50:1812–8.
238. Jeejeebhoy KN, Phillips MJ, Bruce-Robertson A, et al. Biochem J 1972;126:1111–26.
239. Preedy VR, Siddig T, Why H, Alcohol Alcohol 1994;29:141–7.
240. Preedy VR, Marway JS, Siddig T, et al. Drug Alcohol Depend 1993;34:1–10.
241. Baraona E, Leo MA, Borowsky SA, et al. Science 1975; 190:794–5.
242. Crow KE, Cornell NW, Veech RL. Clin Exp Res 1977;1:143–7.
243. Bode JL, Goebell H, Stahler M. Gesampte Exp Med 1970; 152:111–24.
244. Bode JL, Buchwald B, Goebell H. German Med Mon 1971; 1:149–51.
245. Meijer AJ, Van Woebkon GM, Williamson JR, et al. Biochem J 1975;150:205–9.
246. Korsten MA, Matsuzaki S, Feinman L, et al. N Engl J Med 1975;292:386–9.
247. Caballeria J, Baraona E, Rodamilans M, et al. Gastroenterology 1989;96:388–92.
248. Hernandez-Muñoz R, Caballeria J, Baraona E, et al. Alcohol Clin Exp Res 1990;14:946–50.
249. Frezza M, Di Padova C, Pozzato G, et al. N Engl J Med 1990;322:95–9.
250. Lieber CS, Lasker JM, DeCarli LM, et al. Pharmacol Exp Ther 1988;247:791–5.
251. Lieber CS. Alcohol, protein nutrition and liver injury. In: Winick M, ed. Nutrition and drugs. New York: John Wiley & Sons, 1983.
252. Klatskin G, Krehl WA, Conn HO. J Exp Med 1954;100:605.
253. Lieber CS, DeCarli LM. Am J Clin Nutr 1970;23:474.
254. Lieber CS, Spritz, N. J Clin Invest 1966;45:1400.
255. Lieber CS, Spritz N, DeCarli LM. J Lipid Res 1969;10:283.
256. Best CH, Hartroft WS, Lucas CC, et al. Br J Med 1949;11:10001.
257. Iseri OA, Lieber CS, Gottlieb LS. Am J Pathol 1966;48:535.
258. Konrup J, Grunnet N. Biochem J 1973;132:373.
259. Corredor C, Mansbach C, Bressler R. Fed Proc 1967;26:278.
260. Edreira JG, Hirsch RL, Kennedy JA. Q J Stud Alc 1974;35:20.
261. Chalvardian A. Can Biochem J 1970;48:1234.
262. Haines DSM. Can J Biochem 1966;44:45.
263. Baraona E, Lieber CS. J Clin Invest 1970;49:769–78.
264. DiLuzio NR. Am J Physiol 1958;194:453.
265. Lieber CS, DeCarli LM. Gastroenterology 1966;50:316.
266. Lieber CS, Leo MA, Mak KM, et al. Hepatology 1985;5:561.
267. Wood JL, Allison RG. Fed Proc 1982;41:3015.
268. Lederman S. Alcohol, alcoholisme, alcoholisation. Institut national d'études demographiques, travaux, et documents, cahier no. 41. Paris: Presses Universitaires de France, 1964.
269. United States Bureau of the Census. Vital statistics rates in the United States, 1900–1940. Washington, DC: Government Printing Office, 1943.
270. Lelbach WK. Acta Hepatosplenol (Stuttgart) 1967;14:9.
271. Tuyns AJ, Esteban J, Pequinot G. Br J Addict 1984;79:389.
272. Lieber CS, DeCarli LM. J Med Primatol 1974;3:153–63.
273. Lieber CS, DeCarli LM, Rubin E. Proc Natl Acad Sci USA 1975;72:437–41.
274. Rubin E, Lieber CS. N Engl J Med 1974;290:128–35.
275. Rubin E, Lieber CS. N Engl J Med 1968;278:869.
276. Lieber CS, Jones DP, DeCarli LM. J Clin Invest 1965;44: 1009–21.
277. Lane BP, Lieber CS. Am J Pathol 1966;49:593–603.
278. Lieber CS, Rubin E. Am J Med 1968;44:200–6.
279. Rubin E, Lieber CS. Fed Proc 1967;26:1458.

280. Lieber CS. Alcohol and the liver. In: Arias IM, Frenkel MS, Wilson JHP, eds. Liver annual—VI Amsterdam: Excerpta Medica, 1987;163–240.
281. Patek JA, Post J. J Clin Invest 1941;20:481.
282. Patek AJ, Post J, Ratnoff OB, et al. JAMA 1948;138:543.
283. Morrison LM. Ann Intern Med 1946;24:465.
284. Erenoglu E, Dereira JG, Patek AJ Jr. Ann Intern Med 1964; 60:814.
285. Feinman L, Lieber CS. Alcohol Clin Exp Res 1988;12:2–6.
286. Wilkinson P, Santamaria JN, Rankin JG. Aust Ann Med 1969; 18:222.
287. Morgan MY, Sherlock S. Br Med J 1972;2:939.
288. Gill JS, Sezulka V, Shipley MJ, et al. N Engl J Med 1986; 315:1041.
289. Camargo CA Jr. Stroke 1989;20:1611–26.
290. Blackwelder WC, Yano K, Rhoads G, et al. Am J Med 1980;68:164.
291. Klatsky AL, Friedman GD, Siegelaub A, et al. N Engl J Med 1977;296:1194.
292. Witteman JCM, Willet WC, Stampfer MJ, et al. Am J Cardiol 1990;65:633–7.
293. Coates RA, Corey PN, Ashley MJ, et al. Prev Med 1985;14:1.
294. Taylor JR, Combs-Orune T, Anderson E, et al. Clin Exp Res 1984;8:283–5.
295. Wolf PA. N Engl J Med 1986;315:1085.
296. Lang RM, Borrow KM, Neumann A, et al. Ann Intern Med 1985;102:742–7.
297. Kelbaek, H. Prog Cardiovasc Dis 1990;32:347–64.
298. Gould L, Reddy CVR, Becker W, et al. Electrocardiography 1978;11:219–26.
299. Friedman HS, Neal C, Dowd A, et al. Am J Cardiol 1981;47:61.
300. Segel LD, Klausner SC, Gnadt JTH, et al. Med Clin North Am 1984;68:147–61.
301. Anonymous. Lancet 1985;ii:1374.
302. Thornton JR. Lancet 1984;ii:1013.
303. Kagan A, Yano K, Rhoad GG, et al. Gut 1978;19:290.
304. Barboriak JJ, Anderson AJ, Rimm AA, Tristani FE. Alcohol Clin Exp Res 1979;3:29.
305. Colditz GA, Branch LG, Lipnic RJ, et al. Prog Cardiol 1985; 109:886–9.
306. Gordon T, Doyle JT. Am Heart J 1985;110:331–4.
307. Fuchs CS, Stampfer MJ, Colditz GA, et al. N Engl J Med 1995; 332:1245–50.
308. Agatson AS, Snow ME, Samet P. Alcohol Clin Exp Res 1986; 10:386–7.
309. Kupari M. Postgrad Med J 1984;60:151–4.
310. Lindenbaum J, Lieber CS. N Engl J Med 1969;281:333–8.
311. Haut MJ, Cowan DH. Am J Med 1974;56:22–32.
312. Lindenbaum J, Hargrove RL. Ann Intern Med 1968;68: 526–32.

95. Nutrition and Diseases of the Nervous System

DOUGLAS R. JEFFERY

Nutritional deficiencies may result in a variety of disorders that affect either the peripheral nervous system (PNS) or central nervous system (CNS). More commonly, both the CNS and PNS are affected simultaneously. Nutritional diseases of the nervous system have been carefully studied for more than 100 years, and many that were common in the last century now occur infrequently in developed countries. In the 1800s, beriberi occurred in epidemic proportions throughout the world. Similarly, pellagra was once common in the southern United States, but since 1940 the incidence has greatly diminished as a result of supplementing bread with niacin as well as major improvements in the overall diet of the affected population. In some Third World countries, pellagra and beriberi remain common, and these as well as other nutritional deficiencies continue to be a major cause of disease. In contrast, developed countries may encounter a different set of nutritional deficiencies, most often related to alcohol abuse, dietary habits, and impaired absorption of dietary nutrients secondary to intestinal malabsorption syndromes.

PATHOPHYSIOLOGY OF DEFICIENCIES ON THE NERVOUS SYSTEM

Nutritional deficiencies may have a wide variety of effects on both the CNS and PNS (1). Clinical manifestations of vitamin deficiency states may include neuropathy, visual disturbances, or disorders of the spinal cord leading to spastic quadriparesis with disturbances of bowel and bladder function. Other manifestations may include memory loss, dementia, ataxia, coma, and death, depending on the nutritional deficiency. Other deficiency states (e.g., folic acid) may lead to a rise in homocysteine levels that may be associated with increased risk of stroke and other vascular diseases (2). All of the nutritional deficiency states are treatable, and morbidity can be greatly reduced with early recognition and treatment.

Just as deficiency states can produce neurologic dysfunction, excess ingestion of nutrients may also cause nervous system dysfunction. For example, excess pyridoxine intake can be associated with a peripheral neuropathy resulting in severe irreversible ataxia, and excess intake of vitamin A may be associated with pseudotumor cerebri (benign intracranial hypertension) as well as irritability and lethargy.

Most deficiency states affect both the CNS and PNS but may vary in the degree to which they affect different cellular elements. This is a major determinant of the manifestations of the particular nutritional deficiency or, more commonly, constellation of nutritional deficiencies. Cellular elements most commonly affected by nutritional deficiency include the neuron itself and the myelin sheath. In the CNS, the myelin is formed by oligodendrocytes. In the periphery, myelin is formed by Schwann cells. Myelin acts as an insulator along the axon and allows the axon to conduct impulses at very rapid rates in both the PNS and CNS. In vitamin B_{12} deficiency, both CNS and PNS myelin degenerates, resulting in a host of clinical features including neuropathy, myelopathy, dementia, megaloblastic anemia, and behavioral abnormalities.

In deficiency states that affect the neuron, the axon usually shows the first signs of damage and will be most severely affected. The distal ends of longer axons are affected first, since they are most susceptible to nutritional deprivation. The result is a dying-back neuropathy in which the distal ends of the peripheral nerves slowly degenerate. Hence the PNS will be the major site of damage. With continued deprivation the process moves toward the cell body. This type of neuropathic process usually affects the largest and longest myelinated fibers as well as smaller unmyelinated neurons. There may be axonal degeneration as well as demyelination. The usual manifestation is a painful distal neuropathy in which the patient experiences loss of proprioception, touch, temperature, and pain. There is often a sensation of burning in the feet and a hypersensitivity to touch (hyperpathia). This can be extremely painful, and any contact with the affected extremity may be perceived as unpleasant and painful. With continued deprivation of the nutrient (most commonly thiamin), the pathologic process moves closer to the cell body, and the symptoms move proximally. Sensory loss worsens, and weakness may develop with continued damage to the neuron.

The prototypic nutritional polyneuropathy affecting the PNS is dry beriberi (alcoholic nutritional polyneuropathy). This disorder occurs commonly in well-developed countries and is usually seen in alcoholic patients. As with other nutritional deficiency states, this rarely occurs in its pure form as thiamin deficiency alone but is usually associated with other nutritional deficiency states.

Nutritional deficiencies rarely occur in isolation, and this may complicate neurologic syndromes resulting from vitamin deficiency. Far more commonly, deficiency states involve a variety of different vitamins and nutrients. The reasons for this become clear when the most common causes of nutritional deficiencies are considered. In developed countries, the most common cause of nutritional deficiency is alcoholism (see Chapter 94). In severe alcoholics, caloric intake consists largely of alcohol and carbohydrate. In addition, intestinal malabsorption may further compromise the nutritional state of the individual. The result is a polydeficiency state. The same holds true for malabsorption syndromes due to intestinal disease and to surgical procedures involving the gastrointestinal tract. Peculiarities of diet may have the same consequences. In individuals with borderline deficiency states, fully developed clinical disease may be brought about by stress associated with chronic infection, hyperemesis of pregnancy, or other acute illnesses such as trauma. Again, recognition is of great importance because irreversible neurologic damage due to vitamin deficiency can be easily prevented.

NEUROLOGIC DISORDERS ASSOCIATED WITH VITAMIN DEFICIENCY

Wernicke-Korsakoff Syndrome

In the category of neurologic disorders associated with vitamin deficiency, two entities should actually be considered together, Wernicke encephalopathy and Korsakoff psychosis. Wernicke disease refers to a neurologic disorder characterized by nystagmus, ataxia, confusion, paralysis of the abducens nerve, and other disorders of conjugate gaze (3). Korsakoff psychosis refers more specifically to an amnestic state in which there is severe impairment of short-term memory and confabulation. Korsakoff psychosis may be seen in association with other disorders of the nervous system, whereas Wernicke disease is specific to thiamin deficiency. Nevertheless, they often occur together in the setting of thiamin deficiency seen in alcoholism and other states of nutritional deprivation in which reserves of thiamin are exhausted. Wernicke-Korsakoff syndrome remains very common in both developed and underdeveloped countries (4). Furthermore, recognition of the setting in which this disorder may occur is the key to its prevention in those cases in which it has not progressed to enough to cause irreversible damage to the nervous system.

Wernicke-Korsakoff syndrome may be seen in any malnourished individual including elderly patients, particularly those with chronic illnesses predisposing to malnutrition (5). Table 95.1 lists common causes of nonalcoholic Wernicke-Korsakoff syndrome (6). In the hospital setting, Wernicke-Korsakoff syndrome can be precipitated in those with borderline thiamin deficiency by administration of intravenous fluid containing dextrose. Since metabolism of sugars and carbohydrates requires thiamin as a cofactor, the frank deficiency state can be precipitated with dextrose. This is particularly true in the emergency room setting where chronic, poorly nourished alcoholics may be brought for treatment of a variety of illnesses. In addition, thiamin is unstable in parenteral nutrient fluids containing amino acids with bisulfite, and storage time should be limited (see Chapter 101).

Despite the contention of some authors that Wernicke-Korsakoff is uncommon, pathologic changes of Wernicke-Korsakoff were seen in about 2.2% of 3548 random autopsies (77 cases) (7). If this is representative of the entire country, this may represent a very large number of patients. Furthermore, only 20% of cases may be recognized during life (8). Only 16% of patients exhibit the classic triad of ophthalmoplegia, gait ataxia, and confusion, and as many as 19% may have no clinical signs. Nevertheless, pathologic examination of these patients shows clear evidence of Wernicke-Korsakoff syndrome. This suggests that Wernicke-Korsakoff syndrome is underrecognized in both alcoholic and other malnourished patients. Wernicke-Korsakoff syndrome may be gradual or have sudden onset. Again, the classic triad of eye movement abnormalities, ataxia, and a global confusional state is not consistently seen (9). Other symptoms may be present including hypotension, hypothermia, cardiac failure, and coma (10, 11).

Wernicke-Korsakoff syndrome is the result of thiamin deficiency and is probably not due to any direct effect of alcohol on the CNS (4). Alcohol interferes with active transport of thiamin across the intestinal epithelium, and

Table 95.1
Nonalcoholic Conditions Associated with Thiamin Deficiency

Prolonged intravenous feeding with inadequate thiamin
Prolonged fasting
Anorexia nervosa
Refeeding after starvation
Gastric plication

Adapted from Reuler JB, Girad DE, Gooney TG. N Engl J Med 1985;312:1035–9.

formation of thiamin pyrophosphate from thiamin is decreased in severe liver disease (12, 13). In addition, the diseased liver may have a decreased capacity to store thiamin. Thiamin as thiamin pyrophosphate is a coenzyme for transketolase and pyruvate decarboxylase; transketolase is involved in the pentose phosphate shunt and pyruvate decarboxylase is involved in the tricarboxylic acid cycle, which suggests that depletion of thiamin may result in impaired CNS glucose metabolism (14, 15) (see also Chapter 21).

The neuropathologic appearance of Wernicke-Korsakoff disease is necrosis of both neuronal and oligodendroglial elements in the mammillary bodies, superior cerebellar vermis, and hypothalamus (16). Petechial hemorrhages are frequently seen in the mammillary bodies and periaqueductal gray (4). In addition, there may be involvement of the third and sixth nerve nuclei as well as the vestibular nuclei, accounting for the oculomotor palsies and nystagmus. In alcoholic cerebellar degeneration there are very similar pathologic changes, suggesting that it may also be related to thiamin deficiency (17).

Early on, the encephalopathic state is potentially reversible, and because of the risk of cardiac failure and sudden death, Wernicke-Korsakoff should be considered a neurologic emergency. Often the presenting symptoms of Wernicke-Korsakoff syndrome are stupor or coma. In one study, of 28 neuropathologically active cases, the diagnosis was made during life in only one instance (18). Suspected Wernicke-Korsakoff syndrome should be treated with 100 mg of thiamin given intravenously before starting dextrose infusion and periodically thereafter. The ocular manifestations of Wernicke-Korsakoff syndrome may begin to resolve as early as 6 hours after administration of thiamin. The ataxia and the confusional state may also improve rapidly following thiamin administration, but memory deficits are likely to persist.

Alcoholic beverages are not supplemented with thiamin. Though not all cases of Wernicke-Korsakoff syndrome are related to alcohol abuse and coexistent malnutrition, addition of thiamin to alcoholic beverages might go a long way toward prevention of this disorder.

Alcoholic Cerebellar Degeneration

Although alcoholic cerebellar degeneration has not been historically regarded as a vitamin deficiency state, indirect evidence suggests that it may be related to thiamin deficiency (19). Furthermore, it has been suggested to result from the same process as Wernicke-Korsakoff syndrome. This syndrome is usually seen in undernourished alcoholic patients following prolonged nutritional deprivation and weight loss. It has also been observed in nutritionally deprived nonalcoholics (6). Onset may be acute or subacute with stepwise progression. This disorder usually presents with wide-based gait and truncal ataxia. The upper extremities are frequently spared. Pathologically, there is severe atrophy of the anterior and posterior cerebellar vermis. Further research may help clarify the role of nutrition in this disorder.

Nutritional Polyneuropathy of Alcoholism

Another manifestation of poor nutritional status often associated with chronic alcohol abuse is nutritional polyneuropathy. While this disorder is considered to be primarily due to thiamin deficiency, other nutrients may also be involved (20–24). Almost all patients with Wernicke-Korsakoff syndrome have a coexisting polyneuropathy. The converse is not true; many patients with nutritional polyneuropathy may have no evidence of Wernicke-Korsakoff syndrome. In addition, alcohol toxicity may have a more direct role in this neuropathy, as it has been reported in well-nourished alcoholics (21, 22). Although this neuropathy is generally uncommon in routine clinical practice, it is more frequent in inner-city hospitals where poor nutrition in alcoholics is common. As a result, nutritional polyneuropathy is among the most frequently encountered nutritional disorders of the nervous system.

Nutritional polyneuropathy related to alcoholism is a mixed sensory motor polyneuropathy that is symmetric in distribution. Initial manifestations include paresthesias and numbness of the distal lower extremities, although many patients may be initially asymptomatic (23). There may be mild aching over the calf muscles and pain in the soles of the feet. Many patients experience a burning dysesthetic component. The soles of the feet are affected first, and there may be aching pain or stabbing sensation that evolves into an intense burning sensation that is very sensitive to touch. Patients may not be able to sleep with sheets touching their feet as a result. Later, this neuropathy evolves further, and weakness may become apparent in the affected muscles. When weakness is present at the ankles, there will be loss of Achilles tendon reflexes. With further progression, weakness may extend into the proximal muscles of the thigh and leg. In very severe cases, the hands may become involved, and there may also be involvement of the cranial nerves with hoarseness of speech and impaired phonation. Such severe cases are rare. The pathologic findings in alcoholic nutritional neuropathy are consistent with those of a distal axonopathy (25); that is, the axon itself bears the brunt of the damage. Axonal degeneration results in demyelination. The injury can be widespread, with pathologic changes evident in the distal vagus and recurrent laryngeal nerves as well as in anterior horn cells and dorsal root ganglia (21).

The prognosis of this type of neuropathy is generally quite favorable if treatment is instituted in the early stages. The paresthesias may resolve rapidly, but recovery of muscle strength generally takes much longer, and recovery may take as long as a year. Treatment consists of abstinence from alcohol and a good overall diet. In addition, thiamin supplementation should be carried out with parenteral administration at doses of 50 mg/day given intramuscularly for the first week. This is followed by a daily oral supplement in addition to other vitamin supplementation.

Deficiencies of pyridoxine, niacin, pantothenic acid, vitamin B_{12}, folate, and niacin are also associated with polyneuropathies and could play a role in the commonly seen alcoholic nutritional polyneuropathy. In addition, the spinal cord, optic nerves, and cerebellum may also be affected in patients with this disorder, but manifestations of that involvement may be masked by the polyneuropathy. Systemic manifestations leading to the suspicion of nutritional deficiency include weight loss, seborrheic dermatitis, glossitis, cheilosis, angular stomatitis, anemia, and hair loss.

Nutritional Amblyopia (Nutritional Optic Neuropathy)

Nutritional optic neuropathy is a disorder in which nutritional deprivation leads to demyelination and axonal loss in the optic nerves (26). The usual early manifestation is dimness of vision and the presence of blind spots (scotomas) in the visual fields leading to decreased visual acuity. The disorder usually presents with dimness or blurred vision, difficulty with fine print and reading, photophobia, and retrobulbar pain associated with eye movement. Onset is usually insidious, and slow progression is the rule. This disorder is frequently seen in chronically undernourished alcoholics in Western countries, but its nutritional basis was firmly established in World War II and the Korean war, where it was observed in prisoners of war who had no access to alcohol or tobacco (27). It has not been associated with a deficiency state involving only one vitamin but is seen in mixed nutritional deficiency states in which thiamin and other B vitamins are depleted (28). The syndrome has been observed in association with Crohn's disease, as a sequela of intestinal bypass procedures for the treatment of obesity, and in vitamin B_{12} deficiency (28–30).

Examination of the eyes usually reveals erythema at the temporal margins of the optic discs (31). Later, there may be frank optic atrophy that is bilaterally symmetric. On a cellular level, damage is confined to a region of the optic nerve known as the papulomacular bundle (32).

Treatment with high-caloric diets rich in protein and vitamin supplementation leads to rapid improvement in most early cases. Chronic severe deficiency states with severe visual loss may not respond as well to therapy.

Vitamin B_{12} Deficiency

Deficiency of vitamin B_{12} is one of the most commonly encountered isolated deficiency states in clinical practice. The spinal cord, brain, optic nerves, and peripheral nerves may be affected by vitamin B_{12} deficiency (33). The spinal cord may bear the brunt of damage associated with vitamin B_{12} deficiency, but a variety of neurologic manifestations are known to be associated with this deficiency state.

Vitamin B_{12} deficiency states occur in a variety of clinical settings (Table 95.2) (see also Chapters 27 and 88). The prototypic deficiency state (pernicious anemia) occurs when antibodies are produced against intrinsic factor, which is produced in the parietal cells of the gastric antrum. When B_{12} deficiency is due to a lack of intrinsic factor, the Schilling test result is subnormal because of failure to bind B_{12} in the intestinal lumen and consequent poor absorption of B_{12} in the terminal ileum (see Chapters 27 and 55). Proof of this diagnosis requires a normal response when the Schilling test is repeated with intrinsic factor. Regardless of the cause, vitamin B_{12} deficiency should be considered serious; the cause should be investigated, and supplementation should be initiated promptly lest irreversible damage to the CNS continue to progress. Vitamin B_{12} deficiency usually occurs in secondary association with diseases including celiac sprue, gastric or ileal resections, intestinal stasis with blind loop syndrome, and fish tapeworm infestations (Table 95.2)(33). Deficient intake of the vitamin is limited to those who subsist on vegetarian diets (see Chapter 88). At times, the cause may not be readily apparent.

While macrocytic anemia is usually present in patients who exhibit neurologic manifestations of vitamin B_{12} deficiency, the neuropsychiatric manifestations of cobalamin deficiency may precede the appearance of macrocytic anemia by months or even years (34, 35). The likely reason for this is that ingested folate may suffice to prevent the macrocytic anemia even when B_{12} continues to be deficient. The result is continuing damage to the CNS and PNS in the absence of macrocytosis or anemia. In one study, no evidence of anemia or macrocytosis was seen in 28% of patients with neurologic manifestations of vitamin B_{12} deficiency (35).

The clinical manifestations of cobalamin deficiency are referable to disorders of both CNS and PNS myelin. Patients often show manifestations of myelopathy, peripheral neuropathy, dementia, or neuropsychiatric disorders (36–38). The earliest manifestation is often tingling and paresthesias in the lower extremities. This is accompanied by a pins-and-needles sensation and the perception of muscle weakness. Sensory abnormalities may also occur in the hands and take much the same form as those in the legs. These early symptoms may be due to demyelination in either the peripheral nerves or the sensory tracts of the spinal cord. As the disease state progresses, patients typi-

Table 95.2
Etiology of B_{12} Deficiency

Pernicious anemia
Celiac sprue
Gastric or ileal resection
Fish tapeworm infestation
Inadequate diet

cally develop a spastic paraparesis with weakness and greatly increased muscle tone in the lower extremities. At this stage, neurologic examination reveals hyperactive reflexes, muscle weakness, loss of vibration and position sense, extensor plantar responses, and impaired bowel and bladder function. Impaired bladder function is usually manifest by a sense of urinary urgency and urge incontinence. Bowel dysfunction appears as constipation. Symptoms that occur at this stage of the illness are due to demyelination in the posterior and lateral columns of the spinal cord. The motor and sensory changes that take place in subacute combined degeneration of the spinal cord due to vitamin B_{12} deficiency tend to be symmetric, and generally, no sensory level is found.

Neuropsychiatric manifestations may include irritability, apathy, somnolence, excessive fatigue, suspiciousness or paranoia, emotional instability, confusional states, psychosis, and cognitive decline (39, 40). The neuropsychiatric manifestations are very common and may be severe. These symptoms of cobalamin deficiency are due to demyelination in the deep white matter of the cerebral hemispheres.

In addition to the cognitive/neuropsychiatric manifestations of vitamin B_{12} deficiency, patients may also complain of visual loss that is not dissimilar to that seen in nutritional amblyopia. There may be dimness of vision accompanied by central scotomas, and on examination, visual acuity is decreased. In late cases, there is bilateral optic atrophy. Prior to any clinical manifestations, evidence of demyelination in the optic nerves may be detected by visual evoked potentials (41).

Neuropathologic changes associated with vitamin B_{12} deficiency include degeneration of myelin and axon loss in the white matter of the CNS and in the peripheral nerves (42). The deep white matter of the cerebral hemispheres, the optic nerves, the myelinated tracts of the spinal cord and brainstem, and the peripheral nerves are all affected. The earliest changes in the CNS are seen in the lower cervical and upper thoracic spinal cord. The demyelinating process spreads longitudinally and laterally to involve the dorsal and lateral funiculi. In some cases, these pathologic abnormalities are also seen in the optic nerves and cerebral white matter. In the periphery, there is demyelination, but axon loss tends not to be a part of the process. Nonhuman primates require 33 to 45 months to develop neuropathologic changes associated with vitamin B_{12} deficiency (43). This is the same period of time required in humans with pernicious anemia after B_{12} supplementation has ceased.

The biochemical process that leads to the neuropathologic changes associated with vitamin B_{12} deficiency is incompletely understood. Vitamin B_{12} is a cofactor for methylmalonyl-CoA mutase. This enzyme catalyzes the conversion of methylmalonyl-CoA to propionyl-CoA, which enters the Krebs cycle. Decreased activity of methylmalonyl-CoA isomerase leads to accumulation of propionyl-CoA. One theory holds that elevated levels of propionyl-CoA displace succinyl-CoA, which is the starting point for the synthesis of even-chain fatty acids. This may lead to synthesis of abnormal fatty acids that may be inserted into myelin, resulting in impaired metabolism. On the other hand, a hereditary form of vitamin B_{12} deficiency has been described in which the activity of methylmalonyl-CoA mutase is normal despite the presence of the typical neurologic syndrome associated with vitamin B_{12} deficiency (44).

Carmel (45) suggested that decreased activity of methionine synthetase may be responsible for the neuropathologic changes. Methionine synthetase requires methylcobalamin as a cofactor. Evidence supporting this hypothesis is derived from studies showing that prolonged administration of nitrous oxide may cause degeneration of the posterior and lateral columns of the spinal cord not dissimilar to that seen in true B_{12} deficiency (46). In addition, it may also be associated with megaloblastic changes in bone marrow and polyneuropathy. These effects are believed to be mediated through inhibition of methylcobalamin-dependent enzymes.

The diagnosis of vitamin B_{12} deficiency is usually suggested by the presence of low serum vitamin B_{12} levels (see Chapters 27 and 57). The usual normal level is above 200 pg/mL. Levels below 200 are considered abnormal and should be investigated. Levels below 100 pg are very often associated with neurologic abnormalities. Increased levels of urinary methylmalonic acid occur and indicate vitamin B_{12} deficiency (47). If low serum levels of vitamin B_{12} are found, a Schilling test is indicated to determine whether absorption is impaired (see Chapter 57 for test procedures). Since cobalamin is also necessary for conversion of homocysteine to methionine, homocysteine levels may also be elevated (48) (see Chapter 34 and below).

In confirmed vitamin B_{12} deficiency, treatment should be undertaken as soon as possible regardless of the cause. This should be initiated with intramuscular administration of 1 mg of vitamin B_{12} daily for 7 days followed by 1 mg intramuscularly weekly for 1 month. Large doses of B_{12} are required to replace tissue stores that have been depleted over a long period. Treatment should be continued with once-monthly injections of vitamin B_{12} for the remainder of the patient's life if the underlying cause cannot be overcome.

The response to treatment depends mostly on the duration of symptoms prior to diagnosis. Much of the damage present when treatment is initiated will remain, but progression of neurologic impairment will stop. The best response is usually seen in patients who have exhibited symptoms for less than 3 months. While all patients tend to show some improvement with therapy, those with longstanding disease may show little response.

Pellagra

Niacin deficiency produces a variety of systemic manifestations including skin changes (especially in areas exposed to sunlight) and inflammation of mucosal surfaces resulting in glossitis, stomatitis, vaginitis, and achlorhydria (see Chapters 23 and 30). The neurologic manifestations may vary from fatigue and lethargy to outright psychosis and dementia. In the early 1900s, pellagra reached epidemic proportions in the southern United States and was associated with a high case fatality rate because the deficiency state was far advanced at time of recognition (49). The prevalence of pellagra is now greatly diminished in the United States as a result of niacin supplementation in bread and better diets. However, this deficiency state is still common in developing countries where corn is a major staple and where alkaline treatment of the cereal is not routine (see Chapters 23 and 108). In developed countries, the disease is almost entirely restricted to poorly nourished alcoholic populations with multiple other nutritional deficiencies.

The neurologic manifestations of pellagra often appear before the dermatologic signs. The initial stages may be as subtle as fatigue and lethargy. As the deficiency state progresses, patients may become apathetic, depressed, and fearful (50). This is often accompanied by insomnia, dizziness, and headache as well as a number of other nonspecific symptoms including anxiety and inability to concentrate. Later, patients develop an outright psychosis that may be accompanied by a delusional state, disorientation, confusion, and hallucinations. In short, they suffer from a severe metabolic encephalopathy. Eventually, the encephalopathic state gives way to coma and death, though death in pellagra is usually due to complications associated with severe skin lesions and fluid loss from diarrhea. A minority of patients may exhibit spasticity of gait accompanied by ataxia (50). It is not clear whether this aspect of the disorder is due to coexistent deficiencies or to niacin deficiency itself. The most prominent manifestations are referable to the posterior columns of the spinal cord.

Pellagra may also be seen in association with carcinoid syndrome and in Hartnup's disease. In both disorders, tryptophan is depleted. In Hartnup's disease this is due to impaired absorption, and in carcinoid syndrome there is overuse of tryptophan in a pathway that is normally minor. Normal tryptophan metabolism is required for the synthesis of some niacin; hence depletion of this amino acid through an alternate pathway may predispose patients to niacin deficiency (see Chapter 23). In addition, other amino acids (e.g., leucine) may block the synthesis of niacin.

The symptoms of pellagra can be rapidly reversed by administration of niacin. Generally, 10 to 20 mg/day is sufficient in addition to a diet with adequate amounts of tryptophan.

Vitamin E Deficiency

Vitamin E deficiency in clinical practice is uncommon except in disorders with impaired absorption of fat-soluble vitamins because of either transport across the intestinal epithelium or intraluminal factors (see Chapter 19). These disorders include cholestatic liver disease in which there is impaired entry of bile into the lower bowel or ileal dysfunction so that bile salt concentrations fail to reach the critical micellar concentration needed for normal absorption. Diseases include cystic fibrosis, abetalipoproteinemia with defects in lipoprotein secretion, primary biliary cirrhosis, pancreatic insufficiency, short gut syndrome, and celiac sprue. The resulting deficiency depletes vitamin E in nervous tissue and results in a progressive spinocerebellar degeneration and neuropathy. The full symptomatic deficiency state is associated with ataxia, hyporeflexia, ophthalmoplegia, myopathy, retinal degeneration, and a sensory-motor polyneuropathy (51, 52). This constellation of neurologic abnormalities can be quite disabling and may be mistaken for a variety of other syndromes including multiple sclerosis and Friedreich's ataxia (53). There are also adult forms of spinocerebellar degeneration that may be associated with abnormalities of the α-tocopherol transfer protein.

Because vitamin E functions as an antioxidant, it has been studied in Parkinson's disease. In animal studies, vitamin E deficiency resulted in a 19 to 33% loss of tyrosine hydroxylase immunopositive neurons in the substantia nigra (54). While there has been no reported decrease in vitamin E levels in postmortem brain from patients with Parkinson's disease, it has been suggested that it might be useful to slow the progression of disease which may, in part, be related to oxidative injury to the substantia nigra (55).

Vitamin E deficiency states respond to supplementation with oral or parenteral α-tocopherol. In children with chronic cholestasis, large doses of oral tocopherol (70–212 mg/kg/day) are often ineffective in ameliorating development of neurologic symptoms (56). A water-soluble form is available that was effective in improving or stabilizing most previously unresponsive to large doses of regular fat-soluble vitamin E (56).

Pyridoxine Deficiency

Pyridoxine deficiency has been associated with use of isoniazid for antituberculous therapy and with hydralazine treatment of hypertension (57). Its occurrence in the absence of these agents is extremely rare in adults. Hydralazine leads to formation of complexes composed of pyridoxal and isoniazid and a marked increase in pyridoxine excretion. The result is the appearance of a mixed sensory-motor polyneuropathy characterized by paresthesias and burning sensations in the feet and lower legs. With progression, this may be accompanied by weakness and loss of the Achilles tendon reflexes. This neuropathy can be easily prevented by concomitant administration of pyridoxine in doses of 50 mg/day.

Pyridoxine deficiency occasionally occurs in newborns. In infants, this is associated with hyperirritability and seizures (58). There is a familial syndrome in which seizures due to pyridoxine deficiency appear at birth or shortly after birth. The seizures respond to supplementation with pyridoxine, and this is associated with a normalization of the electroencephalographic pattern. The dose required to control seizures is 15 mg/day. Pyridoxine deficiency may also be seen in normal infants whose intake of vitamin B_6 is below 0.1 mg/day. This is rare even in underdeveloped countries but has occurred in infants fed powdered goats' milk devoid of pyridoxine.

NEUROLOGIC DISORDERS ASSOCIATED WITH VITAMIN EXCESS

Pyridoxine Neuropathy

Just as a deficiency of pyridoxine has been associated with a sensory motor polyneuropathy, an excessive intake of pyridoxine has been associated with a sensory neuropathy that can be quite disabling (59, 60). Excessive intake is a far more common occurrence in the age of widespread use of megavitamins, when large doses of vitamin B_6 are used as over-the-counter medicines for a variety problems including fibrocystic breast disease, carpal tunnel syndrome, and premenstrual syndrome and as a general "health supplement." Doses in the range of 500 mg/day and above may cause a severe sensory neuropathy (60) which is generally associated with progressive ataxia that results from a loss of joint position sense and proprioceptive function. There is usually distal sensory loss and paresthesia as well as numbness in the lips and tongue. The neuropathy results from changes in the dorsal root ganglia that lead to degeneration of large axons and small myelinated fibers. The primary mechanism may have a direct toxic effect of pyridoxine on the dorsal root neurons. Withdrawal of excess vitamin B_6 usually results in some improvement.

Vitamin A Intoxication

Excessive intake of vitamin A has long been known to induce a toxicity syndrome characterized by lethargy, malaise, headaches, abdominal pain, and myalgias (61). The syndrome usually begins with irritability, loss of appetite, and myalgias. With continued ingestion, a number of other symptoms appear including desquamation of the skin, fatigue, confusion, lethargy, headache, and vomiting. This may be accompanied by abdominal pain, excessive sweating, and yellowish pigmentation in the soles of the feet, palms of the hands, and the nasolabial folds. Doses in excess of 25,000 IU/day ingested over a period of several months suffice to induce overt toxicity in most individuals, but infants and children are more susceptible. Patients with renal insufficiency and alcoholics are also at greater risk given comparable ingestion. The toxic state begins when the binding capacity of the plasma is exceeded and free retinol is present in relatively high concentration. It may bind to the plasma membrane or other cellular constituents and alter the permeability of the membranes. This is thought to be the case in patients with pseudotumor cerebri. In this condition, patients present with a severe headache syndrome accompanied by papilledema and raised intracranial pressure. This syndrome is not accompanied by focal neurologic deficits, and their presence would indicate another disorder, not pseudotumor cerebri.

Excessive intake of vitamin A during the first trimester of pregnancy has been associated with increased incidence of cleft palate, harelip, macroglossia, developmental abnormalities in the eyes, and hydrocephalus in the newborn (62). More-recent studies suggest an association between a vitamin A intake above 10,000 IU during pregnancy and a greater risk of congenital defects associated with cranial-neural-crest tissue (63). When women taking more than 10,000 IU/day of vitamin A were compared with women taking less than 5000 IU, the prevalence ratio of congenital abnormalities was 4.8. This suggested that in women taking excess vitamin A, 1 in 57 birth defects was attributable to vitamin A.

ROLE OF NUTRITION IN SELECTED NEUROLOGIC DISORDERS

Cerebrovascular Disease and Homocysteine

While dietary fat intake has long been considered a risk factor for atherosclerotic cerebrovascular disease, a newer awareness of other nutritional factors is slowly growing. It has long been appreciated that patients with homocystinuria were at high risk for stroke and other vascular disease despite their young age. This was first described by McCully (63) in a report of an infant who died as a result of an inborn error of cobalamin metabolism. Severe atherosclerotic disease was evident in this patient and appeared similar to that reported in patients dying from cystathionine synthetase deficiency (homocystinuria). Since elevated levels of homocysteine appeared to be the only common metabolic anomaly in these patients, hyperhomocysteinemia was suggested to be an important cause of atherosclerotic vascular disease. Considerable evidence now supports that idea (65–67). Serum concentrations of vitamin B_{12}, folate, and pyridoxine as well as gender, age, and intake of alcohol play a role in determining the levels of homocysteine and the consequent risk of premature cerebrovascular disease (68–71).

The formation and metabolism of homocysteine are described in detail in Chapter 34; the pathophysiology of its excess is also discussed in Chapter 61. In summary, homocysteine is formed by cleavage of *S*-adenosylhomocysteine; it is metabolized by one of two pathways. The first is through transulfuration to cysteine by cystathionine synthetase, which uses pyridoxal phosphate (the active form of pyridoxine) as a cofactor. The second pathway is through remethylation either through betaine-homocysteine methyltransferase or by way of methionine synthetase using folate as a cofactor to form methionine. The second pathway is probably of greater importance (48). Protein-bound homocysteine comprises 70–85% of the total homocysteine in plasma. Free homocysteine is present in three forms: homocysteine, homocystine, and cysteine-homocysteine disulfide conjugate. The total concentration of these metabolites is referred to as homocyst(e)ine (Hcy).

The level of methionine influences homocysteine synthesis and the proportion of homocysteine that is transulfurated or remethylated. Since methyltetrahydrofolate and homocysteine are substrates for methionine synthesis, a deficiency of folate may be associated with increased circulating Hcy, which is now known to be a risk factor for atherosclerotic vascular disease. For example, Selhub et al. (69), in a study of 1041 elderly patients, found that elevated plasma homocysteine concentrations were associated with a higher risk of carotid artery stenosis and that concentrations of folic acid and vitamin B_6 were inversely related to carotid artery stenosis. Furthermore, elevated levels of Hcy and related metabolites are more common in an elderly population than the prevalence of vitamin deficiency, suggesting that Hcy metabolites may rise before B_{12}, folate, or vitamin B_6 levels in serum decrease (76), and administration of vitamin supplements leads to a decrease in the concentration of Hcy metabolites. The proceedings of a major symposium on the relationships of homocyst(e)ine, vitamins, and cerebrovascular occlusive disease have been published recently (73).

These insights into the relationship between nutritional factors and vascular disease led to a number of clinical trials that are under way to determine whether supplementation of stroke patients with folic acid will decrease the risk of subsequent strokes. The cost benefit provided by positive clinical results would be enormous, considering that the average direct lifetime cost after stroke is $60,000 and there are over 400,000 strokes annually in the United States.

Since deficiency of folic acid is a well-recognized risk factor for neural tube defects, anencephaly, and vascular disease through its effect on Hcy levels, it has been suggested that foods be supplemented with folate (73) as well as vitamin B_{12} (75, 76). Addition of vitamin B_{12} has been advocated because folic acid alone may mask the megaloblastic anemia that occurs in vitamin B_{12} deficiency, with resulting progression of undiagnosed vitamin B_{12} deficiency until serious neurologic damage becomes evident. However, as of February 29, 1996, the Food and Drug Administration approved addition of folic acid only in the amount of 0.43 to 1.4 mg/pound to bread and cereals in an effort to keep the daily intake of folic acid below 1 mg (77).

Wilson's Disease (Hepatolenticular Degeneration)

Wilson's disease is a disorder of copper metabolism that is inherited as an autosomal recessive trait (78). The major defect is an impairment in the synthesis or function of ceruloplasmin, which binds copper. As a result, serum copper levels are markedly elevated as is urinary excretion of copper. Neurologic manifestations of the disease include a tremor of the head and limbs and slowness of movement in the initial stages. With progression, there is typically dysarthria, dysphagia, rigidity, dystonic posturing, mutism, and slowed cognitive function. Kayser-Fleischer rings in the eyes are pathognomonic for the disorder and are almost always present when neurologic symptoms manifest. This is accompanied by chronic hepatitis leading eventually to multilobular cirrhosis and hepatosplenomegaly due to deposition of copper in the liver.

Treatment of this disorder relies on limiting copper intake in the diet to less than 1 mg/day. Foods rich in copper include nuts, shellfish, liver, mushrooms, chocolate, cocoa, broccoli, and beans to name only a few. In addition to limiting dietary intake of copper, chelating agents such as D-penicillamine and triethylenetetramine (and more recently, zinc) are used to increase copper excretion (79). In most patients with early disease, treatment is followed by improved neurologic function. At times, there may be a latent period of several weeks before improvement is seen. Some patients worsen despite therapy.

Refsum's Disease

Refsum's disease is a rare neurologic disorder caused by accumulation of phytol. It has autosomal recessive inheritance, and onset is usually in childhood or adolescence. Manifestations include retinitis pigmentosa, cerebellar ataxia, polyneuropathy, cardiomyopathy, neurogenic deafness, cataracts, and ichthyosis (80). Phytol accumulates because of a deficiency of phytanic acid hydroxylase. Phytanic acid is found in a number of foods including coffee, nuts, vegetables, spinach, ruminant fat, and dairy products. Treatment depends on limiting dietary phytanic acid (Table 95.3). When this is accomplished, there is usually slow but steady improvement in neurologic function (81).

Neural Tube Defects

Neural tube defects result from incomplete closure of the neural tube (Fig. 95.1), termed *spina bifida,* which refers to a defect in the bony structure. The underlying neurologic abnormality may take the form of a meningocele or outpouching of the meninges or it can be present as a meningomyelocele in which a portion of the spinal cord is contained with the outpouching of the meninges. This is associated with paralysis and is often accompanied by hydrocephalus. In the most severe form, failure of neural tube closure results in anencephaly or absence of the cerebral hemispheres. Closure of the neural tube takes place by the end of the 4th week of pregnancy, a stage when many women are unaware that they are pregnant.

While the possibility that folic acid may be involved in neural tube defects was raised as far back as 1964, the first

Table 95.3
Inborn Errors of Metabolisms with Neurologic Manifestations

Disease	Defect	Dietary Treatment
Phenylketonuria	Phenylalanine hydroxylase	Restrict phenylalanine
Maple syrup urine disease	Branched-chain ketoacid decarboxylase	Restrict leucine, isoleucine, valine; give thiamin
Urea cycle defects (partial):		
Argininosuccinicaciduria	Argininosuccinate lyase	Restrict protein
Citrullinemia	Argininosuccinic synthetase	
Low citrulline	Ornithine transcarbamylase	
Hyperammonemia	Carbamyl phosphate synthetase	
Homocystinuria	Cystathionine synthetase	Restrict methionine; give pyridoxine, folic acid, vitamin B_{12}
Galactosemia	Galactose-1-phosphate uridyl transferase	Lactose-free diet; low-galactose diet
Wilson's disease	Low serum ceruloplasmin	Low-copper diet; ↑Zn in diet
Refsum's disease	α-Oxidation of phytanic acid to pristanic acid	Phytol-free diet

Adapted and modified from Menkes JH. Textbook of child neurology. 3rd ed. Philadelphia: Lea & Febiger, 1985.

trials suggesting a preventive effect of folic acid supplementation were not carried out until the early 1980s. In 1991, a multicenter double-blind study was reported in which women were randomly assigned to receive to either 4 mg of folic acid or a mixture of vitamins including A, D, B_1, B_2, C, and nicotinamide. Results of this study showed that women receiving folic acid had a relative risk of giving birth to a second child with a neural tube defect of 0.28, a 72% reduction in risk for those taking folic acid supplements (82). Finding that folic acid supplementation reduced the risk of neural tube defects in the offspring led to a recommendation that it be given as a supplement to all women likely to become pregnant (83, 84). An increase of 0.4 mg of folic acid daily could potentially

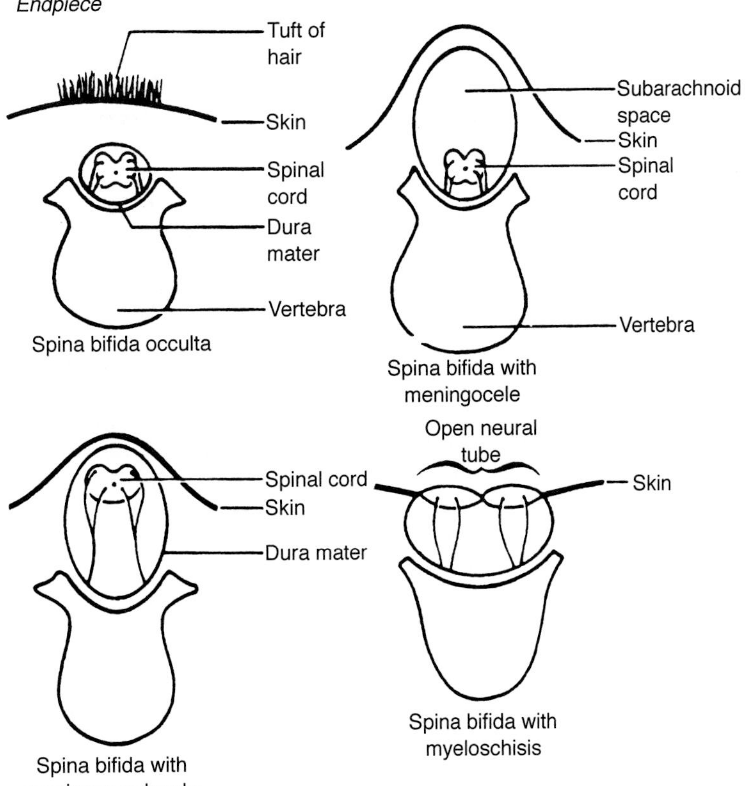

Figure 95.1. Spina bifida terminology. The term *spina bifida* refers to the bony abnormality—defective closure of the vertebral column; the terminology for other abnormalities is shown above. (From Chamberlain G, ed. Turnbull's obstetrics. Edinburgh: Churchill Livingstone, 1995;914, with permission.)

reduce the risk of neural tube defects by as much as 48% (84).

An association has been observed between neural tube defects and impaired activity of methylenetetrahydrofolate reductase, including a mutated form that is susceptible to thermal inactivation (85, 86). The result is decreased enzyme activity and increased concentrations of homocysteine. Levels of homocysteine in serum samples taken during pregnancy are also elevated (87), presumably because of the decreased activity of tetrahydrofolate reductase. Folic acid supplements increase the enzyme activity.

Obesity has also been reported to be a risk factor for neural tube defects (88, 89). Women weighing 80 to 89 kg had a relative risk of 1.9, while those weighing 110 kg had a relative risk of 4. Obese women with a folic acid intake above 0.4 mg did not have the reduction in risk that was seen in women of normal weight. A reduction in the incidence of other fetal anomalies in addition to neural tube defects has also been reported with vitamin supplementation (83). However, a case-control study failed to find a protective effect of supplements taken periconceptually on the risk of orofacial clefts in newborns (90).

Hyperammonemic Disorders (Encephalopathy)

Symptoms of hepatic encephalopathy are increasing confusion, decreased levels of alertness, disorientation, and stupor. In the latter stages of this process, coma may ensue, and death may result. The condition is due to a bilateral disturbance of hemispheric function brought about by unknown metabolic "toxins." The disorder deserves mention in this context because the encephalopathic state may be precipitated by an inability to metabolize branched-chain amino acids (e.g., maple syrup urine disease or those in the urea cycle) (Table 95.3). These are genetic disorders, discussed in detail in Chapter 61. Encephalopathy secondary to cirrhotic liver disease is discussed in Chapter 73.

Protein intake in patients with chronic liver disease should be limited to 30 g/day. With greater intake, bacteria in the gut act on the protein; nitrogen in the form of ammonia is absorbed into the circulation but cannot be converted to urea because of hepatic dysfunction. The result is overt encephalopathy. In recent years, a number of other hypotheses have been proposed to account for the mechanism at play in the encephalopathy. γ-aminobutyric acid (GABA), an inhibitory neurotransmitter, has been suggested to mediate the encephalopathic process on a neurochemical level. Elevated ammonia levels may contribute by providing the nitrogen for conversion of glutamic acid to GABA. Use of branched-chain amino acids in treatment is controversial.

A similar clinical syndrome may be seen in neonates with urea cycle deficits, disorders manifest by onset of an encephalopathic state shortly after feeding begins. These disorders are characterized clinically by mental retardation, seizures, ataxia, stupor, and coma and are inherited as an autosomal recessive trait in which absence of a urea cycle enzyme results in elevated levels of urea nitrogen.

INHERITED VITAMIN-RESPONSIVE NEUROLOGIC DISORDERS

Vitamin-responsive disorders are those that have neurologic manifestations as a result of decreased activity of enzymes requiring vitamins as cofactors (58). In most of these disorders, the enzyme in question is present but in a mutated form that has decreased affinity for its cofactor. When the cofactor or vitamin is provided in a pharmacologic dose, enzyme activity increases, and the concentration of the toxic substrate falls to or toward the normal range. The level of the vitamin in question is not abnormally low prior to supplementation.

An example briefly discussed above is pyridoxine-dependent seizures in the newborn. In this disorder, infants develop status epilepticus that can be reversed by administration of pyridoxine. The disorder results from an abnormal form of glutamic acid decarboxylase with pyridoxal-binding sites of lower affinity than the normal form of the enzyme. When pyridoxine is supplied in supraphysiologic doses, activity of the enzyme increases and the concentration of glutamic acid returns to normal levels. This results in cessation of seizures and normalization of the electroencephalographic pattern. A variety of vitamin-responsive neurologic disorders in the newborn are noted in Chapter 61.

Hartnup's Disease

Hartnup's disease is a rare familial disorder resulting from defective transport of neutral amino acids. The most prominent defect is a lack of absorption of tryptophan across the intestinal wall. Symptoms include photosensitive dermatitis, intermittent cerebellar ataxia, mental disturbances, and renal aminoaciduria. Since the disorder appears similar to pellagra, nicotinic acid (25 mg/day) has been used in the treatment (58). Because the symptoms are intermittent, the effectiveness of this therapy has been difficult to evaluate. In addition, tryptophan may still be absorbed in a di- or tripeptide. As a result, with adequate dietary protein intake, the disorder may at times be asymptomatic.

Anticonvulsant-Induced Vitamin Deficiency

Several drugs commonly used to treat seizure disorders can potentially induce vitamin deficiency states; they include phenytoin, phenobarbital, primidone, and valproic acid (91). Since seizure disorders occur in 1 to 2% of the entire population, the potential impact of such effects is considerable. Phenobarbital, primidone, and phenytoin may interfere with folate metabolism, and during pregnancy, this has been associated with an increased incidence of neural tube defects. Decreased folate levels in blood and cerebrospinal fluid are demonstrable after long-term administration of these agents (92). Consequently, patients being treated with these agents should receive concomitant folic acid as well as a multivitamin supplement.

These same agents have also been associated with decreased production of vitamin K–dependent clotting factors and bleeding in the newborn. The factors affected prothrombin, factor V, and factor VII. To prevent bleeding in the newborns of mothers treated with phenytoin, phenobarbital, or primidone, vitamin K should be administered in the latter stages of pregnancy.

Another anticonvulsant agent that has been associated with diet-responsive neurologic disease is valproic acid. This drug is used in the treatment of primary generalized and partial complex seizures. It has been associated with liver dysfunction and development of hyperammonemia (93, 94), which may occur in the absence of hepatic dysfunction. The syndrome is more common in patients on multiple anticonvulsant agents, though it appears to be dose related and may occur after several years of therapy. Hyperammonemia has been suspected as a cause of lethargy and stupor in patients in whom it is observed. The mechanism may involve inhibition of carbamyl phosphate synthetase, which is involved in conversion of ammonia to urea. As a result, liver function tests and serum ammonia levels should be monitored periodically in patients being treated with valproic acid. Since venous ammonia levels may be artificially elevated due to hemolysis, an elevated level should be confirmed with an arterial blood sample. In patients who develop hyperammonemia, protein intake should be curtailed to decrease serum ammonia levels, and alternative anticonvulsants should be considered.

REFERENCES

1. Victor M, Adams RD, eds. Principles of neurology. 5th ed. New York: McGraw-Hill, 1993.
2. Boushey CJ, Beresford SAA, Omenn GS, et al. JAMA 1995; 274:1049–57.
3. Victor M, Laureno R. Neurologic complications of alcohol abuse: epidemiologic aspects. In: Schoenberg BS, ed. Advances in neurology, vol 19. New York: Raven Press, 1978;603–17.
4. Victor M, Adams RD, Collins GH. The Wernicke-Korsakoff syndrome and related neurologic disorders due to alcoholism and malnutrition. 2nd ed. Philadelphia: FA Davis, 1989.
5. Harper CG, Giles M, Finlay-Jones R. J Neurol Neurosurg Psychiatry 1979;42:226–31.
6. Reuler JB, Girad DE, Gooney TG. N Engl J Med 1985; 312:1035–9.
7. Victor M. Am J Neuroradiol 1990;11:895.
8. Harper CG, Giles M, Finlay-Jones R. J Neurol Neurosurg Psychiatry 1986;49:341–5.
9. Harper C. J Neurol Neurosurg Psychiatry 1983;46:593–8.
10. Birchfield RI. Am J Med 1964;36:404–14.
11. Wallis WE, Willoughby EB. Lancet 1978;2:400–1.
12. Tomasulo PA, Kater RMH, Iber FL. Am J Clin Nutr 1968; 21:1341–4.
13. Camilo ME, Morgan MY, Sherlock S. Scand J Gastroenterol 1981;16:273–9.
14. McCandless DW, Schenker S, Cook M. J Clin Invest 1968; 47:2268–80.
15. Dreyfus PM. Thiamine-deficiency encephalopathy: thoughts on its pathogenesis. In: Gubler CJ, Fujiwara M, Dreyfus PM, eds. Thiamine. New York: John Wiley, 1974.
16. Torvik A, Londboe CF, Rogde S. J Neurol Sci 1982;56:233–48.
17. Victor M, Adams RD, Mancall EL. Arch Neurol 1959;1:577–83.
18. Cravioto H, Korein J, Silberman J. Arch Neurol 1961;4:510–9.
19. Mancall EL, McEntee WJ. Neurology 1981;15:303–13.
20. Mayer RF, Garcia-Mullin R. Peripheral nerve and muscle disorders associated with alcoholism. In: Kissin B, Begleiter H, eds. Biology of alcoholism. New York: Plenum, 1972.
21. Behse F, Buchthal F. Acta Neurol 1977;32:1–29.
22. Claus D, Eggers R, Engelhardt A, et al. Acta Neurol Scand 1985;72:312–6.
23. Schaumburg HH, Spencer PS. Ann NY Acad Sci 1979; 329:116–25.
24. Victor M. Polyneuropathy due to nutritional deficiency and alcoholism. In: Dyck PJ, Thomas PK, Lambert EH, Bunge R, eds. Peripheral neuropathy. 2nd ed. Philadelphia: Saunders, 1984.
25. Shields RW Jr. Muscle Nerve 1985;8:183–87.
26. Dreyfus PM. Amblyopia and other neurological disorders associated with chronic alcoholism. In: Vinken PJ, Bruyn GW eds. Handbook of clinical neurology. Amsterdam: North Holland Publishing, 1976.
27. Fisher CM. Can Serv Med J 1955;11:157–62.
28. Lerman S, Feldman JL. Arch Ophthalmol 1961;65:381–5.
29. Iansek R, Edge CJ. J Neurol Neurosurg Psychiatry 1985; 48:1307–8.
30. Thompson RE, Felton JL. Ann Ophthalmol 1982;14:848–50.
31. Victor M, Mancall EL, Dreyfus PM. Arch Ophthalmol 1960; 64:1–33.
32. Potts AM. Surv Ophthalmol 1973;17:313–39.
33. Carmel R. Arch Intern Med 1982;142:2206–7.
34. Jewesbury ECO. Lancet 1954;2:307–12.
35. Lindenbaum J, Helaton EB, Savage DG, et al. N Engl J Med 1988;318:1720–8.
36. Woltmann HW. Am J Med Sci 1919;157:400–9.
37. Victor M, Lear AA. Am J Med 1956;20:896–911.
38. Reynolds EH. The neurology of vitamin B_{12}: proceedings of the Third European Symposium on Vitamin B_{12} and Intrinsic Factor, University of Zurich, March 5–8, 1979. Berlin: Walter de Gruyter, 1979:1001–8.
39. Holmes JM. Br Med J 1956;4:1394–8.
40. Strachan RW, Henderson JG. Q J Med 1965;34:303–17.
41. Troncoso J, Mancall EL, Schatz JN. Arch Neurol 1982; 36:168–9.
42. Agamanolis DP, Chester EM, Victor M, et al. Neurology 1976;26:905–14.
43. Agamanolis DP, Victor M, Harris JW, et al. J Neuropathol Exp Neurol 1978;37:273–7.
44. Carmel R, Watkins D, Goodman SI, et al. N Engl J Med 1988;318:1738–41.
45. Carmel R. Am J Hematol 1990;34:108–14.
46. Amess JAL, Burman JF, Nancekievill DG, et al. Lancet 1978; 2:339–42.
47. Allen RH, Stabler SP, Savage DG, et al. Am J Hematol 1990; 34:90–8.
48. Kang SS, Wong PW, Malinow MR. Annu Rev Nutr 1992; 12:279–98.
49. Lanska DJ. Neurology 1996;47:829–34.
50. Jolliffe N, Bowman KM, Rosenblum LA, Fein HD. JAMA 1940; 114:307–15.

51. Satya-Murti S, Howard L, Krohel G, Wolf B. Neurology 1986; 36:917–21.
52. Kayden HJ. Neurology 1993;43:2167–9.
53. Muller DP, LLoyd JK, Wolff OH. Lancet 1983;1:225–8.
54. Dexter DT, Nanayakkara I, Goss-Sampson MA, et al. 1994; 5:1773–6.
55. Przedborski S, Jackson-Lewis V, Muthane U. Ann Neurol 1993; 33:5:560–1.
56. Sokol RJ, Butler-Simon N, Conner C, et al. Gastroenterology 1993;104:1727–35.
57. Biehl JP, Vilter RW. Proc Soc Exp Biol Med 1954;85:389–92.
58. Menkes JH. Textbook of child neurology. 3rd ed. Philadelphia: Lea & Febiger, 1985;720–63.
59. Albin RL, Albers JW, Greenberg HS, et al. Neurology 1987; 37:1729–32.
60. Schaumburg H, Kaplan J, Windeband A, et al. N Engl J Med 1983;309:445–8.
61. Rudman D, Williams PJ. N Engl J Med 1983;309:488–90.
62. Rothman KJ, Moore LL, Singer MR, et al. N Engl J Med 1995;21:1369–77.
63. McCully KS. Am J Pathol 1969;56:111–28.
64. Clarke R, Daly L, Robinson K, et al. N Engl J Med 1991; 324:1149–55.
65. Stamler MJ, Malinow MR, Willett WC, et al. JAMA 1992; 268:877–81.
66. Heijer M, Blom HJ, Gerritis WB, et al. Lancet 1995;345:882–5.
67. Miller JW, Ribaya-Mercado JD, Russell RM, et al. Am J Clin Nutr 1992;55:1154–60.
68. Ubbink JB, Vermack WJH, van der Merwe A, et al. J Nutr 1994;124:1927–33.
69. Selhub J, Jaques PF, Bostom AG, et al. N Engl J Med 1995; 332:286–91.
70. Lussier-Cacau S, Xhiguesse M, Piolot A, et al. Am J Clin Nutr 1996;64:587–93.
71. Neurath HJ, Joosten E, Riezler R, et al. Lancet 1995;346:85–9.
72. Cravo ML, Gloria LM, Selhub J, et al. Am J Clin Nutr 1996; 63:220–4.
73. Colloquium. Homocyst(e)ine, vitamins and arterial occlusive diseases. J Nutr 1996:126(Suppl 45):1235S–308S.
74. Tucker KL, Mahnken B, Wilson, PWF, et al. JAMA 1996; 276:1879–85.
75. Herbert V, Bigaouette J. Am J Clin Nutr 1997;65:572–3.
76. Bower C, Wald NJ. Eur J Nutr 1995;49:787–93.
77. McCarthy M. Lancet 1996;347:682.
78. Scheinberg IH. Wilson's disease. Philadelphia: WB Saunders, 1984.
79. Scheinberg IH, Jaffe ME, Sternlieb I. N Engl J Med 1987; 317:209–13.
80. Refsum S. Acta Psychiatr Scand 1946;1(Suppl 38).
81. Steinberg D, Mize CE, Herndon JH Jr, et al. Arch Intern Med 1970;125:75–87.
82. MRC Vitamin Study Research Group. Lancet 1991;338:131–7.
83. Czeizel AE. Br Med J 1993;306:1645–8.
84. Daly LE, Kirke PN, Molloy A, et al. JAMA 1995;274:1698–702.
85. Van der Put N, Steegers-Theunissen RP, Frosst P, et al. Lancet 1995;346:1645–8.
86. Whitehead AS, Gallagher P, Mills JL, et al. Q J Med 1995; 88:763–6.
87. Mills JL, McPartlin JM, Kirke PN, et al. Lancet 1995; 345:145–51.
88. Werler MM, Louik C, Shapiro S, et al. JAMA 1996;275:1089–92.
89. Shaw GM, Velie EM, Schaffer D. JAMA 1996;275:1093–6.
90. Hayes C, Werler MM, Willett WC, et al. Am J Epidemiol 1996; 143:1229–34.
91. Engel J. Antiepileptic drugs. In: Engle J, ed. Seizures and epilepsy. Philadelphia: FA Davis, 1989.
92. Reynolds EH, Mattson RH, Gallagher BB. Neurology 1972; 22:841–4.
93. Coulter DL, Allen RJ. Lancet 1980;1:1310–1.
94. Rawat S, Borkowski WJ, Swick HM. Neurology 1981;31:1173–4.

96. The Hypercatabolic State

MICHELLE K. SMITH and STEPHEN F. LOWRY

The hypercatabolic state is induced by endogenous production of a variety of mediators in response to diverse stimuli including trauma, sepsis, and specific advanced diseases. This state is characterized by progressive severe loss of body protein and lipid that may result in organ failure and which, at present, may be ameliorated to some extent by nutritional support but can be reversed only by major palliation or cure of the underlying disease process. The hypercatabolic state is characterized by hypermetabolism and implies a disruption of normal metabolic homeostasis. Since the pioneering work of Cuthbertson over 50 years ago, much research has focused on mechanisms underlying this often dramatic host metabolic response to injury or disease, as well as the means to modify such responses via direct nutrient intervention or modulation of the inflammatory milieu. This chapter describes the hypermetabolic state, the neuroendocrine and cytokine mediators of this response, the metabolic consequences of prolonged net hypermetabolism to the host, and, briefly, how this condition influences aspects of nutrient use. The clinical features of this response, in general, are qualitatively similar, regardless of the nature of the insult. However, the catabolic response to cancer and HIV are distinct and are reviewed separately.

METABOLIC RESPONSES TO INJURY AND DISEASE

The temporal sequence of postinjury metabolic events is well known from the careful evaluation of many investigators. Cuthbertson initially established the basis for understanding the biologic response to injury. He found that urinary excretion of nitrogen, potassium, and phosphorus was markedly increased in patients with long bone fractures. The relative concentrations of these excreted nutrients were similar to those of muscle, and he concluded that muscle was the source of these losses (1). These and subsequent isotopic dilution studies by Moore and his colleagues (2) characterized the ebb and flow phases of the postinjury response. The early ebb phase occurs immediately postinsult and is characterized by hemodynamic instability with decreased cardiac output and oxygen consumption, low core temperature, and elevated glucagon, catecholamine, and free fatty acid levels. This phase typically lasts from 12 to 24 hours and is modified to some degree by the extent and adequacy of fluid volume resuscitation. The subsequent flow phase is fundamentally a metabolic response that alters energy and protein use to preserve critical organ function and repair damaged tissue. Total body oxygen consumption, metabolic rate, and amino acid efflux from peripheral muscle stores all increase, counterregulatory hormone concentrations are elevated, glucose metabolism is altered, and lactate production, urinary nitrogen losses, and tissue protein catabolism all increase (3) (Table 96.1). Discussion below focuses on the flow phase response and the endogenous mediators that regulate this response.

Energy Expenditure

Injury and Sepsis

During the postinsult flow phase there is increased energy expenditure by the body as well as an increased metabolic rate. Total body oxygen consumption increases because of increased oxidation of fuel sources (carbohydrates, amino acids, and lipids) to provide needed energy. These reactions produce heat, and the increased heat production indicates an increased metabolic rate. To some extent, the elevation of the metabolic rate above basal levels correlates with the cause and/or the severity of the initial injury. Energy expenditure may increase minimally with mild injury (4), 15 to 25% following long bone fractures (1), and as much as double with burn injury over more than 40% of total body surface (5) (Fig. 96.1).

The increased metabolic rate requires mobilizing the body's nutrient stores to provide substrates for the increased energy demand. The body's stores of carbohydrates, primarily glycogen, are quickly depleted in the first 24 hours postinjury. Thereafter, fat and protein serve as the main energy sources. In the hypermetabolic state there is obligatory net protein catabolism in an attempt to

Table 96.1
Metabolic Alterations following Injury

Ebb Phase	Flow Phase
Increased blood glucose	Normal/slightly elevated blood glucose
Increased circulating free fatty acids	Normal/slightly elevated free fatty acids
Decreased insulin	Normal/increased insulin
Increased catecholamines	Increased catecholamines
Decreased cardiac output	Increased cardiac output
Decreased oxygen consumption	Increased oxygen consumption
Decreased core temperature	Elevated core temperature

provide substrates for gluconeogenesis and amino acids for increased synthesis of acute-phase proteins. Stored triglycerides are also mobilized and oxidized to provide substrates for the hypermetabolic state but are unable to prevent protein catabolism. During this state, there is also a marked rise in the counterregulatory hormones: glucocorticoids, catecholamines, and glucagon. These hormones promote a variety of metabolic effects as discussed below. Also important in the response to injury are the cytokines, whose effects are largely mediated by endocrine mechanisms. These acute alterations in metabolic and hormonal responses serve to maintain the vital organs necessary for survival by providing substrates for energy production during the hypermetabolic state (Fig. 96.2).

Cancer

In contrast to the hypermetabolic state universally seen posttrauma, hypermetabolism is not an invariable finding in cancer patients. Because cancer patients in the advanced stages of disease often become cachectic, it was hypothesized that this weight loss was due to increased energy expenditure and net negative energy balance. Studies do not confirm this hypothesis but indicate a variable metabolic response to cancer; some investigators report a hypermetabolic response, while others observe no change or a hypometabolic response (6–8) (Fig. 96.3). One study failed to demonstrate a correlation between resting energy expenditure (REE) and weight loss or tumor burden (9). Other studies demonstrated no significant difference in REE in patients who were losing weight or were weight stable with gastric or colon cancer (7).

Numerous studies show that the variations in REE seen in cancer may be influenced by tumor histology (10–13). One study found that patients with non-small-cell lung cancer had an elevated REE, while patients with gastric or colorectal cancer did not. Another study demonstrated a hypermetabolic state in patients with gastric cancer, while patients with esophageal or colorectal cancers were evenly distributed in their metabolic response, and patients with pancreatic or hepatobiliary neoplasms were mostly hypometabolic (12). In contrast, a recent study of cachectic patients with pancreatic cancer demonstrated an increase in REE (13). Thus the metabolic response to tumor burden varies and may depend in part on tumor type and/or other endogenous mediators involved in the host-tumor interaction.

AIDS

Another patient population in which a hypermetabolic response is often observed are those with HIV infection. Several studies suggest that the REE is elevated in patients with early HIV infection and increases further with subsequent AIDS (14–17). This REE increase may occur in an asymptomatic patient with normal CD4 lymphocyte counts (18). Certain secondary infections may cause even further elevations in the REE, although it appears that even latent HIV infection can cause an increase in REE above basal levels. Other studies have indicated that a small percent-

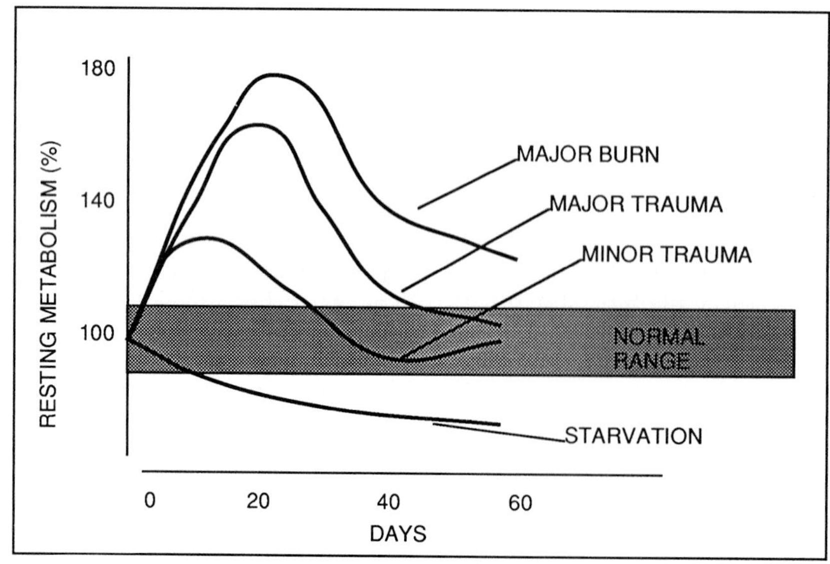

Figure 96.1. Effect of injury on metabolic rate. (Adapted from Wilmore DW. The metabolic management of the critically ill. New York: Plenum Medical Book, 1977.)

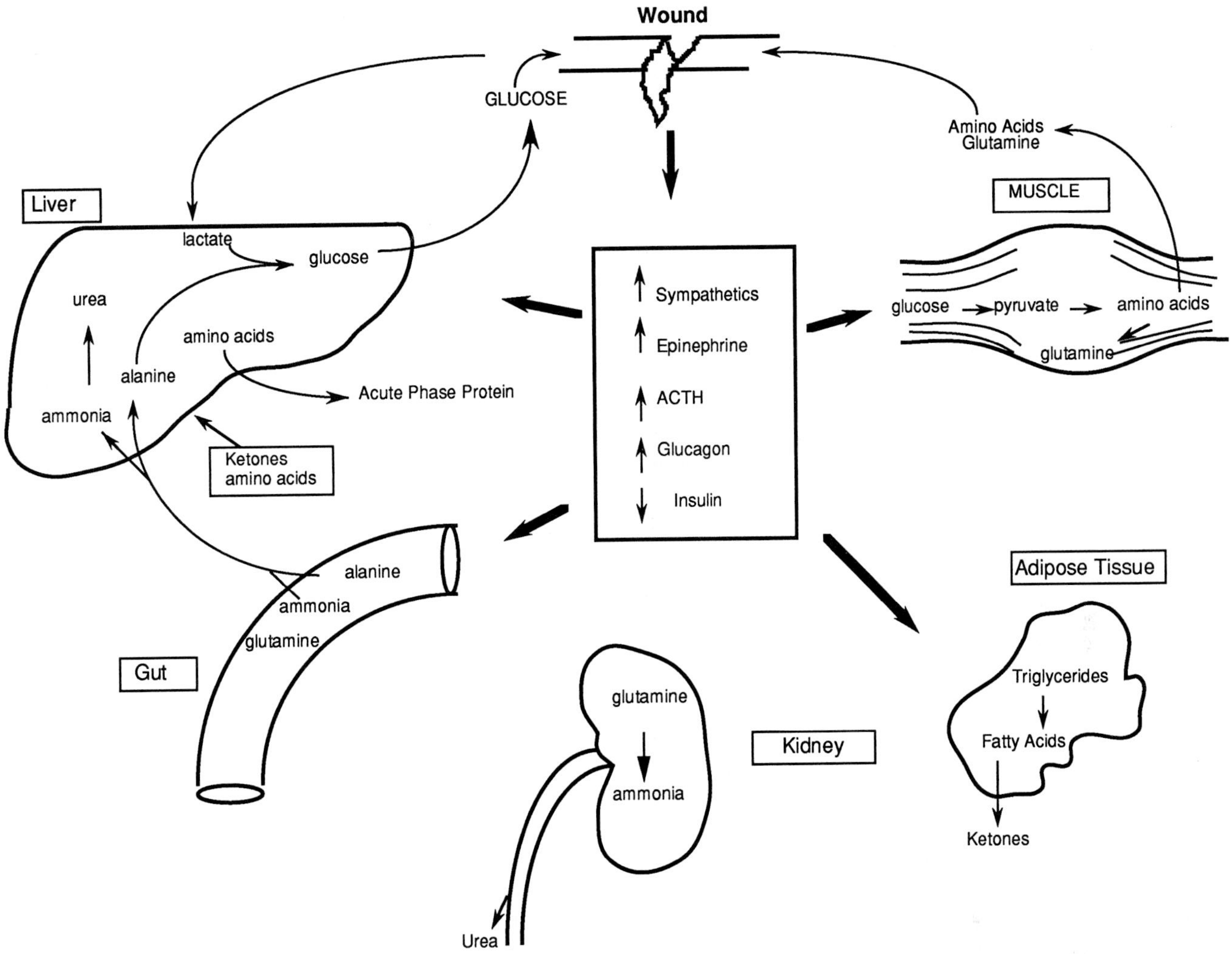

Figure 96.2. Neuroendocrine and metabolic consequences of injury.

age of AIDS patients without secondary infection may in fact be hypometabolic and demonstrate a metabolic response similar to that seen in starvation (15). This response has been strongly associated with oral candidiasis

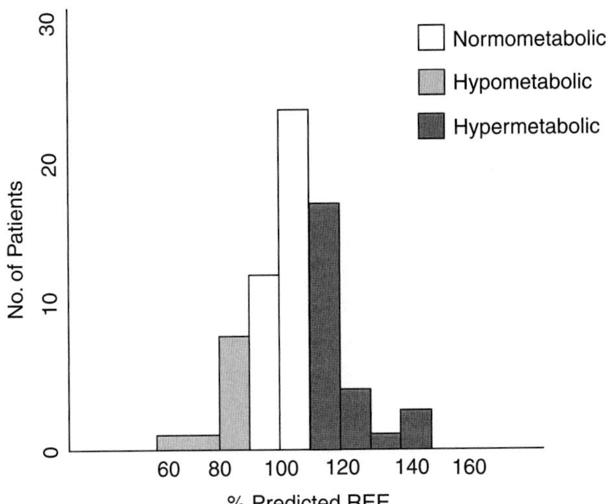

Figure 96.3. Preoperative REE in cancer patients. (Adapted from Luketich JD, Mullen JL, Feurer ID, et al. Arch Surg 1990;125:337–41.)

or odynophagia, which suggests that poor food intake may impose a starvation metabolic response in addition to the hypermetabolic response (19).

Thus the hypermetabolic response in the host can be initiated by a variety of initial insults including trauma, burns, infection (including HIV), and cancer. The increased energy expenditure results in an alteration of fuel metabolism, leading to a breakdown of protein and fat and alterations in glucose metabolism to provide the necessary substrates for these increased energy demands.

Protein Metabolism

Injury and Sepsis

Protein represents a large reserve of body fuel. In response to the increased energy demands after injury, skeletal muscle protein stores are mobilized. This leads to increased amino acid efflux from peripheral stores and increased urinary nitrogen excretion. The extent of this urinary nitrogen loss correlates with the severity of the injury. The result is a net negative nitrogen balance as protein catabolism exceeds protein synthesis by the liver. This acceleration of protein catabolism generally parallels the increase in oxygen consumption and represents a constant fraction of total oxidation following injury (4). If allowed to proceed unabated, the net protein catabolism may result in critical organ failure (20).

The mechanism of muscle catabolism during sepsis involves increased protein breakdown (21), especially of myofibrillar protein, as well as reduced protein synthesis (22) and inhibition of amino acid uptake by muscle (23). In animal models, important mediators of this catabolism during sepsis include glucocorticoids as well as certain cytokines, particularly tumor necrosis factor (TNF) and interleukin-1 (IL-1) (24).

The intracellular mechanism involved in muscle protein breakdown in sepsis and injury is not clearly defined; however, recent animal studies indicate that sepsis induces a nonlysosomal, energy-dependent proteolysis (25). This involves activation of the ubiquitin-proteasome-dependent pathway that increases mRNAs encoding ubiquitin and proteasomes in muscle. In this pathway, proteins destined for degradation are ligated to the polypeptide ubiquitin and then degraded by a protease that acts on ubiquinated proteins (26). Other studies indicate that the mRNA for ubiquitin increases during glucocorticoid excess and acidosis, and may occur in septic states (27). Therefore it is likely that the ubiquitin pathway is important in proteolysis in sepsis, but further studies are needed to delineate other possible mechanisms.

The increased amino acid efflux from peripheral stores postinjury provides substrates for enhanced hepatic gluconeogenesis and acute-phase protein synthesis. It also allows new protein tissue in wounds and proliferation of cellular components involved in the inflammatory response. There is increased splanchnic uptake of glucogenic amino acids, particularly alanine and glutamine. This increase in uptake in burn patients corresponds to the quantity and distribution of peripheral tissue amino acid release (28). The enhanced splanchnic uptake is achieved by increased glutamine uptake in the gut enterocytes while alanine is released by the gastrointestinal tract in increased amounts during stress (32).

During the postinjury response, alanine and glutamine are also preferentially released from muscle stores. While these amino acids make up approximately 6% of protein in muscle stores, they constitute 60 to 80% of the free amino acids released in response to insult (29, 30). This effect may be influenced by glucocorticoid activity; in a study using a canine model, both acute and chronic glucocorticoid excess increased glutamine and alanine release (31).

Despite net peripheral proteolysis, liver mass is usually preserved during injury, often with an increase in total liver protein, RNA, and DNA (33). Preservation of liver mass occurs with sustained or increased hepatic capacity for gluconeogenesis and synthesis of acute-phase proteins (34).

In summary, skeletal protein catabolism may serve three main purposes. First, it provides amino acids that can serve as substrate for protein synthesis by the wound or liver. Secondly, the released amino acids can be converted to glucose by the liver as an energy source during the hypermetabolic response. Thirdly, it provides a source of glutamine to be used as a fuel source by the gut and possibly by other tissues involved in the metabolic response to stress.

Cancer

Cancer patients with significant weight loss demonstrate protein kinetics similar to those seen in traumatized or infected patients. Whole-body protein turnover rates are increased, with increases in protein synthesis as well as catabolism (35–37). Attempts have been made to correlate the increase in protein turnover rates with changes in REE or weight loss. Isotope infusion studies suggest a significant increase in whole-body protein catabolism in cancer patients with cachexia, compared with noncachectic cancer patients or patients with benign disease (38). However, although the protein turnover rate is increased in other studies, it does not appear to correlate with energy expenditure or weight loss in most evaluations of cancer patients (7).

AIDS

By contrast to other patient populations, those infected with HIV show an elevated REE with decreased protein synthesis and catabolism in the absence of secondary infection (39). Preliminary data indicate that protein catabolism and a negative nitrogen balance occur when an AIDS patient becomes secondarily infected (17).

Glucose Metabolism

Injury and Sepsis

Hyperglycemia is a common response to septic or traumatic insult. It results from both increased hepatic gluconeogenesis and decreased glucose uptake by insulin-dependent tissues. In the ebb phase, insulin levels are depressed, but they become normal to elevated during the flow phase, although remaining depressed in relation to the degree of hyperglycemia. The persistent hyperglycemia suggests injury-induced insulin resistance (3). In addition, studies using hepatic vein cannulations in thermally injured patients demonstrate increased uptake of gluconeogenic amino acids by the splanchnic tissues (28). These amino acids are then used for gluconeogenesis, resulting in increased splanchnic production of glucose and further contributing to the hyperglycemic state.

Altered glucose metabolism in response to stress results in decreased skeletal muscle uptake of glucose and decreased glucose incorporation into fatty acids by adipocytes (40). The decreased uptake by skeletal muscle is due to peripheral insulin resistance, which may be mediated in part by excess cortisol and catecholamines (41, 42). Recent evidence also indicates that TNF-α induces insulin resistance ([43] and references therein). In these stressed patients, hyperglycemia fails to suppress hepatic gluconeogenesis or glycogenolysis; administration of a dextrose infusion suppresses gluconeogenesis less effectively in septic or trauma patients than in healthy volunteers (44, 45). Amino acid infusions are also unable to inhibit gluconeogenesis in trauma patients (46). This alteration in glucose metabolism maintains glucose availability to non-insulin-dependent tissues such as the central nervous system (CNS), kidneys, wound tissue, and hematologic cells, which are vital for survival.

During the stress response, another source of glucose results from the change to anaerobic glycolysis in skeletal muscle and hypoxic tissue (i.e., the wound) producing increased amounts of lactate. Lactate can be converted into glucose in the liver via the Cori cycle, which is increased in both burn and trauma patients (47, 48). In burn patients, lactate is the most important gluconeogenic substrate (49). The resultant lacticacidemia may be mediated in part by both catecholamines and cytokines (50, 51).

The efficiency of glucose oxidation is altered by injury (52) and in postoperative (53) and burn patients (54), further contributing to the hyperglycemic state. Maximum glucose oxidative capacity appears to be inversely related to severity of the injury. The decrease in oxidation may be due to reduced activity of intracellular enzymatic metabolic pathways, such as pyruvate dehydrogenase (55).

Cancer

Glucose intolerance has long been observed in association with malignancy and, as early as 1919, was proposed as a means to distinguish patients who were more likely to have gastric carcinoma than peptic ulcer disease (56). Since that initial report, many investigators have confirmed glucose intolerance in diverse cancer populations with advanced disease (57–59). Glucose intolerance results from increased resistance to both exogenous and endogenous insulin (60). The mechanism underlying this insulin resistance is not well defined, but since monocyte insulin receptors from cancer patients are normal, a postreceptor defect has been postulated ([61] and references within). However, this effect may not be cancer induced per se but may be related to the effects of cancer, such as weight loss, since glucose intolerance also occurs in response to weight loss due to calorie deprivation in benign disease (62) as well as in response to sepsis (63, 64).

There are numerous reports of increased endogenous glucose production in cancer patients (57, 58, 65, 66), with an observed increase in glucose turnover rate that is affected by tumor stage (67, 68), histology (58, 66), and type. In a study comparing patients with early (limited to gut wall) and advanced gastrointestinal malignancies (esophagus, stomach, and pancreas), rates of glucose turnover were significantly higher in patients with advanced lesions (67). Similar findings were observed in patients with advanced colon cancer (68), indicating that increased glucose turnover is consistent with an advanced disease stage. Other studies make it evident that tumor histology also affects glucose turnover rates. Studies in sarcoma (66) and leukemic patients (58) indicate a glucose turnover rate two to almost three times that seen in normal volunteers. In contrast, patients with lymphoma demonstrated a glucose turnover rate similar to that of normal volunteers (58). Other studies indicate that the increased glucose turnover is related specifically to the cancer. The increase in glucose turnover rate is significantly higher in cancer patients with weight loss than in a cancer-free population with comparable weight loss (62). Another study demonstrated that cancer patients with progressive weight loss had markedly elevated rates of glucose turnover while weight-stable cancer patients had glucose turnover rates similar to those in normal volunteers (64). These findings contrast with the decreased glucose turnover rates in patients with weight loss due to uncomplicated starvation (69).

Regulation of hepatic glucose production is altered in cancer patients. While infusion of glucose in normal subjects suppresses hepatic gluconeogenesis, glucose infusion reduces glucose production by only 70% in patients with early or advanced gastric cancer (67). In sarcoma or leukemic patients, the hepatic glucose production was decreased by less than a third (58, 66).

Increased gluconeogenesis via the Cori cycle represents a substantial proportion of the observed increase in glucose turnover rate in cancer patients. During this cycle, lactate released from anaerobic glycolysis in peripheral tissue is recycled to glucose in the liver in an energy-requiring reaction. Increased Cori cycle activity occurs in cancer patients, particularly those with weight loss (64). The increase in Cori cycle activity seems to be a specific response to the neoplasm and not directly related to weight loss. The source of the lactate molecules remains a matter of debate. Tumor cells may be one source of lactate production (70). Other studies indicate that the tumor itself may exert distal effects on the host carbohydrate metabolism; the rates of glucose uptake and lactate release from forearm tissue of cancer patients were significantly higher than those in tissue from normal subjects (62, 71). Taken together, it seems probable that increased glycolysis in both the tumor and host tissues contributes to the increased lactate production.

Increased glucose oxidation is also observed in cancer patients with weight loss (64, 72, 73). The increase in oxidation rate is not proportional to the increased glucose availability, which implies a loss of efficiency in the oxidative process (62, 67). The effects of alterations in carbohydrate metabolism incurred by cancer patients on energy balance and use are difficult to quantitate but are likely to influence whole-body kinetics and, to some extent, development of cancer cachexia.

AIDS

Although there are few studies on carbohydrate metabolism in HIV patients, hyperglycemia does not appear to be a prevalent finding in patients who are HIV positive. There is evidence that abnormal glucose metabolism in AIDS patients may be related to pentamidine toxicity. Also HIV infection has been reported to cause islet β cell dysfunction leading to insulin-dependent diabetes mellitus in the absence of islet cell or insulin antibodies (74).

Lipid Metabolism

Injury and Sepsis

Lipid is a major source of fuel for the body, representing 80% of the body's energy reserves. In response to stress, lipid mobilization and use can potentially preserve proteins. Immediately postinsult, there is enhanced lipolysis mediated by sympathetic stimulation of adipose tissue as well as activation of lipase by norepinephrine and glucagon (75). The result is an increase in free fatty acids and glycerol concentration in the circulation.

Several studies have indicated that there may be a preference for oxidation of fat as a source of energy in septic or trauma patients (76). In the nonstressed condition, the normal respiratory quotient (RQ) is 0.85 (77). In the injured patient, the RQ is lower, indicating increased lipid oxidation (5). A decreased RQ is also seen in patients with worsening sepsis, and isotopic studies have corroborated increased fat oxidation in these patients (78, 79). The increased amount of free fatty acids serves as a fuel source for tissues except red blood cells and the CNS.

Cancer

A large body of evidence indicates that most of the weight loss seen in cancer cachexia is due to depletion of body fat (68, 80, 81). Fat is stored mainly as triglyceride in adipocytes, which is hydrolyzed to glycerol and free fatty acid. This is accomplished by the action of specific lipases that are regulated by hormones that may stimulate (e.g., catecholamines) or inhibit (e.g., insulin) lipolysis. The turnover rates of glycerol and free fatty acids have been used in studies as a measurement of lipolysis. The effect that cancer has on lipolysis rate is unclear. Whole-body lipolytic rates in cancer patients have been reported to be both increased and normal (82, 83). In a study using stable isotopes, the turnover rate of glycerol and free fatty acids in weight-stable and weight-losing cancer patients was compared with that seen in healthy volunteers. There were no significant differences in weight-stable patients and normal volunteers, but there was a significant increase in the rate of glycerol and free fatty acid release in the weight-losing cancer patients (84, 85). However, in a similar study using cachectic patients without cancer as a control group for weight loss, the rate of lipolysis was similar in cachectic patients with and without cancer (86). Thus the increased weight loss itself may account for the increased lipolysis.

In their discussion of lipolysis in esophageal cancer patients, Klein and Wolfe propose four possible mechanisms for increased lipolysis in cancer patients: *(a)* increased lipolytic rates caused by decreased food intake and malnutrition; *(b)* increased lipolysis when expressed per kilogram of body weight caused by body fat loss and an increased percentage of body weight as lean body mass; *(c)* stimulation of lipolysis caused by the stress response with adrenal medullary stimulation, increased circulating catecholamines, and insulin resistance; and *(d)* the release of lipolytic factors produced by the tumor or by myeloid tissue cells (86).

An increased rate of fat oxidation has been reported in many cancer patient populations (62, 72, 83). A study of patients with colorectal or gastric cancer found that patients with cancer and weight loss oxidized fat more rapidly than patients with cancer and no weight loss or patients with benign disease and weight loss (73). Therefore, as with stressed patients, it appears that the body responds to the tumor-bearing state with a preference for fat oxidation.

AIDS

In contrast to injury or sepsis, adipose tissue is often conserved in patients with AIDS at the expense of body cell mass (87). Grunfeld and Feingold in their review of metabolic disturbances in AIDS describe alterations in fat metabolism that occur in the disease. There is decreased triglyceride clearance due to decreased lipoprotein lipase activity, with a resultant marked triglyceridemia (17). Hepatic synthesis of fatty acids increases (88), and the levels of circulating free fatty acids are elevated (89). There appears to be no correlation between the alterations in triglyceride metabolism and wasting in AIDS (17, 89).

MEDIATORS OF HYPERMETABOLIC RESPONSE

There is a characteristic postinjury neuroendocrine response, with an increase in catecholamines and glucocorticoids. However, despite extensive investigation of the hormonal milieu and response to injury and stress, hormone increase with normal subjects have not been able to reproduce the amount of protein catabolism seen in severe injury. This indicates that hormonal changes alone cannot account for all the metabolic consequences of severe stress and injury. Therefore, increased attention to other possible mediators of hypercatabolic stress mechanisms has largely focused on the role of immunopeptide regulation of host metabolic response to injury. These endogenous mediators of postinjury hypermetabolism, including the humoral mediators of the neuroendocrine system, the autonomic nervous system, and the cytokines, can integrate and transfer information from the injury site to effect a response beneficial to the host. The next section focuses on the role of these mediators in the postinjury response.

Another recent hypothesis attempts to correlate the amount of protein catabolism observed in the hypermetabolic state with the cellular hydration state (121). This hypothesis postulates that cellular dehydration is the common pathway to signal an antiproliferative and catabolic state. Cellular dehydration is influenced by many factors, including altered nutrition, hormones, cytokines, and oxygen radicals. While it proposes an interesting mechanism for the proteolysis observed in critically ill patients, this hypothesis remains to be substantiated by multiple clinical trials.

Neuroendocrine Response

Early studies by Hume and Egdahl established the importance of an intact CNS in mediating the early response to injury (90). Their original studies demonstrated that the increase in adrenocorticoid steroids after a burn injury could be blocked by sectioning the peripheral nerve, cervical spinal cord, or medulla oblongata in dogs. Other clinical studies show less adrenocorticotropic hormone (ACTH) or growth hormone (GH) release in response to minor tissue injury (herniorrhaphy) in patients receiving spinal anesthesia than in those receiving general anesthesia (91). The CNS also appears instrumental in the hypermetabolic response to injury. One study demonstrated that administration of inert gas anesthesia to hypermetabolic burn patients lowered their core temperatures and metabolic rates (92). A study of patients with head injuries who were in a barbiturate coma established that metabolic rate and nitrogen excretion were reduced to basal levels with administration of the barbiturate (93).

Afferent signals from the site of injury, baroreceptors sensing hypovolemia, and infection can elicit hypothalamic mechanisms to stimulate the anterior pituitary to secrete prolactin, ACTH, antidiuretic hormone (ADH), and GH (29). ACTH release stimulates a increase in adrenal glucocorticoid secretion. Evidence of increased ACTH secretion has been observed following elective operations, extensive trauma (94–96), thermal injury (97, 98), and infection (99, 100). Circulating levels of GH are markedly increased immediately postinjury and tend to decrease to normal levels within 24 to 48 hours.

Thyroid-stimulating hormone (TSH) levels do not appear to be greatly affected by injury. However there is a characteristic pattern of normal T_4, elevated rT_3, and depressed T_3 during prolonged periods of stress, which is related in part to calorie deficiency (101, 102) as well as in response to an inflammatory stimulus (103).

Catecholamines

The catecholamines, specifically epinephrine and norepinephrine, are rapidly produced in response to a variety of insults. Elevated levels are most pronounced during the early postinjury period (48 hours) and decrease during recovery (104, 105). Postinjury levels of catecholamines correlate to some extent with the severity of initial injury (105). Mild injury may elicit a moderate increase in catecholamines, while more severe injuries may be associated with a prolonged rise in urinary or circulating levels of catecholamines ([3] and references within).

The net metabolic influence of catecholamines is to increase energy expenditure, hepatic glycogenolysis, glycolysis, and lipolysis with a resultant increase in free fatty acid concentration. Paradoxically, catecholamine excess acutely decreases the efflux of amino acids from peripheral tissue while increasing lactate release from skeletal muscle. This was confirmed by studies in which epinephrine infusion into healthy subjects resulted in increased energy expenditure, hyperglycemia, lactic acidosis, and decreased amino acid efflux (5, 106, 107). Although the precise effect of adrenergic stimulation on protein kinetics is controversial, studies indicate that β-stimulation promotes gluconeogenesis and may limit skeletal muscle nitrogen loss, whereas α-adrenergic stimulation leads to protein catabolism (108, 109). Taken together these studies indicate appreciable catecholamine influence on the extreme changes in protein metabolism seen in severe stress and injury (see also Chapter 44).

Cortisol

Glucocorticoid excess promotes negative body nitrogen balance (106) but exhibits little influence upon overall energy expenditure (107). Cortisol effects a slight increase in free fatty acid concentration, promotes hepatic gluconeogenesis, and increases peripheral tissue amino acid efflux. In normal subjects, cortisol infusion alone produced the same net sustained nitrogen loss as that produced by combined cortisol, epinephrine, norepinephrine, and glucagon infusion (106). Also, short-term cortisol infusion in high physiologic concentrations in healthy subjects increased plasma amino acid concentration, particularly the branched-chain amino acids (leucine, isoleucine, and valine) (110, 111).

Insulin

Insulin levels are initially decreased during the ebb phase after injury but are mildly to markedly increased during the early flow phase. Hyperglycemia and hyperinsulinemia are characteristic of the early stress response. As stated above, the body becomes resistant to insulin in such tissues as adipocytes and skeletal myocytes (41, 112). The splanchnic tissues also display a relative resistance to insulin, manifested by continued hepatic gluconeogenesis despite elevated glucose levels (112, 113). Insulin resistance may be mediated in part by cortisol (42) as well as by catecholamines (41). The role of the characteristic hyperinsulinemia observed after injury remains unclear, as critical organs, including the CNS, hematogenous cells, wounds, and the kidney, can incorporate glucose in a insulin-independent manner. Nevertheless, continuous infusion of glucose and insulin resulted in decreased urine urea nitrogen excretion as well as decreased amino acid efflux and decreased 3-methylhistidine excretion (a marker of protein catabolism) (114); therefore, the increase in insulin may serve to decrease protein catabolism during the flow phase.

Glucagon

Circulating glucagon levels increase during the hypermetabolic postinjury phase and correlate roughly with the severity of injury (94, 115, 116). Glucagon appears to exert little independent influence on peripheral tissue metabolism (117) but is a potent stimulant of the hepatic cyclic AMP system, facilitating hepatic uptake of amino acids (118) and gluconeogenesis (119). Glucagon is also influenced by the autonomic nervous system (120).

Cytokines

Proinflammatory Cytokine Peptides

Proinflammatory cytokine peptides were originally studied for their effect on immunologic homeostasis in several areas, but they also exert potent activity toward regulation of hemodynamic and metabolic responses (122). During early postinjury or infectious conditions, the initial cytokine response to such insults likely mediates beneficial protective signaling of the immune system. Nevertheless, excessive acute production of some cytokines, such as TNF, may promote septic shock. Prolonged production of tissue cytokines sustains some metabolic effects of the hypercatabolic state.

The proinflammatory cytokine peptides are produced by diverse cell types of both myeloid and nonmyeloid origin. These proteins may function by autocrine (acting on the same cell), paracrine (acting on cells in the immediate area), or systemic mechanisms of action. They produce local tissue responses by cell-to-cell interaction at very low concentrations but also may exert systemic effects in higher concentrations. While many cytokines are now well characterized, those exhibiting the more prominent proinflammatory activities include TNF-α, IL-1, IL-6, and γ-interferon (IFN-γ) have been more widely studied from a metabolic perspective (Table 96.2).

Tumor Necrosis Factor. TNF is a 17-kDa protein primarily secreted from monocytes and macrophages. Although originally isolated as a soluble factor that produced cachexia during infection and (as implied by the name) in vivo necrosis of some solid tumors (123), this cytokine has been implicated as the initiating signal for a variety of cellular and metabolic events seen in critically ill patients. TNF administration to healthy subjects elicits a systemic response resembling that observed during septicemia (124), including increased stress hormone release, temperature elevation, and increased acute-phase protein synthesis (125). The systemic effects of bacterial liposaccharide (endotoxin) are replicated, if not largely mediated, by TNF (125). Indeed endotoxin infusion induces a rapid increase in circulating TNF levels, and blocking TNF with antibodies in animal models alleviates many of the toxic effects of endotoxin (126, 127). TNF may circulate predominately as a complex with its soluble receptors, making detection of the bioactive ligand more difficult. Increased levels of these soluble TNF receptors are seen in response to diverse inflammatory stimuli including sepsis, cancer, and AIDS ([43] and references therein). Nevertheless, elevated TNF levels are detected in many disease states including bacterial infections, infected thermal injury, tumor-bearing states, sepsis, and AIDS ([40] and references therein [128]). The metabolic effects of TNF and perhaps of the proinflammatory cytokines seem to promote redistribution of body protein and lipid stores (124). The result is a net loss of peripheral tissue protein with a concomitant increase in hepatic uptake. Alterations in fat metabolism elicited by TNF resemble the changes seen in infection. They include promotion of cellular lipolysis and hepatic lipogenesis with decreased free fatty acid synthesis and decreased clearance of extracellular lipids (126, 129–131).

Interleukin-1. IL-1 is produced by macrophages/monocytes, neutrophils, lymphocytes, and keratinocytes (122). Its production is stimulated by TNF and endotoxin, and, like TNF, it may represent an early cytokine response to injury. Once released, it exerts multiple immunologic and metabolic effects including stimulation of ACTH (132), induction of fever, hepatic acute-phase protein synthesis, and alteration of energy metabolism (122). Like TNF activity, IL-1 activity is regulated by shedding of soluble

Table 96.2
Major Cytokines Involved in Hypermetabolic Response

Cytokine	Cell Source	Metabolic Effects
Tumor necrosis factor–α	Monocytes/macrophages, lymphocytes, Kupffer cells, glial cells, endothelial cells, natural killer cells, mast cells	Decreased FFA synthesis Increased lipolysis Increased peripheral amino acid loss Increased hepatic amino acid uptake Fever
IL-1	Monocytes/macrophages, neutrophils, lymphocytes, keratinocytes, Kupffer cells	Increased ACTH Increased hepatic acute-phase protein synthesis Fever
IL-6	Monocytes/macrophages, keratinocytes, endothelial cells, fibroblasts, T cells, epithelial cells	Increased acute-phase protein synthesis Fever
IFN-γ	Lymphocytes, pulmonary macrophages	Increased monocyte respiratory burst

receptors, as well as by a unique, naturally occurring receptor antagonist (IL-1ra) (133). IL-1ra binds to the IL-1 receptor without an agonist influence.

Interleukin-6. IL-6 is the most frequently detected cytokine in patients with acute infection (134), injury, and tumor-bearing states (135) and after elective surgical procedures (136). The biologic actions of this protein include regulation of acute-phase protein synthesis after injury (137, 138) and differentiation of lymphocytes (139). It also induces fever via prostaglandin production (140). Administration of IL-6 to humans induced modest changes in the kinetics of glucose and protein. (141)

Interferon-γ. IFN-γ is secreted from lymphocytes and macrophages and exerts antiviral effects as well as protection against bacteria, fungi, and parasites. It enhances TNF production in response to endotoxin (142) and increases the cytotoxicity of monocytes, possibly by increasing their respiratory burst activity (143). A direct role for IFN-γ in directing altered metabolic processes has not been defined in humans, although its administration does induce cachexia and loss of protein and lipid stores in animals (144).

Antiinflammatory Cytokines

Regulation of the various cytokines produced in response to injury or disease is complex and involves counterregulation by antiinflammatory cytokines such as IL-10, which downregulates secretion of proinflammatory cytokines (i.e., TNF and IL-1) as well as suppressing macrophage and T-cell functions.

Neuroendocrines and Cytokines

Recent work indicates that the neuroendocrine system also exerts a significant influence upon production of both pro- and antiinflammatory cytokines. For example, glucocorticoids can inhibit production of TNF or IL-6 (142, 145, 146), and in the case of TNF, the mechanism appears to include altering transcription of the mRNA (147). Cortisol infusion attenuates the endogenous TNF response to endotoxin administration (142, 143). Catecholamine infusion also inhibits endotoxin-induced TNF production while simultaneously increasing release of IL-10 (148). Hence, the neuroendocrine milieu elicited by injury, infection, or other hypermetabolic conditions may serve to alter cytokine mediator activities in a complex manner. It remains to be determined to what extent these parallel signaling pathways direct the human metabolic response.

SYSTEMIC AND ORGAN REACTIONS

Gastrointestinal Tract

The gastrointestinal tract provides important nutrient absorptive and metabolic functions and recently has emerged as an immunologically important organ. TPN and bowel rest are associated with an exaggerated response to injury (152). The etiology of this enhanced response is unclear, but bowel rest or TPN may alter intestinal flora or intestinal mucosal permeability. The gut mucosa normally provides a barrier to foreign material such as bacteria, their products, and other ingested particles. Enteral feeding is essential to maintain the integrity of this mucosal barrier (149, 150). In animal studies, bowel rest and parenteral nutrition produce increased translocation of bacteria to intestinal lymphoid tissue (151). Whether bacterial translocation is an important source of systemic bacteremia and sepsis during disease states in humans is a matter of debate. However, it may be that stimulation of splanchnic immune cells by foreign antigens that have crossed the mucosal barrier influences systemic immunologic and metabolic processes during disease states. Cytokines secreted by splanchnic cells or lymphocytes or macrophages influence both the immune and hemodynamic responses to injury as well as the metabolic response (153, 154). In this way, the intestine may partially regulate the immune response to injury or disease.

Cachexia

The hypermetabolic response may result in cachexia if it is allowed to proceed unabated. The clinical syndrome of cachexia is characterized by anorexia, tissue wasting, and weight loss and can occur in many different disease states such as cancer, chronic infection, and AIDS. Multiple mechanisms appear to be involved in the development of cachexia, including anorexia, decreased physical activity, decreased secretion of host anabolic hormones, and altered host metabolic response with abnormalities in protein, lipid, and carbohydrate metabolism. The degree of wasting is an important prognostic factor, with a weight loss to 66% of ideal body weight being predictive of death regardless of the specific cause of the weight loss (155). Therefore, a more thorough understanding of the pathogenesis of cachexia might lead to further therapeutic options that theoretically could improve survival (see also Chapter 41).

The degree of wasting does not correlate with the infective burden or tumor size; thus it appears to be the host response via endogenous mediators that effects the cachectic response in diseased patients. Much research has focused on possible mediators of the cachexia induced by disease, with much attention on cytokine mediators of anorexia, most notably TNF, but also IL-1, IL-6, IFN-γ, and leukemia-inhibitory factor. TNF can induce weight loss when given in increasing doses or continuous infusion or when secreted from tumors genetically engineered to express TNF (156). However, TNF is not often found in cancer patients with cachexia (157) and generally is not found in patients with chronic infections that lead to wasting, including AIDS (158). In addition, it has been difficult to correlate levels of TNF or IL-6 with the degree of cancer cachexia (157, 159), and leukemic factor itself may be toxic (160).

Other work has focused on the leptin molecule, which appears to play a significant role in weight maintenance. Alterations in the leptin molecule or its receptor result in weight control abnormalities (161). Because leptin expression is increased in response to endotoxin, TNF, and IL-1, it may be an important factor in weight loss in the stress response.

Recent research has identified another potential mediator of cachexia which is a proteoglycan isolated from mice with adenocarcinoma and from the urine of cachectic cancer patients (162). In this study using a murine adenocarcinoma, MAC16, transplantation of tumor cells in mice induced significant cachexia without anorexia. The proteoglycan was isolated from the mice and found to induce cachexia in non-tumor-bearing animals. Also, the proteoglycan was present in cancer patients with weight loss but absent in patients with weight loss attributable to other factors. Further characterization and study of this molecule may yield new insight into the pathogenesis of cachexia.

GENERAL NUTRITION AND ANABOLIC SUPPORT

Macronutrients

Treatment of patients who are hypermetabolic for extended periods of time should in all likelihood include nutrient supplementation. Nutritional management of stressed patients is reviewed in Chapters 92, 98, 100, and 101 of this textbook and is only briefly mentioned here.

The fundamental objectives of nutritional support of the hypermetabolic patient are to provide sufficient nonprotein energy sources and sufficient protein substrate to alleviate or at least minimize catabolism of endogenous energy and protein stores. Enteral and parenteral nutritional support in depleted patients often demonstrably improves nitrogen balance during the catabolic phase of injury (163). Enteral nutrient provision is clearly the preferred route of feeding in the presence of a functional intestinal tract. Recent studies indicate that there may be some clinically demonstrable benefit to enteral feedings in selected patient populations (164–166).

There is also evidence to suggest that some nutrients may become conditionally essential during catabolic illness. Among these are the amino acid glutamine, which is a major component of the tissue free amino acid pool and appears to be rapidly depleted in periods of stress. It is also essential for nucleotide and glutathione biosynthesis, as well as gluconeogenesis. Other studies suggest that other amino acids, such as arginine, may also be limiting to the maintenance of lymphocyte function and wound healing (167, 168) (see also Chapter 35).

Anabolic Therapy

Although nutritional supplementation may improve body nitrogen and calorie balance during hypermetabolic states, progressive depletion of structural protein still continues. Consequently, additional means of adjuvant anabolic therapy, such as insulin, insulin-like growth factor (IGF-1), anabolic steroids, or GH, have been investigated in an effort to decrease muscle protein loss in hypermetabolic patients. Administration of GH or IGF-1 increases skeletal muscle amino acid uptake and muscle mRNA synthesis during full nutritional support (169, 170).

IGF-1 infusion in healthy humans also increases peripheral glucose disposal, reduces lipolysis, and decreases total branched-chain amino acid levels, suggesting a protein-anabolic effect (171, 172). Insulin administration also reduces protein loss in burn and trauma patients, resulting in decreased urinary urea excretion and reduced protein breakdown rates (173, 174). Recent studies using a combination of GH and insulin in cancer patients indicate that this combination therapy may lead to whole-body nitrogen retention and skeletal muscle sparing (175). GH affects nitrogen balance positively by exerting an anabolic effect on proteins (176). In clinical trials, the effect of GH also seems to depend on the severity of injury. In patients under mild-to-moderate stress, GH does promote improved nitrogen balance, with an anabolic effect on protein synthesis. However, in severely stressed patients (those losing more than 1.5 g/kg/day protein), exogenous GH is not demonstrably effective as an anabolic agent (177). While most studies show anabolic effects of GH treatment of patients in mild-to-moderate catabolism, improved clinical outcome has been difficult to document in most hypermetabolic patient populations. A study of ventilator-dependent critically ill patients does suggest that prolonged GH treatment may promote pulmonary function in this group (178).

Micronutrients

The major intracellular elements—potassium, magnesium, and phosphate—follow patterns of nitrogen loss in response to acute infection (183). Zinc as well as iron is sequestered by the liver, with a decrease in circulating plasma levels. This may represent a host survival mechanism during infection by making zinc and iron unavailable to the replicating bacteria. Increases in serum iron concentration during infection may impair the host resistance to infection. Zinc is essential for wound healing, and thus adequate levels must be maintained in the stressed individual to ensure healing. Ceruloplasmin synthesis is increased by the liver with a concomitant rise in copper levels. There is catabolic destruction or urinary loss of many vitamins, most notably vitamin A, which may contribute to morbidity and mortality in some infections.

NUTRITIONAL SUPPORT IN ORGAN FAILURE

The hypermetabolic patient who responds to therapeutic interventions will proceed to an anabolic stage of recovery and, eventually, positive nitrogen balance. However, some patients continue to be hypermetabolic and may develop multiorgan system failure. The pathogenesis of organ system failure remains to be completely clarified, but it is multifactorial. With the onset of multiorgan system failure, nutritional requirements may be modified.

Pulmonary

Respiratory insufficiency may be the end result of protein-energy malnutrition leading to decrease in muscle mass of respiratory muscles as well as disturbances in respiratory drive (179). The net result is increased CO_2 retention and difficulty in oxygenation. This process may be exacerbated by vasoactive factors released during infection that increase pulmonary vascular permeability with an ensuing ventilatory mismatch. It is hypothesized that increased CO_2 production from the carbohydrate provided in supplemental nutrition increases CO_2 retention. Therefore an increased proportion of calories from lipid might be used in these patients (see also Chapter 90).

Kidney

The etiology of acute renal failure in the injured or septic patient is multifactorial and can include shock, nephrotoxic drugs, glomerulonephritis, and urinary tract obstruction. The multiple metabolic consequences of renal failure include fluid and electrolyte abnormalities as well as alterations in protein, carbohydrate, lipid, trace element, and vitamin metabolism (180) with decreased clearance of phosphate, potassium, and magnesium and elevations in their concentrations as the result of impaired glomerular filtration. Acidosis develops from decreased renal excretion of acid and increased tissue catabolism. Uremia ensues due to increased protein breakdown and decreased urea clearance. When renal tubular disorder is present (e.g., as the result of nephrotoxic drugs), renal loss of minerals may occur. Dialysis is initiated to minimize these metabolic disturbances. Traditionally, patients with acute renal failure have been treated with low-protein nutritional support to decrease urea production. However, there are no data to indicate that a low-protein intake can decrease loss of renal function or improve recovery of renal function in acute renal failure (180). Therefore, protein should not be restricted; nutritively sufficient amounts should be given, with increased metabolites and waste products treated by appropriate dialysis. The protein requirements in dialysis patients are higher than normal because of increased catabolism in these patients and loss of nutrients in the dialysate (180). Data suggest that hypercatabolic patients with acute renal failure require 1.25 to 1.5 g/kg/day of protein, with higher requirements for patients receiving dialysis. Close regulation of magnesium, potassium, and phosphate is also necessary in patients with renal failure.

Liver

Hepatic dysfunction in the critically ill patient ranges from mild abnormalities in liver function tests to fulminant liver failure with severe jaundice and wasting. Nutritional requirements in such patients depend upon the primary disease process underlying the liver dysfunction. Infectious processes that affect the liver itself, such as hepatitis, localized abscesses, and pylephlebitis, may result in liver dysfunction. In the presence of encephalopathy, the protein load should be decreased, and parenterally administered amino acids are generally better tolerated than those administered enterally (181). Some have advocated use of solutions high in branched-chain amino acids with no aromatic amino acids, but the benefit of such solutions is controversial (182).

Occasionally, hypoglycemia may occur in end-stage liver failure. More often, minor elevations in liver function tests occur during the course of intravenous feeding. This generally resolves after cessation of parenteral feeding and, in the absence of drastically altered liver function or associated inflammatory processes, is of minimal consequence to the acute recovery process.

Heart

The goal of nutrition in patients with cardiac failure is to provide nutrient requirements in limited fluid volume with restricted sodium intake. This can be achieved parenterally with a concentrated solution of hypertonic dextrose, but as with most patients, enteral feeding is preferred.

REFERENCES

1. Cuthbertson D. Br Med Bull 1945;3:96–102 .
2. Moore F. Metabolic care of the surgical patient. Philadelphia: WB Saunders, 1959.
3. Lowry SF. Host metabolic response to injury. In: Gallin JI, Fauci AS, eds. Advances in host defense mechanisms, vol 6. New York: Raven Press, 1986;169–90.
4. Duke JH, Jorgensen SB, Broell JR, et al. Surgery 1970;68: 168–74.
5. Wilmore D, Long JM, Mason AD, et al. Ann Surg 1974; 180:653–69.
6. Bozzetti F, Pagnoni A, Del Vecchio M. Surg Gynecol Obstet 1980;150:229–34.
7. Fearon KCH, Hansell DT, Preston T, et al. Cancer Res 1988;48:2590–5.
8. Knox CS, Crosby LO, Feuer IB, et al. Ann Surg 1983;197: 152–62.
9. Knox L, Crosby LO, Feurer ID, et al. (Abstract) Clin Res 1980;38:620A.
10. Fredrix EW, Soeters PB, Wouters EFM, et al. Cancer Res 1991;51:6138–41.
11. Fredrix EW, Wouters EFM, Soeters PB, et al. Cancer 1991;68:1612–21.
12. Dempsey DT, Feurer ID, Knox LS, et al. Cancer 1984;53:1265–73.
13. Falconer JS, Fearon KCH, Plester CE, et al. Ann Surg 1994;219:325–31.
14. Hommes MJ, Romijn JA, Godfried MH, et al. Metabolism 1990;39:1186–90.
15. Melchior JC, Salmon D, Rigaud D, et al. Am J Clin Nutr 1991;53:437–41.
16. Melchior JC, Raguin G, Rigaud D, et al. (Abstract) Abstracts

of the Seventh International Conference on AIDS, Florence, Italy, June 16–21, 1991;1:293.
17. Grunfeld C, Feingold KR. N Engl J Med 1992;327:329–37.
18. Hommes MJT, Romijn JA, Endert E, et al. Am J Clin Nutr 1991;54:311–5.
19. Centers for Disease Control. MMWR 1987;36(Suppl 1): 1S–15S.
20. Lowry SF. Nutritional support of the trauma patient. In: Shires GT, ed. Principles of trauma care, vol 3. New York: McGraw-Hill, 1985;592–608.
21. Hasselgren PO, James JH, Benson DW, et al. Metab Clin Exp 1989;38:634–40.
22. Hummel RP, Hasselgren PO, James JH, et al. Metab Clin Exp 1988;37:1120–7.
23. Hasselgen PO, James JH, Fischer JE. Ann Surg 1986;203: 360–5.
24. Zamir O, Hasselgren PO, Higashiguchi T, et al. Mediat Inflam 1992;1:247–50.
25. Tiao G, Fagan JM, Samuels N, et al. J Clin Invest 1994; 94:2255–64.
26. Hershko A, Ciechanover A. Annu Rev Biochem 1992;61: 761–807.
27. Price SR, England BK, Bailey JL, et al. Am J Physiol 1994; 267:C955–60.
28. Wilmore DW, Goodwin CW, Aulick LH, et al. Ann Surg 1980;192:491–504.
29. Bessey PQ. Metabolic response to critical illness. In: Wilmore DS, ed. Care of the surgical patient. Sci Am 1994;(Suppl): 3–31.
30. Shou J. Glutamine. In: Zaloga GP, eds. Nutrition in critical care. Philadelphia: CV Mosby, 1994;123–41.
31. Muhlbacher F, Kapadia CR, Colpoys MF, et al. Am J Physiol 1974;247:E75–83.
32. Souba WW, Wilmore DW. Surgery 1983;94:342–50.
33. Kinney JM, Elwyn DH. Annu Rev Nutr 1983;3:433–66.
34. Wannemacher RW Jr, Pekarek RS, Thompson WL, et al. Endocrinology 1975;96:651–61.
35. Carmichael MJ, Clague MB, Kier MJ, et al. Br J Surg 1980;67:736–9.
36. Eden E, Ekman L, Lindmark L, et al. Metabolism 1984; 33:1020–7.
37. Heber D, Chlebowski RT, Ishibashi DE, et al. Cancer Res 1982;42:4815–9.
38. Shaw JHF, Humberstone DA, Douglas RG, et al. Surgery 1991;109:37–50.
39. Stein TP, Nutinsky C, Condoluci D, et al. Metabolism 1990;39:876–81.
40. Fong Y, Lowry SF. Metabolic consequences of critical illness. In: Barie PS, Shires GT, eds. Surgical intensive care, vol 1. Boston: Little, Brown, and Co, 1993;893–905.
41. Deibert DC, DeFronzo RA. J Clin Invest 1980;65:717–21.
42. Diethelm AG. Ann Surg 1977;185:251–63.
43. Tracey KJ, Cerami A. Annu Rev Cell Biol 1993;9:317–43.
44. Nelson KM, Long CL, Bailey R, et al. Metabolism 1992;41:68–75.
45. Shaw JHF, Januskiewicz J, Horsborough R. Circ Shock 1985;16:77–8.
46. Long CL, Nelson KM, Geiger JW, et al. J Trauma 1996;40:335–41.
47. Wolfe RR, Herndon DN, Jahoor F, et al. Am J Physiol 1977;232:415–8.
48. Wolfe RR, Herndon DN, Jahoor F, et al. N Engl J Med 1987;317:403–8.
49. Warren RS, Starnes HF, Gabrilove JL, et al. Arch Surg 1987;122:1396–400.
50. Bearn AG, Billing B, Sherlock S. J Physiol (London) 1951; 115:430.
51. Shaw JHF, Wolfe RR. Ann Surg 1989;209:63–72.
52. Clowes GHA, O'Donnell TF, Blackburn GF, et al. Surg Clin North Am 1976;56:1169–84.
53. Wolfe RR, O'Donnell TF Jr, Stone MD, et al. Metabolism 1980;29:892–900.
54. Burke JF, Wolfe RR, Mullany CJ, et al. Ann Surg 1979; 190:274–85.
55. Vary TC, Siegal JH, Wakatani T, et al. Am J Physiol 1986; 13:634–40.
56. Rohdenberg GL, Bernhard A, Krehbiel O. JAMA 1919;72: 1528–9.
57. Holroyde CP, Skutches CL, Boden G, et al. Cancer Res 1984; 44:5910–3.
58. Humberstone DA, Shaw JHF. Cancer 1988;207:283–9.
59. Lundholm K, Edstrom S, Karlberg, I. et al. Cancer 1982;50:1142–50.
60. Lawson DH, Richmond A, Nixon DW, et al. Annu Rev Nutr 1982;2:277–301.
61. Douglas RG, Shaw JHF. Br J Surg 1990;77:246–54.
62. Eden E, Edstrom S, Bennegard K, et al. Cancer Res 1984;44:1717–24.
63. Cheblowski RT, Heber D. Surg Clin North Am 1986; 66:957–68.
64. Holroyde CP, Gabuzda TG, Putnam RC, et al. Cancer Res 1975;35:3710–4.
65. Waterhouse C. Cancer 1974;33:66–71.
66. Shaw JHF, Humberstone DM, Wolfe RR. Ann Surg 1988;207:283–9.
67. Shaw JHF, Wolfe RR. Surgery 1987;101:181–91.
68. Kokal WA, McCullough A, Wright PO, et al. Ann Surg 1983;198:146–50.
69. Holroyde CP, Reichard GA. Cancer Treat Rep 1981;65 (Suppl):55–9.
70. Warburg O. The metabolism of tumours. New York: Richard F Smith, 1930.
71. Burt ME, Brennan MF. Semin Oncol 1984;11:127–35.
72. Holroyde CP, Meyers RN, Smink RD, et al. Cancer Res 1977;37:3109–14.
73. Hansell DT, Davies JWL, Burns HJG. Ann Surg 1986;203: 240–5.
74. Vendrell J, Nubiola A, Goday A, et al. (Letter) Lancet 1987;2:1212.
75. Wolfe RR, Bagby GJ. Lipid metabolism in shock. In: Altura BM, Lefer AM, Schumer W, et al., eds. Handbook of shock and trauma. New York: Raven Press, 1983;199–219.
76. Askanazi J, Carpentier YA, Elwyn DH, et al. Ann Surg 1980;191:40–6.
77. Wolfe RR, Allsop JR, Burke JF. Metabolism 1979;28:210–20.
78. Nanni G, Siegel JH, Coleman B, et al. J Trauma 1984;24:14–30.
79. Stoner HB, Little RA, Frayn KN, et al. Br J Surg 1983;70:32–5.
80. Lundholm K. Surg Clin North Am 1986;66:1013–24.
81. Cohn S, Gartenhaus W, Sawitsky A, et al. Metabolism 1980;30:222–9.
82. Jeevanandam M, Horowitz GD, Lowry SF, et al. Metabolism 1986;35:304–10.
83. Legaspi A, Jeevanandam M, Starnes HF, et al. Metabolism 1987;36:958–63.
84. Shaw JHF, Wolfe RR. Ann Surg 1987;205:368–76.
85. Eden E, Edstrom S, Bennegard K, et al. Surgery (St. Louis) 1985;97:176–84.
86. Klein S, Wolfe RR. J Clin Invest 1990;86:1403–8.
87. Kotler DP, Tierney AR, Wang J, et al. Am J Clin Nutr 1989;50:444–7.

88. Hellerstein MK, Grunfeld C, Wu K, et al. J Clin Endocrinol Metab 1993;76:559–65.
89. Grunfeld C, Kotler DP, Hamadeh R, et al. Am J Med 1989;86:27–31.
90. Hume DM, Egdahl RH. Ann Surg 1959;150:697–712.
91. Newsome HH, Rose JC. J Clin Endocrinol Metab 1971;33:481–7.
92. Taylor JW, Hander EW, Skreen R, et al. J Surg Res 1976;20:313–20.
93. Dempsey DT, Guenter P, Mullen JL, et al. Surg Gynecol Obstet 1985;160:128–34.
94. Meguid MM, Brennan MF, Aoki TT, et al. Arch Surg 1978;776–83.
95. Hume DM, Bell CC, Bartter F. Surgery 1962;52:174–87.
96. Carey LC, Cloutier CT, Lowery BD. Ann Surg 1971;174:451–60.
97. Popp MB, Srivastava LS, Knowles HC, et al. Surg Gynecol Obstet 1977;145:517–24.
98. Wise L, Margraf HW, Ballinger WF. Arch Surg 1972;105:213–20.
99. Marchuk JB, Finley RJ, Graces AC, et al. J Surg Res 1977;23:177–82.
100. Beisel WR. Am J Clin Nutr 1977;30:1236–47.
101. O'Brien JT, Bybee DE, Burman BD, et al. Metabolism 1980;29:721–7.
102. Richmand DA, Molitch MD, O'Donnell TF. Metabolism 1980;29:936–42.
103. van der Poll T, Van Zee KJ, Endert E, et al. J Clin Endocrinol Metab 1995;80:1341–6.
104. Jaattela A, Alho A, Avikainen V, et al. Br J Surg 1975;62:177–81.
105. Davies CL, Newman RJ, Molyneux SG, et al. J Trauma 1984;24:99–105.
106. Gelfand RA, Matthews DE, Bier DM, et al. J Clin Invest 1984;74:2238–48.
107. Fong Y, Albert JD, Tracey KJ, et al. J Trauma 1991;31:1467–76.
108. Kraenzlin ME, Keller U, Keller A, et al. J Clin Invest 1989;84:388–93.
109. Shaw JHF, Holdaway CM, Humberstone DA. Surgery 1988;103:520–5.
110. Shamoon HP, Soma V, Sherwin RS. J Clin Endocrinol Metab 1980;50:495–501.
111. Simmons PS, Miles JM, Gerich JE, et al. J Clin Invest 1984;73:412–20.
112. Porte D Jr, Robertson RP. Fed Proc 1973;32:1792–6.
113. Flaim KE, Hutson SM, Lloyd CE, et al. Am J Physiol 1985;249:E447–53.
114. Inculet RI, Finley RI, Duff JH, et al. Surgery 1986;99:752–8.
115. Alberti KGMM, Batstone GF, Foster KJ, et al. JPEN J Parenter Enteral Nutr 1980;4:141–6.
116. Wolfe BM, Culebras JM, Aoki TT, et al. Surgery 1979;86:248–56.
117. Pozefsky T, Tancredi RG, Moxley RT, et al. Diabetes 1976;25:128–35.
118. Warren RS, Donner DB, Starnes HF, et al. Proc Natl Acad Sci USA 1987;84:8619–22.
119. Felig P, Wahren J, Hendler R. J Clin Invest 1976;58:761–5.
120. Iversen J. J Clin Invest 1973;52:2102–16.
121. Haussinger D, Roth E, Lang F, et al. Lancet 1993;341:1330–2.
122. Fong Y, Lowry SF. Cytokines and the cellular response to injury and infection. In: Harken AH, Wilmore DW, eds. Care of the surgical patient. Sci Am 1996;(Suppl)1–21.
123. Carswell EA, Old LJ, Kassel RL, et al. Proc Natl Acad Sci USA 1975;72:3666–70.
124. van der Poll RJA, Endert E, et al. Am J Physiol 1991;261:E457–65.
125. Michie HR, Spriggs DR, Manogue KR, et al. Surgery 1988;1004:280–6.
126. Fong Y, Lowry SF. Clin Immunol Immunopathol 1990;55:157–70.
127. van Zee KJ, Kohno T, Fischer E, et al. Proc Natl Acad Sci USA 1992;89:4845–9.
128. Lahdevirta J, Maury CPJ, Teppo AM, et al. Am J Med 1988;85:289–91.
129. Beutler B, Mahoney J, Le Trang N, et al. J Exp Med 1985;161:984–5.
130. Feingold KR, Grunfeld C. J Clin Invest 1987;80:184–90.
131. Zechner R, Newman TC, Sherry B, et al. Mol Cell Biol 1988;8:2394–401.
132. Tracey KJ, Lowry SF. Adv Surg 1990;23:21–56.
133. Fischer E, Van Zee KJ, Marano MA, et al. Blood 1992;79:2196–200.
134. Helfgott DC, Tatter SB, Santhanam U, et al. J Immunol 1989;142:948–53.
135. Gelin J, Moldawer LL, Lonnroth C, et al. Biochem Biophys Res Commun 1988;157:575–9.
136. Shenkin A, Fraser WD, Series J, et al. Lymphokine Res 1989;8:123–7.
137. Ritchie DG, Fuller GM. Ann NY Acad Sci 1983;408:490–502.
138. Castell JV, Gomez-Lechon MJ, David M, et al. FEBS Lett 1989;242:237–9.
139. Garman RD, Jacobs KA, Clark SC, et al. Proc Natl Acad Sci USA 1987;84:7629–33.
140. Helfgott DC, Fong Y, Moldawer LL, et al. Clin Res 1989;37:564A.
141. Stouthard JML, Romijn JA, van der Poll T, et al. Am J Physiol 1995;268:E813–9.
142. Luedke CE, Cerami A. J Clin Invest 1990;86:1234–40.
143. Nathan CF, Murray HW, Weibe ME, et al. J Exp Med 1983;158:670–89.
144. Matthys P, Duksman R, Proost P, et al. Int J Cancer 1991;49:77–82.
145. Ray A, LaForge KS, Sehgal PB. Mol Cell Biol 1990;10:5736–46.
146. Zuckerman SH, Shellhaas J, Butler LD. Eur J Immunol 1989;19:301–5.
147. Han J, Thompson P, Beutler B. J Exp Med 1990;172:391–4.
148. van der Poll T, Coyle SM, Barbosa K, et al. J Clin Invest 1996;97:713–9.
149. Robin CN, Williamson MB, Chir M. N Engl J Med 1978;298:1393–402.
150. Streilen JW, Stein-Streilen J, Head J. Regional specialization in antigen presentation. In: Phillips SM, Escobar MR, eds. The reticuloendothelial system, vol 9. New York: Plenum, 1986;37–94.
151. Alverdy JC, Aoys E, Moss GS. Surgery 1988;104:185–90.
152. Fong Y, Marano MA, Barber A, et al. Ann Surg 1989;210:449–57.
153. Fong Y, Lowry SF, Cerami A. JPEN J Parenter Enteral Nutr 1988;12:72S–7S.
154. Fong Y, Moldawer LL, Marano M, et al. J Immunol 1989;142:2321–4.
155. Kotler DP. J Nutr 1992;122:723–7.
156. Tracey KJ, Wei H, Manogue KR, et al. J Exp Med 1988;167:1211–27.
157. Socher SH, Martinez D, Craig JB, et al. J Natl Cancer Inst 1988;80:595–8.
158. Grunfeld C, Pang M, Doerrler W, et al. J Clin Endocrinol Metab 1992;74:1045–52.
159. Soda K, Kawakami M, Kashii A, et al. Jpn J Cancer Res 1994;85:1124–30.

160. Metcalf D, Nicola NA, Gearing DP. Blood 1990;76:50–6.
161. Nabel GJ, Grunfeld C. Nature Med 1996;2:397–8.
162. Todorov P, Cariuk P, McDevitt T, et al. Nature 1996;379:739–42.
163. Shenkin A, Neuhauser M, Bergstrom J, et al. Am J Clin Nutr 1980;33:2119–27.
164. Moore FA, Moore EE, Jones TN, et al. J Trauma 1989; 29:916–23.
165. Moore FA, Feliciano DV, Andrassy RJ, et al. Ann Surg 1992; 216:171–83.
166. Kudsk KA, Croce MA, Fabian TC, et al. Ann Surg 1992;215:503–13.
167. Efron D, Kirk SJ, Regan MC, et al. Surgery 1991;110:327–34.
168. Barbul A, Lazarou S, Efron DT, et al. Surgery 1990;108:331–7.
169. Thompson WA, Coyle SM, Lazarus D, et al. Surg Forum 1991;42:23–5.
170. Fong Y, Rosenbaum M, Tracey KJ, et al. Proc Natl Acad Sci USA 1989;86:3371–4.
171. Boulware SD, Tamborlane W, Sherwin R. Am J Physiol 1992;262:130–3.
172. Clemmons DR, Smith-Banks A, Celniker AC, et al. J Clin Endocrinol Metab 1992;75:1192–7.
173. Hinton P, Allison SP, Littlejohn S, et al. Lancet 1971;1:767–9.
174. Woolfson AMJ, Heatley RV, Allison SP. N Engl J Med 1979;300:14–7.
175. Wolf RF, Pearlstone DB, Newman E, et al. Ann Surg 1992;216:280–8.
176. Ziegler TR, Gatzen C, Wilmore DW. Annu Rev Med 1994;45:459–80.
177. Koea JB, Breier BH, Douglas RJ, et al. Br J Surg 1996;83:196–202.
178. Knox JB, Wilmore DW, Demling RH, et al. Am J Surg 1996;171:576–80.
179. Arora NS, Rochester DF. Am Rev Respir Dis 1982;126:5–8.
180. Suleiman MY, Zaloga GP. Renal failure. In: Zaloga G, ed. Nutrition in critical care. St. Louis: CV Mosby, 1993;661–684.
181. Rombeau JL, Rolandelli RH, Wilmore DW, et al. Nutritional support. In: Harken AH, Wilmore DW, eds. Care of the surgical patient. Sci Am 1994;3–35.
182. Wahren J, Denis J, Desurmont P, et al. Hepatology 1983;3:475–80.
183. Beisel WR, Sawyer WD, Ryll ED, et al. Ann Intern Med 1967;67:744–79.
184. Luketich JD, Mullen JL, Feurer ID, et al. Arch Surg 1990;125:337–41.

97. Nutrition and Infection

LUCAS WOLF and GERALD T. KEUSCH

The temporal relationship between nutrition and infection has long been appreciated, and there are many historical references to the concurrence of pestilence and famine (1). Even the catabolic response to infection was known in history, as evidenced by the popular designation of tuberculosis as "consumption." A more recent example of the obvious nature of the interaction of nutrition and infection is acquired immune deficiency syndrome (AIDS), which was first recognized in East Africa by the lay term "slim disease" because of the dramatic wasting in these patients (2).

Slower to develop has been an understanding of the mechanisms involved and an appreciation of the intricate coupling of the altered host metabolism, which underlies catabolic responses, to activation and amplification of host defenses. Much has been learned and many new interventions are being defined and investigated. Nonetheless, much remains to be done to critically assess the impact of individual and combined nutrient deficiencies on immunologic host defense mechanisms. This chapter explores these issues and describes the multifaceted relationships between nutrition, immune responses, and infection. To provide the background needed to understand the complexities involved, host defense mechanisms are reviewed first.

HOST DEFENSE MECHANISMS

The immune system is highly organized, and its function in the host response to infection represents an extraordinary integration of multiple functional components (3). Host defense is not synonymous with immunity, since there are both immunologic and nonimmunologic defense mechanisms. An example of a nonimmunologic defense is the ability of gastric acid to protect against infection with certain enteric pathogens, e.g., *Vibrio cholerae,* the causative agent of cholera, or nontyphoidal salmonellae, common causes of food- or waterborne diarrhea. These organisms are rather acid intolerant, and the typical pH below 1 in gastric contents during a meal more than suffices to lower the viability of an ingested inoculum to a number too low to cause clinical infection. Individuals with defects in gastric acid production for any reason, whether due to prior ulcer surgery or current use of H2 blockers, are thus at increased risk if exposed to the pathogens. This is clearly shown by epidemiologic evidence obtained during the present cholera pandemic. When cholera reached Europe during the 1970s, clinical disease was observed primarily among individuals with hypochlorhydria (4). While protection based on creating a hostile environment (such as low pH) is "nonspecific" in that no specific recognition events are involved, not all pathogens are affected by the gastric acid barrier. For example, no relation has been found between hypochlorhydria and *Shigella* infection, because these organisms have an adaptable acid-resistance response that is turned on as the organisms reach stationary phase (5). These conditions occur as the organism is excreted in the stool; hence, *Shigella* are in an acid-resistant stage when they reach the environment, ready to infect the next host who ingests the organisms.

In contrast, immunologic mechanisms are truly specific in the sense that they depend on stringent receptor-ligand recognition mechanisms. Similar specific recognition also underlies the typical species, organ, and cellular selectivity of infectious agents. On the host side of the equation, specific immune responses are mediated by effector cells, such as T lymphocytes, macrophages, and granulocytes, or soluble molecules, such as antibodies, complement (C)-derived peptides, and cytokines (also see Chapter 45). Given this organization of the immune system, and the *specificity* inherent to both infection and immune responses, it is not surprising that immune defenses exhibit *selectivity* as well; that is, individual responses are specialized for certain classes of infecting agents and not others. Convincing clinical evidence of this level of specialization comes from observations of patients with genetically mediated immunodeficiency states that predispose to some, but not all, types of infection (Table 97.1) (6). In general, humoral defects of antibody or complement predispose to pyogenic systemic bacterial infections; defects

Abbreviations: **AIDS**—acquired immune deficiency syndrome; **CMI**—cell-mediated immune(ity); **HIV**—human immunodeficiency virus; **Ig**—immunoglobulin; **IL**—interleukin; **IFN**—interferon(s); **MHC**—major histocompatibility complex; **NK**—natural killer; **PEM**—protein-energy malnutrition; T_H—helper T cell.

Table 97.1
Infections in Congenital Immunodeficiency Syndromes

	Associated Pathogenic Organisms			
Nature of Defect	Bacteria	Viruses	Protozoa	Fungi
Agammaglobulinemia	Hib, Sp, Sa, Ps	Echo	G1, ?Pc	—
IgA deficiency	—	—	—	—
IgE deficiency	OM, S, CSP			
HyperIgE syndromes[a]	Sa, Hib, Sp	RSV, Pi		
IgG1 deficiency	CSP			
IgG2,4 deficiency	Hib, Sp, CSP			
DiGeorge syndrome[b]	CSP, DD		Pc	Ca
SCID[c]	CSP, BCG	VZV, A, HSV, CMV	Pc	Ca
Bare lymphocytes[d]	DD		Pc	Ca
Wiscott-Aldrich[e]	OM, CSP	VZV, HSV, CMV	Pc	Ca
HAT[f]	CSP	CMV		
CGD[g]	Sa, Psc, Lp, Nc			As
MPO deficiency[h]	—	—	—	—
C3 deficiency	Sp, Hib, Nm, GNB			

Abbreviations: Hib, *H. influenzae* type b; Sp, *S. pneumoniae;* Sa, *S. aureus;* Psc, *Pseudomonas cepacia;* Lp, *Legionella pneumophila;* Nc, *Nocardia* spp; Mc, *N. meningiditis;* GNB, gram-negative bacilli; Echo, echovirus meningoencephalitis; RSV, respiratory syncytial virus; Pi, parainfluenza virus; VZV, varicella-zoster virus; A, adenovirus; H, herpesvirus; GI, *G. lamblia;* Pc, *P. carinii;* Ca, *Candida albicans;* As, *Aspergillus* spp.; OM, otitis media; S, sinusitis; CSP, chronic suppurative pneumonia; RSP, recurrent suppurative pneumonia; DD, diarrheal disease.

[a]Associated with various lymphocyte defects.

[b]Pure T-cell defect.

[c]Severe combined immunodeficiency, combined T- and B-cell defect.

[d]Failure of HLA class I or class II antigen production.

[e]Associated with T-cell defects, hyper IgE, poor antipolysaccharide antibody responses.

[f]Heriditary ataxia telangiectasia—IgA deficiency, poor CMI.

[g]Chronic granulomatous disease—defective neutrophil oxidative response.

[h]Myeloperoxidase deficiency.

of T cells and cell-mediated immunity (CMI) commonly predispose to viral, fungal, and intracellular bacterial infections; and defects of phagocytes increase the prevalence and severity of pyogenic bacterial and certain fungal infections.

For example, X-linked agammaglobulinemic males develop recurrent pyogenic infections of the respiratory tract, middle ear, and skin, beginning in the second year of life after maternally acquired immunity wanes. The most common pathogen is *Haemophilus influenzae;* however, significant problems with *Streptococcus pneumoniae, Streptococcus pyogenes,* and *Pseudomonas* spp. also are found. Yet these children have no difficulty with diarrheal diseases, urinary tract infections, or common childhood viral illnesses.

Congenital deficiency of complement components also results in specific heightened susceptibility to encapsulated bacterial organisms, even though complement activation products are critical to orderly and effective activation of the entire inflammatory response. Deficiencies of the early components of the classical pathway, C1, 2, or 4, are not ordinarily accompanied by increased systemic infections, but when these do occur, they are commonly due to *S. pneumoniae* or other encapsulated bacteria. No doubt the ability to activate complement via the alternative pathway serves an important protective function in these patients. When C3 is deficient, however, neither pathway can be effectively activated, and encapsulated bacteria such as *S. pneumoniae, H. influenzae,* and *Neisseria meningitidis* cause severe and recurrent infections. Deficiency of either late components or properdin of the alternative complement pathway frequently leads to invasive infection with *N. meningitidis* in particular.

Severe combined immunodeficiency is a syndrome with different genetic causes, but all are characterized by marked reduction in T cells and a decrease in CMI competence. Affected children experience AIDS-like opportunistic infections with *Candida albicans* and other skin pathogens, chronic diarrhea, and interstitial pneumonia, commonly due to *Pneumocystis carinii.* If bacillus Calmette-Guérin (BCG) is given as a routine childhood immunization at birth, progressive systemic BCG infection may occur. Whereas varicella, herpesvirus, or adenoviruses cause disseminated and severe infections, the pyogenic bacteria are not especially troublesome.

Defects of phagocytic cell function (e.g., chronic granulomatous disease, in which neutrophils cannot generate normal oxidative bactericidal products) result in excess susceptibility to organisms positive for catalase, the enzyme that breaks down the bactericidal product, hydrogen peroxide, to water and oxygen. Catalase-negative organisms, such as *S. pneumoniae* or *S. pyogenes,* are not a problem because they cannot detoxify the hydrogen peroxide they produce during growth; therefore, these organisms are quickly eliminated. Chronic granulomatous disease (CGD) patients typically develop serious infections with *Staphylococcus aureus,* gram-negative bacilli such as *Pseudomonas aeruginosa* and *Serratia marcescens,* and fungi

Table 97.2
Immune Defects and Infections in Protein Energy Malnutrion

Immune Defect	Associated Microorganisms
T-cell responses	Intracellular bacteria, measles, *Pneumocystis, Candida*
Antibody defects	Mucosal infections, pyogenic bacteria, fungi
Neutrophil defects	Pyogenic bacteria, gram-negative bacilli
Complement defects	Gram-negative bacilli

such as *Aspergillosis,* but not with routine upper respiratory bacterial pathogens or usual childhood viral pathogens.

Based on these correlations between particular immune mechanisms and susceptibility to specific organisms, it should be possible to predict the effects of nutritional immunodeficiencies on clinical susceptibility to infection (Table 97.2). Such predictions are less than perfect, however, because there is a built-in redundancy and capacity for adaptation in the immune system. Thus, specific defects in host responses may be measurable by in vitro functional tests and yet not be associated with increased clinical infections because alternative defense mechanisms are available to the host. Congenital immunoglobulin (Ig)A deficiency is such an example in which production of IgM and IgG antibodies compensate for diminished mucosal immunity due to lack of IgA. Similarly, patients with congenital absence of myeloperoxidase, a neutrophil enzyme involved in generation of bactericidal oxygen radicals, usually do not experience recurrent or unusually severe infections because other bactericidal products are still produced.

FUNCTIONAL ORGANIZATION OF THE IMMUNE SYSTEM

Organization of the immune system is detailed in Chapter 45. This section addresses interactions between components of the immune system and various infectious agents in more general terms. Activation of host responses may involve simply triggering biochemical reactions or proteolytic cascades such as the complement system, which result in production of biologically active products that alter the host-pathogen interaction. The other hallmark of immune responses is the proliferation of specific clones of T and/or B lymphocyte subsets that recognize specific antigens, as well as the division of bone marrow granulocyte precursors. Therefore, it is reasonable to predict that any nutritional deficit that impairs the ability of a host to sustain cellular proliferation can adversely affect host defense. This is particularly important because it is often the *speed* with which host responses are called into play that determines the difference between harmless encounters between host and microorganism and a fatal infection. Indeed, any reduction in the capacity to support growth and expansion of immunologically capable cells caused by nutrient deficiencies (or in some situations, even nutrient excess) can tip the balance toward more dire outcomes.

Once set in motion, however, host defense responses generate products able to damage normal structures, and the host must be able to dampen and control these reactions. For this reason, elaborate mechanisms involving regulatory cells and proteins have evolved for all classes of immune reactions, to modulate responses and ultimately prevent "immunologic runaway." There are also well-characterized situations in which the host response results in clinical pathology that is amplified in the presence of nutritional deficits because normal immunoregulation fails and leads to more extensive immunopathology. In contrast, nutritionally induced immunodeficiency may diminish immunopathology, as in *Schistosoma mansoni* infection. In this disease, granuloma formation and fibrosis are mediated by specific T cells, and nutritional deficiencies that reduce the ability to mount CMI reactions decrease the size of the granuloma formed in response to schistosome eggs deposited in the liver. Nutritional modulation of granuloma size and diminished organ damage and dysfunction have been documented in experimental murine schistosomiasis.

Separating the immune system into its *cellular* compartments (including T lymphocyte and phagocytic cell responses) and *humoral* compartments (including complement, antibody, and cytokine responses), while convenient, nonetheless obscures the extent of the *interactions* among these elements. For example, B lymphocytes are essential but not sufficient for antibody formation, which requires antigen-presenting macrophages and T cells; normal phagocytes cannot function without complement and antibody for opsonization; and various cytokines produced by either lymphocytes or monocyte-macrophages interact with all of these cells to up- or downregulate their function. The term *immune system* should be interpreted literally to suggest that the various "compartments" really do function as an interactive "system" in which communication among the individual parts is critical.

Viruses

Viruses are obligate intracellular pathogens because the number of viral genes is insufficient to encode the necessary life-support "housekeeping" functions for the organism. Therefore, viruses must usurp the metabolic machinery of the host cell to carry out their own life cycle. It is quite remarkable how intricate this simple life form is and how diverse are the habitats and the pathologic processes viruses induce, ranging from acute to chronic or even latent quiescent or relapsing infections of particular organ systems, to induction of tumors and autoimmune diseases, and to infection and destruction of CD4+ helper T lymphocytes, the distinctive feature of human immunodeficiency virus (HIV) infection, which leads to the dramatic immunosuppression of AIDS. Different viruses can enter the host across the skin or mucous membranes by inhalation or via inoculation from infected blood or tissues; viruses are versatile. Viremia or replication within

specific organs or cell types, or both, can result in almost any combination of cellular dysfunction, inflammatory responses, damage, and destruction, which determines the nature of the subsequent clinical disease. Species specificity and both tissue and cell tropism can differ significantly among isolates of the same virus and may result from limited alterations in the virus genome.

As a general rule, soluble antigens produce good humoral immunity and poor lymphocyte-mediated cytotoxic cellular immunity, whereas antigens synthesized within cells and presented as a complex with the major histocompatibility complex (MHC) glycoproteins generally induce cytotoxic cellular immunity. Viruses can stimulate both kinds of response. The MHC antigens in humans are called HLAs, for human leukocyte antigens, and they comprise several distinct groups of molecules. Class I MHC determinants are transplantation antigens and include three loci in humans (HLA-A, -B, and -C) present on the surface of virtually all nucleated cells. Class I molecules act as antigen-presenting sites for molecules from intracellular pathogens and are recognized by CD8+ cytotoxic lymphocytes (CTLs). In this way, virus-infected cells are killed by the CTL response, virus replication is interrupted, and the disease process is controlled. This is accomplished largely by production of a membrane-attack protein complex similar to the terminal complement C7,8,9 complex, which punches holes in the infected target-cell surface. Some viruses also induce suppressor lymphocyte responses among CD8+ cells, thus downregulating both virus-specific CMI and antibody mechanisms, and in a nonspecific manner, responses to unrelated infectious agents as well.

In contrast, MHC class II molecules are more restricted in distribution to macrophages and T and B lymphocytes and are used to present extrinsic soluble antigens to the humoral immune system. Thus, soluble antigens encountered by macrophages are internalized, processed, and placed on the surface of the antigen-presenting cell in association with the class II molecule. The complex is recognized by T-cell receptors on CD4+ helper T cells, which in turn interact with B cells capable of antibody responses. Certain viruses such as poliovirus are effectively neutralized by antibody present in secretions or plasma. Live oral polio vaccine, like natural infection, induces a local immune response in the gut, including neutralizing secretory IgA that inactivates orally ingested virus before it can invade through the intestinal mucosa and systemically spread to the central nervous system. Killed polio vaccine induces only systemic antibodies that to be effective must interact with the virus in the circulation before it reaches target neurons in the spinal cord. Both vaccine approaches work.

Interferons

Some antiviral effects are mediated or conditioned by soluble host products such as interferons (IFNs), a family of immunoregulatory proteins with direct or, more likely, indirect antiviral properties. Three related IFN classes include IFN-α (leukocyte derived), IFN-β (fibroblast derived), and IFN-γ, or "immune" interferon (produced by antigen- or mitogen-activated lymphocytes). These IFNs have diverse biologic effects, but all regulate expression of normally repressed cellular genes. Surprisingly, recent clinical trials of the antiviral effects of recombinant IFNs has shown that IFN-α, not IFN-γ, is of greatest efficacy; however, the underlying mechanism remains uncertain.

Complement

Complement can also contribute to antiviral effects by binding to the agent and preventing attachment to receptors, by opsonizing virus-antibody complexes for phagocytosis and later degradation, or by mediating direct lysis of lipid-enveloped viruses. Typical complement-antibody lysis of virus-infected cells is demonstrable in vitro as well. Viruses can also cause immunologically mediated pathology, and a variety of mechanisms are known. With persistent infections such as hepatitis B, measles, or cytomegalovirus, even normal antibody responses can lead to deposition of circulating antigen-antibody complexes in tissues with fenestrated vessels such as the renal glomerulus, resulting in acute glomerulonephritis. Recent data indicate that IgE virus-specific antibodies to parainfluenza or respiratory syncytial virus cause local mast cell degranulation in the lung and may lead to the severe respiratory symptoms sometimes associated with these agents, especially in children with hyper-IgE responses. Viruses are also suspected as an inciting cause of autoimmune phenomena as in postinfection encephalitis after common viral infections such as measles, mumps, and varicella-zoster.

Bacteria

Bacteria, like viruses, are exceedingly diverse life forms, ranging from strict anaerobes, to facultative anaerobes able to survive in the presence or absence of oxygen, to organisms that absolutely require oxygen. Some can grow at very high temperature (e.g., in hot springs) while others prefer cool temperatures; some tolerate or require high salt concentrations (seawater organisms such as *V. cholerae,* the cause of cholera); most divide rapidly, but some grow very slowly; certain organisms possess polysaccharide capsules, others have a proteinaceous coat; many are motile, and many are not; a few make lethal toxins, and some others produce required nutrients for the host.

A major host defense response against bacteria is ingestion by phagocytic cells, with bacterial killing resulting from alterations in host cell metabolism. Ingestion may require the presence of immunoglobulin or complement-derived opsonins, which bind to the surface of the organism and assist in the close interaction of phagocytic cells and bacteria that is necessary for inducing phagocytosis. This requirement for opsonic help is particularly impor-

tant when the infecting microorganism makes an antiphagocytic carbohydrate capsule, as is the case with *Streptococcus pneumoniae* or gram-negative organisms such as *Klebsiella pneumoniae.* Unless the ingested organism can inhibit the subsequent activation of antibacterial mechanisms within the phagolysosome (e.g., *Legionella pneumophila*), phagocytic ingestion of a microorganism triggers release of bactericidal oxidative and nonoxidative metabolic products. Not only must there be enough host cells able to produce these bactericidal substances (infection is much more likely when there are fewer than 500 neutrophils per mm^3, as seen in neutropenic patients), but they must also be able to migrate to the site of infection and respond to external stimuli in appropriate fashion.

Some bacterial pathogens, termed *facultative intracellular pathogens,* can survive and multiply within phagocytic cells. They use a variety of strategies to accomplish this. Organisms that survive in the intracellular niche in neutrophils or, especially, within macrophages may sense unique signals in the phagolysosome in which they reside, however temporarily, such as low pH or Ca^{2+} concentration. These signals regulate bacterial genes controlling their ability to resist phagocyte antibacterial mechanisms. How to activate the latent bactericidal mechanisms for such "facultative intracellular" organisms remains a frontier question in microbiology. In many examples, later immunologic engagement of T lymphocytes leads ultimately to macrophage activation and production of interferons and other cytokines that induce acquired microbicidal capability.

Specific immunoglobulins serve many functions in the immune response. Immunoglobulins recognizing and binding to bacterial surface structures via their antibody-combining site (Fab region) can opsonize and facilitate attachment of the organism to phagocyte receptors for the other end of the Ig molecule, the Fc portion. Binding of opsonized organisms to Fc receptors also initiates phagocytic uptake. Immunoglobulin on the bacterial surface can also lead to complement activation and assembly of the terminal complex of C7,8,9, directly resulting in bacterial lysis and death. Thus, it is not surprising that bacteria recovered from the bloodstream of septic patients are usually resistant to complement-mediated lysis. In many cases, complement resistance is not due to either the failure of complement activation or its assembly on the bacterial cell surface, but rather to a more fundamental failure in the microbe's response to complement deposition.

Antibody directed to specific virulence attributes of a bacterium can interfere with disease pathogenesis. For example, anti-colonization factor antibodies may prevent initial establishment of infections on mucosal surfaces, and such antigens are targets for vaccine development for mucosal pathogens of the oral, respiratory, intestinal, and genitourinary tracts. A variation of the same theme is to produce antibody to the invasins mediating epithelial cell penetration by invasive bacteria. These antibodies should restrict systemic infection by organisms such as *Salmonella* (including the typhoid bacillus), *Listeria monocytogenes,* and many others.

When disease results from the action of specific bacterial products, such as toxins, antitoxins can prevent symptoms even if the same antibodies arising during infection are too late to affect its course. In fact, this strategy was the first success of applied microbiology almost a century ago, when vaccines were developed for tetanus and diphtheria based on inactivated toxin antigens. Much contemporary research on microbial pathogenesis is therefore designed to identify molecular targets for immunization, although few infections have turned out to be as simple to deal with as tetanus or diphtheria. Protective antibody-mediated immunity can be induced by a proper vaccine even when antibody plays no role in recovery from natural infection. For example, an unimmunized patient surviving clinical tetanus remains susceptible to the disease unless immunized with toxoid because so little antigen is produced during the natural infection that no effective immune response results. Similarly, it is possible to protect against *Salmonella typhi* by immunizing with the Vi polysaccharide antigen of the organism; however, Vi antibodies arising during the course of established typhoid fever have no impact on recovery. This is because preexisting anti-Vi is bactericidal during the initial bacteremia of *S. typhi* infection, and by preventing initial invasion of macrophages by the organism, it prevents the clinical disease. But the antibody has little impact on the course of the intramacrophage phase of the infection.

Complement activation is essential for efficient activation of the inflammatory response and phagocytic cell function, especially for bacterial infections. Thus, products of complement activation are potent chemotactic factors for neutrophils; they increase vascular permeability and facilitate movement of intravascular phagocytic cells to tissue, and they serve as opsonins or mediate bacteriolysis. The complement cascade can be activated by two different pathways (see Chapter 45): the classical pathway, which requires specific antibody to form a complex with the first, second, and fourth components of complement, or an "alternative pathway" that does not require specific antibody and involves a set of distinctive proteins including factors B and D. Once the system gets going, both pathways result in cleavage of C3, which triggers further activation of the system, and from then on, the biologic results are the same. Because specific antibody is not needed for complement activation via the alternative pathway, this system is of particular importance early in infection before antibody develops.

Fungi

Humans are normally rather resistant to systemic fungal invasion, although mucosal yeast infections are common. Severe mucosal yeast infections occur in patients with defects in CMI, as in AIDS. In the presence of severe neutropenia, however, invasive candidiasis becomes prominent. Risk of fungal infection is increased as well in the presence of debilitating illness, especially when patients have tracheal tubes, catheters, and/or multiple indwelling intravenous lines in place, including hyperalimentation lines.

Parasites

Relatively little is known about immune defenses against protozoa and worms. Many disease-causing parasites have evolved strategies to fool the host by turning off immune responses. They can masquerade as "self" by expressing host self-antigens on their surface or evade recognition by continuously shedding surface antigens recognized by the host immune system or by rapidly changing antigens. Some parasites may be able to subvert killing mechanisms directly within phagocytic cells. For example, they may be polyclonal B-cell activators, stimulating production of a large array of irrelevant antibodies instead of protective ones, or they may induce selective immunosuppression. In general, however, defects in CMI responses, but not antibody, complement, or phagocytic cell abnormalities, increase risk of parasitic infection.

NUTRITIONAL INTERACTIONS

Effects of Protein-Energy Malnutrition on Host Defense Mechanisms

The development of laboratory methods to study immune responses of relevance to host defense has permitted studies in patients with protein-energy malnutrition (PEM) (see Chapters 45 and 59). A broad range of abnormalities have been identified, including both cellular and humoral immune defects, suggesting that an immunodeficiency state may be responsible for the high frequency of severe infections in these patients (Table 97.2). However, many subjects have been infected at the time of study, making it difficult to determine cause and effect of immunologic deficits (infection can be immunosuppressive), and few studies have been longitudinal, which would permit determination of the temporal impact of the defect on clinical responses.

PEM has been described as a mosaic of nutrient deficits resulting from diverse dietary inadequacies, complicated by infection-induced anorexia and catabolism (7). It is best understood as a syndrome associated with variable losses of protein, carbohydrate, and fat stores, along with changes in micronutrients such as minerals and vitamins. However, in practice, the physical and biochemical markers of protein and energy depletion are most obvious and most likely to be recorded. The clinical definitions of PEM are broad and cover a range of physiologic abnormalities. Because PEM patients are not metabolically homogeneous, it is surely perilous to describe any associated immunologic abnormalities in general terms. Nevertheless, a common finding in these patients is depletion of lymphocytes from the central and peripheral lymphoid tissues, particularly in T-cell regions of thymus, spleen, and lymph nodes (8). On this basis, PEM has been dubbed the most prevalent acquired immunodeficiency syndrome in the world.

Based on current understanding of normal T-lymphocyte development, the importance of the thymus gland in this process, and the role of thymic peptide hormones, the reduced circulating thymic factor levels described in a few studies in PEM patients suggest that the T-cell defect in PEM may represent maturational arrest secondary to an abnormal thymic environment (9). In one study of severely malnourished Bolivian infants, thymic involution was documented by sonography, with a reduction of over 90% in the size of the thymus gland compared with normally nourished controls (10). The impact is a relative reduction in circulating mature T lymphocytes. Thus, blood samples obtained for study are enriched in immature and functionally defective cells, defined on the basis of lymphocyte cell-surface maturation antigen expression (Table 97.3). In addition, incubation of peripheral blood lymphocytes from these malnourished Bolivian infants with the thymic peptide thymulin dramatically decreased immature circulating CD1a+ T cells and increased mature CD3+ T cells, without a change in the percentage of CD21+ B cells (Table 97.3). The reduction in mature CD4+ helper T cells (T_H) and, to a lesser and more variable extent, an increase in CD8+ cytotoxic-suppressor T cells ($T_{C/S}$) result in impaired delayed-type skin hypersensitivity responses in vivo and inhibited mitogen- and antigen-driven lymphocyte proliferation in vitro. The clinical consequence of this finding is a reduction in the efficacy

Table 97.3
Lymphocyte Subpopulations in Patients with Protein-Energy Malnutrition: Effects of in Vitro Incubation with the Thymic Hormone Thymulin

	% Marker-Positive Cells, Controls			% Marker-Positive Cells, Malnourished Patients		
Antigen	None	With Thymulin	*p*	None	With Thymulin	*P*
CD1a	7.6 ± 0.8	3.0 ± 0.3	<.001	27.7 ± 1.0	15.2 ± 0.8	<.001
CD3	61.7 ± 1.3	65.1 ± 1.2	ns	51.3 ± 1.0	55.6 ± 1.1	<.01
CD4	41.7 ± 1.3	46.4 ± 1.2	<.05	37.8 ± 1.3	43.4 ± 1.4	<.05
CD8	27.3 ± 1.3	29.1 ± 1.1	ns	31.1 ± 1.0	34.9 ± 0.9	<.01
CD21	31.8 ± 0.9	32.2 ± 0.8	ns	33.9 ± 31.8	34.6 ± 1.1	ns

Modified from Parent G, Chevalier P, Zalles L, et al. Am J Clin Nutr 1994;60:274–8.

of host defenses that depend on T-cell function, including macrophage microbicidal mechanisms for intracellular pathogens and T cell–mediated cytotoxic responses to viruses.

Antibody to most protein antigens is T-cell dependent and requires signals from primed antigen-specific T lymphocytes. T cells are also involved in switching antibody production from the first response, low-affinity IgM antibody, to the second response, high-affinity IgG antibody. Because serum Ig levels are usually normal or elevated in PEM, the ability of malnourished hosts to make Ig is unaffected (11), and in fact, in developing countries, very high levels of IgE are frequently detected (7). This finding probably reflects both the effect of helminths as stimulators of IgE production as well as loss of T-cell suppression of IgE, a normal control mechanism for this immunoglobulin (9). One of the current major limitations in our understanding of the effect of malnutrition on the immune system is the dearth of information regarding the mechanism underlying thymic dysfunction and the resulting impairment in T_H-cell maturation and why (and how) $T_{C/S}$ cells are altered in some, but not all, individuals. This most likely reflects multiple levels of control of these processes, with a multiplicity of maturational signals that become disrupted or disturbed and result in altered signaling events.

In the past decade, an additional refinement in our understanding of the biology of T_H cells has been the division of these cells into at least two groups, T_H1 and T_H2, based on the pattern of cytokines produced by T_H clones when they are activated (12). T_H1 cells produce interleukin (IL)-2, tumor necrosis factor, and IFN-γ and are involved in CMI and delayed-type hypersensitivity responses to intracellular pathogens; T_H2 cells produce IL-4 (which stimulates IgG1 and IgE production), IL-5 (an eosinophil-activating cytokine), and IL-10 and IL-13 (which inhibit macrophage functions) and activate phagocyte-independent host defenses. Following the initial description of these distinctive T cells in mice, similar findings were made in humans by cloning T cells with different reactivities (13). Many of the phenotypic changes in immune function that accompany PEM will likely be found to be due to alterations in the normal T_H1:T_H2 ratios induced by different infectious stimuli. For example, T_H2 cells induce production of IgE (in addition to IgM, IgG, and IgA), whereas T_H1 cells provide B-cell help for IgM, IgG, and IgA, but not IgE synthesis and at low T:B cell ratios. The factors that regulate the T_H1:T_H2 cell ratio in vivo are not known; however, some of the signals in vitro include glucocorticoids (enhance T_H2), 25-hydroxy and 1,25-dihydroxy vitamin D_3 (evoke T_H2 responses), and perhaps other nutritional signals as well (14).

In contrast to simple measurement of Ig levels, the effect of PEM on formation of specific functional antibody in humans has not been studied systematically. Available data are derived principally from observing the response to vaccines. These studies are crude because no titration of antigen dose is possible and limited blood sampling precludes assessing the kinetics of the response. However, the results suggest that antibody responses to certain T cell–dependent protein antigens (e.g., tetanus toxoid) may be relatively preserved in PEM, whereas response to polysaccharide antigens (e.g., somatic carbohydrate antigens of *S. typhi*), classical T cell–independent immunogens in mice, is often subpar. Breast-fed Swedish infants receiving "low"-protein cow-milk formula (1.6 g/kg/day) produced levels of serum, salivary, and fecal antibodies to oral poliovirus vaccine or parenteral diphtheria or tetanus toxoids similar to those of infants fed a conventional protein isocaloric formula (2.2 g/kg/day), but both groups were significantly less responsive than comparable breast-fed infants (15). The authors concluded that breast milk promotes antibody responses. However, no mechanism was suggested and the relevance of the observation to the malnourished child is unknown. In most studies, investigators have neither looked at very young infants nor compared breast-fed and formula-fed babies under controlled conditions.

Antipolysaccharide antibodies are mostly of the IgG2 and IgG4 subclasses that are either locally produced in the lungs or transported into respiratory secretions (16). If the difficulty in making antibody to polysaccharide antigens results from a special defect in synthesis of these IgG subclasses in PEM, it could contribute to the frequency and severity of infection by encapsulated bacteria in PEM patients. In addition, when levels and activity of secretory IgA have been evaluated, they typically are depressed in PEM patients. This defect could also be a factor in the frequency of mucosal infections of the gut, respiratory, and urinary tracts in these individuals.

The complement system is a typical proteolytic cascade resulting in formation of biologically active products during sequential proteolysis and activation of complement components. When the cascade is activated, complement proteins are cleaved and consumed. Enhanced production is required to sustain the response, and the normal host does indeed increase complement synthesis as part of the acute-phase response to inflammatory stimuli. In PEM patients, however, active complement levels are depressed, often in the presence of breakdown products of activation, suggesting simultaneous consumption and inadequate replacement of these proteins (17). The deficit is more profound for the less efficient and often early acting alternative pathway, suggesting that early responses to infection are particularly impaired. This deficiency may be significant in predisposing to gram-negative sepsis, a well-described complication during the course of PEM. It is not clear whether the complement deficit is secondary to consumption induced by infection and/or impaired acute-phase response (thus increasing the severity of the process) or whether it precedes and thus predisposes to infection, or possibly both.

When phagocytic cells from PEM patients are studied in vitro, they often display impaired chemotaxis and reduced oxidative metabolic response, while the initial and subsequent events in phagocytosis, including microbial ingestion, fusion of phagocytic vesicles with lysosomes, and degranulation, are preserved. In the presence of normal opsonins, intracellular killing of organisms in vitro by neutrophils from PEM patients remains intact or only mildly impaired. However, because these patients have reduced complement and may not make high-affinity antibody, serum opsonic activity should be depressed in vivo. This has been reported (17, 18), and thus phagocytic host-defense mechanisms are likely to be more impaired in vivo than they appear to be in vitro.

These data imply that PEM patients have the potential for problems in CMI and phagocytosis, as well as in antibody- and complement-mediated defense. Thus, PEM patients should exhibit increased frequency and/or severity of certain bacterial, viral, fungal, and parasitic infections. This is generally consistent with clinical observations and is not only true for pediatric patients in developing countries, but also for hospitalized patients, usually the elderly, in the developed world. For example, in a study conducted in Scotland, 69 consecutive patients admitted to a geriatric ward were examined for nutritional deficits on admission, and the incidence of septic events was followed prospectively (19). The mean age of the group was 82.2 years, and approximately one-fifth were below the 5th percentile in body mass index, compared with a community sample. Episodes of sepsis were significantly more common in the severely undernourished than in better-nourished subjects (73 vs. 39%; $P < .04$). Mortality was also markedly increased in malnourished versus better-nourished patients. In one study of emergency admissions of elderly patients without cancer to a hospital in Sweden, 41 of 205 subjects (20%) were classified as malnourished, and their cumulative mortality increased to 44% over the 9 months of follow-up, compared with 18% in the better-nourished group (20).

Iron

Phlebotomy has a revered place in history as a traditional intervention for treatment of almost any ailment that did not respond to prayer, incantations, herbs, and other available remedies (21). It has been suggested that the apparent benefits of phlebotomy might have been related to removal of enough iron from the host to create a state of iron deficiency (22). In its more modern form, exchange transfusion, blood letting provides a significant benefit in a few specific infections, such as severe falciparum malaria or babesiosis, presumably because the procedure results in rapid and major reduction in the number of circulating parasitized erythrocytes. Whether or not actual removal of iron from the host enhances the response to these or other infectious agents remains controversial. The controversy has even spread to public health decision making, specifically, whether or not it is beneficial (or harmful) to provide iron supplements to repair iron deficiency anemia in malnourished populations at risk for infectious disease morbidity and mortality (23). The suggestion that low iron levels are helpful is based on limited in vivo observations, including the well-described reduction in circulating iron levels during acute infection and inflammation secondary to iron uptake into tissue stores and the susceptibility of patients with iron overload to certain infections (24). In addition, in vitro data show that removing iron from microbiologic culture media reduces microorganism growth (25). Protective responses based on nutrient alterations in the host have been termed “nutritional immunity” (26). In the case of iron, the benefits should theoretically be reversed by administration of iron, and clinical data have been advanced to support this thesis (27).

However, the basic concept has come into question, as other studies have demonstrated just the opposite, i.e., impaired in vitro immune function and increased infectious morbidity in vivo in iron deficiency states (28). These data have fueled the controversy over the impact of iron on susceptibility to infection. This section considers two opposing questions: does iron deficiency impair immune responses and increase susceptibility to infection (and consequently should be corrected by iron administration) and, conversely, does iron deficiency impede infection by withholding a required nutrient from pathogens so that iron replacement favors microbial virulence (29)?

Physiology

Iron (Chapter 10) is a highly reactive transition metal that readily catalyzes oxidative/peroxidative processes and interacts with oxygen to form unstable reactive intermediates able to damage cell membranes or degrade DNA. To prevent such destructive events and still safely deliver oxygen in mammals, virtually all iron is maintained tightly bound to metalloproteins and enzymes involved in oxygen transport and use, energy metabolism, and DNA synthesis; the bound metal is required for their activity (30). Excess free iron is precluded by the normal excess high-affinity iron-binding capacity in transferrin, lactoferrin, and ferritin (31). In normal iron balance, all mammalian hosts, including humans, maintain a highly iron-restricted environment.

Because mammalian pathogens encounter a “low-iron” compartment in the host, they must compete for this tightly bound iron to survive and multiply. They accomplish this primarily by making iron-chelating proteins (siderophores) with extremely high affinities for iron (32) that can strip bound iron from host proteins, as well as by making iron-siderophore receptors and transport proteins to transport the iron into the microorganism (33). A few microorganisms synthesize receptors for transferrin that resemble the natural receptors of the host, enabling them to acquire iron directly from transferrin (34).

Given sufficient environmental iron, microbes do not need to make these siderophores, microbial outer-membrane-protein (OMP) siderophore receptors, or transport proteins. However, human pathogens have evolved mechanisms to turn on synthesis of these same iron-regulated OMPs (or "IROMPs") under conditions of limited iron (32, 33). IROMPs are made by bacteria growing in vivo in mammalian hosts, just as occurs in vitro in experimental conditions of iron deprivation (35). Pathogens should therefore be seen as constitutively adapted to respond to low iron levels. This ability to use low iron concentrations as a critical signal to indicate that the pathogen has found its host and to regulate transcriptionally the proteins needed to obtain iron when supply is limited certainly raises the question of whether additional iron restriction imposed by clinical iron deficiency states or the hypoferremia of infection (nutritional immunity) can affect microbial growth in vivo.

Regulation of Microbial Genes

Many successful pathogens regulate production of virulence factors so that these are made only when needed in the host, and they have evolved mechanisms to monitor environmental signals such as temperature, cyclic nucleotides, or divalent cations such as calcium or iron (36) to determine their presence in a potential host. Only when detection of the signal triggers gene transcription are the needed virulence proteins made. One of the best known of these environmental regulators is an iron-responsive gene called *fur* (ferric uptake regulator) (37). In an iron-dependent manner, *fur* exerts control over the genes for iron acquisition and transport systems, as well as other genes, many of which are involved in disease causation (38). Thus, low iron states are used by disease-causing microorganisms to increase their pathogenic potential, overcoming the putative protection of the host, attributed to iron deficiency by the nutritional immunity hypothesis.

Iron, Iron-Binding Proteins, and the Immune System

Because transferrin-iron is continuously required for all DNA synthesis (39), lymphocytes undergoing clonal expansion in immune responses must take up iron to synthesize ribonucleotide reductase, the rate-limiting iron-metalloenzyme for DNA synthesis. For this reason, receptors for transferrin appear on lymphocytes responding to IL-2 during the period of activation (40). Therefore, at some point during the development of iron deficiency states, cellular proliferation may be impaired.

Immune responses in iron-deficient humans have been studied primarily by testing skin reactivity to recall antigens in vivo or by assessing in vitro incorporation of ^{3}H-thymidine by mitogen-stimulated cells. Reported results are somewhat variable, although a common theme is reduced skin-test reactivity in iron-deficient hosts, with enhanced reactivity after iron therapy (41). In vitro proliferation data are even more variable, more often than not showing decreased mitogen responses (42). It is at least possible in these in vitro studies that enough iron is present in the culture media to sometimes correct defects in cells obtained from iron-deficient subjects. Thus, iron deficiency most likely impedes rapid cell proliferation during lymphocyte activation and in this way may adversely affect the course of an infection.

A more constant finding in iron deficiency is diminished activity of the neutrophil iron-metalloenzyme myeloperoxidase (43). This enzyme generates reactive bactericidal halide radicals during the oxidative burst of phagocytosis. However, this defect alone is not likely to be of clinical significance, because congenital absence of myeloperoxidase does not increase the risk of infection. However, iron is also required to produce oxygen radicals used in phagocytic bactericidal reactions (44). Therefore, iron deficiency may have more pervasive effects on neutrophil function than just reducing myeloperoxidase activity. As evidence of this possibility, reduction of nitroblue tetrazolium by peroxide released from activated neutrophils is abnormal in iron-deficient subjects (45). This deficit predicts abnormal bactericidal activity, and some investigators have found a modest diminution in bacterial killing capacity (46); contradictory data also exist (47). Other neutrophil functions, such as chemotaxis, phagocytosis, and degranulation, are consistently reported to be normal in iron deficiency, as might be expected if the effects of iron deficiency on neutrophils are specific and related to the biologic functions of the metal.

The amount of human data on iron deficiency and macrophage function is small. Animal studies have shown reduced clearance of polyvinyl pyrrolidone and impaired generation of oxygen radicals in iron-deficient mice (48) and diminished IL-1 responses in iron-deficient rat leukocytes (49). If these findings mean that iron deficiency can adversely affect macrophage presentation of antigens, then one consequence may be a negative effect on antibody production. Limited data in animals support this possibility (50).

Effects of Excess Iron

The evidence for nutritional immunity includes finding enhanced microbial growth in vitro or increased infections in vivo in conditions of iron excess (51). Impaired growth of bacteria in the presence of iron-binding proteins in vitro is reversed when excess iron is added back. Serum from hemochromatosis patients supports the growth of *Vibrio vulnificus*, which fails to survive in normal human serum. It also has been suggested that clinical iron overload states (e.g., β-thalassemia, sickle cell anemia with multiple transfusions, idiopathic hemochromatosis, or so-called Bantu hemosiderosis resulting from grossly excessive oral iron loads) are associated with increased infection morbidity (52). In these patients, transferrin is fully saturated with iron, and iron is readily available to pathogens from circulating low-molecular-weight, loose complexes of iron and albumin (53). However, more-careful analysis puts these clinical findings into question, since it is difficult to separate the effects of excess iron itself from associated hepatic or splenic dysfunction or effects of secondary diabetes.

Review of infection deaths in thalassemia patients shows that nearly all occur in splenectomized patients, long before significant transfusion siderosis could develop. When experimental iron overload states in animals are examined, susceptibility is increased, but only to certain organisms that do not produce their own siderophores and depend instead on available environmental iron sources (54, 55). This finding is consistent with the clinical association of human iron excess with severe *Yersinia* infections in both chronic iron overload patients (56) and in patients after acute oral ingestion of iron (57). Many *Yersinia* strains are of low virulence and growth restricted in the normal host (58), except when transport proteins are iron saturated and free iron becomes available. These strains can also obtain iron from iron-desferoxamine chelates, and an association between desferoxamine therapy and *Yersinia* sepsis has been reported (59). Organisms with analogous mechanisms of iron acquisition, including the bacteria *V. vulnificus* (60) and possibly *Listeria* (61), and certain fungi, including *Mucor* (62), *Rhizopus* (63), and *Cunninghamella* spp. (64), seem to be associated with iron excess states.

Immune function is probably impaired as well because of tissue-damaging oxidative and peroxidative reactions associated with iron excess. This decreased function would explain why neutrophils, which use iron-catalyzed reactions to produce bactericidal oxygen radicals, are less able to kill microorganisms when obtained from patients with iron excess. Thus, superoxide and hydrogen peroxide production and nitro blue tetrazolium (NBT) dye reduction are decreased in cells from β-thalassemia or dialysis patients with transfusion siderosis (65, 66). Chemotactic responses and random migration are also said to be reduced in thalassemic cells (67), and peripheral blood monocytes from subjects with β-thalassemia show diminished capacity to kill *Candida pseudotopicalis* (68) or *S. aureus* (69).

Clinical Data in Excess States

The malaria parasite spends most of its lifetime within red blood cells, in close association with an enormous pool of iron in the form of hemoglobin, resulting in lysis of erythrocytes and hemolytic anemia. Malaria, therefore, is a well-recognized cause of iron deficiency. A number of studies in Africa have noted an association between administration of oral or parenteral iron and a marked increase in the prevalence of malaria parasitemia (70–72). However, these studies have been criticized for lack of simultaneous placebo controls, failure to control for the presence of PEM and associated reduced transferrin levels, and lack of proper blinding of the investigators. Subsequently, the association of parenteral iron with increased rates of smear-positive malaria has been confirmed in a carefully designed, properly conducted, double-blind study in Papua New Guinea (73); a 64% increase in parasitemia rate in infants given iron supplements was observed, although the parasite density did not differ from that in the control group. An associated clinical significance was suggested by an increase in malaria-related hospital admissions, measles, otitis media, and pneumonia in the iron group (74). Another study in Papua New Guinea of total-dose iron-dextran infusion in pregnant women, who are at increased risk of malaria morbidity, also found higher risk of malaria parasitemia in treated than in untreated women (75).

Several more-recent studies of oral iron have failed to demonstrate a major clinical or parasitologic effect on malaria (76). In one study of prepubescent school children given 200 mg of ferrous sulfate or placebo, there was no change in parasitemia rate or density, level of antimalarial antibody, spleen size, or clinical episodes of malaria, but iron status improved (77). Another study in patients with malaria being treated with antimalarials confirmed the lack of effect of oral iron on the clinical course of the malaria but found an increase in other causes of morbidity in the iron-supplemented group (78). Since there was no improvement in hemoglobin, the authors concluded that iron was not indicated in acute malaria. In pregnant women, iron supplements did not increase the peripheral blood or placental malaria infection rate but did increase maternal iron and hemoglobin levels and was associated with an increase in birth weight by a mean of 56 g (79).

Because the parasites use the globin portion of hemoglobin for nutrition, relative depletion of hemoglobin in red cells due to iron deficiency may be a key limiting factor for parasite growth, whether or not heme iron is used by the parasite to meet its iron requirements (80). When iron is given to deficient subjects, hemoglobin synthesis and iron uptake are stimulated, providing both protein and iron for parasite development, because parasites too require iron for essential metalloenzymes (81, 82). This is the basis for the strategy of iron chelation for treatment of malaria (83).

Hemolysis is a known risk factor for bacterial infection, particularly salmonellosis, regardless of the cause of erythrocyte lysis (84), but this is not due to the presence of iron-hemoglobin in the circulation. Rather, it is because macrophages ingest the released hemoglobin, which results in a state of reduced macrophage phagocytosis and intracellular microbicidal defects, sometimes termed "reticuloendothelial" or "macrophage blockade." Consistent with this concept, hemolysis induced by the mouse malaria parasite *Plasmodium berghei* or phenylhydrazine administration dramatically increased the virulence of *Salmonella typhimurium,* whereas simple iron deficiency induced by bleeding did not (85).

Clinical Data in Iron Deficiency States

These examples indicate clearly that the relationship between iron and infection depends in part on the causative organism, the metabolism of the pathogen, and its ability and mechanisms used to acquire the iron it needs. Although iron deficiency adversely affects certain host defenses and most pathogens appear to be well equipped to compete for available iron stores, clinical examples in which iron deficiency apparently protects the host have been published (72, 86–88). However, contradictory results have also been reported (89, 90), with no difference being found in iron-supplemented or unsupplemented groups, while other investigators found increased prevalence and severity of infections in treated subjects (91).

Unfortunately, interpretation is difficult because published studies on iron deficiency and susceptibility to infection often are flawed in design, sometimes lack sufficient numbers of subjects to permit statistical analysis, or fail to control for the numerous confounders likely to be encountered in a field study. Thus, differences in the age of subjects, and route and form of the iron administered; failure to include simultaneous controls or to demonstrate the comparability of the control group except for iron status; presence of other nutritional deficiencies such as PEM; lack of laboratory confirmation of infection; use of imprecise criteria to characterize iron nutritional state of the host; and lack of correlation of infectious episodes with the severity of the nutrient deficiency or the effect of the supplement all complicate the final interpretation (92, 93).

Although conclusive proof is lacking, the impression from these various reports is that iron deficiency is likely associated with some increased incidence of common infections in children. Also, iron supplementation by the parenteral route in very young infants or use of iron chelators in disease states with iron excess appears to increase the incidence of some specific infections. There is no longer any justified rationale for use of parenteral iron in very young infants. Newborns normally have excess iron and highly saturated serum iron-binding proteins, they are immunologically immature and susceptible to invasive bacterial infections under any circumstances, and they are the group most likely to experience an adverse effect of the therapy. In addition, because severe PEM is known to result in reduced transferrin levels, it is unwise to administer iron in any form to patients with PEM while their iron-binding capacity is low. An association between low transferrin and severe systemic infection in PEM has been inferred (94), although such patients have multiple defects in all limbs of host defense. For these reasons, nutritional rehabilitation of PEM patients usually does not include iron supplements during the 1st week. This supplementation commonly is delayed until the 2nd week of treatment, when new protein synthesis is actively occurring and the circulating levels of export proteins, such as transferrin, are increasing (95).

Zinc

Like iron, altered distribution of zinc is part of the acute-phase response in infections, with the metal being rapidly removed from the circulation to an intracellular compartment primarily in liver, thymus, and bone marrow. This phenomenon is related to increased synthesis of the intracellular zinc-binding protein metallothionein (96), which is transcriptionally regulated by IL-1 (97), an important cytokine mediator of events during infection and inflammation.

Zinc is critical in the function of some enzymes involved in DNA transcription and RNA translation (see Chapter 11) (98, 99). Thus, shifting zinc to the intracellular compartment of lymphocytes may prime the proliferation of lymphocyte clones involved in immune responses and host defense. These important responses to alterations in zinc distribution may be affected by zinc deficiency, which can restrict rapid multiplication and clonal expansion of critical cell populations in the immune response.

Zinc-binding finger loop domains, known as "zinc fingers," are also involved in conformational stabilization of transcription-factor proteins, permitting sequence-specific DNA recognition and gene expression (100). Zinc deficiency severe enough to impede these regulatory signals further impairs the host response by limiting translation of proteins encoded by genes activated during the acute-phase response to infection.

Certain thymus-derived peptides, postulated to function as thymic hormones in the differentiation of T cells are noted above. These thymic factors are a family of zinc metalloproteins (101, 102), and their decreased production in PEM (which is almost always accompanied by zinc deficiency as well) may well underlie the T-cell maturational arrest seen in this condition. The depletion of mature T cells observed in other zinc deficiency states may be traceable to this defect. Zinc deficiency commonly results in lesions of skin and mucous membranes that disrupt these mechanical barriers and provide a route for both high- and low-virulence microorganisms to invade and initiate infection (103). Thus, in a number of ways, abnormal zinc nutrition can be related to heightened infection susceptibility and/or severity.

Effects on Immune Function

The relationship between zinc status and host defense is not well understood (see also Chapter 45). Whereas IL-1 induces metallothionein and shifts zinc from plasma to tissues, production and/or membrane binding of certain cytokines that regulate the immune system, including IL-1, IL-2, and IFN, may depend on zinc (104–106). However, careful systematic studies of zinc status, cytokines, and immune function have not yet been reported. What seems clear is that zinc deprivation in animals affects the thymus, which undergoes involution associated with splenic atrophy and lymphopenia (107–109). In the early stages of deficiency, cells are preferentially lost from the cortical regions normally populated by glucocorticoid-sensitive immature thymocytes. This change is actually independent of any glucocorticoid effect, because it occurs even when the adrenal glands are removed (110). Similar thymic involution occurs in Friesian cattle, a breed with a genetic defect that impairs zinc absorption and results in severe zinc deficiency, strongly suggesting that the lymphoid organ changes are in fact due to zinc deficiency per se (111, 112).

Despite an unresolved controversy over whether zinc deficiency affects particular T cell subpopulations (113), little doubt remains that the proliferative response to both T-dependent and T-independent mitogens is reduced (114, 115). This may happen in several ways, for example, indirectly by altered cytokine metabolism (116, 117) or directly by affecting lymphocytic DNA synthesis (118, 119). As a consequence of impaired T-cell function, delayed-type hypersensitivity responses are diminished in zinc deficiency (120); whether this is related to lymphocyte abnormalities alone or to additional changes in macrophage functions that are demonstrable in zinc-deficient cells is not clear (121, 122).

Consistent with these abnormalities in the immune system, increased susceptibility to infection has been reported in zinc-deficient animals experimentally infected with a wide variety of pathogens, including bacteria *(Francisella tularensis)*, protozoa *(Trypanosoma cruzi)*, helminths *(Trichinella spiralis)*, and fungi *(C. albicans)* (123, 124). Friesian cattle, nature's own experimental model for zinc deficiency and the equivalent of human acrodermatitis enteropathica (125), are also hypersusceptible to life-threatening infections.

Immunity and Susceptibility to Infection in Humans

Data concerning zinc and infection in humans are still limited. Most of the recent data have come from interventional trials in developing countries, in which zinc supplements have been provided to infants and children at risk of PEM with evidence of limiting zinc in their diet and low measured zinc in hair, nail clippings, or plasma. These trials were based on prior reports associating zinc deficiency, immune defects, and hypersusceptibility to infection. In one of the earliest reports in humans, zinc deficiency associated with geophagia in Iranian children was found to result in growth retardation, hypogonadism, and frequent infections (126). Subsequently, recognition of zinc deficiency in a series of clinical situations associated with immunologic deficits and infections, including acrodermatitis enteropathica, the clinical use of total parenteral nutrition formulas without added zinc, malabsorption states, Down's syndrome, and sickle cell disease, led to trials of zinc administration and have supported the notion that increased infections are associated with the lack of this mineral.

Development of a diet-induced zinc deficiency model in humans has helped establish this relationship (127). Dietary restriction of zinc results in negative zinc balance of about 1 mg/day, with a cumulative loss approaching 180 to 200 mg over a 6-month period. Because most zinc in the body is present in bone and muscle, only 200 to 400 mg is in a mobile exchangeable pool in the liver and the circulation. Because zinc is not stored in quantity, dietary restriction rapidly leads to a deficiency, mostly affecting tissues with high turnover rates such as liver and leukocytes (128). In some instances, abnormalities in zinc deficiency can be reversed by providing zinc supplements. For example, reduced serum thymic hormone activity in zinc-deficient subjects was related to circulation of inactive thymulin protein, and addition of zinc restored biologic activity (129). Similarly, the increase in immature T cells and decreases in the T4:T8 ratio, IL-2 production (129), and natural killer cell (NK) activity (130) are also reversed by correcting the zinc deficiency, as are the abnormalities in patients with acrodermatitis enteropathica.

These findings are consistent with observations in humans with genetic diseases associated with zinc deficiency, in whom thymic atrophy, lymphopenia, diminished NK activity and IL-2 production, decreased serum thymulin levels, and alterations in lymphocyte subpopulations are reported (129, 131–133). Alterations in the zinc-dependent enzyme nucleoside phosphorylase may result in accumulation of toxic levels of nucleotides, leading to impaired cell division or cell death (134). In addition, zinc-reversible chemotaxis and motility abnormalities of granulocytes from zinc-deficient rhesus monkeys and in experimental human zinc deficiency and acrodermatitis enteropathica have been described (135–137). Few data currently attribute immunologic defects in PEM to zinc deficiency, but the concept is plausible (138). These data include enlarging thymic shadows on radiographs or improved granulocytic function in PEM children after zinc therapy or increased skin delayed-type hypersensitivity reactions when topical zinc is applied directly to the test site (139–141). Interestingly, thymus gland thymulin content is diminished in PEM, although zinc levels are high and correlate best with infections (142). Experimental zinc deficiency in mice is associated with decreases in B-lineage cells in bone marrow (143); however, the residual cells respond appropriately to stimuli such as mitogens (144).

Zinc supplementation studies in poorly nourished infants and children in either community studies among low socioeconomic groups or in therapeutic trials in acutely ill subjects suggest decreased susceptibility to infection and/or shortening of the illness duration, primarily of diarrheal disease (145–150). Further trials are under way to evaluate the role of zinc in respiratory disease and malaria. Low levels of zinc have been noted in AIDS patients (151), and initial studies to evaluate the impact of zinc supplements in AIDS show an apparent reduction in infectious complications in one study but an increase in mortality associated with any level of zinc supplementation in another (152, 153). Because zinc may play important roles in HIV replication (154), the effect of zinc intake is clearly complicated and may have more to do with its impact on the virus than on immune responses. Further study is required.

Vitamin A

Animals maintained on low vitamin A diets are more susceptible to a wide variety of infections than those fed adequate diets (155, 156); vitamin A came to be known as the "antiinfective vitamin" soon after its discovery (157). On the basis of several field trials over the past decade, intense interest has focused on the potential use of vitamin A supplementation to reduce morbidity and mortality due to infectious diseases in humans. Vitamin A influences susceptibility to infection by alterations in both nonspecific (non-antigen-specific) and specific antigen-mediated host defense mechanisms. Vitamin A deficiency is associated with metaplasia of mucosal epithelia (see Chapter 17) and replacement of ciliated cells with keratinized cells; these changes reduce the efficacy of the ciliary ladder in clearing bacteria from mucosal surfaces. This is at least partly due to negative transcriptional regulation of keratin synthesis by retinoids. Furthermore, vitamin A deficiency alters production of mucous glycoproteins and/or other glycoconjugates. Thus, in vitamin A deficiency states, mucus-secreting cells are either reduced in number or replaced by multilayered keratinized cells. These changes are associated with a loss of the nonspecific barrier function of the mucosal epithelium.

Vitamin A also appears to be important in the normal functioning of the immune system. Vitamin A deficiency in animal studies has been associated with reduced mitogen-induced lymphocyte proliferation; delayed-type skin hypersensitivity reactions; reduced macrophage, cytotoxic T-cell, and NK cell function; and reduced B-cell proliferation and antibody production (158, 159). Fewer data are available regarding the specific effects of vitamin A deficiency on the human immune system. Abnormalities in T-lymphocyte subset proportions and reduced response to tetanus toxoid in vitamin A–deficient (xerophthalmic) children were demonstrated (160, 161). In South African children with measles, vitamin A–supplemented children had significantly higher total lymphocyte counts and measles-specific IgG antibody than controls (162).

Study of vitamin A and its effects on immune function has been hampered by the complexities of assessing vitamin A nutriture, especially during episodes of infection. Plasma retinol is a relatively poor indicator of vitamin A stores in the best of circumstances (163). During an infectious illness, plasma retinol values become essentially meaningless, as the circulating concentrations of retinol and retinol-binding protein (RBP) are reduced as a part of the acute-phase response to infection and inflammation, similar to the hypoferremia that rapidly develops at the onset of infection (164). Vitamin A–sufficient rats injected with endotoxin exhibit a 30 to 40% reduction in circulating retinol and RBP (165). Both poorly and well-nourished children demonstrate reduced plasma retinol levels during malaria (164). These findings have led to the suggestion that reduction of circulating retinoids and their distribution into extravascular fluids and tissues during acute inflammatory episodes may be an adaptive rather than harmful host response, delivering vitamin A to the sites where it is most needed. Other manifestations of the acute-phase response may contribute to losses of vitamin A, as some adults with acute febrile illnesses excrete almost 10 times more urinary retinol daily than afebrile controls (166).

How should these complex alterations be interpreted? It has been suggested that the acute-phase response may be beneficial overall to the vitamin A–sufficient host, accelerating tissue recovery, but when vitamin A status is poor to begin with, the resulting very low retinol levels may impair recovery and increase mortality (167). This assertion is largely supported by the results of human interventional trials (described below), in which morbidity and mortality benefits of vitamin A supplementation are limited to more severely malnourished subgroups.

Deficiency and Infection Mortality

The concept that vitamin A deficiency exacerbates mortality due to infectious diseases and, therefore, that vitamin A administration can reduce this originated from a large study of deprived Indonesian children over a decade ago (168). The proposition is attractive: a magic bullet to target the malnutrition/infection complex in developing countries. Over 3500 children were enrolled and then evaluated prospectively every 3 months over an 18-month period. Mildly symptomatic vitamin A deficiency was detected by the presence of early xerophthalmia (night blindness or the presence of Bitot's spots on the cornea). Children with severe xerophthalmia were treated immediately and excluded from the study; the remainder were followed. The prevalence of mild xerophthalmia increased during the first 3 years of life to a plateau of 7% and was associated with a fourfold increase in risk of death. This higher mortality was apparent even after controlling for differences in concurrent illnesses and PEM as assessed by weight for height. These findings were supported by a subsequent study among Sudanese children, which demonstrated a strong inverse correlation between vitamin A intake and mortality (169). The effects of "presymptomatic" (subclinical) vitamin A depletion on child mortality have not been studied, despite the availability of newer, more sensitive biochemical tests for measuring vitamin A stores, such as the relative dose-response assay.

On the basis of the observations by Sommer et al. (168), eight large-scale vitamin A supplementation trials involving over 100,000 Asian and African preschool-age children at risk of vitamin A deficiency have been implemented in the last 10 years (Table 97.4). The trial designs varied, and different doses and regimens of vitamin A supplementation were used. Six of the eight trials demonstrated significantly reduced mortality rates in the supple-

Table 97.4
Mortality in Field Trials of Vitamin A Supplementation

Author (Ref no.)	Vitamin A Dose (Age Range)	Country	Observation Period	Change in Mortality
Sommer (168)	200,000 IU 6 monthly × 2 (0–5 years)	Indonesia	1 year	−34%
Daulaire (171)	50–200,000 IU by age, once (1–59 months)	Nepal	6 months	−26%
West (172)	60,000 RE 4 monthly × 3 (6–72 months)	Nepal	1 year	−30%
Ramathullah (173)	8,333 IU weekly (6–60 months)	India	1 year	−54%
Vijayaraghavan (175)	200,000 IU 6 monthly × 2 (1–5 years)	India	1 year	nil

mented children, compared with the unsupplemented controls.

For those studies in which disease-specific mortality data were available, the largest reductions in mortality were seen in diarrhea-associated deaths (170–173). Lesser reductions were also seen in deaths due to measles and respiratory tract infections. Causes of death were determined by "verbal autopsy" methods, which depend on interviews and parental recall of events. While there may not be a better method of assigning causality, the reliability of "verbal autopsies" is less than that of clinical and pathologic methods (174).

It is unclear why the results from two of the trials, one in India (175) and one in the Sudan (176), are discordant. Among the possible explanations are differences in the demographics of the populations studied, including differences in the baseline mortality rates or the prevalence of vitamin A deficiency, other nutrient deficiencies, or diarrheal disease frequency or severity. In addition, the doses of vitamin A used in these trials may have been too small or too infrequent to adequately supplement the children. Finally, the study protocols themselves may have obscured differences between groups, since the most seriously malnourished children were referred for care and dropped from the study. The frequent contacts between field workers and villagers in control villages could have led to transmittal of health advice that may have been heeded; for example, in the Indian study, there was a significantly higher mortality rate among children who did not participate in the trial than among those who did. It may also be explained by basic differences in health-related behavior between those who elect to join a clinical trial and those who opt not to join.

Metaanalysis of these supplementation trials was reported in 1993 (174), prior to completion of the most recent study in Ghana (170), and in 1994 (177) including the Ghana study. Aggregation of all results, with adjustment according to study quality, yielded a highly significant reduction in all-cause mortality by about 30% (odds ratio 0.70; 95% confidence interval 0.62–0.79) (174) and by 23% in the second analysis (177). Figure 97.1 illustrates the results of eight individual studies and the combined results from metaanalysis (177). Overall, the effect of vitamin A was highly significant ($P < 1 \times 10^{-8}$). Recent placebo-controlled studies of vitamin A supplementation and mortality among very young infants in developing countries have produced more variable results. Among a group of 10,000 Nepalese infants under 6 months of age,

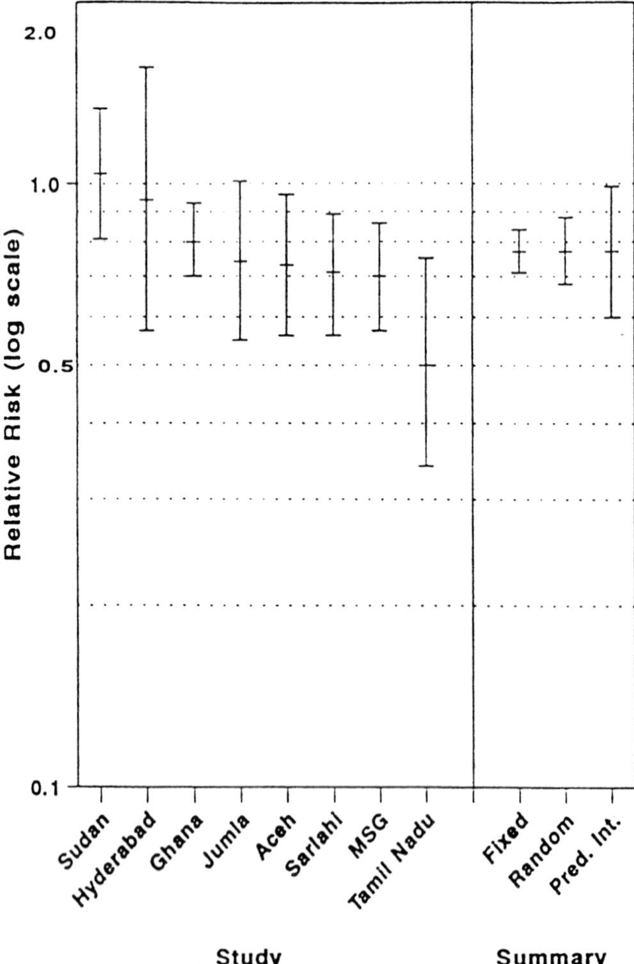

Figure 97.1. Mean change in young child mortality in individual studies and by metaanalysis of eight studies. Bars show the mean ± 95% confidence intervals. The overall effect of vitamin A, a 23% reduction in mortality, was highly significant ($P < 10^{-8}$). (From Beaton GH, Martorell R, Aronson KA, et al. Food Nutr Bull 1994;15:282–9, with permission.)

a single vitamin A dose had no impact on short-term mortality (178). By contrast, vitamin A given once at birth to Indonesian neonates significantly reduced 1-year mortality, although the total number of deaths in the placebo and vitamin A–supplemented groups was small, yielding very wide confidence intervals (179). Prophylactic vitamin A supplementation was of no benefit in preventing mortality due to malaria in Ghanaian children (180), despite the observation that acute malaria almost invariably results in a sharp drop in plasma retinol levels (164).

Deficiency and Infection Morbidity

Paradoxically, despite the marked reduction in mortality seen with vitamin A supplementation in poor children, an impact on infection-related morbidity has been more difficult to demonstrate. In the earlier observational study of Indonesian children, Sommer et al. (168) found that children with mild xerophthalmia had relative risks of 2 and 2.8 for respiratory and diarrheal disease, respectively, compared with children without eye signs. Subsequently, other groups examined the relationship between vitamin A status and morbidity with inconsistent results. Several placebo-controlled trials found no effect on morbidity attributable to vitamin A, even among populations that had significant reductions in mortality and in the same geographic regions where mortality benefits were seen (170, 179, 181–184). A randomized vitamin A supplementation trial was recently completed among a population of preschool-age Indonesian children (185) demographically similar to the group studied by Sommer et al. 10 years earlier (186). In the former study, an increased incidence of respiratory tract infection was found in the vitamin A–supplemented group, especially among adequately nourished children; there was no overall effect on the incidence of diarrheal disease (185). In other studies, vitamin A supplementation reduced morbidity due to diarrheal disease (but not respiratory disease) in children living in urban slums in New Delhi (187) and rural Brazil (188). It may be that vitamin A supplementation can reduce the frequency of severe and life-threatening illness among severely malnourished children without decreasing the frequency of less-severe illness (170).

A few studies have evaluated the role of vitamin A in infection in developed countries. Five small supplementation trials have been carried out, three in the United States and two in Australia—none are comparable to the use of vitamin A in developing countries. Two studies demonstrate modest but significant reductions in morbidity due to bronchopulmonary dysplasia in very low birth weight infants (189) or in preschool-age children prone to recurrent respiratory tract infections (190). Two more-recent studies failed to show a benefit of vitamin A compared with placebo in children with acute respiratory syncytial virus (RSV) infection (191) or a history of RSV in infancy (192). One study conducted among the elderly (193) demonstrated no effect of the supplement on the incidence of bacterial infections among a group of nursing home residents. Taken together, these studies suggest that vitamin A supplementation has little apparent benefit in reducing infectious morbidity in populations that are adequately nourished.

Vitamin A Deficiency and Measles Mortality and Morbidity

Measles remains a major public health problem in the developing world wherever measles immunization rates are low. Measles infects approximately 70 million children annually, and it is estimated that 2 million die each year from the disease itself or its complications. In addition to fever and rash, the consequences of measles include acute diarrhea or dysentery, pneumonia, encephalitis, and blindness due to acute vitamin A deficiency. Thus, in developing countries, case fatality rates may reach 10 to 20% (159). The interaction between measles and vitamin A deficiency was first reported in 1932 (194), and many subsequent reports have documented a synergistic interaction between the two (195–197). It is not clear why there should be a special relationship between measles and vitamin A status. It is possible that the marked disruption of the respiratory mucosal epithelium in measles causes a massive increase in vitamin A requirements. In addition, measles itself is immunosuppressive, and it may act in concert with the adverse immunologic effects of vitamin A deficiency to increase the severity of the infection (198).

Several studies have examined the effect of vitamin A supplementation on measles-associated morbidity and mortality. Two reports from Africa demonstrate that administration of a large bolus of vitamin A to measles patients at the time of admission significantly reduces the associated in-hospital mortality. In one study from Tanzania (199), 12 of 96 controls died, compared with 6 of 88 treated children; the difference reached statistical significance only for children under 2 years of age. However, in another report from Cape Town, South Africa (200), patients with measles seen within 5 days of onset of the rash complicated by pneumonia, diarrhea, or croup were randomly assigned to receive an oral dose of 400,000 IU of retinyl palmitate (equal to 120 mg retinol) or placebo. Twelve (6.3%) children died, nearly all from associated pneumonia; 10 of the 12 deaths were in the placebo group. Vitamin A administration was associated with a significantly reduced risk of death (relative risk, 0.21). In addition, recovery from pneumonia as well as from diarrhea was significantly more rapid in the treated patients. Furthermore, when disease-specific mortality was analyzed in the large-scale community intervention trials in India and Nepal, measles mortality was significantly reduced in one study (172), and a trend in the same direction was noted in a second (173).

The effects of vitamin A supplementation on measles morbidity has been addressed in two trials. In Durban, South Africa, 60 children under 2 years old with measles rash documented for 5 days or less and no history of vitamin A administration in the past month were randomly assigned to receive retinyl palmitate or placebo at the time of hospital admission (197). The baseline data, including reduced plasma retinol levels in over 90%, were comparable in the two groups. Subjects were seen in follow-up at 6 weeks, when another dose of vitamin A or placebo was given, and again 6 months after discharge. A total morbidity score was calculated for each visit, based on cumulative episodes and severity of diarrhea, upper respiratory infections, laryngotracheobronchitis, and pneumonia. Initial in-hospital recovery from pneumonia, diarrhea, and fever was more rapid in the treated group, and the morbidity score was 85% lower than that of the controls. At the 6-week follow-up visit, the morbidity score was 61% lower in the vitamin A group; at 6 months, the morbidity score was 85% lower in the vitamin A group.

Analysis of markers of immune function in a subset of these children revealed significantly higher total lymphocyte counts and measles-specific IgG antibody levels among the vitamin A–supplemented children. These markers correlate most closely with clinical outcome in measles (198). The findings are supported by a randomized placebo-controlled trial of high-dose vitamin A for children hospitalized because of acute measles in Nairobi, Kenya (201). Modest but significant reductions in complications were observed in the vitamin A–supplemented group, with decreased rates of severe tracheobronchitis and otitis media and faster resolution of diarrhea.

Based on these findings, it has been suggested that vitamin A supplementation should be routinely given to children in vitamin A–deficient communities at the time of measles immunization (197). However, another study demonstrated that a large oral dose of vitamin A given at the time of measles immunization actually reduced seroconversion to the vaccine (202). The suggestion was made that the supplement may have impaired the ability of the vaccine strain to replicate in the subject and thus reduced the immune response. In contrast, however, randomized, double-blind, placebo-controlled study of the effect of simultaneous measles vaccination and vitamin A supplementation showed no indication that vitamin A adversely affected measles immunity (203).

Vitamin A and HIV

The emergence of the AIDS epidemic in developing countries has focused attention on the potential of low-cost nutrition-based treatment strategies for populations unable to afford antiretrovirals and multiple drugs to suppress opportunistic infections. Considerable interest has centered around the potential of vitamin A deficiency to exacerbate or accelerate the immunosuppression of AIDS. There are some, albeit limited, in vitro data suggesting that vitamin A or its metabolites play a role in regulation of HIV gene expression and virus replication in human cells. Several laboratories have demonstrated that retinoic acid (the active intracellular metabolite of vitamin A) can inhibit transcription of HIV mRNA and replication of the HIV virion in tissue culture (204–208). However, the effect was not consistent and depended on the cell type studied and the experimental conditions employed. Some workers found that retinoic acid actually increased HIV transcription and replication (209, 210).

Clinical studies have repeatedly shown that plasma retinol levels in HIV-1 seropositive patients are below population norms (211–214). As a follow-up, Semba et al. (215, 216) showed that low plasma retinol levels correlate strongly with low CD4+ counts and mortality. Similarly, in Malawi, HIV-infected pregnant women with low plasma retinol levels transmitted HIV to their fetuses at a much higher rate than women with normal retinol levels (217). However, plasma retinol is neither sensitive nor specific for detection of vitamin A deficiency, especially during an infectious or inflammatory illness. Thus, the low mean plasma retinol levels in the patients with progressing disease or vertically transmitting HIV infection may simply indicate concomitant inflammatory processes (218). Indeed, one small study of 25 HIV-infected patients in the United States that used the relative dose-response test to evaluate vitamin A status determined that all patients except one were normal (219). A randomized, placebo-controlled trial of vitamin A supplementation in South Africa involving infants given placebo or vitamin A found significantly reduced diarrhea-related morbidity in the AIDS patients (220). However, it is unclear if this represents the correction of an interaction between vitamin A and HIV infection or simply a confirmation of previous studies demonstrating the effect of vitamin A on diarrheal disease morbidity in children with diarrhea (159).

At the present time, the amount of data is insufficient to conclude whether vitamin A supplements benefit AIDS patients, have no effect, or are harmful, and more studies are needed to sort this out. In pregnant women, the benefit of reducing maternal-fetal transmission is balanced by the increased risk of major fetal malformations in women given vitamin A supplements during pregnancy (221). A variety of effects of retinoids on viral replication have been shown, presumably related to the effects of retinoids on inflammatory processes.

Recommendations for the Use of Vitamin A for Infection

Although the metabolic changes that occur during infection are complex, vitamin A deficiency compounds the problems and may be crucial in exacerbating morbidity and mortality due to measles and diarrheal disease and possibly respiratory disease as well (159). The need for vitamin A–supplementation programs differs from one country to the next and must be assessed for each population, region by region. Implementation should be undertaken whenever there is clinical evidence of vitamin A deficiency in the population, wherever PEM is common, and wherever there is an excess of measles deaths. Further studies are necessary to evaluate systematically the optimal dose, regimen, and timing of vitamin A supplements in the population for prevention or modulation of infection (222). Most nutritionists will agree that the best long-term measure to improve vitamin A status of a population is to ensure adequate dietary intake. At this time, the benefits and principles for use of supplementary vitamin A remain debatable, awaiting careful and well-planned studies.

REFERENCES

1. Keusch GT, Scrimshaw NS. Rev Infect Dis 1986;8:349–53.
2. Serwadda D, Sewankambo NK, Carswell JW, et al. Lancet 1985;2:849–52.
3. Keusch GT. Immunologic mechanisms in infectious diseases. In: Stiehm ER, ed. Immunologic disorders in infants and children. 4th ed. Philadelphia: WB Saunders, 1996.
4. Gitelson S. Isr J Med Sci 1971;7:663–7.
5. Waterman SR, Small PL. Mol Microbiol 1996;21:925–40.
6. Rosen FS. Semin Hematol 1990;27:333–41.
7. Keusch GT. Semin Infect Dis 1979;2:265–303.
8. Keusch GT, Wilson CS, Waksal SD. Nutrition, host defenses, and the lymphoid system. In: Gallin JD, Fauci AS, eds. Advances in host defense mechanisms. New York: Marcel Dekker, 1983.
9. Keusch GT. Malnutrition and the thymus gland. In: Cunningham-Rundles S, ed. Nutritional modulation of immune response. New York: Marcel Dekker, 1992.
10. Parent G, Chevalier P, Zalles L, et al. Am J Clin Nutr 1994;60: 274–8.
11. Ozkan H, Olgun N, Sasmaz E, et al. J Trop Pediatr 1993;39: 257–60.
12. Mosmann TR, Chervinski H, Bond MW, et al. J Immunol 1986;136:2348–57.
13. Del Prete GF, De Carli M, Mastromauro C, et al. J Clin Invest 1991;88:346–50.
14. Romagnani S. J Clin Immunol 1995;15:121–9.
15. Hahn-zoric M, Fulconis F, Minoli L, et al. Acta Paediatr Scand 1990;79:1137–42.
16. Reynolds HY. Mayo Clin Proc 1988;63:161–74.
17. Keusch GT, Torun B, Johnston RB Jr, et al. J Pediatr 1984;105:434–6.
18. Keusch GT, Urrutia JJ, Guerrero O, et al. Bull WHO 1981; 59:923–9.
19. Potter J, Klipstein K, Reilly JH, et al. Age Ageing 1995;24: 131–6.
20. Cederholdm T, Jargren C, Hellstrom K. Am J Med 1995;98: 67–74.
21. Brain P. S Afr Med J 1979;56:149–54.
22. Weinberg RJ, Weinberg ED. Med Hypotheses 1986;21:441–3.
23. deMaeyer EM. Preventing and controlling iron deficiency anemia through primary health care. A guide for health administrators and programme managers. Geneva: WHO, 1989.
24. Weinberg ED. Physiol Rev 1984;64:65–102.
25. James BW, Mauchline WS, Fitzgeorge RB, et al. Infect Immun 1995;63:4224–30.
26. Kochan I. Curr Top Microbiol Immunol 1973;60:1–30.
27. Murray AM, Murray AB, Murray MB, et al. Br Med J 1978;2:1113–5.
28. Hershko C, Peto TEA, Weatherall DA. Br Med J 1988;296:660–4.
29. Keusch GT, Ann NY Acad Sci 1990;587:181–8.
30. Griffiths E. Iron in biological systems. In: Bullen JJ, Griffiths E, eds. Iron and infection. London: Wiley, 1987.
31. Bothwell TH. Nutr Rev 1995;53:237–45.
32. Neilands JB. J Biol Chem 1995;270:26723–6.
33. Guerinot ML. Annu Rev Microbiol 1994;48:743–72.
34. Gray-Owen SD, Schryvers AB. Trends Microbiol 1996;4: 185–91.
35. Chart H, Stevenson P, Griffiths E. J Gen Microbiol 1988;134: 1549–59.
36. DiRita VJ, Mekalanos JJ. Annu Rev Genet 1989;23:455–82.
37. DeLorenzo V, Wee S, Herrero M, et al. J Bacteriol 1987; 169:2624–30.
38. Wooldrige KG, Williams PH. FEMS Microbiol Rev 1993;12: 325–48.
39. Kay JE, Benzie CR. Immunol Lett 1986;12:55–8.
40. Neckers LM, Cossman J. Proc Natl Acad Sci USA 1983;89: 3494–8.
41. Krantman HJ, Young SR, Ank BJ, et al. Am J Dis Child 1982;136:840–4.
42. Sawitsky B, Kanter R, Sawitsky A. Am J Med Sci 1976;272: 153–60.
43. Yetgin S, Altay C, Ciliv G, et al. Acta Haematol 1979;61:10–4.
44. Fridovich I. Science 1978;201:875–80.
45. Celada A, Herreros V, Pugin P, et al. Br J Haematol 1979;43:457–63.
46. Water T, Arredondo S, Arevalo M, et al. Am J Clin Nutr 1986;44:877–82.
47. Van Heerden C, Oosthuizen R, Van Wyk H, et al. S Afr Med J 1981;24:111–3.
48. Kuvibidila S, Wade S. J Nutr 1987;117:170–6.
49. Helyar L, Sherman AR. Am J Clin Nutr 1987;46:346–52.
50. Kochanowski BA, Sherman AR. Am J Clin Nutr 1985;41:278–84.
51. Chart H, Griffiths E. FEMS Microbiol Lett 1985;26:227–31.
52. Barrett-Connor E. Medicine 1971;50:97–112.
53. Hershko C, Peto TEA. Br J Haematol 1987;66:149–51.
54. Robins-Browne RM, Prpic JK. Infect Immun 1985;47:774–9.
55. Fletcher J, Goldstein E. Br J Exp Pathol 1970;51:280–5.
56. Kelly DA, Price E, Wright V, et al. J Pediatr Gastroenterol Nutr 1987;6:643–5.
57. Mofenson HC, Caraccio TR, Sharieff N. N Engl J Med 1988;316:1092–3.
58. Carniel E, Mercereau-Puijalon O, Bonnefoy S. Infect Immun 1989;57:1211–7.
59. Paitel JF, Guerci AP, Dorvaux V, et al. Rev Med Interne 1995;16:705–7.
60. Amaro C, Biosca EG, Fouz B, et al. Infect Immun 1994;62:759–63.
61. Mossey RT, Sondheimer J. Am J Med 1985;79:397–9.
62. McDonald ML, Weiss PJ, Deloach-Banta LJ, et al. Cutis 1994;54:275–8.
63. deLocht M, Boelaert JR, Schneider YJ. Biochem Pharmacol 1994;47:1843–50.
64. Daly AL, Velazquez LA, Bradley SF, et al. Am J Med 1989;87:468–71.
65. Flament J, Goldman M, Waterlot Y, et al. Clin Nephrol 1987;25:227–30.
66. Cantineaux B, Hariga C, Ferster A. Eur J Haematol 1987; 389:28–34.
67. Khan AJ, Les C, Wolff JA, et al. Pediatrics 1983;60:349–51.
68. Ballart IJ, Estevez ME, Sen L, et al. Blood 1986;67:105–9.
69. Van Asbeck BS, Marx JJM, Struyvenberg A. J Immunol 1984;132:851–6.
70. Byles AB, D'Sa A. Br Med J 1970;3:625–7.
71. Masawe AEJ, Muindi JM, Swai GBR. Lancet 1974;2:314–7.

72. Murray MJ, Murray AB, Murray MB, et al. Br Med J 1978;2:113–5.
73. Oppenheimer SJ, Gibson FD, Macfarlane SB, et al. Trans R Soc Trop Med Hyg 1986;80:603–12.
74. Oppenheimer SJ, Macfarlane SBJ, Moody JB, et al. Trans R Soc Trop Med Hyg 1986;80:596–602.
75. Oppenheimer SJ, Macfarlane SBJ, Moody JB, et al. Trans R Soc Trop Med Hyg 1986;80:818–22.
76. Oppenheimer SJ. Acta Paediatr Scand 1989;361:53–62.
77. Harvey PW, Heywood PF, Nesheim MC. Am J Trop Med Hyg 1989;40:12–8.
78. van den Hombergh J, Dalderop E, Smit Y. J Trop Pediatr 1996;42:220–7.
79. Menendez C, Todd JA, Alonso PL. Trans R Soc Trop Med Hyg 1994;88:590–3.
80. Hershko C, Peto TEA. J Exp Med 1988;168:375–87.
81. Scheibel LW, Sherman IW. Metabolism and organellar function during various stages of the life cycle: proteins, lipids, nucleic acids and vitamins. In: Wernsdorfer W, McGregor I, eds. Malaria: principles and practice of malariology. Edinburgh: Churchill Livingstone, 1988.
82. Scheibel LW. Plasmodium parasite biology: carbohydrate metabolism and related organellar function during various stages of the life cycle. In: Wernsdorfer W, McGregor I, eds. Malaria: principles and practice of malariology. Edinburgh: Churchill Livingstone, 1988.
83. Gordeuk VR, Thuma PE, Brittenham GM. Adv Exp Med Biol 1994;356:371–83.
84. Bennett IL, Hook EW. Annu Rev Med 1959;10:1–20.
85. Kaye D, Gill FA, Hook EW. Am J Med Sci 1967;254:205–15.
86. Murray MJ, Murray AB, Murray MB, et al. Lancet 1975;1:653–4.
87. MacKay HM. Arch Dis Child 1928;3:117–47.
88. Andelman MB, Sered BR. Am J Dis Child 1966;111:45–55.
89. James JA, Combes M. Pediatrics 1960;26:368–73.
90. Damsdaran M, Naidu AN, Sarma KVR. Indian J Med Res 1979;69:448–56.
91. Oppenheimer SJ, Hendrickse R. Nutr Rev 1979;53:585–98.
92. Strauss RG. Am J Clin Nutr 1978;31:660–6.
93. Dhur A, Galan P, Hecberg S. Comp Biochem Physiol 1989;94A:11–19.
94. McFarlane H, Reddy S, Adcock KJ, et al. Br Med J 1970;4:11–19.
95. Torun B, Viteri FE. Protein-energy malnutrition. In: Warren KS, Mahmoud AAF. Tropical and geographical medicine. 2nd ed. New York: McGraw-Hill, 1990.
96. Sobocinski PA, Canterbury WJ Jr, Mapes CA, et al. Am J Physiol 1978;234:E399–406.
97. Cousins RJ, Leinart AS. FASEB J 1988;2:2884–90.
98. Liebeman I, Abrams R, Hunt N. J Biol Chem 1963;238:3955–62.
99. Beisel WR. Am J Clin Nutr 1982;35:417–68.
100. Schwabe JWR, Rhodes D. Trends Biochem Sci 1991;16:291–6.
101. Cuningham-Rundles S, Harbison M, Guirguis S, et al. Ann NY Acad Sci 1994;730:71–83.
102. Dardenne M, Savino W. Immunol Today 1994;15:518–23.
103. Hambridge KM, Casey CE, Krebs NF. Zinc. In: Mertz W, ed. Trace elements in human health and animal nutrition. New York: Academic Press, 1986.
104. Salas M, Kirchner H. Clin Immunol Immunopathol 1987;45:139–42.
105. Winchurch RA, Togo J, Adler WH. Clin Immunol Immunopathol 1988;49:215–22.
106. Driessen C, Hirv K, Rink L, et al. Lymphokine Cytokine Res 1994;13:15–20.
107. Dowd PS, Kelleher J, Guillou PJ. Br J Nutr 1986;55:59–69.
108. Dardenne M, Boukaiba N, Gagnerault MC, et al. Clin Immunol Immunopathol 1993;66:127–35.
109. Mocchegiani E, Santarelli L, Muzzioli M, et al. Int J Immunopharmacol 1995;17:703–18.
110. DePasquale-Jardieu R, Fraker PJ. J Immunol 1980;124:2650–5.
111. Brummerstedt E, Basse A, Flagstad T. Am J Pathol 1977;87:725–8.
112. Ripa S, Ripa R. Minerva Med 1995;86:315–8.
113. Keen CL, Gershwin ME. Annu Rev Nutr 1990;10:415–31.
114. Gross RL, Osdin N, Fong L, et al. Am J Clin Nutr 1979;32:1260–5.
115. Zanzonica P, Fernandez G, Good RA. Cell Immunol 1981;60:203–11.
116. Winchurch RA, Togo J, Adler WH. Eur J Immunol 1987;17:127–32.
117. Winchurch RA. Clin Immunol Immunopathol 1988;47:174–80.
118. Prasad AS. J Am Coll Nutr 1996;15:113–20.
119. Prasad AS, Beck FW, Endre L, et al. J Lab Clin Med 1996;128:51–60.
120. Fraker PJ, Zwicki CM, Luecke RW. J Nutr 1982;112:309–13.
121. Wirth JJ, Fraker PJ, Kierszenbaum F. Immunol 1989;68:114–9.
122. James SJ, Swendseid M, Makinodan T. J Nutr 1987;117:1982–8.
123. Salvin SB, Rabin BS. Cell Immunol 1984;87:546–52.
124. Fenwick PK, Aggett PJ, McDonald D, et al. Am J Clin Nutr 1990;52:166–72.
125. Moynahan EJ. Lancet 1975;2:710.
126. Prasad AS. Am J Clin Nutr 1991;53:403–12.
127. Prasad AS, Rabbani P, Abbasi A, et al. Ann Intern Med 1978;89:483–90.
128. Prasad AS. Ann Intern Med 1996;125:142–4.
129. Prasad AS, Meftah S, Abdallah J, et al. J Clin Invest 1978;82:483–90.
130. Tapazoglou E, Prasad AS, Hill G, et al. J Lab Clin Med 1985;105:19–22.
131. Moynahan EJ. Immunodermatology 1981;30:437–47.
132. Fraker PJ, Gershwin ME, Good RA, et al. Fed Proc 1986;45:1474–9.
133. Ballester OF, Prasad AS. Ann Intern Med 1983;98:180–2.
134. Cossack ZT. Eur J Cancer Clin Oncol 1989;25:973–6.
135. Viruwink KJ, Fletcher MP, Keen CL, et al. J Immunol 1991;146:244–9.
136. Baer MT, King JC, Tamura T, et al. Am J Clin Nutr 1985;41:1220–35.
137. Weston WL, Huff JC, Humbert JR, et al. Arch Dermatol 1977;113:422–5.
138. Woodward B, Filteau SM. Adv Nutr Res 1990;8:11–34.
139. Golden MHN, Golden BE, Jackson AA. Lancet 1977;2:1057–9.
140. Chevalier P, Sevilla R, Zalles L, et al. Sante 1996;6:201–8.
141. Golden MHN, Harland PSEG, Golden BE, et al. Lancet 1978;1:1226–8.
142. Jambon B, Ziegler O, Maire B, et al. Am J Clin Nutr 1988;48:335–42.
143. King LE, Osati-Ashtiani F, Fraker PJ. Immunol 1995;85:69–73.
144. Cook-Mills JM, Fraker PJ. Br J Nutr 1993;69:835–48.
145. Sazawal S, Black RE, Bhan MK, et al. J Nutr 1996;126:443–50.
146. Ninh NX, Thissen JP, Collette L, et al. Am J Clin Nutr 1996;63:514–9.

147. Sazawal S, Black RE, Bhan MK, et al. N Engl J Med 1995; 333:839–44.
148. Alam AN, Sarker SA, Wahed MA, et al. Gut 1994;35:1707–11.
149. Rosado JL, Lopez P, Munoz E, et al. Am J Clin Nutr 1997;65: 13–9.
150. Bandari N, Bahl R, Hambidge KM, et al. Acta Paediatr 1996;85:148–50.
151. Koch J, Neal EA, Schlott MJ, et al. Nutr 1996;12:515–8.
152. Mocchegiani E, Veccia S, Ancarani F, et al. Int J Immunopharmacol 1995;17:719–27.
153. Tang AM, Graham NM, Saah AJ. Am J Epidemiol 1996;143: 1244–56.
154. Zheng R, Jenkins TM, Craigie R. Proc Natl Acad Sci USA 1996;93:13659–64.
155. Cohen BE, Elin RJ. J Infect Dis 1974;129:597–600.
156. Bang FB, Bang BG, Foard M. Am J Pathol 1975;78:417–26.
157. Green HN, Mellanby E. Br Med J 1928;2:691–6.
158. Ross AC. Proc Soc Exp Biol Med 1992;200:303–20.
159. Semba RD. Clin Infect Dis 1994;19:489–99.
160. Semba RD, Muhilal, Scott AL, et al. J Nutr 1992;122:101–7.
161. Semba RD, Muhilal, Ward BJ, et al. Lancet 1993;341:5–8.
162. Coutsoudis A, Kiepiela P, Coovadia HM, et al. Pediatr Infect Dis 1992;11:203–9.
163. Olson JA. J Natl Cancer Inst 1984;73:1439–44.
164. Thurnham DI, Singkamani R. Trans R Soc Trop Med Hyg 1991;85:194–9.
165. Rosales FJ, Ritter SJ, Zolfaghari R, et al. J Lipid Res 1996;37:962–71.
166. Stephensen CB, Alvarez JO, Kohatsu J, et al. Am J Clin Nutr 1994;60:388–92.
167. Thurnham DI. Trans R Soc Trop Med Hyg 1989;83:721–3.
168. Sommer A, Tarwotjo I, Hussaini G, et al. Lancet 1983;2:585–8.
169. Fawzi WW, Herrera MG, Willett WC, et al. Am J Clin Nutr 1994;59:401–8.
170. Ghana VAST Study Team. Lancet 1994;342:7–12.
171. Daulaire NMP, Starbuck ES, Houston RM, et al. Br Med J 1992;304:207–10.
172. West KP, Pokhrel RP, Katz J, et al. Lancet 1991;338:67–71.
173. Rahmathullah L, Underwood BA, Thulasiraj RD, et al. N Engl J Med 1990;323:929–35.
174. Glasziou PP, Mackerras DEM. Br Med J 1993;306:366–70.
175. Vijayaraghavan K, Radhaiah G, Prakasam BS, et al. Lancet 1990;336:1342–5.
176. Herrera MG, Nestel P, el Amin A. Lancet 1992;340:267–71.
177. Beaton GH, Martorell R, Aronson KA, et al. Food Nutr Bull 1994;15:282–9.
178. West KP, Katz J, Shrestha SR. Am J Clin Nutr 1995;62:143–8.
179. Humphrey JH, Agoestina T, Wu L, et al. J Pediatr 1996;128:489–96.
180. Binka FN, Ross DA, Morris SS, et al. Am J Clin Nutr 1995; 61:853–9.
181. Rahmathulla L, Underwood BA, Thulasiraj RD, et al. Am J Clin Nutr 1991;54:568–77.
182. Abdeljaber MH, Monto AS, Tilden RL, et al. Am J Public Health 1991;81:1654–66.
183. Biswas R, Biswas AB, Manna B, et al. Eur J Epidemiol 1994;10:57–61.
184. Ramakrishnan U, Latham MC, Rajaratnam A, et al. Am J Clin Nutr 1995;61:1295–303.
185. Dibley MJ, Sadjimin T, Kjolhede CL, et al. J Nutr 1996;126:434–42.
186. Sommer A, Tarwotjo I, Djunaedi E, et al. Lancet 1986;8491: 1169–73.
187. Bhandari N, Bhan MK, Sazawal S. Br Med J 1994;309: 1404–7.
188. Barreto ML, Santos LM, Assis AM, et al. Lancet 1994;334: 228–31.
189. Shenai JP, Kennedy KA, Chytil F, et al. J Pediatr 1987;111: 269–77.
190. Pinnock CB, Douglas RM, Badcock NR. Aust Paediatr J 1986;22:95–9.
191. Quinlan KP, Hayani KC. Arch Pediatr Adolesc Med 1996;150:25–30.
192. Pinnock CB, Douglas RM, Martin AJ, et al. Aust Paediatr J 1988;24:286–9.
193. Murphy S, West KP, Greenough WB, et al. Age Ageing 1992;21:435–9.
194. Ellison JB. Br Med J 1932;2:8–11.
195. Inua M, Duggan MB, West CE, et al. Ann Trop Paediatr 1983;3:181–91.
196. Reddy V, Bhaskaram P, Raghuramulu N, et al. Am J Clin Nutr 1986;44:924–30.
197. Coutsoudis A. J Nutr Immunol 1991;4:111–23.
198. Coutsoudis A, Broughton M, Coovadia HM. Am J Clin Nutr 1991;54:890–95.
199. Barclay AJG, Foster A, Sommer A. Br Med J 1987;294:294–6.
200. Hussey GD, Klein M. N Engl J Med 1990;323:160–4.
201. Ogaro FO, Orinda VA, Onyango FE, et al. Trop Geogr Med 1993;45:283–6.
202. Semba RD, Munasir Z, Beeler J, et al. Lancet 1995;345: 1330–2.
203. Benn CS, Aaby P, Balé C, et al. Lancet 1997;350:101–5.
204. Towers G, Harris J, Lang G, et al. AIDS 1995;9:129–36.
205. Semmel M, Macho A, Coulaud D, et al. Blood 1994;84: 2480–8.
206. Yamaguchi K, Groopman JE, Byrn RA. AIDS 1994;8:1675–82.
207. Yang Y, Bailey J, Vacchio MS, et al. Proc Natl Acad Sci USA 1995;92:3051–5.
208. Poli G, Kinter A, Justement JS, et al. Proc Natl Acad Sci USA 1992;89:2689–93.
209. Turpin JA, Vargo M, Meltzer MS, et al. J Immunol 1992; 148:2539–46.
210. Maciaszek J, Talmage DA, Viglianti GA. J Virol 1994;68: 6598–604.
211. Sappey C, Leclerq P, Coudray C, et al. Clin Chim Acta 1994; 230:35–42.
212. Beach RS, Mantero-Atienza E, Shor-Posner G, et al. AIDS 1992;6:701–8.
213. Karter DL, Karter AJ, Yarrish R, et al. J Acquired Immune Defic Syndr Hum Retrovirol 1995;8:199–203.
214. Periquet BA, Jammes NM, Lambert WE, et al. AIDS 1995;9:887–93.
215. Semba RD, Graham NMH, Caiaffa WT, et al. Arch Intern Med 1993;153:2149–54.
216. Semba RD, Caiaffa WT, Graham NMH, et al. J Infect Dis 1995;171:1196–1202.
217. Semba RD, Miotti PG, Chipangwi JD, et al. Lancet 1994;343:1593–7.
218. Rosales FJ, Ross AC. J Infect Dis 1996;173:507–8.
219. Ward BJ, Humphrey JH, Clement L, et al. Nutr Res 1994;13:157–66.
220. Coutsoudis A, Bobat RA, Coovadia HM, et al. Am J Public Health 1995;85:1076–81.
221. Rothman KJ, Moore LL, Singer MR, et al. N Engl J Med 1995;333:1369–73.
222. Keusch GT. N Engl J Med 1990;323:985–6.

SELECTED READINGS

Beisel WR. Herman Award Lecture, 1995: infection-induced malnutrition—from cholera to cytokines. Am J Clin Nutr 1995;62:813–9.

Bendich A. Antioxidant vitamins and human immune responses. Vitam Horm 1996;52:35–65.

Chandra RK. Nutrition, immunity and infection: from basic knowledge of dietary manipulation of immune responses to practical application of ameliorating suffering and improving survival. Proc Natl Acad Sci USA 1996;93:14304–7.

Gallagher HJ, Daly JM. Malnutrition, injury, and the host immune response: nutrient substitution. Curr Opin Gen Surg 1993;92–104.

Keusch GT, Scrimshaw NS. Selective primary health care: strategies for control of disease in childhood malnutrition. Rev Infect Dis 1986;8:349–53.

Krenitsky J. Nutrition and the immune system. AACN Clin Issues 1996;7:359–69.

Lunn PG, Northrup-Clewes CA. The impact of gastrointestinal parasites on protein-energy malnutrition in man. Proc Nutr Soc 1993;52:101–11.

Semba RD. Vitamin A, immunity, and infection. Clin Infect Dis 1994;19:489–99.

98. Diet and Nutrition in the Care of the Patient with Surgery, Trauma, and Sepsis

WILEY W. SOUBA and DOUGLAS WILMORE

Nutritional support is defined as provision of nutrients using the enteral (delivery into the gut lumen via a feeding tube) and/or parenteral (intravenous) routes. This expensive and sophisticated technology was not available prior to the 1970s, and many patients who could not eat died from starvation and its associated complications. Today, virtually all patients can be fed because of two important technologies: *(a)* central venous catheterization and infusion of hypertonic nutrient solutions and *(b)* specific enteral formula diets that can be administered intraluminally through a feeding tube. Both parenteral and enteral formulations deliver all essential nutrients, and many patients who cannot eat normally live productive lives while being nourished exclusively by one or both of these routes. The justification for providing nutritional support to patients has been to prevent or reverse host tissue wasting, broaden the spectrum of therapeutic options, improve the clinical course, and prolong survival.

In spite of these advances, definitive indications for use of nutritional support in many patients, however, are unclear, and its efficacy in many circumstances is unproved. Nonetheless, use of enteral and parenteral nutritional therapies is widespread for several reasons (1): *(a)* protein-calorie malnutrition is common in a variety of hospitalized patients; *(b)* documented association between malnutrition and increased morbidity and mortality; *(c)* it seems intuitive that well-nourished patients respond more favorably to therapeutic interventions than malnourished patients; *(d)* nutritional support can be provided safely to most patients; *(e)* several randomized prospective clinical trials suggest that nutritional support benefits selected patients.

Unlike other groups of patients (e.g., cancer patients, patients with AIDS) in which a role for nutrition support remains controversial, use of nutritional support in specific groups of surgical patients is established. This chapter reviews the metabolic alterations that occur in patients undergoing elective operations, in patients with accidental injury, and in those with sepsis. Methods of nutritional assessment of individuals in each of these general groups are provided, along with current knowledge of the nutritional requirements of patients with these illnesses. The basis for selecting the safest and most effective route of nutrient administration is discussed, and newer methods of modifying the catabolic response to critical illness are reviewed.

IDENTIFYING THE PATIENT AT NUTRITIONAL RISK

Nutritional support is used most frequently in surgical patients as short-term adjuvant therapy to treat individuals who have preexisting weight loss or are at risk for developing malnutrition. The most common form of malnutrition in surgical patients is protein-calorie malnutrition (PCM), a state of undernutrition that results in a reduced body cell mass. PCM is common in hospitalized patients (1), and although its evolution during illness frequently reflects the severity of the underlying disease or toxicity associated with certain therapies, a cause-and-effect relationship between malnutrition and a poorer outcome has not been definitely established. Identification of PCM is based on objective measurements including weight loss (2), serum concentrations of proteins produced by the liver (3), anthropometric measurements (4), grip-strength, anergy (5), immunologic functions, body mass index, and nutritional risk index.

Patients become nutritionally “at risk” when their malnutrition reaches a point where they are at increased risk for a poorer clinical outcome than if they were not malnourished. As recently stated, it has been difficult to quantitate “at risk” malnutrition.

> No single measurement is highly sensitive and specific for identifying malnutrition. For example, although serum albumin values are used to predict nutritional risk and a low serum albumin concentration at the time of hospital admission can predict death and length of stay, hypoalbuminemia is not specific for poor nutritional status. In many patients weight loss does not increase their risk for developing treatment-associated complications. There is a strong relationship between the absence of a delayed-type hypersensitivity response and mortality but, despite mild malnutrition in anergic patients, nutrition support failed to correct the response and the cellular immune dysfunction. The clinical assessment (history, physical examination) of the patient is as effective a method for assessing nutritional status as are objective measurements [see also Chapters 54, 55]. The cheapest and simplest way to screen for malnutrition is to ask the patient about unintentional weight loss. If reliable criteria for identifying at risk malnourished patients were established, the value of nutritional intervention could be studied more scientifically. (1)

It has also been difficult to define the role of nutritional support because of the paucity of well-designed rigorous clinical trials. Many published studies suffer from problems with experimental design (inappropriate controls), heterogeneous study populations, small sample size, or inappropriate clinical endpoints or they are retrospective (1). Some studies have included well-nourished or minimally malnourished patients who were unlikely to benefit from nutritional intervention, thus possibly masking therapeutic efficacy.

ELECTIVE OPERATIVE PROCEDURES

Physiologic Responses to Surgery

Although cytokines clearly play an important role in regulating the body's response to stress, their role appears more significant in patients with major injury and infection. Therefore, the importance of cytokines in the cellular response to injury and infection is discussed in the section under trauma (see also Chapters 45 and 96).

Endocrine Changes and Their Metabolic Consequences

One of the earliest consequences of a surgical procedure is the rise in levels of circulating cortisol that occurs in response to a sudden outpouring of adrenocorticotropic hormone (ACTH) from the anterior pituitary gland. The pituitary gland is activated when afferent nervous signals from the operative site reach the hypothalamus to initiate the stress response. The rise in ACTH stimulates the adrenal cortex to elaborate cortisol. This hormone remains at 2 to 5 times normal levels for approximately 24 hours after a major operation (6). Cortisol has generalized effects on tissue catabolism and mobilizes amino acids from skeletal muscle that provide substrates for wound healing and serve as precursors for the hepatic synthesis of acute-phase proteins or new glucose. Associated with the activation of the adrenal cortex is stimulation of the adrenal medulla through the sympathetic nervous system, with elaboration of epinephrine. This circulating neurotransmitter is important in circulatory adjustment, but it may also elicit metabolic responses if the augmented secretion rate continues over a prolonged period.

In addition to increased circulating levels of epinephrine, norepinephrine levels rise during and following elective operative procedures (7). The excitement, pain, fear, and hypovolemia that may accompany the surgical procedure are potent stimulators of the sympathetic nervous system. Urinary catecholamines may be elevated for 24 to 48 hours after operation and may then return to normal. The major catabolic role of this regulatory system may be stimulation of hepatic glycogenolysis and gluconeogenesis in concert with glucagon and glucocorticoids.

The neuroendocrine responses to operation also modify the various mechanisms that regulate salt and water excretion. Alterations in serum osmolarity and tonicity of body fluids secondary to anesthesia and operative stress stimulate secretion of aldosterone and antidiuretic hormone (ADH) (7, 8). Aldosterone is a potent stimulator of renal sodium retention, whereas ADH stimulates renal tubular water reabsorption. Although the neutral and humoral mediators that result from tissue trauma may stimulate aldosterone release, afferent signals from volume receptors appear to be the major stimuli for these hormonal adjustments.

The ability to excrete a water load after elective surgical procedures is restricted (9). The usual postoperative patient concentrates urine to 1 to 2 mL water/mosmol solute excreted, corresponding to a urine osmolarity of 500 to 1000 mosmol/mL, even in the presence of adequate hydration. Hence, weight gain secondary to salt and water retention is usual following operation. Edema occurs to a varying extent in all surgical wounds and is proportional to the extent of tissue dissection and local trauma. Administration of sodium-containing solutions during operation replaces this functional volume loss as extracellular fluid redistributes in the body. This "third-spaced" fluid eventually returns to the circulation as wound edema subsides and diuresis commences 2 to 4 days after the operation.

Following elective operation, the response of the endocrine pancreas is altered. In general, insulin elaboration is diminished, and glucagon concentrations rise (10). This response may be related to increased sympathetic activity or to the rise in levels of circulating epinephrine, which is known to suppress insulin release (11). The increased sympathetic nervous system stimulation results in alterations in circulating mediators. The rise in glucagon and the corresponding fall in insulin are a potent signal to accelerate hepatic glucose production, and with other hormones (epinephrine and glucocorticoids), gluconeogenesis is maintained.

Postoperative hormonal responses are thought to orchestrate physiologic and biochemical changes that benefit the host. Salt and water conservation support the circulating blood volume. Augmented hepatic glucose production provides adequate essential fuel for the nervous system, red and white blood cells, and the healing wound. Skeletal muscle proteolysis provides amino acid precursors for gluconeogenesis and hepatic protein synthesis. Postoperative lipolysis provides abundant quantities of free fatty acids, as an additional energy source. Current techniques of postoperative care minimize, but do not reverse, these responses.

Stage of Surgical Convalescence

The period of catabolism initiated by operation, a combination of inadequate nutrition and alteration of the hormonal environment, has been termed the *adrenergic-corticoid phase.* This period is followed by onset of anabolism, which occurs at a variable time in the patient's convalescence. In general, in the absence of postoperative complications, this phase starts 3 to 6 days after an abdominal operation of the magnitude of a colectomy or gastrectomy, often concomitant with the start of oral feedings. This "turning point" from catabolism to anabolism is referred to as the "corticoid-withdrawal phase" because it is characterized by spontaneous sodium and free-water diuresis, positive potassium balance, and reduced nitrogen excretion. This transitional phase usually lasts only 1 to 2 days.

The patient then enters a prolonged period of early anabolism characterized by positive nitrogen balance and weight gain. Protein synthesis is increased as a result of sustained enteral feedings, and this change is related to the return of lean body mass and muscular strength. The positive nitrogen balance is usually in the range of 2 to 4 g of nitrogen/day in the average adult, representing a daily gain of 60 to 120 g lean tissue. The total amount of nitrogen ultimately gained equals the amount lost, but the rate of gain is much slower than the rate of initial loss.

The fourth and final phase of surgical convalescence is late anabolism, the hallmark of which is much slower weight gain. During this period, the patient is in nitrogen equilibrium but in positive carbon balance, which results from the deposition of body fat.

Effects of Nutritional Support on Postoperative Metabolism

Most patients undergoing elective operations are adequately nourished. Following an operation of the magnitude of cholecystectomy with common duct exploration, aneurysmectomy, or colectomy, oral feeding is generally not tolerated for 2 to 6 days. In a patient without postoperative complications, the duration of postoperative ileus depends on the extent of manipulation of the abdominal viscera and the length of the operation. Nasogastric decompression is frequently required, and the patient is routinely supported by 2 to 4 L intravenous fluids, usually containing 5% dextrose and appropriate electrolytes. Unless the patient has suffered significant preoperative malnutrition, characterized by a weight loss of more than 15%, or has had a major intraoperative or postoperative complication, solutions containing 5% dextrose may be administered for 10 days before initiation of enteral nutrition (EN), with no detrimental effect on outcome. With no dietary nitrogen and with insufficient calories, negative nitrogen balance occurs, in which urinary nitrogen excretion averages 10 to 15 g/day for 2 to 3 days, and then gradually diminishes. This nitrogen excretion is associated with a loss of potassium and phosphorus and indicates a loss of lean body mass.

Early investigators who studied the catabolic responses to operation concluded that the negative nitrogen balance was "obligatory" and an irreversible consequence of the metabolic response to injury. This view was challenged by data from two studies in postoperative patients. Riegel et al. fed patients who had undergone gastrectomy and neurosurgical procedures with tube-feeding techniques and showed that nitrogen equilibrium could be achieved when 0.30 g nitrogen and 30 kcal/kg were provided daily (12). Subsequently, Holden et al. nutritionally supported gastrectomy patients in the early postoperative period with intravenous nutrients and noted that body weight was maintained and near nitrogen balance was achieved when adequate calories and nitrogen were administered (13). These investigators concluded that the catabolic response to operation is largely due to inadequate food intake and is not an obligatory consequence of operative stress.

In general, if the patient is well nourished preoperatively and is expected to eat by the 10th postoperative day, 5% dextrose solutions provide adequate calories to prevent detrimental loss of endogenous body protein. Although a balanced nutrient intake administered in the postoperative period reduces the brief negative nitrogen balance associated with elective surgery and may maintain body weight, such an approach appears to be unwarranted in most patients undergoing elective operations. Such feedings have not accelerated recovery or decreased hospital stays in this group of patients. Therefore, the increased cost of feedings and the potential complications associated with intravenous nutrition cannot be justified. Jejunal feedings in the postoperative period may benefit some patients, especially those undergoing extensive upper gastrointestinal surgery. Such feedings are considerably less expensive than total parenteral nutrition (TPN) and can be administered safely. Studies evaluating the effectiveness of postoperative nutrition are reviewed below.

Nutritional Support of Elective Surgical Patients

Nutritional Assessment

The two major objectives of nutritional assessment are *(a)* to determine the patient's nutritional status and *(b)* to determine energy, protein, and macro- and micronutrient requirements. The nutritional status of a patient is determined by a careful history and physical examination, followed by additional tests to confirm the clinical impression (see Chapter 55). The medical history should include inquiries about associated disease processes, medication, and history of weight loss and dietary habits. The physical examination may establish the diagnosis of cachexia, protein-energy malnutrition, or specific nutrient deficiencies. Weight loss exceeding 10% of the weight before illness may compromise the patient's ability to combat infection or heal wounds.

Anthropometric measurements include measurement of body weight and height. The features are compared with population norms (14). Measurements of skinfold thickness are helpful to determine fat mass, and a 24-hour urine collection with measurement of creatine allows determination of the creatine-height index (CHI), a factor proportional to the size of muscle mass (15). More-sophisticated techniques to determine body composition include isotopic dilution methods, underwater weighing, total-body computerized axial tomography, and γ-neutron activation; these methods are not generally practical in routine screening of most elective surgical patients. Detailed evaluation of assessment procedures is given in Chapters 54–58.

Immunologic status has been used to evaluate nutritional status; total peripheral lymphocyte count, delayed hypersensitivity using a skin-test response to common antigens, and lymphocyte transformation have all been used to indicate immunocompetence in the critically ill patient (16). Depressed immune function often returns to normal with nutritional repletion, but altered immunologic responses are not specific for nutritional deficiencies and are observed in patients with advanced malignant disease or in those who have had a severe injury. Moreover, delayed hypersensitivity may return on resolution of the disease process, despite inadequate nutrient intake.

Laboratory tests are useful to confirm the clinical suspicion of malnutrition (see Chapter 57). Serum albumin and transferrin are the most common serum proteins measured, and they correlate well with body protein deficiency in isolated cases of malnutrition. Most nutritional deficits in surgical patients are secondary to a disease process, however, and the presence may alter these indicators. Other laboratory studies that may be useful in nutritional assessment include red blood cell indices to determine iron and micronutrient deficiencies, plasma glucose to assess insulin resistance, blood urea nitrogen to determine renal status, and liver function tests to evaluate hepatic function.

Determining Nutritional Requirements

Nutritional therapy should be directed to a specific goal; depending on the patient's nutritional status, this goal should be *(a)* to diminish the rate of weight loss and body protein breakdown, *(b)* to maintain body weight and protein stores, and *(c)* to achieve weight gain and anabolism. In general, patients with normal body composition (no major nutritional deficiencies) and who are not hypercatabolic do not develop significant nutritional deficits and tolerate isotonic dextrose solutions for about 10 days. For example, the uncomplicated postoperative patient may receive intravenous infusions of 5% dextrose in water or inadequate oral intake for this period of time without any detrimental effect on recovery or ultimate health. The malnourished patient who has lost more than 15% of normal preillness weight often requires vigorous nutritional support, however. The immediate goal in such an individual is nutritional maintenance; the ultimate goal is restoration of body mass, which generally occurs in the later phases of surgical convalescence.

Total energy requirements are based on several factors: *(a)* the basal metabolic rate, *(b)* the degree of stress imposed by the disease process, and *(c)* the amount of energy expended with activity. Available nomograms relate normal metabolic requirements to a person's age, sex, height, and weight (14). Once basal metabolic requirements of the nonstressed individual have been determined, additional factors such as the stress of the disease and hospital activity should be considered. These relationships are expressed in Table 98.1.

The principal influences on nitrogen balance in surgical patients are total energy intake, nitrogen intake, and the metabolic state of the patient. Energy and nitrogen relationships are altered in nutritionally depleted and hypermetabolic patients. Persons with nutritional deficits have intact protein-conserving mechanisms that allow nitrogen equilibrium when 7 to 8% of total caloric needs are provided as protein. This translates into a calorie:nitrogen ratio of approximately 350:1. Hypermetabolic, catabolic patients, on the other hand, have a diminished protein economy and require much more protein. For example, Duke et al. showed that in injured patients, protein contributes 15 to 20% of the total energy expenditure, such that the optimal calorie:nitrogen ratio is approximately 150:1 (17).

Route of Feeding

For patients who can eat and who have a functional gastrointestinal (GI) tract, adequate nutrition can best be provided by the regular hospital diet. This diet may be supplemented with between-meal snacks if necessary. Daily calorie counts and body weight determinations are necessary to monitor intake and the response to therapy. Some patients with a functional intestinal tract will not or cannot eat. Such patients include neurosurgical patients, those with oropharyngeal or esophageal obstruction, the elderly, and small children. In these patients, nasogastric or nasojejunal feedings may be indicated. Gastric feedings can be delivered five to six times daily by bolus feedings. Jejunal feedings require continuous administration. When permanent feedings are anticipated, a gastrostomy or feeding jejunostomy should be considered (18). A variety

Table 98-1
Formulas for Determinations of Total Energy Requirements

Daily energy requirement for weight maintenance = normal BMR × stress factor × 1.25[a]
Daily energy requirement for weight gain = maintenance energy +1000 kcal[b,c]

Normal BMR (basal metabolic rate, usually 1500 to 1800 kcal/day) can be determined using standard nomograms or formulas. The approximate values of the basal metabolic rate for adults of average size are given below:

Body weight (kg)	50	55	60	65	70	75	80
Normal BMR (kcal/day)	1316	1411	1509	1602	1694	1784	1872

Stress factor is the term used to correct the normal BMR for the effects of a disease process:

Condition	Stress Factor
Mild starvation	0.85–1.00
Postoperative recovery (no complications)	1.00–1.05
Cancer[d]	1.10–1.45
Long-bone fracture	1.25–1.30
Peritonitis	1.05–1.25
Severe infection or multiple trauma[d]	1.30–1.55
Burns >40% body surface area	2.0

[a]The basal caloric requirements of the stressed patient are adjusted upward an additional 20 to 25% for hospital activity and the stress associated with treatment. This adjustment is unnecessary for patients receiving artificial ventilation who are paralyzed or are heavily sedated.

[b]If anabolism and weight gain are the goals, an additional 1000 kcal/day may be added to maintenance requirements to provide for a weight gain of approximately 1 kg (2 lb)/week. Weight maintenance, not weight gain, should be the primary objective in most critically ill patients.

[c]1 kilocalorie (kcal) = 4.18 kilojoules (kJ)

[d]Proportional to the extent of the disease.

of nutrient formulas are now available for enteral feedings. In general, intact or partially hydrolyzed nutrients are most appropriate. These diets should be nutritionally complete and free of lactose (see Chapter 100).

Often, surgical patients require nutritional support but have a diseased or nonfunctional GI tract. These persons are candidates for parenteral nutrition, which can be infused through a peripheral or central vein. Peripheral venous feedings provide dilute nutrients in a large fluid volume and rely on fat emulsions as a principal calorie source. Central venous feedings consist of hypertonic glucose and amino acid solutions infused through a catheter placed in the superior vena cava. Adequate calories can be administered in a small fluid volume, but this method of feeding requires placement and care of a central venous catheter (see Chapter 101).

Formulating a Nutritional Support Plan

Most patients undergoing elective operative procedures recover quickly, resume oral feeding early in the postoperative period, and require no specialized nutritional support. Other surgical patients do not fit this description and require formal nutritional care. This group includes patients with preoperative malnutrition, those with dysfunctional GI tracts (prolonged ileus, inflammatory bowel disease), or those with specific diseases associated with a catabolic course (severe infection, major injury). These patients generally fall into one of these categories. In normally nourished patients, the nutritional goal is to maintain body weight and protein stores. In malnourished, nonstressed patients, weight gain and repletion of lean body tissue are indicated and are usually accomplished by providing an extra 1000 kcal/day. Anabolism is difficult to achieve in stressed catabolic patients, but body mass is generally restored simultaneously on resolution of the disease process. Hence, the nutritional goal in these patients is weight maintenance and treatment of the underlying disease process.

Perioperative Nutritional Support—Is It Beneficial?

Many of the studies undertaken to evaluate the effectiveness of perioperative nutritional support have study design flaws that make interpretation difficult. Collectively, these studies indicate that the vast majority of patients undergoing elective operative procedures do not require formal nutritional support. In those that do, enteral feeding is always the route of choice if feasible. There are specific indications for the use of preoperative and postoperative nutrition. Surgeons should be familiar with these indications and how to monitor during feedings (Fig. 98.1).

Preoperative Nutritional Support

Parenteral Nutrition. Randomized prospective clinical trials (19, 20) and a metaanalysis (21) strongly suggest that use of preoperative parenteral nutrition (PN) in severely malnourished patients, defined as those with weight loss exceeding 10 to 15% and/or serum albumin concentration below 3 g/dL, reduces the rate of postoperative complications. In one study (19), reduction in major postoperative complications (intraabdominal abscess, peritonitis,

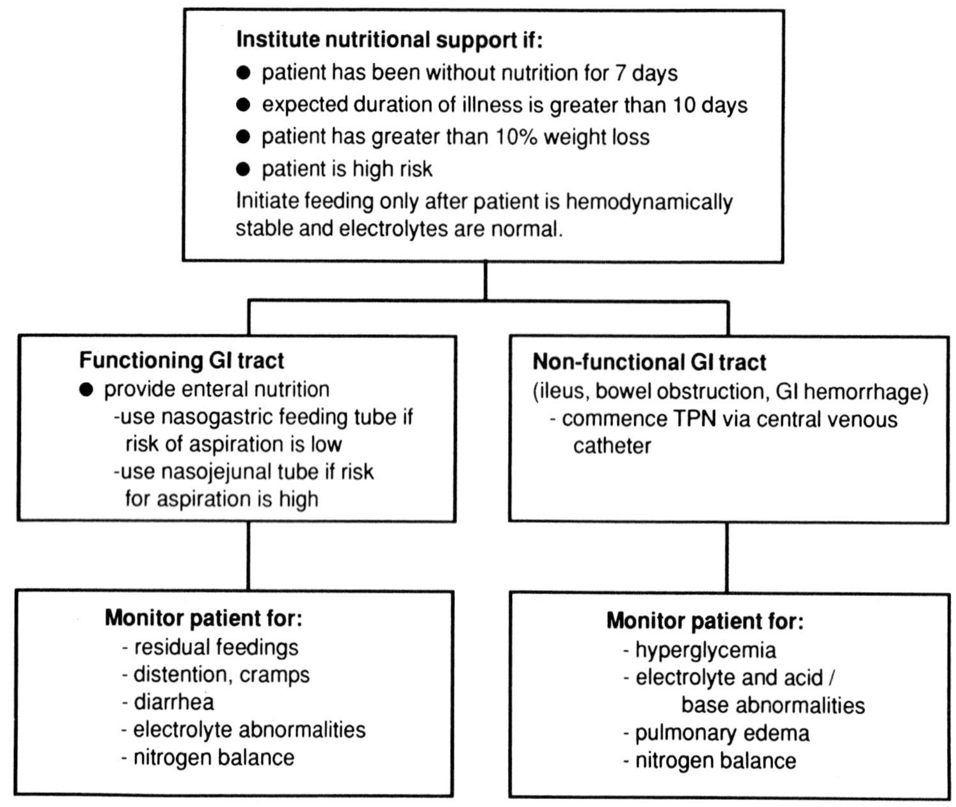

Institute nutritional support if:
● patient has been without nutrition for 7 days
● expected duration of illness is greater than 10 days
● patient has greater than 10% weight loss
● patient is high risk
Initiate feeding only after patient is hemodynamically stable and electrolytes are normal.
Functioning GI tract
● provide enteral nutrition
-use nasogastric feeding tube if risk of aspiration is low
-use nasojejunal tube if risk for aspiration is high
Non-functional GI tract
(ileus, bowel obstruction, GI hemorrhage)
- commence TPN via central venous catheter
Monitor patient for:
- residual feedings
- distention, cramps
- diarrhea
- electrolyte abnormalities
- nitrogen balance
Monitor patient for:
- hyperglycemia
- electrolyte and acid / base abnormalities
- pulmonary edema
- nitrogen balance

Figure 98.1. Nutritional management of the critically ill patient.

anastomotic disruption) was associated with improved serum protein levels and immunologic parameters and reduced mortality. This study has been criticized because it included well-nourished patients and because the actual nutrient intake by the control group was not apparent. The Veterans Administration Cooperative Trial (20) was a large multiinstitutional study, but it has been criticized because the control group (oral intake ad libitum) consumed fewer calories than the PN group. Unfortunately, none of these studies included a preoperative enteral arm.

Enteral Nutrition. Beneficial effects of preoperative nutrition were observed in two trials. The first study demonstrated that 10 days of a preoperative polymeric diet decreased the complication rate, death rate, and length of hospital stay in patients undergoing surgery for a variety of diseases (22). An Italian study by Foschi et al. (23) indicated that preoperative enteral hyperalimentation following percutaneous transhepatic biliary drainage for obstructive jaundice was beneficial. Patients in this study received an average of 20 days of enteral feedings via a feeding tube or were allowed ad libitum intake of a regular hospital diet. The patients receiving the enteral diet had a reduced incidence of complications (anastomotic disruptions and organ failure) and a decreased mortality rate. Although neither of these studies compared EN with PN, in the very small group of severely malnourished patients who may require nutritional support, the enteral route is recommended over the parenteral route.

Postoperative Nutritional Support and Its Indications

Rigorous studies evaluating the use of postoperative nutrition are limited. One study (24) in minimally malnourished patients with hepatomas showed that the combination of preoperative and postoperative PN resulted in a statistically significant reduction in infectious complications (pneumonia) and a decreased diuretic requirement to control ascites, compared with patients who ate ad libitum. The relative contributions of preoperative and postoperative nutrition to the observed benefits were not studied. In contrast, Brennan et al. (25) reported that use of TPN (vs. a 5% dextrose infusion) after pancreatic resection was associated with a statistically significant increase in the incidence of intraabdominal infection. Although the Brennan study had no enteral arm, it is apparent from this and other trials that postoperative undernutrition in the elective surgical patients is well tolerated for as long as 14 days. Sandstrom et al. evaluated the effects of postoperative PN (vs. a 5% dextrose infusion) on outcome in 300 patients undergoing major elective surgery (26). Some 60% of patients were eating normally by postoperative day 9—PN was of no benefit in these individuals. Patients receiving 5% dextrose for more than 2 weeks had a higher mortality rate and more postoperative complications. PN improved outcome in 20% of the group overall, but the authors could not identify these "at risk" patients by preoperative criteria. Thus, surgical patients who develop a postoperative complication that precludes oral intake for more than 10 days are candidates for nutritional support.

High-Risk Surgical Patients. Only an occasional previously healthy patient undergoing elective operation develops complications and subsequently requires nutritional support. Most such surgical patients requiring nutritional support are individuals at increased operative risk. For example, TPN can induce remissions in 60 to 70% of patients with inflammatory bowel disease, but bowel rest alone, as an independent variable from nutritional support, is not a major factor in inducing remission in patients with Crohn's disease, and long-term outcome is unaffected by nutritional support (1). There are no trials comparing EN with PN in patients with active inflammatory bowel disease. Other high-risk patients are those with diabetes, cirrhosis, heart disease, renal failure, or marked obesity and those known to abuse drugs or alcohol. In addition, immunocompromised patients should be carefully evaluated, and their nutritional deficits should be restored before operation.

A major complication observed in the high-risk patient is wound dehiscence. This separation of the wound is most impressive when it occurs following laparotomy. When abdominal evisceration occurs, the patient should be taken to the operating room, and the wound should be debrided and approximated. Because wound disruption is frequently associated with infection and results in a massive inflammatory reaction, caloric and nitrogen demands increase and should be provided by intravenous feedings.

Hepatic failure occurs most commonly in the alcoholic cirrhotic patient who has a major gastrointestinal hemorrhage that requires operative intervention. Although the origin of hepatic encephalopathy is unknown, central nervous system function may be influenced by circulating levels of amino acids (27). The branched-chain amino acids (leucine, isoleucine, and valine) circulate at unusually low levels in patients with liver failure, whereas levels of the aromatic amino acids (phenylalanine, tyrosine, and tryptophan) are elevated. The hypothesis states that branched-chain amino acids compete with neutral amino acids for uptake across the blood-brain barrier. Because of the low blood levels of the branched-chain amino acids, preferential uptake of several of the amino acids that serve as precursors for synthesis of false neurotransmitters may occur (28).

It is has been postulated that nutritional support may have beneficial effects on liver tissue and on the biochemical abnormalities that develop in the livers of patients with hepatic insufficiency and may improve survival. The principal data supporting this contention are from a multicenter study (29) in which the mortality rate in patients receiving PN enriched with branched-chain amino acids was 50% lower than that in persons treated with 25% dextrose and enteral neomycin. Results of other studies (30, 31) and a metaanalysis (32) did not show improved survival in patients receiving nutritional support. Collectively, the studies indicate that branched-chain amino acid–enriched formulas improve mental status in encephalopathic patients. Appropriate nutritional therapy for encephalopathic patients continues to be under investigation (see also Chapters 94 and 96).

When acute renal failure follows a major operation, the kidneys cannot excrete waste solute (nitrogen) or solvent, although occasionally, polyuric renal failure occurs. Provision of the usual amounts of amino acids in the diet exacerbates the already elevated level of blood urea nitrogen. These patients should be provided adequate nonnitrogenous calories to minimize protein breakdown, and nitrogen intake should be restricted if the patient does not require hemodialysis. Potassium, magnesium, and zinc are administered with caution. Solutions of essential amino acids (e.g., Nephramine) may improve protein synthesis and reduce urea generation. These amino acids are mixed with a 50 to 70% dextrose solution to minimize fluid intake and is administered through central venous catheters.

This renal-failure formula has been evaluated in patients with postoperative acute renal failure. Abel et al. reported that such PN improved survival rates and diminished renal dysfunction in patients with acute renal failure following aortic aneurysmectomy (33). In this prospective, randomized, double-blind trial, patients given glucose and essential amino acids had a better chance of surviving acute renal failure than those receiving only glucose (75 vs 44%; $P = .02$). These results may only be applicable to a select group of individuals with postoperative acute renal failure, as other studies have failed to observe similar beneficial effects of essential amino acids in patients with acute renal failure (34, 35) (see also Chapter 89).

What Is the Optimal Route of Delivery of Nutritional Formulations?

The recommendation that the enteral route be preferentially used (when the gut is usable and functional) for nutritional support is based on studies in injured patients (see below). The effects of TPN on the human GI tract include decreased brush border hydrolase activity (36), reduced amino acid transporter activity (37), increased mucosal permeability (38), and a slight decrease in villus height (38). The splanchnic response to endotoxin appears to be exaggerated in volunteers fed parenterally, compared with subjects fed enterally, suggesting that TPN may amplify the metabolic alterations that develop during sepsis (39). Several studies (20, 21) have shown that intravenous nutrition increases the risk of septic complications. Thus, it seems prudent to use the enteral route of feeding unless use of the gut is contraindicated (e.g., bowel obstruction, intractable diarrhea, inadequate surface area, feeding intolerance).

TRAUMA

Usual Response to Injury

General Overview and Time Course

Accidental injury is followed by a well-described pattern of physiologic responses. The events are generally related to the severity of injury; that is, the greater the insult, the more pronounced the specific response (Fig. 98.2). Alterations following injury were first described in the 1860s, but not until the 1930s were changes in injured humans carefully studied and an integrated response pattern described. Cuthbertson studied patients with long-bone fractures and reported that these patients lost large quantities of nitrogen, potassium, and phosphorus in their urine following injury and that this accelerated excretion rate could not be reversed by vigorous oral feeding (40). Cuthbertson also noted that the injured patient's oxygen consumption gradually rose, with simultaneous elevation in body temperature. Because no apparent site of infection was identified, this febrile response was referred to as "posttraumatic fever." Cuthbertson described the time course for many of posttraumatic responses, and two distinct periods were identified. An early ebb or shock phase was usually of short duration (12 to 24 hours) and occurred immediately following injury. Blood pressure, cardiac output, body temperature, and oxygen consumption were reduced. These events were often associated with hemorrhage and resulted in hypoperfusion and lactic acidosis. With restoration of blood volume, ebb-phase alterations gave way to more accelerated responses. The flow phase was then characterized by hypermetabolism, increased cardiac output, increased urinary nitrogen losses, altered glucose metabolism, and accelerated tissue catabolism (Table 98.2).

The flow-phase responses to accidental injury are similar to those seen following elective operation; however, the response to injury is usually much more intensive and extends over a long period of time. For example, following soft tissue injury, patients often have an impaired ability to excrete a water load because of heightened elaboration of aldosterone and ADH. The retention of large quantities of sodium and water that may occur during fluid resuscitation results in a dramatic increase in body weight, which may rise 10 to 20% over the preinjury weight. During recovery, the edema fluid reenters the vascular compartment, and the salt and water load is gradually excreted by the kidneys. Although sodium and water retention may occur following elective operation, the magnitude is much lower, and subsequent events (fluid mobilization followed by volume expansion and diuresis) are much less dramatic than in injured patients.

Characteristics of the Flow Phase of the Injury Response

The flow phase is characterized by hypermetabolism and alterations in the metabolism of glucose, protein, and fat.

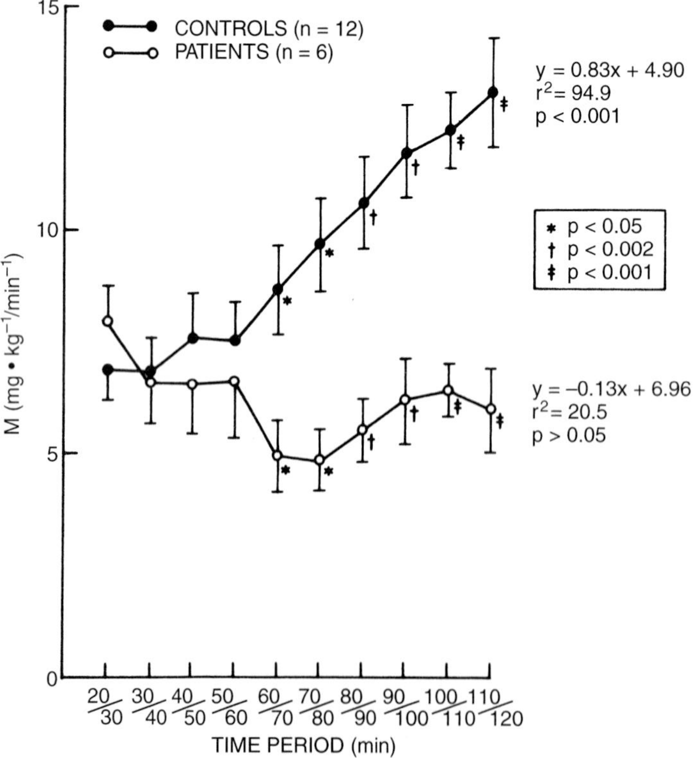

Figure 98.2. With time, the rate of glucose disposal *(M)* progressively increases in the control subjects during the hyperglycemic glucose clamp. In contrast, glucose removal was constant in these patients over the 2 hours of study and averaged approximately 7 mg/kg/min. (From Black PR, Brooks DC, Bessey PQ, et al. Ann Surg 1982;196:420–33, with permission.)

Table 98.2
Metabolic Alterations following Injury

Ebb Phase	Flow Phase
Blood glucose elevated	Glucose normal or slightly elevated
Glucose production normal	Glucose production increased
Free fatty acids elevated	Free fatty acids normal or slightly elevated; flux increased
Insulin concentration low	Insulin concentration normal or elevated
Catecholamines and glucagon elevated	Catecholamines high normal or elevated glucagon elevated
Blood lactate elevated	Blood lactate normal
Oxygen consumption depressed	Oxygen consumption elevated
Cardiac output below normal	Cardiac output increased
Core temperature below normal	Core temperature elevated

Hypermetabolism. Hypermetabolism is defined as an increase in basal metabolic rate (BMR) above that predicted on the basis of age, sex, and body size. Metabolic rate is usually determined by measuring the exchange of respiratory gases and by calculating heat production from oxygen consumption and carbon dioxide production (see Chapter 5). The degree of hypermetabolism (increased oxygen production) is generally related to the severity of the injury. Patients with long-bone fractures have a 15 to 25% increase in metabolic rate, whereas the metabolic needs of patients with multiple injuries increase by 50%. Patients with severe burn injury (more than 50% of body surface area [BSA]) have resting metabolic rates that may reach twice basal levels (14). These rates of heat production in trauma patients are contrasted with those in postoperative patients, who rarely increase their BMR by more than 10 to 15% following operation.

Concomitant with development of hypermetabolism, the trauma patient usually develops a 1 to 2°C elevation in body temperature. This posttraumatic fever is a well-recognized component of the injury response and represents an upward shift in the thermoregulatory setpoint of the brain (41). In general, if the patient is asymptomatic, the fever will rarely be treated.

Altered Glucose Metabolism. Hyperglycemia commonly occurs following injury, and the elevation of fasting blood sugar levels generally parallels the severity of stress in the ebb phase. At that time, insulin levels are low, and glucose production is only slightly elevated (42). Later, during the flow phase, insulin concentrations are normal or elevated; yet, hyperglycemia persists. This phenomenon suggests an alteration in the relationship between insulin sensitivity and glucose disposal. Hepatic glucose production is increased (43), and the accelerated gluconeogenesis is generally related to the extent of the injury. Studies in injured patients show that much of the new glucose generated by the liver arises from 3-carbon precursors (lactate, pyruvate, amino acids, and glycerol) released from peripheral tissues (43).

To determine which peripheral tissues use the large quantity of glucose produced by the liver, investigators measured substrate exchange across injured and uninjured extremities of severely burned patients matched for age, weight, and extent of total-body-surface burn (44). Net glucose flux across uninjured extremities was low, suggesting that fat, not glucose, is the primary fuel for resting skeletal muscle in the postabsorptive state. Similar observations have been made in a study of normal volunteers; however, glucose uptake was increased across the burned extremity. In addition, the injured extremity released large quantities of lactate, which accounted for as much as 80% of the glucose consumed. This finding is consistent with our knowledge of the biochemistry of the specialized cells of the wound and inflammatory tissue (fibroblasts, macrophages, leukocytes), which undergo anaerobic metabolism and have a large capacity for lactate production. Additional measurements of blood flow and substrate concentration differences across the kidney and the brain further characterized the glucose disposal in stable trauma patients. (44, 45). The glucose consumed by the central nervous system in the injured patient is approximately normal (120 g/day), whereas that consumed by kidney is approximately twice normal (75 g/day). Only a small fraction of the glucose is taken up by the resting skeletal muscle, and the remainder is consumed by the wound. The wound converts most of the glucose to lactate, which is recycled to glucose in the liver via the Cori cycle.

These alterations in glucose metabolism have a profound impact on the handling of exogenously administered glucose contained in enteral or parenteral feedings. To characterize glucose disposal during the flow phase of injury, six traumatized patients who did not have sepsis were studied by means of the hyperglycemic glucose "clamp" technique for 5 to 10 days after the injury (46). The results were compared with those from 11 age-matched control subjects. After an overnight fast, a 20% glucose solution was infused intravenously to elevate plasma glucose concentrations suddenly to 125 mg/dL above basal levels. This elevation was maintained for 2 hours with bedside glucose monitoring and negative feedback servocontrol. The results showed a progressive increase in glucose disposal with time in normal control subjects, whereas the injured patients maintained a constant glucose disposal throughout the study (Fig. 98.2). Moreover, the quantity of insulin elaborated in the patients was greater than in control subjects; nonetheless, the rising insulin concentrations failed to increase glucose clearance in these patients.

Other studies have demonstrated a failure to suppress hepatic glucose production in trauma patients during glucose loading or insulin infusion (47). Either of these perturbations usually inhibits hepatic glucose production in normal subjects. Wolfe et al., using tracer methods, found that endogenous suppression comprised only 73% of the infused glucose load in burn patients (2.6 mg/kg/min) (48). This rate of glucose infusion completely suppresses

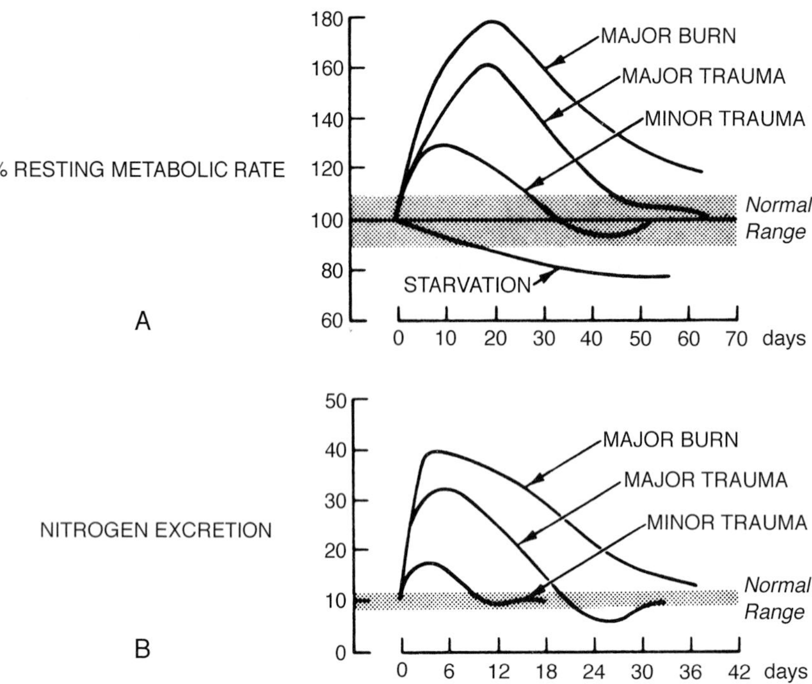

Figure 98.3. Metabolic rate *(A)* and nitrogen excretion *(B)* are related to the extent of injury. The two responses generally parallel each other. Patients received 12 g nitrogen daily. (From Wilmore DW. The metabolic management of the critically ill. New York: Plenum Medical Book, 1977, with permission.)

glucose production in normal subjects. When investigators used the hyperglycemic glucose "clamp" technique combined with tracer methods, endogenous glucose production was only partially reduced in trauma patients, in spite of high concentrations of both glucose and insulin (46).

To quantitate the insulin resistance in peripheral tissues, Brooks et al. measured glucose uptake across the uninjured forearm in conjunction with hyperinsulinemic-euglycemic clamp studies in 11 normal subjects and 5 patients with multiple trauma (49). Glucose uptake by uninjured forearm skeletal muscle of trauma patients was much lower than that observed in control subjects.

Thus, profound insulin insensitivity occurs in injured patients. Direct measurements show that liver and skeletal muscle are resistant tissues, and studies by Carpentier et al. suggest that lipolysis is not attenuated in trauma patients after glucose administration (50). The cause of this marked insensitivity to insulin is unknown; however, similar effects are observed following alterations in the hormonal environment. For example, insulin-mediated forearm glucose uptake is diminished in normal subjects following 2 hours of epinephrine infusion (51). Similarly, 3 days of glucocorticoid administration decreases glucose consumption (52).

Alterations in Protein Metabolism. Extensive urinary nitrogen loss occurs following major injury. Because of the magnitude of these losses and the progressive wasting of skeletal muscle mass and associated muscle weakness, it was originally hypothesized that the nitrogen loss represented a generalized and accelerated breakdown of muscle protein. Like other responses, the loss of nitrogen following injury is related to the extent of the trauma, but it also depends on the previous nutritional status, as well as the age and sex, of the patient, because these factors determine, in part, the size of the muscle mass (Fig. 98.3).

Although nitrogen balance studies demonstrate marked negative nitrogen balance following injury, these studies reflect only net nitrogen catabolism, not the absolute rate of nitrogen breakdown. In normal subjects, nitrogen equilibrium is maintained by a careful balance between rates of protein synthesis and rates of degradation. Negative nitrogen balance occurs if the breakdown rate increases and protein synthesis remains the same or if the breakdown rate remains the same and the rate of synthesis decreases. The use of isotopically labeled, nonradioactive amino acids allows quantification of the alterations in synthesis and breakdown rates associated with many disease processes. Herrmann et al. (53) administered ^{15}N-glycine to achieve a steady state and measured ^{15}N-urea nitrogen enrichment using the two-pool model of Picou and Taylor-Roberts (54). Turnover rates of protein were measured, and rates of synthesis and catabolism were calculated in fed and fasted states in normal subjects. During feeding, synthesis and catabolism were equal. Restriction of food intake caused a marked reduction in synthesis, with minimal impact on rates of protein catabolism. Birkhahn et al. described protein kinetics in four patients following multisystemic injury, including long-bone fractures (55). In contrast to patients undergoing elective orthopaedic operations, these patients had a marked increase in catabolic rate and a slight increase in synthesis; because catabolism exceeded synthesis, the patients were in marked negative nitrogen balance while receiving standard infusions of 5% dextrose and water.

Thus, trauma accelerates nitrogen turnover. In unfed patients, breakdown rates exceed synthesis, and negative balance results. Providing exogenous calories and nitrogen increases synthesis, and when adequate nutrients are provided, the two rates are matched and nitrogen balance is maintained (Table 98.3).

Cuthbertson (56) initially suggested that the nitrogen lost in the urine following extensive injury originates in muscle. In his patients with long-bone fractures, he suggested that this reaction was a uniform response of the entire muscle mass, and nitrogen was not lost solely from damaged muscle at the site of injury. This concept is supported by a variety of studies that measured important markers of muscle catabolism, such as creatinine, creatine, zinc, and 3-methylhistidine. Further evidence of net skeletal muscle breakdown comes from quantification of amino acid loss from extremities of severely injured patients. Aulick and Wilmore used plethysmographic techniques to measure leg blood flow and simultaneously determine arterial and femoral venous amino acid concentrations in traumatized patients (57). They found a three- to fourfold higher amino acid flux from the extremities of injured patients than from normal subjects. Alanine efflux was the most highly elevated of the amino acids measured, but glutamine was not measured. The increase in alanine release from the legs of severely traumatized patients was generally related to the extent of injury and the oxygen consumption of the patient, but it was not related to the size of the limb injury or to blood flow in the leg. The accelerated rate of α-amino nitrogen release from the limbs of these patients appeared to be a generalized catabolic effect of injury, rather than a response to local inflammatory or metabolic events in the injured extremities. This response may be the result of chronic hypercortisolism, which occurs in injury.

Using dogs catheterized on a long-term basis to study hindquarter amino acid metabolism, Muhlbacher et al. observed that long-term administration of dexamethasone (a potent glucocorticoid) resulted in a fourfold increase in glutamine and alanine release from skeletal muscle (58). Although glutamine stores in muscle were reduced by 50% within 10 to 14 days, the accelerated glutamine release was exceeded by an accelerated consumption of this amino acid, and plasma glutamine levels fell by 30%.

Table 98.3
Alterations in Rates of Protein Synthesis and Catabolism That May Affect Hospitalized Patients

	Synthesis[a]	Catabolism
Normal: patient starved	↓	o
Normal: patient fed, during bedrest	↓	o
Elective surgical procedure	↓	o
Injury/sepsis: patient receiving intravenous dextrose	↑↑	↑↑↑
Injury/sepsis: patient fed	↑↑↑	↑↑↑

[a]↓, decrease; 0, no charge; ↑, increase.

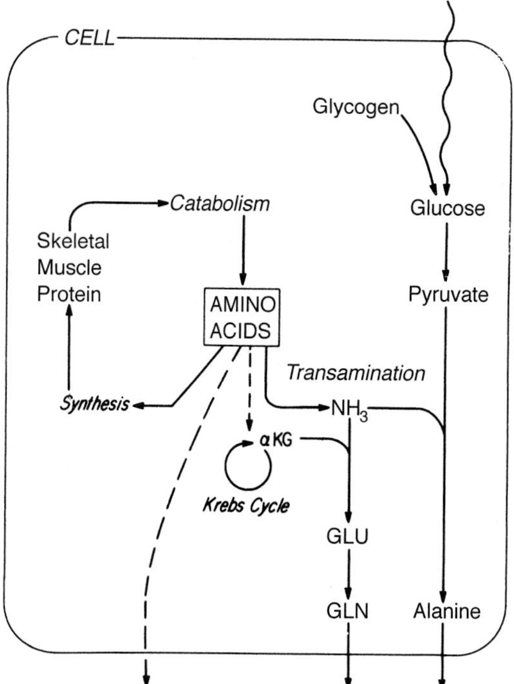

Figure 98.4. Major biochemical reactions that lead to synthesis of glutamine *(GLN)* and alanine in skeletal muscle.

Although it is now recognized that amino acids are released by muscle in increased quantities following injury, it has only recently been appreciated that the composition of amino acid efflux does not reflect the composition of muscle protein. Alanine and glutamine comprise 50 to 60% of amino acids released, whereas each makes up only about 6% of muscle protein. The branched-chain amino acids (valine, leucine, and isoleucine), on the other hand, make up approximately 6% of the released amino acids, but constitute nearly 15% of muscle protein. To explain these observations, Goldberg and Chang proposed that the branched-chain amino acids serve as amino donors for α-ketoglutarate, yielding the corresponding branched-chain ketoacids and glutamate (59). The ketoacids can be converted to tricarboxylic-cycle intermediates in skeletal muscle, or they can be exported through the circulation. Glutamate may be a precursor for glutamine synthesis or an amino donor for alanine synthesis. These coupled reactions could explain the synthesis and increased release of alanine and glutamine as well as the diminished release of branched-chain amino acids (Fig. 98.4). Oxidation of branched-chain amino acids by skeletal muscle is accelerated following injury (60), and skeletal muscle release of glutamine and alanine is increased. (See also Chapter 35.)

Glutamine is also extracted by the kidney, where it contributes ammonium groups for ammonia generation, a process that excretes acid loads (61). This effect can be augmented in the dog by administration of glucocorticoids. Glutamine is taken up by the GI tract and serves as an oxidative fuel (62). The gut enterocytes convert glutamine primarily to ammonia and alanine, and these two substances are released into the portal venous blood. This ammonia is then removed by the liver and is converted to urea; the alanine may also be removed by the liver and may serve as a gluconeogenic precursor. Following elective surgical stress, glutamine consumption by the bowel and kidney is accelerated (63), a reaction that appears to be regulated by increased elaboration of glucocorticoids (64). Although skeletal muscle releases alanine at an accelerated rate, the GI tract and kidney also release increased amounts of alanine. This amino acid is extracted by the liver and used in the synthesis of glucose and acute-phase proteins. Hence glutamine and alanine are important participants in the transfer of nitrogen from skeletal muscle to visceral organs; however, their metabolic pathways favor production of urea and ammonia, both of which are lost from the body (Fig. 98.5).

Alterations in Fat Metabolism. To support hypermetabolism, increased gluconeogenesis, and interorgan substrate flux, stored triglyceride is mobilized and is oxidized at an accelerated rate. Lipolysis is poorly attenuated following glucose administration (50); this phenomenon may result from continuous stimulation of the sympathetic nervous system. Although mobilization and use of free fatty acids are accelerated in injured subjects, ketosis during brief starvation is blunted, and the accelerated protein catabolism remains unchecked (65). Unfed, severely injured patients rapidly deplete their fat and protein stores. Such malnutrition increases their susceptibility to added stresses of hemorrhage, operations, and infection and may contribute to organ system failure, sepsis, and death.

Mediators of the Injury Response

Hormonal Environment Associated with the Injury Response

A variety of hormonal alterations occur in patients following injury; yet, the cause-and-effect relationships have only recently been established. In all phases of injury, one sees a marked rise in the counterregulatory hormones glucagon, glucocorticoids, and catecholamines (66). During the ebb phase of injury, the sympathoadrenal axis primarily maintains the pressure-flow relationships necessary for an intact cardiovascular system. With onset of hypermetabolism, characteristic of the flow phase, these and other hormones exert a variety of metabolic effects. Glucagon has potent glycogenolytic and gluconeogenic effects on the liver, and these effects signal the liver to make new glucose from hepatic glycogen stores and gluconeogenic precursors. Cortisol mobilizes amino acid from skeletal muscle, increases hepatic gluconeogenesis, and maintains body fat stores. The catecholamines stimulate hepatic gluconeogenesis and glycolysis and increase lactate production from peripheral tissues (skeletal muscle). Catecholamines also increase metabolic rate and stimulate lipolysis. The level of growth hormone is ele-

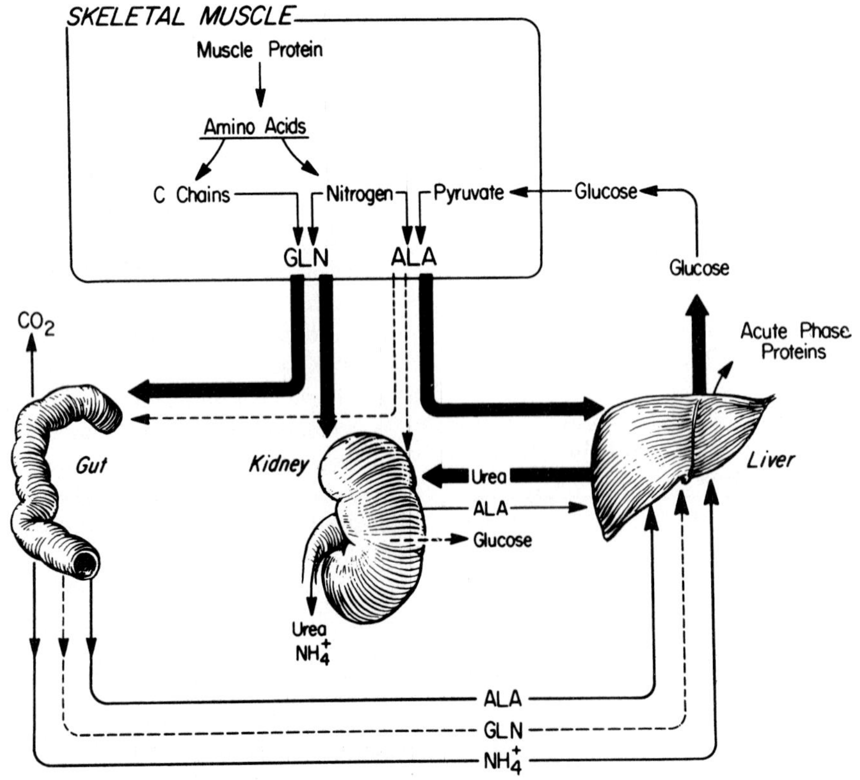

Figure 98.5. Major pathways of "obligatory" loss of nitrogen from the body. *ALA*, alanine; *GLN*, glutamine.

vated, even in the presence of hyperglycemia, and thyroid levels are reduced to low-normal concentrations.

Cytokines and the Metabolic Response to Injury

Although the classic counterregulatory hormones of stress (cortisol, catecholamines, glucagon) are important in mediating the body's response to injury and infection, they exert their influence largely via endocrine mechanisms. Other mediators, peptide compounds known collectively as cytokines, are produced both at the site of injury by endothelial cells and by diverse immune cells throughout the body and also occupy a pivotal position in the stress response (67). The cytokines that have been studied most extensively and appear to play the most important role in the injury response are tumor necrosis factor–α (TNF, cachectin), interleukins 1, 2, and 6 (IL-1, IL-2, and IL-6), and interferon-γ (IFN).

Originally it was thought that cytokines' primary influence was on immune cell function. It is now clear that cytokines are key regulators of the metabolic response to injury and infection (Fig. 98.6). These polypeptide signals, produced by the organism in response to bacteremia or endotoxemia, induce many of the adverse responses following severe infection (68, 69). A large number of these reticuloendothelial cell products have now been described (see Chapters 45, 46, and 96). TNF, IL-1, and IL-6 have been convincingly demonstrated in the circulation of humans following administration of endotoxin (67, 70).

TNF is considered the primary signal that initiates many of the metabolic responses to injury and infection. The host response to endotoxin includes a rapid increase in circulating TNF levels, which are no longer detectable after several hours. Although infusion of TNF to patients results in fever, malaise, tachycardia, and chills indicating an acute-phase response, the potent effects that TNF exerts on body metabolism may in concert benefit the host because they promote mobilization of nitrogen and carbon from the periphery, which are transported to the splanchnic circulation. TNF has no effect on skeletal muscle protein balance or amino acid efflux when it is administered to healthy animals or incubated with skeletal muscle. However, TNF stimulates amino acid uptake by the liver and endothelial cells (71).

IL-1 is a protein with a molecular mass of about 17 kDa. Previously called lymphocyte-activating factor, or endogenous pyrogen, this peptide plays a central role in the acute-phase protein response, including an increase in myofibrillar protein breakdown, and in the release of amino acids from skeletal muscle, in particular glutamine. Like TNF, IL-1 also stimulates glutamine transport by endothelial cells (71) and by the liver. Its effects on intestinal glutamine metabolism are similar to those of endotoxin and include a decrease in glutamine extraction from the blood and a fall in mucosal glutaminase activity (72).

The pattern of appearance of various cytokines in the circulation has been examined in animals receiving intravenous infusions of bacteria. TNF levels peak at about 90 minutes, while IL-1 peaked at 3 hours. IL-6 levels continued to rise for up to 8 hours. Thus, the pattern of cytokinemia appears to be monophasic and probably explains the occasional failure to detect these mediators in the blood of infected patients. In addition, many of the biologic responses to cytokines may be due to tissue levels of cytokines rather than circulating levels. Clearly, cytokines may exert their effects in a paracrine, autocrine, or endocrine fashion (74, 75). They also appear to work in

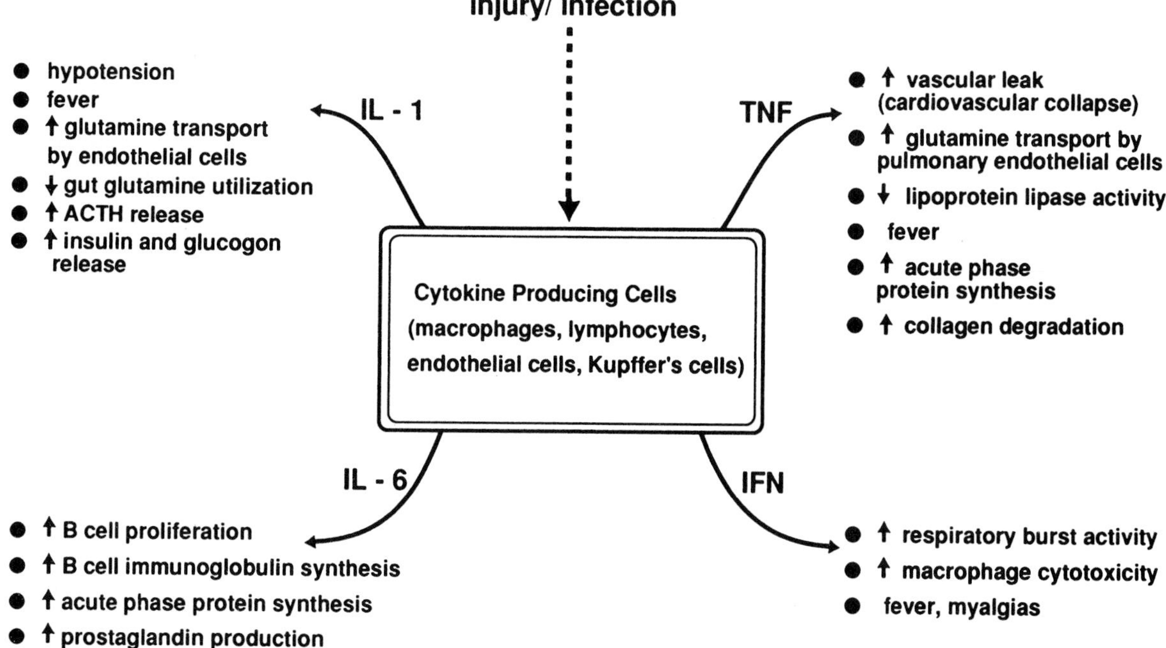

Figure 98.6. Some metabolic activities of selected cytokines as they relate to the body's response to injury and infection.

synergy to produce the metabolic derangements found in traumatized and septic patients.

Nutritional Support of the Injured Patient

Usual Course: Case Example

A 28-year-old, nonobese male (6 ft tall; 170 lb; BSA, 2.0 m^2 is admitted to the hospital with a pelvic fracture and soft tissue injury following a motor vehicle accident. He was always in good health prior to this accident. He is resuscitated without incident with intravenous fluids and blood products. The patient is admitted to the trauma intensive care unit of the hospital, and a nasogastric tube is placed. Over the next 24 hours, his blood volume is restored, and he is given maintenance solutions with 5% dextrose and appropriate electrolytes at the rate of 125 mL/h (3 L/day). His urine output on his first hospital day is 1500 mL, and he gains 5 kg following fluid resuscitation. Because of a prolonged ileus, the patient is not fed, and he continues to receive intravenous fluids. On day 7 of the injury, the ileus resolves, and a spontaneous diuresis of 3000 mL ensues. On day 8 following the accident, the patient starts taking clear liquids and is gradually advanced to regular diet over the next 4 days. He is discharged from the hospital 4 weeks later, when his fractures have stabilized.

Nitrogen balance studies from hospital day 1 through day 7 reveal a cumulative 7-day nitrogen loss of 108 g. During this 7-day period, the patient had 0 nitrogen intake and 600 kcal glucose/day. On the day 8 of hospitalization, the patient lost 5 kg. Approximately half the weight represented loss of lean body mass (108 g nitrogen = 675 g protein = 2.5 kg lean body mass), and the remainder, loss of fat. On discharge from the hospital a month later, the patient had regained his initial body weight (Fig. 98.7).

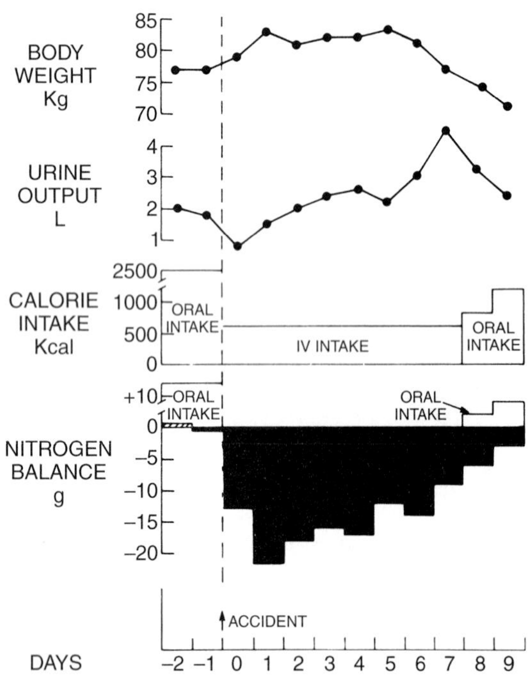

Figure 98.7. Metabolic response of a previously healthy individual to an injury of moderate severity.

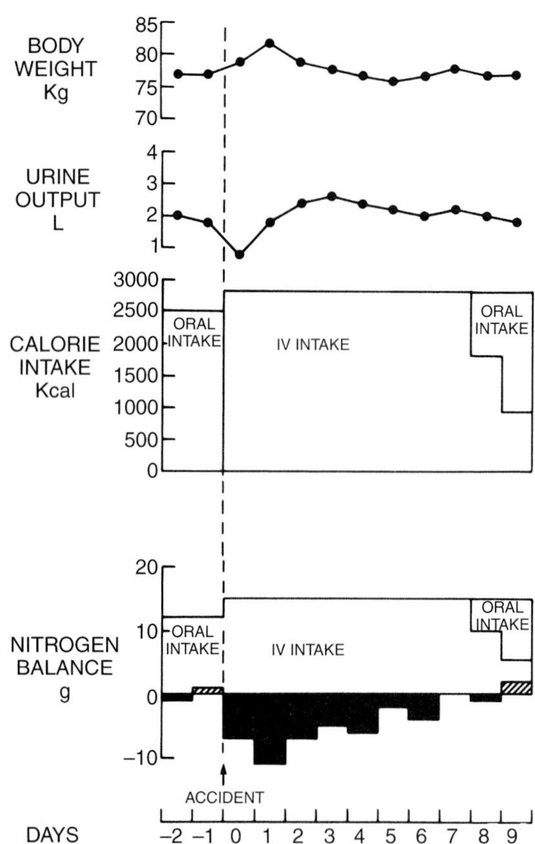

Figure 98.8. Injury response with nutrition provided by central vein infusions.

Response to Fixed Enteral or Parenteral Nutrition

The elective surgical patient can tolerate the mild catabolic responses following operation, with inadequate food intake, but the trauma patient cannot because of accelerated tissue catabolism. This "obligatory" nitrogen loss can, in part, be reversed nutritionally, but the accelerated nitrogen excretion only returns to normal when the wound is closed and the fracture is stabilized and is healing. Nutritional support does not affect the hypermetabolic response associated with severe trauma, but provision of adequate calories and amino acids does reduce the magnitude of net lipogenesis, skeletal muscle proteolysis, and negative nitrogen balance.

Suppose the patient described above sustains the same injury but has his postinjury period modified by administration of all essential nutrients. The patient receives 3 L of a parenteral solution that delivers, 2800 kcal plus 15 g nitrogen/day as a balanced amino acid mixture (Fig. 98.8). This caloric intake is judged adequate to maintain body weight. Nitrogen balance studies show cumulative loss of 140 g from hospital day 1 through hospital day 7, so his net loss for the 7 days equals 35 g. The patient lost 1 kg during this time, primarily lean body tissue.

Administration of nutrients to this patient is designed to combat the negative nitrogen balance and weight loss associated with injury. The benefits of such feedings in patients with extensive injury have been translated into reduced morbidity and mortality rates when nutritional support is combined with other improvements in intensive care.

Consequences of Malnutrition

The metabolic response to injury results in increased energy expenditure. If energy intake is less than expenditure, oxidation of body fat stores and erosion of lean body mass will occur, with resultant loss of weight. Most injured patients can tolerate losing of 10% of their weight prior to injury without a significant increase in the risks of injury. When weight loss exceeds 10% of body weight, the complications of undernutrition interact with the disease process, with increased morbidity and mortality rates. Undernutrition to this extent following injury may impair the body's ability to respond appropriately to the injury and inhibit responses to added stress such as infection.

The major impact of nutritional support in the trauma patient is in aiding host defense. These patients are exposed to a variety of infectious agents in the hospital, and their injuries and requirements of care increase the risk of infection. The normal barrier defense mechanisms are disrupted by multiple indwelling catheters, nasotracheal and nasogastric tubes, and breakdown of skin and mucous membranes. Undernutrition may compromise the available host defense mechanism and may thus increase the likelihood of invasive sepsis, multiple-organ system failure, and death. Additional consequences of malnutrition include poor wound healing, decreased mobility and activity, occurrence of pressure sores and decubitus ulcers, altered GI function, and occurrence of edema secondary to reduced colloid osmotic pressure. Whereas these complications are most frequently observed in patients with severe malnutrition (>15% body weight loss), adequate nutritional support helps prevent them.

Priorities of Care

Nutrition should be integrated into the overall care of the critically ill patient to maximize the benefits of nutritional support yet minimize complications in a complex intensive care setting. Priorities in care should be established at various points following injury. Resuscitation, oxygenation, and arrest of hemorrhage are immediate priorities for survival. Wounds should then be repaired or stabilized as expeditiously as possible. During wound repair, a patient's intensive metabolic demands abate, and nutrients become more effective in achieving anabolism. Early excision and grafting of burns and internal fixation of fractures are examples of early definitive wound care; yet even these procedures may be followed by several weeks of posttraumatic hypermetabolism. While the wound is treated, care should be taken to minimize other potential stresses that heighten metabolic demands in addition to those imposed by the injury alone. Such factors include pain, fever, mild cold exposure, acidosis, and hypovolemia. The greatest acceleration of catabolism occurs with infection, however, and every effort should be made to prevent sepsis.

Nutritional support is an essential part of the metabolic care of the critically ill trauma patient. Adequate nutrition allows normal responses that optimize wound healing and recovery. Nutritional support should be instituted before significant weight loss occurs. Development of techniques for intravenous administration of hypertonic nutrient solutions, the use of peripheral venous feedings with fat emulsions, and the availability of specific enteral diets have made it possible for virtually all injured patients to receive safe and effective nutritional support.

Goals of Nutritional Support

Most injured persons are not malnourished at the time of injury, but the increased metabolic demands following injury will quickly lead to a malnourished state if the patient is not nutritionally supported (Fig. 98.9). Thus,

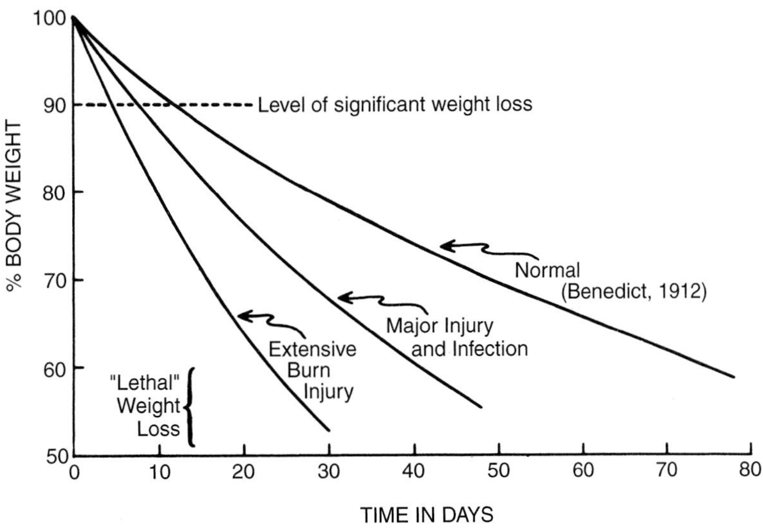

Figure 98.9. Weight loss with starvation is accelerated after major injury and infection.

nutritional support should be considered for all injured patients. Provision of full nutritional support early after injury may be fraught with metabolic complications, however. Hyperglycemia, hyperosmolarity, and electrolyte disorders are frequently observed. Thus, intravenous feedings are not usually begun immediately following the admission of the patient to the hospital. After stabilization of the patient's condition and development of a care plan, nutritional support can be gradually initiated. The goal of nutritional support is maintenance of body cell mass and limitation of weight loss to less than 10% of preinjury weight. Considerations include nutritional evaluation, requirements, monitoring, routes of administration, and specific formulas.

Nutritional Assessment and Requirements. Nutritional assessment of the trauma patient helps to determine energy and protein requirements. A careful medical history and physical examination are essential, but the usual indicators of malnutrition are frequently misleading in the trauma patient. For example, body weight is increased in these patients because of edema, and serum albumin and transferrin decrease in concentration because of an enlarged distribution space. Hence nutritional support should be considered for all injured patients, with the goal to maintain usual (preinjury) body weight and body tissue mass.

Basal energy requirements are determined from standard tables based on age, sex, and BSA (14). These requirements are adjusted for the increase in metabolic rate due to the injury or disease process by multiplication by a stress factor based on the severity of injury (see Table 98.1). An additional 25% is added to account for the energy expenditure associated with treatment and activity, but this addition is not required in inactive patients (e.g., those sedated or paralyzed while receiving artificial ventilation). The product of the factors (BMR times stress factors times 1.25, if needed) is an estimate of the patient's energy requirements.

The next step is to calculate nitrogen requirements. In normal subjects, the ratio of nitrogen to nonprotein caloric intake is usually 1:300 to 350; that is, for every 300 to 350 kcal, 1 g nitrogen is provided. Because of the heightened protein catabolism associated with the posttraumatic response, more dietary protein is required to achieve nitrogen balance. For critically ill patients, the optimal nitrogen:calorie ratio is thought to range between 1:100 and 1:200. This ratio indicates that approximately twice the quantity of protein is required to achieve "balance" in the injured patient than in healthy persons. Approximately 15 to 20% of caloric intake should be protein.

Once energy and nitrogen requirements have been determined, the proportions of fat and carbohydrate must be estimated, to maximize nitrogen retention. Long et al. studied the nitrogen-sparing effects of different isocaloric mixtures of glucose and fat in patients receiving 11.7 g nitrogen/m^2/day (76). They found no additional nitrogen-sparing effects when glucose calories exceeded the measured metabolic rate. Nitrogen equilibrium was approached when glucose made up 60 to 70% of the caloric needs, approximately 7 mg/kg/min. In addition, Wolfe et al. studied oxidation rates of postoperative patients receiving glucose (77). No increase in oxidation of administered glucose was observed when patients received glucose infusions above 7 mg/kg/min. Black et al., using the glucose clamp technique, demonstrated that injured patients had an upper limit to glucose disposal of approximately 6 to 7 mg/kg/min, a value that represented 60 to 70% of the estimated caloric needs (46). In contrast, normal subjects could dispose of increasing quantities of glucose and approached an upper limit of 15 to 17 mg/kg/min. The results of these 3 independent studies using different techniques point to the same conclusion: no clear-cut gain is made in providing glucose calories in excess of 60 to 70% of daily metabolic requirements to injured patients. Administration of larger glucose loads has been associated with increased incidence of complications such as hyperglycemia, hyperosmotic states, hepatic dysfunction, and respiratory insufficiency (78). For patients who tolerate large caloric loads, provision of 60% of caloric needs as glucose and the rest as fat should minimize complications and maximize protein synthesis.

Multivitamins are administered daily (see Chapter 101 for parenteral formulations). Supplemental vitamin C is believed by some to be required in increased amounts following injury (79). Electrolytes are present in standard diets or tube feedings as are trace elements (Chapter 100), and they must be added to parenteral infusions (Chapter 101). Potassium, magnesium, and phosphate supplements in addition to those in tube formulas may be required to maintain normal serum concentrations of these electrolytes. They must be added to parenteral fluids to meet needs, except when present in amino acid–electrolyte combinations. Although the need for zinc has been demonstrated experimentally, clinical reports of zinc replacement therapy in burn patients provide no definitive answers about the benefit of this supplement following injury (80). Zinc supplements should be administered to severely malnourished individuals and those with a history of poor nutrient intake (alcoholic patients) who have a major injury or major intestinal fluid losses.

In summary, the nutritional requirements of the trauma patient can be determined as follows:

1. Determine BMR for age, sex, and BSA from the tables of Fleisch or the Harris-Benedict equation (BMR in kcal/day) (14).
2. Determine the percentage increase in metabolic rate due to the injury (see Table 98.1), multiply by BMR, and add to 1 (% × BMR + BMR).
3. Add 25% × BMR for hospital activity (walking, physical therapy, sitting, treatment).
4. The sum of steps 1 to 3 is an estimated daily caloric requirement for maintenance of body weight.
5. Divide step 4 by 150 to determine nitrogen requirements (protein = 6.25 × nitrogen).

6. Give approximately 60% of caloric requirement (determined in step 4) as glucose.
7. Give remaining caloric requirement as fat (glucose can be used if tolerated by the patient). Glucose is much less expensive, and a central venous catheter will be necessary to administer the glucose solution. If glucose is used as the remaining caloric source, insulin may need to be given to avoid hyperglycemia. Fat emulsion should then be given 2 to 3 times per week to provide essential fatty acid requirements.
8. Reassess energy and nitrogen needs at least twice weekly. Weigh the patient daily.
9. If nutritional support seems unsatisfactory because of progressive weight loss, consider direct measurement of oxygen consumption or measurement of nitrogen loss and calculation of nitrogen balance.

Nutritional Monitoring. Once the trauma patient is nutritionally assessed, feedings can be gradually commenced. Protein and caloric intake should be measured and recorded daily. If nutritional requirements are not met by current therapy, then other feeding techniques should be used. Combined nutritional support techniques may be necessary during the convalescence of a severely injured patient (Fig. 98.10).

If the patient continues to lose more weight than can be attributed to postresuscitation diuresis, then additional nutritional assessment using such techniques as indirect calorimetry or nitrogen balance testing should be performed. Plasma glucose levels should be determined regularly, especially when one is beginning or increasing nutritional support. Insulin should be administered to maintain a plasma glucose level of 100 to 150 mg/dL. Urine sugar content should be evaluated by the hospital nursing staff every 6 to 8 hours. Levels of serum electrolytes, blood urea nitrogen (BUN), and creatinine and liver function should be determined regularly, as consistent with proper care. Serum potassium concentrations may need to be followed more closely because of increased potassium losses after injury and a tendency toward metabolic alkalosis.

Additional Nutritional Assessment Techniques. Energy requirements may be estimated with reasonable accuracy in 85% of hospital patients. If estimated requirements are delivered by current nutritional support but therapy seems inadequate because of persistent weight loss in excess of estimated net fluid losses or an unsatisfactory clinical course, energy requirements may be measured by indirect calorimetry. Oxygen consumption ($\dot{V}O_2$) and carbon dioxide production $\dot{V}CO_2$) are determined under resting, unstressed, basal conditions. These respiratory parameters are interrelated to energy expenditure by the following relationships:

$$\text{Metabolic rate (kcal/h)} = 3.9 \times \dot{V}O_2\ (L/h) + 1.1 \times \dot{V}CO_2\ (L/h)$$

This value, the resting energy expenditure of the patient, should be increased 20 to 30% to account for minimal daily activity when used to determine energy requirements.

Nitrogen balance studies help define the effectiveness of nutritional support. These should be performed in patients whose clinical course is unsatisfactory or in whom nutritional efficacy cannot be estimated on clinical grounds alone. Nitrogen balance is the quantity of nitrogen taken in or administered to the patient minus the quantity of nitrogen lost:

$$N_{bal}\ (g/day) = N_{in} - N_{out}$$

Most nitrogen is lost in the urine, mainly as urea. The urine is collected for 24-hour periods and is stored in acidified containers. Urinary urea nitrogen (UUN) is measured. This represents approximately 80% of urinary nitrogen. Additionally, about 2 g/day are lost in the feces and from the skin. If the BUN changes during the 24-hour period, the whole body changes in urea nitrogen (ΔBUN) in grams per day should be estimated as follows:

$$\Delta BUN = [(BUN_{day\ 2} - BUN_{day\ 1})^{a} \times (0.6 \times \text{body weight})^{b}] \div 1000$$

where term a represents the daily change in concentration in milligrams per deciliter, and term b the estimated quantity of total body water in kilograms.

$$N_{out} = UUN \div 0.8 + 2\ g/day^{c} + d$$

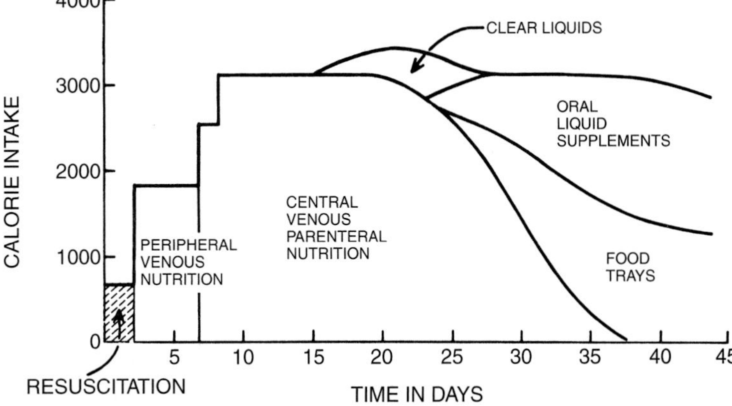

Figure 98.10. Subjects with moderate-to-severe injury require various techniques to provide safe and efficient nutrition.

where *c* is estimated stool and skin losses, *d* is measured nitrogen losses from wounds or drains, and all values are expressed as grams of nitrogen per day. Nitrogen is conventionally taken to be 16% of the total protein intake, thus

$$N_{in}/\text{day} = \text{protein intake (g/day)} \times 0.16.$$

Route of Nutritional Support and Nutrient Formulas. The routes of nutritional support are the same as those described elsewhere: oral, enteral, and parenteral. In general, oral and enteral routes are preferred over intravenous administration. Injured patients rarely take the required quantity of calories spontaneously from their hospital food tray. Hence oral liquid supplements should be administered. Nutrient intake is monitored daily by the dietitian, and each nursing shift is assigned a quantity of supplement to be provided. Free water or low-calorie drinks are not offered. All liquid is a calorie-dense nutrient supplement.

Three different clinical trials (81–83) and a comprehensive metaanalysis (84) documented the superiority of immediate postoperative enteral (jejunal) feedings over PN in patients with blunt and penetrating trauma. EN initiated within 24 hours of injury was well-tolerated and resulted in a statistically significantly lower incidence of postoperative pneumonia, intraabdominal abscess, and catheter sepsis. Other studies in injured patients also suggest benefits of aggressive early EN (85). Burned children who received a high-nitrogen enteral diet displayed improved hepatic synthetic function, fewer bacteremic days, and improved survival (86). Aggressive early nutritional support of patients with severe head injury also improves outcome (87–89). Head injury patients are candidates for TPN only if they exhibit enteral feeding intolerance. Early enteral feeding of injured patients (within 24 h) has established benefits over feeding later in the course of the hospitalization. Tube feeding should discontinue when adequate oral intake is achieved.

The patient's injuries may, however, preclude the use of oral feeding (e.g., patients with facial trauma may have their jaws wired together). Children, older adults, patients with head injuries, and those receiving artificial ventilation are all potential candidates for tube feeding. Retro- or intraperitoneal hematomas, intraabdominal sepsis, severe GI injury and extensive repair, or other factors may lead to reduced intestinal motility (ileus) or intolerance to enteral feedings. Jejunal or duodenal tube feedings are often successful even if the stomach must be continuously decompressed. Thus, for all patients who have undergone abdominal operations, feeding jejunostomy placement should be considered. Alternatively, the jejunum or duodenum can be intubated perorally with special tubes, with or without the aid of fluoroscopy. Development of diarrhea in a patient receiving enteral feedings may limit the caloric load given by these routes. When the nutritional needs of the patient cannot be met by oral and enteral feedings, intravenous techniques can be used.

Enteral formulas are usually balanced mixtures of fat, carbohydrate, and protein. Several recently developed formulas are particularly rich in calories and protein, yet have low osmolarity. In light of the injured patient's nutritional requirements, these formulas would seem particularly advantageous; however, a variety of formulas are available and may be preferred in selected cases.

Intravenous feedings may be necessary to supplement enteral feedings, or they may be required to provide adequate nutritional intake if enteral feedings cannot be tolerated or are inadequate. Peripheral nutrient solution can be given to supplement enteral feedings. These dilute solutions of glucose and amino acids should be minimized and fat infusion should be maximized while high-carbohydrate tube feeding is provided. This approach ensures adequate carbohydrate loads in a minimal fluid volume. Trauma patients, particularly burn patients, are usually young adults without cardiovascular disease and with large daily fluid requirements. Thus, these patients are ideal candidates for peripheral-vein nutrient infusion. Unfortunately, however, adequate carbohydrate calories can rarely be provided solely by this route, and when PN is required, central venous feedings are usually indicated. The hypertonic solution provides glucose, amino acids, and other essential nutrients. Fat emulsion and supplemental fluids are easily administered through a second intravenous access site, usually a peripheral vein.

SEPSIS

Unlike in elective operations and uncomplicated trauma, major infections often have unpredictable response patterns. The variability in metabolic and physiologic responses is related in part to the patient's age, previous state of health, preexisting disease, previous stresses, site of infection, and specific pathogens. Moreover, organ-system failure, such as septic shock or pulmonary insufficiency, may mask the more subtle manifestations of systemic infection. In spite of numerous advances in treatment of infection and a better understanding of its mediators and pathophysiology, mortality and morbidity rates for septicemia remain as high as 50%.

In general, two physiologic response patterns have been described, based on cardiac output (90). The first is characterized by increased cardiac output and heightened systemic perfusion. This state varies, depending on the patient's physiologic compensation and the administered fluid volume. The second response pattern is characterized by cardiac decomposition, inadequate tissue perfusion, and profound acidosis. This pattern is described as "low-flow sepsis." Both these responses reflect the body's reaction to systemic infection. These patterns are also modified by the underlying disease process and the physiologic reserve of the particular patient. This section reviews the metabolic responses to sepsis and the priorities for safe nutritional support. Sepsis is defined as the presence of infection, resulting in systemic signs and symptoms, and diagnosed by bacteremia. Low-flow sepsis is difficult to reverse and usually results in death. Most of this discussion focuses on the metabolic responses that occur during the hyperdynamic high-flow state.

Physiologic Responses to Systemic Infection

General Overview and Time Course

Invasion of the body by microorganisms initiates many host responses. Local penetration of tissues stimulates mobilization of phagocytes, initiates an inflammatory response at the local site, and may activate additional host immunologic mechanisms. If the infection progresses, fever, tachycardia, and other systemic responses occur; these more generalized reactions may reflect direct or indirect effects of the inflammatory response. Systemic events during the hyperdynamic phase of sepsis can be categorized into two general types of responses: *(a)* those related to the host's immunologic defenses and *(b)* those related to the body's general metabolic and circulatory adjustments to infection. The predominant alterations in host defense mechanisms include fever, leukocytosis, changes in acute-phase protein synthesis, and activation of a variety of immunologic reactions. Metabolic changes are related to altered glucose, nitrogen, and fat metabolism, as well as redistribution of trace metals. These events are initiated by invasion of the microorganism and evolve as the infectious disease progresses through its period of incubation, initiation of metabolic responses and fever, and into early convalescence and recovery.

- These responses appear stereotyped and can be produced by administering many microorganisms or their toxins. While the systemic responses to infection are similar in many respects to events that follow injury, these processes are not the same.
- The magnitude of the responses varies with the extent and duration of the infection.
- The complex sequence of systemic events that follows infection appears to change with time, and hence sequential studies must be performed to locate the responses precisely within that time.
- Although the systemic responses to infection are stereotyped, these processes are modulated by the physiologic reserves of the individual. The magnitude of the responses to infection depends on the patient's age and sex, previous nutritional state, function of vital organs, immunologic memory, and associated disease processes. The classic response to infection has been observed in young, previously healthy, well-nourished, active adults with no other medical problems. These patients are rarely admitted to surgical services, however. Surgeons usually see patients at extremes of life or those who are hospitalized because of disease processes and who have additional stress, usually an operation or injury, that limits physiologic, biochemical, or immunologic responses to infection. Thus, infection complicating the recuperative course of a surgical patient may not evoke standard systemic responses. Limitations in the patient's capacity to respond to infection may affect recovery or survival.
- As infection progresses, additional functional limitations may be imposed on one or more specific organs and may further impair the host systemic response. These limitations can be observed in patients with severe pneumonia and marked pulmonary dysfunction causing hypoxemia, associated with circulatory failure and hypotension related to severe gram-negative sepsis.

In spite of the complexities of unraveling and understanding the systemic responses to infection in critically ill surgical patients, a large body of investigative and clinical data is available to aid our understanding of these host defense mechanisms.

Beisel described the time course of metabolic and immunologic responses during the course of a typical febrile illness (91). Phagocytic activity, an early response, occurs shortly after exposure to the pathogen. The febrile period is the hallmark of systemic effects. With the onset of fever, negative nitrogen balance, accelerated loss of potassium, phosphate, and magnesium, and retention of salt and water occur. On resolution of the sepsis, one sees spontaneous diuresis and a return to positive nitrogen balance. Associated with the loss of elements from the body is an internal redistribution of substances, particularly iron and zinc, which are sequestered in the body, presumably to make them unavailable to the invading organisms (Fig. 98.11).

Systemic Metabolic Responses

Because many of the metabolic responses to infection are similar to those observed following injury, investigators have speculated that a final common pathway may apply to all catabolic states. Severe infection is characterized by prolonged fever, hypermetabolism, diminished protein economy, altered glucose dynamics, and accelerated lipolysis. Anorexia is commonly associated with systemic infec-

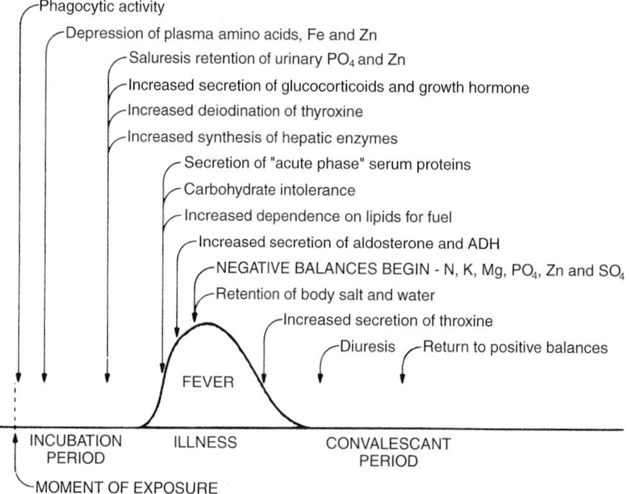

Figure 98.11. Nutritional responses that evolve following a generalized febrile, infectious illness. (From Beisel WR. Am J Clin Nutr 1977;30(1):236, with permission.)

tion and contributes to the loss of body tissue. These effects are compounded in the patient with sepsis by multiorgan system failure, which includes the GI tract, liver, heart, and lungs.

Hypermetabolism. Oxygen consumption is usually elevated in the infected patient. The extent of this increase is related to the severity of infection, with peak elevations reaching 50 to 60% above normal (14). Such responses often occur in the postoperative and postinjury periods secondary to severe pneumonia, intraabdominal infection, or wound invasion. If the patient's metabolic rate is already maximally elevated because of severe injury, no further increase will be observed. In patients with only slightly accelerated rates of oxygen consumption, infection causes a rise in metabolic rate that appears additive to the preexisting state. A portion of the increase in metabolism may be ascribed to the increase in reaction rate associated with fever (Q10 effect) (14). Calculations suggest that the metabolic rate increases 10 to 13% for each elevation of 1°C in central temperature. On resolution of the infection, the metabolic rate returns to normal.

Altered Glucose Dynamics. Blood glucose levels are generally elevated in the infected patient, but the descriptive term *diabetes of infection* is inappropriate because plasma insulin concentrations are generally normal or elevated in previously healthy individuals who develop infection (92). Increased glucose production in infected patients appears to be additive to the augmented gluconeogenesis that occurs following injury. For example, uninfected burn patients have an accelerated glucose production rate approximately 50% above normal; onset of bacteremia in similar individuals increases hepatic glucose production to twice basal levels. Glucose dynamics following infection are complex, and profound hypoglycemia and diminished hepatic glucose production have also been described in both animals and human patients (93, 94). The best clinical example of the imbalance in hepatic glucose production and tissue glucose consumption is found in neonatal hypoglycemia associated with gram-negative septicemia (95). Studies in animals and in human patients show that deterioration in glucogenesis is associated with more-progressive stages of infection and may be related to altered splanchnic blood flow. Hepatic dysfunction this profound is usually associated with other complications of sepsis, such as respiratory insufficiency and renal failure, and usually heralds impending cardiovascular instability and death.

Alterations in Protein Metabolism. Accelerated proteolysis, increased nitrogen excretion, and prolonged negative nitrogen balance occur following infection, and the response pattern is similar to that described for injury. Protein catabolism is increased in infected patients; this enhanced rate of breakdown may be partially offset by vigorous feeding, which can stimulate protein synthesis (96). Amino acid flux from skeletal muscle is accelerated in patients with sepsis (97) and this flux is matched by accelerated visceral amino acid uptake. In infected burn patients, splanchnic uptake of amino acids is increased 50% above rates in uninfected burn patients with injuries of comparable size (14). These amino acids serve as glucose precursors and are used for synthesis of acute-phase proteins. In addition, acidosis frequently occurs in the patient with sepsis, and this stimulus serves as a signal for accelerated glutamine uptake by the kidney. Glutamine liberates an ammonia ion that combines with a hydrogen ion and is excreted in the urine, thus participating in acid-base homeostasis. The amino acid glutamine undergoes marked changes in interorgan metabolism following critical illness and may become conditionally essential. These issues are discussed in Chapter 35.

Alterations in Fat Metabolism. Fat is a major fuel oxidized in infected patients, and increased metabolism of lipids from peripheral fat stores is especially prominent during a period of inadequate nutritional support. Lipolysis is most probably mediated by the heightened sympathetic activity that is a potent stimulus for fat mobilization and accelerated oxidation (14). Serum triglyceride levels reflect the balance between rates of triglyceride production by the liver and use and storage by peripheral tissues. Marked hypertriglyceridemia has been associated with gram-negative infection, but plasma triglyceride concentrations are usually normal or low. The use of free fatty acids is coupled with increased hepatic fat clearance. During starvation, hepatic uptake of free fatty acids is associated with ketosis, and concentrations of β-hydroxybutyrate and acetoacetate rise. This change does not occur in infected patients, and it has been hypothesized that the accelerated proteolysis seen during infection is a consequence of this hypoketonemic state. This hypothesis was tested by infusion of β-hydroxybutyrate into infected animals (98). Following infusion, the accelerated gluconeogenesis and proteolysis were not diminished.

Changes in Mineral Metabolism. Changes in balance of magnesium, inorganic phosphate, zinc, and potassium generally follow alterations in nitrogen balance. Although the iron-binding capacity of transferrin is usually unchanged in early infection, iron disappears from the plasma, especially during severe pyrogenic infections; similar alterations are observed with serum zinc levels. Both iron and zinc accumulate within the liver, and this accumulation appears to be another host defense mechanism (14, 99). Administration of iron to the infected host, especially early in the disease, is contraindicated because increased serum iron concentrations may impair resistance (see Chapter 97). Zinc may be required during a prolonged, infective illness because zinc is both sequestered in body tissues and excreted in the urine. Zinc deficiency, however, is not reflected in serum concentrations, which are usually diminished as an initial host response. Unlike iron and zinc, copper levels generally rise, and the increased plasma concentrations can be ascribed almost entirely to the increase in ceruloplasmin produced by the liver.

Mediators of the Catabolic Response

The hormonal and cytokine responses during the hypermetabolic phase of infection are similar to those described following injury. Serum cortisol levels are elevated and lose their usual circadian rhythm. Glucagon levels are increased, and the insulin:glucagon ratio, a hormonal relationship considered to indicate hepatic stimulation of gluconeogenesis, remains below normal, however. Levels of catecholamines, growth hormone, ADH, and aldosterone are all elevated. The growth hormone level persists into convalescence, presumably to promote anabolism.

Gut Mucosal Barrier Function and Gut-Origin Sepsis

Although the intestinal tract is generally viewed as an organ of digestion and absorption, it also protects the host from intraluminal bacteria and their toxins (Fig. 98.12). Maintenance of an intact brush border and intercellular tight junctions prevents the movement of toxic substances into the intestinal lymphatics and circulation. Bacteria that do translocate appear to do so in small numbers, and the mesenteric lymph nodes effectively dispose of them without deleterious systemic effects. Bacterial endotoxins that are absorbed into the portal venous blood are rapidly detoxified by the Kupffer cells of the liver.

Gut immune function is the term applied to the structural and functional characteristics of the GI tract that make it resistant to the entry of infectious or toxic agents into the systemic circulation (100). This function is a combination of nonimmunologic processes (physical factors, intestinal flora) and the local mucosal immune system function. Immune factors include secretion of secretory IgA (S-IgA) and the function of macrophages and lymphocytes in the Peyer's patches, mesenteric lymph nodes, and lamina propria of the intestinal mucosa. These collections of cells of the immune system within the GI tract are known collectively as the gut-associated lymphoid tissue (GALT). Maintenance of a gut mucosal barrier that effectively excludes luminal bacteria and toxins requires an intact epithelium and normal mucosal immune mechanisms.

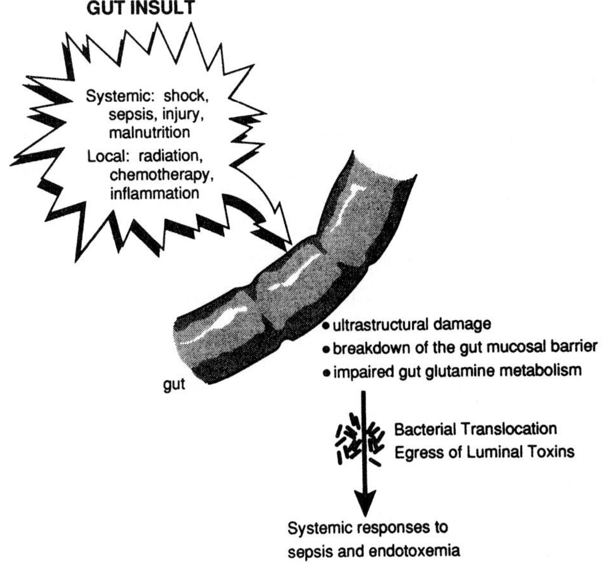

Figure 98.12. The gut hypothesis proposes that local and systemic insults can damage the gut epithelium and allow egress of luminal bacteria and toxins. If systemic responses such as hypermetabolism and persistent catabolism are self-perpetuating, multiple organ failure can develop.

Stimulation of gut S-IgA secretion begins in the Peyer's patches of the small intestine (100). Enteric antigens are presented to immunocompetent cells through M cells, which are specialized epithelial cells overlying the Peyer's patches. The antigens are processed by macrophages and presented to T and B lymphoblasts. The B cells are then committed to production of antigen-specific S-IgA. These cells are released from the Peyer's patch, pass through mesenteric lymph nodes, and eventually enter the systemic circulation via the thoracic duct. The B cells then come to the intestinal lamina propria where they mature and secrete specific S-IgA in response to enteric antigen presentation. B cells are also distributed to other tissues such as the liver, and thus S-IgA is found in bile as well as intestinal succus. In the GI tract, bile appears to contribute about 90% of the S-IgA present in the intestinal lumen. S-IgA prevents the binding of enteric pathogens to the cells of the intestinal mucosa and acts in conjunction with the indigenous intestinal microflora to control enteric pathogenic bacteria.

Bacterial translocation is the process by which microorganisms migrate across the mucosal barrier and invade the host (101). The most extensive work on bacterial translocation has been done in animal models, where the number and pathogenicity of the endogenous flora can be precisely controlled and the microorganisms that invade the host, carefully quantified. Generally, three principal mechanisms promote bacterial translocation: *(a)* altered permeability of the intestinal mucosa (as caused by hemorrhagic shock, sepsis, distant injury, or administration of cell toxins), *(b)* decreased host defense (secondary to glucocorticoid administration, immunosuppression, or protein depletion), and *(c)* an increased number of bacteria within the intestine (as caused by bacterial overgrowth, intestinal stasis, or feeding bacteria to experimental animals). A number of retrospective and epidemiologic studies have associated infection in specific patient populations with bacterial invasion from the gut (102, 103). These reports suggest that bacterial invasion occurs in patients after injury, multiorgan system failure, or severe burns and in cancer patients after chemotherapy or bone marrow transplantation. Nonmetabolizable markers of known size, such as lactulose or mannitol, have also been used to determine permeability. These studies demonstrated an increase in mucosal permeability in normal volunteers receiving endotoxin and in infected burn patients. Because many of the factors that facilitate bacterial translocation occur simultaneously in surgical patients and their effects may be additive or cumulative, patients in an intensive care unit may be extremely vulnerable to invasion by enteric bacteria or to absorption of their toxins (Fig. 98.12). Such patients do not generally receive enteral feedings, and current parenteral therapy results in gut atrophy, and methods currently used to support critically ill patients neither facilitate repair of the intestinal mucosa nor maintain gut barrier function.

Nutritional Assessment and Requirements

As with accidental injury, the onset of sepsis is generally sudden and unplanned. On the other hand, in contrast to trauma victims who are well nourished and healthy prior to their injury, infected patients are often nutritionally depleted when bacteremia develops. Malnutrition is inseparable from the occurrence and effects of infectious diseases, and their interaction is synergistic.

As with all patients, the primary objectives of nutritional assessment are to evaluate the patient's present nutritional status and to determine energy, protein, and macro- and micronutrient requirements. Assessment of patients with sepsis should start with a medical history and physical examination, which is frequently difficult because of the severity of the patient's illness. Use of anthropometric measurements is helpful, but weight may be an inaccurate reflection of nutritional status because of fluid retention. Serum protein concentrations (albumin and transferrin) are low because of redistribution secondary to the infection; hence these values are not useful indicators of malnutrition.

The immediate goal of nutritional therapy is weight maintenance. Weight gain and anabolism are generally difficult to achieve during the septic process, but they do occur once the disease process has abated. Total energy requirements can be calculated using the stress equation; mild-to-moderate infections increase energy requirements 20 to 30%, and severe infection increases caloric needs about 50% above basal levels. The optimal calorie:nitrogen ratio is approximately 150:1, although providing more nitrogen has been proposed.

The following case example illustrates the value of nutritional support in the overall integrated care of a patient with prolonged sepsis. A 65-year old man (6′ tall; 175 lb; BSA, 2.0 m^2) appeared in the hospital emergency ward with right-upper-quadrant pain, a temperature of 103°F, and mild jaundice. A recent ultrasound had shown the presence of gallstones, but the patient was otherwise well nourished and in good health. Initial laboratory studies showed a white blood cell count of 17,000, with a left shift, total bilirubin level of 5 mg/dL, and an alkaline phosphatase level of 550 Bodansky units. Shortly after hospital admission, the patient became confused, and his blood pressure fell to 70 mm Hg systolic. His skin was warm and pink, and a diagnosis of ascending cholangitis and septic shock was made. Intravenous fluid was administered, and the patient's blood pressure returned to normal. Antibiotics were started, and shortly thereafter the patient was taken into the operating suite, where he was found to have an impacted gallstone in the common bile duct. A cholecystectomy and common duct exploration were performed, and the impacted stone was removed. Pus was present in the gallbladder and the biliary tract.

Postoperatively, the patient required ventilatory support. On postoperative day 1, he was no longer dependent on cardiotonic agents to maintain normal blood pressure. He had a marked ileus and remained febrile. He received 5% dextrose solutions containing appropriate electrolytes. He gradually became alert, but remained dependent on the ventilator. On postoperative day 5, the patient's fever increased to 103.6°F, and he had marked leukocytosis. Diagnostic studies showed an intraabdominal abscess, and the patient returned to the operating room for surgical drainage. Postoperatively, the patient received large doses of antibiotics, and 3 days after a second operation, he was weaned from the ventilator. Results of liver function tests gradually returned to normal, and the patient's ileus resolved. On postoperative day 15, the patient started a clear-liquid diet, and he was discharged from the hospital on postoperative day 22. Nitrogen balance studies from postoperative day 1 to day 16 showed a cumulative 15-day negative balance of 225 g (Fig. 98.13). The patient had lost 11 lb by postoperative day 15, half of which was lean tissue, the remainder fat. By day 15, the patient had started oral intake, and by discharge day (day 22), he was clearly afebrile and anabolic, taking adequate quantities of nutrients.

Response to Fixed Nutrient Intake

To evaluate the effect of fixed nutrient intake in sepsis, suppose that the above patient with ascending cholangitis is supported vigorously with PN throughout his course. A combination of sepsis, anesthesia, and tissue trauma increased his metabolic rate by 50%, so his energy needs are approximately 2900 kcal/day. The patient receives 3 L of central venous nutrition, which provides 21 g of nitrogen and 3000 kcal/day. Nitrogen balance studies from postoperative day 1 to 16 show a cumulative loss of 375 g, and cumulative nitrogen balance for this 15-day period is ~60 g. On postoperative day 16, the patient has lost only 4 lb, half of which is body fat, and the remainder lean body mass (Fig. 98.14).

Prompt initiation of nutritional support in patients with sepsis who cannot eat enough or should not eat is mandatory. On the other hand, provision of nutrients requires integration into the patients' management and support plan. The patient in the case example was started gradually on nutritional feedings, to avoid untoward complications of hyperglycemia, and the infusion was diminished

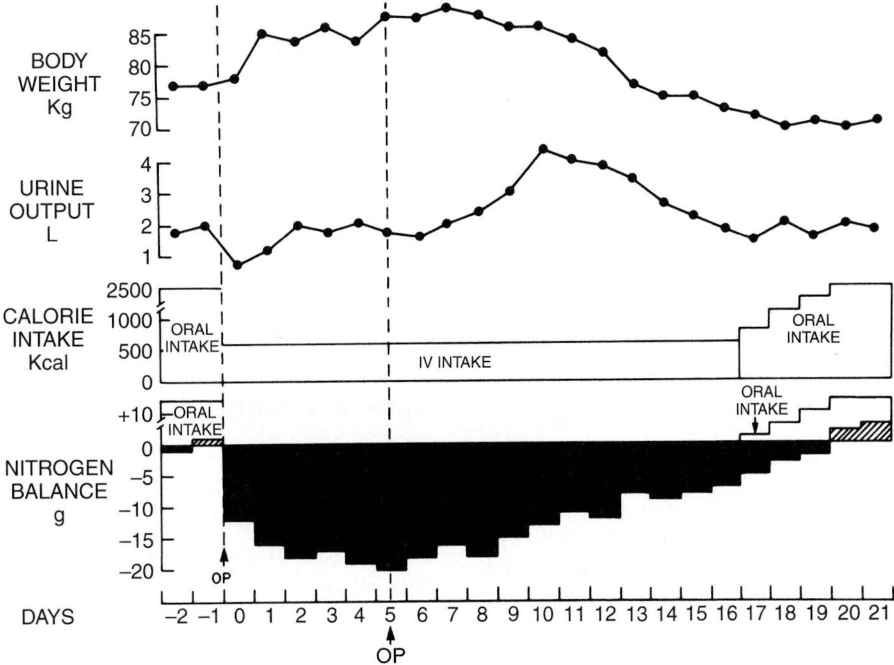

Figure 98.13. Metabolic responses to sepsis.

during the second septic interval. Fat should compose a moderate proportion of the infused energy, to avoid the complications of hyperglycemia and to diminish the possibility of increased carbon dioxide production complicating hypercaloric glucose infusions. Severe erosion of lean body mass is possible in such a patient, and nutritional support helps to diminish such erosion. Provision of calories and nitrogen cannot attenuate the hypermetabolism characteristic of sepsis, but it does reduce accelerated catabolism.

Route of Feeding

The routes of nutrient administration are similar to those for the elective surgical patient and the trauma victim. The enteral route should always be used when possi-

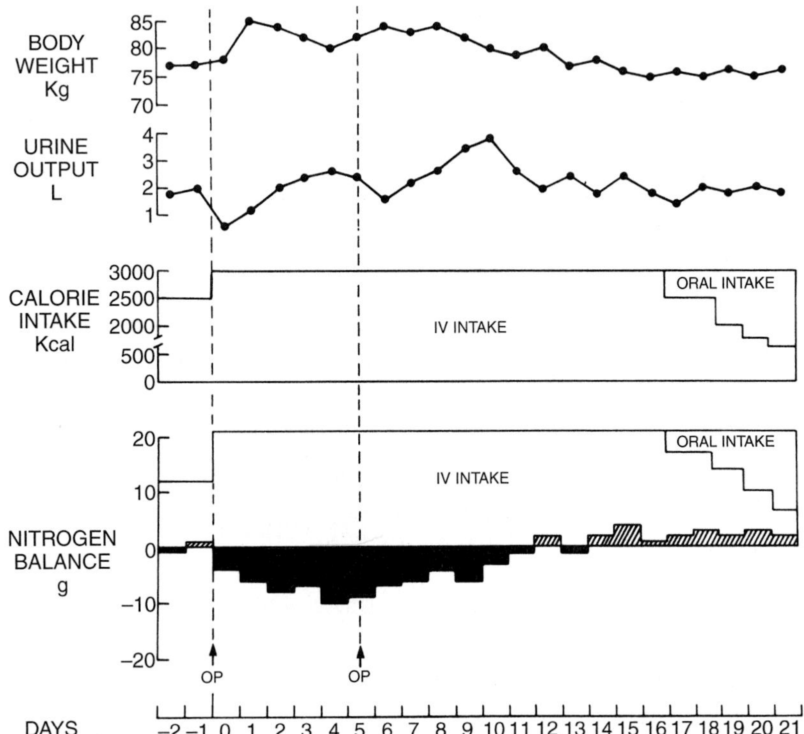

Figure 98.14. Metabolic responses to sepsis with constant intravenous nutrition.

ble, but patients with sepsis usually have an ileus and therefore require PN. In general, this condition requires central venous nutrition because peripheral nutritional support cannot provide adequate calories in a moderately restrictive fluid volume. The risks of catheter sepsis are minimized by dedicating the central line solely to infusion of the hypertonic nutrient solutions and maintaining strict asepsis at the catheter entrance site. In addition, the catheter may be changed over a guide wire using a strict aseptic technique, and the catheter tip may be cultured. This culturing, done at intervals of 3 to 5 days, ensures that the catheter has not become the focus of the septic process.

Nutritional Support in Surgical Patients with Sepsis

A role for nutritional support in septic patients has been difficult to prove because improvements in nutritional markers such as serum proteins, nitrogen balance, and weight gain have generally not translated into clinical benefits (1). In most studies, nutritional support failed to correct multiple biochemical and immune parameters and did not affect outcome. Similarly, provision of nutritional support to critically ill patients with a poor outcome did not alter the plasma amino acid profile (104) and does not appear to prevent muscle protein loss (105).

Nutritional support is often used aggressively in septic patients because erosion of lean body mass will, at some point, have a negative impact on outcome. It is unclear how long such patients can tolerate inadequate nutrition before outcome is adversely affected. Limited data reported to date in patients in intensive care units have not shown an effect of nutritional support on mortality (106). As a general rule, nutritional support should not be withheld in septic or other critically ill patients who are anticipated to be unable to eat for more than 7 to 10 days (1). As mentioned above, the impact of nutritional support on organ function also requires further study (Table 98.4). When nutritional support is used, the enteral route is preferred if the gut is functional and usable. Unfortunately, septic patients often develop an ileus, and advancement to full feedings often demands perseverance and may take several days. Gastric residuals, diarrhea, abdominal distention, and physician practice habits can be barriers to the use of enteral feedings.

Complications, Organ Failure, and Other Special Feeding Problems

The most severe complication of sepsis is the failure of essential organs, which may result in death. The current treatment of systemic infection consists of *(a)* bacteriologic control by removal and drainage or containment of the source; *(b)* use of appropriate antibiotics; *(c)* support of cardiovascular and respiratory function; *(d)* supportive therapy of specific organ failure, whether cardiac, pulmonary, hepatic, renal, or gastrointestinal; and *(e)* vigorous nutritional support of the host.

Respiratory Insufficiency

A common problem associated with systemic infection is oxygenation and elimination of carbon dioxide. A variety of endotoxins and vasoactive factors mediated by the infectious process can alter pulmonary vascular permeability and may lead to pulmonary insufficiency. Patients often require intubation and vigorous ventilatory support with volume-cycle ventilation and positive expiratory pressure. Ongoing problems include development of pneumonia and pulmonary insufficiency secondary to increased capillary permeability. Most of the enteral and

Table 98.4
Nutritional Support (NS) in Patients With Surgery, Trauma, and Sepsis

Problems with establishing recommendations	
Consistently reliable criteria for diagnosing "at risk" malnutrition have not been identified	
Limited number of well-designed prospective, randomized clinical trials	
Nutritional support is indicated	
Indication	*Benefit of nutritional support*
Patients who cannot eat or absorb nutrients for long periods of time or indefinitely (permanent neurologic impairment, premature infant, oropharyngeal dysfunction, short gut syndrome)	Life saving
Severely malnourished patients who require a major surgical procedure	Preoperative nutrition decreases the incidence of major septic complications
Patients sustaining major trauma	Enteral nutrition is superior to parenteral nutrition in decreasing the incidence of septic complications; NS improves outcome in head injury patients
Role of Nutritional support is unclear	
Patient group	*Some areas requiring further study*
Liver failure	Impact of NS on survival
Renal failure	Impact of NS on outcome in patients with acute renal failure and in patients on chronic dialysis
Catabolic patients (ICU, severe pancreatitis) who cannot eat for variable periods of time	How long is too long to go without nutrition?
Solid organ transplantation	Impact of NS on graft survival

Adapted from Souba WW. N Engl J Med 1977;1:49–58.

parenteral formulas used to provide nutritional support for critically ill patients contain large amounts of carbohydrate, which generate large quantities of carbon dioxide following oxidation. A large carbon dioxide load may worsen existing pulmonary dysfunction or may delay weaning from the ventilator (107). If this becomes a problem, the carbohydrate load should be reduced to 50% of metabolic requirements and fat emulsion administered to provide additional calories.

Renal Failure

The origin of renal failure associated with sepsis is unclear. Circulating factors are associated with increasing blood flow to the kidney. However, if cardiac output is inadequate, such a response is not possible, and this failure, coupled with redistribution blood flow, may cause progressive deficiency of the cortical portion of the kidney. In addition, the use of aminoglycoside antibiotics, which are nephrotoxic, may also cause progressive impairment and malfunction. When renal failure becomes progressive, early use of hemodialysis, with or without filtration, minimizes the effects of uremia superimposed on the metabolism of sepsis. Adequate caloric support limits ureagenesis and normalizes alterations in serum electrolyte levels. Because uremia itself is a potent catabolic signal, this condition further impairs the hypercatabolic infected host. Metabolic studies in patients with acute and chronic renal failure have limited intake of nonessential amino acids, in an attempt to lower urea production. Proteins of high biologic value, but in much smaller quantities (<0.5 g/kg/day) than usually given, are administered along with adequate calories, usually in the form of glucose. When enteral feedings are not feasible, a central venous infusion of an essential amino acid solution and hypertonic dextrose provides calories and a small quantity of nitrogen, to reduce protein catabolism while simultaneously controlling the rise in BUN. Whether such nutritional therapy reduces mortality rates for renal failure associated with sepsis remains controversial (33–35). During dialysis, protein intake is liberalized, but the BUN is maintained below 100 mg/dL.

Gut Dysfunction

Sepsis causes marked changes in GI function. The most common abnormality is ileus, which can result from intraabdominal disease or from the effects of bacteria elsewhere. Stress ulcers lead to upper GI bleeding, which may require operative treatment. The factors that promote breakdown of the gut mucosal barrier and lead to translocation of luminal bacteria and their toxins have been discussed. Nutritional support may be necessary in such patients, particularly if the gut dysfunction persists.

TPN increases the spontaneous rate of closure of enterocutaneous fistulae that occur in patients with abdominal sepsis, but reduced mortality rates are due to improved fistula care rather than nutritional intervention (108, 109). Local wound care of the skin site reduces problems such as irritation and wound infection. Similarly, the amount of fistula output can be quantitated and fluid and electrolyte adjustments made accordingly. Fistula closure occurs in 40 to 60% of patients treated with TPN (90% close within 5 weeks). During this period of medical management, TPN will maintain nutritional status should surgical intervention be required.

Although TPN does not alter the clinical course of severe acute pancreatitis and results in a higher rate of catheter sepsis (110, 111) and total hospital costs (111), it is unclear how long nutritional support should be withheld in these individuals. There are no randomized prospective trials comparing enteral with parenteral nutrition in patients with acute pancreatitis, and thus treatment decisions are empiric rather than on based on scientific evidence.

Hepatic Failure

Hepatic dysfunction is a common manifestation of septicemia. The degree of dysfunction varies; it may appear early, as a slight elevation of liver enzymes, or it may cause severe jaundice and hyperbilirubinemia. Specific bacteria overwhelm the reticuloendothelial system of the liver and result in fulminant hepatic failure. Localized infections, such as hepatic abscesses, pyelophlebitis, and hepatitis, may cause profound liver dysfunction because of the direct effect of infection on this organ. Occasionally, hypoglycemia accompanies ascending cholecystitis because of the direct effect of hepatic inflammation. Fulminant hepatic failure in the patient with sepsis has a high mortality rate, especially when hepatic encephalopathy occurs. As discussed in the section on trauma, the effects of normalization of amino acid concentration and reversal of hepatic coma remain controversial. More common, however, are alterations on liver function studies, such as elevations in levels of alkaline phosphatase, hepatic enzymes, and serum bilirubin, which appear secondary to the septic event but may worsen with intravenous feedings. Hepatic dysfunction generally resolves on resolution of the sepsis, but if the inflammatory process persists, adjustments in the feeding formulation are necessary. The carbohydrate load is usually reduced to consist of no more than 50% of metabolic requirements, with the additional calories provided as fat emulsion. A patient whose serum bilirubin level becomes elevated (generally above 12 mg/dL) should be observed for the presence of encephalopathy; if this complication occurs, the protein load should also be reduced.

Cardiac Dysfunction

The myocardial dysfunction that occurs in sepsis may be secondary to the elaboration of cytokines or to heart failure secondary to pulmonary insufficiency. Malnourished patients with sepsis may be sensitive to volume overload, and use of a concentrated solution of hypertonic dextrose

(D-70%) mixed with amino acids may be indicated to maximize calories and minimize volume. In addition, a 20% fat emulsion can be administered to provide additional energy.

Organ Transplantation

The benefits of nutritional support have been established in patients undergoing bone marrow transplantation (BMT) (1), but the role of nutritional intervention in patients undergoing solid organ transplantation is less clear. In one of the BMT studies, 137 patients with normal nutritional status were randomized to receive PN (plus ad libitum oral intake) beginning 1 week prior to and for 4 weeks after transplantation or to receive hydration with 5% dextrose (plus ad libitum oral intake) (112). Patients randomized to prophylactic PN exceeded their basal energy and nitrogen requirements, while those in the dextrose group received only about half of their nutrient requirements. Use of parenteral nutrition was associated with weight gain, increased serum protein concentrations, and improved survival and time to relapse, compared with 5% dextrose. In another study, 61 patients received PN or EN for 4 weeks after BMT (113). EN was well tolerated, but three-quarters of the patients required supplemental peripheral amino acid infusions for an average of 1 week to meet nitrogen needs. Although the enteral feeding program was less effective in maintaining body cell mass, hematopoietic recovery rate, length of hospitalization, and survival did not differ between the groups. Nutrition-related costs were considerably higher in the PN group, suggesting that EN be used if feasible.

Most patients undergoing kidney or heart transplantation can eat within several days of surgery. Therefore, formal nutritional support in these individuals is not generally indicated unless they develop a complication that precludes use of the GI tract. Likewise, many patients undergoing liver transplantation are discharged from the hospital within 1 week of operation and usually do not require nutritional support. When nutritional support is used, the enteral route is preferred (114). As in other patients, provision of nutritional support is based on two different rationales: to prevent starvation-induced complications (e.g., infection) and to alter favorably the natural history (i.e., reduce rejection) of the transplanted organ. This second rationale is based on correcting existing nutritional or metabolic deficiencies in the transplanted patient or organ so that outcome will improve. One study (24) in minimally malnourished patients undergoing major hepatic resection demonstrated the benefits of preoperative and postoperative PN in reducing postoperative complications. Extrapolating from this study, there may be a role for nutritional support in patients undergoing organ transplantation.

Small bowel transplantation continues to pose a challenge in the field, in part because the organ is highly immunogenic. Simultaneously, home parenteral nutrition for patients with the short gut syndrome is expensive (~$100,000/year) and is associated with well-described metabolic complications. A recent study (115) demonstrated that the requirement for TPN could be decreased or even eliminated in patients with short gut syndrome by providing a nutritional regimen consisting of supplemental glutamine, growth hormone, and a modified high-carbohydrate, low-fat diet. There was a marked improvement in absorption of nutrients with this combination therapy, and a decrease in stool output. In addition, the cost associated with care of these individuals was substantially reduced. Discontinuation of growth hormone did not significantly increase TPN needs in these patients once they had undergone successful gut rehabilitation (see also Chapter 101).

The indications for postoperative nutritional support in patients undergoing solid organ transplantation are similar to those for other elective surgical patients. It remains unclear how long transplant patients can tolerate undernutrition without adverse consequences. If the patient develops a posttransplant complication that precludes oral intake, formal nutritional support should be instituted. Such complications include ileus, sepsis, or failure of other organs. Fluid and electrolyte abnormalities must be carefully monitored, as these patients often have substantial fluid requirements, and electrolyte shifts commonly occur.

The potential for nutritional intervention to influence graft rejection is an area of research that is likely to have promise, since it is well established that nutritional status can modulate cytokine production by inflammatory cells.

CHOICE OF NUTRITION IN SURGICAL PATIENTS

Enteral or Parenteral?

Although the physiologic advantage of EN is apparent, preoperative nutritional repletion via the enteral route has not been as extensively studied as preoperative TPN. Although its use can be associated with development of nausea, diarrhea, and distention, we recommend use of EN (via a feeding tube or as between-meal supplements) in malnourished patients who need elective surgery. Candidates must have a functional GI tract and must be able to receive adequate amounts of calories and nitrogen. In general, such preoperative nutritional support should be limited to 7 to 10 days.

Studies in elective surgical patients comparing the efficacy of PN and EN in the postoperative elective surgery setting have failed to show significant differences. However, significant benefits of enteral feeding have been shown in trauma patients; septic complications were significantly reduced in trauma patients fed via feeding tube immediately after blunt trauma. Luminal nutrition is beneficial even when relatively small amounts of the formula, below caloric requirements, are provided.

In an effort to evaluate the cost effectiveness and metabolic consequences of nutritional support, investigators have compared postoperative TPN and EN. The cost of EN is considerably lower than the cost of TPN, and home administration is easier in patients who are nourished enterally. Bower et al. (116) randomized 20 patients undergoing major upper GI or pancreaticobiliary surgery to receive either postoperative TPN or an elemental diet via a needle catheter jejunostomy (NCJ). Early nitrogen balance was improved in the TPN group, but late nitrogen balance was similar between groups. Complications were minimal, and insignificant differences in serum albumin concentration and transaminase levels were noted. The major difference between groups was the estimated cost of nutritional support: $2313 in the TPN group compared with $849 in the NCJ group.

Nutrition and the Gastrointestinal Tract: Supporting the Gut in Critically Ill Patients

The intestinal tract was long considered an organ of inactivity following operation or injury. Ileus is generally present, nasogastric decompression is often necessary, and the gut is usually unused in the immediate postoperative period. Digestion and absorption were thought to be the only physiologic role of the gut. However, studies have shown that the gut functions as a central organ of amino acid metabolism, a role that may become more pronounced during critical illness (117, 118). Disuse of the GI tract, via either starvation or nutritional support by TPN, may lead to numerous physiologic derangements as well as changes in gut microflora, impaired gut immune function, and disruption of the integrity of the mucosal barrier. Thus, maintaining gut function in the perioperative period may be essential to minimize septic complications and organ failure. Treatment strategies designed to support the gut during critical illness should be directed toward provision of appropriate nutrition and maintenance of mucosal structure and function. Presumably, such efforts will assist the gut in its roles as a metabolic processing station and as a barrier.

Nutritional Support: Enteral Feedings

Enteral feedings are probably the best single method of maintaining mucosal structure and function (Table 98.5). The trophic effects of luminal nutrition are key, and the beneficial effects are well documented, even if relatively small amounts of nutrients are provided. Elegant studies using Thiry-Vella loops (119) to study the effects of excluding a segment of small intestine from the nutrient stream demonstrated the superiority of enteral stimulation. On the other hand, potentially detrimental effects of TPN include mucosal atrophy characterized by a fall in mucosal mass and brush border activity (120, 121). Elemental diets provided to rats promote translocation, but the incidence is significantly lower than that observed when an identical solution is administered intravenously for 2 weeks. In rats subjected to an intraperitoneal injection of hemoglobin and *Escherichia coli*, the survival rate was clearly enhanced when the same nutrient solution was given enterally rather than parenterally (122). Mochizuki et al. (123) studied endocrine and gut responses to burn injury in guinea pigs and demonstrated that early EN blunted the catabolic response and helped preserve mucosal integrity.

Table 98.5
Proposed Effects of Lack of Enteral Stimulation on the Gut

Decreased villous height
Decreased cellular mass
Decreased brush border enzyme activities
Increased gut permeability
Changes in gut microflora
Decreased gut immunity

Nutritional Support Using the Gut-Specific Nutrient Glutamine

It is now clear that both the composition of the diet and the route of delivery are important in maintaining gut structure and function. Several gut-specific nutrients have been studied, but glutamine has received the most attention. The role of glutamine as a nutritional supplement is discussed in Chapter 35.

The Use of Growth Factors to Support the Gut Mucosa

Specific growth factors that may promote intestinal mucosal growth have been implicated in a number of physiologic processes including growth, tissue repair, and regeneration. Among these is epidermal growth factor (EGF), a polypeptide secreted by submaxillary glands and by Brunner's glands of the small intestine. The most widespread effect of EGF on the gastrointestinal mucosa is overall stimulation of DNA synthesis as evidenced by thymidine incorporation. Provision of EGF subcutaneously to rats receiving TPN decreases the degree of villous atrophy that otherwise occurs (124).

Adjuncts to Nutritional Support That May Modify the Catabolic Response to Critical Illness

Beside nutritional intervention, several other methods of modifying the physiologic and biochemical responses to an elective operative procedure have been studied in an effort to reduce the stress of operations and to provide insight into mechanisms of these responses. A variety of human studies have shown that many postoperative responses can be ablated following denervation of the wound (125, 126). These studies suggest that regional anesthetic techniques block afferent signals from the wound and interrupt sympathetic nervous efferent signals to the adrenal gland and possibly the liver. The effect of sympathetic blockade is a reduction in the apparent magnitude of the stress response. These techniques have also been used during the postoperative period. Bromage et al. suppressed hyperglycemia and hypercortisolism with maintenance of an epidural anesthetic for the first 24 hours after operation (127). Brandt et al. reported better 5-day cumulative nitrogen balance in patients undergoing elective abdominal hysterectomy with epidural anesthesia than in a similar group receiving general anesthesia (128).

Several investigators have studied stress responses in sympathectomized animals by blocking the efferent limb of the neuroendocrine reflex response. Propranalol has been shown to improve postoperative nitrogen balance and decrease muscle protein breakdown. Herndon et al. reported that administration of propranalol to burned children decreased cardiac work without affecting wound healing or mortality (129). Brandt et al. reported that large doses of morphine (4 mg/kg) given prior to skin incision diminished the normal rise in plasma ACTH, cortisol, growth hormone, and glucose in patients undergoing aortic valve replacement (130). These reports indicate that central nervous system blockade interrupts afferent signals stimulated by operative procedures.

Studies in the 1960s and 1970s demonstrated that short courses of growth hormone (GH) promoted nitrogen retention following thermal injury. More-recent studies have documented the safety of long-term exogenous recombinant GH administration. GH promotes anabolism and favorably affects a number of biochemical parameters (131–136), but it is unclear whether such improvements translate into clinical benefits. Thus, the potential synergistic effects of specialized nutrition in combination with GH require further study.

Cyclooxygenase inhibitors such as aspirin and ibuprofen attenuate the symptoms and endocrine responses that occur in critical illness without altering cytokine elaboration. For example, pretreatment with ibuprofen may attenuate the undesirable symptoms associated with the inflammatory response (137). It is anticipated that researchers will eventually be able to selectively block the deleterious effects of excessive cytokines and preserve their beneficial effects. Specific antibodies are already being used in the clinical setting to block the TNF and IL-1 receptor. Clearly, the type of nutrition used in critically ill patients can influence the metabolic alterations seen with infection (138, 139). No doubt patient care strategies in the future will use combination therapies designed to minimize the undesirable consequences of the body's response to critical illness and simultaneously accelerate wound healing, immune function, and recovery.

REFERENCES

1. Souba WW. N Engl J Med 1977;1:49–58.
2. Windsor JA, Hill GL. Ann Surg 1988;207:290–302.
3. Hermann FR, Safran C, Levkoff SE, et al. Arch Intern Med 1992;152:125–30.
4. Weinser R, Hunker EM, Krumdieck CL, et al. Am J Clin Nutr 1979;32:418–26.
5. Christou NV, Meakins JL, Gordon J, et al. Ann Surg 1995; 222:534–48.
6. Burke G, Francsson C, Plaintin CO. Acta Endocrinol 1955;18:201–9.
7. Traynor C, Hall GM. Br J Anaesth 1981;53:153–60.
8. Deutsch S. Surg Clin North Am 1975;55:775–86.
9. Philbin DM, Coggins CH. Anesthesiology 1978;49:95–8.
10. Russell RC, Walker CJ, Bloom SR. Br Med J 1975;1:10–2.
11. Porte D, Graber AL, Kuzuwa T, et al. J Clin Invest 1966;45:228–36.
12. Riegel C, Koop CE, Drew J, et al. J Clin Invest 1947;26:18–23.
13. Holden WD, Krieger H, Levey S, et al. Ann Surg 1957;146: 563–79.
14. Wilmore DW. The metabolic management of the critically ill. New York: Plenum Medical Book, 1977.
15. Grant A. Nutritional assessment: guidelines for dietitians. 2nd ed. Seattle: 1979.
16. Meakins JH, McLean APH, Kelly R, et al. J Trauma 1978;18:240–7.
17. Duke JH, Jorgensen SB, Broell JR, et al. Surgery 1970; 68:168–74.
18. Page CP, Ryan JA, Haff RC. Surg Gynecol Obstet 1976;142: 184–8.
19. Muller JM, Brenner U, Dienst C, et al. Lancet 1982;1:68–72.
20. The Veterans Affairs Total Parenteral Nutrition Cooperative Study Group. N Engl J Med 1991;325:525–32.
21. Detsky A, Baker JP, O'Rourke K, et al. Ann Intern Med 1987; 107:195–203.
22. Shukla HS, Rao RR, Banu N, et al. Indian J Med Res 1984;80:339–43.
23. Foschi D, Cavagna G, Callioni F, et al. Br J Surg 1986;73:716–9.
24. Fan ST, Lo CM, Lai ECS, et al. N Engl J Med 1994;331: 1547–52.
25. Brennan MF, Pisters PWT, Posner M, et al. Ann Surg 1994; 220:436–44.
26. Sandstrom R, Drott A, Hyltander A, et al. Ann Surg 1993;217:185–95.
27. Fischer JE, Rosen HM, Ebeid AM, et al. Surgery 1976;80: 77–91.
28. Cerra FB, McMillen M, Angelico R, et al. Surgery 1983; 94:612–9.
29. Cerra F, Cheung NK, Fischer JE, et al. JPEN J Parenter Enteral Nutr 1985;9:288–95.
30. Naveau S, Pelletier G, Poynard T, et al. Hepatology 1986;6:270–4.
31. Nasrallah SM, Galambos JT. Lancet 1980;2:1276–8.
32. Naylor CD, O'Rourke K, Detsky AS, et al. Gastroenterology 1989;97:1033–42.
33. Abel RM, Beck CH, Abbott WM, et al. N Engl J Med 1973;288:695–9.
34. Leonard CD, Luke RG, Siegel RR. Urology 1975;6:154–7.
35. Kopple JD. Am J Kidney Dis 1994;24:1002–9.
36. Guedon C, Schmitz J, Lerebours E, et al. Gastroenterology 1986;90:373–8.
37. Inoue Y, Espat NJ, Frohnapple DJ, et al. Ann Surg 1993;217:604–14.
38. Van der Hulst R, Van Kreel BK, Von Meyenfeldt MF, et al. Lancet 1993;341:1363–5.
39. Fong Y, Marano MA, Barber A, et al. Ann Surg 1989;210: 449–57.
40. Cuthbertson DP. Q J Med 1932;1:233–46.
41. Wilmore DW, Orcutt TW, Mason AD, et al. J Trauma 1975;15:697–703.
42. Wilmore DW. In: Alberti KGMM, ed. Clinics in endocrinology and metabolism. Philadelphia: WB Saunders, 1976.
43. Wilmore DW, Goodwin CW, Aulick LH, et al. Ann Surg 1980;192:491–504.

44. Wilmore DW, Aulick LH, Mason AD, et al. Ann Surg 1977;186:444–58.
45. Goodwin C, Aulick L, Powanda M, et al. Eur J Surg Res 1980;12(Suppl 126):126–7.
46. Black PR, Brooks DC, Bessey PQ, et al. Ann Surg 1982;196:420–33.
47. Wilmore DW, Aulick LH, Goodwin CW, et al. Acta Chir Scand 1980;498(Suppl):43–7.
48. Wolfe RR, Durkot MJ, Allsop JR, et al. Metabolism 1979;28:1031–9.
49. Brooks DC, Bessey PQ, Black PR, et al. J Surg Res 1984;34:100–7.
50. Carpentier YA, Askanazi J, Elwyn DH, et al. J Trauma 1979;19:649–54.
51. Bessey PQ, Brooks DC, Black PR, et al. Surgery 1983;94:172–9.
52. Bessey PQ, Watters JM, Aoki TT, et al. Ann Surg 1984;200(3):264–81.
53. Herrmann VM, Clark D, Wilmore DW, et al. Surg Forum 1980;31:92–4.
54. Picou D, Taylor-Roberts T. Clin Sci 1969;36:283–96.
55. Birkhahn RH, Long CL, Fitkin D, et al. Am J Physiol 1981;241:E64–71.
56. Cuthbertson D. Lancet 1942;1:433–7.
57. Aulick LH, Wilmore DW. Surgery 1979;85:560–5.
58. Muhlbacher F, Kapadia CR, Colpoys MF, et al. Am J Physiol 1974;247:E75–83.
59. Goldberg AL, Chang TW. Fed Proc 1978;37:2301–7.
60. Moldawer LL, Echenique MM, Bistrian BR, et al. In: Johnson IDA, ed. Advances in clinical nutrition. Boston: MTP Press, 1983.
61. Pitts RF. Am J Med 1964;36:720–42.
62. Windmueller HG, Spaeth AE. J Biol Chem 1974;249:5070–9.
63. Souba WW, Wilmore DW. Surgery 1983;94:342–50.
64. Souba WW, Kapadia CR, Smith RJ, et al. Surg Forum 1983;34:74–8.
65. Birkhahn RH, Long CL, Fitkin DL, et al. J Trauma 1981;21:513–9.
66. Wilmore DW, Aulick LH, Becker RA. In: Fischer JE, ed. Surgical nutrition. Boston: Little, Brown, 1983.
67. Michie HR, Wilmore DW. Arch Surg 1990;125:531–6.
68. Akira S, Hirano T, Taga T, et al. FASEB J 1990;4:2860–7.
69. Arai K, Lee F, Miyajima A, et al. Annu Rev Biochem 1990;59:783–836.
70. Michie HR, Manogue KR, Spriggs DR. N Engl J Med 1988;318(23):1481–6.
71. Souba WW, Salloum RM, Bode BP, et al. Surgery 1991;110:295–302.
72. Austgen TR, Chen MK, Dudrick PS, et al. Am J Surg 1992;163:174–80.
73. Fong Y, Tracey KJ, Moldawer LL, et al. J Exp Med 1989;170:1627.
74. Fong Y, Moldawer LL, Marano M, et al. J Immunol 1989;142:2321.
75. Fong Y, Marano MA, Moldawer LL, et al. J Clin Invest 1990;85:1896.
76. Long JM III, Wilmore DW, Mason AD, et al. Ann Surg 1977;185:417–22.
77. Wolfe RR, Allsop JR, Burke JF. Metabolism 1979;28:210–20.
78. Askanazi J, Rosenbaum SH, Hyman AI, et al. JAMA 1980;243:1444–7.
79. Levine M. N Engl J Med 1986;314:892–902.
80. Brodribb AJM, Ricketts CR. Injury 1971;3:25–9.
81. Kudsk KA, Croce MA, Fabian TA, et al. Ann Surg 1992;217:503–13.
82. Moore EE, Jones TN. J Trauma 1986;26:874–81.
83. Moore FA, Moore EE, Jones TN, et al. J Trauma 1989;29:916–23.
84. Moore FA, Feliciano DV, Andrassy RJ, et al. Ann Surg 1992;216:172–83.
85. Border JR, Hassett J, LaDuca J, et al. Ann Surg 1987;206:427–45.
86. Alexander JW, MacMillan BG, Stinnett JD, et al. Ann Surg 1980;192:505–17.
87. Hadley MN, Graham TW, Harrington T, et al. Neurosurgery 1986;19:367–73.
88. Grahm TW, Zadrozny DB, Harrington T. Neurosurgery 1989;25:729–35.
89. Clifton GL, Robertson CS, Choi SC. J Neurosurgery 1986;64:895–901.
90. Clowes GHA, Vucinic M, Weidner MG. Ann Surg 1966;163:866–85.
91. Beisel WR. Annu Rev Med 1975;26:9–20.
92. Gump FE, Long C, Killian P, et al. J Trauma 1974;14:378–88.
93. LaNoue KF, Mason AD, Daniels JP. Metabolism 1968;17:606–11.
94. McFadzean AJS, Yeung RTT. Trans R Soc Trop Med Hyg 1965;59:179–85.
95. Yeung CY. J Pediatr 1970;77:812–7.
96. Herrmann V, Clark D, Wilmore DW. Surg Forum 1980;31:92–4.
97. Duff JH, Viidik T, Marchuk JB, et al. Surgery 1979;85:344–8.
98. Radcliffe AG, Wolfe RR, Colpoys MF, et al. Am J Physiol 1983;244:R667–75.
99. Dudrick PS, Souba WW. Cytokines, sepsis, and the surgeon: a perspective. Surgery annual. Norwalk, CT: Appleton-Lange, 1994.
100. Alverdy JC. JPEN J Parenter Enteral Nutr 1990;14(Suppl):109S–13S.
101. Deitch EA. Arch Surg 1990;125:403–4.
102. Hollander D, Vadheim CM, Brettholz E, et al. Ann Intern Med 1986;105:883–5.
103. Jarrett F, Balish E, Moylan JA, et al. Surgery 1978;83:523–7.
104. Cerra FB, Siegel JH, Coleman B, et al. Ann Surg 1980;192:570–81.
105. Monk DN, Plank LD, Franch-Arcas G, et al. Ann Surg 1996;223:395–405.
106. Koretz RL. Am J Resp Crit Care Med 1995;151:570–3.
107. Askanazi J, Elwyn DH, Silverberg PA. Surgery 1980;87:596–603.
108. Rose D, Yarborough MF, Canizaro PC, et al. Surg Gynecol Obstet 1986;163:345–50.
109. Soeters PB, Ebeid AM, Fischer JE. Ann Surg 1979;190:189–202.
110. Grant JP, James S, Grabowski V, et al. Ann Surg 1984;200:627–31.
111. Sax HC, Warner BW, Talamini MA, et al. Am J Surg 1987;153:117–24.
112. Szeluga D, Stuart, RK, Utermohlen V, et al. Cancer Res 1987;47:3309–16.
113. Weisdorf SA, Lysne J, Wind D, et al. Transplantation 1987;43:833–8.
114. Wicks C, Somasundaram S, Bjarnason I, et al. Lancet 1994;344:837–40.
115. Byrne T, Persinger R, Young L, et al. Ann Surg 1995;222:243–55.
116. Bower RH, Talaman MA, Sax HC, et al. Arch Surg 1986;121:1040–5.
117. Souba WW, Klimberg VS, Plumley DA, et al. J Surg Res 1990;48:383–91.
118. Lacey J, Wilmore DW. Nutr Rev 1990;48:297–313.

119. Gleeson MH, Dowling RH, Peters TJ. Clin Sci 1982;43:743–57.
120. Johnson LR, Copeland EM, Dudrick SJ, et al. Gastroenterology 1975;68:1177–83.
121. Levine GM, Deren JJ, Steiger E, et al. Gastroenterology 1974;67:975–82.
122. Kudsk KA, Carpenter G, Petersen S, et al. J Surg Res 1981;31:105–10.
123. Mochizuki H, Trocki O, Dominioni L, et al. Ann Surg 1984;200:297–310.
124. Jacobs DO, Evans DA, Mealy K, et al. Surgery 1988;104(2):358–64.
125. Kehlet H, Brandt RM, Rem J. JPEN J Parenter Enteral Nutr 1980;4:152–5.
126. Engquist A, Brandt MR, Fernandes A, et al. Acta Anaesthesiol Scand 1977;21:330–5.
127. Bromage PR, Shibata HR, Willoughby HW. Surg Gynecol Obstet 1971;132:1051–6.
128. Brandt MR, Fernandes A, Mordhorst R, et al. Br Med J 1978;1:1106–8.
129. Herndon DN, Barrow RE, Rectan TC, et al. Ann Surg 1988;208:484–90.
130. Brandt MR, Korshin J, Hansen AP, et al. Acta Anaesthesiol Scand 1978;22:400–12.
131. Inoue Y, Copeland EM, Souba WW. Ann Surg 1994;219: 715–24.
132. Suchner U, Rothkop, MM, Stanislaus G, et al. Arch Intern Med 1990;150:1225–30.
133. Ziegler TR, Rombeau J, Young LS, et al. J Clin Endocrinol Metab 1992;74:865–73.
134. Voerman HJ, Van Schijndel RJ, Groeneveld AJ, et al. Ann Surg 1992;216:648–55.
135. Ziegler T, Young L, Ferrari-Baliviera E, et al. JPEN J Parenter Enteral Nutr 1990;14:574–81.
136. Ziegler TR, Lazarus JM, Young LS, et al. J Am Soc Nephrol 1991;2:1130–5.
137. Revhaug A, Michie HR, Manson JM, et al. Arch Surg 1988;123:162–70.
138. Fong Y, Marano MA, Barber A, et al. Am Surg 1990;210:449–57.
139. Souba WW. Curr Probl Surg 1994;31(7):577–652.

99. Diet, Nutrition, and Drug Interactions

VIRGINIA UTERMOHLEN

This chapter discusses the interactions among diet, nutritional status, and drugs. It is intended as a general account of these interactions, with illustrative examples. More specific accounts concerning individual drugs, drug preparations, and routes of administration can be found in the references to this chapter. New drugs and drug preparations are coming onto the market constantly and may be administered in new ways or added to new nutrient formulations. In caring for a patient, the practitioner should always consider the literature and experience concerning the specific drugs a patient may be taking.

DEMOGRAPHICS, DISEASE STATE, AND RISK OF DRUG-NUTRIENT AND DRUG-NUTRITIONAL STATUS INTERACTIONS

Medical conditions, age, and gender dictate the drugs a patient may be taking and may influence a person's diet and nutritional status. These medical conditions determine not only the therapeutic drugs prescribed but also the types of over-the-counter drugs patients take for symptom relief.

Patients who are under the care of different specialists for multiple conditions and who are likely to self-medicate for symptoms such as arthritic pain or heartburn are at greatest risk for adverse drug-nutrient and diet interactions, because no single practitioner may be aware of all medications the patient may be taking or the diet the patient may have adopted. Therefore, to estimate the likelihood of drug-nutrient and diet interactions, the practitioner should consider all the patient's medical conditions, their metabolic consequences, and the drugs administered for these conditions; should have a high index of suspicion concerning the possibility of self-medication; and should be aware not only of any prescribed diet but also of the patient's actual dietary habits and the possibility of alcohol or substance abuse.

The complexity of the influences imposed by both medical conditions and age on the risk of drug-nutrient interactions is exemplified by the risk of severe iron deficiency anemia in an elderly diabetic patient with an autonomic neuropathy of the colon (1). If this patient also has osteoarthritis, it is likely he or she will also be taking a nonsteroidal antiinflammatory drug (NSAID), either over the counter or by prescription. Such a patient is at risk for colonic ulceration and secondary NSAID-induced bleeding, which in turn leads to loss of iron and anemia (2). The risk of anemia is further increased if the patient uses anticoagulant drugs concurrently (e.g., to prevent coronary thrombosis) or abuses alcohol (3).

Patients receiving enteral nutrition via a feeding tube are at additional risk, because drugs that are normally administered orally may be added to the nutrient formula. These patients may develop problems because of physical incompatibilities between the drug and the formula, pharmaceutical incompatibilities resulting from the form in which the drug must be administered (e.g., as an elixir of high osmolality, which may render the tube feeding hyperosmolar), and constipation (or, more commonly, diarrhea), which may be erroneously attributed to the tube feeding itself (e.g., diarrhea caused by excess ingestion of sorbitol, a common excipient of syrups).

Given the complexities of these interactions, it is not surprising that adverse consequences of drug-nutrient and drug-diet interactions are sufficiently common for the Joint Commission on Accreditation of Healthcare Organizations, in the 1996 accreditation standards (4), to require that hospitals implement a program to ensure that "patients are educated about the potential for drug-food interactions." At the same time, Lasswell et al. (5) reported that 80% of the family practice residents they surveyed said they had received little or no formal training in drug-nutrient interactions.

EFFECTS OF DIET AND NUTRITIONAL STATUS ON DRUG ABSORPTION, DISPOSITION, METABOLISM, AND ACTION

Pharmacokinetics and Pharmacodynamics

The term *pharmacokinetics* refers to the characteristics of a drug's absorption, distribution, biotransformation, and excretion; the term *pharmacodynamics* refers to the mechanisms of drug action and the relationships between a drug's concentration at the active site and its pharmacologic effects. While drug-nutrient interactions may affect drug pharmacodynamics, the most commonly encountered and best studied interactions concern their effects on pharmacokinetics.

Bioavailability

The term *bioavailability* refers to the extent to which a drug reaches its site of pharmacologic action. For practical purposes, this definition includes the extent to which the drug reaches a fluid (e.g., blood or spinal fluid) that bathes the site of action and via which the drug can readily reach the site of action. The bioavailability of a drug depends directly on the extent to which the drug is absorbed and distributed to the site of action and depends inversely on the extent to which it is metabolized and excreted prior to arriving at the site of action.

Absorption

The term *absorption* refers to the rate at which, and the extent to which, a drug leaves its site of administration. Factors that affect absorption include the route and site of drug administration; the site and area of absorption; the concentration of the drug at that site; the physical form of the drug and the vehicle in which the drug is administered; local conditions that affect the drug's solubility, and therefore its ability to reach a site of entry into the bloodstream or cerebrospinal fluid; and, finally, the circulation at the site of absorption. Drug absorption is influenced by physicochemical processes that influence both the extent and the rate at which the drug crosses the mucosal barrier and enters the bloodstream. Table 99.1 lists factors that specifically enhance absorption of an orally or enterally administered drug.

Table 99.1
Factors That Enhance the Extent and Rate of Absorption of an Orally/Enterally Administered Drug

Lack of complex formation with diet ingredients
Maintenance of drug's chemical stability at stomach/small intestinal pH
Presence of a specific transporter
Small size (<200 Da) for transportation with bulk water flow
Lipid solubility—nonionized at local pH
High circulation to the site of absorption, to maintain concentration gradient
Appropriate stomach-emptying rate
Low small intestinal motility

Routes of Drug Administration

Drugs can be administered orally, enterally, or parenterally. The most common route of drug administration is the oral/enteral route. The main parenteral routes include intravenous, subcutaneous, and intramuscular routes. Drugs can also be administered through the lung, rectum, spinal fluid, artery, and peritoneum. Because drug-food and drug-nutrient interactions at the level of absorption occur primarily when the drug is administered via oral/enteral routes, the following discussion concentrates on these routes. Table 99.2 shows the sites of drug absorption in the gastrointestinal tract and their characteristics.

Effects of Food Components on Drug Absorption and Bioavailability

Food components affect drug absorption and bioavailability through three general mechanisms: physicochemical interactions between the drug and food components in the gut lumen, alterations in gastric emptying time, and competitive inhibition between the drug and food components for absorption. Erratic responses to drugs can often be explained by their administration in a haphazard way in relation to mealtimes, if their bioavailability is

Table 99.2
Sites of Drug Absorption and Their Characteristics

Site	Absorption	Characteristics
Mouth	Poor	Short residence time Drug can make contact only if in solution
Stomach	Poor	Small surface area Thick, mucus-covered, electrically resistant mucosa
Proximal small intestine	Excellent	Large surface area Thin, low-electrical-resistance mucosa can absorb both unionized and ionized drugs

affected by the presence or absence of food in the stomach and intestine. Table 99.3 lists common drugs whose absorption is decreased by concomitant consumption of food. Absorption of the drugs listed in Table 99.4 is significantly enhanced when they are taken with food.

Note that the effect of meals on the absorption of drugs may differ strikingly from one formulation to another. For example, three preparations of controlled-release theophylline differ dramatically in their bioavailability when they are consumed with meals. The bioavailability of Uniphyl almost doubles when taken with a high-fat meal, compared with fasting, while the bioavailability of Theo-Dur Sprinkles in the fed state is half that in the fasting state. The bioavailability of Theo-24, an ultra-long-acting preparation, is also markedly increased with a high-fat meal, and the peak concentration of drug reached is significantly higher. Because the therapeutic window (i.e., the blood levels of the drug that lie between the ineffective and the toxic) for theophylline is narrow, it may be important in fact to take Theo-24 with low-fat meals (<10 g), to prevent the sharp increase in blood levels and to provide a longer-acting, more consistent effect (6, 7).

Given these differences in pharmacokinetics, the reader is strongly cautioned to examine the literature and individual experience concerning different formulations of drugs of interest, particularly of formulations of drugs with narrow therapeutic windows.

Table 99.3
Compounds That Should Be Taken in a Fasting State

Ampicillin	Ketoprofen[g]
Astemizole	Lansoprazole
AzoGantanol/AzoGantrisin	Levodopa[h]
Bacampicillin	Lisinopril
Bethanechol[a]	Lomustil[i]
Bisacodyl	Methotrexate[j]
Calcium carbonate	Methyldopa[h]
Captopril	Nafcillin[k]
Carbenicillin	Nalidixic acid
Castor oil	Naltrexone
Chloramphenicol	Norfloxacin[j]
Cyclosporine (soft gelatin capsule only)[b]	Oxytetracycline[c]
Demeclocycline[c]	Penicillamine[l]
Dicloxacillin	Penicillin
Disopyramide	Phenazine (antipyrine)[m]
Digitalis preparations[d]	Phenytoin[n]
Erythromycin base/ erythromycin estolate	Propantheline
Etidronate	Rifampicin
Folic acid	Sotalol
Ferrous salts[e]	Sulfamethoxazole
Flavoxate	Tetracycline[c]
Furosemide	Theophylline[o]
Isoniazid[f]	Thyroid hormone preparations[p]
Isosorbide dinitrate	Terbutaline sulfate
	Trientene[l]
	Trimethoprim

[a]Nausea and vomiting occurs when taken with food.
[b]Should not be taken with fatty meals.
[c]Should not be consumed with dairy products or foods containing high amounts of calcium.
[d]Should not be taken with high-fiber foods.
[e]Do not take with cereals, fiber, tea, coffee, egg, or milk.
[f]Absorption reduced by calcium carbonate.
[g]If GI distress, may be taken with food.
[h]Should not be consumed with high-protein foods (meat, milk, cheese); meals delay absorption and reduce peak plasma concentration; avoid caffeine.
[i]Should be taken on an empty stomach to decrease nausea—no effect of food on absorption.
[j]Milk/cream/yogurt in food may decrease absorption.
[k]Variably inactivated by stomach acid; variably absorbed, with or without food.
[l]Absorption reduced by antacids and iron as well as food.
[m]Not used in U.S.
[n]Effect of food varies with preparation—take with food to decrease GI distress; bioavailability with enteral formulas decreased; mechanism ill defined.
[o]Absorption of controlled release preparations varies by preparation—see text.
[p]Limit foods containing goitrogens: asparagus, broccoli, Brussels sprouts, cabbage, kale, lettuce, peas, soy beans, spinach, turnip greens, watercress, other leafy green vegetables.

Table 99.4
Clinically Significant Drug-Food Interactions II: Drugs That Should Be Taken with Food Because Absorption/Bioavailability Is Increased

Buspirone
Carbamazepine[a]
Chlorothiazide
Clofazimine
Gemfibrozil
Grisefulvin[b]
Isotretinoin
Labetalol
Lovastatin[b]
Methenamine
Metoprolol
Nifedipine[c]
Nitrofurantoin
Oxcarbazepine
Probucol[b]
Propranolol
Spironolactone
Trazodone
Ursodeoxycholate
Verapamil sustained-release tablets[d]

[a]Absorption erratic.
[b]Fatty meals.
[c]Grapefruit juice increases bioavailability.
[d]Extent of absorption varies by manufacturer; risk of heart block if absorption is too rapid.

Physicochemical Interactions between Diet Ingredients and Drug Ingredients

Physicochemical interactions between diet ingredients and drug ingredients include adsorption, complex formation, precipitation, and the effects of one interactant on another whereby stability of one or both is altered. Physicochemical interactions require the simultaneous presence of the drug and the food component at the site of interaction. Therefore, physicochemical interactions occur in the gut lumen for orally and enterally administered drugs and in the reservoir or tubing containing the nutrient formula when drugs and the formula are administered simultaneously via parenteral or enteral routes.

Physicochemical interactions usually result in reduced absorption of the drug, the nutrient, or both. For orally administered drugs, decreased absorption due to physicochemical incompatibilities occurs primarily because of errors in the timing of food intake with drug intake. When the drug is administered via a feeding tube, incompatibilities can also occur when the drug is added to the feeding formula or when it is administered without adequately flushing the tubes.

Disintegration and Dissolution of Drugs Administered Orally. Common dosage forms of drugs designed for oral administration include solid forms (tablets, capsules, or granules) and liquid forms (suspensions, syrups, elixirs, and solutions). Sublingual tablets (e.g., nitroglycerin) are designed for rapid drug absorption through the oral mucosa and contain very small dosages that are absorbed before hydrolysis can occur. Slow-release formulations contain granules of coated medication designed to dissolve at varying rates and release medication over hours.

When taken orally, solid forms of drugs must disintegrate and dissolve before being absorbed. Most preparations are designed to undergo these processes in the stomach. However, certain drugs that may be destroyed by the pH and enzymes of the stomach or may irritate the stomach mucosa are often administered in enteric-coated preparations designed to resist breakdown at acid pH. By contrast, an acidic environment is required for the dissolution of ketoconazole, so patients with achlorhydria or those taking drugs to diminish stomach acidity (such as antacids, H2 histamine blockers, or proton pump inhibitors) may have problems obtaining therapeutically effective doses of this drug (8).

The rate of dissolution of a pill or capsule is increased by the presence of liquid in the stomach. Solid drugs taken with a beverage dissolve more rapidly and more completely than when taken dry. However, if large amounts of fluid are consumed, the concentration of the drug in solution may decrease, leading to a decrease in the rate of absorption.

Physical Interactions between Enteral Formulas and Drugs. Physical interactions between drugs and enteral formulas in formula reservoirs or feeding tubes lead to sometimes subtle changes in the appearance of the formula, with clouding, curdling, flocculation, phase separations, and changes in the formula's viscosity (sometimes thinning, but more often thickening, coagulation, and gelling). These changes generally clog feeding tubes and decrease delivery of both drug and feeding formula to the patient (9). Table 99.5. lists methods of avoiding incompatibilities due to physical interactions between drugs and enteral formulas.

Pharmaceutical Incompatibility of Drugs and Enteral Formulas. Pharmaceutical incompatibility refers to adverse interactions between drugs and enteral formulas that occur because the form of the drug must be altered (e.g., by crushing) so that it can be administered through a feeding tube. When the form of a drug is altered, safe delivery of the drug to its site of absorption may not occur. For example, drugs that are enterically coated to prevent destruction by stomach acid are not good candidates for crushing and delivery in an enteral formula, because crushing destroys the enteric coat. Similarly, crushing slow-delivery preparations leads to immediate release of the drug in a single dose and the possibility of overdose. Instead, the complete contents of a capsule of slow-release drugs should be administered as intact beads, making certain that the beads pass successfully through the feeding tube. Approaches to avoiding pharmaceutical incompatibilities are listed in Table 99.5.

Chemical Stability. The chemical stability of a drug is affected by pH, enzyme activity, and drug-nutrient binding reactions (chelation). Certain salts of drugs are resistant to acid hydrolysis in the stomach, while other drugs are inactivated in an alkaline environment. For example, erythromycin is available as four different salts: base, stearate, ethylsuccinate, and estolate. To avoid acid hydrolysis, the first two salts are delivered in enteric-coated tablets, while the other two salts (particularly the estolate) are acid stable and can be administered without enteric coating (10). Misoprostol, whose active form is misoprostol acid, is an example of a drug that is less bioavailable in an alkaline environment, although the *rate* of absorption and the peak concentration reached in plasma are not changed by the presence of antacid (11).

Drug-Nutrient Chelation. Certain drugs chelate minerals and render both the drug and the mineral unavailable for absorption. The best-known example of this effect is the chelation of divalent and trivalent cations by tetracycline and its congeners (12). This effect is less pronounced with minocycline (13) and controversial with doxycycline (14,

Table 99.5
Approaches to Avoid Physical and Pharmaceutical Incompatibilities between Drugs and Enteral Formulas

- Avoid mixing the drug and formula
  - No direct mixing of drug and formula
  - Flush tubing with water before and after administering drug
- Change the formula to one compatible with the drug
- Change drug dosage, dosage form, or drug
  - Lower the concentration of the drug in the formula by decreasing or dividing the dosage
  - Use an alternate dosage form
    - Substitute the dosage from an opened capsule rather than from an acidic solution if the carrier of the drug is responsible for the incompatibility
    - Use an elixir, rather than an enteric-coated tablet
    - Use an acid-stable salt that is more amenable to crushing and delivery directly to the stomach
  - Use an alternate route of drug administration (intramuscular, intravenous, subcutaneous, etc.)
  - Substitute a therapeutically equivalent but chemically distinct drug that is compatible with the formula (examples of equivalent drug pairs: loperamide and diphenoxylate for diarrhea; promethazine and prochlorperazine for nausea and vomiting)

Data from Rollins C. Physiological impact of drug-nutrient interactions. Handout for the 20th Clinical Congress, American Society of Parenteral and Enteral Nutrition, January 1996.

15). These drugs should not be taken within 2 hours of consuming foods containing calcium, magnesium, iron, or zinc. The other drugs that interact with iron include the dopa drugs (methyldopa, levodopa, carbidopa), ciprofloxacin, penicillamine, and trientine; thyroxine and captopril form stable complexes with iron (15a).

Gastric Emptying and Drug Absorption Kinetics

A drug leaves the stomach at a rate that depends on gastric emptying. Gastric emptying, in turn, depends on the general functioning of the stomach and gastrointestinal tract (e.g., a person with autonomic neuropathy affecting the gut has very slow gastric emptying), on the physiologic changes in the gastrointestinal tract in the fed versus the fasted state, and on the effects of the drugs themselves on gastric emptying. In the fasted state or when little food is in the stomach, drugs usually leave the stomach rapidly and thus reach the small intestine rapidly. If a drug is formulated as a solid preparation—such that disintegration of drug particles as well as dissolution of the drug in stomach fluid must precede absorption—then rapid stomach emptying militates against rapid drug absorption. The aspects of drug pharmacokinetics that are affected by gastric emptying time include the time to peak plasma level, the number of plasma level peaks (i.e., one or more), the heights of the peak plasma levels, and the area under the curve of plasma drug concentration (AUC).

When a drug or food is delivered to the stomach, the stomach initially empties some of its contents within a few minutes. This emptying, termed the *adaptive phase of gastric emptying,* may be of varying volume (16). When this initial emptying delivers some of the ingested material into the duodenum, hormones are released that decrease antral contractions and increase pyloric contractions, which lead to retention of material in the stomach. Fatty foods are the most potent inducers of these changes in contractions, through the release of cholecystokinin (17). Note that erythromycin counteracts this effect and speeds up gastric emptying (17). Carbohydrates in the ileum can also alter the contraction pattern and decrease gastric emptying, so that carbohydrates ingested in one meal can affect gastric emptying in the next (18).

The initial gastric emptying leads to the first opportunity for a drug to be absorbed by the small intestine and delivered to the bloodstream. This initial absorption results in development of the first plasma drug peak (19). The height of this peak also depends on the transit time through the rest of the gastrointestinal tract, with more rapid transit lowering the height of the peak and decreasing the AUC. Drugs delivered without food but with water have only one peak in plasma concentration (19). The height and duration of the peak depends on the size of the drug particles, the extent to which they are dissolved in the gastric juices and water, the size of the initial emptying, the intestinal transit time, and the rate of drug absorption in the intestine.

While rapid delivery of a drug into the small intestine may increase the initial rate of absorption and the peak concentration of the drug in the bloodstream, the total AUC may be decreased, particularly if the intestinal transit time is also decreased, because the drug's residence time in the small intestine is short (20). Under these circumstances, the drug may be better absorbed after food intake. Coated drugs may also be better absorbed with food because the capsules may disintegrate better in the small intestine after longer residence in the stomach (21).

When drugs are taken with food, there is usually a second peak in the plasma concentration-time curve. The second peak corresponds to absorption of the drug as it is delivered with food to the intestine in the second phase of gastric emptying. The height and duration of the peak depend on the gastrointestinal transit time, the surface area over which the drug can be absorbed, the kinetics of absorption, and the size and timing of the first peak with respect to the second phase of delivery of the drug to the absorptive sites (19). The dependence of the second peak on the first peak reflects the fact that the systemic levels of a drug influence the drug's further absorption from the gastrointestinal tract. This effect can be clearly seen for drugs absorbed by simple diffusion, because the drug concentration *gradient* directly influences the amount of drug absorbed.

Particles up to about 1.1 mm in diameter are emptied from the stomach with food prior to the interdigestive phase, although there is great interindividual variability, and not all particles of the same size may be released with food (22, 23). Larger particles are released from the stomach during the interdigestive phases, with the very largest particles requiring the "housekeeper" phase-three contractions of the stomach that occur well after a meal, when the stomach is empty (24). This phenomenon accounts for the observation that certain drug preparations are not cleared from the stomach until night, even though they may be consumed during the day, if there is not sufficient time between meals and snacks to ensure complete emptying of the stomach (25). There is evidence that taking enteric-coated pills or capsules with meals severely delays their delivery into the duodenum, sometimes as much as 10 to 12 hours (25). If given in multiple doses throughout the day, these drugs may accumulate in the stomach and be dumped into the duodenum at night when the stomach finally empties. This problem, which deserves further investigation, can be prevented by taking these drugs on an empty stomach and avoiding between-meal snacks (25). Release of a drug from the stomach also depends critically on its particle size, with larger particles being retained for longer times.

Note that gastric emptying may differ considerably from individual to individual in the fasting state. These differences may contribute to some of the unpredictability of drug absorption in this state (26). Gastric emptying is delayed in neonates irrespective of fasting (27), so that the oral route for drug administration is unreliable. By contrast, gastric emptying may be normal (28) or prolonged (29) in healthy fit elderly persons. Women may have slower gastric emptying times than men, even when controlled for menstrual stage (29). Pregnancy appears to have no effect on gastric emptying, although intestinal transit time is increased (30). Chronic alcoholics experience striking delays in gastric emptying, which may affect both drug pharmacokinetics and nutrient consumption and absorption (31). Note that gastric emptying is delayed by acute cigarette smoking, although it is not delayed in smokers if they are not smoking at the time of drug administration (32).

A delay in gastric emptying may also enhance drug absorption because the drug is delivered more slowly and efficiently to its intestinal absorption site. This is especially true if drug transport across the intestine is saturable and site specific. This effect may explain the enhanced absorption of chlorothiazide after food intake (33). Hydrochlorothiazide, by contrast, is absorbed equally well whether taken with or without food. Although food slows absorption and decreases the height of the plasma concentration peaks of this drug, the 48-hour dose recovery in the urine is the same whether the person has fasted or not (34).

Transport across the Enterocyte Lipid Membrane

To be absorbed, drugs must be transported across the lipid membrane of the mucosal barrier, either by diffusion or by a specific carrier. Although a drug's pK_a influences its absorption in the stomach, most drugs are absorbed in the small intestine, irrespective of pK_a, because the surface is optimized for absorption. Most drugs are transported across the lipid membrane by simple diffusion that depends on the concentration gradient of the drug across the intestinal mucosa. As a result, food-induced increases in splanchnic blood flow may increase the bioavailability of drugs, although this may not be a simple effect, as noted.

Competitive Inhibition of Absorption. Drugs absorbed through transport mechanisms may be subject to competitive inhibition by the individual nutrients that are the normal substrate for the transport mechanism. For example, L-dopa and methyldopa are transported across the small intestine via the aromatic amino acid transporter. Therefore, absorption of these drugs is reduced when they are taken with a high-protein meal or with an amino acid mixture that contains aromatic amino acids (35, 36).

Transport of L-dopa across the blood-brain barrier also depends on the aromatic amino acid transporter, so consumption of a high-protein meal inhibits entry of the drug into the brain (37, 38). Patients with "on-off" effect, who fluctuate between good function and severe bradykinesia, are particularly sensitive to the interaction between dietary protein and L-dopa efficacy (39). Daytime restriction of protein intake can provide a more acceptable level of function during waking hours (38), provided that the diet consumed before bedtime adequately compensates for any potential deficiencies (40).

Distribution

The term *distribution* refers to the dissemination of the drug via the bloodstream to the interstitial and intracellular fluids. Distribution of a drug depends on *(a)* its lipid solubility and ionization state (e.g., lipid-soluble drugs cross the blood-brain barrier readily, while acidic or basic drugs do not); *(b)* the blood flow to the body compartments from which the drug is absorbed and to which the drug is distributed; *(c)* the size and nature of these compartments; *(d)* the solubility of the drug in the compartment, so that the compartment can act as a drug reservoir (e.g., lipid-soluble drugs are distributed to adipose tissue, where they may be retained for long periods of time); *(e)* the degree to which the drug is bound to the components of the compartment (e.g., the extent of binding to plasma proteins); and, finally, *(f)* the time over which distribution is examined—drugs move from compartment to compartment over time, depending on the local concentration gradients of the drug and the barriers to diffusion.

Neonates have an increased fractional volume of extracellular fluid to total body water, with a resultant increase in drug half-life relative to a similar dosage in adults (27). The effects of edema on the half-life of drugs in adults is not so clear (41).

Protein Binding and Drug Availability at the Site of Pharmacologic Action

To be pharmacologically active, drugs must be in a free, unbound state. However, a proportion of many drugs circulates bound to plasma proteins. The major proteins involved in drug binding are albumin and α_1-acid glycoprotein (AAG), although other proteins, such as the lipoproteins, also bind certain drugs. Albumin has two major drug binding sites, I and II. Site I binds phenylbutazone, oxyphenbutazone, warfarin, and long-chain fatty acids. Site II binds benzodiazepines, indoles, ibuprofen, flufenamic acid, and ethacrynic acid, as well as long-, medium-, and short-chain fatty acids and certain amino acids (42).

In conditions characterized by low plasma albumin levels, such as liver disease, nephrotic syndrome, and renal disease, drug binding is decreased. Thus, overdosing may occur. Glycosylation of albumin, which occurs when blood glucose levels are chronically elevated, as in poorly controlled diabetics, appears to decrease site II binding (43, 44). Disagreement exists on this point, possibly because of the probes used (45). Free fatty acids increase dissociation of drugs from albumin site II, so postprandial elevations of free fatty acids as well as the increased free fatty acid levels in the fasting state and in poorly controlled diabetes mellitus may decrease drug binding and increase drug bioavailability and thus the potential for toxicity (44, 45).

Both albumin and AAG levels change with age: albumin

decreases while AAG increases (46). The effects of these changes on drug pharmacokinetics are unknown.

Biotransformation

Most drugs must undergo biotransformation for excretion and some for activation. Lipophilic drugs are most easily absorbed from the gastrointestinal tract and cross membrane barriers best. However, to terminate drug action through excretion, drugs must be water soluble. Biotransformation reactions, then, generate compounds that are more polar than their parent compounds. In most instances, these compounds are inactive and are readily excreted, primarily through the urine. However, biotransformation occasionally leads to either formation of the active form of the drug or formation of toxic metabolites.

Phases of Biotransformation

Phase I Biotransformation. Phase I transformations either expose a functional group on a parent compound or introduce a functional group to that compound. These transformations are carried out (primarily in the liver) by the cytochrome P450 monooxygenase system, found in the endoplasmic reticulum. Humans have 12 genetically determined cytochrome P450 enzyme families, of which three, the CYP1, CYP2, and CYP3 families, are involved with most drug transformations (8). Large interindividual differences in drug metabolism can be attributed to genetic polymorphisms of the cytochrome P450 enzymes, which lead to classification of individuals as rapid or slow metabolizers for a given class of drugs.

The role of intestinal phase I biotransformation in drug bioavailability and the role of foodstuffs in inducing and reducing cytochrome P450 function have not been well studied. Evidence obtained in rats suggests that the P450 enzymes in the intestine are affected by food and ethanol but that the effects differ from those seen in the liver (47). The clinical importance of any differences in humans remains to be determined.

Phase II Biotransformation. Phase II biotransformations involve the conjugation of a parent compound's functional group with a polar group (acetate, glucuronic acid, sulfate, glutathione, or amino acids). Such transformations inactivate most drugs. Rarely, the more polar compound is the more active form of a drug. The resultant conjugated drug is excreted either in the urine or the feces. When the drug is excreted in the feces, bacteria can deconjugate the drug, which then may be reabsorbed, thus undergoing repeated cycles of activity and prolongation of its effect.

Most compounds undergo phase II biotransformation via glucuronidation. However, the sulfotransferases have a higher affinity than the glucuronyl transferases for their common substrates, so at low doses, given a sufficient quantity of sulfur-containing amino acids, sulfation predominates, while at higher doses, glucuronide formation predominates (8).

A number of drugs, including isoniazid (INH), procainamide, dapsone, and caffeine, are metabolized through acetylation of an amino or hydrazino group, primarily through one of several *N*-acetyl transferases. This acetylation process is under genetic control, with rapid acetylation caused by an autosomal dominant gene. Slow acetylation leads to slow clearance of the drug, so that slow acetylators need lower doses of a drug for therapeutic effects than do rapid acetylators. However, for some drugs, the acetylated form may be less water soluble than its parent compound, which may prolong its residence in the body (8). Rifampin is acetylated to a form that is as potent as the parent drug. However, this form is excreted into the bile. Its reuptake is lower than uptake of the parent drug and is further reduced by food. The result is that bioavailability of rifampin and its active metabolites is highly variable (8).

First-Pass Metabolism

Melander and McLean (48) pointed out that drugs can have low oral bioavailability despite complete gastrointestinal absorption. Their explanation is that some drugs undergo extensive presystemic metabolism during their first passage through the gut mucosa and liver. By decreasing first-pass metabolism, food consumption can increase the bioavailability of certain drugs known to undergo presystemic metabolic clearance, including the lipophilic bases propranolol, metoprolol, labetalol, and hydralazine. With aging, decreases in liver blood flow and liver mass contribute to a decline in biotransformation capacity with a corresponding increase in bioavailability. The decrease in phase I biotransformation is more severely affected than that in phase II.

Dietary Factors That Affect Drug Biotransformation

Drug biotransformation is affected by enzyme induction and inhibition, substrate availability, and phenotypic differences in enzyme expression caused by genetic polymorphisms, disease, and age. Dietary factors can affect both enzyme induction and enzyme inhibition, while overall liver and intestinal function may modulate the effects of enzyme function through changes in tissue mass and perfusion.

Whereas relatively few dietary factors have been examined in human subjects for their effects on drug metabolism, a wide range of macro- and micronutrients, including vitamins and trace elements, have been investigated in rodents (49). The findings in rodents should be extrapolated to humans with caution, however, because of the differences in drug handling between the two species and because many of the studies of diet-drug interaction were performed before we understood the individual P450 enzymes and their functions (49).

Epidemiologic and metabolic studies of effects of diet composition on drug toxicity are greatly needed, particularly in the elderly (50, 51). Studying the roles of diet in drug metabolism in the elderly is difficult because they are usually taking multiple drugs. A number of different drugs act on the phase I transforming enzymes, which may mutually alter their metabolism. However, these inhibitory interactions are usually not the result of drug-nutrient interactions, with the exceptions noted below. By contrast, phase II biotransformation may be inhibited by the lack of necessary cofactors; this lack may be of nutritional origin.

Dietary Components and Drug Biotransformation. The substrates needed for drug biotransformation include a sufficient energy source, because biotransformations are energetically expensive; protein for formation of the enzymes themselves; fatty acids of the appropriate composition for presentation of the enzymes in the microsomal membrane; iron for formation of the cytochromes; and, finally, substrates for phase II biotransformation: glucose, sulfur-containing amino acids, specific amino acids such as taurine (which may be limiting in the neonate), and glutathione. The availability of these dietary components appears to regulate not only the function of the enzymes involved in biotransformation but also their expression, as discussed below.

Starvation. Short-term starvation is a common experience for persons with illness and may occur under other circumstances as well. While the literature contains references to alterations in drug bioavailability in starvation, there is relatively little information on the effects of starvation on phase I and phase II biotransformation (52). Rat studies suggest that short-term (48 hours) starvation leads to induction of a number of different cytochromes and a decrease in the functional amounts of others in the liver (53). The effects of starvation on drug biotransformation in humans has not been adequately studied.

Protein. In rodents, high-protein diets enhance drug metabolism, and protein-deficient diets slow drug metabolism. Humans metabolize theophylline and antipyrine more rapidly when they are on a high-protein diet (49). The rise in metabolism appears to be due to an increase in CYP1A2, as there is an increase in catabolism of 17β-estradiol by 2-hydroxylation, which is a function of CYP1A2, but not by 6-hydroxylation, which does not depend on CYP1A2. This effect of protein is particularly noticeable when a person is placed on total parenteral nutrition (TPN) after receiving dextrose in water for a period of time (49). By contrast, children with kwashiorkor have a generalized decrease in drug metabolism, although this decrease may be associated with the fatty liver and overall liver malfunction seen in this condition. In support of the notion that the changes in kwashiorkor result from liver dysfunction, there is evidence that people with anorexia nervosa do not have altered drug metabolism (49).

With respect to phase II biotransformation, when animals are fed a low-protein diet that is adequate in energy content, glucuronidation increases. Diets low in the sulfur-containing amino acids methionine and cysteine reduce sulfate conjugation rates (54, 55). Whether a similar effect occurs in humans is not known.

Carbohydrate. Short-term carbohydrate restriction leads to depletion of the cofactors needed for oxidation and glucuronide formation, and thereby a decrease in both phase I and phase II biotransformation (56). Chronic high-carbohydrate diets and the high blood glucose levels seen in uncontrolled diabetics decrease phase I biotransformation, probably through inhibition of the synthesis of δ-aminolevulinic acid, a precursor of the heme component of the cytochromes (57). The importance of the carbohydrate and protein effects is underscored in persons (especially children) taking theophylline for asthma. This drug has a very narrow therapeutic range. Increasing the protein:carbohydrate ratio can decrease the effectiveness of a given dose of theophylline; decreasing this ratio may lead to development of toxicity (58). Persons taking theophylline should therefore maintain a consistent diet (with a consistent content of caffeine and other methylxanthines, which compete for theophylline for biotransformation, as well) to establish and maintain therapeutic blood levels of the drug.

Enzyme Induction and Inhibition by Specific Compounds in Food. Exposure to foods, drugs, and environmental pollutants can induce increased synthesis of (usually specific) cytochrome P450 enzymes or can inhibit their induction. Induction of P450 enzymes can be accompanied by induction of the conjugation enzymes. The dietary inducers and inhibitors of these enzymes are usually nonnutritive components of foods, such as heterocyclic amines, flavones, indolic compounds, and terpenoids, as well as ethanol, although the fatty acid composition of the diet may have important effects on P450 enzyme activity.

Fatty acids are metabolized by the cytochrome P450 enzymes and in turn affect enzyme expression. When fat-free diets are fed to laboratory animals, cytochrome P450 function decreases (59, 60). This decrease may be the result of polyunsaturated fatty acid deficiency, which in turn may affect the microsomal membrane's composition, fluidity, and ability to present enzymes (60, 61).

CYP2E1 is responsible for lipid peroxidation, which is enhanced in the presence of highly polyunsaturated fatty acids, such as fish oils. The activity of this enzyme increases with ethanol feeding in rats and may be responsible for the centrilobular fatty liver seen with excessive ethanol consumption (62–65). In fact, Nanji et al. (65) have suggested that consumption of saturated fatty acids may suppress development of a fatty liver in alcoholism. On a parenthetical note, watercress appears to inhibit CYP2E1 activity (66).

Char-broiled meats, which contain large amounts of heterocyclic amines, are highly potent inducers of CYP1A2 (67, 68). Induction of this enzyme increases the oxidation of caffeine, theophylline, antipyrine, bufuralol, acetaminophen, ondansetron, tacrine, and warfarin. The indoles in cruciferous vegetables and their metabolites also activate CYP1A2. This effect may contribute to the presumed anticancer effects of cruciferous vegetables (49). At the same time, the phenylethylisocyanate in cruciferous vegetables acutely decreases CYP2E1 activity in rats (69). Whether a similar effect occurs in humans is not known.

Flavonoids can induce, directly activate, or inhibit P450 enzymes. The targets for this activity are CYP3A4 and CYP1A2 (49, 70, 71). Some interactions of these enzymes with flavones lead to induction and others to inhibition, which makes predictions about the effects of dietary flavones particularly difficult. For example, flavones markedly enhance activation of aflatoxin B1, a carcinogen. By contrast, the flavonoids in grapefruit juice (naringin, naringenin, limonin, obacunone) inhibit CYP3A, as measured by 6β-hydroxylation of testosterone by rat and human liver microsomes (71). Quercetin and kaempferol in grapefruit may also inhibit metabolism of midazolam and quinidine by inhibiting CYP3A4 (71a).

Studies of the interaction of components of grapefruit juice with CYP3A have ascribed the clinically significant inhibition of metabolism of the dihydropyridine calcium channel blockers (nifedipine, felodipine, and nisoldipine) by small quantities of juice to 6′,7′-dihydroxybergamottin, a furanocoumarin (psoralen) (71, 72) present in grapefruit but not in orange juice. Previous studies have ascribed this action to the flavonoids in citrus juices, which are indeed effective in inhibiting liver CYP3A (49, 70). However these compounds are present in grapefruit at too low a concentration to account for the effectiveness of this fruit in CYP3A inhibition (71). Interestingly, the increased bioavailability of the calcium channel blockers following consumption of grapefruit juice appears to be due to inhibition of intestinal, rather than liver, CYP3A4 (73).

Terpenoids, which are plentiful in citrus fruits, increase the total level of P450 enzymes in rat liver, but their role in human P450 activity and drug metabolism has not been established (49).

Acute ethanol consumption reduces the activity of the P450 enzymes by depriving them of the reducing equivalents derived from mitochondrial metabolism. Ethanol also competitively inhibits CYP2E1 (63). Thus, phenytoin metabolism is decreased when it is consumed at the same time as ethanol. Chronic ethanol consumption, by contrast, induces the CYP2E1 family of enzymes, so that when a chronic alcoholic takes phenytoin after a period of abstinence, metabolism of the drug is enhanced. Similar effects occur with metabolism of tolbutamide and related agents. Note that chronic alcohol consumption depletes liver glutathione and thereby decreases phase II biotransformation of a host of drugs (8).

Pyridoxine supplementation decreases the effectiveness of L-dopa in patients with parkinsonism, possibly through increased peripheral decarboxylation of the drug, which results in decreased L-dopa delivery to the brain (74, 75). For this reason, L-dopa is routinely administered in combination with a peripheral decarboxylase inhibitor, such as carbidopa. Pyridoxine supplementation appears to have no effect on the efficacy of L-dopa administered with a peripheral decarboxylase inhibitor (76).

Propranolol, a Drug Whose Pharmacokinetics Are Significantly Affected by Food Consumption

The effect of food consumption in increasing bioavailability of a single dose of propranolol illustrates the complex interactions between drug characteristics and metabolism on one hand and the physiologic alterations induced by food consumption on the other. Propranolol is a highly lipophilic drug that is almost completely absorbed from the intestine on oral administration, with or without the consumption of food (8). In humans, it is metabolized by two different P450 enzyme families, CYP2D and CYP1A2 (77, 78). At least two enzymes are involved in each metabolic transformation (79). On average, only about 25% of a dose of propranolol reaches the systemic circulation, while 75% undergoes first-pass metabolism (8). The drug circulates tightly bound to α_1-acid glycoprotein. The bioavailability of propranolol can vary 20-fold from individual to individual, mostly because of differences in first-pass metabolism (8).

There are numerous reasons for the food-induced decrease in first-pass metabolism of a single dose of propranolol; these run the gamut from alterations in liver function induced by the mere thought of food to changes in phase I and phase II metabolism of the drug. One or more of these effects may be operative in a given individual, which may account for the very large interindividual differences in systemic bioavailability of a single dose of the drug.

Simultaneous oral administration of a dose of propranolol and presentation of an appetizing meal without allowing it to be eaten, significantly increased the bioavailability of propranolol in healthy human volunteers (80). This observation (which was replicated in dogs) suggests preprandial anticipatory changes in splanchnic function—including increased hepatic blood flow and cephalic-phase secretion of insulin and glucagon—which may be responsible, although the exact mechanism is unknown. In experimental animals, propranolol undergoes phase I biotransformation in the small intestine, a process that is diminished when the drug is administered with food (81).

In most (but not all) humans, consumption of a high-protein meal with a single dose of propranolol significantly enhances the bioavailability of the propranolol, whereas a high-carbohydrate meal appears to have little effect (82). This observation appears to be true when volunteers are fed a single high-protein meal. The opposite is true when the volunteers are habituated first to high-carbohydrate meals and then switched to high-protein meals (58). The increased bioavailability following a single high-protein meal appears to be due to decreased first-pass hepatic metabolism, because production of metabolites is delayed rather than reduced (82).

In a nonhabituated person, a high-protein meal increases hepatic blood flow. Initially the increased hepatic blood flow was thought to cause the decreased hepatic extraction of propranolol, because extraction of propranolol by the liver was assumed to be primarily limited by the fact that the P450 enzymes involved in phase I biotransformation of propranolol are saturable and obey Michaelis-Menten kinetics (83), as they do in the rat (84). Under these assumptions, increased flow would be expected to result in *decreased* propranolol extraction per unit blood per unit time (85). However, increasing blood flow to the liver by changing posture does not change propranolol bioavailability, so increased blood flow per se probably is not the only reason for the increased bioavailability of the drug caused by a high-protein meal (86).

In fact, the increased bioavailability with food may be due to the combination of increased blood flow, the lipophilicity and protein binding of the drug, and the effects of meal-induced hormones on phase I and phase II metabolism. The primary site of CYP1A in the healthy liver of a healthy person (and a healthy rat) is the centrilobular area (87, 88), which is also the location of CYP2D in rat liver (89). With increased hepatic blood flow, propranolol is extracted by a larger proportion of the liver, including the periportal areas that do not efficiently metabolize the drug. This extraction is enhanced by the drug's binding to AAG (90) and by its lipophilicity (91).

The sight of a meal induces an anticipatory phase of insulin and glucagon secretion. In rats, glucagon (but not insulin) increases hepatic uptake of propranolol, although it does not affect metabolism (92), so plasma levels of the active drug are higher than without the sight of a meal. By contrast, hepatic uptake of propranolol is decreased with a glucose meal. As a result, plasma propranolol concentration initially decreases because more drug is metabolized when hepatic uptake is relatively low, as noted above (93). Whether a similar effect occurs in humans is not known. If so, this effect could explain the paradoxical differences in propranolol bioavailability between persons who have been habituated or not to high-carbohydrate meals. Habituation to high-carbohydrate meals induces a basal hyperinsulinemia, which dampens the rise in glucagon induced by consumption of a high-protein meal. Because no glucagon-induced decrease in phase I metabolism occurs, first-pass metabolism is unchanged, and a high-protein meal fails to enhance bioavailability of the drug.

Phase II biotransformation may also be decreased by coconsumption of propranolol with food. Liedholm and Melander (94) have shown that in women, administration of propranolol with a meal not only increased the bioavailability but also decreased the ratio of conjugated:unconjugated drug. This decrease was not seen when a slow-release formulation was administered.

Despite the intensive study of propranolol bioavailability and its relationship to meal consumption and the important biologic issues this question engenders, ultimately this question is of relatively little clinical importance for those receiving *maintenance* dosages of the drug. With chronic administration, propranolol decreases its own first-pass metabolism to a maximal extent (95). Its lipophilicity means that adipose tissue can serve as a reservoir to dampen fluctuations in blood levels. Finally, the β-adrenergic blockade induced by propranolol lasts well beyond what would be expected from its approximately 4-hour plasma half-life (8). Therefore, a twice-a-day dosage usually yields adequate clinical effect, regardless of the timing and nature of meals.

Dietary Effects on Drug Function

When a drug acts on processes that involve dietary components, we can anticipate that dietary components may affect that drug's function. The following interactions are probably not the only ones that occur. However, they are either the most common or ones that deserve further study.

Dietary Electrolytes and the Functions and Side Effects of Drugs Used to Treat Cardiovascular Disease

The digitalis glycosides block Na^+-K^+ ATPase. Hypokalemia potentiates the ATPase block and leads to toxicity. Therefore, dietary maintenance of normal plasma potassium levels is critical for prevention of this side effect, particularly if the patient is also taking a potassium-losing diuretic. Note that persons taking potassium-sparing diuretics (e.g., triamterene or amiloride) may develop a life-threatening hyperkalemia if they are given a high-potassium diet, potassium supplements, or drugs with a high potassium content, including potassium penicillin.

A dose-dependent side effect of the thiazide diuretics, which occurs in up to 3% of subjects, is development of glucose intolerance and overt diabetes mellitus, through mechanisms that are not completely elucidated (96, 97). Maintenance of adequate plasma potassium and magnesium levels through diet or, if necessary, supplements may prevent development of this complication (97). Hypomagnesemia may also play a role in development of thiazide-induced glucose intolerance (98), so monitoring of magnesium levels may be indicated with supplementation or dietary change recommended as needed.

Potentiation of MAO Inhibitors

Foods containing tyramine and other phenylethylamines should be avoided by persons taking first-generation monoamine oxidase (MAO) inhibitors. These include not only the antidepressants such as phenelzine, tranylcypromine, pargyline, and selegiline, but also the cancer chemotherapeutic drug procarbazine (8), the antiprotozoal drug furazolidone (99), and the analgesic meperidine (100). Dietary phenylethylamines, including tyramine, are normally oxidatively deaminated via MAO in the gastrointestinal tract and the liver. When a person is taking MAO inhibitors, the phenylethylamines are not deaminated by the gut and liver, so they are absorbed systemically and taken up in the brain, where they displace norepinephrine from storage vesicles. The resulting flood of norepinephrine released into synapses leads to severe acute hypertension with the potential for stroke or myocardial infarction. Attacks of hypertension of short duration are associated with headaches, palpitations, nausea, and vomiting. The newer antidepressant MAO inhibitors such as moclobemide, which act much more selectively in the central nervous system, do not lead to severe reactions with dietary components (101).

Foods accumulate phenylethylamines through the action of bacterial or fungal tyrosine decarboxylase. Thus, fermented foods and protein-rich foods that have begun to spoil contain large amounts of phenylethylamines (8). Table 99.6 lists common foods containing large quantities of tyramine. Note, however, that the amount of phenylethylamines in a food varies from sample to sample and depends on storage method and time since preparation. Those at greatest risk of a hypertensive crisis due to phenylethylamines are vegetarian, have poor appetites, and/or are on a weight-reduction diet, because the phenylethylamines consumed are not "diluted" by other foods. Iron deficiency may increase susceptibility to hypertensive crisis. Consumption of yeast supplements also presents a significant risk. Tyramine consumed with a meal may diminish tyramine absorption (102).

Table 99.6
Tyramine in Foods

Foods that contain significant amounts of tyramine
Broad beans
Raspberries
Banana peel
Cheese (except cream cheese and cottage cheese)
Imitation cheese
Prepared meats: sausage, chopped liver, pate, salami, mortadella
Meat extracts
Concentrated yeast extracts/brewer's yeast
Liquid and powdered protein supplements
Fermented soy products: fermented bean curd, soya bean paste, miso soup
Hydrolyzed protein extracts for sauces, soups, and gravies
Fermented cabbage products: sauerkraut, kimchee
Chianti, vermouth
Nonalcoholic beer
Some non-U.S. brands of beer
Foods that may contain significant amounts of tyramine
Avocado
Yogurt
Cream from fresh pasteurized milk
Soy sauce
Peanuts
Chocolate
Red and white wines, port wines
Distilled spirits

Data from Smith CH, West J. Food medication interactions. Tempe, AZ: Ann Moore Allen, 1991;244.

The amino acid dopa or its amine derivative, dopamine, present in broad beans (fava beans), may also trigger hypertension in patients on MAO inhibitor drugs (103).

Dietary Effects on the Coumarin Anticoagulants

The coumarin anticoagulants (warfarin, Coumadin, dicumarol) act through antagonism of vitamin K. Consumption of vitamin K–enriched foods or supplements may counteract the effects of the anticoagulants. Because the dosage of the coumarin antagonists is based on the patient's prothrombin time rather than on vitamin K levels, it is more important to maintain a steady, consistent intake of vitamin K–containing foods while receiving anticoagulants, than it is to decrease intake.

Certain herbal teas (woodruff, tonka beans, melilot) contain natural coumarins that can augment the effects of Coumadin and should be avoided (104). Large amounts of avocado also appear to augment the effects of warfarin (105). Brussels sprouts and possibly other cruciferous vegetables increase the catabolism of warfarin and thereby decrease its anticoagulant activities (106).

Interactions of Caffeine and Other Methylxanthines with Drug Function

Caffeine and other methylxanthines have numerous effects on the function of other drugs, both through induction of P450 enzymes (as observed in rats [107]) and through other pathways. For example, methylxanthines enhance the cytotoxicity of alkylating agents by hastening passage through the G_2 phase of the cell cycle, thereby decreasing the time for repair of sublethally "hit" DNA (108). In vitro, caffeine binds to DNA-intercalating drugs such as the antitumor drug doxorubicin; in vivo consequences of this binding are not known (109). Caffeine also decreases the effectiveness of a number of antiepileptic drugs, including phenobarbital and valproate, in preventing electroshock seizures in mice, probably through adenosine-mediated inhibition. These findings suggest that persons taking these drugs should probably not take caffeine-containing foods and beverages, or if they do, they should maintain their intake at a constant level (110).

Interactions of Diet with Hypolipidemic Drugs

Although the hypolipidemic effects of the hypolipidemic drugs may be augmented by a lipid-lowering diet, the effects are usually additive and do not result from a specific interaction between diets and the drug (e.g., see [111] and Chapter 75). There may be exceptions to this statement. Fibrates bind to proteins known as peroxisome proliferator-activated receptors (PPARs). PPARs, members of the steroid hormone receptor superfamily, have recently been found to play distinctive roles in the regulation of fat and cholesterol metabolism. Their role in drug function and metabolism and the effects of dietary fatty acids and retinoids on the function of fibrate drugs as mediated through PPARs are just beginning to be elucidated (112).

Drug Excretion

Drugs are primarily excreted via the kidneys and the gastrointestinal tract, with minor excretion via other routes. However, many drugs are excreted into breast milk, and nonelectrolytes (e.g., ethanol) reach the same concentration in breast milk as they do in plasma (8).

Effects of Diet on Drug Excretion

Diet can affect drug excretion by altering either the clearance by the drug's organ of excretion or the drug's volume of distribution. The half-life of a drug in circulation is a direct function of the volume of distribution of the drug and an inverse function of its clearance.

The clearance of a drug depends on the amount of drug delivered to the organ of excretion and the extent to which the drug is extracted from the blood for excretion (the extraction ratio). In the case of renal excretion, clearance of the drug depends on the concentration of free drug in the plasma, on the glomerular filtration rate, and on the amount of drug secreted and/or reabsorbed in the tubules per unit time.

Low-Protein Diets and Hypoalbuminemia. The concentration of free drug in the plasma depends on the chemical characteristics of the drug. For example, if a drug binds to albumin, a decrease in plasma albumin levels (due to inadequate protein intake or disease) may increase the proportion of free drug to bound drug. However, the effect on excretion of an increase in the unbound fraction of the drug may be counteracted by an increase in the drug's volume of distribution. An increase in distribution volume may occur for two reasons. First, hypoalbuminemia leads to an increase in total body water. Second, if the drug binds to particular tissues (e.g., adipose tissue), a larger proportion of the drug is sequestered by these tissues and therefore is unavailable for immediate excretion.

Thus, low-protein diets can in theory affect renal clearance of drugs in potentially opposing ways. Acutely, low-protein meals decrease glomerular filtration rates (113), so less drug is available for excretion per unit time. However, tubular reabsorption may be more efficient, so the clearance of the drug may be decreased out of proportion to the decrease in filtration rate (114). Chronic low-protein consumption with hypoalbuminemia leads to an increase in free drug available for excretion, if the drug is bound to albumin, and to alterations in the volume of distribution, as noted above. However, the result of a low-protein diet on actual clearance varies from drug to drug and depends on the severity and duration of the low-protein intake. For example, dietary protein restriction decreases clearance of the antigout drug allopurinol and promotes renal tubular reabsorption of its chief metabolite, oxypurinol (114). Because high levels of the drug may lead to an acute attack of gout, the protein content of the diet is particularly important in patients with compromised renal function.

Another effect of a low-protein diet, albeit an indirect one, is to increase net renal excretion of base. The increased excretion of base is due to decreased production of acid residues (phosphate, sulfate, and chloride) from protein metabolism, coupled with decreased renal secretion of hydrogen ions due to increased extracellular fluid volume. This effect lessens the rate of excretion of basic drugs such as the antibiotic gentamicin or the antiarrhythmic drugs procainamide and quinidine because less of the ionized form of these drugs is presented in the renal tubule and thus more of the drug is reabsorbed. A similar effect is produced by intake of antacids. In patients receiving basic drugs, urinary pH should be monitored, and if the pH is increasing, the drug dose should be reduced or an alternative drug considered (115).

Dehydration and Starvation. Dehydration, and starvation without hypoproteinemia, may significantly decrease the distribution volume of a drug because of decreases in the size of the aqueous compartment. Glomerular filtration rates may also be decreased. In addition, starvation decreases the distribution volume of lipophilic drugs because of a loss of adipose tissue. By contrast, people who are lean but not starved have a higher proportion of body water per kilogram than nonlean people, so the half-life of drugs that are primarily distributed in the aqueous compartment is prolonged in lean persons (116). The result of these changes in compartment size varies from individual to individual and from drug to drug, so that drug regimens should be individualized and drug levels and clinical effect should be monitored in critically ill or malnourished persons whenever feasible.

Competition between Drugs and Nutrients for a Common Excretory Pathway. Competition between drugs or between drugs and nutrients for a common renal pathway can also change the rate of drug excretion. Renal tubular reabsorption of lithium chloride is increased in sodium depletion. Because of the potential for toxicity, a patient receiving lithium chloride should not be placed on a low-sodium diet unless close attention is paid to blood lithium levels (8).

EFFECTS OF DRUGS ON FOOD INTAKE, BODY WEIGHT, NUTRIENT REQUIREMENTS, AND GROWTH

Alteration in Food Intake

Drugs can alter food intake by causing either a perversion or loss of appetite or an increase in appetite.

Appetite Suppression

Drugs may suppress appetite either as their primary effect (e.g., the anorexigenic drugs used to treat obesity)

Table 99.7
Classification of Anorexigenic Drugs

A. Primary appetite suppression
   1. Centrally acting
      a. Catecholaminergic, e.g., dextroamphetamine
      b. Dopaminergic, e.g., levodopa
      c. Serotoninergic, e.g., fenfluramine
      d. Endorphin modulators, e.g., naloxone
   2. Peripherally acting
      a. Agents that inhibit gastric emptying, e.g., levodopa
      b. Bulking agents, e.g., methylcellulose
B. Secondary (adverse response to food, loss of appetite)
      a. Drugs causing nausea and vomiting, e.g., digoxin
      b. Drugs causing loss of taste, e.g., penicillamine
      c. Drugs causing stomatitis, e.g., 5-fluorouracil
      d. Hepatotoxic agents, e.g., alcohol

Based on Pawan GLS. Proc Nutr Soc 1974;33:239–44.

or as an unwanted side effect. Drugs designed to suppress appetite (Table 99.7) usually act at the level of the central nervous system. Appetite suppression as an unwanted side effect can result from a number of different mechanisms, from development of food aversions because of nausea associated with a drug's action on the central chemoreceptor trigger zone to food avoidance associated with a sore mouth or slow gastric emptying.

Centrally Acting Drugs Used for Appetite Suppression. Appetite-reducing drugs that act centrally include those that act via catecholamine pathways and those that appear to act via serotonin pathways (117). The former include unsubstituted and substituted amphetamines and related compounds (amfepramone, phentermine, mazindol, and phenylpropanolamine). Amphetamines are sometimes used to treat obesity, although tolerance to appetite suppression develops rapidly (117). These drugs are also undesirable because of their stimulant properties. The halogenated amphetamine fenfluramine and dexfenfluramine (its dextrorotatory stereoisomer) act through pathways that are yet unknown, although they profoundly deplete brain serotonin, suggesting a neurotoxic action. However, in experimental animals, fenfluramine's neurotoxic and anorexigenic effects can be distinguished (118), suggesting that the anorexia is not a consequence of neurotoxicity. Fluoxetine, a serotonin reuptake inhibitor, can increase appetite when it is used to relieve depression (119), but generally, this drug is anorexigenic, an effect that has been used clinically in the treatment of obesity (117).

Appetite Change and Decreased Food Intake As an Unwanted Side Effect. Unwanted changes in appetite and, hence, changes in food intake may be caused by nausea and vomiting, development of food aversions, impaired oral function, dysgeusia or ageusia, gastric irritation, and changes in gastrointestinal tract function. The class of drugs most commonly associated with these side effects are the cytotoxic antineoplastic drugs. At effective therapeutic dosages, these drugs commonly have an acute anorectic effect due to their action on the chemoreceptor trigger zone in the brain, which is an integral part of their systemic toxicity. However, food intake may be reduced on a more chronic basis because of changes in taste, oral or intestinal ulcerations, or development of food aversions (120).

Risks Associated with Drug-Induced Loss of Appetite. Risks from the effects of drug-induced loss of appetite depend on both the primary toxicity of the substance and the secondary effects of the loss of desire to eat. The latter includes not only weight loss but also specific nutrient deficiencies that may ensue because of diminished intake of nutrients. For example, dextroamphetamine, which has been used to treat attention deficit hyperactivity disorder in children, causes growth retardation, partly due to appetite suppression (8). Fortunately, rebound growth occurs when the drug is discontinued.

Nausea/Vomiting. Virtually every drug can cause nausea and vomiting, either centrally through activation of the chemoreceptor trigger zone in the area postrema of the brain or, more commonly, peripherally through irritation of the gastrointestinal tract. Drugs that act centrally include cytotoxic drugs (in particular cisplatin, doxorubicin, methchlorethamine, cyclophosphamide, chlorambucil, melphalan, dacarbazine, dactinomycin), opioids, cholinomimetics, L-dopa, bromocriptine, and cardiac glycosides (8). Any drug that induces nausea is likely to reduce food intake and hence contribute to weight loss. For example, digitalis preparations can cause severe wasting (digitalis cachexia) because nausea diminishes the desire for food at dosages below those that lead to cardiac toxicity (121).

Food Aversions. Food aversion develops when eating the food is associated with development of nausea and vomiting, even though the nausea and vomiting may be due to another agent (e.g., a cytotoxic drug). Food aversions develop in more than half of all patients who undergo cancer chemotherapy and usually affect consumption of two to four foods. The aversions are usually transient, however, lasting several weeks to several months after cessation of therapy (121).

Impaired Oral Function. Drugs that cause a dry or sore mouth and make eating difficult or painful lead to avoidance of food intake. Patients may develop sore mouths because of drugs that cause stomatitis (e.g., busulfan and other antineoplastics), gum inflammation and hyperplasia (cyclosporine and phenytoin), delay in wound repair and healing (antineoplastics), gingival bleeding (Coumadin and related drugs), microbial infections (antineoplastics, captopril), and oral candidiasis (broad-spectrum antibiotics). Dry mouth may be caused by drugs that decrease salivary flow, including atropine, amantadine, opioids, phenothiazines, tricyclic antidepressants, and α-adrenergic agents.

Dysgeusia and Ageusia. Drugs can alter the taste of saliva or food by excretion in the saliva, often leading to a metallic taste (e.g., acetazolamide); alteration or decrease in taste receptor function (e.g., captopril—possibly because of decreased salivary magnesium concentration (122); penicillamine—possibly because of decreased zinc availability); and alteration of olfactory function (e.g., chronic use of antihistamines or bronchodilators). Some drugs may not taste good (e.g., potassium preparations, penicillin) or may have a disagreeable texture (e.g., cholestyramine). Antineoplastics may cause dysgeusia and ageusia by inhibiting replication of taste bud cells.

Gastric Irritation. All drugs can potentially cause nausea and vomiting because they all can potentially cause gastric irritation. In a given individual, gastric irritation may not lead to frank nausea but to disagreeable sensations that lead to a loss of appetite. The most commonly consumed drug that causes notable gastric irritation is aspirin.

Altered Gastric Emptying and Intestinal Motility. Alterations in intestinal motility, whether an increase or a decrease, may cause a loss of appetite. Prokinetic agents such as metoclopramide, domperidone, and cisapride as well as erythromycin increase the rate of gastric emptying and the overall motility of the upper and lower gastrointestinal tract. Patients with gastroparesis may exhibit improved appetite because they no longer feel full after small amounts of food (123). However, the increased lower gastrointestinal motility may suffice to cause decreased appetite, which would counteract the improvement due to more rapid gastric emptying.

Opioids cause considerable delays in gastric emptying and marked constipation (124), which may pose problems following a myocardial infarct and for management of cancer pain (125). Morphine coupled with bed rest leads to loss of appetite and constipation, so increasing dietary fiber intake is important to relieve discomfort and, postinfarct, to prevent arrhythmias caused by straining with bowel movements.

Drugs with anticholinergic activity (e.g., atropine, scopolamine, Pro-Banthine, benztropine mesylate, trihexyphenidyl, tricyclic antidepressants, diphenhydramine) or sympathomimetic activity (e.g., epinephrine, β-adrenergic agents) delay gastric emptying. Delayed gastric emptying may lead to discomfort and loss of appetite, which in turn lead to malnutrition, particularly in the elderly and others whose appetite may already be limited.

Anticholinergics also decrease intestinal motility and cause constipation. The constipation caused by antihistamines, antiparkinsonian drugs, phenothiazines, and tricyclic antidepressants is due to their anticholinergic effects. Drugs that may lead to diarrhea or constipation are listed in Table 99.8.

Bezoars. Bezoars, balls of unabsorbed material residing in the stomach, may form from undissolved portions of drugs and from masses of food matter, in particular plant fiber (phytobezoars). Bezoars tend to form in patients with achlorhydria, in whom tablets may not dissolve, and in those with poor gastric emptying, often because of surgical intervention (126); in patients with autonomic neuropathy due to diabetes mellitus (127); or in patients with alcoholism, especially following variceal sclerotherapy (128). Typical drugs found in bezoars include sucralfate, cholestyramine, aluminum hydroxide gel, and iron and antacid tablets. All of these preparations either form precipitates with foods or require stomach acid for dissolution or both. Bezoars may cause feelings of gastric fullness, pain, nausea, vomiting, and gastric outlet obstruction. Bezoar prevention in susceptible persons consists of changing the

Table 99.8
Drugs That Cause Constipation or Diarrhea

Constipation
Antacids
Anticholinergic drugs
Anticholinergic agents
Antihistamines
Phenothiazines
Tricyclic antidepressants
Corticosteroids
Clonidine
Ganglionic blocking agents
Iron supplements
Laxatives when abused
Lithium
MAO inhibitors
Muscle relaxants
Octreotide
Opioids
Prostaglandin synthesis inhibitors
Nonsteroidal antiinflammatory drugs
Diarrhea
Adrenergic neuron blockers: reserpine, guanethidine
Antimicrobials, particularly broad-spectrum agents
Cholinergic agonists and cholinesterase inhibitors
Erythromycin
Osmotic and stimulant laxatives
Prokinetic agents: metoclopramide, domperidone, cisapride
Quinidine

Modified from Hardman JG, Limbird LE, eds. Goodman and Gilman's the pharmacological basis of therapeutics. 9th ed. New York: McGraw Hill, 1996;918.

Table 99.9
Foods to Be Avoided for Prevention of Bezoar Formation

Apples
Berries
Broccoli
Brussels sprouts
Coconuts
Dandelion greens
Figs
Grapes
Kidney beans
Oranges
Grapefruits
Persimmons
Potato skins
Sauerkraut

Data from Thompson KC, Iredale JP. Drug Safety 1996;14:85–93.

drug formulation from solid to liquid when possible; changing the drugs to therapeutically equivalent forms; using drugs to enhance gastric emptying; and using low-fiber diets with restriction of foods listed in Table 99.9 (129).

Appetite Enhancement. Several drugs are used therapeutically to enhance appetite in patients with cancer and AIDS (130–132). Megestrol acetate, a progesterone analogue, may prove significant for management of poor appetite in patients with a good prognosis (130). In double-blind trials, some (but not all) patients respond to treatment with this drug with increased appetite. At high doses, this drug appears to have a positive metabolic effect, increasing lean and particularly fat body mass. Patients taking the drug report increased feelings of well-being, with relatively few side effects, although development of deep-vein thrombosis and emboli may prove to limit the usefulness of this drug (133).

Dronabinol, a metabolite of cannabinol, the active ingredient in marijuana, is an effective antiemetic. At high doses it increases appetite, sense of well-being, and weight but is associated with side effects such as dizziness and sleepiness (131).

The mechanisms whereby corticosteroids increase appetite are unknown, although the increase is associated with euphoria and may be a central effect (132). Unfortunately, corticosteroids increase total body water rather than lean tissue mass. Cyproheptadine, a serotonin blocker, probably acts by decreasing the antiappetitive effects of serotonin in the central nervous system (132). It also appears to interfere with the regulation of growth hormone secretion and thereby leads to weight gain and increased growth in children (8).

The phenothiazine and benzodiazepine tranquilizers and lithium carbonate have appetite enhancement as a side effect. These effects are related to both direct pharmacologic effects and the fact that administration of the drugs reduces mental agitation (134).

Drug-Induced Maldigestion and Malabsorption

Drug-induced maldigestion and malabsorption may be due to interactions between the drug and the nutrient or to global changes in gastrointestinal tract function. Unless a drug causes widespread destruction of the intestinal villi or fat malabsorption, drug-induced maldigestion and malabsorption primarily affect minerals and vitamins, rather than macronutrients. One example of an interaction between drugs and nutrients is that between bile acid sequestrants or mineral oil and fats and fat-soluble vitamins. The clinical importance of this drug-induced malabsorption lies in its potential effects on mineral and vitamin absorption.

Global changes leading to maldigestion and malabsorption include increases or decreases in gut motility and changes in the mucosal surface. For example, cancer chemotherapeutic agents and colchicine, which damage the intestinal mucosa because of their antimitotic effects, may cause generalized malabsorption.

Effects of Drugs on Vitamin and Mineral Status, Requirements, and Activity

Drugs can affect vitamin and mineral status by interfering with absorption, metabolism, and function. The antivitamin or mineral-related effects of drugs may be used intentionally in the treatment of disease or may be an unwanted side effect of drug therapy. Changes in vitamin status that occur as a side effect often have a relatively slow, insidious onset, so the practitioner should anticipate these drug-nutrient interactions by appropriate monitoring.

Antacids

By increasing stomach pH, antacids decrease the bioavailability of vitamin A, folate, thiamin, and phosphate.

Vitamin A and Carotene Malabsorption. Absorption of vitamin A and carotenoids requires release of these compounds from dietary proteins via pepsin proteolysis. Pepsin is rapidly inactivated, and autoactivation of pepsin from pepsinogen is suppressed at pH 5. In addition, aluminum hydroxide adsorbs pepsin above pH 3.

Thiamin Degradation. Thiamin is unstable at high pH and hence is inactivated when taken with antacids.

Folate Malabsorption. When the pH of the upper part of the jejunum is increased after ingestion of sodium bicarbonate, folate absorption is reduced. The clinical significance of this malabsorption is not clear, although it may contribute to the folate deficiency seen in persons who chronically consume alcohol and take sodium bicarbonate for gastrointestinal distress.

Sodium Overload. Sodium overload with development of congestive heart failure can result from intake of antacids containing sodium bicarbonate. The risk is most severe in elderly people with preexisting heart disease who are also consuming high-sodium diets.

Phosphate Depletion. People taking heavy doses of antacids containing aluminum or magnesium hydroxide or mixtures of these substances may develop a phosphate depletion syndrome. Dietary phosphate combines with aluminum and magnesium hydroxide to form insoluble aluminum and magnesium phosphates, which are excreted through the gastrointestinal tract. The risk of phosphate depletion is greatest when the person consumes a low-phosphate diet. Effects of phosphate depletion include muscle weakness (which may be limited to the proximal limb muscles), malaise, paresthesias in the limbs, anorexia, hemolytic anemia, and convulsions (8). Myocardial depression may occur, although not frank congestive heart failure (135). Low-phosphate osteomalacia has developed in a few patients with phosphate depletion (136).

Milk-Alkali Syndrome. The milk-alkali syndrome occurs as a complication of excessive ingestion of soluble, absorbable alkali (e.g., sodium bicarbonate) and milk. It is characterized by hypercalcemia, precipitation of calcium in the kidney, and progressive renal insufficiency. This syndrome occurs in people taking large amounts of sodium bicarbonate or calcium carbonate, particularly those with preexistent renal insufficiency (8).

Use of calcium salt supplements to delay age- or medication (corticosteroid)-related bone loss or to prevent hypertension has the potential to cause the milk-alkali syndrome (137). The current extensive use of calcium carbonate tablets for osteoporosis and hypertension prevention might therefore increase the prevalence of the syndrome, as happened in peptic ulcer patients when the Sippy diet and antacid treatment were in vogue.

Magnesium Overload. Patients with chronic renal failure who are taking magnesium-containing antacids can develop magnesium intoxication. Signs include nausea, vomiting, flushing, impaired respiratory function, and partial or complete heart block.

Iron Malabsorption. Absorption of iron occurs when it is in the ferrous state, at low pH. The elevated pH induced by antacids may lead to iron aggregate formation and conversion of iron to its ferric form. In addition, aluminum hydroxide gels bind iron and thereby decrease its absorption.

H2 Blockers and Proton Pump Inhibitors

Histamine H2-receptor antagonists and proton pump inhibitors can profoundly decrease stomach acid secretion. Histamine H2 blockers give a more inconsistent and variable reduction in acidity than do proton pump inhibitors.

Vitamin B_{12} Malabsorption. In a review of the literature on H2 blockers, Force and Nahata (138) found evidence for a significant effect of histamine H2 receptor antagonists on vitamin B_{12} absorption because stomach acid failed to release the vitamin from dietary protein. The malabsorption may become clinically manifest only 2 or more years after initiation of therapy and is a particular hazard for those who may have low stores of vitamin B_{12} before the initiation of therapy (138).

Omeprazole therapy decreases cyanocobalamin absorption in a dose-dependent manner at both 20 and 40 mg daily (139). This effect of omeprazole may be at least partially counteracted by consuming an acidic drink with meals (140). The clinical importance of this decrease may only become manifest after prolonged (>4 years) administration (141).

Sulfasalazine

Folate Malabsorption. Sulfasalazine is a competitive inhibitor of intestinal folate transport. Folate malabsorption in patients with inflammatory bowel disease who are receiving this drug depends not only on drug intake but also on whether they obtain sufficient dietary folate (142).

Sulfasalazine and other NSAIDs with a carboxylic sidechain inhibit folate-dependent enzymes in vitro, including dihydrofolate reductase and phosphoribosylaminoimidazolecarboxamide formyltransferase. The in vivo significance of this inhibition is unknown, although synthesis of serine from glycine and formate is decreased in vitro in mononuclear cells from persons taking these drugs (143).

Antituberculous Agents

Vitamin D Metabolism. Two drugs used in the treatment of tuberculosis, rifampin and isoniazid, affect vitamin D metabolism, presumably through their effects on the hepatic P450 enzyme, vitamin D 25-hydroxylase (144–146). Although short-term studies of these drugs have shown marked alterations in vitamin D metabolism and calcium status in nontuberculous subjects (146, 147), longer-term studies of patients receiving the drugs for tuberculosis have not shown clinically significant effects on vitamin D status and calcium and phosphate metabolism (148–150). Patients with untreated tuberculosis may have abnormally low levels of vitamin D metabolites, so it may be difficult to distinguish the effects of drugs from the effects of the disease itself (151).

Hydrazone Formation with Pyridoxine. Isoniazid and other carbonyl compounds combine with pyridoxine to form hydrazones. These compounds are potent inhibitors of pyridoxal kinase and place the person at risk for developing peripheral neuritis. The elderly, diabetic, alcoholic, uremic, or pregnant patient is most susceptible to this side effect. Pyridoxine supplementation can prevent development of this complication of isoniazid therapy (8).

Niacin Deficiency. Isoniazid can induce a secondary niacin deficiency with development of pellagra (152); this problem is rare but has been reported in tuberculous patients who have been on a marginal intake of niacin. The deficiency in these patients is thought to result from inhibition of the enzyme kynureninase, which lies in the pathway of nicotinamide nucleotide synthesis from tryptophan. This enzyme is inhibited as a result of complex formation between isoniazid and pyridoxal phosphate (Schiff base formation). Supplementation with nicotinamide may allow chemotherapy to continue.

Interactions of Pyridoxine with Decarboxylases: Effects on l-Dopa and Hydralazine/Cycloserine

Pyridoxine is an essential coenzyme of aromatic L-amino acid decarboxylase. Hydralazine and cycloserine deplete pyridoxine, which leads to defective dopamine production and neurologic signs in persons treated with these drugs. Pyridoxine supplementation can reverse the defect in dopa decarboxylation (8, 153), but sodium excretion is attenuated, which may not be desirable in persons with hypertension (154).

Anticonvulsants

Calcium and Vitamin D Metabolism. The anticonvulsant drugs phenytoin and phenobarbital can cause hypocalcemia, rickets in children, and high-turnover osteoporosis in adults. Phenytoin acts through three mechanisms: decreased calcium absorption, possibly through inhibition of the synthesis of calcium-binding protein; stimulation of the catabolism of 25-hydroxycholecalciferol, with a possible reduction in 24,25-dihydroxycholecalciferol production; and increased catabolism of vitamin K, with reduction in formation of the vitamin K–dependent proteins involved in calcium handling by osteoblasts, in particular osteocalcin (8). Levels of 1,25-dihydroxy cholecalciferol appear to be normal, suggesting that the effects on calcium absorption are probably the major reason for the development of bone disorders with these drugs.

Folate Metabolism. High doses of folic acid may counteract the anticonvulsant effects of phenobarbital, phenytoin, and primidone (155). Patients who develop megaloblastic anemia while taking these drugs may respond to folate supplementation with increased seizure frequency. It may be necessary either to change the drugs the patient is taking or to tolerate a degree of anemia, if a change in drugs is not possible. Note that for phenytoin, part of the mechanism for decreased effectiveness with folate supplementation may lie in increased formation and excretion of hydroxylated metabolites of the drug.

Vitamin K Catabolism. Phenytoin and phenobarbital, probably through their action on hepatic P450 enzymes, increase hepatic catabolism of vitamin K and decrease production of vitamin K–dependent proteins. Infants born to mothers who have taken these drugs in pregnancy are susceptible to neonatal hemorrhage, which may be counteracted by injection of vitamin K (8).

Mineral Oil

Mineral oil acts as both a physical barrier and a lipid solvent and thereby decreases absorption of fat and fat-soluble vitamins.

Bile Acid Sequestrants

Drugs that bind bile acids (e.g., cholestyramine and aluminum-containing antacids) may lead to malabsorption of fats and hence to malabsorption of fat-soluble vitamins, particularly vitamins A and E. Cholestyramine also binds folic acid (156). Although the clinical significance of cholestyramine-induced malabsorption may not be great, patients taking this drug over long periods of time should be monitored for vitamin A and vitamin E status and prothrombin time and should receive folate supplements (157).

Methotrexate and Other Folate Antagonists

The clinical effectiveness of methotrexate and other folate antagonists (e.g., trimethoprim, trimetrexate) depends on their ability to bind tightly to dihydrofolate reductase, displacing folate (see Chapter 26). Drug polyglutamates are formed, and synthesis of folate polyglutamates is diminished. Thymidylate synthetase is inhibited, which in turn leads to inhibition of the synthesis of DNA, RNA, and protein (8). Methotrexate reduces incorporation of deoxyuridine (dU) into DNA and favors incorporation of thymidine into DNA by the alternate pathway. The dU suppression test is abnormal in those who are receiving methotrexate (158).

Methotrexate is used at low dosages for the treatment of rheumatoid arthritis. In this regimen, the risk of antifolate effects is low. Folic acid supplements can further reduce the risk of these side effects (159). Patients with AIDS who are taking trimethoprim for long periods of time are at particular risk for developing folate deficiency. Because bacterial dihydrofolate reductase is a thousand-fold more sensitive to trimethoprim than is the human enzyme (8), folate supplementation may be appropriate for these patients (160). Similarly, patients receiving trimetrexate for *Pneumocystis carinii* infection should also receive leucovorin (161).

Methotrexate has a greater affinity than folate for folate-binding protein at the pH optimum for the radiometric assay for plasma folate. It has therefore been proposed that this assay, which involves competitive protein binding in plasma and erythrocytes, should not be used to measure this vitamin in the plasma or erythrocytes of patients receiving the drug (162).

Nitrous Oxide

Nitrous oxide, long used as an anesthetic and more recently used in the management of patients after cardiac bypass surgery, is a vitamin B_{12} antagonist. Megaloblastic erythropoiesis and neurologic disorders have been reported in both man and laboratory animals after exposures to high concentrations of this gas, especially in persons whose vitamin B_{12} status is marginal (e.g., vegans) (163). Exposure may also present a particular hazard to dentists and others who use this anesthetic in office situations (164).

Nitrous oxide oxidizes vitamin B_{12} and inhibits methionine synthetase. Inactivation of methionine synthetase displaces cobalamin from the enzyme. Furthermore, there is increased formation of inactive cobalamin analogues. In animals exposed to NO_2, the neuropathy can be partially prevented by feeding methionine (165).

Corticosteroids

Corticosteroids administered chronically increase the need for vitamin B_6, calcium, and vitamin D. Table 99.10 shows the nutritionally significant consequences of long-term corticosteroid use.

Antibiotics and Coagulation

Effects of Antibiotic Therapy on Intestinal Synthesis of Vitamin K. In humans, intestinal microbes synthesize vi-

Table 99.10
Nutritionally Significant Consequences of Long-Term Corticosteroid Use

Gastrointestinal system
- Peptic ulceration
- Gastric or intestinal perforation
- Pancreatitis

Endocrine system and metabolism
- Hyperglycemia
- Hyperlipidemia
- Weight gain
- Altered distribution of fat tissue
- Hypertension with renal sodium retention and potassium and zinc loss

Skeletal system
- Osteoporosis
- Growth failure in children
- Spontaneous fractures

Immune system
- Immunosuppression with increased risk of infection leading to hypermetabolism

tamin K in the form of menaquinones. Thus it is theoretically possible for a person taking broad-spectrum antibiotics to become deficient in this vitamin. Indeed, menaquinone levels are diminished in the livers of persons who have taken broad-spectrum antibiotics (166). However, the main sources of liver vitamin K are phylloquinones in the diet (167), and phylloquinone levels were unchanged in the livers of persons taking broad-spectrum antibiotics (166). Conversely, bacterial vitamin K cannot compensate for a dietary deficiency in vitamin K (168).

Cephalosporin Antibiotics. Cephalosporin antibiotics with *N*-methylthiotetrazole sidechains can decrease clotting through inhibition of hepatic vitamin K epoxide reductase, with the appearance of PIVKA II (prothrombin induced in vitamin K absence II) (169). This decrease in vitamin K function is only measurable in persons who are otherwise vitamin K deficient (170) and, in fact, may be only a minor cause (if at all) of clotting problems in persons receiving these antibiotics (171). Prevention is accomplished by providing vitamin K injections to persons receiving these drugs.

Doxorubicin

Doxorubicin produces a dose-dependent cardiomyopathy when the total cumulative dose exceeds 500 mg/m^2. In laboratory animals, the histopathologic aspects of the cardiac lesion are similar to those of vitamin E deficiency and appear to be due to free radical reactions that cause peroxidation of membrane lipids. The incidence and severity of the doxorubicin-induced cardiac damage has been reduced by administration of vitamin E to laboratory animals, but this vitamin has not been effective in preventing doxorubicin cardiotoxicity in man (172).

Drugs That Inhibit Riboflavin Absorption and Metabolism

Psyllium hydrophilic mucilloid decreases absorption of pharmacologic doses of riboflavin (173). The clinical importance of this finding is unknown. Phenothiazines, the tricyclic antidepressants, and quinacrine inhibit conversion of riboflavin to FMN flavokinase. Riboflavin supplementation may reverse this effect (8).

Vitamin B_6 Analogues: Hydralazine and Cycloserine

Hydralazine and cycloserine are analogues of pyridoxine. Concomitant administration of pyridoxine supplements may reduce the incidence of neurotoxicity caused by these drugs (8).

Diuretics

Electrolyte Imbalance. Because diuretics act by altering renal excretion of sodium and potassium, they may lead to the development of electrolyte imbalance. Common drugs that cause potassium deficiency include thiazide, loop-type diuretics, and laxatives. The potassium-losing diuretics deliver large amounts of sodium to the distal tubule, where part of the sodium is exchanged for potassium, with loss of potassium. Drugs that cause potassium depletion may damage the renal tubule and thereby cause secondary depletion of magnesium and zinc (174).

Drugs that can cause hyperkalemia include spironolactone, an aldosterone antagonist, and triamterene and amiloride, which appear to block the luminal sodium channels that drive potassium excretion in the late distal tubule and collecting duct (8). Persons with impaired renal function or those taking a high potassium diet or potassium supplements are particularly prone to develop hyperkalemia when taking these drugs.

Drug-induced mineral depletion is commonly multifactorial. For example, in the elderly, it may result from concurrent use of several drugs that have this side effect, as well as decreased intake of the mineral. Factors predisposing to mineral depletion include prolonged drug intake and renal disorder, including the age-related decline in renal function, and catabolic diseases, including metastatic cancer.

Calcium Status. Thiazide diuretics cause renal calcium retention and can cause hypercalcemia, although this side effect is relatively uncommon and may only be temporary. However, thiazide users do have a greater bone mineral content than age- and sex-matched nonusers. It has been suggested that thiazide drugs might have a therapeutic role in the management of osteoporosis (8).

Nondiuretic Antihypertensive Agents

The antihypertensive agent diazoxide, which increases the proximal tubular reabsorption of sodium, can cause sodium overload (8). Increased serum potassium levels have been reported with use of β-blocking drugs in conjunction with potassium-sparing diuretics (8).

Oral Antiglycemic Agents

The oral antihyperglycemic agent metformin decreases absorption of vitamin B_{12} and folate, although significant hematologic effects appear to be rare (175).

Low-Molecular-Weight Heparin

Low-molecular-weight heparin is commonly used for prevention and treatment of thromboembolism. Heparin inhibits aldosterone biosynthesis. Treatment with low-molecular-weight heparin increases serum potassium levels, so the potassium status of persons treated with this drug should be monitored (176).

Alcohol

For a discussion of the effects of alcohol on vitamin and mineral status and metabolism, see Chapter 94.

DRUG-FOOD AND DRUG-ALCOHOL INCOMPATIBILITIES

Food and drug incompatibilities usually result from drug-induced inhibition of enzymes required in the catabolism of potentially toxic endogenous metabolites. These are outlined in Table 99.11.

EFFECTS OF NONTHERAPEUTIC DRUG COMPONENTS AND NONNUTRITIVE COMPONENTS OF FOODS

Food additives, nonnutritive components of foods, and excipients and preservatives in medications may lead to untoward effects when ingested.

Monosodium Glutamate

Monosodium glutamate (MSG) is added to food to enhance flavor. Although MSG is classically thought of in connection with "Chinese restaurant syndrome," in fact it is found in numerous prepared foods. MSG causes symptoms that mimic those of angina pectoris.

Tartrazine

Tartrazine (Yellow Dye no. 5) is a color additive used in both foods and drugs. Patients may have allergic reactions to this dye, so the Food and Drug Administration requires that its presence be noted on the labels of both foods and drugs.

Sulfites

Sulfites are added to foods, beverages, and drugs as preservatives because of their antioxidant properties. They can cause severe allergic reactions. Sulfites are added as sulfur dioxide, sodium sulfite, sodium and potassium bisulfite, and sodium and potassium metabisulfite.

Licorice

Black licorice contains glycyrrhizic acid, a compound that has mineralocorticoid activity through inhibition of 11-β-hydroxysteroid dehydrogenase (8). It thereby enhances sodium and water retention and increases potassium excretion. Consumption of licorice (as little as "a couple of twists" a day) can counteract the effects of diuretics and increase the mineralocorticoid effects of corticosteroids.

Lactose

Many drugs contain lactose as an excipient. Although the amount per capsule or pill may be small, lactose-intolerant patients taking large amounts of these drugs may experience symptoms, including bloating and diarrhea.

Oxalates

Oxalates are absorbed when they are not bound to calcium or magnesium in the gut. When absorbed, they are

Table 99.11
Drug-Food and Drug-Alcohol Incompatibilities

Reaction	Drug	Food	Signs/Symptoms
"Histamine poisoning," probably due to histaminase/MAO inhibitor activity of drug[a]	Isoniazid	Certain kinds of fish, including tuna and skipjack[b]	Redness of face; itching of eyes, face and palms; severe headache
Tyramine reactions	MAO inhibitors	Tyramine-containing foods	Hypertensive crisis
Disulfiram reaction	All drugs that are aldehyde dehydrogenase inhibitors[c]	Alcohol, in foods or in lotions/ other solutions applied to the skin	Flushing, nausea, vomiting, variable degree of chest and/or abdominal pain
Hypoglycemia	Sulfonylureas	Alcohol, including sweet or semisweet drinks with alcohol	Hypoglycemia, manifesting as weakness, mental confusion, irrational behavior, loss of consciousness

[a]Ref. 177.
[b]Ref. 178.
[c]Including disulfiram (Antabuse), cyanamide, metronidazole, sulfonylureas, animal charcoal, inky-cap mushrooms, griseofulvin, procarbazine, and the β-lactam antibiotics cefamandole, cefotetan, moxalactam, cefoperazone (8).

excreted by the kidney, where they precipitate as calcium or magnesium salts. Excessive oxalate consumption in situations when calcium or magnesium is unavailable (e.g., with consumption of aluminum hydroxide gels that bind calcium and magnesium) may lead to formation of kidney stones and interstitial renal failure.

Aspartame

Certain drugs contain phenylalanine, usually in the form of aspartame, which may be detrimental to persons with phenylketonuria.

Methylxanthines

Caffeine, other methylxanthines, and theophylline are all metabolized by demethylation and xanthine oxidase activity, although the major pathway for theophylline catabolism involves hydroxylation. Because of the common degradative pathways and the fact that the therapeutic range for theophylline is very narrow, methylxanthine consumption by persons receiving theophylline and its congeners should be kept constant. A person taking theophylline who decreases consumption of methylxanthines (caffeine, theobromine in coffee, teas, chocolate, cola drinks) must receive a higher dose of theophylline to maintain therapeutic blood levels. When methylxanthine consumption is decreased, theophylline is metabolized more rapidly and blood levels of the drug cannot be maintained within a therapeutic range unless the dose is increased. Increased methylxanthine consumption would lead to increased blood levels of theophylline and resultant toxicity.

PROBIOTICS

Probiotics is the term given to live bacteria, often coupled with substances that enhance bacterial growth, which are either components of foods or are added to foods to provide a pharmacologic effect. These bacteria (usually *Lactobacillus* spp. and *Bifidobacterium* spp.) multiply in the gastrointestinal tract and displace pathogenic bacteria.

Probiotics have been used for the prevention and treatment of antibiotic-associated diarrhea, acute infantile diarrhea, and recurrent *Clostridium difficile* infection (178). There is reason to believe that they may be effective in peptic ulcers associated with *Helicobacter pylorii* (180).

The lower gastrointestinal tract is critically dependent on bacterial metabolism for provision of specific nutrients, such as short-chain fatty acids. These bacteria require nutrients derived from enterally delivered food. Antibiotics wipe out these essential bacteria, while TPN does not provide the luminal nutrients they require. With antibiotics or TPN, gut mucosal atrophy can occur, with increased bacterial translocation and sepsis (180). Probiotics also stimulate local immunity and thus may prevent bacterial translocation immunologically as well as through trophic effects on the gut (181).

For probiotics to regenerate the gut flora following treatment with antibiotics, the probiotic bacteria must be antibiotic resistant and adhere readily to the gastrointestinal tract mucosa. Probiotics are usually given in a vehicle that enhances bacterial multiplication. Some vehicles are the actual foods created by bacterial action, such as fermented foods (sour milk, yogurt); some probiotic bacteria are added to foods accompanied by galactooligosaccharides, which serve as substrates for their growth (182).

Complex carbohydrates coupled with surfactant lipids and glutamine are important for maintenance of the probiotic flora. In this respect, oat bran appears especially useful because it is high in glutamine, surfactant lipids, and water-soluble, fermentable β-glucans (183). Elemental enteral formulae, which do not contain proteins or complex carbohydrates, are poor substrates for these bacteria, because the components of the formulae are absorbed in the proximal tract and do not reach the lower intestine in any quantity.

There is evidence that probiotics may have beneficial effects on blood cholesterol levels (184), possibly through action of *Lactobacillus*-derived bile salt hydrolases (185), which may help prevent gastrointestinal carcinogenesis (186).

Despite their overall benign profile, lactobacilli do have pathogenic potential in certain populations (187). They are involved in formation of dental caries and in septicemia, rheumatic vascular disease, and infectious endocarditis. Subjects who are immunocompromised or elderly and who are receiving broad-spectrum antibiotics are particularly susceptible to these complications. It appears that the capacity of the lactobacilli to aggregate platelets and to adhere to collagen (particularly type V collagen, which is associated with sites of damage) is indicative of this pathogenic potential (187). However, in general, the pathogenic potential of probiotics appears to be very low (188).

For a review of the status of probiotics, see Elmer et al. (179).

FOOD-DRUG INTERACTIONS AND THE JOINT COMMISSION ON ACCREDITATION OF HEALTHCARE ORGANIZATIONS (JCAHO)

In its 1996 accreditation standards, the JCAHO cited the issue of food-drug interactions as important in the care of patients (4). The commission particularly emphasized the importance of considering food-drug interactions in the safe use of medication, in provision of nutrition care, and in education. Regulation PF.2.2.3 specifically states that the patient should receive "instruction on potential drug-food interactions and counseling on nutrition intervention and/or modified diets, as appropriate."

The JCAHO targeted five drugs for specific monitoring, to ensure that both in-hospital and outpatient administration of these drugs is appropriate. These drugs are captopril, sucralfate, prednisone/dexamethasone, and warfarin. These drugs were chosen by a multidisciplinary group consisting of persons in pharmacy, nursing, dietetics, and nutrition, based on *(a)* the high risk associated with these drugs if they are not prescribed and administered appropriately and *(b)* their high frequency of use and the chronicity with which they are taken. Extensive standards were developed to implement this monitoring, including standards for staff and patient education and standards for administration of these drugs in conjunction with diet and the timing of meals.

ACKNOWLEDGMENTS

This chapter is dedicated to the memory of Daphne A. Roe, M.D., extraordinary colleague and friend. Some of her text has been included in this chapter.

REFERENCES

1. Lamy PP. Adverse drug effects. In: Lamy PP, ed. Clinics in geriatric medicine. Philadelphia: WB Saunders, 1990;293–307.
2. Brown CB. Handbook of drug therapy monitoring. Baltimore: Williams & Wilkins, 1990;165–6.
3. Carson JL, Strom BL, Taragin MI, et al. Arch Intern Med 1987;147:85–8.
4. Joint Commission on Accreditation of Healthcare Organizations. 1996 Comprehensive accreditation manual for hospitals. Oakbrook Terrace, IL: 1995.
5. Lasswell AB, Deforge BR, Sobal J, et al. J Am Coll Nutr 1995; 14:137–43.
6. Karim A, Burns T, Wearley L, et al. Clin Pharm Ther 1985; 38:77–83.
7. Karim A, Burns T, Janky D, et al. Clin Pharm Ther 1985;38: 642–7.
8. Hardman JG, Limbird LE, eds. Goodman and Gilman's the pharmacological basis of therapeutics. 9th ed. New York: McGraw Hill, 1996.
9. Thomson CA, Rollins CJ. Support Line 1991;8:9–11.
10. Rollins C. Physiological impact of drug-nutrient interactions. Handout for the 20th Clinical Congress, American Society of Parenteral and Enteral Nutrition, January 1996.
11. Karim A, Rozek LF, Smith MA, et al. J Clin Pharmacol 1989; 29:439–43.
12. Neovonen P, Gothoni G, Hackman R. Br Med J 1970;4:532–4.
13. Leyden JJ. J Am Acad Dermatol 1985;12:308–12.
14. Saux MC, Mosser J, Pontagnier H, et al. Eur J Metab Pharmacokinet 1983;8:43–9.
15. Meyer FP, Specht H, Quednow B, et al. Infection 1989;17: 245–6.

15a. Campbell NRC, Hasinoff BB. Br J Clin Pharmacol 1991;31: 251–6.

16. Rashid MU, Bateman DN. Br J Clin Pharmacol 1990;30:25–34.
17. Fraser R, Shearer T, Fuller J, et al. Gastroenterology 1992;103: 114–9.
18. Jain NK, Boivin M, Zinsmeister AR, et al. Pancreas 1991;6: 495–505.
19. Suttle AB, Pollack GM, Brouwer KLR. Pharm Res 1992;9: 350–6.
20. Greiff JMC, Rowbotham D. Clin Pharmacokinet 1994;27: 447–61.
21. Kenyon CJ, Cole ET, Wilding IR. Int J Pharm 1994; 112:207–13.
22. Coupe AJ, Davis SS, Evans DF, et al. Int J Pharm 1993; 92:167–75.
23. Sugito K, Ogata H, Goto H, et al. Chem Pharm Bull 1992;40:3343–5.
24. Coupe AJ, Davis SS, Evans DF, et al. Pharm Res 1991;8:1281–5.
25. Ewe K, Press AG, Oestreicher M. Dtsch Med Wochenschr 1992;117:287–90.
26. Dressman JB, Berardi RR, Elta GH, et al. Pharm Res 1992; 9:901–7.
27. Routledge PA. J Antimicrob Chemother 1994;34(Suppl A):19–24.
28. Gainsborough N, Maskrey VL, Nelson ML, et al. Age Ageing 1993;22:37–40.
29. Mojaverian P, Vlasses PH, Kellner PE, et al. Pharm Res 1988;5:639–44.
30. MacFie AG, Magides AD, Richmond MN, et al. Br J Anaesth 1991;67:54–7.
31. Sankaran H, Larkin EC, Rao GA. Med Hypotheses 1994;42:124–8.
32. Scott AM, Kellow JE, Shuter B, et al. Gastroenterology 1993;104:410–6.
33. Welling PG, Barbhaiya RH. J Pharm Sci 1982;71:32–5.
34. Barbhaiya RH, Craig WA, Corrick-West HP, et al. J Pharm Sci 1982;71:245–8.
35. Goldin BR, Goldman P. Fed Proc (Abstract) 1973;32:798.
36. Sved AF, Goldberg IM, Fernstrom JD. J Pharmacol Exp Ther 1980;214:147–51.
37. Brannan T, Martinez-Tica J, Yahr MD. Neuropharmacology 1991;30:1125–8.
38. Eriksson T, Granerus AK, Linde A, Carlsson A. Neurology 1988;38:1245–8.
39. Pincus JH, Barry K. Arch Neurol 1987;44:270–2.
40. Pare S, Barr SI, Ross SE. Am J Clin Nutr 1992;55:701–7.
41. Vrhovac B, Sarapa N, Bakran I, et al. Clin Pharmacokinet 1995;28:405–18.
42. Aki H, Yamamoto M. J Pharm Sci 1994;83:1712–6.
43. Okabe N, Hashizume N. Biol Pharm Bull 1994;17:16–21.
44. Woerner W, Preissner A, Rietbock N. Eur J Clin Pharmacol 1992;43:97–100.
45. Bohney JP, Feldhoff RC. Biochem Pharmacol 1992;43: 1829–34.
46. Woo J, Chang HS, Or KH, et al. Clin Biochem 1994;27: 289–92.
47. Hakkak R, Ronis MJJ, Badger TM. Gastroenterology 1993; 104:1611–8.
48. Melander A, McLean AEM. Clin Pharmacokinet 1983;8: 286–96.
49. Guengerich FP. Am J Clin Nutr 1995;61(Suppl):651S–8S.
50. Pampori NA, Shapiro BH. Biochem Pharmacol 1994;47: 121–9.
51. Anonymous. Drug Nutr Interact 1985;4:251–63.
52. Wanwimolauk S, Levy G. J Pharmacol Exp Ther 1987; 242:166–72.
53. Imaoka S, Terrano Y, Funae Y. Arch Biochem Biophys 1990;278:168–78.
54. Woodcock BG, Wood GC. Biochem Pharmacol 1971;20:2703.
55. Krjjgsheld KR, Scholtens E, Mulder GJ. Biochem Pharmacol 1981;30:1973–81
56. Kwei GY, Zaleski J, Thurman RG, et al. J Nutr 1991;121: 131–7.
57. Giger U, Meyer UA. J Biol Chem 1981;42:4875–917.
58. Fagan TC, Walle T, Oexmann MJ, et al. Clin Pharmacol Ther 1987;41:402–6.
59. Kim HJ, Choi ES, Wade AE. Biochem Pharmacol 1990;39:1423–30.
60. Dinh L, Dumont D, Durand G. Biochem Mol Biol Int 1994; 32:869–78.

61. Christon R, Fernandez Y, Cambon-Gros C, et al. J Nutr 1988; 118:1311–8.
62. Hu Y, Ingelman-Sundberg M, Lindros KO. Biochem Pharmacol 1995;50:155–61.
63. Morimoto M, Zern MA, Hagbjoerk AL, et al. Proc Soc Exp Biol Med 1994;107:197–205.
64. Morimoto M, Reitz RC, Morin RJ, et al. J Nutr 1995;125: 2953–64.
65. Nanji AA, Sadrzadeh SMH, Yang EK, et al. Gastroenterology 1995;109:547–54.
66. Kim RB, Wilkinson GR. Clin Pharm Ther 1996;59:170.
67. Kall MA, Clausen J. Hum Exp Toxicol 1995;14:801–7.
68. Sinha R, Rothman N, Brown ED, et al. Cancer Res 1994; 54:6154–9.
69. Guo Z, Smith TJ, Wang E, et al. Carcinogenesis 1992;13: 2205–10.
70. Fuhr U, Klittich K, Staib AH. Br J Clin Pharmacol 1993;35: 431–6.
71. Fukuda K, Ohta T, Yamazoe Y. Biol Pharm Bull 1997;20:560–4.
71a. Ha HR, Chen J, Leuenberger PM, et al. Eur J Clin Pharm 1995;48:367–71.
72. Edwards DJ, Bellevue FH III, Woster PM. Drug Metab Dispos 1996;24:1287–90.
73. Lown KS, Bailey DG, Fontana RJ, et al. J Clin Invest 1997; 99:2545–53.
74. Siow YL, Dakshinamurti K. Ann NY Acad Sci (Vitamin B6: International Multidisciplinary Conference) 1990;585: 173–88.
75. Pfeiffer R, Ebadi M. J Neurochem 1972;19:2175–81.
76. Klawans HL, Ringel SP, Shenker DM. J Neurol Neurosurg Psychiatry 1971;34:682–6.
77. Masubichi Y, Hosakawa S, Horie T, et al. Drug Metab Dispos 1994;22:909–15.
78. Yoshimoto K, Echizen H, Chiba K, et al. Br J Clin Pharmacol 1995;39:421–31.
79. Marathe PH, Shen DD, Nelson WL. Drug Metab Dispos 1994;22:237–47.
80. Power JM, Morgan DJ, McLean AJ. Biopharm Drug Dispos 1995;16:579–89.
81. DuSouich P, Maurice H, Heroux, L. Drug Metab Dispos 1995;23:279–84.
82. Liedholm H, Wahlin-Boll E, Melander A. Eur J Clin Pharm 1990;38:469–76.
83. Semple HA, Tam YK, Coutts RT. Biopharm Drug Dispos 1990;11:61–7.
84. Ishida R, Suzuki K, Masubichi Y, et al. Biochem Pharmacol 1992;44:2281–8.
85. Olanoff LS, Walle T, Cowart TD, et al. Clin Pharmacol Ther 1986;40:408–14.
86. Modi MW, Hassett JM, Lalka D. Clin Pharmacol Ther 1988;44:268–74.
87. Murray GI, Foster CO, Barnes TS, et al. Carcinogenesis 1992;13:165–9.
88. Tritscher AM, Goldstein JA, Portier CJ, et al. Cancer Res 1992;52:3436–42.
89. Waguri S, Iyanagi, Uchiyama Y. Histochemistry 1992;97: 247–53.
90. Gariepy L, Fenyves D, Villeneuve JP. J Pharm Sci 1992;81: 255–8.
91. Rivory LP, Roberts MS, Pond SM. J Pharmacokinet Biopharm 1992;20:19–61.
92. Semple HA, Xia F. Drug Metab Dispos 1994;22:822–6.
93. Ogisa T, Iwaki M, Tanino T, et al. Biol Pharmacol Bull 1994;17:112–6.
94. Liedholm H, Melander A. Clin Pharmacol Ther 1986;40: 29–36.
95. Kagimoto N, Masubichi Y, Fujita S, et al. J Pharm Pharmacol 1994;46:528–30.
96. Pollare T, Lithell H, Berne C. N Engl J Med 1989;321: 868–73.
97. Helderman JH, Elahi D, Andersen DK, et al. Diabetes 1983;32:106–11.
98. Tannen R. Kidney Int 1985;28:988–1000.
99. Zheng ZT, Wang YB. J Gastroenterol Hepatol 1992;7:533–7.
100. Clark RF, Wei EM, Anderson PO. J Emerg Med 1995;13: 797–802.
101. Mayersohn M, Guentert TW. Clin Pharmacokinet 1995; 29:292–332.
102. Korn A, Da Prada M, Raffesberg W, et al. J Cardiovasc Pharmacol 1988;11:17–23.
103. Blomley BJ. Lancet 1964;2:1181–2.
104. Tyler VE. The new honest herbal. Philadelphia: George F. Stickley, 1988.
105. Wells PS, Holbrook AM, Crowther NR, et al. Ann Intern Med 1994;121:676–83.
106. Ovesen L, Lyduch S, Idorn ML. Eur J Clin Pharmacol 1988;34:521–4.
107. Berthou F, Goosduff T, Dreana Y, et al. Life Sci 1995;57:541–9.
108. Fingert HJ, Chang JD, Pardee AB. Cancer Res 1986;46: 2463–7.
109. Traganos F, Kapuscinski J, Darzynkiewicz Z. Cancer Res 1991; 51:3682–9.
110. Czuczwar SJ, Gasior M, Janusz W, et al. Epilepsia 1990; 31:318–23.
111. Hunninghake DB, Stein EA, DuJoune CA, et al. N Engl J Med 1993;328:1213–9.
112. Green S. Mutat Res 1995;333:101–9.
113. Kitt TM, Park GD, Spector R, et al. Clin Pharmacol Ther 1988;43:681–7.
114. Berlinger WA, Park GD, Spector R. N Engl J Med 1985; 313:771–6.
115. Reidenberg MM. N Engl J Med 1985;313:816–8.
116. Jameson JP, Munyika A. Ther Drug Monit 1990;12:54–8.
117. Silverstone T. Drugs,1992;43:820–36.
118. McCann UD, Yuan J, Ricaurte GA. Eur J Pharmacol 1995; 283:R5–7.
119. Worthington J, Fava M, Davidson K, et al. Psychopharmacol Bull 1995;31:223–6.
120. Ovesen L. Int J Oncol 1994;5:889–99.
121. Pawan GLS. Proc Nutr Soc 1974;33:239–44.
122. Musumeci V, DiSalvo S, Zappacosta B, et al. Clin Exp Hypertens 1993;15:245–56.
123. Sturm A, von der Ohe M, Rosein U, et al. Dtsch Med Wochenschr 1996;121:402–5.
124. Manara L, Bianchetti A. Annu Rev Pharmacol Toxicol 1985; 25:249–73.
125. Duthie DJR, Nimmo WS. Br J Anaesth 1987;59:61–77.
126. Cifuentes-Tebar J, Robles-Campos R, Parrilla-Paricio P, et al. Dig Dis Sci 1992;37:1694–6.
127. Ahn YH, Maturu P, Steinheber FU, et al. Arch Intern Med 1987;147:527–8.
128. Davion T, Delamarre J, Reix N, et al. Scand J Gastroenterol 1989;24:818–20.
129. Thompson KC, Iredale JP. Drug Safety 1996;14:85–93.
130. Strang P. Anticancer Res 1997;17:657–62.
131. Gorter R. Oncology 1991;5(Suppl):13–7.
132. LoPrinzi CL, Goldberg RM, Burnham NL. Drugs 1992;43: 499–506.

133. Tchekmedyian NS, Hickman M, Heber D. Semin Oncol 1991;18:35–42.
134. Stanton JM. Schizophrenia Bulletin 1995;21:463–72.
135. Davis SV, Olichwier KK, Chakko SC. Am J Med Sci 1988;295:183–7.
136. Boutsen Y, Devogelaer JP, Malghem J, et al. 1996;15:75–80.
137. Abreo K, Adlakha A, Kilpatrick S, et al. Arch Intern Med 1993;153:1005–10.
138. Force AW, Nahata MC. Ann Pharmacother 1992;26:1283–6.
139. Marcuard SP, Albernaz L, Khazanie PG. Ann Intern Med 1994;120:211–5.
140. Saltzman JR, Kemp JA, Glover BB, et al. J Am Coll Nutr 1994;13:584–91.
141. Koop H. Aliment Pharmacol Ther 1992;6:399–406.
142. Hanauer SB. N Engl J Med 1996;334:841–8.
143. Bagott JE, Morgan SL, Ha T, et al. Biochem J 1992;282: 197–202.
144. Davies PDO, Brown RC, Woodhead JS. Br J Clin Pharmacol 1985;20:303P–4P.
145. Bengoa JM, Bolt MJ, Rosenberg IH. J Lab Clin Med 1984;104:546–52
146. Brodie MJ, Boobis AR, Hillyard CJ, et al. Clin Pharmacol Ther 1981;30:363–7.
147. Brodie MJ, Boobis AR, Dollery CT, et al. Clin Pharmacol Ther 1980;27:810–4.
148. Brodie MJ, Boobis AR, Hillyard CJ, et al. Clin Pharmacol Ther 1982;32:525–30.
149. Perry W, Erooga MA, Brown J, et al. J R Soc Med 1982;75:533–6.
150. Williams SE, Wardman AG, Taylor GA, et al. Tubercle 1985;66:49–54.
151. Davies PD, Brown RC, Woodhead JS. Thorax 1985;40:187–90.
152. Ishii N, Nishihara Y. J Neurol Neurosurg Psychiatry 1985;48:628–34.
153. Cohen AC. Ann NY Acad Sci 1969;166:436–9.
154. Shigetomi S, Kuchel O. Am J Hypertens 1993;6:33–40.
155. Reynolds EH. Brain 1968;29:837–51.
156. Hoppner K, Lampi B. Int J Vitam Nutr Res 1991;61:130–4.
157. West RJ, Lloyd JK. Gut 1975;16:93–8.
158. Wickramasinghe SN, Saunders JE. Acta Haematol 1977; 58:193–206.
159. Morgan SL, Baggott JE, Vaughn WH, et al. Arthritis Rheum 1990;33:9–18.
160. Fong IW, Mastali K, Chin T. 35th Interscience Conference on Antimicrobial Agents and Chemotherapy, San Francisco, California, September 17–20, 1995. Abstracts. 1995;35:245.
161. Marshall JL, Delap RJ. Clin Pharmacol 1994;26:190–200.
162. Waxman S. The value of measurement of folate levels by radioassay. In: Botez MI, Reynolds EH, eds. Folic acid in neurology, psychiatry, and internal medicine. New York: Raven Press, 1979;47–53.
163. Roesener M, Dichgans J. J Neurol Neurosurg Psychiatry 1996;60:354.
164. Layzer RB. Lancet 1978;2:1227–30.
165. Chanarin I, Deacon R, Lamb M, et al. Blood 1985;66: 479–89.
166. Conly J, Stein K. Clin Invest Med 1994;17:531–9.
167. Lipsky JJ. Mayo Clin Proc 1994;69:462–6.
168. Allison PM, Mummah-Schendel LL, Kindberg C. J Lab Clin Med 1987;110:180–8.
169. Shearer MJ, Bechthold H, Andrassy K, et al. J Clin Pharmacol 1988;28:88–95.
170. Cohen H, Scott SD, Mackie IJ, et al. Br J Haematol 1988;6 8:63–6.
171. Goss TF, Walawander CA, Grasela TH Jr, et al. Pharmacotherapy 1992;12:283–91.
172. Legha SS, Wang YM, MacKay B, et al. Ann NY Acad Sci 1982;393:411–8.
173. Roe DA, Kalkwarf H, Stevens J. J Am Diet Assoc 1988;88: 211–3.
174. Roe DA. Clin Lab Med 1981;1:647–64.
175. Melchior WR, Jaber LA. Ann Pharmacother 1996;30:158–64.
176. Curnova CR, Fischler MP, Reinhart WH. Lancet 1997;349: 1447–8.
177. Hui JY, Taylor SL. Toxicol Appl Pharmacol 1985;81:241–9.
178. Diao Y, et al. Chin J Tuberc Respir Dis 1986;9:267–9, 317–8.
179. Elmer GW, Surawicz CM, McFarland LV. JAMA 1996;275: 870–6.
180. Bengmark S. Clin Nutr 1996;15:1–10.
181. Salminen S, Isolauri E, Onnela T. Chemotherapy 1995;41 (Suppl 1):5–15.
182. Yang ST, Silva EM. J Dairy Sci 1995;78:2541–62.
183. Bengmark S, Jeppsson B. JPEN J Parenter Enteral Nutr 1995;19:410–5.
184. Mital BK, Garg SK. Crit Rev Microbiol 1995;21:175–214.
185. De Smet I, Van Hoorde L, De Saeyer N, et al. Microb Ecol Health Dis 1994;7:315–29.
186. Perdigon G, Alvarez S, Rachid M, et al. J Dairy Sci 1995;78: 1597–606.
187. Harty DWS, Oakey HJ, Patrikakis M, et al. Int J Food Microbiol 1994;24:179–89.
188. Saxelin M. Food Rev Int 1997;13:293–313.

100. Enteral Feeding

MOSHE SHIKE

Enteral feeding is a method of providing nutrient solutions into the gastrointestinal (GI) tract through a tube. This method is used for nutritional support in patients who cannot ingest or digest sufficient amounts of food but have adequate intestinal absorptive capacity. The increasing popularity of enteral feeding in various clinical states can be attributed to a number of factors:

1. Development of simple, low-risk procedures for placement of tubes in the GI tract, particularly percutaneous endoscopic gastrostomies and jejunostomies
2. Availability of a wide variety of commercial enteral feeding formulas with diverse nutrient components that allow a choice of suitable formulas for patients with limitations in GI function or those who require special nutrition
3. Advantages of enteral feeding over the alternative of parenteral feeding: preservation of the structure and function of the GI tract (absence of nutrients in the intestines is associated with atrophy of the intestinal mucosa and decreased function of the pancreatic-biliary system), more efficient nutrient use, fewer infectious and metabolic complications, greater ease of administration, and lower cost

HISTORY

The history of enteral feeding has been reviewed by Randall (1). The practice of placing nutrients into the GI tract while bypassing the mouth originated in ancient times with the Egyptians, who used nutrient enemas for preservation of general health. Greek physicians used enemas containing wine, whey, milk, and barley broth to treat diarrhea and provide nutrients. In the 19th century, European physicians installed various foods and liquids in patients' rectums, including beef extracts, milk, and whiskey. Rectal feeding was widely used until the beginning of the 20th century, when Einhorn pointed out its inadequacies (2). Capivacceus, a Venetian physician, is considered the first (in 1598) to use a hollow tube attached to an animal's bladder for feeding into the esophagus. The use of a small silver tube passed from the nose to the esophagus was reported in 1617 for feeding patients suffering from tetanus. A major development in provision of nutrition through tubes occurred at the end of the 18th century, when John Hunter, a famous surgeon at the time, proposed that a nasogastric tube be made from eel skin to feed a patient suffering from neurogenic dysphagia. The tube was made and used successfully for 5 weeks, after which the patient regained his ability to swallow. The use of nasogastric tubes both for feeding and for emptying the stomach became widespread in the 19th century.

The concept of early postoperative enteral feeding was introduced by Andresen in 1918 when he started jejunal feeding in a patient following a gastrojejunostomy (3). This practice gained increasing popularity because of the realization that following an operation, small bowel peristalsis is preserved, although the stomach remains nonmotile for a few days. Regular foodstuffs were mixed and ground or blenderized into a fine solution, which was instilled into the stomach through a tube. In 1959, Barron reported on enteral feeding in the postoperative period in a few hundred patients who had undergone various surgical procedures (4). He used natural juices and foods in finely dispersed solutions. He also infused GI secretions collected from drainage from biliary, pancreatic, gastric, and intestinal fistulas; these were introduced through polyethylene tubes passed through the nose.

Specialized enteral feeding formulas appeared in the 1930s with the introduction of casein hydrolysate for use in both enteral and parenteral feeding. Subsequently, crystalline amino acids were used in combination with various amounts of carbohydrates, fats, minerals, and vitamins. The first commercial enteral feeding formula was Nutramigen, introduced to the market in 1942 for treatment of children with intestinal diseases and allergies. A major advance in knowledge and use of chemically defined formulas was achieved through studies sponsored by the National Aeronautics and Space Administration

(5). These studies demonstrated that normal volunteers could be maintained in a normal nutritional and physical status while being fed solely with chemically defined solutions during a 6-month period. Based on the results of these studies, Randall and colleagues started a series of studies using commercial chemically defined diets (1) and demonstrated the usefulness of these diets given to patients with a variety of GI diseases.

FEEDING TUBES

Enteral feeding requires administration of the nutrient solutions (or more properly, liquid formulas, because they are rarely true solutions) through a tube into the upper GI tract. (The ancient practice of feeding through the rectum has been abandoned.) At present, enteral feeding devices can be divided into two major categories—those entering the GI tract through the nose (nasogastric or nasoenteral tubes) and those entering through the abdominal wall (gastrostomies, duodenostomies, or jejunostomies). Occasionally, feedings are given through a pharyngostomy or an esophagostomy.

Nasogastric and Nasoenteral Tubes

Numerous types of nasogastric and nasoenteral tubes are available commercially. Most are made of silicone or polyurethane. Tubes used in adults vary in length from 30 to 43 inches, with diameters from 5 to 16 French. The shorter tubes are used for nasogastric feeding and the longer tubes are used for nasoduodenal or nasojejunal feeding, usually in patients who are at an increased risk from aspiration.

Most tubes have tips containing tungsten or silicone to facilitate passage through the GI tract. However, whether a weighted tip is necessary for placement or maintenance of the tube in the GI tract has been questioned, and tubes without weighted tips are now available. The tubes come with a stylet that facilitates insertion through the nose and into the GI tract. Nasogastric tubes are generally used for short-term enteral feeding, mostly in the hospital. They are placed at the bedside by health professionals, and verification of the location of the tip of the tube in the stomach or small intestine is required. This verification can be made by obtaining a radiograph of the abdomen. Listening for airflow over the upper abdomen can provide misleading information and is not recommended. Airflow can be heard over the epigastrium even if the tip of the tube is in the chest (6) and can thus lead to serious complications. Color, pH, and quantity of aspirated fluid are also inadequate for determining the location of the feeding tube tip. Nasojejunal rather than nasogastric tubes should be used whenever there is risk for aspiration or gastric motility is impaired. Advancement of such tubes from the stomach into the small bowel may be facilitated by administering prokinetic drugs: erythromycin, metoclopramide, or Cisapride (7). Placement of the tubes in the duodenum or jejunum can also be assisted by endoscopic (8) or radiographic techniques (9).

Complications related to nasogastric and nasoenteral tubes can be divided into two categories: those resulting from insertion of the tube and those arising thereafter. Insertion-related complications include trauma and bleeding from the nose and upper GI tract, perforation, misplacement of the tube into the respiratory tract (particularly in unconscious patients), respiratory compromise caused by coiling of the tube in the nasopharynx, aspiration pneumonia, and vomiting of gastric contents as a result of pharyngeal irritation. Postinsertion complications include migration of the tube (especially into the esophagus), aspiration of infused solutions, erosion of the GI tract mucosa by the tip of the tube, and ear and nose infections.

Malfunction of nasogastric and nasoenteral tubes occurs commonly because of clogging with nutrition solutions or medications, kinking, or bursting (secondary to forceful injection of solutions). These malfunctions can be avoided with appropriate care of the tube. Complication rates of feeding tubes vary, depending on the experience of the person inserting the tube and on the care of the tube after it is inserted. The reported complication rate varies between 7.6 and 19% (10, 11). The average time of use of nasogastric and nasoenteral tubes is 10 days (8). A comprehensive review of nasogastric and nasoenteral feeding tubes, techniques, complications, and recommendations for practice has been published recently (12).

Gastrostomy and Jejunostomy Tubes

For long-term enteral feeding (more than 2 weeks), gastrostomy or jejunostomy tubes are advantageous for the following reasons: *(a)* they have a larger diameter (15–24 French) and thus do not tend to clog, and wider tubes also allow easier and more rapid administration of feeding solution and medications; *(b)* the risk of aspiration is considerably decreased because they are fixed in the stomach or upper intestines and do not migrate into the esophagus (as may happen with nasogastric tubes; and *(c)* they are more convenient and aesthetically acceptable to the patient. A recent randomized study demonstrated that feeding patients with acute strokes through a gastrostomy tube was associated with more optimal provision of nutrients, a better nutritional state, and less mortality than feeding through a nasogastric tube (13). The various methods of placement of gastrostomy and jejunostomy tubes have been reviewed extensively (14). In a prospective study comparing nasogastric tube feeding with percutaneous endoscopic gastrostomy (PEG) feeding in patients with neurologic dysphagia, the PEG group received 93% of the prescribed feeding compared with 55% in the nasogastric tube group. Most of the failures in the nasogastric tube group were attributed to tube dislodgement (15).

Gastrostomy and jejunostomy tubes can be placed surgically, endoscopically, or radiologically. For many years only the surgical technique was used. Although the operation is relatively minor, it requires a laparotomy, which has a complication rate of 2.5 to 16% and a mortality rate of 1 to 6% (16–18). An alternative surgical technique for placement of gastrostomy and jejunostomy tubes uses the laparoscope for access into the abdomen. Experience with this technique is still limited (19). Radiologic techniques have been developed for placement of percutaneous gastrostomies and jejunostomies (20). The advantage is the more aseptic procedure; however, the radiologically placed tubes are usually of small diameter and tend to clog. The radiologic techniques are also considerably more expensive than the endoscopic techniques (21).

In recent years, the PEG has become the most commonly used method because of the ease of the procedure, its safety, and the ability to perform the procedure on an outpatient basis. The technical aspects of the procedure have been reported (22, 23). In patients with gastric resection and those with increased risk for aspiration, (e.g., gastroparesis, severe reflux, neurologic disorders) jejunal tubes can be placed using a modification of the technique of endoscopic gastrostomy tube placement (24). Such percutaneous endoscopic jejunostomy (PEJ) tubes can be placed directly into a jejunal loop. This technique requires a high level of expertise because of the small diameter of the jejunum compared with that of the stomach. An alternative technique is to place a wide PEG tube (28 French) through which a small-diameter (usually 8 French) jejunal tube is passed into the stomach and carried into the jejunum by forceps passed through the endoscope. However, the narrow jejunal feeding tube tends to clog and to migrate.

Endoscopic placement of PEG and PEJ tubes is associated with a morbidity rate of 5 to 15% and a mortality rate of 0.3 to 1% (22–24). The tubes function well in the long term, with few complications (23). Active patients who require long-term enteral feeding can benefit from a skin-level button gastrostomy or jejunostomy (25), which is less obtrusive and more convenient than the regular PEG or PEJ tubes.

ENTERAL FEEDING SOLUTIONS

More than 100 commercial solutions are available for enteral feeding. The names and types of various enteral feeding products and the companies that produce them are listed in the Appendix Table VI-A-40-a. The composition of different solutions varies greatly, with some intended for general nutrition and others designed for specific metabolic or clinical conditions. In addition to, or instead of, using commercial products, patients can blenderize regular foods and use them for enteral feeding. Such foods can be easily administered through PEGs and PEJs because of the wide diameter of the tubes.

Solutions used for enteral feeding have been classified according to various criteria. The names given to different classes of solutions have not always been consistent and often overlap, thus leading to lack of clarity and confusion. The general term *medical foods* has been used since 1989 by the United States Food and Drug Administration (FDA) to define enteral nutrition products (2):

> Medical foods (MF) are distinguished from other foods for special dietary purposes or foods which make health claims (e.g., fiber in relation to cancer) by the requirement that they (MF) be used under medical supervision. In general, in order to be considered a MF a product must, at a minimum, meet the following criteria:
>
> - The product is labeled for the dietary management of a medical disorder, disease, or condition.
> - The product is labeled for the dietary management of a medical disorder, disease or condition.

The definitions and regulatory aspects of enteral feeding products have been summarized by Talbot (27).

The term *defined formula diets* was suggested as a general term to indicate that the ingredients (including nutrients processed from foods and/or relatively purified compounds, simple or complex) are prepared commercially by designated procedures so that their composition is established fairly well, although not necessarily with chemical precision (28).

The term *elemental* has been used mostly to indicate formulas containing predigested protein. Most of the so-called elemental solutions, however, are not elemental in the chemical sense (see below).

As stated above, solutions for enteral feeding can be classified in different ways. The following classification is based on practical considerations according to the clinical indications for the solution:

> Blenderized foods: Natural foods, semiliquified in a blender, which can be used to provide nutrition by the oral route or through a tube
>
> Polymeric solutions: Solutions containing macronutrients in the form of isolates of intact protein, triglycerides, and carbohydrate polymers, which can be used orally or through a tube and provide complete nutrition
>
> Monomeric solutions: Solutions usually containing proteins as peptides and/or amino acids, fat as long-chain triglycerides (LCTs) or a mixture of LCTs and medium-chain triglycerides (MCTs), and carbohydrates as partially hydrolyzed starch maltodextrins and glucose oligosaccharides; these solutions are often used for patients with impaired digestion or absorption, but it is questionable whether they are necessary or more advantageous than polymeric solutions
>
> Solutions for specific metabolic needs: Solutions intended for patients who have unique metabolic requirements—inborn errors of metabolism, renal failure, hepatic failure, etc.
>
> Modular solutions: Nutritional components that can be given by themselves or be mixed with other enteral products to provide solutions that meet special nutritional or metabolic needs of a given patient (e.g., increased calories, increased minerals)
>
> Hydration solutions: Solutions providing minerals, water, and small amounts of carbohydrates.

Natural Foods

Blenderized natural foods are available commercially or can be prepared at home. Commercial blenderized food solutions are prepared from milk, beef, fruits, vegetables, and fiber; hence their nutrient content is not determined precisely. Although they have the advantage of being "natural foods," they are prepared from a limited number of food items, and thus, their nutritional completeness is not ensured. Commercial blenderized food products are usually more expensive than others. Currently the use of blenderized products is limited. The ranges of the nutrient contents are listed in Table 100.1.

Patients who use enteral feeding in the home can prepare blenderized foods from regular foods in the household. If this practice is used, nutritional adequacy of the blenderized foods must be ensured.

Polymeric Solutions

The term *polymeric formulas* refers to those that contain macronutrients in the form of isolates of intact protein, triglycerides, and carbohydrate polymers. A wide variety of polymeric commercial enteral feeding solutions is available. In most of them, protein constitutes 12 to 20% of total calories; carbohydrates, 40 to 60%; and fats, 30 to 40%. In the standard formulas, the ratio of nonprotein calories:nitrogen is about 150 kcal/g nitrogen. In the high-nitrogen polymeric solutions, this ratio can be as low as 75 kcal/g nitrogen.

Table 100.1
Ranges of Nutrient Content of Enteral Feeding Products

Nutrients	Blenderized Foods or Milk-Base Formulas: Complete	Polymeric Formulas: Complete	Polymeric Formulas with Fiber: Complete	Monomeric Formulas	Disease-Specific Formulations
kcal/mL	0.7–1.0	0.5–2.0	1.0–1.2	1.0–1.33	1.0–2.0
Protein g/L					
Intact	42.0–84.0	17.5–83.7	39.7–53.0	0	30.0–83.0
Hydrolyzed	0	0	0	31.5–58.1	0
Amino acids	0	0	0	20.6–38.2	19.4–69.7
Carbohydrate g/L	82.8–192.0	68.0–250.0	123.0–162.0	127.0–226.3	93.7–365.6
Fat g/L	20.0–42.8	17.5–106.0	35.0–46.0	1.45–52.0	7.4–96.0
MCT:LCT ratio	NA	20:80–73:27[a]	NA	40:60–70:30[a]	25:75–70:30[a]
Fiber g/L	4.24	NA	5.9–14.4	NA	NA
Osmolality	300–450	120–710	303–480	270–650	320–910
Volume to meet 100% RDA	—	750–2000	1250–1800	1500–2250	947–3000
Nonprotein calorie:N ratio	131:1	75:1–167:1	116:1–148:1	125:1–284:1	NA
Vitamin A (IU)	3332–9000	1250–10,000	3300–5000	2500–5000	735–6700[a]
Vitamin D (IU)	266.8–800.0	100.0–560.0	267.0–420.0	140.0–280.0	84.5–423.0[a]
Vitamin E (IU)	24–42	15–75	21–64	15–40	10–60[a]
Vitamin K (μg)	66.8–80.0	38.0–320.0	48.0–160.0	22.3–160.0	35.0–160.0[a]
Vitamin C (mg)	60.0–120.0	56.0–317.0	120.0–254.0	33.3–200.0	30.0–317[a]
Thiamin (mg)	1.48–2.12	0.75–4.0	1.2–3.22	0.83–2.00	0.69–3.17[a]
Riboflavin (mg)	1.68–4.76	0.85–4.8	1.36–3.64	0.94–2.4	0.7–3.59[a]
Niacin (mg)	16.0–28.0	10.0–56.0	16.0–42.4	11.1–28.0	8.82–42.0[a]
Vitamin B_6 (mg)	2.0–2.8	1.0–8.0	1.6–4.24	1.11–4.0	1.07–8.61[a]
Folate (μg)	266.8–560.0	200.0–1,080.0	270.0–540.0	210.0–540.0	47.6–1056.0[a]
Pantothenic acid (mg)	6.68–14.0	5.0–28.0	8.0–21.2	5.00–14.0	2.62–21.1[a]
Vitamin B_{12} (μg)	4.8–12.0	3.0–16.0	4.8–12.7	2.0–8.0	2.94–12.7[a]
Biotin (μg)	49.2–440.0	150.0–800.0	240.0–400.0	100.0–400.0	142.5–634.0[a]
Sodium (mg)	760–1320	350–1184	500–930	460–1000	235–1310[a]
Potassium (mg)	1400–3640	600–2500	1250–1800	782–1661	882–1902[a]
Chloride (mg)	1132–3600	500–2000	1000–1440	819–2501	677–1691[a]
Calcium (mg)	668–2320	250–1400	667–910	451–800	491–1284[a]
Phosphorus (mg)	868–2000	250–1400	667–850	499–700	491–1056[a]
Magnesium (mg)	240–560	100–680	267–340	200–400	192–423[a]
Iron (mg)	12.0–25.2	4.5–24.0	12.0–15.0	9.0–13.3	8.82–19.0[a]
Iodine (μg)	100.0–212.0	37.5–200.0	100.0–127.0	74.7–101.3	73.5–158.4[a]
Copper (mg)	1.32–2.8	0.5–3.0	1.3–1.7	1.0–1.6	0.96–2.11[a]
Zinc (mg)	12.0–21.2	3.75–30.0	12.0–20.0	8.33–15.0	7.35–23.8[a]
Manganese (mg)	0.16–4.0	1.0–5.4	1.77–3.8	0.94–3.33	1.23–5.3[a]

NA, Not available.
[a]Information available only on some of the solutions.

Polymeric solutions contain whole proteins isolated from casein, lactalbumin, whey, egg white, or a combination of these. Carbohydrates are usually glucose polymers in the form of starch and its hydrolysates. The fats are of vegetable origin, such as corn oil, safflower oil, sunflower oil, and others. Vitamins and essential trace elements are present in adequate quantities so that a daily intake of 1500 to 2000 kcal provides the necessary recommended daily allowances of these nutrients. The amounts of such minerals as sodium and potassium vary considerably among the various solutions, thus allowing a choice when intake of these minerals is restricted. Polymeric solutions are lactose free. The osmolality varies between 300 and 450 mosm/kg in solutions that contain 1 kcal/mL. In solutions that contain more than 1 kcal/mL, however, the osmolality is higher and may reach 650 mosm/kg. Some polymeric solutions contain fiber in the form of complex nondigestible carbohydrates. The amounts of fiber range between 6 and 14 g/1000 kcal. The caloric density is between 1 and 2 kcal/mL. The high-caloric formulas allow provision of large amounts of calories in a smaller volume and are particularly suitable for patients who require fluid restriction. Administration of these formulas requires close follow-up, however, because they can be associated with dehydration and electrolyte abnormalities. The ranges of the nutrient contents of polymeric solutions are listed in Table 100.1.

Monomeric Solutions

The main feature of monomeric solutions is that they require less digestion than do regular foods or polymeric solutions. The protein in these solutions is in the form of peptides and/or free amino acids and is derived from hydrolysis of casein, whey, and other proteins. Net absorption of dipeptides and tripeptides and the amino acids generated from their digestion is more rapid and efficient than absorption of equivalent amounts of free amino acids (29). In addition, di- and tripeptides create a lower osmotic load than the corresponding amounts of amino acids. Therefore, monomeric solutions containing partially digested protein have physiologic advantages over those containing only free amino acids.

The carbohydrates are in the form of partially hydrolyzed starch (maltidextrins and glucose oligosaccharides). Fat is frequently a mixture of MCTs and LCTs of plant origin. Most calories are present as carbohydrates (as much as 80%), whereas only 1 to 5% are in the form of fat. Protein contributes 12 to 20% of the total calories. The caloric density of monomeric formulas varies between 1 and 1.5 kcal/mL. The solutions contain sufficient minerals, trace elements, and vitamins; 2000 kcal may provide the daily requirements of these nutrients. Some of the micronutrients, however, may be inadequate for a patient with increased needs.

Monomeric formulas are lactose free and do not contain fiber. The partially digested macronutrients in monomeric solutions contribute to the higher osmolality than that of polymeric solutions. The osmolality of monomeric solutions ranges between 270 and 650 mosm/kg (Table 100.1).

Based on physiologic considerations, these solutions might be regarded as suitable for patients with impaired digestion, such as those with pancreatic insufficiency or short bowel syndrome (in which case time for digestion and absorption is insufficient because of the shortened bowel). Clinical trials to demonstrate such an advantage, however, have not been adequate.

When the osmolality of such solutions is above 300 mosm/kg, they tend to shift free water into the intestinal space and thus can induce rapid transit and diarrhea. Some polymeric solutions have a high osmolality; however, these are the more concentrated solutions that contain more than 1.5 kcal/mL. The osmolality of monomeric solutions is higher than that of polymeric solutions with the same caloric density.

Solutions for Specific Metabolic Needs

Solutions for specific metabolic needs are mostly complete nutritional solutions with specific nutrients either added or removed to meet special requirements. These can be divided into two categories:

1. Solutions designed for use in patients with inherited metabolic disorders (Chapter 61). They are low in, or devoid of, specific nutrients (e.g., phenylalanine or other amino acids) that cannot be properly metabolized because of enzymatic defects or deficiencies.
2. Solutions designed for use in patients with specific medical conditions, such as liver failure, renal failure, or critical illness with multiple organ failure. Feeding solutions in this category are designed to lessen the metabolic burden on the failing organ or to correct metabolic abnormalities that result from the organ dysfunction.

Branched-Chain Amino Acid (BCAA) Solutions

BCAA solutions contain about 40 to 50% of the amino acids as leucine, isoleucine, and valine. Concentrations of the aromatic amino acids (AAA) tryptophan, tyrosine, and phenylalanine are low. Solutions high in BCAAs have been designed for use in two conditions: *(a)* hepatic failure and encephalopathy and *(b)* severe illness and stress with multiple organ failure, such as sepsis and major injury.

Patients with hepatic encephalopathy tend to have decreased levels of BCAAs and increased levels of AAAs in blood and cerebrospinal fluid. AAAs were postulated to act as false neurotransmitters in the central nervous system, contributing to hepatic encephalopathy (30). Thus, providing a nutritional solution containing high levels of BCAAs and low levels of AAAs was designed to reverse or improve the hepatic encephalopathy induced by the AAA false neurotransmitters. Randomized studies examining the use of solutions high in BCAAs in patients with hepatic encephalopathy, however, have not shown a clear benefit, and their role in these patients is controversial (31, 32) (for a detailed discussion see Chapter 73).

Major acute illnesses with severe metabolic stress, such as sepsis, severe trauma, major operations, and burns, are associated with accelerated muscle catabolism (see Chapters 96 and 98). Because BCAAs are used extensively by muscles, providing solutions high in BCAA was proposed to be beneficial for muscle preservation in severely ill and catabolic patients. Some clinical trials have shown improved nitrogen balance with enteral or parenteral solutions high in BCAAs in critically ill patients (33); however, other studies have not shown such benefit or any clinically relevant benefit in decreasing morbidity or mortality (34, 35) (see Chapter 98). At present, no decisive information supports routine use of solutions high in BCAAs in patients who either are suffering from liver failure or are critically ill.

Essential Amino Acid Solutions

Essential amino acid (EAA) solutions are designed for feeding patients with renal failure (Chapter 89), many of whom have trauma and/or sepsis. Failing kidneys have a reduced capacity for clearance of various metabolites (urea, creatinine, uric acid) and minerals (potassium, phosphate, magnesium). Serum levels of some nonessential amino acids are elevated, and levels of essential amino acids, such as leucine, isoleucine, and valine, are decreased. The objectives of nutritional support in patients with renal failure are to provide optimal nutrition while minimizing the load of metabolites presented for handling by the compromised kidneys. The latter objective is particularly important when an effort is being made to avoid dialysis in patients with compromised renal function. However, optimal nutrition should not be compromised because of a need for dialysis. Renal enteral feeding solutions contain EAAs, histidine, small amounts of fat, and electrolytes. They do not contain vitamins or trace elements, which must be supplemented as needed. The low content of electrolytes allows flexibility—electrolytes can be added on an individual basis as needed. Most of the clinical studies on the role of high-EAA feeding regimens have been performed with parenteral nutrition, and although some metabolic benefits have been noted, a clear clinical advantage has not been documented. The few studies in which enteral nutrition was examined suggest that administration of EAAs is associated with improved nitrogen balance and attenuation of the rise in BUN (for detailed discussion see Chapter 89).

High-Fat/Low-Carbohydrate Solutions for Pulmonary Insufficiency

In pulmonary insufficiency formulas, fat content is increased to 50 to 55% of the total calories, with a corresponding decrease in carbohydrate content. Calories provided from any source increase O_2 consumption and CO_2 production and thus present an added burden to the failing lungs. Carbohydrate calories require more O_2 consumption and produce more CO_2 than do fat calories. Hence, the notion that replacing carbohydrate calories by fat calories presents a lighter burden on the respiratory system. In most patients, the difference is not clinically significant; however, in those with borderline pulmonary function (36, 37) the difference may be important, especially when excess calories are given (see Chapter 90).

Immune-Modulating Solutions

Specific nutrients can influence the immune response (Chapter 45). The immune-enhancing role of zinc and the immune-inhibiting effect of certain fatty acids have long been known. Experimental studies suggest that substances that have not been considered essential nutrients for adults, such as derivatives of ω-3 polyunsaturated fatty acids (38), ribonucleic acid (RNA) (39), and arginine (40), may also have beneficial effects on the immune response. These observations prompted formulation of enteral feeding solutions containing these nutrients in addition to the regular nutrients. A randomized study in surgical cancer patients found that compared with a standard enteral feeding solution, the immune-modulating solution administered postoperatively resulted in better immunologic and metabolic outcomes, with a decrease in infectious and wound complications and a decrease in postoperative hospitalization (41). However, a subsequent study in a large group of surgical cancer patients comparing the immune-modulating solution with routine intravenous fluids postoperatively did not demonstrate a benefit (42). In the critically ill patient, immune-modulating solution was observed to decrease major septic complications (43).

Modular Solutions

Modular solutions provide each of the macronutrients or micronutrients in suitable combinations or singly and can be used to prepare specialized formulas or to augment regular enteral or oral feeding. Protein modular products are usually available as powder that has to be mixed with water prior to administration. Carbohydrates are available as glucose polymers; fat is supplied as triglycerides of long-chain polyunsaturated or medium-chain fatty acids. These nutrients can be added when extra calories or protein are needed. They are particularly useful when the patient cannot receive the required macronutrient by increasing the amount of enteral feeding formula because of limited tolerance to fluids or to other components present in the regular feeding solution. The use of these solutions to modify commercial solutions or to prepare a special solution is limited by the difficulty they present and the lack of specific indication for their use. For instance, fat emulsions require an emulsifier to keep them dispersed in solutions after they have been mixed with other enteral solutions. Glucose polymers added to solutions can increase the osmolality and induce diarrhea once they are digested to glucose. Protein powder is hard to mix and tends to clump, thereby creating mechanical difficulties when administered.

When requirements increase for certain micronutrient solutions, those available for oral intake and parenteral use can also be used for enteral feeding; thus, in patients needing additional potassium, an oral potassium solution can be added to regular enteral feeding to increase potassium intake. However, when adding nutrients to enteral feedings, caution must be exercised to prevent precipitation that will decrease absorption. For instance, phosphate added to enteral feedings may cause precipitation of calcium, which can clog small-diameter tubes and may not be absorbed in the intestines. Such problems can be avoided, preferably by administering additives separately from the enteral feeding solutions unless advance testing has been adequate.

Hydration Solutions

Hydration solutions have been designed mostly to provide fluid and minerals to children and adults with acute diarrhea to prevent dehydration. The solutions contain sodium and glucose. The osmolarity varies from 224 to 311 mmol/L (44). Glucose facilitates sodium absorption in the small bowel (see Chapter 39). Hydration solutions have been used successfully in underdeveloped countries during epidemics of infectious diarrhea to treat or to prevent dehydration (45). These solutions can be administered through tubes to patients with excessive fluid and mineral requirements, such as patients with certain types of short bowel syndrome.

INDICATIONS

Enteral feeding is indicated in patients who cannot ingest adequate amounts of food but have enough GI function to allow digestion and absorption of feeding solutions delivered into the GI tract through tubes. Choice of appropriate feeding solutions and method of administration based on sound pathophysiologic considerations of the GI tract are essential to maximize digestion and absorption of enteral feeding in the compromised GI tract. Specific indications for enteral feeding:

1. Severe dysphagia from obstruction or dysfunction of the oropharynx or esophagus
2. Coma or delirious state
3. Persistent anorexia
4. Nausea or vomiting; patients whose nausea and vomiting arise from a gastric disorder (e.g., gastroparesis, gastritis, gastric outlet obstruction) can be safely fed enterally into the jejunum; in those whose symptoms result from intestinal obstruction, enteral feeding should be avoided
5. Partial obstruction of the stomach or small bowel
6. Fistulas of the distal small bowel or colon
7. Severe malabsorption secondary to decreased absorption capacity of the GI tract, such as a short bowel or inflammatory disease of the bowel; in these conditions, a pump-controlled slow drip of enteral feeding solution can maximize use of the limited absorption capacity, which may be overwhelmed by the large volume of food and fluids delivered to the intestines in oral feeding
8. Recurrent aspiration; in this condition, feeding solutions should be delivered through a jejunostomy; feeding into the stomach must be avoided
9. Diseases or disorders that require administration of specific solutions that cannot be taken orally for prolonged periods (see Chapter 61)
10. Increased nutritional requirements that cannot be met by oral intake; this indication applies mostly to burn patients who have high nutritional requirements
11. Growth induction in children with Crohn's disease (Chapter 69)

The clinical efficacy of enteral feeding in specific clinical conditions is reviewed in the various chapters dealing with these conditions.

Enteral feeding is contraindicated in patients with complete intestinal obstruction, paralytic ileus, severe pseudo-intestinal obstruction, severe diarrhea, or extreme malabsorption. In patients with a proximal intestinal fistula, enteral feeding can be attempted only if the tip of the feeding tube is distal to the fistula. In these conditions, however, enteral feeding may still aggravate the fistula by increasing the amount of fluid secreted into the GI tract (from stomach, pancreas, and bile). Enhanced secretion can occur even if the enteral feedings enter the GI tract distal to the duodenum.

A general indication for enteral feeding relates to maintaining the GI tract mucosa in a healthy state and preventing its atrophy, particularly in patients with trauma, postsurgical patients, or those for whom prolonged fasting is associated with a lengthy illness. Atrophy of the intestinal mucosa can occur rapidly after trauma and major illness (45). In an experimental setting, these disorders may lead to bacterial translocation from the gut (45). The presence of nutrients in the GI tract can serve as trophic factors both in the short bowel syndrome (Chapter 68) and in the presence of severe trauma. Thus, oral or enteral feeding early in the course of trauma or severe illness has been advocated not only to provide nutrition, but also to maintain a healthy GI mucosa and prevent bacterial translocation and sepsis (45). Whether such a benefit can be achieved in humans remains to be seen.

METHODS OF INFUSION

Enteral feedings can be administered by either bolus (17) or continuous drip (18). When possible, the bolus method is preferable because it takes less time, gives the patient more freedom, and is easier to use. It does not require pump control. The bolus of feeding solution can be given by administering as much as 500 mL over 10 to 15 minutes. The solution can be administered through a syringe with a slow push or by gravity-driven drip from a bag.

Bolus feeding is suitable when the tip of the feeding tube is in the stomach. The bolus of feeding solution is delivered into the stomach, and outflow of the solution into the duodenum is regulated by the stomach and the pyloric sphincter. Thus, a bolus containing one-third of the daily volume can be delivered without causing dumping in a patient with a normal stomach. When the tip of the feeding tube is in the duodenum or jejunum, the feeding solution must be delivered in a continuous drip (preferably pump controlled) to avoid intestinal distention and dumping. Feeding into the small bowel usually can be tolerated at a rate as high as 150 mL/h, and some patients can tolerate higher rates.

When bolus feeding is used (e.g., in patients with dysphagia who are fed with gastrostomy tubes), daily intake of about 2000 mL can be given in 3 to 5 boluses administered every 3 to 5 hours (23). The bolus must be administered with the patient sitting or reclining 45° to prevent aspiration. When feeding into the stomach, isoosmolar and hyperosmolar solutions can be used because the pylorus prevents passage of a large volume of solution into the duodenum. When feeding into the small bowel, isoosmolar solutions usually are preferable to avoid passage of free water from the intestinal wall into the lumen.

COMPONENTS AND ABSORPTION

Protein

Protein is digested in the proximal intestinal tract and absorbed through the intestinal mucosa as dipeptides, tripeptides, or single amino acids (Chapters 2 and 39). With enteral feeding solutions containing intact protein, the process of digestion and absorption of protein does not differ from that of regular foods. An important issue regarding protein is whether incorporating it in enteral solutions as small peptides or amino acids presents any advantage, particularly in the compromised GI tract where digestion may be impaired or inadequate. In certain conditions there are theoretical physiologic advantages to predigested protein.

1. Pancreatic proteolytic enzymes are not required for hydrolysis of small oligopeptides; this hydrolysis occurs by mucosal peptide hydrolysis. Hence, small peptides would be absorbed in severe pancreatic insufficiency, whereas intact protein hydrolysis would be less efficient.
2. Patients with the short bowel syndrome may not have adequate time for proteolytic enzymes to break down whole protein. Dipeptides and tripeptides may be advantageous because they can be absorbed at once. However, predigested protein presents a higher osmotic load in the GI tract and thus may decrease tolerance to infusion.

In perfusion studies in persons with a normal GI tract, administration into the jejunum of lactalbumin as hydrolysates (dipeptides to pentapeptides) resulted in better absorption than administration of the corresponding large proteins or free amino acids (46). Another study showed that ovalbumin hydrolysates that contained mostly di- and tripeptides were absorbed better than those containing mainly tetra- and pentapeptides (47). Other observations have not confirmed these results (48). Results of the British studies comparing absorption of free amino acids, small and larger peptides, and various intact proteins are complex (46–48).

Various studies have addressed the question of whether administration of peptides or free amino acids as part of an enteral feeding solution rather than as a single nutrient (as in the above studies) offers an advantage. Undernourished patients with no malabsorption who were fed by a tube positioned in the proximal jejunum absorbed nitrogen as effectively from a solution with intact protein (Isocal) as from an isocaloric isonitrogenous solution containing protein hydrolysates (Criticare HN) (49). Better nitrogen retention was observed in subjects given Criticare HN than in those given a free amino acid formula (Vivonex) (50, 51). Jones et al. found only small differences between a solution containing free amino acids (Vivonex) and an intact protein diet (Clinifeed 400) infused by tube over 24 hours in a randomized fashion in 70 malnourished patients needing nutritional support after a period of inadequate intake (52). With similar nitrogen and caloric intakes, nutritional parameters were about the same, but the intact protein formula was associated with a better nitrogen balance. Other studies have shown that feeding a peptide-based formula (Reabilen) resulted in higher levels of serum transferrin and prealbumin than those attained by feeding a solution with intact protein (53, 54).

The same question about comparative value arises in patients with compromised absorptive and digestive capacity. A randomized crossover study in four malnourished patients with short bowel syndrome compared the nutritional and metabolic effects of isonitrogenous isocaloric enteral solutions containing a free amino acid mixture or hydrolyzed casein. Protein turnover was studied by leucine kinetics. There was no significant difference in the rates of protein flux, synthesis, breakdown, or oxidation during the period of administration of free amino acids compared with the period of casein hydrolysate (55). A crossover study in seven patients with the short bowel syndrome (less than 150 cm of residual jejunum ending in a stoma) examined absorption from a defined-formula diet with a protein isolate, a defined-formula diet with a protein hydrolysate (15 to 20% free amino acids, 80 to 85% 2- to 6-amino acid peptides), and three solid diets (56). The diets varied in fat, fiber, and carbohydrate. Although variations in absorption among patients were marked, almost all had similar percentages of caloric and nitrogen absorption when receiving the two defined-formula diets. Caloric and nitrogen absorption was generally better with the defined-formula diets than with the solid diets. The investigators concluded that a liquid diet consisting of peptides, oligosaccharides, and MCTs is not more beneficial than a polymeric diet in a patient with the short bowel syndrome. A randomized study comparing tolerance of polymeric solutions with that of elemental solutions in patients receiving enteral feeding following GI operations found no significant difference (57).

The various enteral feeding solutions differ not only in their sources and amounts of amino acids, but also in their content of carbohydrates, fats, and other nutrients. This point should be considered in evaluating results of comparative experiments, because these variables are essentially uncontrolled. Furthermore, in most comparison experiments that have been reported, the amino acid composition of the free amino acid formulation differed from that of the protein hydrolysate or protein in the respective formulations (58).

The comparative value of enterally and parenterally fed amino acid mixtures regarding protein accretion was investigated in healthy dogs by use of a multilabeled leucine tracer. The study demonstrated that enteral administration of an amino acid mixture resulted in more-efficient protein anabolism in the gut and the splanchnic region. Overall whole-body leucine use was similar in the enterally and parenterally fed groups. The authors concluded that enteral feeding was superior to total parenteral nutrition (TPN) in this situation (59).

At present, no clear, consistent clinical data support the use of solutions containing protein in the form of hydrolysates or free amino acids. One reason for the lack of clear superiority of these forms of protein may be the great reserve and adaptive capacity of the absorptive mucosa of the small bowel (see Chapter 39). Even when a large percentage of the small bowel mucosa is injured or resected, the remaining parts may still process adequate amounts of nutrients. Although some patients with malabsorption might benefit from a peptide enteral feeding solution, this possibility must be clearly demonstrated in clinical trials. Because of the high cost of enteral solutions with free amino acids or peptides, their routine use cannot be supported at present.

Glutamine

Glutamine, a nonessential amino acid, is the most abundant free amino acid in the body (Chapters 2 and 35). It is synthesized mostly in muscle and used as the primary fuel in the small intestine. In recent years, glutamine has become increasingly recognized as important for maintenance of healthy intestinal mucosa, and it may protect the mucosa from injury induced by chemotherapy, radiation, and other injurious factors (60, 61). In addition, glutamine helps maintain acid-base equilibrium through generation of ammonia. Glutamine is unstable in aqueous solutions, spontaneously breaking down to ammonia and pyroglutamic acid; thus, including glutamine in nutritional solutions poses a manufacturing hurdle.

In rats with the short bowel syndrome, addition of glutamine (25% of total amino acids) to a defined-formula diet resulted in a trophic effect on the mucosa of the remaining small bowel, with increased villous height and greater hyperplasia (63). Glutamine in combination with growth hormone administration and a dietary regimen containing fiber was reported to enhance absorption in patients with short bowel syndrome (64).

In catabolic states, both release of glutamine from muscle and use of glutamine by the GI mucosa seem to increase (65, 66) (see Chapter 35). This increase may result in severe loss of muscle tissue. When catabolism is prolonged, glutamine synthesis and release from muscle decrease and may not cover the increased use by various tissues, especially the GI mucosa. Thus, glutamine deficiency may ensue. Glutamine consequently has been suggested to be essential for the intestinal mucosa and other organs of patients in catabolic states and thus may need to be added to nutritional regimens for patients with catabolic illnesses (67). Provision of adequate glutamine in nutritional regimens results in better immune response in the GI mucosa and in maintenance of mucosal mass and its barrier function against bacteria (68). Such maintenance may provide protection against bacterial translocation and sepsis. However, such an advantage has not been demonstrated in humans. Before large amounts of glutamine are added to enteral feedings, its safety and efficacy must be studied. Some investigators are concerned that glutamine, a primary nutrient in some tumors, may act as a tumor stimulator (69). Therefore, any potentially adverse effects of glutamine must be carefully evaluated, particularly in cancer patients.

Proteins in enteral feeding solutions contain glutamine, but it is protein based. Determining the glutamine content is difficult because it requires hydrolyzing the protein with heat and acid, which also converts glutamine to glutamate. The data on the beneficial effect of glutamine on the small intestinal mucosa have been derived from studies in which free glutamine was administered. It is not clear that protein-bound glutamine has the same beneficial effects as the free form. Commercial enteral feeding solutions with intact protein contain glutamine in quantities of less than 14% of the total protein amino acids. However, solutions are available with added glutamine (Vivonex, Alitraq).

Carbohydrates

The various starches in commercial enteral feeding solutions are eventually hydrolyzed to glucose in the small intestine. Starches vary in their glucose units, from 400 to many thousands. Hydrolysis forms polymers with decreasing numbers of glucose units (see Chapter 3). The osmolality of a formula is influenced to a major extent by the sources and amounts of glucose, sucrose, and the shorter-chain glucose units and to a lesser extent by free amino acid and electrolyte concentrations.

The patient with normal GI function hydrolyzes starch and long-chain glucose polymers rapidly. Most of the glucose is absorbed in the proximal small bowel. In patients with marked pancreatic insufficiency, oligosaccharides may be useful because they are hydrolyzed to glucose by the intestinal brush-border enzyme α-dextrinase.

Initial rapid infusion of large volumes of high osmolality into the stomach or jejunum should be avoided in patients with vagotomy (which also occurs with esophagectomy), gastrectomy, and intestinal dysfunction, because this infusion can induce rapid transit, glucose malabsorption, abdominal discomfort, and diarrhea. Hyperosmolar nonketotic coma can occur with high-carbohydrate feedings; coma is most likely to develop in the diabetic patient who is infected and dehydrated. Excess carbohydrate calories in enteral feeding can result in hypercarbia in patients with respiratory insufficiency and in a rise in metabolic rate.

Lipids

The fat content of enteral feeding solutions varies from less than 2% to 45% of the total calories. The lipids, usually corn oil or soy oil, contain large amounts of polyunsaturated fatty acids; some contain lecithin (added as an emulsifier). Others have MCTs in small or large proportions. The rationale for adding MCTs is that they are easily hydrolyzed and absorbed in various states of malabsorption (70, 71); however, absorption of enteral feeding solutions containing MCTs has not been proved superior to that of LCT-based solutions. Because MCTs are ketogenic, they should be avoided in patients with diabetes, ketosis, or acidosis (71). The relatively large amounts of polyunsaturated fat in most formulas provide more than enough essential fatty acids; the need is approximately 3 to 4.5% of total calories (see Chapter 4). An enteral feeding solution (Impact) has been introduced that contains part of the fat as fish oil. Fish oil has a high content of ω-3 fatty acids and has been reported superior to vegetable oil in its effect on the immune response (38).

As for other nutrients, the efficiency of absorption of lipids depends on the rate of infusion, the concentration of the nutrient, and the digestive and absorptive capacities of the GI tract. (Lipid characteristics and other factors affecting digestion, absorption, and metabolism are reviewed in detail in Chapter 4). Patients with exocrine pancreatic insufficiency may absorb more than 50% of dietary fat despite the absence of measurable pancreatic lipase activity. This absorption appears to be related lingual and gastric lipases (72). Nevertheless, administration of pancreatic extracts is useful in patients with pancreatic insufficiency. Patients with the short bowel syndrome have been reported to absorb 54% of the fat from a diet containing 46% of the calories as fat (73). Fat did not adversely affect absorption of magnesium, calcium, and zinc. This finding dispels the notion that patients with the short bowel syndrome require a low-fat diet and has an important implication for the use of enteral feeding in such patients. A high-fat enteral feeding solution administered by continuous drip can provide a large number of calories and thus ensure absorption of adequate calories despite the malabsorption. A report compared the effectiveness of five different levels of fat (from 10 to 50% of nonprotein calories) in enteral feeding solutions given to guinea pigs with full-thickness burns over 30% of the total body surface (63). Fat content between 5 and 15% of nonprotein calories was deemed optimal for nutritional support.

Enteral feeding solutions are available with fat providing up to 55% of the calories. The value of such formulas in patients with impaired pulmonary function has been reviewed above in this chapter and in chapter 90.

Vitamins and Trace Elements

Enteral feeding solutions were designed to provide the recommended dietary allowance (RDA) of vitamins and trace elements with an intake of 1500 to 2000 calories. Patients maintained on enteral feeding for periods exceeding 6 months had normal or high blood levels of the various vitamins (75).

The stability of vitamins in commercial enteral feeding solutions has been determined only to a limited extent. Short- and long-term studies demonstrated stability of vitamins A and E and riboflavin for as long as 3 months. Specific data regarding absorption of vitamins from enteral feeding solutions are lacking. However, the adequate or high levels of vitamins in the blood of patients who received long-term enteral feeding suggest that both stability and absorption are adequate and, consequently, that current enteral feeding solutions contain adequate vitamins (75).

Most enteral feeding formulas contain sufficient amounts of trace elements, including iron, zinc, copper, and iodine, so that intake of 1500 to 2000 calories per day provides adequate amounts of these nutrients. However, deficiencies of zinc and other micronutrients can occur when the caloric intake from enteral feeding is low or when GI loss of zinc persistently exceeds intake, as can happen in patients with active Crohn's disease.

Fiber

Enteral feeding formulas initially were fiber free, except for those prepared by blenderizing natural foods. There has been increasing recognition that dietary fiber offers numerous physiologic and metabolic benefits (Chapter 43). Most Americans ingest 8 to 12 g of dietary fiber daily (78). The recommended amounts for healthy Americans are 10 to 13 g of fiber per 1000 calories (77).

Some enteral feeding solutions are now prepared with fiber. Blenderized enteral feeding solutions contain 1.9 to 3.3 g fiber per 250 mL (79). Some polymeric enteral solutions are manufactured with fiber from different sources, including soy polysaccharide fiber, oat fiber, and others. Soy polysaccharide is a tasteless and odorless material that is easily added to enteral feeding solutions because it can be suspended in liquid. Only about 6% of soy polysaccharide is water soluble. It can improve lipid metabolism and diabetic control in hyperlipidemic patients (80). The amounts of soy polysaccharide added to enteral feeding solutions vary between 2.5 and 5.9 g per 250 mL (79).

Pectin and gum are poor candidates as fibers in enteral feeding solutions because they have high viscosity. Some enteral feeding solutions contain a combination of fibers including oat, pectin, gum arabic, and hydrolyzed gums, providing both soluble and insoluble fibers. Fiber derived from oats may have a cholesterol-lowering effect, whereas most insoluble fibers, such as cellulose and hemicellulose, act mostly as laxatives.

If a solution without fiber is used, fiber can be administered separately in other forms, such as natural bran or Metamucil. In spite of the physiologic considerations pointing to gastrointestinal and metabolic functions of dietary fiber, results of investigations on its role in enteral feeding have been inconsistent. The effects of different fibers in enteral feedings were studied in a randomized study in healthy subjects. Compared with a fiber-free polyremic enteral feeding solution, supplementation with 30 g of oat fiber, soy oliogosaccharide fiber, or a soy polysaccharide had a negligent effects on bowel function (81). Other studies showed similar results with soy polysaccharides (82, 83).

A study of healthy young male subjects compared the effects of adding 0, 30, or 60 g/day of soy fiber to a feeding solution (Ensure). The results showed that dietary fiber increased daily fecal weights and frequency of bowel movements. All dosages of fiber resulted in decreased transit time in the GI tract (84).

The effects on bowel function of a fiber-containing enteral feeding solution (Enrich, 12.8 g fiber/1000 kcal) were compared in a crossover randomized study to the effects of a solution without fiber (Ensure)(85). Mean daily fecal weight and frequency of bowel movements were similar during administration of the two solutions; however, patients fed Ensure required more laxatives and had more diarrhea. Constipation was similar in both groups. The authors reported that the fiber-containing solution was associated with improved GI function. Because the patients fed Ensure received more laxatives, their worsened GI function (i.e., more diarrhea) could have been caused by the laxative use. Most of the patients in this study were comatose, and thus these results are of limited clinical application in other groups of patients.

A concern was raised that fiber in enteral feeding solutions would decrease absorption of minerals and vitamins (86). Addition of 120 g/day of soy polysaccharides to an elemental solution did reduce the overall absorption rate of magnesium, zinc, and phosphorus but did not affect potassium and calcium absorption. The balance for all five minerals was still positive, however (87). Others studied the effect of adding 20, 30, and 40 g of soy polysaccharides; 40 g of fiber caused negative balances for copper and iron, whereas zinc, calcium, and magnesium were in positive balance (88).

Administration of enteral feeding solutions containing soy polysaccharide apparently does not result in malabsorption and deficiency of major minerals and vitamins in the short term. The effects, however, in patients receiving long-term enteral feeding with fiber as the primary or sole diet are unclear. Appropriate monitoring for these nutrients is recommended.

COMPLICATIONS

Enteral feeding can be a safe and effective nutritional support method. Its safety depends on *(a)* choice of the appropriate formula and infusion method, *(b)* delivery of the formulas into the appropriate part of the GI tract, and *(c)* clinical and metabolic evaluation of the patient prior to and during enteral feeding.

The most severe potential complication of enteral feeding is aspiration. Numerous factors can predispose to aspiration, including misplacement of the tip of the feeding tube in the esophagus or upper stomach, impaired gastric emptying, decreased lower esophageal sphincter pressure, large feeding volume, patient's position during feeding, and various medications that decrease GI peristalsis. The risk of aspiration can be reduced by appropriately positioning the feeding tube, elevating the upper body to 30 to 45°, and avoiding enteral feeding when contraindicated. Placement of a gastrotomy tube per se does not affect the lower esophageal pressure. However, gastric distention caused by rapid delivery of an intragastric bolus of enteral feeding can relax the sphincter (89) and may predispose to reflux, heartburn, and aspiration. In the presence of impaired gastric emptying or in the absence of gag reflex, the feeding solution is best delivered into the jejunum. The incidence of aspiration depends on how vigorously it is sought and the type of patient. Severe aspiration was reported in 1% of patients receiving an average of 10 days of enteral feeding (90). In a prospective study, the incidence of aspiration was 2.4 per 1000 enteral feeding days. Little morbidity and no mortality resulted from aspiration (91). However, other studies reported aspiration rates between 17 and 32% in patients receiving gastric feeding (92–94).

Bacterial contamination of enteral feeding formulas can occur easily because the solutions are an ideal growth medium for bacteria. Occasional case reports of sepsis associated with feeding contaminated enteral solutions have surfaced.

Nausea and vomiting have been reported to occur in as many as 20% of patients (95). Nonspecific symptoms of abdominal cramps, distention, and bloating can occur and are usually caused by too-rapid infusion or an underlying intestinal disorder.

Diarrhea has been reported in 5 to 30% of patients receiving enteral feeding (96). Defining diarrhea and determining its cause in patients receiving enteral feeding may be difficult, however, and the method of reporting may significantly alter the reported incidence of this complication (95). Tolerance to enteral feeding depends on several factors, including the functional capacity of the GI tract, the rate of infusion, the type of formula, and concomitant medications. The healthy GI tract can easily handle bolus feedings of as much as 500 mL given over 10 to 15 minutes. This feeding method has been used successfully in patients with dysphagia secondary to cancer of the head and neck (23).

Patients with GI diseases may require a slow rate of infusion. Those with a short bowel or with small bowel mucosal disease (e.g., radiation enteritis or Crohn's disease) may require a pump-controlled continuous feeding over 10 to 15 hours with a rate not exceeding 100 mL/hour. Isoosmolar solutions are better tolerated by patients prone to diarrhea because hyperosmolar solutions tend to draw fluids into the upper intestine, thereby increasing the load that must be absorbed distally. Solutions with an osmolality of approximately 300 mosm/kg do not require dilution to enhance tolerance and decrease diarrhea.

One of the most important factors in causing diarrhea during enteral feeding is concomitant use of medications, particularly antibiotics and magnesium-containing antacids. In some reports, as many as half of the patients on enteral feeding who were receiving antibiotics developed diarrhea; these two factors seem to work synergistically to induce diarrhea (97). Studies in healthy volunteers demonstrated that significant colonic secretion of water, sodium, and chloride occurs during enteral feeding (98). This may contribute to diarrhea, especially in patients with compromised intestinal function or when antibiotics are administered concomitantly. Infusion of short-chain fatty acids into the cecum prevented net fluid secretion into the colon. When these fatty acids are absorbed in t he colon, they enhance water and electrolyte absorption (98).

Constipation occurs in as many as 15% of patients receiving long-term enteral feedings. As mentioned above, there is no clear evidence from clinical trials that fiber-containing enteral feeding solutions alleviate this problem.

Metabolic abnormalities can occur in patients receiving enteral feeding. Their frequency and severity depend mostly on the general medical condition of the patient. Thus, patients with renal failure are at risk for developing increased azotemia, hyperkalemia, hypermagnesemia, and hyperphosphatemia, and the diabetic patient is at risk for hyperglycemia. These potential complications are not inherent to enteral feeding and can be avoided by careful attention to the medical condition of the patient.

Dehydration is a potential complication in patients given high-osmolality enteral feeding solutions. When such solutions are administered, close observation is necessary to prevent dehydration and metabolic complications.

ENTERAL FEEDING IN VARIOUS MEDICAL CONDITIONS

The role of enteral feeding in specific medical conditions is presented in the various chapters as follows: inherited metabolic diseases, Chapters 61 and 62; inflammatory bowl disease, Chapter 69; pancreatic disorders, Chapter 72; cancer, Chapter 82; renal disorders, Chapter 89; pulmonary disorders, Chapter 90; the hypercatabolic state, Chapter 96; infection, Chapter 97; and surgery, Chapter 98.

HOME ENTERAL NUTRITION (HEN)

HEN is used increasingly to provide nutrients and fluids outside the hospital. In 1992, an estimated 152,000 patients used HEN (99). The National Registry of Home TPN and HEN reported clinical data on 3931 patients (99). The two most common diagnoses of patients receiving HEN were cancer, which accounted for 42%, and swallowing disorders, 30%. The later group included mostly patients with strokes. The therapy was safe in the home. HEN complications requiring hospitalization ocurred at an annual rate of 0.4 and 0.3% in the cancer and swallowing disorders groups, respectively. The 1-year survival was 30% for cancer patients and 55% for the neurologic disorders patients; 30% of the cancer patients and 15% of the neurologic patients were able to resume full oral nutrition. In patients with cancer of the head and neck whose tumors are successfully treated, HEN has been used for periods exceeding 7 years, providing good nutrition and rehabilitation with minimal impact on quality of life (23, 100). Regular medical follow-up is essential to ensure appropriate functioning of the feeding tube and optimization of the nutrition regimen.

REFERENCES

1. Randall HT. JPEN J Parenter Enteral Nutr 1984;8:113–36.
2. Einhorn M. Med Rec 1910;78:92–5.
3. Andresen AFR. Ann Surg 1918;67:565–6.
4. Barron J. Surg Clin North Am 1959;39:1481–91.
5. Winitz M, Seedman, DA, Graff J. Am J Clin Nutr 1970;23:525–45.
6. Rubenoff R, Ravich W. Arch Intern Med 1989;149:184–8.
7. American Gastroenterological Association Technical Review of the Feeding for Enteral Nutrition. Gastroenterology 1995;108:1282–90.
8. Mathers-Vliegen EMH, Tytgat GNJ, Merkus MD. Gastrointest Endosc 1993;39:537–42.
9. Gutierrez ED, Balfe DM. Radiology 1991;178:759–62.
10. Benya R, Langer S, Mobrahan S. JPEN J Parenter Enteral Nutr 1990;14:108–9.
11. Ghahremani GG. Dig Dis Sci 1981;31:574–8.
12. Rakel AB, Titlen M, Goode C, et al. AAEN Clin Issues 1994;5(2):194–201.
13. Norton B, Homer-Ward M, Donnelly MT, et al. Br Med J 1996;312:13–6.
14. Minard G. Nutr Clin Pract 1994;9:172–82.
15. DiLorenzo C, Lachman R, Hyman PE. J Pediatr Gastroenterol Nutr 1990;11:45–7.
16. Shellito M. Ann Surg 1985;201:763–7.
17. Gallagher MW, Tyson KRT, Ashcraft KW. Surgery 1973;74: 536–9.
18. Holder TM, Leape LL, Ashcraft KW. N Engl J Med 1972;286: 1345–7.
19. Collins JB, Georgeson KE, Vicente Y. J Pediatr Surg 1995;32: 1065–71.
20. Ho CS, Young EY. AJR 1992;158:251–7.
21. Wollman B, D'Agostino WB, Walus-Wigle JR, et al. Radiology 1995;197:699–704.

22. Ponsky JL, Gauderer MWL, Stellato TA. Arch Surg 1983;118: 913–4.
23. Shike M, Berner YN, Gerdes H. Otolaryngol Head Neck Surg 1989;101:549–54.
24. Shike M, Latkany L, Gerdes H. Gastrointest Endosc 1996; 37:62–5.
25. Shike M, Wallach C, Herman-Zaidins M. JPEN J Parenter Enteral Nutr 1989;13:648–50.
26. U.S. Food and Drug Administration. Compliance program guidance manual, chap. 21, program no. 7321.002. Washington, DC: 1989–1991.
27. Talbot JM. Guidelines for the scientific review of enteral food products for medicinal purposes. Bethesda, MD: Life Sciences Research Office, Federation of American Societies for Experimental Biology, 1990.
28. Shils ME, ed. Introduction to proceedings of conference: defined-formula diets for medical purposes. Chicago: American Medical Association, 1977.
29. Grimble GK, Silk DBA. Nutr Clin Pract 1990;5:227–30.
30. Fischer JE, Yoshimura N, Aqueri A, et al. Am J Surg 1974; 127:40–7.
31. Eciksson LS, Conn HO. Hepatology 1989;10:228–46.
32. Riordan SM, Williams RW. N Engl J Med 1997;337:472–9.
33. Cerra FB, Shronts EP, Raup S, et al. Crit Care Med 1989;17: 619–22.
34. Yu YM, Wagner DA, Walesrewski JC, et al. Ann Surg 1988;207:421–9.
35. Von Meyenfeldt MF, Soeters PB, Vente JP, et al. Br J Surg 1990;77:924–9.
36. Kwan R, Min MA. Am J Med 1987;82:751–8.
37. Weisman C, Askanazi J, Rosenblum SH, et al. Ann Intern Med 1983;98:41–4.
38. Alexander JW, Saito H, Ogle CK, et al. Ann Surg 1986;204: 1–8.
39. Kulkarnic AD, Fanslow WC, Drath DB, et al. Arch Surg 1986;121:169–72.
40. Kirk SJ, Barbul A. JPEN J Parenter Enteral Nutr 1990;14: 226S–9S.
41. Daly JM, Lieberman MD, Goldfine J, et al. Surgery 1992;112: 56–67.
42. Heslin MJ, Latkany L, Leung D, et al. Ann Surg 1997;226: 567–80.
43. Kudok KA, Minard G, Croce MA, et al. Ann Surg 1996;224: 531–43.
44. International Study Group on ORS Solutions. Lancet 1995; 282–5.
45. Alexander JW. JPEN J Parenter Enteral Nutr 1990;14:170S–4S.
46. Grimble GK, Keohane PP, Higgins BE, et al. Clin Sci 1986; 71:65–9.
47. Grimble GK, Silk DBA. Nutr Res Rev 1989;2:87–108.
48. Moriarty KJ, Hegarty JE, Fairclough PD, et al. Gastroenterology 1985;26:694–9.
49. Heymsfield SB, Bleir J, Whitmir L, et al. Am J Clin Nutr 1985;39:234–50.
50. Smith JL, Arteaga C, Heymsfield SB. N Engl J Med 1982; 306:1013–8.
51. Beer WH, Halsted CH. Am J Clin Nutr (Abstract) 1984;39: 689.
52. Jones BJM, Lees R, Andrews J, et al. Gut 1983;24:78–84.
53. Meridith JW, Ditesheim JA, Zeluga GP. J Trauma 1990;30: 825–9.
54. Heimburger DC. Nutr Clin Pract 1990;5:225–6.
55. Rees RG, Grimble GK, Halliday D. Gut 1988;28:A1397.
56. McIntyre PB, Fitchew M, Lennard-Jones JE. Gastroenterology 1986;91:25–33.
57. Ford EG, Jull SF, Jennings LM, et al. J Am Coll Nutr 1992;11: 11–6.
58. Trocki O, Mochizuki H, Dominion L. JPEN J Parenter Enteral Nutr 1986;10:139–45.
59. Yu Yong-Ming, Young VR, Tompkins RG, et al. JPEN J Parenter Enteral Nutr 1995;19:209–15.
60. Souba WW, Herskowitz K, Salloum RM. JPEN J Parenter Enteral Nutr 1990;14:45S–50S.
61. Klimberg VS, Souba WW, Dolson DJ, et al. Cancer 1990;66: 62–8.
62. Fox AD, Kriple SA, Depauler JA, et al. JPEN J Parenter Enteral Nutr 1988;12:324–31.
63. Smith RJ, O'Dwyer T, Wang XO. Report of the 8th Conference on Medical Research. Columbus, OH: Ross Laboratories, 1988.
64. Bryne TA, Morrissey TB, Nutatkan TV, et al. JPEN J Parenter Enteral Nutr 1995;19:296–302.
65. Souba WW, Smith RJ, Wilmore DW. JPEN J Parenter Enteral Nutr 1985;9:608–17.
66. Stehle P, Zonder J, Merters N. Lancet 1989;1:231–5.
67. Smith FR. JPEN J Parenter Enteral Nutr 1990;14:40S–4S.
68. Alverdy JC. JPEN J Parenter Enteral Nutr 1990;14:109S–13S.
69. Fischer J, Chance WT. JPEN J Parenter Enteral Nutr 1990;14:86S–9S.
70. Jandacek RJ, Whiteside JA, Holcombs BN, et al. Am J Clin Nutr 1987;45:940–5.
71. Bach AC, Babeyan VK. Am J Clin Nutr 1982;36:950–62.
72. Abrams CK, Hamosh M, Dutta SK, et al. Gastroenterology 1987;92:125–9.
73. Woolf GM, Miller C, Kurian R, et al. Dig Dis Sci 1987;32:8–15.
74. Mochizuki H, Trocki O, Dominioni L, et al. JPEN J Parenter Enteral Nutr 1984;8:638–46.
75. Berner YN, Morse R, Frank O, et al. JPEN J Parenter Enteral Nutr 1989;13:525–8.
76. Lanza E, Jones Y, Block G, et al. Am J Clin Nutr 1987;46: 790–7.
77. Pilch SM, ed. Physiological effects and healthy consequences of dietary fiber. Washington, DC: U.S. Food & Drug Administration, Federation of American Societies of Experimental Biology, 1987.
78. Slavin J. Nutr Clin Pract 1990;5:247–9.
79. Fredstron SB, Baglien KS, Lampe JW, et al. JPEN J Parenter Enteral Nutr 1991;15:450–3.
80. Lo GS, Goldberg AP, Lim A, et al. Atherosclerosis 1986;622:239–44.
81. Kapadia SA, Raimundo AH, Grimble GK, et al. J Pediatr Gastroenterol Nutr 1985;19:63–68.
82. Lamje JW, Effertz M, Larson JL, et al. J Pediatr Gastroenterol Nutr 1992;16:538–44.
83. Patel DH, Grimble GK, Keohane P, et al. Hum Nutr Clin Nutr 1985;4:67–71.
84. Slavin JL, Nelson NL, McNamara EA, et al. JPEN J Parenter Enteral Nutr 1985;9:317–21.
85. Shankardass K, Chuchmach S, Chelswick K, et al. JPEN J Parenter Enteral Nutr 1990;14:508–12.
86. Scheppach W, Burghardt W, Bartram P, et al. JPEN J Parenter Enteral Nutr 1990;14:204–9.
87. Heymsfield SB, Roongspisuthipong C, Evert M, et al. JPEN J Parenter Enteral Nutr 1988;12:265–73.
88. Taper LJ, Milam RS, McCallister MS, et al. Am J Clin Nutr 1988;48:305–11.
89. Coben RM, Weintraub A, DeMarino AJ, et al. Gastroenterol 1994;106:13–8.
90. Kohane PP, Attecill H, Silk DBA. J Clin Nutr Gastroenterol 1986;1:189–93.

91. Mullen H, Roubenoff RA, Roubenoff RJ. JPEN J Parenter Enteral Nutr 1992;16:160–4.
92. Strong RM, Condon SC, Salinger MR, et al. JPEN J Parenter Enteral Nutr 1992;16:59–63.
93. Montealuo MA, Steger KA, Farber HW, et al. Crit Care Med 1992;20:1377–87.
94. Kearns PJ, Cusato K, Jensen B, et al. Gastroenterology (Abstract) 1994;106:A612.
95. Keohane PP, Attcill H, Love M. Br Med J 1984;288:678–81.
96. Bliss DZ, Guenter PA, Settle RG. Am J Clin Nutr 1992;55:753–9.
97. Silk DBA. Clin Nutr 1987;6:61–74.
98. Bowling TE, Raimundo AH, Grimble GK, et al. Lancet 1993;342:1266–88.
99. Howard L, Ament M, Fleming CR, et al. Gastroenterology 1995;109:355–365.
100. Shike M, unpublished data.

101. Parenteral Nutrition

MAURICE E. SHILS and REX O. BROWN

The efforts to introduce fluid, salt, and food directly into the bloodstream began with Sir Christopher Wren in 1658 and the intervening history has been summarized (1–3). The scientific groundwork resulting in successful parenteral nutrition was laid in the third to fifth decades of the 20th century. Such developments included *(a)* the ability to provide pyrogen-free fluids as a result of Seibert's work (4), *(b)* elucidation by many investigators of the chemical nature of essential nutrients and their eventual availability in safe intravenous forms, *(c)* increased understanding of fluid and electrolyte needs and the importance of acid-base balance, all of which were aided by advances in analytic instrumentation, and *(d)* recognition of the metabolic and nutritional changes and needs associated with disease (5, 6).

World War II stimulated further research into the metabolic changes induced by trauma and infection, led to wider recognition of the importance of nutrition in these and other clinical states (7), and furthered the use of parenteral nutrition (PN) in the seriously ill (8, 9). Peripheral (and occasionally central) parenteral feedings using 5 or 10% glucose, protein hydrolysates, intravenous fat (Lipomul), electrolytes, and multivitamins were used from 1955 to 1965 by various clinicians for limited periods (3). Serious side effects led to withdrawal of intravenous Lipomul from the United States market in the early 1960s. This created a serious problem requiring that glucose be given either in large, relatively isotonic volumes for peripheral vein infusion or else in hyperosmolar form requiring infusion into a major vein. Although central catheters threaded into veins had been used as early as 1944 (3), they were uncommon. A safe and effective intravenous lipid preparation (Intralipid) had been developed by Schuberth and Wretlind, tested by 1961 in Sweden (10), and approved for use in most European countries by 1963; it was not approved for use in Canada or in the United States until 1977. Intralipid availability in Europe in the early 1960s led to increased use of PN through peripheral veins.

Widespread interest and increased use of PN occurred after publication of reports by Dudrick et al. (11). Using percutaneous central catheters to deliver nutrient solutions with glucose as the source of nonprotein calories, these investigators demonstrated convincingly that PN as the sole source of nutrients resulted in good growth in malnourished infants and positive nitrogen balance and nutritional and clinical improvement in malnourished adults over periods of many weeks.

Development of PN has been marked by replacement of hydrolyzed casein or blood fibrin by free amino acid mixtures and by the advent of safe lipid formulations and the availability of improved formulations of parenteral vitamins and trace elements (3, 10, 12, 13). Sophisticated pumps with programed metering controls have increased safety and simplified the care of these patients.

All parenteral solutions and emulsions are classified as drugs and must meet the standards of the United States Food and Drug Administration (FDA) for sterility, safety, and efficacy. Accordingly, these agents are appreciably more expensive than enteral products, with consequent limitations on development of new items or modifications of older ones. Nutrients of poor solubility or stability in aqueous solutions still present problems in formulations.

The major physiologic difference between parenteral and enteral products is the direct entry of parenteral solutions into the systemic circulation, bypassing the alimentary tract and the first circulatory pass through the liver by nutrients entering the portal vein. Other problems related to the parenteral route involve venous access, sterile and stable solutions, technique in administration, nutritional adequacy, and presence of an indwelling catheter in the vascular system.

NOMENCLATURE

Nutritional needs may be high (e.g., in the hypercatabolic patient) or relatively restricted (i.e., primarily water, electrolytes, and/or micronutrients). Various descriptive terms have been applied to the procedure used in supplying these requirements. The term *hyperalimentation* entered the clinical nutritional lexicon in various ways to indicate the need for large amounts of calories and certain other nutrients. Co Tui et al. used the term in 1944 and 1945 in describing large amounts of casein hydrolysate and carbohydrates given postoperatively by tube to patients who had undergone gastrectomy (14) and orally or by tube to patients with peptic ulcer (15). In 1965, the same term was used by others to describe supplementary intravenous lipid feeding given to cancer patients. (16). The term was reintroduced by the University of Pennsylvania group (11) to describe techniques for supplying total nutritional support by the intravenous route. *Hyperalimentation* became widely used in the context of high caloric formulation and was often shortened to *hyperal.* Because it was applied also to tube feeding, *intravenous hyperalimentation* and *enteral hyperalimentation* appeared in the literature.

Both historically and etymologically, the term *hyperalimentation* has implied needing and providing amounts of nutrients that exceeded normal requirements (particularly for energy and amino acids). It is now clear that used in this way, the term has a potentially misleading connotation because provision of excess energy and certain nutrients is often undesirable. For this reason, the term is little used now. It was replaced by the designation *total parenteral nutrition* (TPN) and more recently by the general designation of *parenteral nutrition* (PN), with appropriate qualifiers such as total or supplementary, central or peripheral, to designate amount and route.

INDICATIONS

The primary objective of PN is maintaining or improving the nutritional and metabolic status of patients who, for a critical period of time, cannot be adequately nourished by oral or tube feeding (Table 101.1). The value and use of this treatment method in the management of patients with specific clinical problems are discussed in this book and elsewhere: the short bowel syndromes (Chapter 68), other types of bowel dysfunction (Chapter 70), pediatric disorders (Chapter 64), cancer (Chapter 82), obstetric problems (17), neurologic injuries (18), and other hypermetabolic states, surgery, sepsis, and AIDS (Chapter 96). Use of PN in the perioperative period has been evaluated and is discussed further in Chapter 98 and elsewhere (20–22).

For those individuals who are well nourished or minimally malnourished before undergoing elective surgery and who are likely to be eating again in 5 to 7 days, adequate postoperative nutritional support usually consists of hypocaloric glucose, electrolytes, and micronutrients.

Table 101.1
Clinical States Likely to Benefit from Parenteral Nutrition

1. Malabsorptive syndromes (intestinal, renal tubular, or combined) with severe food, electrolyte and fluid losses not adequately managed by oral or enteral nutrition
   a. Severe short bowel syndrome
   b. Those induced by infection, inflammatory, and immunologic disorders, drugs, or radiation
   c. High-output gastrointestinal fistulas unable to be bypassed by enteral intubation
   d. Severe renal tubular defects with large fluid and ion losses
2. Motility disorders
   a. Persistent ileus (postoperative or disease related)
   b. Severe intestinal pseudoobstruction
   c. Severe persistent vomiting induced by medication, brain tumor, or other disease (e.g., hyperemesis gravidarum)
3. Mechanical intestinal obstruction not immediately remediable by surgery
4. Perioperative state with severe undernutrition
5. Critically ill patients, especially those with hypermetabolism, when enteral nutrition is contraindicated or has failed
6. Very low birth weight premature infants when enteral feeding is inappropriate

Preexisting serious undernutrition, however, increases the likelihood of postoperative complications, especially with major surgery (Chapter 98) (20–22).

The decision to undertake PN requires weighing various factors and considering the patient's diagnosis and prognosis as discussed in appropriate chapters. It is not a defensible substitute for oral or tube feeding when adequate provision by either of these methods is feasible. Issues related to its use in the hopelessly ill are reviewed in Chapter 102.

The conditions for PN listed in Table 101.1 are widely accepted as noncontroversial indications. However, its use in a variety of other conditions listed in the chapters enumerated above is often controversial, because of the paucity of appropriate studies that give statistically valid data supporting or negating the value of PN. The many reasons for the lack of information to serve as acceptable clinical guidelines have been discussed often and recently (Chapter 98, [23]). They include the variability of severity of disease, level of malnutrition in patients, complication rates, varying medication schedules, and other interventions, as well as differences in quality of management and protocol. The variable and changing healthcare system and payment practices have added to the pressures to justify use of PN. Answers will not be found easily or quickly. The purpose of this chapter is to help ensure that when PN is used, it will be done well, by considering the many aspects of this complex and potentially lifesaving procedure, including its potential for serious complications (Chapter 98, [23]).

VENOUS ACCESS: PERIPHERAL AND CENTRAL

Infusion of nutrient solution directly into a peripheral vein has an advantage over central infusion in avoiding insertion and maintenance of a central catheter. Peripheral parenteral nutrition (PPN) with a short cannula reduces peripheral vein damage by substituting 10 or 20% isotonic lipid emulsions with their large caloric content for the hypertonic glucose solutions used in central PN. For example, a preparation composed of 1 L each of 6% amino acids, 10% lipid, and 18% dextrose provides 9 g of nitrogen and 1620 nonprotein calories, with an osmolality of 680 mosm/L (24). Infusion for 8 hours, cannula removal, and using the opposite arm the next day, minimized thrombophlebitis (24). Such PPN may be useful (although the restricted carbohydrate may present some problems) for the patient who needs nutritional support for 5 to 10 days and has ample patent peripheral vessels. Many patients requiring intravenous nutrition have had numerous prior peripheral infusions and venesections, with consequent vessel sclerosis. Critically ill patients whose condition is unstable must have reliable venous access at all times, and a central catheter is a necessity.

Providing sufficient energy by the central route without providing a large percentage as lipid necessitates infusing hypertonic glucose solutions. Consequently, the catheter tip must be in a vessel with high blood flow causing rapid dilution; this minimizes the occurrence of phlebitis and thrombosis. Numerous routes for such vascular access have been used (Table 101.2) (25–36). Popularized by Dudrick et al., the percutaneous subclavian vein approach in adults and the jugular approach in infants were widely adopted (10, 11, 26). Arteriovenous fistulas of the internal type have been prepared, usually with a bovine graft, and external fistulas have been used; some of the early patients discharged home on PN had one or another of these fistulas. Other vascular approaches have been adopted when the usual vessels were not patent or were otherwise unavailable.

Occasionally, peripherally inserted central catheters (PICC lines) are used for long-term PN. If these types of catheters are used for PN, the tip of the catheter *must* be positioned in a central vein such as the superior or inferior vena cava. Kearns et al. have reported a significantly higher incidence of thrombosis and infection and decreased catheter survival when the tip of a PICC resided in the axillosubclavian-innominate vein compared with use of the superior vena cava (25).

Table 101.2
Vascular Access Routes for Parenteral Nutrition

Route	Reference
Peripheral vein: percutaneous approach	24, 25
Jugular vein (internal or external): percutaneous approach	26
Jugular vein (internal or external): surgical approach[a]	*27*
Subclavian vein or tributary: percutaneous approach	26
Subclavian vein or tributary: surgical approach[a,b]	28
Portal vein	29
Arteriovenous fistulas	
Internal	30, 31
External	32
Femoral or iliac vein	
Azygos vein (via right thoracotomy)	33
Common facial vein	27
Inferior epigastric vein	34
Saphenous vein	35
Right atrium	36

[a]Used in placement of tunneled catheter.
[b]Used in placement of tunneled or subcutaneous port.

In an effort to reduce the incidence of infection, tunneled central catheters were introduced in 1973. These are usually placed surgically within the subclavian or jugular vein, with the tip in the superior vena cava. The extravascular portion of the catheter is tunneled under the skin for a variable distance before being taken through the skin. The catheter is often anchored at the skin exit with a Dacron cuff to eliminate the need for sutures in the skin. More recently, subcutaneously placed chambers of silicone or other elastomer, termed *ports,* have been developed; the chamber is connected by a catheter, usually placed into the subclavian vein with its tip in the superior vena cava (35). Nutrient solution is infused into the chamber via special needles inserted through the skin.

Insertion and use of an indwelling central venous catheter pose various risks to the patient, including pneumothorax, hemothorax, hematuria, aneurysms, venous or nerve injury, hypersensitivity-like reactions, and microbial contamination. Reported complication rates range from 0.3 to 12%, according to different definitions and physician expertise (38). Thrombogenicity varies with the catheter material; the earlier and stiffer polyvinyl and polyethylene catheters were associated with more thrombus formation than silicone or polyurethane elastomers. Multilumen catheters have increased in use that provide additional access for infusing medications and blood and for blood sampling without interfering with PN administration. There are conflicting reports about the relative amount of catheter-related sepsis (39, 40). Placement site is related to infection rates; e.g., femoral and jugular sites tend to have higher rates than the subclavian site (40). Similarly, catheter tunneling (e.g., jugular) reduces percutaneous cannulation sepsis (41) and also reduces other problems such as dislodgement.

Complications tend be less frequent when experienced surgical and other personnel (preferably members of a clinical nutritional team) exercise necessary precautions, including using aseptic technique in catheter insertion and maintenance, checking proper placement by x-ray study before use, and adequately caring for the insertion site. Recommendations for infection control in association with PN have been published (42, 43).

Ultrasound, recommended as a means of determining vein position and/or catheter placement, was evaluated by comparing ultrasound-guided location of the subclavian vein by marking the site before the attempt with standard insertion procedures. The two methods did not differ in catheterization failures or complication rates (9.7%). Complications increased with failed attempts: 28% with placement failure versus 7.2% with successful placement. The complication rate increased from 4.3% with one-pass failure to 24.0% with more than two passes. Realtime ultrasound guidance during actual placement and/or placement only by very experienced physicians would presumably reduce such complications (38).

In general, a diagnosis of bacteremia or fungemia with the possibility of catheter colonization should be seriously considered when the patient experiences sudden spiking fever and/or shaking chills. A sustained fever is more likely to be related to an abscess somewhere, often without catheter colonization. With onset of fever, sources of infection should be sought, and material taken from both the catheter and a peripheral vein for appropriate culture. Appropriate antibiotic treatment should be instituted as indicated.

When microbial colonization is suspected in a percutaneously placed catheter, a modified Seldinger technique may be useful. This involves rapid replacement of a central catheter over a flexible wire using appropriate sterile technique without another venipuncture (44, 45). The tip and/or subcutaneous portion of the removed catheter should be cultured in addition to other relevant cultures. The modified Seldinger technique greatly reduces the need for further venipunctures and possible complications and is particularly valuable for the patient considered a candidate for long-term PN, for whom continued vascular access is critical. Most catheters removed on suspicion of sepsis are found to be sterile. When an endoluminal brush is used to sample the catheter, the acridine orange leukocyte cytospin test may be useful for detecting infected catheters in situ (46).

Experience indicates that with good technique in both catheter placement and solution preparation and with proper maintenance, indwelling catheters of the percutaneous or tunneled type may remain safely in place for months and years without infection or disruption (47, 48). Several comprehensive reports have been published regarding the catheter-related sepsis rate in patients who have long-term catheters for intravenous access. Buchman et al. reported on 527 patients receiving home PN (HPN) who were followed for a median time of 206 days (range, 7–6344 days) (49). Some 81% of the adults and 3% of the children were never infected. Thirty-six of these patients were infection free for more than 10 years. The catheter-related sepsis rate was 0.37/patient-year for all patients and 0.51/patient-year for children. Patients having catheters for more than 10 years had a catheter-related sepsis rate of 0.28/patient-year (49). Risk factors for sepsis were Crohn's disease, presence of jejunostomy, smoking, and central vein thrombosis (50).

Randomized large-scale hospital trials comparing standard central catheters with those either impregnated with chlorhexidine and silver sulfadiazine (50a) or with minocycline and rifampin (50b) found that the antiseptic or antibiotic-treated catheters significantly reduced the rates of catheter colonization and bloodstream infection with no apparent side effects.

The use of subcutaneously placed ports has been increasing, presumably on the assumption that the risk of infection is reduced during the 8 to 16 hours of infusion by having a fine needle as the only external vascular access. No controlled comparative data are available for comparison of this technique with other types of catheters. These devices are expensive and are not without infection and maintenance problems.

The designation "fibrin sheath" for the thin, white, adherent covering on chronically implanted catheters is incorrect. At this stage, the coating is vascularized fibrous connective tissue not likely to be dissolved by fibrinolytic agents such as urokinase, streptokinase, or tissue plasminogen activator (51).

DELIVERY SYSTEMS

Nutrient solutions for PN are usually delivered from bottles or plastic bags via electronic pumps without drop counters. Central PN solutions are generally delivered using peristaltic pumps of various types. These have become increasingly sophisticated, automated, and expensive. They ensure even flow rates, overcome the increased resistance of filters of small porosity (especially with continued use), minimize the likelihood of clotting at the catheter tip, and reduce the need for frequent nursing surveillance.

There has been a resurgence in the use of filters, especially after the two deaths reported from improper admixing of calcium and phosphorus into a total nutrient admixture (52). Many practitioners are now using 0.22-μm filters for patients receiving 2-in-1 PN solutions (dextrose + amino acids), and 1.2- or 5-μm filters for those receiving total nutrient admixtures (53).

The use of pliable plastic bags of various sizes eliminates the danger of breakage, simplifies transportation and storage, and reduces storage space requirements before and after filling, compared with use of glass or formed-plastic bottles. The usual water solutions of nutrient formulations do not extract measurable amounts of phthalate plasticizer used in the manufacture of polyvinyl chloride (PVC) bags; however, albumin, lipids, and blood take up the plasticizer (54). The amount of plasticizer eluted from PVC administration sets by lipid emulsions is relatively small compared with that from the bags. Plasticizer-free ethylene vinyl acetate tubing and bags are available. Another elastomer contains the plasticizer trioctyl trimellitate, which is not extracted by lipid. These are useful with certain lipid formulas.

Dual-chambered plastic bags have been marketed (55) that allow admixture of macronutrients immediately before infusion of PN admixtures. These are very convenient for HPN, especially for patients who receive intravenous lipid on a regular basis. Dual-chambered bags are manufactured either empty or with the macronutrients in them (i.e., dextrose in one chamber and amino acids in the other chamber). When lipid is used, the dextrose, amino acids, and electrolytes are added to the bottom chamber of the empty bag and the desired intravenous lipid dose to the upper chamber. This increases stability, because the total nutrient admixture is not prepared until just before infusion.

Insulin adsorption varies appreciably, depending on the binding characteristics of the nutrients present, the type of plastic in the delivery system, the presence of filters, and the concentration of insulin added (56). When insulin is added to parenteral solutions for diabetic patients, the dosage must be closely monitored until properly adjusted (56, 57). An in vitro study simulating the clinical setting showed that 90% of regular insulin added to admixtures with and without lipid was available after infusion through tubing (58). This requires confirmation.

Because of adherence and loss of vitamins A and E (particularly the former) when solutions are infused very slowly to very low birth weight infants, a delivery system using minimal tubing and more rapid infusion has been recommended (59).

PARENTERAL COMPONENTS AND REQUIREMENTS

General Requirements

The weight of a relatively unstressed middle-aged patient with restricted activity, who has no fever or other hypermetabolic condition, should be maintained in an acceptable range by approximately 30 kcal (7.2 kJ) per kg of body weight per day. A ratio of grams of nitrogen to kilocalories (N:kcal) of approximately 1:130 to 150 (1:31–36 N/kJ) is an appropriate formula for such a patient (60). Malnourished nonhypercatabolic adults can be placed in positive nitrogen balance on a caloric intake of approximately 1.3 times resting energy expenditure (REE) or 29 kcal/kg while receiving PN supplying 1.13 g of amino acids/kg (180 mg N/kg) per day (61). When twice this amount of amino acids per kilogram was given, nitrogen retention was better; such patients appear to behave like growing children in this respect. More calories are required for weight gain, depending on the weight gain desired. Shaw et al. developed a graphic presentation of the effects of nitrogen and energy intakes on nitrogen and fat balance in depleted patients (61). The amount of additional protein needed is usually proportionally higher than that of energy; e.g., for adult patients acutely stressed by trauma, burns, or infection, the N:kcal ratio is generally increased (1:100) (Chapter 98), with such patients receiving as much as 40 to 45 total kcal/kg or occasionally more. Care must be taken not to exceed caloric expenditure. The goals for infants and children are reviewed in Chapter 64.

All essential and sufficient nonessential amino acids should be provided in amounts needed to sustain adequate protein synthesis and intermediary metabolism. Essential fatty acids should be supplied regularly. Macromineral, trace element, and vitamin intakes should meet individual requirements without excessive wastage or toxicity. No matter how adequate the formula is in other respects, a deficiency of any essential nutrient may lead to negative balance in nitrogen and other nutrients. A single deficiency of either potassium, sodium, phosphate, or nitrogen impaired or abolished retention of other elements (63), and zinc depletion also caused negative nitrogen balance (64).

Water

The fluid component must meet individual needs and avoid the twin dangers of over- and underhydration in patients who may have difficulty in excreting or retaining needed water. The close interrelationships of water, electrolytes, hormonal factors, and the kidney are considered in Chapter 6. Proper management of fluid and electrolyte status is a most important aspect of nutritional support. In addition, clinical factors that could cause excessive retention or loss, consideration must be given to fluid intake with medications and "keep-vein-open" infusions, as well as changes in insensible water loss. As noted in Table 101.3, formation of sodium-free water from the metabolism of nutrients may add a volume of approximately 18%. Daily weighing and meticulous recording of intakes and outputs are mandatory.

Standard PN admixtures can be administered to the patient with increased fluid needs, especially when extrarenal losses are involved, with a supplemental intravenous solution to meet needs in the acute care setting. In the home setting, the extra intravenous solution can be added to the PN admixture in one plastic bag, in most situations. For the patient who is fluid overloaded, the PN prescription should use the most concentrated macronu-

Table 101.3
Water Formed in the Metabolism of Tissue and Calorie Sources

Sources	Amount
Muscle	1 g yields 0.85 mL (0.1 mL from protein + 0.75 mL cellular water)
Mixed tissue	100 kcal yields 10 mL
Fat	1 g yields 1.0 mL
Protein	1 g yields 0.4 mL
Glucose	1 g yields 0.64 mL
Glucose · H_2O	1 g yields 0.60 mL
Mixed diet	100 kcal yields 20 mL
Example: high-glucose PN solution	
750 mL 10% amino acids	300 kcal yields 30 mL H_2O
1175 mL 50% glucose/water	2000 kcal yields 353 mL H_2O
143 mL 10% lipid	157 kcal yields 14 mL H_2O
Total: 2068 mL	2457 kcal yields 397 mL H_2O
Example: glucose-lipid PN solution	
750 mL 10% amino acids	300 kcal yields 30 mL H_2O
750 mL 50% glucose/water	1275 kcal yields 225 mL H_2O
500 mL 20% lipid	1000 kcal yields 100 mL H_2O
Total: 2000 mL	2575 kcal yields 355 mL H_2O

trients (D70W, amino acids 15%, and intravenous lipid 30%) to minimize intake.

Expansion of extracellular fluid (ECF) is common in hospitalized patients with malnutrition, and this increases body weight and decreases serum albumin levels. Starker et al. described different patterns of change in body weight and serum albumin in various clinical situations during the first week of PN (65). Severe malnutrition and inflammatory processes are associated with sodium and fluid retention in the early period of nutritional rehabilitation.

Carbohydrates

Glucose is the commonly used carbohydrate for caloric replacement in PN and is usually the major source of energy. Parenteral glucose is in the form of the monohydrate, with 1 g providing about 3.4 kcal. It is readily available in various concentrations in liquid form, is relatively inexpensive, and is rapidly metabolized by most patients. Using primarily glucose to meet large energy needs within a tolerable fluid volume requires an extremely hypertonic solution (Table 101.4).

Other carbohydrates given intravenously are metabolized wholly or in part. Fructose is converted to glucose in the liver and requires insulin for use of the formed glucose. Use of even small amounts of exogenous fructose is seriously impaired in hypoinsulinemic conditions (66). Fructose given in large quantities increases serum lactate, urate, and bilirubin and depresses hepatic adenosine triphosphate (ATP) and serum phosphate concentrations (67). It has a low renal threshold, with resultant urinary loss when given in high concentration. Sorbitol, a hexose hydroxyalcohol, is used in some countries other than the United States; it is converted to fructose. Xylitol is a pentose hydroxyalcohol that bypasses insulin-dependent glucose pathways (68); like sorbitol, it is not available in the United States. Neither intravenous maltose (69) nor oligosaccharide (70) is hydrolyzed sufficiently to be useful as a source of carbohydrate energy in PN. A solution containing 3% glycerol, amino acids (3%), and electrolytes (Procalamine, McGaw) is available for use in PPN. The glycerol is a good energy source in traumatized patients when it is given with 10% lipid (71). Compared with glucose, glycerol required only about half the amount of insulin to maintain the glycemia of diabetics in the range of 150 to 200 mg/dL (72).

Table 101.4
Osmolalities and Energy Values of Intravenous Glucose and Lipid Preparations

Solution	Percentage (%)	mosm/kg H_2O^a	kcal/L
Glucose[b]	5	278	170
Glucose	10	523	340
Glucose	20	1250	680
Glucose	30	1569	1020
Glucose	40	2092	1360
Glucose	50	2615	1700
Glucose	70	3660	2330
Lipid[c]	10	280	1100
Lipid	20	330	2000
Lipid	30	330	3000

[a]Plasma, 290; 0.9% NaCl, 308 mosm/kg H_2O.
[b]Monohydrate form.
[c]Intravenous lipid contains glycerol adding approximately 100 kcal/L.

Glucose Metabolism and Hormonal Changes

Adaptation to increasing loads of parenteral glucose and other nutrients decreased as the duration of infusion was shortened in test subjects who were relatively stable adults being prepared for or already receiving HPN (73) (Fig. 101.1). Glucose and various hormone concentrations were measured in the course of 24-, 17-, and 12-h infusions of the same PN formulas and volumes and during the postinfusion period. Tapering the 24- and 17-hour infusions resulted in a fall of glucose to fasting levels in less than 30 minutes, together with a decline in insulin. No significant changes in glucagon, cortisol, or growth hormone were noted. With the 12-hour infusion, one of the five patients developed marked hyperglycemia, hyperinsulinemia, hyperglucagonemia, and increased growth hormone and cortisol levels; the elevated hormone levels persisted into and beyond the tapering period. Because such patients are not uncommon, tolerance to glucose must be checked before large amounts are infused in cyclic fashion. Other studies in adults found that abrupt termination of PN was rarely associated with significant hypoglycemia or its symptoms (74, 75). The literature on the effects of abrupt termination in young children is contradictory, but symptoms (when they occurred) were mild (reviewed in [76]), perhaps because the children remained in bed for a time following termination. Sudden increases or decreases in glucose infusion can be averted by the use of infusion pumps that can gradually increase infusion of the admixture and taper it automatically, without changing the pump settings.

Altered Substrate Metabolism in Hypercatabolic Patients

Glucose metabolism in patients with trauma, injury, burns, and sepsis or advanced cancer that induces weight loss differs markedly from that of normal individuals. This is discussed in some detail in Chapters 82, 96, and 98 and elsewhere (77–79), and some aspects that relate directly to PN use are summarized here.

The reasonably stable patient can oxidize infused glucose to CO_2 efficiently up to approximately 14 mg/kg/min, whereas the critically ill patient has only about half that capacity: 5 mg/kg/min in burn patients and 6 to 7 mg/kg/min in postoperative patients. Infusion above the limiting rate results in conversion of glucose to fat, with a rise in energy expenditure and a rise above 1.0 in the respiratory quotient (RQ). Conversion of excess glucose to fat is energy dependent; after oxidation of the resultant fat, the derived energy (as ATP sources) is 30% of that the-

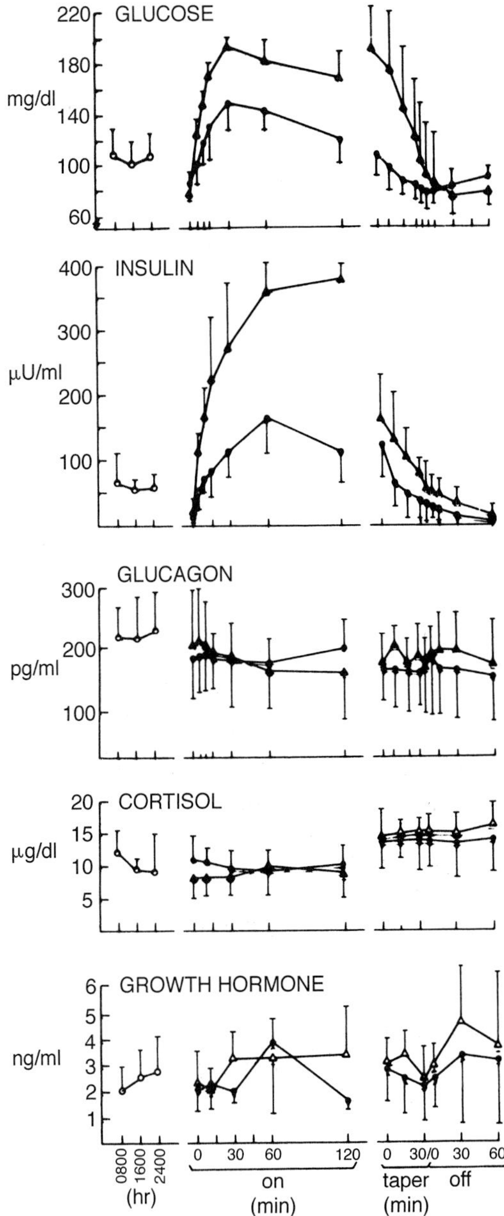

Figure 101.1. Responses of glucose, insulin, glucagon, cortisol, and growth hormone to infusions of TPN solution in the same five adapted patients over 24 hours *(open circles)*, 17 hours *(closed circles)*, and 12 hours *(open triangles)* and over a 30-min period during which the infusions were tapered and stopped and over the first 60 min following cessation of infusion. Mean ± SEM is depicted for all 5 patients at 24 and 17 hours and for 4 patients at 12 hours. (Reprinted from Byrne WJ, Lippe BM, Strobel CT, et al. Gastroenterology 1981;80:947–56, with permission.)

oretically obtained by direct oxidation of the converted glucose (80). Other potentially detrimental effects of providing glucose in excess exist. Wolfe et al. have calculated that at an infusion rate of 9 mg/kg/min into the stressed patient, 206 g/day of triglyceride were synthesized in the liver. Only a small fraction of newly synthesized fat would have to remain in the liver for fatty liver to develop (77). Other undesirable effects of excess glucose relate to the risk of hyperglycemia and glycosuria, with resultant water and sodium losses and, particularly in the dehydrated and infected diabetic patient, the danger of hyperosmolar nonketotic coma.

The value of pharmacologic treatment to normalize the elevated rate of glucose production in severely hypermetabolic patients (e.g., burns) has been questioned. Lowering glucagon had no effect, and somatostatin infusion was not justified because of effort and cost, but exogenous insulin was beneficial in controlling hyperglycemia and increasing the anabolic response in muscle (79).

Elwyn et al. demonstrated that malnourished individuals had no increase in REE with increasing glucose intake in amounts below those needed for energy equilibrium; however, with excess glucose, REE increased by 1 kcal for each 5 kcal of intake in association with fat deposition and rise in RQ above 1.0 (81). In contrast, the injured and/or septic patient given a large amount of glucose with lipid-free PN exhibited major increases in both resting CO_2 production and O_2 consumption; however, the nonprotein RQ remained below 1.0 (82). This finding is compatible with other evidence indicating that some fat oxidation persists despite a glucose intake that normally abolishes fat oxidation (77).

Differences in energy expenditure were apparent when surgical patients receiving a high-glucose PN formula were compared with those receiving an isocaloric glucose-fat formula with 69% of nonnitrogen calories as fat. When the high-glucose formula was given at an infusion rate that provided carbohydrate at 4 mg/kg/min, the energy increase was 11% of the mean daily energy intake and 21% of the mean REE; those receiving the glucose-fat formula had increases of 3 and 7%, respectively (83).

As would be expected from the absence of lipids and their phospholipids, PN solutions with glucose as the nonnitrogen energy source have been associated with low serum cholesterol and triglyceride levels (see below). A 26% increase occurred in the fractional catabolic rate of low-density lipoprotein (LDL) with an associated reduction of plasma cholesterol levels through changes in both LDL and high-density lipoprotein (HDL) (84).

The diabetic patient who has been on insulin prehospitalization and is to be placed on PN presents a special problem in glucose control. A tested procedure for estimating insulin requirement has been published (85).

Ventilatory Response to Glucose

When malnourished individuals were given glucose infusion in amounts exceeding the REE, with resultant lipogenesis, minute ventilation at rest increased by about 32%; it increased appreciably more in hypermetabolic patients who had an elevated resting ventilation before PN (86). In patients with decreased sensitivity to CO_2 or those with compromised lung function or who are already hyperventilating, the added ventilatory stimulus of high-glucose PN may aggravate preexisting pulmonary dysfunction. This is discussed in detail in Chapter 90.

Lipids

Composition

Lipid emulsions consist of tiny droplets (≤0.5 μm) with triglyceride as the core and cholesterol derived from egg yolk phosphatides surrounded by a solubilizing and stabilizing surface layer of the emulsifying phospholipids. Several intravenous lipid preparations are available as 10, 20, and 30% concentrations that serve as a source of calories and essential fatty acids (EFA) (Table 101.5).

The cholesterol content per liter of Intralipid is appreciably higher than that of Liposyn II and III, presumably because of the phosphatide used. Per kilocalorie, the 20% emulsion has only half and the 30% only one-third, as much cholesterol as the 10% preparation. The rise in serum cholesterol concentration after a single infusion of lipid emulsion is transient and usually reverts to near preinfusion concentrations within 4 to 6 hours. As noted below, however, more-frequent use of lipid infusions is associated with elevated plasma phospholipid and free cholesterol levels.

Glycerin (glycerol) makes the emulsions isotonic and is also a carbohydrate source. The isotonicity and tolerance of the endothelium of small vessels for the intravenous lipid preparation permit peripheral infusion of a large number of calories. The 2000 kcal in 1 L of 20% lipid emulsion is the caloric equivalent of 1 L of 59% glucose solution, and the 3000 kcal in 1 L of 30% lipid is that of 1 L of 88% glucose solution. In the United States, the 30% intravenous lipid emulsion can only be used as part of a total nutrient admixture; in Europe, it can be directly infused into patients.

As noted in Table 101.5, Intralipid and Liposyn III contain more linolenic acid (C18:3,n-3) than Liposyn II because of soy oil, whereas Liposyn II has more linoleic acid (C18:2,n-6) because of incorporation of safflower oil. The nutritional role of these EFAs and their metabolism and requirements are discussed in Chapter 4 and elsewhere in this book. EFA deficiency is prevented by average daily provision of about 3.2% of total calories as highly unsaturated intravenous fat in adults (87). Requirements for infants and children are noted below in this discussion and reviewed in Chapter 64. Newer lipid formulations under clinical study are reviewed below.

Metabolism

Although the particle sizes of lipid emulsions are within the range of those of chylomicrons, significant differences exist between the two types of particles (88). In emulsions, phospholipids (PLs) are in excess; some serve as surface emulsifiers of the triglycerides (TGs) and the rest is present as liposomes (89). The latter take up from the circulation free cholesterol, various lipoproteins (in particular apoliproprotein E (apoE) and albumin (90) to yield the abnormal lipoprotein X (LpX) (91).

On short-term ultracentrifugation in saline, two-thirds of the PLs separate from TGs in 10% Intralipid, whereas only one-third separated in the 20% emulsion. The former would contribute four times the amount of liposomal LpX of the 20% emulsion when expressed per gram of TG. The significance of this difference is illustrated by a study in which 1.75 g/kg/day of long-chain TGs was infused into postoperative patients as one of two 10% emulsions with

Table 101.5
Comparison of Parenteral Lipid Emulsion Fat Sources

	Soybean Oil					Soybean Plus Safflower Oil (Equal Parts)	
	Intralipid[a]			Liposyn III[b]		Liposyn II[b]	
Total fat (%)	10	20	30	10	20	10	20
kcal/mL	1.1	2	3	1.1	2	1.1	2
Glycerin (%)	2.25			2.5		2.5	
Egg phosphatides (%)	1.2			1.2		1.2	
Linoleic acid (%)[c]	49[d]			55		66	
Oleic acid (%)	21[d]					18	
Palmitic acid (%)	11[d]					9	
Linolenic acid (%)	6.5[d]			8.3		4	
Cholesterol (mg/L)	250–300			19–21		13–22	
Phosphorus (mg/L)	150–200			267–500		267–500	
mosm/L	300			284–292		260–280	
pH	8			8.3		8.3	8.0
α-tocopherol mg/L[e]	8–12	16–24	24–36	8–12	16–24		
Vitamin K μg/L[f]	308	680				132	270

[a]Baxter, Deerfield, IL.
[b]Abbott Laboratories, Abbott Park, IL.
[c]As percentage of total fatty acid.
[d]Data from Ito Y, Hudgens LC, Hirsch J, et al. Am J Clin Nutr 1991;53:1487–92.
[e]Tocopherol isomer data (mg/L of 10% soybean lipid): (*a*) alpha = 7.7, delta = 38.3, alpha and beta = 51.1 (Gutscher et al. J Parenter Enteral Nutr 1984;8:269–73 (*b*) alpha = 12, gamma = 92, delta = 44 (Steephen et al. JPEN J Parenter Enteral Nutr 1991;15:647–52. See also Chapter 19 for discussion of relative isomer antioxidant activities.
[f]Data from Lennon, et al. JPEN J Parenter Enteral Nutr 1993;17:142–4.

PL:TG ratios of either 0.12 or 0.06. Over an infusion period of 5 days, plasma PL, free cholesterol and apoE levels increased progressively only when the PL:TG ratio was 0.06. Free fatty acids (FFAs) and TGs remained constant with all formulations (92).

The LpX level is appreciably higher in the plasma of patients receiving 10% Intralipid than in those receiving 20% Intralipid, presumably because of the higher PL content per kilocalories infused in the 10% preparation. The half-life of LpX appears to be 2 to 4 days, with small amounts still present 7 days after termination of the lipid infusion (93). Excess PL induces alterations of plasma lipids even in a few days; use of lipid emulsions with a PL:TG weight ratio of 0.06 is preferable (i.e., 20% or 30%).

Tolerance

When the concentration of lipid increases to the level at which binding sites on lipoprotein lipase (LPL) are saturated, a maximum elimination capacity has been reached. In normal adults, this maximum rate is about 3.8 g of fat/kg/24 hours, which corresponds to about 35 kcal/kg/24 hours. It increases in starvation (approximately 50%) and even more in trauma (94).

Daily infusion of fat emulsion over a week or more is associated with increased tolerance, as indicated by decreased preinfusion serum TGs. Serum FFAs are cleared more rapidly with simultaneously administered carbohydrate. The clearance rate from plasma is not equivalent to the oxidative rate of lipid.

Effect of Lipid Infusion with PN

When lipid (supplying one-third of the calories) is infused for approximately 8 hours, together with a glucose-based PN formula given over 24 hours, fat oxidation is approximately 6 kcal/kg/min; it falls to about 3 kcal/kg/min after cessation of lipid. A PN formula with glucose and no lipid is associated with a fat oxidation rate of about 2 kcal/kg/min, decreasing to approximately 0 by the end of 24 hours (95).

Hypermetabolic patients with sepsis and/or trauma in the basal state have increased rates of lipolysis, as indicated by higher glycerol flux and fat oxidation than in normal individuals (e.g., 5.3 vs. 2.2 μmol/kg/min and 2 versus 1 mg/kg/min, respectively) (78, 96). In patients with sepsis who were given PN with lipid, most of the fat oxidized was from endogenous fat stores rather than from infused cleared lipid (96).

Nonnitrogen Caloric Sources and Nitrogen Retention

Solid evidence exists for the nitrogen-sparing effect of carbohydrate (including glycerol), with and without amino acids (see Chapters 2 and 41). In the absence of amino acids, fat appears not to spare nitrogen beyond its glycerol content released on hydrolysis and its metabolism as a carbohydrate precursor. At low energy intakes, the effects of carbohydrate on nitrogen balance are much greater than those of fat. Increasing amounts of carbohydrate from 0 up to about 100 to 150 g intake (400 to 600 kcal) increase nitrogen balance by approximately 7.5 mg of N per added kcal (1.8 mg N/kJ). This effect is not shared by fat. Above this amount, however, the effect of added carbohydrate on increased nitrogen balance is only about 1.5 mg N per added kcal; this effect is thought to be shared by fat (97).

Investigators have disagreed on the nitrogen-sparing effect of fat in the presence of amino acids in hypercatabolic subjects. Long et al. were unable to achieve nitrogen equilibrium or positive balance when fat was supplied as the nonnitrogen energy source in burn or trauma patients. Calories from carbohydrate were required in an amount equal to the resting metabolic rate to achieve maximum nitrogen retention (98). A review of nitrogen balance studies in patients with various inflammatory diseases, however, indicated that fat and carbohydrate were comparable in promoting nitrogen balance (99), presumably after the minimum of 100 g glucose had been met (97).

Total Nutrient Admixture

Use of lipid emulsions has increased as their cost has decreased and their clinical efficacy has been appreciated. They have been infused by piggybacking the tubing from the separate emulsion container into the tubing from the water-based PN solution. Admixtures of amino acids, dextrose, minerals, vitamins, and a fat emulsion are also used frequently; these are designated total nutrient admixture (TNA) or triple mix.

Stability and Safety Factor. The admixture system is potentially unstable. The relevant properties of the phosphatide emulsifiers and various factors influencing stability of the fat emulsions in the presence of various additives in the admixture have been reviewed (100–103). The cumulative effects on aggregation of various cations of different charge can be predicted from an equation defining the critical aggregation number (CAN) at and above which neutralization of anionic surface groups results in lipid particle aggregation.

Driscoll et al. found that iron dextran was the most disruptive component of TNAs (102). They studied the effects of many additives, including amino acids, lipids, dextrose, and mono-, di-, and trivalent ions. TNAs were assessed for stability by particle-size analysis, done by light obscuration and dynamic light-scattering methods. Based on these results, using more sophisticated analysis, addition of any iron dextran to a TNA is discouraged.

Microbial Growth. Less microbial growth over 24 hours occurs in TNAs than in fat emulsions per se (103). This finding led the Centers for Disease Control of the United States Public Health Service to recommend a 12-hour maximal infusion time for fat emulsions not in TNAs (104). The major advantages and disadvantages of the TNA system are listed in Table 101.6.

Catheter Occlusion

Various investigators have reported blockage of catheters in patients receiving TNA for periods of 37 to 206 days, with deposition of a soft, creamy material on the internal catheter surface (105). Such material obtained after filtration (5-μm filter) of a specific TNA formulation stored for 7 days at 4°C in four different commercial EVA bags averaged 99.4% fat and less than 0.5% mineral salts (105). Of concern was finding plasticizer particles (means of 2,890 to 16,204 from different bags) with a size range of 1.4 to 43.8 μm that had been flushed out of the bags with saline before adding the TNA solution. As indicated above, filters are advised with such solutions (53). Sterile 70% ethanol has been used successfully by some investigators to unclog catheters that were occluded with fat from a TNA (106, 107). In fact, if urokinase is unsuccessful, ethanol should be used to attempt to clear the catheter, especially in patients who have been receiving TNAs.

Complications of Lipid Infusions

Because the ability to metabolize these emulsions is related directly to infant maturity, the risk of lipid accumulation in blood and its sequelae is greatest in the premature infant, the small-for-age gestational low-birthweight (LBW) infant, and the nutritionally depleted older child (see Chapter 64).

Possible Altered Pulmonary Function. Lipid accumulation in the hepatic reticuloendothelial system (RES) with the likelihood of depressed immune responses and its competition with bilirubin and other substances for albumin binding have been described. Cases have been reported, primarily in young children, of bleeding dyscrasia in association with high plasma lipid levels and platelets engorged with lipid (108). Reports of altered pulmonary function during acute hyperlipidemia have varied; whereas decreased pulmonary diffusion capacity has been noted by some (109); other investigators have found no change in lung dynamics, but rather, decreased arterial oxygenation (110). Still others have not found oxygen impairment in neonates with hyperlipidemia (94) or in healthy men (111). Patients with acute respiratory distress syndrome who received 500 mL of 20% intravenous fat emulsion over 8 hours (maximum rate suggested in package inserts) demonstrated a significant decrease in PaO_2/FiO_2 and mean pulmonary arterial pressure and a significant increase in pulmonary vascular resistance and pulmonary venous admixture (112). Intravenous lipid emulsions should be administered cautiously to patients with adult respiratory distress syndrome and at lower doses infused over longer periods of time than those noted above by Venus et al. (112). While recognizing the toxic potential of lipid infusions in infants, biochemical evidence of EFA deficiency occurred in more than half of premature infants at 7 days of age (113). A progressive program of lipid infusion for such infants has been described (113).

Fat Overload Syndrome. The fat overload syndrome, a rare complication of intravenous administration of fat, is characterized by sudden elevation of serum TGs in association with fever, hepatosplenomegaly, coagulopathy, and variable end-organ dysfunction. Fat sludging occurs within the microvasculature in spleen, liver, kidney, lungs, and brain. Plasma exchange benefited one patient who did not respond to conservative medical therapy (114).

Various fat emulsions given intravenously are known to elicit lipid particles and deposition of a ceroid pigment in the RES of the bone marrow, lymph nodes, and spleen, and the Kupffer cells and hepatocytes of the liver of adults, children, and laboratory animals (115, 116). To date, no deleterious effect of these histologic changes on hepatic function has been discovered.

Effects on Immunity. The increased uptake of long-chain lipids by the RES in patients with hepatosplenomegaly and decreased clearance of lipid have led to concern about possible depression of immune responses with such infusions and increased susceptibility to infection. Mice injected with streptococci demonstrated higher mortality rates and incidence of bacteremia and decreased neutrophil chemotaxis when Intralipid was given (115). In healthy and in burned guinea pigs, intravenous long-chain triglyceride (LCT) infusion at 75% or more of total nonprotein calories resulted in RES overload and an altered pattern of intravenously administered pseudomonas

Table 101.6
Advantages and Disadvantages of the Total Nutrient Admixture (TNA) System

Advantages
1. Decreased nursing personnel time and subsequent cost savings because of simplified administration
2. Increased compliance in home patients because of ease of administration
3. Decreased training time for home patients requiring daily lipid emulsion
4. Potential decrease in rate of extrinsic contamination because of fewer manipulations of i.v. delivery system by nursing personnel
5. Less likelihood of lipid toxicity by increased dilution and duration of lipid infusion; better tolerance by neonates
6. Decreased pharmacy preparation time

Disadvantages
1. Supports growth of a variety of microorganisms significantly better than conventional dextrose/amino acid solutions but less than fat emulsions per se
2. Undesired effects (i.e., oiling out) when base solution ratios and/or additives exceed the amounts tested under stipulated controlled conditions
3. Inability of TNA systems to be filtered with a 0.22-μm bacterial-retention filter
4. Inability to use total membrane sampling of TNA systems for a pharmacy quality assurance sterility testing program
5. Unknown consequences of long-term administration of larger particle size (>4 μm) in TNA system

(117). In vitro studies of neutrophil chemotaxis have given variable results reflecting different dosages and conditions.

Using clearance of sulfur colloid technetium-99 as a marker of RES function, 3 days of administration of long-chain intravenous fat emulsion resulted in significant impairment in humans receiving PN at a dose of 0.13 g/kg/h for 10 hours daily. It took 3 days of lipid administration for this impairment to occur (118). A follow-up study demonstrated little change in the clearance of sulfur colloid technetium-99 when a lipid emulsion containing both LCTs and medium-chain TGs (MCTs) was used (119).

What has been observed with respect to infection rates in patients receiving PN? Various immune functions were studied in malnourished cancer patients maintained on either a glucose PN formula or one with both glucose and lipid; depressed cell-mediated immunity was noted before starting PN, and no alteration in these parameters was observed with fat infusion (120). In a randomized trial, preoperative PN patients who received 50% of their caloric intake as lipid experienced more major complications and deaths than control subjects receiving lipid-free PN (121). A metaanalysis of randomized studies showed that cancer patients receiving chemotherapy and PN had a fourfold greater risk of significant infection than control subjects who did not receive PN (122). Meta-analysis of the same data by another group revealed that the infection rate for patients receiving PN who did not receive intravenous lipid did not differ from that of the control subjects, and those receiving lipid one to three times per week had a risk of infection ($P < .02$) 2.3 times that of controls, while those given lipid daily had 6.3 times the risk ($P < .01$) (123). Freeman et al. analyzed risk factors associated with bacteremia due to coagulase-negative staphylococci in neonatal intensive care units; this organism was the most common blood-culture isolate in this situation (124). Infants with this type of bacteremia were 5.8 times as likely as control subjects to have received intravenous lipid emulsion before the onset of bacteremia; because lipid infusions were common, 56.6% of all cases of nosocomial infections were attributed to lipid administration. Although such data are suggestive, whether intravenous lipid is immunosuppressive in humans and whether it leads to increased infection remain unresolved (125).

Newer Intravenous Lipids

Beyond providing the small basic needs for linoleic and linolenic acids, are there lipids suitable for intravenous use that are metabolically and nutritionally more efficacious than the present vegetable oil–derived LCTs? MCTs derived from coconut oil, mixed LCTs and MCTs, short-chain fatty acids, and ω-3 fatty acids are all under current study as lipid fuels in PN (126).

Medium-Chain Triglycerides and MCT-LCT Mixtures. MCTs (see Chapter 4) have an established role given enterally by tube and orally in the management of malabsorptive disorders (see Chapters 64 and 65). Experimental laboratory animal studies have indicated that MCT is cleared and oxidized more rapidly than LCT and is equivalent in providing energy and supporting protein synthesis. MCT (with octanoic acid as the main fatty acid) has been tested experimentally in laboratory animals as physical mixtures of MCT and LCT and as chemically structured TGs (127). The latter has fatty acids of various chain lengths (short, medium, or long) esterified on the same glycerol backbone; the amounts of the different fatty acids depend on the starting proportions of the types of fatty acids in their preparation.

Physical mixtures of MCT and LCT (as soybean oil) in equal amounts have been given intravenously to patients in Europe and elsewhere (89, 119, 127). Clinical investigations have been conducted in the United States with 75/25 physical mixtures of MCT and LCT (119). Long-term studies were conducted in Belgium in patients with inflammatory bowel disease with 20% LCT or a 20% MCT-LCT mixture (equal amounts), with glucose providing an equal proportion of energy; each emulsion was infused for 3 months, followed by the other in random order (89). None of the patients receiving an MCT-LCT mixture developed abnormal liver function tests; three of eight patients receiving LCT developed abnormal liver function tests that regressed to normal when LCT was replaced by an MCT-LCT mixture. MCFAs released in high amounts during MCT-LCT infusion were oxidized in greater proportions than LCFAs and produced more ketone bodies. LCT infusion led to a significant increase in the LDL:HDL cholesteryl ester ratio, whereas MCT-LCT infusion did not; LCT infusion caused an imbalance in the fatty acid pattern of erythrocyte PLs, which was corrected by MCT-LCT infusion (89).

Ultrasonic comparison of liver size and gray-scale value (which relates to liver density and incorporation of fat and connective tissue) was done before and after patients were given PN with either 10% Intralipid or a 10% mixture of MCT and LCT in equal amounts; no changes were noted in either parameter with the MCT-LCT infusion, whereas both rose significantly with LCT (128). Although the rates and amounts of MCT infused in these and other studies appear to be safe (129), infusion of octanoate as the salt or as MCT in various laboratory species at higher doses can produce lactic acidosis and encephalopathy (130).

Structured TG (40:60, MCT:LCT by weight) emulsions have been shown to be well tolerated at 1 g/kg/day by postoperative patients in short-term studies (5–7 days), when compared with 20% Intralipid (131). One-day repeated crossover studies comparing this structured TG preparation with 20% Intralipid at 1.0 and 1.5 g/kg/day indicated similar tolerance in postoperative patients, and the former was associated with greater whole-body fat oxidation (132). It has been suggested that such structured TGs may be less toxic and less likely to promote acidosis (131).

One reason given for favoring MCT over LCT has been the belief that unlike LCFA transport, carnitine is not required for MCFA transport into the mitochondria (133). Measurements of the levels of the various plasma carnitine fractions in healthy subjects before and during infusion of glucose or amino acids, LCT, and 1:1 MCT-LCT revealed significant differences in the carnitine fractions between the LCT and MCT-LCT infusions; such data support the hypothesis that MCFA metabolism involves carnitine in some manner and suggest the need for more study of these interactions (133).

ω-3 (n-3) Fatty Acids. Important physiologic differences among the prostanoids and leukotrienes, derived from linoleic and linolenic acids (see Chapters 4 and 45), have directed attention to the possible advantages of including n-3 fatty acids and/or dihomo-γ-linolenic acid as TGs or PLs in intravenous fat emulsions to allow conversion to their eicosanoids (134). Eicosanoid synthesis must be carefully regulated to provide their various mediators in appropriate quantities in response to appropriate stimuli while avoiding harmful excesses of these potent compounds.

Mashima et al. developed and originally tested in rats a fish oil emulsion (FOE) containing purified fish oil (1.5%) that supplied EPA and DHA and soybean oil (8.5%) that supplied linoleic and linolenic acids. FOE was reportedly well tolerated by patients for up to 6 weeks and raised their low EPA and DHA serum levels to normal. The preparation was contained in a double shielded plastic bag with an oxygen absorbent between the layers to prevent oxidation (135).

Twenty postoperative trauma patients who received isonitrogenous and isocaloric PN were randomized to either soybean oil 1 g/kg/day or a combination of soybean oil 0.85 g/kg/day and fish oil 0.15 g/kg/day as part of the PN formula (135a). After 5 days of PN administration, patients receiving the FOE demonstrated a 2.5-fold increase in eicosapentanoic acid, a 1.5-fold increase in leukotriene B(5), and a 7-fold increase in leukotriene C(5). In the group receiving the soybean oil fat emulsion, eicosapentanoic acid and leukotriene B(5) remained unchanged while leukotriene C(5) doubled (135a). Such data demonstrate the usefulness of modified lipids in elevating levels of desired eicosanoids and leukotrienes.

Short-Chain Fatty Acids. Supplementation of PN solutions with short-chain fatty acids (SCFAs) prevents PN-associated mucosal atrophy and facilitates morphologic adaptation to small bowel resection in rats (136). Rats with 80% small bowel resection had better ileal glucose absorption and higher expression of glucose transporter 2 messenger RNA, glucose transporter 1, and Na^+,K^+ ATPase RNA when receiving a glucose-lipid PN formulation with sodium acetate, propionate, and butyrate than with non-SCFA PN (137).

Lipids As Pharmacologic Vehicles. Some drugs are now marketed in intravenous fat emulsion. One example is propofol, originally marketed for induction of anesthesia, but used more often for sedation in the critical care setting. It is prepared by the manufacturer in 10% fat emulsion, and some patients who needed large doses of propofol have more than 1000 kcal/day from fat (137a). Also, several lipid formulations of amphotericin B have been marketed in the United States (138), including amphotericin B in liposomes, lipid complex, or colloidal dispersion. Preliminary data suggest that these lipid-based preparations are equivalent in efficacy to amphotericin B deoxycholate, with reduced toxicity, especially nephrotoxicity, mainly because of the lower renal concentrations observed with lipid-based amphotericin B preparations. The caloric contribution of lipid formulations of amphotericin B is negligible (138a).

Amino Acids

Intravenous amino acid solutions have evolved from the original hydrolysates of casein or blood fibrin to formulations of crystalline L-amino acids of different compositions and varying concentrations based in part on the amino acid composition of high-quality dietary proteins. This history has been reviewed (3, 12). Formulations of crystalline L-amino acids have been developed for specific clinical problems, with varying claims for superiority over more-general formulas for use in renal and hepatic failure, in trauma, and for growth of infants (see Chapters 51, 89, 94, and 98 for discussion of their value in such clinical situations). The compositions of some commercially available pediatric solutions are given in Chapter 64 and Appendix Table V-A-40-b. The reader is referred to the *Handbook of Injectable Drugs* for adult solution content (138a). Commercial formulations differ between and within manufacturers in amino acid composition and concentrations, depending on clinical purpose; in addition, they may have added electrolytes and/or glucose. Concentrated standard amino acids in a 15% solution are now available for patients who are fluid overloaded and require PN.

The eight amino acids essential for normal adults are present in all formulas, as are histidine and arginine, which are needed for young children. Glycine, alanine, and proline are present in moderately high concentration in the general adult formulations as sources of nonessential amino nitrogen. Some manufacturers add serine, tyrosine, glutamic acid, and aspartic acid in variable amounts, and a few have taurine in small amounts. The ratio by weight of essential to total amino acids in the pediatric and standard adult solutions varies between 0.41 and 0.54; higher ratios are present in formulas designed for patients with renal or hepatic failure.

Amino acid infusion during surgery has been noted to increase body temperature, which otherwise falls customarily during anesthesia and surgery because of heat loss to the environment and a reduced threshold to initiate heat conservation (139). Hypothermia (core temperature

<35°C) can adversely affect coagulation, drug action, metabolism, and healing (139a). The thermic effect of amino acid infusion is high and may account for 30 to 40% of the energy infused. Although effective, use of amino acids for this purpose not only increases cost but also requires caution in patients unable to tolerate the extra fluid load and without the pulmonary and cardiac reserve needed for the resulting increased oxygen uptake and cardiac output. Use of intravenous fluids warmed to 38°C reduces hypothermia (139a).

Calculating the Energy Contribution of Amino Acids

Should the amino acids in PN be included in the total energy calculations of the formulation? This question is raised periodically, and a recent discussion states two opposing positions (140). The basic issue is whether the amino acids avoid oxidation by being incorporated in significant amounts of newly synthesized protein, being lost as such in urine or through the gut, or else being diverted into carbohydrate stores. In fact, the amounts of new protein laid down in successfully renourishing a child or an adult are a small proportion of the amino acid equivalent given (e.g., 3 to 4 g/protein/day or 60–90 g of protein-equivalent given to adults). Even though the energy cost of protein synthesis from amino acids is high, this is a small factor in terms of daily synthesis, even in growing, malnourished, and hypercatabolic individuals. Finally, accumulation of stored glucose (as glycogen) derived from gluconeogenesis from amino acids is limited, and the amino acids are mostly metabolized if hyperglycemia is minimized. It is our opinion that the energy contributed by the amino acids in the PN formulation should be included in the total calculation.

Achieving nitrogen equilibrium or positive nitrogen balance requires sufficient essential amino acids and sufficient nonessential amino nitrogen, adequate nonnitrogen energy, and other nutrients (such as potassium and phosphorus) essential for nitrogen use. Recent research on amino acids or their derivatives of interest in PN usage is summarized below.

Branched-Chain Amino Acids

Muscle uptake and metabolism of the essential amino acids isoleucine, leucine, and valine are reviewed in Chapter 2, and their clinical applications are discussed in Chapters 35, 44, 96, and 98. The role of these branched-chain amino acids (BCAAs) as amino group donors in accelerated protein catabolism in muscle of hypermetabolic patients is noted in Chapter 98. Do injured and/or septic patients need more BCAAs than are usually present in general PN formulations? Claims have been contradictory concerning beneficial effects (e.g., improved nitrogen balance with higher BCAA levels than the 19 to 25% in standard United States amino acid formulations). An expert panel concluded: "In clinical studies, while some positive results in parameters of nitrogen metabolism have been noted using BCAA-enriched solutions in the most severely ill patients, little or no major effect on outcome has yet been demonstrated" (141). Additional negative effects have been published (142).

Taurine

Metabolism and formulation of taurine, which has a sulfuric acid group replacing the carboxyl group of what would otherwise be alanine, is discussed in Chapter 34. Considered a nonessential amino acid for humans, taurine is of nutritional interest with respect to PN because its plasma, platelet, and urine levels are depressed in children and adults maintained on long-term PN. No other substantial evidence for deficiency has been forthcoming. In fact, the low levels in adult and pediatric patients receiving long-term PN did not appear to be correlated with any index of visual function (143). Because of limited ability of LBW infants to synthesize taurine, the low levels of its precursor cysteine in PN solutions, and the reduced capacity to reabsorb taurine, this amino acid is added to some pediatric formulas (see Chapter 64).

Glutamic Acid and Glutamine

The central role of glutamic acid and glutamine in metabolism is reviewed in Chapters 2 and 35. Although glutamic acid was present in the early parenteral protein hydrolysates, it was omitted from the later free amino acid formulations because it is synthesized in the body and glutamine synthetase catalyzes its reaction with ammonia to form glutamine. Interest in the clinical importance of glutamine has increased in recent years, partly because of its role as an energy and nitrogen source in rapidly dividing cells (e.g., intestine and stimulated lymphocytes) and because under conditions that include hypercatabolic disease states, glutamine levels can decrease markedly. These conditions are discussed briefly in their various aspects in Chapters 35, 96, and 98.

The issues for PN concern proof of stability in solutions, safety, and evidence of efficacy of glutamine in improving nitrogen balance, muscle protein kinetics, and other metabolic parameters when added to standard formulas given to hypercatabolic patients. Concern about the stability of glutamine stored with PN components was alleviated; glutamine was stable for 22 days at 40°C when dissolved in sterile water and added to various TPN solutions at concentrations of 1 and 1.5% wt/vol with cold sterilization using two membrane filters (144). Infusing 20 to 57 g (136 to 390 mmol) of glutamine in PN solutions for more than 5 days did not significantly change serum ammonia and glutamate concentrations (145). (See also Chapter 35).

In an increasing number of clinical studies in stressed patients, L-glutamine has been given intravenously in PN solutions as such (146, 147), as the dipeptide L-alanyl-L-glutamine (148–150), or as its α-keto precursors, α-ketoglutarate or ornithine α-ketoglutarate (148). In these studies, glutamine in its various forms was provided in daily amounts ranging from approximately 0.19 g (1.3 mmol)/kg body weight (148) to 0.57 g/kg (146). Given to postoperative patients in short 3- to 5-studies, glutamine decreased the negative nitrogen balance noted in the control subjects, increased intramuscular free glutamine concentration (148, 150), and maintained skeletal muscle ribosome concentrations (150). After bone marrow transplantation, glutamine significantly decreased the negative nitrogen balance of the subjects during posttransplant days 7 to 11; over 3 weeks, glutamine infusion raised plasma glutamine without increasing plasma glutamate or changing the ammonia concentration gradient between the groups. Fewer patients given glutamine developed clinical infection and microbial colonization, and their hospital stay was shortened (146). Villus height was maintained and intestinal permeability was lower in patients receiving PN plus glycyl L-glutamine than in patients receiving PN alone (151). As noted above, glutamine in a protocol with growth hormone enhanced nutrient absorption. (The role of glutamine in intestinal translocation is discussed in Chapter 35.)

Issues remain to be resolved concerning the reported beneficial effects of glutamine in hypercatabolic patients. How much glutamine is necessary and safe for optimum results? On the basis of their work and that of others, Fürst et al. suggest that in routine postoperative patients, about 13 g (89 mmol) of glutamine daily meets the intestinal mucosal need for cell replication plus increased muscle needs, whereas severely injured or stressed patients may need 27 to 40 g (187 to 237 mmol) per day (149).

How valid are the nitrogen balance data? Walser has pointed out that gains or losses of body free glutamine nitrogen should be included in overall nitrogen balance data, just as a net change in body urea nitrogen must be included in patients with renal disease (152). Furthermore, changes in free glutamine nitrogen pools do not represent modification of protein nitrogen. While this issue has raised some controversy (153, 154), Ziegler et al. acknowledge that about 25% of the improved nitrogen balance may represent a relative increase in the free glutamine pool within skeletal muscle; these investigators point out that direct measurement of intracellular glutamine concentrations in biopsy specimens is needed for confirmation (146). Further data are needed on the effect of glutamine on quantitative changes in net protein synthesis in muscle in hypercatabolic states.

Short-Chain Peptide Use

Adibi has summarized the advantages of using short-chain peptides in place of free amino acids in PN solutions: *(a)* increased usable nitrogen sources in more concentrated form (minimizing fluid volume), *(b)* decreased osmolality with its advantage for PPN, and *(c)* perhaps most important, the increased solubility as dipeptides of poorly soluble amino acids or the increased stability of unstable free forms (155). How well used are small peptides given intravenously? Adibi summarized his studies in baboons, in which a series of free amino acids and their dipeptides as the relevant nitrogen sources were infused as the only nitrogen sources, and his studies of glutamine in peptide form (155). In a 1-week crossover study and in 4-week studies comparing free amino acids and dipeptides, no significant differences were noted with respect to nitrogen balance, plasma and muscle amino acid concentrations, urinary losses, plasma concentration of insulin, glucose, and lipids, and other parameters (156).

Minerals

Sodium, potassium, calcium, magnesium, phosphate, and chloride are essential nutrients. Because a significant proportion of patients receiving or needing PN have malabsorption of the alimentary tract or impaired renal reabsorption or both, often associated with large fluid ionic losses, a continuing concern in the care of such patients is the adequacy of fluid and electrolyte balance. (These and related important issues are considered in some detail in Chapters 6 through 9 and elsewhere in this book.)

The basic daily needs of patients with reasonably normal cardiovascular, intestinal, renal, hormonal, and hydration status are 50 to 60 meq (mmol) of sodium, 40 meq (mmol) of chloride and bicarbonate (including those associated with amino acids as acetate), and 40 to 60 meq (mmol) of potassium. Excessive losses from the intestine or kidney and abnormal retention require appropriate changes, with suitable monitoring as needed.

Calcium, Phosphorus, and Magnesium

Calcium and phosphorus (as inorganic phosphate) are needed in relatively large amounts by infants; however, when both are present in relatively large concentrations, solubility in the PN solution becomes a problem. It has been recommended that glycerophosphate or glucose phosphate be given together with calcium gluconate (157) or calcium glycerophosphate (158) as more soluble forms of these nutrients. Reference curves have been developed to estimate calcium and phosphate compatibility in commonly used neonatal PN solutions (159). The electrolyte needs of infants and children per kilogram per day are given in Chapter 64. Recommended pediatric concentrations of calcium, phosphorus, and magnesium per liter of PN solution are given in reference 160 and for children and adults in Table 101.7 (161).

Negative calcium balance related to hypercalciuria may occur in adults receiving PN, especially during the infusion period of cyclic PN; supplementation with either sodium or potassium acetate (replacing equimolar amounts of NaCl or KCl) resulted in major decreases in urinary calcium in patients receiving 24-hour and cyclic PN, primarily because of increased renal tubular reabsorption with reduced excretion to near-infusion levels (162). Reports are contradictory

Table 101.7
Recommended Levels for Calcium, Phosphorus, and Magnesium in PN Formulations

	Pediatric[b]			
Minerals[a]	Preterm Infants (mg/L[c])	Term Infants (mg/L[c])	Children <1 year (mg/L)	Adults (meq/day)
Ca	500–600	500–600	200–400	10–25
P	400–450	400–450	150–300	20–30[d]
Mg	50–70	50–70	20–40	12–20[d]

[a]Equivalents: Ca, 100 mg = 2.5 mmol = 5 meq; P, 100 mg = 3.3 mmol; Mg, 12 mg = 0.5 mmol = 1 meq.
[b]Data from Greene HL, Hambidge M, Schanier R, et al. Am J Clin Nutr 1988;48:1324–1342 (rev. reprint issued Dec 1990).
[c]To avoid Ca-P precipitation, recommended intakes are given per liter and assume an average fluid intake of approximately 120–150 mL/kg/day with 25 g amino acids/L of a pediatric formulation. Dosages for preterm infants are to be given in a central vein infusion.
[d]P and Mg needs vary from these ranges, depending on the extent of intestinal losses and renal retention or losses.

concerning whether urinary calcium excretion with 12-hour cyclic PN is greater than that with continuous 24-hour infusion (161). While this may not be a significant issue for the short-term patient, it may be important for those on prolonged PN because of skeletal calcium loss.

Hypophosphatemia has multiple causes; however, in PN patients it is often associated with sudden provision of glucose, the metabolism of which stimulates transfer of phosphate from plasma to cells (see Chapter 8). Hypophosphatemia was treated during provision of PN by using a graduated dosing scheme based on the serum phosphorus concentration in patients with normal renal function (163). For serum phosphorus concentrations below 1.5 mg/dL, 0.64 mmol/kg was given over 8 hours; doses of 0.32 mmol/kg over 4 to 6 hours and 0.16 mmol/kg over 4 hours were given for serum phosphorus concentrations of 1.6 to 2.2 mg/dL and 2.3 to 3.0 mg/dL, respectively (163).

The importance of magnesium and magnesium balance is being appreciated more, especially in the critical care setting where serum magnesium concentrations are being assessed with increased frequency and risk factors for magnesium depletion are now well recognized (see Chapter 9). Although the serum magnesium concentration does not always accurately reflect magnesium status, a low concentration usually indicates magnesium deficiency. Doses for management of moderate-to-severe deficiency in various clinical situations for various age groups are given in Chapter 9 and elsewhere (164, 165). Hypermagnesemia may occur with fluctuating or progressively deteriorating renal function or decreasing intestinal or renal magnesium loss; periodic monitoring of serum magnesium is necessary.

Fluid and electrolyte disorders are particularly prone to occur soon after discharge of patients on HPN, either because of inadequate testing in the hospital; fluctuating cardiac, renal, and intestinal functions; or variation in supplementary intake at home (166).

Trace Elements

Currently, acceptable direct evidence indicates that iron, iodide, zinc, copper, chromium (Cr^{3+}), and selenium are essential human nutrients. Manganese (Mn^{2+}) has been found essential for all experimental species studied, but clear evidence for manganese deficiency in man is lacking. A single well-documented case of molybdenum deficiency was noted in a patient receiving long-term PN. (The biochemical and physiologic roles of these trace elements and the effects of their depletion in humans and other species are reviewed in Chapters 10 through 16.)

Several generalizations about essential trace elements are in order. The cationic trace elements (Fe, Zn, Cu, Cr^{3+}, and Mn) in their salt forms are highly regulated and tend to be absorbed in small amounts from food by the normal intestine. When in excess in the body, all these elements may be toxic. Giving them intravenously risks excessive retention, because intestinal controls are bypassed. Iron, particularly, is poorly excreted in the urine after PN or blood infusion. Copper, manganese, and (to a much smaller extent) molybdate, are excreted through the bile into the intestinal tract; hence continued administration of the usual amounts of copper and manganese in the presence of excretory liver dysfunction imposes a risk (see below). In contrast, all the anionic forms of trace elements (iodide, selenite, or molybdate) are well absorbed and excreted in the urine; again, excess imposes a risk of toxicity. Many trace elements are present as contaminants in PN components and so contribute variably to the input. Finally, nonessential and potentially toxic trace elements, which may be contaminants, must be considered.

Iron. The intravenous requirement for the term infant is estimated to be about 100 μg/kg/day; the premature infant probably needs double that amount intravenously (160). Older children need 1 to 2 mg/day. Nonmenstruating females and men whose condition is stable need about 1 mg, and menstruating females double that amount. Iron loss through frequent venipuncture for various tests may be estimated on the basis of 1 mg of iron lost for every 1 mL of packed red cells removed (see Chapter 10).

Contamination of various PN additives with iron varies by item and by manufacturer; the amounts found in complete formulations with free amino acids vary from 0.025 to 1.4 mg/L (167). On average, the needs of children and adults who have no significant blood loss and are receiving their normal fluid and energy requirements are met by these contaminants. When evidence indicates iron depletion, iron may be given intravenously as dilute iron dextran solution in varying amounts, after ensuring that the patient has no hypersensitivity to a test dose; ferrous citrate may be used (168). As noted above, addition of iron dextran and other iron salts disrupts TNA stability (100).

Patients who receive chronic PN without iron and eat very little invariably become iron deficient over time. Iron should be added to the PN solution (preferably a dextrose/amino acid PN) to either prevent or treat iron deficiency in this situation. This can be accomplished by adding small daily doses of iron dextran to the PN solution (e.g., 1–2 mg/day) or by giving regular doses of therapeutic iron dextran via PN (e.g., 25–50 mg/day for 2–4 weeks). Patients who have a duodenum and proximal jejunum and eat a normal diet during chronic PN usually absorb enough iron to prevent deficiency; These patients may never need supplemental iron via PN. Regular measurement of serum iron, mean corpuscular volume, and serum ferritin helps in assessing iron stores. During acute stress such as infections, measuring serum iron and ferritin concentrations may not be helpful in the diagnosis of iron deficiency, because serum iron concentration decreases while serum ferritin concentration increases (169) (see Chapters 10 and 96).

Iodide. Serum iodide often remains normal in infants (170) and adults (171) with no added iodide in PN. Over 4 or more years of observation in adult patients receiving long-term PN at home without added iodide, the various parameters of thyroid function have remained within normal limits (171). This is explained by iodide contamination of various mineral additives, by efficient absorption in the upper gastrointestinal tract of iodides from any ingested diet, and by the use of iodide-containing topical antimicrobial solutions. For the occasional previously depleted adult patient with malabsorption who may have a low serum iodide level, 1 μg/kg appears adequate during the repletion period. The same amount has been recommended for infants, to avoid any risk of deficiency or toxicity (160).

Following the recommendation of an expert committee of the Nutrition Advisory Group of the American Medical Association (AMA) to the FDA in 1979 (172), commercial intravenous solutions of zinc, copper, manganese, and chromium became available, ending a period in which such solutions were available only to physicians and pharmacists who personally prepared them. We have modified the 1979 suggested intakes on the basis of newer information (Table 101.8). Some data relevant to PN are reviewed briefly below.

Zinc. Pediatric dosages of zinc have been more precisely defined by Greene et al. (160) (see Table 101.8). The original recommendations of the AMA committee (172) for stable and for hypermetabolic patients is deemed reasonable (167). As in adults, severe diarrhea secondary to infectious disease and the short bowel syndrome in children are associated with increased zinc losses and increased need (173). The guidelines in the appropriate footnote for zinc in Table 101.8 are helpful in estimating intestinal losses. Periodic checks of serum levels in such circumstances are essential. Zinc contamination of PN additives is variable, depending on the specific sources. As a result, total zinc in the formulation may be as high as 0.3 to 0.4 mg/L (174). Data on specific components have been published (172, 175).

Copper. The pediatric copper dose recommendations in Table 101.8 are the same as the AMA recommendations (172). The work of Shike et al. showed that unlike zinc, increased stool volume is not associated with a major increase in copper excretion, and urinary losses tend to be low; thus, copper accumulates in the body when infused in amounts needed for maintenance or growth (176). On

Table 101.8
Recommended Levels for Trace Elements

	Infants (μg/kg/day)		Children[b] (μg/kg/day)[c]		Adult (per day)		
Trace element[a]	Preterm[b]	Term[b]			Stable	Acute Hypermetabolic	With Intestinal Losses
Zinc	400	>3 month-250 <3 month-100	50[d]	[5000]	2.5–4.0 mg[e]	Add 2.0 mg[e]	Add[f]
Copper[g]	20[e]	20[e]	20[e]	[300]	0.3–0.5 mg[d,h,i]	—	Total 0.5 mg[h]
Chromium	0.2[e]	0.2[e]	0.2[e] 0.05[l]	[50]	10–15 μg[e]	—	Add 20 μg[k]
Manganese[g]	1.0	1.0	1.0[d]	[50]	60–100 μg[d]	—	—
Selenium[j]	2.0	2.0	2.0	[30]	40–80 μg[k]		
Molybdenum[j]	0.25	0.25	0.25	[5]	0 (see text)		

[a]Conversion factors: Zn, 1 μg = 0.0153 μmol, Cu, 1 μg = 0.0157 μmol; Cr, 1 μg = 0.0192 μmol; Mn, 1 μg = 0.0182 μmol; Se, 1 μg = 0.0127 μmol; Mo, 1 μg = 0.0104 μmol.
[b]Data from Greene HL, Hmbidge M, Schanler R, et al. Am J Clin Nutr 1988;48:1324–42 (rev. reprint issued Dec 1990).
[c]Maximum in micrograms per day in brackets.
[d]Lower range than in 1979 AMA recommendations; data from Shils ME, Burke AW, Greene HL, et al. JAMA 1979;241:2051–4.
[e]Unchanged from 1979 AMA recommendations; data from Shils ME, Burke AW, Greene HL, et al. JAMA 1979;241:2051–4.
[f]Add 12 mg/L of small bowel losses and 17 mg/kg of stool or ileostomy losses; data from Shils ME, Burke AW, Greene HL, et al. JAMA 1979;241:2051–4.
[g]Decrease or omit with increasing severity of obstructive jaundice.
[h]Data from Phillip GD, Garnys VP. JPEN J Parenter Enteral Nutr 1981;5:11–8.
[i]Data from Shike M, Roulet M, Kurlan R, et al. Gastroenterology 1981;81:291–7.
[j]Decrease or omit with increasing severity of renal dysfunction.
[k]Data from Berkelhammer CH, Wood RJ, Sitrin MD. Am J Clin Nutr 1988;48:1482–9.
[l]Data from Moukarzel AA, Son MK, Buchman AL, et al. Am J Clin Nutr 1992;339:385–8.

the basis of these and other findings, it is suggested that the range for copper be lowered to 0.3 to 0.5 mg/day for stable patients; hence the upper limit of the recommendation in Table 101.8 is at the lower limit of the AMA recommendation. Caution in copper administration in obstructive jaundice is emphasized because the major excretory route is through bile. The copper content of PN additives varies.

Manganese. The manganese content in PN components (177) and the blood levels found in PN patients given varying amounts of Mn^{2+} (178) suggested an appreciable reduction in the AMA recommendations. The current pediatric recommendations of 1 μg/kg/day with a total of 50 μg/day for older children in Table 101.8 are below the AMA recommendation of 2 to 10 μg/kg/day.

Manganese contamination of various PN additives produced in the United States may result in an adult receiving 8 to 22 μg/day (177). HPN patients receiving 60 to 120 μg/day (~1.5–3.0 μg/kg/day) of added Mn^{2+} had normal serum levels (178). As suggested above, it appears wise to provide only 60 to 100 μg/day to adults (Table 101.8) (179) rather than the 150 to 180 μg/day supplement of the AMA recommendations.

The potential for excessive retention escalates when cholestasis is present (which interferes with manganese elimination from the body) and there is continued provision of the amount of manganese listed in Table 101.8 in PN. Even with normal liver function, higher dosages in infants and children (180, 181) and in a few adults (182) on long-term PN resulted in high blood levels associated with high signal intensity in T1-weighted imaging in the basal ganglia (180–182a). Levels of plasma (183) or whole-blood (180) manganese in children showed a significant positive correlation with bilirubin levels. Reducing or omitting supplementary Mn^{2+} resulted in major decreases in blood manganese over periods varying from weeks to months (180–182) in children and adults, and the high-intensity signal on magnetic resonance brain imaging disappeared in one adult (184) and in a child (181) and was markedly reduced in another adult (182). The amounts of manganese given to patients who developed high blood levels and imaging changes (180–184) were appreciably greater than those in either the AMA recommendations or Table 101.8.

The exact relation of manganese to the high-intensity signal in the basal ganglia is uncertain. Some authors postulate deposition of a paramagnetic metal (i.e., manganese) (180, 184); others suggest that the disappearance with cessation of manganese infusion is more likely to be related to manganese-induced reversible changes in the ultrastructural membrane composition (185). Also uncertain is the possible role of high levels of blood manganese per se as one of the many factors in PN that can lead to hepatotoxicity (180).

Neurologic signs were present in one adult on long-term PN containing 1 to 2 mg/day of Mn^{2+}; these improved, and serum and urinary Mn^{2+} decreased when manganese was omitted from PN. Nine months later the patient died from a massive GI hemorrhage secondary to her cancer. At autopsy, the Mn^{2+} content of the caudate nucleus and centrum ovale was two to three times that found in some non-PN patients (182a).

Chromium (Cr^{3+}). As noted in the 1979 AMA report, quantitative data on chromium requirements were lacking at that time, and the qualitative suggestions were based on estimates from balance data on healthy individuals (172). The current situation is not appreciably clearer, largely because of the difficulty of measuring plasma chromium levels (normally very low), lack of information on tissue levels of this ion, and lack of controlled studies on very low Cr^{3+} intake.

The relatively few cases of well-documented symptomatic chromium depletion have occurred in long-term adult PN patients receiving little or no supplementary Cr^{3+}. It has been associated with sudden occurrence of glucose intolerance, glycosuria, weight loss, and neurologic symptoms, especially peripheral neuropathy. Development of symptoms appeared to be related to prolonged glucose infusions and intestinal fluid losses—both of which increase Cr^{3+} need. The patients responded well to Cr^{3+}, often 250 μg Cr^{3+} infused daily for weeks ([186], Chapter 15). Cr^{3+} toxicity has not been observed, even with doses above 250 μg/day.

More analytic data on Cr^{3+} content of PN additives are now available. The total daily Cr^{3+} content of high-glucose PN formulas using a variety of PN additives from different batches and sources ranged from 2.4 to 8.1 μg, and that of a high-lipid formula, from 2.6 to 10.5 μg (187). Amino acids, especially those containing phosphate or with phosphate additives, accounted for 85 to 90% of the Cr^{3+}. British investigators found 4 to 11 μg in 3 L of a PN solution (188).

A pediatric formula containing 4 μg of Cr^{3+} as a contaminant, given over 16 months, did not produce signs or symptoms suggesting chromium deficiency (189). Children aged 1.3 to 14 years who were receiving chromium during long-term PN at 0.15 ± 0.09 μg/kg/day had higher serum chromium concentrations than control subjects (2.1 ± 1.2 vs. 0.10 ± 0.03 μg/L). Supplementation was discontinued for 1 year (during which time the Cr^{3+} intake was estimated to be 0.05 ± 0.01 μg/kg/day), at which time the serum Cr^{3+} concentration was 0.5 ± 0.3 μg/L, and no signs of deficiency were observed (190). It was suggested that the parenteral Cr^{3+} pediatric intake should be lowered to 0.05 μg/kg and that current values of Cr^{3+} as contaminants may be sufficient for adults. A period of 1 year of reduced Cr^{3+} intake following a period of high intake without signs or symptoms may not be an adequate test of need in long-term patients. We believe that for children and adults on long-term PN, the recommendations given in Table 101.8 are still valid pending further studies. However, for periods of 1 year or less, the recommendations of Moukarzel et al. (190) may be tried with adequate precautions.

Selenium. Recommendations for selenium were not made in the 1979 AMA report. That year saw the first reports in English relating selenium deficiency to Keshan disease in China (see Chapter 14) and the report of Van Rijn et al. of a case of selenium deficiency in a patient receiving PN (191). Considerable clinical and biochemical information has accrued since then, including selenium deficiency in patients receiving PN, with some deaths associated with cardiomyopathy and reports of muscle tenderness and weakness (see Chapter 14). As noted in Chapter 14, serious deficiency in mice is associated with increased virulence of coxsackievirus.

Although deaths may occur, low plasma levels of selenium (<10 μg/mL or <0.13 μmol/L) may be present without symptoms. Cohen et al. followed five patients on HPN without added selenium for an average of 18.6 months (192). Selenium-dependent glutathione peroxidase (GSHPx) in plasma reached very low levels (<15% of normal values, 0.32 U/mL) in approximately 1 year; GSHPx in red cells reached that level (24 U/g Hb) in 1 to 2 years. At the time plasma GSHPx was at this level, plasma selenium was 0.19 ± 0.07 pmol/mL. There was no evidence of either cardiac or skeletal muscle dysfunction in this (192) or another depletion study (193). Following infusion of 400 μg of selenium as selenite, plasma GSHPx rose within 6 hours; that in red cells did not reach normal levels until 3 to 4 months later—the time required for new red cells to appear (192).

Selenious acid (as selenite salts) is available for intravenous use. Use of 40 μg/day in PN usually maintains normal plasma levels; 100 μg/day in the infusate will raise low levels in previously depleted patients receiving PN into a control range of 100 μg/mL (1.3 μmol/L) (191).

Selenoprotein P levels in plasma (measured by radioimmunoassay) correlated well with extracellular glutathione peroxidase and selenium as markers for selenium status in deficient patients on long-term PN (194).

Molybdenum. Whether a true molybdenum deficiency has been observed in several species of experimental laboratory animals is controversial because tungsten must be added to the diet as an antagonist to molybdenum uptake to induce depletion (195). A single documented case of molybdenum deficiency was reported in a patient with Crohn's disease receiving long-term PN; clinical and biochemical abnormalities were reversed by daily supplementation with 300 μg of ammonium molybdate (196, 197). Tissue levels of molybdenum and balance data were not obtained, nor were molybdenum-dependent enzyme activities measured. Two patients with active Crohn's disease and malabsorption had ileostomy losses of 560 and 300 to 350 μg/day of this ion.

In view of a time lapse of at least 6 months from the initiation of PN to development of symptoms in the single reported patient, the availability of simple biochemical criteria as diagnostic clues, and the reportedly high molybdenum content of PN solutions, it is recommended that molybdenum not be added at present to PN infusions in adults and that it be withheld in children with the following consideration for those receiving long-term PN (160). Serum urate and urine sulfate measurements should be made periodically to monitor a need to initiate this element. If deficiency is suspected in adults, a dose of 200 to 300 μg as ammonium molybdate appears to be safe. More data on levels of molybdenum contamination of PN solutions and its serum and urine levels in long-term PN patients are needed.

Multi–Trace Element Additives. The most commonly used commercially available trace element combination products, which contain four to five individual metals, are listed in Tables 101.9 (adults) and 101.10 (pediatric). A combination product containing six trace elements (molybdenum plus zinc, copper, manganese, chromium, and selenium) and one containing seven trace elements (iodine plus the six mentioned above) are also commercially available.

Use of multiple trace elements in a fixed formula poses

Table 101.9
Trace Element Combination Products for Adults (Contents per mL)

Category	Product (Manufacturer)	Zn (mg as sulfate)	Cu (mg as sulfate)	Cr (μg as chloride)	Mn (μg as sulfate)	Se (μg as selenious acid)
Four-element product[a]	MTE-4 (Lymphomed) MulTE-PAK-4 (Smith & Nephew Solopak) Multiple Trace Element (American Regent)	1	0.4	4	100	
Four-element product[+] concentrated	MTE-4 Concentrated (Lymphomed) ConTE-PAK-4 (Smith & Nephew Solopak) Multiple Trace Element Concentrated (American Regent)	5	1	10	500	
Five-element product[a]	MTE-5 (Lymphomed) MulTE-PAK-5 (Smith & Nephew Solopak) Multiple Trace Element with Selenium (American Regent)	1	0.4	4	100	20
Five-element product[+] concentrated	MTE-5 concentrated (Lymphomed) Multiple Trace Element with Selenium Concentrated (American Regent)	5	1	10	500	60

[a]Usual adult dose is 3 mL/day; daily dose of manganese exceeds suggested dose in Table 101.8.
[+]Usual adult dose is 1 mL/day; daily dose of manganese exceeds suggested dose in Table 101.8.

Table 101.10
Trace Element Combination Products for Pediatrics and Neonates (Content per mL)

Category	Product (Manufacturer)	Zn (mg as sulfate)	Cu (mg as sulfate)	Cr (μg as chloride)	Mn (μg as sulfate)	Se (μg as selenious acid)
Neonatal	Multiple Trace Element Neonatal (American Regent)	1.5	0.1	0.85	25	
	Neotrace-4	1.5	0.1	0.85	25	
	Pedtrace-4	0.5	0.1	0.85	25	
Pediatric	PedTE-PAK-4 (Smith & Nephew Solopak)	1	0.1	1	25	
	P.T.E.-4 (Lyphomed)	1	0.1	1	25	
	Multiple Trace Element Pediatric (American Regent)	0.5	0.1	1	30	
	P.T.E.-5 (Lyphomed)	1	0.1	1	25	15

[a]The volumes used in practice may exceed recommended levels in Table 101.8. See text for toxicity related to dosage with hepatic cholestasis.

the risk of excessive dosage of one or more of the constituents to long-term patients with metabolic abnormalities who require restriction or omission. Furthermore, evidence reviewed in this chapter and recommendations in Table 101.8 suggest that routine needs for some trace elements are appreciably lower than those recommended in the AMA-FDA report (172). A combination of individual trace elements or decreased volume of a given multitrace element formulation may be necessary when restriction of one or more of the latter is indicated.

Ultratrace Elements. Ultratrace elements are reviewed in detail in Chapter 16. Data are available on the contamination levels in PN additives of boron, nickel, and vanadium (197a). At present, evidence is insufficient to warrant their addition to PN solutions.

Potential Toxicity of Other Trace Elements. The issue of toxicity of parenterally administered lead, cadmium, mercury, and aluminum present as contaminants merits consideration because they bypass the normal barriers of the gastrointestinal tract (198). Twenty components of a PN solution were individually analyzed for mercury; all values were at or below the lowest quantitative detection limit (198a). The complete formulations had 0.001 μg/mL of mercury (the lower detection limit), 0.08 ng/mL of cadmium, and 2 ng/mL of lead. Potassium chloride and phosphate solutions contained 135 and 77 ng/mL of lead, respectively. Some 22 μg of cadmium was measured in a daily PN formula (198), approximately the amount estimated not to exceed reported amounts absorbed daily by normal individuals.

Aluminum. Aluminum is of special concern because its toxicity was well delineated in patients with renal disease who were treated with aluminum-containing phosphate-binding antacids and/or received aluminum-contaminated water in hemodialysis. Neurologic changes include apraxic motor abnormalities involving speech, myoclonus, seizures and dementia. Also seen is an osteomalacia refractory to therapy with vitamin D analogues, calcium or phosphate; bone pain; pathologic fractures; aluminum deposition on bone osteoid front; and a microcytic anemia without evidence of iron deficiency (199, 200).

Reports of serious metabolic bone disease in a group of patients receiving HPN for 6 to 72 months were followed by the discovery that the casein hydrolysate used as the source of amino acids contained relatively large amounts of aluminum (2313 ± 149 μg/L) (201). Aluminum concentrations in plasma, urine, and bone were markedly elevated in all patients studied, and the bone morphology was that of osteomalacia, ranging from mild to severe. Intense periarticular and lower extremity pain in long bones and weight-bearing joints developed within 5 months in 5 of the initial 11 patients despite improvement in their overall nutritional state. Patients with impaired renal clearance are at increased risk. As noted below, use of casein hydrolysate at this institution was discontinued, and the patients' bone status improved.

Even though free amino acid solutions have much smaller amounts of aluminum (e.g., 26 ± 20 μg/L of 10% solution), other PN ingredients may have significant amounts and may contribute to the total burden. Premature infants are at increased risk because of their poor renal clearance (160). Widely varying concentrations of aluminum have been found in the same component from different manufacturers or in different salts of the same mineral; careful selection can reduce aluminum contamination from 288 μg/L of PN solution to 10.9 μg/L (202). There is evidence from a study conducted in Cambridge in the U.K. that preterm infants given PN for a median period of 9.5 days (range, 5–15) with a solution providing 45 μg/kg/day of aluminum had dose-related reduced developmental attainment at the postterm age of 18 months, compared with a control group who were given a solution containing only 4 to 5 μg/kg/day of aluminum (202a).

A joint working group on standards for aluminum content of PN solutions supported the FDA proposal to set an upper limit of 25 μg Al/L (0.93 μmol/L) in large-volume parenteral infusions; it recommended that salts of calcium, phosphate, and magnesium; trace element and multivitamin solutions; and heparin state the amount of aluminum on their label and that pharmacists and physicians be educated about the risk of aluminum (203). As noted by Klein, the FDA has not implemented action despite the recommendations of its advisory panel in 1986 and its proposed regulations published in 1990 (200). The FDA in early 1998 again requested comments on proposed regulations.

Vitamins

Formulations

The current parenteral multivitamin formulations in the United States are based on those proposed in 1975 by the Nutrition Advisory Group of the AMA for intravenous vitamin formulations (204). Its adult formulation was approved by the FDA in 1979 and is designated here as the AMA-FDA adult formula. In 1984, its recommended pediatric formula was approved. The vitamin content of the formulations per unit in the U.S. are the same regardless of manufacturer (Table 101.11). The pediatric formula provides all known essential vitamins; the adult formula omits vitamin K, which must be added separately to the PN solution at a recommended dose of 5 mg once weekly or daily at a dose of 1 mg/day. Manufacturers add excess nutrients at production time (within limits set by the FDA) to meet label requirements at the expiration date.

Provision of lipid-soluble vitamins in aqueous suspension requires one or more synthetic solubilizing agents. In addition, these parenteral multivitamins contain a variety of excipients serving as stabilizers, antioxidants, buffers, and preservatives. Their presence and concentrations in various commercial preparations of the AMA-FDA formulas are given in Table 101.12. The American Academy of Pediatrics has reviewed the issue of excipients as inactive ingredients in pharmaceutical products with particular reference to infants and children (205).

In many other countries, other formulations are available. One (Vitalipid, adult and infant) contains fat-soluble vitamins dissolved in fractionated soybean oil emulsified with egg phospholipids similar to that used in Intralipid; accordingly, it can be infused with intravenous fat emulsions (Table 101.11). The other (Soluvit) is a solution of nine water-soluble vitamins; the pediatric formulation has the same vitamins and content as the AMA-FDA pediatric formula (Table 101.11).

Stability. Some absorption and/or destruction of individual vitamins may occur through contact with plastic containers and tubes and in passage through filters, exposure to light and heat, and interactions with other substances present in solutions. Factors affecting the solubility and stability of vitamins in various pharmaceutical preparations have been reviewed (206).

Appreciable amounts of retinol appear to be lost from solution by a combination of adsorption and photodegradation when flow through tubing is slow. This is particularly true with the increased light intensity used in neonatal nurseries (160). With exposure to bright sunlight, 100% of retinol in PN solutions can be lost in 3 hours (207). Use of polyolefin tubing rather than polyvinyl tubing reduces vitamin A loss (160). Little loss of vitamin D occurs in plastic delivery systems. DL-α-tocopherol is stable to sunlight, but 50% of vitamin K can be lost from PN solutions in 3 hours (207). Riboflavin and pyridoxine are also

Table 101.11
Composition of Parenteral Multivitamin Formulations

	Children				Adult (per unit dose)		
Vitamin[a]	Very Low Birth Weight (per kg)[b]	Term to 11 years: AMA FDA (per day)	Soluvit Infant[c] (per day)	Vitalipid Infant[c] (per day)	AMA-FDA[d]	Soluvit	Vitalipid
A[e] (μg)[IU]	500 [167]	700 [2300]	—	690 [2270]	990 [3300]	—	750 [2500]
D_2(μg) [IU]	4 [160]	10 [400]	—	10 [400]	5 [200]	—	3 [120]
E[f](mg) [IU]	2.8 [2.8]	7 [7]	—	6.4 [6.4]	10 [10]	—	[g]
K_1(μg)	80	200	—	200	0	—	150
Thiamin[h] (mg)	0.35	1.2	1.2	—	3	1.24	—
Riboflavin[i] (mg)	0.15	1.4	1.4	—	3.6	2.47	—
Pyridoxine[h] (mg)	0.18	1	1	—	4	2.43	—
Niacin[j] (mg)	6.8	17	17	—	40	10	—
Pantothenate (mg)	2[k]	5[k]	5	—	15[k]	10	—
Biotin (μg)	6	20	20	—	60	300	—
Folate (μg)	56	140	140	—	400	200	—
Cobalamin (B_{12})(μg)	0.3	1	1	—	5	2	—
Ascorbate (mg)	25	80	80	—	100	34	—

[a]For International System equivalent units, see Appendix Table A-1a.

[b]Proposed by Greene HL, Hambidge M, Schanler R, et al. Am J Clin Nutr 1988;48:1324–42 (rev. reprint issued Dec 1990); not commercially available.

[c]Kabi-Pharmacia. Data from Dahl GB, Svensson L, Kinnander NJG, et al. JPEN 1994;18:235, Table 1. The daily unit dose of Vitalipid Infant contains soybean oil 1000 mg, phospholipids 120 mg, glycerol 225 mg, NaOH to pH 8, water to 10 mL.

[d]May be in divided form and different volumes.

[e]As retinol or retinyl palmitate.

[f]As DL-α-tocopherol acetate.

[g]Vitamin E from soybean oil.

[h]As the hydrochloride.

[i]As the phosphate.

[j]As niacinamide.

[k]As dexpanthenol.

Table 101.12
Excipients and Their Distribution in Commercial Parenteral Multivitamin Solutions (per daily dose) in the United States

Ingredient	Function	Pediatric MVI-Pediatric[a] 5 mL[b]	Adult MVI-12[a] 10 mL[c]
Polysorbate 80	Surfactant; emulsifier	50 mg	1.6[d]
Polysorbate 20	Surfactant; emulsifier	0.8 mg	0.28%
Gentisic acid ethanolamide	Solubilizer; stabilizer; preservative	—	2%[e]
Propylene glycol	Stabilizer	—	30%[d]
Butylated hydroxytoluene	Lipid antioxidant	0.058 mg	0.002%
Butylated hydroxyanisole	Lipid antioxidant	0.014 mg	0.0005%
Citric acid, sodium citrate, and/or sodium hydroxide	Buffer	Present	Present
Mannitol	Lyophilization aid	375 (mg)	—

[a]Manufactured by Armour, Kankakee, IL, for Astra Pharmaceutical Products, Westborough, MA.
[b]On reconstitution of lyophilized product.
[c]In two vials of 5 mL: vial 2 contains biotin, folate, and B_{12}; vial 1 has the other vitamins (see Table 101.11). Also available as two chambers and single-dose vial, and as multi-dose vial with the same excipients.
[d]In vials 1 and 2
[e]In vial 1 only.

unstable when exposed to direct sunlight for a matter of hours (208). Thiamin, folate, riboflavin, and pyridoxine are stable under fluorescent light.

Addition of the multivitamin solution to other PN constituents presents the possibility of some loss of specific vitamins. Thiamin is split and so loses biologic activity in the presence of sulfite compounds (209) that are components of amino acid solutions in the United States; hence, multivitamin solutions should not be added directly to undiluted amino acid solutions but rather to the ultimate solution shortly before infusion into the patient. Ascorbic acid is progressively lost in the presence of Cu^{2+} and oxygen (210). Folate is stable when the PN solution has the usual pH between 5.0 and 6.0 (211).

Adult Needs

The issue of vitamin needs for the sick and injured has long been of concern. Varying amounts of vitamins have been administered to postoperative and other patients who are receiving PN, with differing intervals between the times of vitamin infusion and those of blood sampling; blood levels have been the usual criteria, although some investigators have used enzymatic methods. Few investigators have completely surveyed all 13 vitamins. Much of the published data obtained in seriously ill adult patients is based on information gathered from a few weeks to a few months, the critical time range for most patients. These data indicate a relatively narrow range of requirements for certain of these nutrients, and adequate blood levels or related enzyme activities may be attained in hypercatabolic patients with daily infusion dosages for some that are appreciably below the old MVI concentrate formula and in some cases, below, at, or not far above, the AMA-FDA adult dosages (212–214).

The adequacy of the adult AMA-FDA formulation was tested in 16 adults with severe malabsorption or intestinal obstruction who had been receiving HPN for 1 to 9 years. These patients were studied serially over many months on this formulation (MVI-12) (210). Blood was sampled at least 36 hours after the preceding infusion of vitamins was terminated. Mean values for plasma vitamin A were near or above the upper limit of reference values, in part because five subjects had renal insufficiency; the high values were associated with elevated retinol-binding protein levels. Thiamin, pyridoxine, niacin, biotin, riboflavin, vitamin B_{12}, and folate levels were within the reference ranges for all subjects; pantothenate levels tended to be within or above the reference ranges, thiamin tended to be toward the lower half of the reference range, as did vitamin E levels. In addition to the label amount of 10 mg/dL α-tocopherol acetate, additional vitamin E was given as a constituent of the intravenous lipid. The low plasma lipid levels of these patients tended to decrease circulating vitamin E levels. A few subjects had ascorbic acid values persistently below 0.3 mg/dL, which may have been caused by loss of this vitamin during storage for 30 hours. Levels of 25-OH vitamin D and $1,25(OH)_2$ vitamin D in eight individuals over 430 to 588 days on MVI-12 were within reference range, as were parathormone levels. Prothrombin times were normal, with 5 mg of vitamin K oxide added once per week (210).

In another study, the plasma vitamin E levels measured in patients over 28 to 250 days on this formulation rose from 2.1 ± 4.6 to 16.5 ± 4.6 μmol/L (mean ± SD) (208). In a study using some of the same patients as in ref. 210 on HPN, the same multivitamins, and twice the volume of Intralipid, plasma α-tocopherol levels of 17.5 ± 6.6 μmol in seven patients were not statistically different from values in controls (215). When a different source of vitamin E was given to patients on long-term HPN, the average plasma α-tocopherol level was 11.14 μmol/L (normal, 18.11 μmol/L), and there were significantly higher breath pentane levels (a measure of lipid peroxidation) than in controls (216).

The amounts of vitamin E present in Intralipid as α-tocopherol are given in Table 101.5 together with concentrations of other isomers. (See Chapter 19 for a discussion of vitamin E isomer activities.) In addition, as noted in this table, lipid emulsions contain appreciable amounts of vitamin K, with roughly twice as much in those containing soybean oil only. Consequently, with regular lipid infusions, separate vitamin K infusions may be reduced or eliminated (217, 218).

A major function of vitamin D is improved efficiency of absorption of calcium and phosphate by the small intestine. PN bypasses this route, so why is this vitamin included in parenteral solutions? Calcitriol, as the active form of vitamin D, plays an intimate role with parathyroid hormone in bone turnover; the vitamin also plays a role in cellular differentiation (see Chapter 18). Whether the current parenteral dosage recommendations are higher than necessary for these functions remains to be demonstrated.

Pediatric Needs

Greene et al. summarized research on vitamin levels in term-gestation infants and children and problems related to the needs of preterm and underweight newborn infants (160, 219). They concluded that the vitamin dosages suggested for children in the 1975 AMA report were adequate for continued use in term infants and children up to 11 years of age. This formulation is commercially available as MVI-Pediatric (Table 101.11). Use of this formulation for underweight infants was found to increase blood tocopherol to a high level; the manufacturer and the FDA then recommended that the daily dose be reduced successively to 65% and then to one-third of a vial for infants weighing less than 1000 g. The last level may prove too low. Further problems have surfaced in providing this formulation to very LBW infants, including large losses of retinol through the delivery sets and elevated riboflavin and vitamin B_6 plasma concentrations (219). Greene et al. recommended a revised formulation for the very LBW infant (160) (Table 101.11); currently, this is not in production. When a European pediatric fat-soluble multivitamin formulation (Vitalipid Infant) and a water-soluble multivitamin formula (Soluvit Infant) (Table 101.11) were administered as part of Intralipid 10%, the vitamins had good stability for up to 24 hours, except for ascorbic acid (50% loss); the emulsion was stable for 24 hours (220).

Thiamin Deficiency

There continue to be reports of severe thiamin deficiency in adult patients receiving PN. This occurs despite *(a)* the availability and safety of its parenteral preparation in multivitamin or individual form, *(b)* widespread knowledge of its increased need with use of high-glucose formulas, *(c)* its demonstrated instability in contact with the sulfite in amino acids, necessitating minimum storage at room temperature before use (220a) and *(d)* the fairly rapid onset (1–2 months) of life-threatening metabolic changes characteristic of its deficiency. Unfortunately, the problem has been complicated by periodic production difficulties in the U.S. resulting in nationwide shortages (221, 221a). In six published reports in a period of 3 years, 15 cases have been described (221–225) with four deaths (221, 225); 14 patients had severe lactic acidosis (221, 221a, 224), and 4 had peripheral neuropathy and/or ataxia (221a, 225).

COMPLICATIONS OF ORGAN FUNCTION

Complications related to vascular access, catheter-related sepsis, concentration problems resulting from formula composition, and underlying diseases are discussed above. They can be prevented or minimized by having responsibility vested in experienced physicians, nurses, dietitians, and pharmacists working as a team that closely supervises their inpatients and outpatients (226). Here we discuss certain disorders related directly to intravenous feeding, including liver dysfunction, gallstones, and decreased bone mass.

Hepatic Dysfunction

Children

Since the first description of PN-associated cholestasis and early cirrhosis in 1971 in a premature infant (227), a large and continuing literature has confirmed PN as a contributing risk factor for hepatobiliary dysfunction of varying degree and incidence. Reviews of the biochemical, clinical, and histopathologic changes in adults and children have emphasized the multifactorial nature of the problem (228, 229). In children, the degree of prematurity, infection, inability to consume food orally, extent of intestinal dysfunction, number of surgical procedures, duration of PN, and long-term administration of excessive calories are associated risk factors (228–231). Immaturity of the hepatic excretory function and the enterohepatic circulation, particularly in the neonate, is one reason for development of cholestasis. Cholestasis has been reported in various series to occur in 7.4 to 42.1% of infants, with wide variations among differing populations, criteria, hospital practices, and clinical conditions (232).

Intravenous lipid emulsions with their endogenous content of phytosterols from vegetable oils were addressed as a potential cause of cholestatic liver disease in a preliminary study of children (233). Five of 29 patients who were receiving PN and had severe cholestatic liver disease had significantly increased concentrations of campesterol, stigmasterol, sitosterol, and isofucosterol (all phytosterols); they also had elevated concentrations of cholestanol and sitostanol (a phytostanol). The 24 patients receiving PN who did not have severe cholestatic disease had normal or slightly elevated phytosterol levels. Thrombocytopenia, a common complication in patients with hereditary phytosterolemia, was clearly evident in the 5 patients with severe cholestatic liver disease. The dose of intravenous fat emulsion was substantially higher in the 5 patients with liver disease than in the other 24 patients (233). Possible relationship of high blood manganese to the development of cholestasis was mentioned above (180).

Fatty liver (steatosis), intrahepatic cholestasis, and portal inflammation can occur, particularly in children, but also in adults. It can progress to portal tract fibrosis and infiltration, liver failure, and death.

Adults

In adults, preexisting liver and other diseases, sepsis, preexisting malnutrition, extent of bowel resection and/or damage (such as from radiation), excess nonprotein calories, little or no oral intake, and duration on PN are also associated risk factors. Increases may occur in serum transaminase, alkaline phosphatase, γ-glutamyltransferase (GGT) and, less frequently, bilirubin as indicators of hepatic dysfunction.

Adult patients receiving long-term PN (median, 18 months) who were given relative excesses of carbohydrate, fat, and amino acids showed abnormal hepatic function and cholestatic changes. When the amounts of these macronutrients were reduced, jaundice was reversed and liver function tests and histologic features improved (234). Other investigators noted increasing steatosis with administration of excess calories as carbohydrate or lipid or both (235, 236). Forty-three patients who received PN were randomized to receive either glucose as the sole nonprotein calorie source or a combination of glucose and fat. The dose of nonprotein energy used in this study was moderate compared with that in many of the previous studies. Even though the patients were not dramatically overfed (1.5 times calculated basal energy expenditure), alkaline phosphatase and GGT increased significantly in both groups. Aspartate aminotransferase (AST), alanine aminotransferase (ALT), and direct bilirubin increased more in the group receiving only glucose as nonprotein calories. It appears that liver enzyme laboratory tests are affected by administration of PN, even when used in moderate doses and when part of the energy dose is given as intravenous lipid emulsion (237).

Data from various studies strongly suggest that patients with little or no remaining small intestine are at increased risk of developing serious hepatic dysfunction with fibrotic changes; the rapidity of development and the severity of the disease vary among series (data and literature review in ref. 238). Unlike in children, actual liver failure in adults is uncommon.

Amelioration or Prevention

A variety of agents have been tested on patients receiving PN who have developed evidence of associated significant hepatic dysfunction and who require continued PN. Giving a mixture of MCT and LCT to PN patients as the intravenous lipid source did not cause a change in liver size or gray-scale value, whereas LCT infusion increased both (128). On the grounds that metronidazole could depress formation by intestinal bacteria of potentially damaging bile acids, this drug has been tested in patients receiving PN and has been reported by some to reduce increases in liver enzymes compared with untreated control subjects (229, 239). Ursodeoxycholic acid (UDCA), an epimer of chenodeoxycholic acid, has been given with benefit to adults (240) and children (241) on long-term PN who developed cholestatic liver disease. Jaundice and enzyme abnormalities regressed, and their clinical condition improved. Discontinuance of the UDCA resulted in an increase in liver enzymes, which again regressed when this drug was administered. UDCA given intravenously for 3 weeks to newborn piglets on PN was effective in reducing cholestasis by normalizing bile flow, bile acid secretion, and the bilirubin content of liver and serum; bile composition remained abnormal (242).

Cholecystokinin in synthetic form was given intravenously twice daily from onset of PN for at least 14 days to 26 neonates on PN in a case-matched study; its use was associated with a significant trend toward lower serum direct bilirubin levels (242a). Choline as such or as lecithin has been reported to decrease hepatic steatosis, (243 and Chapter 32). Treatment of hepatic complications of PN has been reviewed recently (244).

Gallstones

Sludge in the gallbladder has been observed repeatedly as a PN- and bowel rest–associated risk factor; this situation can progress to gallstone formation as the duration of PN increases. Patients who receive long-term PN maintenance because of resection or disease of the terminal ileum usually malabsorb bile salts. Thus, the bile salt pool decreases, and lower levels of bile salts are present in the gallbladder. This situation, in turn, increases the tendency of cholesterol to precipitate in the bile forming the nidus of gallstones. There is also an increase in unconjugated bilirubin and calcium, which are present in the stones that form from the accumulated sludge in the gallbladder (245). Impaired gallbladder contraction is important. Ultrasonography indicated development of biliary sludge within 12 days of starting PN in 14 of 23 patients. By 6 weeks, all had sludge, with 6 developing stones and 3 requiring surgery. The sludge disappeared 4 weeks after instituting oral feeding (246). Stasis and resulting sludge were prevented in the PN prairie dog model given daily injections of cholecystokinin (247a). When chenodeoxycholate was given intravenously to a group of prairie dogs on PN for about 40 days, they did not develop gallstone or calcium bilirubinate crystals; the controls on TPN only had gallstones (5 of 6) or crystals (6 of 6) (247b).

Gallstones are a significant problem in adults, but even more so in children on PN. For example, 9 of 29 children developed cholelithiasis; 64% of these with ileal disorders or resections developed stones (248); 6 of 13 children with less than 38 cm of small bowel remaining required a cholecystectomy (249). In a Paris hospital, the frequency of gallstones led to a policy of routine cholecystectomy whenever total or subtotal resection of the terminal ileum was performed (250). Emergency cholecystectomy in PN patients is not a benign procedure; for example, the operative morbidity was 54% and hospital mortality was 11% in 35 patients (23 adult, 12 children) with PN-associated gallbladder disease (251).

These potential problems have led to the following suggestions for management of such patients at risk: if food can be ingested safely, it should be taken orally or by tube routinely in an effort to decrease biliary stasis; ultrasonic examination should be performed periodically to detect development of biliary sludge and stones; when stones are first detected, elective cholecystectomy should be considered; if laparotomy is to be done for any reason, cholecystectomy should be considered at that time. Meanwhile, clinical studies continue on UDCA.

Metabolic Bone Disease

Rickets has been described in infants receiving PN (252). The causative factor appeared to be a need for more calcium and phosphate in the small fluid volume required by the neonate, rather than more vitamin D.

Reference has been made above to the effects of aluminum contamination on bone (200). When contaminated casein hydrolysate was replaced by crystalline amino acids, increased bone formation occurred with reduced osteoid area, decreased amounts of aluminum at the bone surface and in plasma, and reduced calcium excretion (253).

The histomorphologic features of bone were examined in relation to formula composition in patients receiving long-term HPN who were not subsisting on aluminum-contaminated casein hydrolysate. In a prospective study in Toronto by Shike et al., bone biopsies of HPN patients initially showed a hyperkinetic pattern, possibly resulting from initial malnutrition; at 6 to 73 months on HPN, the histologic features changed, with 12 of 16 patients having some degree of osteomalacia (254). In this study, 500 IU (12.5 μg, or 32.5 nmol) of vitamin D_2 were given every other day; all other vitamins were supplied, except biotin. Because 7 of these patients were hypercalcemic and 6 had elevated 25(OH) vitamin D levels, further studies were performed on 11 patients before and after withdrawal of vitamin D_2 (and, by necessity, the accompanying vitamin A) for 6 months (255). Six of 10 patients had less osteoid and increased tetracycline uptake with the vitamin modification, but there was continuing evidence of a high turnover rate. In the three symptomatic patients, bone pain subsided, fractures healed, and urinary loss of calcium and phosphate was decreased. It was recommended that vitamin D solutions not be added to PN solutions of home patients (255). The mechanism of the postulated adverse role of this vitamin was not delineated.

Others have noted improvement in HPN patients with respect to bone fractures and pain following withdrawal of vitamin D from the PN formulations (literature review and new data in [256]). Withdrawal of vitamin D for 4.5 ± 0.2 years from nine HPN patients with low parathyroid hormone (PTH) and calcitriol levels was associated with normalization of these values and some increase in lumbar spine bone mineral; there was no decrease in the mean level of calcidiol (256).

In a study in New York City of 12 HPN patients given crystalline amino acids (with the exception of two who had been transferred from casein hydrolysate 6 years earlier), the average daily vitamin D intake over the years had been 284 IU (7.1 μg) replaced 3 to 10 months earlier by 200 IU (5 μg) daily. Histomorphometry with tetracycline labeling revealed osteopenia, subnormal osteoid volume, and normal trabecular osteoid seam width; the calcification rate was normal. Of the seven women, four were in the 66- to 77-year range, and at least one had been a heavy cigarette smoker for many years. Six patients had minor bone complaints associated with osteoarthritis or postmenopausal osteoporosis (257). Serum calcium, PTH, and calcitriol values were normal. The reasons for the marked difference in the histologic features of bone between the Toronto and New York studies are not apparent, but there were some formula differences. The PN formulas in the New York study had appreciably fewer fat calories, proportionately more glucose calories, and a different vitamin formulation, including biotin.

A longitudinal study of bone with regional densitometry and bone biopsy was performed in 14 patients on long-term PN who had either never been on protein hydrolysate or not for at least 7 years (258). Most subjects had osteopenia with heterogeneity in bone status, complaints of bone pain, and some documented fractures while on HPN; all 11 females were amenorrheic. In the follow-up period (27 ± 14 months), some patients had improved bone mass, some had no change, and others lost bone. Serum calcium, which had been low at baseline in six, normalized in most; PTH was high in five; calcitriol was normal.

It has been suggested that PN patients lose a significant amount of bone mass early as a result of hypocalcemia that then stabilizes. Amenorrhea and/or smoking are also factors. The conclusion is that osteopenia is characteristic of long-term PN patients but that present PN formulations do not necessarily cause deterioration of bone health and may benefit some (258). A trial of antiresorptive therapy is indicated.

COMPATIBILITY OF DRUGS WITH PN SOLUTIONS

The frequency of drug interventions for coexistent illnesses or complications of PN requires ensuring that administering a drug as part of the PN solution or in conjunction with that solution will not produce incompatibility or an adverse reaction. Significant information on this issue has been summarized (259, 259a). Table 101.13 contains compatibility information for PN solutions and many

Table 101.13
Compatibilities of Selected Drugs in Parenteral Nutrition Solutions

Drugs compatible with PN solutions		
Dextrose/amino acids		*Total nutrient admixtures*
Albumin		Albumin
Cimetidine		Cimetidine
Famotidine		Famotidine
Folic acid		Heparin
Heparin		Regular human insulin
Hydrochloric acid		Metoclopramide
Regular human insulin		Phytonadione
Iron dextran		Ranitidine
Metoclopramide		Thiamin
Phytonadione		
Ranitidine		
Thiamin		
Drugs incompatible with PN solutions		
Dextrose/amino acids		*Total nutrient admixtures*
Amphotericin B		Amphotericin B
Ampicillin		Hydrochloric acid
Metronidazole (with $NaHCO_3$)		Iron dextran
Phenytoin		Methyldopa
		Phenytoin
Drugs incompatible with PN solutions with simulated Y-site administration		
Acyclovir	Doxorubicin	Minocycline
Amphotericin B	Fluorouracil	Mitoxantrone
Cefazolin	Furosemide	Potassium phosphate
Ciprofloxacin	Ganciclovir	Promethazine
Cisplatin	Methotrexate	Sodium bicarbonate
Cyclosporine	Metoclopramide	
Cytarabine	Midazolam	

commonly used drugs. Both dextrose/amino acid PN solutions and TNAs are listed in this table. Drugs that can or should be administered as continous infusions and that are compatible with PN solutions are ideal additives, especially in the critical care setting where fluid intake often must be regulated. Not all combinations of drugs and different PN solutions have been studied. Also, some drugs are compatible in traditional dextrose/amino acid PN solutions but not in TNAs (e.g., iron dextran). Still other drugs are compatible in PN solutions because they are diluted in a large volume of fluid and are incompatible when given during Y-site administration with the same PN solution. This problem undoubtedly occurs because the drug concentration is high when coinfused with PN through the same tubing. Trissel et al. (259a) found that 82 of 102 drugs were compatible during Y-site administration with PN solutions; the 20 incompatible drugs are listed in Table 101.13.

HOME PARENTERAL NUTRITION

Since the first patients were discharged from hospital to home on PN in 1969 and the early 1970s, in the United States and Canada (260–262), HPN as primary outpatient nutritional support has mushroomed. An HPN registry for the United States and Canada was established at the New York Academy of Medicine during the years 1978 to 1983 to collect and compile the data being accrued by an increasing number of medical centers who discharged patients on HPN. Data were distributed regularly to participants and interested parties (263, 264). In 1984, this registry became a joint effort of the Oley Foundation and the American Society for Enteral and Parenteral Nutrition, originally designated the OASIS Registry and, more recently, the North American Home Parenteral and Enteral Nutrition Patient Registry (HPRN Registry) produced by the Oley Foundation.

Issues related to suitability, training, formulations, and home support have been extensively studied (265), and standards on organization, patient selection, and management have been developed (266). Benefits and current issues are discussed in this and other chapters.

Patient Numbers and Categories

Because Medicare in the U.S. is the largest single payer for HPN, its data provide useful information on national use, growth, and costs (267, 268). In 1992, an estimated 10,035 Medicare beneficiaries were on HPN of the total Medicare enrollment of 34,853,000, at an expenditure of $156 million. Based on the figures for patients in the HPEN Registry in 1992, with 25% covered by Medicare, it was estimated that 40,000 patients used HPN therapy in that year, with 54% percent supported by private insurance (267). The age distribution of HPN changed over the period 1978 to 1988: the percentage of those 10 years of age or less roughly doubled, and the percentage of those over 65 years tripled.

Of the 5481 HPN patients entering the registry during their first year on therapy between 1985 and 1992, the 10 top specific diagnoses in percentages were neoplasm 40.4, Crohn's disease 10.8, ischemic bowel 6.2, motility disorders 5.7, AIDS 5.5, congenital bowel disease 3.3, chronic pancreatitis 3.0, radiation enteritis 2.7, chronic obstruction 2.3, and cystic fibrosis 1.0 (267, 268).

Patient Outcome

Detailed data have been published for 11 diagnoses concerning survival, likelihood of rehabilitation to full and to partial function, and frequency of HPN and non-HPN complications (268). Annual survival rates of those with gastrointestinal (GI) diseases were 87% or better, with a 50 to 73% likelihood of complete rehabilitation in 1 year except for those with radiation enteritis or obstruction with chronic adhesions. In the three most common GI diseases (Crohn's disease, ischemic bowel disease, and motility disorders), survival rates over 1 year for patients 18 years or less was about 95%; for those 35 to 55, 90%; and for those 65 and older, about 70%. Younger patients were more likely to resume full oral nutrition and have more complete rehabilitation, but they had more septic admissions. The registry to 1992 lists 66 patients with these three GI diseases plus radiation enteritis who have survived 15 to 20 years on HPN. Only about 30% of cancer patients on HPN were alive at 6 months, and 20% at 1 year (268). The mortality of AIDS patients at 1 year was 90%; decreased use of HPN is likely if the reported effectiveness of newer medications in HIV patients continues.

The frequency of HPN-related complications was similar in all diagnostic groups: one to two rehospitalizations per year, one-half because of sepsis (268). Complications associated with HPN accounted for only 5% of deaths. If earlier experience continues to be true (263), a minority of patients account for a majority of rehospitalizations.

The organization, care, and outcome of PN in European countries has been summarized (269, 270). In certain European countries, France, Italy, Denmark, and probably others, care of HPN is restricted to approved specialist centers, and in the U.K., two adult centers managed one-half the number of registered patients (269). Adult patients (n = 217) with nonmalignant non-HIV chronic intestinal failure in HPN programs in approved programs in Belgium (n = 2) and France (n = 7) from 1980 through 1989 had survival probabilities of 91% at 1 year, 70% at 3 years, and 62% at 5 years, with better survival after 1987, with younger age, and with no chronic intestinal obstruction (270). In the U.K. in 1994, 4 to 5 patients per million received HPN at any one time in the course of a year. The actual number is approximately two or three times greater.

One of the more dramatic successes of HPN is the much better outcome of the newborn with abnormalities of the gastrointestinal tract requiring extensive intestinal resection. In a Los Angeles HPN program for the years 1977 to 1984, 13 children were left with less than 38 cm of remaining jejunum and ileum (JI) beginning in the first month of life; of these, 69% survived, compared with 23% previously (248). Five of these had HPN discontinued after 4 to 32 months and had normal growth and development; whereas two remained on partial HPN after 9 and 55 months, and two required PN after 66 and 68 months; these four children have grown normally. Of those with 15 to 38 cm without an ileocecal valve (ICV) and those with less than 15 cm with and without an ICV, 70% survived (compared with none in Wilmore's review of 1972 [270a]); 3 of the 10 discontinued HPN. Ultimate survival with normal growth and without HPN is now possible with as little as 11 cm residual JI and an intact ICV and as little as 25 cm JI without an ICV (248).

The course of 87 children with major resections managed from 1970 to 1988 in a Paris hospital have been analyzed. HPN was introduced in 1980. Fourteen of the 16 deaths occurred before 1980. Of those with less than 40 cm of JI who were born before 1980, 42% survived. Of those born after 1980, 94% in this category survived. The presence of an ICV did not significantly affect survival. The average time needed for adequate bowel adaptation was 27.3 months for those with less than 40 cm and 14 months for those with 40 to 80 cm (249).

Quality of Life and Support Needs

HPN presents various stresses to the patient and family members (271), including the sudden need to cope with the technical aspects, time demands, and safety issues of HPN after hospital discharge; management of handicaps resulting from primary and secondary illness and their treatments; concerns about meeting costs; patient dependency; and excessive dependence on others. A smooth transition to home care requires *(a)* adequate predischarge assessment and training of the patient and family in HPN management and *(b)* close support by the health-care team via telephone contact and follow-up at home or in the physician's office to ensure that the patient's condition remains satisfactory. Dietary intake and other factors at home may require modification of the PN formulation from that deemed satisfactory in the hospital setting.

Data are available from a survey of 178 randomly selected families with a member on HPN for an average of 4.6 years, with 116 follow-up questionnaires (272). Patient and caregiver mean family scores for quality-of-life, self-esteem, life satisfaction, family cohesion, and quality of patient-caregiver relationship were similar to published norms for other healthy populations and other groups of chronically ill patients. HPN family adaptability and coping scores were higher. There were problems associated with financial strain and mild depression in patients related to increasing duration of PN and being barred from work (although able to) because of their disability classification.

Issues concerning nutritional support decision making for the competent and incompetent patient and for the terminally ill are reviewed in Chapter 102 and elsewhere (265, 266, 273).

Cost-Effectiveness

Estimates of the cost of HPN vary from $75,000 to $150,000 per patient-year (273). Many factors enter into the total cost of maintaining a patient on HPN; such charges vary considerably, depending in part on the method used in their estimations and on differences in the perspectives chosen for the analyses, particularly the matter of estimating benefits gained and/or the effectiveness gained. Goel has discussed these issues and has reviewed the pertinent literature relating to hospital PN and to HPN (274). Daily costs of HPN were estimated to be 60 to 70% lower than those of hospital PN. Goel has also summarized factors involved in cost-effectiveness analysis, the variability in determining precise costs, and the inclusion of effectiveness as measured by quality-adjusted life-year (QALY)—a composite measure of life expectancy and morbidity.

A cost-effectiveness analysis of HPN in a cohort of 72 patients from 1970 to 1982 in Toronto was compared with the alternative costs that would have accrued from intermittent hospital care, including PN on each admission for the same patients not receiving HPN. It was concluded that HPN was cost-effective (275). In commenting on his study (275) and others, Detsky said, "Home Parenteral Nutrition is indeed a mature technology that almost certainly provides considerable survival benefit and reasonable quality of life. The estimated incremental cost-effectiveness ratio for this technology is attractive when it is delivered in patients without disseminated cancer or advanced HIV disease" (276).

SMALL BOWEL TRANSPLANTATION

Successful small bowel transplantation was demonstrated to be technically feasible in laboratory animals in the late 1950s (277). Until the late 1980s, attempts were unsuccessful in patients because the immunosuppressive drugs available in that period could not prevent rejection of the transplanted intestine (277, 278). With the availability of cyclosporine and tacrolimus, single successful transplants (of several or more attempts) of isolated bowel were reported from Kiev and Paris (278), and a successful combined liver–small bowel transplantation was performed in London, Ontario (279). Three types of intestinal allografts are now being performed. For example, between May 1990 and February 1995, the University of Pittsburgh's transplantation group performed 71 small bowel transplantations in 67 patients: 23 received an isolate intestine, 32 a combined intestine and liver, and 23 a multivisceral transplant (280, 281).

A series of recent reviews summarize techniques, problems, advances, and results in the U.S. (280–283), and internationally (284). Of the 62 intestinal transplant patients reviewed by Lee et al., only 36 (58%) were alive at a median follow-up of 594 days, and only 31 (50%) were alive and retaining a functioning graft (281). In Grant's review of 180 intestinal transplantations performed between 1985 and June 1995, in 170 patients (two-thirds of whom were children), graft/patient survival (%) at 1 and 3 years with cyclosporine immunosuppression was, respectively, 17/57 and 11/50 for small bowel only, 44/44 and 28/28 for intestine plus liver, and 41/41 for multiviscera (284). With the use of tacrolimus the corresponding figures were 65/83 and 29/47, 64/66 and 38/40, and 51/59 and 37/43. Of the 86 survivors, 67 had stopped PN and resumed oral nutrition, 10 required partial PN, and 9 were on PN after removal of their graft. Successful small-bowel grafts can absorb oral nutrients, including fat, despite denervation and disruption of lymphatics at the time of surgery.

The review of the International Intestinal Transplant Registry concludes: "to become the standard treatment for intestinal failure, transplantation must offer greater safety, lower costs, and a better quality of life than PN." While progress has been made, "further refinements are needed before bowel transplantation becomes a routine surgical procedure" (284). Intestinal transplantation to date has been considered and performed in the context of serious hepatobiliary disease or loss of venous access, both secondary to PN complications (282–284).

EFFECTS OF TROPHIC AGENTS

Standard PN solutions cannot adequately support patients whose catabolic state is so advanced that they cannot develop a net positive peripheral uptake of amino acids despite adequate provision of energy and known essential nutrients (285, 287) (see also Chapter 96). Strategies that have been adopted to try to improve this situation have included *(a)* having the patient perform regular exercise (285); *(b)* providing increased amounts of such nutrients such as arginine, BCAAs, n-3 polyunsaturated fatty acids (286), glutamine (Chapters 35 and 98); *(c)* blocking the signals of interleukins, which initiate responses to inflammation (286, 287); *(d)* providing hormones and related growth factors that appear to enhance protein retention, such as recombinant human growth hormone (Chapter 96), insulin-like growth factor–1 (IGF-1) (Chapter 96), the β-adrenergic agonist clenbuterol, and low-dose bradykinin (288); and *(e)* a combination of the above (see Chapters 35, 96, and 98).

The concept of using trophic agents with modified diet

has now been applied in an open study to selected patients with short bowel syndrome requiring HPN, in an effort to increase hyperplasia and hypertrophy. Some 47 long-term patients who had no cancer, diabetes, dysmotility, inflammatory obstructive symptoms, or active inflammatory bowel disease were hospitalized on a regimen of diet (60% carbohydrate, 20% fat, 20% protein), glutamine (0.6 g/kg/day) orally and r methionyl growth hormone (0.14 mg/kg/day) parenterally for 26 days (289). They were discharged on 30 g glutamine/day and the diet. After 4 weeks, 27 of the subjects were off PN, 14 were on reduced PN, and 6 were continued on PN. After 5 months to 5 years, 19 patients (40%) were off PN, an equal number were on reduced PN, and 9 (20%) were on their original PN formula. Multicenter trials of this therapy are under way (289).

A more-recent study of eight long-term HPN patients compared the effects on bowel function of a similar triple regimen with those of placebo in a randomized, double-blind, crossover format (289a). Although the treated patients had modest improvements in sodium and potassium absorption and in gastric emptying delay, there were no consistent improvements in small bowel morphology, stool losses, or macronutrient absorption. The two studies (289, 289a) differed with respect to duration, degree of bowel resection, hospital stay and supervision, and routes of medication administration; nevertheless, the very different outcomes indicate the need for additional well-controlled studies (289b).

Exogenous epidermal growth factor (EGF) (290, 291), glucagon-like peptide 2 (GLP-2) (292), IGF-1 (293), and TNF-α (294) have induced mucosal or mucosal cell proliferation of small animals. These peptides may prove to have value in improving human intestinal proliferation in patients with the short bowel syndrome.

REFERENCES

1. Elman R. Parenteral alimentation in surgery. New York: Paul B. Hoeber, 1947.
2. Gamble JL. Pediatrics 1953;11:554–67.
3. Levenson SM, Hopkin BS, Waldron M, et al. Fed Proc 1984;43:1391–406.
4. Seibert FB. Am J Physiol 1923;67:90–104.
5. DuBois EF. Basal metabolism in health and disease. Philadelphia: Lea & Febiger, 1924;237–88.
6. Cuthbertson DP. Q J Med 1932;1:233–46.
7. Spies TD, ed. Med Clin North Am 1943;27:273–600.
8. Levenson SM, Green RW, Lund CC. Ann Surg 1946;124: 840–56.
9. Ellison EH, McCleery RS, Zollinger RM, et al. Surgery 1949;26:374–83.
10. Schuberth O, Wretlind A. Acta Chir Scand 1961;278 (Suppl):1–21.
11. Dudrick S, Wilmore DW, Vars HM, et al. Surgery 1968;64: 134–42.
12. Winters RW, Heird WC, Dell RB. Fed Proc 1984;43:1407–11.
13. Shils ME. Fed Proc 1984;43:1412–6.
14. Co Tui, Wright AM, Mulholland JH, et al. Ann Surg 1944;120:99–122.
15. Co Tui, Wright AM, Mulholland JH, et al. Gastroenterology 1945;5:5–17.
16. Watkin DM, Steinfeld JL. Am J Clin Nutr 1965;16:182–212.
17. Wolk RA, Rayburn WF. Nutr Clin Pract 1990;5:139–52.
18. Chin DE, Kearns P. Nutr Clin Pract 1991;6:213–22.
19. Ott L, Young B. Nutr Clin Pract 1991;6:223–9.
20. Veterans Affairs Total Parenteral Nutrition Cooperative Study Group. N Engl J Med 1991;325:525–32.
21. Detsky AS. Editorial. N Engl J Med 1991;325:573–5.
22. Campos AC, Meguid MM. Am J Clin Nutr 1992;55:117–30.
23. Wolfe BM, Mathiesen KA. JPEN J Parenter Enteral Nutr 1997;21:1–6.
24. Stokes MA, Hill GL. JPEN J Parenter Enteral Nutr 1993; 17:145–7.
25. Kearns PJ, Coleman S, Wehner JH. JPEN J Parenter Enteral Nutr 1996;20:20–4.
26. Dudrick SJ, Wilmore DW, Vars HM, et al. Ann Surg 1969;169:974–84.
27. Jeejeebhoy KN, Zohrab WJ, Langer B, et al. Gastroenterology 1973;65:811–20.
28. Broviac JW, Cole JJ, Scribner BH. Surg Gynecol Obstet 1973;136:602–6.
29. Joyeux J, Astruc B, Martin G, et al. J Chir (Paris) 1974;107:335–66.
30. Zincke H, Hirsche BL, Amamoo DG, et al. Surg Gynecol Obstet 1974;139:350–2.
31. Heizer WD, Orringer EP. Gastroenterology 1977;72:527–32.
32. Shils ME, Wright WL, Turnbull A, et al. N Engl J Med 1970;283:341–4.
33. Malt RA, Kempter M. JPEN J Parenter Enteral Nutr 1983;7:580–1.
34. Krog M, Gerdin B. JPEN J Parenter Enteral Nutr 1989;13: 666–7.
35. Fonkalsrud EW, Berquist W, Burke M, et al. Am J Surg 1982;143:209–11.
36. Oram-Smith JC, Muller JL, Harken AH, et al. Surgery 1979;83:274–6.
37. Lokich JJ, Bothe A, Benotti P. J Clin Oncol 1985;3:710–7.
38. Mansfield PF. Hohn DC, Fornage BD, et al. N Engl J Med 1994;331:1735–38.
39. Clark-Christoff N, Watters VA, Sparks W, et al. JPEN J Parenter Enteral Nutr 1992;16:403–7.
40. Kemp L, Burge J, Choban P, et al. JPEN J Parenter Enteral Nutr 1994;18:71–4.
41. Timsit JF, Sebille V, Farkas JC, et al. JAMA 1996;276:1416–20.
42. Williams WW. JPEN J Parenter Enteral Nutr 1985;9:735–46.
43. Savage AP, Picard M, Hopkins CC, et al. Br J Surg 1993;80:1287–90.
44. Shils ME. Am J Clin Nutr 1975;28:1429–35.
45. Newsome HH, Armstrong CW, Mayhall GC, et al. JPEN J Parenter Enteral Nutr 1984;8:560–2.
46. Tighe MJ, Kite P, Thomas D, et al. JPEN J Parenter Enteral Nutr 1996;20:215–18.
47. Press OW, Ramsey PG, Larson EB, et al. Medicine 1984;63:189–200.
48. Peterson FB, Clift RA, Hickman RO, et al. JPEN J Parenter Enteral Nutr 1986;10:58–62.
49. Buchman AL, Moukarzel A, Goodman B, et al. JPEN J Parenter Enteral Nutr 1994;18:297–302.
50. O'Keefe SJ, Burnes JU, Thompson RL, JPEN J Parenter Enteral Nutr 1994;18:256–63.

50a. Maki DG, Stolz SM, Wheeler S, et al. Ann Intern Med 1997;127:257–66.

50b. Raad I, Darouiche R, Dupuis J, et al. Ann Intern Med 1997;127:267–74.

51. O'Farrell L, Griffith JW, Lang M. JPEN J Parenter Enteral Nutr 1996;20:156–8.

52. Hill SE, Heldman S, Goo ED, et al. JPEN J Parenteral Enteral Nutr 1996;20:81–7.
53. Food and Drug Administration. Am J Hosp Pharm 1994;51: 1427–8.
54. Allwood MC. Int J Pharm 1986;29:233–6.
55. Tripp MG, Menon SK, Mikrut BA. Am J Hosp Pharm 1990;47: 2496–503.
56. Seres DS. Nutr Clin Pract 1990;5:111–7.
57. McMahon M, Manji N, Driscoll DF, et al. JPEN J Parenter Enteral Nutr 1989;13:545–53.
58. Marcuard SP, Dunham B, Hobbs A, et al. JPEN J Parenter Enteral Nutr 1990;14:262–4.
59. Inder TE, Carr AC, Winterbourn CC, et al. J Pediatr 1995;126:128–31.
60. Smith RC, Burkinshaw L, Hill GL. Gastroenterology 1982;82:445–52.
61. Shaw SN, Elwyn DH, Askanazi J, et al. Am J Clin Nutr 1983;37:930–40.
62. Bessey PQ. Parenteral nutrition in trauma. In: Rombeau JL, Caldwell MD, eds. Parenteral nutrition. 2nd ed. Philadelphia: WB Saunders, 1993;538–65.
63. Rudman E, Millikan WJ, Richardson TJ, et al. J Clin Invest 1975;55:94–104.
64. Wolman SL, Anderson GH, Marliss EB, et al. Gastroenterology 1979;76:458–67.
65. Starker PM, LaSala PA, Forse A, et al. JPEN J Parenter Enteral Nutr 1985;9:300–2.
66. Fryburg DA, Gelfand RA. JPEN J Parenter Enteral Nutr 1990;14:535–7.
67. Woods HF, Alberti KG. Lancet 1972:2:1354–7.
68. Georgieff M, Moldawer LL, Bistrian BR, et al. JPEN J Parenter Enteral Nutr 1985;9:199–209.
69. Young EA, Drummond A, Cool DA, et al. J Clin Endocrinol Metab 1980;50:764–72.
70. Young EA, Fletcher JT, Cioletti LA, et al. JPEN J Parenter Enteral Nutr 1981;5:369–77.
71. Waxman K, Day AT, Stellin GP, et al. JPEN J Parenter Enteral Nutr 1992;16:374–8.
72. Lev-Ram A, Johnson J, Hwang DL, et al. JPEN J Parenter Enteral Nutr 1987;11:271–4.
73. Byrne WJ, Lippe BM, Strobel CT, et al. Gastroenterology 1981;80:947–56.
74. Wagman LD, Miller KB, Thomas RB, et al. Ann Surg 1986;204:524–29.
75. Krzywda A, Andris DA, Whipple JK, et al. JPEN J Parenter Enteral Nutr 1993;17:64–7.
76. Bendorf K, Friesen CA, Roberts CC. JPEN J Parenter Enteral Nutr 1996;20:120–2.
77. Wolfe R, ODonnell TF, Stone MD, et al. Metabolism 1980;29:892–900.
78. Shaw JH, Wolfe RR. Ann Surg 1989;209:63–72.
79. Wolfe RR. Am J Clin Nutr 1996;64:800–8.
80. Flatt JP. The biochemistry of energy expenditure. In: Bray G, ed. Recent advances in obesity research. London: Newman 1978;211–28.
81. Elwyn DH, Gump FE, Munroe HN, et al. Am J Clin Nutr 1979;32:1597–611.
82. Askanazi J, Carpentier YA, Elwyn DH, et al. Ann Surg 1980;191:40–6.
83. MacFie J, Halmfield JH, King RF, et al. JPEN J Parenter Enteral Nutr 1983;7:1–5.
84. Chait A, Foster D, Miller DG, et al. Proc Soc Exp Biol Med 1981;168:97–104.
85. Hongsermeier T, Bistrian BR. JPEN J Parenter Enteral Nutr 1993;17:16–9.
86. Askanazi J, Rosenbaum SH, Hyman AI, et al. JAMA 1980; 243:1444–7.
87. Barr LH, Dunn GD, Brennan MF. Surgery 1981;193:304–11.
88. Carlsson LA. Scand Lab Invest 1980;40:139–44.
89. Carpentier YA. Clin Nutr 1989;8:115–25.
90. Mendez AJ, He LJ, Huang HS, et al. Lipids 1988;23:961–7.
91. Griffin E, Breckenridge C, Kuksis A, et al. J Clin Invest 1979;64:1703–12.
92. Roulet M, Wiesel PH, Pilet M, et al. JPEN J Parenter Enteral Nutr 1993;17:107–12.
93. Rigaud D, Serog P, Legrand A, et al. JPEN J Parenter Enteral Nutr 1984;8:529–34.
94. Adamkin DH, Gelke KN, Andrews BF. JPEN J Parenter Enteral Nutr 1984;8:563–7.
95. Elwyn DH, Kinney JM, Gump FE, et al. Metabolism 1980;29:125–32.
96. Goodenough RD, Wolfe RR. JPEN J Parenter Enteral Nutr 1984;8:357–60.
97. Elwyn DH. Repletion of the malnourished patient. In: Blackburn GL, Grant JP, Young VR, et al., eds. Amino acids: metabolism and medical application. Boston: P.S.G., 1983:359–75.
98. Long JM, Wilmore DW, Mason AD, et al. Ann Surg 1977;185:417–22.
99. Jeejeebhoy KN: Lipid emulsions. In: Fischer JE, ed. Total parenteral nutrition. 2nd ed. Boston: Little, Brown, 1991;410–3.
100. Davis SS. The stability of fat emulsions for intravenous administration. In: Johnson ID, ed. Advances in clinical nutrition. Boston: MTP Press, 1983;214–39.
101. Driscoll DF. Nutr Clin Pract 1995;10:114–9.
102. Driscoll DF, Bhargava HN, Li L, et al. Am J Hosp Pharm 1995;52:623–34.
103. Bullock L, Fitzgerald JF, Walter WV. JPEN J Parenter Enteral Nutr 1992;16:64–8.
104. Simmons BP, Hooten TM, Wang ES, et al. J Natl Intrav Ther Assoc 1982;5:40–6.
105. Rubin M, Bilik R, Aserin A, et al. JPEN J Parenter Enteral Nutr 1989;13:641–3.
106. Pennington CR, Pithie AD. JPEN J Parenter Enteral Nutr 1987;11:507–8.
107. Holcombe BJ, Forloines-Lynn S, Garmhausen LW. J Intrav Nurs 1992;15:36–41.
108. Campbell AN, Freedman MH, Pencharz PB, et al. JPEN J Parenter Enteral Nutr 1984;8:447–9
109. Greene HC, Hazlett D, Demaree R. Am J Clin Nutr 1975;29:127–35.
110. Pereira GR, Fox WW, Stanley CA, et al. Pediatrics 1980;66: 26–30.
111. Sundstrom G, Zaunder CW, Arborelius M. J Appl Physiol 1973;34:816–20.
112. Venus B, Smith RA, Patel C, et al. Chest 1989;95:1278–81.
113. Gutcher GR, Farrell PM. Am J Clin Nutr 1991;54:1024–8.
114. Kollef MH, McCormack MT, Caras WE, et al. Ann Intern Med 1990;112:545–6.
115. Fischer GW, Hunter KW, Wilson SR, et al. Lancet 1980,1: 819–20.
116. Cleary TG, Pickering LK. J Clin Lab Immunol 1983;11:21–6.
117. Sobrado J, Moldawer L, Pomposelli J, et al. Am J Clin Nutr 1985;42:855–63.
118. Seidner DL, Mascioli EA, Istfan NW, et al. JPEN J Parenter Enteral Nutr 1987;13:614–9.
119. Jensen GL, Mascioli EA, Seidner DL, et al. JPEN J Parenter Enteral Nutr 1990;14:467–71
120. Ota DM, Jessup JM, Babcock GE, et al. JPEN J Parenter Enteral Nutr 1985;9:23–7.

121. Muller JM, Keller HW, Brenner U, et al. World J Surg 1986;10:53–63.
122. American College of Physicians position paper. Ann Intern Med 1989;110:734–6.
123. Desai TK, Kinzie J. JPEN J Parenter Enteral Nutr (Abstract) 1990;14:75.
124. Freeman J, Goldmann DA, Smith NE, et al. (Letter) N Engl J Med 1990;323:301–8; 1991;324:268.
125. Pomposelli JJ, Bistrian BR. New Horizons 1994;2:224–9.
126. Furst P. Eur J Clin Nutr 1994;48:681–91.
127. Hyltander A, Sandstorm R, Lundholm K. Nutr Clin Pract 1995;10:91–7.
128. Baldermann H, Wicklmayr M, Rett K, et al. JPEN J Parenter Enteral Nutr 1991;15:601–3.
129. Ball MJ. Am J Clin Nutr 1991;53:916–22.
130. Miles JM, Cattalini M, Sharbrough FW, et al. JPEN J Parenter Enteral Nutr 1991;15:37–41.
131. Sandstorm R, Hyltander A, Krner V, et al. JPEN J Parenter Enteral Nutr 1993;17:153–7.
132. Sandstorm R, Hyltander A, Krner V, et al. JPEN J Parenter Enteral Nutr 1995;19:381–6.
133. Rossle C, Carpentier YA, Richelle M, et al. Am J Physiol 1990;258:E944–7.
134. Wan JM, Teo TC, Babayan VK, et al. JPEN J Parenter Enteral Nutr 1988;12:43S–8S.
135. Mashima Y, Tashiro T, Yamamori H, et al. Advances in polyunsaturated fatty acid research. New York: Elsevier Science Publications, 1993;239–40.
135a. Morlion BJ, Torwesten E, Lessire H, et al. Metabolism—clinical and experimental 1996;45:1208–13.
136. Koruda MJ, Rolandelli RH, Settle RG, et al. Gastroenterology 1988;95:715–20.
137. Tappenden KA, Thomson ABR, Wild GE, et al. Gastroenterology 1997;112;792–802.
137a. Lowrey TS, Dulap AW, Brown RO, et al. Nutr Clin Pract 1996;11:147–9.
138. Graybill JR. Ann Intern Med 1996;124:921–3.
138a. Trissel LA, ed. Handbook of injectable drugs. 9th ed. Bethesda, MD: American Society of Health System Pharmacists, 1996;26–7.
139. Duthie DJR. (Commentary) Lancet 1996;347:1199.
139a. Sessler KI. N Engl J Med 1997; 336:1730–7.
140. Miles JM, Klein JA. Nutr Clin Pract 1996;11:204–6.
141. Brennan MF, Cerra F, Daly JM, et al. JPEN J Parenter Enteral Nutr 1986;10:446–52.
142. Brown RO, Buonpane EA, Vehe KL, et al. Crit Care Med 1990;18:1096–101.
143. Vinton NE, Heckenlively JR, Laidlaw SA, et al. Am J Clin Nutr 1990;52:895–902.
144. Hornsby-Lewis L, Shike M, Brown P, et al. JPEN J Parenter Enteral Nutr 1994;18:266–7.
145. Lowe DK, Benfell K, Smith RJ, et al. Am J Clin Nutr 1990;52:1101–1106.
146. Ziegler TR, Young LS, Benfell K, et al. Ann Intern Med 1992;116:821–8.
147. Schloerb PR, Amare M. JPEN J Parenter Enteral Nutr 1993;17:407–13.
148. Stehle P, Zander J, Merten N, et al. Lancet 1989;1:231–3.
149. Fürst P, Albers S, Stehle P. JPEN J Parenter Enteral Nutr 1990;14:118S–24S.
150. Hamarqvist F, Wernerman J, von der Decken A, et al. Ann Surg 1990;212:637–44.
151. van der Hulst R, van Kreel BK, von Meyenfeldt MF, et al. Lancet 1993;341:363–5.
152. Walser M. Am J Clin Nutr (Editorial) 1991;53:1337–8.
153. Fürst P, Stehle P, Rennie MJ. Am J Clin Nutr1992;56:959–60.
154. Walser M. Am J Clin Nutr (Letter) 1992;56:960.
155. Adibi SA. Metab Clin Exp 1987;36:1001–11.
156. Vazquez JA, Paleos GA, Steinhardt HJ, et al. Am J Clin Nutr 1986;44:24–32.
157. Raupp P, Dries R, Pfahl HG, et al. JPEN J Parenter Enteral Nutr 1991;15:469–73.
158. Hanning RM, Atkinson SA, Whyte RK. Am J Clin Nutr 1991;54:903–8.
159. Dunham B, Marcuard S, Khazanie PG, et al. JPEN J Parenter Enteral Nutr 1991;15:608–11.
160. Greene HL, Hambidge M, Schanler R, et al. Am J Clin Nutr 1988;48:1324–42. (Rev. reprint issued Dec 1990).
161. Klein GL, Coburn JW. Annu Rev Nutr 1991;11:93–119.
162. Berkelhammer CH, Wood RJ, Sitrin MD. Am J Clin Nutr 1988;48:1482–9.
163. Clark CL, Sacks GS, Dickerson RN, et al. Crit Care Med 1995;23:1504–11.
164. Sacks GS, Brown RO, Dickerson RN, et al. Nutrition 1997;13:303–8.
165. Whang R, Hampton EM, Whang DD. Ann Pharmacother 1994;28:220–6.
166. Herfindal ET, Bernstein LR, Wong AF, et al. Clin Pharm 1992;11:543–8.
167. Fleming CR. Am J Clin Nutr 1989;49:573–9.
168. Sayers MH, Johnson KD, Schumann LA, et al. JPEN J Parenter Enteral Nutr 1983;7:117–20.
169. Finch CA, Huebers H. N Engl J Med 1982;306:1520–8.
170. Greene HL. Personal communication.
171. Shils ME, Jacobs DH. Unpublished data.
172. Shils ME, Burke AW, Greene HL, et al. JAMA 1979;241: 2051–4.
173. Schwarz K, Peden VH. Nutr Rev 1982;40:81–3.
174. Solomons NW, Layden TJ, Rosenberg IH, et al. Gastroenterology 1976;70:1022–5.
175. Phillips GD, Garnys VP. JPEN J Parenter Enteral Nutr 1981;5:11–8.
176. Shike M, Roulet M, Kurian R, et al. Gastroenterology 1981; 81:290–7.
177. Kurkus J, Alcock NW, Shils ME. JPEN J Parenter Enteral Nutr 1984;8:254–7.
178. Shike M, Ritchie ME, Shils ME. Clin Res (Abstract) 1986; 34:804A.
179. Shils ME. Parenteral nutrition. In: Shils ME, Olson JA, Shike M, eds. Modern nutrition in health and disease. 8th ed. Philadelphia: Lea & Febiger, 1994;1445(Table 80.8).
180. Fell JME, Reynolds AP, Meadows N, et al. Lancet 1996;347:1218–21.
181. Ono J, Harada K, Kodaka R, et al. JPEN J Parenter Enteral Nutr 1995;19:310–2.
182. Ejima A, Imanura T, Nakamura S, et al. Lancet (Letter) 1992;339:426.
182a. Alves G, Thiebot J, Tracqui A, et al. JPEN J Parenter Enteral Nutr 1997;21:41–5.
183. Hambidge KM, Sokol RJ, Fidanze SJ, et al. JPEN J Parenter Enteral Nutr 1989;13:168–71.
184. Mirowitz SA, Westrich TJ, Hirsch JD. Radiology 1991;181: 117–20.
185. Mirowitz SA, Westrich TJ. Radiology 1992;185:535–6.
186. Verhage AH, Cheong WK, Jeejeebhoy KN. JPEN J Parenter Enteral Nutr 1996;20:123–7.
187. Ito Y, Alcock NW, Shils ME. JPEN J Parenter Enteral Nutr 1990;14:610–4.
188. Shenkin A, Fell GS, Halls DG. Selenium and chromium requirements during intravenous nutrition. In: Prasad AS,

ed. Essential and toxic trace elements in health and disease. New York: Alan R Liss, 1988;479–88.
189. Kien CL, Veillon C, Patterson KY, et al. JPEN J Parenter Enteral Nutr 1986;10:662–4.
190. Moukarzel AA, Song MK, Buchman AL, et al. Lancet 1992;339:385–8.
191. Van Rijn AM, Thompson CD, McKenzie JM, et al. Am J Clin Nutr 1979;43:2076–85.
192. Cohen HJ, Brown MR, Hamilton D, et al. Am J Clin Nutr 1989;49:132–9.
193. Rannem T, Ladefoged K, Hylander T, et al. JPEN J Parenter Enteral Nutr 1995;19:351–5.
194. Rannem T, Persson-Moschos M, Huang W, et al. JPEN J Parenter Enteral Nutr 1996;20:287–91.
195. Rajagopalan KV. Annu Rev Nutr 1988;8:401–27.
196. Abumrad NN, Schneider AJ, Steel D, et al. Am J Clin Nutr 1981;34:2551–9.
197. Abumrad NN. Bull NY Acad Med 1984;60:163–71.
197a. Berner YN, Schuler TR, Nielsen FJ, et al. Am J Clin Nutr 1989;50:1079–83.
198. Mahaffey KR. Bull NY Acad Med 1984;60:196–209.
198a. Mahaffey KR. Personal communication, 1984.
199. Swartz RD. Fluid, electrolyte, and acid-base changes during renal failure. In: Kokko JP, Tannen RL eds. Fluids and electrolytes. 3rd ed. Philadelphia: WB Saunders, 1996;510.
200. Klein GA. Am J Clin Nutr 1995;61:449–56.
201. Klein GL, Alfrey AC, Miller NL, et al. Am J Clin Nutr 1982; 35:1425–9.
202. Wu WW, Kaplan LA, Horn J, et al. JPEN J Parenter Enteral Nutr 1986;10:591–5.
202a. Bishop NJ, Morley R, Day JP, et al. N Engl J Med 1997;336:1557–61.
203. Klein GL, Alfrey AA, Shike M, et al. Am J Clin Nutr 1991; 53:399–402.
204. Vanamee P, Shils ME, Burke AW, et al. JPEN J Parenter Enteral Nutr 1979;3:258–62.
205. American Academy of Pediatrics Committee on Drugs. Pediatrics 1985;76:635–43.
206. De Ritter E. J Pharm Sci 1982;71:1073–96.
207. Billion-Ray F, Guillaumont M, Frederich A, et al. JPEN J Parenter Enteral Nutr 1993;17:56–61.
208. Chen F, Boyce HW, Tripiett L. JPEN J Parenter Enteral Nutr 1983;7:462–4.
209. Scheiner JM, Aranjo MM, DeRitter E. Am J Hosp Pharm 1982;38:1911–3.
210. Shils ME, Baker H, Frank O. JPEN J Parenter Enteral Nutr 1985;9:179–88.
211. Barker A, Hebron BS, Beck PR, et al. JPEN J Parenter Enteral Nutr 1984;8:3–7.
212. Stromberg P, Shenkin A, Campbell RA, et al. JPEN J Parenter Enteral Nutr 1981;5:295–9.
213. Kirkemo AK, Burt ME, Brennan M. Am J Clin Nutr 1982;35:1003–9.
214. Jeppson B, Gimmon Z. Vitamins. In: Fischer JE, ed. Surgical nutrition. Boston: Little, Brown, 1983.
215. Steephen AC, Traber MG, Ito Y, et al. JPEN J Parenter Enteral Nutr 1991;15:647–52.
216. Lemoyne M, Gossum AV, Kurian R, et al. Am J Clin Nutr 1988;48:1310–5.
217. Lennon C, Davidson KW, Sadowski JA. JPEN J Parenter Enteral Nutr 1993;17:142–4.
218. Drittij-Reijnders MJ, Sels JP, Rouflart M, et al. Eur J Clin Nutr 1994;48:525–7.
219. Greene HL, Smith R, Pollack P, et al. J Am Coll Nutr 1991;10:281–8.
220. Dahl GB, Svensson L, Kinnander NJG, et al. JPEN J Parenter Enteral Nutr 1994;18:234–9.
220a. Baumgartner TG. Henderson GN, Fox J, et al. Nutrition 1997;13:547–53.
221. Centers for Disease Control. MMWR 1989;38:43–6.
221a. Center for Disease Control, MMWR 1997;46:523–8.
222. Wilmanns H, Witzigmann H, Schlag P, et al. Chirurgie 1990;61:183–6.
223. Klein G, Behne M, Probst S, et al. Dtsch Med Wochenschr 1990;115:254–6.
224. Oriot D, Wood C, Gottesman R, et al. JPEN J Parenter Enteral Nutr 1991;15:105–9.
225. Zak J, Burns D, Lingenfelser T, et al. JPEN J Parenter Enteral Nutr 1991;15:200–1.
226. Chris-Anderson D, Heimberger DC, Morgan SL, et al. JPEN J Parenter Enteral Nutr 1996;20:206–10.
227. Peden Y, Witzleben C, Shelton M, et al. J Pediatr (Letter) 1971;78:180.
228. Bowyer BA, Fleming CR, Ludwig J, et al. JPEN J Parenter Enteral Nutr 1985;9:11–7.
229. Payne-James JJ, Silk DB. Dig Dis 1991;9:106–24.
230. Kubota A, Okada A, Nezu R, et al. JPEN J Parenter Enteral Nutr 1988;12:602–6.
231. Drongowski RA, Coran AG. JPEN J Parenter Enteral Nutr 1989;13:586–9.
232. Bell RL, Ferry GD, Smith EO, et al. JPEN J Parenter Enteral Nutr 1986;10:356–9.
233. Clayton PT, Bowron A, Mills KA, et al. Gastroenterology 1993;105:1806–13.
234. Messing B, Colombel JF, Heresbach D, et al. Nutrition 1992;8:30–6.
235. Buzby GP, Mullen JL, Stein PT, et al. J Surg Res 1981; 31:46–54.
236. Wagner WH, Lowry AC, Silberman H. Am J Gastroenterol 1983;78:199–202.
237. Buchmiller CE, Kleiman-Wexler RL, Ephgrave KS, et al. JPEN J Parenter Enteral Nutr 1993;17:301–6.
238. Ito Y, Shils ME. JPEN J Parenter Enteral Nutr 1989;15:271–6.
239. Lambert JP, Thomas SM. JPEN J Parenter Enteral Nutr 1985;9:501–3.
240. Lindor KD, Burnes J. Gastroenterology 1991;101:250–3.
241. Spagnuolo MM, Iorio R, Vegnente A, et al. Gastroenterology 1996;111:716–9.
242. Duerksen DR, van Aerde JE, Gramlich L, et al. Gastroenterology 1996;111:1111–17
242a. Teitelbaum DH, Han-Marker T, Drongowski RA, et al. JPEN J Parenter Enteral Nutr 1997;21:100–3.
243. Buchman AL, Dubin M, Venden D, et al. Gastroenterology 1992;102:1363–70.
244. Spiliotis JD, Kalfarentzos F. Nutrition 1994;10:255–60.
245. Muller EL, Grace PA, Pitt HA. J Surg Res 1986;40:55–62.
246. Messing B, Bories C, Kustlinger F, et al. Gastroenterology 1983;84:1012–9.
247a. Doty JE, Pitt HA, Porter-Fink V, et al. Ann Surg 1985;201: 76–80.
247b. Broughton G II, Fitzgibbons RJ Jr, Geiss RW, et al. JPEN J Parenter Enteral Nutr 1996;20:187–93.
248. Roslyn JJ, Berquist WE, Pitt HA, et al. Pediatrics 1983;71: 784–9.
249. Dorney SF, Ament ME, Berquist WE, et al. J Pediatr 1985;107:521–5.
250. Goulet ON, Revillion Y, Jan D, et al. J Pediatr 1991;119:18–23.
251. Roslyn JJ, Pitt HA, Mann LL. Am J Surg 1984;148:58–63.
252. Kien CL, Browring C, Jona J, et al. JPEN J Parenter Enteral Nutr 1982;6:152–6.

253. Vargas JH, Klein GL, Ament ME, et al. Am J Clin Nutr 1988;48:1070–8.
254. Shike M, Harrison JE, Sturtridge WC, et al. Ann Intern Med 1980;92:343–50.
255. Shike M, Sturtridge WC, Tam CS, et al. Ann Intern Med 1981;95:560–8.
256. Verhage AH, Cheong WK, Allard JP, et al. JPEN J Parenter Enteral Nutr 1995;19:431–6.
257. Shike M, Shils ME, Heller A, et al. Am J Clin Nutr 1986;44:89–98.
258. Saitta JC, Ott SM, Sherrard DJ, et al. JPEN J Parenter Enteral Nutr 1993;17:214–9.
259. Dickerson RN, Brown RO, White KG. Parenteral nutrition solutions. In: Rombeau JL, Caldwell MJ, eds. Parenteral nutrition. 2nd ed. Philadelphia: WB Saunders, 1993;310–33.
259a. Trissel LA, Gilbert DL, Martinez JF, et al. Am J Health Syst Pharm 1997;54:1295–300.
260. Shils ME, Wright WL, Turnbull A, et al. N Engl J Med 1970;283:341–4.
261. Scribner BH, Cole JJ, Christopher TG, et al. JAMA 1970; 212:457–63.
262. Jeejeebhoy KN, Zohrab WJ, Langer B, et al. Gastroenterology 1973;65:811–20.
263. Shils ME. (Unpublished) Home TPN Registry Annual Reports New York City: NY Acad Med 1978–1983.
264. Howard L, Michalek AV. Annu Rev Nutr 1984;4:69–99.
265. Grant JP, ed. Home total parenteral nutrition. Handbook of total parenteral nutrition. 2nd ed. Philadelphia: WB Saunders, 1992.
266. American Society for Parenteral and Enteral Nutrition. Nutr Clin Pract 1992;7:65–9.
267. Howard L, Ament M, Fleming CR, et al. Gastroenterology 1995;109:355–65.
268. North American Home Parenteral and Enteral Nutrition Patient Registry Annual Report 1985–1992. Data. Albany, NY: Oley Foundation, 1994.
269. Elia M. Lancet 1995;345:1345–9.
270. Messing B, Lemann M, Landais P, et al. Gastroenterology 1995;108:1005–10.
270a. Wilmore DW. J Pediatr 1972;80:88–95.
271. Gulledge AD, Srp F, Sharp JW, et al. Nutr Clin Pract 1987; 2:183–94.
272. Smith CE. JPEN J Parenter Enteral Nutr 1993;17:501–6.
273. Howard L, Heaphey L, Fleming CR, et al. JPEN J Parenter Enteral Nutr 1991;15:384–93.
274. Goel V. The economics of total parenteral nutrition in evaluating total parenteral nutrition. Program in technology and health care. Washington, DC: Georgetown University School of Medicine, 1989;41–51.
275. Detsky AS, McLaughlin JR, Abrams HB, et al. JPEN J Parenter Enteral Nutr 1986;10:49–57.
276. Detsky AS. Gastroenterology (Editorial) 1995;108:1302–4.
277. Schraut WH. Gastroenterology 1988;94:525–38.
278. Wood RF, Ingraham-Clark CL. Br Med J 1992;304:1453–4.
279. Grant D, Wall W, Mimeault R, et al. Lancet 1990;335:181–4.
280. Reyes J, Todo S, Starzl TE. Immunol Allergy Clin North Am 1996;16:299–312.
281. Lee RG, Nakamura K, Tsamandas AC, et al. Gastroenterology 1996;110:1820–34.
282. Langnas AN, Shaw PW Jr, Antonson DL, et al. Pediatrics 1996;97:443–8.
283. Quigley EMM. Gastroenterology (Editorial) 1996;110: 2009–12.
284. Grant D, on behalf of the International Intestinal Transplant Registry. Lancet 1996;347:1801–3.
285. Ng EH, Lowry SF. Hematol Oncol Clin North Am 1991; 5:162–84.
286. Wilmore DW. N Engl J Med 1991;325:695–702.
287. Gruenfeld C, Feingold KR. N Engl J Med 1992;327:328–37.
288. Hartl WH, Jauch KW, Herndon DN, et al. Lancet 1990;335:69–71.
289. Byrne TA, Persinger RL, Young LS, et al. Ann Surg 1995;222:243–55.
289a. Scolapio JS, Camilleri M, Fleming CR, et al. Gastroenterology 1997;113:1074–81.
289b. Thompson JS. Gastroenterology (Editorial) 1997;113: 1402–5.
290. Goodlad RA, Playford RJ. Gastroenterology (Letter) 1995; 108:1330–1.
291. O'Loughlin E, Shur A, Wintermetal. Gastroenterology (Letter) 1995;108:1331.
292. Drucker DJ, Ehrlich P, Asa SL, et al. Proc Nat Acad Sci USA 1996;93:7911–6.
293. Burrin DG, Wester TJ, Davis TA, et al. Am J Physiol 1996;270:R1085–91.
294. Kaiser GC, Polk DB. Gastroenterology 1997;112:1231–40.

102. Nutrition and Medical Ethics: The Interplay of Medical Decisions, Patients' Rights, and the Judicial System

MAURICE E. SHILS

The widespread availability of essential nutrients in stable and safe forms and the means to administer them, by enteral tube or vein, have made nutritional support an effective therapy in many clinical situations. Much attention has been devoted in recent years to the ethical, medical, and legal aspects of providing or withholding nutrition and fluids to patients with advanced and often incurable diseases, especially those unable to make such critical decisions for themselves. These issues are considered in some detail in this chapter. First, however, consideration is given to bioethical issues related to nutritional support for other types of patients.

NUTRITIONAL SUPPORT AS AN ETHICAL ISSUE

Without clinical craftsmanship, the physician-humanist is without authenticity. Incompetence is inhumane because it betrays the trust the patient places in the physician's capacity to help and not harm.

Edmund D. Pellegrino (1)

Prevention of Undernutrition

Physicians have become significantly more sensitive to the need for remedial attention to the problem of disease-related malnutrition. However, many physicians still either overlook development of serious undernutrition in their patients or delay proper therapy in the hope that the underlying disease will soon be controlled and the "patient will again eat well"—a hope often delayed. At intervals over many years, reports of the prevalence of such hospital-based malnutrition resurface with notations of increased morbidity, delayed convalescence, and increased mortality (2). In addition to failing to recognize the need to institute adequate nutritional support, some physicians fail to oversee these modalities adequately (particularly total parenteral nutrition), with resultant adverse consequences.

Serious undernutrition has many sequelae, discussed in various chapters in this book. An ethical issue arises when the risks of serious undernutrition are either not anticipated or not treated in a potentially curable patient. One way to help such patients is to try to prevent serious undernutrition and aggressively treat existing malnutrition.

The sick may refuse food for many reasons, including the anorexia of illness, chronic nausea, depression exacerbated by fear, generalized or localized pain, medication effects, obstruction, and malabsorption. Noting and tending to relevant problems may be helpful. Food intake can be enhanced directly in a number of ways, such as making the food more acceptable in taste and appearance, providing more familiar and desirable foods, minimizing skipped meals, providing regular assistance in hand feeding when needed, and making palatable liquid supplements easily available. When indicated, tube feeding or parenteral nutrition may be necessary.

Prevention of Chronic Illness

Chronic diseases, particularly cardiovascular diseases, cancer, osteoporosis, hypertension, and diabetes, are major causes of morbidity and mortality. In recent years, it has become apparent that certain diets instituted at appropriate times and maintained can play an important role as preventive or ameliorating factors. This is clearly the case with management of hyperlipidemias in controlling coronary artery disease (see Chapter 75), efforts to minimize or delay serious osteoporosis (see Chapter 85), optimum management of insulin-independent diabetes mellitus (see Chapter 86), and assistance in controlling hypertension (see Chapter 76). In addition, because many of these diseases are exacerbated by overweight, weight control is important (see Chapter 87). Some evidence indicates that restricted protein intake can slow progression of renal disease in some groups (see Chapter 89). Increasing data from epidemiologic and intervention studies show promise for certain diets in preventing or controlling cancer (see Chapter 79).

With such information, "doing good" for the individual requires the physician's attention to the possible need for dietary and other interventions to delay, ameliorate, or prevent one or more diet-sensitive chronic illnesses. Neglect in obtaining the proper history (e.g., patient family history and dietary characteristics), in doing an adequate physical examination, or in ordering relevant laboratory studies is as much a professional failure as is failure to diagnose an existing illness or to prescribe a correct medication. The traditional responsibilities of the physician expand as biomedical knowledge advances.

CHANGING VIEWS ABOUT MEDICAL ETHICS

> *Clinical ethics deals with situations in which there are strong reasons both for and against a course of action. Decisions often are difficult because ethical guidelines conflict and people of integrity and good will may disagree over what to do.*
>
> *Bernard Lo (3)*

Hippocratic Tradition

The moral principles to which medical professionals are exposed during their training and in their professional organizations have a long history. The Hippocratic tradition of some 2500 years developed from interactions of ancient Greek philosophic schools and medicine with modifications of Stoic attitudes to duty and virtue. These were further modified by the views of the Galen, with subsequent religious Christian input to remove pagan influences (4). Ethical precepts from the Hippocratic tradition include beneficence and maleficence (the obligation to promote the patient's welfare while balancing benefits and harm), duty, compassion, and confidentiality as well as such prohibitions as abortion and euthanesia. The tradition combined precepts on gentlemanly conduct, education, and practical judgment including a good physician-patient relationship. These would lead physicians toward right and good decisions for their patients in situations of moral choice. Inherent in this system of medical practice and ethics was the authoritarian role of the physician; this long era has been termed one of paternalism (5) or the quiescent period (6).

"Principalism"

The traditional Hippocratic system of professional ethics was increasingly questioned in the United States in the mid-1960s in conjunction with many professional and societal changes that included depersonalization and fragmentation in many physician-patient relationships and challenges to governmental authority with the rise in the civil rights, antiwar, feminist, and consumer rights movements in a multiethnic pluralistic democratic society. As physician-patient relationships came under increasing scrutiny with claims for more patient rights, a series of principles of medical ethics were advanced (designated by some as "principalism"). These were effectively set out by Beauchamp and Childress in the first edition of *Principles of Biomedical Ethics* (7) and its successors. Its first two principles (nonmaleficence and beneficence) were similar to those in the Hippocratic ethic; the third concept, patient *autonomy,* contravened paternalism; while the fourth, *justice* (an area of diverse views often involving elements of fairness and entitlement for individuals), was completely at odds with the old tradition.

The term *autonomy* signifies the right of the competent individual to make choices freely about medical care and denotes the obligation of the healthcare provider to communicate effectively with the patient and solicit those decisions. As detailed by Beauchamp and Childress, autonomous actions require that definitions be available including criteria so that someone could give or refuse informed consent and make other decisions. Furthermore, the principle of respect for autonomy must be evaluated in given situations in competition with the other principles (7). Widespread acceptance of principalism in the United States was circumscribed to a period of about 20 years from the mid-1960s, as other ethical concepts became more prominent (4).

Alternative Ethical Approaches

There has been increased advocacy in the past decade for alternative ethical approaches that place more emphasis on the value of a more personal decision-making interaction of physician and patient (8–12). Alternative ethical approaches include casuistry (analysis of a specific case in relation to a system of principles) and cross-cultural, narrative, and virtue ethics. These gained advocacy as changes continued in society and in medical practice and care. Key examples of the latter are institution of diagnosis-related groups (DRGs) in 1983 and, more recently, the widespread movement toward managed care systems owned or directed by for-profit corporations and nonprofit organizations vying competitively, which raised serious concerns, divided physician loyalties, and imposed limitations on medical care (10).

In addition to secular ethical positions, some bioethicists have formulated their positions on the basis of particular religious traditions (13, 14) and some attempt to construct a basis for secular ethics for those "who do not share a contentful moral vision" (15).

ISSUES IN NUTRITIONAL SUPPORT OF THE COMPETENT PATIENT

Many of the ethical and legal issues concerning medical practice and patient-physician relations relate to provision of nutrition and hydration. Prior to the practical application of forced-feeding techniques, the inability to maintain adequate nutrition by mouth meant progressive body wasting until death. Except for deaths occurring very rapidly from violence, trauma, or acute overwhelming infection, the more usual direct causes of death were dehydration and starvation associated with more chronic illness. Under these circumstances, there was relatively little that a physician could do in restoring health while maintaining a good nutritional state. This situation began to change significantly in the late 19th century as effective therapies (initially surgical) and other advances in diagnosis and treatment enhanced the societal importance of the physician.

Concerning oversight of medical care in general, the prevailing judicial position in the past was that of "compelling state interest" such as preservation of life, prevention of suicide, and certification of physician education. This legal position in conjunction with the paternalistic role of the physician eventually led to contentious legal issues.

The patient's right to refuse medical treatment was not established until 1891, in a case in which the United States Supreme Court upheld the right of a personal injury plaintiff to refuse a medical examination (16). This decision established the general rights of individuals to make choices regarding bodily examination and treatment under the principle that common law guards the right of every individual to the possession and control of his or her own person on the basis of the doctrine of informed consent. However, this only began to establish judicial decisions that more specifically defined the laws of informed consent and the rights of the incompetent patient.

In the past, the issue of provision of nutrition and fluids has caused the most controversy among adult patients, their surrogates, physicians, hospital administrators, and state courts. The right of the competent individual to decide whether or not to receive medical therapy (autonomy) was not automatically granted. Withholding or withdrawal of artificial nutrition and hydration became a contentious issue because some physicians, ethicists, theologians, and "right-to-life" groups considered such acts assisted suicide or euthanasia (and hence likely to involve criminal penalties) or were cessation of "ordinary" medical procedure.

The Bouvia Case

The Bouvia case posed the issue of the right of a competent individual to starve to death. Elizabeth Bouvia, a quadriplegic in her mid-20s, was hospitalized in California with severe cerebral palsy and arthritic pain requiring morphine injection. While able to ingest food orally with assistance, she asked that such feeding be stopped. The hospital refused to accede to her wishes, and a lower court ruling in 1984 supported the hospital (17). When her condition deteriorated to the point that feeding by nasogastric tube was necessary, the appellate court ruled in 1986 that her refusal of treatment was not a form of suicide, thus rejecting the arguments of hospital officials that removing the tube would make them a party to suicide (18). With the additional support given later by the United States Supreme Court decision in the Cruzan case (see below), the right of an irreversibly ill but competent patient to refuse artificial feeding is unlikely to be seriously challenged again.

Bouvia's condition was classified as a state of severe and permanent paralysis, which may acutely or progressively result in a "permanent locked-in state." This was first described as a medical condition in 1966 by Cranford, as irreversible loss of motor function with preservation of normal consciousness, possible long-term survival of years or even decades, and physical and psychologic suffering of a degree that may become extreme because of the patient's awareness of the condition (19). Eleven years later Bouvia was still alive, totally dependent on others for her care and, despite several half-hearted attempts, unable to bring herself to insist on actual discontinuation of artificial feeding (19a).

Patient-Physician Interaction and Decision Making

In an incisive essay, Pellegrino stated "that a more sensitive and compelling guide to the care of the sick is to be found in the fact of illness as a human experience rather than in the assigned role of the profession. Without supplanting traditional professional ethics, the intrinsic dehumanizing nature of illness imposes additional obligations of greater sensitivity" (20). Individuals with "illness as an acute event or as a chronic accompaniment of life are deprived in varying degrees of those things which distinguish humanity from other forms of existence." These include loss of freedom of action, freedom to make choices, and freedom from the power of others as well as threats to personal self-image. These disabilities "must be the infrangible base for the obligations of physicians and all others who profess to heal . . . , these obligations constitute the substance of professional medical ethics, . . . Its rooting in the existential situation is more authentic and more human . . . than the traditional one in the self declared duties of the profession . . . The professional can make a valid claim for technical authority but this no longer extends to moral authority . . . The patient has the human right to his own moral agency if he or she wishes to exercise it. The physician has the moral obligation to ascertain the degree to which the patient wishes to exercise his moral prerogatives and to provide the fullest exposition which will enable the privilege to be exercised" (20).

The principle of respect for autonomy of the competent patient may result in tension between a patient or the parent of a minor and the physician when the patient's decision seems inappropriate. What appears legally to be a clear-cut situation, i.e., the rights of a competent patient, may be a complex and difficult situation for all concerned with the welfare of the individual. The old Spanish proverb quoted elsewhere in this context is apt: "The appearance of the bull changes as one leaves the grandstand and enters the ring" (21). The patient's viewpoint may reflect a lucid and rational decision or an undisclosed or undiagnosed problem(s) such as depression, other mental difficulty, side effect of medication (22, 23), an unspoken complicating social problem, strong opposing family influence, misunderstanding the physician's intentions, or the patient's failure to know, comprehend, or accept the severity or irreversibility of the disease.

Disagreement may occur, for example, when the patient wishes parenteral or enteral feeding stopped and the physician believes that continued feeding is in the patient's best interest. An even more difficult situation pertains to stopping parenteral feeding in an intestinally obstructed cancer patient who has failed all therapy but is still competent and ambulatory, and for whom such continued support at home could conceivably extend life for months.

Recommendations of the President's Commission

Several recommendations on this issue were considered by the President's Commission for the Study of Ethical Problems in Medicine and Biomedical and Behavioral Research (24). It held that "health care professionals serve patients best by maintaining a presumption in favor of sustaining life while recognizing that competent patients are entitled to choose to forgo any treatments, including those that sustain life" and "the voluntary choice of a competent and informed patient should determine whether or not life-sustaining therapy will be undertaken, while healthcare institutions and professionals should try to enhance patients' abilities to make decisions on their own behalf and to promote understanding of the available options." In such situations, members of the hospital nutritional support team, who are often and intimately involved in a major aspect of the patient's care, may be helpful in affording insight into the patient's status and expressed position. The physician's discussion of the medical situation with patient and family, the basis for the medical recommendations, the therapeutic alternatives with their probabilities of success, and the offer of a second opinion are all essential to the decision-making process.

This commission also examined the role of traditional moral distinctions as they relate to decisions about medical care and whether they are acceptable or unacceptable. It noted that from the viewpoint of most competent patients, decisions about alternative available courses of treatment are made on the basis of factors that include treatment benefits in terms of extension of life, the nature and quality of that life, the degree of suffering involved, and the various costs to themselves and to others (24). It noted that other criteria have been used in judging the acceptability or unacceptability of life-and-death decisions and stated (24):

> these bases are traditionally presented in the form of opposing categories. Athough the categories causing death—by acting versus by omitting the act; withholding versus withdrawing treatment; the intended versus the unintended but foreseeable consequences of a choice; and ordinary versus extraordinary treatment—do reflect factors that can be important in assessing the moral and legal acceptability of decisions to forego life sustaining treatment, they are inherently unclear. Worse, their invocation is often so mechanical that it neither illuminates an actual case nor provides an ethically persuasive argument.

Several of the commission's conclusions about such distinctions are relevant to the issue of nutrition and hydration and have, in fact, had a significant influence on the attitudes of physicians and the courts. For example (24):

> The distinction between acting and omitting to act provides a useful rule-of-thumb by separating cases that probably deserve more scrutiny from those that are likely not to need it. Nonetheless, the mere difference between acts and omissions—which is often hard to draw in any case—never by itself determines what is morally acceptable. Rather, the acceptability of particular actions or omissions turns on other morally significant considerations, such as the balance of harms and benefits likely to be achieved, the duties owed by others to a dying person, the risks imposed on others in acting or refraining, and the certainty of outcome . . . A justification that is adequate for not commencing a treatment is also sufficient for ceasing it. Moreover, erecting a higher requirement for cessation might unjustifiably discourage vigorous initial attempts to treat seriously ill patients that sometimes succeed.

The guidelines of the Hastings Center also expressed concern that the terms *ordinary* and *extraordinary* "obscure ethically important questions rather than helping to resolve them. Prevalence of a treatment or its degree of technological complexity is sometimes used to make the distinction between 'ordinary' and 'extraordinary'. We reject the distinction. No treatment is intrinsically 'ordinary' or 'extraordinary'. All treatments that impose undue burdens on the patient without overriding benefits or that simply provide no benefits may justifiably be withheld or withdrawn. While traditional definitions of `extraordinary' hinged on this comparison of benefits and burdens, the term has become so confusing that it is no longer useful" (25).

The Law Reform Commission of Canada, an official agency for evaluating and recommending reform of Canadian federal law, issued in 1983 a series of principles and recommendations for amendments to the criminal code. These amendments suggested changing existing laws so that they would not be interpreted as requiring a physician to initiate medical treatment against the wishes of the patient or to continue such treatments when they have become therapeutically useless and not in the best interest of the patient (26). These and related amendments have not been adopted as of early 1996 (27).

Resolving Differences between Patient and Physician

When all the stated precautions and efforts have been honored in decision making but the choice of the competent and informed patient is contrary to the judgment of the physician, where does this leave the physician? "The physician too has a set of values to which he owes allegiance. He has a double obligation, to protect those of the patient and to be faithful to his own" (19). To deal humanely with the conflicts that must occasionally arise, "the physician must know enough about his own beliefs to decide when he can compromise, when he cannot, and when he must give the patient the opportunity to transfer his care to another physician whose values more closely coincide" (20). In this situation, the President's Commission took the position that "health care professionals or institutions may decline to provide a particular option because that choice would violate their conscience or professional judgment, though in doing so they may not abandon a patient" (24). In the case of the attending physician, responsibility for the care of the patient must be transferred to another physician who accepts the patient's decision and acts accordingly. Abandonment means leaving the patient without care, a serious and punishable infraction of both the legal and ethical obligations of the physician. There has been a recent emphasis on nonabandonment "as an open-ended commitment over time" (28) of the physician to the patient (28, 29); examples include accepting competent patient decisions on demanding or stopping artificial feeding. Objection has been raised to the apparent elevation of nonabandonment to a principle rather than considering it one of the essential derivatives of medical ethics (30).

When the patient's request is opposed by the hospital administration, the solutions open to the hospital are to yield to staff pressure on behalf of the patient, to transfer the patient to another hospital willing to accept the patient, or to yield to a court order when it supports the patient. Often in the past and continuing to some degree today, it has been the reluctance of the hospital administration to discontinue tube feeding or some other life support—usually because of fear of civil or criminal penalties or on religious grounds—that has led to legal actions by patients or family members.

Distinguishing Patient Refusal from Requests

Physicians may differentiate between the competent patient's refusal of a recommended treatment and the request for a nonrecommended treatment (31). Refusals must be honored even when the physician knows that death will result. In contrast, a physician may feel that there is no moral or legal obligation to honor a request that the physician firmly believes will have an undesirable effect or result in death. This is a matter of judgment focusing on the issue of treatments deemed useless or futile by the physicians or hospital.

Denial of Treatment as Medically Futile

Statements such as those made by the President's Commission (24) and the chief counsel for the American Medical Association (AMA) (32) supporting the physician's right to deny futile treatments have been under increasing scrutiny and criticism as being too simplistic. This area has considerable relevance to artificial nutrition, especially by the intravenous route, because of its expense, increased risk of infection, and evidence of little or no benefit in advanced disease, particularly cancer unresponsive to disease-specific therapy.

Justifications for physician refusal of futile interventions for the competent patient include *(a)* the specific intervention proposed has no physiologic rationale; *(b)* the intervention has already been tried and failed to achieve any apparent benefit; *(c)* maximal treatment for the underlying advanced disease is a failure; and *(d)* the intervention(s) will not help achieve the goal of care, is burdensome, and may worsen the quality of life (3).

With respect to nutrition, how valid are these justifications? Item *(a)* above is obviously questionable or incorrect in the case of intravenous feeding, because it does provide essential nutrition and hydration; *(b)* would not hold if nutrition has not previously been given; arguments *(c)* and *(d)* may hold true. However the challenge to statement *(d)* rests on the answer to the question: whose goal or value is most valid—the physician's or the patient's? If the patient wishes to continue the requested treatment—even for a limited period—to achieve his or her goal (e.g., survival and additional months to see an only child married or the first grandchild born), what is the justification for saying "nay"?

Even if the likelihood of success, in the opinion of the physician, is very small, how can one know if a particular patient will or will not respond? Furthermore, can the patient be certain that the physician is fully conversant with the medical literature on this point, or has not misinterpreted the situation, or that other physicians in the same hospital or elsewhere will be in agreement? Uncertainty and changes of therapeutic options in medicine are hardly uncommon (33, 34).

The basis of physician opinion may be that the prospective benefit for the patient does not justify the required resources. However, futility is not to be confused with resource allocation (which requires well-tested clinical data plus administrative and societal decisions for acceptability), even though they do share a common purpose (35, 36). A continuum of conditions and situations extends from those that are obviously futile, to those that produce an effect but are deemed by the physician to be of no net benefit, to those in which the physician is believed to be in error by other physicians or by the patient. In the case of the incompetent patient, the same issues about futile treatments arise in the physician-surrogate relationship.

This issue has resulted in a large number of papers, letters, editorials, and conferences in the medical and bioethics literature (e.g., 32–40), to the point where the question has been posed: "Is futility a futile concept?" This is based on the argument that its proponents have not paid sufficient attention to the problematic nature of the data supporting the use of their definitions (40).

It is not surprising that strongly held differences of opinion may arise between and among physicians, patients, families, and surrogates about treatment that arguably is futile. Collaborative procedures have been advocated or instituted to help solve such problems and settle such differences constructively, short of the courts (41, 42).

Caring for the Hunger Striker

The hunger striker "is a mentally competent person who has indicated that he/she has decided to embark on a hunger strike and has refused to take food and/or fluids for a significant interval" (43). Once the physician agrees to attend a hunger striker, that person becomes his or her patient. Guidelines of the World Medical Association (WMA) include thorough examination of the patient, daily visits, information on the clinical consequences of a hunger strike, treatment of trauma and infection, and advice on fluid intake; any treatment must have the patient's approval. "Treatment or care of the hunger striker must not be conditional upon his suspending his hunger-strike" (43). Autonomy must be respected. In Israel, however, a district judge authorized force-feeding of a political prisoner on a hunger strike (43a).

Serious moral dilemmas arise when the patient is comatose when first seen and the person's wishes are not known. In that situation, the WMA, the British Medical Association, and other medical societies hold that treatment should be initiated until resuscitation has occurred and the patient's wishes are known. In the instance of a hunger striker becoming severely confused or comatose during medical observation, "the physician shall be free to make the decisions for his patient which he considers to be in the best interest of the patient taking into account the decision he has arrived at during his preceding care of the patient" (43). The problems related to management of asylum seekers on hunger strike has been reviewed (43b, 43c).

The Patient Self-Determination Act

As a result of the recommendation of the President's Commission and other similar suggestions, federal legislation (the Patient Self-Determination Act of 1990) was enacted and became law on December 1, 1991 (44). This law applies to hospitals, nursing homes, hospices, healthcare maintenance organizations, and healthcare companies receiving Medicare and Medicaid funds. At the time of admission, enrollment, or on initiating home care, they are required to inform patients about their legal rights in that specific state and assist them in making decisions concerning their medical care and formulating advance directives. Such a directive must be in the patient's medical record, indicating whether life support has been rejected. This federal law, as well as most state laws and court decisions on this subject, also allows hospitals and nursing homes to express their administrative positions on these subjects to the patient before or at admission. One goal of the statute is to encourage (but not require) adults to complete advanced directives in the form of treatment directives, a proxy appointment, or both while they are competent. Another goal is to influence both healthcare givers and institutions to honor advance directives.

As a result of the majority decision of the United States Supreme Court on the Cruzan case (see later) and the Patient Self-Determination Act now in force, advance directives must be based on the legal requirement of individual states. Thus, standards in the United States have been established in varying degrees for truth in prognosis (45), informed consent, and advanced care directives.

The existence of advanced care directives has stimulated a number of empirical studies. It has been noted that most patients do not execute directives in part because physicians frequently fail to discuss this issue (32) or because patients fail to see the directive when it is presumably distributed on admission (46). Even when executed, only about 39% in one study wished to have the directives observed strictly by the physician (47). In addition, a significant number of directives are either ignored or overridden by the physician; sometimes more treatment is given than requested and sometimes less (32, 48).

Attitudes toward executing directives, especially by older individuals, are significantly influenced by a number of factors including dependence on family decisions, educational and economic status, religious views, ethnic backgrounds, and national origins. For example, Korean Americans and Mexican Americans were more likely to hold a family-centered model of medical decision making, rather than the patient autonomy model favored by most African American and European American respondents (49). The great majority of Navajo informants considered advance care planning a dangerous violation of their traditional values (50). To develop the understanding of and respect for cultural differences that will help avoid inappropriately paternalistic judgments, physicians do well to seek assistance from family members and others who are knowledgeable in this area (51).

Recently, a series of survey reports introduced another view of the purpose of advanced directive and planning, namely, its intent to limit life-sustaining treatments and reduce healthcare costs. Such an approach creates the potential conflict between the original purpose of advanced directives (stimulating informed consent and patient autonomy) to that of reducing medical care (51a).

Patient Choices for Life-Sustaining Treatments

Studies have been done on the process of decision making concerning medical intervention and life support of the seriously ill and the issue of quality-of-life and its expected duration. Earlier studies used measures of physiologic competence (e.g., organ function or metabolic indices), economic or environmental factors, or overall individual performance to ascertain whether any of these factors are improved by specific therapies. More recently, efforts have been spent in obtaining information on the relative importance patients assign to the value of their lives and how it may be influenced by their therapies (52, 53). The subjective health values and ratings of 1438 seriously ill but competent patients with at least one of nine diseases with a projected overall mortality rate of 50% were compared with similar ratings obtained from the patients' surrogates and their physicians. The health values of the patients varied greatly from one to another, but the individual patient showed excellent test-retest reliability. Their preferences for living at current health levels compared with living in excellent health correlated strongly with their preferences for care that extended life even though it was at the expense of pain and discomfort. Furthermore, their individual health values and ratings were generally higher than those postulated by their surrogates and physicians. The study concluded that when it comes to the issue of resource allocation for care, the patient is the true "expert on the values of living," whereas the value of society is that of taxpayers or insurance premium payers who often foot the healthcare bill (54).

There are important differences in the responses of elderly individuals about the use of living wills and desire for life-sustaining treatments between those who have chosen to forgo life-sustaining treatments and those who have not indicated such a preference. Those with living wills were less likely to change their expressed wishes (14%) over a 2-year period than those without (41%) (55). During the study period, patients who had been hospitalized, had an accident, become more immobile or depressed, or had less social support showed appreciable change in the stability of choice and now wanted increased treatment. Such data indicate the need for periodic review of preferences for life-sustaining treatments.

NUTRITIONAL SUPPORT OF THE INCOMPETENT PATIENT

The major medical, ethical, and legal issues on cessation of involuntary nutritional support have involved incompetent patients. More than 30 separate state court decisions on this issue between 1983 and 1995 have been summarized (56).

There are a number of causes of incompetence, ranging from serious memory loss without other physical disability, through progressive loss of cognitive ability requiring hand feeding, to one of several forms of persistent unconsciousness. The patient in the last category requires artificial nutrition and hydration to avert starvation or dehydration. Until physicians have had sufficient time to develop a firm prognosis of the individual who is unable to take sufficient food and fluid by mouth, nutrition and hydration are indicated.

Traditionally, the right of the state to preserve the life of the incompetent patient has been manifest in the requirement for a court-appointed guardian or surrogate to act on behalf of the adult patient. In the case of minors, courts have almost always affirmed the authority of the parents or (if needed) a surrogate to make decisions.

The Persistent Vegetative State (PVS)

The Multi-Society Task Force on PVS has summarized current knowledge of this state, which it defined as a "clinical condition of complete unawareness of the self and the environment accompanied by sleep wake cycles with partial preservation of hypothalamic and brain stem autonomic functions" (57). Seven diagnostic criteria were given. Facial and reflex movements, groans, and cries may occur, and small amounts of food placed in the mouth may be swallowed (19, 57). Clinical observation, the results of positron-emission tomographic (PET) studies, and neuropathologic examination support the belief that these patients are unaware and insensate and lack the cerebral cortical capacity to be conscious of pain (58).

When this "wakeful unconscious" state persists for a month in a patient with an acute traumatic or nontraumatic brain injury (e.g., from stroke or cardiorespiratory arrest) or with one of a number of degenerative or metabolic disorders or developmental malformations, the term *persistent vegetative state* is in order. Of 257 patients, the cumulative mortality rate at 3 years was 70%, and at 5 years, 84% (58a); survival beyond 10 years was unusual, but some lived for 30 years (19, 58). Progressive spasticity and bed rest lead to muscle atrophy and limb, hand, and foot contraction (13). The term *permanent vegetative state* is prognostic, because the outcome cannot be known with absolute accuracy. It may be used after the time lapses noted, which strongly indicate that recovery is very unlikely.

The task force noted that few patients in PVS had verified recovery of consciousness after 12 months following traumatic injury, or more than 3 months after a nontraumatic injury; the few who recovered were left with severe disability (58). A British unit specializing in neurodisability reported that 40 (41%) of 97 patients with profound brain damage admitted from 1992 to 1995 had been diagnosed by the referring physician as being in a vegetative state; of these 40, 17 (43%) were considered misdiagnosed because all but one responded in some manner to a command within 16 days of admission (59). An accompanying editorial questioned the diagnosis of vegetative state in 9 of the patients and emphasized the severity of their physical, neurologic, and cognitive states despite some responsiveness (60). The need for competent and persistent serial evaluation of all vegetative patients and use of additional evaluation techniques is emphasized (60, 60a).

The prevalence of PVS is not known because it was not a codable diagnosis until recently in ID-9-CM and elsewhere. The task force referred to estimates of PVS in the

United States of 10,000 to 25,000 adults and 4,000 to 10,000 children (57).

Guidelines were published recently by a multidisciplinary group convened by the Royal College of Physicians, working on the diagnostic criteria and terminology of PVS (61). This group preferred the general term "vegetative state: to describe the condition which may be transient with recovery/or which might persist to death." The term *continuing vegetative state* (CVS) was applied when the condition persisted for more than 4 weeks and recovery from coma became unlikely. A "permanent" state exists "when the diagnosis of irreversibility can be established with a high degree of clinical certainty." The working group accepted the U.S. Multi-Society Task Force on PVS (52) suggestion for use of the term *permanent* for adults and children with traumatic injury of 12 months duration, and 3 months for those with nontraumatic injuries.

In contrast to incompetent adults with PVS, forgoing medically provided nutrition and hydration in children has received less discussion and legal review. The current status of this aspect has been reviewed recently (62). Nelson et al. noted that pediatricians were more likely than internists to continue artificial nutrition and hydration in PVS against parental desires, even though other life-support systems had been discontinued. They listed three major medical categories of children for whom consider it is ethically permissible to forgo such nutrition and hydration: neurologic devastation, such as PVS from severe brain injury or anencephaly; irreversible total intestinal failure, such as total bowel necrosis or neural dysplasia; and proximate death (days or weeks) in conditions such as advanced unresponsive cancer. The issue of total intestinal failure is discussed in light of the possibility of a successful bowel transplant and the presence of other serious disease in recipient and donor. Various judicial decisions concerned with cessation of artificial feeding (in the great majority of which the courts have upheld the desire by the parents for termination) are reviewed as well as federal statutory law and state laws (62).

Forgoing nutritional support in children with severe intestinal dysfunction requires careful consideration because most of these children are not in the terminal state or in PVS. Total parenteral nutrition, despite the cost and probability of complications, has proven effective in improving and maintaining adequate nutrition and a reasonably good quality of life. Despite major intestinal loss, in a number of patients the remaining bowel can often adapt to the point that parenteral nutrition can eventually be discontinued (see Chapter 101). For those who may develop severe hepatic insufficiency, bowel transplant is an increasingly successful option (Chapter 101).

The impact of PVS on the patient's family and friends is one of distress and helplessness. Psychologic consequences of seeing the loved one remain unresponsive with increasing atrophy and contractures as weeks and months pass are exacerbated by developing monetary and social problems. As noted above, a large number of such cases have led to court decisions that have focused the attention of the public, other courts, and medical societies on biomedical and ethical issues related to the requests for withdrawal of life-sustaining treatments including withdrawal of artificial nutrition and hydration. Some instructive cases and decisions affecting adults are summarized below.

The Quinlan Case

The case of Karen Ann Quinlan was a landmark effort to discontinue life support. She was a young woman in New Jersey who was in PVS on a respirator. The state's supreme court, on a reversal of a lower court decision, made medical legal history in 1976 when, at the request of the parents and despite the opposition of the patient's physician and hospital, it ruled that the respirator could be discontinued (63). When this was done, the patient was found to be able to breathe spontaneously, and she survived for 9 years on tube feeding until she died from overwhelming infection. Withdrawal of tube feeding was not considered an option by the parents. This position reflected a view then widely held, namely, that food and hydration were not in the category of a special life-support system but rather a humanitarian action necessary for the comfort of the patient.

The Barber-Nejde Case. Another troubling judicial issue was the legal liability of physicians when nutrition was withheld from an incompetent patient who was not terminally ill and who, while competent, had not clearly indicated in writing or verbally to a reliable witness a desire not to be force fed when terminally or incurably ill. This concern is illustrated by the legal developments resulting from the medical management of Clarence Herbert, who had suffered respiratory arrest in association with routine intestinal surgery (64, 65). Following resuscitation, he remained comatose over the following several days. On the advice of physicians that prognosis for recovery was poor and with consent of family, use of the respirator was stopped. The patient then breathed spontaneously but without change in his comatose state. Two days later, again after consultation with the family, the attending physicians ordered removal of the nasogastric tube, intravenous nutrition, and air mist. The patient died 6 days later. He had not previously executed a formal directive under the California Natural Death Act, nor had he written anything concerning his wishes in such circumstances; however, he had stated to his wife that he did not want to be kept alive by machine or "become another Karen Ann Quinlan."

A nurse reported the actions of the physicians to local authorities, who then filed criminal charges for murder against both attending physicians, Drs. Barber and Nejde. Despite a municipal court magistrate ruling that death had resulted from brain damage secondary to anoxia and that the conduct of the physicians was not "unlawful," the district attorney appealed the case to Los Angeles Superior Court. The murder charge was reinstated by a judge who decided that there was no legal justification for the physicians' action. The physicians then appealed to the California Court of Appeals, which dismissed the criminal charges.

The Conroy Case

Another case, occurring at the same time, further delineated the complex medicolegal issues that arise when the status of an incurably ill patient is presented to different jurists. Claire Conroy was an 84-year-old woman severely ill with advanced atherosclerosis, diabetes, and organic brain syndrome (66, 67). Although the case description stated that she was not in PVS, her described behavior approximated closely the clinical description of this state. A nephew filed a petition to authorize removal of the nasogastric feeding tube from the patient, although there was no clear evidence of what the patient would have desired. A trial judge authorized removal of the feeding tube but not cessation of any voluntary or assisted oral feeding. The decision was appealed by the institution, and pending the hearing, tube feeding was continued to the patient's death.

Despite Conroy's death, the New Jersey Appellate Court heard the appeal and reversed the earlier trial judge's decision. It held that *(a)* she was neither comatose nor terminally ill, *(b)* the feeding tube was not a particularly invasive treatment as was the respirator in the Quinlan case, and *(c)* if the nasogastric tube had been removed in accordance with the trial judge's decision, Mrs. Conroy would have died not as a result of her condition but from a "new and independent condition: dehydration and starvation and that this would constitute murder (euthanasia)." The case was appealed to the New Jersey Supreme Court, which sanctioned withdrawal of artificial nutrition and hydration in this type of case, but with a time constraint of expected survival of 1 year or less (66).

This final decision in the Conroy case is of special interest in the context of criteria established by judges as guidelines for decisions in terminating medical care of incompetent patients. Emanuel noted that the court laid down three standards for terminating such care and stipulated that one of them be satisfied before treatment could be stopped (67). The court designated the first a "subjective standard," which permits termination of treatment when an incompetent patient left clear indication, such as a living will, that he or she would have refused that treatment. It called the second a "pure objective standard," which permits termination of life-sustaining treatment for patients if the burden of the care outweighs the benefits, although they have not left indication of their preferences about life-sustaining care. For example, administering life-sustaining care would be inhumane because it would perpetuate severe pain. Others label this the "best interests standard," in which the patient's surrogate objectively evaluates the benefits and risks of a treatment and decides what most benefits the patient. In the Conroy Case, the court, acting as surrogate, accepted this standard. The third standard, called by the court a "limited objective standard," is a combination of the first two and permits termination of care if there is some evidence (such as remarks made during a conversation) or opinion of the surrogate that the patient would not want the treatment and if the burden and pain of continued life outweigh the benefits; this is similar to the substituted judgment standard.

The Jobes Case

A subsequent ruling by the same court involved the case of Nancy Jobes, who was in PVS following hemorrhage (68). Her husband and parents requested that a feeding tube be removed and that she be allowed to die. The nursing home refused to honor this request. When the case was brought before the New Jersey Supreme Court, the court sanctioned removal of the feeding tube but rejected as "remote," "general," and "casual conversation" statements by the patient's friends and relatives that she had said in conversation that she did not wish to be dependent on a respirator. The court eliminated its previous "Conroy" criterion and instead, based its ruling on the Quinlan case, ruled that the "substituted judgment standard" exercised by the family should apply to patients in a PVS, and therefore, the feeding tube could be removed. In reviewing this case, Emanuel noted that the substituted judgment standard means, in effect, that the surrogate for an incompetent patient is put into position of attempting to make a decision for the patient as if that individual were competent; this standard thus differs from the best interest standard, which is based on an objective standard of benefits and burdens (68).

The judicial and legislative history and endorsement of decision making for incompetent patients by proxy or surrogate and their ethical justification have been briefly reviewed by Emanuel and Emanuel (69). They summarize objections to proxy making on the grounds that "proxy decision makers cannot divine or implement the incompetent patient's wishes regarding the termination of life sustaining care." Alternative solutions are suggested, with recognition that each has limitations. While agreeing with the array of concerns about proxy decision making, Lynn, in an accompanying editorial, takes the position that "a morally justifiably and pragmatic policy for decision making for incompetent adults, at this point, will have to rely heavily on appointed and family proxies, with a morally defensible and practical plan" (70) which provides options similar to those suggested by the Coordinating Council on Life Sustaining Medical Treatment Decision-Making by the Courts (71).

AMA Statement of 1986

In the midst of these and other pertinent judicial decisions, the AMA, through its Council on Ethical and Judicial, issued in 1984 (and in revised form in 1986) statements on withholding or withdrawing life-prolonging medical treatment. The 1986 statement consists of four short paragraphs that include the following, which also relate to food and fluids (72):

> In the absence of the patient's choice or an authorized proxy, the physician must act in the best interest of the patient . . . For humane reasons, with informed consent, a physician may do what is medically necessary to alleviate severe pain, or cease or omit treatment to permit a terminally ill patient whose death is imminent to die. Even if death is not imminent but a patient's coma is beyond doubt irreversible and there are adequate safeguards to confirm the accuracy of the diagnosis and with the concurrence of those with responsibility for the care of the patient, it is not unethical to discontinue all means of life prolonging medical treatment. Life prolonging medical treatment includes medication and artificially or technologically supplied respiration, nutrition or hydration.

The changed physician attitudes resulting from the widespread interest and discussion of these issues is evidenced by significant differences in the 1984 and 1986 statements. For example, the first version refers only to terminally ill patients, while the later one includes those in irreversible coma; the 1984 version did not define "life prolonging medical treatment," whereas in 1986, these are specifically designated and include nutrition or hydration.

The Cruzan Case

This case was the first to involve the United States Supreme Court in the issue of discontinuance of tube feeding an incompetent patient. Like the Quinlan case, it aroused widespread public and professional interest and resulted in a decision with far-reaching implications. In January 1983, at the age of 25 years, Nancy Cruzan suffered irreversible brain damage secondary to prolonged hypoxia following an automobile accident. She was then supported in the hospital by food and fluid fed through a tube. In 1986 her parents requested discontinuance of the feedings but had to resort to legal action at the insistence of the Missouri state hospital administration. In July 1988, a trial court ruled that tube feeding could be withheld; however on appeal, the Missouri Supreme Court, by a 4 to 3 decision, reversed the trial court on the grounds that no reliable evidence was presented indicating that Cruzan would have refused artificial feeding (73).

On June 25, 1990, the United States Supreme Court affirmed the reversal by a vote of 5 to 4 (74). Five justices stated that the Constitution did not prohibit Missouri from choosing to rule as it did. Three of the four dissenting justices stated that incompetent as well as competent patients had the constitutional right to be free of unwanted medical treatment and the fourth stated that the Constitution required that the best interest of the patient be followed. Six of the nine justices explicitly found no distinction between fluids and nutrition delivered artificially and other medical treatments; none of the other three found a constitutionally relevant distinction (74, 75). Six months later, nearly 8 years after the parents' first request, a judge in Missouri Circuit Court, in a brief order, authorized the parents as coguardians "to cause the removal of nutrition and hydration from our ward, Nancy Beth Cruzan" (76). This was done, and Cruzan died 12 days later.

While some bioethicists felt that the Supreme Court's opinion would make a constitutional right to refuse artificial nutrition more difficult to achieve in the future (77, 78), others believed that the decision had important positive aspects. These were summarized in a statement by physicians, nurses, lawyers, and bioethicists (79). The best evidence of the impact of the Supreme Court's decision was the rapid collapse of the medical, institutional, surrogate, and legal opposition in Missouri to discontinuing Cruzan's feedings. Another effect of the Cruzan decision was the speed with which many states enacted health proxy legislation (80). Problems still remained, however, because of the variability in important requirements among state laws. As a result of publicity about the Cruzan case and variability of relevant state laws, some families in similar situations have requested that physicians not start artificial feedings because they and the patient may become prisoners of technology and state law (19). This type of request presents a professional problem for physicians who are hesitant to start or to stop such treatment before the prognosis seems certain. To help resolve this dilemma, Cranford proposed that the family be assured that once a diagnosis and prognosis were established with great certainty, physicians would be willing to discontinue artificial nutrition and hydration, thus freeing the family of the fear that the patient and family would be held hostage by medical technology (19).

The problem is further complicated by family members or surrogates who, despite physicians' recommendations, insist that life-support systems be continued in patients in a PVS (e.g., cases of Wanglie [81] and of Baby K [82]). While various recommendations have been offered in an effort to increase legal support for medical decisions, in the United States, the legal outcome in a suit depends on state court decisions as they arise.

In some other countries, the highest national courts have upheld the right of physicians to withdraw lifesaving treatment in specific instances of patients in PVS. In the United Kingdom, the House of Lords made that decison on February 4, 1993, in the case of Anthony Bland, who had suffered severe brain damage in 1989 (83); the wording of this decision led the Royal College of Physicians to provide standards for decision making by physicians that will have High Court or Parliamentary approval (58).

The Irish Supreme Court by a 4 to 1 majority ruled that a gastrostomy feeding system could be withdrawn from a 45-year-old woman in "near permanent" vegetative state for 23 years and that she be allowed to die (84). In recent years, courts in New Zealand and South Africa have ruled it lawful to discontinue treating PVS patients (85).

Patients with Progressive Neurologic Deterioration

In addition to the state of severe and permanent paralysis ("locked-in syndrome" described above in the Bouvia case) and PVS, a third syndrome, dementia, is in the category of disabling neurologic conditions with the potential for prolonged survival and the resulting issue of life-sustaining medical treatment. Dementia includes Alzheimer's disease, the most common cause in the elderly, with its variable destruction of the neocortex; multiinfarct and other vascular dementias with variable cognitive deficits (19, 23); and the variants of Creutzfeldt-Jakob disease and dementias associated with parkinsonism and progressive supranuclear palsy (85a). These disorders are characterized by gradual onset of progressive neurologic deterioration occurring over years to decades, with time to prognostic certainty usually months to years, and with suffering decreasing with increasing impairment of cortical function.

The PVS is the ultimate and terminal form of dementia as the result of complete loss of neocortical function (19, 57). An estimated 4 million patients in the United States have various stages of dementia, of whom 1.3 to 1.9 million have Alzheimer's disease (23).

The President's Commission (24), the American College of Physicians (86), the AMA (87), and other relevant organizations draw a distinction between the incompetent patient in PVS and one in a "conscious" state but with severe, irreversible, and deteriorating mental impairment. The critical difference between these states is retention until late in the disease of self-awareness, motor function, and feelings of pain and suffering (57). At what stage and on what grounds is the family or surrogate to make the decision to accept or forgo further life-sustaining treatments?

There are major differences in the judgmental criteria of various medical ethicists. One opinion is that the decision should be that which the patient when fully rational would have made, based on what Dworkin calls "critical interests" (88–90), which is equivalent to the "substituted judgment" standard mentioned above. An opposing opinion is based on the proposition of an existing awareness on the part of the patient and the possibility that his or her interests and wishes might have changed. In this situation, the family, surrogate, and physician should attempt to understand the experiential world of the patient by observation and testing so as to better weigh the benefits and burdens of current treatment (88–90). This is essentially the "best interest," "objective," or "benefit burden" judgment standard.

The situation changes when the patient becomes unable to eat voluntarily and swallow adequately when hand fed and has minimal consciousness. In such circumstances, some bioethicists have favored withholding nutrition and hydration (19, 68, 90). Undoubtedly, this issue will receive increasing medicolegal scrutiny as long as such conditions remain irreversible and family members or surrogates continue efforts to erase the distinction between PVS and severe dementia.

Attitudes and Beliefs Influencing Decisions

The major professional societies, most bioethicists, and many state legislatures and courts support withholding or terminating artificial feeding for the competent patient who requests it. Some states still limit parental authority or advance directives for the incompetent terminally ill patient or for children and adults in a PVS (reviewed in 62 and 93). The attitudes of physicians about artificial feeding vary. As mentioned above, physicians may be unaware of advance directives or do not make serious efforts to obtain them or may undertreat or overtreat despite directives, and pediatricians are believed to be more reluctant than internists to discontinue feeding with PVS (62).

Long-term comparative data are not available on attitudes and behavior of large numbers of physicians concerning the issue of artificial feeding. However, some data on physician attitudes are at hand. A national survey of 169 neurologists and 150 nursing home medical directors indicated general concurrence (89%) that it was ethical to withdraw artificial nutrition and hydration from patients with PVS in an irreversible stage (94). In a survey of 32 internists familiar with tube feeding, 80% favored withdrawing tube feeding and the remaining 20% opposed it when presented with a case of a woman in PVS for 1 year who was being fed via gastrostomy (95).

A more complex study was conducted with 456 university internists presented with the issue of withdrawing life support; preferences were obtained on withdrawal of eight different life-support systems including TPN, enteral feeding, and intravenous fluids in relation to 13 attributes including cost, invasiveness, patient discomfort, rapidity of death. The order of preferences of withdrawal of specific supports was marked. Physicians were much more likely to withdraw TPN before tube feeding before intravenous fluids—the latter two being classed with artificial ventilation. Older physicians were less likely than younger ones to prefer withdrawing a number of such supports. The authors concluded that "even when physicians may have agreed that life support should be withdrawn, the choices that they make about the manner of withdrawing life support reflect other moral, social, and clinical goals" (96). A study of actual patterns in withdrawing life-support systems for dying patients indicated a stepwise retreat in forgoing different types of support until death occurred; enteral and parenteral nutrition and, finally, ventilatory support were the last to be withdrawn (97).

Patients, surrogates, and physicians may hold religious beliefs that influence their decisions on terminating artificial nutrition. Leading church figures and other theologic scholars have stated their opinions. The Archbishop of Canterbury concluded in 1977 that extending life by artificial means was distinct from euthanasia and that removal of life support was acceptable if it would be better for the patient to be allowed to die (98). The National Conference of United States Catholic Bishops in 1992 restated the Pope's earlier view that Catholics are not obliged to use extraordinary or disproportionate means when there is no hope for recovery and only the burden of care remains (99).

For Orthodox Jews, the legal ethical system known as halacha governs most aspects of daily life, including the medical ethic that the "Sanctify of life, the halachic, the imperative to preserve life, supersedes, with a few exceptions, quality-of-life-considerations" (100). Freedman states that the concept of duty and obligation rather than rights is important and that Halachic Judaism has a concept of informed consent and guidelines for individual medical decision making (14). In his review of relevant rabbinical decisions, an Orthodox Jewish theologian-ethicist has noted differing positions on artificial feeding and concludes that "the question of withholding and withdrawing artificial nutrition and hydration—tube feeding—is not clear cut in halacha" (100). His own opinion is that in geriatric patients, advance directives should be limited to withholding nutrition and hydration as opposed to withdrawing it. In Israel, the preservation of life in the sick has been embodied in parliamentary legislation that empowers hospital ethics committees that can overrule a patient's expressed will (43a). At the same time, its Supreme Court has recognized the right of a terminally ill suffering patient to reject intrusive and uncomfortable therapy that cannot cure the basic illness (43a).

The physician and hospital must each make their positions clear to patients and surrogates concerning such end-of-life issues so that, if necessary, alternatives can be found without rancor and undue distress. It is equally important that physicians, nurses, and other members of the healthcare team "be skilled in the two essential aspects of good clinical care of dying patients—technical issues in the compassionate withdrawal of life-prolonging therapy and counseling and emotional support for patients, families, and staff during this process" (101).

Physiologic Responses to Restriction

Young, healthy, active individuals in negative water balance develop thirst, dry mouth, and headache, followed by fatigue; cognitive impairment occurs as dehydration progresses and becomes severe with abnormal electrolytes, rising blood urea, and hemoconcentration. Renal failure ensues unless water is available. In healthy elderly people, in contrast, reduced thirst may occur with water deprivation (102).

Those involved in palliative care of terminally ill patients have reported frequently that the conscious competent patient with an advancing severe illness unresponsive to therapy and in little or no pain becomes progressively weaker, with decreasing communication, increasing anorexia, decreased desire for fluids, and progressive apathy. In such patients with little intake of fluids, signs and symptoms of dehydration appear: dryness of skin and mouth, decreased urinary output, and occasional thirst. Nausea, vomiting, or cramps are reportedly rare in this situation, and the dehydrated patient rarely needs oral pharyngeal suction; this is in contrast to the hydrated patient (19, 103–106). Obtundation usually progresses to a peaceful death.

There are a significant number of reports (summarized in ref. 92) that many terminally ill patients have relatively few of the changes in blood and urine chemistry that indicate clinical dehydration and that thirst is usually absent. In a brief report about terminally ill patients, no differences were noted in biochemical parameters and state of consciousness in those given intravenous fluids and those given only oral fluids (107). In their detailed study of 32 competent terminally ill cancer patients, McCann et al. concluded that "food and fluid administered beyond the specific requests of patients may play a minimal role in providing comfort to terminally ill patients"; 97% either did not experience hunger at all or only initially, 66% either did not experience thirst or only initially, and the rest were comfortable with mouth care and sips of water (108). The relationships among symptoms, laboratory evidence of dehydration, and medications were studied in 82 individuals dying of cancer in a hospice; none were given artificial fluid therapy, and the time from entry into the study to death ranged from 1 to 5 days (median, 2 days). Fifty percent had normal serum osmolalities below the upper limit of normal and a urea concentration below 11.0 mmol/L, which was not considered evidence of dehydration. The others had evidence of dehydration. There was no statistically significant relationship between hydration status and the symptoms of dry mouth and thirst noted by about 85% of those able to respond clearly to questions. Almost all of the latter group were on medications known to cause dry mouth and/or had other causes for this condition such as mouth breathing, candidiasis, and past treatment with chemotherapeutic agents and radiotherapy (109). Such reports put into question the use of tube and orally administered fluids to the dying patient.

The common use of intravenous isotonic glucose—with or without electrolytes or vitamin additives—in this situation also seems less defensible because this prevents ketosis and inhibits some dehydration, thereby overcoming their contribution to comfort and prolonging the dying process.

In the management of such patients with the stated goal of comfort, one must also consider some of the undesirable effects of tube feeding, whether via nasal or gastrostomy tube. These include increased agitation, accidental or self-extubation often requiring restraints, and aspiration pneumonia (110, 111); in addition, leakage, diarrhea, or impaction may occur. As Cranford has stated "to a large extent limiting nutrition and hydration is more a medical than a moral issue" (19).

Management of symptoms that may arise when artificial

Table 102.1
Management of Symptoms That Occasionally Complicate Withdrawal of Artificial Nutrition and Hydration

Symptom	Management
Thirst (rare)	Sips of fluids (patients commonly take much less than required for physiologic volume replacement)
Dry mouth (common)	Glycerine swabs, ice chips, sips of fluid; review medication list for any that cause dry mouth
Dry mouth (if aggravated by glycerine or lemon swabs)	Artificial saliva, petroleum jelly, lip balm
Mouth debris or poor hygiene	Nonalcoholic mouthwashes, dilute hydrogen peroxide
Oral inflammation	Diphenhydramine liquid, viscous lidocaine; antimonilial therapy
Pain, restlessness (rare)	Morphine or benzodiazepines in titrated doses
Nausea (rare)	Antiemetic drugs

From Brody H, Campbell ML, Faber-Langendoen K, et al. N Engl J Med 1997;336:652–7, with permission.

nutrition and hydration are withheld or withdrawn is outlined in Table 102.1.

REFERENCES

Note: The references to judicial decisions follow the form generally used in legal writing. Following the case name, the first number refers to the volume of the reporter series for the decisional court; the reported series follows as an abbreviation, then the number of the first page of the printed judicial decision, and finally the year of the decision. For example, *Smith v Jones,* 261 F2d448 (1990) can be found in vol. 261 of the second series of the Federal Reporter beginning on page 448.
Published court decisions are generally available to the public through state, county, or city bar association libraries or law school libraries. West Publishing Company and Mead Data Services also provide case text databases on a fee-for-service basis to libraries and law firms.

1. Pellegrino ED. JAMA 1974;227:1288–94.
2. Pennington CR. Nutrition 1996;12:56–7.
3. Lo B. Resolving ethical dilemmas. A guide for clinicians. Baltimore: Williams & Wilkins 1995.
4. Conrad LI, Neve M, Nutton V, et al. The western medical tradition: 800 BC–1800 AD. New York: Cambridge University Press, 1995, chapter 1.
5. Siegler M. Mayo Clinic Proc 1993;68:461–7.
6. Pellegrino ED. JAMA 1993;269:1158–62.
7. Beauchamp TL, Childress JF. Principles of biomedical ethics. 1st ed. New York: Oxford University Press, 1979.
8. Mahowald MD. Clin Geriatr Med 1994;10:403–18.
9. Wolf SM. Am J Law Med 1994;20:395–487.
10. Pellegrino ED. JAMA 1994;271:1668–70.
11. Beauchamp TL, Childress JF. Principles of biomedical ethics. 4th ed. New York: Oxford University Press, 1994.
12. Jones AH. Lancet 1997;349:1243–6.
13. Pellegrino ED, Thomasma DC. The Christian virtues in medical practice. Washington, DC: Georgetown University Press, 1996.
14. Freedman F. Duty and healing foundation of a Jewish bioethics. Available only on the World Wide Web at http://www.mcgill.ca/CTRG/bfreed/.
15. Engelhardt HT Jr. The foundations of bioethics. 2nd ed. New York: Oxford University Press, 1996.
16. *Union Pacific Ry v Botsford,* 141 US 250, 251 (1891).
17. *Bouvia v county of Riverside,* 159780 Riverside Co. CA. Sup. Ct. 1984.
18. *Bouvia v Superior Court (Glenchur),* 179 cal. App. 3d 1127 1986;225 cal. Rpts. 297.
19. Cranford RD. Law Med Health Care 1991;19:13–22.
19a. Columbia Broadcasting Co. Sixty Minutes. Interview with Mike Wallace broadcast Sept 8, 1997.
20. Pellegrino ED. NY State J Med 1977;77:1456–2.
21. Nevins M. Am Coll Physicians Observer 1986;Mar:13–16.
22. Applebaum PS, Grisso T. N Engl J Med 1988;319:1635–8.
23. Howe EG, Gordon DS, Valentin M. Law Med Health Care 1991;19:27–33.
24. President's Commission for the Study of Ethical Problems in Medicine and Biomedical and Behavioral Research. Deciding to forego life-sustaining treatment. A report on the ethical, medical, and legal issues in treatment decisions. Washington, DC: United States Government Printing Office, 1983;3, 61–62.
25. Hastings Center. Guidelines on the termination of life sustaining treatment and the care of the dying. Briarcliff Manor, NY: Hastings Center 1987;50.
26. Law Reform Commission of Canada. Report on euthanasia, aiding suicide and cessation of treatment. Report 20 to the Minister of Justice and Attorney General. Ottawa 1983;11–12, 32, 35.
27. Personal communication from Y. Roy, Senior General Counsel, Criminal Law Policy Section, Department of Justice, Canada, March 28, 1996.
28. Quill TE, Cassel CK. Ann Intern Med 1995;122:368–74.
29. Cimino JE. Topics Clin Nutr 1993;9:29–34.
30. Pellegrino ED. Ann Intern Med 1995;122:377–8.
31. Gert B, Bernat JL, Mogulnicki RP. Hastings Cent Rep 1994;24(4):13–5.
32. Orentlicher D. JAMA 1992;267:2101–4.
33. Tiemstra JD. J Clin Ethics 1995;6:163–5.
34. Logan RL, Scott PJ. Lancet 1996;347:595–8.
35. Veach RM, Spicer CM. Am J Law Med 1992;18:15–56.
36. Gatter RA Jr, Moskop JC. J Med Philos 1995;20:191–205.
37. Lantos JD, Singer PA, Walker RM, et al. Am J Med 1989;87:81–4.
38. J Med Philos 1995;20:109–21, 145–63.
38a. J Clin Ethics 1995;6:112–26, 128–32, 138–48.
39. Schneiderman LJ, Jecker NS. Doctors, patients, and futile treatment. Baltimore: Johns Hopkins University Press, 1995.
40. Brody AB, Halevy A. J Med Philos 1995;20:123–44.
41. Spielman BJ. Law Med Ethics 1995;23:136–42.
42. Halevy A, Brody B. JAMA 1996;276:571–74.
43. British Medical Association. World Medical Association declaration on hunger strikers in medicine betrayed. The participation of doctors in human rights abuse. London: Zed Books, 1992:212–4, 119–31.
43a. Glick SM. N Engl J Med 1997;336:954–6.
43b. Silove D, Curtis J, Mason C, et al. JAMA 1996;276:410–5.
43c. Annas GJ. (Editorial) Br Med J 1995;311:1114–5.
44. The Patient Self-Determination Act, sections 4206 and 4751 of the Omnibus Budget Reconciliation Act of 1960; P.L. 101-508 Nov 5, 1990.
45. Annas GJ. N Engl J Med 1994;330:223–5.
46. Cugliari AM, Miller T, Sokal J. Arch Intern Med 1995;155:1893–8.
47. Sehyal A, Gallbraith A, Chesney M, et al. JAMA 1992;267:59–63.

48. Danis M, Southerland LI, Barrett JM, et al. N Engl J Med 1991;324:882–8.
49. Blackhall LJ, Murphy ST, Frank G, et al. JAMA 1955;274: 820–5.
50. Carrese JA, Rhodes LA. JAMA 1995;274:826–9.
51. Gostin LO. JAMA 1995;274:844–5.
51a. Levinsky NG. N Engl J Med 1996;335:741–3.
52. Gill TM, Feinstein AR. JAMA 1994;272:619–26.
53. Guyatt GH, Feeny DH, Patrick DL. Ann Intern Med 1993;118:622–9.
54. Tsevat J, Cook EF, Green ML, et al. Ann Intern Med 1995;122:514–20.
55. Danis M, Garrett J, Harris R, et al. Ann Intern Med 1994;120:567–73.
56. American Medical Association Council on Ethical and Judicial Affairs. Code of medical ethics. Current opinions with annotations, 1996–1997 ed. Chicago: American Medical Association, 1996;41–51.
57. The Multi-Society Task Force on PVS. N Engl J Med 1994;330:1499–508.
58. The Multi-Society Task Force on PVS. N Engl J Med 1994;330;1572–9.
58a. Ashwell S, Cranford R. N Engl J Med 1995;333:130 (correction).
59. Andrews K, Murphy L, Munday R, et al. Br Med J 1996;313:13–6.
60. Cranford R. Br Med J (Editorial) 1996;313:5–6.
60a. Zeman A. Lancet 1997;350:795–9.
61. Royal College of Physicians Working Group. J R Coll Physicians (London) 1996;30:119–21.
62. Nelson LJ, Rushton CH, Cranford RE, et al. J Law Med Ethics 1995;23:33–46.
63. *In re Quinlan* 70 NJ 10, 355 A2d; 647, 1976.
64. *People v Barber* A025586 Los Angeles Sup. Ct. 1983.
64a. *Barber v Superior Ct.* 147 CA 3d 1006 Ca, 1983.
65. Myers DW. Arch Intern Med 1985;145:125–7.
66. *Matter of Claire Conroy* 453, 464 A 2d 303 (NJ App. 1983).
66a. *Matter of Claire Conroy* rev'd cf also 98 NJ 321, 486A 2d 1209 (1985).
67. Emanuel EJ. Lancet 1988;1:170–71.
68. Emanuel EJ. Lancet 1988;1:106–07.
69. Emanuel EJ, Emanuel LL. JAMA 1992;267:2067–71.
70. Lynn J. JAMA 1992;267:2082–84.
71. Coordinating Council on Life-Sustaining Medical Treatment Decision-Making by the Courts. Guidelines for state court decision-making in authorizing or withholding life sustaining medical treatment. Williamsburg, VA: National Center for State Courts, 1991.
72. Council on Ethical and Judicial Affairs of the American Medical Association. Withholding or withdrawing life prolonging medical treatment. Chicago: American Medical Association, 1986.
73. *Cruzan v Harmon* 760 SW 2d 408 (MO 1988).
74. *Cruzan v Missouri Department of Health* 760 sw 2d 408 aff 110 S. Ct. 2841 (1990).
75. Annas GJ. Law Med Health Care 1991;19:52–9.
76. *Cruzan v Mouton Estate* No CV 384-9P (Circ. Ct Jasper Co, filed Dec. 14, 1990 (Teel).
77. Lo B, Steinbrook R. Ann Intern Med 1991;114:895–901.
78. Annas GJ. N Engl J Med 1990;323:670–3.
79. Bioethicists' statement on the US Supreme Court's Cruzan decision. N Engl J Med 1990;323:686.
80. King PA. Law Med Health Care 1991;325:511–2.
81. Angell M. N Engl J Med 1991;325:511–2.
82. Annas CJ. N Engl J Med 1994;330:1542–5.
83. Lancet (Editorial) 1993;341:41.
84. Wall M. Lancet 1995;346:368.
85. Brahams D. Lancet 1992;340:1534–5.
85a. Case Records of the Massachusetts General Hospital—Case 26-1997. N Engl J Med 1997;337:549–56.
86. American College of Physicians ethics manual. Ann Intern Med 1992;117:947–60.
87. Council on Scientific Affairs American Medical Association. JAMA 1990;263:426–30.
88. Dworkin R. Life's dominion: an argument about abortion, euthanasia, and individual freedom. New York: Alfred A Knopf, 1993:195.
89. Nelson JL. J Law Med Ethics 1995;23:143–8.
90. Callahan D. Hastings Center Rep 1995;25(6):25–31.
91. Dresser R, Whitehouse PJ. Hastings Center Rep 1994;24:6–12.
92. Fletcher JC, Spencer EM. Lancet 1995;345:271–2.
93. Kapp MB. J Am Geriatr Soc 1992;40:722–6.
94. Payne K, Taylor RM, Stocking C, et al. Ann Intern Med 1996;125:104–10.
95. Hodges MO, Tolle SW, Stocking C, et al. Arch Intern Med 1994;154:1013–20.
96. Asch DA, Cristakis NA. Med Care 1996;34:103–11.
97. Faber-Langendoen K. Arch Intern Med 1996;156:2130–6.
98. Coggan F. Proc R Soc Med 1977;70:75–81.
99. Maillet JO. J Am Diet Assoc 1995;95:231–4.
100. Schostak Z. J Med Ethics 1994;20:93–100.
101. Brody H, Campbell ML, Faber-Langendoen K, et al. N Engl J Med 1997;336:652–7.
102. Phillips P, Rolls BJ, Ledingham GG Jr, et al. N Engl J Med 1984;311:753–9.
103. Zerwekh JV. Nursing 1983;83:47–51.
104. Printz LA. Geriatrics 1988;43:84–8.
105. Schmitz P. Law Med Health Care 1991;19;19:23–6.
106. Dunlop RJ, Ellershaw JE, Baines MJ. J Med Ethics 1995; 21:141–3.
107. Waller A, Adunski A, Hershkowitz J. Lancet 1991;337:745.
108. McCann RM, Hall WJ, Groth-Juncker A. JAMA 1994; 272:1263–6.
109. Ellershaw JE, Sutcliffe JM, Saunders CM. J Pain Symptom Manage 1995;10:192–7.
110. Giocon JO, Silverstone FA, Graner LM, et al. Arch Intern Med 1988;148:429–3.
111. Quill TE. Arch Intern Med 1989;149:1937–41.

SELECTED READINGS

Beauchamp TL, Childress JF. Principles of biomedical ethics. 4th ed. New York: Oxford University Press, 1994.

Lo B. Resolving ethical dilemmas. A guide for clinicians. Baltimore: Williams & Wilkins, 1995.

Pellegrino E, Mazzarella P, Corsi P, eds. Transcultural dimensions in medical ethics. Frederick, MD: University Publishing, 1992.

Pellegrino ED, Thomasma DC. The virtues in medical practice. New York: Oxford University Press, 1993.

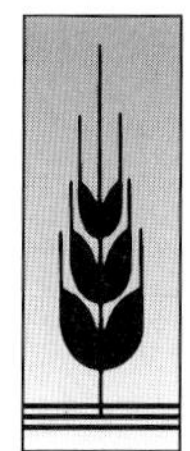

PART V.

Diet and Nutrition in Health of Populations

103. Recommended Dietary Intakes: Individuals and Populations

GEORGE H. BEATON

We know accurately only when we know little; with knowledge doubt increases.

(Goethe)

That which is sure is not sure; as things are they shall not remain.

(Bertolt Brecht)

EVOLUTION OF THINKING AND UNDERSTANDING

Perceived Purposes of Standards

From ancient times man has known that health and physical well-being depend on diet and that particular foods have special virtue for curing diseases (1). More than 2000 years ago, liver was known to cure night blindness. There was, and still is, an abundance of information about diet and disease in the folklore of almost every culture. Unfortunately, in modern times in North America, that folklore continues to expand. The work of Lind (1753) was a milestone for human nutrition for it is perhaps one of the earliest recognized applications of the methods of science to the claims of folklore. Lind, with his now-famous treatise (2), established the relationship between diet and scurvy, validating what had been folklore. The first "dietary standard" given any sort of official status was created in 1862 at the request of the British Privy Council (3). That standard was intended "to prevent starvation diseases" and was to serve the purpose of evaluating estimated intakes in the first dietary surveys conducted in Britain shortly thereafter. Table 103.1 provides a brief summary of some markers of the changes in perceived purposes of dietary standards.

Since these early works, much has changed, slowly at first and then with ever-increasing speed. Today that speed is feverish. Even as this chapter is being written, it is being superseded by events. The changes have been in many areas. First, our knowledge concerning the diverse functions of nutrients has increased phenomenally. However, this rapid progress has not necessarily improved our ability to estimate human nutrient needs; rather, it has fostered an evolving concept of what we hope to achieve (the markers of "inadequacy" are changing). Change is also evident in shifts in the type of evidence used in attempts to estimate human needs. The earliest requirement estimates were based on epidemiologic observation—the intakes of healthy versus sick people. Gradually this gave way to experimental approaches seen as more respectable—balance studies, planned deprivation and repletion studies, and theoretical modeling based on experimentally established functions of nutrients. It was soon recognized that estimates based on experiments conducted under controlled conditions had to be confirmed under field conditions; thus, epidemiologic evidence came back into its own.

We have now gone full circle and are starting again. Epidemiologic evidence currently suggests relationships between consumption of certain types of foods and some forms of cancer, cardiovascular disease, and other noncommunicable chronic diseases. Unfortunately, although the dietary associations seem clear, identifying the active factors in the foods is not clear. For that reason, attempts to develop estimates of human needs for fat, specific fatty acids, carotenoids, tocopherols, ascorbic acid, and "antioxidant substances," and to incorporate this knowledge into public health policy has faced many difficulties and much controversy. It is not necessarily that we know too little; perhaps we know too much. Yet we cannot seem to put all the pieces together into a coherent whole (for discussion of these issues, see Garza et al. [17]).

Another phenomenal and highly problematic evolution, particularly since World War II, has been in the scope and sheer divergence of applications of the recommended dietary allowances (RDAs). A few years ago, the Food and Nutrition Board (FNB) established a committee to identify and catalogue the then-current uses of the RDAs. The 1983 report of that committee was never published, though a summary of the findings was included in the FNB 1994 report (18) "How Should the Recommended Dietary Allowances be Revised?" That summary (reproduced verbatim as Table 103.2) did not imply endorsement by the FNB of these uses and, as stated, they certainly are not all endorsed by the present author. What is not

Table 103.1
Changing Purposes of Dietary Standards—Some Markers

Year and Author	Described Purpose of Report
1753 Lind (2)	To prevent scurvy
1862 Smith (3)	To prevent starvation diseases (for evaluation of a dietary survey)
1881 Voit (5) (later modified by Rubner)	A description of observed group mean intakes of apparently healthy men, described as a "normal diet"
1918 Lusk (U.S.) (6)	To feed the army and the nation (an energy standard used to calculate the total food needs of a large population group or total nation)
1933 British Medical Association (7)	To maintain health and working capacity and to determine minimum weekly food expenditure
1933 Stiebling (U.S.) (8)	To marry health and agriculture; Stiebling described this in terms of an informed consumer getting the most for his or her money and an informed producer knowing what was going to be consumed
1933–36 League of Nations (a series of reports) (9)	To be used in the evaluation of national diets (aggregate supply) and agricultural planning
1938 Canadian Council on Nutrition (10)	To be used as a basis for evaluation of observed intakes
1941 Food and Nutrition Board (11)	"Tentative goal toward which to aim in planning practical dietaries". A presidential conference adopted the numeric estimates as appropriate to *maintain perfect health* (existing intakes to be evaluated in relation to the goal); the 1941 RDAs were adopted by Canada in 1942 (continued for a period of 6 years)
1943 Food and Nutrition Board	"To serve as a guide for planning an adequate diet for every normal person of the population and not for the average member of the group categories . . . the allowances should be demographically weighted to estimate per caput needs of the population"; the committee purposefully included some Canadians since Canada had officially adopted the 1941 report
1948 Canadian Council on Nutrition (13)	To plan food supplies for individuals or groups and to evaluate estimated intakes of individuals or groups; the issue dividing U.S. and Canadian committees was related to how individual variability was to be treated, particularly in the planning and assessment of food supplies for populations and large groups; from 1948 until today, the U.S. and Canadian reports have been separate, though there has often been overlapping membership on the committees
1990 WHO (14)	To provide *dietary* (food-based) recommendations that could help to prevent chronic diseases; this report took pains to emphasize that its recommendations referred to population mean intakes, not to the intakes of particular individuals; the WHO report is representative of a large number of national or regional reports that emerged to the 1970s and 1980s offering food-based advice; there was (and is) considerable confusion about whether numeric recommendations were intended to apply to group/population mean intakes or to the diets of individuals
1993 FAO/WHO (15)	To examine the role of fats and oils in human nutrition; this group appeared to take little heed of the report of the earlier WHO committee; its recommendations about acceptable fat intakes were said to refer to individuals rather than groups and in that sense represented a major scientific disagreement with the earlier WHO committee; no explanation was offered
1996 WHO/FAO/IAEA (16)	To reevaluate the role of trace elements in human health and nutrition; the committee broke new ground in producing the first report (other than the WHO report on chronic disease) to actually include estimates of required group mean intakes rather than addressing only individual intakes; this report placed the important distinction between groups and individuals squarely on the table in a manner that can no longer be ignored

Based on Leitch (1), Young (4), and statements in the published reports.

apparent from the table is that many of these applications have been given a legal dimension by being incorporated into regulations issued by federal and state bodies. This has further complicated a tangled situation. For example, the Food and Drug Administration (FDA) established the U.S. recommended *daily* allowances, derived from the 1968 recommended *dietary* allowances, as a reference point for food labeling. Numerically and conceptually these two sets of numbers are very different, although they were, at one time, related. The most confusing aspect is that the abbreviation *RDA* applies to both. In fact the name used by the FDA is identical to the name used in the first FNB report on RDAs (19).

With the growth of scientific knowledge about the function of nutrients as well as about factors likely to affect requirements, inevitable pressure developed to alter the criteria of adequacy, the specification of "requirement for what?" The nutrition community adopted the vague and unmeasurable goal of establishing "optimal intake." The North American public has monumental expectations of the relationship between diet and all aspects of their health and well being. Although these expectations may be unrealistic, they are now a part of the climate (and folklore?) in which the nutritional scientist must work. This phenomenal belief in the power of nutrients has led to massive growth in the use of nutritional supplements and pressure to allow health claims for dietary supplements (20). As criteria of adequacy shifted, requirement estimates tended to increase. In some cases, as the base of knowledge increased, requirement estimates actually decreased, either because previously accepted evidence was found inappropriate or incorrectly interpreted or because committees felt comfortable in lowering the "margin of safety," sometimes called the "margin of doubt."

Another rapidly evolving feature of the estimation, description, and application of human nutrient require-

Table 103.2
Reported Uses of the RDAs

Use	Examples	Comments on the Use of the RDAs
Food planning and procurement	Use to develop plans for feeding groups of healthy people	Use as an appropriate nutrient standard for a period of at least a week, but also the use as one of many food-planning criteria; should be adjusted as group varies from RDA reference individual
	Use for food purchasing, cost control, and budgeting	Use as an appropriate nutrient standard with knowledge of such factors as food composition, availability, acceptability, and storage changes and losses
Food programs	Serve as basis for nutritional goal for feeding programs	Use as a standard for nutritional quality of meals along with other food-selection criteria
	Provide the nutritional standard for the thrift food plan, the basis of allotments in the food stamp program	Use as a guideline along with other selection criteria
	Provide national guidelines for food distribution programs	Use as a standard for nutritional quality of food packages
Evaluating dietary survey data	Evaluate dietary intake of individuals	Use as a standard for evaluating dietary status, but not for evaluating individual nutritional status
	Evaluate household food use	Use as a bench mark to compare households and to identify nutrient shortfalls
	Evaluate national food supply (food disappearance data)	Use only as a bench mark for comparison over time and to identify nutrient shortfalls
Guides for food selection	Develop and evaluate food guides and family food plans	Use along with other food-selection criteria
Food and nutritional information and education	Provide guidelines for obtaining nutritious diets	Use as a point of reference; becomes more useful to consumers when translated into food-selection goals
	Use as a basis for educators to discuss individuals' nutrient needs	Use in combination with information in the text accompanying the RDA table and with recognition that the RDAs are for reference individuals
	Evaluate an individual's diet as a basis for recommending specific changes in food patterns and/or dietary supplements	Use to identify nutrient shortfalls and as a tool to assess nutrient contribution of diet; do not use in a prescriptive manner
Food labeling	Provide basis for nutritional labeling of foods	Use as a basis for labeling standards (U.S. RDA); such standards should not be used to evaluate nutritional intake of individuals or groups
Food fortification	Serve as a guide for fortification for the general population	Use as a guide, but such other factors as food consumption patterns and contribution to the total diet must also be considered
Developing new or modified foods	Provide guidance in establishing nutritional levels for new food products	Use in combination with information on probable product use within the context of the total diet
Clinical dietetics	Develop therapeutic diet manuals	Use to assess the nutritional quality of modified diets
	Plan modified diets	Use as a starting point along with information on the patient's nutritional status and individual needs
	Counsel patients requiring modified diets	Use as one basis of food selection
	Plan menus and food served in institutions for the developmentally disabled	Use as a starting point, but modify for individual's developmental status and body size
Nutrient supplements and special dietary foods	Use as a basis to formulate supplements and special dietary foods	Use as a basis in developing infant formulas and other oral supplements or foods, but also consider nutrient bioavailability and nutrient balance; cannot be used as the only guide for parenteral feeding products

This table is based on an unpublished 1983 report "Uses of the Recommended Dietary Allowances" prepared by a special Food and Nutritional Board committee. Reproduced from Food and Nutrition Board. How should the recommended dietary allowances be revised? Washington, DC: National Academy Press, 1994.

ment estimates is the use of statistical concepts. The need to address the distribution of both requirements and intakes has been progressively realized. When assembling evidence to estimate human requirements, one must be aware of exactly what each type of evidence actually estimates. It could be the average of individual requirements for a class of individuals; it could be the required concentration of nutrient in a diet consumed ad libitum by subjects in an experimental study; it could be a necessary group mean intake in an epidemiologic study. These estimates are not the same conceptually or numerically. Nevertheless, they can all be related by proper application of statistical concepts concerning univariate and bivariate (joint) distributions of intakes and requirements. In parallel, given the appropriate construct and the relevant information, one can move from estimating human nutrient requirements to specifying the necessary concentration of nutrients in the diet or to estimating necessary group mean intakes.

Only relatively recently (in the last 20–25 years) has there been a real effort to merge the evolving biologic and statistical knowledge bases concerning estimation and application of human nutrient requirements. Most experimental scientists and even many epidemiologists, consider statistics a tool used to test hypotheses about effects or associations, which it is. Statistics can also be used to understand and describe relationships; in the past this has received too little recognition. The Food and Agriculture (FAO)/World Health Organization (WHO) series of reports on nutrient requirements, and the report of the eighth Joint Expert Committee on Nutrition (21) chronicle the progressive integration of statistical concepts into the estimation, description, and application of nutrient requirement estimates. Specifically, one can follow the attempts to describe and work with distributions of nutrient requirements and gradually see conceptual development of approaches to concurrently dealing with distributions of requirements and of intakes. At first this involved assessing the apparent adequacy of diets in population groups. Gradually, merging of nutrition and statistics led to estimation of necessary nutrient:energy ratios and, in 1996, to estimation of necessary group mean intakes (16).

In 1945, when Canadian and U.S. committees charged with developing a Dietary Standard and Recommended Dietary Allowances, respectively, disagreed and went their own ways, a major issue was the stated goal and suggested interpretation of the 1945 revision of the U.S. RDAs (22):

> The allowances are intended to serve as a guide for planning an adequate diet *for every normal person* of the population and not for the average member of the group categories . . . In order to meet the needs of the whole population it is necessary to satisfy the requirements of those with less efficient usage. Because the allowances take into consideration the requirements of those at the upper level of the normal range of requirements, they allow a factor of safety for persons who have an average or less than average requirement. In most categories this factor of safety is approximately 30%, but for many persons the allowances cover only the amounts needed for maintenance . . . When the tables are used to estimate the per capita needs of population groups and the agricultural production required to supply such groups, the allowances should be weighted by the composition of the population according to the categories and ages. When the allowances are weighted in this manner the average allowance for each individual [the per capita allowance] is lower than that for a man for all factors except calcium. . . . Even when weighted in this manner, the allowances are greater than the average or the mode of the need for many factors because the allowances are planned to be sufficiently high to meet the needs of normal persons who are less efficient in utilization.

The apparent disagreement between Canadian and U.S. committees at that time appeared to relate more to a difference in philosophy and approach than to any real difference in scientific judgment. In the United States, strong emphasis was placed on the individual and ensuring adequacy for every individual. In Canada, greater emphasis was and, until relatively recently, continued to be, placed on the group or population. Parallel differences between U.S. and Canadian perspectives and approaches can be seen in aspects of their respective healthcare systems and, for example, approaches to asymptomatic hypercholesterolemia screening (favored in the U.S. and opposed, except for high-risk individuals, in Canada). The open debate appears to have centered on how the U.S. RDAs were to be applied to population groups. Both Canada and the U.S. accepted the reality of variation in need among individuals, but the Canadian group felt that a more realistic estimate of needs could be developed if factors believed to affect requirement (and hence explaining part of the variation among individuals) were built into the dietary standard (13). Unfortunately, that Canadian report (13) described the figures as representing a "nutritional floor beneath which maintenance of health in people cannot be assumed." That phraseology generated major reaction and for years split the two communities. Had the report, instead, said that the numbers "indicate a nutritional floor above which maintenance of health [with reference to the tabulated nutrients] could be assumed," the debate might have been much less acrimonious, and harmonization of standards might have followed many years ago instead of still being discussed today.

What is interesting and important is that, by 1945, the major issues that have plagued the development, interpretation, and application of the RDAs were already on the table. A paper written in that era captures the crux of one of the major issues—the need to marry statistical and biologic concepts. In 1945 Pett et al. (23) noted four basic uses of dietary and nutritional standards:

i) for use in calculating the nutrient requirements of a population in connection with a national food and nutrition policy for health.
ii) for use in evaluating the dietary status of a group of people from the total and average quantities of foods eaten, or providing foods for such a group.
iii) for use in establishing regulations under the Foods and Drugs Act [a Canadian Act] governing the contents of foods, dietary supplements or drugs and of allowable claims for them.
iv) for use in evaluating the dietary status of an individual person from the foods eaten, or from the foods purchased.

The authors commented (13) (absolutely correctly), "it is not likely that a single set of figures in a table could be used properly for all these purposes . . . Nevertheless it is possible to marshal information about requirements in a manner that forms a uniform basis for various calculations suited to different purposes . . . It is thus apparent that the problem of arranging and interpreting figures for human requirements is basically statistical." The paper went on to speak of "the probability of the individual's suffering from a serious deficiency or from a suboptimal state of nutrition" and "the likelihood of finding specific medical signs in any particular individual."

They pointed out that "Medical evidence is necessary before the story is known about any individual. However, if the [intake and requirement] curves are properly determined it would indeed be possible and correct to estimate the proportions of the population receiving an insufficient amount of any nutrient." Those authors had the elements of the puzzle in hand and mapped out a solution. However, at the time, the story fell on "stony ground" (L.B. Pett, personal communication, 1989), and there was little or no follow-up.

It has taken the rest of us 50 years to reachieve the insights expressed in that paper. We are finally there, this time equipped with more complete scientific knowledge and statistical concepts and tools that are more widely accepted and applied. We still have a long road to follow before the nutrition community and other users of the RDA reports are ready to use the new insights and new techniques they bring. The FNB (18) has indicated that in the current revision of the RDAs, under way as this chapter is being written, the board will direct major effort to developing a guidelines report relating to interpretation and application of whatever Dietary Reference Intakes (DRIs) or RDAs it chooses to publish. Perhaps the dream of Pett and his colleagues will finally be realized. Perhaps also we will see a much greater willingness to harmonize nutrient requirement reports around the world. It is amazing that in an international community of knowledgeable scientists, misunderstandings rather than true scientific disagreements have persisted for so long.

This chapter attempts to document and illustrate some of the major evolutions mentioned above. In so doing, the author hopes that the reader will recognize that while new concepts and approaches at first seem complicated and nonintuitive, the benefits of understanding and applying them correctly are great, and before long they become the accepted norm, and old approaches are forgotten.

Scientific Basis of Estimated Human Nutrient Requirements and RDAs

In the 8th edition of this book, Harper (24), who formerly chaired an FNB/RDA committee, reviewed the progressive increase in the scope and scientific security of estimates of human nutrient requirements. In Table 103.1, the first report cited (Lind, 1753), concerned only one food factor, and its chemical identity was unknown. When Smith (3) prepared his report for the British Privy Council, human needs were described in terms of energy, carbon, and nitrogen. von Voit (5) believed that a complete diet was supplied by protein, fat, and carbohydrate, reflecting the advances in chemistry and proximate analyses. Much later, classical nutritional science began exploring and identifying the "accessory food factors," which included first the essential minerals and then the vitamins. This began the era of true experimental nutrition that characterized the mid-20th century. Much of this work was initially conducted in small animals, then confirmed in humans. Some was initially based on observation of now-classic deficiency diseases in farm animals.

In its 1943 report on recommended dietary allowances (12), the FNB commented: "The difficulty [in establishing goals for good nutrition and a yardstick to measure progress toward these goals] lies in the lack of sufficient experimental evidence on which to estimate requirements for various nutrients with any great degree of accuracy. Judgments as to requirements are necessarily based on incomplete and often conflicting reports of research and clinical observations and from data derived from work on animals. Experiments with the various vitamins also differ with regard to procedure and interpretation. These variables explain the wide divergence in 'requirements' as set forth in current literature in nutrition".

Earlier, the National Research Council's (NRC) Committee on Food and Nutrition arranged for a critical appraisal of the literature on each of the recognized dietary essentials, formulated tentative allowances, subjected them to review by the original contributors, and then presented them for comment and criticism to the larger community of nutrition scientists. A final, slightly revised version was adopted in May 1941 (11, 19). The report addressed allowances for energy, protein, two minerals (calcium and iron), and six vitamins (vitamin A, thiamin, riboflavin, niacin, ascorbic acid, and vitamin D), a total of 10 nutritional variables. The tabulated allowances were related to 12 age/sex/physiologic state categories, and for adults, three levels of physical activity were considered. In the 10th revision of the RDAs (25), the tables present numeric estimates of RDAs "designed for the maintenance of good nutrition in practically all healthy people in the United States" for energy, protein, four fat-soluble vitamins, seven water-soluble vitamins, and seven minerals. In addition, "Safe and Adequate Daily Dietary Intakes" were offered for two vitamins and five trace elements. The text of the report also addressed needs for nine amino acids, dietary guidelines for fat and cholesterol, the function and role of linoleic, linolenic, and arachidonic acids, dietary guidelines for carbohydrate and fiber, and needs for water and three electrolytes, a total of at least 45 nutritional variables. The age/sex/physiologic state categories had grown to 16, and energy needs were exemplified (for adults) by five categories of activity. This is an amazing change in only 48 years!

By 1989, the science base supporting estimated human nutrient requirements was clearly becoming very strong. This did not mean an end to disagreements on judgments about how *dietary allowances* should relate to *nutrient requirement estimates* or about what information justified changes in allowances from one revision of the RDAs to the next; such controversy was a prominent feature of the 10th revision. The 1989 report (25) also directed major attention to possible upper limits of desirable or safe intakes. In the revision of the RDAs now under way, the FNB has established a special subcommittee to look explicitly at safe or desirable upper limits of nutrient intakes, since this has become important both in establishing fortification guidelines and policies and in considering the safety of the ever-increasing use of minimally controlled, and often high-potency, pharmaceutical supplements and food extracts and concentrates. Historically, the greatest demand for knowledge related to preventing inadequate intake; today, in North America, the demand for knowledge is increasingly directed toward safe upper limits of intake, whether of macronutrients such as fat or of vitamin and mineral micronutrients (18). What the 1941 RDA report said about nutrient requirements might today be said about nutrient excesses. It is to be hoped that we will see an equally encouraging growth of knowledge in this area. Perhaps not too long after the turn of the century we will finally be able to describe safe and suitable ranges of nutrient intakes, will have dropped the search for the nebulous "optimal intake," and indeed may be able, with good evidence, to restore the public's faith that one can obtain "good nutrition" from reasonable and acceptable dietary practices—certainly a goal well worth achieving.

The above discussion has centered on the increasing volume and quality of evidence and the evolution of focal issues. However, the scope of evidence brought to bear in the final estimation process has also changed. We no longer rely on isolated pieces of information about a specific nutrient. Rather, we look for congruence of information arising from several lines of evidence. That congruence (Fig. 103.1) gives confidence to our judgments.

Terminology and Concepts

As successive committees in different countries have attempted to deal with evolving concepts, they have often changed terminology in hopes of persuading users to check their text to see the intended meaning. The changed terminology has not necessarily added clarity. For many years, the term *recommended intake* was applied to what in the United States has been called *recommended dietary allowance*, even within the RDA reports. Recently, there has been growing disavowal that the tabulated numbers are actually "recommended" as intakes for all citizens.

Conceptual Development

In its 1969 report, the U.K. Panel on Recommended Allowances of Nutrients (26) again identified and described very clearly the conceptual issue that was then emerging for many committees; in essence, the same issue raised by Pett et al. (23) a quarter century earlier. The U.K. report states:

> For nutrients, distributions of intake may be quite unrelated to distributions of need. The recommended intakes, which are judged to be sufficient for practically all individual members of population, must of necessity be in excess of the requirements of most of them. If an individual is taking more than the recommended intake, he is almost certainly obtaining more than he requires; but if the average intake of a group is greater that the recommendation, one cannot be sure that there is no malnutrition because of uncertainty about the distribution of intakes within the group. Equally, it is not legitimate to deduce the presence of malnutrition in a population merely on the basis of a survey in which the average intake of nutrient is less than the recommendation. But malnutrition is more likely to be present the further average intake falls below the recommendations.

That paragraph touched upon three distinct issues, each of which has been addressed in the 25 years since it was written:

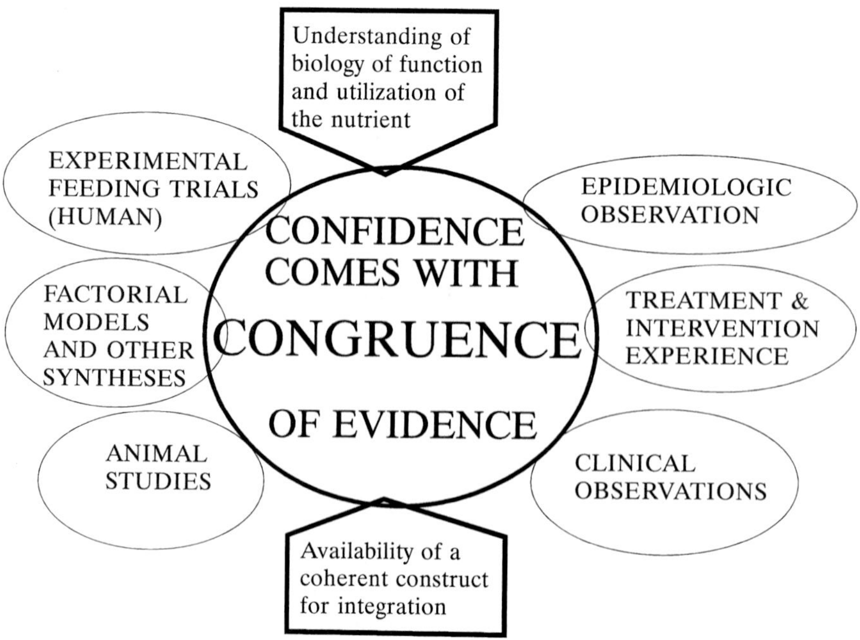

Figure 103.1. Nutrient requirements and recommended intakes are based on multiple types of evidence. Congruence of lines of evidence gives confidence in the estimates. However, such a blending and synthesis of evidence is feasible only when there is an understanding of the function and use of the nutrient and a coherent theoretical construct for integration that has strong statistical components. (From Beaton GH. J Nutr 1996;126:2320S–8S, with permission.)

1. Almost all committees have addressed requirements of *individuals,* not populations. The numeric recommendations relate to usual intakes of individuals. Terminology changes were intended to better reflect actual meanings, not to mark conceptual shifts. An FAO/WHO committee (27) had already followed that route, encouraging others to rethink the nomenclature.
2. Since one can only estimate the precise requirements of a particular individual by intensive study, the published requirement estimates can be applied to a particular person only on a probability basis, and observed intake can only be assessed on a probability or risk basis. This was finally examined in detail in a seminal report issued by an FNB committee in 1986. That report (28) merged biologic and statistical concepts and fostered development of theory-grounded approaches to resolution of issues that had fomented for nearly 50 years.
3. Setting guidelines for population mean intakes requires considering the distribution of both requirements and usual intakes among individuals. This issue was identified earlier by the Joint FAOWHO Committee on Nutrition in its eighth report (21). Procedures have since been developed and were applied in a 1996 FAO/WHO/International Atomic Energy Agency (IAEA) report on trace elements (16).

Terminology Shifts

In 1973, an FAO/WHO committee (27) dealing with protein and energy requirements expressed concern that its recommendations for protein intake were well *below* usual intakes and noted that it did not intend to *recommend lowering* intakes to these levels. That committee abandoned use of the term *recommended intake* and adopted the term *safe level of protein intake,* which elicited strong objection from those concerned with food safety from the perspective of toxicity rather than inadequacy. A Canadian committee used a terminology shift to address another issue that had gained prominence in assessment of nutrient intakes. It had been the practice in Canada to publish "Recommended Daily Nutrient Intakes" (RDNIs), but these were being taken too literally, as an intake to be achieved *each* day rather than persisting over time, as intended. In 1983, the name was changed to *Recommended Nutrient Intake (RNI)* (29) (see Appendix Table II-A-3). In 1989, the United States dropped the word *daily,* which had been introduced in the 1953 revision of the RDAs (see Appendix Table II-A-2-b). Between those editions, the summary tables carried the heading "Recommended Daily Dietary Allowance," itself a revision from the much earlier "Recommended Daily Allowance" (19), a term that is identical with the current U.S. recommended daily allowance used by the FDA. Another change, reflecting new British terminology, has been proposed for the RDA revisions in progress (18) (see Appendix Table II-A-4).

Perhaps the most heretical shift in terminology was introduced in the United Kingdom in 1991. The U.K. committee (30) abolished the use of "recommended" as part of the name and adopted instead the concept and terminology of reference values. It went a step further and formally incorporated the probability concept. In the U.K. approach (30), the "Reference Nutrient Intake" (RNI) represents the upper tail of the nutrient requirement distribution "that is enough for almost every individual, even someone who has high needs for the nutrient. This level of intake is, therefore, considerably higher than most people *need.* If individuals are consuming the RNI of a nutrient, they are most unlikely to be deficient in that nutrient." The British group then defined a "Lower Reference Nutrient Intake" (LRNI), representing the lower tail of the requirement distribution, as "the amount of the nutrient that is enough for only a small number of people with *low* needs. Most people will need more than the LRNI if they are to eat enough. If individuals are habitually eating less than the LRNI they will almost certainly be deficient." The report also defined the "Estimated Average Requirement" (EAR), noting that "clearly many people will need more than the EAR and many people will need less." Unfortunately, as discussed below, the U.K. committee did not probe deeply enough into how these reference values should relate to groups rather than individuals. In that regard, they shared the shortcomings of U.S. (25) and Canadian (31) reports.

The reader must recognize that these name changes have no direct bearing on the scientific basis of nutrient requirements estimates. The choice of points on the distribution of requirements reflects judgments about desirable levels of intake *for a randomly chosen individual whose true requirement is unknown* and about how best to incorporate the concept of a distribution of requirements among seemingly similar individuals.

The U.S. (25) and U.K. (30) committees accepted the scientific basis of the estimation of human adult protein requirements presented by the earlier FAO/WHO/United Nations University (UNU) committee (32). The most recent Canadian committee (31) found it necessary to make some adjustments in the FAO/WHO/UNU approach (32) and also adjusted for the estimated quality of Canadian diets. Figure 103.2 portrays the estimated distributions of adult protein requirements, expressed per kilogram body weight, and the points on the distributions singled out by the respective committees; the nomenclature used is shown. All of the names (except the British LRNI and EAR) are based upon the same scientific (evidence and are clearly supposed to carry identical conceptual meanings in the eyes of the parent committees. In choosing names, each committee was attempting to address either what it saw as a particular application of the numbers or a frequent misuse of previous reports (the stated purpose of the U.K. change [30]). If one were to consider something other than protein, there might be some major differences among the committees, relating more to judgments than to science. None of the committees is entirely consistent in its approach across nutrients.

Further, there is an unfortunate similarity of names with very different intended meanings. The U.K. com-

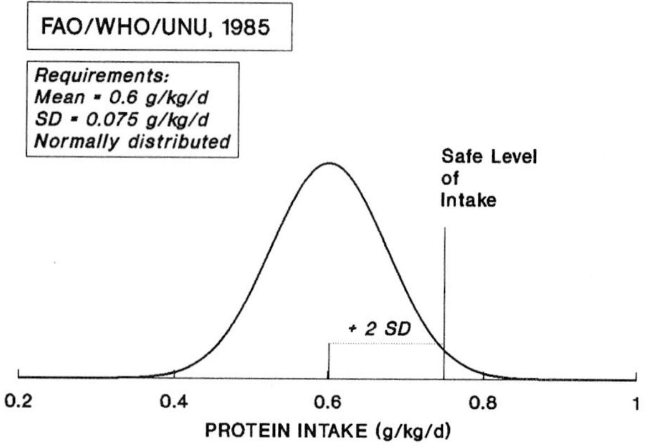

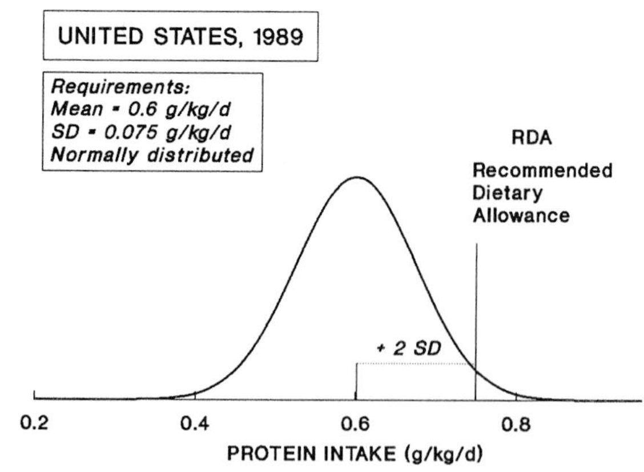

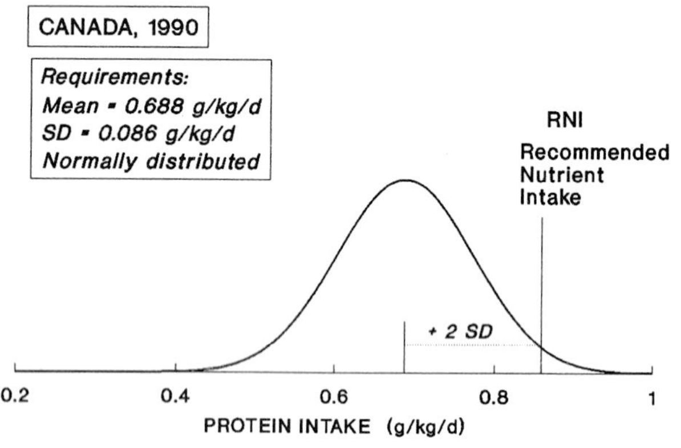

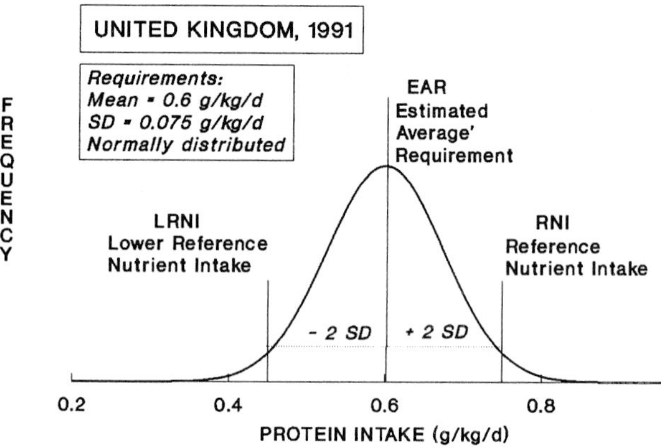

Figure 103.2. Existing descriptions of adult protein requirements and recommendations. The figure shows the estimated distributions of requirement per kilogram (identical for FAO/WHO/UNU, the U.S., and the U.K. but slightly different for Canada) and the levels singled out for tabulation in the respective reports. In spite of differences in names, the "Safe Level of Intake," "Recommended Dietary Allowance," "Recommended Nutrient Intake," and "Reference Nutrient Intake" have identical conceptual meanings.

mittee (30) decided to use "Safe Intake" to indicate that there was not enough information to estimate requirements (the term is unhappily close to the "Safe Level of Intake" applied by FAO/WHO committees (27, 40) to describe well-grounded requirement estimates. In the U.K. report, "a Safe Intake is one which is judged to be adequate for almost everyone's needs but not so large as to cause undesirable effects." The U.S. committee (25) chose a different term for the same sort of situation; it refers to "Safe and Adequate Daily Dietary Intakes," often expressed as a range. The notes make it clear that this is intended to be treated as a safe range of intake and that chronic intake above this range should be avoided. FAO/WHO/UNU presented a conceptual framework for a "safe range of protein intakes" referred to the individual but did not provide estimates of the upper limit of the safe range. It appears that the current U.S. committee may attempt to define such a range or at least to present estimates of safe upper limits to intakes (18); a separate subcommittee was established to address this.

Other Modes of Expression of Requirements

For some purposes, it may be desirable to consider protein:energy ratios, a diet quality measure, rather than absolute protein intakes. Many uses for such ratios have been proposed, but there has not always been consistency about how the reference value (i.e., a level "adequate" or "safe" for almost all individuals) should be computed (32). Two requirement distributions must be estimated and combined in a joint distribution of nutrient and energy requirements. The FAO/WHO/UNU report (32) presents a mathematical probability-based formula (developed by committee member Will Rand, a statistician) for computing the "safe protein:energy ratio." There is a distribution of required P:E ratios, and the safe ratio is a point in the upper tail of that distribution (a conceptual parallel to the portrayals in Fig. 103.2). Since many have difficulty internalizing the equation presented in the FAO/WHO/UNU report (32), an empirical example of computation of the distribution of P:E ratios is presented below.

The 1994 phase of the most recent U.S. Department of Agriculture (USDA) survey (33) reported the body weights of 2269 adults. For each of these subjects, an energy requirement was computed as a random member of the distribution of requirements for persons of that age, sex, and weight as described in the 1989 revision of the U.S. RDAs (25). This required computing an average basal metabolic rate (BMR) for a person of the specified age, weight, and sex, using the FAO/WHO/UNU prediction equations (32). The estimated BMR was multiplied by the activity factors specified in the U.S. report (25) (between 1.55 and 1.67 depending on age and sex). To this was added a random normal deviate with SD equal to 440 kcal for women and 580 kcal for men (variabilities taken from the U.S. report [25]). These estimates of daily energy need were then converted to kilocalories per kilogram by dividing by weight, yielding

Simulated energy requirements:

Adult males ($n = 1145$)	37.15 ± 7.93 kcal/kg/day
Adult women ($n = 1124$)	33.32 ± 7.87 kcal/kg/day

In the case of protein, the simulation was simpler. For each subject, a protein requirement was generated as 0.6 plus a random normal deviate, with SD equal to 0.075. The resultant distributions were

Simulated protein requirements:

Adult males ($n = 1145$)	0.60 ± 0.075 g/kg/day
Adult women ($n = 1124$)	0.60 ± 0.076 g/kg/day

In this simulation, each of the 2269 adult subjects was assigned an energy requirement and a protein requirement. The plot of the joint distribution of these requirements is shown in the upper panel of Figure 103.3. To convert this into the distribution of P:E ratios, the protein requirement was multiplied by 4 kcal/g, divided by the energy requirement, and then multiplied by 100 to express the ratio as the more familiar term, protein energy as a percentage of total energy need. The derived distributions are portrayed in the lower panel of Fig 103.3. Mean values plus SD

Simulated distribution of required P:E ratios

Adult men ($n = 1145$)	6.78 ± 1.78 % energy as protein
Adult women ($n = 1124$)	7.68 ± 2.39 % energy as protein

The distribution of the ratios is skewed. In this situation one might set the equivalent of the RDA as the level that meets or exceeds the expected needs of 95% of individuals (the 95th centile of the distribution). For men, for women, and for the two sexes combined, the 95th centile is about 11% energy as protein.

The point of this exercise is simply to illustrate that for special purposes, other modes of estimating and describing requirements can be applied. Because the derived requirements expressed a new way still constitute a distribution, it is still necessary to establish how best to apply the distribution to the purpose at hand.

ESTIMATING AND DESCRIBING GROUP NEEDS

Most of the above discussion has related to estimation and description of the requirements of individuals. However, as noted, confusion and controversy exist about how the numbers should be related to large groups or whole populations. The most common suggestion is that the mean (or median) intake of a group of persons of one sex and about the same age should approximate the RDA or RNI. For groups heterogeneous with regard to sex, age, or other variables affecting the requirement, it has been suggested that the demographically weighted average of the RDAs or RNIs should serve as a reference for comparison of the observed or planned mean intake. Although these approaches are specifically suggested or implied in several recent national reports, they are scientifically flawed approaches as illustrated below.

Homogeneous Groups

Consider first the simpler case of a homogeneous group (e.g., young adult men). The task is to estimate the average protein intake to offer the group (e.g., in an institutional setting). In the 1994 round of the USDA Continuing Survey of Food Intake by Individuals (CSFII) (34), the distribution of estimated usual protein intakes (35) is associated with an expected prevalence of about 1% of individuals with usual intakes below their actual (but unknown) requirements, as estimated by the probability approach (28) (top panels, Fig. 103.4). Almost all those interested in public nutrition and certainly health planners would consider this acceptable. However, the estimated requirement distribution has a mean of 0.6 ± SD 0.075 g/kg/day, and this distribution is taken as Gaussian. In contrast, the estimated intake distribution has a mean of 1.39, a median of 1.34, and an SD of 0.42 g/kg/day. That is, the mean and median intakes are *well above the RDA* of 0.75 g/kg/day.

According to the principle that characterized the early RDA reports and is said to still hold for nutrient RDA figures, each individual should be at low risk of having an intake below his or her actual requirement. Thus, many users of the RDA report, particularly those involved in one-on-one dietary counseling, seem to feel that the goal is to have *every individual* achieve an intake at or above the RDA. To establish this condition, the intake distribution would be shifted upward until there is very little, if any, overlap between the distributions of intakes and requirements (middle panels of Fig. 103.4) (intake distribution: mean, 1.53; median, 1.48; SD, 0.42 g/kg/day). Here the expected prevalence of inadequate intakes is only 0.1%.

A moment's consideration, however, reveals that this is very wasteful. Almost all individuals would have protein

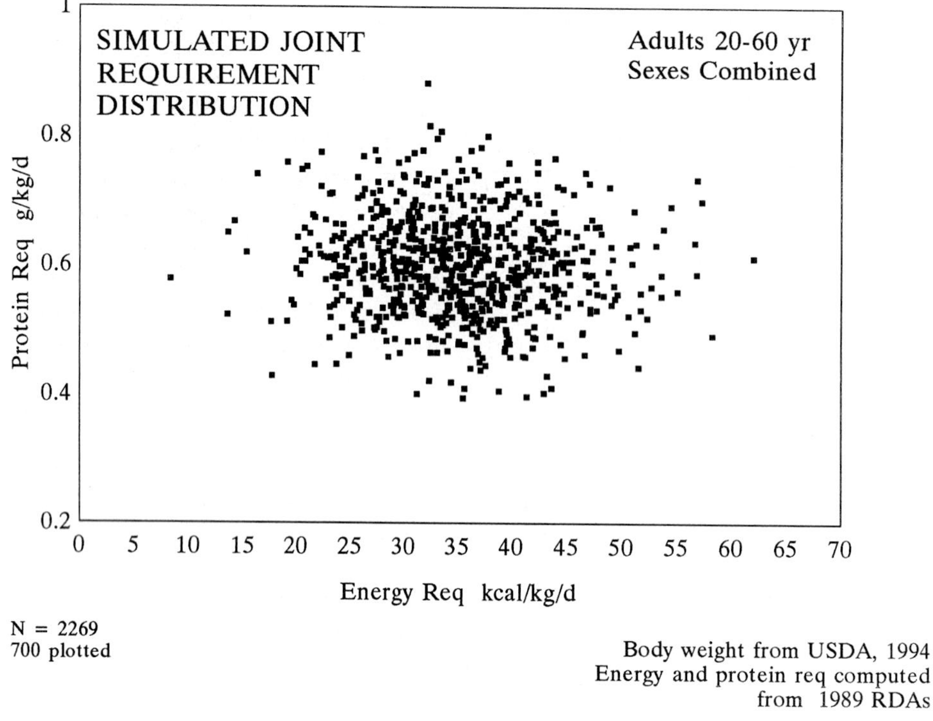

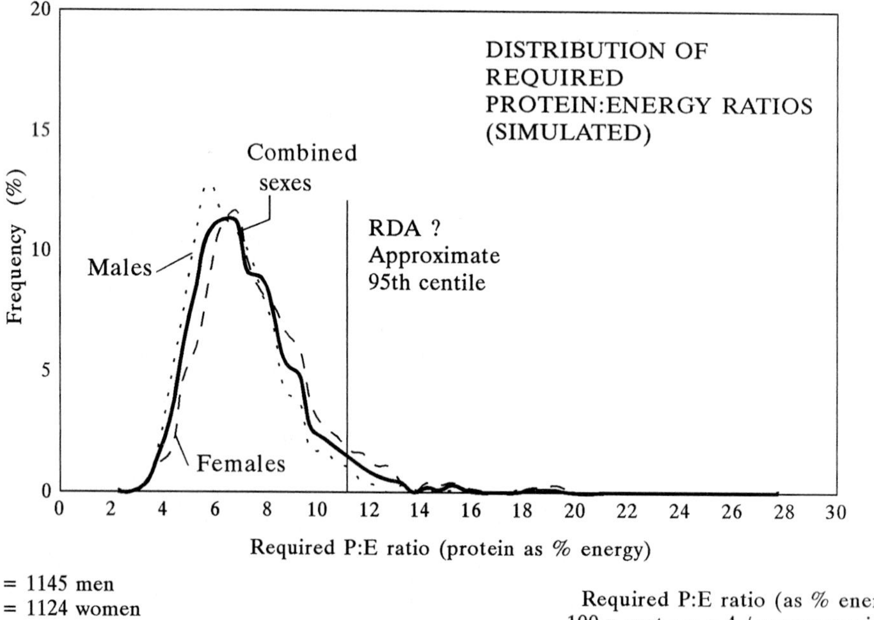

Figure 103.3. Derivation of required protein:energy ratios. The *upper panel* displays a simulation of the joint distribution of protein and energy requirements for 2269 U.S. adults, assuming that energy and protein requirements per unit body weight are essentially independent (low correlation) and that energy and protein requirements were correctly estimated and described in the most recent U.S. RDA report (25). The *lower panel* simply converts the joint distribution to a univariate distribution of the ratio of protein:energy requirements, expressed in the familiar form of protein as % energy. The 95th centile of that distribution is identified as the likely RDA recommended under existing practices. Note that both panels refer to the needs of individuals.

intakes that greatly exceed their actual requirements. *The 1986 FNB report (28) shows that the proportion of intakes falling below the average requirement gives a good empirical estimate of the proportion of individuals expected to have intakes below their own true (but unknown) requirements.* (The empirical observation has been supported on theoretical grounds by A. Carriquiry and colleagues at Iowa State University in a presentation to the FNB, 1995). This approach does not identify the individuals with inadequate intakes, only the proportion or expected prevalence of inadequate intakes in the group. If covering all but 2.5% is taken as satisfactory (the arbitrary value adopted when looking at individual

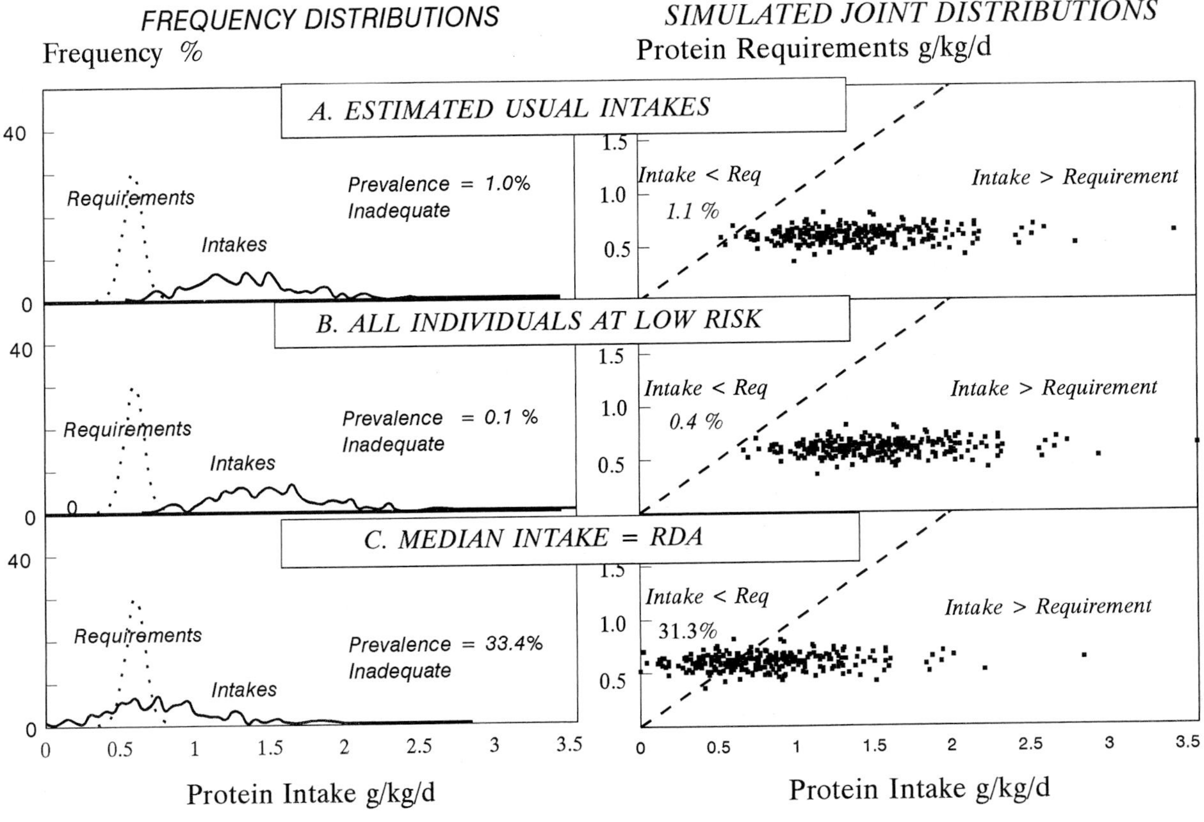

Figure 103.4. Illustration of the relationship among requirement distributions, intake distributions, and numbers of individuals with intakes below their own requirement (protein used as the example). Figures on the *left* present frequency distributions and the estimated prevalence of inadequate intakes (probability assessment [28]); those on the *right* portray simulated joint distributions and counts of individuals with intakes below their requirements. The two sets of prevalence estimates are very close but not identical. *Top panels* portray the apparent current situation in the United States. In the *next panel,* the intake distribution has been shifted slightly so that inadequate intakes have been virtually eliminated. The *bottom panel* portrays the erroneous advice offered for many decades, namely, that the mean or median intake should approximate the RDA (here, median intake = RDA). Clearly this is not a satisfactory or desirable situation for the group; existing advice must be wrong.

needs and setting an RDA), the required group mean or median intake is defined by positioning the intake distribution so that the 2.5 centile approximates the average protein requirement. If the intake distribution is approximately Gaussian, the satisfactory group mean intake would be *mean requirement plus 2 SD of intake.* In the examples at hand, that might suggest 1.44 g/kg/day (0.6 + 2 × 0.42) as a group mean intake target. In fact, because of the skewed distribution, this is a bit higher than necessary, but in the absence of detailed knowledge of the actual usual intake distribution, it remains a useful approximation.

In contrast, the recommendation offered frequently in national reports and formerly in FAO/WHO reports was that "the group mean intake should approximate the RDA." This situation is illustrated in the bottom panels of Figure 103.4. The median intake has been set equal to the RDA, 0.75 g/kg/day, the generated mean intake is 0.80 with an SD of 0.42 g/kg/day. Here the estimated prevalence of individuals with intakes below their actual requirements is 33.4%. This situation is vastly different from the assumption made by the authors of the recommendation. *The common advice that the group mean intake should approximate the RDA is seriously flawed.* As Pett et al. (23) pointed out 50 years ago, no single number published in a table can possibly serve both applications.

The illustrations in Figure 103.4 contain no assumption about normality of the distribution of usual intakes. The top panel represents an estimate of the existing situation in young adult males. The intake distribution has been adjusted using the Iowa State University (ISU) methodology (35) to reduce the effect of day-to-day variation on the apparent distribution of usual intakes. This distribution was then shifted by addition or subtraction of constants to generate the examples shown in the other panels. In Figure 103.4, the panels on the left side portray frequency distribution curves (intake and requirement). The panels on the right portray simulated joint distributions of intakes and requirements under the assumption that protein intake and protein requirement per unit body size, are essentially unrelated (very low correlation).

There is no excuse for continuing to misinterpret and misuse the RDAs, *when they have been based on estimates of actual requirements.* However, the arguments presented within specific sections of the reports indicate that for some nutrients, the published numbers refer to group mean intakes not intakes of individuals; individual requirements were not estimated (Beaton, unpublished report to the FNB, 1995). That is the case for the early FAO/WHO group that examined calcium requirements and proposed "Suggested Practical Allowances" (36). These practical allowances were ranges of group mean intakes deemed appropriate for four different age groups. The Canadian RNI for calcium is explicitly described as related to the group mean intake (31, 33). Of course, for energy, all reports worldwide seem to be in agreement that the published numbers refer to group mean intakes or expenditures of adequately nourished groups (also assuming that for energy, and for energy alone, there is high correlation between chronic intake and chronic expenditure or requirement such that energy balance is closely approximated on a chronic basis).

Heterogeneous Populations

Just as there has been monumental confusion about applying the RDAs to individuals versus applying them to groups, there is an even more serious potential for misunderstanding and major error in applying requirement estimates and RDAs to heterogeneous groups (males and females, adults and children, etc).

It had been common practice to estimate population per capita nutritional needs as a weighted average of the recommended intakes (RDAs). This approach came from approaches developed for estimating per capita energy needs. Although commonly applied during the past 50 years, such an approach for nutrients (but not for energy) is seriously flawed. The limitation was pointed out in the applied section of the FAO/WHO report on iron requirements (37). That report acknowledged the then-conventional approach to estimating population needs but noted that "studies in many countries . . . have shown that although national per capita intake of iron is usually above the average national recommended allowance, iron deficiency often remains an important public health problem." As the report pointed out, the reason for this apparent contradiction lies in the great disparity between the iron requirements of men and women. In practice, iron intakes are likely to be distributed within households in roughly the same manner as the total supply of calories is distributed. In most populations, women probably receive less iron than men, since they eat less food. Requirements for iron are unaffected by caloric intakes. Thus, even though the per capita supply of iron may seem adequate, individuals with high iron needs (women) can be expected to have lower intakes than men, who have low requirements. Iron deficiency continues to be a prominent problem in certain population groups.

Table 103.3, taken directly from that FAO/WHO report, illustrates this issue. Although one can question the estimates of energy and iron needs that existed in 1970, the point of the table is clear. Conventional approaches to estimating and applying a demographically weighted per capita nutrient requirement completely ignored issues of the distribution of intakes. Serious errors resulted. If the iron intakes were adjusted to levels expected to meet the needs of the persons with the highest needs (here, adult women), obviously, the iron intakes of adult men would greatly exceed estimated needs.

This issue was picked up again by the FAO/WHO Joint Expert Committee on Nutrition in its eighth report (21) the following year. As noted above, the FAO/WHO/UNU committee that considered protein and energy requirements directly addressed the joint distribution of energy and nutrient needs and its implication for estimating the "safe protein:energy ratio." A conceptual framework now existed to allow examination of the sort of problem that the iron committee had identified. We can estimate a nutrient:energy ratio need for the heterogeneous population, and through this, we can begin to estimate per capita nutrient needs. This is illustrated below.

Recently, Beaton ("Fortification of Foods for Refugee

Table 103.3
A Theoretical Example of Iron Distribution in the Family (A Comparison of the Inequities in Distributions of Intakes and Needs)

	Family Member						
	Reference Male	Reference Female	14 years Male	10 years Female	6 years (either sex)	19 months (either sex)	Average
Caloric allowance (kcal)[a]	3200	2400	2200	2000	1300	1000	2020
Recommended iron intake (mg)[b]	5	14	12	5	5	5	7.7
Distribution of iron intakes (mg)[c]							
Population A[d]	12.2	10.2	8.4	7.5	5.0	3.8	7.7
Population B[e]	18.6	14	12.6	11.6	7.5	5.8	11.7

From FAO/WHO. Requirements of ascorbic acid, vitamin D, vitamin B_{12}, folate and iron. WHO Tech Rep Ser no. 452. Geneva: World Health Organization, 1970.

[a]Based on FAO (38). 1 kcal = 4.184 kJ.

[b]Based on FAO/WHO (37), assuming a diet rich in animal foods.

[c]Assuming iron intake is distributed in proportion to caloric intake.

[d]Probable iron intakes if average family intake equals per capita recommended intake.

[e]Probable iron intakes if the intake of the adult woman equals the recommended intake of the reference woman.

Feeding," unpublished report to the Canadian International Development Agency, 1995) conducted such an analysis for a very specific situation. In the early stages of establishing a refugee camp, the refugees may depend almost totally on food made available through the World Food Program and the United Nations High Commission for Refugees. These food packages barely contain enough total energy to meet the estimated per capita needs for sedentary activity (39). Beaton estimated that provision of nutrients fell grossly below estimated requirements. Classic deficiency diseases were periodically reported. Major interest existed in improving micronutrient intakes, and one possible approach was fortification of the staple cereal being distributed. Consideration of this approach required developing a profile of needs for extra nutrient, which implied the need for a reference requirement pattern, applicable to the demographically mixed population, with which per capita supplies could be compared.

Under the unusual circumstances of the refugees, it was reasonable to assume that food distribution within a "household unit" would parallel energy needs of the individuals. Hence the germane question became "what is the profile of required nutrient densities in the distributed food ration so that almost all individuals in the household (and, by analogy, in a heterogeneous population) meet their individual nutrient needs when consuming the available food in proportion to energy needs?" This query follows directly from, but goes well beyond, the iron committee model. In essence, the approach taken by Beaton was to estimate the average nutrient:energy ratio required in the ration for each class of individuals, with the proviso that the expected prevalence of inadequate intakes in that age and sex group would be below 5%. This is the calculation that was developed in the FAO/WHO/UNU report (32). The estimation was repeated for each of 12 different age and sex reference groups (excluding infants and children under 2, who really require a different diet and would not be expected to share the ration in the same sense as others). Then, selecting the highest of these ratios as a reference for the refugee ration would give reasonable assurance that nutrient intakes would be adequate for all age/sex groups. Although calculations were made for pregnant and lactating women, pregnant women were not included in selecting the final reference nutrient density. It was unreasonable to attempt to meet estimated iron and folate needs of pregnant women by diet alone. If direct supplementation was needed, then the requirements of pregnant women clearly should not drive the dietary nutrient density reference. Below, Beaton's approach for iron is described; the original report considered 16 nutrients.

To implement this approach, iterative models were developed such that the mean and variability of requirements for iron and for energy and the expected variability of the nutrient:energy ratio in the diets of individuals could all be taken into account. With each iteration, the test nutrient density was increased until the target condition (≤5% individuals at risk of inadequate intake) was met. These models were run using the estimates of need for usable iron described by the FAO/WHO committee (40). Table 103.4 shows that excluding pregnant and lactating women, adolescent females who were still growing but had started menstruation required the highest-quality diet. If their needs were met, the needs of the other groups would also be met. The apparently necessary 1.35 mg of usable iron per 1000 kcal of the total mix of foods offered to refugees could be translated to dietary iron by using FAO/WHO estimates of iron availability in different diets. Beaton's report recommended dietary fortification with sodium iron EDTA. This chelated iron is well absorbed, and EDTA is believed to strongly enhance absorption of iron from other dietary sources (41). Beaton suggested that iron availability of the total diet (added an indigenous iron) might be in the range designated "moderate availability" by the FAO/WHO committee (i.e., about 15%), which yielded an estimate of the necessary average iron density of about 9 mg/1000 kcal. This was expected to prevent anemia in the menstruating females and to meet all functional needs in the other groups; it would *not* meet the estimated needs of pregnant women,

Table 103.4
Estimating a "Safe" Nutrient-Energy Ratio for a Heterogeneous Population: Reference Iron:Energy Ratios for Refugee Rations

Sex and Age Group	Estimated Requirements (Mean): Usable Iron (mg)[a]	Estimated Requirements (Mean): Energy (kcal)[b]	Necessary Average Iron:Energy Ratio[c] as Usable Iron (mg/1000 kcal)
M 2.5 years	0.55	1300	0.55
M 7 y	0.95	1465	0.85
M 12 y	1.5	1855	1.06
M 15 y	1.5	2050	1.03
M 17 y	0.9	2450	0.48
M 25 y	0.9	2400	0.50
F 2.5 y	0.55	1250	0.58
F 7 y	0.95	1425	0.87
F 12 y	1.6[d]	1700	1.23
F 15 y	1.6[d]	1900	1.35[e]
F 17 y	1.25[d]	2050	1.25
F 25 y	1.25[d]	2400	1.32

Based on material in an unpublished report (Beaton GH. "Fortification of Foods for Refugee Feeding," 1995) to the Canadian International Development Agency.

[a]Based on FAO/WHO (40). CV of requirement is taken as 15% except for menstruating females. Here the distribution of needs was taken as log normal, and models of requirement distributions were built using the framework of the FAO/WHO report (40). Approaches similar to those presented in the Food and Nutrition Board report (28), are used in the assessment of intake.

[b]Based on FAO/WHO/UNU (32), adopting estimated body sizes typical of populations in Africa. For older children, adolescents, and adults, energy need was estimated as 1.5 × calculated BMR. The CV of requirement per unit body weight was taken as 10%. 1 kcal = 4.184 kJ.

[c]A diet with this average nutrient density would be adequate to meet the iron needs of all but 5% of individuals of the specified age and sex. For method of computation, see text. It is not the often-reported simple ratio of nutrient requirement:energy requirement; instead, the computation takes into account variation in requirement and expected variation in intake.

[d]Median shown. Distribution of requirement is taken as log normal.

[e]This is the highest nutrient density needed by any of the age-sex groups. If the diet contained this concentration, it would be expected to be adequate for all other groups.

but would suffice for lactating females. The point of this example is simply to indicate that while not easy, we do have conceptual and methodologic frameworks that allow us to develop reasonable (not perfect) approaches to estimating per capita nutrient intake targets for heterogeneous population groups.

For many years, committees charged with estimating human nutrient needs and "recommended intakes" have worried about estimating the requirement variability when there are too few data to provide reliable estimates. In the absence of data-based estimates, they have adopted judgments, sometimes referred to as the "margin of safety" or even "margin of ignorance." In the 10 years since the FNB report on assessment of nutrient adequacy (28), the variability of requirement has become much less important for many applications than the variability of usual intakes. The mean or median requirement is the critical estimate, along with the knowledge (or reasonable assumption) that the requirement distribution is approximately symmetric, not necessarily Gaussian. This implies that we have ample data and well-advanced methodology for estimating the distribution of usual intakes, for the examination of intake variability (35). It is reasonable to expect that the next 10 years will see major development of methods related to application of requirement estimates in human population groups, small and large, with further integration of biologic and statistical principles. As we refine application procedures, we also open the door for new ways to "test" requirement estimates (47). We increase the scope of evidence that can be brought to bear on requirement estimation. Thus, for example, tentative requirement estimates can be applied to population data. If they suggest a major problem of inadequate intakes in the population, but there is no such evidence, there is reasonable basis for at least questioning the requirement evidence. Thus, development of the constructs and approaches for application can and will also offer the opportunity to improve nutrient requirement estimates (the generation of congruent evidence enhances reassurance; see Fig. 103.1). Again, by shifting attention from the variability of requirement to the variability of intake, we can gradually replace a remaining area of opinion and judgment with data and science.

ADDRESSING UPPER LIMITS TO NUTRIENT INTAKE

The concept of a safe range of intakes is not new. It has long been recognized that excessive intakes of many nutrients are detrimental to health and well-being if not blatantly toxic. We know, for example, that very high doses of iron, vitamin D, and vitamin A can cause acute and/or chronic toxicity. In Canada, steps were taken to limit possible excessive exposure to vitamin A and vitamin D by limiting the degree of fortification of multiple foods with these nutrients and/or by regulating the levels that could be included in nonprescription over-the-counter nutrient supplements. Excessive intakes of a number of other nutrients over long periods can have detrimental effects. Furthermore, because of known nutrient:nutrient interactions, excessive intake of one nutrient may have a negative impact on the absorption or use of another. When the FAO/WHO/IAEA committee was established to consider trace elements in human health (16), therefore, both "requirement" and "toxicity" were to be considered in framing recommendations and guidelines. Traditionally, concern about high intakes of trace elements has been left mostly in the hands of food toxicologists.

A potentially serious conflict was on the horizon. The nutrition community had a strong tendency to increase what it perceived as a margin of safety and to recommend higher and higher levels of intake. At the same time, there was also a tendency among toxicologists to increase what they saw as a margin of safety and to talk about lowering the acceptable intake levels. There was a very real possibility that the two groups would come into direct conflict, with intakes recommended by nutritionists approaching or exceeding levels deemed unsafe by toxicologists. This situation did not actually emerge but it set in motion a serious attempt to consider both ends of the spectrum (inadequacy and excess) concurrently and within a common conceptual framework. The U.S. FNB has now taken up the challenge and will attempt to offer guidance on suitable intakes. Merging concepts from nutrition and toxicology will not be easy; persons working in these fields generally come from quite different backgrounds, have quite different concerns, and perhaps work with quite different conceptual frameworks.

Given the propensity of the North American consumer to purchase and use high-potency nutrient supplements, there is growing concern about safe upper limits of intake. Conceptually there should be a direct parallel between establishing reference levels that define "undesirably high" and reference levels that ensure nutrient needs. That is, there is every reason to believe that the biologic mechanisms associated with the detrimental effects of high doses exhibit variable individual tolerances just as biologic mechanisms lead to variable individual requirements. Conceptually, we then have risk or probability curves relating to both risk of inadequacy and risk of excess. Such theoretical curves, applied to usual intakes of individuals, were presented by the FAO/WHO/UNU committee (32) and have since been widely reproduced. That committee also coined the phrase "safe range of intake."

The FAO/WHO/IAEA committee (16) took the conceptual framework a step further. They were interested in establishing reference levels for populations and large groups as well as for intakes of individuals. In many parts of the world, where inadequate trace element intakes were presumed to exist, only group mean intake data (at best) were available. The FAO/WHO/IAEA report (16) provides approaches to estimating both a *safe range of intakes* (individuals) and a *safe range of population mean intakes.* From the discussions above in this chapter, it should be apparent that the safe range of population mean intakes is numerically narrower than the safe range of intakes for individuals.

If conceptual frameworks already exist, then what challenge do we face in the coming decades when attention focuses upon these upper limits? First, we will need a much stronger database relating to detrimental effects of high intakes, and we shall have to bridge concepts. As mentioned above, we are entering the domain of toxicology, which has operated with its own conceptual frameworks. Originally, much of that work derived from studies with mortality as an endpoint. This has changed to include concern about detrimental, but nonfatal, effects. Much of the toxicology literature is conceptually based on "dose-response curves," and the notion that subjects vary in response to the same dose is a relatively recent entry into that literature. In nutrition, the dose-response curve was historically very important and remains important today, but once the criterion of requirement has been set, the nutrition community's interest turns more to the issue of variability in the intakes necessary to meet that criterion. The toxicology community has not really addressed such issues as the relationship between fat intake and heart disease. They might correctly consider that this is not really a "toxic effect" and thus not their concern. Nevertheless, the nutrition community is concerned about safe upper limits of fat intake as related to chronic diseases. For effective bridging to develop between the nutrition and toxicology communities, both communities must give careful consideration to definitions of "requirement for what function" and "detrimental to what function." In essence, we *must* get rid of the nebulous concept of optimal intakes and begin to think about *ranges* of "acceptable intakes," "desirable intakes," "safe intakes," or whatever other term we apply. Intakes falling in these ranges carry low risk of detrimental effects attributable to either inadequacy or excess. One of the greatest challenges will be to eliminate the notion of "margin of safety" from our thinking and replace it with meaningful and estimable variables. Unless this is done, many in the nutrition community will continue to argue that the "optimal" intake is likely to be *higher*, often much higher, than existing intakes, while some in the toxicology community are more likely to think of "optimal" as *lower* than existing intakes. We need conceptually consistent frameworks if we are going to be able to draw on science in resolving these emerging issues.

CRITERIA OF REQUIREMENT AND ADAPTATION

Whether considering intakes required to prevent manifestations of inadequacy or intakes likely to generate effects of excess, one *must* clearly define the physiologic criteria of adequacy or excess. Failure to do so leads to irresolvable debate about requirements (42). This was illustrated in a recent commentary by V. R. Young (43) on the RDA for vitamin C. This was written in response to a pharmacokinetic analysis indicating that measures of body levels of ascorbic acid continued to respond to intakes well above the published RDA, suggesting that since this might be important, the RDA should be as high as 200 mg. In responding, Young illustrated the expected prevalence of inadequate intakes in the U.S. population if the mean requirement was set at different levels. If the FNB truly believes that the requirement for vitamin C should be defined by the highest achievable level of any measure of body vitamin C, then it must also believe that the suggested prevalence of inadequacy in the U.S. population also marks a health problem that warrants immediate and drastic public health action. That is, not only is there a scientific need to carefully set meaningful criteria of requirement (or of excess), there is also an ethical responsibility to do so before advising whole populations about nutritional needs. Young's closing sentences were "Only in this way [by examining the population implications of a requirement estimate] can a sound judgement be reached on the RDA for ascorbic acid for use by health policy makers and for the design of effective national nutrition programs. Regardless of what policy decisions are made, it is essential that the requirement values provided for this purpose are based on rigorous scientific evidence and critical thought."

A parallel picture holds when one rereads the long-standing debates about the importance of *nutritional adaptation* and asks how it affects the estimation of human nutritional requirements. In a 1984 symposium on nutritional adaptation, John Waterlow (44) tried to present his concept of nutritional adaptation as a range of dietary situations over which physiologic mechanisms allow adjustments that serve to preserve a body function (not necessarily all body functions). To make this concept operational, he was forced to accept that there must be other (external?) criteria to mark the limits of adaptive capacity. At these limits, the function(s) declared important is no longer maintained. Seemingly, this parallels the concepts embodied in setting criteria for "deficiency" (perhaps a lower limit to adaptation in the Waterlow schema) or "excess" (the upper limit of adaptation?). In both instances, the estimation of "safe" ranges of intake and the discussion of ranges of human adaptability, one must carefully define the functions to be preserved (the criteria to be met). Dr. Waterlow emphasized that the adaptation and functional markers he discussed were physiologic, recognizing that there are also behavioral adjustments that can, for example, reestablish or maintain energy balance if intake is altered. Setting limits on these sorts of adjustments requires assigning value judgments to certain human behaviors and even modification of social structures (45). The need to address normative desirable activity levels before estimating human energy requirements was presented in the report of the FAO/WHO/UNU committee (32) and immediately became a topic of considerable controversy. In general, nutritionists and physiologists prefer to avoid discussing behavioral adaptations to dietary change because they lack self-assurance in judging meaningful limits to those adaptations. Thus, any discussion of energy *requirements* evokes a great deal of ambivalence and hedging.

Perhaps iron represents a classic example of nutritional adaptation, with associated implications for estimation of requirements. There are well-described physiologic processes by which the human organism adjusts to, adapts to, or accommodates, different levels of chronic iron intake. These mechanisms can be seen as increasing the efficiency of dietary iron use at the low end of the intake range (protecting against loss of a function) and decreasing the efficiency of iron use, increasing waste, at the upper end (protecting against toxic manifestations). With iron, hematopoiesis has gained the greatest attention as the function to be preserved. An FAO/WHO committee (40) judged that maintaining this physiologic function would preserve all other physiologically important functions. Of course, health consequences might not become apparent until anemia developed, so one could use the appearance of anemia to mark the limit of adaptation to low intake. In the case of high intake, the concern is the effects of high concentrations of iron in tissues and necrotic changes in those tissues. The most frequently cited manifestation of iron overload is hemochromatosis, but in dealing with safe upper limits, criteria related to the beginning of a detrimental process are preferable to presentation of overt clinical disease.

The nutrition community has long argued that it is "desirable" to maintain substantial stores of body iron. They may have no immediate functional importance, but they serve as a reserve against future need (e.g., to offset the heavy iron demands of pregnancy [37]). Clearly, movement of iron into and out of storage is a central adaptive mechanism. So far no evidence suggests that a specific level of iron storage has particular physiologic advantage. Stores approach zero before the hematopoietic function is compromised (40). The second major adaptive mechanism is alteration of dietary iron absorption efficiency (conditioned by the nature of the diet and its effect upon bioavailability).

Faced with this situation, it is impossible to estimate iron requirements without first clearly defining the criterion of adequacy, the "requirement for what?" Once this is done, one has also defined the lower limit to adaptation in John Waterlow's scheme. For example, if it is judged important to maintain iron stores of at least *x* amount, then reduction of stores below *x* cannot be considered an "adaptation"—it marks the failure of adaptation. Adaptation to higher levels still continues. An important feature of the adaptive processes involved in iron homeostasis is the rapidity of their response to change in diet or in the internal milieu (e.g., response of iron absorption to phlebotomy).

The FAO/WHO committee (40) addressed the problem of adaptation in iron metabolism by defining three levels of iron requirement: a normative level that maintained a desirable level of iron stores without functional markers; a basal level that preserved the hematopoietic function; and a level that prevented anemia as defined by WHO. In fact, they estimated and published requirement estimates for only the last two classes of requirement, noting that for many populations, it was unrealistic to advocate dietary intakes high enough to support iron storage levels that were often suggested to be desirable but that were nearly impossible for most women living in developing countries to achieve and of questionable benefit if achieved.

More recently the FAO/WHO/IAEA committee (16) had to address adaptation in the context of zinc requirements. They developed two levels of requirement estimates, one relating to the "adapted" state and the other to the nonadapted state. In the judgment of that group, there was no immediate functional difference between the two states but as for iron, the normative requirement estimate (nonadapted state) was consistent with temporary protection against future intake shortfalls or increased need.

The early literature suggests a different sort of "adaptation" for calcium. People maintained chronically on different levels of calcium intake show a capacity to alter their efficiency of calcium absorption and retention. Also, when intakes are changed under controlled experimental conditions, compensatory adjustments require a long time to become established. It was once thought that perhaps this adjustment of absorption efficiency was not fully reversible or that populations exposed to high calcium intake in early childhood might persist in exhibiting lower absorption efficiencies as adults, even when on a low calcium intake. Malm (46), working with Norwegian prisoners, placed 26 adult male subjects on a diet providing 450 mg of calcium per day. Prior to this, the men had been maintained on a high-calcium diet providing 950 mg/day for an average of 7 months. The low-calcium regimen was continued for as long as 1.5 years (average, 240 days). Of the 26 apparently healthy men age 20 to 69 years, Malm found 10 with a faculty for rapid adaptation (38%); 12 with a much slower and less marked faculty (46%); 1 with evidence of adaptive capability but not sufficient to establish zero balance (4%); and 3 with no evidence of adaptation (12%). The important feature to note is the large variation in the time required to reestablish equilibrium (to adapt) with the new lower intake.

Many reviewers have commented, as did an FAO/WHO committee (36), that the major determinant of calcium requirement is the habitual intake of calcium. In populations where intakes are high at all ages, calcium requirements (to preserve balance) also appear high; conversely, where intakes are habitually low at all ages, evidence suggests that very low intakes suffice to maintain calcium balance. We have then what appears to be a direct impact of "adaptation" on nutrient requirement. Exposure to high intakes for long periods results in changes in body processes to establish equilibrium among intake, absorption, and excretion to maintain body calcium metabolism within physiologic norms. However, because we also have evidence that these changes are reversed slowly to adjust to lower intakes or may even be irreversible in terms of accommodating very low intakes, we can reasonably state that the process of "adaptation" has influenced nutrient requirement.

Perhaps the only generalization that can be made is that offered in the opening of this section. To set nutrient requirements we must first decide on the criterion of adequacy (requirement for what?). Having done this, we have also defined the limit to adaptation and, with few exceptions, have set aside concerns about the impact of adaptation in setting nutrient requirements.

DIETARY REFERENCE INTAKES

In August 1997, after this chapter had been submitted for publication, prepublication copies of the uncorrected proofs of the first volume of the new dietary reference intakes (54) were released. This volume addresses calcium, phosphorus, magnesium, vitamin D, and fluoride. It is understood that changes will be made (particularly in the calcium chapter) prior to release of the final version of the report (see Appendix Table II-A-2-b). Nevertheless, it is relevant to compare aspects of the DRI report with discussion in the present chapter. The report follows very closely the structure and conceptual framework of the United Kingdom report (30), although terminology is not identical, and the DRI report extends further. The DRI report deals with four different estimates, with the following definitions:

Estimated average requirement (EAR): "the nutrient intake value that is estimated to meet the requirement defined by a specific indicator of adequacy in 50 percent of the individuals in a life-stage and gender group." Note that this actually describes the median requirement, but if the requirement distribution is symmetric, mean and median are the same (they can be expected to differ for iron requirements of menstruating women [40]).

Recommended dietary allowance (RDA): "the daily intake level that is sufficient to meet the nutrient requirements of nearly all (97 or 98 percent) individuals in the life-stage and gender group. The RDA applies to individuals and not to groups. The EAR serves as the foundation for setting the RDA."

Adequate intake (AI): "If sufficient evidence is not available to calculate an EAR, a value called an AI is used instead. The AI is based on observed or experimentally determined approximations of the average nutrient intake, by a defined population or subgroup, that appears to sustain a defined nutritional state, such as normal circulating nutrient values or growth . . . The AI is expected to exceed the RDA for the same specified end points of nutritional adequacy."

Tolerable upper intake level (UL): "the maximal level of nutrient intake that is unlikely to pose risks of adverse health effects to almost all individuals in the target group. The term *tolerable intake* was chosen to avoid implying a possible beneficial effect . . . The UL applies to chronic daily use." The important feature to note is that as described and derived in the DRI report, the UL is an estimate of the lower tail of the distribution of individual susceptibilities—it has conceptual parallelism to the RDA (an estimate of the upper tail of the distribution of individual requirements) in this regard.

The EAR and RDA are entirely consistent in concept with the portrayal presented in Figure 103.2 and hence with prior U.S., Canadian, and U.N. reports. The other two estimates are unique to the DRI report although the ideas are not.

As defined, the AI is similar to the concept of the early German standards developed by Voit and Rubner—descriptions of existing diets believed to be adequate and estimated as the group mean intake (Table 103.1). The AI is also conceptually similar to the necessary group mean intake discussed above in this chapter but differs in one very important feature. While the necessary group mean intake is derived from knowledge of the EAR and characteristics of the intake distribution, the AI will more often be based on observation of adequate intakes (descriptive epidemiology) and could exceed the necessary group mean intake. It is possible (but not likely) that experimental data could lead to an estimate of the AI without allowing estimation of an EAR. From the first volume of the DRI reports, it is clear that there will be major inconsistencies in the approach to derivation, and hence interpretation, of the AI. Perhaps its most important attribute is that it represents a clear declaration that the body of scientific evidence does not yet support estimation of requirements for that nutrient in the particular life-stage gender group. Prior reports have tended to overlook the demand for explicit evidence and instead offered informed judgments under the heading of an RDA. Creation of the AI can be hoped to end that practice, even though it declares the existence of major problems for interpretation and application. Meaning and intended interpretation of the AI are heavily clouded by the suggestion within the DRI report that the AI, derived as an estimate of the adequate group mean intake, "may be used as a goal for nutrient intake for individuals." Seemingly, with the AI, the DRI report has gone full circle and has again suggested that a single numeric estimate can serve all purposes (see early critique by Pett et al. [23]).

The truly unique and evolutionary step of the DRI reports (and the feature that in the end may cause the greatest trouble for the authors) is that there is a concerted attempt to describe nutrient requirements for the prevention or delay of chronic diseases, many of which are multifactorial. In such a venture, epidemiology should constitute a major cornerstone of the evidence linking nutrient and disease. Unfortunately, the DRI process seems to continue to place the major emphasis and greatest weight on experimental studies, sometimes to the exclusion of epidemiologic evidence. As the reports on other nutrients emerge, it will be interesting to see if the committees become more successful in linking what can be studied under controlled experimental conditions with what happens in free-living populations where chronic diseases actually develop.

The introduction to this volume of the DRIs again offers assurance that "the DRI committee intends to issue a subsequent report that will focus on the uses of the DRIs in various settings." At the time of writing, it is understood that funding for the preparation of such a report has not been identified, and it remains more a hope than an actual plan. In the meantime, some suggestions about possible applications of the EAR, RDA, AI, and UL are included, but these do not go into the depth necessary to achieve a change in understanding and use of what many will see as merely another iteration in the series of RDA reports. In fact, the DRI reports represent a major evolutionary step in thinking and approach to the derivation and application of human nutrient requirement estimates. We can hope that the aspirations of those in charge of the DRI process come to fruition and that a detailed applications report will emerge. It is desperately needed.

A welcome change in these DRI reports is the presentation for each nutrient of a detailed review and assessment of the evidence used to derive the presented estimates. This allows others to evaluate the evidence and, more importantly, offers the opportunity to identify gaps or weaknesses that require future research—an incentive for progress in nutritional science. The authors of this first DRI report are to be congratulated for breaking new ground and opening new vistas.

A second DRI volume in prepublication form was distributed in April 1998 and covers 8 B vitamins and choline (55) (see Appendix Table II-A-2-c-1 to 5).

EPILOGUE: POSSIBILITIES AND LIMITATIONS FOR APPLICATION

This chapter emphasizes conceptual issues. Statistically based approaches to facilitate application of biologic concepts and knowledge to populations and individuals are a part of nutritional science both today and tomorrow. However, one must not ignore valid criticisms and limitations of these approaches. The most serious criticisms are not conceptual; they relate to our limited ability to estimate dietary intakes. Numeric estimates of desirable intakes may be formulated with great scientific accuracy and precision and may be used in recommending what people should do. However, we must be able to estimate and evaluate existing food and nutrient intakes more effectively to know what people are doing and progress toward scientifically defined nutritional goals. Our limited ability to estimate dietary intakes limits application of our scientific knowledge and the use of any statistical model.

The 1970s saw a sudden upsurge in interest in the "day-to-day variation" in intake (47–49) that prompted committees around the world to emphasize that their estimates of requirements referred to usual intakes (the average intake persisting over moderate periods of time). At that time approaches to population assessments (counting the proportion of persons with intakes below some cutoff, often using 1-day data) yielded estimates of the magnitude of problems that were potentially seriously biased, simply because the "tails" of the intake distribution were inflated by the day-to-day variation (50). In 1986, the FNB (28) issued a report that proposed, in addition to a probability assessment approach to evaluation, a statistical approach to adjusting the distribution of observed intakes, to eliminate or at least attenuate the impact of day-to-day variation. This methodology has since been greatly improved by a team at Iowa State University (35). Consequently, we have new methodologies to overcome one of the perceived limitations in estimating and assessing the distribution of intakes of populations or large groups.

But, no available methodology can reliably estimate the usual intake of a particular individual. It may become possible to estimate intake for a finite period of time without error, but unless that period extends for a long time, an important error remains in estimating an individual's *usual* intake. This is illustrated in Table 103.5. To appreciate the impact of this factor, recognize that human protein requirement is thought to have a coefficient of variation of about 12.5% (25, 30–32). Thus, the 95% confidence interval in estimating the true protein requirement of an individual approximates the average requirement ± 25%. Table 103.5 suggests that with 1 day of intake data, the confidence interval of apparent protein intake as an estimate of the individual's usual intake might be about ± 50%. If the observed intake equaled the RDA (0.75 g/kg), then the individual's usual intake could be as low as 0.38 or as high as 1.12 g/kg/day, i.e., the confidence band associated with the intake estimate encompasses the whole range of estimated requirements. One could not assign any confident assessment to the observed intake. With more days of data (Table 103.5), the situation improves, but even with the equivalent of 2 weeks of data and a mean intake equal to the RDA, one could only say that the usual intake is likely to lie between 0.55 and 0.965 g/kg/day. Hence, the assessed risk of the intake being inadequate would lie between 0 and 0.5. As a consequence of this characteristic of dietary data, severe limitations exist in our ability to assess the intake of particular individuals,

Table 103.5
Impact of Number of Days of Data Collection on the 95% Confidence Interval of the Estimate of Usual Intake[a]

Number of Days of Intake Data Pooled	Expected 95% Confidence Interval for Estimate of Usual Intake of the Individual[b]
1	Observed ± 50%
3	Mean ± 29%
7	Mean ± 19%
14	Mean ± 13.3%
21	Mean ± 10.9%
28	Mean ± 9.5%

[a]Assumes that days of data collection are independent of one another.
[b]Assumes that within person CV of estimated protein intake is 25%, a variability estimate consistent with many published reports but not necessarily applicable to all situations.

although these limitations have been largely overcome for group assessments.

What has reemerged as a potentially serious limitation to assessment of observed intakes is an alleged and almost certain bias toward underreporting or undercapture of actual intake. This can be documented only for total energy intake (51, 52). If total intake is underestimated, at least some nutrient intakes are certainly underreported as well. Unfortunately, even if we can use external validity measures to estimate the possible overall degree of underestimation of energy intake, we cannot assume proportional underreporting of all aspects of the diet. We would have to know what components of the diet are missing or underreported. Without question, this is a serious problem. There are some potentially encouraging signs. One "external validity" check is to compute the expected BMR from age, weight, and gender data for each individual. The observed energy intake may then be expressed as a ratio to BMR. The group mean energy:BMR ratio may then be computed and compared with the expected ratio (believed to be a function of physical activity). Beaton et al. (48) computed these ratios for young adult females in the 1985 USDA survey and in a recent Dutch national survey. He then reported the data on the basis of weight (BMI) status (Table 103.6). The approach has now been applied to data from adults of both sexes included in the 1994 wave of the most recent USDA Continuing Survey of Individual Food Intakes (34). The results are shown in Table 103.7. Group mean ratios are compared with the ratios assumed to apply when the RDAs for energy were being developed (25). The values for males are low, albeit reasonably close to expected group means. The means for females are far below those expected. The 1985 and 1994 data, therefore, indicate that underreporting of food and energy intake may be a serious issue for adult females but perhaps not for adult males, at least by use of current USDA dietary methodology. Because of the high prevalence of dieting among American women, part of the apparent underreporting is likely to be true low intake on the days sampled. Based on analyses of USDA data, Ballard-Barbash and colleagues (personal communication) have convincingly argued that this practice explains part of the low intakes seen among overweight women.

Table 103.6
Apparent Ratio of Energy Intake: BMR in Adult Women in Two National Surveys: An Approach to External Validation?

	BMI Status		
	Thin	Normal	Overweight
USDA			
n	23	376	198
BMR kJ/day	4466	5182	6275
Energy:BMR	1.67	1.28	0.97
Dutch			
n	52	915	218
BMR kJ/day	5316	5768	6379
Energy:BMR	1.85	1.58	1.37

From Beaton GH, Burema J, Ritenbaugh C. Am J Clin Nutr 1997;65(Suppl):1100S–7S, with permission.

Table 103.7
Computed Ratio of Energy Intake:BMR in Adults Included in the 1994 Wave of the USDA Survey

	Females		Males	
Age Group (years)	*n*	Ratio Energy Intake:BMR[a]	*n*	Ratio Energy Intake:BMR[a]
20–29	270	1.28 (*1.60*)	267	1.52 (*1.67*)
30–39	287	1.17 (*1.55*)	309	1.45 (*1.60*)
40–49	288	1.15 (*1.55*)	303	1.31 (*1.60*)
50–59	278	1.09 (*1.50*)	266	1.18 (*1.50*)

[a]Values in parentheses are the expected ratios, as proposed in the RDA calculations, for light-to-moderate physical activity (25).

It is to be hoped that continuing refinement of data collection methods will yield high-quality data in national surveys. Until data quality can be documented (e.g., through comparative studies of energy expenditure and estimated energy intake, using doubly labeled water), application of the approaches discussed in this chapter (or any other application of the RDAs) is seriously constrained.

Do these constraints imply that we should not worry about getting our conceptual frameworks and approaches to application correct? Certainly not. We must be optimistic about successfully addressing the problems of dietary intake estimation and be ready. Further, only some of the applications of the RDAs are compromised by problems of intake estimation. The other applications also require the basic conceptual framework in the formulation of RDAs or RDIs. Finally, only with the availability of scientifically valid and coherent conceptual frameworks can we identify the sources and potential impact of existing constraints. We must continue to move forward.

DEDICATION

This chapter is dedicated to Lionel Bradley Pett and his counterparts in many other countries who attempted to struggle with conceptual frameworks and consistent approaches to application of the RDAs in the early stages of this evolution. Their work may not have had the immediate impact it deserved, but it has come to fruition. The chapter acknowledges also the many scientists who participated in national and international nutrient requirement estimation and application committees and, through their work, contributed to the evolution of the concepts.

REFERENCES

1. Leitch I. Nutr Abstr Rev 1942;11:509–21
2. Lind J. A treatise of the scurvy. London: A Millar, 1753. (Republished as Lind's treatise on scurvy. Edinburgh: University Press, 1953.)
3. Smith E. Fifth report of the medical officer of the Privy Council. London: Her Majesty's Stationery Office, 1863.
4. Young EG. Dietary standards. In: Beaton GH, McHenry EW, eds. Nutrition: a comprehensive treatise, vol 2. New York: Academic Press, 1964;299–350.

5. von Voit C. öber die ErnÑhrung des Menschen in vershiedenen Klimaten. Munich: M Rieger, 1881.
6. Lusk G. J Am Med Assoc 1918;70:821.
7. British Medical Association. Report of the Committee on Nutrition. London: British Medical Association, 1933.
8. Stiebling HK. Food budgets for nutrition and production programs. U.S. misc. publ. no. 183. Washington, DC: U.S. Department of Agriculture, 1933.
9. League of Nations. Report on the physiological bases of nutrition. The problem of nutrition, vol II. Geneva: League of Nations, 1936.
10. Canadian Council of Nutrition. Canadian dietary standards. Ottawa: Department of Pensions and National Health, 1938.
11. National Research Council, Committee on Food and Nutrition. Recommended daily allowances. Washington: National Research Council, 1941.
12. Food and Nutrition Board. Recommended dietary allowances. National Research Council reprint and circular series no. 115. Washington, DC: National Research Council, 1943.
13. Canadian Council on Nutrition. A dietary standard for Canada. Ottawa: Department of National Health and Welfare (Released in mimeographed form). 1948; (later published in slightly modified form in Can Bull Nutr 2:1. Ottawa: Department of National Health and Welfare, 1950.)
14. WHO. Diet, nutrition and the prevention of chronic diseases. WHO tech. report series no. 797. Geneva: World Health Organization, 1990.
15. FAO/WHO. Fats and oils in human nutrition. FAO food and nutrition paper no. 57. Rome: Food and Agriculture Organization of the United Nations. 1993.
16. WHO/FAO/IAEA. Trace elements in human nutrition and health. Geneva: World Health Organization. 1996.
17. Garza C, Haas, JD, Habicht J-P, Pelletier Dl, eds. Beyond nutrition recommendations: implementing science for healthier populations. Proc 14th annual Bristol-Myers Squibb-Mead Johnson Nutrition Research Symposium. Ithaca, NY: Nutritional Sciences, Cornell University, 1996.
18. Food and Nutrition Board. How should the recommended dietary allowances be revised? Washington, DC: National Academy Press, 1994.
19. Roberts LJ. NY State J Med 1944;44:59–60.
20. Forbes AL. National nutrition policy, food labeling, and health claims. In: Shils ME, Olson JA, Shike M, eds. Modern nutrition in health and disease. 8th ed. Philadelphia: Lea & Febiger, 1994;1626–57.
21. FAO/WHO. Eighth report of the joint FAO/WHO Expert Committee on Nutrition. WHO tech. report series no. 477. Geneva: World Health Organization, 1971.
22. Food and Nutrition Board. Recommended dietary allowances. National Research Council reprint and circular series no. 122. Washington, DC: National Research Council, 1945.
23. Pett LB, Morrell CA, Hanley FW. Can J Public Health 1945; 36:232–9.
24. Harper AE. Recommended dietary intakes: current and future approaches. In: Shils ME, Olson JA, Shike M, eds. Modern nutrition in health and disease. 8th ed. Philadelphia: Lea & Febiger, 1994;1475–90.
25. Food and Nutrition Board. Recommended dietary allowances. 10th ed. Washington, DC: National Academy Press, 1989.
26. Panel on Recommended Allowances of Nutrients. Recommended intakes of nutrients for the United Kingdom. Department of Health and Social Security reports on public health and medical subjects, no. 120. London: Her Majesty's Stationery Office, 1969.
27. FAO/WHO. Energy and protein requirements. WHO tech. report series no. 522. Geneva: World Health Organization, 1973.
28. Food and Nutrition Board. Nutrient adequacy: assessment using food consumption surveys. Washington, DC: National Academy Press, 1986.
29. Bureau of Nutritional Sciences, Health and Welfare Canada. Recommended nutrient intakes for Canadians. Ottawa: Canadian Government Publishing Centre, 1983.
30. Committee on Medical Aspects of Food Policy (COMA). Dietary reference values for food energy and nutrients for the United Kingdom. Department of Health report on health and social subjects, no. 41. London: Her Majesty's Stationery Office, 1991. (See also Department of Health. Dietary reference values: a guide. London: Her Majesty's Stationery Office, 1991.)
31. Health and Welfare Canada. Nutrition recommendations. Ottawa: Canadian Government Publishing Centre, 1990.
32. FAO/WHO/UNU. Energy and protein requirements. WHO tech. report series no. 724. Geneva: World Health Organization, 1985.
33. Department of National Health and Welfare. Recommended nutrient intakes for Canadians. Ottawa: Canadian Government Publishing Center, 1983.
34. Food Surveys Research Group, Agricultural Research Service. 1994 Continuing survey of food intakes by individuals and diet and health knowledge survey on CD-ROM. Riverdale, MD: US Department of Agriculture, 1996.
35. Department of Statistics, Iowa State University. A user's guide to software for intake distribution estimation (SIDE), version 1.0. Ames: Iowa State University Statistical Laboratory, 1996.
36. FAO/WHO. Calcium requirements. WHO tech. report series no. 230. Geneva: World Health Organization, 1962.
37. FAO/WHO. Requirements of ascorbic acid, vitamin D, vitamin B_{12}, folate and iron. WHO tech. report series no. 452. Geneva; World Health Organization, 1970.
38. FAO Second Committee on Calorie Requirements. FAO nutritional studies series no. 15. Rome: Food and Agriculture Organization of the United Nations, 1957.
39. Allen LH, Howson CP, eds. Estimated mean per capita energy requirement for planning emergency aid rations. Washington, DC: National Academy Press, 1995.
40. FAO/WHO. Requirements of vitamin A, iron, folate and vitamin B_{12}. FAO food and nutrition series no. 23. Rome: Food and Agriculture Organization of the United Nations, 1988.
41. Lynch SR, Bothwell TH, Hurrell RF, MacPhail AP. Iron EDTA for food fortification: a report of the International Anemia Consultative Group. Washington, DC: The Nutrition Foundation, 1993.
42. Beaton GH. The significance of adaptation in the definition of nutrient requirements and for nutrition policy. In: Blaxter K, Waterlow JC, eds. Nutritional adaptation in man. London: John Libbey, 1985;219–32.
43. Young VR. Proc Natl Acad Sci USA 1996;93:14344–8.
44. Waterlow JC. What do we mean by adaptation? In: Blaxter K, Waterlow JC, eds. Nutritional adaptation in man. London: John Libbey, 1985;1–11.
45. Payne P, Lipton M. How third world rural households adapt to dietary energy stress: the evidence and the issues. Food policy review 2. Washington, DC: International Food Policy Research Institute, 1994.
46. Malm OJ. Calcium requirement and adaptation in adult men. Scand J Clin Lab Invest 1958;10(Suppl).
47. Beaton GH. Am J Clin Nutr 1994;59(Suppl):253S–61S
48. Beaton GH, Burema J, Ritenbaugh C. Am J Clin Nutr 1997; 65(Suppl):1100S–7S.

49. Tarasuk V, Beaton GH. Am J Clin Nutr 1991;54:464–70
50. Hegsted DM. Ecol Food Nutr 1972;1:255–65
51. Mertz W, Tsui JC, Judd JT, et al. Am J Clin Nutr 1991;54:291–5.
52. Schoeller DA. Nutr Rev 1990;48:373–9.
53. Beaton GH. J Nutr 1996;126:2320S–8S.
54. Food and Nutrition Board. Dietary reference intakes for calcium, phosphorus, magnesium, vitamin D and fluoride, prepublication copy. Washington, DC: National Academy Press, 1997.
55. Food and Nutrition Board—Institute of Medicine. Dietary reference intakes. Thiamin, riboflavin, niacin, Vitamin B_6, folate, vitamin B_{12}, pantothenic acid, biotin, and choline. Prepublication copy. Washington, DC: national Academy Press, 1998.

SELECTED READINGS

Beaton GH. Criteria of an adequate diet. In: Shils ME, Olson JA, Shike M, eds. Modern nutrition in health and disease. 8th ed. Philadelphia: Lea & Febiger, 1994;1491–505.

Food and Nutrition Board. How should the recommended dietary allowances be revised? Washington, DC: National Academy Press, 1994.

Garza C, Haas, JD, Habicht J-P, Pelletier Dl, eds. Beyond nutrition recommendations: implementing science for healthier populations. Proc 14th Annual Bristol-Myers SquibbMead Johnson Nutrition Research Symposium. Ithaca, NY: Nutritional Sciences, Cornell University, 1996.

104. Dietary Goals and Guidelines: National and International Perspectives

A. STEWART TRUSWELL

THE NEED FOR DIETARY GUIDELINES

Nutrition research is ultimately paid for by taxpayers (if it is funded by national research institutes or councils or public universities) or by consumers (if funded by food or pharmaceutical companies). In other words, it is paid for by the great majority of men and women in the community. They are not scientifically trained in nutrition, but the politicians and administrators who allocate money to nutritional research on their behalf must believe that nutritional science has three objectives:

- Healthier foods
- Healthier food choices
- Healthier food consumption

All the research results and interpretations in this book and in the reference lists for each chapter, and in the wider literature of nutritional science cannot help the great majority of people in our countries until this mass of data is translated into information that most people can understand and accept.

Food consumption patterns can become healthier in two ways: from change in the foods that are available and affordable or from change in the foods people choose to eat and in the way they prepare them. What is needed ideally as the foundation of nutritional education and national food policy is a set of nutritional recommendations or dietary guidelines that are evidence-based, authoritative, and comprehensible.

Evidence Based

Scientific communication to the nonscientific majority of people often consists of "breakthroughs" and news snippets on television or radio, in newspapers and women's magazines. These items of news—and documentaries as well—are selected by producers and editors because of newsworthiness (1), not because they are good for you. Mere statement of an unsubstantiated hypothesis or a pilot case-control study, being new, is more likely to be in the news than completion of a systematic review or meta-analysis. News about nutrition is often negative, undermining confidence in traditional foods (2) rather than emphasizing the principles of a sensible diet. We have to live with a Tower of Babel of nutrition breakthroughs and threats.

Nutritional recommendations for a nation should therefore be based on objective, unbiased, and thorough reviews of all the evidence relating the nutrients, food components, and foods to health or disease risk. Evidence-based medicine is now encouraged (3), and metaanalysis is a recent powerful method in epidemiology (4), but systematic reviews of nutrition and health have been appearing since the 1960s (5), at first focused on diet and heart disease.

Authoritative

Food and drink companies advertise their products, and most advertising is for products that make the largest profit (e.g., carbonated soft drinks and alcoholic beverages). Food companies and associations defend products that nutrition scientists consider less healthy. Vested interests are academic as well as commercial. Some nutrition researchers like to publicize their new results and opinions; this may help them obtain funding for more research. Specialized journalists with some background for interpreting nutrition news are rare. In the postmodern world there is no longer universal agreement that there is one truth waiting to be revealed: it is constructed by people, always provisional, and influenced by context and power (6). As well as orthodox, scientific nutritionists, who read this book, there are alternative nutritionists, naturopaths, and herbalists (see Chapter 110). Alongside the mainline grocery supermarket is the "health food" store. In all cities, there are many different ethnic restaurants alongside fast food chain outlets.

For most people to take notice of and accept national dietary recommendations, the recommendations have to be credible and be prepared by a committee of experts convened by a government department, national academy of science, or professional association. Membership of the committee should have broad coverage (of scientific area and constituency), adequate independence, and minimal commercial bias. The best model is the committee that prepared the "Diet and Health" report for the U.S. National Research Council (NRC) in 1989 (7). It had 33 experts on the main committee and another 76 specialists recorded as providing input.

Comprehensible

Every branch of knowledge and every occupation has its technical terms. Nutrition is the same. But everyone has to eat, and everyone has an opinion about which foods are good for them. Dietary guidelines have to be comprehensible to the general public (8), who are confused about terms like *cholesterol, fat, fiber, polyunsaturated,* and *energy.* Guidelines must also be available in language meaningful to health professionals who can explain the above and other technical terms and the meanings of *moderate in, low in,* and *plenty of* for individuals.

In public health nutrition, two major sets of messages are sent from a consensus of nutritional scientists to the rest of the population—politicians, government departments, food industry, farmers, health professionals, economists, journalists, school teachers, supermarkets, caterers, shoppers, and consumers. *Recommended dietary intakes* (RDIs; see Chapter 103 and Appendix Tables II-A-2 to A-8) are the first and older set. They advise the quantities of the essential nutrients that people ought to consume. These technical numbers have to be converted for ordinary people to educational devices such as food groups, meal plans, or exchange lists, or to food enrichment, subsidies etc. In underdeveloped countries and communities, food and nutritional policy must concentrate on striving to reach the RDIs for as many people and as many nutrients as possible.

In affluent countries, intakes near the RDIs can be taken for granted for most people. Other sets of authoritative statements, *dietary guidelines,* have emerged since the late 1960s and advise how to select from the many combinations of foods in adequate diets to give the best chances of long-term health. The variety of food products is bewildering, and the whole food system needs signposts—guidelines to healthier diets that can be used in nutritional education, planning by food companies, and national nutrition policy.

FEATURES OF DIETARY GUIDELINES OR GOALS

Dietary guidelines aim to reduce the chances of developing chronic degenerative diseases rather than to provide enough of the essential nutrients (that is the purpose of RDIs). While there is never more than one RDI (or RDA, recommended dietary allowance) committee and report in a country, there can be several sets of dietary guidelines at a time (5).

Dietary goals or guidelines start not from zero intake (as RDIs do) but from the present estimated national average diet. They deal with the optimal proportions of the energy-yielding macronutrients: how much carbohydrate? fat? protein? alcohol? and which types? They are not usually expressed as nutrients, but as food components, food groups, or even eating behavior. So, they are often a hybrid collection of recommendations.

Dietary goals or guidelines are not usually expressed as weight of nutrient per day; but as semiquantitative advice on consumption of a food component or on people's eating behavior. If expressed quantitatively, this is mostly as a percentage of total energy, that is, nutrient density (e.g., total fat intake should be 30 to 35% of total energy).

Dietary guidelines are targets for the population to aim for some time in the future. In some sets, the year is given or goals are progressive (e.g., total fat: intermediate goal, 35% energy; ultimate goal, 20–30% [9]). RDIs by contrast are needed now and every day (although there are reserves in the body—large for some nutrients, small for others).

A few sets of dietary guidelines draw a distinction between general advice for the whole population and (usually more radical) advice for groups at risk. For example, the U.S. Surgeon General's report (10) has five recommendations for most people and another four for some people. The recommendations of the World Health Organization (WHO) Europe (9) give intermediate goals separately for the general population and for the cardiovascular high-risk group.

Although most RDIs are relatively well established scientifically, guidelines are more provisional, being based on indirect evidence about the complex role of food components in causing multifactorial diseases with very long incubation periods. Dietary goals and guidelines, which primarily examine macronutrients, rely more on epidemiologic data than RDIs do. In addition, they depend on using food consumption patterns. The NRC Committee on Diet and Health (7) observed that

> the term *insufficient data* could perhaps be applied to most issues concerning nutrition and health. In particular it characterizes many of the relationships between diet and certain chronic diseases. The lack of certainty about causal associations and mechanisms of action is common and stems in part from attempts to relate a complex mixture such as diet to complex, multifactorial chronic diseases for which the pathophysiological, environmental, and genetic predisposing factors are imprecisely understood . . . Despite such limitations, a large body of evidence has emerged in the past four decades concerning chronic diseases and their relationship to general dietary patterns or specific dietary components (7).

Unlike RDIs, which give separate numbers for males and females and for different age groups and physiologic states, dietary guidelines have usually appeared to be the same for every man, woman, and child. Of course adjustments have to be made at the implementation stage. An international WHO symposium in Japan (11) concluded that while countries could usually share their RDIs, dietary guidelines are most effective if the target group is defined. New Zealand has different dietary guidelines reports for infants (12), children (13), adolescents (14), most adults (15), healthy pregnant women (16), and healthy older people (17). (Most of these reports [except ref. 15] do not appear to be the work of a large, representative committee). In Australia, there is a general dietary guidelines report (18) and a separate report for infants, children, and adolescents (19). Canada has a separate report on fat recommendations for children (40).

Although they are more recent than RDIs, dietary guidelines are better known by the general public. Their summary recommendations, written in deliberately simple language about major food components or food habits appeal to journalists, consumer organizations, and cookbook writers.

GOALS OR GUIDELINES?

The classic *Dietary Goals for the United States* (20) was addressed to the nation, and the recommendations were expressed in such technical terms as "increase the consumption of complex carbohydrates and naturally occurring sugars from about 28% of energy intake to about 48% of energy intake" (20)—not a calculation the shopper can manage in the aisle of a supermarket! These dietary goals were followed by *Dietary Guidelines for Americans,* published by the departments of Agriculture and Health, in which the corresponding recommendation in the 1995 edition (21) is headed "Choose a diet with plenty of grain products, vegetables and fruits." In Australia, "dietary goals" was also used for statements on nutritional policy, "Increase consumption of complex carbohydrates and dietary fibre . . ." (22), while dietary guidelines came later in a mass-produced booklet, written in less technical language for consumers, "Eat more bread and cereals (preferably wholegrain), vegetables and fruit" (23). Helsing (24) has suggested that recommendations are needed at three levels: quantitative nutrient goals for scientists and health professionals, quantitative food goals for politicians and food producers, and dietary guidelines expressed as advice to individual consumers. The report *Diet, Nutrition and the Prevention of Chronic Diseases* by a WHO committee (25) defines population nutrient goals as the range in which population average intakes are judged to be consistent with a low prevalence of diet-related diseases in the population. The report sets out goals for 11 nutrients in numerical terms, e.g., total average carbohydrate for a population should be between 55 and 75% of energy. It stresses the difference between population nutrient goals and individual nutrient intakes, e.g., if the population's total carbohydrate intake is 60% of energy, individual intakes might range from 45% to 75% of energy (see Appendix Table II-A-9). The contrasting concept of dietary guidelines was well explained by Robbins (26) in a commentary on the first proposed nutritional guidelines for Britain: "Guidelines express the goals in terms of foods (or combinations of foods) which are to be eaten by individuals . . . Guidelines need not be quantified but need to be based on goals. Many different dietary patterns can be compatible with a given set of dietary goals." For instance, the goal of reducing total fat intake can be achieved by drinking skimmed milk, by eating less fatty meat, or by reducing hard cheese and biscuits.

HISTORY OF DIETARY GOALS AND GUIDELINES

Nordic *Synpunkter* (1968)

The first set of dietary goals were *Mediciniska synpunkter pa folkkosten i de Nordiska landerna* (medical viewpoints on people's food in the Nordic countries). "Nordic" and "Scandinavian" are often used interchangeably, but the original meaning of "Scandinavia" was the peninsula comprising Norway and Sweden. "Nordic" includes Denmark, Finland, and Iceland. These goals were developed by Professsor Arvid Wretlind and other nutrition professors in Sweden, Finland, Norway, and Denmark and published in 1968 (27, 28) (Table 104.1). Ancel Keys arranged for an English translation to be printed in *Nutrition Reviews* 4 months later (29).

The first idea behind these recommendations was that mechanization had reduced physical work and with it, caloric consumption. Consumers with low caloric intakes needed to increase the density of iron, calcium, and other critical nutrients per 1000 kcal if they are to obtain their RDIs. Meanwhile, the proportion of dietary fat had risen in Sweden from 29% of energy at the end of the 19th century to 42% in the mid-1960s (30). "Simple calculations showed that a diet ensuring the requirements of the low

Table 104.1
Medical Viewpoints on People's Food in the Nordic Countries (1968)

The calorie supply in the diet should in many cases be reduced to prevent overweight.

The total fat consumption should be reduced from the present around 40% to between 25 and 35% of total calories.

The use of saturated fat should be reduced and consumption of polyunsaturated fat increased simultaneously.

Consumption of sugar and sugar-containing products should be reduced.

One should increase consumption of vegetables, fruit, potatoes, skimmed milk, fish, lean meat, and cereal products.

From the medical and nutritional standpoint it is essential to emphasize the importance of regular exercise habits from childhood for all individuals with mainly sedentary work.

Translated by the author from Mediciniska synpunkter på folkkosten ′ı de Noridska länderna. Var föda 1968;20:3–5 and Mediciniska synpunkter på folkkosten i de Noridska länderna. Läkartidningen 1968;65:2102–3.

calorie groups is practically impossible to achieve without reduction of the fat consumption . . . to, at most, 35% of calories" (31). In addition, replacement of saturated fats by polyunsaturated fats should lower plasma cholesterol levels, and reduction of sugar and confectionery should help reduce dental caries. The Nordic viewpoints met considerable local opposition from conservative professionals and food companies, but they were the foundation for the 1972 "Diet and Exercise" campaign in Sweden and the Norwegian nutrition policy (32).

Meanwhile, evidence was accumulating for the dietary fat hypothesis of coronary heart disease that Ancel Keys started to develop in 1952 (33, 34). The American Heart Association has been publishing diet-heart statements since 1961, and these statements have become progressively less tentative, with a stronger scientific infrastructure. Since 1970, other scientific and professional bodies in the United States, Australia, New Zealand, the Netherlands, the United Kingdom, Germany, and Canada (in temporal order) have published expert committee statements on diet and coronary heart disease. So, by the mid-1970s, there were two lines of reasoning for general dietary advice to the public in affluent countries. The Nordic recommendations aimed primarily to replace empty-calorie foods (fats and refined sugars) with a mixture of nutrient-dense foods because people were expending less energy and, as a consequence, eating less food than their grandparents. The followers of Ancel Keys aimed primarily to bring down the plasma (total) cholesterol concentration. Their advice concentrated on eating less saturated fat and cholesterol.

Dietary Goals for the United States (1977)

Dietary Goals for the United States (1977) was a pivotal document. It added to the above two concepts a third group of miscellaneous ideas: the dietary fiber hypothesis; the possible relationship of high fat intake to breast and large bowel cancer, and the possible role of sodium salt in causing essential hypertension. *Dietary Goals* was written by a group of staff members and associates without specialized nutritional experience under committee chairman, Senator George McGovern. Some expert input was provided by Professor Mark Hegsted before publication. The report contains no major blunders, although the references are few and some of them, unconventional. The first edition (20) was revised before the end of 1977 (35) (Table 104.2) in response to objections cited in group 8 of Table 104.3. The other objections were of a more political or philosophical nature. Committees that draft dietary guidelines have to keep these possible objections in mind (Table 104.3) and work to minimize them. Never again have there been so many published comments and criticisms of nutrition recommendations as followed the first edition of *Dietary Goals for the United States*. One collection of commentaries runs to 889 pages (36).

Nevertheless, the first independent comment overseas, an editorial in *The Lancet* (37), generally welcomed *Dietary Goals*. The goals were never an official U.S. government statement, although most nutritionists outside the country did not realize this. The ideas in *Dietary Goals* have been modified and reused—or rediscovered—in subsequent official or authoritative sets of guidelines in the U.S. and in many national sets of nutritional recommendations around the world.

Table 104.2
Recommendations from Dietary Goals for the United States, 1st and 2nd editions, in Abbreviated Form and Original Order

Dietary Goals, Feb. 1997 (20)		Dietary Goals, Dec. 1997 (35)	
		Avoid overweight	
↑ Carbohydrate		↑ Complex carbohydrates	
↓ Total fat		↓ Sugars	
↓ Saturated fatty acids	↑ PUFA	↓ Total fat	
↓ Dietary cholesterol		↓ Saturated fatty acids	↑ PUFA
↓ Sugar		↓ Dietary cholesterol	
↓ Salt to 3 g/day		↓ Salt to 5 g/day	

PUFA, Polyunsaturated fatty acids.

Table 104.3
Objections to *Dietary Goals for the United States* (1st Edition)

Reasoning not scientific enough; based more on intuition than scientific reasoning; not a scientifically sound review; should be reexamined by expert bodies: NIH, FDA, USDA, NAS, etc.

Not needed; America's health is improving; the committee has perpetrated a hoax by claiming that Americans are suffering from an epidemic of killer diseases

We need more research; too soon; the lipid hypothesis of coronary heart disease not yet proven; the relation between salt and hypertension not yet proven; we are only on the threshold of discovery in nutrition; it's unwise to base recommendations on food-disappearance data; promises too much; the politicians are over-selling nutrition

Political; politically motivated; a puritanical, "big brother" approach; it's unwise to tamper with the diets of the great majority of people; for high-risk groups, diets should be individually prescribed by medical practitioners or dietitians

Problem of recommending for all age-sex groups; these look like guidelines for food intake by overweight middle-aged men; neglects children, pediatrics

Vested interests; my advice wasn't asked or that of our professional association; our industry may be affected (salt, dairy, sugar, egg, cattlemen)

There could be adverse effects; we are concerned that increased intake of polyunsaturated fat could have side effects; if less meat is eaten, iron deficiency may increase

Major issues were omitted and corrections are required; left out alcohol (although prohibitionist in tone); should add a goal about obesity; should add encouragement of water fluoridation; the goal of 3 g NaCl per day is far too low

Based mainly on reference (36), on commentaries in Nutrition Today November/December, 1977, and on Harper AE. Am J Clin Nutr 1978;31:310–321.

Note: Many of the commentaries were a mixture of positive and (some of the above) negative comments. Individual commentators often made criticisms in several of the above groups.

CURRENT GUIDELINES IN THE UNITED STATES

Dietary Guidelines for Americans

Now in its fourth revised edition (21), *Dietary Guidelines for Americans* first appeared in 1980. The fourth edition is a 43-page booklet, 10 × 22.5 cm, which can conveniently slip into a handbag or pocket. It is published with the joint authority of the U.S. Departments of Agriculture and Health and Human Services. It is intended for all healthy Americans over 2 years of age and is written, as far as possible, in nontechnical, reader-friendly language. Table 104.4 shows the headings of the seven guidelines. They are similar to the 1977 dietary goals (Table 104.2) except that variety of food consumption has been added as a first principle plus a guideline on alcohol consumption. *Dietary Guidelines for Americans* has been revised and updated about every 5 years. It is instructive to compare the wording of headings in the fourth (1995) edition with those of the first (1980) edition (Table 104.4). Much care has gone into the wording, which must be brief as well as clear. "Avoid too much fat" turned out to be rather meaningless and has been replaced by "Choose a diet low in fat and saturated fat and cholesterol," with simple semiquantitative advice in the body of the booklet. *Dietary Guidelines* is Home and Garden bulletin no. 232, widely distributed and written for ordinary consumers. It is not written for health professionals, but they should have a copy and note how simply it presents the main conclusions of modern nutritional research.

The Surgeon General's Report on Nutrition and Health

The Surgeon General's Report on Nutrition and Health (of 1988) is a large review (10) of 727 pages, which had 90 contributors and 171 reviewers. There are five recommendations for most people:

- Reduce consumption of fat (especially saturated) and cholesterol
- Energy and weight control
- Increase consumption of whole-grain cereal foods, vegetables, and fruits (complex carbohydrates and fiber)
- Reduce intake of sodium
- Take alcohol only in moderation (no more than two drinks per day), if at all

There are another four recommendations *for some people:*

- Community water systems should be fluoridated
- Children should limit consumption and frequency of use of foods high in sugars
- Adolescent girls and adult women should increase consumption of foods high in calcium
- Children, adolescents, and women of childbearing age should be sure to eat foods that are good sources of iron

Table 104.4
Headings from *Dietary Guidelines for Americans*

1980 (1st edition)	1995 (4th edition)
Eat a variety of foods	Eat a variety of foods
Maintain ideal weight	Balance the food you eat with physical activity—maintain or improve your weight
Avoid too much fat, saturated fat, and cholesterol	Choose a diet with plenty of grain products, vegetables, and fruits
Eat foods with adequate starch and fiber	Choose a diet low in fat, unsaturated fat, and cholesterol
Avoid too much sugar	Choose a diet moderate in sugars
Avoid too much sodium	Choose a diet moderate in salt and sodium
If you drink alcohol, do so in moderation	If you drink alcoholic beverages, do so in moderation

The National Research Council's 1989 *Diet and Health* Review

A substantial, large book (7) of 750 pages, *Diet and Health* was written by a committee of 33 persons, with contributions or advice of a further 76 specialists acknowledged. It is the most thorough review of the evidence on which dietary guidelines are based. Its recommendations are

- Reduce total fat intakes to 30% of calories or less. Reduce saturated fatty acid intake to less than 10% of calories and dietary cholesterol to less than 300 mg daily. Polyunsaturated fatty acid intake should stay at about the present 7% of calories (and not be above 10% of calories in individuals). Concentrated fish oils are not recommended (for the general public).
- Eat five or more servings of a combination of vegetables and fruits each day (especially green and yellow vegetables and citrus fruits). Also, increase intake of starches and complex carbohydrates by eating six or more servings of a combination of breads, cereals, and legumes. Increase of added sugars is not recommended.
- Maintain protein intake at moderate levels, i.e., less than twice the RDA.
- Balance food intake and physical activity to maintain appropriate body weight. Increased abdominal fat carries a higher risk for chronic diseases than comparable fat deposits in the hips or thighs. All healthy people should maintain physical activity at a moderate level. Neither large fluctuations in body weight nor extreme restrictions in food intake are desirable.
- The committee does not recommend alcohol consumption. For those who do drink, limit consumption to two standard drinks a day. Pregnant women and women attempting to conceive should avoid alcoholic beverages.
- Limit total daily salt intake to 6 g (sodium chloride) or less.
- Maintain adequate calcium intake, but the potential benefits of calcium above the RDA are not well documented.
- Avoid taking dietary supplements in excess of the RDA.
- Maintain an optimum intake of fluoride, particularly during the years of primary and secondary tooth formation and growth, i.e., fluoridated water or (if not available) fluoride supplements.

Guidelines to Prevent Cancer

To reduce dietary factors that appear to contribute to development of cancer, recommendations in a large review by an NRC committee (38) were initially published in 1982 and updated in 1989. Summarized briefly these are

1. Reduce fat (unsaturated as well as saturated) to 30% total energy or less
2. Frequently consume fruits (e.g., citrus) and vegetables (especially carotene-rich and cruciferous)
3. Reduce consumption of salt-cured and smoked foods
4. Continue efforts to minimize contamination of foods with carcinogens from any source
5. Make further efforts to identify mutagens in foods, test them for carcinogenicity, and minimize their concentration
6. If alcoholic beverages are consumed, do so in moderation.

The American Cancer Society's 1997 guidelines are compatible with these, but they add encouragement to eat grain products and to be physically active. Consumption of meats (especially high-fat meats) should be limited (38A).

The United States is a large country with by far the largest investment in nutritional research in the world. It is not surprising that there have been more than one set of authoritative dietary guidelines in the country since 1977. There are other important sets not reviewed here, such as those of the American Heart Association and of the American Dietetic Association (guidelines for women). The different sets of recommendations agree closely, with no serious conflict.

DIETARY GUIDELINES IN OTHER COUNTRIES

Most major countries formulated authoritative sets of dietary guidelines following the 1977 appearance of *Dietary Goals for the United States*. Dietary guidelines are popular with governments. They are inexpensive, involving only a few committee meetings and a small secretariat. Nutritional scientists are pleased to be asked their opinions. Most food companies accept guidelines if they are seen to be balanced and objective; they can assist companies in developing new products and forward planning. The expectation must be that if a country has dietary guidelines agreed on by representative experts, they will be used in school education programs for the nation's future shoppers and food preparers. Nutrition and food professionals will use them in advising members of the general public, and when there is a query or dispute about nutritional messages or the nutritiousness of a food, the guidelines are there for reference.

Table 104.5 lists sets of authoritative dietary guidelines known at the time of writing this chapter (9, 15, 18, 19, 39–62). There may be others, and certainly other sets of guidelines have been proposed by individual nutritionists that have not been through the full process of committee, consultation, and approval by a government department.

A Selection of Guidelines for Developed Countries

There is only space to record the headings and add a few brief notes.

Table 104.5
Authoritative Dietary Guidelines Outside the United States

Australia	1992 (18)	1995 (19)
Canada	1990 (39)	1995 (40)
China	1989 (41)	
Denmark	1984 (42)	
Europe (WHO)	1988 (9)	
Fiji	1988 (43)	
Finland	1989 (44)	
France	1992 (45)	
Germany	1985 (46)	
Hungary	1988 (47)	
Iceland	1989 (48)	
India	1988 (49)	
Italy	1988 (50)	
Japan	1985 (51)	
Korea (South)	1987 (52)	
Latin America	1988 (53)	
Malta	1986 (54)	
Netherlands	1986 (55)	
New Zealand	1991 (15)	
Nordic countries	1989 (56)	
Norway	1981 (57)	
Philippines	1990 (57A)	
Portugal	1982 (58)	
Singapore	1989 (59)	
Sweden	1985 (60)	
United Kingdom	1990 (61)	1991 (62)

Australia (1979, Revised 1992)

The first set of dietary guidelines, published in 1979 (23), were well accepted by nutritionists, health authorities, and the food industry. In the 1992 revised set of guidelines (18), the elements have been reordered and reworded with more emphasis on a low-fat diet, and two guidelines on specific nutrients have been added. The ten guidelines are *(a)* enjoy a wide variety of nutritious foods; *(b)* eat plenty of breads and cereals (preferably wholegrain), vegetables (including legumes), and fruits; *(c)* eat a diet low in fat and, in particular, low in saturated fat; *(d)* maintain a healthy body weight by balancing food intake and regular physical activity; *(e)* if you drink alcohol, limit your intake; *(f)* eat only a moderate amount of sugars and foods containing added sugars; *(g)* use salt sparingly and choose foods with little added salt; *(h)* encourage and support breast-feeding; *(i)* eat foods containing calcium; this is particularly important for girls and women; and *(j)* eat foods containing iron; this is particularly important for girls, women, vegetarians, and athletes.

Canada (1990)

The Canadian diet (39) should *(a)* provide energy consistent with maintenance of body weight within the recommended range; *(b)* include essential nutrients in amounts recommended; *(c)* include no more than 30% of energy as fat and no more than 10% as saturated fat; *(d)* provide 55% of energy as carbohydrate from a variety of sources; *(e)* contain reduced sodium; *(f)* include no more than 5% of total energy as alcohol, or two drinks daily, whichever is less; *(g)* contain no more caffeine than the equivalent of four regular cups of coffee per day; and *(h)* community water supplies containing less than 1 mg/L should be fluoridated to that level.

For children (40) from the age of 2 until the end of linear growth there should be a transition from the high-fat diet of infancy to a diet that includes no more than 30% of energy as fat and no more than 10% of energy as saturated fat.

Europe (1988)

In a report for WHO Europe (9), goals (not guidelines) are given for the general population; (intermediate goals) and ultimate goals: complex carbohydrates (>40 en%) 45 to 55 en%; protein 12 to 13 en%; sugar 10 en%; total fat (35 en%) 20 to 30 en%; saturated fat (15 en%) 10 en%; P:S ratio (≤0.5) ≤1.0; dietary fiber (30 g/day) >30 g/day; salt (7 to 8 g/day) 5 g/day; dietary cholesterol <100 mg per 4.2 MJ (1000 kcal); fluoride 0.7 to 1.2 mg/L. (For cardiovascular high-risk groups, the intermediate goal for fat and saturated fat is the same as the ultimate goal for the general population).

Germany (1985)

In *Ten Guidelines for Sensible Nutrition* (1985) (46) recommendations are to *(a)* use variety in the choice of foods; *(b)* eat not too much and not too little; *(c)* eat small meals more often; *(d)* eat sufficient protein; *(e)* avoid too much fat; *(f)* eat sweets seldom; *(g)* eat fresh food (fruits, juices, vegetables, milk) and whole grain products daily; *(h)* prepare foods properly; *(i)* use salt sparingly; and *(j)* use restraint with alcohol.

Hungary (1988)

Recommendations (47) are to *(a)* eat a variety of foods; *(b)* avoid too much fat; use vegetable oil and margarine; *(c)* avoid too much salt; *(d)* reduce sugary snacks; *(e)* drink half a liter of low-fat milk per day; *(f)* eat fresh fruits, vegetables, and salads more often; *(g)* always have whole-grain bread on the table; choose potatoes over rice; *(h)* eat four or five meals daily, none too rich or too light; *(i)* quench thirst with water; it's best to avoid alcohol and it is forbidden for children and pregnant women; and *(j)* good nutrition means a balanced diet—in other words, no food is prohibited, but some are to be preferred and others to be eaten less frequently.

Italy (1988)

Guidelines for a healthy Italian "alimentation" (50) are headed *(a)* watch your weight; *(b)* less fat and cholesterol; *(c)* more starch and more fiber; *(d)* sweet foods: not too much; *(e)* salt? much less; *(f)* alcohol: with moderation; *(g)* variety of foods and six food groups.

Japan (1985)

Recommendations (51) are *(a)* obtain well-balanced nutrition with a variety of foods; eat 30 foodstuffs a day; take staple food, main dish, and side dish together; *(b)* take energy corresponding to daily life activity; *(c)* consider the amount and quality of the fats and oils you eat: avoid too much; eat more vegetable oils than animal fat; *(d)* avoid too much salt, not more than 10 g a day; *(e)* happy eating makes for happy family life; sit down and eat together and talk; treasure family taste and home cooking.

South Korea (1986)

Korean recommendations (52) are *(a)* eat a variety of foods; *(b)* keep ideal body weight; *(c)* consume enough protein; *(d)* keep fat consumption at 20% of energy intake; *(e)* drink milk every day; *(f)* reduce salt intake; *(g)* keep in good dental health; *(h)* moderate alcohol and caffeine consumption; *(i)* keep the harmony between diet and daily life; and *(j)* enjoy meals. (Those in Western countries who think a target of 30% energy from total fat too stringent should ponder the fourth Korean recommendation.)

Netherlands (1986)

The Dutch recommendations (55) are *(a)* achieve or maintain a normal body weight; *(b)* diet should be balanced and supply adequate amounts of all essential nutrients; *(c)* average total fat intake of 30 to 35% dietary energy; *(d)* saturated fat should be around 10% total energy, and polyunsaturated fat 50 to 100% of saturated fat; *(e)* dietary cholesterol should not exceed 33 mg/MJ; *(f)* carbohydrates (total), 50 to 60% of energy; sugars, 15 to 25% of energy; *(g)* protein, 10 to 15% of energy (as at present); *(h)* dietary fiber target, 3 g/MJ; *(i)* current alcohol consumption is far too high in many cases; *(j)* salt, upper level 8 g/day.

There is also advice for special groups, e.g., about vitamin D and fluoride for children.

New Zealand (1991)

The food and nutrition guidelines (15) are *(a)* eat a variety of foods from each of the four major food groups each day; at least three servings of vegetables, two of fruit, six of bread and cereals, two of milk and dairy products (especially low fat), one of lean meats or poultry, fish, eggs, nuts, or pulses; *(b)* prepare meals with minimal added fat (especially saturated fat) and salt; *(c)* choose preprepared foods and snacks that are low in fat (especially saturated fat), salt, and sugar; *(d)* maintain a healthy body weight by regular physical activity and by healthy eating; *(e)* drink plenty of liquids each day; *(f)* if you drink alcohol, do so in moderation.

Nordic Countries (1989)

These are the first set of guidelines (56) agreed for the countries of a region, *Denmark, Finland, Norway,* and *Sweden.* The report contains RDIs as well as guidelines. For adults and children over 3 years *(a)* protein ought to provide 10 to 15% of the total energy intake; *(b)* fat should not provide more than 30% of the total energy intake. The decrease from most people's present intake should be primarily by reducing saturated fat, which will generally be accompanied by a desirable decrease in dietary cholesterol. Total fat should not, however, be below 20 to 25% energy. Essential fatty acids should contribute 3 to 10% (at least 4.5% for pregnancy and 6% for lactation). Both linoleic (ω-6) and linolenic (ω-3) are essential, but requirement of the former is greater. Linolenic and long-chain ω-3 acids should provide at least 0.5% of energy; *(c)* carbohydrates should provide 55 to 60% of energy. Sugar should not provide more than 10% of energy (i.e., refined, not naturally occurring sugar). The intake of dietary fiber should be at least 3 g/MJ (12.5 g/1000 kcal), which for adults is 25 to 30 g/day. *(d)* It is desirable that the sodium intake gradually decrease to a level corresponding to 5 g NaCl per day; *(e)* consumption of alcohol should be avoided or be moderate. During pregnancy alcohol should be avoided entirely.

Singapore (1989)

Recommendations (59) are to *(a)* eat a variety of foods; *(b)* maintain desirable body weight; *(c)* restrict total fat intake to 20 to 30% of total energy intake; *(d)* modify composition of fat in the diet to one-third polyunsaturated, one-third monounsaturated, and one-third saturated; *(e)* reduce cholesterol intake to less than 300 mg/day; *(f)* maintain intakes of complex carbohydrates at about 50% of total energy intake; *(g)* reduce salt intake to less than 4.5 g a day (1800 mg Na); *(h)* reduce intake of salt-cured, preserved, and smoked foods; *(i)* reduce intake of refined and processed sugar to less than 10% of energy; *(j)* increase intake of fruit and vegetables and whole-grain cereal products, thereby increasing vitamins A and C and fiber; *(k)* for those who drink, not more than two to three standard drinks (about 40 g alcohol) per day; *(l)* encourage breast-feeding of infants until at least 6 months of age.

United Kingdom (1990, 1991)

After considerable earlier controversy (63–66), dietary guidelines and goals are now accepted by the British establishment. The Ministry of Agriculture published in 1990 a thin book (61) for the general public (without scientific background). The eight guidelines are *(a)* enjoy your food; *(b)* eat a variety of different foods; *(c)* eat the right amount to be a healthy weight; *(d)* eat plenty of foods rich in starch and fiber; *(e)* don't eat too much fat (we don't need saturates at all); *(f)* don't eat sugary foods too often; *(g)* look after the vitamins and minerals in your food; *(h)* if you drink, keep within sensible limits.

The next year, quantitative population goals for fats and carbohydrates were included in the new report on dietary reference values (62). Of the population's average percentage of total energy (including alcohol), total fat should be 33%. Of total fatty acids, saturated fatty acids should be 10%; *cis* polyunsaturated fatty acids, 6% (not more than 10%); and *trans* fatty acids not more than 2%. Nonstarch polysaccharides should be 18 to 24 g/day (corresponding to around 30–35 g/day dietary fiber) and "nonmilk extrinsic sugars" should average 60 g/day ("data in support of any specific quantified targets for non-milk extrinsic sugars were scanty").

Guidelines for Less-Industrialized Countries

Dietary guidelines were originally introduced to meet the nutritional problems of affluent communities. Until the end of the 1980s, there were no (published) proposals to apply them in developing countries, where the dominating nutritional problem is that many people can't afford or grow all the food they need. However, in these developing countries, *(a)* coronary heart disease and cancers are increasing their share of mortality as infections come under control (67); *(b)* the affluent middle class in a country like India may only be 5% of the population, but it comprises 40 million individuals who play a major part in the development of the country (49); *(c)* developing countries had a bad experience when they followed industrial countries and abandoned breast-feeding; *(d)* now is a good time to try to prevent the consequences of further increases in fat intake; and *(e)* low-income countries cannot afford to add the burden of medical care of degenerative diseases to their health budgets.

Dietary guidelines are a low-cost measure. If they have official status they can be written into nutritional material, adopted by multinational companies for their staff, and accepted by voluntary and international agencies as well as by national health workers. Two conditions that make formulation of dietary guidelines specially challenging in low-income countries are the scarcity of food composition data (food analysis is very expensive) and the wide range of nutritional status, from undernutrition among the poor to overnutrition in the affluent class.

For India, Gopalan proposes two sets of guidelines (49). For the relatively poor, diets should be least expensive and conform to tradition and cultural practices as far as possible. Some pulses (legumes) should be eaten along with the high-cereal diet, and at least 150 mL/day of milk and 150 g/day of leafy vegetables. Energy from fat and oil need not exceed 15%, and that from sugar need not exceed 5% of total calories.

For affluent Indians, he proposes (49, 68) restricting energy intake to levels commensurate with sedentary occupations; giving preference to undermilled cereals; including green leafy vegetables in the diet; limiting edible fat to no more than 20% of total energy and restricting ghee (clarified butter) to special occasions; restricting intake of sugar and sweets; and avoiding high salt intake, especially by those prone to hypertension.

For Latin America, Bengoa et al. (53) propose an alternative model, dietary goals that can apply to all, rich and poor, "metas nutricionales." These then have to be converted into focused guidelines for different segments of the population. Energy and protein requirements are derived from the FAO/WHO/UNU report (69). Fat should be 20 to 25% of dietary energy, with the ratio of fatty acids, saturated:monounsaturated:polyunsaturated, equal to 1:1:1. Omega-3 fatty acids should be 10% of total polyunsaturated fatty acids. Carbohydrate should provide 60 to 70% of total energy, with the emphasis on less-refined cereals and products. Sugar contributes to dental caries, but it can be useful for increasing the caloric density of diets, particularly for young children. Most adults in Latin America can only take moderate amounts of milk because of lactase insufficiency. Fiber (recommendation, 8 to 10 g/1000 kcal) only needs to be encouraged for the more affluent. Attention to biologic interactions among nutrients can enhance availability of limited micronutrients. Salt intake should be below 10 g/day. There are separate recommendations for different age groups, including of course breast-feeding for infants and adequate calcium for adolescents and pregnant women.

With goals like this, some people need to be helped to eat more fat, while other sections of society should bring their fat intake down to 20 to 25% energy that Bengoa, and Scrimshaw and colleagues think are the optimal range for health. Dietary goals like this might eventually be developed, after wide consultation, into international dietary goals. A WHO Study Group (25) has proposed *population* nutrient goals for the whole world, expressed as ranges, including: total fat between 15% of energy (lower limit) and 30% of energy (interim goal); saturated fatty acids between 0% (lower limit) and 10% (upper limit); polyunsaturated fatty acids, 3 to 7% of energy; total protein, 10 to 15% of energy; total carbohydrate, 55 to 75% of energy; "complex" carbohydrates, 50 to 70% of energy; "free sugars," 0 to 10% of energy; dietary fiber (expressed as nonstarch polysaccharides) 16 to 24 g/day; fruits and vegetables (lower limit), 400 g/day; salt, 0 to 6 g/day (25).

WHERE SETS OF GUIDELINES AGREE AND WHERE THEY DISAGREE

There is *almost complete agreement* on the following six recommendations:

1. Eat a nutritionally adequate diet from a variety of foods
2. Eat less fat, particularly saturated fat
3. Adjust energy intake and/or physical activity to maintain or achieve healthy body weight
4. Eat more complex carbohydrates and fiber *or* eat more cereals/grains, vegetables, and fruits
5. Reduce salt intake
6. Drink alcohol in moderation, if at all

The Japanese recommendations (51) suggest 30 different foods a day to give a numerical expression to the concept of *variety*. A more usual way to explain variety is advice to eat foods from each of the five (three to seven in different countries) nutritional food groups each day and to make regular changes of foods within each group.

The target for *total fat* is sometimes not quantitative. If a number is stated, it ranges between 35 (62) and 20% (52) of total energy. (Note that fat percent energy is a somewhat lower number if total energy includes alcoholic drinks as well as food, and it is also lower if fat is expressed as fatty acids, instead of fatty acids plus glycerol.) The recommendation to increase complex *carbohydrates* and fiber is stated in different ways and is less likely to be expressed quantitatively.

The recommendation to reduce *salt* is often not expressed quantitatively, but when it is, the target upper limit ranges between 4.5 (59) and 10 g/day (51). The NRC (7) sets 6 g salt per day, which corresponds in Australia to the upper end of the RDI range of 100 mmol sodium (70).

Where the quantity of *alcohol* is stated (for those not pregnant), it has usually been two drinks per day.

A *second group* of recommendations is more controversial; these give advice about polyunsaturated fats, dietary cholesterol, and sugar. When polyunsaturated fats are mentioned, the usual upper limit for individuals is 10% of energy (7, 18, 56, 62), but guidelines more often concentrate only on reduction of saturated fat, usually to 10% of energy. A few guidelines mention ω-3 and ω-6 polyunsaturated fatty acids.

Some U.S. guidelines and Singapore recommend reducing dietary cholesterol (to less than 300 mg day) (7, 59), but most committees do not mention dietary cholesterol in their headings. Indeed, the U.K. committee states that "dietary cholesterol has a small effect on serum cholesterol levels. The effect of dietary cholesterol in raising serum cholesterol is minimized when saturated fatty acid intake represents a small proportion of energy" (62).

On sugar(s) (other than those naturally occurring in milk and fruits, etc.), there appears to be the largest difference of opinion. Canada (39) recommends 55% of energy from carbohydrates from a variety of sources and does not mention sugar. Japan (51) and Korea (52) do not mention sugar either. At the other extreme, the Nordic recommendations (56) and Singapore (59) advise restricting refined sugar to less than 10% of energy. In between are several different opinions: "Do not increase sugar consumption" (7), "decrease sugar intake" (not quantified) (42), "limit total sugar intake to 15–25% of energy" (55), "cut down sugary snacks and sweets between meals" (46, 47), and "eat only a moderate amount of sugars and sugary foods" (18, 21).

A *third group* of recommendations appears only in a small number of guideline sets: encourage breast-feeding (18, 59); do not ingest too much protein (7); preserve (by good preparation) the nutritive value of foods (46, 61); drink fluoridated water (or use fluoride tablets) (7, 10, 39); make sure you get enough calcium (or milk) (7, 10, 47, 52); reduce intake of salt-cured and smoked foods (59); limit the intake of *trans*-unsaturated fatty acids (62); limit caffeine intake (39); foster happy eating for happy family life (51); enjoy your food (61).

SCIENTIFIC BASES OF GUIDELINES

The original hypotheses underlying dietary guidelines were mentioned in describing their history. After 30 years of evolution, how well are current guidelines justified by scientific knowledge? The six guidelines on which there is general agreement have clearly been reasoned by large numbers of experienced scientists, independently, in more than 20 different countries, and examined at greater length than is possible in this chapter. The evidence they used is, of course, also discussed in different places in this textbook. The following brief notes are intended to help link the six major guidelines with these scientific bases.

Eat a Nutritionally Adequate Diet from a Variety of Foods

A nutritionally adequate diet means eating all (or nearly all) the RDAs of those nutrients for which there is an RDA. A varied diet, if built around the food groups of nutritional education, is a fundamental principle of nutrition, older than dietary guidelines. It maximizes the probability of eating all the RDAs as well as minor nutrients that lack an RDA. At the same time, variety minimizes the risk of toxins and pathogens from food and drink. Food variety, how to quantify it, and associated health experience is the subject of a small but growing literature (71–73).

Eat Less Fat, Particularly Saturated Fat

Fats in food provide more calories than any other food component, and much of this is hidden in attractive dishes and products. Reducing fat is the most important way of reducing excess energy intake. Many fatty ingredients in foods contain few other nutrients. If they are replaced by lean meat, low-fat milk, and vegetable foods, the intake of essential nutrients is improved. Saturated fat raises plasma total and LDL (low-density lipoprotein) cholesterol. The importance of limiting these is explained in Chapters 74 and 75.

Adjust Energy (Calorie) Intake to Expenditure and Avoid Overweight and Underweight

"Don't eat too much or too little" (46) is the fundamental quantitative principle of nutrition; it long antedates dietary guidelines. Mortality and morbidity are increased in people who are too thin (see Chapters 41 and 59) or too fat (see Chapters 63 and 87).

Eat More Food Containing Complex Carbohydrates and Fiber

The terms *complex carbohydrates* and *fiber* are both imprecise. "Complex carbohydrates" is presumably used here to mean starchy foods and naturally occuring sugars (as in milk and fruits). "Fiber" presumably covers nonstarch polysaccharides and resistant starch. While this heading reflected the thinking in nutrition science in the 1970s, it is now realized that foods containing complex carbohydrates and fiber very likely contain a cocktail of other potentially protective substances: carotenoids other than β-carotene, folate, flavonoids, phytoestrogens, glucosinolates, alliin and allicin, limonoids, etc. (74) (see Chapter 81). The older heading is therefore being replaced by "Choose a Diet with Plenty of Grain Products, Vegetables and Fruits" (18, 21) (Table 104.4).

From the preceding guidelines, these plant foods should of course be eaten in variety and without added fat. They should also be eaten as whole foods (i.e., not refined), because they are intended not only to replace fat-rich foods but also to provide generous intakes of essential nutrients and a mixture of apparently protective other substances (mentioned above).

Reduce Salt Intake

Reducing salt intake is recommended in an attempt to reduce the prevalence of essential hypertension and (a firmer epidemiologic index) mortality from cerebral hemorrhage (see Chapter 76). The evidence may not be as strong as that for saturated fat and plasma cholesterol, but a taste for salty food is an acquired one, handed down from the era before refrigerators. Most societies consume several times more sodium than people need; no harm, and possibly some benefit, could result from intakes of 50 to 100 mmol sodium per day (3–6 g NaCl). In explaining this guideline, it is important to stress that "most sodium or salt intake comes from foods to which salt has already been added during processing or preparation" (21).

Drink Alcohol in Moderation, if at All

Drinking alcohol in excess causes road accidents, domestic violence, raised blood pressure, cirrhosis of the liver, fetal alcohol syndrome, and many other complications (see Chapter 94). While it appears that two or three standard drinks per day give some protection against coronary heart disease, this benefit is only of value in older adults and in communities with high risk of coronary heart disease. It has a smaller beneficial impact on the whole population than the adverse impact of alcohol in young people, since more person-years are lost from alcohol among people less than 35 years old than are saved in the older age group (75).

PRODUCTS OF DIETARY GUIDELINES

Dietary goals and guidelines have most impact on peoples' lives when they are incorporated into policies, nutrition education handbooks, food labeling, modified foods, and health claims.

A National Food and Nutrition Policy. The Plan of Action of the World Declaration of Nutrition adopted by ministers of 159 states at the FAO/WHO International Conference on Nutrition (Rome, December 1992) states as the first of the strategies, "incorporating nutritional objectives, considerations and components into development policies and programmes" (76). For "nutritional objectives," read dietary goals.

There is a big difference between a government report that induces no action and a policy that is followed through and supported with education, subsidies, tariffs, etc. The best-worked policy has been the Norwegian Nutrition and Food Policy (77).

In Britain a major government "white paper," "Health of the Nation" (78) has four nutrition targets among its 10 risk-factor targets. These are to reduce saturated fat consumption, to reduce total fat consumption, to reduce the prevalence of obesity, and to reduce the proportion of people who drink too much alcohol. Ways of achieving these objectives are proposed. Healthier nutrition also is featured in the cancer section. These nutritional targets are naturally derived from the nation's dietary goals.

In the United States, there are 21 nutrition targets in the large volume of national health promotion and disease prevention objectives (79). The first group of these relate to dietary guidelines and the later ones to services.

Food Guides. FAO and WHO have produced a recent report, *The Preparation and Use of Food-Based Dietary Guidelines* (8). The underlying idea of the consultation that prepared the report is that dietary guidelines need to be expressed in terms of foods and in ordinary language. Meanwhile, new food guides, centered on a colored diagram or poster have been produced (Fig. 104.1) in Canada (a quarter rainbow) (80), in the U.K. (a plate with food sectors) (81), and in the U.S. (the black pyramid [82], which is similar to the earlier Australian pyramid (83). These food guides use a simple visual form to show the groups of foods that provide the RDAs and, in the same picture, to show the dietary guidelines.

Nutrition Labeling. The food components in dietary guidelines—calories, fat, saturated fat, cholesterol, carbohydrate, sugar, fiber, and sodium (salt) are the main items in nutrition labeling of processed foods ("Nutrition Facts").

Modified Foods. Special foods have been developed to help consumers follow dietary guidelines, namely, foods with reduced calories, reduced fat, reduced saturated fat, reduced sugar, increased fiber, increased calcium, reduced salt, or increased iron. Food standards have to be revised to include *standards* for these foods modified in line with dietary guidelines (i.e., definitions of "reduced fat," "low fat," "reduced salt," "low salt," etc.).

Health Claims. Eight health claims are allowed by the U.S. FDA in 1997 under the Nutrition Labeling and Education Act (1990) (NLEA) (see Chapter 115). The wording is regulated and so is the definition of appropriate foods. A typical claim essentially states the dietary guideline in its first sentence and, in the second sentence, states that this product is appropriate. For example, "Diets low in sodium may reduce the risk of high blood pressure, a disease associated with many factors. This product can be part of a low-sodium, low-salt diet that might reduce the risk of high blood pressure (hypertension)" (84).

Only one of the permitted health claims on foods in the United States is not based on a current dietary guideline, the claim about folate and prevention of neural tube defects. This is not yet a dietary guideline because the conclusive evidence was accumulated after the last major review for *Diet and Health* (1989) (7). This folate function will presumably belong with dietary guidelines in the future. In March 1996 the FDA authorized a health claim for folic acid and neural tube defects (see Chapter 115). Some other countries are discussing whether to adopt similar sorts of health claims.

SOME PROBLEMS AND QUESTIONS ABOUT DIETARY GUIDELINES

Keeping up to Date

As illustrated by folate, *trans*-unsaturated fatty acids, coffee (kahweol and cafestol) and plasma cholesterol, glycemic index of foods, resistant starch, phytoestrogens and bovine spongiform encephalopathy—none of which feature in most 1996 sets of dietary guidelines—nutritional research rolls on, and practitioners have to modify and add to authoritative guidelines, while committees should regularly revise (or at least add to) the last set of guidelines.

How Much Should I Eat?

Defining the amounts of food components and the foods that contain them in dietary guidelines is difficult. These recommendations are not medical prescriptions or diets for sick people but are intended for the healthy majority, people with a wide range of energy expenditures and intakes. Thus, it is almost impossible to hit the happy medium between being too vague and too detailed. *Servings* are being used as a semiquantitative indicator (85), but they work better for discrete foods than for mixed dishes.

Consider Sustainability, the Environment, and the World Food Problem

Two of the four principal objectives of the Norwegian Food and Nutrition Policy (1975 to 76)(32) were far ahead of their time: "the policy should aim at increased production and consumption of domestic food and at strengthening the ability to increase rapidly the degree of self-sufficiency in the food supply" and "for regional policy reasons the highest priority should be placed on utilizing the food production resources of the economically weaker areas" (of Norway).

Sooner or later national food and nutrition policies will have to consider the costs in energy and water consumption of the different dietary recommendations. It costs much more energy to ship fruit by air, to catch deep-sea

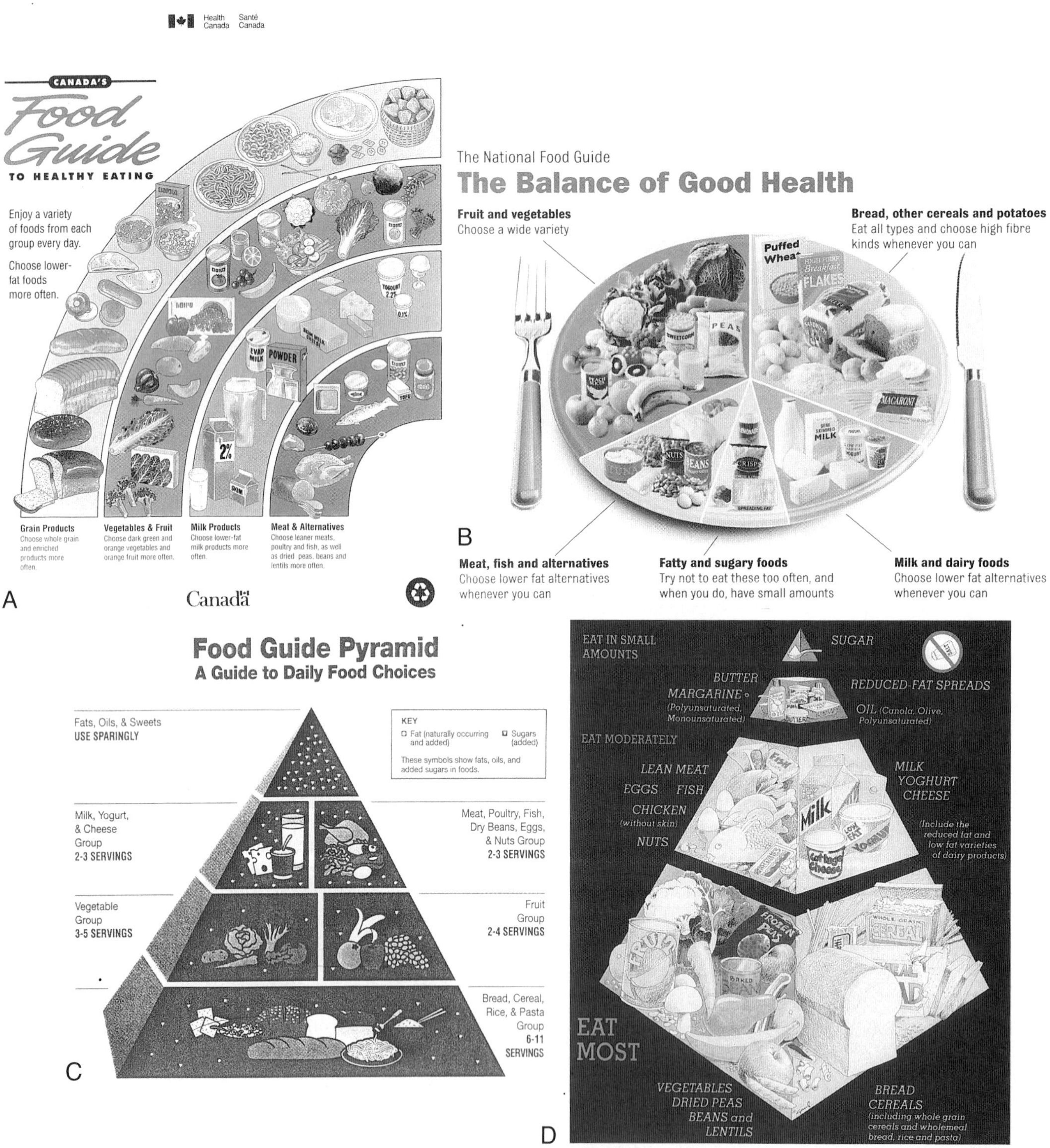

Figure 104.1. Recent food guides for nutrition education. *A.* Canada (Health Canada): quarter rainbow (80); *B.* United Kingdom (Health Education Authority): plate (81); *C.* United States (U.S. Department of Agriculture): black pyramid (82); *D.* Australia (Australian Nutrition Foundation).

fish, and to produce stall-fed beef than to grow plant foods in open fields (86, 87). It costs much more water to produce a kilogram of beef than a kilogram of chicken and more water to produce rice than wheat, maize, or potatoes. Gussow has written about dietary guidelines for sustainability (88, 89). A widely supported nutritional recommendation is to eat "five servings a day of fruit and vegetables." Many do not eat this at present (90). If everyone did, the impact on agriculture, including the increased demands on ground water and for agrochemicals, would be enormous (91).

Dietary Guidelines or Idealized Traditional Cuisine(s)

Dr Elizabeth Helsing, who directed the WHO Nutrition Office for Europe in Copenhagen, declared at the 7th

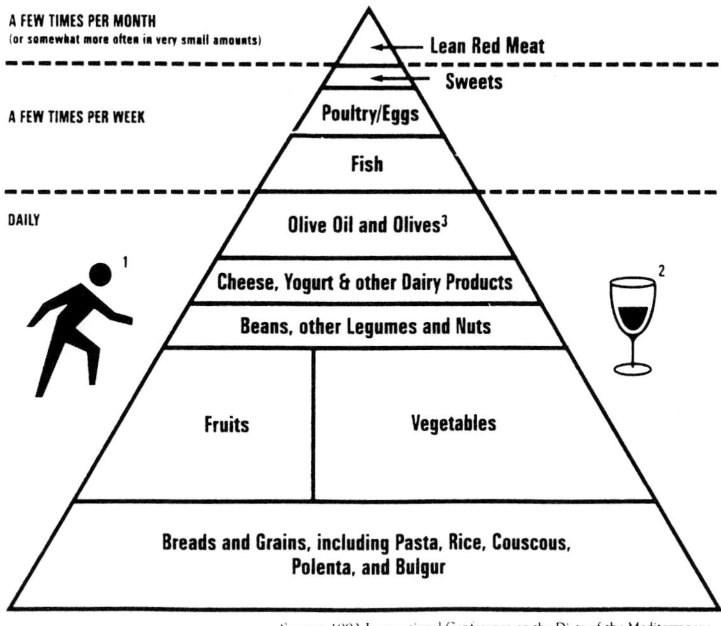

Figure 104.2. Alternative nutritional education pyramid, designed by Willet et al. (92), based on an ideal traditional Mediterranean diet.

European Nutrition Conference in Vienna in 1995 that the "Mediterranean diet" is a more effective educational concept than dietary guidelines. Professor Willett of Harvard also prefers the concept of an idealized Mediterranean diet to the NRC's dietary guidelines (92), and he has collaborated in designing a different pyramid from the U.S. Department of Agriculture black pyramid (Fig. 104.2). An ideal, traditional Mediterranean diet has interested many nutritional scientists in recent years, and excellent symposia have been published on it (93–95).

Two other traditional diets should be considered in helping to make the results of nutritional research more palatable. One is the Japanese diet, initially a variant of classical Chinese cuisine, but now distinct and associated with the world's best life expectancy. Its fish consumption would not be sustainable for wider adoption, however, and the traditional salt content is too high.

The third ideal diet concept is the hunter-gatherer's diet. Our human ancestors' bodies presumably had time (50,000 generations) for genetic adaptation to diets of this type, which all humans ate until agriculture started only 10,000 years ago. These hunter-gatherers' diets contained a great range of parts of plants and animals but did not contain cereals or milk (after early childhood), sugar, salt, or alcohol (96, 97). To look backward at such diets is probably of more philosophic than practical value.

CHECKLIST FOR DIETARY GUIDELINES

- Dietary guidelines are recommendations about foods or food components other than essential nutrients. Are standards for essential nutrients included as well?
- Are dietary guidelines defined solely in terms of food components and foods (usually food groups) or do they also include eating behavior and food habits?
- Are recommendations expressed as *change* from the estimated present average diet in the country ("eat less ———") or in absolute terms ("choose a diet low in ———")?
- Are the recommendations qualitative, quantitative, or mixed? If quantitative, are the limits intended for individuals or for the population's average intake?
- Are they published by an authoritative group (e.g., the Ministry [Department] of Health) with minimal likelihood of commercial or other bias?
- Are they for a single country, for a region, or for the whole world (including low-income countries)?
- Are the goals and guidelines for now or for some date in the future?
- Are they addressed to everyone in the population or are some recommendations for one subgroup?
- Are they written in technical language and/or in language that ordinary people can understand?
- Are they ranked in order of importance or priority? This may vary between different subgroups of the population.
- Do they include special advice for at-risk subgroups (e.g., people with atherosclerotic diseases, overweight and obese people)?
- Are they focused on the general population or on prevention of specific diseases (e.g., heart disease, cancer, diabetes)?

REFERENCES

1. Chapman S, Lupton D. The fight for public health. Principles and practice of media advocacy. London: BMJ Publishing, 1994;31–7.
2. McGlashan A. Lancet 1971;2:812.
3. Sackett DL, Rosenberg WMC, Gray JAM, et al. Br Med J 1996;312:71–2.
4. Dickersin K, Berlin JA. Epidemiol Rev 1992;14:154–76.
5. Cannon G. Food and health: the experts agree. An analysis of 100 authoritative scientific reports on food, nutrition and public health published throughout the world in 30 years, between 1961 and 1991. London: Consumers' Association, 1992.
6. Hodgkin P. Br Med J 1996;313:1568–9.
7. Committee on Diet and Health, Food and Nutrition Board,

National Research Council. Diet and health: implications for reducing chronic disease risk. Washington, DC: National Academy Press, 1989.
8. World Health Organization and Food and Agriculture Organization of the United Nations. Preparation and use of food-based dietary guidelines. Report of a joint FAO/WHO consultation, Nicosia, Cyprus. WHO/Nut/96.6 Geneva: WHO Nutrition Programme, 1996.
9. James WPT, Ferro-Luzzi A, Isaksson B, et al. Healthy nutrition. Preventing nutrition-related diseases in Europe. Copenhagen: WHO Regional Office for Europe, 1988.
10. Surgeon General's Report on Nutrition and Health. U.S. Department of Health and Human Services publ. PHS 88-50210. Washington, DC: U.S. Government Printing Office, 1988.
11. Highlights from the second WHO symposium on health issues for the 21st century: nutrition and quality of life. (November 1993, Kobe, Japan). Geneva: World Health Organization Nutrition Programme, 1994.
12. New Zealand Department of Health. Food and nutrition guidelines for infants and toddlers. Wellington, NZ: Department of Health, 1994.
13. Reid J, George J, Pears R. Food and nutrition guidelines for children aged 2 to 12 years. Wellington, NZ: Department of Health, 1992
14. Public Health Commission. Food and nutrition guidelines for New Zealand adolescents. Wellington, NZ: Public Health Commission, 1993.
15. Report of the nutrition taskforce. Food for health. Wellington, NZ: Department of Health, 1991.
16. Guidelines for healthy pregnant women. A background paper. Wellington, NZ: Public Health Commission, 1995.
17. Guidelines for healthy older people. A background paper. 2nd ed. Wellington, NZ: Ministry of Health, 1996.
18. National Health Medical Research Council. Dietary guidelines for Australians. 2nd ed. Canberra: Australian Government Publishing Service, 1992.
19. National Health and Medical Research Council. Dietary guidelines for children and adolescents. Canberra: Australian Government Publishing Service, 1995.
20. Select Committee on Human Needs, U.S. Senate. Dietary goals for the United States. Washington, DC: U.S. Government Printing Office, February 1977.
21. U.S. Department of Agriculture and U.S. Department of Health and Human Services. Dietary guidelines for Americans. 4th ed. Home and garden bull. no. 232. Washington, DC: U.S. Government Publishing Office, 1995.
22. Langsford WA. Food and Nutrition Notes and Reviews (Australian Commonwealth Department of Health) 1979;36:100–3.
23. Commonwealth Department of Health. Dietary guidelines for Australians. Canberra: Australian Government Publishing Service, 1982.
24. Helsing E (rapporteur). Nutrition targets in the EEC. In: Important components for a food and nutrition policy in the EEC (Corfu, Greece, 6–8 October 1988). Report of a workshop. Athens: School of Public Health, Department of Nutrition and Biochemistry, 1988;15.
25. Report of a WHO study group. Diet, nutrition and the prevention of chronic diseases. Tech Rep Ser 797. Geneva: World Health Organization, 1990.
26. Robbins C. Lancet 1983;2:1351–3.
27. Mediciniska synpunkter på folkkosten i de Noridska länderna. Var föda 1968;20:3–5.
28. Mediciniska synpunkter på folkkosten i de Noridska länderna. Läkartidningen 1968;65:2012–3.
29. Keys A. Nutr Rev 1968;26:259–63.
30. Wretlind A. Nutrition problems in healthy adults with low activity and low caloric consumption. In: Blix G, ed. Nutrition and physical activity. Symposia of the Swedish Nutrition Foundation No. 6. 1967:114–30.
31. Blix G, Isaksson B, Wretlind A. Bibl Nutr Diet 1973;19:154–65.
32. On Norwegian nutrition and food policy. Report no. 32 to the Storting (1975-76). Oslo: Royal Norwegian Ministry of Agriculture, 1976.
33. Keys A. Voeding 1952;13:535–56.
34. Keys A. JAMA 1957;164:1912–9.
35. Select Committee on Nutrition and Human Needs, United States Senate. Dietary goals for the United States. 2nd ed. Washington, DC: US Government Printing Office, December 1977.
36. Select Committee on Nutrition and Human Needs, United States Senate. Dietary goals for the United States: supplemental views. Washington, DC: US Government Printing Office, 1977.
37. Editorial. Dietary goals. Lancet 1977;1:887–8.
38. Committee on Diet, Nutrition and Cancer. National Research Council. Diet, nutrition and cancer. Washington, DC: National Academy Press, 1982.
38a. New American Cancer Society guidelines on diet, nutrition and cancer prevention. J Natl Cancer Inst 1997;89:198.
39. Health and Welfare Canada. Report of the scientific committee. Nutrition recommendations. Ottawa: Canadian Government Publishing Centre, 1990.
40. Joint working group of the Canadian Paediatric Society & Health Canada. Nutr Rev 1995;53:367–75.
41. Chinese Nutrition Society. Dietary guidelines for China. Beijing: Chinese Nutrition Society, 1989.
42. The National Food Agency. Nutrition and food policy of the Danish Government. Copenhagen: National Food Authority, 1984.
43. National dietary guidelines for Fiji. Fiji Food Nutr Newsletter 1988;9:2.
44. Résumé of the committee report of the State Advisory Board on Nutrition 1987:3. Dietary guidelines and their scientific principles. Helsinki: Government Printing Centre, 1989.
45. Dupin H, Abraham J, Giachetti I. Apports nutritionnels conseillés pour la population française, deuxième édition. Paris Cedex: TEC & DOC-Lavoisier, 1992.
46. Ten guidelines for sensible nutrition (translated by C. Leitzmann). Frankfurt am Main: Deutsche Gesellschaft für Ernährung, 1985.
47. Complex Committee on Food Science of the Hungarian Academy of Sciences and the Ministry of Food and Agriculture; National Institute of Food Hygiene and Nutrition. Dietary guidelines for Hungarians. Budapest: Hungarian Society of Nutrition, 1988.
48. Ministry of Health and Social Security. A parliamentary resolution on an Icelandic nutrition policy. Reykjavik: Ministry of Health & Social Security, 1989.
49. Gopalan C. Dietary guidelines from the perspective of developing countries. In: Latham MC, van Veen MS, eds. Dietary guidelines: Proceedings of an international conference, Toronto, Canada, June 1988. Cornell Int Nutr Monogr ser no. 21, 1989;88–111.
50. Instituto Nazionale della Nutrizione. Linee guida per una alimentazione Italiana. Rome: Instituto Nazionale della Nutrizione, 1988.

51. Ministry of Health and Welfare. Dietary guidelines for health promotion in Japan (English translation). Tokyo: Ministry of Health & Welfare, 1985.
52. Korean RDA and dietary guidelines. Seoul: Korean Nutrition Society, 1986.
53. Bengoa JM, Torún B, Scrimshaw NS, et al. Guias de alimentacion bases para su desarrollo en America Latina. Caracas, Venezuela: Fundación Cavendes, 1988.
54. Helsing E. Formulation of a nutrition policy. Report of the first conference on nutrition in Malta. Copenhagen: World Health Organization Regional Office for Europe, 1986.
55. Guidelines for a Healthy Diet (in English). The Hague: Netherlands Nutrition Council, 1986.
56. Nordisk Ministerråd. Nordic Nutrition Recommendations. 2nd ed. (English version). Uppsala: National Food Administration, 1989.
57. Report No. 11 to the Storting (1981–82). On the follow-up of Norwegian nutrition policy. Oslo: Royal Ministry of Health and Social Affairs, 1981.
57a. Food and Nutrition Research Institute, Department of Science and Technology. Nutritional guidelines for Filipinos. Manila: Food and Nutrition Research Institute, 1990.
58. National Institute of Health. Portuguese national dietary guidelines and nutrient goals. Lisbon: National Institute of Health, 1982.
59. Recommendations of the National Advisory Committee on Food & Nutrition. Guidelines for a healthy diet. Singapore: Ministry of Health, 1989.
60. The Food Committee of 1983. A Swedish diet and health (adapted and translated by Conrod G, Bruce Å). Uppsala: National Food Administration, 1985.
61. Ministry of Agriculture, Fisheries & Food. Eight guidelines for a healthy diet. Advice for healthy eating from H.M. Government. London: Food Sense, 1990.
62. Report of the Panel on Dietary Reference Values of the Committee on Medical Aspects of Food Policy (COMA). Dietary reference values for food energy and nutrients for the United Kingdom. London: H.M. Stationery Office, 1991.
63. Anonymous. Nutrition: the changing scene. Implementing the NACNE report. Lancet 1983;2:1351–6.
64. Walker C, Cannon G. The food scandal. London: Century Publishing, 1984.
65. Passmore R. J R Coll Gen Pract 1985;35:387–9.
66. Anderson D, ed. A diet of reason. London: The Social Affairs Unit, 1986.
67. Solon MA. Dietary guidelines for non-industrialized countries. In: Latham MC, van Veen MS, eds. Dietary guidelines: proceedings of an international conference, Toronto, June 1988. Cornell Int Nutr Monogr ser. no. 21, 1989;45–68.
68. Gopalan C. Bull Nutr Found India 1988:9:3.
69. Report of a Joint FAO/WHO/UNU Expert Consultation. Energy and protein requirements. Tech Rep Ser 724. Geneva: World Health Organization, 1985.
70. National Health and Medical Research Council. Recommended dietary intakes for use in Australia. Canberra: Australian Government Publishing Service, 1991.
71. Smiciklas-Wright H, Krebs-Smith SM, Krebs-Smith J. Variety in foods. In: What is American eating? Food and Nutrition Board, National Research Council Symposium. Washington, DC: National Academy Press, 1986;126–40.
72. Wahlqvist ML, Lo CS, Myers KA. J Am Coll Nutr 1989;6:515–23.
73. Kant AK, Shatzkin A, Harris TB, et al. Am J Clin Nutr 1993;57:434–40.
74. Truswell AS. Protective plant foods: new opportunities for health and nutrition. Food Aust 1997;49:40–3.
75. Scragg R. Aust NZ J Med 1995;25:5–11.
76. World Declaration on Nutrition. Plan of Action. Adopted by the International Conference on Nutrition, jointly sponsored by the Food and Agriculture Organization of the United Nations and the World Health Organization on 11 December 1992. Geneva: World Health Organization, 1993.
77. Norum K, Bjørneboe GEA. The Norwegian Nutrition and Food Policy. In Wahlqvist ML, Truswell AS, Smith R, et al., eds. Nutrition in a sustainable environment. Proc XV International Nutrition Congress, Adelaide. London: Smith Gordon, 1994;179–82.
78. The health of the nation. A strategy for health in England. Presented to Parliament by the Secretary of State for Health, July 1992. London: H.M. Stationery Office (reprinted) 1993.
79. U.S. Department of Health and Human Services, Public Health Service. Healthy people 2000. National health promotion and disease prevention objectives. DHHS publ. PHS 91-50212. Washington, DC: U.S. Government Printing Office, 1991.
80. Using the food guide. Health & Welfare, Canada, 1992.
81. Hunt P, Gatenby S, Rayner M. J Hum Nutr Diet 1995;8:335–51.
82. U.S. Department of Agriculture, Human Information Service. The food guide pyramid. Home & garden bull no. 252. Washington, DC: U.S. Government Printing Office, 1992.
83. Truswell AS. Am J Clin Nutr 1987;45:1060–72.
84. The Keystone national policy dialogue on food, nutrition & health. Final report. Keystone, CO, and Washington, DC: The Keystone Center, 1996.
85. Williams C. Br Med J 1995;310:1453–5.
86. Leach G. Energy & food production. Guildford (Surrey, UK): IPC Science & Technology Press, 1976.
87. von Koerber K, Männle T, Leitzmann C. Vollwert-ernährung. Konzeption einer zeitgemässen Ernährungsweise. Heidelberg (Germany): K.F. Haug, 1981;123.
88. Gussow JD, Clancy KL. J Nutr Educ 1986;18:1–5.
89. Herrin M, Gussow JD. J Nutr Educ 1989;21:270–5.
90. Nuemarksztainer D, Story M, Resnick MD, et al. Prev Med 1996;25:497–505.
91. O'Brien P. Am J Clin Nutr 1995;61:1390–6.
92. Willett WC. Science 1994;264:532–7.
93. Symposium: Mediterranean food and health (Truswell AS, chairman). Proc Nutr Soc 1991;50:513–26.
94. Helsing E, Trichopoulou A, eds. The Mediterranean diet and food culture—a symposium. Eur J Clin Nutr 1989;43(Suppl 2):1–92.
95. Nestle M, ed. Mediterranean diets and policy implications. Am J Clin Nutr 1995;61(Suppl):1313S–427S.
96. Truswell AS, Hansen JDL. Medical research among the !Kung. In: Lee RB, De Vore I, eds. Kalahari hunter gatherers. Cambridge, MA: Harvard University Press, 1976;169–95.
97. Eaton SB, Konner J. N Engl J Med 1985;312:283–9.

105. Nutrition Monitoring in the United States

MARIE FANELLI KUCZMARSKI and ROBERT J. KUCZMARSKI

The nutrition-monitoring program in the United States is considered the most comprehensive in the world. A model national nutritional program has been described as one that possesses such features as a coordinated set of activities that responds to the diverse needs of its data users, provides data on a continuous basis, supports reliable inferences about all population groups and geographic areas, and assists state and local nutrition-monitoring activities (1). The present National Nutrition Monitoring and Related Research Program (NNMRRP) in the United States is continually evolving. Yet, it has known limitations with respect to these model features. For example, it does not completely describe the current dietary and nutritional status of selected subgroups of the United States population, such as Native Americans residing on Indian reservations, Alaska natives, persons without a place of residence (homeless persons), institutionalized persons, and persons with particular physiologic and nutritional characteristics. National nutritional surveys provide data representative of the entire country and of major geographic regions but not of states, counties, and cities.

Although various national surveys have been conducted since the 1930s, Congress and the executive branch of government did not mandate a comprehensive strategy for a coordinated program to strengthen existing national monitoring efforts until 1990. This strategy was designed to review and integrate the various federal surveys to provide timely, useful information that systematically addresses questions concerning the dietary and nutritional status of the American population. Thus, the National Nutrition Monitoring and Related Research Act of 1990, a public law (PL 101-445), was enacted to place the existing monitoring system composed of interacting federal groups under an expanded program that includes related research. This program was designated to be guided by a specific 10-year plan under which action would be taken toward a goal of comprehensive national nutrition monitoring.

The National Nutrition Monitoring and Related Research Act defines nutrition monitoring as "the set of activities necessary to provide timely information about the role and status of factors that bear on the contribution that nutrition makes to the health of the people in the United States" (2). Nutrition monitoring is characterized by regular data collection, analysis, and interpretation to provide a description of nutritional conditions in the population, and linkages with policy making and research. Monitoring provides a database for public policy decisions related to such issues as public health intervention programs, fortification, safety and labeling of the food supply, food assistance programs, and federally supported food service programs (3). It also assists in identifying health and nutritional research priorities of public health significance such as food security/insecurity, thereby strengthening the research base for monitoring and policy making.

The five components of the United States National Nutrition Monitoring System (NNMS) were specified in the 1987 Operational Plan as follows: *(a)* nutritional and health status measurements; *(b)* food consumption measurements; *(c)* food composition measurements and nutrient data banks; *(d)* dietary knowledge and attitude measurements; and *(e)* food supply and demand determinations (4). Although the titles of these components have been modified slightly in the 10-year plan for the NNMRRP, the content of these components remains essentially the same (see Table 105.1 for revised names).

This chapter provides a brief account of the historical

Abbreviations: **ARS**—Agricultural Research Service; **CDC**—Centers for Disease Control and Prevention; **CSFII**—Continuing Survey of Food Intakes by Individuals; **DHHS**—Department of Health and Human Services; **FASEB**—Federation of American Societies for Experimental Biology; **IBNMRR**—Interagency Board for Nutrition Monitoring and Related Research; **ICNM**—Interagency Committee on Nutrition Monitoring; **JNMEC**—Joint Nutrition Monitoring Evaluation Committee; **LSRO**—Life Sciences Research Office; **NFCS**—Nationwide Food Consumption Survey; **NHANES**—National Health and Nutrition Examination Survey; **NHES**—National Health Examination Survey; **NNMRRP**—National Nutrition Monitoring and Related Research Program; **NNMS**—National Nutrition Monitoring System; **PedNSS**—Pediatric Nutrition Surveillance System; **PregNSS**—Pregnancy Nutrition Surveillance System; **USDA**—United States Department of Agriculture; **WIC**—Women, Infants and Children.

Table 105.1
Principal NNMRRP Activities, Sponsoring Federal Agencies, and Survey Designs

Activity	Agency	Survey Design
Nutritional and related health measurements		
National Ambulatory Medical Care Survey	NCHS, CDC	Multistage, stratified, probability sample of licensed physicians in office based patient care
National Health and Nutrition Examination Survey	NCHS, CDC	Complex, multistage, stratified, probability cluster sample of individuals in households
NHANES I Epidemiologic Follow-up Study	NCHS, CDC	Follow-up on NHANES I participants, aged 25 to 74 years in 1971–1975
Pediatric Nutrition Surveillance System	NCCDPHP, CDC	Convenience population of low-income children, 0–17 years of age, who participate in publicly funded health, nutrition, and food assistance programs
Pregnancy Nutrition Surveillance System	NCCDPHP, CDC	Convenience population of low-income, high-risk pregnant women who participate in publicly funded prenatal nutrition and food assistance programs
Vital Statistics Program	NCHS, CDC	Vital registration system
Food and nutrient consumption measurements		
Continuing Survey of Food Intakes by Individuals	BHNRC, ARS	Multistage, stratified area probability sample of defined populations
Military feeding systems and military populations	USARIEM, MND	Varies with specific study
Knowledge, attitudes, and behavior assessments		
Behavioral Risk Factor Surveillance System	NCCDPHP, CDC	Multistage, cluster telephone survey based on Waksberg method
Youth Risk Behavior Surveillance System	NCCDPHP, CDC	Representative sample of 9–12th grade students and national household survey of a representative sample of persons 12–21 years of age
Diet-Health Knowledge Survey	BHNRC, ARS	Follow-up of CSFII meal planners using telephone interview
Health and Diet Survey	DMS, FDA	Telephone interviews with a national probability Waksberg sample selected by random digit dialing method
National Health Interview Survey	NCHS, CDC	Complex, multistage, stratified, probability cluster sample of households
Food composition and nutrient databases		
Food Label and Package Survey	CFSAN, FDA	Biennial probability survey of retail packaged foods using commercial market research data bases (A.C. Nielsen Scantrack)
National Nutrient Data Bank	BHNRC, ARS	NA
Nutrient Composition Laboratory	BHNRC, ARS	NA
Survey Nutrient Data Base	BHNRC, ARS	NA
Food supply determinations		
A.C. Nielsen Scantrack	ERS[a]	NA
Total Diet Study	CFSAN, FDA	NA
United States Food and Nutrition Supply Series	CNPP	NA

[a]Primary sponsor.
Acronyms and abbreviations: NCHS, National Center for Health Statistics; CDC, Centers for Disease Control and Prevention; NCCDPHP, National Center for Chronic Disease Prevention and Health Promotion; BHNRC, Beltsville Human Nutrition Research Center; ARS, Agricultural Research Service; USARIEM, United States Army Research Institute of Environmental Medicine; MND, Military Nutrition Division; DMS, Division of Market Studies; FDA, Food and Drug Administration; CFSAN, Center for Food Safety and Applied Nutrition; ERS, Economic Research Service; CNPP, Center for Nutrition Policy and Promotion.

development of the NNMS and the current NNMRRP (Table 105.2); describes the cornerstone surveys of the NNMS, giving special attention to survey design; discusses some of the limitations of the current program; and recognizes provisions in PL 101-445 that may enhance the program. In the context of nutrition monitoring, related health status refers to health conditions that may be associated with nutritional variables, such as diabetes and obesity, or osteoporosis and calcium. The terms *dietary status* and *nutritional status,* although often used interchangeably, have different connotations. Nutritional status encompasses anthropometric, biochemical, clinical, dietary, and sociodemographic factors. Dietary status is a more limited term that refers to intake of foods, beverages (nonalcoholic and alcoholic), and nutrients, including supplements.

HISTORICAL OVERVIEW

In the late 1960s, concerns about the nutritional status of the United States population emerged as reports about the existence of hunger and malnutrition were released (5). Between 1969 and 1977, the Senate Select Committee on Nutrition and Human Needs investigated not only the extent to which hunger existed in the United States but also how effective the federal government was in measuring this problem. Recognizing serious deficiencies in federal nutrition-monitoring efforts and identifying the need

Table 105.2
History of Nutrition Monitoring in the United States

1977	Food and Agriculture Act (PL 95-113)
1978	Proposal to Congress for a comprehensive nutritional status monitoring system
1981	Joint Implementation Plan for a comprehensive national nutrition monitoring system
1986	First report to Congress: *Nutrition Monitoring in the United States: A Progress Report from the Joint Nutrition Monitoring Evaluation Committee*
1987	Operational plan for the National Nutrition Monitoring System
1988	Interagency Committee on Nutrition Monitoring formed
1989	Second report to Congress: *Nutrition Monitoring in the United States: An Update Report on Nutrition Monitoring*
1990	National Nutrition Monitoring and Related Research Act (PL 101-445)
1991	Interagency Board for Nutrition Monitoring and Related Research formed, Draft comprehensive plan published in the Federal Register on October 29th
1992	National Nutrition Monitoring Advisory Council formed
1993	Comprehensive plan for the National Nutrition Monitoring and Related Research program signed by the president and transmitted to Congress
1993	First nutrition monitoring *Chartbook*
1995	Third report to Congress: *Third Report on Nutrition Monitoring in the United States*

for a coordinated comprehensive national nutrition monitoring system, Congress sought to remedy the situation by legislative action.

The Food and Agriculture Act of 1977 (PL 95-113) (6) required the secretaries of agriculture and of health, education and welfare (currently health and human services) to

> formulate and submit to Congress . . . a proposal for a comprehensive nutritional status monitoring system, to include: (1) an assessment of a system consisting of periodic surveys and continuous monitoring to determine: the extent of risk of nutrition-related health problems in the United States; which population groups or areas of the country face greatest risk; and the likely causes of risk and changes in risk factors over time; (2) a surveillance system to identify remediable nutrition-related health risks to individuals or for local areas, in such a manner as to tie detection to direct intervention and treatment . . . ; and (3) program evaluations to determine the adequacy, efficiency, effectiveness and side effects of nutrition-related programs in reducing health risks to individuals and populations.

The proposal for a comprehensive national nutrition monitoring system was submitted by the Department of Health, Education and Welfare and the United States Department of Agriculture (USDA) to Congress in 1978 (7). This proposal reviewed current federal, state, and local agency activities in the areas of nutritional and dietary status assessment, nutritional quality of foods, dietary practices and knowledge, and the impact of nutritional intervention programs. It acknowledged the deficiencies in existing nutritional and dietary assessment methods, recognized delays in data analysis and the publication of results, pointed out the inadequate coverage of certain target groups and geographic areas, and recognized the inadequate evaluation of nutritional intervention programs. Although the proposal contained a series of recommendations for improving and expanding the scope of federal nutrition-monitoring activities, it lacked a set of priorities; assignment of tasks and a timetable for completion; a prospective plan; a reporting component to monitor progress of the NNMS; a timetable for publications; assignment of responsibility for implementation; identification of costs; and identification of the relationship to the Joint Subcommittee on Human Nutrition Research (8).

At the request of the Committee on Science and Technology, the proposal was reviewed by the General Accounting Office, which recommended that the departments develop an implementation plan for a national nutrition monitoring system to provide specific information on how and when the system could be implemented and on its cost. The Department of Health and Human Services and the Department of Agriculture (DHHS-USDA) Joint Implementation Plan for a Comprehensive NNMS was submitted to Congress in 1981 (9). The plan made the assistant secretary for food and consumer services, USDA, and the assistant secretary for health, DHHS, responsible for implementing compatible survey plans. It also identified and described the current efforts in nutrition monitoring conducted by the USDA and DHHS and proposed major goals and objectives for the NNMS. The two major objectives were *(a)* to achieve the best possible coordination of the National Health and Nutrition Examination Survey (NHANES) and the Nationwide Food Consumption Survey (NFCS) and *(b)* to develop a reporting system to translate the findings from these two national surveys and other monitoring activities into periodic reports to Congress on the nutritional status of the American population. The plan described how to implement the first coordinated NHANES-NFCS survey in 1987. However, certain critical features were never fully addressed, which inhibited achieving a comprehensive system (8).

In 1982 and 1983, the Subcommittee on Science, Research, and Technology and the Subcommittee on Department Operations, Research, and Foreign Agriculture jointly held hearings to review the system. They noted that coordination had improved but was still inadequate. The NNMS lacked a central focus, a provision for continuous monitoring, and a mechanism for evaluating food assistance programs.

In 1983, the Joint Nutrition Monitoring Evaluation Committee (JNMEC) was appointed. This federal advisory committee, jointly sponsored by the USDA and DHHS, was responsible for the first progress report to the Congress, as stipulated in the Joint Implementation Plan. The report, published in 1986, contained information on the nutritional status of the United States population and made specific recommendations to improve the monitoring system (10). The JNMEC reported that the principal nutrition-related health problems experienced by Americans arose from overconsumption of fat, saturated fat, cholesterol, and sodium. Intakes of iron and vitamin C were low in certain population groups. In addition to reviewing available data, the committee made 14 recommendations on how to improve nutrition monitoring efforts.

In 1987, the DHHS and the USDA published an operational plan for the NNMS, a revision of the 1981 Joint Implementation Plan (4). The operational plan described the goals of the operational phase, progress during the implementation phase (1981 to 1986), and proposed activities for the operational phase (1987 to 1996), including a calendar of events. The specific goals were to achieve a comprehensive system through coordination among NNMS components, thereby improving both information dissemination and exchange between data generators and users and Congress, as well as the research base for nutrition monitoring.

The operational plan did not stipulate a time for implementation of the comprehensive, coordinated system sought by the Congress. Given the lack of legislative mandate to establish such a system, it was unclear how this operational plan would be any more successful than the 1981 Joint Implementation Plan. In 1988, the Interagency Committee on Nutrition Monitoring (ICNM) was formed (11). The committee was cochaired by the assistant secretary for health, DHHS, and the assistant secretary for food and consumer services, USDA. The purpose of this committee was to increase the effectiveness and productivity of federal nutrition-monitoring efforts by improving planning, coordination, and communication among the agencies engaged in nutrition monitoring. The membership included representatives from Public Health Service (DHHS) agencies, USDA agencies, the Agency for International Development, the Bureau of Labor Statistics, the Census Bureau, the Department of Defense, and the Veterans Administration.

In 1989, the second progress report on nutrition monitoring, prepared by an ad hoc expert panel, was transmitted to Congress. This report provided *(a)* an update to the 1986 report on the dietary and nutritional status of the United States population and *(b)* an in-depth analysis of the contributions of the NNMS to the assessment of iron nutriture and of dietary and nutritional factors related to cardiovascular disease (12). The expert panel concluded that the principal nutrition-related health problems experienced by Americans were related to overconsumption of selected nutrients, particularly food energy, fat, saturated fatty acids, cholesterol, sodium, and alcohol. Iron deficiency was cited as the most common single nutrient deficiency. The expert panel also made several recommendations to improve the NNMS.

Between 1984 and 1990, several attempts were made to pass a legislative bill to establish a coordinated national nutrition-monitoring and related research program (8, 13). This proposed legislation included developing a comprehensive plan to assess both the nutritional status and dietary intake of the United States population and the nutritional quality of the food supply. Provisions for conducting scientific research were also included. Finally, on October 22, 1990, the National Nutrition Monitoring and Related Research Act (PL 101-445) was signed into law (2).

The key monitoring provisions of this bill (Titles I and II) were

1. To establish an Interagency Board for Nutrition Monitoring and Related Research (IBNMRR) jointly chaired by an assistant secretary from the USDA and an assistant secretary from the DHHS.
2. To establish a National Nutrition Monitoring Advisory Council of nine voting members who are not federal employees.
3. To develop and implement a 10-year comprehensive plan for a coordinated program designed to assess and report on a continuous basis the dietary and nutritional status of the United States population, particularly infants and children, the aged, disadvantaged persons, minorities, and women; to develop and update nutrient data banks; to sponsor and conduct research to develop uniform indicators and methods for conducting and reporting nutrition-monitoring activities; and to assist state and local government agencies in developing procedures and networks for nutrition monitoring and surveillance.
4. To publish at least once every 5 years or sooner a report to the Congress on the dietary, nutritional, and health-related status of the American population and the nutritional quality of food consumed in the United States.

In 1991, the IBNMRR was established through expansion of the Interagency Committee on Nutrition Monitoring. As shown in Figure 105.1, the IBNMRR is the central coordination point for the federal government's nutrition-monitoring program. About 20 agencies are members of the board (14). Board responsibilities include coordinating scientific reports that describe the nutritional and health status of the U.S. population, providing mechanisms for increased communication and collaboration among member agencies, and developing the annual budget report.

The National Nutrition Monitoring Advisory Council, composed of nine nonfederal members with expertise in the areas of public health, nutrition-monitoring research, and food production and distribution, was established in 1992. The cochairpersons of the IBNMRR are ex officio nonvoting members of the council. The council is charged with providing scientific and technical advice on the development and implementation of the coordinated NNMRR Program and advising the secretaries of the USDA and DHHS. It is required to report to the secretaries annually on the effectiveness of the NNMRR Program and to offer recommendations for enhancing the program's effectiveness. Since its formation, the council has identified six priorities for the NNMRRP: identifying ways to include high-risk subgroups of the population; integrating federal, state, and private data needs; determining the cost-effec-

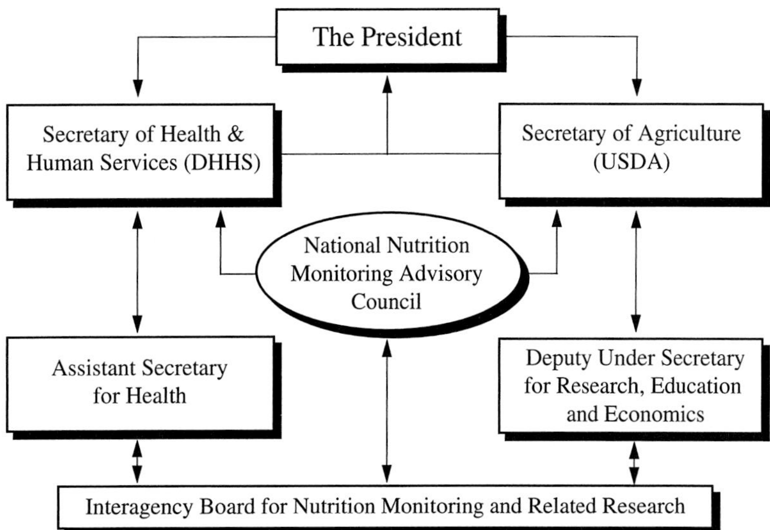

Figure 105.1. Structure of federal coordination of the National Nutrition Monitoring and Related Research Program.

tiveness of the NNMRRP; providing timely data dissemination; assessing nutrition-monitoring research activities; and determining trends in NNMRRP data, especially those relating to measures of the food supply and to consumers' knowledge and attitudes toward nutritional and dietary guidance (15).

The Ten-Year Comprehensive Plan for the NNMRR Program describes national nutrition-monitoring activities for the period 1992 to 2002. A proposed plan was compiled by members of a DHHS/USDA working group and published on October 29, 1991 (16). After subsequent public comment and departmental revision periods, the plan was finalized. It was signed by the president and forwarded to Congress in January 1993 and published in the *Federal Register* on June 11, 1993 (17). This plan is intended to be the guidance mechanism to provide direction to the federal and state agencies participating in the national nutrition monitoring program. It discusses a tentative course of action designed to address some of the recognized deficiencies in the NNMS. For a detailed presentation of the proposed national nutrition monitoring activities and the agencies responsible, the reader is encouraged to refer to the 10-year comprehensive plan (17).

The plan includes three objectives at the national level and three at the state and local levels. The national objectives are to provide for a comprehensive NNMRR Program through continuous and coordinated data collection, to improve the comparability and quality of data across the NNMRR Program, and to improve the research base for nutrition monitoring. For each national objective, activities within the five components are delineated. The state and local objectives are to develop and strengthen state and local capacity for continuous and coordinated data collection that complements national nutritional surveys; to improve methodologies to enhance comparability of NNMRR Program data across federal, state, and local levels; and to improve the quality of state and local nutrition monitoring data.

Chartbook I: Selected Findings from the National Nutrition Monitoring and Related Research Program was published in 1993. This resource highlighted dietary intake data from the Hispanic HANES and the 1989 and 1990 Continuing Survey of Food Intakes by Individuals (CSFII), changes in the food supply, progress in developing food composition analysis methods, and selected dietary knowledge and attitudes of the U.S. population (18). Chartbooks that display data with graphics and brief narratives are proposed intermediates to the scientific reports to Congress by DHHS and USDA. They are designed to keep users of nutrition-monitoring data up to date on the latest findings and research of the NNMRR Program.

In 1995, the third report on nutrition monitoring prepared by the Life Sciences Research Office (LSRO) and a group of expert consultants was transmitted to the president and Congress (19). This two-volume report updated the 1989 report. Special emphasis was placed on the dietary and nutrition-related health status of Americans, and concerns for low-income and high-risk population subgroups were expressed. The expert consultants noted that a considerable gap existed between what Americans eat and what they should eat and that some Americans do not get enough to eat. The increasing prevalence of overweight and the high proportion of the population with high serum cholesterol levels and hypertension are cause for public health concern. The expert consultants also provided recommendations for strengthening each component of the NNMRR Program and indicated ways to overcome some of the limitations of the present program.

NATIONAL NUTRITION-MONITORING CORNERSTONE SURVEYS

Between 1896, when the first food composition tables were published, and 1991, over 100 federal nutritional surveys and surveillance activities have been conducted. A chronologic listing categorized by measurement components was published in the comprehensive plan for national nutrition monitoring and related research (16, 17). Although many surveys and surveillance activities have been sponsored by a variety of agencies in the federal government, three in particular, the NFCS, the CSFII, and the NHANES, were regarded as the cornerstones of national nutrition monitoring. Because the NFCS was discontinued in the early 1990s, the two cornerstone NNMRRP surveys are the CSFII, sponsored by the Agricultural Research Service (ARS) of the USDA and the NHANES, sponsored by the National Center for Health Statistics of the DHHS.

Nationwide Food Consumption Survey

The involvement of the federal government in nutrition monitoring actually dates back to 1893, when the USDA received the first appropriation to conduct human nutritional research. The first national survey of household food consumption and dietary levels was conducted in 1936 to 1937 as part of the Consumer Purchases Study (20). Between 1942 and 1955, three nationwide studies on household food consumption (NFCS) were conducted by the Human Nutrition Information Service (21). These surveys included collecting information on household food use over 7 days and reflected food use from an economic perspective; that is, it included food used, whether it is eaten, discarded, or fed to pets. The person primarily responsible for food preparation in a given household provided this information. Food distribution among members of the household was not taken into account. In the 1965 and subsequent NFCS (1977–78 and 1987–88), data were obtained on dietary intakes and patterns of individuals as well as on household food use. Information on food consumed by individuals both at and away from home was collected for 1 day in the 1965 NFCS and for 3 consecutive days in the 1977–78 and 1987–88 NFCS. Nutrient content of food used by households and of food consumed by individuals was estimated from food composition data files developed from the National Nutrient Data Bank (22).

The objectives of the NFCS were to describe current food consumption behavior, to identify changes in diet since the previous NFCS, and to assess the nutritional content of diets for their implications on policies relating to food production and marketing, food safety, food assistance, and nutritional education. More specifically, data from the NFCS have been used to develop the *Dietary Guidelines for Americans* (23) and the "Thrifty Food Plan" (24), which is used as the statutory basis for the Food Stamp Program; to evaluate the achievement of the 1990 Health Objectives for the Nation (25): and to help develop the nutritional objectives included in *Healthy People 2000* (26).

The NFCS was designed to provide a multistage stratified area probability sample representative of the 48 conterminous states (22). The stratification plan takes into account geographic location and degree of urbanization. In the 1987–88 NFCS, households were drawn from nine geographic divisions and three urbanization classes as defined by the Bureau of the Census (27). This NFCS included two probability samples—one for the basic survey of the general population (households and individuals with all incomes), and one for the low-income survey (households with incomes consistent with eligibility for the Food Stamp Program).

The 1987–88 NFCS involved three visits with participants (28). The initial visit identified respondents and provided them with materials needed to keep notes on household food used during the survey period. The next visit, 7 days later, consisted of a 2- to 3-hour personal interview to conduct the household phase of the survey, to obtain a 1-day dietary recall from individual members, and to leave these individuals a 2-day dietary record to complete. The final contact with respondents was 2 days later, to collect the 2-day dietary record. In addition to obtaining information on food use/intake, questions were asked about household characteristics; individual characteristics such as self-reported height, weight, and health status; participation in food assistance programs; and diet-related topics such as supplement use, alcohol consumption, use of salt at the table, and dieting (27). To reduce data processing time and make NFCS results more readily available, laptop computers were used in these household interviews.

The target sample for the basic 1987–88 survey was about 6000 households and their approximately 15,000 individual members. The low-income survey targeted 2500 households and about 6000 individual members (22, 29). The household response rate was 38% for the basic sample and 42% for the low-income sample (30). The individual response rate for the basic sample was 31% for individuals completing 1 day of intake and 25% for individuals who completed all 3 days of intake (29).

A national survey is designed to represent the United States population; if response rates are extremely low, it is questionable whether the data provide an unbiased estimate of the dietary and nutritional status of the nation. USDA contracted with the LSRO of the Federation of American Societies for Experimental Biology (FASEB) to conduct an independent review of the impact of nonresponse on the estimates of food and nutrient intakes. LSRO convened an expert panel of statisticians who noted that it was impossible to determine the extent to which nonresponse bias influenced the interpretation of the data. This panel consequently recommended that persons using the 1987–88 NFCS data should exercise great caution and should recognize that the respondents might not be completely representative of subgroups when group comparisons are made. Comprehensive evaluations of the possible effects of nonresponse in the NFCS and of potential limitations in using the collected data have been published (29, 31).

Continuing Survey of Food Intakes by Individuals

The first CSFII was conducted in 1985, the second in 1986. These two surveys constitute series I. Series II began in 1989 and includes the 1990 and 1991 CSFIIs. Series III began in 1994 and continued through 1996. This 3-year survey is popularly known as the "What We Eat in America Survey." The purpose of these surveys is to provide information on the dietary status of the United States population and to monitor changes in dietary intakes. In addition, individuals identified as main meal planners/preparers in the 1989 to 1991 CSFIIs were contacted to participate in the Diet and Health Knowledge Survey, another NNMRRP activity sponsored by the USDA. The dietary data collected in the CSFII was then linked to an individual's nutritional knowledge and attitudes.

"Usual" intakes were assessed in the 1985 and 1986 CSFII by multiple 24-hour dietary recalls over a 1-year period. A 1-day dietary recall in an in-person interview and a self-administered 2-day dietary record were used in the second CSFII series (32). As in the NFCS, nutrient intakes were calculated from the National Nutrient Data Bank. The dietary data collection method for the 1994–96 CSFII consisted of two nonconsecutive 1-day recalls of food intake through in-person interviews.

The target population for series I and II CSFII consisted of individuals selected by sex and age residing in the 48 conterminous states in households with incomes at all levels (basic sample) and with incomes at or below 130% of poverty guidelines (low-income sample). The 1985 CSFII included men and women aged 19 to 50 years and children 1 to 5 years of age (33–35), whereas the 1986 CSFII included women 19 to 50 years of age and children 1 to 5 years of age (36, 37). For the series I CSFII, the basic sample included approximately 1300 households and their 2000 individual members. The 1985 low-income sample included about 1900 households and their 3400 individual members, whereas the 1986 low-income sample had about 1200 households and 2100 individual members. Individual response rates for women and children completing 1-day recalls were 71% for the basic sample and 65% for the low-income sample in 1985 and 66% for the basic sample and 75% for the low-income sample in 1986 (38).

The 1989 to 1991 CSFIIs were designed to obtain information on food intakes from all household members (men, women, and children of all ages). Like the 1985 and 1986 CSFII, they had basic and low-income samples. Approximately 6700 households and their 15000 individual members were included in the samples. Overall household response rate for the 1989 to 1991 CSFII was 67%. Individual response rates were 58% for those completing 1 day of dietary recall and 45% for those completing 3 days (19).

The sample size for the 1994–96 CSFII was projected to include approximately 15,000 to 16,000 respondents, about 5,500 individuals each year. In 1994, 5,540 individuals completed 1 day of intake recall, and 5,263 completed both days of intake recall (39). Notable design changes from the first two series include a target population of noninstitutionalized persons in all 50 states, oversampling of the low-income population rather than a separate low-income survey, larger samples of young children and older adults, subsampling within households, and collection of 2 nonconsecutive days of food intake data through in-person interviews rather than 3 consecutive days of food intake data using a 1-day recall and a 2-day record (39, 40).

National Health and Nutrition Examination Survey

In 1967, the Senate Subcommittee on Employment, Manpower, and Poverty of the Committee on Labor and Public Welfare noted in a letter to President Lyndon Johnson that malnutrition and widespread hunger had reached emergency proportions. In response to these concerns and the lack of a monitoring system to determine the magnitude of the problem, Congress mandated, in Section 14 of the Partnership for Health Amendments of 1967, that the secretary of health, education, and welfare, in collaboration with other federal government and state officials, was to conduct a comprehensive survey to assess the incidence and location of serious hunger, malnutrition, and health problems. This action authorized the National Nutrition Survey, better known as the Ten State Nutrition Survey.

The Ten State Nutrition Survey, 1968 to 1970, was designed to select families randomly from the 1960 Bureau of Census enumeration districts, where the highest percentage of families had incomes below the Orshansky Poverty Index in the states of California, Kentucky, Louisiana, Massachusetts, Michigan, New York, South Carolina, Texas, Washington, and West Virginia. The sample population included middle- and upper-income persons who, because of changes in residential patterns subsequent to 1960, were living in selected enumeration districts. Nutritional status was assessed on the basis of dietary intakes and food patterns, dental examinations, and anthropometric and biochemical measurements. Information on nonnutritional factors that affect food intake (e.g., socioeconomic characteristics, health status, and income) was also gathered. The findings indicated nutritional problems in selected age and sex groups (41).

While the Ten State Survey was still under way, in 1969, President Richard Nixon asked the secretary of the Department of Health, Education, and Welfare to expand it to describe the extent of hunger and malnutrition in the entire United States. In response, a Task Force on Nutritional Surveillance at the National Center for Health Statistics (NCHS) was formed and asked to plan and implement a survey to provide an effective nutritional surveillance system. To minimize duplication with other surveys conducted by the NCHS and to permit nutritional variables to be correlated with other health status measurements already being collected in the National Health Examination Survey (NHES), a nutritional assessment component was added to the NHES to create the first NHANES. Conducted between 1971 and 1974, NHANES I was the first health survey to assess dietary intake and other measures of nutritional status in a nationally representative sample of persons aged 1 to 74 years in the civilian, noninstitutionalized population in the United States (42, 43).

A major objective of the NHANES is the periodic assessment of the health and nutritional status of the United States population and monitoring changes in status over time. The second NHANES was conducted from 1976 to 1980 (44), and the third NHANES, from 1988 to 1994. The Hispanic HANES (HHANES) was conducted from 1982 to 1984 (45). This special survey included three Hispanic groups: Mexican Americans residing in five southwestern states; Cubans in Dade County, Florida; and Puerto Ricans in the New York City metropolitan area.

Each of the NHANES surveys has used complex, multistage, probability, cluster sampling to select a representative sample of the civilian noninstitutionalized population residing in households in the United States. Special oversampling techniques were used to ensure adequate representation of subgroups considered at high risk of malnutrition. NHANES II statistically selected a sample of 27,805 individuals to represent the entire United States population and selected subgroups. About 91% of those selected agreed to be interviewed, and 73% agreed to be interviewed and examined (38). In the full 6 years of data collection for the NHANES III, 1988 to 1994, approximately 40,000 individuals were selected, of whom 86% were interviewed and 78% were examined. The age range for NHANES III was expanded to begin at 2 months with no upper age limit.

The NHANES is unique because it collects data on the health and nutritional status of Americans through interviews and direct physical examinations. The household interview is administered in four parts:

1. A household screener questionnaire is used to determine household eligibility and select sample persons.
2. An adult household questionnaire is used to assess health status and practices, including reported health conditions, use of health and dental services, meal program participation, and use of vitamin/mineral supplements and medications.
3. A child household questionnaire contains items similar to those asked of adults plus questions on infant feeding practices, weight status, breast-feeding history and status, and other nutrition-related questions.
4. A family questionnaire is used to determine relationships of persons in the household, to obtain basic demographic data, and to assess participation in income assistance programs, including the Food Stamp Program and Women, Infants and Children (WIC) Program.

After completing the household interview, sample persons are invited to Mobile Examination Centers where the NHANES staff administer standardized examination and laboratory tests.

Nutritional status is evaluated from data generated through interviews and direct physical examinations. Listings of the major parameters measured by sex and age have been published (46). Briefly, the interviews include a single 24-hour dietary recall; a food frequency questionnaire for persons 12 years of age or older; questions related to eating habits, lifestyle, and other nutrition-related practices; and a medical history. NHANES III includes a quantitative measure of intake of vitamins and minerals from supplements and a series of food sufficiency questions. Physical examinations include such components as anthropometric measurements, hematologic and biochemical assessments, and physical and dental examinations. The survey design and implementation strategies have been described in various reports (46, 47), and a compendium of all data collection instruments for the NHANES III has been published (48).

The NHANES is designed as a multipurpose survey. Some examples of the major uses of the data include assessment of selected conditions (e.g., growth retardation, exposure to lead, prevalence of overweight [49], hypertension [50], and high blood cholesterol level [51]), evaluation and development of nutritional policy (e.g., *Healthy People 2000* [26] and the *Dietary Guidelines for Americans* [23]), and assessment of food fortification policies.

OTHER NUTRITION-MONITORING ACTIVITIES

In addition to the core components, CSFII and NHANES, several other survey and surveillance activities constitute the NNMRRP. Approximately 50 monitoring activities that will provide information on the five measurement components are planned between 1992 and 2002 (17). The activities conducted on a regular basis and their sponsoring federal agencies are shown in Table 105.1. The periodicity of the activities varies. For example, food supply estimates are conducted annually, whereas the Food Label and Package Survey is done biennially. Many special surveys, such as the Vitamin and Mineral Intake Survey, the Navajo Health and Nutrition Survey, and the National Maternal and Infant Health Survey, are also conducted periodically as needs arise. A comprehensive compilation of all NNMRRP activities with descriptions about survey design and objectives, sample sizes, and response rates is provided in the *Directory of Federal and State Nutrition Monitoring Activities* (30) and the comprehensive plan for national nutrition monitoring and related research (17).

LIMITATIONS OF THE NATIONAL NUTRITION-MONITORING SYSTEM

The five components of the NNMRRP provide much valuable information. Recommendations for strengthening each component of the NNMRRP are published in the

Third Report on Nutrition Monitoring in the United States (52). In general, there is a need for improvement, especially with regard to components that have not been functionally integrated into a coordinated and comprehensive system. Both the USDA and the DHHS have made serious efforts to improve and coordinate their individual nutrition-monitoring activities. To improve communication and coordination among the NNMRRP member agencies as well as to oversee the activities delineated in the 10-year comprehensive plan, three staff working groups in the areas of survey comparability, food composition data, and federal-state relations and information dissemination and exchange, were established.

In 1992, a report on comparability of selected population descriptors was published (53). The purpose of this report was to standardize collection and reporting of key socioeconomic variables and to enhance data linkages across NNMRPP surveys and surveillance systems. With completion of the population descriptors report, the Survey Comparability Working Group has focused on documenting selected nutritional and nutrition-related health variables across the NNMRRP and identifying specific assessments that would constitute a minimum set of indicators for nutritional status.

USDA and DHHS are continually collaborating to improve dietary information and linkage of dietary data. The same food codes and nutrient database were used to analyze data collected in the NHANES III and the 1994–96 CSFII. Development of automated procedures for tracking food composition changes to facilitate analysis of trends in nutrient intakes and expansion of the Survey Nutrient Data Base to include foods reported in national dietary intake surveys is planned. Additionally, the Food Composition Working Group has started evaluating the effectiveness of the food composition data component in meeting the needs of the NNMRRP.

A survey of primary users of NNMRRP data, including persons in federal, state, and local government, academic institutions, and for-profit businesses such as food industries and hospitals, indicated that most were satisfied with the quality of NNMRRP data and the degree to which these data meet their needs. Despite their satisfaction, the respondents noted changes that would increase their confidence in, or substantially increase their use of, NNMRRP data. Common themes for improvement were more detailed information on racial, ethnic, and age groups; data that can support estimates for small geographic areas; improved timeliness and documentation of data; continuous or more-frequent data collection; and increased dissemination of the data in general formats that facilitate access and analysis (54). Some of these shortcomings are discussed below.

Population Subgroup Coverage

The core components (CSFII and NHANES) provide data representative of the civilian, noninstitutionalized population in the United States. Groups excluded from these surveys include active-duty military personnel residing on military installations and persons in institutions, such as long-term care hospitals, homes for the aged, convents, monasteries, and penal and mental institutions. Homeless people with no address are excluded from all household surveys because lists of addresses within census tracts are used as the basic unit for sampling.

As shown in Table 105.1, a complex, multistaged, stratified probability method of sampling is used in the core national surveys. This method either limits or eliminates the sample size of some subgroups that may be at higher risk for nutritional problems. For example, selected subgroups (e.g., pregnant or lactating women) and ethnic minority groups (e.g., Asians and selected Hispanic subgroups) do not occur in the population in sufficient numbers to yield adequate representation in the survey sample for reliable detailed estimates of their nutritional and health status. To capture all population subgroups, other approaches need to be implemented (55). Special surveys, such as the Hispanic HANES or the CSFII low-income sample, can be conducted. Oversampling, a technique used to increase sample size, can help improve the precision of estimates for nutritional and health variables. For example, NHANES III oversampled African American and Mexican American persons, children under 6 years of age, and adults aged 60 years or older.

The nutrition objectives in *Healthy People 2000,* give a high priority to obtaining more data on the nutritional status of seven selected groups: people in hospitals, nursing homes, convalescent centers, and institutions such as those for the developmentally disabled; physically, mentally, and developmentally disabled individuals in community settings; children in child care facilities; Native Americans on reservations; old and very old individuals living independently; people in correctional facilities; and the homeless (26). PL 101-445 also cited the need to gather data on these groups (2). More specifically, this current legislation mandates that the comprehensive plan include components to incorporate, in survey design, military and (where appropriate) institutionalized populations; to sample representative subsets of identifiable low-income populations such as Native Americans and the homeless; and to collect dietary and nutritional status measurements on preschool and school-age children, pregnant and lactating women, elderly individuals, low-income populations, blacks, and Hispanics. The *Third Report on Nutrition Monitoring,* prepared by the LSRO with input from expert consultants, recommended focused studies of these high-risk populations using data collection techniques comparable to national surveys. This approach seems to be the most economical way to assess these groups (52).

Geographic Coverage

Many users of NNMRRP data request that federal agencies provide information on defined geographic areas, such as cities, counties, and individual states. The design of federal surveys uses primary sampling units consisting of a county or a contiguous group of small counties that are stratified by characteristics such as urbanization and income. However, confidentiality restrictions prohibit release of data with identification of limited geographic areas. Areas are selected randomly within regions to provide the most representative sample while minimizing operational costs. Both NHANES and CSFII are designed to provide a picture of the nation. The USDA also reports the findings from CSFII by the four major geographic regions of the country (Northeast, North Central, South, and West), as defined by the Bureau of the Census. Data from NHANES III can be analyzed and reported by these four regions. Data from the NHANES I and II were available by region; however, the regions were not identical to those defined by the Census Bureau (44). Although regional data are available, representative state and local (city) data cannot be obtained from the core surveys.

Surveillance activities at the Centers for Disease Control and Prevention (CDC) effectively target high-risk populations in narrow geographic areas. These activities include the Pediatric Nutrition Surveillance System (PedNSS) and the Pregnancy Nutrition Surveillance System (PregNSS), whose target populations consist of a convenience sample of low-income children and pregnant women, respectively, who participate in publicly funded health, nutrition, and food assistance programs. Participation in the CDC system is voluntary. In 1995, 43 states, 5 Indian tribes, the Intertribal Council of Arizona, and Washington, DC, and Puerto Rico participated in the PedNSS, and 26 states, Washington, DC, the Navajo Nation, the Intertribal Council of Arizona, and American Samoa participated in the PregNSS. The states involved in these two surveillance activities receive the data analysis results on a monthly, quarterly, or annual basis for use in program planning, management, and evaluation.

The comprehensive plan for the NNMRRP in PL 101-445 requires that the federal government provide scientific and technical assistance, training, and consultation to state and local governments for the purposes of obtaining dietary and nutritional status data; developing related databases; and promoting development of regional, state, and local data collection services so they might become integral components of a national nutritional status network. A grant program to encourage and assist state and local governments in developing their capacity to monitor and oversee nutritional status, food consumption, and nutritional knowledge and to enhance nutritional services is also a provision of PL 101-445 (2). However, this legislation has no statutory provision for additional funds to establish such programs. Therefore, as part of the related research provision of this law, innovative ways must be developed to help smaller areas meet their needs for information about the nutritional status and health of their residents.

Timeliness of Data

Timely data are essential for both policy makers and researchers. National surveys involve large sample sizes and oftentimes relatively long periods for data collection. In the past, one of the major limitations of the NNMS was inordinate delays in processing and release of data from both the core and ancillary surveys (56). With improved technology and use of automated data collection systems, such as an automated system for assigning food codes that was used in the NHANES III, data from future NNMRRP activities should be disseminated faster. Indeed, some results from NHANES III, a 6-year survey conducted from 1988 to 1994, were analyzed and published after the first 3 years of data collection (49–50, 57–59). The full 6-year data were available for public release and analysis on a CD-ROM in 1997. Electronic bulletin boards are used to distribute nutrition-monitoring publications and survey data, and CD-ROMs are used to distribute survey data. The data from the 1994 series III CSFII was released in March 1996 on a CD-ROM at a USDA-sponsored users conference. Although progress has been made toward more timely release of survey data, further improvements are needed to meet the needs of public health administrators and nutritional policy makers.

CONCLUSIONS

The future direction of the NNMRRP will continue to be largely determined by the interpretation of PL 101-445 and by the various federal agencies that sponsor monitoring activities and contribute to the 10-year comprehensive plan. The law provides many windows of opportunity to enhance the current NNMRRP by increasing involvement at the state and local levels. The law authorizes carrying nutrition-monitoring activities into nonfederal areas, with the potential to expand monitoring beyond the core components of DHHS and USDA. The 10-year plan is ambitious and includes new activities. The extent to which these proposed initiatives are carried out and realized will largely depend on adequate allocation of resources.

Organizations and programs are currently changing both to become more efficient and effective in conducting their activities and to minimize duplication of efforts. Although the impact that reorganization, program restructuring, and resource reallocation will ultimately have on the NNMRRP is uncertain, such changes can have potentially far-reaching implications. With governmental reorganization, some agency units inevitably disappear as they are combined with other divisions for greater efficiency. Other units are selected to reorient their ongoing nutrition-monitoring activities. For example, at the time of this writing, discussions are under way within the IBNMRR by representatives of USDA and DHHS to explore implementing a joint survey and research project that would incorporate CSFII and NHANES components into a single national survey. Although the outcomes of these discussions are not yet final, these are precisely the type of negotiations that the NNMRR Act of 1990 was designed to foster.

With potential decentralization of programs from the federal government and increasing empowerment of the states through block grants and other financial and administrative mechanisms, current nutrition-monitoring approaches may need reevaluation. Because of potential changes in the methods used to administer food assistance programs and the movement toward managed health care, nutrition-monitoring activities may increasingly focus on providing information that can be better applied and interpreted at the state and local levels.

Finally, some monitoring activities have become more sophisticated. Nutrition-monitoring databases, for example, are becoming much larger, and computerized methods allow rapid, selective retrieval of desired information. However, the full potential of these advances may not be realized if fiscal constraints restrict their use. The 10-year plan was ambitious, optimistic, and visionary. A review of the plan was scheduled to begin in 1997. To what extent the goals and objectives of this plan will be met by the year 2002, when it is scheduled to be completed, depends largely on the availability and judicious allocation of adequate resources to support the activities and projects described in it.

The NNMRRP is still evolving and probably still surpasses the nutrition-monitoring activities in any other nation. Taken together, the many national nutrition-monitoring components provide an opportunity for comprehensive and coordinated evaluation of the dietary status and the nutritional status of the U.S. population and of selected subgroups considered at high-risk for developing nutrition-related health problems.

REFERENCES

1. U.S. General Accounting Office. Nutrition monitoring: establishing a model program. GAO/PEMD 95-19. Washington, DC: U.S. General Accounting Office, 1995;1–88.
2. National Nutrition Monitoring and Related Research Act of 1990 (PL 101-445). Cong Rec 136, Oct 22, 1990.
3. Forbes AL, Stephenson MG. J Am Diet Assoc 1984;84:1189–93.
4. Departments of Health and Human Services and of Agriculture. Operational plan for the national nutrition monitoring system. Unpublished government report, 1987;1–47.
5. Ostenso GL. J Am Diet Assoc 1984;84:1181–5.
6. Food and Agriculture Act of 1977 (PL 95-113). Sec. 1428. Cong Rec 123, September 29, 1977.
7. Departments of Health, Education and Welfare and of Agriculture. Proposal—a comprehensive nutritional status monitoring system. Unpublished government report, 1978.
8. Porter D. A national nutrition monitoring system: brief background and bill review. CRS report for Congress no. 88-199 SPR. Washington, DC: Congressional Research Service, 1988; 1–50.
9. Departments of Health and Human Services and of Agriculture. Joint implementation plan for a comprehensive national nutrition monitoring system. Unpublished government report, 1981;1–59.
10. Departments of Health and Human Services and of Agriculture. Nutrition monitoring in the United States: a progress report from the Joint Nutrition Monitoring Evaluation Committee. DHHS publ no. (PHS) 86-1255. Washington, DC: U.S. Government Printing Office, 1986;1–356.
11. Department of Health and Human Services, Interagency Committee on Nutrition Monitoring. Announcement of committee formation. 53 FR 26505 no. 134. Washington, DC: U.S. Government Printing Office, 1988.
12. Life Sciences Research Office, Federation of American Societies for Experimental Biology. Nutrition monitoring in the United States: an update report on nutrition monitoring. DHHS publ no. (PHS) 89-1255. Washington, DC: U.S. Government Printing Office, 1989;1–158 plus 247 pp of appendices.
13. Nestle M. J Nutr Educ 1990;22:141–4.
14. Kuczmarski MF, Moshfegh A, Briefel R. J Am Diet Assoc 1994; 94:753–60.
15. Briefel RR. Nutrition monitoring in the United States. In: Ziegler EE, Filer LJ, eds. Present knowledge in nutrition. 7th ed. Washington, DC: International Life Sciences Institute, 1996;517–29.
16. Departments of Health and Human Services and of Agriculture. Ten-year comprehensive plan for the National Nutrition Monitoring and Related Research Program. Fed Regist 1991;56:55716–67.
17. Departments of Health and Human Services and of Agriculture. Ten-year comprehensive plan for the National Nutrition Monitoring and Related Research Program. Fed Regist 1993;58:32752–806.
18. Interagency Board for Nutrition Monitoring and Related Research. Nutrition monitoring in the United States. Chartbook I: selected findings from the National Nutrition and Related Research Program. Ervin B, Reed D, eds. DHHS publ no. (PHS) 93-1255-1. Hyattsville, MD: Public Health Service, 1993;1–136.
19. Life Sciences Research Office, Federation of American Societies for Experimental Biology. Third report on nutrition monitoring in the United States (Executive summary, 51 pp; vol 1, 365 pp; and vol 2, 354 pp). Prepared for the Interagency Board for Nutrition Monitoring and Related Research. Washington, DC: U.S. Government Printing Office, 1995.
20. Stiebeling HK, Monroe D, Coons CM, et al. Family food consumption and dietary levels: five regions. Consumer Purchases Study. USDA misc publ no. 405. Washington, DC: U.S. Government Printing Office, 1941.
21. Woteki CE, Fanelli-Kuczmarski MT. The national nutrition monitoring system. In: Brown ML, ed. Present knowledge in nutrition. 6th ed. Washington, DC: International Life Sciences Institute, 1990;415–29.
22. Peterkin BB, Rizek RL, Tippett KS. Nutr Today 1988;23:18–24.
23. Departments of Agriculture and of Health and Human Services. Nutrition and your health: dietary guidelines for Americans, 4th ed. Home and garden bull no. 232. Washington, DC: U.S. Government Printing Office, 1995;1–43.
24. Cleveland LE, Peterkin BB. Fam Econ Rev 1983;2:12–21.
25. Department of Health and Human Services. The 1990 health objectives for the nation: a midcourse review. Washington, DC: U.S. Government Printing Office, 1986;1–253.
26. Department of Health and Human Services. Healthy people 2000: national health promotion and disease prevention objectives. DHHS publ no. (PHS) 91-50212. Washington, DC: U.S. Government Printing Office, 1991;1–692.
27. Hamma MY, Riddick HA. Fam Econ Rev 1988;2:24–7.
28. National Analysts. Nationwide Food Consumption Survey 1987/88, Survey operations report. Philadelphia: National Analysts, 1991.

29. Life Sciences Research Office, Federation of American Societies for Experimental Biology. Impact of nonresponse on dietary data from the 1987–88 Nationwide Food Consumption Survey. Bethesda, MD: LSRO/FASEB, 1991;1–39.
30. Interagency Board for Nutrition Monitoring and Related Research. Nutrition monitoring in the United States: the directory of federal and state nutrition monitoring activities. DHHS publ no. (PHS) 92-1255-1. Washington, DC: U.S. Government Printing Office, 1992;1–117.
31. U.S. General Accounting Office. Nutrition monitoring: mismanagement of nutrition survey has resulted in questionable data. GAO/RCED 91-117. Gaithersburg, MD: U.S. General Accounting Office, 1991.
32. National Analysts. The Continuing Survey of Food Intakes by Individuals and the Diet and Health Knowledge Survey: 1989, survey operations reports. Philadelphia: National Analysts, 1991.
33. Department of Agriculture. Nationwide Food Consumption Survey: Continuing Survey of Food Intakes by Individuals, women 19–50 years and their children 1–5 years, 1 day, 1985. NFCS, CSFII rep no. 85-1. Washington, DC: U.S. Government Printing Office, 1985;1–102.
34. Department of Agriculture. Nationwide Food Consumption Survey: Continuing Survey of Food Intakes by Individuals, low-income women 19–50 years and their children 1–5 years, 1 day, 1985. NFCS, CSFII rep no. 85-2. Washington, DC: U.S. Government Printing Office, 1986;1–186.
35. Department of Agriculture. Nationwide Food Consumption Survey: Continuing Survey of Food Intakes by Individuals, men 19–50 years, 1 day, 1985. NFCS, CSFII rep no. 85-3. Washington, DC: U.S. Government Printing Office, 1986;1–94.
36. Department of Agriculture. Nationwide Food Consumption Survey: Continuing Survey of Food Intakes by Individuals, women 19–50 years and their children 1-5 years, 1 day, 1986. NFCS, CSFII rep no. 86-1. Washington, DC: U.S. Government Printing Office, 1987;1–98.
37. Department of Agriculture. Nationwide Food Consumption Survey: Continuing Survey of Food Intakes by Individuals, low-income women 19–50 years and their children 1–5 years, 1 day, 1986. NFCS, CSFII rep no. 86-2. Washington, DC: U.S. Government Printing Office, 1987;1–166.
38. Interagency Committee on Nutrition Monitoring. Nutrition monitoring in the United States: the directory of federal nutrition monitoring activities. DHHS publ no. (PHS) 89-1255-1. Washington, DC: U.S. Government Printing Office, 1989;1–64.
39. Cleveland LE, Goldman JD, Borrud LG. Nutr Today 1997;32: 37–40.
40. U.S. General Accounting Office. Nutrition monitoring: progress in developing a coordinated program. GAO/PEMD 94-23. Washington, DC: U.S. General Accounting Office, 1994; 1–50.
41. Department of Health, Education and Welfare. Ten-State Nutrition Survey 1968–1970. DHEW publ no. (HSM) 72-8130–72-8133. Washington, DC: U.S. Government Printing Office, 1972.
42. National Center for Health Statistics. Plan and operation of the Health and Nutrition Examination Survey, United States, 1971–1973 (pt A, Development, plan, and operation) Vital and Health Statistics. Series 1, no. 10a. DHEW publ no. (PHS) 79-1310. Washington, DC: U.S. Government Printing Office, 1973;1–46.
43. National Center for Health Statistics. Plan and operation of the Health and Nutrition Examination Survey, United States, 1971–1973 (pt B, Data collection forms of the survey) Vital and Health Statistics. Series 1, no. 10b. DHEW publ no. (PHS) 79-1310. Washington, DC: U.S. Government Printing Office, 1977;1–77.
44. National Center for Health Statistics. Plan and operation of the Second National Health and Nutrition Examination Survey, 1976–80. Vital and Health Statistics. Series 1, no. 15. DHHS publ no. (PHS) 81-1317. Washington, DC: U.S. Government Printing Office, 1981;1–144.
45. National Center for Health Statistics. Plan and operation of the Hispanic Health and Nutrition Examination Survey, 1982–1984. Vital and Health Statistics. Series 1, no. 19. DHHS publ no. (PHS) 85-1321. Washington, DC: U.S. Government Printing Office, 1985;1–429.
46. Woteki CE, Briefel RB, Kuczmarski R. Am J Clin Nutr 1988;47:320–8.
47. Woteki CE, Briefel RB, Hitchcock D, et al. J Nutr 1990;120:1440–5.
48. National Center for Health Statistics. National Health and Nutrition Examination Survey III data collection forms. Hyattsville, MD, 1990;1–310.
49. Kuczmarski RJ, Flegal KM, Campbell SM, et al. JAMA 1994;272:205–11.
50. Burt VL, Whelton P, Roccella EJ, et al. Hypertension 1995;25: 305–13.
51. Johnson CL, Rifkind BM, Sempos CT, et al. JAMA 1993;269: 3002–8.
52. Life Sciences Research Office, Federation of American Societies for Experimental Biology. Executive summary from the third report on nutrition monitoring in the United States. J Nutr 1996;126:1907S–36S.
53. Interagency Board for Nutrition Monitoring and Related Research, Survey Comparability Working Group. Improving comparability in the National Nutrition Monitoring and Related Research program: population descriptors. Hyattsville, MD: National Center for Health Statistics, 1992;1–135.
54. U.S. General Accounting Office. Nutrition monitoring: data serve many purposes; users recommend improvements. GAO/PEMD 95–15. Washington, DC: U.S. General Accounting Office, 1995;1–62.
55. Lepkowski JM. J Nutr 1991;121:416–23.
56. Callaway CW. J Am Diet Assoc 1984;84:1179–8.
57. Brody DJ, Pirkle JL, Kramer RA, et al. JAMA 1994;272:277–83.
58. Looker AC, Johnson CC, Wahner HW, et al. J Bone Miner Res 1995;10:796–802.
59. Looker AC, Wahner HW, Dunn WL, et al. Osteoporosis Int 1995;5:389–409.

SELECTED READINGS

Briefel RR. Nutrition monitoring in the United States. In: Ziegler EE, Filer LJ, eds. Present knowledge in nutrition. 7th ed. Washington, DC: International Life Sciences Institute, 1996; 517–29.

Department of Health and Human Services and Department of Agriculture. Ten-year comprehensive plan for the National Nutrition Monitoring and Related Research Program. Fed Regist 1993;58:32752–806.

Findings and implications of the Navajo Health and Nutrition Survey. J Nutr 1997;127:2075S–2133S.

Life Sciences Research Office, Federation of American Societies for Experimental Biology. Third report on nutrition monitoring in the United States (Executive summary, vols 1 and 2). Prepared for the Interagency Board for Nutrition Monitoring and Related Research. Washington, DC: U.S. Government Printing Office, 1995.

National Nutrition Monitoring and Related Research Act of 1990 (PL 101-445). Cong Rec, October 20, 1990.

106. Nutritional Implications of Vegetarian Diets

PATRICIA K. JOHNSTON

HISTORICAL CONTEXT

For centuries, vegetarian diets have been used to meet nutritional needs, perhaps most often out of economic necessity in underdeveloped countries. Nonetheless, even in ancient times some advocated such diets for a variety of health-related, religious, or ethical reasons. Pythagoras is considered the founder of the vegetarian movement; advocates included other ancient Greeks. Eastern religions, including Buddhism, Zainism, and Hinduism, also promoted vegetarian diets and continue to urge preservation of animal life; vegetarians are found among their adherents.

In the 18th century, Benjamin Franklin was perhaps the most famous of the scientists, physicians, and philosophers who supported vegetarian diets. The vegetarian movement expanded considerably in the 19th century with the formation of societies, establishment of health care facilities, publication of books, and opening of restaurants, all promoting vegetarian diets. The 20th century witnessed a further expansion of interest and knowledge. Details of the history of vegetarian dietary practices can be found in recent reviews (1, 2).

A 1994 survey reported that some 12.4 million people in the United States call themselves vegetarians (3). This represents approximately 7% of the population and a near doubling in number of reported vegetarians over an 8-year period. It is predicted that 10% of all Americans will consider themselves vegetarians by the year 2000 (4).

The growing vegetarian population necessitates that health professionals be informed about the potential benefits and risks associated with these dietary practices. Position papers and scientific reviews have been published, as well as the proceedings from two international congresses addressing this topic (5–8); proceedings from the third, held in 1997, are under review. A recent monograph addresses virtually all topics related to the nutritional status of vegetarians and provides useful summaries of the literature as well as dietary suggestions for different conditions (9).

DEFINITIONS AND RATIONALE FOR VEGETARIAN DIETARY PRACTICES

The term *vegetarian* encompasses a wide range of dietary practices with potentially differing implications for health. It is not uncommon for individuals who call themselves vegetarians to consume meat. It was recently reported that 20% of vegetarians said they ate meat at least once a month (4). Consumption of fish or poultry is even more common.

The varied dietary practices result in differing nutritional intakes and necessitate that health professionals ascertain what actually is eaten rather than depend on what persons call themselves. Unfortunately, there is no consistent definition for vegetarian in the various scientific studies, although researchers may classify subjects on reported dietary intake rather than on what the subjects call themselves or their diets.

Cereal grains, fruits, vegetables, legumes, nuts, and seeds form the basis of vegetarian diets, with varying amounts of dairy products, with or without eggs. The types of animal products included frequently are used to identify the kind of vegetarian diet. Lactoovovegetarians (LOVs), sometimes called ovolactovegetarians, and lactovegetarians are the largest subgroups. Both exclude meat, poultry, fish, and other seafood.

It is quite common for nonvegetarians to believe that vegetarians eat fish; while this may be true in some cases, it is not true of all vegetarians. Those who include fish may be called pescovegetarians, and those who include poultry may be called pollovegetarians; however, they are more commonly classified as semivegetarians, with individuals who are occasional or infrequent meat eaters.

Persons who exclude all animal products may be called strict, total, or pure vegetarians. However, these descriptors are also sometimes used, albeit inaccurately, to mean simply exclusion of flesh foods. The term *vegan* is explicitly used to define individuals who do not use any animal products. Some vegans also refrain from using honey and animal products such as leather or wool. Only 4% of vegetarians report they are vegans (4).

Additional subgroups of vegetarians or near vegetarians have been reported in recent years. In the 1970s, individuals who did not belong to vegetarian groups common at the time and who did not fit the usual definitions for vegetarians were classified as "new" vegetarians. The rationales for their dietary practices and actual food choices differed considerably among them.

Macrobiotic diets are often classified as vegetarian, although they may include fish. The macrobiotic diets of today are an outgrowth of a 10-step approach to eating that culminated in a diet composed almost exclusively of brown rice. This diet resulted in severe nutritional deficiencies and has since been modified. Although it still emphasizes brown rice and other whole grains, it also includes sea vegetables, legumes, and root vegetables. Animal foods are limited to white-meat fish, once or twice a week. Standard macrobiotic diet recommendations include 50 to 60% whole grains, 20 to 25% vegetables, 10% beans and sea vegetables, and 5% soups. Locally grown fruit may be consumed occasionally in season. Meat, poultry, eggs, dairy products, butter, yogurt, sugar, honey, and artificial sweeteners are to be avoided.

Occasionally, a fruitarian may be encountered or an individual who consumes only raw foods. The fruitarian diet consists of fruits (including those vegetables botanically classified as such), nuts, and seeds. A raw food diet, also called "living food diet," includes uncooked, fermented, or sprouted plant foods and the juice made from sprouts.

Thus a broad spectrum of dietary practices may be classified as vegetarian. Regardless of how persons identify themselves, so far as dietary practices are concerned, actual dietary intake must be ascertained before effective nutritional intervention can take place. Knowledge of why an individual follows particular dietary practices is also helpful in developing an appropriate counseling approach.

Although, historically, vegetarian diets were associated with certain religious practices, currently, health appears to be the primary reason for adopting a vegetarian diet (4). The second reason encompasses ecologic and environmental issues relating to the large differences in resources necessary to support animal- and plant-based diets. The third currently most common reason relates to ethical concerns about the treatment of animals and may extend to the use of animals for clothing or research. In many cases, however, multiple reasons underlie vegetarian dietary practices.

The differing reasons for adopting a vegetarian diet may affect food choices and subsequently nutritional status. In addition, the rationale for a particular diet may be associated with other lifestyle practices that can affect health. Thus, ascertaining these reasons and associated practices is an important aspect of a patient's history.

DIETARY INTAKE AND NUTRITIONAL STATUS AMONG VEGETARIANS

There are many and varied ways to meet nutrient needs, and the adequacy of a diet depends not on what it is called but on the foods that are included. A vegetarian diet need not be deficient in nutrients; however, the more foods eliminated from any diet, the greater the risk of deficiency.

Most vegetarians ingest an adequate diet; however, those following restrictive dietary patterns may not, and these engender significant concern, especially when they include pregnant and lactating women, infants, children, and the elderly. As our understanding of both beneficial and problematic aspects of vegetarian dietary practices grows, it allows us to focus our attention on those issues of greatest consequence for preventing disease and promoting health. Thus, our attention here addresses those questions that are most frequently raised.

Dietary Intake

Energy

Energy Intake and Weight Status. Some, but not all, investigators report that vegetarians weigh less than nonvegetarians, with the difference being least among the LOVs and greatest among the vegans. The lower weight among vegetarians is consistent with the lower intake of calories often reported. The energy-yielding nutrients of protein and fat are generally consumed in somewhat greater amounts by nonvegetarians, while larger amounts of carbohydrates are consumed by vegetarians. The result of this difference is that vegetarians may more closely approximate dietary recommendations for the distribution of macronutrients than do omnivores, and they may be closer to desirable weight.

A variety of other reasons have been suggested for the weight difference. In addition to the higher intake of carbohydrates, which may be less efficiently converted to body fat, they include perhaps greater control of food intake, possibly greater physical activity, and greater intake of fiber, which may enhance satiation (10).

Although overweight is a frequent concern in the general population, maintaining adequate weight through appropriate caloric intake may be a concern to some vegetarians. Those at risk include children, adolescents, the elderly, and those who include no added oils or fat in the diet.

Vegetarian Diets and Weight Loss. The general understanding that vegetarian diets are associated with lower weight status may be the rationale for some females to adopt such a diet in hope of weight loss. Vegetarian dietary practices have been found among anorexia nervosa patients, although most were not vegetarians prior to the anorexia. It was suggested that vegetarian diets are a convenient and socially acceptable way to reduce caloric intake (11). A recent study of eating behavior found that vegetarian women had lower dietary restraint scores, indicating they were not motivated by weight loss to adopt the vegetarian diet (12). Thus, it is inappropriate to conclude that vegetarians are more prone to eating disorders than the general population.

Protein

One of the most frequent questions regarding the nutritional adequacy of vegetarian diets relates to protein, yet there is little supporting evidence for such concerns with usual dietary intake in healthy vegetarians. However, the inadequate energy intake seen in some vegetarians may compromise protein status.

Nutritional Quality of Plant Proteins. The nutritional quality of plant proteins may be underestimated in studies of animals, because animals have greater protein needs than humans. More relevant human data confirm the adequacy of plant proteins to meet the needs of both adults and children. Plant foods are often said to lack certain indispensable amino acids and thus be of lesser quality than animal foods. Although a certain plant food may be low in a specific amino acid, it is inaccurate to say it is incomplete. A single plant food, if fed as the only protein source, may prove inadequate; however, this is likely to occur only in a research setting. Appropriate mixtures of plant foods are equivalent to animal protein in quality and are commonly consumed.

Limiting Amino Acids. Two amino acids are of particular interest in vegetarian diets: lysine, the limiting amino acid in cereal grains, and methionine, the limiting amino acid in legumes. Lysine occurs in significant amounts in the intracellular spaces of the skeletal musculature where it is deposited after a protein-rich meal (13). Subsequently, it is available to buffer a low-lysine amino acid mixture resulting from consumption of a meal deficient in this amino acid.

Methionine is of interest because it is the limiting amino acid in soy and other legumes, often a major source of protein in vegetarian diets. Soy protein isolates have been used successfully to refeed children recovering from malnutrition; they provide a protein quality comparable to that of milk. They may be used as the sole source of protein for adults and children; however, modest supplementation with methionine may be appropriate for soy-based infant formulas, although the amount needed is lower than predicted from rat studies (13).

Complementation. Protein complementation occurs when a food low in a particular amino acid is combined with a food containing an adequate amount of that amino acid. Animal studies have influenced our attitudes toward combining complementary proteins within one meal. In these studies, an amino acid otherwise absent from the diet was added several hours later. Such a delay in providing a supplementary amino acid to rapidly growing rats and pigs affects protein use. Similar effects were not seen in human adults when the plant protein was distributed among several meals. The supplementary effect was somewhat lower in young children when the proteins were fed at intervals longer than 6 hours; however, this is a longer period than usual in young children, and meals are not entirely devoid of an amino acid as in the laboratory studies (13). It can be concluded that combinations of plant foods consumed throughout the day provide adequate amino acids for nitrogen retention and use.

Digestibility. Plant proteins in their natural form are, in general, less digestible than animal protein sources. Well-processed soy isolates, however, are as digestible as egg protein (13). Processing methods may have beneficial or detrimental effects on the nutritional quality of plant proteins. Consuming a broad variety of foods prepared in many different ways ensures adequate intake of amino acids.

Protein Intake. Vegetarians, in general, consume less total protein and even less animal protein than omnivores; however, studies consistently show they more than meet the recommended dietary allowances (RDA) and the recommended 10% of calories as protein. In addition, they more than meet the needs for the indispensable amino acids. Current evidence suggests that lower animal protein intake is beneficial and may lower urinary calcium excretion and slow the progression of renal disease. In addition, compared with animal protein, plant sources contribute less total fat, saturated fat, and cholesterol and more carbohydrate and fiber. In more restrictive diets, where variety or energy intake is limited, greater attention must be given to providing an adequate protein intake, especially in pregnant women, infants, growing children, and the elderly.

Hematologic Status

Iron

Nonheme iron from plant foods is less available than heme iron, and plant foods contain a variety of substances known to reduce iron availability; thus, the iron status of vegetarians is often questioned. However, plant foods also contain other substances that enhance iron uptake, and well-planned vegetarian diets often contain more iron than omnivorous diets.

Some studies suggest that long-term LOVs, even with a higher fiber intake, maintain iron status no different from omnivores (14). Other studies, however, indicate vegetarians may have reduced iron stores, even though iron deficiency anemia as determined by hemoglobin levels is no more prevalent than among omnivores (15). However, although there was no significant difference in iron intake, a recent study found significantly lower hemoglobin levels in vegetarian children in England (15a). The authors suggested dietary advice was needed to ensure optimal absorption of iron. Another recent study found lower serum ferritin levels in both male and female vegetarians than in omnivorous controls, although the vegetarians consumed significantly more iron (16). Although lower iron stores increase risk of deficiency, the optimal storage level continues to be debated, particularly in view of evidence of an association between elevated iron stores and coronary heart disease.

The high levels of iron in well-planned vegetarian diets combined with the frequent intake of vitamin C–rich fruits and vegetables appear to protect against iron deficiency, which is more likely to be encountered among those on restrictive vegetarian diets, such as macrobiotic. Iron deficiency is also more prevalent in developing countries where dietary choices are limited and there is greater reliance on unleavened and unrefined cereal products (14).

Folate

Intake and blood levels of folate are often higher in vegetarians than omnivores because of their greater use of fruits and vegetables. Elevated folate is of concern in individuals whose vitamin B_{12} intake is low because folate may delay the appearance of megaloblastic anemia and thus mask a developing vitamin B_{12} deficiency with its potentially irreversible neurologic effects (17).

Vitamin B_{12}

Vitamin B_{12} is of particular interest because the usual dietary sources of this vitamin are animal products. Persons who include only plant foods in their diet, such as vegans, are at increased risk of deficiency unless care is taken to include a reliable source of vitamin B_{12}. Vitamin B_{12} deficiency can result in serious and irreversible neurologic and neuropsychiatric abnormalities, and these potentially significant consequences necessitate giving attention to this vitamin in any discussion of vegetarian diets.

In addition, inactive analogues of this vitamin occur in foods and are found in the body. However, they are not differentiated in the usual microbiologic assays used to assess either vitamin B_{12} status or its content in foods, which are likely overestimated unless a method specific for cobalamin, the active form, is used (18).

Sources. Plants do not synthesize or store vitamin B_{12}. The ultimate source of this vitamin is microbial synthesis. Vitamin B_{12} occurs in plants only if they are contaminated by bacteria producing it (18). Such contamination is more likely where sanitary procedures are not followed in handling food and may be a reasonable explanation for the limited vitamin B_{12} deficiency occurring among vegan populations in developing countries. Animals either ingest the vitamin or absorb what is produced by bacteria in their intestines, thus becoming a source of vitamin B_{12} for those who consume animal products.

As noted, the microbiologic assays often used to assess vitamin B_{12} content determine the inactive vitamin B_{12} analogues, as well as cobalamin, the active form of the vitamin. Labels on many food products give values for the nonactive analogues rather than for cobalamin. This is misleading and causes confusion for the consumer. Assays specific for cobalamin indicate that many food products commonly thought to be sources of vitamin B_{12} in actuality contain mostly inactive analogues (18); these include spirulina, tempeh, other fermented foods, and most sea algae. It was suggested that individuals relying on spirulina as a source of vitamin B_{12} might develop a deficiency more rapidly because some of the analogues contained in it actually block vitamin B_{12} metabolism (18).

Intake and Status. Serum vitamin B_{12} levels in vegans are generally lower than those in omnivores, with intermediate levels found in LOVs. Recently, individuals adopting a vegan diet showed a more rapid drop in serum vitamin B_{12} levels than anticipated, and those using vitamin B_{12} supplements or vitamin B_{12} fortified foods had higher mean serum levels over time (19). Similarly, serum vitamin B_{12} levels declined over a 2-year period in six of nine subjects adhering to a "living food diet" (20).

It is remarkable that there are so few reported cases of vitamin B_{12} deficiency even among vegans. Observations, however, suggest that suboptimal vitamin B_{12} status may occur well before the deficiency is discovered. Reasons for the low incidence of vitamin B_{12} deficiency include the very small requirement, relatively large stores, and a very efficient enterohepatic circulation that recovers most of the vitamin B_{12} excreted in the bile. Intestinal bacteria produce vitamin B_{12}; however, most of this occurs below the ileal site for vitamin B_{12} absorption and it is excreted in the feces (18). Some evidence indicates that small amounts are produced in the small intestine; however, it is unclear how much of this is the active form (18). Some vegans may consume the vitamin in foods eaten outside their homes. In developing countries, food and water contaminated with vitamin B_{12}–producing bacteria, in conjunction with poor hygienic practices, may contribute to vitamin B_{12} intake.

There is limited evidence that some seaweeds may contribute active vitamin B_{12}, presumably from contamination with plankton. Vegans consuming *Chlorella* or Nori seaweed had serum vitamin B_{12} concentrations twice as high as those not consuming these seaweeds (20). In another study, increased consumption of seaweeds by a mother led to normalization of urinary methylmalonic acid (MMA) in her breast-fed infant (21). In contrast, ample consumption of seaweed by vitamin B_{12}–deficient infants did not improve their abnormal hematologic indexes and there was no relationship between algae consumption by macrobiotic adults and their vitamin B_{12} status (22, 23). Reliable sources of vitamin B_{12} must be ensured to prevent deficiency in individuals who consume no animal foods.

Other Nutrients

Calcium and Vitamin D

Adequate calcium and vitamin D intakes are important to ensure optimal bone status over the lifetime. Recent evidence suggests that calcium also may be important in regulating blood pressure and preventing colon cancer. Milk and dairy products supply 70% of calcium in U.S. diets, and questions regarding adequacy are often expressed when intake of these foods is limited, as in vegan diets.

Intake. Calcium intake among LOVs appears to be similar to that of omnivores, whereas vegans take in less. The long-term impact of this lower intake on bone health is not yet known, although some evidence warrants concern (24). In addition to the lower intake of calcium, vegans also consume lower levels of vitamin D. The low consumption of vitamin D may be further exacerbated in some cases by limited exposure to sunlight. Low vitamin D concentrations and secondary hyperparathyroidism were documented during the winter in vegans living at northern latitudes (25). Vitamin D deficiency was also documented in British Asian vegetarians and is a frequent concern among macrobiotic children (26, 27). The Institute of Medicine recently released new recommendations for intake of nutrients related to bone health (27a).

Factors Affecting Calcium Status. Besides vitamin D, a variety of other dietary factors also influences calcium status. A consistently lower intake of protein, as often seen among vegetarians, may decrease calcium requirements (28). Numerous studies demonstrate that increases in animal protein intake result in increased urinary calcium excretion. This relationship is not seen with plant protein (28). In addition, the ratio of dietary calcium to protein is thought to be important (29). This ratio in milk and dairy products is very favorable to a positive calcium balance (29). It is higher in LOVs than in omnivores and even higher than in vegans.

Similarly, a high intake of sodium increases calcium excretion (29a). There is some evidence that vegans consume less sodium than LOVs or omnivores. However, it was suggested that the characteristically increased consumption by vegans of oxalate- and phytate-containing foods may offset the benefits of their lower intake of protein and sodium (24).

Although lower rates of hip fracture are reported in populations worldwide with much less calcium intake than the United States where fracture rates are higher, genetic and lifestyle factors may play important roles. Optimal calcium intake under different dietary and lifestyle conditions remains to be determined.

Sources. Obtaining adequate calcium intake, as with all nutrients, depends on food choices. Individuals consuming relatively large amounts of animal protein, even though dairy products are not excluded, may need to give special attention to calcium intake. Vegans also may need to give attention to supplying an appropriate intake, especially during periods of growth. In general, few other foods provide as concentrated a calcium source as dairy products; however, it is relatively widely distributed among plant foods. The bioavailable calcium from various food sources has been calculated and may be useful in guiding food choices (24). The calcium in high-oxalate vegetables such as spinach, Swiss chard, and beet greens is largely unavailable; however, kale, broccoli, Chinese cabbage, and mustard and turnip greens provide substantial amounts of available calcium. Legumes and some nuts and seeds also contribute to calcium intake. Unfortified soy beverages provide negligible amounts, whereas calcium-set tofu and fortified soy milks are rich sources.

Zinc

Meat, fish, and poultry provide 40 to 45% of the zinc in the U.S. diet; dairy foods and grain products each contribute a little less than 20%. Nonetheless, reported zinc intake among vegetarians is similar to that of omnivores. However, its lesser availability from plant foods may result in somewhat lower zinc status among vegetarians than among nonvegetarians. A lower zinc intake was found among vegetarian children and adolescents, but it did not affect their growth; vegetarians were slightly taller than nonvegetarian controls (30). A recent study of adolescent female vegetarians found no difference in dietary zinc intake by LOVs, semivegetarians, or omnivores (31). Further, the investigators found no differences in mean values for any indicator of zinc status among the groups. Nonetheless, 24% of LOVs, 33% of semivegetarians, and 18% of omnivores had low serum zinc levels. Attention should be given to ensuring an adequate intake of foods that supply this nutrient.

VEGETARIAN DIETS IN THE LIFE CYCLE

Risk of nutritional deficiencies is greatest during periods of growth and adequate intake of all nutrients should be ensured at these times. The impact of vegetarian diets on various stages of the life cycle was recently reviewed (6).

Pregnancy and Lactation

LOV diets provide adequate nutritional support during pregnancy and lactation, but special attention is needed to obtaining certain nutrients when following a vegan or macrobiotic diet. These include energy, iron, vitamin B_{12}, calcium, and vitamin D. Vegetarians are more likely to breast-feed their infants and to do so longer than the general population. This necessitates continued attention to dietary intake. Guidelines for counseling pregnant vegetarians also have broader application to other groups (32).

The few reports of pregnant vegetarians suggest a possible increased risk of earlier labor and lower birth weight in those following a more limited diet, although no difference in incidence of pregnancy complications was seen (33). More-concentrated energy sources may be necessary than are usually consumed on a vegan diet to ensure appropriate weight gain. Low serum ferritin levels are associated with increased risk of prematurity and low birth weight, and therefore care should be taken to ensure adequate iron intake for all pregnant women.

Normally, enough vitamin B_{12} is deposited in the fetus to last from 6 to 12 months after birth, yet a number of cases of vitamin B_{12} deficiency have been reported in infants of vegan mothers, with the deficiency frequently developing before 6 months of age (34, 34a, 34b). The infants were totally breast-fed by vegan mothers who showed no clinical signs of deficiency, although later testing confirmed they had low vitamin B_{12} status. Low maternal serum vitamin B_{12} levels were reflected in low values in milk (35). It is suggested that it is currently ingested vitamin B_{12} that is available for placental transport and secretion in the breast milk (36). Thus, totally breast-fed infants born to vegan mothers are at increased risk of vitamin B_{12} deficiency because of decreased stores at birth and low milk values.

Certain features are characteristic of infants developing a vitamin B_{12} deficiency: increased fretfulness and apathy, decreased socialization and activity, and regression in motor control. The infants are generally very small for their age and show serious neurologic deficits. Upon testing, the vitamin B_{12} deficiency is apparent. The usefulness of MRI (magnetic resonance imaging) in diagnosis and follow-up of patients with suspected diseases of myelination was recently emphasized (34a). In most cases there is rapid improvement with administration of vitamin B_{12}. Unfortunately, however, there appear to be long-term neurologic deficits in some cases (37). Vegan women *must* understand the importance of consuming a reliable source of vitamin B_{12}, at least during pregnancy and lactation, and it must be included in the diets of infants and children.

Low vitamin D status and low calcium intake were found in lactating macrobiotic women (35). In view of the increased calcium needs in pregnancy and lactation, this could result in maternal bone demineralization. Adequate calcium and vitamin D must be ensured at these critical stages of the life cycle.

Essential fatty acids and their derivatives play important roles in fetal development, especially of the retina and central nervous system, and parturition (33). Docosahexanoic acid (DHA, 22:6n-3), while found in fish, occurs in only small amounts in eggs and is absent from commonly consumed plant foods. In contrast to the low level of DHA, vegetarian diets contain high amounts of linoleic acid (18:2, n-6). DHA can be synthesized in the body from linolenic acid (18:3, n-3); however, high levels of linoleic acid inhibit this process.

In comparison to omnivores, a lower proportion of DHA was found in plasma and cord artery phospholipids, as well as in the milk of vegan mothers (33). As expected, the erythrocyte lipids of their infants contained a lower proportion of DHA than those of infants breast-fed by omnivorous mothers or fed cow's milk formula. It was suggested that vegans use soybean or canola oils, which have a lower ratio of linoleic:linolenic acid, to facilitate the body's synthesis of DHA.

Infancy and Childhood

Concerns have been expressed regarding vegetarian diets for children whose vulnerability is great for nutrient deficiency, yet there is little evidence that physical or intellectual growth has been harmed (6). The growth of Seventh-day Adventist LOV children is the same as that of omnivores, with no greater evidence of nutritional deficiencies (30). While vegan children weighed less and were shorter than controls, their growth was within normal ranges and catch-up occurred by about age 10 (38). The lower growth appeared related to the high bulk and low energy density of some vegetarian diets combined with the small stomach capacity of young children. Recently, investigators reported significant catch-up in height and arm circumference for age in boys and girls combined who had followed a macrobiotic diet in early childhood. However, both boys and girls were still significantly below reference values for height, and girls were below reference for weight-for-height and arm circumference for age (38a). Multiple regression analysis showed that inclusion of moderate amounts of dairy products improved growth of vegan children.

Inadequate weaning foods deficient in calories, vitamin D, calcium, iron, and vitamin B_{12} may be used by some vegan or macrobiotic parents, resulting in low growth and nutritional deficiencies. Similar diets continued into preschool years resulted in impaired growth, rickets, iron deficiency anemia, and vitamin B_{12} deficiency (39). Vegetarian food guides are available and can be helpful in planning diets for children and other age groups (40).

Adolescents

The few studies describing the nutritional status of vegetarian adolescents were recently reviewed, and suggestions were made for dietary management (41). Not everyone adopting a vegetarian diet understands the nutritional implications of excluding animal products, and care must be taken to ensure adequate intake, especially of vitamin B_{12}, calcium, and vitamin D, as well as iron and other trace elements.

Preadolescent LOV females were shorter than omnivores, but were taller than omnivores later in adolescence (30). This suggests a delay in the pubertal growth spurt. They were also reported to experience a 6-month delay in onset of menarche. These findings appear to represent a delay in physical maturation that may be of benefit in adult life, particularly in relation to decreased risk of breast cancer (30). Recent investigations in Europe also found that vegetarian children grow at least as well as omnivorous children, and both were close to the 50th percentiles for both height and weight (41a).

Compared with omnivores, LOV adolescents reported significantly greater intake of fruits, vegetables, and starchy foods and lower intake of dairy products, junk foods, and (as expected) meat (30). Thus, their dietary pattern more closely approximated current recommendations than that of the omnivorous controls. As noted previously, a larger proportion of LOVs and semivegetarians had low serum zinc levels than omnivores, although there was no difference in intake (31). Similarly, more LOVs and semivegetarians than omnivores had low iron stores. They were, however, more likely to consume greater amounts of antioxidants and other protective phytochemicals.

Adult and Elderly Vegetarians

Adults may adopt vegetarian diets to lose weight, to decrease risk of chronic disease, or as part of a therapeutic regimen to control disease. As noted, vegetarians, and especially vegans, generally weigh less and have lower serum cholesterol levels and lower blood pressure. If no animal products are included in the diet, attention is warranted for those nutrients noted above as at risk. Low vitamin D levels were reported in some elderly vegetarians as well as marginal iron and zinc status (6, 16, 42). Adequate vitamin D is particularly important in maintaining bone health in aging women and care must be taken to ensure an adequate intake and/or exposure to sunshine.

Impaired absorption makes vitamin B_{12} deficiency increasingly common with advancing age in both vegetarians and omnivores. Possibly, vegetarians, if they have reduced stores, may be at risk for earlier manifestation of the deficiency. Further, vitamin B_{12} deficiency in the elderly is rarely accompanied by anemia or megaloblastosis, and serum vitamin B_{12} levels in the elderly are often within the currently defined normal range (43). It was suggested that the cutoff for suspecting a vitamin B_{12} deficiency should be below 258 pmol/L (<350 pg/mL) rather than below 148 pmol/L (<200 pg/mL). Because there is a limited window of time for effective intervention in a vitamin B_{12} deficiency, attention must be directed to the status of this vitamin in elderly persons.

HEALTH IMPLICATIONS OF VEGETARIAN DIETARY PRACTICES

The association of vegetarian diets with lower risk for several chronic diseases is well documented, and various studies investigating the relationships have been reviewed (10, 44). The standardized mortality ratio (SMR) for all-cause mortality is greatly reduced among vegetarians who are known to consume more fruits, vegetables, and polyunsaturated fatty acids and less saturated fatty acids, cholesterol, and alcohol than the general population (5–9, 44, 44a). They also smoke less, have a lower body mass index (BMI), and may exercise more.

The specific health-promoting factors associated with a vegetarian lifestyle continue to be investigated, with particular attention currently focused on phytochemicals and the foods that contain them. These nonnutritive substances include a wide range of chemicals found in plant foods and are reviewed elsewhere (45, 45a). These substances can alter various hormone actions and metabolic paths in beneficial ways. The advantages of fruits and vegetables are so well accepted that recommendations to include more of them in the diet are heard with increasing frequency. Some of the positive health effects of vegetarian diets may be due to the increased intake of these foods.

Several major epidemiologic studies focus on Seventh-day Adventists, a conservative religious denomination. Adventists follow a broad range of dietary practices, from total vegetarian to usual American diets. Approximately half are vegetarians, with the great majority of these being LOVs. Certain lifestyle characteristics, such as smoking and alcohol consumption, which can confound or modify the effects of other factors, are largely absent from this population. The Adventist Health Study provides opportunity to compare vegetarian and omnivorous dietary practices within a population with great similarity of other lifestyle factors. Overall mortality rates are lower among Adventists than in the general population. Although they die of similar diseases, they appear to develop these diseases at a later age (46).

Cancer

The German Vegetarian Study found death from all cancers in vegetarians was reduced by 52% in men and 26% in women compared with expectations (47). More specifically, the SMR for colon cancer was found to be 44 in men and 78 in women. Longer duration of vegetarian practices decreased risk of cancer mortality.

The risk of death from cancer is considerably lower among Adventists as a whole than in an appropriate reference population (48). Lower risk would be expected for those sites associated with cigarette smoking or alcohol; however, the reduction in risk included nearly all major cancer sites, with a greater reduction for males than for females.

The relationships between dietary components and specific cancer sites were investigated in the Adventist population and recently reviewed (46). Multivariate analysis was used to control for factors other than the variable of interest.

Frequent consumption of fruit (>1/day vs. <3/week) was associated with a 75% reduction in risk of lung cancer, independent of past smoking status. The risk of stomach cancer was also greatly reduced in those who consumed fruit frequently. Raisins, dates, and other dried fruit provided significant protection against prostate cancer. Frequent consumption of tomatoes and dried beans also may protect against prostate cancer, while consumption of fish more than once a week may increase risk. No association with dietary factors, including animal fat, was found for breast cancer.

Striking protection against pancreatic cancer was afforded by frequent consumption of legumes, with those consuming dried beans and peas more than twice a week having only 1/30th the risk of those who consumed these foods rarely or not at all. An 80% reduction in risk of this cancer was associated with frequent consumption of raisins, dates, and other dried fruit.

Individuals who ate beans more than twice a week had a 42% lower risk of developing colon cancer than those who ate beans less than once a week. A similar reduction was seen in those who consumed more fiber. In contrast, a somewhat greater risk was associated with eating meat, fish, or fowl several times each week. After adjusting for age, sex, and smoking history, frequent consumption of beef was associated with a more than twofold increase in risk of bladder cancer.

These results suggest that, with the exception of bladder and perhaps colon cancer, dietary factors other than the absence of meat are the protective agents in the reduced risk of cancer seen among vegetarians (46). Others reported an inverse relationship between milk intake and incidence of breast cancer (49). Thus, increasing attention is being focused on foods commonly consumed by vegetarians and the protective compounds they contain.

Coronary Heart Disease

Lower risk of death from coronary heart disease (CHD) among vegetarian populations is well established and not surprising given their dietary and lifestyle characteristics resulting in lower body weight, lower blood pressure, and lower serum lipid levels (6–9). An LOV vegetarian diet in an African American population was also associated with a more favorable profile of blood lipid risk factors for premature CHD than the omnivorous diet (50). Multiple factors undoubtedly play roles in decreasing the risk seen among vegetarians.

An association of meat consumption and fatal ischemic heart disease was described in the Adventist Mortality Study, and more recently, data from the Adventist Health Study confirmed that relationship (51). Risk of fatal CHD was nearly twice as great in men who ate beef up to three times a week than in men who never ate any, and in men consuming beef three times a week or more, risk was more than twofold greater. Meat eating did not change the risk of CHD for women.

The same analysis revealed other intriguing relationships. The risk of both nonfatal and fatal CHD was lower in those who consumed mainly whole wheat bread than in those who ate mainly white bread (51). Similarly, the risk of both nonfatal and fatal CHD was lower in those who ate nuts frequently than in those who ate nuts less than once a week. The protective effect of frequent consumption of nuts was found consistently among various subgroups including both vegetarians and nonvegetarians.

A carefully controlled dietary trial was subsequently conducted to investigate these relationships further (52). Moderate quantities of walnuts were incorporated into a National Cholesterol Education Program Step 1 isocaloric diet in place of fatty foods, meat, and visible oils, while maintaining fat at 30%. This resulted in a more favorable lipoprotein profile. The possible mechanisms mediating the beneficial effect of nuts have been reviewed (53).

To date much of the research investigating the relationships between diet and CHD has focused on dietary factors related to modifying serum lipids. Rapid expansion over the last decade of our understanding of various plant constituents has led to rethinking the relationship of diet to heart disease (54). Whereas great emphasis was placed on dietary fat, it is now suggested that other factors, such as higher intake of antioxidants, may play important, if not deciding, roles. This is not to suggest fat intake should be ignored, but other factors should also receive attention.

Hypertension

Cross-sectional studies often report that vegetarians have lower blood pressure and lower incidence of hypertension than omnivores. This was also documented in African Americans, a population with a well-recognized increased risk of hypertension (50). Confirmed hypertension occurred in significantly fewer vegetarians than semi-vegetarians and omnivores. Mean systolic blood pressure was significantly lower in black vegetarians than in black nonvegetarians but was higher than in white vegetarians or nonvegetarians, suggesting that vegetarian dietary practices do not completely offset the risk of hypertension in the black population (50).

In contrast, the Health Food Shop Users cross-sectional study found no difference in blood pressure between vegetarians and omnivores (44). It was suggested that lifestyle factors other than avoidance of meat may be shared by vegetarians and other health conscious individuals and may affect blood pressure.

Randomized controlled trials introducing an LOV diet to meat eaters were reviewed (55). The review indicated that the reported blood-pressure-lowering effect of vegetarian diets is between 5 and 10 mm Hg in systolic blood pressure and is independent of effects of changes in body weight.

The relationships between vegetarian diets and decreased risk of hypertension are complex because of the myriad dietary and lifestyle components that interact in this, as in other, chronic diseases. None of the characteristics of the vegetarian diet alone—absence of meat, type of protein, high polyunsaturated:saturated fat ratio, or high fiber, potassium, or magnesium intakes—has been identified as the active agent (56). The combined effect of several specific foods and/or nutrients may be responsible for the lower blood pressure seen in vegetarians.

Diabetes

Vegetarians may be at less risk for developing diabetes than omnivores. Among Adventist Health Study volunteers, vegetarians have lower rates of diabetes than omnivores. Nonvegetarian men, after adjusting for age and weight, were 1.8 times more likely to die from diabetes than vegetarian men. No difference, however, was seen among women (56). Further, an increased risk of diabetes appearing on the death certificate was seen with increased meat consumption in men, i.e., there was a dose response; in women, increased risk was seen only with meat consumption more than six times a week.

Various factors found among vegetarians have been suggested as protective for diabetes. Among these are lower body weight, lower serum cholesterol levels, high complex carbohydrate and fiber intake, and lower fat and animal protein intake. The benefits of high-carbohydrate, high-fiber diets in treating diabetes have been demonstrated (57).

Osteoporosis

Studies of bone mineral status in vegetarians and omnivores were reviewed (58). No differences were found in either cortical or trabecular bone in recent studies. However, an earlier report suggested postmenopausal vegetarian women were protected against bone loss and that their lower protein intake might be a major beneficial factor (58). A recent prospective study reported a small but significant increase in risk of forearm fracture for women who consumed more than 95 g/day of total protein, compared with those who consumed less than 68 g (59). A similar increase in risk was seen for animal protein, but no association was found with vegetable protein. Those who ate five or more servings per week of red meat had a higher risk of forearm fracture than those eating fewer than one serving a week.

Concern was expressed about the bone status of vegans (24). Recent reports lend support to that concern, although to date there are few studies specifically of vegans. Obese postmenopausal omnivorous subjects placed on a low-calorie, high-fiber diet for 6 months lost significantly more bone from the lumbar spine than nondieting obese controls (60). Whether the loss of bone was due to the loss in weight, dietary factors, or a combination is not known. However, the fiber, calcium, and protein intakes reported in this study would not be uncommon among vegans. Since leanness is also a risk factor for osteoporosis and since vegans are often leaner than the general population, it would be wise to give attention to their bone status. Investigators recently reported a higher risk of exceeding the lumbar spine fracture threshold and of being classified as osteopenic in vegan than in lactovegetarian postmenopausal Taiwanese women (60a). Others reported significantly lower bone mass at several sites in Dutch adolescents who had followed a vegan macrobiotic diet in childhood (60b).

Bone density was compared with dietary intake in five counties in China with widely differing calcium intakes (61). Bone density was approximately 20% higher from the fourth to well into the eighth decade of life in areas where dairy products were consumed (Ca intake 724 mg/day) compared with those where dairy products were not used (Ca intake 230–359 mg/day). Protein intake in the former was 75 g/day versus 49 to 57 g/day in the latter counties. The lower protein intake reported in these Chinese did not confer protection against low bone density when the calcium intake was very low.

The dietary and lifestyle factors related to risk of osteoporosis have been reviewed (62). Many factors other than calcium affect bone status and risk of fractures; however, a consistently low calcium intake combined with low vitamin D status and high fiber intake may place vegans at greater risk for low bone density. On the other hand, their lower protein intake, and common consumption of soy foods that contribute phytoestrogens may be protective. Studies are needed to clarify these issues.

PHYSIOLOGIC RESPONSE TO VEGETARIAN DIETS

Metabolic Rate

The reduced risk of disease found among vegetarians suggests biologic processes are influenced by the diet. Vegetarians generally weigh less and have less body fat than omnivores. However, the exact reason for the differences remains to be resolved. Possibilities include lower total energy consumption or differences in resting metabolic rate (RMR) and the thermic effect of a meal (TEM) that could ultimately affect energy expenditure. High fiber intake and meditation, both possibly observed more frequently among vegetarians, appear to decrease postprandial thermogenesis, a finding that would not, however, contribute to the lower weight in vegetarians (63, 64). Vegetarians had a higher RMR than nonvegetarians, as well as a higher plasma norepinephrine concentration and a faster rate of norepinephrine appearance (65). The investigators concluded that macronutrient composition and plasma norepinephrine may be independent modulators of RMR, but the effect appears to be small.

The Colonic Milieu

Lower cancer incidence among vegetarians has led investigators to study various factors thought to be related to particular cancers. Some, but not all, reports suggest vegetarians have a lower concentration of total bile acids in their stools than nonvegetarians. A recent investigation found no difference in bile acid concentration in total feces of vegetarians and omnivores, but the vegetarians did have a lower concentration in fecal water (66). The latter may be of greater significance, because it is the fecal water that is in contact with the colonic mucosa. Further, vegetarians had a higher ratio of primary to secondary bile acids and a lower concentration of deoxycholic acid in fecal water. These findings are similar to those of other studies comparing populations at low and high risk of colon cancer. Deoxycholic acid is thought to be a promoting factor for colon cancer, and its concentration appears to be influenced by dietary saturated fat (66). Vegetarians also have higher wet fecal weight and a higher defecation frequency. In addition, a significant decrease in mutagenic activity in urine and feces was recently reported after shifting from an omnivorous to a lactovegetarian diet (66a). Similarly, switching from a diet rich in fat and meat and poor in dietary fiber to a vegetarian diet poor in fat and rich in dietary fiber resulted in a marked decrease in formation of hydroxyl radicals in the feces (66b). All of these factors may contribute to the lower frequency of colon cancer found among vegetarians.

Colonic epithelial cell proliferation was investigated in populations at differing risk for colon cancer. Compared with omnivores, vegetarians had a lower rate of cell proliferation (67). The possible association between cell proliferation and various dietary factors was investigated in healthy vegetarians and omnivores (68). Increased intake of calcium appeared to be associated with a reduced rate of cell proliferation, although not all studies agree.

Hormonal Effects

The relationship between dietary fat intake and breast cancer has prompted numerous studies, some among vegetarians, many looking at various hormonal associations. Results of studies investigating menstrual differences among vegetarians are inconclusive, with some showing more ovulatory disturbances and some reporting less (69). These differences are likely due to different study designs. Some were of short duration; dietary components including fat, fiber, and carbohydrate differed; and the definition of vegetarian was not consistent.

An inverse relationship between dehydroepiandrosterone sulfate (DHS) and breast cancer has been suggested in premenopausal women. A study of adolescents found higher DHS levels in vegetarians than in omnivores (70). However, no association was found with any nutrient, and caution was urged until more definitive data are available.

The biologic effects of soy protein, a common ingredient in vegetarian diets, were investigated in premenopausal women (71). The menstrual changes found in response to the inclusion of soy protein may be beneficial with respect to risk of breast cancer and may help to explain the lower risk in populations who consume significant amounts of soy.

Antioxidant Status

Much attention is currently focused on the benefits of dietary antioxidants. It is not surprising that vegetarians, in view of their diet, are reported to have higher blood levels of β-carotene, vitamin C, and vitamin E, nutrients thought to play important roles in the prevention of chronic disease (72).

The various modifications to the physiologic milieu will continue to be investigated as reasons are sought for the beneficial effects of vegetarian diets.

VEGETARIAN DIETS IN THE TREATMENT OF DISEASE

Vegetarian diets have been proposed, and used, as treatment for various disease conditions. Macrobiotic diets are claimed to be helpful in treatment of serious disease; however, evidence supporting the claims is limited (6).

Coronary Heart Disease

A number of clinical trials have investigated diet and lifestyle changes in the treatment of coronary heart disease, with or without drug intervention. Regression of atherosclerosis has now been shown in patients with advanced disease in multiple studies, which were recently reviewed (73). Generally, the diets used were similar to vegetarian diets, viz., low in fat, saturated fat, and cholesterol, and high in fiber. Lifestyle factors were often incorporated in the treatment and included exercise and stress management. Recently, a very low fat, vegetarian diet was used as part of a comprehensive treatment approach. Quantitative coronary angiography demonstrated regression of atherosclerosis in subjects after a year, but progression in controls (74). Frequency, duration, and severity of angina were reduced in subjects, while controls experienced increases. Just as vegetarian diets appear to provide primary prevention against coronary heart disease, they also contribute to secondary prevention and the reversal of CHD.

Diabetes

A vegetarian diet may be helpful in managing diabetes. Current recommendations for diabetics include reducing total fat, saturated fat, and cholesterol, as well as increasing fiber intake. This may result in a food pattern similar to a vegetarian diet, especially if significant sources of plant proteins are included. Because diabetics are prone to diabetic nephropathy, this may be particularly appropriate. Evidence from insulin-dependent diabetics suggests that isocaloric substitution of vegetable for animal protein results in beneficial effects on renal function (75).

Low-fat, high-fiber diets effectively reduced serum glucose and cholesterol levels in diabetics (57). In addition, such diets may help control weight. Thus, evidence indicates that vegetarian diets are not only compatible with therapeutic diabetic regimens but may be beneficial in controlling the metabolic aberrations associated with diabetes. The Diabetes Care and Education Dietetic Practice Group of the American Dietetic Association recently published a comprehensive resource for diabetes management in vegetarians (75a).

Renal Disease

The importance of protein in the management of renal disease is recognized. Although a low-protein intake is desirable, the use of vegetarian diets is often questioned because of their high phosphorus content relative to the quality and quantity of protein they contain. However, a recent review of the impact of vegetarian diets on renal disease provides evidence from both animal and human studies of potential benefits from such diets (76).

Plant proteins exert significantly different renal effects from animal proteins; the effects seem comparable to those achieved by reducing the total amount of dietary protein. In subtotally nephrectomized rats, soy protein resulted in less proteinuria, reduced glomerular filtration rate, milder renal histologic damage, and longer survival than casein. In patients with diabetic nephropathy, an LOV diet that provided 1 g protein/kg/day reduced proteinuria while maintaining good nutritional status over 8 weeks. In addition, plant-based diets exert beneficial effects on the hyperlipidemias associated with renal disease, and soy-based diets reduce serum cholesterol independent of dietary fat (76). A carefully designed vegan diet used successfully to manage mild chronic renal failure may be the diet of choice when the conventional low-protein diet is poorly tolerated (76a).

Because plant foods provide more nonessential amino acids than do animal proteins, they generate more urea. Consequently, it may be more difficult to minimize uremic toxicity on a strictly plant-based diet in severe chronic renal insufficiency (76). Fewer problems will be encountered on an LOV diet. In addition, a vegetarian diet may require an increase in phosphate binders in end-stage renal disease or dialysis, and attention should be directed to using lower potassium fruits, vegetables, and grains to compensate for the higher potassium content of some legumes, nuts, and seeds. Guidelines for planning a vegetarian renal diet are available (77).

Other Conditions

Rheumatoid Arthritis

Claims are frequently made that special diets, including vegan or LOV diets, can alleviate the symptoms of rheumatoid arthritis. A recent review suggested this is part of "the folklore of the disease" (78). Although a number of studies have been reported, most were poorly designed, did not include controls, and were not adequately blinded. Often the subjects held a strong belief in the intervention. Clinically demonstrable improvements rather than subjective responses were not always used. Nonetheless, some patients may benefit from a vegetarian diet (79).

Cancer

Claims continue to abound that a macrobiotic diet can cure cancer. Unfortunately, there is little supportive scientific evidence; however, recent reports suggest survival may be greater in some cases (80). Considerable concern exists that individuals may delay appropriate treatment for their disease and that the diet may contribute to malnutrition and weight loss (81).

COUNSELING ISSUES AND DIETARY GUIDELINES

Careful investigation of the dietary practices of individuals calling themselves vegetarians is essential for the health professional to provide optimal counseling, and general lifestyle practices that may affect health should be evaluated as well. The beliefs and attitudes that support these practices may affect a patient's willingness to follow suggestions. Those adhering to more restrictive dietary practices, such as macrobiotics, may be less willing to seek or follow the advice of health care professionals. The attitude of the health professional will be perceived quickly, and a nonjudgmental approach is of utmost importance in establishing a productive relationship.

Issues to be considered in counseling pregnant vegetarians are described above and are applicable to others as well (32). Vegetarian food guides are available, as are specific applications for vegetarian adolescents (40, 41). Food sources for the nutrients most likely at risk are included in these guides. Bioavailable sources of calcium are also described (24). A vegetarian diet manual is available for use in various clinical conditions (82).

The basic principles for planning a vegetarian diet are the same as those for planning any other diet, with variety a key component. A diet restricted in either variety or amount can limit the intake of essential nutrients. Energy intake to maintain appropriate weight must be considered. Obtaining adequate calories may be a challenge on a vegan or macrobiotic diet, while avoiding excess calories may be equally challenging on an LOV diet that relies on full-fat dairy products (40). An emphasis is appropriately placed on unrefined foods in any diet.

There are many different ways to obtain the essential nutrients, and the health care provider should be aware of alternate sources for those nutrients commonly supplied by foods excluded from a given diet. A registered dietitian can be very helpful in providing guidance, information, and counsel. An adaptable, creative, and sensitive approach will be most successful in providing dietary suggestions for individuals whose dietary patterns and beliefs differ from our own.

CONCLUSION

Current dietary recommendations call for increased consumption of plant foods in all diets. Evidence from populations consuming plant-based diets supports these recommendations. As one researcher said, "vegetables and fruits . . . are chemical powerhouses that produce dozens if not hundreds of unique and complex organic compounds, many of which are biologically active" (54). The potential health benefits, as well as issues of concern regarding vegetarian diets, have been described. The health professional has a responsibility to be informed regarding both, to encourage those dietary and lifestyle practices that promote health, and to provide alternatives to those that may be detrimental.

ACKNOWLEDGMENTS

The generous reading of the manuscript and insightful suggestions of Ella Haddad and Joan SabatÇ are gratefully acknowledged.

REFERENCES

1. Roe DA. J Nutr 1986;116:1355–63.
2. Whorton JC. Am J Clin Nutr 1994;59(Suppl):1103S–9S.
3. Stahler C. Vegetarian J 1994;13:6–9.
4. Murray J. FoodService Dir 1993;6:74.
5. Messina VK, Burke KI. J Am Diet Assoc 1997;97:1317–21.
6. Dwyer JT. Annu Rev Nutr 1991;11:61–91.
7. Mutch PB, Johnston PK, guest eds. Am J Clin Nutr 1988;48(Suppl):707–927.
8. Johnston PK, guest ed. Am J Clin Nutr 1994;59(Suppl): 1099S–262S.
9. Messina M, Messina V. The dietitian's guide to vegetarian diets. Gaithersburg, MD: Aspen, 1996;1–511.
10. Dwyer JT. Am J Clin Nutr 1988;48:712–38.
11. O'Conner MA, Touyz SW, Dunn SM, et al. Med J Aust 1987;147:540–2.
12. Janelle KC, Barr SI. J Am Diet Assoc 1995;95:180–6, 189.
13. Young VR, Pellett PL. Am J Clin Nutr 1994;59(Suppl): 1203S–12S.
14. Craig WJ. Am J Clin Nutr 1994;59(Supppl):1233S–37S.
15. Nelson M, Bakaliou F, Trivedi A. Br J Nutr 1994;72:427–33.
15a. Nathan I, Hackett AF, Kirby S. Br J Nutr 1996;75:533–44.
16. Alexander D, Ball MJ, Mann J. Eur J Clin Nutr 1994;48:538–46.
17. Herbert V. Am J Clin Nutr 1994;59(Suppl):1213S–22S.
18. Herbert V. Am J Clin Nutr 1988;48:852–8.
19. Crane MG, Sample C, Patchett S, et al. J Nutr Med 1994;4: 419–30.
20. Rauma AL, Törrönen R, Hänninen O, et al. J Nutr 1995; 125:2511–5.
21. Specker BL, Miller D, Norman EJ, et al. Am J Clin Nutr 1988;47:89–92.
22. Dagnelie PC, van Staveren WA, van den Berg H. Am J Clin Nutr 1991;53:695–7.
23. Miller DR, Specker BL, Ho ML, et al. Am J Clin Nutr 1991;53:524–9.
24. Weaver CM, Plawecki KL. Am J Clin Nutr 1994;59 (Suppl):1238S–41S.
25. Lamberg-Allardt C, Kärkkäinen M, Seppänen R, et al. Am J Clin Nutr 1993;58:684–9.
26. Iq-bal SJ. J Hum Nutr Diet 1994;7:47–52.
27. Dagnelie PC, van Staveren WA. Am J Clin Nutr 1994;59 (Suppl):1187S–96S.
27a. Food and Nutrition Board, Institute of Medicine. Dietary reference intakes: calcium, phosphorus, magnesium, vitamin D, and fluoride. Washington, DC: National Academy Press, 1997.
28. Zemel MB. Am J Clin Nutr 1988;48:880–3.
29. Heaney RP. J Am Diet Assoc 1993;93:1259–60.
29a. Evans CEL, Chughtai AY, Blumsohn A, et al. Eur J Clin Nutr 1997;51:394–9.
30. Johnston PK, Haddad E, Sabate J. Adolesc Med 1992;3:417–37.
31. Donovon UM, Gibson RS. J Am Coll Nutr 1995;14:463–72.
32. Johnston PK. Am J Clin Nutr 1988;48:901–5.
33. Reddy S, Sanders TAB, Obeid O. Eur J Clin Nutr 1994;48: 358–68.
34. Michaud JL, Lemieux B, Ogier H, et al. Eur J Pediatr 1992;151:218–20.
34a. Lovblad K, Ramelli G, Remonda L, et al. Pediatr Radiol 1997;27:155–8.
34b. Grattan-Smith PJ, Wilcken B, Procopis PG, et al. Mov Disord 1997;12;39–46.
35. Specker BL. Am J Clin Nutr 1994;59(Suppl):1182S–6S.
36. Higginbottom MC, Sweetman L, Nyhan WL. N Engl J Med 1978;299:317–23.
37. Graham SM, Arvela OM, Wise G. J Pediatr 1992;121:710–4.
38. Sanders TAB. Pediatr Clin North Am 1995;42:955–65 .
38a. van Dusseldorp M, Arts IC, Bergsma JS, et al. J Nutr 1996;126:2977–83.
39. Dagnelie PC, van Staveren WA. Am J Clin Nutr 1994;59 (Suppl):1187S–96S.
40. Haddad EH. Top Clin Nutr 1995;10:7–16.
41. Johnston PK, Haddad EH. Vegetarian and other dietary practices. In: Richert VI, ed. Adolescent nutrition: assessment and management. New York: Chapman Hall, 1995;57–88; 637–45.
41a. Nathan I, Hackett AF, Kirby S. Eur J Clin Nutr 1997;51:20–5.
42. Brants HAM, Lowik RH, Westenbrink S, et al. J Am Coll Nutr 1990;9:292–302.
43. Allen LH, Casterline J. Am J Clin Nutr 1994;60:12–4.
44. Thorogood M. Nutr Res Rev 1995;8:179–92.
44a. Key TJ, Thorogood M, Appleby PN, et al. Br Med J 1996;313:775–9.
45. Steinmetz KA, Potter JD. Cancer Causes Control 1991;2: 427–42.
45a. Knight D, Eden JA. Obstet Gynecol 1996;87:897–904.
46. Adventist Health Study slide show. University Relations, Loma Linda University. Loma Linda, CA, 1995.
47. Frentzel-Beyme R, Chang-Claude J. Am J Clin Nutr 1994;59(Suppl):1143S–52S.
48. Mills PK, Beeson WL, Phillips R, et al. Am J Clin Nutr 1994;59(Suppl):1136S–42S.
49. Knekt P, Järvinen R, Seppänen R, et al. Br J Cancer 1996;73:687–91.
50. Melby CL, Toohey ML, Cebrick J. Am J Clin Nutr 1994;59: 103–9.
51. Fraser GE, Sabate J, Beeson WL, et al. Arch Intern Med 1992;152:1416–24.
52. Sabate J, Fraser GE, Burke K, et al. N Engl J Med 1993;328:603–7.
53. Sabate J, Fraser GE. Curr Opin Lipidol 1994;5:11–6.
54. Fraser GE. Am J Clin Nutr 1994;59(Suppl):1117S–23S.
55. Beilin LJ. Am J Clin Nutr 1994;59(Suppl):1130S–5S.
56. Snowdon DA, Phillips RL. Am J Public Health 1985;75:507–12.
57. Anderson JW, Zeigler JA, Deakins DA, et al. Am J Clin Nutr 1991;54:936–43.
58. Hunt IF. Bone mineral content in postmenopausal vegetarians and omnivores. In: Draper HH, ed. Advances in nutritional research, vol 9. New York: Plenum Press, 1994;245–55.

59. Feskanich D, Willett WC, Stampfer MJ, et al. Am J Epidemiol 1996;143:472–9.
60. Avenell A, Richmond PR, Lean MEJ, et al. Eur J Clin Nutr 1994;48:561–6.
60a. Chiu JF, Lan SJ, Yang CY, et al. Calcif Tissue Int 1997;60:245–9.
60b. Parsons TJ, van Dusseldorp M, van der Vliet M, et al. J Bone Miner Res 1997;12:1486–94.
61. Hu JF, Zhao XH, Jia JB, et al. Am J Clin Nutr 1993;58:219–27.
62. Burckhardt P, Heaney RP. Nutritional aspects of osteoporosis '94. Rome: Ares-Serono Symposia, 1995;1–435.
63. Contaldo F, Coltorti A. JAMA 1987;257:1330.
64. Poehlman ET, Arciero PJ, Melby CL, et al. Am J Clin Nutr 1988;48:209–13.
65. Toth MJ, Poehlman ET. Metabolism 1994;43:621–5.
66. van Faassen A, Hazen MJ, van den Brandt PA, et al. Am J Clin Nutr 1993;58:917–22.
66a. Johansson G, Holmen A, Persson L, et al. Cancer Detect Prev 1997;21:258–66.
66b. Erhardt JG, Lim SS, Ghode JC, et al. J Nutr 1997;127:706–9.
67. Lipkin M, Uehara K, Winawer S, et al. Cancer Lett 1985;26: 139–44.
68. Morgan JW, Singh PN. Nutr Cancer 1995;23:247–57.
69. Barr SI, Janelle KC, Prior JC. Am J Clin Nutr 1994;60:887–94.
70. Persky VW, Chatterton RT, Van Horn LV, et al. Cancer Res 1992;52:578–83.
71. Cassidy A, Bingham S, Setchell KDR. Am J Clin Nutr 1994; 60:333–40.
72. Rauma AL, Törrönen R, Hänninen O, et al. Am J Clin Nutr 1995;62:1221–7.
73. Superko HR, Krauss RM. Circulation 1994;90:1056–69.
74. Ornish D, Brown SE, Scherwitz LW, et al. Lancet 1993;336: 129–33.
75. Kontessis P, Bossinakou I, Sarika L, et al. Diabetes Care 1995;18:1233–40.
75a. Holzmeister LA, ed. On the Cutting Edge 1997;18:1–38.
76. Paggenkamper J. Top Clin Nutr 1995;10:22–6.
76a. Barsotti G, Morelli E, Cupisti A, et al. Nephron 1996;74:390–4.
77. Paggenkamper J. J Renal Nutr 1995;5:234–8.
78. Darlington LG, Ramsey NW. Br J Rheumatol 1993;32:507–14.
79. Kjeldsen-Kragh J, Mellbye OJ, Haugen M, et al. Scand J Rheumatol 1995;24:85–93.
80. Carter JP, Saxe GP, Newbold V, et al. J Am Coll Nutr 1993;12:209–26.
81. Dwyer J. Nutr Forum 1990;7:9–11.
82. Hodgkin G, Maloney S, eds. Seventh-day Adventist diet manual including a vegetarian plan. 7th ed. Loma Linda, CA: Seventh-day Adventist Dietetic Association, 1995;1–559.

SELECTED READINGS

Hodgkin G, Maloney S, eds. Seventh-day Adventist diet manual including a vegetarian plan. 7th ed. Loma Linda, CA: Seventh-day Adventist Dietetic Association, 1995;1–559.
Johnston PK, ed. Vegetarian nutrition; proceedings of a symposium held in Arlington, VA. Am J Clin Nutr 1994;59 (Suppl):1099S–262S.
Melina V, Davis B, Harrison V. Becoming vegetarian. Summertown, TN: Book Publishing Group, 1995.
Messina M, Messina V. The dietitian's guide to vegetarian diets. Gaithersburg, MD: Aspen, 1996;1–511.
Mutch PB, Johnston PK, eds. Proceedings of the First International Congress on Vegetarian Nutrition. Am J Clin Nutr 1988;48 (Suppl):707–927.

107. International Priorities for Clinical and Therapeutic Nutrition in the Context of Public Health Realities

NOEL W. SOLOMONS

INTRODUCTION AND CONCEPTUAL FRAMEWORK

Modern Nutrition in Health and Disease (MNHD) is an influential textbook, frequently updated to absorb and distill the avalanche of ongoing discovery in the areas of human and clinical nutrition. Nutrition is a discipline that has derived from various influences, including biochemistry, animal sciences, dietetics, clinical medicine, epidemiology, and public health. Table 107.1 provides a convenient working outline of the hierarchy of levels of nutritional concern—both basic and applied—when the issue is primarily the nutritional health of *human beings*. Both implicitly and explicitly, the body of information in textbooks such as *MNHD* is based upon these interacting levels. However, in planning space allowances and selecting topics and contributors, this and other texts must make choices of emphasis. The extent to which these choices make the contents more or less useful for different readerships is a legitimate concern of editors.

This author has commented on a breach between the center of gravity of the selections in this textbook and the center of gravity of nutrition and health for the practitioners and populations of developing countries (1). For instance, acute gastroenteritides accost toddlers and preschoolers in billions of episodes annually, but *MNHD VIII* devoted much more text to nutritional management of celiac sprue and Crohn's disease (1). This chapter represents both a practical and conceptual approach, which tries to harmonize the emphases in *MNHD* with a profile of priorities for the so-called developing countries of the world at the dawn of the 21st century.

DEFINITIONS AND APPROACHES

This is not the first time that a commentary on nutritional priorities for developing countries has come forth. A commission of the U.S. National Research Council published the *World Food and Nutrition Study* (2) in 1977. This panel cited the highest priority research areas for developing countries as the relationship of nutritional status to performance, the role of dietary components in health and nutrition, nutritional interventions, and policy aspects of nutrition. Philip R. Payne (3), in a symposium titled Strategy for Nutrition Research at the 324th scientific meeting of the Nutrition Society in 1978, whose paper was subsequently published in the *Proceedings of the Nutrition Society*, was assigned the topic nutrition research priorities for the Third World. This was no doubt a daunting challenge for someone occupying a chair at the London School of Tropical Medicine and Hygiene in the capital city of an affluent Western democracy. He concluded that the highest priorities were estimating the magnitude of and trends in malnutrition, determining the relationship of malnutrition to infectious diseases, and orienting research in food science and agriculture to the problems of the neediest. It is no less daunting to attempt a similar exercise from a capital in the highlands of Central America. As discussed below, the diversity of national realities and the dynamics of social, demographic, and environmental change do not permit any single individual's perspective to encompass the entire problem. If this contribution can serve as a framework for discussion and analysis of how nutritional knowledge can be produced and can be applied to meet the concerns of different international regions, it will have begun the appropriate process.

Developing countries is a term used to designate a set of nations situated primarily in a belt bounded by the Tropics of Cancer and Capricorn and located in Africa, Asia, Latin America, and Oceania. They are characterized by high fertility rates; low levels of education and literacy; unequal distribution of wealth, with large sectors living in poverty; and underdeveloped infrastructure and public services. Classically, manufacturing and service industries in urban centers have been rare. Thus, most populations have been dedicated to agricultural pursuits (subsistence, commercial, or both), to nomadic pastoral lifestyles, or to tribal hunter-gathering activities. Developing countries have historically had high infant and under-5 mortality rates, alarming morbidity statistics for acute and infectious diseases, and life expectancies grossly inferior to those of the industrialized nations.

This chapter is based on a number of premises. One is that there is only one fundamental nutritional science for all geography and all humanity. The scientific methodology applies equally in the north and in the south. Stated another way, the first heading of Table 107.1, "Basic Nutrition," is universal. Globalization of communication reaches toward globalization of information; a core body of nutritional knowledge receives and incorporates contributions from all over the globe. This chapter's focus also recognizes that clinical and therapeutic concerns in nutrition must be understood and addressed in the context of Third World nations; to the extent that these considerations have been neglected, the utility of *MNHD* in addressing these issues is diminished.

However, there is a valid need for geographic differentiation; this chapter is also predicated on that need. Distinctions between developed and developing countries are based on the relative wealth, political history, and climate and ecology of each of the regions. Table 107.2 outlines the sources of differentiation and diversity across countries that tend to produce different realities in nutrition and health. These, in turn, influence the priorities for research and application in all branches of human-related nutrition. Although the *principles* of nutrition are universal, the *prescriptions,* as we shall see, may require regional distinctions.

Table 107.1
Outline of Various Interacting Levels of Concern in Understanding Nutrition of Human Beings and Promotion of Nutritional Health

- Basic Nutrition
  - Nutritional biology, biochemistry, physiology
  - Normative human nutrition
- Clinical nutrition
  - Effect of patients' disease on nutritional status
    - Producing deficiency
    - Producing excess
  - Effect of imbalance of individual's nutrient intake and use
    - Producing deficiency states
    - Producing excess states
  - Nutritional and dietary therapeutics
- Public health nutrition (public nutrition)
  - Effects of endemic diseases and environmental conditions on nutritional status
  - Effects of subadequate dietary nutrient intake in producing endemic nutritional deficiency states
  - Effects of excess dietary nutrient intake in producing endemic nutritional excess states
  - Interaction of dietary patterns and prevention and production of chronic diseases
  - Prophylactic and remedial public health interventions

Table 107.2
Sources of Diversity That Differentiate Developing and Developed Countries, and Developing Countries from One Another

- Genetic and ethnic makeup
- Infrastructure and natural resources
- Academic institutions and traditions
- Dietary patterns
- Climate and physical environment
- Cultural beliefs and practices
- Economic status and distribution of wealth
- Degree of urbanization and industrialization

A few examples can illustrate the different textures in human nutrition. For instance, the most often reported parable about the influence of parasites on human nutrition is that of human vitamin B_{12} deficiency caused by the fish tapeworm *Diphyllobothrium latum.* This, however, is a cold-water marine fish, irrelevant to tropical climates. On the other hand, various species of parasitic flukes that reside in human visceral organs, such as *Fasciola* and *Schistosoma,* worms unknown in temperate latitudes, can produce nutritional disturbances in the tropics and subtropics. The dietary issues of cystic fibrosis, celiac sprue, and inflammatory bowel disease are relevant in industrialized countries with populations of European ancestry, but the genetic makeup of most developing countries makes these topics irrelevant. Dietary management of patients with persistent diarrhea and visceral leishmaniasis (Chagas' disease) are more relevant in the tropics. Tuberculosis and HIV infection are present in both industrialized and preindustrialized regions, but ecologic—and even genetic—factors, as distributed in different regions, characterize the clinical and public health dissemination of these two pandemics as well as their mutual interaction.

Not only is diversity across countries important in international nutrition, but diversity *within* communities is an important reality. There has been a prevailing myth of the monolith. It is common to characterize the diets of the Third World's poor as "monotonous"; we tend to see uniformity in the levels of poverty. Table 107.3 highlights variables that differ *within* communities and are often even more polarized than in affluent populations. A seminal contribution to the eventual understanding is the concept of "positive deviance" (4), which notes that not all of the poor are malnourished or ill. It seeks to characterize the coping strategies and other factors that allow some to do better than others in situations of deprivation.

Table 107.3
Interindividual Variables That Can Differentiate and Characterize Nutritional Status within Poor Communities

Height
Body weight
Respiratory infections
Enteric infections
Geohelminthic infestations
Dietary pattern
Nutrient intake

From a pragmatic, utilitarian perspective, findings made in developing countries have often served to unravel clinical mysteries in affluent settings. Manifestations of human copper deficiency described in children recovering from kwashiorkor in 1964 (5) led to recognition of an iatrogenic form of this deficiency in patients undergoing total parenteral nutrition (TPN) (6, 7). Similarly, Keshan disease is endemic to parts of China. Linkage of its selenium deficiency manifestations with problems occurring in TPN patients led to the recognition that this nutrient was deficient in human cardiomyopathies (8, 9).

From a humanistic point of view, making the benefits of nutritional knowledge available to most of the world's population—not only to an affluent elite—has intrinsic merit. From an intellectual and academic standpoint, the huge number of individuals interacting with various climates, diets, environments, and endemic disease patterns will provide new insights. The sphere of the nutrition community that produces and traditionally uses *MNHD* would be expanded and enriched by a better understanding of the issues of the tropics.

PUBLIC HEALTH NUTRITION (PUBLIC NUTRITION)

In the balance among the topics in Table 107.1, it is virtually self-evident that the public health aspects of nutrition have been the dominant concern. Epidemiologic and community nutrition remain the principal focus of nutritional research, at least as expressed in the international English-language literature. How developing country priorities are considered in developed countries can be viewed, in part, from the perspectives of scientific offerings in nutrition journals. In 1992, the *Journal of Nutrition (JN)* created a subcategory of "Community and International Nutrition." Over the ensuing 4 years, 37 papers from developing countries were published under that heading. Ten of these related to vitamin A in terms of prevalences of hypovitaminosis A or its consequences, deficiency manifestations, or dosing. Eight papers related to growth or body composition, and two additional papers to energy expenditure. Five papers considered topics in dietary intake. Minerals were the topic of five papers: three principally about iron and two about zinc, with folic acid, vitamin B_{12}, and other trace elements variously included. Individual papers on the prevalence of lactose maldigestion, the impact of breakfasting on cognitive function, and indicators of food security rounded out the 4-year roster of contributions. Four papers included geohelminths as an interactive factor, three from Kenya and one from Jamaica. Most papers were exclusively about children (n = 23) or women of childbearing age (n = 7), including the pregnant and lactating; seven papers covered other adult segments of the population.

The *American Journal of Clinical Nutrition (AJCN)*, by virtue of its name and its being the official organ of the American Society for Clinical Nutrition, would be expected to attract clinical and metabolic studies to a greater extent than the *JN*. The *AJCN* reestablished a category of "international nutrition" with its June issue in 1994. Through the end of 1996, 20 original articles appeared under that heading. All were community-based field surveys in nature; none was clinical. Eight publications concerned vitamin A; four were about iron; three related to growth, body composition, or both; two were about iodine; and one each concerned zinc, vitamin B_{12}, and energy expenditure. All but two were focused exclusively on women (in three instances, pregnant women) or children. Thus, nutrition in *populations*—and in the groups relevant to maternal and child health—continue to be the expressed priority of researchers in this field.

Fads and fashions will always dominate scientific interest during a defined era. The relative frequency of topics considered under "international nutrition" in the 1990s suggests an emphasis on micronutrients in general and on vitamin A in particular. Since the end of World War II, so-called international nutrition has gone through a series of topical concerns. The first was protein-energy malnutrition and the "protein gap"; the United Nations' major permanent nutrition panel was the Protein Advisory Group. In the 1970s, when the factual pillars about a worldwide protein shortage were corroded by evidence (10), the new concern became the issue of total food and a potential "energy gap" (11), which reigned from the mid-1970s to the mid-1980s. This gave rise to the Nutrition Collaborative Research Study Project (12). In the mid-1980s, a field study in Indonesia reported that administration of oral vitamin A produced a 34% reduction in juvenile death from childhood illnesses (13). On the basis of their minute weight in the daily diet, the term *hidden hunger* (14) was coined at the Micronutrient Conference in Montreal in 1991 (which emerged from the World Summit on Children in 1990) for a constellation of micronutrient deficiencies common to preschool children. With this development, the last decade of the 20th century had identified its dominant nutritional paradigm. Child growth and development and maternal and child health seems to be an enduring context.

These consensus agendas are set by academics and agencies on the basis of legitimate advances in new knowledge. Generally, the loudest voices in a given era affix their personal discoveries to the central agenda. The topics become "fads" when consolidated and maintained by the donor community. In an international context, these donations have generally originated in United Nations organizations such as the World Health Organization (WHO), Food and Agriculture Organization (FAO), and United Nations Children's Fund (UNICEF). Bilateral assistance from the foreign-assistance or research-fomenting agencies of specific donor nations has followed in lock step with the dominant consensuses. Fads and trends are not necessarily totally negative, as they provide for an intensive burst of research and focus the discussion of an entire professional community into a common idiom. Such intense scrutiny should eventually separate the myths from the realities, as has occurred with the "protein gap" theory. On the debit side, fashions can delay the diversification and broadening of interests toward other important areas. For developing countries, these narrowly focused mandates within the confines of public health concerns have undoubtedly retarded development, expression of other clinical and therapeutic concerns, and application of advanced biologic concepts and technology to community problems in nutrition and health.

Effects of Endemic Diseases and Environmental Conditions on Nutritional Status

As noted, Third World countries are characterized by poor health statistics, poor sanitation, and widespread and common infections. There is a well-known synergistic interaction of infection and malnutrition (15). The clinical syndrome of kwashiorkor, conventionally ascribed to protein deficiency, is most often precipitated by a single attack or a series of infectious episodes.

Based on data from the early 1980s, Walsh (16) estimated the burden of tropical disease in terms of the prevalences (or incidences) and mortality from communicable illnesses in Africa, Asia, and Latin America, a population of about 4.5 billion people. She estimated that 1.5 billion of them are infected with tuberculosis (seropositive), with malaria affecting close to 1 million persons annually in these zones. The roundworms, *Ascaris* and hookworm, infect close to 1 billion people each, but with a low mortality. In terms of cumulative annual mortality, Walsh estimated that diarrheal disease, respiratory infections, malaria, schistosomiasis, and pertussis each cause a million or more deaths. The second tier comprised tuberculosis, hepatitis B infection, and tetanus, with about half a million deaths from each annually. Following the humanistic imperative, linkage of these very common and widespread diseases to their nutritional consequences would have greater impact than more esoteric concerns. The linkage to malnutrition is well understood for hookworm, and malaria and tuberculosis are also understood to impair nutrition.

The acquired immunodeficiency syndrome (AIDS) was barely recognized in the era for which the above estimates of worldwide mortality and morbidity were calculated. The AIDS pandemic is now over 15 years old, and the greatest rates of increase in incidence now occur in the developing countries of Africa, Asia, and Latin America. Since wasting is such a dominant feature of AIDS, mediated by inappetence, malabsorption, and catabolic reactions, Tomkins (17) suggested that we shall have to unlearn all of the conventional epidemiologic lessons about underweight and wasting in populations of developing countries and relearn them in the context of the AIDS factor.

Growth deficit, reflected in short stature and stunting, has been treated as synonymous with "chronic malnutrition." However, any deficit accumulates largely prior to 36 months of age, after which growth rates parallel those in affluent societies. Poor growth can only be explained in part on a dietary basis and further by recurrent infections such as diarrhea. Solomons et al. (18) postulated that an important factor in growth deficit is chronic stimulation of the immune system. Thus, the constant low-grade activation of the acute-phase response by the sheer number of microbes in the environment signals white cells to activate catabolic processes, thereby increasing nutrient requirements and enhancing nutrient deficits.

The interplay of pollution and nutrition is an emerging paradigm. As populations grow, environmental regulations get set aside, and long-lived and poorly degradable compounds increase in our environment (19). Soil, water, and air are the vectors for contaminants. Even forms of radiation such as solar and ionizing radiation and noise are polluting the environment. Some formats for understanding the interaction of contaminants and nutrition exist. The influence of lead on hematologic status by interfering with iron metabolism is the classic example. A committee of the International Union of Nutritional Sciences is beginning to explore paradigms to examine and understand the interrelation of pollution and nutrition.

Effects of Subadequate Dietary Nutrient Intake in Producing Endemic Nutritional Deficiency States

Public health nutrition has traditionally dealt with endemic nutrient *deficiencies*. In view of the shift away from interest in protein and energy undernutrition and the rise of the "hidden hunger" paradigm, recent concern has focused on micronutrients. The principal micronutrient deficiencies of interest have been those of vitamin A, iron, and iodine. Those of zinc, selenium, riboflavin, and vitamin B_{12} have become the subject of more recent research in developing countries.

In the past decade, no micronutrient has received more attention than vitamin A. After the protective effect of this vitamin in toddlers and preschoolers was established, questions about mortality in relation to marginal vitamin A deficiency were extended to younger ages (20). The relationship of morbidity to both vitamin A supplementation (21, 22) and vitamin A deficiency and growth (23, 24) has been explored. The picture is not consistent, and there are various textures; specific ecologic features of each geographic region may characterize the response to vitamin A. Better diagnostic assessment tools are being sought, among them the conjunctival impression cytology test (25, 26) and the modified relative dose-response test (27, 28). The field still suffers from the lack of a definitive diagnostic test for vitamin A status of the individual (29).

Iron deficiency is the most widespread of all nutritional deficiencies (30). Recent interest in iron has focused on its relation to growth. Studies from Tanzania suggest that iron has a trophic effect on growth (31). On the other hand, supplementing iron to children in Indonesia with a normal iron status tended to reduce their ponderal growth (32). Serum ferritin has been the indicator of iron status for two decades, but it is sensitive to confounding by infection and inflammation. Soluble transferrin receptor in serum appears to be an alternative index (33).

What had earlier been classified as "endemic goiter" was reclassified as iodine deficiency disorder (IDD) in 1987 (34). IDD has a negative impact on learning ability and cognitive function (35). Refinements in assessing iodine status have been explored. The use of creatinine measurement to normalize for urinary iodine was discarded in favor of simply assaying its elemental concentration (36). Ultrasound measurements can assess thyroid size by use of portable units, as an alternative to visual inspection and manual palpation. In recent years, the threshold for declaring a public health problem with IDD has been lowered to a rate of five goiters detected per 100 persons examined.

Zinc is a nutrient involved in both growth and host defenses. Shrimpton (37) has queried whether zinc deficiency is endemic in developing countries. The approaches have largely consisted of population intervention trials to see whether zinc is associated with growth (38). A byproduct has been a reduced incidence of diarrheal episodes in the zinc-treated wings of the trials (39, 40).

Vitamin B_{12} is uniquely associated with foods of animal origin in the human diet, as plants are devoid of this vitamin. For reasons of both economics and culture, flesh and dairy products are absent from the diets of a large number of individuals in developing societies. Allen et al. (41) uncovered an unexpected prevalence of B_{12} deficiency in a central Mexican rural population.

Riboflavin deficiency, reaching the stage of showing the overt manifestations of hyporiboflavinosis, rarely occurs in free-living people in the community. On the other hand, submaximal saturation of tissues with flavin coenzymes is widespread in developing nations (42, 43). Whether low riboflavin status interacts with iron metabolism to the detriment of hematologic status remains unanswered.

Effects of Excess Dietary Nutrient Intake in Producing Endemic Overnutrition (Nutrient Excess)

Poverty is more likely to produce scarcity than excess. However, a few endemic excessive nutritional states are recognized as unique to specific regions of the developing world, such as African-type hemosiderosis (44) and Indian childhood cirrhosis (45). Excessive iron intake causes the former, but a specific genetic predisposition interacts with the custom of consuming iron-laden home-brewed beer for expression of this iron overload condition (44). Just drinking the beer will not produce the syndrome. Excessive exposure to copper, presumably in the diet because of the use of copper cookware, is the precipitating factor in the juvenile cirrhosis observed in parts of the Indian subcontinent (45); whether any genetic component is involved has not been determined.

Prof. Barry Popkin, a nutritionist and epidemiologist, has characterized a phenomenon associated with demographic transition and globalization that he terms *nutrition transition.* It is defined as a situation in which "problems of under- and overnutrition often coexist, reflecting the trend in which an increasing proportion of people consume the types of diets associated with a number of chronic diseases" (46). It is the irony of the poor and powerless that, when the lowest end of the totem pole is one of scarcity, their lot is undernutrition, but when the bottom of the barrel contains high-energy foods with empty calories, the consequences of their consumption also befalls the lowest social strata.

The 1992 International Conference on Nutrition in Rome (47) yielded enlightening statistics on worldwide obesity in the preschool years. Of the 34 countries included in the analysis, 15 had a rate greater than the 2.7% expected in the standard reference population. These included Italy and Canada in the developed world, and in ascending order of prevalence in the developing world: Zambia, Venezuela, Panama, Peru, Barbados, Honduras, Lesotho, Bolivia, Trinidad-Tobago, Iran, Mauritius, and Jamaica. In the last two nations, the obesity rate for preschoolers was over 10%. Again, insights from Popkin et al. (48) may be relevant. In examining large survey data sets from countries in the developing world, he found that the risk of fatness was highest in persons of shortest stature. As the process of stunting continues apace, but nutritional transition transforms the pattern of diet, overweight may be accentuated in persons of short stature in the developing regions of the world.

Interaction of Dietary Patterns and the Prevention and Promotion of Chronic Diseases

In the context of public health nutrition in developing countries, deficiency and undernutrition have been emphasized to the virtual exclusion of overnutrition, dietary excess, and substances potentially active in preventing chronic diseases. In 1990, the National Research Council published the committee report *Diet and Health: Implications for Chronic Disease* (49). Its 28 chapters contain 5951 references, of which less than 0.2% derive from research or observations in developing countries. Either research performed in the Third World was ignored as irrelevant to conclusions for U.S. populations, or there is a paucity of dietary and disease research on these issues from developing societies; the latter is more likely.

The falling of trade barriers will allow a major influx of Western processed foods, bringing a very different macronutrient balance to less-institutional countries. The effect of drastic and dramatic changes in the nature of foods and food patterns, especially in individuals who began life in the setting of poverty and scarcity, is of concern. The "virginal" nature of some populations relative to both the dietary and environmental risk factors of chronic diseases provides a unique setting to verify theories about the multifactorial determination of degenerative conditions. Are the same dietary correlates for diabetes and hypertension found in Bangkok as in Boston, in Singapore as in Salzburg?

The "diet and disease" paradigm, however, should be broadened beyond *chronic* disease to include acute illnesses as well. The work of Fawzi et al. (50, 51) in the Sudan is seminal. In this study, involving a randomized trial of retinyl palmitate or placebo, the chemically pure vitamin had no effect on diarrheal or respiratory disease risk or mortality, but the patterns of the underlying diets were strong predictors of well-being and survival.

Prophylactic and Remedial Public Health Interventions

Just as clinical nutrition goes beyond description and diagnosis to therapy, public health nutrition is concerned with interventions at the population level that promote adequate nutrition. For vitamin A, a primary issue is delivering more of the vitamin to populations with endemic hypovitaminosis A. A strictly food-based strategy is limited by poverty. The major sources of the vitamin are edible plants, and the efficiency of conversion of provitamin A in foods to the active vitamin has probably been overestimated (52, 53). Fortification of a common vehicle, such as sugar, with vitamin A is practiced in Central America with promising results.

Periodic supplementation of vitamin A, either in special "campaigns" or as part of the routine immunization series, has been advocated to break the cycle of marginal vitamin A deficiency and child mortality (54, 55). The younger the child, the lower the apparent benefit and the greater the risk of adverse reactions and consequences. Simultaneous vitamin A administration may interfere with developing immunity with some vaccines. Supplementation of the lactating *mother* can potentially enhance the vitamin A intake during the first 6 months of life (56).

Public health delivery has focused on two modalities: fortification and supplementation. Some of the adverse characteristics of inorganic salts, such as metallic taste, oxidation of food, and poor absorption, may be eliminated by the iron chelate iron-sodium EDTA, which can be added to table sugar (57). Pregnant women usually receive high-dose iron supplements. Compliance is a problem due to intolerance. Several approaches exist: the "gastric delivery system," in which the ferrous salt is combined with a hydrocolloid matrix that dissolves after ingestion and floats on the gastric contents (58), and weekly—rather than daily—prescription of two or three times the usual daily dose (59). In areas endemic for hookworm infections, antihelminthic treatment may complement iron-folate tablets to control anemia (60).

Most authorities feel that universal iodization of salt would be a panacea, eliminating IDD throughout the world. However, the will to enforce fortification laws is often absent. Alternatives to salt fortification include placing iodine in water or fertilizers and either injecting iodine intramuscularly or administering it orally. The role of chemical goitrogens in goitrogenesis is still not clear. The effect of some goitrogens can be overcome competitively by additional iodine, but those that are noncompetitive can produce goiter regardless of the level of iodine intake.

Environmental pollution may play an important role in nutritional health and in the interaction of diet and health (19). Some elements of contamination that influence nutrition are both well known and relatively constant. Some agents that have traditionally been absent are now increasing. Some agents are common to ecosystems in industrialized nations, whereas others are uniquely endemic to tropical, developing regions.

Breast-feeding and its relationship to complementary weaning foods represent a public health concern, especially in developing countries in which early and improper artificial feeding can prejudice both health and nutritional status. The WHO recommends exclusive breast-feeding for 4 to 6 months. When exclusive breast-feeding ends, weaning begins. The timing (when), content (what), and pattern (how) of complementary feeding have occupied the attention of scientists, technologists, and public health professionals. The age at which weaning begins has always been multifactorial. It is generally believed that in more traditional times, a community consensus based on cultural norms governed the transition from the breast or bottle to nonliquid foods. Factors such as family composition, religion, household income, use of health services, mother's age, parental literacy, and maternal work outside the home clearly influence the age at which complementary foods are introduced (61). These foods consist both of items especially concocted for the weanling, such as gruels and porridges, and scaled-down versions of the adult diet. Issues of microbiologic safety, nutrient content, and nutrient density are predominant concerns (62). The bulkiness in terms of fibrous matrix or hydration of adult foods often means that the infant cannot consume sufficient volume to meet his or her macro- and micronutrient needs. Two strategies—more frequent feedings or greater nutrient density—are debated as programmatic options (63).

Finally, however, some nutritional public health concerns in affluent countries may *not* be reflected in developing countries. A case in point is increased folic acid intake and prevention of spina bifida and neural tube defects in the developing fetus. In the United States, a call has been made to increase folic acid intakes (64). The genetic makeup of nonwhite ethnic groups may make them less susceptible to poor folate transport to the fetus, making the ambient folic acid intake sufficiently protective.

BASIC NUTRITION

Nutritional Biology, Biochemistry, and Physiology

The basic biology of nutrition advanced along the lines of nutritional biochemistry (i.e., the chemistry of the nutrients) until the date of publication of the previous edition of *MNHD*. Since then, the decade of progress in molecular biology and biotechnology has caught on in the nutritional sciences. Prof. Ed Harris (65), commenting on the differential display polymerase chain reaction (PCR) technique, stated: "A missing dietary component can leave an indelible mark on biologic systems, such as a failed enzyme or an impaired physiologic function. Today, nutrition science has a new tool for spotting effects caused by missing nutrients. [It can be] put to the task of examining which genes are and which are not being expressed." Important fruits of genetic probes have been insights into the cellular regulation of nutrient metabolism. The iron regulatory element is a mechanism at the level of the messenger RNA for proteins, specifically ferritin and membrane transferrin receptors, which themselves regulate the systemic and cellular metabolism of iron (66, 67). A metal regulatory element that involves zinc regulates metallothionein expression (68). "Zinc finger" proteins, dependent on adequate zinc status of the host, are a class of transcriptional modifiers, with over 100 thus far identified in the human genome. Some act to regulate transcription whereas others serve as nuclear membrane receptors for steroid and thyroid hormones (67). When a pathway is regulated, the tools to uncover how the information is transmitted are available to the nutritionist. Animal models with dietary manipulation represent the current locus of nutritional molecular biology. At the level of human research, Third World populations may come into play because of the spontaneous occurrence of deficiency states.

The same technology has brought the interaction of nutrients into the regulation and metabolism of individual cells. The acute-phase response (APR) to injury, a complex component of the immune response, is responsible for a catabolic nutritional response (69). That the APR is relevant to populations in developing countries is evident from the high incidence of microbial contamination of the environment and recurrent infections. The APR is mediated by hormones known as "cytokines," produced by monocytes and tissue macrophages. How nutrients influence cytokine production and activity is an important new vista (70). What basic biology may contribute to nutrition in poor countries is an understanding of how nutritional status influences the acute-phase response.

A third example of basic biology is the inquiry into free radicals and oxygen-reactive species (71, 72). Nutrients are involved both in oxidation and free-radical generation (Cu, Fe) and in antioxidant protection and free-radical quenching (carotenoids, tocopherol, ascorbic acid, Mn, Zn, Cu). The issue is the balance between free-radical generation and their control (73). How cellular hydration and metabolism are influenced by the balance between oxidative and antioxidant actions is an important consideration for developing country populations, as the additional stresses of infection and microbial contamination are superimposed. A challenge to basic nutritional science with profound implications for developing countries is the linkage from systemic to cellular levels of the immune response and oxidative processes.

The topic of biomarkers is a final area of basic science development with profound, medium-term ramifications for developing countries. Since the final, pathologic outcomes in chronic disease, morbidity and mortality are prolonged in their evolution, epidemiologists seek to measure the earliest changes that herald eventual illness. These are called biomarkers. As discussed, the role of chronic disease in the profile of Third World pathology is increasing. Linking advances in biomarker identification to the demographic transition carries the potential for predicting and monitoring the emergence of chronic diseases that are not yet seen as endemic in regions of the developing world.

Normative Human Nutrition

Normative human nutrition relates to free-living populations without nutritional disease or other forms of pathology. Whereas the *principles* of nutritional science are universal, the *prescriptions* may not be universal or general, and what is prudent for affluent nations may not be so for poor populations. This may find its validation in the area of nutrient requirements.

One area in which prescriptions from one region may not be applicable to another is that of recommended dietary intakes. Recommended nutrient intakes have traditionally been linked to nutrient requirements. While nutrient requirements have been touted as universal for all people—at least this is the message of the recommendations of the UN agencies (74, 75)—what is probably correct, within certain limits, is that the effect on pool size or tissue reserves of a given nutrient intake is similar from population to population. To the extent that environmental stressors cause wastage and poor utilization of nutrients, more than the usual amounts of the nutrients may be needed in tissues. However, the circumstances of genetic constitution and environmental conditions set up a tradeoff situation in developing countries.

Adaptation is the concept that has been lost in the equations for analysis of nutritional recommendations

(76). This concept has been discussed with respect to trace elements (77). "We must confront the nutritionally heretical hypothesis that sometimes lower intakes or stores of nutrients are adaptively favorable for the species in process of evolution." Weinberg (78) introduced the concept of "nutritional immunity," based on an antagonistic interaction of malnutrition and infection. Especially, with iron (but also with other trace elements), deprivation of the mineral blunts proliferation of intracellular pathogens. Selenium deficiency retards *Salmonella* infections, and a low antioxidant state may reduce the parasitemia of malaria by causing infected host red cells to collapse.

Adaptive responses apply not only to trace elements and vitamins but to macronutrients as well. Nutritionists and biological anthropologists tend to diverge. Whereas the former see growth as the end, the latter see growth as the means to the end (76, 79). When being smaller is adaptive, nutritional deficiency may mediate modulation of size. A classic quandary is the issue of promoting in utero growth for babies in wombs of small mothers. Low birth weight has recognized adverse implications for survival, health, and development of infants (80). On the other hand, fetal-pelvic disproportion can lead to obstetric complications difficult for traditional midwives to resolve. In summary, recommended intakes might be better set to maximize the adaptation to group survival than to achieve a given size, tissue concentration, or body store.

The relations of body composition, nutrition, and health is an important area. Traditionally, such physical measurements of the body as height, weight, skinfold thickness, and circumferences have been the tools of body composition assessment. New models for the levels of composition of the body from that of its elements to that of its organs are important to body composition evaluation. Change in the "quality" of lean tissue may be a marker for ill health (81). A host of tools—isotope dilution, multifrequency bioelectric impedance spectroscopy, imaging techniques, and in vivo neutron activation—are being developed. The former two approaches have already been applied in developing countries to move assessment of body composition beyond anthropometry (82). Two imaging techniques may eventually make assessment of nutritional anemia a matter of noninvasive imaging. The *Erlangen* microlight-guided photometer (EMPHO) technology, from Germany, has already been explored in Indonesia to provide a functional index of oxygen transport (83). Magnetic resonance imaging (MRI) can differentiate metals in vivo, and it is a matter of time before iron reserves can be determined by this form of diagnostic radiology. Metal concentrations in other tissues may likely also be accessible by MRI.

The effect of aging is an aspect of normative nutrition. It is latent in developing countries in which 5% or less of the population is over 60 years of age. The elderly in the Third World, born in 1938 or before, are survivors from an era of high infant mortality rates; they have endured pestilence and famine and have witnessed major social and political changes, such as decolonization of their nations. Much is to be learned about what is intrinsic senescence (chronobiology) and what is an accumulation of insult (pathology). Comparative study of elderly from different regions may well provide insight into this issue. This process has begun to embrace preindustrialized and emerging nations in large multicenter studies (84, 85).

CLINICAL NUTRITION

It is appropriate, given limited resources and widespread and endemic diseases, that the dominant strategy in developing countries has been at the public health level. Nonetheless, individuals contract exotic diseases or show severe manifestations of common diseases. More than its relationship to disease, I view clinical nutrition as a process based on the interaction between an individual and a health practitioner. The aforementioned resource constraints have produced a dearth of hospitals, a paucity of physicians trained in clinical nutrition, and a shortage of diagnostic and therapeutic modalities. For this reason, the focus of *MNHD* must be linked with the health circumstances of the vast majority of the world's population. Following the outline in Table 107.1, we can examine priority loci for this interfacing.

Effect of Patients' Disease on Induction of Nutritional Deficiency

Many of the diseases discussed in detail in *MNHD* are rare or nonexistent in developing countries because they are genetically linked to European ancestry, they occur in extreme age, or they are related to a lavish and affluent lifestyle. Some diseases such as cancer, renal disease, tuberculosis, and AIDS are found in both developed and developing countries. But many diseases that come to a physician's attention in the Third World have not been discussed in detail in the present volume of *MNHD*.

For those diseases that are universal, both north and south, some factors in Table 107.2 intercede to differentiate the situation. Different dietary patterns and ethnic makeup may precipitate or protect against the collapse of adequate nutriture in the face of acute and chronic infirmities. Diseases specific to tropic regions are a matter for research, either library inquiry or direct clinical studies with patients.

Effect of Patients' Disease on Induction of Nutritional Excesses

In industrialized nations, clinical entities such as Prader-Willi syndrome and acromegaly would cause excess accumulation of tissue. Wilson's disease, a hereditary disturbance of copper storage, and hemochromatosis are also rare outside European populations. The ethnic makeup and associated genetic constitution in developing nations make the specific aforementioned entities and others of their class rare to nonexistent. Only by careful prospective research might pathologic conditions that lead to nutrient accumulations in nonwhite populations be identified. We would tentatively conclude, however, that this issue is of disproportionately greater concern in the north than in the south.

Effect of Imbalances of Individual's Nutrient Intake and Use in Producing Clinical Deficiency States

As noted, nutrient deficiency has been the obsessive concern of nutritionists in developing countries, but only in the *public health* context. In clinical contact with health practitioners, individual deficiencies may be identified in consulting individuals. Such recognition calls for therapy, and the practitioner must then decide whether "general" factors for endemicity are at play or more specific and exotic causes are present. Anorexia nervosa and fear-of-food syndromes (86) are recognized causes of weight loss and marasmus. With a "westernization" of culture, especially in urban areas, such psychogenic eating disorders may emerge in developing countries. Diets that are essentially vegetarian (vegan) in composition are a consequence of poverty, religious practice, or both. Consequences such as macrocytic anemia may result.

Aside from the aforementioned psychogenic or culturally based causes of undereating, the appearance in one's office of patients with specific nutrient deficiencies should be viewed by the medical practitioner as a potential warning. Occasional abnormal cases of clinical deficiency imply the existence of a potentially vast submerged problem at the preclinical, endemic stage.

Effect of Imbalances of Individual's Nutrient Intake and Use in Producing States of Overnutrition

In Western nations, obesity—rather than underweight—is the major issue of primary malnutrition. If indeed, as noted above, short stature is a factor for obesity in urban settings, practitioners should begin seeing overweight and obese patients in increasing numbers in developing countries. Moreover, the iron (44) and copper (45) overload conditions mentioned above have environmental causes, but practically speaking, the solution is in case finding and treatment in the clinical context.

NUTRITIONAL AND DIETARY THERAPEUTICS

In earlier editions of this textbook, *MNHD* was subtitled "Dietotherapy," which implied the modification of diet as an adjunct in treatment of diseases. That dietary prescription is an essential feature of overall therapy in clinical medicine can be proven from a litany of conditions common in affluent nations: diabetes mellitus, chronic renal insufficiency, hypertension, obesity, allergy, and peptic disease. In the area of therapeutics, the question of whether the prescriptions for affluent countries are *feasible* or *prudent* for less-industrial countries, is joined.

Feasibility and Prudence

The *feasibility* of concocting diets as a prescription for the aforementioned conditions in most developing societies is high. The required tolerances for sodium, carbohydrates, protein, stimulant substances, liquid volume, and total energy can be achieved with almost any combination of regional foods. In fact, the traditional rural diets in most regions of the world are closer to those prescribed in industrialized countries for all of the mentioned conditions—with the exception of those for allergies and peptic diseases—than is the usual fare of affluent societies. What is needed for precise adjustments is an understanding of local cuisines and data on their nutrient and chemical composition. In the latter respect, modern data on food composition are often lacking for diets in developing countries. An initiative of the United Nations University's Food and Nutrition Programme, called INFOODS, has been working to create or update food composition data on regional diets throughout the world.

In terms of *prudence* in prescribing therapeutic diets based on Western medical practices, the differences between regions (Table 107.2) are influential. The situation of the nutritional management of a patient with a malignant tumor is illustrative. Much has been written recently about whether to deprive the tumor of certain nutrients, at the risk of undernutrition to the host, or whether to counteract the effects of the tumor on host nutrition with compensatory nutrition (87). The former option is relevant when modern chemotherapy is being brought to bear on malignancies, and a short-term nutrient deficit for the host might be a reasonable tradeoff to allow a remission. When aggressive palliative or curative therapy is not available, as is the situation for most cancer patients in low-income nations, then supporting the nutrition of the patient—irrespective of its proliferative effect on the tumor—would be the situational option.

Nutritional and dietary therapy for AIDS is another illustration. In recent years, in North America and Europe, combined antiviral therapy has extended survival and improved the quality-of-life of persons infected with HIV. The logistics and expense involved in antiviral therapy limit its accessibility to AIDS patients in developing countries. Malnutrition is a major mediator and predictor of death from AIDS (88). Another interesting therapeutic aspect of AIDS management relating to nutrients is the report that vertical transmission of the virus in pregnant, seropositive women can be attenuated by supplementation with vitamin A (89).

Parenteral and Enteral Nutrition

Use of parenteral and enteral nutrition in nutritional therapy is fraught with difficulties. The nutritive solutions for both modalities can either be created from primary materials in hospital pharmacies or be purchased from commercial pharmaceutical houses. The high cost of commercial purchase limits this source of parenteral and enteral solutions. This raises the temptation to attempt individualized production of media for artificial nutrition in the kitchens and pharmacies of local healthcare facilities in developing countries.

A sensible aphorism is "If the gut works, use it." Hence, when either parenteral or enteral approaches could be used in a patient's situation, the latter is the practical option for reasons of both physiology and safety. Enteral nutrition can be less safe where resources are scarce. Scarcity may begin with the nonavailability of appropriate low-irritant, small-bore feeding tubes or with the difficulty of maintaining tubes securely in place via the nasal and percutaneous (gastroscopy, jejunostomy) routes that permit long-term enteral feeding. Formulation of enteral fluids should minimize cost, minimize osmolarity, provide adequate macro- and micronutrient nutrition, and respond to the digestive and absorptive capabilities of specific patients. For this reason, formulations from elemental to polymeric to liquified food exist in the pharmaceutical marketplace. When made in dietary kitchens of individual hospitals, quality control from osmolarity to nutrient balance can become an issue. Milk powder as the protein base may be inappropriate in most Africa and Asian countries because of the high prevalence of lactase nonpersistence (90, 91). Moreover, bacterial contamination increases with the amount of time the bags or bottles of liquid formula are left hanging. In hot, humid, and contaminated environments, microbiologic safety is even more rapidly compromised. In developing countries, the solution is encouraging local or regional commercialization of low-cost, high-quality, *prepackaged* products that can be fed orally or by tube.

When the gut does not work, the parenteral route is sought. In TPN, all nutrients are delivered by large-bore intravenous catheters into central veins. This approach magnifies the limitations discussed for the enteral route. The products are more expensive per calorie delivered; the premium on sterility and antisepsis is much higher; the paraphernalia for administration are expensive and uncommon; and the appropriate osmolarity and nutrient and electrolyte composition are critical. It is tempting to use parenteral nutrition in common situations such as protein-energy malnutrition (PEM) and persistent diarrhea. Experience with TPN in PEM has produced disastrous results (92), and most cases of kwashiorkor and marasmus can be managed much better by oral and tube feeding (93). Experience in noninvestigative settings in persistent diarrhea is not well characterized.

Oral Rehydration Therapy

Clinical nutritionists in developing countries must recognize that managing infantile diarrheal disease is more than just using fluids to replete and maintain the fluid and electrolyte balance until the purging subsides. Issues of *nutritive* feedings during the episode are important. Both conventional and folk wisdom often recommend "starving" the diarrhea. Without oral intake, there would be little fecal output. Modern concepts of the pathophysiology of secretory and invasive diarrheas give no credence to this notion.

Conventional oral rehydration solution (ORS) based on glucose and salts provides only 80 kcal of metabolizable energy per liter. This falls far short of meeting the basal energy needs of the small child or the superimposed stress of infection in a diarrheal episode. Brown (94) has reviewed the concepts behind introducing semisolids and solid foods early in the course of treatment and the progress that has been made in producing hypercaloric diets based on rice or other cereals as the source of glucose to promote absorption of fluids for rehydration. These prevalences have advantages both in lowering osmolalities and in protecting the general nutriture. Indeed, there might be something unique about rice as a carbohydrate source. Recently, Macleod et al. (95) isolated a low-molecular-weight antisecretory substance in extracts of rice that actively inhibits chloride secretion by blocking cyclic AMP channels. Such substances may provide the mechanistic basis of the positive effects of rice-based oral rehydration solutions on childhood diarrhea. Finally, micronutrients (specifically, zinc) added to ORS may also reduce the rate of fluid secretion and speed recovery in secretory diarrheal episodes (96).

DISCIPLINARY ORGANIZATION AND PROFESSIONAL TRAINING IN NUTRITION

For nutritional science and practice to progress in developing countries, the local nutritional communities and their constituent professionals must have the tools to guide such progress. Specifically, with respect to the perceived needs of low-income populations, debate has arisen about what format for professional training should be emphasized and what type of professional produced in the area of nutrition. It is a most timely discussion.

The Western academic model has been experienced by many contemporary faculty leaders from low-income countries, who have subsequently devised curricula modeled on the nutritional training in *developed* countries. Dietetics and public health epidemiology applied to nutrition are prominent in these curricula. Indeed, this combination is often offered under the title "community nutrition." Laboratory research and clinical nutrition are represented to a lesser extent. All of these diverse components, however, are based on nutritional biology, quantitative analysis, or both.

Nutritional Engineers and Public Nutrition

The first salvo of a reconsideration came from Alan Berg in 1993 (97). In an indictment of the present direction of training and investment in nutritional research in, and for, developing countries entitled "Sliding towards Nutritional Malpractice. Time to Reconsider and Redeploy," he called for creation of "nutritional engineers." He argued that the balance between research and applied investment had been overly shifted toward the former. A sector of opinion went so far as to assert that all of the knowledge needed to alleviate and eradicate undernutrition problems afflicting the Third World had already been gathered (98, 99). The same individuals later met in Bellagio, Italy, where they forged a programmatic definition for a "new" discipline of training and professional development in nutrition in developing societies (100). Programs in "Public Nutrition" have emerged as the suggested focus for training nutritional professionals in and for developing countries (101). The main argument is to drop "health" from the title and reach beyond the academic forum of nutrition departments in schools of public health or tropical medicine and hygiene.

A central premise of this new program is that nutrition goes beyond the biologic and health issues. Agricultural production, distribution of the food supply, and aspects of food security are consistently prominent. Advocacy and mobilization of opinion for change is a major role of the new public nutritionist. Breadth (rather than depth) and application (rather than inquiry) should be the tenets of training and of the professional mission. In my opinion, this discussion merits continuation.

Nonetheless, I see a danger in the margination of the health focus of nutrition and its fundamental scientific underpinnings with an excessive broadening and diffusion of the scope. What this chapter demonstrates, however, is how neglected the clinical and biologic aspects of nutrition for developing country populations have been. An exclusive focus on *under*nutrition, as populations are urbanizing and undergoing nutrition transition, is not without peril, as one can miss the already manifest health problems derived from nutrient excess and overload. The fact that undernutrition in early life may condition susceptibility to chronic disease in later life is another reason to broaden the focus beyond one strictly adhering to macro- and micronutrient *deficits*. Thus, whether it is in the context of a new program or in the present format of training, it is urgent to strengthen the ability of professionals serving low-income countries to adapt to, and to adopt, modern clinical nutrition. Grounding in the scientific method, a fund of basic nutritional biology, and experience in research activities are as vital to the progress of clinical nutrition in developing nations as they are in more affluent ones.

New Realities in Nutrition and Health Care

When it comes to applied nutrition, many public health nutritionists have been laboring with a model of action that is somewhat a relic of the past. The current "working" model for intervention features both a postulated universal common solution and the presumed need for a highly centralized administration. National ministries of health had prevailed as the exclusive loci for action on health initiatives; they envision investing public funds into operations conducted by public servants of the central governments. For crop and food initiatives, a similar model existed, centralized in ministries of agriculture. Coordination and logistical support from U.N. or bilateral sources was part of the model.

The phenomenon of economic structural readjustment has rendered such centralized and concerted actions somewhat unrealistic and obsolete. With disincorporation of state projects and decentralization of resources and responsibilities, modalities such as private insurance, fee-for-service, and nongovernmental organizations become part of a mosaic for nutritional action in developing countries. These *new* realities point to clinical nutrition and therapeutics as an important part of the emerging picture and lead to the diametrically opposite conclusion of those (98, 99) who would place a moratorium on research in and for the Third World.

CONCLUSION

It is said that armies are always trained and equipped to fight the *last* war. If we can extend this metaphor to the science of nutrition, in both its investigative and applied facets, nutrition for the developing countries may be based on past realities that have ceased to be true or that were false perceptions that were never really valid.

There is only one humanity and only one nutritional biology. Progress in relieving suffering and maximizing human and social development is tied to the extent to which nutritional science is brought to bear on the problems in low-income nations. Past nutritional activities have been expressed primarily in public health and epidemiologic terms; most research publications reflect this context. While population diagnosis and collective prevention and redress will remain important, differentiation of individual health problems and recognition of disease in the clinical setting make clinical nutrition and therapeutics an increasingly important focus for developing and transitional nations.

The advances in basic biology provide tools to unlock new information relating nutrition to health and disease. This is true in both the north and the south. The principles and lessons in clinical nutrition in this textbook are universal and relevant across the globe. But, populations in the world possess much genetic polymorphism, great variety in dietary habits, and substantial diversity in disease patterns, and most of this diversity is expressed in the 70% of the earth's population living in low-income countries. This diversity is truly a challenge, as it makes populations in developing countries different from the reference groups in affluent nations upon which many diagnostic and therapeutic norms are based. Clearly, much work needs to be done to adapt modern nutritional concepts and the insights of clinical nutritional research and service to the needs of the developing world.

REFERENCES

1. Solomons NW. Am J Clin Nutr 1994;60:643–4.
2. National Research Council. World food and nutrition study. Washington, DC: National Academy of Sciences Press, 1977.
3. Payne PR. Proc Nutr Soc 1979;38:207–11.
4 Zeitlin M, Ghassemi H, Mansour M. Positive deviance in child nutrition. Tokyo: UNU Press, 1990.
5. Cordano A, Graham GG. Pediatrics 1964;34:324–6.
6. Dunlap WM, James GW III, Hume DM. Ann Intern Med 1974;80:470–6.
7. Vilter RW, Bozian RC, Hess EV, et al. N Engl J Med 1974; 291:188–91.
8. Johnson RA, Baker SS, Fallon JT, et al. N Engl J Med 1981;384;1210–2.
9. Kien CL, Ganther HE. Am J Clin Nutr 1983;37:319–28.
10. Payne PR. Am J Clin Nutr 1975;28:281–6.
11. Ashworth A, Draper A. The potential of traditional technologies for increasing the energy density of weaning foods. Geneva: World Health Organization, 1992.
12. Calloway DH, Murphy S, Balderston J, et al. Functional implications of malnutrition. Village nutrition in Egypt, Kenya, and Mexico: Looking across the CRSP Project. Human Nutrition Collaborative Research Support Program (final report). University of California at Berkeley, 1992.
13. Sommer A, Tarwojto I, Djunaedi E, et al. Lancet 1986;1: 1169–72.
14. Scrimshaw NS. Food Nutr Bull 1994;15:3–24.
15. Scrimshaw NS, Taylor CE, Gordon JE. Interaction of nutrition and infection. WHO Monogr Ser no. 57. Geneva: WHO, 1968.
16. Walsh JA. Estimating the burden of illness in the tropics. In: Warren KS, Mahmoud AAF, eds. Tropical and geographic medicine. 1st ed. New York: McGraw-Hill, 1984;1073–85.
17. Tomkins A. Malnutrition and risk of infection. In: Wahlqvist ML, Truswell AS, Smith R, Nestel PJ, eds. Nutrition in a sustainable environment. Proc XV Int Cong Nutr. London: Smith-Gordon, 1994;655–8.
18. Solomons NW, Mazariegos M, Brown KH, et al. Nutr Rev 1993;51:327–32.
19. Rerat AA. Nutrition, food and the environment. In: Wahlqvist ML, Truswell AS, Smith R, Nestel PJ, eds. Nutrition in a sustainable environment. Proc XV Int Cong Nutr. London: Smith-Gordon, 1994;1–16.
20. Sommer A, West KP Jr. Vitamin A deficiency: health, survival, and vision. Oxford: Oxford University Press, 1996.
21. Underwood BA. Nutr Rev 1994;52:140–2.
22. Binka FN, Ross DA, Morris SS, et al. Am J Clin Nutr 1996;63:61:853–9.
23. Kirkwood BR, Ross DA, Arthur P, et al. Am J Clin Nutr 1996;63:773–81.
24. Ramakrishanan U, Latham MC, Abel R, et al. J Nutr 1995;125:202–12.
25. Rahman MM, Mahalanabis D, Wahed MA, et al. J Nutr 1995;125:1869–74.
26. Fuchs GJ, Ausayakhun S, Ruckphaopunt S, et al. Am J Clin Nutr 1994;60:293–8.
27. Tanumihardjo SA, Permaesih D, Dahro AM, et al. Am J Clin Nutr 1994;60:136–41.
28. Tanumihardjo SA, Muherdiyantiningsih, Permaesih D, et al. Am J Clin Nutr 1994;60:142–7.
29. World Health Organization/UNICEF. Indicators for assessing vitamin A deficiency and their application in monitoring and evaluating intervention programmes. Geneva: World Health Organization, 1996;45–56.
30. Yip R. J Nutr 1994;124:1279S–90S.
31. Lawless JW, Latham MC, Stephenson LS, et al. J Nutr 1994;124:645–54.
32. Idjradinata P, Watkins W, Pollitt E. Lancet 1993;341:1–4.
33. Kuvibidila S, Yu LC, Ode DL, et al. Am J Clin Nutr 1994;60:603–9.
34. Hetzel BS, Dunn JT, Stanbury JB, eds. The prevention and control of iodine deficiency disorders. Amsterdam: Elsevier Science Publishers, 1987.
35. Tiwari BD, Godbole MM, Chattapadhyuy N, et al. Am J Clin Nutr 1996;63:782–91.
36 Furnee CA, van der Haar F, West CE, et al. Am J Clin Nutr 1994;59:1415–7.
37. Shrimpton R. SCN News 1992;9;24–7.
38. Brown KH. Proc Nutr Soc 1997;56:139–48.
39. Ruel MT, Rivera J, Brown K, et al. (Abstract 917) FASEB J 1995;9:A157.
40. Rosado JL, Allen LH, Lopez P, et al. (Abstract 918) FASEB J 1995;9:A157.
41. Allen LH, Rosado JL, Casterline JE, et al. Am J Clin Nutr 1995;62:1013–9.
42. Bates CJ, Powers HJ, Downes R, et al. Am J Clin Nutr 1989;50:825–9.
43. Boisvert WA, Castañeda C, Mendoza I, et al. Am J Clin Nutr 1993;58:85–90.
44. Gordeuk V, Mikiibi J, Hestedt SJ, et al. N Engl J Med 1992;326;95–100.
45. Bhave SA. J Pediatr Gastroenterol Nutr 1987;6:562–7.
46. Popkin B. Nutr Rev 1994;52:285–98.
47. Food and Agriculture Organization/World Health Organization. International conference on nutrition. Rome: FAO, 1992.
48. Popkin B, Richards MK, Montieno CA. J Nutr 1996;126: 3009–16.
49. National Research Council. Diet and health: implications for chronic disease risk. Washington, DC: National Academy Sciences Press, 1990.
50. Fawzi WW, Herrera MG, Willett WC, et al. Am J Clin Nutr 1994;59:401–8.
51. Fawzi WW, Herrera MG, Willett WC, et al. J Nutr 1995;125:1211–21.
52. Solomons NW, Bulux J. Nutr Rev 1994;52:62–4.
53. de Pee S, West CE, Muhilal, et al. Lancet 1995;346:75–81.
54. Humphrey JH, West KP Jr, Muhilal, et al. J Nutr 1993;123: 1363–9.
55. Humphrey JH, Natadisastra G, Muhilal, et al. J Nutr 1994;124: 1172–8.
56. Stoltzfus RJ, Hakimi M, Miller KW, et al. J Nutr 1993;123: 666–75.
57. Viteri FE, Alvarez E, Batres R, et al. Am J Clin Nutr 1995;61:1153–63.
58. Ekström E-CM, Kavishe FW, Habicht J-P, et al. Am J Clin Nutr 64:368–74.
59. Viteri FE. Int Child Health 1995;6:49–61.
60. Adams EJ, Stephenson LS, Latham MC, et al. J Nutr 1994;124:1199–206.
61. Subbulakshmi G, Udipi SA. Food Nutr Bull 1990;12:318–22.
62. Desikachar HSR. Food Nutr Bull 1982;4:57–9.
63. Brown KB, Creed-Kanashiro H, Dewey KG. Food Nutr Bull 1995;16:320–9.
64. Centers for Disease Control and Prevention. Recommendations for the use of folic acid to reduce the number of cases of spina bifida and other neural tube defects. MMWR 1992;41:1–7.
65. Harris ED. Nutr Rev 1996;54:287–9.

66. Uchida T. Int J Hematol 1995;62:193–202.
67. Chesters JK. Nutr Rev 1992;50:217–23.
68. Cousins RJ. Annu Rev Nutr 1994;14:449–69.
69. Keusch GT, Farthing MJG. Annu Rev Nutr 1986;6:131–54.
70. Grimble GK. Eur J Clin Nutr 1991;45:413–7.
71. Halliwell B, Gutteridge JMC, Cross CE, et al. J Lab Clin Med 1992;119:598–620.
72. Nutritional immunomodulation in disease and health promotion. Report of the 15th Ross conference on medical research. Columbus, OH: Ross Products Division, Abbott Laboratories, 1996.
73. Fürst P, Stehle P. Parenteral nutrition substrates. In: Payne-James JJ, Grimble GK, Silk DBA, eds. Artificial nutrition in clinical practice. London: Arnold Publishers, 1994;301–22.
74. World Health Organization/Food and Agriculture Organization/ United Nations University. Protein and energy requirements. Geneva: WHO, 1985.
75. World Health Organization. Trace elements in human health and nutrition. Geneva: WHO, 1996.
76. Frisancho AR, ed. Human adaptation and accommodation. Ann Arbor: University of Michigan Press, 1996.
77. Solomons NW. Social environmental and biological bases of trace element 'deficiencies' in underprivileged populations. In: Wahlqvist ML, Truswell AS, Smith R, Nestel PJ, eds. Nutrition in a sustainable environment. Proc XV Int Cong Nutr. London: Smith-Gordon, 1994;292–5.
78. Weinberg ED. Physiol Rev 1984;64:65–102.
79. Mascie-Taylor CGN, Bogin B, eds. Human variability and plasticity, Cambridge studies in biological anthropology. Cambridge: Cambridge University Press, 1995.
80. Beaton GH. Eur J Clin Nutr 1989;43:863–75.
81. Pierson RN, Wang J. The quality of lean body mass: implications for clinical medicine. In: Ellis KJ, Yasamura S, Morgan WD, eds. In vivo body comoposition studies. London: IPSM Publication, 1987;123–30.
82. Solomons NW, Mazariegos M. Asia Pac J Clin Nutr 1995;4:19–22.
83. Gross R, Gliwitzki M, Gross P, et al. Food Nutr Bull 1996;17:27–36.
84. Andrews GR, Esterman AS, Braunack-Mayer AJ, Rungie CM. Ageing in the Western Pacific—a four country study. Western Pacific reports and studies no 1. Manila: WHO Regional Office for the Western Pacific, 1986.
85. Wahlqvist ML, Davies L, Hsu-Hage BH-H, et al., eds. Food habits in later life: a cross-cultural approach. Melbourne: United Nations University and Asia Pac J Clin Nutr, 1996.
86. Lifshitz FA. Ann NY Acad Sci 1993;699:230–6.
87. Laviano A, Meguid MM. Nutrition 1996;12:358–71.
88. Kotler D, Tierney AR, Brenner SK, et al. Am J Clin Nutr 1990;51:7–15.
89. Semba RD, Miotti PG, Chiphangwi JD, et al. Lancet 1994;343:1593–7.
90. O'Keefe SJD, O'Keefe EA, Burke E, et al. Am J Clin Nutr 1991;54:130–5.
91. Rosado JL, Morales M, Pasquetti A. JPEN J Parenter Enteral Nutr 1989;13:157–61.
92. Vis HL. Ann Soc Belg Med Trop 1976;56:233–52.
93. Solomons NW, Torún B. Ann Pediatr 1982;11:911–1002.
94. Brown KH. J Nutr 1994;124:1455S–60S.
95. Macleod R, Bennet H, Hamilton J. Lancet 1995;346:90–2.
96. Sazawai S, Black R, Bhan KN, et al. N Engl J Med 1995; 333:839–44.
97. Berg A. Annu Rev Nutr 1993;13:1–15.
98. Jonsson U. Am J Clin Nutr 1993;58:579–80.
99. Grant JP. Halving child malnutrition by the year 2000: an ethical imperative. In: Wahlqvist NL, Truswell AS, Smith R, Nestel PJ, eds. Nutrition in a sustainable environment. Proc XV Int Cong Nutr. London: Smith-Gordon, 1994;xxxi–xli.
100. Overcoming malnutrition: a new global initiative: a Bellagio declaration. SCN News 1995;12:insert.
101. Mason J, Habicht J-P, Greaves J, et al. Am J Clin Nutr 1996;63:399–400.

SELECTED READINGS

Berg A. Sliding toward nutrition malpractice: time to reconsider and deploy. Annu Rev Nutr 1993;13:1–16.

Solomons NW, Gross R. Urban nutrition in developing countries. Nutr Rev 1995;53:90–5.

Sommer A, West KP Jr. Vitamin A deficiency: health, survival, and vision. Oxford: Oxford University Press, 1996.

Wahlquist NL, Truswell AS, Smith R, Nestel PJ, eds. Nutrition in a sustainable environment. London: Smith-Gordon, 1994.

108. Social and Cultural Influences on Food Consumption and Nutritional Status

SARA A. QUANDT

The social sciences' approach to human nutrition complements those of the biologic and physical sciences. The latter approaches have been used in other chapters of this book to describe the biologic mechanisms by which hunger and satiety are regulated in the organism, as well as the nutrient levels required for health and function. Despite a fair degree of uniformity among humans in these regulatory pathways and in nutrient needs, there is considerable variety in *what* humans eat and the extent to which they are *successful* in meeting their nutrient needs. Social sciences focus on these issues.

This chapter describes social and cultural approaches to explaining why people eat what they eat. The goal is to show that understanding the social and cultural aspects of food consumption is critically important if nutritional scientists are to understand why groups of humans differ in nutritional status and how dietary change can be effected to correct problems of under- and overnutrition. Attempts to change dietary habits cannot depend solely on nutrition education. Rather, they must recognize the way dietary habits are embedded in the social structure and culture of groups and design interventions that are culturally appropriate.

This presentation begins by expanding the contrast between nutritional and social science approaches to food consumption and then gives an overview of the theoretical approaches used to study human dietary choices: materialist, ideationist, and social interactionist approaches. Data collection and analysis methods particular to such approaches are briefly summarized. The perspective then changes to an examination of the effects of social and cultural factors on food consumption and nutritional status. Whether social groups are defined at the level of family, social class, or world system, the patterning of these is evident in nutritional measures ranging from dietary quality to obesity to stature.

CONTRASTING NUTRITIONAL AND SOCIAL SCIENCES APPROACHES TO FOOD CONSUMPTION

Humans achieve and regulate their nutritional status by consuming *foods*, substances (vegetable, animal, mineral, or combination) that supply *nutrients*. Although food is composed of nutrients, cognizance of these nutrients and their relationship to health and biologic functioning is neither necessary nor usual. What is—and what is *not*—food is defined socially and culturally. Thus, while some societies consider insects good to eat, others view them with disgust; some societies relegate maize to cattle feed, and others celebrate its harvest as a food for people. Nutritional science and the social sciences differ considerably in their approach to food consumption and the importance they attribute to contrasts such as these. The social science approach goes beyond food to focus on patterning of foods into meals and the meanings (both social and biologic) of such patterning (1–5).

The nutritional approach, which has been dominant in most research on food consumption, views food and eating in relation to the nutrient composition of foods and their instrumental roles in the physiologic functioning of the human body. Eating practices either promote development and function and should be encouraged or they impair these processes and should be discouraged. The nutritional perspective is functionally oriented, viewing food consumption as a means to an end. This perspective makes food habits and preferences secondary to the biologic activity of foods. The social and cultural factors surrounding food consumption become, thus, a barrier to the objectives of nutrition, consumption of a health-promoting diet.

Conceptually, the approach of social scientists (both anthropologists and sociologists of food) is quite different. Anthropologists and sociologists view food consumption as the "completion (most usually) of a culturally appropriate sequence of interpersonal cooking, feeding, and eating, involving social intercourse that leads towards culturally recognized consequences on bodily and mental life" (6). Thus, food consumption is a considerably more complex act than a nutritional/biologic perspective implies. Analytically removing it from social and cultural contexts eliminates the nonbiologic qualities it embodies and transmits to the consumer.

While the anthropologic and sociologic perspectives are not important to understanding the biology of nutrition, they are central to addressing questions that bear on the nutritional status and health of populations: How do food preferences and food habits arise? How do they become established in a society? How are they transmitted and changed? What role do such diverse factors as gender and economics play in determining food consumption patterns? How do the symbolic aspects of food relate to consumption patterns? Why do variations in cultural or social factors correlate with variations in nutritional status?

UNDERSTANDING WHY PEOPLE EAT WHAT THEY EAT: THEORETICAL APPROACHES IN THE SOCIAL SCIENCES

As social and behavioral scientists have studied food consumption, it has become clear that many interconnected factors influence consumption. To help make sense of them, they have been organized into logically connected groups that constitute theoretical approaches. As in any science, the value of these theoretical approaches is in their power to generate predictions and hypotheses concerning food consumption in diverse circumstances, as well as to explain observations. For nutritionists, familiarity with some of the major theoretical approaches can be useful in understanding the causes of food consumption patterns they observe, as well as for predicting the outcome of interventions to change food behavior. Table 108.1 shows these approaches, as well as their key concepts.

Materialist Approaches to Food Consumption

Materialist approaches to food consumption are grounded in cultural ecology theory. Cultural ecology takes a systems approach to food consumption, modeling the interactions of the physical, cultural, and historical environments in producing food consumption patterns. Its focus on the physical environment leads some to classify it as *geographic* (7). Cultural ecology sets food consumption within the broader concept of "foodways." These characterize populations and consist of all information surrounding the ways food is obtained, distributed, and processed, as well as consumed by a particular population (8, 9). Foodways are limited by the resources available within a specific environment. They can be considered adaptive to the extent that they promote health and functioning or maladaptive to the extent they prevent this. The history of maize consumption and deficiency disease provides illustration.

Table 108.1
Theoretical Approaches to Food Consumption

Name	Approach	Key Concepts
Materialism	Interactions of physical, cultural, social, and historical environments predict food consumption	Foodways
Ideationism	Food consumption reflects the way people conceptually organize the world and their social relations	Social order, rules
Social constructionism	Food-related discourse produces subjective knowledge and self-understanding	Subjectivity, power

Katz et al. documented cross-cultural patterns in the techniques used to process maize for human consumption (10). They showed that dependence on maize as a primary staple occurs only when alkali processing techniques are used (e.g., soaking the kernels in lye or a wood ash solution before drying and grinding). Viewed biologically, this process alters the amino acid balance by enhancing the bioavailability of niacin. However, from a cultural standpoint, the importance for the consumer lies in the ability of the altered maize to be satisfactorily shaped into tortillas and other culturally preferred forms.

Katz et al. could find no examples of maize dependence without alkali processing. However, historians of medicine have identified significant health consequences of failure to carry out such processing under conditions in which economic deprivation rendered foods other than maize unavailable. The pellagra epidemic in the southeastern United States in the early 20th century is a case in point (11). Mill workers and tenant farmers who were forced by poverty to subsist on a diet of maize (made palatable by small amounts of salt pork and molasses) had high levels of pellagra as a result of niacin deficiency. Goldberger's studies of pellagra made possible the ecologic analysis, situating the pellagra-inducing food consumption pattern in the economic context of cash-cropping (cotton) in lieu of subsistence cropping (gardening) (12). The cultural ecology analysis of pellagra in the South links food consumption to the socioeconomic environment of social stratification and poverty.

Other food consumption patterns analyzed from the perspective of cultural ecology include such food taboos as the Hindu proscription of beef consumption and the Jewish and Moslem, of pork (13), as well as the prohibition of fish consumption in Africa (14).

Differing somewhat by drawing on world systems theory, but still squarely in the materialist domain is Mintz's analysis of the remarkable increase in British sugar consumption in the 18th and 19th centuries (15). He links the system of indentured servitude on the sugar plantations of the Caribbean to changes in work and income in England. Sugar consumption, he argues, increased not so much because of a desire for sweets, but because of the working class's need for affordable calories.

Despite their utility in placing food consumption in context, materialist approaches have been criticized as overly functional explanations, relying too heavily on an attribution of rationality to human societies and better suited to post hoc explanation than prediction. Other theoretical perspectives focus far less on linking cultural practices to favorable biologic outcomes and center more on how societies *think* about food.

Ideationist Approaches

Rejecting functionalist or economic explanations for food consumption patterns, many anthropologists and sociologists have approached food consumption as a complex set of rules corresponding to the ways people organize their thinking about the world as a whole and reflecting the social interactions in which they engage. Such explanations avoid the pitfalls of teleologic thinking inherent in many materialist analyses, but their tendency to focus on aesthetic aspects of food or mundane details of eating sometimes results in their importance being overlooked by nutritionists.

Mary Douglas's studies of British meal patterns are classic structural analyses connecting the ordering of foods into daily, weekly, and annual cycles with ordering of social systems (16, 17). Based on observations carried out in British households of varying social class, Douglas declared meal consumption to be a ritual activity with rules regulating the order in which foods of different tastes, temperatures, and textures were permitted. Changes to the pattern (e.g., a single food for the evening meal rather than a central meat with starch and vegetable) create disharmony and unease for the participants, challenging their sense of order. From the most basic units of eating—tea and biscuits—Douglas showed how meals are used to symbolize and order social interactions. Principles of inclusion or exclusion and of hierarchy operated. In British households, beverages were shared with strangers and casual acquaintances, in contrast to meals, which were shared with family and close friends. Thus, to be invited into a home for a meal encoded a high degree of affiliation (literal or figurative kinship). To be offered only a drink excluded a guest from this circle and signified a social threshold that the guest had not crossed (16). By maintaining social boundaries, food consumption patterns helped create and reinforce the social order (17). Similar analyses differentiating "proper meals" from snacks and other eating events have been conducted more recently by Murcott (18) in South Wales and by Quandt, Roos, and colleagues in the United States (19, 20). They too found that meals are defined by where and with whom food is eaten, in addition to by what is eaten.

Other ideationist analyses of food consumption patterns point to how the history of a people shapes present eating by providing organizing codes (21). Some show that the past is not so much a blueprint for present eating as a source of symbols or meanings that can be called upon in a somewhat arbitrary way. One example of this is the use of African foods by contemporary African Americans in the U.S. in the context of Kwanzaa to enhance the sense of African heritage and reinforce their separateness from European Americans. Few if any of the African dishes have been retained through time in the Americas. Rather, they have been researched and reintroduced for their symbolic value. Another example is the popularity of large "country" breakfasts in the U.S. Though often consumed in relatively anonymous urban settings, they give the consumers a link to the agrarian past, with its connotations (accurate or not) of family, abundance, and a simpler, easier life. Quandt, Roos, and colleagues have studied older adults in the southeastern U.S. and noted the meanings attached to such meal patterns and the sense of loss often experienced as women living alone shift to a cold, uncooked breakfast (19, 20).

Even within meals, there are rules by which foods are combined or separated. A recent study by Drewnowski demonstrated the cognitive categories within which American adults think about common vegetables (22). Asking subjects to judge the similarity of pairs of vegetables as well as to rate the vegetables along attribute scales (e.g., weak to strong flavored, nutritious to nonnutritious) Drewnowski discovered that adults use the dimensions of calories, color, and convenience to think about vegetables. Vegetable preference is most closely linked to convenience, but compatibility of vegetables is associated with color contrast. Thus, vegetable combinations such as broccoli and cauliflower were more acceptable than broccoli and brussels sprouts.

The ideationist approaches to uncovering the grammar of food consumption patterns show that unwritten rules govern the seemingly mundane, everyday activity of eating. These rules vary from culture to culture, and indeed, they are often maintained by subgroups (e.g., ethnic groups) as a way of creating and reinforcing group identity. Social scientists using ideationist approaches to study food point to the implications this has for attempting dietary change (22). While substitution of one type of food for another might create what more biologically oriented nutritionists would consider a better meal (e.g., replacing meat with fish or vegetables), such a change may be met with resistance because it violates the eater's sense of propriety (23), unless an effort is made to find cognitively acceptable substitutes.

Social Constructionist Approaches

Recently, the analysis of food consumption has shifted to one that views preferences and choices as more fluid, marked by discontinuities and paradoxes. This "social constructionist" approach, like the ideationist approach, recognizes the importance of food as a domain in which individuals define who they are in contrast to others. However, it focuses less on fixed patterns of food use and their reinforcement of social hierarchy and more on the way discourse, the patterning of language and behavior, around food produces meaning for individual consumers. Two concepts stand out in this approach. The first is *subjectivity,* the ways individuals use experiences in their lives to understand themselves. This understanding is flexible, less rigid than "identity," depending on experiences with food and eating over time to create a subjective understanding of oneself. The second concept is *power,* a property that runs through food-related interactions between individuals and groups, creating subjective knowledge and self-understanding. Both these result, among other things, in foods having relationships to gender, to age, and to life histories.

Gendered Foods

Contemporary Western society as well as many non-Western societies has a large body of assumptions about what foods are appropriate for men and what are appropriate for women. Women are expected to like sweets more than men do and to use them to achieve certain ends (e.g., to make children behave [24]). The concept of "light" foods is also used to describe women's foods, so that salads, rather than potatoes, and chicken, rather than red meat, should be consumed (23–25). Bourdieu highlights gender differences in preferences for fish among the working class in France (26). He notes that fish is considered women's food, as it has to be eaten in small mouthfuls, in the front of the mouth rather than the back, and with considerable restraint to avoid bones. Such an eating style is antithetical to the understanding of a male body as powerful and large. Red meat and strong cheeses are considered more manly. By serving these to men and taking only small portions or eating fish or salads herself, women reinforce gender identities in the context of food. Such gender differences in foods are frequently and consistently reported by lay persons. Lupton, for example, surveyed residents of Great Britain and found a consistent association of "lighter" foods for women and "heavier" for men (23).

The notion of gendered foods is borne out in food consumption surveys (27). Women eat more fruit, more sweets, and less meat than men. Men also tend to eat larger quantities and frequently exaggerate their food consumption in surveys, while women underreport theirs.

Such patterns of gendered food ideology and consumption develop in the day-to-day interactions in which people engage. Mealtimes in Western households center on the serving of food, usually by women, in ways that meet expectations of men and children. DeVault in her study of American families documented the "invisible, caring work" women, particularly wives and mothers, do in catering to tastes, preferences, and schedules of family members (28). Hers and numerous other studies have shown that women often subordinated their own preferences to those of men (24, 29–31a). Gittelsohn's detailed observations of intrahousehold food distribution patterns in Nepal extended the concept of gendered food interactions beyond Western cultures (32). He showed that at an early age, girls learn to eat only when served from the common pot, while boys learn to ask for more. As adults, these females eat last after the largest and choicest portions have gone to men and boys.

This pattern of social interactions over food shaping female and males notions of relative power and status is replicated across many cultures. While studies tend to emphasize the normality and uniformity of such interactions, their linkage to gender relations is highlighted in the exceptions, domestic disputes. Several studies of divorced couples and of domestic violence note the role played in precipitating problems by discontinuities between male and female behaviors and expectations related to food. In these studies, women not subordinating their own tastes to husbands' or not preparing foods as expected evoked violence on the part of husbands (33, 34).

The social interactions surrounding food and the way that notions of gender are conveyed through them have been linked in Western society to the preponderance of eating disorders in women, compared with men. Susan Bordo argues that Western culture demands self-control for all adults, but especially for women. Girls learn this through interactions concerning food and its relationship to their body shape from an early age. Bordo contends that their bodies come to symbolize the arena in which control must be maintained, and women who are not thin embody a lack of self-control. Self-starvation gives women a strategy for establishing control of the feminine emotions and appetites (35).

Age-Appropriate Foods

The domain of food is also used to differentiate age groups. Several studies have examined the interaction of parents and adolescents over food and the way adolescents use this interaction to declare their independence. Although many dictums about feeding children have changed (e.g., forcing children to clean their plates is now recognized as creating the potential for overeating in adulthood), parents in Western societies are still expected to control their children's food intake. Through the discourse surrounding this control, children learn to define themselves within families and relative to adults (36, 37). Because eating is a domain used to reinforce relationships, it becomes one in which to redefine them. Hence, adolescents, particularly females, resist parents by such acts as becoming vegetarian, skipping meals, and preparing their own food (23, 24, 38). Prättälä studied Finnish teenagers and found that they used "junk" food to differentiate themselves from adults (39). While they knew well the nutritional benefits of the food served at family meals, they opted for "junk" food when with friends. This dual food preference was articulated in the contrast between parents and peers, and it helped to establish teens' subjective knowledge of themselves as leaving childhood. Roos studied preadolescents in the U.S. and found that they used age as the primary distinction around which to group food; "kid" food was always their stated preference, not "adult" food (40).

Food and Life History

Social constructionist approaches have also been used to study the transmission of food habits from one generation to the next. Sharman studied dietary choices and allocation of resources in low-income African American households, with special attention paid to the effects of federal food programs (41). After analyzing life histories from the women in these households, Sharman found that differences between women in the use of food derived in part from their experiences with it. In particular, she noted that the birth order of a woman—whether she was the oldest daughter or one of the youngest children of her mother—determined how much she was taught about food shopping, preparation, and meal formats. Eldest daughters knew more about these because they had been taught to assist their mothers; younger children had not needed to know these things and came to adulthood with a different set of food-related knowledge, skills, and values. These formed the basis for food habits in households but were modified in the context of current activity patterns related to strategies for survival. For example, even women who preferred traditional cooked meals resorted to processed and quickly prepared foods when the demands of holding multiple low-wage jobs made it impossible to prepare the traditional meal. Such studies demonstrate that even within the same family, there are differences in what ideas about food are transmitted. In addition, they show that dietary intake may not reflect nutritional knowledge or food preference, a finding of importance to nutrition educators.

Another study of the transmission of dietary practices through time focused on Italian American communities (42–44). In this ethnic group, the interactions of social networks composed of adult sisters produced continuity of some food traditions, particularly for holiday or communally prepared meals. However, outside this continuity, the experiences of members of individual households contributed to change in meal patterns consumed at everyday meals. A major factor determining dietary intake was the tradition of food exchange and regularly feeding persons besides household residents. In households monitored by the researchers, guests were present at meals or other food events from 30 to 50 times per month, and food exchanges between households occurred 16 to 29 times per month. For nutritionists this study is important in demonstrating how households overlap in determining the dietary intake and nutritional status of residents. Understanding the history of households as well as ethnic-specific values related to reciprocity and obligations helps to make sense of these food consumption patterns.

Ethnic Foods

Foods and cuisines are frequently categorized popularly or by nutritionists into "ethnic" or "regional" food patterns (e.g., Mexican food or Southern cuisine). Such labeling creates expectations of what foods will be eaten by members of a particular group or in a certain locale, expectations that are frequently not met as foodways change. Social scientists' current view of ethnicity as a *process* rather than a *thing* is useful in understanding why ethnic and regional foods are maintained and why they may change over time (45). Social scientists view self-ascribed membership in an ethnic group or in a regional population as a means by which individuals establish an identity (46). This identity can be reinforced by any number of symbols or behaviors, from eating particular foods, to wearing characteristic clothing, to proclaiming one's allegiance to a particular sports team. As individuals or groups choose to invest in a particular ethnic identity or reject it, they frequently do so through the symbols of food (47).

For this reason, those studying the changes in foodways with immigration note generational differences in food consumption patterns that are not necessarily a continuum from native to American cuisine (48). While members of the immigrant generation frequently try to maintain their foodways, the second generation rejects them in favor of newly available foods as they attempt to differentiate themselves from their parents. Then, in third and subsequent generations, there may be a conscious return to foods that provide identity with the original group or homeland. The content and context of such foods are often quite different from those of the immigrant generation, however. Substitutions are made on the basis of available ingredients, ethnic foods may be consumed only on special occasions or as an accompaniment to foods of the dominant culture, or higher status foods of the ethnic group may be substituted for those actually consumed by the immigrant generation.

Two factors complicate attempts to predict the food use of groups on the basis of presumed ethnicity. First, ethnicity is frequently confounded by such variables as income, occupation, and education, making it impossible to know if an ethnic group's consumption of a particular diet represents choices made to symbolize identity or simply limitations dictated by what is affordable. Epidemiologists currently argue that one must exclude the possibility that health-related behaviors do not reflect economic constraints before categorizing them as products of ethnicity (49). Those studying food use would do well to use similar caution.

The second factor complicating the prediction of food use on the basis of ethnicity is that choosing so-called ethnic foods is a behavior readily open to anyone. In their analysis of eating in America, Root and de Rochemont argue that American eating reflects social relations (50). Ethnic foods (with the exception of perhaps German, Dutch, and British) have not melted into a single pot. Rather, they remain distinct and highly available. Consumption of foods from different ethnic groups (e.g., the spread of Vietnamese restaurants in the U.S. in the past two decades) symbolizes acceptance of the ethnic group, rather than membership in the group.

Methods for Studying Social and Cultural Influences on Food Consumption

Methods used by social scientists to study food consumption differ substantially from those in which most nutritionists are trained (51). In the studies cited above, the two principal data collection methods are open-ended interviewing and participant observation. Both methods rely heavily on qualitative data, rather than the quantitative data familiar to most nutritionists.

Open-ended interviewing is a technique designed to reveal how persons talk about a particular subject, the meaning they attach to it, and how they relate it to other aspects of their lives (52, 53). These are topics that when approached directly, most people cannot articulate. Thus, the analysis and interpretation of the text a person produces in response to open-ended questioning becomes the source of such insight. Open-ended interviewing can be conducted with one informant at a time or with groups. One-on-one interviewing is usually called "key-informant interviewing" because the informant has been chosen for being particularly knowledgeable about a specific domain of information. For example, a midwife with years of experience in a town might be interviewed about infant feeding practices, rather than a new mother. In key-informant interviews, one can delve into how that person thinks about food without their responses being influenced by others.

It is important to conduct a number of such interviews and to be aware of the type of sample such persons comprise. In contrast to most quantitative research, which depends on a random or probability sample, most qualitative work uses an ethnographic sample. In such a sample, persons are chosen to provide breadth. Hence, the data produced are designed to give a better idea of the range of variation than of the central tendency (Fig. 108.1) (54, 55). For example, qualitative interviewing with an ethnographic sample can uncover the range of foods people

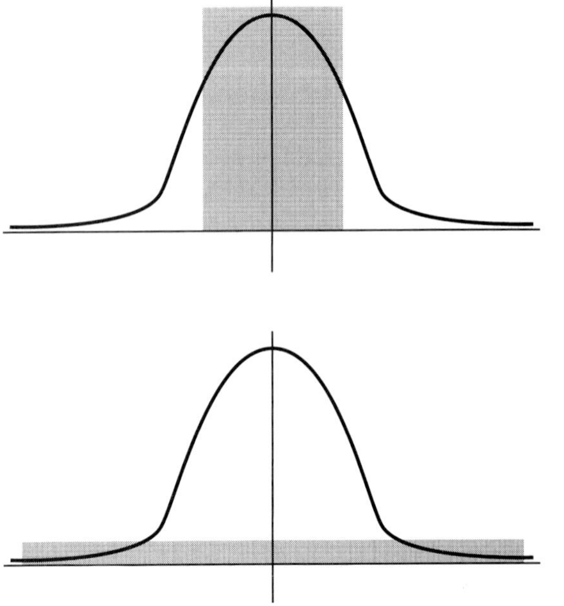

Figure 108.1. A comparison of the portion of variation *(shaded area)* in a group's food behavior that will be detected from research using a probability sample *(top)* and an ethnographic sample *(bottom)*. (Based on information in Werner O, Bernard HR. Cult Anthropol Methods 1994;(June):7–9; and Arcury TA, Quandt SA. Arthritis Care Res 1998;11:66–73.

classify as being for males versus those for females. A statistical sample would be necessary to then measure how these ideas about food are distributed in the population.

Group interviews are an increasingly popular alternative to key-informant interviewing for qualitative research. Group interviews about food consumption can be conducted with natural groups (e.g., neighbors or members of a class or club), expert groups (e.g., home economics extension agents for a group of counties), or focus groups (56). Focus groups are unacquainted persons who are brought together to participate in a facilitated discussion of a particular issue (57, 58). For example, the Best Start breast-feeding promotion intervention used focus groups of women to identify barriers to breast-feeding among low-income and minority group mothers (59, 60). Focus groups were also used to critique possible media messages for breast-feeding promotion. Group interviews, unlike key-informant interviews, have the potential for reactive effects as participants listen to others and shape their responses to topics introduced by the facilitator. For example, it may be more difficult for a participant to state a socially unacceptable opinion in a group than when alone. For this reason, it is important to conduct multiple group interviews with groups defined on theoretically relevant characteristics. In Best Start, separate groups were conducted with members of different ethnic groups, and mothers were interviewed separately from pregnant women because ethnicity and parity were expected to be linked to contrasting ideas about infant feeding. This made it possible to link different sets of ideas or beliefs with different groups, as well as ensuring that participants were not suppressing their opinions because of contrasting ideas from persons different from themselves.

Participant observation is a research method in which the researcher tries to fit into the group under study, to systematically interpret the interviews conducted and observations made in such a role (61, 62). In several of the studies described above (16, 42), researchers lived in homes of research subjects to observe and participate in meals.

Qualitative methods appear deceptively simple to those not trained in their use (63). However, they are extremely time-consuming and subject to established conventions of scientific rigor for their use within the social sciences that are analogous to the standards used in laboratory-based nutrition methods (64). These include such aspects of research design as sampling, measurement, and analysis. Despite the lack of familiarity with these methods, their use by nutritionists in studies of food and nutrition, either alone or in combination with other quantitative or nutritional methods (65, 66), can produce understanding of food consumption behaviors.

IMPACT OF SOCIAL FACTORS ON NUTRITIONAL STATUS

In addition to explaining the social and cultural patternings of food consumption, social science provides ways of examining the impact of social structures on nutritional status. Such an approach can help identify points for intervention for both under- and overnutrition.

Families and Food

The family is the basic social unit in which individuals are socialized into eating and which is organized to reflect larger societal patterns, such as age and gender roles. Some distinct patterns of nutritional status are attributable to variations in families (37). Several studies have examined the family environment's effect. Such indicators of family environment as levels of conflict and suppression of independence predict less-adequate dietary intake among adult family members (67). For children, poor parenting skills, family conflict, and marital instability predict failure to thrive (68), as does a family environment with little physical contact and verbal interaction from mothers (69).

Other studies of families indicate that family size and birth order affect nutritional status. Their results support the "dilution model" of family resources (70). This model argues that greater numbers of children necessitate stretching resources (money, time, food) so that the quality of the family's end product is lower. This end product can range from educational attainment of children to nutritional status. In general, children from large families are more likely to be stunted (short for age) than those from smaller families (71). The risk is particularly high for last-born children in large families (72). Such children have lower intakes of individual nutrients, and their diets are nutritionally inadequate overall compared with a standard such as the recommended dietary allowances (73). This pattern of poorer nutritional status of children in large families (74–76) or of high birth order (77–81), particularly in the context of poverty, has been documented in many populations, both Western and non-Western.

The effects of birth order sometimes differ when specific groups are examined, so that it is the oldest child who is most at risk. Cecily Williams was the first to describe acute protein energy malnutrition (82). She proposed the term "kwashiorkor," the name for the disease used by the Ga people of Ghana among whom she worked (83). Translated, kwashiorkor is literally the disease of the first born. Even without understanding the specific nutritional effects of abrupt weaning and transition to low-nutrient-density gruels, the Ga recognized the adverse consequences for the weanling (82).

Because mothers and wives are responsible for feeding families in virtually all societies, it has been argued that women's participation in the labor force has a deleterious effect on the nutritional status of family members. However, there is little support for this argument. In the United States, a comparison of diets of children of mothers employed outside the home with those not employed (84) found no evidence of either inadequate intake of nutrients or excessive intakes of fats. This lack of difference may be explained by other research that shows that working outside the home simply makes production of family meals more difficult. Women simplify such meals (85), but they continue to produce them (29).

The evidence from research in the Third World linking maternal employment and nutritional status demonstrates that children's nutritional status frequently improves as a result of their mothers' income-generating activities (86), particularly when women control the income. Women are more likely than men to direct extra cash income to feeding children, and in many cases, it can smooth out the highs and lows of the agricultural cycles (87, 88). Hence, many developing country interventions aimed at improving child nutritional status take advantage of circumstances such as those in West Africa, where spousal incomes are customarily separated, by introducing income-generating activities for women. However, maternal employment can sometimes impair child nutrition by diverting time from food preparation and child care activities (89, 90), so assessments of its impact are situation dependent.

Social Stratification and Nutritional Status

Whether measured by income, education, ethnic group, occupation, or composites of these, social stratification has a pronounced effect on nutrition-related health. Persons of higher social rank live longer and enjoy lower morbidity than do those of lower social rank. Recent sociologic analysis showed that the effect of social rank on mortality is continuous, not just a difference between those of the highest and lowest ranks. Even within higher social classes, there are health and mortality differences that parallel wealth and other measures (91, 92). These associations of social rank and health reflect the differences between groups in life course experience and are manifest in lifestyle differences.

In general, high social classes have greater access to high-quality diets, education, health care, and employment in higher-paying occupations that are not physically hazardous. These are associated with a lifestyle of more health-promoting behaviors, including more healthful diets, less smoking and other substance abuse, and lower rates of both chronic and infectious disease (93).

Class effects on nutritional status and dietary practices are evident in both historic and contemporary populations (94, 95). Persons of higher social class are taller. The secular trend in increasing stature correlates with social class, as stature increased earlier in upper than lower classes. Today, diminished nutritional status can be linked to poverty.

The social class distribution of obesity, another measure of nutritional status, is marked in women in the United States and other developed countries. Women in lower-income groups, those with lower educational attainment, and those of minority status are on average the most obese (96). This is reinforced by preference for fatter body shape (97) or greater acceptance of various body shapes (98) among lower class and minority women.

There are conflicting explanations for the social stratification of nutritional status. Economic and social explanations point to the greater cost of a high-quality diet and the limits on opportunities for physical activity in poor neighborhoods (98, 99). In contrast, cultural explanations suggest that obesity has historically symbolized wealth and plenty. This may continue among lower social classes, just as it predominates in many developing countries to the present (96, 99–102).

There is recent evidence that class differences in dietary intake among adults may be decreasing. In a comparison of national food consumption surveys in the United States from 1965 to 1991, socioeconomic and racial differences in dietary quality decreased over time (103). However, this leveling of dietary quality may not be occurring in children, the most vulnerable age group, or it may not suffice to offset factors such as disease and stress that depress nutritional status (104).

International Perspectives on Malnutrition

Moving from national or population contexts to a worldwide perspective, social scientists have attempted to explain and to help alleviate overwhelming inequalities in nutritional status (105, 106). One approach is to note the association of numerous nutrition indicators (e.g., nutritional deficiency diseases, stunting, starvation, dietary quality) with a country's gross national product (GNP). The association of better nutritional status with higher GNP and greater evidence of malnutrition with lower GNP is clear (107, 108). Two contrasting perspectives have been taken to interpret this association. The first has predicted that increasing GNP will improve nutrition; the second has taken a historical approach to explore the interconnections of national economies and to predict the likelihood of ameliorating worldwide nutrition problems.

The idea that increasing GNP will lead to improvements in nutrition has produced a massive international economic development effort to raise the economic productivity of lower-GNP countries (109, 110). Some early nutritional research challenged the utility of this approach. In a classic study of the transition from subsistence agricultural production to cash cropping, the latter was found to result in a decline in nutritional status as workers expended larger amounts of energy for lower nutrient intake (111). Likewise, a study in Mexico exemplifies those that demonstrated that dietary shifts to a poor-quality diet accompanied participation in commercial agriculture (112). More recent studies suggest a more positive effect on nutrition, caused by the increased income being applied to family food purchases (113), resulting in improved nutritional status (114).

To explain these contradictory findings, other social scientists have been critical of the economic development approach to improving worldwide nutrition. They contend that such an approach may improve the GNP of countries, but with similar gains for developed countries, thus maintaining the same power relations and flow of resources from poor to rich countries. They present a much less hopeful outlook for improving nutrition worldwide. This approach is referred to as a world systems perspective (115). Adherents argue that current inequalities between nations that lead to high levels of malnutrition in some countries with overnutrition in others reflect centuries old patterns in which western Europe represented a core that economically exploited other peripheral countries with resources necessary for European lifestyles.

In recent years, countries at the periphery (those with the lowest GNPs) have become dependent on imported foods from core countries (often surplus grain production) as they either exported their food or turned to industrial production of goods to be sold to core countries. Dependence on fluctuating supplies and prices, as well as the necessity of having cash to purchase food has reduced food security and increased the likelihood of hunger (116).

World systems theory suggests that nations at the periphery will have lower standards of living and greater nutrition problems. Data compiled from international sources (117, 118) bear this out. Ranking countries on the basis of GNP and other aspects of development from periphery (e.g., Tanzania, Bangladesh, El Salvador) to semiperiphery (e.g., Egypt, Philippines, Mexico) to semicore (e.g., Brazil, Korea) to core (e.g, United States, Japan) results in a gradient in such measures as wasting, stunting, and prevalence of anemia in pregnant women (37). Both the economic development and world systems perspectives link nutritional status to such measures of national economic well-being as GNP. The latter, however, stress the interdependence of economies and suggest that alleviating hunger and malnutrition around the world is far from simple.

Many of the concepts and findings presented in this chapter may seem, at first glance, self-evident. This is because all persons (including nutritionists) are members of families, communities, and societies, giving them ample opportunity to make observations related to the social and cultural aspects of food and nutrition. The value of social and behavioral sciences to modern nutrition lies in the rigorous methodology that they can employ. This methodology, usually based on commonplace behaviors of observation and conversation, can be used to examine ideas about food and their distribution, as well as the relationship of nutritional status to social and cultural variation.

REFERENCES

1. Jerome NW, Kandel RF, Pelto GH, eds. Nutritional anthropology. Pleasantville, NY: Redgrave, 1980.
2. Messer E. Annu Rev Anthropol 1984;13:204–49.
3. Quandt SA, Ritenbaugh C. Training manual in nutritional anthropology. Washington DC: American Anthropological Association, Special Publication No. 20, 1986.
4. Ritenbaugh C. J Nutr Educ 1982;13:S12–7.
5. Jerome NW, Pelto GH. Fed Proc 1981;40:2601–5.
6. Khare R. Soc Sci Inf 1980;19:519–42.

7. Grivetti LE. Annu Rev Nutr 1981;1:47–68.
8. Harris M, Ross EB, eds. Food and evolution: toward a theory of human food habits. Philadelphia: Temple University Press, 1987;1–633.
9. Ritenbaugh C. Human foodways: a window on evolution. In: Bauwens EE, ed. The anthropology of health. St. Louis: CV Mosby, 1978;111–20.
10. Katz SH, Hediger M, Valleroy L. Science 1974;184:765–73.
11. Etheridge EW. Pellagra: an unappreciated reminder of southern distinctiveness. In: Savitt TL, Young JH, eds. Disease and distinctiveness in the American South. Knoxville: University of Tennessee Press, 1988;100–19.
12. Goldberger J, Wheeler GA, Sydenstricker E. Public Health Rep 1920;35:2693–701.
13. Harris M. Cows, pigs, wars and witches. New York: Vintage Books, 1974.
14. Simoons FJ. Ecol Food Nutr 1974;3:185–201.
15. Mintz S. Sweetness and power: the place of sugar in modern history. New York: Penguin, 1986.
16. Douglas M, Nicod M. New Society 1974;30:744–7.
17. Douglas M. Daedalus 1972;101:61–81.
18. Murcott A. 'It's a pleasure to cook for him': food, mealtimes and gender in some South Wales households. In: Gamarnikow E, Morgan D, Purvis J, et al., eds. The public and the private. London: Heinemann, 1983;78–90.
19. Quandt SA, Vitolins MZ, DeWalt KM, et al. J Appl Gerontol 1997;16:152–71.
20. Roos G, Quandt SA, DeWalt KM. Appetite 1993;21:295–8.
21. Barthes R. Toward a psychosociology of contemporary food consumption. In: Forster R, Ranum O, eds. Food and drink in history: selections from the Annales E-S-C. Baltimore: Johns Hopkins University Press, 1979;166–73.
22. Drewnowski A. J Am Coll Nutr 1996;15:147–53.
23. Lupton D. Food, the body and the self. London: Sage Publications, 1996.
24. Charles N, Kerr M. Women, food and families. Manchester: Manchester University Press, 1988.
25. Visser M. Much depends on dinner: the extraordinary history and mythology, allure and obsessions, perils and taboos, of an ordinary meal. London: Penguin, 1986.
26. Bourdieu P. Distinction: a social science critique of the judgment of taste. Cambridge: Harvard University Press, 1984.
27. Patterson BH, Harlan LC, Block G, et al. Nutr Cancer 1996:23:105–19.
28. DeVault M. Feeding the family: the social organization of caring as gendered work. Chicago IL: University of Chicago Press, 1991.
29. Mennell S, Murcott A, van Otterloo AH. The sociology of food: eating, diet and culture. London: Sage Publications, 1992.
30. McIntosh WA, Zey M. Food Foodways 1989;3:317–32.
31. Schafer RB, Bohlen JM. Home Econ Res J 1977;6:131–40.
31a. Messer E. Soc Sci Med 1997;44:1675–84.
32. Gittelsohn J. Soc Sci Med 1991;33:1141–54.
33. Burgoyle J, Charles D. You are what you eat: food and family reconstitution. In: Murcott A, ed. The sociology of food and eating. Aldershot: Gower, 1983;152–63.
34. Ellis R. The way to a man's heart: food in the violent home. In: Murcott A, ed. The sociology of food and eating. Aldershot: Gower, 1983;164–71.
35. Bordo S. Anorexia nervosa: psychopathology as the crystallization of culture. In: Curt D, Heldke L, eds. Cooking, eating, thinking: transformative philosophies of food. Bloomington, IN: Indiana University Press, 1992;28–55.
36. DeGarine I. Ecol Food Nutr 1972;1:143–63.
37. McIntosh WA. Sociologies of food and nutrition. New York: Plenum, 1996.
38. Brannen J, Dodd K, Oakley A, et al. Young people, health and family life. Buckingham: Open University Press, 1994.
39. Prättälä R. Young people and food: socio-cultural studies of food consumption patterns. Dissertation, Helsinki: University of Helsinki, 1989.
40. Roos G. Cultural analysis of children, food and gender in the United States. Ann Arbor, MI: University Microfilms, 1995.
41. Sharman A. From generation to generation: resources, experience, and orientation in the dietary patterns of selected urban American households. In: Sharman A, Theophano J, Curtis K, et al., eds. Diet and domestic life in society. Philadelphia: Temple University Press, 1991:173–204.
42. Theophano J, Curtis K. Sisters, mothers, and daughters: food exchange and reciprocity in an Italian-American community. In: Sharman A, Theophano J, Curtis K, et al., eds. Diet and domestic life in society. Philadelphia: Temple University Press, 1991:147–72.
43. Theophano JS. "It's really tomato sauce but we call it gravy": a study of food and women's work among Italian-American families. Ann Arbor, MI: University Microfilms, 1982.
44. Curtis K. "I can never go anywhere empty handed": food exchange and reciprocity in an Italian American community. Ann Arbor, MI: University Microfilms, 1983.
45. Barth F. Ethnic groups and boundaries. Boston: Little, Brown and Co, 1969.
46. Alba R. Ethnic identity: the transformation of white America. New Haven: Yale University Press, 1990.
47. van den Berghe PL. Racial Ethnic Studies 1984;7:387–97.
48. Kalcik S. Ethnic foodways in America: symbol and the performance of identity. In: Brown LK, Mussell K, eds. Ethnic and regional foodways in the United States. Knoxville: University of Tennessee Press, 1985:37–65.
49. Kaufman JS, Cooper RS. Public Health Rep 1996;110:662–666.
50. Root W, de Rochemont R. Eating in America. Hopewell, NJ: Ecco Press, 1995.
51. Pelto GH, Pelto PJ, Messer E. Research methods in nutritional anthropology. Food and Nutrition Bulletin Supplement 11. Tokyo: United Nations University, 1989.
52. Quandt SA, Arcury TA. Arthritis Care Res 1997;10:273–81.
53. Denzin NK and Lincoln TS, eds. Handbook of qualitative research. Thousand Oaks, CA: Sage, 1994;1–643.
54. Werner O, Bernard HR. Cult Anthropol Methods 1994;(June):7–9.
55. Arcury TA, Quandt SA. Arthritis Care Res, 1998;11:66–73.
56. Coreil J. Med Anthropol 1995;16:193–210.
57. Krueger RA. Focus groups: a practical guide for applied research. Newbury Park, CA: Sage, 1988.
58. Morgan DL, ed. Successful focus groups: advancing the state of the art. Newbury Park, CA: Sage, 1993.
59. Bryant CA, Coreil J, D'Angelo SL, et al. NAACOGS Clin Issues Perinatal Women's Health Nurs 1992:3:723–30.
60. Coreil J, Bryant CA, Westover BJ, et al. J Hum Lact 1991;11:265–71.
61. Kolasa KM, Bass MA. J Nutr Educ 1974;6:89–92.
62. Bernard HR: Research methods in anthropology: qualitative and quantitative approaches. 2nd ed. Thousand Oaks, CA: Sage, 1994.
63. Gubrium JF. Gerontologist 1992;32:581–2.
64. Luborsky MR, Rubinstein RL. Res Aging 1995;17:89–113.
65. Steckler A, McLeroy KR, Goodman RM, et al. Health Educ Q 1992;19:1–8.
66. Stange KC, Miller WL, Crabtree BF, et al. J Gen Intern Med 1994;9:278–82.

67. Kintner M, Boss P, Johnson N. J Marriage Fam 1978;43: 633–41.
68. Chase P, Martin HP. N Engl J Med 1970;282:934–9.
69. Pollitt E, Leibel R. Biological and social correlates of failure to thrive. In: Greene LS, Johnston FE, eds., Social and biological predictors of nutritional status, physical growth and neurological development. New York: Academic Press, 1980:173–200.
70. Blake J. Demography 1981;18:421–8.
71. Wray JD. Population pressure on families: family size and child spacing. In: Study Committee of the Office of the Foreign Secretary, ed. Rapid population growth: consequences and policy implications. Washington, DC: National Academy of Sciences, 1971:403–61.
72. Grant MW. Br J Prev Soc Med 1964;18:35–9.
73. Kucera B, McIntosh WA. Ecol Food Nutr 1991;25:1–12.
74. Ighogboja SI. East Afr Med J 1992;69(10):566–71.
75. MacCorquodale DW, de Nova HR. Public Health Rep 1977;92(5):453–7.
76. Margo G, Lipschitz S, Joseph E, et al. S Afr Med J 1976; 50:67–74.
77. Vella V, Tomkins A, Nviku J, et al. J Trop Pediatr 1995; 41:89–98.
78. Reddaiah VP, Kapoor SK. Indian J Pediatr 1992;59:567–71.
79. Herold P, Sanjur D. Arch Latinoam Nutr 1986;36:599–624.
80. Hearst N. Int J Epidemiol 1985;14:575–81.
81. Grantham-McGregor SM, Desai P, Buchanan E. Trop Geogr Med 1977;29:165–71.
82. Williams CD. Arch Dis Child 1933;8:423–33.
83. Williams CD. Lancet 1935;2:1151–2.
84. Johnson RK, Smiciklas-Wright H, Croutier AC, et al. Pediatrics 1992;90:245–9.
85. Kinsey J. Am J Agricul Econ 1983;65:10–9.
86. Wandel M, Holmboe-Otterson G. Food Nutr Bull 1992;14: 49–54.
87. Krieger J. Women, men and household food in Cameroon. Ann Arbor, MI: University Microfilms, 1994.
88. Tripp R. J Trop Pediatr 1981;27:1407–16.
89. Popkin B, Solon FS. J Trop Pediatr 1976;6:156–66.
90. Kumar S. The role of the household economy in child nutrition at low incomes: a case study in Kerala. Cornell University Occasional Paper no. 95. 1978.
91. Hertzman C, Frank J, Evans RG. Heterogeneities in health status and the determinants of population health. In: Evans RG, Barer ML, Marmor TR, eds. Why are some people healthy and others not? Hawthorne, NY: Aldine de Gruyter, 1994;67–92.
92. Marmot MG. Social inequalities in mortality: the social environment. In: Wilkinson RG, ed. Class and health: research and longitudinal data. London: Tavistock, 1986;21–33.
93. Link BG, Phelan JC. Am J Public Health 1996;86:471–2.
94. Komlos J. On the significance of anthropometric history. In: Komlos J, ed. Stature, living standards and economic development. Chicago: University of Chicago Press, 1994:210–20.
95. Crooks DL. Yearb Phys Anthropol 1995;38:57–86.
96. Sobal J, Stunkard AJ. Psychol Bull 1989;105:260–75.
97. Massara EB. Que Gordita: a study of weight among women in a Puerto Rican community. New York: AMS Press, 1989.
98. Okamoto E, Davidson LL, Conner DR. Am J Dis Child 1993;147:155–9.
99. Greenwood MRC, Johnson PR, Karp RJ, et al. Obesity in disadvantaged children. In: Karp RJ, ed. Malnourished children in the United States: caught in the cycle of poverty. New York: Springer, 1993.
100. Brown PJ, Konner M. Ann NY Acad Sci 1987;499:29–46.
101. Ritenbaugh C. Cult Med Psychiatry 1982;6:347–61.
102. Bryant C. Soc Sci Med 1982;16:1757–65.
103. Popkin BM, Siega-Riz AM, Haines PS. N Engl J Med 1996;335:716–20.
104. Miller JE, Korenman S. Am J Epidemiol 1994;140:233–43.
105. Berg A. The nutrition factor. Washington, DC: Brookings Institution, 1973.
106. Chambers R. Longhurst R, Pacey A, eds. Seasonal dimensions of rural poverty. Totowa, NJ: Allanheld-Osmun, 1981.
107. Périssé K, Sizaret F, François P. FAO Nutr Newslett 1969;7:2.
108. Timmer CP, Falcon WP, Pearson SR. Food policy analysis. Baltimore: Johns Hopkins University Press, 1983.
109. World Bank. The assault on world poverty: problems in rural development, education and health. Baltimore: Johns Hopkins University Press, 1975.
110. Hoben A. Annu Rev Anthropol 1982;11:349–75.
111. Gross DR, Underwood BA. Am Anthropol 1971;72:725–40.
112. DeWalt KM. Nutritional strategies and agricultural change in a Mexican community. Ann Arbor, MI: UMI Research Press, 1983.
113. von Braun J. Production, employment, and income effects of commercialization of agriculture. In: von Braun J, Kennedy E, eds. Agricultural commercialization, economic development, and nutrition. Baltimore: Johns Hopkins University Press, 1994;37–64.
114. Pinstrup-Anderson P, Pelletier D, Alderman H, eds. Child growth and nutrition in developing countries: priorities for action. Ithaca, NY: Cornell University Press. 1995.
115. Wallerstein I. The modern world system. Capitalist agriculture and the origins of the European world economy in the sixteen century. New York: Academic Press, 1975.
116. Bernstein H, Crow B, Mackintosh M et al., eds. The food question: profits vs. people. New York: Monthly Review Press, 1990.
117. World Bank. World development report 1993. Investing in health. New York: Oxford University Press. 1993.
118. Levin HM, Pollitt E, Galloway R, et al. Micronutrient deficiency disorders. In: Jamison DT, Mosley WH, Measham AR, et al., eds. Disease control priorities in developing countries. New York: Oxford University Press, 1993:421–51.

109. Fads, Frauds, and Quackery

STEPHEN BARRETT and VICTOR HERBERT

Food faddism can be defined as an unusual pattern of food behavior enthusiastically adopted by its adherents (1). It is commonly expressed by *(a)* beliefs that particular foods or food substances can cure diseases, *(b)* elimination of certain foods from the diet without adequate reason, and/or *(c)* emphasis on "natural" foods. Many aspects of food faddism become social movements that represent symbolic rebellions against authority, society-at-large, or some imagined enemy.

Quackery can be defined as the promotion for profit of a medical scheme or remedy that is unproven or known to be false. This definition seeks to distinguish folk practices and neighborly advice from practices for financial gain. "Health fraud" has been defined in a similar way. However, since most people regard *fraud* as a deliberate attempt to deceive, the term *health fraud* is most appropriate when deliberate deception is involved.

Quack methods are sometimes referred to as "alternatives." Since ineffective methods are not true alternatives to effective ones, the terms *unscientific* or *dubious* are preferable. "Alternative" methods related to nutrition are discussed in Chapter 110.

Faddists and quacks urge everyone to distrust large food companies, government regulators, and scientific health professionals (2). This negative philosophy is essential because without it, there would be no reason to buy health-food-industry products or consult "alternative" practitioners.

VULNERABILITY TO QUACKERY

Victims of quackery usually have one or more of the following characteristics:

1. *They are unsuspecting.* Many people believe that if something appears in print or in a broadcast, it must be true or somehow it wouldn't be allowed. People also tend to believe what others tell them about personal experience.
2. *They believe in magic.* Some people are easily taken in by the promise of an easy solution to their problem. Those who buy one fad diet book after another fall into this category.
3. *They are desperate.* Many people faced with a serious health problem that doctors cannot solve become desperate enough to try almost anything that arouses hope. Many victims of cancer, arthritis, multiple sclerosis, and AIDS are vulnerable in this regard.
4. *They are alienated.* Some people feel deeply antagonistic toward scientific medicine but are attracted to methods that are "natural" or otherwise unorthodox. They may also harbor extreme distrust of the medical profession, the food industry, drug companies, and government agencies.

MISLEADING CLAIMS

Nutritional faddism and quackery are promoted with five basic fallacies:

1. *Our food supply is nutritionally inadequate because our soils are depleted and important nutrients are removed by food processing.* These claims encourage purchase of "organic," "natural," and "health" foods. A typical example is this passage from a book by Earl Mindell (3), cofounder of the Great Earth chain of health-food stores: "Much of our soil our food is grown in has been depleted of many vitamins and minerals, thanks to the overuse of fertilizers and chemicals. Then the food takes a long time to get to the supermarket . . . The longer these foods are stored the more vitamins they lose. Many of the foods we eat have been heavily processed, meaning they have been crushed, heated, bleached, extracted, chemicalized and preserved . . . Then we cook the food, destroying valuable enzymes and what's left of many vitamins. It's a wonder there's any nutrition at all left in our food by the time it gets to our tables (3)!"
2. *Vitamin and mineral deficiencies are common.* This claim is used to persuade people that everyone should take supplements. A typical example is this passage from *Prescription for Nutritional Healing* (4), a book that recommends supplements and/or herbs for more than 250 health problems: "The problem with most of us is that we do not get what we need from our modern diet. Even if you are not sick, you may not necessarily be healthy. By understanding the principles of wholistic nutrition and knowing what nutrients we need, we can improve the state of our health, stave off disease, and maintain a harmonious balance in the way nature intended."
3. *Most health problems are due to faulty diet and can be treated by nutritional methods.* These types of claims are used to market "food supplements," "health foods," and quack dietary methods.
4. *Americans are in danger of being poisoned by food additives and pesticide residues.* This claim, along with accusations that the food industry and government regulators are untrustworthy, is used to promote the sale of "organic" and "natural" foods.
5. *Personal experience is the best way to tell whether a health-related action is effective.* This claim encourages people to rely on

testimonial evidence rather than scientific studies and prevailing medical beliefs.

Table 109.1 lists ways to help spot food quacks.

Misleading Claims for Foods

Many foods are promoted with slogans suggesting that they are safer, more nutritious, or have special therapeutic value. "Organically grown" foods are said to be grown without use of "artificial" fertilizers or pesticides. The foods themselves are usually indistinguishable from "ordinary" foods but cost significantly more. Studies comparing organically grown and conventionally grown foods have found that their pesticide content is similar (5). U.S. Food and Drug Administration (FDA) market-basket studies indicate that pesticide residues are insignificant in the overall diet (6). Nutrients are absorbed by the plant in their inorganic chemical state regardless of whether the soil has been prepared with manure, compost, or manufactured fertilizer. Plants grow only if they receive enough nutrients, and their vitamin content is determined by their genes. Fertilizers can influence the mineral composition of plants, but these variations are rarely significant in the overall diet. A recent study encompassing 460 assessments of nine different fruits and vegetables found no significant difference in taste quality between "organic" and conventionally grown samples (7). Despite such facts, a federal law passed in 1990 requires the U.S. Department of Agriculture to establish standards for organic food "certification."

The word *natural* is said by its proponents to designate foods that are minimally processed and contain no artificial additives or preservatives, implying that these substances pose a health risk. Actually, they help make our food supply safe, abundant, and palatable. Although one is occasionally found to pose a health hazard (e.g., sulfites), the vast majority appear safe, and the overall level in our food supply should not cause concern—or be a reason to buy "natural" foods. The health-food industry also circulates unfounded criticisms of food irradiation, milk pasteurization, and genetically engineered foods (8).

Although the term *health food* cannot actually be defined, it is used to suggest that certain foods have special health-giving properties not found in "ordinary" foods. Some "health" foods are rich in various nutrients and can be a valuable part of a balanced diet. But no food has any special health-promoting property beyond those of its components. FDA regulations permit food labels and packages to contain truthful and nonmisleading claims related to *(a)* calcium and osteoporosis, *(b)* sodium and high blood pressure, *(c)* dietary fats and heart disease, *(d)* dietary fats and cancer, *(e)* dietary fiber and cancer, *(f)* fiber and cardiovascular diseases, and *(g)* oatmeal or oat bran and heart disease. The claims must be limited to the relationship between these conditions and a particular food component, rather than the specific product. The recommendation must also be consistent with sound total diet (9, 10). Food advertising is primarily regulated by the Federal Trade Commission (FTC), which plans to apply similar criteria (11).

Promotion of Supplements

Americans waste several billion dollars a year on worthless or unnecessary "dietary supplements." These products are promoted with scare tactics and false promises. The most common sales pitch is "nutrition insurance," the idea

Table 109.1
Thirty Tips to Help Spot Vitamin Pushers and Food Quacks

1. When talking about nutrients, they tell only part of the relevant story.
2. They claim that most Americans are poorly nourished.
3. They recommend "nutrition insurance" for everyone.
4. They say that if you eat badly, you'll be ok as long as you take supplements.
5. They say that most diseases are due to faulty diet and can be treated with "nutritional" methods.
6. They allege that modern processing methods and storage remove all nutritive value from our food.
7. They claim that diet is a major factor in behavior.
8. They claim that fluoridation is dangerous.
9. They claim that soil depletion and the use of pesticides and "chemical" fertilizers result in food that is less safe and less nourishing.
10. They claim you are in danger of being "poisoned" by ordinary food additives and preservatives.
11. They charge that the recommended dietary allowances (RDAs) have been set too low.
12. They claim that under stress, and in certain diseases, your need for nutrients is increased.
13. They recommend "supplements" and "health foods" for everyone.
14. They say it is easy to lose weight.
15. They claim that sugar is a deadly poison.
16. They oppose pasteurization of milk and fluoridation of water.
17. They recommend a wide variety of substances similar to those found in your body.
18. They claim that "natural" vitamins are better than "synthetic" ones.
19. They suggest that a questionnaire can be used to indicate whether you need dietary supplements.
20. They promise quick, dramatic, miraculous results.
21. They routinely sell vitamins and other "dietary supplements" as part of their practice.
22. They use disclaimers couched in pseudomedical jargon.
23. They use anecdotes and testimonials to support their claims.
24. They offer phony "vitamins."
25. They display credentials not recognized by responsible scientists or educators.
26. They offer to determine your body's nutritional state with a single laboratory test.
27. They claim they are being persecuted by orthodox medicine and that their work is being suppressed because it's controversial.
28. They warn you not to trust your doctor.
29. They sue to intimidate their critics.
30. They encourage patients to lend political support to their treatment methods.

From Barrett S, Herbert V. The vitamin pushers: how the "health food" industry is selling America a bill of goods. Amherst, NY: Prometheus Books, 1994.

that everyone needs vitamin and mineral supplements to be sure of getting enough. Some promoters falsely suggest that it is difficult to balance one's diet, while others insist that our food supply is inadequate.

Another common ploy is the suggestion that supplementation is advisable to help deal with "stress." This idea was commercialized by distorting a 1952 National Academy of Sciences report (12). The report merely stated that people who are seriously ill or injured (some of whom have impaired appetite) might benefit from supplementation to prevent depletion of water-soluble vitamins, which have limited storage. However, in 1976, a major vitamin manufacturer began falsely advertising that "stress robs the body of vitamins" and that water-soluble vitamins must be replaced *daily* because the body cannot store them. Other manufacturers embellished further, suggesting that extra vitamins are needed to cope with emotional stress, the stress of a busy lifestyle, or life's other stressful events. Some manufacturers made no claims for their "stress" products but assumed that consumers would understand the implications. Several manufacturers falsely suggest that being active and elderly creates special needs that their products supposedly meet.

In the mid-1980s, the New York State attorney general secured consent agreements with two major "stress supplement" manufacturers to stop misrepresenting the need for their products. Since that time, the amount of direct advertising of "stress supplements" has greatly decreased. However, the Council for Responsible Nutrition (CRN), a trade organization that represents major supplement manufacturers and suppliers, has advertised that a busy lifestyle places Americans at nutritional risk. The ad included a narrowly worded "Vitamin Gap Test" suggesting that virtually everyone may have one or more "gaps." CRN representatives maintain that virtually everyone needs supplements (13). In 1990, the FTC secured a consent agreement barring another large manufacturer from making unsubstantiated claims that any vitamin product is needed to replace nutrients lost as a result of athletic activities or "the stress of daily living." Such "stress" is not a true hypercatabolic state in which increased amounts of calories and nutrients are needed (see Chapter 96).

During the past few years, many health-food manufacturers have developed "ergogenic aids"—amino acid supplements falsely claimed to increase stamina, endurance, and muscle development. Some of these products are claimed to be "natural steroids" that release growth hormone (14). There is no scientific evidence that these products actually release growth hormone—which is fortunate, because if they did, acromegaly might result. David Lightsey, who coordinates the National Council Against Health Fraud's Task Force on Ergogenic Aids, has requested documentation from more than 80 companies that market "ergogenic aids." Fewer than half sent anything, and the rest submitted studies that were poorly designed or did not actually support product claims. Lightsey also checked statements that various teams were using certain products and found that management had neither endorsed the products nor encouraged their use (15).

The Federation of American Societies for Experimental Biology (FASEB) has criticized the widespread use of amino acids in supplements. Following extensive review, FASEB experts concluded that *(a)* single- or multiple-ingredient capsules, tablets, and liquid products are used primarily for pharmacologic purposes or enhancement of physiologic functions rather than for nutritional purposes, *(b)* little scientific literature exists on most amino acids ingested for these purposes, *(c)* no scientific rationale has been presented to justify use of amino acid supplements by healthy individuals, *(d)* safety levels for amino acid supplement use have not been established, and *(e)* a systematic approach to safety testing is needed (16).

Vitamin C, vitamin E, and β-carotene are being vigorously promoted with claims that their antioxidant properties can help prevent various diseases by blocking the harmful action of free radicals. Epidemiologic evidence indicates that diets containing significant amounts of fruits, vegetables, and grains are associated with a lower incidence of heart disease and certain cancers (17). But it is not known which, if any, specific substances in the diet are responsible or whether taking above-RDA doses of supplements will do more good than harm. Evidence exists, for example, that vitamin E can help prevent atherosclerosis by interfering with oxidation of low-density lipoproteins (LDL). However, this vitamin can also exert an anticoagulant effect. The issue can be settled scientifically by conducting long-term double-blind clinical studies that compare vitamin users and nonusers and measure death rates from all causes.

So far, four large clinical trials have been reported. The first compared the effects of vitamin E, β-carotene, and a placebo among heavy smokers. The researchers found no benefit from vitamin E and 18% *more* lung cancer among those who received β-carotene. In addition, the overall death rate of β-carotene recipients was 8% higher, and those who took vitamin E had a higher frequency of hemorrhagic stroke (18). The second study found no evidence that supplementing with vitamin C, vitamin E, or β-carotene prevented colorectal cancer (19). The third study, which followed 22,000 physicians for 12 years, found no difference in cancer or cardiovascular disease rates between users and nonusers of β-carotene (20). The fourth trial, which tested a combination of β-carotene and vitamin A, was terminated after 4 years because it appeared that the supplement-takers who smoked had a 28% higher incidence of lung cancer and a 17% higher death rate (21).

In addition to marketing antioxidants, many companies are marketing products said to be concentrates of fruits and/or vegetables. Critics note, however, that it is not possible to condense large amounts of produce into a pill without losing fiber, nutrients, and many other phytochemicals (22). Although some products contain significant amounts of nutrients, these nutrients are readily obtainable at lower cost from foods.

Advice from Retailers

Health Foods Business estimates that in 1996 there were 9789 "health food" stores in America with total gross sales of $7.6 billion, including $3 billion for vitamins and other supplements, up from 1992 figures of 7500, $3.8 billion, and $1.5 billion, respectively (23). No special knowledge or training is required to become a salesperson at a health-food store. Personnel in these stores typically obtain information by reading books and magazines that promote supplements and herbs for treatment of virtually all health problems. Retailers also get information from manufacturers and can attend seminars at trade shows sponsored by industry groups and trade magazines (13). Several large studies have demonstrated that their proprietors often give advice that is irrational, unsafe, and illegal:

- In 1983, investigators from the American Council on Science and Health (ACSH) made 105 inquiries at stores in New York, New Jersey, and Connecticut. Asked about eye symptoms characteristic of glaucoma, 17 of 24 suggested a wide variety of products for a person not seen; none recognized that urgent medical care was needed. Asked over the telephone about sudden, unexplained 15-pound weight loss in 1 month's time, 9 of 17 recommended products sold in their store; only 7 suggested medical evaluation. Seven of 10 stores carried "starch blockers" despite an FDA ban. Nine stores contacted made false claims of effectiveness for bee pollen, and 10 stores did so for RNA (24).
- In 1987, a registered dietitian posed five similar questions to 10 health-food-store proprietors in eastern Pennsylvania and concluded that only 23 of 50 responses (46%) were correct (25).
- In 1989, volunteers of the Consumer Health Education Council telephoned 41 Houston-area health-food stores and asked to speak with the person who provided nutritional advice. The callers explained that they had a brother with AIDS who was seeking an effective alternative against the HIV virus. The caller also explained that the brother's wife was still having sex with her husband and wanted to reduce or eliminate her risk of being infected. All 41 retailers offered products they said could benefit the brother's immune system, improve the woman's immunity, and protect her against harm from the HIV virus. Thirty said they sold products that would cure AIDS. None recommended abstinence or using a condom (26).

In 1993, posing as prospective customers, FDA agents visited local health-food stores throughout the United States. The investigators asked, "What do you sell to help high blood pressure?" "Do you have anything to help fight infection or help my immune system?" and/or "Do you have anything that works on cancer?" Of 129 requests for information, 120 resulted in recommendations of specific dietary supplements (27). Retailers who recommend products when customers describe symptoms violate state laws against the unlicensed practice of medicine or pharmacy, but they are rarely prosecuted.

Several dozen companies market supplements through person-to-person (multilevel) sales. Virtually anyone can become a distributor by filling out a one-page application and buying a distributor kit for less than $50. Most multilevel companies claim their products can prevent or cure a wide range of diseases. A few companies merely suggest that people will feel better, look better, or have more energy if they use supplements.

Although pharmacists receive scientific training in nutrition, a study by *Consumer Reports* has cast considerable doubt on the ability of community pharmacists to give appropriate advice about supplements. When 30 pharmacists were asked by undercover reporters whether vitamins could relieve their nervousness or fatigue, 17 recommended vitamins, one recommended L-tryptophan, and only 9 mentioned seeing a doctor (28).

A large percentage of supplement products are irrationally formulated. Several years ago, two dietitians examined the labels of vitamin products at five pharmacies, three groceries, and three health-food stores in New Haven. Products were judged appropriate if they contained between 50 and 200% of the U.S. RDA and no more than 100% of others for which "Estimated Safe and Adequate Daily Dietary Intakes" exist. Only 16 of 105 (15%) multivitamin/mineral products met these criteria (29).

Few supplement products have any usefulness against disease, and most that do (e.g., niacin for cholesterol or triglyceride control and folic acid for lowering abnormal blood levels of homocysteine) should not be taken without competent medical supervision.

DUBIOUS CREDENTIALS

Since the early 1980s, many individuals and groups have developed credentials intended to resemble those of established medical and nutritional organizations (13, 30). During this period, unaccredited correspondence schools and other organizations have issued a steady stream of "degrees" and other certificates intended to suggest that the recipient is a qualified expert in nutrition. The schools typically issue B.S., M.S., and/or Ph.D. "degrees" based on study of unscientific writings plus open-book tests that are scored quite liberally. The professional organizations typically grant immediate "professional memberships" and a fancy certificate for a modest fee. Household pets and nonexistent individuals have achieved membership in several of these groups. Some organizations offer "certification" based on correspondence courses that invariably include unscientific teachings. The most significant of these is the C.N. (Certified Nutritionist) issued by the nonaccredited National Institute for Nutrition Education (NINE). Such credentials have no legal or scientific standing but can be advertised or displayed in most states that do not regulate nutritionists. The American Dietetic Association is striving for increased regulation of nutritional practice and by 1996 had gained passage of laws in 38 states.

In 1993, a 32-state survey sponsored by the National

Council Against Health Fraud found that 286 (46%) of 618 "Yellow Pages" listings under the heading "Nutritionists" were spurious, and 72 (12%) were suspicious. Listings were considered "spurious" if the advertiser used an invalid method of diagnosis, treatment, or nutritional assessment. Listings were rated "suspicious" if the practitioner did not comply with a request for information on credentials or methods used. Dubious nutrition practitioners were also found under the headings "Acupuncture," "Health & Diet Products," "Health, Fitness & Nutrition Consultants," "Herbs," "Holistic Practitioners," "Weight Control Services," and "Wellness Programs." Many such listings were for chiropractors, homeopaths, naturopaths, "holistic" physicians, health-food stores, and multilevel distributors for such companies as Herbalife International, Nu Skin International, Shaklee Corporation, and Sunrider International. The credentials used included CCN (certified clinical nutritionist), CN (certified nutritionist), CCT (certified colon therapist), CMT (certified massage therapist), CNC (certified nutrition consultant), HMD (homeopathic medical doctor), L.Ac. (licensed acupuncturist), MLD (manual lymph drainage), NC (nutrition counselor), ND (doctor of naturopathy), NMD (doctor of nutrimedicine), and OMD (oriental medical doctor). Of 24 individuals identified as "Ph.D." in their ad, 17 had spurious credentials. Of 231 listings under the heading "Dietitians," 21 (9%) were spurious, including several from GNC stores (31).

The best strategy to avoid entanglement with an unqualified nutritionist is to avoid *all* practitioners who sell supplements in their offices or espouse the statements listed in Table 109.1.

DUBIOUS DIAGNOSTIC TESTS

Unscientific practitioners use a variety of tests as a basis for prescribing supplements and/or making dietary recommendations. The most common such test is hair analysis, which is purported to detect "mineral imbalances" or the presence of "toxic minerals." The test is usually obtained by sending a small amount of hair from the nape of the neck to a commercial laboratory for analysis. The laboratory then issues a computerized report suggesting what supplements might be prescribed. When 52 hair samples from two healthy teenagers were sent under assumed names to 13 commercial hair-analysis laboratories, the reported levels of minerals varied considerably between identical samples sent to the same laboratory and from laboratory to laboratory. The laboratories also disagreed about what was "normal" or "usual" for many of the minerals. Literature from most of the laboratories suggested falsely that their reports were useful against a wide variety of diseases and supposed nutrient imbalances (32). Properly performed, hair analysis has limited value as a research tool but little if any clinical application (33).

Supplement purveyors sometimes use "nutrient deficiency tests" to help them decide what their customers need. One type involves completion of a dietary history; another involves completion of a questionnaire about common symptoms that supposedly are signs of deficiency. The answers are then fed into a computer programed to recommend supplements for everyone. Some manufacturers issue a self-administered questionnaire that invariably recommends supplements.

Functional intracellular analysis (FIA), formerly called essential metabolics analysis, is performed by a laboratory that claims that most Americans have nutrient deficiencies and that "intracellular nutrient deficiencies" even occur in over 40% of Americans who take multivitamins as "insurance." The test is performed by placing isolated lymphocytes from the patient's blood into petri dishes containing various concentrations of nutrients. Properly performed lymphocyte cultures have a legitimate role in testing for concentrations of certain nutrients, but they are not appropriate for general screening or for diagnosing nutrient deficiencies (13).

Some practitioners use data from legitimate laboratory tests but misrepresent their meaning. Chemistry profiles, which measure many different chemical characteristics of the blood, are a valuable screening test in scientific medical practice. But dubious practitioners misuse the test by narrowing the normal ranges so that healthy individuals appear to have abnormalities, which are then used to recommend expensive supplements or special diets (13).

Some practitioners claim that food allergies may be responsible for virtually any symptom and can be treated with vitamin supplementation plus dietary restriction. To detect the alleged offenders, they assess the levels of various immune responses to foods. These levels, however, are not necessarily related to allergy and have nothing whatsoever to do with a person's need for supplements (13).

Although thousands of practitioners (mostly chiropractors) use the above procedures, government regulatory agencies rarely attempt to stop them. Chapter 110 addresses this problem further.

OBESITY QUACKERY

Many weight-reduction schemes are promoted to the public as a solution to obesity. Fad diet books typically have several things in common. They claim to offer a revolutionary new idea based on the author's personal experience. They suggest that certain nutrients, foods, or food combinations are either the key to weight reduction or villains that prevent it. And, they contain inaccurate biochemical information. Many fad diets are unbalanced and lack important nutrients. During the past two decades, many best-selling diet plans have emphasized proteins, some recommending "unlimited" amounts and others using small amounts. "Food-combining" schemes also have been popular. *Fit for Life,* which sold over 3 million copies, claims that obesity caused accumulation of "toxic waste" from incomplete assimilation of foods eaten in the wrong combinations.

Mail-order diet pills are typically "guaranteed" to produce effortless, rapid, and permanent weight loss. Dozens of such pills are offered each year through direct mail solicitations and newspaper advertising. Some of these, as well as others sold over the counter, contain phenylpropanolamine (PPA), a nasal decongestant that can have a temporary effect on appetite. However, there is no evidence that PPA offers any long-term benefit for weight control, many users have experienced severe anxiety reactions, and several cases have been reported of young adults who suffered a stroke after using products containing PPA (34).

Other mail-order pills have been falsely claimed to block absorption of starch, fat, or calories; to flush fat out of the body; or to step up the body's "fat-burning system." Some contain a fiber (e.g., glucomannan or guar gum) that is claimed to curb appetite by absorbing water and swelling to fill the stomach. However, the amount of fiber is too small to actually fill the stomach, and even if it could, that would not necessarily curb a person's appetite. In 1990, guar gum was banned as a diet aid after the FDA received 17 reports of individuals whose esophagus became blocked as a result of using tablets of Cal-Ban 3000, a widely promoted guar gum product (35).

Spirulina, a dark-green powder or pill derived from algae, is said by its promoters to suppress appetite. However, there is no scientific evidence to support this claim.

Products containing *Gymnema sylvestre* are being touted as weight-control aids with claims that they block absorption of sugar. The leaves of this plant, when chewed, can prevent the taste sensation of sweetness. But there is no evidence that *Gymnema sylvestre* blocks absorption of sugar into the body.

Supplements containing chromium picolinate are promoted with unsubstantiated claims that it promotes fat loss and increases lean muscle mass. The FTC has stopped two companies from making such claims, but others have continued to do so.

Products containing ma huang are marketed as weight-loss aids even though they have not been proven safe or effective for this purpose. Ma huang is an herb that contains ephedrine, a nasal decongestant and nervous-system stimulant. Ephedrine can raise blood pressure and therefore is hazardous to individuals with high blood pressure. Deaths have been reported among users of stimulants containing ephedrine and caffeine.

In a study of 653 sick babies, every infant with colic had low blood potassium. "Improvement was dramatic," and the colic disappeared immediately, when physicians gave 500 to 1,000 milligrams of potassium chloride intravenously or 1,000 to 2,000 milligrams by mouth. These doctors found that most babies needed 3,000 milligrams of potassium chloride (⅔ teaspoon) before colic was corrected. They suggested that potassium be given to prevent colic, especially during diarrhea, when much of this nutrient is lost in the feces. Potassium is also lost when too much salt (sodium) is allowed a baby, and/or when pantothenic acid is so deficient that the adrenals become exhausted.

Figure 109.1. Fatal advice. In 1979, this passage from Adelle Davis's *Let's Have Healthy Children* persuaded the mother of 2-month-old Ryan Pitzer to administer potassium drops when he developed colic and became dehydrated. The potassium caused Ryan's heart to stop beating. Davis's advice was based on misrepresentation of a scientific study of infants hospitalized for severe gastroenteritis. The article had nothing do with colic and even warned that giving potassium to dehydrated infants could produce cardiac arrest. Ryan's parents sued Adelle Davis's estate, the book's publisher, and the manufacturer of the potassium drops and won out-of-court settlements totaling $160,000.

DANGERS OF QUACKERY

Quackery's harm can be classified as economic, indirect, direct, psychologic, and societal (36). Individual economic damage can range from a few dollars a year for "nutrition insurance" to many thousands of dollars wasted on quack remedies for serious disease. Since everyone must eat, the potential market for nutritional quackery is immense. Indirect harm occurs when the use of an ineffective approach diverts someone from effective care. Direct harm occurs when a dubious method causes death (Fig. 109.1), serious injury, or unnecessary suffering. Psychologic harm arises when individuals blame themselves for the failure of an ineffective remedy or when they mistakenly conclude they have been helped and become more vulnerable to future deception. Quackery can also harm our democratic society when large numbers of people hold erroneous beliefs about the nature of disease and the best way to deal with it. Limited resources can be wasted if funds are used to follow leads based on inadequate or faked data. Between 1986 and 1990, the American Dietetic Association documented more than 500 cases of people harmed by inappropriate nutritional advice from bogus "nutritionists," health-food-store operators, and others. Privacy considerations, however, have prevented the association from publishing a detailed analysis.

The recent tryptophan tragedy illustrates how inappropriate use of supplements can lead to disaster. In 1989, a form of L-tryptophan was implicated in an outbreak of eosinophilia-myalgia syndrome, a previously rare disorder characterized by severe muscle and joint pain, weakness, swelling of the arms and legs, fever, and rash. This amino acid had been promoted by the health-food industry to treat insomnia, depression, premenstrual syndrome, and overweight, although it had not been proven safe and effective for these purposes. Within a year, more than 1500 cases were reported, with 27 deaths and many hospitalizations (37). When the outbreak's cause was identified, the FDA banned the sale of L-tryptophan products. The outbreak was traced to a Japanese bulk wholesaler that had used a new bacterial strain to produce the L-tryptophan sold to American manufacturers. Attorneys handling the resultant lawsuits state that more than 5000 users were injured and total damages paid by the errant producer have exceeded $1 billion (38).

CONSUMER PROTECTION

Three federal agencies have responsibility for fighting quackery. The Postal Service has jurisdiction over products sold through the mail with false claims. When a scheme is detected, the Postal Service can use an administrative procedure to block transfer of money and orders through the mail. The Postal Service has a vigorous enforcement program but is hampered by loopholes in its law.

The FTC has jurisdiction over the advertising of nonprescription products and services. It files complaints and negotiates settlements, going to court when necessary. It has a very powerful law but insufficient manpower to act against most violations it encounters. The FTC's most notable recent action was a 1994 consent agreement under which General Nutrition, Inc., paid $2.4 million dollars to settle charges that it had falsely advertised 41 products, most of which had been packaged by other manufacturers. The products included 15 alleged weight-control products, 18 alleged "ergogenic aids," 5 bogus hair-loss preventers, 2 alleged antifatigue products, and 2 purported disease-related products (13).

The FDA has jurisdiction over the labeling of foods and drugs. Under federal law, any product "intended for use in the cure, mitigation, treatment or prevention of disease" is a drug. If a product is marketed with drug claims that lack FDA approval, the agency can issue a warning letter, initiate a seizure, obtain an injunction, and/or seek criminal penalties. The claim does not have to be on the product label itself. Any claim traceable to the manufacturer is considered part of the label. The FDA's enforcement ability has been weakened by passage of the Dietary Supplement Health Education Act of 1994 (see Chapter 115), which defines the term *dietary supplement* to include not only vitamins and minerals but also herbs, amino acids, and other substances intended "for use to supplement the diet by increasing total dietary intake." The law also shifted the burden of proof of product safety from manufacturers to the FDA and permits sellers to use third-party literature as sales aids.

Several state attorneys general have been active in combating quackery. But their actions may not stop promoters from continuing their schemes out of state. State and federal laws pertaining to quackery need strengthening (39).

The primary antiquackery force in the United States is the National Council Against Health Fraud (NCAHF), Inc., P.O. Box 1276, Loma Linda, CA 92354. NCAHF is a nonprofit organization of about 1300 health and nutrition professionals, educators, researchers, attorneys, and other concerned citizens wishing to actively oppose misinformation, fraud, and quackery in the health marketplace. Financed primarily by membership dues, it conducts research, publishes a newsletter and task force reports, serves as a clearinghouse, and helps victims of quackery file lawsuits. Table 109.2 advises where to complain about nutrition-related wrongdoing.

Table 109.2
Where to Complain about Nutrition-Related Wrongdoing

Problem	Agencies to Contact[a]
False advertising	FTC Bureau of Consumer Protection or regional office National Advertising Division, Council of Better Business Bureaus
Product marketed with false or misleading claims	Editor or manager of media outlet where ad appeared National or regional FDA office State attorney general State health department Local Better Business Bureau Congressional representatives
Bogus mail-order promotion	Chief postal inspector U.S. Postal Service regional postal inspector State attorney general
Dubious telemarketing	State attorney general FTC Bureau of Consumer Protection or regional office National Fraud Information Center hotline
Improper treatment by licensed practitioner	Editor or station manager of media outlet where ad appeared Local or state professional society (if practitioner is a member) Local hospital (if practitioner is a staff member) State professional licensing board National Council Against Health Fraud Task Force on Victim Redress
Improper treatment by unlicensed individual	Local district attorney State attorney general National Council Against Health Fraud Task Force on Victim Redress

[a]When more than one regulatory agency appears to have jurisdiction, contact each of them:

Chief Postal Inspector, U.S. Postal Service, Washington, DC 20260.

FDA, 5600 Fishers Lane, Rockville, MD 20857.

FTC Bureau of Consumer Protection, Washington, DC 20580.

National Advertising Division, Council of Better Business Bureaus, 845 Third Ave, New York, NY 10022.

National Council Against Health Fraud Task Force on Victim Redress, P.O. Box 1747, Allentown, PA 18105. Tel. (610)437-1795.

National Fraud Information Center hotline: (800)876-7060.

For regional offices of federal agencies consult the telephone directory under U.S. Government.

REFERENCES

1. Schafer R, Yetley EA. J Am Diet Assoc 1975;66:129–33.
2. Barrett S, Jarvis WT, eds. The health robbers: a close look at quackery in America. Amherst, NY: Prometheus Books, 1993.
3. Mindell E. Dr. Earl Mindell's live longer & feel better with vitamins & minerals. New Canaan, CT: Keats Publishing, 1994.
4. Balch JF, Balch PA. Prescription for nutritional healing: a practical A–Z guide to drug-free remedies using vitamins, minerals, herbs & food supplements. Garden City Park, NY: Avery Publishing Group, 1990.
5. Institute of Food Technologists Expert Panel on Food Safety and Nutrition. Food Technol 1990;44(12):123–30.
6. Food and Drug Administration Pesticide Program. Residues monitoring 1994. Washington, DC: Food and Drug Administration, 1995.

7. Basker D. Am J Alternative Agric 1992;7:129–36.
8. Whelan EM, Stare FJ. Panic in the pantry. 2nd ed. Amherst, NY: Prometheus Books, 1992.
9. Federal Register 1993;58(3):631–91,2065–964. (For summary, see Barrett S. Nutr Forum 1993;10:25–30.)
10. Federal Register 1996;61:296–337.
11. Enforcement policy statement on food advertising. Washington, DC: Federal Trade Commission, May 1994.
12. Pollack H, Halpern SL. Therapeutic nutrition. Washington, DC: National Research Council, 1952.
13. Barrett S, Herbert V. The vitamin pushers: how the health food industry is selling America a bill of goods. Amherst, NY: Prometheus Books, 1994.
14. Friedl KE. Performance-enhancing substances: effects, risks, and appropriate alternatives. In: Baechle TR, ed. Essentials of strength training and conditioning. Champaign, IL: Human Kinetics Press, 1994:188–209.
15. Lightsey D, Attaway JR. Natl Strength Conditioning J 1992;14(2):26–31.
16. Anderson SA, Raiten DJ, eds. Safety of amino acids used as dietary supplements. Bethesda, MD: Federation of American Societies for Experimental Biology, 1992.
17. Jha P, Flather M, Lonn E, et al. Ann Intern Med 1995;123(11):860–72.
18. Alpha-Tocopherol, Beta Carotene Cancer Prevention Study Group. N Engl J Med 1994;330:1029–35.
19. Greenberg RE, Baron JA, Tosteson TD, et al. N Engl J Med 1994;331:141–7.
20. Hennekens CH, Buring JE, Manson JE, et al. N Engl J Med 1996;334:1145–9.
21. Omenn GS, Goodman GE, Thornquist MD, et al. N Engl J Med 1996;334:1150–5.
22. Consumer Reports on Health 1995;7:133–5.
23. Geslewitz G. Health Foods Business 1996;42(4):36.
24. Stookey HE, Miller B, Meister K. ACSH News Views 1983;4(3):1, 8–9, 13–4.
25. Aigner C. Nutr Forum 1988;5:1–3.
26. Martin N. Nutr Forum 1990;7:16.
27. Unsubstantiated claims and documented health hazards in the dietary supplement marketplace. Rockville, MD: Food and Drug Administration, 1993.
28. Consumer Reports 1986;51:170–5.
29. Bell LS, Fairchild M. J Am Diet Assoc 1987;87:341–3.
30. Raso J. Nutr Forum 1995;12:13–9.
31. Milner I. Nutr Forum 1995;11:19–22.
32. Barrett S. JAMA 1985;254:1041–5.
33. Hambidge KM. Am J Clin Nutr 1982;36:943–9.
34. Glick R, Hoying J, Cerullo L, et al. Neurosurgery 1987;20: 969–74.
35. Barrett S. Nutr Today 1990;25(6):24–8.
36. Jarvis W. How quackery harms. In: Barrett S, Cassileth BR, eds. Dubious cancer treatment. Tampa: American Cancer Society, Florida Division, 1991:85–92
37. Swygert LA, Maes EF, Sewell LE, et al. JAMA 1990;264: 1698–703.
38. Barrett S. Skeptical Inquirer 1995;19(4):6–9.
39. Barrett S. Priorities 1990;Fall:35–6.

SELECTED READINGS

Barrett S, Herbert V. The vitamin pushers: how the health food industry is selling Americans a bill of goods. Amherst, NY: Prometheus Books, 1994.

Herbert V. Separating food facts from myths. In: Herbert V, Suback-Sharpe GJ, eds. Total nutrition: the only guide you'll ever need. New York: St. Martin's Press, 1995;24–34.

Nutrition Forum, a bimonthly newsletter that forcuses on nutrition quackery and alternative health methods, edited by Jack Raso, and Manfred Kroger; published by Prometheus Books, 59 John Glenn Drive, Amherst, NY 14228.

Yetiv J. Popular nutritional practices: sense and nonsense. San Carlos, CA: Popular Nutritional Press, 1987.

For additional information see Barrett S. Quackwatch (http://www.quackwatch.com)

110. Alternative Nutrition Therapies

VICTOR HERBERT and STEPHEN BARRETT

The dictionary definition of the noun *alternative* is a choice between mutually exclusive possibilities. Until the late 1980s, in standard medical usage, it referred to choices among effective treatments. In some cases, they were equally effective (e.g., the use of radiation or surgery for certain cancers); in others, the expected outcome differed, but there were reasonable tradeoffs between risks and benefits. During recent years, however, the word *alternative* has been applied to a multitude of unsubstantiated approaches that differ from standard medical ones.

To avoid confusion, alternative methods should be classified as genuine, experimental, or questionable. *Genuine* alternatives are comparable methods that have met science-based criteria for safety and effectiveness. Under the rules of science (and federal law), proponents who make health claims bear the burden of proof. It is their responsibility to conduct suitable studies and report them in sufficient detail to permit evaluation and confirmation by others. Methods can be evaluated by addressing four questions: *(a)* Has the method shown potential for benefit that clearly exceeds the potential for harm? *(b)* Have safety and efficacy been demonstrated by objective studies using adequate controls? *(c)* Have the methodology and results been published in peer-reviewed scientific journals? and *(d)* Have the results been replicated by others? Peer review is a process in which work is reviewed by others, usually with equivalent or superior knowledge. The best scientific journals use experts for this purpose. Detailed standards for reporting and evaluating studies have been published (1).

Experimental alternatives are unproven but have a plausible rationale and are undergoing responsible investigation. The most noteworthy is the use of a 10%-fat diet for treating coronary heart disease. *Questionable* alternatives are groundless because they lack a scientifically plausible rationale or have been disproved. The archetype is homeopathy, which claims that "remedies" so dilute that they contain no active ingredient can exert powerful therapeutic effects. When the three types of alternatives are lumped together, promoters of questionable methods can argue that because some have merit, the rest deserve equal consideration and respect. This chapter uses the word *alternative* in its "questionable" sense.

When someone feels better after using a product or procedure, it is natural to credit whatever was done. This can mislead, however, because most ailments resolve spontaneously, and those that persist can have symptoms that wax and wane. Even serious conditions can have sufficient month-to-month variation to enable spurious methods to gain large followings. In addition, taking action often temporarily relieves symptoms via the placebo effect. This effect is a beneficial change in a person's condition that occurs in response to a treatment but is not due to the pharmacologic or physical aspects of the treatment. Belief in the treatment is not essential, but the placebo effect may be enhanced by such factors as faith, sympathetic attention, sensational claims, testimonials, and the use of scientific-looking charts, devices, and terminology. Another drawback of individual success stories is that they don't indicate how many failures might occur for each success. (In other words, no score is kept.) People unaware of these facts often give undeserved credit to "alternative" methods.

"Complementary medicine" is described by its proponents as a synthesis of standard and "alternative" methods that uses the best of both. However, no published data indicate the extent to which "complementary" practitioners actually use proven therapies or the extent to which they burden patients with medically useless methods. These practitioners typically claim credit for any improvement experienced by the patient and blame standard treatments for any negative effects. The result may be to undermine the patient's confidence in standard care, reducing compliance or causing the patient to abandon it altogether (2).

"Alternative" nutrition therapies appeal to people who would like to take an active role in their treatment. The products used are claimed to be safer and more effective than medically prescribed drugs. Government regulation of these products and the practitioners who prescribe them is minimal.

UNSUBSTANTIATED CLAIMS

When challenged about the lack of scientific evidence supporting what they espouse, "alternative" promoters may claim that *(a)* scientific reports (whose meaning they distort) back them up, *(b)* research isn't necessary because they have seen with their own eyes that their methods are effective, *(c)* funds are not available for them to perform research, *(d)* the scientific establishment is unwilling to test their methods or look at their data, and *(e)* scientific journals are unwilling to consider their research because it poses a threat to the establishment. Each of these claims is incorrect. Preliminary research does not require funding or even take much effort. The principal ingredients are careful clinical observations, detailed record keeping, and long-term follow-up to "keep score." Proponents of "alternative" methods almost never do any of these things. Some even claim their concepts cannot be tested by scientific methods.

A study involving vitamin C illustrates why anecdotal evidence is not an appropriate substitute for carefully designed clinical trials. The study compared the effect of administering vitamin C supplements and placebo before and during colds. Although the experiment was supposed to be double blind, half the subjects were able to guess which pill they were getting. When the results were tabulated with all subjects lumped together, the vitamin group reported fewer colds per person over a 9-month period. But among the half who hadn't guessed which pill they had been taking, no difference in the incidence or severity was found (3). This demonstrates how people who think they are doing something effective can report a favorable result even when none exists.

Each of the approaches described in this chapter has one or more of the following characteristics: *(a)* its rationale or underlying theory has no scientific basis, *(b)* it has not been demonstrated safe and/or effective by well-designed studies, *(c)* it is deceptively promoted, or *(d)* its practitioners are not qualified to make appropriate medical diagnoses.

"ALTERNATIVE" SYSTEMS

Many "alternative" approaches involve nutrition-related methods. Proponents of these methods typically claim that *(a)* certain foods or nutrients have special ability to cure specific diseases; *(b)* certain foods are harmful and should be eliminated from the diet; and *(c)* "natural foods" are best. Most systems described in this section are also rooted in *vitalism,* the concept that bodily functions are due to a "vital force" that cannot be explained by the laws of physics and chemistry. Vitalistic proponents maintain that diseases should be treated by stimulating the body to heal itself rather than by "treating symptoms." Naturopaths, for example, claim that illness is due to a disturbance of the body's natural healing force, which they can augment by "detoxification." Some vitalists assert that food can be "dead" or "living" and that "live" foods contain a dormant or primitive "life force" that humans can assimilate. None of these "energies" can be measured by scientific methods.

Chinese Medicine

Traditional Chinese medicine (TCM), also called Oriental medicine, is based on beliefs that the body's vital energy (*Chi* or *Qi*) circulates through 14 hypothetical channels called meridians, which have branches connected to bodily organs and functions (4). Illness and disease are attributed to imbalance or interruption of *Chi.* Acupuncture, herbs, and various other modalities are claimed to restore balance. After extensive study of published reports, a National Council Against Health Fraud task force concluded that *(a)* acupuncture has not been proven effective for the treatment of any disease; *(b)* the greater the benefit claimed in a research report, the worse the experimental design, and *(c)* the best-designed experiments—those with the highest number of controls on variables—found no difference between acupuncture and control groups (5).

Many TCM practitioners are licensed acupuncturists. They are not permitted to prescribe drugs, but they are free to recommend dietary supplements and herbs. The diagnostic process they use may include questioning (medical history, lifestyle), observations (skin, tongue, color), listening (breath sounds), and pulse taking. Medical science recognizes only one pulse, corresponding to the heartbeat, which can be felt in the wrist, neck, feet, and various other places throughout the body. TCM practitioners check six alleged pulse aspects at each wrist and identify more than 25 alleged pulse qualities such as "sinking," "slippery," "soggy," "tight," and "wiry." TCM's "pulses" supposedly reflect the type of imbalance, the condition of each organ system, and the status of the patient's *Chi.* The herbs they prescribe are not regulated for safety, potency, or effectiveness. Although some cases of adverse effects from herbs have been reported (6), no systematic assessment of this problem has been published.

Maharishi Ayur-Ved

Proponents state that ayurvedic medicine originated in ancient times but was reconstituted in the early 1980s by the Maharishi Mahesh Yogi, who also popularized transcendental meditation (TM). Its origin is traced to four Sanskrit books called the *Vedas*—the oldest and most important scriptures of India, shaped sometime before 200 BCE. These books attributed most disease and bad luck to demons, devils, and the influence of stars and planets. Ayurveda's basic theory states that the body's functions are regulated by three "irreducible physiologic principles" called *doshas,* whose Sanskrit names are *vata, pitta,* and *kapha.* Like the "sun signs" of astrology, these terms are used to designate body types as well as the traits that typify them. Like astrologic writings, ayurvedic writings contain long lists of supposed physical and mental characteristics of each constitutional type. Through various combinations of *vata, pitta,* and *kapha,* 10 body types are possible. However, one's *doshas* (and therefore one's body type) can vary from hour to hour and season to season.

Ayurvedic proponents state that the symptoms of disease are always related to balance of the *doshas,* which can be determined by feeling the patient's wrist pulse or completing a questionnaire (7). Balance is supposedly achieved through "pacifying" diets, "purification" (to remove "impurities due to faulty diet and behavioral patterns"), TM, and a long list of procedures and ayurvedic products, many of which are said to be formulated for specific body types. Most of these cost several hundred dollars, but some cost thousands and require the services of an ayurvedic practitioner. Although many ayurvedic herbal products have been marketed with illegal claims, FDA regulatory action has been minimal.

Macrobiotics

Macrobiotics is a quasireligious system that advocates a semivegetarian diet. Macrobiotic diets have been promoted for maintaining general health and for preventing and treating cancer, AIDS, and other diseases. The optimal diet is said to balance "yin" and "yang" foods. It is composed of whole grains (50–60% of each meal), vegetables (25–30% of each meal), whole beans or soybean-based products (5–10% of daily food), nuts and seeds (small amounts as snacks), miso soup, herbal teas, and small amounts of white meat or seafood once or twice weekly (8). The yin/yang classification is not related to nutrient content but is based on the food's color, pH, shape, size, taste, temperature, texture, water content, and weight; the region and season in which the food was grown; and how it is prepared and eaten. Some macrobiotic diets contain inadequate amounts of certain nutrients. Infants on macrobiotic diets have developed rickets and had deficiencies of vitamin B_{12} and iron (9, 10).

Macrobiotics is promoted through books, local organizations, health-food stores, unlicensed practitioners, and a few physicians. Practitioners typically base their recommendations on "pulse" diagnosis and other unscientific procedures related to Chinese medicine. These include "ancestral diagnosis," "astrologic diagnosis," "aura and vibrational diagnosis," "environmental diagnosis" (including consideration of "celestial influences" and tidal motions), and "spiritual diagnosis" (an evaluation of "atmospheric vibrational conditions" to identify spiritual influences, including "visions of the future") (11).

Today's leading proponent is Michio Kushi, founder and president of the Kushi Institute in Becket, Massachusetts. Institute publications state that the macrobiotic way of life should include chewing food at least 50 times per mouthful (or until it becomes liquid), not wearing synthetic or woolen clothing next to the skin, avoiding long hot baths or showers, having large green plants in your house to enrich the oxygen content of the air, and singing a happy song every day (12). Kushi claims that cancer is largely due to improper diet, thinking, and way of life, and can be influenced by changing these factors. He recommends yin foods (such as tropical fruits) for cancers due to excess yang, and yang foods (such as eggs and meat) for tumors that are predominantly yin (13). His books contain case histories of people whose cancers have supposedly disappeared after they adopted macrobiotic eating. However, the only reports of efficacy are testimonials by patients, many of whom also received standard medical treatment (14). The high-fiber diet can cause cancer patients to undergo serious weight loss (15).

Naturopathy

Naturopaths claim to remove the underlying cause(s) of disease and to stimulate the body's natural healing processes (16). They maintain that diseases are the body's effort to purify itself and that cures result from increasing the patient's "vital force" by ridding the body of waste products and "toxins." However, they do not specify the chemical names of the "toxins," indicate how to measure them, or demonstrate that "detoxification" reduces the quantity in the body.

Although naturopaths say they emphasize prevention, they tend to oppose immunization. The doctor of naturopathy (N.D.) degree is available from three full-time naturopathy schools and a few correspondence schools. Naturopaths are licensed as independent practitioners in 11 states and may legally practice in a few others.

Most naturopaths believe that virtually all diseases are within the scope of their practice. Their methods include fasting, "natural food" diets, vitamins, herbs, tissue minerals, cell salts, manipulation, massage, exercise, colonic irrigation (see below), acupuncture, natural childbirth, minor surgery, and applications of water, heat, cold, air, sunlight, and electricity. They may use radiation for diagnosis but not for treatment. "Detoxification" plays a prominent role. The most comprehensive naturopathic textbook recommends special diets, vitamins, minerals, and/or herbs for more than 70 health problems ranging from acne to AIDS (17). For many of these conditions, daily administration of 10 or more products is recommended, some in dosages high enough to be toxic.

Natural Hygiene

Natural Hygiene, an offshoot of naturopathy, is a "philosophy" of health and "natural living" that advocates a "raw food" diet of vegetables, fruits, and nuts. It also advocates periodic fasting and "food combining" (avoiding food combinations it considers detrimental) (18). Natural

Hygienists oppose immunization, fluoridation, and food irradiation and eschew most forms of medical treatment.

Orthomolecular Therapy

During the early 1950s, a few psychiatrists began adding massive doses of nutrients to the treatment of severe mental problems. The original substance used was niacin, and the therapy was termed *megavitamin therapy.* Since that time, the treatment regimen has been expanded to include other vitamins, minerals, hormones, and diets, any of which may be combined with mainstream drug therapy or electroconvulsive therapy.

Current proponents now call this system *orthomolecular psychiatry,* a term meaning "the treatment of mental disease by providing an optimum molecular environment for the mind, especially substances normally present in the human body." Proponents claim that abnormal conditions are caused by molecular imbalances that can be corrected by administration of the "right" nutrient molecules at the right time. (*Ortho* is Greek for "right.") They also claim that their treatment is effective against many diseases. Their evaluations usually include laboratory tests that most physicians would consider questionable.

In 1973, an American Psychiatric Association task force report noted that megavitamin proponents used unconventional methods not only in treatment, but also in diagnosis. The report concluded that "the credibility of the megavitamin proponents is low" and "is further diminished by a consistent refusal over the past decade to perform controlled experiments and to report their new results in a scientifically acceptable fashion" (19). In 1979, the Research Advisory Committee of the National Institute of Mental Health concluded that megavitamin therapy was ineffective and could be harmful. Additional claims that megavitamins and megaminerals are effective against psychosis, learning disorders, and mental retardation in children were debunked in reports by the nutrition committees of the American Academy of Pediatrics in 1976 and 1981 and by the Canadian Academy of Pediatrics in 1990 (20). Both groups warned that there was no proven benefit in any of these conditions and that megadoses can have serious toxic effects. The 1976 report concluded that a cult had developed among followers of megavitamin therapy (21).

Iridology

Iridology is based on the notion that each area of the body is represented by a corresponding area in the iris of the eye (the colored area surrounding the pupil). Many of its practitioners are chiropractors or naturopaths, but it is also used by bogus nutritionists and by laypersons involved in multilevel marketing (22). Iridologists claim that states of health and disease can be diagnosed from the color, texture, and location of various pigment flecks in the eye. Iridology practitioners purport to diagnose "imbalances" and treat them with vitamins, minerals, herbs, and similar products. They may also claim that the eye markings can reveal a complete history of past illnesses as well as previous treatment. Two large objective trials involving prominent iridologists found that they could not distinguish between patients who had a disease (kidney or gallbladder disease) and those who were healthy. Nor did they agree with each other about who was ill (23–24).

Metabolic Therapy

Proponents of "metabolic therapy" claim to diagnose abnormalities at the cellular level and correct them by normalizing the patient's metabolism. They regard cancer, arthritis, multiple sclerosis, and other "degenerative" diseases as the result of metabolic imbalance caused by a buildup of "toxic" substances in the body. They claim that scientific practitioners merely treat the symptoms of the disease while they treat the cause by removing "toxins" and strengthening the immune system so the body can heal itself. The "toxins" are neither defined nor objectively measurable. "Metabolic" treatment regimens vary from practitioner to practitioner and may include a "natural food" diet, coffee enemas, vitamins, minerals, "glandulars," enzymes, laetrile, and various other nostrums that are not legally marketable in the United States. The components of metabolic therapy vary from practitioner to practitioner. No controlled study has shown that any of its components has any value against cancer or any other chronic disease. However, many people find its concepts appealing because they do not seem far removed from scientific medicine's concerns with diet, lifestyle, and the relationship between emotions and bodily responses.

The most visible proponent of metabolic therapy was Harold Manner, Ph.D., a biology professor who announced in 1977 that he had cured cancer in mice with injections of laetrile, enzymes, and vitamin A. In fact, he had digested the tumors by injecting them with digestive enzymes, which cannot cure cancers that have metastasized. During the early 1980s, Manner left his teaching position and became affiliated with a clinic in Tijuana, Mexico. Although he claimed a high success rate in treating cancers, there is no evidence that he kept track of patients after they left his clinic (25). He died in 1988, but the clinic is still operating.

"Chiropractic Nutrition"

Chiropractic nutrition is based on beliefs that most ailments are the result of spinal problems (26). Chiropractors can be divided into two main types: "straights" and "mixers." Straights tend to cling to the doctrine that most illness is caused by misaligned vertebrae ("subluxations") that can be corrected by "spinal adjustment." Mixers acknowledge that germs, hormones, and other factors play a role in disease, but they tend to regard mechanical disturbances of the nervous system as the underlying cause (through "lowered resistance"). In addition to spinal manipulation, mixers may use nutritional methods and various types of physiotherapy (heat, cold, traction, exercise, massage, and ultrasound). Chiropractors are licensed in all 50 states. They are not permitted to prescribe drugs or perform surgery, but most states permit them to prescribe dietary supplements, herbs, and homeopathic products.

Chiropractors who give nutritional advice typically recommend supplements that are unnecessary or are inappropriate for treating health problems. One such product is Spine Align, which, according to its manufacturer, can help repair, regenerate, correct, and normalize the spine. Its ingredients include "whole spinal column" (from cows), bone meal, silica, boron aminoate, copper gluconate, aromatic root beer, and potassium iodide. Many chiropractors espouse nutrition-related systems of diagnosis and treatment that lack scientific validity. The most noteworthy are applied kinesiology (AK), bioenergetic synchronization technique (B.E.S.T.), and contact reflex analysis (CRA).

AK is a pseudoscientific system of muscle testing and therapy based on assertions that specific muscle weaknesses are signs of disease in body organs. AK practitioners—most of whom are chiropractors—claim that nutritional deficiencies, allergies, and other adverse reactions to food substances can be detected by placing substances in the mouth or hand and testing muscle strength. "Good" substances supposedly make specific muscles stronger, whereas "bad" substances cause specific weaknesses. "Treatment" typically includes dietary modification, food supplements, acupressure, and spinal manipulation. Controlled studies of AK muscle-testing procedures have found no difference between results with test substances and those with placebos (27). Differences from one test to another may be due to suggestibility, variations in the amount of force or leverage involved, and/or muscle fatigue.

B.E.S.T. practitioners claim that an imbalance in the patient's electromagnetic field causes unequal leg length, which the chiropractor can instantly correct by applying his or her own electromagnetic energy to proper points on the body. According to this notion, two fingers on each of the chiropractor's hands are "North poles," two are "South poles," and the thumbs are electromagnetically neutral. When imbalance is detected, the hands are held for a few seconds at "contact points" on the patient's body until "pulsation" is felt and the patient's legs test equally long. Proponents recommend that such testing be started early in infancy and continued at least monthly throughout life.

B.E.S.T.'s "nutritional" component is based on the notion that "patients can maintain life and vitality by consuming four times as much alkaline-forming as acid-forming foods." Proponents claim that saliva pH can reveal whether a person's symptoms are nutritionally or emotionally based and indicates whether the most effective method of care is nutritional supplementation and/or adjustive. The recommended supplements include a barley juice concentrate, a weight-reduction formula, an alleged digestive aid, and various herbs. For babies, a mixture of raw goat milk, carrot juice, and distilled water is said to be "an excellent replacement for infant formulas."

CRA resembles aspects of applied kinesiology and B.E.S.T. To diagnose a patient, the practitioner pulls on the patient's outstretched arm while placing a finger or hand on one of about 75 "reflex" points on the patient's body. If the patient's arm can be pulled downward, the disease corresponding to the reflex is said to be present. Large numbers of pills containing vitamins, minerals, dehydrated vegetables, and/or freeze-dried animal organs are then prescribed to correct the alleged problems.

Many companies market supplements exclusively or primarily through chiropractic offices, where they are sold for at least twice their wholesale cost. Thousands of these products are intended for the treatment of disease, even though they are questionable and lack FDA approval for this use.

The percentage of chiropractors engaging in unscientific nutritional practices is unknown but appears to be substantial. A 1991 survey by the National Board of Chiropractic Examiners found that 83.5% of 4835 full-time practitioners who responded said they had used "nutritional counseling, therapy or supplements," and 37.2% said they had used AK within the previous 2 years. Chiropractors who prescribe supplements usually sell them to their patients for two to three times their wholesale cost. A typical regimen costs the patient several dollars per day. Chiropractic licensing authorities have not attempted to curtail inappropriate "chiropractic nutrition."

Colonic Irrigation

Some chiropractors and naturopaths advocate colonic irrigation as part of their treatment system. In this procedure, a rubber tube is passed into the rectum for a distance of up to 20 or 30 inches, and warm water is pumped in and out, a few pints at a time, typically using 20 or more gallons. Some practitioners add herbs, coffee, or other substances to the water. The procedure is said to "detoxify" the body. Its advocates claim that as a result of intestinal stasis, intestinal contents putrefy, and toxins are formed and absorbed, which causes chronic poisoning of the body.

This "autointoxication" theory was popular around the turn of the century but was abandoned by the scientific community during the 1930s. No such "toxins" have ever been identified, and careful observations have shown that individuals in good health can vary greatly in bowel habits. Proponents may also suggest that fecal material collects on the lining of the intestine and causes trouble unless removed by laxatives, colonic irrigation, special diets, and/or various herbs or food supplements that "cleanse" the body. The falsity of this notion is obvious to doctors who perform intestinal surgery or peer within the large intestine with a diagnostic instrument. Fecal material does not adhere to the intestinal lining.

Colonic irrigation is not only therapeutically worthless but can cause fatal electrolyte imbalance. Cases of death due to intestinal perforation and infection (from contaminated equipment) have also been reported (28).

"Electrodiagnosis"

Hundreds of "alternative" practitioners use devices purported to detect and treat "energy imbalances" said to signify organ dysfunctions, allergies, and other problems. This approach, called electrodiagnosis or Electroacupuncture according to Voll (EAV), was initiated during the 1970s by a German physician who developed the first model of the device (29). Subsequent models include the Vega, Dermatron, Accupath 1000, and Interro. Proponents claim these devices measure disturbances in the body's flow of "electro-magnetic energy" along "acupuncture meridians." Actually, they measure electrical resistance of the patient's skin when touched by a probe. One wire from the device goes to a brass cylinder covered by moist gauze, which the patient holds in one hand. A second wire is connected to a probe, which the operator touches to "acupuncture points" on the patient's other hand or foot. This completes a low-voltage circuit, and the device registers the flow of current. The information is then relayed to a gauge that provides a numerical readout. The size of the number actually depends on how hard the probe is pressed against the patient's skin. The "treatment" selected depends on the scope of the practitioner's practice and may include acupuncture, dietary change (to avoid supposed allergens), vitamin supplements, and/or homeopathic remedies.

FAD DIAGNOSES

Some practitioners misdiagnose large numbers of their patients with one or more conditions considered rare or even nonexistent by scientific practitioners. Some of these diagnoses are based on the patient's history (typically including fatigue and other common emotionally related symptoms), while others are based on inappropriate or misinterpreted laboratory tests.

Hypoglycemia

Many "alternative" practitioners diagnose "hypoglycemia" in large numbers of patients who report symptoms of nervousness or fatigue. It is actually quite rare, however. The diagnosis of functional hypoglycemia should not be made unless a person on a balanced diet gets symptoms 2 to 4 hours after eating, has a blood glucose level below 45 mg/100 mL whenever symptoms occur, and is immediately relieved of symptoms when the blood glucose level is raised. The glucose tolerance test is not reliable for evaluating most cases of suspected hypoglycemia (30). Low blood sugar levels without symptoms occur commonly in normal individuals fed large amounts of sugar and are of no diagnostic significance.

"Environmental Illness"

"Clinical ecologists" claim that hypersensitivity to common foods and chemicals triggers dozens of symptoms that they label "environmental illness," or "multiple chemical sensitivity." They speculate that *(a)* although various substances alone may not cause trouble, low doses of different substances can add to or multiply each other's effects; *(b)* hypersensitivity develops when the total load of physical and psychologic stresses exceeds a person's tolerance; *(c)* hypersensitivities may be related to "immune system dysregulation" that can be difficult to diagnose and treat; *(d)* potential stressors include practically everything that modern humans encounter; and *(e)* the resultant symptoms can mimic almost any other condition (31). They base their diagnoses primarily on the results of "provocation" and "neutralization" tests, which are performed by having the patient report symptoms that occur within a specified period of time after suspected harmful substances are placed under the tongue or injected into the skin. If any symptoms occur, the test is considered positive, and lower concentrations are given until a dose is found that "neutralizes" the symptoms. Double-blind testing conducted by researchers at the University of California demonstrated that these procedures are not valid (32).

The American Academy of Allergy and Immunology (AAAI), the nation's largest professional organization of allergists, has warned that "although the idea that the environment is responsible for a multitude of health problems is very appealing, to present such ideas as facts, conclusions, or even likely mechanisms without adequate support, is poor medical practice" (33). Chapter 92 describes the appropriate diagnosis of food allergies.

"Yeast Infections"

"Candidiasis hypersensitivity" is an alleged condition with multiple symptoms similar to those of "environmental illness." The AAAI regards this diagnosis as "speculative and unproven." Nevertheless, proponents claim that if a careful checkup does not reveal a cause for such symptoms and a medical history includes antibiotic usage, a "yeast" problem is likely (34). The proposed treatment program includes food supplements, special diets, and treatment with antifungal drugs. In 1990, a double-blind trial found the antifungal drug nystatin was no better than a placebo for relieving systemic or psychologic symptoms attributed to "candidiasis hypersensitivity syndrome" (35).

"Mercury-Amalgam Toxicity"

The alleged condition "mercury-amalgam toxicity" is diagnosed by a few hundred dentists and physicians who claim that the mercury in silver-mercury fillings is toxic and causes a wide range of illnesses. They recommend replacing these fillings with other materials, which can cost thousands of dollars. Some recommend an elaborate program of supplements to minimize negative effects said to occur when the mercury-containing fillings are removed. The ADA Council on Ethics, Bylaws, and Judicial Affairs considers the unnecessary removal of silver-amalgam fillings improper and unethical (36). The leading antiamalgamist, a dentist, had his license revoked in 1996.

Many physicians accustomed to rendering the above "fad diagnoses" have added chronic fatigue syndrome, Lyme disease, food allergies, and "parasites" to their list of overdiagnosed conditions.

QUESTIONABLE CANCER THERAPIES

The American Cancer Society (ACS) defines questionable methods as lifestyle practices, clinical tests, or therapeutic modalities that are promoted for *general* use for the prevention, diagnosis, or treatment of cancer and which are, on the basis of careful review by scientists and/or clinicians, deemed to have no real evidence of value (37). These methods include corrosive agents, plant products, special diets and "dietary supplements," drugs, correction of "imbalances," biologic methods, devices, miscellaneous concoctions, psychologic approaches, and worthless diagnostic tests. Many promoters combine methods to make themselves more marketable. A 1987 ACS investigation found that 452 (9%) of 5047 cancer patients identified through a telephone survey had used questionable treatments. Of these, 49% had used "mind therapies" (mental imagery, hypnosis, or psychic therapy), and 38% had used diets (38).

Promoters of questionable cancer treatment typically explain their approach in commonsense terms that appear to offer patients an active role: *(a)* cancer is a symptom, not a disease; *(b)* symptoms are caused by diet, stress, or environment; and *(c)* proper fitness, nutrition, and mental attitude allow biologic and mental defense against cancer. Nutrition-related methods are compatible with each of these "selling points" and therefore are highly marketable. They include fasting, megadoses of nutrients, consumption of raw foods, "detoxification," organ extracts, and various dietary regimens. The ACS advises that although dietary measures (e.g., eating more vegetables) may help prevent certain cancers, there is no scientific evidence that any dietary regimen is appropriate as a primary *treatment* for cancer (39).

Laetrile

Laetrile, which achieved great notoriety during the 1970s and early 1980s, is the trade name for a synthetic relative of amygdalin, a chemical in the kernels of apricot pits, apple seeds, bitter almonds, and some other stone fruits and nuts. Some promoters have called it "vitamin B_{17}" and falsely claimed that cancer is a vitamin deficiency disease that laetrile can cure. When subjected to enzymatic breakdown in the body, amygdalin forms glucose, benzaldehyde, and hydrogen cyanide. Some cancer patients treated with laetrile have suffered nausea, vomiting, headache, and dizziness, and a few have died from cyanide poisoning (40). Laetrile has been tested in at least 20 animal tumor models and found to have no benefit either alone or together with other substances. Studies of case reports of humans have also been uniformly negative, as has a clinical trial sponsored by the National Cancer Institute (NCI) (41–43).

In 1975 a patient sued in federal court to try to stop the FDA from interfering with the sale and distribution of laetrile. Early in the case, a sympathetic judge issued orders allowing cancer patients to import a 6-month supply of laetrile for personal use if they could obtain a physician's affidavit that they were "terminal." A higher court partially upheld this ruling, but in 1979, the U.S. Supreme Court ruled that it is not possible to be certain who is terminal and that even if it were possible, both terminally ill patients and the general public deserve protection from fraudulent cures. In 1987, after further appeals were denied, the judge who set up the affidavit system finally yielded to the higher courts and terminated it (44). Today few sources of laetrile are available within the United States, but it still is used at Mexican clinics (45).

Gerson Method

Proponents of the Gerson diet claim that cancer can be cured only if toxins are eliminated from the body. They recommend "detoxification" with frequent coffee enemas and a low-sodium diet that includes more than a gallon a day of juices made from fruits, vegetables, and raw calf's liver. This method was developed by Max Gerson, a German-born physician who emigrated to the United States in 1936 and practiced in New York City until his death in 1959. Still available at a Mexican clinic, Gerson therapy is actively promoted by his daughter, Charlotte Gerson, through lectures, talk show appearances, and publications. Gerson protocols have included liver extract injections, ozone and coffee enemas, "live cell therapy," thyroid tablets, royal jelly capsules, linseed oil, castor oil enemas, clay packs, laetrile, and vaccines made from influenza virus and killed *Staphylococcus aureus* bacteria.

Charlotte Gerson claims that treatment at the clinic has produced high cure rates for many cancers. In 1986, however, a Gerson publicist admitted that patients were not monitored after they left the facility (46). Three naturopaths who visited the Gerson Clinic in 1983 were able to track 18 patients over a 5-year period (or until death) through annual letters or phone calls. At the 5-year mark, only one was still alive (but not cancer free); the rest had succumbed to their cancer (47).

A review of the Gerson rationale has concluded that *(a)* the "poisons" Gerson claimed were present in processed foods have never been identified, *(b)* frequent coffee enemas have never been shown to mobilize and remove poisons from the liver and intestines of cancer patients, *(c)* there is no evidence that any such poisons are related to the onset of cancer, *(d)* there is no evidence that a "healing" inflammatory reaction exists that can seek out and kill cancer cells (48).

Kelley Metabolic Therapy

In the 1960s, William Donald Kelley, D.D.S., developed a program for cancer patients that involved dietary measures, vitamin and enzyme supplements, and computerized "metabolic typing." Kelley classified people as "sympathetic dominant," "parasympathetic dominant," or "metabolically balanced" and made dietary recommendations for each type. He claimed that his "Protein Metabolism Evaluation Index" could diagnose cancer before it was clinically apparent and that his "Kelley Malignancy Index" could detect "the presence or absence of cancer, the growth rate of the tumor, the location of the tumor mass, prognosis of the treatment, age of the tumor and the regulation of medication for treatment" (49).

In 1970, Kelley was convicted of practicing medicine without a license after witnesses testified that he had diagnosed lung cancer on the basis of blood from a patient's finger and prescribed dietary supplements, enzymes, and a diet as treatment. In 1976, following court appeals, his dental license was suspended for 5 years. However, he continued to promote his methods until the mid-1980s through his Dallas-based International Health Institute. Under the institute's umbrella, licensed professionals and "certified metabolic technicians" throughout the United States would administer a 3200-item questionnaire and send the answers to Dallas. The resultant computer printout provided a lengthy report on "metabolic status" plus detailed instructions covering foods, supplements (typically 100–200 pills per day), "detoxification" techniques, and lifestyle changes.

Treatment said to be similar is still provided today by Nicholas Gonzales, M.D., of New York City, who claims to have analyzed Kelley's records and drafted a book about his findings. The manuscript was never published, but experts who evaluated its chapter on 50 cases found no evidence of benefit (50). Gonzales says that he offers "10 basic diets with 90 variations" and typically prescribes coffee enemas and up to "150 pills a day in 10 to 12 divided doses."

In 1997, a jury awarded $2.65 million in damages to a former Gonzales patient. The woman had consulted Gonzales after having surgery for early uterine cancer. She testified that he encouraged her to rely on his treatment instead of medically recommended follow-up radiation and chemotherapy. The cancer progressed, damaging her spine and leaving her blind (49a).

Livingston-Wheeler Regimen

Virginia C. Livingston, M.D., who died in 1990, postulated that cancer is caused by a bacterium she called *Progenitor cryptocides,* which invades the body when "immunity is stressed or weakened." She claimed to combat this by strengthening the body's immune system with vaccines (including one made from the patient's urine); "detoxification" with enemas; digestive enzymes; a vegetarian diet that avoided chicken, eggs, and sugar; vitamin and mineral supplements; visualization; and stress reduction. She claimed to have a very high recovery rate but published no clinical data to support this (51). Scientists who attempted to isolate the organism she postulated found that it was a common skin bacterium. Researchers compared 78 patients treated at the University of Pennsylvania Cancer Center with similar patients treated at the Livingston-Wheeler Clinic. All had advanced cancers for which no proven treatment was known. As expected, the study found no difference in average survival time of the two groups. However, Livingston-Wheeler patients reported more appetite difficulties and pain (52).

Shark Cartilage

Powdered shark cartilage is purported to contain a protein that inhibits the growth of new blood vessels needed for the spread of cancer. Although a modest effect has been observed in laboratory experiments, it has not been demonstrated that feeding shark cartilage to humans significantly inhibits blood-vessel formation in patients with cancer. Even if direct applications were effective, oral administration would not work because the protein would be digested rather than absorbed intact into the body. Nevertheless, in 1993 CBS-TV's "60 Minutes" aired a program promoting the claims of biochemist/entrepreneur I. William Lane, Ph.D., coauthor of *Sharks Don't Get Cancer.* The program highlighted a Cuban study of 29 "terminal" cancer patients who received shark-cartilage preparations. Narrator Mike Wallace filmed several of the patients doing exercises and reported that most of them felt better several weeks after the treatment had begun. The fact that "feeling better" does not indicate whether a cancer treatment is effective was not mentioned. Nor was the fact that sharks do get cancer, even of their cartilage (53). NCI officials who reviewed the Cuban data called them "incomplete and unimpressive" (54). Proponents claim to be doing additional research, but none of it has been published in a significant scientific journal.

Vitamin C

The claim that vitamin C is useful for treating cancer is largely attributable to Linus Pauling, Ph.D. During the mid-1970s, Pauling began claiming that high doses of vitamin C are effective in preventing and curing cancer. In 1976 and 1978, he and a Scottish physician, Ewan Cameron, reported that a group of 100 terminal cancer patients treated with 10,000 mg of vitamin C daily had survived three to four times longer than historically matched patients who did not receive vitamin C supplements. However, Dr. William DeWys, chief of clinical investigations at the NCI, found that the patient groups were not comparable (55). The vitamin C patients were Cameron's, while the other patients were managed by other physicians. Cameron's patients were started on vitamin C when he labeled them "untreatable" by other methods, and their subsequent survival was compared with the survival of the "control" patients after they were labeled "untreatable" by their doctors. DeWys found that Cameron's patients were labeled untreatable much earlier in the course of their disease, which meant that they entered the hospital before they were as sick as the other doctors' patients and would naturally be expected to live longer. Nevertheless, to test whether Pauling might be correct, the Mayo Clinic conducted three double-blind studies involving a total of 367 patients with advanced cancer. All three studies found that patients given 10 g of vitamin C daily did no better than those given a placebo (56–58).

POLITICAL CONSIDERATIONS

The "alternative movement" is part of a general societal trend toward rejection of science as a method of determining truth. This movement embraces the postmodernist doctrine that science is not necessarily more valid than pseudoscience (59). In line with this philosophy, "alternative" proponents assert that scientific medicine (which they mislabel as allopathic, conventional, or traditional medicine) is but one of a vast array of healthcare options. Instead of subjecting their work to scientific standards, they would like to change the rules by which they are judged and regulated.

Research proposals normally get funded by competing on the basis of merit. A federal law passed in 1991 ordered the National Institutes of Health (NIH) to foster research into unconventional practices. The law was passed after proponents of questionable cancer treatments convinced several congressmen that they deserved more study than they had been getting. To carry out the law's intent, NIH established what is now called the Office of Alternative Medicine (OAM). It also appointed an advisory committee that included the former congressman and advocates of acupuncture, "energy medicine," homeopathy, ayurvedic medicine, and questionable cancer therapies. A few qualified researchers have served on the panel but have had little influence on its output. Some advisory committee members have used their NIH affiliation for promotional purposes.

In 1992, about 200 "alternative" proponents attended a workshop to help develop a research agenda for OAM. The outcome was a 420-page report, published in 1995, that promotes a large number of questionable methods plus a few that have scientific support (60). The report states that NIH has not endorsed the practices it describes and warns that "many of the therapies described have not been subjected to rigorous scientific investigation to prove safety or efficacy."

The OAM has distributed 42 grants of about $30,000 each for research projects, two $840,000 grants to set up research centers at Bastyr University (a naturopathic institution) and at a mental health facility that treats drug abusers with acupuncture, and eight grants averaging about $1 million to set up research centers affiliated with medical schools (61). Many academic scientists have criticized these awards and doubt that they will generate significant research results (62). The OAM's first director resigned in 1994, charging that a prominent senator and others had interfered with his ability to carry out the OAM's mission in a scientific manner (63).

"Alternative" proponents trumpet the OAM's existence as evidence that whatever they espouse is valid. Most press reports—even in medical publications—have contained little criticism and featured the views of proponents and their satisfied clients. Few reporters make any effort to determine whether the "alternative" methods they mention are useful, promising, or nonsensical. Even if the OAM generates some useful research, the benefit is unlikely to outweigh the publicity bonanza already given to worthless methods (64).

Additional publicity has been generated by a *New England Journal of Medicine* report of a telephone survey concerning 16 types of "unconventional therapy." The authors concluded that 34% of the respondents had used at least one unconventional therapy during the previous year and that Americans had made an estimated 425 million visits to providers of such therapy during 1990 (65). However, the methods they selected included some that are medically appropriate (e.g., self-help groups) and some that are appropriate under proper circumstances (e.g., relaxation therapy, biofeedback, hypnosis, massage, and commercial weight-loss clinics). Although the numbers of those using "alternative" methods were thus inflated, most commentators now accept as gospel the idea that "One out of three Americans uses alternative therapies."

"Alternative" promoters would like to weaken or overturn the laws that protect against methods that are ineffective or are promoted with misinformation. During the height of the laetrile controversy, 27 states legalized the manufacture and sale of laetrile within their borders. Within the past few years, 6 states have passed "Medical Freedom of Choice" bills. These prevent or make it difficult for their licensing boards to discipline practitioners who use an inappropriate treatment, as long as it does not directly threaten the life or health of the patient. A federal "Access to Medical Treatment" Act has been introduced to prevent the FDA from protecting the public against the sale and distribution of questionable drugs and devices. The 1976 Proxmire Amendment to the Food, Drug, and Cosmetic Act and the 1994 Dietary Supplement Health Education Act prevent the FDA from regulating the dosage of vitamin, mineral, amino acid, and herbal products unless it can prove in court that a product is inherently unsafe (see also Chapter 115).

Proponents claim that such laws increase individual freedom without increasing consumer risk. This is untrue. The basic principle of health-related consumer-protection law is that products cannot be marketed until demonstrated safe and effective by appropriate testing. Physicians and pharmaceutical companies who wish to test a new product can obtain FDA permission by showing reasonable preliminary evidence of safety and potential usefulness. This policy is not oppressive; it simply requires that studies be carried out as outlined in the front section of this chapter. "Medical freedom" laws facilitate the sale of worthless treatments and make it difficult to prevent unscientific practitioners from exploiting patients.

REFERENCES

1. Standards of Reporting Trials Group. JAMA 1994;272:1926–31.
2. Zwicky JF, Hafner AW, Barrett S, Jarvis WT. Reader's guide to alternative health methods. Chicago: American Medical Association, 1993.
3. Karlowski TR, Chalmers TC, Frenkel LD, et al. JAMA 1975; 246:2235–7.
4. Tai D. Acupuncture & moxibustion. St. Louis: CV Mosby, 1987.
5. NCAHF Task Force on Acupuncture. Clin J Pain 1991;7:162–6.
6. Okada F. Lancet 1996;348:5–6.
7. Lad V. Ayurveda: the science of self-healing. Santa Fe, NM: Lotus Press, 1984.
8. Kushi M, Blauer B. The macrobiotic way. Wayne, NJ: Avery Publishing, 1985.
9. Dagnelie PC, van Staveren WA. Am J Clin Nutr 1989;50: 818–24.
10. Anon. Am J Clin Nutr 1990;51:202–8.
11. Raso J. Nutr Forum 1990;7:17–21.
12. Anon. Macrobiotics: standard dietary and way of life suggestions (flyer). Brookline, MA: Kushi Institute, 1986.
13. Kushi M, Esko E. The macrobiotic approach to cancer. Garden City Park, NY: Avery Publishing Group, 1991,
14. American Cancer Society. CA Cancer J Clin 1989;39:248–251.
15. Dwyer J. Nutr Forum 1990;7:9–11.
16. Pizzorno JE Jr. Let's Live 1988;56(2):64.
17. Pizzorno JE Jr, Murray MT, eds. A textbook of natural medicine. Seattle: John Bastyr College Publications, 1985–1996.
18. Raso J. Nutr Forum 1990;7:33–6.
19. Lipton M, Ban TA, Kane FJ, et al. Task Force report on megavitamin and orthomolecular therapy in psychiatry. Washington, DC: American Psychiatric Association, 1973.
20. Nutrition Committee, Canadian Paediatric Society. Can Med Assoc J 1990;143:1009–13.
21. Committee on Nutrition, American Academy of Pediatrics. Pediatrics 1976;58:910–2.
22. Raso J. Nutr Forum 1992;9:17–23.
23. Simon A, Worthen DM, Mitas JA II. JAMA 1979;242:1385–7.
24. Knipschild P. Br Med J 1988;297:1578–81.
25. South J. Nutr Forum 1988;5:61–7.
26. Magner G. Chiropractic: the victim's perspective. Amherst, NY: Prometheus Books, 1995.
27. Kenny JJ, Clemens R. J Am Diet Assoc 1988;88:698–704.
28. Istre GR, Kreiss K, Hopkins RS, et al. N Engl J Med 1982;307: 339–42.
29. Katelaris CH, Weiner JM, Stuckey MS, Yan KW. Med J Aust 1991;155:113–4.
30. Nelson RL. Mayo Clin Proc 1988;63:263–9.
31. Barrett S. Nutr Today 1989;24(2):6–11.
32. Jewett DL, Fein G, Greenberg MH. N Engl J Med 1990;323: 429–33.
33. American Academy of Allergy and Immunology. J Allergy Clin Immunol 1986;78:269–73.
34. Crook W. The yeast connection: a medical breakthrough. Jackson, TN: Professional Books, 1985.
35. Dismukes W. N Engl J Med 1990;323:1717–23.
36. Berry JH. J Am Dental Assoc 1987;115:679–85..
37. Anon. Questionable methods of cancer management. New York: American Cancer Society, 1992.
38. Lerner IJ, Kennedy BJ. CA Cancer J Clin 1992;42:181–91.
39. American Cancer Society. CA Cancer J Clin 1993;43:309–19.
40. Herbert VD. In: Shils ME, Young VR, eds. Modern nutrition in health and disease. 7th ed. Philadelphia: Lea & Febiger, 1988: 475–7.
41. American Cancer Society. CA Cancer J Clin 1991;41:187–92.
42. Wilson B. Nutr Forum 1988;5:33–40.
43. Moertel C, Fleming TR, Rubin J, et al. N Engl J Med 1982; 306:201–6.
44. *United States et al. v Rutherford et al.* Certiorari to the United States Court of Appeals for the Tenth Circuit. No. 78-605. Decided June 18, 1979.
45. American Cancer Society. CA Cancer J Clin 1991;41:310–9.
46. Lowell J. Nutr Forum 1986;3:9–12.
47. Austin S, Dale EB, DeKadt S. J Naturopathic Med 1994;5 (1):74–6.
48. Green S. JAMA 1992;268:3224–7.
49. American Cancer Society. Kelley malignancy index and ecology therapy. In: Unproven methods of cancer management. New York: American Cancer Society, 1971.
49a. Arena S. New York Daily News 1997;Mar 31, p 19.
50. Congress, Office of Technology Assessment. Unconventional cancer treatments, OTA-H-405. Washington, DC: U.S. Government Printing Office, 1990.
51. American Cancer Society. CA Cancer J Clin 1990;40:103–7.
52. Cassileth BR, Lusk EJ, Guerry D, et al. N Engl J Med 1991;324: 1180–5.
53. Barrett S, Herbert V. The vitamin pushers: how the health food industry is selling America a bill of goods. Amherst, NY: Prometheus Books, 1994;370–5.
54. Mathews J. J Natl Cancer Inst 1993;85:1190–1.
55. DeWys WD. Your Patient Cancer 1982;2(5):31–6.
56. Creagan ET, Moertel CG, O'Fallon JR, et al. N Engl J Med 1979;301:687–90.
57. Anon. Proc Am Soc Clin Oncol 1983;2:92.
58. Moertel CG, Fleming TR, Creagan E, et al. N Engl J Med 1985;312:137–41.
59. Sampson W. In: Gross PR, Levitt N, Lewis MW, eds. The flight from science and reason. New York: New York Academy of Sciences, 1996;188–97.
60. Berman BM, Larson DB, et al. Alternative medicine: expanding medical horizons. A report to the National Institutes of Health on alternative medical systems and practices in the United States. Washington, DC: U.S. Government Printing Office, 1995.
61. Villaire M. Alternative Ther 1996;2(2):20, 22, 90.
62. Kolata G. New York Times, June 18, 1966;Al, B7.
63. Marshall E. Science 1994;265:2000–2.
64. Barrett S. Nutr Forum 1993;10:1–5.
65. Eisenberg DM, Kessler RC, Foster C, et al. N Engl J Med 1993;328:246–52.

SELECTED READINGS

Barrett S, Herbert V. The vitamin pushers: how the health food industry is selling America a bill of goods. Amherst, NY: Prometheus Books, 1994.

Barrett S, Jarvis WT, eds. The health robbers: a close look at quackery in America. Amherst, NY: Prometheus Books, 1993.

Barrett S, Jarvis WT, London WM, Kroger M. Consumer health: a guide to intelligent decisions. 6th ed. Madison, WI: Brown & Benchmark, 1997.

Magner G. Chiropractic: the victim's perspective. Amherst, NY: Prometheus Books, 1995.

Zwicky JF, Hafner AW, Barrett S, et al. Reader's guide to alternative health methods. Chicago: American Medical Association, 1993.

Quackwatch (http://www.quackwatch.com).

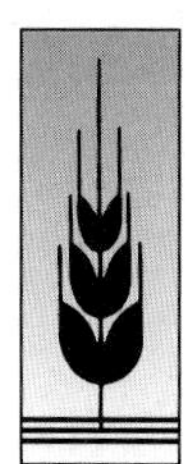

PART VI.

Adequacy, Safety, and Oversight of the Food Supply

111. Food Processing: Nutrition, Safety, and Quality Balances

ALEXA W. WILLIAMS and JOHN W. ERDMAN, JR.

Mankind's attempts to preserve food go back for centuries. One of the earliest examples is the curing of meat, which involves drying, salting, and smoking. This practice dates from 1500 BC. A more recent advancement in food preservation came in the late 18th century in France. Napoleon's armies were hindered by inadequate supplies of food, and prizes were offered as an incentive to develop useful methods for preserving food for soldiers. In this competition, Nicholas Appert showed that food sufficiently heated in a sealed container and stored unopened could be preserved. For this, he was awarded 12,000 francs in 1809, and canning was born. The work of Louis Pasteur 50 years later helped explain the effectiveness of Appert's canning by showing that growth of microorganisms was the major cause of food spoilage (1).

Today's society has evolved from a largely rural way of life to modern urban living. Relatively few people live on farms, because of improvements in farm production and development of the food-processing industry. Processing, storage, and transportation systems are critical to provide food for urban populations. Additionally, the number of dual-income families has grown, leaving less time for home food preparation and creating increased demand for convenience foods.

Consumers are health conscious and insist that even convenience foods be nutritious. Although foods are processed to increase the storage time for which a food is safe with minimal nutrient and quality losses, some losses are inevitable. There will always be a need to reevaluate processing techniques and to look for ways to improve nutrient retention and food quality. As technology continues to advance, it will be possible to produce processed foods with even greater nutritive value.

OVERVIEW OF FOOD PROCESSING

Foods are processed for several beneficial reasons: to preserve and extend shelf life, to increase digestibility, to increase bioavailability of some nutrients, to improve palatability and texture, to prepare foods for serving, to eliminate microorganisms, to destroy toxins, to remove inedible parts, to destroy antinutritional factors, and to create new types of foods. Food processing can also increase consumer convenience and availability of a variety of foods year-round. Of these reasons, perhaps the most important is safety. Although processing may decrease the overall nutrient content of a food, it is a small price to pay for increased safety.

There are three major causes of food spoilage: microbial growth, chemical changes, and enzymatic changes. Raw foods are living systems containing enzymes that may contribute to rapid spoilage. Additionally, microorganisms are ubiquitous and can multiply under certain conditions. Inactivation of these enzymes or microorganisms by a thermal process can greatly extend the shelf life and quality of a food. This is especially important for foods with a high moisture content, because they deteriorate more rapidly than those with a low moisture content or low water activity.

Food-borne illnesses can occur because of *(a)* microorganisms, including bacteria, molds, viruses, and parasites; *(b)* chemicals or additives added to food intentionally or unintentionally as the result of their use in the processing or distribution; or *(c)* poisonous plants or animals. It has been reported that the public is most concerned about *(b)*, although microorganisms are a larger safety issue. Effective food processing can reduce the risk of food-borne illnesses.

Environmental conditions such as pH, temperature, light, and oxygen can affect the shelf life and nutrient retention of a stored food. Manipulation of these environmental conditions can minimize spoilage and nutrient damage. For example, riboflavin is greatly affected by environmental conditions. It is very sensitive to light, and its rate of destruction increases as the temperature and pH increase. Milk is sold in cardboard or opaque plastic containers to minimize riboflavin degradation.

Food processing can have both positive and negative effects on nutrient retention. An example of a positive effect is the lime-[$Ca(OH)_2$] treatment of corn during tortilla or corn chip production. Unfortunately, the added calcium is not highly bioavailable (2), but the process increases the bioavailability of niacin. Niacin is tightly bound to corn proteins as niacytin but can be liberated under alkaline conditions (3). Alkaline treatment of corn helps eliminate pellagra in populations where corn is the mainstay of the diet (4). Unfortunately, the alkaline conditions associated with lime treatment are damaging to another B vitamin, thiamin.

An example of a negative effect of food processing is nutrient destruction during extrusion of food materials. Heat-labile nutrients such as thiamin and ascorbic acid can be destroyed in the extrusion process. Significant losses of the amino acids lysine and methionine can occur as well. Appropriate processing of foods is always a question of balance. Some nutrient loss is inevitable, especially with certain vitamins. In a breakfast cereal, one wants sufficient heat treatment to maximize digestibility of the cereal and destruction of heat-labile antinutrients, while minimizing the loss of heat-labile vitamins and amino acids.

Are nutrient losses in food processing significant or a cause for concern? This depends on whether the nutrient in question is abundant or scarce in the total average diet and whether the food is generally relied on as a major source of that nutrient. About 15% of the vitamin C in milk is destroyed in pasteurization, but milk is not an important source of this vitamin, compared with citrus fruits and juices. Conversely, milk is an important source of riboflavin; thus, its destruction due to light or heat would be a concern to populations consuming low levels of riboflavin.

A common misconception is that commercially processed foods are always nutritionally inferior to freshly prepared foods. In fact, nutrient losses in commercially processed products are often comparable to those in preparation of "fresh produce" in the home (5). Unprotected raw food can rapidly lose nutritional value after harvest if not preserved. The procedures used during harvesting and the ensuing handling and storage period can dramatically affect both nutritional value and sensory properties of fruits and vegetables. Ascorbic acid, thiamin, and folic acid are especially susceptible to both enzymatic and nonenzymatic oxidation during this period. Enzymatic destruction of ascorbic acid can begin as soon as a crop is harvested. Storage under both cool and humid conditions reduces wilting and improves retention of ascorbic acid during storage. Other preprocessing conditions that influence nutrient content of the final prepared food are genetic variation, soil composition, fertilizer use, type of feed, and degree of maturity when picked or killed (6).

Vitamin C and thiamin are readily lost in the processing of foods because they are thermally labile and water soluble (susceptible to leaching during processing). It is generally assumed that if these two vitamins are well retained during processing and storage, other nutrients also are well retained (7). Vitamin stability during processing is largely related to heat, pH, oxygen, and light. The presence of trace elements can also accelerate the loss of some vitamins. Factors that affect vitamin loss are presented in Table 111.1.

Table 111.1
Factors Affecting Vitamin Loss

Nutrient	Main Causes of Loss
Ascorbic acid[a]	Water leaching, oxidation-accelerated by heat, light, copper, iron
Biotin	Alkaline conditions
Carotenoids	Oxidation, isomerization; accelerated by heat, light
Cobalamin (B_{12})	Alkaline and acid conditions, oxidation
Folic acid	Light and heat
Niacin	Water leaching
Pantothenic acid	Alkaline and acidic conditions; accelerated by heat
Pyridoxine (B_6)	Light; accelerated by alkaline conditions
Riboflavin (B_2)	Light and heat; accelerated by alkaline conditions
Thiamin (B_1)[a]	Alkaline conditions, water leaching, oxidation; accelerated by heat and light
Vitamin E	Oxidation
Vitamin A	Oxidation and isomerization; accelerated by heat and light
Vitamin D	Alkaline conditions; accelerated by light and oxygen
Vitamin K	Light and alkaline conditions

[a]Considered one of the more heat-labile vitamins.

Minerals are relatively heat stable, but many of them are easily leached from food exposed to excess water. During processing, their bioavailability may be altered both positively and negatively by interactions with other components of the food.

Of the amino acids, lysine is the most labile, but all amino acids are sensitive to dry heat. Thus, in roasting and toasting legumes, cereals, and prepared dry mixtures of foodstuffs, the biologic value of proteins may be significantly reduced (8).

Essential fatty acids can isomerize when heated in alkali and are sensitive to oxygen and light, especially at high temperatures. When oxidized, they become biologically inactive and can produce off flavors and free radicals.

THERMAL PROCESSING

Heat processing is one of the most important methods of food preservation. The sections below detail some of the advantages and disadvantages of blanching, pasteurization, canning, extrusion, microwaving, and baking. In general, for any thermal process, exposure to high temperature for a short time is less damaging to nutrients than a moderate temperature for a longer time. Heat increases the digestibility of protein, carbohydrates, and other nutrients in many foods, thereby enhancing their nutritive value. Heat treatment can also inactivate some naturally occurring spoilage enzymes, such as pectinase and lipoxygenase, in fruits and vegetables, thereby protecting against off flavors, color loss, and poor texture. The bioavailability of vitamins B_6, niacin, folacin, and certain carotenoids can be enhanced by thermal processing, because heat can release these nutrients from poorly digested complexes. Another advantage of thermal processing is inactivation of antinutritional factors in certain foods. In these foods, nutritional

Table 111.2
Heat-Labile Antinutritional Factors Inactivated by Thermal Processing

Antinutritional Factor	Common Food Sources	Effects of Antinutritional Factor
Avidin	Egg whites	Binds biotin, making it biologically unavailable
Hemagglutinins	Red kidney beans, yellow wax beans	Induces red blood cell clumping
Lathyrogens	Chick peas	Disrupts collagen structure
Goitrogens	Sweet potatoes, beans, cabbage, turnips	Causes goiters by limiting iodine absorption
α-Amylase inhibitors	Cereal grains, peas, beans	Slows starch digestion
Trypsin inhibitor	Legumes, egg whites, potatoes	Inhibits activity of trypsin
Thiaminases	Fish, shellfish, brussel sprouts, red cabbage	Destroys thiamin

value is greatly enhanced by processing (Table 111.2) (9). On the other hand, thermal processing does have several adverse effects. During thermal processing and subsequent storage, thiamin and ascorbic acid are especially susceptible to leaching and thermal degradation. Carotenoids and folacin are also heat labile. Lipids, minerals, vitamin K, biotin, and niacin are normally stable during heating.

Maillard browning (nonenzymatic browning) is commonly accelerated during thermal processing conditions. It can occur in foods containing reducing sugars (glucose, fructose, lactose) and protein. Foods that undergo Maillard browning include bread and other baked items, dried fruits, gravy mixes, maple syrup, dried milk, cocoa, and extruded products (e.g., cereals). During heat processing, the free aldehyde or ketone groups of sugars can react with amino groups of certain amino acids to create poorly digested complexes. Maillard browning can destroy many of the amino acids, in particular the basic amino acids. Lysine is one of the most labile of the amino acids because of its ϵ-amino group. Loss of arginine and methionine also occur. Thus, Maillard browning reduces the protein quality of plant foods (10). Overall, the Maillard reaction can decrease caloric content, increase color and flavor, and reduce essential amino acids and total nitrogen digestibility. For foods such as breads, cocoa, and maple syrup, a certain amount of Maillard browning is desirable to improve appearance and flavor. On the other hand, for a food such as milk, Maillard browning is undesirable because it produces a "cooked" flavor and undesirable color. The Maillard reaction can be minimized by decreasing the concentration of reducing sugars, increasing the moisture content, reducing heat, and lowering pH.

In addition to the Maillard reaction, thermal processing at high temperatures for extended periods can also cause other undesirable reactions with protein. Such reactions include oxidation of amino acids (particularly sulfur amino acids), altered peptide linkages between amino acids that delay or impair amino acid release during digestion, and formation of new amino acid structures or dipeptides that are not subject to normal digestion and absorption processes.

Blanching

Blanching is the heat treatment typically applied to fruits and vegetables prior to canning, freezing, or drying. Before canning, blanching can activate desirable enzymes such as pectin methyl esterase or can inactivate such undesirable enzymes as catalase and peroxidase, but it is mainly used to wilt food tissue prior to can closure and to remove tissue gases. Further enzymatic and microbial inactivation occurs during commercial sterilization. The primary purpose of blanching before freezing or drying is to inactivate enzymes that cause undesirable changes in color (browning), texture, flavor, aroma, or nutritive value during storage. Microbial destruction is not a primary objective of blanching.

The nutritive value of fruits and vegetables can vary, depending on the plant variety, maturity, and time of harvest. Harvest, transport, and storage conditions prior to processing can also influence the vitamin content. Blanching helps maintain the harvest quality of a product until it is prepared at home.

Blanching typically uses temperatures around 75 to 95°C for 1 to 10 minutes, depending on the product, and involves water, steam, microwaves, or hot gas. Water blanching is most common because the initial capital investment and running costs are lower. It also allows addition of processing aids. For example, acidification of blanching water improves vegetable color and retention of vitamin C (ascorbic acid). Trace minerals found in processing water also enhance the nutritional quality of the product. However, some processing aids can be detrimental to the nutritional quality. Sulfite in blanching water can destroy thiamin (11).

Overall, the effects of blanching are predictable. Loss of water-soluble vitamins increases with contact time in water blanching, because of increased leaching, while fat-soluble vitamins are relatively stable. Vitamin C loss ranges from about 10 to 50%, and about 9 to 60% of thiamin is lost (7). Steam blanching retains more of the water-soluble vitamins, but not enough to make the process cost-effective (12). The three vitamins most affected by blanching are thiamin (vitamin B_1), vitamin C, and folate. The extent of loss depends on the vegetable and the location of the vitamin within it. For example, more vitamin C is lost from broccoli than from green beans in blanching because vitamin C is stored in the green bean seed and is protected by the pod. In blanching, thermal destruction and enzymatic oxidation can explain a small portion of the disappearance of vitamin C, thiamin, and folate; however, most is lost by leaching (11). Finally, microwave blanching results in even smaller losses of nutrients than steam blanching (7); however, this method is relatively expensive (12).

Generally, blanching is a pretreatment for freezing, drying, or canning. With the exception of freezing, these further processing methods can also affect the nutritive value of the food as described below.

Pasteurization

The main objectives of pasteurization are to reduce the populations of spoilage microorganisms and enzymes and to inactivate pathogenic microorganisms. The food is not rendered sterile, so pasteurization must be used in conjunction with another preservation method like refrigeration (e.g., milk). It may be used alone if the food is highly acidic (e.g., jams, jellies, or wine) and packaging is adequate. Nutrient losses during pasteurization of acidic products are minor, because most heat-labile nutrients are relatively stable under acidic conditions (13).

Milk is pasteurized by one of three methods: *(a)* Low temperature–long time (LTLT), 63°C (145°F) for 30 minutes; *(b)* high temperature–short time (HTST), 72°C (161°F) for 15 seconds; and *(c)* ultra-high temperature (UHT, sterilization), 135°C (275°F) for less than 10 seconds, an aseptic process. UHT milk is commercially sterile and does not require refrigeration. As can be seen above, a higher processing temperature requires a dramatically shorter processing time. This results in a product with greater nutrient retention because, as Lund noted, "an increase in process temperature (with an appropriate decrease in process time) will have a greater effect in increasing the rate of microbial destruction than it will on the rate of nutrient destruction" (13). For example, the Institute of Food Technologists' Expert Panel on Food Safety and Nutrition stated, "An 18°F rise in processing temperature usually produces a tenfold increase in bacterial destruction, while only doubling the chemical reactions which lead to the destruction of certain nutrients and flavors" (12). So theoretically, a higher processing temperature results in better quality and nutrient retention. However, in the United States, where most families have refrigerators, UHT milk has not become popular. HTST milk is comparable to UHT milk in nutritional quality and is considerably less expensive. Therefore, in the U.S., milk is most frequently processed by HTST (12).

Pasteurization of milk is geared toward elimination of the most heat-resistant pathogen, *Coxiella burnetti,* the rickettsial organism responsible for Q fever. Both HTST and UHT processes destroy harmful microorganisms without adversely affecting most nutrients to a great extent. All the fat-soluble vitamins and certain water-soluble vitamins such as riboflavin, pantothenic acid, biotin, and nicotinic acid are stable during pasteurization. On the other hand, folic acid, thiamin, and vitamins B_6, B_{12}, and C are susceptible to heat and oxidative degradation. Methods that exclude oxygen during processing and storage protect folic acid and vitamins C and B_{12} (14).

UHT is also used for juices and other low-viscosity products such as pudding. The products are heated in thin layers by heat exchangers or direct steam injection, cooled, and packaged into sterile containers (15). Aseptic processing provides products that are superior to retorted versions in flavor, texture, and nutrition. In particular, retention of vitamin B_6 and thiamin is significantly improved (12).

Canning

Canning, also known as commercial sterilization or retorting, produces shelf-stable foods with longer shelf lives than pasteurized products. The thermal heat treatment varies with the type of food but usually exceeds 80°C (176°F). Canning destroys most pathogenic and toxin-forming organisms, with a maximum allowable level of 1×10^{-12} organisms per can. Because some nonpathogenic microorganisms and spores are extremely heat resistant, it is impossible to render a food completely sterile without unacceptably altering its sensory qualities and nutritive value (13). On the other hand, foods are not always processed solely on the bases of safety and optimal nutrient retention. In terms of food quality, UHT milk can be commercially sterile and still contain active enzymes that cause "lipase taint." Additionally, beans can be sterilized without being fully cooked. A balance between safety, nutrition, and quality must be achieved (15).

Retorting is an in-package thermal process in which the package can be a metal can, glass jar, or flat retortable pouch. The rate and mechanism of heat transfer determine the processing time. For example, a solid food such as pumpkin heats by conduction. To heat the center of the can adequately, the outer layer receives a more severe heat treatment, and fewer nutrients are retained. Similarly, uneven heat transfer occurs when still retorts are used.

A product processed in an agitating retort or by flame sterilization heats more quickly, because of convection currents within the can. Flame sterilization, an HTST process in which cans rotate over gas burners, is used for particulate canned food such as mushrooms (15). Nutrient retention is better in agitating systems than in still retorts.

Retort pouches are flexible, heat-sealable, flat containers made of polymeric laminates capable of withstanding the high temperatures of thermal processing. Polymeric laminates are thinly layered materials such as plastics, paper, or aluminum that are tightly joined together (10). The thin slablike retort pouch has a higher surface:volume ratio than glass containers or metal cans. Because of the pouch geometry, the product temperature increases more rapidly than it does in a traditional container, typically decreasing process time by one-third to one-half. As in HTST processing, retention of heat-labile vitamins is significantly enhanced because of the shorter processing time. For example, one study showed that retorted sweet potato puree had a thiamin retention of 77%, whereas heated cans with equal volume retained only 60% of the thiamin (10).

Canning is widely used for many fruits, vegetables, and juices. Unpeeled fruit retains more nutrients during canning. In canned vegetables, water-soluble vitamins and minerals are distributed between the solids and liquids. The liquid, usually discarded by the consumer, contains significant quantities of nutrients. For example, approximately 30% of the available thiamin is found in the liquid portion of canned vegetables (16). Also, more than 50% of the manganese, cobalt, and zinc may end up in the liquid portion of canned spinach, beans, and tomatoes (12). The consumer can avoid these losses by incorporating the liquid into soups, sauces, and gravies

Baking

Baking is a common heat-processing technique used by the food industry and in the home. It results in some destruction of nutrients, especially water-soluble vitamins (particularly thiamin) and basic amino acids because of Maillard browning. Thermal destruction is most pronounced in the crust portion of baked foods, where temperature exposure is highest. As one would predict, baking time, pH, trace metals, enzymes, and moisture content also affect the degree of destruction. Added milk solids or milk protein concentrates containing lactose intensify the Maillard reaction.

On the other hand, yeast fermentation followed by baking can improve the absorption and use of nutrients by inactivating or destroying antinutrients and mineral complexes. Proteins become more digestible as the heat of baking denatures them. During fermentation of a yeast dough, microbial enzymes cause chemical changes. The loss of nutrients due to this fermentation is small. In fact, the nutrient level may even increase through vitamin and protein synthesis by the yeast and liberation of nutrients bound in indigestible plant materials (17).

Conversely, chemical leavening can have a negative impact on at least one nutrient. Thiamin is relatively stable during fermentation of a yeast dough because the pH is mildly acidic. However, in chemically leavened goods (such as some cookies and crackers), the pH can rise above 6, destroying nearly all the thiamin (18, 19). One study on high-protein cookies revealed thiamin losses of more than 90%, whereas losses of riboflavin and niacin were only modest. Lower baking temperatures may improve thiamin retention in baked goods.

Much of the niacin in grain products, especially those from unrefined flours, is present as bound niacin, which is essentially unutilizable by humans. Baking appears to release bound niacin; the proportion of free niacin was found to be higher in bread, cakes, and crackers than from the flours from which they were made (18, 19). As stated above, alkali treatment of corn in the making of tortillas improves niacin availability, probably through release of bound niacin during baking. In the United States, many breads are made with flour to which thiamin, riboflavin, niacin, iron, and possibly calcium are added. No significant losses of these added vitamins occur during bread making (18).

Baking is unlikely to have an adverse effect on the mineral content of foods (19). The enzymes present during fermentation of bread dough and the heat of baking may increase mineral bioavailability by breaking up organic complexes of minerals, such as phytate (18). Phytic acid, a much-studied organic chemical, is a chief storage form of phosphate and inositol in such whole-grain cereals as corn and wheat. It is a strong chelating agent that binds monovalent and divalent metal ions to form complex phytates. Unfortunately, phytate is not degraded when chemical leaveners are used.

Extrusion

Extrusion cooking is a modern HTST processing method applied primarily to grain. Raw materials can be converted to finished products in as little as 30 seconds. Extruded foods include breakfast cereals, snack foods, flat breads, textured vegetable proteins (TVPs), infant food formulas, modified starches and flours, and pet foods. Extrusion has both desirable and undesirable effects on nutritional quality. Benefits include increased digestibility, increased mineral availability, and destruction of heat-labile antinutritional factors such as trypsin inhibitors. Undesirable effects include reduced protein quality due to Maillard browning, destruction of polyunsaturated fatty acids (PUFAs), inactivation of amylase and phytase, and loss of heat-labile vitamins. The effects of extrusion on thiamin (vitamin B_1), riboflavin (vitamin B_2), vitamin C, and vitamin A have been investigated, but few or no data are available for extrusional effects on other B vitamins or vitamins E, D, or K (20).

Extruders can be classified into single-screw or twin-screw systems. Solids are fed into the hopper and conveyed forward by rotation of the screw(s) at temperatures between 115 and 200°C for 10 to 90 seconds. Liquid or steam is added to create a continuous dough. During this process, starch granules are disrupted, and protein is denatured. At the barrel exit, water vaporization because of the pressure drop leads to product expansion. A spinning blade can be used to cut the product to appropriate lengths (10).

Vitamin retention can be negatively affected by higher process temperatures, increased screw speed, decreased moisture, decreased throughput, smaller die diameter, and higher specific energy input. Vitamin stability decreases with higher barrel temperatures or longer residence time in the extruder. Increasing the initial moisture content of the product improves retention of thiamin, vitamin B_6, vitamin B_{12}, and folate, potentially because higher moisture lowers the dough viscosity, resulting in less shear (20).

The effects of extrusion cooking and the processing

parameters on vitamins have been investigated since the late 1960s. Pertinent references are available from the Killeit review (20). These studies showed that degradation of thiamin and β-carotene, a provitamin A carotenoid, follows first-order kinetics. Retention of nutrients could be improved with less-stringent processing conditions; however, products with high sensory appeal, such as some breakfast cereals and snacks, are unlikely to be changed. Instead, the industry has chosen to supplement the premixes with more thermally stable forms of the vitamins or to apply nutrients after extrusion.

In model systems for extrusion processing, extensive loss of lysine occurs before product browning is seen (21). Loss of lysine was comparable to or worse than losses that occur during baking. Lysine losses usually increase with increased extrusion temperature or decreased moisture content (10). For example, retention of available lysine was 93% at a processing temperature of 170°C, but only 63% at 210°C (10). Arginine and tryptophan retention also decreases as processing conditions become more severe.

Microwave Cooking

In conventional cooking, heat is applied to the exterior of the food and is conducted toward the interior. During microwave processing, heat is generated within the food product by microwave-induced molecular vibrations. The oscillation creates intermolecular friction that generates heat (22). Microwave cooking can be used for pasteurization, sterilization, precooking, dehydration, baking, blanching, and tempering (used to raise temperature in frozen foods to just below the freezing point of water). Combining traditional heating methods with microwave exposure can offer both sensory and nutritional benefits. In conventional ovens, microwaves are used to achieve internal heating, while conventional heating methods are used to produce the desired surface browning and crispness. The most highly developed commercial applications include tempering frozen foods (frozen meat and fish blocks), precooking meat products (bacon, poultry, and beef patties), and dehydrating low-moisture solids (pasta) (23).

Generally, microwave cooking can be as good as the best conventional processes for a food product. However, "drip" loss during microwave cooking of meats can result in higher losses of minerals, protein, water-soluble vitamins, and some fats than with conventional methods (10).

Generally, less ascorbic acid is lost in microwave cooking than in conventional methods (24). In 1987, the Institute of Food Technologists' Expert Panel on Food Safety and Nutrition reported that vitamin retention in microwave foods is improved because cooking time is shorter than with conventional methods (23). Similarly, the use of microwaves for reheating minimizes the need for "warmholding," which is a nutritional advantage (22). However, retention varies with cooking time, internal temperature, product type, oven size, oven design, power input, and cooking method. A cooking method that uses water will typically retain lower levels of water-soluble nutrients than one that does not.

FREEZING

Freezing is considered the best method of food preservation with regard to sensory qualities and retention of nutrients. Nutrient losses from fruits and vegetables can be minimized if blanching procedures are adequate, proper packaging is provided, and storage temperatures are low and constant. Any nutrient loss that occurs usually takes place during blanching or frozen storage, not during the actual freezing process. In general, low stable storage temperatures result in greater nutrient retention and product quality. Loss of vitamins during frozen storage varies, depending on the product and packaging. For example, ascorbic acid loss is influenced by the oxygen permeability of the packaging material. Vitamin C retention is greater when the oxygen permeability of the package is lower.

Storage temperature significantly affects nutrient retention. In one study, vegetables stored at −7°C lost more vitamin C, β-carotene, folic acid, and pantothenic acid than those stored at −18°C. No significant effect on niacin, riboflavin, thiamin, vitamin B_6, nor minerals was observed (7). For excellent nutrient retention, storage temperatures should remain below −18°C.

As discussed above, blanching is responsible for most water-soluble nutrient loss in vegetables prior to freezing (7). This loss could be significantly reduced if vegetables were blanched and cooled without water, by processes like microwaving or steaming. For fruits and meats, the biggest losses of vitamins occur during prolonged storage and thawing.

MOISTURE REMOVAL

Methods of moisture removal include both dehydration and concentration processes. Multiple factors prior to drying or concentration will influence ultimate nutrient retention. For example, the presence of sulfur dioxide adversely affects thiamin but protects ascorbic acid. However, the presence of copper, iron, light, or dissolved oxygen can decrease ascorbic acid concentration. Also, metals can catalyze oxidation of carotenes (25). Temperatures during moisture removal vary, depending on the process and the product, and can range from −30°C to above 100°C. Generally, low-temperature processing such as freeze-drying produces the least chemical deterioration. However, low-temperature processing is usually more expensive because of the longer processing times (25).

Dehydration

Methods for dehydration include sun drying, tunnel drying, spray drying, drum drying, and freeze drying. Microbial metabolism and growth require free (not bound) water. Removing available water prevents microbial growth and reduces the rates of enzymatic activity and chemical reactions if the product is stored under proper conditions.

For most types of drying, heat is supplied to the food and vaporized moisture is removed. Dehydrated foods are susceptible to loss of vitamin A and provitamin A activity during storage when oxygen is present. Vitamin C may also be lost during drying.

Sun Drying

Sun drying is one of the least expensive methods of drying. It is used to dry grapes, prunes, apricots, dates, figs, spices, grain, and other foods. This is a time-consuming method that usually takes 3 to 4 days, and it is often accompanied by large vitamin losses. Additional problems such as mold growth can occur if rain or high humidity is present. An increase in mold toxins such as aflatoxin can be an issue. For best results, a warm, dry climate is necessary.

Tunnel Drying

Tunnel driers are an important class of driers used for pasta, fruits, and vegetables. The food is placed on trays or conveyors and passed through a stream of high-velocity air.

Spray Drying

Spray drying is an HTST process used for nonfat dry milk, eggs, tea, and coffee. It is more expensive than tunnel drying, but product quality is better. Little or no vitamin A or D is lost during the spray drying of milk. Additionally, spray-dried milk powder has negligible loss of available lysine. Most dried milk available to the consumer is further processed by rewetting and drying to produce an instant powder that dissolves well in water. During this rewetting and drying process, amino acid losses are minimal (25).

Drum Drying

A fairly inexpensive process, drum drying is generally used for foods that are relatively heat insensitive, such as potatoes. Mashed potatoes are processed by drum drying to produce "instant" potatoes. Most of the vitamin C in potatoes is lost during drum drying and subsequent storage of the product (5). Milk can also be processed by drum drying, which results in lysine losses of 3 to 16% (25). Little or no loss of vitamin A or D occurs during the drum drying of milk (25). Deterioration of heat-sensitive nutrients is greater in spray drying or tunnel drying because of the high temperature and the direct contact between the food and the hot drum.

Freeze Drying

Freeze drying is the most expensive drying process, but it results in foods of very high quality. The food is frozen in sheets and placed in chambers with low atmospheric pressure. Water evaporates directly from the ice phase (sublimation) in about 6 to 8 hours. The effect of temperature on product quality and nutrient retention is minimal. Even vitamin C is retained in this process, because the process is carried out in the absence of oxygen (25).

Concentration

Evaporation, freeze concentration, and membrane processes are commonly used by the food industry to concentrate foods and juices.

Evaporation

Evaporation is the most common method of concentrating food products and the least expensive. Basically, this process consists of boiling off water at temperatures that depend on the product and process. Foods processed by this method include condensed milk, fruit juice, candy, jam, and jelly. The processing times should be short to minimize nutrient destruction. Some lysine is lost due to nonenzymatic browning. One study showed a 20% reduction in lysine when evaporated milk was retorted at 113°C for 15 minutes. However, when sweetened condensed milk was evaporated at 50 to 55°C, only 3% of the lysine was destroyed (25). Evaporation under partial vacuum can improve nutrient retention because of the lower boiling temperatures and lower concentration of atmospheric oxygen.

Freeze Concentration

Freeze concentration is a low-temperature moisture-removal method used commercially for the manufacture of orange juice concentrate. This process involves freezing water to produce large ice crystals, which are then separated from the orange concentrate. Excellent nutrient retention is expected because it is a low-temperature process. Only adhering solutes that are removed with the ice are lost (25).

Membrane Processes

Ultrafiltration and reverse osmosis are nonthermal food processing methods that use membranes. Reverse osmosis is a concentration process designed to remove only water, whereas ultrafiltration is a less-specific concentration and purification process. With both processes, the liquid solution to be concentrated is passed through equipment holding a membrane. The membrane allows selective passage of water, with or without other compounds of low molecular weight (25). Ultrafiltration results in a substantial loss of water-soluble vitamins and minerals along with the water. Reverse osmosis uses a much smaller pore size, so fewer nutrients are lost.

Of the concentration methods discussed, ultrafiltration shows the highest nutrient losses (particularly of water-soluble vitamins and minerals). Drying processes generally offer good nutrient retention, with the exception of β-carotene and ascorbic acid. Losses of water-soluble vitamins, other than ascorbic acid, during drying average approximately 5%. Fat-soluble vitamins are not lost to any significant degree during spray drying, drum drying, or evaporation of milk. Loss of ascorbic acid during concentration is minimal. Freeze concentration offers excellent nutrient retention (25).

OTHER PROCESSES

Irradiation

Food irradiation is used to destroy microorganisms, to eliminate insect infestations, and to inhibit ripening and sprouting in a number of food products. The process uses high-energy ionizing radiation to create free radicals that can react with the DNA of insects or microorganisms to kill them (26).

The ionizing radiation used for food products comes from one of two sources. Most commonly, γ-radiation or x-rays are used, which are generated from cobalt-60 (^{60}Co). The ^{60}Co is encapsulated in several layers of stainless steel and raised into an irradiation chamber with the food. γ-Rays are effective because of their high penetration power; the γ-ray source never contacts the food directly. This makes γ-rays suitable for irradiation of bulk items such as chickens or drums of food. Ionizing radiation can also be generated by machines. The electron beams produced can only penetrate about 8 cm into food, which limits their use to low-density foods such as spices or grains. However, this system is more suited to in-line processing because it can be used with conveyors and can be switched on and off (26).

Irradiation doses are measured in kilograys (kGy), with a maximum dose of 10 kGy recommended by the World Health Organization and legalized in Europe. Doses below 1 kGy are effective in inhibiting potato sprouting or in preventing insect breeding in grains and citrus fruits. A slightly higher dose, 1 to 3 kGy, reduces both spoilage and food poisoning microorganisms in soft fruit, meat, and fish. It has been reported that the O157:H57 *Escherichia coli* bacterium is highly sensitive to irradiation and can be eliminated from ground meat with a dose of only 0.16 to 0.44 kGy (27). Decontamination of dry spices requires the highest irradiation dose, 10 kGy (26).

The changes in food caused by irradiation are small. As with the other thermal processes, thiamin and vitamin C are the most sensitive nutrients. However, beef sterilized by irradiation is reported to retain more thiamin than that canned and thermally processed. Additionally, reported vitamin C losses in irradiated fruits and vegetables are small relative to the natural variance in vitamin C content. The effect of ionizing irradiation on the nutrient content of food is comparable to that of conventional heat processing (12). Irradiating food at low temperatures without oxygen further improves retention of nutritional quality.

Even though irradiation of food has been shown to be safe, approval for its use in foods has been limited. Consumer mistrust of the process and difficulties in gaining Food and Drug Administration (FDA) clearances have prevented substantial commercial use in the United States (29). However, because irradiation is a promising replacement for hazardous chemical fumigants such as methyl bromide and can effectively prevent food-borne illnesses, it will gradually become a more widespread food processing tool.

Milling

Milling is a process by which bran and germ are removed from cereal grains. It is commonly used to refine wheat to make white flour. In the United States, milling wheat to produce white flour results in a 40 to 60% loss of vitamins and minerals. Most wheat flour and breads are enriched with thiamin, niacin, riboflavin, and iron (addition of calcium and other nutrients is optional) in accordance with a standard defined by the FDA (12, 30). Degermination of grains also results in loss of vitamin E.

Milling is used to remove bran and germ from rice. The outer husk is broken and separated from the grain by winnowing, although some of the germ and pericarp are removed at the same time. Traditionally, rice was extracted from the husk by pounding it in a stone or wooden mortar. Today, machine milling can produce an even more refined product with an even greater loss of bran. Brown rice may contain about 15.0 nmol/g (4 μg/g) thiamin, whereas highly polished rice may contain as little as 2.6 nmol/g (0.7 μg/g). Other B vitamins are also lost. The Asian practice of washing the rice before cooking results in additional loss of water-soluble thiamin. Thiamin losses are of most concern in areas of the world where polished rice is the staple food. Thiamin deficiency can result in beriberi, which at one time was a major cause of death in many countries (5). Now, white rice is usually enriched with niacin, thiamin, and iron.

Home Cooking

A discussion of nutrient loss during processing would not be complete without mentioning the losses that occur in the home or food service establishment. The greatest nutrient losses are due to excess heat, leaching into cooking water, and "cook-drip." Thus, the cooking methods ultimately determine nutrient retention. Substantial vitamin and mineral losses often occur in the final preparation steps.

The final vitamin content of home-cooked foods may be similar to that of commercially processed foods, because vitamin losses are inevitable with cooking. Vitamin retention can be improved by using less cooking water, minimally trimming fruits and vegetables, chopping coarsely, covering pans to lessen cooking time, cooking vegetables only until tender, and using cooking water for soups. For example, baked or unpeeled boiled potatoes were reported to have almost total vitamin retention, whereas boiled peeled potatoes retained as little as 63% of the initial nutrients (20). In general, steaming or stir-frying result in greater nutrient retention than boiling or typical pan frying (12, 31).

Overall, there are a few things that both the industrial food processor and home cook must remember. Steaming retains more nutrients than boiling. Boiling with minimal water is better than boiling with larger amounts of water. Finally, vitamin losses increase with surface contact area. In more practical terms, this means that more nutrients are lost from leafy vegetables than from root vegetables (20).

In conclusion, the most common food-processing methods generally do not cause major loss of nutrients. Some loss of nutrients will accompany the process used to ensure product safety and quality. Major nutrient losses are incurred with excessive use of heat and water during cooking. Extreme or prolonged conditions of food storage, distribution, and food preparation can also influence nutrient retention. As more sophisticated food-processing methods are perfected, even greater nutrient retention during commercial processing will be possible.

REFERENCES

1. Potter NN. Food science. 3rd ed. Westport, CT: AVI Publishing, 1978.
2. Rosado JL, Lopez P, Morales M, et al. Br J Nutr 1992;68:45–58.
3. Darby WJ, McNutt KW, Todhunter EN. Nutr Rev 1975;33: 289–97.
4. Wall JS, Carpenter KJ. Food Technol 1988;42:98–204.
5. Bender AE. Food processing and nutrition. New York: Academic Press, 1978.
6. Committee on Nutritional Misinformation. Nutr Rev 1976; 34:316–7.
7. Fennema O. Effects of freeze preservation on nutrients. In: Karmas E, Harris RS, eds. Nutritional evaluation of food processing. 3rd ed. New York: AVI Publishing, 1988;269–317.
8. Harris RS. General discussion on the stability of nutrients. In: Karmas E, Harris RS, eds. Nutritional evaluation of food processing. 3rd ed. New York: AVI Publishing, 1988;3–5.
9. Nelson PE. Hortscience 1972;7:13–5.
10. Dietz JM, Erdman JW Jr. Nutr Today 1989;24:6–15.
11. Selman JD. Food Chem 1994;49:137–47.
12. IFT. Food Technol 1986;40:109–16.
13. Lund D. Effects of heat processing on nutrients. In: Karmas E, Harris RS, eds. Nutritional evaluation of food processing. 3rd ed. New York: AVI Publishing, 1988;319–54.
14. Swaisgood HE. Characteristics of edible fluids of animal origin. In: Fennema OR, ed. Food chemistry. New York: Marcel Dekker, 1985; 791–827.
15. Ryley J, Kajda P. Food Chem 1994;49:119–29.
16. Borenstein B, LaChance PA. Effects of processing and preparation on the nutritive value of foods. In: Shils ME, Young VR, eds. Modern nutrition in health and disease. 7th ed. Philadelphia: Lea & Febiger, 1988;672–84.
17. Adams CE, Erdman JW Jr. Effects of home food preparation practices on nutrient content of foods. In: Karmas E, Harris RS, eds. Nutritional evaluation of food processing. 3rd ed. New York: AVI Publishing, 1988;557–95.
18. Ranhotra GS, Bock MA. Effects of baking on nutrients. In: Karmas E, Harris RS, eds. Nutritional evaluation of food processing. 3rd ed. New York: AVI Publishing, 1988;355–64.
19. Ranhotra GS, Gelroth JA. Cereal Chem 1986;63:401–3.
20. Killeit U. Food Chem 1994;49:149–55.
21. Harper JM. Effects of extrusion processing on nutrients. In: Karmas E, Harris RS, eds. Nutritional evaluation of food processing. 3rd ed. New York: AVI Publishing, 1988;365–91.
22. Hill MA. Food Chemistry 1994;49:131–6.
23. IFT. Food Technol 1989;43:117–26.
24. Klein BP. Contemp Nutr 1989;14:1–2.
25. Bluestein PM, Labuza TP. Effects of moisture removal on nutrients. In: Karmas E, Harris RS,eds. Nutritional evaluation of food processing. 3rd ed. New York: AVI Publishing, 1988; 393–422.
26. Kilcast D. Food Chemistry 1994;49:157–64.
27. Loaharanu P. Food Technol 1994:124–31.
28. Karmas E. The major food groups, their nutrient content, and principles of food processing. In: Karmas E, Harris RS, eds. Nutritional evaluation of food processing. 3rd ed. New York: AVI Publishing, 1988;7–19.
29. Thomas MH. Use of ionizing radiation to preserve food. In: Karmas E, Harris RS, eds. Nutritional evaluation of food processing. 3rd ed. New York: AVI Publishing, 1988;457–90.
30. Tannenbaum SR, Young VR. Vitamins and minerals. In: Food chemistry. New York: Marcel Dekker, 1985;477–544.
31. Erdman JW Jr. Food Technol 1979;33:38–48.

SELECTED READINGS

Bender AE. Food processing and nutrition. London: Academic Press, 1978.

Karmas E, Harris RS, eds. Nutritional evaluation of food processing. 3rd ed. New York: AVI Publishing, 1988.

Labuza TP, Erdman JW Jr. Food science and nutritional health. St. Paul: West Publishing, 1984.

Rechcigl M Jr, ed. Handbook of nutritive value of processed food. Boca Raton, FL: CRC Press, 1982.

Vangard SJ, Woodburn M. Food preservation and safety: principles and practice. Ames: Iowa State University Press, 1994.

112. Designing Functional Foods

WAYNE R. BIDLACK and WEI WANG

Throughout evolution, each species, whether single cell or multicellular, has sought sustenance to provide nutrients for survival, growth, and reproduction. Humans have selected a broader variety of foods of animal and vegetable origin than most other species to provide the nutrients needed for their existence (1). As a complex mixture of chemicals, food provides essential nutrients, requisite calories, and other physiologically active constituents needed for life and health. Yet, very little is known about most substances found in foods.

The amount and composition of food consumed at various stages of life may affect the expression of certain diseases. During the past 25 years, epidemiologic studies have consistently implicated diet with the five leading causes of death in the United States: coronary heart disease (CHD), certain types of cancer, stroke, non-insulin-dependent diabetes mellitus (NIDDM), and atherosclerosis (2). In this century alone, nutrition and food sciences have enhanced development of an abundant, nutritious, safe food supply that has contributed to better health for people around the world.

A new paradigm for "optimal nutrition" may be evolving that would emphasize the positive aspects of diet, identifying physiologically active components that contribute to disease prevention. Understanding how individual nutrients and nonnutrient constituents function physiologically should allow food scientists actually to design food products for a healthy diet. Thus, even though genetic predisposition increases susceptible persons' risk for some of these chronic diseases (especially with advancing age), optimal nutrition should enable persons to achieve their maximum genetic potential and decrease their susceptibility to disease.

From the beginnings of recorded history, plant components (leaves, flowers, roots, and bark) have been used to treat specific diseases. Hippocrates, the father of medicine, included food as a basic part of treatment to cure disease. Taken from many cultures, herbs and plants commonly used for treatment of specific disorders have been carefully identified. Modern analytic methods have identified numerous physiologically active constituents, many of which have been developed into pharmaceutical agents.

Epidemiologic evidence continues to correlate positive effects of fruits, vegetables, and grains with a lower incidence of cancer, CHD, and other diseases (3, 4), although the correlations do not always agree solely with nutrient content. Nonnutrient constituents have been identified with beneficial physiologic effects that may retard or prevent disease (5). Foods that combine these properties have been called "designer foods," "functional foods," "nutraceuticals," and other related names.

The new diet-health paradigm acknowledges the nutritious and healthful aspects of food but goes beyond the role of food constituents as dietary essentials for sustaining life and growth to one of preventing or delaying the premature onset of chronic disease later in life. The promise of functional foods has emerged at a time when consumer interest in diet and health are at an all-time high (6).

FUNCTIONAL FOODS

The functional foods concept has unified the medical, nutritional, and food sciences. Over the past decade, new technologies, such as biotechnology, genetic engineering, food processing, product innovations, and mass production have enabled food scientists to design new healthful products. Initially, the term *designer foods* was developed by the National Cancer Institute to describe foods that naturally contained, or were enriched with, nonnutritive, biologically active chemical components of plants (phytochemicals) that were potentially effective in reducing cancer risk (7). The Institute of Medicine of the U.S. National Academy of Sciences defined functional foods as those that encompass potentially healthful products, including any modified food or food ingredients that may provide a health benefit beyond the traditional nutrients it contains.

Nutraceutical was the term first described by the Foundation for Innovation in Medicine (8, 9) to identify "any substance considered a food or part of a food that provides medical or health benefits, including the prevention and treatment of disease." Nutraceuticals may range from isolated nutrients, dietary supplements, and diets to genetically engineered "designer" foods, herbal products, and processed products such as cereals, soups, and beverages.

The term *functional food* may prove to be the best name

for the category of physiologically active foods. The response of consumers to the different names suggests that "ceutical" reminds people of medicine, while "designer" suggests artificial or synthetic.

In 1988, the orphan drugs amendment to the federal Food, Drug, and Cosmetic Act provided the term *medical foods* with a legal definition: "A food which is formulated to be consumed or administered enterally under the supervision of a physician and which is intended for the specific dietary management of a disease or condition for which distinctive nutritional requirements, based on recognized scientific principles, are established by medical evaluation." Thus, medical foods are complex, formulated products designed to provide complete or supplemental nutritional support to individuals who cannot ingest adequate amounts of food in a conventional form or to provide specialized nutritional support to patients who have special physiologic and nutritional needs associated with their conditions (10).

Medical foods differ from the general food supply, since these foods frequently serve as the sole source of nutrition. Generally, medical foods require sophisticated and exacting science and technology in their design and manufacture, comparable to that used in the manufacture of infant formulas and drugs. Yet, medical foods are subject to much less scrutiny by the Food and Drug Administration (FDA) than virtually all other foods categories. The 1990 National Labeling Education Act (NLEA) specifically exempted medical foods from the NLEA labeling provisions (11). There are no specific requirements for label information or substantiation of claims, formulations, and compositional characteristics; manufacturing quality controls; or notification to the FDA of intent to market medical foods.

Each of these terms, *functional foods, nutraceuticals, designer foods,* and *medical foods,* should be carefully defined so that consumers and health practitioners do not become confused. The significance and relevance of any definition of functional foods depend totally on an adequate description of these foods and substantiation of their health benefits (12).

REGULATORY ISSUES

The United States has established two new labeling laws in an effort to regulate functional foods, medical foods, and designer foods: the 1990 National Labeling Education Act (NLEA) and the 1994 Dietary Supplement Health and Education Act (DSHEA). These changes will affect the development of functional food products (13).

A major dilemma in considering functional foods, is that they exist at the interface between foods and drugs (14). Compounds exerting this type of physiologic effect have been classified by the federal Food, Drug, and Cosmetic Act of 1938 (15) as drugs, that is "articles intended for the diagnosis, cure, mitigation, treatment or prevention of disease." Thus, the legal display on a label referring to disease prevention or risk reduction associated with consuming a particular functional food is extremely limited at this time. Currently four categories exist (16):

1. Ordinary foods and nutrients. Health claims can be made on labels only when they are supported by the totality of publicly available scientific evidence, and then only after receiving regulatory approval from the FDA.
2. Dietary supplements. Health claims are based only on "evidence that the statement is truthful and not misleading." The FDA must be notified of the statement, and the label must include a disclaimer stating that the agency has not evaluated the claim and that the product is not intended to diagnose, treat, cure, or prevent any disease.
3. Medical foods. Health claims must be based on a somewhat higher standard than that for dietary supplements; namely, being backed by "sound scientific evidence." Medical foods do not require FDA approval for claims, though their packages must include disclaimers similar to those of dietary supplements.
4. Drugs. Drug claims have the strictest standards. Drugs must be proven safe and effective in FDA-approved and reviewed clinical trials.

NLEA

The NLEA (17) allows health or disease prevention claims on a food label. A health claim is a statement that asserts or implies a relationship of a substance to a disease or health-related condition within the context of a total daily diet (18). The NLEA requires a prominent panel of nutrition facts, daily reference values, ingredients, nutrient content, and health claims. The Institute of Medicine provided a working definition for functional foods, indicating that they were "foods in which the concentrations of one or more ingredients have been manipulated to enhance contributions to a healthful diet." Eight health claims for foods are currently approved by the FDA (19) (Table 112.1).

New regulations might be needed to ensure some kind of limited patent or copyright on a health claim for companies willing to make the research commitment. Otherwise, because of the time delay and costs involved in

Table 112.1
Eight Health Claims for Foods Currently Approved by the FDA

- Fiber-containing grain products, fruits, and vegetables and cancer
- Fruit, vegetables, and grain products containing fiber, particularly soluble fiber, and risk of cardiovascular disease
- Fruits and vegetables and cancer
- Calcium and osteoporosis
- Dietary saturated fat and cholesterol and risk of cardiovascular disease
- Dietary fat and cancer
- Sodium and hypertension
- Sugar alcohols and dental caries

From Department of Health and Human Services, Food and Drug Administration, 1993. Food labeling: general requirements for health claims for food. Fed Reg 58:2478–536.

achieving approval, companies may well not bother with clinical trials and simply avoid label claims. Although a strong claim for health or longevity would be very marketable in the long term, functional foods may be promoted in other ways first. If handled through advertising with satisfied customer statements, only the Federal Trade Commission (FTC) would be involved, and they only require that the advertising not be misleading.

DSHEA

The DSHEA (20) broadly defined a dietary supplement as a product "intended to supplement the diet that bears or contains a vitamin, a mineral, an herb or other botanical, an amino acid, a dietary substance for use by man to supplement the diet by increasing the total dietary intake, or a concentrate, metabolite, constituent, extract or combination [of any ingredient described above]." Under the DSHEA, dietary supplements are exempt from regulation as drugs and, for the most part, as food additives. Unfortunately, the DSHEA puts the burden of proof for safety of dietary supplements directly on the FDA and limits the agency's authority over labeling. With regard to functional foods, DSHEA allows the use of structure/function claims and dissemination of third-party literature.

The description of a dietary supplement in the DSHEA specifically includes *(a)* a product intended for ingestion in tablet, capsule, liquid, powder, soft gel, or gelcap or (if not in such form) not represented as a conventional food or sole item of a meal or of the diet, and labeled as a dietary supplement; *(b)* a drug, antibiotic, or biologic marketed as a dietary supplement prior to such approval; *(c)* a food, but one not considered a food additive; *(d)* a preparation other than tobacco, intended to supplement the diet by increasing total intake, which bears or contains one or more of the following dietary ingredients: a vitamin, a mineral, an herb or botanical, an amino acid, a dietary substance for use by man to supplement the diet by increasing the total dietary intake, or a concentrate, metabolite, constituent, extract, or any combination of these ingredients (21). A definition of dietary supplement as broad as this allows the addition of many ingredients with functional effects that span the food-drug spectrum.

The DSHEA provides for statements of nutritional support, which can be applied to a wide variety of dietary ingredients. Specifically, one is permitted (20, 21):

- to claim a benefit related to a classical nutrient deficiency disease and disclose the prevalence of such a disease in the United States
- to describe the role of a nutrient or dietary ingredient intended to affect structure or function in humans
- to characterize the mechanism by which a nutrient or dietary ingredient acts to maintain such structure or function
- to describe the general well-being derived from the consumption of a nutrient or dietary ingredient.

Structure/function claims do not require prior approval. The FDA must be notified that such a statement is being made, and the product label must include the following: "This statement has not been evaluated by the FDA. This product is not intended to diagnose, treat, cure, or prevent any disease." The tone of this message will deter consumer acceptance and thus diminish industry use.

Dietary supplements have been drastically redefined by the DSHEA in terms of what they are and may contain. They are permitted to contain ingredients based on a lesser safety standard than that which applies to those in conventional foods. The use of such components in different food products and their suitability for claims in labeling depend on the application of appropriate standards for safety of use and for labeling criteria of a particular product category. In the general food supply, an inherent constituent of the food can be marketed unless it has been found to be "ordinarily injurious to health." As an intentional additive, a functional food component can be used to fortify a processed food, but it requires a stricter condition of "reasonable certainty of no harm" within the context of the total estimated exposure of the "additive." According to the DSHEA, a dietary supplement is considered an unapproved food additive in terms of conventional food use, since the supplement might be considered adulterated. A functional food component used in a supplement could be less safe than one that occurred naturally or that was intentionally added to a conventional food.

Additional regulations may be needed to clarify the product and label descriptions. There has not been a systematic approach to categorization and documentation for a role in health promotion or disease prevention. Some potential categories suggested by Glinsmann (21) are listed in Table 112.2. Although further modification may be necessary, these categories can serve as an excellent starting point.

The changes described in the DSHEA appear to favor development of functional food products in the form of dietary supplements. In the long term, this legislation may do little to stimulate scientific investigation into the potential role of functional food products in health promotion and disease prevention.

Table 112.2
Potential Categorization of Functional Dietary Supplements

- Antioxidants, modifiers of oxidative damage, and defense mechanisms related to oxidative stress
- Antimutagens, anticarcinogens, and inducers of enzymes of xenobiotic metabolism
- Antimicrobial and antiviral substances
- Enhancers of GI function, including dietary fibers, probiotics, prebiotics, and colonic microflora
- Immunomodulators and antiinflammatory agents
- Neuroregulatory substances
- Phytoestrogens
- Antihypertensives
- Hypocholesterolemic agents
- Food components with diminished allergenicity

Modified from Glinsmann WH. Nutr Rev 1996;54:S33–7.

OPPORTUNITY FOR DEVELOPMENT

The key change in the new health paradigm is prevention rather than treatment. With the recent economic history of nutritional supplements, natural products, sports drinks, and health foods, all food companies have contemplated, or have already entered into, the functional foods arena.

Consumers are making more healthcare decisions for themselves than ever before, including lower-cost alternative healthcare and use of unconventional medical therapies. These consumers also select healthy foods that are low in fat, vitamin fortified, and high in fiber. Sales of vitamin supplements, "health" foods, and "natural" foods continue to grow. Functional foods, food products, and supplements that deliver a possible physiologic benefit in the management or prevention of disease represent an opportunity for future new product growth in the food and beverage industries.

Market in the United States

By 1988, the health product market was growing at an annual rate of 18 to 20%, with annual sales of $2.5 billion. The functional food market should remain a high-growth business and reach $7.5 to 9.0 billion within a few years (22–24). If the market value were expanded to include all health-benefit products, including natural and organic foods, the market might exceed $71 billion (24). The inability of state and federal agencies to work with industry to develop equitable regulations hampers the development of functional foods.

If market interest in new products was stimulated by a health proclamation like that which accompanied oat bran, perhaps for a presumed anticancer component of phytochemicals, the market could easily increase at an annual rate of 30%. The specialty market may mature as the worldwide functional food market grows.

International Perspective

Japan. Functional food markets highlight cultural differences between regions in the global marketplace. For example, products that appeal to the Japanese consumer (e.g., lactic acid–containing beverages) may not appeal to the Western consumer. The Japanese can be credited with advancing the functional food market from its infant stage as functional isotonic beverages to the more advanced stages of functional sweeteners and natural sources of edible fiber. Beyond the organoleptic qualities, the potential therapeutic benefits offered by functional products will vary with the consumer desires within that market. Japanese functional food products are aimed at every market segment and include every age group. These products claim to improve intestinal health through inclusion of oligosaccharides or active bacterial cultures, whereas the functional food market in the United States has emphasized products related to reducing the incidence of CHD or cancer. Thus, the functional food market is influenced by both health interests and consumer acceptability within each culture.

To date, the Ministry of Health and Welfare (MHW) of Japan has viewed the functional food industry as benefiting the general well-being of the Japanese populace. A wide variety of products exist, including chewing gums with oligosaccharides, drinks containing high levels of soluble fiber, and infant formulas developed to be analogous to mother's milk. Until recently, these products were developed and sold with little concern, but the Japanese regulatory agencies are considering standards for these products and the claims that are made (25).

The functional food market in Japan is mature, but the annual growth rate has slowed to 8%, totaling about $4.5 billion in 1995. Product development and market growth continues because of a favorable government regulatory attitude and significant investment in ingredient and product development. Although the MHW has increased efforts to monitor and regulate the functional food industry, it has not inhibited innovation and commercialization.

China. Currently, more than 10,000 varieties of functional food products identified as "health" foods exist in China, and annual sales of such foods totals about U.S. $2.5 billion. Twenty different categories of these "new source foods" were approved in 1987, with the following characteristics: *(a)* most are based on compound formulas (mix of herb extracts); *(b)* all are claimed to have multiple health effects on various body systems; *(c)* in most cases, experimental evidence of their safety and efficacy is weak; *(d)* the active compounds of most of these mixtures derived from animals and plants are unknown; and *(e)* the mechanisms of their health effects are basically unknown (26). The Chinese populace differentiates little between foods used for traditional Chinese medicine and functional foods (27). Both are assumed to promote health.

Recently, the Chinese government has announced its intention to improve the standards for these products, including restricting the use of "curative" claims. The immediate result would be a major reduction in health food products in the market place (13).

Europe and the United Kingdom. The European diet, already high in fiber, is considered to be of natural origin. Many products already exist, but the functional food categories are limited to fiber-based products, yogurt and cultured milk products, and products that enhance intestinal function (28).

A large number of functional foods exist in the United Kingdom as well. Product claims are aimed at preventing heart disease, reducing blood cholesterol, promoting a healthy nervous system, and maintaining a healthy cardiovascular system. Food labeling regulations prohibit express or implied claims that a food can prevent, treat, or cure a disease unless the product has a medical license. No prior approval system exists, however; thus enforcement is difficult.

Regulatory Issues

The major concerns within the industry are *(a)* the inconsistency of regulatory guidelines for functional food products and *(b)* the lack of direction in promoting development of products and ingredients that actually can have a positive impact on the health of the consumer. The major regulatory agencies of the world may eventually adopt a more positive position in regard to certain classes of these products. However, the health goals of these agencies are *(a)* to protect the consumer from harm, including suppression of misleading health claims; *(b)* to ensure product safety, particularly in regard to high concentrations of specific constituents; and *(c)* to minimize the potential negative impact of such products on the maintenance of a nutritious diet. The consumer should be able to trust the safety and efficacy controls placed on these health products, which in turn will promote the quality of the food industry's products.

Market Overview

The functional foods market began with the introduction of isotonic sports beverages in the United States and Japan that offered a benefit beyond the nutritional content of traditional products. These products were not classed as functional foods, and they received little regulatory attention. The advent of functional food products occurred in the United States and Japan with promotion of high-fiber products. These products received international attention through their claim to provide a physiologic and therapeutic activity. Fiber-based products set the stage for development of other types of functional products—low fat, low cholesterol, or low sodium—based on consumer demand for healthier products.

Functional foods are focused to meet the needs of different market segments; for example, new infant formulas, women's health, increased mental alertness and well-being, and maintenance of the physical condition of elderly persons. Functional foods represent an interesting challenge for the food industry, which must constantly adjust its products to meet the needs and demands of our ever-changing society.

PHYSIOLOGICALLY ACTIVE COMPOUNDS

There has been no evolutionary pressure on plants to cause development of food components that protect man from diseases and cancer; yet, diets rich in fruits and vegetables appear to do just that. Most likely, these compounds developed as part of the plants' own defense mechanisms against environmental insult and only fortuitously benefit man. Similar positive effects are being identified for a few specific proteins isolated from animal sources.

The number of physiologically active food chemicals has increased dramatically in the last decade. A few of the studied compounds are listed in Table 112.3 (29–62). Most were identified by epidemiologic surveys that correlated a positive health benefit with specific food groups; then the focus narrowed to determining the dietary intake of individual foods. Researchers have examined the compositions of these foods, isolating and identifying chemical structures and suggesting possible functions for these agents. In many cases, animal experiments have tested the hypotheses of health benefits and mechanisms of action, while in others, some human testing has been initiated. Experiments needed to identify and characterize the physiologically active phytochemicals are described in Table 112.4. Very few phytochemicals have been examined as thoroughly as necessary.

It will be many years before we clearly understand whether these agents offer significant health benefits as either natural ingredients, food additives, or dietary supplements. In many cases, benefits may result from additive or synergistic effects. In all cases, safety must be ensured. Only a few examples of research are presented here to represent the exciting potential of some of these agents as future physiologically active agents that might be incorporated into functional foods. A decision on efficacy must consider the lowest doses that produce their effects, since higher doses increase the risk for toxicity. In addition, it is important to determine whether the dose of agent in the food has the same efficacy as the isolated compound. Each of the following examples has physiologic effects at levels found naturally in foods.

Catechins. Jasmine green tea is an excellent source of natural polyphenol antioxidants, specifically including (−)-epicatechin (EC), (−)-epicatechin-3-gallate (ECG), (−)-epigallocatechin (EGC), and (−)-epigallocatechin-3-gallate (EGCG). The purified catechins exhibited strong protection against red blood cell (RBC) hemolysis induced chemically by an azo free-radical initiator. The effective dose for antioxidant activity was between 2.5 and 40 μM. EGCG and ECG were most effective. Only EGC and EC were found in the circulation after a gavage dose of jasmine tea, suggesting selective absorption. However, the tea also reduced RBC hemolysis (33).

The effects of green tea as a chemopreventive agent in multiple animal models is of great interest. Either green tea infusion or isolated tea catechins express a broad spectrum of anticarcinogenic activity. EGCG inhibits proliferation of leukemic blast cells from patients with acute myeloblastic leukemia. EGCG did not inhibit granulocyte-macrophage colony-stimulating factor (GM-CSF) but did block stimulation of GM-CSF release by tumor necrosis factor (TNF)-α or tetradecanoylphorbol acetate (TPA) and blocked modulation of c-kit, a receptor for stem cell factor on leukemic cells (34).

Catechins can inhibit every stage of the carcinogenic process, including development of tumors at different sites and in different organs, a wide array of enzymes involved in cell proliferation (such as protein kinase C, DNA polymerase, RNA polymerase, lipoxygenase, orni-

Table 112.3
Physiologically Active Food Chemicals That May Prevent Disease

Active Compounds	Food Source	Potential Health Benefit	Possible Mechanisms and Functions	Reference
Sulforaphane and other organic isothiocyanates	Cruciferous vegetables	Chemoprevention of cancer	Mediation of chemopreventive activity in animal models by modulating drug-metabolizing enzymes	29, 30, 31
Epigallocatechin and epigallocatechin gallate	Green tea	Reduction of cancer and heart disease	Inhibition of the initiation, promotion and progression of cancer Antioxidant activity; reduces free radical/ oxidative damage; protects RBC membrane from free radical–induced oxidation	32, 33, 34
Carotenoids	Tomatoes, carrots, yams, cantaloupe, spinach, sweet potatoes, citrus fruits	Reduction of coronary heart disease and cancer	Antioxidant activity; free radical scavenger; induction of cell-cell communication; growth control; inhibition of the proliferation of acute myeloblastic leukemia	35, 36
Lactoferrin	Milk	Stimulation of the immune system; antimicrobial agent; healing of gastrointestinal wounds	Stimulation of the release of neutrophil-activating polypeptide interleukin 8 from human PMN; endogenous antibiotic molecule that helps leukocytes destroy invading microorganisms; augmentation of T-cell-dependent NK cell activity; inhibition of the cell migration of certain gastrointestinal cell lines	37, 38, 39, 40
Conjugated linoleic acid	Dairy products	Chemoprevention of cancer; and atherosclerosis	Inhibition of cancer cell growth by interfering with the hormone regulated mitogenic pathway; reduction of the LDL-cholesterol: HDL-cholesterol ratio and total cholesterol to HDL-cholesterol ratio in rabbits	41, 42
Genestein, daidzein, and other isoflavones	Soybeans, soy foods	Reduction in menopausal symptoms, osteoporosis cancer, and heart disease	Inhibition of the growth of human breast cancer cell lines; decrease in total plasma cholesterol, LDL-cholesterol, and triglycerides	43, 44, 45
Diallyl disulfide and allicin	Garlic, onions	Chemoprevention of cancer stimulation of immune function; free radical scavenger; and reduction of serum cholesterol and serum triglyceride	Inhibition of the proliferation of human tumor cells in culture, the metabolic activation of toxicants and carcinogens, and cholesterol biosynthesis	46, 47, 48, 49
Limonene	Citrus fruits	Chemoprevention of cancer	Regulation of malignant cell proliferation; inhibition of posttranslational isoprenylation of cell growth–regulatory proteins	50, 51
Nondigestible but fermentable oligosaccharides	Garlic, asparagus, chicory	Stimulation of immune function; inhibition of tumorigenesis; reduction of serum cholesterol	Probiotics—effective substrate for bifidobacteria; stimulation of the immune system; reduction in infection; modulation of lipid metabolism	52, 53, 54
ω-3 Fatty acids	Algae, fish	Reduction of serum cholesterol and heart disease; immunosuppressant activity	Reduction in the total and LDL-cholesterol: HDL-cholesterol ratios; increase in serum HDL-cholesterol; inhibition of arachidonic acid-derived products, such as prostaglandins and leukotrienes	55, 56, 57
Coumarins	Vegetables, citrus fruits	Reduction in blood clotting; anticarcinogenic activity	Anticoagulants; inhibitors and inactivators of carcinogens and mutagens; scavengers of superoxide anion radicals	58, 59, 60, 61, 62

thine decarboxylase, cytochrome P450, and the induction of phase II enzymes), and a variety of indirect and direct chemical carcinogens and tumor promoters. The results of animal experiments consistently indicate that the effective concentrations of these phenolic compounds equal the levels found naturally in brewed tea (63).

Phytoestrogens. Phytoestrogens are present in the human diet in substantial amounts, especially in soybeans and soy foods (43–45). They have been shown to have many biologic effects in cell culture and in animals and humans. Most of these effects are considered positive, although a few harmful effects have been reported.

Phytoestrogens, estrogenic compounds found in plants, exert estrogenic effects on the central nervous system, induce estrus, and stimulate growth of the female genital tract in animals (43). Three main classes of phytoestrogens exist: isoflavones, coumestans, and lignans. All are

Table 112.4
Research Needed to Clarify Possible Roles of Phytochemicals in Health

- Identify the specific types of phytochemicals that provide health benefits
  - Determine the strength of association
  - Characterize the sources, dietary or supplemental, of phytochemicals that are beneficial or harmful
- Define the effective dose of phytochemicals that provides protection against cancer
  - Determine dose response
  - Determine effect of intervention on precancerous stage vs. existing tumors
  - Evaluate chemically induced model vs. spontaneous tumor model
- Determine the type of cancer most responsive to specific phytochemicals
  - Evaluate timing of dose to the onset of cancer
- Determine the effective dose of phytochemicals that protects against disease
  - Coronary heart disease
  - Diabetes
  - Osteoporosis
- Determine the concentrations at which pharmacologic doses become a toxicologic problem
- Identify new mechanisms by which the phytochemicals produce protective effects
  - Gap junction communication
  - Effects on cell differentiation
  - Immunomodulation
- Characterize the factors that affect absorption and bioavailability of phytochemicals
- Determine the metabolic fate of absorbed phytochemicals
- Establish the levels of phytochemicals identified with specific tissues
  - Determine specific functions of the phytochemicals in these tissues
  - Identify specific binding proteins
  - Identify selective uptake mechanisms
  - Determine species specificity
  - Identify differences in metabolic pathways in tissues accumulating different forms
- Identify and characterize metabolites of phytochemical metabolism
  - Determine physiologic activities of metabolic products
- Characterize effects of phytochemicals on cell-to-cell communication
  - Determine effects at various concentrations
  - Determine effects of specific carotenoids
  - Determine specificity relative to other lipophilic agents (e.g., tocotrienols)
- Determine effects of phytochemicals on cell differentiation
  - Determine effect at various concentrations
  - Determine effect of specific isomers
  - Determine specificity relative to other agents
- Determine optimal phytochemical mixtures
  - Determine composition
  - Determine duration of feeding
  - Determine amounts to be fed
- Identify the proportion of the population likely to respond positively to phytochemicals
- Establish the pharmacokinetics of delivered doses
  - Evaluate single and combined doses
  - Evaluate with and without food sources present
- Examine more closely the dietary components associated with health and with disease prevention relative to the diet as a whole

diphenolic compounds with structural similarities to natural estrogens and antiestrogens.

Although the amount of phytoestrogen absorbed may be low, the level circulating in the blood may be 100 to 500 times that of naturally occurring β-estradiol. Absorption is facilitated by hydrolysis of the sugar moiety by intestinal bacterial β-glucosidases, gastric hydrochloric acid, and β-glucosidases in foods. When the diet is supplemented with soy products, the level of phytoestrogens can reach 1000 times the level of β-estradiol. Soy food processing appears to affect isoflavone bioavailability (e.g., fermented tempeh appears to enhance their absorption).

After absorption, isoflavones and lignans are conjugated with glucuronic acid and sulfate by hepatic phase II enzymes (UDP-glucuronosyltransferases and sulfotransferases). These metabolic changes make the lipophilic compounds more water soluble and enhance their excretion. Glucuronic acid derivatives are the primary excretory products in urine.

Phytoestrogens can affect the menstrual cycle and the concentration of reproductive hormones in the blood of premenopausal women but less so in postmenopausal women. Natural flavones, such as daidzein or coumestrol, inhibit the (placental) aromatase enzyme in vitro. Aromatase catalyzes the rate-limiting step in estrogen synthesis in humans.

Genistein, the most abundant phytoestrogen, and coumestrol enhance bone calcium retention in rats. They inhibit bone resorption and stimulate bone mineralization. Similar effects are noted after consuming soy protein, which still contains the phytoestrogens. The protective effects are also observed in osteoporotic patients. Soy foods also contain a good source of dietary calcium, which enhances the effect.

Isoflavones (e.g., genistein) inhibit protein tyrosine kinase (PTK), an oncogene product that catalyzes tyrosine phosphorylation involved in tumor cell signal transduction and proliferation. Genistein inhibits growth of various human cancer cells, including melanoma cells and leukemic cells. Similarly, phytoestogens inhibit endothelial cell proliferation in capillaries.

Genistein also increases the activities of such antioxidant enzymes as superoxide dismutase, glutathione peroxidase, glutathione reductase, and liver cumene hydroperoxidase. Thus, genistein might work together with other phytochemicals with antioxidant activities to provide a broader cellular defense against free-radical attack and oxidative damage.

Thus, studies in humans, animals, and cell culture all indicate a positive role for phytoestrogens in prevention of menopausal symptoms, osteoporosis, cancer, and heart disease, and dietary supplementation with soy foods produces a response similar to that of the isolated phytoestrogen.

Lactoferrin. Lactoferrin (LF) represents a physiologically active animal product (LF) (37–40). Similar to transferrin, it has been assumed to be an iron transport protein that delivers iron to the infant gut. Lactoferrin binding sites have been identified on a variety of cells and tissues, but a high pI makes it difficult to determine whether these "receptors" are specific or nonspecific. Several functions have been hypothesized LF: enhancing bioavailability of breast milk iron, antimicrobial activity, and enhancing immune responses, including antibody production, complement activation, and natural killer cell function (64). The broad-spectrum antimicrobial properties of LF highlight the potential application of this protein as an enteral and parenteral antimicrobial factor, as well as a potential food additive.

The bacteriostatic effect of orally administered bovine LF (bLF) was evaluated on intestinal bacteria in the gut of mice fed bovine milk. Bovine milk feeding increased proliferation of Enterobacteriaceae, but added bLF suppressed this proliferation. Similar effects were noted when the gut was seeded with *Clostridium ramosum* and other *Clostridium* spp. Compared with other proteins, only bLF demonstrated this effect. Partial hydrolysis of bLF with pepsin—similar to digestive hydrolysis—did not alter the bacteriostatic effect; bLF still protected infant animals from gastrointestinal infections (64).

Recombinant human LF (rhLF) has been produced and characterized. Addition of rhLF to infant formula awaits further research to ensure stability during processing and to further evaluate biologic activity through studies on intestinal microflora from large numbers of infants. Before implementing a new product with increased cost, the biologic effect must be confirmed and shown of clear benefit to the infant. Mature human milk contains 2 to 3 mg/mL of hLF, although most infant formulas currently contain no LF. At this level, benefits can be seen after 3 months of feeding, although not all studies indicate a need for LF supplementation.

The potential exists for use of LF as a food additive. As a natural antimicrobial agent, many uses can be identified, such as decreasing microbial contamination and decreasing risk for toxicity from ground meat used in fast food restaurants.

Carotenoids. Understanding the use and function of phytochemicals requires understanding the bioavailability, absorption, metabolism, transport, and distribution of carotenoids, as well as determining their mechanism of action (65) (see also Chapter 33 on carotenoids).

The term *carotenoids* encompasses both carotene, which identifies the hydrocarbon forms, and the xanthophylls, which include carotenoid derivatives with one or more oxygen-containing functional groups (66). With more than 600 distinct carotenoids and their glycosides identified, it is curious that most research has focused on β-carotene. Other carotenoids may better support health in certain instances than β-carotene. Use of β-carotene as a model carotenoid because of its availability and relative safety, however, provides an opportunity to establish methods for studying other carotenoids and phytochemicals in general.

Important factors affecting carotenoid availability include the release of carotenoids from the physical food matrix in which they are ingested. Heating food improves bioavailability by disassociating the protein-carotenoid complexes and enhancing dispersion of the crystalline carotenoid to form multilamellar lipid vesicles with the lipid droplets resulting from bile salt and pancreatic lipase action. Nondigested lipids such as sucrose polyesters and some dietary fibers interfere with carotenoid absorption.

Movement of the carotenoid micelle into the mucosal cells of the duodenum appears to occur via passive diffusion but may be species specific (67). An intracellular binding protein was recently identified for β-carotene (68), as was previously reported for α-tocopherol, retinol, and cholecalciferol.

Transport of the carotenoids in plasma occurs exclusively by lipoproteins. β-Carotene, α-carotene, and lycopene are primarily found in low-density lipoproteins (LDLs), as is cholesterol. Some 40 to 50% of the dihydroxy carotenoids (lutein and zeaxanthin) are distributed in HDLs, which is more similar to the distribution pattern of α-tocopherol (35, 67). Differential uptake and retention of different carotenoid species has been confirmed for several tissues. The specificity of tissue distribution may contribute to further understanding of the physiologic role of carotenoids in biologic processes.

The source of dietary carotenoid affects transport from the intestine to the circulation. In one study, carotenoids were fed to 30 men over a 6-week period; either of two supplementary doses of β-carotene (30 and 12 mg) was compared with dietary intake of carrots, broccoli, or tomato juice. Purified β-carotene produced greater plasma response than did similar quantities of carotenoids provided from the food sources, suggesting a difference in bioavailability or interference by other dietary components (69).

Intestinal absorption, serum clearance, and interactions between β-carotene and lutein have been evaluated in human subjects (70). Individual variance included 9-fold differences for lutein and 6-fold differences for β-carotene. Comparison of individual and combined doses indicated that β-carotene significantly reduced lutein absorption by 40 to 45%, while lutein had mixed results on β-carotene levels in the same patients (half were increased, half decreased).

The role of β-carotene, and other carotenoids, in relation to other antioxidants has been examined. Tocopherols, tocotrienols, ascorbic acid, and carotenoids react with free radicals (specifically, peroxyl radicals) and with singlet oxygen (71). *RRR-α*-Tocopherol is the primary peroxyl radical scavenger in biologic lipid phases, such as membranes or LDL. Ascorbic acid is present in aqueous compartments, such as cytosol or plasma and other body fluids, and can reduce the tocopheroxyl radical. These biologic agents are regenerated via coupling to nonradical reducing systems such as glutathione peroxidase. Carotenoids such as β-carotene, lycopene, and some oxycarotenoids (e.g. zeaxanthin and lutein) can exert antioxidant actions as well as quench singlet oxygen and interact with free radicals.

Carotenoids may also interact with α-tocopherol and ascorbic acid. Using peroxidation of a microsomal membrane suspension as a model, β-carotene was an effective antioxidant at low oxygen tension (150 mm Hg pO_2); however, at higher oxygen tension (760 mm pO_2), β-carotene became a prooxidant (72). Oxygen binds to the carotene radical to form peroxy radicals, which then become part of the propagation reaction stimulating lipid peroxidation. α-Tocopherol prevents the prooxidant effect of β-carotene in a dose-dependent manner.

Recent studies involving β-carotene supplementation of smokers has indicated that there is no "magic bullet." In reviewing these human experiments, Mayne (73) indicated that most carotenoids had either no effect on cancer expression or actually enhanced it in lung and possibly enhanced cardiovascular disease as well. These studies suggest that other carotenoids and other substances in fruits and vegetables may be more protective than β-carotene. However, the enhanced lung cancer in males who smoke heavily may also be related to the high dose of β-carotene provided as a supplement (see Chapter 33 on carotenoids).

To date, dietary levels of the carotenoids have not been shown to cause adverse effects. However, the other dietary phytochemicals cannot be ignored. Since diets rich in fruits and vegetables correlate highly with health benefits, any one phytochemical may not be protective alone but may enhance protection in concert with other dietary components.

DESIGNING FUNCTIONAL FOODS

The new generation of functional foods represents an opportunity to apply food technology to production of specific functional ingredients by using gene transfer, genetic engineering, bioengineering, cell culture, and specialized breeding programs. Many of these processes have been used over the last decade in an effort to enhance the nutritional quality of the food supply. Examples are breeding meat animals for lower body fat content, altering plant fatty acid content to achieve desired ratios of beneficial fatty acids in the extracted oil, and improving the nutritional quality of plant proteins. These efforts continue as a means of improving the diet without labeling them as functional foods.

The examples of functional food products provided here only represent a larger effort to provide a healthy and safe diet. Some are in existence; others are being developed.

- Soyfoods are food sources containing naturally occurring phytochemicals such as isoflavones that may provide health benefits. In addition, tofu and other products are prepared by calcium coagulation of the protein, thus providing the food products with a ready source of calcium. Potential functional food areas include postmenopausal treatment to prevent osteoporosis, heart disease, or cancer.
- Milk and dairy products provide high-quality protein with a good source of calcium. Partial hydrolysis of casein has yielded phosphorylated peptides that enhance calcium absorption and may also enhance other physiologic responses. These peptides have been added to beverages as natural products that enhance calcium absorption.
- A nutraceutical milk has been developed, replacing fat with β-glucan + Oatrim (USDA) to lower cholesterol. A similar fiber-based drink has been popular in Japan.
- Yogurt and bifidobacteria cultures are promoted as beneficial for intestinal function. One aspect of this claim is the use of live cultures to compete with pathogenic or unfavorable microbial growth in the intestine.
- Lactoferrin, a milk protein, has several unique properties including antimicrobial functions. It has excellent potential of serving as a natural food additive, replacing other chemically derived agents. Use in sausages or canned meats would not only protect the food supply but also provide a biologically active protein that could also diminish gastrointestinal pathogens. Expansion into enteral and parenteral medical products is possible.
- The dairy cow can be used as a bioincubator. If the cow is challenged with specific microorganisms, production of specific gamma globulins is induced. These natural antimicrobial agents can then be isolated from the milk and used in therapeutic situations.
- Modified cheese starter cultures are being created in an effort to find a strain that will diminish cholesterol, reduce fat, and reduce sodium. Using the natural culture to change the cheese composition might well provide a health benefit and produce a product that could be used in a variety of new functional food products.
- Recovery of blood from slaughterhouses has provided an opportunity to isolate several blood proteins for food use. For example, albumin can be used as an egg white substitute. The crude gamma globulin fraction fed to newborn animals can serve as a natural antimicrobial agent to maintain their growth. Other blood components might also be isolated, purified, and developed into usable products.
- Calcium fortification of beverages, such as orange juice and snack foods, can contribute to prevention of osteoporosis.
- Chewing gum has been used to deliver specific functional ingredients. Inclusion of zinc allows coating of the throat and supposedly decreases colds significantly (42%).
- Chewing gum has been used to deliver oligosaccharides (in Japan) to promote maintenance of beneficial bacteria in the gastrointestinal tract.
- Ready-to-eat breakfast cereals are one of the early functional foods. Whole grains were processed to deliver fiber and nutrient value in a palatable form. Milk and fruit are consumed with the product as well. Today the cereal is coated with vitamins and some minerals, thereby acting as a convenient nutrient delivery system. This medium will most likely provide an early delivery system for other functional food ingredients. "Breakfast" bars might subsequently develop.
- ω-3 Fatty acids have been promoted for numerous properties primarily in prevention of CHD. Originally, the products were sold as supplements; namely, oil that had been extracted from fish livers. The same positive effects were provided by eating modest portions of fish two to three times weekly. The primary source of the fish ω-3 fatty acids is algae consumed by the fish. A better delivery system is sought to provide general access to this functional food ingredient; for example, an ω-3 fatty acid–containing margarine might be developed.

- Growth incubators have been designed for continuous growth of the algae, which are actively recovered for isolation of the ω-3 fatty acids.
- Plant species are also being developed through breeding and biotechnology programs that will contain ω-3 fatty acids for use in an ever-increasing product category.
- "Designer" oils containing eicosapentanoic acid and docosahexanoic acid can be created. These oils could be mixed with other oils as ingredients to create specialty products.
- Adding cholestyramine to the diet of poultry reduces the cholesterol content of eggs. Eggs with a lower cholesterol level might further enhance the use of these inexpensive, nutritionally rich foods.
- If chickens are fed higher levels of dietary carotenoids, the dietary carotenoids are incorporated into egg yolks. Incorporating phytochemicals in this way essentially transforms eggs into a functional food.

To date, the average consumer has seemed willing to pay a higher price for health foods and supplement products. How much the consumer will consistently pay for these and future "value-added" products remains unknown.

CONCLUSIONS

In view of the consumers' preference for more convenient and healthful foods, the U.S. food industry, armed with improved knowledge of human nutritional and physiologic needs and more sophisticated technology, has developed a wider variety of products. These include fortified foods, low-fat and low-calorie foods, functional foods (in which the concentrations of one or more food constituents have been manipulated to enhance their contributions to a healthful diet), and, most recently, foods produced by the emerging techniques of biotechnology (cereal grains with greater nutritional value). Taking a raw commodity, such as wheat or soybeans, and making it more nutritious, safer, more convenient, more acceptable, easier to prepare, or more appropriate for the needs of special population groups adds immense value to the commodity.

Techniques of adding value to foods in the future also include improved methods of manufacture, preservation, and packaging. Our ability to prepare high-quality, value-added foods will increase as we learn more about the physical properties of food, develop better technologies to prepare food ingredients, and make greater use of computers and biosensors in food-processing systems. As a result, product quality and safety and process efficiency will improve, while minimizing waste. Beneficial effects on health will depend on integration of a well-balanced diet, good lifestyle habits, environmental factors, and heredity. This context must be stressed; otherwise, the designer-functional foods concept might be misinterpreted as a kind of "magic bullet."

Better health through improved diet and nutrition, together with the factors just mentioned, can improve the quality of life, enhance productivity, and maximize learning potential. Functional foods can help reduce health-care costs by preventing or delaying the onset of chronic disease. The food industry should be recognized for its contribution to a healthier, safer diet that benefits everyone.

REFERENCES

1. Bidlack WR. J Am Coll Nutr 1996;15:422–33.
2. National Research Council, Committee on Diet and Health. Diet and health: implications for reducing chronic disease risk. Washington, DC: National Academy of Science, 1989.
3. Block G, Patterson B, Subar A. Nutr Cancer 1992;18:1–29.
4. Committee on Diet, Nutrition, and Cancer, National Research Council. Executive summary. In: Diet, nutrition and cancer. Washington, DC: National Academy Press, 1982;1–16.
5. Steinmetz KA, Potter JD. Cancer Causes Control 1991;2:325–57, 427–42.
6. Wrick KL. Crit Rev Food Sci Nutr 1995;35:167–73.
7. Caragay AB. Food Technol 1992;46:65–8.
8. Anon. The nutraceutical initiative: a proposal for economic and regulatory reform (white paper). New York: Foundation for Innovative Medicine, 1991.
9. DeFelice SL. Trends Food Sci Technol 1995;6:59–61.
10. Anon. Medical food. A scientific status summary by the Institute of Food Technologists' Expert Panel on Food Safety and Nutrition. Food Technol 1992;46:87–96.
11. Yetley EA, Moore RJ. Food Technol 1997;51:136.
12. Head RJ, Record IR, King RA. Nutr Rev 1996;54:S17–20.
13. Silverglade BA, Heller IR. Food Drug Law J 1997;52:313–21.
14. Wrick KL. Cereal Foods World 1993;38:205–14.
15. Federal Food, Drug and Cosmetic Act of 1938. Publ. no. 75-717, 52 Stat 1040, 1938.
16. Neff J, Holman JR. Food Process 1997;23:25–8.
17. House of Representatives. Nutrition Labeling and Education Act of 1990. Washington, DC: House Report 101-538, 1990.
18. Department of Health and Human Services, Food and Drug Administration. 1993. Food labeling: general requirements for health claims for food. Fed reg. 58:2478–536.
19. Anon. Nutr Rev 1993;51:90–3.
20. Dietary Supplement Health and Education Act of 1994. Publ. no. 103-417, 108 Stat 4325–35, 1994.
21. Glinsmann WH. Nutr Rev 1996;54:S33–7.
22. Mongelsdorf ME, Bianchi A. Inc. Magazine, June 1994;33.
23. Stibel GM, Devilbiss K. SPECTRUM Food Ind 1993;30:1–12.
24. Hasler CM. Nutr Rev 1996;54:S6–10.
25. Nutriceutical Products and Functional Food Additives. Falls Church, VA: Technology Catalysts, 1991;1–237.
26. Dai Y, Luo X. Nutr Rev 1996;54:S21–3.
27. Weng W, Chen J. Nutr Rev 1996;54:S11–6.
28. Pascal G. Nutr Rev 1996;54:S29–32.
29. Gerhauser C, You M, Liu J, et al. Cancer Res 1997;57:272–8.
30. Zhang Y, Kensler TW, Cho CG, et al. Proc Natl Acad Sci USA 1994;91:3147–50.
31. Zhang Y, Talalay P, Cho CG, et al. Proc Natl Acad Sci USA 1992;89:2399–403.
32. Dreosti IE. Nutr Rev 1996;54:S51–8.
33. Zhang A, Zhu QY, Luk YS, et al. Life Sci 1997;61:383–94.
34. Asano Y, Okamura S, Ogo T, et al. life Sci 1997;60:135–42.
35. Stahl W, Sies H. Arch Biochem Biophys 1996;336:1–9.
36. Tyurin VA, Carta G, Tyurin YY, et al. Lipids 1997;32:131–42.
37. Shinoda I, Takase M, Fukuwatari Y, et al. Biosci Biotechnol Biochem 1996;60:521–3.
38. Ganz T, Lehrer RI. Curr Opin Hematol 1997;4:53–8.
39. Shimizu K, Matsuzuwa H, Okada K, et al. Arch Virol 1996;141:1875–89.

40. Nakajima M, Shinoda I, Samejima Y, et al. J Cell Physiol 1997;170:101–5.
41. Durgam VR, Fernandes G. Cancer Lett 1997;116:121–30.
42. Lee KN, Kritchevsky D, Pariza MW. Atherosclerosis 1994;108: 19–25.
43. Kurzer MS, Xu X. Annu Rev Nutr 1997;17:353–81.
44. Perterson G, Barnes S. Biochem Biophys Res Commun 1991;179:661–7.
45. Anderson JW, Johnstone BM. N Engl J Med 1995;333:276–82.
46. Sundaram SG, Milner JA. Biochim Biophys Acta 1996;1315: 15–20.
47. Milner JA. Nutr Rev 1996;54:S82–6.
48. Hong JY, Wang ZY, Smith TJ, et al. Carcinogenesis 1992;13: 901–4.
49. Gebhardt R, Bech H. Lipids 1996;31:1269–76.
50. Hohl RJ. Adv Exp Med Biol 1996;401:137–46.
51. Crowell PL, Siar Ayoubi A, Burke YD. Adv Exp Med Biol 1996; 401:131–6.
52. Gibson GR, Roberfroid MB. J Nutr 1995;125:1401–12.
53. Roberfroid MB. Nutr Rev 1996;54:S38–42.
54. Oku T. Nutr Rev 1996;54:S59–66.
55. Conquer JA, Holub BJ. J Nutr 1996;126:3032–9.
56. Sacks FM, Cutler JA, Kirchner KA, et al. J Hypertens 1994;12: 209–13.
57. Uauy-Dagach R, Valenzuela A. Nutr Rev 1996;54:S102–8.
58. Booth SL, Charnley JM, Sadowski JA, et al, Thromb Haemost 1997;77:504–9.
59. Hoult JR, Paya M. Gen Pharmacol 1996;27:713–22.
60. Cai Y, Baer-Dubowska W, Ashwood-Smith M, et al. Carcinogenesis 1997;18:215–22.
61. Ednharder R, Tang X. Food Chem Toxicol 1997;35:357–72.
62. Paya M, Goodwin PA, De Las Heras B, et al. Biochem Pharmacol 1994;48:445–51.
63. Ho CT, Ferraro T, Chen Q, et al. Phytochemicals in teas and rosemary and their cancer-preventive properties. In: Ho CT, Osawa T, Huang MT, Rosen RT, eds. Food phytochemicals for cancer prevention II. ACS symposium series. Washington, DC: American Chemical Society, 1992;2–19.
64. Hutchens TW, Lonnerdal B, eds. Lactoferrin: interactions and biological functions. Totowa, NJ: Humana Press 1997.
65. Omaye ST, Krinsky NI, Kagan VE, et al. Fundam Appl Toxicol, 1997;40:163–74.
66. Armstrong GA, Hearst JE. FASEB J 1996;10:228–37.
67. Parker RS. FASEB J 1996;10:542–51.
68. Rao MN, Ghosh P, Lakshman MR. J Biol Chem 1997;272: 24455–60.
69. Micozzi MS, Brown ED, Edwards BK, et al. Am J Clin Nutr 1992;55:1120–5.
70. Kostie D, White WS, Olson JA. Am J Clin Nutr 1995;62:604–10.
71. Handelman GJ, Packer L, Cross CE. Am J Clin Nutr 1996;63:559–65.
72. Palozza P, Calviello G, Bartoli GM. Free Radical Biol Med 1995;19:887–92.
73. Mayne ST. FASEB J 1996;10:690–701.

SELECTED READINGS

Anon. Functional Foods: commercial and technical trends and developments. Symposium proceedings, no. 60. British Food Manufactoring Industries Research Association Leatherhead, Surrey, England.

Bidlack WR, Omaye ST, Meskin MS, Jahner D, eds. Phytochemicals: a new paradigm. Technomics Inc., in press.

First International Conference on East-West Perspectives on Functional Foods. Nutr Rev 1996;54:S1–202.

Goldberg I. Functional foods: designer foods, pharmafoods and nutraceuticals. New York: Chapman & Hall, 1994.

Goldberg I, Willaims R. Biotechnology and food ingredients. New York: Van Nostrand Reinhold, 1991.

Huang MT, Ho CT, Lee CY, eds. Phenolic compounds in food and their effect on health II. Antioxidants and cancer prevention. Symposium series 507. Washington, DC: American Chemical Society, 1996.

Huang MT, Osawa T, Ho CT, Rosen RT, eds. Food phytochemicals for cancer prevention I. Symposium series 546. Washington, DC: American Chemical Society, 1994.

Huang MT, Osawa T, Ho CT, Rosen RT, eds. Food phytochemicals for cancer prevention II. Symposium series 547. Washington, DC: American Chemical Society, 1995.

Knorr D, ed. Food biotechnology. New York: Marcel Dekker, 1987.

National Research Council, Committee on Technological Options to Improve the Nutritional Attributes of Animal Products. Designing foods: animal product options in the marketplace. Washington, DC: National Academy Press, 1988.

Tabeska GR, Teranishi R, Williams PJ, Kobayasbi A, eds. Biotechnology for improved foods and flavors. Symposium series 637. Washington, DC: American Chemical Society, 1996.

113. Food Additives, Contaminants, and Natural Toxins

JOHN N. HATHCOCK and JEANNE I. RADER

Human foods contain a wide variety of chemicals with the potential for adverse effects if consumed in excess. These substances may occur naturally in foods, may be added directly or indirectly during food processing, or may contaminate foods as a result of their use in agricultural or livestock production (1). Direct food additives are intentionally added to foods to perform a variety of technical functions. Other chemicals (indirect food additives) are present in foods as a result of their use in some phase of food production, processing, storage, etc. Contaminants such as mercury, lead, arsenic, selenium, and cadmium enter foods or forages via the soil or the marine environment in which they occur naturally or to which they have been added as a result of human agricultural or industrial activities. Proteinase inhibitors, goitrogens, alkaloids, allergens, oxalates, phytates, and other such substances are natural innate components of particular foods, whereas other compounds (e.g., aflatoxins, paralytic shellfish toxins) are products of the metabolism of fungi, molds, or marine dinoflagellates. Some of these toxicants or contaminants are found in foods that are common in the human diet, whereas others are found only in unusual food sources. As might be expected, the potential hazard to human health posed by such varied compounds ranges from virtually nil to substantial.

FOOD ADDITIVES

Categories

The broadest use of the term *food additive* would include all natural or synthetic, nutritive or nonnutritive, physiologically active or inert chemicals added directly or indirectly to foods. Such a definition is far more inclusive than the legal definition of food additive used in the Food Additive Amendment to the Federal Food, Drug, and Cosmetic Act (FDCA). For regulatory purposes, distinctions are made between *direct* and *indirect* food additives and between food additives and *generally recognized as safe (GRAS) substances* (1). *Direct* food additives include chemicals added to foods during processing to perform a specific function. From a functional viewpoint, examples of direct additives include antioxidants, antispoilage agents, vitamins, minerals, flavoring agents, coloring agents, emulsifiers, stabilizers, bleaching agents, acidulants, nutritive and nonnutritive sweeteners, fat substitutes, and leavening agents; some of these food additives are GRAS substances and others are not. Indirect additives include chemicals that become components of foods indirectly or unintentionally via, for example, contact of food with processing equipment or packaging containers. Food contaminants include substances such as products of molds (e.g., aflatoxins), agricultural chemicals (e.g., pesticide residues), and environmental chemicals (e.g., dioxin and lead).

Safety considerations for food chemicals begin with the axiom that any substance can be toxic if consumed in sufficiently high quantity. The intake necessary to generate a toxic response, however, varies greatly from one substance to another. Some substances, such as sucrose, have such low toxic potential and such a long history of widespread use as direct food additives that they are known as GRAS substances for defined uses, with the amount limited only by good manufacturing practice. Contaminants such as aflatoxins and dioxin have such high toxicity that they are stringently regulated in foods.

Certain categories of food chemicals have generated much interest and debate because of their widespread use, their relatively common occurrence in foods, or the uncertain degree of health risk associated with them.

Dr. Rader's contribution to this chapter was made in her private capacity. No official support or endorsement by the Food and Drug Administration is intended or should be inferred.

Selected categories that meet these criteria are discussed in detail below.

Nutrients

Interest is growing in the value of treating specific diseases with vitamins and minerals in larger than nutritionally required quantities. Clinical uses of iron, iodine, and fluoride have long been recognized and are well described (2). The safety of vitamins and minerals, whether used as food ingredients, dietary supplements, or, in some cases, drugs depends on *(a)* the inherent toxicodynamic potency of the specific compound, *(b)* its chemical form, *(c)* total daily intake, *(d)* the duration and regularity of consumption, and *(e)* the biologic characteristics of the person consuming the compound (2, 3).

Fat-soluble vitamins are usually considered more toxic than those that are water soluble. This generality is not valid: vitamin E (tocopherols and tocotrienols) is fat soluble but quite nontoxic, and niacin and pyridoxine are water soluble but have demonstrated toxicities. There are large differences in inherent toxic potency within each category.

Vitamin A

Among the vitamins, vitamin A is one of few for which substantial numbers of human cases of intoxication have been reported (4–6). To assess toxic potential, the total intake of preformed vitamin A from all sources must be considered; these include foods with naturally high levels (e.g., eggs and liver), foods fortified with vitamin A (milk and many ready-to-eat cereals), and nutrient supplements. Although vitamin A toxicity from excessive consumption of liver has been reported, most reports have associated vitamin A toxicity with prolonged consumption of very high potency single-nutrient supplements. The toxicity of vitamin A is discussed in Chapter 17.

Vitamin E

Vitamin E is added to food as a nutrient and as an antioxidant. Vitamin E is considered relatively innocuous, with no side effects at intakes up to 300 IU (201 mg *RRR*-α-tocopherol or its equivalent) per day (20 times the adult male recommended dietary allowance, or RDA) (7, 7a) and with few side effects at intakes of 3200 IU (2148 mg *RRR*-α-tocopherol or its equivalent) per day (8). Food additive uses of vitamin E are not known to generate intakes near the possibly adverse range. The potential toxicity of vitamin E is discussed in Chapter 19.

Pyridoxine

Water-soluble vitamins usually have been considered virtually nontoxic because of their solubility and rapid excretion. Reports of toxic effects of pyridoxine have proven such assumptions to be unjustified (6). No toxicity has been reported from food-ingredient uses of pyridoxine. The toxicity of pyridoxine is discussed in Chapter 24.

Vitamin C

Vitamin C is used in foods as a nutrient and as an antioxidant. Intakes resulting from such uses of vitamin C are modest compared with those that can cause adverse effects (2, 7, 8–16). Most high intakes result from supplement use (8). Apparently, vitamin C has low toxicity, or intoxications would be common because of the widespread use of supplements. Although large intakes may cause adverse effects in some individuals, some of the widely reported and often-cited adverse effects have little apparent basis. High intakes of vitamin C can make a small contribution to oxalate excretion but such intakes are not known to increase the risk of oxalate renal stones. The toxicity of vitamin C is discussed in Chapter 29.

Niacin

Niacin (nicotinic acid or nicotinamide) is nutritionally essential. At high dosages, it is an effective drug for lowering blood cholesterol levels (17, 18), and this use of niacin has led to nearly all cases of niacin toxicity. An error in preparation of niacin-containing bagel dough resulted in accidental overfortification, with undesirable reactions (skin flushing) in consumers (19). Niacin toxicity is discussed in Chapter 23.

Copper

Copper in single massive doses is among the most inherently toxic of the essential trace elements. At the low levels found naturally in foods or added by food-additive (GRAS substance) uses, dietary copper causes no known toxicity, except in persons with Wilson's disease (15). In general, humans are less sensitive to copper intoxication than are some animals, such as sheep. The toxicity of specific levels of copper is affected by dietary iron and zinc as well as protein. Copper toxicity is discussed in Chapter 12.

Iron

Iron oxides are used as food-coloring agents. Ferric phosphate and pyrophosphate, ferrous gluconate, lactate, sulfate, and reduced iron are classified as GRAS substances for use as food ingredients in the United States. Absorption of nonheme iron is closely regulated by the intestinal mucosa. Diets high in heme iron or high in promoters of nonheme iron absorption may occasionally lead to iron overload and resulting disease (20–22). The contribution of dietary iron to iron overload in some individuals is uncertain. Accidental, massive, acute ingestion of multiple units of high-potency iron supplements for adults can result in severe injury or death in young children. To help prevent this problem, the Food and Drug Administration (FDA) has recently required warnings on iron-containing dietary supplement and drug products and on individual unit-dose ("blister") packaging for products with more than 30 mg of iron per dosage unit. The toxicity of iron is discussed in Chapter 10.

Zinc

Several zinc compounds are used as food additives. Prophylactic supplementation of poultry and livestock feeds with zinc is common. Individual tolerances for zinc sulfate vary widely (3). Chronic ingestion of large doses of supplements may have adverse effects, but no toxicity seems to have resulted from ingestion of the moderate levels from food-additive uses (3, 23, 24). Zinc toxicity is discussed in Chapter 11.

Selenium

Selenium is one of the most toxic of the essential elements. Intoxications have been caused by incorrectly formulated supplements and may be caused by high dietary intakes in some geographic areas (15, 24–26). There are currently no approved selenium compounds for use as food additives in human foods in the United States, although the FDA has set a reference daily intake as a standard for food labeling (27). The toxicity of selenium is discussed in detail in Chapter 14.

Artificial Sweeteners

Much of the use of nonnutritive sweeteners is prompted by the accompanying reductions in calorie intake. Also, some consumers may be motivated by the absence of a procariogenic effect. Safety concerns center around possible carcinogenicity of some artificial sweeteners and neurologic effects of others.

Saccharin

Saccharin is 300 to 500 times sweeter than sucrose. There is no apparent tissue accumulation or metabolism, and ingested saccharin is excreted unchanged in the feces or urine. Mutagenicity studies have been all negative. Carcinogenicity studies in animals have produced positive results in certain experimental designs (28, 29). Saccharin produced bladder cancer in two-generation studies in which exposure began in utero by dietary treatment of the pregnant rat and continued through the diet for 2 years following birth. The doses used ranged up to 7.5% of the diet. No adverse effects have been observed with less than 1% dietary saccharin. Epidemiologic studies have given relative risk ratios close to unity (no significant risk).

Cyclamate

The metabolism of cyclamate depends on the intestinal microflora. It is excreted largely unaltered in test animals treated for the first time. Pretreatment with cyclamate, however, may alter the microflora by selection of microbes capable of converting cyclamate to cyclohexylamine, dicyclohexylamine, and cyclohexanone. These metabolites have been found in rats, dogs, guinea pigs, monkeys, and humans. The results of toxicity studies with cyclamate have been largely negative (27, 29). In the rat, bladder tumors have occurred when cyclamate and saccharin were fed in a 10:1 ratio in conjunction with cyclohexylamine. Also, dietary cyclamate appears to promote bladder cancer initiated by intravenous doses of methylnitrosourea (MNU) in the rat. The results of carcinogenicity studies in mice, dogs, hamsters, and primates have been negative. The FDA banned food use of cyclamate in 1969.

Aspartame

Considering its structure and constituent parts, there are many hypothetical possibilities for adverse effects by aspartame. Extensive investigation has not shown side effects from aspartame (28, 29), but research and further interpretation of possible adverse effects continues. Aspartame is metabolized to several products, including phenylalanine and aspartic acid. Thus, aspartame is a very low calorie sweetener, not a zero-calorie sweetener. Diketopiperazine occurs as a contaminant in aspartame, at about 1%. Since aspartame is metabolized to phenylalanine, it carries a risk for persons with phenylketonuria (PKU) proportional to consumption of equivalent amounts of phenylalanine. Claims of risk for other consumers, however, have not been substantiated. Such claims relate mainly to purported adverse neurologic effects of phenylalanine or aspartame. Phenylalanine is a precursor of the neuroactive substances norepinephrine and epinephrine. Adverse neurologic effects might logically be related to overproduction of either or both of these compounds. Concrete evidence for such effects, however, has not been found.

Fat Substitutes

Fat substitutes are substances that have one or more of the technical effects of fat in foods but are not metabolized as fats and thus may be used in low-fat foods and diets. At present, two types of fat substitutes have been approved for use in human food: *(a)* microparticulated proteins that have the functional properties of fat (viscosity and organoleptic properties) only at low temperatures and *(b)* heat-stable sucrose polyesters that are not hydrolyzed by digestive enzymes and thus make no contribution to dietary (digestible) fat.

Microparticulated Proteins

A microparticulated protein product (*Simplesse*) has been affirmed by FDA as a GRAS ingredient for use as a fat substitute in low temperature products such as ice cream (30). The proteins come from egg or milk or both and can be digested and metabolized as dietary protein. The microparticulation process does not provide heat stability; thus, this fat substitute may be used as a fat substitute in low-fat foods and diets but not in cooking and frying. Because this fat substitute is composed of microparticulated edible proteins, safety questions mainly relate to possible antigenicity and allergenicity. Individuals who consumed a microparticulated product with protein from both eggs and milk had normal clinical signs and chemistries (31) and no evidence of immunologic sensitivity to "novel" protein fractions (32).

Sucrose Polyesters

Olestra is the common name for a mixture of sucrose polyesters used as a food additive. The additive may have six, seven, or eight fatty acid molecules esterified to the hydroxy groups of sucrose. The fatty acids used are commonly found in foods (as triacylglycerols). The chain length and degree of unsaturation of the fatty acids affects the physical characteristics of the product. Olestra has organoleptic properties similar to those of ordinary lipids. It is heat-stable and is not hydrolyzed or otherwise metabolized. In food products it behaves as a dietary fat, but it is not digested and thus yields no fatty acids or energy. From the viewpoint of nutritional effects, it is not a dietary fat.

Toxicologic research has shown no systemic uptake, storage, or direct toxicologic effects of olestra. Sucrose polyesters present a different set of safety issues than most food additives. Since olestra is not digested or absorbed, it raises unique issues for a food additive. Because it becomes an ever-larger fraction of intestinal contents as it passes through the intestine, it raises safety issues related to effects on the intestine and its functions, including possible interference with normal digestion and absorption.

After extensive review of a petition for food-additive approval of olestra, the FDA approved use of olestra as a replacement for fats and oils in certain types of foods (33). The data evaluated came from studies on absorption, distribution, metabolism, and elimination; genetic toxicity; animal toxicity; effects on absorption of fat-soluble drugs; effects on gastrointestinal health and function; and nutritional studies. The potentially adverse effects observed included antinutritive effects on the fat-soluble vitamins and carotenoids. To compensate for these effects, the FDA's approval required addition of the following vitamins to foods containing olestra (quantity per gram of olestra): 1.9 mg α-tocopherol, 51 μg retinol equivalents of vitamin A as retinyl acetate or retinyl palmitate, 12 IU vitamin D, and 8 μg vitamin K_1. The FDA determined that current scientific evidence does not justify or indicate a need for fortifying olestra-containing foods with any carotenoid. Although consumption of olestra lowered the serum concentration of β-carotene more than that of the fat-soluble vitamins, the decision not to require fortification of olestra-containing foods was based on the absence of recognized direct benefits from consumption of carotenoids.

Based on review by their own scientists and with the advice of outside experts, the FDA found that all potentially adverse effects of olestra could be ameliorated by the specified additions of fat-soluble vitamins to food that contain olestra and concluded that with these additions, the required "reasonable certainty of no harm" had been demonstrated.

Food-Color Additives

Food colorants include both natural substances and synthetic compounds (34). Natural substances that have been used as food colorants include carmine, paprika, saffron, and turmeric. When used to impart color, certain nutrients (e.g., β-carotene and riboflavin) are regarded as color additives, as are fruit or vegetable juices, carrot oil, and beet extract. Synthetic compounds permitted for food use under good manufacturing practices and subject to certification by the FDA include FD&C (Food, Drug & Cosmetic Act) Yellow No. 5 (tartrazine), Red No. 3 (erythrosine), Red No. 40, Blue No. 1, and Citrus Red No. 2. Provisionally listed colors include FD&C Blue No. 2, Yellow No. 6, and Green No. 3.

The safety evaluation and history of use and regulation for food colors are complex (34). For several food colors, such as FD&C Red No. 2 (amaranth) and FD&C Red No. 3, the crucial safety issue is possible carcinogenicity. Use of FD&C Red No. 2 was banned because concerns about carcinogenicity were not addressed by available data. For FD&C Red No. 3 (a synthetic compound with a high content of iodine), the possibility of indirect carcinogenicity has provoked much controversy about whether this should be sufficient reason to ban it from use in food. Erythrosine causes hypertrophy, hyperplasia, adenomas, and carcinomas of the thyroid glands. These changes may be associated with secondary (indirect) oncogenesis. Whether hypertrophy and hyperplasia from any cause in any organ would carry risk for increased tumors remains an unanswered question. The FDA concluded there were insufficient data to determine that erythrosine-induced carcinogenicity was caused by an indirect mechanism.

Synthetic food colors and some flavoring agents such as methyl salicylate (oil of wintergreen) have been alleged to cause hyperactivity in some children (35). This concept, promoted by Feingold in 1975, stimulated research in hyperactivity in both humans and animals. Various chemical insults to the central nervous system can result in hyperactivity in brain-damaged animals. Some dyes (e.g., FD&C Red No. 3) inhibit uptake of neurotransmitters in rat striatal synaptosomes, but this effect may be nonspecific and may not account for any selective behavioral effects. The ease with which hyperactivity can be induced in brain-damaged rats suggests that this model should not be used to evaluate the hyperactive child. Clinical trials of salicylates and other food additives in children have yielded little or no information concerning the cause of hyperactivity or therapy for it.

The viewpoint that the only function of food colors is to add aesthetic appeal overlooks the psychologic value of food color in diet therapy. Alteration of the average American diet to meet the dietary goals in the *Surgeon General's Report on Nutrition and Health* (35a) is a difficult objective. Food colors may have a positive role in dietary management (35), but few argue that this role is essential.

Preservatives

Chemical preservatives include both antioxidants and antimicrobial agents. Antioxidants are used to inhibit changes in flavor, nutritive value, and appearance that result from oxidation of fatty acids, amino acids, and vitamins. Antimicrobial agents are used to prevent the growth of bacteria, yeasts, and molds that may generate foodborne intoxications or infections or cause undesirable alterations in flavor, appearance, or nutritive value. Although refrigeration obviates the need for some preservatives, it is comparatively expensive and is not available under many circumstances. Food irradiation as an alternative to chemical preservatives has received relatively little acceptance because of technical requirements and public controversy.

Antioxidants

Common antioxidant food additives include ascorbic acid, ascorbyl palmitate, tocopherols, butylated hydroxyanisole (BHA), butylated hydroxytoluene (BHT), ethoxyquin, propyl gallate, and *t*-butylhydroquinone (TBHQ). The common antimicrobial agents nitrite and sulfite have antioxidant activity as well as other properties.

BHA and BHT. Considerable controversy has existed about the safety of BHA and BHT. Both are lipid-soluble antioxidants capable of inducing increased concentrations and activities of several liver enzymes involved in detoxifying foreign compounds. Each of these roles, antioxidant and inducing agent, can provide protection against chemically induced carcinogenesis under certain experimental conditions.

Antioxidants can protect against the reactivity of electrophilic chemicals that may bind to DNA and cause mutations and initiate carcinogenesis. Many carcinogens are actually procarcinogens that are metabolized to electrophilic carcinogens. Some carcinogens are electrophilic and do not require metabolic activation. Inducers of liver enzymes that metabolize foreign compounds may have either anticarcinogenic or procarcinogenic activities, depending on the dose and timing in relation to exposure to the initiating carcinogen. If treatment with the inducer precedes treatment with the carcinogen, the resulting induction usually results in more-rapid metabolism of the carcinogen to inactive forms and decreased net carcinogenicity. If exposure to the carcinogen precedes treatment with high doses of the inducing agent, the resulting hyperplasia and hypertrophy can promote the carcinogenesis caused by the carcinogen. With certain carcinogens, late treatment with high doses of inducing antioxidants may inhibit carcinogenesis.

BHA treatment alone in high doses (2% of the diet) has produced hyperplasia, papilloma, and squamous cell carcinoma in the forestomachs of rats and hamsters (36). No evidence of carcinogenicity was found when BHT was included in diets of male and female mice at a level of 0.5% in one study (36). Both BHA and BHT protect against the early neoplastic changes in the liver caused by diethylinitrosourea.

The importance of early administration of BHA or BHT in studies of their potential anticarcinogenic actions is well established (37, 38). It is widely thought that lung cancer requires two decades for development from the first initiation events to clinically obvious cancer. Indeed, with the most powerful known protective action against lung cancer, cessation of smoking, decreases in risk become significant only over a 10- to 15-year period (39).

The relationships between antioxidants and carcinogenesis are complex, and no generalization can be completely accurate. The effect of antioxidants on cancer depend on the carcinogen, organ and tumor types, and timing and dose of both antioxidant and carcinogen.

Nitrite

Sodium nitrite is used as an antimicrobial preservative, a flavoring agent, and a color-fixing agent (via its reactivity with myoglobin). Nitrite is effective in preventing growth of *Clostridium botulinum,* thereby decreasing the risk of botulism.

Nitrite reacts with secondary amines and amides to form the corresponding N-nitroso derivatives (40, 41). Many but not all N-nitroso compounds are carcinogenic. Ascorbic acid and other reducing agents inhibit the nitrosation reactions of nitrite; ascorbic acid is an especially effective inhibitor in the acid environment of the stomach where much nitrosation takes place. Some nitrosamines are formed in foods during processing, but the largest part of nitrosamine exposure occurs via the nitrosation reactions in the stomach. Food-additive sources of nitrite are significant, but a substantial portion of total nitrite exposure comes from bacterial reduction of nitrate to nitrite in the mouth. Food nitrate, principally from vegetables, is absorbed and then slowly released into saliva. This slow reconsumption of nitrate allows ample time for reduction to nitrite in the mouth and subsequent nitrosation reactions in the stomach. Safety evaluation of nitrite as a food additive must take into account this major additional endogenous source.

The question of possible direct carcinogenicity by nitrite has been addressed through studies of nitrite "alone." Biologic systems, however, always contain a variety of amines, and any studies comparing the carcinogenicity of nitrite with that of nitrosamines must take this into account.

Nitrite is capable of causing some toxic reactions not related to carcinogenesis, but the dose required is relatively large. Persons chronically exposed to large amounts of nitrite may develop methemoglobinemia, but this problem is not common.

Sulfite and Sulfur Dioxide

Sulfur dioxide and its salts are commonly used as inhibitors of enzymatic and nonenzymatic browning, broad-spectrum antimicrobial agents, dough conditioners, bleaching agents for certain products, and antioxidants. Sulfites are very reactive, and consequently little free sulfite remains in foods. Sulfites have been used for centuries with little evidence of adverse reactions in consumers.

Asthma is the most common and severe adverse reaction attributed to sulfite ingestion (42, 43). An association has been recognized between sulfite ingestion and the onset of asthma in sensitive individuals. To date, more than 20 deaths have been attributed to this idiosyncratic reaction. Sensitive individuals are more likely to respond to acidified sulfited beverages than to sulfited foods, perhaps because sulfur dioxide is volatilized in the beverages. Challenge tests indicate that only 1 to 2% of asthmatics are sensitive to sulfite. In one large test, none of the mild asthmatics was sensitive to sulfite.

The pathogenesis of sulfite-induced asthma is not understood. The mechanisms may involve IgE-mediated reactions, hyperreactivity to inhaled sulfur dioxide, or sulfite oxidase deficiency. Sulfite-sensitive individuals are especially sensitive to sulfite-containing acidified beverages and sulfite-treated lettuce. Lettuce contains a preponderance of free sulfite. Regulations limiting sulfite concentrations and labeling requirements have been strengthened in recent years.

Toxicity studies in animals indicate rapid metabolism to sulfate by sulfite oxidase and excretion. At high concentrations in vitro, sulfite causes some mutations and sister chromatid exchanges in Chinese hamster ovary cells. At high doses (more than 600 mg/kg), there is no evidence of sulfite genotoxicity in Chinese hamsters.

GRAS Substances

The Food, Drug and Cosmetic Act has been much amended since its passage in 1938 (44). One of these amendments, the Food Additives Amendment of 1958, used the phrase "generally recognized as safe," from which the term *GRAS* arose. The amendment required prior approval from the FDA for all substances intended to be added to foods. When this amendment was passed, several hundred substances that were previously sanctioned or that were already in common use as food additives were exempted from its requirements. A listing of "Substances Generally Recognized as Safe" for their intended use was first published in the early 1960s. Among the several hundred substances on the diverse GRAS list were a variety of nutrients, general purpose food chemicals, emulsifying agents, anticaking agents, stabilizers, spices, and flavorings.

The Food Additives Amendment of 1958 exempted GRAS substances from the premarketing clearance required for food additives; thus GRAS substances are not officially food additives. In presuming GRAS substances to be safe when used in the amounts and manner intended and in accordance with good manufacturing practice, the Food Additives Amendment effectively negated the need for the FDA to require a demonstration of safety before these ingredients could be used in food. Consequently, the 1958 amendment required the FDA to demonstrate that a GRAS substance was no longer generally recognized as safe before its use in food could be prohibited. In 1972, a Select Committee on GRAS Substances, in coordination with the FDA and the Federation of American Societies for Experimental Biology (FASEB) reevaluated the safety data available on GRAS substances. The committee supported continued GRAS status for many substances, suggested further studies for some, and rescinded the GRAS status for others. Because the safety and toxic potential of any substance depends on intake, the GRAS reviews have prompted considerable study of the consumption levels for many substances in food.

CONTAMINANTS

Food contaminants may include minerals and heavy metals, mycotoxins, shellfish toxins, pesticide residues, and environmental organic chemicals.

Minerals and Heavy Metals

A number of minerals present in foods are of concern because of their potential toxicity. Because plant materials are the primary source of minerals for both animals and humans, the complex factors influencing the mineral content of plants are also important as major determinants of dietary intakes of certain elements. The literature relating to the metabolism of essential and nonessential minerals, the interrelationships among environmental factors and plant and seafood content of minerals, and the toxic and carcinogenic effects of excessive mineral intake is extensive (45–47). Only a few examples of toxicities related to high levels of specific minerals in foods are described here.

Arsenic

Arsenic (As) is ubiquitous in the environment and occurs in inorganic and organic compounds in the trivalent or pentavalent form (48, 49). Levels of arsenic in most foods are low (normally below 0.25 mg/kg) (50). Meats, poultry, and fish contribute most of the arsenic consumed by humans. Analysis of a special diet excluding seafood gave a calculated average intake of 0.04 mg As/day whereas a more typical diet contributed 0.19 mg As/day (51). Arsenic uptake by plants is related to the type of plant, chemical composition of the soil, and concentration of soluble arsenic in the soil. Arsenic concentrations in marine organisms and seaweed, in which arsenic occurs in a variety of organic methylated forms, are generally much higher than those in other foods. These methylated compounds are considerably less toxic than inorganic arsenic compounds. Symptoms from acute and chronic arsenic toxicity from various arsenic compounds have been reviewed by Anke (48) and Nielsen (49). Carcinogenic effects of arsenic were recognized more than 100 years ago through examination of workers in the smelting industry. It has been suggested that arsenic alone cannot produce malignant changes and should therefore be considered a cocarcinogen (52, 53).

Selenium

Selenium (Se) is among the most toxic of the essential trace elements. It is ubiquitous in the environment but is unevenly distributed over the earth's surface. Areas of both selenium deficiency (e.g., New Zealand and parts of China) and selenium excess (e.g., North Dakota and parts of China) are now recognized. "Accumulator" (or "converter") plants play major roles in determining the effects of soil conditions on selenium availability to livestock in selenium-rich areas. These plants absorb selenium from soils containing selenium in forms that are relatively unavailable to other plants. The absorbed selenium is converted to organic forms that are returned to the soil and then become available to other plants. Cereal grains may accumulate high levels of selenium in selenium-rich areas. Excess selenium intake due to consumption of seleniferous plants by animals produces a wide range of adverse effects (54). Well-defined symptoms and lesions following acute or chronic ingestion of high-selenium forages are now recognized. Chronic toxicity signs in livestock include cirrhosis, lameness, hoof malformations, hair loss, and emaciation. In laboratory animals, the signs most commonly include cirrhosis. The minimum dietary level of selenium recognized to produce adverse effects in farm animals is 4 to 5 μg/g dry weight of diet.

The discovery of selenium as the cause of the "blind stagger" syndrome and "alkali disease" in livestock led to concerns about possible deleterious effects of human dietary overexposure to selenium. Liver dysfunction resulting from excessive selenium intake was proposed as a possible cause of a high incidence of gastrointestinal disturbances and skin discolorations reported in a group of people living in a high-selenium area of North Dakota (55, 56).

Endemic human selenium intoxication has been reported in a high-selenium area of China (57). This syndrome involves adverse effects on nails, skin, the nervous system, and teeth. The adverse effects occurred in susceptible persons with intakes of 910 μg/day or more. No adverse effects have been associated with lower levels, but the ratio of plasma selenium to erythrocyte selenium increases with dietary intakes of 750 μg/day or more (58). Human surveys in seleniferous areas of the United States have failed to find any signs of selenium intoxication with intakes up to slightly more than 700 μg/day (59). Because the chemical forms of selenium in foods grown in seleniferous areas are not known, the human data on adverse effects from chronically high intakes apply only to total dietary selenium and not to any specific form. During the peak prevalence years of 1961 to 1964, morbidity approached 50% in the most severely affected Chinese villages. No adverse effects were observed, however, in the 8- to 10-year clinical trial at daily supplemental intakes of 200 μg selenium in yeast (60, 61).

Signs and symptoms similar to those in China have been reported among persons living in a seleniferous area of Venezuela (62).

Mercury

With the exception of fish, food products generally contain inorganic mercury (Hg) at levels below 50 ng/g. Fish can contain 10 to 1500 ng/g in the form of methyl mercury (63). Even higher levels can be found in fish following ingestion of methylmercury formed from mercury released into lakes from chloroalkali plants (64). The hazardous nature of residues of mercury in fish is well recognized. Recent episodes of serious poisonings include those of Minamata Bay (1953 to 1960) (65) and the Niigata area (1965) in Japan. In 1971 to 1972, ingestion of bread prepared from alkyl mercury–treated wheat seed caused widespread mercury intoxication in Iraq. These acute poisonings were widely publicized. However, chronic effects of low-level exposure are harder to identify and evaluate. "Late-onset" symptoms have been recognized in individuals not thought to have been affected in the original poisonings in the Niigata area in Japan, for example, which raises concern about injuries that are not detectable using current procedures and about determination of "lowest-effect" levels. Marketing limits of 0.4 to 1.0 mg/kg for mercury in fish have been established in several countries including the United States, Canada, Finland, Sweden, and Japan.

Lead

Lead is a toxic element but cannot be completely avoided because it occurs naturally in soil and foods. Exposure from lead in water, food, and insecticides has decreased since antiquity, but exposure from paints, automobile exhaust, and workplace environment increased in this century (66). In recent decades, concern about lead exposure and toxicity caused uses to decrease and blood levels to decline (67). Entry of lead into the food chain depends strongly on human activities. Significant and irreducible background amounts, however, originate from the lead in the earth's crust and soil.

The concentration of lead in a food depends on the type of food and the human activities in the geographic location of its origin. Bread, cereals, and beverages account for about 35% of the daily intake of lead, with the remainder coming from a wide variety of other foods; daily ingestions of lead are thought to range from 9 to 278 μg for children and 20 to 282 μg for adults (67). The concentration of lead in milk may vary as much as tenfold across geographic locations (68). The lead content of calcium dietary supplements also varies widely, with bone meal usually having higher concentrations than other sources (69).

Lead is poorly absorbed, but high blood levels can cause a variety of toxic effects including adverse neurologic, neurobehavioral, and developmental effects, decreased erythrocyte life span, inhibition of heme synthesis, renal tubular dysfunction, and increased blood pressure (67).

Because most dietary lead occurs as a divalent cation, this element strongly interacts with chemically similar nutrients such as calcium and iron (70, 71). Much of the absorbed lead deposits in bone, perhaps replacing calcium in the mineral matrix. Accordingly, increased dietary concentrations of calcium or iron inhibit intestinal absorption of lead, thereby limiting its toxic potential. Moreover, low calcium intake would be expected to cause mobilization of lead as well as calcium from the skeleton; thus, low dietary calcium levels may increase the risk of lead toxicity, and high calcium intakes may decrease the risk, even if the better calcium sources contain more lead than other foods in the diet.

Cadmium

Cadmium (Cd) is a highly toxic element that accumulates in biologic systems and has a long half-life. There is increasing concern regarding the potential for renal damage from long-term, low-level exposure to cadmium. The kidney is a critical target organ for cadmium accumulation, and the half-life of cadmium in this tissue is about 30 years (72). Food is one of the principal environmental sources of cadmium. Cadmium in soil can be increased by application of sewage sludge and phosphatidic fertilizers, all of which contain some cadmium. Wheat and the edible portions of fruits and vegetables grown on soil heavily fertilized with superphosphate have higher levels of cadmium than those grown on less heavily treated soil. Atmospheric cadmium contamination may also increase the cadmium content of foods. Daily intake of 25 to 60 μg of cadmium for a 70-kg individual has been estimated for typical diets in Europe and the United States (73). Cadmium accumulates primarily in the kidney, liver, lungs, and pancreas; the kidney is the organ most sensitive to long-term, low-level exposures.

Cadmium toxicity results in a variety of syndromes. Effects include kidney dysfunction, hypertension, hepatic injury, reproductive toxicity, lung damage after inhalation exposure, and bone effects (72, 74). Itai-itai ("ouch-ouch") disease, first reported in Japan in 1955, resulted from industrial contamination of the food and water supply (75). The poisoning occurred primarily in postmenopausal, multiparous women who consumed diets poor in calcium and protein. Symptoms included bone pain, lumbago, and a ducklike gait. Pathologic changes associated with the progressive disease included osteomalacia, osteoporosis, and renal atrophy and degeneration. The disease appeared to be caused by a combination of low dietary calcium, mobilization of bone calcium during pregnancy, and a cadmium-induced calciuria. Cadmium-induced calciuria and radiologic signs of osteomalacia have been reported in occupationally exposed workers (76). The bone changes caused by ingestion of cadmium in rats are more severe when the animals are fed calcium-deficient diets low in protein (77).

Ikeda (1992) reported the results of cadmium analysis of more than 2000 blood samples and about 1000 24-hour total food duplicates collected in nonpolluted regions of Japan between 1977 and 1981 (78). The levels of cadmium in blood correlated significantly with levels of cadmium in foods when results were compared on a regional basis. Boiled rice was the major food source of cadmium. A preliminary follow-up in 1989 suggested a decrease of about 30% in blood cadmium levels among the Japanese population. The decrease may have been due to a reduction in the cadmium concentration in rice and a decreased rice intake.

Louekari (1992) has reviewed the strengths and weaknesses of methods used to estimate dietary intake of cadmium, emphasizing the importance of representative sampling of foods, quality assurance of analytical methods, selection of adequate food consumption data, and combining food consumption data with concentrations of heavy metals in foods. He also emphasized the importance of intake estimations for possible risk groups such as children, those living in contaminated areas, lactating women, and smokers (79).

Information on background levels of elements in U.S. shellfish is of interest since shellfish may be collected from chemically contaminated waters and the contaminants may enter into the commercial food chain; shellfish can accumulate toxic elements from environments contaminated from natural or industrial sources (80). Background levels of elements can also be used as baselines for future comparisons. A recently reported FDA survey provided the agency with extensive baseline data on cadmium, lead, and 19 other elements in shellfish (80). The FDA continues to monitor shellfish and other types of seafood for elements to identify potential public health hazards.

Pesticides

The most common types of pesticides are fungicides, herbicides, insecticides, and rodenticides. Pesticides may also be classified by chemical type, such as organochlorine, organophosphorus, pyrethrins, and carbamates.

Pesticides are, by definition, toxic to living organisms, which raises the possibility that nontarget organisms, including humans, will also be harmed (80–83). Pesticides are deliberately introduced into the environment, in contrast to other types of environmental and food contaminants. Humans may be exposed through air, water, or direct contact, as well as through residues in foods.

Selective Exposure

Because it is not usually feasible to administer a pesticide directly to organisms of the pest species, the pesticide is applied to the particular part of the environment that a pest is likely to occupy. Most pesticides are quite unstable in the environment, thereby allowing application of the substance at higher concentrations when the pest is likely to be present and at much lower concentrations when the food is harvested (84). This strategy is highly effective for most pesticides in current use. In contrast, the organochlorine insecticides, such as dichlorodiphenyltrichloroethane (DDT) and lindane, are environmentally persistent pesticides for which this strategy is not very successful. For these substances, selective exposure is helpful but not sufficient to prevent harm to nontarget species.

Selective Toxicity

Selective toxicity may be based on species differences in either toxicokinetic or toxicodynamic characteristics, or both. These changes influence the distribution of the substance into tissues, rate of elimination, type of toxic reactivity, and toxicodynamic potency of the molecule (81, 82).

When humans or other inadvertently exposed species have responsive systems or receptors essentially identical to those for the pesticide in the target species, the relationships of toxicity and potency to the effective exposure (tissue concentration) may be similar, even though responsiveness to the total exposure may differ. Toxicity in humans may also involve effects on structures and systems not found in the target species.

Most pesticides are active as the parent compound; metabolic changes generally result in detoxification. Phase I metabolism usually introduces functional groups into the pesticide molecule or exposes existing functional groups. Toxicity and potency may or may not be decreased, but responsiveness to phase II metabolism is dramatically increased. Phase II (i.e., conjugation with another substance) ordinarily causes markedly decreased reactivity and large increases in water solubility and rate of excretion.

The difference between pest species and humans or other nontarget species in rate of metabolism of the pesticide chemical is a common basis of selective toxicity. Rapid metabolism in most instances decreases toxic potency. If the rate of metabolism is high enough, the compound may never reach the threshold toxic concentration in the exposed organism. In general, organophosphorus insecticides are hydrolyzed much faster by mammals than by insects, causing mammals to be relatively resistant to these toxicants. Some compounds such as aldicarb are exceptions to this generalization.

Because of resistance to metabolic degradation and excretion some substances bioaccumulate. These substances may also be resistant to environmental breakdown, that is, resistant to light, heat, water, oxygen, and other factors. Also, highly bioaccumulative substances usually are lipid soluble and readily absorbed by organisms ingesting them. Bioaccumulation involves gradual increases in the concentration of a substance in an organism with continuing exposure. This is reflected in magnification of the concentration at succeeding steps in the food chain. The environmental behavior of DDT is an excellent example of bioaccumulation and food-chain magnification with resulting toxicity in the species at the top of the exposed food chain.

Acute Effects. Organophosphate and carbamate insecticides produce their lethal effects in insects by inhibiting acetylcholine esterase, an enzyme essential to the function of nerves that use the neurotransmitter acetylcholine (62, 63). Humans and other mammals also have essential nerve functions based on acetylcholine; thus, organophosphorus and carbamate pesticides are potent toxicants in these nontarget species. Toxicity in humans is limited by selective (lower) exposure and by more-rapid metabolism, not by any inherent resistance to these pesticides. Both types of cholinesterase-inhibiting pesticides can be powerful acute toxicants in vertebrate species. The most important difference between organophosphorus and carbamate pesticides is the rate at which the phosphoryl and carbamoyl groups are released from the active site of acetylcholine esterase. The release step, which occurs rapidly (milliseconds) with the natural substrate acetylcholine, proceeds at a moderate rate (seconds or minutes) for carbamates, but very slowly (hours or days) for organophosphorus compounds. Thus, carbamate poisoning is a reversible inhibition, whereas organophosphorus poisoning is essentially irreversible, even though both result from competitive inhibition of the active center of the enzyme. Although a crisis phase in poisoning may be reached rapidly following exposure to a high level of either type of insecticide, the more-rapid recovery of acetylcholine esterase from carbamate inhibition makes this type of poisoning more survivable.

Pyrethroid compounds, notably the natural pyrethrum extracted from certain chrysanthemums, have multiple toxic actions (81). The effect on neuron Na^+ channels is similar to that of DDT, and ATPases and Cl^- uptake are inhibited in much the same way as they are by the organochlorine insecticides.

A wide variety of other compounds have been used as pesticides, and they produce numerous types of toxicity. In general, the herbicides, being designed for toxicity to plants, are relatively nontoxic to humans. Notable exceptions are paraquat and diquat, which have high toxic potency in mammals (LD_{50} values of 100 to 250 mg/kg).

The practical importance of food-borne pesticides as a cause of acute toxicity seems to be limited to occasional heavy contamination related to a spill, not to the usual residue levels in foods.

Neurotoxicity. Chronic neurotoxicity of gradually increasing severity may be caused by continued exposure to pesticides. Also, many pesticides causing chronic toxicity are bioaccumulative and can be accumulated in nerve and adipose tissues. If dietary energy intake is suddenly reduced to a level substantially below expenditures, mobilization of energy stores from body fat may increase blood levels of stored fat-soluble pesticides enough to cause toxicity (85).

Gradual accumulation of alkylmercury compounds in nerve tissue may cause gradual-onset central nervous system toxicity with symptoms of tremors, incoordination, paralysis, and behavioral/emotional changes. For example, ingestion of wheat treated with a methylmercury fungicide resulted in an outbreak of methylmercury poisoning among Iraqi farmers (81).

Certain organophosphorus compounds cause a delayed toxic response (82). In experimental animals, the toxic symptoms are irreversible and may start 10 days or more after a single dose of certain phenylphosphonothioates. The mechanism of this delayed neurotoxicity is uncertain but may involve inhibition of the synthesis of microtubules in neurons. Thus, neurotoxicity is delayed until deficits in microtubule replacement impair function.

The significance of pesticide residues in foods as a cause of neurotoxicity is intensely debated, but the preponderance of available scientific evidence indicates that they are not a problem for most individuals. Some individuals are claimed to be extremely sensitive to such effects, but evidence of such susceptibility is lacking.

Mutagenicity. Many pesticides are mutagenic in various tests (81). Mechanisms of these changes in genetic information include DNA alkylation, base substitution, intercalation of the mutagen molecule into the DNA helix, chromosome breakage, and chromosome cross-linking. Some pesticides are directly mutagenic, whereas others require activation through formation of a derivative that reacts with nucleic acids. Although mutagenesis itself may be considered a toxic effect, a major concern is the possibility that carcinogenesis may result from exposure to a mutagen. The significance, if any, of mutagenesis caused by pesticide residues in food and the clinical importance of such mutagenicity are not known.

Carcinogenicity. Some organochlorine pesticides cause malignant tumors in mammals (81, 82, 86). Carcinogenic nitrosamine contaminants occur in nitroaniline herbicides. The potent carcinogen ethylene thiourea is a degradation product of the ethylene bisdithiocarbamate fungicides. The pesticides mirex, aminotriazole, and daminozide (Alar) produce positive results in multiple carcinogenesis test systems. The degree of threat to the public health generated by exposure to carcinogenic pesticides in foods is the subject of continuing debate over both exposure estimates and risk assessment methods.

Teratogenicity. Adverse effects on embryonic and fetal development caused by maternal exposure have been experimentally demonstrated for a wide variety of pesticides (81, 82). The chlorinated hydrocarbons mirex, Kepone, and DDT have teratogenic activity. Some organophosphorus pesticides, notably dimethoate and monocrotophos, have some teratogenic potency. The teratogenic effects of pesticides include impaired growth, neurologic defects, biochemical abnormalities, and deformed structures of the skeleton, skull, and viscera. Pesticide residues in foods are not known to cause such effects.

Reproductive Toxicity. Adverse reproductive effects, other than teratogenesis, can result from high exposure to some pesticides. The effects include fetotoxicity, decreased female fertility, lowered sperm count, and decreased male libido (81, 82). Some chlorinated hydrocarbons or related compounds, such as methoxychlor and *o,p'*-DDT, have estrogenic activity, thereby altering reproduction. The fumigant dibromochloropropane (DBCP) has caused spermatogenesis to fail in factory workers and experimental animals. A variety of other toxic reproductive effects may be caused by a few pesticides. Reproductive problems associated with pesticides relate to pesticide workers and have not been associated with the pesticide residues in foods.

Behavioral Toxicity. As might be expected for substances that are neurotoxic or concentrated in nerve tissue, many pesticides can cause behavioral alterations (81). Very low levels of exposure can cause decreased learning and memory functions, hyperactivity, altered aggressive and defensive behaviors, and other behavioral changes. Two main issues are of importance: *(a)* alterations in higher-order functions such as memory and learning and *(b)* the extremely low dose threshold for behavioral effects.

Impairments in physical behavioral tests such as swimming, walking, and balance seem directly attributable to neurotoxic effects. The importance of behavioral effects in evaluating the safety of pesticide residues at levels commonly found in foods is not established.

Enzyme Induction. Pesticides can induce increased enzyme activity in many species. Different types of enzymes are affected, but most commonly affected are those involved in detoxification processes, namely, the cytochrome P450-dependent mixed-function oxidases (monooxygenases) and the transferases (conjugating enzymes) (81, 82). The effects include increased cellular concentrations of the endoplasmic reticulum membrane, the most common location for cytochrome P450 and some of the transferases, and increased expression of the genes for these enzymes. Enzyme induction not only increases rates of pesticide metabolism (and hence usually increases rates of pesticide detoxification) but also increases metabolism of essential substances such as hormones.

Enzyme induction cannot be categorically considered harmful because it is often protective, but it does indicate that exposure suffices to elicit a response. Whether any enzyme induction whatever should be considered evidence of excessive exposure is an unsettled issue, but the usual conclusion is that it should not.

Sources of Exposure

The total exposure to pesticides may occur through air, water, food, or direct contact. Determination of the risk associated with a specific level of exposure through food must take account of the additional contributions of the other routes of exposure. In some instances, the contribution of food to the total may be relatively small compared with exposure through the other routes, especially for pesticide workers (87).

There are few basic sources of pesticide residues in foods; these include approved applications in registered uses, unapproved applications (use of an approved pesticide in excessive amounts or at times too near harvest), and environmental contamination (accidental spillage, contamination from a source such as nearby application or a manufacturing facility in the vicinity, and persistence from previous use). In general, accidents cause massive and possibly highly toxic contamination in localized areas, inappropriate applications cause higher-than-normal and perhaps higher-than-permitted residue levels, and environmental persistence can result in low levels of residues of substances no longer in use.

Risk Assessment

The term *risk assessment,* although seemingly general, is most often used to mean quantitative assessment of cancer risk. The science of assessment of carcinogenic risk is well developed, compared with that of risk assessment for other types of toxicity such as reproductive effects and neurotoxicity. A recent National Research Council report titled "Regulating Pesticides in Food" focuses specifically on carcinogenic risk from herbicides, insecticides, and fungicides that the Environmental Protection Agency (EPA) has found to be oncogenic.

The basic steps in risk assessment are *(a)* determination of carcinogenicity and the dose-response relationship in animal studies, *(b)* estimation of human exposure, and *(c)* calculation of the human risk from human exposure data and animal dose-response data (86, 88). After these steps are completed, a decision must be made as to whether the calculated risk is at an acceptable level. Although the basics of risk assessment may be conceptually defined in simple terms, the actual process is complex.

Carcinogenicity and Dose-Response Studies. The validity of extrapolation from animal data to humans is uncertain because of possible species differences in reactivity and the potency of the carcinogen. Calculation of equivalent dosages for different body sizes may be performed on several bases, including dose per weight and dose per surface area. Animal studies of practical size (tens to no more than hundreds of animals per treatment group) must use dosage levels that will give statistically significant results with the numbers of animals used. In practice, a treatment group of about 50 is needed to detect a tumor rate of about 10%; the specific number depends on the background tumor rate and the uniformity of response. Tumor induction rates far below 10% would, of course, be important in assessing the impact of the pesticide on human health. Thus, high doses far in excess of anticipated human exposure levels are necessary in animal studies.

Estimation of Risk to Humans. Many procedures have been proposed for extrapolation from the high-dose, high-response range in test animals to the low-dose, low-response range of interest in human health and pesticide regulation. Although the mathematical models and procedures used to estimate carcinogenic potency in humans assume that effects seen at higher doses in animals extend to lower doses in humans, the data do not exclude the possibility that a threshold exists. The assumption is usually made in risk assessment that there is no threshold or (if it is concluded that one logically must exist) that it cannot be identified with present data and methods (86, 89). This is one of several conservative assumptions used to preclude underestimating risk. Thus, a risk assessment usually does not attempt to assess actual risk, but maximum risk. Risk assessment may be used to estimate the risk that may be associated with a specific residue intake. Conversely, risk assessment may be used to calculate the dose associated with an agreed-to upper limit of acceptable risk, for example, 1×10^{-6} in a lifetime.

Elimination of the "Delaney Paradox" for Pesticides. The so-called Delaney Amendment to the food additive provisions of the Federal FDCA (sec. 409(c)(3)(A)), passed in 1958, stipulated that "no food additive shall be deemed to be safe if it is found to induce cancer when ingested by man or animals." Although this provision seems to apply only to food additives, the EPA and FDA have applied it to pesticide residues in a processed food when those residues occurred in concentrations above those found in the raw (and unprocessed) food (88). In essence, the pesticide residue with increased concentration in a processed food was regulated as a food additive. This regulatory scheme sometimes produced an illogical and paradoxical outcome: Any measurable residue whatever of a carcinogenic pesticide with increased concentration in a processed food was prohibited, even though a larger amount might be permissible, under carcinogenic risk assessment methods and regulatory standards, in another food product if the concentration were not increased in that product through processing of the raw agricultural commodity. This long-lasting focus on the possible carcinogenicity of synthetic pesticides may have had a perverse effect by diverting attention from other factors making substantial contributions to the population's cancer rate (90).

A recently passed law, the Food Quality Protection Act, amended the FDCA in relation to pesticides (91). Among other provisions, this amendment imposed the same standards for pesticide residues in processed foods as for raw agricultural commodities, thereby preventing the regulation of pesticides with increased concentration in processed foods as "food additives" and thus eliminating the "Delaney paradox" for processed foods. The new law made no change, however, in application of the "Delaney clause" to substances properly considered to be food additives and regulated as such.

Synthetic Environmental Organic Chemicals

Several types of synthetic organic chemicals in addition to pesticides are present in the environment at detectable concentrations and may become incorporated into food. Dioxin is a contaminant in certain chlorinated pesticides, combustion products, and bleached paper. Polyaromatic hydrocarbons occur in soot, diesel smoke, and many coal tar–derived chemicals. Polychlorinated biphenyls (PCBs) and polybrominated biphenyls (PBBs) are used in a wide variety of industrial applications, and spillage may result in their entry into the food chain (92).

Polychlorinated Biphenyls (PCBs)

PCBs caused food contamination problems after their use became widespread as heat-transfer liquids in applications such as electrical transformers. Because PCBs are environmentally stable, resistant to metabolism, lipid soluble, and readily absorbed, they bioaccumulate strongly. The environmental contamination and migration patterns of these substances caused the greatest exposure to persons who consumed fresh water fish. Few adverse health effects have been clearly related to PCB exposure. In the late 1960s in Japan, a heat exchanger leaked PCB into rice oil, resulting in massive contamination and heavy exposure of consumers (92). Many exposed persons, including newborn babies exposed in utero, developed a variety of symptoms, including chloracne, increased skin pigmentation, eye discharges, transient visual disturbances, lethargy, tactile sensory loss in extremities, and decreased liver function. The affected adults showed protracted effects and slow regression of symptoms.

A significant factor in estimating human intake of PCBs from fish consumption is determining the loss of PCBs that may occur during cooking. Although several studies have investigated the extent of such loss, perceived inconsistencies in the data precluded determining the extent to which cooking alters contaminant levels (93). Sherer and Price reviewed the available literature and concluded that expressing the degrees of PCB loss on a mass basis greatly reduced the apparent variability in the existing data and allowed concluding that PCBs are preferentially removed by cooking processes that involve higher temperatures, longer cooking times, and separation of fat from the cooked fish (93).

Spontaneous fetal death has been observed in some mammalian species following exposure to PCBs. As a consequence, the relationship between consumption of PCB-contaminated Lake Ontario sport fish and spontaneous fetal death among more than 1820 women was examined in a recent exposure-based cohort study (94). The results of the study suggested that consumption of PCB-contaminated sport fish did not increase the risk of spontaneous fetal death.

Polybrominated Biphenyls (PBBs)

A major contamination of food occurred in Michigan in 1972 when a PBB-containing flame retardant sold under the trade name FireMaster was mistakenly used in place of a dairy-feed supplement containing magnesium oxide sold under the trade name NutriMaster (92). Both products contained the same level of magnesium, which may have contributed to the mixup. The contamination was first noticed when cows in several dairy herds refused to eat, produced less milk, lost body weight, and developed abnormal hoof growth and lameness. Affected cattle and swine aborted. No acute human intoxications occurred, but contamination of humans was confirmed by blood analysis. Long-term effects of exposure include some alterations in liver functions and a decrease in immune competence.

Toxicants Produced during Cooking of Foods

Poly(cyclic) aromatic hydrocarbons (PAHs) represent one of the most important classes of organic contaminants in food. Human exposure to these compounds occurs via air, water, and food. One pathway is contamination resulting from environmental pollution (e.g., air, water, soil), and a second is contamination resulting from food processing (e.g., smoking, roasting, grilling, broiling, and frying) due to the pyrolysis of lipids, proteins, carbohydrates, and other food components. Contamination of foods with PAHs may occur during processing and home cooking.

Smoking, charcoal-broiling, grilling, frying, and roasting are primarily responsible for PAH-contamination of meat, meat products, fish, coffee, tea, certain kinds of cheese, and cereal products. PAHs originating from the smoking of meats may be a particularly important source of secondary contamination. Smoke and smoke flavor contain various PAHs that are deposited on the surface of smoked products. The distribution of PAH in smoked meats is not homogeneous, with about 60 to 70% of benzo(a)pyrene formed in the surface layer (95). In addition to smoked meats, smoked cereal products may also be a source of PAHs. For example, foods prepared from smoked oats, barley, and peas, widely consumed in some Finnish and Russian localities, may add significantly to intake of PAHs (96).

Many cooking methods involve intense heat and limited availability of oxygen at the site of highest heat, conditions that cause pyrolytic decomposition of some food components. Major pyrolytic products are the PAHs (97) and the heterocyclic amines (HCAs) (98). PAHs are produced during cooking mainly by pyrolysis of fats, and

HCAs are pyrolysis products of amino acids, especially tryptophan. PAHs also originate from environmental sources such as wood-burning stoves, diesel exhaust, oil-burning heaters, and boilers.

A high rate of food component pyrolysis occurs during charbroiling of meats. In addition to direct pyrolysis of the fats or amino acids in the meat, melted fat and water drip into the flame or onto the hot charcoal where oxygen supplies probably are low, and the searing heat pyrolyses the fat and any amino acids in the water. Steam from the water steam-distills the pyrolysis products, which may then come in contact with the meat.

A large number of PAHs have been identified as pyrolysis products in foods; those most likely to pose problems are benzo[a]pyrene (BP) and 7,12-dimethylbenzanthrene (DMBA). These PAHs and many others are potent carcinogens that are active after metabolic conversion to electrophilic epoxide derivatives.

HCAs produced by food pyrolysis include several carbolines, quinolines, and quinoxalines. The carbolines Trp-P-2 and Trp-P-1 are tryptophan pyrolysis products, and they are considerably more potent in mutagenesis test systems than are BP and DMBA. The quinolines IQ and MeIQ and the quinoxalines MeIQx and two dimethyl MeIQx derivatives have mutagenic potencies similar to those of the Trp-P compounds.

These HCAs occur in very small quantities, but their mutagenic potencies raise concerns about their possible carcinogenicity (99). For several years after their discovery, the HCAs were not available in sufficient amounts to permit carcinogenesis bioassays. Carcinogenicity of several of the HCAs has been confirmed in animal test systems. An epidemiologic survey indicated a higher risk of stomach cancer in people who frequently ate broiled fish. Thus, HCAs may be related to some types of cancer in humans.

Polycyclic aromatic compounds (PACs) comprise the largest class of known environmental carcinogens. Some PACs and PAHs are constituents of some coals, asphaltic rocks, and petroleum and are obtained from these matrices by distillation or extraction. Incomplete combustion of organic matter yields complex mixtures of many types of PACs. Mixtures of PACs are also found in smoke from motors, heating units, and cigarettes and from industrial emissions (e.g., the iron, aluminum, and steel industries), coke ovens, and incinerating plants. Possible sources of PACs found in processed food include environmental contamination and possible accidental contamination during food processing (e.g., as a result of thermal processes used during food manufacture). Several reliable methods may be used for separation and quantitative determination of PACs from foods (100).

Contaminants from Natural Sources

Diseases associated with consumption of contaminated seafood include hepatitis A, Norwalk virus gastroenteritis, cholera (*Vibrio* species), *Campylobacter* gastroenteritis, botulism, and various parasitic infections. Additional diseases are caused by ingestion of seafood toxins. Seafood toxins are becomingly increasingly important as causative agents of food-borne illnesses around the world. There is increasing awareness of potential problems with paralytic shellfish poisoning (PSP), neurotoxic shellfish poisoning, diarrheic shellfish poisoning, and more recently, a new type of shellfish poisoning called amnesic shellfish poisoning (101). Discussions of seafood-borne viral, bacterial, and parasitic illnesses are beyond the scope of this chapter.

Areas of particular concern and interest include development of standardized methods for detecting and quantifying seafood toxins, the importance of economic losses resulting from their presence, and the importance of establishing regular chemical monitoring for them.

Fishing industries dealing with affected fish species from endemic areas face major problems as they try to expand their market worldwide. To deal with the problems, it has become necessary to develop practical and sensitive detection methods for the wide range of seafood toxins (102).

In the past, assays have relied heavily on use of experimental animals such as mice for detection of toxins. The mouse bioassay involves injecting mice with fish or shellfish extracts and observing them for a set of defined symptoms against control mice over a given period of time. The bioassay requires large numbers of test animals, uses relatively large amounts of tissue extracts, relies on subjective interpretation of results, and lacks specificity (102). Because of these problems, the evolution of marine toxin detection assays have moved in the direction of analytical high-performance liquid chromatography (HPLC) and immunologic analysis. The ideal characteristics of toxin detection assays are within the capabilities of immunologic technology. Development of reliable and practical toxin detection will allow expansion of various fishing industries, increase the food supply, and prevent marine food poisonings on an individual level.

Mycotoxins

A wide variety of fungal toxins are now recognized as contaminants of human foods and animal forages. These include aflatoxins, patulin, ochratoxin, penicillic acid, trichothecene toxins, zearalenone, slaframine, and swainsonine (103–107).

Aflatoxins. The first reports of aflatoxin contamination of plant products followed large-scale poisonings of turkeys in the early 1960s (108). The birds had consumed Brazilian ground nut meal contaminated with the mold *Aspergillus flavus*. The responsible fungal metabolites were identified and collectively termed *aflatoxins*. These highly substituted coumarins were further classified as B or G, depending on their fluorescence (blue or green, respectively) in ultraviolet light. Aflatoxin B_1 is the most potent hepatocarcinogen known, and the Fischer 344 rat is the most sensitive to aflatoxin-induced carcinogenesis among the wide variety of species tested.

Acute poisonings in man by foodstuffs contaminated with aflatoxin-producing *A. flavus* and *Aspergillus parasiticum* have been described, with primary effects relating to hepatotoxicity. One study showed that feeding contaminated ground nut meal to rats resulted in formation of liver tumors (109). A role for aflatoxin as a human liver carcinogen is based on epidemiologic data. Epidemiologic associations between the level of staple food contamination by aflatoxin-producing molds and the incidence of primary liver cancer have been found in parts of Africa and Asia but not in the United States (110, 111). Because epidemiologic studies have also indicated a high correlation between primary hepatocellular carcinoma and exposure to hepatitis B virus, a combined role for aflatoxin and hepatitis B virus in hepatic carcinogenesis has also been suggested.

In the United States, the major commodities affected by aflatoxin contamination are corn, peanuts, and cottonseed meal. Given the potential significance of a role for aflatoxins in human hepatic carcinogenesis, it is important that measures be established and used to remove or reduce possible risks posed by the consumption of aflatoxin-contaminated products (112). Ammoniation processes can effectively reduce aflatoxin levels in corn (113). Under the conditions used, the inactivated aflatoxin does not revert to the parent compound following treatment. Studies are in progress to evaluate the potential uses of ammonia-treated aflatoxin-decontaminated corn in products for animal feed as well as for human consumption.

Studies of storage of products in controlled environments are important because they can help identify conditions that may be necessary to minimize growth of *Aspergillus*. Recent studies with sorghum seeds showed that each of the aflatoxin components B_1, B_2, G_1, and G_2 has a well-defined range of temperature and humidity for optimal production, and these in turn depend on the specific substrate and the fungal strain (114).

Hundreds of different metabolites are produced by *Penicillium* species (115). These include the nephrotoxins citrinin and ochratoxin A (produced by various species of *Aspergillus* and *Penicillium*) and patulin and penicillic acid (produced by *P. expansum* and *P. aurantiogriseum*, respectively).

Patulin. Patulin, a mycotoxin produced by species of *Penicillium, Aspergillus,* and *Byssochlamys*, is found in apples and other fruits subject to soft rot (116). *Penicillium* spp. are the predominant sources of patulin, whose structure (4-hydroxy-4H-furo[3,2-c]pyran-2(6*H*)-one) is that of a highly reactive unsaturated lactone. Patulin was initially intended for use as an antibiotic because it was found to be bacteriostatic to *Staphylococcus,* Streptococcus, Corynebacterium, Neisseria, and *Haemophilus.* Its antibiotic activity was eliminated when patulin was treated with cysteine. Subsequent toxicologic studies concluded that the compound was too toxic for therapeutic use (117). Patulin was found to be carcinogenic in 100-g rats (118), but a later study apparently did not confirm this result (119).

Ochratoxins. Ochratoxins are produced by several *Penicillium* and *Aspergillus* spp. and may be found in grains and related foodstuffs. Ochratoxin A is the major causative factor in outbreaks of porcine nephropathy in Denmark, which occur in association with unusually wet climatic conditions. Histologic similarity between the nephropathy described in pigs and "Balkan nephropathy" in humans suggests a role for ochratoxin in the latter (120). Balkan nephropathy occurs endemically in Bulgaria, Romania, and Yugoslavia. Levels of ochratoxins in foodstuffs, like those of other mycotoxins, are affected by heavy rainfall, especially during harvest. A significant association between the number of individuals dying of nephropathy over a 2-year period and excess rainfall during two previous harvest periods has been reported (121). Ochratoxin levels of 3 to 5 ng/g of serum were measured in 6.5% of blood samples obtained from individuals living in an endemic area (122). These data together with epidemiologic data linking rainfall and death rates from the nephropathy support a possible link between ochratoxin contamination and the disease. Ochratoxin produces a similar renal disease in animals (123). The nephrotoxicity of other metabolites of some *Penicillium* strains was recognized in the course of studies of endemic Balkan nephropathy (123, 124). The role of other mycotoxins (e.g., penicillic acid) in the disease remains to be determined.

In Tunisia, many cereals, olives, and mixed feed for fish are contaminated by ochratoxin A and other aflatoxins. Ochratoxin A has been detected in high concentrations in human blood samples collected in nephrology departments in Tunisia from nephrology patients undergoing dialysis, particularly those categorized as having a chronic interstitial nephropathy of unknown origin (125). To clarify the situation, food and blood samples were collected from nephropathy patients and controls (i.e., those with no familial cases of nephropathy). The disease appeared to be related to ochratoxin A blood levels and food contamination, since the control group had significantly lower levels of ochratoxin A contamination in both food and blood than did the nephropathy group. A correlation exists between ochratoxin A in human food, blood contamination, and chronic interstitial nephropathy. Because biologic, biochemical, clinical, and radiologic parameters in Tunisian patients seem very similar to those of Balkan nephropathy, it is likely that human nephropathy related to ochratoxins is occurring in Tunisia and possibly in other parts of northern Africa with the same climate and eating patterns.

Vomitoxins. Many *Fusarium* species produce trichothecene toxins, all of which have a tetracyclic 12,13-

epoxytrichothec-9-ene skeleton. Moldy barley may contain the trichothecene "vomitoxin" (deoxynivalenol), which causes vomiting in pigs, deaths with hemorrhagic lesions in the gut in cattle, and necrosis of the mucosa of the esophagus and gizzard in ducks and geese.

Zearalenone. Zearalenone, a fungal metabolite found in feed grains, maize, and soybeans, is related to periodic infection of the plants by *Fusarium roseum.* Estrogenic syndromes in pigs fed moldy grains have been described for many years (126). Enlargement of the mammary glands and vulva are the primary signs of the disorder. Feeding studies in animals have confirmed these findings. There are at present no confirmed reports of effects in man.

Slaframine. "Slobbers" in ruminants is caused by consumption of forage that has been infected with *Rhizoctonia leguminocola.* Various clovers, soybean, kudzu, blue lupine, cow peas, and alfalfa may be infected. Conditions favoring the growth of *R. leguminicola* include wet weather and high humidity. Outbreaks of the disease have been reported in the northwestern, midwestern, and southeastern United States. Pathologic effects of ingestion of the fungus include excessive salivation, lacrimation, diarrhea, and frequent urination. The structure of the toxin is L-acetoxy-6-aminooctahydroindolizine, and total synthesis of the compound has been achieved (126). Slaframine is activated in the liver following ingestion; a ketoimine derivative is thought to be the active metabolite (127).

Swainsonine. Consumption of legumes of the genus *Swainsonia* by cattle, horses, and sheep produces a chronic disease characterized by neurologic disturbances, weight loss, and addiction to the plant (128). Mortality is high among young animals; older animals may survive for months in poor condition. Swainsonine, the active toxicant of the plant, is a strong inhibitor of mannosidase. Swainsonine has been identified in hays that are known to cause slobbers. Its role, if any, in sporadic outbreaks of the slobber syndrome is unknown.

Tremorgenic Mycotoxins. A number of potent neurotoxins, termed *tremorgenic* mycotoxins, have been identified as metabolites of *A. flavus, Penicillium crustosum,* and *Paspalum dilatatum* (103). These metabolites at low doses cause sustained, incapacitating whole-body trembling in susceptible animals. Higher doses can lead to convulsive seizures that may be fatal.

Fumonisins. Equine leukoencephalomalacia (ELEM) is a readily diagnosed toxicosis of horses, historically referred to as "moldy corn poisoning" because it was associated with consumption of corn infested with *Fusarium moniliforme.* The etiologic agent of ELEM was identified as fumonisin B_1 and characterized in 1988.

Numerous reports of a syndrome of pulmonary edema and hydrothorax in swine (PPE) and of ELEM in horses occurred following the 1989 U.S. corn harvest (129). Reports of outbreaks continued into the first half of 1990 as corn was moved from storage into animal feeds. Studies clearly implicated feed containing fumonisin-contaminated corn or corn screenings as the cause of the toxicosis. Investigations demonstrated fumonisins in almost all corn and corn-related products harvested in 1989. The significance of the outbreak has been difficult to determine because of a lack of toxicologic data and/or data on incidence and levels of the disease. Subsequent corn harvests have not been associated with widespread toxicoses (129), but survey data have shown fumonisins in corn each year.

Fumonisins are structurally similar to sphingosine, which forms the long-chain base backbone of sphingolipids, prompting speculation that they may be biosynthetically related. Fumonisin B_1 is a potent inhibitor of de novo sphingolipid biosynthesis in vitro, which led to the hypothesis that consumption of feed containing fumonisins should cause an increase in the free sphinganine:free sphingosine ratio in tissues and serum. Use of the free sphinganine:free sphingosine ratio has been suggested as a presumptive test for identifying animals consuming fumonisin-contaminated feed (130). Since their discovery and characterization in 1988, the fumonisins have been extensively studied because of their toxic effects in animals, their cancer-promoting potential, their occurrence in corn-based human food, and the worldwide occurrence of fumonisin-producing fungi (131).

Seafood Toxins

Several marine illnesses may result from consumption of toxic fish and shellfish. Such illnesses are being increasingly recognized and reported in the United States as consumption of seafood increases. Almost one-fourth of the cases of food poisoning reported to the Centers for Disease Control from 1978 to 1982 resulted from ingestion of toxic fish or shellfish (132).

Ciguatera Toxins. Ciguatera poisoning is a serious human intoxication that can be caused by ingestion of any one of over 400 species of marine fishes, many of which are highly valued as food (133). The poisoning results from eating certain tropical and subtropical fish that consume marine bacteria and dinoflagellates associated with coral reefs and nearby coastal waters. Various species of dinoflagellates from the Caribbean have been grown in large-scale culture and assayed for toxicity (134). Five of nine species examined produced one or more toxin fractions that killed mice within 48 hours. Okadaic acid has been isolated and characterized from the Caribbean dinoflagellates *Pfiesteria concavum* and *P. lima* (135). Signs and symptoms observed in humans following ingestion of contaminated fish vary but generally include moderate-to-severe gastrointestinal disorders, moderate-to-severe neurologic problems and, in extreme cases, death due to respiratory failure. Gastrointestinal symptoms are of relatively short duration, but the neurologic problems may persist for weeks or months.

As a consequence of these toxins in the food chain,

ciguatera poisoning is the most commonly reported fish-borne illness worldwide and the most common type of nonbacterial food poisoning reported in the U.S. The most commonly implicated human food species are large predatory reef fish such as barracuda, grouper, snapper, and sea bass (136). Important amounts of the toxin or toxins are produced by the dinoflagellate *Gambierdiscus toxicus* and transmitted up the food chain, although the toxin is harmless to the fish.

Significant differences in the stable carbon and nitrogen isotope contents of the meat tissues of identifiable fish have been found in the gut contents of ciguatoxic and nonciguatoxic barracuda caught along the coast of Puerto Rico (137). Stable isotopic ratios (^{13}C:^{12}C and ^{15}N:^{14}N) have been used successfully to trace trophic levels and pathways in terrestrial and aquatic organisms, and measurement of such ratios may be a potentially powerful tool for tracing ciguatoxins through the food chain and possibly for identifying ciguatoxic fish. Such studies provide a means to address the unresolved question of the origins of ciguatoxins and their relationship with toxins isolated from presumed benthic microalgal and/or bacterial vectors (137).

Paralytic Shellfish Toxins. Poisonings of shellfish have been recorded in Atlantic and Pacific coastal waters and in waters around South Africa, New Zealand, and a number of Western European countries for many years. The poisonings, which primarily affect mussels and clams, are associated with the growth of dinoflagellates in the waters. The dinoflagellates produce a toxin that is retained in the hepatopancreas of the shellfish. The toxic principle, "saxitoxin," has been isolated from Alaskan butter clams and from cultured dinoflagellates and appears to block nerve transmission in the motor axon. Hazardous levels of toxin accumulate in shellfish feeding in waters in which the dinoflagellates are undergoing rapid growth ("blooms"). The associated conditions are referred to as "red tides." Symptoms of toxicity, which develop within several hours of eating infected shellfish, include numbness of the lips and fingertips and an ascending paralysis. Death from respiratory paralysis may occur in as many as 8.5% of cases (138, 139).

Contamination of bivalves with paralytic shellfish poison (PSP) poses a serious problem to the shellfish-culture industry and to public health in various parts of the world. In late March to May of 1993, monitoring for toxins in commercial shellfish in Hiroshima Bay, one of the largest oyster-culture areas in Japan, showed that clams, mussels, and oysters were contaminated with paralytic toxins associated with appearance of the toxic dinoflagellate *Alexandrium tamarense.* Although no cases of food poisoning were associated with the infestation, the incident provided an opportunity to determine the PSP profiles of the causative dinoflagellate and the infested bivalves (140).

The alkaloid neurotoxins, or saxitoxins, are estimated to be 50 times more potent than curare (141). Until recently, outbreaks were thought to occur principally along cold temperate coastlines. In July to August 1987, however, a major outbreak of PSP occurred along the Pacific coast of Guatemala, in which 26 of 187 persons affected with the poisoning died. The case-fatality rate was 50% in children under 6 years of age. This poisoning represented the first large outbreak of PSP in Guatemala. The illness can occur with little or no warning and can have disastrous outcomes, particularly for children (141).

Four significant PSP incidents occurred in the Philippines between 1983 and 1991. Because there is no specific antidote to the poison, clinical management has largely remained symptomatic (142). Thus, the best approach to the problem of PSP is prevention, with strict adherence to public health quarantine guidelines regarding harvesting areas, conduct of intensive education campaigns, and provision of economic alternatives for affected fishermen and vendors.

In November, 1993, 188 people were hospitalized in Madagascar after eating the meat of a single shark. Clinical signs appeared 5 to 10 hours after ingestion of the shark flesh and liver and consisted almost exclusively of neurologic dysfunction (e.g., stinging or burning sensations in the mouth and lips, paraesthesia, ataxia with hypotonia and predominant involvement of the lower limbs, and severe gait impairment). The agent of this outbreak was remarkably toxic, and every individual whose consumption of the shark could be confirmed became ill. Case mortality was close to 30%. The extent and seriousness of this mass poisoning were uncommon for an incident of fish poisoning and differed in several significant aspects from ciguatera poisonings. Two potent heat-stable lipid-soluble toxins tentatively named "carchatoxin-A" and "carchatoxin-B" were isolated; differences observed in biologic and chromatographic properties between these two new toxins and ciguatoxin may explain the differences observed in clinical aspects and mortality (143).

Domoic Acid. Domoic acid intoxication in humans (also called amnesic shellfish poisoning) is a recently recognized entity. The first reported outbreak occurred in November 1987, when 145 individuals developed gastrointestinal and neurologic symptoms following consumption of cultured mussels from Prince Edward Island in Canada. Domoic acid, an excitatory neurotoxin, was subsequently detected in the mussels associated with this mass intoxication.

Toxic material isolated from mussels caused death with some highly characteristic and unusual neurotoxic symptoms, very different from those of paralytic shellfish toxin and other known toxins. Probably the most remarkable finding was that approximately 25% of those affected reported some memory loss (144). Subsequent studies determined that the toxin, a potent heat-stable neurotoxin, had been produced by a marine diatom *Nitzschia pungens* forma multiseries (145).

NATURAL TOXINS INNATE IN CERTAIN FOODS

The literature on naturally occurring toxicants of the types mentioned above is extensive, and it was necessary to select specific topics to be covered. The toxicities of specific foods can arise from lipids, antivitamins, plant phenolics, estrogens, hallucinogens, and a variety of other components (146–153). Two National Research Council volumes review the available information on the carcinogenicity of a variety of naturally occurring toxicants (146, 154).

Proteinase Inhibitors

Legumes are the source of compounds that inhibit the proteolytic activity of enzymes such as trypsin and chymotrypsin. Proteinase inhibitors have been found in many varieties of beans, peas, and peanuts as well as potatoes and sweet potatoes. The trypsin inhibitor found in soybeans is perhaps the best studied of this type of compound (155). Soybeans contain two major types of trypsin inhibitors: the Kunitz inhibitor (molecular weight ~20,000) and the smaller, extensively disulfide cross-linked Bowman-Birk inhibitor (molecular weight ~8000). Enzyme activity assays for trypsin inhibitors do not distinguish between the two types of inhibitors. Progress is being made in development and application of an enzyme-linked immunosorbent assay that should permit rapid determination of the amounts of the two types of inhibitors in raw and processed soy products (156).

Chicks, rats, and mice fed raw soy meal experience reduced growth, decreased fat absorption, enlarged pancreas, and hypersecretion of pancreatic enzymes. Metabolizable energy from the diet is also reduced. The nutritive value of soy protein is enhanced by heat treatment, with increased nutritive value paralleling the loss of trypsin inhibitor activity (155). The observation that feeding raw soybeans or trypsin inhibitor concentrates led to hypertrophy and hyperplasia of the pancreas and increased output of proteolytic enzymes explained the effects of trypsin inhibitors on protein nutrition: fecal loss of nitrogen as digestive enzymes would be a substantial drain on protein supply. Although heat treatment improves the nutritional quality of soybean products through destruction of trypsin inhibitor activity, standard heat processing methods often leave 5 to 20% of the original trypsin inhibitor content (157).

The rat responds to treatment with trypsin inhibitor with increased secretion of trypsin and chymotrypsin. Continued treatment with trypsin inhibitor leads to hypertrophy and hyperplasia of the pancreas (158, 159). No overtly neoplastic changes are observed unless the animals are also treated with a pancreatic carcinogen such as azaserine (158, 160). Both adenomas and adenocarcinomas have been observed in the pancreas after about a year of trypsin inhibitor treatment following azaserine initiation. In these studies, trypsin inhibitor appears to promote azaserine-initiated pancreatic cancer. Long-term feeding of trypsin inhibitor (1–2 years) without treatment with azaserine or other initiators may result in progression of hypertrophy and atypical acinar cell foci to adenoma and carcinoma (158).

The relationship between trypsin inhibitors and pancreatic carcinogenesis and the species differences in response to such inhibitors are not fully understood. Species that respond to trypsin inhibitor with increased pancreatic enzyme secretion, hypertrophy, and hyperplasia include rats, mice, and chickens; species reported to be unresponsive include the calf, pig, dog, rhesus monkey, cebus monkey, and marmoset (160). A recent study with humans indicated that a single dose of the soybean Bowman-Birk inhibitor elicited increased pancreatic secretion of trypsin and chymotrypsin (161). Present knowledge is insufficient for risk assessment of residual trypsin inhibitors in foods (162).

In a review of the biochemical properties, physiologic effects, mode of action, and nutritional significance for humans of soybean proteinase inhibitors, Liener noted that with increasing use of soybean products for human consumption, it is increasingly important to assess, if possible, the risk to human health that may be associated with consumption of soybean preparations in which trypsin inhibitors may not be fully inactivated (163). Because of the need to achieve a balance between the amount of heat necessary to destroy the trypsin inhibitors and that which may damage the nutritional or functional properties of the protein, commercially available edible-grade soybean products retain 5 to 20% of the trypsin inhibitors originally present in the raw soybeans from which they were prepared (164).

The question remains whether chronic ingestion of low levels of trypsin inhibitor remaining in some soybean products constitutes a risk to human health (163). In considering means of eliminating trypsin inhibitors from foods, Liener notes that some efforts have been directed at the search for varieties and cultivars of soybeans that are low in trypsin inhibitor (165). Two cell lines devoid of the Kunitz inhibitor were found, and although soybeans without the Kunitz inhibitor still retained about 50% of the trypsin inhibitor activity of most commercial varieties of soybeans (presumably because of the presence of the Bowman-Birk inhibitor), a milder heat treatment than that used with standard varieties of soybeans achieved near-zero levels of trypsin inhibitor (163).

Trypsin inhibitor activity is usually measured by inhibition of the hydrolytic activity of bovine trypsin on *N*-α-DL-arginine-*p*-nitroanilide, a synthetic substrate, or on casein. Specific quantification of the two inhibitors by an immunochemical approach has also been described (166, 167).

Differences in the responses of various species of animals to the physiologic effects of trypsin inhibitors have been mentioned above. Differences have also been observed in the in vitro inhibition of proteases by pancreatic juice of different species of animals as well as in the amount of activity that the protease inhibitors retain after exposure to gastric juice (163). Thus, caution must be observed in attempting to extrapolate the results of in vitro assays for protease inhibitor activity to their physiologic effects in a specific animal species (163).

Hemagglutinins

The terms *phytohemagglutinins, phytagglutinins,* and *lectins* are used interchangeably to refer to plant proteins that can agglutinate red blood cells. Plant sources of hemagglutinins include castor beans (ricin), soybeans, peanuts, red kidney beans (phytohemagglutinin A), black beans (phaseolatoxin, phaseotoxin A), yellow wax beans (hemagglutinin), and jack beans (concanavalin A) (148, 168). Rats fed purified kidney bean agglutinin at 0.5% of the diet died within 2 weeks in one study (169). Differences in oral toxicity among various hemagglutinins may be related to susceptibility of some (but not others) to inactivation by pepsin or other proteolytic enzymes. Most purified plant hemagglutinins are carbohydrate-containing proteins. Concanavalin A from jack beans is free of sugars (170). The phytohemagglutinins have marked effects on cell division: lymphocytes respond with induction of mitosis. Some phytohemagglutinins have become useful tools in studies related to immunocompetence in which exposure to specific lectins causes increased DNA synthesis.

Although protease inhibitors are generally regarded as the primary antinutritional factor in soybeans, they may account for only about 40% of the growth inhibition observed in animals fed untreated raw soybeans. Research into other factors in soybeans responsible for growth inhibition led to identification of the class of proteins called lectins. Lectins are widely distributed in the plant kingdom and have high specificity in binding to carbohydrate-containing molecules. Lectins can agglutinate red blood cells and interact strongly with specific glycoconjugate receptors on other types of cell membranes.

Soybean lectin, or soybean agglutinin, accounts for about 25% of the growth inhibition produced by feeding raw soybeans. A significant portion of the lectin survives intestinal transit, becomes bound to the intestinal epithelium, and causes disruption of the brush border, atrophy of the microvilli, and reduced viability of epithelial cells. Although the mechanism(s) whereby soybean lectin causes its effects are not understood, they are related to the ability of the lectin to interact with specific glycoprotein receptors on the cell membranes of organs involved in metabolism (163).

Aminonitriles and Related Compounds

Seeds of various vetches (*Lathyrus sativus, L. cicera,* and *L. clymenum*) contain potent toxic compounds that cause neurologic diseases in humans, cattle, and horses, thereby limiting food use of these plants (171). Toxic compounds isolated from *Lathyrus* species include various diaminobutyric acids, diaminopropionic acid, oxalylaminoalanine, and β-cyanoalanine (150). Neurolathyrism, characterized by progressive muscle weakness and irreversible paralysis of the legs, may be fatal. Outbreaks of neurolathyrism are generally associated with periods of famine during which large quantities of *Lathyrus* meal are eaten for lack of other food (172).

The condition of osteolathyrism, as distinct from neurolathyrism, is observed in domestic fowl (chickens, turkeys) and experimental animals (rats) following ingestion of *L. odoratus* and is characterized by significant disturbances in development of bones and connective tissue. The toxic component responsible for this disease has been isolated from seeds of *L. odoratus* and *L. pusillus* and identified as β-*N*-(L-glutamyl)-aminopropionitrile. The β-aminopropionitrile (BAPN) moiety is thought to be the active component of this toxicant (173).

Osteolathyrism results from inhibition by BAPN (which occurs naturally in several *Lathyrus* species) of lysyl oxidase. The enzyme is required for formation of lysine-derived cross-links in structural proteins, including those of eggshell membranes (174). Adverse effects of lathyrogens on egg quality (e.g., increase in misshapen eggs, soft or thin-shelled eggs) contribute to increased breakage and economic loss. This disorder has been induced experimentally in laboratory animals by feeding seeds of *L. odoratus* (sweet pea). The disorder involves defective collagen and elastin metabolism induced by BAPN and its γ-glutamyl derivative. These compounds lack toxic effects on the nervous systems and have no known relationship to human neurolathyrism (175).

Levels of β-*N*-oxalyamino-L-alanine (BOAA), one of the neurotoxic amino acids formed from β-cyano-L-alanine, may be reduced by plant breeding, but a safe level has not been defined. While repeated cooking, draining, soaking, and steeping may reduce the BOAA content of seeds by up to 80%, this reduction may not suffice to prevent long-term toxic effects of ingestion (175).

Alkaloids

A wide variety of alkaloids, some very toxic, are found in plants that have considerable economic and food value. For example, glycoalkaloids occur in potato, tomato, and eggplant. Quinolizidine and/or piperidine alkaloids are found in lupine *(Lupinus albus, L. luteus, L. angustifolius)* seeds, a food crop in South America and a valuable oilseed crop in temperate climates. Purine alkaloids are found in coffee, tea, cola beverages, cocoa, and chocolate; and quinine and alkaloids in black and red peppers are important flavoring ingredients.

***Solanum* Glycoalkaloids.** Glycoalkaloids are the naturally occurring toxicants of potato tubers, and consumption of potatoes high in glycoalkaloids has caused severe illness and death (176). The two major potato glycoalkaloids are α-solanine and α-chaconine. α-Solanine inhibits blood and brain cholinesterases and injures membranes in the gastrointestinal tract and elsewhere (177).

The current toxicologic status of the glycoalkaloids present in potatoes is poorly defined, a conclusion that can also be drawn for many natural dietary constituents (178). Although a no-observed-adverse-effect level (NOAEL) has not been established, the traditionally held view is that potatoes can contain up to 200 mg of glycoalkaloids per kg of whole raw unpeeled potato and still be fit for human consumption.

The potential toxic effects of consumption of potato leaves, which form part of the diets of certain ethnic communities, has been less well studied. Although potato leaves contain several highly toxic alkaloids, it is unlikely that moderate consumption of potato tops would result in intake of high enough concentrations of the alkaloids to cause injury (179).

Ingestion of ripened nightshade berries, *Solanum dulcamara,* is one of the commonest poisonous plant exposures reported (180). Nightshade is in the same genus as the potato *(Solanum tuberosum),* which is known to contain a variety of toxic glycoalkaloids and alkamines, collectively known as solanine (181).

Pyrrolizidine Alkaloids from *Senecio* Species

A large number of inedible plants may contaminate animal forages and human food grains. For example, a variety of *Senecio* spp. produce toxic alkaloids, and "Senecio disease" has been reported in human populations eating breads containing seeds from the poisonous plants (182). A major feature of pyrrolizidine alkaloid intoxication in man and animals is delayed liver damage (183). Venoocclusive disease and cirrhosis have been reported in humans, and induction of liver cancer has been reported in animals (184, 185). The genera *Senecio* (ragworts), *Crotalaria* (rattleboxes), and *Heliotropium* (heliotropes) contain specific alkaloids in amounts ranging from traces to as much as 5% of the dry weight of the plant.

Consumption of teas prepared from plants of the *Senecio* genus has been associated with several forms of cancer, but data are not conclusive. Seneciphylline and senkirkine, two pyrrolizidine alkaloids that occur in animal forages and medicinal teas, respectively, appeared to act as indirect mutagens (186). Transfer of mutagenic activity via milk following treatment of lactating rats with seneciphylline was also reported (186). The hepatocarcinogenicity of the pyrrolizidine alkaloids may be due to promoting effects on initiated hepatocytes rather than to their weak initiating activity (187).

Little research has been directed toward elucidating the natural toxicants or their metabolites that may enter the food chain through milk, milk products, or meat. With the increasing concern for food safety, it is important to broaden research in these areas. Factors that need to be considered are consumption of milk by infants or young children who are more susceptible to plant toxicants, consumption of milk produced by lactating mothers who use natural product remedies with potential toxicity, and availability of toxic plants to lactating animals. Currently, few methods have been developed for monitoring natural toxicants (particularly those of plant origin) in milk, milk products, and meat products. Research is needed to identify toxins in poisonous plants ingested by livestock, to determine the ability of the products of such plants to pass into the food chain, and finally, to assess their potential danger to human health.

Determining the disposition of xenobiotics, including natural plant toxicants, in milk and other natural products, is important. It is generally believed that the human health risk from plant toxicants in milk is minimal because of current practices of bulk milk handling, which dilutes possible plant toxicants, and intense range-land management, which eliminates opportunities for dairy animals to graze on poisonous plants.

Milk is an emulsion of lipids in an aqueous solution of proteins. For this reason, it may contain a mixture of virtually any toxins or compounds that are in solution in the animal's body water (188). Many natural plant toxicants are known to be present in milk from lactating animals grazing on plants that contain them. These include tremetol from *Eupatorium* and *Haplopappus,* pyrrolizidine alkaloids from *Senecio,* piperidine alkaloids, quinolizidine alkaloids, glucosinolates in *Brassica* and *Limnanthes,* indolizidine alkaloids in *Astragalus* and *Oxytropis,* and seleno compounds known to accumulate in grasses and some cereal grains. In the western United States, the pyrrolizidine alkaloid–containing plants of greatest concern to livestock are various *Senecio* species; in the southern U.S., various *Crotalaria* species are of major concern.

The principal effects of pyrrolizidine alkaloids on the liver are acute necrosis, venoocclusive disease, and megalocytosis. It has been postulated that effects on lungs and kidneys may occur from excess pyrrolic metabolites generated in the liver. The alkaloids themselves are not hepatotoxic, but after they are ingested, they undergo microsomal enzyme oxidation to the corresponding pyrrole and subsequent hydrolysis to the hepatotoxin. The pyrrolizidine alkaloids are carcinogens and mutagens. Carcinogenic effects in livestock are limited because most animals are slaughtered relatively early in their lives. Carcinogenicity becomes a greater issue in milk-transmitted pyrrolizidine alkaloids and presents a potential risk to the human population.

Some plants that produce pyrrolizidine alkaloids are consumed directly by humans. *Symphytum officinale* (comfrey) is commonly used as a salad vegetable and tea. Pyrrolizidine-containing herbs are also in use. The flower stalks of *Petasites japonicus,* a type of coltsfoot that has been shown to be carcinogenic in rats (189), are used as a vegetable in Japan.

Accidental consumption of pyrrolizidine alkaloids may occur when seeds from pyrrolizidine alkaloid–containing plants contaminate grain crops. This has been reported in underdeveloped countries when drought situations have caused weed species to flourish at the expense of cultivated crops or when famine has forced populations to consume poor-quality commodities.

Goitrogens

A number of food-borne compounds interfere with utilization of iodine or functioning of the thyroid gland (190). The type of goiter induced by goitrogens results from inhibition of iodine incorporation into thyroid hormones. Goiter induced by goitrogenic compounds is not prevented or alleviated by high iodine intake. Vegetables and fruits containing goitrogens were shown to reduce the rate of uptake of radioactive iodine by human thyroid glands (191). Seeds of various vetches *(Lathyrus sativus, L. cicera,* and *L. clymenum)* contain potent goitrogenic compounds. Goitrogens such as sinigrin (allylthioglucoside), glucobrassicin (3-indoylmethylthioglucoside), progoitrin (2-hydroxy-3-butenylthioglucoside), and gluconapin (3-butenylthioglucoside) are among the compounds isolated and characterized from various *Brassica* species (cabbage, kale, Brussels sprouts, cauliflower, broccoli, and kohlrabi).

Mimosine, a nonprotein free amino acid, and its ruminal degradation product 3,4-dihydroxypyridine (3,4-DHP) are the major toxic constituents of *Lucaena leucocephala* and closely related species with limited food and forage uses. Mimosine is an antimitotic and depilatory agent, and 3,4-DHP is a potent goitrogen. Signs of *lucaena* toxicosis in ruminants, which can be acute or chronic, include alopecia, reduced weight gain or weight loss, enlarged thyroid, and low circulating concentrations of thyroid hormones (192). *Lucaena* toxicosis does not occur in all geographic areas where ruminants are fed the crop; the lack of toxicosis in such areas is due to the ability of rumen bacteria in unaffected ruminants to degrade and detoxify 3,4-DHP. Important steps are being taken to control *lucaena* toxicosis in ruminants by inoculating ruminal contents from "adapted" ruminants into those susceptible to intoxication. The availability of viable approaches to controlling *lucaena* toxicosis makes exploitation of *lucaena's* potential as a high-quality legume for tropical and subtropical areas possible (192).

The prevalence of goiter in rural areas of western Sudan, where the staple food is millet, is significantly higher than in urban areas, where less millet is consumed. Millet diets are rich in *C*-glycosylflavones, the three most abundant of which are glycosylvitexin, glycosylorientin, and vitexin. Vitexin has significant antithyroid activity when fed to rats (193), and like the potent antithyroid drug methimazole, vitexin inhibits thyroid peroxidase–catalyzed protein iodination. These results directly implicate the *C*-glycosylflavones as the goitrogens in millet (194).

Allergens

In some individuals, complex interactions among ingested food antigens, the digestive tract, tissue mast cells, circulating basophils, and food antigen–specific IgE lead to food hypersensitivity (195–197). Foods such as peanuts, nuts, eggs, milk, soy, fish and other seafood, bananas, and chicken have been implicated in immediate hypersensitivity reactions in children. Symptoms may include atopic eczema, asthma, and rhinitis (198–200). The numerous foods studied in attempts to characterize specific food allergens include codfish (201), peanuts (202), shrimp (203), and eggs (204).

Gluten, a protein found in wheat, rye, barley, and oats, elicits a severe enteropathy ("gluten-sensitive-enteropathy" or "nontropical sprue") in sensitive individuals. The complex and heterogeneous nature of wheat proteins has hindered attempts to identify the component of gluten responsible for the intestinal damage that occurs in sensitive individuals. Gliadin, an alcohol-soluble component of gluten, appears to be the primary toxic component (205).

Oxalates

High levels of oxalates are found in a number of vegetables. Oxalates generally occur as soluble sodium or potassium salts or as insoluble calcium salts (206). Leafy portions of plants usually contain higher concentrations of oxalates than do stalks. Insoluble calcium oxalate crystals are readily visible on microscopic examination of leaves of high-oxalate plants (207). The percentage oxalate content of some plant foods is as follows (fresh-weight basis): beet tops and cocoa leaves, 0.3 to 0.9%; spinach and rhubarb, 0.2 to 1.3%; and tea leaves, 0.3 to 2.0%. Ingestion of oxalate-containing plants can cause acute poisoning; plants of the rhubarb and sorrel grass species are particularly harmful. Symptoms of mild oxalate poisoning (e.g., following ingestion of rhubarb) include abdominal pain and gastroenteritis. Symptoms of severe poisoning include diarrhea, vomiting, convulsions, noncoagulability of the blood, and coma (207). Calcium oxalate kidney stones have been found in Thai children consuming native plants of high oxalate content (208).

Since urinary oxalate is considered an important determinant for formation of calcium oxalate kidney stones, it has been customary to recommend restricting oxalate-rich foods in persons with calcium oxalate nephrolithiasis. In considering the stone-forming potential of various oxalate-rich foods, the bioavailability of oxalate from foods may be calculated by expressing oxalate absorption as a percentage of the total oxalate contained in specific foods (209). The ability of different food items to increase urinary oxalate excretion varies significantly. Based on activity in increasing urinary oxalate, spinach was rated as a "high-risk" food item; peanuts, instant tea, almonds, chocolate, and pecans were rated as "moderate-risk" items; and turnip greens, brewed tea with milk, and okra were rated as "negligible-risk" items. The authors noted that these results were derived from studies with normal subjects and may not apply to certain patients with nephrolithiasis (209).

Phytates

Phytate (myoinositol hexaphosphate) is widely distributed in plants. Its location in specific plants varies; for example, the phytate of seed plants such as corn is contained primarily in the bran and germ. The primary adverse effects of dietary phytate are due to its activity in decreasing the bioavailability of such essential minerals as zinc, calcium, iron, and manganese (210). The bioavailability of zinc appears to be most severely affected. Extensive studies in the Middle East resulted in recognition of the seriousness of this effect in humans. Zinc deficiency with delayed sexual development and growth retardation observed in certain populations was attributable to the high amounts of phytate ingested in whole-grain bread that served as the main dietary staple.

Much of the phytate of plants goes into the byproducts of flour milling and may become concentrated in high-protein flours (211). The concentration of protein from seeds, particularly soybeans, and the use of plant protein to supplement or replace meat products is an important activity of the food industry. The processes used to obtain plant protein from seeds include adjustments in pH, aqueous washes, drying, and hot pressure extrusion to yield a wide range of products varying in protein, fiber, phytic acid, and essential mineral content. Other food processes result in hydrolysis of phytate to yield lower-inositol phosphates or inorganic phosphate and myoinositol. Processing seeds to prepare protein concentrates and isolates results in some mineral loss and sometimes decreased bioavailability of the remaining minerals. The decreased bioavailability of minerals resulting from food processing can be counterbalanced to some extent by the large amount of minerals occurring in most whole seeds. Areas of current interest in relation to phytates in foods include *(a)* methods of removing phytate, *(b)* beneficial and adverse effects of smaller inositol phosphates, *(c)* differences in sensitivity among varying age groups, and *(d)* adaptation to dietary phytates.

The deleterious effects of phytates on growth and mineral status have led to attempts to reduce the phytate content of soybeans. One of the most effective means of reducing phytate takes advantage of endogenous phytase (212). For example, autolysis of an aqueous suspension of soy flour results in a low-phytate soybean protein isolate. Ultrafiltration, ion-exchange chromatography, and close control of such variables as pH, salt concentration, and temperature during extraction of the protein from the bean have also been used to remove phytate.

Cycad

High-incidence foci of amyotrophic lateral sclerosis (ALS) and parkinsonism dementia (PD) occur on Guam, the Kii peninsula of Japan, and southern West New Guinea in the western Pacific. The original incidence rates of ALS in the foci on Guam and in West New Guinea were 50 and 1300 per 100,000 population, respectively, versus a rate of 1 per 100,000 population in the United States (213). These foci have provided unique opportunities to study the cause and mechanisms of pathogenesis of fatal neurodegenerative disorders. Attempts to identify an infectious agent in ALS and PD have been unsuccessful. Several studies have attempted to identify a relationship between the high incidence of ALS and ingestion of cycad plant material. In tropical and subtropical regions, including the foci mentioned above, nuts of the palmlike cycad trees provide food for humans and livestock. Because ingestion of cycad fruits was known to produce motor neuron toxicity in foraging domestic animals, the cycad became a major candidate for a causative role in the human disorders. Rats fed diets containing 2% of a crude flour prepared from unwashed cycad nuts developed liver and kidney tumors (214, 215). A neurologic disease was not observed (216). Extensive efforts to implicate cycad in neurologic disease have been unsuccessful (213).

A toxic substance was extracted from cycad nuts and identified as methylazoxymethanol-β-glucoside (cycasin). Cycasin is one of the most potent carcinogens found in plants. Macrozamin, a related glucoside, is also found in cycad nuts. Because liver cancer also occurs at high rates in Guam and Okinawa, ingestion of cycasin in cycad nuts has been proposed as an etiologic factor in this disease. The available information does not allow a definitive conclusion (217). In contrast, studies with experimental animals support the hypothesis that a basic metabolic defect, provoked by a chronic nutritional deficiency of calcium, leads to increased absorption of toxic minerals and deposition of calcium, aluminum, and silicon in neurons of patients with ALS (147). Although deposition of toxic minerals in neurons of patients with ALS is now recognized, the process by which neuronal degeneration occurs is not understood.

Cycad flours from various geographic areas of Guam and Rota were found to contain the neurotoxins previously found in cycad seeds. Consumption of food products prepared from these flours would expose consumers to numerous cycad chemicals, including the known neurotoxins. The body burden of these chemicals may also be increased by percutaneous exposures to unprocessed cycad seed, since in some areas, crushed raw cycad seed kernel is used to poultice open wounds (218).

While washing cycad seed may potentially remove all traces of cycasin, the Chamarro methods of seed kernel detoxification are variable and incomplete in this regard. Differential processing of cycad seed in the islands of the western Pacific may be related to the respective presence and absence of western Pacific ALS/PD among different cycad-consuming populations (219). The findings provide evidence for discontinuing cycad consumption on Guam. If the contaminated cycad flour is a major etiologic factor for ALS/PD on Guam, then cessation of cycad use should lead to the eventual disappearance of the disease.

Bracken Fern Toxins

Bracken fern is consumed by both humans and animals in several parts of the world. Damage to the bone marrow and intestinal mucosa of cattle has been associated with ingestion of this plant. In one study, a high risk of esophageal cancer was associated with daily intake of bracken fern (146). Rats fed fresh or powdered milk from cows that had consumed bracken fern daily (1 g/kg body weight) for about 2 years developed carcinomas of the intestine, urinary bladder, and kidney (220). In another study, however, dietary administration of quercetin, which occurs as a conjugate in the fern, did not lead to increased incidence of tumors in ACI rats (126). A highly mutagenic substance has been isolated from bracken fern and identified as aquilide-A (221).

Phytoalexins

Several plants, including the sweet potato, can produce "stress metabolites" (phytoalexins) in response to fungal infections, mechanical damage, and insect invasion. These compounds accumulate at fungitoxic levels at sites of infection and are thought to be part of the mechanisms by which potatoes resist disease. Some of these metabolites are toxic to animals consuming infected roots. Because sweet potatoes are a food staple for large numbers of people, the toxicities of these metabolites are of considerable importance (103, 148). One of the most abundant of these metabolites, ipomeamarone, produces liver necrosis in mice when fed or injected intraperitoneally. In large-scale outbreaks of moldy sweet potato poisoning, however, the predominant manifestation is lung edema, leading to death from asphyxiation rather than liver damage. The fatal pulmonary disease has been described as acute interstitial pneumonia, acute bovine pulmonary emphysema (ABPE), or pulmonary edema (222). Components of moldy sweet potatoes other than ipomeamarone, when fed to mice, reproduce certain features of the bovine disease and cause death of the animals from asphyxiation within 24 hours.

ABPE can be caused by other toxic plant components (223). Outbreaks of ABPE occur in animals grazing on pastures that contain a variety of plant species, but no single plant type or combination of plants has been consistently associated with the disease (224). The most common observation associated with outbreaks of the disease is a sudden change from relatively dry to lush forage. Ruminal microorganisms can convert L-tryptophan via indoleacetic acid to 3-methylindole, which can cause pulmonary lesions in cattle, goats, and sheep. Presumably, tryptophan contained in pasture plants can be converted to enough 3-methylindole to induce ABPE. Observations that ABPE is associated with changes from dry to wetter pastures may also support a role for mycotoxins or stress metabolites.

Vasoactive Amines

Certain foods, notably aged cheeses, contain vasoactive amines such as tyramine, dopamine, norepinephrine, serotonin, and histamine. These compounds can cause large increases in blood pressure when administered intravenously to humans. Levels of tyramine may be as high as 2000 μg/g in Camembert cheese; somewhat lower levels have been reported in cheddar (120–1500 μg/g) and Emmenthaler (225–1000 μg/g) cheeses. Pickled herring may contain as much as 3000 μg tyramine/g (225). The foregoing amines are normally metabolized rapidly in the human body by monamine oxidase (MAO). Tyramine has been found to produce serious effects in persons taking drugs that inhibit MAO, often prescribed for depressive illnesses. Episodes of hypertension, intense headaches, and intracerebral hemorrhage have been reported following ingestion of high-tyramine food by individuals taking MAO inhibitors. Hypertensive reactions are not limited to cheese or to ingestion of tyramine only and have been reported in persons taking MAO inhibitors following ingestion of pickled herring, chicken liver, stewed bananas, and beef liver. Other chemically effective antidepressants without the "cheese effect" have been described (226, 227).

REFERENCES

1. Gilchrist A. Foodborne disease & food safety. Chicago: American Medical Association, 1981.
2. Hathcock JN, Rader JI. Ann NY Acad Sci 1990;587:257–66.
3. Hathcock JN. J Nutr 1989;119:1779–84.
4. Hathcock JN, Hattan DG, Jenkins MY, et al. Am J Clin Nutr 1990;52:183–202.
5. Krasinski SD, Russell RM, Otradovec CL, et al. Am J Clin Nutr 1989;49:112–20.
6. Bendich A, Langseth L. Am J Clin Nutr 1989;49:358–71.
7. Miller D, Hayes KC. Vitamin excess and toxicity. In: Hathcock J, ed. Nutritional toxicology, vol 1. New York: Academic Press, 1982;81–133.

7a. Hathcock J. Vitamin and mineral safety. Washington, DC: Council for Responsible Nutrition, 1997.

8. Stewart ML, McDonald JT, Levy AS, et al. J Am Diet Assoc 1985;85:1585–90.
9. Cochrane WA. Can Med Assoc J 1965;93:893–9.
10. Siegel C, Barker B, Kunstadter M. J Periodontol 1982;53: 453–5.
11. Hoffer A. Can Med Assoc J 1985;132:320.
12. Ringsdorf WM, Cheraskin E. South Med J 1981;74:41–6.
13. Schrauzer, GN, Ishmael D, Kiefer, GW. Ann NY Acad Sci 1975;258:377–81.
14. Guinta JL. J Am Diet Assoc 1983;107:253–6.
15. National Nutrition Consortium. Vitamin-mineral safety, toxicity, and misuse. Chicago: American Dietetic Association, 1978.
16. Metz J, Hundertmark U, Pevny I. Contact Dermatitis 1980;6: 172–4.
17. Henkin Y, Johnson KC, Segrest JP. JAMA 1990;264:241–3.
18. Hodis HN. JAMA 1990;264:181.
19. Patterson DJ, Dew EW, Gorkey F, et al. South Med J 1983;76:239–41.

20. Cantinieaux B, Boelaert J, Hariga C, et al. J Lab Clin Med 1988;111:524–8.
21. Akbar AN, Fitzgerald-Bocarsly PA, DeSousa M, et al. J Immunol 1986;136:1635–40.
22. McEnery JT. Clin Toxicol 1971;4:603–10.
23. Chandra RK. JAMA 1984;252:1443–6.
24. Beisel WR. Am J Clin Nutr 1982;35:417–68.
25. National Research Council. Selenium. Washington, DC: National Academy of Sciences, 1976;110–1.
26. Food and Nutrition Board, National Research Council. Recommended dietary allowances. 10th ed. Washington, DC: National Academy Press, 1989.
27. Food and Drug Administration. Food labeling: reference daily intakes. Fed Regist 1995;60:67164–75.
28. Conning DM. Artificial sweeteners—a long running saga. In: Gibson GG, Walker R, eds. Food toxicology—real or imaginary problems? London: Taylor and Francis, 1985;11–4.
29. Munro IC. A case study: the safety evaluation of artificial sweeteners. In: Taylor SL, Scanlan RA, eds. Food toxicology: a perspective on the relative risks. New York: Marcel Dekker, 1989;151–67.
30. Food and Drug Administration. Direct food substance affirmed as generally recognized as safe: microparticulated protein. Fed Regist 1990;37:8384–91.
31. Widhalm K, Stargel WW, Burns TS, Tschanz C. J Am Coll Nutr 1994;13:392–6.
32. Sampson HA, Cooke S. Clin Exp Allergy 1992;22:963–9.
33. Food and Drug Administration. Food additives permitted for direct addition to food for human consumption: olestra. Fed Regist 1996;61:3118–73.
34. Berdick M. Safety of food colors. In: Hathcock JN, ed. Nutritional toxicology, vol 1. New York: Academic Press, 1982;383–434.
35. Norton S. Effects of food chemicals on behavior of experimental animals. In: Hathcock JN, ed. Nutritional toxicology, vol 1. New York: Academic Press, 1982;451–72.
35a. Department of Health and Human Services. The surgeon general's report on nutrition and health. Washington, DC: Government Printing Office, 1988.
36. Ito N, Fukushima S, Tsuda H, et al. Antioxidants: carcinogenicity and modifying activity in tumorigenesis. In: Gibson GG, Walker R, eds. Food toxicology—real or imaginary problems? London: Taylor and Francis, 1985;181–98.
37. Tatsuta M, Mikuni T, Taniguchi H. Int J Cancer 1983;32:253–4.
38. Williams GM. Inhibition of chemical-induced experimental cancer by synthetic phenolic antioxidants. In: Williams GM, Sies S, Baker GT, et al., eds. Antioxidants: chemical, physiological, nutritional and toxicological aspects. Princeton, NJ: Henry Prenceton Scientific Press, 1993:303–8.
39. Miller YE. Pulmonary neoplasms. In: Bennett JC, Plum F, eds. Textbook of medicine. Philadelphia: WB Saunders, 1996; 436–42.
40. Archer MC. Hazards of nitrate, nitrite and N-nitroso compounds in human nutrition. In: Hathcock JN, ed. Nutritional toxicology, vol 1. New York: Academic Press, 1982;328–82.
41. Hotchkiss JH. Relative exposure to nitrite, nitrate, and N-nitroso compounds from endogenous and exogenous sources. In: Taylor SL, Scanlan RA, eds. Food toxicology: a perspective on the relative risks. New York: Marcel Dekker, 1989;57–100.
42. Taylor SL. Allergic and sensitivity reactions to food components. In: Hathcock JN, ed. Nutritional toxicology, vol 2. New York: Academic Press, 1987;173–98.
43. Taylor SL, Nordlee JA, Rupnow JH. Food allergies and sensitivities. In: Taylor SL, Scanlan RA, eds. Food toxicology: a perspective on the relative risks. New York: Marcel Dekker, 1989;255–96.
44. Irving GW Jr. Determination of the GRAS status of food ingredients. In: Hathcock JN, ed. Nutritional toxicology, vol 1. New York: Academic Press, 1982;435–50.
45. Oehme FW. Toxicity of heavy metals in the environment, pts 1 and 2. New York: Marcel Dekker, 1978 and 1979.
46. Mertz W. Trace elements in human and animal nutrition, 5th ed., vols. I and II. New York: Academic Press, 1986 and 1987.
47. Smith KT. Trace minerals in foods. New York: Marcel Dekker, 1988.
48. Anke M. Arsenic. In: Mertz W, ed. Trace elements in human and animal nutrition, 5th ed. New York: Academic Press, 1986;347–72.
49. Nielsen FH. The ultratrace elements. In: Smith KT, ed. Trace minerals in foods. New York: Marcel Dekker, 1988;357–428.
50. Jelinek CF, Comeliussen PE. Environ Health Perspect 1977;19:83–7.
51. Schroeder HA, Balassa JJ. J Chronic Dis 1966;19:85–106.
52. Axelson O, Dahlgren E, Jansson C.-D, et al. Br J Ind Med 1978;35:8–15.
53. Mabuchi K, Lilienfeld AM, Snell LM. Arch Environ Health 1979;34:312–9.
54. National Research Council. Selenium in nutrition. Washington, DC: National Academy Press, 1983.
55. Smith MJ, Franke KW, Westfall BB. Public Health Rep 1936;51:1496.
56. Smith MJ, Westfall BB. Public Health Rep 1937;152:1375.
57. Yang G, Wang S, Zhou R, Sun S. Am J Clin Nutr 1983;37: 872–81.
58. Yang G, Yin S, Zhou R, et al. J Trace Elem Electrolytes Health Dis 1989;3:123–30.
59. Longnecker MP, Taylor PR, Levander OA, et al. Am J Clin Nutr 1991;53:1288–94.
60. Clark LC, Combs GF Jr, Turnbull BW, et al. JAMA 1996;276:1957–63.
61. Combs GF Jr, Clark LC. Selenium. In: Garewal HS, ed. Antioxidant nutrients and disease prevention. New York: CRC Press, in press.
62. Jaffee WG. In: Proceedings of the symposium on selenium-tellurium in the environment. South Bend, IN: University of Notre Dame, 1976;188–193.
63. Bennett BG. Exposure commitment assessments of environmental pollutants, vol 1, no. 2. London: Monitoring and Assessment Research Center, 1981.
64. Environmental Protection Agency. Mercury health effects update. Research Triangle Park, NC: U.S. Environmental Protection Agency, 1984.
65. Tsubaki T, Irukuyama K. Minamata disease. Tokyo: Kodansha, 1977.
66. Underwood EJ. Trace elements. In: Toxicants occurring naturally in foods. 2nd ed. Washington, DC: National Academy of Sciences, 1973;43–87.
67. World Health Organization. Trace elements in human nutrition and health. Geneva: World Health Organization, 1996.
68. Carrington CD, Bolger PM. Regul Toxicol Pharmacol 1992; 16:265–72.
69. Burgoin BP, Evans DR, Cornett JR, et al. Am J Public Health 1993;83:1155–60.
70. Goyer RA. Am J Clin Nutr 1995;61:646S–50S.
71. Mushak P, Corcetti AF. Nutr Today 1996;31:12–7.
72. Friberg L, Kjellstrom T, Nordberg G. Cadmium. In: Friberg L,

Nordberg GF, Vouk VB, eds. Handbook of the toxicology of metals, vol. 2. 2nd ed. New York: Elsevier, 1986;130–83.
73. Dunnick JK, Fowler BA. Cadmium. In: Seiler HG, Sigal H, Sigal A, eds. Handbook on toxicity of inorganic compounds. New York: Marcel Dekker, 1988;155–74.
74. Kostial K. Cadmium. In: Mertz W, ed. Trace elements in human and animal nutrition. New York: Academic Press, 1986;319–45.
75. Kobayashi J, Morii F, Muramoto S, et al. Jpn J Hyg 1970;25:364–7.
76. Kazantzis G. Environ Health Perspect 1979;28:155–60.
77. Itokawa Y, Tomoko A, Tanaka S. Arch Environ Health 1973;26:241–7.
78. Ikeda M. Biological monitoring of the general population for cadmium. In: Nordberg GF, Herber RFM, Alessio L, eds. Cadmium in the human environment: toxicity and carcinogenicity. Lyon, France: International Agency for Research on Cancer (IARC), 1992;65–72.
79. Louekari K. Estimation of dietary intake of cadmium: reliability of methods. In: Nordberg GF, Herber RFM, Alessio L, eds. Cadmium in the human environment: toxicity and carcinogenicity. Lyon, France: International Agency for Research on Cancer (IARC), 1992;163–7.
80. Capar SG, Yess NJ. Food Addit Contam 1996:13:553–60.
81. Coats JR. Toxicology of pesticide residues in food. In: Hathcock JN, ed. Nutritional toxicology, vol 2. Orlando, FL: Academic Press, 1987;249–80.
82. Ecobichon DJ. Toxic effects of pesticides. In: Klaassen CD, ed. Casarett's and Doull's toxicology. 5th ed. New York: McGraw-Hill, 1996;643–90.
83. Bülchel KH. Regul Toxicol Pharmacol 1984;4:174–91.
84. Turnbull GJ. J R Soc Med 1984;77:932–5.
85. Ariens EJ, Simonis AM. General principles of nutritional toxicology. In: Hathcock JN, ed. Nutritional toxicology, vol 1. New York: Academic Press, 1982;17–80.
86. Roberts L. Science 1989;243:1430.
87. Hathcock JN, Zarba-Vary A. Standards for pesticide residues in foods. In: Taylor TG, Jenkins NK, eds. Proceedings XIII Intern Congr Nutr. London: John Libby, 1986;819–22.
88. National Research Council. Regulating pesticides in foods—the Delaney paradox. Washington, DC: National Academy Press, 1987.
89. Fan AM, Jackson RJ. Regul Toxicol Pharmacol 1989;9:158–74.
90. Abelson PH. Science 1993;259:1235.
91. The Food Quality Protection Act. Public Law 104-170, Aug. 3, 1996.
92. Cordle F, Kolbye AC. Environmental contaminants in food. In: Hathcock JN, ed. Nutritional toxicology, vol 1. New York: Academic Press, 1982;303–27.
93. Sherer RA, Price PS. The effect of cooking processes on PCB levels in edible fish tissue. Qual Assur: Good Pract Regul Law 1993;2:396–407.
94. Mendola P, Buck GM, Vena JE, et al. Environ Health Perspect 1995;103:498–502.
95. Davidek J, ed. Natural toxic compounds of foods: formation and change during processing and storage. Boca Raton, FL: CRC Press, 1995.
96. Tuominen JP, Pyysalo HSM, Sauri M. J Agric Food Chem 1988;36:118–20.
97. Santodonato J, Howard P, Basu D. J Environ Pathol Toxicol 1981;5:1–364.
98. Hargraves WA. Mutagens in cooked foods. In: Hathcock JN, ed. Nutritional toxicology, vol 2. Orlando, FL: Academic Press, 1987;157–72.
99. Sugimura T, Wakabayashi K, Nagao M, et al. Heterocyclic amines in food. In: Taylor SL, Scanlan RA, eds. Food toxicology: a perspective on the relative risks. New York: Marcel Dekker, 1989;31–56.
100. Guillen MD. Food Addit Contam 1994;11:669–84.
101. Scoging AC. Communicable Dis Rep 1991;1(Review 11):R117–22.
102. Hokama Y. Food Addit Contam 1993;10:71–82.
103. Wilson BJ. Mycotoxins and toxic stress metabolites of fungus-infected sweet potatoes. In: Hathcock JN, ed. Nutritional toxicology, vol 1. New York: Academic Press, 1982;239–302.
104. Berry CL. J Pathol 1988;154:301–11.
105. Schiatter C. Bibl Nutr Dieta 1988;41:55–65.
106. Krogh P. J Appl Bacteriol 1989;(Symp Suppl):99S–104S.
107. Mantle PG. J Appl Bacteriol 1989;(Symp Suppl):83S–8S.
108. Sargent K, Sheridan K, Sheridan A, et al. Toxicity associated with certain samples of groundnuts. Nature 1961;192: 1096.
109. Goldblatt LA. Aflatoxin. New York: Academic Press, 1969.
110. National Research Council. Diet, nutrition and cancer. Washington, DC: National Academy Press, 1982.
111. Stoloff L. Nutr Cancer 1983;5:165–86.
112. Henry SH, Scheuplein RJ, Bowers J, Tollefson L. Qual Assur: Good Pract Regul Law 1993;2:271–7.
113. Weng CY, Martinez AJ, Park DL. Food Addit Contam 1994;11:649–58.
114. Mukherjee K, Lakshminarasimham AV. Zentralbl Bakteriol 1995;282:237–43.
115. Lee LS, Bayman P, Benett JW. Mycotoxins. Biotechnology 1992;21:463–503.
116. Doores S. CRC Crit Rev Food Sci Nutr 1983;19:133–49.
117. Broom WA, Buibring E, Chapman CJ, et al. Br J Exp Pathol 1944;25:95–100.
118. Dickens F, Jones HEH. Br J Cancer 1961;15:85–92.
119. Anonymous. Food Chem News 1980;22:9.
120. Szczech GM, Carlton WW, Tuite J. Vet Pathol 1973;10:219–31.
121. Austwick PKC, Carter RL, Greig JM, et al. Contrib Nephrol 1979;16:154–60.
122. Hult K, Plestina R, Hzbazin-Novak et al. Arch Toxicol 1982;51:313–21.
123. Barnes JM, Austwick PKC, Carter RL, et al. Lancet 1977;1:671–5.
124. Yeulet SF, Mantle PG, Rudge MS, Greig JB. Mycopathologia 1988;102:21–30.
125. Maaroufi K, Achour A, Betbeder AM, et al. Arch Toxicol 1995;69:552–8.
126. Broquist H. Annu Rev Nutr 1985;5:391–409.
127. Aust SD, Broquist HP, Rinehart KL Jr. Biotechnol Bioeng 1968;10:408–12.
128. Hartley WJ. A comparative study of Darling pea (*Swainsona* spp.) poisoning in Australia with locoweed (*Astragalus* and *Oxytropis* spp.) poisoning in North America. In: Keeler RF, VanKampen KR, James LF, eds. Effects of poisonous plants on livestock. New York: Academic Press, 1978;363–9.
129. Ross PF. J Assoc Off Anal Chem Int 1994;77:491–4.
130. Riley RT, Wang E, Merrill AH Jr. J Assoc Off Anal Chem Int 1994;77:533–40.
131. Bennett GA, Richard JL. J Assoc Off Anal Chem Int 1994;77:501–6.
132. Engleberg N, Morris J, Lewis J, et al. Ann Intern Med 1983;98:336–7.
133. Halstead B. Poisonous and venomous marine animals of the world, vol 2. Washington, DC: U.S. Government Printing Office, 1967.
134. Tindall DR, Dickey RW, Carlson RD, et al. Ciguatoxigenic dinoflagellates from the Caribbean Sea. In: Ragelis EP, ed.

Seafood toxins. Washington, DC: American Chemical Society, 1984;225–40.
135. Dickey RW, Bobzin SC, Faulkner DJ, et al. Toxicon 1990;28:371–7.
136. Eastaugh J, Shepherd S. Arch Intern Med 1989;149:1735–40.
137. Winter A, Tosteson TR. Bull Soc Pathol Exot 1992;85: 510–3.
138. Gessner BD, Middaugh JP. Am J Epidemiol 1995;141:766–70.
139. Baden DG. Int Rev Cytol 1983;82:99–150.
140. Asakawa M, Miyazawa K, Takayama H, Noguchi T. Toxicon 1995;33:691–7.
141. Rodrigue DC, Etzel RA, Hall S, et al. Am J Trop Med Hyg 1990;42:267–71.
142. Hartigan-Go K, Bateman DN. Hum Exp Toxicol 1994; 13:824–30.
143. Boisier P, Ranaivoson G, Rasolofonirina N, et al. Toxicon 1995;33:1359–64.
144. Zatorre RJ. Can Dis Weekly Rep 1990;16(Suppl):101–4.
145. Wright JLC, Bird CJ, deFreitas ASW, et al. Can Dis Weekly Rep 1990;16(Suppl):21–6.
146. National Research Council. Toxicants occurring naturally in foods. Washington, DC: National Academy of Sciences, 1973.
147. Morton ID. J Hum Nutr 1977;31:53–60.
148. Salunkhe DK, Wu MR. CRC Crit Rev Food Sci Nutr 1977;12:265–324.
149. Somogyi JC. Bibl Nutr Dieta 1980;29:110–27.
150. Furihata C, Matsushima T. Annu Rev Nutr 1986;6:67–94.
151. Ory RL, ed. Antinutrients and natural toxicants in foods. Westport, CT: Food and Nutrition Press, 1981.
152. deWolff FA. Hum Toxicol 1988;7:443–7.
153. Newberne PM. Naturally occurring food-borne toxicants. In: Shils ME, Young VR, eds. Modern nutrition in health and disease. 7th ed. Philadelphia: Lea & Febiger, 1988;685–771.
154. National Research Council. Diet and health: implications for reducing chronic disease risk. Washington, DC: National Academy Press, 1989.
155. Rackis JJ. Biologically active components. In: Smith AK, Circle SJ, eds. Soybeans: chemistry and technology, vol 1. Westport, CT: Avi Publishing, 1978;158–202.
156. Brandon DL, Bates AH, Friedman M. J Food Sci 1988;53: 102–6.
157. Rackis JJ, Gumbmann MR. Protease inhibitors: physiological properties and nutritional significance. In: Ory RL, ed. Antinutrients and natural toxicants in foods. Westport, CT: Food and Nutrition Press, 1981;203–37.
158. Roebuck B. J Nutr 1987;117:398–404.
159. Smith JC, Wilson FU, Alle, PV, et al. J Appl Toxicol 1989;9:175–9.
160. Liener IE. J Nutr 1986;116:920–3.
161. Liener IE, Goodale RL, Desmukh A, et al. Gastroenterol 1988;94:419–27.
162. Hathcock JN. Residual trypsin inhibitor. In: Friedman M, ed. Nutritional and toxicological consequences of food processing. New York: Plenum Press 1991;273–9.
163. Liener IE. Crit Rev Food Sci Nutr 1994;34:31–67.
164. Rackis JJ, Gumbmann MR. Protease inhibitors: physiological properties and nutritional significance. In: Ory RL, ed. Antinutrients and natural toxicants in foods. Westport, CT: Food and Nutrition Press, 1982;203–37.
165. Friedman M, Brandon DL, Bates AH, Hymowitz T. J Agric Food Chem 1991;39:326–34.
166. Brandon DL, Bates AH, Friedman M. J Agric Food Chem 1989;37:1192–5.
167. Brandon DL, Bates AH, Friedman M. J Food Sci 1988;53: 102–6.
168. Grant G, Dorward PM, Buchan WC, et al. Br J Nutr 1995;73:17–29.
169. Honavar PM, Shih CV, Liener IE. J Nutr 1962;77:109–14.
170. Olsen MOJ, Liener IE. Biochemistry 1967;6:105–11.
171. Chowdhury SD. World's Poult Sci J 1988;44:7–16.
172. Bell EA. Amino nitriles and amino acids not derived from proteins. In: National Research Council. Toxicants occurring naturally in foods. Washington, DC: National Academy of Sciences, 1973;153–69.
173. Dasler W. Science 1954;120:307–8.
174. Chowdhury SD, Davis RH. Br Poult Sci 1995;36:575–83.
175. Gupta YP. Plant Foods Hum Nutr 1987;37:201–28.
176. Morris SC, Lee TH. Food Technol Aust 1984;36:118–24.
177. Slanina P. Food Chem Toxicol 1990;28:759–61.
178. Hopkins J. Food Chem Toxicol 1995;33:323–9.
179. Phillips BJ, Hughes JA, Phillips JC, et al. Food Chem Toxicol 1996;34:439–48.
180. Hornfeldt CS, Collins JE. Clin Toxicol 1990;28:185–92.
181. Strong FM. Can Med Assoc J 1966;94:568–73.
182. Selzer G, Parker GF. Am J Pathol 1951;27:S85.
183. Bull L, Culvenor I, Dick AT. The pyrrolizidine alkaloids. New York: John Wiley & Sons, 1968.
184. Schoental R. Cancer Res 1968;28:2237–46.
185. Hirono I, Ueno I, Hosaka S, et al. Cancer Lett 1981;13:15–21.
186. Canadrian U, Luthy J, Graf U, et al. Food Chem Toxicol 1984;22:223–5.
187. Hayes MA, Roberts E, Farber E. Cancer Res 1985;45:3726–34.
188. Panter KE, James LF. J Anim Sci 1990;68:892–904.
189. Hirono I. CRC Crit Rev Toxicol 1981;11:235–77.
190. Tookey HL, VanEtten CH, Daxenbichler MR. Glucosinolates. In: Liener IE, ed. Toxic constituents of plant foodstuffs. 2nd ed. New York: Academic Press, 1980;103–42.
191. Greer MA, Astwood EB. Endocrinology 1948;43:105–9.
192. Hammond AC. J Anim Sci 1995;73:1487–92.
193. Gaitan E, Cooksey RC, Legan J, Lindsay RH. J Clin Endocrinol Metab 1995;80:1144–7.
194. Gaitan E. Annu Rev Nutr 1990;10:21–39.
195. Berrens L. Monogr Allergy 1971;13:164–93.
196. Spies JRL. J Agric Food Chem 1974;22:30–6.
197. Metcalfe DD. Clin Rev Allergy 1985;3:331–49.
198. Van Metre TE, Anderson SA, Barnard JH, et al. J Allergy 1968;41:195–208.
199. Taylor SL, Lemanske RF Jr, Bush RK, Busse WW. Ann Allergy 1987;55:93–9.
200. Sampson H. J Allergy Clin Immunol 1983;71:473–80.
201. Aas K. Int Arch Allergy Appl Immunol 1967;31:239–60.
202. Sachs MI, Jones RT, Yunginger JW. J Allergy Clin Immunol 1981;67:27–34.
203. Hoffman DR, Day ED, Miller JS. Ann Allergy 1981;47:17–22.
204. Langeland T, Harbitz O. Allergy 1983;38:131–9.
205. Jos J, Charbonnier L, Mosse J, et al. Clin Chim Acta 1982;119:263–74.
206. Gleason MN, Gosselin RE, Hodge HC. Clinical toxicology of commercial products. Baltimore: Williams & Wilkins, 1963.
207. Jeghers H, Murphy R. N Engl J Med 1945;233:208–15.
208. Valyesevi A, Dhanamitta S. Am J Clin Nutr 1974;27:877–82.
209. Brinkley J, Gregory J, Pak CYC. J Urol 1990;144:94–6.
210. Fox MRS, Tao S-H. Antinutritive effects of phytate and other phosphorylated derivatives. In: Hathcock JN, ed. Nutritional toxicology, vol 3. Orlando, FL: Academic Press, 1989;59–96.
211. Ferrell RE, Wheeler EL, Pence JW. Cereal Sci Today 1969;14: 110.
212. Liener IE. Control of antinutritional and toxic factors in oilseeds and legumes. In: Lucas EW, Erickson DR, Nip W-K,

eds. Food uses of a whole oil and protein seeds. Champaign, IL: American Oil Chemists Society, 1989;344.
213. Garruto RM, Yanagihara R, Gajdusek DC. Environ Geochem Health 1990;12:137–51.
214. Hirono I. CRC Crit Rev Toxicol 1981;8:235–77.
215. Yang MG, Sanger VL, Mickelsen O, Laqueur GL. Proc Soc Exp Biol Med 1968;127:1171–5.
216. Laqueur GL, Spatz M. Cancer Res 1968:28:2262–7.
217. Hirono I, Kachi H, Kato C. Acta Pathol Jpn 1970;20:327–37.
218. Spencer PS, Palmer V, Herman A, Asmedi A. Lancet 1987;2:1273–4.
219. Kisby GE, Ellison M, Spencer PS. Neurology 1992;42:1336–40.
220. Pamukcu AM, Yalciner S, Hatcher JF, et al. Cancer Res 1980;40:3468–72.
221. Van der Hoeven JCM, Lagerweg WJ, et al. Carcinogenesis 1983;4:1587–90.
222. Peckham JC, Mitchell FE, Jones OH, et al. J Am Vet Med Assoc 1972;160:169–72.
223. Linnabary RD, TarTier MP. Vet Hum Toxicol 1988;30:255–6.
224. Hammond AC, Bradley BJ, Yokoyama MT, et al. Am J Vet Res 1978;40:1398–401.
225. Kuhn DM, Lovenberg W. Psychoactive and vasoactive substances in food. In: Hathcock JN, ed. Nutritional toxicology, vol 1. New York: Academic Press, 1982;473–95.
226. Larochelle P, Hamet P, Enjalberg M. Clin Pharmacol Ther 1979;26:24–30.
227. Marley E. Monamine-oxidase inhibitors and drug interactions. In: Grahame-Smith DG, ed. Drug interactions. Baltimore: University Park Press, 1977;171–94.

SELECTED READINGS

Archer MC. Hazards of nitrate, nitrite and N-nitroso compounds in human nutrition. In: Hathcock JN, ed. Nutritional toxicology, vol 1. New York: Academic Press, 1982;328–81.

Ariens J, Simonis AM. General principles of nutritional toxicology. In: Hathcock JN, ed. Nutritional toxicology, vol 1. New York: Academic Press, 1982:17–80.

Hathcock JN. Nutritional toxicology: basic principles and actual problems. Food Addit Contam 1990;7:S12–8.

Hathcock JN. Toxicology of pesticide residues in foods. In: Encyclopedia of human biology, vol 7. San Diego: Academic Press, 1991;559–66.

Hathcock JN, Rader JI. Micronutrient safety. Ann NY Acad Sci 1990;587:257–66.

Mertz W, ed. Trace elements in human and animal nutrition. 5th ed. New York: Academic Press, 1986.

National Research Council. Toxicants occurring naturally in foods. Washington, DC: National Academy Press, 1973.

Rackis JJ, Gumbmann MR. Antinutrients and natural toxicants in foods. In: Ory RL, ed. Antinutrients and natural toxicants in foods. Westport, CT: Food and Nutrition Press, 1981.

Ragelis, EP. Seafood toxins. Washington, DC: Chemical Society, 1984.

Salunke DK, Wu MR. Toxicants in plant and plant products. CRC Crit Rev Food Sci Nutr 1977;12:265–32.

Sugimura T, Wakabayashi K, Nagao M, et al. Heterocyclic amines in food. In: Taylor SL, Scanlan RA, eds. Food toxicology: a perspective on the relative risks. New York: Marcel Dekker, 1989;31–55.

114. Risk Assessment of Environmental Chemicals in Food

A. M. FAN and R. S. TOMAR

In the past three decades, the public has become increasingly aware of and concerned about health risks associated with the chemical products and byproducts of modern industrial society, as well as naturally occurring substances, that may be present as chemical contaminants in food. Potential health hazards from food may result from microbiologic contaminants, pesticide residues, excessive preservatives or additives, nutritional imbalances, overconsumption, and other chemicals (natural or synthetic) accumulated from the environment. The present discussion focuses on health issues associated with environmental chemicals found in, but not intentionally added to, food (pesticides and direct additives are excluded and are reviewed in Chapter 113), plus other current and emerging issues relating to dietary risk. Regulatory agencies use the risk assessment process for safety assessment and to establish regulatory limits in media such as air, water, soil, and food. For food, the process involves special considerations and complexities not found in other media.

REGULATORY AGENCIES AND SCIENTIFIC BODIES

In the United States, the U.S. Food and Drug Administration (FDA) is primarily responsible for assessment and management of chemical contaminants in food. The process and responsibilities involved (described in [1]) are summarized below. The Center for Food Safety and Applied Nutrition (CFSAN) within the FDA is charged with protecting the public from chemical hazards in foods. Although the present discussion is focused on environmental contaminants, excluding substances intentionally added to foods, some indirect food additives may become contaminants in food. Thus, a brief description on additives as regulated by the FDA is in order. *Direct additives* are substances added deliberately in limited amounts (usually at very low concentrations) for a special technical purpose and consumed because they remain in the food. *Secondary direct additives* are substances added to food during manufacturing or processing that are removed before the final product is consumed, but low levels may still remain. *Indirect food additives* are substances that may unintentionally become components of food because they migrate from food contact surfaces during production, packaging, transporting, preparing, or storing (e.g., lead in ceramic ware and diethylhexylphthalate [DEHP] from plastic wraps).

The FDA uses a formal risk assessment process to estimate the hazard posed by food contaminants, color additives, and residues of animal drugs in animal food products (1). These procedures are also used under the general safety clause included in the FDA's impurities or constituents policy published in 1982 as an advanced notice of proposed rule making (ANPR). Under this clause, if a food or color additive itself is found to induce cancer, it is subject to the Delaney clause. However, if the additive itself is not a carcinogen, but a contaminant or

---

Abbreviations: **ADI**—acceptable daily intake; **CPF**—carcinogenic potency factor; **DEHP**—diethylhexylphthalate; **ESADDI**—estimated safe and adequate daily dietary intake; **FAO**—Food and Agriculture Organization; **GRAS**—generally recognized as safe; **IARC**—International Agency for Research on Cancer; **IPCS**—International Program on Chemical Safety; **JECFA**—Joint Expert Committee on Food Additives; **JMPR**—Joint Meeting on Pesticide Residues; **LOAEL**—lowest-observed-adverse-effect level; **NOAEL**—no-observed-adverse-effect level; **PCBs**—polychlorinated biphenyls; **PCDDs**—polychlorinated dibenzo-*p*-dioxins; **PCDFs**—polychlorinated dibenzofurans; **PTTI**—provisional and tolerable total intake; **PTWI**—provisional tolerable weekly intake; **RDA**—recommended dietary allowance; **REL**—reference exposure level; **RfD**—reference dose; **TCDD**—2,3,7,8-tetrachlorodibenzo-*p*-dioxin; **TDI**—tolerable daily intake; **TEF**—toxicity equivalent factor; **TEQ**—total toxicity equivalent; **U.S. EPA**—United States Environmental Protection Agency; **U.S. FDA**—United States Food and Drug Administration; **UF**—uncertainty factor; **WHO**—World Health Organization constituent of the additive is found to be a carcinogen, then the risk assessment procedure is used, as appropriate, to determine the upper limit of risk to the consumer from a contaminant or chemical constituent of the food additive.

At CFSAN, the Cancer Assessment Committee (CAC) performs hazard identification with information from various scientific disciplines such as toxicology, pathology, and epidemiology. A Quantitative Risk Assessment Committee (QRAC) performs dose-response assessment, exposure assessment, and risk characterization—the steps in the traditional risk assessment process, further described below. The first two steps (hazard identification and dose-response assessment) are common to all risk assessment procedures for carcinogens and noncarcinogens, whether they are used to evaluate chemicals in food, water, air, or soil. The data most appropriate for the route of exposure under assessment are used (e.g., dietary data rather than inhalation data in experimental animals would be used to assess risk in humans from food). The third and fourth steps, exposure assessment and risk characterization, may differ more widely for different chemicals because the exposure pattern varies depending on the medium of primary exposure.

FDA evaluations of food are applicable nationwide, but food safety evaluations also occur at the state level. For example, regulatory actions related to commercial fish are addressed by the FDA, but state government agencies have taken the responsibility of evaluating and issuing health advisories concerning contamination of sport fish. The U.S. Environmental Protection Agency (EPA) also addresses sport fish contamination by providing general guidance on fish sampling, risk management, and risk communication. However, this guidance does not apply to commercial fish, nor does the EPA issue site-specific advisories. In addition to the FDA, the agency responsible for the safety of animal, poultry, and dairy products is the U.S. Department of Food and Agriculture (USDA).

Many states depend on the federal agencies for risk assessment support in food contamination situations. Other states have their own resources and capabilities. Since the food distribution system and interstate commerce often involve various states, food contamination situations often require coordination among the affected states and with the federal agencies.

At the international level, the International Program on Chemical Safety (IPCS) of the World Health Organization (WHO) evaluates the effects of chemicals on human health and the environment (2). Two other joint committees of the Food and Agriculture Organization (FAO) and the WHO are responsible for evaluation of food additives, contaminants, and pesticides. The Joint Expert Committee on Food Additives (JECFA) evaluates food additives and contaminants and the Joint Meeting on Pesticide Residues (JMPR) evaluates pesticide residues in food. These committees serve as scientific advisory bodies to the Codex Alimentarius Commission, a subsidiary body of FAO and WHO. The Codex primarily promotes harmony in international trade of food commodities by establishing standards with consensus views based upon safety evaluations conducted by JECFA and JMPR. The JECFA has evaluated more than 700 different substances, primarily food additives but also numerous chemical contaminants. JECFA sets provisional endpoints for food contaminants, subject to revaluation if new data become available. Health benefits of limiting exposure to contaminants are balanced against the impact of limiting intake of a nutritious food supply.

PRINCIPLES AND APPROACHES IN RISK ASSESSMENT

Response to the increasing concern regarding health risks from environmental chemicals has led to new legislation and regulations aimed at reducing human exposure to these chemicals. Risk assessment is either specified or may be assumed as the methodology to be used to predict health risks and establish regulatory limits. In the 1960s, qualitative methods were developed to estimate risks from carcinogens, and these methods and the underlying science evolved during the 1970s and 1980s. In 1986, the EPA issued guidelines for assessing the risk of carcinogens, mutagens, developmental toxicants, and chemical mixtures. They include default options and various assumptions for assessing exposure and risk. Several of these guidelines and new guidelines for emerging issues are being revised. (For an update on the status and trend of risk assessment see Fan et al. [3].)

The principles of risk assessment were identified by the National Academy of Sciences and recently updated by Roberts and Abernathy (4). Risk assessment of a chemical estimates the possibility of a health-related event occurring in a population following exposure to that chemical. The basic elements include hazard identification, dose-response assessment, exposure assessment, and risk characterization. *Hazard identification* is the evaluation and determination of the toxic or hazardous properties of a chemical, based on all available human, animal, and in vitro data. Animal studies examine acute, subacute, or chronic toxicity (e.g., any target organ toxicity such as toxicity of the liver or lung, reproductive or development toxicity, neurotoxicity, genotoxicity, immunotoxicity, and carcinogenicity). The *dose-response assessment* determines the relationship between changes in exposure levels and specific effects that result. *Exposure assessment* determines the extent of exposure to a chemical (in this case, the amount of food ingested and the concentration of chemical in or on that food). *Risk characterization* is the qualitative and quantitative description of risk, with the attendant limitations and uncertainties, after integration of all factors involved.

In practice, hazard identification may identify one or more toxic endpoints of concern from experimental animal studies or human studies. Human studies generally are preferred, if they are of adequate quality. The FDA publishes guidelines for experimental animal studies for food additives and contaminants (5). The use of human data is described by Ames (6), and extrapolation of animal data to humans, by Brown and Salmon (7). Extrapolation of animal experimental data to humans requires many assumptions to compensate for differences in size, life span, metabolic rate, and absorption and to relate the high doses used in animal studies to the expected low-dose exposures in humans. For the carcinogenic endpoint, a carcinogenic potency factor (CPF) is developed for a specific chemical based on suitable data sets using appropriate mathematical models, from the slope of the dose-response curve. The CPF can be used to estimate cancer risk, by incorporating information on exposure using the following formula:

$$\text{Cancer risk} = \text{CPF (mg/kg-day)}^{-1} \times \text{exposure (mg/kg-day)}$$

Overall assessment of carcinogenic risk and future trends in the field are described by Velazquez et al. (8). To assess the risk from ingestion of a specific environmental chemical from food, the known or estimated exposure (i.e., amount of chemical ingested) is used to calculate the risk level if the chemical is considered a carcinogen.

For noncarcinogens, the no-observed-adverse-effect level (NOAEL) and lowest-observed-adverse-effect level (LOAEL) for a toxicity endpoint specific to a chemical are determined. These are then divided by an uncertainty factor (UF) as shown below to account for one or more of the following: quality of data, intraspecies differences, and interspecies differences. The value obtained represents the total health protective reference exposure level (REL), with a reasonable safety margin, at which no appreciable adverse health effects are anticipated. A more detailed description of the method is provided by Cicmanec et al. (9). The REL may be referred to as the reference ingested level (RIL), the acceptable daily intake (ADI), or the the reference dose (RfD), depending upon the scientific body.

$$\frac{\text{NOAEL or LOAEL (mg/kg-day)}}{\text{UF}} = \text{RIL (mg/kg-day)}$$

The RIL obtained can also be used to establish an exposure limit for an environmental chemical in food, based on the same information on NOAEL/LOAEL and use of the UF. Setting such limits has been described for pesticides in food (10). The general formula can be expressed as

$$[\text{RIL (mg/kg-day)} \times \text{body weight (kg)}]/\text{Food consumption rate (kg/day)} = \text{level of chemical in food (mg/kg)}$$

One major difficulty in setting a limit for a chemical in food or in assessing total exposure for a chemical in foods, is that a specific chemical may be present in more than one type of food item, and one food item or category of food may be composed of different individual food items (e.g., egg and cheese in cake and pizza). A total assessment would require considering the consumption rate for each food item. Assessing ingestion of a chemical from the consumption of various food items and setting a limit for that chemical in each of those food items complicate the risk assessment process and are further described below.

SPECIAL CONSIDERATIONS

Diet Composition and Food Consumption Rate

A major component of risk assessment of chemicals in food is estimation of chemical exposure based on food consumption. This can be difficult, since an individual's diet contains a variety of items, and the food composition and dietary intake, or food consumption rate, can vary in relation to individual variability, age, seasonal differences, and geographic, cultural, and economical conditions.

Various studies have been conducted to collect food consumption information. Nationwide food consumption surveys include those conducted by the USDA (11, 12), which give consumption rates by age and sex for dietary items either for the United States as a whole, or for various populations based on regional differences (northern, southern, western, eastern regions). Special studies have been conducted that consider ethnic differences, income level, women, and infants. Each of these studies has certain limitations that require careful consideration before the information collected can be used for risk assessment.

The USDA has used the available food consumption data to estimate intake of various substances in food in the annual total diet study (13), based on information on the diet of the U.S. population, sampling and analysis of food purchased in supermarkets and consumed as prepared, and chemical residue levels in food sample analyses. The chemical intakes are then compared with the WHO's ADIs and the EPA's RfDs for the chemicals.

Chemical Intake Estimates

As described by Rees and Tennant (14), the accuracy of chemical intake estimates is important for optimal balance of the potential risk from an environmental chemical contaminant and the potential benefits to be achieved. Such dietary intake assessments can be done by estimating actual or potential intakes. Different systems have been used to assess risk to "average," "nonaverage," or "critical" groups of consumers, the latter being those who may be more susceptible to the specific toxic effects of a chemical, who consume greater quantities, or who regularly consume foods with higher concentrations of the specific contaminant. Estimates can be averaged for consumers (eaters) or noneaters or averaged over a study period as actual number of consuming days. Chemical intake can also be expressed as a percentile of the range of intakes or by body weight. Methodologies used for food intake assessment include the following: per capita, total diet study, modeling scenarios, surveillance, duplicate diet, and post-marketing surveillance. One must know how the food intake data were generated to determine their appropriateness for use in risk assessment.

Toxicity versus Essentiality

Some trace metals that occur as environmental contaminants also play an important role in human nutrition, creating a delicate balance between chemical toxicity and nutritional essentiality. Usually, the nutritional role involves comparatively low levels of intake, and the potential for toxicity increases as the intake increases beyond the nutritional needs. For some metals (e.g., selenium), the margin between nutritional intake level and toxicity level is very narrow. For others (e.g., zinc), estimated ranges of nutritional and toxicity levels actually overlap. Therefore, risk assessment for these substances has to consider both the toxicity and nutritional aspects.

In environmental toxicology, risk assessment is used to establish a limit of exposure to prevent or protect from chemical toxicity, based on the RIL or RfD. For nutritional essentiality, a level of intake is established to meet the nutritional requirement based on the recommended dietary allowances (RDAs) (15). An estimated safe and adequate daily dietary intake (ESADDI) may be established for micronutrients when the scientific database is not adequate to establish a RDA, but available information suggests that a range of intakes will meet nutritional requirements and represent no threat of toxicity. Performing risk assessment requires understanding the concepts underlying these terms and the associated chemical intake values.

Chemical Forms and Effect of Food Processing, Food Preparation, or Metabolic Conversion

The chemical and physical properties are important determinants of a chemical's toxicity and bioavailability. For example, the inorganic form of arsenic is more toxic in humans, whereas in fish, the organic form of mercury is the toxic form. In addition, the toxicity of dioxins and polychlorinated biphenyls (PCBs) varies greatly among the different congeners. These examples are further discussed below under the specific chemicals.

Food processing may also affect the final concentration and form of chemicals found in food as consumed, but this information for environmental contaminants is limited. However, to better characterize the risk, it is important to know if the parent compound or a breakdown product is of concern and should be targeted for risk assessment. The issue of chemical mutagens (i.e., agents that cause genetic effects) resulting from cooking (such as charbroiling) has been extensively studied and discussed but this information has not been regularly used for risk assessment purposes.

Other examples in which a breakdown or conversion product should be the major chemical form used for risk assessment (rather than the parent chemical) include the 1,1-unsymmetrical dimethylhydrazine (1,1-UDMH) that is a hydrolysis product of daminozide, and nitrite, which is converted from nitrate by microorganisms in contaminated water or in the body.

Bioaccumulation, Bioconcentration, and Biomagnification

Increased concentration of a chemical in various dietary items can result from bioaccumulation, bioconcentration, or biomagnification. Lipophilic chemicals such as PCBs, dioxins, and other chlorinated pesticides can accumulate in fatty tissues and breast milk. Chemicals in the aquatic environment (e.g., selenium) can bioconcentrate in fish; the degree of bioconcentration depends on the bioconcentration factor (the ratio of the concentration in tissue to concentration in water). Chemical concentration can also increase with biomagnification up the food chain, such that fish at higher trophic levels contain more of the chemical than fish at the lower trophic level (as with mercury in fish).

RISK ASSESSMENT OF SELECTED CHEMICALS

Inorganics

Lead (Pb)

The major concern regarding lead exposure is neurotoxicity, both in adults and children (16, 17). In children, lead toxicity can be seen as impaired neurobehavioral development and other effects on red blood cells and their stem cells, the central and peripheral nervous system, and the kidneys. In adults, the effects are peripheral nerve dysfunction, red blood cell protoporphyrin elevation, and elevated blood pressure. In male adults, hypertension occurs at about the same level of lead exposure that affects cognitive function, the most sensitive endpoint in children.

The index of lead exposure is the concentration of lead in blood. A 1991 report from the Centers for Disease Control (CDC) (16) suggests that as little as 10 μg lead/dL of blood may be of concern. Each incremental increase in lead intake is expected to result in an incremental increase in blood level. The relationship between lead ingestion and blood lead levels is estimated to be 0.16 and 0.04 μg lead/dL blood for each microgram of lead ingested daily by children and adults, respectively.

Humans are exposed to lead in air, water, soil, and food. Environmental exposure to lead in the United States has decreased significantly since the early 1970s, when the use of lead in gasoline and paint was restricted. Dietary exposure to lead in the United States has also declined since the reduction in the use of lead solder in cans.

Human dietary intake in various age groups is estimated to be in the range of 1 to 5 μg of Pb daily (17).

Because safe levels of lead exposure have not been identified, the FDA has derived provisional and tolerable total intake (PTTI) levels (17) based on the relationship between lead ingestion and blood lead levels. The levels for children 0 to 6 years old, children 7+ years, pregnant and lactating women, and adults are 6, 15, 25, and 75 μg Pb/day, respectively. The PTTI level derived for adults was based on a blood lead level of 30 μg/dL associated with hypertension. On the basis of recent data reported by the CDC (16), the authors indicated that it would be appropriate to adjust the PTTI level to 25 μg Pb/day for adults. Most of the U.S. population has a blood lead level below 10 μg/dL (18). The fetus, pregnant women, children (for neurotoxicity), and adult males (for hypertension) are identified as sensitive populations.

Zinc (Zn)

Zinc, an essential trace nutrient, is a cofactor for approximately 200 enzymes. On the other hand, gastrointestinal distress resulted from intake of high levels of zinc from improper storage of acidic foods in zinc-containing vessels, acute ingestion of 2000 mg of zinc sulfate (455 mg Zn), and zinc supplementation of 50 to 150 mg/day over a period of 6 weeks to 2 years (19). Consumption of zinc as a dietary supplement at moderate levels for several months to several years has also been reported to have adverse effects on immune function, serum lipoprotein levels, and copper and iron homeostasis. In the study of Yadrick et al. (20), nine healthy adult females received supplementation with 50 mg zinc as zinc gluconate and nine were given 50 mg Zn plus 50 mg Fe as ferrous sulfate monohydrate. After 10 weeks, erythrocyte copper-zinc superoxide dismutase (ESOD) decreased significantly in both groups. The LOAEL was 60 mg/day for effect on copper homeostasis. The EPA used this to develop an RfD, using an uncertainty factor of 3 for a minimally adverse effect in a moderate-duration study of the most sensitive humans and a substance that is an essential nutrient (19). Supplementation provided 50 mg of zinc and approximately 10 mg was from the diet. The reference female body weight was 60 kg.

Humans can be exposed to zinc through environmental sources or dietary supplements (19). Americans were reported to consume 4.5 to 7.0 mg of zinc per 1000 kcal. Approximately 70% of the zinc consumed by Americans is from animal products; thus, zinc intake is lower in the elderly, dieters, and vegetarians than in those who consume meat. A review of 12 studies published worldwide from 1969 to 1988 showed zinc intakes of 1.90 to 20.30 mg/kg for individuals aged 1 month to 85.5 years. Among these studies, six conducted in the U.S. (1969–1988) showed intakes of 5 to 96 mg/day for individuals aged 2 to 81.7 years. Pregnant women were reported to take in less than 20 mg/day. Intake from breast milk varied from 3 mg/day for week 2 of lactation to 0.36 mg/day for week 36. The 1989 RDA of the Food and Nutrition Board, National Academy of Sciences ranged from 5 mg/day for infants up to 19 mg/day for lactating women (15) (see Appendices Table II A-2a-2.)

Selenium (Se)

Selenium toxicity can be described in terms of clinical manifestation of acute, subacute, and chronic selenosis (21). Acute selenosis in animals was associated with unsteady walking, cyanosis of the mucous membranes, labored breathing, and sometimes death. Pathologic findings revealed liver congestion, endocarditis and hypocarditis, degeneration of the smooth musculature of the gastrointestinal tract, gall bladder, and urinary bladder, and erosion of the long bones. Subacute selenosis resulted in neurologic dysfunction (impaired vision, ataxia, disorientation) and respiratory distress typically seen in grazing livestock feeding upon Se-accumulating plants. Chronic selenosis in animals resulted in skin lesions, alopecia, hoof necrosis and loss, emaciation, and increased serum transaminase and alkaline phosphatase levels.

In humans, selenosis is characterized by chronic dermatitis, anorexia, gastroenteritis, increased concentrations of selenium in the hair and nails, hair changes, nail and hair loss, "garlic odor" in the breath, and central nervous system abnormalities (peripheral acute anesthesia, acroparesthesia, and pain in the extremities). These were reported in some of the case studies worldwide and in an epidemiologic study in China. In the U.S., selenosis (gastroenteritis, nail changes, hair loss) and sour-milk breath odor were found in individuals who had taken superpotent supplements that resulted from a manufacturing error.

Animal experiments showed reproductive toxicity in rats and mice following administration of selenium in a seleniferous diet or drinking water. Teratogenicity was not seen in experiments using rodents and nonhuman primates, but deformities were seen in avian species (waterfowl) following environmental and laboratory exposure. Selenium has both mutagenic and antimutagenic properties, depending on the concentration and chemical form used.

The EPA's oral reference dose is 0.005 mg/kg-day, or 350 μg/day, using an uncertainty factor of 3 (21), based on observation of clinical selenosis in a human epidemiologic study (22). In this study of 400 individuals from three separate geographic areas in China with low, medium, and high selenium levels in soil and food, persistent clinical signs of selenosis (changes in fingernail morphology) were seen at an intake of 1261 μg/day, and no signs of significant biochemical changes or selenosis were found at 853 μg/day. A regression equation relating selenium intake to blood selenium concentrations yielded an NOAEL of 853 μg/day or 16 μg/kg-day (for a 55-kg person). Supporting work included an epidemiologic study in the U.S. that showed no selenosis with intake of up to 724 μg/day, reported in 1990, earlier data on endemic selenosis in China reported in 1983, and data on human intoxication in the U.S. from selenium supplements, reported in the late 1980s.

Selenium occurs naturally in rock, shale, sandstone, limestone, coal, soil, surface water, and vegetation. The primary sources of human exposure to environmental levels of selenium are food and drinking water. Dietary selenium intake levels for various human populations range from 20 to 300 μg/day worldwide, or 60 to 240 for the U.S. (23). The common dietary sources are cereal grains and grain products, poultry, meat, vegetables, and seafood. The levels of selenium in plants (e.g., vegetables) are often directly correlated with the levels in soil. Selenium is also used as a dietary supplement for some farm animals and is taken as a nutritional supplement by humans. It has various industrial and commercial uses such as those in semiconductor research, glass manufacturing, photoconductors, veterinary remedies, and biologic tracers. Occupational exposures may involve forms of selenium not present in the diet. The RDAs for selenium are 70 μg for men (79 kg) and 55 μg for women (63 kg) (or 0.87 μg Se/kg body weight/day) (15). No toxicity or deficiency has been reported in the U.S. from regular dietary intake of selenium, suggesting that intake has been adequate and not excessive.

Arsenic (As)

Organic arsenic is virtually nontoxic (24, 25). Arsenobetaine at 10 g/kg given to mice depressed mobility and respiration, but the symptoms disappeared within an hour. In contrast, the acute LD_{50} for inorganic arsenic is in the range of 1 to 4 mg/kg for humans, 9 mg/kg for the guinea pig, and 40 mg/kg for the rat (for sodium arsenite). Short-term exposures affected the heart, liver, kidney, and nervous system. Subacute and chronic exposure of humans to high concentrations of inorganic arsenic produced signs of dermatosis, hematopoietic depression, liver damage, sensory disturbances, peripheral neuritis, anorexia, and weight loss. Animal studies showed developmental toxicity following arsenic exposures. In humans, inorganic arsenic can cause cancer of the skin, lung, and kidney. Peripheral vascular effects leading to gangrene of the extremities (blackfoot disease) have been reported in Taiwan following ingestion of well water containing arsenic.

The EPA evaluated various human studies on the effects of subchronic-to-chronic exposure of arsenic from drinking water (26) and determined that the work reported by Tseng and coworkers (27, 28), which surveyed over 40,000 residents on the southwest coast of Taiwan, was the best available study for deriving an RfD. Arsenic is unique in that animal experiments have not shown the carcinogenic potential seen in humans. Skin cancer has been reported in South America, India, and Taiwan from ingestion of arsenic from drinking water, but studies in the U.S. did not show similar responses.

The study population in Taiwan had various signs of arsenic exposure, including skin cancer, blackfoot disease, hypo- and hyperpigmentation, and keratosis. The critical noncancer effect used is blackfoot disease, a peripheral vascular disorder causing gangrene of the extremities. The critical effects for RfD derivation were limited to hyperpigmentation, keratosis, and possible vascular problems. The calculated NOAEL is 0.8 μg/kg-day and LOAEL is 14 μg/kg-day. An uncertainty factor of 3 is used to derive the RfD of 0.0003 mg/kg-day. However, any value from 0.0001 to 0.0008 mg/kg-day could be used for the RfD, depending on the scientific justification. For cancer, a unit risk estimate of 5.0×10^{-5}/μg/L was developed by the EPA for ingestion of arsenic from drinking water.

In general, arsenic occurs in inorganic forms in water and organic forms in food. The average daily dietary intake of arsenic in humans ranges from 12 to 40 μg, with seafood, grains, and cereal products as the primary dietary sources (24). Studies in rats, hamsters, chicks, goats, and minipigs have supported the essentiality of arsenic. The requirement for growing rats and chicks eating a diet containing approximately 4000 kcal/kg is suggested to be 25 and 50 ng/g diet, respectively. The corresponding requirement for humans eating 2000 kcal is calculated to be 12 to 25 μg/day. However, presently there is no conclusive evidence of human arsenic essentiality. Given the lack of arsenic deficiency as a practical nutritional problem in humans and the derived requirement, it would seem that current dietary intakes satisfy the needs for arsenic. Thus, the ESADDI of arsenic by adults is suggested to be 12 to 40 μg/day for a 70-kg person. The ESADDI for infants 0 to 0.5 years of age (6 kg) is 1 to 4 μg; children 1 to 3 years (13 kg), 3 to 8 μg; children 4 to 6 years (20 kg), 4 to 12 μg; and children 7 to 10 years (28 kg), 5 to 16 μg. The FAO/WHO maximum acceptable daily load of arsenic for humans is 2 μg/kg, or 140 μg for a 70-kg person. The upper limit of the safe and adequate range probably could be higher than 140 μg/day, because in vivo reduction of As^{5+} to As^{3+} must also occur for toxicity. However, the closeness of the nutritional requirement and reported average intake may be of concern if the need for arsenic is enhanced by nutritional stressors that upset sulfur amino acid or labile methyl metabolism.

Although the carcinogenicity of inorganic arsenic from drinking water has been extensively studied, information on the carcinogenicity of arsenic in food is limited. Arsenic levels are generally high in seafood (0.39–42 ppm), and most of the dietary arsenic intake is organic and obtained from eating fish and shellfish (24). The health significance of the small fraction of inorganic arsenic in fish has not been clearly determined. Cancer risk estimated from drinking water at the current drinking water standard of 50 ppb is approximately 1/1000. More research has been proposed to reduce uncertainties in the database for risk assessment.

In vivo methylation of inorganic arsenic was considered a detoxification pathway because the acute toxicity of methyl and dimethyl arsenic acids is less than that of arsenite (As^{3+}) or arsenate (As^{5+}). More recently, a question has been raised as to whether some of the toxicity associated with inorganic arsenic exposure is due to the methylated metabolic product of inorganic arsenic or even the process by which these products are formed. Overall, the toxicity of arsenic appears to depend on the chemical form, and knowledge of the chemical form is important for risk assessment.

Organics

Methylmercury

Human exposure to methylmercury is primarily through fish consumption. Inorganic mercury is methylated by microorganisms in the aquatic environment and taken up by fish. The human health concerns from ingesting fish containing methylmercury are the potential neurologic and developmental/behavioral effects that characterize methylmercury toxicity. These can be seen as paresthesia, ataxia, impaired mental and motor development, coma, and even death.

The toxicity data for methylmercury are primarily derived from two poisoning episodes that occurred in Minamata, Japan, and Iraq (29–31). The former involved eating fish contaminated with methylmercury as a result of industrial discharge of mercury, and the latter involved eating bread made from phenylmercury-treated grains. Various estimates of exposure to methylmercury have been based on measurements of mercury in hair and blood and modeling of dietary intake based on several studies of the poisoning outbreaks. The LOEL estimated by WHO corresponds to a blood mercury level of 200 to 500 μg/L (29). Extrapolation to average daily intakes was based on the biokinetics of methylmercury distribution among body compartments. The intake of methylmercury associated with the earliest effects in the most sensitive group in the adult population was estimated to be in the range of 3 to 7 μg/kg-day, based on the most conservative (linear) relationship of steady-state blood concentrations to daily intake of methylmercury among data from numerous studies.

Several epidemiologic studies have attempted to determine a threshold for maternal exposure to methylmercury. The effects on offspring were the more sensitive endpoints. Since exposure estimates were made after the actual exposures had occurred, mercury concentrations were measured in hair and extrapolated to blood concentrations at the time of past exposures. Women with 10.0 to 19.9 μg/g of mercury in hair were twice as likely to have offspring with neurologic abnormalities as those with less than 10.0 μg/g (30). Based on all the studies combined, a maternal hair level of about 10 to 20 μg/g was considered to be associated with subtle neurologic effects in offspring. This level is also the best estimate of an effective maternal threshold dose for a developmental neurologic endpoint.

In experimental studies, methylmercury affected spermatogenesis and was fetotoxic in mice. It was teratogenic in rats and adversely affected the behavior of offspring of monkeys administered the chemical before and during pregnancy. A number of the animal studies on the reproductive or developmental effects showed effects at 1 mg/kg-day or above, while some effects on development/behavior functions were observed at dose levels below 1 mg/kg-day. The lowest no-observed-effect level (NOEL) was 5 μg/kg/day given prenatally to rats; 10 μg/kg-day caused decrements in operant behavior performance (32). Pregnant rats were treated during days 6 to 9 after conception, and the offspring were tested at 4 months of age.

The FDA's ADI for methylmercury is 30 μg/day (0.4 μg/kg-day with a 10-fold uncertainty factor) (33). The EPA's reference dose is 0.3 μg/kg-day (34). The FDA's ADI is based on a linear relationship between ingested methylmercury and blood mercury level that yielded a blood level of 200 μg/L at steady state in a study of high fish consumers with an intake of 300 μg/day in 70-kg persons. Both values are within the range calculated by the WHO.

Methylmercury is the only contaminant that has resulted in known human fatalities as a result of dramatic biomagnification in the aquatic food chain following industrial discharge. The WHO (30) concluded that the general population does not face a significant health risk from methylmercury. However, groups with high fish consumption may attain blood methylmercury levels that are associated with a low (5%) risk of neurologic damage in adults. Fetuses and children are the sensitive subpopulations.

Dioxins

Polychlorinated dibenzo-*p*-dioxins (PCDDs) and polychlorinated dibenzofurans (PCDFs) (commonly known as dioxins) are ubiquitous environmental contaminants formed as byproducts in combustion of chlorine-containing compounds (ATSDR) (35). Of the possible 75 congeners of PCDDs and 135 congeners of PCDFs, 2,3,7,8-tetrachlorodibenzo-*p*-dioxin (TCDD) is the most toxic and most extensively studied. Assessing the potential health implications of these individual compounds in various media including food is difficult because they are present as complex mixtures of PCDD and PCDF congeners with varying toxicity. Because of the presumed common mechanism of action and qualitative similarity of the toxic effects of various congeners, exposure estimates are based on toxicity estimates of each congener in a mixture and are expressed as total toxicity equivalent (TEQs). The relative toxic potential of each congener is expressed as a toxicity equivalent factor (TEF). TEF is expressed as the ratio of toxic potency of a congener to the toxic potency of TCDD, which is assigned a TEF of 1. The total TEQ of a sample is calculated by multiplying the amount of each congener present in the sample by its TEF value and then adding the products for all congeners in the mixture. Depending on the availability of toxicity data, TEFs may be based on carcinogenic, reproductive, immunotoxic, subchronic or acute effects, Ah-receptor binding, or in vitro toxicity data.

Most of the toxic effects of dioxins are attributed to a mechanism involving cytosolic receptor (Ah receptor) binding and subsequent regulation of the transcription of specific genes. The most commonly known responses include P450 enzyme induction, weight loss, thymic atrophy, immunotoxicity, teratogenicity, reproductive effects, endocrine effects, and carcinogenicity. The toxicity of dioxins varies with the species, strain, age, and sex.

TCDD has been shown to be a multisite carcinogen in both sexes and in several species, including the rat, mouse, Syrian hamster, and fish (36). In a two-stage model for liver and skin cancer, TCDD was a promoter with limited initiating activity. The EPA has estimated an NOAEL of 1 ng/kg-day based on liver cancer in female rats; using the linearized multistage model, the cancer potency was calculated to be 1.56×10^{-5}/mg/kg-day. The EPA's safe dose estimate of 0.006 pg/kg-day is based on an upper-bound excess lifetime cancer risk of 1×10^{-6} (37). The TCDD regulations of European countries and Health Canada are based on determination of the tolerable daily intake (TDI), an absence of firm scientific evidence of human carcinogenicity, and equivocal evidence on genotoxicity. Using an NOAEL of 0.001 μg/kg-day from a rat reproductive study and a safety factor of 100, Health Canada derived a TDI of 10 pg/kg-day (38).

There have been a number of human exposures to dioxins from accidental (Missouri, U.S.A., and Seveso, Italy; Yusho disease in Japan and Taiwan from contaminated rice oil) or occupational (use of Agent Orange in Vietnam by military personnel) exposure. To date, chloracne is the only proven consequence of human exposure to TCDD and related compounds. However, other toxic endpoints such as cancer, immunotoxicity, and reproductive and developmental toxicity have been suggested. A number of reports involving weight loss, digestive disorders, neurologic and psychiatric disturbances, and other nonspecific effects have also been reported. Due to the extreme toxicity of TCDD and some other congeners in various animal species, reported human exposure levels are close to Health Canada's TDI or exceed the EPA's safe dose estimate.

Most human exposure to dioxins is through contaminated food, primarily meat, dairy products, milk, eggs, and fish (35, 36). Exposure estimates from various European countries average about 120 pg/day, expressed as a TEQ. The estimated exposure of 119 pg/day in the United States is similar (36). Most daily intake (>90%) is from food (beef, 31%; dairy products, 20%; milk, 15%; fish 7%; eggs 3.4%). Small amounts are accounted for by inhalation (1.8%), soil ingestion (0.7%), and water ingestion (0.01%) (35). Children and certain subpopulations may receive a higher dose because of higher intake of such foods as milk or fish.

Polychlorinated Biphenyls

PCBs are a group of 209 chemicals containing 1 to 10 chlorine atoms attached to a biphenyl backbone. PCBs (trade name, Aroclor) were widely used as lubricants and hydraulic and cooling fluids before being banned in the mid-1970s because of their toxicity and environmental persistence. The number of chlorine atoms and their positions in PCBs are the principal determinants of their physical (vapor pressure and stability in the environment) and biologic (metabolism, receptor binding, toxicity) properties. The different Aroclor preparations contained variable mixtures of congeners and isomers, which were commercially differentiated by the average number of chlorine atoms per molecule. Thus, Aroclor 1248 contains about 48% chlorine atoms and Aroaclor 1260 contains about 60% chlorine atoms. Their large-scale use and long half-life resulted in widespread contamination of the environment.

A number of reviews on the health effects of PCBs have been published (39–41). The main effects of PCBs are hepatic enzyme induction, potential carcinogenicity, immunotoxicity, neurodevelopmental toxicity, and possible reproductive effects in experimental animals and humans. Epidemiologic studies in occupationally exposed individuals have suggested that PCBs may cause dermal lesions, changes in cytochrome P450 metabolism, respiratory effects, reproductive effects, liver function changes, malignant melanoma, and low birth weight. People consuming fish from the Great Lakes containing high concentrations of PCBs have been evaluated for reproductive effects, neurologic effects on infants, child growth and cognitive functioning, breast cancer, and immune functions. Infants born to mothers who consumed a greater amount of fish from the Great Lakes had smaller head circumference and lower birth weight than those in a low-fish-consuming population. Because many confounding factors were not properly controlled for in data analysis in these epidemiologic studies, a recent critical review suggested that the association of effects with PCB consumption was generally either negative or inconclusive (42).

Studies conducted in experimental animals show more definite toxic effects of these chemicals. A number of rat studies with Aroclor 1260 suggest increased hepatocellular carcinoma and neoplastic nodules. Aroclor 1254 and related Kanechlor 500 promote cancer development in animals exposed to another carcinogenic initiator. PCBs decrease fertility and litter size in many laboratory animals. Developmental effects such as impaired learning, decreased activity, and delayed reflex development have been reported in monkeys. Immunotoxicity has been shown in various animal species. In monkeys, an increased antibody response of IgM and IgG to sheep red blood cells was observed after 23 months of exposure to 5 μg/kg-day of Aroclor 1254.

Certain planar PCB congeners have been reported to have toxicities similar to those of TCDD, such as immunotoxicity, reproductive effects, teratogenicity, endocrine effects, and carcinogenicity (43). The binding of these compounds to the Ah receptor suggests a mechanism of action similar to that of TCDD. Thus, to simplify risk assessment, TEQs are used for these "dioxin-like" PCBs. A recent EPA draft document on dioxins recommends using international PCB TEF values (44) for risk assessment.

Because of the characteristic toxic effects of each Aroclor mixture, different toxic endpoints have been identified for PCB-induced toxicity. The EPA (45) has determined a cancer potency factor of 7.7 mg/kg-day for Aroclor 1260 based on an increased incidence of hepatocellular carcinoma. An RfD of 2×10^{-5} mg/kg-day for Aroclor 1254 is based on immunotoxicity, and a RfD of 7×10^{-5} mg/kg-day for Aroclor 1016 is based on reproductive toxicity.

Humans are exposed to PCBs from air, water, soil, and food. However, most exposure is thought to be from meat, dairy products, eggs, and fish, because of bioconcentration of PCBs in fat. Concentrations of PCBs in various media have been decreasing over the years because of restricted use since 1972. To decrease exposure to these compounds in food products, FDA set tolerances for various foods; for example, milk, 1.5 ppm; manufactured dairy products, 3 ppm; eggs, 0.3 ppm. Because of bioaccumulation of PCBs in aquatic organisms, fish consumption could be a major source of PCB exposure. Based on the FDA's total diet study survey, human exposures in 1989 were estimated to be 0.05 μg/day, compared with 6.9 μg/day in 1970 (40). Estimated human exposure from soil, air, and drinking water was 0.48 μg/day in the 1980s. Thus, the total exposure to PCBs was estimated to be 0.53 μg/day, or 0.008 μg/kg-day, based on a 70-kg human. Considering the overall human exposure to combined PCBs of 0.008 μg/kg-day and the lowest noncarcinogenic RfD of 0.02 μg/kg-day, exposure estimates are very close to the RfD.

Diethylhexylphthalate (DEHP)

Phthalate esters are added to plastics to make them flexible. Because phthalates are not part of the plastic polymer, they are easily released from the product. DEHP, one of the major phthalates, has been most studied, but usually a mixture of congeners is used. The chemicals enter the environment by vaporization from plastics in use, burning of plastic products, disposal of plastic waste in landfills, and groundwater leaching from landfills.

The oral LD_{50} for DEHP in rats exceeds 25 g/kg, suggesting a low order of acute human toxicity (49, 50). The metabolite monethylhexyl phthalate (MEHP) has a lower LD_{50}, about 1.5 g/kg, suggesting a relatively higher acute toxicity. Hepatomegaly and increased relative kidney weights have been reported in long-term animal studies. DEHP produced reproductive and developmental effects in a variety of mammalian and nonmammalian species. Several studies have shown that DEHP and MEHP cause testicular atrophy. The suggested mechanism for testicular toxicity is a membrane alteration that leads to separation of germ cells (spermatocytes and spermatids) from the underlying Sertoli cells. Younger rats seem to be more susceptible than older ones, and susceptibility seems to differ among species. MEHP also has a toxic effect on Sertoli cells in vitro. Teratogenicity studies have reported malformations in mice at dietary levels of 0.5 to 2 g/kg. Embryotoxic effects were observed at dietary levels above 10 g/kg. DEHP was negative in most genotoxicity studies; however, it induces cell transformation and is carcinogenic in rats and mice. DEHP is a strong peroxisome proliferator and its liver carcinogenicity is associated with peroxisome proliferation. Very limited information is available on the toxicity of DEHP to humans. Only gastric disturbances were reported in humans given 5 or 10 g of DEHP (49)

Morgenroth (51) determined a TDI of 1 mg/kg based on peroxisome proliferation, assuming a positive association with carcinogenicity. Based on teratogenicity, a TDI of 0.04 mg/kg was determined.

Humans may be exposed to DEHP from air, water, soil, and food (49, 50). The main source of DEHP and other phthalates in food products is from plastic used in food packaging. Persons who undergo repeated blood transfusion or dialysis may be exposed to a higher level of DEHP leached from polyvinyl chloride tubing. DEHP and other phthalate esters were reported in Canadian butter and margarine as migrating from laminated aluminum foil–paper. DEHP concentrations were estimated to be 11.9 μg/g of butter. A mean DEHP concentration below 50 μg/L in retail whole milk was observed in 1 German and 14 Danish dairy samples. A TDI of 25 μg/kg body weight is set by the EEC Scientific Committee for Food. This suggests that intake of whole milk does not constitute a health hazard for the Danish population. Migration of DEHP from plasticized tubing was found in a commercial milking operation. Concentration in the milking chamber for each individual cow averaged 30 μg/kg; this rose to 50 μg/kg in the central collecting tank. Two retail cream samples contained 1200 and 1400 μg/kg of DEHP, reflecting the association of plasticizer with the fat phase. Hand milking resulted in a DEHP concentration below 5 μg/kg. The WHO working group (49) estimated an average daily exposure to DEHP of about 300 μg/person in the U.S. in 1974 and 20 μg/person in the U.K. in 1986. Levels ranging from 13.4 to 91.5 mg/kg (dry weight) have been detected in lung tissues of patients receiving blood transfusions.

Naturally Occurring Substances

Aflatoxin and Mycrocystin

Mycotoxins are naturally occurring unintentional environmental contaminants in food. Among the mycotoxins are aflatoxins, which are fungal metabolites produced by *Aspergillus flavus* and *A. parasiticus*. Four major metabolites have been identified: aflatoxin B_1 (AFB_1), aflatoxin B_2 (AFB_2), aflatoxin G_1 (AFG_1), and aflatoxin G_2 (AFG_2). The predominant metabolite, AFB_1, is the most studied and of most public health concern. However, depending upon the environmental conditions, several metabolites may be present in different proportions in any contaminated food sample.

Aflatoxin is produced by these fungi in nut crops (peanuts, almonds, pecan, pistachios, walnuts), corn, cotton, sorghum, and millet, either in field conditions or during storage. Commercial peanuts and peanut butter are the major sources of aflatoxin exposure for consumers in the United States. FDA samples from 1984, 1985, and 1986 had average aflatoxin levels of 2.4, 1.6, and 8.3 ppb for shelled roasted peanuts and 2.1, 1.7, and 3.1 ppb for peanut butter, respectively. American Peanut Product Manufacturers Association (APPMI) samples in 1985, 1986, 1987, and 1988 had average aflatoxin levels of 1.1, 1.3, 1.3, and 1.1 ppb for roasted peanuts and 3.1, 4.0, 2.5, and 1.9 ppb, for peanut butter, respectively (46). In addition to aflatoxin exposure from contaminated or moldy food, occupational exposure may occur from inhalation of contaminated dust from milling operations.

Aflatoxin is a well-understood hepatotoxicant and hepatocarcinogen, and there is considerable evidence of its carcinogenicity from both human and animal studies (46). Accordingly, the International Agency for Research on Cancer (IARC) classified aflatoxin as a human carcinogen. Many epidemiologic studies from Asia and Africa have shown a relationship between aflatoxin exposure and development of liver cancer. However, the role of such confounding factors as hepatitis B viral (HBV) infection and alcohol consumption, which are also known to cause liver cancer, were not addressed in these studies. A recent prospective study of about 8000 people in Guangxi, China, indicated a causal relationship between aflatoxin exposure and primary hepatocellular carcinoma. Aflatoxin exposure estimates were based on the aflatoxin content of staple foods sampled twice per year over several years. The HBV status was determined by testing for hepatitis B surface antigens (HbsAg) in sera of 25% of the cohort. From this study, a cancer potency factor of 46 $(mg/kg\text{-}day)^{-1}$ is estimated based on subjects who are negative for HbsAg (47). Using epidemiologic data obtained in various countries, Kuifer-Goodman (48) estimated the TDI for total aflatoxin B_1 to be 0.11 to 0.19 ng/kg-day for a risk level of 1×10^{-5}. The author suggested that in the absence of endemic HBV infection, the TDI would be about one order of magnitude higher. It was not possible to consider confounding factors in these studies.

In experimental studies, aflatoxin induced liver tumors in mice, rats, hamsters, and primates. The rat appears to be the most sensitive species tested. The cancer potency for humans, estimated from a study in which male Fisher rats were treated with AFB_1 for 109 weeks at concentrations ranging from 1 ppb to 100 ppb, would be 2700 (mg/kg-day) (46).

In addition to liver toxicity, aflatoxin affects the reproductive, renal, and gastrointestinal systems. Both cellular and humoral parameters of immune responses were altered by doses of aflatoxin that caused no overt toxicity. Aflatoxin was genotoxic and positive in gene mutation, chromosomal aberration, unscheduled DNA synthesis, and neoplastic transformation assays. Exogenous activation is required for in vitro studies.

Using the cancer potency value of 50 $(mg/kg\text{-}day)^{-1}$ derived from the human study in China, the cancer risk associated with consumption of peanut butter at 2.5 ppb (the APPMI average value, 1985–1988) is 6×10^{-6}, assuming a lifetime average dose in the range of 1.1×10^{-7} to 1.4×10^{-7} mg/kg-day.

Mycrocystin is an algal toxin, commonly found in ditch and pond water in China. In the laboratory, this toxin can cause severe liver damage and promote hepatocellular carcinoma. Epidemiologic studies in southern China found an association between liver cancer and drinking pond and ditch water (52).

GENERALLY RECOGNIZED AS SAFE (GRAS) COMPOUNDS

A good historical perspective on GRAS compounds is given by Kilgore and Li (53). The amendment to the Food, Drug and Cosmetic (FD&C) Act in 1958 to regulate food additives recognized a category of additives presumed to be safe by the absence of toxic effects after long use. These chemicals were designated generally recognized as safe (GRAS). GRAS status can also be given to compounds determined safe by experts qualified by scientific training and experience to evaluate food safety. Additions to the GRAS list were proposed by the Flavor and Extract Manufacturers Association (FEMA) for flavoring ingredients, based on the approval of experts qualified by scientific training and experience.

Originally, GRAS status was not based on the relative toxicity or potency of the compounds, but on the assumed or apparent safety of the compounds under conditions of use. New toxicology data subsequently revealed that some GRAS compounds might have toxic potential in foods. For example, cyclamate, which had GRAS status, was later found to cause bladder cancer in rats and was banned from food. In 1970, the FDA started a review of GRAS compounds by a select committee. Based on the committee recommendations, GRAS compounds were either reaffirmed, allowed while additional data were sought, or changed to a food additive requiring toxicologic data for safety assessment. Thus, GRAS status is not permanent, and compounds can be added to or taken off the list on the basis of newly available toxicity data. Risk assessment of GRAS compounds follows the same principles and methodologies used for other chemicals.

EMERGING ISSUES

Biotechnology

Biotechnology has been practiced from ancient days to improve plants and animals, first by a simple process of selection and then by breeding and selection for desired qualities in plants or animals. Recombinant DNA techniques (genetic engineering) not only speed the process but also allow introduction of desired characteristics in plants or animals, which was not possible by traditional means. Thus, the process has a great potential to increase quality, yield, and disease resistance and to produce novel foods for specific needs. Current examples are the slow-rotting genetically engineered tomato and the administration of recombinant bovine somatotropin (r-BST) to increase milk production in cows.

However, along with desired characteristics, undesirable characteristics may also be introduced in this process. For example, introduction of an albumin from Brazil nuts into soybeans to improve the content of the sulfur-containing amino acids methionine and cysteine also transferred a main source of Brazil nut allergenic protein (54). Originally, the FDA statement of policy of 1992 dealt with such situations by requiring notification and premarket testing and labeling of foods when gene transfer is from commonly allergenic foods (54a). However, this fails to address the potential for rare protein allergies not previously known by requiring that consumers be informed of all cross-species protein transfer in the food they purchase. Gene expression depends upon the genetic makeup of the organism, and introduction of new genetic material may modify the characteristic of an existing gene and create a potential hazard for some consuming the product. Therefore, when genetic material is transferred to a product from a species not commonly used for food purposes, toxicity testing of the product would help provide data for risk assessment.

Dietary Estrogens

There is growing concern about environmental toxicants that could alter endocrine regulation, called *endocrine disrupters*. Some environmental chemicals with estrogenic activity have been associated with sexual, behavioral, and reproductive problems and carcinogenesis (55). While most of the evidence comes from domestic and wildlife species, there are recent reports of reduced sperm count in human populations over the last 40 years and increases in breast cancer incidence and endometriosis. The potential for long-term effects of endocrine disruption in humans is well recognized in the classic example of daughters who developed cervical cancer because of prenatal exposure to diethylstilbestrol after their mothers took the drug to avoid miscarriage. Another example is eggshell thinning in birds exposed to high levels of DDE, a metabolite of DDT (56). Other epidemiologic reports appear to associate human cancer of the prostate and testicles with exposure to environmental estrogenic compounds (57).

Humans are exposed to a wide variety of synthetic and naturally occurring estrogenic and antiandrogenic compounds, and the results of such exposures are difficult to predict. The final outcome depends on the complex interactions among all the factors including genetic susceptibility, duration of exposure, and stage of development during exposure. For example, neonatal exposure of rat pups through milk of dams fed either a plant isoflavonoid, coumestrol, a control, or a soy-based diet for the initial 10 days had no effect on estrous cycle, but 21-day treatment resulted in a persistent estrous state by 132 days of age. In contrast, 10-day treatment in males produced a significant defect in sexual behavior suggesting variability in endpoints. Immature females treated with natural dietary concentrations of coumestrol demonstrated estrogenic effects in the reproductive tract, brain, and pituitary. Some low-potency estrogenic environmental chemicals may have little effect on biologic systems. However, a combination of such chemicals may have synergistic effects.

Low-level exposure to environmental toxicants such as dioxins, which showed no overt toxicity, altered mating behavior and induced structural abnormalities in the external genitalia of the female rat and altered sperm count and delayed puberty in male rats. Prenatal exposure to PCBs can also delay puberty. Some dioxin-like PCBs can cause endocrine effects similar to those of dioxin. Many of these estrogenic compounds are lipophilic and are stored in the body. They can be excreted with the milk during lactation, exposing infants to very high levels. Since their developmental and reproductive effects can be delayed for a long time, it may be difficult to associate exposure to the developmental effects. Thus, the greatest uncertainty in risk assessment of endocrine disrupters is in the unborn fetus, nursing infants, and the young, who would be at greatest risk (because of their immature development) of such adverse effects.

PUBLIC HEALTH PERSPECTIVE, CURRENT METHODOLOGY AND FUTURE DIRECTIONS

Risk assessment is an important tool used by regulatory agencies to control the use of harmful substances and exposure to environmental hazards thought to be harmful to human health (59). More frequently, environmental substances or hazards are of concern in air, water, and soil rather than in food. However, many of these substances are also found in food, and thus they should be assessed in combination with all environmental exposures. Also, most essential trace elements are released into the environment in minute quantities so that no immediate effect is observed; yet they can accumulate in the environment and bioaccumulate up the food chain, and total exposure can involve multimedia exposure.

Different health agencies may have either separate or combined risk assessment and risk management practices. The overall public health perspective is gained only when agencies balance health hazards against health benefits, with a goal of providing a wholesome, nutritious, affordable food supply safe from environmental contaminants. Thus, the results of risk assessment are useful in providing information for the risk-benefit analysis that may follow.

There is an opinion that it is unrealistic to set exposure limits so low that they are unattainable in the diets of a large proportion of the population. The situation with methylmercury in fish is an example of a case in which the toxicity of a contaminant must be balanced against the health impact of severely restricting intake of the food that may contain it. At the 1988 JECFA reevaluation of methylmercury, the committee confirmed the provisional tolerable weekly intake (PTWI) of 3.3 μg/kg, noting that this weekly value could be exceeded easily, as some species of fish contain methylmercury at levels of up to several parts per million (2). However, JECFA did not strongly recommend limiting consumption of fish because of the nutritional value of fish, and efforts are under way in many countries to increase fish consumption as an integral part of a well-balanced diet. The adverse health impact of too-restrictive intake of fish may include undernutrition and lowered intake of essential nutrients. However, the committee did recommend that efforts be made to minimize industrial exposure to methylmercury. Others may hold that restricting industrial exposure is necessary to prevent methylmercury exposure. Under such circumstances, information on risk assessment of various dietary components or habits would be useful for the general public. With such information, people can make comparisons and informed decisions themselves and, at the same time, have confidence in the risk assessments performed by professionals who understand the associated health implications.

Risk communication is important to give the public confidence in risk assessment and associated decision-making processes. This activity reaches out to educate the public. To support this communication, risk analysis must describe the health risk, quality of the database, strength and weaknesses of the evidence compiled, assumptions, limitations, and uncertainties. In interpreting the results of risk assessment, one must note that the risks predicted by extrapolation from animal data are theoretical risks. In general, regulatory agencies adopt a conservative approach to ensure public health protection. Current awareness and evolving risk assessment techniques permit prediction of potential health risks to assist in developing and implementing such public health protection measures as issuing health advisories and setting exposure limits for environmental chemicals.

The current methodology in risk assessment has been considerably refined during the last 10 years, but the process still carries some limitations and uncertainties. Default assumptions are adopted to overcome data limitations in performing risk assessment. Some common uncertainties and limitations include inadequate toxicology data, extrapolation from high- to low-dose exposure, extrapolation from animal data to human situations, and the uncertainty of results produced by the theoretical modeling of exposures used in the absence of actual monitoring data. The following issues are being examined to improve the risk assessment process and the accuracy of the results: default options (e.g., conversion factors for extrapolating from animal data to humans) and the related principles for modifying and deviating from them, scientifically plausible exposure data considering human activity patterns, validation and update of methods and models for generating and analyzing data, consideration of uncertainties in methods and data obtained, variations among individuals based on sex, age, or ethnicity in their exposures to chemicals and the associated susceptibility to specific toxicity of chemicals, interactions among chemicals, and multipathway and multimedia exposures.

Although dietary exposure estimates for food contaminants should be based on the consideration of all routes of exposure, such estimates are limited by the availability of the database for food consumption rates, contaminant concentrations in various food items, and contributions from other sources of exposure, food preparation methods, bioavailability, bioactivity, monitoring data on chemical or reactive breakdown product, and chemical forms in food. With such limitations and uncertainties in mind, the question arises whether the present methodology produces relevant findings with regard to risk in foods. First, much of the limitation and uncertainty is associated with the database. As the database is strengthened, the findings will become more relevant. Second, the results of risk assessment may be applied to prevent adverse health outcomes, and an adverse health outcome will not be observed if it is prevented from occurring (e.g., risk assessment is used to set exposure limits.) Third, the results of a risk assessment may be used to predict an adverse outcome, but that outcome may take a long time to manifest itself (e.g., cancer), making it difficult to associate the outcome with exposure to a particular chemical in food ingested at a certain stage in life, unless other data and evidence exist. Fourth, an adverse effect that occurs later in life may also be masked by exposure to other possible etiologic agents. So a major question is whether data are being generated to build a database that will permit adequate assessment with current methodology. There are additional questions: What chemicals are present in our food supply and at what levels? How much of the food is monitored for chemical residues and how representative are the monitoring data of the overall food supply? What do we know of the toxicology of the chemicals and their breakdown products? As for the current methodology, guidelines provide a reasonable certainty that the conclusions drawn from risk assessment can be used to make health-protecting decisions. However, the current methodology conducts risk assessment for single chemicals, not for all chemicals that humans are simultaneously exposed to. It does permit consideration of multiple chemicals and thus allows additivity when dealing with the same health-effect endpoint. It does not usually consider synergism or antagonism between chemicals. The lack of information on other parameters of chemicals as noted above also poses a major limitation on consideration of multiple chemical exposure in risk assessment.

The FDA's total diet study (TDS) can be used to illustrate how risk assessment can help provide relevant information about risk in food. This major program provides systemic evaluation of chemicals in food in the United States. Although the TDS does not specifically conduct risk assessments, the dietary intake estimates derived for individual chemicals provide a database for comparison with health-protective values previously determined by risk assessment. No health risk is anticipated when an intake estimate is lower than a chemical's health-protective value (e.g., the WHO's ADI or the EPA's RfD).

In most cases, adults have been used for risk assessment, and thus infants and children, who may be more sensitive than adults to certain toxic properties of chemicals, may not have been adequately considered. In this regard, the recent Food Quality Protection Act of 1996 requires that the EPA address human variability and risk to infants and children and publish a specific safety finding before pesticide tolerances in food are established. It also provides for an additional safety factor (up to 10-fold) to ensure that pesticide tolerances are safe for infants and children. The EPA has been using a negligible-risk standard for chemicals that pose a carcinogenic risk, except in cases where the Delaney clause of the FFDCA applied. Prior to 1996 the FFDCA authorized pesticide residue tolerances for raw commodities under Section 408, based on risk-benefit standards, and for processed foods under Section 409, which contains the Delaney clause that prohibits carcinogens that concentrate in processed foods. This new law repeals the Delaney clause and provides for setting tolerances for pesticide residues in both raw and processed foods on the basis of a determination that the tolerances are safe. *Safe* is defined as "a reasonable certainty that no harm will result from aggregate exposure," including all dietary exposure and that from other nonoccupational sources including drinking water.

Future recognition of a health concern relating to environmental contaminants in food will rely on the availability of new toxicologic and exposure data and state-of -the-art techniques. Therefore, continued efforts in conducting food consumption surveys, total diet studies, and food residue monitoring, combined with development of our knowledge of the toxic properties of chemicals and refinement of risk assessment techniques, are necessary to provide early warning of any potential problem with chemicals in our food supply. Recent activities by the EPA, which include issuing the cancer-risk-assessment guidelines, issuing the risk-characterization guidelines, reevaluating the cancer potency of PCBs, the national forum on chemicals in fish and advisories issues, and developing a screening and testing program for endocrine disrupters, plus the passage by Congress of the Food Quality Protection Act of 1996 all point to current and future efforts in providing new developments to support risk assessment in ensuring a safe food supply. Increasing effort is also being expended to evaluate multiple chemical exposures or complex mixtures and human variability in response to chemical exposure. The variations in the kind, number, levels, intake, and combination of chemicals in any one medium, particularly food, make risk assessment of environmental chemicals in our food a very challenging task.

REFERENCES

1. Bolger PM, Carrington CD, Henry SH. Risk assessment for risk management and regulatory decision-making at the U.S. Food and Drug Administration. In: Fan AM, Chang LW, eds. Toxicology and risk assessment. Principles, methods and applications. New York: Marcel Dekker, 1995;791–8.
2. Hermal JL. Use of intake data in risk assessment by JECFA/JMPR and in Codex decisions. In: MacDonal I, ed. Monitoring dietary intakes, Washington, DC: ILSI, 1991;90–8.
3. Fan AM, Howd R, Davis B. Annu Rev Pharmacol Toxicol 1995;35:341–68.
4. Roberts WC, Abernathy CO. Risk assessment: principles and methodologies. In: Fan AM, Chang LW, eds. Toxicology and risk assessment. Principles, methods and applications. New York: Marcel Dekker, 1995;245–70.
5. U.S. FDA. Toxicological principles for the safety assessment of direct food additives and color additives used in foods. Washington, DC: U.S. Food and Drug Administration, Bureau of Foods, 1982.
6. Ames R. Epidemiology: general principles, methodological issues and applications in environmental toxicology. In: Fan AM, Chang LW, eds. Toxicology and risk assessment. Principles, methods and applications. New York: Marcel Dekker, 1995;559–72.
7. Brown JP, Salmon AG. Issues in data extrapolation. In: Fan AM, Chang LW, eds. Toxicology and risk assessment. Principles, methods and applications. New York: Marcel Dekker, 1995; 601–18.
8. Velazquez SF, Schoeny R, Cogliano VJ, et al. Cancer risk assessment: historical perspectives, current issues, and future directions. In: Fan AM, Chang LW, eds. Toxicology and risk assessment. Principles, methods and applications. New York: Marcel Dekker, 1995;219–44.
9. Cicmanec JL, Dourson ML, Hertzberg RC. Noncancer risk assessment: principles and methodologies. In: Fan AM, Chang LW, eds. Toxicology and risk assessment. Principles, methods and applications. New York: Marcel Dekker, 1995; 245–70.
10. Fan AM. Pesticides and food safety. In: Handbook of hazardous marterials. San Diego: Academic Press, 1993;563–76.
11. U.S. Department of Agriculture. Food intakes: individuals in 48 states, year 1977–78. Nationwide food consumption survey 1977–78, rep. no. 1-1. Hyattsville, MD: U.S. Department of Agriculture, 1983;1–617.
12. USDA (U.S. Department of Agriculture) 1993. Food and nutrient intake by individuals in the United States, 1 Day, 1987–88:

Nationwide Food Consumption survey, rep. no. 87-I-1. Hyattsville, MD: Human Nutrition Information Service, U.S. Department of Agriculture.

13. Gunderson EL. FDA total diet study, April 1982–April 1994: dietary intake of pesticides, selected elements, and other chemicals. J Assoc Off Anal Chem 1988;71:1200–9.
14. Rees N, Tennant D. Estimation of food chemical intake. In: Kotsonis FN, Mackey M, Hjelle J, eds. Nutritional toxicology. New York: Raven Press, 1994;199–221.
15. National Research Council. Recommended dietary allowances, 10th ed. Washington, DC: National Academy Press, 1989.
16. CDC. Preventing lead poisoning in young children. Atlanta, GA: Centers for Disease Control, 1991.
17. Carrington CD, Bolger PM. Regul Toxicol Pharmacol 1992; 16:265–72.
18. Pirkle J, Brody D, Gunter E, et al. JAMA 1994;272:284–91.
19. Cantilli R, Abernathy CO, Donohue JM. Derivation of the reference dose for zinc. In: Mertz W, Abernathy CO, Olin SS, eds. Risk assessment of essential elements. Washington, DC: International Life Sciences Institute (ILSI), 1994;113–26.
20. Yadrick MK, Kenney MA, Winterfeldt ZA. Am J Clin Nutr 1989;49:145–50.
21. Environmental Protection Agency. Selenium. Cincinnati, OH: Integrated Risk Information Service (IRIS), updated 1992, printed 1996.
22. Yang GS, Yin S, Zhon R, et al. J Trace Elem Electrolytes Health Dis 1989;3(2):123–30.
23. Fan AM, Kizer KW. West J Med 1990;153:160–7.
24. Uthus EO. Estimation of safe and adequate daily intake for arsenic. In: Mertz W, Abernathy CO, Olin SS, eds. Risk assessment of essential elements. Washington, DC: International Life Sciences Institute, 1994;273–82.
25. ATSDR. Toxicology profile for arsenic. Atlanta: Agency for Toxic Substances Disease Registry, 1994.
26. Abernathy C. The arsenic reference dose. In: Mertz W, Abernathy CO, Olin SS, eds. Risk assessment of essential elements. Washington, DC: International Life Sciences Institute, 1994;283–93.
27. Tseng WP, Chu HM, How SW, et al. J Natl Cancer Inst 1968;40:453–61.
28. Tseng WP. Environ Health Perspect 1977;19:109–19.
29. WHO. Environmental health criteria no. 1. Mercury. Geneva: World Health Organization. 1976.
30. WHO. Environmental health criteria doc. no. 101. Methylmercury. Geneva: World Health Organization, 1990.
31. Fan AM, Chang LW. In: Dillon HK, Ho MH, eds. Biological monitoring of exposures to chemicals: metals. New York: John Wiley & Sons, 1991;223–39.
32. Bornhausen M, Musch HR, Grem H. Toxicol Appl Pharmacol 1980;56:305–10.
33. Tollefson L, Cordle F. Environ Health Perspect 1986;68:203–8.
34. EPA. Methylmercury. Integrated Risk Information Service (IRIS). Last evaluated 1996. Printed 1996. Cincinnati, OH: U.S. Environmental Protection Agency.
35. ATSDR (Agency for Toxic Substances and Disease Registry) Toxicology profile for 2,3,7,8-tetrachlorodibenzo-*p*-dioxin. Prepared by Syracuse Research Corporation for ATSDR. Atlanta: ATSDR/TP-99/23. NTIS PB89-214522, 1989.
36. U.S. EPA. Estimating exposure to dioxin-like compounds, vol 1: Executive summary (EPA/600/6-88/005). Washington, DC: Office of Research and Development, 1994;1–112.
37. Kociba RJ, Keyes DG, Beyer JE, et al. Toxicol Appl Pharmacol 1978;46:279–303.
38. Feeley MM, Grant DL. Regul Toxicol Pharmacol 1993;18: 428–37.
39. ASTDR. Toxicological profile for elected PCBs (Aroclor-1260, -1254, -1248, -1242, -1232, -1221 and 1016). Atlanta, GA: Agency for Toxic Substances and Disease Registry, U.S. Department of Health and Human Services, 1993.
40. Expert Panel. Regul Toxicol Pharmacol 1994;20:S187–307.
41. Safe S. Crit Rev Toxicol 1994;24:87–149.
42. Swanson GM, Ratcliffe HE, Fischer J. Regul Toxicol Pharmacol 1995;21:136–50.
43. Davis D, Safe S. Toxicol Appl Pharmacol 1988;94:141–9.
44. Ahlborg UG, Becking CC, Birnbaum LS, et al. Chemosphere 1994;1049–67.
45. EPA PCB. Integrated Risk Information Service (IRIS) printed 1996. Cincinnati, OH: U.S. Environmental Protection Agency.
46. Cal/EPA. Risk specific intake levels for the proposition 65 carcinogen aflatoxin. Berkeley, CA: California Environmental Protection Agency, 1990;1–182.
47. Wu-Williams AH, Zeise L, Thomas D. Risk Analysis 1992;12: 559–67.
48. Kuifer-Goodman T. Prevention of human mycotoxicoses through risk assessment and risk management. In: Miller JD, Trenholm ML, eds. Mycotoxins in grains: compounds other than aflatoxins. St. Paul, MN: Eager Press, 1994;439–69.
49. WHO. Dielhylhexyl phthale. Environmental health criteria doc. no. 131 Geneva: World Health Organization, 1992.
50. Woodward KN, Smith AM, Mariscotti SP, et al. HSE toxicity review 1985;1–183.
51. Morgenroth V. Food Addit Contam 1993;3:363–73.
52. Skolnick AA. JAMA 1996;276:1458–9.
53. Kilgore WW, Li M. Food additives and contaminants . In: Doul J, Klassen C, Amdur MO, eds. Casarett & Doull's toxicology. The basic science of poisons. 2nd ed. New York: Macmillan, 1986.
54. Nordlee JA, Steve MS, Taylor L, et al. N Engl J Med 1996;334:688–92.

54a. FDA. Fed Register 1992;57:22984.

55. Whitten PL, Lewis C, Russel E, Naftolin F. J Nutr 1995;125(3 Suppl):7715–65.
56. Calborn T, Frederick S, Saal V, et al. Environ Health Prospect 1993;101:378–84.
57. Birnbanm LS. Environ Health Prospect 1994;102:676–9.
58. Arnold SF, Klotz DM, Bridgette M, et al. Science 1996;272:1498–2.
59. Johnson BL, Ademoyero A. A public health perspective on risk assessment of essential elements. In: Mertz W, Abernathy CO, Olin SS, eds. Risk assessment of essential elements. Washington, DC: International Life Sciences Institute, 1994; 3–12.

SUGGESTED READINGS

ASTDR. Toxicological profile for selected PCBs (Aroclor-1260, -1254, -1248, -1242, -1232, -1221 and 1016). Atlanta, GA: Agency for Toxic Substances and Disease Registry, U.S. Department of Health and Human Services, 1993.

Fan AM, Chang L, eds. Toxicology and risk assessment. New York: Marcel Dekker, 1995.

Mertz W, Abernathy CO, Olin SS, eds. Risk assessment of essential elements. Washington, DC: International Life Sciences Institute (ILSI), 1994.

U.S. EPA. Estimating exposure to dioxin-like compounds, vol 1: Executive summary (EPA/600/6-88/005). Washington, DC: Office of Research and Development, 1994;1–112.

WHO. Environmental health criteria doc. no. 101. Methylmercury. Geneva: World Health Organization, 1990.

115. Food Labeling, Health Claims, and Dietary Supplement Legislation

ALLAN L. FORBES and STEPHEN H. MCNAMARA

Chapter 94 in the 8th edition of this textbook, entitled "National Nutrition Policy, Food Labeling and Health Claims," discussed food labeling and health claims and reviewed three aspects of national nutrition policy: the key players, the system, and the policy (1). This chapter updates events related to food labeling and health claims from early 1993 to the spring of 1996 and reviews the Dietary Supplement Health and Education Act of 1996.

FOOD LABELING AND HEALTH CLAIMS: AN UPDATE

The Congress has become the leader in establishing national nutritional policy. On November 8, 1990, President Bush signed into law the Nutrition Labeling and Education Act of 1990, which in general became operational law as of November 8, 1992 (2). Much of the first part of this chapter pertains to implementation of the 1990 act. On October 25, 1994, President Clinton signed into law the Dietary Supplement Health and Education Act of 1994 (3); from a nutrition science point of view, this is one of the most unusual pieces of "health" legislation ever passed and certainly the most important nutritional event at the federal level over the past 4 years.

Despite the debates in the 104th Congress, little has changed on such matters as food stamps, school breakfast and lunch programs, other nutrition-related "entitlement" programs and nutritional research funding. The scientifically based nutrition infrastructure remains intact at the federal level at this time. This infrastructure provides the base for evolution of food labeling and health claims and implementation of the dietary supplement legislation.

Federal Agencies

National Institutes of Health (NIH)

In fiscal year (FY) 1988, support for nutritional research and training at the NIH was $276 million (1), and in FY 1993, it had increased to $373 million (4). This total represents the combined individual contribution of 17 NIH institutes and two centers. As in the past, NIH provides about three-quarters of support for nutritional research at the federal level, and the two biggest contributors continue to be the National Cancer Institute (NCI) and the National Heart, Lung and Blood Institute (NHLBI). Administration of the NIH Nutrition Coordinating Committee (NCC) has been moved from the Office of the Director of NIH to the Division of Nutrition Research Coordination, National Institute of Diabetes and Digestive and Kidney Diseases (NIDDK). The functions of the NCC remain the same, and NIH continues to be a very active participant in governmentwide coordinating committees.

Department of Agriculture (USDA)

Since FY 1991, there has been a dramatic shift in USDA resources toward food and nutritional programs (5). In FY 1991, 47% of the total USDA budget went to support such programs. In FY 1996, this rose to 60%, specifically to $39.8 billion, administered by the USDA Food and Consumer Service. As in the past, the lion's share of the total is now distributed as follows: *(a)* Food Stamp Program: $27.6 billion; *(b)* School Lunch Program: $4.4 billion; *(c)* School Breakfast Program: $1.2 billion; and *(d)* Special Supplemental Nutrition Program for Women, Infants and Children (WIC): $3.5 billion. There have been no fundamental policy changes at the USDA. Unfortunately, the Congress has only extended USDA's efforts in nutritional research, education, and economics for 2 years, so the fate of these programs remains unclear, and the matter will be a major policy issue for the next several years. In 1994, USDA established their internal Nutrition Education and Research Coordinating Council.

USDA plays a major role in the interdepartmental committees known as the Interagency Board on Nutrition Monitoring and Related Research and the Interagency Committee on Human Nutrition Research. The total USDA support for human nutritional research, monitoring, and education in FY 1993 was $343.5 million, somewhat higher than that of NIH (6). The Agricultural Research Service (ARS) continues to support its five nutrition research centers, and has added a new one recently:

the Arkansas Children's Hospital Research Institute in Little Rock. USDA's Continuing Survey of Food Intakes by Individuals (CSFII) remains ongoing under its 1994–96 plan. In 1995, USDA in collaboration with the Department of Health and Human Services (DHHS) published the 4th edition of *Nutrition and Your Health: Dietary Guidelines for Americans* (7). The seven basic guidelines remain much the same as in the 1st edition issued in 1980 (which one of us, ALF, coauthored). USDA's approach to food labeling is discussed further below.

Food and Drug Administration (FDA)

Most of this chapter is devoted to recent activities of the FDA; hence, comments here are limited. The food and nutritional activities of FDA continue to be administered by the FDA Center for Food Safety and Applied Nutrition (CFSAN). CFSAN has begun to go "outside" for advice and counsel, particularly by establishing the FDA Food Advisory Committee. This committee has already had a significant impact on nutrition policies, e.g., recommending approval of the nonabsorbable fat substitute olestra. This recommendation was accepted by CFSAN, and a final rule approving olestra as a food additive was issued on January 30, 1996 (8). The science base at CFSAN has been modified in the last several years as the focus has shifted from in-house nutritional research and development to purely regulatory issues. On April 15, 1996, FDA and the University of Maryland announced formation of a unique partnership program, the Joint Institute for Food Safety and Applied Nutrition (JIFSAN). FDA issues are discussed further below.

Centers for Disease Control (CDC)

In February 1996, the National Health and Nutrition Examination Survey (NHANES-IV) was nearly cancelled by Congress (9). It now appears that it has survived and will start in 1998. The NHANES surveys (including food labeling) are fundamental to our entire nutritional efforts at the national level, as operated by the National Center for Health Statistics (NCHS), which is part of CDC, located in Hyattsville, Maryland, and further supported by the Nutritional Biochemistry Branch at CDC in Atlanta.

Life Sciences Research Office (LSRO), Federation of American Societies for Experimental Biology (FASEB)

In December 1995, LSRO published a very extensive report entitled "Third Report on Nutrition Monitoring in the United States" (10). The report was prepared under a joint contract with USDA and DHHS and is required by Congress at least every 5 years under the provisions of the National Nutrition Monitoring and Related Research Act of 1990. The report is based on national data through June 1994. It provides the foundation for current nutritional status, covering nutrition-related health status (e.g., lipid status, obesity, hypertension, osteoporosis, maternal and child health), food consumption, nutrient intakes from food, dietary supplement use, household food expenditures, etc. The report provides information of major importance for the evolution of nutrition labeling. LSRO also has two major efforts under way currently under FDA contract that will affect food labeling: *(a)* criteria required to establish safety decisions about new food ingredients and *(b)* assessment of nutrient requirements for infant formulas.

Food and Nutrition Board (FNB), Institute of Medicine (IOM), National Academy of Sciences (NAS).

The FNB has one major current activity that will have a direct impact on food labeling. The board is updating their classic series of texts on recommended dietary allowances. The first publication has been issued (10a), cosponsored by NIH, FDA, and USDA (see Appendix Tables II-A-2-b).

Implementation of the Nutritional Labeling and Education Act of 1990 (NLEA)

A "Primer" on Terminology

Before getting into the specifics of implementation, a brief "primer" on terminology seems in order because of a general lack of understanding of certain terms that govern implementation of acts such as the NLEA. *Content claims* in labeling refer to such adjectival descriptors of food characteristics as "low fat," "reduced calorie," and "healthy." No mention of diseases is involved. *Health claims* is a bit of a misnomer because it involves label claims referring to specific diseases or conditions such as "osteoporosis," "cardiovascular disease," and "hypertension." Such claims are better categorized as *disease-specific claims.*

The Federal Register (FR) is distinct from the Code of Federal Regulations (CFR). The FR, published every working day of the year, provides an enormous array of notices by every segment of the federal government. Further, the FR provides details of why a specific regulation is being proposed or finalized, including the history of the idea, the science base, responses to comments received, cost analyses, and potential environmental impacts. All regulatory concepts must first be proposed in the FR for public comment before a final order is issued. The downside is that for practical purposes, these scholarly discussions are lost. Few libraries and fewer individuals can store and easily retrieve specific items in the FR because of its enormous size. (References to the FR are usually in a form such as 58 FR January 6, 1993, page 2066 where "58" refers to the volume, and the page listed is the first page for the notice.)

The CFR is exactly what it says it is—a compilation of actual finalized regulations, usually short, and without any of the justification for the regulations provided in the FR. All effective regulations governmentwide are published once a year in a massive collection of volumes, usually in April. All FDA regulations are in Title (or volume) 21; USDA nutrition-related regulations are in Title 9. (References to the CFR are usually in a form such as 21 CFR 101.12, where "21" refers to the title, and 101.12 refers to the specific section in the CFR.) The regulation is easy to find; how it got there is not.

Implementation of the NLEA

On January 6, 1993, FDA issued in the FR the core final rules to implement the NLEA. In that one issue, 897 pages were devoted to the task—obviously a massive effort by FDA (11). Since then, FDA has issued over 40 major regulations for NLEA and many more minor regulations to revise existing regulations for such things as standardized foods and food additive regulations. There are four consequences of all this: *(a)* nutrition labeling is now virtually universal on packaged foods; *(b)* new nomenclature for declaring nutrient contents has been implemented, specifically, reference daily intakes (RDIs) and daily reference values (DRVs) have replaced the former USRDAs, and are combined as "Daily Values" (DVs) on labels; *(c)* the format of the nutrition label has been simplified, standardized, and made more flexible; and *(d)* a series of disease-specific claims are now authorized. Review of each regulatory proposal and final order would be information overload, so comment is limited to regulations of particular interest to the nutrition community.

The January 6, 1993 FR provided the general rules for implementation of the NLEA as a preamble (12). It then established the mandatory status of nutrition labeling (12) (now 21 CFR 101.9), revised the format (13) (now 21 CFR 101.9), and established effective dates for implementation by industry (February 14 and May 8, 1994) (13, 14).

This same issue of the FR contained the final rule to replace the USRDAs with the new RDIs and DRVs (15), now universally used. Also, an enormous final rule on serving sizes of foods was issued, covering hundreds of individual foods ([16], now 21 CFR 101.12). Simultaneously, a final order was issued on nutrient content claims (17), including general principles (now 21 CFR 101.13); definitions of terms such as *low, good source of, light, reduced,* and *fresh;* voluntary nutritional labeling of restaurant foods (now 21 CFR 101.10); and revision of a long series of new regulations governing label statements for foods for special dietary use (now 21 CFR part 105), e.g., weight reduction products.

Also, in the same issue of the FR, USDA published its final rules governing labeling of meat and poultry products (18) (now 9 CFR parts 317, 320, and 381), stating "FSIS's (Food Safety and Inspection Service) nutrition labeling final regulations for meat and poultry products will parallel to the extent possible, as authorized by the Federal Meat Inspection Act and the Poultry Products Inspection Act, FDA's nutrition labeling regulations promulgated under the Nutrition Labeling and Education Act."

USDA did in fact do precisely that. Consequently, USDA labeling in the marketplace is almost identical to that of FDA-labeled products. USDA's regulations provide for "voluntary nutrition labeling on single-ingredient, raw meat and poultry products, and by establishing mandatory nutrition labeling for all other meat and poultry products, with certain exceptions." USDA accepted most of FDA's nutrient-content claim definitions but had a problem with lipids, simply because meat and poultry by nature contribute significantly to lipid intake. USDA therefore emphasized additional adjectival descriptors such as "lean" and "extra lean." For example, the regulation 9 CFR 317.362 states, "The term 'lean' may be used on the label or in labeling of a meat product, provided that the product contains less than 10 grams fat, less than 4 grams saturated fat, and less than 95 milligrams cholesterol per 100 grams and Reference Amount Customarily Consumed (RACC) for individual foods, and per 100 grams and labeled serving size for meal-type products."

FDA Rules for Disease-Specific Claims

Starting on January 6, 1993, FDA's initial final rules for disease-specific claims were issued as required by Congress (briefly reviewed in [1]). Because they are fundamental parts of the current scheme for food labeling they deserve iteration. (The general requirements for disease-specific claims are now 21 CFR 101.14.) Specific claims and their status are:

1. Fiber and cancer: *not authorized,* but a claim is authorized for diets low in fat and high in fiber and containing grain products, fruits, and vegetables. (Now 21 CFR 101.76.)
2. Fiber and cardiovascular disease: *not authorized,* but a claim is authorized for diets low in saturated fat and cholesterol and high in fruits, vegetables, and grain products. (Now 21 CFR 101.77.)
3. Folic acid and neural tube defects: *not authorized in 1993, but recently authorized.* In the March 5, 1996, issue of the FR, FDA finalized authorization of a health claim for folic acid and neural tube defects for both conventional foods and dietary supplements (now 21 CFR 101.79) (19). In addition, in this same FR issue (61 FR 8781), FDA mandated that standardized enriched grain products such as enriched bread, rolls, and buns add folate and amended a long series of standards of identity accordingly.
4. Antioxidant vitamins and cancer: *not authorized,* but a claim is authorized re substances in diets low in fat and high in fruits and vegetables. (Now 21 CFR 101.71.)
5. Zinc and immune function in the elderly; *not authorized.* (Now 21 CFR 101.71.)
6. Calcium and osteoporosis: *authorized.* (Now 21 CFR 101.72.)
7. ω-3 Fatty acids and coronary heart disease: *not authorized.* (Now 21 CFR 101.71.)
8. Dietary saturated fat and cholesterol and coronary heart disease: *authorized.* (Now 21 CFR 101.75.)
9. Dietary fat and cancer: *authorized.* (Now 21 CFR 101.73.)
10. Sodium and hypertension: *authorized.* (Now 21 CFR 101.74.)

Currently, there are two new proposals by the FDA to add to the list of authorized disease-specific claims: *(a)* On

July 20, 1995, FDA proposed authorizing a health claim on the association between sugar alcohols and nonpromotion of dental caries (20), referring particularly to xylitol, sorbitol, mannitol, maltitol, isomalt, lactitol, hydrogenated starch hydrolysates, and hydrogenated glucose syrups and *(b)* on January 4, 1996, FDA proposed authorizing a health claim on the association between oat products (i.e., oat bran and oatmeal) and reduced risk of coronary heart disease (21).

As pointed out above, FDA has issued a huge number of regulations to implement the NLEA. Many are technical corrections or additions, but one more deserves mention. On December 28, 1995, FDA issued a final order (22) establishing new RDIs for vitamin K, selenium, manganese, chromium, molybdenum, and chloride but not for fluoride. This action amends 21 CFR 101.9. The new regulation has one unfortunate drawback—on the label, it separates chloride from the other classic electrolytes, i.e., sodium and potassium. Appeals have been made in this regard.

As reported in *Food Labeling & Nutrition News* of May 2, 1996 (23), a number of consumer studies have been conducted recently by FDA and the private sector on the relative success of the new food labeling approach. Most consumers find the new labels easier to understand, but considerable concern about label accuracy remains, and in many cases, consumers are downright suspicious of health claims, particularly because of the plethora of often-conflicting health claims they confront from the media. Many believe that the label information is at the discretion of the manufacturer, and that such information is not strictly regulated by FDA. At best, one can reasonably conclude that implementation of the NLEA has been only a modest success, in spite of the enormous efforts devoted to its implementation.

In some regards, FDA has been a bit overzealous in implementing labeling for disease-specific claims. For example, consider the regulation for calcium and osteoporosis. Most manufacturers would simply like to claim that "calcium helps prevent osteoporosis," when their food product contains a reasonable amount of calcium. However, the FDA regulation (21 CFR 101.72) provides several model label statements that they anticipate being used. For example, one such model for foods exceptionally high in calcium and most calcium supplements states: "Regular exercise and a healthy diet with enough calcium helps teen and young adult white and Asian women maintain good bone health and may reduce their high rate of osteoporosis later in life. Adequate calcium intake is important, but daily intakes above about 2,000 mg are not likely to provide any additional benefit." Given the limited space on food labels, that is too long. Thus, there are not a lot of disease-specific claims being made in the marketplace at present.

For the most part, the American public seems nutritionally illiterate, and they will remain so until our schools make nutritional education an integral part of health and science education. The food label does not substitute for such education.

DIETARY SUPPLEMENT HEALTH AND EDUCATION ACT OF 1994

Regulation of Dietary Supplements

During the period 1992–1994, there was extensive pressure on Congress to amend the Federal Food, Drug, and Cosmetic Act (FDCA) to reduce the regulatory burdens on dietary supplements. Many senators and representatives claimed to be receiving more mail, more phone calls, and generally more constituent pressure on this subject than on anything else—including healthcare reform, abortion, or the deficit.

Not surprisingly, given all of this pressure, Congress eventually passed the Dietary Supplement Health and Education Act of 1994 (DSHEA) (24). The House of Representatives approved the measure by unanimous consent on October 7, 1994, and the Senate approved it, also by unanimous consent, on October 8, 1994. The president signed it into law on October 25, 1994.

The new law, like virtually all legislation, is a compromise. It does not include all of the restraints on FDA regulation of dietary supplements that the sponsors had originally wanted. Furthermore, it imposes some significant new requirements for such products. Nevertheless, viewed as a whole, this legislation is a very favorable development for those who want to sell or consume a free range of dietary supplements of vitamins, minerals, herbs, other botanicals, amino acids, and other similar substances.

Expanded Definition of "Dietary Supplement"

For many years, there has been a substantial business in the selling of "dietary supplements" in the United States (25). These products, usually tablets or capsules, have provided not only vitamins or minerals viewed as "essential" by the mainstream community of nutritionists, such as vitamin A or iron, but also other substances that FDA personnel often have regarded as being of dubious usefulness—substances ranging from rutin and other bioflavonoids to herbs to shark cartilage.

Until the DSHEA was passed, agency personnel often maintained that it was "misleading" and improper to distribute as a "dietary supplement" a substance that the agency regarded as lacking in nutritional usefulness. Agency personnel sometimes also asserted that a substance that did not provide "taste, aroma, or nutritional value" in its dietary supplement (pill-type) form could not properly be sold as a food product (26).

The new DSHEA deals with this fundamental definitional matter by unequivocally providing a broad, expansive definition of *dietary supplement* that includes a "product . . . intended to supplement the diet that bears or contains . . . a vitamin; . . . a mineral; . . . an herb or other botanical; . . . an amino acid; . . . a dietary substance for use by man to supplement the diet by increasing the total dietary intake; or . . . a concentrate, metabolite, constituent, extract, or combination [of any ingredient described above]" (27). The practical effect of this definition makes it clear that the new provisions of the DSHEA for dietary supplements apply broadly to a wide class of products, including products that FDA nutritionists might regard as having no nutritional value.

Exemption of Dietary Ingredients in Dietary Supplements from "Food Additive" Status

One of the most important provisions of the new law, from the perspective of manufacturers of dietary supplement products, is the explicit amendment of the FDCA to be clear that the term *food additive* does not apply to a dietary ingredient in, or intended for use in, a dietary supplement (28)

Previously, FDA had argued that substances added to dietary supplement products were much like substances added to any other food product, i.e., that if such a substance was not "generally recognized as safe" (not GRAS) by "experts," based on published scientific literature, it would be subject to regulation as a "food additive" (29). Under the FDCA, if a substance is a food additive, it may not be added to food products unless a food additive regulation, issued by FDA, explicitly permits such addition (30). Typically, preparation of a food additive petition, including needed research (often involving extensive animal feeding studies) and participation in the ensuing administrative proceedings, can cost a petitioner $1 million or more; and after receiving even a well-founded food additive petition, it often takes FDA 5 years or more to issue an approving food additive regulation (31).

The "bottom line" of all of this for dietary supplements had been that alleged "food additive" status and the absence of a food additive regulation approving use as a dietary supplement meant alleged *illegality* and ended or curtailed marketing of many products. Based on allegations of "unapproved food additive" status, before the DSHEA, FDA had pursued regulatory actions against numbers of popular dietary supplement ingredients—including, for example, calcium acetate, orotate compounds such as magnesium orotate, evening primrose oil, black currant oil, borage seed oil, linseed/flaxseed oil, chlorella, lobelia, St. Johnswort, and coenzyme Q10.

The new law, thus, frees dietary supplement ingredients from the continuing risk that at any time, FDA might assert that its scientists did not believe that a particular dietary ingredient was GRAS for use in dietary supplements, and therefore, the ingredient was an unapproved food additive and illegal.

New Safety Standards

As a quid pro quo, however, the new law replaces the voided food additive provisions with some new safety standards. In general, the DSHEA provides that a dietary supplement will be deemed to be adulterated if it "presents a *significant or unreasonable risk of illness or injury*" [emphasis added] ("under . . . conditions of use recommended or suggested in labeling, or . . . if no conditions of use are suggested or recommended in the labeling, under ordinary conditions of use") (32). The new law is also clear, however, that FDA shall bear the burden of proof in court if it asserts that a dietary supplement is adulterated under this standard (33).

There are additional requirements with respect to a *new* dietary ingredient, i.e., an ingredient that "was not marketed in the United States before October 15, 1994" (34). A dietary supplement that contains a *new* dietary ingredient is deemed to be adulterated unless either *(a)* the supplement "contains only dietary ingredients which have been present in the food supply as an article used for food in a form in which the food has not been chemically altered," or *(b)* there is a "history of use or other evidence of safety establishing that the dietary ingredient when used under the conditions recommended or suggested in the labeling . . . will reasonably be expected to be safe" (35). In the latter case, "at least 75 days before being introduced or delivered for introduction into interstate commerce," the manufacturer or distributor of the dietary ingredient or dietary supplement must provide "the Secretary [of Health and Human Services] with information, including any citation to published articles, which is the basis on which the manufacturer or distributor has concluded that a dietary supplement containing such dietary ingredient will reasonably be expected to be safe" (36).

In addition, the new legislation provides that the secretary of health and human services may declare a dietary supplement "to pose an imminent hazard to public health or safety," in which case it immediately becomes illegal to market the product, although the secretary must promptly hold a formal hearing to assemble data "to affirm or withdraw the declaration" (37). The new law gives the authority to declare a dietary supplement an "imminent hazard" only to the secretary, and it *may not be delegated to the FDA.*

In sum, under the new law, with respect to safety, the FDA-asserted "food additive" requirement for agency *preclearance* of dietary ingredients not believed by FDA to be GRAS was deleted, but FDA and the secretary were granted substantial new *policing* authority to stop distribution of a dietary supplement if government personnel believe they can show that the product is not safe.

The amendment to the food additive definition that exempts ingredients in dietary supplement products only applies to "dietary ingredients," that is, an ingredient that is a vitamin, a mineral, an herb or other botanical, an amino acid, a "dietary substance for use by man to supplement the diet by increasing the total dietary intake," or a "concentrate, metabolite, constituent, extract, or combination" of any of these (38). This means that an ingredient added to a dietary supplement product as a binder, diluent, or preservative or for any other nondietary purpose remains subject to the food additive provisions of the FDCA and, if not "generally recognized as safe" for its intended use, may require approval of a food additive regulation prior to use (39). Furthermore, if an ingredient is added to a dietary supplement product for use as a color, it would be subject to the "color additive" approval requirements of the FDCA (40).

It may take some time for FDA to develop a consistent policy and practice concerning the nature and degree of risk to human health that will elicit regulatory action against an allegedly adulterated dietary supplement product under the new safety standards in the DSHEA. Nevertheless, it seems clear already that FDA has not abandoned safety-related enforcement actions against dietary supplement products that contain ingredients it believes present unreasonable risk to the public health. FDA has issued at least one warning letter and a related public warning asserting that a dietary supplement containing a particular combination of herbs was unsafe and adulterated within the meaning of the new standards of the DSHEA (41).

New Rights for Sellers to Convey Information about Usefulness of Dietary Supplements

Some of the most intriguing, and potentially important, changes brought about by the new legislation relate to new freedoms for sellers of dietary supplements to use published literature to convey information to potential customers about the usefulness of dietary ingredients. Prior to enactment of the new legislation, FDA routinely asserted that a book, article, or other publication used in connection with the sale of a dietary supplement to customers could be regulated as "labeling" for the product, and if the publication included information to the effect that an ingredient present in the product might be useful in the cure, mitigation, treatment, or prevention of any disease, the product itself was subject to regulation as a *drug*. For example, FDA would assert that someone selling a dietary supplement product could not promote that product to customers by showing them (in connection with selling the product) copies of books or articles that claimed disease prevention benefits for nutrients in the supplement (42).

The new law greatly restricts the FDA's ability to object to the use of books and other publications in connection with the sale of dietary supplement products. In a significant new provision, the law provides that a "publication," including "an article, a chapter in a book, or an official abstract of a peer-reviewed scientific publication that appears in an article and was prepared by the author or the editors of the publication," "shall not be defined as labeling" and may be "used in connection with the sale of a dietary supplement to consumers" *if* the publication is "reprinted in its entirety" *and* meets certain specific criteria. Among these criteria: *(a)* the publication must not be "false or misleading," *(b)* it must not "promote a particular manufacturer or brand of a dietary supplement," *(c)* it must be "displayed or presented . . . so as to present a balanced view of the available scientific information," *(d) if* "displayed in an establishment," it must be "physically separate from the dietary supplements," and *(e)* it must *not* "have appended to it any information by sticker or any other method" (43).

So long as these criteria are met, the new law would appear to allow a salesperson to show a potential customer published nutritional or other scientific literature that describes the health benefits of a dietary supplement's ingredients. Furthermore, an additional, explicit provision in the new legislation states that it shall *not* "restrict a retailer or wholesaler of dietary supplements in any way whatsoever in the sale of books or other publications as a part of the business of such retailer or wholesaler" (44). This is the first affirmative provision in the FDCA that protects the right of those selling dietary supplements to sell "books or other publications" as well—publications that would, of course, be expected to describe the health-related benefits of nutrients and to help sell dietary supplements as well as educate customers.

FDA Statements of Nutritional Support

FDA regulations published pursuant to the NLEA provide that *no* "health claim" may appear on the label or in other labeling (including brochures) for food products, *including dietary supplements,* unless FDA has first approved use of the claim in a final regulation (45). As a new exception to the general requirement for FDA approval of health claims in food labeling, under the DSHEA dietary supplements are *allowed* to have four types of "statements of nutritional support" on labels or in other labeling *without* obtaining FDA approval (46):

1. A statement that "claims a benefit related to a classical nutrient deficiency disease and discloses the prevalence of such disease in the United States"
2. A statement that "describes the role of a nutrient or dietary ingredient intended to affect the structure or function in humans"
3. A statement that "characterizes the documented mechanism by which a nutrient or dietary ingredient acts to maintain such structure or function"
4. A statement that "describes general well-being from consumption of a nutrient or dietary ingredient"

The legislation provides that such a statement may be made in labeling for a dietary supplement *if* (47)

1. The manufacturer "has substantiation that such statement is truthful and not misleading"
2. The labeling contains, prominently displayed, the following additional text: "This statement has not been evaluated by the Food and Drug Administration. This product is not intended to diagnose, treat, cure, or prevent any disease"
3. The manufacturer notifies FDA "no later than 30 days after the first marketing of the dietary supplement with such statement that such a statement is being made"

Summary Effect of DSHEA

In summary, the new legislation will substantially change the way FDA regulates dietary supplements. As discussed above, in general, the legislation:

1. Creates a broad, new definition of "dietary supplement" products

2. Moderates the regulatory burdens for use of dietary ingredients in dietary supplements, both *(a)* changing the safety standards for use of an ingredient and *(b)* generally changing the regulating procedure from preclearance to policing
3. Permits additional use of information about the putative benefits of dietary supplements, *both* through the use of "statements of nutritional support" on labels or in other labeling *and* by enabling sellers to refer customers to books, articles, and other publications that provide health-related information

REFERENCES

1. Forbes AL. National nutrition policy, food labeling and health claims. In: Shils ME, Olson JA, Shike M, eds. Modern nutrition in health and disease. 8th ed. Philadelphia: Lea & Febiger, 1994.
2. Nutrition Labeling and Education Act of 1990. PL 101-535, November 8, 1990, 104 Stat. 2353, 21 USC.
3. Dietary Supplement Health and Education Act of 1994. PL 103-417; 108 Stat/4325-4335; 103d Congress, 2d sess. (October 25, 1994).
4. U.S. Department of Health and Human Services. Nutrition Research at NIH. NIH publ. no. 95-2611, 1995.
5. U.S. Department of Agriculture. Nutrition program facts, food and consumer service. (3101 Park Center Drive, Alexandria, VA 22302), 1995.
6. U.S. Department of Agriculture. 1993 report on USDA human nutrition research and education activities—a report to Congress covering the period January—December 1993. 1995.
7. U.S. Department of Agriculture. Nutrition and your health: dietary guidelines for Americans. 4th ed. USDA home and garden bull. no. 232. (1996-402-519) Washington, DC: Government Printing Office, 1995.
8. Food additives permitted for direct addition to food for human consumption; olestra; final rule. Fed Register 1996;61:3118.
9. Squires S. Washington Post (Feb 12)1996;A17.
10. U.S. Department of Health and Human Services and US Department of Agriculture. Third report on nutrition monitoring in the United States, vols 1 and 2, 365 pp. Washington, DC: Government Printing Office, 1995.

10a. Food and Nutrition Board, Institute of Medicine. Dietary reference intakes for calcium, phosphorus, magnesium, vitamin D and fluoride. Washington, DC: National Academy Press, 1997.

11. Food labeling regulations implementing the Nutrition Labeling and Education Act of 1990, final rule, opportunity for comments. Fed Register 1993;58:2066.
12. Nutrition labeling of food. Title 21, Code of Federal Regulations, sect. 101.9.
13. Food labeling; mandatory status of nutrition labeling and nutrient content revision; format for nutrition label. Fed Register 1993;58:2079.
14. Food labeling; establishment of date of application. Fed Register 1993;58:2070.
15. Food labeling; reference daily intakes and daily reference values. Final rule. Fed Register 1993;58:2206.
16. Food labeling; serving sizes. Final rule. Fed Register 1993;58: 2229.
17. Food labeling; nutrient content claims, general principles, petitions, definition of terms; definitions of nutrient content claims for the fat, fatty acid, and cholesterol content of food. Fed Register 1993;58:2302.
18. Nutrition labeling of meat and poultry products, food safety and inspection service, and USDA, final rule. Fed Register 1993;58:632.
19. Food labeling; health claims and label statements; folate and neural tube defects, final rule. Fed Register 1996;61:8752.
20. Food labeling; health claims; sugar alcohols and dental caries, proposed rule. Fed Register 1995;60:37507.
21. Food labeling; health claims; oats and coronary artery disease, proposed rule. Fed Register 1996;61:296.
22. Food labeling; reference daily intakes, final rule. Fed Register 1995;60:67164.
23. Food Industry Associations, FDA Offer Mixed Reviews on Impact of NLEA. Food Labeling Nutr News 1996;3–5.
24. PL 103-417; 108 Stat. 4325-4335; 103d Cong. 2d sess. (October 25, 1994).
25. FDA has long regarded dietary supplements as a type of *food* intended for "special dietary uses." Section 403(j) of the FDCA, which has been part of the Act since its original passage in 1938, provides that a food shall be deemed to be "misbranded" (and therefore illegal) "[i]f it purports to be or is represented for special dietary uses, unless its label bears such information concerning its vitamin, mineral, and other dietary properties as the Secretary determines to be, and by regulations prescribes as, necessary in order fully to inform purchasers as to its value for such uses." 21 USC 343(j). This section of the FDCA recognizes that a product that is intended "for special dietary uses" because of "its vitamin, mineral, and other dietary properties" is a type of *food.* Note that section 403(j) authorizes but does not require the issuance of regulations to prescribe mandatory label information. The authority of the secretary of DHHS to issue regulations under the FDCA has been delegated to the Commissioner of Food and Drugs, who directs the FDA. 21 CFR 5.10(a)(1). FDA regulations issued pursuant to section 403(j) of the Act state that the term "special dietary uses" includes "[u]ses for *supplementing* or fortifying the ordinary or usual *diet* with any vitamin, mineral, or other dietary property." 21 CFR 105.3(a)(1)(iii) (hence "dietary supplement"). (Emphasis added.)
26. Judicial rulings that FDA personnel have cited as supportive of this proposition include *Nutrilab, Inc. V. Schweiker,* 713 F.2d 335 (7th Cir. 1983) and *American Health Products Co. V. Hayes,* 574 F. Supp. 1498 (S.D.N.Y. 1983), aff'd, 744 F.2d 912 (2d Cir. 1984). However, perhaps inconsistently, FDA also has long accepted that, "Ingredients or products such as rutin, other bioflavonoids, para-amino-benzoic acid, inositol, and similar substances which have in the past been represented as having nutritional properties but which have not been shown to be essential in human nutrition...may be marketed as individual products or mixtures thereof: *Provided,* That the possibility of nutritional, dietary, or therapeutic value is not stated or implied. . ." 21 CFR 101.9(i)(5) (April 1, 1993 ed.). Tablets or capsules of such products might have no taste, aroma, or nutritional value, but nevertheless the agency acknowledged that they could properly be sold as foods (provided that no misleading nutritional or therapeutic claims were made). (This particular statement no longer appears in FDA's revised regulations on nutrition labeling. 21 CFR 101.9 (April 1, 194 ed.). However, when the FDA revised its nutrition labeling regulations to delete this statement, it explicitly said that it was not intending to change its policy that permitted sale, as food, of a substance that offered no nutritional value (in FDA's judgment). For example, *see generally* 58 FR 2166 (January 6, 1993).)
27. New section 201(ff)(1) of the FDCA, 21 USC 321(ff)(1). There are additional criteria. The product must either be intended for ingestion in tablet, capsule, powder, softgel, gelcap, or liquid droplet form, or, if not intended for ingestion in such a form, not be "represented for use as a conventional food or as a sole item of a meal or the diet." New section

201(ff)(2) of the FDCA, 21 USC 321(ff)(2). In addition, it must be labeled as a "dietary supplement." New section 201(ff)(2)(C) of the FDCA, 21 USC 321(ff)(2)(C); new section 403(s)(2)B) of the FDCA, 21 USC 343(s)(2)(B).

The new definition includes some highly technical provisions about the situation where an ingredient in a supplement is also approved by FDA for use as a drug. In general, if "an article" has been "marketed as a dietary supplement or as a food" *before* it is approved by FDA as a new drug, certified by FDA as an antibiotic, or licensed by FDA as a biologic, it may continue to be marketed as a dietary supplement unless FDA publishes a prohibitory regulation (which would be subject to judicial review. New section 201(ff)(3)(A) of the FDCA, 21 USC 321(ff)(3)(A).

On the other hand, in general, if, *before* "an article" is "marketed as a dietary supplement or as a food," *either* (1) FDA has approved the article as a new drug, certified the article as an antibiotic, or licensed the article as a biologic, *or* (2) FDA has authorized the article for investigation as a new drug, antibiotic, or biologic, *and* "substantial clinical investigations have been instituted," *and* "the existence of such investigations has been made public," under these circumstances the article may *not* be marketed as a dietary supplement unless FDA first issues an approving regulation. New section 201(ff)(3)(B) of the FDCA, 21 USC 321(ff)(3)(B).

28. New section 201(s)(6) of the FDCA, 21 USC 321(s)(6).
29. Section 201(s) of the FDCA, 21 USC 321(s). As an example of FDA's use of the food additive allegation for dietary ingredients in dietary supplement products prior to enactment of the DSHEA, *see* FDA Compliance Policy Guide No. 7117.04, "Botanical Products for Use as Food' (as issued on July 1, 1986). Even before enactment of the DSHEA, however, the courts had expressed the view that FDA had sometimes overreached in its attempts to regulate dietary ingredients in dietary supplement products as "food additives." *See*, for example, *United States v. Two Plastic Drums...Black Currant Oil,* 984 F.2d 814 (7th Cir. 1993) (ruling that black currant oil in a gelatin capsule was not subject to regulation as a "food additive," and that FDA's allegations of food additive status constituted an "Alice-in-Wonderland approach...to make an end-run around the statutory scheme and shift to the processors the burden of proving the safety of a substance in all circumstance," 984 F.2d at 819) and *United States v. 29 Cartons...Oakmont Investment Co.,* 987 F.2d 33 (1st Cir. 1993) ("The [i.e., FDA's] proposition that placing a single-ingredient food product into an inert capsule as a convenient method of ingestion converts that food into a food additive perverts the statutory text, undermines legislative intent, and defenestrates common sense. We cannot accept such anfractuous reasoning." 987 F.2d at 39.).
30. 21 USC 342(a)(2)(C), 348(a).
31. Kutak, Rock, Campbell. Food Chem News 1991;33:67.
32. New section 402(f)(1)(A) of the FDCA, 21 USC 342(f)(1)(A).
33. New section 402(f)(1) of the FDCA, 21 USC 342(f)(1).
34. New section 413(c) of the FDCA, 21 USC 350b(c).
35. New section 413(a) of the FDCA, 21 USC 350b(a).
36. Id.
37. New section 402(f)(1)(C) of the FDCA, 21 USC 342(f)(1)(C).
38. New section 201(s)(6) of the FDCA, 21 USC 321(s)(6), which cross-references the ingredients described in new section 201(ff) of the FDCA, 21 USC 321(ff).
39. 21 USC 321(s), 342(a)(2)(C), 348.
40. 21 USC 321(t), 342(c), 379e.
41. FDA. Warning letter no. 95-DAL-WL-04 (November 22, 1994) issued to Alliance U.S.A., Richardson, Texas (asserting that the company's "Nature's Nutrition Formula One" product was "in violation of Sections 402(a)(1) and 402(f)(1)(A) of the Federal Food, Drug, and Cosmetic Act," i.e., 21 USC 342(a)(1) and (f)(1)(A), because the product allegedly "contain[ed] an added poisonous or deleterious substance, namely ephedrine and other alkaloids which may render it injurious to health") and FDA news release dated February 28, 1995 entitled "FDA Warns Consumers Against Nature's Nutrition Formula One" (warning the public not to consume the "Formula One" product described in the warning letter). More recently, FDA has consulted with its national food advisory committee about how best to regulate dietary supplements of the herb ma huang.
42. For a judicial ruling upholding FDA assertions of this type, *see United States v. Articles of Drug...Honey,* 344 F.2d 288 (6th Cir. 1965) (ruling that a jar of honey became subject to regulation as a drug when a book that made drug claims for honey was used in "immediate connection...with the sale of the product" by the retailer). Cf. *United States v."Sterling Vinegar and Honey"...Balanced Foods,* 338 F.2d 157 (2d Cir. 1964) (ruling that a book that made drug-type claims for a vinegar-honey combination did *not* create drug status for a vinegar-honey product, although the book was available for sale in the same store as the product, when there was "no evidence of any joint promotion" of the book and the product).
43. New section 403B(a) of the FDCA, 21 USC 343-2(a).
44. Section 403B(b) of the FDCA, 21 USC 343-2(b).
45. 21 CFR 101.14(e)(1).
46. New section 403(r)(6) of the FDCA, 21 USC 343(r)(6).
47. *Id.* It would appear that labeling claims that come within the four types of "statements of nutritional support" described in new section 403(r)(6) will *not* always come within FDA's definition of a "health claim." *See* 21 CFR 101.14(a)(1)–(6). For example, a label claim that "calcium helps build strong bones" is a claim that "describes the role" of calcium "to affect the structure or function in humans." Yet, such a claim does *not* come within the FDA's definition of a "health claim." *See* 21 CFR 101.14(a)(6). In such circumstances, it would appear that *neither* the approval of a health claim regulation *nor* compliance with the DSHEA's requirements for the new "statements of nutritional support" exception from health claim requirements would be applicable or needed.

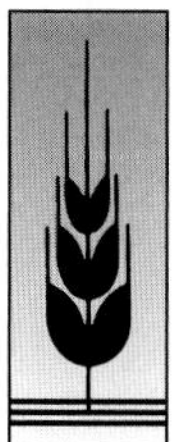

PART VII.

Appendix

Appendix Contents

ABBY S. BLOCH and MAURICE E. SHILS

Section IV.
NUTRIENTS, LIPIDS, AND OTHER ORGANIC COMPOUNDS IN BEVERAGES AND SELECTED FOODS / A-117

Section V.
EXCHANGE LISTS AND THERAPEUTIC DIETS / A-137

SECTION I. CONVERSION FACTORS, WEIGHTS AND MEASURES, AND METABOLIC WATER FORMATION

Table A-1-a
Conversion Factors Between Traditional and SI Units

Factors for converting nutrients expressed in metric or milliequivalent units into International System (SI) units.

1. Definitions
  a. Equivalent weight (EW) = atomic weight of element/valence of ionic form. Example with magnesium: atomic wt = 24, valence = 2+; therefore EW = 12
  b. Quantity of an electrolyte in milliequivalents per liter (meq/L) = mg of electrolyte/L/EW. Example: 48 mg of magnesium/L/12 = 4 meq/L
  c. Quantity of an electrolyte in mg/dL = (meq/L × EW)/10
  d. To convert mg/dL (= mg%) of an electrolyte to meq/L: mg/dL × 10/EW = meq/L
  e. 1 mol = 1 molecular or atomic weight of element or compound in grams (GMWt). In solutions this is usually expressed as moles per liter; i.e., 1 mol/L = 1 M; 1 mM (mmol) = 1 mol × 10^{-3}, 1 μM (μmol) = 1 mol × 10^{-6}; 1 nM (nmol) = 1 mol × 10^{-9}
  f.
    (1) To convert meq/L of an electrolyte or other ions in solution to mmol/L: meq/L divided by valence = mmol/L; e.g., (a) 2 meq/L of magnesium (Mg^{2+}) = 2/2 = 1 mmol/L; e.g., (b) 140 meq Na^+/L = 140/1 = 140 mmol/L
    (2) To convert mg/dL to mmol/L: (mg/dL × 10/EW) divided by valence = mmol/L; e.g., 2 mg/dL of magnesium = (2 × 10/12) divided by 2 = 0.83 mmol/L
    (3) For organic substances: mmol/L = wt in mg/L/MW (in mg)

2. SI units for expressing clinical laboratory data

These units are now widely used and are increasingly required for publication of scientific data in physical, biologic, and biomedical publication. Extensive SI conversion tables have been published together with an explanation of the rationale for their use and technical aspects of usage (1–3) (see Table 3).

  a. The base units of interest in physical quantities used in clinical chemistry are

Quantity	Base Unit
mass	kilogram
time	second
amount	mole
length	meter

A derived unit for energy is the kjoule (kJ) 4.18 kJ = 1 kcal
1 MJ = 239 kcal

  b. Prefixes and symbols for decimal multiples and submultiples include

Factor	Prefix	Symbol	Factor	Prefix	Symbol
10^9	giga	G	10^{-3}	milli	m
10^6	mega	M	10^{-6}	micro	μ
10^3	kilo	k	10^{-9}	nano	n
10^2	hecto	h	10^{-12}	pico	p
10^1	deca	da	10^{-15}	femto	f
10^{-1}	deci	d	10^{-18}	atto	a
10^{-2}	centi	c			

3. Conversion factors for selected compounds of nutrition interest[a]

	(1)	(2)	(3)	(4)
Component	Present Unit	Conversion Factor	SI Unit Symbol	Mass Conversion Factor
Albumin (s)	g/dL	10	g/L	—
Aluminum (s)	μg/L	37.04	nmol/L	μg/27 = mol
Amino acids	(see ref. 3. p. 119 for individual amino acids)			
Amino acid nitrogen (p)	mg/dL	0.714	mmol/L	mg/14 = mmol
Ascorbic acid (p)	mg/dL	56.78	μmol/L	mg/176 = mmol
Calcium (s)	mg/dL	0.250	mmol/L	mg/40 = mmol
Calcium (s)	meq/dL	0.500	mmol/L	meq/2 = mmol
β-Carotene[b] (s)	μ/dL	0.0186	μmol/L	μg/536.85 μmol
Chloride (s)	meq/L	1.00	mmol/L	meq = mmol
Cholesterol (p)	mg/dL	0.0259	mmol/L	mg/386.6 = mmol
Cobalamin (B_{12})	pg/mL	0.738	pmol/L	pg/1355 = pmol
Copper (s)	μg/dL	0.157	μmol/L	μg/63.5 = μmol
Ethanol (p)	mg/dL	0.217	mmol/L	mg/46 = mmol
Folic acid	ng/mL	2.265	nmol/L	ng/441.4 = nmol
Glucose (p)	mg/dL	0.0555	mmol/L	mg/180.2 = mmol
Iron (s)	μg/dL	0.179	μmol/L	μg/55.9 = μmol
Phosphate (p) (as phosphorus)	mg/dL	0.323	mmol/L	mg/31 = mmol
Potassium (s)	meq/L	1.000	mmol/L	meq = mmol
Potassium	mg/dL	0.256	mmol/L	mg/39.1 = mmol
Magnesium (s)	mg/dL	0.411	mmol/L	mg/24.3 = mmol
Pyridoxal (B)	ng/mL	5.981	nmol/L	ng/167 = nmol
Retinol[b] (p,s)	μg/dL	0.0349	μmol/L	μg/286 = μmol
Riboflavfin (s)	μg/dL	26.57	nmol/L	μg/376 = nmol
Sodium (s)	meq/L	1.00	mmol/L	meq = mmol
Thiamin HCl (U)	μg/24 h	0.00298	μmol/d	μg/337 = μmol
α-Tocopherol (p)	mg/dL	23.22	μmol/L	μg/431 = μmol
Vitamin D_3	μg/dL	26.01	nmol/L	μg/384 = μmol
Calcidiol	ng/mL	2.498	nmol/L	ng/400 = nmol
Zinc (s)	μg/dL	0.153	μmol/L	μg/65.4 = μmol

[a]To convert metric or equivalent unit per unit volume (column 1) to SI units per liter (column 3), multiply by the conversion factor in column 2. p, plasma; s, serum; B, blood; U, urine.

[b]See Appendix Table I-A-1-b for detailed conversion figures for retinol and carotene.

References

1. Young DS. Ann Intern Med 1987; 106:114.
2. Lundberg GD, Iberson C, Radulescu G: JAMA *255:* 2329, 1986; 255:2329.
3. Monsen ER: J Am Diet Assoc *87*:356, 1987.

Table A-1-b
Factors and Formulas Used in Interconverting Units of Vitamin A and Carotenoids

Factors
1 nmol retinol = 286.42 ng
1 nmol retinoic acid = 300.42 ng
1 nmol β-carotene = 536.85 ng
1 μg retinol equivalent (μg RE)
= 1 μg all-*trans* retinol
= 3.49 nmol all-*trans* retinol
= 6 μg all-*trans* β-carotene
= 11.18 nmol all-*trans* β-carotene
= 12 μg other all-*trans* provitamin A carotenoids
= 3.33 IU_a (the international unit of all-*trans* retinol)
= 10 IU_c (the international unit of all-*trans* β-carotene)
1 IU_a
= 0.3 μg all-*trans* retinol
= 0.3 μg RE
= 1.05 nmol all-*trans* retinol
= 1.8 μg all-*trans* β-carotene
= 3.35 nmol all-*trans* β-carotene
= 3 IU_c
= 3.6 μg other all-*trans* provitamin A cartoneoids
1 IU_c
= 0.6 μg all-*trans* β-carotene
= 1.12 nmol all-*trans* β-carotene
= 0.1 μg RE
= 0.33 IU_a
= 1.2 μg other all-*trans* provitamin A carotenoids

Formulas and examples: all-*trans* configurations of retinol and carotenoids are assumed

1. μg RE = μg retinol + μg β-carotene/6
A diet contains 500 μg retinol and 1800 μg β-carotene. Then,

$$\mu g\ RE = 500 + 1800/6 = 800\ \mu g\ RE$$

2. μg RE = IU_a/3.33 + IU_c/10
A diet contains 1667 IU_a of retinol and 3000 IU_c of β-carotene, Then,

$$\mu g\ RE = 1667/3.33 + 3000/10 = 800\ \mu g\ RE$$

3. μg RE = μg β-carotene/6 + μg other provitamin A carotenoids/12
A serving of sweet potato contains 2400 μg of β-carotene and 480 μg of other provitamin A carotenoids. Then,

$$\mu g\ RE = 2400/6 + 480/12 = 440\ \mu g\ RE$$

4.
$$\%\ \mu g\ RE\ \text{as retinol} = \left[1.5 - \frac{0.15\ \text{total IU}}{\text{total RE}}\right] \times 100$$

$$\%\ \mu g\ RE\ \text{as carotenoids} = \left[\frac{0.15\ \text{total IU}}{\text{total RE}} - 0.5\right] \times 100$$

A 100-g portion of cheese contains a total of 300 μg RE and a total of 1200 IU, in which 1 IU_a has been *assumed* to equal 1 IU_c. Then,

$$\%\ RE\ \text{as retinol} = \left[1.5 - \frac{0.15 \times 1200}{300}\right] \times 100 = 90\%$$

$$\%RE\ \text{as carotenoids} = \left[\frac{0.15 \times 1200}{300} - 0.5\right] \times 100 = 10\%$$

In this sample of cheese, therefore, 270 μg (270 μg RE) is present as retinol and 180 μg, or 30 μg RE is present as β-carotene or its equivalent of other provitamin A carotenoids.

5.
$$IU_a = \frac{10\ \mu g\ RE - \text{total IU}}{2}$$

$$IU_c = \frac{3\ \text{total IU} - 10\ \mu g\ RE}{2}$$

In a cheese sample containing a total of 300 μg RE and a total of 1200 IU, in which 1 IU_a is *assumed* to equal 1 IU_c,

$$IU_a = \frac{10 \times 300 - 1200}{2} = 900$$

$$IU_c = \frac{3 \times 1200 - 10 \times 300}{2} = 300$$

Note: Assumptions used from revised sections of the United States Department of Agriculture's *Handbook* 8 (i.e., 8.1–8.10) are (*a*) that 1 IU_a = 1 IU_c and (*b*) that 1 RE = 1 μg of retinol = 6 μg of β-carotene = 12 μg of other provitamin A carotenoids.

In some cases, small negative values for IU_c are obtained when the values for total IU and total RE are given for foods containing only performed vitamin A_1 particularly in fortified foods like margarine. This aberrant calculation results from the rounding of analytic values. Similarly, small negative values for IU_a may result for foods containing only carotenoids. In both cases, the negative values should be taken as zero.

Prepared by J. A. Olson.

Table A-1-c-1
Atomic Weights (Alphabetical Order)

Element	Symbol	Atomic Number	Atomic Weight	Element	Symbol	Atomic Number	Atomic Weight
Actinium	Ac	89	227.0278[a]	Neodymium	Nd	60	144.24
Aluminum	Al	13	26.981539	Neon	Ne	10	20.1797
Americium	Am	95	243.0614[a]	Neptunium	Np	93	237.0482[a]
Antimony	Sb	51	121.760	Nickel	Ni	28	58.6934
Argon	Ar	18	39.948	Niobium	Nb	41	92.90638
Arsenic	As	33	74.92159	Nitrogen	N	7	14.00674
Astatine	At	85	209.9871[a]	Nobelium	No	102	259.1009[a]
Barium	Ba	56	137.327	Osmium	Os	76	190.23
Berkelium	Bk	97	247.0703[a]	Oxygen	O	8	15.9994
Beryllium	Be	4	9.012182	Palladium	Pd	46	106.42
Bismuth	Bi	83	208.98037	Phosphorus	P	15	30.973762
Boron	B	5	10.811	Platinum	Pt	78	195.08
Bromine	Br	35	79.904	Plutonium	Pu	94	244.0642[a]
Cadmium	Cd	48	112.411	Polonium	Po	84	208.9824[a]
Calcium	Ca	20	40.078	Potassium	K	19	39.0983
Californium	Cf	98	251.0796[a]	Praseodymium	Pr	59	140.90765
Carbon	C	6	12.011	Promethium	Pm	61	144.9127[a]
Cerium	Ce	58	140.115	Protactinium	Pa	91	231.0388[a]
Cesium	Cs	55	132.90543	Radium	Ra	88	226.0254[a]
Chlorine	Cl	17	35.4527	Radon	Rn	86	222.0176[a]
Chromium	Cr	24	51.9961	Rhenium	Re	75	186.207
Cobalt	Co	27	58.93320	Rhodium	Rh	45	102.90550
Copper	Cu	29	63.546	Rubidium	Rb	37	85.4678
Curium	Cm	96	247.0703[a]	Ruthenium	Ru	44	101.07
Dysprosium	Dy	66	162.50	Samarium	Sm	62	150.36
Einsteinium	Es	99	252.083[a]	Scandium	Sc	21	44.955910
Erbium	Er	68	167.26	Selenium	Se	34	78.96[a]
Europium	Eu	63	151.965	Silicon	Si	14	28.0855
Fermium	Fm	100	257.0951[a]	Silver	Ag	47	107.8682
Fluorine	F	9	18.9984032	Sodium	Na	11	22.989768
Francium	Fr	87	223.0197[a]	Strontium	Sr	38	87.62
Gadolinium	Gd	64	157.25	Sulfur	S	16	32.066
Gallium	Ga	31	69.723	Tantalum	Ta	73	180.9479
Germanium	Ge	32	72.61	Technetium	Tc	43	97.9072[a]
Gold	Au	79	196.96654	Tellurium	Te	52	127.60
Hafnium	Hf	72	178.49	Terbium	Tb	65	158.92534
Helium	He	2	4.002602	Thallium	Tl	81	204.3833
Holmium	Ho	67	164.93032	Thorium	Th	90	232.0381
Hydrogen	H	1	1.00794	Thulium	Tm	69	168.93421
Indium	In	49	114.818	Tin	Sn	50	118.710
Iodine	I	53	126.90447	Titanium	Ti	22	47.867
Iridium	Ir	77	192.217	Tungsten	W	74	183.84
Iron	Fe	26	55.845	Unnilquadium	Unq	104	261.11[a]
Krypton	Kr	36	83.80	Unnilpentium	Unp	105	262.114[a]
Lanthanum	La	57	138.9055	Unnilhexium	Unh	106	263.118[a]
Lawrencium	Lr	103	262.11[a]	Unnilseptium	Uns	107	262.12[a]
Lead	Pb	82	207.2	Uranium	U	92	238.0289
Lithium	Li	3	6.941	Vanadium	V	23	50.9415
Lutetium	Lu	71	174.967	Xenon	Xe	54	131.29
Magnesium	Mg	12	24.3050	Ytterbium	Yb	70	173.04
Manganese	Mn	25	54.93805	Yttrium	Y	39	88.90585
Mendelevium	Md	101	258.10[a]	Zinc	Zn	30	65.39
Mercury	Hg	80	200.59	Zirconium	Zr	40	91.224
Molybdenum	Mo	42	95.94				

Based on 1993 IUPAC Table of Standard Atomic Weights of the Elements.

[a]Relative atomic mass of the isotope of that element with the longest known half-life.

Table A-1-c-2
Atomic Weights (Order of Atomic Number)

Atomic Number	Element	Symbol	Atomic Weight	Atomic Number	Element	Symbol	Atomic Weight
1	Hydrogen	H	1.00794	55	Cesium	Cs	132.90543
2	Helium	He	4.002602	56	Barium	Ba	137.327
3	Lithium	Li	6.941	57	Lanthanum	La	138.9055
4	Beryllium	Be	9.012182	58	Cerium	Ce	140.115
5	Boron	B	10.811	59	Praseodymium	Pr	140.90765
6	Carbon	C	12.011	60	Neodymium	Nd	144.24
7	Nitrogen	N	14.00674	61	Promethium	Pm	144.9127[a]
8	Oxygen	O	15.9994	62	Samarium	Sm	150.36
9	Fluorine	F	18.9984032	63	Europium	Eu	151.965
10	Neon	Ne	20.1797	64	Gadolinium	Gd	157.25
11	Sodium	Na	22.989768	65	Terbium	Tb	158.92534
12	Magnesium	Mg	24.3050	66	Dysprosium	Dy	162.50
13	Aluminum	Al	26.981539	67	Holmium	Ho	164.93032
14	Silicon	Si	28.0855	68	Erbium	Er	167.26
15	Phosphorus	P	30.973762	69	Thulium	Tm	168.93421
16	Sulfur	S	32.066	70	Ytterbium	Yb	173.04
17	Chlorine	Cl	35.4527	71	Lutetium	Lu	174.967
18	Argon	Ar	39.948	72	Hafnium	Hf	178.49
19	Potassium	K	39.0983	73	Tantalum	Ta	180.9479
20	Calcium	Ca	40.078	74	Tungsten	W	183.84
21	Scandium	Sc	44.955910	75	Rhenium	Re	186.207
22	Titanium	Ti	47.867	76	Osmium	Os	190.23
23	Vanadium	V	50.9415	77	Iridium	Ir	192.217
24	Chromium	Cr	51.9961	78	Platinum	Pt	195.08
25	Manganese	Mn	54.93805	79	Gold	Au	196.96654
26	Iron	Fe	55.845	80	Mercury	Hg	200.59
27	Cobalt	Co	58.93320	81	Thallium	Tl	204.3833
28	Nickel	Ni	58.6934	82	Lead	Pb	207.2
29	Copper	Cu	63.546	83	Bismuth	Bi	208.98037
30	Zinc	Zn	65.39	84	Polonium	Po	208.9824[a]
31	Gallium	Ga	69.723	85	Astatine	At	209.9871[a]
32	Germanium	Ge	72.61	86	Radon	Rn	222.0176[a]
33	Arsenic	As	74.92159	87	Francium	Fr	223.0197[a]
34	Selenium	Se	78.96	88	Radium	Ra	226.0254[a]
35	Bromine	Br	79.904	89	Actinium	Ac	227.0278[a]
36	Krypton	Kr	83.80	90	Thorium	Th	232.0381[a]
37	Rubidium	Rb	85.4678	91	Protactinium	Pa	231.0388[a]
38	Strontium	Sr	87.62	92	Uranium	U	238.0289
39	Yttrium	Y	88.90585	93	Neptunium	Np	237.0482[a]
40	Zirconium	Zr	91.224	94	Plutonium	Pu	244.0642[a]
41	Niobium	Nb	92.90638	95	Americium	Am	243.0614[a]
42	Molybdenum	Mo	95.94	96	Curium	Cm	247.0703[a]
43	Technetium	Tc	97.9072[a]	97	Berkelium	Bk	247.0703[a]
44	Ruthenium	Ru	101.07	98	Californium	Cf	251.0796[a]
45	Rhodium	Rh	102.90550	99	Einsteinium	Es	252.083[a]
46	Palladium	Pd	106.42	100	Fermium	Fm	257.0951[a]
47	Silver	Ag	107.8682	101	Mendelevium	Md	258.10[a]
48	Cadmium	Cd	112.411	102	Nobelium	No	259.1009[a]
49	Indium	In	114.818	103	Lawrencium	Lr	262.11[a]
50	Tin	Sn	118.710	104	Unnilquadium	Unq	261.11[a]
51	Antimony	Sb	121.760	105	Unnilpentium	Unp	262.114[a]
52	Tellurium	Te	127.60	106	Unnilhexium	Unh	263.118[a]
53	Iodine	I	126.90447	107	Unnilseptium	Uns	262.12[a]
54	Xenon	Xe	131.29				

From *The Merck Index: An Encyclopedia of Chemicals, Drugs, and Biologicals*, Twelfth Edition. Susan Budavari, Maryadele J. O'Neil, Ann Smith, Patricia E. Heckelman, Joanne F. Kinneary, Eds. (Merck & Co., Inc., Whitehouse Station, NJ: USA, 1996.)

Based on 1993 IUPAC Table of Standard Atomic Weights of the Elements.

[a]Relative atomic mass of the isotope of that element of longest known half-life as indicated in Table A-1-c-1.

Table A-1-d
Weights and Measures

Volumes: Apothecaries' Measure	Metric	Household
1 fluid dram (fl dr)	4 milliliter (mL)	1 teaspoon (tsp)
2 fl dr	8 mL	1 dessert spoonful
½ fluid ounce (fl oz)	15 mL	1 tablespoon (Tbsp) (3 tsp)
1 fl oz	30 mL	2 Tbsp (⅛ cup)
1-½ fl oz	45 mL	1 jigger
2 fl oz	59 mL	4 Tbsp (¼ cup)
2-⅔ fl oz	80 mL	5-⅓ Tbsp (⅓ cup)
4 fl oz	118 mL	8 Tbsp (½ cup)
8 fl oz	237 mL	1 cup
16 fl oz	473 mL	1 pint (pt)
32 fl oz	947 mL	1 quart (qt)
128 fl oz	3785 mL	1 gallon (gal)
3.38 fl oz	1 deciliter (dL) (100 mL)	
2.11 pt	1 liter (L) (1,000 mL)	

Weights: Avoirdupois	Metric
	1 femtogram (fg) (10^{-15} g)
	1 picogram (pg) (10^{-12} g)
	1 nanogram (ng) (10^{-9} g)
	1 microgram (μg) (10^{-6} g)
1 grain (gr)	0.065 g (65 mg)
1 gram (0.035 oz)	15.432 gr
1 scruple (20 gr)	1.296 g
1 dram (dr) (= drachm) (27.3 gr)	1.77 g
1 oz (16 dr)	28.35 g
1 lb (16 oz)	453.59 g
1 ton (2000 lb)	0.91 metric tons
1.015 gr	1 milligram (mg) (10^{-3} g)
	1 centigram (cg) (10^{-2} g)
	1 decigram (dg) (10^{-1} g)
15.4 gr (0.035 oz)	1 gram (g)
2.2 lb	1 kilogram (kg) (10^{3} g)

Length/Area:	Metric
1 angstrom (Å)	10 millimeter (mm)
1/2500 inch (in)	1 micron (μ) (10^{-3} mm) = micrometer (μm)
0.039 in	1 mm
0.39 in	1 centimeter (cm)
1 in	2.54 cm
1 foot (ft) (12 in)	30.5 cm
39.4 in	1 meter (m)
1 yard (yd) (3 ft)	0.9 m
1 rod (5.5 yd)	4.95 m
1093.6 yd (0.62 mile)	1 kilometer (km)
1 mile (mi) (5280 ft)	1.61 km
1 acre (160 square rods)	0.4 hectare

Temperature Conversions:

F to C: 5/9 (F − 32)
C to F: (9.5 × C) + 32

Electrolyte Data:

Ion		Atomic Wt (1)	Valence (2)	Equivalent Wt[a] 1 ÷ 2
Bicarbonate	HCO_3^-	61.0	1	61.0
Calcium	Ca^{2+}	40.1	2	20.0
Chloride	Cl^-	35.5	1	35.5
Magnesium	Mg^{2+}	24.3	2	12.2
Phosphate[b]	HPO_4^{2-}	96.0	2	48.0[b]
Potassium	K^+	39.1	1	39.1
Sodium	Na^+	23.0	1	23.0
Sulfate	SO_4^{2+}	96.1	2	48.0

continued

Table A-1-d—*continued*
Weights and Measures

[a]Milliequivalent (meq) = equivalent weight in milligrams (mg). To convert mg quantities of all electrolytes to meq:

$$\frac{\text{mg of electrolyte}}{\text{equivalent weight in mg}} = \text{meq}$$

To convert meq quantities of all electrolytes to mg:

$$\text{meq} \times \text{equivalent wt} = \text{mg}$$

To convert mg/dL to meq/L:

$$\frac{\text{mg/dL} \times 10}{\text{equivalent wt in mg}} = \text{meq/L}$$

To convert meq/L to mg/dL: meq/L × equivalent wt in mg × 0.1

[b]At the normal pH of plasma, 20% of the total inorganic phosphate radical is combined with one equivalent of base as BH_2PO_4, and 80% with two equivalents of base as B_2HPO_4. Under these conditions, base equivalence is therefore 0.2 + (0.8 × 2) = 1.8, and the equivalent weight of 53.3 is obtained by dividing the ionic weight by 1.8 instead of by 2. For phosphorus content of phosphate solutions, 1 meq provides approximately 15 mg, and 1 mmol provides approximately 31 mg.

Table A-1-e
Water Formed in the Metabolism of Tissue and Caloric Sources

Source	Amount
Muscle	1 g yields 0.85 mL (0.1 mL from protein + 0.75 mL cellular water)
Mixed tissue	100 kcal yields 10 mL
Fat	1 g yields 1.0 mL
Protein	1 g yields 0.4 mL
Glucose	1 g yields 0.64 mL
Glucose • H_2O	1 g yields 0.60 mL
Mixed diet	100 kcal yields 20 mL
Example: High-glucose TPN solution	
750 mL 10% amino acids	= 300 kcal yields 30 mL H_2O
1175 mL 50% glucose/water	= 2000 kcal yields 353 mL H_2O
143 mL 10% lipid	= 157 kcal yields 14 mL H_2O
Total: 2068 mL	= 2457 kcal yields 397 mL H_2O
Example: Glucose-lipid TPN solution	
750 mL 10% amino acids	= 300 kcal yields 30 mL H_2O
750 mL 50% glucose/water	= 1275 kcal yields 225 mL H_2O
500 mL 20% lipid	= 1000 kcal yields 100 mL H_2O
Total: 2000 mL	= 2575 kcal yields 355 mL H_2O

See Chapter 101. Courtesy of M. E. Shils.

INTRODUCTION TO SECTION II

Chapter 103 of the 9th edition of *Modern Nutrition in Health and Disease,* authored by George H. Beaton, Ph.D., is a comprehensive review of the historical development of nutritional standards and current controversial issues. It provides pertinent comments and recommendations concerning key national and international standards.

Key tables from the various national and international reports are included in this section. The reader is referred to the original reports for background statements and ancillary tables. Because the United Kingdom report is unlikely to be easily available to readers in the United States, significant excerpts have been included in Table II-A-4-a.

The tables from the first two volumes of the new Food and Nutrition Board—Institute of Medicine Dietary Reference Values are given in Tables A-2-b-1 to 6 and A-2-c-1 to 5 following the excerpts from the reports preceeding Table A-2-b.

—The Appendix Editors

A-2-a. Revised 1989 Recommendations—United States

Table A-2-a-1
Median Heights and Weights and Recommended Energy Intake in the United States[a]

		Weight		Height				Average Energy Allowance (kcal)[c]	
Category	Age (years) or Condition	(kg)	(lb)	(cm)	(in)	REE[b] (kcal/day)	Multiples of REE	Per kg	Per day[d]
Infants	0.0–0.5	6	13	60	24	320		108	650
	0.5–1.0	9	20	71	28	500		98	850
Children	1–3	13	29	90	35	740		102	1300
	4–6	20	44	112	44	950		90	1800
	7–10	28	62	132	52	1130		70	2000
Males	11–14	45	99	157	62	1440	1.70	55	2500
	15–18	66	145	176	69	1760	1.67	45	3000
	19–24	72	160	177	70	1780	1.67	40	2900
	25–50	79	174	176	70	1800	1.60	37	2900
	51+	77	170	173	68	1530	1.50	30	2300
Females	11–14	46	101	157	62	1310	1.67	47	2200
	15–18	55	120	163	64	1370	1.60	40	2200
	19–24	58	128	164	65	1350	1.60	38	2200
	25–50	63	138	163	64	1380	1.55	36	2200
	51+	65	143	160	63	1280	1.50	30	1900
Pregnant	1st trimester					—			+0
	2nd trimester								+300
	3rd trimester								+300
Lactating	1st 6 months								+500
	2nd 6 months								+500

From Food and Nutrition Board, National Research Council. Recommended dietary allowances. 10th ed. Washington, DC: National Academy Press, 1989:33.

[a]Median height/weight used by the RDA are those which are the medians for the U.S. population of designated age as reported in NHANES III.

[b]Calculations based on WHO equation derived from BMR data (Table II-A-10-b), then rounded.

[c]In the range of light to moderate activity, the coefficient of variation is ±20%.

[d]Figure is rounded.

Table A-2-a-2
Recommended Dietary Allowances,[a] Revised 1989 (Designed for the Maintenance of Good Nutrition of Practically All Healthy People in the United States)

Category	Age (years) or Condition	Weight[b] (kg)	Weight[b] (lb)	Height[b] (cm)	Height[b] (in)	Protein (G)	Fat-Soluble Vitamins: Vitamin A (μg RE)[c]	Vitamin D (μgx)[d]	Vitamin E (mg α-TE)[a]	Vitamin K (μg)
Infants	0.0–0.5	6	13	60	24	13	375	7.5	3	5
	0.5–1.0	9	20	71	28	14	375	10	4	10
Children	1–3	13	29	90	35	16	400	10	6	15
	4–6	20	44	112	44	24	500	10	7	20
	7–10	28	62	132	52	28	700	10	7	30
Males	11–14	45	99	157	62	45	1000	10	10	45
	15–18	66	145	176	69	59	1000	10	10	65
	19–24	72	160	177	70	58	1000	10	10	70
	25–50	79	174	176	70	63	1000	5	10	80
	51+	77	170	173	68	63	1000	5	10	80
Females	11–14	46	101	157	62	46	800	10	8	45
	15–18	55	120	163	64	44	800	10	8	55
	19–24	58	128	164	65	46	800	10	8	60
	25–50	63	138	163	64	50	800	5	8	65
	51+	65	143	160	63	50	800	5	8	65
Pregnant						60	800	10	10	65
Lactating	1st 6 months					65	1300	10	12	65
	2nd 6 months					62	1200	10	11	65

From Food and Nutrition Board, National Research Council. Recommended dietary allowances. 10th ed. Washington, DC: National Academy Press, 1989.

[a]The allowances, expressed as average daily intakes over time, are intended to provide for individual variations among most normal persons as they live in the United States under usual environmental stresses. Diets should be based on a variety of common foods in order to provide their nutrients for which human requirements have been less well defined. See text for detailed discussion of allowances and of nutrients not tabulated.

[b]Weights and heights of reference adults are actual medians for the U.S. population of the designated age, as reported by NHANES II. The median weights and heights of those under 19 years of age were taken from Hamill et al. (1979). The use of these figures does not imply that the height:weight ratios are ideal.

continued on next page

Table A-2-a-3
Estimated Safe and Adequate Daily Dietary Intakes of Selected Vitamins and Minerals[a]

Category	Age (years)	Vitamins: Biotin (μg)	Pantothenic Acid (mg)
Infants	0–0.5	10	2
	0.5–1	15	3
Children and adolescents	1–3	20	3
	4–6	25	3–4
	7–10	30	4–5
	11+	30–100	4–7
Adults		30–100	4–7

Category	Age (years)	Trace Elements[b]: Copper (mg)	Manganese (mg)	Fluoride (mg)	Chromium (μg)	Molybdenum (μg)
Infants	0–0.5	0.4–0.6	0.3–0.6	0.1–0.5	10–40	15–30
	0.5–1	0.6–0.7	0.6–1.0	0.2–1.0	20–60	20–40
Children and adolescents	1–3	0.7–1.0	1.0–1.5	0.5–1.5	20–80	25–50
	4–6	1.0–1.5	1.5–2.0	1.0–2.5	30–120	30–75
	7–10	1.0–2.0	2.0–3.0	1.5–2.5	50–200	50–150
	11+	1.5–2.5	2.0–5.0	1.5–2.5	50–200	75–250
Adults		1.5–3.0	2.0–5.0	1.5–4.0	50–200	75–250

From Food and Nutrition Board, National Research Council. Recommended dietary allowances. 10th ed. Washington, DC: National Academy Press, 1989:284.

[a]Because there is less information on which to base allowances, these figures are not given in the main table of RDA and are provided here in the form of ranges of recommended intakes.

[b]Because the toxic levels for many trace elements may be only several times usual intakes, the upper levels for the trace elements given in this table should not be habitually exceeded.

Table A-2-a-2
Continued

Water-Soluble Vitamins							Minerals						
Vitamin C (mg)	Thiamin (mg)	Riboflavin (mg)	Niacin (mg NE)[f]	Vitamin B_6 (mg)	Folate (μg)	Vitamin B_{12} (μg)	Calcium (mg)	Phosphorus (mg)	Magnesium (mg)	Iron (mg)	Zinc (mg)	Iodine (μg)	Selenium (μg)
30	0.3	0.4	5	0.3	25	0.3	400	300	40	6	5	40	10
35	0.4	0.5	6	0.6	35	0.5	600	500	60	10	5	50	15
40	0.7	0.8	9	1.0	50	0.7	800	800	80	10	10	70	20
45	0.9	1.1	12	1.1	75	1.0	800	800	120	10	10	90	20
45	1.0	1.2	13	1.4	100	1.4	800	800	170	10	10	120	30
50	1.3	1.5	17	1.7	150	2.0	1200	1200	270	12	15	150	40
60	1.5	1.8	20	2.0	200	2.0	1200	1200	400	12	15	150	50
60	1.5	1.7	19	2.0	200	2.0	1200	1200	350	10	15	150	70
60	1.5	1.7	19	2.0	200	2.0	800	800	350	10	15	150	70
60	1.2	1.4	15	2.0	200	2.0	800	800	350	10	15	150	70
50	1.1	1.3	15	1.4	150	2.0	1200	1200	280	15	12	150	45
60	1.1	1.3	15	1.5	180	2.0	1200	1200	300	15	12	150	50
60	1.1	1.3	15	1.6	180	2.0	1200	1200	280	15	12	150	55
60	1.1	1.3	15	1.6	180	2.0	800	800	280	15	12	150	55
60	1.0	1.2	13	1.6	180	2.0	800	800	280	10	12	150	55
70	1.5	1.6	17	2.2	400	2.2	1200	1200	320	30	15	175	65
95	1.6	1.8	20	2.1	280	2.6	1200	1200	355	15	19	200	75
90	1.6	1.7	20	2.1	260	2.6	1200	1200	340	15	16	200	75

[c]Retinol equivalents. 1 retinol equivalent = 1 μg retinol or 6 μg β-carotene. See text for calculation of vitamin A activity of diets as retinol equivalents.

[d]As cholecalciferol. 10 μg cholecalciferol = 400 IU of vitamin D.

[e]α-Tocopherol equivalents. 1 mg *d*-α tocopherol = 1 α-TE. See text for variation in allowances and calculation of vitamin E activity of the diet as α-tocopherol equivalents.

[f]1 NE (niacin equivalent) is equal to 1 mg of niacin or 60 mg of dietary tryptophan.

A-2-b. DIETARY REFERENCE INTAKES FOR CALCIUM, PHOSPHORUS, MAGNESIUM, VITAMIN D, AND FLUORIDE BY LIFE-STAGE GROUP, 1997 (1). DIETARY REFERENCE INTAKES (DRIs) FOR THIAMIN, RIBOFLAVIN, NIACIN, VITAMIN B_6, FOLATE, VITAMIN B_{12}, PANTOTHENIC ACID, BIOTIN, AND CHOLINE (2). EXCERPTS FROM THE REPORTS.

DRIs replace the Food and Nutrition Board's previous RDAs for healthy individuals (3). Four levels of intake values are documented.

The *Estimated Average Requirement (EAR)* is the nutrient intake value that is estimated to meet the requirement defined by a specified indicator of adequacy (e.g., balance studies) in 50 percent of the individuals in a life stage and gender group. Hence, it is a median rather than an average. At this level of intake, the remaining 50 percent of the specified group would not have its nutrient needs met. For some groups, data had to be extrapolated to estimate the value. In deriving the EARs, contemporary concepts of reduction of disease risk were among the factors considered, rather than basing reference values solely upon prevention of nutrient deficiencies. Because the EAR is a dietary intake value, it includes an adjustment for an assumed bioavailability of the nutrient. The EAR is used in setting the RDA.

The *Recommended Dietary Allowance (RDA)* is the daily dietary intake level that is sufficient to meet the nutrient requirements of nearly all (97 to 98%) individuals in the life stage and gender group. The RDA applies to individuals, not to groups. The EAR serves as the foundation for setting the RDA. If the standard deviation (SD) of the EAR is known, the RDA is set at two SDs above the EAR. If the data are insufficient to calculate an SD, a coefficient of variation of 10% is assumed, and the RDA = 1.2 × EAR.

The RDA for a nutrient is a value to be used as a goal for dietary intake by individuals and is not intended for use in assessing the diets of either individuals or groups or for planning for groups. [The 1989 RDAs are listed for comparison with the new RDA in Appendix Table II-A-2-a-2.]

Adequate intake (AI). This is a value for a nutrient used when there is insufficient evidence to calculate an EAR. It is based on observed or experimentally determined approximations of the average intake of a defined population that appears to sustain a defined nutritional state such as normal circulating nutrient values or growth. AIs rather than EARs and RDAs are being proposed for all nutrients for infants to age 1 year (1,2) and for calcium, vitamin D, and fluoride (1) and for pantothenic acid, biotin, and choline (2) for all life stages. The methods used in deriving the AIs are reviewed in the basic document.

The *Tolerable Upper Intake Level (UL)* is the maximal level of nutrient intake that is unlikely to pose risks of adverse health effects to almost all individuals in the target group. The term was chosen to avoid implying a possible beneficial effect and is not intended to be a recommended intake level. For most nutrients, the UL refers to total intakes—from food, fortified food, and nutrient supplements. In some instances, it may refer only to intakes from pharmacologic agents. The UL applies to chronic daily use.

The relations of these four dietary reference intakes is depicted in the following figure.

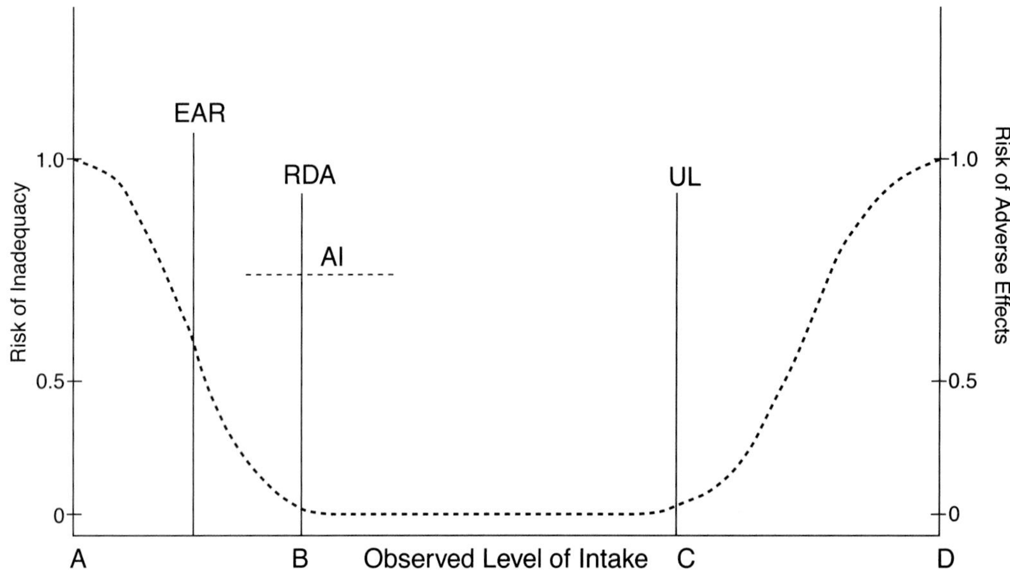

Dietary reference intakes. This figure shows that the Estimated Average Requirement *(EAR)* is the intake at which the risk of inadequacy is 0.5 (50%). The Recommended Dietary Allowance *(RDA)* is the intake at which the risk of inadequacy is very small—only 0.02 to 0.03 (2 to 3%). The Adequate Intake *(AI)* does not bear a consistent relationship to the EAR or the RDA because it is set without being able to estimate the requirement. At intakes between the RDA and the Tolerable Upper Intake Level *(UL)*, the risks of inadequacy and of adverse effects are both close to 0. The UL is the highest level of daily nutrient intake that is likely to pose no risks of adverse health effects to almost all individuals in the general population. At intakes above the UL, the risk of adverse effects increases. A *dashed line* is used because the actual shape of the curve has not been determined experimentally. The distances between points *A* and *B, B* and *C,* and *C* and *D* may differ much more than is depicted in this figure. (This is Figure S-1 in reference 2 below.)

Table A-2-b-1
Criteria and Dietary Reference Intake Values for Calcium by Life-Stage Group

Life-Stage Group[a]	Criterion	AI (mg/day)[b]
0 to 6 months	Human milk content	210
6 to 12 months	Human milk + solid food	270
1 through 3 years	Extrapolation of maximal calcium retention from 4 through 8 years	500
4 through 8 years	Maximal calcium retention	800
9 through 13 years	Maximal calcium retention	1300
14 through 18 years	Maximal calcium retention	1300
19 through 30 years	Maximal calcium retention	1000
31 through 50 years	Calcium balance	1000
51 through 70 years	Maximal calcium retention	1200
>70 years	Extrapolation of maximal calcium retention from 51 through 70 years	1200
Pregnancy		
≤18 years	Bone mineral mass	1300
19 through 50 years	Bone mineral mass	1000
Lactation		
≤18 years	Bone mineral mass	1300
19 through 50 years	Bone mineral mass	1000

From Food and Nutrition Board, Institute of Medicine. Dietary reference intakes for calcium, phosphorus, magnesium, vitamin D, and fluoride. Washington, DC: National Academy Press, 1997 (prepublication copy). Table S-1 in original.

[a]All groups except Pregnancy and Lactation are males and females.

[b]AI = Adequate Intake. The observed average or experimentally set intake by a defined population or subgroup that appears to sustain a defined nutritional state, such as growth rate, normal circulating nutrient values, or other functional indicators of health. AI is used if sufficient scientific evidence is not available to derive an EAR. For healthy breast-fed infants, AI is the mean intake. Some seemingly healthy individuals may require higher calcium intakes to minimize risk of osteopenia, and some individuals may be at low risk on even lower intakes. **The AI is not equivalent to an RDA.**

REFERENCES

1. Food and Nutrition Board—Institute of Medicine. Dietary reference intakes for calcium, phosphorus, magnesium, vitamin D, and fluoride. Washington, DC: National Academy Press, 1997.
2. Food and Nutrition Board—Institute of Medicine. Dietary reference intakes for thiamin, riboflavin, niacin, vitamin B_6, folate, vitamin B_{12}, pantothenic acid, biotin, and choline. Washington, DC: National Academy Press, 1998.
3. Food and Nutrition Board—National Research Council. Recommended Dietary Allowances. 10th ed. Washington, DC: National Academy Press, 1989.

Table A-2-b-2
Criteria and Dietary Reference Intake Values for Phosphorus by Life-Stage Group

Life-Stage Group[a]	Criterion	EAR (mg/day)[b]	RDA (mg/day)[c]	AI (mg/day)[d]
0 to 6 months	Human milk content	—	—	100
6 to 12 months	Human milk + solid food	—	—	275
1 through 3 years	Factorial approach	380	460	—
4 through 8 years	Factorial approach	405	500	—
9 through 13 years	Factorial approach	1055	1250	—
14 through 18 years	Factorial approach	1055	1250	—
19 through 30 years	Serum P_i[e]	580	700	—
31 through 50 years	Serum P_i	580	700	—
51 through 70 years	Extrapolation of serum P_i from 19 through 50 years	580	700	—
>70 years	Extrapolation of serum P_i from 19 through 50 years	580	700	—
Pregnancy				
≤18 years	Factorial approach	1055	1250	—
19 through 50 years	Serum P_i	580	700	—
Lactation				
≤18 years	Factorial approach	1055	1250	—
19 through 50 years	Serum P_i	580	700	—

From Food and Nutrition Board, Institute of Medicine. Dietary reference intakes for calcium, phosphorus, magnesium, vitamin D, and fluoride. Washington, DC: National Academy Press, 1997 (prepublication copy). Table S-2 in original.

[a]All groups except Pregnancy and Lactation are males and females.

[b]EAR, estimated average requirement. The intake that meets the estimated nutrient needs of 50% of the individuals in a group.

[c]RDA, recommended dietary allowance. The intake that meets the nutrient need of almost all (97–98%) of individuals in a group.

[d]AI, adequate intake. The observed average or experimentally set intake by a defined population or subgroup that appears to sustain a defined nutritional status, such as growth rate, normal circulating nutrient values, or other functional indicators of health. AI is used if sufficient scientific evidence is not available to derive an EAR. For healthy breast-fed infants, AI is the mean intake. **The AI is not equivalent to an RDA.**

[e]P_i, Serum inorganic phosphate concentration.

Table A-2-b-3
Criteria and Dietary Reference Intake Values for Magnesium by Life-Stage Group

Life-Stage Group	Criterion	EAR (mg/day)[a]		RDA (mg/day)[b]		AI (mg/day)[c]	
		Male	Female	Male	Female	Male	Female
0 to 6 months	Human milk content	—	—	—	—	30	30
6 to 12 months	Human milk + solid food	—	—	—	—	75	75
1 through 3 years	Extrapolation of balance from older children	65	65	80	80		
4 through 8 years	Extrapolation of balance from older children	110	110	130	130		
9 through 13 years	Balance studies	200	200	240	240		
14 through 18 years	Balance studies	340	300	410	360		
19 through 30 years	Balance studies	330	255	400	310		
31 through 50 years	Balance studies	350	265	420	320		
51 through 70 years	Balance studies	350	265	420	320		
>70 years	Intracellular studies; decreases in absorption	350	265	420	320		
Pregnancy							
≤18 years	Gain in lean mass		335	—	400	—	—
19 through 30 years	Gain in lean mass		290		350	—	
31 through 50 years	Gain in lean mass		300		360		
Lactation							
≤18 years	Balance studies		300		360	—	—
19 through 30 years	Balance studies		255		310	—	—
31 through 50 years	Balance studies		265		320		

From Food and Nutrition Board, Institute of Medicine. Dietary reference intakes for calcium, phosphorus, magnesium, vitamin D, and fluoride. Washington, DC: National Academy Press, 1997 (prepublication copy). Table S-3 in original.

[a]EAR = Estimated Average Requirement. The intake that meets the estimated nutrient needs of 50% of the individuals in a group.

[b]RDA = Recommended Dietary Allowance. The intake that meets the nutrient need of almost all (97–98%) of individuals in a group.

[c]AI = Adequate Intake. The observed average or experimentally set intake by a defined population or subgroup that appears to sustain a defined nutritional status, such as growth rate, normal circulating nutrient values, or other funcitonal indicators of health. AI is used if sufficient scientific evidence is not available to derive an EAR. For healthy breast-fed infants, AI is the mean intake. **The AI is not equivalent to an RDA.**

Table A-2-b-4
Criteria and Dietary Reference Intake Values for Vitamin D by Life-Stage Group

Life-Stage Group[a]	Criterion	AI (μg/day)[b,c,d]
0 to 6 months	Serum 25(OH)D	5
6 to 12 months	Serum 25(OH)D	5
1 through 3 years	Serum 25(OH)D	5
4 through 8 years	Serum 25(OH)D	5
9 through 13 years	Serum 25(OH)D	5
14 through 18 years	Serum 25(OH)D	5
19 through 30 years	Serum 25(OH)D	5
31 through 50 years	Serum 25(OH)D	5
51 through 70 years	Serum 25(OH)D	10
>70 years	Serum 25(OH)D	15
Pregnancy		
≤18 years	Serum 25(OH)D	5
19 through 50 years	Serum 25(OH)D	
Lactation		
≤18 years	Serum 25(OH)D	5
19 through 50 years	Serum 25(OH)D	

From Food and Nutrition Board, Institute of Medicine. Dietary reference intakes for calcium, phosphorus, magnesium, vitamin D, and fluoride. Washington, DC: National Academy Press, 1997 (prepublication copy). Table S-4 in original.

[a]All groups except Pregnancy and Lactation are males and females.

[b]As cholecalciferol, 1 μg cholecalciferol = 40 IU vitamin D.

[c]AI = Adequate Intake. The observed average or experimentally set intake by a defined population or subgroup that appears to sustain a defined nutritional status, such as growth rate, normal circulating nutrient values, or other functional indicators of health. AI is utilized if sufficient scientific evidence is not available to drive an EAR. For healthy breast-fed infants, AI is the mean intake. All other life-stage groups should be covered at the AI value. **The AI is not equivalent to an RDA.**

[d]In the absence of adequate exposure to sunlight.

Table A-2-b-5
Criteria and Dietary Reference Intake Values for Fluoride by Life-Stage Group

Life-Stage Group	Criterion	AI (mg/day)[a] Male	Female
0 to 6 months	Human milk content	0.01	0.01
6 to 12 months	Caries prevention	0.5	0.5
1 through 3 years	Caries prevention	0.7	0.7
4 through 8 years	Caries prevention	1.1	1.1
9 through 13 years	Caries prevention	2.0	2.0
14 through 18 years	Caries prevention	3.2	2.9
19 through 30 years	Caries prevention	3.8	3.1
31 through 50 years	Caries prevention	3.8	3.1
51 through 70 years	Caries prevention	3.8	3.1
>70 years	Caries prevention	3.8	3.1
Pregnancy			
≤18 years	Caries prevention	—	2.9
19 through 50 years	Caries prevention	—	3.1
Lactation			
≤18 years	Caries prevention	—	2.9
19 through 50 years	Caries prevention	—	3.1

From Food and Nutrition Board, Institute of Medicine. Dietary reference intakes for calcium, phosphorus, magnesium, vitamin D, and fluoride. Washington, DC: National Academy Press, 1997 (prepublication copy). Table S-5 in original.

[a]AI = Adequate intake. The observed average or experimentally set intake by a defined population or subgroup that appears to sustain a defined nutritional status, such as growth rate, caries-resistant teeth, normal circulating nutrient values, or other functional indicators of health. AI is used if sufficient scientific evidence is not available to derive an EAR. For healthy breast-fed infants, AI is the mean intake. All other life-stage groups should be covered at the AI value. **The AI is not equivalent to an RDA.**

Table A-2-b-6
Tolerable Upper Intake Levels (UL[a]), by Life-Stage Group

Life-Stage Group	Calcium (g/day)	Phosphorus (g/day)	Magnesium[b] (mg/day)	Vitamin D (μg/day)[c]	Fluoride (mg/day)
0 to 6 months	ND[d]	ND	ND	25	0.7
6 to 12 months	ND	ND	ND	25	0.9
1 through 3 years	2.5	3	65	50	1.3
4 through 8 years	2.5	3	110	50	2.2
9 through 18 years	2.5	4	350	50	10
19 through 70 years	2.5	4	350	50	10
>70 years	2.5	3	350	50	10
Pregnancy					
≤18 years	2.5	3.5	350	50	10
19 through 50 years	2.5	3.5	350	50	10
Lactation					
≤18 years	2.5	4	350	50	10
19 through 50 years	2.5	4	350	50	10

From Food and Nutrition Board, Institute of Medicine. Dietary reference intakes for calcium, phosphorus, magnesium, vitamin D, and fluoride. Washington, DC: National Academy Press, 1997 (prepublication copy). Table S-6 in original.

[a]UL = tolerable upper intake level. The maximum level of daily nutrient intake that is unlikely to pose risks of adverse effects to members of the general population. Unless specified otherwise, the Ul represents total nutrient intake from food, water and supplements.

[b]The UL for magnesium represents intake from a pharmacological agent only and does not include intake from food and water.

[c]As cholecalciferol. 1 μg cholecalciferol = 40 IU vitamin D.

[d]ND = Not determinable due to lack of data of adverse effects in this age group and concern with regard to lack of ability to handle excess amounts. Source of intake should be from food only in order to prevent high levels of intake.

Table A-2-c-1

Food and Nutrition Board, National Academy of Sciences, Institute of Medicine Recommended Levels for Individual Intake, 1998, B Vitamins and Choline

Life-Stage Group	Thiamin (mg/day)	Riboflavin (mg/day)	Niacin (mg/day)[a]	B_6 (mg/day)	Folate (μg/day)[b]	B_{12} (μg/day)[b]	Pantothenic Acid (mg/day)	Biotin (μg/day)	Choline[c] (mg/day)
Infants									
0–5 months	0.2*	0.3*	2*	0.1*	65*	0.4*	1.7*	5*	125*
6–11 months	0.3*	0.4*	3*	0.3*	80*	0.5*	1.8*	6*	150*
Children									
1–3 years	**0.5**	**0.5**	**6**	**0.5**	**150**	**0.9**	2*	8*	200*
4–8 years	**0.6**	**0.6**	**8**	**0.6**	**200**	**1.2**	3*	12*	250*
Males									
9–13 years	**0.9**	**0.9**	**12**	**1.0**	**300**	**1.8**	4*	20*	375*
14–18 years	**1.2**	**1.3**	**16**	**1.3**	**400**	**2.4**	5*	25*	550*
19–30 years	**1.2**	**1.3**	**16**	**1.3**	**400**	**2.4**	5*	30*	550*
31–50 years	**1.2**	**1.3**	**16**	**1.3**	**400**	**2.4**	5*	30*	550*
51–70 years	**1.2**	**1.3**	**16**	**1.7**	**400**	**2.4**[d]	5*	30*	550*
>70 years	**1.2**	**1.3**	**16**	**1.7**	**400**	**2.4**[d]	5*	30*	550*
Females									
9–13 years	**0.9**	**0.9**	**12**	**1.0**	**300**	**1.8**	4*	20*	375*
14–18 years	**1.0**	**1.0**	**14**	**1.2**	**400**[e]	**2.4**	5*	25*	400*
19–30 years	**1.1**	**1.1**	**14**	**1.3**	**400**[e]	**2.4**	5*	30*	425*
31–50 years	**1.1**	**1.1**	**14**	**1.3**	**400**[e]	**2.4**	5*	30*	425*
51–70 years	**1.1**	**1.1**	**14**	**1.5**	**400**[e]	**2.4**[d]	5*	30*	425*
>70 years	**1.1**	**1.1**	**14**	**1.5**	**400**	**2.4**[d]	5*	30*	425*
Pregnancy (all ages)	**1.4**	**1.4**	**18**	**1.9**	**600**[f]	**2.6**	6*	30*	450*
Lactation (all ages)	**1.5**	**1.6**	**17**	**2.0**	**500**	**2.8**	7*	35*	550*

From Food and Nutrition Board, Institute of Medicine. Dietary reference intakes. Thiamin, riboflavin, niacin, vitamin B_6, folate, vitamin B_{12}, pantothenic acid, biotin, and choline. Washington, DC: National Academy Press, 1998 (prepublication copy).

Note: This table presents Recommended Dietary Allowances (RDAs) in bold type and Adequate Intakes (AIs) in ordinary type followed by an asterisk (*). RDAs and AIs may both be used as goals for individual intake. RDAs are set to meet the needs of almost all (97 to 98%) individuals in a group. For healthy breast-fed infants, the AI is the mean intake. The AI for other life-stage groups is believed to cover their needs, but lack of data or uncertainty in the data prevent clear specification of this coverage.

[a]As niacin equivalents. 1 mg of niacin = 60 mg of tryptophan.

[b]As dietary folate equivalents (DFE). 1 DFE = 1 μg food folate = 0.6 μg of folic acid (from fortified food or supplement) consumed with food = 0.5 mg of synthetic (supplemental) folic acid taken on an empty stomach.

[c]Although AIs have been set for choline, there are few data to assess whether a dietary supply of choline is needed at all stages of the life cycle, and it may be that the choline requirement can be met by endogenous synthesis at some of these stages.

[d]Since 10 to 30 percent of older people may malabsorb food-bound B_{12}, it is advisable for those older than 50 years to meet their RDA mainly by taking foods fortified with B_{12} or a B_{12}-containing supplement.

[e]In view of evidence linking folate intake with neural tube defects in the fetus, it is recommended that all women capable of becoming pregnant consume 400 μg of synthetic folic acid from fortified foods and/or supplements in addition to intake of food folate from a varied diet.

[f]It is assumed that women will continue taking 400 μg of folic acid until their pregnancy is confirmed and they enter prenatal care, which ordinarily occurs after the end of the periconceptional period–the critical time for formation of the neural tube.

Table A-2-c-2
Estimated Average Requirements for B Vitamins

Life-Stage Group	Thiamin (mg/day)	Riboflavin (mg/day)	Niacin (mg/day)[a]	Vitamin B_6 (mg/day)	Folate (μg/day)[b]	Vitamin B_{12} (μg/day)[b]
Children						
1–3 years	0.5	0.4	5	0.4	120	0.7
4–8 years	0.6	0.5	6	0.5	160	1.0
Males						
9–13 years	0.7	0.8	9	0.8	250	1.5
14–18 years	1.0	1.1	12	1.1	330	2
19–30 years	1.0	1.1	12	1.1	320	2
31–50 years	1.0	1.1	12	1.1	320	2
51–70 years	1.0	1.1	12	1.4	320	2
>70 years	1.0	1.1	12	1.4	320	2
Females						
9–13 years	0.7	0.8	9	0.8	250	1.5
14–18 years	0.9	0.9	11	1.0	330	2
19–30 years	0.9	0.9	11	1.1	320	2
31–50 years	0.9	0.9	11	1.1	320	2
51–70 years	0.9	0.9	11	1.3	320	2
>70 years	0.9	0.9	11	1.3	320	2
Pregnancy (all ages)	1.2	1.2	14	1.6	520	2.2
Lactation (all ages)	1.2	1.3	13	1.7	450	2.4

From Food and Nutrition Board, Institute of Medicine. Dietary reference intakes. Thiamin, riboflavin, niacin, vitamin B_6, folate, vitamin B_{12}, pantothenic acid, biotin, and choline. Washington, DC: National Academy Press, 1998 (prepublication copy). This is Table 13-1 in the original report.

Note: Estimated Average Requirements (EARs) have not been set for infants or for pantothenic acid, biotin, or choline.

[a]As niacin equivalents. 1 mg of niacin = 60 mg of tryptophan.

[b]As dietary folate equivalents. 1 dietary folate equivalent = 1 μg food folate = 0.7 μg of folic acid (from fortified food or supplement) consumed with food = 0.5 μg of synthetic (supplemental) folic acid taken on an empty stomach.

Table A-2-c-3
Estimated Average Requirements and Reported Dietary Intakes of Six B Complex Vitamins by Gender for Young and Elderly Adults

Life-Stage Group	Thiamin (mg/day)	Riboflavin (mg/day)	Niacin (mg/day)	B_6 (mg/day)	Folate (μg/day)[a]	B_{12} (μg/day)
Males						
19–30 years						
EAR[b]	**1.0**	**1.1**	**12**	**1.1**	**320**	**2.0**
CSFII Median Dietary Intake,[c]	1.95,	2.33,	30.5,	2.31,	297,	5.60,
Range (5th–95th percentiles)	1.16–3.14	1.32–4.00	17.60–50.60	1.25–4.01	148–584	2.90–13.10
NHANES III Median Dietary Intake,[d]	1.78,	2.09,	25.30,	2.02,	277,	5.22,
Range (5th–95th percentiles)	1.07–3.41	1.18–3.90	15.00–45.60	1.16–3.91	163–564	4.42–7.56
>70 years						
EAR	**1.0**	**1.1**	**12**	**1.4**	**320**	**2.0**
CSFII Median Dietary Intake,[c]	1.64,	1.97,	21.7,	1.89,	276,	5.10,
Range (5th–95th percentiles)	0.97–2.62	1.09–3.30	12.60–35.30	1.01–3.29	137–527	2.40–10.30
NHANES III Median Dietary Intake,[d]	1.56,	1.84,	20.8,	1.72,	269,	4.99,
Range (5th–95th percentiles)	1.03–2.68	1.13–3.28	13.84–35.67	1.02–3.22	163–542	4.45–6.81
Females						
19–30 years						
EAR	**0.9**	**0.9**	**11**	**1.1**	**320**	**2.0**
CSFII Median Dietary Intake,[c]	1.22,	1.49,	17.5,	1.38,	200,	3.45,
Range (5th–95th percentiles)	0.80–1.99	0.80–2.55	9.50–29.10	0.76–2.31	100–374	1.67–6.47
NHANES III Median Dietary Intake,[d]	1.45,	1.63,	19.69,	1.54,	223,	4.77,
Range (5th–95th percentiles)	0.94–2.49	0.99–2.85	13.23–33.56	0.93–2.77	145–497	4.27–6.23
>70 years						
EAR	**0.9**	**0.9**	**11**	**1.3**	**320**	**2.0**
CSFII Median Dietary Intake,[c]	1.18,	1.40,	16.8,	1.41,	212,	3.32,
Range (5th–95th percentiles)	0.68–1.86	0.83–2.34	9.70–26.60	0.76–2.35	105–383	1.49–11.63
NHANES III Median Dietary Intake,[d]	1.38,	1.60,	18.78,	1.53,	252,	4.74
Range (5th–95th percentiles)	0.94–2.21	1.01–2.71	12.74–30.30	0.92–2.76	152–474	4.37–5.99

From Food and Nutrition Board–Institute of Medicine. Dietary reference intakes. Thiamin, riboflavin, niacin, vitamin B_6, folate, vitamin B_{12}, pantothenic acid, biotin, and choline. Washington, DC: National Academy Press, 1998 (prepublication copy). This is Table 5-1 in the original report.

Note: The Estimated Average Requirements (EAR) can be used to assess the adequacy of nutrient intakes by groups. To do this, one determines the percentage of individuals whose usual intakes are less than the EAR. From this table it can be seen that less than 5% of young men have thiamin intakes less than the EAR, but more than half of young women have reported folate intakes less than the EAR. Appendixes C and D allow more accurate estimates of percentages for all age groups than does this excerpted table.

[a]As dietary folate equivalents for the Estimated Average Requirement but not for reported dietary intakes. Reported intakes are likely to underestimate true intakes because of limitations of the methods used to analyze the folate content of food (see Chapter 8) and because adjustment has not been made for the higher bioavailability of the folic acid consumed in fortified foods and supplements: 1 dietary folate equivalent = 1 μg food folate = 0.6 μg of folic acid (from fortified food or supplement) consumed with food = 0.5 μg of synthetic (supplemental) folic acid taken on an empty stomach.

[b]EAR = Estimated Average Requirement.

[c]SOURCE: CSFII data on B vitamin intake from food, A. Carriquiry, Iowa State University, unpublished, 1997.

[d]SOURCE: NHANES III, 1988–1994, unpublished data on B vitamin intake from food, C. Johnson, National Center for Health Statistics, 1997.

Table A-2-c-4
Tolerable Upper Intake Levels

Life-Stage Group (years)	Niacin (mg/day)	Vitamin B_6 (mg/day)	Synthetic Folic Acid (μg/day)	Choline (g/day)
1–3	10	30	300	1.0
4–8	15	40	400	1.0
9–13	20	60	600	2.0
14–18	30	80	800	3.0
≥19	35	100	1000	3.5
Pregnant	35	100	1000	3.5
Lactating	35	100	1000	3.5

From Food and Nutrition Board–Institute of Medicine. Dietary reference intakes. Thiamin, riboflavin, niacin, vitamin B_6, folate, vitamin B_{12}, pantothenic acid, biotin, and choline. Washington, DC: National Academy Press, 1998 (prepublication copy).

Table A-2-c-5
Reference Heights and Weights for Children and Adults in the United States[a]

Gender	Age	Median Body Mass Index (kg/m²)	Reference Height in cm (in.)	Reference Weight[b] in kg (lb)
Male, female	2–6 months	—	64 (25)	7 (16)
	7–11 months	—	72 (28)	9 (20)
	1–3 years	—	91 (36)	13 (29)
	4–8 years	15.8	118 (46)	22 (48)
Male	9–13 years	18.5	147 (58)	40 (88)
	14–18 years	21.3	174 (68)	64 (142)
	19–30 years	24.4	176 (69)	76 (166)
Female	9–13 years	18.3	148 (58)	40 (88)
	14–18 years	21.3	163 (64)	57 (125)
	19–30 years	22.8	163 (64)	61 (133)

From Food and Nutrition Board–Institute of Medicine. Dietary reference intakes. Thiamin, riboflavin, niacin, vitamin B_6, folate, vitamin B_{12}, pantothenic acid, biotin, and choline. Washington, DC: National Academy Press, 1998 (prepublication copy). This is Table 1-1 in the original report.

[a]Based on data from the Third National Health and Nutritional Examination Survey, 1988–1994 (Briefer, U.S. Department of Health and Human Services, 1997, personal communication).

[b]Calculated from median body mass index and median heights for ages 4–8 years and older.

Table A-3-a
Summary of Examples of Recommended Nutrients Based on Energy Expressed As Daily Rates, Canada

Age	Sex	Energy (kcal)	Thiamin (mg)	Riboflavin (mg)	Niacin (ne[a])	n-3 PUFA[b] (g)	n-6 PUFA (g)
Months							
0–4	Both	600	0.3	0.3	4	0.5	3
5–12	Both	900	0.4	0.5	7	0.5	3
Years							
1	Both	1100	0.5	0.6	8	0.6	4
2–3	Both	1300	0.6	0.7	9	0.7	4
4–6	Both	1800	0.7	0.9	13	1.0	6
7–9	M	2200	0.9	1.1	16	1.2	7
	F	1900	0.8	1.0	14	1.0	6
10–12	M	2500	1.0	1.3	18	1.4	8
	F	2200	0.9	1.1	16	1.2	7
13–15	M	2800	1.1	1.4	20	1.5	9
	F	2200	0.9	1.1	16	1.2	7
16–18	M	3200	1.3	1.6	23	1.8	11
	F	2100	0.8	1.1	15	1.2	7
19–24	M	3000	1.2	1.5	22	1.6	10
	F	2100	0.8	1.1	15	1.2	7
25–49	M	2700	1.1	1.4	19	1.5	9
	F	1900	0.8[c]	1.0[c]	14[c]	1.1[c]	7[c]
50–74	M	2300	0.9	1.2	16	1.3	8
	F	1800	0.8[c]	1.0[c]	14[c]	1.1[c]	7[c]
75+	M	2000	0.8	1.0	14	1.1	7
	F[d]	1700	0.8[c]	1.0[c]	14[c]	1.1[c]	7[c]
Pregnancy (additional)							
1st trimester		100	0.1	0.1	1	0.05	0.3
2nd trimester		300	0.1	0.3	2	0.16	0.9
3rd trimester		300	0.1	0.3	2	0.16	0.9
Lactation (additional)		450	0.2	0.4	3	0.25	1.5

From Health and Welfare Canada. Nutrition recommendations. The report of the Scientific Review Committee. Ottawa: Supply and Services Canada, 1990. Reproduced with permission of the Minister of Public Works and Government Services Canada 1996.

[a]NE, Niacin equivalents.

[b]PUFA, Polyunsaturated fatty acids.

[c]Level below which intake should not fall.

[d]Assumes moderate (more than average) physical activity.

Table A-3-b
Summary of Examples of Recommended Nutrient Intake Based on Age and Body Weight Expressed as Daily Rates, Canada

Age	Sex	Weight (kg)	Protein (g)	Vit. A (RE)[a]	Vit. D (μg)	Vit. E (mg)	Vit. C (mg)	Folate (μg)	Vit. B_{12} (μg)	Calcium (mg)	Phosphorus (mg)	Magnesium (mg)	Iron (mg)	Iodine (μg)	Zinc (mg)
Months															
0–4	Both	6.0	12[b]	400	10	3	20	25	0.3	250[c]	150	20	0.3[d]	30	2[d]
5–12	Both	9.0	12	400	10	3	20	40	0.4	400	200	32	7	40	3
Years															
1	Both	11	13	400	10	3	20	40	0.5	500	300	40	6	55	4
2–3	Both	14	16	400	5	4	20	50	0.6	550	350	50	6	65	4
4–6	Both	18	19	500	5	5	25	70	0.8	600	400	65	8	85	5
7–9	M	25	26	700	2.5	7	25	90	1.0	700	500	100	8	110	7
	F	25	26	700	2.5	6	25	90	1.0	700	500	100	8	95	7
10–12	M	34	34	800	2.5	8	25	120	1.0	900	700	130	8	125	9
	F	36	36	800	2.5	7	25	130	1.0	1100	800	135	8	110	9
13–15	M	50	49	900	2.5	9	30[e]	175	1.0	1100	900	185	10	160	12
	F	48	46	800	2.5	7	30[e]	170	1.0	1000	850	180	13	160	9
16–18	M	62	58	1000	2.5	10	40[e]	220	1.0	900	1000	230	10	160	12
	F	53	47	800	2.5	7	30[e]	190	1.0	700	850	200	12	160	9
19–24	M	71	61	1000	2.5	10	40[e]	220	1.0	800	1000	240	9	160	12
	F	58	50	800	2.5	7	30[e]	180	1.0	700	850	200	13	160	9
25–49	M	74	64	1000	2.5	9	40[e]	230	1.0	800	1000	250	9	160	12
	F	59	51	800	2.5	6	30[e]	185	1.0	700	850	200	13	160	9
50–74	M	73	63	1000	5	7	40[e]	230	1.0	800	1000	250	9	160	12
	F	63	54	800	5	6	30[e]	195	1.0	800	850	210	8	160	9
75+	M	69	59	1000	5	6	40[e]	215	1.0	800	1000	230	9	160	12
	F	64	55	800	5	5	30[e]	200	1.0	800	850	210	8	160	9
Pregnancy (additional)															
1st trimester			5	0	2.5	2	0	200	0.2	500	200	15	0	25	6
2nd trimester			20	0	2.5	2	10	200	0.2	500	200	45	5	25	6
3rd trimester			24	0	2.5	2	10	200	0.2	500	200	45	10	25	6
Lactation (additional)			20	400	2.5	3	25	100	0.2	500	200	65	0	50	6

From Health and Welfare Canada. Nutrition recommendations. The report of the Scientific Review Committee. Ottawa: Supply and Services Canada, 1990. Reproduced with permission of the Minister of Public Works and Government Services Canada 1996.

[a]Retinol equivalents.

[b]Protein is assumed to be from breast milk and must be adjusted for infant formula.

[c]Infant formula with high phosphorus should contain 375 mg calcium.

[d]Breast milk is assumed to be the source of the mineral.

[e]Smokers should increase vitamin C by 50%.

A-4. DIETARY REFERENCE VALUES FOR FOOD ENERGY AND NUTRIENTS FOR THE UNITED KINGDOM (1)

Comments: To assist the reader in understanding the following tables taken from this Dietary Reference Values report, excerpts from its Introduction are given here. We make special note of the following:

1. The abbreviation RDA for nutrients differs from the RDA of the 10th RDA (1989) (Table II-A-2-a) and the recent Dietary Reference Intakes of the United States Food and Nutrition Board of the Institute of Medicine (Table II-A-2-b). The UK RDA refers to a group mean (see their paragraph 1.3 below).
2. The UK report defines three different sets of reference values as indicated in 1.3.8.
3. The figures in the various tables for individuals and groups are designated Dietary Reference Values (DRVs) rather than recommendations.
4. The values for protein, vitamins, and minerals given in the following tables are at the RNI level as defined in 1.3.8 below. These are statistically equivalent in derivation to the U.S. 1989 10th RDA and new U.S. dietary reference intakes. With the exception of the figures for energy (given as EAR), only the RNI values are included in these tables.

—The Appendix Editors

A-4-a. Excerpts from the Report's Introduction (1)

1.3 Interpretation of the Terms of Reference

1.3.1 The definition of the Recommended Daily Amount (RDA) for a nutrient which was used in the previous Report of the Committee on Medical Aspects of Food Policy is "the average amount of the nutrient which should be provided per head in a group of people if the needs of practically all members of the group are to be met." This was framed in an attempt to make it clear that the amounts referred to are averages for a group of people and not amounts which individuals must consume . . .

1.3.7 The Panel found no single criterion to define requirements for all nutrients. Some nutrients may have a variety of physiological effects at different levels of intake. Which of these effects should form the parameter of adequacy is therefore to some extent arbitrary. For each nutrient the particular parameter or parameters which were used to define adequacy are given in the text . . .

1.3.8 *Definition of Dietary Reference Values* Although information is usually inadequate to calculate the precise distribution of requirements in a group of individuals for a nutrient, it has been assumed to be normally distributed . . . This gives a notional mean requirement or Estimated Average Requirement (EAR) . . . The Panel has defined the Reference Nutrient Intake (RNI) as a point in the distribution, that is two notional standard deviations above the (EAR) . . . Intakes above this amount will almost certainly be adequate. At a point, two notional standard deviations (2 SD) below the mean, the Lower Reference Nutrient Intake (LNRI), represents the lowest intakes which will meet the needs of some individuals in the group. Intakes below this level are almost certainly inadequate for most individuals. For some nutrients the derivation of DRVs was not possible from these principles, and this is stated in the text. In particular, for those nutrients where no requirement could be defined (starches, sugars, fat and fatty acids), the DRVs are not derived on these principles, although analogous figures based on pragmatic judgements have been proposed (see original report).

1.3.9 At higher levels of consumption there may be evidence of undesirable effects. Guidance on such high levels of consumption is given in the text. The RNI . . . is the amount sufficient or more than sufficient to meet the nutritional needs of practically all healthy persons in a population, and therefore exceeds the requirements of most.

1.3.11 *Interpretation of Dietary Reference Values* For most nutrients the Panel found insufficient data to establish any of the DRVs with great confidence. There are inherent errors in some of the data, for instance in individuals' reports of their food intake, and the day-to-day variation in nutrient intakes also complicates interpretation. Even given complete accuracy of a dietary record, its relation to habitual intake remains uncertain, however long the recording period. The food composition tables normally used to determine nutrient intake from dietary records contain a number of assumptions and imperfections. Furthermore, there is uncertainty about the relevance of many biological markers, such as serum concentrations of a nutrient, as evidence of an individual's 'status' for that nutrient . . .

1.3.14 *Weights and standard age ranges* As requirements for most nutrients vary with both age and sex, the Panel has attempted to set DRVs for all such groups of the population. The Panel has sought new weight data for use in calculating DRVs for people of all ages in the UK . . . These weights are given in the table below for each of the standard age groups.

Children		Males		Females	
Age	Weight (kg)	Age	Weight (kg)	Age	Weight (kg)
0–3 months (formula fed)	5.9	11–14 years	43.1	11–14 years	43.8
4–6 months	7.7	15–18 years	64.5	15–18 years	55.5
7–9 months	8.9	19–50 years	74.0	19–50 years	60.0
10–12 months	9.8	50+ years	71.0	50+ years	62.0
1–3 years	12.6				
4–6 years	17.8			Pregnancy	
7–10 years	28.3			Lactation: 0–4 months	
				4+ months	

1.3.18 *Safe intakes* For some nutrients, which are known to have important functions in humans, the Panel found insufficient reliable data on human requirements and were unable to set any DRVs for these. However, they decided on grounds of prudence to set a safe intake, particularly for infants and children, and these are given in [Report] Table 1.6 [Appendix Table II-A-4-f]. The safe intake was judged to be a level or range of intake at which there is no risk of deficiency, and below a level where there is a risk of undesirable effects.

1.4 *Uses of Dietary Reference Values* These DRVs apply to groups of healthy people and are not necessarily appropriate for those with different needs arising from disease, such as infections, disorders of the gastro-intestinal tract or metabolic abnormalities. **The DRVs for any one nutrient presuppose that requirements for energy and all other nutrients are met** . . .

1.4.1 *For assessing diets of individuals*

1.4.1.1 The impression of most estimates both of individuals' nutrient intakes and of nutritional status, and thus of the estimation of the DRVs themselves, means that utmost caution should be used in applying the figures to the interpretation (or assessment) of individual diets. Even with a perfect measure of an individuals's habitual intake of a nutrient (a difficult goal), the DRVs can give no more than a guide to the adequacy of diet for that individual.

1.4.1.2 If the habitual intake is below the LRNI it is likely that the individual will not be consuming sufficient of the nutrient to maintain the function selected by the Panel as an appropriate parameter of nutritional status for that nutrient, and further investigation, including biological measures, may be appropriate.

1.4.1.3 If the habitual intake is above the RNI, then it is extremely unlikely that the individual will not be consuming sufficient.

1.4.1.4 If the intake lies between the two, then the chances of the diet being inadequate (in respect of the chosen function parameter for any nutrient) fall as the intake approaches the RNI . . . It is impossible to say with any certainty whether an individual's nutrient intake, if it lies between the LRNI and the RNI, is or is not adequate, without some biological measure in that individual.

1.4.2 *For assessing diets of groups of individuals*

1.4.2.1 When measures of individual diets are aggregated, one of the sources of imprecision is attenuated—that is intraindividual day to day variability. Assuming that the interindividual variability is random, then in a sufficiently large group, this source of imprecision is also diminished. Thus the group mean intake will more precisely represent the habitual group mean intake than any of the individual measures will represent individual intakes.

1.5 DRV for energy

1.5.1 . . . RNIs for all nutrients, but not energy, can be set at the upper end of the range of requirements because an intake moderately in excess of requirements has no adverse effects, but reduces the risk of deficiency. For energy, however, this is not the case. Recommendations for energy have therefore always been set as the average of energy requirements for any population group. The Panel has therefore calculated EARs for energy, but not LRNIs or RNIs.

1.7 DRVs for protein . . . The approach derived from estimates of basic nitrogen requirements with additions for specific situations such as growth and pregnancy, which was adopted by joint FAO/WHO/UNU Expert Consultation in 1985, has formed the basis of the Panel's deliberations and enabled calculations of DRVs including EARs shown in [Report] Table 1-3 [Appendix Table II-A-4-c].

REFERENCE

1. Report on Health and Social Subjects No. 41. Dietary Reference Values for Food Energy and Nutrients for the United Kingdom. Report of the Panel on Dietary Reference Values of the Committee on Medical Aspects of Food Policy. London: Her Majesty's Stationery Office, 1991.

Table A-4-b
Estimated Average Requirements (EARs) for Energy, United Kingdom[a]

Age	EARs MJ/d (kcal/day)	
	Males	Females
0–3 months	2.28 (545)	2.16 (515)
4–6 months	2.89 (690)	2.69 (645)
7–9 months	3.44 (825)	3.20 (765)
10–12 months	3.85 (920)	3.61 (865)
1–3 years	5.15 (1230)	4.86 (1165)
4–6 years	7.16 (1715)	6.46 (1545)
7–10 years	8.24 (1970)	7.28 (1740)
11–14 years	9.27 (2220)	7.72 (1845)
15–18 years	11.51 (2755)	8.83 (2110)
19–50 years	10.60 (2550)	8.10 (1940)
51–59 years	10.60 (2550)	8.00 (1900)
60–64 years	9.93 (2380)	7.99 (1900)
65–74 years	9.71 (2330)	7.96 (1900)
75+ years	8.77 (2100)	7.61 (1810)
Pregnancy		+0.80[b] (200)
Lactation		
1 month		+1.90 (450)
2 months		+2.20 (530)
3 months		+2.40 (570)
4–6 months (group 1)[c]		+2.00 (480)
4–6 months (group 2)		+2.40 (570)
> 6 months (group 1)		+1.00 (240)
> 6 months (group 2)		+2.30 (550)

From Report on Health and Social Subjects: no. 41, Dietary reference values for food energy and nutrients for the United Kingdom. Report of the Panel on Dietary Reference Values of the Committee on Medical Aspects of Food Policy. London: Her Majesty's Stationery Office, 1991. This is the U.K.'s Report Table 1.1.

[a]See paragraph 1.5 in Table II-A-4-a.

[b]Last trimester only.

[c]See original text for comments.

Table A-4-c
Reference Nutrient Intakes for Protein, United Kingdom[a]

Age	Reference Nutrient Intake[b] (g/day)
0–3 months	12.5[c]
4–6 months	12.7
7–9 months	13.7
10–12 months	14.9
1–3 years	14.5
4–6 years	19.7
7–10 years	28.3
Males	
11–14 years	42.1
15–18 years	55.2
19–50 years	55.5
50+ years	53.3
Females	
11–14 years	41.2
15–18 years	45.0
19–50 years	45.0
50+ years	46.5
Pregnancy[d]	+6
Lactation[d]	
0–4 months	+11
4+ months	+8

From Report on Health and Social Subjects: no. 41, Dietary reference values for food energy and nutrients for the United Kingdom. Report of the Panel on Dietary Reference Values of the Committee on Medical Aspects of Food Policy. London: Her Majesty's Stationery Office, 1991. This is the U.K.'s Report Table 1.3.

[a]See paragraph 1.7 in Table II-A-4-a.

[b]These figures, based on egg and milk protein, assume complete digestibility.

[c]No values for infants 0–3 months are given by WHO. The RNI is calculated from the recommendations of Committee on Medical Aspects of Food Policy (COMA).

[d]To be added to adult requirement through all stages of pregnancy and lactation.

Table A-4-d
Reference Nutrient Intakes for Vitamins, United Kingdom[a]

Age	Thiamin (mg/day)	Riboflavin (mg/day)	Niacin (nicotinic acid equivalent) (mg/day)	Vitamin B_6 (mg/day)[b]	Vitamin B_{12} (μg/day)	Folate (μg/day)	Vitamin C (mg/day)	Vitamin A (μg/day)	Vitamin D (μg/day)
0–3 months	0.2	0.4	3	0.2	0.3	50	25	350	8.5
4–6 months	0.2	0.4	3	0.2	0.3	50	25	350	8.5
7–9 months	0.2	0.4	4	0.3	0.4	50	25	350	7
10–12 months	0.3	0.4	5	0.4	0.4	50	25	350	7
1–3 years	0.5	0.6	8	0.7	0.5	70	30	400	7
4–6 years	0.7	0.8	11	0.9	0.8	100	30	400	—
7–10 years	0.7	1.0	12	1.0	1.0	150	30	500	—
Males									
11–14 years	0.9	1.2	15	1.2	1.2	200	35	600	—
15–18 years	1.1	1.3	18	1.5	1.5	200	40	700	—
19–50 years	1.0	1.3	17	1.4	1.5	200	40	700	—
50+ years	0.9	1.3	16	1.4	1.5	200	40	700	—[c]
Females									
11–14 years	0.7	1.1	12	1.0	1.2	200	35	600	—
15–18 years	0.8	1.1	14	1.2	1.5	200	40	600	—
19–50 years	0.8	1.1	13	1.2	1.5	200	40	600	—
50+ years	0.8	1.1	12	1.2	1.5	200	40	600	—[c]
Pregnancy	+0.1[d]	+0.3	—[e]	—[e]	—[e]	+100	+10[d]	+100	10
Lactation									
0–4 months	+0.2	+0.5	+2	—[e]	+0.5	+60	+30	+350	10
4+ months	+0.2	+0.5	+2	—[e]	+0.5	+60	+30	+350	10

From Report on Health and Social Subjects: no. 41. Dietary reference values for food energy and nutrients for the United Kingdom. Report of the Panel on Dietary Reference Values of the Committee on Medical Aspects of Food Policy. London: Her Majesty's Stationery Office, 1991. This is the U.K.'s Report Table 1-4.

[a]See Table II-A-4-a for definition.

[b]Based on protein providing 14.7% of EAR for energy.

[c]After age 65 the RNI is 10 μg/day for men and women.

[d]For last trimester only.

[e]No increment.

Table A-4-e-1
Reference Nutrient Intakes for Minerals (SI Units) United Kingdom[a]

Age	Calcium (mmol/day)	Phosphorus[b] (mmol/day)	Magnesium (mmol/day)	Sodium[c] (mmol/day)	Potassium[d] (mmol/day)	Chloride[e] (mmol/day)	Iron (μmol/day)	Zinc (μmol/day)	Copper (μmol/day)	Selenium (μmol/day)	Iodine (μmol/day)
0–3 months	13.1	13.1	2.2	9	20	9	30	60	5	0.1	0.4
4–6 months	13.1	13.1	2.5	12	22	12	80	60	5	0.2	0.5
7–9 months	13.1	13.1	3.2	14	18	14	140	75	5	0.1	0.5
10–12 months	13.1	13.1	3.3	15	18	15	140	75	5	0.1	0.5
1–3 years	8.8	8.8	3.5	22	20	22	120	75	6	0.2	0.6
4–6 years	11.3	11.3	4.8	30	28	30	110	100	9	0.3	0.8
7–10 years	13.8	13.8	8.0	50	50	50	160	110	11	0.4	0.9
Males											
11–14 years	25.0	25.0	11.5	70	80	70	200	140	13	0.6	1.0
15–18 years	25.0	25.0	12.3	70	90	70	200	145	16	0.9	1.0
19–50 years	17.5	17.5	12.3	70	90	70	160	145	19	0.9	1.0
50+ years	17.5	17.5	12.3	70	90	70	160	145	19	0.9	1.0
Females											
11–14 years	20.0	20.0	11.5	70	80	70	260[f]	140	13	0.6	1.0
15–18 years	20.0	20.0	12.3	70	90	70	260[f]	110	16	0.8	1.1
19–50 years	17.5	17.5	10.9	70	90	70	260[f]	110	19	0.8	1.1
50+ years	17.5	17.5	10.9	70	90	70	160	110	19	0.8	1.1
Pregnancy	[c,f,e]	—[f]	—[f]	—[f]	—[f]	—[f]	*	*	*	*	*
Lactation											
0–4 months	+14.3	+14.3	+2.1	*	*	*	*	+90	+5	+0.2	*
4+ months	+14.3	+14.3	+2.1	*	*	*	*	+40	+5	+0.2	*

From Report on Health and Social Subjects: no. 41. Dietary reference values for food energy and nutrients for the United Kingdom. Report of the Panel on Dietary Reference Values of the Committee on Medical Aspects of Food Policy. London: Her Majesty's Stationery Office, 1991. This is the U.K.'s Report Table 15.

*No increment.

[a]See Table II-A-4-a for definition.

[b]Phosphorus RNI is set equal to calcium in molar terms.

[c]1 mmol sodium = 23 mg.

[d]1 mmol potassium = 39 mg.

[e]Corresponds to sodium 1 mmol = 35.5 mg.

[f]Insufficient for women with high menstrual losses where the most practical way of meeting iron requirements is to take iron supplements (see Table 28-2 in original report).

Table A-4-e-2
Reference Nutrient Intakes for Minerals (Traditional Units), United Kingdom[a]

Age	Calcium (mg/day)	Phosphorus[b] (mg/day)	Magnesium (mg/day)	Sodium (mg/day)[c]	Potassium (mgl/day)[d]	Chloride[e] (mg/day)	Iron (mg/day)	Zinc (mg/day)	Copper (mg/day)	Selenium (µg/day)	Iodine (µg/day)
0–3 months	525	400	55	210	800	320	1.7	4.0	0.2	10	50
4–6 months	525	400	60	280	850	400	4.3	4.0	0.3	13	60
7–9 months	525	400	75	320	700	500	7.8	5.0	0.3	10	60
10–12 months	525	400	80	350	700	500	7.8	5.0	0.3	10	60
1–3 years	350	270	85	500	800	800	6.9	5.0	0.4	15	70
4–6 years	450	350	120	700	1100	1100	6.1	6.5	0.6	20	100
7–10 years	550	450	200	1200	2000	1800	8.7	7.0	0.7	30	110
Males											
11–14 years	1000	775	280	1600	3100	2500	11.3	9.0	0.8	45	130
15–18 years	1000	775	300	1600	3500	2500	11.3	9.5	1.0	70	140
19–50 years	700	550	300	1600	3500	2500	8.7	9.5	1.2	75	140
50+ years	700	550	300	1600	3500	2500	8.7	9.5	1.2	75	140
Females											
11–14 years	800	625	280	1600	3100	2500	14.8[f]	9.0	0.8	45	130
15–18 years	800	625	300	1600	3500	2500	14.8[f]	7.0	1.0	60	140
19–50 years	700	550	270	1600	3500	2500	14.8[f]	7.0	1.2	60	140
50+ years	700	550	270	1600	3500	2500	8.7	7.0	1.2	60	140
Pregnancy	—*	—*	—*	—*	—*	—*	—*	—*	—*	—*	—*
Lactation											
0–4 months	+550	+440	+50	—*	—*	—*	*	+6.0	+0.3	+15	—*
4+ months	+550	+440	+50	—*	—*	—*	*	+2.5	+0.3	+15	—*

From Report on Health and Social Subjects: no. 41. Dietary reference values for food energy and nutrients for the United Kingdom. Report of the Panel on Dietary Reference Values of the Committee on Medical Aspects of Food Policy. London: Her Majesty's Stationery Office, 1991. This is the U.K.'s Report Table 1.5.

*No increment.

[a]See Table II-A-4-a for definition.

[b]Phosphorus RNI is set equal to calcium in molar terms.

[c]1 mmol sodium = 23 mg.

[d]1 mmol potassium = 39 mg.

[e]Corresponds to sodium 1 mmol = 35.5 mg.

[f]Insufficient for women with high menstrual losses where the most practical way of meeting iron requirements is to take iron supplements (see Table 28.2 in original report).

Table A-4-f
Safe Intakes, United Kingdom[a]

Nutrient	Safe Intake[b]
Vitamins	
Pantothenic acid	
Adults	3–7 mg/day
Infants	1.7 mg/day
Biotin	10–200 μg/day
Vitamin E	
Men	Above 4 mg/day
Women	Above 3 mg/day
Infants	0.4 mg/g polyunsaturated fatty acids
Vitamin K	
Adults	1 μg/kg/day
Infants	10 μg/day
Minerals	
Manganese	
Adults	Above 1.4 mg (26 μmol)/day
Infants and children	Above 16 μg (0.3 μmol)/kg/day
Molybdenum	
Adults	50–400 μg/day
Infants, children, and adolescents	0.5–1.5 μg/kg/day
Chromium	
Adults	Above 25 μg (0.5 μmol)/day
Children and adolescents	0.1–1.0 μg (2–20 nmol)/kg/day
Fluoride	
Children over 6 years and adults	0.5 mg/kg/day (3 μmol/kg/day)
Children over 6 months	0.12 mg/kg/day (6 μmol/kg/day)
Infants under 6 months	0.22 mg/kg/day (12 μmol/kg/day)

From Report on Health and Social Subjects: no. 41. Dietary reference values for food energy and nutrients for the United Kingdom. Report of the Panel on Dietary Reference Values of the Committee on Medical Aspects of Food Policy. London: Her Majesty's Stationery Office, 1991.) This is the U.K.'s Report Table 1.6.

[a]See Table II-A-4-a for definition.

[b]For some nutrients, which are known to have important functions in humans, the Panel found insufficient reliable data on human requirements and were unable to set any dietary reference values for these. However, they decided on grounds of prudence to set a safe intake, particularly for infants and children. The safe intake was judged to be a level or range of intake at which there is no risk of deficiency and below a level where there is risk of undesirable effects. They are not therefore intended as a "toxic level," and although exceeding these safe intakes would not necessarily result in undesirable effects, equally there is no evidence for any benefits. The Panel agreed that the safe range of intakes set for the nutrients need not be exceeded.

Table A-5-a

Recommended Dietary Allowances for the Japanese: Dietary Allowances for Growth Period and Moderate Level (II) of Physical Activity, Japan

Age (years)	Reference Height (cm) Male	Female	Reference Body Weight (kg) Male	Female	Energy (kcal) Male	Female	Protein (g) Male	Female	Fat Energy Ratio (%)	Calcium (g) Male	Female	Iron (mg) Male	Female	Vitamin A (IU) Male	Female	Vitamin B_1 (mg) Male	Female	Vitamin B_2 (mg) Male	Female	Niacin (mg) Male	Female	Vitamin C (mg)	Vitamin D (IU)
0 month					120/kg		3.0/kg		45	0.5		6		1300		0.2		0.3		4			
2 month					110/kg		2.4/kg		45	0.5		6		1300		0.3		0.4		6			
6 month					100/kg		2.8/kg		30–40	0.5		6		1000		0.4		0.5		6			
1	80.2	79.1	10.57	10.07	960	920	30	30				7	7	1000	1000	0.4	0.4	0.5	0.5	6	6		400
2	89.6	88.4	12.85	12.36	1200	1150	35	35				7	7	1000	1000	0.5	0.5	0.7	0.6	8	8		
3	97.6	96.4	15.00	14.57	1400	1350	40	40				8	8	1000	1000	0.6	0.5	0.8	0.7	9	9		
4	104.7	103.6	17.12	16.74	1550	1500	45	45			0.5	8	8	1000	1000	0.6	0.6	0.9	0.8	10	10	40	
5	111.2	110.2	19.34	18.97	1650	1550	50	50				8	8	1000	1000	0.7	0.6	0.9	0.9	11	10		
6	117.2	116.2	21.70	21.25	1700	1600	55	50				9	9	1200	1200	0.7	0.6	0.9	0.9	11	11		
7	123.0	121.9	24.40	23.75	1800	1650	60	55				9	9	1200	1200	0.7	0.7	1.0	0.9	12	11		
8	128.6	127.5	27.42	26.60	1900	1750	65	60				9	9	1200	1200	0.8	0.7	1.0	1.0	13	12		
9	133.9	133.2	30.69	29.95	1950	1850	70	65	25–30			10	10	1500	1500	0.8	0.7	1.1	1.0	13	12		
10	139.2	139.7	34.34	34.23	2050	1950	75	70		0.6	0.6	10	10	1500	1500	0.8	0.8	1.1	1.1	14	13		
11	145.4	146.5	38.73	39.28	2200	2100	80	75		0.7		10	10	1500	1500	0.9	0.8	1.2	1.2	15	14		
12	153.0	151.6	44.31	43.92	2350	2250	85	75		0.8		12	12	1500	1500	0.9	0.9	1.3	1.2	16	15		
13	160.5	154.7	50.39	47.60	2550	2300	90	75		0.9	0.7	12	12	2000	1800	1.0	0.9	1.4	1.3	17	15		
14	166.0	156.5	55.69	50.38	2650	2300	90	75		0.9		12	12	2000	1800	1.1	0.9	1.5	1.3	17	15		
15	169.3	157.4	59.62	52.08	2700	2250	90	70		0.8		12	12	2000	1800	1.1	0.9	1.5	1.2	18	15		
16	171.0	158.0	61.93	52.92	2750	2200	80	65		0.8		12	12	2000	1800	1.1	0.9	1.5	1.2	18	15		
17	171.9	158.3	63.15	52.95	2700	2150	75	65		0.7		12	12	2000	1800	1.1	0.9	1.5	1.2	18	14		100
18	172.3	158.5	63.53	52.53	2700	2100	75	60		0.7		12	12	2000	1800	1.1	0.8	1.5	1.2	18	14		
19	172.3	158.5	63.53	51.93	2600	2050	70	60				12	12	2000	1800	1.0	0.8	1.4	1.1	17	14		
20–29	171.3	158.1	64.69	51.31	2550	2000	70	60				10	12	2000	1800	1.0	0.8	1.4	1.1	17	13	50	
30–39	170.8	157.3	66.62	54.02	2500	2000	70	60				10	12	2000	1800	1.0	0.8	1.4	1.1	17	13		
40–49	168.8	155.9	66.19	55.49	2400	1950	70	60				10	12	2000	1800	1.0	0.8	1.3	1.1	16	13		
50–59	165.9	153.0	63.66	53.95	2300	1850	70	60	20–25	0.6	0.6	10	12 (postmenopausal 10)	2000	1800	0.9	0.7	1.3	1.0	15	12		
60–64	163.4	150.6	61.12	51.28	2100	1750	70	60				10	10	2000	1800	0.8	0.7	1.2	1.0	14	12		
65–69	162.1	149.1	59.28	49.53	2100	1700	70	60				10	10	2000	1800	0.8	0.7	1.2	1.0	14	12		
70–74	160.7	147.6	57.28	47.69	1850	1600	70	60				10	10	2000	1800	0.8	0.7	1.2	1.0	14	12		
75–79	159.3	146.1	55.30	45.83	1800	1500	65	55				10	10	2000	1800	0.8	0.7	1.2	1.0	14	12		
80–	157.3	143.9	52.85	43.67	1650	1400	65	55				10	10	2000	1800	0.8	0.7	1.2	1.0	14	12		

From Recommended Dietary Allowances for the Japanese, 5th rev. Supervised by Health and Nutrition Division, Health Service Bureau, Ministry of Health and Welfare, 1996. With permission.

Notes to "Dietary allowances for the Japanese" (table)

1. The dietary allowances shown in Tables A-5-a-d are not to be applied to individuals without modification. Reference should be made to original report for application.
2. As for determination of the intensity of living activity, reference should be made to the "classification" for intensities of living activities as viewed from daily life (standards). Those falling under "I (light)" in the degree of intensity of living activities are recommended to expend calories equivalent to "II (moderate)" degree of intensity as listed in Table A-5-a by either changing the daily activities or engaging in additional physical activities.
3. The daily salt intake is recommended to be 10 g/day/person or less as previously.
4. Vitamin E (α-tocopherol equivalent) intake should preferably be 8 mg for adult males and 7 mg for adult females.

Table A-5-b
Dietary Allowances for Light Level (I) of Physical Activity

Age (years)	Energy (kcal) Men	Energy (kcal) Women	Protein (g) Men	Protein (g) Women	Fat Energy Ratio (%)	Calcium (g) Men	Calcium (g) Women	Iron (mg) Men	Iron (mg) Women	Vitamin A (IU) Men	Vitamin A (IU) Women	Vitamin B_1 (mg) Men	Vitamin B_1 (mg) Women	Vitamin B_2 (mg) Men	Vitamin B_2 (mg) Women	Niacin (mg) Men	Niacin (mg) Women	Vitamin C (mg)	Vitamin D (IU)
15	2400	2000	90	70		0.8		12	12	2000	1800	1.0	0.8	1.3	1.1	16	13		
16	2400	1950	80	65	25-30	0.8	0.7	12	12	2000	1800	1.0	0.8	1.3	1.1	16	13		
17	2400	1900	75	65		0.7		12	12	2000	1800	1.0	0.8	1.3	1.0	16	13		
18	2400	1850	75	60		0.7		12	12	2000	1800	1.0	0.7	1.3	1.0	16	12		
19	2350	1850	70	60				12	12	2000	1800	0.9	0.7	1.3	1.0	16	12		
20–29	2250	1800	70	60				10	12	2000	1800	0.9	0.7	1.2	1.0	15	12		
30–39	2200	1750	70	60				10	12	2000	1800	0.9	0.7	1.2	1.0	15	12		
40–49	2150	1700	70	60				10	12 (PM 10)	2000	1800	0.9	0.7	1.2	0.9	14	11	50	100
50–59	2050	1650	70	60	20-25	0.6	0.6	10	12	2000	1800	0.8	0.7	1.1	0.9	14	11		
60–64	1900	1550	70	60				10	10	2000	1800	0.8	0.6	1.0	0.9	13	10		
65–69	1800	1500	70	60				10	10	2000	1800	0.7	0.6	1.0	0.9	12	10		
70–74	1700	1400	70	60				10	10	2000	1800	0.7	0.6	0.9	0.9	12	10		
75–79	1600	1350	65	55				10	10	2000	1800	0.7	0.6	0.9	0.9	12	10		
80	1500	1250	65	55				10	10	2000	1800	0.7	0.6	0.9	0.9	12	10		
Additions: Pregnancy 1–5 months		+150		+10			+0.3		+3		+0		+0.1		+0.1		+1	+10	+300
Additions: Pregnancy 6–10 months		+350		+20	25-30		+0.3		+8		+200		+0.2		+0.2		+2	+10	+300
Additions: Lactation		+700		+20			+0.5		+8		+1400		+0.3		+0.4		+5	+40	+300

Note: Additions for pregnant and lactating women are shown for convenience. Their levels of physical activity should not be regarded uniformly as falling subject to the light level (I).

Table A-5-c
Dietary Allowances for Light-Heavy Level (III) of Physical Activity

Age (years)	Energy (kcal)		Protein (g)		Fat Energy Ratio (%)	Calcium (g)		Iron (mg)		Vitamin A (IU)		Vitamin B_1 (mg)		Vitamin B_2 (mg)		Niacin (mg)		Vitamin C (mg)	Vitamin D (IU)
	Men	Women	Men	Women		Men	Women	Men	Women	Men	Women	Men	Women	Men	Women	Men	Women		
15	3250	2650	105	85		0.8		12	12	2000	1800	1.3	1.1	1.8	1.5	21	17		
16	3250	2600	95	80		0.8	0.7	12	12	2000	1800	1.3	1.0	1.8	1.4	21	17		
17	3250	2550	90	80		0.7		12	12	2000	1800	1.3	1.0	1.8	1.4	21	17		
18	3200	2500	90	75		0.7		12	12	2000	1800	1.3	1.0	1.8	1.4	21	17		
19	3150	2450	85	70				12	12	2000	1800	1.3	1.0	1.7	1.3	21	16		
20–29	3050	2400	85	70	25–30			10	12 (PM10)	2000	1800	1.2	1.0	1.7	1.3	20	16	50	100
30–39	3000	2350	85	70				10	12	2000	1800	1.2	0.9	1.7	1.3	20	16		
40–49	2900	2300	85	70		0.6	0.6	10	12	2000	1800	1.2	0.9	1.6	1.3	19	15		
50–59	2750	2250	85	70				10	12	2000	1800	1.1	0.9	1.5	1.2	18	15		
60–64	2500	2050	80	70				10	10	2000	1800	1.0	0.8	1.4	1.1	17	14		
65–69	2400	2000	80	70				10	10	2000	1800	1.0	0.8	1.4	1.1	17	14		

Table A-5-d
Dietary Allowances for Heavy Level (IV) of Physical Activity

Age (years)	Energy (kcal)		Protein (g)		Fat Energy Ratio (%)	Calcium (g)		Iron (mg)		Vitamin A (IU)		Vitamin B_1 (mg)		Vitamin B_2 (mg)		Niacin (mg)		Vitamin C (mg)	Vitamin D (IU)
	Men	Women	Men	Women		Men	Women	Men	Women	Men	Women	Men	Women	Men	Women	Men	Women		
15	3800	3100	115	95		0.8		12	12	2000	1800	1.5	1.2	2.1	1.7	25	20		
16	3800	3050	115	95		0.8	0.7	12	12	2000	1800	1.5	1.2	2.1	1.7	25	20		
17	3800	2950	110	90		0.7		12	12	2000	1800	1.5	1.2	2.1	1.6	25	19		
18	3750	2950	110	90		0.7		12	12	2000	1800	1.5	1.2	2.1	1.6	25	19		
19	3700	2850	105	85				12	12	2000	1800	1.5	1.1	2.0	1.6	24	19		
20–29	3550	2800	100	85	25–30			10	12 (PM10)	2000	1800	1.4	1.1	2.0	1.5	23	18	50	100
30–39	3500	2750	100	85				10	12	2000	1800	1.4	1.1	1.9	1.5	23	18		
40–49	3400	2700	100	85		0.6	0.6	10	12	2000	1800	1.4	1.1	1.9	1.5	22	18		
50–59	3200	2600	100	85				10	12	2000	1800	1.3	1.0	1.8	1.4	21	17		
60–64	2900	2350	95	80				10	10	2000	1800	1.2	1.0	1.6	1.3	19	16		
65–69	2800	2300	95	80				10	10	2000	1800	1.1	1.0	1.6	1.3	19	16		

Table A-6
Recommended Daily Dietary Allowances, Korea[a]

Category	Age (years)	Weight (kg)	Height (cm)	Energy (kcal)	Protein (g)	Vitamin A (re)[b]	Vitamin B_1 (mg)	Vitamin B_2 (mg)	Niacin (mg)	Vitamin C (mg)	Vitamin D (μg)[c]	Calcium (mg)	Iron (mg)[d]
Infants													
	0–3 months	5.5	58.5	800	25	350	0.40	0.48	6.4	35	10	400	10
	4–6 months	8.4	67.5	900	25	350	0.45	0.54	7.2	35	10	400	10
	7–9 months	9.5	76.0	1000	30	350	0.50	0.60	8.0	35	10	400	15
	10–12 months	10.4	79.0	1100	30	350	0.55	0.66	8.0	35	10	400	15
Children													
	1–3	12.6	87.0	1200	35	350	0.60	0.72	8.0	40	10	500	15
	4–6	19.0	110.0	1300	40	400	0.75	0.90	10.0	40	10	600	10
	7–9	26.0	130.0	1800	50	500	0.90	1.08	12.0	40	10	700	10
Males													
	10–12	36.0	144.0	2100	60	600	1.05	1.26	14.0	50	10	800	15
	13–15	51.0	161.0	2600	80	700	1.30	1.36	17.0	50	10	800	18
	16–19	59.0	169.0	2500	75	700	1.25	1.50	16.5	55	10	800	18
	20–29	64.0	170.5	2500	70	700	1.25	1.50	16.5	55	5	600	10
	30–49	65.0	168.5	2500	70	700	1.25	1.50	16.5	55	5	600	10
	50–64	63.0	168.0	2200	70	700	1.10	1.32	14.5	55	5	600	10
	65 or older	61.0	167.0	1900	70	700	1.00	1.20	13.0	55	5	600	10
Females													
	10–12	37.0	145.0	2000	60	600	1.00	1.20	13.0	50	10	800	18
	13–15	48.0	155.0	2300	65	700	1.15	1.38	15.0	50	10	800	18
	16–19	52.0	158.0	2200	60	700	1.10	1.32	14.5	55	10	700	18
	20–29	52.5	159.5	2000	60	700	1.00	1.20	13.0	55	5	600	18
	30–49	55.0	158.0	2000	60	700	1.00	1.20	13.0	55	5	600	18
	50–64	54.0	156.0	1900	60	700	1.00	1.20	13.0	55	5	600	10
	65 or older	53.0	156.0	1600	60	700	1.00	1.20	13.0	55	5	600	10
Pregnancy		First half		+150	+30	+0	+0.40	+0.30	+2.0	+15	+5	+400	+2
		Second half		+350	+30	+100	+0.40	+0.30	+2.0	+15	+5	+400	+2
Lactation				+700	+30	+300	+0.60	+0.50	+6.0	+35	+5	+500	+2

From the Ministry of Health and Social Affairs, Kyonggi, Korea, 1989.

[a]Allowances for energy are based on individuals of moderate activity. Data in this table are intended to provide only a standard figure under usual environment and given conditions.

[b]Retinol equivalent: 1 RE = 1 μg retinol = 6 μg β-carotene.

[c]Vitamin D: 10 μg = 400 IU.

[d]Supplemental iron should be taken to meet the increased requirement during pregnancy and lactation.

A-7. NOTES ACCOMPANYING AUSTRALIAN RDIs (1)

1. Amounts of nutrients which should be available per head of a population group if the needs of practically all members of the population group are to be met.
2. Recommendations for all nutrients were revised between 1982 and 1988, energy revised 1989.
3. All RDIs are based upon estimates of requirements with a generous "safety factor" added.
4. Recommendations for dietary intakes of vitamin D were not considered necessary unless people are house bound, since the vitamin D status of Australians is determined by exposure to UV light from the sun.
5. RDIs for thiamin, riboflavin, niacin, and vitamin B_6 are based on energy requirements in existence when these B vitamin recommendations were revised (NHMRC 1986).
6. The following factors were used:

   Thiamin, 0.1 mg/1000 kJ

   Riboflavin, 0.15 mg/1000 kJ

   Niacin, 1.6 mg/1000 kJ

   Vitamin B_6, 0.02 mg/g protein (based on protein as 10–15% of recommended energy uptake).

7. Niacin values are presented as a single figure, the midpoint of the range adopted in 1984.
8. Iron is expressed as a range to allow for differences in bioavailability of iron from different Australian foods. The RDIs for pregnancy are for the 2nd and 3rd trimesters.
9. Selenium intake should not exceed 600 μg/day.
10. Background documents to these recommendations are included in the bibliography to this report.

Table A-7-a
Recommended Dietary Intakes for Children Under 7 Years (Expressed as Mean Daily Intake)

	Infants			Young Children	
	0–6 months				
	Breast-Fed	Bottle-Fed	7–12 months	1–3 years	4–7 years
Vitamin A (μg retinol equivalents)	425	425	300	300	350
Thiamin (mg)	0.15	0.25	0.35	0.5	0.7
Riboflavin (mg)	0.4	0.4	0.6	0.8	1.1
Niacin (mg niacin equivalents)	4	4	7	10	12
Vitamin B_6 (mg)	0.25	0.25	0.45	0.6–0.9	0.8–1.3
Total folate (μg)	50	50	75	100	100
Vitamin B_{12} (μg)	0.3	0.3	0.7	1.0	1.5
Vitamin C (mg)	25	25	30	30	30
Vitamin E (mg α-tocopheral equivalents)	2.5	4.0	4.0	5.0	6.0
Zinc (mg)	3	3–6	4.5	4.5	6
Iron (mg)	0.5	3.0	9.0	6–8	6–8
Iodine (μg)	50	50	60	70	90
Magnesium (mg)	40	40	60	80	110
Calcium (mg)	300	500	550	700	800
Phosphorus (mg)	150	150	300	500	700
Selenium (μg)	10	10	15	25	30
Sodium (mmol)	6–12	6–12	14–25	14–50	20–75
(mg)	140–280	140–280	320–580	320–1150	460–1730
Potassium (mmol)	10–15	10–15	12–35	25–70	40–100
(mg)	390–580	390–580	470–1370	980–2730	1560–3900
Protein (g)	[a]	2.0/kg body wt	1.6/kg body wt	14–18	18–24

National Health and Medical Research Council. Recommended dietary intakes for use in Australia. Canberra: Australian Government Publishing Service, 1991.

[a]No recommendation has been made for protein for breast-fed infants under the age of 6 months. Many observations show that infants breast-fed by healthy well-nourished mothers will grow at a satisfactory rate for the first 4–6 months. It can therefore be assumed that protein requirements are met if the volume of milk maintains growth at an acceptable rate.

Table A-7-b
Recommended Dietary Intakes for Children Over 7 Years (Expressed as Mean Daily Intake)

	Boys			Girls		
	8–11 years	12–15 years	16–18 years	8–11 years	12–15 years	16–18 years
Vitamin A (μg retinol equivalents)	500	725	750	500	725	750
Thiamin (mg)	0.9	1.2	1.2	0.8	1.0	0.9
Riboflavin (mg)	1.4	1.8	1.9	1.3	1.6	1.4
Niacin (mg niacin equivalents)	15	20	21	15	18	16
Vitamin B_6 (mg)	1.1–1.6	1.4–2.1	1.5–2.2	1.0–1.5	1.2–1.8	1.1–1.6
Total folate (μg)	150	200	200	150	200	200
Vitamin B_{12} (μg)	1.5	2.0	2.0	1.5	2.0	2.0
Vitamin C (mg)	30	30	40	30	30	30
Vitamin E (mg α-tocopheral equivalents)	8.0	10.5	11.0	8.0	9.0	8.0
Zinc (mg)	9	12	12	9	12	12
Iron (mg)	6–8	10–13	10–13	6–8	10–13	10–13
Iodine (μg)	120	150	150	120	120	120
Magnesium (mg)	180	260	320	160	240	270
Calcium (mg)	800	1200	1000	900	1000	800
Phosphorus (mg)	800	1200	1100	800	1200	1100
Selenium (μg)	50	85	85	50	70	70
Sodium (mmol)	26–100	40–100	40–100	26–100	40–100	40–100
(mg)	600–2300	920–2300	920–2300	600–2300	920–2300	920–2300
Potassium (mmol)	50–140	50–140	50–140	50–140	50–140	50–140
(mg)	1950–5460	1950–5460	1950–5460	1950–5460	1950–5460	1950–5460
Protein (g)	27–38	42–60	64–70	27–39	44–55	57

Table A-7-c
Recommended Dietary Intakes for Adults (Expressed as Mean Daily Intake)

	Men		Women			
	19–64 years	64 years	19–54 years	54+ years	Pregnant	Lactating
Vitamin A (μg retinol equivalents)	750	750	750	750	+0	+450
Thiamin (mg)	1.1	0.9	0.8	0.7	+0.2	+0.4
Riboflavin (mg)	1.7	1.3	1.2	1.0	+0.3	+0.5
Niacin (mg niacin equivalents)	19	16	13	11	+2	+5
Vitamin B_6 (mg)	1.3–1.9	1.0–1.5	0.9–1.4	0.8–1.1	+0.1	+0.7–0.8
Total folate (μg)	200	200	200	200	+200	+150
Vitamin B_{12} (μg)	2.0	2.0	2.0	2.0	+1.0	+0.5
Vitamin C (mg)	40	40	30	30	+30	+45
Vitamin E (mg α-tocopheral equivalents)	10.0	10.0	7.0	7.0	+0	+2.5
Zinc (mg)	12	12	12	12	+4	+6
Iron (mg)	7	7	12–16	5–7	+10–20	+0
Iodine (μg)	150	150	120	120	+30	+50
Magnesium (mg)	320	320	270	270	+30	+70
Calcium (mg)	800	800	800	1000	+300	+400
Phosphorus (mg)	1000	1000	1000	1000	+200	+200
Selenium (μg)	85	85	70	70	+10	+15
Sodium (mmol)	40–100	40–100	40–100	40–100	+0	+0
(mg)	920–2300	920–2300	920–2300	920–2300	+0	+0
Potassium (mmol)	50–140	50–140	50–140	50–140	+0	+0
(mg)	1950–5460	1950–5460	1950–5460	1950–5460	+0	+0
Protein (g)	55	55	45	45	+6	+16

A-7-d. METHODS FOR ESTIMATING ENERGY REQUIREMENTS (1)

A method for estimating energy requirements for individual adults and older children is given below.

Infants and Children Less Than 10 Years Old

The 1981 FAO/WHO/UNU Consultation estimated energy requirements from birth to 10 years by extrapolating from intakes of healthy children growing normally. Doubly-labeled water studies by Prentice et al. in children up to 3 years of age suggest that these estimates may be too high for this age group.

The FAO/WHO/UNU Consultation took the NCHS charts to represent "normal growth" with 2 standard deviations from the median as the "normal range."

Summary of Method to Estimate Food Energy Requirements from Estimates of Energy Expenditure in Adults and Children Aged 10–18 Years

The method summarized below may be applied to both groups and individuals. However, estimates of food energy requirements obtained by this method are only approximate, especially for individuals in whom variations in energy requirements can be very large, even in individuals of the same age, sex and body weight, and apparently similar levels of activity.

Method

1. Determine the basal metabolic rate (BMR) of the group or individual. BMR may be measured using indirect calorimetry, or predicted from the equations in Table 2. (See Appendix Table II-A-7-d-1.)
2. Determine the approximate level of activity (expressed as a multiple of BMR) of the group or the individual, from estimates of the amount of time spent in different activities, or from the values listed in Table 3. (See Appendix Table II-A-7-d-2.)
3. Determine daily energy expenditure by multiplying the BMR by the level of activity (expressed as a multiple of BMR).
4. Add to the estimate of energy expenditure any extra energy requirements for growth, pregnancy, or lactation, as appropriate.
   a. The energy cost of growth may be taken as 8 kJ/kg body weight for children aged 10 to 14 years, 4 kJ/kg at 15 years, and 2 kJ/kg at age 16 to 18 years.
   b. The average additional energy requirement in pregnancy may be taken as 0.85 to 1.1 MJ/day, assuming a weight gain of 10 to 12 kg and no change in level of activity.
   c. The average additional energy requirement in lactation may be taken as 2.0 to 2.4 MJ/day in the first 6 months, assuming no change in level of activity and a maternal fat loss of 2 kg over 6 months.
5. Correct the estimate of energy requirement obtained from #4 above for the metabolizable energy content of the diet to be eaten, if appropriate. For the "typical" Australian diet that contains about 20 g/day of dietary fiber, no correction is necessary. For high-fiber diets, the estimate of energy requirement should be increased by about 5%.

Example

Prediction of the food energy required to maintain energy balance in a group of nonpregnant, nonlactating women aged 45 years, with a mean body weight of 60 kg and a light activity level.

a. Predicted BMR (from Table 2 in original or Appendix Table II-A-7-d-1) is 5.6 MJ/day.
b. Energy expenditure in light activity is 1.5 × BMR (Table 3; Appendix Table II-A-7-d-2).
c. Daily energy expenditure = BMR × activity level
   = 5.6 × 1.5
   = 8.4 MJ/day
d. No adjustments are necessary for growth, pregnancy, or lactation in this case.
e. No correction is needed to the energy requirement obtained if the women are consuming a "typical" Australian diet containing approximately 20 g/day of dietary fibre. If these women are consuming a high-fibre diet, the food energy requirement obtained in (d) above should be increased by 5% (i.e., from 8.4 MJ/day to 8.8 MJ/day).

Tables A-7-d-1 and A-7-d-2 may be used as a guide to energy expenditure for use with groups of people.

REFERENCE

1. National Health and Medical Research Council. Recommended dietary intakes for use in Australia. Canberra: Australian Government Publishing Service, 1991.

Table A-7-d-1
Equations for Estimating Basal Metabolic Rate (BMR)[a] in MJ/Day from Body Weight (kg) of Adults and Children over the Age of 10 Years

	Age (years)	Equation
Males	10–18	0.074wt + 2.754
	18–30	0.063wt + 2.896
	30–60	0.048wt + 3.653
	over 60	0.049wt + 2.459
Females	10–18	0.056wt + 2.898
	18–30	0.062wt + 2.036
	30–60	0.034wt + 3.538
	over 60	0.038wt + 2.755

Equations are taken from Schofield WN, Schofield C, James WPT. Basal metabolic rate—review and prediction, together with an annotated bibliography of source material. Hum Nutr Clin Nutr 1985; 39C(Suppl 1):1–96.

[a]Wt is body weight in kg; BMR value is in MJ/day.

Table A-7-d-2
Average Daily Energy Expenditure of Adults and Children over the Age of 10 at Different Levels of Activity Expressed as Multiples of Basal Metabolic Rate (BMR)

	Daily Energy Expenditure as Multiples of BMR			
	Males		Females	
Activity Level	Average	(Range)	Average	(Range)
Bed rest	1.2	(1.1–1.3)	1.2	(1.1–1.3)
Very sedentary	1.3	(1.2–1.4)	1.3	(1.2–1.4)
Sedentary/maintenance	1.4	(1.3–1.5)	1.4	(1.3–1.5)
Light	1.5	(1.4–1.6)	1.5	(1.4–1.6)
Light–moderate	1.7	(1.6–1.8)	1.6	(1.5–1.7)
Moderate	1.8	(1.7–1.9)	1.7	(1.6–1.8)
Heavy	2.1	(1.9–2.3)	1.8	(1.7–1.9)
Very heavy	2.3	(2.0–2.6)	2.0	(1.8–2.2)

Table A-7-d-3
Recommended Energy Intakes for Infants

Age (months)	kJ/kg	Age (months)	kJ/kg
0–0.9	520	6–7	395
1–2	485	7–8	395
2–3	455	8–9	395
3–4	430	9–10	415
4–5	415	10–11	420
5–6	405	11–12	435

From FAO/WHO/UNU, 1985.

Table A-7-d-4
Recommended Energy Intakes for Children 1 to 10 Years

	MJ/Day	
Age (years)	Males	Females
1–2	5.0	4.8
2–3	5.9	5.5
3–4	6.5	6.0
4–5	7.1	6.4
5–6	7.6	6.8
6–7	7.9	7.1
7–8	8.3	7.4
8–9	8.7	7.7
9–10	9.0	7.9

From FAO/WHO/UNU, 1985.

Table A-7-d-5
Recommended Energy Intakes for Adolescents 10 to 18 Years

	MJ/Day	
Age (years)	Males	Females
10–11	8.1–9.1	7.3–8.2
11–12	8.7–9.8	7.7–8.7
12–13	9.2–10.3	8.1–9.1
13–14	9.8–11.0	8.4–9.5
14–15	10.5–11.8	8.6–9.8
15–16	11.1–12.5	8.7–9.9
16–17	11.7–13.2	8.8–10.0
17–18	12.0–13.5	8.8–10.0

From FAO, WHO, UNU. Energy and protein requirements. Report of a joint FAO-WHO-UNU meeting. Geneva: WHO, 1985; (Tech rep ser no. 274).

Note: Level of energy expenditure: males 1.6–1.8 BMR; females 1.5–1.7 BMR.

BMR estimated from Schofield WN, Schofield C, James WPT. Basal metabolic rate—review and prediction, together with an annotated bibliography of source material. Hum Nutr Clin Nutr 1985;39C(Suppl 1):1–96.

Table A-7-d-6
Recommended Energy Intakes for Adults

Age Group (years)		MJ/Day	
		Males	Females
18–30			
Height (cm)	**Weight (kg)**		
150	50.6	—	7.2–8.3
160	57.6	9.1–10.4	7.9–9.0
170	65.0	9.8–11.2	8.5–9.7
180	72.9	10.5–12.0	9.2–10.5
190	81.2	11.2–12.8	9.9–11.3
200	90.0	12.0–13.7	—
30–60			
Height (cm)	**Weight (kg)**		
150	50.6	—	7.2–8.3
160	57.6	9.0–10.3	7.7–8.8
170	65.0	9.5–10.8	8.0–9.2
180	72.9	10.0–11.4	8.4–9.6
190	81.2	10.6–12.1	8.8–10.1
200	90.0	11.2–12.8	—
Over 60			
Height (cm)	**Weight (kg)**		
150	50.6	—	6.5–7.5
160	57.6	7.4–8.5	6.9–7.9
170	65.0	7.9–9.0	7.3–8.4
180	72.9	8.4–9.6	7.7–8.8
190	81.2	9.0–10.3	8.2–9.3
200	90.0	9.6–11.0	—

From BMI at midpoint of acceptable range (22.5); NHMRC (1984) table of acceptable weight-for-height. Report of the 98th session. National Health and Medical Research Council, AGPS, Canberra. Level of energy expenditure, 1.4–1.6 BMR. BMR estimated from Schofield WN, Schofield C, James WPT. Basal metabolic rate—review and prediction, together with an annotated bibliography of source material. Hum Nutr Clin Nutr 1985;39C(Suppl 1):1–96.

Table A-8-a-1
Values for the Digestibility of Protein in Man[a]

Protein Source	True Digestibility (mean ±SD)	Digestibility Relative to Reference Proteins
Egg	97 ± 3	
Milk, cheese	95 ± 3 91	100
Meat, fish	94 ± 3	
Maize	85 ± 6	89
Rice, polished	88 ± 4	93
Wheat, whole	86 ± 5	90
Wheat, refined	96 ± 4	101
Oatmeal	86 ± 7	90
Millet	79	83
Peas, mature	88	93
Peanut butter	95	100
Soyflour	86 ± 7	90
Beans	78	82
Maize + beans	78	82
Maize + beans + milk	84	88
Indian rice diet	77	81
Indian rice diet + milk	87	92
Chinese mixed diet	96	98[b]
Brazilian mixed diet	78	82
Filipino mixed diet	88[c]	93
American mixed diet	96[c]	101
Indian rice + bean diet	78[c]	82

From Energy and Protein requirements: report of a Joint FAO/WHO/UNU Expert Consultation. Technical report series no. 724, Geneva: World Health Organization, 1985:119.

[a]See original reference for data sources.

[b]Relative to egg measured in the same study.

[c]Recalculated from apparent digestibility, using F_K = 12 mg N/kg (see original text).

Table A-8-a-2-a
Daily Average (per kg) Energy Requirements and Safe Level of Protein Intake for Infants and Children Aged 3 Months to 10 Years (Sexes Combined up to 5 Years)

Age	Median Weight (kg)	Energy Requirement (kcal$_{th}$/kg)		Energy Requirement (kJ/kg)		Safe Level of Protein Intake (g/kg)[a]
Months						
3–6	7.0	100		418		1.85
6–9	8.5	95		397		1.65
9–12	9.5	100		418		1.50
Years						
1–2	11.0	105		439		1.20
2–3	13.5	100		418		1.15
3–5	16.5	95		397		1.10
		Boys	Girls	Boys	Girls	
5–7	20.5	90	85	377	356	1.00
7–10	27.0	78	67	326	280	1.00

From Diet, nutrition and the prevention of chronic diseases: report of a WHO Study Group. Technical report series no. 797. Geneva: World Health Organization, 1990:167–168.

[a]Minimum level considered safe.

Table A-8-a-2-b
Daily Average Energy Requirements and Safe Level of Protein Intake for Adolescents Aged 10 to 18 Years

Age (years)	Median Weight (kg)	Energy Requirement (kcal$_{th}$)	Energy Requirement (kJ)	Safe Level of Protein Intake (g/kg)[a]
Boys				
10–12	34.5	2200	9200	1.00
12–14	44.0	2400	10,000	1.00
14–16	55.5	2650	11,100	0.95
16–18	64.0	2850	11,900	0.90
Girls				
10–12	36.0	1950	8200	1.00
12–14	46.5	2100	8800	0.95
14–16	52.0	2150	9000	0.90
16–18	54.0	2150	9000	0.80

From Diet, nutrition and the prevention of chronic diseases: report of a WHO Study Group. Technical report series no. 797. Geneva: World Health Organization, 1990:167–168.

[a]Minimum level considered safe.

Table A-8-a-2-c
Daily Average Energy Requirements and Safe Level of Protein Intake for Adults[a]

Weight (kg)	Energy Requirement 18–30 years (kcal$_{th}$)	(kJ)	30–60 years (kcal$_{th}$)	(kJ)	Over 60 years (kcal$_{th}$)	(kJ)	Safe Level of Protein Intake (g/day)[b]
Men							
50	2300	9700	2350	9700	1850	7700	37.5
55	2400	10,100	2450	10,100	1950	8300	41.0
60	2550	10,600	2500	10,400	2100	8600	45.0
65	2700	11,300	2600	10,900	2200	9100	49.0
70	2800	11,700	2700	11,200	2300	9600	52.5
75	2900	12,300	2800	11,800	2400	10,000	56.0
80	3050	12,900	2900	12,000	2500	10,400	60.0
Women							
40	1700	7200	1900	7900	1650	6800	30.0
45	1850	7700	1950	8300	1700	7100	34.0
50	1950	8200	2050	8500	1800	7500	37.5
55	2100	8600	2100	8800	1900	7900	41.0
60	2200	9200	2200	9000	1950	8200	45.0
65	2300	9800	2250	9400	2050	8500	49.0
70	2450	10,300	2300	9600	2150	8900	52.5
75	2550	10,800	2400	10,000	2200	9300	56.0

From Diet, nutrition and the prevention of chronic diseases: report of a WHO Study Group. Technical report series no. 797. Geneva: World Health Organization, 1990:167–168.

[a]For a basal metabolic rate factor of 1.6.

[b]Minimum level considered safe.

Table A-8-a-3
Recommended Dietary Allowances of Vitamins and Minerals

Age	Vitamin A[a,b] Safe Level (μg retinol/day) M	F	Folate[a] (μg/day) M	F	Vitamin B_{12}[a] (μg/day) M	F	Vitamin C[c] (mg/day) M	F	Vitamin D[c] (μg/day) M	F	Iron[a,d] Absorbed (μg/kg per day) M	F	Zinc[e] (mg/day) M	F
Infants (months)														
0–3	350		16		0.1		20		10		120		3.1	
4–6	350		24		0.1		20		10		120		3.1	
7–9	350		32		0.1		20		10		120		2.8	
10–12	350		32		0.1		20		10		120		2.8	
Children and adults (years)														
1–2	400		50		1.0		20		10		56		4.0	3.9
3–4	400		50		1.0		20		10		44		4.0	3.9
5–6	400		102		1.0		20		10		40		4.0	3.9
7–10	400		102		1.0		20		2.5		40		4.0	3.9
11–12	500		102		1.0		20		2.5		40		7.0	6.6
13–14	600		170		1.0		30		2.5		34	40	7.0	6.6
15–16	600	500	170		1.0		30		2.5		34	40	7.0	5.5
17–18	600	500	200	170	1.0		30		2.5		34	40	7.0	5.5
19+	600	500	200	170	1.0		30		2.5		18	43	5.5	5.5
Pregnant women		600	370 to 470		1.4		50		10					6.4 to 7.5
Lactating women		850	270		1.3		50		10		24			13.7
Postmenopausal women		500	170		1.0		30		2.5		18			5.5

From Diet, nutrition and the prevention of chronic diseases; report of a WHO Study Group. Technical report series no. 797. Geneva: World Health Organization, 1990:169.

Note: A detailed exposition has been published by the WHO on trace elements and nutrition entitled "Trace elements in human nutrition and health." World Health Organization, Geneva, 343;1996.

[a]Adapted from reference 1.

[b]Minimum level considered safe.

[c]Adapted from reference 2; 2.5 μg of cholecalciferol is equivalent to 100 IU of vitamin D.

[d]The amount of absorbed iron is a variable proportion of the intake, depending on the type of diet.

[e]Adapted from reference 3.

[f]Requirements during pregnancy depend on the woman's iron status before pregnancy.

See references on next page

REFERENCES

1. FAO Food and Nutrition Series no. 23. Rome: Food and Agriculture Organization, 1988.
2. WHO Technical report series no. 452. Geneva: World Health Organization, 1970.
3. WHO technical report series no. 532. Geneva: World Health Organization, 1973.

A-8-b. European Community Nutrient and Energy Intakes

A-8-b-1. Recommendations and Nomenclature: Excerpts from the Report (1)

. . . This Committee is attempting to give, as far as possible, three values to indicate the spread of needs.

. . . This Committee will call the intake that is enough for virtually all healthy people in a group the Population Reference Intake (PRI). [This corresponds with the traditional RDA of the United States and includes the nutritional needs 2 standard deviation's above the mean requirement of the group—The Appendix Editors]

The Average Requirement (AR), the mean nutrient requirement of the group, according to the criterion chosen.

The Lowest Threshold Intake (LTI) is that which is 2 standard deviations below the mean. This is the intake below which, on the basis of our current knowledge, almost all individuals will be unlikely to maintain metabolic integrity according to the criterion chosen for each nutrient.

. . . In this report LTIs are often set on the prudent side, being not those intakes below which frank deficiency is almost certain, but rather those intakes below which there may be cause for concern for a substantial section of the population. Consequently, the PRI and LTI values are not always the means plus and minus two standard deviations.

For nutrients where the requirements are given in terms of energy intake, . . . the convention adopted in this report [gives] the PRIs and LTIs for average energy intakes.

The Committee has given only one value for increases during pregnancy or lactation; it considers it has inadequate information to give more with any confidence.

REFERENCE

1. Reports of the Scientific Committee for Food (31st Series: December 11, 1992). Published by the Commission of the European Communities. Luxembourg, 1993.

Table A-8-b-2[a]
Multiple Values Proposed for Adults (Amounts Per Day, Unless Given in Other Terms. If That for Women is Different From That for Men, It Is Given in Parentheses)

Nutrient	Average Requirement	Population Reference Intake	Lowest Threshold Intake
Protein (g)	0.6/kg body wt	0.75/kg body wt	0.45/kg body wt
Vitamin A (μg)	500 (400[c])	700 (600)	300 (250)
Thiamin (μg)	72/MJ	100/MJ	50/MJ
Riboflavin (mg)	1.3 (1.1[c])	1.6 (1.3[c])	0.6
Niacin (mg niacin equivalents)	1.3/MJ	1.6/MJ	1.0/MJ
Vitamin B_6 (μg)	13/g protein	15/g protein	—
Folate (μg)	140	200	85
Vitamin B_{12} (μg)	1.0	1.4	0.6
Vitamin C (mg)	30	45	12
Vitamin E (mg α-tocopherol equivalents)		0.4/g PUFA[b]	4 (3[c])/day regardless of PUFA[b] intakes
n-6 PUFA[b] (as percentage of dietary energy)	1	2	0.5
n-3 PUFA[b] (as percentage of dietary energy)	0.2	0.5	0.1
Calcium (mg)	550	700	400
Phosphorus (mg)	400	550	300
Potassium (mg)	—	3100	1600
Iron (mg)	7 (10[d], 6[c])	9 (16[d], 8[c])	5 (7[d], 4[c])
Zinc (mg)	7.5 (5.5[c])	9.5 (7[c])	5 (4)
Copper (mg)	0.8	1.1	0.6
Selenium (μg)	40	55	20
Iodine (μg)	100	130	70

[a]This is Table 37.1 in the original report.
[b]Pufa, polyunsaturated fatty acids.
[c]Postmenopausal women.
[d]PRI to cover 90% of women.

Table A-8-b-2-a[a]
Nutrients with Acceptable Ranges of Intake

Nutrient	Range
Pantothenic acid (mg)	3–12
Biotin (μg)	15–100
Vitamin D (μg)	0–10
Sodium (g)	0.575–3.5
Magnesium (mg)	150–500
Manganese (mg)	1–10

[a]This is Table 37.1 in the original report.

Table A-8-b-3[a]
Population Reference Intakes

Age Group	Protein	n-6 PUFA[b]	n-3 PUFA[b]	Vitamin A	Thiamin	Riboflavin	Niacin	Vitamin B_6	Folate	Vitamin B_{12}	Vitamin C	Calcium	Phosphorus	Potassium	Iron	Zinc	Copper	Selenium	Iodine
	(g/kg body wt/day)	(% of dietary energy)	(% of dietary energy)	(μg/day)	(μg/MJ)	(mg/day)	(mg/MJ)	(μg/g protein)	(μg/day)	(μg/day)	(mg/day	(mg/day)	(mg/day)	(mg/day)	(mg/day)	(mg/day)	(mg/day)	(μg/day)	(μg/day)
6–11 months	1.6	4.5	0.5	350	100	0.4	1.6	15	50	0.5	20	400	300	800	6	4	0.3	8	50
1–3 years	1.1	3	0.5	400	100	0.8	1.6	15	100	0.7	25	400	300	800	4	4	0.4	10	70
4–6 years	1.0	2	0.5	400	100	1.0	1.6	15	130	0.9	25	450	350	1100	4	6	0.6	15	90
7–10 years	1.0	2	0.5	500	100	1.2	1.6	15	150	1.0	30	550	450	2000	6	7	0.7	25	100
Males																			
11–14 years	1.0	2	0.5	600	100	1.4	1.6	15	180	1.3	35	1000	775	3100	10	9	0.8	35	120
15–17 years	0.9	2	0.5	700	100	1.6	1.6	15	200	1.4	40	1000	775	3100	13	9	1.0	45	130
18+ years	0.75	2	0.5	700	100	1.6	1.6	15	200	1.4	45	700	550	3100	9	9.5	1.1	55	130
Females																			
11–14 years	0.95	2	0.5	600	100	1.2	1.6	15	180	1.3	35	800	625	3100	22[d] 18[e]	9	0.8	35	120
15–17 years	0.85	2	0.5	600	100	1.3	1.6	15	200	1.4	40	800	625	3100	21[d] 17[e]	7	1.0	45	130
18+ years	0.75	2	0.5	600	100	1.3	1.6	15	200[c]	1.4	45	700	550	3100	20[d] 16[e] 8[f]	7	1.1	55	130
Pregnancy	0.75 (+10 g/day)	2	0.5	700	100	1.6	1.6	15	400	1.6	55	700	550	3100	[g]	7	1.1	55	130
Lactation	0.75 (+16 g/day)	2	0.5	950	100	1.7	1.6 (+2 mg/day)	15	350	1.9	70	1200	950	3100	10	12	1.4	70	160

[a]Table 37.2 in the original report.

[b]Polyunsaturated fatty acids.

[c]Neural tube defects have been shown to be prevented in offspring by periconceptual ingestion of 400 μg folic acid per day in the form of supplements.

[d]To cover 95% of population.

[e]To cover 90% of population.

[f]Postmenopausal.

[g]Supplementation necessary.

Table A-8-b-4[a]
Daily Intakes of Those Nutrients for Which the Recommendations Are Given in Relation to Body Weight, Energy, or Protein Intakes[b]

Age Group	Protein (g)	n-6 PUFA[c] (g)	n-3 PUFA[c] (g)	Thiamin (mg)	Niacin (mg)	Vitamin B_6 (mg)
6–11 months	15	4	0.5	0.3	5	0.4
1–3 years	15	4	0.7	0.5	9	0.7
4–6 years	20	4	1	0.7	11	0.9
7–10 years	29	4	1	0.8	13	1.1
Males						
11–14 years	44	5	1	1.0	15	1.3
15–17 years	55	6	1.5	1.2	18	1.5
18+ years (PRI)	56	6	1.5	1.1	18	1.5
(AR)	45	3	0.6	0.8	15	1.3
Females						
11–14 years	42	4	1	0.9	14	1.1
15–17 years	46	5	1	0.9	14	1.1
18+ years (PRI)	47	4.5	1	0.9	14	1.1
(AR)	37	2.5	0.5	0.6	11	1.0
Pregnancy	57	5[d]	~1	1.0[d]	14	1.3[e]
Lactation	63	5.5	1	1.1	16	1.4[e]

[a]Table 37.3 in the original report.

[b]Population reference intakes (PRIs) except where indicated as average requirements (ARs) (calculated as mean group intake × PRI or AR).

[c]Polyunsaturated fatty acids.

[d]From 10th week of pregnancy.

[e]Based on protein increments in pregnancy and lactation.

Table A-9-a
Dietary Recommendations in Industrialized and Developing Countries, 1977 to 1989[a,b]

Country/Region or Source of Recommendation	Target Group(s)	Maintain Appropriate Body Weight, Exercise	Limit or Reduce Total Fat (% Energy)	Reduce Saturated Fatty Acids (% energy)	Increase Polyunsaturated Fatty Acids (% energy)	Limit Cholesterol (mg/day)	Limit Free Sugars (% Energy)	Increase Complex Carbohydrates (% energy for total carbohydrates)	Increase Dietary Fiber (g/day)	Restrict Sodium Chloride (g/day)	Moderate Alcohol Intake (% energy)	Other Recommendations
Australia 1983	GP	Yes	Yes	NC	NC	NC	Yes	Yes	Yes	Yes	Yes	Promote breast-feeding; variety
1987, targets for 1995	GP	Reduce obesity prevalence to 30%	35%	NS	NS	NS	<14%	Indirectly	25	130 mmol/day	<5%	Promote water fluoridation, increase prevalence of breast-feeding
1987, targets for 2000	GP	To 25%	33%	NS	NS	NS	<12%	Indirectly	30	100 mmol/day	<5%	
Canada 1982	GP	Yes	35%	Yes	Yes	No	Yes	Yes	Yes	Yes	Yes	Exercise
Czechoslovakia 1988	GP	Yes, reduce by 10–15%	Yes, reduce by 15 g/day	Yes	No	NS	Yes	Yes, more plant foods, vegetables, cereals, legumes	Yes	Yes	Yes	Increase vitamin C intake; more plant foods; nutrition education; variety
France 1981	GP	Yes	30–35%	Yes	NS	NS	Yes	50–55%	Yes	Yes	<10%	Water fluoridation
Germany, Federal Republic of, 1995	GP	Yes	Yes	NS	NS	NS	Avoid excess	Yes; fresh fruits and vegetables, whole-grain cereals	Yes	Yes	Yes	Variety; small, frequent meals, proper cooking; sufficient protein
Hungary 1988	GP	Yes	Avoid too much	Use vegetable oil	NS	NS	Yes	Yes; fresh vegetables, salads, whole grains	Yes	Yes	Yes	Variety; focus on cooking methods; consume milk and cheese as skimmed-milk products; 4 or 5 even meals daily, food labeling
India 1988	HR (affluent people)	Yes	15–20%	NC	Balance $(n-3)/(n-6)$ ratio	NC	Yes	Yes; avoid refined and polished grains	Include grains, leafy vegetables, and whole grains	Yes	NC	Breast-feeding; water fluoridation upper limit 1 mg/L; different recommendation for general, poorer population
Ireland 1984	GP	Yes	≤35%	Yes	NC	NC	Moderation; ≤7 g/day for weight reduction	Yes	To 20–35	<9	<5%	Reduce protein to 1 g/kg of body weight daily; more vegetable protein
Japan 1985	GP	Yes	20–25%	Yes	Use vegetables, and fish oils	NC	NC	NC	NC	<10	NC	Varied diet (at least 30 different foods daily); home cooking; pleasant eating environment
Latin America 1988	GP	Yes	20–25%	≤8	P/S = 1.0	<100 mg/1000 $kcal_{th}$ in children, up to 300 mg/day	Yes	Yes	>8 g/1000 $kcal_{th}$	≤5; in profuse sweating, up to 10	NC	Protein 10–12% energy; variety; dietary interactions; vitamin C with iron-containing foods; calcium intake
Netherlands												
1983–1984	GP	Yes	30–35%	Yes	Maximum 10%	Yes	Yes	NS	NC	NC	Yes	Variety
1986	GP	Yes	30–35%	Yes	P/S = 1.0	<30 mg/MJ	Mono- and disaccharides 15–25%	45–55%	3 g/MJ	Yes	<9 g/day	Variety
New Zealand 1982	GP HR	Yes	Yes	Yes	NS	NS	Yes	Yes	Yes	Yes	Yes	Variety; less animal protein; water fluoridation

continued

Table A-9-a—*continued*

Dietary Recommendations in Industrialized and Developing Countries, 1977 to 1989[a,b]

Country/Region or Source of Recommendation	Target Group(s)	Maintain Appropriate Body Weight, Exercise	Limit or Reduce Total Fat (% Energy)	Reduce Saturated Fatty Acids (% energy)	Increase Polyunsaturated Fatty Acids (% energy)	Limit Cholesterol (mg/day)	Limit Free Sugars (% Energy)	Increase Complex Carbohydrates (% energy for total carbohydrates)	Increase Dietary Fiber (g/day)	Restrict Sodium Chloride (g/day)	Moderate Alcohol Intake (% energy)	Other Recommendations
Norway 1981–1982	GP	NC	<35%	Yes	P/S = 0.5	NS	<10%	Yes; 50–60%	Yes	NC	NC	Maintain adequate nutrient intake
Poland 1988	GP	Yes	≈30%	Yes	NS	Yes, <300 mg	<10%	Yes	Yes	?	?	?
Sweden 1981	GP	Yes	25–35%	Yes	P/S = 0.5	Yes	<10%	Yes; 50–60%	>30	≈7–8	Yes	Varied diet, exercise, regular meals
1985	GP	Yes	Reduce by 5% energy by 1990; to ≈30% by 2000	NS	P/S = >0.5	NS	Decrease by 3% energy by 1990	Yes; increase starch to 45–50% energy by 2000	Increase by 7–8 g/day by 1990 and to 30–35 g by 2000	Reduce by 1–2 g/day by 1990 to 7–8 g by 2000	Yes	Year 1990 and year 2000 goals
United Kingdom 1983	GP	Yes	30%	10	NS	No	To 20 kg/year	Through whole grains, vegetables cereals, fruit	To 30	Decrease by 3 g/day	<4%	Long-term proposals; food labeling; nutrition education; greater proportion of vegetable protein
United States of America[b] 1977	GP	Yes	27–33%	Yes	Yes	250–350	Yes	Yes	Yes	<8	Yes	Limit additives and processed foods
1979	GP	Yes	Yes	Yes	NS	Yes	Yes	Yes	NS	Yes	Yes	More fish, poultry, legumes; less red meat
1985	GP	Yes	Yes	Yes	No	Yes	Yes	Adequate starch and fiber	Yes	Yes	Yes	Variety in diet; consider high-risk groups
1988	GP HR	Yes	Yes	Yes	No	Yes	Yes	Yes	Yes	Yes	Yes	Fluoridation of water; adolescent girls and women increase intake of calcium-rich foods; children, adolescents, and women of child-bearing age increase intake of iron-rich foods
1989	GP	Balance energy intake and expenditure	≤30%	<10% for individuals, 7–8% population mean	Up to 10 for individuals and ≈7 population mean	<300	Yes	≥55%; ≥5 servings/day vegetables and fruits; ≥6 daily servings cereals, breads, and legumes	Indirectly through vegetables, fruits and cereals	≤6 with a goal of 4.5	<30 g of ethanol or < 2 drinks/day	Population and individual goals; avoid dietary supplements in excess of RDAs; drink fluorinated water; limit protein intake to less than twice the RDA; comments on future goals
WHO 1988 Intermediate goals	GP	BMI	35%	15%	P/S ≥0.5	<100 mg/1000 $kcal_{th}$	10%	>40%	>30	7–8	Yes	Increase nutrient density of food; water fluoridation; iodine prophylaxis
Ultimate goals		20–25	20–30%	10–15%	P/S = 1.0			45–55%		5		

From Diet, nutrition and the prevention of chronic diseases. Report of a WHO Study Group. Technical report series no. 797. Geneva: WHO, 1990:180–181.

[a]BMI, body-mass index; GP, general population; HR, high-risk groups, NC, no comment; NS, not specified; PS, ratio of polyunsaturated to saturated fatty acids; RDA, recommended dietary allowance.

[b]See updated USDA/US DHHS publication, *Nutrition and Your Health: Dietary Guidelines for Americans*, 4th ed., 1995.

Table A-9-b

Dietary Recommendations to Reduce Coronary Heart Disease Risk in Industrialized Countries[a]

Country/Region or Source of Recommendation	Target Group(s)	Body Weight/ Exercise	Total Fat (% Energy)	Saturated Fat (% energy)	Polyunsaturated Fat (% energy)	Cholesterol (mg/day)	Complex Carbohydrates and Fiber	Free Sugars	Sodium Chloride (g/day)	Alcohol Intake	Ohter Recommendations
Australia											
1979	HR	Avoid obesity	Reduce to 30–35	P:S = 1.0	P:S = 1.0	Restrict	Eat enough	Use less	Restrict	Moderation	Focus on HR groups; food labeling, recommendations safe for GP
Canada											
1977	GP	Maintain appropriate body weight	Reduce to 35	10	10	NC	Increase	NC	Restrict	NC	Variety of foods
1988	GP HR	Adjust energy intake and expenditure	<30	<10	<10	Restrict through less meats and egg yolks; for HR <300	Increase	NC	Limit	Limit	Focus on HR groups; limit protein to 10–15% energy
Europe											
1987	GP HR	Control obesity; increase exercise	≤30	<10	Increase oleic acid linoleic acids	<300	Increase, especially vegetables, fruits, cereals, legumes	Reduce	Moderation	Moderation, <25–30 g/day	Nutrition education; collaboration among government and other groups; food labeling
Finland											
1987	GP HR	Avoid excess weight; exercise	<30	<10	P:S >0.5	Reduce	NC	NC	Reduce; for HR <5	Moderation	Avoid trace element deficiencies; food labeling; focus on HR groups
Finland, Norway, Sweden											
1968	GP	Reduce energy intake to avoid obesity;	Reduce to 25–35	Reduce	Increase	NC	Increase vegetables, fruits, potatoes	Decrease	NC	NC	10–12% of energy from protein; 30–50% of animal origin
Germany, Federal Republic of											
1975	GP	NC	Reduce	Reduce	Increase	Reduce	NC	NC	NC	NC	NC
Japan											
1983	GP	NC	20–25	NC	Cook with vegetable oil	NC	Increase	Reduce	Limit to <10	Avoid too much	Variety; eat enough protein, half from vegetables and half from animal sources; eat enough potassium, especially from green vegetables; eat lean meat and fish and fewer sweets
Netherlands											
1973	GP	Maintain appropriate body weight	33	Restrict	10–13	250–300	Increase to make up energy need	Use little	NC	NC	NC
New Zealand											
1976	GP HR	Maintain appropriate body weight	35	Reduce especially for HR	HR should substitute for saturated fatty acids	Reduce	NC	Restrict to reduce weight	NC	Restrict to reduce weight	NC
United Kingdom											
1982	GP	Avoid obesity; increase exercise	30	<10	NC	NC	Increase	NC	NC	NC	Special attention to children
1984	GP	Avoid obesity; exercise	Reduce to 35	Reduce to 15	P/S = 0.45	NS	Increase breads, cereals, vegetables, fruits	Do not increase	Decrease	Avoid excess; <90 mL/day men; ≤65 mL/day women	Special recommendations for governments, professionals, industry

continued

Table A-9-b—*continued*

Dietary Recommendations to Reduce Coronary Heart Disease Risk in Industrialized Countries[a]

Country/Region or Source of Recommendation	Target Group(s)	Body Weight/ Exercise	Total Fat (% Energy)	Saturated Fat (% energy)	Polyunsaturated Fat (% energy)	Cholesterol (mg/day)	Complex Carbohydrates and Fiber	Free Sugars	Sodium Chloride (g/day)	Alcohol Intake	Other Recommendations
United States of America											
1984	GP	Control obesity	<30	8	<10	<250	Increase to make up energy loss	NC	5	NC	NC
1985	GP HR	Maintain appropriate body weight	<30	10	Up to 10	250–300	Endorsed earlier recommendations		NC	NC	Guidelines for health professionals, industry, and public
1988	GP	Maintain appropriate body weight	<30	<10	Up to 10	<300	Increase, ≥50% energy from total carbohydrates	NS	<3 (as sodium)	30–50 g ethanol/day	Protein to make up remainder of energy; wide variety of foods
WHO											
1982	GP	Avoid obesity	Reduce to 20–30	≤10	Up to 10	<300	Increase	NC	<5	Drink less	Emphasis on plant foods, fish, poultry, lean meats, low-fat dairy products, and fewer whole eggs
1988	HR	BMI 20–25, regular exercise	20–30	10	Up to 10 P/S >1.0	<100 mg/1000 $kcal_{th}$	45–55% energy <30 g fiber/day	10% energy	<5	Limit	Increase nutrient density; water fluoridation 0.7–1.2 mg/L; iodine prophylaxis; intermediate and ultimate goals

From Diet, nutrition and the prevention of chronic diseases. Report of a WHO Study Group. Technical report series no. 797. Geneva, WHO, 1990:182–183. With permission.

[a]BMI, body-mass index; GP, general population; HR, high-risk groups; NC, no comment; NS, not specified; P:S, ratio of polyunsaturated to saturated fatty foods.

Table A-9-c
Dietary Recommendations to Reduce Cancer Risk in Industrialized Countries

Country/ Region	Maintain Appropriate Body Weight, Exercise[a]	Limit or Reduce Total Fat (% Energy)	Modify Ratio of Dietary Fats[a]	Promote Fruit and Vegetable Intake	Increase Complex Carbohydrate/ Fiber Intake	Restrict Sodium Chloride[a]	Food Preparation Methods	Alcohol Intake	Other Recommendations[a]
Canada									
1985	Yes	Reduce	Decrease saturated fatty acids and cholesterol	Yes	More fiber-containing foods	NS	Minimize cured, pickled, and smoked foods	Two or fewer drinks per day, if any	NC
Europe									
1986	Yes	To ≈ 30	NC	Yes	Yes	To <5 g/day	As above; avoid frying and high-temperature cooking	Drink less, if at all	Varied diet; no food supplements; recommendations to government, scientists, and industry
Japan									
1983	NC	Avoid excess	NC	Especially green/ yellow vegetables oranges, carotene, and fungi	Unrefined cereal, seafood, fiber-rich legumes	Yes	Avoid hot drinks and burned foods	Drink less, if at all	Varied diet; chew food well
United States of America[b]									
1982	NC	To ≈ 30	NC	Especially citrus fruits, green and yellow and cruciferous vegetables	Whole-grain products, vegetables, and fruits	Minimize cured and pickled foods	Minimize cured, pickled, and smoked foods	Drink less, if at all	Avoid food supplements; monitor and test mutagens and carcinogens; recommendations to government, scientists, and industry
1984	Yes	To ≈ 30	NC	Especially vitamin A- and C-rich foods and cruciferous vegetables	High-fiber foods, whole-grain cereals	NS	As above	As above	NC
1987	Yes	To ≈ 30	NC	Vitamin A-rich, green and yellow vegetables, citrus fruits	Whole-grain products, 20–30 g fiber/day	NS	As above, avoid frying and high-temperature cooking	As above	Balanced diet; read labels

From Diet, nutrition and the prevention of chronic diseases. Report of a WHO Study Group. Technical report series no. 797. Geneva; World Health Organization, 1990:184–185.

[a]NC, no comment; NS, not specified.

[b]The American Cancer Society recently published "Guidelines on Diet, Nutrition, and Cancer Prevention: Reducing the Risk of Cancer with Healthy Food Choices and Physical Activity." American Cancer Society 1996 Advisory Committee on Diet, Nutrition, and Cancer Prevention. CA-A Cancer Journal for Clinicians 1996; 46:325–341.

A-9-d. NATIONAL NUTRITION OBJECTIVES (USA)

Table A-9-d-1
Objectives for the Year 2000

A. *Health Status*

1. Reduce deaths from coronary heart disease to no more than 100 per 100,000 persons (age-adjusted baseline: 135 per 100,000 in 1987).

2. Reverse the rise in deaths from cancer to achieve a rate of no more than 130 per 100,000 persons (age-adjusted baseline: 133 per 100,000 in 1987).

3. Reduce the overweight population to no more than 20% among adults aged 20 years and older and no more than 15% among adolescents aged 12 through 19 years (baseline: 26% for adults aged 20 through 74 years in 1976 to 1980, 24% for men and 27% for women; 15% for adolescents aged 12 through 19 years in 1976 to 1980).

4. Reduce growth retardation among low-income children aged 5 years and younger to less than 10% (baseline; up to 16% among low-income children in 1988, depending on age and race/ethnicity).

B. *Risk Reduction Objectives*

5. Reduce dietary fat intake to an average of 30% of calories or less and reduce average saturated fat intake to less than 10% of calories among persons aged 2 years and older (baseline: 36% of calories from total fat and 13% from saturated fat for persons aged 20 through 74 years in 1976 to 1980; 36% and 13% for women aged 19 through 50 years in 1985).

6. Increase complex carbohydrates and fiber-containing foods in the diets of adults to 5 or more daily servings for vegetables (including legumes) and fruits, and to 6 or more daily servings for grain products (baseline: 2.5 servings of vegetables and fruits and 3 servings of grain products for women aged 19 through 50 years in 1985).

7. Increase to at least 50% the proportion of overweight persons aged 12 years and older who have adopted sound dietary practices combined with regular physical activity to attain an appropriate body weight (baseline: 30% of overweight women and 25% of overweight men for people aged 18 years and older in 1985).

8. Increase calcium intake so that at least 50% of youth aged 12 through 24 years and at least 50% of pregnant and lactating women are consuming 3 or more servings daily of foods rich in calcium, and at least 50% of adults aged 25 years and older are consuming 2 or more servings daily (baseline: 7% of women and 14% of men aged 19 through 24 years and 24% of pregnant and lactating women consumed 3 or more servings daily, and 15% of women and 23% of men aged 25 through 50 years consumed 2 or more servings daily in 1985 to 1986).

9. Decrease salt and sodium intake so that at least 65% of those who prepare home-cooked meals do so without adding salt, at least 80% of persons avoid using salt at the table, and at least 40% of adults regularly purchase foods modified or lower in sodium (baseline: 54% of women aged 19 through 50 years did not use salt at the table in 1985; 20% of all persons aged 18 years and older regularly purchased foods with reduced salt and sodium content in 1988).

10. Reduce iron deficiency to less than 3% among children aged 1 through 4 years and among women of childbearing age (baseline: 9% for children aged 1 through 2 years, 4% for children aged 3 through 4 years, and 5% for women aged 20 through 44 years in 1976 to 1980).

11. Increase to at least 75% the proprotion of mothers who breast-feed their babies in the early postpartum period and to at least 50% the proportion who continue to breast-feed until their babies are 5 to 6 months old (baseline: 54% at discharge from birth site and 21% at 5 to 6 months in 1988).

12. Increase to at least 75% the proportion of parents and caregivers who use feeding practices that prevent baby-bottle tooth decay.

13. Increase to at least 85% the proportion of persons aged 18 years and older who use food labels to make nutritious food selections (baseline: 74% used labels to make food selections in 1988).

C. *Service and Protection Objectives*

14. Achieve useful and informative nutrition labeling for virtually all processed foods and for at least 40% of fresh meats, poultry, fish, fruits, vegetables, baked foods, and ready-to-eat carry-out foods (baseline: 60% of processed foods regulated by the Food and Drug Administration had nutrition labeling in 1988; baseline data on fresh and carry-out foods are unavailable).

15. Increase the available processed food products that are reduced in fat and saturated fat to at least 5000 brand items (baseline: 2500 brand items reduced in fat in 1986).

16. Increase to at least 90% the proportion of restaurants and institutional service operations than offer identifiable low-fat, low-calorie food choices, consistent with the nutrition principles in the *Dietary Guidelines for Americans.*

17. Increase to at least 90% the proportion of school lunch and breakfast services and child-care food services that offer menus consistent with the nutrition principles in the *Dietary Guidelines for Americans.*

18. Increase to at least 80% the receipt of home food services by people aged 65 years and older who cannot prepare their own meals or are otherwise in need of home-delivered meals.

19. Increase to at least 75% the proportion of schools in the United States that provide nutrition education from preschool through 12th grade, preferably as part of quality school health education.

20. Increase to at least 50% the proportion of worksites with 50 or more employees that offer nutrition education and/or weight management programs for employees (baseline: 17% offered nutrition education activities and 15% offered weight-control activities in 1985).

21. Increase to at least 75% the proportion of primary care providers who provide nutrition assessment and counseling and/or referral to qualified nutritionists or dietitians (baseline: physicians provided diet counseling for an estimated 40 to 50% of patients in 1988).

From Nutrition in healthy people 2000. In National health promotion and disease prevention objectives. Washington, DC: U.S. Government Printing Office. 1991.

A-9-d-2. Midcourse Review in 1995

A midcourse review and revisions in 1995 indicated that many challenges remain in preventing premature death and in improving health as the next century approaches (Table A-9-d-2-a) (1).

Summary of progress indicated that of the 27 objectives in this area (nutrition), 5 objectives (2.2, 2.4, 2.15, 2.23, and 2.25) have met the target. Progress toward the targets has been made on 11 objectives (2.1, 2.5, 2.6, 2.11, 2.13, 2.14, 2.16, 2.19, 2.22, 2.26, and 2.27). Five objectives moved away from the target (2.3, 2.7–2.9, and 2.24). Objectives 2.10 (for anemia prevalence) and 2.20 (for worksite nutrition or weight management programs) show mixed results. Four objectives have no new data beyond the baseline with which to measure progress (2.12, 2.17, 2.18, and 2.21) (2).

A-9-d-3. Objectives for Healthy People for the Year 2010. Excerpts from The Report (3)

A-9-d-3-a Nutrition–Health Status Objectives

2.1 Reduce coronary heart disease deaths to no more than 100 per 100,000 people. (Age-adjusted baseline: 135 per 100,000 in 1987.)

2.2. Reverse the rise in cancer deaths to achieve a rate of no more than 130 per 100,000 people. (Age-adjusted baseline: 134 per 100,000 in 1987.)

2.3 Reduce overweight to a prevalence of no more than 20% among people aged 20 and older and no more than 15% among adolescents aged 12–19. (Baseline: 26% for people aged 20–74 in 1976–80, 24% for men and 27% for women; 15% for adolescents aged 12–19 in 1976–80.)

2.4 Reduce growth retardation among low-income children aged 5 and younger to less than 10 percent. . . .

A-9-d-3-b Risk Reduction Objectives

2.5 Reduce dietary fat intake to an average of 30% of calories or less and average saturated fat intake to less than 10% of calories among people aged 2 and older. . . . Increase to at least 50% the proportion of people aged 2 and older who meet the *Dietary Guidelines'* average daily goal of no more than 30% of calories from fat, and increase to at least 50% the proportion of people aged 2 and older who meet the average daily goal of less than 10% of calories from saturated fat. . . .

2.6 Increase complex carbohydrate and fiber-containing foods in the diets of people aged 2 and older to an average of 5 or more daily servings for vegetables (including legumes) and fruits, and to an average of 6 or more daily servings for grain products. . . . Increase to at least 50% the proportion of people aged 2 and older who meet the *Dietary Guidelines'* average daily goal of 5 or more servings of vegetables/fruits, and increase to at least 50% the proportion who meet the goal of 6 or more servings of grain products. . . .

2.7 Increase to at least 50% the proportion of overweight people aged 12 and older who have adopted sound dietary practices, combined with regular physical activity, to attain an appropriate body weight. . . .

2.8 Increase calcium intake so at least 50% of people aged 11–24 and 50% of pregnant and lactating women consume an average of 3 or more daily servings of foods rich in calcium, and at least 75% of children aged 2–10 and 50% of people aged 25 and older consume an average of 2 or more servings daily. . . .

2.9 Decrease salt and sodium intake so at least 65% of home meal planners prepare foods without adding salt, at least 80% of people avoid using salt at the table, and at least 40% of adults regularly purchase foods modified or lower in sodium. . . .

2.10 Reduce iron deficiency to less than 3% among children aged 1–4 and among women of childbearing age. . . .

2.11 Increase to at least 75% the proportion of mothers who breastfeed their babies in the early postpartum period and to at least 50% the proportion who continue breastfeeding until their babies are 5–6 months old. . . .

2.12 Increase to at least 75% the proportion of parents and caregivers who use feeding practices that prevent baby bottle tooth decay. . . .

2.13 Increase to at least 85% the proportion of people aged 18 and older who use food labels to make nutritious food selections. . . .

A-9-d-3-c Services and Protection Objectives

2.14 Achieve useful and informative nutrition labeling for virtually all processed foods and at least 40% of ready-to-eat carry-away foods. Achieve compliance by at least 90% of retailers with the voluntary labeling of fresh meats, poultry, seafood, fruits, and vegetables. . . .

2.15 Increase to at least 5000 brand items the availability of processed food products that are reduced in fat and saturated fat. . . .

2.16 Increase to at least 90% the proportion of restaurants and institutional food service operations that offer identifiable low-fat, low-calorie food choices, consistent with the *Dietary Guidelines for Americans*. . . .

2.17 Increase to at least 90% the proportion of school lunch and breakfast services and child care food services with menus that are consistent with the nutrition principles in the *Dietary Guidelines for Americans*. . . .

2.18 Increase to at least 80% the receipt of home food services by people aged 65 and older who have difficulty in preparing their own meals or are otherwise in need of home-delivered meals. . . .

2.19 Increase to at least 75% the proportion of the Nation's schools that provide nutrition education from preschool–12th grade, preferably as part of comprehensive school health education. . . .

2.20 Increase to at least 50% the proportion of worksites with 50 or more employees that offer nutrition education and/or weight management programs for employees. . . .

2.21 Increase to at least 75% the proportion of primary care providers who provide nutrition assessment and counseling and/or referral to qualified nutritionists or dietitians. . . .

A-9-d-3-d 1995 Additions

In the 1995 midcourse review, additonal health status objectives were introduced as follows (3).

A-9-d-3-d-1 Health Status Objectives

2.22 Reduce stroke deaths to no more than 20 per 100,000 people. . . .

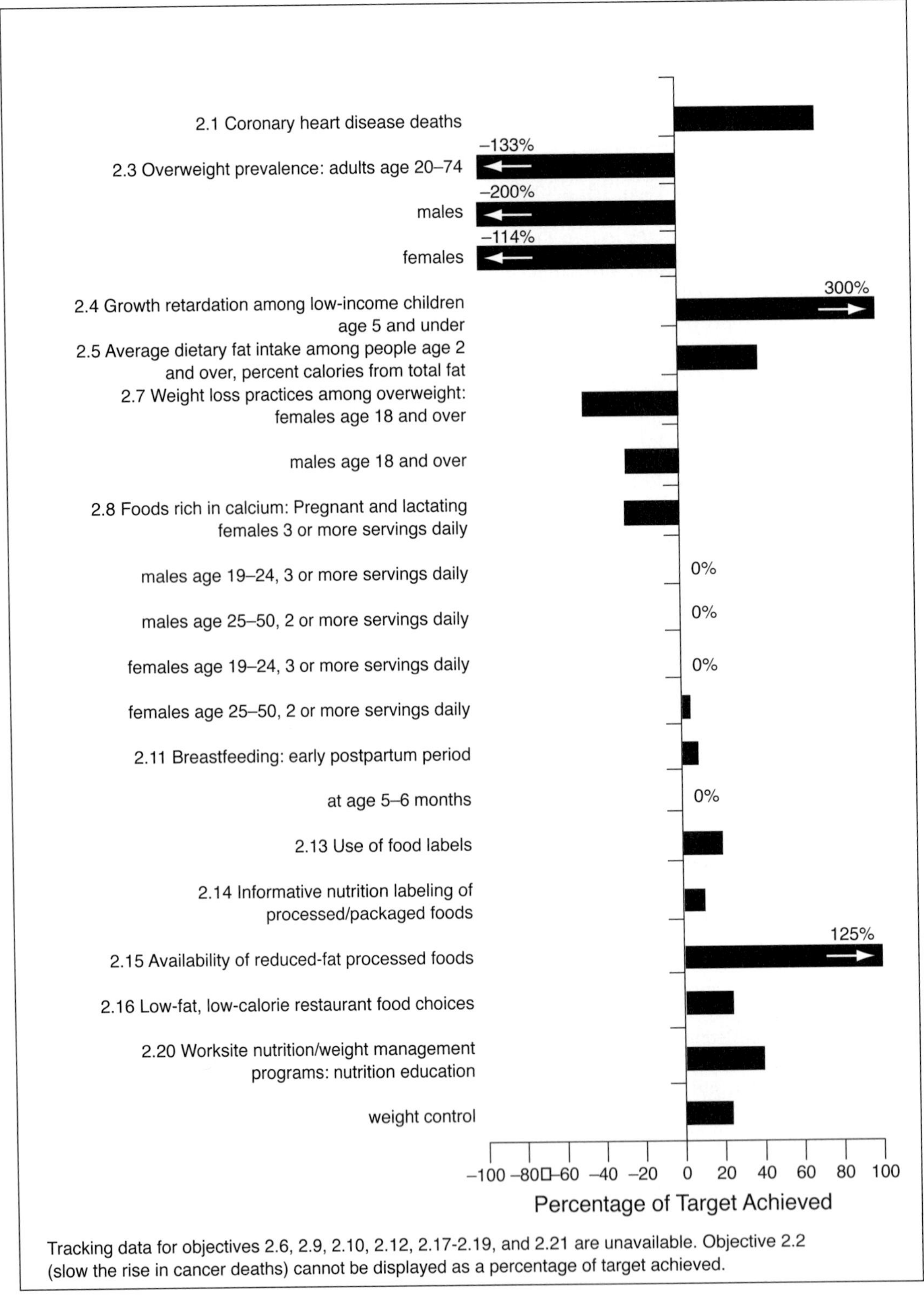

Table A-9-d-2-a. Status of nutrition objectives for the year 2000 at the time of midcourse review (1) in terms of the percentage of target achieved.

2.23 Reduce colorectal cancer deaths to no more than 13.2 per 100,000 people. . . .

2.24 Reduce diabetes to an incidence of no more than 2.5 per 1000 people and a prevalence of no more than 25 per 1000 people. . . .

A-9-d-3-d-2 Risk Reduction Objectives

2.25 Reduce the prevalence of blood cholesterol levels of 240 mg/dL or greater to no more than 20% among adults. . . .

2.26 Increase to at least 50% the proportion of people with high blood pressure whose blood pressure is under control. . . .

2.27 Reduce the mean serum cholesterol level among adults to no more than 200 mg/dL . . .

REFERENCES

1. Healthy People 2000 Midcourse Review and 1995 Revisions. US DHHS, Public Health Service. http://odphp.osophs.dhhs.gov/pubs/hp2000 or http://web.health.gove/healthypeople

2. Healthy People 2000 Review 1997, National Health Promotion and Disease Prevention Objectives, US DHHS, Centers for Disease Control and Prevention, National Center for Health Statistics, DHHS Publ no. (PHS) 98-1256, Hyattsville, MD: Public Health Service, 1997.

3. Developing Objectives for Healthy People 2010. US DHHS, Office of Disease Prevention and Health Promotion, Sept 1997.http://odphp.osophs.dhhs.gov/pubs/hp2000 or http://web.health.gov/healthypeople/

A-9-e. Approaches to Management of High Blood Cholesterol Levels

A-9-e-1. Excerpts from the NCEP Report (1*)

A-9-e-1-a General and Specific Approaches

The underlying theme of this report is specific therapy for high blood cholesterol, particularly elevated LDL-cholesterol, and dietary therapy is the cornerstone of cholesterol lowering. Three major dietary factors contribute to high levels of blood cholesterol: a high intake of saturated fat, a high intake of dietary cholesterol, and an imbalance between calorie intake and energy expenditure leading to obesity.

The first goal of dietary therapy is to reduce LDL-cholesterol levels, but dietary modification and increased physical activity may decrease risk for CHD in other ways as well. For example, weight reduction and increased physical activity will reduce VLDL and raise HDL levels, both of which may decrease CHD risk. Weight reduction (combined with decreased salt and alcohol intake) will often lower blood pressure and improve glucose tolerance, also decreasing CHD risk. Beyond these well-known effects, some epidemiologic and experimental data indicate that low intakes of saturated fats and cholesterol lessen risks for CHD beyond LDL-cholesterol lowering. . . .

Diet modification is presented in two steps (Table II-A-9-e-1-b). The Step I Diet is similar in nutrient composition to the eating pattern recommended by the NCEP for the population at large. For patients who have not adopted this eating pattern prior to treatment, the Step I Diet is the initial therapy. For those already on the Step I Diet, further reductions in saturated fat and dietary cholesterol—the Step II Diet—should achieve more LDL-cholesterol lowering. Step I and Step II diets are given in Table V-A-30.

These changes in diet composition should be carried out simultaneously with regular physical activity in all patients and weight reduction in the overweight.

The first task in dietary therapy is to assess current eating habits. This assessment determines whether to start with the Step I Diet or to move directly to Step II. The Step I Diet calls for 8 to 10% of calories from saturated fat, 30% or less of calories from total fat, and less than 300 mg/day of cholesterol. The serum cholesterol response to this diet should be determined at 4–6 weeks and at 3 months. Failure to obtain expected serum cholesterol lowering fre-

Table A-9-e-1-b
Dietary Therapy of High Blood Cholesterol: General Recommendations

Nutrient[a]	Recommended Intake		
	Step I Diet[b]		Step II Diet[b]
Total fat		30% or less of total calories	
Saturated fatty acids	8–10% of Total calories		Less than 7% of total calories
Polyunsaturated fatty acids		Up to 10% of total calories	
Monounsaturated fatty acids		Up to 15% of total calories	
Carbohydrates		55% or more of total calories	
Protein		Approximately 15% of total calories	
Cholesterol	Less than 300 mg/day		Less than 200 mg/day
Total calories		To achieve and maintain desirable weight	

[a]Calories from alcohol not included.

[b]Step I and II diets are presented in Table V-A-30.

*The original report is very well documented with references; review of the original report is recommended.
—The Appendix Editors.

quently indicates inadequate dietary compliance; therefore, reassessment of dietary adherence is needed at follow-up visits.

If the goals of therapy are not achieved after 3 months on a Step I Diet, it is important to reassess adoption of an adherence to this diet. If the goals are not achieved in spite of adherence, the patient should advance to the more intensive Step II Diet. This diet reduces saturated fat to *less than* 7% of calories and cholesterol to *less than* 200 mg/day. The decision to adopt a Step II Diet should be reinforced and encouraged through discussion of its feasibility between physician and patient and in consultation with other health professionals involved in the patient's management.

A-9-e-2. Primary Prevention

A-9-e-2-a High-Risk LDL-Cholesterol (≥160 mg/dL) and Fewer than Two Other CHD Risk Factors (Table A-9-e-2-a)

The goal of therapy for this category of patients is an LDL-cholesterol below 160 mg/dL; and, in the absence of severe hypercholesterolemia, dietary change combined with exercise is the mainstay of therapy. As indicated before, the initial step of dietary therapy depends on the patient's prior eating habits. If the Step I Diet is adopted and does not reduce the LDL-cholesterol level to <160 md/dL after 3 months, the Step II Diet should be initiated. If the LDL-cholesterol level still exceeds 190 mg/dL after 6 months of dietary therapy, drug treatment can be considered according to the general guidelines developed in this report. Patients with LDL-cholesterol levels well above 220 mg/dL can proceed to drug treatment once dietary therapy is underway, but they should progress to the Step II Diet and remain on this diet while on drug therapy.

A-9-e-2-b LDL-Cholesterol >130 mg/dL and Two (or More) CHD Risk Factors (Table A-9-e-2-a)

The goal for LDL-cholesterol lowering in patients with two (or more) CHD risk factors is a level below 130 mg/dL. When LDL-cholesterol is 130 to 159 mg/dL, dietary therapy and exercise should achieve the goal of therapy in most patients. Even if an LDL-cholesterol level of <130 mg/dL is not reached, drug therapy rarely is necessary unless a patient is at very high risk from other risk factors that cannot be controlled.

When LDL-cholesterol is greater than 160 mg/dL and multiple other risk factors are present, diet and exercise should be instituted first, but drug therapy may be required to reach the target of <130 mg/dL. Drug therapy can be considered if the other risk factors are difficult to modify or if the LDL-choelsterol level is especially high. On the other hand, if obesity underlies high LDL-cholesterol and other risk factors (e.g., low HDL-cholesterol, hypertension, and diabetes mellitus), weight reduction alone may eliminate all these factors.

Table A-9-e-2-a
Initial Cholesterol Levels and Therapeutic Goals

	Initiation Level	Goal of Therapy	Monitoring Goal
	LDL-Cholesterol		Total Cholesterol
Without CHD and with fewer than 2 risk factors	≥160 mg/dL	<160 mg/dL	<240 mg/dL
Without CHD and with 2 or more risk factors	≤130 mg/dL	<130mg/dL	<200 mg/dL
With CHD	>100 mg/dL	≤100 mg/dL	≤160 mg/dL

A-9-e-3. Secondary Prevention: CHD (or Other Atherosclerotic Disease) and LDL-Cholesterol >100 mg/dL (Table A-9-e-2-a)

The goal here is to reduce LDL-cholesterol to 100 mg/dL or below. In most patients dietary therapy should begin with the Step II Diet, combined appropriately with weight reduction and exercise. If the goal of therapy is not reached in 6 to 12 weeks, drug therapy can be considered. When LDL-cholesterol falls to 100 to 129 mg/dL on dietary therapy alone, the decision to proceed to drug therapy requires weighing the benefits of further LDL-cholesterol lowering versus the costs and potential side effects of drugs.

The degree of reduction of LDL-cholesterol levels achieved by dietary therapy depends on dietary habits before starting the diet, the degree of compliance, and inherent biological responsiveness. . . . It is not possible to determine the inherent responsiveness of an individual short of a trial of diety therapy. The response of many patients to a change in diet composition, however, may be considerably enhanced by weight reduction.

REFERENCE

1. Detection, Evaluation, and Treatment of High Blood Cholesterol in Adults. 2nd Report of the Expert Panel: Adult Treatment, National Cholesterol Education Program and National Institutes of Health, National Heart, Lung, and Blood Institute NIH Publ. #93-3095 Sept 1993.

A-10. BASAL METABOLIC RATE DATA

Table A-10—a
Nomograph for Estimation of Caloric Needs and Surface Area

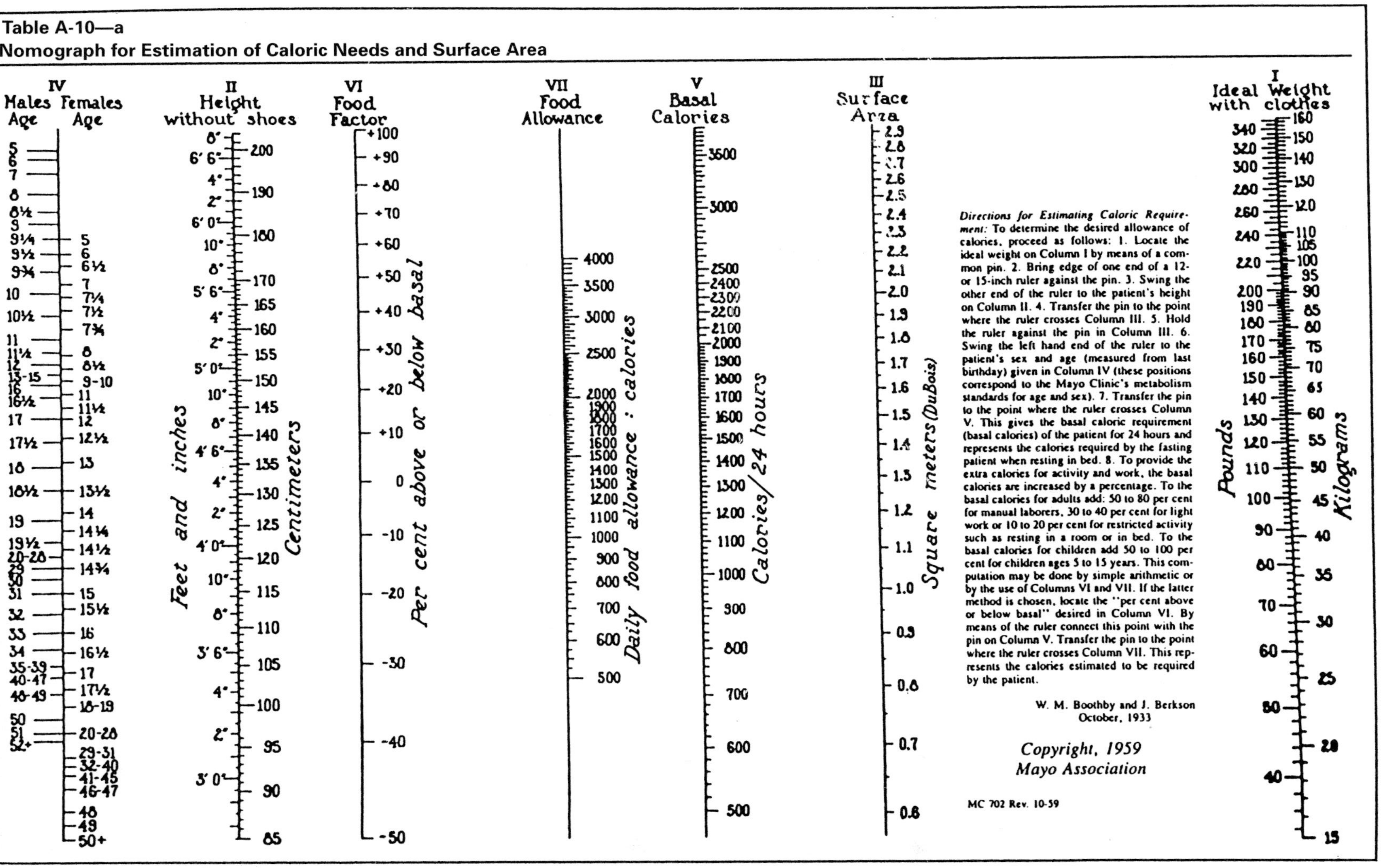

IV Males Age Females Age
II Height without shoes
Feet and inches
Centimeters
VI Food Factor
Per cent above or below basal
VII Food Allowance
Daily food allowance : calories
V Basal Calories
Calories/24 hours
III Surface Area
Square meters (DuBois)
I Ideal Weight with clothes
Pounds
Kilograms
Directions for Estimating Caloric Requirement: To determine the desired allowance of calories, proceed as follows: 1. Locate the ideal weight on Column I by means of a common pin. 2. Bring edge of one end of a 12- or 15-inch ruler against the pin. 3. Swing the other end of the ruler to the patient's height on Column II. 4. Transfer the pin to the point where the ruler crosses Column III. 5. Hold the ruler against the pin in Column III. 6. Swing the left hand end of the ruler to the patient's sex and age (measured from last birthday) given in Column IV (these positions correspond to the Mayo Clinic's metabolism standards for age and sex). 7. Transfer the pin to the point where the ruler crosses Column V. This gives the basal caloric requirement (basal calories) of the patient for 24 hours and represents the calories required by the fasting patient when resting in bed. 8. To provide the extra calories for activity and work, the basal calories are increased by a percentage. To the basal calories for adults add: 50 to 80 per cent for manual laborers, 30 to 40 per cent for light work or 10 to 20 per cent for restricted activity such as resting in a room or in bed. To the basal calories for children add 50 to 100 per cent for children ages 5 to 15 years. This computation may be done by simple arithmetic or by the use of Columns VI and VII. If the latter method is chosen, locate the "per cent above or below basal" desired in Column VI. By means of the ruler connect this point with the pin on Column V. Transfer the pin to the point where the ruler crosses Column VII. This represents the calories estimated to be required by the patient.
W. M. Boothby and J. Berkson
October, 1933
Copyright, 1959
Mayo Association
MC 702 Rev. 10-59

(From Pemberton, C.M., Gastineau, C.F.: Mayo Clinic Diet Manual. 5th Ed. Philadelphia, W.B. Saunders, 1981.)

Table A-10-b
Equations for Predicting Basal Metabolic Rate from Body Weight (W)[a]

Age Range (years)	Kcal$_{th}$/day	Correlation Coefficient	SD[b]	MJ/Day	Correlation Coefficient	SD
Males						
0–3	60.9 W − 54	0.97	53	0.255 W − 0.226	0.97	0.222
3–10	22.7 W + 495	0.86	62	0.0949 W + 2.07	0.86	0.259
10–18	17.5 W + 651	0.90	100	0.0732 W + 2.72	0.90	0.418
18–30	15.3 W + 679	0.65	151	0.0640 W + 2.84	0.65	0.632
30–60	11.6 W + 879	0.60	164	0.0485 W + 3.67	0.60	0.686
>60	13.5 W + 487	0.79	148	0.0565 W + 2.04	0.79	0.619
Females						
0–3	61.0 W − 51	0.97	61	0.255 W − 0.214	0.97	0.255
3–10	22.5 W + 499	0.85	63	0.0941 W + 2.09	0.85	0.264
10–18	12.2 W + 746	0.75	117	0.0510 W + 3.12	0.75	0.489
18–30	14.7 W + 496	0.72	121	0.0615 W + 2.08	0.72	0.506
30–60	8.7 W + 829	0.70	108	0.0364 W + 3.47	0.70	0.452
>60	10.5 W + 596	0.74	108	0.0439 W + 2.49	0.74	0.452

From Energy and protein requirements: report of a Joint FAO/WHO/UNU Expert Consultation. Technical report series no. 724. Geneva: World Health Organization, 1985:71.
[a]Since the present report was compiled, the database for the equations contained in Schofield et al. Hum Nutr Clin Nutr 1985; 39(Suppl), has been slightly expanded. They therefore differ from the equations shown in this table, but the differences are negligible.
[b]Standard deviation of differences between actual BMR and predicted estimates.

Table A-10-c
Examples of Predicted Basal Metabolic Rate (BMR) in Subjects of the Same Height but Different Weights, Predicted from Actual Weight and from Median Acceptable Weight for Height

	Man, Age 40, Height 1.8 m			Woman, Age 25, Height 1.5 m		
	Position in Range[a]			Position in Range[a]		
	Upper	Median	Lower	Upper	Median	Lower
BMI[b]	25	22	20	24	21	19
Wt (kg)	81.0	71.3	64.8	54.0	47.2	42.7
BMR[c] from actual wt						
kcal$_{th}$/day	1,820	1,710	1,630	1,290	1,190	1,120
MJ/day	7.61	7.15	6.82	5.39	4.98	4.68
BMR from median wt						
kcal$_{th}$/day	1,710	1,710	1,710	1,190	1,190	1,190
MJ/day	7.15	7.15	7.15	4.97	4.97	4.97

From Energy and protein requirements: report of a Joint FAO/WHO/UNU Expert Consultation. Technical report series no. 724. Geneva: World Health Organization, 1985:72.
[a]Acceptable range of BMI (see Annex 2A in original reference).
[b]Body mass index = wt(kg)/ht^2(m).
[c]Predicted from equations in Table A-10-b.

Table A-10-d
Basal Metabolic Rates of Adolescent Boys and Girls

			BMR[c]			
			Total		per kg	
Age (years)	Height[a] (cm)	Weight[b] (kg)	(kcal$_{th}$/day)	(MJ/day)	(kcal$_{th}$/day)	(MJ/day)
Boys						
10–11	140	32.2	1215	5.08	37.7	0.16
11–12	147	37.0	1300	5.43	35.1	0.15
12–13	153	40.9	1370	5.73	33.4	0.14
13–14	160	47.0	1465	6.12	31.4	0.13
14–15	166	52.6	1570	6.57	29.9	0.12
15–16	171	58.0	1665	6.96	28.7	0.12
16–17	175	62.7	1750	7.32	27.9	0.12
17–18	177	65.0	1790	7.48	27.5	0.12
Girls						
10–11	142	33.7	1160	4.85	34.3	0.14
11–12	148	38.7	1220	5.10	31.5	0.13
12–13	155	44.0	1280	5.38	29.1	0.12
13–14	159	48.8	1340	5.60	27.5	0.12
14–15	161	51.4	1375	5.75	26.7	0.11
15–16	162	53.0	1395	5.83	26.3	0.11
16–17	163	54.0	1405	5.87	26.0	0.11
17–18	164	54.4	1410	5.89	25.9	0.11

From Energy and protein requirements: report of a Joint FAO/WHO/UNU Expert Consultation. Technical report series no. 724. Geneva: World Health Organization, 1985:72.
[a]Median height for age from NCHS standards.
[b]Median weight for height and age from Baldwin's standards (Annex 2(B) of original reference.)
[c]Boys: BMR = 17.5 W + 651 kcal$_{th}$/day (2.72 MJ/day); girls: 12.2 W + 746 kcal$_{th}$/day (3.12 MJ/day).

Table A-10-e
Basal Metabolic Rate in Adult Men and Women in Relation to Height and Median Acceptable Weight for Height[a] (values given in $kcal_{th}$ with MJ in parentheses)

Height (m)	Weightb (kg)	18–30 Years Per kg per Day	18–30 Years Per Day	30–60 Years Per kg per Day	30–60 Years Per day	>60 Years Per kg per Day	>60 Years Per Day
Men							
1.5	49.5	29.0 (121)	1440 (6.03)	29.4 (123)	1450 (6.07)	23.3 (98)	1150 (4.81)
1.6	56.5	27.4 (115)	1540 (6.44)	27.2 (114)	1530 (6.40)	22.2 (93)	1250 (5.23)
1.7	63.5	26.0 (109)	1650 (6.90)	25.4 (106)	1620 (6.78)	21.2 (89)	1350 (5.65)
1.8	71.5	24.8 (104)	1770 (7.41)	23.9 (99)	1710 (7.15)	20.3 (85)	1450 (6.07)
1.9	79.5	23.9 (100)	1890 (7.91)	22.7 (95)	1800 (7.53)	19.6 (82)	1560 (6.53)
2.0	88	23.0 (96)	2030 (8.49)	21.6 (90)	1900 (7.95)	19.0 (80)	1670 (6.99)
Women							
1.4	41	26.7 (112)	1100 (4.60)	28.8 (120)	1190 (4.98)	25.0 (105)	1030 (4.31)
1.5	47	25.2 (105)	1190 (4.98)	26.3 (110)	1240 (5.19)	23.1 (97)	1090 (4.56)
1.6	54	23.9 (100)	1290 (5.40)	24.1 (101)	1300 (5.44)	21.6 (90)	1160 (4.85)
1.7	61	22.9 (96)	1390 (5.82)	22.4 (94)	1360 (5.69)	20.3 (85)	1230 (5.15)
1.8	68	22.0 (92)	1500 (6.28)	20.9 (87)	1420 (5.94)	19.3 (81)	1310 (5.48)

From Energy and protein requirements: report of a Joint FAO/WHO/UNU Expert Consultation. Technical report series no. 724. Geneva: World Health Organization, 1985:72.

[a]BMR from equations in Table A-10-b rounded to 10 $kcal_{th}$.

[b]Weight taken as median acceptable weight for height: body mass index (wt/ht^2) = 22 in men, 21 in women.

A-11. ENERGY EXPENDITURE AND REQUIREMENTS: WHO—1985

Table A-11-a
Calculated Energy Requirements of Infants From Birth to 1 Year

Age (months)	Intake[a] ($kcal_{th}$/kg per day)	Intake[a] (kJ/kg per day)	Calculated Energy Requirement[b] ($kcal_{th}$/kg per day)	Calculated Energy Requirement[b] (kJ/kg per day)	Median Body Weight[c] Boys (kg)	Median Body Weight[c] Girls (kg)	Total Requirement Boys ($kcal_{th}$/day)	Total Requirement Boys (kJ/day)	Total Requirement Girls ($kcal_{th}$/day)	Total Requirement Girls (kJ/day)
0.5	118	494	124	519	3.8	3.6	470	1965	445	1860
1–2	114	477	116	485	4.75	4.35	550	2300	505	2115
2–3	107	448	109	456	5.6	5.05	610	2550	545	2280
3–4	101	423	103	431	6.35	5.7	655	2740	590	2470
4–5	96	402	99	414	7.0	6.35	695	2910	630	2635
5–6	93	389	96.5	404	7.55	6.95	730	3055	670	2800
6–7	91	381	95	397	8.05	7.55	765	3220	720	3010
7–8	90	377	94.5	395	8.55	7.95	810	3390	750	3140
8–9	90	377	95	397	9.0	8.4	855	3580	800	3350
9–10	91	381	99	414	9.35	8.75	925	3870	865	3620
10–11	93	389	100	418	9.7	9.05	970	4060	905	3790
11–12	97	406	104.5	437	10.05	9.35	1050	4395	975	4080
12	102	427								

From Energy and protein requirements: report of a Joint FAO/WHO/UNU Expert Consultation. Technical report series no. 724. Geneva: World Health Organization, 1985:91.

[a]Observed intakes at ages indicated, from data of sources given in original publication. Average intake predicted from equation (age in months); 1 ($kcal_{th}$/kg) = 123 − 8.9 age + 0.59 age. See original reference.

[b]Requirement over interval indicated, calculated as predicted intake + 5%. See original reference.

[c]NCHS median weights at midpoint of month.

Table A-11-b
Estimated Average Daily Energy Intakes and Requirements, Ages 1 to 10 Years

Age (years)	Boys			
	Intake[a]		Requirement[b]	
	(kcal$_{th}$/day)	(MJ/day)	(kcal$_{th}$/day)	(MJ/day)
1–2	1140	4.76	1200	5.02
2–3	1340	5.60	1410	5.89
3–4	1490	6.23	1560	6.52
4–5	1610	6.73	1690	7.07
5–6	1720	7.19	1810	7.57
6–7	1810	7.57	1900	7.94
7–8	1895	7.92	1990	8.32
8–9	1970	8.24	2070	8.66
9–10	2045	8.55	2150	8.99

Age (years)	Girls				Requirement by Weight[c]			
					Boys		Girls	
	Intake[a]		Requirement[b]					
	(kcal$_{th}$/day)	(MJ/day)	(kca$_{th}$/day)	(MJ/day)	(kcal$_{th}$/kg per day)	(kJ/kg per day)	(kcal$_{th}$/kg per day)	(kJ/kg per day)
1–2	1090	4.56	1140	4.76	104	435	108	452
2–3	1250	5.23	1310	5.48	104	410	102	427
3–4	1370	5.73	1440	6.02	99	414	95	397
4–5	1465	6.12	1540	6.44	95	397	92	385
5–6	1550	6.48	1630	6.81	92	385	88	368
6–7	1620	6.77	1700	7.11	88	368	83	347
7–8	1685	7.05	1770	7.40	83	347	76	318
8–9	1740	7.28	1830	7.65	77	322	69	268
9–10	1795	7.51	1880	7.86	72	301	62	259

From Energy and protein requirements: report of a Joint FAO/WHO/UNU Expert Consultation. Technical report series no. 724. Geneva: World Health Organization, 1985:94–95.
[a]From data of Ferro-Luzzi and Durnin, Rome: FAO, 1981 (Document ESN: FAO/WHO/UNU/EPR/81/9).
[b]Intakes +5%. See original reference.
[c]From NCHS median weights at midyear.

Table A-11-c
Calculated Average Energy Expenditure and Observed Intakes and Comparison With Recommendations of 1971 Committee, Ages 10 to 18 Years

Age (years)	Expenditure (× BMR)[a]	Expenditure		Intake[b]		1971 Committee[c] Recommended Requirement	
		(kcal$_{th}$/day)	(MJ/day)	(kcal$_{th}$/day)	(MJ/day)	(kcal$_{th}$/day)	(MJ/day)
Boys							
10–11	1.76	2140	8.95	2110	8.82	2500	10.46
11–12	1.73	2240	9.37	2170	9.07	2600	10.87
12–13	1.69	2310	9.66	2200	9.20	2700	11.29
13–14	1.67	2440	10.20	2280	9.53	2800	11.71
14–15	1.65	2590	10.83	2340	9.79	2900	12.13
15–16	1.62	2700	11.29	2390	9.99	3000	12.55
16–17	1.60	2800	11.71	2440	10.20	3050	12.76
17–18	1.60	2870	12.0	2490	10.41	3100	12.97
Girls							
10–11	1.65	1910	7.99	1850	7.74	2300	9.62
11–12	1.63	1980	8.28	1890	7.90	2350	9.83
12–13	1.60	2050	8.57	1930	8.07	2400	10.04
13–14	1.58	2120	8.87	1970	8.24	2450	10.25
14–15	1.57	2160	9.03	2010	8.40	2500	10.46
15–16	1.54	2140	8.95	2050	8.57	2500	10.46
16–17	1.53	2130	8.91	2080	8.70	2420	10.12
17–18	1.52	2140	8.95	2120	8.87	2340	9.79

From Energy and protein requirements: report of a Joint FAO/WHO/UNU Expert Consultation. Technical report series no. 724. Geneva: World Health Organization, 1985:98.
[a]Expenditure calculated as in original publication.
[b]Intakes from reference in original publication.
[c]Reference in original 1971 publication. (cf ref. d)

Table A-11-d
Derivation of Average Values of the Energy Cost of Three Grades of Physical Activity at Work for Women and Men[a]

	Women[b]				Men[c]			
	Cost/Min ($kcal_{th}$)	(kJ)	Average cost × BMR (gross)	(net)	Cost/Min ($kcal_{th}$)	(kJ)	Average cost × BMR (gross)	(net)
Light work								
75% of time sitting or standing	1.51	6.3			1.79	7.5		
25% of time standing and moving	1.70	7.1			2.51	10.5		
Average	1.56	6.5	1.7	0.7	1.99	8.3	1.7	0.7
Moderate work								
25% of time sitting or standing	1.51	6.3			1.79	7.5		
75% of time spent on specific occupational activity	2.20	9.2			3.61	15.1		
Average	2.03	8.5	2.2	1.2	3.16	13.2	2.7	1.7
Heavy work								
40% of time sitting or standing	1.51	6.3			1.79	7.5		
60% of time spent on specific occupational activity	3.21	13.4			6.22	26.0		
Average	2.54	10.6	2.8	1.8	4.45	18.6	3.8	2.8

From Energy and protein requirements: report of a Joint FAO/WHO/UNU Expert Consultation. Technical report series no. 724. Geneva: World Health Organization, 1985:76.
[a]Times and energy costs of sitting, standing, moving around, and work tasks are composite values derived from published and unpublished data (Annex 5) in original reference.
[b]Based on young adult females (18–30 years). Wt 55 kg, BMR 0.90 $kcal_{th}$ (3.8 kJ)/min (Table A-10-b.)
[c]Based on young adult males (18–30 years). Wt 65 kg, BMR 1.16 $kcal_{th}$ (4.9 kJ)/min (Table A-10-b.)

Table A-11-e
Average Daily Energy Requirement of Adults Whose Occupational Work is Classified as Light, Moderate, or Heavy, Expressed as a Multiple of Basal Metabolic Rate

	Light	Moderate	Heavy
Men	1.55	1.78	2.10
Women	1.56	1.64	1.82

From Energy and protein requirements: report of a Joint FAO/WHO/UNU Expert Consultation. Technical report series no. 724. Geneva: World Health Organization, 1985:78.

Table A-11-f
Estimates of Energy Cost of Weight Gain[a]

Subjects		Energy Cost ($kcal_{th}$/g)	(kJ/g)
Premature infants		4.9	20.5
Premature infants		5.7	23.8
Normal infants		5.6	23.4
Infants recovering from malnutrition		5.55	23.2
		4.6	19.2
		3.5	14.6
		4.4	18.4
		7.1	29.7
Adults recovering from anorexia nervosa		6.4	26.7
Adults, intentional overfeeding		8.2	34.3
Pregnancy	Theoretic estimate[b]	6.4	26.7

From Energy and protein requirements: report of a Joint FAO/WHO/UNU Expert Consultation. Technical report series no. 724. Geneva: World Health Organization, 1985:185.
[a]See original references for data sources.
[b]Calculated as 80,000 $kcal_{th}$ (335 mJ) stored for 12.5 kg of weight gain.

A-12-a. HEIGHT-WEIGHT TABLES: THEIR SOURCES AND DEVELOPMENT (SIDNEY ABRAHAM)

The Metropolitan Life Insurance Company presented their height and weight tables derived from data of the Build Study, 1979 (1). Metropolitan Life had previously utilized data from life insurance mortality studies compiled in the early 1900s and late 1950s to develop desirable weight tables in 1942 (2), 1943 (3) and 1959 (4). These studies reported the prevalence of mortality among insured persons according to variations in body build (height and weight) and also presented the average weight for height of persons by age. Such studies were designed to determine which groups (those underweight or overweight) showed a proportionately higher prevalence of mortality to yield information for underwriting purposes and for warranting changes in insurance policy premiums.

Average Weight By Height Tables and Age-Group

Mortality Studies

In the American life insurance industry, interest in build (height and weight) as factors that influence mortality dates back to 1885. In that year, the Union Mutual Life Insurance Company published a pamphlet containing the results of a study of the company's records on mortality in relation to build (5). The first indepth study on the subject was presented in 1901 by a representative of the New York Life Insurance Company at the twelfth annual meeting of the Association of Life Insurance Medical Directors of America (6). In this presentation it was pointed out that a certain amount of overweight had previously been looked on favorably. Nonetheless, the summary of this report noted that: "First among life insurance risks [is that] the [health] hazard increases in proportion to the degree of over- or underweight, second, whereas among overweights the mortality to be expected increases with [the] increased age of [the] applicant, among underweights the mortality decreases with advancing years."

Height-Weight Tables

The first height-weight table based on a considerable volume of statistics and taking age into account was the

"Shepherd Table." This table was prepared in 1897 and was based on 74,162 male applicants accepted for life insurance in the United States and Canada (7).

The basic study of height and weight based on life insurance statistics, however, was made as part of the study and the tables derived therefrom were the bases of the height-weight tables prepared for the general population. In addition to the study of the prevalence of mortality of certain groups of the insured population, the 1912 investigation included a study of the height and weight of a sample of persons insured from 1885 to 1900 (8). The height and weight were recorded with the subjects wearing shoes and street clothes. A total of 221,819 men residing in the United States and Canada were included in this sample. At least 40% of the weights were estimated by the medical examiners. The data as tabulated were then smoothed to provide the figures for the height-weight age tables, and the adjusted tables became the basis for height-weight tables for males in the United States at this time.

Substantially the same procedure was employed to develop height-weight tables for women, but to secure enough cases for the preparation of tables it was necessary to add 126,504 policies issued after 1900 to the 10,000 included in the 1885 to 1900 sample.

In the Medical Impairment Study of 1929 (9), height-weight data were again collected on 667,000 men and 85,000 women. The average weights of both men and women in the 1929 study were not significantly different from those observed in the Medico-Actuarial Mortality Investigation (8). In fact, differences were so small that it was decided not to revise the standard height-weight tables except for those individuals younger than age 15.

Tables of "Ideal" or "Desirable" Weights

An article presented in 1920, "Is the 'Average' the Same as the 'Normal' for Weight and Blood Pressure?" (10) illustrates an important development in the preparation of height-weight tables. In this paper the "normal" weight group is defined as that having the lowest mortality rates. The article presented a table of "normal" weights, so defined, for medium-sized men averaging 68 inches in height, and several discussants added their tables of similarly defined normal weights for men of small, medium, and tall height. In 1922, complete height-weight tables were presented that showed this normal weight for each inch of height and for each age group (11). In general, all such tables of normal weight indicated that the ideal weight in terms of mortality was the average weight for height at age 30.

Metropolitan Life Develops "Ideal" Height-Weight Tables

Desirable Weight Tables, 1942 and 1943

The concept of a "normal" weight, represented by the average weight of men at age 30, plus an awareness of the shortcomings of height and weight alone as complete indications of obesity, led to the development of "ideal" weight tables by the Metropolitan Life Insurance Company (2, 3). Although employed for many purposes, these tables were originally intended for use in health education. The basic data were derived from the standard height-weight tables of the Medico-Actuarial Study of 1912, using the average weight for each inch of height at age 30 for men and at age 25 for women. Arbitrary ranges were then developed, using the base figures as reference points. These ranges are approximately the standard deviation of average weights for a given height and include the lightest weight for persons with small frames to the heaviest weight for persons with large frames. The total was then arbitrarily divided into three overlapping ranges, and the resulting figures represented ideal weights for individuals of small, medium, and large frames. However, no definition of frame size was presented.

These tables were intended to aid people in achieving a weight below the average for their height. Before these tables were developed, only average weights for each inch of height by age and sex were available. The new approach represented a change in concept between average weight (assuming that the average value is optimal for health) and desirable weight (weight based on the criterion of longevity). The concept underlying these tables deemphasized the use of a single average at each height and refuted the popular notion that weight increments attendant with advancing age were normal and therefore not harmful.

Desirable Weight Tables, 1959

The next study of build in relation to mortality was made in conjunction with the Build and Blood Pressure Study of 1959 (4). This investigation was based on the combined experience of 26 life insurance companies in the United States and Canada from 1935 to 1954 and involved observation of nearly 5 million insured persons for periods up to 20 years. Only those insured persons ages 15 through 69 were included. The height and weight data were recorded with the subjects wearing street shoes and indoor clothing. More than 90% of the insured persons were reported to have been actually weighed and measured at the time of examination for life insurance. The study presented average weights for men and women for each inch of height, ranging from 62 to 76 inches for men and from 58 to 72 inches for women. To provide some indication of the sole effect of weight on mortality, persons with heart disease, cancer, or diabetes were excluded.

When the Build and Blood Pressure Study was completed, the "ideal weight" table, originally developed by the Metropolitan Life Insurance Company in 1942 and 1943, was revised to conform to the latest data. The new table, called the "desirable weight" table (Table A-12-a-1) was derived directly from weights associated with lowest mortality. Ranges of "desirable weight" for individuals 25 years and older with small, medium, and large frames were given, but again, no definition of frame size was included.

Metropolitan Height-Weight Tables

Data published by the Society of Actuaries and the Association of Life Insurance Medical Directors of American in the Build Study, 1979 (1), are the source for the 1983 Metropolitan Life Insurance Height-Weight Tables (Table A-12-a-2). The data are from 25 life insurance companies in the United States and Canada and show the prevalence of mortality from 1954 to 1972 of approximately 4.2 million insured men and women. Almost 90% of the recorded weights submitted for the study was obtained by actually weighing the applicants. As in the 1959 Build and Blood Pressure Study, applicants with major disease conditions at the time of policy issuance were excluded from the study. The terms "ideal body weight" and "desirable body weight," used in the earlier tables were not applied to the new height and weight tables because of the various misinterpretations of their meaning.

The findings from the Build Study, 1979, showed that the gap between the weights based on lowest mortality and average weights had narrowed considerably since the 1959 Build and Blood Pressure Study. Metropolitan Life considered this factor in developing the 1983 height-weight tables. Weight for height has increased in contrast to the 1959 tables, but the increased weights are still less than the average weights (Table A-12-a-5). Additionally, the increases in weight are not uniformly distributed throughout the 1983 height-weight tables. For each frame size, the weight increases for tall men or women were not as large as those for short men or women or for those of medium height.

In conjunction with investigations based on the life insurance data previously enumerated, long-term studies such as the Framingham Heart Study (12) and the Manitoba Study (13) all indicate that the weight associated with the greatest longevity tends to be below the average weight of the population under consideration and that "slimmer is better," provided that the underweight is not associated with a medical history of significant impairment.

Frame Size

The 1983 Metropolitan height-weight tables related weight to body frame size. A distinction is made among persons with small, medium, and large frames. The previous Metropolitan height-weight tables also related weight to body frame size, but although the body frame sizes were statistically defined, no generally accepted method of measuring frame size was provided. Body frame size is an integral factor in considering variation in weight, assuming that persons with larger frames have larger lean body mass and therefore weigh more. In the 1983 tables, elbow breadth is now used to determine frame size in men and women (Table A-12-a-3). The frame sizes were developed from elbow breadth measurements taken from the first National Health and Nutrition Examination Survey, 1971 to 1975 (14), and were distributed so that 50% of the population falls within the medium frame and 25% each falls within the small and large frames.

Summary

Major insurance mortality studies on insured populations in the United States and Canada conducted in 1912 by the Actuarial Society of America (8) and in 1959 and 1979 by the Society of Actuaries and the Association of Life Insurance Medical Directors of America (1, 4) analyzed the mortality experience among insured persons according to variations of weight by height. The studies also presented data on the distribution of weight and height. The earliest study showed that the lowest mortality by build (weight for height) was found for those somewhat overweight at younger ages and among those underweight at older ages. In later mortality studies, it was generally found that insured persons whose weight was below average lived longer than those whose weights were above average.

Since 1942, the Metropolitan Life Insurance Company has developed weight tables from data derived from each of the three major studies. The weights in each of the tables at given heights for men and women are classified according to frame size and refer to the weights associated with lowest mortality of policyholders. The weights were those obtained when the individual was originally insured. Because it is recognized that height and weight alone are incomplete indicators of excess weight, the weight tables also considered measurements of body build. In the tables issued in the 1940s (2, 3), 1959 (4), and 1983, three groups of frame size were identified. In each frame size, weight was given as a range rather than as a single value. However, no objective method was presented to estimate frame size in the earlier two tables. In the 1983 Metropolitan Height-Weight Tables, elbow breadth, unaffected by degree of adiposity and closely representative of bony dimension, was suggested to estimate frame size in the three categories of body build.

The views herein are solely those of the author and do not necessarily represent those of the National Center for Health Statistics.

REFERENCES

1. Build Study, 1979: Society of Actuaries and Association of Life Insurance Medical Directors of America. Philadelphia: Recording and Statistical Corporation, 1980.
2. Ideal weight for men. Stat Bull Metropol Life Insur Co 1942;23:6.
3. Ideal weights for women. Stat Bull Metropol Life Insur Co 1943;24:6.
4. New weight standards for men and women. Stat Bull Metropol Life Insur Co 1959;40:1.
5. Grant FS: Proc Assoc Life Insur Med Dir Am 1902;2:323–7.

6. Rogers OH: Proc Assoc Life Insur Med Dir Am 1901;1:280–8.
7. Shepherd GR: Proc Assoc Life Insur Med Dir Am, 1912;6:46–58.
8. Medico-Actuarial Mortality Investigation. New York: Actuarial Society of America, 1912.
9. Medical Impairment Study, 1929. New York: the Association of Life Insurance Medical Directors of America and the Actuarial Society of America, 1931.
10. Hunger A. Trans Actuar Soc Am 1920;21:365–70.
11. Knight AS. Proc Assoc Life Insur Med Dir Am 1922;9:193–9.
12. Huberg HB, Feinleig M, McNamara PM, et al. Circulation 1983;5:968–77.
13. Rabkin SW, Mathewson FAL, HSU PH: Am J Cardiol 1977;39: 452–8.
14. Public Use Data Tape, NHANES I—Anthropometry, goniometry, skeletal age, bone density, and cortical thickness, ages 1–74. Tape no. 4111, National Health and Nutrition Examination Survey, 1971–1975. Hyattsville, MD: National Center for Health Statistics.

Table A-12-a-1
Desirable Weights for Men and Women Aged 25 and Over (in Pounds by Height and Frame, in Indoor Clothing), 1959

Men (in shoes, 1-inch heels)					Women (in shoes, 2-inch heels)				
Height					Height				
Feet	Inches	Small Frame	Medium Frame	Large Frame	Feet	Inches	Small Frame	Medium Frame	Large Frame
5	2	112–120	118–129	126–141	4	10	92–98	96–107	104–119
5	3	115–123	121–133	129–144	4	11	94–101	98–110	106–122
5	4	118–126	124–136	132–148	5	0	96–104	101–113	109–125
5	5	121–129	127–139	135–152	5	1	99–107	104–116	112–128
5	6	124–133	130–143	138–156	5	2	102–110	107–119	115–131
5	7	128–137	134–147	142–161	5	3	105–113	110–122	118–134
5	8	132–141	138–152	147–166	5	4	108–116	113–126	121–138
5	9	136–145	142–156	151–170	5	5	111–119	116–130	125–142
5	10	140–150	146–160	155–174	5	6	114–123	120–135	129–146
5	11	144–154	150–165	159–179	5	7	118–127	124–139	133–150
6	0	148–158	154–170	164–184	5	8	122–131	128–143	137–154
6	1	152–162	158–175	168–189	5	9	126–135	132–147	141–158
6	2	156–167	162–180	173–194	5	10	130–140	136–151	145–163
6	3	160–171	167–185	178–199	5	11	134–144	140–155	149–168
6	4	164–175	172–190	182–204	6	0	138–148	144–159	153–173

Data adapted from new weight standards for men and women. Stat Bull Metropol Life Insur Co. 1959;40:1.

Table A-12-a-2
Height-Weight Tables, 1983[a]

Men					Women				
Height					Height				
Feet	Inches	Small Frame	Medium Frame	Large Frame	Feet	Inches	Small Frame	Medium Frame	Large Frame
5	2	128–134	131–141	138–150	4	10	102–111	109–121	118–131
5	3	130–136	133–143	140–153	4	11	103–113	111–123	120–134
5	4	132–138	135–145	142–156	5	0	104–115	113–126	122–137
5	5	134–140	137–148	144–160	5	1	106–118	115–129	125–140
5	6	136–142	139–151	146–164	5	2	108–121	118–132	128–143
5	7	138–145	142–154	149–168	5	3	111–124	121–135	131–147
5	8	140–148	145–157	152–172	5	4	114–127	124–138	134–151
5	9	142–151	148–160	155–176	5	5	117–130	127–141	137–155
5	10	144–154	151–163	158–180	5	6	120–133	130–144	140–159
5	11	146–157	154–166	161–184	5	7	123–136	133–147	143–163
6	0	149–160	157–170	164–188	5	8	126–139	136–150	146–167
6	1	152–164	160–174	168–192	5	9	129–142	139–153	149–170
6	2	155–168	164–178	172–197	5	10	132–145	142–156	152–173
6	3	158–172	167–182	176–202	5	11	135–148	145–159	155–176
6	4	162–176	171–187	181–207	6	0	138–151	148–162	158–179

Reprinted with permission from the Metropolitan Life Insurance Company, New York.
[a]Weight according to frame (ages 25 to 59) for men wearing indoor clothing weighing 5 lb shoes with 1-inch heels; for women, indoor clothing weighing 3 lb shoes with 1-inch heels.

Table A-12-a-3
Height and Elbow Breadth for Men and Women[a]

Height in 1-Inch Heels	Elbow Breadth[b]
Men	
5'2"–5'3"	2½"–2⅞"
5'4"–5'7"	2⅝"–2⅞"
5'8"–5'11"	2¾"–3"
6'0"–6'3"	2¾"–3⅛"
6'4"	2⅞"–3¼"
Women	
4'10"–4'11"	2¼"–2½"
5'0"–5'3"	2¼"–2½"
5'4"–5'7"	2⅜"–2⅝"
5'8"–5'11"	2⅜"–2⅝"
6'0"	2½"–2¾"

Reprinted with permission from Metropolitan Life Insurance Company, New York.

[a]See our Table A-12-b for other data on frame size by elbow breadth from NHANES I and II.

[b]Procedure: Extend your arm and bend the forearm upward at a 90° angle. Keep fingers straight and turn the inside of your wrist toward your body. If you have a caliper, use it to measure the space between the two prominent bones on either side of your elbow. Without a caliper, place thumb and index finger of your other hand on these two bones. Measure the space between your fingers against a ruler or tape measure. Compare it with these tables that list elbow measurements for medium-frame men and women. Measurements lower than those listed indicate you have a small frame. Higher measurements indicate a larger frame.

Table A-12-a-4
Height-Weight Tables (Metric Units), 1983[a]

	Men				Women		
Height (cm)	Small Frame (kg)	Medium Frame (kg)	Large Frame (kg)	Height (cm)	Small Frame (kg)	Medium Frame (kg)	Large Frame (kg)
157.5	58.2–60.9	59.4–64.1	62.7–68.2	147.5	46.4–50.5	49.5–50.5	53.6–59.5
160	59.1–61.8	60.5–65.0	63.6–69.5	150	46.8–51.4	50.5–55.9	54.5–60.9
162.5	60.0–62.7	61.4–65.9	64.5–70.9	152.5	47.3–52.3	51.4–57.3	55.5–62.3
165	60.9–63.7	62.3–67.3	65.5–72.7	155	48.2–53.6	52.3–58.6	56.8–63.6
167.5	61.8–64.5	63.2–68.6	66.4–74.5	157.5	49.1–55.0	53.6–60.0	58.2–65.0
170	62.7–65.9	64.5–70.0	67.7–76.4	160	50.5–56.4	55.0–61.4	59.5–66.8
173	63.6–67.3	65.9–71.4	69.1–78.2	162.5	51.8–57.7	56.4–62.7	60.9–68.6
175	64.5–68.6	67.3–72.7	70.5–80.0	165	53.2–59.1	57.7–64.1	62.3–70.5
178	65.4–70.0	68.6–74.1	71.8–81.8	167.5	54.5–60.5	59.1–65.5	63.6–72.3
180	66.4–71.4	70.0–75.5	73.2–83.6	170	55.9–61.8	60.5–66.8	65.0–74.1
183	67.7–72.7	71.4–77.3	74.5–85.6	173	57.3–63.2	61.8–68.2	66.4–75.9
185.5	69.1–74.5	72.7–79.1	76.4–87.3	175	58.6–64.5	63.2–69.5	67.7–77.3
188	70..5–76.4	74.5–80.9	78.2–89.5	178	60.0–65.9	64.5–70.9	69.1–78.6
190.5	71.8–78.2	75.9–82.7	80.0–91.8	180	61.4–67.3	65.9–72.3	70.5–80.0
193	73.6–80.0	77.7–85.0	82.3–94.1	183	62.3–68.6	67.3–73.6	71.8–81.4

Reprinted with permission from the Metropolitan Life Insurance Company, New York.

[a]The 1983 Metropolitan Height-Weight Tables are based on the 1979 Build Study. The values are statistical computations from individuals ranging from 25 to 59 years of weights by height and body frame at which mortality has been found to be lowest or longevity the highest. Metropolitan Life does not advocate the use of the term *ideal*, which has different meanings to various individuals, because the term was used originally in their 1942 to 1943 tables. If one wishes to use these tables in the sense that they are "ideal" in terms of lowest mortality, they are "appropriate" in that context. These tables do not provide weights related to minimizing illness, optimizing job performance, or creating the best appearance.

Table A-12-a-5
Average Weights by Height and Age Group: 1959 and 1979 Build and Blood Pressure Studies[a]

	Height														
Men	5'2"	5'3"	5'4"	5'5"	5'6"	5'7"	5'8"	5'9"	5'10"	5'11"	6'0"	6'1"	6'2"	6'3"	6'4"
15–16 Years															
1959 study	107	112	117	122	127	132	137	142	146	150	154	159	164	169	[b]
1979 study	112	116	121	127	133	137	143	148	153	159	162	168	173	178	184
Weight change	+5	+4	+4	+5	+6	+5	+6	+6	+7	+9	+8	+9	+9	+9	—
17–19 Years															
1959 study	119	123	127	131	135	139	143	147	151	155	160	164	168	172	176
1979 study	124	129	132	137	141	145	150	155	159	164	168	174	179	185	190
Weight change	+5	+6	+5	+6	+6	+6	+7	+8	+8	+9	+8	+10	+11	+13	+14
20–24 Years															
1959 study	128	132	136	139	142	145	149	153	157	161	166	170	174	178	181
1979 study	130	136	139	143	148	153	157	163	167	171	176	182	187	193	198
Weight change	+2	+4	+3	+4	+6	+8	+8	+10	+10	+10	+10	+12	+13	+15	+17
25–29 Years															
1959 study	134	138	141	144	148	151	155	159	163	167	172	177	182	186	190
1979 study	134	140	143	147	152	156	161	166	171	175	181	186	191	197	202
Weight change	+0	+2	+2	+3	+4	+5	+6	+7	+8	+8	+9	+9	+9	+11	+12
30–39 Years															
1959 study	137	141	145	149	153	157	161	165	170	174	179	183	188	193	199
1979 study	138	143	147	151	156	160	165	170	174	179	184	190	195	201	206
Weight change	+1	+2	+2	+2	+3	+3	+4	+5	+4	+5	+5	+7	+7	+8	+7
40–49 Years															
1959 study	140	144	148	152	156	161	165	169	174	178	183	187	192	197	203
1979 study	140	144	149	154	158	163	167	172	176	181	186	192	197	203	208
Weight change	+0	+0	+1	+2	+2	+2	+2	+3	+2	+3	+3	+5	+5	+6	+5
50–59 Years															
1959 study	142	145	149	153	157	162	166	170	175	180	185	189	194	199	205
1979 study	141	145	150	155	159	164	168	173	177	182	187	193	198	204	209
Weight change	−1	+0	+1	+2	+2	+2	+2	+3	+2	+2	+2	+4	+4	+5	+4
60–69 Years															
1959 study	139	142	146	150	154	159	163	168	173	178	183	188	193	198	204
1979 study	140	144	149	153	158	163	167	172	176	181	186	191	196	200	207
Weight change	+1	+2	+3	+3	+4	+4	+4	+4	+3	+3	+3	+3	+3	+2	+3

	Height														
Women	4'10"	4'11"	5'0"	5'1"	5'2"	5'3"	5'4"	5'5"	5'6"	5'7"	5'8"	5'9"	5'10"	5'11"	6'0"
15–16 Years															
1959 study	97	100	103	107	111	114	117	121	125	128	132	136	[b]	[b]	[b]
1979 study	101	105	109	112	117	121	123	128	131	135	138	142	146	149	152
Weight change	+4	+5	+6	+5	+6	+7	+6	+7	+6	+7	+6	+6	—	—	—
17–19 Years															
1959 study	99	102	105	109	113	116	120	124	127	130	134	138	142	147	152
1979 study	103	108	111	115	119	123	126	129	132	136	140	145	148	150	154
Weight change	+4	+6	+6	+6	+6	+7	+6	+5	+5	+6	+6	+7	+6	+3	+2
20–24 Years															
1959 study	102	105	108	112	115	118	121	125	129	132	136	140	144	149	154
1979 study	105	110	112	116	120	124	127	130	133	137	141	146	149	155	157
Weight change	+3	+5	+4	+4	+5	+6	+6	+5	+4	+5	+5	+6	+5	+6	+3
25–29 Years															
1959 study	107	110	113	116	119	122	125	129	133	136	140	144	148	153	158
1979 study	110	112	114	119	121	125	128	132	134	138	142	148	150	156	159
Weight change	+3	+2	+1	+3	+2	+3	+3	+3	+1	+2	+2	+4	+2	+3	+1
30–39 Years															
1959 study	115	117	120	123	126	129	132	135	139	142	146	150	154	159	164
1979 study	113	115	118	121	124	128	131	134	137	141	145	150	153	159	164
Weight change	−2	−2	−2	−2	−2	−1	−1	−1	−2	−1	−1	0	−1	0	0
40–49 Years															
1959 study	122	124	127	130	133	136	140	143	147	151	155	159	164	169	174
1979 study	118	121	123	127	129	133	136	139	143	147	150	155	158	162	168
Weight change	−4	−3	−4	−3	−4	−3	−4	−4	−4	−4	−5	−4	−6	−7	−6
50–59 Years															
1959 study	125	127	130	133	136	140	144	148	152	156	160	164	169	174	180
1979 study	121	125	127	131	133	137	141	144	147	152	156	159	162	166	171
Weight change	−4	−2	−3	−2	−3	−3	−3	−4	−5	−4	−4	−5	−7	−8	−9
60–69 Years															
1959 study	127	129	131	134	137	141	145	149	153	157	161	165	[b]	[b]	[b]
1979 study	123	127	130	133	136	140	143	147	150	155	158	161	163	167	172
Weight change	−4	−2	−1	−1	−1	−1	−2	−2	−3	−2	−3	−4	—	—	—

Data from Association of Life Insurance Medical Directors of America and Society of Actuaries. Compiled by Seltzer F. Dietetic Currents 1983; 10:17–22. Reprinted with permission of Ross Laboratories, Columbus, Ohio.

[a]Height in shores (feet and inches) and weight in indoor clothing (pounds).

[b]Average weights omitted in classes with too few cases for analysis.

Table A-12-b
Comparison of the Weight-for-Height Tables from Actuarial Data (Build Study): Non-Age-Corrected Metropolitan Life Insurance Company and Age-Specific Gerontology Research Center Recommendations[a]

Height	Metropolitan 1983 Weights for Ages 25–59[b]		Gerontology Research Center Weight Range for Men and Women by Age (Years)				
	Men	Women	25	35	45	55	65
(ft–in)	lb						
4–10	—	100–131	84–111	92–119	99–127	107–135	115–142
4–11	—	101–134	87–115	95–123	103–131	111–139	119–147
5–0	—	103–137	90–119	98–127	106–135	114–143	123–152
5–1	123–145	105–140	93–123	101–131	110–140	118–148	127–157
5–2	125–148	108–144	96–127	105–136	113–144	122–153	131–163
5–3	127–151	111–148	99–131	108–140	117–149	126–158	135–168
5–4	129–155	114–152	102–135	112–145	121–154	130–163	140–173
5–5	131–159	117–156	106–140	115–149	125–159	134–168	144–179
5–6	133–163	120–160	109–144	119–154	129–164	138–174	148–184
5–7	135–167	123–164	112–148	122–159	133–169	143–179	153–190
5–8	137–171	126–167	116–153	126–163	137–174	147–184	158–196
5–9	139–175	129–170	119–157	130–168	141–179	151–190	162–201
5–10	141–179	132–173	122–162	134–173	145–184	156–195	167–207
5–11	144–183	135–176	126–167	137–178	149–190	160–201	172–213
6–0	147–187	—	129–171	141–183	153–195	165–207	177–219
6–1	150–192	—	133–176	145–188	157–200	169–213	182–225
6–2	153–197	—	137–181	149–194	162–206	174–219	187–232
6–3	157–202	—	141–186	153–199	166–212	179–225	192–238
6–4	—	—	144–191	157–205	171–218	184–231	197–244

Gerontology Research Center data from Andres R. Mortality and obesity: the rationale for age-specific height-weight tables. In: Principles of Geriatric Medicine. Andres R, Bierman E, Hazzard WR, eds. New York: McGraw-Hill, 1985:311–318.

[a]Values in this table are for height without shoes and weight without clothes. To convert inches to centimeters, multiply by 2.54; to convert pounds to kilograms, multiply by 0.455.

[b]The weight range is the lower weight for small frame and the upper weight for large frame.

A-12-c, FRAME SIZE AND ELBOW BREADTH

A-12-c-1. . . . three frame size categories, age- and sex-specific percentiles of Frame Index 2 were determined. Three categories of frame size were established—small, medium, and large—corresponding respectively to values below the 25th, from the 25th to the 75th, and above the 75th sex- and age-specific percentiles of Frame Index 2 [see original Table II.5 in Frisancho]. With these percentile cutoffs, 25%, 50%, and 75% of the sample of both males and females were classified as either small, medium, or large frame, respectively.

We decided to base the frame size classification on Frame Index 2 rather than on elbow breadth alone [because] weight increases until about the fifth decade in males and the sixth decade in females, while height starts declining by the fourth decade (see Table A-12-e) (1).

Weight not only varies with height and age but it is also influenced by factors such as body width, bone thickness, muscularity, and length of trunk relative to total height . . . An appropriate evaluation of frame size requires a reliable measurement of elbow breadth . . . it should be measured accurately, not by simple manual touch as suggested by the Metropolitan Life Insurance Co., but with a broad faced calipers or other appropriate measuring devices. Otherwise estimations of desirable weight based on inappropriate frame size estimation may be unrealistic and subject to large errors.

REFERENCE

1. Frisancho AR. Anthropometric standards for the assessment of growth and nutritional status. Ann Arbor: University of Michigan Press, 1990.

Categories of Frame Size: Excerpts from Comments of A. R. Frisancho (1)

The present classification is based upon a new index hereafter referred to as *Frame Index 2,* which is derived from measurements *of elbow breadth, height,* and *age*. The formula for calculating Frame Index 2 is:

$$\text{Frame Index 2} = [\text{elbow breadth (mm)}/\text{stature (cm)}] \times 100$$

Table A-12-c-2
Means, Standard Deviations, and Percentiles of Weight (kg) by Age for Adult Males of Small, Medium, and Large Frames

Age (years)	N	Mean	SD	Percentiles 5	10	15	25	50	75	85	90	95
Males with small frames												
18.0–24.9	444	69.9	11.5	54.5	57.4	59.0	62.3	68.3	76.1	80.5	83.8	89.8
25.0–29.9	318	73.4	12.0	56.7	60.3	61.9	65.1	71.8	79.4	84.7	87.5	97.9
30.0–34.9	239	75.7	12.5	57.9	61.6	63.2	67.0	74.6	83.1	87.8	92.9	98.0
35.0–39.9	212	75.5	12.0	56.0	59.9	62.1	66.6	75.9	83.5	87.8	91.4	96.0
40.0–44.9	210	78.3	12.4	58.8	62.8	65.4	70.3	76.1	86.3	92.3	94.8	101.0
45.0–49.9	220	76.3	11.7	57.7	60.9	63.2	67.6	76.2	83.6	89.0	92.1	95.8
50.0–54.9	225	75.4	11.9	57.3	60.2	64.5	67.1	74.7	82.8	88.2	90.5	99.3
55.0–59.9	204	74.5	12.0	54.7	58.2	61.5	66.7	74.8	81.9	87.2	90.6	94.7
60.0–64.9	318	74.0	12.3	54.2	59.2	62.5	65.9	73.4	80.7	85.7	88.4	93.8
65.0–69.9	446	70.7	12.1	50.8	55.4	57.8	61.9	70.3	79.0	83.3	86.8	92.4
70.0–74.9	315	70.5	12.5	49.9	54.4	57.3	61.9	70.1	78.4	83.0	85.5	92.8
Males with medium frames												
18.0–24.9	877	74.0	12.7	57.5	60.6	62.3	65.3	71.5	80.3	86.0	91.6	99.6
25.0–29.9	627	77.0	13.2	58.5	61.8	64.5	68.4	75.9	84.1	88.3	92.4	100.4
30.0–34.9	473	78.5	12.9	59.8	63.0	65.9	69.5	77.8	85.8	91.1	93.8	98.8
35.0–39.9	419	80.5	12.8	58.7	64.8	68.4	72.9	80.4	87.4	91.5	95.9	102.5
40.0–44.9	414	80.1	12.4	60.8	64.2	67.9	71.9	79.3	88.1	92.4	96.8	102.6
45.0–49.9	436	80.7	13.0	60.3	65.1	67.1	71.9	79.8	88.7	93.3	96.7	101.3
50.0–54.9	441	79.0	13.7	58.4	62.5	65.8	70.0	78.3	86.3	91.7	96.6	103.1
55.0–59.9	404	78.8	12.7	59.9	64.5	66.7	70.5	77.9	85.3	91.1	95.4	102.2
60.0–64.9	629	76.7	11.9	58.3	61.5	64.5	68.7	76.3	84.4	88.4	91.6	97.8
65.0–69.9	886	75.0	12.2	56.1	59.5	62.5	66.9	74.5	82.9	86.9	90.8	97.2
70.0–74.9	627	73.6	12.2	54.3	58.3	61.1	65.5	72.6	81.0	86.1	89.8	93.9
Males with large frames												
18.0–24.9	433	77.5	15.4	58.2	61.3	62.6	67.4	74.7	85.0	91.2	95.0	104.9
25.0–29.9	310	84.3	17.4	61.2	66.0	68.4	72.6	82.2	91.6	99.8	102.8	115.2
30.0–34.9	233	86.5	16.6	65.5	68.4	70.2	75.2	85.4	94.0	101.6	106.7	116.7
35.0–39.9	206	85.0	15.0	59.6	67.4	71.8	75.4	84.1	93.1	98.9	104.1	113.3
40.0–44.9	205	85.8	16.4	63.7	67.7	68.8	74.3	84.9	94.5	100.3	107.4	113.3
45.0–49.9	215	85.5	16.5	62.7	67.0	69.4	74.0	84.0	94.0	101.3	105.9	119.2
50.0–54.9	216	84.7	14.7	64.4	66.9	68.8	73.3	83.1	94.3	101.7	103.6	108.4
55.0–59.9	199	85.7	15.7	64.5	67.1	70.3	74.8	84.5	93.5	100.5	103.5	121.1
60.0–64.9	313	82.1	14.6	61.5	66.6	69.3	73.1	80.7	89.4	94.5	98.9	107.7
65.0–69.9	440	79.5	13.8	57.0	61.5	64.9	70.4	78.9	87.8	93.0	96.3	104.0
70.0–74.9	310	77.1	13.8	55.3	59.9	63.6	67.9	76.7	84.1	90.5	95.8	101.4

From Frisancho AR. Anthropometric standards for the assessment of growth and nutritional status. Ann Arbor: University of Michigan Press, 1990, Table IV.22. With permission.

Table A-12-c-3
Means, Standard Deviations, and Percentiles of Weight (kg) by Age for Adult Females of Small, Medium, and Large Frames

Age (years)	N	Mean	SD	Percentiles 5	10	15	25	50	75	85	90	95
Females with small frames												
18.0–24.9	652	56.2	8.7	44.0	46.1	48.0	50.3	55.1	60.9	64.4	66.9	71.5
25.0–29.9	487	56.9	9.5	44.1	47.3	48.6	50.9	55.6	61.1	64.5	67.6	72.6
30.0–34.9	413	59.1	10.0	45.7	48.2	50.0	52.7	57.6	63.4	68.1	71.8	77.7
35.0–39.9	369	61.1	11.4	45.8	48.2	50.8	53.4	59.5	66.7	71.9	76.0	79.5
40.0–44.9	353	60.6	9.4	48.1	50.3	51.8	54.5	59.1	66.1	70.0	73.6	80.3
45.0–49.9	244	61.4	11.1	46.3	47.8	50.8	53.6	60.3	67.3	71.4	75.1	80.8
50.0–54.9	257	61.3	10.8	46.3	49.1	51.7	54.5	60.3	66.9	71.0	73.1	78.4
55.0–59.9	224	61.3	11.1	47.3	49.5	52.2	54.7	59.9	65.3	70.2	73.6	81.5
60.0–64.9	351	61.9	11.0	46.4	48.9	50.6	54.2	60.9	68.5	71.7	74.0	82.2
65.0–69.9	491	61.1	10.7	44.9	48.4	50.7	53.6	60.2	67.4	71.7	74.0	79.3
70.0–74.9	369	60.6	12.1	42.6	45.9	48.5	51.6	60.2	67.0	72.3	75.4	81.0
Females with medium frames												
18.0–24.9	1297	59.5	10.4	46.0	48.4	50.0	52.5	58.1	64.4	69.5	72.8	78.4
25.0–29.9	967	60.9	11.5	46.9	49.1	50.6	53.0	58.6	66.3	72.2	76.9	83.0
30.0–34.9	815	63.5	13.4	47.2	50.0	51.7	54.3	60.7	69.3	76.7	80.6	87.2
35.0–39.9	730	64.1	12.1	49.2	51.7	53.0	56.1	61.8	69.8	74.7	79.4	87.9
40.0–44.9	700	65.6	13.3	48.8	51.3	53.6	57.0	62.8	71.8	77.3	82.4	92.1
45.0–49.9	484	65.8	13.4	48.3	51.4	53.3	56.4	63.4	72.2	77.8	83.1	91.6
50.0–54.9	504	66.4	12.2	48.9	52.0	54.4	57.7	64.4	73.1	79.3	82.8	89.7
55.0–59.9	444	68.0	15.3	48.2	51.1	54.3	58.1	66.3	74.8	81.0	86.2	92.1
60.0–64.9	695	66.2	12.4	49.1	52.3	54.0	57.5	64.5	73.5	78.1	82.2	89.0
65.0–69.9	973	66.2	12.7	48.1	51.4	53.6	57.1	64.9	73.1	78.7	82.4	88.8
70.0–74.9	731	64.3	11.9	46.8	50.5	52.5	56.8	62.9	70.8	76.9	80.2	84.7
Females with large frames												
18.0–24.9	642	68.0	17.2	48.9	51.3	53.1	56.3	62.9	76.2	83.8	89.0	102.7
25.0–29.9	480	72.6	17.7	49.9	53.4	55.6	59.3	68.7	82.9	90.9	98.8	105.0
30.0–34.9	402	76.4	19.7	51.1	54.9	57.7	61.1	72.7	88.4	97.3	102.8	111.9
35.0–39.9	361	79.1	19.5	52.8	56.1	59.1	64.5	76.7	90.4	98.1	106.0	117.9
40.0–44.9	346	79.7	19.8	53.4	57.3	60.7	65.7	77.1	91.3	99.2	104.9	114.2
45.0–49.9	240	80.1	19.6	54.5	60.1	63.2	66.7	76.8	86.6	97.6	105.0	116.9
50.0–54.9	250	79.4	16.9	55.6	60.0	63.0	67.8	77.7	88.8	97.1	103.3	112.1
55.0–59.9	218	79.8	17.5	56.4	60.2	62.5	67.6	77.6	89.9	97.0	101.6	111.3
60.0–64.9	346	77.8	15.6	56.0	59.4	62.8	66.8	76.8	85.7	92.8	100.0	104.8
65.0–69.9	484	76.6	15.4	55.3	59.4	62.0	65.8	74.5	84.6	91.7	97.8	105.0
70.0–74.9	363	74.9	14.0	53.5	57.9	60.9	65.8	74.5	82.7	87.9	91.3	99.1

From Frisancho AR. Anthropometric standards for the assessment of growth and nutritional status. Ann Arbor: University of Michigan Press, 1990, Table IV.23. With permission.

Table A-12-d
Means, Standard Deviations, and Percentiles of Elbow Breadth (mm) by Age for Males and Females 1 to 74 Years

Age (years)	N	Mean	SD	Percentiles 5	10	15	25	50	75	85	90	95
Males												
1.0–1.9	681	40.4	2.9	36.0	37.0	37.0	39.0	40.0	42.0	43.0	44.0	45.0
2.0–2.9	677	42.5	2.7	38.0	39.0	40.0	41.0	42.0	44.0	45.0	46.0	47.0
3.0–3.9	717	44.5	2.8	40.0	41.0	42.0	43.0	44.0	46.0	47.0	48.0	50.0
4.0–4.9	709	46.4	3.0	42.0	43.0	43.0	44.0	46.0	48.0	50.0	50.0	52.0
5.0–5.9	676	48.3	3.3	43.0	44.0	45.0	46.0	48.0	50.0	51.0	52.0	53.0
6.0–6.9	298	50.4	3.3	45.0	46.0	47.0	48.0	51.0	52.0	54.0	55.0	56.0
7.0–7.9	312	51.9	3.6	47.0	48.0	49.0	49.0	52.0	54.0	56.0	56.0	57.0
8.0–8.9	296	53.7	3.7	48.0	49.0	50.0	51.0	54.0	56.0	57.0	59.0	60.0
9.0–9.9	322	55.7	3.8	50.0	51.0	52.0	53.0	56.0	58.0	60.0	61.0	62.0
10.0–10.9	334	58.1	4.2	52.0	53.0	54.0	55.0	58.0	61.0	62.0	64.0	65.0
11.0–11.9	324	59.9	4.4	53.0	55.0	56.0	57.0	60.0	62.0	64.0	65.0	67.0
12.0–12.9	349	62.8	5.0	55.0	57.0	58.0	60.0	63.0	66.0	68.0	69.0	72.0
13.0–13.9	350	65.8	4.8	58.0	60.0	61.0	62.0	66.0	69.0	71.0	72.0	74.0
14.0–14.9	358	68.4	4.4	61.0	63.0	64.0	66.0	68.0	71.0	73.0	74.0	76.0
15.0–15.9	359	69.8	4.1	63.0	64.0	65.0	67.0	70.0	72.0	74.0	75.0	77.0
16.0–16.9	350	70.5	4.0	64.0	66.0	66.0	68.0	71.0	73.0	74.0	76.0	77.0
17.0–17.9	339	70.7	4.0	64.0	66.0	67.0	68.0	71.0	73.0	75.0	76.0	77.0
18.0–24.9	1757	71.2	4.1	64.0	66.0	67.0	69.0	71.0	74.0	75.0	76.0	78.0
25.0–29.9	1256	71.6	4.1	65.0	67.0	67.0	69.0	71.0	74.0	76.0	77.0	79.0
30.0–34.9	946	71.8	4.2	65.0	67.0	68.0	69.0	72.0	74.0	76.0	77.0	79.0
35.0–39.9	838	72.3	4.2	65.0	67.0	68.0	70.0	72.0	75.0	77.0	77.0	80.0
40.0–44.9	830	72.8	4.0	66.0	68.0	69.0	70.0	73.0	75.0	77.0	78.0	80.0
45.0–49.9	871	73.1	4.3	66.0	68.0	69.0	70.0	73.0	76.0	78.0	79.0	80.0
50.0–54.9	882	73.3	4.2	66.0	68.0	69.0	71.0	73.0	76.0	77.0	78.0	80.0
55.0–59.9	809	73.7	4.5	67.0	68.0	69.0	71.0	73.0	77.0	78.0	80.0	81.0
60.0–64.9	1263	73.5	4.3	67.0	68.0	69.0	71.0	73.0	76.0	78.0	79.0	81.0
65.0–69.9	1774	73.2	4.4	66.0	68.0	69.0	70.0	73.0	76.0	78.0	79.0	81.0
70.0–74.9	1252	73.5	4.3	67.0	68.0	69.0	71.0	73.0	76.0	78.0	79.0	81.0
Females												
1.0–1.9	622	38.7	2.8	34.0	35.0	36.0	37.0	39.0	41.0	42.0	42.0	43.0
2.0–2.9	615	40.7	2.8	36.0	37.0	38.0	39.0	41.0	42.0	44.0	44.0	45.0
3.0–3.9	652	42.5	2.9	38.0	39.0	40.0	41.0	42.0	44.0	45.0	46.0	47.0
4.0–4.9	681	44.2	2.9	40.0	41.0	41.0	42.0	44.0	46.0	47.0	48.0	49.0
5.0–5.9	674	46.4	3.1	42.0	43.0	43.0	44.0	46.0	48.0	50.0	50.0	52.0
6.0–6.9	296	47.9	3.2	43.0	44.0	45.0	46.0	48.0	50.0	51.0	52.0	53.0
7.0–7.9	331	50.1	3.4	45.0	46.0	47.0	48.0	50.0	52.0	53.0	54.0	55.0
8.0–8.9	276	51.5	3.7	46.0	47.0	48.0	49.0	51.0	54.0	55.0	56.0	58.0
9.0–9.9	322	54.0	3.9	48.0	50.0	50.0	51.0	54.0	56.0	57.0	59.0	60.0
10.0–10.9	330	55.6	3.9	50.0	51.0	52.0	53.0	56.0	58.0	60.0	61.0	62.0
11.0–11.9	302	57.8	4.0	52.0	53.0	54.0	55.0	58.0	60.0	62.0	63.0	64.0
12.0–12.9	324	59.2	3.7	53.0	55.0	55.0	57.0	59.0	62.0	63.0	64.0	66.0
13.0–13.9	361	60.1	3.8	54.0	56.0	56.0	58.0	60.0	62.0	64.0	65.0	66.0
14.0–14.9	370	60.4	3.5	54.0	56.0	57.0	58.0	60.0	63.0	64.0	65.0	66.0
15.0–15.9	309	60.7	4.0	54.0	56.0	57.0	58.0	61.0	63.0	65.0	66.0	67.0
16.0–16.9	343	61.0	3.8	55.0	56.0	57.0	59.0	61.0	64.0	65.0	66.0	67.0
17.0–17.9	293	61.3	4.0	55.0	56.0	57.0	59.0	61.0	64.0	65.0	66.0	68.0
18.0–24.9	2591	61.0	3.8	55.0	56.0	57.0	59.0	61.0	63.0	65.0	66.0	67.0
25.0–29.9	1934	61.5	3.9	56.0	57.0	58.0	59.0	61.0	64.0	65.0	66.0	68.0
30.0–34.9	1630	62.1	4.3	56.0	57.0	58.0	59.0	62.0	64.0	66.0	67.0	70.0
35.0–39.9	1460	62.7	4.4	56.0	58.0	59.0	60.0	62.0	65.0	67.0	68.0	71.0
40.0–44.9	1399	63.2	4.4	57.0	58.0	59.0	60.0	63.0	66.0	67.0	69.0	71.0
45.0–49.9	968	63.7	4.4	57.0	59.0	59.0	61.0	63.0	66.0	68.0	69.0	72.0
50.0–54.9	1011	64.1	4.7	57.0	59.0	60.0	61.0	64.0	67.0	69.0	70.0	73.0
55.0–59.9	887	64.7	4.8	58.0	59.0	60.0	61.0	64.0	67.0	70.0	71.0	73.0
60.0–64.9	1394	64.6	4.4	58.0	60.0	61.0	62.0	64.0	67.0	69.0	70.0	72.0
65.0–69.9	1950	64.7	4.5	58.0	59.0	60.0	62.0	64.0	67.0	69.0	71.0	73.0
70.0–74.9	1464	64.8	4.4	58.0	60.0	60.0	62.0	64.0	68.0	69.0	71.0	72.0

From Frisancho AR. Anthropometric standards for the assessment of growth and nutritional status. Ann Arbor: University of Michigan Press, 1990, Table IV.9. With permission.

Table A-12-e
Changes in Weight and Height With Age

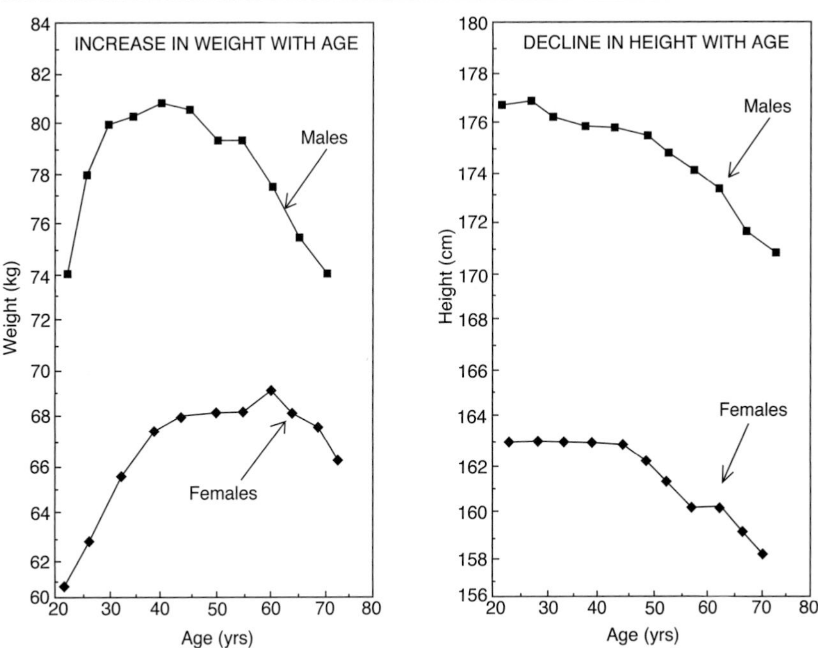

Relationship of weight and height to age among adults. Note that weight increases until about the fifth decade in males and sixth decade in females, while height begins to decline after the age of 40 years in both males and females. From Frisancho AR. Anthropometric standards for the assessment of growth and nutritional status. University of Michigan Press, Ann Arbor, 1990. Figure II.15.

Table A-13-a
Means, Standard Deviations, and Percentiles of Body Mass Index (w/s²) by Age for Males and Females 1 to 74 Years

Age (years)	N	Mean	SD	Percentiles 5	10	15	25	50	75	85	90	95
Males												
1.0–1.9	366	17.3	2.4	15.2	15.6	15.9	16.4	17.1	18.0	18.6	19.0	19.6
2.0–2.9	664	16.2	1.3	14.3	14.6	15.0	15.4	16.2	17.1	17.5	17.8	18.4
3.0–3.9	716	16.0	1.4	14.2	14.6	14.8	15.1	15.8	16.6	17.1	17.5	18.2
4.0–4.9	709	15.7	1.3	13.9	14.2	14.5	14.9	15.6	16.4	16.8	17.2	17.8
5.0–5.9	675	15.6	1.5	13.8	14.1	14.3	14.7	15.5	16.3	16.8	17.2	18.1
6.0–6.9	298	15.8	1.9	13.7	14.1	14.3	14.8	15.3	16.4	17.2	18.0	19.3
7.0–7.9	312	16.0	1.8	13.7	14.1	14.3	14.9	15.6	16.7	17.5	18.2	19.5
8.0–8.9	296	16.3	2.2	13.8	14.3	14.6	15.0	15.9	17.1	18.0	19.1	20.1
9.0–9.9	322	16.9	2.4	14.1	14.6	14.8	15.3	16.3	17.7	19.0	19.9	21.8
10.0–10.9	334	17.7	2.8	14.6	15.0	15.3	15.8	17.1	18.7	19.8	21.2	23.4
11.0–11.9	324	18.4	3.6	14.7	15.1	15.7	16.2	17.4	19.8	21.5	22.5	25.3
12.0–12.9	349	18.9	3.5	15.2	15.7	16.1	16.7	17.9	20.2	21.7	23.7	25.8
13.0–13.9	348	19.5	3.5	15.6	16.4	16.6	17.2	18.7	20.7	22.2	24.0	25.9
14.0–14.9	359	20.3	3.3	16.5	17.0	17.5	18.1	19.5	21.6	23.1	24.2	26.4
15.0–15.9	359	20.8	3.1	16.8	17.5	18.0	19.0	20.4	22.0	23.4	24.1	26.6
16.0–16.9	349	21.9	3.3	18.0	18.5	19.0	19.6	21.3	23.0	24.8	25.9	27.3
17.0–17.9	338	21.8	3.5	17.8	18.4	18.9	19.5	21.1	23.4	24.9	26.1	28.3
18.0–24.9	1755	23.6	3.8	18.8	19.6	20.1	21.0	23.0	25.5	27.2	28.5	31.0
25.0–29.9	1255	24.9	4.3	19.5	20.4	21.1	21.9	24.3	27.0	28.5	30.0	32.8
30.0–34.9	947	25.7	4.2	19.9	21.0	21.9	23.0	25.1	27.8	29.3	30.5	32.9
35.0–39.9	839	25.9	4.0	19.7	21.0	21.9	23.3	25.6	28.0	29.5	30.6	32.8
40.0–44.9	829	26.2	4.0	20.4	21.5	22.2	23.4	26.0	28.5	29.9	31.0	32.5
45.0–49.9	871	26.3	4.2	20.1	21.5	22.4	23.5	26.0	28.6	30.1	31.2	33.4
50.0–54.9	882	26.1	4.2	19.9	21.1	22.0	23.3	25.9	28.2	30.1	31.3	33.3
55.0–59.9	807	26.2	4.3	19.8	21.3	22.1	23.5	26.1	28.5	30.2	31.6	33.6
60.0–64.9	1261	28.8	3.8	20.1	21.3	22.0	23.4	25.6	28.0	29.4	30.4	32.4
65.0–69.9	1773	25.5	4.0	19.1	20.5	21.4	22.7	25.5	27.8	29.6	30.7	32.3
70.0–74.9	1257	25.3	4.0	19.0	20.3	21.4	22.6	25.1	27.7	29.3	30.5	32.3
Females												
1.0–1.9	333	16.7	1.5	14.4	14.9	15.2	15.7	16.7	17.6	18.2	18.6	19.3
2.0–2.9	610	16.0	1.5	14.1	14.4	14.7	15.1	15.9	16.8	17.3	17.8	18.4
3.0–3.9	651	15.7	1.4	13.6	14.1	14.4	14.7	15.5	16.4	17.0	17.5	18.0
4.0–4.9	678	15.5	1.4	13.6	13.9	14.2	14.6	15.3	16.2	16.7	17.2	18.0
5.0–5.9	673	15.5	1.7	13.3	13.7	14.0	14.5	15.2	16.3	16.9	17.5	18.6
6.0–6.9	296	15.5	1.7	13.5	13.7	13.9	14.3	15.2	16.2	17.0	17.5	18.7
7.0–7.9	331	15.9	1.9	13.7	14.1	14.2	14.7	15.4	16.8	17.5	18.3	19.6
8.0–8.9	276	16.5	2.7	13.8	14.1	14.4	14.9	15.8	17.4	18.7	19.8	21.7
9.0–9.9	322	17.3	3.1	14.0	14.6	14.8	15.3	16.5	18.1	19.8	21.5	23.3
10.0–10.9	330	17.7	3.1	14.0	14.5	15.0	15.6	16.9	18.9	20.7	22.0	24.1
11.0–11.9	303	18.9	3.8	14.8	15.3	15.6	16.3	18.1	20.3	21.8	23.4	26.2
12.0–12.9	324	19.6	3.7	15.0	15.6	16.2	17.0	18.9	21.2	23.1	24.6	27.0
13.0–13.9	361	20.4	4.1	15.4	16.3	16.7	17.7	19.4	22.2	23.8	25.2	28.6
14.0–14.9	370	21.1	3.9	16.5	17.1	17.7	18.4	20.3	22.8	24.7	26.2	28.9
15.0–15.9	309	21.1	3.8	17.0	17.5	18.0	18.8	20.3	22.4	24.1	25.6	28.7
16.0–16.9	343	22.1	4.0	17.7	18.3	18.7	19.3	21.1	23.5	25.7	26.8	30.1
17.0–17.9	293	22.5	4.7	17.1	17.9	18.7	19.6	21.4	24.0	26.2	27.5	32.1
18.0–24.9	2592	22.9	4.6	17.7	18.4	19.0	19.9	21.8	24.5	26.5	28.6	32.1
25.0–29.9	1935	23.7	5.2	18.0	18.8	19.2	20.1	22.3	25.6	28.4	30.8	34.3
30.0–34.9	1633	24.8	5.9	18.5	19.4	19.9	20.8	23.1	27.2	30.4	33.0	36.6
35.0–39.9	1461	25.3	5.8	18.7	19.5	20.2	21.3	23.8	28.0	31.0	33.1	36.9
40.0–44.9	1399	25.7	5.9	18.8	19.8	20.5	21.5	24.2	28.3	31.6	33.7	36.6
45.0–49.9	969	26.0	6.2	19.0	20.1	20.8	21.9	24.5	28.6	31.4	33.4	37.1
50.0–54.9	1012	26.3	5.5	19.2	20.3	21.0	22.4	25.2	29.2	32.1	33.8	36.5
55.0–59.9	887	26.9	6.1	19.2	20.5	21.3	22.8	25.7	30.1	32.7	34.7	38.2
60.0–64.9	1392	26.7	5.5	19.3	20.7	21.4	22.9	25.8	29.7	32.1	33.8	36.6
65.0–69.9	1952	26.8	5.5	19.5	20.7	21.7	23.0	26.0	29.6	32.0	33.8	36.6
70.0–74.9	1467	26.6	5.3	19.3	20.5	21.5	23.0	26.0	29.5	31.7	33.1	35.8

From Frisancho AR. Anthropometric standards for the assessment of growth and nutritional status. Ann Arbor: University of Michigan Press, 1990. Table IV.5. With permission.

A-13-b
Nomograph for Estimating Body Mass Index (kg/m²)*

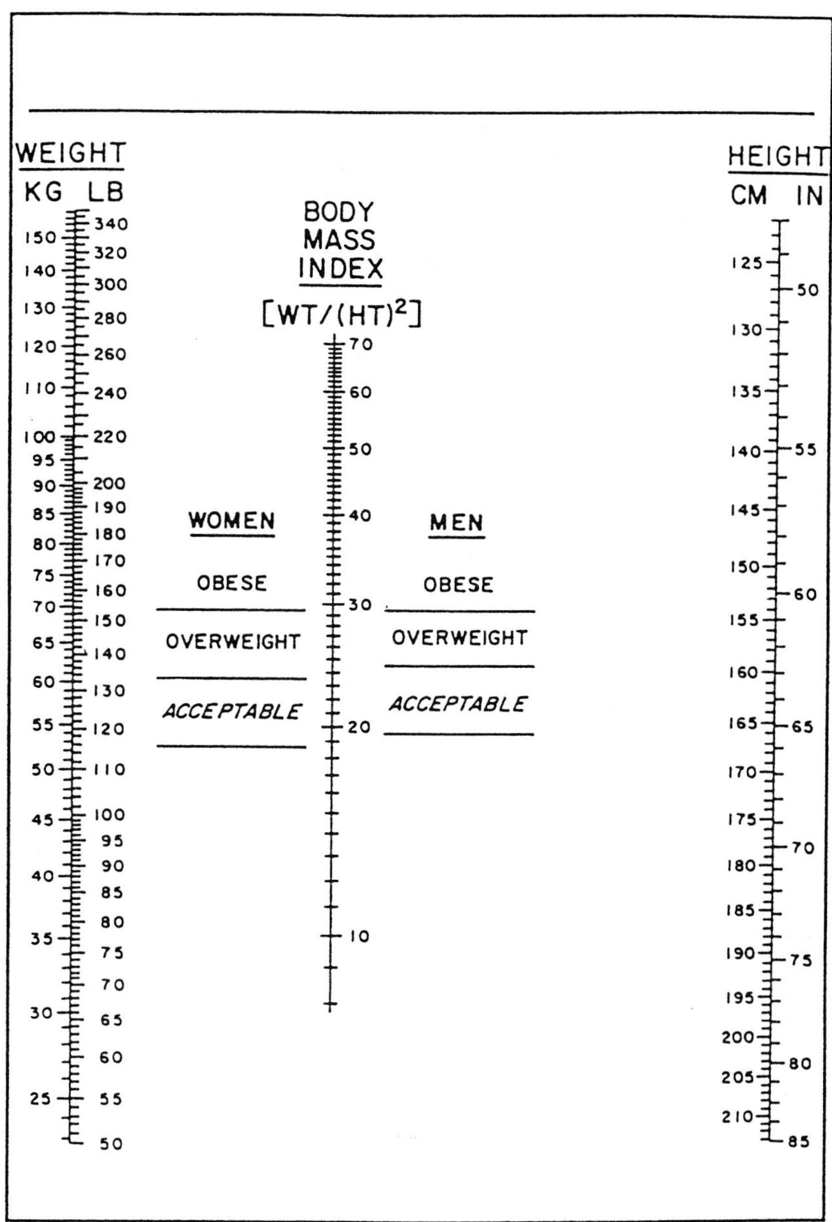

*The ratio of weight/height² emerges from varied epidemiologic studies as the most generally useful index of relative body mass in adults. This nomograph facilitates use of this relationship in clinical situations. While showing the range of weight given as desirable in life insurance studies, the scale expresses relative weight as a continuous variable. This method encourages use of clinical judgment in interpreting "overweight" and "underweight" and in accounting for muscular and skeletal contributions to measured mass. From G. A. Bray, 1978.

A-14-a
Fetal Growth Standards: Intrauterine Weight[1] and Length[2] Charts

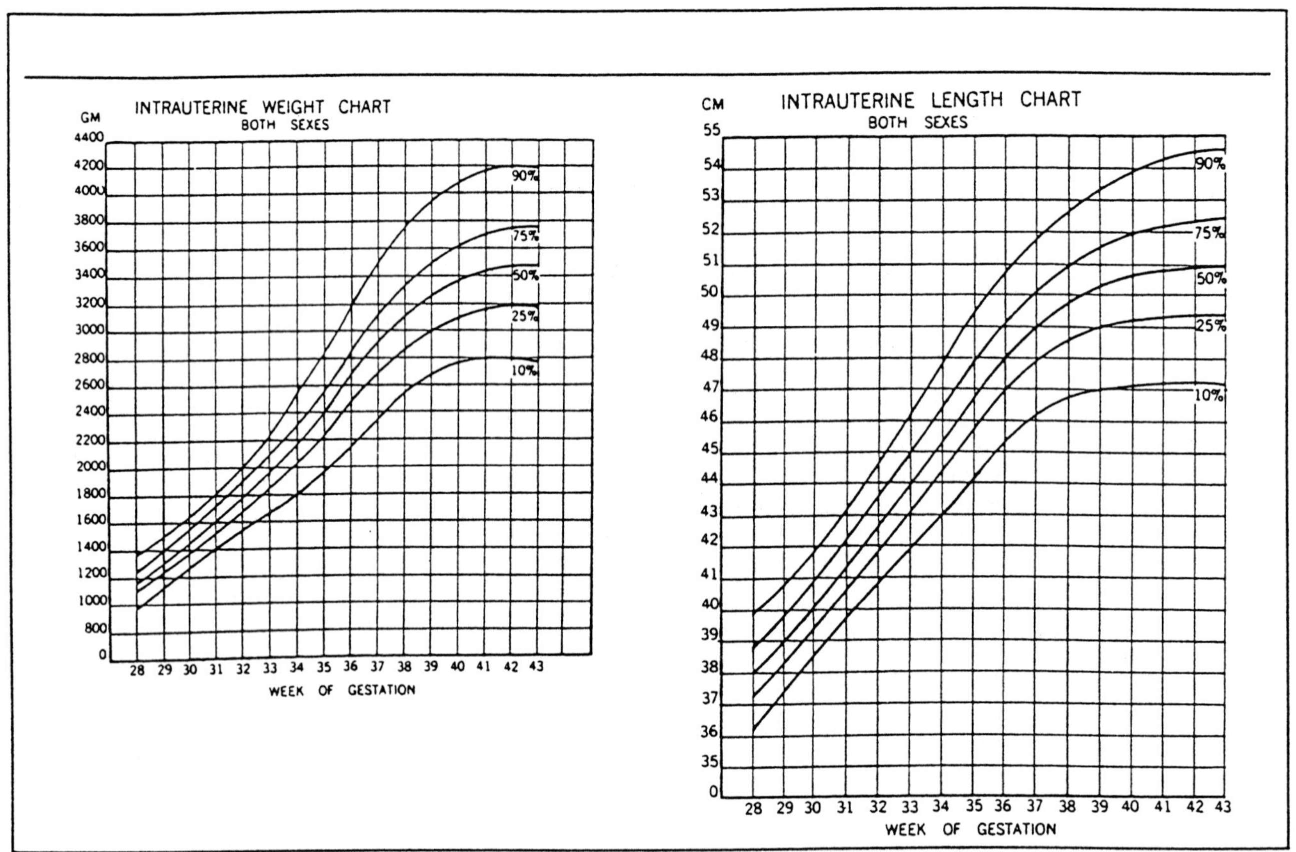

From Naeye RL, Dixon JB. Pediatr Res 1978;12:989.
[1]Fetal body weight percentiles from 28 to 43 weeks of gestation.
[2]Fetal body length percentiles from 28 to 43 weeks of gestation.

A-14-b-1
Physical Growth NCHS Percentiles: Girls from Birth to 36 Months

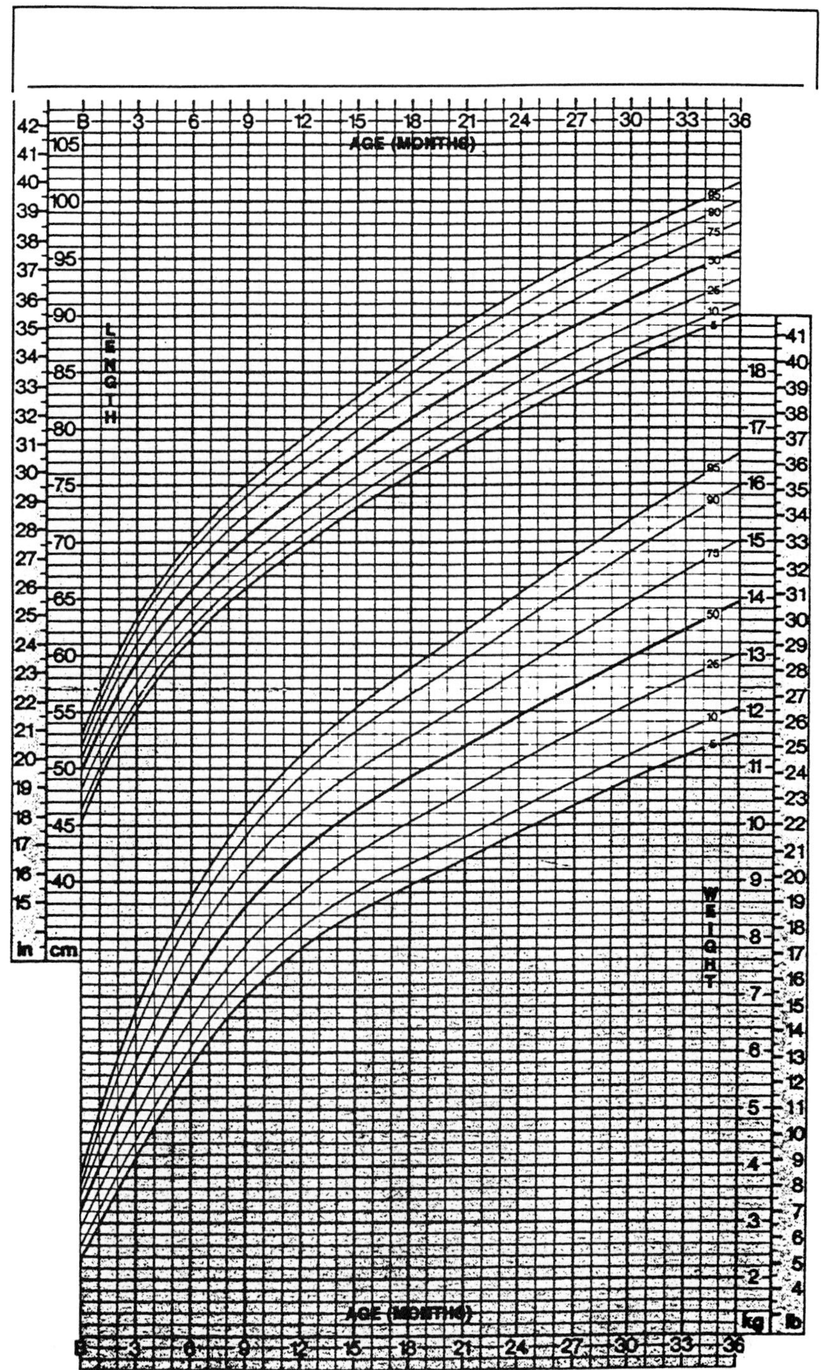

Courtesy of Ross Laboratories, who adapted the growth curves from the original data: National Center for Health Statistics, NCHS Growth Charts, 1976. Monthly Vital Statistics Report, Vol. 25, No. 3, Suppl. (HRA) 76–1120. Rockville, MD, Health Resources Administration, June 1976. Data from the Fels Research Institute, Yellow Springs, Ohio.

A-14-b-2
Physical Growth NCHS Percentiles: Boys from Birth to 36 Months

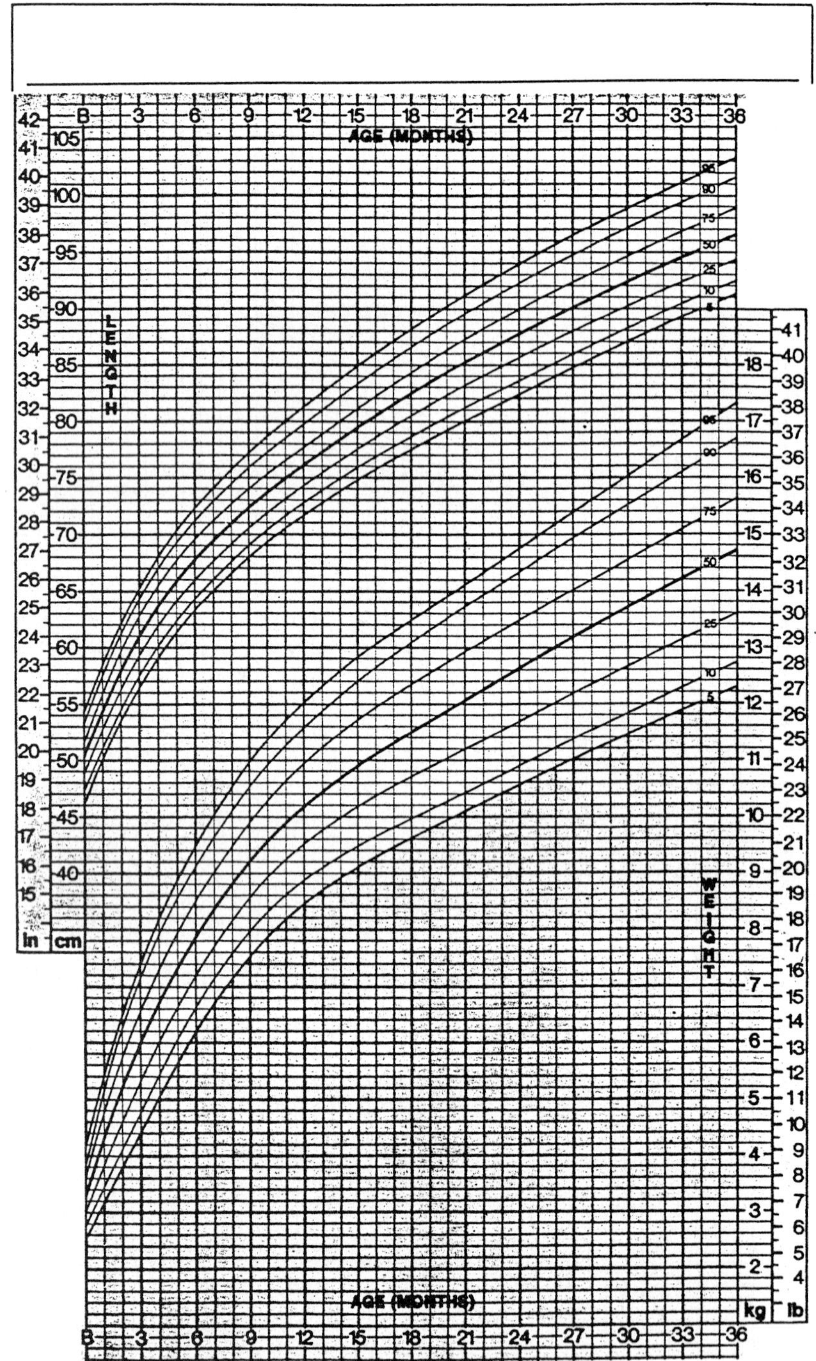

Courtesy of Ross Laboratories, who adapted the growth curves from the original data: National Center for Health Statistics, NCHS Growth Charts, 1976. Monthly Vital Statistics Report, Vol. 25, No. 3, Suppl. (HRA) 76–1120. Rockville, MD, Health Resources Administration, June 1976. Data from the Fels Research Institute, Yellow Springs, Ohio.

A-14-c-1-a

Percentiles of Stature in cm (and in.) by Age for Girls Ranging in Age from 1 to 10 Years

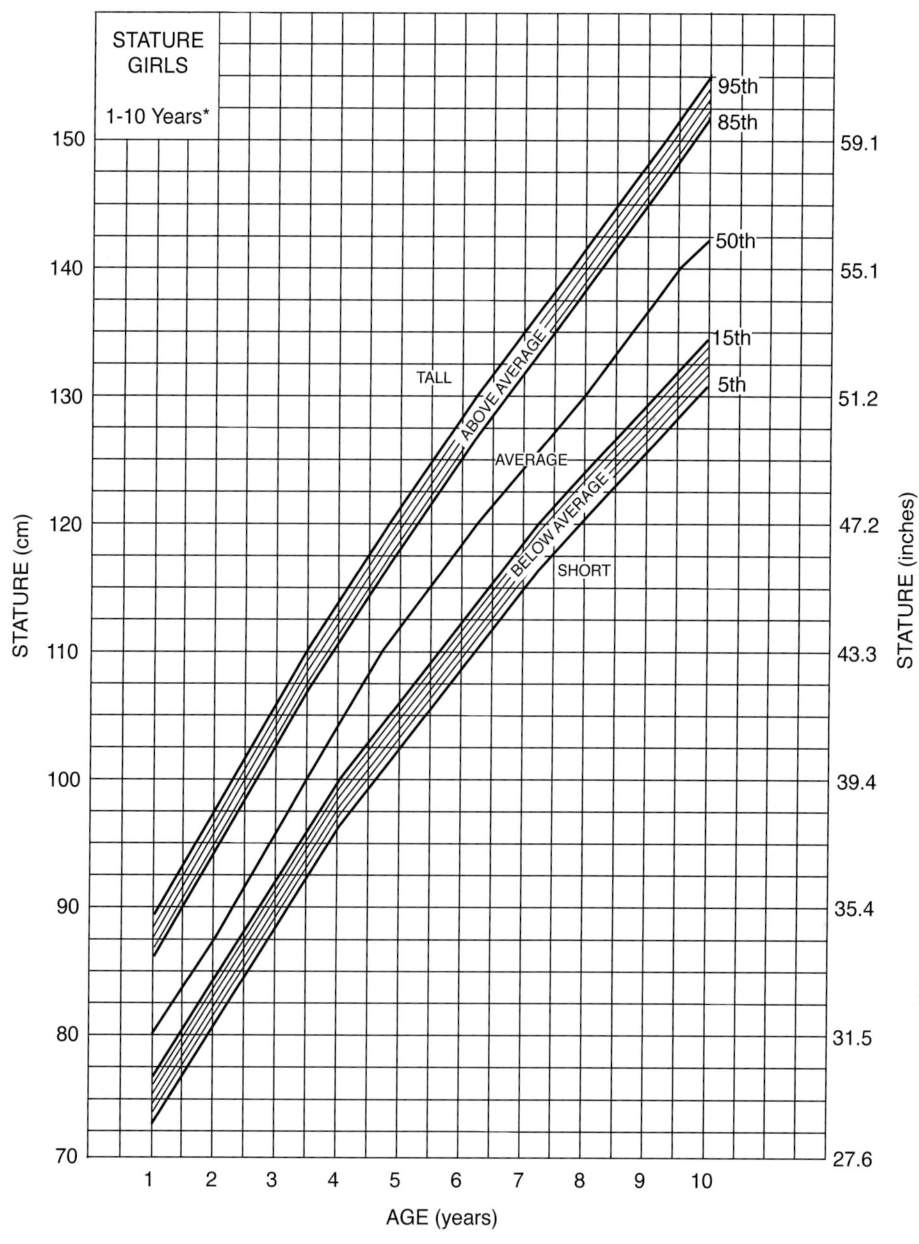

*From Frisancho AR. Anthropometric standards for the assessment of growth and nutritional status. Ann Arbor: University of Michigan Press, 1990. Figure IV.3.

A-14-c-1-b
Percentiles of Stature in cm (and in.) by Age for Girls Ranging in Age from 11 to 17 Years

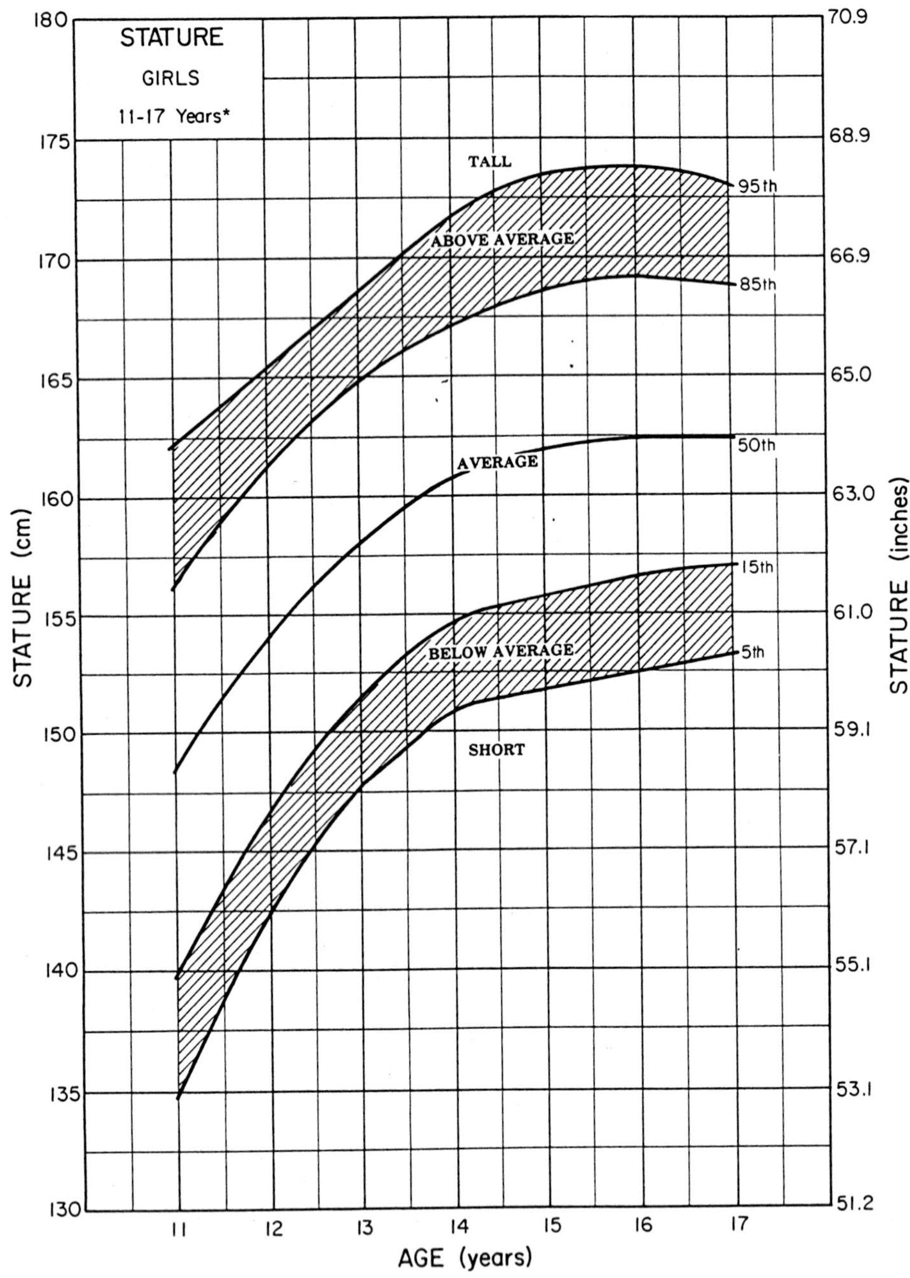

*From Frisancho AR. Anthropometric standards for the assessment of growth and nutritional status. Ann Arbor: University of Michigan Press, 1990. Figure IV.4.

A-14-c-2-a
Percentiles of Stature in cm (and in.) by Age for Boys Ranging in Age from 1 to 11 Years

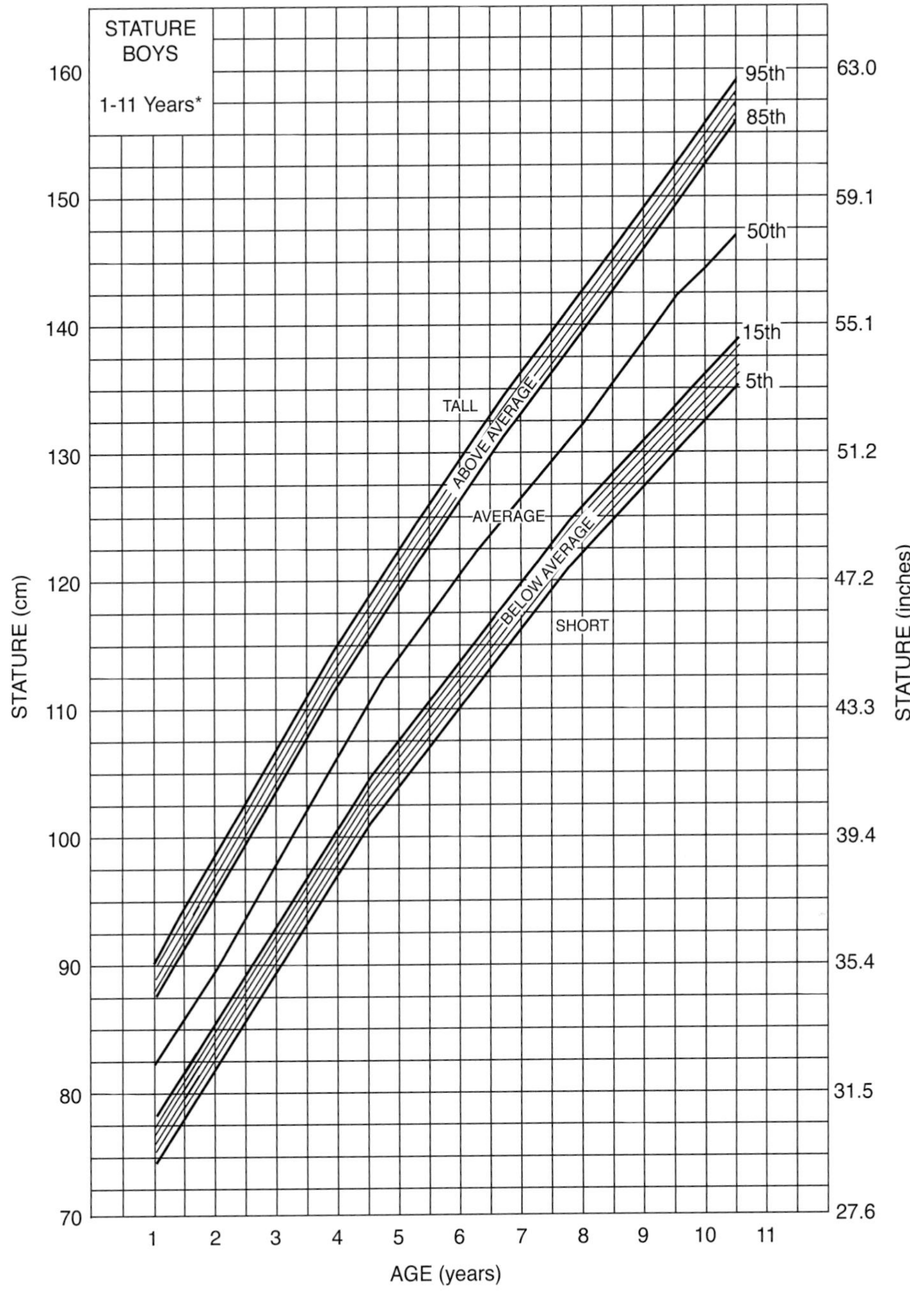

*From Frisancho AR. Anthropometric standards for the assessment of growth and nutritional status. Ann Arbor: University of Michigan Press, 1990. Figure IV.1.

A-14-c-2-b
Percentiles of Stature in cm (and in.) by Age for Boys Ranging in Age from 12 to 17 Years

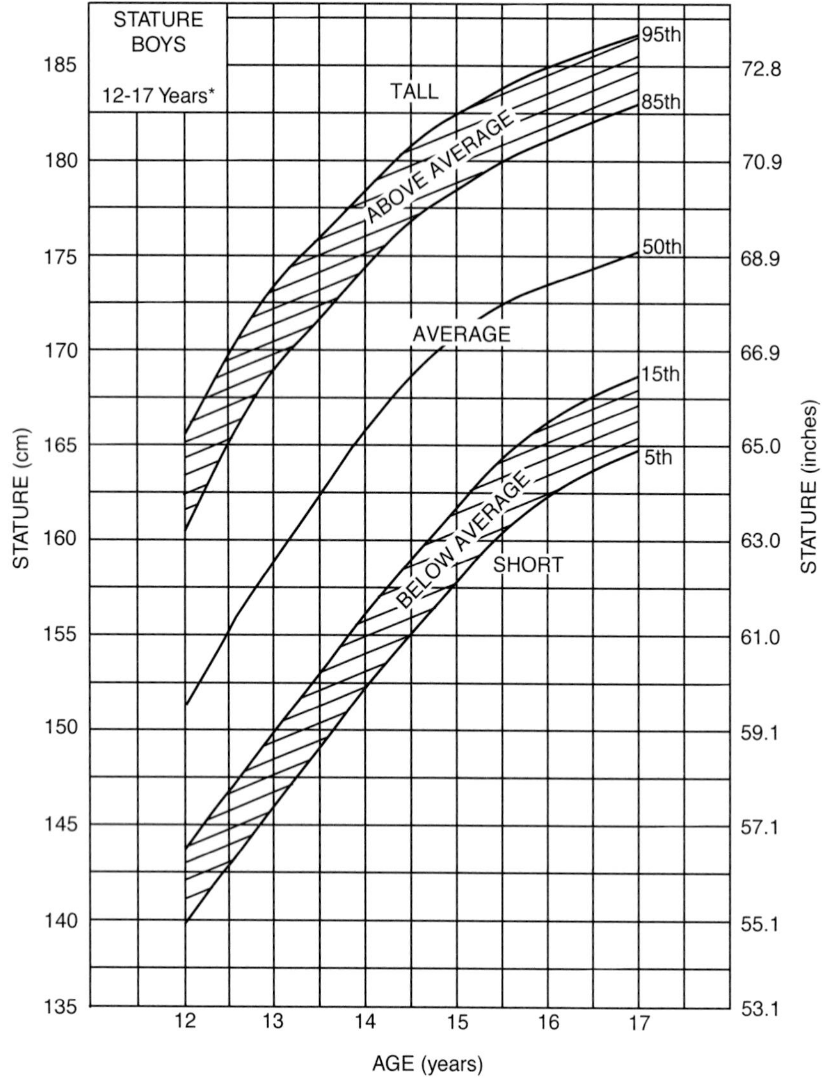

*From Frisancho AR. Anthropometric standards for the assessment of growth and nutritional status. Ann Arbor: University of Michigan Press, 1990. Figure IV.2.

A-14-d-1-a
Percentiles of Weight in kg (and lb.) by Age for Girls Ranging in Age from 1 to 10 Years

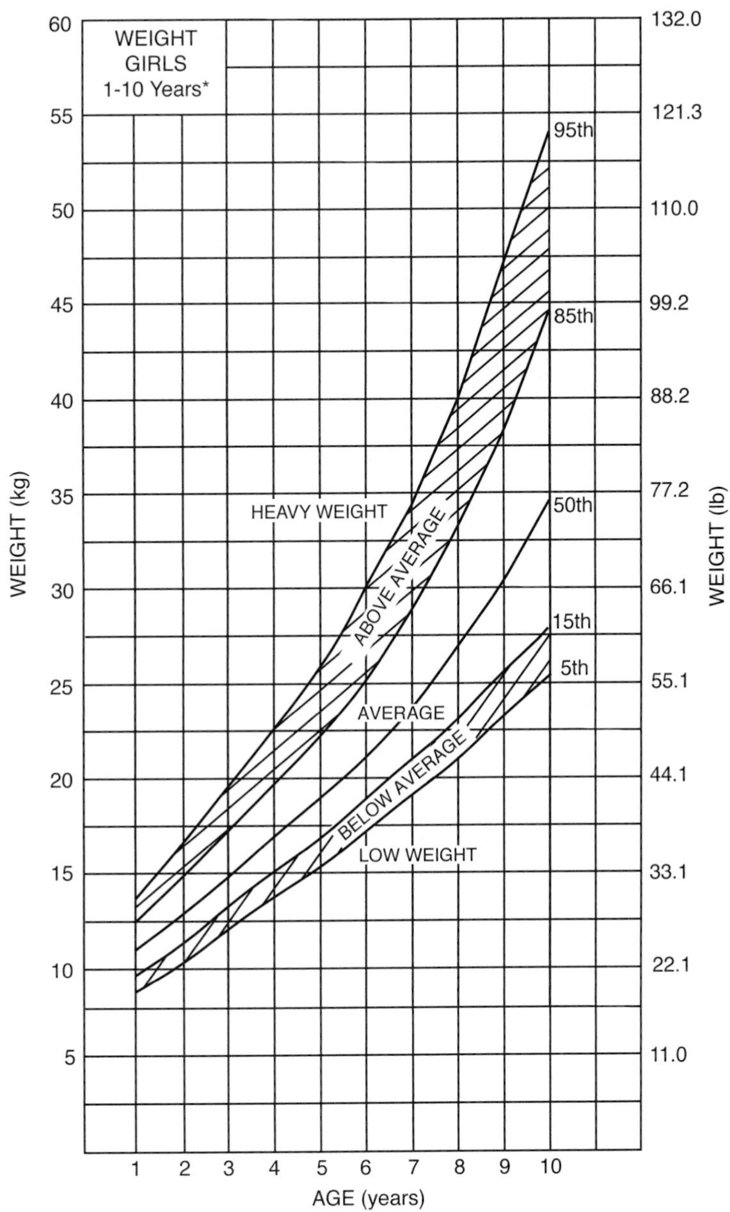

*From Frisancho AR. Anthropometric standards for the assessment of growth and nutritional status. Ann Arbor: University of Michigan Press, 1990. Figure IV.8.

A-14-d-1-b
Percentiles of Weight in kg (and lb.) by Age for Girls Ranging in Age from 11 to 17 Years

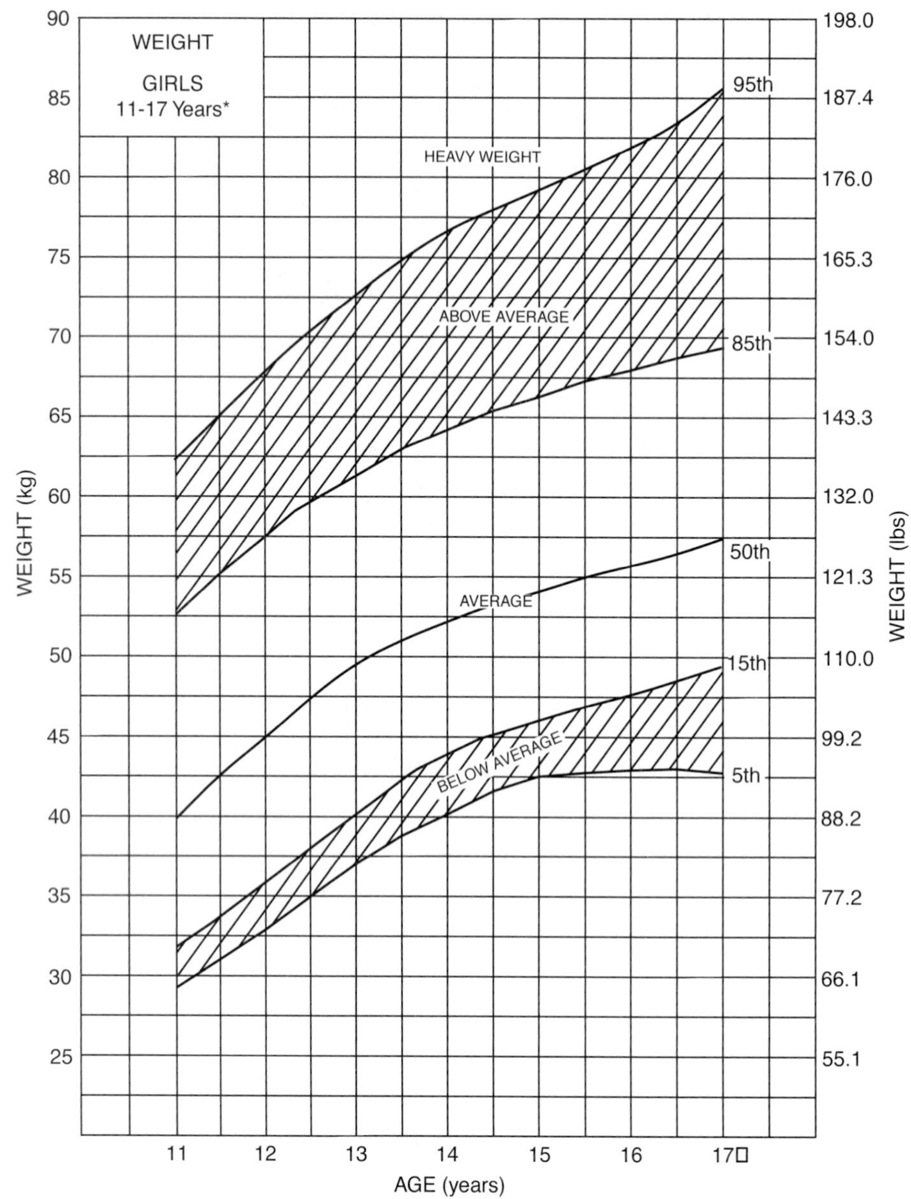

*From Frisancho AR. Anthropometric standards for the assessment of growth and nutritional status. Ann Arbor: University of Michigan Press, 1990. Figure IV.9.

A-14-d-2-a
Percentiles of Weight in kg (and lb.) by Age for Boys Ranging in Age from 1 to 11 Years

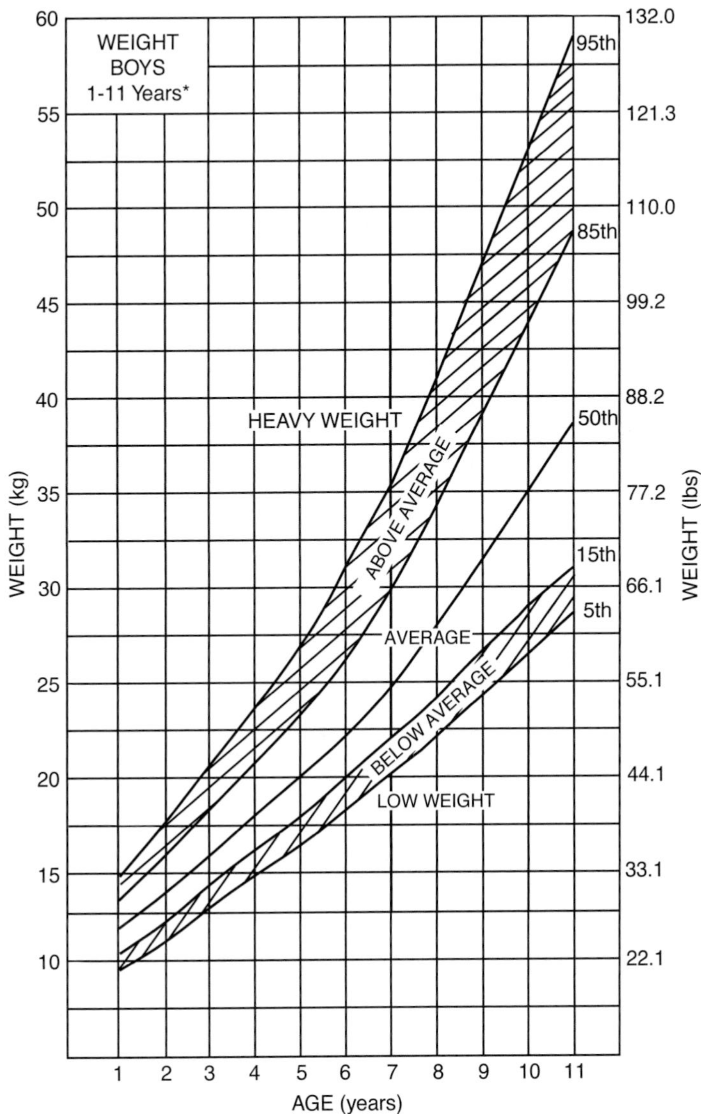

*From Frisancho AR. Anthropometric standards for the assessment of growth and nutritional status. Ann Arbor: University of Michigan Press, 1990. Figure IV.5.

A-14-d-2-b
Percentiles of Weight in kg (and lb.) by Age for Girls Ranging in Age from 12 to 17 Years

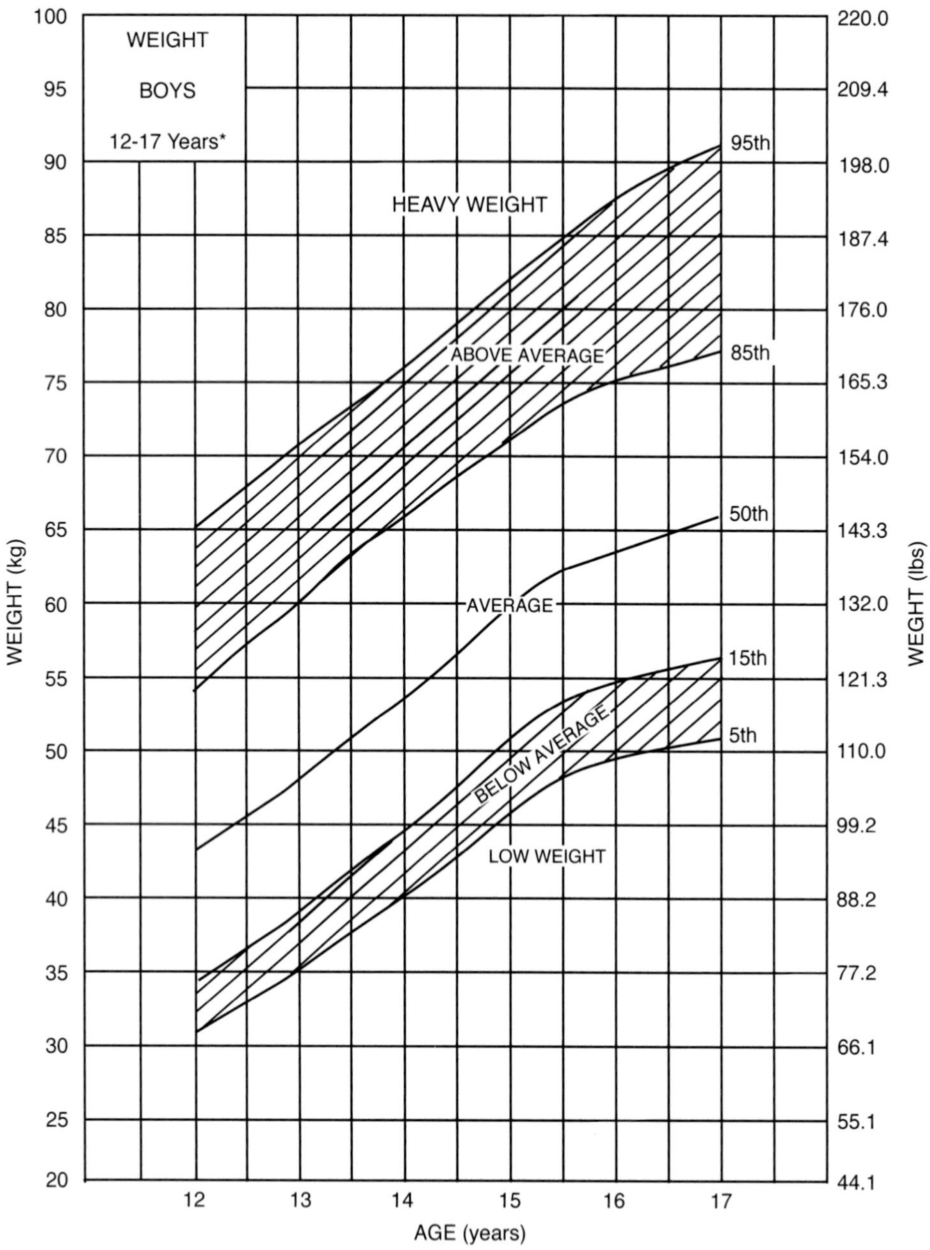

*From Frisancho AR. Anthropometric standards for the assessment of growth and nutritional status. Ann Arbor: University of Michigan Press, 1990. Figure IV.6.

A-14-e-1

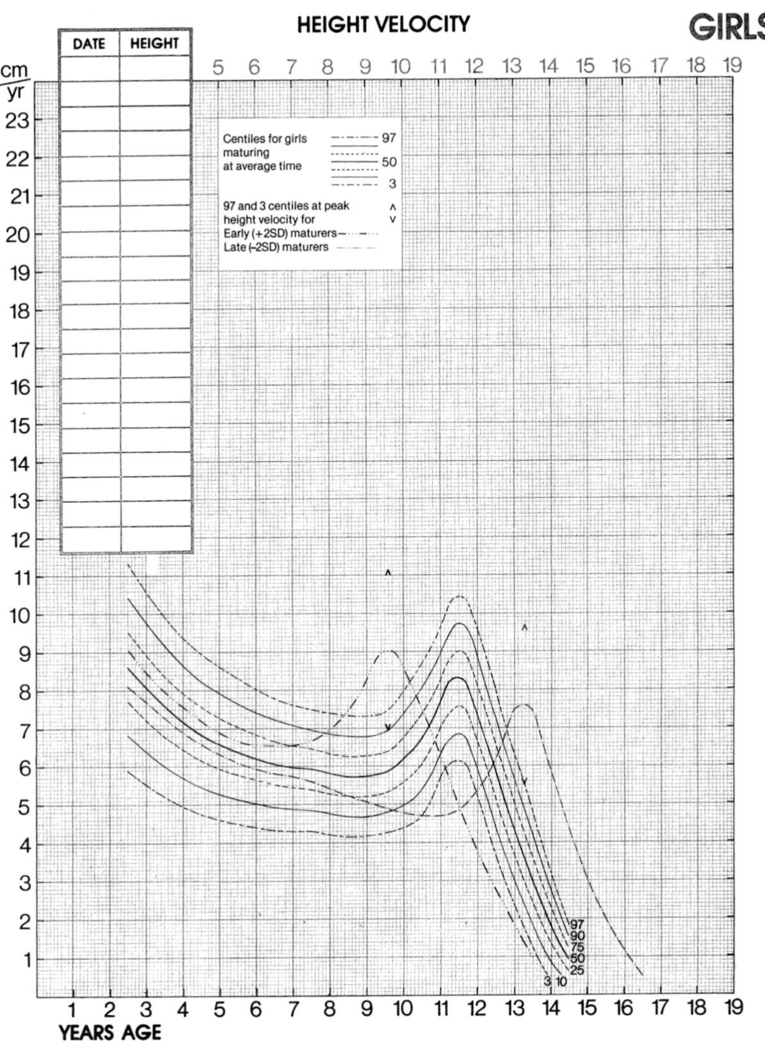

From Tanner JM, Davies PSW. Journal of Pediatrics 1985:107.

A-14-e-2

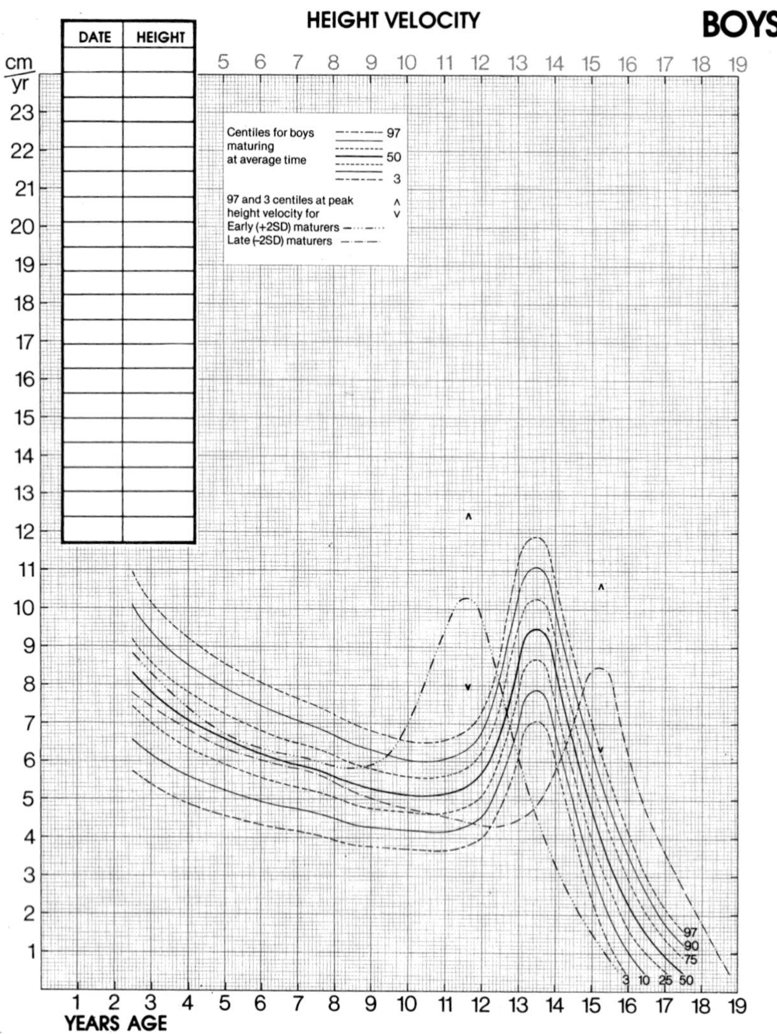

From Tanner JM, Davies PSW. Journal of Pediatrics 1985:107.

A-14-f-1

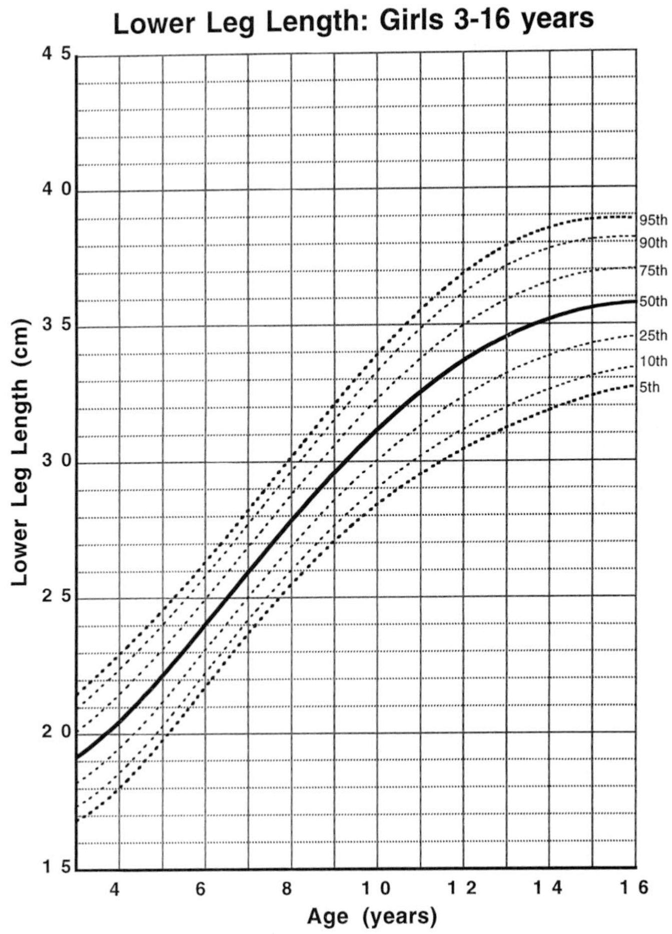

Published in: Stallings VA, Zemel BS. Nutritional assessment of the disabled child. In: Sullivan PB, Rosenbloom L, eds. Feeding the disabled Child. London: Cambridge University Press 1996:62–76.

A-14-f-2

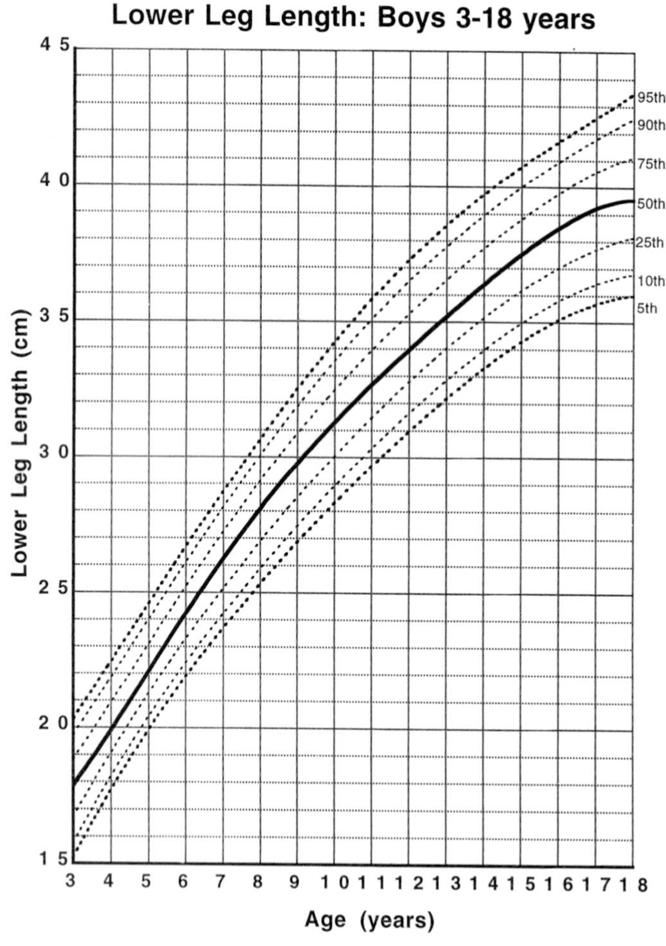

Published in: Stallings VA, Zemel BS. Nutritional assessment of the disabled child. In: Sullivan PB, Rosenbloom L, eds. Feeding the disabled Child. London: Cambridge University Press 1996:62–76.

A-14-g-1

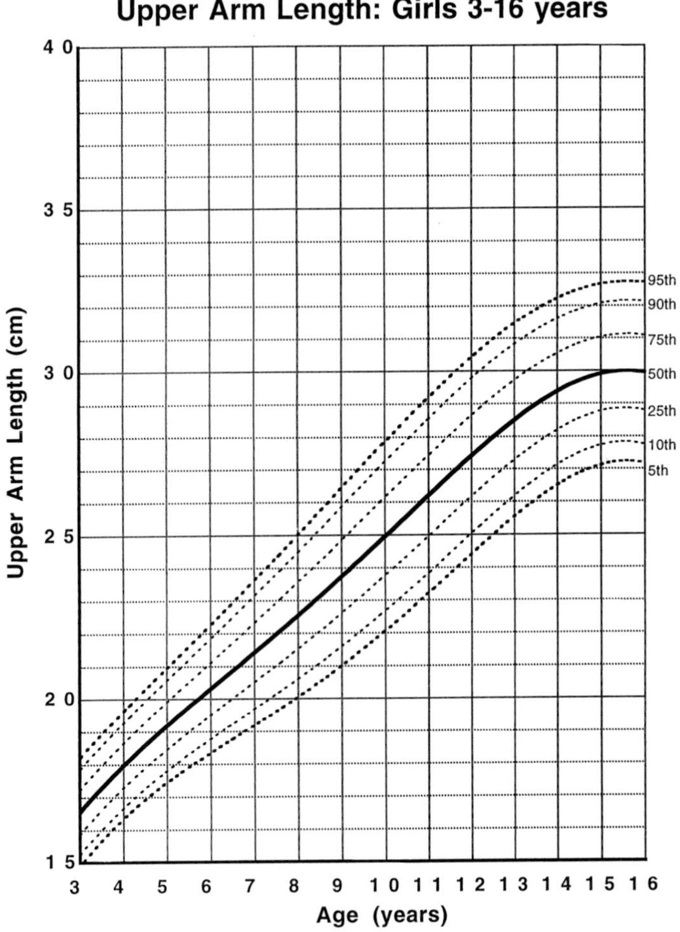

Published in: Stallings VA, Zemel BS. Nutritional assessment of the disabled child. In: Sullivan PB, Rosenbloom L, eds. Feeding the disabled Child. London: Cambridge University Press 1996:62–76.

A-14-g-2

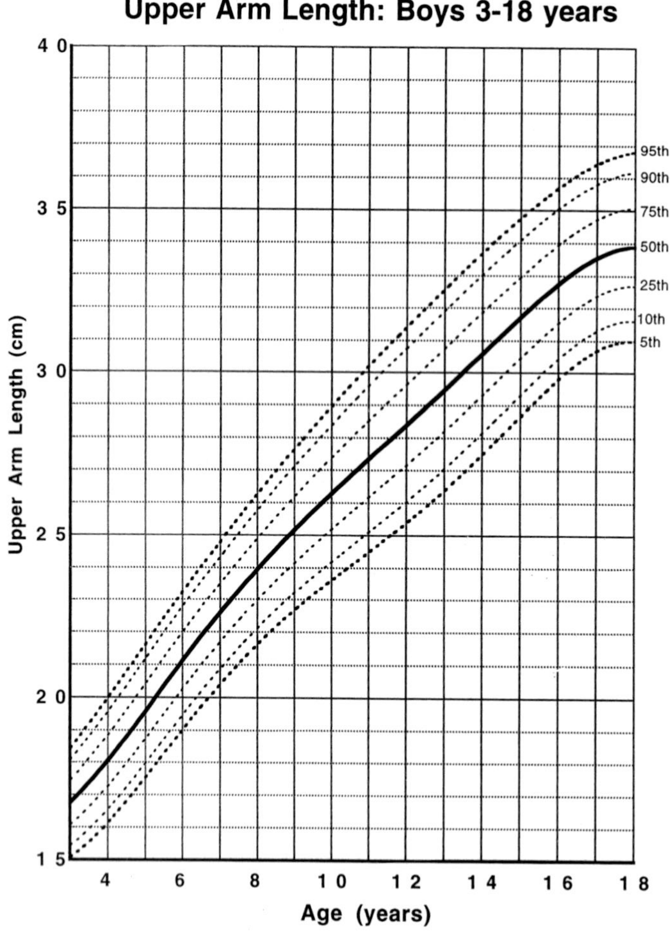

Published in: Stallings VA, Zemel BS. Nutritional assessment of the disabled child. In: Sullivan PB, Rosenbloom L, eds. Feeding the disabled Child. London: Cambridge University Press 1996:62–76.

Table A-15-a
Means, Standard Deviations, and Percentiles of Stature (cm) by Age for Males and Females, 1 to 74 Years

Age (years)	N	Mean	SD	Percentiles								
				5	10	15	25	50	75	85	90	95
Males												
1.0–1.9	366	82.5	5.1	75.5	76.7	77.8	79.3	82.1	85.6	87.2	88.0	89.8
2.0–2.9	664	91.4	4.3	84.9	86.3	87.2	88.4	91.4	94.4	95.8	96.9	98.0
3.0–3.9	716	99.1	4.7	91.6	93.7	94.7	96.1	98.7	102.0	103.9	104.9	107.0
4.0–4.9	709	106.0	5.1	98.1	99.5	100.5	102.7	106.1	109.3	111.2	112.3	114.1
5.0–5.9	675	112.6	5.3	103.9	105.9	107.4	109.3	112.7	115.7	118.1	119.2	121.2
6.0–6.9	298	119.2	5.4	109.4	112.0	113.3	115.7	119.4	122.8	124.9	126.0	127.7
7.0–7.9	312	125.1	5.7	115.6	118.2	119.6	121.5	125.4	128.5	130.6	131.6	133.5
8.0–8.9	296	129.8	6.3	120.0	122.6	123.9	125.9	130.1	133.7	136.0	137.5	140.0
9.0–9.9	322	135.8	5.8	126.0	128.7	129.7	131.4	135.8	139.9	142.0	143.0	145.0
10.0–10.9	334	140.9	6.9	130.2	132.3	133.8	136.1	140.9	145.8	148.2	150.1	152.7
11.0–11.9	324	146.4	7.4	134.3	136.6	138.8	141.6	146.4	151.5	154.0	155.0	158.1
12.0–12.9	349	152.2	8.1	139.7	141.9	143.6	146.4	151.4	157.9	160.4	162.3	166.0
13.0–13.9	350	159.2	8.8	145.1	147.8	149.6	152.8	159.3	165.6	168.9	170.7	173.2
14.0–14.9	359	167.1	8.2	153.3	156.3	158.6	161.7	166.9	172.8	175.9	178.2	179.9
15.0–15.9	359	170.8	7.3	158.5	161.5	162.9	165.6	171.2	176.2	177.9	179.8	182.5
16.0–16.9	349	174.5	7.1	163.4	165.0	167.3	169.8	174.1	178.7	182.0	183.8	186.7
17.0–17.9	338	175.5	6.9	164.4	166.9	168.6	170.7	175.1	180.5	183.0	184.5	187.3
18.0–24.9	1755	176.6	7.0	165.4	167.8	169.5	171.9	176.6	181.2	183.7	185.5	188.6
25.0–29.9	1255	176.7	7.0	165.1	167.8	169.4	172.0	176.6	181.5	184.0	185.7	188.0
30.0–34.9	947	176.2	6.9	164.8	167.4	169.0	171.5	176.2	180.9	183.3	184.8	187.2
35.0–39.9	839	176.1	7.2	164.0	166.8	168.8	171.9	176.1	181.0	183.5	185.0	187.7
40.0–44.9	829	175.9	6.7	165.0	167.2	168.9	171.4	176.0	180.3	182.7	184.2	186.9
45.0–49.9	871	175.2	7.1	163.8	166.5	168.0	170.6	174.8	180.2	182.9	184.5	186.6
50.0–54.9	882	174.6	6.5	164.2	166.4	167.8	170.1	174.6	178.8	181.4	183.2	185.3
55.0–59.9	807	173.9	6.8	163.2	165.0	166.8	169.3	173.8	178.7	181.0	182.3	184.6
60.0–64.9	1261	173.0	6.6	161.9	165.0	166.4	168.7	173.0	177.4	179.8	181.3	183.7
65.0–69.9	1773	171.5	6.9	159.7	162.9	164.5	166.7	171.6	176.3	178.6	180.1	182.5
70.0–74.9	1257	170.6	6.8	159.5	162.0	163.6	165.8	170.7	175.0	177.4	179.4	182.0
Females												
1.0–1.9	333	80.6	4.8	73.2	74.7	75.6	77.4	80.5	83.6	85.9	86.8	88.6
2.0–2.9	610	90.1	4.5	83.1	84.9	85.6	86.8	90.1	93.0	94.6	95.7	97.4
3.0–3.9	651	97.7	4.5	90.3	92.1	92.9	94.8	97.5	100.6	102.4	103.4	105.0
4.0–4.9	678	105.0	4.9	97.0	98.5	99.6	101.6	104.9	108.3	110.0	111.2	113.6
5.0–5.9	673	112.0	5.4	103.1	105.3	106.7	108.6	111.9	115.4	117.4	119.0	120.6
6.0–6.9	296	118.3	5.6	109.9	111.4	112.4	114.2	118.5	122.2	124.2	125.2	127.6
7.0–7.9	331	124.2	6.0	115.3	117.0	118.3	120.3	124.3	128.4	130.1	131.7	134.5
8.0–8.9	276	129.8	6.0	120.1	122.1	123.7	125.5	129.7	133.5	135.6	137.8	140.1
9.0–9.9	322	135.7	7.2	125.7	127.5	128.4	130.5	135.6	140.4	142.5	143.9	147.2
10.0–10.9	330	141.5	7.4	129.5	132.2	133.9	136.3	141.6	146.0	148.3	150.9	154.4
11.0–11.9	303	148.1	8.2	134.7	138.1	139.8	142.3	148.4	153.4	156.1	158.0	162.1
12.0–12.9	324	154.6	7.2	143.0	145.2	147.0	149.6	154.6	159.3	162.5	164.0	165.5
13.0–13.9	361	158.8	6.2	149.1	151.1	152.8	155.1	158.8	162.8	164.8	165.7	168.3
14.0–14.9	370	160.9	6.2	151.0	153.0	154.5	156.8	160.8	164.9	167.0	168.8	171.7
15.0–15.9	309	163.2	6.5	152.8	155.2	157.1	158.8	162.7	167.2	169.7	172.0	175.4
16.0–16.9	343	162.2	6.6	151.4	153.6	155.5	157.7	162.3	166.4	169.1	171.6	173.2
17.0–17.9	293	162.7	6.0	153.2	155.5	156.9	159.2	162.3	166.4	168.7	169.9	172.8
18.0–24.9	2592	163.0	6.5	152.3	154.8	156.4	158.8	163.1	167.1	169.6	171.0	173.6
25.0–29.9	1935	162.9	6.3	152.6	155.2	156.6	158.6	162.8	167.1	169.5	170.9	173.3
30.0–34.9	1633	162.6	6.2	152.9	155.2	156.4	158.4	162.4	166.8	169.2	171.2	173.1
35.0–39.9	1461	162.8	6.5	152.0	155.0	156.4	158.6	162.7	167.0	169.4	171.0	173.5
40.0–44.9	1399	162.6	6.4	151.6	154.3	156.2	158.1	162.7	166.7	168.8	170.5	173.2
45.0–49.9	969	162.0	6.3	151.7	154.0	155.4	157.9	162.0	166.3	168.4	169.9	172.2
50.0–54.9	1012	161.2	6.0	151.3	153.8	155.3	156.9	161.1	165.1	167.3	169.2	171.0
55.0–59.9	887	160.3	6.2	149.8	152.7	154.1	156.7	160.3	164.4	166.6	167.8	170.1
60.0–64.9	1392	159.6	6.4	149.2	151.4	153.0	155.6	160.0	163.7	166.1	167.3	169.8
65.0–69.9	1952	158.6	6.1	148.5	150.7	152.4	154.8	158.8	162.6	164.8	166.2	168.1
70.0–74.9	1467	157.6	6.1	147.2	150.0	151.7	153.7	157.4	161.5	163.8	165.5	167.5

From Frisancho AR. Anthropometric standards for the assessment of growth and nutritional status. Ann Arbor: University of Michigan Press, 1990, Table IV.1. With permission.

Table A-15-b
Means, Standard Deviations, and Percentiles of Weight (kg) by Age for Males and Females, 1 to 74 Years

Age (years)	N	Mean	SD	Percentiles 5	10	15	25	50	75	85	90	95
Males												
1.0–1.9	681	11.8	1.7	9.6	10.0	10.3	10.7	11.6	12.6	13.1	13.7	14.4
2.0–2.9	677	13.6	1.7	11.1	11.6	11.9	12.5	13.6	14.6	15.2	15.8	16.6
3.0–3.9	717	15.7	2.1	12.8	13.4	13.8	14.4	15.5	16.8	17.5	18.1	19.4
4.0–4.9	709	17.7	2.4	14.1	15.0	15.4	16.1	17.5	19.0	20.0	20.6	21.5
5.0–5.9	676	19.9	3.0	16.0	16.7	17.1	17.8	19.6	21.4	22.4	23.5	25.4
6.0–6.9	298	22.6	3.7	17.5	18.8	19.4	20.2	21.9	24.0	26.0	27.7	30.0
7.0–7.9	312	25.1	4.2	19.0	20.4	21.2	22.2	24.7	27.2	28.7	29.9	33.1
8.0–8.9	296	27.7	5.2	21.5	22.7	23.5	24.5	26.8	29.7	31.8	33.6	37.3
9.0–9.9	322	31.3	6.3	23.6	24.7	25.7	27.1	30.3	33.6	37.1	40.3	43.2
10.0–10.9	334	35.4	7.8	26.2	27.7	28.5	30.2	33.8	38.6	42.1	45.6	53.1
11.0–11.9	324	39.8	10.0	28.3	30.0	31.5	33.4	37.6	43.3	48.6	52.3	58.6
12.0–12.9	349	44.2	11.1	30.8	32.8	34.4	36.6	42.2	49.0	53.9	59.0	66.9
13.0–13.9	348	49.8	11.6	34.6	37.1	38.7	41.6	48.5	56.1	60.3	65.2	69.6
14.0–14.9	359	56.9	11.9	41.3	44.0	45.9	49.2	55.3	63.0	66.4	70.1	76.9
15.0–15.9	359	61.0	11.2	44.7	48.6	50.8	54.2	60.0	66.2	70.4	74.4	81.3
16.0–16.9	349	66.8	11.9	51.7	54.2	55.7	59.0	64.8	72.9	77.8	81.6	89.0
17.0–17.9	339	67.5	12.2	51.1	54.1	56.5	59.3	65.7	72.5	78.0	83.3	91.4
18.0–24.9	1758	73.9	13.4	56.4	59.8	61.6	64.8	71.4	80.5	86.3	91.5	99.9
25.0–29.9	1256	77.9	14.6	58.7	61.8	64.5	68.1	76.0	84.8	90.6	95.1	103.4
30.0–34.9	948	79.8	14.4	59.8	63.3	66.3	69.8	78.4	87.4	93.4	96.8	103.0
35.0–39.9	840	80.3	13.6	58.4	62.9	66.6	72.2	79.8	87.8	92.4	96.7	102.8
40.0–44.9	830	81.0	13.8	60.7	64.3	67.9	71.9	79.6	89.4	94.3	98.8	104.8
45.0–49.9	871	80.8	14.0	60.0	64.0	66.8	71.4	79.7	89.2	94.0	97.2	103.6
50.0–54.9	882	79.5	13.9	58.7	93.3	66.2	70.0	78.0	87.4	93.3	99.3	103.6
55.0–59.9	808	79.4	13.9	58.2	63.0	66.4	70.2	78.5	86.8	92.9	97.1	103.5
60.0–64.9	1263	77.3	13.1	57.9	61.8	64.5	68.8	76.8	84.9	89.3	92.5	100.0
65.0–69.9	1774	75.0	13.0	55.1	58.5	61.5	66.4	74.5	83.2	88.0	91.8	97.2
70.0–74.9	1257	73.7	12.9	53.9	57.5	60.4	65.2	73.0	81.3	86.3	90.4	95.9
Females												
1.0–1.9	622	10.9	1.4	8.7	9.2	9.5	9.9	10.8	11.8	12.4	12.8	13.4
2.0–2.9	615	13.0	1.6	10.8	11.2	11.6	12.0	12.8	13.9	14.6	15.1	15.9
3.0–3.9	653	15.0	2.1	11.8	12.6	13.0	13.6	14.7	16.2	17.1	17.6	18.6
4.0–4.9	682	17.1	2.4	13.7	14.3	14.7	15.5	16.8	18.4	19.4	20.1	21.3
5.0–5.9	674	19.5	3.2	15.3	16.2	16.8	17.3	19.0	21.0	22.4	23.6	25.3
6.0–6.9	296	21.8	3.6	17.0	17.7	18.6	19.4	21.3	23.7	24.8	26.5	28.9
7.0–7.9	331	24.7	4.5	19.2	19.8	20.6	21.9	23.8	26.5	28.7	29.9	32.7
8.0–8.9	276	28.1	6.3	20.9	21.9	22.6	24.0	26.9	30.4	33.3	35.1	39.9
9.0–9.9	322	32.0	7.5	23.7	24.8	25.6	26.8	30.7	34.7	38.9	41.7	46.5
10.0–10.9	330	35.7	8.4	25.6	27.0	27.9	29.6	33.9	39.2	44.1	46.5	52.4
11.0–11.9	303	41.8	11.0	29.1	30.5	31.6	34.3	39.8	46.3	52.8	56.9	61.9
12.0–12.9	324	47.1	10.7	32.5	34.3	36.3	39.1	45.9	53.0	58.5	61.2	66.7
13.0–13.9	361	51.5	11.7	37.2	39.3	40.6	44.3	49.6	55.7	61.6	66.8	76.2
14.0–14.9	370	54.7	11.2	40.3	42.9	44.8	47.3	52.7	60.0	64.9	69.5	75.6
15.0–15.9	309	56.4	11.6	43.4	45.3	46.6	48.6	54.2	60.3	65.2	69.5	79.4
16.0–16.9	343	58.2	11.7	43.4	46.1	47.5	50.8	55.7	62.8	68.9	73.1	80.8
17.0–17.9	293	59.7	13.3	43.2	46.4	49.2	51.9	57.4	63.3	69.4	74.7	86.0
18.0–24.9	2592	60.8	12.8	45.6	48.4	50.0	52.6	58.3	65.4	71.5	76.1	84.3
25.0–29.9	1935	62.8	14.2	46.6	49.0	50.7	53.4	59.4	68.4	76.1	81.6	90.8
30.0–34.9	1633	65.6	16.1	47.5	50.1	52.0	54.9	61.5	72.2	80.5	86.5	97.9
35.0–39.9	1461	67.1	15.8	48.6	51.7	53.1	56.4	63.3	73.7	82.0	88.1	98.2
40.0–44.9	1399	67.8	16.1	49.2	51.8	54.0	57.0	64.0	75.1	83.3	89.8	99.1
45.0–49.9	969	68.2	16.3	47.8	51.4	53.5	57.1	64.9	75.9	83.0	87.4	98.4
50.0–54.9	1012	68.3	14.8	48.8	51.9	54.4	58.1	65.8	75.8	83.1	88.4	97.1
55.0–59.9	888	69.2	16.3	48.6	52.2	54.5	58.2	66.3	77.2	85.2	89.4	98.5
60.0–64.9	1393	68.0	14.2	48.5	51.7	54.1	58.1	66.0	75.8	82.1	86.0	94.1
65.0–69.9	1954	67.5	14.2	47.8	51.4	53.9	57.7	65.7	74.8	80.8	86.1	93.9
70.0–74.9	1468	66.0	13.6	46.5	50.1	52.4	57.0	64.5	74.4	79.7	83.3	88.8

From Frisancho AR. Anthropometric standards for the assessment of growth and nutritional status. Ann Arbor: University of Michigan Press, 1990, Table IV.2. With permission.

Table A-15-c
Means, Standard Deviations, and Percentiles of Weight (kg) by Height (cm) for Males, 2 to 74 Years

Height (cm)	N	Mean	SD	Percentiles 5	10	15	25	50	75	85	90	95
Boys: 2 to 11 years												
84–86	75	12.1	1.1	10.7	10.9	11.1	11.3	11.9	12.8	13.1	13.5	14.3
87–89	170	12.8	1.1	11.2	11.4	11.7	12.0	12.7	13.4	13.8	14.2	14.6
90–92	207	13.5	1.0	11.9	12.1	12.5	12.8	13.6	14.2	14.6	14.9	15.2
93–95	278	14.4	1.2	12.7	13.0	13.4	13.6	14.3	15.1	15.5	15.8	16.3
96–98	310	15.0	1.3	13.3	13.6	13.8	14.2	15.0	15.6	16.1	16.4	17.0
99–101	300	16.0	1.3	13.9	14.4	14.7	15.1	15.9	16.7	17.2	17.6	18.3
102–104	290	16.9	1.4	15.1	15.4	15.6	15.9	16.8	17.7	18.0	18.5	19.3
105–107	291	17.6	1.6	15.4	15.9	16.2	16.6	17.5	18.4	19.0	19.4	19.8
108–110	298	18.7	1.7	16.7	17.0	17.1	17.6	18.5	19.6	20.1	20.5	21.3
111–113	274	20.0	2.2	17.0	17.8	18.1	18.7	19.6	21.0	21.7	22.4	23.4
114–116	223	20.9	2.2	18.6	19.0	19.2	19.6	20.5	21.7	22.3	22.7	23.6
117–119	199	21.9	2.3	19.0	19.6	20.2	20.5	21.5	23.0	23.8	24.3	26.0
120–122	177	23.3	2.4	19.8	20.8	21.2	21.9	23.1	24.5	25.4	26.0	27.3
123–125	174	25.0	2.8	21.5	22.0	22.7	23.4	24.5	26.2	27.0	28.2	30.0
126–128	185	26.5	3.8	22.6	23.1	23.8	24.3	25.9	27.8	29.4	30.6	32.0
129–131	174	27.6	3.1	23.5	24.4	24.7	25.6	27.3	28.9	30.0	31.0	32.9
132–134	180	29.3	3.5	25.1	25.7	25.8	26.8	28.5	31.0	33.0	34.4	35.4
135–137	175	31.4	4.6	26.2	27.1	27.6	28.5	30.4	33.0	34.9	37.4	41.5
138–140	150	33.5	4.7	28.2	28.9	29.4	30.5	32.3	35.1	37.8	39.9	42.0
141–143	153	36.1	5.0	30.4	31.3	31.8	33.0	34.9	38.2	40.5	43.3	45.4
144–146	114	38.9	6.6	31.6	32.7	33.1	35.1	37.6	41.2	43.9	46.3	50.7
147–149	87	40.9	6.8	33.6	34.3	35.3	35.9	39.2	43.8	47.3	51.5	56.7
Boys: 12 to 17 years												
144–146	59	38.1	5.5	31.1	32.4	33.6	34.6	36.5	40.3	42.1	46.1	53.0
147–149	77	40.9	7.1	33.6	34.0	34.7	36.5	38.3	43.8	47.4	49.4	59.8
150–152	103	43.4	6.6	36.3	37.2	38.0	38.7	41.4	46.5	51.5	54.7	56.7
153–155	106	45.9	7.9	36.5	38.1	39.1	40.6	43.7	49.7	51.9	55.2	60.9
156–158	113	48.5	9.2	39.9	40.7	41.3	42.5	45.8	50.0	57.9	62.0	67.3
159–161	146	51.1	9.2	40.8	42.9	43.9	45.6	48.6	53.6	60.9	65.4	68.4
162–164	177	54.8	8.9	44.7	45.9	46.9	49.1	53.2	58.4	61.8	64.3	69.1
165–167	197	57.3	9.2	47.1	48.8	49.9	51.3	55.3	61.0	64.8	68.6	73.3
168–170	235	61.4	10.4	49.2	51.4	52.4	55.0	59.9	65.5	69.6	72.5	79.1
171–173	233	62.8	8.8	51.4	53.4	54.8	56.9	61.3	66.1	71.2	73.7	78.2
174–176	202	66.7	10.9	52.3	55.7	57.4	60.0	64.8	71.2	75.5	81.4	89.9
177–179	166	68.8	12.0	55.8	58.7	59.6	61.6	66.3	72.3	75.5	79.6	88.0
180–182	103	71.8	9.7	60.2	60.9	62.1	64.0	70.1	79.5	82.2	85.2	88.7
183–185	64	73.5	9.1	62.4	63.6	65.4	67.8	72.1	77.3	79.4	89.9	91.1
Males: 18 to 74 years												
153–155	56	64.6	13.0	48.6	51.3	54.5	57.1	62.0	66.8	76.8	80.6	83.5
156–158	140	65.5	11.2	48.3	51.4	54.0	57.4	64.9	72.0	77.3	79.3	86.0
159–161	292	66.2	10.8	49.1	53.8	56.4	59.2	66.0	71.2	76.9	80.2	84.3
162–164	643	68.0	10.5	52.2	55.2	57.0	60.4	67.3	74.5	79.1	81.6	86.9
165–167	1147	70.8	11.6	53.0	56.6	59.6	62.7	70.3	77.6	82.3	85.2	90.1
168–170	1582	73.5	12.0	55.9	58.6	61.3	65.9	72.7	80.2	84.5	87.9	93.4
171–173	2047	76.1	12.5	58.2	61.3	63.6	67.6	75.1	83.2	88.1	92.0	97.8
174–176	2053	78.3	12.7	60.0	63.8	66.1	69.5	77.3	84.9	90.1	93.8	99.7
177–179	1750	80.3	12.8	61.9	65.1	67.5	71.4	79.4	87.3	92.6	96.5	102.6
180–182	1252	82.6	13.6	63.4	67.3	69.6	72.9	81.4	90.1	95.0	99.4	105.7
183–185	833	85.2	13.9	65.1	69.2	71.5	75.3	83.3	93.4	99.1	103.2	110.4
186–188	398	88.0	13.3	68.9	72.3	74.8	79.4	86.6	95.1	100.4	103.5	109.8
189–191	161	92.0	16.0	71.3	75.3	77.8	80.7	89.9	99.4	105.0	110.8	123.7
191–194	66	95.9	15.8	71.8	78.6	80.2	84.8	94.2	105.2	109.1	111.8	123.8

From Frisancho AR. Anthropometric standards for the assessment of growth and nutritional status. Ann Arbor: University of Michigan Press, 1990, Table IV.3. With permission.

Table A-15-d
Means, Standard Deviations, and Percentiles of Weight (kg) by Height (cm) for Females, 2 to 74 Years

Height (cm)	N	Mean	SD	Percentiles 5	10	15	25	50	75	85	90	95
Girls: 2 to 10 years												
81–83	36	11.2	.8	10.1	10.2	10.3	10.4	11.0	11.7	12.1	12.6	12.6
84–86	118	11.9	.9	10.5	10.8	11.0	11.3	12.0	12.5	12.7	13.0	13.6
87–89	156	12.5	1.2	11.0	11.3	11.6	11.8	12.4	13.0	13.6	13.8	14.6
90–92	229	13.2	1.2	11.6	11.8	12.0	12.3	13.0	13.8	14.3	14.6	15.2
93–95	259	13.9	1.2	12.0	12.6	12.8	13.1	13.8	14.6	15.1	15.5	16.1
96–98	275	15.0	1.3	13.1	13.5	13.7	14.1	14.9	15.6	16.3	16.7	17.2
99–101	272	15.8	1.6	13.8	14.1	14.3	14.6	15.5	16.6	17.2	17.6	18.4
102–104	278	16.6	2.0	14.2	14.6	15.0	15.5	16.4	17.3	18.0	18.5	19.4
105–107	270	17.6	1.6	15.3	15.8	16.1	16.6	17.3	18.4	19.2	19.4	20.1
108–110	275	18.3	1.6	15.9	16.6	16.8	17.2	18.1	19.2	20.0	20.4	21.1
111–113	251	19.4	1.9	16.6	17.1	17.3	17.9	19.4	20.4	21.2	21.8	22.8
114–116	215	20.7	2.5	17.5	18.3	18.6	19.0	20.2	21.8	22.9	23.9	25.7
117–119	191	21.9	2.6	19.0	19.4	19.5	20.2	21.4	23.0	24.0	24.8	26.6
120–122	181	23.1	2.5	20.1	20.4	20.9	21.5	22.6	24.0	25.3	26.2	27.7
123–125	162	24.5	2.5	21.2	21.8	22.3	22.8	24.0	25.9	26.5	27.2	29.0
126–128	172	26.2	3.1	22.6	23.0	23.4	23.9	25.6	27.7	29.4	30.0	31.5
129–131	157	28.0	3.8	23.6	24.3	24.8	25.6	27.3	29.4	31.1	33.4	36.6
132–134	148	30.3	4.4	25.1	25.8	26.2	27.0	29.4	32.3	34.5	37.2	39.9
135–137	135	32.1	5.4	25.6	27.2	27.7	28.3	30.8	33.9	35.8	41.6	44.1
138–140	124	34.6	7.3	27.6	28.8	29.1	30.6	32.5	35.5	40.9	43.5	47.5
141–143	97	36.0	6.3	28.8	29.8	30.7	32.2	34.8	37.9	41.3	45.6	49.9
144–146	65	39.2	7.0	31.0	31.9	32.9	34.5	37.6	42.9	45.3	48.4	51.8
147–149	45	40.0	7.3	30.7	32.3	34.0	35.0	38.3	44.2	48.0	50.8	54.8
Girls: 11 to 17 years												
141–143	54	37.1	7.8	28.9	29.8	31.1	32.2	34.9	38.6	42.4	45.7	59.5
144–146	67	38.5	6.8	30.4	30.8	31.6	32.9	38.4	41.4	44.1	46.5	52.4
147–149	127	43.4	10.0	32.7	34.3	35.4	37.0	40.7	46.7	51.3	56.4	61.2
150–152	180	45.8	9.1	34.7	36.3	37.4	39.5	44.1	49.9	54.3	56.1	61.9
153–155	235	48.8	8.9	38.0	39.5	40.6	43.1	46.7	53.6	56.5	60.0	66.3
156–158	352	52.3	10.4	39.7	41.7	43.1	45.1	49.9	57.5	62.5	66.0	72.3
159–161	372	55.1	11.0	42.2	44.3	46.0	48.3	52.8	59.2	62.9	68.4	77.6
162–164	344	56.6	9.9	44.9	46.6	47.5	50.2	54.4	60.6	65.3	68.6	73.8
165–167	243	60.0	12.5	46.3	48.8	50.1	52.8	57.6	62.7	69.4	74.7	84.7
168–170	124	61.2	10.8	48.9	49.2	51.1	53.5	59.0	65.7	73.4	75.1	82.4
171–173	74	67.5	15.0	53.0	54.3	54.9	57.7	62.1	72.3	80.1	89.1	104.2
Females: 18 to 74 years												
141–143	64	55.9	10.2	39.2	41.3	43.9	49.0	56.5	63.3	64.9	67.7	76.6
144–146	178	57.1	14.2	38.7	42.0	44.3	48.1	54.3	64.4	71.3	74.6	82.0
147–149	430	59.4	13.2	41.5	44.6	46.8	50.1	56.9	66.9	71.9	76.1	84.8
150–152	928	61.1	13.2	43.1	46.5	48.1	51.5	59.0	68.3	74.3	78.4	86.2
153–155	1685	63.0	13.7	45.3	47.5	49.8	53.2	60.7	70.2	77.3	81.6	88.6
156–158	2670	63.8	14.6	46.6	49.1	50.8	53.5	60.7	70.9	77.1	82.3	90.0
159–161	3041	65.3	14.5	47.7	50.2	52.0	55.2	62.3	72.6	79.4	84.6	92.9
162–164	2849	66.9	14.6	49.4	51.5	53.4	56.6	63.5	74.2	81.4	86.0	94.9
165–167	2327	68.2	15.3	50.3	52.8	54.9	57.8	64.5	74.7	82.4	88.6	98.2
168–170	1327	69.5	15.1	52.5	54.7	56.5	59.2	65.4	76.1	83.5	90.1	99.4
171–173	685	71.8	15.8	54.1	55.9	57.9	60.5	67.6	78.9	86.1	93.9	105.0
174–176	334	72.9	17.3	56.1	57.9	59.6	62.3	68.4	77.6	85.7	93.1	106.9
177–179	97	75.3	16.5	57.6	59.9	60.7	64.4	71.2	81.8	89.6	102.1	112.8

From Frisancho AR. Anthropometric standards for the assessment of growth and nutritional status. Ann Arbor: University of Michigan Press, 1990, Table IV. 4. With permission.

Table A-15-e
Provisional Age- and Sex-Specific Reference Values for Weight in Kilograms (pounds) in Elderly Subjects[a,b]

Age Group (years)	5%	50%	95%
Men			
65	62.6 (138.0)	79.5 (175.0)	102.0 (224.9)
70	59.7 (131.6)	76.5 (168.7)	99.1 (218.5)
75	56.8 (125.2)	73.6 (162.3)	96.3 (212.3)
80	53.9 (118.8)	70.7 (155.9)	93.4 (205.9)
85	51.0 (112.4)	67.8 (149.5)	90.5 (199.5)
90	48.1 (106.0)	64.9 (143.1)	87.6 (193.1)
Women			
65	51.2 (112.9)	66.8 (147.3)	87.1 (192.0)
70	49.0 (108.0)	64.6 (142.4)	84.9 (187.2)
75	46.8 (103.2)	62.4 (137.6)	82.8 (182.5)
80	44.7 (98.5)	60.2 (132.7)	80.6 (177.7)
85	42.5 (93.7)	58.0 (127.9)	78.4 (172.8)
90	40.3 (88.8)	55.9 (123.2)	76.2 (168.0)

From Chumlea WC, Roche AF, Mukherjee D. Nutritional assessment of the elderly through anthropometry. Dayton, Ohio, Wright State University School of Medicine, 1984. With permission.
[a]Data from 119 men and 150 women. The subjects were all ambulatory.
[b]From data compiled by Frisancho from NHANES I and II data.

A-16. ANTHROPOMETRIC DATA

Anthropometric data are multiple and changing. Included here is basic material derived from Dr. Frisancho's publication *Anthropometric Standards for the Assessment of Growth and Nutritional Status,* Ann Arbor: University of Michigan Press, 1990. The interested reader is referred to this comprehensive publication for numerous other tables, graphs, and detailed text.

—The Appendix Editors

Table A-16-a-1
Triceps Skinfold Thickness (mm) in Percentiles by Age (years) for White Males and Females, 1 to 74 Years

Age				Percentiles								
(years)	N	Mean	SD	5	10	15	25	50	75	85	90	95
Males												
1.0–1.9	508	10.5	2.8	6.5	7.0	7.5	8.5	10.0	12.0	13.5	14.0	15.5
2.0–2.9	513	10.1	2.8	6.0	7.0	7.0	8.0	10.0	12.0	13.0	14.0	15.0
3.0–3.9	541	10.1	2.7	6.5	7.0	7.5	8.0	10.0	12.0	13.0	14.0	15.0
4.0–4.9	547	9.6	2.7	6.0	7.0	7.0	8.0	9.0	11.0	12.0	13.0	14.5
5.0–5.9	535	9.3	3.0	5.5	6.5	6.5	7.0	8.5	10.5	12.0	13.0	14.5
6.0–6.9	231	9.3	3.6	5.0	6.0	6.0	6.5	8.5	10.5	12.0	13.0	16.0
7.0–7.9	240	9.6	4.0	5.0	6.0	6.0	7.0	9.0	11.0	13.0	15.0	17.5
8.0–8.9	240	9.9	4.3	5.0	6.0	6.0	7.0	9.0	11.5	13.0	16.0	18.5
9.0–9.9	242	11.1	5.3	5.5	6.0	6.5	7.0	10.0	13.0	16.5	17.0	21.0
10.0–10.9	269	12.0	5.7	5.5	6.0	7.0	8.0	10.5	14.5	18.0	20.0	24.0
11.0–11.9	248	13.2	7.1	5.5	6.0	7.0	8.0	11.5	16.0	20.0	24.0	30.0
12.0–12.9	272	12.8	6.7	5.5	6.0	7.0	8.0	11.0	14.5	20.0	23.0	28.5
13.0–13.9	268	11.9	7.0	5.0	5.5	6.5	7.0	10.0	14.0	18.5	22.0	26.0
14.0–14.9	286	11.1	6.9	4.5	5.0	6.0	6.6	9.0	14.0	16.0	20.0	24.0
15.0–15.9	286	10.0	6.5	5.0	5.0	5.0	6.0	7.5	11.5	15.0	18.0	22.0
16.0–16.9	279	10.4	6.1	4.0	5.0	5.5	6.5	8.5	12.5	15.5	18.5	24.0
17.0–17.9	266	9.3	5.2	4.5	5.0	5.5	6.0	7.5	11.5	14.0	16.0	19.0
18.0–24.9	1463	11.6	6.3	4.5	5.0	6.0	7.0	10.0	15.0	18.0	20.0	24.0
25.0–29.9	1070	12.5	6.5	5.0	5.5	6.0	7.5	11.0	16.0	19.0	21.0	25.0
30.0–34.9	794	13.4	6.5	5.0	6.0	7.0	8.5	12.0	16.5	20.0	22.0	25.5
35.0–39.9	732	13.1	6.0	5.0	6.0	7.0	8.5	12.0	16.0	19.0	21.0	24.5
40.0–44.9	722	13.2	6.4	5.0	6.0	7.0	8.5	12.0	16.0	19.0	22.0	26.0
45.0–49.9	745	13.1	6.2	5.5	6.5	7.0	9.0	12.0	16.0	19.0	21.0	24.5
50.0–54.9	764	12.8	6.0	5.5	6.5	7.5	8.5	12.0	15.5	19.0	20.5	25.0
55.0–59.9	694	12.6	5.7	5.0	6.0	7.0	8.5	11.5	15.0	18.0	20.5	24.0
60.0–64.9	1120	12.6	5.9	5.0	6.5	7.0	8.5	11.5	15.5	18.0	20.0	23.5
65.0–69.9	1489	12.4	5.8	5.0	6.0	6.5	8.0	11.5	15.0	18.0	20.0	23.0
70.0–74.9	1051	12.4	5.7	5.0	6.0	7.0	8.0	11.5	15.0	18.0	20.0	23.0
Females												
1.0–1.9	470	10.5	3.1	6.0	7.0	7.5	8.0	10.0	12.0	13.5	15.0	16.5
2.0–2.9	482	10.7	2.9	6.5	7.0	8.0	9.0	10.5	12.5	14.0	15.0	16.0
3.0–3.9	509	10.6	2.8	6.5	7.0	8.0	8.5	10.5	12.0	13.0	14.0	16.0
4.0–4.9	522	10.5	2.9	6.0	7.0	7.5	8.5	10.0	12.0	13.0	14.0	15.5
5.0–5.9	504	10.6	3.3	6.0	7.0	8.0	8.5	10.0	12.0	14.0	15.0	16.5
6.0–6.9	218	10.8	3.6	6.0	7.0	7.5	8.0	10.5	12.0	13.5	15.0	17.0
7.0–7.9	244	11.4	4.0	6.0	7.0	8.0	9.0	11.0	13.0	15.0	17.0	19.0
8.0–8.9	221	12.5	5.5	6.5	7.0	8.0	9.0	11.5	15.0	17.0	18.0	22.5
9.0–9.9	248	14.1	5.8	7.0	8.0	8.5	10.0	13.0	16.5	19.5	22.0	25.5
10.0–10.9	266	14.2	5.9	7.0	8.0	8.0	10.0	13.0	17.5	20.0	22.5	27.0
11.0–11.9	229	15.4	6.6	7.0	8.5	9.0	11.0	13.0	18.5	21.5	24.5	29.0
12.0–12.9	247	15.2	5.9	8.0	9.0	9.5	11.0	14.0	18.0	20.5	23.0	27.0
13.0–13.9	275	16.4	7.2	7.0	8.0	9.5	11.0	15.0	20.0	24.0	25.0	30.0
14.0–14.9	287	17.5	7.1	9.0	10.0	10.5	12.0	17.0	21.0	23.5	27.0	31.0
15.0–15.9	234	17.6	6.8	8.5	10.0	11.0	12.5	17.0	20.5	23.0	26.0	32.0
16.0–16.9	284	19.4	6.9	10.5	12.0	13.0	14.5	18.0	22.5	26.0	29.0	32.5
17.0–17.9	223	20.0	8.1	10.0	11.5	12.0	14.0	19.0	24.0	26.5	30.0	35.0
18.0–24.9	2058	20.2	8.1	10.0	11.0	12.0	14.5	19.0	24.5	28.0	31.0	35.5
25.0–29.9	1608	21.5	8.5	10.0	12.0	13.0	15.0	20.0	26.0	30.5	33.5	38.0
30.0–34.9	1362	23.5	8.8	11.0	13.0	15.0	17.0	22.5	29.0	32.5	35.0	40.0
35.0–39.9	1194	24.3	9.0	12.0	13.5	15.5	18.0	23.0	30.0	34.0	36.0	40.5
40.0–44.9	1136	24.7	8.7	12.0	14.0	16.0	18.5	24.0	30.0	34.0	36.5	40.0
45.0–49.9	826	25.9	8.9	12.5	15.0	16.5	20.0	25.5	31.0	35.5	37.5	42.0
50.0–54.9	858	26.1	8.6	12.0	15.5	17.5	20.5	25.5	31.5	35.5	37.5	40.5
55.0–59.9	754	26.3	8.8	12.0	15.0	17.0	20.5	26.0	32.0	35.0	37.5	42.0
60.0–64.9	1223	26.5	8.7	13.0	16.0	17.5	20.5	26.0	32.0	35.5	38.0	42.0
65.0–69.9	1644	25.0	8.3	12.0	15.0	16.0	19.0	24.5	30.0	33.0	35.5	39.0
70.0–74.9	1260	24.0	8.3	11.5	14.0	15.5	18.0	24.0	29.5	32.0	34.5	38.0

From Frisancho AR. Anthropometric standards for the assessment of growth and nutritional status. Ann Arbor: University of Michigan Press, 1990, Appendix B, Table 16. With permission.

Table A-16-a-2
Means, Standard Deviations, and Percentiles of Triceps Skinfold Thickness (mm) by Age (years) for Black Males and Females, 1 to 74 Years

Age (years)	N	Mean	SD	Percentiles								
				5	10	15	25	50	75	85	90	95
Males												
1.0–1.9	157	10.2	3.0	6.0	7.0	7.0	8.0	10.0	12.0	12.5	13.5	15.0
2.0–2.9	142	9.6	3.1	5.0	6.0	6.5	7.0	10.0	11.0	13.0	14.0	15.0
3.0–3.9	151	9.0	2.6	6.0	6.0	6.5	7.0	9.0	10.5	12.0	12.0	13.5
4.0–4.9	150	8.2	2.4	5.0	5.5	6.0	7.0	7.5	9.5	11.0	11.0	12.0
5.0–5.9	122	7.5	3.0	4.5	5.0	5.0	5.5	7.0	8.5	10.0	11.0	13.0
6.0–6.9	60	7.4	4.1	4.0	4.0	5.0	5.0	6.5	8.0	9.5	10.0	13.0
7.0–7.9	67	7.1	3.6	4.0	4.0	5.0	5.0	6.0	8.0	9.0	11.0	13.0
8.0–8.9	49	7.8	3.9	4.0	4.0	5.0	6.0	7.0	8.0	10.0	11.5	15.0
9.0–9.9	74	7.6	3.5	3.5	4.0	5.0	6.0	6.5	9.0	10.5	12.0	17.0
10.0–10.9	60	9.5	5.5	5.0	5.0	5.5	6.0	7.5	11.0	13.0	16.5	20.0
11.0–11.9	71	9.8	6.0	4.0	5.0	5.0	6.0	8.0	11.0	15.0	18.0	25.0
12.0–12.9	71	10.0	6.9	4.0	4.0	4.5	6.0	8.0	11.0	17.0	18.0	24.0
13.0–13.9	74	8.0	4.2	3.0	4.0	5.0	5.0	6.5	9.0	11.5	14.0	19.0
14.0–14.9	68	7.6	3.9	3.5	4.0	4.5	5.0	7.0	8.5	10.0	12.5	17.0
15.0–15.9	64	9.3	6.9	4.5	5.0	5.0	6.0	6.7	9.0	12.0	18.0	28.0
16.0–16.9	66	8.0	5.1	4.0	4.0	4.5	5.5	6.5	9.0	11.0	12.0	17.0
17.0–17.9	62	7.8	5.1	4.0	4.0	4.5	5.0	6.5	8.5	10.0	12.0	20.0
18.0–24.9	253	9.6	7.0	3.0	4.0	4.5	5.0	7.0	12.0	15.0	18.5	23.5
25.0–29.9	160	10.3	7.7	3.5	4.0	4.3	5.0	8.0	12.0	17.0	21.0	24.0
30.0–34.9	120	11.8	7.4	3.5	4.0	5.0	6.0	11.0	15.5	18.5	20.0	23.5
35.0–39.9	83	11.7	7.7	4.0	4.5	5.0	7.0	10.0	15.0	17.0	19.0	24.0
40.0–44.9	89	11.7	7.1	4.0	5.0	6.0	6.0	10.0	14.2	17.0	20.5	25.5
45.0–49.9	112	11.8	7.5	3.0	4.5	5.5	6.0	10.0	15.0	18.0	21.0	30.0
50.0–54.9	105	11.2	6.4	3.5	4.0	5.0	6.0	10.0	15.0	16.0	19.0	25.5
55.0–59.9	104	11.2	7.2	3.0	4.0	5.0	5.5	10.0	14.0	19.0	22.0	28.0
60.0–64.9	126	11.8	7.0	4.0	5.0	5.5	7.0	10.0	16.0	20.0	22.0	24.5
65.0–69.9	254	10.7	6.8	4.0	4.5	5.0	6.0	9.0	13.0	15.0	19.0	25.0
70.0–74.9	186	9.8	5.3	4.0	4.5	5.0	6.0	9.0	12.0	15.0	16.0	19.0
Females												
1.0–1.9	134	10.2	2.9	6.0	6.0	7.0	8.0	10.0	12.0	13.0	14.0	15.0
2.0–2.9	119	9.8	2.7	6.0	6.5	7.0	8.0	10.0	11.0	12.0	13.0	16.0
3.0–3.9	127	9.4	3.2	5.5	6.0	7.0	7.0	9.0	11.0	12.0	13.0	15.0
4.0–4.9	147	9.4	3.2	5.0	6.0	6.5	7.0	9.0	11.0	12.0	13.5	16.0
5.0–5.9	163	9.6	4.0	5.0	5.5	6.5	7.0	8.5	11.5	13.0	15.0	18.0
6.0–6.9	72	9.1	3.9	4.5	5.5	6.0	7.0	8.0	10.0	12.0	12.0	18.5
7.0–7.9	81	10.0	4.4	5.0	6.0	6.5	7.5	9.0	12.0	13.0	15.0	18.0
8.0–8.9	54	10.4	4.5	5.0	6.0	7.0	7.0	9.0	12.0	15.0	17.5	19.0
9.0–9.9	71	11.1	5.7	5.5	6.0	6.5	7.0	10.0	13.0	17.0	20.0	21.0
10.0–10.9	61	13.0	7.0	5.5	6.5	7.5	8.0	10.0	17.5	19.5	22.0	24.5
11.0–11.9	67	13.6	7.7	5.0	6.5	7.5	8.0	11.5	17.5	22.0	23.0	30.0
12.0–12.9	71	14.7	7.6	6.0	7.0	7.0	9.0	12.5	19.0	25.0	26.0	31.0
13.0–13.9	82	16.3	8.1	6.0	8.0	8.5	10.5	15.5	20.5	24.0	25.0	34.0
14.0–14.9	79	15.5	7.7	6.5	8.0	9.0	10.5	13.5	19.0	24.0	27.0	32.0
15.0–15.9	73	16.1	8.8	6.0	8.0	9.0	10.0	14.0	20.0	23.0	27.5	40.0
16.0–16.9	54	18.9	7.5	8.0	11.0	11.5	12.0	18.5	24.0	26.0	31.0	33.0
17.0–17.9	66	15.9	6.9	7.0	9.0	9.0	12.0	14.0	20.0	24.0	27.0	28.0
18.0–24.9	473	19.3	8.9	8.0	9.0	10.5	12.5	17.0	25.0	30.0	32.0	36.0
25.0–29.9	275	22.8	10.2	8.5	10.5	12.0	15.0	22.0	29.0	32.2	35.0	40.5
30.0–34.9	236	25.0	11.0	8.0	10.0	13.0	16.0	24.0	32.0	35.5	40.0	45.0
35.0–39.9	235	26.6	10.7	10.0	12.0	15.0	18.0	26.0	33.5	37.0	40.8	46.0
40.0–44.9	231	26.8	10.0	11.0	14.0	15.5	20.0	27.0	35.0	37.0	40.5	42.0
45.0–49.9	125	27.1	11.7	10.0	12.0	14.0	19.0	26.0	34.0	40.0	42.0	50.0
50.0–54.9	135	29.5	10.9	10.0	13.5	16.5	22.0	30.5	37.5	41.0	42.5	46.0
55.0–59.9	119	28.7	12.0	8.5	13.0	15.0	20.0	28.0	37.5	41.0	43.0	50.0
60.0–64.9	152	27.7	10.1	12.0	15.0	17.0	21.0	27.0	34.5	39.5	40.5	46.0
65.0–69.9	282	25.6	9.6	10.0	13.0	15.5	18.5	25.5	31.0	35.0	38.0	44.0
70.0–74.9	196	24.3	9.3	10.0	13.0	15.0	17.0	24.0	30.0	33.0	37.0	40.5

From Frisancho AR. Anthropometric standards for the assessment of growth and nutritional status. Ann Arbor: University of Michigan Press, 1990, Appendix A, Table 16. With permission.

Table A-16-b-1
Means, Standard Deviations, and Percentiles of Subscapular Skinfold Thickness (mm) by Age (years) for White Males and Females, 1 to 74 Years

Age (years)	N	Mean	SD	Percentiles								
				5	10	15	25	50	75	85	90	95
Males												
1.0–1.9	508	6.3	1.9	4.0	4.0	4.5	5.0	6.0	7.0	8.0	8.5	10.0
2.0–2.9	513	5.8	2.0	3.5	4.0	4.0	4.5	5.5	6.5	7.5	8.5	9.5
3.0–3.9	540	5.5	1.8	3.5	4.0	4.0	4.5	5.0	6.0	7.0	7.0	9.0
4.0–4.9	546	5.3	2.0	3.0	3.5	4.0	4.0	5.0	6.0	6.5	7.0	8.5
5.0–5.9	535	5.2	2.3	3.0	3.5	4.0	4.0	5.0	5.5	6.5	7.0	8.0
6.0–6.9	231	5.6	3.3	3.0	3.5	3.5	4.0	4.5	6.0	7.0	8.0	13.0
7.0–7.9	240	5.9	3.4	3.0	3.5	4.0	4.0	5.0	6.0	7.0	9.0	12.0
8.0–8.9	240	6.0	3.9	3.0	3.5	4.0	4.0	5.0	6.0	7.5	9.0	12.0
9.0–9.9	242	7.1	5.1	3.5	4.0	4.0	4.0	5.5	7.5	10.5	12.5	15.0
10.0–10.9	269	7.7	5.4	3.5	4.0	4.0	4.5	6.0	8.0	11.0	14.0	19.5
11.0–11.9	248	9.3	8.1	4.0	4.0	4.0	5.0	6.0	10.0	15.0	20.0	27.0
12.0–12.9	273	9.1	7.1	4.0	4.0	4.5	5.0	6.5	10.0	14.0	19.0	24.0
13.0–13.9	268	9.3	7.6	4.0	4.0	5.0	5.0	7.0	10.0	14.0	17.0	26.0
14.0–14.9	286	9.4	6.9	4.0	5.0	5.0	5.5	7.0	10.0	13.0	16.0	23.0
15.0–15.9	286	9.2	6.5	5.0	5.0	5.5	6.0	7.0	10.0	12.0	15.5	22.0
16.0–16.9	278	10.2	6.5	5.0	6.0	6.0	6.5	8.0	11.0	14.0	17.0	23.5
17.0–17.9	267	10.1	5.7	5.0	6.0	6.5	7.0	8.0	11.5	14.0	17.0	20.5
18.0–24.9	1461	13.5	7.5	6.0	7.0	7.0	8.0	11.0	16.0	20.0	24.0	30.0
25.0–29.9	1067	15.6	8.0	7.0	7.5	8.0	10.0	13.5	20.0	24.5	26.5	30.5
30.0–34.9	791	17.3	8.2	7.0	8.0	9.0	11.0	16.0	22.0	25.5	28.0	32.5
35.0–39.9	730	17.4	8.0	7.0	8.0	10.0	11.0	16.0	22.0	25.0	27.5	32.0
40.0–44.9	714	17.3	8.0	7.0	8.0	9.5	11.5	16.0	21.5	25.5	28.0	33.0
45.0–49.9	739	18.2	8.2	7.5	9.0	10.0	12.0	17.0	23.0	26.5	30.0	34.0
50.0–54.9	759	17.7	8.1	7.0	8.0	9.0	12.0	16.0	22.5	26.0	30.0	34.0
55.0–59.9	691	17.6	7.8	7.0	8.5	10.0	11.5	16.5	22.5	25.5	28.0	31.0
60.0–64.9	1112	18.1	8.3	7.0	8.0	10.0	12.0	17.0	23.0	26.0	29.0	33.5
65.0–69.9	1486	16.9	8.0	6.0	8.0	9.0	11.0	15.5	21.5	25.0	28.0	32.0
70.0–74.9	1048	16.4	7.6	6.5	7.5	9.0	11.0	15.0	21.0	25.0	27.5	30.5
Females												
1.0–1.9	470	6.4	2.0	4.0	4.0	4.5	5.0	6.0	7.5	8.5	9.0	10.0
2.0–2.9	483	6.3	2.1	4.0	4.0	4.5	5.0	6.0	7.0	8.0	9.0	10.5
3.0–3.9	509	6.2	2.2	3.5	4.0	4.5	5.0	6.0	7.0	8.0	9.0	10.0
4.0–4.9	522	6.0	2.1	3.5	4.0	4.0	4.5	5.5	7.0	8.0	8.5	10.0
5.0–5.9	503	6.2	2.9	3.5	4.0	4.0	4.5	5.5	7.0	8.0	9.0	12.0
6.0–6.9	218	6.4	3.2	3.5	4.0	4.0	4.5	5.5	7.0	9.0	10.0	11.5
7.0–7.9	244	6.8	3.6	4.0	4.0	4.0	4.5	6.0	7.0	9.5	11.0	13.0
8.0–8.9	221	8.0	6.0	3.5	4.0	4.0	5.0	6.0	8.0	11.5	14.5	21.0
9.0–9.9	248	9.4	6.8	4.0	4.5	5.0	5.0	7.0	10.0	14.0	18.5	24.5
10.0–10.9	266	9.8	6.4	4.0	4.5	5.0	5.5	7.0	11.5	16.0	19.5	24.0
11.0–11.9	227	10.7	7.4	4.5	5.0	5.0	6.0	8.0	12.0	16.0	21.0	28.5
12.0–12.9	247	10.9	6.9	5.0	5.5	6.0	6.0	9.0	12.5	15.5	19.5	29.0
13.0–13.9	275	11.9	7.8	5.0	5.5	6.0	7.0	9.5	15.0	19.0	22.0	26.5
14.0–14.9	287	13.0	7.7	6.0	6.5	7.0	7.5	10.5	16.0	21.0	24.5	30.0
15.0–15.9	234	12.7	7.0	6.0	7.0	7.5	8.0	10.0	15.0	20.0	22.0	27.0
16.0–16.9	284	14.2	8.5	6.5	7.5	8.0	9.0	11.5	16.0	22.5	25.5	32.0
17.0–17.9	223	15.4	9.1	6.0	7.0	7.5	9.0	12.5	19.0	24.5	28.0	34.0
18.0–24.9	2058	15.7	9.1	6.0	7.0	8.0	9.0	13.0	19.5	25.0	28.0	35.0
25.0–29.9	1603	16.8	10.1	6.0	7.0	8.0	9.0	14.0	21.5	27.0	32.0	38.0
30.0–34.9	1359	18.6	11.1	6.5	7.0	8.0	10.0	15.5	25.0	30.5	35.5	41.0
35.0–39.9	1189	19.5	11.2	7.0	8.0	9.0	10.8	16.0	26.0	32.0	35.5	43.0
40.0–44.9	1131	19.6	10.7	6.5	7.5	9.0	11.0	17.0	26.0	32.0	35.0	39.5
45.0–49.9	823	20.9	10.8	7.0	8.5	10.0	12.0	19.0	28.0	33.0	35.5	41.5
50.0–54.9	852	21.8	10.8	7.0	9.0	10.0	13.0	20.5	28.0	34.0	37.0	42.0
55.0–59.9	745	22.2	11.2	7.0	9.0	10.5	13.0	20.5	30.0	34.5	36.5	41.5
60.0–64.9	1213	22.2	11.0	7.5	9.0	10.5	13.5	20.5	30.0	34.0	37.5	42.5
65.0–69.9	1636	20.7	10.3	7.0	8.0	10.0	12.5	19.0	27.0	31.5	35.0	40.0
70.0–74.9	1256	20.2	10.0	6.5	8.5	10.0	12.0	19.0	26.0	31.0	35.0	38.0

From Frisancho AR. Anthropometric standards for the assessment of growth and nutritional status. Ann Arbor: University of Michigan Press, 1990, Appendix B, Table 17. With permission.

Table A-16-b-2
Means, Standard Deviations, and Percentiles of Subscapular Skinfold Thickness (mm) by Age (years) for Black Males and Females, 1 to 74 Years

Age (years)	N	Mean	SD	Percentiles 5	10	15	25	50	75	85	90	95
Males												
1.0–1.9	157	6.6	2.0	4.0	4.0	4.5	5.0	6.0	8.0	8.5	9.0	10.5
2.0–2.9	142	6.1	2.1	4.0	4.0	4.5	5.0	6.0	7.0	8.0	9.0	10.0
3.0–3.9	151	5.4	1.7	3.5	4.0	4.0	4.5	5.0	6.0	6.5	7.0	8.5
4.0–4.9	151	5.0	1.4	3.0	3.5	4.0	4.0	5.0	5.5	6.0	6.5	7.5
5.0–5.9	122	5.0	2.2	3.0	3.0	3.5	4.0	4.5	5.0	6.0	7.0	8.0
6.0–6.9	60	5.1	3.5	3.0	3.0	3.0	4.0	4.0	5.0	5.5	6.5	11.0
7.0–7.9	67	5.2	3.0	3.0	3.5	3.5	4.0	4.5	5.0	6.0	7.0	10.0
8.0–8.9	49	5.7	3.0	3.5	3.5	4.0	4.0	5.0	6.0	7.5	9.0	11.0
9.0–9.9	74	5.6	3.6	3.0	3.5	3.7	4.0	5.0	6.0	7.0	8.0	11.0
10.0–10.9	60	7.3	5.7	4.0	4.0	4.0	4.5	5.0	7.0	8.0	12.0	19.0
11.0–11.9	71	7.6	5.9	4.0	4.0	4.5	5.0	5.5	7.0	10.5	14.5	21.0
12.0–12.9	71	8.3	7.3	4.0	4.0	4.0	4.5	5.5	7.0	16.0	18.0	22.0
13.0–13.9	74	6.9	3.8	3.0	4.5	5.0	5.0	6.0	8.0	8.5	9.5	17.0
14.0–14.9	68	7.4	4.6	4.0	4.5	5.0	5.0	6.0	8.0	8.0	11.0	16.0
15.0–15.9	65	10.4	8.4	5.0	5.0	6.0	6.5	8.0	10.0	14.5	17.0	24.0
16.0–16.9	66	9.6	4.7	5.5	6.5	7.0	7.0	8.0	10.0	13.0	14.5	17.5
17.0–17.9	63	9.5	4.9	5.0	6.0	6.0	6.5	8.0	10.5	12.0	14.0	16.0
18.0–24.9	253	12.7	7.9	6.0	6.5	7.0	8.0	10.0	15.0	18.5	22.5	29.0
25.0–29.9	159	14.5	9.4	6.5	7.0	7.5	8.0	11.0	17.0	24.0	28.0	38.0
30.0–34.9	120	17.4	9.9	6.0	8.0	9.0	10.0	15.0	22.0	25.0	30.0	36.0
35.0–39.9	88	19.0	10.1	7.0	8.0	10.0	11.0	17.0	24.0	26.5	33.0	35.5
40.0–44.9	87	17.2	9.4	6.5	7.5	8.5	10.0	15.0	22.0	25.0	30.0	35.0
45.0–49.9	111	17.9	10.7	5.0	6.5	7.0	9.0	16.0	25.0	29.0	31.5	35.0
50.0–54.9	103	17.4	10.1	6.0	7.0	7.5	9.0	15.0	25.0	28.0	30.0	36.0
55.0–59.9	103	17.7	10.0	5.0	6.5	7.0	9.5	15.0	24.0	27.0	30.5	35.0
60.0–64.9	126	18.0	9.6	6.0	7.5	8.0	10.5	16.0	24.0	27.0	30.5	39.5
65.0–69.9	253	16.3	9.6	5.0	6.0	7.0	9.0	14.0	21.0	25.5	30.0	37.5
70.0–74.9	185	15.8	9.2	6.0	6.0	7.0	8.0	13.5	21.0	26.0	30.5	35.0
Females												
1.0–1.9	134	6.6	1.9	4.0	5.0	5.0	5.0	6.5	8.0	8.5	9.0	10.0
2.0–2.9	119	6.4	2.9	4.0	4.0	4.5	5.0	6.0	7.0	8.5	9.5	12.0
3.0–3.9	127	5.7	2.2	3.0	4.0	4.0	4.5	5.0	6.5	7.0	7.5	9.0
4.0–4.9	147	6.0	2.7	3.5	4.0	4.0	4.5	5.0	7.0	8.0	9.0	11.0
5.0–5.9	163	6.0	3.1	3.5	4.0	4.0	4.0	5.0	6.5	8.0	10.0	12.0
6.0–6.9	72	6.1	4.1	3.0	4.0	4.0	4.0	5.0	6.5	7.0	7.5	12.0
7.0–7.9	81	6.4	2.9	3.5	4.0	4.0	5.0	5.5	7.0	8.0	10.0	12.0
8.0–8.9	54	7.1	4.7	4.0	4.0	4.0	4.5	5.0	7.0	11.5	14.0	16.0
9.0–9.9	71	7.9	5.5	4.0	4.0	4.5	5.0	6.0	8.0	10.0	13.5	24.0
10.0–10.9	61	9.5	6.8	4.0	4.5	5.0	5.5	6.5	11.0	16.0	17.0	23.6
11.0–11.9	67	10.8	8.4	5.0	5.0	5.0	6.0	8.0	12.0	15.0	20.0	30.5
12.0–12.9	71	13.4	10.1	5.0	5.5	5.5	6.5	9.0	16.0	26.5	30.0	36.0
13.0–13.9	82	13.5	7.6	5.5	6.5	7.0	8.0	12.0	16.5	20.0	25.0	28.4
14.0–14.9	79	13.1	8.1	6.0	6.0	6.0	7.5	10.0	17.0	19.5	27.0	33.5
15.0–15.9	72	13.8	9.1	6.0	7.0	7.5	8.0	10.0	16.5	20.0	26.5	35.0
16.0–16.9	54	17.1	10.0	7.0	8.0	9.0	10.5	14.0	20.0	27.0	33.0	40.5
17.0–17.9	66	14.9	7.9	6.5	7.0	8.0	9.0	12.0	20.0	24.0	27.0	30.0
18.0–24.9	472	17.9	10.2	6.5	7.5	8.0	10.0	15.0	24.0	29.0	32.0	38.0
25.0–29.9	272	21.6	11.3	7.0	8.5	10.0	12.0	20.5	28.0	34.5	37.0	41.5
30.0–34.9	235	25.2	13.1	7.0	9.0	11.0	14.5	25.0	34.5	40.0	43.0	49.0
35.0–39.9	233	26.1	11.9	7.0	9.5	12.0	16.5	27.5	34.0	38.0	40.6	45.0
40.0–44.9	227	27.2	12.3	8.0	11.0	13.0	18.0	27.5	35.0	40.0	44.0	48.0
45.0–49.9	122	27.8	12.9	9.5	11.0	12.5	17.0	28.0	37.0	41.0	44.0	50.0
50.0–54.9	131	30.7	12.5	10.0	13.5	16.0	22.0	30.5	38.0	43.1	47.8	52.5
55.0–59.9	118	28.8	13.1	7.0	9.0	13.0	21.0	28.0	37.0	44.0	47.5	54.5
60.0–64.9	149	28.0	12.0	8.5	12.0	14.0	20.0	28.0	35.5	39.0	44.0	50.0
65.0–69.9	277	25.1	11.5	7.5	9.5	11.0	16.0	25.0	32.0	37.0	40.4	45.5
70.0–74.9	197	22.9	10.5	7.5	9.9	11.0	14.0	22.0	31.0	35.0	37.0	40.0

From Frisancho AR. Anthropometric standards for the assessment of growth and nutritional status. Ann Arbor: University of Michigan Press, 1990, Appendix A, Table 17. With permission.

Table A-16-c-1
Means, Standard Deviations, and Percentiles of Upper Arm Circumference (cm) by Age (years) for White Males and Females, 1 to 74 Years

Age (years)	N	Mean	SD	Percentiles 5	10	15	25	50	75	85	90	95
Males												
1.0–1.9	508	16.1	1.2	14.3	14.7	14.9	15.2	16.0	16.9	17.4	17.8	18.2
2.0–2.9	508	16.4	1.5	14.3	14.8	15.2	15.5	16.3	17.2	17.6	18.0	18.6
3.0–3.9	539	16.9	1.5	15.1	15.3	15.6	16.0	16.8	17.6	18.1	18.4	19.0
4.0–4.9	547	17.3	1.4	15.3	15.6	15.9	16.2	17.2	18.0	18.5	19.0	19.4
5.0–5.9	534	17.7	1.8	15.4	15.9	16.1	16.6	17.5	18.6	19.1	19.6	20.5
6.0–6.9	231	18.3	2.1	15.8	16.1	16.4	16.9	18.0	19.1	19.8	20.6	22.7
7.0–7.9	240	19.1	2.0	16.2	16.8	17.1	17.7	18.8	20.1	21.0	22.1	22.9
8.0–8.9	240	19.7	2.3	16.5	17.2	17.6	18.3	19.3	20.5	21.6	22.8	24.4
9.0–9.9	242	20.9	2.8	17.5	18.0	18.4	19.1	20.3	22.1	23.5	24.9	26.0
10.0–10.9	268	22.0	3.0	18.2	18.7	19.1	19.8	21.4	23.2	24.9	26.2	27.9
11.0–11.9	248	23.0	3.5	18.6	19.3	19.8	20.5	22.3	24.6	26.1	27.8	29.8
12.0–12.9	273	23.9	3.3	19.4	20.1	20.7	21.6	23.2	25.5	27.3	28.5	30.5
13.0–13.9	268	25.0	3.3	20.0	21.3	22.0	22.8	24.7	26.7	28.2	29.5	31.0
14.0–14.9	286	26.4	3.5	21.8	22.7	23.3	23.9	26.0	28.3	29.2	30.2	32.3
15.0–15.9	288	27.2	3.2	22.3	23.2	23.8	25.1	27.1	28.9	30.1	31.2	32.5
16.0–16.9	279	28.7	3.3	24.0	24.8	25.6	26.6	28.1	30.8	32.2	33.3	34.7
17.0–17.9	267	29.1	3.3	24.5	25.1	26.1	27.0	28.7	30.8	32.3	33.3	34.5
18.0–24.9	1467	31.1	3.4	26.2	27.2	27.8	28.8	30.8	33.1	34.4	35.5	37.2
25.0–29.9	1072	32.1	3.4	27.1	28.2	28.8	29.9	31.9	34.2	35.4	36.5	38.1
30.0–34.9	797	32.7	3.2	27.8	28.8	29.4	30.5	32.5	34.9	35.8	36.6	38.2
35.0–39.9	733	32.9	3.2	27.9	28.9	29.7	30.7	32.8	34.9	36.1	36.7	37.9
40.0–44.9	723	32.9	3.1	28.2	29.0	29.8	31.0	32.8	34.8	35.9	36.6	37.9
45.0–49.9	748	32.7	3.3	27.4	28.7	29.5	30.7	32.7	34.8	36.0	36.8	38.1
50.0–54.9	767	32.3	3.2	27.2	28.4	29.2	30.2	32.3	34.3	35.6	36.5	37.8
55.0–59.9	695	32.2	3.2	26.8	28.1	29.2	30.4	32.3	34.2	35.2	36.1	37.4
60.0–64.9	1123	31.9	3.3	26.7	27.8	28.6	29.7	32.0	34.0	35.1	35.8	37.1
65.0–69.9	1488	31.1	3.3	25.3	26.8	27.8	29.1	31.2	33.2	34.4	35.1	36.5
70.0–74.9	1051	30.6	3.3	25.1	26.3	27.3	28.6	30.7	32.6	33.7	34.6	35.9
Females												
1.0–1.9	470	15.7	1.3	13.7	14.2	14.4	14.9	15.7	16.5	17.0	17.3	17.9
2.0–2.9	483	16.2	1.3	14.3	14.7	15.0	15.4	16.1	17.0	17.4	18.0	18.5
3.0–3.9	509	16.7	1.4	14.5	15.1	15.3	15.8	16.6	17.5	18.1	18.4	19.0
4.0–4.9	521	17.1	1.4	15.1	15.5	15.8	16.2	17.1	18.0	18.5	18.9	19.4
5.0–5.9	504	17.8	1.7	15.4	15.8	16.2	16.6	17.5	18.5	19.3	20.0	20.8
6.0–6.9	218	18.2	1.9	15.7	16.2	16.5	17.0	17.9	19.1	20.0	20.6	22.1
7.0–7.9	245	19.1	2.3	16.4	16.7	17.1	17.5	18.6	20.1	21.1	21.8	23.4
8.0–8.9	220	20.1	2.7	16.9	17.2	17.6	18.4	19.5	21.3	22.4	23.3	25.3
9.0–9.9	247	21.3	2.8	17.8	18.3	18.8	19.4	21.0	22.3	24.3	25.3	26.9
10.0–10.9	266	21.7	3.0	17.8	18.4	18.9	19.6	21.2	23.4	24.7	25.7	27.2
11.0–11.9	229	23.2	3.5	18.8	19.6	20.0	20.7	22.4	25.2	26.5	27.9	30.3
12.0–12.9	247	23.9	3.1	19.5	20.3	20.8	21.6	23.7	25.7	27.2	28.1	29.4
13.0–13.9	276	25.0	3.8	20.0	20.8	21.5	22.3	24.3	26.7	28.5	30.1	33.4
14.0–14.9	287	26.0	3.4	21.2	22.2	23.0	23.9	25.2	27.6	29.6	30.9	32.2
15.0–15.9	234	25.9	3.3	21.4	22.3	23.0	23.9	25.3	27.7	28.8	30.0	32.0
16.0–16.9	284	26.7	3.3	22.1	23.0	23.6	24.3	26.1	28.4	29.9	31.4	32.8
17.0–17.9	223	27.3	4.0	22.2	23.1	23.7	24.5	27.0	29.1	30.7	32.4	34.7
18.0–24.9	2060	27.4	3.8	22.5	23.3	24.0	24.9	26.8	29.1	30.8	32.1	34.7
25.0–29.9	1617	28.3	4.1	23.1	23.9	24.5	25.4	27.4	30.2	32.1	33.8	36.5
30.0–34.9	1371	29.3	4.5	23.8	24.7	25.4	26.3	28.4	31.3	33.5	35.4	37.9
35.0–39.9	1197	29.8	4.5	24.2	25.2	25.7	26.5	29.0	31.8	34.2	35.9	38.4
40.0–44.9	1141	30.1	4.5	24.2	25.4	26.1	27.0	29.3	32.4	34.9	36.4	38.1
45.0–49.9	831	30.6	4.7	24.2	25.5	26.2	27.3	29.9	33.2	35.2	37.0	39.3
50.0–54.9	862	30.8	4.3	24.8	26.0	26.7	27.9	30.3	33.1	35.3	36.8	38.5
55.0–59.9	756	31.2	4.6	24.8	26.0	26.7	28.1	30.6	33.8	36.3	37.4	39.5
60.0–64.9	1227	31.2	4.5	25.0	26.1	27.1	28.3	30.6	33.8	35.5	37.1	39.4
65.0–69.9	1648	30.7	4.4	24.3	25.7	26.6	27.8	30.3	33.1	34.9	36.2	38.3
70.0–74.9	1261	30.4	4.3	23.8	25.3	26.3	27.6	30.2	33.0	34.5	35.8	37.3

From Frisancho AR. Anthropometric standards for the assessment of growth and nutritional status. Ann Arbor: University of Michigan Press, 1990, Appendix B, Table 10. With permission.

Table A-16-c-2
Means, Standard Deviations, and Percentiles of Upper Arm Circumference (cm) iby Age (years) for Black Males and Females, 1 to 74 Years

Age (years)	N	Mean	SD	Percentiles 5	10	15	25	50	75	85	90	95
Males												
1.0–1.9	157	16.0	1.3	14.0	14.3	14.8	15.3	16.0	16.9	17.2	17.6	18.6
2.0–2.9	142	16.3	1.2	14.4	14.7	14.9	15.4	16.3	17.1	17.5	17.8	18.2
3.0–3.9	151	16.6	1.4	14.6	15.1	15.2	15.7	16.5	17.4	18.0	18.2	18.9
4.0–4.9	150	16.8	1.4	14.3	15.2	15.5	16.0	16.9	17.8	18.5	18.6	18.9
5.0–5.9	122	17.6	1.6	15.8	16.0	16.2	16.6	17.3	18.2	19.0	19.5	20.2
6.0–6.9	60	18.3	2.2	16.0	16.2	16.5	17.0	17.7	18.6	19.6	20.7	23.0
7.0–7.9	67	18.7	2.4	15.6	16.6	17.0	17.3	18.4	19.7	20.3	21.0	22.6
8.0–8.9	49	19.2	1.9	17.1	17.1	17.3	17.6	19.0	20.3	20.9	21.8	23.1
9.0–9.9	74	20.0	2.3	17.0	17.5	18.4	18.7	19.6	21.0	21.9	22.2	25.0
10.0–10.9	60	21.3	3.0	18.0	18.5	19.1	19.7	20.4	21.8	23.3	25.0	27.3
11.0–11.9	71	22.2	3.2	18.2	19.2	19.4	20.5	21.3	22.8	26.0	27.2	28.7
12.0–12.9	71	23.3	4.1	19.2	20.1	20.4	20.8	22.3	24.0	27.1	27.9	29.0
13.0–13.9	74	24.2	3.4	19.8	20.3	20.9	21.7	23.4	25.9	28.1	28.8	29.9
14.0–14.9	68	25.5	2.9	21.5	22.2	22.5	23.4	25.4	26.9	28.2	28.7	31.5
15.0–15.9	65	27.6	3.2	23.0	24.0	24.7	25.4	27.3	29.0	30.9	31.1	33.2
16.0–16.9	66	28.8	2.6	25.2	25.7	25.9	27.2	28.6	30.1	31.5	32.5	34.0
17.0–17.9	63	28.5	3.2	24.3	25.3	25.6	26.4	28.0	29.8	32.0	32.6	36.2
18.0–24.9	254	30.8	3.8	25.9	27.0	27.4	28.2	30.2	32.6	33.8	34.8	38.0
25.0–29.9	162	32.3	4.3	26.8	28.0	28.5	29.5	31.7	34.5	36.2	37.2	39.8
30.0–34.9	121	33.4	4.1	28.0	29.4	29.9	31.0	32.6	35.3	36.8	38.0	39.3
35.0–39.9	88	33.8	3.9	27.2	27.7	29.6	31.1	33.9	36.5	37.6	38.2	39.3
40.0–44.9	90	33.2	3.9	26.3	28.0	29.0	30.3	33.2	36.1	37.1	37.7	40.0
45.0–49.9	113	33.0	4.1	26.8	27.8	28.8	30.1	32.7	35.6	37.2	38.5	40.1
50.0–54.9	105	33.1	4.5	26.5	27.9	28.3	29.9	32.7	35.7	38.6	39.4	40.1
55.0–59.9	105	32.9	4.1	26.9	27.9	28.7	30.0	32.3	35.3	37.4	38.1	39.1
60.0–64.9	127	32.4	3.8	26.0	27.8	28.8	30.0	32.8	34.1	36.1	37.9	39.0
65.0–69.9	254	31.3	4.0	25.7	26.6	27.4	28.5	31.0	34.0	35.5	36.5	38.6
70.0–74.9	186	30.4	3.7	25.1	25.9	26.5	27.5	30.3	32.5	34.3	35.2	37.0
Females												
1.0–1.9	134	15.5	1.3	13.5	14.0	14.3	14.7	15.6	16.3	16.7	17.0	17.6
2.0–2.9	119	16.1	1.4	13.8	14.3	14.7	15.2	16.0	17.0	17.5	17.8	18.4
3.0–3.9	126	16.3	1.4	14.3	14.7	14.9	15.4	16.2	17.1	17.5	18.4	19.0
4.0–4.9	147	16.9	1.7	14.1	14.8	15.2	15.8	16.8	17.8	18.6	19.1	19.8
5.0–5.9	163	17.6	2.0	14.8	15.5	16.0	16.3	17.2	18.5	19.4	20.2	21.6
6.0–6.9	72	18.2	2.4	15.7	16.0	16.3	16.8	17.5	18.8	19.9	20.2	22.0
7.0–7.9	80	18.8	2.0	16.4	16.7	16.8	17.3	18.6	19.9	20.3	21.0	22.0
8.0–8.9	54	19.3	2.2	16.0	17.0	17.4	17.9	19.0	20.0	21.6	22.5	23.6
9.0–9.9	71	20.2	2.5	16.9	17.8	17.9	18.6	19.6	21.3	23.1	23.7	25.1
10.0–10.9	62	22.1	3.5	18.3	18.7	19.0	19.5	21.2	23.8	26.0	26.8	28.9
11.0–11.9	67	23.3	4.0	18.8	19.6	20.1	20.7	22.1	25.1	26.6	29.6	30.0
12.0–12.9	72	24.2	4.5	17.9	19.1	19.3	20.7	23.9	26.3	29.0	30.1	33.0
13.0–13.9	82	25.1	3.5	20.5	21.3	21.8	22.8	24.5	26.7	27.8	30.1	31.3
14.0–14.9	79	25.6	4.4	20.8	21.2	21.8	22.3	24.7	27.2	29.5	31.6	33.4
15.0–15.9	73	26.0	4.1	21.7	22.3	22.6	23.2	25.0	27.8	29.1	31.2	37.1
16.0–16.9	54	27.6	4.3	22.8	23.3	23.9	24.7	26.4	29.3	31.4	33.8	38.3
17.0–17.9	68	26.9	4.3	21.8	22.5	23.6	24.2	26.0	28.2	30.1	34.6	35.6
18.0–24.9	474	28.0	4.6	22.4	23.2	24.0	24.9	27.0	30.2	32.2	34.5	37.3
25.0–29.9	279	29.9	5.0	23.4	24.3	25.1	26.0	29.3	32.3	34.6	37.2	40.1
30.0–34.9	237	31.2	5.3	23.9	25.0	25.9	27.2	30.9	34.5	36.5	37.8	41.4
35.0–39.9	239	32.5	5.7	24.0	25.1	26.5	28.4	32.0	36.0	37.7	39.5	43.7
40.0–44.9	232	32.7	5.7	24.6	25.6	27.4	29.1	32.1	35.9	37.8	39.7	41.1
45.0–49.9	126	33.0	6.2	24.8	26.4	27.2	29.2	31.6	35.8	38.4	41.0	44.2
50.0–54.9	135	33.7	5.2	24.8	27.2	28.4	30.7	33.7	36.7	39.3	40.2	43.6
55.0–59.9	124	34.2	7.0	24.0	27.3	28.4	29.5	33.5	36.8	39.5	42.9	48.2
60.0–64.9	153	33.0	5.0	25.1	26.3	28.1	29.3	32.7	36.0	38.0	39.1	41.8
65.0–69.9	282	32.0	4.7	24.0	26.1	27.6	29.0	31.8	35.1	36.8	37.7	39.4
70.0–74.9	197	31.0	4.4	23.3	25.5	26.3	27.7	31.5	34.0	35.0	36.2	39.0

From Frisancho AR. Anthropometric standards for the assessment of growth and nutritional status. Ann Arbor: University of Michigan Press, 1990, Appendix A, Table 10. With permission.

A-16-d-1
Percentiles of Upper Arm Muscle Area (cm^2) by Age for Males Ranging in Age from 18 to 74 Years

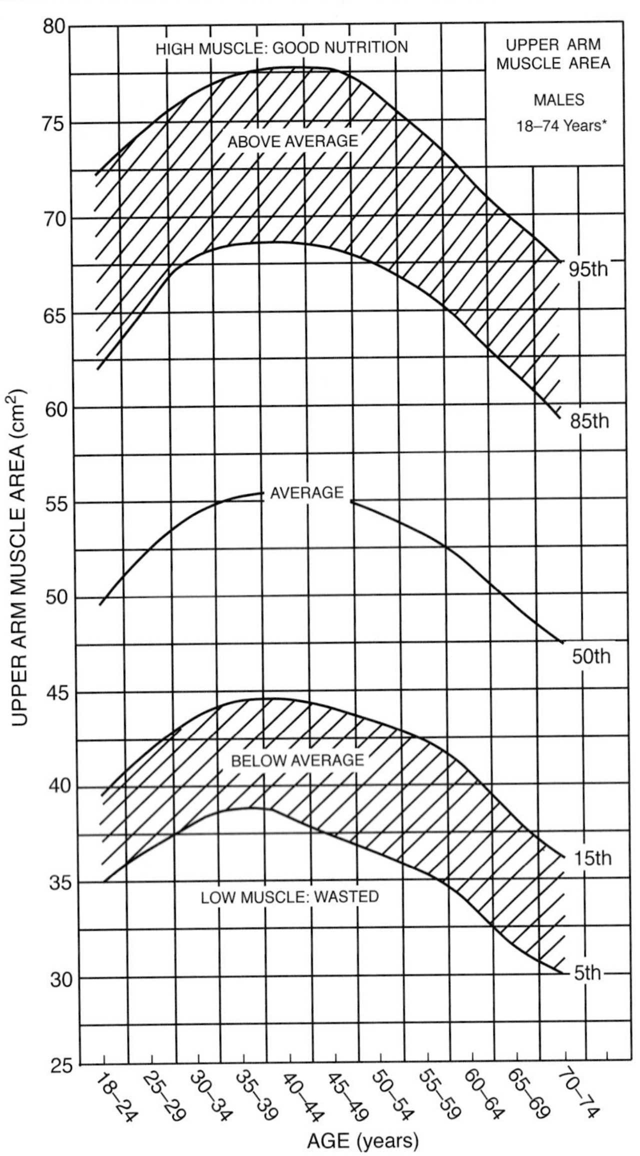

Note: Values for males aged 18 years and older have been adjusted for bone area by subtracting 10.0 cm^2 from the calculated muscle area. From Frisancho AR. Anthropometric standards for the assessment of growth and nutritional status. Ann Arbor: University of Michigan Press, 1990. Figure IV.23.

A-16-d-2
Percentiles of Upper Arm Muscle Area (cm^2) by Age for Females Ranging in Age from 18 to 74 Years

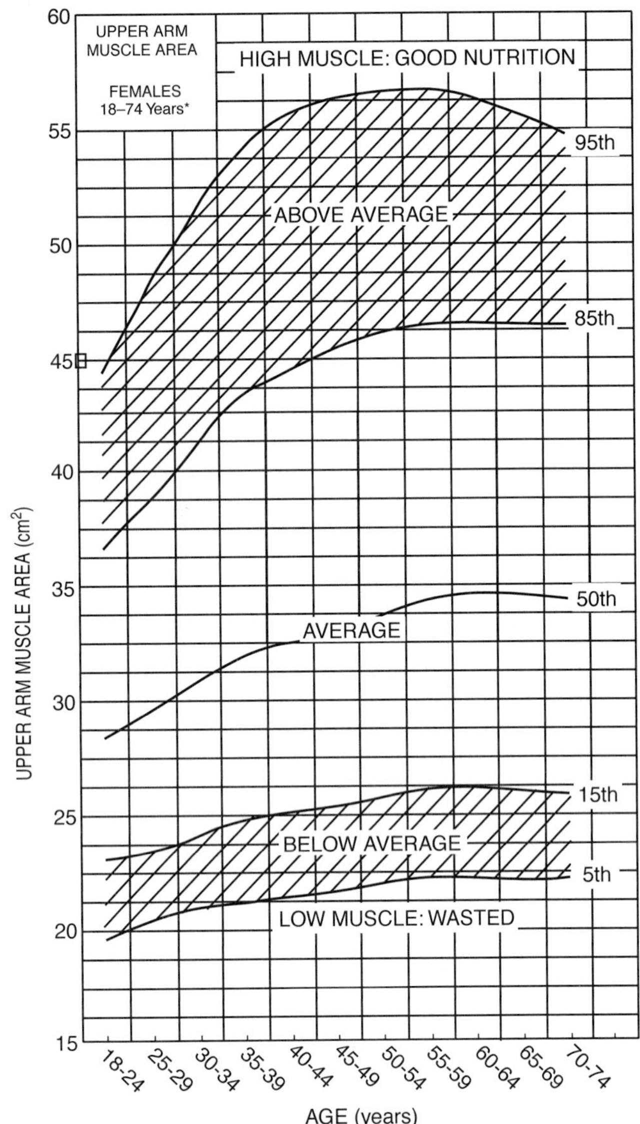

Note: Values for females aged 18 years and older have been adjusted for bone area by subtracting 6.5 cm^2 from the calculated muscle area. From Frisancho AR. Anthropometric standards for the assessment of growth and nutritional status. Ann Arbor: University of Michigan Press, 1990. Figure IV.26.

A-16-e-1

Percentiles of Sum of Triceps and Subscapular Skinfold Thicknesses by Age for Males Ranging in Age from 18 to 74 Years

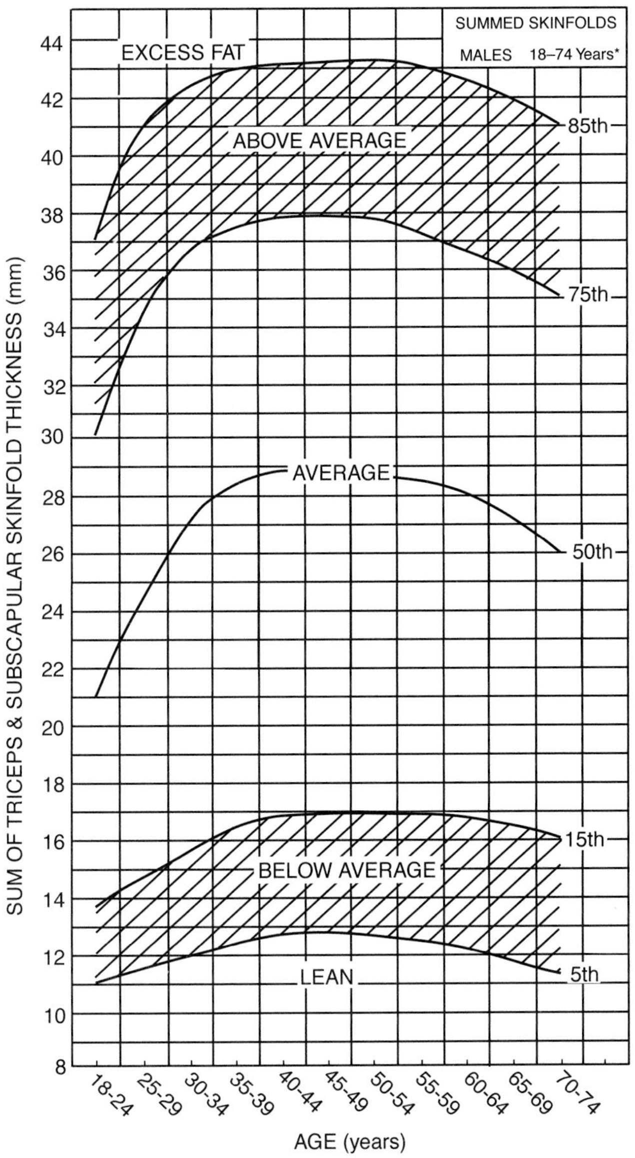

*From Frisancho AR. Anthropometric standards for the assessment of growth and nutritional status. Ann Arbor: University of Michigan Press, 1990. Figure IV.39.

A-16-e-2

Percentiles of Sum of Triceps and Subscapular Skinfold Thicknesses by Age for Females Ranging in Age from 18 to 74 Years

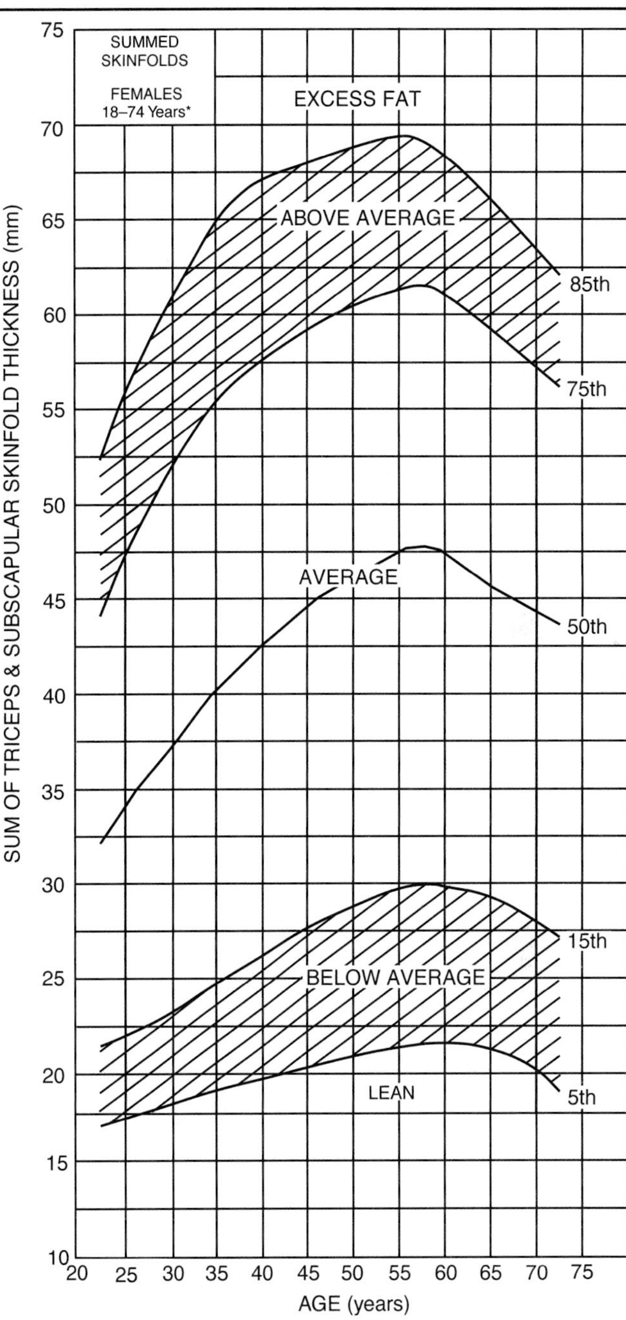

*From Frisancho AR. Anthropometric standards for the assessment of growth and nutritional status. Ann Arbor: University of Michigan Press, 1990. Figure IV.42.

Table A-16-f-1
Provisional Percentiles for Triceps Skinfold Thickness in the Elderly[a,b]

Age Group (years)	Percentile 5th	50th	95th
Men			
65	8.6	13.8	27.0
70	7.7	12.9	26.1
75	6.8	12.0	25.2
80	6.0	11.2	24.3
85	5.1	10.3	23.4
90	4.2	9.4	22.6
Women			
65	13.5	21.6	33.0
70	12.5	20.6	32.0
75	11.5	19.6	31.0
80	10.5	18.6	30.0
85	9.5	17.6	29.0
90	8.5	16.6	28.0

From Chumlea WC, Roche AF, Mukherjee D. Nutritional assessment of the elderly through anthropometry. Dayton, Ohio, Wright State University School of Medicine, 1984. With permission.

[a]Data are from 119 men and 150 women. All subjects were ambulatory, and measurements were made in the recumbent position on the left side.

[b]See Tables A-16-a for data compiled by Frisancho from NHANES I and II.

Table A-16-f-2
Provisional Percentiles for Midarm Muscle Area (cm^2) in the Elderly[a,b]

Age Group (years)	Percentile 5th	50th	95th
Men			
65	43.2	59.4	77.1
70	41.4	57.7	75.3
75	39.6	55.9	73.5
80	37.8	54.1	71.7
85	36.0	52.3	69.9
90	34.3	50.5	68.2
Women			
65	33.5	44.5	66.4
70	33.0	44.1	65.9
75	32.6	43.6	65.5
80	32.2	43.2	65.1
85	31.8	42.8	64.7
90	31.3	42.4	64.2

From Chumlea WC, Roche AF, Mukherjee D. Nutritional assessment of the elderly through anthropometry. Dayton, Ohio, Wright State University School of Medicine, 1984. With permission.

[a]Data are from 119 men and 150 women. All subjects were ambulatory, and measurements were made in the recumbent position on the left side.

[b]See Tables A-16-d for data compiled by Frisancho from NHANES I and II.

Table A-16-g
Means, Standard Deviations of Percent Fat Weight (%) in Percentiles by Age for Males and Females, 18 to 74 Years

Age (years)	N	Mean	SD	Percentiles 5	10	15	25	50	75	85	90	95
Males												
18.0–24.9	1708	16.5	6.2	8.0	9.0	10.0	12.0	16.0	20.0	23.0	25.0	28.0
25.0–29.9	1217	18.2	6.2	9.0	10.0	11.0	13.0	18.0	23.0	25.0	26.0	29.0
30.0–34.9	916	22.6	4.2	16.0	17.0	18.0	20.0	23.0	26.0	27.0	28.0	30.0
35.0–39.9	817	22.5	4.1	15.0	17.0	18.0	20.0	23.0	25.0	27.0	27.0	29.0
40.0–44.9	805	25.3	6.6	14.0	16.0	18.0	21.0	26.0	30.0	32.0	34.0	36.0
45.0–49.9	842	25.7	6.6	15.0	17.0	19.0	21.0	26.0	30.0	32.0	34.0	36.0
50.0–54.9	858	26.4	6.7	15.0	17.0	19.0	22.0	27.0	31.0	33.0	35.0	37.0
55.0–59.9	780	26.6	6.4	15.0	18.0	20.0	22.0	27.0	31.0	33.0	35.0	37.0
60.0–64.9	1228	26.8	6.5	16.0	18.0	20.0	22.0	27.0	31.0	33.0	35.0	37.0
65.0–69.9	1725	25.8	6.9	13.0	16.0	18.0	21.0	26.0	30.0	33.0	35.0	37.0
70.0–74.9	1229	25.4	6.7	13.0	16.0	18.0	21.0	26.0	30.0	33.0	34.0	36.0
Females												
18.0–24.9	2585	27.9	7.0	17.0	19.0	21.0	23.0	27.0	33.0	35.0	37.0	40.0
25.0–29.9	1905	29.1	7.3	18.0	20.0	21.0	24.0	29.0	34.0	37.0	39.0	41.0
30.0–34.9	1613	31.4	6.4	21.0	23.0	25.0	27.0	31.0	36.0	38.0	40.0	42.0
35.0–39.9	1442	32.1	6.2	22.0	24.0	25.0	28.0	32.0	37.0	39.0	40.0	42.0
40.0–44.9	1376	34.9	5.7	25.0	28.0	29.0	31.0	35.0	39.0	41.0	42.0	43.0
45.0–49.9	952	35.5	5.6	26.0	28.0	29.0	32.0	36.0	39.0	41.0	42.0	44.0
50.0–54.9	991	38.9	6.4	27.0	30.0	32.0	35.0	39.0	43.0	46.0	47.0	48.0
55.0–59.9	867	38.9	6.5	27.0	30.0	32.0	35.0	39.0	44.0	45.0	47.0	49.0
60.0–64.9	1370	39.0	6.2	28.0	31.0	32.0	35.0	40.0	43.0	45.0	46.0	48.0
65.0–69.9	1927	38.0	6.2	27.0	30.0	32.0	34.0	38.0	42.0	44.0	46.0	47.0
70.0–74.9	1454	37.3	6.4	26.0	29.0	31.0	34.0	38.0	42.0	44.0	45.0	47.0

From Frisancho AR. Anthropometric standards for the assessment of growth and nutritional status. Ann Arbor: University of Michigan Press, 1990, Table IV, 19. With permission.

A-17. BODY FAT ESTIMATIONS FROM SKINFOLD DATA

Various investigators have developed equations for predicting the proportions of body fat by anthropometric measures of specific regions. Durnin and Womersley used four different skinfolds (Table A-17-a). Pollock, Schmidt, and Jackson have prepared tables based on three sites, including thigh skinfolds (Tables A-17-b and A-17-c). Because some technicians have difficulty obtaining consistent results with thigh skinfold measurements, data also are available based on equations that do not use this skinfold. These data are included in the following sources:

Golding LA, Meyers CR, Sinning WE. Y's way to physical fitness: the complete guide to fitness testing and instruction. 3rd ed. Champaign, IL: Human Kinetics Publishers, 1989.

Pollock ML, Schmidt DH, Jackson AS. Compr Ther 1980;6:12–27.

Jackson AS, Pollock ML. Phys Sportsmed 1985;13:76–90.

—The Appendix Editors

Table A-17-a
Equivalent Fat Content, as Percentage of Body Weight, for a Range of Values for the Sum of Four Skinfolds[a]

Skinfolds (mm)	Men (age in years)				Women (age in years)			
	17–29	30–39	40–49	50+	16–29	30–39	40–49	50+
15	4.8				10.5			
20	8.1	12.2	12.2	12.6	14.1	17.0	19.8	21.4
25	10.5	14.2	15.0	15.6	16.8	19.4	22.2	24.0
30	12.9	16.2	17.7	18.6	19.5	21.8	24.5	26.6
35	14.7	17.7	19.6	20.8	21.5	23.7	26.4	28.5
40	16.4	19.2	21.4	22.9	23.4	25.5	28.2	30.3
45	17.7	20.4	23.0	24.7	25.0	26.9	29.6	31.9
50	19.0	21.5	24.6	26.5	26.5	28.2	31.0	33.4
55	20.1	22.5	25.9	27.9	27.8	29.4	32.1	34.6
60	21.2	23.5	27.1	29.2	29.1	30.6	33.2	35.7
65	22.2	24.3	28.2	30.4	30.2	31.6	34.1	36.7
70	23.1	25.1	29.3	31.6	31.2	32.5	35.0	37.7
75	24.0	25.9	30.3	32.7	32.2	33.4	35.9	38.7
80	24.8	26.6	31.2	33.8	33.1	34.3	36.7	39.6
85	25.5	27.2	32.1	34.8	34.0	35.1	37.5	40.4
90	26.2	27.8	33.0	35.8	34.8	35.8	38.3	41.2
95	26.9	28.4	33.7	36.6	35.6	36.5	39.0	41.9
100	27.6	29.0	34.4	37.4	36.4	37.2	39.7	42.6
105	28.2	29.6	35.1	38.2	37.1	37.9	40.4	43.3
110	28.8	30.1	35.8	39.0	37.8	38.6	41.0	43.9
115	29.4	30.6	36.4	39.7	38.4	39.1	41.5	44.5
120	30.0	31.1	37.0	40.4	39.0	39.6	42.0	45.1
125	31.0	31.5	37.6	41.1	39.6	40.1	42.5	45.7
130	31.5	31.9	38.2	41.8	40.2	40.6	43.0	46.2
135	32.0	32.3	38.7	42.4	40.8	41.1	43.5	46.7
140	32.5	32.7	39.2	43.0	41.3	41.6	44.0	47.2
145	32.9	33.1	39.7	43.6	41.8	42.1	44.5	47.7
150	33.3	33.5	40.2	44.1	42.3	42.6	45.0	48.2
155	33.7	33.9	40.7	44.6	42.8	43.1	45.4	48.7
160	34.1	34.3	41.2	45.1	43.3	43.6	45.8	49.2
165	34.5	34.6	41.6	45.6	43.7	44.0	46.2	49.6
170	34.9	34.8	42.0	46.1	44.1	44.4	46.6	50.0
175	35.3					44.8	47.0	50.4
180	35.6					45.2	47.4	50.8
185	35.9					45.6	47.8	51.2
190						45.9	48.2	51.6
195						46.2	48.5	52.0
200						46.5	48.8	52.4
205							49.1	52.7
210							49.4	53.0

From Durnin JVGA, Womersley J. Br J Nutr 1974; 32:77–97, with permission.

[a]Biceps, triceps, subscapular, and suprailiac of men and women of different ages.

Table A-17-b
Percentage of Body Fat Estimation for Women From Age and Triceps, Supralium, and Thigh Skinfolds[a]

Sum of Skinfolds (mm)	Age to the last year								
	Under 22	23 to 27	28 to 32	33 to 37	38 to 42	43 to 47	48 to 52	53 to 57	Over 58
23–25	9.7	9.9	10.2	10.4	10.7	10.9	11.2	11.4	11.7
26–28	11.0	11.2	11.5	11.7	12.0	12.3	12.5	12.7	13.0
29–31	12.3	12.5	12.8	13.0	13.3	13.5	13.8	14.0	14.3
32–34	13.6	13.8	14.0	14.3	14.5	14.8	15.0	15.3	15.5
35–37	14.8	15.0	15.3	15.5	15.8	16.0	16.3	16.5	16.8
38–40	16.0	16.3	16.5	16.7	17.0	17.2	17.5	17.7	18.0
41–43	17.2	17.4	17.7	17.9	18.2	18.4	18.7	18.9	19.2
44–46	18.3	18.6	18.8	19.1	19.3	19.6	19.8	20.1	20.3
47–49	19.5	19.7	20.0	20.2	20.5	20.7	21.0	21.2	21.5
50–52	20.6	20.8	21.1	21.3	21.6	21.8	22.1	22.3	22.6
53–55	21.7	21.9	22.1	22.4	22.6	22.9	23.1	23.4	23.6
56–58	22.7	23.0	23.2	23.4	23.7	23.9	24.2	24.4	24.7
59–61	23.7	24.0	24.2	24.5	24.7	25.0	25.2	25.5	25.7
62–64	24.7	25.0	25.2	25.5	25.7	26.0	26.7	26.4	26.7
65–67	25.7	25.9	26.2	26.4	26.7	26.9	27.2	27.4	27.7
68–70	26.6	26.9	27.1	27.4	27.6	27.9	28.1	28.4	28.6
71–73	27.5	27.8	28.0	28.3	28.5	28.8	28.0	29.3	29.5
74–76	28.4	28.7	28.9	29.2	29.4	29.7	29.9	30.2	30.4
77–79	29.3	29.5	29.8	30.0	30.3	30.5	30.8	31.0	31.3
80–82	30.1	30.4	30.6	30.9	31.1	31.4	31.6	31.9	32.1
83–85	30.9	31.2	31.4	31.7	31.9	32.2	32.4	32.7	32.9
86–88	31.7	32.0	32.2	32.5	32.7	32.9	33.2	33.4	33.7
89–91	32.5	32.7	33.0	33.2	33.5	33.7	33.9	34.2	34.4
92–94	33.2	33.4	33.7	33.9	34.2	34.4	34.7	34.9	35.2
95–97	33.9	34.1	34.4	34.6	34.9	35.1	35.4	35.6	35.9
98–100	34.6	34.8	35.1	35.3	35.5	35.8	36.0	36.3	36.5
101–103	35.3	35.4	35.7	35.9	36.2	36.4	36.7	36.9	37.2
104–106	35.8	36.1	36.3	36.6	36.8	37.1	37.3	37.5	37.8
107–109	36.4	36.7	36.9	37.1	37.4	37.6	37.9	38.1	38.4
110–112	37.0	37.2	37.5	37.7	38.0	38.2	38.5	38.7	38.9
113–115	37.5	37.8	38.0	38.2	38.5	38.7	39.0	39.2	39.5
116–118	38.0	38.3	38.5	38.8	39.0	39.3	39.5	39.7	40.0
119–121	38.5	38.7	39.0	39.2	39.5	39.7	40.0	40.2	40.5
122–124	39.0	39.2	39.4	39.7	39.9	40.2	40.4	40.7	40.9
125–127	39.4	39.6	39.9	40.1	40.4	40.6	40.9	41.1	41.4
128–130	39.8	40.0	40.3	40.5	40.8	41.0	41.3	41.5	41.8

Reprinted with permission from Pollock ML, Schmidt DH, Jackson AS. Measurement of cardiorespiratory fitness and body composition in the clinical setting. Compr Ther 1980; 6:12–27.

[a]Percentage of fat calculated by the formula of Siri: percentage of fat = $(4.95/D_b - 4.5) \times 100$, where Db = body density.

Table A-17-c
Percentage of Body Fat Estimation for Men From Age and the Sum of Chest, Abdominal, and Thigh Skinfolds[a]

Sum of Skinfolds (mm)	Age to the last year								
	Under 22	23 to 27	28 to 32	33 to 37	38 to 42	43 to 47	48 to 52	53 to 57	Over 58
23–25	9.7	9.9	10.2	10.4	10.7	10.9	11.2	11.4	11.7
26–28	11.0	11.2	11.5	11.7	12.0	12.3	12.5	12.7	13.0
29–31	12.3	12.5	12.8	13.0	13.3	13.5	13.8	14.0	14.3
32–34	13.6	13.8	14.0	14.3	14.5	14.8	15.0	15.3	15.5
35–37	14.8	15.0	15.3	15.5	15.8	16.0	16.3	16.5	16.8
38–40	16.0	16.3	16.5	16.7	17.0	17.2	17.5	17.7	18.0
41–43	17.2	17.4	17.7	17.9	18.2	18.4	18.7	18.9	19.2
44–46	18.3	18.6	18.8	19.1	19.3	19.6	19.8	20.1	20.3
47–49	19.5	19.7	20.0	20.2	20.5	20.7	21.0	21.2	21.5
50–52	20.6	20.8	21.1	21.3	21.6	21.8	22.1	22.3	22.6
53–55	21.7	21.9	22.1	22.4	22.6	22.9	23.1	23.4	23.6
56–58	22.7	23.0	23.2	23.4	23.7	23.9	24.2	24.4	24.7
59–61	23.7	24.0	24.2	24.5	24.7	25.0	25.2	25.5	25.7
62–64	24.7	25.0	25.2	25.5	25.7	26.0	26.7	26.4	26.7
65–67	25.7	25.9	26.2	26.4	26.7	26.9	27.2	27.4	27.7
68–70	26.6	26.9	27.1	27.4	27.6	27.9	28.1	28.4	28.6
71–73	27.5	27.8	28.0	28.3	28.5	28.8	29.0	29.3	29.5
74–76	28.4	28.7	28.9	29.2	29.4	29.7	29.9	30.2	30.4
77–79	29.3	29.5	29.8	30.0	30.3	30.5	30.8	31.0	31.3
80–82	30.1	30.4	30.6	30.9	31.1	31.4	31.6	31.9	32.1
83–85	30.9	31.2	31.4	31.7	31.9	32.2	32.4	32.7	32.9
86–88	31.7	32.0	32.2	32.5	32.7	32.9	33.2	33.4	33.7
89–91	32.5	32.7	33.0	33.2	33.5	33.7	33.9	34.2	34.4
92–94	33.2	33.4	33.7	33.9	34.2	34.4	34.7	34.9	35.2
95–97	33.9	34.1	34.4	34.6	34.9	35.1	35.4	35.6	35.9
98–100	34.6	34.8	35.1	35.3	35.5	35.8	36.0	36.3	36.5
101–103	35.3	35.4	35.7	35.9	36.2	36.4	36.7	36.9	37.2
104–106	35.8	36.1	36.3	36.6	36.8	37.1	37.3	37.5	37.8
107–109	36.4	36.7	36.9	37.1	37.4	37.6	37.9	38.1	38.4
110–112	37.0	37.2	37.5	37.7	38.0	38.2	38.5	38.7	38.9
113–115	37.5	37.8	38.0	38.2	38.5	38.7	39.0	39.2	39.5
116–118	38.0	38.3	38.5	38.8	39.0	39.3	39.5	39.7	40.0
119–121	38.5	38.7	39.0	39.2	39.5	39.7	40.0	40.2	40.5
122–124	39.0	39.2	39.4	39.7	39.9	40.2	40.4	40.7	40.9
125–127	39.4	39.6	39.9	40.1	40.4	40.6	40.9	41.1	41.4
128–130	39.8	40.0	40.3	40.5	40.8	41.0	41.3	41.5	41.8

Reprinted with permission from Pollock ML, Schmidt DH, Jackson AS. Measurement of cardiorespiratory fitness and body composition in the clinical setting. Compr Ther 1980;6:12–27.

[a]Percentage of fat calculated by the formula of Siri: percentage of fat = $(4.95/D_b - 4.5) \times 100$, where D_b = body density.

Table A-17-d-1
Mean Percentage Body Fat Weight by Sum of Triceps and Subscapular Skinfold Thicknesses for Adults Ranging in Age from 18 to 49 Years

Males		Females	
Summed Skinfold Thicknesses Range (mm)	Percentage Fat Weight (Mean ± SD)	Summed Skinfold Thicknesses Range (mm)	Percentage Fat Weight (Mean ± SD)
Age group: 18 to 24 years			
9 to 11	6.8 ± 1.0	8 to 17	15.5 ± 2.3
12 to 13	9.3 ± 0.7	18 to 21	19.8 ± 1.1
14 to 30	15.2 ± 3.1	22 to 44	27.0 ± 3.2
31 to 37	22.1 ± 0.8	45 to 52	34.1 ± 0.8
38 to 113	27.2 ± 3.0	53 to 130	39.5 ± 3.0
Age group: 25 to 29 years			
9 to 12	7.9 ± 1.2	9 to 17	15.3 ± 2.2
13 to 14	10.2 ± 0.4	18 to 22	20.1 ± 1.2
15 to 35	17.1 ± 3.3	23 to 48	28.1 ± 3.5
36 to 42	23.9 ± 0.7	49 to 58	35.9 ± 0.9
43 to 100	28.2 ± 2.6	59 to 116	40.9 ± 2.7
Age group: 30 to 34 years			
9 to 13	14.4 ± 1.1	9 to 18	18.4 ± 2.2
14 to 17	17.2 ± 0.9	19 to 24	23.3 ± 1.0
18 to 38	22.2 ± 2.1	25 to 55	30.6 ± 3.1
39 to 44	26.3 ± 0.5	56 to 64	37.2 ± 0.7
45 to 104	29.1 ± 1.7	65 to 117	41.3 ± 2.1
Age group: 35 to 39 years			
8 to 12	13.9 ± 1.1	8 to 19	19.5 ± 2.3
13 to 17	16.7 ± 0.9	20 to 25	23.8 ± 1.1
18 to 37	22.3 ± 2.0	26 to 57	31.4 ± 3.1
38 to 42	26.0 ± 0.4	58 to 66	37.7 ± 0.6
43 to 114	28.6 ± 1.8	67 to 112	41.3 ± 2.0
Age group: 40 to 44 years			
8 to 13	12.6 ± 1.6	8 to 20	22.9 ± 2.8
14 to 17	16.6 ± 1.1	21 to 27	27.8 ± 1.2
18 to 37	24.7 ± 3.1	28 to 58	34.5 ± 2.8
38 to 43	31.0 ± 0.8	59 to 67	40.2 ± 0.6
44 to 92	35.5 ± 2.7	68 to 115	43.2 ± 1.7
Age group: 45 to 49 years			
9 to 14	12.8 ± 2.0	8 to 21	23.4 ± 2.5
15 to 18	17.5 ± 1.1	22 to 27	27.8 ± 1.0
19 to 39	25.3 ± 3.3	28 to 59	35.0 ± 2.8
40 to 44	31.7 ± 0.6	60 to 69	40.5 ± 0.6
45 to 98	35.6 ± 2.7	70 to 117	43.6 ± 1.6

From Frisancho AR. Anthropometric standards for the assessment of growth and nutritional status. Ann Arbor: University of Michigan Press, 1990, Table IV. 20. With permission.

Table A-17-d-2
Mean Percentage Body Fat Weight by Sum of Triceps and Subscapular Skinfold Thicknesses for Adults Ranging in Age from 50 to 74 Years

Males		Females	
Summed Skinfold Thicknesses Range (mm)	Percentage Fat Weight (Mean ± SD)	Summed Skinfold Thicknesses Range (mm)	Percentage Fat Weight (Mean ± SD)
Age group: 50 to 54 years			
8 to 13	12.9 ± 2.2	10 to 21	24.1 ± 3.1
14 to 17	17.5 ± 1.1	22 to 30	30.5 ± 1.5
18 to 37	25.7 ± 3.2	31 to 61	38.7 ± 3.0
38 to 43	32.3 ± 0.8	62 to 70	44.7 ± 0.7
44 to 94	36.8 ± 2.5	71 to 114	48.1 ± 1.8
Age group: 55 to 59 years			
9 to 13	13.2 ± 1.5	12 to 21	24.5 ± 2.2
14 to 18	18.5 ± 1.3	22 to 29	30.3 ± 1.4
19 to 37	26.2 ± 3.0	30 to 62	38.6 ± 3.2
38 to 43	32.3 ± 0.8	63 to 69	44.6 ± 0.5
44 to 86	36.4 ± 2.4	70 to 125	48.1 ± 2.2
Age group: 60 to 64 years			
9 to 14	14.1 ± 1.9	8 to 22	25.2 ± 2.7
15 to 18	18.6 ± 1.1	23 to 30	30.8 ± 1.3
19 to 37	26.1 ± 3.1	31 to 61	38.6 ± 3.0
38 to 43	32.2 ± 0.7	62 to 68	44.4 ± 0.5
44 to 94	36.9 ± 2.7	69 to 120	47.9 ± 1.9
Age group: 65 to 69 years			
8 to 12	12.0 ± 1.6	8 to 21	24.0 ± 2.9
13 to 16	16.6 ± 1.1	22 to 29	30.1 ± 1.4
17 to 36	25.2 ± 3.4	30 to 57	37.7 ± 2.8
37 to 42	31.9 ± 0.8	58 to 64	43.4 ± 0.5
43 to 102	36.4 ± 2.7	65 to 118	46.9 ± 2.1
Age group: 70 to 74 years			
9 to 12	12.0 ± 1.3	8 to 19	22.5 ± 2.9
13 to 16	16.6 ± 1.1	20 to 27	29.1 ± 1.4
17 to 35	24.7 ± 3.2	28 to 56	37.2 ± 3.1
36 to 41	31.3 ± 0.9	57 to 62	43.0 ± 0.6
42 to 90	35.8 ± 2.6	63 to 122	46.3 ± 2.0

From Frisancho, AR. Anthropometric standards for the assessment of growth and nutritional status. Ann Arbor, University of Michigan Press, 1990. Table IV. 21. With permission.

A-18. GROWTH AND ANTHROPOMETRIC DATA FOR CLINICAL CONDITIONS

Table A-18-a-1

Classification of Overweight and Obesity by BMI, Waist Circumference, and Associated Disease Risks

			Disease Risk[a] Relative to Normal Weight and Waist Circumference[b]	
	BMI (kg/m2)	Obesity Class	Men ≤ 102 cm (≤40 in) Women ≤ 88 cm (≤35 in)	>102 cm (>40 in) >88 cm (>35 in)
Underweight	<18.5		—	—
Normal	18.5–24.9		—	—
Overweight	25.0–29.9		Increased	High
Obesity	30.0–34.9	I	High	Very High
	35.0–39.9	II	Very High	Very High
Extreme Obesity	≥40	III	Extremely High	Extremely High

From U.S. Department of Health and Human Services, National Institutes of Health, National Heart, Lung, and Blood Institute. Clinical guidelines on the identification, evaluation, and treatment of overweight and obesity in adults. The evidence report. Bethesda, MD; Preprint June 1998:228pp. This is Table ES-4 in the original report.

[a]Disease risk for type 2 diabetes, hypertension, and CVD.

[b]Increased waist circumference can also be a marker for increased risk, even in persons of normal weight.

Table A-18-a-2

Selected BMI Units Categorized by Inches (cm) and Pounds (kg)

	BMI 25 kg/m^2	BMI 27 kg/m^2	BMI 30 kg/m^2
Height in Inches (cm)	Body Weight in Pounds (kg)		
58 (147.32)	119 (53.98)	129 (58.51)	143 (64.86)
59 (149.86)	124 (56.25)	133 (60.33)	148 (67.13)
60 (152.40)	128 (58.06)	138 (62.60)	153 (69.40)
61 (154.94)	132 (59.87)	143 (64.86)	158 (71.67)
62 (157.48)	136 (61.69)	147 (66.68)	164 (74.39)
63 (160.02)	141 (63.96)	152 (68.95)	169 (76.66)
64 (162.56)	145 (65.77)	157 (71.22)	174 (78.93)
65 (165.10)	150 (68.04)	162 (73.48)	180 (81.65)
66 (167.64)	155 (70.31)	167 (75.75)	186 (84.37)
67 (170.18)	159 (72.12)	172 (78.02)	191 (86.64)
68 (172.72)	164 (74.39)	177 (80.29)	197 (89.36)
69 (175.26)	169 (76.66)	182 (82.56)	203 (92.08)
70 (177.80)	174 (78.93)	188 (85.28)	207 (93.90)
71 (180.34)	179 (81.19)	193 (87.54)	215 (97.52)
72 (182.88)	184 (83.46)	199 (90.27)	221 (100.25)
73 (185.42)	189 (85.73)	204 (92.53)	227 (102.97)
74 (187.96)	194 (88.00)	210 (95.26)	233 (105.69)
75 (190.50)	200 (90.72)	216 (97.98)	240 (108.86)
76 (193.04)	205 (92.99)	221 (100.25)	246 (111.59)

Metric conversion formula = weight (kg)/height (m)^2

Example of BMI calculation:
A person who weighs 78.93 kilograms and is 177 centimeters tall has a BMI of 25:
weight (78.93 kg)/height (1.77 m)^2 = 25

Non-metric conversion formula = [weight (pounds)/height (inches)^2] × 704.5

Example of BMI calculation:
A person who weighs 164 pounds and is 68 inches (or 5′8″) tall has a BMI of 25:
[weight (164 pounds)/height (68 inches)^2] × 704.5 = 25

From U.S. Department of Health and Human Services, National Institutes of Health, National Heart, Lung, and Blood Institute. Clinical guidelines on the identification, evaluation, and treatment of overweight and obesity in adults. The evidence report. Bethesda, MD; Preprint June 1998:228pp.

Table A-18-a-3
Age-Adjusted Prevalence of Overweight (BMI 25–29.9) and Obesity (BMI ≥30), Years 20–74

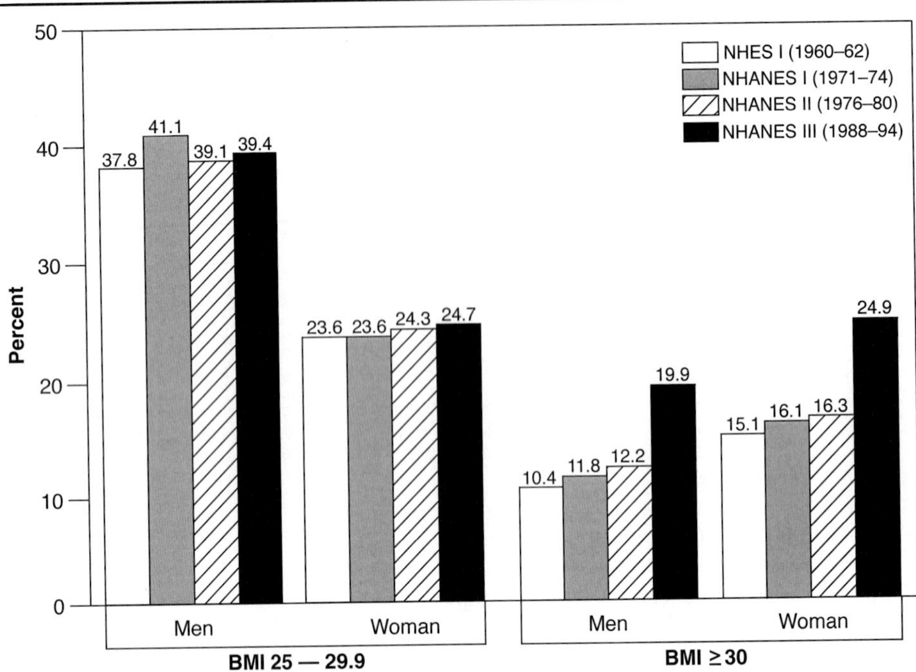

From Centers for Disease Control and Prevention. National center for Health Statistics. United States 1960–94. This is Figure 1 in reference of Table A-18-a-1.

A-18-b-1
Defining Obesity and Superobesity Using 85th and 95th Percentiles for Body Mass Index and Triceps Skinfold Thickness

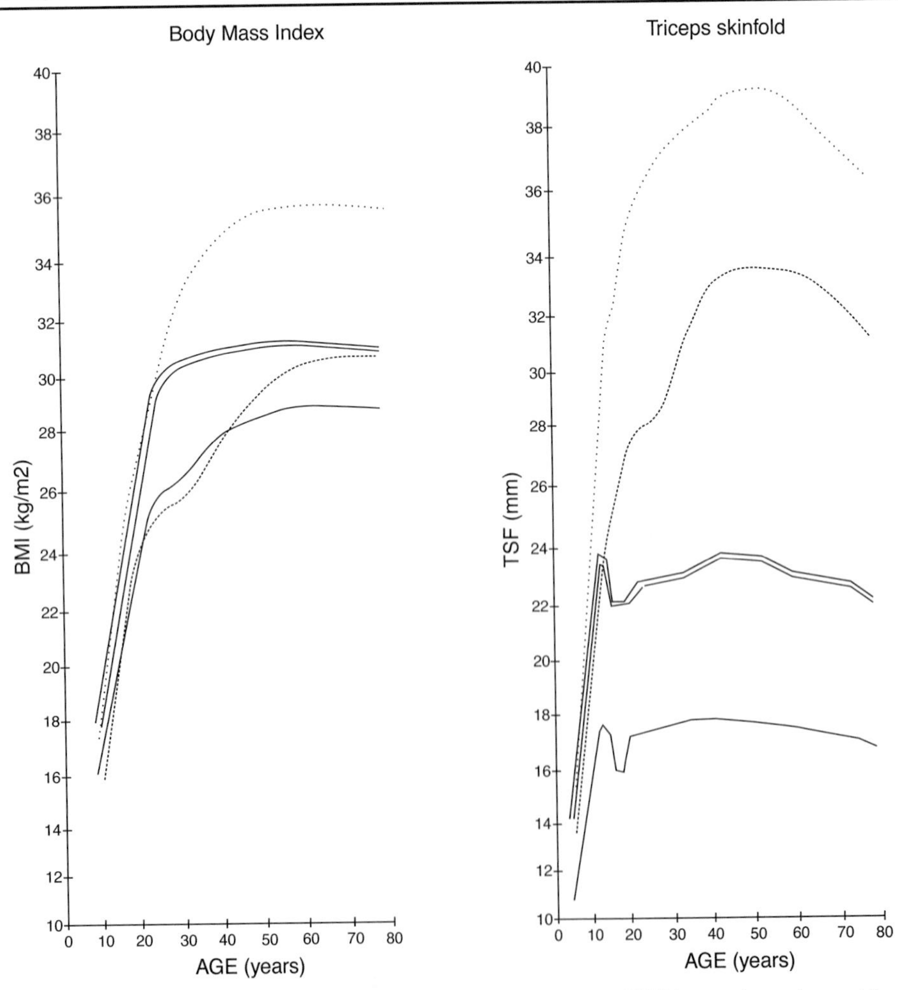

Smoothed 85th- and 95th-percentile body mass index (BMI) and triceps skinfold thickness (TSF) by age for males and females. —— , 85th percentile for males; ········ , 85th percentile for females; ═ , 95th percentile for males; ······ , 95th percentile for females. From Must A, Dallal GE, Dietz WH. Am J Clin Nutr 1991;53:839–846. These data were based on NHANES I data collected between 1971–1974 on 20,839 participants aged 6–74 years.

Table A-18-b-2
Smoothed 85th and 95th Percentiles of Body Mass Index (in kg/m²)

	Whites						Blacks						Population					
Age (y)	*n*	5th	15th	50th	85th	95th	*n*	5th	15th	50th	85th	95th	*n*	5th	15th	50th	85th	95th
Males																		
6	117	12.93	13.46	14.62	16.52	17.75	47	12.68	13.66	14.49	16.83	18.58	165	12.86	13.43	14.54	16.64	18.02
7	122	13.30	13.88	15.15	17.31	18.98	40	13.11	14.03	14.98	17.29	19.56	164	13.24	13.85	15.07	17.37	19.18
8	117	13.67	14.31	15.70	18.10	20.22	30	13.54	14.41	15.49	17.76	20.51	149	13.63	14.28	15.62	18.11	20.33
9	121	14.04	14.75	16.24	18.88	21.45	55	13.98	14.81	16.00	18.26	21.45	177	14.03	14.71	16.17	18.85	21.47
10	146	14.42	15.19	16.79	19.67	22.66	29	14.41	15.21	16.53	18.78	22.41	177	14.42	15.15	16.72	19.60	22.60
11	122	14.81	15.64	17.35	20.47	23.87	44	14.86	15.62	17.06	19.32	23.42	169	14.83	15.59	17.28	20.35	23.73
12	153	15.21	16.11	17.93	21.28	25.01	50	15.36	16.06	17.61	19.85	24.39	204	15.24	16.06	17.87	21.12	24.89
13	134	15.69	16.65	18.57	22.12	26.06	42	15.89	16.64	18.28	20.62	25.26	177	15.73	16.62	18.53	21.93	25.93
14	131	16.16	17.22	19.25	22.97	27.02	42	16.43	17.22	18.94	21.54	26.13	173	16.18	17.20	19.22	22.77	26.93
15	128	16.57	17.79	19.94	23.82	27.86	43	16.97	17.79	19.56	22.50	27.05	175	16.59	17.76	19.92	23.63	27.76
16	131	17.00	18.35	20.63	24.63	28.69	40	17.51	18.37	20.19	23.45	27.95	172	17.01	18.32	20.63	24.45	28.53
17	133	17.29	18.72	21.13	25.44	29.50	33	17.86	18.77	20.70	24.41	28.89	167	17.31	18.68	21.12	25.28	29.32
18	91	17.50	18.95	21.46	26.08	29.89	28	18.05	19.03	21.09	25.06	29.35	120	17.54	18.89	21.45	25.92	30.02
19	108	17.77	19.25	21.88	26.53	29.98	24	18.32	19.35	21.51	25.38	29.62	137	17.80	19.20	21.86	26.36	30.66
20–24	423	18.62	20.26	23.09	27.02	31.43	82	18.43	19.84	22.59	25.76	32.00	514	18.66	20.21	23.07	26.87	31.26
25–29	582	19.10	21.02	24.17	28.15	31.89	81	18.48	20.26	23.87	27.81	32.68	671	19.11	20.98	24.19	28.08	31.72
30–34	390	19.45	21.58	24.90	28.76	32.04	63	18.44	20.75	24.49	29.34	32.95	466	19.52	21.51	24.90	28.75	31.99
35–39	394	19.44	21.82	25.29	29.17	32.12	49	18.58	20.90	24.47	29.99	33.09	451	19.55	21.71	25.25	29.18	32.23
40–44	412	19.44	21.87	25.54	29.34	32.21	58	18.67	20.91	24.66	30.61	33.27	474	19.52	21.75	25.49	29.37	32.41
45–49	466	19.39	21.84	25.61	29.36	32.15	81	18.73	20.90	24.70	30.83	33.45	532	19.45	21.72	25.55	29.39	32.40
50–54	452	19.31	21.78	25.60	29.29	32.04	75	18.82	20.87	24.61	30.62	33.52	531	19.35	21.66	25.54	29.31	32.27
55–59	406	19.23	21.70	25.58	29.23	31.95	57	18.92	20.81	24.47	30.40	33.59	468	19.25	21.58	25.51	29.24	32.18
60–64	327	19.14	21.60	25.54	29.17	31.87	46	19.02	20.75	24.32	30.16	33.67	378	19.15	21.49	25.47	19.17	32.08
65–69	888	19.06	21.50	25.49	29.10	31.78	184	19.12	20.67	24.15	29.90	33.77	1084	19.05	21.39	25.41	29.08	31.98
70–74	616	18.98	21.39	25.41	29.01	31.69	129	19.21	20.60	23.97	29.60	33.86	752	18.94	21.29	25.33	28.99	31.87
Females																		
6	118	12.81	13.37	14.33	16.14	17.59	42	12.52	13.40	13.83	16.24	16.06	161	12.83	13.37	14.31	16.17	17.49
7	126	13.18	13.82	15.00	17.16	18.99	47	12.88	13.79	14.55	17.36	17.95	174	13.17	13.79	14.98	17.17	18.93
8	118	13.57	14.27	15.68	18.19	20.39	35	13.25	14.17	15.26	18.49	19.84	153	13.51	14.22	15.66	18.18	20.36
9	125	13.96	14.72	16.35	19.21	21.78	47	13.63	14.57	15.98	19.64	21.71	173	13.87	14.66	16.33	19.19	21.78
10	152	14.36	15.18	17.02	20.23	23.15	41	14.02	14.96	16.69	20.79	23.57	194	14.23	15.09	17.00	20.19	23.20
11	117	14.76	15.64	17.69	21.24	24.48	43	14.41	15.36	17.39	21.96	25.44	163	14.60	15.53	17.67	21.18	24.59
12	129	15.17	16.11	18.36	22.25	25.53	47	14.83	15.77	18.11	23.15	27.27	177	14.98	15.98	18.35	22.17	25.95
13	151	15.59	16.55	18.91	23.13	26.46	47	15.33	16.23	18.78	24.41	28.90	199	15.36	16.43	18.95	23.08	27.07
14	141	15.89	16.89	19.29	23.87	27.31	49	15.77	16.66	19.24	25.46	30.29	192	15.67	16.79	19.32	23.88	27.97
15	117	16.21	17.23	19.69	24.28	27.89	47	16.20	17.07	19.67	26.04	31.40	164	16.01	17.16	19.69	24.29	28.51
16	142	16.55	17.59	20.11	24.68	28.45	30	16.65	17.48	20.11	26.68	32.51	173	16.37	17.54	20.09	24.74	29.10
17	114	16.76	17.84	20.39	25.07	28.95	44	16.92	17.81	20.45	27.38	33.38	159	16.59	17.81	20.36	25.23	29.72
18	109	16.87	18.01	20.58	25.34	29.23	29	17.04	18.06	20.78	27.92	33.18	140	16.71	17.99	20.57	25.56	30.22
19	104	17.00	18.20	20.80	25.58	29.37	37	17.20	18.35	21.11	28.40	33.27	142	16.87	18.20	20.80	25.85	30.72
20–24	956	17.47	18.61	21.38	25.78	31.25	261	17.26	18.97	22.38	28.81	35.19	1244	17.38	18.64	21.46	26.14	31.20
25–29	1093	17.90	19.05	21.94	27.16	32.79	191	17.64	19.70	23.88	31.03	36.82	1307	17.84	19.09	22.10	27.68	33.16
30–34	900	18.21	19.48	22.47	28.38	34.07	180	18.23	20.41	25.06	32.28	37.79	1092	18.23	19.54	22.69	28.87	34.58
35–39	815	18.48	19.84	22.99	29.25	34.77	185	18.66	21.00	25.87	32.98	38.45	1017	18.51	19.91	23.25	29.54	35.35
40–44	799	18.61	20.13	23.48	29.90	35.04	183	18.76	21.60	26.61	34.06	39.12	999	18.65	20.20	23.74	30.11	35.85
45–49	519	18.67	20.40	23.91	30.38	35.09	79	18.66	21.97	27.07	34.75	39.26	603	18.71	20.45	24.17	30.56	36.02
50–54	529	18.76	20.62	24.30	30.66	35.09	83	18.52	22.19	27.32	35.11	39.35	615	18.79	20.66	24.54	30.79	35.95
55–59	416	18.84	20.83	24.69	30.93	35.08	74	18.38	22.40	27.52	35.50	39.49	492	18.88	20.86	24.92	31.00	35.88
60–64	394	18.92	21.04	25.08	31.20	35.04	68	18.21	22.60	27.71	35.92	39.64	463	18.96	21.06	25.29	31.21	35.80
65–69	958	18.99	21.25	25.46	31.46	34.98	194	18.01	22.79	27.87	36.32	39.77	1157	19.03	21.25	25.66	31.40	35.70
70–74	711	19.06	21.45	25.84	31.70	34.91	134	17.78	22.93	28.00	36.67	39.88	848	19.09	21.44	26.01	31.58	35.58

From Must A, Dallal GE, Dietz WH. Am J Clin Nutr 1991; 54:773. Data source: NHANES I. With permission.

Table A-18-b-3
Smoothed 85th and 95th Percentiles of Triceps Skinfold Thickness

Age (y)	Whites						Blacks						Population					
	n	5th	15th	50th (*mm*)	85th	95th	*n*	5th	15th	50th (*mm*)	85th	95th	*n*	5th	15th	50th (*mm*)	85th	95th
Males																		
6	117	5.26	6.09	8.74	11.63	14.47	47	4.01	4.86	6.85	9.35	12.86	165	5.04	6.19	8.36	11.10	14.12
7	122	5.28	6.12	8.94	12.78	15.95	40	4.01	4.88	6.85	10.09	14.11	164	5.01	6.14	8.59	12.38	15.61
8	117	5.28	6.15	9.12	13.95	17.51	30	4.00	4.88	6.84	10.76	15.35	149	4.96	6.08	8.79	13.66	17.18
9	121	5.27	6.17	9.27	15.10	19.11	55	3.99	4.88	6.83	11.37	16.50	177	4.91	6.02	8.96	14.93	18.81
10	146	5.24	6.18	9.40	16.29	20.96	29	3.98	4.88	6.81	11.52	17.79	177	4.84	5.95	9.10	16.02	20.68
11	122	5.20	6.20	9.51	17.32	22.53	44	3.97	4.89	6.81	11.31	18.68	169	4.78	5.88	9.23	16.87	22.20
12	153	5.15	6.23	9.59	17.79	23.53	50	3.97	4.91	6.80	10.79	18.74	204	4.69	5.79	9.35	17.26	23.25
13	134	5.01	6.21	9.42	17.63	23.87	42	3.94	4.88	6.72	10.23	18.67	177	4.56	5.65	9.17	17.12	23.71
14	131	4.91	6.15	9.26	16.88	23.42	42	3.86	4.84	6.66	9.92	18.58	173	4.47	5.60	8.93	16.35	23.46
15	128	4.81	6.10	9.12	16.11	22.42	43	3.81	4.80	6.62	9.96	18.99	175	4.40	5.59	8.70	15.75	22.34
16	131	4.69	6.05	8.95	15.81	22.05	40	3.76	4.77	6.58	10.30	20.18	172	4.33	5.55	8.45	15.75	21.53
17	133	4.61	6.02	8.92	15.95	21.99	33	3.69	4.72	6.63	10.73	21.12	167	4.29	5.58	8.38	15.95	21.51
18	91	4.53	6.01	9.02	16.69	22.28	28	3.60	4.64	6.79	11.34	21.95	120	4.25	5.63	8.53	16.59	21.83
19	108	4.48	6.00	9.09	17.53	22.65	24	3.52	4.57	6.92	11.95	22.88	137	4.22	5.69	8.63	17.33	22.12
20–24	423	4.67	6.00	9.90	18.11	23.00	82	3.55	4.38	6.95	12.29	22.90	514	4.21	5.97	9.70	17.84	22.53
25–29	582	4.80	6.30	10.72	18.28	23.47	81	3.55	4.55	7.79	12.22	20.17	671	4.23	6.35	10.68	18.21	23.53
30–34	389	4.88	6.53	11.23	18.27	23.30	63	3.72	4.71	8.55	14.28	21.70	465	4.39	6.60	11.11	18.24	23.49
35–39	394	4.99	6.69	11.38	18.20	23.08	49	3.83	4.76	8.86	15.34	22.38	451	4.56	6.76	11.25	18.14	23.19
40–44	412	5.06	6.87	11.42	18.13	23.55	59	3.79	4.77	9.04	15.57	21.96	474	4.69	6.86	11.29	18.03	23.27
45–49	446	5.07	6.98	11.36	17.88	23.44	81	3.82	4.76	9.08	15.99	22.06	532	4.75	6.85	11.21	17.79	23.18
50–54	452	5.07	7.01	11.29	17.55	23.26	75	3.88	4.76	9.07	16.17	22.24	531	4.77	6.83	11.09	17.50	23.01
55–59	406	5.07	7.04	11.20	17.25	22.99	57	3.94	4.76	9.05	15.70	22.04	467	4.78	6.81	10.96	17.26	22.78
60–64	328	5.06	7.07	11.11	16.99	22.40	46	3.98	4.74	8.99	15.17	21.73	378	4.79	6.79	10.82	17.04	22.21
65–69	888	5.06	7.09	11.01	16.71	21.79	184	4.03	4.73	8.92	14.67	21.40	1084	4.78	6.76	10.68	16.81	21.59
70–74	615	5.05	7.10	10.91	16.48	21.23	129	4.07	4.72	8.85	14.04	20.92	751	4.76	6.72	10.54	16.61	20.96
Females																		
6	118	5.65	6.96	10.19	13.48	15.47	42	4.90	6.10	7.99	13.71	14.94	161	6.00	6.76	10.01	13.44	15.57
7	126	6.09	7.42	10.89	14.93	18.08	47	5.09	6.33	8.60	15.27	17.20	174	6.24	7.17	10.68	14.94	17.89
8	118	6.52	7.86	11.60	16.35	20.60	35	5.29	6.57	9.22	16.82	19.41	153	6.47	7.58	11.36	16.41	20.18
9	125	6.94	8.31	12.31	17.74	23.07	47	5.51	6.83	9.85	18.40	21.65	173	6.71	8.01	12.05	17.85	22.47
10	152	7.37	8.77	13.02	18.84	24.84	41	5.73	7.09	10.47	19.63	23.76	194	6.95	8.44	12.74	19.01	24.38
11	117	7.80	9.23	13.74	19.82	26.23	43	5.96	7.36	11.08	20.72	25.84	163	7.20	8.87	13.43	20.13	26.15
12	129	8.17	9.68	14.44	20.97	27.73	47	6.21	7.62	11.68	21.58	27.53	177	7.45	9.31	14.13	21.25	27.98
13	151	8.49	10.19	15.14	22.00	29.08	47	6.50	8.05	12.22	21.86	29.17	199	7.78	9.84	14.87	22.25	29.51
14	141	8.78	10.76	15.77	22.99	30.22	49	6.81	8.53	12.56	21.71	30.48	192	8.15	10.37	15.47	23.27	30.86
15	117	9.06	11.29	16.39	24.08	31.48	47	7.11	8.94	12.95	21.77	30.54	164	8.46	10.85	16.03	24.32	32.22
16	142	9.34	11.83	17.03	24.85	32.35	30	7.41	9.35	13.36	22.06	30.07	173	8.78	11.34	16.62	25.12	33.22
17	114	9.55	12.18	17.45	25.48	32.95	44	7.67	9.70	13.75	23.03	30.46	159	9.03	11.66	17.02	25.80	33.83
18	109	9.66	12.29	17.67	26.22	33.51	29	7.87	10.03	14.19	24.94	31.42	140	9.21	11.79	17.24	26.51	34.26
19	104	9.79	12.46	17.95	26.95	34.07	37	8.08	10.37	14.59	26.92	32.32	142	9.41	11.97	17.50	27.23	34.74
20–24	956	10.29	12.86	19.02	27.52	34.45	261	8.20	11.20	17.59	28.48	33.54	1244	9.91	12.54	18.75	27.80	35.01
25–29	1090	10.77	13.73	20.18	29.34	36.09	190	8.65	12.25	20.31	31.25	38.39	1307	10.44	13.45	20.02	29.58	36.43
30–34	897	11.23	14.47	21.18	30.72	37.41	180	9.05	13.36	22.26	33.41	40.44	1089	11.00	14.30	21.25	31.03	37.70
35–39	815	11.50	15.19	22.17	31.59	38.35	185	9.62	14.19	23.71	34.04	41.44	1017	11.36	15.08	22.35	32.00	38.55
40–44	799	11.56	15.66	22.74	31.98	38.81	183	9.89	14.55	24.90	34.92	42.00	999	11.46	15.53	23.02	32.69	39.16
45–49	519	11.56	15.92	23.04	32.25	38.94	79	9.96	14.65	25.28	35.52	42.42	603	11.47	15.78	23.41	33.11	39.43
50–54	528	11.53	16.04	23.22	32.34	38.68	83	10.00	14.68	25.51	35.23	42.75	615	11.43	15.92	23.65	33.21	39.12
55–59	416	11.49	16.15	23.40	32.23	38.10	73	10.03	14.69	25.78	34.77	42.40	491	11.38	16.05	23.89	32.98	38.51
60–64	393	11.44	16.23	23.56	31.74	37.14	68	10.02	14.67	26.05	33.68	41.27	462	11.31	16.16	24.10	32.30	37.44
65–69	959	11.38	16.29	23.70	31.21	36.13	194	9.97	14.60	26.30	32.47	40.22	1157	11.23	16.24	24.28	31.59	36.31
70–74	711	11.32	16.33	23.80	30.65	35.09	134	9.88	14.50	26.51	31.12	39.03	848	11.13	16.30	24.42	30.83	35.12

From Must A, Dallal GE, Dietz WH. Am J Clin Nutr 1991; 53:839–46. Data source: NHANES I. With permission.

A-18-c
Human Body Proportions for Assessing Amputees

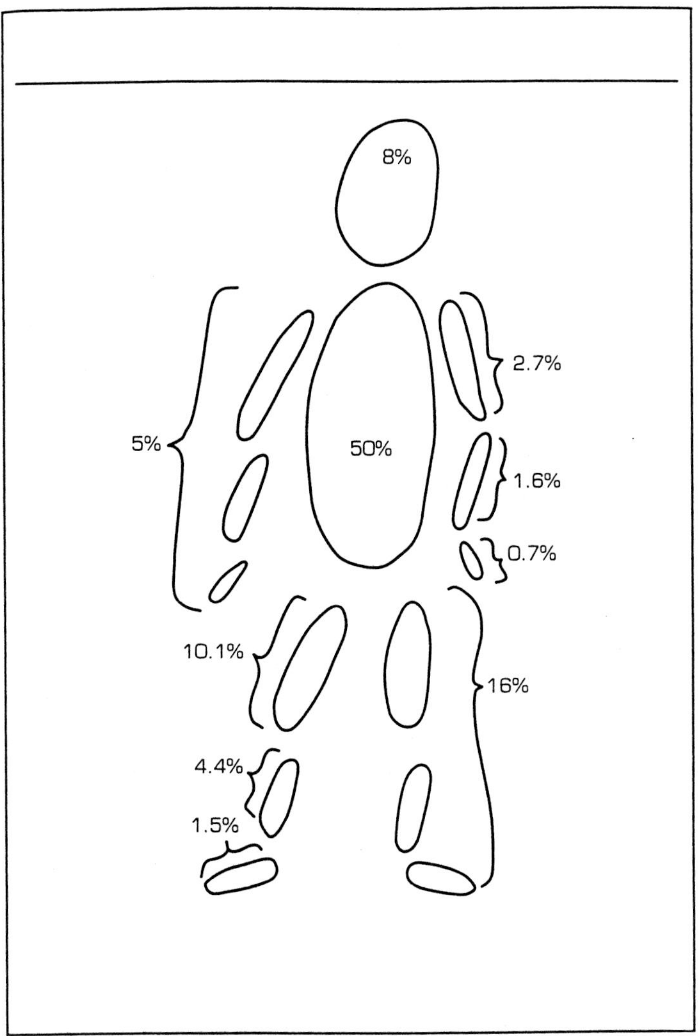

Ratio of segment weight to body weight based on 1955 data of Dempster and the 1969 data of Clauser et al (N = 21). From Osterkamp LK. J Am Dietetic Assn 1995;95:215–218. Current perspective on assessment of human body proportions of relevance to amputees.

Table A-18-d
Recommended Equations for Predicting Stature in Individuals Unable to Stand

Group	Age Group	Equation
White men	18–60	Stature = 1.88 (knee height) + 71.85
	17–67	Stature = 2.31 (knee height) + 51.1
	60–80	Stature = 2.08 (knee height) + 59.01
	17–67	Stature = 2.30 (knee height) − 0.063 (age) + 54.9
	17–67	Stature = 0.762 (arm span) + 40.7
Black men	18–60	Stature = 1.79 (knee height) + 73.42
	60–80	Stature = 1.37 (knee height) + 95.79
White women	18–60	Stature = 1.87 (knee height) − 0.06 (age) + 70.25
	22–71	Stature = 1.84 (knee height) + 70.2
	22–71	Stature = 1.91 (knee height) − 0.098 (age) + 71.3
	60–80	Stature = 1.91 (knee height) − 0.17 (age) + 75.00
	22–71	Stature = 0.693 (arm span) + 50.3
Black women	18–60	Stature = 1.86 (knee height) − 0.06 (age) + 68.10
	60–80	Stature = 1.96 (knee height) + 58.72
White boys	6–18	Stature = 2.22 (knee height) + 40.54
Black boys	6–18	Stature = 2.18 (knee height) + 39.60
Chinese boys	4–16	Stature = 1.75 (lower segment) + 26.56
	4–16	Stature = 0.92 (arm span) + 10.84
White girls	6–18	Stature = 2.15 (knee height) + 43.21
Black girls	6–18	Stature = 2.02 (knee height) + 46.59
Chinese girls	4–16	Stature = 1.81 (lower segment) + 22.75
	4–16	Stature = 0.93 (arm span) + 10.34

From Chapter 56, see text for references, use, and source. With permission.

[a]Arm span, knee height, and stature are in cm; lower segment (subischial leg length) in cm = standing height minus sitting height; and age in years.

Table A-19
Beverages and Alcoholic Drinks: Calories and Selected Electrolytes (per 100 mL)

Beverage	Calories	Sodium (mg)	Sodium (meq)	Potassium (mg)	Potassium (meq)	Phosphorus (mg)
Coffee, brewed	2.0	2.0	0.1	54.0	1.4	1.0
expresso	9.0	14.0	0.6	115.0	3.0	7.0
Tea, brewed	1.0	3.0	0.1	37.0	1.0	1.0
herbal	1.0	1.0	<0.1	9.0	0.2	0.0
Cola (avg)	41.0	4.0	0.2	1.0	<0.1	12.0
Diet cola (avg)	1.0	6.0	0.3	0.0	—	9.0
Grape/orange	43.0	15.0	0.7	1.0	<0.1	0.0
Lemon-lime	40.0	11.0	0.5	1.0	<0.1	0.0
Root beer	41.0	13.0	0.6	1.0	<0.1	0.0
Club soda	0.0	21.0	0.9	2.0	0.1	0.0
Tonic	34.0	4.0	0.2	0.0	—	0.0
Orange	48.0	12.0	0.5	2.0	0.1	1.0
Ginger ale	34.0	7.0	0.3	1.0	<0.1	0.0
Pepper-type/diet	41.0/0	10.0/16.0	0.4/0.7	1.0/2.0	<0.1/0.1	11.0/11.0
Apple juice	47.0	3.0	0.1	119.0	3.1	7.0
Apricot nectar	56.0	3.0	0.1	114.0	2.9	9.0
Cranberry juice, cocktail	57.0	2.0	0.1	18.0	0.5	2.0
Grape juice, canned	61.0	3.0	0.1	132.0	3.4	11.0
Grape juice, unsweetened (pink, raw)	39.0	1.0	Tr	162.0	4.2	15.0
Orange juice, unsweetened, or fresh	45.0	1.0	<0.1	200.0	5.1	17.0
Peach nectar	54.0	7.0	0.3	40.0	1.0	6.0
Pear nectar	60.0	4.0	0.2	13.0	0.3	3.0
Pineapple juice, unsweetened	56.0	1.0	<0.1	134.0	3.4	8.0
Tomato juice w/ w/o salt	17.0/17.0	361.0/10.0	15.7/0.4	220.0/220.0	5.6/5.6	19.0/19.0
Punch, frozen	50.0	5.0	0.2	77.0	2.0	0.0
Beer, regular	41.0	5.0	0.2	25.0	0.6	12.0
Beer, light	28.0	3.0	0.1	18.0	0.5	12.0
Gin, rum, vodka, whiskey (86 proof)	250.0	1.0	<0.1	2.0	0.1	4.0
Table wine	70	8.0	0.3	89.0	2.3	14.0
Dessert wine sweet/dry	153.0/126.0	9.0/9.0	0.4/0.4	92.0/92.0	2.4/2.4	9.0/9.0

Data from U.S. Department of Agriculture, Agricultural Research Service. 1996. USDA nutrient database for standard reference, release 11. Nutrient Data Laboratory home page, http://www.nal.usda.gov/fnic/foodcomp. Release 11-1 as of August 29, 1997 was used.
Note: Alcoholic beverages are customarily served in special glassware, the size of which tends to standardize the alcoholic content.

1 cordial glass = 20 mL
1 brandy glass = 30 mL
1 jigger = 45 mL
1 sherry glass = 60 mL
1 cocktail glass = 90 mL
1 burgundy glass = 120 mL
1 champagne glass = 150 mL
1 tumbler = 240–360 mL
1 mixing glass = 360 mL

Table A-20
Dietary Fiber Content of Common Foods

Food Item	Serving Size	Total Fiber per Serving (g)	Soluble Fiber per Serving (g)	Insoluble Fiber per Serving (g)
Cereals				
All Bran	⅓ cup	8.6	1.4	7.2
Benefit	¾ cup	5.0	2.8	2.2
Cheerios	1¼ cups	2.5	1.2	1.3
Corn flakes	1 cup	0.5	0.1	0.4
Cream of wheat, regular, uncooked	2½ tbsp	1.1	0.4	0.7
Fiber One	½ cup	11.9	0.8	11.1
40% Bran Flakes	⅔ cup	4.3	0.4	3.9
Grapenuts	¼ cup	2.8	0.8	2.0
Grits, corn, quick, uncooked	3 tbsp	0.6	0.1	0.5
Heartwise	1 cup	5.7	2.9	2.8
Nutri-Grain wheat	⅔ cup	2.7	0.7	2.0
Oat bran, cooked	¾ cup	4.0	2.2	1.8
Oat bran flakes	½ cup	2.1	0.8	0.3
Oat flakes	⅔ cup	2.1	1.0	1.1
Oatmeal, uncooked	⅓ cup	2.7	1.4	1.3
Product 19	1 cup	1.2	0.3	0.9
Puffed Rice	1 cup	0.2	0.1	0.1
Puffed Wheat	1 cup	1.0	0.5	0.5
Quaker Oat Squares	½ cup	2.2	0.8	1.4
Raisin Bran	¾ cup	5.3	0.9	4.4
Rice Krispies	1 cup	0.3	0.1	0.2
Shredded Wheat	⅔ cup	3.5	0.5	3.0
Shredded Wheat and Bran	⅔ cup	2.5	0.6	1.9
Special K	1 cup	0.9	0.2	0.7
Total, whole wheat	1 cup	2.6	0.6	2.0
Wheat flakes	¾ cup	2.3	0.4	1.9
Wheaties	⅔ cup	2.3	0.7	1.6
Grains				
Cornmeal	2½ tbsp	0.4	0.1	0.3
Flour, oat	2½ tbsp	1.8	1.0	0.8
rye	2½ tbsp	2.6	0.8	1.8
white	2½ tbsp	0.6	0.3	0.3
whole wheat	2½ tbsp	2.1	0.3	1.8
Macaroni, white, cooked	½ cup	0.7	0.4	0.3
whole wheat, cooked	½ cup	2.1	0.4	1.7
Noodles, egg, cooked	½ cup	1.4	0.4	1.0
spinach, cooked	½ cup	1.1	0.5	0.6
Popcorn, popped	3 cups	2.0	0.1	1.9
Rice, white, cooked	⅓ cup	0.5	trace	0.5
wild, cooked	⅓ cup	0.4	0.1	0.3

continued

Table A-20
Dietary Fiber Content of Common Foods

Food Item	Serving Size	Total Fiber per Serving (g)	Soluble Fiber per Serving (g)	Insoluble Fiber per Serving (g)
Spaghetti, white, cooked	½ cup	0.9	0.4	0.5
whole wheat, cooked	½ cup	2.7	0.6	2.1
Wheat bran	½ cup	12.3	1.0	11.3
Wheat germ	3 tbsp	3.9	0.7	3.2
Breads and Crackers				
Bagel, plain	½	0.7	0.3	0.4
Biscuit, baked	1	0.5	0.3	0.2
Bread, bran	1 slice	1.5	0.2	1.3
cornbread	1–2-in cube	1.4	0.3	1.1
cracked wheat	1 slice	1.9	0.3	1.6
French	1 slice	0.9	0.3	0.6
mixed grain	1 slice	1.9	0.3	1.6
oatmeal	½ slice	1.2	0.3	0.9
pita, white	½ pocket	0.5	0.2	0.3
pumpernickel	1 slice	2.7	1.2	1.5
raisin	1 slice	1.2	0.3	0.9
rye	1 slice	1.8	0.8	1.0
sourdough	1 slice	0.8	0.3	0.5
white	1 slice	0.6	0.3	0.3
whole wheat	1 slice	1.5	0.3	1.2
Bread sticks	2	0.6	0.2	0.4
Bun, hamburger	½	0.7	0.2	0.5
Crackers, matzo	1	1.0	0.5	0.5
saltine	6	0.5	0.3	0.2
saltine, wheat	5	0.5	0.2	0.3
snack, whole wheat	4	2.0	0.3	1.7
wheat	5	0.6	0.2	0.4
English muffin	½	0.8	0.2	0.6
Melba toast, wheat	5 slices	1.8	0.4	1.4
Pretzels, hard	¾ oz	0.8	0.2	0.6
Roll, brown-and-serve	1 roll	0.8	0.3	0.5
Taco shell	2	1.4	0.2	1.2
Tortilla, corn	1	1.4	0.2	1.2
Tortilla, flour	1	0.7	0.3	0.4
Waffle, toasted	1	0.7	0.3	0.4
Fruits				
Apple, red, fresh w/skin	1 sml	2.8	1.0	1.8
Applesauce, canned, unswt	½ cup	2.0	0.7	1.3
Apricots, canned, drained	4 halves	1.2	0.5	0.7
dried	7 halves	2.0	1.1	0.9
fresh w/skin	4	3.5	1.8	1.7
Avocado, fresh, flesh only	⅛	1.2	0.5	0.7
Banana, fresh	½ sml	1.1	0.3	0.8
Blueberries, fresh	¾ cup	1.4	0.3	1.1

continued

Table A-20
Dietary Fiber Content of Common Foods

Food Item	Serving Size	Total Fiber per Serving (g)	Soluble Fiber per Serving (g)	Insoluble Fiber per Serving (g)
Cherries, black, fresh	12 lrg	1.3	0.6	0.7
Cherries, red, canned	½ cup	1.8	0.9	0.9
Currants, dried	2 tbsp	0.4	0.2	0.2
Dates, dried	2½ med	0.9	0.3	0.6
Figs, dried	1½	2.3	1.1	1.2
Fruit cocktail, canned	½ cup	2.0	0.7	1.3
Grapefruit, fresh	½ med	1.6	1.1	0.5
Grapes, red, fresh w/skin	15 sml	0.4	0.2	0.2
Grapes, white, fresh w/skin	15 sml	0.6	0.3	0.3
Kiwifruit, fresh flesh only	1 lrg	1.7	0.7	1.0
Mango, fresh, flesh only	½ sml	2.9	1.7	1.2
Melon, cantaloupe	1 cup cubed	1.1	0.3	0.8
honeydew	1 cup cubed	0.9	0.3	0.6
watermelon	1¼ cups cubed	0.6	0.4	0.2
Nectarine, fresh	1 sml	1.8	0.8	1.0
Orange, fresh, flesh only	1 sml	2.9	1.8	1.1
Peaches, canned, unswt	½ cup	2.0	0.7	1.3
fresh, w/skin	1 med	2.0	1.0	1.0
Pear, canned	½ cup	3.7	0.7	3.0
fresh, w skin	½ lrg or 1 sml	2.9	1.1	1.8
Pineapple, canned	⅓ cup	1.4	0.2	1.2
fresh	¾ cup	1.4	0.1	1.3
Plum, red, fresh	2 med	2.4	1.1	1.3
Prunes, dried	3 med	1.7	1.0	0.7
stewed, unswt, drained	¼ cup	1.6	0.9	0.7
Raisins, dried	2 tbsp	0.4	0.2	0.2
Raspberries, fresh	1 cup	3.3	0.9	2.4
Strawberries, fresh	1¼ cups	2.8	1.1	1.7
Vegetables				
Asparagus, cooked	½ cup	1.8	1.7	1.1
Bean sprouts, fresh	1 cup	1.6	0.6	1.0
Beets, flesh only, cooked	½ cup	1.8	0.8	1.0
Broccoli, cooked	½ cup	2.4	1.2	1.2
Brussel sprouts, cooked	½ cup	3.8	2.0	1.8
Cabbage, fresh	1 cup	1.5	0.6	0.9
red, cooked	½ cup	2.6	1.1	1.5

continued

Table A-20
Dietary Fiber Content of Common Foods

Food Item	Serving Size	Total Fiber per Serving (g)	Soluble Fiber per Serving (g)	Insoluble Fiber per Serving (g)
Carrots, canned	½ cup	1.5	0.7	0.8
fresh	1 7½-in long	2.3	1.1	1.2
sliced, cooked	½ cup	2.0	1.1	0.9
Cauliflower, cooked	½ cup	1.0	0.4	0.6
Celery, fresh	1 cup chopped	1.7	0.7	1.0
Corn, whole kernel, canned	½ cup	1.6	0.2	1.4
Cucumber, fresh	1 cup	0.5	0.2	0.3
Green beans, canned	½ cup	2.0	0.5	1.5
French style, cooked	½ cup	2.8	1.1	1.7
Kale, chopped, frozen	½ cup	2.5	0.7	1.8
Lettuce iceberg	1 cup	0.5	0.1	0.4
Mushrooms, fresh	1 cup pieces	0.8	0.1	0.7
Okra, frozen, cooked	½ cup	4.1	1.0	3.1
Olives, canned	10 sml	1.0	0.1	0.9
Onion, cooked	½ cup chopped	2.0	1.1	0.9
fresh	½ cup chopped	1.7	0.9	0.8
Peas, green, canned	½ cup	3.2	0.4	2.8
green, frozen, cooked	½ cup	4.3	1.3	3.0
Pepper, green, fresh	1 cup chopped	1.7	0.7	1.0
Potato, sweet, canned	⅓ cup	0.8	0.3	0.5
sweet, flesh only, cooked	⅓ cup	2.7	1.2	1.5
Pumpkin, fresh, cooked	1 cup	1.2	0.4	0.8
Snow peas, fresh, cooked	½ cup	1.4	0.6	0.8
Spinach, cooked	½ cup	1.6	0.5	1.1
Squash, yellow, crookneck, frozen	½ cup	0.7	0.3	0.4
Tomato, canned	½ cup	1.3	0.5	0.8
fresh	1 med	1.0	0.1	0.9
sauce	⅓ cup	1.1	0.5	0.6
Turnip, cooked	½ cup	4.8	1.7	3.1
V-8 Juice	½ cup	0.7	0.2	0.5
Zucchini, sliced, cooked	½ cup	1.2	0.5	0.7
Legumes				
Black beans, cooked	½ cup	6.1	2.4	3.7
Black-eyed peas, canned	½ cup	4.7	0.5	4.2
Broad beans, no pods, cooked	½ cup	5.1	1.0	4.1
Butter beans, dried, cooked	½ cup	6.9	2.7	4.2

continued

Table A-20
Dietary Fiber Content of Common Foods

Food Item	Serving Size	Total Fiber per Serving (g)	Soluble Fiber per Serving (g)	Insoluble Fiber per Serving (g)
Chick peas, dried, cooked	½ cup	4.3	1.3	3.0
Garbanzo beans, canned	⅓ cup	2.8	0.3	2.5
Kidney beans, dk red, dried, cooked	½ cup	6.9	2.8	4.1
lt red, canned	½ cup	7.9	2.0	5.9
Lentils, dried, cooked	½ cup	5.2	0.6	4.6
Lima beans, canned	½ cup	4.3	1.1	3.2
Mung beans, dried, cooked	½ cup	3.3	0.7	2.6
Navy beans, dried, cooked	½ cup	6.5	2.2	4.3
Pinto beans, canned	½ cup	6.1	1.4	4.7
dried, cooked	½ cup	5.9	1.9	4.0
Split peas, dried, cooked	½ cup	3.1	1.1	2.0
White beans, Great Northern, canned	½ cup	7.2	2.2	5.0
Great Northern, dried, cooked	½ cup	5.0	1.4	3.6
Nuts and Seeds				
Almonds	6 whole	0.6	0.1	0.5
Brazil nuts	1 tbsp	0.5	0.1	0.4
Coconut, dried	1½ tbsp	1.5	0.1	1.4
fresh	2 tbsp	1.1	0.1	1.0
Hazlenuts (filberts)	1 tbsp	0.5	0.2	0.3
Peanut butter, smooth	1 tbsp	1.0	0.3	0.7
Peanuts, roasted	10 lrg	0.6	0.2	0.4
Sesame seeds	1 tbsp	0.8	0.2	0.6
Sunflower seeds	1 tbsp	0.5	0.2	0.3
Walnuts	2 whole	0.3	0.1	0.2

From the Manual of Clinical Dietetics. 5th ed. Chicago: American Dietetic Association, 1996; 847–51, with permission.

Adapted from Anderson JW. Plant Fiber in Foods. 2nd ed. HCF Nutrition Research Foundation Inc., PO Box 22124, Lexington, KY 40522, 1990.

Data from

Anderson JW, Bridges SR. Dietary fiber content of selected foods. Am J Clin Nutr 1988;47:440–447.

Food items analyzed by Anderson JW, Bridges SR, Siesel AE, 1989–1990.

Englyst HN, Bingham SA, Runswick SA, et al. Dietary fibre (non-starch polysaccharides) in fruit, vegetables, and nuts. J Hum Nutr Diet 1988;1:247–286.

Englyst HN, Bingham SA, Runswick SA, et al. Dietary fibre (non-starch polysaccharides) in cereal products. J Hum Nutr Diet 1989;2:257–276.

Ranhotra GS, Gelroth JA, Astroth K. Total and soluble fiber in selected bakery and other cereal products. Cereal Chem 1990;67:499–501.

Note: For additional information on fiber in foods, please see Marlett JA, Cheung T-F. Database and quick methods of assessing typical dietary fiber intakes using data for 228 commonly consumed foods. J Am Diet Assoc 1997; 97;1139–1148. and Marlett JA, Slavin JL. Position of the American Dietetic Association: health implications of dietary fiber. J Am Diet Assoc 1997; 97:1157–1159.

Table A-21-a
Average Values for Triglycerides, Fatty Acids (FA) (Including Omega-3-FA), and Cholesterol in Selected Foods and Oils (per 100 g Edible Portion)[a]

	FAT (g)	SFA (g)	MFA (g)	PFA (g)	M18:1 (g)	P18:2 (g)	P18:3 (g)	P:S	CHOL. (mg)	S14:0 (g)	S16:0 (g)	S18:0 (g)	P20:5 (g)	P22:5 (g)	P22:6 (g)
Meats															
Liver, calf, cooked	6.90	2.56	1.49	1.09	1.28	0.61	0.08	0.43	561.00	0.00	1.40	1.16	0.00	0.00	0.00
Liver, pork, cooked	4.40	1.41	0.63	1.05	0.56	0.42	0.04	0.74	355.00	0.02	0.53	0.84	0.00	0.04	0.03
Kidney, beef, cooked	3.44	1.09	0.74	0.74	0.61	0.40	0.01	0.68	387.00	0.06	0.47	0.51	0.00	0.00	0.00
Kidney, pork, cooked	4.70	1.51	1.55	0.38	1.40	0.25	0.01	0.25	480.00	0.05	0.85	0.60	0.00	0.00	0.00
Brains, beef, cooked	12.53	2.92	2.50	1.44	2.00	0.03	0.00	0.49	2054.00	0.06	1.51	1.27	0.00	0.30	0.67
Brains, pork, cooked	9.51	2.15	1.72	1.47	1.10	0.09	0.12	0.68	2552.00	0.04	1.06	1.03	0.00	0.22	0.46
Beef, roast, chuck, cooked	25.98	10.52	11.16	0.90	10.04	0.61	0.27	0.09	84.00	0.85	6.45	3.07	0.00	0.00	0.00
Beef, steak, sirloin, cooked	14.92	5.63	6.59	0.57	5.85	0.39	0.14	0.10	80.00	0.44	3.58	1.54	0.00	0.00	0.00
Beef, steak, tenderloin, T-bone, ribeye, cooked	19.76	7.82	8.31	0.71	7.49	0.48	0.19	0.09	79.00	0.63	4.79	2.31	0.00	0.00	0.00
Beef, steak, prime rib, cooked	29.77	12.01	12.75	1.04	11.45	0.69	0.32	0.09	85.00	0.97	7.35	3.52	0.00	0.00	0.00
Lamb, chop or roast, cooked	19.97	8.44	8.17	1.62	7.34	1.19	0.34	0.20	92.00	0.75	4.30	2.68	0.00	0.00	0.00
Lamb, leg, cooked	13.31	4.76	5.83	0.87	5.40	0.71	0.08	0.18	88.00	0.42	2.56	1.64	0.00	0.00	0.00
Pork, fresh, chop or roast, cooked	15.15	5.35	6.68	1.30	6.00	1.12	0.03	0.24	81.00	0.18	3.32	1.70	0.00	0.00	0.00
Veal, cutlet, chop, cooked	10.45	4.51	4.08	0.68	3.49	0.52	0.07	0.15	102.00	0.45	2.36	1.48	0.00	0.00	0.00
Poultry, light meat, unknown part, skin removed, cooked	3.86	1.15	1.05	0.92	0.88	0.66	0.02	0.80	77.00	0.03	0.67	0.32	0.00	0.02	0.03
Poultry, light meat, unknown part, with skin, cooked	9.59	2.70	3.55	2.16	2.90	1.81	0.10	0.80	80.00	0.08	1.85	0.58	0.00	0.02	0.03
Poultry, dark meat, unknown part, skin removed, cooked	8.48	2.54	2.60	2.21	2.16	1.81	0.08	0.87	89.00	0.06	1.56	0.68	0.00	0.04	0.06
Poultry, dark meat, unknown part, with skin, cooked	13.66	3.93	4.92	3.29	4.04	2.82	0.14	0.84	90.00	0.10	2.64	0.90	0.01	0.03	0.05
Duck, domestic, with skin, light meat, cooked	10.50	2.75	4.40	1.58	4.76	1.51	0.07	0.57	135.00	0.06	2.21	0.59	0.00	0.00	0.00
Duck, domestic, with skin, dark meat, cooked	11.07	2.82	4.70	1.85	5.01	1.78	0.35	0.66	113.00	0.07	2.28	0.60	0.00	0.00	0.00
Ground beef, unknown % fat, cooked	22.56	8.86	9.88	0.85	8.63	0.62	0.09	0.09	89.00	0.64	5.10	2.66	0.00	0.00	0.00
Bologna, beef, regular	28.50	12.07	13.80	1.09	12.16	0.85	0.24	0.09	58.00	0.87	6.64	4.05	0.00	0.00	0.00
Frankfurter, all beef (Kosher), regular	28.50	12.05	13.62	1.38	11.99	1.11	0.27	0.11	61.00	0.94	6.52	3.96	0.00	0.00	0.00
Frankfurter, chicken	17.70	5.89	5.58	5.00	5.30	4.64	0.36	0.85	107.00	0.30	3.62	1.83	0.00	0.00	0.00
Frankfurter, regular, beef and pork	29.15	10.76	13.67	2.73	12.36	2.34	0.39	0.25	50.00	0.53	6.45	3.65	0.00	0.00	0.00
Ham, cured	15.20	5.04	7.07	1.78	6.61	1.62	0.16	0.35	62.00	0.16	3.19	1.65	0.00	0.00	0.00
Salami, hard or dry, pork	33.72	11.89	16.00	3.74	14.67	3.27	0.28	0.31	79.00	0.52	7.64	3.56	0.00	0.00	0.00
Bacon, regular cut	49.24	17.42	23.69	5.81	21.96	4.89	0.79	0.33	85.00	0.62	10.98	5.67	0.00	0.00	0.00
Fish															
Cod, cooked	1.53	0.36	0.31	0.63	0.15	0.01	0.02	1.75	68.00	0.06	0.23	0.06	0.24	0.05	0.26
Trout, cooked	4.86	1.43	1.38	0.92	0.20	0.09	0.00	1.01	73.00	0.06	0.29	0.10	0.18	0.09	0.15
Salmon, sockeye, cooked	10.97	1.92	5.29	2.41	1.34	0.11	0.06	1.26	87.00	0.26	1.01	0.16	0.53	0.13	0.70
Herring, smoked/kippered, canned and drained	12.37	2.79	5.11	2.92	2.07	0.18	0.14	1.05	82.00	0.76	1.85	0.15	0.97	0.08	1.18
Salmon, canned, drained, with salt	6.05	1.54	1.81	2.05	1.07	0.06	0.06	1.33	55.00	0.05	1.35	0.14	0.84	0.05	0.81

continued

Table A-21-a
Average Values for Triglycerides, Fatty Acids (FA) (Including Omega-3-FA), and Cholesterol in Selected Foods and Oils (per 100 g Edible Portion)[a]

	FAT (g)	SFA (g)	MFA (g)	PFA (g)	M18:1 (g)	P18:2 (g)	P18:3 (g)	P:S	CHOL. (mg)	S14:0 (g)	S16:0 (g)	S18:0 (g)	P20:5 (g)	P22:5 (g)	P22:6 (g)
Sardines, canned in oil, drained	11.45	1.53	3.87	5.15	2.14	3.54	0.50	3.37	142.00	0.19	0.99	0.34	0.47	0.00	0.51
Tuna, canned oil pack, regular, drained	8.21	1.53	2.95	2.88	2.84	2.68	0.07	1.88	18.00	0.03	1.42	0.09	0.03	0.00	0.10
Tuna, canned, water pack, regular, drained, not rinsed	0.82	0.23	0.16	0.34	0.09	0.01	0.00	1.48	30.00	0.02	0.16	0.06	0.05	0.01	0.22
Clams and mussels, cooked from fresh or frozen	1.95	0.19	0.17	0.55	0.07	0.03	0.01	2.89	67.00	0.03	0.12	0.04	0.14	0.10	0.15
Crab, hard-shell, Alaskan King, cooked	1.77	0.23	0.28	0.68	0.15	0.03	0.02	2.96	100.00	0.02	0.14	0.06	0.24	0.05	0.23
Lobster, cooked	0.59	0.11	0.16	0.09	0.10	0.00	0.00	0.82	72.00	0.01	0.08	0.02	0.05	0.00	0.03
Oyster, cooked, Pacific	4.91	1.54	0.63	1.94	0.24	0.12	0.10	1.26	105.00	0.25	1.07	0.15	0.54	0.12	0.58
Scallops, cooked	1.40	0.15	0.07	0.48	0.03	0.01	0.00	3.20	31.81	0.02	0.10	0.02	0.17	0.03	0.20
Shrimp, cooked	1.08	0.29	0.20	0.44	0.11	0.02	0.01	1.52	195.00	0.02	0.14	0.10	0.17	0.02	0.14
Caviar	17.90	4.21	5.86	5.66	2.94	0.99	0.55	1.34	588.00	0.90	1.87	0.72	1.03	0.81	1.35
Eggs/Dairy															
Eggs, whole, cooked	10.02	3.10	3.81	1.36	3.47	1.15	0.03	0.44	425.00	0.03	2.23	0.78	0.00	0.00	0.04
Eggs, yolk only, cooked	30.87	9.55	11.74	4.20	10.70	3.54	0.10	0.44	1281.00	0.10	6.86	2.42	0.01	0.00	0.11
Eggs, white only, cooked	0.00	0.00	0.00	0.00	0.00	0.00	0.00	0.00	0.00	0.00	0.00	0.00	0.00	0.00	0.00
Cream, coffee creamer, liquid/frozen	7.13	1.93	3.87	1.00	3.87	0.93	0.07	0.52	0.00	0.00	1.27	0.60	0.00	0.00	0.00
Cream, coffee creamer, powder, regular	35.48	32.52	0.97	0.01	0.97	0.00	0.01	0.00	0.00	5.99	3.75	6.34	0.00	0.00	0.00
Cream, half and half, 10 to 12% fat	11.50	7.16	3.32	0.43	2.89	0.26	0.17	0.06	36.90	1.16	3.02	1.39	0.00	0.00	0.00
Cream, light/coffee cream 20% fat	19.31	12.02	5.58	0.72	4.86	0.44	0.28	0.06	66.10	1.94	5.08	2.34	0.00	0.00	0.00
Milk, buttermilk, 1% fat	0.88	0.55	0.25	0.03	0.22	0.02	0.01	0.05	3.50	0.09	0.23	0.11	0.00	0.00	0.00
Milk, skim	0.18	0.12	0.05	0.01	0.04	0.00	0.00	0.08	1.80	0.02	0.05	0.02	0.00	0.00	0.00
Milk, 1% fat	1.06	0.66	0.31	0.04	0.27	0.02	0.02	0.06	4.00	0.11	0.28	0.13	0.00	0.00	0.00
Milk, 2% fat	1.92	1.20	0.56	0.07	0.48	0.04	0.03	0.06	7.50	0.19	0.51	0.23	0.00	0.00	0.00
Milk, whole, 3.5 to 4% fat	3.34	2.08	0.96	0.12	0.84	0.08	0.05	0.06	13.60	0.34	0.88	0.40	0.00	0.00	0.00
Parmesan cheese, dry	30.02	19.07	8.73	0.66	7.74	0.32	0.34	0.03	78.70	3.38	8.10	2.68	0.00	0.00	0.00
American cheese, processed	31.25	19.69	8.95	0.99	7.51	0.61	0.38	0.05	94.40	3.21	9.10	3.80	0.00	0.00	0.00
Cottage cheese, low fat, 2% fat	1.93	1.22	0.55	0.06	0.45	0.04	0.02	0.05	8.40	0.20	0.58	0.22	0.00	0.00	0.00
Cottage cheese, regular or creamed, 4% fat	4.51	2.85	1.28	0.14	1.06	0.10	0.04	0.05	14.90	0.47	1.36	0.52	0.00	0.00	0.00
Cream cheese, Neufchatel	23.43	14.80	6.77	0.65	5.66	0.45	0.20	0.04	76.10	2.35	6.88	2.98	0.00	0.00	0.00
Cheddar cheese, natural	33.14	21.09	9.39	0.94	7.90	0.58	0.36	0.04	104.90	3.33	9.80	4.01	0.00	0.00	0.00
Cheddar cheese, low-fat	17.12	10.88	4.85	0.51	4.17	0.36	0.15	0.05	54.00	1.72	5.22	2.08	0.00	0.00	0.00
Swiss cheese, natural	27.45	17.78	7.27	0.97	6.02	0.62	0.35	0.05	91.70	3.06	7.79	3.25	0.00	0.00	0.00
Swiss cheese, low-fat	10.58	6.63	3.08	0.33	2.65	0.22	0.12	0.05	52.91	1.19	3.05	1.29	0.00	0.00	0.00
Monterey Jack cheese, natural	30.04	19.11	8.71	0.66	7.34	0.43	0.23	0.03	95.60	3.07	9.22	3.57	0.00	0.00	0.00
Mozzarella cheese, part skim milk	17.12	10.88	4.85	0.51	4.17	0.36	0.15	0.05	54.00	1.72	5.22	2.08	0.00	0.00	0.00
Brie cheese	24.26	15.26	7.02	0.72	5.75	0.45	0.27	0.05	72.00	2.69	7.23	2.52	0.00	0.00	0.00
American flavor cheese, low-fat	15.50	9.77	4.44	0.49	3.73	0.30	0.19	0.05	52.91	1.59	4.51	1.88	0.00	0.00	0.00

continued

Table A-21-a
Average Values for Triglycerides, Fatty Acids (FA) (Including Omega-3-FA), and Cholesterol in Selected Foods and Oils (per 100 g Edible Portion)[a]

	FAT (g)	SFA (g)	MFA (g)	PFA (g)	M18:1 (g)	P18:2 (g)	P18:3 (g)	P:S	CHOL. (mg)	S14:0 (g)	S16:0 (g)	S18:0 (g)	P20:5 (g)	P22:5 (g)	P22:6 (g)
Yogurt, frozen, fruit or vanilla, whole milk 3 to 4% fat	3.24	2.10	0.90	0.09	0.75	0.06	0.03	0.04	9.74	0.33	0.87	0.30	0.00	0.00	0.00
Yogurt, frozen, fruit or vanilla, low-fat, 1 to 2%	1.08	0.70	0.30	0.03	0.25	0.02	0.01	0.04	4.20	0.11	0.29	0.10	0.00	0.00	0.00
Yogurt, plain, low-fat, 1 to 2% fat	1.55	1.00	0.43	0.04	0.35	0.03	0.01	0.04	6.10	0.16	0.42	0.15	0.00	0.00	0.00
Yogurt, fruit, non-fat <1% fat	0.20	0.12	0.05	0.01	0.02	0.00	0.00	0.08	2.00	0.01	0.03	0.01	0.00	0.00	0.00
Yogurt, fruit, whole milk, 3 to 4% fat	3.24	2.10	0.90	0.09	0.75	0.06	0.03	0.04	9.74	0.33	0.87	0.30	0.00	0.00	0.00
Ice cream, regular, 11% fat, flavors except chocolate	11.00	6.79	3.17	0.41	2.93	0.25	0.16	0.06	44.00	1.13	3.06	1.33	0.00	0.00	0.00
Ice cream, light, 7% fat, except chocolate	7.65	4.70	2.20	0.27	2.03	0.17	0.11	0.06	28.99	0.78	2.12	0.93	0.00	0.00	0.00
Ice milk, 4% fat, flavors except chocolate	4.30	2.63	1.23	0.16	1.13	0.10	0.06	0.06	14.00	0.44	1.18	0.52	0.00	0.00	0.00
Sherbet, plain	2.00	1.16	0.53	0.08	0.49	0.05	0.03	0.07	5.00	0.20	0.51	0.23	0.00	0.00	0.00
Fats/Oils															
Oils, canola	100.00	7.10	58.90	29.60	56.10	20.30	9.30	4.17	0.00	0.00	4.00	1.80	0.00	0.00	0.00
Oils, corn	100.00	12.70	24.20	58.70	24.20	58.00	0.00	4.62	0.00	0.00	10.90	1.80	0.00	0.00	0.00
Oils, sunflower	100.00	10.30	19.50	65.70	19.50	65.70	0.00	6.38	0.00	0.00	5.90	4.50	0.00	0.00	0.00
Oils, cottonseed	100.00	25.90	17.80	51.90	17.00	51.50	0.20	2.00	0.00	0.80	22.70	2.30	0.00	0.00	0.00
Oils, safflower	100.00	9.10	12.10	74.50	11.70	74.10	0.40	8.19	0.00	0.10	6.20	2.20	0.00	0.00	0.00
Oils, sesame	100.00	14.20	39.70	41.70	39.30	41.30	0.30	2.94	0.00	0.00	8.90	4.80	0.00	0.00	0.00
Oils, soybean (partially hydrogenated)	100.00	14.90	43.00	37.60	42.50	34.90	2.60	2.52	0.00	0.10	9.80	5.00	0.00	0.00	0.00
Oils, olive	100.00	13.50	73.70	8.40	72.50	7.90	0.60	0.62	0.00	0.00	11.00	2.20	0.00	0.00	0.00
Oils, peanut	100.00	16.90	46.20	32.00	44.80	32.00	0.00	1.89	0.00	0.10	9.50	2.20	0.00	0.00	0.00
Oils, coconut	100.00	86.50	5.80	1.80	5.80	1.80	0.00	0.02	0.00	16.80	8.30	2.80	0.00	0.00	0.00
Oils, palm	100.00	49.30	37.00	9.30	36.60	9.10	0.20	0.19	0.00	1.00	43.50	4.30	0.00	0.00	0.00
Oils, palm kernel	100.00	81.50	11.40	1.60	11.40	1.60	0.00	0.02	0.00	16.40	8.10	2.80	0.00	0.00	0.00
Shortening, vegetable	100.00	25.00	44.50	26.10	44.50	24.50	1.60	1.04	0.00	0.40	14.10	10.60	0.00	0.00	0.00
Margarine, regular, stick, salted, soybean oil	80.50	16.70	39.30	20.90	39.10	19.40	1.50	1.25	0.00	0.20	9.60	6.90	0.00	0.00	0.00
Margarine, spread, soybean oil	52.00	7.23	26.66	15.82	26.66	13.33	2.49	2.19	0.00	0.00	5.14	2.04	0.00	0.00	0.00
Margarine, diet, soybean oil	38.80	6.81	17.59	12.95	17.59	12.51	0.43	1.90	0.00	0.05	4.16	2.27	0.00	0.00	0.00
Lard	100.00	39.20	45.10	11.20	41.20	10.20	1.00	0.29	95.00	1.30	23.80	13.50	0.00	0.00	0.00
Butter, regular, salted	81.11	50.49	23.43	3.01	20.40	1.83	1.18	0.06	218.90	8.16	21.33	9.83	0.00	0.00	0.00
Oils, medium chain triglyceride	100.00	94.50	0.00	0.00	0.00	0.00	0.00	0.00	0.00	0.00	0.00	0.00	0.00	0.00	0.00
Mayonnaise, regular, commercial	79.40	11.80	22.70	41.30	22.50	37.10	4.20	3.50	59.00	0.10	8.50	3.10	0.00	0.00	0.00
Mayonnaise, low-fat, no cholesterol	32.99	4.92	14.18	12.40	14.01	11.51	0.86	2.52	0.00	0.03	3.23	1.65	0.00	0.00	0.00

continued

Table A-21-a
Average Values for Triglycerides, Fatty Acids (FA) (Including Omega-3-FA), and Cholesterol in Selected Foods and Oils (per 100 g Edible Portion)[a]

	FAT (g)	SFA (g)	MFA (g)	PFA (g)	M18:1 (g)	P18:2 (g)	P18:3 (g)	P:S	CHOL. (mg)	S14:0 (g)	S16:0 (g)	S18:0 (g)	P20:5 (g)	P22:5 (g)	P22:6 (g)
Mayonnaise type dressing, regular	48.90	7.45	20.97	18.13	20.69	16.82	1.24	2.43	43.00	0.05	4.92	2.47	0.00	0.00	0.00
Mayonnaise type dressing, low-fat	33.40	4.90	9.00	18.00	9.00	16.00	2.00	3.67	26.00	0.00	3.50	1.40	0.00	0.00	0.00
Salad dressing, french, regular	37.50	5.40	8.73	21.69	8.54	19.11	2.54	4.02	0.00	0.04	3.86	1.42	0.00	0.00	0.00
Salad dressing, italian, regular	33.31	4.80	7.77	19.29	7.60	16.99	2.27	4.02	0.00	0.03	3.43	1.27	0.00	0.00	0.00
Salad dressing, 1000 island, regular	29.99	4.48	7.10	16.99	6.93	14.95	1.98	3.79	30.36	0.04	3.20	1.18	0.00	0.00	0.00
Salad dressing, french, reduced calorie	5.00	0.39	2.92	1.46	2.79	1.00	0.46	3.74	1.72	0.01	0.22	0.10	0.00	0.00	0.00
Salad dressing, italian, reduced calorie	22.59	3.25	5.26	13.07	5.15	11.51	1.53	4.02	0.00	0.02	2.32	0.86	0.00	0.00	0.00
Salad dressing, 1000 island, reduced calorie	10.04	0.73	5.90	2.96	5.62	2.03	0.93	4.05	0.50	0.00	0.42	0.18	0.00	0.00	0.00
Miscellaneous															
Almonds, roasted, salted	56.53	5.27	36.71	11.86	36.03	11.36	0.40	2.25	0.00	0.32	3.74	1.11	0.00	0.00	0.00
Cashews, roasted, salted	48.21	9.70	28.42	8.15	27.89	7.97	0.17	0.84	0.00	0.36	4.53	3.09	0.00	0.00	0.00
Peanuts, roasted, salted	49.30	6.84	24.46	15.58	23.79	15.58	0.00	2.28	0.00	0.02	5.16	1.10	0.00	0.00	0.00
Walnuts	61.87	5.59	14.18	39.13	13.30	31.76	6.81	7.00	0.00	0.19	4.24	1.08	0.00	0.00	0.00
Peanut butter w/salt, creamy or chunky	51.03	10.34	24.28	13.91	23.84	13.71	0.00	1.35	0.00	0.22	5.71	2.69	0.00	0.00	0.00
Olives, black	10.68	1.42	7.89	0.91	7.77	0.85	0.06	0.64	0.00	0.00	1.18	0.24	0.00	0.00	0.00
Candy bar or chips, dark chocolate, sweet or semisweet	30.00	17.75	9.97	0.97	9.89	0.91	0.06	0.05	0.00	0.15	7.72	9.47	0.00	0.00	0.00
Avocado	15.32	2.44	9.67	1.96	8.96	1.84	0.11	0.80	0.00	0.00	2.40	0.03	0.00	0.00	0.00
Coconut, fresh	33.49	29.70	1.42	0.37	1.42	0.37	0.00	0.01	0.00	5.87	2.84	1.73	0.00	0.00	0.00
Soybeans, cooked from dried	8.97	1.30	1.98	5.06	1.96	4.46	0.60	3.89	0.00	0.02	0.95	0.32	0.00	0.00	0.00
Peas, black-eyed, cooked from dried	0.53	0.14	0.04	0.22	0.04	0.14	0.08	1.57	0.00	0.00	0.11	0.02	0.00	0.00	0.00
Split peas, yellow or green, cooked from dried	0.39	0.05	0.08	0.16	0.08	0.14	0.03	3.20	0.00	0.00	0.04	0.01	0.00	0.00	0.00

With appreciation to the Nutrition Coordinating Center, University of Minnesota, Minneapolis, MN for the compilation and preparation of these tables. Data are based on version 26 of the NCC Nutrient Database 1997, with permission.

[a]SFA, saturated fatty acid; MFA, monounsaturated fatty acid; PFA, polyunsaturated fatty acid; M18:1, oleic acid; P18:2, linoleic acid; P18:3, linolenic acid; S14.0, myristic acid; S16:0, palmitic acid; S18:0, stearic acid; P20:5, omega-3 (eicosapentaenoic acid); P22:5, omega-3 (docosapentaenoic acid); P22:6, omega-3 (docosahexaeonic acid).

Table A-21-b
Average Values for Triglycerides, Fatty Acids (FA) (Including Omega-3 Fatty Acids)[a], and Cholesterol of Marine Foods and Oils

Fish (100 g)	FAT (g)	CHOL (mg)	SFA (g)	MFA (g)	PFA (g)	M18:1 (g)	P18:2 (g)	P18:3 (g)	P20:5 (g)	P22:5 (g)	P22:6 (g)
Anchovy, European, raw	4.84	60.00	1.28	1.18	1.64	0.62	0.10	—[b]	0.54	0.03	0.91
Bass, striped, raw	2.33	80.00	0.51	0.66	0.78	0.45	0.02	0.02	0.17	0.00	0.58
Bluefish, raw	4.24	59.00	0.92	1.79	1.06	0.68	0.06	0.00	0.25	0.06	0.52
Burbot, raw	0.81	60.00	0.16	0.13	0.30	0.10	0.01	—[b]	0.07	0.03	0.10
Carp, raw	5.60	66.00	1.08	2.33	1.43	1.15	0.52	0.27	0.24	0.08	0.11
Catfish, wild, raw	2.82	58.00	0.72	0.84	0.86	0.59	0.10	0.07	0.13	0.10	0.23
Catfish, farmed, raw	7.59	47.00	1.77	3.59	1.57	3.17	0.88	0.10	0.07	0.09	0.21
Cod, Atlantic, raw	0.67	43.00	0.13	0.09	0.23	0.06	trace[c]	trace[c]	0.06	0.01	0.12
Eel, all varieties, raw	11.66	126.00	2.36	7.19	0.95	2.77	0.20	0.43	0.08	0.07	0.06
Flounder, unspecified, raw	1.19	48.00	0.28	0.23	0.33	0.12	0.01	0.01	0.09	0.05	0.11
Haddock, raw	0.72	57.00	0.13	0.12	0.24	0.07	0.01	trace[c]	0.06	0.02	0.13
Halibut, raw	2.29	32.00	0.32	0.75	0.73	0.36	0.03	0.06	0.07	0.09	0.29
Herring, Atlantic, raw	9.04	60.00	2.04	3.74	2.13	1.52	0.13	0.10	0.71	0.06	0.86
Mackerel, Atlantic, raw	13.89	70.00	3.26	5.46	3.35	2.28	0.22	0.16	0.90	0.21	1.40
Mussel, blue, raw	2.24	28.00	0.42	0.51	0.61	0.20	0.02	0.02	0.19	0.02	0.25
Octopus, raw	1.04	48.00	0.23	0.16	0.24	0.06	0.01	0.00	0.08	0.01	0.08
Oyster, Eastern, wild, raw	2.46	53.00	0.77	0.31	0.97	0.12	0.06	0.05	0.27	0.06	0.29
Oyster, Eastern, farmed, raw	1.55	25.00	0.44	0.15	0.59	0.07	0.03	0.04	0.19	—[b]	0.20
Perch, all varieties, raw	0.92	90.00	0.18	0.15	0.37	0.07	0.01	0.10	0.08	0.03	0.17
Pike, walleye, raw	1.22	86.00	0.25	0.29	0.45	0.20	0.03	0.01	0.09	0.04	0.22
Pollock, Atlantic, raw	0.98	71.00	0.14	0.11	0.48	0.07	0.01	0.00	0.07	0.02	0.35
Sablefish, raw	15.30	49.00	3.20	8.06	2.04	4.07	0.16	0.10	0.68	0.17	0.72
Salmon, Chinook, raw	10.44	66.00	2.51	4.48	2.08	2.80	0.11	0.09	0.79	0.23	0.57
Salmon, coho, wild, raw	5.93	45.00	1.26	2.13	1.99	1.20	0.21	0.16	0.43	0.23	0.66
Salmon, coho, farmed, raw	7.67	51.00	1.82	3.33	1.86	1.72	0.35	0.08	0.38	—[b]	0.82
Sea bass, all varieties, raw	2.00	41.00	0.51	0.42	0.74	0.29	0.02	0.00	0.16	0.08	0.43
Smelt, rainbow, raw	2.42	70.00	0.45	0.64	0.88	0.41	0.04	0.05	0.28	0.02	0.42
Squid, all varieties, raw	1.38	233.00	0.36	0.11	0.52	0.05	trace[c]	trace[c]	0.15	trace[c]	0.34
Red snapper, all varieties, raw	1.34	37.00	0.28	0.25	0.46	0.16	0.02	trace[c]	0.05	0.06	0.26
Sole, raw	1.19	48.00	0.28	0.23	0.33	0.12	0.01	0.01	0.09	0.05	0.11
Sturgeon, all varieties, raw	4.04	60.00	0.92	1.94	0.69	1.43	0.07	0.10	0.19	0.04	0.09
Swordfish, raw	4.01	39.00	1.10	1.54	0.92	1.09	0.03	0.19	0.11	0.00	0.53
Trout, rainbow, wild, raw	3.46	59.00	0.72	1.13	1.24	0.61	0.24	0.12	0.17	0.11	0.42
Trout, rainbow, farmed, raw	5.40	59.00	1.55	1.54	1.80	1.06	0.71	0.06	0.26	0.00	0.67
Tuna, bluefin, fresh, raw	4.90	38.00	1.26	1.60	1.43	0.92	0.05	0.00	0.28	0.12	0.89
Whitefish, all varieties, raw	5.86	60.00	0.91	2.00	2.15	1.35	0.27	0.18	0.32	0.16	0.94
Cod liver oil	100.00	570.00	22.61	46.71	22.54	20.65	0.94	0.94	6.90	0.94	10.97
Herring oil	100.00	766.00	21.29	56.56	15.60	11.96	1.15	0.76	6.27	0.62	4.21
Menhaden oil	100.00	521.00	30.43	26.69	34.20	14.53	2.15	1.49	13.17	4.92	8.56
Max EPA conc fish body oil	100.00	600.00	25.00	28.00	41.00	7.00	2.00	5.00	18.00	0.00	12.00
Salmon oil	100.00	485.00	19.87	29.04	40.32	16.98	1.54	1.06	13.02	2.99	18.23

Data compiled from U.S. Department of Agriculture nutrient database for standard reference, release 11-1 and the Nutrition Coordinating Center, University of Minnesota, Nutrient database, version 28. Table compiled by the Nutrition Coordinating Center, University of Minnesota, 1997,with permission.

[a]CHOL, cholesterol; SFA, saturated fatty acid; MFA, monounsaturated fatty acid; PFA, polyunsaturated fatty acid; M18:1, oleic acid; P18:2, linoleic acid; P18:3, linolenic acid; P20:5, eicosapentaenoic acid (EPA); P22:5, docosapentaenoic acid (DPA); P22:6, docosahexaenoic acid (DHA). The omega-3 fatty acids are P20:5, P22:5, and P22:6.

[b]Denotes lack of reliable data for nutrient.

[c]Trace is $\leq$ 0.005 g/100 g food.

Table A-21-c
Names, Codes, and Formulas of Various Fatty Acids

Common Name	Geneva Nomenclature	Code	Formula[a]
Short-chain saturated fatty acids			
butyric acid	butanoic acid	C4:0	$CH_3(CH_2)_2COOH$
Medium-chain saturated fatty acids			
caproic acid	hexanoic acid	C6:0	$CH_3(CH_2)_4COOH$
caprylic acid	octanoic acid	C8:0	$CH_3(CH_2)_6COOH$
capric acid	decanoic acid	C10:0	$CH_3(CH_2)_8COOH$
lauric acid	dodecanoic acid	C12:0	$CH_3(CH_2)_{10}COOH$
Long-chain fatty acids			
myristic acid	tetradecanoic acid	C14:0	$CH_3(CH_2)_{12}COOH$
palmitic acid	hexadecanoic acid	C16:0	$CH_3(CH_2)_{14}COOH$
stearic acid	octadecanoic acid	C18:0	$CH_3(CH_2)_{16}COOH$
palmitoleic acid	9-hexadecaenoic acid	C16:1, n-7 *cis*	$CH_3(CH_2)_5CH=\copyright CH(CH_2)_7COOH$
oleic acid	9-octadecaenoic acid	C18:1, n-9 *cis*	$CH_3(CH_2)_7CH=\copyright CH(CH_2)_7COOH$
elaidic acid	9-octadecaenoic acid	C18:1, n-9 *trans*	$CH_3(CH_2)_7CH=\copyright CH(CH_2)_7COOH$
linoleic acid	9, 12-octadecadienoic acid	C18:2, n-6, 9 all *cis*	$CH_3(CH_2)_4CH=\copyright CHCH_2CH=\copyright CH(CH_2)_7COOH$
α-linolenic acid	9, 12, 15-octadecatrienoic acid	C18:3, n-3, 6, 9 all *cis*	$CH_3CH_2CH=\copyright CHCH_2CH=\copyright CHCH_2CH=\copyright CH(CH_2)_7COOH$
γ-linolenic acid	6, 9, 12-octadecatrienoic acid	C18:3, n-6, 9, 12 all *cis*	$CH_3(CH_2)_4CH=\copyright CHCH_2CH=\copyright CHCH_2CH=\copyright CH(CH_2)_4COOH$
columbinic acid	5, 9, 12-octatrienoic acid	C18: n-6, cis, 9 cis, 13 *trans*	$CH_3(CH_2)_4CH=\copyright CHCH_2CH=\copyright CHCH_2CH_2CH=tCH(CH_2)_3COOH$
Very long chain fatty acids			
arachidic acid	eicosanoic acid	C20:0	$CH_3(CH_2)_{18}COOH$
behenic acid	docosanoic acid	C22:0	$CH_3(CH_2)_{20}COOH$
eicosenoic acid	11-eicosenoic acid	C20:1, n-9 *cis*	$CH_3(CH_2)_7CH=\copyright CH(CH_2)_9COOH$
erucic acid	13-docosaenoic acid	C22:1, n-9 *cis*	$CH_3(CH_2)_7CH=\copyright CH(CH_2)_{11}COOH$
brassidic acid	13-docosaenoic acid	C22:1, n-9 *trans*	$CH_3(CH_2)_7CH=tCH(CH_2)_{11}COOH$
cetoleic acid	11-docosaenoic acid	C22:1, n-11 *cis*	$CH_3(CH_2)_9CH=\copyright CH(CH_2)_9COOH$
nervonic acid	15-tetracosaenoic acid	C24:1, n-9 *cis*	$CH_3(CH_2)_7CH=\copyright CH(CH_2)_{13}COOH$
"Mead" acid	5, 8, 11-eicosatrienoic acid	C20:3, n-9, 12, 15 all *cis*	$CH_3(CH_2)_7CH=\copyright CHCH_2CH=\copyright CHCH_2CH=\copyright CH(CH_2)_3COOH$
dihomo-γ-linolenic acid	8, 11, 14-eicosatrienoic acid	C20:3, n-6, 9, 12 all *cis*	$CH_3(CH_2)_4CH=\copyright CHCH_2CH=\copyright CHCH_2CH=\copyright CH(CH_2)_6COOH$
arachidonic acid	5, 8, 11, 14-eicosatetraenoic acid	C20:4, n-6, 9, 12, 15 all *cis*	$CH_3(CH_2)_4CH=\copyright CHCH_2CH=\copyright CHCH_2CH=\copyright CHCH_2CH=\copyright CH(CH_2)_3COOH$
timnodonic acid	5, 8, 11, 14, 17-eicosapentaenoic acid	C20:5, n-3, 6, 9, 12, 15 all cis	$CH_3(CH_2CH=\copyright CH)_5(CH_2)_3COOH$
clupanodonic acid	7, 10, 13, 16, 19-docosapentaenoic acid	C22:5, n-3, 6, 9, 12, 15 all cis	$CH_3(CH_2CH=\copyright CH)_5(CH_2)_5COOH$
docosahexaeonic acid	4, 7, 10, 13, 16, 19-docosahexaenoic acid	C22:6, n-3, 6, 9, 12, 15, 18 all cis	$CH_3(CH_2CH=\copyright CH)_6(CH_2)_2COOH$

[a]t, trans; ©, cis.

Table A-22-a
Protein, Sodium, Potassium, Calcium, Phosphorus, and Magnesium Content of Selected Common Foods per Serving Portion[a]

Food Name	Serving Portion	Pro (g)	Na (mg)	K (mg)	Ca (mg)	P (mg)	Mg (mg)
Dairy products							
Egg, whole, hard boiled, large	1.0 item	6.29	62.00	63.00	25.00	86.00	5.00
Cheese, cottage, uncreamed	1.0 oz	4.88	3.62	9.15	8.96	29.38	1.11
Cream, coffee, table, light	1.0 tbsp	0.40	5.94	18.26	14.43	11.98	1.30
Cream, sour, cultured	1.0 tbsp	0.38	6.40	17.28	13.97	10.19	1.35
Milk, buttermilk, fluid	1.0 cup	8.11	257.00	370.68	285.18	218.54	26.83
Milk, whole, 3.3% fat, fluid	1.0 cup	8.03	119.56	369.66	291.34	227.90	32.79
Milk, nonfat/skim, fluid	1.0 cup	8.35	126.18	405.72	302.33	247.20	27.83
Milk, whole, low sodium	1.0 cup	7.56	6.10	616.83	245.95	208.62	12.20
Fats							
Butter, regular	1.0 tbsp	0.12	117.29	3.69	3.41	3.27	0.28
Vegetable oil, corn	1.0 tsp	0.00	0.00	0.00	0.00	0.00	0.00
Vegetable oil, olive	1.0 tsp	0.00	trace	0.00	0.01	0.06	0.00
Shortening, veg, soybean/cottonseed	1.0 tsp	0.00	0.00	0.00	0.00	0.00	0.00
Margarine, regular, hard, unsalted	1.0 tsp	0.02	0.10	1.16	0.82	0.62	0.07
Mayonnaise, soy, commercial	1.0 tsp	0.05	26.15	1.56	0.83	1.29	0.05
Cereals							
Bran flakes, Kellogg's	0.75 cup	3.02	226.20	175.16	13.92	149.93	60.03
Corn flakes, Kellogg's	1.0 Cup	1.84	297.92	25.48	1.12	10.92	3.36
Cream of rice, cooked	1.0 cup	2.20	2.44	48.80	7.32	41.48	7.32
Cream of Wheat, instant	1.0 cup	4.34	7.23	48.20	60.25	43.38	14.46
Farina, cooked, enriched	1.0 cup	3.26	0.00	30.29	4.66	27.96	4.66
Oatmeal, cooked	1.0 cup	6.08	2.34	131.04	18.72	177.84	56.16
Wheat, puffed, plain	1.25 cup	2.44	0.75	54.6	3.60	49.65	19.95
Wheat, shredded, biscuit	1.0 item	2.57	0.47	77.17	9.68	85.67	40.12
Rice Krispies, Kellogg's	1.25 cup	2.08	353.76	42.24	3.30	43.56	15.84
Breads, cookies, crackers							
Bread, white, soft	1.0 slice	2.05	134.50	29.75	27.00	23.50	6.00
Bread, whole-wheat, soft	1.0 slice	2.72	147.56	70.56	20.16	64.12	24.08
Crackers, graham, plain	1.0 cracker	0.48	42.35	9.45	1.68	7.28	2.10
Crackers, low sodium/whole-wheat	1.0 cracker	0.35	9.88	11.88	2.00	11.80	3.96
Crackers, saltines	1.0 cracker	0.28	39.06	3.84	3.57	3.15	0.81
Muffin, English, plain	0.5 item	2.19	132.24	37.34	49.59	37.90	5.98
Bread, Italian, enriched	1.0 slice	1.76	116.80	22.00	15.60	20.60	5.40
Roll, hard, enriched	0.5 item	2.82	155.04	30.78	27.08	28.50	7.70
Roll, hamburger/hot dog	1.0 item	3.66	240.80	60.63	59.77	37.84	8.60
Cookies, vanilla wafer, lower fat	5.0 items	1.00	62.40	19.40	9.60	20.80	2.80
Meat/Fish							
Pot roast, arm, beef, cooked	1.0 oz	9.36	18.70	81.88	2.55	75.93	6.80
Hamburger patty, beef/lean, broiled	1.0 oz	7.00	21.82	85.28	3.12	44.77	5.95
Steak, sirloin, lean, broiled	1.0 oz	8.60	18.70	114.18	3.12	69.13	9.07
Chicken, leg, no skin, roasted	1.0 oz	7.66	25.80	68.61	3.40	51.88	6.80
Chicken, breast, no skin, roasted	1.0 oz	8.79	20.98	72.58	4.25	64.64	8.22
Lamb, all cuts, lean/fat, cooked	1.0 oz	6.95	20.40	87.83	4.82	53.27	6.52
Turkey, dark meat, no skin, roasted	1.0 oz	8.10	22.40	82.22	9.07	57.83	6.80
Turkey, light meat, no skin, roasted	1.0 oz	8.48	18.14	86.47	5.39	62.09	7.94
Veal, all cuts, lean, cooked	1.0 oz	9.04	25.22	95.77	6.80	70.83	7.93
Bluefish, cooked, dry heat	1.0 oz	7.28	21.82	135.15	2.55	82.45	11.90
Flatfish, cooked, dry heat	1.0 oz	6.85	29.75	97.47	5.10	81.88	16.43
Cod, cooked, dry heat	1.0 oz	6.47	22.10	69.13	3.97	39.10	11.90
Halibut, cooked, dry heat	1.0 oz	7.56	19.55	163.20	17.00	80.75	30.32
Shrimp, mixed species, cooked	1.0 oz	5.92	63.47	51.57	11.05	38.82	9.63
Tuna, can/oil, drained	1.0 oz	8.26	100.36	58.68	3.69	88.17	8.79
Tuna, can/water, low sodium	1.0 oz	7.23	14.17	67.15	3.12	46.18	7.65
Sweets							
Honey, strained/extracted	1.0 tbsp	0.06	0.84	10.92	1.26	0.84	0.42
Ice milk, vanilla, hard, 4% fat	0.5 cup	2.51	56.10	139.26	91.74	71.94	9.90
Ice cream, vanilla, hard, 11% fat	0.5 cup	2.31	52.80	131.34	84.48	69.30	9.24
Ice cream, van, rich, 16% fat	0.5 cup	2.59	41.44	177.66	86.58	70.30	8.14
Jams/ preserves, regular	1.0 tbsp	0.14	8.00	15.40	4.00	2.20	0.80
Sherbet, orange, 2% fat	0.5 cup	1.09	45.54	95.04	53.46	39.60	7.92
Sugar, brown, pressed down	0.5 cup	0.00	42.90	380.60	93.50	24.20	31.90
Sugar, white granulated	1.0 tbsp	0.00	0.12	0.25	0.12	0.25	0.00

continued

Table A-22-a
Protein, Sodium, Potassium, Calcium, Phosphorus, and Magnesium Content of Selected Common Foods per Serving Portion[a]

Food Name	Serving Portion	Pro (g)	Na (mg)	K (mg)	Ca (mg)	P (mg)	Mg (mg)
Juices							
Apple juice, can and bottle	1.0 fl oz	0.02	0.93	36.89	2.17	2.17	0.93
Apricot nectar, can	1.0 fl oz	0.12	0.94	35.80	2.20	2.83	1.57
Cranberry juice cocktail, bottle	1.0 fl oz	0.00	0.63	5.69	0.95	0.63	0.63
Grape juice, can and bottle	1.0 fl oz	0.18	0.95	41.71	2.84	3.48	3.16
Grapefruit juice, can, unsweetened	1.0 fl oz	0.16	0.31	47.28	2.16	3.40	3.09
Lemon juice, can and bottle	1.0 tbsp	0.06	3.19	15.50	1.67	1.37	1.22
Orange juice, prep from frozen conc	1.0 fl oz	0.21	0.31	59.09	2.80	4.98	3.11
Pear nectar, can	1.0 fl oz	0.03	1.25	4.06	1.56	0.94	0.94
Pineapple juice, can	1.0 fl oz	0.10	0.31	41.94	5.32	2.50	4.07
Prune juice, can	1.0 fl oz	0.20	1.28	88.32	3.84	8.00	4.48
Tomato juice, can	1.0 fl oz	0.23	109.50	66.73	2.73	5.76	3.34
Tomato juice, can, low sodium	1.0 fl oz	0.23	3.04	66.88	2.74	5.78	3.34
Vegetables, pasta, rice							
Asparagus, can, spears	0.5 cup	2.59	347.27	208.12	19.36	52.03	12.10
Asparagus, cooked from frozen	0.5 cup	2.66	3.60	196.20	20.70	49.50	11.70
Beans, snap, green, can	0.5 cup	0.78	176.85	73.58	17.55	12.82	8.78
Beans, snap, green, boiled, drained	0.5 cup	1.01	6.08	85.05	33.08	20.92	16.20
Beans, snap, wax, boiled	0.5 cup	1.18	1.88	186.88	28.75	24.38	15.62
Beets, can, whole	0.5 cup	0.74	158.11	120.62	12.22	13.86	13.86
Beets, boiled, drained	0.5 cup	1.43	65.45	259.25	13.60	32.30	19.55
Broccoli, boiled, drained	0.5 cup	2.32	20.28	227.76	35.88	46.02	18.72
Cabbage, common, boiled, drained	0.5 cup	0.76	6.00	72.75	23.25	11.25	6.00
Carrots, can, sliced, drained	0.5 cup	0.47	176.66	130.67	18.25	17.52	5.84
Carrots, boiled, drained	0.5 cup	0.85	51.48	117.06	24.18	23.40	10.14
Carrot, raw, whole, scraped	1.0 item	0.63	21.35	197.03	16.47	26.84	9.15
Cauliflower, boiled, drained	0.5 cup	1.14	9.30	88.04	9.92	19.84	5.58
Celery, raw, stalk	1.0 item	0.30	34.80	114.80	16.00	10.00	4.40
Corn, sweet, can, drained	0.5 cup	2.15	175.48	159.90	4.10	53.30	16.40
Corn, sweet, boiled, drained	0.5 cup	2.26	4.10	120.54	3.28	46.74	15.58
Cucumber, raw, sliced, with peel	0.5 cup	0.36	1.04	74.88	7.28	10.40	5.72
Peas, green, can, drained	0.5 cup	3.76	214.20	147.05	17.00	56.95	14.45
Peas, green, boiled, drained	0.5 cup	4.29	2.40	216.80	21.60	93.60	31.20
Potato, baked, with skin	1.0 item	4.65	16.16	844.36	20.20	115.14	54.54
Potato, boiled, peeled before cooked	1.0 item	2.31	6.75	442.80	10.80	54.00	27.00
Tomato, raw, red, ripe	1.0 item	1.04	11.07	273.06	6.15	29.52	13.53
Tomato, red, can, stewed	0.5 cup	1.21	281.78	303.45	42.08	25.50	15.30
Tomato, can, no salt added	0.5 cup	1.10	12.00	272.40	36.00	22.80	14.40
Noodles, egg, enriched, cooked	0.5 cup	3.80	5.60	22.40	9.60	55.20	15.20
Rice, white, enriched, parboiled, cooked	0.5 cup	2.00	2.62	32.38	16.62	36.75	10.50
Fruits							
Apples, raw, unpeeled	1.0 item	0.26	0.00	158.70	9.66	9.66	6.90
Apples, raw, peeled	1.0 item	0.19	0.00	144.64	5.12	8.96	3.84
Applesauce, can, unsweetened	0.5 cup	0.21	2.44	91.50	3.66	8.54	3.66
Apricots, can, light syrup	0.5 cup	0.67	5.06	174.57	13.92	16.44	10.12
Bananas, raw, peeled	1.0 item	1.22	1.18	467.28	7.08	23.60	34.22
Blueberries, raw	0.5 cup	0.49	4.35	64.52	4.35	7.25	3.62
Cherries, sweet, can/juice pack	0.5 cup	1.14	3.75	163.75	17.50	27.50	15.00
Grapefruit, raw, all varieties	0.5 item	0.81	0.00	177.92	15.36	10.24	10.24
Oranges, raw, all varieties	1.0 item	1.23	0.00	237.11	52.40	18.34	13.10
Peaches, raw, whole	1.0 item	0.69	0.00	193.06	4.90	11.76	6.86
Peaches, can, light syrup	0.5 cup	0.56	6.28	121.74	3.76	13.80	6.28
Pears, raw, unpeeled	1.0 item	0.65	0.00	207.50	18.26	18.26	9.96
Pineapple, can/juice pack	0.5 cup	0.52	1.24	151.89	17.43	7.47	17.43
Strawberries, raw, whole	0.5 cup	0.44	0.72	119.52	10.08	13.68	7.20

Data compiled from U.S. Department of Agriculture nutrient database for standard reference, release 11-1, and the Nutrition Coordinating Center, University of Minnesota, Nutrient database, version 28. Table compiled by the Nutrition Coordinating Center, University of Minnesota, 1997, with permission.

[a]Pro, protein; Na, sodium; K, potassium; Ca, calcium; P, phosphorus; Mg, magnesium.

Table A-22-b
Iron, Zinc, Copper, Selenium, and Manganese Content of Selected Foods per 100 Grams[a]

Food Name	Fe (mg)	Zn (mg)	Cu (mg)	Se (μg)	Mn (mg)
Dairy products					
Egg, whole, hard boiled, large	1.19	1.05	0.01	30.80	0.03
Cheese, cottage, uncreamed	0.23	0.47	0.03	9.00	trace
Cream, coffee, table, light	0.04	0.27	0.01	0.60	trace
Cream, sour, cultured	0.06	0.27	0.02	0.60	trace
Milk, buttermilk, fluid	0.05	0.42	0.01	2.00	trace
Milk, whole, 3.3% fat, fluid	0.05	0.38	0.01	2.00	trace
Milk, nonfat/skim, fluid	0.04	0.40	0.01	2.10	trace
Milk, whole, low sodium	0.05	0.38	0.01	2.00	trace
Fats					
Butter, regular	0.16	0.05	0.02	1.60	trace
Vegetable oil, corn	0.00	0.00	0.00	0.00	0.00
Vegetable oil, olive	0.38	0.06	0.00	21.20	—
Shortening, veg, soybean/cottonseed	0.00	0.00	0.00	0.00	—
Margarine, regular, hard, unsalted	0.00	0.00	0.00	1.60	0.00
Mayonnaise, soy, commercial	0.50	0.16	0.01	1.70	0.01
Cereals					
Bran flakes, Kellogg's	28.00	12.93	0.40	55.50	4.22
Corn flakes, Kellogg's	31.00	0.60	0.10	10.82	0.24
Cream of Rice, cooked	0.20	0.16	0.03	4.15	0.14
Cream of Wheat, instant	5.00	0.17	0.04	2.75	0.00
Farina, cooked, enriched	0.50	0.07	0.01	2.75	0.09
Oatmeal, cooked	0.68	0.49	0.06	5.48	0.58
Wheat, puffed, plain	4.68	3.07	0.61	123.10	2.00
Wheat, shredded, biscuit	3.15	2.51	0.50	5.90	3.07
Rice Krispies, Kellogg's	6.00	1.81	0.20	20.32	1.05
Breads, cookies, crackers					
Bread, white, soft	3.03	0.62	0.13	28.20	0.38
Bread, whole-wheat, soft	3.30	1.94	0.28	36.60	2.32
Crackers, graham, plain	3.73	0.81	0.20	13.79	0.80
Crackers, low sodium/whole-wheat	3.08	2.15	0.44	23.56	2.25
Crackers, saltines	5.40	0.77	0.20	27.95	0.70
Muffin, English, plain	2.50	0.70	0.13	20.10	0.36
Bread, Italian, enriched	2.94	0.86	0.19	27.20	0.46
Roll, hard, enriched	3.28	0.94	0.16	39.10	0.46
Roll, hamburger/hot dog	3.17	0.62	0.11	26.50	0.33
Cookies, vanilla wafer, lower fat	2.38	0.36	0.10	18.45	0.26
Meat/Fish					
Pot roast, arm, beef, cooked	3.79	8.66	0.16	17.80	0.02
Hamburger patty, beef/lean, broiled	2.11	5.36	0.07	18.00	0.01
Steak, sirloin, lean, broiled	3.36	6.52	0.15	28.10	0.02
Chicken, leg, no skin, roasted	1.31	2.86	0.08	29.00	0.02
Chicken, breast, no skin, roasted	1.04	1.00	0.05	27.60	0.02
Lamb, all cuts, lean/fat, cooked	1.88	4.46	0.12	17.00	0.02
Turkey, dark meat, no skin, roasted	2.33	4.46	0.16	40.90	0.02
Turkey, light meat, no skin, roasted	1.35	2.04	0.04	32.10	0.02
Veal, all cuts, lean, cooked	1.16	5.10	0.12	13.00	0.04
Bluefish, cooked, dry heat	0.62	1.04	0.07	51.60	0.03
Flatfish, cooked, dry heat	0.34	0.63	0.03	58.20	0.02
Cod, cooked, dry heat	0.49	0.58	0.04	37.60	0.02
Halibut, cooked, dry heat	1.07	0.53	0.04	58.20	0.02
Shrimp, mixed species, cooked	3.09	1.56	0.19	39.60	0.03
Tuna, can/oil, drained	1.39	0.90	0.07	76.00	0.02
Tuna, can/water, low sodium	1.53	0.77	0.05	80.40	0.11
Sweets					
Honey, strained/extracted	0.42	0.22	0.04	0.80	0.08
Ice milk, vanilla, hard, 4% fat	0.10	0.44	0.01	2.80	0.01
Ice cream, vanilla, hard, 11% fat	0.09	0.69	0.02	2.50	0.01
Ice cream, van, rich, 16% fat	0.05	0.40	0.02	2.50	0.01
Jams/ preserves, regular	0.49	0.60	0.10	2.00	0.04
Sherbet, orange, 2% fat	0.14	0.48	0.03	0.84	0.01
Sugar, brown, pressed down	1.91	0.18	0.30	1.20	0.32
Sugar, white granulated	0.06	0.03	0.04	0.60	0.01

continued

Table A-22-b
Iron, Zinc, Copper, Selenium, and Manganese Content of Selected Foods per 100 Grams[a]

Food Name	Fe (mg)	Zn (mg)	Cu (mg)	Se (μg)	Mn (mg)
Juices					
Apple juice, can and bottle	0.37	0.03	0.02	0.10	0.11
Apricot nectar, can	0.38	0.09	0.07	0.03	0.03
Cranberry juice cocktail, bottle	0.15	0.07	0.02	0.06	0.19
Grape juice, can and bottle	0.24	0.05	0.03	0.00	0.36
Grapefruit juice, can, unsweetened	0.20	0.09	0.04	0.00	0.02
Lemon juice, can and bottle	0.13	0.06	0.04	0.00	0.02
Orange juice, prep from frozen conc	0.10	0.05	0.04	0.10	0.01
Pear nectar, can	0.26	0.07	0.07	0.27	0.03
Pineapple juice, can	0.26	0.11	0.09	0.00	0.99
Prune juice, can	1.18	0.21	0.07	0.00	0.15
Tomato juice, can	0.58	0.14	0.10	0.50	0.08
Tomato juice, can, low sodium	0.58	0.14	0.10	0.50	0.40
Vegetables, pasta, rice					
Asparagus, can, spears	1.83	0.40	0.10	1.70	0.17
Asparagus, cooked from frozen	0.64	0.56	0.17	1.70	0.18
Beans, snap, green, can	0.90	0.29	0.04	0.40	0.20
Beans, snap, green, boiled, drained	0.88	0.48	0.06	0.40	0.32
Beans, snap, wax, boiled, drained	1.28	0.36	0.10	0.40	0.29
Beets, can, whole	1.82	0.21	0.06	0.90	0.29
Beets, boiled, drained	0.79	0.35	0.07	0.90	0.33
Broccoli, boiled, drained	0.84	0.38	0.04	1.90	0.22
Cabbage, common, boiled, drained	0.17	0.09	0.01	0.60	0.12
Carrots, can, sliced, drained	0.64	0.26	0.10	0.80	0.45
Carrots, boiled, drained	0.62	0.30	0.13	0.80	0.75
Carrot, raw, whole, scraped	0.50	0.20	0.05	1.10	0.14
Cauliflower, boiled, drained	0.33	0.18	0.03	0.80	0.14
Celery, raw, stalk	0.40	0.13	0.03	0.90	0.10
Corn, sweet, can, drained	0.86	0.39	0.06	0.70	0.17
Corn, sweet, boiled, drained	0.35	0.40	0.04	0.70	0.13
Cucumber, raw, sliced, with peel	0.26	0.20	0.03	6.30	0.08
Peas, green, can, drained	0.95	0.71	0.08	1.70	0.30
Peas, green, boiled, drained	1.54	1.19	0.17	1.00	0.52
Potato, baked, with skin	1.36	0.32	0.30	0.80	0.23
Potato, boiled, peeled before cooked	0.31	0.27	0.17	1.04	0.14
Tomato, raw, red, ripe	0.45	0.09	0.07	0.40	0.10
Tomato, red, can, stewed	0.73	0.17	0.11	0.70	0.06
Tomato, can, no salt added	0.55	0.16	0.11	0.70	0.13
Noodles, egg, enriched, cooked	1.59	0.62	0.09	21.70	0.26
Rice, white, enriched, parboiled, cooked	1.13	0.31	0.09	7.50	0.26
Fruits					
Apples, raw, unpeeled	0.18	0.04	0.04	0.30	0.04
Apples, raw, peeled	0.07	0.04	0.03	0.30	0.02
Applesauce, can, unsweetened	0.12	0.03	0.03	0.30	0.08
Apricots, can, light syrup	0.39	0.11	0.08	0.20	0.05
Bananas, raw, peeled	0.31	0.16	0.10	1.10	0.15
Blueberries, raw	0.17	0.11	0.06	0.00	0.28
Cherries, sweet, can/juice pack	0.58	0.10	0.07	0.22	0.06
Grapefruit, raw, all varieties	0.09	0.07	0.05	0.87	0.01
Oranges, raw, all varieties	0.10	0.07	0.04	0.50	0.02
Peaches, raw, whole	0.11	0.14	0.07	0.40	0.05
Peaches, can, light syrup	0.36	0.09	0.05	0.30	0.05
Pears, raw, unpeeled	0.25	0.12	0.11	1.00	0.08
Pineapple, can/juice pack	0.28	0.10	0.09	0.40	1.12
Strawberries, raw, whole	0.38	0.13	0.05	0.20	0.29

Data compiled from U.S. Department of Agriculture nutrient database for standard reference, release 11-1, and the Nutrition Coordinating Center, University of Minnesota, Nutrient database, version 28. Table compiled by the Nutrition Coordinating Center, University of Minnesota, 1997, with permission.

[a]Fe, iron; Zn, zinc; Cu, copper; Se, selenium; Mn, manganese.

[b]Trace is ≤ 0.005 g/100 g food.

Table A-23-a
Vitamin A, Vitamin E, α-Tocopherol (TOC), Vitamin C, Thiamin, Riboflavin, Niacin, Vitamin B_6, Vitamin B_{12}, and Folate Content of Selected Common Foods per Serving Portion

Food Name	Serving Portion	A[a] (RE)	E[b] (mg)	α-TOC (mg)	C (mg)	Thiamin (mg)	Ribo (mg)	Niacin (mg)	B_6 (mg)	B_{12} (μg)	Folate (μg)
Dairy products											
Egg, whole, hard boiled, large	1.0 item	84.00	0.52	0.50	0.00	0.03	0.26	0.03	0.06	0.56	22.0
Cheese, cottage, uncreamed	1.0 oz	2.26	0.03	0.03	0.00	0.01	0.04	0.04	0.02	0.23	4.1
Cream, coffee, table, light	1.0 tbsp	27.30	0.02	0.02	0.11	trace[c]	0.02	0.01	trace[c]	0.03	0.3
Cream, sour, cultured	1.0 tbsp	23.40	0.07	0.07	0.10	trace[c]	0.02	0.01	trace[c]	0.04	1.3
Milk, buttermilk, fluid	1.0 cup	19.60	0.15	0.15	2.40	0.08	0.38	0.14	0.08	0.54	12.2
Milk, whole, 3.3% fat, fluid	1.0 cup	75.64	0.24	0.24	2.29	0.09	0.40	0.20	0.10	0.87	12.2
Milk, nonfat/skim, fluid	1.0 cup	149.45	0.10	0.10	2.40	0.09	0.34	0.22	0.10	0.93	12.7
Milk, whole, low sodium	1.0 cup	78.08	0.24	0.24	2.29	0.05	0.26	0.10	0.08	0.88	12.2
Fats											
Butter, regular	1.0 tbsp	107.07	0.22	0.22	0.00	trace[c]	trace[c]	0.01	0.00	0.02	0.4
Vegetable oil, corn	1.0 tsp	0.00	0.96	0.66	0.00	0.00	0.00	0.00	0.00	0.00	0.0
Vegetable oil, olive	1.0 tsp	0.00	0.56	0.51	0.00	0.00	0.00	0.00	0.00	0.00	0.0
Shortening, veg, soybean/ cottonseed	1.0 tsp	0.00	0.35	0.14	0.00	0.00	0.00	0.00	0.00	0.00	0.0
Margarine, reg, hard, unsalted	1.0 tsp	37.55	0.52	0.36	trace[c]	0.00	trace[c]	trace[c]	0.00	trace[c]	0.0
Mayonnaise, soy, commercial	1.0 tsp	3.86	0.54	0.50	0.00	0.00	0.00	trace[c]	0.03	0.01	0.3
Cereals											
Bran flakes, Kellogg's	0.75 cup	362.79	5.36	5.28	14.99	0.38	0.44	5.00	0.49	1.45	102.3
Corn flakes, Kellogg's	1.0 cup	210.28	0.04	0.03	14.00	0.36	0.39	4.68	0.48	0.00	98.8
Cream of Rice, cooked	1.0 cup	0.00	0.05	0.05	0.00	0.00	0.00	0.98	0.07	0.00	7.3
Cream of Wheat, instant	1.0 cup	0.00	0.03	0.03	0.00	0.24	0.00	1.69	0.03	0.00	9.6
Farina, cooked, enriched	1.0 cup	0.00	0.03	0.03	0.00	0.19	0.12	1.28	0.02	0.00	4.6
Oatmeal, cooked	1.0 cup	4.68	0.23	0.19	0.00	0.26	0.05	0.30	0.05	0.00	9.3
Wheat, puffed, plain	1.25 cup	0.15	0.10	0.09	0.00	0.06	0.04	1.79	0.02	0.06	5.1
Wheat, shredded, biscuit	1 item	0.00	0.12	0.08	0.00	0.07	0.07	1.08	0.06	0.00	11.8
Rice Krispies, Kellogg's	1.25 cup	247.83	0.04	0.04	16.50	0.43	0.46	5.51	0.56	0.00	116.4
Breads, cookies, crackers											
Bread, white, soft	1.0 slice	0.00	0.07	0.06	0.00	0.12	0.08	0.99	0.02	trace[c]	8.5
Bread, whole-wheat, soft	1.0 slice	0.00	0.29	0.27	0.00	0.10	0.06	1.07	0.05	trace[c]	14.0
Crackers, graham, plain	1.0 cracker	0.00	0.13	0.07	0.00	0.02	0.02	0.29	trace[c]	0.00	1.1
Crackers, low sodium, whole-wheat	1.0 cracker	0.00	0.16	0.09	0.00	0.01	trace[c]	0.18	0.01	0.00	1.1
Crackers, saltines	1.0 cracker	0.00	0.05	0.03	0.00	0.02	0.01	0.16	trace[c]	0.00	0.9
Muffin, English, plain	0.5 item	0.00	0.03	0.02	0.03	0.13	0.08	1.11	0.01	0.01	10.5
Bread, Italian, enriched	1.0 slice	0.00	0.06	0.02	0.00	0.10	0.06	0.88	0.01	0.01	6.0
Roll, hard, enriched	0.5 item	0.00	0.05	0.05	0.00	0.14	0.10	1.21	0.02	0.00	4.2
Roll, hamburger/hot dog	1.0 item	0.00	0.20	0.19	0.00	0.21	0.13	1.69	0.02	0.01	11.6
Cookies, vanilla wafer, lower fat	5.0 items	3.60	0.27	0.15	0.00	0.06	0.06	0.62	0.02	0.02	1.8
Meat/fish											
Pot roast, arm, beef, cooked	1.0 oz	0.00	0.04	0.04	0.00	0.02	0.08	1.05	0.09	0.96	3.1
Hamburger patty, beef, lean, broiled	1.0 oz	0.00	0.06	0.06	0.00	0.01	0.06	1.46	0.07	0.67	2.5
Steak, sirloin, lean, broiled	1.0 oz	0.00	0.04	0.04	0.00	0.04	0.08	1.21	0.13	0.81	2.8
Chicken, leg, no skin, roasted	1.0 oz	5.39	0.08	0.08	0.00	0.02	0.07	1.79	0.10	0.09	2.2
Chicken, breast, no skin, roasted	1.0 oz	1.70	0.08	0.08	0.00	0.02	0.03	3.89	0.17	0.10	1.1
Lamb, all cuts, lean/fat, cooked	1.0 oz	0.00	0.04	0.04	0.00	0.03	0.07	1.89	0.04	0.72	5.1
Turkey, dark meat, no skin, roasted	1.0 oz	0.00	0.18	0.18	0.00	0.02	0.07	1.03	0.10	0.10	2.5
Turkey, light meat, no skin, roasted	1.0 oz	0.00	0.03	0.03	0.00	0.02	0.04	1.94	0.15	0.10	1.7
Veal, all cuts, lean, cooked	1.0 oz	0.00	0.12	0.12	0.00	0.02	0.10	2.39	0.09	0.47	4.5
Bluefish, cooked, dry heat	1.0 oz	39.10	—[d]	—[d]	0.00	0.02	0.03	2.05	0.13	1.76	0.5
Flatfish, cooked, dry heat	1.0 oz	3.12	0.54	0.54	0.00	0.02	0.03	0.62	0.07	0.71	2.6
Cod, cooked, dry heat	1.0 oz	3.97	0.08	0.08	0.28	0.02	0.02	0.71	0.08	0.30	2.3
Halibut, cooked, dry heat	1.0 oz	15.30	0.31	0.31	0.00	0.02	0.03	2.02	0.11	0.39	3.9
Shrimp, mixed species, cooked	1.0 oz	18.70	0.14	0.14	0.62	0.01	0.01	0.73	0.04	0.42	0.9
Tuna, can/oil, drained	1.0 oz	6.52	0.34	0.34	0.00	0.01	0.03	3.52	0.03	0.62	1.5
Tuna, can/water, low sodium	1.0 oz	4.82	0.15	0.15	0.00	0.01	0.02	3.76	0.10	0.85	1.1

continued

Table A-23-a
Vitamin A, Vitamin E, α-Tocopherol (TOC), Vitamin C, Thiamin, Riboflavin, Niacin, Vitamin B_6, Vitamin B_{12} and Folate Content of Selected Common Foods per Serving Portion

Food Name	Serving Portion	A[a] (RE)	E[b] (mg)	α-TOC (mg)	C (mg)	Thiamin (mg)	Ribo (mg)	Niacin (mg)	B_6 (mg)	B_{12} (μg)	Folate (μg)
Sweets											
Honey, strained/extracted	1.0 tbsp	0.00	0.00	0.00	0.10	0.00	0.01	0.02	trace	0.00	0.4
Ice milk, vanilla, hard, 4% fat	0.5 cup	31.02	0.00	0.00	0.53	0.04	0.18	0.06	0.04	0.44	3.9
Ice cream, vanilla, hard, 11% fat	0.5 cup	77.22	0.00	0.00	0.40	0.03	0.16	0.08	0.03	0.26	3.3
Ice cream, vanilla, rich, 16% fat	0.5 cup	136.16	0.00	0.00	0.52	0.03	0.12	0.06	0.03	0.27	3.7
Jams/preserves, regular	1.0 tbsp	0.20	0.00	0.00	1.76	0.00	trace[c]	0.01	trace	0.00	6.6
Sherbet, orange, 2% fat	0.5 cup	13.86	0.06	0.06	4.26	0.02	0.07	0.10	0.03	0.13	3.9
Sugar, brown, pressed down	0.5 cup	0.00	0.00	0.00	0.00	0.01	0.01	0.09	0.03	0.00	1.1
Sugar, white, granulated	1.0 tbsp	0.00	0.00	0.00	0.00	0.00	trace[c]	0.00	0.00	0.00	0.0
Juices											
Apple juice, can and bottle	1.0 fl oz	0.00	trace[c]	trace[c]	0.28	0.01	trace[c]	0.03	0.01	0.00	0.0
Apricot nectar, can	1.0 fl oz	41.45	0.02	0.01	0.19	trace[c]	trace[c]	0.08	0.01	0.00	0.4
Cranberry juice cocktail, bottle	1.0 fl oz	0.00	0.00	0.00	11.19	trace[c]	trace[c]	0.01	0.01	0.00	0.0
Grape juice, can and bottle	1.0 fl oz	0.32	0.00	0.00	0.03	0.01	0.01	0.08	0.02	0.00	0.8
Grapefruit juice can, unsweetened	1.0 fl oz	0.31	0.02	0.02	9.02	0.01	0.01	0.07	0.01	0.00	3.2
Lemon juice, can and bottle	1 tbsp	0.30	0.01	0.01	3.77	0.01	trace[c]	0.03	0.01	0.00	1.5
Orange juice, prep from frozen concentrate	1.0 fl oz	2.49	0.06	0.06	12.10	0.02	0.01	0.06	0.01	0.00	13.6
Pear nectar, can	1.0 fl oz	0.00	0.03	0.03	0.34	trace[c]	trace[c]	0.04	trace[c]	0.00	0.3
Pineapple juice, can	1.0 fl oz	0.00	0.01	0.01	3.35	0.02	0.01	0.08	0.03	0.00	7.2
Prune juice, can	1.0 fl oz	0.00	trace[c]	trace[c]	1.31	trace[c]	0.02	0.25	0.07	0.00	0.1
Tomato juice, can	1.0 fl oz	16.99	0.28	0.28	5.55	0.01	0.01	0.20	0.03	0.00	6.0
Tomato juice, can, low sodium	1.0 fl oz	17.02	0.28	0.28	5.56	0.01	0.01	0.20	0.03	0.00	6.0
Vegetables, pasta, rice											
Asparagus, can, spears	0.5 cup	64.13	0.52	0.51	22.26	0.07	0.12	1.15	0.13	0.00	115.6
Asparagus, cooked from frozen	0.5 cup	73.80	1.12	1.08	21.96	0.06	0.09	0.93	0.02	0.00	121.2
Beans, snap, green, can	0.5 cup	23.62	0.09	0.09	3.24	0.01	0.04	0.14	0.02	0.00	21.4
Beans, green, boiled, drained	0.5 cup	27.00	0.09	0.08	2.77	0.02	0.06	0.26	0.04	0.00	15.5
Beans, snap, wax, boiled, drained	0.5 cup	5.00	0.18	0.18	6.06	0.05	0.06	0.38	0.04	0.00	20.8
Beets, can, whole	0.5 cup	0.82	0.24	0.19	3.34	0.01	0.03	0.13	0.05	0.00	24.6
Beets, boiled, drained	0.5 cup	3.40	0.26	0.21	3.06	0.02	0.03	0.28	0.06	0.00	68.0
Broccoli, boiled, drained	0.5 cup	108.42	1.32	1.30	58.19	0.04	0.09	0.45	0.11	0.00	39.0
Cabbage, common, boiled, drained	0.5 cup	9.75	0.08	0.08	15.08	0.04	0.04	0.21	0.08	0.00	15.0
Carrots, can, sliced, drained	0.5 cup	1005.21	0.31	0.31	1.97	0.01	0.02	0.40	0.08	0.00	6.7
Carrots, boiled, drained	0.5 cup	1914.90	0.33	0.33	1.79	0.03	0.04	0.40	0.19	0.00	10.8
Carrot, raw, whole, scraped	1.0 item	1715.93	0.28	0.27	5.67	0.06	0.04	0.57	0.09	0.00	8.5
Cauliflower, boiled, drained	0.5 cup	1.24	0.02	0.02	27.47	0.03	0.03	0.25	0.11	0.00	27.2
Celery, raw, stalk	1.0 item	5.20	0.14	0.14	2.80	0.02	0.02	0.13	0.04	0.00	11.2
Corn, sweet, can, drained	0.5 cup	13.12	0.12	0.10	6.97	0.03	0.06	0.98	0.04	0.00	39.8
Corn, sweet, boiled, drained	0.5 cup	18.04	0.07	0.04	2.54	0.7	0.06	1.06	0.11	0.00	25.4
Cucumber, raw, sliced, with peel	0.5 cup	10.92	0.04	0.04	2.76	0.01	0.01	0.12	0.02	0.00	6.7
Peas, green, can, drained	0.5 cup	65.45	0.32	0.32	8.16	0.10	0.07	0.62	0.05	0.00	37.6
Peas, green, boiled, drained	0.5 cup	48.00	0.31	0.04	11.36	0.21	0.12	1.62	0.17	0.00	50.6
Potato baked with skin	1.0 item	0.00	0.10	0.10	26.06	0.22	0.07	3.32	0.70	0.00	22.2
Potato, boiled, peeled before cooked	1.0 item	0.00	0.07	0.07	9.99	0.13	0.03	1.77	0.36	0.00	12.0
Tomato, raw, red, ripe	1.0 item	76.26	0.47	0.43	23.49	0.07	0.06	0.77	0.10	0.00	18.4
Tomato, red, can, stewed	0.5 cup	68.85	0.48	0.45	14.54	0.06	0.04	0.91	0.02	0.00	6.8
Tomato, can, no salt added	0.5 cup	72.00	0.46	0.44	17.04	0.05	0.04	0.88	0.11	0.00	9.8
Noodles, egg, enriched, cooked	0.5 cup	4.80	0.04	0.02	0.00	0.15	0.07	1.19	0.03	0.07	5.6
Rice, white, enriched, parboiled, cooked	0.5 cup	0.00	0.04	0.04	0.00	0.22	0.02	1.22	0.02	0.00	3.5
Fruit											
Apple, raw, unpeeled	1.0 item	6.90	0.44	0.44	7.87	0.02	0.02	0.11	0.07	0.00	3.8
Apple, raw, peeled	1.0 item	5.12	0.10	0.10	5.12	0.02	0.01	0.12	0.06	0.00	0.5
Applesauce, can, unsweetened	0.5 cup	3.66	0.01	0.01	1.46	0.02	0.03	0.23	0.03	0.00	0.7
Apricots, can, light syrup	0.5 cup	166.98	1.13	1.09	3.42	0.02	0.03	0.38	0.07	0.00	2.1
Bananas, raw, peeled	1.0 item	9.44	0.32	0.32	10.74	0.05	0.12	0.64	0.68	0.00	22.5

continued

Table A-23-a
Vitamin A, Vitamin E, α-Tocopherol (TOC), Vitamin C, Thiamin, Riboflavin, Niacin, Vitamin B_6, Vitamin B_{12}, and Folate Content of Selected Common Foods per Serving Portion (Continued)

Food Name	Serving Portion	A[a] (RE)	E[b] (mg)	α-TOC (mg)	C (mg)	Thiamin (mg)	Ribo (mg)	Niacin (mg)	B_6 (mg)	B_{12} (μg)	Folate (μg)
Blueberries, raw	0.5 cup	7.25	0.72	0.63	9.42	0.03	0.04	0.26	0.03	0.00	4.6
Cherries, sweet, can/juice pack	0.5 cup	16.25	0.12	0.12	3.12	0.02	0.03	0.51	0.04	0.00	5.2
Grapefruit, raw, all varieties	0.5 item	15.36	0.32	0.32	44.03	0.05	0.03	0.32	0.05	0.00	13.0
Oranges, raw, all varieties	1.0 item	27.51	0.31	0.31	69.69	0.11	0.05	0.37	0.08	0.00	39.6
Peaches, raw, whole	1.0 item	52.92	0.69	0.67	6.47	0.02	0.04	0.97	0.02	0.00	3.3
Peaches, can, light syrup	0.5 cup	43.92	1.12	1.11	3.01	0.01	0.03	0.74	0.02	0.00	4.1
Pears, raw, unpeeled	1.0 item	3.32	0.83	0.80	6.64	0.03	0.07	0.17	0.03	0.00	12.1
Pineapple, can/juice pack	0.5 cup	4.98	0.12	0.12	11.83	0.12	0.02	0.35	0.09	0.00	5.9
Strawberries, raw, whole	0.5 cup	2.16	0.10	0.09	40.82	0.01	0.05	0.17	0.04	0.00	12.7

Data compiled from U.S. Department of Agriculture nutrient database for standard reference, release 11-1 and the Nutrition Coordinating Center, University of Minnesota, Nutrient database, version 28. Table compiled by the Nutrition Coordinating Center, University of Minnesota, 1997, with permission.

[a]1 RE is equal to 1 μg retinol or 6 μg β-carotene.

[b]mg of vitamin E represents total tocopherol activity, including α-tocopherol.

[c]Trace is a value ≤ 0.005/serving portion.

[d]Denotes lack of reliable data.

Table A-23-b
Average Vitamin K Content (μg/100 g) of Ordinary Foods

Food	Vitamin K	Food	Vitamin K
Milk and milk products		Vegetables	
Butter	30.0	Asparagus	70
Cheese	2.8	Beans, green	46
Milk (cow)	1.0	Broccoli	147
Milk (human)	0.2	Brussels sprouts	250
Eggs		Cabbage	110
Hens (whole)	11.0	Celery	5
Meat and meat products		Collards	440
Bacon	0.1	Kale	726
Beef liver	3.0	Lettuce	75
Chicken liver	0.3	Peas, green	33
Ground beef	2.4	Potato	1
Ham	0.1	Spinach	413
Lamb chop	4.6	Tomato	5
Pork tenderloin	0.1	Turnip	1
Fats		Turnip greens	650
Olive oil	56	Fruits	
Soy bean oil	198	Applesauce	0.6
Corn oil	3	Banana	0.2
Safflower oil	10	Orange	0.1
Margarine	30	Peach	2.5
Cereal and grain products		Pear	4.0
Bread	2.5	Strawberry	1.5
Maize	0.1	Beverages	
Oatmeal	2.0	Coffee	<0.1
Rice	0.1	Cola	<0.1
Cornflakes	0.1	Tea	<0.1
Granola	1.8	Lemonade	0.1
Shredded wheat	1.5	Beer	<0.1
		Tobacco	
		Cigarettes	5000

Data from Shearer, Bach, Kohlmeier. J Nutrition 1996; 126 (Suppl): 1181S–86S; Booth, Sadowski, Pennington. J Agric Food Chem 1995; 43:1574–9; Ferland, MacDonald, Sadowski. J Am Diet Assoc 1992; 92:593–7. Courtesy of RE Olson (See Chapter 20).

Table A-23-c
Retention of Nutrients in Cooked Vegetables[a]

	Ascorbic Acid (%)	Thiamin (%)	Riboflavin (%)	Niacin (%)	Pantothenic Acid[b] (%)	Vitamin B_6 (%)	Folate[c] (%)	Vitamin A (%)
Potatoes								
Prepared from raw								
Baked in skin	80	85	95	95	90	95	90	—[d]
Boiled in skin	75	80	95	95	90	95	90	—
Boiled without skin	75	80	95	95	90	95	75	—
Fried	80	80	95	95	90	95	75	—
Hashed-brown[e]	25	40	85	80	—	—	65	—
Mashed	75	80	95	95	90	95	75	—
Scalloped and au gratin	80	80	95	95	90	95	75	—
Prepared from frozen								
French fried, heated	50	75	95	95	90	95	75	—
Baked, stuffed, heated	80	85	95	95	90	95	80	—
Hashed-brown	80	80	95	95	90	95	80	—
Sweet Potatoes								
Prepared from raw								
Baked in skin	80	85	95	95	90	95	90	90
Boiled in skin	75	80	95	95	90	95	90	85
Prepared from frozen								
Baked	80	80	95	95	90	95	80	90
Boiled	75	80	95	95	90	95	80	85
Tomatoes (prepared from raw, baked, boiled, or stewed)	95	95	95	95	95	95	70	95
Other vegetables (cooked in small or moderate amount of water until tender)								
Prepared from raw, drained								
Greens, dark and leafy[f]	60	85	95	90	95	90	65	95
Roots, bulbs, other vegetables of high starch and/or sugar content[g]	70	85	95	95	90	95	70	90
Other[h]	80	85	95	90	90	90	70	90
Prepared from frozen, drained								
Greens, dark and leafy[f]	60	90	95	90	95	90	55	95
Roots, bulbs, other vegetables of high starch and/or sugar content[g]	70	90	95	95	90	95	70	90
Other[h]	80	90	95	90	90	90	70	90

From Composition of foods, raw, processed, prepared. 1990 Supplement. Washington, DC: U.S. Department of Agriculture. Human Nutrition Information Service, Agriculture handbook no. 8.

[a] $\% \text{ True retention} = \frac{\text{Nutrient content per g of cooked food} \times \text{g of food after cooking}}{\text{Nutrient content per g of raw food} \times \text{g of food before cooking}} \times 100$

[b] Because of limited data, values are based on nutrient retention data from other cooked plant products.

[c] Values are based on limited data.

[d] Dashes denote lack of reliable data.

[e] Potatoes were pared, boiled, and held overnight before hashed-browning.

[f] Vegetables such as beet greens, Chinese cabbage, collards, mustard greens, spinach, Swiss chard, turnip greens, and other wild greens.

[g] Vegetables such as beets, carrots, green peas, lima beans, onions, parsnips, rutabagas, salsify, turnips, summer and winter squash, and other immature seeds of the legume group.

[h] Vegetables such as asparagus, bean sprouts, broccoli, brussels sprouts, cabbage, cauliflower, eggplant, kohlrabi, okra, and sweet peppers.

Table A-24-a
Caffeine Content of Selected Common Foods per Serving Portion

Food Name	Serving Portion	Caffeine (mg)
Candy, milk chocolate	1.0 oz	7.24
Candy, semisweet chocolate	1.0 oz	17.58
Candy, sweet chocolate	1.0 oz	18.71
Chocolate, unsweetened, baking type	1.0 oz	57.83
Chocolate beverage mix, prepared	8.0 fl oz	7.98
Cocoa mix, prepared	6.0 fl oz	4.12
Cocoa powder, unsweetened	1.0 tbsp	12.42
Coffee, brewed, regular	6.0 fl oz	103.24
Coffee, brewed, espresso	6.0 fl oz	377.54
Coffee, instant, regular, prepared	6.0 fl oz	57.28
Coffee, instant, decaffeinated, prepared	6.0 fl oz	1.79
Coffee, instant, cappuccino flavor, prepared	6.0 fl oz	74.88
Coffee, instant, french flavor, prepared	6.0 fl oz	51.03
Coffee, instant, mocha flavor, prepared	6.0 fl oz	33.84
Cola beverage, regular	12.0 fl oz	37.00
Cola beverage, diet	12.0 fl oz	49.70
Ice cream, chocolate	0.5 cup	40.92
Milk, chocolate	8.0 fl oz	5.00
Pudding, chocolate	0.5 cup	5.65
Tea, brewed	6.0 fl oz	35.60
Tea, instant, unsweetened, prepared	6.0 fl oz	23.14
Tea, instant, unsweetened, lemon flavored, prepared	6.0 fl oz	19.64
Topping, chocolate, fudge type	1.0 tbsp	1.89
Topping, chocolate, syrup	1.0 tbsp	2.63

Data compiled from U.S. Department of Agriculture Nutrient database for standard reference, release 11-1, and the Nutrition Coordinating Center, University of Minnesota, Nutrient database, version 28. Table compiled by the Nutrition Coordinating Center, University of Minnesota, 1997, with permission.

Table A-24-b
Carnitine Content of Selected Foods

Food Item	Carnitine Content[a]	Food Item	Carnitine Content
Meat products		*Fruits*	
Beef steak	592 ± 260 (4)	Bananas	0.0056
Ground beef	582 ± 32 (3)	Apples	0.0002
Pork	172 ± 32 (3)	Strawberries	ND
Canadian bacon	146 ± 52 (3)	Peaches	0.0060
Bacon	145 ± 24 (3)	Pineapple	0.0063
Fish (cod)	34.6 ± 11.7 (3)	Pears	0.0107
Chicken breast	24.3 ± 8.0 (3)		
Dairy products		*Grains*	
Whole milk	20.4	White bread	0.912
American cheese	23.2	Whole-wheat bread	2.26
Ice cream	23.0	Rice (cooked)	0.090
Butter	3.07	Macaroni	0.780
Cottage cheese	6.96	Corn Flakes	0.078
Vegetables		*Nondairy beverages*	
Broccoli (fresh)	0.0228	Grapefruit juice	ND
(cooked)	0.0111	Orange juice	0.012
Carrots (fresh)	0.0408	Tomato juice	0.030
(cooked)	0.0393	Coffee	0.009
Green beans (cooked)	0.0189	Cola	ND
Green peas (cooked)	0.0369	Grape juice	0.093
Asparagus (cooked)	1.21	*Miscellaneous*	
Beets (cooked)	0.0195	Eggs	0.075
Potato (baked)	0.0800	Peanut butter	0.516
Lettuce	0.0066		

Adapted from Rebouche CJ, Engel AG. J Clin Invest 1984; 73:857–67.

[a]Units are μmol/100 g (solid foods) or μmol/100 mL (liquids). ND, not detectable. Values for meat products are mean ± SD (number of observations in parentheses) and are based on precooked weight. Values reported are for total (nonesterified plus esterified) carnitine.

With appreciation to CJ Rebouche (see Chapter 31).

Table A-24-c
Choline Content of Some Common Foods

	Concentration (μmol/kg)[a]		
Food	Choline	Phosphatidylcholine	Sphingomyelin
Apple	27	280	15
Banana	240	37	20
Beef liver	5831	43500	1850
Beef steak	75	6030	506
Butter	42	1760	460
Cauliflower	1306	2770	183
Corn oil	3	12	5
Coffee	90	34	23
Cucumber	218	76	27
Egg	42	52000	2250
Ginger ale	2	4	3
Grape juice	475	15	5
Iceberg lettuce	2930	132	50
Margarine	30	450	15
Milk (bovine, whole)	150	148	82
Orange	200	490	24
Peanut butter	3895	3937	9
Peanuts	4546	4960	78
Potato	511	300	26
Tomato	430	52	32
Whole wheat bread	968	340	11

Modified from Zeisel SH. Biological consequences of choline deficiency. In: Wurtman R, Wurtman J, eds. Choline metabolism and Brain Function. New York: Raven Press, 1990; 75–99.

[a]Choline, phosphatidylcholine and sphingomyelin were measured using a gas chromatography/mass spectrometry assay in foods prepared in the form that they would normally be consumed.

Courtesy of SH Zeisel (see Chapter 32).

Table A-25-a
Standard Exchange Lists for Meal Planning

STARCH LIST

Cereals, grains, pasta, breads, crackers, snacks, starchy vegetables, and cooked beans, peas, and lentils are starches. In general, one starch is equivalent to:

- ½ cup of cereal, grain, pasta, or starchy vegetable
- 1 oz of a bread product, such as 1 slice of bread
- ¾ to 1 oz of most snack foods (Some snack foods may also have added fat.)

Selection Notes

1. Starchy vegetables prepared with fat count as one starch and one fat.
2. Bagels or muffins can be 2 oz, 3 oz, or 4 oz in size, and can, therefore, count as two, three, or four starch choices.
3. Beans, peas, and lentils are often found on the Meat and Meat Substitutes list.
4. Regular potato chips and tortilla chips are found on the Other Carbohydrates list.
5. Most of the serving sizes are measured after cooking.

One starch exchange equals 15 g carbohydrate, 3 g protein, 0–1 g fat, and 80 calories.

Bread

Bagel	½ (1 oz)	Pita, 6 in. across	½
Bread, reduced-calorie	2 slices (1½ oz)	Raisin bread, unfrosted	1 slice (1 oz)
Bread, white, whole-wheat, pumpernickel, rye	1 slice (1 oz)	Roll, plain, small	1 (1 oz)
Bread sticks, crisp, 4 in. long × ½ in.	2 (⅔ oz)	Tortilla, corn, 6 in. across	1
English muffin	½	Tortilla, flour, 7–8 in. across	1
Hot dog or hamburger bun	½ (1 oz)	Waffle, 4½ in. square, reduced fat	1

Cereals and Grains

Bran cereals	½ cup	Millet	¼ cup
Bulgur	½ cup	Muesli	¼ cup
Cereals	½ cup	Oats	½ cup
Cereals, unsweetened, ready-to-eat	¾ cup	Pasta	½ cup
Cornmeal (dry)	3 tbsp	Puffed cereal	1½ cups
Couscous	⅓ cup	Rice milk	½ cup
Flour (dry)	3 tbsp	Rice, white or brown	⅓ cup
Granola, low-fat	¼ cup	Shredded Wheat	½ cup
Grape-Nuts	¼ cup	Sugar-frosted cereal	½ cup
Grits	½ cup	Wheat germ	3 tbsp
Kasha	½ cup		

Starchy Vegetables

Baked beans	⅓ cup	Potato, baked or boiled	1 small (3 oz)
Corn	½ cup	Potato, mashed	½ cup
Corn on cob, medium	1 (5 oz)	Squash, winter (acorn, butternut)	1 cup
Mixed vegetables with corn, peas, or pasta	1 cup	Yam, sweet potato, plain	½ cup
Peas, green	½ cup		
Plantain	½ cup		

Crackers and Snacks

Animal crackers	8	Pretzels	¾ oz
Graham crackers, 2½ in. square	3	Rice cakes, 4 in. across	2
Matzoh	¾ oz	Saltine-type crackers	6
Melba toast	4 slices	Snack chips, fat-free (tortilla, potato)	15–20 (¾ oz)
Oyster crackers	24	Whole-wheat crackers, no fat added	2–5 (¾ oz)
Popcorn (popped, no fat added or low-fat microwave)	3 cups		

continued

Table A-25-a—*continued*
Standard Exchange Lists for Meal Planning

Beans, Peas, and Lentils
(Count as 1 starch exchange, plus 1 very lean meat exchange.)

Beans and peas (garbanzo, pinto, kidney, white, split, black-eyed)	½ cup	Lima beans	⅔ cup
		Lentils	½ cup
		Miso[a]	3 tbsp

[a]Equals 400 mg or more sodium per exchange.

Starchy Foods Prepared with Fat
(Count as 1 starch exchange, plus 1 fat exchange.)

Biscuit, 2½ in. across	1	Pancake, 4 in. across	2
Chow mein noodles	½ cup	Popcorn, microwave	3 cups
Corn bread, 2 in. cube	1 (2 oz)	Sandwich crackers, cheese or peanut butter filling	3
Crackers, round butter type	6	Stuffing, bread (prepared)	⅓ cup
Croutons	1 cup	Taco shell, 6 in. across	2
French-fried potatoes	16-25 (3 oz)	Waffle, 4½ in. square	1
Granola	¼ cup	Whole-wheat crackers, fat added	4–6 (1 oz)
Muffin, small	1 (1½ oz)		

FRUIT LIST

Fresh, frozen, canned, and dried fruits and fruit juices are on this list. In general, one fruit exchange is equivalent to

- 1 small to medium fresh fruit
- ½ cup of canned or fresh fruit or fruit juice
- ¼ cup of dried fruit

One fruit exchange equals 15 g carbohydrate and 60 calories.
The weight includes skin, core, seeds, and rind.

Fruit

Apple, unpeeled, small	1 (4 oz)	Kiwi	1 (3½ oz)
Applesauce, unsweetened	½ cup	Mandarin oranges, canned	¾ cup
Apples, dried	4 rings	Mango, small	½ fruit (5½ oz) or ½ cup
Apricots, fresh	4 whole (5½ oz)	Nectarine, small	1 (5 oz)
Apricots, dried	8 halves	Orange, small	1 (6½ oz)
Apricots, canned	½ cup	Papaya	½ fruit (8 oz) or 1 cup cubes
Banana, small	1 (4 oz)	Peach, medium, fresh	1 (6 oz)
Blackberries	¾ cup	Peaches, canned	½ cup
Blueberries	¾ cup	Pear, large, fresh	½ (4 oz)
Cantaloupe, small	⅓ melon (11 oz) or 1 cup cubes	Pears, canned	½ cup
Cherries, sweet, fresh	12 (3 oz)	Pineapple, fresh	¾ cup
Cherries, sweet, canned	½ cup	Pineapple, canned	½ cup
Dates	3	Plums, small	2 (5 oz)
Figs, fresh	1½ large or 2 medium (3½ oz)	Plums, canned	½ cup
Figs, dried	1½	Prunes, dried	3
Fruit cocktail	½ cup	Raisins	2 tbsp
Grapefruit, large	½ (11 oz)	Raspberries	1 cup
Grapefruit sections, canned	¾ cup	Strawberries	1¼ cup whole berries
Grapes, small	17 (3 oz)	Tangerines, small	2 (8 oz)
Honeydew melon	1 slice (10 oz) or 1 cup cubes	Watermelon	1 slice (13½ oz) or 1¼ cup cubes

Fruit Juice

Apple juice/cider	½ cup	Grapefruit juice	½ cup
Cranberry juice cocktail	⅓ cup	Orange juice	½ cup
Cranberry juice cocktail, reduced-calorie	1 cup	Pineapple juice	½ cup
Fruit juice blends, 100% juice	⅓ cup	Prune juice	⅓ cup
Grape juice	⅓ cup		

Selection Notes

1. Count ½ cup cranberries or rhubarb sweetened with sugar substitutes as free foods.
2. Encourage clients to read the Nutrition Facts on the food

continued

Table A-25-a—*continued*
Standard Exchange Lists for Meal Planning

label. If one serving has more than 15 g of carbohydrate, the size of the serving will need to be adjusted.
3. Fresh, frozen, and dried fruits have about 2 g of fiber per choice.
4. Portion sizes for canned fruits are for the fruit and a small amount of juice.
5. Whole fruit is more filling than fruit juice and may be a better choice.
6. Food labels for fruits may contain the words "no sugar added" or "unsweetened." This means that no sucrose (table sugar) has been added.
7. Generally, fruit canned in extra light syrup has the same amount of carbohydrate per serving as the "no sugar added" or the juice pack. All canned fruits on the fruit list are based on one of these three types of pack.

MILK LIST

Different types of milk and milk products are on this list. Cheeses are on the Meat list and cream and other dairy fats are on the Fat list. Based on the amount of fat they contain, milks are divided into fat-free/low-fat milk, reduced-fat milk, and whole milk. One choice of these includes

	Carbohydrate (g)	Protein (g)	Fat (g)	Calories
Fat-free/low-fat	12	8	0–3	90
Reduced-fat	12	8	5	120
Whole	12	8	8	150

Selection Notes

1. One cup equals 8 fl oz or ½ pt.
2. Chocolate milk, frozen yogurt, and ice cream are on the other carbohydrates list.
3. Nondairy creamers are on the Free Foods list.
4. Rice milk is on the Starch list.
5. Soy milk is on the Medium-fat Meat list.

One milk exchange equals 12 g carbohydrate and 8 g protein.

Fat free and Reduced-fat Milk (0–3 g fat per serving)

Fat-free milk	1 cup	Fat-free dry milk	⅓ cup dry
½% milk	1 cup	Plain nonfat yogurt	¾ cup
1% milk	1 cup	Nonfat or low-fat fruit-flavored yogurt sweetened with aspartame or with a nonnutritive sweetener	1 cup
Fat-free or reduced-fat buttermilk	1 cup		
Evaporated fat-free milk	½ cup		

Reduced-fat Milk (5 g fat per serving)

2% milk	1 cup
Plain low-fat yogurt	¾ cup
Sweet acidophilus milk	1 cup

Whole Milk (8 g fat per serving)

Whole milk	1 cup
Evaporated whole milk	½ cup
Goat's milk	1 cup
Kefir	1 cup

OTHER CARBOHYDRATES LIST

Food choices from this list can be substituted for a starch, fruit, or milk choice. However, they do not contain as many important vitamins and minerals as the choices on the Starch, Fruit, or Milk list. Some choices will also count as one or more fat choices.

continued

Table A-25-a—*continued*
Standard Exchange Lists for Meal Planning

Selection Notes

1. Because many of these foods are concentrated sources of carbohydrate and fat, the portion sizes are often very small.
2. Many fat-free or reduced-fat products made with fat replacers contain carbohydrate. When eaten in large amounts, they may need to be counted.
3. Fat-free salad dressings can be found in smaller amounts on the Free Foods list.

One exchange equals 15 g carbohydrate, or 1 starch, or 1 fruit, or 1 milk.

Food	Serving Size	Exchanges per Serving
Angel food cake, unfrosted	1/12 cake	2 carbohydrates
Brownie, small, unfrosted	2 in. square	1 carbohydrate, 1 fat
Cake, unfrosted	2 in. square	1 carbohydrate, 1 fat
Cake, frosted	2 in. square	2 carbohydrates, 1 fat
Cookie, fat-free	2 small	1 carbohydrate
Cookie or sandwich cookie with cream filling	2 small	1 carbohydrate, 1 fat
Cranberry sauce, jellied	¼ cup	1½ carbohydrates
Cupcake, frosted	1 small	2 carbohydrates, 1 fat
Doughnut, plain cake	1 medium (1½ oz)	1½ carbohydrates, 2 fats
Doughnut, glazed	3¾ in. across (2 oz)	2 carbohydrates, 2 fats
Fruit juice bars, frozen, 100% juice	1 bar (3 oz)	1 carbohydrate
Fruit snacks, chewy (pureed fruit concentrate)	1 roll (¾ oz)	1 carbohydrate
Fruit spreads, 100% fruit	1 tbsp	1 carbohydrate
Gelatin, regular	½ cup	1 carbohydrate
Gingersnaps	3	1 carbohydrate
Granola bar	1 bar	1 carbohydrate, 1 fat
Granola bar, fat-free	1 bar	2 carbohydrates
Honey	1 tbsp	1 carbohydrate
Hummus	⅓ cup	1 carbohydrate, 1 fat
Ice cream	½ cup	1 carbohydrate, 2 fats
Ice cream, light	½ cup	1 carbohydrate, 1 fat
Ice cream, fat-free, no sugar added	½ cup	1 carbohydrate
Jam or jelly, regular	1 tbsp	1 carbohydrate
Milk, chocolate, whole	1 cup	2 carbohydrates, 1 fat
Pie, fruit, 2 crusts	⅙ pie	3 carbohydrates, 2 fats
Pie, pumpkin or custard	⅛ pie	2 carbohydrates, 2 fats
Potato chips	12–18 (1 oz)	1 carbohydrate, 2 fats
Pudding, regular (made with low-fat milk)	½ cup	2 carbohydrates
Pudding, sugar-free (made with low-fat milk)	½ cup	1 carbohydrate
Salad dressing, fat-free[a]	¼ cup	1 carbohydrate
Sherbet, sorbet	½ cup	2 carbohydrates
Spaghetti or pasta sauce, canned[a]	½ cup	1 carbohydrate, 1 fat
Sugar	1 tbsp	1 carbohydrate
Sweet roll or Danish	1 (2½ oz)	2½ carbohydrates, 2 fats
Syrup, light	2 tbsp	1 carbohydrate
Syrup, regular	1 tbsp	1 carbohydrate
Syrup, regular	¼ cup	4 carbohydrates
Tortilla chips	6–12 (1 oz)	1 carbohydrate, 2 fats
Vanilla wafers	5	1 carbohydrate, 1 fat
Yogurt, frozen, low-fat, fat-free	⅓ cup	1 carbohydrate, 0–1 fat
Yogurt, frozen, fat-free, no sugar added	½ cup	1 carbohydrate
Yogurt, low-fat, with fruit	1 cup	3 carbohydrate, 0–1 fat

[a]Equals 400 mg or more sodium per exchange.

continued

Table A-25-a—*continued*
Standard Exchange Lists for Meal Planning

VEGETABLE LIST

In general, one vegetable exchange is equivalent to

- ½ cup of cooked vegetables or vegetable juice
- 1 cup of raw vegetables

SELECTION NOTES

1. One to two vegetable choices at a meal or snack do not have to be counted because they contain only small amounts of calories or carbohydrates.
2. Three cups or more of raw vegetables or 1½ cups of cooked vegetables at one meal count as 1 carbohydrate choice.
3. Starchy vegetables such as corn, peas, winter squash, and potatoes that contain larger amounts of calories and carbohydrates are on the Starch list.
4. Tomato sauce is different from spaghetti sauce, which is on the Other Carbohydrates list.

One vegetable exchange equals 5 g carbohydrates, 2 g protein, 0 g fat, and 25 calories.

Artichoke	Eggplant	Salad greens (endive, escarole, lettuce, romaine, spinach)
Artichoke hearts	Green onions or scallions	
Asparagus	Greens (collard, kale, mustard, turnip)	Sauerkraut[a]
Beans (green, wax, Italian)		Spinach
Bean sprouts	Kohlrabi	Summer squash
Beets	Leeks	Tomato
Broccoli	Mixed vegetables (without corn, peas, or pasta)	Tomatoes, canned
Brussel sprouts		Tomato sauce[a]
Cabbage	Mushrooms	Tomato/vegetable juice[a]
Carrots	Okra	Turnips
Cauliflower	Onions	Water chestnuts
Celery	Pea pods	Watercress
Cucumber	Peppers (all varieties)	Zucchini
	Radishes	

[a]Equals 400 mg or more sodium per exchange.

MEAT AND MEAT SUBSTITUTES LIST

Meat and meat substitutes that contain both protein and fat are on this list. In general, one meat exchange is equivalent to

- 1 oz meat, fish, poultry, or cheese
- ½ cup beans, peas, and lentils

Based on the amount of fat they contain, meats are divided into very lean, lean, medium-fat, and high-fat lists. One ounce (one exchange) of each of these includes

	Carbohydrate (g)	Protein (g)	Fat (g)	Calories
Very lean	0	7	0–1	35
Lean	0	7	3	55
Medium-fat	0	7	5	75
High-fat	0	7	8	100

continued

Table A-25-a—*continued*
Standard Exchange Lists for Meal Planning

Selection Notes

1. Meat should be weighed after cooking and removing bones and fat. Four oz of raw meat is equal to 3 oz of cooked meat. Following are some examples of meat portions:
   1 oz cheese = 1 meat choice and is about the size of a 1-in. cube
   2 oz meat = 2 meat choices, such as
   1 small chicken leg or thigh
   ½ cup cottage cheese or tuna
   3 oz meat = 3 meat choices and is about the size of a deck of cards, such as
   1 medium pork chop
   1 small hamburger
   ½ of a whole chicken breast
   1 unbreaded fish fillet
2. Limit choices from the high-fat group to three times per week or less.
3. Most grocery stores stock Select and Choice grades of meat. Select grades of meat are the leanest meats. Choice grades contain a moderate amount of fat, and Prime cuts of meat have the highest amounts of fat. Restaurants usually serve Prime cuts of meat.
4. "Hamburger" may contain added seasoning and fat, but ground beef does not.
5. Encourage clients to read labels to find products that are low in fat and cholesterol (5 g or less of fat per serving).
6. Beans, peas, and lentils are also found on the Starch list.
7. Peanut butter, in smaller amounts, is also found on the Fat list.
8. Bacon, in smaller amounts, is also found on the Fat list.
9. Some processed meats, seafood, and soy products may contain carbohydrate when consumed in large amounts. If so, these should be counted as a carbohydrate choice as well as a meat choice.

Meal Planning Tips

1. Bake, roast, grill, poach, steam, or boil these foods rather than frying them.
2. Place meat on a rack so the fat will drain off during cooking.
3. Use a nonstick spray and a nonstick pan to brown or fry foods.
4. Trim off visible fat before or after cooking.
5. If flour, bread crumbs, coating mixes, fat, or marinades are added when cooking, these may need to be counted in the meal plan.

Very Lean Meat and Substitutes List
One exchange equals 0 g carbohydrate, 7 g protein, 0–1 g fat, and 35 calories.

One very lean meat exchange is equal to any one of the following items:	
Poultry: Chicken or turkey (white meat, no skin), Cornish hen (no skin)	1 oz
Fish: Fresh or frozen cod, flounder, haddock, halibut, trout; tuna fresh or canned in water	1 oz
Shellfish: Clams, crab, lobster, scallops, shrimp, imitation shellfish	1 oz
Game: Duck or pheasant (no skin), venison, buffalo, ostrich	1 oz
Cheese with 1 g or less fat per ounce:	
Nonfat or low-fat cottage cheese	¼ cup
Fat-free cheese	1 oz

continued

Table A-25-a—*continued*
Standard Exchange Lists for Meal Planning

Other: Processed sandwich meats with 1 g or less fat per ounce, such as deli thin, shaved meats, chipped beef,[a] turkey ham	1 oz
Egg whites	2
Egg substitutes, plain	¼ cup
Hot dogs with 1 g or less fat per ounce[a]	1 oz
Kidney (high in cholesterol)	1 oz
Sausage with 1 g or less fat per ounce	1 oz
Count as one very lean meat and one starch exchange.	
Beans, peas, lentils (cooked)	½ cup

[a]Equals 400 mg or more sodium per exchange.

Lean Meat and Substitutes List
One exchange equals 0 g carbohydrate, 7 g protein, 3 g fat, and 55 calories.

One lean meat exchange is equal to any one of the following items:	
Beef: USDA Select or Choice grades of lean beef trimmed of fat, such as round, sirloin, and flank steak; tenderloin, roast (rib, chuck, rump); steak (T-bone, porterhouse, cubed), ground round	1 oz
Pork: Lean pork, such as fresh ham; canned, cured, or boiled ham; Canadian bacon[a]; tenderloin, center loin chop	1 oz
Lamb: Roast, chop, leg	1 oz
Veal: Lean chop, roast	1 oz
Poultry: chicken, turkey (dark meat, no skin), chicken (white meat, with skin), domestic duck or goose (well-drained of fat, no skin)	1 oz
Fish:	
Herring (uncreamed or smoked)	1 oz
Oysters	6 medium
Salmon (fresh or canned), catfish	1 oz
Sardines (canned)	2 medium
Tuna (canned in oil, drained)	1 oz
Game: Goose (no skin), rabbit	1 oz
Cheese:	
4.5%-fat cottage cheese	¼ cup
Grated Parmesan	2 tbsp
Cheeses with 3 g or less fat per ounce	1 oz
Other:	
Hot dogs with 3 g or less fat per ounce[a]	1½ oz
Processed sandwich meat with 3 g or less fat per ounce, such as turkey pastrami or kielbasa	1 oz
Liver, heart (high in cholesterol)	1 oz

[a]Equals 400 mg or more sodium per exchange.

Medium-Fat Meat and Substitutes List
One exchange equals 0 g carbohydrate, 7 g protein, 5 g fat, and 75 calories.

One medium-fat meat exchange is equal to any one of the following items:	
Beef: Most beef products fall into this category (ground beef, meat loaf, corned beef, short ribs, Prime grades of meat trimmed of fat, such as prime rib	1 oz
Pork: Top loin, chop, Boston butt, cutlet	1 oz
Lamb: Rib roast, ground	1 oz
Veal: Cutlet (ground or cubed, unbreaded)	1 oz
Poultry: Chicken (dark meat, with skin), ground turkey or ground chicken, fried chicken (with skin)	1 oz
Fish: Any fried fish product	1 oz
Cheese: With 5 g or less fat per ounce	
Feta	1 oz
Mozzarella	1 oz
Ricotta	¼ cup (2 oz)

continued

Table A-25-a—*continued*
Standard Exchange Lists for Meal Planning

Other:	
Egg (high in cholesterol, limit to 3 per week)	1
Sausage with 5 g or less fat per ounce	1 oz
Soy milk	1 cup
Tempeh	¼ cup
Tofu	4 oz or ½ cup

[a]Equals 400 mg or more sodium per exchange.

High-Fat Meat and Substitutes List
One exchange equals 0 g carbohydrate, 7 g protein, 8 g fat, and 100 calories.

One high-fat meat exchange is equal to any one of the following items:	
Pork: Spareribs, ground pork, pork sausage	1 oz
Cheese: All regular cheeses, such as American,[a] cheddar, Monterey Jack, Swiss	1 oz
Other: Processed sandwich meats with 8 g or less fat per ounce, such as bologna, pimento loaf, salami	1 oz
Sausage, such as bratwurst, Italian, knockwurst, Polish, smoked	1 oz
Hot dog (turkey or chicken)[a]	1 (10/lb)
Bacon	3 slices (20 slices/lb)
Count as one high-fat meat plus one fat exchange:	
Hot dog (beef, pork, or combination)[a]	1 (10/lb)
Count as one high-fat meat plus two fat exchanges:	
Peanut butter (contains unsaturated fat)	2 tbsp

[a]Equals 400 mg or more sodium per exchange.

FAT LIST

Fats are divided into three groups, based on the main type of fat they contain: monounsaturated, polyunsaturated, and saturated. Saturated fats are linked with heart disease and cancer. In general, one fat exchange is equivalent to

- 1 tsp of regular margarine or vegetable oil
- 1 tsp of regular salad dressings

Selection Notes

1. One fat exchange is based on a serving size containing 5 g of fat.
2. Fat-free salad dressings are on the Other Carbohydrates list and the Free Foods list.
3. See the Free Foods list for nondairy coffee creamers, whipped topping, and fat-free products, such as margarines, salad dressings, mayonnaise, sour cream, cream cheese, and non-stick cooking spray.

Monosaturated Fats List
One fat exchange equals 5 g fat and 45 calories.

Avocado, medium	⅛ (1 oz)
Oil (canola, olive, peanut)	1 tsp
Olives: ripe (black)	8 large
green, stuffed*	10 large
Nuts	
Almonds, cashews	6 nuts
Mixed (50% peanuts)	6 nuts
Peanuts	10 nuts
Pecans	4 halves
Peanut butter, smooth or crunchy	2 tsp
Sesame seeds	1 tsbp
Tahini paste	2 tsp

[a]Equals 400 mg or more sodium per exchange.

continued

Table A-25-a—*continued*
Standard Exchange Lists for Meal Planning

Polyunsaturated Fats List **One fat exchange equals 5 g fat and 45 calories.**	
Margarine: stick, tub, or squeeze	1 tsp
Lower-fat (30% to 50% vegetable oil)	1 tbsp
Mayonnaise: regular	1 tsp
Reduced-fat	1 tbsp
Nuts, walnuts, English	4 halves
Oil (corn, safflower, soybean)	1 tsp
Salad dressing: regular[a]	1 tbsp
Reduced-fat	2 tbsp
Miracle Whip Salad Dressing: regular	2 tsp
Reduced-fat	1 tbsp
Seeds: pumpkin, sunflower	1 tbsp

Saturated Fats List **One fat exchange equals 5 g of fat and 45 calories.**	
Bacon, cooked	1 slice (20 slices/lb)
Bacon, grease	1 tsp
Butter: stick	1 tsp
Whipped	2 tsp
Reduced-fat	1 tbsp
Chitterlings, boiled	2 tbsp (½ oz)
Coconut, sweetened, shredded	2 tbsp
Cream, half and half	2 tbsp
Cream cheese: regular	1 tbsp (½ oz)
Reduced-fat	2 tbsp (1 oz)
Fatback or salt pork[b]	
Shortening or lard	1 tsp
Sour cream: regular	2 tbsp
Reduced-fat	3 tbsp

[a]Equals 400 mg or more sodium per exchange.

[b]Use a piece 1 in. × 1 in. × ¼ in. when eating the fatback cooked with vegetables. Use a piece 2 in. × 1 in. × ½ in. when eating only the vegetables with the fatback removed.

FREE-FOODS LIST

A free food is any food or drink that contains fewer than 20 calories or less than 5 g of carbohydrate per serving. Foods with a serving size listed should be limited to three servings per day, spread throughout the day. Foods listed without a serving size can be eaten as often as desired.

Fat-free or Reduced-fat Foods	
Cream cheese, fat-free	1 tbsp
Creamers, nondairy, liquid	1 tbsp
Creamers, nondairy, powdered	2 tsp
Mayonnaise, fat-free	1 tbsp
Mayonnaise, reduced-fat	1 tsp
Margarine, fat-free	4 tbsp
Margarine, reduced-fat	1 tsp
Miracle Whip, nonfat	1 tbsp
Miracle Whip, reduced-fat	1 tsp
Nonstick cooking spray	
Salad dressing, fat-free	1 tbsp
Salad dressing, fat-free, Italian	2 tbsp
Salsa	1/4 cup
Sour cream, fat-free, reduced-fat	1 tbsp
Whipped topping, regular or light	2 tbsp

continued

Table A-25-a—*continued*
Standard Exchange Lists for Meal Planning

Sugar-free or Low-sugar Foods	
Candy, hard, sugar-free	1 candy
Gelatin dessert, sugar-free	
Gelatin, unflavored	
Gum, sugar-free	
Jam or jelly, low-sugar or light	2 tsp
Sugar substitutes[a]	
Syrup, sugar-free	2 tbsp

[a]Sugar substitutes, alternatives, or replacements that are approved by the Food and Drug Administration (FDA) are safe to use. Common brand names include Equal (aspartame), Sprinkle Sweet (saccharin), Sweet One (acesulfame K), Sweet-10 (saccharin), Sugar Twin (saccharin), Sweet 'n Low (saccharin).

Drinks	
Bouillon, broth, consommé[a]	
Bouillon or broth, low-sodium	
Carbonated or mineral water	
Club soda	
Cocoa powder, unsweetened	1 tbsp
Coffee	
Diet soft drinks, sugar-free	
Drink mixes, sugar-free	
Tea	
Tonic water, sugar-free	

Condiments	
Catsup	1 tbsp
Horseradish	
Lemon juice	
Lime juice	
Mustard	
Pickles, dill[a]	1½ large
Soy sauce, regular or light[a]	
Taco sauce	1 tbsp
Vinegar	

Seasonings
Some seasonings contain sodium or are salts, including garlic or celery salt, and lemon pepper
Flavoring extracts
Garlic
Herbs, fresh or dried
Pimento
Spices
Tabasco or hot pepper sauce
Wine, used in cooking
Worcestershire sauce

[a]Equals 400 mg or more of sodium per exchange.

Table A-25-a—*continued*
Standard Exchange Lists for Meal Planning

Combination Foods List

Combination foods do not fit into any one exchange list. This is a list of exchanges for some typical combination foods.

Food	Serving Size	Exchanges per Serving
Entrees		
Tuna noodle casserole, lasagna, spaghetti with meatballs, chili with beans, macaroni and cheese*	1 cup (8 oz)	2 carbohydrates, 2 medium-fat meats
Chow mein (without noodles or rice)*	2 cups (16 oz)	1 carbohydrate, 2 lean meats
Pizza, cheese, thin crust†	¼ of 10 in. (5 oz)	2 carbohydrates, 2 medium-fat meats, 1 fat
Pizza, meat topping, thin crust*	¼ of 10 in. (5 oz)	2 carbohydrates, 2 medium-fat meats, 2 fats
Pot pie*	1 (7 oz)	2 carbohydrates, 1 medium-fat meat, 4 fats
Frozen entrees		
Salisbury steak with gravy, mashed potato*	1 (11 oz)	2 carbohydrates, 3 medium-fat meats, 3–4 fats
Turkey with gravy, mashed potato, dressing*	1 (11 oz)	2 carbohydrates, 2 medium-fat meats, 2 fats
Entree with less than 300 calories*	1 (8 oz)	2 carbohydrates, 3 lean meats
Soups		
Bean*	1 cup	1 carbohydrate, 1 very lean meat
Cream (made with water)*	1 cup (8 oz)	1 carbohydrate, 1 fat
Split pea (made with water)*	½ cup (4 oz)	1 carbohydrate
Tomato (made with water)*	1 cup (8 oz)	1 carbohydrate
Vegetable beef, chicken noodle, or other broth-type*	1 cup (8 oz)	1 carbohydrate

Fast Foods

Food	Serving Size	Exchanges per Serving
Burritos with beef*	2	4 carbohydrates, 2 medium-fat meats, 2 fats
Chicken nuggets*	6	1 carbohydrate, 2 medium-fat meats, 1 fat
Chicken breast and wing, breaded and fried*	1 each	1 carbohydrate, 4 medium-fat meats, 2 fats
Fish sandwich/tartar sauce*	1	3 carbohydrates, 1 medium-fat meats, 3 fats
French fries, thin*	20–25	2 carbohydrates, 2 fats
Hamburger, regular	1	2 carbohydrates, 2 medium-fat meats
Hamburger, large*	1	2 carbohydrates, 3 medium-fat meats, 1 fat
Hot dog with bun*	1	1 carbohydrate, 1 high-fat meat, 1 fat
Individual pan pizza*	1	5 carbohydrates, 3 medium-fat meats, 3 fats
Soft-serve cone	1 medium	2 carbohydrates, 1 fat
Submarine sandwich*	1 sub (6 in.)	3 carbohydrates, 1 vegetable, 2 medium-fat meats, 1 fat
Taco, hard shell*	1 (6 oz)	2 carbohydrates, 2 medium-fat meats, 2 fats
Taco, soft shell*	1 (3 oz)	1 carbohydrate, 1 medium-fat meat, 1 fat

From the American Dietetic Association and the American Diabetes Association Exchange Lists for Meal Planning, 1996; reprinted with permission from the American Dietetic Association Manual of Clinical Dietetics, 5th ed, © 1996, Chicago, IL.

* Equals 400 mg or more sodium per exchange

Table A-25-b
Supplementary Exchange Lists for Traditional Alaskan Native Foods[a]

Food Group	Food	Portion
Starch/bread	Pilot bread, 4-in diameter	1
Meats and substitutes		
Lean meats	Caribou	1 oz
	Gumboots (leathery chiton)	2 oz
	Halibut	1 oz
	Herring eggs, plain	½ cup
	Moose	1 oz
	Pike	1 oz
	Venison	1 oz
	Walrus	1 oz
	Whale	1 oz
Medium-fat meats	Dried fish	½ oz
	Muskrat	1 oz
	Salmon	1 oz
High-fat meats	Smoked hooligan (eulachon)	1 oz
High-fat meat + 1 fat	Muktuk	1 × 1 × 2 in
Vegetables	Seaweed, dried	
(½ cup cooked	Fiddlehead fern	
or 1 cup raw)	Willow greens	
	Sour dock	
Fruits	Highbush cranberries	1¼ cup
	Huckleberries	1 cup
	Salmonberries	1¼ cup
Fat	Seal oil	1 tsp
Free food	Beach asparagus	

From the American Dietetic Association and the American Diabetes Association, Inc. Ethnic and regional food practices: a series. Alaska native food practices, customs, and holidays, 1993, with permission. Currently being revised to reflect updated information based on the American Diabetes Association's 1994 recommendations for nutrition management of diabetes.

*Nutrition practitioners who work with Alaska Native clients with NIDDM do not often use the Exchange system in client education sessions. This listing is presented for the few occasions when supplementary Exchange values may be needed.

Table A-25-c
Supplementary Exchange List for Traditional Cajun Creole Foods

Food Group	Food	Portion
Starch	Peas, crowder/purple hull	½ cup
	Couche-couche, no fat added	½ cup
Meats and substitutes		
Very lean meat	Alligator	1 oz
	Crawfish	2 oz
	Shrimp, dried	36 small
	Frog legs	2
	Guinea	1 oz
Lean meat	Beef tasso	1 oz
	Goat	1 oz
	Dove	1 oz
	Turtle	1.5 oz
	Squab	1 oz
	Tripe	2 oz
Medium-fat meat	Hogshead cheese	¼ cup
	Tongue, beef	1 oz
	Lamb	1 oz
High-fat meat	Pork sausage	1 oz
	Smoked pork sausage	1 oz
	Smoked beef sausage	1 oz
	Pickled pigs feet	½ foot
High-fat meat + 1 fat	Cracklins	¼ cup
Vegetable	Pumpkin, cooked, no fat	½ cup
	Mirliton/chayote, cooked	½ cup
	Cushaw squash	½ cup
Fruit	Muscadines (scuppernongs)	17
	Dewberries/blackberries	¾ cup
	Satsuma/mandarin	2 small
	Kumquats	5
	Passionfruit (maypops)	3
	Persimmons (Japanese)	½ of 2.5" diameter
½ milk, whole	Cafe au lait (4 oz coffee, 4 oz whole milk)	1 cup
Fat	Salt pork (fatback)	½ cubic inch
	Remoulade sauce	1 tbsp
Free foods	Italian parsley	10 sprigs
	Green onions	2 tbsp
	Tabasco	5 drops
	Hot pepper vinegar	5 drops
	Cocktail sauce	1 tbsp

From the American Dietetic Association and the American Diabetes Association, Inc. Ethnic and regional food practices: a series. Cajun and Creole food practices, customs, and holidays, 1996. With permission.

In general, people who consume Cajun/Creole food eat a variety of foods, many of which can be found in the *Exchange Lists for Meal Planning*, published by the American Dietetic Association and the American Diabetes Association (see Table A-25-a).

Table A-25-d
Supplementary Exchange Lists for Chinese American Foods

Food Exchange Group	Food	Portion
Starch/bread	Cellophane or mung bean noodles (cooked)	¾ cup
	Ginkgo seeds	½ cup
	Lotus root, ¼"-thick slice, 2½" diameter	10 slices
	Mung beans or green gram beans (cooked)	⅓ cup
	Red beans (cooked)	⅓ cup
	Rice congee or soup	¾ cup
	Rice vermicelli or noodles (cooked)	½ cup
	Taro (cooked)	⅓ cup
Meat and meat substitutes		
Lean meat	Beef jerky, 3½" × 1[a]	½ oz
	Dried scallop	1 large
	Dried shrimp	1 Tbsp or 10 medium shrimp
	Soybeans (cooked)	3 Tbsp
	Squid	2 oz
	Tripe (beef)	2 oz
Medium-fat meat and substitutes	Beef tongue	1 oz
	Tofu or soybean curd, 2½" × 2¾" × 1"[b]	4 oz or ½ cup
High-fat meat	Salted duck egg,[c,d]	1
	Thousand-year-old or preserved limed duck eggs[c,d]	1
High-fat meat + 1 fat	Chinese sausage (pork and spices and/or liver)[a,d]	1 (2 oz)
Vegetables (½ cup cooked or 1 cup raw unless indicated otherwise)	Amaranth or Chinese spinach (cooked)	
	Arrowheads, or fresh corms (raw), 3½" diameter	
	Baby corn (canned)[a]	
	Bamboo shoots	
	Bitter melon or bitter gourd	
	Chayote	
	Chinese celery	
	Chinese eggplant (white or purple)	
	Chinese or black mushroom (dried)	2 medium
	Hairy melon or hairy cucumber	
	Leeks[b]	
	Luffa (angled or smooth)	
	Mung bean sprouts	
	Mustard greens[b]	
	Peapods or sugar peas[b]	
	Soybean sprouts (cooked or raw)	½ cup
	Straw mushrooms	
	Turnip[b]	
	Water chestnuts (canned)[b]	½ cup
	Winter melon or wax gourd	
	Yard-long beans	
Fruits	Carambola or star fruit (raw)	2 medium
	Chinese banana (raw)	1 dwarf
	Guava (raw)	1 medium
	Kumquats (raw)	5 medium
	Litchi or lychee (raw)	10
	Litchi or lychee (canned, drained)	½ cup
	Longan (raw)	30
	Longan (canned, drained)	¾ cup
	Mango (raw)[b]	½ small
	Papaya (raw), 3½" diameter, 5⅛" high[b]	½
	Persimmon, Japanese (soft type) (raw)	½
	Pummelo (raw)	¾ cup
Milk	Soybean milk (unsweetened)	1 cup
Fats	Coconut milk	1 Tbsp
	Sesame paste	1½ tsp
	Sesame seeds (whole, dried)	1 Tbsp
Free Foods	Amaranth or Chinese spinach	
	Bok choy	
	Chili pepper (raw)[b]	1
	Chinese or Peking cabbage[b]	
	Choy sum or Chinese flowering cabbage	
	Coriander	
	Garland chrysanthemum	
	Ginger	¼ cup
	Mustard greens (salted and soured)	2 Tbsp

continued

Table A-25-d—*continued*
Supplementary Exchange Lists for Chinese American Foods

Food Exchange Group	Food	Portion
	Oriental radish or daikon	
	Watercress	
Combination	Mock duck or wheat gluten (canned)	½ cup (equals ½ starch/ bread, 1 lean meat)

(From the American Dietetic Association and The American Diabetes Association, Inc. Ethnic and regional food practices: a series, Chinese food practices, customs and holidays. 1990. With permission. Currently being revised to reflect updated information based on the American Diabetes Association's 1994 recommendations for nutrition management of diabetes.

[a]400 mg or more of sodium per serving.

[b]Foods are included in *Exchange Lists for Meal Planning,* 1986. © American Diabetes Association and the American Dietetic Association.

[c]Probably 400 mg or more of sodium per serving, based on original author's estimate.

[d]Limit high-fat meat choices to 3 times per week.

Table A-25-e
Supplementary Exchange List for Traditional Filipino Native Foods

Food Group (Food Exchange)	Food	Portion per Exchange (Measure)
Starch/bread	Cassava tuber, cooked	½ cup
	Kamoteng kahoy	
	Mung bean, cooked	⅓ cup
	Munggo[a]	
	Mung bean noodles, cooked	¾ cup
	Sotanghon	
	Plantain, cooked[b]	½ cup
	Saging saba	
	Rice sticks, boiled	¾ cup
	Bihon	
	Taro, cooked	⅓ cup
	Gabi	
Lean meat	Beef shank, cooked, lean	1 oz
	Chicken gizzard, cooked	1 oz
	Balunbalunan	
	Clam, cooked, 3 med[c]	1 oz
	Halaan	
	Long-jawed anchovy[d], dried, raw	2 tbsp
	Dilis	
	Oyster,[a] cooked, 1 medium[c]	1 oz
	Talaba	
	Indian sardines, dried, raw	1 oz
	Tamban tuyo[d]	
Medium-fat meat	Corned beef, cured[d], cn[3]	1 oz
	Beef tongue	1 oz
	Sausage, simulated, frozen	1 oz
	Soy bean curd[b]	½ cup
	Tofu (2¼ × 1¾ × 1½ in.)	
High-fat meat	Vienna sausage[d]	2 sm pc
	Chinese sausage	1 oz
	Macao longganisa	
High-fat meat + 1 fat	Native sausage[d]	1 oz
	Filipino longganisa	
	Spanish sausage[d]	1 oz
	Chorizo bilbao	
Vegetable	Bamboo shoots, canned	½ cup
	Labong	
	Banana squash, cooked	½ cup
	Kalabasa	
	Bittermelon, cooked	½ cup
	Ampalaya	
	Bottle gourd, cooked	½ cup
	Upo	
	Chayote, cooked	½ cup
	Chinese celery—raw[a]	1 cup
	Kintsay	

continued

Table A-25-e—*continued*
Supplementary Exchange List for Traditional Filipino Native Foods

Food Group (Food Exchange)	Food	Portion per Exchange (Measure)
	Horseradish leaves, cooked[a]	½ cup
	Malunggay	
	Jicama, cooked	½ cup
	Singkamas	
	Papaya, unripe, cooked	½ cup
	Pea pods, cooked[b]	½ cup
	Sitsaro	
	Stringbeans, yardlong, cooked[a]	½ cup
	Sitaw	
	Swamp cabbage, cooked[a]	½ cup
	Kangkong	
Fruit	Banana, native *latundan* 4" long, 1" diameter	1 sm
	Guava, medium[a]	1½ fruit
	Mango, small[b]	½ fruit
	Papaya, ripe[b]	1 cup
	Pummelo	¾ cup
	Suha	
Milk[c]	Caribou's milk	1 cup
3 fat exchanges		
Fat	Coconut milk, canned	1 tbsp
	Niyog, gata	
	Cracklings, crushed	2 tbsp
	Sitsaron	
	Sesame seeds, whole, dried	1 tbsp
	Linga	
	Watermelon seeds, dried[d]	1 tbsp
	Butong pakwan	
Free foods	Banana sauce	1 tsp
	Saging salsa	
	Ceylon moss bar	¼ bar =
	Gulaman	½ cup
	Chinese spinach, raw[a]	1 cup
	Kulitis	
	Papaya, unripe, cooked	1 cup
	Papaya, berde	
	Fish sauce[d]	1 tbsp
	Patis	
	Oriental radish or daikon , raw	1 cup
	Labanos	
	Small shrimp, salted & fermented[d]	1 tbsp
	Bagoong	
	Cafe au lait (4 oz coffee, 4 oz whole milk)	1 cup

continued

Table A-25-e—*continued*
Supplementary Exchange List for Traditional Filipino Native Foods

Food Group (Food Exchange)	Food	Portion per Exchange (Measure)
Fat	Salt pork (fatback)	½ cubic inch
	Remoulade sauce	1 tbsp
Free foods	Italian parsley	10 sprigs
	Green onions	2 tbsp
	Tabasco	5 drops
	Hot pepper vinegar	5 drops
	Cocktail sauce	1 tbsp

From the American Dietetic Association and The American Diabetes Association, Inc.; Ethnic and regional food practices: a series. Filipino American food practices, customs, and holidays, 1994 used by permission.

[a]3 or more g fiber per exchange.

[b]Foods are included in *Exchange Lists for Meal Planning*, 1986.

[c]Food, amount, and/or exchange category differ from the 1986 *Exchange Lists for Meal Planning* because of new information.

[d]400 mg or more of sodium per exchange.

Table A-25-f
Supplementary Exchange Lists for Hmong American Foods

Food Exchange Group	Food	Portion
Starch/bread	Cellophane or mung bean noodles (cooked)	¾ cup
	Rice vermicelli or noodles (cooked)	½ cup
	Rice soup	¾ cup
Meat and meat substitutes		
Lean meat	Pheasant[a]	1 oz
	Squirrel[a]	1 oz
	Venison[a]	1 oz
Medium-fat meat and substitutes	Pig's feet	2½ oz (equals 2 exchanges)
	Tofu or soybean curd, 2½" × 2¾" × 1"	4 oz or ½ cup
High-fat meat	Ground pork[a,b]	1 oz
Vegetables (½ cup cooked or 1 cup raw unless indicated otherwise)	Bamboo shoots	
	Bitter melon or bitter gourd	
	Chinese onion (leeks[b])	
	Cucuzzi squash (spaghetti squash)	
	Luffa gourd/squash	
	Mustard greens[a]	
	Mung bean sprouts	
	Pumpkin	
	Sugar peas, snow peas, sweet peas, peapods[a]	
	Yard-long beans, pod and seeds	½ cup
Fruits	Apple pear, Asian pear (raw), 2¼" high, 2½" diameter	1
	Guava (raw)	1½ medium
	Jackfruit (raw)	½ cup
	Mango (raw)[a]	½ small
	Papaya (raw), 5⅛" high, 3½' diameter[a]	½ or 1 cup
Fats	Beef fat	1 tsp
	Chicken fat	1 tsp
	Coconut cream or milk	1 Tbsp
	Coconut (raw)[a]	2 Tbsp
	Pork lard	1 tsp
	Pork intestine, chitterlings[a]	½ oz
Free foods	Fish sauce[c]	
	Pumpkin or squash blossom	
	Soy sauce[a,c]	
	Tender vines and leaves of pumpkin, squash, luffa gourd, and pea plants	
Occasional foods	Condensed milk, sweetened	1 oz (equals 1½ starch/bread)

From the American Dietetic Association and The American Diabetes Association, Inc.: Ethnic and regional food practices, a series. Hmong food practices, customs and holidays, 1992 with permission. Currently being revised to reflect updated information based on the American Diabetes Association's 1994 recommendations for nutrition management of diabetes.

[a]Foods are included in *Exchange Lists for Meal Planning*, 1986. © American Diabetes Association and The American Dietetic Association.

[b]Limit high-fat meat choice to 3 times per week.

[c]400 mg or more of sodium per serving.

Table A-25-g
Supplementary Exchange List for Traditional Indian and Pakistani Foods

Food Group (Food Exchange)	Food	Portion
Starch	*Aviyal*	½ cup
	Idli, plain, steamed	3" round
	Naan	¼ of 8" × 2"
	Phulka/sookhi roti	6" round
	Plantain, green[a,b]	⅓ cup
	Rice (plain, cooked) (regular/basmati/jasmine)[a,b]	⅓ cup
	Sambar	½ cup
Starch + 1 fat	*Dhansak*[c]	½ cup
	Dhokla, khaman[c]	1" square
	Matki usal[c]	½ cup
	Pesrattu[c]	9" round
	Poha[c]	½ cup
	Puri[c]	5" round
Meats and meat substitutes		
Very lean meat + 1 starch	Tomato *dhal*	½ cup
	Plain, cooked *toor* (red gram/split pigeon pea) *dhal*[d]	½ cup
	Plain, cooked *mung dhal* (green gram)[d]	½ cup
	Plain, cooked garbanzo and most other beans[d]	½ cup
Lean meat	Baked, spiced chicken (no skin)[a]	1 oz
	Chicken *tikka* (skinless)	3 1" pieces
	Tandoori chicken (skinless) (combination of light and dark meat)	1 oz
Vegetables (cooked plain; when stir-fried, make allowance for added fat)	*Brinjal* (eggplant)	½ cup
	Cucumber *raita*	½ cup
	Karela (bittermelon/gourd)	½ cup
	Lady's fingers (okra)[a]	½ cup
	Mung bean sprouts	½ cup
Fruits	Mango, small[a]	½
	Guava, medium, raw	1½
Skim and very low-fat milk	*Lassi* (blended nonfat yogurt)[e]	1 cup
	Paneer (from 1% milk)[f]	1 oz
Fats/ oils	Coconut, fresh, shredded	3 tbsp
	Ghee (clarified butter)	1 tsp
	Sesame oil (others including coconut, mustard, peanut)	1 tsp
Free foods	*Chai masala* (spiced tea)[g]	½ cup
	Fresh coriander (raw)	
	Ginger, fresh and dried	
	Jherra pani	½ cup
	Rasam	1 cup

From the American Dietetic Association and The American Diabetes Association, Inc. Ethnic and regional food practices: a series. Indian and Pakistani food practices, customs, and holidays, 1996, with permission.

[a]*Exchange Lists for Meal Planning* (1995).

[b]Other versions may be prepared with a large amount of added oil or *ghee*, as in *pulao*, fried rice, and *biryani*.

[c]Often prepared in a way that is higher in added fat.

[d]May be cooked in various forms with vegetables, seasoning, and added fat.

[e]May be high in added salt or sugar.

[f]Eaten in many forms, eg., deep-fried and mixed in other dishes or soaked in reduced milk with added sugar.

[g]Can become high in calories and carbohydrates if prepared with whole milk and added sugar.

Table A-25-h
Supplementary Exchange List for Jewish Foods

Food Exchange Group	Food	Portion
Starch/bread	Bagel[a] or bialy	½ small, 1 oz
	Bulgur (cooked)[a]	½ cup
	Bulke	½ medium
	Farfel (dry)	½ cup
	Hallah	1 slice, 1 oz
	Kasha (cooked)	½ cup
	Kasha (raw)	2 Tbsp
	Lentils[a]	⅓ cup
	Matzoh[a]	¾ oz
	Matzoh meal	2½ Tbsp
	Potato starch (flour)	2 Tbsp
	Pumpernickel bread[a]	1 slice, 1 oz
	Rye bread[a]	1 slice, 1 oz
	Split peas[a]	⅓ cup
Starch/bread prepared with fat	Matzoh ball[b]	3 balls, 1½ oz (equals 1 starch/bread + 1 fat)
	Potato pancake	½ pancake (equals 1 starch/bread + 1 fat)
Meat		
Lean meat	Flanken[a]	1 oz
	Gefilte fish	2 oz
	Herring[a] (smoked, uncreamed)	1 oz
	Lox[a]	1 oz
	Sardines[a] (canned, drained)	2 medium
	Smelts	1 oz
Medium-fat meat	Beef tongue	1 oz
	Brisket	1 oz
	Chopped livers[c]	¼ cup
	Corned beef[a]	1 oz
	Sablefish (smoked)	1 oz
	Salmon[a] (canned)	¼ cup
High-fat meat	Pastrami	1 oz
Vegetables	Borscht (no sugar or sour cream)	½ cup
	Sorrel	½ cup
Fats	Cream cheese[a]	1 Tbsp
	Nondairy creamer[a] (liquid)	2 Tbsp
	Nondairy creamer[a] (powder)	4 tsp
	Schmaltz	1 tsp
	Sour cream[a]	2 Tbsp
Free foods (in reasonable amounts)	Horseradish[a]	
	Pickels, dill[a]	
Occasional foods	Sweet kosher wine	½ cup (equals 2 fat)

From The American Dietetic Association and The American Diabetes Association, Inc. Ethnic and regional food practices, a series. Jewish food practices, customs and holidays, 1989. With permission. Currently being revised to reflect updated information based on the American Diabetes Association's 1994 recommendations for nutrition management of diabetes.

Unless otherwise specified, all foods are 1 exchange.

[a]Foods are included on the American Diabetes Association and American Dietetic Association Exchange Lists for Meal Planning. 1986. © American Diabetes Association and the American Dietetic Association (see Table A-25-a).

[b]High in sodium.

[c]No additional salt in recipe.

Table A-25-i
Supplementary Exchange Lists for Mexican American Foods[a]

Food Exchange Group	Food	Portion
Starch/bread	Bolillo (French roll), 4½" to 5" long	¼
	Frijoles cocidos[b] (cooked beans)	⅓ cup
	Frijoles cocidos	1 cup (equals 2 starch/bread + 1 lean meat)
	Frijoles refritos (refried beans) (no fat added)	⅓ cup
	Tortilla, corn, 7½" across (ready to bake)[c]	1
	Tortilla, flour, 7" across (ready to bake)[c]	1 (equals 1½ starch/bread)
	Tortilla, flour, 9" across (ready to bake)[c]	⅓
Starch/bread prepared with fat	Frijoles refritos (fat added)	⅓ cup (equals 1 starch/bread + 1 fat)
	Taco shell, 5" across (ready to use)	2 (equals 1 starch/bread + 1 fat)
	Tortilla, flour, 7" across (fried with added fat)	1 (equals 1½ starch/bread + 1 fat)
	Tortilla, corn, 7½" across (fried with added fat)	1 equals 1 starch/bread + 1 fat)
	Tortilla, flour, 9" across (fried with added fat)	1 (equals 3 starch/bread + 2 fat)
Meat		
Lean meat	Menudo (tripe soup)	½ cup
Medium-fat meat	Queso fresco (cheese made with skim milk)	¼ cup (2 oz)
High-fat meat	Chorizo (Mexican sausage)	1 oz (equals 1 high-fat meat + 1 fat)
Vegetables	Chayote (squash) (cooked)	½ cup
	Jícama (yambean root) (raw)	½ cup
	Nopales (cactus) (raw)	½ cup
Fruits	Mango[b]	½ small
	Papaya[b]	1 cup
Fats	Avocado[b]	⅛ medium
Free foods	Jalapeño chillis	
	Salsa de chile (chili/taco sauce)	
	Verdolagas (purslane)	
Occasional foods	Pan dulce (sweet bread), 4½" across	1 (equals 4 starch/bread + 1 fat)

From the American Dietetic Association and the American Diabetes Association, Inc. Ethnic and regional food practices, a series. Mexican food practices, customs and holidays, 1989. With permission. Currently being revised to reflect updated information based on the American Diabetes Association's 1994 recommendations for nutrition management of diabetes.

[a]Unless otherwise specified, all foods are 1 exchange.

[b]Food and amount are same as in 1986 *Exchange Lists for Meal Planning.* © American Diabetes Association, Inc., The American Dietetic Association.

[c]Food, amount, or both differ from 1986 *Exchange Lists for Meal Planning* because of new information.

Table A-25-j
Supplemental Exchange List for Traditional Soul Foods*

Food Group (Food Exchange)	Food	Portion
Starch/bread	Hominy	¾ cup
	Succotash	½ cup
Lean meat	*Pork:* Brains	1 oz
	Ham hock	1 oz
	Hog maw	1 oz
	Pig ear	1 oz or ¼ ear
	Beef: Tripe	2 oz
	Opossum	1 oz
Medium-fat meat	*Pork:* Neck bones	1 oz meat removed from bones after cooking
	Pig feet	½ foot
	Sousemeat	½ oz or 4 × 4 × ⅒" slice
	Tongue	1 oz or ⅓ tongue
	Beef: Oxtail	1 oz meat removed from bones after cooking
High-fat meat	*Pork:* Pig tails	1 oz or ⅓ tail
	Vienna sausages	2 small
Vegetables	All vegetables should be cooked fat free	
	Kale	½ cup cooked
	Poke salad	½ cup cooked (If vegetables are prepared with fat, ½ cup serving equals 1 vegetable and 1 fat exchange.)
Fruit	Muscadines	17
Saturated fat	Lard	1 tsp
	Fatback	¼ oz
	Hog jowls	1 oz
	Pork cracklings	1 round tsp

*From The American Dietetic Association and The American Diabetes Association, Inc. Ethnic and regional food practices: a series. Soul and traditional southern food practices, customs, and holidays, 1995. With permission.

In general, people who consume soul food eat a variety of foods, many of which can be found in the Exchange Lists for Meal Planning, published by the American Dietetic Association and the American Diabetes Association (see Table A-25-a).

Table A-25-k
Supplementary Exchange Lists for Traditional Navajo Foods[a]

Food Exchange Group	Food	Portion
Starch/bread	Blue corn mush	¾ cup
	Flour tortilla, 8" diameter	¼
	Steamed corn hominy (cooked)	½ cup
Meat		
Lean meat	Mutton, flesh (lean only) (cooked without added fat)	1 oz
High-fat meat	Mutton, flesh (lean and fat) (cooked without added fat)	1 oz
Fats	Piñon nuts	1 Tbsp (about 25 nuts)

From The American Dietetic Association and the American Diabetes Association, Inc. Ethnic and regional food practices, a series. Navajo food practices, customs and holidays, 1991. With permission. Currently being revised to reflect updated information based on the American Diabetes Association's 1994 recommendations for nutrition management of diabetes.

[a]Nutrition practitioners who work with Navajo clients with non-insulin-dependent diabetes mellitus do not often use the exchange system in client education sessions. This listing is presented for the few occasions when supplementary exchange values may be needed.

Table A-26-a
Glycemic Index Values Adjusted To White Bread of 100[a,b]

Food	Mean	Food	Mean
Breads		Legumes	
Rye (crispbread)	95	Baked beans (canned)	70
Rye (wholemeal)	89	Bengal gram dal	12
Rye (whole grain, i.e., pumpernickel)	88	Butter beans	46
Wheat (white)	100	Chick peas (dried)	47
Wheat (wholemeal)	100	Chick peas (canned)	60
Pasta		Green peas (canned)	50
Macaroni (white, boiled 5 min)	64	Green peas (dried)	85
Spaghetti (brown, boiled 15 min)	61	Garden peas (frozen)	85
Spaghetti (white, boiled 15 min)	67	Haricot beans (white, dried)	54
Star pasta (white, boiled 5 min)	54	Kidney beans (dried)	43
Cereal grains		Kidney beans (canned)	74
Barley (pearled)	36	Lentils (green, dried)	36
Buckwheat	78	Lentils (green, canned)	74
Bulgur	65	Lentils (red, dried)	38
Millet	103	Pinto beans (dried)	60
Rice (brown)	81	Pinto beans (canned)	64
Rice (instant, boiled 1 min)	65	Peanuts	15
Rice (polished, boiled 5 min)	58	Soya beans (dried)	20
Rice (polished, boiled 10–25 min)	81	Soya beans (canned)	22
Rice (parboiled, boiled 5 min)	54	Fruit	
Rice (parboiled, boiled 15 min)	68	Apple	52
Rye kernels	47	Apple juice	45
Sweet corn	80	Banana	84
Wheat kernels	63	Orange	59
Breakfast cereals		Orange juice	71
All Bran	74	Raisins	93
Cornflakes	121	Sugars	
Muesli	96	Fructose	26
Porridge oats	88	Glucose	138
Puffed Rice	132	Honey	126
Puffed Wheat	110	Lactose	57
Shredded Wheat	97	Maltose	152
Weetabix	109	Sucrose	83
Cookies		Dairy products	
Digestive	82	Custard	59
Oatmeal	78	Ice cream	69
Rich tea	80	Skim milk	46
Plain crackers (water biscuits)	100	Whole milk	44
Shortbread cookies	88	Yogurt	52
Root vegetables		Snack foods	
Potato (instant)	120	Corn chips	99
Potato (mashed)	98	Potato chips	77
Potato (new/white boiled)	80		
Potato (russett, baked)	116		
Potato (sweet)	70		
Yam	74		

[a]Glycemic index is defined as the blood glucose response to a 50-g available carbohydrate portion of a food expressed as a percentage of the response to the same amount of carbohydrate from a standard food, in this case white bread (From Wolever TMS. World Rev Nutr Diet 1990;62:120–185.

[b]See also Foster-Powell K, Miller JR. International tables of glycemic index. Am J Clin Nutr 1995;62:871S–893S. This documents almost 600 separate entities with values for the most common Western foods, many indigenous foods, and pure suger solutions. Values are given for both white bread and a glucose standard.

Table A-26-b
Diets for Weight Management

	Total Daily Intake (kcal)			
Nutrient Class	800	1200	1800	2250
Carbohydrate (g)	109 (54%)	154 (51%)	249 (55%)	309 (55%)
Protein	54 (27%)	60 (20%)	84 (19%)	107 (19%)
Fat (g)	17 (19%)	40 (29%)	54 (27%)	65 (26%)
Food Group	Total Exchanges for one Day (see Table A-25-a)			
Skim milk	2	2	2	2
Vegetable	2	2	3	6
Fruit	3	4	5	7
Bread[a]	2	4	9	10
Meat	4[b]	4	5	7
Unsaturated fat	1	4	4	4
Meal	Sample Meal Pattern (servings based on exchanges)			
Breakfast				
Skim milk	½	1	1	1
Fruit	1	1	1	1 + 1 midmeal
Bread	1	1	2	2 + 1 midmeal
Meat	0	0	0	1
Unsaturated fat	1	1	1	1
Lunch				
Skim milk	1	½	0	0
Vegetable	0	1	1	2 + 2 midmeal
Fruit	1	1	2	1 + 1 midmeal
Bread	½	1	3	2
Meat	1	1	2	2
Unsaturated fat	0	1	1	1
Dinner				
Skim milk	½	0	0	0
Vegetable	2	1	2	2
Fruit	1	1	1	2
Bread	½	1	2	3
Meat	3	3	3	4
Unsaturated fat	0	1	1	1
Evening				
Skim milk	0	½	1	1
Vegetable	0	0	0	0
Fruit	0	1	1	1
Bread	0	1	2	2
Meat	0	0	0	0
Unsaturated fat	0	1	1	1

This table, prepared by us with assistance from Ms. Lori Cohen, R.D., is based on the dietary recommendations in Nutrition Guide for Professionals: Diabetes Education and Meal Planning. Powers M, ed. American Diabetes Association, Inc., and the American Dietetic Association, 1988. See Table A-27 for nutrition guidelines.

[a]In exchange lists, trace fat is listed for breads. For calculation purposes, 1 g fat can be used when amount of breads contribute significantly to diet (i.e., >6 servings per day).

[b]Lean meat exchanges are used to calculate the 800-kcal meal pattern. All other meal patterns are based on medium-fat meat exchange.

Table A-27
Nutrition Guidelines for Persons with Non-Insulin-Dependent Diabetes Mellitus (NIDDM)

	Lean Persons	Obese Persons
Energy	Enough to maintain desirable body weight	Enough to achieve reasonable body weight[a]
	Men and physically active women require 30 kcal/kg desirable body weight	20 kcal/kg desirable body weight
	Sedentary persons and persons older than 55 years require 28 kcal/kg desirable body weight	20 kcal/kg desirable body weight
Carbohydrate	Up to 55 to 60% of total energy	Same
Sucrose	Can be included with an individualized diet plan[b]	Low nutrient density; limit on low-calorie diets
Fiber	Up to 40 g/day, with emphasis on water-soluble fiber	25 g/1000 kcal
Protein	Recommended dietary allowance is 0.8 g/kg body weight	Minimum of 60 g when restricted to ≤1200-kcal diet[c]
Fat	Ideally <30% of energy	Same
Polyunsaturated fats	Up to 10% of energy	
Saturated fats	<10% of energy	
Monounsaturated fats	10 to 15% of energy	
Cholesterol	<300 mg/day	
Alternative sweeteners	Use is acceptable	Same
Sodium	Not to exceed 3000 mg/day	Same
Alcohol	Occasional or no use; limit to 1 to 2 alcohol equivalents 1 to 2 times per week	Same
Vitamins/minerals	No evidence that diabetes causes increased need	
Snacks	Individualized on the basis of preferences and glucose patterns; snack should be coordinated with insulin schedule if on insulin	Not necessary; if desired, should be included in total day's meal plan; if on insulin, coordinate with insulin schedule or adjust insulin as needed

From Beebe CA, Pastors JG, Powers MA, et al. Nutrition management for individuals with noninsulin-dependent diabetes mellitus in the 1990's: a review by the Diabetes Care and Educaiton Dietetic Practice Group. J Am Diet Assoc 1991;91:199. With permission.

[a]Reasonable body weight is that which is achievable and maintainable for the patient, although it may not be in the range considered desirable. For example, a reasonable weight goal for a patient weighing 105 kg may be 95 kg, although desirable body weight may actually be closer to 84 kg. Losing 4.5 to 9 kg may dramatically improve a person's glucose intolerance and may be a maintainable weight loss. Individual weight goals should be discussed and set.

[b]Individualization should be based on nutritional adequacy, promotion of diet adherence, and glucose and lipid control. Postprandial glucose response to a high-sucrose snack or meal should be evaluated; use of food and glucose records is helpful.

[c]For example, 12% of a 1200-kcal diet is only 36 g protein, which is less than the recommended dietary allowance (9) for a 163-cm-tall woman; 20% of a 1200-kcal diet will provide the recommended 60 g protein.

Note: See Chapter 86 for an extensive discussion of nutritional management of patients with diabetes mellitus.

A-28. NUTRITION MANAGEMENT OF CHRONIC RENAL INSUFFICIENCY

A-28a Purpose, Use, and Modifications

Chronic renal insufficiency (CRI) is characterized by a decrease in the kidney's ability to remove waste products as reflected by an increased serum creatinine level. Goals for nutritional management of chronic renal insufficiency include the following:

- Prevent or minimize uremic symptoms by reducing the accumulation of nitrogenous waste products
- Slow the progression of renal failure and possibly delay the need for maintenance dialysis
- Control hypertension by minimizing fluid and electrolyte disturbances
- Maintain nutritional status
- Translate the nutritional modifications into a meal plan that is understandable and practical for the patient

This diet (often called the predialysis diet) is indicated for patients with chronic renal insufficiency who do not yet require dialysis. This diet has two major restrictions—protein and phosphorus. The levels of sodium, potassium, fluid, and calories are based on individual needs. General recommendations are outlined in Table A-28-a-1.

Adequacy

Chronic uremic patients are prone to develop deficiency of water-soluble vitamins because of the restrictive diet, decreased consumption associated with anorexia and uremia, and altered metabolism of certain vitamins. Therefore, supplementation with water-soluble vitamins is advisable. Dietary supplementation of iron, calcium, vitamin D analogue, and zinc might be beneficial and should be individualized.

A-28b. Meal Planning

Table A-28-b-1-a presents a sample menu for a 70-kg man with chronic renal insufficiency. It summarizes the average energy, protein, sodium, and phosphorus content of the food group lists in Table A-28-b-2. These food lists were developed specifically for use in meal planning for patients with kidney disease not requiring dialysis. Food lists for patients receiving hemodialysis can be found in the chapter "Nutrition Management of Chronic Renal Failure." Additional food lists for patients receiving peritoneal dialysis and for patients with diabetes and renal disease are also available.

Table A-28-a-1
Nutrient Recommendations for Adult Patients with Chronic Renal Insufficiency

Nutrient	Modification
Protein	0.6–0.8 g/kg desirable body weight (DBW)[a] or adjusted body weight (ABW)[b,c]
Energy	
Normal weight	35 kcal/kg
Obese	20–30 kcal/kg DBW or ABW
Underweight or catabolic	45 kcal/kg
Fat (% of total energy intake)	30–40
Polyunsaturated:saturated fatty acid ratio	1.0:1.0
Carbohydrate	Remaining nonprotein calories (primarily complex)
Phosphorus	8–12 mg/kg DBW[a,d]
Calcium	1200–1600 mg/day
Sodium	1000–3000 mg/day; additional sodium may be required with salt-losing nephropathies
Potassium	Generally not restricted unless serum potassium is elevated and urine output is less than 1 L/day
Fluid	Generally unrestricted; balance fluid intake with urine output in patients with edema or congestive heart failure

[a]Based on "standard" or desirable body weight (DBW) as determined from weight-for-height tables by frame size and as used during the MDRD Study.

[b]Adjusted body weight (ABW).

[c]The upper end of this range is preferred for patients with diabetes mellitus or malnutrition. Suggested protein intake for patients with nephrotic syndrome is 0.8–1.0 g/kg.

[d]Intake of 5–10 mg phosphorus per kilogram IBW is frequently quoted in the scientific literature, but 5–10 mg phosphorus per kilogram IBW is practical only when used in conjunction with a very low protein diet supplemented with amino acids or keto analogues.

Table A-28-b-1-a
Sample Menu for Chronic Renal Insufficiency (70-kg man: 40 g protein, 2400 kcal, 600 mg phosphorus)

Breakfast	Lunch	Dinner	Snack
Orange juice (½ cup)	Roast beef (1 oz)	Baked chicken thigh (1½ oz)	Apple pie (1 slice)
Cinnamon applesauce (½ cup)	Bread (2 slices)	White rice (½ cup)	Lemon-lime soda (1 can)
Frosted cereal (1 cup)	Mayonnaise (1 tbsp)	Green beans (½ cup)	
Toast (1 slice)	Lettuce salad (1 cup)	Margarine (1 tbsp)	
Margarine (1 tsp)	Vinegar & oil dressing (2 tbsp)	Strawberries (1 cup)	
Jelly or jam (1 tbsp)	Sliced canned peaches (½ cup)	Lemonade (1 cup)	
Liquid nondairy creamer (½ cup)	Lemon-lime soda (1 can)	Tea with sugar	
Coffee or tea with sugar		Sherbet (½ cup)	

Approximate Nutrient Analysis

Energy (kcal)	2495.0	Phosphorus (mg)	456.7
Protein (g)	38.2	Potassium (mg)	1685.2
(6.1% of kcal)		Sodium (mg)	1623.2
Carbohydrate (g)	425.8	Zinc (mg)	5.8
(68.3% of kcal)		Vitamin A (μg RE)	683.9
Total fat (g)	78.4	Vitamin C (mg)	184.3
(28.3% of kcal)		Thiamin (mg)	1.5
Saturated fatty acids (g)	19.2	Riboflavin (mg)	1.6
Monounsaturated fatty acids (g)	30.3	Niacin (mg)	18.3
Polyunsaturated fatty acids (g)	23.7	Folate (μg)	339.4
Cholesterol (mg)	80.7	Vitamin B_6 (mg)	1.5
Calcium (mg)	301.9	Vitamin B_{12} (μg)	1.1
Iron (mg)	12.1	Dietary fiber (g)	16.1
Magnesium (mg)	149.0	Water-insoluble fiber (g)	10.3

Table A-28-b-1-b
Average Calculation Figures for Planning Chronic Renal Insufficiency (CRI) Diet[a]

Food Choices	kcal	Protein (g)	Na (mg)	P (mg)
Milk and dairy	120	4.0	80	110
Milk substitutes[b]	140	0.5	40	30
Meats	65	7.0	25	65
Starches	90	2.0	80	35
Vegetables[c]	25	1.0	15	20
Fruits	70	0.5	Trace	15
Fats	45	Trace	55	5
High-calorie choices[d]	100	Trace	15	5
Salt choices	—	—	250	—

From Renal Dietitians Dietetic Practice Group. National renal diet. Chicago, IL: the American Dietetic Association; 1993.

[a]Serving sizes for each food choice are shown in the food lists in Table A-28-b-2.

[b]Milk substitute choices are nondairy products, which can be used in lieu of milk and milk products.

[c]Average sodium level values do not include canned vegetables. Add 250 mg sodium for canned vegetables with added salt.

[d]High-calorie choices are foods high in carbohydrates that contain only a trace of protein and minimal electrolytes. These should be used to raise calorie intake to the desired level.

National Renal Diet Choices

1 milk

1 nondairy

2½ meat

5 starch

2 vegetable

4 fruit

5 high-calorie sources

7 fat

Table A-28-b-2
Food Lists for Chronic Renal Insufficiency Diet

Milk and Dairy Choices

Average per choice: 4 g protein, 120 kcal, 80 mg sodium, 110 mg phosphorus

Milk (nonfat, low-fat, whole)	½ cup
Alterna	1 cup
Buttermilk, cultured	½ cup
Chocolate milk	½ cup
Light cream or half and half	½ cup
Ice milk or ice cream	½ cup
Yogurt, plain or fruit-flavored	½ cup
Evaporated milk	¼ cup
Cream cheese	3 tbsp
Sour cream	4 tbsp
Sherbet	1 cup
Sweetened condensed milk	¼ cup

Nondairy Milk Substitutes

Average per ounce: 0.5 g protein, 140 kcal, 40 mg sodium, 30 mg phosphorus

Dessert, nondairy frozen	½ cup
Dessert topping, nondairy frozen	½ cup
Liquid nondairy creamer, polyunsaturated	½ cup

continued

Table A-28-b-2—*continued*
Food Lists for Chronic Renal Insufficiency Diet

Meat Choices

Average per ounce: 7 g protein, 65 kcal, 25 mg sodium, 65 mg phosphorus

Prepared without added salt	
Beef	
Round, sirloin, flank, cubed, T-bone, and porterhouse steak; tenderloin, rib, chuck, and rump roast; ground beef and ground chuck	1 oz
Pork	
Fresh ham, tenderloin, chop, loin roast, cutlet	1 oz
Lamb	
Chop, leg, roast	1 oz
Veal	
Chop, roast, cutlet	1 oz
Poultry	
Chicken, turkey, Cornish hen, domestic duck and goose	1 oz
Fish	
All fresh and frozen fish	1 oz
Lobster, scallops, shrimp, clams	1 oz
Crab, oysters	1½ oz
Canned tuna, canned salmon (unsalted)	1 oz
Sardines[a] (unsalted)	1 oz
Wild game	
Venison, rabbit, squirrel, pheasant, duck, goose	1 oz
Egg	
Whole	1 large
Egg white or yolk	2 large
Low-cholesterol egg product	¼ cup
Chitterlings	2 oz
Organ meats[a]	1 oz
Prepared with added salt	
Beef	
Deli-style[b]	1 oz
Pork	
Boiled or deli-style ham[b]	1 oz
Poultry	
Deli-style chicken or turkey[b]	1 oz
Fish	
Canned tuna, canned salmon[b]	1 oz
Sardines[a,b]	
Cheese	
Cottage[b]	¼ cup
High in sodium, phosphorus, and/or saturated fat—should be used in limited quantities	
Bacon	
Frankfurters, bratwurst, Polish sausage	
Lunch meats including bologna, braunschweiger, liverwurst, picnic loaf, salami, summer sausage	
All cheeses except cottage cheese	

Starch Choices

Average per choice: 2 g protein, 90 kcal, 80 mg sodium, 35 mg phosphorus

Breads and rolls	
Bread (French, Italian, raisin, light rye, sourdough white)	1 slice (1 oz)
Bagel	½ small (1 oz)
Bun, hamburger or hot dog type	½
Danish pastry or sweet roll, no nuts	½ small
Dinner roll or hard roll	1 small
Doughnut	1 small
English muffin	½
Muffin, no nuts, bran, or whole wheat	1 small (1 oz)
Pancake[b,c]	1 small
Pita, or pocket bread	½ 6-in

continued

Table A-28-b-2—*continued*
Food Lists for Chronic Renal Insufficiency Diet

Tortilla, corn or	2 6-in
flour	1 6-in
Waffle[c,d]	1 small (1 oz)
Cereals and grains	
Cereals, ready to eat, most brands[c]	¾ cup
Puffed rice	2 cups
Puffed wheat	1 cup
Cooked cereal	
Cream of rice or wheat, farina, Malt-O-Meal	½ cup
Oat bran or oatmeal, Ralston	⅓ cup
Corn meal, cooked	¾ cup
Grits, cooked	½ cup
Flour, all-purpose	2½ tbsp
Pasta (noodles, macaroni, spaghetti), cooked	½ cup
Pasta made with egg (egg noodles), cooked	⅓ cup
Rice, white or brown, cooked	½ cup
Starchy vegetables	
Corn	⅓ cup or ½ ear
Green peas	¼ cup
Potatoes, boiled, mashed	½ cup
Potatoes, baked, white or sweet	1 small (3 oz)
Potatoes, french fried	½ cup or 10 small
Potatoes, hash brown	½ cup
Squash, butternut, mashed	½ cup
Squash, winter, baked (all other varieties), cubed	1 cup
Crackers and snacks	
Crackers (saltines, round butter)	4
Graham crackers	3 squares
Melba toast	3 oblong
RyKrisp[c]	3
Popcorn, plain	1½ cups popped
Potato chips	1 oz (14 chips)
Tortilla chips	¾ oz (9 chips)
Pretzels,[c] sticks or rings	¾ oz (10 sticks)
Desserts	
Cake, angel food	1/20 cake or 1 oz
Cake	2 × 2-in square or 1½ oz
Sandwich cookies[b,c]	4
Shortbread cookies	4
Sugar cookies	4
Sugar wafers	4
Vanilla wafers	10
Fruit pie (apple, berry, cherry, peach)	⅛ pie
Sweetened gelatin	½ cup

High in poor-quality protein and phosphorus—should be used rarely and in limited quantities
Bran cereal or muffins, Grape-Nuts, granola cereal or bars
Boxed, frozen, or canned meals, entrees, or side dishes
Pumpernickel, dark rye, whole-wheat, or oatmeal breads
Whole-wheat crackers
Whole-wheat cereals

Vegetable Choices

Average per choice: 1 g protein, 25 kcal, 15 mg sodium, 20 mg phosphorus
See Starch List for other vegetables. Prepared or canned without added salt.[e]

1 cup serving

Alfalfa sprouts	Escarole
Cabbage	Lettuce, all varieties
Celery	Pepper, green, sweet
Cucumber (or ½ whole)	Radishes, sliced (or 15 small)
Eggplant	Turnip
Endive	Watercress

continued

Table A-28-b-2—*continued*
Food Lists for Chronic Renal Insufficiency Diet

½ cup serving

Artichoke	Mushrooms, fresh (or 4 medium)
Bamboo shoots	Onions
Bean sprouts	Parsnips[f]
Beans, green or wax	Pumpkin
Beets	Rutabagas[f]
Carrots (or 1 small)	Squash, summer
Cauliflower	Tomato (or 1 medium)
Chard	Tomato juice, unsalted
Chinese cabbage	Tomato juice, regular[g]
Collard greens	Tomato puree
Kale	Turnip greens
Kohlrabi	Vegetable juice cocktail, regular[g]

¼ cup serving

Asparagus (or 2 spears)	Mushrooms, cooked
Avocado (¼ whole)	Mustard greens
Beet greens	Okra
Broccoli	Snow peas
Brussels sprouts	Spinach
Chili pepper	Tomato sauce

Fruit Choices

Average per choice: 0.5 g protein, 70 kcal, 15 mg phosphorus

1 cup serving

Apple (1 medium)	Papaya nectar
Apple juice	Peach nectar
Applesauce	Pear nectar
Cranberries	Pear, canned or fresh (1 medium)
Cranberry juice cocktail	Tangerine (1 medium)

½ cup serving

Apricot nectar	Lemon (½ medium)
Banana (½ small)	Lemon juice
Blueberries	Mango (½ medium)
Figs, canned	Nectarine (½ medium)
Fruit cocktail	Orange (½ medium)
Grapes (15 small)	Peach, canned or fresh (½ medium)
Grape juice	Pineapple
Grapefruit (½ medium)	Plums, canned or fresh (1 medium)
Grapefruit juice	Rhubarb
Gooseberries	Strawberries
Kiwifruit (½ medium)	Watermelon

¼ cup serving

Apricots (2 halves)	Honeydew melon (⅛ small)
Apricots, dried (2)	Orange juice
Blackberries	Papaya (¼ medium)
Cantaloupe (⅛ small)	Prune juice
Cherries	Prunes, cooked (5)
Dates (2 tbsp)	Raisins (2 tbsp)
Figs, dried (1 whole)	Raspberries

Fat Choices

Average per choice: trace protein, 45 kcal, 55 mg sodium, 5 mg phosphorus

Unsaturated fats	
Margarine	1 tsp
Reduced-calorie margarine	1 tbsp
Mayonnaise	1 tsp
Low-calorie mayonnaise	1 tbsp
Oil	
Safflower, sunflower, corn, soybean, olive, peanut, canola	1 tsp
Salad dressing, mayonnaise-type	2 tbsp
Salad dressing, oil-type	1 tbsp
Low-calorie salad dressing (mayonnaise-type)[h]	2 tbsp
Low-calorie salad dressing (oil-type)[h]	2 tbsp
Tartar sauce	1½ tsp

continued

Table A-28-b-2—*continued*
Food Lists for Chronic Renal Insufficiency Diet

Saturated fats	
Butter	1 tsp
Coconut	2 tbsp
Powdered coffee whitener	1 tbsp
Solid shortening	1 tsp

High-Calorie Choices

Average per choice: trace protein, 100 kcal, 15 mg sodium, 5 mg phosphorus

Beverages			
Carbonated beverages Fruit flavors, root beer, colas[i] or pepper type	1 cup	Kool-Aid	1 cup
		Limeade	1 cup
		Lemonade	1 cup
Cranberry juice cocktail	1 cup	Tang	1 cup
Fruit-flavored drink	1 cup	Wine[j]	½ cup
Frozen desserts			
Fruit ice	½ cup	Popsicle (3 oz)	1 bar
Juice bar (3 oz)	1 bar	Sorbet	½ cup
Candy and sweets			
Candy corn	20 or 1 oz	Butter mints	14
Gumdrops	15 small	Fruit chews	4
Hard candy	4 pieces	Chewy fruit snacks	1 pouch
Jelly beans	10	Fruit Roll-Ups	2
LifeSavers or cough drops	12	Cranberry sauce or relish	¼ cup
Marshmallows	5 large		
Honey	2 tbsp	Sugar, powdered	3 tbsp
Sugar, brown or white	2 tbsp	Marmalade	2 tbsp
Jam or jelly	2 tbsp	Syrup	2 tbsp
Special low-protein products			
Low-protein gelled dessert	½ cup		
Low-protein bread	1 slice		
Low-protein cookies	2		
Low-protein pasta	½ cup		
Low-protein rusk	2 slices		

Salt Choices

Average per choice: 250 mg sodium

Salt	⅛ tsp
Seasoned salts (onion, garlic)	⅛ tsp
Accent	¼ tsp
Barbecue sauce	2 tbsp
Bouillon	⅓ cup
Ketchup	1½ tbsp
Chili sauce	1½ tbsp
Dill pickle	⅙ large or ½ oz
Mustard	4 tsp
Olives, green	2 medium or ⅓ oz
Olives, black	3 large or 1 oz
Soy sauce	¾ tsp
Steak sauce	2½ tsp
Sweet pickle relish	2½ tbsp
Taco sauce	2 tbsp
Tamari sauce	¾ tsp
Teriyaki sauce	1¼ tsp
Worcestershire sauce	1 tbsp

From Renal Dietitians Dietetic Practice Group. National renal diet. Chicago, IL: the American Dietetic Association, 1993. See references there.

[a]High phosphorus ≥100 mg/serving.

[b]High sodium, each serving counts as 1 meat choice and 1 salt choice.

[c]High sodium, each serving counts as 1 starch choice and 1 salt choice.

[d]High phosphorus, ≥70 mg/serving.

[e]For vegetables canned with salt, add 250 mg sodium and count as 1 vegetable choice and 1 salt choice.

continued

[f]High phosphorus, ≥40 mg/serving.

[g]Very high sodium; each serving counts as 1 vegetable choice and 2 salt choices.

[h]High sodium; each serving counts as 1 fat choice and 1 salt choice.

[i]High phosphorus, ≥20 mg/serving.

[j]Check with physician for recommendation regarding alcohol.

Commercial Sources: Alterna, Ross Laboratories, Columbus, OH 43216; Malt-O-Meal, Malt-O-Meal Co, Minneapolis, MN 55402; Ralston, RyKrisp, Ralston Purina Co, St Louis, MO 63164; Grape-Nuts, Kool-Aid, Tang, General Foods Corp, White Plains, NY 10625; Popsicle, Popsicle Industries Inc, Englewood, NJ 07631; LifeSavers, Nabisco Brands, Inc, East Hanover, NJ 07936; Fruit Roll-Ups, General Mills, Inc, Minneapolis, MN 55440; Accent, Pet, Inc, St Louis, Mo 63102

A-29. GUIDELINES FOR DIETARY SODIUM RESTRICTION

A-29-a. Purpose and Modifications

The goal of a sodium-restricted meal plan is to manage hypertension in sodium-sensitive persons and to promote the loss of excess fluids in edema and ascites. Numerous national health agencies concur that Americans should limit daily sodium intake to less than 3000 mg/day. This is based on findings from epidemiologic studies and clinical trials that support the correlation between reduced sodium intake and blood pressure lowering. The National Research Council recommends that the daily intake of sodium be limited to 2400 mg or less. The National High Blood Pressure Education Program (NHBPEP) recommends that sodium intake be reduced below 2300 mg sodium per day. A public health recommendation is not a mandate; instead, it provides guidelines for menu planning and offers directions for persons who wish to exercise free choice in selecting more healthful alternatives. The Nutrition Facts panel of food labels lists the Daily Value for sodium at 2400 mg/day.

A therapeutic sodium-restricted meal plan should be prescribed in terms of milligrams or milliequivalents of sodium desired on a daily basis. Depending on the severity of cardiac or vascular disease, the amount of edema, and the type of drug therapy, varying degrees of sodium restriction are prescribed. Traditionally, more liberal sodium-restricted diets have allowed up to 4000 to 5000 mg of sodium daily. However, this is inconsistent with public policy recommendations.

Diets containing less than 2000 mg of sodium per day may be used in the hospital setting on a short-term basis but are considered impractical on an outpatient basis. Special low-sodium food products are often expensive and unpalatable, leading to poor patient compliance. The following levels of sodium restriction may be prescribed.

- 3000 mg sodium (130 meq): Eliminate or eat sparingly high-sodium processed foods and beverages such as fast foods; salad dressings; smoked, salted, and "koshered" meats; regular canned foods; pickled vegetables; luncheon meats; and commercially softened water. Allow up to 1/4 tsp of table salt in cooking or at the table.

- 2000 mg sodium (87 meq): Eliminate processed and prepared foods and beverages high in sodium. Do not allow any salt in the preparation of foods or at the table. Limit milk and milk products to 16 oz daily. Check labels of canned and instant products for sodium content and replace with low-sodium versions when available. Table A-29-a-1 lists standard definitions for sodium claims on food labels.
- 1000 mg sodium (45 meq): Eliminate processed and prepared foods and beverages high in sodium. Omit the following regular items: canned foods, cheeses, margarines, and salad dressings. Look for low-sodium or low-salt varieties of these foods (check the label). Omit many frozen foods, deli foods, and fast foods. Limit regular breads to two servings per day. Limit milk and milk products to 16 oz daily. Do not allow any salt in food preparation or for table use. This meal plan is used in the inpatient setting on a short-term basis only.
- 500 mg sodium (22 meq): Omit canned or processed foods containing salt. Do not use any salt in food preparation or at the table. Omit vegetables containing high amounts of natural sodium. Limit meat to 5 oz daily and milk and milk products to 16 oz daily. Use low-sodium bread in place of regular bread, and distilled water for cooking and drinking. This meal plan is used in the inpatient setting on a short-term basis only.

Table A-29-a-1
Sodium Claims on Food Labels (FDA)

Sodium free	Less than 5 mg sodium per serving
Salt free	Meets requirements for sodium free
Low sodium	140 mg sodium or less per serving
Very low sodium	35 mg or less sodium per serving
Reduced sodium	At least 25% less sodium than in a reference food[a]
Light in sodium	50% less sodium per serving; restricted to foods with more than 40 calories per serving or more than 3 g of fat per serving (if pertaining to sodium content)
Unsalted, Without added salt, No salt added	(1) No salt is added during processing; (2) the product it resembles and substitutes for is normally processed with salt; and (3) the label bears the statement "not a sodium-free food" or "not for control of sodium" in the diet if the food is not sodium free

[a]A reference food is the regular version of the labeled product. It may be either a group of foods, such as an average of the three market leaders, or an individual food product.

Adequacy

Depending on individual food choices, sodium-restricted meal plans (1000 mg or more) are adequate in all nutrients, based on the 1989 Recommended Dietary Allowances. Meal plans with daily sodium intakes below 1000 mg may be inadequate in calcium because of the restriction of milk and milk products. However, this level of restriction is not recommended for long-term use.

From the American Dietetic Association Manual of Clinical Dietetics, 5th ed. © 1996, with permission, pp. 495–509; references on p. 509.

Table A-29-b-1
Guidelines for Food Selection for 3000-mg Sodium Diet[a]

Food Category	Recommended	Excluded
Beverages	Milk, buttermilk (limit to 1 cup daily); eggnog; all fruit juices; low-sodium, salt-free vegetable juices; regular vegetable or tomato juices (limit to ½ cup daily); low-sodium carbonated beverages	Regular vegetable or tomato juices used in excessive amounts; commercially softened water used for drinking or cooking
Breads and cereals	Enriched white, wheat, rye, and pumpernickel bread; hard rolls and dinner rolls; muffins, cornbread, light biscuits, waffles, and pancakes; most dry and hot cereals; unsalted crackers and breadsticks	Breads, rolls, and crackers with salted tops; instant hot cereals
Desserts and sweets	All	None
Fats	Butter or margarine; vegetable oils; low-sodium salad dressing, other salad dressings in limited amounts; light, sour, and heavy cream	Salad dressings containing bacon fat, bacon bits, and salt pork; snack dips made with instant soup mixes or processed cheese
Fruits	All	None
Meats and meat substitutes	Any fresh or frozen beef, lamb, pork, poultry, fish, and most shellfish; canned tuna or salmon, rinsed; eggs and egg substitutes; regular cheese, ricotta, and cream cheese (2 oz daily); low-sodium cheese as desired; cottage cheese, drained; regular yogurt; regular peanut butter (3 times weekly); dried peas and beans; frozen dinners (<600 mg sodium)	Any smoked, cured, salted, koshered, or canned meat, fish, or poultry including bacon, chipped beef, cold cuts, ham, hot dogs, sausage, sardines, anchovies, marinated herring, and pickled meats; frozen breaded meats; pickled eggs; processed cheese, cheese spreads and sauces; salted nuts
Potatoes and potato substitutes	White or sweet potatoes; squash; enriched rice, barley, noodles, spaghetti, macaroni, and other pastas; homemade bread stuffing	Commercially prepared potato, rice, or pasta mixes; commercial bread stuffing
Soups	Commercially canned and dehydrated soups, broths, and boullions (once per week); homemade broth, soups without added salt and made with allowed vegetables; reduced-sodium canned soups and broths	Canned or dehydrated regular soups (more than once per week)

continued

Table A-29-b-1—*continued*
Guidelines for Food Selection for 3000-mg Sodium Diet[a]

Food Category	Recommended	Excluded
Vegetables	All fresh and frozen vegetables; canned, drained vegetables	Sauerkraut, pickled vegetables, and others prepared in brine; vegetables seasoned with ham, bacon, or salt pork
Miscellaneous	Limit added salt to ¼ tsp/day used at the table or in cooking; salt substitute with physician's approval; pepper, herbs, spices; vinegar, ketchup (1 tbsp), mustard (1 tbsp), lemon, or lime juice; hot pepper sauce; low-sodium soy sauce (1 tbsp); unsalted tortilla chips, pretzels, potato chips, popcorn, salsa (¼ cup)	Any seasoning made with salt including garlic salt, celery salt, onion salt, and seasoned salt; sea salt, rock salt, kosher salt; meat tenderizers; monosodium glutamate; regular soy sauce, teriyaki sauce, most flavored vinegars; regular snack chips, olives

Sample Menu for 3000-mg Sodium Diet[a]

Breakfast	Lunch	Dinner
Orange juice (½ cup)	Vegetable soup (1 cup)	Green salad (3½ oz)
Whole-grain cereal (¾ cup)	Unsalted crackers (4)	Vinegar and oil dressing (1 tbsp)
Banana (½)	Lean beef patty (3 oz)	Broiled skinless chicken breast (3 oz)
Whole-wheat toast (2 slices)	Hamburger bun (1)	Herbed brown rice (½ cup)
Margarine (2 tsp)	Mustard (1 tbsp)	Steamed broccoli (½ cup)
Jelly or jam (1 tbsp)	Ketchup (1 tbsp)	Whole-grain roll (1)
Skim milk (1 cup)	Sliced tomato (2 oz) and lettuce	Margarine (2 tsp)
Coffee/tea	Fresh fruit salad (½ cup)	Low-fat frozen yogurt (½ cup)
	Graham crackers (4)	Medium apple (1)
	2% milk (1 cup)	Coffee/tea
	Coffee/tea	

Approximate Nutrient Analysis

Nutrient	Amount	Nutrient	Amount
Energy (kcal)	2113.9	Phosphorus (mg)	1720.9
Protein (g)	103.5	Potassium (mg)	3763.2
(19.6% of kcal)		Sodium (mg)	2945.8
Carbohydrate (g)	281.6	Zinc (mg)	16.0
(53.3% of kcal)		Vitamin A (μg RE)	845.7
Total fat (g)	70.7	Vitamin C (mg)	145.4
(30.1% of kcal)		Thiamin (mg)	2.0
Saturated fatty acids (g)	22.8	Riboflavin (mg)	2.6
Monounsaturated fatty acids (g)	26.7	Niacin (mg)	32.5
Polyunsaturated fatty acids (g)	14.1	Folate (μg)	474.2
Cholesterol (mg)	180.8	Vitamin B_6 (mg)	3.0
Calcium (mg)	1065.3	Vitamin B_{12} (μg)	7.4
Iron (mg)	15.6	Dietary fiber (g)	30.6
Magnesium (mg)	466.0	Water-insoluble fiber (g)	23.0

[a]May use up to ¼ tsp salt per day in cooking and at the table (500 mg sodium).

Table A-29-b-2
Guidelines for Food Selection for 2000-mg Sodium Diet[a]

Food Category	Recommended	Excluded
Beverages	Milk (limit to 16 oz daily); buttermilk (limit to 1 cup/week); eggnog; all fruit juices; low-sodium, salt-free vegetable juices; low-sodium, carbonated beverages	Malted milk, milkshake, chocolate milk; regular vegetable or tomato juices; commercially softened water used for drinking or cooking
Breads and cereals	Enriched white, wheat, rye, and pumpernickel bread, hard rolls, and dinner rolls; muffins, cornbread, and waffles, most dry cereals, cooked cereal without added salt; unsalted crackers and breadsticks; low-sodium or homemade bread crumbs	Breads, rolls, and crackers with salted tops; quick breads; instant hot cereals; pancakes; commercial bread stuffing; self-rising flour and biscuit mixes; regular bread crumbs or cracker crumbs
Desserts and sweets	All; desserts and sweets made with milk should be within allowance	Instant pudding mixes and cake mixes
Fats	Butter or margarine; vegetable oils; unsalted salad dressings, regular salad dressings, limited to 1 tbsp; light, sour, and heavy cream	Regular salad dressings containing bacon fat, bacon bits, and salt pork; snack dips made with instant soup mixes or processed cheese
Fruits	Most fresh, frozen, and canned fruits	Fruits processed with salt or sodium-containing compounds (i.e., some dried fruits)

continued

Table A-29-b-2—*continued*
Guidelines for Food Selection for 2000-mg Sodium Diet[a]

Food Category	Recommended	Excluded
Meats and meat substitutes	Any fresh or frozen beef, lamb, pork, poultry, fish, and shrimp; canned tuna or salmon, rinsed; eggs and egg substitutes; low-sodium cheese including low-sodium ricotta and cream cheese; low-sodium cottage cheese; regular yogurt; low-sodium peanut butter; dried peas and beans; frozen dinners (<500 mg sodium)	Any smoked, cured, salted, "koshered," or canned meat, fish, or poultry including bacon, chipped beef, cold cuts, ham, hot dogs, sausage, sardines, anchovies, crab, lobster, imitation seafood, marinated herring, and pickled meats; frozen breaded meats; pickled eggs; regular hard and processed cheese, cheese spreads and sauces; salted nuts
Potatoes and potato substitutes	White or sweet potatoes; squash; enriched rice, barley, noodles, spaghetti, macaroni, and other pastas cooked without salt; homemade bread stuffing	Commercially prepared potato, rice, or pasta mixes; commercial bread stuffing
Soups	Low-sodium commercially canned and dehydrated soups, broths, and boullions; homemade broth, and soups without added salt and made with allowed vegetables; cream soups within milk allowance	Regular canned or dehydrated soups, broths, or bouillon
Vegetables	Fresh, frozen vegetables and low-sodium canned, vegetables	Regular canned vegetables, sauerkraut, pickled vegetables, and others prepared in brine; frozen vegetables in sauces; vegetables seasoned with ham, bacon, or salt pork
Miscellaneous	Salt substitute with physician's approval; pepper, herbs, spices; vinegar, lemon or lime juice; hot pepper sauce; low-sodium soy sauce (1 tbsp); hot pepper sauce; low-sodium condiments (ketchup, chili sauce, mustard) in limited amount (1 tsp); fresh ground horseradish; unsalted tortilla chips, pretzels, potato chips, popcorn, salsa (¼ cup)	Any seasoning made with salt including garlic salt, celery salt, onion salt, and, seasoned salt; sea salt, rock salt, kosher salt; meat tenderizers, monosodium glutamate; regular soy sauce, barbecue sauce, teriyaki sauce, steak sauce, Worcestershire sauce, and most flavored vinegars; canned gravy and mixes; regular condiments; salted snack foods, olives

Sample Menu for 2000-mg Sodium Diet[a]

Breakfast	Lunch	Dinner
Orange juice (½ cup)	Low-sodium vegetable soup (1 cup)	Green salad (3½ oz)
Whole-grain cereal (¾ cup)	Unsalted crackers (4)	Vinegar and oil dressing (1 tbsp)
Banana (½)	Lean beef patty (3 oz)	Broiled skinless chicken breast (3 oz)
Whole-wheat toast (2 slices)	Hamburger bun (1)	Herbed brown rice (½ cup)
Margarine (2 tsp)	Mustard (1 tsp)	Steamed broccoli (½ cup)
Jelly or jam (1 tbsp)	Mayonnaise (2 tsp)	Whole-grain roll (1)
2% milk (1 cup)	Sliced tomato (2 oz) and lettuce	Margarine (2 tsp)
Coffee/tea	Fresh fruit salad (½ cup)	Fruit sorbet (½ cup)
	Graham crackers (2)	Medium apple (1)
	2% milk (1 cup)	Coffee/tea
	Coffee/tea	

Approximate Nutrient Analysis

Energy (kcal)	2160.4	Phosphorus (mg)	1585.7
Protein (g)	103.3	Potassium (mg)	3619.3
(19.1% of kcal)		Sodium (mg)	1693.1
Carbohydrate (g)	282.4	Zinc (mg)	16.1
(52.3% of kcal)		Vitamin A (μg RE)	885.5
Total fat (g)	75.3	Vitamin C (mg)	125.2
(31.4% of kcal)		Thiamin (mg)	2.0
Saturated fatty acids (g)	22.4	Riboflavin (mg)	2.6
Monounsaturated fatty acids (g)	28.0	Niacin (mg)	34.9
Polyunsaturated fatty acids (g)	17.7	Folate (μg)	444.8
Cholesterol (mg)	195.5	Vitamin B_6 (mg)	2.9
Calcium (mg)	896.1	Vitamin B_{12} (μg)	7.1
Iron (mg)	15.6	Dietary fiber (g)	28.9
Magnesium (mg)	445.9	Water-insoluble fiber (g)	22.2

[a]No salt added in cooking.

Table A-29-b-3
Guidelines for Food Selection for 1000-mg Sodium Diet[a]

Food Category	Recommended	Excluded
Beverages	Milk (limit to 16 oz daily); eggnog; all fruit juices; low-sodium, salt-free vegetable juices; low-sodium carbonated beverages	Malted milk, milkshake, buttermilk, chocolate milk; regular vegetable or tomato juices; commercially softened water used for drinking or cooking

continued

Table A-29-b-3—*continued*
Guidelines for Food Selection for 1000-mg Sodium Diet[a]

Food Category	Recommended	Excluded
Breads and cereals	Enriched white, wheat, rye, and pumpernickel bread; hard rolls, and dinner rolls (2 servings/day); low-sodium bread, crackers, matzo, and melba toast; muffins, cornbread, pancakes, and waffles made with low-sodium baking powder; cooked cereal without added salt; low-sodium dry cereals including puffed rice, puffed wheat, and shredded wheat, unsalted crackers and breadsticks; low-sodium or homemade bread crumbs and cracker crumbs	Breads, rolls, and crackers with salted tops or made with regular baking powder; quick breads; instant hot cereals; self-rising flour and biscuit mixes; regular bread crumbs or cracker crumbs
Desserts and sweets	Ice cream, pudding, and custard made with milk should be within allowance; fruit ice; unsalted bakery goods, homemade or commercial; sherbet and flavored gelatin (not to exceed ½ cup/day)	All candies made with sweet chocolate, nuts, or coconut; desserts made with rennin or rennin tablets; instant pudding mixes; commercial cake, cookie, and brownie mixes
Fats	Unsalted butter or margarine; vegetable oils; unsalted salad dressings, low-sodium mayonnaise; nondairy cream (up to 1 oz daily)	Salted butter and margarine; regular salad dressings, bacon bits, and salt pork; snack dips made with instant soup mixes or processed cheese
Fruits	Most fresh, frozen, and canned fruits	Fruits processed with salt or sodium-containing compounds
Meats and meat substitutes	Any fresh or frozen beef, lamb, pork, poultry, fish; low-sodium canned tuna or salmon, eggs; low-sodium cheese, cottage cheese, ricotta, and cream cheese; regular yogurt; low-sodium peanut butter; dried peas and beans; frozen dinners (<150 mg sodium)	Any smoked, cured, salted, "koshered," or canned meat, fish, or poultry including bacon, chipped beef, cold cuts, ham, hot dogs, sausage, sardines, anchovies, marinated herring, and pickled meats; all shellfish; frozen breaded meats; pickled eggs, egg substitutes; regular hard and processed cheese, cheese spreads and sauces; salted nuts
Potatoes and potato substitutes	White or sweet potatoes; squash; unsalted enriched rice, barley, noodles, spaghetti, macaroni, and other pastas cooked without salt; homemade bread stuffing	Commercially prepared potato, rice, or pasta mixes; commercial bread stuffing
Soups	Low-sodium commercially canned and dehydrated soups, broths, and bouillons; homemade broth, soups without added salt and made with allowed vegetables; low-sodium cream soups within milk allowance	Regular canned or dehydrated soups, broths, or bouillon
Vegetables	Fresh, unsalted frozen vegetables and low-sodium canned vegetables	Regular canned vegetables, sauerkraut, pickled vegetables, and others prepared in brine; frozen peas, lima beans, and mixed vegetables; all frozen vegetables in sauces; vegetables seasoned with ham, bacon, or salt pork
Miscellaneous	Salt substitute with physician's approval; pepper, herbs, spices; vinegar, lemon, or lime juice; hot pepper sauce; low-sodium condiments (ketchup, chili sauce, mustard); fresh ground horseradish; unsalted tortilla chips, pretzels, potato chips, popcorn	Salt and any seasoning made with salt including garlic salt, celery salt, onion salt, and seasoned salt; sea salt, rock salt, kosher salt; meat tenderizers; monosodium glutamate; regular and low-sodium soy sauce (check label), barbecue sauce, teriyaki sauce, steak sauce, Worcestershire sauce, and most flavored vinegars; canned gravy and mixes; regular condiments including olives, horseradish, pickles, relish, ketchup, mustard, and commercial salsa

Sample Menu for 1000-mg Sodium Diet[a]

Breakfast	Lunch	Dinner
Orange juice (½ cup)	Low-sodium vegetable soup (1 cup)	Green salad (3½ oz)
Shredded wheat cereal (¾ cup)	Unsalted crackers (4)	Salt-free vinegar and oil dressing (1 tbsp)
Banana (½)	Lean beef patty (3 oz)	Broiled skinless chicken breast (3 oz)
Low-sodium whole-wheat toast (2 slices)	Low-sodium bread (2 slices)	Herbed brown rice (½ cup)
Unsalted margarine (2 tsp)	Low-sodium mayonnaise (1 tbsp)	Steamed broccoli (½ cup)
Jelly or jam (1 tbsp)	Sliced tomato (2 oz) and lettuce	Whole-grain roll (1)
2% milk (1 cup)	Fresh fruit salad (½ cup)	Unsalted margarine (1 tsp)
Coffee/tea	Graham crackers (2)	Fruit sorbet (½ cup)
	2% milk (1 cup)	Medium apple (1)
	Coffee/tea	Coffee/tea

continued

Table A-29-b-3—*continued*
Guidelines for Food Selection for 1000-mg Sodium Diet[a]

Approximate Nutrient Analysis			
Energy (kcal)	2213.4	Phosphorus (mg)	1628.6
Protein (g)	105.9	Potassium (mg)	3718.1
(19.1% of kcal)		Sodium (mg)	904.1
Carbohydrate (g)	290.6	Zinc (mg)	14.3
(52.5% of kcal)		Vitamin A (μg RE)	931.0
Total fat (g)	76.8	Vitamin C (mg)	145.6
(31.2% of kcal)		Thiamin (mg)	1.6
Saturated fatty acids (g)	21.8	Riboflavin (mg)	2.1
Monounsaturated fatty acids (g)	29.5	Niacin (mg)	30.2
Polyunsaturated fatty acids (g)	18.8	Folate (μg)	361.5
Cholesterol (mg)	197.8	Vitamin B_6 (mg)	2.4
Calcium (mg)	904.8	Vitamin B_{12} (μg)	4.1
Iron (mg)	15.4	Dietary fiber (g)	30.7
Magnesium (mg)	462.2	Water-insoluble fiber (g)	23.3

[a]No salt added in cooking

Guidelines for Food Selection for 500-mg Sodium Diet

Use the 1000-mg sodium diet guidelines (Table A-29-b-3) with the following modifications:

- Use low-sodium bread only
- Omit sherbet and flavored gelatin
- Limit meat to 5 oz per day; one egg may be used daily in place of 1 oz of meat
- Omit the following vegetables: beets, beet greens, carrots, kale, spinach, celery, white turnips, rutabagas, mustard greens, chard, peas, and dandelion greens
- Use distilled water
- Limit milk and milk products to 16 oz daily

Table A-29-b-4
Sample Menu for 500-mg Sodium Diet

Breakfast	Lunch	Dinner
Orange juice (½ cup)	Low-sodium vegetable soup (1 cup)	Green salad (3½ oz)
Shredded wheat cereal (¾ cup)	Unsalted crackers (4)	Salf-free vinegar and oil dressing (1 tbsp)
Banana (½)	Lean beef patty (2 oz)	Broiled skinless chicken breast (3 oz)
Low-sodium whole-wheat toast (2 slices)	Low-sodium bread (2 slices)	Herbed brown rice (½ cup)
Unsalted margarine (2 tsp)	Low-sodium mayonnaise (2 tsp)	Steamed broccoli (½ cup)
Jelly or jam (1 tbsp)	Sliced tomato (2 oz) and lettuce	Low-sodium bread (1 slice)
2% milk (1 cup)	Graham crackers (2)	Fruit sorbet (½ cup)
Coffee/tea	Fresh fruit salad (½ cup)	2% milk (½ cup)
	Fruit juice (1 cup)	Medium apple (1)
	Coffee/tea	Coffee/tea

Approximate Nutrient Analysis			
Energy (kcal)	2080.9	Phosphorus (mg)	1492.6
Protein (g)	96.3	Potassium (mg)	3431.9
(18.0% of kcal)		Sodium (mg)	555.5
Carbohydrate (g)	310.5	Zinc (mg)	11.8
(58.0% of kcal)		Vitamin A (μg RE)	858.3
Total fat (g)	59.7	Vitamin C (mg)	146.2
(25.4% of kcal)		Thiamin (mg)	1.6
Saturated fatty acids (g)	18.3	Riboflavin (mg)	2.2
Monounsaturated fatty acids (g)	23.8	Niacin (mg)	28.5
Polyunsaturated fatty acids (g)	15.1	Folate (μg)	338.2
Cholesterol (mg)	173.5	Vitamin B_6 (mg)	2.1
Calcium (mg)	809.0	Vitamin B_{12} (μg)	3.5
Iron (mg)	14.2	Dietary fiber (g)	26.3
Magnesium (mg)	400.7	Water-insoluble fiber (g)	19.2

A-30. DIETARY THERAPY OF HIGH BLOOD CHOLESTEROL

(From Detection, Evaluation and Treatment of High Blood Cholesterol in Adults. Second Report of the Expert Panel: Adult Treatment, National Cholesterol Education Program. NIH publ. no. 93-3095, September, 1993.)

A-30-a. Step I and Step II Diets—Nutrients and Rationale

The Step I Diet emphasizes the choice of fruits, vegetables, grains, cereals, and legumes, as well as poultry, fish, lean meats, and low-fat dairy products instead of foods high in saturated fat and cholesterol, such as whole milk dairy products and high-fat meats. For many patients this diet can be achieved with a moderate change in dietary habits. The Step II Diet further reduces saturated fat and cholesterol; neither of these is an essential nutrient, and they can be reduced to very low intakes without harm . . . Any therapeutic diet must be nutritionally adequate and meet Recommended Dietary Allowances . . .

[The original report reviews the roles of various nutrients and alcohol as they affect risk factors for hypercholesterolemia. The following tables reflect the text in terms of specific recommendations for foods. The Appendix editors]

Table A-30-b
Examples of Foods to Choose or Decrease for the Step I and Step II Diets[a]

Food Group	Choose	Decrease
Lean meat, poultry, and fish ≤5–6 oz per day	Beef, pork, lamb—lean cuts well trimmed before cooking	Beef, pork, lamb—regular ground beef, fatty cuts, spare ribs, organ meats
	Poultry without skin	Poultry with skin, fried chicken
	Fish, shellfish	Fried fish, fried shellfish
	Processed meat—prepared from lean meat, e.g., lean ham, lean frankfurters, lean meat with soy protein or carrageenan	Regular luncheon meat, e.g., bologna, salami, sausage, frankfurters
Eggs ≤4 yolks per week, Step I ≤2 yolks per week, Step II	Egg whites (two whites, can be substituted for one whole egg in recipes), cholesterol-free egg substitute	Egg yolks (if more than four per week on Step I or if more than two per week on Step II); includes eggs used in cooking and baking
Low-fat dairy products 2–3 servings per day	Milk—skim, ½%, or 1% fat (fliud, powdered, evaporated), buttermilk	Whole milk (fluid, evaporated, condensed), 2% fat milk (lowfat milk), imitation milk
	Yogurt—nonfat or low-fat yogurt or yogurt beverages	Whole milk yogurt, whole milk yogurt beverages
	Cheese—low-fat natural or processed cheese	Regular cheeses (American, blue, Brie, cheddar, Colby, Edam, Monterey Jack, whole-milk mozzarella, Parmesan, Swiss), cream cheese, Neufchatel cheese
	Low-fat or nonfat varieties, e.g., cottage cheese—low-fat, nonfat, or dry curd (0 to 2% fat)	Cottage cheese (4% fat)
	Frozen dairy dessert—ice milk, frozen yogurt (low fat or nonfat)	Ice cream
	Low-fat coffee creamer, low-fat or nonfat sour cream	Cream, half & half, whipping cream, nondairy creamer, whipped topping, sour cream
Fats and oils ≤6–8 teaspoons per day	Unsaturated oils—safflower, sunflower, corn, soybean, cottonseed, canola, olive, peanut	Coconut oil, palm kernel oil, palm oil
	Margarine—made from unsaturated oils listed above, light or diet margarine, especially soft or liquid forms	Butter, lard, shortening, bacon fat, hard margarine
	Salad dressings—made with unsaturated oils listed above, low-fat or fat free	Dressings made with egg yolk, cheese, sour cream, whole milk
	Seeds and nuts—peanut butter, other nut butters	Coconut
	Cocoa powder	Milk chocolate
Breads and cereals 6 or more servings per day	Breads—whole-grain bread, English muffins, bagels, buns, corn or flour tortilla	Bread in which eggs, fat, and/or butter are a major ingredient; croissants
	Cereals—oat, wheat, corn, multigrain	Most granolas
	Pasta	
	Rice	
	Dry beans and peas	
	Crackers, low-fat—animal-type, graham, soda crackers, breadsticks, melba toast	High-fat crackers
	Homemade baked goods using unsaturated oil, skim or 1% milk, and egg substitute—quick breads, biscuits, cornbread muffins, bran muffins, pancakes, waffles	Commercial baked pastries, muffins, biscuits
Soups	Reduced- or low-fat and reduced-sodium varieties, e.g., chicken or beef noodle, minestrone, tomato, vegetable, potato, reduced-fat soups made with skim milk	Soup containing whole milk, cream, meat fat, poultry fat, or poultry skin
Vegetables 3–5 servings per day	Fresh, frozen, or canned, without added fat or sauce	Vegetables fried or prepared with butter, cheese, or cream sauce

continued

Table A-30-b—*continued*

Examples of Foods to Choose or Decrease for the Step I and Step II Diets[a]

Food Group	Choose	Decrease
Fruits 2–4 servings per day	Fruit—fresh, frozen, canned, or dried Fruit juice—fresh, frozen, or canned	Fried fruit or fruit served with butter or cream sauce
Sweets and modified-fat desserts	Beverages—fruit-flavored drinks, lemonade, fruit punch Sweets—sugar, syrup, honey, jam, preserves, candy made without fat (candy corn, gumdrops, hard candy), fruit-flavored gelatin	Candy made with milk chocolate, coconut oil, palm kernel oil, palm oil
	Frozen desserts—low-fat and nonfat yogurt, ice milk, sherbet, sorbet, fruit ice, popsicles	Ice cream and frozen treats made with ice cream
	Cookies, cake, pie, pudding—prepared with egg whites, egg substitute, skim milk or 1% milk, and unsaturated oil or margarine; ginger snaps, fig and other fruit bar cookies, fat-free cookies; angel food cake	Commercial baked pies, cakes, doughnuts, high-fat cookies, cream pies

Examples of Daily Food Choices

Food Group	No of Servings	Serving Size	Some Suggested Foods
Vegetables	3–5	1 cup leafy/raw	Leafy greens, lettuce
		½ cup other	Corn, peas, green beans, broccoli, carrots, cabbage, celery, tomato, spinach, squash, bok choy, mushrooms, eggplant, collard and mustard greens
		¾ cup juice	Tomato juice, vegetable juice
Fruits	2–4	1 piece fruit ½ cup diced fruit	Orange, apple, applesauce, pear, banana, grapes, grapefruit, tangerine, plum, peach, strawberries and other berries, melons, kiwi, papaya, mango, lychee
		¾ cup fruit juice	Orange juice, apple juice, grapefruit juice, grape juice, prune juice
Breads, cereals, pasta, grains, dry beans, peas, potatoes, and rice	6–11	1 slice	Wheat, rye or enriched breads/rolls, corn and flour tortillas
		½ bun, bagel, muffin	English muffin, bagel, muffin, cornbread
		1 oz. dry cereal	Wheat, corn, oat, rice, bran cereal, or mixed grain cereal
		½ cup cooked cereal	Oatmeal, cream of wheat, grits
		½ cup dry beans or peas	Kidney beans, lentils, split peas, black-eyed peas
		½ cup potatoes	Potato, sweet potato
		½ cup rice, noodles, barley, or other grains	Pasta, rice, macaroni, barley, tabbouli
		½ cup bean curd	Tofu
Skim/low-fat dairy products	2–3	1 cup skim, 1% milk	Low/nonfat yogurt, skim milk, 1% milk, buttermilk
		1.0 oz low-fat, fat-free cheese	Low-fat cheeses
Lean meat, poultry, and fish		≤6 oz/day Step I Diet ≤5 oz/day Step II Diet	Lean and extra lean cuts of meat, fish, and skinless poultry, such as sirloin, round steak, skinless chicken, haddock, cod
Fats and oils	≤6–8	1 teaspoon soft margarine 1 Tablespoon salad dressing	Soft or liquid margarine, vegetable oils
		1 oz nuts	Walnuts, peanuts, almonds, pecans
Eggs		≤4 yolks/week—Step I ≤2 yolks/week—Step II	Used in preparation of baked products
Sweets and snack foods		In moderation	Cookies, fortune cookies, pudding, bread pudding, rice pudding, angel food cake, frozen yogurt, candy, punch, carbonated beverages Low-fat crackers and popcorn, pretzels, fat-free chips, rice cakes

[a]Careful selection of processed foods is necessary to stay within the sodium <2400 mg guideline.

[b]Includes fats and oils used in food preparation, also salad dressings and nuts.

Table A-30-c-1
Step I Sample Menus[a] Traditional American Cuisine Males 25 to 49 Years

Breakfast
Bagel, plain (1 medium)
Cream cheese, low-fat (2 tsp)
Cereal, shredded wheat (1½ cups)
Banana (1 small)
Milk, **1%** (1 cup)
Orange juice (¾ cup)
Coffee (1 cup)
Milk, **1%** (1 oz)
Lunch
Minestrone soup, canned, low sodium (1 cup)
Roast beef sandwich
Whole wheat bread (2 slices)
Lean roast beef, unseasoned **(3 oz)**[a]
American cheese, low-fat and low sodium (¾ oz)
Lettuce (1 leaf)
Tomato (3 slices)
Mayonnaise, low-fat and low sodium (2 tsp)
Fruit and cottage cheese salad
Cottage cheese, **2%** and low sodium (½ cup)
Peaches, canned in juice (½ cup)
Apple juice, unsweetened (1 cup)
Dinner
Salmon (3 oz)[b]
Vegetable oil (1 tsp)
Baked potato (1 medium)[b]
Margarine (2 tsp)
Green beans (½ cup), seasoned with margarine (½ tsp)[b]
Carrots (½ cup), seasoned with margarine (½ tsp)[b]
White dinner rolls (1 medium)
Margarine (1 tsp)
Ice milk (1 cup)
Iced tea, unsweetened (1 cup)
Snack
Popcorn (3 cups)[b]
Margarine (1 T)

Calories	2518	Total carb, % kcals	53
Total fat, % kcals	29	Simple carb, % carb	36
SFA, % kcals	8.6	Complex carb, % carb	64
Cholesterol, mg	181	Sodium[b], mg	1821
Protein, % kcals	18		

[a]100% RDA met for all nutrients except zinc 90%; boldface food items represent differences between the Step I and Step II Diets. See companion menu.

[b]No salt is added in recipe preparation or as seasoning. All margarine is low sodium.

Table A-30-c-2
Step I Sample Menus[a] Traditional American Cuisine Females 25 to 49 Years

Breakfast
Bagel, plain (½ medium)
Cream cheese, low-fat (1 tsp)
Cereal, shredded wheat (1 cup)
Banana (1 small)
Milk, **1%** (1 cup)
Orange juice **(¾ cup)**
Coffee (1 cup)
Milk, **1%** (1 oz)
Lunch
Minestrone soup, canned, low sodium (½ cup)
Roast beef sandwich
Whole wheat bread (2 slices)
Lean roast beef, unseasoned **(3 oz)**[b]
American cheese, low-fat and low sodium (¾ oz)
Lettuce (1 leaf)
Tomato (3 slices)
Mayonnaise, low-fat and low sodium (2 tsp)
Apple (1 medium)
Water (1 cup)
Dinner
Salmon (3 oz)[b]
Vegetable oil (1 tsp)
Baked potato (½ medium)[b]
Margarine (1 tsp)
Green beans (½ cup), seasoned with margarine (½ tsp)[b]
Carrots (½ cup), seasoned with margarine (½ tsp)[b]
White dinner roll (1 medium)
Margarine (1 tsp)
Ice milk (½ cup)
Iced tea, unsweetened (1 cup)
Snack
Popcorn (2 cups)[b]
Margarine (**1 tsp**)

Calories	1831	Total carb, % kcals	52
Total fat, % kcals	30	Simple carb, % carb	37
SFA, % kcals	8.7	Complex carb, % carb	63
Cholesterol, mg	156	Sodium[b], mg	1415
Protein, % kcals	18		

[a]100% RDA met for all nutrients except zinc 90%; boldface food items represent differences between the Step I and Step II Diets. See companion menu.

[b]No salt is added in recipe preparation or as seasoning. All margarine is low sodium.

Table A-30-d-1
Step II Sample Menus[a] Traditional American Cuisine Males 25 to 49 Years

Breakfast
Bagel, plain (1 medium)
Margarine (2 tsp)
Jelly (2 tsp)
Cereal, shredded wheat (1½ cups)
Banana (1 small)
Milk, **skim** (1 cup)
Orange juice (¾ cup)
Coffee (1 cup)
Milk, **skim** (1 oz)
Lunch
Minestrone soup, canned, low sodium (1½ cups)
Roast beef sandwich
Whole wheat bread (2 slices)
Lean roast beef, unseasoned **(2 oz)**[b]
American cheese, low-fat and low sodium (¾ oz)
Lettuce (1 leaf)
Tomato (3 slices)
Margarine (2 tsp)
Fruit and cottage cheese salad
Cottage cheese, **1%** and low sodium (½ cup)
Peaches, canned in juice (½ cup)
Apple juice, unsweetened (1 cup)
Dinner
Flounder (3 oz)[b]
Vegetable oil (1 tsp)
Baked potato (1 medium)[b]
Margarine (2 tsp)
Green beans (½ cup), seasoned with margarine (½ tsp)[b]
Carrots (½ cup), seasoned with margarine (½ tsp)[b]
White dinner roll (1 medium)
Margarine (1 tsp)
Frozen yogurt (1 cup)
Iced tea, unsweetened (1 cup)
Snack
Popcorn (3 cups)[b]
Margarine (1 T)

Calories	2533	Total carb, % kcals	55
Total fat, % kcals	28	Simple carb, % carb	36
SFA, % kcals	6.6	Complex carb, % carb	64
Cholesterol, mg	150	Sodium[b], mg	1803
Protein, % kcals	17		

[a]100% RDA met for all nutrients except zinc 90%; boldface food items represent differences between the Step I and Step II Diets. See companion menu.
[b]No salt is added in recipe preparation or as seasoning. All margarine is low sodium.

Table A-30-d-2
Step II Sample Menus[a] Traditional American Cuisine Females 25 to 49 Years

Breakfast
Bagel, plain (½ medium)
Margarine (1 tsp)
Jelly (1 tsp)
Cereal, shredded wheat (1 cup)
Banana (1 small)
Milk, **skim** (1 cup)
Orange juice (**1 cup**)
Coffee (1 cup)
Milk, **skim** (1 oz)
Lunch
Minestrone soup, canned, low sodium (½ cup)
Roast beef sandwich
Whole wheat bread (2 slices)
Lean roast beef, unseasoned **(2 oz)**[b]
American cheese, low-fat and low sodium (¾ oz)
Lettuce (1 leaf)
Tomato (3 slices)
Margarine (2 tsp)
Apple (1 medium)
Water (1 cup)
Dinner
Flounder (3 oz)[b]
Vegetable oil (1 tsp)
Baked potato (½ medium)[b]
Margarine (1 tsp)
Green beans (½ cup), seasoned with margarine (½ tsp)[b]
Carrots (½ cup), seasoned with margarine (½ tsp)[b]
White dinner roll (1 medium)
Margarine (1 tsp)
Frozen yogurt (½ cup)
Iced tea, unsweetened (1 cup)
Snack
Popcorn (3 cups)[b]
Margarine (**2 tsp**)

Calories	1867	Total carb, % kcals	55
Total fat, % kcals	29	Simple carb, % carb	38
SFA, % kcals	6.8	Complex carb, % carb	62
Cholesterol, mg	134	Sodium[b], mg	1417
Protein, % kcals	16		

[a]100% RDA met for all nutrients except zinc 90%; boldface food items represent differences between the Step I and Step II Diets. See companion menu.
[b]No salt is added in recipe preparation or as seasoning. All margarine is low sodium.

A-31. FAT-CONTROLLED DIET (25 OR 50G)

A-31-a. Purpose, Use, and Modifications

A fat-controlled diet is used to relieve symptoms of diarrhea, steatorrhea, flatulence, abdominal pain, and/or to control nutrient losses caused by the ingestion of excess dietary fat.

This diet may be used in the treatment of diseases of the hepatobiliary tract, pancreas, intestinal mucosa, and the lymphatic system as well as in malabsorption syndromes in which digestion, absorption, or utilization and transport of dietary fat is impaired. The latter include small bowel resection, intestinal lymphangiectasia, abetalipoproteinemia, chronic pancreatitis, Crohn's disease, malabsorption in the elderly, and patients with acquired immune deficiency syndrome (AIDS). The excretion of more than 6 g to 8 g of fat (or over 10% of fat consumed) per day over a 3-day period following a fecal fat assay indicates overall fat malabsorption. Further testing is needed to determine whether the steatorrhea is caused by small intestinal, pancreatic, or hepatobiliary disease. This diet is not designed for use in lowering serum lipid levels. Refer to the chapter on Nutrition Management of Hyperlipidemias in Adults in the original reference for further information.

A low-fat diet may also be useful in the treatment of patients with gastroesophageal reflux. A decreased fat intake will increase lower esophageal sphincter pressure, thus reducing symptoms of heartburn and dysphagia. Although steatorrhea is often a presenting symptom in celiac sprue (gluten-sensitive enteropathy), adherence to a strict gluten-free diet often brings about an end to steatorrhea, thus obviating the need for a low-fat diet. Refer to chapter on Gluten-Restricted, Gliadin-Free Diet for further information.

In individuals with cystic fibrosis, generally a low-fat diet is no longer recommended since the advent of enteric-coated pancreatic enzymes. Adequate doses of these supplements can normalize fat excretion in these individuals. Liberalizing fat intake may increase the likelihood that a nutritionally adequate diet will be consumed.

Many persons with malabsorption also may have difficulty tolerating excess dietary fiber and/or lactose. Refer to the chapters on Lactose-Controlled Diet, and Fiber- and Residue-Restricted Diet for further information.

In general, the 50-g-fat diet allows 6 oz of lean meat or meat substitutes and three to five fat equivalents per day. A 25-g-fat diet allows 4 oz of lean meat or meat substitutes per day and one fat equivalent per day (Table A-31-b). The food plan should be adjusted and individualized based on food preferences and a person's ability to monitor total fat intake. Individual tolerance should be monitored closely and the level of fat restriction adjusted if symptoms persist. Medium-chain triglycerides may be substituted for some fat in the diet. Additional carbohydrates in the form of starches and sugars also may be indicated for some patients to meet caloric requirements. Protein intake can be increased with the use of nonfat dairy products, as tolerated. Low-fat dietary supplements also may prove useful to increase nutrient intake. Pancreatic enzyme replacements may be prescribed by the physician. Mean fat excretion may be significantly decreased when enzymes are given prior to meals.

In patients with acquired immune deficiency syndrome (AIDS) who present with steatorrhea, dietary restriction of fat may be ordered. Since weight gain is often difficult to achieve, however, these individuals should also receive nutritional supplementation, with particular emphasis on protein.

(From The Manual of Clinical Dietetics. 5th ed. Chicago: the American Dietetic Association, 1996:431–439. With permission. *Note:* For references, see original diet, p. 439.)

Table A-31-b
Guidelines for Food Selection for Fat-Restricted Diet (25 or 50 g of fat)

Food Group	Foods Recommended	Foods to Avoid
Beverages To be taken as desired (fat/serving: trace)	Cocoa made with cocoa powder and skim milk; coffee; tea; soft drinks; fat-free powdered drinks; juices	Whole-milk beverages; added cream or chocolate
Breads and cereals 6–11 servings/day (fat/servings ≤1 g)	Whole-grain breads, enriched breads; saltines, soda crackers, other low-fat crackers; cooked cereals, whole-grain cereal except granola type; plain corn or flour tortillas; bagels	Biscuits; breads containing egg or cheese; sweet rolls; pancakes; French toast; doughnuts; waffles; fritters; muffins; granola-type cereals and breads to which extra fat is added; popovers; snack crackers with added fat; snack chips; stuffing; fried tortillas
Desserts In moderation (fat/serving: trace)	Skim-milk sherbet, fruit ice; gelatin; angel food cake; vanilla wafers; graham crackers; meringues; skim-milk pudding; fat-free commercial baked products; nonfat ice cream and frozen yogurt; fruit whips with gelatin	All other cakes, cookies, pies, and pastries; puddings made with whole milk or eggs; cream puffs and eclairs; ice cream

continued

Table A-31-b—*continued*
Guidelines for Food Selection for Fat-Restricted Diet (25 or 50 g of fat)

Food Group	Foods Recommended	Foods to Avoid
Fats Amount listed equals 1 fat equivalent; 3–5 equivalents/day allowed for 50 g fat; 1 equivalent/day allowed for 25 g fat; unsaturated fats are recommended (fat/serving: 5 g)	***Unsaturated Fats*** Margarine (1 tsp) Diet margarine (1 tbsp) Fat-free margarine[a] Mayonnaise Reduced-calorie (1 tbsp) Regular (1 tsp) Fat-free[a] Creamy salad dressings Reduced-calorie (1 tbsp) Regular (2 tsp) Fat-free[a] Vegetable oils (1 tsp) Nuts Cashews (1 tbsp) or 2 Whole almonds (6 whole) Peanuts (20 small or 10 large) Peanut butter (2 tsp) Cashew butter (2 tsp) Walnuts (2 whole) Pistachios (18 whole) Other nuts (1 tbsp) Seeds Sesame (1 tbsp) Sunflower (1 tbsp) Pumpkin (2 tsp) Avocado, med (1 oz) Olives (10)	Any in excess of recommended amounts
	Saturated Fats Bacon (1 slice) Bacon fat (1 tsp) Butter (1 tsp) Whipped butter (2 tsp) Chitterlings (½ oz) Shredded coconut (1 tbsp) Cream Light, coffee, table (2 tbsp) Heavy whipping (1 tbsp) Sour cream (2 tbsp) Cream cheese Light (2 tbsp) Regular (1 tbsp) Coffee whitener Liquid (2 tbsp) Powder (4 tsp) Lard (1 tsp) Shortening (1 tsp) Salt pork (¼ oz) Oils Coconut (1 tsp) Palm (1 tsp)	Any in excess of recommended amounts
Fruits 2–4 servings/day (fat/serving: trace)	Fresh, frozen, canned, or dried fruit; fruit juices	Avocado in excess of amount allowed on fat list
Lean meat and meat substitutes For 50-g-fat diet, 6 oz/day For 25-g-fat diet, 4 oz/day (fat serving: 3 g) Recommended preparation methods are broiling, roasting, grilling, or boiling; weigh meat after cooking *Note:* All visible fat and poultry skin should be trimmed prior to eating; amount stated denotes cooked portion		

continued

Table A-31-b—*continued*
Guidelines for Food Selection for Fat-Restricted Diet (25 or 50 g of fat)

Food Group	Foods Recommended	Foods to Avoid
Fish	All fresh, frozen, or canned in water: crab, lobster, scallops, shrimp, clams, oysters, tuna; herring (uncreamed or smoked); sardines (canned, drained); salmon (canned in water)	Tuna (packed in oil), salmon (packed in oil)
Poultry	Chicken, turkey, Cornish hen	Duck, goose
Veal	All cuts are lean except those listed under foods to avoid	Cutlets (ground or cubed)
Lean beef	USDA select or choice grades such as round, sirloin, and flank steak; tenderloin; chopped beef	Most USDA prime cuts, such as ribs, corned beef, ground beef, roasts (rib, chuck, rump); most steaks including cubed, T-bone, and Porterhouse; meatloaf
Lean pork	Fresh, canned, cured, or boiled ham; Canadian bacon; tenderloin	Spareribs; ground pork; pork sausage (patty or link); chops; loin roast; Boston butt; cutlets; ham hocks; pigs' feet; chitterlings
Lean lamb	Arm, foreshank, leg, loin, and shank cuts	Patties (ground lamb), blade, rib, and shoulder cuts
Luncheon meats	95% fat-free; lean ham, turkey, or beef	Luncheon meats such as bologna, salami, pimento loaf
Legumes	Cooked or canned without added fat	Legumes cooked with added fat
Soy products	Natto (3½ oz = 11 g fat); tempeh (3½ oz = 8 g fat); tofu (3½ oz = 9 g fat)	
Cheese	Any cottage cheese; low-fat cheeses made with skim milk and containing 3 g of fat or less per oz; parmesan cheese, grated (2 tbsp = 1 oz), ricotta cheese, part skim	All regular cheeses including American, blue, brie, cheddar, colby, Monterey jack, and Swiss
Milk 2 or more servings/day (fat/serving: trace)	Skim milk, skim buttermilk, powdered and evaporated skim milk; nonfat yogurt	1%, 2%, whole milks, buttermilk made with whole milk; chocolate milk; cream; regular evaporated milk; whole milk yogurt
Eggs In moderation (fat/serving: trace)	Egg whites and fat-free egg substitutes	Egg yolks
Potatoes and potato substitutes As desired (fat/serving: trace)	Potatoes; rice; barley; noodles without yolks; spaghetti, macaroni, and other pastas	Fried potatoes; fried rice; potato chips; chow mein noodles; items prepared with added fat, such as au gratin potatoes, unless fat is deduced from fat allowance
Soups As desired (fat/serving: trace)	Fat-free broth; fat-free vegetable soup; cream soup made with skim milk and allowed fat; packaged dehydrated soups	All others
Sweets In moderation (fat/serving: trace)	Sugar; honey; jelly, jam; marmalade; molasses; maple syrup; sour balls; gum drops; jelly beans; marshmallows; hard candy; cocoa powder	Candies made with butter, coconut, chocolate, or cream
Vegetables 3–5 servings/day (fat/serving: trace)	All fresh, frozen, or canned vegetables prepared without fats or sauces containing fat	Buttered, au gratin, creamed, or fried vegetables unless made with allowed fat
Miscellaneous In moderation (fat/serving: trace)	Ketchup; chili sauce; vinegar; pickles; vanilla; unbuttered popcorn; white sauce made with skim milk, and allowed fat; mustard; all herbs and seasonings; apple butter	Olives and nuts in excess of specified portions; cream sauces; gravies; buttered popcorn

[a]Some "fat-free" items contain trace amounts of fat and should not be eaten indiscriminately. Check food labels and/or consult food manufacturer for individual items.

Adequacy

The diet is adequate in all nutrients based on the 1989 Recommended Dietary Allowances. Prolonged diarrhea or steatorrhea may lead to nutrient deficiencies including calcium, iron, magnesium, potassium, zinc, fat-soluble vitamins (A, D, E, and K), folic acid, and vitamin B_{12}. While other water-soluble vitamin deficiency states are rarely associated with malabsorption, the vitamin B complex is also sometimes supplemented.

Vitamin and mineral deficiencies can be treated with supplements and control of causative factors. Medium-chain triglycerides can be incorporated to provide additional calories.

Table A-31-c-1
Sample Menu for Fat-Restricted Diet (25 g of fat)

Breakfast	Lunch	Dinner	Snack
Orange juice (1 cup) Whole-grain cereal (¾ cup) Banana (1 medium) Whole-wheat toast (1 slice) Diet margarine (½ tsp) Jelly or jam (2 tbsp) Skim milk (1 cup) Coffee or tea	Fat-free vegetable soup (1 cup) Saltine crackers (4) Sliced turkey breast (2 oz) Whole-wheat bread (2 slices) Mustard (½ tbsp) Fat-free mayonnaise (1 tbsp) Sliced tomato (½ medium) and lettuce Fresh fruit salad (½ cup) Graham crackers (4) Skim milk (1 cup) Coffee/tea	Tossed green salad (3½ oz) Fat-free salad dressing (1 tbsp) Broiled boneless skinless chicken breast (3 oz) Herbed brown rice (½ cup) Steamed broccoli (½ cup) Whole-grain roll (1) Diet margarine (½ tsp) Jelly or jam (1 tbsp) Fruit ice (½ cup) Medium apple (1) Coffee/tea	Canned peaches (1 cup) Nonfat plain yogurt (½ cup)

Approximate Nutrient Analysis

Nutrient	Amount	Nutrient	Amount
Energy (kcal)	2173.7	Phosphorus (mg)	1888.4
Protein (g)	100.2	Potassium (mg)	5256.9
(18.4% of kcal)		Sodium (mg)	3100.4
Carbohydrate (g)	414.2	Zinc (mg)	13.9
(76.2% of kcal)		Vitamin A (μg RE)	2863.7
Total fat (g)	24.1	Vitamin C (mg)	223.5
(10.0% of kcal)		Thiamin (mg)	2.3
Saturated fatty acids (g)	6.6	Riboflavin (mg)	2.8
Monounsaturated fatty acids (g)	8.0	Niacin (mg)	33.2
Polyunsaturated fatty acids (g)	5.8	Folate (μg)	670.1
Cholesterol (mg)	111.1	Vitamin B_6 (mg)	3.7
Calcium (mg)	1237.5	Vitamin B_{12} (μg)	6.0
Iron (mg)	16.2	Dietary fiber (g)	43.7
Magnesium (mg)	560.1	Water-insoluble fiber (g)	31.2

Table A-31-c-2
Sample Menu for Fat-Restricted Diet (50 g of fat)

Breakfast	Lunch	Dinner	Snack
Orange juice (½ cup) Whole-grain cereal (¾ cup) Banana (½ medium) Whole-wheat toast (2 slices) Margarine (1 tsp) Jelly or jam (1 tbsp) Skim milk (1 cup) Coffee or tea	Vegetable soup (1 cup) Saltine crackers (4) Lean roast beef (3 oz) Whole-wheat bread (2 slices) Mustard (1 tbsp) Reduced-calorie mayonnaise (1 tbsp) Sliced tomato (½ medium) and lettuce Fresh fruit salad (½ cup) Graham crackers (4) Skim milk (1 cup) Coffee/tea	Tossed green salad (3½ oz) Fat-free salad dressing (1 tbsp) Broiled boneless skinless chicken breast (3 oz) Herbed brown rice (½ cup) Steamed broccoli (½ cup) Whole-grain roll (1) Margarine (1 tsp) Fruit ice (½ cup) Medium apple (1) Coffee/tea	Canned peaches (½ cup) Nonfat plain yogurt (½ cup)

Approximate Nutrient Analysis

Nutrient	Amount	Nutrient	Amount
Energy (kcal)	2139.7	Phosphorus (mg)	1959.9
Protein (g)	108.9	Potassium (mg)	4458.1
(20.4% of kcal)		Sodium (mg)	2589.7
Carbohydrate (g)	337.5	Zinc (mg)	18.1
(63.1% of kcal)		Vitamin A (μg RE)	1182.5
Total fat (g)	47.0	Vitamin C (mg)	155.3
(19.8% of kcal)		Thiamin (mg)	2.2
Saturated fatty acids (g)	12.5	Riboflavin (mg)	2.7
Monounsaturated fatty acids (g)	18.8	Niacin (mg)	33.0
Polyunsaturated fatty acids (g)	10.1	Folate (μg)	523.9
Cholesterol (mg)	150.8	Vitamin B_6 (mg)	3.1
Calcium (mg)	1204.6	Vitamin B_{12} (μg)	8.1
Iron (mg)	17.3	Dietary fiber (g)	35.1
Magnesium (mg)	519.6	Water-insoluble fiber (g)	26.5

A-32. FIBER MODIFIED DIETS

A-32-a. Fiber- and Residue-Restricted Diet

(From The Manual of Clinical Dietetics, 5th ed. Chicago: the American Dietetic Association, 1996:397–401, with permission. *Note:* For references, see original diet, pp. 400–1.)

Purpose and Modifications

The fiber- and residue-restricted diet is designed to prevent blockage of a stenosed gastrointestinal tract and to reduce the frequency and volume of fecal output while prolonging intestinal transit time.

In planning a fiber-restricted diet, indigestible carbohydrate intake is reduced by using limited amounts of well-cooked or canned vegetables and canned, cooked, or very ripe fruits, and by replacing whole-grain breads and cereals with refined products. Legumes, seeds, and nuts are omitted.

A low-fiber diet is not synonymous with a low-residue diet. Fiber is the portion of carbohydrates not capable of being digested by enzymes in the human digestive tract, thus contributing to increased fecal output. Residue is the unabsorbed dietary elements and total postdigestive luminal contents present following digestion. Residue-containing foods tend to increase the fecal residue and stool weight despite their low-fiber contents. However, since low-residue diets are based on old literature, tradition, and studies on laboratory animals, tolerance to residue-containing foods should be assessed on an individual basis. Limited data are available on the actual residue content of foods and the efficacy of the low-residue diet.

The fiber content of some common foods can be found in Table A-20-a. Adherence to the guidelines in Table A-32-a-2 generally results in a diet that contains less than 20 g of fiber per day.

Adequacy

Depending on individual food choices, the diet is adequate in all nutrients based on the 1989 Recommended Dietary Allowances (RDA). However, the diet does not meet the RDA for iron in pregnant, lactating, and premenopausal women. Vitamin and mineral supplementation may be indicated for these individuals or for those with suboptimal intakes and increased requirements resulting from illness. The potential risks and benefits of long-term restriction of dietary fiber should be addressed before using the diet for any extended period. Strict reductions in vegetables and fruits may necessitate supplementation of ascorbic acid, folate, and others depending on actual intake. In persons with lactase deficiency who do not tolerate milk, calcium also may need to be supplemented. Individual response, particularly in the patient with ulcerative colitis and Crohn's disease, must be monitored to avoid an overly restrictive regimen and to determine continued indications for using the diet.

Table A-32-a-2 and 3 provide guides to meal planning and to a sample menu for restricted diets.

Table A-32-a-1
Fiber Components and Food Sources

Fiber Type	Components	Food Sources
Soluble fibers		
Hydrated, resulting in gellike viscous substance, and fermented by colonic bacteria	Gums, mucilages, pectin, some hemicelluloses, β-glucan	Fruits, vegetables, barley, legumes, oats and oat bran
Insoluble fibers		
Remain essentially unchanged during digestion	Cellulose, lignin, some hemicelluloses	Fruits, vegetables, cereals, whole-wheat products, wheat bran

Table A-32-a-2
Guidelines for Food Selection for Fiber- and Residue-Restricted Diet

Food Category	Recommended	May Cause Distress
Beverages	Coffee, tea, carbonated beverages, strained fruit drinks; milk as tolerated[a]	Any containing fruit or vegetable pulp; prune juice[b]
Breads	Refined breads, rolls, biscuits, muffins, crackers; pancakes or waffles; plain pastries	Any made with whole-grain flour, bran, seeds, nuts, coconut, or raw or dried fruits; cornbread, graham crackers
Cereals	Refined cooked cereals including grits and farina; refined cereals including puffed rice and puffed wheat	Oatmeal; any whole-grain, bran, or granola cereal; any containing seeds, nuts, coconut, or dried fruit
Desserts and sweets	Plain cakes and cookies; pie made with allowed fruits; plain sherbet, fruit ice, frozen pops, yogurt, gelatin, and custard; jelly; plain hard candy; marshmallows; ice cream as tolerated[a]	Any made with whole-grain flour, bran, seeds, nuts, coconut, or dried fruit
Fats	Margarine, butter, salad oils and dressings, mayonnaise; bacon; plain gravies	Any containing whole-grain flour, bran, seeds, nuts, coconut, or dried fruit
Fruits	Most canned or cooked fruits[b]; applesauce[b]; fruit cocktail[b]; ripe banana[b]	Dried fruit; all berries; most raw fruit
Meats and meat substitutes	Ground or well-cooked, tender beef, lamb, ham, veal, pork, poultry, fish, organ meats; eggs and cheese	Tough, fibrous meats with gristle[b]; any made with whole-grain ingredients, seeds, or nuts; dried beans, peas, lentils, legumes; peanut butter
Potato and potato substitutes	Cooked white and sweet potatoes without skin; white rice; refined pasta	All others
Soups	Bouillon, broth, or cream soups made with allowed vegetables, noodles, rice, or flour	All others
Vegetables	Most well-cooked and canned vegetables without seeds[b] except those excluded; lettuce if tolerated; strained vegetable juice	Sauerkraut, winter squash, peas, and corn; most raw vegetables and vegetables with seeds
Miscellaneous	Salt, pepper, sugar, spices, herbs, vinegar, ketchup, mustard	Nuts, coconut, seeds, and popcorn

[a]Mixed consensus exists regarding the inclusion of milk on a low-residue diet. It has been suggested that because milk is not considered a high-residue food, it should not be eliminated from the low-residue diet unless an individual has lactase deficiency. Some practitioners continue to limit milk and products containing milk to 2 cups per day, as suggested in previous literature.

[b]These foods are not necessarily high in fiber but may increase colonic residue; assess patient food tolerance and limit as needed. Residue may be further reduced by excluding all fruits and vegetables with the exception of strained juices and white potatoes without skin.

Table A-32-a-3
Sample Menu for Fiber- and Residue-Restricted Diet

Breakfast	Lunch	Dinner
Cranberry juice (½ cup)	Vegetable broth (1 cup)	Strained tomato juice (½ cup)
Puffed rice cereal (¾ cup)	Saltine crackers (4)	Broiled skinless chicken breast (3 oz)
Canned peaches (½ cup)	Lean beef patty (3 oz)	White rice (½ cup)
White-bread toast (2 slices)	Hamburger bun without seeds (1)	Cooked spinach (½ cup)
Margarine (2 tsp)	Mustard (1 tbsp)	White roll (1)
Jelly (1 tbsp)	Ketchup (1 tbsp)	Margarine (2 tsp)
2% milk (1 cup)	Canned fruit cocktail (½ cup)	Low-fat frozen yogurt (½ cup)
Coffee or tea	Vanilla wafer cookies (2)	Applesauce (½ cup)
	2% milk (1 cup)	Coffee/tea
	Coffee/tea	

Approximate Nutrient Analysis

Energy (kcal)	1929.7	Phosphorus (mg)	1349.5
Protein (g)	96.7	Potassium (mg)	3454.7
(20.1% of kcal)		Sodium (mg)	2725.7
Carbohydrate (g)	274.4	Zinc (mg)	14.1
(56.9% of kcal)		Vitamin A (μg RE)	2013.8
Total fat (g)	51.9	Vitamin C (mg)	72.1
(24.2% of kcal)		Thiamin (mg)	1.8
Saturated fatty acids (g)	17.7	Riboflavin (mg)	2.5
Monounsaturated fatty acids (g)	18.9	Niacin (mg)	28.8
Polyunsaturated fatty acids (g)	10.4	Folate (μg)	324.5
Cholesterol (mg)	171.6	Vitamin B_6 (mg)	2.3
Calcium (mg)	1191.8	Vitamin B_{12} (μg)	4.3
Iron (mg)	15.2	Dietary fiber (g)	16.2
Magnesium (mg)	318.4	Water-insoluble fiber (g)	10.6

A-32-b. High-Fiber Diet

(From The Manual of Clinical Dietetics, 5th ed. Chicago: the American Dietetic Association, 1996:403–9, with permission. *Note:* For references, see original diet, pp. 408–9.)

Purpose and Modifications

A high-fiber diet is designed to exert a variety of physiologic and metabolic effects depending on the physical properties, chemical composition, and form in which the fiber is consumed. Both soluble and insoluble fibers exert physiologic effects, whereas only soluble fibers exert metabolic effects.

The high-fiber diet is a general diet with an emphasis on fiber-rich food sources including fruits, legumes, vegetables, whole-grain breads, and cereals. To date there is no Recommended Dietary Allowances for fiber. Actual intake data indicate that the average fiber intake for all persons is approximately 7 g per 1000 kcal, which translates into approximately 10 g for children, 12 g for women, and 18 g for men.

The American Dietetic Association recommends a daily dietary fiber intake of 20 g to 35 g from a variety of sources, combined with a low-fat, high-carbohydrate diet. Increased fiber intake should come from a variety of food sources, rather than from dietary fiber supplements, to ensure adequate intake of vitamins, minerals, and other nutrients. Consumption of adequate amounts of liquid (at least eight 8-oz glasses per day) in conjunction with high-fiber intake is recommended.

Fiber intake should be increased gradually to minimize potentially adverse side effects such as abdominal distress, bloating, flatulence, cramps, and diarrhea. These effects are usually temporary and subside within several days; however, if they persist, the fiber content of the diet should be reduced and a physician consulted. High-fiber diets may be inappropriate for persons with autonomic neuropathy. Table A-32-b-1 offers a guide to meal planning for a high-fiber diet. When combined with a general diet, this plan provides approximately 25 g to 30 g of dietary fiber depending on actual foods chosen. The diet can also be planned using the food composition table of fiber contents found in A-20-a.

Adequacy

Depending on individual food selection, the high-fiber diet is adequate in all nutrients (Table 32-b-2). Some studies suggest that excessive (>30 g per day) intakes of some dietary fiber sources may bind and interfere with the absorption of calcium, copper, iron, magnesium, selenium, and zinc. However, it is hypothesized that long-term adaptation to high-fiber intakes may occur; therefore, consumption of a varied high-fiber diet may not cause mineral or nutrient imbalances in the general population. Limiting total dietary fiber intake to 35 g per day so that mineral absorption is not inhibited appears to be an adequate safeguard while obtaining the benefits of a high-fiber diet. Intake of adequate fluid is necessary due to the hygroscopic nature of fiber.

Table A-32-b-1
Guide to Meal Planning for a High-Fiber Diet

Food and Serving Size	Approximate Amount of Dietary Fiber (g)	Recommended Daily Servings
Breads and Starches	2	6 (plus ≤5 additional servings of refined breads and starches)
Whole-grain or rye bread (1 slice)		
Whole-grain bagel or pita bread (½)		
Oat bran muffin (½)		
Whole-wheat crackers, crisp breads (4)		
Whole-wheat pasta, corn, or peas (½ cup)		
Popcorn, air-popped (3 cups)		
Wheat germ (1½ tbsp)		
Cereals	4–8	
Whole-grain or bran cereals, cold (1 oz)		
Oatmeal, oat bran, or grits (½ cup dry)		
Vegetables	2	3 (plus ≤2 additional servings of other vegetables or juices)
Cooked—asparagus, green beans, broccoli, cabbage, carrots, cauliflower, greens, onions, snow peas, spinach, squash, canned tomatoes (½ cup); potato with skin (1 small)		
Raw—broccoli, cabbage, carrots, cauliflower, tomatoes, celery, green peppers, zucchini (1 cup)		
Fruits	2	2 (plus ≤2 or additional servings of other fruits or juices)
Apple, nectarine, orange, peach, banana (1 medium)		
Grapefruit, pear (½)		
Berries (1 cup)		
Beans	5	Optional
Garbanzo beans, kidney beans, lentils, lima beans, split peas, pinto beans, other beans and peas (½ cup cooked)		
Nuts and Seeds	2	Optional
Almonds (10 whole), walnuts (6 whole), peanut butter (1 tbsp), peanuts (15), sesame seeds (1 tbsp), sunflower seeds (2 tbsp)		

Table A-32-b-2
Sample Menu for a High-Fiber Diet

Breakfast	Lunch	Dinner
Orange juice (½ cup)	Split pea soup (1 cup)	Green salad (3½ oz)
Oatmeal (1 cup)	Whole-wheat crackers (4)	Vinegar and oil dressing (1 tbsp)
Raisins (2 tbsp)	Lean beef patty (3 oz)	Broiled boneless skinless chicken breast (3 oz)
Whole-wheat toast (2 slices)	Hamburger bun (1)	Herbed brown rice (½ cup)
Margarine (2 tsp)	Mustard (1 tbsp)	Steamed broccoli (½ cup)
Jelly or jam (1 tbsp)	Ketchup (1 tbsp)	Whole-grain roll (1)
2% milk (1 cup)	Sliced tomato (2 oz) and lettuce	Margarine (2 tsp)
Coffee or tea	Fresh fruit salad (½ cup)	Low-fat frozen yogurt (½ cup)
	Bran muffin (1)	Medium pear (1)
	2% milk (1 cup)	Coffee/tea
	Coffee/tea	

Approximate Nutrient Analysis

Energy (kcal)	2238.6	Phosphorus (mg)	1816.0
Protein (g)	109.9	Potassium (mg)	3760.3
(19.6% of kcal)		Sodium (mg)	2375.9
Carbohydrate (g)	294.0	Zinc (mg)	15.2
(52.5% of kcal)		Vitamin A (μg RE)	828.4
Total fat (g)	74.9	Vitamin C (mg)	139.4
(30.1% of kcal)		Thiamin (mg)	1.9
Saturated fatty acids (g)	23.8	Riboflavin (mg)	2.1
Monounsaturated fatty acids (g)	28.3	Niacin (mg)	25.3
Polyunsaturated fatty acids (g)	15.4	Folate (μg)	345.5
Cholesterol (mg)	201.4	Vitamin B_6 (mg)	1.9
Calcium (mg)	1109.1	Vitamin B_{12} (μg)	4.3
Iron (mg)	15.5	Dietary fiber (g)	28.8
Magnesium (mg)	475.3	Water-insoluble fiber (g)	19.9

A-33. SOFT DIET

(From The Manual of Clinical Dietetics, 5th ed. Chicago: the American Dietetic Association, 1996:141–3, with permission. *Note:* For references, see original diet, p. 143.)

A-33-a. Purpose and Related Physiology

The soft diet is designed for patients who are unable to tolerate a general diet. It has traditionally been used to prevent nausea, vomiting, gas, and distension in the postsurgical patient. However, the rationale for this premise is poorly documented, since symptoms of nausea, vomiting, gas, and distension are more likely to be caused by anesthesia and gut immobility than by diet. If gas or distension is a problem, smaller, frequent meals may provide some relief. If nausea or vomiting interferes with food intake, it may be helpful to provide dry foods in small quantities and to progress to frequent, small feedings of simple palatable foods. Hot beverages (tea, clear broths) and cold beverages (iced tea, carbonated liquids, especially ginger ale) are usually well tolerated.

Adequacy

Based on individual food choices, the diet is adequate in all nutrients according to the 1989 Recommended Dietary allowances. Table A-33-a-1 lists recommended foods, and Table A-33-a-2 presents a sample meal plan.

Table A-33-a-1
Soft-Diet Foods

Food Group	Recommended	May Cause Distress
Beverages	Milk and milk products; all other beverages	Alcoholic beverages
Breads and cereals	White, refined-wheat, or light-rye enriched breads, soft rolls, and crackers; cooked or ready-to-eat cereals	Coarse cereals (e.g., bran); whole-grain breads or crackers with seeds; bread or bread products with nuts or dried fruits
Desserts	Cakes, cookies, pies, pudding, custard, ice cream, sherbet, and gelatin made with allowed foods; fruit ice and frozen pops	All sweets and desserts containing nuts, coconut, or dried fruits not allowed; fried pastries (e.g., doughnuts)
Fats	Butter or fortified margarine; salad dressings; all fats and oils	Highly seasoned salad dressings
Fruits	All fruit juices; cooked or canned fruit; avocado, banana, melon, grapefruit and orange sections without membrane; other ripe, soft fruits without seeds	Other fresh and dried fruits
Meats and meat substitutes	All lean, tender meats, poultry, fish, and shellfish; eggs; mild-flavored cheeses; creamy peanut butter; soybean and other meat substitutes; plain or flavored yogurt	Strong-smelling or highly seasoned meats, cheeses, or fish (e.g., luncheon meats; frankfurters, sausage); yogurt with nuts or dried fruits
Potatoes and potato substitutes	Potatoes; enriched rice, barley, spaghetti, macaroni, and other pasta	Potato chips, fried potatoes
Vegetables	All vegetable juices; cooked vegetables and lettuce as tolerated; salads made from allowed foods	Raw and fried vegetables; whole kernel corn; gas-producing vegetables (e.g., broccoli, brussels sprouts, cabbage, onions, leeks, cauliflower, cucumber, green pepper, rutabagas, turnips, sauerkraut, dried peas, dried beans)
Soups	Soups made with allowed foods	Highly seasoned soups and soups made with gas-producing vegetables
Sweets	Sugar, syrup; honey; jelly, and seedless jam; hard candies; plain chocolate candies; molasses; marshmallows	Any with nuts or coconut
Miscellaneous	Iodized salt; flavorings; mildly flavored gravies and sauces; pepper, herbs, spices, ketchup, mustard, vinegar in moderation	Strongly flavored seasonings and condiments (e.g., garlic, chili sauce, chili pepper, horseradish); pickles; popcorn; nuts and coconut

Table A-33-a-2
Sample Menu for Soft Diet

Breakfast	Lunch	Dinner
Orange juice (½ cup)	Vegetable soup (1 cup)	Tomato juice (6 oz)
Cornflake cereal (¾ cup)	Saltine crackers (4)	Broiled, skinless chicken breast (3 oz)
Banana slices (½ cup)	Lean beef patty (3 oz)	Enriched rice (½ cup)
White toast (2 slices)	Hamburger bun (1)	Steamed green beans (½ cup)
Margarine (2 tsp)	Mustard (1 tbsp)	Soft dinner roll (1)
Jelly (1 tbsp)	Mayonnaise (1 tbsp)	Margarine (2 tsp)
2% milk (1 cup)	Lettuce leaf	Low-fat frozen yogurt (½ cup)
Coffee or tea	Canned fruit cocktail (½ cup)	Applesauce (½ cup)
	Graham crackers (4)	Coffee/tea
	2% milk (1 cup)	
	Coffee/tea	

Approximate Nutrient Analysis

Energy (kcal)	2156.9	Phosphorus (mg)	1341.9
Protein (g)	96.7	Potassium (mg)	3454.3
(18.0% of kcal)		Sodium (mg)	4024.1
Carbohydrate (g)	284.3	Zinc (mg)	12.4
(52.7% of kcal)		Vitamin A (μg RE)	915.8
Total fat (g)	73.0	Vitamin C (mg)	115.6
(30.4% of kcal)		Thiamin (mg)	1.9
Saturated fatty acids (g)	23.4	Riboflavin (mg)	2.5
Monounsaturated fatty acids (g)	28.5	Niacin (mg)	29.6
Polyunsaturated fatty acids (g)	14.3	Folate (μg)	324.0
Cholesterol (mg)	189.4	Vitamin B_6 (mg)	2.5
Calcium (mg)	1067.9	Vitamin B_{12} (μg)	4.4
Iron (mg)	15.6	Dietary fiber (g)	15.1
Magnesium (mg)	304.3	Water-insoluble fiber (g)	9.1

A-34. NUTRITIONAL MANAGEMENT OF DYSPHAGIA

A-34-a. Purpose, Use, and Modifications

The goal of the dysphagia diet is to provide adequate calories, protein, vitamins, minerals, and fluids in a consistency best tolerated by the patient. Dysphagia connotes a disturbance in the normal transfer of food from the oral cavity to the stomach and refers to difficulty in swallowing liquids, solids, or both. The nutritional implications of dysphagia result from inadequate dietary intake. They can include weight loss, dehydration, and vitamin and mineral deficiencies. Untreated, these problems can result in protein-energy malnutrition, which can be a significant complication in otherwise healthy people and especially devastating for debilitated patients.

Dysphagia refers to a swallowing impairment that results from an anatomic or physiologic abnormality. Neurologic illnesses, surgical procedures involving mechanical and anatomic alterations, anticancer therapy, and aging may lead to dysphagia and risk of aspiration. Psychologic factors may exacerbate, but rarely cause, dysphagia.

Diagnosis or conditions of patients who may have swallowing problems include

Alzheimer's disease/ dementia	Myotonic dystonia
Amyotrophic lateral sclerosis (ALS)	Parkinson's disease
Cerebral palsy	Poliomyelitis
Closed head injury	Sjögren's disease
Dermatomyositis	Stroke/cerebrovascular accident
Dysautonomia	Torticollis
Head or neck cancer	Guillain-Barré syndrome
Huntington's chorea	Inflammation of the pharynx or esophagus
Multiple sclerosis	Throat webs
Muscular dystrophy	History of aspiration or pneumonia
Myasthenia gravis	History of nonspecific respiratory problems

Warning signs of swallowing problems include

Pocketing of food under tongue, in cheeks, or on the hard palate

Spitting food out of the mouth, tongue thrusting

Poor tongue control

Facial weakness

Excessive tongue movement

Slow oral transit time

Delay or absence of elevation of the larynx (Adam's apple/ thyroid cartilage)

Coughing before, during, or after swallowing

Choking

Excessive secretions, drooling

"Gurgly" (wet) voice after eating or drinking

Hoarse, harsh, or breathy voice

Slurred speech

Regurgitation of material through nose, mouth, or tracheostomy tube

Inadequate intake of food or fluid; weight loss

Excessive eating time

Mealtime resistance—clenching teeth, pushing food away, or clenching throat

Recurrent pneumonia (due to aspiration)

No two patients with dysphagia are alike; thus, diets must be individualized on the basis of swallowing ability and patient preference. A dysphagia menu plan should

- Provide foods and beverages that reduce the risk of choking and aspiration
- Be modified when the impairment level changes, as assessed by the speech-language pathologist or designated clinician
- Provide foods that stimulate the swallowing reflex
- Promote positive nutritional balance to achieve or maintain a desirable weight and optimal nutritional status
- Facilitate independent eating and swallowing, if appropriate
- Provide a variety of foods that are visually appealing and nutrient dense
- Provide moist foods or thickened beverages as needed for adequate hydration

(From The Manual of Clinical Dietetics, 5th ed. Chicago: the American Dietetic Association, 1996:145-163, with permission. *Note:* For references, see original diet on p. 163.)

Table A-34-a-1
Review of Dysphagic Problems and Dietary Management Strategies

Problem/Condition	Effect	Dietary Considerations
Oral preparation phase		
Reduced buccal (cheek) and/or lip tension	Food falls into the lateral sulcus during chewing and is difficult to retrieve; food or liquid leaks from the mouth	Maintain semisolid consistencies that form a cohesive bolus; use lighter-density foods; avoid thin liquids
Reduced oral sensation	Food lodges or becomes pocketed in areas of reduced sensitivity; particles may fall over base of tongue, causing aspiration before the swallow	Position food in the most sensitivie area; avoid foods with more than one texture; use foods at colder temperatures and highly seasoned, flavorful foods; try dense foods to provide stimulation
Reduced tongue movement; partial glossectomy	Limited ability to form a food bolus and propel it to the back of the throat results in separation of food particles and increased risk for food to fall into the pharynx before initiation of the swallow	Maintain semisolid consistencies that form a cohesive bolus; use moist, well-lubricated foods
Mucositis	Severe mouth soreness associated with chewing and swallowing; difficulty manipulating food in the mouth	Use soft, bland foods; avoid acidic foods, temperature extremes, and rough, raw, salty, and spicy foods
Dry mouth/xerostomia; associated with cancer treatment and Sjögren's disease	Difficulty lubricating and manipulating food; thick saliva; gagging	Use moist, well-lubricated foods; add gravies, margarine, and sauces; use artificial salivas, sugarless lemon drops, papain, or citrus juices to thin secretions; avoid dry, crumbly foods; ensure adequate fluid intake Some patients may benefit from avoidance of, or dilution of, fresh dairy products if secretions become thick or unmanageable with milk products
Total glossectomy; floor of mouth resection; palate resection	Effects vary depending on extent of resection; may result in varying levels of difficulty in forming and propelling the food bolus	Modifications are individualized and require close supervision to assess ability to manipulate foods and swallow safely
Oral transit phase		
Delayed or absent swallow reflex; associated with progressive neuromuscular disease	Aspiration before the swallow is initiated due to pooling and overflow of food and liquid into the airway	Use cohesive foods; density depends on the level of oral sensation; temperature extremes and highly seasoned foods may help to excite nerves; use thickened liquids
Incomplete sealing of the nasal airway during passage of food and beverage	Material enters the nasal cavity and increases risk of nasal regurgitation	Use cohesive, semisolid foods and thickened liquids; avoid dry, crumbly foods
Reduced coordination during preparation for swallowing	Foods fall behind the base of the tongue into the valleculae	Use highly textured foods (e.g., diced, cooked vegetables and diced fruit); try dense, cohesive foods; include highly seasoned foods served at very warm or very cold temperatures; avoid sticky or bulky foods; assess ability to control liquids
Pharyngeal transit phase		
Reduced laryngeal closure; associated with supraglottic laryngectomy	Airway protection is nonexistent or incomplete, resulting in risk for aspiration before the swallow	Use cohesive foods that do not fall apart and thickened liquids
Reduced or slowed movement of bolus through the pharynx	Food residue remains at the base of the tongue and high in throat, resulting in aspiration after the swallow if particles fall into the airway	Use moist, well-lubricated foods that maintain a cohesive bolus
Decreased laryngeal elevation	Food remains on top of the larynx and may result in aspiration after the swallow when the larynx opens to restore breathing	Use soft solids and thick to spoon-thick liquids; avoid sticky and bulky foods that tend to fall apart.
Dysfunctional cricopharyngeal flap	Food may collect in the pyriform sinuses and overflow into the airway, resulting in risk for aspiration after the swallow	Use thickened liquids and pureed foods
Esophageal transit phase		
Weakened or lazy cricopharyngeus	Food material returns from the esophagus into the pharynx and may spill into the airway, resulting in aspiration after the swallow	Use semisolid, moist foods that maintain a cohesive bolus
Reduced esophageal peristalsis	Food bolus remains in the esophagus	Avoid sticky and dry foods; try dense foods followed by liquids
Esophageal obstruction from fistulas, soft bone growth, or tissue growth	Narrowing of esophageal passage	Use thin liquids and pureed or soft solids; avoid sticky, dry foods

Note: Use dietary modifications in conjunction with positioning and safe swallowing techniques recommended by a swallowing therapist.

Table A-34-a-2
Food Consistencies and Representative Foods

Consistency	Example
Semisolid, traditionally prepared foods that are cohesive	Baked egg dishes (e.g., souffles, quiches, custards) Salads with mayonnaise or other binding agents (e.g., egg, tuna, macaroni, or meat salad) Cheese that is soft (cream cheese) or melted Pasta or rice casseroles with thick binders Meat loaf or fish loaf made with bread and binders (eggs) Aspic Pudding, cheesecake, mousse, and gelatin Thick hot cereals
Soft foods that tend to fall apart or separate and may be difficult to control	Whole-grain breads Foods that separate into liquid and pulp (e.g., thin pureed fruits and vegetables) Dry cottage cheese Plain rice; ground meats Thin hot cereals Foods of two or more consistencies (e.g., canned fruits in juice or syrup and soups with whole vegetables, pasta, or grains)
Foods that are sticky, bulky, and dense	Moist white bread Peanut butter Plain mashed potatoes Bananas Refried beans
Thin liquids	Apple, cranberry, citrus, and grape juices Milk Broth and thin cream soups Coffee, tea, and hot chocolate Frozen pops, fruit ices[a] Water, soda, and alcohol Most 1-kcal/mL oral supplements
Thin-to-medium liquids	Vegetable juice Fruit nectars
Thick liquids	Blenderized or cream soups Eggnog, buttermilk Ice cream, sherbet[a] Milkshakes, malts, and yogurt shakes[a] Most 1.5 to 2.0-kcal/mL oral supplements
Spoon-thick liquids	Yogurt drink (kefir) Gelatin

[a]Unstable liquids (e.g., milkshakes, ice cream, sherbets, ice slushes, and frozen pops) separate into a thin liquid food mass or melt completely when allowed to stand at room temperature or when placed in the mouth. For a patient with delayed swallow, these foods should be stabilized with thickening agents. (see Table A-34-b-1-a).

Table A-34-a-3
Compensatory Techniques

- Eliminate distractions
- Do not use liquids to clear the mouth of food; use liquids only after the food has been cleared
- Encourage small bites, especially if the ability to manage food is impaired
- Allow frequent dry swallows to help clear the mouth of food between bites
- Watch for the rise of the Adam's apple; make sure food is being swallowed and not pocketed in the cheeks
- Check frequently for voice quality; a wet or gurgling voice indicates that food may be resting on the vocal cords
- Have patient rest before meals since mealtime can be very tiring
- Ensure correct positioning; the patient should be sitting upright with the hips at a 90° angle, shoulders slightly forward, and feet flat on the floor or firmly supported

A-34-b. Dysphagia Diet Levels

A-34-b-1. Dysphagia Diet Level I

Rationale This diet is designed for patients just beginning to eat by mouth or who need maximum restriction due to dysphagia and cannot swallow chewable foods and thin liquids safely. Foods that are sticky or require bolus formation or controlled manipulation in the mouth (e.g., melted cheese, peanut butter) are omitted. This diet is mechanically nonirritating and low in fiber. It is based on modifications of pureed diets, except that all thin liquids are omitted or thickened. This diet consists of thick, smooth, semiliquid textures and may be appropriate for persons with severely reduced oral preparatory stage abilities, impaired lip and tongue control, delayed swallow reflex triggering, oral hypersensitivity, reduced pharyngeal peristalsis, and/or cricopharyngeal dysfunction.

Description

- Thick, homogeneous textures are emphasized
- No coarse textures, nuts, raw fruits, or raw vegetables are allowed
- Liquid or crushed medications are required and may be mixed with pureed fruits
- No water is allowed
- All liquids are thickened with a commercial thickening agent (see Table A-34-b-1-a)

Table A-34-b-1-a
Clinically Appropriate Thickening Combinations

Type of Thickener	Comments
Gelatin[a]	*Inexpensive*—provides a light density and moisture; stabilizes viscosity of liquids held at body temperature; forms a soft gel when used with cakes, cookies, and crackers; can be used flavored or unflavored; often utilized with pureed chilled fruits, juices, broths, aspics, frozen beverages, regular beverages, pureed cold vegetables, salads
Commercial thickeners[b]	*Moderate- to high-cost*—provides a smooth texture; can be used in hot foods; provides an excellent thickener at the high-viscosity level but not at lower-viscosity levels; best used with meats, soups, beverages, breakfast and dinner breads; commercial thickeners can usually be obtained through community pharmacies
Pureed thick vegetables	*Inexpensive*—can alter flavor depending on the pureed vegetable used; best used with soups and meat-based dishes
Pureed fruits or applesauce	*Inexpensive*—alters the flavor; separates when used with thin liquids; best used with fruit juices; more appropriately used as a flavoring agent with thickened products
Baby rice cereal	*Inexpensive*—excellent thickener at high-viscosity level but not at low-viscosity level; fortified cereals may be a significant source of iron
Baby apple flakes	*Expensive*—excellent thickener at all viscosity levels

[a]Gelatin made with NutraSweet (NutraSweet Co, Deerfield, IL 60015) is kelp-based, does not melt at room temperature, and can congeal fruits that standard gelatins cannot.

[b]High-quality commercial thickeners do not leave an aftertaste, do not continue to thicken after they set (1–2 min), and are fully digestible. Thickening agents that are gum based, such as guar gum or pectin, are not recommended as they will bind fluid so it is unavailable for hydration.

Table A-34-b-1-b
Dysphagia Diet Level I: Recommended Foods

Food Group	Recommended Foods
Breads and cereals	Cream of wheat, cream of rice
Eggs	Soft poached
Milk products	Yogurt without fruit; thickened milk
Fruits	Pureed fruits without seeds or skins; thickened juices
Vegetables	Pureed vegetables without seeds or skins; thickened juices
Fats	Gravy; margarine; thickened sauces or broths
Meats and meat substitutes	Pureed, tender meats or casseroles with gravy or broth to moisten
Soups	Pureed, strained soups; thicken as needed
Desserts	Shakes, custard, pudding, ice cream, sherbet; Pudding Pops, Jello if tolerated
Beverages	All liquids must be cold and thickened with a commercial thickening agent; no water

Table A-34-b-1-c
Sample Menu for Dysphagia Diet Level I

Breakfast	Lunch	Dinner
Thickened orange juice (½ cup)	Strained pureed pea soup (1 cup)	Strained pureed chicken noodle soup (1 cup)
Cream of wheat (1 cup)	Pureed chicken (2 oz) or pureed casserole (1 cup)	Pureed beef (3 oz) or pureed casserole (1½ cup)
Soft, poached egg (1)	Gravy (1 tbsp)	Gravy (1 tbsp)
Butter or margarine (1 tsp)	Pureed carrots (½ cup)	Pureed green beans (½ cup)
Sugar (1–2 tsp)	Pudding or custard (½ cup)	Sherbet (½ cup) or yogurt without fruit (1 cup)
Thickened coffee/tea	Pureed pears (½ cup)	Pureed peaches (½ cup)
Thickened 2% milk (1 cup)	Thickened coffee/tea	Thickened coffee/tea
	Sugar (1–2 tsp)	Sugar (1–2 tsp)
	Thickened 2% milk (1 cup)	Thickened 2% milk (1 cup)

Approximate Nutrient Analysis

Energy (kcal)	2004.6	Phosphorus (mg)	1767.2
Protein (g)	98.8	Potassium (mg)	4103.1
(19.7% of kcal)		Sodium (mg)	1647.8
Carbohydrate	274.9	Zinc (mg)	14.1
(54.9% of kcal)		Vitamin A (μg RE)	2670.4
Total fat (g)	59.5	Vitamin C (mg)	221.8
(26.7% of kcal)		Thiamin (mg)	1.3
Saturated fatty acids (g)	25.4	Riboflavin (mg)	2.7
Monounsaturated fatty acids (g)	21.6	Niacin (mg)	19.0
Polyunsaturated fatty acids (g)	6.3	Folate (μg)	364.0
Cholesterol (mg)	418.1	Vitamin B_6 (mg)	1.5
Calcium (mg)	1357.8	Vitamin B_{12} (μg)	6.4
Iron (mg)	19.3	Dietary fiber (g)	14.6
Magnesium (mg)	344.3	Water-insoluble fiber (g)	9.2

Nutritional Adequacy This diet does not meet the 1989 Recommended Dietary Allowances (RDAs). Amount of intake may be limited because of the increased time required for eating and swallowing. Additional tube feeding or a vitamin and mineral supplement is recommended. Fluid intake should be monitored.

A-34-b-2. Dysphagia Diet Level II

Rationale This diet is designed for patients who can tolerate a minimum amount of easily chewed foods but cannot swallow thin liquids safely. This diet has a pureed base with the addition of *some* texture, flavor, and variety. Small amounts of liquids may be added to achieve the appropriate consistency for the food. This diet may be appropriate for persons with moderately impaired oral preparatory-phase abilities, edentulous oral cavity, decreased pharyngeal peristalsis, and/or cricopharyngeal muscle dysfunction.

Description

- Liquids are thickened only as needed with a commercial thickening agent (see Table A-34-b-1-a)
- The patient may begin to drink beverages such as very thick juices and milk products without thickeners, if tolerated
- No coarse textures, nuts, raw fruits, or vegetables are allowed
- Liquid or crushed medications may still be required
- No water is allowed

Nutritional Adequacy Depending on individual selection and amounts consumed, this diet is designed to provide an adequate quantity of nutrients as indicated by the RDA. More-frequent feedings are recommended, and fluid intake should be monitored.

Table A-34-b-2-a lists recommended foods for the dysphagia diet level II. Table A-34-b-2-b shows a sample menu.

Table A-34-b-2-a
Recommended Foods for Diet Level II

Food Group	Recommended Foods
Breads and cereals	Cream of wheat, cream of rice, thinned oatmeal; pancakes with syrup if tolerated
Eggs	Soft poached, soft scrambled
Milk products	Yogurt; cottage cheese
Fruits	Pureed fruits without seeds or skins; applesauce; ripe, mashed bananas; thickened juices or nectars
Vegetables	Pureed vegetables without seeds or skins; moist mashed potatoes; mashed winter squash; thickened juices
Fats	Gravy, sauces, margarine, seasonings as tolerated
Meats and meat substitutes	Pureed, tender meats or casseroles with gravy or broth to moisten; macaroni and cheese if tolerated
Soups	Pureed or, strained creamed soups
Desserts	Shakes; custard, pudding; ice cream, sherbet; Pudding Pops, Jello if tolerated; avoid hard candies and nuts
Beverages	Very thick juices, nectars, and milk products if tolerated; all other liquids must be cold and thickened with a commercial thickening agent; no water
Miscellaneous	Syrup if tolerated

Table A-34-b-2-b
Sample Menu for Diet Level II

Breakfast	Lunch	Dinner
Thickened orange juice (½ cup)	Strained cream pea soup (1 cup)	Strained cream of chicken noodle soup (1 cup)
Thinned oatmeal (1 cup)	Pureed chicken (2 oz) or pureed casserole (1 cup)	Pureed beef (3 oz) or pureed casserole (1½ cup)
Soft, scrambled egg (1)	Moist mashed potato (½ cup)	Moist mashed potato (½ cup)
Butter or margarine (1–2 tsp)	Gravy (1 tbsp)	Gravy (1 tbsp)
Sugar (1–2 tsp)	Pureed carrots (½ cup)	Pureed green beans (½ cup)
Thickened coffee/tea	Pudding or custard (½ cup)	Sherbet (½ cup) or yogurt without fruit (1 cup)
Thickened 2% milk (1 cup)	Pureed pears (½ cup)	Pureed peaches (½ cup)
	Thickened coffee/tea	Thickened coffee/tea
	Sugar (1–2 tsp)	Sugar (1–2 tsp)
	Thickened 2% milk (1 cup)	Thickened 2% milk (1 cup)

Approximate Nutrient Analysis

Nutrient	Amount	Nutrient	Amount
Energy (kcal)	2146.2	Phosphorus (mg)	1797.0
Protein (g)	106.3	Potassium (mg)	4128.6
(19.8% of kcal)		Sodium (mg)	1499.7
Carbohydrate	262.3	Zinc (mg)	15.5
(48.9% of kcal)		Vitamin A (μg RE)	2847.0
Total fat (g)	77.2	Vitamin C (mg)	89.5
(32.4% of kcal)		Thiamin (mg)	1.3
Saturated fatty acids (g)	32.0	Riboflavin (mg)	2.8
Monounsaturated fatty acids (g)	28.9	Niacin (mg)	20.0
Polyunsaturated fatty acids (g)	8.9	Folate (μg)	220.1
Cholesterol (mg)	563.1	Vitamin B_6 (mg)	1.9
Calcium (mg)	1371.8	Vitamin B_{12} (μg)	6.8
Iron (mg)	11.8	Dietary fiber (g)	19.6
Magnesium (mg)	390.5	Water-insoluble fiber (g)	11.3

A-34-b-3. Dysphagia Diet Level III

Rationale This diet is designed for patients who may have difficulty chewing, manipulating, and swallowing certain foods. It is based on a mechanically altered or edentulous diet and consists of soft food items prepared without blenderizing or pureeing. It may be apropriate for persons beginning to chew or with mild oral preparatory-phase deficits.

Description

- Textures are soft, with no tough skins
- No nuts or dry, crispy, raw, or stringy foods are allowed
- Meats should be minced or cut into small pieces
- Liquids can be used as tolerated
- Liquid or crushed medications may still be required

Nutritional Adequacy Depending on individual selection and amounts consumed, this diet is designed to provide an adequate quantity of nutrients as indicated by the RDA. Table A-34-b-3-a lists recommended foods for the dysphagia diet level III. Table A-34-b-3-b suggests a sample menu.

Table A-34-b-3-a
Recommended Foods for Diet Level III

Food Group	Recommended Foods
Breads and cereals	Soft breads and graham crackers only; cooked and cold cereals in milk; waffles, pancakes; rice, pasta; avoid Grape Nuts, granola, and whole-grain crackers or crackers with seeds
Eggs	Poached, scrambled; egg salad
Milk products	Yogurt; cottage cheese; American or processed cheese; ricotta; cream cheese
Fruits	Any fresh or canned fruit without seeds, coarse skins, or fibers such as peeled apples, applesauce, bananas, canned seedless cherries, canned apricots, peeled or canned peaches and pears; juices, nectars
Vegetables	Well-cooked or canned vegetables; avoid spinach, lettuce, and peas
Fats	Gravy, sauces, margarine, seasonings as tolerated
Meats and meat substitutes	Small pieces with gravy, meat salads; macaroni and cheese; soft sandwiches; casseroles made with allowed foods; smooth peanut butter if tolerated
Soups	Mixed textures if well-cooked with small pieces
Desserts	Soft desserts; avoid nuts and hard candies
Beverages	Juices, nectars, milk products if tolerated; hot liquids and water may be attempted in small amounts (½ tsp); thicken as needed with a commercial thickening agent
Miscellaneous	Syrup; honey

Table A-34-b-3-b
Sample Menu for Diet Level III

Breakfast	Lunch	Dinner
Banana, small (1)	Vegetable soup (1 cup) with 6 saltine-type crackers (no seeds)	Chicken noodle soup (1 cup) with 6 saltine-type crackers (no seeds)
Cold, crisped rice cereal (¾ cup)	Finely chopped chicken (2 oz) or finely chopped casserole (1 cup)	Finely chopped beef (2 oz) or finely chopped casserole (1 cup)
Soft, scrambled egg (1)	Rice (⅓ cup)	Mashed potato (½ cup)
White bread (1 slice)	Gravy (1 tbsp)	Gravy (1 tbsp)
Butter or margarine (1–2 tsp)	Cooked carrots (½ cup)	Cooked green beans (½ cup)
Sugar (1–2 tsp)	Pudding or custard (½ cup)	Sherbet (½ cup) or yogurt without fruit (1 cup)
Coffee/tea	Canned pears (½ cup)	Canned peaches (½ cup)
2% milk (1 cup)	Coffee/tea	Coffee/tea
	Sugar (1–2 tsp)	Sugar (1–2 tsp)
	2% milk (1 cup)	2% milk (1 cup)

Approximate Nutrient Analysis

Nutrient	Amount	Nutrient	Amount
Energy (kcal)	2028.2	Phosphorus (mg)	1651.7
Protein (g)	89.6	Potassium (mg)	3930.3
(17.7% of kcal)		Sodium (mg)	2711.5
Carbohydrate	286.0	Zinc (mg)	13.9
(56.4% of kcal)		Vitamin A (μg RE)	3223.9
Total fat (g)	61.0	Vitamin C (mg)	45.9
(27.1% of kcal)		Thiamin (mg)	1.3
Saturated fatty acids (g)	23.9	Riboflavin (mg)	2.8
Monounsaturated fatty acids (g)	23.0	Niacin (mg)	20.7
Polyunsaturated fatty acids (g)	8.3	Folate (μg)	178.0
Cholesterol (mg)	395.0	Vitamin B_6 (mg)	2.1
Calcium (mg)	1369.0	Vitamin B_{12} (μg)	5.8
Iron (mg)	11.2	Dietary fiber (g)	16.0
Magnesium (mg)	310.1	Water-insoluble fiber (g)	9.2

Table A-34-b-4-a
Recommended Foods for Diet Level IV

Food Group	Recommended Foods
Breads and cereals	Soft or lightly toasted breads and crackers; cooked or cold cereals in milk; waffles, pancakes; pasta; avoid crunchy or chewy foods such as hard bagels or English muffins, hard breadsticks, unleavened bread, or Melba toast
Eggs	All eggs
Milk products	Any milk and dairy products if tolerated; cheeses
Fruits	Canned, cooked, or overripe fruits; juices, nectars; peeled fresh fruits in small pieces; soft dried fruits if tolerated
Vegetables	Tender, cooked vegetables
Fats	Any as tolerated
Meats and meat substitutes	Fine, moist meats; meat loaf; meat salads; any other soft foods; small amounts of smooth peanut butter if tolerated
Soups	Any soups
Desserts	Soft desserts and candies; avoid chewy desserts such as hard marshmallow or caramel
Beverages	All beverages
Miscellaneous	Any as tolerated; avoid chips, popcorn, chewing gum

A-34-b-4. Dysphagia Diet Level IV

Rationale This diet is designed for patients who chew soft textures and swallow all liquids safely. This is based on a soft diet and may be appropriate for persons with mild oral preparatory-stage deficits. The patient may progress from level IV to a soft or general hospital diet.

Description

- Soft textures that do not require grinding or chopping are used
- No nuts; no raw, crisp, or deep-fried foods are allowed
- All liquids and medications are used as tolerated

Nutritional Adequacy Depending on individual selection and amounts consumed, this diet is designed to provide an adequate quantity of nutrients as indicated by the RDA. Table 34-b-4-a suggests foods recommended for the dysphagia diet level IV. Table 34-b-4-b presents a sample menu.

A-34-c. Special Considerations

Food Preparation The diet can be adequate in all nutrients if it is chosen and prepared appropriately. The use of blenders and food processors assists in altering solid foods to an acceptable consistency. Blenders require the addition of fluids for processing, resulting in increased volume, which may be a concern for appetite-depressed patients. Food processors, on the other hand, do not

Table A-34-b-4-b
Sample Menu for Diet Level IV

Breakfast	Lunch	Dinner
Banana, small (1)	Vegetable soup (1 cup) with 6 saltine-type crackers (no seeds)	Chicken noodle soup (1 cup) with 6 saltine-type crackers (no seeds)
Cold, crisped rice cereal (¾ cup)	Soft baked chicken (2 oz) or casserole (1 cup)	Soft roast beef (3 oz) or casserole (1½ cup)
Soft, scrambled egg (1)	Rice (⅓ cup)	Mashed potato (½ cup)
White bread (1 slice)	Gravy (1 tbsp)	Gravy (1 tbsp)
Butter or margarine (1–2 tsp)	Cooked carrots (½ cup)	Cooked green beans (½ cup)
Sugar (1 tsp)	Pudding or custard (½ cup)	Sherbet (½ cup) or yogurt without fruit (1 cup)
Coffee/tea	Canned pears (½ cup)	Canned peaches (½ cup)
2% milk (1 cup)	Coffee/tea	Coffee/tea
	Sugar (1–2 tsp)	Sugar (1–2 tsp)
	2% milk (1 cup)	2% milk (1 cup)

Approximate Nutrient Analysis

Nutrient	Amount	Nutrient	Amount
Energy (kcal)	2169.4	Phosphorus (mg)	1744.4
Protein (g)	99.0	Potassium (mg)	3849.0
(18.3% of kcal)		Sodium (mg)	3201.3
Carbohydrate (g)	284.8	Zinc (mg)	14.6
(52.5% of kcal)		Vitamin A (μg RE)	2783.4
Total fat (g)	73.2	Vitamin C (mg)	41.6
(30.4% of kcal)		Thiamin (mg)	1.3
Saturated fatty acids (g)	28.4	Riboflavin (mg)	2.9
Monounsaturated fatty acids (g)	28.6	Niacin (mg)	22.5
Polyunsaturated fatty acids (g)	9.4	Folate (μg)	171.5
Cholesterol (mg)	425.3	Vitamin B_6 (mg)	2.1
Calcium (mg)	1344.6	Vitamin B_{12} (μg)	6.7
Iron (mg)	12.0	Dietary fiber (g)	16.2
Magnesium (mg)	322.7	Water-insoluble fiber (g)	9.4

require the addition of liquid to alter the consistency of food and, therefore, may be preferred.

Thickened liquids can be used in any stage of the dysphagia diet. Table A-34-b-1-a provides some clinically appropriate thickening combinations for foods and liquids. The following is a list of some commercially available thickeners:

- THICK-IT by Milani Foods, a division of Diafood, Melrose Park, IL
- NUTRA-THICK by Menu Magic, a division of NALCO, Indianapolis, IN
- THICK'N EASE by American Institutional Products, Lancaster, PA
- THIXX by Bernard Foods, Evanston, IL
- THICKENUP by Delmark, a division of Novartis Nutrition, Minneapolis, MN.
- INSTANT FOOD THICKENER by Diamond Crystal Specialty Foods, Inc., Wilmington, MA

The following are some common food thickeners:

Instant cereal	Unflavored/flavored gelatin
Baby strained bananas or banana flakes	Powdered skim milk
	Cottage cheese
Potato flakes	Cream cheese
Finely chopped crackers	Heavy cream
Flavored plain yogurt	Bread crumbs

Slurry Preparation The term *slurry* refers to thickener dissolved in liquid. Pureed fruits and vegetable salads, cakes, cookies, sandwiches, and other items that are served chilled can be softened, thickened, or made cohesive with gelatin. Gelatin is generally used in a ratio of 1 tbsp to 2 cups of liquid.

Any hot item can be softened, thickened, or made cohesive with a commercial thickener. Thickeners are used in varying ratios depending on the density of the original product.

- Gelatin slurry: To soften or stiffen bread, cake, or cookies, 1 tbsp of gelatin is dissolved in 2 cups of the liquid to be poured over the food item.
- To stiffen or gel purees: 1 tbsp of gelatin is dissolved in 1 cup of liquid and added to 1 cup of a pureed item for a total volume of 2 cups.
- Commercial thickener slurry: To thicken or gel meat, chicken, and fish purees, 2 tbsp, 3 tbsp, and 4 tbsp, respectively, of commercial thickener are dissolved in 4 oz of liquid. One tablespoon of this preparation is used for every 1 oz of meat, chicken, or fish puree. To soften or gel bread, cake, and cookies, 1 tbsp of thickener is dissolved in 4 oz of liquid.

Mucus Problems Although the association between milk products and mucus production is poorly documented in the literature, it is frequently cited by some health professionals. It may be that the opaque quality of milk makes mucus more apparent and that milk does not actually stimulate mucus production. However, patient tolerance should be assessed on an individual basis. For patients with thick mucus, citrus juices and cranberry juice may be helpful in cutting or thinning the mucus. Papain, either on a swab or in tablet form, can be given before mealtime in severe cases.

Hydration Thin liquids, such as water and similar liquids, are usually the most difficult consistency for dysphagic patients to control, especially in the oral phase of the swallow. Therefore, adequate hydration must be ensured in the patient with dysphagia. Thickening these liquids will assist with increased control and optimize the intake of fluids for hydration. Typically, liquids are thickened to the consistency of honey, using a variety of substances. Thickening agents change the caloric and carbohydrate content of foods, which must be noted particularly in monitoring the intake of patients with diabetes. Patients who are unable to maintain adequate hydration status through diet modification may require hydration by an alternate method.

Nutrition Support Patients undergoing chewing and swallowing rehabilitation while making the transition from tube feedings to oral feedings should be tube-fed at a time that is least likely to interfere with their desire to eat orally, such as overnight. Oral intake should be documented to determine how quickly the tube feeding rate can be decreased. Increasing the nutrient density of mealtime foods can help a patient reach an oral intake goal more rapidly. For some patients it may be necessary to continue a tube feeding to provide adequate nutrition and hydration.

A-35. POSTGASTRECTOMY DIET

A-35-a. Purpose, Use, Modifications and General Guidelines

The postgastrectomy diet is designed to provide adequate calories and nutrients to support tissue healing and prevent weight loss and dumping syndrome after gastric surgery.

A postgastrectomy diet is used for persons who undergo a surgical procedure involving bypass or excision of the pyloric sphincter, resulting in an inability to regulate normal emptying of the stomach. Surgical procedures include vagotomy, pyloroplasty, hemigastrectomy involving Billroth I and II anastomosis, total gastrectomy, esophagogastrectomy, Whipple's procedure, gastroenterostomy, gastrojejunostomy, Roux-en-Y procedure, and gastric resection.

The diet limits beverages and liquids at meals, limits the intake of simple carbohydrates, and is high in protein and moderate in fat (Table A-35-b). Small, frequent feedings should be provided daily. If no complications occur, additional foods are added as tolerated.

After surgery, the diet generally progresses as follows:

1. All fluids and foods by mouth are withheld for 3 to 5 days and the patient is fed by nasogastric tube.
2. Next, ice chips are held in mouth or small, infrequent sips of water are given. Some people tolerate warm water better than ice chips or cold water.

3. Then, low-carbohydrate, clear liquids such as broth, bouillon, unsweetened gelatin, or diluted unsweetened fruit juices are given.
4. The postgastrecomy diet then begins, with gradual progression to a general diet as tolerated. Bland foods are usually started first, but a more important priority is offering the patient foods he or she likes and can tolerate. By the 5th to 7th day, most patients can tolerate solid foods.

It is important to note that the stated guidelines must be tailored to each patient's surgery, food tolerances, and nutrition problems and deficiencies.

Dumping Syndrome

- Avoid taking liquids with meals. Liquids should be taken 30 to 60 minutes after meals and limited to 0.5- to 1-cup servings. However, at least 6 cups of fluid should be consumed daily to replace losses resulting from diarrhea. Carbonated beverages and milk are not recommended in the initial stages of the diet.
- Small, frequent feedings should be provided. The number of feedings depends on the patient's tolerance to specific portions of food. Foods should be eaten slowly and chewed well. Avoid foods known to cause individual problems.
- The diet should be low in simple carbohydrates, high in complex carbohydrates and protein, and moderate in fat. For persons near desirable body weight, about 1.5 g to 2 g protein per kilogram should be given and 35 kcal to 45 kcal per kilogram.
- All food and drink should be moderate in temperature. Cold drinks tend to cause increased gastric motility.
- If "dumping" is a problem, it may be helpful to lie down 20 to 30 minutes after meals, or even up to an hour, to retard transit to the small bowel.
- Introduce small amounts of milk to determine tolerance. If milk intolerance is found to be caused by a lactase deficiency, a lactose-restricted diet may be necessary.
- If adequate caloric intake cannot be provided due to steatorrhea, use of medium-chain triglyceride products (e.g., Lipisorb [Mead Johnson Enteral Nutritionals, Evansville, IN 47721, USA], Nutrisource Lipid [Novartis Nutrition, Minneapolis, MN 55440, USA]) may be needed.
- Pectin, a dietary fiber found in fruits and vegetables, may be helpful for treating dumping syndrome. Pectin delays emptying, slows carbohydrate absorption, and reduces the glycemic response, though small dry meals are of more benefit.

Alimentary Hypoglycemia

- Avoid concentrated sweets such as candy, sugar, cola drinks, cookies, cakes, and ice cream unless made with sugar substitutes.
- Have concentrated forms of sugar available *only* for treatment of hypoglycemia.
- Eat small meals six times each day.

Adequacy

The adequacy of the diet depends on the extent of surgery as well as individual food tolerances. With careful selection, this diet is adequate in all nutrients (Table A-35-c). After gastric surgery, some patients experience malabsorption, which may be specific for macronutrients (e.g., carbohydrates, proteins, and fats) or micronutrients (e.g., folate, vitamin B_{12}, iron, vitamin D, and calcium). Vitamin and mineral supplementation may be necessary depending on the extent of surgery and whether the symptoms of dumping syndrome persist.

(From The Manual of Clinical Dietetics, 5th ed. Chicago: the American Dietetic Association, 1996:411–7, with permission. *Note:* For references, see original diet, p. 417.)

Table A-35-b
Guidelines for Food Selection for Postgastrectomy Diet

Food Groups	Recommended	May Cause Distress[a]
Beverages[b]	Milk as tolerated; coffee, tea; unsweetened or diluted fruit drinks; unsweetened carbonated beverages	Alcohol; chocolate milk drinks, milk shakes; sweetened fruit drinks; sweetened carbonated beverages
Breads and cereals	Whole-grain or enriched breads and cereals; English muffins and bagels; unsweetened cooked cereals	Breads made with dried fruits, nuts and seeds; pastries, doughnuts, muffins
Cereals	Unsweetened dry and cooked cereals	Sugar-coated cereals; coarse cereals (e.g., bran)
Desserts	Plain cakes, cookies; sugar-free pudding, gelatin dessert, custard, yogurt, frozen yogurt	All sweets and desserts made with chocolate or dried fruits; sweetened gelatin dessert; fried pastries; ice cream, ice milk; regular fruited or frozen yogurt
Fats	Butter, margarine; salad dressings; mayonnaise; vegetable oils; sour cream; cream cheese as tolerated	None
Fruits	Unsweetened canned fruits and fruit juice[b]; fresh fruits	All dried fruits; sweetened fruit juice; fruits canned in heavy syrup
Meats and meat substitutes	Lean tender meats; fish; poultry; shellfish; eggs; peanut butter; cottage cheese; mild cheeses; highly seasoned and spicy meats	Fried meats or eggs
Potatoes and substitutes	Potatoes; enriched rice; barley; noodles, spaghetti, macaroni, and other pastas	Any to which sugar has been added (e.g., candied sweet potatoes)
Soups	Soups made with allowed foods; spicy soups as tolerated	Soups prepared with heavy cream or high-fat ingredients

Table A-35-b—*continued*
Guidelines for Food Selection for Postgastrectomy Diet

Sweets	Sugar substitutes and sweets made with sugar substitutes	Sugar; syrup; honey; jelly, jam, molasses; marshmallows
Vegetables	Cooked (fresh, frozen, canned) vegetables or vegetable juice[b]; raw vegetables as tolerated	Any to which sugar has been added
Miscellaneous	Iodized salt; pepper; mildly flavored sauces and gravies; strongly flavored seasonings as tolerated	None

[a]If no adverse symptoms occur, these foods can be added as tolerated.

[b]All fluids should be consumed 30 to 60 minutes after meals and limited to ½- to 1-cup servings.

Table A-35-c
Sample Menu for Postgastrectomy Diet[a]

Breakfast	Lunch	Dinner
Grapefruit (½) Oatmeal (½ cup) Whole-wheat toast (2 slices) Margarine (1 tsp) 2% milk[b] (½ cup) Coffee/tea[b] (½ cup)	Lean hamburger patty (2 oz) Hamburger bun (1) Mayonnaise (1 tbsp) Sliced tomato (2 oz) and lettuce Fresh fruit salad (½ cup) 2% milk[b] (½ cup) Coffee/tea[b] (½ cup)	Broiled skinless chicken breast (3 oz) Herbed brown rice (½ cup) Steamed broccoli (½ cup) Margarine (2 tsp) Unsweetened applesauce (½ cup) 2% milk[b] (½ cup) Coffee/tea[b] (½ cup)
Midmorning Snack	**Midafternoon Snack**	**Bedtime Snack**
Cheese (1 oz) Saltine crackers (4) Banana (½)	Roast beef (1 oz) Bread (1 slice) Mustard (1 tsp) Vegetable soup[b] (1 cup)	Peanut butter (2 tbsp) Graham crackers (4) 2% milk[b] (½ cup)

Approximate Nutrient Analysis

Energy (kcal)	2186.4	Phosphorus (mg)	1708.5
Protein (g)	111.4	Potassium (mg)	3475.0
(20.4% of kcal)		Sodium (mg)	3792.8
Carbohydrate (g)	239.1	Zinc (mg)	16.8
(43.7% of kcal)		Vitamin A (μg RE)	1263.1
Total fat (g)	92.4	Vitamin C (mg)	136.7
(38.0% of kcal)		Thiamin (mg)	1.6
Saturated fatty acids (g)	29.8	Riboflavin (mg)	2.1
Monounsaturated fatty acids (g)	35.8	Niacin (mg)	29.2
Polyunsaturated fatty acids (g)	19.5	Folacin (μg)	269.3
Cholesterol (mg)	206.1	Vitamin B_6 (mg)	2.4
Calcium (mg)	1088.6	Vitamin B_{12} (μg)	4.1
Iron (mg)	14.8	Dietary fiber (g)	25.1
Magnesium (mg)	420.2	Water-insoluble fiber (g)	16.6

[a]The sample menu incorporates 6 meals per day. The number of feedings depends on the patient's tolerance to food portions and, therefore, should be adjusted accordingly.

[b]Liquids should be given 30 to 60 minutes after the meal and limited to ½- to 1-cup servings.

A.36. GLUTEN-RESTRICTED AND GLIADIN- AND PROLAMIN-FREE (WHEAT-, RYE-, OAT-, AND BARLEY-FREE) DIET

This menu pattern is designed to provide adequate nutrition while eliminating wheat, rye, oats, and barley from the diet. The fraction of gluten protein in wheat that injures the intestine of susceptible persons is gliadin. The equivalent toxic protein fractions in barley, rye, and oats are prolamins. When all sources of gliadin and prolamin are removed from the diet, the intestine is able to regenerate, and normal function is usually restored.

Gliadin and prolamin may be either present in foods as a basic ingredient (i.e., listed as wheat, rye, oats, or barley) or added as a derivative when a food is processed or prepared. Thus, reading labels carefully is very important! A great deal of confusion occurs about the presence of gliadin- and prolamin-containing additives in foods. This table includes lists of both nebulous ingredients and common additives.

Since flour and cereal products are quite often used in the preparation of foods, it is important to be aware of the methods of preparation used, as well as the foods themselves. This is especially true when dining out.

Table A-36-a
Food Group with Suggested Daily Intake

	Foods Allowed	Foods to Avoid
Milk (2 or more cups)	Fresh, dry, evaporated, or condensed milk; cream; sour cream;[a] whipping cream; yogurt[a]	Malted milk; some commercial chocolate drinks; some nondairy creamers[b]
Meat, fish, poultry	All kinds of fresh meats, fish, other seafood, poultry; fish canned in oil, brine, or vegetable broth; some meat products, such as hot dogs and lunch meats[b]	Prepared meats containing wheat, rye, oats, or barley, such as some sausages[b], hot dogs[b], bologna[b]; luncheon meats[b]; ground beef and pork with oat bran added in the form of "Oatrim" or "LeanMaker"; chili con carne[b]; bread-containing products, such as swiss steak, meat loaf, and croquettes; tuna canned with hydrolyzed protein[b]; turkey with hydrolyzed vegetable protein (HVP) injected as part of the basting solution; "imitation crab" containing wheat starch or other unacceptable filler
Cheeses (Can be used for meat and milk groups)	All aged cheeses, such as cheddar, swiss, edam, parmesan; cottage cheese[a]; cream cheese[b]; pasteurized processed cheese[a,b]	Any cheese product containing oat gum as an ingredient
Eggs	Plain or in cooking	Eggs in sauce made from wheat, rye, oats, or barley. Usually wheat flour is used in white sauce
Potato or other starch	White and sweet potatoes; yams; hominy; rice; wild rice; special pasta made from rice, soy, or corn[c]; some oriental rice and bean thread noodles	Regular noodles; spaghetti or macaroni (semolina = wheat); most packaged rice mixes and frozen rice side dishes; frozen potato products with wheat starch or wheat flour added
Vegetables (2 or more servings)	All plain, fresh, frozen, or canned; dried peas, beans, and lentils; some commercially prepared vegetables[b]	Creamed vegetables[b]; vegetables canned in sauce[b]; some canned baked beans[b]; commercially prepared vegetables and salads[b]
Fruits	All fresh, frozen, canned, or dried; all fruit juices; some canned pie fillings	Thickened or prepared fruits; some pie fillings[b]
Breads (3 or more servings)	Specially prepared breads using only allowed flours. Breads may be purchased ready-to-eat or as mixes to prepare at home. Recipes have been developed for home use and for use in automatic bread machines[c]	Those containing wheat, rye, oats, and/or barley flours. Avoid those with buckwheat[c]; millet[c]; amaranth[c]; quinoa[c]; spelt[c]; or teff[c]. *Beware: wheat-free* does not always mean gliadin- and prolamin-free! Breads made from "carob-soy flour" may contain 80% wheat flour!
Cereals (1 or more servings)	*Hot cereals* Corn meal Cream of Rice Hominy Rice *Cold cereals* Puffed Rice Corn Pops Fruity and Choc. Pebbles Kenmei Special cereals made without malt or malt flavoring	Those containing wheat, rye, oats, barley, graham, wheat germ, malt or malt flavoring, kasha, bulgar, buckwheat[c], millet[c], amaranth[c], quinoa[c], spelt[c], teff[c] New products with "unusual" grains are constantly being introduced; do not use them until you can clear them with a reliable source
Crackers and snack foods	Rice wafers; rice crackers; plain corn and potato chips; rice cakes[b]; pure cornmeal tortillas; popcorn; caramel corn[b]	Those with wheat, rye, barley, oats, or other questionable (grainlike) ingredients; *Read labels carefully*; some coating mixes used on chips contain wheat flour! If the product shows "brown rice syrup," contact the manufacturer to check for "barley malt enzymes" used in processing.
Soups	Homemade broth and soup using allowed ingredients; a few canned soups[b]; specialty dry soup mixes[c]	Most canned soups[b] and soup mixes[b]; bouillon and bouillon cubes with hydrolyzed vegetable protein (HVP). HVP may appear as "flavoring" or "natural flavoring" ingredient
Flours and thickening agents[e]	Arrowroot starch (A) Corn bean (B) Corn flour[c] (B, C, D) Corn germ (B) Corn meal (B, C, D) Potato flour (B, C, E) Potato starch flour (B, C, E) Rice bran (B) Rice flours Plain (B, C, D, E) Brown (B, C, D, E) Sweet (A, B, C, F) Rice polish[c] (B, C, G) Rice starch (A) Soy flour[c] (B, C, G) Tapioca starch (A)	Wheat starch Wheat germ, bran Wheat flour Rye Oats Barley Buckwheat[d] Amaranth[d] Quinoa[d] Spelt[d] Teff[d] "Carob-soy" flour containing 80% wheat flour

continued

Table A-36-a—*continued*
Food Group with Suggested Daily Intake

	Foods Allowed	Foods to Avoid
Fats	Butter; margarine; vegetable oil; hydrogenated vegetable oil; nuts; peanut butter; some salad dressings[b]; mayonnaise[b] (mayonnaise made with cider or wine vinegar is found at Kosher delis)	Some commercial salad dressings[b,f]
Desserts	Cakes; quick breads; pastries; puddings made with allowed ingredients; cornstarch; tapioca; rice puddings; gelatin desserts; cook and serve puddings; "expensive" ice cream with a few simple ingredients; sorbet; frozen yogurt[b]; sherbet[b]	Commercial cakes, cookies, pies, made with wheat, rye, oats, barley, millet, amaranth, buckwheat, quinoa, spelt, teff; some "instant" pudding; products containing brown rice syrup made with barley malt enzyme
Beverages	Instant and ground coffee; instant tea; carbonated beverages[b]; pure cocoa powder; wines made in United States; rums; some root beers[b]; vodka distilled from grapes or potatoes	Grain beverages; malted milk; ale; beer; gin; whiskeys[f]; vodka distilled from grain; flavored coffees[b]; some herbal teas with barley or barley malt added[b]
Sweets	Jelly; jam; honey; brown and white sugar; molasses; most syrups[b]; some candy[b]; chocolate; pure cocoa; coconut; marshmallows[b]	Some commercial candies; foods with malt/malt flavoring or "natural flavoring"[b]; chocolate-coated nuts, which may be rolled in wheat flour[b]; brown rice syrup made with barley malt enzyme[b]
Miscellaneous	Spices (salt, pure pepper, cloves, ginger, nutmeg, cinnamon, allspice, etc.); herbs (oregano, rosemary, etc.); food coloring; alcohol-free extracts; yeast; baking soda; baking powder; cream of tartar; dry mustard; cider, rice and wine vinegars; olives; monosodium glutamate (MSG) made in United States	Condiments made with wheat-derived distilled white vinegar[f]; alcohol-based extracts[b,f]; some curry powders[b]; some dry seasoning mixes[b]; some gravy extracts[b]; some meat sauces[b]; most soy sauces[b]; some chewing gum[b]; communion wafers/bread[g]

[a]Check vegetable gum used.

[b]Consult label and contact manufacturer to clarify questionable ingredients.

[c]See Special Products List for availability and ordering information.

[d]These cereals should be avoided due to the high risk of cross-contamination by gluten-containing grains.

[e]A, good thickening agent; B, good combined with other flours; C, best combined with milk and eggs in baked products; D, grainy-textured products; E, drier product than with other flours; F, moister product than with other flours; G, adds distinct flavor to product, use with moderation.

[f]Distilled white vinegar uses grain as a starting material. Most often the grain mash includes wheat. Whiskies, including "corn whiskey," use wheat, rye, oats, or barley in their mash. According to chemistry professors consulted, in large-scale distillation processes, such as those used in the manufacture of whiskey and vinegar, it is possible that a very small amount of protein may be carried over into the distillate. The presence of such a small amount of gliadin and/or prolamin must be tested via immunoassay. Currently, we are advising gliadin- and prolamin-intolerant individuals to use cider, wine, or rice vinegar in such food preparation as making salad dressings, pickles, and in cooking. To be 100% safe, purchase or make condiments with cider, wine, or rice vinegar. These condiments (ketchup, mustard, mayonnaise, pickles) are usually available in kosher delis. Foods with nongrain vinegars are produced for Passover.

[g]Contact the Gluten Intolerance Group of North America to obtain instructions for making communion wafers from acceptable ingredients. *Note:* In Catholic communion, host crumbs are often added to the wine before it is served. A workable solution is to arrange to use a goblet of your own.

Table A-36-b
Nebulous Ingredients

Nebulous Ingredients[a]	Include	Avoid
"Hydrolyzed vegetable protein" or "hydrolyzed protein"	Those from soy, corn, or milk	Mixtures of wheat, corn, and soy[b]
"Flour" or "cereal products"	Rice flour, corn flour, corn meal, potato flour, soy flour	Wheat, rye, oats, barley, amaranth, quinoa, spelt, teff, millet, buckwheat
"Vegetable protein"	Soy, corn	Wheat, rye, oats, barley
"Vegetable broth"	In the United States, this must contain two or more of the following: beans, cabbage, carrots, celery, garlic, onions, parsley, peas, potatoes, green bell pepper, red bell pepper, spinach, or tomatoes; it cannot contain any other ingredients; *it can be used*	
"Malt" or "malt flavoring"	Those derived from corn	Those derived from barley or barley malt syrup
"Brown rice syrup"	Rice only	Rice plus barley malt enzyme
"Starch"	In the United States, it must be *cornstarch*	
"Modified starch" or "modified food starch"	Arrowroot, corn, potato waxy maize, maize	Wheat starch
"Vegetable gum"	Carob bean, locust bean, cellulose, guar, gum arabic, gum acacia, gum tragacanth, xanthan gum	Oat gum
"Soy sauce" or "soy sauce solids"	Those that *do not* contain wheat (*soy only*)	Those brewed from wheat and soy
"Mono-" and "diglycerides"	Those using *non*-wheat-based carrier	Those using a wheat starch carrier

[a]These questionable ingredients must be cleared with the manufacturer before they are eaten. A sample letter requesting information on starting materials and packaging and processing ingredients is available in Table A-36-f.

[b]Hydrolyzed vegetable protein: A combination of wheat, corn, and soy is primarily used as starting material for hydolyzed vegetable protein (HVP). When wheat protein is "hydrolyzed," its large amino acid chains are broken down into smaller chains. Some protein researchers believe the same sequence of amino acids found in these smaller chains contain the same toxicity as the intact gliadin subfraction of the gluten protein. Thus, HVP made from wheat is not recommended for use on a gliadin-free diet.

Table A-36-c
Additives That Are Gliadin- and Prolamin-Free[a]

Adipic acid Ascorbic acid BHA BHT Beta carotene Biotin Calcium chloride Calcium pantothenate Calcium phosphate Carboxymethylcellulose Carrageenan Citric acid Corn sweetener Corn syrup solids Demineralized whey Dextrimaltose Dextrose—dextrins Dioctyl sodium sulfosuccinate Folic acid—folacin Fructose Fumaric acid	Gums: acacia, arabic, carob bean, cellulose, guar, locust bean, tragacanth, xanthan Invert sugar Lactic acid Lactose Lecithin Magnesium hydroxide Malic acid Microcrystalline cellulose Monosodium glutamate (MSG) made in United States Niacin—niacinamide Polyglycerol Polysorbate 60; 80 Potassium citrate Potassium iodide Propylene glycol monostearate Propylgallate Pyridoxine hydrochloride	Riboflavin Sodium acid pyrophosphate Sodium ascorbate Sodium benzoate Sodium caseinate Sodium citrate Sodium hexametaphosphate Sodium nitrate Sodium silico aluminate Sorbitol—mannitol Sucrose Sulfosuccinate Tartaric acid Thiamin hydrochloride Tri-calcium phosphate Vanillan Vitamin A (palmitate) Vitamins and minerals

[a]This is not an exhaustive list.

Table A-36-d
Medications

All medications have fillers/dispersing agents added. These are usually lactose or corn starch. Wheat starch may also be used. *Before you take any medication, take the following precautions.*

Over-the-counter drug: Read the list of active and inactive ingredients carefully. Use the list of "Nebulous Ingredients" in Table A-36-b to spot potential problems. Ask your pharmacist to "translate" the terms you do not know.

Prescription drug: Inactive ingredients are *not* listed. Even your pharmacist must call the drug company to obtain this information! When the pharmaceutical company is contacted, they will need the lot number of the product so they can check the formulation of the batch you will be taking. A list of drug companies with addresses and phone numbers can be found in the Physicians' Desk Reference.

Liquid cold and flu medications: These medications often contain alcohol. Check source.

Table A-36-e
Special Products List

AlpineAire Foods P.O. Box 926 Nevada City, CA 95959 916-272-1971	Freeze-dried foods for backpacking. Vacuumed packed. No preservatives, no added sugar, no artificial flavors or colors. *Note:* The "vegetable pasta" in Pasta Roma and Vegetable Pasta Stew *contains wheat flour.* Mail orders accepted.
Bickford Laboratories 282 S. Main Street Akron, OH 44308 216-762-4666	Forty-nine varieties of alcohol-free flavorings. Selection ranges from common flavorings, like vanilla and almond to exotic. Mail orders accepted.
DeBoles Garden City Park, NY 11040	Corn pasta products, including ribbon noodles, macaroni, and spaghetti.
Dietary Specialties P.O. Box 227 Rochester, NY 14601 1-800-544-0099	A wide assortment of mixes, crackers, cookies, and pasta. Many exclusive imported items. Mail orders accepted.
Ener-G Foods, Inc. P.O. Box 84487 Seattle, WA 98124-5787 1-800-331-5222	Excellent assortment of flours and flour mixes. Will ship in bulk (20# boxes). Variety of baked products, dry soup mixes, flavorings. Mail orders accepted.
Lundberg Family Farms Box 369 Richvale, CA 95974 916-882-4551	Interesting variety of combination rices. Brown rice cereals and rice cakes. *Note:* Sweet Dreams Brown Rice Syrup is made using barley malt enzyme. Products made with this syrup should be avoided. Soups contain wheat-derived soy sauce. Mail orders accepted.

continued

Table A-36-e—*continued*
Special Products List

Med-Diet Inc. 3050 Ranchview Lane Plymouth, MN 55447 1-800-med-diet	Carries various brands of breads, crackers, cookies, cake and muffin mixes, and pasta. *Note:* Their order blank is not designed for those who must eliminate gliadin and prolamin. Request their list of "wheat/gluten-free foods that contain no wheat starch" so you'll know what to order!
Red Mill Farms, Inc. 290 S. 5th Street Brooklyn, NY 11211 718-384-2150	Three suitable products that are also lactose free: Dutch Chocolate Cake, Banana-Nut Cake, and Coconut Macaroons. All vacuumed packed. Mail orders accepted.
Tad Enterprizes 9356 Pleasant Tinley Park, IL 60477 708-429-2101	Carry a variety of flours for gliadin- and prolamin-free baking. Mail orders accepted.
Van Brode's Milling Clinton, MA 01510	Carries some cold breakfast cereals (malt free). Write for complete product information.

A-37. LACTOSE-CONTROLLED DIET

A-37-a. Purpose, Modifications and Related Physiology

The lactose-controlled diet is designed to prevent or reduce gastrointestinal symptoms of bloating, flatulence, cramping, nausea, and diarrhea associated with consumption of the disaccharide lactose.

The diet is a general one that restricts or eliminates lactose-containing foods. Lactose is primarily found in dairy products but may be present as an ingredient or component of various food products. (See Table A-37-b for lactose content of common foods and beverages.) Depending on individual tolerance, limiting products with lactose may help to alleviate symptoms.

Labels should be read carefully to identify sources of lactose. Dairy products that include milk, milk solids, whey, lactose, curds, skim milk powder, skim milk solids, sweet or sour cream, buttermilk, or malted milk are sources of lactose. Other possible sources of lactose are breads, candy, cookies, cold cuts, hot dogs, bologna, commercial sauces and gravies, dessert mixes, cream soups, some ready-to-eat cereals, frostings, chocolate drink mixes, salad dressings, sugar substitutes, and medications.

Dairy products can be consumed depending on individual tolerance. Most persons with lactase nonpersistence can consume milk without the development of symptoms, particularly if small portions of milk (4 fl oz to 6 fl oz) or lactose-containing foods are eaten at separate times during the day. The ingestion of solid food with lactose-

Table A-36-f
Writing Effective Letters to Food Manufacturers[a]

Clarifying questionable ingredients on product labels and in medications is essential for those following this diet. Manufacturers are usually courteous and prompt when answering questions regarding their products. The usefulness of their reply, however, often depends on how the question is posed. Use the following letter format when you need to contact a manufacturer.

Your Address
Date

Dear Sir/Madam:

I am on a gluten-restricted, gliadin- and prolamin-free diet for the treatment of a celiac sprue (dermatitis herpetiformis). I must avoid the protein found in wheat, rye, oats, and barley, since they cause an immune response that damages the lining of my intestine.

Although I would like to use your product, (insert name), your ingredient listing does not give adequate information for me to determine if it would be suitable. Specifically, I need to know

examples would be:
the source of your "food starch modified"
whether your "soy sauce solids" are derived from wheat
what "natural flavorings" you use in this product
from what source your "vegetable gum" is derived
the inactive ingredients used in the medication, including those used in the coatings and capsules

Another likely source of gliadin and prolamin contamination is the incidental ingredients which are used in the packaging and processing of your product. Since these incidental ingredients are not listed on the packaging, I am relying on your thoroughness to clarify these substances.

If it would be possible, I would appreciate a copy of your response to be forwarded to: The Gluten Intolerance Group of North America
P.O. Box 23053
Seattle, WA 98102-0353

This will allow your efforts to be shared with others through our national organization which reaches health-care personnel as well as persons with celiac sprue and dermatitis herpetiformis. If you have questions regarding these disorders and the required dietary restrictions, please direct them to our national office.

Thank you for your efforts on my behalf.

Sincerely,
Your Signature

[a]Additional information on celiac sprue and dermatitis herpetiformis may be obtained from The Gluten Intolerance Group of North America, P.O. Box 23053, Seattle WA 98102-0353.

Table A-37-b
Lactose Content of Common Foods and Beverages

Product	Lactose (g)
Milk (1 cup)	
Whole	11
1% and 2% low-fat	9–13
Skim	12–14
Evaporated	24
Sweetened, condensed	30
Chocolate	10–12
Buttermilk	9–11
Yogurt, low-fat (1 cup)	11–15
Cottage cheese (1 cup)	5–8
Pasteurized processed cheese food (1 oz)	0.5–2
Other cheeses (1 oz)	0.4–0.8
Ice cream (1 cup)	9
Ice milk (1 cup)	10
Sherbet, orange (1 cup)	4
Half and half, light cream, whipped cream topping (1 tbsp)	0.5
Sour cream (1 tbsp)	<1

containing beverages modifies lactose malabsorption. Food solids delay gastric emptying and/or provide endogenous lactase additional time to digest lactose. Cocoa and chocolate milk have a suppressive effect on human lactose intolerance as evidenced by significantly lowered mean breath hydrogen, bloating, and cramping.

Adequacy

Lactose-reduced dairy products are available and are suitable substitutions for conventional lactose-containing products. Commercial products are available with varying degrees of lactose reduction. A 50% reduction in lactose may be adequate to relieve signs and symptoms of milk intolerance in most healthy adults with lactose malabsorption. Individuals may choose to use conventional dairy products and reduce the lactose levels themselves with commercially available lactase enzyme drops or tablets. It has been suggested that yogurt is as effective as hydrolyzed lactose milk in alleviating symptoms of lactose intolerance. Lactase activity in yogurt may vary across brands. Yogurt that has endogenous cultures added postpasteurization has more lactase activity.

Primary lactase deficiency, a condition in which lactase enzyme activity falls postweaning, is a common develop-

Table A-37-c
Guidelines for Food Selection for Lactose-Controlled Diet

Food Category	Recommended	May Cause Distress
Beverages	All beverages with allowed ingredients, soybean milks, other lactose-free supplements, lactose-hydrolyzed milk	Milk, milk products, or acidophilus milk as tolerance dictates
Breads and cereals	Whole-grain or enriched breads and cereals	Depending on tolerance, some breads and cereals prepared with milk or milk products may need to be avoided
Desserts	Cakes, cookies, pies; flavored gelatin desserts; water ices made with allowed foods	Any prepared with milk or milk products (e.g., sherbet, ice cream, ice milk, custard, pudding commercial desserts, and mixes)
Fats	Butter or margarine; salad dressings; nondairy creamer; all oils	Any prepared with lactose-containing ingredients
Fruits	All fruits and juices	None
Meats and meat substitutes	All meats, poultry; fish; eggs; peanut butter; dried peas and beans; hard, aged, and processed cheese, if tolerated; yogurt as tolerated	Cold cuts and frankfurters that contain lactose filler; cottage cheese
Potatoes and potato substitutes	Potatoes; enriched rice; barley; noodles, spaghetti, macaroni, and other pastas	Potatoes or substitutes prepared with milk or milk, products; mixes prepared with lactose-containing ingredients
Soups	Broth, bouillon; soups made with allowed ingredients	Soups made with milk or milk products
Sweets	Sugar; corn syrup; pure maple syrup; honey; jellies, jams; pure sugar candies; marshmallows	Chocolate; caramels; any candies made with lactose-containing ingredients
Vegetables	All	Vegetables prepared with milk or milk products
Miscellaneous	All spices, seasonings, flavorings	Any prepared with milk or milk products

ment with aging. It is most commonly seen in African Americans, Hispanics, Native Americans, Asians, and people of Jewish descent. Adult lactase deficiency is the most common of all enzyme deficiencies; well over half the world's adults are lactose intolerant. Secondary lactase deficiency can be attributed to mucosal injury from a condition or disease process such as regional enteritis, ulcerative colitis, Crohn's disease, gluten-induced enteropathy, and parasitic infections or following antibiotic therapy and surgical procedures, including gastrectomy, extensive bowel resection, and gastric bypass.

Lactose tolerance is variable; if an individual is asymptomatic, no restrictions are indicated. If an individual experiences adverse reactions to lactose, following a lactose-controlled diet is advisable. Symptoms associated with lactose intolerance usually subside within 3 to 5 days on a lactose-controlled diet.

Individuals can often identify discomfort associated with digesting lactose; however, true lactase deficiency can be diagnosed clinically with a breath hydrogen test. The breath hydrogen test measures hydrogen produced by colonic bacteria in the presence of unabsorbed sugars.

Depending on individual choices, the diet can provide adequate amounts of all essential nutrients. When dairy products are limited, intake of calcium, phosphorus, vitamins A and D, and riboflavin may be deficient. Use of dairy products within individual tolerance level and/or use of lactose hydrolyzed milk and milk products could satisfy these nutrient needs. Calcium supplementation is indicated if the diet does not provide adequate calcium.

Special Product Information

Lactaid can be purchased in tablets, drops, or as lactase-treated milk and cheese products. Lactaid products are distributed by
McNeil CPC
7050 Camp Hill Road
Fort Washington, PA 19034
Lactaid Hotline: 800/LACTAID, 9 AM–5 PM Eastern time, Monday through Friday

Dairy Ease products including tablets, drops, and lactase-treated milk are produced by
Sterling Health
Division of Sterling Winthrop
90 Park Avenue
New York, NY 10016

Check at a grocery and read labels for other lactose-reduced, lactose-free, and lactase-treated products. Other brands may be available.
(From The Manual of Clinical Dietetics, 5th ed. Chicago: the American Dietetic Association, 1996:419–24, with permission. *Note:* For references, see original diet, p. 424.)

Table A-37-d
Sample Menu for Lactose-Controlled Diet

Breakfast	Lunch	Dinner
Orange juice (½ cup)	Vegetable soup (1 cup)	Green salad (3½ oz)
Whole-grain cereal (1 cup)	Crackers (4)	Vinegar and oil dressing (1 tbsp)
Banana (½)	Lean beef patty (3 oz)	Broiled skinless chicken breast (3 oz)
Whole-wheat toast (2 slices)	Hamburger bun (1)	Baked potato (1 medium)
Margarine (2 tsp)	Sliced tomato (2 oz) and lettuce	Whole-grain roll (1)
Jelly or jam (1 tbsp)	Fresh fruit salad (½ cup)	Steamed broccoli (½ cup)
Lactose-reduced 1% milk[a] (1 cup)	Graham crackers (4)	Lemon ice (½ cup)
Coffee/tea	Lactose-reduce 1% milk[a] (1 cup)	Margarine (1 tsp)
	Coffee/tea	Coffee/tea

Approximate Nutrient Analysis

Nutrient	Amount	Nutrient	Amount
Energy (kcal)	1940.1	Phosphorus (mg)	1509.7
Protein (g)	97.1	Potassium (mg)	3587.2
(20.0% of kcal)		Sodium (mg)	2621.1
Carbohydrate (g)	267.3	Zinc (mg)	14.4
(55.1% of kcal)		Vitamin A (μg RE)	738.4
Total fat (g)	59.0	Vitamin C (mg)	136.3
(27.4% of kcal)		Thiamin (mg)	2.0
Saturated fatty acids (g)	18.5	Riboflavin (mg)	2.5
Monounsaturated fatty acids (g)	22.8	Niacin (mg)	31.6
Polyunsaturated fatty acids (g)	11.8	Folate (μg)	459.4
Cholesterol (mg)	159.4	Vitamin B_6 (mg)	2.9
Calcium (mg)	910.3	Vitamin B_{12} (μg)	7.0
Iron (mg)	15.0	Dietary fiber (g)	24.1
Magnesium (mg)	406.9	Water-insoluble fiber (g)	17.2

[a]If lactose-reduced milk is not tolerated, substitute ½ cup nondairy creamer at breakfast and fruit juice at lunch. A calcium supplement should be provided if this substitution is made.

A-38. OXALATE CONTENT OF SELECTED FOODS

Table A-38-a
Oxalate Content by Food Group

Foods	**Little or no Oxalate** *<2 mg oxalate/serving* Eat as desired	**Moderate-Oxalate Content** *2–10 mg oxalate/serving* Limit: two (1/2 cup) servings/day or two servings of the stated serving size	**High-Oxalate Foods** *>10 mg oxalate/serving* Avoid completely
Beverages/ juices	Apple juice Beer, bottled Black coffee (brewed 5 min) Cranberry juice Diet Coke Grapefruit juice Lemonade or limeade Wine, red, rosé Pineapple juice Tap water (preferred for extra calcium) Orange soda (12 fl oz Minute Maid) Ginger ale (Schweppes) Root beer (Borg's and A&W) Aloe vera juice	Beer, Budweiser (12 fl oz) Coffee, any kind (8 oz serving) Cranberry juice (4 oz serving) Cocoa, Carnation dry Nescafe powder (1 tsp) Tomato juice (4 oz serving) Lipton tea (steeped 5 min)	Beer; Stout, Guiness, Draft, Lager, Tuborg, Pilsner Juices containing berries not allowed Ovaltine and other beverage mixes Tea, cocoa
Milk (2 or more cups)	Buttermilk Low-fat milk Low-fat yogurt with allowed fruit Skim milk Whole milk	Yogurt plain, nonfat (1 cup)	
Meat group	Eggs Cheese, cheddar Lean lamb, beef, or pork Poultry Seafood	Sardines	Baked beans canned in tomato sauce Peanut butter Soybean curd (tofu)
Vegetables	Avocado Broccoli, boiled Brussels sprouts, boiled Cabbage, boiled Chive Potatoes, white, boiled Radishes Turnips, boiled Waterchestnuts	Asparagus Carrots, canned Cauliflower, boiled Corn, sweet white and yellow Cucumbers, peeled raw Onions, raw, boiled Green peas, boiled, canned Lettuce, iceberg, fresh Lima beans, cooked Parsnips Tomato, fresh, 1 small Mushrooms, fresh Escarole Kale, raw	Beans, boiled or raw: green, wax, dried Beets, boiled; tops, roots, and green Celery Chard, Swiss Collards Dandelion greens Eggplant, raw Leeks Mustard greens Okra Parsley, raw Peppers, green Pokeweed Potatoes, sweet Rutabagas Spinach Summer squash Watercress
Fruits	Avocado Banana Cherries, bing or sour Cranberries, canned Grapes, Thompson seedless Mangoes Melons: cantaloupe casaba honeydew watermelon Nectarines Peaches, Hiley, canned Pineapple, canned, stewed Plums, green or Golden age Pear, Bartlett, canned Orange juice fresh Papaya, Hawaiian Strawberries, fresh	Apple Apricots Black currants Cranberries, dried Grapefruit Orange Peaches, Alberta Pears, raw Plums, stewed Prunes, Italian Pineapple, Dole's Coconut Kiwi	Berries Concord grapes Red currants Fruit cocktail Gooseberries Lemon peel Lime peel Orange peel Raspberries Rhubarb, canned, stewed Strawberries, canned Tangerine Plums, Damson
Bread/ starches	Cornflakes Macaroni, boiled Noodles, egg boiled	Cornbread Sponge cake Spaghetti, canned in tomato sauce	Fruit cake Grits, white corn Soybean crackers

continued

Table A-38-a—*continued*
Oxalate Content by Food Group

Foods	Little or no Oxalate *<2 mg oxalate/serving* Eat as desired	Moderate-Oxalate Content *2–10 mg oxalate/serving* Limit: two (1/2 cup) servings/day or two servings of the stated serving size	High-Oxalate Foods *>10 mg oxalate/serving* Avoid completely
	Oatmeal, porridge Rice, boiled Wild rice, cooked Bread, white Barley, cooked	Cornmeal, yellow, dry Cheerios (1 cup) Bagel (1 medium; 2 oz) Brown rice, cooked Garbanzo beans, canned Lentils, cooked Split peas, cooked Macaroni, cooked Spaghetti, cooked Corn tortilla (1 medium; 1.5 oz) English muffin (1 medium; 2 oz) Bread, whole wheat	Wheat germ Fig Newtons Graham crackers Popcorn (4 cups popped) Whole wheat flour
Fats & oils	Mayonnaise Salad dressing Vegetable oils Butter Margarine	Bacon	Nuts: Peanuts and pecans Sunflower seeds Mayonnaise (Heinz)
Miscellaneous	Jelly or preserves, made with allowable fruits Lemon/lime juice, fresh Salt, pepper (1 tsp/day) Soups with allowed ingredients Sugar Honey (1 tbsp) Corn syrup (Karo) Unflavored gelatin (Knox), 1 pkt Maple syrup, pure Vanilla extract Oregano, dried (1 tsp) Apple cider vinegar (1 tsp. Ralph's Supermarket) Nutmeg, dry (1 tsp) Cornstarch (1 tbsp)	Vegetable soup Tomato soup Tofu (firm) Malt (1 tbsp) Basil, fresh (1 tbsp) Mustard, Dijon style (1 tbsp) Ginger, raw (1 tbsp sliced)	Chocolate, plain Dry cocoa, plain Pepper (in excess of 1 tsp/day) Cinnamon, ground (1 tsp)

From Brzezinski E, Durning AM, Grasse B, Fusselman E, Ciaraldi T. Oxalate content of selected foods. The General Clinical Research Center, University of California, San Diego Medical Center. 1996:1–53. With permission. There is now a 1998 edition available.

Table A-38-b
Foods to Use and Avoid

These contain small amounts of oxalate
0–2 mg oxalate per serving (½ cup)

Vegetables	Fruits	Beverages	Miscellaneous
Broccoli Brussels sprouts Cabbage Cauliflower Chives Cucumber Lettuce Mushrooms Onions Peas Potato white Radishes Rice Turnips	Avocado Banana Cherries Grapes, seedless Mangoes Melons Peaches; canned Hiley Stokes Pineapple Plums: Golden Gage Green Gage Oxtail soup Red plum jam Sweets, boiled	Apple juice Barley water Beer, bottled Cider Coca-Cola Grapefruit juice Lemonade Lucozade, bottled Milk Orange juice Pepsi-Cola Pineapple juice Sherry, dry Wine	Butter Cheese, cheddar Chicken noodle soup Cornflakes Eggs Egg noodle (chow mein) Fish (except sardines) Jelly with allowed fruit Lemon juice Lime juice Macaroni Margarine Meats Oatmeal, porridge Poultry

continued

Table A-38-b—*continued*
Foods to Use and Avoid

These are high in oxalate
>15 mg oxalate per serving (½ cup)

Vegetables	Fruits	Beverages	Miscellaneous
Beans in tomato sauce	Berries;	Chocolate	Cocoa, dry
Beets	Black	Tuborg, Pilsner	Grits, white corn
Celery	Blue	Ovaltine (24 mg/8 oz)	Peanuts
Chard, Swiss	Green goose	Tea (132–181.2 mg/8 oz)	Pecans
Collards	Raspberries		Soybean crackers
Dandelion greens	Currants, red		Wheat germ
Eggplant	Grapes, concord		
Escarole	Lemon peel		
Leeks			
Okra			
Parsley			
Pepper, green			
Pokeweed			
Potato, sweet			
Rutabagas			
Spinach			
Squash, summer			

From Brzezinski E, Durning AM, Grasse B, Fusselman E, Ciaraldi T. Oxalate content of selected foods. The General Clinical Research Center, University of California, San Diego Medical Center. 1996:1–53. With permission. There is now a 1998 edition available.

Table A-38-c
Oxalate Content of Foods per 100 Grams (~½ cup) and per Portion

Food	Portion	mg/100 g	mg/Portion
Cereals, grains, and ceral products			
Bagel, plain	1 medium; 55 g	12.37	6.804
Barley, cooked	1 cup: 156.25 g	3.46	5.404
Bread, white	1 slice; 25 g	4.9	1.225
Bread, whole wheat	1 slice; 25 g	20.9	5.225
Cake, fruit	1 slice; 15 g	11.8	1.77
Cake, sponge	1 slice; 66 g	7.4	4.884
Cheerios	1 cup; 22.6 g	20.66	4.67
Corn tortilla	1 medium; 21.3 g	11.51	2.45
Cornflakes	1 cup; 22.7 g	2	0.454
Cornmeal, yellow	1 cup dry; 138 g	6.25	8.624
Cornstarch	1 tbsp; 8 g	14.51	1.61
Crackers, soybean	1 ounce; 28.35 g	204	58.685
Egg noodle (chow mein)	1 cup; 45 g	1	0.45
English muffin, white	1 each; 58 g	10.22	5.93
Graham crackers (Keebler)	2 crackers; 14 g	12.41	1.74
Fig Newtons	1 each; 14.7 g	14.05	2.07
Garbanzo beans, canned	1 cup; 164 g	11.18	18.34
Grits, white corn	1 cup cooked; 242 g	41	99.22
Grits, white corn	1 cup dry; 156 g	41	63.96
Lentils, cooked	1 cup; 198 g	8.48	16.795
Macaroni, boiled	1 cup boil tender; 140 g	1	1.4
Macaroni, cooked soft	1 cup; 140 g	5.44	7.62
Oatmeal porridge	1 cup; 234 g	1	2.34
Popcorn, Orville Redenbacker, popped	single-serving bag; 4 cups = 50.39 g	33.29	16.777
Rice, brown, cooked	1 cup; 195 g	6.54	12.76
Rice, boiled	1 cup; 175 g	0	0
Spaghetti, boiled	1 cup boil tender; 140 g	1.5	2.1
Spaghetti, cooked soft	1 cup; 140 g	6.24	8.73
Spaghetti in tomato sauce	1 cup; 250 g	4	10
Split peas, cooked	1 cup; 196 g	4.83	9.48
Wheat germ	1 Tbsp; 7.2 g	299	19.37
Wild rice, cooked	1 cup; 164 g	1.65	2.71
Whole wheat flour	1 cup; 120 g	25.03	30.031
Milk and milk products			
Butter	1 Tbsp; 14 g	0	0
Cheddar cheese	1 ounce; 28.35 g	0	0
Margarine	1 Tbsp; 14.1 g	0	0
Milk	1 cup; 244 g	0.15	0.366
Milk, whole	1 cup; 244 g	0.54	1.31
Yogurt, natural, nonfat plain	1 cup; 227 g	1	2.266

continued

Table A-38-c—*continued*
Oxalate Content of Foods per 100 Grams (~½ cup) and per Portion

Food	Portion	mg/100 g	mg/Portion
Meats, eggs and meat alternates			
Bacon, streaky, fried	1 strip; 6.3 g	3.3	0.21
Beef, canned, corned	3 oz; 85 g	0	0
Beef, topside roast	4 oz; 113.4 g	0	0
Chicken roast	4 oz; 113.4 g	0	0
Egg, boiled	1 medium; 50 g	0	0
Fish: haddock	4 oz; 113.4 g	0.2	0.23
plaice	4 oz; 113.4 g	0.3	0.34
sardines	4 oz: 113.4 g	4.8	5.42
Ham	4 oz; 113.4 g	1.6	1.81
Hamburger, grilled	4 oz; 113.4 g	0	0
Lamb, roast	4 oz; 113.4 g	trace	trace
Liver	4 oz; 113.4 g	7.1	8.02
Pork, roast	4 oz; 113.4 g	1.7	1.92
Tofu, raw firm	125 g	5.08	6.35
Vegetables			
Asparagus	1 cup; 180 g	5.2	9.36
Green beans, boiled	1 cup; 135 g	15	20.25
Beans in tomato sauce	1 cup	19	
Beetroot, boiled	1 cup; 170 g	675	1147.5
Beetroot, pickled	1 cup; 227 g	500	1135
Broccoli, boiled	1 cup; 155 g	trace	trace
Brussels sprouts, boiled	1 cup; 156 g	0	0
Cabbage, boiled	1 cup common; 70 g	0	0
Carrots, canned	1 cup; 146 g	4	5.84
Cauliflower, boiled	1 cup; 124 g	1	1.24
Celery	1 cup diced; 120 g	20	24
Chard, Swiss	1 cup raw; 36 g	645	232.2
Chard, Swiss	1 cup boiled; 175 g	645	1128.75
Chive	1 cup raw; 48 g	1.1	0.53
Collards	1 cup raw/boil; 128 g	74	94.72
Corn, yellow	1 cup; 165 g	5.2	8.58
Cucumber, raw	1 med whole; 301 g	1	3.01
Dandelion greens	1 cup raw; 55 g	24.6	13.53
Dandelion greens	1 cup boiled; 105 g	24.6	25.83
Eggplant	1 cup boiled; 96 g	18	17.28
Escarole	1 cup raw; 28 g	31	8.68
Kale	1 cup raw/boil; 130 g	13	16.9
Leek	1 cup raw/boil; 124 g	89	110.36
Lettuce	1 cup; 55 g	3	1.65
Lima beans	1 cup canned; 248 g	4.3	10.66
Mushrooms	1 cup raw/chopped; 70 g	2	1.4
Okra	1 cup boiled; 160 g	146	233.6
Onion, boiled	1 cup; 210 g	3	6.3
Parsley, raw	1 cup; 64 g	100	64
Parsnips	1 cup sliced/boil; 156 g	10	15.6
Peas, canned	1 cup; 170 g	1	1.7
Pepper, green	1 item; 74 g	16	11.84
Pokeweed	1 item; 136 g	476	
Potatoes, white boiled	1 item; 136 g	0	0
Potato, sweet	1 cup boil/mashed; 238 g	56	183.68
Radishes	1 each; 4.5 g	0.3	0.014
Rutabagas	1 cup boil; 170 g	19	32.3
Spinach, boiled	1 cup; 56 g	750	420
Spinach, frozen	1 cup frozen/boil; 205 g	600	1230
Squash, summer	1 cup sliced; 180 g	22	39.6
Tomato, raw	1 cup diced; 240 g	2	4.8
Turnips, boiled	1 cup; 156 g	1	1.56
Waterchestnut canned, whole slices	½ cup; 70 g	1.22	0.86
Watercress early, fine curled	1 cup raw; 34 g	10	3.4
Fruits			
Apple, raw	1 medium; 138 g	3	4.14
Apricot, w/o pit	1 each; 35.3 g	2.8	0.99
Avocado	1 California; 173 g	0	0
Avocado	1 Florida; 173 g	0	0
Banana, raw	1 medium peeled; 114 g	trace	trace
Berries: black	1 cup; 144 g	18	25.92
blue	1 cup; 145 g	15	21.75

continued

Table A-38-c—*continued*
Oxalate Content of Foods per 100 Grams (~½ cup) and per Portion

Food	Portion	mg/100 g	mg/Portion
Berries: dew	1 cup; 144 g	14	20.16
Berries: green goose	1 cup; 150 g	88	132
raspberries, black	1 cup; 123 g	53	65.19
raspberries, red	1 cup; 123 g	15	18.45
Coconut fresh (flesh only)	45 g; 1.5 oz	2.14	0.96
Cranberries, dried	½ cup; 25 g	3.07	0.77
Cranberries, canned Ocean Spray	½ cup; 138 g	0.71	0.98
Cherries: bing	1 cup; 150 g	0	0
Cherries: sour	1 cup; 155 g	1.1	1.705
Currants: black	1 cup; 112 g	4.3	4.82
red	1 cup; 112 g	19	21.28
Fruit salad, canned	1 cup; 249 g	12	29.88
Grapes, red, fresh	1 cup; 92 g	0.52	0.475
Grapes: concord	1 cup; 160 g	25	40
Thompson seedless	1 cup; 160 g	0	0
Kiwi, fresh	1 medium; 76 g	2.6	1.97
Lemon, peel	1 Tbsp; 6 g	83	4.98
Lime, peel	1 Tbsp; 6 g	100	6
Melons: cantaloupe	1 cup; 160 g	0	0
casaba	1 cup; 170 g	0	0
honeydew	1 cup; 170 g	0	0
Mangoes	1 medium; 207 g	0	0
Mango, fresh	1 medium; 207 g	1.06	2.19
Nectarines	1 medium; 136 g	0	0
Orange, raw	1 medium; 131 g	4	5.24
Orange, Navel	1 medium; 140 g	2.18	3.06
Papaya, Hawaiian, fresh	1 medium; 304 g	1.99	6.065
Peaches: Alberta	1 medium; 87 g	5	4.35
canned	1 cup; 250 g	1.2	3
Hiley	1 medium; 87 g	0	0
stokes	1 medium; 87 g	1.2	1.044
Pears, Bartlett, canned	1 cup; 248 g	1.7	4.22
Pineapple, canned	1 cup; 252 g	1	2.52
Pineapple, Dole's (chunks, canned)	½ cup; 125 g	3.07	4.86
Plums: Damson	1 medium; 66 g	10	6.6
Golden Gage	1 medium; 66 g	1.1	0.73
Green Gage	1 medium; 66 g	0	0
Preserves: red plum, jam	1 Tbsp: 20 g	0.5	0.1
strawberry, jam	1 Tbsp; 20 g	9.4	1.88
Rhubarb: canned	1 cup; 240 g	600	1440
stewed, no sugar	1 cup; 242 g	860	2081.2
Strawberries, fresh	1 cup; 149 g	0.7	1.04
Strawberries, canned	1 cup; 254 g	15	38.1
Strawberries, raw	1 cup whole; 149 g	10	14.9
Watermelon	1 cup; 160 g	0	0
Nuts			
Peanuts, roasted	1 cup; 146 g	187	273
Pecans	1 cup; 110 g	202	222.2
Sunflower seeds, hulled, dry roasted, unsalted	1 oz; 28 g	18.9	5.29
Confectionery			
Chocolate, plain	1 oz; 28.35 g	117	33.17
Jelly with allowed fruit	1 Tbsp; 20 g	0	0
Marmalade	1 Tbsp; 20 g	10.8	2.16
Preserves: red plum jam	1 Tbsp; 20 g	0.5	0.1
strawberry jam	1 Tbsp; 20 g	9.4	1.88
Sweets, boiled (plain candies)	Hard candy 1 oz	0	
Beverages			
Barley water, bottled	1 cup; 237 g	0	0
Beer:	12 fl oz; 356 g		
bottled	12 fl oz	0	0
draft	12 fl oz	1	3.56
lager, draft, Tuborg, Pisner	12 fl oz	4	14.24
stout, Guiness draft	12 fl oz	2	7.12
Beer Budweiser	12 fl oz; 355 g	1.05	3.73
Cider	1 cup; 248 g	0	0
Coca-Cola	12 fl oz; 370 g	trace	trace
Coke	12 fl oz; 370 g	0.12	0.444

continued

Table A-38-c—*continued*
Oxalate Content of Foods per 100 Grams (~½ cup) and per Portion

Food	Portion	mg/100 g	mg/Portion
Coke, diet	12 fl oz; 354 g	0.1	0.35
Coffee (0.5 g Nescafe/100 mL)	1 tsp powder; 1.8 g	3.2	11.52
Coffee, black, brewed (brewed 4 min)	1 cup; 236 g	0.61	1.44
Coffee infusion:			
2 g per 100 mL infused 5 min		1	
4.4 g (1 tsp) per 100 mL infused 13 min		7.3	
Cocoa, Carnation Dry	1 pkt; 1 oz	7.69	2.184
Ginger Ale (Schweppes)	12 fl oz; 366 g	0.05	0.196
Lemon squash drink (lemonade)	12 fl oz; 349 g	1	3.49
Lucozade, bottled (soda)	12 fl oz; 350 g	0	0
Orange soda (Minute Maid)	12 fl oz; 372 g	0.24	0.91
Orange squash drink (orangeade)	12 fl oz; 372 g	2.5	9.3
Ovaltine drink, 2 g in 100 mL	1 tsp powder; 2.67 g	10	13.35
Pepsi Cola	12 fl oz; 370 g	trace	trace
Ribena concentrate (black currant drink)	12 fl oz; 360 g	2	7.2
Root beer (Borgs and A&W)	12 fl oz; 370 g	0.19	0.696
Sherry dry	1 cup; 240 g	trace	trace
Tea Indian:			
2-min infusion	1 cup; 237 g	55	130.35
4-min infusion	1 cup; 237 g	72	170.64
6-min infusion	1 cup; 237 g	78	184.86
Tea rosehip	1 cup; 237 g	4	9.48
Tea Lipton, steeped 5 min	1 cup; 237 g	3.74	8.86
Teas (steeped for 5 min w/o stirring, the tea bag then removed)			
Celestial Seasoning teas	1 cup; 250 mL		
Sleepytime	250 mL	0.99	
Peppermint	250 mL	1.71	
Wild Forest Blackberry	250 mL	0.9	
Mandarin Orange Spice	250 mL	0.9	
Cinnamon Apple Spice	250 mL	1.17	
R.C. Bigelow			
Cranberry Apple	250 mL	0.9	
Red Raspberry	250 mL	0.72	
I Love Lemon	250 mL	0.81	
Orange and Spice	250 mL	0.81	
Mint Medley	250 mL	1.71	
Sweet Dreams	250 mL	1.53	
Thomas J. Lipton			
Gentle Orange	250 mL	1.08	
Lemon Soother	250 mL	0.63	
Chamomile Flowers	250 mL	1.26	
Lyons Tetley Black Tea			
Tetley Tea (5-min steep)	250 mL	20.79	
Tetley Tea (1-min steep)	250 mL	10.8	
Tetley Tea (1-min steep with stirring	250 mL	19.26	
Thomas J. Lipton			
Red Rose Classic Tea (5-min steep)	250 mL	11.97	
Red Rose Classic Tea (1-min steep)	250 mL	10.8	
Red Rose Classic Tea (1-min steep with stirring)	250 mL	15.75	
Green Tea R. Twining & Co.			
China Oolong Tea	250 mL	6.84	
Coffee			
Maxwell House (extra fine) coffee	250 mL	1.44	
Tomato juice	1 cup; 244 g	5	12.2
Wine:	1 cup; 236 g		
port	1 cup	trace	trace
rose	1 cup	1.5	3.54
white	1 cup	0	0
Fruit juices			
Aloe vera juice	1 cup; 250 g	0.83	2.07
Apple juice from concentrate	1 cup; 248 g	0.51	1.26
Apple juice	1 cup; 248 g	trace	trace
Cranberry juice	1 cup; 253 g	6.6	16.7
Cranberry juice from concentrate	1 cup; 252 g	0.31	0.78
Grapefruit juice	1 cup; 247 g	0	0
Orange juice	1 cup; 249 g	0.5	1.245
Pineapple juice	1 cup; 250 g	0	0

continued

Table A-38-c—*continued*
Oxalate Content of Foods per 100 Grams (~½ cup) and per Portion

Food	Portion	mg/100 g	mg/Portion
Miscellaneous			
Basil, fresh	1 Tbsp; 2.5 g	115.6	2.89
Cinnamon, ground	1 tsp; 2 g	362.74	7.255
Cocoa, dry powder	1 cup; 86 g	623	535.78
Coffee, powder (Nescafe)	1 tsp; 1.8 g	33	11.52
Corn syrup, Karo	1 Tbsp; 21 g	0.32	0.07
Chicken noodle soup	1 cup; 241 g	1	2.41
Gelatin, unflavored Knox	1 pkt; 7 g	11.73	0.82
Ginger, raw	1 Tbsp sliced; 6 g	115.03	6.902
Honey (clover)	1 Tbsp; 21 g	1.51	0.32
Lemon juice	1 cup; 244 g	1	2.44
Lime juice	1 cup; 246 g	0	0
Malt, powder	1 Tbsp; 12.25 g	19.97	2.447
Maple syrup, pure	1 Tbsp; 20 g	0.7	0.14
Mayonnaise, Heinz	1 Tbsp; 14 g	11.98	1.677
Mustard, Dijon style	1 Tbsp; 15 g	6.57	0.985
Nutmeg, dry	1 tsp; 2 g	63.76	1.275
Oregano, dried	1 tsp; 1.5 g	8.58	0.13
Ovaltine powder, canned	1 tsp; 2.67 g	10	13.35
Oxtail soup	1 cup; 376 g	1	3.76
Pepper	1 tsp; 2.1 g	419	8.8
Tomato soup	1 cup; 244 g	3	7.32
Vanilla extract, imitation	1 tsp; 5 g	0.42	0.021
Vegetable soup	1 cup; 241 g	5	12.05
Vinegar, apple cider Ralph's brand	1 tsp; 5 g	1.31	0.066

From Brzezinski E, Durning AM, Grasse B, Fusselman E, Ciaraldi T. Oxalate content of selected foods. The General Clinical Research Center, University of California, San Diego Medical Center. 1996:1–53. With permission. There is now a 1998 edition available.

Note: For references see original table, pp. 15–26.

Table A-38-d
Low-Oxalate Meal Suggestions

Select any one breakfast, lunch, dinner and snack/dessert combination from the meals/snack options below. Total oxalate will be less than 50 mg.

Oxalate values for meals rounded to nearest whole number.

Breakfast options	**Oxalate (mg)**
1. Banana Smoothie*	15
1 standard slice white toast	
1 tsp margarine	
Bigelow Red Raspberry herbal tea	
2. 1 cup plain yogurt w/1 cup fresh strawberries	12
Toasted plain medium bagel	
1 tsp margarine	
1 cup orange juice	
3. Two scrambled eggs (mixed with water)	8
Three slices bacon, broiled or fried	
Whole English muffin with 1 tsp jelly	
1 cup cantaloupe chunks	
1 cup 1% or 2% lowfat milk	
4. 1 cup Cheerios	8
1 cup 1% or 2% lowfat milk	
1 medium banana	
1 standard slice of white toast	
1 tsp margarine	
5. ½ fresh grapefruit	7
1 poached egg	
1 standard slice white toast	
1 tsp margarine	
1¼ cup cornflakes	
1 cup 1% or 2% lowfat milk	
6. French Toast Bake* with 2 Tbsp maple syrup	12
Fresh kiwi (1 medium) and ½ cup cantaloupe	
1 cup 1% or 2% lowfat milk	
7. 1 whole English muffin with ½ cup cottage cheese and tomato sliced (½ cup)	11

continued

Table A-38-d—*continued*
Low-Oxalate Meal Suggestions

1 cup orange juice	
1 cup 1% or 2% lowfat milk	
Lunch Options	**Oxalate (mg)**
1. California Chicken Sandwich*	9
Picnic Potato Salad*	
1 cup Thompson seedless grapes	
12 fl oz Diet Coke	
2. Turkey burger: 3 oz ground turkey patty, grilled	13
1 white hamburger bun	
1 Tbsp catsup	
1 Tbsp mustard	
Sweet n Sour Cabbage*	
1 cup apple juice	
3. Cauliflower Curry*	11
½ cup steamed white rice	
1 medium fresh mango	
1 cup cranberry juice	
1 small white dinner roll	
4. 1 cup spaghetti in tomato sauce	13
1 slice Italian bread with 1 tsp margarine	
Marinated Cucumbers*	
1 cup 1% or 2% lowfat milk	
5. Lettuce (1 cup) w/avocado slices (¼ avocado)	12
1 Tbsp mayonnaise style salad dressing	
1 cup beef noodle soup	
Roast turkey sandwich: 3 oz roast turkey,	
1 Tbsp mayonnaise	
2 slices white bread	
20 fresh bing cherries	
1 cup 1% or 2% lowfat milk	
6. Chef's salad: 2 cups iceberg lettuce	12
tomato wedges (½)	
hardboiled egg	
½ cup water chestnuts,	

continued

Table A-38-d—*continued*
Low-Oxalate Meal Suggestions

	Oxalate (mg)
3 oz ham slices	
2 oz grated cheese	
½ cup cucumber slices	
½ medium carrot grated	
1 Tbsp mayonnaise-style salad dressing	
1 standard slice white bread	
1 tsp margarine	
1 cup honeydew melon	
12 oz diet soda	
7. Tuna salad sandwich: ½ cup tuna salad (made from tuna and mayonnaise), 2 standard slices white bread	11
Radishes (5 each) and 1 cup cucumber slices	
1 cup Thompson seedless grapes	
1 cup buttermilk	
Dinner Options	**Oxalate (mg)**
1. ½ roasted Cornish game hen	11
California Wild Rice Salad*	
½ cup green peas w/mushrooms	
1 small white dinner roll	
1 tsp margarine	
1 cup 1% or 2% lowfat milk	
2. Chicken Adobo*	10
1 cup white rice boiled	
Salad: 1 cup iceberg lettuce	
½ cucumber	
½ carrot	
1 Tbsp mayonnaise-style salad dressing	
12 fl oz diet soda	
1 small plain white roll	
1 tsp margarine	
3. 4 oz poached salmon	16
Angel Hair Sauté*	
Watermelon Salad*	
1 cup sparkling water	
4. Sandra's Curry Chicken*	13
1 cup steamed white rice	
½ cup cooked carrots	
1 small white dinner roll	
1 tsp margarine	
1 cup apple juice	
5. 1 cup macaroni and cheese	6
Tomato wedges (1 medium tomato)	
1 cup honeydew melon	
1 cup 1% or 2% lowfat milk	
6. Fish taco: 3 oz baked fish, ¼ cup shredded iceberg lettuce, ½ medium tomato, avocado slices (¼), 1 tsp lime juice, 2 small corn tortillas	11
1 small corn on the cob	
1 tsp margarine	
12 fl oz diet soda	
7. 4 oz broiled steak	4
1 medium baked potato	
½ cup cooked cauliflower	
Small french roll	
2 tsp margarine	
8 fl oz lemonade without peel	
Snack/Desserts	**Oxalate (mg)**
Watermelon Ice*	0
Banana Ice Cream*	0
Fruit Kabobs*	6
Graham crackers, 2 each	1.7
Sponge cake, 1 slice	4.9
Fig Newtons, 2 each	4.2
Popcorn, Orville Redenbacker popped, 2 cups	4.2

From Brzezinski E, Durning AM, Grasse B, Fusselman E, Ciaraldi T. Oxalate content of selected foods. The General Clinical Research Center, University of California, San Diego Medical Center. 1996:1–53. With permission. There is now a 1998 edition available.

*Recipe in original document.

A-38-e. National Organizations

National Kidney Foundation
30 E. 33rd Street, Suite 1100
New York, NY 10016
800-622-9010
212-889-2210

American Dietetic Association
216 W. Jackson Blvd.
Chicago, IL 60606-6995
800-877-1600

Oxalosis Foundation
24815 144th Place S.E.
Kent, WA 98042
206-631-0386

National Institutes of Health
One Rockledge Centre
6705 Rockledge Drive MSC 7965
Bethesda, MD 20892-7965

The Vulvar Pain Foundation
Post Office Drawer 177
Graham, NC 27253
336-226-0704
336-226-8518 facsimile

General Clinical Research Center Nutrition Unit
200 West Arbor Drive
San Diego, CA 92103-8203
619-543-6795

A-39. VEGETARIAN DIETS

A-39-a. Purpose, Use and Modifications

The vegetarian diet is composed predominantly of plant foods and may or may not include eggs and dairy products. Vegetarian diets should provide a variety of foods that supply adequate amounts of all required nutrients to allow for tissue maintenance, repair, and growth.

Vegetarian diets are used by any person who chooses to omit animal products for religious preferences, health concerns, environmental considerations, humanitarian issues, ethical concerns, or economic or political reasons.

Although the term *vegetarian* encompasses a variety of eating patterns, it generally involves mainly plant foods. Traditionally, vegetarian diets have been classified by the extent to which animal products are excluded (Table 39-a-1). However, the term *vegetarian* is often used loosely and may involve a variety of animal food exclusions/inclusions among individuals. Many people who occasionally consume beef, fish, or poultry consider themselves to be vegetarians. Therefore, a careful diet history is required to determine the specific food practices of individual vegetarians.

(From The Manual of Clinical Dietetics, 5th ed. Chicago: the American Dietetic Association, 1996:43–59, with permission. *Note:* For references, see original diet, p. 57–9.)

Table A-39-a-1
Traditional Classification of Vegetarian Diets[a]

Classification	Foods Included	Foods Excluded
Lacto-ovovegetarian	Fruits, grains, legumes, nuts, seeds, vegetables, milk and milk products, eggs	Meat, poultry, fish
Lactovegetarian	Fruits, grains, legumes, nuts, seeds, vegetables, milk and milk products	Meat, poultry, fish eggs
Ovovegetarian	Fruits, grains, legumes, nuts, seeds, vegetables, eggs	Meat, poultry, fish, milk, and milk products
Vegan	Fruits, grains, legumes, nuts, seeds, vegetables	Meat, poultry, fish, eggs, milk, and milk products

[a]See Chapter 106 for a comprehensive review of such diets including issues related to ensuring nutrient adequacy.

Table A-39-b
Daily Food Guide for Vegetarians

Food Group	Suggested Daily Servings	Serving Sizes
Breads, cereals, rice, and pasta	6 or more	1 slice bread, ½ bun, bagel, or English muffin; ½ cup cooked cereal, rice, or pasta; 1 oz dry cereal
Vegetables	4 or more	½ cup cooked or 1 cup raw; ¾ cup vegetable juice
Fruits	3 or more	1 piece fresh fruit, ¾ cup fruit juice, ½ cup canned or cooked fruit
Legumes and other meat substitutes	2–3	½ cup cooked beans; 4 oz tofu or tempeh; 8 oz soy milk, 1½ oz soy cheese; 2 tablespoons nuts or seeds, 2 tablespoons peanut butter; 3 oz vegetarian burger patty or 1 vegetarian hot dog
Dairy products (optional)	up to 3 servings	1 cup milk or yogurt, 1½ oz natural cheese, 2 oz processed cheese
Eggs (optional)	limit to 3–4 yolks per week	1 egg or 2 egg whites, ¼ cup egg substitute
Fats, sweets, and alcohol	Go easy on these foods and beverages	Oil, margarine, and mayonnaise; salad dressings; soft drinks; candies; beer, wine, and distilled spirits

Table A-39-c
Guidelines for Vegetarian Diets

Food Groups	Choose More Often	Choose Less Often[a]
Beverages	Juices, water, low-fat milk, soy milk	Whole milk, sweetened beverages, alcohol
Breads and cereals	Whole-grain and enriched breads, whole-grain cereals, muffins, bagels, tortillas; enriched or whole grains (e.g., brown rice, cracked wheat, bulgur, oats, buckwheat); enriched or whole-grain pastas	Fried snacks; biscuits; pancakes; high-fat baked goods (e.g., croissants, pastries)
Desserts	Lightly sweetened and moderate in fat, e.g., puddings made from skim milk, angel food cake, graham crackers, vegetable-based gelatin	High-fat, high-sugar desserts, such as candy, pastries, cakes, pies, cookies; whole-milk puddings, ice cream; candies or sweets containing animal-based gelatin, e.g., marshmallows
Fats	Margarine and salad dressings made from polyunsaturated and monounsaturated oils	Animal fat (butter, lard, sour cream, cream cheese), other saturated fats, coconut and palm oils, hydrogenated shortenings; gravies with meat base
Fruit	All except avocado; at least one vitamin C source daily	Avocado
Legumes and other meat substitutes	Low-fat cheeses, eggs; tofu; legumes, meat analogues made from soy protein; limited amounts of nuts, seeds, and nut and seed butters (e.g., tahini)	High-fat cheeses and eggs; commercial refried beans containing lard
Soups	Made from vegetable stock, low-fat milk, or soy milk	High-sodium canned or dried soups made from meat stock or that contain ham and bacon
Vegetables	Fresh or frozen; include dark-green leafy or deep-yellow daily	Deep-fried or pickled vegetables; high-sodium juices
Miscellaneous	Herbs; low-sodium seasonings	Salt; high-sodium seasonings

[a]Persons with increased energy needs, such as pregnant and lactating women and infants and children, may require some calorie-dense foods listed in this column to achieve an adequate energy intake.

Table A-39-d-1
Sample Menu for Lacto-Ovovegetarian Diet

Breakfast	Lunch	Dinner
Orange juice (½ cup) Whole-grain cereal (¾ cup) Banana (½) Peanut butter (2 tbsp) Enriched whole-wheat toast (2 slices) Jelly or jam (1 tbsp) 2% milk (1 cup) Coffee/tea	Vegetarian lentil soup (1½ cup) Saltine crackers (4) Enriched whole-wheat bread (2 slices) Spinach salad (raw spincach, 1 cup; shredded carrot, ¼ cup; chopped mushrooms, 2 tsp) 1% low-fat cottage cheese (¼ cup) Vinegar and oil dressing (1 tbsp) Fresh fruit salad (½ cup) Graham crackers (4) 2% milk (1 cup) Coffee/tea	Burritos (2): soft corn tortillas (2), fat-free refried beans (½ cup), shredded lettuce (½ cup), diced tomato (½ cup), chopped onions (2 tbsp), tomato salsa (¼ cup) Spanish rice (½ cup) Low-fat frozen yogurt (½ cup) Medium apple (1) Coffee/tea

Approximate Nutrient Analysis

Energy (kcal)	2039.9	Phosphorus (mg)	1672.1
Protein (g)	80.5	Potassium (mg)	4682.4
(15.8% of kcal)		Sodium (mg)	2450.6
Carbohydrate (g)	334.5	Zinc (mg)	12.8
(65.6% of kcal)		Vitamin A (μg RE)	1519.9
Total fat (g)	52.3	Vitamin C (mg)	174.5
(23.1% of kcal)		Thiamin (mg)	2.1
Saturated fatty acids (g)	16.8	Riboflavin (mg)	2.7
Monounsaturated fatty acids (g)	18.7	Niacin (mg)	26.0
Polyunsaturated fatty acids (g)	12.8	Folate (μg)	551.4
Cholesterol (mg)	62.9	Vitamin B_6 (mg)	2.7
Calcium (mg)	1237.4	Vitamin B_{12} (μg)	5.6
Iron (mg)	18.3	Dietary fiber (g)	42.5
Magnesium (mg)	586.2	Water-insoluble fiber (g)	30.7

Table A-39-d-2
Sample Menu for Vegan Diet

Breakfast	Lunch	Dinner	Snack
Orange juice (½ cup) Dry cereal, fortified with vitamin B_{12} (¾ cup) Banana (½) Peanut butter (2 tbsp) Enriched whole-wheat toast (2 slices) Jelly or jam (1 tbsp) Soy milk (½ cup) Coffee/tea	Vegetarian lentil soup (1 cup) with brown rice (½ cup) Enriched whole-wheat bread (1 slice) Spinach salad (raw spinach, 1 cup; shredded carrot, ¼ cup; chopped mushrooms, 2 tsp; tofu, 4 oz) Vinegar and oil dressing (1 tbsp) Graham crackers (4) Fresh fruit salad (½ cup) Coffee/tea	Burritos (2): soft corn tortillas (2), fat-free refried beans (½ cup), shredded lettuce (½ cup), diced tomato (½ cup), chopped onions (2 tbsp), tomato salsa (¼ cup) Spanish rice (½ cup) Collard greens, cooked (½ cup) Margarine (1 tsp) Medium apple (1) Coffee/tea	Trail mix; raisins (1 tbsp), chopped dried apricot (1), pretzels (½ oz)

Approximate Nutrient Analysis

Energy (kcal)	1982.5	Phosphorus (mg)	1386.3
Protein (g)	67.0	Potassium (mg)	4402.7
(13.5% of kcal)		Sodium (mg)	3136.0
Carbohydrate (g)	335.5	Zinc (mg)	26.7
(67.7% of kcal)		Vitamin A (μg RE)	2350.1
Total fat (g)	54.3	Vitamin C (mg)	224.9
(24.7% of kcal)		Thiamin (mg)	3.3
Saturated fatty acids (g)	10.3	Riboflavin (mg)	3.0
Monounsaturated fatty acids (g)	19.2	Niacin (mg)	40.2
Polyunsaturated fatty acids (g)	19.4	Folate (μg)	826.4
Cholesterol (mg)	12.4	Vitamin B_6 (mg)	4.2
Calcium (mg)	638.1	Vitamin B_{12} (μg)	6.8
Iron (mg)	56.6	Dietary fiber (g)	49.3
Magnesium (mg)	688.6	Water-insoluble fiber (g)	34.4

Note: See Chapter 106 for a comprehensive review of such diets including issues related to ensuring nutrient adequacy.

A-40. ENTERAL AND PARENTERAL FORMULAS: CATEGORIES AND SOURCES

A-40-a. Commercial Nutrition Formulations for Oral and Tube Feeding

Most companies making commercial formulas provide updated information in reprints that are widely distributed. These reprints often contain the composition of formulas produced by other companies as well as their own. Additionally, new and revised commercial preparations appear on the market in increasing numbers, whereas some older formulas have been removed. These commercial reference guides make continued publication of detailed formulations unnecessary and actually undesirable in this volume. Thus, outdated information can be avoided.

A list is provided below of the companies currently producing and marketing such formulations. Addresses and telephone numbers are included to help the reader obtain the most current information on a specific product. Each company also produces an enteral product reference list that provides nutrient analysis on each product as well as other relevant information needed to make informed choices. They may be contacted for such publications or for other educational materials they provide. In addition, a list is included of the names of current formulations by dietary use characteristics.

A-40-a-1. Company Lists with Identification Code

McGaw, Inc. (Mc)
2525 McGaw Avenue
P.O. Box 19791
Irvine, CA 92713-9791
1-800-854-6851 (Technical Assistance)

Mead Johnson Nutritionals (M)
A Bristol Myers Squibb Company
2400 West Lloyd Expressway
Evansville, IN 47721
1-800-457-3550

Nestle Clinical Nutrition (Nes)
Three Parkway North, Suite 500
P.O. Box 760
Deerfield, IL 60015-0760
1-800-422-2752

Novartis Nutrition (formerly Sandoz) (Nov)
5100 Gamble Drive
St. Louis Park, MN 55416
1-800-999-9978

Nutrition Medical (Nut)
9850 51st Avenue North
Minneapolis, MN 55442-2283
1-800-569-7828
e-mail: info@nutritionmed.com

Ross Laboratories (R)
Division of Abbott Laboratories
625 Cleveland Avenue
Columbus, OH 43215
1-800-544-7495
(614)624-7677

A-40-a-2. Current List of Formulations for Oral and/or Enteral Feeding by Dietary Use Characteristics

Complete diet formulations containing some natural foods with varying residue

- Carnation Instant Breakfast (Nes)
- Carnation Instant Breakfast, no sugar (Nes)
- Compleat Regular (Nov)
- Compleat Modified (Nov)
- Compleat Pediatric (Nov)
- Meritene (Nov)

Complete defined-formula diets with intact purified protein, low residue, and no lactose

- Citrotein (Nov)
- Comply (M)
- Ensure (R)
- Ensure Light (R)
- Ensure High Protein (R)
- Ensure Plus (R)
- Ensure Plus HN (R)
- Entrition 0.5 (Nes)
- Entrition HN (Nes)
- Introlite (R)
- Isocal (M)
- Isocal HCN (M)
- Isocal HN (M)
- Iso-Pro (Nut)
- Isosource (Nov)
- Isosource HN (Nov)
- Isotein HN (Nov)
- Nitro-Pro (Nut)
- Nutren 1.0 (Nes)

Nutren 1.5 (Nes)

Nutren 2.0 (Nes)

Nutren Junior (Nes)

Osmolite (R)

Osmolite HN (R)

Osmolite HN Plus (R)

Pediasure (for children 1–10 years of age) (R)

Portagen (M)

Promote (R)

Replete (Nes)

Resource Fruit Beverage (Nov)

Resource Just for Kids (Nov)

Resource Liquid (Nov)

Resource Plus Liquid (Nov)

Sustacal Basic (M)

Susta Liquid (M)

Sustacal Plus (M)

Travasorb MCT (Nes)

Two Cal HN (R)

Ultra-Pro (Nut)

Complete defined-formula diets with intact purified protein, no lactose-containing fiber

Ensure with Fiber (R)

Fiber-Pro (Nut)

Fibersource (Nov)

Fibersource HN (Nov)

Isosource VHN (Nov)

Jevity (R)

Jevity Plus (R)

Nutren Junior with Fiber (Nes)

Nutren with Fiber (Nes)

Pediasure with Fiber (for children 1–10 years of age) (R)

Probalance (Nes)

Promote with Fiber (R)

Replete with Fiber (Nes)

Sustacal with Fiber (M)

Ultracal (M)

Defined-formula diets with hydrolyzed protein or amino acids, low residue, and no lactose

Alimentum [for infants] (R)

Alitraq (R)

Criticare HN (M)

Crucial (Nes)

L-Emental (Nut)

L-Emental Pediatric (Nut)

L-Emental Plus (Nut)

Nutramigen [for infants] (M)

Optimental (R)

Peptamen (Nes)

Peptamen Junior (Nes)

Peptamen VHP (Nes)

Pregestamil [for infants] (M)

Pro-Peptide (Nut)

Pro-Peptide for Kids (for children 1–10 years of age) (Nut)

Pro-Peptide VHN (Nut)

Reabilan (Nes)

Reabilan HN (Nes)

Sandosource Peptide (Nov)

Tolerex (Nov)

Travasorb HN (Nes)

Travasorb STD (Nes)

Vital HN (R)

Vivonex Pediatric (Nov)

Vivonex Plus (Nov)

Vivonex T.E.N. (Nov)

Disease-specific formulations

Advera (R)

Alterna (R)

Aminess Essential Amino Acid Tablets (Nes)

Amin-Aid (Mc)[a]

Choice DM (M)

Diabetisource (Nov)

Glytrol (Nes)

Glucerna (R)

Hepatic-Aid II (Mc)

Immun-Aid (Mc)

Impact (Nov)

Impact 1.5 (Nov)

Impact with Fiber (Nov)

L-Emental Hepatic (Nut)

Lipisorb (M)

Magnacal Renal (M)

Nepro (R)

Novasource Renal (Nov)

NutriHep (Nes)

Nutrivent (Nes)

Oxepa (R)

Perative (R)

Protain XL (M)

Pulmocare (R)

RCF (for infants—contains no carbohydrate) (R)

Renalcal (Nes)

Replete (Nes)

Resource Diabetic (Nov)

Respalar (M)

Suplena (R)

TraumaCal (M)

[a] Amin-Aid is manufactured by McGaw, Inc. and distributed by R&D Laboratories, Inc. of Marina del Rey, CA.

Table A-40-b
Amino Acid Content (mg/2.5 g) of Commercially Available Amino Acid Formulations

Amino Acid	Aminosyn[a]	Aminosyn-PF[b]	Travasol (B)[b]	Novamine[b]	Freamine III[d]	Trophamine[d]
Isoleucine	180	191	120	124	175	204
Leucine	235	297	155	174	228	350
Lysine	180	170	145	198	182	204
Methionine	100	45	145	124	132	83
Phenylalanine	110	107	155	174	140	121
Threonine	130	129	105	124	100	104
Tryptophan	40	45	45	41	38	50
Valine	200	161	115	162	165	196
Histidine	75	79	109	147	71	121
Cystine	0	0	0	<12	<6	<8
Tyrosine	11	16	10	9	0	58
Taurine	0	18	0	0	0	6
Alanine	320	175	518	353	178	133
Aspartic acid	0	132	0	74	0	79
Glutamic acid	0	206	0	124	0	125
Glycine	320	96	518	174	350	92
Proline	215	204	104	147	280	171
Serine	105	124	0	100	148	96
Arginine	245	308	258	247	238	304

[a]Abbott Laboratories, N. Chicago, IL.

[b]Clintec, Deerfield, IL.

[c]Clintec

[d]McGaw Laboratories, Irvine, CA.

A-41. WEB SITES OF INTEREST TO THE HEALTH PROFESSIONAL

The following is a list of web sites offering nutrition and healthcare information that might be of interest and helpful to healthcare professionals.

A-41-a. Agencies and Organizations

American Dietetic Association	http://www.eatright.org
American Medical Association	http://www.ama-assn.org
American Society for Clinical Nutrition	http://www.faseb.org/ascn
American Society for Parenteral and Enteral Nutrition	http://www.clinnutr.org
Centers for Disease Control and Prevention	http://www.cdc.gov
Department of Health and Human Services	http://www.dhhs.gov
Food and Drug Administration	http://www.fda.gov
FDA's Center for Food Safety & Applied Nutrition	http://www.vm.cfsan.fda.gov/list.html
Food and Nutrition Information Center	http://www.nalusda.gov/fnic.html
Government Consumer Education materials	http://www.pueblo.gsa.gov
International Food Information Council	http://www.ificinfo.health.org
National Health Information Center	http://www.nhic-nt.health.org
National Heart, Lung, and Blood Institute	http://www.nhlbi.nih.gov/nhlbi/nhlbi.htm
National Library of Medicine (free Medline search service)	http://www.nlm.nih.gov/databases/freemedl.html
Oncology Nursing Society	http://www.ons.org
US Department of Agriculture	http://www.usda.gov/
US Department of Agriculture Database of Release 11-1. (Nutrient analysis for over 5900 foods)	http://www.nal.usda.gov/fnic/foodcomp/
World Health Organization (WHO) World Wide Server	http://www.who.ch/Welcome.html

A-41-b. Medical Journals

Querying any search engine available on Internet for medical journals produces a huge array of options. For example, using Yahoo and selecting health as the topic, after typing in "medical journals" in the search box, categories of journals are displayed. Another source for accessing on-line journals, in addition to free MEDLINE and Pre-MEDLINE citations is PubMed

PubMed	http://www.ncbi.nlm.nih.gov/PubMed/
American Journal of Clinical Nutrition	http://www.faseb.org/ajcn
Annals of Internal Medicine	http://www.acponline.org/journals/annals/ annaltoc.htm
Blood	http://www.bloodjournal.org
British Journal of Nutrition	http://www.cup.org/Journals/JNLSCAT/nut/nut.html
British Medical Journal	http://www.bmj.com/bmj/index.html
Journal of the American Dietetic Association	htpp://www.eatright.org/journaltoc.html
Journal of the American Medical Association	http://www.ama-assn.org/public/journals/jama/
Journal of Clinical Investigation	http://www.jci.org/
Journal of Clinical Oncology	http://www.jcojournal.org
Journal of the National Cancer Institute	http://cancernet.nci.nih.gov/jnci/jncihome.html
Journal of Parenteral and Enteral Nutrition	http://www.clinnutr.org
Lancet	http://www.thelancet.com
McGill University listing of e-journals	http://www.medcor.mcgill.ca/EXPMED/DOCS/on-linej.html
Nature Medicine	http://medicine.nature.com
New England Journal of Medicine	http://www.nejm.org
Proceedings of the National Academy of Sciences USA	http://www.pnas.org

A-41-c. Oncology Information

American Cancer Society	http://www.cancer.org
American Institute for Cancer Research	http://www.aicr.org
CancerNet (National Cancer Institute)	http://cancernet.nci.nih.gov
OncoLink (University of Pennsylvania)	http://www.oncolink.upenn.edu
OncoWeb (European School of Oncology)	http://www.oncoweb.com

A-42. Recent U.S. and Government Publications

Energy and macronutrient intakes of persons ages 2 months and over in the United States: Third National Health and Nutrition Examination Survey, phase 1, 1988–91. US Department of Health and Human Services, Centers for Disease Control and Prevention, National Center for Health Statistics, no. 255, 1994.

Dietary intake of vitamins, minerals, and fiber of persons ages 2 months and over in the United States: Third National Health and Nutrition Examination Survey, phase 1, 1988–91. US Department of Health and Human Services, Centers for Disease Control and Prevention, National Center for Health Statistics, no. 258, 1994.

Krauss RM, Deckelbaum RJ, Ernst N, et al. Dietary guidelines for healthy American adults: a statement for health professionals from the Nutrition Committee, American Heart Association. Circulation 1996;94:1795–1800.

Nutrition and your health: dietary guidelines for Americans. 4th ed. Home and Garden Bulletin no. 232. Washington, DC: US Government Printing Office, 1995.

Report of the Dietary Guidelines Advisory Committee on the Dietary Guidelines for Americans, 1995, to the Secretary of Health and Human Services and the Secretary of Agriculture. Beltsville, MD: US Department of Agriculture, Agriculture Research Service, 1995.

Cleveland LE, Goldman JD, Borrud LG. Data tables: continuing survey from USDA 1994 continuing survey food intakes by individuals in 1994. Diet and Health Knowledge Survey. Riverdale, MD: Agriculture Research Service, USDA.

Pennington JAT, Wilkening VL. Final regulations for the nutrition labeling of raw fruits, vegetables, and fish. J Am Diet Assoc 1997;97:1299–1305.

Moss AJ, Levy AS, Kim I, et al. Use of vitamin and mineral supplements in the US: current use, types of products and nutrients. Advance data from Vital and Health Statistics no. 174, 1989. Hyattsville, MD: National Center for Health Statistics.

Guidelines on diet, nutrition, and cancer prevention: reducing the risk of cancer with healthy food choices and physical activity. The American Cancer Society 1996 Advisory Committee on Diet, Nutrition, and Cancer Prevention.

Food and Nutrition Board, Institute of Medicine. Dietary reference intakes for calcium, phosphorus, magnesium, vitamin D, and fluoride. Washington DC: National Academy Press, 1997.

Food and Nutrition Board, Institute of Medicine. Dietary reference intakes. Thiamin, riboflavin, niacin, vitamin B_6, folate, vitamin B_{12}, pantothenic acid, biotin, and choline. Washington DC: National Academy Press, 1998.

US Department of Health and Human Sciences. National Institutes of Health. National Heart, Lung, and Blood Insitute. Clinical guidelines on the identification, evaluation, and treatment of overweight and obesity in adults. The evidence report. Bethesda, MD. Preprint June 1998.

Index

Page numbers in *italics* denote figures; those followed by t denote tables; and those followed by A denote Appendix page.